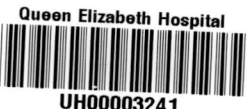

This book is due for return on or before the last date shown below.

DeVita, Hellman, and Rosenberg's

Cancer

Principles & Practice of Oncology

EDITORS

Vincent T. DeVita, Jr., MD

Amy & Joseph Perella Professor of Medicine, Yale Comprehensive Cancer Center and Smilow Cancer Hospital at Yale-New Haven, Yale University School of Medicine, Professor of Epidemiology and Public Health, Yale University School of Public Health, New Haven, Connecticut

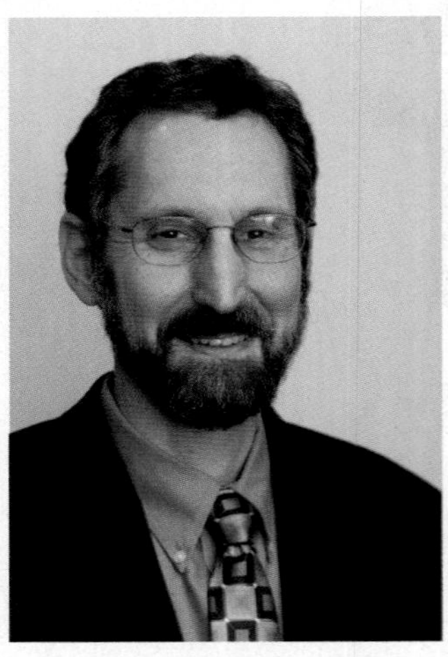

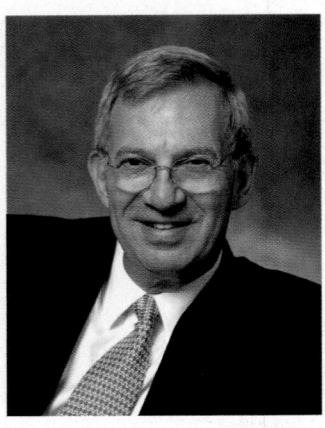

Theodore S. Lawrence, MD, PhD

Isadore Lampe Professor and Chair, Department of Radiation Oncology, University of Michigan, Ann Arbor, Michigan

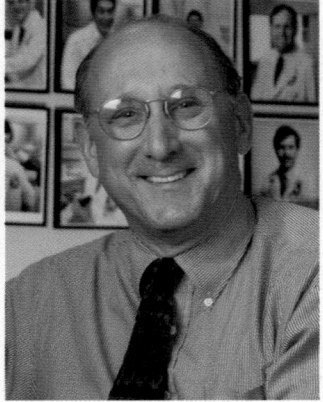

Steven A. Rosenberg, MD, PhD

Chief of Surgery, National Cancer Institute, National Institutes of Health; Professor of Surgery, Uniformed Services University of the Health Sciences School of Medicine, Bethesda, Maryland; Professor of Surgery, George Washington University School of Medicine, Washington, DC

ASSOCIATE SCIENTIFIC ADVISORS

Robert A. Weinberg, PhD

Member, Whitehead Institute for Biomedical Research, Daniel K. Ludwig Professor of Biology, Massachusetts Institute of Technology, Cambridge, Massachusetts

Ronald A. DePinho, MD

Director, Center for Applied Cancer Science, Belfer Institute for Innovative Cancer Science, Dana-Farber Cancer Institute; American Cancer Society Research Professor; Professor of Medicine and Genetics, Harvard Medical School, Boston, Massachusetts

With 431 Contributing Authors

DeVita, Hellman, and Rosenberg's

Cancer

Principles & Practice of Oncology

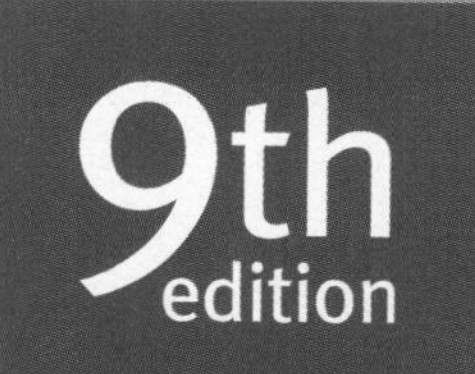

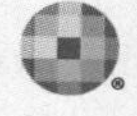
Wolters Kluwer | Lippincott Williams & Wilkins
Health

Philadelphia • Baltimore • New York • London
Buenos Aires • Hong Kong • Sydney • Tokyo

Executive Editor: Jonathan W. Pine, Jr.
Senior Managing Editor: Emilie Moyer
Vendor Manager: Alicia Jackson
Senior Manufacturing Manager: Benjamin Rivera
Senior Marketing Manager: Angela Panetta
Senior Designer: Stephen Druding
Cover Designer: Stephen Druding
Production Service: Aptara, Inc.

Two Commerce Square
2001 Market Street
Philadelphia, PA 19103 USA

LWW.com

First Edition: J.B. Lippincott Company, 1982, Second Edition: J.B. Lippincott Company, 1985. Third Edition: J.B. Lippincott Company, 1989. Fourth Edition: J.B. Lippincott Company, 1993. Fifth Edition: Lippincott-Raven, 1997. Sixth Edition: Lippincott Williams & Wilkins, 2001. Seventh Edition: Lippincott Williams & Wilkins, 2005. Eighth Edition: Lippincott Williams & Wilkins, 2008.

Printed in the USA

Not authorised for sale in the United States, Canada, Australia, or New Zealand

Library of Congress Cataloging-in-Publication Data

[ISBN: 978-1-4511-1813-1]

To purchase additional copies of this book, call our customer service department at (800) 638-3030 or fax orders to (301) 223-2320. International customers should call (301) 223-2300.

Visit Lippincott Williams & Wilkins on the Internet: at LWW.com. Lippincott Williams & Wilkins customer service representatives are available from 8:30 am to 6 pm, EST.

10 9 8 7 6 5 4 3 2 1

To

Mary Kay

Wendy

Alice

CONTRIBUTING AUTHORS

Sumaira Z. Aasi, MD
Yale Surgical Dermatology
Yale New Haven Hospital
New Haven, Connecticut

Amy P. Abernathy, MD
Associate Professor of Medicine
Division of Medical Oncology
Department of Medicine
Associate Director
Duke Comprehensive Cancer Center
Duke University
Durham, North Carolina

Janet L. Abrahm, MD
Associate Professor of Medicine
Harvard Medical School
Staff Physician
Department of Medicine
Psychosocial Oncology and Palliative Care
Dana-Farber Cancer Institute
Brigham and Women's Hospital
Boston, Massachusetts

Maysa M. Abu-Khalaf, MD, MBBS
Assistant Professor
Division of Medical Oncology
Yale University School of Medicine
Yale Comprehensive Cancer Center
New Haven, Connecticut

Gregory P. Adams, PhD
Associate Professor
Developmental Therapeutics Program
Fox Chase Cancer Center
Philadelphia, Pennsylvania

Anupriya Agarwal, PhD
Postdoctoral Fellow
Department of Hematology/Oncology
Center for Hematologic Malignancies
Oregon Health & Science University
Portland, Oregon

Nishant Agrawal, MD
Department of Otolaryngology-Head and Neck Surgery
Johns Hopkins Medical Institutions
Baltimore, Maryland

Jaffer Ajani, MD
Professor of Medicine
Department of Gastrointestinal Medical Oncology
The University of Texas MD Anderson Cancer Center
Houston, Texas

Daniel M. Albert, MD, MS
RRF Emmett A. Humble Distinguished Director of the University of Wisconsin Eye Research Institute
F. A. Davis Professor
Department of Ophthamology and Visual Sciences
University of Wisconsin, Madison
Madison, Wisconsin

Peter C. Albertson, MD, MS
Professor
Department of Surgery
University of Connecticut Health Center
Farmington, Connecticut

H. Richard Alexander, Jr., MD
Professor and Associate Chair for Clinical Research
Department of Surgery
University of Maryland School of Medicine
Baltimore, Maryland

James M. Allan, DPhil
Faculty of Medical Sciences
Newcastle University
Newcastle-Upon-Tyne, United Kingdom

Kenneth C. Anderson, MD
Kraft Family Professor of Medicine
Department of Medicine
Harvard Medical School
Chief
Division of Hematologic Neoplasms
Department of Medical Oncology
Dana-Farber Cancer Institute
Boston, Massachusetts

Matthew L. Anderson, MD, PhD
Assistant Professor
Division of Gynecologic Oncology
Baylor College of Medicine
Attending Surgeon
Texas Cancer Institute
Saint Luke's Episcopal Hospital
Houston, Texas

Smith Apisarnthanarax, MD
Assistant Professor
Department of Radiation Oncology
University of Pennsylvania
Philadelphia, Pennsylvania

Alicia Y. Armstrong, MD, MHSCR
Professor
Department of Obstetrics and Gyneology
Uniformed Services University
Chief, Clinical Services
Program in Reproductive and Adult Endocrinology
National Institue of Child Health and Human Development
National Institutes of Health
Bethesda, Maryland

Vivek K. Arora, MD, PhD
Fellow
Human Oncology & Pathogenesis Program
Memorial Sloan-Kettering Cancer Center
New York, New York

Alan Ashworth, PhD, FRS
Chief Executive
Institute of Cancer Research
London, United Kingdom

Cristina R. Antonescu, MD
Department of Pathology
Memorial Sloan-Kettering Cancer Center
New York, New York

Itzhak Avital, MD
Senior Investigator and Staff Clinician, Assistant Professor of Surgery
Surgery Branch
National Cancer Institute/National Institute of Health
Uniformed University of the Health Sciences
Bethesda, Maryland

Joachim M. Baehring, MD
Associate Professor
Attending Physician
Department of Neurology, Medicine, and Neurosurgery
Yale University School of Medicine
Yale-New Haven Hospital
New Haven, Connecticut

Dean F. Bajorin, MD, FACP
Attending Physician and Member
Department of Medicine
Memorial Sloan-Kettering Cancer Center
Professor
Department of Medicine
Weill Cornell Medical College
New York, New York

Igor J. Barani, MD
Assistant Professor in Residence
Attending Physician
Department of Radiation Oncology
University of California, San Francisco
San Francisco, California

David A. Barbie, MD
Department of Medical Oncology
Massachusetts General Hospital
Boston, Massachusetts

Alberto Bardelli, PhD
Laboratory of Molecular Genetics
Institute for Cancer Research and Treatment
University of Torino Medical School
Candiolo, Italy

David L. Bartlett, MD
Bernard Fisher Professor of Surgery
Department of Surgery
University of Pittsburgh
Chief
Department of Surgery
University of Pittsburgh Medical Center
Pittsburgh, Pennsylvania

Susan Elaine Bates, MD
Senior Investigator
Medical Oncology Branch
National Cancer Institute
Bethesda, Maryland

Steven B. Baylin, MD
Virginia and D.K. Ludwig Professor for Cancer Research
Professor of Oncology and Medicine
Deputy Director
The Sidney Kimmel Comprehensive Cancer Center at Johns Hopkins
Johns Hopkins School of Medicine
Baltimore, Maryland

J. Robert Beck, MD
Professor and Senior Vice President
Chief Academic and Medical Officer
Fox Chase Cancer Center
Philadelphia, Pennsylvania

Jürgen C. Becker, MD, PhD
Professor
Department of General Dermatology
Medical University of Graz (MUG)
Chief
Department of Dermatology
University Hospital-Graz
Graz, Austria

Kevin P. Becker, MD, PhD
Clinical Instructor
Department of Neurology
Yale University School of Medicine
New Haven, Connecticut

David J. Beddy, MD, FRCS
Fellow
Division of Colon and Rectal Surgery
Mayo Clinic
Rochester, Minnesota

Claudio Belluco, MD
Attending Surgeon
Department of Surgical Oncology
Centro di Riferimento Oncologico, National Cancer Institue
Aviano (PN), Italy

Edgar Ben-Josef, MD
Professor
Department of Radiation Oncology
University of Michigan
University of Michigan Hospital
Ann Arbor, Michigan

Andrew Berchuck, MD
Director
Division of Gynecological Oncology
Duke University Medical Center
Durham, North Carolina

Jonathan S. Berek, MD, MMS
Professor and Director
Women's Cancer Center
Stanford Cancer Center
Chair, Department of Obstetrics and Gynecology
Stanford University School of Medicine
Stanford, California

Alice Hawley Berger, BS
Graduate Student
Department of Cancer Biology
Weill Graduate School of Medical Sciences of Cornell University
Cancer Center Genetics Program
Beth Israel Deaconess Cancer Center
Boston, Massachusetts

Ann M. Berger MSN, MD
Bethesda, Maryland

Ross S. Berkowitz, MD
William H. Baker Professor of Gynecology
Department of Obstetrics and Gyncology
Harvard Medical School
Director of Gynecologic Oncology and Gynecology
Department of Obstetrics and Gynecology
Brigham and Women's Hospital and Dana-Farber Cancer Institute
Boston, Massachusetts

Jordan D. Berlin, MD
Associate Professor of Medicine
Clinical Director, GI Oncology Program
Director, Phase I Program
Medical Director, Clinical Trials Shared Resources
Member
Vanderbilt Ingram Cancer Center
Medical Oncologist
Nashville, Tennessee

Leslie Bernstein, PhD
Professor and Director
Division of Cancer Etiology, Department of Population Sciences
Beckman Research Institute of the City of Hope
Dean for Faculty Affairs
City of Hope Medical Center and Beckman Research Institute
Duarte, California

Ravi Bhatia, MD
Director
Hematopoietic Stem Cell & Leukemia Research
Co-Director
Hematological Malignancies Program
City of Hope
Duarte, California

Smita Bhatia, MD, MPH
Professor and Chair
Department of Population Sciences
City of Hope
Professor
Department of Pediatrics
City of Hope National Medical Center
Duarte, California

Adrian M. Di Bisceglie, MD, FACP
Professor and Chair
Department of Internal Medicine
St. Louis University
St. Louis, Missouri

Dale Bixby, MD, PhD
Clinical Assistant Professor
Department of Internal Medicine
University of Michigan
Ann Arbor, Michigan

Elizabeth M. Blanchard, MD
Medical Oncologist
Southcoast Center for Cancer Care
Southcoast Hospital Group
North Dartmouth, Massachusetts

Sharon L. Bober, PhD
Clinical Instructor
Department of Psychology
Harvard Medical School
Director
Sexual Health Program
Dana-Farber Cancer Institute
Boston, Massachusetts

Danielle Campfield Bonadies, MS
Genetic Counselor
Yale Cancer Center
Yale School of Medicine
New Haven, Connecticut

Hossein Borghaei, DO, MS
Assistant Professor
Department of Medical Oncology
Fox Chase Cancer Center
Philadelphia, Pennsylvania

George J. Bosl, MD
Professor of Medicine
Department of Medicine
Weill Cornell Medical College
Chair
Department of Medicine
The Patrick M Byrne Chair in Clinical Oncology
Memorial Sloan-Keetering Cancer Center
New York, New York

Michael Boyiadzis, MD
Division of Hematology/Oncology
University of Pittsburgh School of Medicine
Pittsburgh, Pennsylvania

Dean E. Brenner, MD
Kutsche Family Professor of Internal Medicine
Professor of Pharmacology
University of Michigan and VA Medical Center
Ann Arbor, Michigan

Paul D. Brown, MD
Professor
Department of Radiation Oncology
The University of Texas MD Anderson Cancer Center
Houston, Texas

Gary L. Buchschacher, Jr., MD, PhD
Assistant Clinical Professor of Medicine
David Geffen School of Medicine
University of California, Los Angeles
Staff Physician
Department of Hematology/Oncology
Los Angeles Medical Center, Kaiser Foundation/SCPMG
Los Angeles, California

Harold J. Burstein, MD, PhD
Associate Professor of Medicine
Harvard Medical School
Breat Oncology Center
Dana-Farber Cancer Institute
Boston, Massachusetts

Tim E. Byers, MD, MPH
Associate Dean
Colorado School of Public Health
Aurora, Colorado

John C. Byrd, MD
Division of Hematology and Comprehensive Cancer Center
The Ohio State University
Columbus, Ohio

Joseph Califano, MD
Department of Otolaryngology-Head and Neck Surgery
Johns Hopkins Medical Institutions
Milton J. Dance Head and Neck Center
Greater Baltimore Medical Center
Baltimore, Maryland

Robert B. Cameron, MD
Professor of Cardiothoracic Surgery and Surgical Oncology
Department of Surgery
David Geffen School of Medicine at University of California
Los Angeles, California

Stephen A. Cannistra, MD
Professor of Medicine
Department of Medicine
Harvard Medical School
Director
Department of Gynecological Medical Oncology
Beth Israel Deaconess Medical Center
Boston, Massachusetts

Lewis C. Cantley, PhD
Clinical Oncology
Merck Research Laboratories
Upper Gwynned, Pennsylvania

David P. Carbone, MD, PhD
Professor of Medicine & Cancer Biology
Department of Medicine/ Hematology & Oncology
Vanderbilt University
Nashville, Tennessee

Michele Carbone, MD, PhD
Professor and Chair
Department of Pathology
John A. Burns School of Medicine
Director
Cancer Research Center of Hawaii
University of Hawaii
Honolulu, Hawaii

Tobias Carling, MD, PhD
Assistant Professor of Surgery
Attending Surgeon
Department of Surgery
Yale University School of Medicine
Yale New Haven Hospital
New Haven, Connecticut

Chris L. Carpenter, PhD
Division of Signal Transduction
Department of Medicine
Beth Israel Deaconess Medical Center
Boston, Massachusetts

Darryl Carter, MD
Professor of Pathology, Emeritus
Yale University
New Haven, Connecticut

Eric J. Cassell, MD, MACP
Emeritus Professor of Public Medicine
Weill Cornell Medical College
New York, New York
Adjunt Professor of Medicine
Faculty of Medicine
McGill University
Montreal, Canada
Attending Physician
Department of Medicine
New York Presbyterian Hospital
Cornell Medical Center
New York, New York

Webster K. Cavenee, PhD
Director and Distinguished Professor
Ludwig Institute for Cancer Research
University of California, San Diego
La Jolla, California

Keith A. Cengel, MD, PhD
Assistant Professor
Department of Radiation Oncology
University of Pennsylvania
Director, Photodynamic Therapy Program
Hospital of the University of Pennsylvania
Philadelphia, Pennsylvania

Jan Cerny, MD, PhD
Assistant Professor of Medicine
Department of Medicine
Division of Hematology and Oncology
University of Massachusetts
University of Massachusetts Memorial Medical Center
Worchester, Massachusetts

Raju S. K. Chaganti, PhD
Member and Professor
Cell Biology Program
Member and Attending
Department of Medicine
Memorial Sloan-Kettering Cancer Center
New York, New York

Richard Champlin, MD
Departments of Leukemia and Stem Cell Transplantation and Cellular Therapy
The University of Texas MD Anderson Cancer Center
Houston, Texas

Susan M. Chang, MD
Professor
Attending Physician
Department of Neurological Surgery
University of California, San Francisco
San Francisco, California

Cindy H. Chau, PharmD, PhD
Scientist
Medical Oncology Branch
National Cancer Institute
Bethesda, Maryland

Yu Chen, MD, PhD
Fellow
Human Oncology & Pathogenesis Program
Fellow
Department of Medicine
Memorial Sloan-Kettering Cancer Center
New York, New York

Douglas Brian Chepeha, MD, MSPH, FRCS(C)
Associate Professor
Otolaryngology–Head and Neck Surgery
University of Michigan
Director, Microvascular Reconstructive Surgery
Otolaryngology–Head and Neck Surgery
University of Michigan
Ann Arbor, Michigan

Nathan I. Cherny MBBS, FRACP, FRCP
Cancer Pain and Palliative Medicine Service
Department of Oncology
Shaare Zedek Medical Center
Jerusalem, Israel

Richard W. Childs, MD
Senior Investigator
Hematology Branch
National Heart, Lung, and Blood Institute
National Institutes of Health
Bethesda, Maryland

Lynda Chin, MD
Professor of Dermatology
Department of Medical Oncology
Dana-Farber Cancer Institute
Boston, Massachusetts

Murali Chintagumpala, MD
Professor of Pediatrics
Department of Pediatrics
Baylor College of Medicine
Professor of Pediatrics
Department of Hematology/Oncology, Pediatrics
Texas Children's Hospital
Houston, Texas

Edward Chow, MD
Professor
Department of Radiation Oncology
University of Toronto
Radiation Oncologist
Department of Radiation Oncology
Sunnybrook Health Sciences Centre
Toronto, Canada

Edward Chu, MD
Professor of Medicine
Chief, Division of Hematology-Oncology
Department of Medicine
University of Pittsburgh Cancer Institute
University of Pittsburgh School of Medicine
Pittsburgh, Pennsylvania

Gina G. Chung, MD
Assistant Professor
Department of Internal Medicine
Yale Cancer Center
Yale University School of Medicine
Smilow Cancer Hospital
Yale-New Haven Hospital
New Haven, Connecticut

Timothy R. Church, PhD, MS
Professor
Division of Environmental Health Sciences
University of Minnesota School of Public Health
Minneapolis, Minnesota

Lorenzo Cohen, PhD
Professor
Department of Behavioral Science, Cancer Prevention and Population Sciences
The University of Texas MD Anderson Cancer Center
Houston, Texas

Robert E. Coleman, MD, FRCP, FRCPE
Yorkshire Cancer Research Professor of Medical Oncology
Academic Unit of Clinical Oncology
University of Sheffield
Honorary Consultant
Academic Unit of Clinical Oncology
Weston Park Hospital
Sheffield, United Kingdom

Louis S. Constine, MD, FASTRO
Professor of Radiation Oncology and Pediatrics
Vice Chair
Department of Radiation Oncology
James P. Wilmot Cancer Center
University of Rochester Medical Center
Attending Physician
Department of Radiation Oncology
Strong Memorial Hospital
Rochester, New York

M. Sitki Copur MD, FACP
Associate Professor
Department of Internal Medicine
University of Nebraska Medical Center
Medical Director
Department of Oncology
Saint Francis Cancer Center
Omaha, Nebraska

Christopher Crane, MD
Professor
Program Director and Section Chief, Gastrointestinal Section
Department of Radiation Oncology
The University of Texas MD Anderson Cancer Center
Houston, Texas

Craig M. Crews, PhD
Lewis B. Cullman Professor
Department of Molecular, Cellular, and Developmental Biology
Yale University
New Haven, Connecticut

Douglas M. Dahl, MD, FACS
Associate Professor of Surgery
Harvard Medical School
Chief, Division of Urologic Oncology
Department of Urology
Massachusetts General Hospital
Boston, Massachuesetts

Riccardo Dalla-Favera, MD
Professor and Director
Institute for Cancer Genetics
Columbia University
New York, New York

Mary B. Daly, MD, PhD
Chairperson
Department of Clinical Genetics
Fox Chase Cancer Center
Philadelphia, Pennsylvania

Alan D. D'Andrea, MD
Dana-Farber Cancer Institute
Boston, Massachusetts

Laura A. Dawson, FRCPC, MD
Radiation Medicine Program
Princess Margaret Hospital
Toronto, Ontario, Canada

Lisa M. DeAngelis, MD
Professor of Neurology
Weill Cornell Medical College
Chair
Department of Neurology
Memorial Sloan-Kettering Cancer Center
New York, New York

Alan H. DeCherney, MD
Head
Program in Reproductive and Adult Endocrinology
National Institute of Child Health and Human Development
National Institutes of Health
Bethesda, Maryland

Michael W. Deininger, MD, PhD
Maxwell M. Wintrobe, MD Presidential Endowed Chair in Internal Medicine
Chief, Division of Hematology and Hematologic Malignancies
Department of Internal Medicine
University of Utah/Huntsman Cancer Institute
Salt Lake City, Utah

Marcos De Lima, MD
Departments of Leukemia and Stem Cell Transplantation and Cellular Therapy
The University of Texas MD Anderson Cancer Center
Houston, Texas

George D. Demetri, MD
Senior Vice President for Experimental Therapeutics
Ludwig Center
Medical Oncology
Dana-Farber Cancer Institute
Harvard Medical School
Boston, Massachusetts

Ronald A. DePinho, MD
Director
Belfer Institute for Applied Cancer Science
Dana-Farber Cancer Institute
Harvard Medical School
Professor
Department of Medicine
Brigham & Women's Hospital
Boston, Massachusetts

Marcello Deraco, MD
Professor
Department of Postgraduation on Digestive Surgery
Tor Vergata University
Rome, Italy
Responsible for Perotineal Surface Malignancies
Department of Surgery
IRCCS National Insutute of Tumors Foundation
Milan, Italy

Vincent T. DeVita, Jr., MD
Amy & Joseph Perella Professor of Medicine
Yale Comprehensive Cancer Center and Smilow Cancer Hospital at Yale-New Haven
Yale University School of Medicine
Professor of Epidemiology and Public Health
Yale University School of Public Health
New Haven, Connecticut

John E. Dick, PhD
Professor
Department of Molecular Biology
University of Toronto
Canada Research Chair in Stem Cell Biology, Senior Scientist
Department of Cellular and Molecular Biology
University Health Network
Toronto, Ontario, Canada

Volker Diehl, MD
University Hospital of Cologne
Cologne, Germany

Gerard M. Doherty, MD
N. W. Thompson Professor and Vice Chair
Department of Surgery
University of Michigan
Chief, General Surgery
University of Michigan Hospitals and Health Centers
Ann Arbor, Michigan

Brian J. Druker, MD
Professor
Department of Medicine
Division of Hematolgy and Medical Oncology
Oregon Health & Science University
Investigator
Howard Hughes Medical Institute
Director
Oregon Health & Sciences University Knight Cancer Institute
Portland, Oregon

Craig C. Earle, MD
Associate Professor
Department of Medicine
University of Toronto
Medical Oncologist
Odette Cancer Centre
Sunnybrook Health Sciences Centre
Toronto, Ontario, Canada

James A. Eastham, MD
Professor of Urology
Department of Surgery
Chief, Urology Service
Department of Surgery
Memorial Sloan-Kettering Cancer Center
New York, New York

Richard L. Edelson, MD
Professor and Chairman
Department of Dermatology
Yale School of Medicine
Chief, Dermatology Service
Department of Dermatology
Yale-New Haven Hospital
New Haven, Connecticut

Dennis A. Eichenauer, MD
Resident, Department of Internal Medicine
University Hospital of Cologne
Cologne, Germany

Patricia J. Eifel, MD
Professor
Department of Radiation Oncology
The University of Texas MD Anderson Cancer Center
Houston, Texas

Dominique Elias, MD, PhD
Chief
Department of Surgical Oncology
Gustave Roussy Institute
Villejuif, France

Anthony El-Khoueiry, MD
Assistant Professor of Medicine
Department of Medicine/Medical Oncology
University of Southern California, Norris Comprehensive Cancer Center
Los Angeles, California

Lee M. Ellis, MD
Professor of Surgery and Cancer Biology
Department of Surgical Oncology and Cancer Biology
The University of Texas MD Anderson Cancer Center
Houston, Texas

Andreas Engert, MD
Department of Internal Medicine
University Hospital of Cologne
Cologne, Germany

Charles Erlichman, MD
Consultant, Professor of Oncology
Department of Oncology, Division of Medical Oncology
Mayo Clinic College of Medicine
Rochester, Minnesota

Virginia Espina, MS
Research Assistant Professor
George Mason University
Center for Applied Proteomics and Molecular Medicine
Manassas, Virginia

Laura J. Esserman, MD, MBA
Director
Carol Franc Buck Breast Care Center
Department of Surgery
University of California, San Francisco
San Francisco, California

Eli Estey, MD
Division of Hematology
University of Washington and
Fred Hutchinson Cancer Research Center
Seattle, Washington

Douglas B. Evans, MD
Department of Surgery
Medical College of Wisconsin
Milwaukee, Wisconsin

Stefan Faderl, MD
Associate Professor
Department of Leukemia
The University of Texas MD Anderson Cancer Center
Houston, Texas

Jane M. Fall-Dickson, PhD, RN, AOCN
National Institute of Nursing Research
Bethesda, Maryland

Ann Theresa Farrell, MD
Deputy Division Director
Division of Drug Oncology Products
Office of Oncology Drug Products
Center for Drug Evaluation and Research
Silver Spring, Maryland

Eve C. Feinberg, MD
Fertility Centers of Illinois
Highland Park, Illinois

Darren R. Feldman, MD
Instructor
Department of Medicine
Weill Medical College of Cornell University
Assistant Attending
Department of Medicine
Memorial Sloan-Kettering Cancer Center
New York, New York

James L. M. Ferrara, MD, ScD
Professor
Department of Pediatrics and Internal Medicine
University of Michigan Medical School
Director, Blood and Marrow Transplant Program
Department of Pediatrics, Hematology/Oncology
University of Michigan Comprehensive Cancer Center
Ann Arbor, Michigan

William D. Figg, PharmD, MBA
Senior Investigator
Medical Oncology Branch
National Cancer Institute
National Institute of Health
Bethesda, Maryland

Michelle Cororve Fingeret, PhD
Assistant Professor
Department of Behavioral Science
The University of Texas MD Anderson Cancer Center
Houston, Texas

Joel Finkelstein, MSc, MD, FRCS(C)
Associate Professor
Department of Surgery
University of Toronto
Consultant Orthopaedic Surgeon
Division of Orthopaedics
Sunnybrook Health Sciences Center
Toronto, Ontario

Richard I. Fisher, MD
Senior Associate Dean for Clinical Affairs
Department of Hematology-Oncology
Director
James P. Wilmot Cancer Center
Strong Memorial Hospital
Rochester, New York

Keith Thomas Flaherty, MD
Associate Professor
Harvard School of Medicine
Director of Developmental Therapeutics
Department of Medicine
Massachusetts General Hospital
Boston, Massachusetts

Chris I. Flowers, MBBS, FRCR
Associate Professor
Department of Radiology and Biomedical Imaging
University of California, San Francisco
San Francisco, California

Antonio Tito Fojo, MD, PhD
Senior Investigator
Medical Oncology Branch
National Cancer Institute
Bethesda, Maryland

Kathleen M. Foley, MD
Professor of Nuerology, Neuroscience & Clinical Pharmacology
School of Medicine and Public Health
Department of Neurology
Weill Medical College of Cornell University
Attending Neurologist
Memorial Sloan-Kettering Cancer Center
New York, New York

Kenneth A. Foon, MD
Chief
Department of Hematologic Malignance
Nevada Cancer Institute
Las Vegas, Nevada

Francine Foss, MD
Professor of Medicine
Department of Medical Oncology and and Bone Marrow Transplantion
Yale University School of Medicine
New Haven, Connecticut

Harold P. Freeman, MD
Professor Emeritus
Department of Surgery
Columbia University
Attending Surgeon
Department of Surgery
Memorial Hospital for Cancer and Allied Diseases
New York, New York

Jonathan W. Friedberg, MD, MMSc
Professor, Department of Medicine
Chief, Hematology/Oncology Division
James P. Wilmot Cancer Center
Rochester University Medical Center
Rochester, New York

Sheryl G. A. Gabram, MD, MBA
Professor
Department of Surgery
Emory University
Director
Avon Comprehensive Breast Center
Grady Memorial Hospital
Atlanta, Georgia

Craig J. Galbán, PhD
Professor
Department of Radiology and Biomedical Engineering
University of Michigan
Ann Arbor, Michigan

Don Ganem, MD
Departments of Medicine and of Microbiology and Immunology
University of California, San Francisco School of Medicine
San Francisco, California

Patricia A. Ganz, MD
Professor
School of Medicine and Public Health
Director
Division of Cancer Prevention and Control Research
Jonsson Comprehensive Cancer Center
University of California
Los Angeles, California

Levi A. Garraway, MD, PhD
Assistant Professor of Medicine, Harvard Medical School
Department of Medical Oncology
Dana-Farber Cancer Institute
Boston, Massachusetts
Senior Associate Member, The Broad Institute of Harvard and MIT
Cambridge, Massachusetts

Juan C. Gea-Banacloche, MD
Chief
Infectious Diseases Consultation Service
Experimental Transplantation and Immunology Branch
National Cancer Institute
National Institutes of Health
Bethesda, Maryland

Christos S. Georgiades, PhD, MD, FSIR
Associate Professor
Department of Radiology
Johns Hopkins University
Clinical Director
Department of Vascular and Interventional Radiology
Johns Hopkins Hospital
Baltimore, Maryland

David M. Gershenson, MD
J. Taylor Wharton, MD Distinguished Chair in Gynecological Oncology
Professor & Chairman
Department of Gynecologic Oncology
The University of Texas MD Anderson Cancer Center
Houston, Texas

Jean-Francois H. Geschwind, MD
Professor
Department of Radiology
Johns Hopkins University
Chief
Department of Vascular and Interventional Radiology
Johns Hopkins Hospital
Baltimore, Maryland

Larisa J. Geskin, MD
Director, Cutaneous Oncology Center
Department of Dermatology
University of Pittsburgh Medical Center
Pittsburgh, Pennsylvania

Scott Gettinger, MD
Assistant Professor of Medicine
Yale University School of Medicine
Yale Cancer Center
New Haven, Connecticut

Giuseppe Giaccone, MD, PhD
Chief
Medical Oncology Branch
National Cancer Institute
Bethesda, Maryland

Edward L. Giovannucci, MD, ScD
Professor
Department of Nutrition and Epidemiology
Harvard School of Public Health
Associate Professor
Department of Medicine
Brigham and Women's Hospital
Havard Medical School
Boston, Massachusetts

Olivier Glehen, MD, PhD
Professor
Equipe Accueil
Université Claude Bernard Lyon 1
Oullins, France
Professor
Department of Surgical Oncology
Centre Hospitalier Lyon Sud
Pierre Bénite, France

Matthew P. Goetz, MD
Consultant, Associate Professor of Oncology
Department of Oncology, Division of Medical Oncology
Mayo Clinic College of Medicine
Rochester, Minnesota

Donald P. Goldstein, MD
Professor
Department of Obstetrics, Gyncology, and Reproductive Biology
Harvard Medical School
Attending Gynecologist
Department of Obstetrics and Gynecology
Brigham and Women's Hospital
Boston, Massachusetts

Leonard G. Gomella, MD, FACS
Chairman
Department of Urology
Kimmel Cancer Center, Thomas Jefferson University Hospital
Philadelphia, Pennsylvania

David J. Gordon, MD, PhD
Instructor
Department of Pediatrics
Harvard Medical School
Department of Hematology/Oncology
Dana-Farber Cancer Institute
Boston, Massachusetts

Steven D. Gore, MD
Sidney Kimmel Comprehensive Cancer Center at Johns Hopkins
Baltimore, Maryland

F. Anthony Greco, MD
Director
Sarah Cannon Cancer Center
Centennial Medical Center
Nashville, Tennessee

Jan Grimm, MD, PhD
Department of Radiology
Memorial Sloan-Kettering Cancer Center
New York, New York

Joe W. Grisham, MD
Senior Scientist
Laboratory of Experimental Carcinogenesis
Center for Cancer Research, NCI, National Institutes of Health
Bethesda, Maryland

Ellen R. Gritz, PhD
Professor and Chair
Department of Behavioral Science
The University of Texas MD Anderson Cancer Center
Houston, Texas

José G. Guillem, MD
Department of Surgery
Memorial Sloan-Kettering Cancer Center
New York, New York

Patrick K. Ha, MD
Department of Otolaryngology-Head and Neck Surgery
Johns Hopkins Medical Institutions
Milton J. Dance Head and Neck Center
Greater Baltimore Medical Center
Baltimore, Maryland

Stephen M. Hahn, MD
Professor and Chair
Department of Radiation Oncology
University of Pennsylvania School of Medicine
Philadelphia, Pennsylvania

William C. Hahn, MD, PhD
Associate Professor
Department of Medicine
Harvard Medical School
Division Chief
Department of Molecular and Cellular Oncology
Dana-Farber Cancer Institute
Boston, Massachusetts

John D. Hainsworth, MD
Chief Scientific Officer
Sarah Cannon Cancer Center
Centennial Medical Center
Nashville, Tennessee

Lyndsay N. Harris, MD
Associate Professor
Yale Cancer Center, Section of Medical Oncology
Co-Director Breast Disease Unit
Smilow Cancer Hospital
Yale-New Haven Hospital
New Haven, Connecticut

Jay R. Harris, MD
Professor
Department of Radiation Oncology
Harvard Medical School
Chair
Department of Radiation Oncology
Dana-Farber Cancer Institute
Brigham and Women's Hospital
Boston, Massachusetts

Nancy Lee Harris, MD
Austin L. Vickery Professor
Department of Pathology
Harvard Medical School
Pathologist; Editor, Case Records of the Massachusetts General Hospital
Department of Pathology
Massachusetts General Hospital
Boston, Massachusetts

Axel Hauschild, MD
Professor of Dermatology
Department of Dermatology, Campus Kiel
University Hospital (UKSH)
Kiel, Germany

Marc J. Haxer, MA, CCC-SLP
Speech–Language Pathologist
Departments of Speech–Pathology and Otolaryngology—Head and Neck Surgery
University of Michigan
Ann Arbor, Michigan

Daniel F. Hayes, MD
Professor
Department of Internal Medicine
University of Michgan School of Medicine
Co- Director
Breast Oncology Program
University of Michigan Comprehensive Cancer Center
Ann Arbor, Michigan

Stephen S. Hecht, PhD
Wallin Professor of Cancer Prevention
Masonic Cancer Center
University of Minnesota
Minneapolis, Minnesota

Matthew T. Heller, MD
Assistant Professor of Radiology
Division of Abdominal Imaging
University of Pittsburgh Medical Center
Pittsburgh, Pennsylvania

Lee J. Helman, MD
Scientific Director for Clinical Research
Center for Cancer Research
National Cancer Institute
Bethesda, Maryland

C. William Helm, MB, BChir
Professor
Division of Gynecologic Oncology
Department of Obstetrics, Gynecology and Women's Health
Division of Gynecologic Oncology, Cancer Center
St. Louis University Hospital
St. Louis, Missouri

Katherine D. Henderson, PhD
Assistant Research Professor
Division of Cancer Etiology, Department of Population Sciences
Beckman Research Institute of the City of Hope
Duarte, California

James G. Herman, MD
Department of Hematology/Medical Oncology
Johns Hopkins University
Sidney Kimmel Comprehensive Cancer Center
Baltimore, Maryland

Paul J. Hesketh, MD
Professor
Department of Medicine
Tufts University School of Medicine
Boston, Massachusetts
Director
Thoracic Oncology
Division of Hematology/Oncology
Lahey Clinic Medical Center
Burlington, Massachusetts

Erin W. Hofstatter, MD
Assistant Professor
Yale Cancer Center, Section of Medical Oncology
Yale University
Smilow Cancer Hospital
Yale-New Haven Hospital
New Haven, Connecticut

Leora Horn, MD, MS
Assistant Professor
Department of Internal Medicine
Vanderbilt University
Nashville, Tennessee

Yoshinori Hosoya, MD, PhD
Associate Professor
Department of Surgery
Jichi Medical University
Tochigi, Japan

Peter M. Howley, MD
Professor
Department of Pathology
Harvard Medical School
Boston, Massachusetts

Ralph H. Hruban, MD
Department of Pathology
Johns Hopkins University
Baltimore, Maryland

Melissa M. Hudson, MD
Director, Cancer Survivorship Division
Department of Oncology
St. Jude Children's Research Hospital
Memphis, Tennessee

David H. Ilson, MD, PhD
Professor
Department of Medicine
Weill Medical College of Cornell University
Attending Physician
Department of Medicine
Memorial Sloan-Kettering Cancer Center
New York, New York

Bonnie A. Indeck, MSW, LCSW
Clinical Instructor
Department of Internal Medicine
Yale Cancer Center
Manager, Oncology Social Worker
Department of Social Work
Yale-New Haven Hospital
New Haven, Connecticut

C. David James, PhD
Professor
Department of Neurological Surgery
University of California, San Francisco
San Francisco, California

Ahmedin Jemal
American Cancer Society
Atlanta, Georgia

James R. Jett, MD
Professor of Medicine
Staff Physician
Department of Pulmonary Medicine
Mayo Clinic
Rochester, Minnesota

Yixing Jiang, MD
Assitant Professor
Department of Medicine
Penn State College of Medicine
Hershey, Pennsylvania

Peter A. Jones, MD
Distinguished Professor
Department of Urology, Biochemistry and Molecular Biology
Keck School of Medicine of University of Southern California
Director, Cancer Center
University of Southern California/ Norris Comprehensive Cancer Center
Los Angeles, California

Lisa A. Kachnic, MD
Associate Professor
Chief
Department of Radiation Oncology
Boston Medical Center
Boston, Massachusetts

Madhuri Kakarala, MD, PhD
Clinical Lecturer
University of Michigan and VA Medical Center
Ann Arbor, Michigan

Udai S. Kammula, MD
Senior Investigator
Surgery Branch
National Cancer Institute
National Institutes of Health
Bethesda, Maryland

Hagop M. Kantarjian, MD
Department of Leukemia
The University of Texas MD Anderson Cancer Center
Houston, Texas

Joyson J. Karakunnel, MD, FACP
Bethesda, MD

Vassiliki Karantza, MD, PhD
Assistant Professor
Department of Medicine-Medical Oncology
Cancer Institute of New Jersey
Attending Physician
Robert Wood Johnson University Hospital
New Brunswick, New Jersey

Michael G. Kauffman, MD, PhD
Onyx Pharmaceuticals

Donald S. Kaufman, MD
Clinical Professor of Medicine
Department of Medicine
Harvard Medical School
Director of Education, The John and Claire Bertucci Center for Genitourinary Cancers
Division of Hematology/Oncology
Massachusetts General Hospital
Boston, Massachusetts

Jacob Kaufman
Vanderbilt University Medical Center
Nashville, Tennessee

Electron Kebebew, MD
Senior Investigator, Head of Endocrine Oncology
Surgery Branch
National Cancer Institute
Bethesda, Maryland

Partow Kebriaei, MD
Associate Professor
Department of Stem Cell Transplant and Cellular Therapy
The University of Texas MD Anderson Cancer Center
Houston, Texas

David P. Kelsen, MD
Chief, Gastrointestinal Oncology
Department of Medicine
Memorial Sloan Kettering Cancer Center
Edward S. Gordon Chair in Medical Oncology
Professor of Medicine
Weill School of Medicine of Cornell University
New York, New York

Christopher R. Kelsey, MD
Assistant Professor
Department of Radiation Oncology
Duke Cancer Institute
Duke University Medical Center
Durham, North Carolina

Robert S. Kerbel, PhD
Professor
Department of Biophysics
Senior Scientist
Department of Molecular & Cellular Biology Research
Sunnybrook Health Sciences Centre
Toronto, Ontario, Canada

Scott E. Kern, MD
Professor
Department of Oncology
Johns Hopkins University
Baltimore, Maryland

Alok Anand Khorana, MD, FACP
Associate Professor of Medicine and Oncology
Division of Hematology/Oncology
Department of Medicine
James P. Wilmot Cancer Center
University of Rochester Medical Center
Rochester, New York

Elliott Kieff, MD, PhD
Departments of Medicine and of Microbiology and Molecular Genetics
Harvard Medical School
Boston, Massachusetts

Christopher J. Kirk, PhD
Onyx Pharmaceuticals

Mio Kitano, MD
Surgery Branch
National Cancer Institute, Center for Cancer Research
National Institutes of Health, Bethesda, Maryland

Margaret A. Knowles, PhD
Professor of Experimental Cancer Research
Section of Experimental Oncology
Leeds Institute of Molecular Medicine
St. James's University Hospital
University of Leeds
Leeds, United Kingdom

Manish Kohli, MD
Associate Professor of Oncology
Department of Oncology
Mayo Clinic, College of Medicine
Chief, Genitourinary Medical Oncology
Department of Oncology
Mayo Clinic
Rochester, Minnesota

Marisa A. Kollmeier, MD
Assistant Professor and Assistant Attending
Department of Radiation Oncology
Memorial Sloan-Kettering Cancer Center
New York, New York

Mark G. Kris, MD
Professor of Medicine
Department of Medicine
Weill Medical College of Cornell University
Chief
Department of Thoracic Medicine
Memorial Sloan-Kettering Cancer Center
New York, New York

Lee M. Krug, MD
Associate Member
Associate Attending Physician
Department of Medicine
Memorial Sloan-Kettering Cancer Center
New York, New York

Raju Kucherlapati, PhD
Paul C. Cabot Professor of Genetics
Department of Genetics
Havard Medical School
Professor of Medicine
Departments of Medicine and Genetics
Brigham and Women's Hospital
Boston, Massachusetts

Amol D. Kulkarni, MD
Resident Physician
Department of Ophthamology
University of Wisconsin, Madison
Madison, Wisconsin

Carla Kurkjian, MD
Assistant Professor
Section of Hematology/Oncology
Department of Medicine
University of Oklahoma Health Sciences Center
Oklahoma City, Oklahoma

King F. Kwong, MD
Principle Investigator
Department of Thoracic Oncology, Surgery Branch
Attending Thoracic Surgeon
Surgery Branch, Center for Cancer Research
National Cancer Institute
National Institutes of Health
Bethesda, Maryland

Nadia N. Issa Laack, MD, MS
Assistant Professor
Department of Radiation Oncology
Mayo Clinic
Rochester, Minnesota

Cho Lam, PhD
Assistant Professor
Department of Behavioral Science
The University of Texas MD Anderson Cancer Center
Houston, Texas

Wendy Landier, RN, MSN
Clinical Director
Center for Cancer Survivorship
Department of Population Sciences
City of Hope
Duarte, California

David A. Larson, MD, PhD
Professor
Department of Radiation Oncology
University of California, San Francisco
San Francisco, California

Steven M. Larson, MD, FACNP, FACR
Chief of Nuclear Medicine
Department of Nuclear Medicine
Memorial Sloan-Kettering Cancer Center
New York, New York

Alessandro Laviano, MD
Associate Professor
Department of Clinical Medicine
Sapienza University of Rome
Dirigente Medico I Livello
Department of Internal Medicine, Clinical Immunology, Clinical Nutrition and Endocrinology
Umberto I, Policlinico di Roma
Rome, Italy

Theodore S. Lawrence, MD, PhD
Isadore Lampe Professor and Chair
Department of Radiation Oncology
University of Michigan
Ann Arbor, Michigan

Agnes Yuet Ying Lee, MD, MSc, FRCPC
Associate Professor
Department of Medicine
University of British Columbia
Medical Director, Thrombosis Program
Department of Medicine, Division of Hematology
Vancouver Acute, Vancouver Coastal Health
Vancouver, British Columbia, Canada

Richard Lee, MD
Assistant Professor
Department of General Oncology
The University of Texas MD Anderson Cancer Center
Houston, Texas

David J. Leffell, MD
Section Director
Department of Dermatology
Yale University
New Haven, Connecticut

Alan T. Lefor, MD, MPH
Professor
Department of Surgery
Jichi Medical University
Tochigi, Japan

Heinz-Josef Lenz, MD
Professor of Medicine
Department of Medicine/Medical Oncology
University of Southern California, Norris Comprehensive Cancer Center
Los Angeles, California

Steven K. Libutti, MD
Professor
Department of Surgery and Genetics
Albert Einstein College of Medicine
Vice Chairman
Department of Surgery
Montefiore Medical Center
Bronx, New York

Frank S. Lieberman, MD
Director, Adult Neurooncology Program
Department of Neurology
University of Pittsburgh School of Medicine
Pittsburgh, Pennsylvania

W. Marston Linehan, MD
Chief
Urologic Oncology Branch
National Cancer Institute
National Institutes of Health
Bethesda, Maryland

Lance A. Liotta, MD
Professor, Life Science
George Mason University
Center for Applied Proteomics and Molecular Medicine
Manassas, Virginia

Scott M. Lippman, MD
Professor
Chairman
Department of Thoracic Head & Neck Medical Oncology
The University of Texas MD Anderson Cancer Center
Houston, Texas

Richard F. Little, MD, MPH
Head, Blood and AIDS-related Cancers and Hematopoietic Stem Cell Transplant
Clinical Investigations Branch, Cancer Therapy Evaluation Program
Division of Cancer Therapy and Diagnosis
National Cancer Institute
Bethesda, Maryland

Mats Ljungman, PhD
Associate Professor
Department of Radiation Oncology
University of Michigan
Ann Arbor, Michigan

Patrick J. Loehrer, Sr., MD
H. H. Gregg Professor of Medicine
Department of Medicine
Indiana University
Director
Indiana University School of Medicine
Indiana University Melvin and Bren Simon Cancer Center
Indianapolis, Indiana

Carlos López-Otín
Departamento de Bioquímica y Biología Molecular
Instituto Universitario de Oncología (IUOPA)
Universidad de Oviedo
Oviedo, Spain

Charles L. Loprinzi, MD
Regis Professor of Breast Cancer Research
Department of Oncology
Mayo Clinic
Rochester, Minnesota

Michael T. Lotze, MD
Vice Chair Research
Department of Surgery
University of Pittsburgh School of Medicine
Pittsburg, Pennsylvania

Chrystal Louis, MD, MPH
Assistant Professor
Department of Pediatrics
Baylor College of Medicine
Houston, Texas

David N. Louis, MD
James Homer Wright Pathology Laboratories
Massachusetts General Hospital and Harvard Medical School
Pathology
Massachusetts General Hospital
Boston, Massachusetts

Douglas R. Lowy, MD
Deputy Director, National Cancer Institute
Chief, Laboratory of Cellular Oncology
National Cancer Institute
National Institutes of Health
Bethesda, Maryland

Yani Lu, MD, PhD
Postdoctoral Fellow
Department of Population Sciences
City of Hope National Medical Center
Beckman Research Institute
Duarte, California

Teresa H. Lyden, MA, CCC-SLP
Speech–Language Pathologist
Departments of Speech–Pathology and Otolaryngology—Head and Neck Surgery
University of Michigan
Ann Arbor, Michigan

Xiaomei Ma, PhD
Associate Professor
Department of Epidemiology and Public Health
Yale University
New Haven, Connecticut

John M. Magenau, MD
Department of Hematology/Oncology
University of Michigan
Ann Arbor, Michigan

Robert G. Maki, MD
Departments of Medicine and Pediatrics
Mount Sinai School of Medicine
New York, New York

Martin M. Malawer, MD
Professor (Clinical Scholar)
Professor of Pediatrics (Hematology and Oncology)
Department of Orthopedic Surgery and Pediatrics
Professor of Orthopedic Surgery
Director of Othopedic Oncology
Department of Orthopedic Surgery
George Washington University School of Medicine
Washington, DC

David Malkin, MD, FRCPC
Professor
Department of Pediatrics
Universtiy of Toronto
Senior Staff Oncologist
Division of Hematology/Oncology
The Hospital for Sick Children
Toronto, Ontario, Canada

Jack S. Mandel, PhD, MPH
Chief Science Officer
Exponent, Inc
Menlo Park, California

Judith F. Margolin, MD
Associate Professor of Pediatrics
Department of Pediatrics
Baylor College of Medicine
Attending Physician
Texas Children's Cancer Center
Texas Children's Hospital
Houston, Texas

Maurie A. Markman, MD
Vice President
Department of Clinical Research
Chairman
Department of Gynecological Medical Oncology
The University of Texas MD Anderson Cancer Center
Houston, Texas

Lawrence B. Marks, MD
Professor and Chair
Department of Radiation Oncology
University of North Carolina at Chapel Hill School of Medicine
North Carolina Cancer Hospital
Chapel Hill, North Carolina

Joan Massagué, PhD
Member and Chair
Cancer Biology and Genetics Program
Memorial Sloan-Kettering Cancer Center
New York, New York

Ellen T. Matloff, MS
Research Scientist
Department of Genetics
Director, Cancer Genetic Counseling
Yale Cancer Center
Yale School of Medicine
New Haven, Connecticut

Peter M. Mauch, MD
Professor
Department of Radiation Oncology
Harvard Medical School
Brigham and Women's Hospital
Boston, Massachusetts

Susan T. Mayne, PhD
Professor of Epidemiology
Department of Epidemiology and Public Health
Yale School of Medicine
New Haven, Connecticut

Michael W. McDermott, MD, FRCSC
Professor
Department of Neurosurgery
University of California, San Francisco
Robert & Ruth Halperin Chair
Department of Neurosurgery
Moffitt Hospital
San Francisco, California

W. Scott McDougal, MD
Professor of Urology
Harvard Medical School
Chief of Urology
Department of Urology
Massachusetts General Hospital
Boston, Massachusetts

Michael M. Meguid, MD
Surgical Metabolism and Nutrition Laboratory
Neurosciences Program
Department of Surgery
University Hospital
SUNY Upstate Medical University
Syracuse, New York

Robert A. Meguid, MD, MPH
Chief Resident
Department of Surgery
Johns Hopkins University, School of Medicine
House Staff
Department of Surgery
Johns Hopkins Hospital
Baltimore, Maryland

Minesh P. Mehta, MD
Professor of Human Oncology
Department of Human Oncology
University of Wisconsin School of Medicine and Public Health
Physician
Department of Radiation Therapy
Wisconsin Hospitals and Clinics
Madison, Wisconsin

William M. Mendenhall, MD
Professor
Department of Radiation Oncology
University of Florida
Physician
Department of Radiation Oncology
Shands Hospital at University of Florida
Gainesville, Florida

Matthew Meyerson, PhD
Departeent of Medical Oncology and Center for Genome Discovery
Dana-Farber Cancer Institute
Boston, Massachusetts
Broad Institute of Cambridge, Massachusetts
Broad Institute of Harvard and M.I.T.
Cambridge, Massachusetts

M. Dror Michaelson, MD, PhD
Assistant Professor of Medicine
Department of Medicine
Harvard Medical School
Assistant in Medicine
Massachusetts General Hospital Cancer Center
Massachusetts General Hospital
Boston, Massachusetts

Karin B. Michels, ScD, PhD
Associate Professor
Harvard Medical School
Co-Director
Obstetrics and Gynecology Epidemiology Center
Brigham and Women's Hospital
Boston, Massachusetts

David E. Midthun, MD
Professor of Medicine
Division of Pulmonary and Critical Care Medicine
College of Medicine, Mayo Clinic
Rochester, Minnesota

Andy J. Minn, MD, PhD
Assistant Professor, Assistant Investigator
Department of Radiation Oncology
Abramson Family Cancer Research Institute
University of Pennsylvania
Philadelphia, Pennsylvania

Bruce D. Minsky, MD
Associate Dean and Professor of Radiation and Cellular Oncology
Division of Biological Sciences
University of Chicago
Chief Quality Officer
University of Chicago Medical Center
Chicago, Illinois

Sandra A. Mitchell, PhD, CRNP, AOCN
Research Scientist, Program Director
Outcomes Research Branch
National Camcer Institute
Bethesda, Maryland

Fred Moeslein, MD, PhD
Assistant Professor
Division of Vascular and Interventional Radiology
University of Maryland School of Medicine
Baltimore, Maryland

Jeffrey F. Moley, MD
Professor of Surgery
Department of Surgery
Washington University
Surgeon
Department of Surgery
Barnes Jewish Hospital
St. Louis, Missouri

Christopher J. Molineaux, PhD
CJM Consulting

Meredith A. Morgan, PhD
Research Assistant Professor
Department of Radiation Oncology
University of Michigan
Ann Arbor, Michigan

Monica Morrow, MD
Professor
Department of Surgery Weill Medical College of Cornell University
Chief, Breast Service
Anne Burnett Windfohr Chair of Clinical Oncology
Department of Surgery
Memorial Sloan-Kettering Cancer Center
New York, New York

Robert J. Motzer, MD
Professor of Medicine
Weill Cornell Medical College
Attending Physician
Department of Medicine
Memorial Sloan-Keetering Cancer Center
New York, New York

Franco Muggia, MD
Professor of Medicine
Division of Medical Oncology
New York University
New York University Langone Medical Center
New York, New York

Arno J. Mundt, MD
Department of Radiology and Cellular Oncology
University of Chicago Hospitals
Chicago, Illinois

Nikhil C. Munshi, MD
Associate Professor of Medicine
Harvard Medical School
Associate Director/Jerome Lipper Multiple Myeloma Center
Department of Medical Oncology
VA Boston Healthcare Systems
Dana-Farber Cancer Institute
Boston, Massachusetts

Heidi Nelson, MD
Professor of Surgery
Division of Colon and Rectal Surgery
Mayo Clinic
Rochester, Minnesota

Christian J. Nelson, PhD
Assistant Attending Psychologist
Psychiatry and Behavioral Sciences
Memorial Sloan-Kettering Cancer Center
New York, New York

Andrea K. Ng, MD, PhD
Associate Professor
Department of Radiation Oncology
Harvard Medical School
Attending Physician
Department of Radiation Oncology
Dana-Farber Cancer Institute
Brigham and Women's Hospital
Boston, Massachusetts

Chee M. Ng, PharmD, PhD
Research Assistant Professor
Department of Pediatrics
Department of Pharmacology and Therapeutics
Children's Hospital of Philadelphia
Philadelphia, Pennsylvania

Dao Minh Nguyen, MD
Professor
Department of Surgery
University of Miami
Chief
Section of Thoracic Surgery
Jackson Memorial Hospital
Miami, Florida

Torsten O. Nielsen, MD, PhD, FRCPC
Associate Professor
Department of Pathology and Laboratory Medicine
University of British Columbia
Pathologist
Provincial Pathology Program
British Columbia Cancer Agency
Vancouver, Canada

John M. Norian, MD
Clinical Instructor
Department of Gynecology and Obstetrics
Loma Linda University
Divsion of Reproductive Endocrinology and Infertility
Department Gynecology and Obstetrics
Loma Linda University Health Care
Loma Linda, California

Jeffrey Norton, MD
Department of Surgery
Stanford University School of Medicine
Stanford, California

Urban Novak, MD
Research Scientist
Institute for Cancer Genetics
Columbia University
New York, New York
Klinik und Poliklinik für Medizinische Onkologie
INSELSPITAL, Universitätsspital Bern
Freiburgstrasse
Switzerland

Jed G. Nuchtern, MD, FACS, FAAP
Pediatric Surgery
Baylor College of Medicine
Houston, Texas

Susan O'Brien, MD
Professor of Medicine
Department of Leukemia
The University of Texas MD Anderson Cancer Center
Houston, Texas

Kunle Odunsi, MD, PhD
Professor and Chairman
Department of Gynecologic Oncology
Roswell Park Cancer Institute
Buffalo, New York

Kevin C. Oeffinger, MD
Attending and Member
Director, MSKCC Adult LTFU Program
Departments of Pediatrics and Medicine
Memorial Sloan-Kettering Cancer Center
New York, New York

Brian O'Sullivan, MD, FRCPI, FRCPC, FFRRCS (Hon)
Professor
Department of Radiation Oncology
University of Toronto
Associate Director
Radiation Medicine Program
Princess Margaret Hospital
Toronto, Ontario, Canada

Howard Ozer, MD, PhD
Heidrick Professor of Medicine
Chief
Department of Hematology and Oncology
Associate Director
University of Illinois at Chicago Cancer Center
University of Illinois at Chicago
Chicago, Illinois

Pier Paolo Pandolfi, MD, PhD
George C. Reisman Professor of Medicine
Department of Pathology
Harvard Medical School
Director, Cancer Genetics Program
Beth Israel Deaconess Cancer Center
Associate Director of Research
Chief, Division of Genetics
Department of Medicine
Beth Israel Deaconess Medical Center
Boston, Massachusetts

Alberto S. Pappo, MD
Professor
Division of Pediatrics
University of Tennesee Health Science Center
Member
Department of Hematology and Oncology
St. Jude Children's Research Hospital
Memphis, Tennessee

Laura Pasqualucci, MD
Associate Professor
Department of Pathology and Cell Biology
Institute for Caner Genetics
Columbia University
New York, New York

Harvey I. Pass, MD
Professor of Surgery and Cardiothoracic Surgery
Director, Division of Thoracic Surgery and Thoracic Oncology
Department of Cardiothoracic Surgery
NYU Langone Medical Center
New York, New York

Neha J. Patel, MD
Assistant Professor
Division of Pediatric Hematology and Oncology
University of Wisconsin
Director, Neurocutaneous Clinic
Department of Pediatrics
American Family Children's Hospital
Madison, Wisconsin

Erin Patterson, PhD
Surgery Branch
National Cancer Institute, Center for Cancer Research
National Institutes of Health
Bethesda, Maryland

Arnold C. Paulino, MD
Professor
Vice Chair for Education
Department of Radiation Oncology
Weill-Cornell Medical College/The Methodist Hospital
Houston, Texas

Richard Pazdur, MD
Director
Office of Oncology Drug Products
United States Food and Drug Administration
Silver Spring, Maryland

Tanja B. Pejovic, MD, PhD, FACOG
Assistant Professor, Division Chief
Gynecological Oncologist
Department of Obstetrics and Gynecology
Kinght Cancer Institute
Oregon Health & Science University
Portland, Oregon

David Pellman, MD
Massachusetts General Hospital
Boston, Massachusetts

Emanuel F. Petricoin, III, PhD
Professor, Life Science
George Mason University
Center for Applied Proteomics and Molecular Medicine
Manassas, Virginia

David G. Pfister, MD
Attending Physician and Member
Chief, Head and Neck Oncology Service
Division of Solid Tumor Oncology
Department of Medicine
Co-Leader, Head and Neck Cancer Disease Management Team
Memorial Sloan-Kettering Cancer Center
New York, New York

Maria Catherine Pietanza, MD
Assistant Member, Level I
Department of Medicine
Memorial Sloan-Kettering Cancer Center
Assistant Attending Physician
Department of Medicine
Memorial Hospital for Cancer & Allied Diseases
New York, New York

James F. Pingpank, MD
Division of Surgical Oncology
University of Pittsburgh Medical Center
Pittsburgh, Pennsylvania

Peter W. T. Pisters, MD, FACS
Professor of Surgery
Department of Surgical Oncology
The University of Texas MD Anderson Cancer Center
Houston, Texas

Sherri L. Place, MSLIS
Fox Chase Cancer Center
Philadelphia, Pennsylvania

David G. Poplack, MD
Elise C. Young Professor of Pediatric Oncology
Head, Hematology-Oncology Section
Baylor College of Medicine
Director, Texas Children's Cancer Center
Texas Children's Hospital
Houston, Texas

Carol S. Portlock, MD
Professor of Clinical Medicine
Department of Medicine
Weill Medical College of Cornell University
Attending Physician
Department of Medicine/Lymphoma Service
Memorial Sloan-Kettering Medical Center
New York, New York

Mitchell C. Posner, MD
Thomas D. Jones Professor of Surgery
Chief, Section of General Surgery
Chief, Surgical Oncology
University of Chicago Medical Center
Chicago, Illinois

Thomas A. Puchalski, PharmD
Director, Oncology PK/PD
Department of Biological Clinical Pharmacology
Malvern, Pennsylvania

Karen R. Rabin, MD, PhD
Assistant Professor
Department of Pediatric Hematolog/Oncology
Baylor College of Medicine
Attending Physician
Department of Pediatrics
Texas Children's Hospital
Houston, Texas

Janet S. Rader, MD
Professor
Department of Obstetrics and Gynecology
Medical College of Wisconsin
Chairman
Department of Obstetrics and Gynecology
Froedtert Hospital
Milwaukee, Wisconsin

Glen D. Raffel, MD, PhD
Assistant Professor of Medicine
Department of Medicine
Division of Hematology and Oncology
University of Massachusetts Medical School
Worchester, Massachusetts

Reza Rahbari, MD
Clinical Fellow
Surgery Branch
National Cancer Institute
Bethesda, Maryland
House Officer
Department of Surgery
Universtiy of California San Francisco East Bay
Oakland, California

Ramesh K. Ramanathan, MD
Clinical Professor of Medicine
College of Medicine, Phoenix Campus
University of Arizona
Medical Director
TGen Clinical Research Service
Virginia G. Piper Cancer Center
Scottsdale Health Care
Scottsdale, Arizona

Pedro T. Ramirez, MD
Associate Professor
Director of Minimally Invasive Surgical Research & Education
Department of Gynecological Oncology
The University of Texas MD Anderson Cancer Center
Houston, Texas

Zeshaan Rasheed, MD, PhD
Fellow
Department of Medical Oncology
Johns Hopkins University School of Medicine
Baltimore, Maryland

Paul W. Read, MD, PhD
Associate Professor
Vice Chairman
Department of Radiation Oncology
University of Virginia Medical Center
Charlottesville, Virginia

Abram Recht, MD
Professor
Department of Radiation Oncology
Harvard Medical School
Deputy Chief
Department of Radiation Oncology
Beth Israel Deaconess Medical Center
Boston, Massachusetts

Steven I. Reed, PhD
Professor
Department of Molecular Biology
The Scripps Research Institute
La Jolla, California

Eddie Reed, MD
Professor
Department of Oncologic Sciences
University of South Alabama
Clinical Director
Point Clear Charities Chair
Abraham Mitchell Distinguished Investigator
Mitchell Cancer Institute
Mobile, Alabama

Alnawaz Rehemtulla, PhD
Professor
Department of Radiation Oncology and Radiology
University of Michigan
Ann Arbor, Michigan

Nicholas P. Restifo, MD
Principal Investigator
Surgery Branch
National Cancer Institute
Bethesda, Maryland

Anetta Reszko, MD, PhD
Clinical Instructor
Department of Dermatology
Yale University
New Haven, Connecticut

Victor E. Reuter, MD
Professor
Department of Pathology
Weill Medical College of Cornell University
Vice Chairman
Department of Pathology
Memorial Sloan-Kettering Cancer Center
New York, New York

Michelle B. Riba, MD, MS
Professor of Psychiatry
Associate Chair for Integrated Medicine and Psychiatric Services
Department of Psychiatry
University of Michigan
Ann Arbor, Michigan

Nora C. Rightmer, MSW, LCSW
Oncology Social Worker
Department of Social Work
Smilow Cancer Hospital at Yale-New Haven
New Haven, Connecticut

Lisa M. Rimsza, MD
Professor of Pathology
The Arizona Cancer Center
Tucson, Arizona

Guido Rindi, MD, PhD
Professor
Institute of Anatomic Pathology
Università Cattolica del Sacro Cuore
Chief
Histopathology and Cytodiagnosis Service
Policlinico A. Gemelli
Rome, Italy

Brian I. Rini, MD, FACP
Associate Professor
Department of Medicine
CCF/Lerner College of Medicine
Case Western Reserve University
Staff
Department of Solid Tumor Oncology/Urology
Cleveland Clinic, Taussig Cancer Institute
Cleveland, Ohio

Paul F. Robbins, PhD
Staff Scientist
Surgery Branch
National Cancer Institute
National Institutes of Health
Bethesda, Maryland

Matthew K. Robinson, MD
Assistant Professor
Department of Developmental Therapeutics
Fox Chase Cancer Center
Philadelphia, Pennsylvania

Michal G. Rose, MD
Associate Professor
Department of Medicine
Yale University School of Medicine
New Haven, Connecticut
Director, Cancer Center
VA Connecticut Healthcare System
West Haven, Connecticut

Steven A. Rosenberg, MD, PhD
Chief of Surgery
National Cancer Institute
National Institutes of Health
Professor of Surgery
Uniformed Services University of the Health Sciences School of Medicine
Bethesda, Maryland
Professor of Surgery
George Washington University School of Medicine
Washington, DC

Kenneth Rosenzweig, MD
Professor
Chairman
Department of Radiation Oncology
Mount Sinai Medical Center
New York, New York

Brian D. Ross, PhD
Professor
Department of Radiology and Biological Chemistry
University of Michigan
Ann Arbor, Michigan

Richard E. Royal, MD
Associate Professor
Department of Surgical Oncology
The University of Texas MD Anderson Cancer Center
Houston, Texas

James Louis Rubenstein, MD, PhD
Associate Professor of Medicine
Attending Physician
Department of Medicine
University of California, San Francisco
San Francisco, California

Eric H. Rubin, MD
Therapeutic Area Head, Vice-President
Merck Research Labratories
North Wales, Pennsylvania

Heidi V. Russell, MD
Texas Children's Cancer Center
Baylor College of Medicine
Houston, Texas

Anil K. Rustgi, MD
T. Grier Miller Professor of Medicine and Genetics
Chief of Gastroenterology
University of Pennsylvania
Philadelphia, Pennsylvania

Arjun Sahgal, MD
Assistant Professor
Department of Radiation Oncology
University of Toronto
Radiation Oncologist
Department of Radiation Oncology
Sunnybrook Health Sciences Centre
Toronto, Canada

M. Wasif Saif, MD, MBBS
Professor of Clinical Medicine
Director, Section of Gastrointestinal Cancers
Medical Director, Pancreas Center
Columbia University College of Physicians and Surgeons & New York Presbyterian Hospital
New York, New York

Leonard B. Saltz, MD
Head, Colorectal Oncology Section
Department of Medicine
Memorial-Sloan Kettering Cancer Center
Professor
Department of Medicine
Cornell University Medical College
New York, New York

Yardena Samuels, PhD
Assistant Professor
Cancer Genetics Branch
National Human Genome Research Institute
National Institutes of Health
Bethesda, Maryland

Alton Oliver Sartor, MD
Plitz Professor for Cancer Research
Departments of Medicine and Urology
Tulane Medical School
Tulane University Hospital
New Orleans, Louisiana

Charles L. Sawyers, MD
Investigator
Howard Hughes Medical Institute
Chairman
Human Oncology & Pathogenesis Program
Memorial Sloan-Kettering Cancer Center
New York, New York

Kristen G. Schaefer, MD
Instructor
Department of Psychosocial Oncology and Palliative Care
Harvard Medical School
Attending
Department of Psychosocial Oncology and Palliative Care
Dana-Farber Cancer Institute
Boston, Massachusetts

John T. Schiller, PhD
Laboratory of Cellular Oncology
Center for Cancer Research, National Cancer Institute
National Institutes of Health
Bethesda, Maryland

Laura S. Schmidt, PhD
Principal Scientist
SAIC-Frederick, Inc.
NCI-Frederick
National Cancer Institute
National Institutes of Health
Bethesda, Maryland

Heiko Schöder, MD
Department of Radiology
Memorial Sloan-Kettering Cancer Center
New York, New York

Deborah Schrag, MD, MPH
Associate Professor
Department of Medicine/Oncology
Harvard Medical School
Oncologist
Department of GI/Medical Oncology
Dana-Farber Cancer Institute
Boston, Massachusetts

David S. Schrump, MD
Head, Thoracic Oncology Section
Surgery Branch
National Cancer Institute
Bethesda, Maryland

Brahm H. Segal, MD
Professor
Department of Medicine
University of Buffalo School of Medicine
Chief, Division of Infectious Diseases
Department of Medicine
Roswell Park Cancer Institute
Buffalo, New York

Kathy J. Selvaggi, MD
Associate Professor of Medicine
Harvard Medical School
Staff Physician
Medicine: Psychosocial Oncology and Palliative Care
Dana-Farber Cancer Institute
Brigham and Women's Hospital
Boston, Massachusetts

Norman E. Sharpless, MD
Associate Professor
Department of Medicine and Genetics
The University of North Carolina
Chapel Hill, North Carolina

Joel Sheinfeld, MD
Professor of Urology
Weill Medical College of Cornell University
Deputy Chief
Department of Urology
Memorial Sloan-Kettering Cancer Center
New York, New York

Peter G. Shields, MD
Carcinogenesis, Biomarkers, and Epidemiology Program
Lombardi Comprehensive Cancer Center
Georgetown University Medical Center
Washington, DC

William U. Shipley, MD
Soriano Professor of Radiaiton Oncology
Department of Radiation Oncology
Harvard Medical School
Head, Radiation Therapy Oncology Group Research
Department of Radiation Oncology
Masschusetts General Hospital
Boston, Massachusetts

Ramesh A. Shivdasani, MD, PhD
Associate Professor
Department of Medicine
Harvard Medical School
Associate Professor
Department of Medical Oncology
Dana-Farber Cancer Institute
Boston, Massachusetts

Richard M. Simon, DSc
Chief
Biometric Research Branch
National Cancer Institute
Bethesda, Maryland

Samuel Singer, MD
Professor of Surgery
Department of Surgery
Weill Cornell Medical College
Member with Tenure-of-Title
Chief, Gastric and Mixed Tumor Service
Department of Surgery
Memorial Sloan-Kettering Cancer Center
New York, New York

Craig L. Slingluff, MD
Associate Professor
Department of Radiation Oncology
University of Virginia
Vice Chairman
Department of Radiation Oncology
University of Virginia Medical Center
Charlottesville, Virginia

Robert A. Smith, PhD
Director – Cancer Screening
American Cancer Society
Atlanta, Georgia

Harris S. Soifer, PhD
Assistant Professor of Medicine
Albert Einstein College of Medicine
Bronx, New York

Vernon K. Sondak, MD
Professor
Department of Surgery and Oncologic Sciences
University of Southern Florida
Chair
Department of Cutaneous Oncology
H. Lee Moffitt Cancer Center & Research Institute
Tampa, Florida

Eliezer Soto, MD
Pain and Palliative Care Service
Bethesda, Maryland

David Spiegel, MD
Willson Professor and Associate Chair
Department of Psychiatry and Behavioral Sciences
Stanford University School of Medicine
Medical Director
Center for Integrative Medicine
Stanford Hospital and Clinics
Stanford, California

Cy A. Stein, MD, PhD
Professor
Department of Medicine and Molecular Pharmacology
Albert Einstein College of Medicine
Director, Medical Genitourinary Oncology
Department of Medicine
Montefiore Medical Center
Bronx, New York

Diane E. Stover, MD
Professor of Clinical Medicine
Department of Medicine
Weill Medical College of Cornell University
Head of General Medicine
Chief Pulmonary Service
Department of Medicine
Memorial Sloan-Kettering Medical Center
New York, New York

Michael D. Stubblefield, MD
Assistant Professor of Rehabilitation Medicine
Department of Physical Medicine and Rehabilitation
Weill Medical College of Cornell University
Assistant Attending Psychiatrist
Rehabilitation Medicine Service
Department of Neurology
Memorial Sloan-Kettering Cancer Center
New York, New York

Paul H. Sugarbaker, MD, FACS, FRCS
Director of Programs
Peritoneal Surface Oncology
Cancer Institute
Washington Hospital Center
Washington, DC

Chris H. Takimoto, MD, PhD
Vice President
Department of Translational Medicine
Janssen Research and Development
Radnor, Pennsylvania

Randall K. Ten Haken, PhD
Professor of Radiation Oncology
Co-Director, Radiation Physics Division
Department of Radiation Oncology
University of Michigan
Ann Arbor, Michigan

Kenneth D. Tew, PhD, DSc
Professor and Chairman
Department of Cell and Molecular Pharmacology
Medical University of South Carolina
Charleston, South Carolina

Charles R. Thomas, Jr., MD
Professor and Chair
Department of Radiation Medicine
Knight Cancer Institute, Oregon Health and Sciences University
Service Chief
Department of Radiation Medicine
Oregon Health and Sciences University Hospitals and Clinics
Portland, Oregon

Snorri S. Thorgeirsson, MD, PhD
Chief
Laboratory of Experimental Carcinogenesis
Center for Cancer Research
National Cancer Institute
Bethesda, Maryland

Michael J. Thun, MD
American Cancer Society
Atlanta, Georgia

Robert Timmerman, MD
Professor of Radiation Oncology and Neurosurgery
Department of Radiation Oncology
University of Texas Southwestern Medical Center
Director
Annette Simmons Stereotactic Radiation Center
Zale Lipshy University Hospital
Dallas, Texas

Edouard J. Trabulsi, MD
Associate Professor
Department of Urology
Kimmel Cancer, Thomas Jefferson University Hospital
Philadelphia, Pennsylvania

William D. Travis, MD
Professor of Pathology
Attanding Thoracic Pathologist
Department of Pathology
Weill Medical College of Cornell Univeristy
Memorial Sloan-Kettering Cancer Center
New York, New York

Lois B. Travis, MD, ScD
Director
Ruben Center for Cancer Survivorship
Professor
Department of Radiation Oncology
James P. Wilmot Cancer Center
University of Rochester Medical Center
Rochester, New York

Giorgio Trinchieri, MD
Director
Cancer and Inflammation Program
Center for Cancer Research
National Cancer Institute - Frederick
Frederick, Maryland

Robert Udelsman, MD, MBA
William H. Carmalt Professor and Chairman
Department of Surgery
Yale University School of Medicine
New Haven, Connecticut

Catherine E. Ulbricht, PharmD, MBA(c)
Founder, Editor in Chief
Natural Standard Research Collaboration
Sommerville, Massachusetts
Senior Attending Pharmacist
Massachusetts General Hospital
Boston, Massachusetts

Thomas S. Uldrick, MD, MS
Staff Clinician
HIV and AIDS Malignancy Branch
Center for Cancer Research, National Cancer Institutes
Bethesda, Maryland

Matthew G. Vander Heiden, MD
Koch Institute for Integrative Cancer Research at M.I.T.
Dana-Farber Cancer Institute
Boston, Massachusetts

Veronic Sanchez Varela, PhD
Research Fellow
Department of Psychosocial Oncology and Palliative Care
Harvard Medical School
Dana-Farber Cancer Institute
Boston, Massachusetts

Vic J. Verwaal, MD
Surgeon
Department of Surgery
The Netherlands Cancer Institute
Amsterdam, the Netherlands

Damon J. Vidrine, PhD
Assistant Professor
Department of Behavioral Science
The University of Texas MD Anderson Cancer Center
Houston, Texas

Michael Vogelbaum, MD, PhD
Associate Director
Brain Tumor and Neuro-Oncology Center
Cleveland Clinic
Cleveland, Ohio

Nicholas J. Vogelzang, MD
Chair and Medical Director
Developmental Therapeutics
Member GU Committee
US Oncology Research
Vice chair SWOG GU Committee
Professor of Medicine University of Nevada School of Medicine
Comprehensive Cancer Centers NV
Las Vegas, Nevada

Jean C.Y. Wang, MD, PhD
Assistant Professor
Department of Medicine
University of Toronto
Affiliate Scientist
Division of Stem Cell and Developmental Biology
Ontario Cancer Institute
Toronto, Ontario, Canada

Lisa L. Wang, MD
Assistant Professor
Department of Pediatrics
Baylor College of Medicine
Houston, Texas

Elizabeth Ward, PhD
American Cancer Society
Atlanta, Georgia

Jeffrey S. Wefel, PhD
Assistant Professor
Department of Neuro-oncology
The University of Texas MD Anderson Cancer Center
Houston, Texas

Louis M. Weiner, MD
Director
Lombardt Comprehensive Cancer Center
Georgetown University
Washington, DC

Samuel A. Wells, Jr., MD
Senior Clinician
Medical Oncology Branch
National Cancer Institute
Center for Cancer Research
National Institutes of Health
Bethesda, Maryland

John W. Werning, MD
Associate Professor
Department of Otolaryngology
University of Florida
Head and Neck Surgical Oncologist
Department of Otolaryngology
Shands Hospital at University of Florida
Gainesville, Florida

Eileen White, PhD
Professor
Department of Molecular Biology and Biochemistry
Rutgers University
Associate Director for Basic Science
Cancer Institute of New Jersey
New Brunswick, New Jersey

William Wierda, MD, PhD
Associate Professor
Department of Leukemia
The University of Texas MD Anderson Cancer Center
Houston, Texas

Walter C. Willett, MD, PhD
Professor and Chair
Department of Nutrition
Harvard School of Public Health
Associate Physician
Department of Medicine
Brigham and Women's Hospital
Boston, Massachusetts

Christopher G. Willett, MD
Professor and Chair
Department of Radiation Oncology
Duke University Medical Center
Durham, North Carolina

Grant A. Williams, MD
Division of Oncology Drug Products
Center for Drug Evaluation and Research
United States Food and Drug Administration
Rockville, Maryland

Lynn D. Wilson, MD, MPH
Professor
Department of Therapeutic Radiology
Yale School of Medicine
New Haven, Connecticut

Robert A. Wolff, MD
Medical Oncology
The University of Texas MD Anderson Cancer Center
Houston, Texas

Kwok-Kin Wong, MD, PhD
Associate Professor
Department of Medical Oncology
Dana-Farber Cancer Institute
Harvard Medical School
Attending Physician
Department of Medicine
Brigham & Women's Hospital
Boston, Massachusetts

Flossie Wong-Staal, PhD
Professor Emeritus
Department of Medicine
University of California, San Diego
La Jolla, California

Joachim Yahalom, MD, FACR
Professor of Radiation Oncology
Department of Radiation
Weill Medical College of Cornell University
Attending and Member
Department of Radiation Oncology
Memorial Sloan-Kettering Cancer Center
New York, New York

James C. Yang, MD
Surgery Branch
Center for Cancer Research
National Cancer Institute
Bethesda, Maryland

James C. Yao, MD
Associate Professor
Department of Gastrointestinal Medical Oncology
University of Texas
Deputy Chairman
Department of Gastrointestinal Medical Oncology
The University of Texas MD Anderson Cancer Center
Houston, Texas

Robert Yarchoan, MD
Branch Chief
HIV and AIDS Malignancy Branch
Center for Cancer Research
Attending Physician
National Cancer Institute
NIH Clinical Center
Bethesda, Maryland

Herbert Yu, MD, PhD
Associate Professor
Department of Epidemiology and Public Health
Yale University
New Haven, Connecticut

Stuart H. Yuspa, MD
Laboratory Chief
Laboratory of Cancer Biology and Genetics
National Institutes of Health
Bethesda, Maryland

Jason Todd Yustein, MD, PhD
Assistant Professor
Department of Pediatrics, Hematology/Oncology
Baylor College of Medicine
Houston, Texas

Herbert J. Zeh, III, MD
Assistant Professor of Surgery
Department of Surgical Oncology
University of Pittsburgh Medical Center
Pittsburgh, Pennsylvania

Michael J. Zelefsky, MD
Member, Chief of Brachytherapy Service
Department of Radiation Oncology
Memorial Sloan-Kettering Cancer Center
Professor of Radiation Oncology
Department of Radiation Oncology
New York Cornell Hospital
New York, New York

Anthony L. Zietman, MD
Jenot and William Shipley Professor of Radiation Oncology
Department of Radiation Oncology
Harvard Medical School
Massachusetts General Hospital
Boston, Massachusetts

Amer H. Zureikat, MD
Assistant Professor of Surgery,
Department of Surgical Oncology
University of Pittsburgh Medical Center
Pittsburgh, Pennsylvania

PREFACE

It seems that we are now overloaded every day with new information suggesting that we should be changing our treatments to a new (and, by definition, better?) drug or device. We all want to practice with the best and newest data. Yet which of the new studies we read about each day will actually change practice and which will turn out to be no better, or possibly worse, than current standard practice? Going to the Internet simply produces a list of references, without any ability to distinguish the trustworthy study from the one that my lead us down the wrong path. Where can the general practitioner or oncologist turn to find information that is reliable, practical, and comprehensive?

We feel that the 9th edition of *Cancer: Principles & Practice of Oncology* is that place. As with the 8th edition, we wanted to maintain a 3-year cycle so that the printed book fulfills the needs of the oncologist. In addition, beginning with this 9th edition, the electronic version of the book will be continuously revised to incorporate the most recent practice-changing information. We will be searching the literature for substantiated improvements in treatment while avoiding the speculative and unproven. These changes will be highlighted in the electronic text to permit easy identification. We are excited that this combination of accelerated print editions with a continuously updated electronic version revised by experts should meet the needs of both the specialist and the generalist in oncology.

This new edition also builds on many of the changes we made in the 8th edition. We have continued to work with Drs. Ronald DePinho and Robert Weinberg of Harvard and MIT, respectively, to substantially revise and improve the first section of the book that focuses on the Molecular Biology of Cancer. This section of the book (and the chapters on the molecular biology of specific cancers) has become more and more important in understanding the recent explosion of targeted therapies. Several new chapters, particularly those on personalized medicine and on tyrosine kinase inhibitors, bridge the science of the first section directly to the clinic. The parts covering the principles and the practice of oncology have also been extensively revised so that each chapter reflects the most recent clinical findings.

In addition to these improvements in the book, we have also continued to use *The Cancer Journal: Journal of the Principles & Practice of Oncology* to carry out in-depth multimodality analyses of topical subjects. Each issue contains a set of papers that approach a topic (such as Hepatocellular Cancer or Sexuality and the Cancer Patient) from multiple viewpoints that complements and updates the material found in the book. *Principles & Practice of Oncology Updates* cover more focused topics in detail.

We have attempted to make *Cancer: Principles and Practice of Oncology* and its companions the antidote for information overload. Taken together, the printed and electronic book, the journal and the updates provide a complete package of printed and electronic media that will be permit the busy practitioner to have a suite of materials that is both a comprehensive and usable resource for their patients.

Vincent T. DeVita, Jr., MD
Theodore S. Lawrence, MD, PhD
Steven A. Rosenberg, MD, PhD

ACKNOWLEDGMENTS

The Editors would like to acknowledge the extraordinary contributions of Zia Raven, who played a vital role in the preparation of this edition. Ms. Raven assumed responsibility for the organization and compilation of all of the chapters in this text. We are also grateful to Jonathan W. Pine, Jr., Senior Executive Editor at Lippincott Williams & Wilkins, for his excellent help in the production of this text.

VTD
TSL
SAR

CONTENTS

PART TWO

ETIOLOGY AND EPIDEMIOLOGY OF CANCER

Section 1: Etiology of Cancer

Section 2: Epidemiology of Cancer

PART THREE

PRINCIPLES OF CANCER TREATMENT

PART FOUR

PHARMACOLOGY OF CANCER THERAPEUTICS

Section 1: Chemotherapy Agents

Section 2: Biotherapeutics

PART FIVE

CANCER PREVENTION

PART SIX

CANCER SCREENING

PART SEVEN

SPECIALIZED TECHNIQUES IN CANCER MANAGEMENT

PART EIGHT

PRACTICE OF ONCOLOGY

Section 1: Cancer of the Head and Neck

Section 18: Stem Cell Transplantation

Section 19: Management of Adverse Effects of Treatment

Effects of Cytotoxic Agents on Children 2378

171. Nutritional Support 2448

PART ONE
MOLECULAR BIOLOGY OF CANCER

CHAPTER 1 THE CANCER GENOME

YARDENA SAMUELS, ALBERTO BARDELLI, AND CARLOS LÓPEZ-OTÍN

There is a broad consensus that cancer is, in essence, a genetic disease, and that accumulation of molecular alterations in the genome of somatic cells is the basis of cancer progression (Fig. 1.1).[1] In the past 5 years the availability of the human genome sequence and progress in DNA sequencing technologies has dramatically improved knowledge of this disease. These new insights are transforming the field of oncology at multiple levels:

1. The genomic maps are redesigning the tumor taxonomy by moving it from a histologic- to a genetic-based level.
2. The success of cancer drugs designed to target the molecular alterations underlying tumorigenesis has proven that somatic genetic alterations are legitimate targets for therapy.
3. Tumor genotyping is helping clinicians to individualize treatments by matching patients with the best treatment for their tumors.
4. Tumor-specific DNA alterations represent highly sensitive biomarkers for disease detection and monitoring.
5. Finally, the ongoing analyses of multiple cancer genomes will identify additional targets, whose pharmacological exploitation will undoubtedly result in new therapeutic approaches.

This chapter will review the progress that has been made in understanding the genetic basis of sporadic cancers. The topic of familial cancer is covered in Chapter 12. The emphasis of this chapter is an introduction to novel integrated genomic approaches that allow a comprehensive and systematic evaluation of genetic alterations that occur during the progression of cancer. Using these powerful tools, cancer research, diagnosis, and treatment are poised for a transformation in the next decade.

CANCER GENES AND THEIR MUTATIONS

Cancer genes are broadly grouped into oncogenes and tumor suppressor genes. Using a classical analogy, oncogenes can be considered as the car accelerator, so that a mutation in an oncogene would be the equivalent of having the accelerator continuously pressed.[2] Tumor suppressor genes, in contrast, act as "brakes,"[2] so that when they are not mutated they function to inhibit tumorigenesis. Oncogene and tumor suppressor genes may be classified by the nature of their somatic mutations in tumors.[1] Mutations in oncogenes typically occur at specific hotspots, often affecting the same codon or clustered at neighboring codons in different tumors. Furthermore, mutations in oncogenes are almost always missense, and the mutations usually affect only one allele, making them heterozygous. In contrast, tumor suppressor genes are usually mutated throughout the gene; a large number of the mutations may truncate the encoded protein and generally affect both alleles, causing loss of heterozygosity. Major types of somatic mutations present in malignant tumors include nucleotide substitutions, small insertions and deletions (*indels*), chromosomal rearrangements, and copy number alterations (further described in Chapter 2).

IDENTIFICATION OF CANCER GENES

The completion of the human genome project has marked a new era in biomedical sciences.[3] Knowledge of the sequence and organization of the human genome allows the systematic analysis of the genetic alterations underlying the origin and evolution of tumors. Before elucidation of the human genome, several cancer genes, such as *KRAS*, *TP53*, and *APC*, were successfully discovered using approaches based on oncovirus analysis, linkage studies, loss of heterozygosity, and cytogenetics.[4,5] The completion of the Human Genome Project in 2004,[3] which provided a sequence-based map of the normal human genome, together with the construction of the HapMap, containing single nucleotide polymorphisms (SNPs), and the underlying genomic structure of natural human genomic variation,[6,7] allowed an extraordinary throughput in cataloging somatic mutations in cancer. These projects now offer an unprecedented opportunity: the identification of all the genetic changes associated with a human cancer. This ambitious goal is for the first time within reach of the scientific community. Already a number of studies have demonstrated the usefulness of strategies aimed at the systematic identification of somatic mutations associated with cancer progression. Notably, the Human Genome Project, the HapMap project, as well as the candidate and family gene approaches described below, utilized capillary-based DNA sequencing (first-generation sequencing, also known as Sanger sequencing).[8] Figure 1.2 clearly illustrates the developments in the search of cancer genes, its increased pace, as well as the most relevant findings in this field.

CANCER GENOME INVESTIGATION: TOOLS AND QUALITY CONTROLS

In order to perform mutational analysis of cancer genomes it is imperative to acquire high-quality reagents and to perform several quality controls to verify that the derived data are reliable. To detect somatic (i.e., tumor-specific) mutations in cancer both the tumor DNA and the germline DNA from the same individual are required, especially because knowledge of the variations in the normal human genome is as yet incomplete.

A metastatic cancer genome requires decades to develop

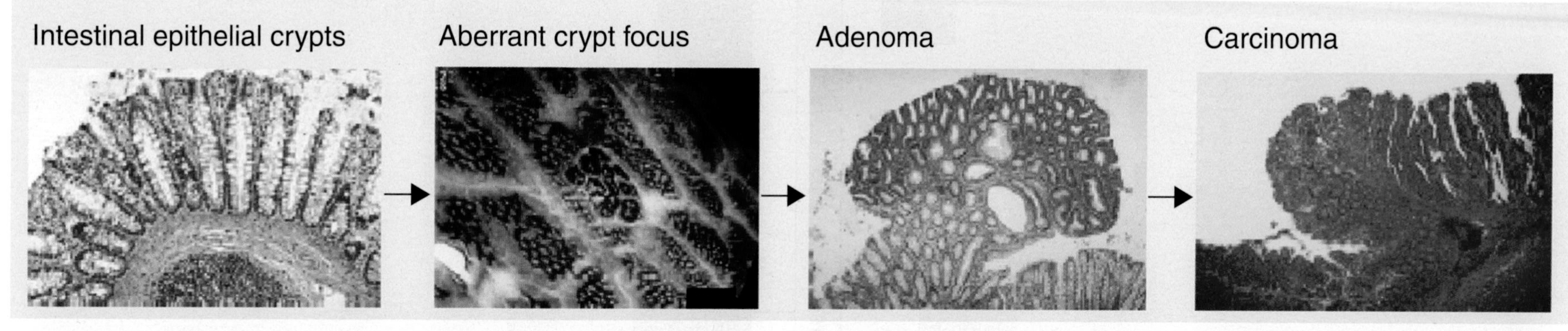

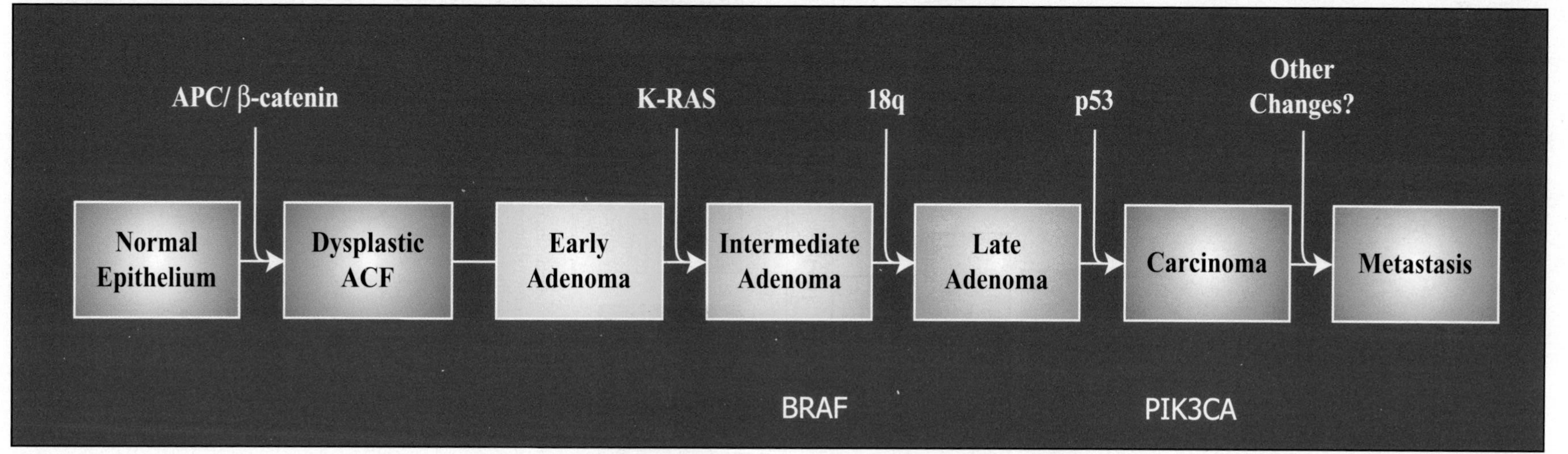

FIGURE 1.1 Schematic representation of the genomic and histopathological steps associated to tumor progression: from the occurrence of the initiating mutation in the founder cell to metastasis formation. It has been convincingly shown that the genomic landscape of solid tumors such as that of pancreatic and colorectal requires the accumulation of many genetic events, a process which requires decades to complete This timeline offers an incredible window of opportunity for the early detection (often associated to excellent prognosis) of this disease.

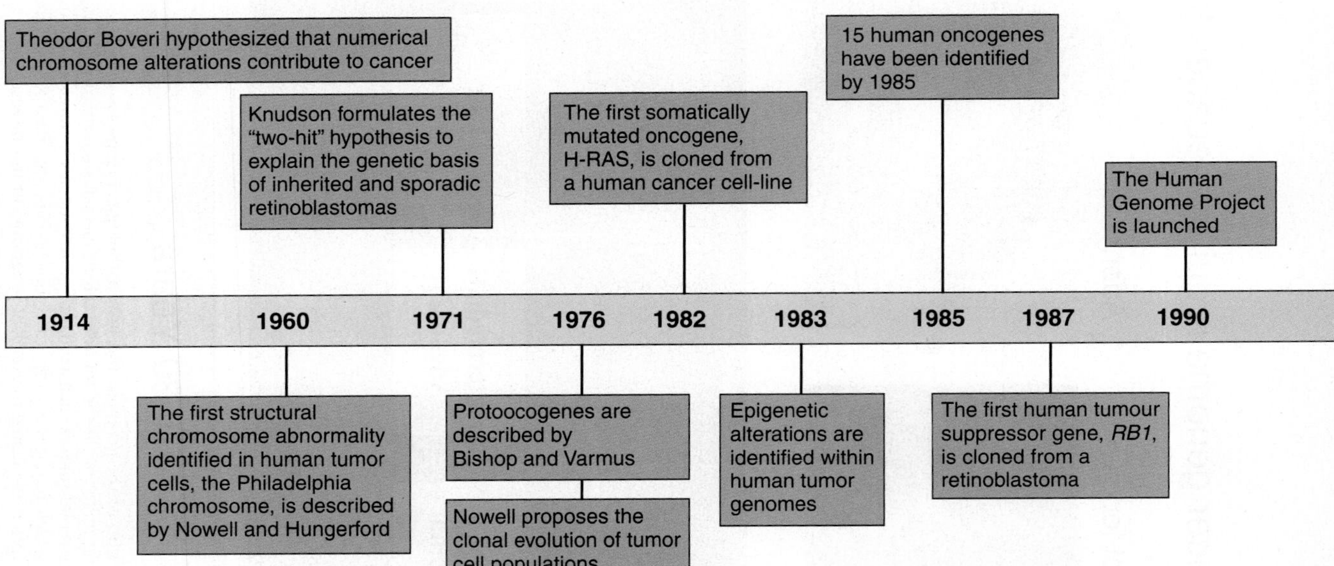

FIGURE 1.2 Timeline of seminal hypotheses, research discoveries, and research initiatives that have led to an improved understanding of the genetic etiology of human tumorigenesis within the past century. The consensus cancer gene data were obtained from the Wellcome Trust Sanger Institute Cancer Genome Project website (http://www.sanger.ac.uk/genetics/CGP). Redrawn from ref. 80.

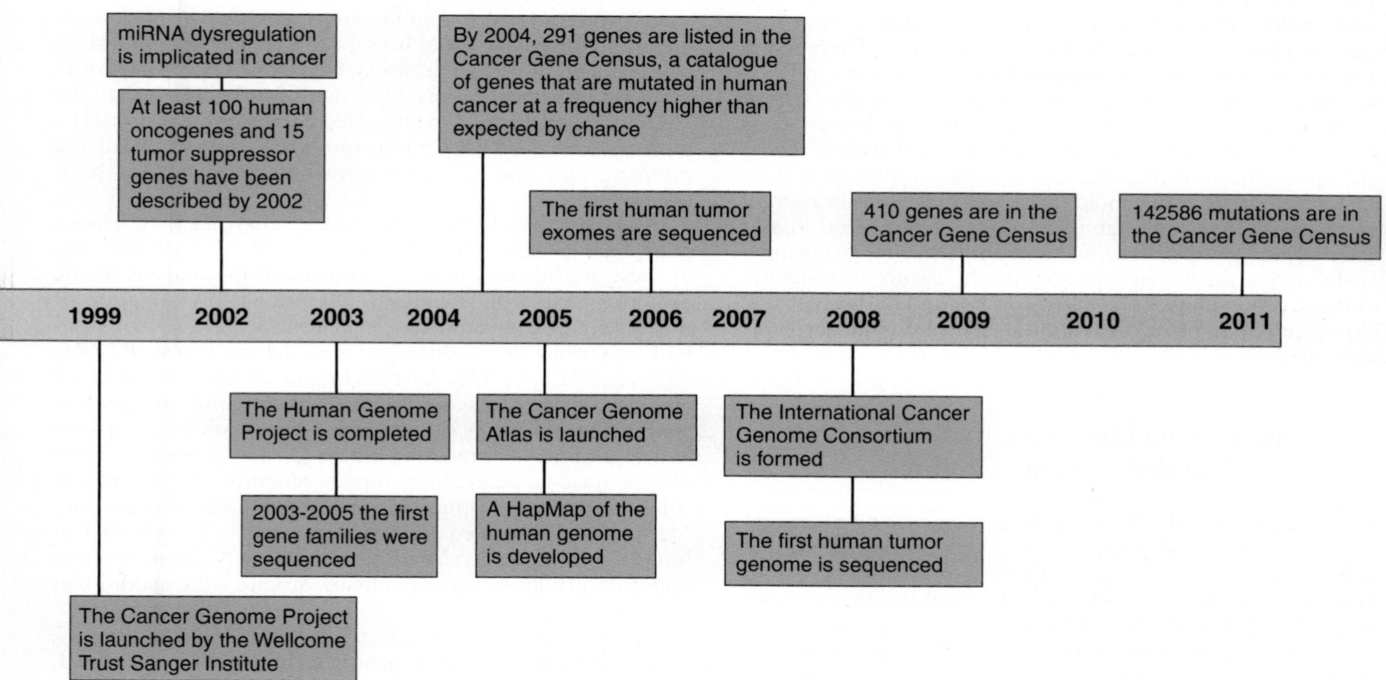
miRNA dysregulation is implicated in cancer
At least 100 human oncogenes and 15 tumor suppressor genes have been described by 2002
By 2004, 291 genes are listed in the Cancer Gene Census, a catalogue of genes that are mutated in human cancer at a frequency higher than expected by chance
The first human tumor exomes are sequenced
410 genes are in the Cancer Gene Census
142586 mutations are in the Cancer Gene Census
1999
2002
2003
2004
2005
2006
2007
2008
2009
2010
2011
The Human Genome Project is completed
2003-2005 the first gene families were sequenced
The Cancer Genome Atlas is launched
A HapMap of the human genome is developed
The International Cancer Genome Consortium is formed
The first human tumor genome is sequenced
The Cancer Genome Project is launched by the Wellcome Trust Sanger Institute

Normal genomic DNA from the same individual may be derived either from blood or from tumor neighboring tissue in cases where solid tumors are investigated.

A cancer sample (either from bioptic or surgical origin) typically contains both malignant and nonmalignant (stromal) cells. Most genomic analyses require that samples are highly enriched for tumor tissue. These can either be generated by deriving early passage tumor cell lines, mouse xenografts, or through a pathologist-guided selective macro- or microdissection of neoplastic tissue. This allows the isolation of tumor-derived genomic DNA and sensitive detection of somatic mutations that would otherwise be masked by contamination of normal tissue. Importantly, the quality of the derived genomic DNA may be affected by its source. Surgical resection specimens are usually large and therefore appropriate for these studies. However, biopsies from patients usually contain few cells, thus reducing the quantity of genomic DNA available. Although whole-genome amplification may be a possibility when low genomic DNA amounts are available, this method can give rise to artifactual genetic alterations.[9] Another reason that negatively affects the quality of genomic DNA is that cancer samples (for example, liver metastases) often contain significant numbers of necrotic or apoptotic cells. These issues might also be resolved by increased genetic coverage utilizing second-generation sequencing approaches,[10] as detailed below.

Prior to genomic analysis multiple key quality controls should be applied to the tumor and normal tissues. These include verification that the tumor sample contains at least 75% cancer cells, a threshold that allows the identification of homozygous and hemizygous deletions, copy-neutral loss of heterozygosity, duplication, and amplification.[11–13] To unequivocally assess the somatic tumor-specific nature of sequence changes, genotyping of SNPs in the tumor and normal tissue is also required to prove that both are derived from the same individual.

Cancer Gene Discovery by Sequencing Candidate Gene Families

The availability of the human genome sequence provides new opportunities to comprehensively search for somatic mutations in cancer on a larger scale than previously possible. Progress in the field has been closely linked to improvements in the throughput of DNA analysis and the continuous reduction in sequencing costs. Below some of the achievements in this research area are described, as well as how they affected knowledge of the cancer genome.

A seminal work in the field was the systematic mutational profiling of the genes involved in the RAF-RAS pathway in multiple tumors. This candidate gene approach led to the discovery that *BRAF* is frequently mutated in melanomas and is mutated at a lower frequency in other tumor types.[14] Follow-up studies quickly revealed that mutations in *BRAF* are mutually exclusive with alterations in *KRAS*,[14,15] genetically emphasizing that these genes function in the same pathway, a concept that had been previously demonstrated in lower organisms such as *Caenorhabditis elegans* and *Drosophila melanogaster.*[16,17]

In 2003, identification of cancer genes shifted from a candidate gene approach to the mutational analyses of gene families. The first gene families to be completely sequenced were those that involved protein[18,19] and lipid phosphorylation.[20] The rationale for focusing initially on these gene families was threefold:

1. The corresponding proteins were already known at that time to play a pivotal role in signaling and proliferation of normal and cancerous cells.
2. Multiple members of the protein kinases family had already been linked to tumorigenesis.
3. Kinases are clearly amenable to pharmacological inhibition, making them attractive drug targets.

The mutational analysis of all the tyrosine kinase domains in colorectal cancers revealed that 30% of cases had a mutation in at least one tyrosine kinase gene, and overall mutations were identified in eight different kinases, most of which had not previously been linked to cancer.[18] An additional mutational analysis of the coding exons of 518 protein kinase genes in 210 diverse human cancers, including breast, lung, gastric, ovarian, renal, and acute lymphoblastic leukemia, identified approximately 120 mutated genes that probably contribute to oncogenesis.[19] A recent somatic mutations interrogation of the protein tyrosine kinases in cutaneous melanoma identified *ERBB4* to be mutated in 19% of cases, making it the most highly mutated protein tyrosine kinase in melanoma.[21] *ERBB4* is a member of the ERBB/HER family of receptor tyrosine kinases. Other family members, including *ERBB1* (EGFR) and *ERBB2* (HER-2), have been implicated by mutations or amplifications in a number of cancers, including lung, colon, and breast cancers. The high mutation frequency as well as the nonsynonymous (NS) to synonymous (S) ratio, which was 24:3, significantly higher than the NS:S ratio predicted for non-selected mutations ($P < .01$)[22] indicated that *ERBB4* mutations are selected for during tumorigenesis and therefore contribute to melanoma tumorigenesis.

As kinase activity is attenuated by enzymes that remove phosphate groups called phosphatases, the rational next step in these studies was to perform a mutation analysis of the protein tyrosine phosphatases. Mutational investigation of this family in colorectal cancer identified that 25% of cases had mutations in six different phosphatase genes (*PTPRF, PTPRG, PTPRT, PTPN3, PTPN13,* or *PTPN14*).[23] Combined analysis of the protein tyrosine kinases and the protein tyrosine phosphatases showed that 50% of colorectal cancers had mutations in a tyrosine kinase gene, a protein tyrosine phosphatase gene, or both, further emphasizing the pivotal role of protein phosphorylation in neoplastic progression. Many of the identified genes had previously been linked to human cancer, thus validating the unbiased comprehensive mutation profiling. These landmark studies led to additional gene family surveys.

The phosphatidylinositol 3-kinase (*PI3K*) gene family, which also plays a role in proliferation, adhesion, survival, and motility, was also comprehensively investigated.[24] Sequencing of the exons encoding the kinase domain of all 16 members belonging to this family pinpointed *PIK3CA* as the only gene to harbor somatic mutations. When the entire coding region was analyzed, *PIK3CA* was found somatically mutated in 32% of colorectal cancers. At that time, the *PIK3CA* gene was certainly not a newcomer in the cancer arena, as it had previously been shown to be involved in cell transformation and metastasis.[24] Strikingly, its staggering high mutation frequency was discovered only through systematic sequencing of the corresponding gene family.[20] Subsequent analysis of *PIK3CA* in other tumor types identified somatic mutations in this gene in additional cancer types, including 36% of hepatocellular carcinomas, 36% of endometrial carcinomas, 25% of breast carcinomas, 15% of anaplastic oligodendrogliomas, 5% of medulloblastomas and anaplastic astrocytomas, and 27% of glioblastomas.[25–29] It is known that *PIK3CA* is one of the two (the other being *KRAS*) most commonly mutated oncogenes in human cancers. Further investigation of the *PI3K* pathway in colorectal cancer showed that 40% of tumors had genetic alterations in one of the *PI3K* pathway genes, emphasizing the central role of this pathway in colorectal cancer pathogenesis.[30] The relevance and the functional role of the PI3K pathway in tumorigenesis is further described in Chapter 5.

Although most cancer genome studies of large gene families have focused on the kinome, recent analyses have revealed that members of other families highly represented in the human genome are also a target of mutational events in cancer. This is the case of proteases, a complex group of enzymes consisting of at least 569 components that constitute the so-called human degradome.[31] Proteases exhibit an elaborate interplay with kinases and have traditionally been associated with cancer progression because of their ability to degrade extracellular matrices, thus facilitating tumor invasion and metastasis.[32,33] However, recent studies have shown that these enzymes hydrolyze a wide variety of substrates and influence many different steps of cancer, including early stages of tumor evolution.[34] These functional studies have also revealed that beyond their initial recognition as prometastatic enzymes, they play dual roles in cancer, as assessed by the identification of a growing number of tumor-suppressive proteases.[35]

These findings emphasized the possibility that mutational activation or inactivation of protease genes occurs in cancer. The first clear evidence of this is derived from systematic analysis of genetic alterations in breast and colorectal cancers, which revealed that proteases from different catalytic classes were candidate cancer genes that had somatically mutated in cancer.[36] These results have prompted the mutational analysis of entire protease families such as MMPs (matrix metalloproteinases), ADAMs (a disintegrin and metalloproteinase) and ADAMTSs (ADAMs with thromsbospondin domains) in different tumors. These studies led to identification of protease genes frequently mutated in cancer, such as *MMP8*, which is mutated and functionally inactivated in 6.3% of human melanomas.[37,38] Other MMP genes, including *MMP2*, *MMP9*, *MMP14*, and *MMP27*, are also somatically mutated in melanomas and other malignant tumors, albeit at low frequency.[37,39] Systematic mutational analysis of all members of the ADAM family of membrane-bound metalloproteases has shown that *ADAM7* and *ADAM29* are also often mutated in melanoma, whereas parallel studies of the ADAMTS family have revealed that *ADAMTS15* is mutated in colorectal carcinomas and *ADAMTS18* and *ADAMTS20* in melanomas.[40,41] Functional analyses have indicated that *ADAM7*, *ADAM29*, and *ADAMTS18* mutations affect adhesion of melanoma cells to specific extracellular matrix proteins and in some cases increase their migrating and invasive properties, suggesting that these mutated genes play a role in melanoma progression.[41,42] In contrast, functional studies of *ADAMTS15* mutations in colorectal cancer cells have revealed that this metalloprotease restrains tumor growth and invasion, further validating the concept that secreted proteases may have tumor-suppressor properties.[40]

The mutational status of caspases has also been extensively analyzed in different tumors as these proteases play a fundamental role in execution of apoptosis, one of the hallmarks of cancer.[43] These studies demonstrated that *CASP8* is deleted in neuroblastomas and inactivated by somatic mutations in a variety of human malignancies, including head and neck, colorectal, lung, and gastric carcinomas.[44–46] Likewise *CASP3*, *CASP4*, *CASP5*, *CASP6*, *CASP7*, *CASP10*, and *CASP14* are occasionally inactivated by mutation in different human cancers.[47–54] Other large protease families whose components are often mutated in cancer are the deubiquitylating enzymes (DUBs), which catalyze the removal of ubiquitin and ubiquitinlike modifiers of their target proteins.[55] Some DUBs were initially identified as oncogenic proteins, but recent work has shown that other deubiquitylases such as CYLD, A20, and BAP1 are tumor suppressors inactivated in cancer. *CYLD* is mutated in patients with familial cylindromatosis, a disease characterized by the formation of multiple tumors of skin appendages.[56] A20 is a DUB family member encoded by the *TNFAIP3* gene, which is mutated in a large number of Hodgkin's lymphomas and primary mediastinal B-cell lymphomas.[57–60] Finally, the *BAP1* gene, encoding an ubiquitin C-terminal hydrolase, has been found to be somatically mutated in 86% metastasizing uveal melanomas of the eye.[61]

Mutational Analysis of Exomes Using Sanger Sequencing

Although the gene family approach for the identification of cancer genes has proven extremely valuable, it still is a candidate approach and thus biased in its nature. The next step forward in the mutational profiling of cancer has been the sequencing of exomes, which is the entire coding portion of the human genome (18,000 protein-encoding genes). As of today the exomes of breast, colorectal, pancreatic, and ovarian clear cell carcinomas, glioblastoma multiforme, and medulloblastoma have been analyzed using Sanger sequencing. These large-scale analyses for the first time allowed researchers to describe and understand the genetic complexity of human cancers.[22,36,62–65] The declared goals of these exome studies were to provide for the first time methods for exome-wide mutational analyses in human tumors, to characterize their spectrum and quantity of somatic mutations, and, finally, to discover new genes involved in tumorigenesis as well as novel pathways that have a role in these tumors. In these studies, sequencing data were complemented with gene expression and copy number analyses, thus providing for the first time a comprehensive view of the genetic complexity of human tumors.[62–65] A number of conclusions can be drawn from these analyses:

1. Cancer genomes have an average of 30 to 100 somatic alterations per tumor, which was a higher number than previously thought. Although the alterations included point mutations, small insertions, deletions, or amplifications, the great majority of the mutations observed were single-base substitutions.[62,63]
2. Even within a single cancer type, there is a significant intertumor heterogeneity. This means that multiple mutational patterns (encompassing different mutant genes) are present in tumors that cannot be distinguished based on histological analysis. The concept that individual tumors have a unique genetic milieu is highly relevant for personalized medicine, a concept that will be discussed below.
3. The spectrum and nucleotide contexts of mutations differ between different tumor types. For example, over 50% of mutations in colorectal cancer were C:G to T:A transitions, and 10% were C:G to G:C transversions. In contrast, in breast cancers, only 35% of the mutations were C:G to T:A transitions, and 29% were C:G to G:C transversions. Knowledge of mutation spectra is vital as it allows insight into the mechanisms underlying mutagenesis and repair in the various cancers investigated.
4. A considerably larger number of genes that had not been previously reported to be involved in cancer were found to play a role in the disease.
5. Solid tumors arising in children, such as medulloblastoma, harbor on average five to ten times less gene alterations compared to a typical adult solid tumor. These pediatric tumors also harbor fewer amplifications and homozygous deletions within coding genes compared to adult solid tumors.

Importantly, to deal with the large amount of data generated in these genomic projects, it was necessary to develop new statistical and bioinformatic tools. Furthermore, examination of the overall distribution of the identified mutations allowed the development of a novel view of cancer genome landscapes and a novel definition of cancer genes. These new concepts in the understanding of cancer genetics are further discussed below. The compiled conclusions derived from these analyses have led to a paradigm shift in the understanding of cancer genetics.

A clear indication of the power of the unbiased nature of the whole exome surveys was revealed by the discovery of recurrent mutations in the active site of *IDH1*, a gene with no known link to gliomas, in 12% of tumors analyzed.[63] As malignant gliomas are the most common and lethal tumors of the central nervous system, and glioblastoma multiforme (GBM; World Health Organization grade IV astrocytoma) is the most biologically aggressive subtype, the unveiling of *IDH1* as a novel GBM gene is extremely significant. Importantly, mutations of *IDH1* predominantly occurred in younger patients (median age of 34 versus 56 years for anaplastic astrocytomas and 32 versus 59 years for GBMs) and were associated with a better prognosis, as patients with *IDH* mutations have a median overall survival of 31 months, and patients with wild type *IDH1* and *IDH2* have a median 15-month survival.[66] Follow-up studies showed that mutations of *IDH1* occur early in glioma progression, the R132 somatic mutation is harbored by the majority (greater than 70%) of grades II and III astrocytomas and oligodendrogliomas, as well as in secondary GBMs that develop from these lower grade lesions.[66–72] In contrast, less than 10% of primary GBMs harbor these alterations. Furthermore, analysis of the associated *IDH2* revealed recurrent somatic mutations in the R172 residue, which is the exact analog of the frequently mutated R132 residue of *IDH1*. These mutations occur mostly in a mutually exclusive manner with *IDH1* mutations,[66,68] suggesting that they have equivalent phenotypic effects. Subsequently, *IDH1* mutations have been reported in additional cancer types such as myeloid leukemia samples,[73–75] a single case of colorectal cancer, two prostate carcinomas,[71] one melanoma case,[76] and a few cases of adult supratentorial primitive neuroectodermal tumors.[69] Further description of the function of *IDH1* and *IDH2* mutations in cancer is found in Chapter 8.

Next-Generation Sequencing and Cancer Genome Analysis

The introduction in 1977 of the Sanger method for DNA sequencing with chain-terminating inhibitors has transformed biomedical research.[8] Over the past 30 years, this first-generation technology has been universally used for elucidating the nucleotide sequence of DNA molecules. However, the launching of new large-scale projects, including those implicating whole-genome sequencing of cancer samples, has made necessary the development of new methods that are widely known as next-generation sequencing technologies.[77–79] These approaches have significantly lowered the cost and the time required to determine the sequence of the 3×10^9 nucleotides present in the human genome. Moreover, they have a series of advantages over Sanger sequencing, which are of special interest for the analysis of cancer genomes.[80] First, next-generation sequencing approaches are more sensitive than Sanger methods and can detect somatic mutations even when they are present only in a subset of tumor cells.[81] Moreover, these new sequencing strategies are quantitative and can be used to simultaneously determine both nucleotide sequence and copy number variations.[82] They can also be coupled to other procedures such as those involving paired-end reads, allowing the identification of multiple structural alterations, such as insertions, deletions, and rearrangements, commonly occurring in cancer genomes.[81] Nonetheless, next-generation sequencing still presents some limitations mainly derived from the relatively high error rate in the short reads generated during the sequencing process. In addition, these short reads make the task of *de novo* assembly of the generated sequences and the mapping of the reads to a reference genome extremely complex. To overcome some of these current limitations, deep coverage of each analyzed genome is required and a careful validation of the identified variants must be performed, typically using Sanger sequencing. As a consequence, there is a substantial increase in both cost of the process and time of analysis. Therefore, it can be concluded that whole-genome sequencing of cancer samples is already a feasible task but not yet a routine process. Further technical improvements will be required before the task of decoding the entire genome of any malignant tumor of any cancer patient can be applied to clinical practice.

The number of next-generation sequencing platforms has substantially grown over the past few years and currently includes technologies from Roche/454, Illumina/Solexa, Life/APG's SOLiD3, Helicos BioSciences/HeliScope, and Pacific Biosciences/PacBio RS.[79] Noteworthy also are the recent introduction of the Polonator G.007 instrument, an open source platform with freely available software and protocols, the Ion Torrent's semiconductor sequencer, as well as those involving self-assembling DNA nanoballs or nanopore technologies.[83–85] These new machines are driving the field toward the era of third-generation sequencing, which brings enormous clinical interest as it can substantially increase speed and accuracy of analysis at reduced costs and facilitate the possibility of single-molecule sequencing of human genomes. A comparison of next-generation sequencing platforms is shown in Table 1.1. These various platforms differ in the method utilized for template preparation and in the nucleotide sequencing and imaging strategy, which finally result in their different performance. Ultimately, the most suitable approach depends on the specific genome sequencing projects.[79]

Current methods of template preparation first involve randomly shearing genomic DNA into smaller fragments from which a library of either fragment templates or mate-pair templates are generated. Then, clonally amplified templates from single DNA molecules are prepared by either emulsion polymerase chain reaction (PCR) or solid-phase amplification.[86,87] Alternatively, it is possible to prepare single-molecule templates through methods that require less starting material and do not involve PCR amplification reactions, which can be the source of artifactual mutations.[88] Once prepared, templates are attached to a solid surface in spatially separated sites, allowing thousands to billions of nucleotide sequencing reactions to be performed simultaneously.

The sequencing methods currently used by the different next-generation sequencing platforms are diverse and have been classified into four groups: cyclic reversible termination, single-nucleotide addition, real-time sequencing, and sequencing by ligation[79,89] (Fig. 1.3). These sequencing strategies are coupled with different imaging methods, including those based on measuring bioluminescent signals or involving four-color imaging of single molecular events. Finally, the extraordinary amount of data released from these nucleotide sequencing platforms is stored, assembled, and analyzed using powerful bioinformatic tools that have been developed in parallel with next-generation sequencing technologies.[90]

Next-generation sequencing approaches represent the newest entry into the cancer genome decoding arena and have already been applied to cancer analysis. The first research group to apply these methodologies to whole cancer genomes was that of Ley et al.,[91] who reported in 2008 the sequencing of the entire genome of a patient with acute myeloid leukemia (AML) and its comparison with the normal tissue from the same patient, using the Illumina/Solexa platform. As further described below, this work has allowed the identification of

TABLE 1.1

COMPARATIVE ANALYSIS OF NEXT-GENERATION SEQUENCING PLATFORMS

Platform	Library/Template Preparation	Sequencing Method	Average Read-Length (Bases)	Run Time (Days)	Gb Per Run	Instrument Cost (US$)	Comments
Roche 454 GS FLX	Fragment, Mate-pair Emulsion PCR	Pyrosequencing	400	0.35	0.45	500,000	Fast run times High reagent cost
Illumina HiSeq2000	Fragment, Mate-pair Solid-phase	Reversible terminator	100–125	8 (mate-pair run)	150–200	540,000	Most widely used platform Low multiplexing capability
Life/APG's SOLiD 5500xl	Fragment, Mate-pair Emulsion PCR	Cleavable probe, sequencing by ligation	35–75	7 (mate-pair run)	180–300	595,000	Inherent error correction Long run times
Helicos BioSciences HeliScope	Fragment, Mate-pair Single molecule	Reversible terminator	32	8 (fragment run)	37	999,000	Non-bias template representation Expensive, high error rates
Pacific Biosciences PacBio RS	Fragment Single molecule	Real-time sequencing	1,000	1	0.075	NA	Greatest potential for long reads Highest error rates
Polonator G.007	Mate-pair Emulsion PCR	Non-cleavable probe, sequencing by ligation	26	5 (mate-pair run)	12	170,000	Least expensive platform Shortest read lengths

NA, not available.
(Data represent an update of information provided in ref. 78.)

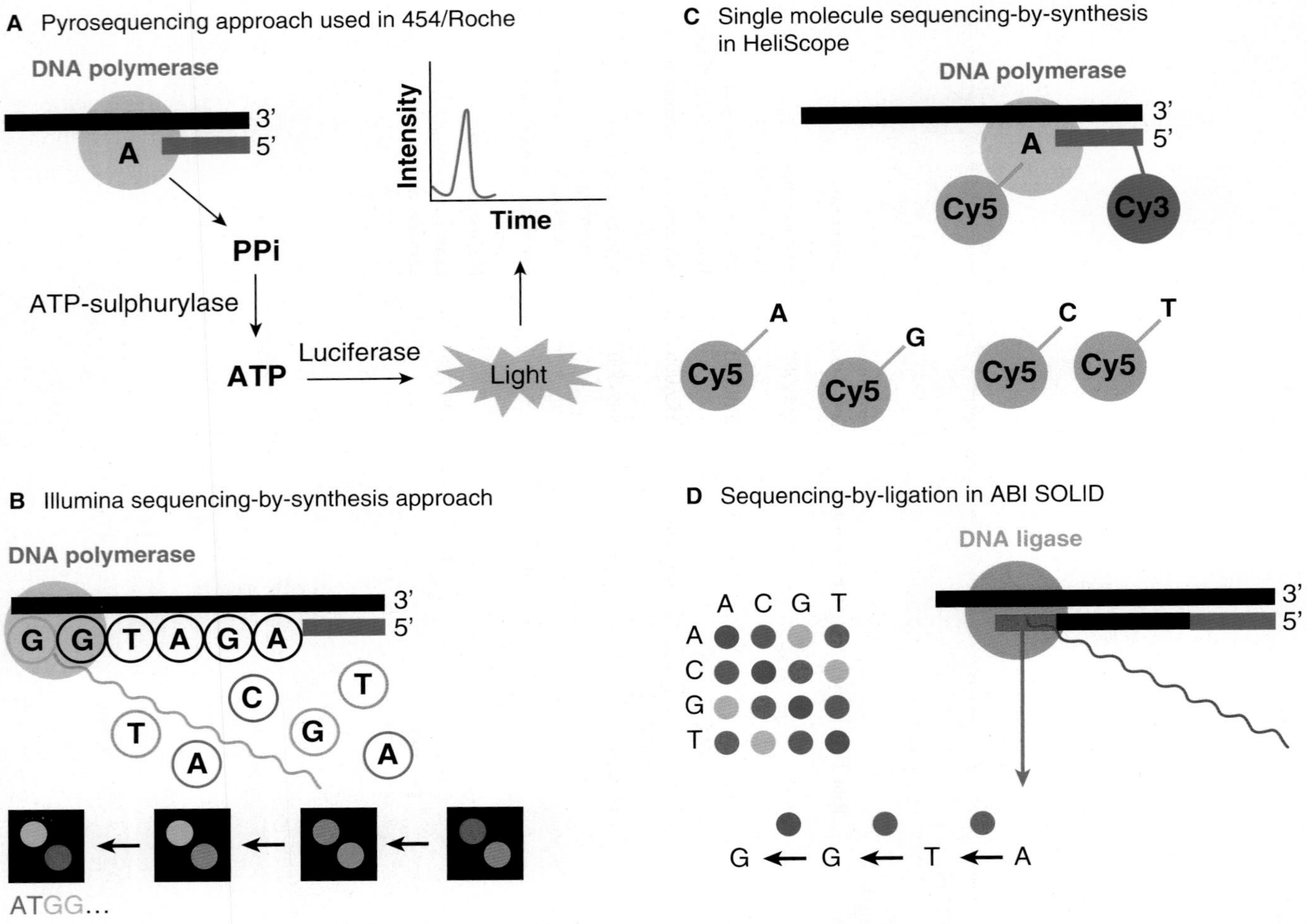

FIGURE 1.3 Advances in sequencing chemistry implemented in next-generation sequencers. **A:** The pyrosequencing approach implemented in 454/Roche sequencing technology detects incorporated nucleotides by chemiluminescence resulting from PPi release. **B:** The Illumina method utilizes sequencing-by-synthesis in the presence of fluorescently labeled nucleotide analogs that serve as reversible reaction terminators. **C:** The single-molecule sequencing-by-synthesis approach detects template extension using Cy3 and Cy5 labels attached to the sequencing primer and the incoming nucleotides, respectively. **D:** The SOLiD method sequences templates by sequential ligation of labeled degenerate probes. Two-base encoding implemented in the SOLiD instrument allows for probing each nucleotide position twice. (From ref. 88.)

point mutations and structural alterations of putative oncogenic relevance in AML and represents proof-of-principle of the relevance of next-generation sequencing for cancer research.

Whole-Genome Analysis Utilizing Second-Generation Sequencing

The sequence of the first whole cancer genome was reported in 2008, where an AML and skin from the same patient were described.[91] Numerous additional whole-genomes, together with the corresponding normal genomes of patients with a variety of malignant tumors, have been reported since then.[73,92–95] The first available whole-genome of a cytogenetically normal AML subtype M1 (AML-M1) revealed eight genes with novel mutations along with another 500 to 1,000 additional mutations found in noncoding regions of the genome. Most of the identified genes were not previously associated with cancer. Validation of the novel mutations identified no novel recurring mutations.[91] Concomitantly, with the expansion in the use of next-generation sequencers, other whole-genomes have been evaluated in a similar manner, including malignant melanoma, small cell lung cancer bone metastasis, lung adenocarcinoma, and a second AML.

In contrast to the first AML whole genome, the second did observe a recurrent mutation in *IDH1*, encoding isocitrate dehydrogenase.[73] Follow-up studies extended this finding and reported that mutations in *IDH1* and the related gene *IDH2* occur at a 20% to 30% frequency in AML patients and are associated with a poor prognosis in some subgroups of patients.[96–98] A good example illustrating the high pace at which second-generation technologies and their accompanying analytical tools are found is demonstrated by the following finding derived from reanalysis of the first AML whole genome. Thus, when improvements in sequencing techniques were available, the first AML whole genome described above, which identified no recurring mutations and had a 91.2% diploid coverage, was re-evaluated by deeper sequence coverage, yielding 99.6% diploid coverage of the genome. This improvement together with more advanced mutation naming algorithms allowed the discovery of several nonsynonymous mutations that had not been identified in the initial sequencing. This included a frameshift mutation in the DNA methyltransferase gene *DNMT3A*. Validation of *DNMT3A* in 280 additional *de novo* AML patients to define recurring mutations led to the significant discovery that a total of 22.1% of AML cases had mutations in *DNMT3A* that were predicted to affect translation. The median overall survival among patients with *DNMT3A* mutations was significantly shorter than that among patients without such mutations (12.3 months vs. 41.1 months; $P < .001$).

Shortly after this study, complete sequences of a series of cancer genomes together with matched normal genomes of the same patients have been reported.[73,92,93,99] These works have opened the way to more ambitious initiatives, including those involving large international consortia, aimed at decoding the genome of malignant tumors from thousands of cancer patients. In addition to these direct applications of next-generation sequencing technologies for the mutational analysis of cancer genomes, these methods have an additional range of applications in cancer research. Thus, genome sequencing efforts have begun to elucidate the genomic changes that accompany metastasis evolution through comparative analysis of primary and metastatic lesions from breast and pancreatic cancer patients.[94,100–102] Likewise, massively parallel sequencing has been used to analyze the evolution of a tongue adenocarcinoma in response to selection by targeted kinase inhibitors.[103] Detailed information of several of these whole genome projects is found below.

The first solid cancer to undergo whole-genome sequencing was a malignant melanoma that was compared to a lymphoblastoid cell line from the same person.[92] Impressively, a total of 33,345 somatic base substitutions were identified, with 187 nonsynonymous substitutions in protein-coding sequences, at least one order of magnitude higher than any other cancer type. Most somatic base substitutions were C:G greater than T:A transitions and of the 510 dinucleotide substitutions, 360 were CC.TT/GG.AA changes, which is consistent with ultraviolet light exposure mutation signatures previously reported in melanoma.[19] Such results from the most comprehensive catalog of somatic mutations not only provide insight into the DNA damage signature in this cancer type but can also be useful in determining the relative order of some acquired mutations. Indeed, this study shows that a significant correlation exists between the presence of a higher proportion of C.A/G.T transitions in early (82%) compared to late mutations (53%). Another important aspect that the comprehensive nature of this melanoma study provided was that cancer mutations are spread out unevenly throughout the genome, with a lower prevalence in regions of transcribed genes, suggesting that DNA repair occurs mainly in these areas.

An interesting example of the power of whole-genome sequencing in deciphering the mutation evolution in carcinogenesis was seen in a study in which a basal-like breast cancer tumor, a brain metastasis, a tumor xenograft derived from the primary tumor, and the peripheral blood from the same patient were compared (Fig. 1.4).[94] This analysis showed a wide range of mutant allele frequencies in the primary tumor, which was narrowed in the metastasis and xenograft samples. This suggested that the primary tumor was significantly more heterogeneous in its cell populations compared to its matched metastasis and xenograft samples as these underwent selection processes whether during metastasis or transplantation. The clear overlap in mutation incidence between the metastatic and xenograft cases suggests that xenografts undergo similar selection as metastatic lesions and are therefore a reliable source for genomic analyses. The main conclusion of this whole-genome study was that although metastatic tumors harbor an increased number of genetic alterations, the majority of the alterations found in the primary tumor are preserved.

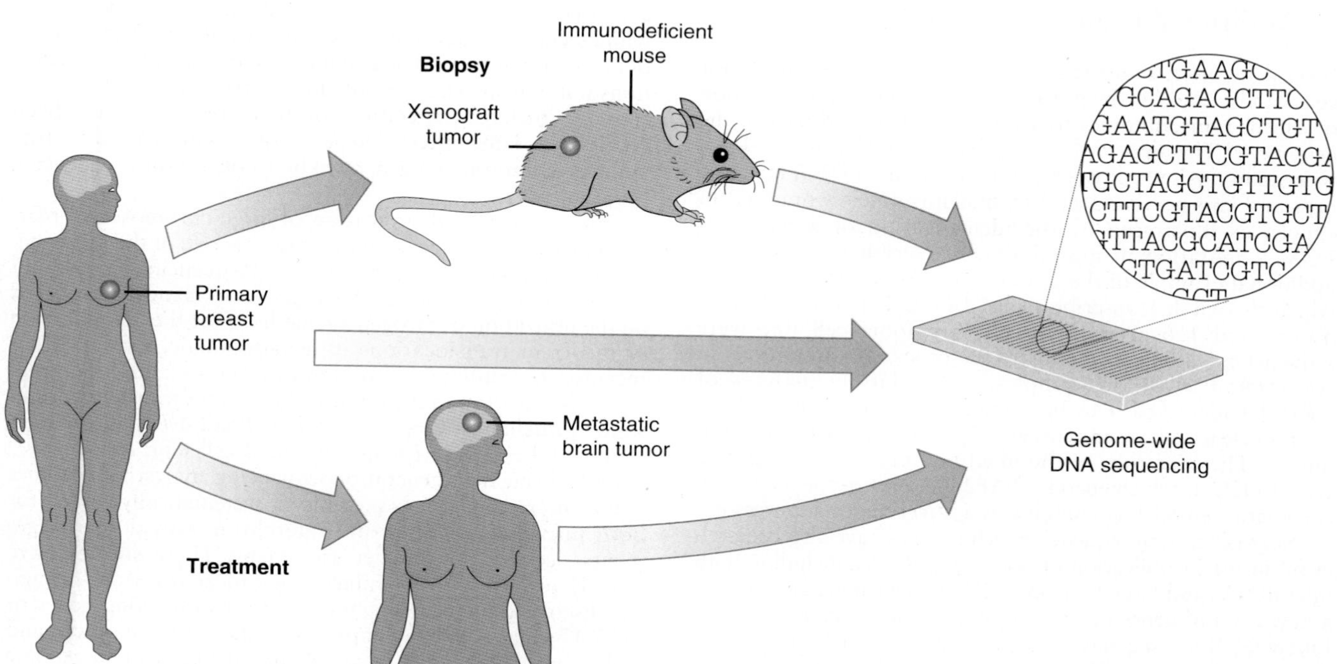

FIGURE 1.4 Covering all the bases in metastatic assessment. Ding et al.[94] performed genome-wide analysis on three tumor samples: a patient's primary breast tumor; her metastatic brain tumor, which formed despite therapy; and a xenograft tumor in a mouse, originating from the patient's breast tumor. They find that the primary tumor differs from the metastatic and xenograft tumors mainly in the prevalence of genomic mutations (permission from Gray et al. Nature 2010).

Whole-Exome Analysis Utilizing Second-Generation Sequencing

Another application of second-generation sequencing involves utilizing nucleic acid "baits" to capture regions of interest in the total pool of nucleic acids. These could either be DNA, as described above,[104,105] or RNA.[106] Indeed, most areas of interest in the genome can be targeted, including exons and noncoding RNAs. Despite inefficiencies in the exome targeting process, including the uneven capture efficiency across exons, which results in not all exons being sequenced, and the occurrence of some off-target hybridization events, the higher coverage of the exome makes it highly suitable for mutation discovery in cancer samples.

A recent study using exome capture followed by massively parallel sequencing surveyed somatic mutations in metastasizing uveal melanoma,[61] which is the most common primary cancer of the eye and is at high risk for fatal metastasis.[107] In this impressive study only two class II uveal melanoma tumors and their matching normal DNA were investigated. Although not much is known about the genetic basis of uveal melanoma, class II tumors are strongly associated with monosomy 3.[108] The authors therefore chose to specifically survey tumors that were monosomic for chromosome 3 to see whether loss of one copy of chromosome 3 could unmask a mutant gene on the remaining copy that promotes metastasis. This strategy was extremely fruitful as it allowed the identification of inactivating somatic mutations in *BAP1*, located at chromosome 3p21.1 and encoding a deubiquitylating enzyme. Further functional studies have implicated mutational inactivation of *BAP1* as a key event in uveal melanoma metastasis, thus expanding the relevance of DUBs as potential therapeutic targets in cancer.[61]

Use of Next-Generation Sequencing for Additional Cancer Genome Applications

Next-generation sequencing of RNA extracted from tumor cells can be used for the precise and complete characterization of cancer transcriptomes to sample the expressed part of the genome.[109] This approach, called RNA-seq, has higher sensitivity than methods of RNA profiling based on DNA microarrays and can be also useful to find novel genes mutated in cancer, as illustrated by the identification of a recurrent *FOXL2* mutation in granulose-cell ovarian tumors.[109] An additional example of the power of RNA-seq was a survey in which the whole transcriptome of 18 ovarian clear-cell carcinomas and 1 ovarian clear-cell carcinoma cell line were sequenced, leading to the discovery of somatic mutations in *ARID1A* in 6 of the samples.[110] Validation analyses of *ARID1A* identified it to be somatically mutated in 46% of ovarian clear-cell carcinomas and 30% of endometrioid carcinomas. The spectrum of the identified mutations suggested that *ARID1A*, which encodes BAF250a, part of the SWI–SNF chromatin remodeling complex, is a novel tumor suppressor.

Next-generation sequencing technologies have also been relevant in the identification of noncoding RNAs, including both microRNAs and large noncoding RNAs, which are encoded by a new class of genes of growing importance in cancer.[89,111,112] Likewise, RNA-seq data have also proven to be useful for detecting alternative splicing events or novel fusion transcripts in cancer samples.[113,114] Finally, several large-scale approaches such as ChIP-seq, which involves chromatin immunoprecipitation coupled with massively parallel sequencing, have facilitated the genome-wide identification of epigenetic alterations in cancer cells.[115,116]

SOMATIC ALTERATION CLASSES DETECTED BY CANCER GENOME ANALYSIS

Whole-genome sequencing of cancer genomes has an enormous potential to detect all major types of somatic mutations present in malignant tumors. This large repertoire of genomic abnormalities includes single nucleotide changes, small insertions and deletions, large chromosomal reorganizations, and copy number variations (Fig. 1.5).

Nucleotide substitutions are the most frequent somatic mutations detected in malignant tumors, although there is a substantial variability in the mutational frequency among different cancers.[78] On average, human malignancies have one nucleotide change per million bases, but melanomas reach mutational rates tenfold higher and tumors with mutator phenotype caused by DNA mismatch repair deficiencies may accumulate tens of mutations per million nucleotides. By contrast, tumors of hematopoietic origin have less than one base substitution per million. Several bioinformatic tools and pipelines have been developed to efficiently detect somatic nucleotide substitutions through comparison of the genomic information obtained from paired normal and tumor samples from the same patient. Likewise, there are a number of publicly available computational methods to predict the functional relevance of the identified mutations in cancer specimens.[78] Most of these bioinformatic tools exclusively deal with nucleotide changes in protein coding regions and evaluate the putative structural or functional effect of an amino acid substitution in a determined protein, thus obviating changes in other genomic regions, which can also be of crucial interest in cancer. In any case, current computational methods used in this regard are far from being optimal, and experimental validation is finally required to assess the functional relevance of nucleotide substitutions found in cancer genomes.

Small insertions and deletions (*indels*) represent a second category of somatic mutations that can be discovered by whole-genome sequencing of cancer specimens. These mutations are about tenfold less frequent than nucleotide substitutions but may also have an obvious impact in cancer progression. Accordingly, specific bioinformatic tools have been created to detect these *indels* in the context of the large amount of information generated by whole-genome sequencing projects.[117]

The systematic identification of large chromosomal rearrangements in cancer genomes represents one of the most successful applications of next-generation sequencing methodologies. Previous strategies in this regard had mainly been based on the utilization of cytogenetic methods for the identification of recurrent translocations in hematopoietic tumors. More recently, a combination of bioinformatics and functional methods has allowed the finding of recurrent translocations in solid epithelial tumors such as *TMPRSS2–ERG* in prostate cancer and *EML4–ALK* in non–small cell lung cancer.[118,119] Now, by using next-generation sequencing analysis of genomes and transcriptomes, it is possible to systematically search for both intrachromosomal and interchromosomal rearrangements occurring in cancer specimens. These studies have already proven their usefulness for cancer research through the discovery of recurrent translocations involving genes of the *RAF* kinase pathway in prostate cancer, gastric cancer, and melanoma.[120] Likewise, massively parallel paired-end genome and transcriptome sequencing has already been used to detect new gene fusions in cancer and to catalog all major structural rearrangements present in some tumors and cancer cell lines.[81,113,121,122] The ongoing cancer genome projects involving thousands of tumor samples will likely lead to the detection of

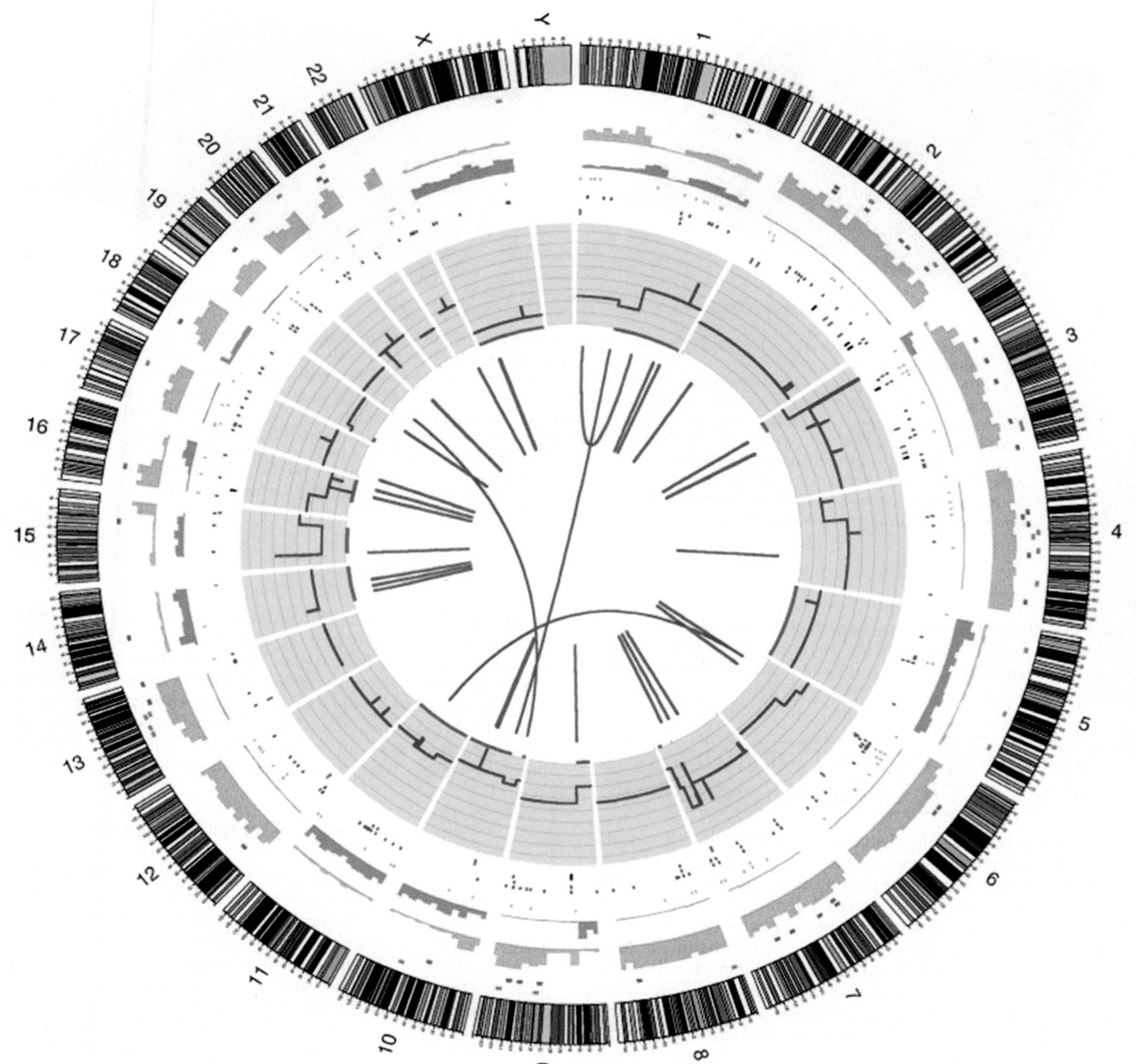

FIGURE 1.5 The catalog of somatic mutations in COLO-829. Chromosome ideograms are shown around the outer ring and are oriented pter–qter in a clockwise direction with centromeres indicated in red. Other tracks contain somatic alterations (*from outside to inside*): validated insertions (*light green rectangles*); validated deletions (*dark green rectangles*); heterozygous (*light orange bars*), and homozygous (*dark orange bars*) substitutions shown by density per 10 megabases; coding substitutions (*colored squares: silent in gray, missense in purple, nonsense in red, and splice site in black*); copy number (*blue lines*); regions of loss of heterozygosity (LOH) (*red lines*); validated intrachromosomal rearrangements (*green lines*); validated interchromosomal rearrangements (*purple lines*). (From ref. 92.)

many other chromosomal rearrangements of relevance in specific subsets of cancers. It is also remarkable that whole-genome sequencing may also facilitate the identification of other types of genomic alterations, including rearrangements of repetitive elements, such as active retrotransposons or insertions of foreign gene sequences, such as viral genomes, which can contribute to cancer development. Indeed, next-generation sequencing analysis of the transcriptome of Merkell cell carcinoma samples has revealed the clonal integration within the tumor genome of a previously unknown polyomavirus likely implicated in the pathogenesis of this rare but aggressive skin cancer.[123]

Finally, next-generation sequencing approaches have also demonstrated their feasibility to analyze the pattern of copy number alterations in cancer, as they allow researchers to count the number of reads in both tumor and normal samples at any given genomic region and then to evaluate the tumor-to-normal copy number ratio at this particular region. These new methods offer some advantages when compared with those based on microarrays, including much better resolution,

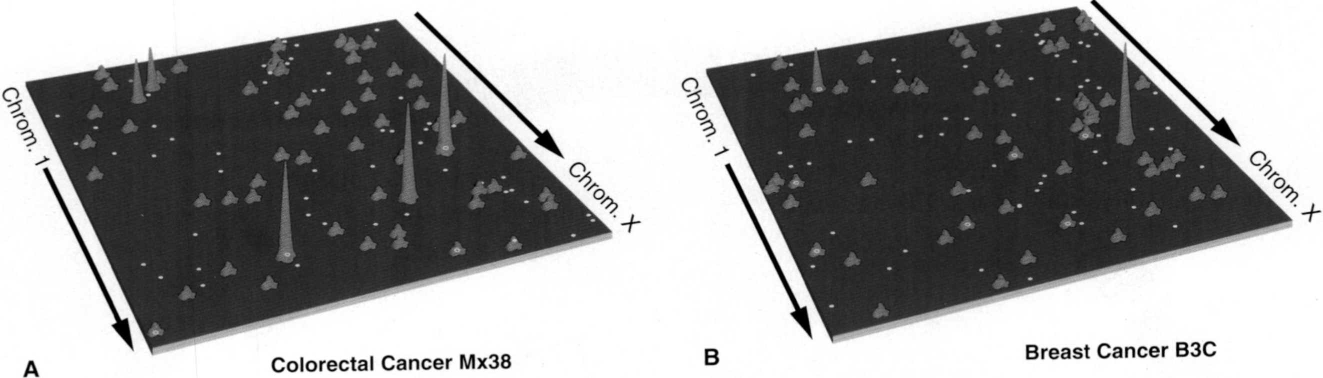

FIGURE 1.6 Cancer genome landscapes. Nonsilent somatic mutations are plotted in two-dimensional space representing chromosomal positions of RefSeq genes. The telomere of the short arm of chromosome 1 is represented in the rear left corner of the green plane and ascending chromosomal positions continue in the direction of the arrow. Chromosomal positions that follow the front edge of the plane are continued at the back edge of the plane of the adjacent row, and chromosomes are appended end to end. Peaks indicate the 60 highest-ranking CAN-genes for each tumor type, with peak heights reflecting CaMP scores (7). The dots represent genes that were somatically mutated in the individual colorectal (Mx38) (**A**) or breast tumor (B3C) (**B**) displayed. The dots corresponding to mutated genes that coincided with hills or mountains are black with white rims; the remaining dots are white with red rims. The mountain on the right of both landscapes represents TP53 (chromosome 17), and the other mountain shared by both breast and colorectal cancers is PIK3CA (upper left, chromosome 3). (Redrawn from ref. 36. Reprinted with permission from AAAS.)

precise definition of the involved breakpoints, and absence of saturation, which facilitates the accurate estimation of high-copy number levels occurring in some genomic loci of malignant tumors.[78]

PATHWAY-ORIENTED MODELS OF CANCER GENOME ANALYSIS

Genome-wide mutational analyses suggest that the mutational landscape of cancer is made up of a handful of genes that are mutated in a high fraction of tumors, otherwise know as "mountains," and most mutated genes are altered at relatively low frequencies, otherwise known as "hills"[36] (Fig. 1.6). The mountains probably give a high selective advantage to the mutated cell, and the hills might provide a lower advantage, making it hard to distinguish them from passenger mutations. As the hills differ between cancer types, it seems that the cancer genome is more complex and heterogeneous than anticipated. Although highly heterogeneous, bioinformatic studies suggest that the mountains and hills can be grouped into sets of pathways and biologic processes. Some of these pathways are affected by mutations in a few pathway members and others by numerous members. For example, pathway analyses have allowed the stratification of mutated genes in pancreatic adenocarcinomas to 12 core pathways that have at least one member mutated in 67% to 100% of the tumors analyzed[62] (Fig. 1.7). These core pathways deviated to some that harbored one single highly mutated gene, such as in *KRAS* in the G_1/S cell cycle transition pathway and pathways where a few mutated genes were found, such as the transforming growth factor (TGF-β) signaling pathway. Finally, there were pathways in which many different genes were mutated, such as invasion regulation molecules, cell adhesion molecules, and integrin signaling. Importantly, independent of how many genes in the same pathway are affected, if they are found to occur in a mutually exclusive fashion in a single tumor, they most likely give the same selective pressure for clonal expansion.

The idea of genetically analyzing pathways rather than individual genes has been applied previously, revealing the concept of mutual exclusivity. Mutual exclusivity has been shown elegantly in the case of *KRAS* and *BRAF* where a *KRAS* mutated cancer generally does not also harbor a *BRAF* mutation, as *KRAS* is upstream of *BRAF* in the same pathway.[14] A similar concept was applied for *PIK3CA* and *PTEN*, where both mutations do not usually occur in the same tumor.[30]

"Passenger" and "Driver" Mutations

By the time a cancer is diagnosed, it is comprised of billions of cells carrying DNA abnormalities, some of which have a functional role in malignant proliferation but also many genetic lesions acquired along the way that have no functional role in tumorigenesis.[19] The emerging landscapes of cancer genomes include thousands of genes that were not previously linked to tumorigenesis but are found to be somatically mutated. Many of these changes are likely to be "passengers" or neutral in that they have no functional effects on the growth of the tumor.[19] Only a small fraction of the genetic alterations are expected to drive cancer evolution by giving cells a selective advantage over their neighbors. Passenger mutations occur incidentally in a cell that later or in parallel develops a "driver" mutation, but are not ultimately pathogenic.[124] Although neutral, cataloging passengers mutations is important as they incorporate the signatures of previous exposures the cancer cell underwent as well as DNA repair defects the cancer cell has. As in many cases passenger and driver mutations occur at similar frequencies, and identification of drivers versus the passenger is of utmost relevance and remains a pressing challenge in cancer genetics.[125–127] This goal will eventually be achieved through a combination of genetic and functional approaches, some of which are listed below.

The most reliable indicator that a gene was selected for and therefore is highly likely to be pathogenic is identification of recurrent mutations, whether at the same exact amino acid position or in neighboring amino acid positions in different patients. Further than that, if somatic alterations in the same

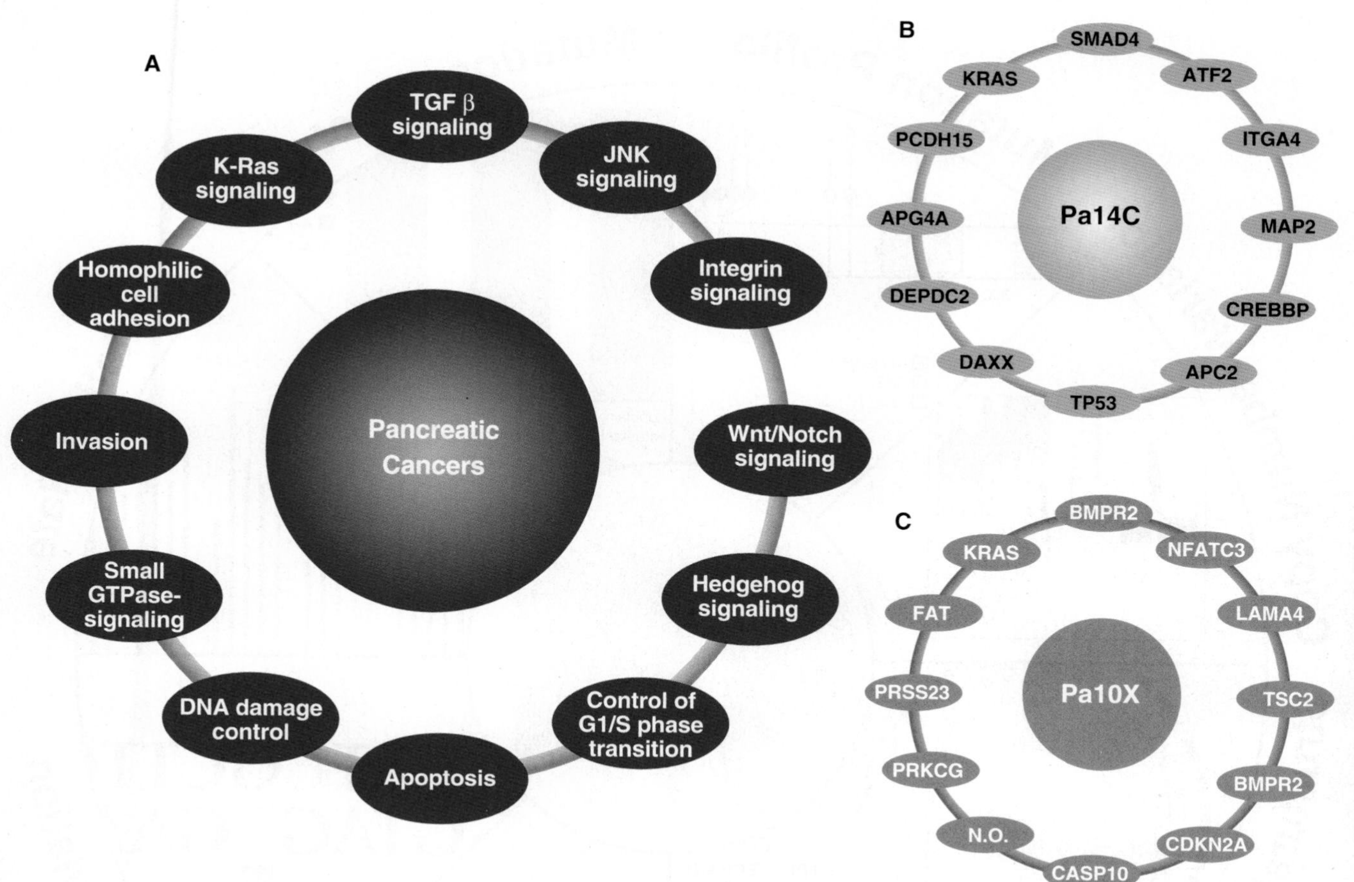

FIGURE 1.7 Signaling pathways and processes. **A:** The 12 pathways and processes whose component genes were genetically altered in most pancreatic cancers. **B, C:** Two pancreatic cancers (Pa14C and Pa10X) and the specific genes that are mutated in them. The positions around the circles in (B) and (C) correspond to the pathways and processes in (A). Several pathway components overlapped, as illustrated by the BMPR2 mutation that presumably disrupted both the SMAD4 and hedgehog signaling pathways in Pa10X. Additionally, not all 12 processes and pathways were altered in every pancreatic cancer, as exemplified by the fact that no mutations known to affect DNA damage control were observed in Pa10X. NO, not observed. (Redrawn from ref. 61. Reprinted with permission from AAAS.)

gene occur very frequently (mountains in the tumor genome landscape), these can be confidently classified as drivers. For example, cancer alleles that are identified in multiple patients and different tumors types such as those found in *KRAS, TP53, PTEN,* and *PIK3CA* are clearly selected for during tumorigenesis.

However, most genes discovered thus far are mutated in a relatively small fraction of tumors (hills), and it has been clearly shown that genes that are mutated in less than 1% of patients can still act as drivers.[128] The systematic sequencing of newly identified putative cancer genes in the vast number of specimens from cancer patients will help in this regard. However, even if examination of large numbers of samples can provide helpful information to classify drivers versus passengers, this approach alone is limited by the marked variation in mutation frequency among individual tumors and individual genes. The statistical test utilized in this case calculates the probability that the number of mutations in a given gene reflects a mutation frequency that is greater than expected from the nonfunctional background mutation rate,[36,129] which is different between different cancer types. These analyses incorporate the number of somatic alterations observed, the number of tumors studied, and the number of nucleotides that were successfully sequenced and analyzed.

Another approach often used to distinguish driver from passenger mutations exploits statistical analysis of synonymous versus nonsynonymous changes.[130] In contrast to nonsynonymous mutations, synonymous mutations do not alter the protein sequence. Therefore, they do not usually apply a growth advantage and would not be expected to be selected during tumorigenesis. This strategy works by comparing the observed-to-expected ratio of synonymous with that of nonsynonymous mutation. An increased proportion of nonsynonymous mutations from the expected two-to-one ratio implies selection pressure during tumorigenesis.

Other approaches are based on the concept that driver mutations may have characteristics similar to those causing Mendelian disease when inherited in the germ line and may be identifiable by constraints on tolerated amino acid residues at the mutated positions. In contrast, passenger mutations may have characteristics more similar to those of nonsynonymous SNPs with high minor allele frequencies. Based on these premises, supervised machine learning methods have been used to predict which missense mutations are drivers.[131] Additional approaches to decipher drivers from passengers include identification of mutations that affect locations that have previously been shown to be cancer causing in protein members of the same gene family. Enrichment for mutations in evolutionarily

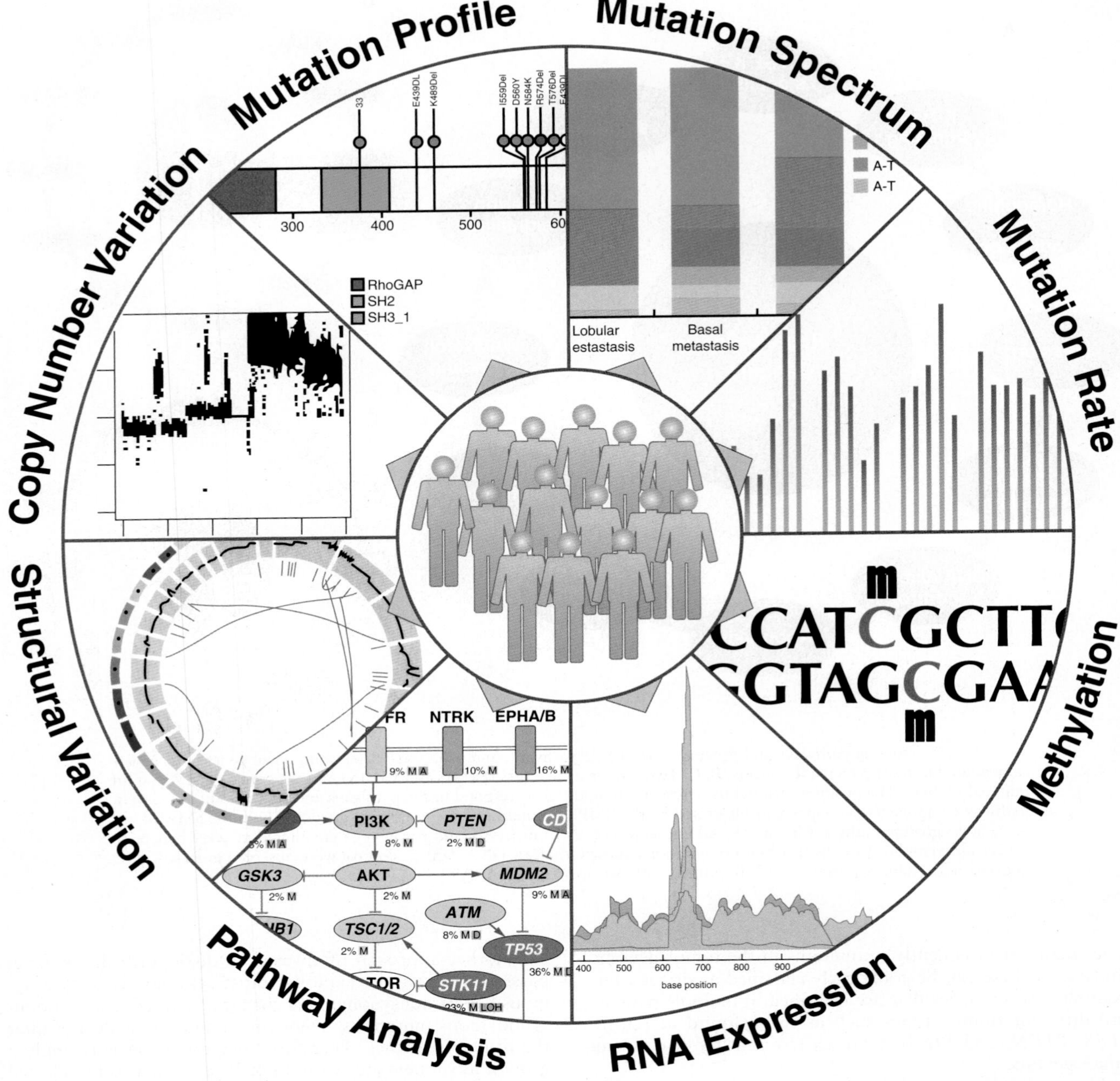

FIGURE 1.8 Landscape of cancer genomics analyses. NGS data will be generated for hundreds of tumors from all major cancer types in the near future. The integrated analysis of DNA, RNA and methylation sequencing data will help elucidate all relevant genetic changes in cancers. (Permission from ref. 94.)

conserved residues and algorithms, such as SIFT (sorting intolerant from tolerant),[132] estimate the effects of the different mutations identified.

Probably the most conclusive methods to identify driver mutations will be rigorous functional studies using biochemical assays as well as model organisms or cultured cells, using knock-out and knock-in of individual cancer alleles.[133] Unfortunately, these methods are not well suited to the analysis of the hundreds of gene candidates that arise from every large-scale cancer genome project. In conclusion, it is fair to say that sequencing cancer genomes is only the beginning of a journey that will ultimately be completed when the thousands of the newly discovered alleles are annotated as being the drivers of this disease. A summary of the various next-generation applications and approaches for their analysis is summarized in Figure 1.8 and Table 1.2.

NETWORKS OF CANCER GENOME PROJECTS

The first large-scale studies of genes mutated in malignant tumors have allowed the identification of new cancer genes that represent potential targets for therapy in different types of cancer. However, these analyses have also demonstrated that the repertoire of oncogenic mutations is extremely heterogeneous, suggesting that it would be difficult for independent

TABLE 1.2

COMPUTATIONAL TOOLS AND DATABASES USEFUL FOR CANCER GENOME ANALYSIS

Category	Tool/Database	URL	Refs.
Alignment	MAQ	http://maq.sourceforge.net	1
	BWA	http://bio-bwa.sourceforge.net	2
Mutation calling	SNVMix	http://www.bcgsc.ca/platform/bioinfo/software/SNVMix	3
	Samtools	http://samtools.sourceforge.net	4
	VarScan	http://varscan.sourceforge.net	5
Indel calling	Pindel	http://www.ebi.ac.uk/-kye/pindel	6
Copy number analysis	CBS	http://www.bioconductor.org	7
	SegSeq	http://www.broadinstitute.org/cgi-bin/cancer/publications/ pub_paper.cgi?mode=view&paper_id=182	8
Functional effect	SIFT	http://blocks.fhcrc.org/sift/SIFT.html	9
	Polyphen-2	http://genetics.bwh.harvard.edu/pph2	10
Visualization	CIRCOS	http://mkweb.bcgsc.ca/circos	11
	IGV	http://www.broadinstitute.org/igv	12
Repository	Cosmic	http://www.sanger.ac.uk/genetics/CGP/cosmic	13
	CGP	http://www.sanger.ac.uk/genetics/CGP	14
	dbSNP	http://www.ncbi.nlm.nih.gov/SNP	15
	Gene Ranker	http://cbio.mskcc.org/tcga-generanker/	16

(Table based on Table 2 from Meyerson M, Stacey G, and Getz G. Advances in understanding cancer genomes through second generation sequencing. *Nature Rev Genet* 2010;11:685–696.)

1. Li H, Durbin R. Fast and accurate short read alignment with Burrows–Wheeler transform. *Bioinformatics* **2009;25:**1754–1760.
2. Li H, Durbin R. Fast and accurate long-read alignment with Burrows–Wheeler transform. *Bioinformatics* 2010;26:589–595.
3. Goya R, et al. SNVMix: predicting single nucleotide variants from next-generation sequencing of tumors. *Bioinformatics* 2010;26:730–736.
4. Li H, et al. The Sequence Alignment/Map format and SAMtools. *Bioinformatics* 2009;25:2078–2079.
5. Koboldt DC, Chen K, Wylie T, et al. VarScan: variant detection in massively parallel sequencing of individual and pooled samples. *Bioinformatics* 2009;25(17):2283–2285.
6. Ye K, Schulz MH, Long Q, et al. Pindel: a pattern growth approach to detect break points of large deletions and medium sized insertions from paired-end short reads. *Bioinformatics* 2009;25:2865–2871.
7. Venkatraman ES, Olshen AB. A faster circular binary segmentation algorithm for the analysis of array CGH data. *Bioinformatics* 2007;23:657–663.
8. Chiang DY, et al. High-resolution mapping of copy-number alterations with massively parallel sequencing. *Nature Methods* 2009;6:99–103.
9. Ng PC, Henikoff S. Predicting deleterious amino acid substitutions. *Genome Res.* 2001;11:863–874.
10. Idzhubei IA, et al. A method and server for predicting damaging missense mutations. *Nature Methods* 2010;7:248–249.
11. Krzywinski M, et al. Circos: an information aesthetic for comparative genomics. *Genome Res.* 2009;19:1639–1645.
12. Robinson JT, Thorvaldsdóttir H, Winckler W, et al. Integrative Genomics Viewer. *Nature Biotechnol* 2010 (In Press).
13. Forbes SA, Bhamra S, Dawson E, et al. The catalogue of somatic mutations in cancer (COSMIC). *Curr Protoc Hum Genet.* 2008; Chapter 10:Unit 10.11
14. Futreal PA, Coin L, Marshall M, et al. A census of human cancer genes. *Nat Rev Cancer.* 2004;4;177–183.
15. Sherry ST, Ward MH, Kholodov M, et al. dbSNP: The NCBI Database of genetic variation. *Nucleic Acids Res.* 2001;29(1):308–311.
16. The Cancer Genome Atlas Research Network. Comprehensive genomic characterization defines human glioblastoma genes and core pathways. *Nature* 2008;455:1061–1068.

cancer genome initiatives to address the generation of comprehensive catalogs of mutations in the wide spectrum of human malignancies. Accordingly, there have been different efforts to coordinate the cancer genome sequencing projects being carried out around the world. The first initiative in this regard was the Cancer Genome Project (CGP) of the Wellcome Trust Sanger Institute launched in the United Kingdom, which has been followed by two large and ambitious projects called the Cancer Genome Atlas (TCGA) and the International Cancer Genome Consortium (ICGC). Besides these three large cancer genome projects, there are other initiatives that are more focused on specific tumors, such as that lead by scientists at St. Jude Children's Research Hospital in Memphis, and Washington University, which aims at sequencing 600 pediatric-cancer genomes.

The CGP initially focused on the systematic search for somatic alterations in human tumors and cancer cell lines, analyzing large sets of candidate cancer genes as well as whole genomes. This project has already completed the whole-genome sequencing of several cancer patients and tumor-derived cell lines, including lung carcinomas and melanomas,[92,93] and intends to extend these studies to a total of 2,000 to 3,000 cases over the next 5 years.

TCGA began in 2006 at the United States as a comprehensive program in cancer genomics supported by the U.S. National Institutes of Health (NIH). The initial project focused on three tumors: glioblastoma multiforme, serous cystadenocarcinoma of the ovary, and lung squamous carcinoma. These studies have already generated novel and interesting information regarding genes mutated in these malignancies.[134] On the basis of these positive results, the NIH has recently announced an expansion of the TCGA program with the aim to produce genomic data sets for at least 10 additional cancers by the end of 2011 and 20 to 25 cancers over the next 5 years.

The ICGC was formed in 2008 to coordinate the generation of comprehensive catalogs of genomic abnormalities in tumors from 50 different cancer types or subtypes that are of clinical and societal importance across the world.[135] The project aims to perform systematic studies of over 25,000 cancer genomes at the genomic level and integrate this information with epigenomic and transcriptomic studies of the same cases as well as with clinical features of patients. At present, ten countries and two European consortia have already initiated cancer genome projects coordinated by the ICGC. These projects will deal with at least 500 samples per cancer type from cancers affecting a variety of human organs and tissues, including blood, brain, breast, kidney, liver, pancreas, stomach, oral cavity, and ovary.[135] All participating countries and scientists have adhered to a series of predetermined procedures for ethical approval, sample quality, clinical annotation, study design, statistical issues, data storage, and intellectual property. In this regard, the ICGC has made the commitment to make the data available to the entire research community as rapidly as possible to accelerate the understanding of cancer biology and translate these discoveries into clinical practice.

All these coordinated projects have already provided new insights into the catalog of genes mutated in cancer and have unveiled specific signatures of the mutagenic mechanisms, including carcinogen exposures or DNA-repair defects, implicated in the development of different malignant tumors.[92,93,136] Furthermore, these cancer genome studies have also contributed to define clinically relevant subtypes of tumors for prognosis and therapeutic management, and in some cases have identified new targets and strategies for cancer treatment.[66,73,95,137,138] Nevertheless, and similar to the doubts raised at the first stages of the Human Genome Project, the proposal to sequence large numbers of cancer genomes has also generated some controversy because of the high cost of these projects, the lack of novel functional hypotheses driving these projects, or their failure to characterize the mutational heterogeneity within individual tumors.[139,140] However, the rapid technological advances in DNA sequencing will likely drop the costs of sequencing cancer genomes to a small fraction of the current price and will allow researchers to overcome some of the current limitations of these global sequencing efforts. Hopefully, worldwide coordination of cancer genome projects with those involving large-scale functional analysis of genes in both cellular and animal models will likely provide us with the most comprehensive collection of information generated to date into the causes and molecular mechanisms of cancer.

THE GENOMIC LANDSCAPE OF CANCERS

Examination of the overall distribution of the identified mutations redefined the cancer genome landscapes whereby the mountains are the handful of commonly mutated genes and the hills represent the vast majority of genes that are infrequently mutated. One of the most striking features of tumor genomic landscape is that it involves different sets of cancer genes that are mutated in a tissue-specific fashion.[141,142] To continue with the analogy, the scenery is very different if we observe a colorectal, a lung, or a breast tumor. This indicates that mutations in specific genes cause tumors at specific sites, or are associated with specific stages of development, cell differentiation, or tumorigenesis, despite many of those genes being expressed in various fetal and adult tissues. Moreover, different types of tumors follow specific genetic pathways in terms of the combination of genetic alterations that it must acquire. For example, no cancer outside the bowel has been shown to follow the classic genetic pathway of colorectal tumorigenesis. Additionally, *KRAS* mutations are almost always present in pancreatic cancers but are very rare or absent in breast cancers. Similarly, *BRAF* mutations are present in 60% of melanomas but are very infrequent in lung cancers.[1] Another intriguing feature is that alterations in ubiquitous housekeeping genes, such as those involved in DNA repair or energy production, occur only in particular types of tumors.

In addition to tissue specificity, the genomic landscape of tumors can also be associated with the gender and the hormonal status. For example *HER-2* amplification and *PIK3C2A* mutations, two genetic alterations associated with breast cancer development, are correlated with the estrogen-receptor hormonal status.[143] The molecular basis for the occurrence of cancer mutations in tissue- and gender-specific profiles is still largely unknown. Organ-specific expression profiles and cell-specific neoplastic transformation requirements are often mentioned as possible causes for this phenomenon. Identifying tissue and gender cancer mutations patterns is relevant as it may allow the definition of individualized therapeutic avenues.

THE CANCER GENOME AND THE NEW TAXONOMY OF TUMORS

The deciphering of the cancer genome has already impacted clinical practice at multiple levels. On the one hand, it allowed the identification of new cancer genes such as *IDH1*, a gene involved in glioma, which was discovered recently (see above), and on the other hand, it is redesigning the taxonomy of tumors.

Until the genomic revolution, tumors had been classified based on two criteria: their localization (site of occurrence) and their appearance (histology). These criteria are also currently used as primary determinants of prognosis and to establish the best treatments. For many decades it has been known that patients with histologically similar tumors have different clinical outcomes. Furthermore, tumors that cannot be distinguished based on histological analysis can respond very differently to identical therapies.[144]

It is becoming increasingly manifest that the frequency and distribution of mutations affecting cancer genes can be used to redefine the histology-based taxonomy of a given tumor type. Lung and colorectal tumors represent paradigmatic examples. Genomic analysis led to the identification of activating mutations in the receptor tyrosine kinase *EGFR* in lung adenocarcinomas.[145] The occurrence of *EGFR* mutations molecularly defines a subtype of non–small cell lung cancer (NSCLC) that occur mainly in nonsmoker women, tend to have a distinctly enhanced prognosis, and typically respond to EGFR-targeted therapies.[146–148] Similarly, the recent discovery of the *EML4-ALK* fusion identifies yet another subset of NSCLC that is clearly distinct from those that harbor *EGFR* mutations, have distinct epidemiologic and biological features, and respond to ALK inhibitors.[119,149]

The second example is colorectal cancers (CRC), the tumor type for which the genomic landscape has been refined with the highest accuracy. CRCs can be clearly categorized according to the mutational profile of the genes involved in the *KRAS* pathway (Fig. 1.9). It is now known that *KRAS* mutations occur in approximately 40% of CRCs. Another subtype of

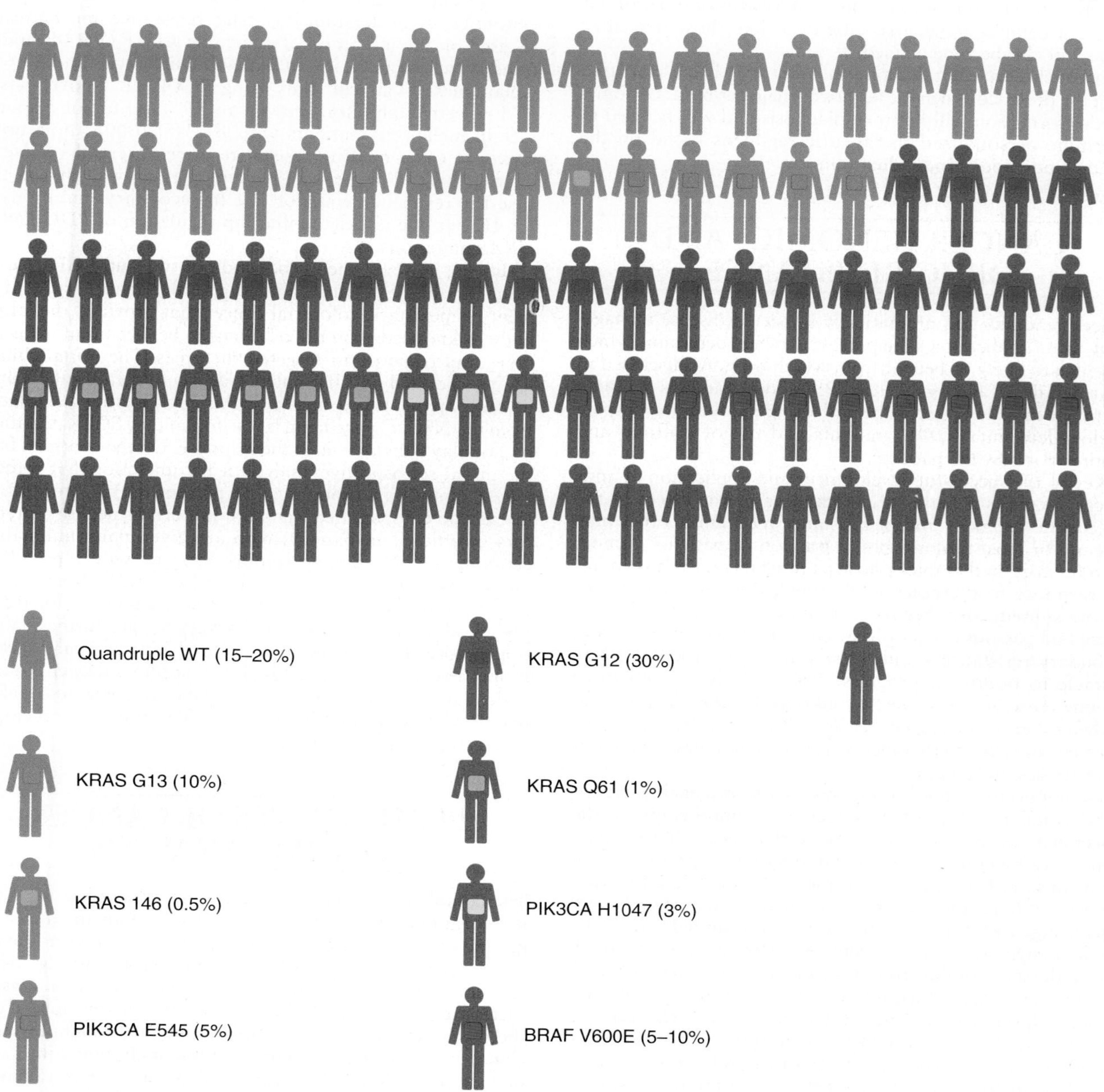

FIGURE 1.9 Graphic representation of a cohort of 100 patients with colorectal cancer treated with cetuximab or panitumumab. The genetic milieu of individual tumors and their impacts on the clinical response are listed. *KRAS*, *BRAF*, and *PIK3CA* somatic mutations as well as loss of PTEN protein expression are indicated according to different color codes. Molecular alterations mutually exclusive or coexisting in individual tumors are indicated using different color variants. The relative frequencies at which the molecular alterations occur in colorectal cancers are described. (Redrawn from Bardelli A, Siena S. Molecular mechanisms of resistance to cetuximab and panitumumab in colorectal cancer. *J Clin Oncol* 2009;22:6043.)

CRC (approximately 10%) harbors mutations in *BRAF*, the immediate downstream effectors of *KRAS*.[15]

In CRC and other tumor types, *KRAS* and *BRAF* mutations are known to be mutually exclusive. The mutual exclusivity pattern indicates that these genes operate in the same signaling pathway. Large epidemiologic studies have shown that the prognosis of tumors harboring wild type *KRAS/BRAF* genes is distinct, typically more favorable, than that of the mutated ones.[150,151] Of note, *KRAS* and *BRAF* mutations have been recently shown to impair responsiveness to the anti-EGFR monoclonal antibodies therapies in CRC patients.[152–154] Clearly distinct subgroups can be genetically identified in both NSCLC and CRC with respect to prognosis and response to therapy. It is likely that, as soon as the genomic landscapes of other tumor types are defined, molecular subgroups like those described above will also become defined.

In conclusion, the taxonomy of tumors is being rewritten using the presence of genetic lesions as major criteria. Genome-based information will improve diagnosis and will be used to determine personalized therapeutic regimens based on the genetic landscape of individual tumors.

CANCER GENOMICS AND DRUG RESISTANCE

Cancer genomics has dramatically impacted disease management, as its application is helping researchers determine which patients are likely to benefit from which drug. As discussed in great detail in Chapters 12 and 39, good examples for such treatment include targeted therapy using imatinib for chronic myeloid leukemia (CML) patients and use of gefitinib and erlotinib for NSCLC patients.

Key to the successful development and application of anticancer agents is a better understanding of the effect of the therapeutic regimens and of resistance mechanisms that may develop. In most tumor types, a fraction of patients' tumors are refractory to therapies (intrinsic resistance). Even if an initial response to therapies is obtained, the vast majority of tumors subsequently become refractory (i.e., acquired resistance) and patients eventually succumb to disease progression. Secondary resistance should therefore be regarded as a key obstacle to treatment progress. The analysis of the cancer genome represents a powerful tool both for the identification of chemotherapeutic signatures as well as to understand resistance mechanisms to therapeutic agents. Examples for each of these are described below.

An important application of systematic sequencing experiments is identification of the effects of chemotherapy on the cancer genome. For example, gliomas that recur after temozolomide treatment have been shown to harbor large numbers of mutations with a signature typical of a DNA alkylating agent.[155,156] Since these alterations were detected using Sanger sequencing, which as described above has limited sensitivity, the data suggested that the detected alterations were clonal. The model that unfolds from this study indicates that although temozolomide has limited efficacy, almost all of the cells in a glioma respond to the drug. However, a single cell that was resistant to the chemotherapy proliferated and formed a cell clone. Later genomic analyses of the cell clone allowed the identification of the underlying mutated resistance genes.[155,156]

Single-molecule targeted therapy is almost always followed by acquired drug resistance.[157–159] Genomic analyses can be successfully exploited to decipher resistance mechanisms to such inhibitors. Below a few paradigmatic examples are presented that will be discussed extensively in other chapters. Despite the effectiveness of gefitinib and erlotinib in EGFR mutant cases of NSCLC,[160] drug resistance develops within 6 to 12 months after initiation of therapy. The underlying reason for this resistance was identified as a secondary mutation in *EGFR* exon 20, T790M, detectable in 50% of patients who relapse.[161–163] Importantly, some studies have shown the mutation to be present before the patient was treated with the drug,[164,165] suggesting that exposure to the drug selected for these cells.[166] As the drug resistant *EGFR* mutation is structurally analogous to the mutated gatekeeper residue T315I in BCR-ABL, T670I in c-KIT, and L1196M in EML4-ALK, which have been shown previously to confer resistance to imatinib and other kinase inhibitors,[158,167,168] this mechanism of resistance represent a general problem that needs to be overcome.

A recent elegant study, which also represents the use of genomics in understanding drug resistance mechanisms, focused on the inhibition of activating *BRAF* (V600E) mutations, which occur in 7% of human malignancies and 60% of melanomas.[14] Clinical trials using PLX4032, a novel class I RAF-selective inhibitor, showed an 80% antitumor response rate in melanoma patients with *BRAF* (V600E) mutations, however, cases of drug resistance were observed.[169] Use of microarray and sequencing technologies showed that in this case the resistance was not due to secondary mutations in *BRAF*, but due rather to either up-regulation of *PDGFRB* or *NRAS* mutations.[170]

It was, however, the introduction of two anti-EGFR monoclonal antibodies, cetuximab and panitumumab, for the treatment of metastatic colorectal cancer that provided the largest body of knowledge on the relationship between tumors' genotypes and response to targeted therapies. The initial clinical analysis pointed out that only a fraction of metastatic colorectal cancer patients benefited from this novel treatment. Different from the NSCLC paradigm, it was found that EGFR mutations do not play a major role in the response. On the contrary, from the initial retrospective analysis it became clear that somatic *KRAS* mutations, thought to be present in 35% to 45% of metastatic colorectal cancers, are important negative predictors of efficacy in patients who are given panitumumab or cetuximab.[152–154] Among tumors carrying wild type *KRAS*, mutations of *BRAF* or *PIK3CA*, or loss of PTEN expression may also predict resistance to EGFR-targeted monoclonal antibodies, although the latter biomarkers require further validation before they can be incorporated into clinical practice. From these few examples, it is clear that future deeper genomic understanding of targeted drug resistance is crucial to the effective development of additional as well as alternative therapies to overcome this resistance.

PERSPECTIVES OF CANCER GENOME ANALYSIS

The completion of the human genome project has marked a new beginning in biomedical sciences. As human cancer is a genetic disease, the field of oncology has been one of the first to be impacted by this historic revolution. Knowledge of the sequence and organization of the human genome allows the systematic analysis of the genetic alterations underlying the origin and evolution of tumors. High throughput mutational profiling of common tumors, including lung, skin, breast, and colorectal cancers, and the application of next-generation sequencing to whole genome, whole exome, and whole transcriptome of cancer samples has allowed substantial advances in the understanding of this disease by facilitating the detection of all main types of somatic cancer genome alterations. These have also led to historical results such as the identification of genetic alterations that are likely to be the major drivers of these diseases.

However, the genetic landscape of cancers is by no means complete, and what has been learned so far has raised new and exciting questions that must be addressed. There are still important technical challenges for the detection of somatic mutations.[78] Clinical tumor samples often contain large amounts of nonmalignant cells, which makes the identification of mutations in cancer genomes more challenging when compared with similar analyses of peripheral blood samples for germline genome studies. Moreover, the genomic instability inherent to cancer development and progression largely increases the complexity and diversity of genomic alterations of malignant tumors, making it necessary to distinguish between driver and passenger mutations. Likewise, the fact that malignant tumors are genetically heterogeneous and contain several clones simultaneously growing within the same tumor mass raises additional questions regarding the quality of the information currently derived from cancer genomes. Hopefully, in the near future, advances in third-generation sequencing technologies will make it feasible to obtain high-quality sequence data of a genome isolated from a single cell, an aspect of crucial relevance for cancer research.

One of the next imperatives is the definition of the oncogenomic profile of all tumor types. Particularly the less common—though not less lethal—ones are still largely mysterious to scientists and untreatable to clinicians. For some of these diseases few new therapeutically amenable molecular targets have been discovered in the past years. For example, identification of druggable genetic lesions associated with pancreatic and ovarian cancers could help define new therapeutic strategies for these aggressive diseases. To achieve this, detailed oncogenomic maps of the corresponding tumors must be drafted. The latter will hopefully be completed in the coming years, thanks to the systematic cancer genome projects that are presently being performed.

Even in the case of common cancers, a lot of genomic profiling efforts still lay ahead. For example, in a significant fraction of breast and lung tumors the mutations that are likely to be drivers have not yet been found. This is not surprising considering that even in these tumor types only a limited number of samples have been systematically analyzed so far. Therefore, low incidence mutations that could represent potentially key therapeutic targets in a subset of tumors might have escaped detection. Consequently, the scaling up of the mutational profiling to large number of specimens for each tumor type is warranted.

Finally, understanding the cellular properties imparted by the hundreds of recently discovered cancer alleles is another area that must be developed. As a matter of fact, compared to the genomic discovery stage, the functional validation of putative novel cancer alleles, despite their potential clinical relevance, is substantially lagging behind. To achieve this, high-throughput functional studies in model systems that accurately recapitulate the genetic alterations found in human cancer must be developed.

To conclude, the eventual goal of profiling the cancer genome is not only to further understand the molecular basis of the disease, but also to discover novel diagnostic and drug targets. One might anticipate that the most immediate application of these new technologies will be noninvasive strategies for early cancer detection. Considering that oncogenic mutations are present only in cancer cells, screening for tumor-derived mutant DNA in patients' blood holds great potential and will progressively substitute current biomarkers, which have poor sensitivity and lack specificity.[171] Further improvements in next-generation sequencing technologies are likely to reduce their cost as well as make these analyses more facile in the future. Once this happens, most cancer patients will undergo in-depth genomic analyses as part of their initial evaluation and throughout their treatment. This will offer more precise diagnostic and prognostic information, which will affect treatment decisions. Although many challenges remain, the information gained from next-generation sequencing platforms is laying a foundation for personalized medicine, in which patients are managed with therapies that are tailored to the specific gene mutations found in their tumors. Ultimately, these should lead to therapeutic successes similar to the ones attained for chronic myelogenous leukemia patients with imatinib,[172,173] melanoma patients with PLX4032,[169] and NSCLC patients with gefitinib and erlotinib.[160] Clearly, this is the absolute goal for all of this work.

MOLECULAR BIOLOGY OF CANCER

Selected References

The full list of references for this chapter appears in the online version.

1. Vogelstein B, Kinzler KW. Cancer genes and the pathways they control. *Nat Med* 2004;10(8):789.
2. Kinzler KW, Vogelstein B. Lessons from hereditary colon cancer. *Cell* 1996;87(2):159.
3. International Human Genome Sequencing Consortium. Finishing the euchromatic sequence of the human genome. *Nature* 2004;431(7011): 931.
5. Rous P. Transmission of a malignant new growth by means of a cell-free filtrate. *JAMA* 1911;56:198.
7. International HapMap Consortium. A haplotype map of the human genome. *Nature* 2005;437(7063):1299.
14. Davies H, Bignell GR, Cox C, et al. Mutations of the BRAF gene in human cancer. *Nature* 2002;417(6892):949.
18. Bardelli A, Parsons DW, Silliman N, et al. Mutational analysis of the tyrosine kinome in colorectal cancers. *Science* 2003;300(5621):949.
19. Greenman C, Stephens P, Smith R, et al. Patterns of somatic mutation in human cancer genomes. *Nature* 2007;446(7132):153.
20. Samuels Y, Wang Z, Bardelli A, et al. High frequency of mutations of the PIK3CA gene in human cancers. *Science* 2004;304(5670):554.
21. Prickett TD, Agrawal NS, Wei X, et al. Analysis of the tyrosine kinome in melanoma reveals recurrent mutations in ERBB4. *Nat Genet* 2009;41(10): 1127.
22. Sjoblom T, Jones S, Wood LD, et al. The consensus coding sequences of human breast and colorectal cancers. *Science* 2006;314(5797):268.
23. Wang Z, Shen D, Parsons DW, et al. Mutational analysis of the tyrosine phosphatome in colorectal cancers. *Science* 2004;304(5674):1164.
33. López-Otín C, Hunter T. The regulatory crosstalk between kinases and proteases in cancer. *Nat Rev Cancer* 2010;10(4):278.
35. López-Otín C, Matrisian LM. Emerging roles of proteases in tumour suppression. *Nat Rev Cancer* 2007;7(10):800.
36. Wood LD, Parsons DW, Jones S, et al. The genomic landscapes of human breast and colorectal cancers. *Science* 2007;318(5853):1108.
37. Palavalli LH, Prickett TD, Wunderlich JR, et al. Analysis of the matrix metalloproteinase family reveals that MMP8 is often mutated in melanoma. *Nat Genet* 2009;41(5):518.
43. Hanahan D, Weinberg RA The hallmarks of cancer. *Cell* 2000;100(1): 57.
44. Teitz T, Wei T, Valentine MB, et al. Caspase 8 is deleted or silenced preferentially in childhood neuroblastomas with amplification of MYCN. *Nat Med* 2000;6(5):529.
54. Ghavami S, Hashemi M, Ande SR, et al. Apoptosis and cancer: mutations within caspase genes. *J Med Genet* 2009;46(8):497.
56. Bignell GR, Warren W, Seal S, et al. Identification of the familial cylindromatosis tumour-suppressor gene. *Nat Genet* 2000;25(2):160.
59. Kato M, Sanada M, Kato I, et al. Frequent inactivation of A20 in B-cell lymphomas. *Nature* 2009;459(7247):712.
61. Harbour JW, Onken MD, Roberson ED, et al. Frequent mutation of BAP1 in metastasizing uveal melanomas. *Science* 2010;330(6009):1410.
62. Jones S, Zhang X, Parsons DW, et al. Core signaling pathways in human pancreatic cancers revealed by global genomic analyses. *Science* 2008;321 (5897):1801.
63. Parsons DW, Jones S, Zhang X, et al. An integrated genomic analysis of human glioblastoma multiforme. *Science* 2008;321(5897):1807.

64. Jones S, Wang TL, Shih Ie M, et al. Frequent mutations of chromatin remodeling gene ARID1A in ovarian clear cell carcinoma. *Science* 2010; 330(6001):228.
65. Parsons DW, Li M, Zhang X, et al. The genetic landscape of the childhood cancer medulloblastoma. *Science* 2010; (in press).
66. Yan H, Parsons DW, Jin G, et al. IDH1 and IDH2 mutations in gliomas. *N Engl J Med* 2009;360(8):765.
73. Mardis ER, Ding L, Dooling DJ, et al. Recurring mutations found by sequencing an acute myeloid leukemia genome. *N Engl J Med* 2009;361(11): 1058.
77. Mardis ER, Wilson RK. Cancer genome sequencing: a review. *Hum Mol Genet* 2009;18(R2):R163.
78. Meyerson M, Gabriel S, Getz G. Advances in understanding cancer genomes through second-generation sequencing. *Nat Rev Genet* 2010;11 (10):685.
79. Metzker ML. Sequencing technologies—the next generation. *Nat Rev Genet* 2010;11(1):31.
80. Bell DW. Our changing view of the genomic landscape of cancer. *J Pathol* 2010;220(2):231.
81. Campbell PJ, Pleasance ED, Stephens PJ, et al. Subclonal phylogenetic structures in cancer revealed by ultra-deep sequencing. *Proc Natl Acad Sci U S A* 2008;105(35):13081.
82. Kidd JM, Cooper GM, Donahue WF, et al. Mapping and sequencing of structural variation from eight human genomes. *Nature* 2008;453(7191): 56.
85. Schadt EE, Turner S, Kasarskis A. A window into third-generation sequencing. *Hum Mol Genet* 2010;19(R2):R227.
89. Morozova O, Hirst M, Marra MA. Applications of new sequencing technologies for transcriptome analysis. *Annu Rev Genomics Hum Genet* 2009;10:135.
91. Ley TJ, Mardis ER, Ding L, et al. DNA sequencing of a cytogenetically normal acute myeloid leukaemia genome. *Nature* 2008;456(7218):66.
92. Pleasance ED, Cheetham RK, Stephens PJ, et al. A comprehensive catalogue of somatic mutations from a human cancer genome. *Nature* 2010; 463(7278):191.
93. Pleasance ED, Stephens PJ, O'Meara S, et al. A small-cell lung cancer genome with complex signatures of tobacco exposure. *Nature* 2010;463 (7278):184.
94. Ding L, Ellis MJ, Li S, et al. Genome remodelling in a basal-like breast cancer metastasis and xenograft. *Nature* 2010;464(7291):999.
95. Ley TJ, Ding L, Walter MJ, et al. DNMT3A mutations in acute myeloid leukemia. *N Engl J Med* 2010;363(25):2424.
99. Lee W, Jiang Z, Liu J, et al. The mutation spectrum revealed by paired genome sequences from a lung cancer patient. *Nature* 2010;465(7297):473.
100. Yachida S, Jones S, Bozic I, et al. Distant metastasis occurs late during the genetic evolution of pancreatic cancer. *Nature* 2010;467(7319):1114.
101. Shah SP, Morin RD, Khattra J, et al. Mutational evolution in a lobular breast tumour profiled at single nucleotide resolution. *Nature* 2009;461 (7265):809.
102. Campbell PJ, Yachida S, Mudie LJ, et al. The patterns and dynamics of genomic instability in metastatic pancreatic cancer. *Nature* 2010;467(7319): 1109.
110. Wiegand KC, Shah SP, Al-Agha OM, et al. ARID1A mutations in endometriosis-associated ovarian carcinomas. *N Engl J Med* 2010;363(16):1532.
111. Farazi TA, Spitzer JI, Morozov P, et al. miRNAs in human cancer. *J Pathol* 2011;223(2):102.
112. Huarte M, Rinn JL. Large non-coding RNAs: missing links in cancer? *Hum Mol Genet* 2010;19(R2):R152.
113. Maher CA, Kumar-Sinha C, Cao X, et al. Transcriptome sequencing to detect gene fusions in cancer. *Nature* 2009;458(7234):97.
115. Park PJ. ChIP-seq: advantages and challenges of a maturing technology. *Nat Rev Genet* 2009;10(10):669.
116. Laird PW. Principles and challenges of genome-wide DNA methylation analysis. *Nat Rev Genet* 2010;11(3):191.
118. Tomlins SA, Rhodes DS, Perner S, et al. Recurrent fusion of TMPRSS2 and ETS transcription factor genes in prostate cancer. *Science* 2005;310(5748): 644.
119. Soda M, Choi YL, Enomoto M, et al. Identification of the transforming EML4-ALK fusion gene in non-small-cell lung cancer. *Nature* 2007; 448 (7153):561.
120. Palanisamy N, Ateeq B, Kalyana-Sundaram S, et al. Rearrangements of the RAF kinase pathway in prostate cancer, gastric cancer and melanoma. *Nat Med* 2010;16(7):793.
121. Leary RJ, Kinde I, Diehl F, et al. Development of personalized tumor biomarkers using massively parallel sequencing. *Sci Transl Med* 2010;2(20): 20ra14.
122. Stephens PJ, McBride DJ, Lin ML, et al. Complex landscapes of somatic rearrangement in human breast cancer genomes. *Nature* 2009;462(7276): 1005.
123. Feng H, Shuda M, Chang Y, et al. Clonal integration of a polyomavirus in human Merkel cell carcinoma. *Science* 2008;319(5866):1096.
127. Kaminker JS, Zhang Y, Waugh A, et al. Distinguishing cancer-associated missense mutations from common polymorphisms. *Cancer Res* 2007;67(2): 465.
128. Futreal PA. Backseat drivers take the wheel. *Cancer Cell* 2007;12(6):493.
129. Greenman C, Wooster R, Futreal PA, et al. Statistical analysis of pathogenicity of somatic mutations in cancer. *Genetics* 2006;173(4):2187.
134. The Cancer Genome Atlas Research Network. Comprehensive genomic characterization defines human glioblastoma genes and core pathways. *Nature* 2008;455(7216):1061.
135. Hudson TJ, Anderson W, Artez A, et al. International network of cancer genome projects. *Nature* 2010;464(7291):993.
136. Bignell GR, Greenman CD, Davies H, et al. Signatures of mutation and selection in the cancer genome. *Nature* 2010;463(7283):893.
137. Dalgliesh GL, Furge K, Greenman C, et al. Systematic sequencing of renal carcinoma reveals inactivation of histone modifying genes. *Nature* 2010;463(7279):360.
142. Benvenuti S, Frattini M, Arena S, et al. PIK3CA cancer mutations display gender and tissue specificity patterns. *Hum Mutat* 2008;29(2):284.
144. Bleeker FE, Bardelli A. Genomic landscapes of cancers: prospects for targeted therapies. *Pharmacogenomics* 2007;8(12):1629.
145. Paez JG, Janne PA, Lee JC, et al. EGFR mutations in lung cancer: correlation with clinical response to gefitinib therapy. *Science* 2004;304(5676):1497.
146. Ciardiello F, Tortora G. EGFR antagonists in cancer treatment. *N Engl J Med* 2008;358(11):1160.
149. Gerber DE, Minna JD. ALK inhibition for non-small cell lung cancer: from discovery to therapy in record time. *Cancer Cell* 2010;18(6):548.
152. Bardelli A, Siena S. Molecular mechanisms of resistance to cetuximab and panitumumab in colorectal cancer. *J Clin Oncol* 2010;28(7):1254.
153. Siena S, Sartore-Bianchi A, Di Nicolantonio F, et al. Biomarkers predicting clinical outcome of epidermal growth factor receptor-targeted therapy in metastatic colorectal cancer. *J Natl Cancer Inst* 2009;101(19):1308.
158. Gorre ME, Mohammed M, Ellwood K, et al. Clinical resistance to STI-571 cancer therapy caused by BCR-ABL gene mutation or amplification. *Science* 2001;293(5531):876.
169. Flaherty KT, Puzanov I, Kim KB, et al. Inhibition of mutated, activated BRAF in metastatic melanoma. *N Engl J Med* 2010;363(9):809.
173. Druker BJ, Guilhot F, O'Brien SG, et al. Five-year follow-up of patients receiving imatinib for chronic myeloid leukemia. *N Engl J Med* 2006;355(23): 2408.

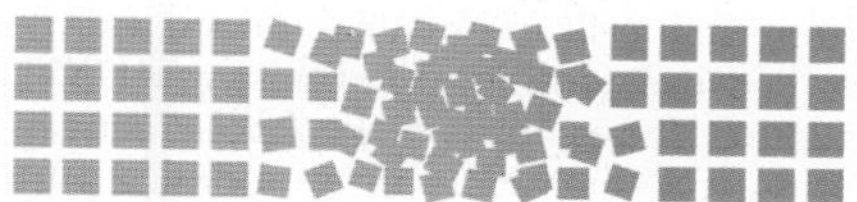

CHAPTER 2 MECHANISMS OF GENOMIC INSTABILITY

DAVID J. GORDON, DAVID A. BARBIE, ALAN D. D'ANDREA, AND DAVID PELLMAN

Cancer arises from a series of genetic alterations that promote resistance to apoptosis, self-sufficiency in growth, cellular immortalization and escape from cell-cycle exit. The acquisition of these properties ultimately facilitates angiogenesis, invasion, and metastasis.[1] It has been recognized for more than a century that genetic instability might represent an important pathway for the development of these disease characteristics. Von Hansemann[2] identified abnormal mitotic figures in cancers, leading Boveri[3] to propose that genetic instability, manifest in his experiments as whole-chromosome aneuploidy, could have a causal role in tumor development. The recognition that mutation of genes involved in monitoring genomic integrity underlies inherited cancer syndromes such as hereditary nonpolyposis colon cancer (HNPCC) and familial *BRCA*-mutant breast cancer provides clear evidence that genomic instability due to a so-called mutator phenotype can be the starting point for tumor development.[4,5]

However, many important questions remain. Does genomic instability play a central role in oncogenesis in common sporadic tumors? When during tumorigenesis does genetic instability develop, and what are the dominant mechanisms in specific cancer types? Why do inherited mutations in caretaker genes such as *BRCA1* and *BRCA2* lead to breast and ovarian cancer when their repair function is presumed to be ubiquitous? What is the relative contribution of telomere shortening to the development of genomic instability? Finally, what is the specific role of aneuploidy in cancer development, and what are the defects that promote chromosomal instability?

This chapter will outline the basic mechanisms involved in the maintenance of genomic integrity and will address these questions. One theme that has emerged from recent work in this area is that the development of genomic instability during cancer progression involves evolutionary tradeoffs.[6–8] Loss of genetic stability is expected to increase the rate of growth-promoting or survival-promoting mutations that could drive tumor growth. However, genomic instability will also increase the rate of deleterious mutations that could kill cells before they develop into tumors. Understanding how these factors balance out will ultimately be the key to understanding tumor development via genome destabilization. Perhaps most importantly, understanding this balance may also have implications for cancer therapeutics. If deleterious, genome-destabilizing mutations are found in the population of developing cancer cells, these defects may provide an "Achilles heel" for therapeutic attack.

BASIC DEFENSES AGAINST GENOMIC INSTABILITY

The roughly 10^{14} cells in the human body are continually exposed to sources of genomic injury, both spontaneous injury accompanying normal cell division and metabolism and external sources of damage. In addition to the oxidative stresses that are a by-product of cellular metabolism, cell populations that undergo constant turnover are subject to errors that may arise during the processes of DNA replication, mitosis, and telomere maintenance. Cells are also exposed to a variety of exogenous genotoxic insults. Examples include ultraviolet and gamma irradiation and certain chemicals (as detailed in other chapters). As a result, mechanisms have evolved at a number of different levels to guard against genomic instability and prevent the propagation of cancer-promoting and/or deleterious mutations.

At an organismal level, tissues are designed to prevent the accumulation of cells with sustained disruption of genomic integrity.[4] For example, those cell types in constant contact with the outside world, including the skin, gastrointestinal tract, and bronchial epithelium, undergo continuous self-renewal, with shedding of those differentiated cells that are exposed most directly to a potentially deleterious environment. In addition to being shielded from this stress, the stem cell compartment undergoes cell division fairly infrequently, with the bulk of exponential growth occurring in transit-amplifying cells that are ultimately discarded at the surface. Thus, in tissues such as the colon, stem cells are normally protected within the crypts, and those cells that proliferate and migrate toward the lumen are ultimately eliminated. Nevertheless, this process is imperfect and subject to persistence of dysplastic clones if a cell sustains a mutation that affords a proliferative advantage.

Many cells also possess physiologic characteristics that can shield them from genotoxic injury.[4,9] For example, melanin in the skin absorbs ultraviolet radiation, while antioxidants and enzymes such as catalase and superoxide dismutase reduce concentrations of reactive oxygen species generated as a result of cell metabolism. In addition, cytochrome P-450 enzymes detoxify a variety of chemicals, and glutathione-S-transferases (GSTs) conjugate glutathione with electrophilic compounds, neutralizing their mutagenic potential. Defective GST function has been observed in lung, breast, and prostate cancer and has been shown to predispose patients to myelodysplastic syndrome. Conversely, drugs that inhibit GST function are being tested in combination with chemotherapy in an attempt to enhance toxicity to cancer cells.

BARRIERS TO GENOMIC INSTABILITY

Cell Cycle Checkpoints

Coordinated progression through the cell cycle is crucial for the maintenance of genome stability.[4,10,11] This is particularly the case for the main tasks of the cell cycle—DNA replication and mitosis. Either incomplete DNA replication or overreplication of DNA would generate lesions that could lead to chromosome breaks and rearrangements. Mitotic errors produce chromosome mis-segregation and whole-chromosome aneuploidy. These types of errors do not occur in isolation; a defect in one process can lead to a cascade of downstream events. Chromosome breaks can lead to translocations, chromosomes with two centromeres (dicentric chromosomes), anaphase bridges, and chromosome mis-segregation. Likewise, mitotic errors leading to aneuploidy will generate gene expression imbalances that could, in principle, compromise DNA replication, telomere maintenance, or DNA repair. Both DNA replication/repair and mitotic errors can cause cytokinesis to fail, resulting in tetraploid cells that contain extra centrosomes and are themselves genetically unstable. Although an extensive review of the cell cycle is beyond the scope of this chapter, selected features of the normal cell cycle that are crucial for preventing genome instability and cancer are described here. In particular, the following sections will focus on the restriction point, the DNA damage checkpoint, and the spindle assembly checkpoint. More extensive summaries of the eucaryotic cell cycle can be found in other chapters and in recent reviews.

Restriction Point

The decision to commit to cell division is controlled by a complex signaling system, the retinoblastoma protein (RB) pathway, that is the major target of human cancer-causing mutations.[11,12] RB represses the transcription of genes involved in cell cycle progression by binding to the E2F family of transcription factors and altering the expression of E2F target genes, blocking E2F-mediated transactivation and recruiting active repressor complexes to promoters.[13,14] E2F target genes include components of the nucleotide synthesis and DNA replication machinery that are essential for S phase entry and transit. In response to mitogenic signals during G1 phase of the cell cycle, RB is phosphorylated and inactivated by cyclin D/CDK (cyclin-dependent kinase) 4/6 complexes, followed by cyclin E/CDK2 and cyclinA/CDK2 complexes, resulting in E2F-target gene expression and S phase transit. Cyclin E/CDK2 regulates a number of other processes involved in the duplication of chromosomes, including the activation of histone gene transcription, as well as promoting the initiation of DNA replication and centrosome duplication.[15,16] Deletion of cyclin E in mice results in defective endoreduplication, while constitutive overexpression of cyclin E has been linked to the generation of polyploidy and chromosomal instability. Thus, the RB pathway integrates intrinsic and external growth signals and is a key mediator of cyclin/CDK complexes that drive cell cycle progression.

CDK inhibitors and phosphatases provide other important mechanisms for counteracting the activity of CDKs and restricting cell cycle progression.[4,11,16] CDK inhibitors fall into two general categories, including specific *in*hibitors of CD*K4* such as p16[INK4A], and those that target CDK activity more broadly such as p21 or p27. CDK2 is also targeted by inhibitory phosphorylation at its active site by the Wee1 family of protein kinases. Activation of cyclin E(A)/CDK2 during the normal G1/S phase transition thus requires the activity of the CDC25A phosphatase. Phosphorylation of CDC25A itself leads to its subsequent ubiquitin-mediated proteasomal degradation and inhibition of S phase progression. Thus, expression of CDK inhibitors and down-regulation of CDC25A phosphatase activity are means by which checkpoint signals are able to mediate downstream cell cycle arrest. Furthermore, PP2A, a protein phosphatase that is also critical to the process of oncogenic transformation, has been shown to regulate an S phase checkpoint by dephosphorylating pRB and licensing recruitment of pRB to chromatin to suppress DNA replication.[17]

Heralded as the guardian of the genome, *p53* integrates the response to DNA damage, replication stress, hypoxia, telomere dysfunction, and activated oncogenes and mediates downstream checkpoint activation.[4,18–20] Inherited mutations in *p53* or its direct upstream activator *CHK2* result in the Li Fraumeni cancer predisposition syndrome, and sporadic inactivation of p53 is one of the most frequent events observed in tumor development. Tumors lacking p53 exhibit widespread genomic instability resulting from an inability to arrest the cell cycle or trigger apoptosis in the setting of DNA damage and the cellular stresses previously described. In normal cells, p53 is maintained at low levels in the cytoplasm because of ubiquitination by MDM2 and proteasomal degradation. In response to checkpoint activation and phosphorylation, p53 increases in abundance and translocates to the nucleus, where it activates a transcriptional program that promotes cell cycle arrest, senescence, or apoptosis, depending on the cell type and conditions. The CDK inhibitor p21 is a key transcriptional target of p53 that mediates checkpoint arrest while repair is attempted. In response to a variety of signals p53 can trigger an apoptotic program, in part via transcriptional activation of proapoptotic targets such as NOXA and BAX.[21]

DNA Damage Checkpoints

Activation of cell cycle checkpoints occurs as part of a larger DNA damage response pathway.[22,23] There are three major DNA damage checkpoints, with two of the checkpoints occurring at the boundaries between G1/S and G2/M. The third checkpoint, however, occurs intra-S phase. In addition to promoting cell cycle arrest through the mechanisms described earlier, these pathways coordinate recruitment of repair proteins to the sites of DNA damage, modulation of transcription, activation of subsequent repair, and apoptosis. The signaling network that controls this response is initiated by the key DNA damage sensors, the ataxia-telangiectasia mutated (ATM) and AT and Rad3-related (ATR) protein kinases.[10,11,24,25] ATM is principally activated in response to double-strand breaks, while ATR is activated by replication fork collapse and by bulky DNA lesions. As will be described in more detail later, both proteins phosphorylate multiple targets in coordinating the subsequent DNA damage response. Key signal transducers in this process include CHK2 (activated by ATM) and CHK1 (activated by ATR). p53 is a major substrate for ATM/CHK2 and ATR/CHK1 phosphorylation, and subsequent activation of p53 represents a principal mechanism by which cell cycle checkpoints are activated in response to DNA damage. Replication stress and hypoxia also appear to activate p53 through ATR signaling, while telomere dysfunction contributes to p53 activation through ATM (Fig. 2.1).[18] In addition, a variety of stress responses have been shown to activate p38MAPK, which can promote checkpoint activation through both p53-dependent and -independent pathways.[26,27] CHK2 activation also leads to phosphorylation and degradation of the phosphatase CDC25A, resulting in activation of an S phase checkpoint.[28]

Spindle Assembly Checkpoint

Errors that occur during mitosis are similarly monitored by a spindle checkpoint, which prevents progression into anaphase when chromosomes are improperly attached to the mitotic spindle.[29] Key sensors of this response include the spindle checkpoint proteins, which assemble onto unattached kinetochores and generate a "wait anaphase" signal that prevents activation of anaphase effector proteins. This pathway is outlined in further detail later.

Cellular Senescence and Crisis

Cellular senescence is another mechanism that limits the progressive accumulation of cells with impaired genomic integrity

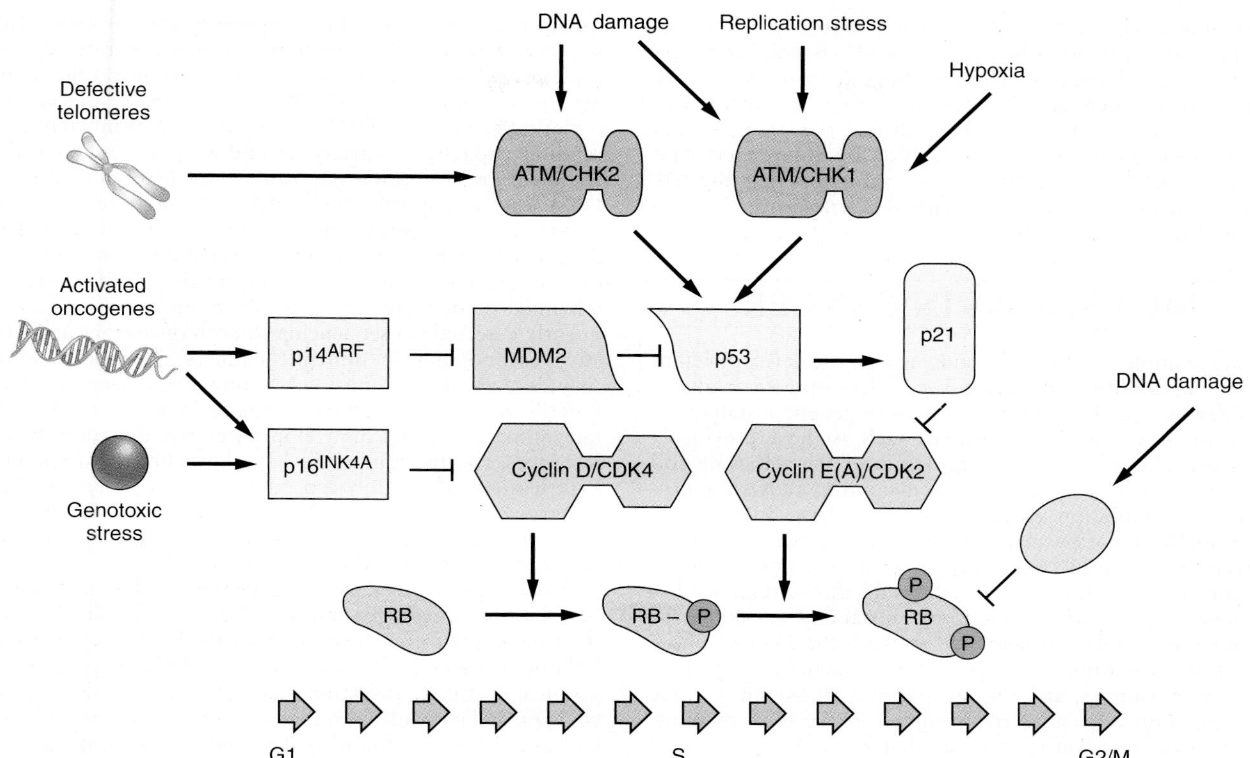

FIGURE 2.1 G1 pathways that can trigger cell cycle arrest, senescence, or apoptosis. A variety of threats to genomic integrity lead to activation of pathways that result in cell cycle arrest. Signaling via ATM/CHK2 and ATR/CHK1 leads to p53 activation, among other effects. One of the principle downstream effects of p53 is activation of p21 expression, with resultant cyclin E(A)/CDK2 inhibition and cell cycle arrest. Senescence, which results in a more sustained cell cycle exit, also involves the up-regulation of p14^{ARF} and p16^{INK4A}. Both proteins ultimately lead to retinoblastoma protein (RB) activation and G1 arrest via cyclin/CDK inhibition. In response to DNA damage during S phase, activation of PP2A can lead to dephosphorylation of RB and inhibition of DNA synthesis.

and oncogenic potential.[4,30–32] Originally described as an irreversible state of cell cycle exit in response to exhausted replicative potential of cultured cells, cellular senescence also occurs as a response to oncogene activation, oxidative stress, suboptimal culture conditions, and chemotherapy. The RB and p53 pathways have been shown to mediate the arrest by replicative senescence, whereby progressive telomere attrition elicits a DNA damage response similar to that induced by other genotoxic stresses (Fig. 2.1). In the setting of RB and p53 pathway inactivation, cells can bypass replicative senescence, but progressive telomere shortening results in the accumulation of massive genetic instability and a state of "crisis." Most cells in crisis will die, but rare malignant clones can emerge. In humans, activation of the enzyme telomerase and subsequent maintenance of telomere length allows such cells to bypass crisis, resulting in cellular immortalization. By contrast, in mice, in which telomeres start out long and seldom shorten to a critical length, a similar but less well understood crisis event occurs that is, at least in part, related to differential sensitivity of mouse cells to oxidative damage in culture.

Senescence induced by oncogene activation, also known as oncogene-induced senescence, results from expression of p16^{INK4A} and p14^{ARF} (note that p14^{ARF} in humans is p19^{ARF} in the mouse), which exists in an *a*lternative *r*eading *f*rame within the *p16^{INK4A}* locus.[33,34] p14^{ARF} inhibits MDM2 function, in part by sequestering it in the nucleolus, resulting in the accumulation and activation of p53. p16^{INK4A} expression is associated with both oncogene activation and genotoxic stress, promoting activation of RB and, in conjunction with HMGA chromatin proteins, the formation of stable heterochromatic foci that envelop and silence E2F target genes.[35] Cellular senescence induced by this latter program is refractory to RB and p53 inactivation, although it can be bypassed by inactivation of p16^{INK4A} and HMGA proteins. Oncogene-induced senescence is also triggered by DNA replication stress, including prematurely terminated DNA replication forks, DNA double-strand breaks, and DNA hyperreplication.[36,37] In a mouse model, inhibiting the DNA double-strand break response kinase ATM suppressed the induction of senescence and led to increased tumor size and invasiveness.

Oncogene-induced senescence has been shown to occur *in vivo*, limiting tumor progression in models of lung and prostate cancer, melanoma, and lymphoma.[33] Whereas inactivation of the PTEN tumor suppressor and resultant activation of the AKT signaling pathway in prostate epithelial cells appears to promote senescence through p14^{ARF}, inappropriate activation of RAS signaling in other tissues results in p16^{INK4A}-mediated senescence. Nonetheless, targeted activation of oncogenic *K-RAS* alleles in somatic tissues in mice predisposes to a wide variety of tumor types, including early-onset lung cancer, suggesting that this barrier may be readily overcome or that the consequence of RAS expression may vary depending on the context.[38,39] Moreover, expression of endogenous levels of oncogenic K-RAS can promote proliferation, and it has been demonstrated that oncogene-induced senescence due to RAS activation can be dose-dependent.[40–42]

RAS-induced senescence in lymphocytes depends on heterochromatin formation via the Suv39h1 histone methyltransferase, the disruption of which facilitates lymphoma development in response to RAS activation.[33] Furthermore, disruption of Suv39h1 by itself has been shown to disrupt heterochromatin formation and to promote genetic instability, contributing to lymphomagenesis.[43] This may occur at least in part through cell division failure and the generation of unstable tetraploid cells (see later discussion). These findings confirm the *in vitro* observations that changes in chromatin structure contribute to cell cycle exit by senescence. In addition, they suggest that emerging epigenetic therapies such as histone deacetylase inhibitors and DNA methyltransferase inhibitors that interfere with chromatin silencing may disrupt this senescence barrier, a potential caveat to their use.

MUTATIONS IN CANCER

Despite multiple levels of protection against the development of genomic instability, with age, cells can develop genetic alterations that escape detection.[4] One path to genetic instability is inactivation of checkpoint proteins such as those previously described. The subsequent deregulation of the cell cycle and impairment of the response to genomic injury allows the progressive accumulation of lesions that can drive oncogenesis. Additionally, mutations can also occur in genes encoding the proteins that repair DNA damage and protect against the development of chromosome abnormalities. In this setting, accelerated mutation rates and chromosomal instability destabilize the genome and facilitate progression through the steps of oncogenic transformation. The basic types of genetic alterations observed in tumors, and the mechanisms by which genome destabilization can occur, are outlined in the next sections. Cancer predisposition syndromes that result from inherited defects in genome maintenance are highlighted in Table 2.1.

Point Mutations

Changes in the nucleotide sequence can arise from spontaneous mutation, exposure to endogenous or exogenous mutagens, or defects in the ability to detect and/or repair simple sequence errors.[4,21] The spontaneous mutation rate per nucleotide per cell division has been estimated to be on the order of 10^{-9} in somatic cells and 10^{-11} in stem cells.[44] Despite the remarkable fidelity of DNA polymerase and its inherent proofreading capacity, a variety of endogenous and exogenous chemical and radiation exposures can introduce additional DNA lesions, requiring the presence of multiple repair pathways for further protection of genomic integrity. Mutations arise when such errors are not detected and repaired by this machinery, which can occur when repair pathways are overwhelmed or defective. As a result, point mutations are frequently detected via sequencing of both oncogenes and tumor suppressor genes in multiple cancers. Notable examples include activating mutations in oncogenic kinases such as K-RAS in colorectal, pancreatic, and lung cancer, B-RAF in melanoma, and JAK2 in myeloproliferative disorders. In some instances, specific mutations have been linked to epidemiologic features such as tobacco exposure, with oncogenic K-RAS mutations in non–small cell lung cancer (NSCLC) occurring more frequently in smokers and epidermal growth factor receptor (EGFR) mutations in nonsmokers.[45]

Next-generation sequencing technology has ushered in a new era in cancer genomics.[46,47] Massively parallel DNA sequencing platforms now allow for the routine sequencing of billions of bases of DNA per week and the identification of point mutations, insertions and deletions, copy number changes, and genomic rearrangements on a genome-wide basis. Large-scale sequencing of coding sequences from a panel of colorectal and breast tumors, for example, revealed that these cancers harbor approximately 100 mutant genes, with computational methods predicting that 14 to 20 of these mutations will be bona fide tumor suppressor genes or oncogenes.[48] In this unbiased effort, both known and unknown mutations were identified, with each tumor possessing a relatively unique cancer gene mutational signature. In another study, sequencing of

TABLE 2.1

INHERITED GENOME MAINTENANCE DEFECTS WITH CANCER PREDISPOSITION

Maintenance Mechanism	Syndrome	Gene Defect
Checkpoint response	Li Fraumeni Familial breast cancer	*p53*, *CHK2*
	Retinoblastoma	*BRCA1*, *CHK2*
	Familial melanoma	*RB*
		$p16^{INK4A}$
Mismatch repair	HNPCC/Lynch syndrome	*MLH1*, *MSH2*, *PMS2*, *MSH6*
Nucleotide excision repair	Xeroderma pigmentosa	*XP* genes
DSB response/repair	Ataxia telangiectasia	*ATM*
	AT-like disorder	*MRE11*
	Nijmegen breakage	*NBS1*
	Fanconia anemia	*Fanc* genes
	Familial breast cancer	*BRCA1*, *BRCA2* *CHK2*, *PALB2*
	SCID, rare lymphoma	*Artemis*
	SCID, rare leukemia	*Ligase IV*
Helicase activity	Bloom	*BLM*
	Werner	*WRN*
	Rothmund Thomson	*RECQ4*
Mitotic checkpoint	Mosaic variegated aneuploidy	*BUB1B*

HNPCC, hereditary nonpolyposis colorectal cancer; DSB, double-strand break; AT, ataxia telangiectasia; SCID, severe combined immunodeficiency.

coding regions of protein kinases in a large number of cancers identified "driver" mutations in approximately 120 genes across all samples.[49] Although these studies identified a greater number of mutational events associated with oncogenesis than previously thought (the "state" of genome integrity), they do not necessarily imply a high "rate" of mutation, which remains low in most mature tumors.[21]

In two early studies, targeted gene resequencing was also applied to lung adenocarcinoma and glioblastoma multiforme (GBM) tumor samples.[50,51] Both studies integrated the somatic mutation data with other genome-wide characterizations and clinical data. In the lung adenocarcinoma samples, for example, the sequencing data were used to identify multiple pathways, including MAPK signaling, p53 signaling, and the mTOR pathway, that are targeted by a combination of point mutations, copy number amplifications and deletions, and loss of heterozygosity (LOH). In a different study of GBM tumor samples, the sequencing of approximately 20,000 protein coding genes led to the discovery of a variety of genes that were not known to be altered in GBM, including the enzyme isocitrate dehydrogenase (*IDH1*).[52] The cancer-associated *IDH1* mutations result in the novel ability of the enzyme to catalyze the NADPH-dependent reduction of alpha-ketoglutarate to R(-)-2-hydroxyglutarate (2HG), which has been shown to lead to an elevated risk of malignant brain tumors.[53] Subsequently, mutations in *IDH1* have also been identified in acute myeloid leukemia (AML) genomes.[54,55]

More recently, there has been a rapid progression from targeted gene sequencing to targeted whole-genome and whole-transcriptome sequencing. The first sequencing of a whole cancer genome was reported for AML.[56] Acquired mutations in coding sequences of annotated genes were identified in ten genes in the AML genome by comparing the genomic DNA of leukemia cells with normal skin cells obtained from a patient with FAB M1 AML. Two of the identified mutations were in genes previously described to have a role in leukemogenesis, *FLT3* and *NPM1*. The other eight mutations, however, were in genes that were not previously implicated in the pathogenesis of AML. Four of the affected genes (*PTPRT, CDH24, PCLKC,* and *SLC15A1*), though, are in gene families that are strongly implicated in cancer pathogenesis. Intriguingly, the remaining genes (*KNDC1, GPR123, EBI2,* and *GRINL1B*) are involved in metabolic pathways.

The genomes of a small cell lung cancer, melanoma, and breast tumor have also been described.[57–59] Interestingly, the mutations in both the lung cancer and melanoma genomes were not distributed evenly throughout the genome—many were present outside the gene-coding regions, suggesting that cells had repaired damaged DNA in those key regions. Sequencing of the melanoma genome, for example, revealed multiple levels of selective DNA repair, including the preferential targeting of repair to transcribed regions compared with nontranscribed regions, to exons compared with introns, to transcribed DNA strands compared with nontranscribed strands, and to the 5′ end of genes compared with the 3′ end.

Next-generation sequencing has also been applied to RNA ("RNA-Seq") extracted from tumor cells for complete transcriptome characterization.[60,61] This approach is more sensitive than microarrays and also provides data that can be used to evaluate for allele-specific expression, structural and copy-number alterations, alternative splice isoforms, fusion transcripts, and single nucleotide mutations.[60] RNA-Seq, for example, was applied to four granulosa-cell tumors and identified missense point mutations in the *FOXL2* gene, which encodes a transcription factor known to be crucial in granulosa cell development.[62] In a different study, RNA-Seq was used to identify both known and novel fusion transcripts in prostate cancer samples.[63] RNA-Seq has also been used to study the role of microRNAs in the regulation of gene expression in both normal and cancerous cells.

The number of sequenced cancer genomes is likely to expand substantially in coming years. The Cancer Genome Atlas Program of the U.S. National Cancer Institute, for example, initially focused its large-scale genomic analysis on only three tumor types, GBM, ovarian serous cystadenocarcinoma, and lung squamous carcinoma. The scope of the Cancer Genome Atlas Research Network, however, has now expanded to include more than 20 tumor types and thousands of samples. The clinical and translational implications of routine cancer genome sequencing are profound and include the identification of new drug targets, as well as the generation of new insights into the genetic patterns of disease phenotype, prognosis, and therapeutic response. One shortcoming of direct sequencing, though, is its failure to detect epigenetic changes, such as DNA methylation, which may alter gene expression indirectly.

Although the role of 2HG in cancer development remains unclear, the identification of this unexpected class of mutations validates the high-throughput cancer genome sequencing approach. Also, because the mutations in *IDH1* result in a gain of function, there is much excitement about developing small molecule inhibitors of mutant *IDH1*. Although major clinical impact of large-scale sequencing projects is yet to be realized, the discovery of *IDH1* illustrates the potential of this approach.

Translocations

Unlike point mutations, small insertions, or deletions of nucleotides, larger chromosomal changes such as translocations, amplifications, and deletions may be observed using cytogenetic analysis[4,21] (Fig. 2.2). Chromosome translocation involves juxtaposition of two different chromosome segments, resulting in fusion of two different genes or placement of a

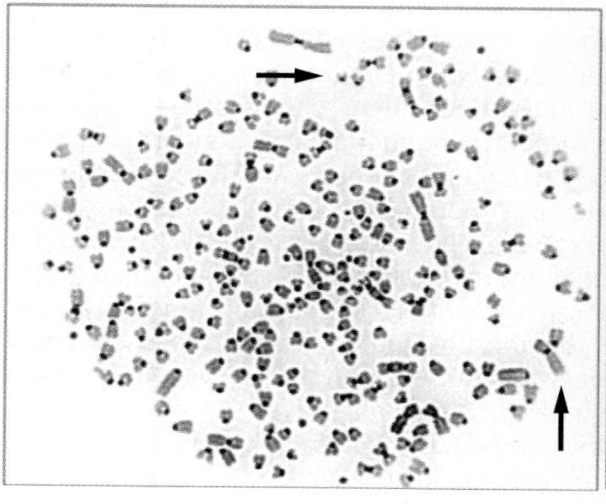
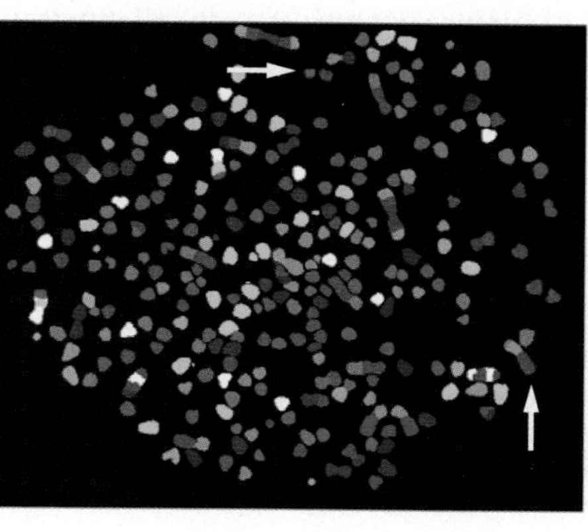

FIGURE 2.2 Common cytogenetic abnormalities. Metaphase spread derived from a mouse tumor model (combined telomerase and p53 deficiency). Individual chromosomes are highlighted by spectral karyotyping (SKY) using fluorescent chromosome probes (**right panel**). Normal mouse cells contain a diploid complement of 40 chromosomes. In this sample, more than 260 chromosomes are observed, with multiple dicentric chromosomes and nonreciprocal translocations.

gene next to an inappropriate regulatory element. Examples include t(9;22) in chronic myelogenous leukemia, resulting in expression of the growth promoting *BCR-ABL* gene product, and t(14;18) in follicular lymphoma, resulting in overexpression of the antiapoptotic protein BCL2 as a result of its fusion with the immunoglobulin heavy chain promoter. Recent work has also identified a translocation between the immunoglobulin heavy chain and the cytokine receptor CRLF2 in a subset of precursor B-cell acute lymphoblastic leukemia associated with a poor outcome and activating *JAK* mutations.[64,65]

One exciting recent development is that translocations not only create chimeric genes or alter promoter sequences, but can also affect the expression of microRNAs.[66,67] MicroRNAs are short regulatory RNAs that control mRNA stability and/or translation, and changes in microRNA expression have been linked to prognostic factors and progression in diseases such as chronic lymphocytic leukemia.[68]

Although translocations and gene fusions are a hallmark of cancer, the mechanisms underlying their genesis are unclear. Recent work, however, has begun to elucidate the mechanisms of some tissue-specific translocations, such as *TMPRSS2* to *ERG* and *ETV1* in prostate cancer.[69,70] A clever bioinformatics approach, termed *cancer outlier profile analysis*, was used to first identify this recurrent translocation in prostate cancer.[71] This approach was used to successfully identify recurrent gene fusions of *TMPRSS2* to *ERG* or *ETV1* in prostate cancer. Further mechanistic work has shown that this translocation requires two roles of the androgen receptor.[69] First, ligand-dependent binding of the androgen receptor to intronic binding sites near the tumor translocation sites creates specific intra- and interchromosomal interactions that result in the spatial proximity of tumor translocation partners. Second, the intron-bound androgen receptor alters local chromatin architecture and recruits the ligand and genotoxic stress-induced enzymes, including the activation-induced cytidine deaminase and LINE-1 repeat-encoded ORF2 endonuclease, to these regions, which results in the generation of DNA double-stranded breaks (DSB). The DSB are subsequently ligated by the nonhomologous end-joining (NHEJ) machinery to create translocations. Further elucidation of the mechanisms leading to gene- and tissue-specific translocations will advance the understanding of basic mechanisms of cancer, as well as possibly facilitating the development of new therapeutic strategies.

Amplifications and Deletions

Amplifications can be detected cytogenetically as double-minute chromosomes or regions of excess signal intensity using fluorescence *in situ* hybridization. Such "amplicons" may range in size from 0.5 to 10 megabases of DNA, resulting in multiple copies of both oncogenes and their neighboring sequences. Conversely, deletions result in loss of chromosomal regions, and can involve small interstitial segments or entire chromosome arms. Genetic alteration of tumor suppressor genes frequently involves mutation in one allele and deletion of the second allele as part of a larger chromosomal segment, resulting in regions of uniform sequence with LOH.

A recent study reported the high-resolution analysis of somatic copy-number alterations (SCNAs) from 3,131 cancer specimens belonging to 26 histologic types.[72] The most prevalent SCNAs were either very short (focal) or almost the length of a chromosome arm or whole chromosome (arm level). The focal SCNAs occurred at a frequency inversely related to their lengths, with a median length of 1.8 megabases. Arm-level SCNAs occurred approximately 30 times more frequently than expected by the inverse-length distribution associated with focal SCNAs. This observation was seen across all cancer types and applied to both copy gains and losses. The study also identified 158 regions of focal SCNAs that were altered at significant frequency across several cancer types, of which 122 could not be explained by the presence of an oncogene located within the region. Several gene families were enriched among the regions of focal SCNA, including the *BCL2* family of apoptosis regulators and the *NF-kB* pathway. Interestingly, the finding that most of the SCNAs were found in multiple cancer types suggests that the diversity across cancer genomes may reflect the combinations of a limited number of functionally relevant events.

Whole-Chromosome Loss/Gain

Nearly all solid tumor types exhibit whole-chromosome loss or gain, resulting in alterations in chromosome number or aneuploidy.[21,73] As will be described later, such defects are generally the result of chromosomal mis-segregation during mitosis. Glioblastomas, for example, frequently exhibit loss of chromosome 10, inactivating the tumor suppressor *PTEN*, while melanomas often show gain of chromosome 7, from which *B-RAF* is expressed. Monosomy 7 and trisomy 8 are associated with myelodysplasia and AML. Whole-chromosome loss may be underestimated by karyotypic analysis, as loss of one parental chromosome may be accompanied by duplication of the other parental chromosome, resulting in an abnormal "allelotype" with accompanying LOH, or copy neutral loss of heterozygosity (CN-LOH).[74]

CN-LOH, also referred to as uniparental disomy, is common in cancer and has been described in AML, breast cancer, multiple myeloma, basal cell carcinoma, childhood acute lymphoblastic leukemia, chronic lymphocytic lymphoma, myelodysplastic syndrome, and glioblastoma.[75] Furthermore, CN-LOH has been shown to have prognostic significance in a number of these cancer types, including primary and secondary AML.[76] The specific role of CN-LOH in tumorigenesis remains undefined, but possible mechanisms include the duplication of oncogenes, loss of tumor suppressors, or acquisition of improper epigenetic patterns.[77] In mice, it has been demonstrated that Bub1 insufficiency can drive tumor formation through tumor suppressor gene *LOH*.[78] Specifically, Bub1 insufficiency predisposed $p53^{+/-}$ mice to thymic lymphomas and $Apc^{Min/+}$ mice to colonic tumors. These tumors demonstrated CN-LOH and lacked the nonmutated tumor suppressor allele, but had gained a copy of the mutant allele.

Epigenetics

Significant evidence now indicates that epigenetic modifications, or heritable changes in gene expression that are not caused by changes in DNA sequence, are critical factors in the pathogenesis of cancer.[79] Although beyond the scope of this chapter, epigenetic mechanisms controlling the transcription of genes involved in cell differentiation, proliferation, and survival are often targets for deregulation in the development of cancer. These epigenetic alterations include DNA methylation, covalent modifications of histones, and noncovalent changes in nucleosome position. The role of epigenetic modifications in cancer pathogenesis is illustrated by the tumor suppressor *SNF5*, which regulates the epigenome as a member of the SWI/SNF chromatin remodeling complex.[80] Biallelic inactivation of *SNF5* is found in the majority of malignant rhabdoid tumors. Most human *SNF5*-deficient cancers are diploid, lack genomic amplifications/deletions, and are genomically stable.[81] Furthermore, the epigenetically based changes in transcription that occur following loss of *SNF5* correlate with the tumor phenotype.

Recent work with an NSCLC cell line, PC9, has also identified a novel role for epigenetics in acquired drug resistance.[82]

Treatment of PC9 cells, which have an activating mutation in the EGFR, with the drug erlotinib results in the death of nearly all of the parental cells. A small percentage of the PC9 cells, however, demonstrate significantly reduced drug sensitivity and remain viable through activation of IGF-1 receptor signaling and an altered chromatin state that requires the histone demethylase RBP2. This drug-tolerant phenotype is transiently acquired at low frequency by individual cells within the population. The drug-tolerant subpopulation can be selectively ablated by treatment with IGF-1 receptor inhibitors or chromatin-modifying agents, such as HDAC inhibitors. There has been much discussion and controversy about the existence of drug-resistant cancer stem cells; the epigenetic effects described in this work provide a potential mechanism for the generation of some "cancer stem cells." Furthermore, this research suggests that the potentially reversible nature of epigenetic changes, unlike genetic mutations, may provide a unique therapeutic avenue in the treatment of cancer.

MECHANISMS OF GENOME DESTABILIZATION IN HUMAN TUMORS

Microsatellite Instability

One of the earliest insights into the contribution of genome destabilization to carcinogenesis came from the study of the familial cancer syndrome HNPCC.[4,11,83] It had been recognized that a subset of sporadic colon cancers and a majority of cancers derived from patients with HNPCC exhibited frequent mutations, particularly in regions of simple repeat sequences known as microsatellites. This type of genetic instability, termed *microsatellite instability* (MIN), had been described in bacteria and yeast mutants defective in mismatch repair. Linkage analysis in kindreds with HNPCC revealed germ line mutations in *hMSH2* and *hMLH1*, which are human homologues of the *mutL* and *mutS* mismatch repair genes in *Escherichia coli*. It is now known that mutations in other components of the human mismatch repair process, *hPMS2*, and *hMSH6*, are also observed in families with HNPCC.

Mismatch repair corrects mispaired bases that can result from errors during DNA replication, as well as mismatched bases occurring in recombination intermediates or occurring as a result of some types of chemical damage to DNA.[84] Mismatched bases are recognized by a complex of MSH2 and MSH6, recruiting MLH1 and PMS2 to the site to initiate the subsequent steps of repair, including excision, DNA synthesis, and ligation (Fig. 2.3). Larger insertion/deletion mispairs due to slippage of the replication machinery in repetitive sequences or recombination errors form a loop structure that is alternatively recognized by a complex of MSH2 and MSH3, with recruitment of an MLH1/MLH3 complex promoting subsequent repair. Cancer cells that exhibit MIN from defects in these components have a nucleotide mutation rate that has been estimated at two to three orders greater than that of normal cells. MLH1 and MSH2 have also been shown to have functions outside mismatch repair, as defects in these proteins have been associated with an impaired G2/M cell cycle checkpoint in response to alkylating agents as well as abnormalities in meiotic recombination in mouse knockout models.[9]

HNPCC is associated with a 60% to 80% lifetime risk of developing colorectal cancer and is responsible for 2% to 5% of all cases of colorectal cancer.[85] Nearly 85% of HNPCC patients have mutations in *MLH1* or *MSH2*, with median age at colon cancer diagnosis being significantly lower in *MLH1* mutation carriers and in males, and with more frequent extracolonic tumors observed in *MSH2* carriers. The MIN phenotype is also observed in 15% of sporadic colon cancers, often due to epigenetic silencing of mismatch repair genes such as *MLH1*. Colorectal cancers exhibiting MIN are typically diploid, in contrast to the remaining 85% of cases, which are associated with chromosomal instability (CIN).[86] Experimental evidence supports the idea that MIN occurs very early in sporadic colorectal cancer formation, prior to

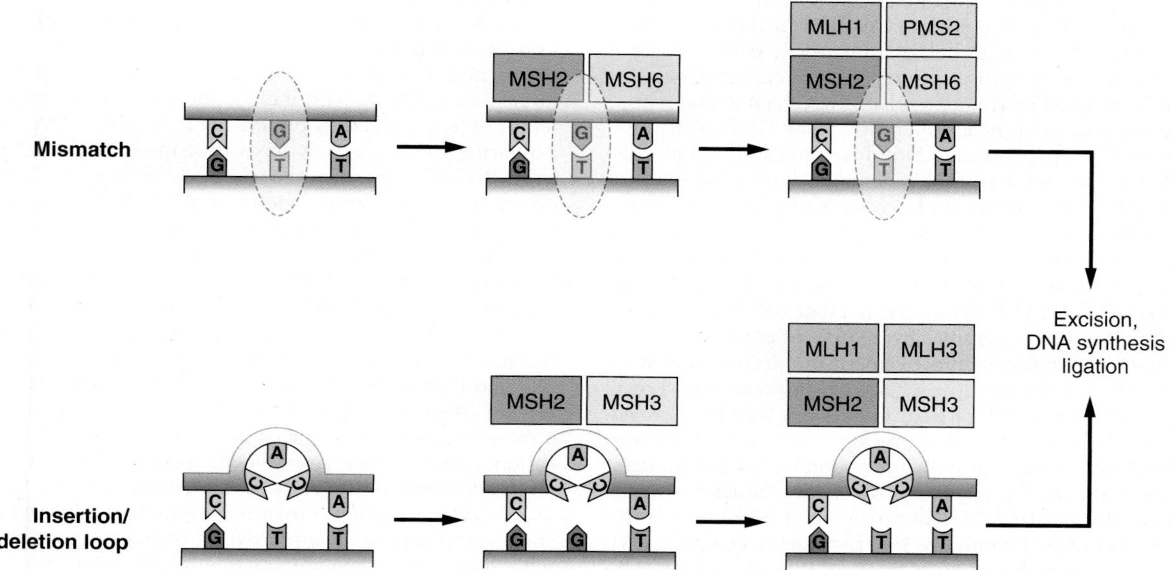

FIGURE 2.3 Mismatch repair pathways. Mispaired bases due to errors in DNA replication or other causes are recognized by the mismatch repair machinery. The initial step involves recognition of simple mismatches by MSH2 and MSH6 (**upper panel**), or recognition of insertion/deletion loops by MSH2 and MSH3 (**lower panel**). Subsequent steps involve recruitment of MLH1 and PMS2 to mismatch sites, or MLH1 and MLH3 to insertion/deletion loop sites. This is followed by excision of the respective lesions, DNA synthesis, and ligation to complete the repair.

anaphase-promoting complex (APC) inactivation, increasing genomic instability and thus obviating the selection pressure to develop another mechanism of genomic instability, CIN. In both sporadic cases and HNPCC, MIN has been associated with more favorable prognosis, lack of *p53* mutation, and a potential resistance to 5-fluorouracil chemotherapy. These observations are in accordance with the hypothesis that the accelerated mutation rate facilitates cancer evolution, but at the same time compromises fitness of cells, presumably by the accumulation of deleterious mutations.

Nucleotide Excision Repair/Base Excision Repair Defects

Whereas the mismatch repair pathway functions primarily in the recognition of and repair of replication errors, the nucleotide excision repair (NER) and base excision repair (BER) pathways respond principally to lesions created by exogenous or endogenous DNA damaging agents.[4,9,84,87] It is becoming apparent that defects in components of these repair pathways have impacts on both cancer pathogenesis and the efficacy of cancer therapy.[88] Ultraviolet radiation or exogenous chemicals such as polycyclic aromatic hydrocarbons and platinum chemotherapeutic drugs can result in bulky, helix-distorting lesions that are recognized by the NER machinery. Components of the NER pathway were in part discovered by mutation in the genetic syndromes xeroderma pigmentosa (*XPA-XPG*) and Cockayne syndrome (*CSA* and *CSB*).[89] Mutation of *XP* genes can also be seen in the related disorder trichothiodystrophy. Whereas all three disorders exhibit dramatic sun sensitivity, only xeroderma pigmentosa is associated with a marked incidence of sun-induced skin cancer.[90] Deletion of *CSB* has been shown to impair tumor formation in cancer-prone mice, and it has been hypothesized that the lack of cancer in Cockayne syndrome may be related to a particular sensitivity of cells to apoptosis or impairment of transcription.[91]

Two separate NER pathways have been identified, one that involves scanning the entire genome for lesions (global genome NER) and another that detects lesions that interfere with elongating RNA polymerases (transcription coupled repair or TCR)[9,87] (Fig. 2.4). *XP* genes are involved in the recognition and repair of lesions in global genome NER, while *CS* genes play a specific role in transcription coupled repair. Subsequent stages of NER are similar and involve ERCC1, an endonuclease involved in excision of the lesion, followed by DNA replication to complete the repair process. Notably, mutant mice defective in NER also accumulate DNA damage, with a more pronounced cancer phenotype and evidence of premature aging. Furthermore, reduced expression of *ERCC1* in NSCLC has been associated with response to cisplatin-based adjuvant chemotherapy.[92] A subgroup analysis of the International Adjuvant Lung Cancer Trial (IALT) demonstrated that *ERCC1* deficiency was observed in tumor samples from 56% of patients and correlated with a significant improvement in survival following cisplatin-based chemotherapy, whereas no benefit was seen in tumors in which normal *ERCC1* expression was maintained. Thus, while reduced *ERCC1* expression may promote genetic instability and facilitate NSCLC development in a significant fraction of patients, the resulting cancers are "stuck" with the deleterious effects of *ERCC1* deficiency and become sensitive to certain therapies. Potentially, this provides a general model for targeted therapy based on fixation of mutations that compromise genomic integrity during tumorigenesis.

BER is primarily involved in the response to damage caused by small chemical alterations and x-rays, as well as spontaneous reactions such as base loss from hydrolysis of glycosyl DNA bonds, which has been estimated to occur on the order of 10^4 times per day per cell.[9,24] Damaged bases are removed by DNA glycosylases, and abasic sites are recognized by a complex that includes the APEX1 endonuclease, poly(ADP-ribose) polymerase (PARP), DNA polymerase and ligase, and XRCC1, a scaffolding protein that interacts with most of the core components (Fig. 2.4). Disruption of any of these genes in the BER pathway results in the cellular accumulation of oxidative DNA damage.

Despite being integrally important to the maintenance of genome stability, human disorders or inherited cancer susceptibility syndromes due to mutation of components of the BER machinery have yet to be described. This may be because of partial redundancy of DNA glycosylases, the fact that mutation of core BER components (in mice) results in embryonic lethality, or simply to the need for additional investigation. As described later, pharmacologic inhibition of PARP may selectively sensitize cancer cells with a pre-existing defect in another repair pathway to death by DNA damage.[93,94]

DNA Damage Response to Double-Strand Breaks

DNA DSBs represent a significant threat to genomic integrity.[4,9] They can occur during DNA replication at sites of stalled replication forks, or after ionizing radiation or oxidative damage.[24] In addition, single-strand nicks can be converted into DSBs by DNA replication. Even a single DSB in budding yeast can trigger a DNA damage response checkpoint, a finding that is not surprising as DSBs can promote major cytogenetic abnormalities such as chromosome translocations, amplifications, and deletions. DSBs are detected and repaired by an intricate cascade of proteins, ultimately involving the processes of homologous recombination (HR) or NHEJ. Defects in multiple components of this process have been linked to genomic instability and cancer predisposition.

The initial detection and activation of signal transduction pathways mediating repair of DNA DSBs involves the PI(3) K-like kinases, ATM and ATR.[10,11,24,95] DSBs induced by DNA damage activate ATM, while regions of single-stranded DNA at stalled replication forks recruit and activate ATR. Once activated, ATM and ATR kinase activity results in phosphorylation of multiple targets, including histone H2AX, resulting in the local alteration of chromatin structure. Key downstream targets of ATM and ATR include the checkpoint mediator proteins (CHK), with ATM principally activating CHK2 and ATR activating CHK1. As previously described, ATM/CHK2 as well as ATR/CHK1 can phosphorylate and activate p53, mediating downstream checkpoint activation. ATM/CHK2 and ATR/CHK1 have also been shown to slow progression through S phase by down-regulating CDC25A.[28]

ATM was identified by virtue of its association with the neurodegenerative disorder ataxia telangiectasia, in which patients are also predisposed to malignancies such as acute lymphoblastic leukemia and lymphoma.[9,10] Inactivating mutations in ATR (AT and Rad3-related) result in embryonic lethality in mice and are not observed in familial human cancer syndromes, presumably reflecting the key role of this kinase in normal DNA replication. However, hypomorphic alleles of ATR that result in low levels of expression have been associated with the Seckel syndrome, which results in dwarfism, microcephaly, and chromosome instability in cells treated with mitomycin C.[96] Patients with Seckel syndrome are not significantly predisposed to cancer development, perhaps reflecting the general balancing of fitness effects and oncogenic potential; in Seckel syndrome the disadvantages of compromised ATR for cell viability may outweigh the potential for an increase in cancer-causing mutations. As previously described, the important caretaker function of

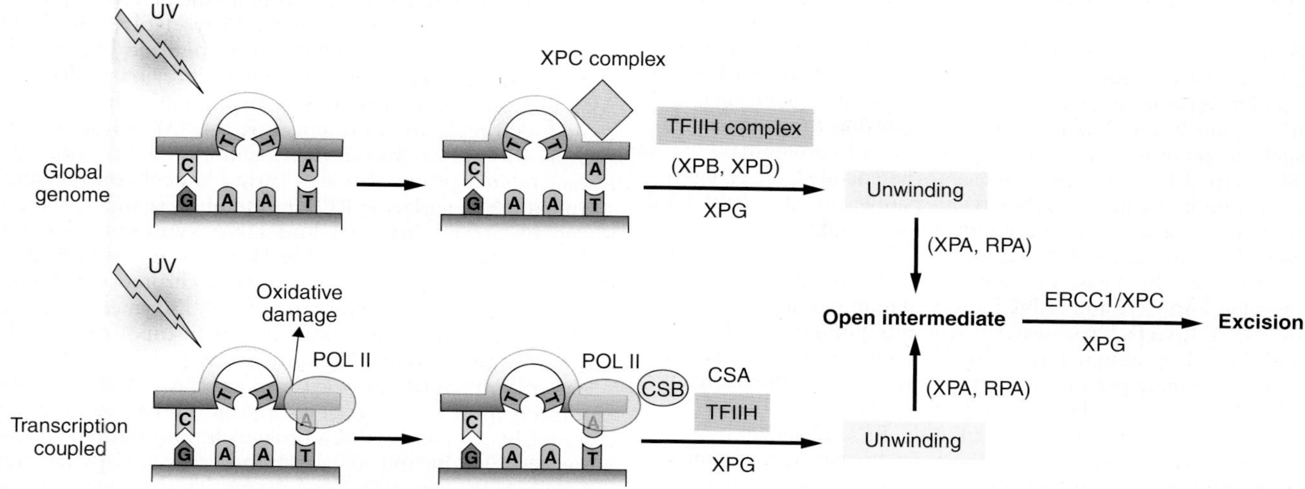

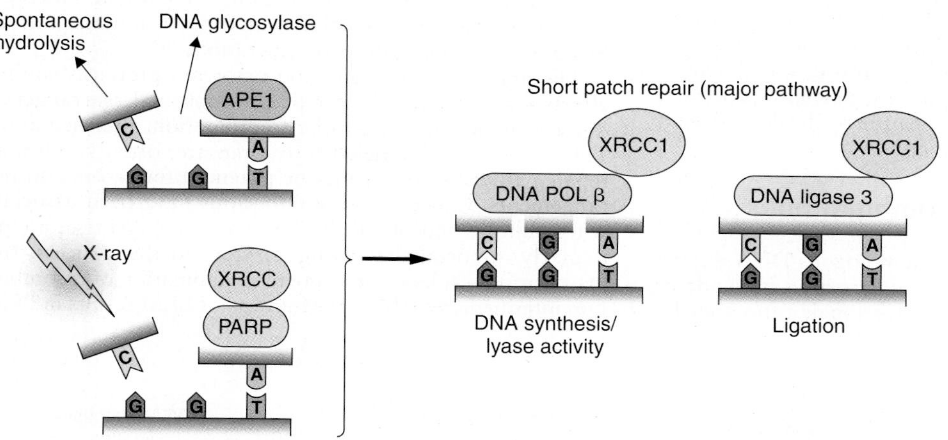

FIGURE 2.4 Nucleotide excision repair and base excision repair. Nucleotide excision repair (NER) is activated in response to bulky lesions that are generated, for example, by UV irradiation (**upper panels**). Global genome (GG) repair involves proteins identified by complementation groups in patients with xeroderma pigmentosa (XP proteins). Initial recognition of lesions occurs by a complex containing xeroderma pigmentosa C (XPC). Transcription coupled repair (TCR) also involves proteins identified by mutation in Cockayne syndrome (CS proteins), and occurs when RNA polymerase II stalls at the site of lesions. Stalled RNA polymerase II recruits Cockayne syndrome B (CSB) to the site of damage. Subsequently, DNA is locally unwound around the injured site by a TFIIH complex containing XPB and XPD. This process also involves XPG, CSA, and other proteins for TCR. Once unwound, XPA and replication protein A (RPA) contribute to stabilization of an open intermediate and recruitment of the ERCC1 and XPF endonucleases that excise the lesion. Subsequent steps involve DNA synthesis and ligation to complete the repair. In base excision repair (BER) (**lower panels**), abasic sites generated by spontaneous hydrolysis, action of DNA glycosylases, or x-ray–induced single-strand breaks are recognized by the APE1 endonuclease, as well as PARP and XRCC1. Subsequent repair is influenced by PARP-mediated ADP ribosylation of histones and other proteins, while XRCC1 serves as a scaffold for recruitment of DNA polymerase β and DNA ligase 3. These latter enzymes catalyze nucleotide reinsertion and ligation into the injured strand as part of the short patch repair pathway (major BER pathway).

CHK2 is evidenced by its mutation in a subset of patients with Li Fraumeni syndrome. *CHK2* mutation has also been observed in familial breast cancer, and in multiple sporadic tumor types.[97] Mutation of *CHK1* is observed less frequently in tumors, which, similar to ATR, could reflect strongly disadvantageous effects of *CHK1* loss on viability.

The initiation of the repair process itself involves recruitment of multiple other proteins to sites of DSBs in conjunction with ATM and ATR.[4,9] DSBs are recognized by the MRN complex, consisting of MRE11 (meiotic recombination 11)/RAD50/NBS1 (Nimjen breakage syndrome 1).[98] Mutations in MRE11 result in an ataxia telangiectasia-like disorder, while NBS1 is mutated in the Nijmegen breakage syndrome, and both diseases are characterized by immunodeficiency, cellular sensitivity to ionizing radiation, chromosomal instability, and a high frequency of malignancies. In addition to their role in DSB repair by HR, the MRN proteins have important roles in telomere maintenance, and, at least in yeast, in NHEJ. ATR/CHK1 signaling is linked with activation of the Fanconi anemia pathway and *BRCA2*.

DNA Repair of Insterstrand DNA Crosslinks

Fanconi anemia is another autosomal recessive human disease characterized by bone marrow failure, congenital abnormalities, cellular hypersensitivity to DNA cross-linking agents such as mitomycin C and cisplatin, and predisposition to malignancies such as acute leukemia and squamous cell carcinomas.[99,100] There are 13 known FA genes, and the encoded FA proteins cooperate in a common DNA repair pathway. Eight of the FA proteins are assembled in a multisubunit ubiquitin ligase complex. In response to DNA damage, or during normal S phase progression, this ligase monoubiquitinates two additional FA proteins, FANCD2 and FANCI. Monoubiquitination is activated by the ATR/CHK1 pathway.[101] Monoubiquitinated FANCD2 and FANCI are required for normal homologous recombination repair, and these proteins further interact with the downstream FA proteins, FANCD1, FANCJ, and FANCN/PALB2.[102,103] Interestingly, FANCD1 is identical to the *BRCA2* gene.[104]

The three downstream FA genes are breast/ovarian cancer susceptibility genes, and heterozygote carriers, with mutations in a single copy of FANCJ, FANCD1, or FANCN have an increased cancer risk. Biochemical functions of monoubiquitinated FANCD2/FANCI were recently elucidated. In a cell-free system, this complex was required for nucleolytic incisions near an interstrand cross-link and for translesion DNA synthesis past the cross-link. Thus, the FA pathway was shown to be required for the generation of a new, partially processed DNA substrate that can be further repaired by the downstream homologous recombination machinery.[105]

Homologous Recombination

In repair by HR, sequences from a homologous DNA duplex are used to provide a template for reconstruction of the damaged DNA segment.[4,9] The template for repair can either be the identical sister chromatid (the preferred substrate in mitotic cells) or the homologous chromosome (the preferred substrate during meiosis). The classic HR pathway involves the following basic steps (Fig. 2.5). DSBs are recognized by the MRN complex and by checkpoint proteins as previously described. A 5′-3 exonuclease generates 3′ overhangs, which are then coated with replication protein A (RPA). "Mediator" proteins such as BRCA2 or Rad52 then facilitate the recruitment of Rad51-related proteins, which form filaments on the single-stranded DNA, replacing RPA. A homology search ensues, followed by strand invasion and DNA synthesis. The links between DNA strands (double Holliday junctions) can be resolved to produce exchange between chromosomes (crossovers) or no exchange (non-crossovers). Enzymes such as the RecQ helicase BLM, in conjunction with topoisomerase IIIα can resolve these double Holliday junctions.[106]

Several other HR pathways also exist. A potentially important mechanism for cancer development is break-induced replication (BIR).[107] During BIR a broken chromosome end invades a homologous site and replication proceeds to copy the entire sequence of the template chromosome. This is relevant to cancer because it can result in large-scale LOH. Furthermore, BIR is an important mechanism for healing breaks at chromosome ends resulting from telomere attrition.[108] Finally, in yeast, aging is accompanied by a switchlike increase in mutagenesis and BIR after a certain number of generations.[109]

Disruption of recombination pathways produces complex effects that pose the danger of chromosomal rearrangement due to the accumulation of recombination intermediates.[4,9] These are then channeled into alternate, often suboptimal, repair pathways, increasing the potential for errors and rearrangements. Cancer-causing mutations have been associated with multiple steps in HR. Given that RecQ helicases are particularly important resolving enzymes in this process, their inactivation results in widespread accumulation of recombination intermediates.[106,110,111] Mutation of BLM results in Bloom

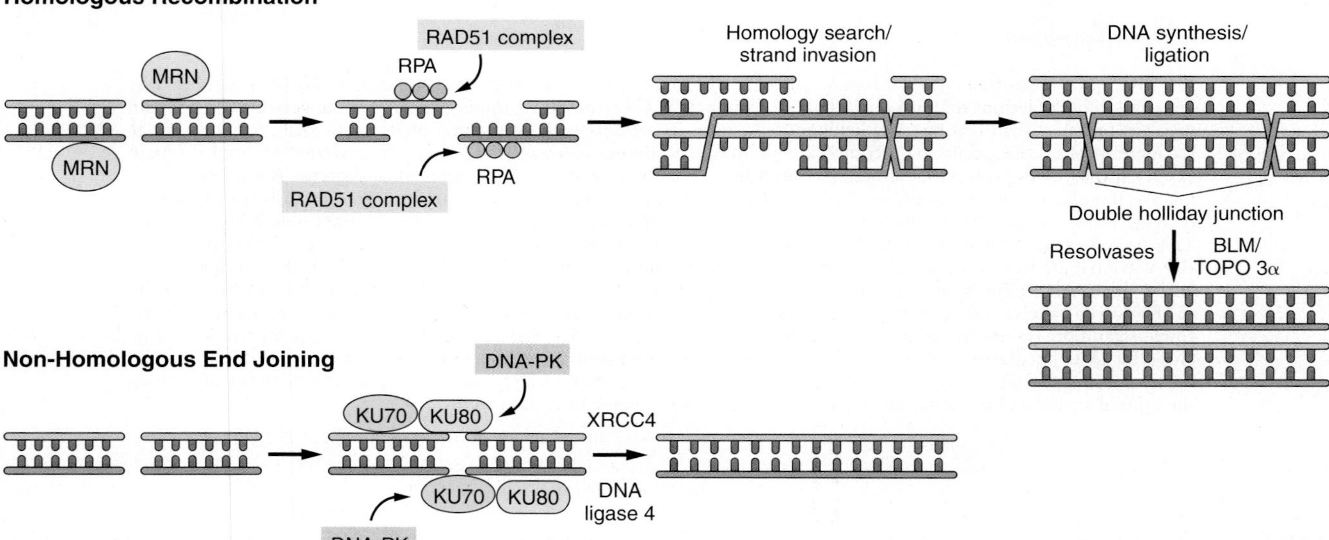

FIGURE 2.5 Double-strand break (DSB) repair by homologous recombination and nonhomologous end-joining (NHEJ). In homologous recombination (HR), DSBs are recognized by the MRN complex, among other proteins. 5′-3′ exonuclease activity results in the generation of single-strand overhangs that are coated with RPA. Mediator proteins such as BRCA2 and RAD52 stimulate assembly of a RAD51 nucleoprotein filament complex that guides subsequent homology search and strand invasion into the homologous strand (e.g., the identical sister chromatid in late S/G2 phase and mitosis). Subsequent DNA synthesis and ligation results in the formation of recombination intermediates that contain double Holliday junctions. These are resolved by resolving enzymes such as the RecQ helicase BLM, in conjunction with topoisomerase 3α. The process of NHEJ involves recognition of DSB ends by the Ku70-Ku80 heterodimer, with subsequent recruitment of DNA-dependent protein kinase. DNA ends are then ligated following recruitment of XRCC4 and DNA ligase 4.

syndrome, a disease characterized by immunodeficiency, male sterility, dwarfism, skin disorders, and a high incidence of both leukemia and solid tumors. In addition, the WRN helicase was identified by virtue of its mutation in Werner syndrome, a disorder characterized by premature aging, with early atherosclerosis, type 2 diabetes, osteoporosis, and age-associated malignancies. Rothmund-Thomson syndrome is associated with mutation in the related RecQ helicase RECQ4, and affected patients exhibit characteristic photosensitivity with poikilodermatous skin changes, early alopecia and hair graying, juvenile cataracts, growth deficiency, and an elevated frequency of malignancies such as osteogenic sarcomas. RecQ helicases have also been shown to facilitate NHEJ, interact with components of the MMR and BER machinery, and play an important role in telomere maintenance. The combination of aging and cancer predisposition phenotypes associated with RecQ lesions provides yet another example of the balance between the deleterious and growth-promoting effects of genomic instability on developing cancer cells.

BRCA1 and *BRCA2* are perhaps the most extensively studied cancer susceptibility genes required for HR. They are mutated in familial breast and ovarian cancer syndromes and represent key components of the response to DSBs and subsequent repair by HR.[112–114] BRCA1 forms a heterodimer with the structurally related protein BARD1, and as previously described, forms a complex together with BRCA2, RAD51, and other proteins involved in the regulation of repair by HR. Another large, multiprotein complex termed BASC (*BRCA1*-associated genome surveillance complex) has been identified, containing tumor suppressors, mismatch repair proteins, ATM, MRN, and BLM, with a presumed role in the global sensing and coordinated response to DNA damage. *BRCA1* has also been implicated in S phase and G2/M checkpoint control, and in the organization of heterochromatin.

Mutations in *BRCA1* and *BRCA2* are associated with a 60% to 85% lifetime risk of developing breast cancer and a 15% to 40% lifetime risk of developing ovarian cancer, although only 2% to 3% of all breast cancer cases are associated with mutation in one of these genes.[113] They account for approximately 40% of cases of familial breast cancer, with mutations in *CHK2* and *p53* responsible for an additional 5% and 1% of cases, respectively. Recently, mutation in *PALB2*, which encodes a BRCA2-binding partner, has also been described in familial breast cancer, and may contribute to inherited prostate cancer as well.[115] *PALB2* is also identical to the Fanconi anemia gene *FANCN*.[116] Germ line biallelic mutations in *PALB2* or *BRCA2* (*FANCD1*) result in Fanconi anemia.[117]

Although it is clear that mutations in *BRCA1* and *BRCA2* can destabilize the genome and promote cancer susceptibility, it remains poorly understood which roles of these proteins are specifically involved in tumor suppression and why patients with germ line defects primarily develop breast and ovarian cancer. Somatic inactivation of *BRCA1* and *BRCA2* has been reported in other tumor types such as colorectal cancer, as have defects in other components of DSB repair such as *ATM* and *FANC* genes. A subset of sporadic breast cancer, defined by lack of expression of the estrogen and progesterone receptors and absence of *HER2* amplification (termed *triple-negative breast cancer*) and a "basal-like" phenotype shares strong similarities with the tumors that develop in patients with germ line *BRCA1* and *BRCA2* mutations. These sporadic basal-like cancers also exhibit defects in X chromosome inactivation,[118] and co-cluster with *BRCA10*-deficient breast cancers on transcriptional arrays. Although these sporadic triple-negative breast cancers appear to have normal *BRCA1*, these similarities have led to the suggestion that they may be defective at another point within the *BRCA1* pathway. Another possibility is that breast tissue selectively accumulates genotoxins that induce a heightened requirement for *BRCA1* and *BRCA2*. Further study is needed to elucidate the mechanism behind the tissue-specific nature of *BRCA1* and *BRCA2* mutant cancer.

Nonhomologous End-Joining

Given that HR uses an identical sister chromatid as template to guide repair, in principle it should be error-free.[4,95,119,120] In yeast, where the genome lacks extensive repetitive sequences, HR is indeed mostly error-free. However, in humans, where the genome contains extensive repetitive sequences, HR poses the danger of repeat sequence recombination resulting in gross chromosomal rearrangements. One factor that prevents this type of error is that repair by HR is limited to late S and G2 phases of the cell cycle, after DNA replication. Thus, HR predominantly occurs when a homologous template sequence is held in close physical proximity to the break by the cohesion between sister chromatids. In humans and other higher eukaryotes it appears that NHEJ is relatively more important than in other organisms such as fungi. It seems that, at least in G1 cells, the small-scale errors generated by NHEJ are less detrimental than the potential large-scale errors (deletions or translocations) that could arise from HR. NHEJ involves direct end-joining of the broken double-strand DNA ends, without a template for repair. Thus, NHEJ can occur during any phase of the cell cycle, although it primarily occurs during G1 phase.

In the process of NHEJ, broken DNA ends are recognized by a heterodimer of Ku70/Ku80, which recruits the catalytic subunit of DNA-dependent protein kinase (DNA-PK) and the Artemis nuclease[120–122] (Fig. 2.5). DNA-PK–mediated phosphorylation of Artemis facilitates its activation and results in the processing of DNA ends in a subset of DSBs, contributing to the error-prone nature of NHEJ. DNA ligation is subsequently mediated by a complex that contains XRCC4 and DNA ligase IV. NHEJ is integrally involved in the V(D)J recombination and class switching that occurs during normal lymphocyte maturation. During V(D)J recombination and certain other physiologic settings, cleavage induced by the RAG nuclease may generate regions of microhomology that allow for relatively precise end-joining.

While mutations in these core NHEJ components in mice cause severe immunologic defects, apoptosis, and premature senescence of cultured fibroblasts, concomitant p53 inactivation results in a high frequency of lymphomas with recurrent, clonal rearrangements.[123] Certain chromosome regions, such as the *c-myc* and the immunoglobulin heavy chain (IgH) loci, are targeted in a recurrent fashion in these lymphomas, similar to common translocations observed human lymphomas. These regions may contain specific sites that are recognized by the RAG nuclease, and the initial cleavage combined with defective NHEJ may be responsible for these aberrant chromosome fusions. Alternatively, NHEJ deficiency has been linked to impaired telomere capping and end-to-end fusions, with so-called breakage-fusion-bridge cycles (see later discussion) promoting translocations and gene amplifications. It is also possible that fragile sites within these chromosomal loci and elsewhere throughout the genome may account for the particular susceptibility of certain chromosome regions to breakage and rearrangement.

Although there is abundant evidence that NHEJ defects can promote tumorigenesis in mouse models—at least in the setting of concomitant *p53* deficiency—there are few reports that implicate NHEJ deficiency in human cancer. The reasons for this are unclear. Loss of NHEJ may be cell-lethal in humans. Consistent with this idea, Artemis deficiency, which results in a very restricted NHEJ defect, is observed in rare lymphoma-prone patients. Similarly, there is a report of a ligase IV mutation in a leukemia patient.[124] However, it may also be the case that more human tumors need to be carefully characterized for subtle mutations, haploinsufficiency, and epigenetic silencing.

Telomere Maintenance

Telomeres, the structures at the ends of chromosomes composed of repetitive sequences and a 3′ G-strand overhang, are key mediators of genomic instability.[125] In humans, telomerase is expressed at low to undetectable levels in somatic tissues, leading to an age-dependent compromise of telomere integrity and resultant telomere dysfunction. By contrast, telomerase is expressed in many tumors, resulting in stabilization of telomere length and restoration of capping function. The activation of telomerase expression during cancer progression supports the idea that telomere dysfunction contributes to chromosome instability during a specific window in oncogenesis.[126,127] For example, telomerase activity is low in small and intermediate-sized colon polyps, and high in late adenomas and colorectal carcinomas, consistent with the observation that CIN arises early during colorectal tumorigenesis, at a time of short telomere length. Furthermore, telomere shortening as a consequence of cell turnover in the setting of chronic inflammatory states such as hepatocellular cirrhosis may contribute to chromosome instability and carcinogenesis in these settings. Conversely, the lack of complex karyotypes in many lymphomas may be related to early activation of telomerase in the setting of the frequent dysregulation of *Myc,* a positive regulator of telomerase expression.[128]

Studies of mice deficient in telomerase activity have yielded powerful evidence that telomere dysfunction can drive chromosomal instability and epithelial carcinogenesis. Strongly reminiscent of the shift in tumor spectrum to epithelial malignancies on aging humans, aging mice deficient in telomerase and heterozygous for mutant *p53* exhibit carcinomas of the breast, colon, and skin.[128] Such tumors are exceedingly rare in wild type mice, which primarily develop sarcomas and hematopoietic malignancies. Moreover, the presence of cytogenetic profiles similar to human carcinomas supports a role for telomere dysfunction in epithelial carcinogenesis. A breakage-fusion-bridge cycle is believed to be responsible for chromosomal fragmentation and the nonreciprocal translocations observed in such tumors (Fig. 2.6). With progressive erosion of telomeres, unprotected chromatid ends can undergo end-to-end fusion, with the formation of a dicentric chromosome. During mitosis, the fused chromosome ends form anaphase bridges as sister centromeres are pulled to opposite centrosomes, resulting in chromosome breakage. The further generation of atelomeric chromosomes by this process can result in propagation of breakage-fusion-bridge mechanisms and continued chromosome instability. In addition to generating translocations, this form of genetic instability can also result in amplifications and deletions.[129,130] The observation that mouse epithelial tumors in this model exhibit amplified and deleted regions syntenic to those seen in human carcinomas lends further support to the notion of chromosomal fragile sites that may be conserved between species.

More recently, key regulatory elements of telomere structure have been implicated in genomic instability and

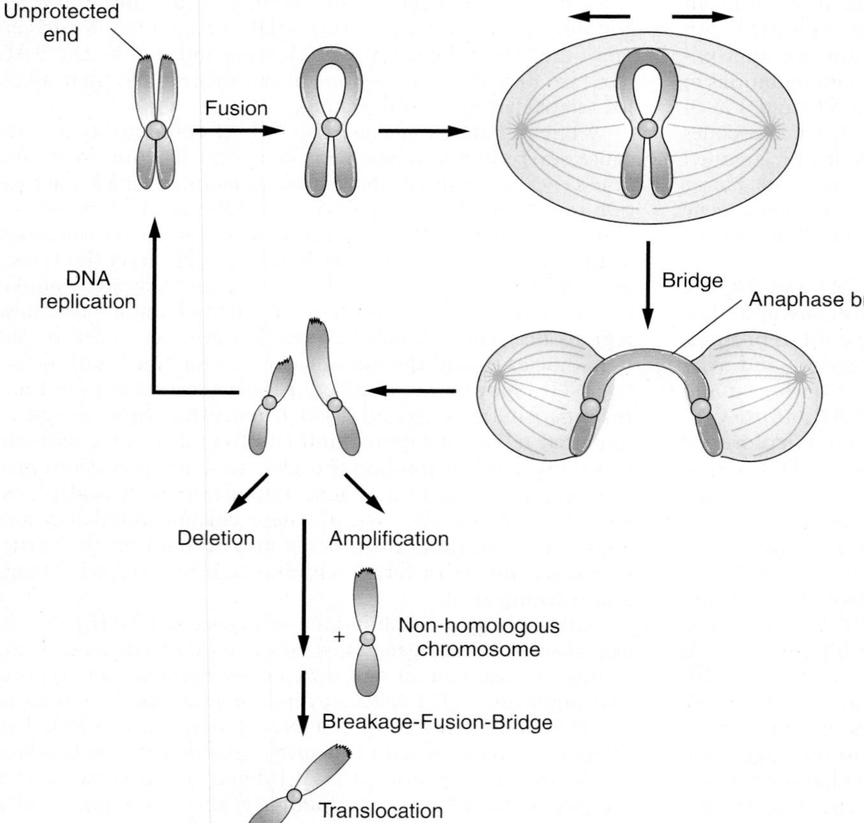

FIGURE 2.6 Breakage-fusion-bridge cycle. In the setting of telomere dysfunction and uncapping of chromosome ends, telomeric fusions may occur between identical sister chromatids or between different chromosomes (dicentrics). During anaphase, as sister chromatids are pulled to opposite poles, the fused chromosome ends are placed under tension and form anaphase bridges. These pulling forces result in chromosome breaks that contribute to deletions, amplifications, and translocations. In addition, because of the further generation of unprotected chromosome ends, the cycle may be repeated.

tumorigenesis.[131,132] TRF2, an important regulator of telomere protection and telomere length, is overexpressed in a variety of epithelial malignancies, including lung, skin, and breast cancer, and has been shown to interact with a number of DNA repair proteins, such as the MRN complex, the WRN and BLM helicases, DNA-PK, PARP, and ERCC1/XPF. Moreover, mice develop an XP-like syndrome when TRF2 is expressed in the skin at high levels, with UV-induced skin cancer, severe telomere shortening, and chromosomal instability.[133] Concomitant telomerase inactivation in these mice dramatically accelerates carcinogenesis, with TRF2 promoting recombination at telomeres and de-repression of pathways that lead to alternative lengthening of telomeres (ALT).[131] ALT involves recombination between telomeres as an alternative means of telomere extension and is operative in a small minority of tumors that are telomerase-negative. Taken together, these studies identify a fundamental role for telomeres and their regulatory proteins in the genesis of chromosome abnormalities and epithelial malignancies.

Telomerase may also play important roles beyond telomere maintenance in the regulation of genome stability.[134] It is expressed at low levels during S phase in normal cells, and targeted disruption of hTERT, the catalytic subunit of telomerase, has been shown to impair heterochromatin formation on a global level and to disrupt the response to DNA damage in normal human fibroblasts.[134,135] These results are consistent with the emerging ties between regulators of telomere maintenance, heterochromatin structure, and components of DNA damage response.[136–138] In addition, they lend further support to the idea that stem cells, which express higher levels of telomerase than their differentiated progeny, are protected from genomic injury. It is important to note, however, that telomerase-deficient mice are viable and do not exhibit significant phenotypic defects until later generations. The specific role of telomerase in chromatin maintenance and the DNA damage response remains to be elucidated, and the reason it is down-regulated in association with cell differentiation remains to be determined.

The role of telomere dysfunction in promoting cancer is further supported by findings in a rare genetic disorder, dyskeratosis congenita (DC). DC is a progressive bone marrow failure syndrome that is classically associated with the clinical triad of abnormal skin pigmentation, leukoplakia, and nail dystrophy. X-linked DC is caused by mutations in dyskerin, which leads to reduced levels of TERC and telomerase activity. Autosomal dominant DC can be caused by mutations in *TERT*, *TERC*, or the telomere binding protein TRF1-interacting nuclear factor 2. Autosomal recessive DC can be caused by mutations in the dyskerin-associated proteins NHP2 and NOP10. In all cases, patients have very short germ line telomeres. In addition to bone marrow failure, patients with DC are also prone to develop myelodysplastic syndrome, leukemia, and solid tumors. Thus, telomere-shortening syndromes in humans recapitulate the impaired maintenance of proliferative tissues and the tumor predisposition seen in telomerase-knockout mice.

WHAT CAUSES CHROMOSOMAL INSTABILITY AND WHOLE-CHROMOSOME ANEUPLOIDY?

Chromosomal instability (CIN), defined as a persistently high rate of loss and gain of whole chromosomes, is a common characteristic of many cancers. CIN, or the "rate" of karyotypic change, should be distinguished from aneuploidy, or the "state" of the karyotype. Although CIN leads to aneuploidy, not all aneuploid tumors exhibit CIN; some tumors are aneuploid with a uniform, stable karyotype. The first breakthrough in understanding the mechanisms of CIN came from studying different colon cancer cell lines that exhibited either a CIN or MIN phenotype.[139] In a single-cell cloning assay, the colon cancer cell lines with MIN maintained a stable chromosome content, but the aneuploid colon carcinoma cells exhibited deviations from the modal chromosome number, indicating the presence of CIN. The fusion of MIN and CIN cells resulted in hybrid cells that retained the CIN phenotype, suggesting that the mechanisms that cause CIN act in dominant fashion. Subsequent work demonstrated that a compromised spindle assembly checkpoint could result in CIN.[140]

Chromosome Cohesion Defects

Accurate chromosome segregation is achieved through carefully orchestrated interactions between the mitotic spindle, kinetochores, and cohesin.[11,29] Replicated chromosomes attach to the spindle microtubules via the kinetochore, an organelle that is assembled onto centromeric chromatin. Prior to anaphase, replicated sister chromatids are held together by cohesin, a protein ring that physically links the sisters.[141,142] The detailed molecular mechanism of how cohesin holds sisters together is a topic of much current research.[143] Most cohesin is lost from chromosome arms prior to metaphase in a manner that requires the Polo and Aurora B kinase. Centromere cohesion is then lost after anaphase onset, a direct consequence of the protease separase cleaving a cohesin subunit (Fig. 2.7). Recently, mutations in genes involved in sister chromatid cohesion, including subunits of the cohesion complex, were identified in colorectal tumors through the sequencing of human homologues of genes known to cause CIN in budding yeast.[144] The frequency and functional consequences of these mutations has not yet been tested experimentally. Additional evidence suggesting a role for the disruption of cohesion in the development of CIN comes from data demonstrating that some breast cancer tumors, as well as osteosarcoma and prostate tumors, express high levels of separase.[145–147] Although, in theory, excessive separase could cause premature chromatid disjunction and subsequent chromosome mis-segregation events, the significance of this mechanism in generation of CIN has not been definitively established.

Spindle Assembly Checkpoint Defects

Attachment of kinetochores to microtubules is monitored by the spindle checkpoint (Fig. 2.7).[29,148,149] A number of spindle checkpoint proteins have been identified, initially via screens in budding yeast, and include MAD1, MAD2, BUB1, BUBR1, BUB3, and a BUB3-related protein RAE1. Although mutations in these spindle assembly checkpoint proteins do occur in human tumors it appears to be a relatively rare event, as discussed in the next section.[150] To prevent chromosome mis-segregation, the spindle checkpoint proteins bind to kinetochores that are improperly attached to the spindle and form a "stop" or "wait" anaphase signal. Ultimately the wait anaphase signal prevents cleavage of cohesin by separase. This involves a cascade of events that include activation of spindle checkpoint proteins at the kinetochore, diffusion of the activated signal throughout the cell, and binding of spindle checkpoint proteins to CDC20, which is the key activator of the E3 ubiquitin ligase complex, the APC. Once all kinetochores are attached to the spindle, the wait anaphase signal is lost and CDC20 is released. Activated APC then triggers mitotic cyclin degradation, separase activation, and cohesin cleavage. How this checkpoint signal is rapidly reversed is poorly understood.

It is important to note that although some CIN cell lines have a defective spindle assembly checkpoint (SAC), several live-cell imaging studies have demonstrated that most CIN cells actually have an intact and functional checkpoint.[151–153] Likewise, in another study, both diploid and CIN cells underwent mitotic arrest in response to spindle poisons with equal efficiency.[151]

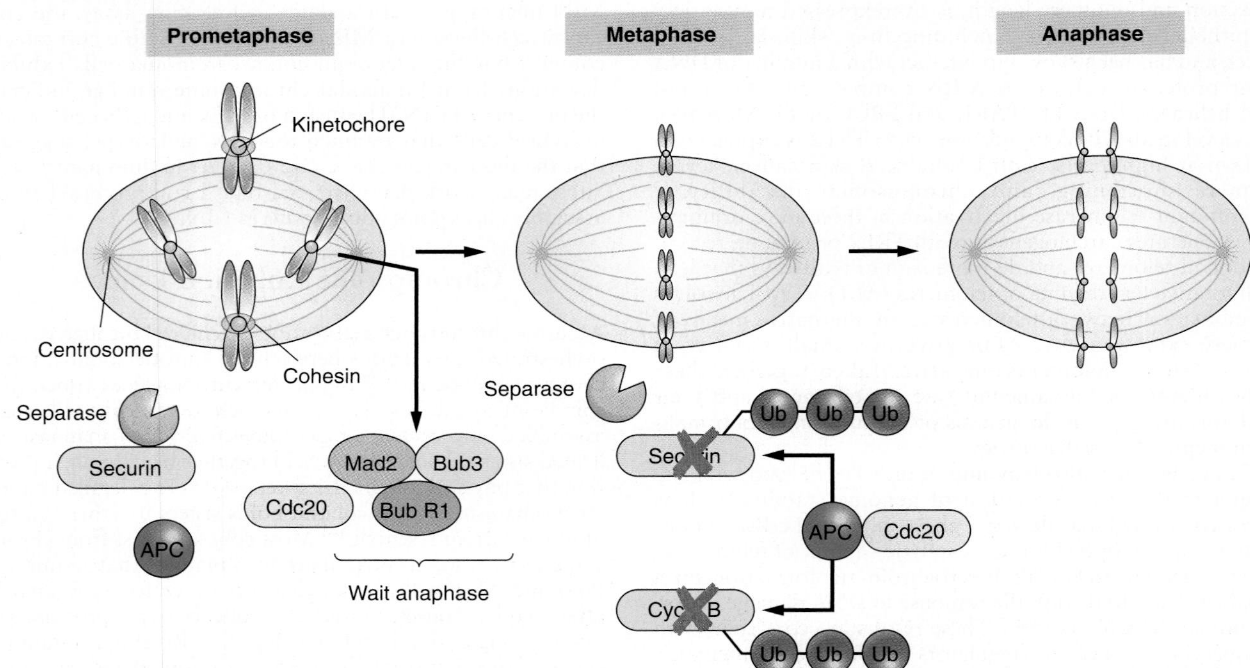

FIGURE 2.7 Spindle checkpoint. During metaphase, paired sister chromatids attach to the bipolar mitotic spindle apparatus at kinetochores, organelles that are assembled onto centromeric chromatin. Sister chromatids are held together by a cohesin, a protein ring that physically links them together. Kinetochores that remain unattached to the spindle catalyze the formation of an active MAD2 complex ("wait" anaphase signal) that binds and inhibits CDC20. Once the final kinetochore is occupied by the spindle, the wait anaphase signal is lost, and CDC20 activates the anaphase-promoting complex to ubiquitinate substrates such as cyclin B and securin. The resultant proteasomal degradation of securin releases the enzyme separase to cleave cohesin and allow for sister chromatid separation under the tension of the mitotic spindle.

Kinetochore-Microtubule Attachment Defects

Attachment of kinetochores to microtubules is necessary but not sufficient for proper chromosome segregation. The spindle checkpoint is also activated if kinetochores are attached but not under proper tension, an indication of successful biorientation.[154] Improper kinetochore-microtubule attachments that are not under normal tension are disassembled by a mechanism involving phosphorylation of kinetochore proteins by the Aurora B kinase.[155,156] Recent work has shown that phosphorylation of an Aurora B substrate at the kinetochore depends on its distance from the kinase at the inner centromere. Repositioning Aurora B closer to the kinetochore prevents stabilization of bioriented attachments and activates the spindle checkpoint. Thus, centromere tension can be sensed by increased spatial separation of Aurora B from kinetochore substrates, which reduces phosphorylation and stabilizes kinetochore microtubules.[157]

The efficient correction of microtubule-kinetochore attachment errors requires the release of incorrectly attached microtubules. Thus, interactions that inappropriately stabilize microtubule attachments might be expected to increase chromosome mis-segregation errors and generate CIN. In fact, recent work demonstrated that kinetochore-microtubule attachments were more stable in cancer cells with CIN than in a noncancerous, diploid cell line.[158] Furthermore, increasing the stability of kinetochore-microtubule attachments in the diploid cell line was sufficient to cause chromosome segregation defects at levels comparable to those in cancer cells with CIN. Conversely, overexpression of proteins that cause increased kinetochore-microtubule dynamics was sufficient to restore stability to chromosomally unstable tumor cell lines.[159] This work demonstrates that the temporal control of microtubule attachments to chromosomes during mitosis is central to genome stability in human cells.

Supernumerary Centrosomes

CIN is also known to be correlated with extra centrosomes. Although this relationship was long-standing, it was not until recently that a mechanism was proposed to link these two common characteristics of cancer cells. Early theories hypothesized that extra centrosomes generate CIN by promoting a multipolar anaphase, which results in three or more aneuploid daughter cells. Recent long-term, live-cell imaging experiments, however, revealed that cells with extra chromosomes typically cluster the extra chromosomes during mitosis to ensure that anaphase occurs with a bipolar spindle.[160–164] The imaging also demonstrated, though, that these cells with extra centrosomes had a significantly increased frequency of lagging chromosomes during anaphase. Further analysis revealed that these segregation errors were a result of the cells with supernumerary centrosomes passing through a transient "multipolar spindle intermediate" in which merotelic kinetochore-microtubule attachment errors accumulated before centrosome clustering and anaphase (Fig. 2.8). Merotely, a conformation where a single kinetochore is attached to microtubules arising from opposite spindle poles, was previously known to generate lagging chromosomes during anaphase and cause chromosome segregation errors.[165,166] The results of these live-cell imaging experiments, consequently, provide a direct mechanistic link between extra centrosomes and CIN, two common

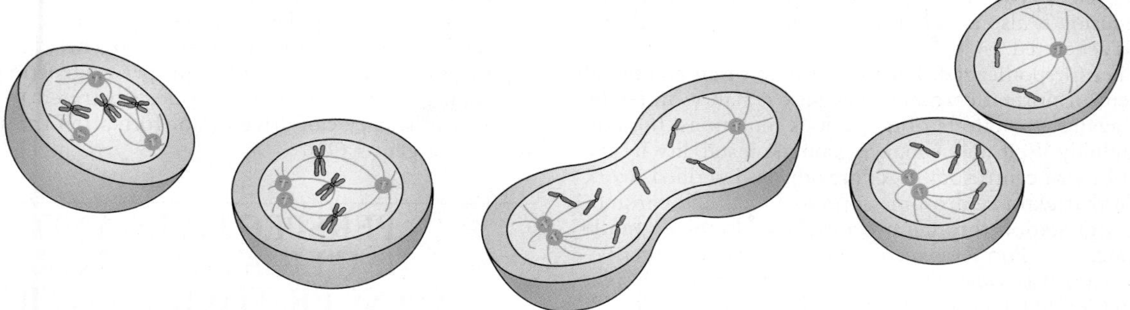

FIGURE 2.8 A mechanism linking extra centrosomes to chromosomal instability. The first cell illustrates a cancer cell with extra centrosomes undergoing a multipolar metaphase. Note that the geometry predisposes to "merotelic" attachments (see chromosome in the middle) where a single chromatid forms attachments to different spindle poles. The second cell illustrates the clustering of centrosomes, which is required for cancer cell survival. Note that the merotelic attachment persists and does not activate the spindle assembly checkpoint. Cell three has undergone anaphase and the merotelic attachment results in a lagging chromosome. Lastly, daughter cells are illustrated with resulting aneuploidy. (Figure provided by L. Kelley and J. DiGianni.)

characteristics of solid tumors. Thus, for chromosome segregation, "CIN geometry" may be as important as "CIN genes."

DOES WHOLE-CHROMOSOME ANEUPLOIDY CAUSE CANCER?

Whole chromosome losses or gains are very common in human cancer.[73] Although the specific gains or losses vary from tumor to tumor, some changes are recurrent in a given tumor type. For example, the gain of chromosome 3 or 3q is reportedly as common in cervical cancer as the Philadelphia chromosome is in chronic myelogenous leukemia.[167] Likewise, glioblastomas frequently exhibit loss of chromosome 10 and melanomas often show gain of chromosome 7. Despite the fact that whole chromosome loss or gain is frequently observed in both solid and hematologic malignancies, a causal role for aneuploidy in cancer progression has been controversial.[168,169]

The identification of germ line mutations in the gene encoding BUBR1 in the disease mosaic variegated aneuploidy has provided the strongest evidence for a causal link between aneuploidy and cancer in humans because patients with this disorder exhibit growth retardation, microcephaly, and multiple childhood malignancies. Premature chromatid separation is frequently seen in more than 50% of lymphocytes from patients with mosaic variegated aneuploidy and many tissues exhibit more than 25% aneuploid cells. Mutations in other components of the spindle assembly checkpoint, including MAD1 and MAD2, have also been described in sporadic cancers and cell lines. Deregulated expression of spindle checkpoint proteins is potentially more common in tumors, but it is always difficult to know which cells to compare with the tumor cells.

Mouse models support the notion that spindle checkpoint misregulation can contribute to tumorigenesis.[150,170–172] However, they also illustrate that there is no simple one-to-one correspondence between checkpoint defects and cancer. Homozygous null mutations in spindle checkpoint genes are early embryonic-lethal. Heterozygous wild type/null animals are viable, but display increased aneuploidy. This illustrates an important point that partial loss of spindle checkpoint function is biologically significant. Although heterozygous checkpoint mouse models do not display a dramatic increase in spontaneous tumors, many models display an increase in tumors after carcinogen exposure. Overexpression of *MAD2*, which is commonly observed in sporadic tumors and can result from RB inactivation, causes extensive chromosomal abnormalities associated with a wide variety of tumors in mice.[173,174] Over 50% of mice engineered to overexpress *MAD2* exhibit tumors including hepatocellular carcinomas, lung adenomas, fibrosarcomas, and lymphomas. Furthermore, *MAD2* is not required for tumor maintenance in this setting, as restoration of normal *MAD2* levels had no effect on subsequent tumor progression. This observation is consistent with the idea that *MAD2* overexpression triggers genetic instability during an early phase of tumor development, promoting subsequent self-sufficiency in tumor growth.

However, at least in theory, spindle checkpoint genes, including *MAD2*, may have additional functions outside mitosis, making it difficult to isolate a primary mitotic defect as the cause of tumor formation in these mice. This issue has been addressed by targeted deletion of CENP-E, a kinetochore-associated motor protein that is specifically expressed during mitosis. Heterozygous loss of CENP-E results in an age-dependent increase in aneuploidy in mice, with associated formation of splenic lymphomas and benign lung tumors.[175] Nonetheless, CENP-E heterozygosity also inhibits tumor formation in the setting of p19^{ARF} loss, suggesting that aneuploidy can act both oncogenically and as a tumor suppressor depending on the genetic context. The tumor-suppressing effect of aneuploidy likely reflects the fitness cost from gene expression imbalance.[176,177] Consistent with this idea, mice with significantly reduced BUBR1 display an array of early aging phenotypes: reduced lifespan, cachectic dwarfism, muscle atrophy, cataracts, and infertility.[170]

An additional, facile way to accumulate whole-chromosome aneuploidy is via a tetraploid intermediate.[178–180] Interestingly, many studies have linked tetraploidy to tumorigenesis. A number of cell-division defects can lead to cytokinesis failure and tetraploidy: errors in DNA replication or repair, or errors in spindle function and chromosome segregation. Mitotic defects lead to spindle checkpoint activation, but cells eventually recover and fail cytokinesis in the face of persistent chromosome segregation errors. This phenomenon is known as *mitotic slippage*. Recent work has also identified a pathway linking telomere damage to tetrapoloidy.[181] Persistent telomere dysfunction in *p53*-deficient cells activates an ATM/ATR and Chk1/Chk2 signaling cascade that blocks entry into mitosis and extends G2. Eventually, the cells switch to a state resembling G1 in which the DNA replication inhibitor geminin, which prevents re-replication in G2, is degraded and Cdt1, which is required for origin licensing, is re-expressed. Thus, in the face of persistent telomere or other DNA damage, cells skip mitosis entirely and "endocycle" between G1 and S phase, producing tetraploid cells. Cell fusion is also an additional mechanism by which tetraploidy is generated.

It has been hypothesized that the presence of an additional complement of normal chromosomes may enhance fitness by buffering against the effects of deleterious mutations. In addition, tetraploidy itself may enhance genomic instability by the presence of extra centrosomes. As previously described, work has shown that extra centrosomes promote CIN and chromosome mis-segregation through a transient multipolar spindle intermediate.[161,162] Further evidence for this tetraploid intermediate model has also come from the study of progressive dysplasia in Barrett's esophagus, which reveals that early loss of *p53* is correlated with the development of tetraploidy and subsequent aneuploidy.[182] Moreover, experimental inhibition of cytokinesis in *p53*-null cells results in the generation of whole-chromosome aneuploidy, chromosome rearrangements, and rapid tumor formation in a mouse breast cancer model.[179] Finally, recent studies suggest that genetic inhibition of cytokinesis or viral induction of cell fusion can promote tumorigenesis.

Finally, aneuploidy associated with APC loss has been shown to result from a combination of defects in mitosis and apoptosis that results in an early stage of tetraploidy and polyploidy.[183,184] Given that APC loss occurs early in colorectal cancer development and is associated with the majority of the 85% of sporadic cancers with CIN, it is possible that genomic instability in this setting is related to the formation of a tetraploid intermediates.[86] However, this remains an open issue because little genomic instability has been detected at early stages in APC-deficient mouse models.[185] Finally, the mechanism by which *MAD2* overexpression generates aneuploidy appears to involve mitotic slippage, resulting in the formation of tetraploid cells.[173] Because RB pathway inactivation is fundamental to tumorigenesis, it is possible that associated up-regulation of *MAD2* promotes aneuploidy more generally in cancer cells via the production of unstable tetraploid cells.

What is the Mechanism of Tumorigenesis?

There are multiple theories of how whole-chromosome aneuploidy could promote tumorigenesis. Extra copies of chromosomes could provide an advantage under certain selective pressures by increasing the expression of a single gene, or a combination of multiple genes on the aneuploid chromosome. This type of mechanism has been described for budding yeast to adapt to defects in cytokinesis, as well as the acquisition of drug resistance by *Candida albicans*.[186,187] An alternative explanation for the tumor-promoting activity of aneuploidy is that the extra chromosomes buffer cancer cells against the effects of deleterious mutations in essential and haploinsufficient genes.

Another theory proposes that the driving force of tumorigenesis is the inherent instability of aneuploid karyotypes.[169] According to this theory, a chromosome mis-segregation event, which is initiated by either a carcinogen or spontaneously, generates additional karyotypic evolution by destabilizing the proteins that segregate, synthesize, and repair chromosomes. Sporadically, such evolutions generate new cancer-causing karyotypes, which are stabilized by selection for their oncogenic function. Thus, in this model, CIN is generated in an autocatalytic fashion. A variation on this theme suggests that aneuploidy can cause protein imbalances that generate additional, non–whole-chromosome genomic instability, such as the acquisition of transforming mutations. In support of this model, structural chromosome abnormalities, such as nonreciprocal translocations, dicentric chromosomes, and double-minute chromosomes, are often noted alongside numerical chromosome abnormalities.[179] It is unclear, though, whether these structural rearrangements are directly linked to the mis-segregation events.

Aneuploidy may also contribute to tumorigenesis through loss of heterozygosity. The possible roles for LOH in tumorigenesis include the duplication of oncogenes, loss of tumor suppressors, or acquisition of improper epigenetic patterns.[77] As discussed earlier, it has been demonstrated in mice that Bub1 insufficiency can drive tumor formation through tumor suppressor gene *LOH*.[78]

PERSPECTIVES AND IMPLICATIONS FOR CANCER THERAPEUTICS

Oncogenesis represents an evolutionary process by which cells acquire successive genetic alterations that facilitate growth, survival, and ultimately properties that allow for dissemination to distant sites. Genomic instability can facilitate tumor development by accelerating the accumulation of such growth-promoting mutations, but this potentially comes with the cost of acquiring deleterious mutations that can impair fitness. Thus, the outcome of genomic instability can be cancer, but it can also be tissue degeneration, cell death, and aging. As detailed in this chapter, a wide variety of mechanisms can result in the generation of genomic instability. At one end of the spectrum, mutations in proteins such as the RecQ helicases, which play critical roles in normal genome maintenance, result in predominantly degenerative disease, manifesting premature aging phenotypes in addition to cancer development. On the other hand, mutations in mismatch repair genes, such as *MLH1*, *MSH2*, and *BRCA*, which have more limited and overlapping roles in the DNA damage response, result in normal development but a tissue-specific predisposition to cancer. Thus, destabilization of the genome can vary in the degree to which cancer promotion or tissue degeneration is favored. A major challenge for the field now is to elucidate the specific mechanisms and genetic interactions that tip the balance in one direction or the other.

Another important consideration is whether conditions leading to genomic instability are present in cancers at diagnosis or are transient, hit-and-run events. For example, inherited cancer syndrome mutations such as mismatch repair gene defects in HNPCC can speed up the acquisition of critical growth-promoting mutations, but, once transformed, the fitness of the tumor cells may be compromised by the ongoing mutator phenotype. Likewise, in sporadic tumors, loss of repair proteins such as ERCC1 in NSCLC may initially promote tumorigenesis, but the presence of these defects in mature tumors may provide a point of attack for certain chemotherapeutic agents. For instance, recent studies suggest the ERCC1-deficient lung tumors are more sensitive to the cytotoxic agent cisplatin.[92] However, some genome-destabilizing events are transient. For instance, some *FANC* genes are methylated and silenced early in cancer progression, leading to genomic instability.[188] However, later in tumorigenesis, these genes may be reactivated, resulting in a tumor with a stable genome. Also, although short telomeres can produce a crisis accompanied by gross chromosomal rearrangements, rampant aneuploidy is suppressed by telomerase re-expression. Similarly, cytokinesis failure and tetraploidy may be transient early events. If the major genome destabilization is transient, cancer cells may be aneuploid, but stably aneuploid. Indeed, it is fairly common for every cell in an aneuploid tumor to have the same abnormal karyotype; metastases and recurrences can have the same abnormal karyotype as the primary tumor. Ill-defined adaptations may enable many tumors to tolerate their altered genomes.

Understanding the mechanisms of genome destabilization that are operative in specific tumors will likely have important consequences for cancer therapeutics. Traditional cytotoxic chemotherapy combinations have largely been derived empirically. Many cytotoxic agents, such as platinum chemotherapies, induce cancer cell killing through DNA damage, with a therapeutic window that is relatively narrow. Tumor cell killing is at least in part correlated with *p53* expression and the ability of cancer cells to undergo apoptosis in response to damaging agents. Indeed, the recent observation that restoration of wild type *p53* function in mouse models of oncogenesis induces spontaneous tumor regression highlights the fact that some tumors become "addicted" to *p53* loss.[18,189] However, the heterogeneity of response within tumor types also suggests that genome-destabilizing mutations present in the cancer genome may sensitize certain subtypes to specific cytotoxic agents. The apparent sensitivity of ERCC1-deficient NSCLC to platinum-based chemotherapy highlights this point.[92] Moreover, topoisomerase I inhibitors such as the camptothecins have been shown to have enhanced sensitivity in the setting of defects in the multiple protein components that respond to DSBs.[190] Similarly, spindle checkpoint defects, if they become fixed in cancer cell populations, may modulate the response to microtubule-based agents such as taxanes and vinca alkaloids.[191,192]

This idea, in which defects in one pathway facilitate sensitivity to DNA-damaging agents, or alternatively, predispose to cell death in response to targeted inhibition of another pathway, relates to the concept of synthetic lethality.[193,194] Originally defined in yeast, extension of this concept to targeted cancer therapy may ultimately result in improved selective cancer cell killing with a wider therapeutic window. An elegant example of this approach has been demonstrated *in vitro* for *BRCA1*- and *BRCA2*-deficient cells.[93,94] Deficiency or inhibition of PARP1 in normal cells results in impairment of the BER response, causing lesions that would normally be repaired by BER to be channeled into the HR pathway. Exposure of cells lacking *BRCA1* and *BRCA2* to PARP inhibition results in the lethal accumulation of DNA damage. Thus, PARP inhibition appears to be selectively toxic for *BRCA*-deficient cancer cells, with potential efficacy in other contexts in which HR or even other types of DNA damage responses are impaired.

The profound sensitivity of *BRCA* mutant cells to PARP inhibition has led to the development of a number of clinical trials to test the efficiency of this approach.[195] A recent phase 1 study reported that the orally active PARP inhibitor olaparib (AZD2281) is well tolerated and has few of the adverse effects associated with conventional chemotherapy.[196] Furthermore, objective antitumor activity was reported in patients with *BRCA1* or *BRCA2* mutations, all of whom had ovarian, breast, or prostate cancer. PARP inhibitors are also being used in combination regimens, as inhibition of PARP can potentiate the effects of numerous DNA-damaging agents, such as temozolomide and irinotecan.

The concept of synthetic lethality has also been applied to tumors harboring mutations in PTEN, MSH2, VHL, and RAS.[197–201] The work with RAS, for example, suggests that targeting the NF-κB signaling pathway might be one strategy to treat K-RAS mutant tumors.[200] Furthermore, this concept might be further generalizable. For example, certain genes in yeast are required for the survival of polyploid cells, with deletion of these genes resulting in so-called ploidy-specific lethality.[202] Identification of similar targets in human cancer cells may facilitate the design of targeted agents that selectively impair the growth of tumors with increased numbers of chromosomes or centrosomes.[203]

Finally, the advent of genomic technologies and large-scale characterization of cancer genomes will allow for a more refined view of carcinogenesis and enhanced subclassification of tumors. Knowledge of genome-destabilizing pathways that promote oncogenesis but impair fitness in specific tumors may eventually allow better tailoring of therapies in individual patients.

Selected References

The full list of references for this chapter appears in the online version.

1. Hanahan D, Weinberg RA. The hallmarks of cancer. *Cell* 2000;100:57.
4. Weinberg R. *The Biology of Cancer*. New York: Garland Science; 2006.
10. Kastan MB, Bartek J. Cell-cycle checkpoints and cancer. *Nature* 2004; 432:316–323.
16. Malumbres M, Barbacid M. Cell cycle, CDKs and cancer: a changing paradigm. *Nat Rev Cancer* 2009;9:153–166.
23. Jackson SP, Bartek J. The DNA-damage response in human biology and disease. *Nature* 2009;461:1071–1078.
32. Collado M, Serrano M. Senescence in tumours: evidence from mice and humans. *Nat Rev Cancer* 2010;10:51–57.
36. Bartkova J, Rezaei N, Liontos M, et al. Oncogene-induced senescence is part of the tumorigenesis barrier imposed by DNA damage checkpoints. *Nature* 2006;444: 633–637.
38. Johnson L, Mercer K, Greenbaum D, et al. Somatic activation of the K-ras oncogene causes early onset lung cancer in mice. *Nature* 2001;410: 1111–1116.
46. Stratton MR, Campbell PJ, Futreal PA. The cancer genome. *Nature* 2009;458:719–724.
49. Greenman C, Stephens P, Smith R, et al. Patterns of somatic mutation in human cancer genomes. *Nature* 2007;446:153–158.
50. Comprehensive genomic characterization defines human glioblastoma genes and core pathways. *Nature* 2008;455:1061–1068.
53. Dang L, White DW, Gross S, et al. Cancer-associated IDH1 mutations produce 2-hydroxyglutarate. *Nature* 2009;462:739–744.
55. Ward PS, Patel J, Wise DR, et al. The common feature of leukemia-associated IDH1 and IDH2 mutations is a neomorphic enzyme activity converting alpha-ketoglutarate to 2-hydroxyglutarate. *Cancer Cell* 2010; 17:225–234.
56. Ley TJ, Mardis ER, Ding L, et al. DNA sequencing of a cytogenetically normal acute myeloid leukaemia genome. *Nature* 2008;456:66–72.
59. Pleasance ED, Cheetham RK, Stephens PJ, et al. A comprehensive catalogue of somatic mutations from a human cancer genome. *Nature* 2010; 463:191–196.
60. Wang Z, Gerstein M, Snyder M. RNA-Seq: a revolutionary tool for transcriptomics. *Nat Rev Genet* 2009;10:57–63.
63. Maher CA, Kumar-Sinha C, Cao X, et al. Transcriptome sequencing to detect gene fusions in cancer. *Nature* 2009;458:97–101.
68. Garzon R, Calin GA, Croce CM. MicroRNAs in Cancer. *Annu Rev Med* 2009;60:167–179.
69. Lin C, Yang L, Tanasa B, et al. Nuclear receptor-induced chromosomal proximity and DNA breaks underlie specific translocations in cancer. *Cell* 2009;139:1069–1083.
72. Beroukhim R, Mermel CH, Porter D, et al. The landscape of somatic copy-number alteration across human cancers. *Nature* 2010;463:899–905.
75. Tuna M, Knuutila S, Mills GB. Uniparental disomy in cancer. *Trends Mol Med* 2009;15:120–128.
78. Baker DJ, Jin F, Jeganathan KB, van Deursen JM. Whole chromosome instability caused by Bub1 insufficiency drives tumorigenesis through tumor suppressor gene loss of heterozygosity. *Cancer Cell* 2009;16: 475–486.
80. McKenna ES, Roberts CW. Epigenetics and cancer without genomic instability. *Cell Cycle* 2009;8:23–26.
82. Sharma SV, Lee DY, Li B, et al. A chromatin-mediated reversible drug-tolerant state in cancer cell subpopulations. *Cell* 2010;141:69–80.
89. Cleaver JE, Lam ET, Revet I. Disorders of nucleotide excision repair: the genetic and molecular basis of heterogeneity. *Nat Rev Genet* 2009;10: 756–768.
92. Olaussen KA, Dunant A, Fouret P, et al. DNA repair by ERCC1 in non-small-cell lung cancer and cisplatin-based adjuvant chemotherapy. *N Engl J Med* 2006;355:983–991.
94. Bryant HE, Schultz N, Thomas HD, et al. Specific killing of BRCA2-deficient tumours with inhibitors of poly(ADP-ribose) polymerase. *Nature* 2005;434:913–917.
100. Moldovan GL, D'Andrea AD. How the Fanconi anemia pathway guards the genome. *Annu Rev Genet* 2009;43:223–249.
105. Knipscheer P, Raschle M, Smogorzewska A, et al. The Fanconi anemia pathway promotes replication-dependent DNA interstrand cross-link repair. *Science* 2009;326:1698–1701.

110. Chu WK, Hickson ID. RecQ helicases: multifunctional genome caretakers. *Nat Rev Cancer* 2009;9:644–654.
121. Lieber MR, Ma Y, Pannicke U, Schwarz K. Mechanism and regulation of human non-homologous DNA end-joining. *Nat Rev Mol Cell Biol* 2003; 4:712–720.
127. Artandi SE, DePinho RA. Telomeres and telomerase in cancer. *Carcinogenesis* 2010;31:9–18.
128. Artandi SE, Chang S, Lee SL, et al. Telomere dysfunction promotes non-reciprocal translocations and epithelial cancers in mice. *Nature* 2000;406: 641–645.
130. Maser RS, Choudhury B, Campbell PJ, et al. Chromosomally unstable mouse tumours have genomic alterations similar to diverse human cancers. *Nature* 2007;447:966–971.
139. Lengauer C, Kinzler KW, Vogelstein B. Genetic instability in colorectal cancers. *Nature* 1997;386:623–627.
150. Schvartzman JM, Sotillo R, Benezra R. Mitotic chromosomal instability and cancer: mouse modelling of the human disease. *Nat Rev Cancer* 2010;10:102.
151. Gascoigne KE, Taylor SS. Cancer cells display profound intra- and inter-line variation following prolonged exposure to antimitotic drugs. *Cancer Cell* 2008;14:111–122.
157. Liu D, Vader G, Vromans MJ, et al. Sensing chromosome bi-orientation by spatial separation of aurora B kinase from kinetochore substrates. *Science* 2009;323:1350–1353.
161. Ganem NJ, Godinho SA, Pellman D. A mechanism linking extra centrosomes to chromosomal instability. *Nature* 2009;460:278–282.
162. Silkworth WT, Nardi IK, Scholl LM, Cimini D. Multipolar spindle pole coalescence is a major source of kinetochore mis-attachment and chromosome mis-segregation in cancer cells. *PLoS One* 2009;4: e6564.
165. Cimini D, Howell B, Maddox P, et al. Merotelic kinetochore orientation is a major mechanism of aneuploidy in mitotic mammalian tissue cells. *J Cell Biol* 2001;153:517–527.
175. Weaver BA, Silk AD, Montagna C, et al. Aneuploidy acts both oncogenically and as a tumor suppressor. *Cancer Cell* 2007;11:25–36.
177. Williams BR, Prabhu VR, Hunter KE, et al. Aneuploidy affects proliferation and spontaneous immortalization in mammalian cells. *Science* 2008; 322:703–709.
179. Fujiwara T, Bandi M, Nitta M, et al. Cytokinesis failure generating tetraploids promotes tumorigenesis in p53-null cells. *Nature* 2005;437: 1043–1047.
189. Luo J, Solimini NL, Elledge SJ. Principles of cancer therapy: oncogene and non-oncogene addiction. *Cell* 2009;136:823–837.
193. Kaelin WG Jr. The concept of synthetic lethality in the context of anticancer therapy. *Nat Rev Cancer* 2005;5:689–698.
195. Ashworth A. A synthetic lethal therapeutic approach:poly(ADP) ribose polymerase inhibitors for the treatment of cancers deficient in DNA double-strand break repair. *J Clin Oncol* 2008;26:3785–3790.
200. Barbie DA, Tamayo P, Boehm JS, et al. Systematic RNA interference reveals that oncogenic KRAS-driven cancers require TBK1. *Nature* 2009;462:108–112.
201. Scholl C, Frohling S, Dunn IF, et al. Synthetic lethal interaction between oncogenic KRAS dependency and STK33 suppression in human cancer cells. *Cell* 2009;137:821–834.
202. Storchova Z, Breneman A, Cande J, et al. Genome-wide genetic analysis of polyploidy in yeast. *Nature* 2006;443:541–547.

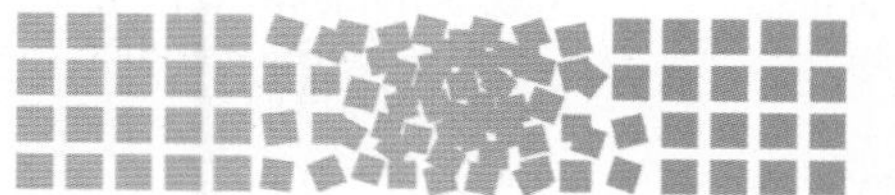

CHAPTER 3 EPIGENETICS OF CANCER

PETER A. JONES AND KARIN B. MICHELS

Cancer is a disease involving the failure of function of regulatory genes that control normal cellular homeostasis. The key roles of mutational processes in the generation of human cancer have been identified in the past decades. More recently the potential for epigenetic processes to complement genetic changes has been realized. In addition to multiple mutations, almost all human cancers contain substantial epigenetic abnormalities that cooperate with genetic lesions to generate the cancer phenotype. Epigenetic aberrations arise early in carcinogenesis preceding gene mutations and therefore provide targets for early detection. Epimutations may be reversed by drug treatments, providing the opportunity to design epigenetic therapies. This chapter will describe the role of epigenetic processes in cancer etiology and discuss their potential as biomarkers for early detection of cancer and precancerous lesions and their promise for drug development.

EPIGENETIC PROCESSES

Epigenetic processes are essential to ensure the appropriate packaging of the genome to fit within the confines of the mammalian nucleus, while maintaining its functionality. DNA is not found as a naked molecule in the nucleus but is wrapped up in nucleosomes composed of histone octamers and 146 base pairs (bp) of DNA, which are the fundamental building blocks of chromatin. Epigenetics is fundamental to organismal development: pluripotent cells arising at fertilization progressively lose their plasticity as they move through the consecutive differentiation steps necessary for embryogenesis. The recent development of whole epigenome approaches allows for the appreciation of the plethora of epigenomic processes that occur during development and the understanding of their role in activation and silencing of regulatory pathways.

The development of "next generation" sequencing approaches coupled with chromatin immunoprecipitation permits assessment of the distribution of the chemical "marks" imparted on the chromatin proteins and DNA. These epigenetic marks include DNA methylation and histone modifications (Table 3.1) and allow the orchestration of activation and silencing pathways. The marks or chemical modifications are placed on the chromatin components by enzymes such as methyltransferases and some of them can be removed by other enzymes (Table 3.1). While we are just beginning to understand the potential roles of specific chemical marks in ensuring the mitotically heritable variation in cell metabolism, which does not involve direct changes in the DNA sequence itself, the key role of a subset of these marks in controlling the potential for gene expression is becoming apparent (Table 3.1).

The fundamental process of DNA methylation applies methyl groups to cytosine residues in CpG dinucleotides to form 5-methylcytosine catalyzed by three DNA methyltransferase enzymes (DNMT1, DNMT3a, DNMT3b).[1] Methylation patterns, once established, can be faithfully copied over a protracted period of time. The CpG dinucleotide is asymmetrically distributed in human DNA with about half of human genes containing CpG-rich regions termed "CpG islands" at their transcriptional start sites (TSS). Mostly, CpG islands are not methylated and genes are switched on or off without changing the methylation status of the CpG sites within islands. However, in certain physiologic situations such as X-chromosome inactivation or genomic imprinting, the CpG islands do become methylated in a manner that ensures permanent silencing due to the inherent mitotic heritability of the DNA methylation patterns. In contrast, embryonic stem cells keep genes quiet but poised for later expression during differentiation by using histone marks that are easier to reverse than DNA methylation to accomplish this purpose.[2]

The histone tails that protrude from the histone octamer, containing 146 bp of DNA in the nucleosome, are also modulated by enzymes and have functional significance for gene expression.[3] Acetylation of the lysine residues (particularly lysines 9 and 14) is strongly associated with gene expression and is highly localized to the TSS of genes. The overall level of lysine modification in chromatin is dictated by opposing enzyme functions involving histone acetyltransferases (HATs) and histone deacetylases (HDACs), which apply or remove acetyl groups on lysine residues, respectively. The level of acetylation correlates with the level of expression, and HDACs have received considerable attention as potential drug targets. The TSS of human genes are also marked by the presence of three methyl groups on the lysine 4 residue of histone H3 (H3K4me3). Overexpression of enzymes that attach the methyl groups to this residue has profound implications for human cancer development. Trimethylation of histone H3 lysine 9 (H3K9me3) or lysine 27 (H3K27me3) is associated with gene repression (Table 3.1). The H3K9me3 is applied by several different methyltransferases, including G9a, and is associated with abnormally silenced methylated CpG islands. The H3K27me3 mark is applied by an enzyme of the polycomb repression complex 2, histone-lysine *N*-methyltransferase (EZH2), and aberrant activity of this enzyme is associated with human cancer development.

Figure 3.1 depicts the positions of a small subset of the possible modifications on the histone H3 protein in the context of nucleosomes. Although there are other modifications such as phosphorylation, ubiquitination, and sumolation of this and other histones, the discussion here is restricted to methylation and acetylation, since their function and potential for drug development is currently best understood. The various modifications can be interpreted by other proteins (not shown) sometimes called "readers," which modify local chromatin structure to either stimulate or repress gene expression. Still other proteins (also not shown), such as histone deacetylases or histone demethylases, can remove the modifications in response to cellular and environmental signals, resulting in a dynamic state.

TABLE 3.1

SOME EPIGENETIC MODIFICATIONS AND THEIR ROLES IN GENE ACTIVITIES

Macromolecule	Modification	Enzymes	Function	Drug
DNA	Cytosine methylation	DNMT1 DNMT3A DNMT3B	Gene silencing	5-azacytidine (5-Aza-CR) 5-aza-2′-deoxycytidine (5-Aza-CdR)
Histone H3/H4	Lysine 9 acetylation (H3K9ac) Lysine 16 acetylation (H4K16ac)	HAT HDAC	Gene activation Gene repression	None Histone deacetylase inhibitors (SAHA, depsipeptide) and many others
Histone H3	Lysine 4 methylation (H3K4me3)	MLL and several others	Gene activation	None
Histone H3	Lysine 9 methylation (H3K9me3)	G9a SUV39h	Gene repression	BIX-01294
Histone H3	Lysine 27 methylation (H3K27me3)	EZH2	Gene repression	3-deazaneplanocin A (DZNep)
Histone H2AZ	Replacement histone		Gene activation	None

The macromolecules that constitute chromatin undergo various covalent modifications, which result in cellular memory of transcriptional competency. The table lists only a subset of these marks and covalent modifications and focuses on those that are mainly localized to the start sites of human genes. The table also lists drugs that are currently in the clinic or are known to modify these processes, thus providing avenues for epigenetic therapies. DNMT, DNA methyltransferase; HAT, histone acetyltransferase; DHAC, histone deacetylases; SAHA, suberoylanilide hydroxamic acid; SUV39h, histone 3 lysine 9 trimethyltransferase; MLL, histone 3 lysine 4 trimethyltransferase; G9a, histone 3 lysine 9 trimethyltransferase, EZH2, histone 3 lysine 27 trimethyltransferase.

The positioning of the modifications relative to the TSS of genes is also critical for their function: Figure 3.2 shows the start site of a hypothetical gene with a CpG island in its promoter, which is normally free of DNA cytosine methylation. Active genes attach the activating H3K4me3 and H3K9ac modifications to the nucleosomes flanking the TSS. These may serve as "beacons," allowing the transcriptional apparatus to "find" the start site and begin producing mRNA.

The silencing of the gene can be brought about in several ways, such as the removal of the activating H3K4me3 and H3K9ac modifications and application of the H3K27me3 mark (Fig. 3.2). Insertion of a nucleosome into the nucleosome-free region characteristic for CpG island–containing genes may also facilitate the silencing process. Genes silenced through DNA cytosine methylation also have nucleosomes at the start site of the gene but include the H3K9me3 modification rather than the H3K27me3 modification as a distinguishing feature.[4] This more permanent mitotically heritable silencing process is used to ensure the long-term silencing of X-chromosome–linked genes and other important genes such as imprinted genes throughout the life of a human. These silencing mechanisms are all essential for mammalian

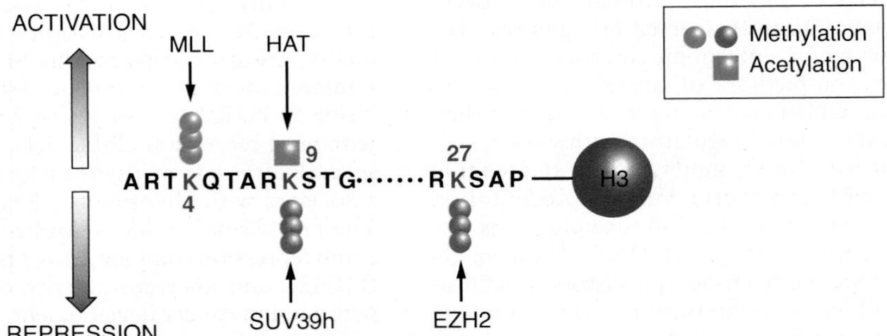

FIGURE 3.1 Covalent modifications of histones can regulate gene activity. The location of activating and repressive marks on histone H3 are shown as an example. These covalent modifications, including trimethylation of lysine 4 (K4me3) and acetylation of lysine 9 (K9ac), are highly localized in start sites of genes and associated with active gene transcription. Conversely, methylation of lysine 9 (K9me3) or lysine 27 (K27me3) is associated with gene inactivity. It is the balance between these marks that define the transcriptional competence of a given gene. Unlike the two activating marks shown (*green*), the two repressive marks (*red*) tend to be more widely distributed on chromatin and potential drug targets. The figure is not intended to be comprehensive, and many additional modifications on histone H3 and other histones are known to participate in the structure of the epigenome. MLL, histone 3 lysine 4 trimethyltransferase; HAT, histone acetyltransferase; SUV39h, histone 3 lysine 9 trimethyltransferase; EZH2, histone 3 lysine 27 trimethyltransferase.

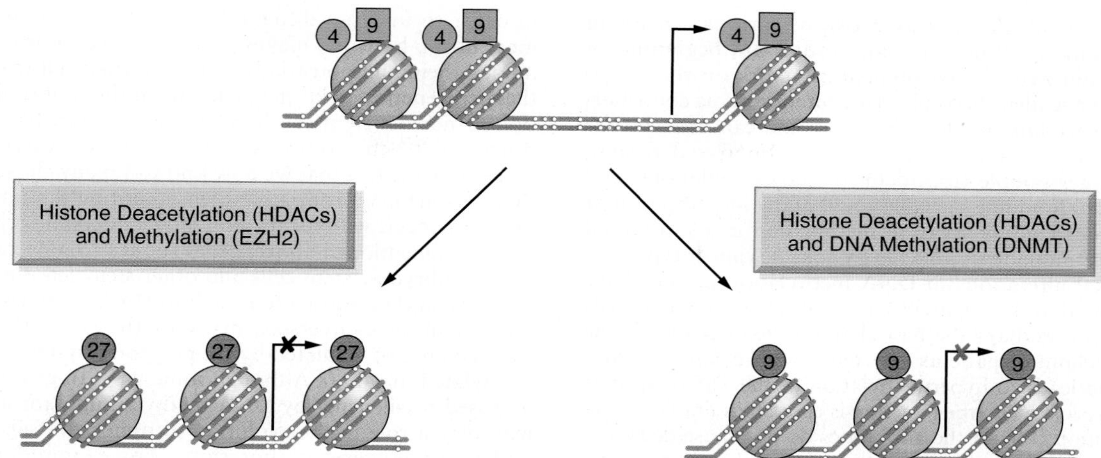

FIGURE 3.2 DNA methylation, histone modifications, and nucleosome occupancy define active and silenced states. The figure depicts a hypothetical CpG island that is active in gene expression and contains unmethylated CpG sites (*white dots*) within the CpG island and the presence of active histone H3 marks, including lysine 4 methylation (H3K4me3) (*green circles*) and lysine 9 acetylation (H3K9Ac) (*green squares*). Genes repressed by histone deacetylation and methylation by EZH2 show the insertion of a nucleosome (*large orange circles*) into the transcriptional start site and the application of lysine 27 trimethylation (H3K27me3) (*red circles*). This state is commonly observed in embryonic stem cells and holds genes in a poised silent state so that they can be called upon later for expression during embryogenesis and cell differentiation. The CpG island can also become silenced in a more permanent manner by histone deacetylation and DNA methylation, resulting in the presence of 5-methylcytosine (*red dots*) near the transcriptional start site. The histone mark associated with this state is often (but not exclusively) lysine 9 methylation (*red circles*). Genes silenced by this mechanism tend to be permanently silenced, and examples include genes on the inactive X-chromosome in mammalian cells.

development and maintenance of normal physiologic functions and can become pathologically altered in cancer and precancerous conditions, leading to widespread mitotically heritable aberrations in gene expression that characterize the cancer state.

Epigenetic processes such as those discussed above not only play important roles during development, but also are involved in maintaining tissue-specific patterns of gene expression in differentiated cells. In particular, DNA methylation patterns vary in different cell types, particularly at the transcription start sites of genes that do not contain CpG islands. Although the exact relations between these methylation patterns and control of gene expression have not been completely worked out, they probably assist in mitotic maintenance of differentiated states.

EPIGENOMIC CHANGES IN CANCER

DNA methylation patterns and histone modifications are essential for physiologic processes yet their dysregulation contributes to the cancer process. Epigenomic changes tend to be self-reinforcing and progressive and arise in normal cellular processes such as aging, which is one of the strongest risk factors for cancer. Several elements such as key genes that control the integrity of the genome (e.g., tumor suppressor genes, the adhesiveness of cells, the regulation of cell division, and the execution of apoptotic pathways) are all subject to inappropriate epigenetic silencing in cancer cells.

The field of cancer epigenetics started more than three decades ago with the observation that DNA methylation levels were profoundly altered in cancer cells relative to their normal counterparts.[5] Subsequently, it became clear that the overall hypomethylation of the genome observed in cancer relative to normal cells was accompanied by focal hypermethylation near the TSS of key regulatory genes such as tumor suppressor genes.[6] This focal hypermethylation of the CpG island regions at the TSS of the genes is associated with mitotically heritable silencing. Because of the inherent ability of DNA methylation patterns to be copied over a protracted time period, it was soon realized that these methylation changes could result in a molecular pathway that satisfies Knudson's hypothesis for the inactivation of tumor suppressor genes. Knudson hypothesized that at least two hits were required for the inactivation of tumor suppressor genes in familial cancers such as retinoblastoma (RB).[7] He proposed that mutations in the coding regions of genes such as the *RB* gene, followed by a loss of the wild-type copy through various pathways, could give rise to the cancer phenotype. However, we now know that inappropriate methylation of the TSS of a gene can also result in its mitotically heritable silencing and give rise to the cancer phenotype.[6] This hypothesis has been confirmed in several human cancers, including gastric cancers in Pacific Islanders. In these cases, families bearing a germline mutation in one allele of the E-cadherin gene show a high propensity for developing gastric cancer at later stages in their lives.[8] In many cases, the wild-type allele of the gene had become inappropriately silenced by aberrant DNA methylation, therefore leading to the initiation of the carcinogenic process in the stomach epithelium.

Widespread alterations in DNA methylation patterns in specific genes known to participate in human carcinogenesis have been identified in numerous studies. In addition, methylation-induced dysregulation of genomic imprinting is also found in cancer. Loss of imprinting of *IGF2* and other imprinted genes have been associated with various childhood and adult cancers. The development of new high-throughput sequencing technologies has resulted in the discovery of even more loci that undergo epigenetic changes, some of which are relevant to the cancer phenotype. This has allowed identification of specific epigenetic cancer signatures such as the CpG island methylator phenotype (CIMP) in sporadic colorectal cancer.[9] Many of these changes occur as a function of aging, which may explain the increased risk of various cancers in older individuals.[10] Epidemiologic studies are beginning to reveal the influence of environmental factors on the epigenome[11] and have identified epigenetic alterations as contributing mechanisms, linking lifestyle factors and cancer incidence and prognosis.[12,13] Future studies with improved design, including larger sample sizes, defined study populations, and control for confounding variables, will allow identification of the key loci affected by aberrant methylation in a substantial proportion of individuals affected by specific cancer types.[14]

Substantial alterations in DNA methylation pattern have also been found in the apparently normal tissues of individuals with infections. Perhaps the best characterized example is the gastric epithelium of patients infected by *Helicobacter pylori*. The infection leads to hypermethylation of the TSS of specific genes that are lost when the infection is cured by suitable antibiotic intervention.[15] Since the antibiotics do not cause demethylation directly, the loss of hypermethylation in these individuals is probably due to the loss of chronic inflammation. Since infections such as *H. pylori*, human papilloma virus, and other viral infections are causal players in carcinogenesis, these changes suggest that epigenetic alterations may play pivotal roles in the formation of cancers in infected individuals.

More recently with the development of chromatin immunoprecipitation (ChIP), coupled with high-throughput sequencing (ChIP-Seq), it has been realized that changes in DNA methylation are only part of the epigenomic alterations in cancer cells. Widespread alterations in the chromatin of cancer cells include genes that, although not silenced by DNA methylation, are repressed by histone modifications such as the application of aberrant patterns of H3K27me3 by the enzyme EZH2.[16] Although these changes may not be as mitotically stable as those induced by DNA hypermethylation, they nevertheless represent important therapeutic targets. Likewise, genes silenced by histone acetylation can be reactivated by treatment with histone deacetylase drugs. Thus, the field of cancer epigenetics is moving into a more holistic appreciation of epigenome-wide changes that occur in human cancer and an understanding of how these dysregulations contribute to cancer pathology.

THE TIMING OF EPIGENETIC ALTERATIONS

Aberrant epigenetic gene silencing probably occurs at a very early stage in neoplastic development. Epimutations may therefore be initiators in carcinogenesis, allowing for the early clonal expansion of cells subsequently at risk for additional alterations. The abnormal silencing of epigenetic "gatekeepers" might be induced by risk factors such as aging and inflammation.[17] Such gatekeepers normally restrict the division potential of stem cells to balance stem or precursor cell hierarchies. Silencing of genes such as *p16*, *SFRPs*, *GATA4* and *GATA5*, and *APC* in the colon, for example, may lock these cells into a proliferative state, thus creating a population of cells at increased risk for additional epigenetic and genetic aberrations.

Recent epigenomic analyses have suggested that genes that control the growth and differentiation of stem cells are often suppressed by the polycomb repressive complex and that their activation results in the cessation of growth in stem cell populations. An early epigenetic alteration that could involve a switch from one type of silencing mechanism to another may be pivotal in moving the genes from a repressed but reversible configuration into a permanently locked state. Indeed, genes silenced by the polycomb repressive complex that involves H3K27me3 are at a much increased risk of switching to a DNA methylation state.[16] Locking these genes may make it difficult for cells to express them at key developmental times in order to undergo differentiation. The change in silencing mechanism, however, makes genes sensitive to drugs that can unlock them and potentially restore normal cell regulation. If these epigenetic gatekeeper genes are at the root of the disruption of normal stem cell homeostasis in epithelia, epigenetic drugs may be able to reverse the early steps of carcinogenesis.

Despite the fact that we now know of many classes of genes that become inappropriately silenced during the formation of human cancer, we still do not fully understand the mechanisms. As mentioned above, genes subject to polycomb silencing in embryonic stem cells and other stem cell types seem to be particularly disposed to switch to DNA methylation silencing in cancer. Conversely, many of the genes that become silenced are not regulated by the polycomb system yet become methylated in cancer. Although some types of genes seem predisposed to silencing by DNA methylation, natural selection may play a role in the evolution of tumors in cells that have undergone epigenetic alterations. For example, epigenetic silencing of a gene (such as *p16*) that restricts cellular growth might allow for the progressive selection of cells that have gradually begun to silence the gene. Evidence for the role of selection comes from studies in which tumors harboring *p16* gene mutations show expression of the mutant but not the wild-type allele.[18] Since the promoters of both the wild-type and mutant allele are identical, yet only one undergoes DNA methylation silencing, epigenetic processes in cancer cells may be selected for in the host by giving a cell a growth advantage in an evolving process.[19]

The role of the polycomb repressive complex 2 (PRC2) in preventing cellular differentiation in embryonic stem cells and its subsequent dysregulation in cancer provides a basis for understanding these two processes. Levels of the histone methyltransferase (EZH2), which is part of the polycomb complex and another protein BMI1, are significantly up-regulated in cancer.[20] The normal function of PRC2 is to control genes in embryonic stem cells and differentiated cells; up-regulation of these proteins may repress genes controlling cell division. The mechanisms responsible for the up-regulation of EZH2 have remained obscure; however, a particular miRNA (mir101) has recently been found to down-regulate the level of EZH2 in physiologic states.[21] Since mir101 is commonly down-regulated in cancer, this may lead to an increase in the EZH2 protein followed by down-regulation of genes, decreasing differentiation and increasing cell growth. This type of dysregulation may be important in the regulation of stem cells and possibly cancer progenitor cells and thus represent an excellent drug target.

Inappropriate gene activation is also a hallmark of cancer, and this process can have an epigenetic basis as well. Hypomethylation of the genome is common in most human neoplasms and leads to demethylation of repetitive elements such as Alus and long interspersed nuclear elements (LINEs), resulting in genome instability. Alternatively it might lead to ectopic gene expression if it occurs in a potentially functional Alu or LINE promoter.[22] Hypomethylation of CpG-poor promoters may also activate cancer-related genes such as oncogenes. Translocations may also reprogram epigenetic modifiers such as in the *MLL* fusion gene, which is a histone methyltransfease resulting in decreased levels of H3K4me3 (Table 3.1, Fig. 3.1) and decreased gene expression.

EPIGENETIC BIOMARKERS FOR EARLY DETECTION OF CANCER

Since aberrant DNA hypermethylation is among the most common molecular alterations in human neoplasia and involved in the early stages of tumorigenesis, it lends itself as a biomarker for early detection with the ultimate goal of preventing advanced stages of cancer and death. Attributes of a good biomarker include high sensitivity and specificity. DNA hypermethylation of gatekeeper genes such as tumor-suppressor genes is highly specific to neoplastic cells, and methylation microarrays have revealed tissue- and tumor-type-specific patterns. A panel of genes with a high frequency of hypermethylation in cancer can probably be identified,[23] and sensitive methods for the detection of DNA methylation are available. Easy accessibility of DNA from tumor cells is essential for the successful population-based application. As tumor tissue cannot always be easily obtained, sophisticated techniques are available to capture circulating tumor cells in blood, urine, and other bodily fluids[24] may be coupled with highly sensitive DNA methylation methods. Alternatively, DNA from peripheral blood lymphocytes or whole blood cells has shown aberrant methylation correlated with patterns found in tumor tissues and is easily accessible.[25]

A number of studies support the potential of DNA methylation markers for the early detection of various cancers, including prostate,[26] bladder,[27] breast,[28] lung,[29] and others. Some of these studies have demonstrated that aberrant methylation changes can be observed several years prior to cancer diagnosis. Additional studies with improved design, including larger samples size, appropriate selection of the case and control population with prediagnostic samples, adjustment for confounding variables, and use of standardized DNA methylation techniques, will be necessary to establish and validate reference panels of characteristically methylated genes.[30,31]

EPIGENETIC THERAPIES

The occurrence of widespread epigenetic alterations, particularly aberrant DNA methylation in human cancers, has encouraged the development of drugs that can reverse these epimutations and restore normal gene expression patterns to cancer cells. The fact that epigenetic alterations can be observed early in the process of carcinogenesis makes this process an attractive target for chemoprevention. Currently there are four drugs that have been approved by the U.S. Food and Drug Administration (FDA) for the treatment of hematologic malignancies (Fig. 3.3). The nucleoside analogues 5-azacytidine (5-aza-CR) and 5-aza-2′-deoxycytidine (5-aza-CdR) were initially developed in Czechoslovakia in the 1960s as cancer chemotherapy agents.[32] These drugs have unstable pyrimidine rings and it was thought that they might be effective cytotoxins following incorporation into DNA and the subsequent hydrolysis of the azanucleoside ring. The azanucleoside ring, however, is quite stable once incorporated into the DNA helix and acts as a powerful mechanism-based inhibitor of DNMTs.[33] These enzymes, responsible for epigenetic maintenance of transcriptional memory, extract the cytosine ring from the DNA molecule, form a covalent bond with the six position of the pyrimidine, and reinsert the base into the helix

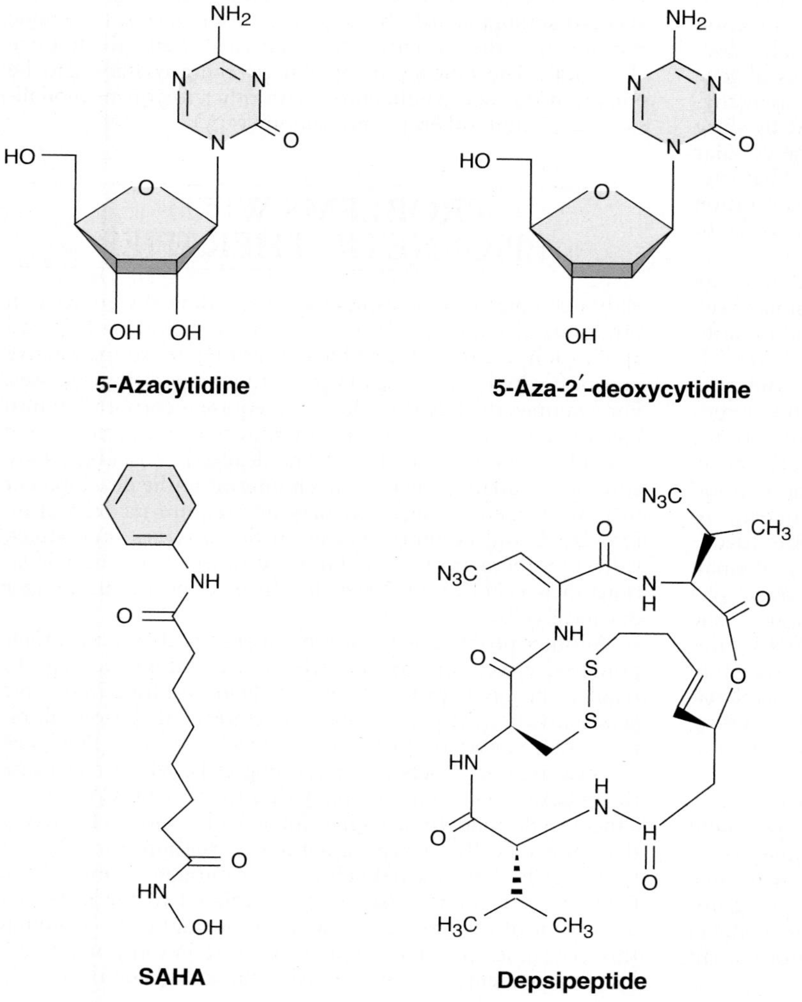

FIGURE 3.3 Structures of epigenetic drugs currently approved for use in humans by the U.S. Food and Drug Administration. The DNA methylation inhibitors (5-aza-CR and 5-aza-CdR) are both approved for use with myeloid dysplastic syndrome (MDS), and the two histone deacetylase inhibitors, suberoylanilide hydroxamic acid (SAHA) and depsipeptide, are approved for use in cutaneous T-cell lymphoma.

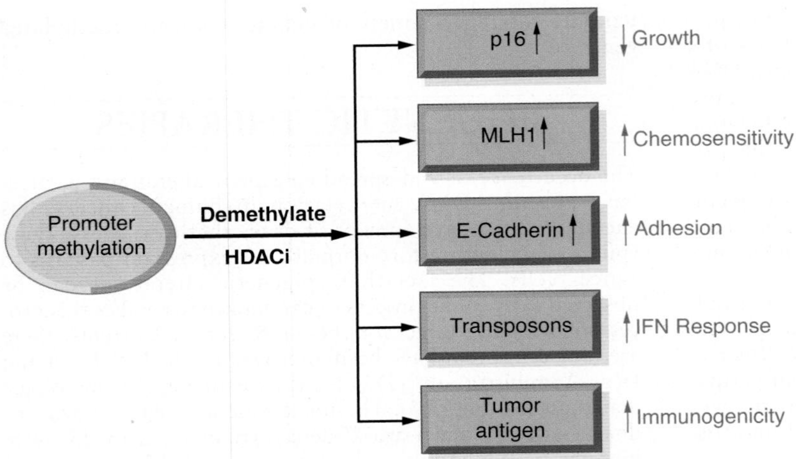

FIGURE 3.4 Combination therapies with DNA methylation inhibitors and histone deacetylase inhibitors can lead to the activation of genes inappropriately silenced in multiple pathways relevant for the generation of human cancer. Activation of these pathways by a drug regimen can result in many properties relevant to normal cell function such as decreased growth rate, increase in chemosensitivity, increased adhesion, and increased response to immunologic activities.

following the transfer of a methyl group to the five position of the cytosine. DNMTs become attached to DNA containing 5-azacytosine, which leads to proteolytic destruction of the enzymes and a pharmacologic knockdown of DNMT activity.[34] Thus, both drugs require incorporation into DNA, and the ribose analogue (5-aza-CR) needs to be reduced by ribonucleotide reductase in order to enter the DNA during DNA synthesis. Although both drugs are cytotoxic at high doses, their optimal biological effects in inducing gene expression are at lower concentrations. They are both extraordinarily effective at removing DNA methylation from newly synthesized DNA resulting in gene reactivation. Once a hypomethylation pattern has been induced, it can be carried over through subsequent cell divisions, resulting in prolonged alterations of gene expression. Unfortunately, cells show a tendency to remethylate DNA sequences that have been demethylated by drug treatment, resulting in the gradual blunting of the cellular response.[35] This problem requires understanding of what triggers remethylation and the development of a new generation of therapeutics that can be repeatedly administered in order to prevent the remethylation process.

Although the causal relation between the chemically induced DNA hypomethylation and gene expression has been well established in cell culture models, it has been more difficult to demonstrate this causality in patients. The 5-Aza-CR prolonged life expectancy of myeloid dysplastic syndrome (MDS) patients in a phase 3 clinical trial[36] and this hypomethylating agent has now become the standard of care for this type of premalignant condition. Global demethylation occurs in the cells of treated patients; however, the relation between the demethylation and a clinical response remains to be demonstrated.[37] The deoxy analogue 5-aza-CdR (decitabine) has also shown good responses in a variety of small clinical trials; however, a large trial failed to show a survival benefit for patients.[38] This result was surprising, since the deoxy analogue is more directly incorporated into DNA without concomitant incorporation into RNA and would therefore be expected to be more effective in the clinic. Possible explanations include a suboptimal study design regarding drug dosing and scheduling, and future trials will directly compare the efficacies of the two analogues.

The two histone deacetylase inhibitors suberoylanilide hydroxamic acid (SAHA) and depsipeptide have been found effective in the treatment of cutaneous T-cell lymphomas.[39] These agents are relatively nonspecific inhibitors of histone deacetylase enzymes. As with the DNA demethylation agents, the clinical efficacy of the drugs have been demonstrated, yet the causal relation between histone acetylation and patient outcome remains to be shown.

Because epigenetic processes are highly interactive and reinforce one another, there is considerable interest in the development of combination therapies, in particular combinations between DNA demethylation and histone deacetylase inhibitors. Since gene expression requires both demethylation and histone acetylation, combinations of drugs that alter both processes may be more effective in treating cancer. Several clinical trials have been designed to test this hypothesis in an attempt to increase the reach of epigenetic therapies beyond the hematological arena into the treatment of solid tumors. Since many pathways relevant to cancer development are silenced simultaneously by epigenetic mechanisms, epigenetic therapy has the potential to reactivate them all at once (Fig. 3.4). The efficacy of epigenetic therapy may also be enhanced through combination with other treatment modalities (e.g., immunotherapy or chemotherapy).

PROBLEMS WITH EPIGENETIC THERAPIES

Although epigenetic therapies have been clinically effective in randomized trials, problems remain with the widespread application to cancer care. One concern relates to the relative nonspecificity of the drugs in inhibiting epigenetic processes. For example, the DNMT inhibitors require incorporation into DNA where they are effective inhibitors of all three known DNMTs. Also, few specific histone deacetylase inhibitors are currently available. There is much interest in the development of more targeted drugs that may not require incorporation into DNA and be more specific in the enzymes they affect. Currently there are few inhibitors of other histone modifications such as H3K27me3, which is likely to be a critical target in cancer cells.

Another problem with current epigenetic therapies is their potential effects on normal cells and collateral damage to regular epigenetic processes within them, resulting in ectopic gene activation. However, since the DNA methylation inhibitors require incorporation into DNA to be effective, they have no measureable effects on noncycling cells, which constitute the bulk of the cell population within the patient. Conversely, cancer cells tend to scavenge nucleosides more effectively than normal cells, incorporating more drug into the DNA of cancer cells than normal cells, which mitigates some of the concern.[40] There are also concerns related to the potential activation of oncogenic pathways in normal cells, although this does not appear to be as serious as initially imagined. However, patients currently receiving these drugs unfortunately do not have their lives extended to the point where secondary carcinogenic effects might become manifest. The remaining uncertainty makes it unlikely for these agents to find application in diseases that are not life-threatening. In the future, nonnucleoside inhibitors of DNA methylation that can be repeatedly administered may have the potential to reverse epimutations and significantly decrease the manifestation of cancer.

Selected References

1. Jones PA, Liang G. Rethinking how DNA methylation patterns are maintained. *Nat Rev Genet* 2009;10:805.
2. Bernstein BE, Mikkelsen TS, Xie X, et al. A bivalent chromatin structure marks key developmental genes in embryonic stem cells. *Cell* 2006;125:315.
3. Campos EI, Reinberg D. Histones: annotating chromatin. *Annu Rev Genet* 2009;43:559.
4. Lin JC, Jeong S, Liang G, et al. Role of nucleosomal occupancy in the epigenetic silencing of the MLH1 CpG island. *Cancer Cell* 2007;12:432.
5. Riggs AD, Jones PA. 5-methylcytosine, gene regulation, and cancer. *Adv Cancer Res* 1983;40:1.
6. Jones PA, Laird PW. Cancer epigenetics comes of age. *Nat Genet* 1999;21:163.
7. Knudson AG Jr. Mutation and cancer: statistical study of retinoblastoma. *Proc Natl Acad Sci U S A* 1971;68:820.
8. Grady WM, Willis J, Guilford PJ, et al. Methylation of the CDH1 promoter as the second genetic hit in hereditary diffuse gastric cancer. *Nat Genet* 2000;26:16.
9. Toyota M, Ahuja N, Ohe-Toyota M, et al. CpG island methylator phenotype in colorectal cancer. *Proc Natl Acad Sci U S A* 1999;96:8681.
10. Issa JP. Epigenetic variation and human disease. *J Nutr* 2002;132:2388S.
11. Christensen BC, Houseman EA, Marsit CJ, et al. Aging and environmental exposures alter tissue-specific DNA methylation dependent upon CpG island context. *PLoS Genet* 2009;5:e1000602.
12. Waterland RA, Michels KB. Epigenetic epidemiology of the developmental origins hypothesis. *Annu Rev Nutr* 2007;27:363.
13. Marsit CJ, Houseman EA, Schned AR, et al. Promoter hypermethylation is associated with current smoking, age, gender and survival in bladder cancer. *Carcinogenesis* 2007;28:1745.
14. Michels KB. The promises and challenges of epigenetic epidemiology. *Exp Gerontol* 2010;45:297.
15. Niwa T, Tsukamoto T, Toyoda T, et al. Inflammatory processes triggered by Helicobacter pylori infection cause aberrant DNA methylation in gastric epithelial cells. *Cancer Res* 2010;70:1430.
16. Gal-Yam EN, Egger G, Iniguez L, et al. Frequent switching of polycomb repressive marks and DNA hypermethylation in the PC3 prostate cancer cell line. *Proc Natl Acad Sci U S A* 2008;105:12979.
17. Jones PA, Baylin SB. The fundamental role of epigenetic events in cancer. *Nat Rev Genet* 2002;3:415.
18. Myohanen SK, Baylin SB, Herman JG. Hypermethylation can selectively silence individual p16ink4A alleles in neoplasia. *Cancer Res* 1998;58:591.
19. Varambally S, Cao Q, Mani RS, et al. Genomic loss of microRNA-101 leads to overexpression of histone methyltransferase EZH2 in cancer. *Science* 2008;322:1695.
20. Varambally S, Dhanasekaran SM, Zhou M, et al. The polycomb group protein EZH2 is involved in progression of prostate cancer. *Nature* 2002;419:624.
21. Friedman JM, Liang G, Liu CC, et al. The putative tumor suppressor microRNA-101 modulates the cancer epigenome by repressing the polycomb group protein EZH2. *Cancer Res* 2009;69:2623.
22. Wolff EM, Byun HM, Han HF, et al. Hypomethylation of a LINE-1 promoter activates an alternate transcript of the MET oncogene in bladders with cancer. *PLoS Genet* 2010;6(4):e1000917.
23. Laird PW. The power and the promise of DNA methylation markers. *Nat Rev Cancer* 2003;3:253.
24. Nagrath S, Sequist LV, Maheswaran S, et al. Isolation of rare circulating tumour cells in cancer patients by microchip technology. *Nature* 2007;450:1235.
25. Sharma G, Mirza S, Prasad CP, et al. Promoter hypermethylation of p16INK4A, p14ARF, CyclinD2 and Slit2 in serum and tumor DNA from breast cancer patients. *Life Sci* 2007;80:1873.
26. Cairns P, Esteller M, Herman JG, et al. Molecular detection of prostate cancer in urine by GSTP1 hypermethylation. *Clin Cancer Res* 2001;7:2727.
27. Hoque MO, Begum S, Topaloglu O, et al. Quantitation of promoter methylation of multiple genes in urine DNA and bladder cancer detection. *J Natl Cancer Inst* 2006;98:996.
28. Novak P, Jensen TJ, Garbe JC, et al. Stepwise DNA methylation changes are linked to escape from defined proliferation barriers and mammary epithelial cell immortalization. *Cancer Res* 2009;69:5251.
29. Palmisano WA, Divine KK, Saccomanno G, et al. Predicting lung cancer by detecting aberrant promoter methylation in sputum. *Cancer Res* 2000;60:5954.
30. Brooks J, Cairns P, Zeleniuch-Jacquotte A. Promoter methylation and the detection of breast cancer. *Cancer Causes Control* 2009;20:1539.
31. Cairns P. Gene methylation and early detection of genitourinary cancer: the road ahead. *Nat Rev Cancer* 2007;7:531.
32. Vesely J, Cihak A. 5-Azacytidine: mechanism of action and biological effects in mammalian cells. *Pharmac Ther A* 1978;2:813.
33. Jones PA, Taylor SM. Cellular differentiation, cytidine analogs and DNA methylation. *Cell* 1980;20:85.
34. Ghoshal K, Datta J, Majumder S, et al. 5-Aza-deoxycytidine induces selective degradation of DNA methyltransferase 1 by a proteasomal pathway that requires the KEN box, bromo-adjacent homology domain, and nuclear localization signal. *Mol Cell Biol* 2005;25:4727.
35. Bender CM, Gonzalgo ML, Gonzales FA, et al. Roles of cell division and gene transcription in the methylation of CpG islands. *Mol Cell Biol* 1999;19:6690.
36. Fenaux P, Mufti GJ, Hellstrom-Lindberg E, et al. Efficacy of azacitidine compared with that of conventional care regimens in the treatment of higher-risk myelodysplastic syndromes: a randomised, open-label, phase III study. *Lancet Oncol* 2009;10:223.
37. Yang AS, Doshi KD, Choi SW, et al. DNA methylation changes after 5-aza-2′-deoxycytidine therapy in patients with leukemia. *Cancer Res* 2006;66:5495.
38. Lübbert M. Epigenetic therapy for myelodysplastic syndromes has entered center stage. *Leuk Res* 2009;33(Suppl 2):S27.
39. Marks PA, Xu WS. Histone deacetylase inhibitors: potential in cancer therapy. *J Cell Biochem* 2009;107:600.
40. Cheng JC, Yoo CB, Weisenberger DJ, et al. Preferential response of cancer cells to zebularine. *Cancer Cell* 2004;6:151.

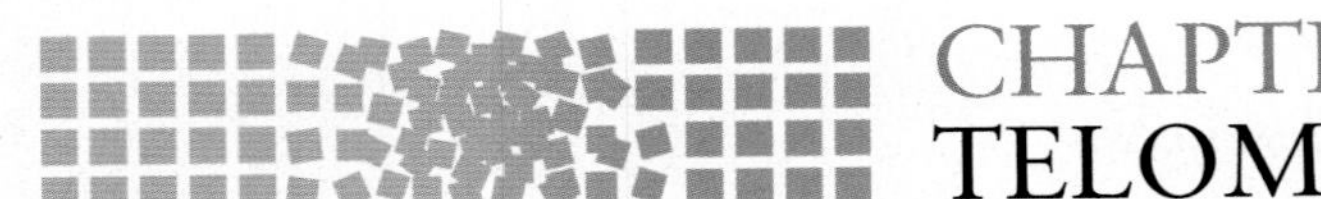

CHAPTER 4 TELOMERES, TELOMERASE, AND CANCER

KWOK-KIN WONG, NORMAN E. SHARPLESS, AND RONALD A. DEPINHO

Maintenance of most adult organ systems requires extensive cell renewal, typified most strikingly by the replacement of the intestinal lining on a weekly basis and the production of trillions of new blood cells daily. Yet a lifetime of factors including continual telomere erosion, errors in DNA replication, intrinsic and carcinogen-induced somatic mutations, cancer-relevant germline variants, and epigenetic insults conspire to endow cells with the large number of changes needed for malignant transformation. How is it that replicating tissues, showered with myriad cancer-relevant somatic alterations, resist malignant transformation? That these mutations are indeed present in normal human tissues is reflected by the remarkable observations that roughly 1% of neonatal cord blood collections contain significant numbers of myeloid clones harboring oncogenic fusions such as the AML1-ETO fusion associated with acute leukemia,[1] and that approximately one-third of adults possess the *IgH-BCL2* translocation associated with follicular lymphomagenesis.[2] As the prevalence of these cancers is far lower in the general population, these observations imply that potent tumor suppressor mechanisms must be operating to constrain the growth and survival of these aspiring cancer cells.

The most prominent biologic manifestations of an activated tumor suppressor response are apoptosis (cell death) and senescence (permanent cell cycle arrest). These biologic processes are linked to powerful checkpoint effector molecules involving the $p16^{INK4a}$-Rb pathway, the ARF-p53 pathway, and specialized chromosomal DNA ends termed *telomeres*. These genetic elements comprise powerful tumor suppressor barriers and act cooperatively to eliminate or to place a limit on the replicative lifespan of rogue would-be cells. The importance of apoptosis in preventing cancer is further discussed in Chapter 7. The focus of this chapter will be on the role of telomere dynamics and associated telomere-related cellular checkpoint processes, particularly senescence, in the regulation of neoplastic transformation. A significant body of clinical and translational science now supports such a role for telomeres and cellular senescence, and in this chapter, we present rapidly increasing clinical data pointing to the relevance of these processes in human disease, particularly cancer. Indeed, it is worth noting that the Nobel Prize for physiology or medicine in 2009 was awarded to Blackburn, Greider, and Szostak for their pioneering and seminal work in telomere biology that advanced our present understanding of aging and cancer.

TELOMERES AND TELOMERASE

Telomere dysfunction is a principal tumor suppressor mechanism manifesting most prominently as apoptosis and senescence. At the same time, when accompanied by functional p53 loss, the genome-destabilizing impact of telomere dysfunction can cause widespread mutations that propel normal cells toward malignant transformation. Thus, the telomere-based anticancer mechanism can actually fuel tumorigenesis in certain contexts. The knowledge of the basic biology of telomeres and telomerase has yielded fundamental insights into both cancer prevention and cancer promotion. The powerful and complex impact of telomere dynamics in model organisms and humans reflects the crucial role of telomere function in processes of genomic instability, organ homeostasis, chronic diseases, aging, and tumorigenesis. With respect to tumorigenesis, the study of telomeres in the mouse has provided insight into how advancing age in humans fuels the development of epithelial cancers as well as how chronic inflammation and degeneration may engender increased cancer risk in affected organs. These advances in the basic understanding of telomere maintenance are now being translated into clinically relevant applications that may have an impact on the diagnosis and management of a broad spectrum of cancers as well as aging, age-related disorders, and degenerative conditions. The important role of telomere biology in aging and degenerative diseases has been reviewed elsewhere.[3,4]

Telomeres

Telomeres are specialized nucleoprotein complexes at the ends of linear chromosomes consisting of long arrays of double-stranded TTAGGG repeats, a G-rich 3′ single-strand overhang, and associated telomeric repeat binding[5–7] (Fig. 4.1). The work of Muller and McClintock in the 1930s led to the concept that telomeres function to "cap" chromosomal termini and prevent end-to-end recombination, thereby maintaining chromosomal integrity. Subsequent work has substantiated this model across the animal and plant kingdom, underscoring the critical roles served by the telomere complex.

Telomere structure and function have been studied extensively in mammals. Although the overall structural features of telomeres are preserved among different mammalian organisms, lengths can vary considerably from species to species: for example, 5 to 15 kb for humans versus 20 to 80 kb for the laboratory mouse. On the structural level, electron microscopy and other studies have shown that telomeres form complex secondary and tertiary structures via DNA-DNA interactions between the telomeric repeats, DNA-protein interactions between the telomeric DNA and the telomeric repeat binding proteins (shelterins or telosomes[8,9]), and protein-protein interactions between the telomeric repeat binding proteins themselves and other associated proteins (Fig. 4.1). The formation of this well-documented, higher-order DNA-protein complex has provided a working model of how the telomere functions as a capping structure, preventing the ends of linear chromosomal

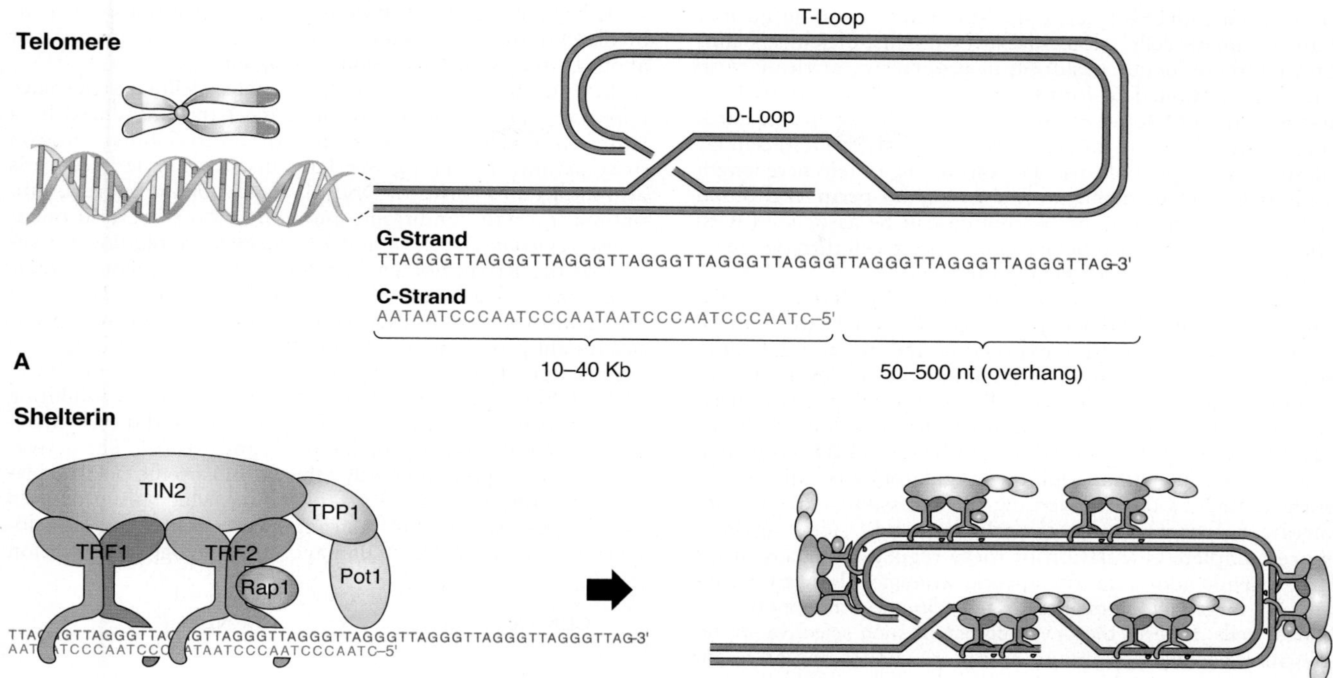

FIGURE 4.1. Human telomere structure. **A:** Human telomeres form telomere loop (T loop) and displacement loop (D loop) secondary structures. Long stretches of telomeric repeats create a loop-back structure (T loop), completed by the invasion of the single GT-rich 3′ overhang into the double-stranded DNA molecule (D loop), thus protecting the chromosome terminus. **B:** In human cells, double-stranded telomeric repeats are bound directly by two proteins, TRF1 (TTAGG repeat binding factor 1) and TRF2. Cell culture studies have suggested that the main function of TRF1 is to regulate telomere length, whereas TRF2 functions to protect telomeres from activating nonhomologous end-joining (NHEJ) and other DNA repair or DNA damage response pathways. TRF2 also interacts with the human Rap1 protein (hRap). Biochemical studies also suggest that the formation of the T loop depends on TRF2. Another protein, POT1 (protection of telomere 1), has been shown to bind to the single-stranded human telomeric 3′ overhang. Two shelterin proteins, TIN2 and TPP1, connect POT1 to TRF1 and TRF2. POT1 has been proposed to interact with TRF1 complexes to regulate telomere length. Thus, there is significant interplay between telomeric binding proteins and the formation of the secondary/tertiary structures that protect the ends of chromosomes.

DNA from being recognized as either a DNA double-strand break (DSB) or DNA single-strand break, thereby avoiding activation of the DNA damage response and the formation of chromosomal end-to-end fusions through the DNA repair machinery.[7]

Many proteins involved in DNA DSB repair, including nonhomologous end-joining and homologous recombination processes, have been found to be physically associated with the telomeres.[7–10] These findings have fueled speculation that DSB repair proteins provide a protective role at the telomere; for example, by sequestering the telomere end from the DNA damage surveillance/repair machinery. Experimental support for this hypothesis has emerged from the mouse, in which germ line inactivation of various repair proteins (e.g., Ku and DNA-PK) results in reduced telomere length or loss of capping function, or both, leading to increased end-to-end fusions.[11] Correspondingly, in cultured human cells, experimental disruption of telomere-binding proteins results in the unraveling of higher-order nucleoprotein structure and telomere localization of DNA DSB surveillance/repair proteins (e.g., 53BP1, gamma-H2AX, Rad17, ATM, and Mre11), establishing that dysfunctional telomeres can indeed serve as substrates for the classic DNA repair machinery.[12] Recently, elegant *in vitro* and mouse genetic experiments have shown that subunits of the shelterin complex actively repress the ATM and ATR DNA damage signaling pathways.[7,13]

A further understanding of the molecular mechanisms governing the repression versus activation of the DNA DSB surveillance/repair apparatus at the telomere could lead to the development of novel cancer therapeutic options. For example, the design of agents that can uncap telomeres while preserving the DNA damage checkpoint response yet neutralize the actual DNA damage repair process would be ideal because they would produce unrepaired DSBs and elicit cell-cycle arrest or apoptosis responses. Lastly, in the near future, agents designed to uncap the telomeres could be used in combination with conventional chemotherapeutic agents that create DSB for cancer treatment, thereby simultaneously targeting these intertwined pathways.

Telomerase

Conventional DNA polymerases operating in the S phase of the cell cycle require an RNA primer for reverse-strand synthesis, resulting in incomplete DNA replication of telomeres during each cell division. The solution to this "end-replication problem" is the telomere-synthesizing telomerase enzyme, a specialized ribonucleoprotein complex with reverse transcriptase activity. The functional telomerase holoenzyme is a large multisubunit complex that includes an essential telomerase RNA (hTERC) component serving as a template for the addition of telomere repeats and a telomerase reverse transcriptase (hTERT) catalytic subunit.[14] In some normal human somatic cells, telomerase levels are insufficient to maintain telomere length, resulting in progressive attrition with each cell division. This forms the basis for the theory that the metered loss of telomeres can serve as a cellular mitotic clock that ultimately limits the number of cell divisions and cellular lifespan. In support of this view, shortening of telomere length with aging can be demonstrated in human peripheral blood cells,[15–17] and the rate of shortening can be associated with conditions of increased hematopoietic stem cell turnover (e.g., in paroxysmal nocturnal hemoglobinuria).[18]

Many normal somatic human cells and differentiated tissues express readily detectable levels of the hTERC component. In contrast, hTERT expression and activity are more restricted because of stringent regulation on the levels of transcriptional initiation, alternative RNA processing, posttranslational modification, and subcellular localization. With the identification of an increasing number of TERT-associated proteins, it is likely that additional regulatory mechanisms will surface, such as those governing the accessibility of the telomerase holoenzyme onto the telomere end.[19] Here again, a more complete elucidation of these regulatory mechanisms may provide additional therapeutic strategies that can preferentially target telomerase-mediated telomere maintenance in cancer cells. Indeed, the development of such selective strategies may become paramount and more challenging as recent studies have revealed low telomerase levels in cycling somatic human cells that were previously thought to have no telomerase activity.[20] Eradication of residual telomerase function in these primary cells alters the maintenance of the 3′ single-strand telomeric overhang without changing the rate of overall telomere shortening, resulting in diminished proliferation rates and overall reduction in proliferative capacity. These studies support an additional protective function of telomerase at the telomeres[21] and raise concerns that generalized antitelomerase therapy could lead to the immediate uncapping of telomeres in normal cells, thus limiting the use of antitelomerase therapy in cancer patients.

Lastly, in addition to forming the telomerase holoenzyme complex with TERC, TERT was recently shown to be able to interact with the RNA component of mitochondrial RNA processing endoribonuclease (RMRP). This distinct TERT/RMRP ribonucleoprotein complex has RNA-dependent RNA polymerase activity and produces double-stranded RNAs that can be processed into small interfering RNAs.[22] Also, there is compelling experimental evidence that TERT can interact and engage the Wnt signaling pathway.[23,24] These results suggest that TERT contributes to cell physiology independently of its ability to elongate telomeres, a fact that further complicates efforts to specifically target telomerase enzymatic activity as an anticancer therapy.

SENESCENCE

Primary human cells, even when cultured under optimal conditions, will eventually encounter a cell division barrier, termed *cellular senescence,* triggered by critically shortened telomeres. Senescence is a specific cell biologic phenotype composed of a permanent and durable growth arrest, alterations in cellular morphology, expression of characteristic markers of senescence such as senescence-associated (SA) β-galactosidase activity, and alterations of chromatin structure to a growth-repressive state.[25] Induction of senescence is intimately associated with p16^{INK4a} and p53 activation, and when induced *in vitro* as a result of telomere dysfunction, this barrier is termed the *Hayflick limit* (M1) in honor of the discoverer of senescence.[26] Because loss of p16^{INK4a}-RB and/or p53 pathway function in primary human cells permits additional cell divisions beyond the Hayflick limit, these pathways appear to be involved in the activation of this senescence program brought about by the "shortened telomere" signal.

Beyond the connection with telomeres, cellular senescence appears to be a general anticancer mechanism, induced by a variety of oncogenic stresses. In addition to telomere erosion or structural uncapping (see later discussion), senescence is also induced by forms of DNA damage, oxidative stress, suboptimal growth conditions, and activation of certain oncogenes (reviewed in refs. 8 and 13). Senescence requires activation of the Rb and/or p53 protein; and expression of their regulators such as p16^{INK4a}, p21^{CIP}, and ARF (Fig. 4.2).[27–30] An important form of senescence is induced by p53, which has several antiproliferative activities including stimulation of the expression of p21^{CIP}, a cyclin-dependent kinase inhibitor. These inhibit progression through the cell cycle by inhibiting cyclin-dependent kinases that phosphorylate and thereby inactivate Rb and related proteins p107 and p130.[31] The activation of p53 is predominantly effected by specific posttranslational modifications and its stabilization, which are prompted by the same stimuli that induce its expression, including telomere dysfunction, DNA damage, and oncogene activation

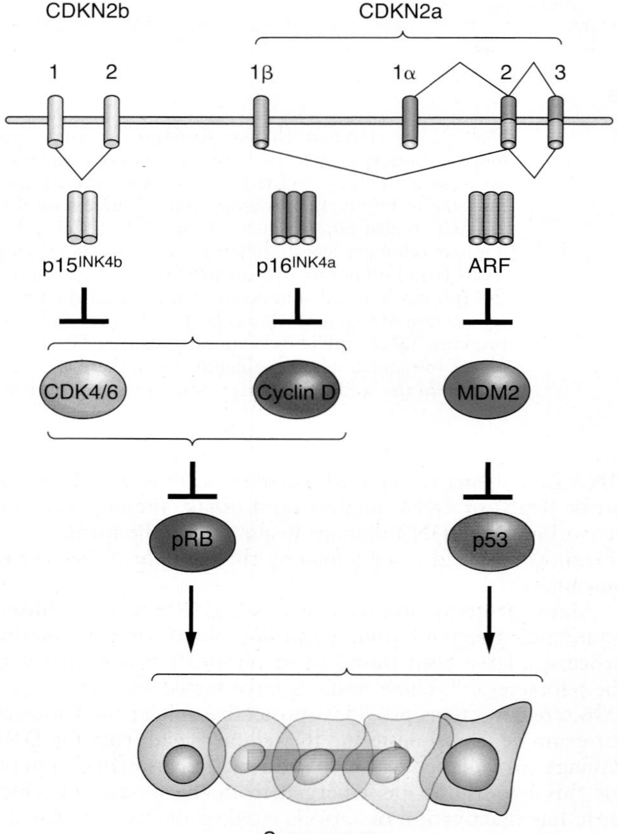

FIGURE 4.2. The *INK4a/ARF/INK4b* locus (also called *CDKN2a* and *CDKN2b*) and downstream pathways. The locus contains three open reading frames encoding the ARF, p15^{INK4b}, and p16^{INK4a} tumor suppressor proteins. p16^{INK4a} and p15^{INK4b} inhibit the activity of the proliferative kinases CDK4/6, which phosphorylate RB and related proteins p107 and p130. Therefore, *INK4* expression induces RB-family hypophosphorylation, which in turn represses E2F-regulated transcription and cell-cycle arrest. ARF inhibits the MDM2-mediated degradation of p53; and p53 stabilization in turn induces a number of targets including many proteins involved in cell-cycle arrest or apoptosis. The entire locus spans a mere 35 kb in the human genome, and inactivation of all three genes by a single genetic deletion is common in many human and murine cancers.

(reviewed in refs. 18 through 20), as well as inappropriate cell cycle entry.[32,33] A major sensor of oncogene activation and inappropriate cell cycle entry is ARF (also designated p14^{ARF} in the human or p19^{ARF} in the mouse), which binds to and blocks MDM2-mediated degradation of p53.[33–36]

Another prominent molecular correlate of senescence is upregulation of the cyclin-dependent kinase inhibitor, p16^{INK4a}, which increases markedly in senescent cells on passage in culture or advancing age in tissues.[37] Correspondingly, ectopic expression of p16^{INK4a} is sufficient to induce senescence in some cell types,[38] and senescence can be delayed or prevented in some cell types by p16^{INK4a} silencing or neutralization by antisense or siRNA.[39–43] The regulation of p16^{INK4a} is not as well understood as that of p53, although it appears to be induced by several stimuli, including oncogene activation and growth in culture.[37] Activation of p53 (and hence p21^{CIP1}) and/or accumulating levels of p16^{INK4a} is able to produce Rb-family member protein hypophosphorylation and activation, which leads to repression of cell-cycle progression,[27,30] enabling initiation of the senescence process. Recent data have suggested that Rb may be of particular importance in the promotion of senescence compared with its related family members p107 and p130, likely explaining the frequent inactivation of Rb in human cancers relative to the other Rb-family members.[44]

Senescence as a Cancer Prevention Mechanism

Several lines of evidence have suggested an important role for senescence in the prevention of cancer *in vivo*. It is important to note that the field has been limited by the lack of robust *in vivo* biomarkers of senescence. Although (SA)-β-galactosidase and p16^{INK4a} expression have been used as markers of *in vivo* senescence, both have certain limitations and neither can be considered unequivocal proof of senescent state *in vivo*. These technical shortcomings notwithstanding, a growth arrest important for the prevention of tumorigenesis with characteristic features of senescence (p16^{INK4a} expression and (SA)-β-galactosidase expression) has been noted in several murine and human *in vivo* tumor systems, and we believe the data suggest bona fide senescence occurs in the intact organism.

The lines of evidence for senescence as a tumor suppressor mechanism are quite strong. First, the aforementioned minimal residual disease data showing frequent oncogenic translocations and other mutagenic events demonstrate a constant need for tumor suppression, even in young animals. Additionally, several of the initially described "tumor suppressor" proteins that are mutated in familial cancer syndromes (e.g., p16^{INK4a}, p53, Rb) are intimately involved in the induction of senescence. Mice lacking p16^{INK4a} or p53 are prone to spontaneous cancers,[45–47] and mice with severe compromise of the senescence pathway due to combined p16^{INK4a} and p53 inactivation die of cancer, often harboring multiple synchronous primary tumors, with a median age of 8 weeks (compared with a normal murine lifespan of more than 100 weeks).[19] Importantly, mice and humans with impaired p16^{INK4a} and/or p53 function develop with only modest phenotypic alterations other than an age-dependent increase in cancer and an increased susceptibility to cancer following carcinogen exposure. Several groups have demonstrated a senescencelike growth arrest in murine and human tissues in association with somatic oncogenic events.[48–54] For example, some forms of benign cutaneous nevi appear to be collections of senescent melanocytes, suggesting that these common benign neoplasms would transform into melanomas were it not for the successful interdiction of this process by the senescence tumor suppressor mechanism. In aggregate, these data establish that senescence-promoting molecules are critical to the prevention of mammalian cancer with advancing age.

Lastly, although the concept of "tumor maintenance" is becoming well established with regard to oncogene-activation,[55] a similarly important role for the persistent inactivation of the senescence checkpoint has been established in cancer. Several groups have established in genetically engineered murine models, for example, that persistent p53 inactivation is required for tumor maintenance.[51,52,56] Therefore, just as the finding that tumors in murine models require persistent RAS activation presaged the successful development of therapeutic compounds such as epidermal growth factor receptor inhibitors that target pathways required for tumor maintenance *in vivo*, similarly, these data support the notion that reactivation of senescence-promoting mechanisms such as p53 could be of therapeutic benefit in some cancers. In fact, it is likely that certain chemotherapeutics exert their therapeutic effects through the promotion of senescence by activating p53 and related senescence-inducing pathways.[57]

Dysfunction of self-renewing somatic stem cell compartments has also been suggested to play a role in organismal aging.[25,58] In this model, the activation of p16^{INK4a} and p53 in response to cellular stresses including telomere dysfunction causes a decline in tissue-regenerative capacity (Fig 4.3). This model is supported by murine studies[59–63] and makes several predictions relevant to human disease. For example, this hypothesis suggests that heritable differences in regulation of the senescence-promoting machinery should alter individual susceptibility to human age-associated diseases, a concept that has been supported by a plethora of recent genomewide association studies.[64] With regard to oncology, this model predicts that some agents and ionizing radiation used to treat cancer, for example, by inducing DNA damage, also can potentially induce senescence of important self-renewing cells of nonmalignant tissues such as the bone marrow. Studies in irradiated or chemotherapy-treated mice support such a role of senescence in the long-term hematopoietic toxicities of these therapeutic approaches.[65,66] Likewise, somatic attrition of regenerative self-renewing cells as a result of senescence activation may place an increased replicative demand on the remaining functional cells of a given tissue, which may increase the rate of telomere dysfunction and speed transformation in other stem cells of a tissue in a cell nonautonomous manner (see later discussion).

In aggregate, these genetic and *in vivo* data support the view that senescence prevents cancer in the intact organism on a near-daily basis and that reactivation of this mechanism in fully established cancers can effect dramatically beneficial responses, but also has the potential to produce long-term toxicity in nonmalignant tissues. It stands to reason that an improved understanding of the molecular basis of senescence could lead to therapeutic approaches designed to beneficially reawaken this potent tumor suppressor mechanism.

The *INK4a/ARF/INK4b* Senescence-Promoting Locus

Senescence is intimately associated with activation of the *INK4a/ARF* locus (also known as *CDKN2a*). This locus possesses an unusual gene structure that dually encodes p16^{INK4a} and ARF (or p14^{ARF} in humans and p19^{ARF} in mice) in nonoverlapping open reading frames (Fig. 4.2). The locus also harbors the neighboring *CDKN2b* gene, which encodes p15^{INK4b}, a protein highly related to p16^{INK4a} that also activates Rb, which is located a short physical distance (10 kb) from the first exon of ARF. In addition to the links of p15^{INK4b}/p16^{INK4a} and ARF to Rb and p53 pathways, respectively, data showing that these proteins play prominent roles in the prevention of human

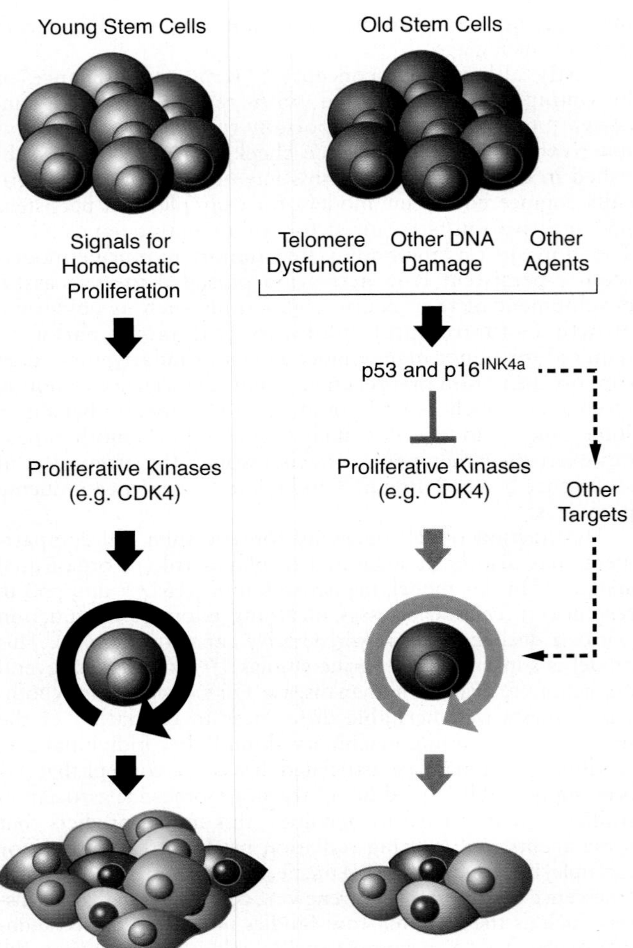

FIGURE 4.3. Senescence and aging. Activation of p53- and/or p16^{INK4a}-mediated senescence pathways in stem cell compartments in response to DNA damage, telomere dysfunction, or other unknown stimuli leads to attrition of tissue-specific stem cells (e.g., hematopoietic stem cell and pancreatic β-cells) with attendant compromise of organ function and aging.

cancer are strong. Activation of the locus in response to stimuli, which may be both independent and dependent on telomere dysfunction, is thought to promote tumor suppression through induction of senescence.

As the *INK4a/ARF/INK4b* locus at chromosome 9p21 is the most frequent site of single copy or homozygous deletion in human cancers,[67,68] extensive analysis of this cytogenetic region has been performed. As somatic deletions in cancer frequently abrogate expression of all three *INK4a/ARF/INK4b* proteins (p15^{INK4b}, p16^{INK4a}, and ARF), debate has focused on which member or members of the locus represents the principal tumor suppressor activity located at human chromosome 9p21. A substantial body of human and murine data has now unequivocally shown that all three proteins are human tumor suppressors.[37] For example, p15^{INK4b} appears mainly important in the suppression of hematopoietic malignancies, whereas p16^{INK4a} and ARF appear to play more general anticancer roles in several tumor types. Elegant murine studies[69] have further shown that these tumor suppressor genes can play "backup" roles to each other, suggesting that combined inactivation of the locus is more oncogenic than deletion of any single member. Therefore, although the human and murine genetic data considered as a whole establish that the *INK4a/ARF/INK4b* locus encodes three major human tumor suppressor proteins, their relative and combinatorial importance in a particular tumor type is a subject of ongoing study.

Crisis, Telomerase Reactivation, and Alternative Lengthening of Telomeres

Under circumstances of extended cell divisions beyond the Hayflick limit with inactivation of the p16^{INK4a} and p53 pathway, progressive telomere erosion ultimately leads to loss of telomere capping function, resulting in increasing chromosomal instability. This leads to progressive loss of cell viability and proliferative capacity across the cell population, ultimately resulting in "cellular crisis." The cellular phenotypes of massive cell death and growth arrest are likely by-products of DNA damage checkpoint responses and rampant chromosomal instability with associated loss of essential genetic material. Emergence from crisis is a rare event in human cell culture and requires restoration of telomere function either by up-regulation of telomerase activity or activation of the alternative lengthening of telomeres (ALT) mechanism.[70] The restoration of functional telomeres serves to quell DNA damage signaling and high levels of chromosomal instability, thereby enhancing the viability of cells with procancer genotypes. Finally, the extent to which normal tissues experience telomere-associated Hayflick and crisis transitions continues to be an area of ongoing investigation. Nevertheless, although clear evidence of the presence of these events is still lacking, strong support is mounting for telomere-based crisis, particularly during early stages of neoplastic development.

Transcriptional up-regulation of the *TERT* gene seems to be a key rate-limiting step in telomerase reactivation, whereas the telomerase-independent ALT pathway appears to be executed via a poorly understood process involving activation of the homologous recombination pathway.[71,72] The analysis of pathways regulating *TERT* gene transcription has forged links to well-known oncoproteins and tumor suppressors including Myc, Mad, and Menin, among others, demonstrating the capacity of these proteins to engage the *TERT* gene promoter directly.[73–75] In contrast, the enigmatic ALT process has been variously associated with p53 deficiency and with tumors of mesenchymal origin.[76]

Studies in yeast have also shown that ALT is enhanced in mismatch repair-deficient cells, owing to increased homologous recombination between chromosomes. The rare use of ALT by epithelial-derived tumors, coupled with functional comparisons of telomerase versus ALT-mediated telomere maintenance, has shown that ALT may not be as biologically robust in advancing malignancy, a finding that diminishes the theoretical concern that ALT may provide a robust resistance mechanism to antitelomerase therapy in advanced malignancy.[77] The idea that ALT may be a less effective telomere maintenance mechanism derives additional support from studies in human cell culture and the mouse revealing that telomerase per se is needed for full malignant transformation, including metastatic potential.[78] The fundamental mechanistic differences between ALT and telomerase reactivation in telomere maintenance may provide an explanation for the report of more favorable clinical outcomes for ALT-positive compared with telomerase-positive glioblastomas,[79] although analysis of 71 human osteosarcoma cases failed to show a more favorable clinical outcome for the ALT-positive subset.[80] However, it should be noted that, in the latter, the absence of any telomere maintenance mechanism was more associated with improved survival than stage or response to chemotherapy, further emphasizing the general importance of telomere maintenance in cancer.

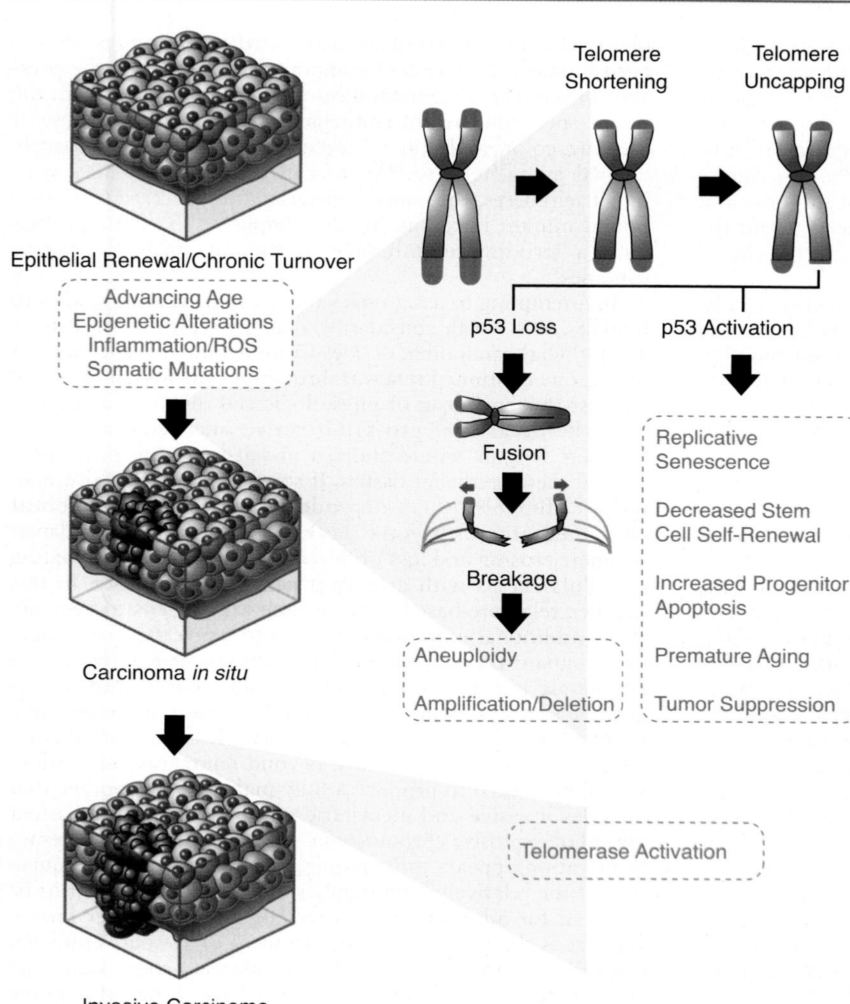

FIGURE 4.4. Dysfunctional telomere-induced genomic instability model of epithelial carcinogenesis. Continuous epithelial turnover during aging coupled with somatic mutations inactivating checkpoint responses is thought to lead to critical telomere erosion, resulting in telomere uncapping and the initiation of breakage-fusion-bridge (BFB) cycles. The double-strand breaks created by the BFB cycles are nidi for amplifications and deletions for the resulting daughter cells. The broken chromosome may become fused to another chromosome, generating a second dicentric chromosome and perpetuating the BFB cycle. This facilitation of the accumulation of genetic changes (via aneuploidy, nonreciprocal translocations, amplifications, and deletions) by the BFB cycles coupled with the reactivation of telomerase enables cells to emerge from crisis and proceed to malignancy.

TELOMERE MAINTENANCE AND CANCER

Robust telomerase activity is observed in more than 80% of all human cancers,[81] a profile consistent with its role in promoting malignant progression. However, another side to the telomerase-cancer connection has emerged from mouse models and correlative data in staged human tumors. These data have indicated that a lack of telomerase and associated telomere attrition during the early stages of neoplastic growth provides a potent mutator mechanism that enables would-be cancer cells to achieve the high threshold of cancer-promoting changes required to traverse the benign to malignant transition.

Indeed, telomeres of human cancer cells are often significantly shorter than their normal tissue counterparts, suggesting that telomere attrition has occurred during the life history of these cancer cells, apparently at very early phases of the transformation process when telomerase activity is low. The subsequent reactivation of telomerase restores telomere function, albeit at a shorter set length. Thus, although reactivation of telomerase is critical to the emergence of immortal human cells, this preceding and transient period of telomere shortening and dysfunction promotes the carcinogenic process through the generation of chromosomal rearrangements. These chromosomal rearrangements are brought about through breakage-fusion-bridge (BFB) cycles (Fig. 4.4). A DSB created by these BFB cycles is now known to provide a nidus for amplification and/or deletion at the site of breakage for the resulting daughter cells. The broken chromosome may become fused to another chromosome, generating a second dicentric chromosome and perpetuating the BFB cycle. The accumulation of wholesale genetic changes via aneuploidy, nonreciprocal translocations, amplifications, and deletions by the BFB cycles coupled with the reactivation of telomerase enables rare cells incurring a threshold number of carcinogenic changes needed to initiate the transformation process.

Although at first glance the cancer-promoting effects of telomere-based crisis seem to counter the established role of telomerase activation in cancer progression, this mechanism is less paradoxical if one considers that many early-stage cancers deactivate pathways essential for telomere checkpoint responses, thus increasing the survival and proliferation of cells experiencing increasing chromosomal instability.[75,82] This hypothesis of "episodic instability" derives additional support from genetic studies in the mouse showing that telomere-based crisis coupled with loss of the p53-dependent DNA damage response can act cooperatively to effect malignant transformation. In humans, the accumulation of oncogenic lesions during normal aging or accelerated accumulation of DNA damage (e.g., environmental carcinogen exposure or oxidative damage) may deactivate the telomere checkpoint response, accelerate telomere attrition, and drive the affected premalignant cells into crisis. It is the rare transformed cell that emerges from this process, often with reactivated telomerase. Thus, telomeric shortening can be viewed as a barrier to cancer development in the presence of intact checkpoint response and as a facilitator for numerous genetic changes necessary for the emergence of nascent cancer cells in the absence of the checkpoint response pathways.

It has also been suggested that telomere dysfunction can be oncogenic in a cell nonautonomous process.[83] Murine data in the hematopoietic system suggest that telomere dysfunction leads to stem cell dysfunction.[84,85] Therefore, telomere dysfunction could induce premature loss of stem cells (as described in Fig. 4.3), which might induce a compensatory hyperproliferation of remaining functional stem cells. This increased proliferative drive might facilitate mutagenesis in the remaining functional self-renewing cells, and in turn select for clones with damaged genomes, in particular those harboring defects in the senesce-promoting machinery.

Several recent lines of evidence have suggested that the oncogenic effects of telomere dysfunction are an important determinant of susceptibility to human cancer. For example, several human kindreds have been identified with congenital telomerase deficiency syndromes due to inactivating mutations of *TERT* or other members of the shelterin complex.[4] Such patients exhibit age-associated pathologies such as bone marrow failure and pulmonary fibrosis, but also appear to be at increased risk for several cancers including acute myelogenous leukemia and cutaneous carcinomas.[4,83,86–88] Likewise, human genomewide association studies of large human cohorts have pointed to sequence variants in the chromosome 5p15.33 locus as a susceptibility locus for many types of cancer, including tumors of the skin, lung, bladder, prostate, and cervix.[89] The single nucleotide polymorphisms associated with these cancers are near to both the *CLPTM1L* (cisplatin resistance-related protein CRRP9) gene and the *TERT* gene. It is unclear whether one or both of these genes are responsible for the association as there is limited functional biological validation. These human data suggest that telomere dysfunction could be oncogenic, and that hypomorphic alleles of TERT could contribute to human cancer susceptibility on a population basis.

Telomere-Induced Chromosomal Instability

The study of senescence and telomeres has provided some insights into the link between advancing age and increased cancer risk. In humans, there is a dramatic escalation in cancer risk between the ages of 40 and 80, resulting primarily from a marked increase in epithelial malignancies such as carcinomas of the breast, lung, colon, and prostate. A conventional view is that the cancer-prone phenotype of older humans reflects the combined effects of cumulative mutational load, decreased DNA repair capabilities, increased epigenetic gene silencing, and altered hormonal and stromal milieus. Although these factors are almost certain to contribute to increasing cancer incidence in aged humans, it is less evident why such processes would spur the preferential development of epithelial cancers. Moreover, these mechanisms do not readily explain one of the cardinal features of adult epithelial carcinomas—namely, a radically altered genome typified by marked aneuploidy and complex nonreciprocal chromosomal translocations.

The study of telomere dynamics in normal and neoplastic cells of the mouse has provided a potential explanation for the observed tumor spectrum and associated cytogenetic profiles in aged humans. In *Terc p53* compound mutant mice, the presence of telomere dysfunction results in a dramatic shift in the tumor spectrum toward epithelial cancers, including those of the lung, colon, and skin.[90] Moreover, in contrast to the largely normal cytogenetic profiles of cancers arising in mice with intact telomeres, the cancers generated in the *Terc p53* compound mutant mice had highly complex cytogenetic profiles with a striking resemblance to human epithelial cancer genomes.

In attempting to assign relevance of these murine studies to humans, it is worth considering that the typical adult cancer, an epithelial carcinoma, derives from a compartment that has undergone continued renewal throughout the human lifespan. Against this backdrop of physiologic cell turnover, combined with the occasional pro-proliferative oncogenic mutation, telomere lengths would shorten in self-renewing progenitor cells of these epithelial tissues. If somatic mutations also neutralize Rb/p16^{INK4a}/p53-dependent senescence checkpoints, continued growth beyond the Hayflick limit further drives telomere erosion and loss of the capping function, culminating in cellular crisis with attendant genomic instability. In this manner, telomere-based crisis provides the means to generate many additional mutations required to reach the early stages of malignant transformation. The subsequent reactivation of telomerase in transformed clones would serve to stabilize the genome to a level compatible with cell viability, allowing these initiated neoplasms to mature further.[91] It is unclear whether additional somatic mutations, beyond telomerase activation, would be needed to produce a fully malignant phenotype that includes invasive and metastatic potential. Thus, a transient period of explosive chromosomal instability before telomerase reactivation appears to be required for the stochastic acquisition of the relatively high number of mutations thought to be required for adult epithelial carcinogenesis. Another line of support is the fact that a proportion of early-stage epithelial cancers are hardwired for lethal metastatic progression, suggesting that many cancers acquire a full profile of genome change early in their life history.

The episodic instability model of epithelial carcinogenesis fits well with current knowledge regarding the timing of telomerase activation and evolving genomic changes during various stages of human carcinoma development, particularly those of the breast, esophagus, and colon. Comparative genome hybridization has demonstrated that dysplastic human breast, esophageal, and colon lesions sustain widespread gains and losses of regions of chromosomes early in their development, often well before these tissues exhibit carcinoma *in situ* or invasive growth.[92–94] The ploidy changes detected by comparative genome hybridization appear to correlate tightly with the presence of complex chromosomal rearrangements, and these markers of genomic instability are evident in the stages of advanced dysplasia of these tissues (e.g., ductal carcinoma *in situ*, Barrett's esophagus). As these cancers progress through invasive and metastatic stages, genomic instability continues, apparently at a moderate rate, but further mutations would be predicted to derive from non–telomere-based mechanisms. Correspondingly, the measurement of telomerase activity in adenomatous polyps and colorectal cancers has established that telomerase activity is low or undetectable in small and intermediate-sized polyps, reflecting less intact telomere function. In contrast, telomerase increases markedly in large adenomas and colorectal carcinomas, reflecting stabilization of telomere function.[95] Therefore, it appears that widespread and severe chromosomal instability is present early on during human tumorigenesis at a time when telomerase activity is low.

Additional support for this episodic instability model derives from the documentation of anaphase bridging (a correlate of telomere-based crisis) in evolving human colorectal cancers and in genomically unstable pancreatic cancers.[96,97] This suggests that the DSB-induced conditions (including but not limited to telomere dysfunction), coupled with mutations that allow survival in the face of a DSB, could provide amplification/deletion mechanisms across the genome. Biologic selection forces would in turn lead to the emergence of clones with the amplifications and deletions that target cancer-relevant loci. Studies in the telomerase mutant mouse have begun to provide mechanistic insight into how BFB leads to cancer-relevant changes. In particular, telomerase-p53 compound mutant mice with telomere dysfunction have increased end-to-end fusions, and the ensuing BFB process is associated with chromosomal regional gains and losses that appear linked to nonreciprocal translocations.[55,75]

In future human studies, it will be important to document telomere attrition in renewing epithelial stem cells and to perform a simultaneous comparison of telomere status, telomerase activity, and chromosomal instability in the same tumor samples, particularly during the earliest stages of human epithelial cell transformation. Defining the temporal point at which telomerase is reactivated in the genesis and progression of the different cancers may also lead to the development of biomarkers for diagnosis, prognosis, and outcomes prediction. Such studies are needed to more firmly establish a causal link between telomere dysfunction and early chromosomal instability in human neoplasms.

Telomere Dynamics, Inflammatory Diseases, and Cancer

The telomere dysfunction-induced genomic instability model also suggests some unanticipated opportunities for the therapies of other human diseases. For example, this model provides a potential explanation for the high cancer incidence associated with diseases characterized by chronic cell destruction and renewal as well as inflammation. One of the most notable examples of this tight link is the high incidence of hepatocellular carcinoma in late-stage cirrhotic livers. Cirrhosis is the phenotypic end point of prolonged cycles of hepatocyte destruction and regeneration, and cirrhotic livers show a documented reduction in telomere length over time. Humans with congenital telomerase deficiency may be predisposed to fibrotic liver disease, including cirrhosis.[87] Mouse models involving the telomerase-deficient mouse have shown that critical reductions in telomere length and function can accelerate the development of cirrhosis and hepatocellular carcinoma in chronic liver injury experiments.[98–100] Another example of a telomere-based pathogenic relationship between chronic tissue turnover, telomere-based crisis, and increased cancer risk is ulcerative colitis, a condition characterized by rapid cell turnover and oxidative injury to the intestines, and a high incidence of intestinal dysplasia or cancer.[97] In addition to the progressive telomere attrition resulting from the cell turnover, accelerated telomere attrition might occur via increased oxidative stress and from the altered inflammatory microenvironment milieu. Together, such observations suggest the intriguing possibility that early somatic reconstitution of telomerase could attenuate telomere attrition and paradoxically reduce the occurrence of cancers in these high-turnover disease states, a theory that requires additional preclinical studies. In addition, serial analyses of telomere length from these tissues may provide prognostic information regarding the rising risk of cancer development. Thus, progress in our understanding of telomere biology has mechanistically connected diverse fields in medicine involving chronic inflammatory diseases, degenerative diseases, geriatrics, and oncology.

Telomerase and Telomere Maintenance As Therapeutic Targets

Some evidence supports the view that telomerase-mediated telomere maintenance represents a near-universal therapeutic target for cancer. Indeed, cell culture–based studies of human cancer cells have established that inhibition of telomerase culminates in cell death after extended cell divisions. The past few years have witnessed intense efforts to design therapeutic strategies capable of targeting telomere structure and the telomerase holoenzyme function.[14,101,102] Unfortunately, most of these compounds and agents are still in preclinical and early clinical development and thus their safety and efficacy profiles in human patients are not fully known.

Presently, the only clinically advanced telomerase-related cancer treatment strategy is immunotherapy, targeting immune recognition and the destruction of cells that express telomerase. Immune responses, specifically cytotoxic T-cell responses, have been generated against peptide sequences of the hTERT protein, and it has been demonstrated that these cytotoxic T cells are capable of selectively lysing target cells that express TERT peptides presented on the cell surface in the context of major histocompatibility complex class I molecules. There have been several promising completed phase 1/2 trials using peptides from telomerase as vaccines.[103,104] A large randomized phase 3 trial comparing gemcitabine alone versus gemcitabine with a telomerase peptide vaccine (GV1001) showed no difference in survival benefit in the first 360 enrolled patients, and the trial was stopped. A second large 1,110 pancreatic cancer patient trial comparing gemcitabine/capecitabine combination therapy with concurrent and sequential gemcitabine/capecitabine therapy with GV1001 is still ongoing. Lastly, other TERT-based immune approaches, such as infusion of patient's primed antigen-presenting dendritic cells *ex vivo* with TERT mRNA, are also currently in early clinical trials.[105]

As for the ongoing design of rational clinical trials of telomere-based therapeutics, such efforts will be informed by the considerable body of knowledge accumulated in telomere biology. Experience with the telomerase mutant mouse model and human cell culture systems should serve to guide the design of human clinical trials. These studies suggest that inhibitors of telomerase activity might be expected to exhibit a long lag time and might promote malignancy in some circumstances, but also may be particularly useful in the setting of minimal residual disease after the administration of standard chemotherapeutic agents and surgery. In addition, pharmacodynamic assays capable of assessing inhibition of telomerase activity in individual patients are needed. Moreover, given that the activation of senescence-promoting mechanisms such as p53 and p16^{INK4a} has been associated with aging-like pathologies in several tissues,[59–63] some caution is warranted regarding the toxicity resulting from the induction of premature senescence in nondiseased tissues. This potential is underlined by evidence of germ cell defects, defects in proliferative homeostasis of certain tissues, and an increased rate of spontaneous malignancy in mice with telomere dysfunction, suggesting that clinical trials of such agents will need to be actively monitoring patients for these sequelae.

Furthermore, it seems prudent that the genetic profile of tumors enlisted into clinical trials should be determined to assess the integrity of p53. This caution relates to mouse models showing that the combination of p53 deficiency and telomere dysfunction drives greater genomic instability and thus potential for emergence of therapeutic resistance. In contrast, when p53 responses are intact, critical telomere shortening should induce p53-dependent senescence and apoptosis. The final answers to these safety questions reside in the analyses of current and future clinical trials with humans.

Conversely, the telomerase-deficient mouse model has also informed that cells and animals with telomere dysfunction are more sensitive to ionizing radiation and DNA DSB chemotherapeutic agents; thus, telomerase activity inhibitors may be more effective when paired with radiation or certain classes of chemotherapy that produce DSBs, as they might produce synergistic cytogenetic catastrophe. Again, however, particular care is warranted here as the combination of increased DNA damage with reduced capacity for normal repair may also produce marked increases in the toxicity of chemoradiotherapy.

Recent years have witnessed significant progress in the telomere biology field that is now maturing into new opportunities for improved diagnostics and novel therapeutic applications in human diseases, including cancer. Discoveries in telomere biology, rewarded with the 2009 Nobel Prize, have provided new mechanistic insights into the pathogenesis of human cancer and of inherited and acquired degenerative disorders. The role of telomere dysfunction driving episodic genomic instability in epithelial cancers—first seen in the telomerase-deficient mouse—has now been substantiated in the study of several human cancer types, with further support from genomewide association studies and kindreds with congenital telomerase deficiency. The pivotal role of telomere attrition in the pathogenesis of cancer and tissue aging provides potential avenues for the development of cancer risk biomarkers, diagnostics, and rationally designed therapeutics.

Selected References

The full list of references for this chapter appears in the online version.

3. Sahin E, Depinho RA. Linking functional decline of telomeres, mitochondria and stem cells during ageing. *Nature.* 2010;464:520.
4. Calado RT, Young NS. Telomere diseases. *N Engl J Med.* 2009;361:2353.
6. O'Sullivan RJ, Karlseder J. Telomeres: protecting chromosomes against genome instability. *Nature Rev.* 2010;11:171.
7. de Lange T. How telomeres solve the end-protection problem. *Science.* 2009;326:948.
8. de Lange T. Shelterin: the protein complex that shapes and safeguards human telomeres. *Genes Dev.* 2005;19:2100.
10. Zhu XD, Kuster B, Mann M, Petrini JH, de Lange T. Cell-cycle-regulated association of RAD50/MRE11/NBS1 with TRF2 and human telomeres. *Nat Genet.* 2000;25:347.
12. Takai H, Smogorzewska A, de Lange T. DNA damage foci at dysfunctional telomeres. *Curr Biol.* 2003;13:1549.
13. Deng Y, Chan SS, Chang S. Telomere dysfunction and tumour suppression: the senescence connection. *Nat Rev Cancer.* 2008;8:450.
16. Valdes AM, Andrew T, Gardner JP, et al. Obesity, cigarette smoking, and telomere length in women. *Lancet.* 2005;366:662.
19. Artandi SE, DePinho RA. Telomeres and telomerase in cancer. *Carcinogenesis.* 2010;31:9.
20. Masutomi K, Yu EY, Khurts S, et al. Telomerase maintains telomere structure in normal human cells. *Cell.* 2003;114:241.
22. Maida Y, Yasukawa M, Furuuchi M, et al. An RNA-dependent RNA polymerase formed by TERT and the RMRP RNA. *Nature.* 2009;461:230.
24. Park JI, Venteicher AS, Hong JY, et al. Telomerase modulates Wnt signalling by association with target gene chromatin. *Nature.* 2009;460:66.
25. Sharpless NE, DePinho RA. Telomeres, stem cells, senescence, and cancer. *J Clin Invest.* 2004;113:160.
26. Hayflick L, Moorhead P. The serial cultivation of human diploid cell strains. *Exp Cell Res.* 1961;25:585.
28. Kamijo T, Zindy F, Roussel MF, et al. Tumor suppression at the mouse INK4a locus mediated by the alternative reading frame product p19ARF. *Cell.* 1997;91:649.
29. Sage J, Miller AL, Perez-Mancera PA, Wysocki JM, Jacks T. Acute mutation of retinoblastoma gene function is sufficient for cell cycle re-entry. *Nature.* 2003;424:223.
31. Classon M, Harlow E. The retinoblastoma tumour suppressor in development and cancer. *Nat Rev Cancer.* 2002;2:910.
36. Zhang Y, Xiong Y, Yarbrough WG. ARF promotes MDM2 degradation and stabilizes p53: ARF-INK4a locus deletion impairs both the Rb and p53 tumor suppression pathways. *Cell.* 1998;92:725.
37. Kim WY, Sharpless NE. The regulation of INK4/ARF in cancer and aging. *Cell.* 2006;127:265.
43. Jacobs JJ, de Lange T. Significant role for p16INK4a in p53-independent telomere-directed senescence. *Curr Biol.* 2004;14:2302.
44. Chicas A, Wang X, Zhang C, et al. Dissecting the unique role of the retinoblastoma tumor suppressor during cellular senescence. *Cancer Cell.* 2010;17:376.
45. Donehower LA, Harvey M, Slagle BL, et al. Mice deficient for p53 are developmentally normal but susceptible to spontaneous tumours. *Nature.* 1992;356:215.
47. Sharpless NE, Bardeesy N, Lee KH, et al. Loss of p16Ink4a with retention of p19Arf predisposes mice to tumorigenesis. *Nature.* 2001;413:86.
48. Braig M, Lee S, Loddenkemper C, et al. Oncogene-induced senescence as an initial barrier in lymphoma development. *Nature.* 2005;436:660.
49. Collado M, Gil J, Efeyan A, et al. Tumour biology: senescence in premalignant tumours. *Nature.* 2005;436:642.
50. Chen Z, Trotman LC, Shaffer D, et al. Crucial role of p53-dependent cellular senescence in suppression of Pten-deficient tumorigenesis. *Nature.* 2005;436:725.
51. Ventura A, Kirsch DG, McLaughlin ME, et al. Restoration of p53 function leads to tumour regression in vivo. *Nature.* 2007;445:661.
52. Xue W, Zender L, Miething C, et al. Senescence and tumour clearance is triggered by p53 restoration in murine liver carcinomas. *Nature.* 2007;445:656.
53. Michaloglou C, Vredeveld LC, Soengas MS, et al. BRAFE600-associated senescence-like cell cycle arrest of human naevi. *Nature.* 2005;436:720.
55. Chin L, Artandi SE, Shen Q, et al. p53 deficiency rescues the adverse effects of telomere loss and cooperates with telomere dysfunction to accelerate carcinogenesis. *Cell.* 1999;97:527.
56. Martins CP, Brown-Swigart L, Evan GI. Modeling the therapeutic efficacy of p53 restoration in tumors. *Cell.* 2006;127:1323.
57. Schmitt CA, Fridman JS, Yang M, Baranov E, Hoffman RM, Lowe SW. Dissecting p53 tumor suppressor functions in vivo. *Cancer Cell.* 2002;1:289.
58. Campisi J. Suppressing cancer: the importance of being senescent. *Science.* 2005;309:886.
61. Krishnamurthy J, Ramsey MR, Ligon KL, et al. p16INK4a induces an age-dependent decline in islet regenerative potential. *Nature.* 2006;443:453.
64. Sharpless NE, DePinho RA. How stem cells age and why this makes us grow old. *Nature Rev.* 2007;8:703.
68. Beroukhim R, Mermel CH, Porter D, et al. The landscape of somatic copy-number alteration across human cancers. *Nature.* 2010;463:899.
69. Krimpenfort P, Ijpenberg A, Song JY, et al. p15Ink4b is a critical tumour suppressor in the absence of p16Ink4a. *Nature.* 2007;448:943.
73. Blasco MA. Telomerase beyond telomeres. *Nat Rev Cancer.* 2002;2:627.
74. Lin SY, Elledge SJ. Multiple tumor suppressor pathways negatively regulate telomerase. *Cell.* 2003;113:881.
75. O'Hagan RC, Chang S, Maser RS, et al. Telomere dysfunction provokes regional amplification and deletion in cancer genomes. *Cancer Cell.* 2002;2:149.
78. Chang S, Khoo CM, Naylor ML, Maser RS, DePinho RA. Telomere-based crisis: functional differences between telomerase activation and ALT in tumor progression. *Genes Dev.* 2003;17:88.
81. Shay JW, Bacchetti S. A survey of telomerase activity in human cancer. *Eur J Cancer.* 1997;33:787.
85. Rossi DJ, Bryder D, Seita J, Nussenzweig A, Hoeijmakers J, Weissman IL. Deficiencies in DNA damage repair limit the function of haematopoietic stem cells with age. *Nature.* 2007;447:725.
89. Rafnar T, Sulem P, Stacey SN, et al. Sequence variants at the TERT-CLPTM1L locus associate with many cancer types. *Nat Genet.* 2009;41:221.
90. Artandi SE, Chang S, Lee SL, et al. Telomere dysfunction promotes non-reciprocal translocations and epithelial cancers in mice. *Nature.* 2000;406:641.
97. O'Sullivan JN, Bronner MP, Brentnall TA, et al. Chromosomal instability in ulcerative colitis is related to telomere shortening. *Nat Genet.* 2002;32:280.
99. Farazi PA, Glickman J, Jiang S, Yu A, Rudolph KL, DePinho RA. Differential impact of telomere dysfunction on initiation and progression of hepatocellular carcinoma. *Cancer Res.* 2003;63:5021.
100. Rudolph KL, Chang S, Millard M, Schreiber-Agus N, DePinho RA. Inhibition of experimental liver cirrhosis in mice by telomerase gene delivery. *Science.* 2000;287:1253.
102. Shay JW, Wright WE. Telomerase therapeutics for cancer: challenges and new directions. *Nat Rev Drug Discov.* 2006;5:577.

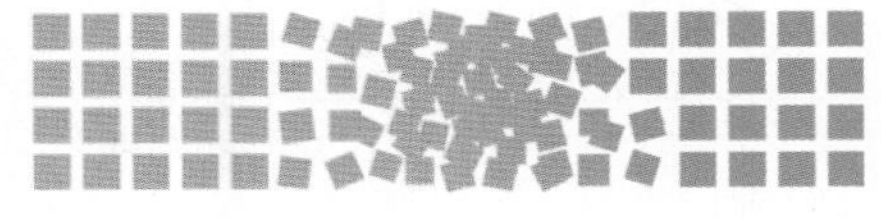

CHAPTER 5 CELL SIGNALING, GROWTH FACTORS AND THEIR RECEPTORS

LEWIS C. CANTLEY, CHRIS L. CARPENTER, WILLIAM C. HAHN, AND MATTHEW MEYERSON

SIGNAL TRANSDUCTION SYSTEMS

Signal transduction is the chemistry that allows communication at the cellular level. Cells sense signals from the extracellular and intracellular environments, as well as directly from other cells. Cells respond to these signals in a variety of ways, primarily by modifying protein levels, activities, and locations. Protein levels are controlled by rates of transcription, translation, and proteolysis, whereas protein activities are affected by covalent modifications and noncovalent interactions with other proteins and small molecules. Signal transduction pathways regulate differentiation, division, and death in the mature and developing organisms. Some pathways are common to all cells, but others are specific to specialized cells (e.g., synthesis and secretion of insulin by the pancreas, migration and phagocytosis by neutrophils). Disruption or alterations of signal transduction pathways plays a key causative role in disease. Indeed, mutations in nearly all of these signaling pathways are found in a wide range of cancers.

To emphasize the essentials of signal transduction, the focus in this chapter is on the variety of solutions to the two common problems faced by cells and organisms in signal transduction:

1. How is a signal sensed?
2. How are the levels, activities, and locations of proteins modified in response to the signal?

Most signals are initiated by ligands and are sensed by the receptors to which they bind. Binding of a ligand to a receptor stimulates the activities of proteins necessary to continue the transmission of the signal through the formation of multiprotein complexes and the generation of small-molecule second messengers. Integration of signals from multiple pathways determines the cell's ultimate response to competing and complementary signals. In addition, cell signaling pathways are highly interconnected to permit dynamic regulation of the strength, duration, and timing of cell responses.

SENSORY MACHINERY: LIGANDS AND RECEPTORS

Signals

Signal transduction pathways have evolved to respond to an enormous variety of stimuli. Molecules that initiate signaling cascades include proteins, amino acids, lipids, nucleotides, gases, and light (Table 5.1). Most extracellular signals, such as growth factors, bind to receptors on the plasma membrane, but others such as androgens or estrogen, diffuse into the cell and bind to receptors in the cytoplasm and nucleus. Some signals are continuous, such as those sent by the extracellular matrix, whereas others are episodic, like the secretion of insulin by pancreatic β cells in response to increases in blood glucose. Signaling molecules originate from a variety of sources. Some, such as neurotransmitters, are stored in the cell and are released to provide communication with other cells under specific conditions. Other ligands are stored outside the cell (e.g., in the extracellular matrix) and become accessible in response to tissue damage or remodeling. Traditionally, signals have been divided based on the cell of origin into those that affect distant cells (endocrine), nearby cells (paracrine), or the same cell (autocrine). Cells also respond to signals that arise from within. Important examples include the checkpoint pathways that ensure the orderly progression of the cell cycle and the pathways that sense and repair damaged DNA.[1]

Receptors

The plasma membrane of eukaryotic cells serves to insulate the cell from the outside environment, but this barrier must be breached to transmit signals of extracellular origin. This fundamental problem of transmitting extracellular signals is solved in two ways. Signals cross the plasma membrane either by activating transmembrane receptors or by using ligands that are membrane permeable (Table 5.2). Cells are exquisitely sensitive to most ligands. The affinity of receptors for ligands generally is in the picomolar to nanomolar range, and very few receptors need to be occupied to transmit a signal. For example, it has been estimated that activation of ten T-cell receptors is sufficient to send a maximal signal. Cytokine-responsive cells may express only a few hundred receptors on the cell surface. Given the small number of receptors that are activated, amplification of most signals is necessary for cellular responses. A requirement for signal amplification also allows opposing or complementary pathways to affect signal strength more efficiently.[2] As a result of ligand binding, receptors undergo conformational changes or oligomerization, or both, and the intrinsic activity of the receptor or of associated proteins is stimulated. Receptors may bind and respond to more than one ligand. For example, the epidermal growth factor (EGF) receptor binds to transforming growth factor-alpha (TGF-α), EGF, heparin-binding EGF (HB-EGF), beta-cellulin, epiregulin, epigen, and amphiregulin. The stimulation of most receptors leads to the activation of several downstream pathways that either function cooperatively to activate a common target or stimulate distinct targets. Generally, some of the pathways activated are counter-regulatory and serve to attenuate the signal. Receptors may also activate other receptors. A well-studied example is the activation of the EGF receptor by G protein-coupled receptors (GPCR), which occurs as a result of protease cleavage and activation of HB-EGF.

TABLE 5.1

LIGANDS THAT STIMULATE SIGNAL TRANSDUCTION PATHWAYS

Types of Ligands	Examples
PROTEIN	
Soluble	Insulin
Matrix	Fibronectin
Bound to other cells	Ephrines
AMINO ACIDS	
Nucleotides	
Soluble	Adenosine triphosphate
DNA	Double-strand breaks
LIPIDS	Prostaglandins
GASES	Nitric oxide
LIGHT	Rhodopsin, visual system

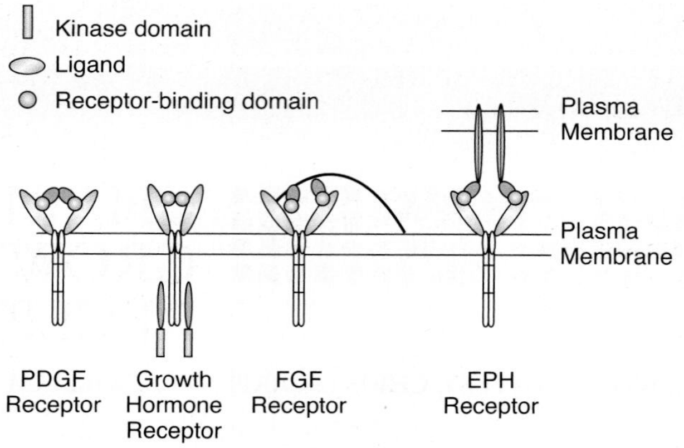

FIGURE 5.1 Dimerization of tyrosine kinase receptors. Most tyrosine kinase receptors are activated by ligand-induced dimerization. Some ligands, such as platelet-derived growth factor (PDGF), are dimeric and induce dimerization using the two receptor-binding domains. Other ligands, such as growth hormone, contain two receptor-binding domains in the same molecule. The fibroblast growth factors (FGFs) relay on proteoglycans to aid the formation of ligand dimmers. Some ligands, such as the ephrins (EPHs), are present on nearby cells and, when the cells come into contact, bind to the receptors and promote clustering.

There are a number of transmembrane receptor families. This chapter will discuss several of them to illustrate distinct signaling mechanisms.

Receptor Tyrosine Kinases

Receptor tyrosine kinases are transmembrane proteins that have an extracellular ligand-binding domain, a transmembrane domain, and a cytoplasmic tyrosine kinase domain.[3] The ligands for these receptors are proteins or peptides. Most receptor tyrosine kinases are monomeric, but members of the insulin-receptor family are heterotetramers in which the subunits are linked by disulfide bonds. Receptor tyrosine kinases have been divided into six classes, primarily on the basis of the sequence of the extracytoplasmic domain. Examples of tyrosine kinase receptors include the insulin receptor, the platelet-derived growth factor (PDGF) receptor, the EGF receptor family, and the fibroblast growth factor (FGF) receptor family.

Activation of receptor tyrosine kinases is generally believed to require tyrosine phosphorylation of the receptor. In the case of the insulin receptor, an insulin-stimulated conformational change activates the kinase. Most of the tyrosine kinases are activated by oligomerization, which brings the kinase domains of distinct molecules into close proximity so that they cross-phosphorylate. Autotransphosphorylation of tyrosine in the activation loop of the kinase domain locks the kinase into a high-activity conformation, stimulating phosphorylation of other sites on the receptor, as well as other substrates. However, cancer-derived mutants of the EGF receptor may be activated without receptor autophosphorylation.[4]

Ligands stimulate receptor oligomerization in a variety of ways (Fig. 5.1). Some ligands, such as PDGF, are dimeric, so that the ligand is able to bind two receptors simultaneously.[5] Other ligands, such as growth hormone, are monomeric but have two receptor-binding sites that allow them to induce receptor dimerization.[6] FGFs are also monomeric but have only a single receptor-building site. FGF molecules bind to heparin sulfate proteoglycans, which concentrates FGF and facilitates dimerization of the FGF receptor.[7] EGF is also monomeric, but binding of EGF to the receptor changes the receptor conformation and promotes interaction with a second ligand or receptor dimmer, leading to activation.[8] Some ligand-receptor interactions result in signaling by the ligand, in addition to the receptor. Ephrins are ligands for EPH tyrosine kinase activity in the

TABLE 5.2

RECEPTORS IN SIGNAL TRANSDUCTION

Types of Receptors	Examples	Types of Ligands
Tyrosine kinase	PDGF, EGF, FGF, and insulin receptors	Peptide growth factors
Serine kinase	TGF-β receptor	Activin
Heterotrimeric G protein	Thrombin, smell receptors	Thrombin
Receptors bound to tyrosine kinases	IL-2, interferon receptors	IL-2
TNF family	Fas receptor	Fas
Notch	Notch	Delta-Serrate-LAG-2
Guanylate cyclase	Atrial naturic factor receptor	Atrial natriuretic factor
Tyrosine phosphatase	CD45, LAR	Contactin
Nuclear receptors	Estrogen, androgen receptors	Estrogen
Adhesion receptors	Integrins, CD44	Fibronectin, hyaluronic acid

PDGF, platelet-derived growth factor; EGF, epidermal growth factor; FGF, fibroblast growth factor; TGF-β, transforming growth factor-β; IL-2, interleukin-2; TNF, tumor necrosis factor.

target cell, but they also stimulate signaling by ephrins in the ephrin-presenting cell.[9]

Studies of the EGF receptor-family illustrate some important concepts. The EGF-signaling pathways involve four receptors (EGF receptor, ERB2, ERB3, and ERB4) and many ligands.[10] EGF stimulates homodimerization of the EGF receptor, but, under certain conditions, heterodimerization with other family members also occurs. Activation of EGFR proceeds via asymmetric dimerization of the receptor. Ligand causes extracellular dimerization, which then causes the kinase domains to form an intracellular head-to-tail dimer, which activates the receptor.[11,12]

Receptors that Activate Tyrosine Kinases

A number of receptors do not have intrinsic enzymatic activity but stimulate associated tyrosine kinases. Important examples of this type of receptor include the cytokine and interferon receptors that associate constitutively with members of the Jak family of tyrosine kinases[13] and the multichain immune recognition receptors that activate SKF and Syk family tyrosine kinases.[14,15] The kinase appears to be inactive in the absence of ligand, but, as happens in receptors with intrinsic tyrosine kinase activity, signaling is initiated by ligand-stimulated heterodimerization and conformational changes of the receptors.

Serine-Threonine Kinase Receptors

The TGF-β family of receptors are transmembrane proteins with intrinsic serine-threonine kinase activity.[16] TGF-β ligands are dimmers that bind to and oligomerize type I and type II receptors. The type I and type II receptors homologous but distinctly regulated. The type II receptors seem to be constitutively active but do not normally phosphorylate substrates, whereas the type I receptors are normally inactive. Ligand-mediated dimerization of the type I and type II receptors causes the type II receptor to phosphorylate the type I receptor, converting it to an active kinase. Subsequent signal propagation is dependent on the kinase activity of the type I receptor and the phosphorylation of downstream substrates.

Receptor Phosphotyrosine Phosphatases

Receptor protein tyrosine phosphatases (RPTPs) have an extracellular domain, a single transmembrane-spanning domain, and cytoplasmic catalytic domains.[17] The extracellular domains of some receptor tyrosine phosphatases contain fibronectin and immunoglobulin repeats, suggesting that these receptors may recognize adhesion molecules as ligands. Several RPTPs are capable of homotypic interaction, but no true ligands are yet known for RPTPs. Most receptor tyrosine phosphatases have two catalytic domains, and both are active in at least some receptors. Functional and structural evidence suggests that the phosphatase activity of some of these receptors is inhibited by dimerization. Ligand-dependent dimerization could cause constitutively active tyrosine phosphatases to lose activity, enhancing signals emanating from tyrosine kinases. RPTPs do not always function in strict opposition to tyrosine kinases, however. For example, CD45 is necessary for signaling by the B-cell receptor, which also requires tyrosine kinase activity.[18] Since some Tyr-phosphorylation events, such as phosphorylation of a Tyr near the C-terminus of src-family protein-Tyr kinases, can be inhibitory to the Tyr kinase activity, activation of certain phospho-Tyr phosphatases can paradoxically cause an increase in global tyrosine phosphorylation (discussed in more detail below).

G Protein-Coupled Receptors

GPCRs are by far the most numerous receptors.[19] Almost 700 GPCRs are present in the human genome.[20] The number of GPCRs is so high because they encode the light, smell, and taste receptors, all of which require great diversity. These receptors have seven membrane-spanning domains: The N-terminus and three of the loops are extracellular, whereas the other three loops and the C-terminus are cytoplasmic. A wide variety of ligands bind GPCRs, including proteins and peptides, lipids, amino acids, and nucleotides. No common binding domain exists for all ligands, and interactions of ligands with GPCRs are fairly distinct.[21] In the case of the thrombin receptor, thrombin cleaves the N-terminus of the receptor, freeing a new N-terminus that self-associates with the ligand pocket, leading to activation. Amines and eicosanioids bind to the transmembrane domains of their GPCRs, whereas peptide ligands bind to the transmembrane domains of their GPCRs, and peptide ligands bind to the transmembrane domains and the extracellular loops of their GPCRs. Neurotransmitters and some peptide hormones require the N-terminus for binding and activation.

Intramolecular bonds that involve residues in the transmembrane or juxtamembrane regions keep GPCRs in an inactive conformation.[22] In the inactive state, the receptor is bound to a heterotrimeric G protein, which is also inactive. Agonist binding causes a conformational change that stimulates the guanine nucleotide exchange activity of the receptor. Exchange of guanosine triphosphate (GTP) for guanosine diphosphate (GDP) on the α-subunit of the heterotrimeric G proteins initiates signaling. Ultimately, GPCRs stimulate the same downstream pathways as other receptor types, including ion channels, cytosolic protein tyrosine and serine kinases, and enzymes that phosphorylate or hydrolyze membrane lipids.[19] Certain GPCRs also activate receptor tyrosine kinases. As mentioned earlier, GPCR-dependent cleavage of HB-EGF stimulates the EGF receptor, which is necessary for the GPCR to activate the mitogen-activated protein kinase (MAP kinase) pathway.

Notch Family of Receptors

The Notch receptor has a large extracellular domain, a single transmembrane domain, and a cytoplasmic domain.[23] Ligands for the Notch receptor are proteins expressed on the surface of adjacent cells, and activation results in two proteolytic cleavages of Notch. Initial cleavage by ADAM family proteases removes the extracellular domain and causes endocytosis. Subsequent proteolysis by the preselinin protease family releases the cytoplasmic region of Notch as a soluble signal. This fragment moves to the nucleus, where it complexes with the transcriptional repressor CBFI, relieving its inhibitory effects and stimulating transcription.

Guanylate Cyclases

Guanylate cyclases (GCs) convert guanosine triphosphate to cyclic guanosine monophosphate (cGMP) upon activation.[24] There are both transmembrane and soluble forms of GCs. The membrane GCs are receptors for atrial natriuretic hormone, peptides that regulate intestinal secretion and are necessary for regulating cGMP levels for vision. In addition to the catalytic domain, the cytoplasmic tail includes a protein kinase homology domain that lacks kinase activity. Soluble GCs are activated by nitrous oxide. These receptors are widely expressed and regulate vascular tone and neuron function. They are heterodimers and each subunit has catalytic activity.

Tumor Necrosis Factor Receptor Family

The tumor necrosis factor family of receptors has a conserved cysteine-rich region in the extracellular domain, a transmembrane domain, and a domain called the *death domain* in the

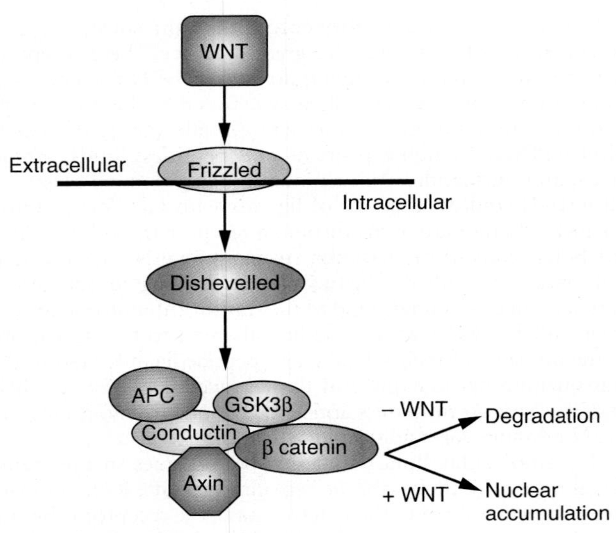

FIGURE 5.2 Wingless (Wnt)/β catenin signaling. Wnt extracellular ligands bind Frizzled receptors and regulate the phosphorylation status of axin. Axin functions as part of the destruction complex that regulates the stability of β-catenin, a transcriptional regulator.

cytoplasmic tail.[25] The receptors undergo oligomerization after ligand binding, which is necessary for signaling. These receptors are distinct in several respects. Stimulation of the receptor leads to recruitment of cytoplasmic proteins that bind to each other and the receptor through death domains, thereby activating a protease, caspase 8, that initiates apoptosis. Under some conditions, however, tumor necrosis factor receptors (TNFRs) stimulate antiapoptotic signals. This family of receptors also includes "decoys" or receptors that are missing all or part of the cytoplasmic tail and thus cannot transmit a signal. This feature provides a unique mechanism for inhibiting and further regulating signaling. A second class of TNFRs lack death domains but bind to TNFR-associated factors.

WNT Receptors

The Wnt family of growth and differentiation factors are small proteins that bind to cell surface receptors of the Frizzled family.[26] These receptors resemble GPCRs but utilize a unique mechanism of signal transduction (Fig. 5.2). Binding of Wnt to the receptor suppresses a kinase cascade involving the protein Ser/Thr kinases casein kinase I (CK I) and glycogen synthase kinase 3 (GSK3) and the low-density lipoprotein-related protein (LRP). Active Wnt signaling requires inactivation of Axin and the adenomatous polyposis coli (APC) protein. This complex mediates phosphorylation and ultimately proteosome-dependent degradation of β-catenin. Suppression of β-catenin degradation in response to Wnt allows β-catenin to accumulate to higher levels in the cell and to migrate into the nucleus where it regulates genes involved in cell growth regulation, acting as a heterodimer with the T-cell factor (TCF) transcription factors.

Nuclear Receptors

Ligands for nuclear hormone receptors diffuse into the cell and bind their receptors either in the cytoplasm or the nucleus. The ligands include steroids, eicosanoids, retinoids, and thyroid hormone. The sex steroids, androgens such as testosterone and estrogen and progesterone, are ligands for the androgen receptor, estrogen receptor, and progesterone receptor, respectively. Inhibition of androgen receptor is central to treatment of prostate cancer, while inhibition of estrogen receptor is central to treatment of estrogen receptor–positive breast cancer. The receptors are transcription factors that have both DNA- and ligand-binding domains. The unliganded receptor is bound to heat shock proteins that are dissociated after ligand binding. Release from the chaperone complex and ligand association lead to binding of the receptor to cofactors and DNA to regulate transcription.

Adhesion Receptors

Cell adherence, either to the extracellular matrix or to other cells, is mediated by receptors that function mechanically and stimulate intracellular signaling pathways, primarily through tyrosine kinases.[27] Integrins mediate adherence to extracellular matrix and are composed of heterodimers of α and β subunits. They bind to an arginine/glycine/aspartate or leucine/aspartate/valine motif found in matrix molecules. Binding to ligand leads to integrin clustering and activation. Structural studies show that inactive integrins adopt a conformation that inhibits ligand binding. In this conformation the intracellular regions are also hindered from binding effector molecules.[28] Binding of ligand opens the intracellular regions so that they bind to the molecules required to transmit integrin-dependent signals. Similarly, modification of the intercellular region, such as phosphorylation, affects the conformation of the extracellular region to favor ligand binding. This is an example of a receptor that signals both "outside-in" and "inside-out." Integrin signaling is necessary for cell movement, but, in contrast to other pathways, adherence in nonmotile cells provides a continuous signal. This signal is necessary for survival of most cells. The ability to circumvent the requirement for adherence-dependent survival plays a major role in the development of human cancers by allowing tumor survival in inappropriate locations.

Propagation of Signals to the Cell Interior

Although the structures and mechanisms of the various receptors and ligands that initiate cell signaling are very different, most receptors activate a set of common downstream molecules to transmit their signals. The molecules that transmit signals include protein and lipid kinases, GTPases, phospholipases, proteases, adaptors, and adenylate cyclases (Table 5.3). These pathways lead to a broad array of responses, including changes in transcription and translation, enzymatic activities, and cell motility.

REGULATION OF PROTEIN KINASES

The balance between protein kinase and phosphatase activity controls protein phosphorylation. Protein kinases themselves, transcription factors, and cytoskeletal components are a few examples of proteins regulated by phosphorylation (Fig. 5.3). Protein kinases are classified by the residues they phosphorylate. Eukaryotic cells have protein tyrosine kinases, protein serine-threonine kinases, and dual-specificity kinases that phosphorylate serine, threonine, and tyrosine residues. Important issues in understanding the role and regulation of protein phosphorylation are how specificities or kinases and phosphatases are determined and how phosphorylation alters the function of substrates. Work at the structural and functional levels has provided preliminary answers to these questions.

Most signal transduction pathways require protein tyrosine kinases. Receptors that are not themselves tyrosine kinases use

TABLE 5.3

ENZYME CLASSES STIMULATED BY ACTIVATED RECEPTORS

Enzyme Classes	Examples
PROTEIN KINASES	
Tyrosine	Jak
Serine, threonine	ERKs
PROTEIN PHOSPHATASES	
Tyrosine	SHP-2
Serine, threonine	Calcineurin
LIPID KINASES	
Phosphatidylinositol	PI3-kinase
LIPID PHOSPHATASES	
Phosphatidylinositol	SHIP, PTEN
PHOSPHOLIPASES	
A	CPLA2
C	PLCγ
D	
G PROTEINS	
Heterotrimeric	Gs, Gi
Ras-like	Ras, Rac
NUCLEOTIDE CYCLASES	
Adenylate	
Guanylate	

ERKs, Extracellular signaling-regulated kinases; PI3-kinase, phosphoinositide 3 kinase; PLC, phospholipase C.

several cytoplasmic tyrosine kinases, including the Src, Syk, and Jak families. Phosphorylation of proteins on tyrosine can either stimulate or inhibit enzymatic activity. In addition, phosphorylation of proteins on Tyr can lead to new protein-protein interaction. An example of how tyrosine phosphorylation regulates enzymatic activity is found in the Src family of protein tyrosine kinases, which are regulated positively and negatively by tyrosine phosphorylation.[29] Phosphorylation of a tyrosine residue in the C-phosphotyrosine and the Src homology 2 (SH2) domain blocks access of substrate to the catalytic domain. In contrast, phosphorylation of a tyrosine in the transactivation loop (T loop) of the catalytic domain stimulates the kinase activity by stabilizing the catalytic pocket in an active conformation.

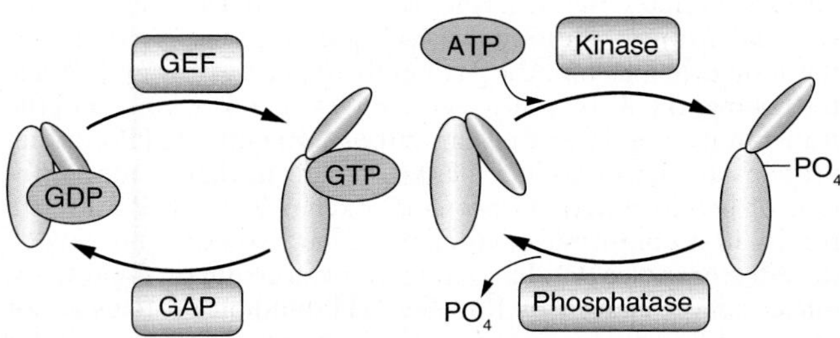

FIGURE 5.3 Regulation of protein activity by phosphate. The exchange of guanosine triphosphate (GTP) for guanosine diphosphate (GDP) bound to G proteins induces an activating conformational change dependent on the additional γ phosphate of GTP. Guanine nucleotide exchange factors catalyze GDP/GTP exchange. GTPase-activating proteins (GAPs) accelerate the hydrolysis of GTP to GDP to remove the γ phosphate and attenuate G-protein signaling. Protein kinases add phosphate to proteins, resulting in conformational changes and changes in enzymatic activity. Protein phosphatases remove the phosphate to inhibit the signal. G proteins and protein kinase substrates undergo a similar cycle of phosphate addition and removal to regulate their activity. ATP, adenosine triphosphate; GEF, guanine nucleotide exchange factor.

The activity of many other tyrosine and serine-threonine protein kinases is regulated by phosphorylation of the activation, or T, loop. The T loop forms a lip of the catalytic pocket and may occlude the active site, preventing access of the substrate. In the case of the insulin receptor, the unphosphorylated T loop also appears to interfere with adenosine triphosphate (ATP) binding.[30] Crystallographic studies indicate that the T loop is mobile and thus is probably not always in an inhibitory confirmation, providing kinases with some constitutive activity. Low basal activity is sufficient to phosphorylate a nearby kinase (e.g., autotransphosphorylation of a partner in a dimeric receptor). After phosphorylation, the T loop undergoes a conformational change that provides much more efficient substrate access to the catalytic site.

Once a protein kinase is active, only specific substrates are phosphorylated. Specificity is determined on two properties: colocalization of the kinase with the substrate (discussed later in this chapter) and the presence of particular motifs in a substrate that can be phosphorylated by the kinase. A proline following the serine or threonine residue to be phosphorylated is absolutely required for MAP kinase substrates. In other cases, particular motifs are favored as phosphorylation sites. These motifs probably fit best into the catalytic cleft of the kinase. In some cases, sequences distant from the site of phosphorylation mediate low-affinity association of a kinase with its substrate and thereby enhance phosphorylation.

Most signaling pathways activate serine kinases, but there is also a high level of constitutive phosphorylation of proteins on serine and threonine residues. The relevance of this basal phosphorylation is still unclear. Myriad cellular functions are regulated by serine phosphorylation, ranging from the activity of transcription factors and enzymes to the polymerization of actin. Serine kinases themselves are regulated in a variety of ways. Mammalian serine-threonine kinases have been subdivided into 11 subfamilies based on primary sequence homology, which has also been predictive of related function.[31] Localization, phosphorylation, and ligand binding regulate serine kinases. Activation by ligand binding characterizes some classes of serine protein kinases. For example, cyclic nucleotides (e.g., cyclic adenosine monophosphate [cAMP]) activate the protein kinase A superfamily. Calcium and diacylglycerol (DAG) activate members of the protein kinase C (PKC) family. The protein kinase B or Akt family is activated by phosphatidylinositol (PtdIns) phosphate products of phosphoinositide-dependent kinase 1 (PDK1) to phosphorylate the activation, or T, loop. Association with cyclins activates the cyclin-dependent kinase family, and the calcium-calmodulin–dependent kinases are activated by calcium. Kinase cascades also are important in providing multiple levels of regulation and amplification of serine kinase activity. For example, MAP kinases are activated by phosphorylation of the T loop after activation of upstream kinases: Activation of Raf leads to phosphorylation and activation of MEK1, which phosphorylates and activates the extracellular signaling-regulated kinases (ERKs) (Fig. 5.4).

Protein kinase signals are generally attenuated by phosphatases, metabolism of activating second messengers, or both. Dephosphorylation of the T-loop site markedly reduces the activity of most kinases, and dephosphorylation of motifs required for protein-protein binding prevents kinases from interacting with their substrates. Phosphatases also counteract the phosphorylation of substrate molecules, reversing the effects of the kinases.

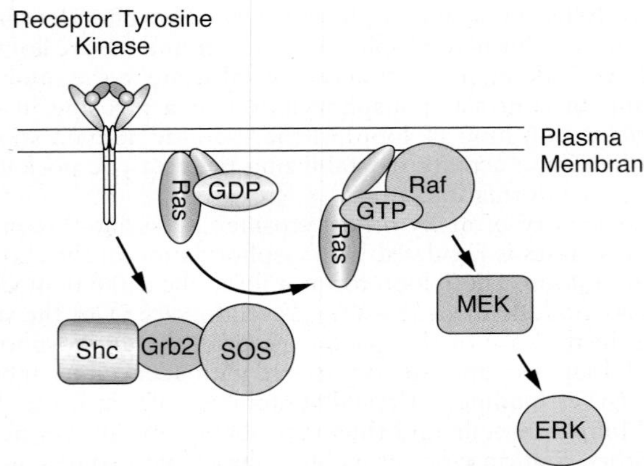

FIGURE 5.4 Activation of the extracellular signaling-regulated kinases (ERK) pathway. Many receptors activate the ERKs. Most receptor tyrosine kinases stimulate the activity of the Ras guanine nucleotide exchange factor son of sevenless (SOS), which associates with the linker proteins Shc and Grb2. The activation of Ras by SOS stimulates a protein serine kinase cascade initiated by Raf, which stimulates MEK. MEK then activates the ERKs. ERKs phosphorylate transcription factors to regulate gene expression. GDP, guanosine diphosphate; GPT, guanosine triphosphate.

Regulation of Protein Phosphatases

Protein phosphatases remove the phosphate residues from proteins, which can either activate or inhibit signaling pathways. Protein phosphatases are divided into the same three groups as the kinases on the basis of their substrates: tyrosine phosphatases, serine-threonine phosphatases, and dual-specificity phosphatases, which use a cysteinylphosphate intermediate, whereas the serine-threonine phosphatases are metal-requiring enzymes that dephosphorylate in a single step.[32]

Structural work has revealed how the activity of some nonreceptor tyrosine phosphatases is regulated.[33] The SHP2 phosphatase has, in addition to the catalytic domain, two SH2 domains. These domains (discussed later in this chapter) mediate binding to other proteins by direct association with phosphorylated tyrosine residues. In the inactive state, the catalytic cleft of SHP2 is blocked by the N-terminal SH2 domain. Binding of the N-terminal SH2 domain to a phosphotyrosine residue of a target protein induces a conformational change that allows substrate access to the catalytic domain. Tyrosine phosphatases act to attenuate signals that require tyrosine phosphorylation and to activate pathways inhibited by tyrosine phosphorylation. An example of the negative regulatory function of tyrosine phosphatases is the role of SHP1 (a homologue of SHP2) in inhibiting cytokine and B-cell receptor signaling. In contrast, SHP2 is necessary for cytokine stimulation of cells. On the basis of the ability of phosphatase inhibitors (e.g., vanadate) to activate tyrosine kinase-dependent signaling in the absence of ligands, acute inactivation of specific tyrosine phosphatases may play an important role in regulating the balance of tyrosine phosphorylation and dephosphorylation that controls signaling pathways. Reactive oxygen generated in response to many signals can inhibit tyrosine phosphatases by oxidizing the catalytic cysteine.

Protein phosphatase 1 (PP1), PP2, PP2B, and PP2C are the major serine-threonine phosphatases; PP1 and PP2A are composed of catalytic and regulatory subunits. PP1 affects many pathways from glycogen metabolism to the cell cycle. PP2B binds to calmodulin and is regulated by calcium. Phosphorylation of either the regulatory or catalytic subunit affects the activity of serine phosphatases. More than 100 PP1 regulatory subunits function to target the catalytic domain to different cellular locations and mediate activation or inhibition. This illustrates how a single catalytic activity can perform multiple specific functions as a result of targeting by a regulatory subunit.

Guanosine Triphosphate-Binding Proteins

Protein-protein interaction is also an important mechanism of signal transduction. G proteins, which bind GTP, are the best-studied protein mediators that regulate other proteins by direct binding.[21] GTP-binding proteins function as digital switches. GTP binding results in a conformational change that allows G proteins to bind to effector molecules and transmit a signal (Fig. 5.3). GTP hydrolysis to GDP ultimately returns the protein to its inactive conformation. GTP-binding proteins regulate the same molecules activated by receptors: protein and lipid kinases, phosphatases, and phospholipases. GTP-binding proteins are categorized into two large classes: the heterotrimeric GTP-binding proteins and the Ras-like GTP-binding proteins. Activation of GTP-binding proteins is regulated by guanine nucleotide exchange factors that catalyze the release of GDP and allow GTP to bind. Since the concentration of GTP in the cell far exceeds that of GDP, proteins (GAPs) accelerate GTP hydrolysis, inactivating GTP-binding proteins. All GTP-binding proteins have lipid modifications that promote membrane association.

Heterotrimeric GTP-binding proteins have three subunits and are activated by GPCRs. In the inactive state, the α, β, and γ subunits form a heterotrimer. In mammalian cells, 20 α subunits, 6 β subunits, and 12 γ subunits are known. The heterotrimeric forms are divided into four classes on the basis of function. Gαs stimulates adenylate cyclase, Gαi inhibits adenylate cyclase, and Gαq activates PLC β. G12 and G13 form a related group. In general they activate the small GTPase RhoA. GPCRs have GDP/GTP exchange activity, and binding of ligand stimulates GTP binding to the subunit of heterotrimeric G proteins. In response to GTP loading, the α and β/γ subunits dissociate. The α subunits and the β/γ complex each send signals. Release of the β/γ dimmer from the α subunit exposes surfaces that allow β/γ to bind to effectors. The α and β/γ subunits regulate a wide range of downstream effectors, including ion channels, protein kinases, and phospholipases. Domains termed *regulators of G-protein signaling* act as GAPs toward the α subunit and attenuate the signal by catalyzing hydrolysis of GTP to GDP.

Ras-like GTP-binding proteins are monomeric and usually of lower molecular weight than are the heterotrimeric GTP-binding proteins. Ras-like GTP-binding proteins are classified into five families: the Ras, Rho, Rab, Arf, and Ran families. The Ras and Rho families regulate cell growth, transcription, and the actin cytoskeleton; the Arf family regulates PLD and vesicle trafficking; the Rab family regulates vesicle trafficking; and the Ran family regulates nuclear import. Ras-like GTP-binding proteins are activated in a manner similar to that of the α subunit of heterotrimeric G proteins. Exchange of GTP for GDP results in a conformational change that promotes binding to the effector molecules. In contrast to heterotrimeric G proteins, nucleotide exchange for Ras-like GTP-binding proteins is not catalyzed directly by receptor or in response to specific cellular events. Signals are attenuated by the action of GAPs, analogous to regulators of the G protein-signaling domain-containing proteins that catalyze GTP hydrolysis.

GTP-binding proteins affect the activity of their targets by causing conformational changes and perhaps by serving to localize the target. Crystal structures of the catalytic domain of adenylate cyclase bound to G proteins illustrate the conformational change.[34] Gαs binds to the C2a domain of adenylate cyclase, causing rotation of the C1a domain, which positions the catalytic residues more favorably for conversion of ATP to cAMP. Although crystal structures of small G proteins bound to portions of their targets also have been solved, the effect on the activity of target molecules as a result of binding has not yet been explained. Studies of the role in Ras in the interaction of Raf suggest that an important role of Ras is localization of Raf to the membrane, but Ras also may help to activate Raf directly.[35]

SMALL-MOLECULE SECOND MESSENGERS

Small molecules transmit signals by binding noncovalently to protein targets and affecting their function. These molecules are called *second messengers* because they are generated within the call in response to a first messenger, such as a growth factor, binding to a cell surface receptor.

cAMP was the first of the second messengers discovered. Adenylate cyclase, activated by heterotrimeric G proteins, catalyzed the synthesis of cAMP from ATP.[36] The primary target of cAMP is protein kinase A, and the activation of protein kinase A by cAMP demonstrates how second messengers function. The inactive form of protein kinase A is a tetramer of two catalytic and two regulatory subunits; the regulatory subunit contains two cAMP-binding sites. Binding of cAMP to the first site causes a conformational change that exposes the second site. Binding of cAMP to the second site results in dissociation of the regulatory and catalytic subunits. The free catalytic subunits are then active.

Phospholipase C proteins (PLCs) are common downstream effectors of signaling.[37] They cleave PtdIns-4,5-P_2 to generate two small molecule signals: inositol-1,4,5-trisphosphate (IP_3) and diaclyglycerol (DAG). All three families of PLC-β, -γ, and -δ are activated by calcium. PLC-β is also activated by the α and β/γ subunits of heterotrimeric G proteins, and PLC-γ is activated by tyrosine phosphorylation. DAG interacts with the C1 domain of PKCs to mediate their membrane localization and activation. IP_3 binds to a calcium channel in the endoplasmic reticulum (ER) and stimulates the release in cytoplasmic calcium from intracellular stores.[38] The initial increase in cytoplasmic calcium is followed by an influx of extracellular calcium via capacitive calcium channels at the plasma membrane. In unstimulated cells, cytosolic calcium is much lower than in the extracellular space of ER (100 nM vs. 1 mM), and, therefore, opening channels in the ER or plasma membrane allows calcium to flood into the cytoplasm, temporarily raising the cytoplasmic calcium to micromolar concentrations. Ultimately, calcium returns to basal levels as a result of the channels closing and removal of cytosolic calcium by both extracellular transport and pumping calcium into intracellular compartments. Calcium has a multitude of cellular effects, including directly regulating enzymatic activities, ion channels, and transcription. Several calcium-binding domains are known, including the C2 domain and EF hands. Calcium binds directly to enzymes and regulates their activity or to regulatory subunits, such as calmodulin.

Eicosanoids are ubiquitous signaling molecules that bind to GPCRs and transcription factors.[39] Eicosanoid synthesis occurs in response to a number of stimuli and is an example of rapid cell-to-cell signaling. Unlike most second messengers, eicosanoids produced in one cell escape that cell and diffuse to nearby cells and either bind to receptors or are metabolized further. Eicosanoid synthesis is regulated by the production of arachidonic acid, which is produced from DAG via diglyceride lipases or from phospholipids by PLA. PLA2s clear the sn-2 acyl group of phospholipids to produce a free fatty acid and a lysophospholipid. The calcium-regulated form of PL2 shows a preference for substrates containing arachidonic acid. The further metabolism of arachidonic acid results in the synthesis of prostaglandins and leukotrienes.

The Phosphatidyl Inositol 3′ Kinase Pathway

The phosphatidyl inositol 3 (PI3)-kinase pathway is central to intracellular signaling.[40,41] The intracellular messenger PIP3 is produced by PI3-kinase proteins, encoded by the *PIK3CA* and *PIK3R1* genes for the catalytic and regulatory subunits, respectively. PIP3 is cleaved by the lipid phosphatase protein, PTEN. PI3 signaling leads to activation of the Akt kinase and the related PDK1 kinase, and then signals through the tuberous sclerosis 1 and 2 (TSC1/TSC2) complex to the mammalian target of rapamycin (mTOR) protein (Fig. 5.5).

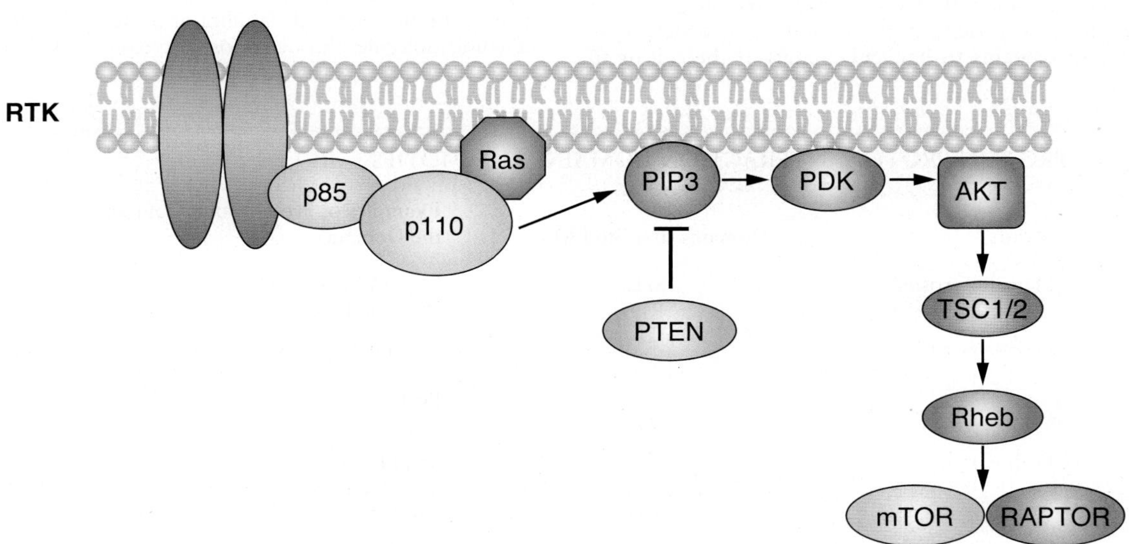

FIGURE 5.5 The phosphoinositide 3 kinase (PI3-kinase) pathway. PI3-kinase is activated by many growth factor receptors and leads to the formation of the intracellular messenger PI3. The lipid phosphatase tumor suppressor PTEN dephosphorylates PI3K. Downstream effectors include the mammalian target of rapamycin (mTOR) kinase.

EFFICIENCY AND SPECIFICITY: FORMATION OF MULTIPROTEIN SIGNALING COMPLEXES

Compartmentalization

The ability of a signal transduction pathway to transmit a signal is dependent on the probability that a protein finds its target. The likelihood of any two proteins coming into contact is proportional to their concentrations. Recruiting a protein to a specific compartment in a cell markedly increases the local concentration of that protein, thereby enhancing the probability that it will interact with other proteins or small molecules that are recruited to or generated in the same compartment. Colocalization of proteins in a signaling pathway is achieved by recruitment to the same membrane surface or organelle (e.g., plasma membrane vs. ER) and by protein-protein interactions. Conversely, separating proteins or second messengers (or both) into distinct compartments runs off signaling pathways.

Transport of signaling proteins into the nucleus is important in a number of signal transduction pathways, and it illustrates the concept of colocalization in the same organelle.[42] Nuclear transport proceeds through nuclear pores. Proteins of less than about 40 kD cross by simple diffusion, but transport of larger molecules requires a nuclear localization signal to which the importin proteins bind. The importins target the protein to the nuclear pore, and the complex is transported into the nucleus. The Ran G protein dissociates the importins from their cargo once they are in the nucleus. Regulated export of proteins from the nucleus is similar to import. A nuclear export signal is recognized by the protein exportin, which then transports the cargo out of the nucleus. A specific example is nuclear localization of the transcription factor nuclear factor of activated T cells (NFAT), which is required for its transcriptional activity.[43] In response to T-cell activation and a rise in intracellular calcium, NFAT is dephosphorylated by the calcium-responsive phosphatase calcineurin. Dephosphorylation allows the nuclear localization signal in NFAT to bind to the importins, and NFAT, along with calcineurin, is imported into the nucleus. NFAT also contains a nuclear export signal, and phosphorylation appears to allow the nuclear export signal to bind to exportin, resulting in transport to the cytoplasm.

Protein compartmentalization also occurs on a smaller scale in the form of protein-protein complexes, which serve either to target proteins to particular parts of the cell or to promote efficient signal transmission. Well-studied examples of the use of protein-protein interaction to determine the localization of enzymes include the A kinase anchoring proteins that bind to protein kinase A, a family of proteins that bind to PCK, and the subunits of PP2A.[44]

Lipid rafts are regions where sphingolipids and cholesterol are concentrated in the outer leaflet of the plasma membrane and are important sites for signaling.[45] The lipid composition provides structural cohesiveness. Rafts both concentrate and exclude proteins, promoting the formation of signaling complexes. Glycosylphosphatidylinositol-linked proteins on the extracellular surface of the plasma membrane concentrate in lipid rafts, as do acylated proteins on the intracellular surface. Transmembrane receptors can be recruited into rafts following their activation, along with their targets, leading to efficient signal generation.

Domains that Mediate Protein-Protein Binding

The regulated assembly of protein-protein complexes has several functions in signal transduction, including the formation of complexes allowing proteins to signal to each other, forming a "solid state" module that does not require diffusion to transmit a signal. Protein-protein interactions also localize an enzyme near its substrate: the binding of PLC $\gamma 1$ to the PDGF receptor brings the enzyme to the plasma membrane where its substrate, PtdIns-4, 5-P_2, is concentrated. These interactions are often mediated by conserved domains that recognize phosphorylated tyrosine or serine residues or proline-rich sequences (Table 5.4).

SH2 and phosphotyrosine-binding domain bind to motifs that contain phosphorylated tyrosine residues.[46] The crystal structures of several SH2 domains have been determined and reveal a pocket that binds the phosphotyrosine and a groove that determines binding specificity based on the fit of the residue's C-terminal (or, in a few cases, N-terminal) to the phosphotyrosine. Tyrosine kinases and phosphatases regulate the formation of complexes involving these domains. Tyrosine kinases themselves serve as docking sites for other proteins, which is most evident with tyrosine kinase receptors that recruit PI3-kinase, p120 Ras GAP, PLCγ, and SHP-2 through SH2 domain–dependent interactions. Tyrosine kinases phosphorylate adaptors such as the IRS and Gab families of proteins also recruit other signaling molecules through phosphotyrosine-based interactions.

TABLE 5.4

PROTEIN-PROTEIN INTERACTION DOMAINS AND MOTIFS

Motifs	Domains that Bind Motif	Examples of Proteins that Contain the Domain
Phosphotyrosine	SH2	Scr, PI3-kinase, SHP-2
	PTB	IRS Family, SHC
Phosphoserine	WD40	Telomerase, APAF-1, Coatamer
	14-3-3	
	WW	Pin1
	FHA	Rad53
Proline-rich	SH3	Src, PI3-kinase
	WW	YAP, Dystrophin
	EVH1	VASP, ENA, WASp
C-terminal sequences	PDZ	ZO-1, lim kinase

PI3-kinase, phosphoinositide 3 kinase; SH2, src homology 2; SH3, src homology 3.

In addition to mediating protein-protein interactions, binding of SH2 domains also bind to intramolecular phosphotyrosines, as in the case of Src, to inhibit catalytic activity.

Phosphotyrosine-binding domains are functionally analogous to SH2 domains in that they bind phosphotyrosine sequence or structural similarity to SH2 domains. Thus, they represent an independent evolutionary solution to phosphoty-photyrosine-binding, and SH2 domains bind to a tyrosine-containing motif in the absence of phosphorylation.

Recognition of phosphoserine motifs is also an important means of protein-protein interaction. Forkhead-associated domains, 14-3-3 proteins, and some WD40 and WW domains bind to regions of proteins containing phosphothreonine or phosphoserine.[47] WD40 domains in members of the F-box and ubiquitination and subsequent proteolysis of proteins. A prominent example of this pathway is degradation of the inhibitor of κB (IκB), which regulates the activity of the transcription factor nuclear factor κB (NF-κB). The 14-3-3 proteins are a family of small proteins whose primary function is binding to phosphoserine or phosphothreonine motifs. An example of the importance of this interaction is the role of 14-3-3 in regulating the nuclear location of the phosphatase Cdc25 that regulates the cell cycle. Binding of 14-3-3 to phosphorylated Cdc25 leads to its export from the nucleus and blocks the cell cycle.

Src homology 3 (SH3), WW, and ena-vasp homology domains are structurally distinct, but all bind to proline-rich sequences. Many proteins that contain SH3 domains also have proline-rich regions that could be involved in intramolecular binding, suggesting that a conformational change in the protein could disrupt intramolecular binding and allow the SH3 domain to interact with other proteins. Similarly, the accessibility of proline-rich regions to SH3 domains may be regulated by conformational changes that expose the proline-rich region or disrupt an intramolecular interaction.

PDZ domains recognize motifs in the C-termini of proteins and bind to each other and lipids.[48] These C-terminal motifs are found in cytoplasmic proteins, many of which also contain multiple PDZ domains. PDZ domain-containing proteins function to aggregate transmembrane proteins, such as the glutamate receptor. Group I PDZ domains bind to a consensus sequence, T/S-X-V/I, where V/I is the C-terminus of the protein. In some cases, phosphorylation of the S or T in this motif disrupts PDZ domain binding. For example, phosphorylation of this serine in the β_2-adrenergic receptor was shown to lead to a loss of PDZ domain–mediated binding to EBP50, which regulates endocytic sorting of receptor.

Domains that Mediate Protein Binding to Membrane Lipids

Localization of proteins to membranes greatly limits the space in which they can diffuse and increases the probability that enzymes and substrates will contact each other. A variety of domains have evolved to bind phospholipids as a means of membrane localization (Table 5.5). C1 domains present in PKCs and some other signaling molecules bind to DAG, thereby recruiting PKCs to the membrane.[49] Membrane recruitment of PKCs is also aided by the C2 domain, which binds to anionic phospholipids in the presence of calcium. This pathway is controlled by DAG production by PLC-dependent hydrolysis of PtdIns-4,5-P_2.

Several different domains bind to phosphoinositides, localizing the proteins that contain them to membranes.[50] These domains include pleckstrin homology (PH), Phox, FYVE, FERM, and ENTH domains. Particular PH domains bind specific phosphoinositides, including PtdIns-3-P, PtdIns-4,5-P_2, PtdIns-3,4-P_2, and PtdIns-3,4,5-P_3. Phox and FYVE domains typically bind to PtdIns-3-P. FERM and ENTH domains bind to PtdIns-4,5-P_2. The accessibility of the domain and the availability of PtdIns phosphates regulate these interactions. Phosphoinositide kinases synthesize phosphoinositides. PtdIns4-kinases synthesize PtdIns-4-P from PtdIns. Type I PtdIns phosphate kinases phosphorylate PtdIns-4-P at the 5 position to make PtdIns-4,5-P_2. Phosphoinositide levels are also regulated by phosphatases. PTEN and related phosphatases remove the phosphate from the 3 position of the PtdIns-3,4,5-P_3. PtdIns-3,4-P_2, and PtdIns-3-P.[51] PTEN thus counteracts PI3-kinase signals, and cells lacking PTEN expression have increased signaling through PI3-kinase–dependent pathways. A family of phosphatases that removes the phosphate from the 5 position of PtdIns-3,4,5-P_3, the SH2 inositol phosphatases (SHIP1 and SHIP2), also regulates phosphoinositide signaling pathways.[52]

TABLE 5.5

DOMAINS THAT BIND PHOSPHOLIPIDS

Phospholipid	Domains that Bind
Diacylglycerol	C1
Phosphatidic acid	PX
PtdIns-4-P	PH
PtdIns-3-P	PX, PH, FYVE
PtdIns-3,4-P_2	PH, PX
PtdIns-3,5-P_2	PH
PtdIns-4,5-P_2	PH, Tubby, FERM, Sprouty, ENTH, ANTH
PtdIns-3,4,5-P_3	PH

PH, pleckstrin homology.

Acute production of specific phosphoinositides in a membrane compartment results in the recruitment of proteins containing PH domains that recognize that phosphoinositide. Colocalization of a subset of proteins allows them to interact more efficiently. An example of the role of PH domains in such a pathway is the activation of Akt by PDK1.[53] PDK1 and Akt are protein serine-threonine kinases that contain PH domains that bind PtdIns-3,4-P_2 or PtdIns-3,4,5-P_3. Activation of PI3-kinase leads to local synthesis of PtdIns-3,4-P_2 and PtdIns-3,4,5-P_3, which causes recruitment of Akt and PDK1 to the same membrane location. This localization facilitates phosphorylation and activation of Akt by PDK1.

Regulation of Protein Levels: Transcription, Translation, and Proteolysis

In addition to influencing the activity of proteins in the cell, signal transduction pathways also regulate the type and levels of proteins expressed in cells. This sort of regulation is necessary for development, differentiation, and the specific function of distinct cell types. Whether a protein is expressed at all in a cell is regulated at the transcriptional level, whereas transcription, translation, and proteolysis have a role in determining the concentration of a protein in a cell.

Ultimately, most signal transduction pathways regulate gene transcription and, thus, the level and type of proteins expressed in the cell. Analysis of the effects of stimuli on gene expression profiles using microarray analysis has shown that a single stimulus affects the transcription of hundreds of genes. The ability to transcribe a gene is regulated at multiple levels, including the structure of chromatin in the region of the gene, modifications of the promoter regions, and the activity of transcription factors and coactivators. Signal transduction pathways regulate histone acetylases and deacetylases that determine the accessibility of chromatin to the transcriptional apparatus. Recent work has shown that a number of signals lead to histone hyperacetylation that disrupts the nucleosome to allow transcription. These pathways cooperate with the activation of transcription factors.

Signal transduction pathways regulate transcription factors in numerous ways. The binding of ligands to the nuclear receptor family of transcription factors causes dissociation of the receptor from a complex with heat shock proteins and allows the receptor to bind to DNA. Tyrosine phosphorylation of the STAT family of transcription factors by Jak kinases in response to stimulation of cytokine receptors allows them to dimerize through their SH2 domains, enter the nucleus, and bind to DNA.[54] TGF-β receptors activate transcription by phosphorylating SMAD proteins on serine residues. Phosphorylation of SMAD proteins promotes heterodimerization with SMAD4 and exposes the DNA-binding domain. Activated SMADs translocate to the nucleus complex with a protein called Fast1 and bind to DNA to regulate transcription.

Activation of transcription factors also occurs much farther downstream from the receptor. Stimulation of the transcriptional activity of Elk-1 by EGF requires a Ras exchange factor, which leads to activation of Ras. Active Ras stimulates Raf. Raf in turn phosphorylates and activates MEK1, which phosphorylates and activates ERK. Active ERK translocates to the nucleus and phosphorylates Elk-1.

Translation is controlled at several levels.[55] The sequences of some RNAs result in stable tertiary structures that bind proteins to regulate location or translation. The ability of these types of RNAs to be translated is regulated by protein kinase cascades. A common mechanism is phosphorylation of initiation factor eIF-4E. $p70^{S6}$ kinase regulates the translation of specific RNAs containing a 5′ terminal oligopyrimidine tract by phosphorylation of the ribosomal S6 protein. This increases the ability of the ribosome to process such messages.

The levels of some proteins are regulated by proteolysis, which occurs either via the proteosome or the lysosome. Ubiquitination targets proteins to the proteosome but can also regulate other aspects of protein function.[56] An example of the role of ubiquitination is the regulation of IκB levels (introduced previously). Phosphorylation of IκB is stimulated by a number of receptor-mediated signaling pathways and leads to its dissociation from NF-κB and allows NF-κB to enter the nucleus and bind DNA. After phosphorylation, the β-transducin repeat-containing protein binds to IκB, recruiting ubiquitin ligase that catalyzes the ubiquitination of IκB and leads to its recognition and degradation by the proteosome.

The second major pathway of protein degradation is the lysosomal pathway. An early response to the stimulation of receptors is their internalization into endosomes. Some receptors continue to signal following endocytosis.[57] In the case of receptor tyrosine kinases, ligand-dependent kinase activity is necessary for endocytosis, mediated by clathrin-coated pits. After endocytosis, receptors recycle to the plasma membrane of the endosomes and fuse with lysosomes, leading to degradation of the receptor.

SIGNALING NETWORKS

Although signaling pathways are usually depicted as linear cascades, nearly all signaling pathways are highly interconnected and form networks that allow dynamic regulation of the timing, strength, and duration of signaling. In addition, both feed forward and feed backward loops provide the means to self-regulate signaling or to integrate signaling from multiple signals simultaneously.

As a consequence, the same signal may induce different outcomes depending on the particular cell or cell state. For example, TGFβ can stimulate cell proliferation or arrest in different cells. With the development of small molecule and antibody inhibitors that show exquisite specificity for their targets, inhibition of one part of a signaling cascade may lead to cell death in some contexts and paradoxical proliferation in others. For example, a small molecule inhibitor of the serine-threonine kinase BRAF in some melanomas that harbor an activated mutant BRAF leads to cell death, while this same inhibitor can lead to increased proliferation in tumor cells that contain a normal *BRAF* gene but instead have an activating mutation in *KRAS*.[58–60] Thus, deciphering specific pathways as well as their interconnections is necessary to understand how cells and tissues respond to physiologic and pathologic stimuli as well as to predict the response to therapy.

Selected References

The full list of references for this chapter appears in the online version.

1. Kao J, Rosenstein BS, Peters S, Milano MT, Kron SJ. Cellular response to DNA damage. *Ann N Y Acad Sci* 2005;1066:243.
2. Ferrell JE Jr. Self-perpetuating states in signal transduction: positive feedback, double-negative feedback and bistability. *Curr Opin Cell Biol* 2002; 14:140.
3. Schlessinger J. Cell signaling by receptor tyrosine kinases. *Cell* 2000; 103:211.
4. Rothenberg SM, Engelman JA, Le S, et al. Modeling oncogene addiction using RNA interference. *Proc Natl Acad Sci U S A* 2008;105:12480.
5. Fretto LJ, Snape AJ, Tomlinson JE, et al. Mechanism of platelet-derived growth factor (PDGF) AA, AB, and BB binding to alpha and beta PDGF receptor. *J Biol Chem* 1993;268:3625.
6. de Vos AM, Ultsch M, Kossiakoff AA. Human growth hormone and extracellular domain of its receptor: crystal structure of the complex. *Science* 1992;255:306.
7. Spivak-Kroizman T, Lemmon A, Dikic A, et al. Heparin-induced oligomerization of FGF molecules is responsible for FGF receptor dimerization, activation, and cell proliferation. *Cell* 1994;79:1015.
8. Schlessinger J. Ligand-induced, receptor-mediated dimerization and activation of EGF receptor. *Cell* 2002;110:669.
10. Harris RC, Chung E, Coffey RJ. EGF receptor ligands. *Exp Cell Res* 2003; 284:2.
11. Zhang X, Pickin KA, Bose R, et al. Inhibition of the EGF receptor by binding of MIG6 to an activating kinase domain interface. *Nature* 2007; 450:741.
12. Zhang X, Gureasko J, Shen K, Cole PA, Kuriyan J. An allosteric mechanism for activation of the kinase domain of epidermal growth factor receptor. *Cell* 2006;125:1137.
13. Kerr IM, Costa-Pereira AP, Lillemeier BF, Strobl B. Of JAKs, STATs, blind watchmakers, jeeps and trains. *FEBS Lett* 2003;546:1.
14. Mustelin T, Abraham RT, Rudd CE, Alonso A, Merlo JJ. Protein tyrosine phosphorylation in T cell signaling. *Front Biosci* 2002;7:d918.
15. Gauld SB, Dal Porto JM, Cambier JC. B cell antigen receptor signaling: roles in cell development and disease. *Science* 2002;296:1641.
16. Shi Y, Massague J. Mechanisms of TGF-beta signaling from cell membrane to the nucleus. *Cell* 2003;113:685.
17. Tonks NK. Protein tyrosine phosphatases: from genes, to function, to disease. *Nat Rev Mol Cell Biol* 2006;7:833.
19. Pierce KL, Premont RT, Lefkowitz RJ. Seven-transmembrane receptors. *Nat Rev Mol Cell Biol* 2002;3:639.
21. Wettschureck N, Offermanns S. Mammalian G proteins and their cell type specific functions. *Physiol Rev* 2005;85:1159.
24. Murad F. Shattuck lecture. Nitric oxide and cyclic GMP in cell signaling and drug development. *N Engl J Med* 2006;355:2003.
26. van Amerongen R, Nusse R. Towards an integrated view of Wnt signaling in development. *Development* 2009;136:3205.

27. Arnaout MA, Mahalingam B, Xiong JP. Integrin structure, allostery, and bidirectional signaling. *Annu Rev Cell Dev Biol* 2005;21:381.
29. Bjorge JD, Jakymiw A, Fujita DJ. Selected glimpses into the activation and function of Src kinase. *Oncogene* 2000;19:5620.
30. Hubbard SR. Protein tyrosine kinases: autoregulation and small-molecule inhibition. *Curr Opin Struct Biol* 2002;12:735.
31. Manning G, Whyte DB, Martinez R, Hunter T, Sudarsanam S. The protein kinase complement of the human genome. *Science* 2002;298:1912.
32. Barford D, Das AK, Egloff MP. The structure and mechanism of protein phosphatases: insights into catalysis and regulation. *Annu Rev Biophys Biomol Struct* 1998;27:133.
33. Barford D, Neel BG. Revealing mechanisms for SH2 domain mediated regulation of the protein tyrosine phosphatase SHP-2. *Structure* 1998;6:249.
34. Simonds WF. G protein regulation of adenylate cyclase. *Trends Pharmacol Sci* 1999;20:66.
35. Chong H, Vikis HG, Guan KL. Mechanisms of regulating the Raf kinase family. *Cell Signal* 2003;15:463.
37. Rhee SG. Regulation of phosphoinositide-specific phospholipase C. *Annu Rev Biochem* 2001;70:281.
39. Soberman RJ, Christmas P. The organization and consequences of eicosanoid signaling. *J Clin Invest* 2003;111:1107.
40. Bunney TD, Katan M. Phosphoinositide signalling in cancer: beyond PI3K and PTEN. *Nat Rev Cancer* 2010;10:342.
41. Grant S. Cotargeting survival signaling pathways in cancer. *J Clin Invest* 2008;118:3003.
42. Lei EP, Silver PA. Protein and RNA export from the nucleus. *Dev Cell* 2002;2:261.
43. Hogan PG, Chen L, Nardone J, Rao A. Transcriptional regulation by calcium, calcineurin, and NFAT. *Genes Dev* 2003;17:2205.
44. Virshup DM. Protein phosphatase 2A: a panoply of enzymes. *Curr Opin Cell Biol* 2000;12:180.
46. Schlessinger J, Lemmon MA. SH2 and PTB domains in tyrosine kinase signaling. *Sci STKE* 2003;2003(191):RE12.
47. Yaffe MB, Elia AE. Phosphoserine/threonine-binding domains. *Curr Opin Cell Biol* 2001;13:131.
48. Nourry C, Grant SG, Borg JP. PDZ domain proteins: plug and play! *Sci STKE* 2003;2003(179):RE7.
50. Hurley JH. Membrane binding domains. *Biochim Biophys Acta* 2006;1761: 805.
51. Maehama T, Taylor GS, Dixon JE. PTEN and myotubularin: novel phosphoinositide phosphatases. *Annu Rev Biochem* 2001;70:247.
52. Rohrschneider LR, Fuller JF, Wolf I, Liu Y, Lucas DM. Structure, function, and biology of SHIP proteins. *Genes Dev* 2000;14:505.
53. Mora A, Komander D, van Aalten DM, Alessi DR. PDK1, the master regulator of AGC kinase signal transduction. *Semin Cell Dev Biol* 2004;15:161.
54. Levy DE, Darnell JE Jr. Stats: transcriptional control and biological impact. *Nat Rev Mol Cell Biol* 2002;3:651.
55. Dever TE. Gene-specific regulation by general translation factors. *Cell* 2002;108:545.
56. Kerscher O, Felberbaum R, Hochstrasser M. Modification of proteins by ubiquitin and ubiquitin-like proteins. *Annu Rev Cell Dev Biol* 2006;22:159.
57. Di Fiore PP, De Camilli P. Endocytosis and signaling. an inseparable partnership. *Cell* 2001;106:1.
58. Hatzivassiliou G, Song K, Yen I, et al. RAF inhibitors prime wild-type RAF to activate the MAPK pathway and enhance growth. *Nature* 2010;464: 431.
59. Poulikakos PI, Zhang C, Bollag G, Shokat KM, Rosen N. RAF inhibitors transactivate RAF dimers and ERK signalling in cells with wild-type BRAF. *Nature* 2010;464:427.
60. Heidorn SJ, Milagre C, Whittaker S, et al. Kinase-dead BRAF and oncogenic RAS cooperate to drive tumor progression through CRAF. *Cell* 2010;140:209.

CHAPTER 6 CELL CYCLE

STEVEN I. REED

Cell division is a process that must be carried out with absolute fidelity. The program of generating an adult organism from a single zygote involves countless cell duplications, each requiring the precise partitioning of genetic material and most other cellular components to daughter cells. The division process then continues during adult life to replenish essential cells restricted to a limited lifespan. As a result, organisms have evolved cell-duplication strategies that include redundant safeguards to prevent errors or, if errors occur, to correct them. Nevertheless, errors do occur at a measurable frequency, and mutations accumulated over time can weaken protective mechanisms, rendering the genome increasingly vulnerable to challenges. The resulting loss of genetic and genomic stability has serious implications for survival in that it is a major contributing factor to the development of malignancy. Indeed, cancer is one of the leading causes of mortality in humans.

In this chapter, the basic principles of mammalian cell division and the mechanisms that have evolved to safeguard the integrity of the process are reviewed. Then there is a discussion of how the normal control mechanisms of cell division and protective safeguards become subverted in cancer cells. It is hoped that, ultimately, detailed knowledge of cell division in normal and cancer cells will lead to rational effective therapeutic approaches.

CELL-CYCLE ENGINE

Although the details of cell division vary considerably across phylogenetic lines and even in different cell types within the same organism, the underlying infrastructure that mediates and controls the cell division process is remarkably conserved. If one compares yeast cells and mammalian cells in culture, perhaps the two most aggressively studied model cell division systems are not only the respective cell division cycles organized along a similar scheme, but many of the proteins used in the cell division pathway are easily recognizable as being evolutionarily related. Indeed, some of these proteins are so highly conserved that they are functional in the heterologous organism despite a billion years of divergent evolution.

Phases of the Cell Cycle

As alluded to previously, the basic organization of the cell cycle is highly conserved in eukaryotic evolution. In 1951, Howard and Pelc,[1] studying the division of plant root cells, separated the process into four phases eventually referred to as *GAP1*, *synthetic phase*, *GAP2*, and *mitosis*. The shorthand that emerged from this descriptive work (G_1, S phase, G_2, and M phase or mitosis) has been the lens through which all subsequent dividing cells have been observed, and the four successive phases are referred to collectively as the *cell cycle*. The key observation made by these investigators was that the events that together make up the cell division process do not all occur continuously. Specifically, although growth and protein synthesis occur constantly for the most part, synthesis of DNA occurs only during a discrete interval. The preceding phase was designated *GAP1* or G_1, and the subsequent phase before cell division was referred to as *GAP2* or G_2. Although at the time little could be said concerning what a cell did during these silent "gap" phases, it is now known that these are not idle periods in a cell's life but the intervals in which most regulation of the cell cycle is specifically exerted. A large amount of information, originating from the external environment and the cell's internal milieu, is integrated during the G_1 and G_2 intervals and used to determine whether and when to proceed into S phase and M phase, respectively.

Mitosis, the most visibly dynamic interval of the cell cycle, has itself been traditionally subdivided into five phases: prophase, prometaphase, metaphase, anaphase, and telophase. In metazoans and plants (as opposed to fungi) mitosis entails a particularly dramatic change of state for the cell. During prophase most of the internal membranous compartments of the cell, including the nucleus, are disassembled and dispersed. Replicated chromosomes (chromatids) are condensed into paired compact rods, and a bipolar microtubule spindle is assembled. Biosynthesis of proteins (transcription and translation) largely ceases. During prometaphase, chromosomes form bivalent attachments to the spindle, driving them to the cellular equator. Proper alignment of paired chromatids on the spindle is indicative of metaphase. During anaphase, the paired sister chromatids lose cohesion and microtubule forces separate the chromatids and pull them to opposite poles of the cell. During telophase, the events of prophase are reversed: The nuclei and other membrane structures reassemble, the chromosomes decondense, and protein synthesis resumes. After mitosis, the two daughter cells pull apart and separate in a process known as *cytokinesis*.

Current knowledge of the cell cycle has accrued historically from a number of different experimental approaches and systems. In the early 1970s, experiments carried out by fusing mammalian cells in different cell-cycle phases revealed the existence of dominant inductive activities for the S phase and the M phase.[2,3] Shortly thereafter, similar inductive activities were isolated from mature frog eggs arrested at meiotic metaphase II and shown to be capable of inducing G_2 oocytes to enter into meiotic divisions,[4] equivalent in many respects to mitosis. At the same time, genetic analysis of cell division in yeast revealed that the products of individual genes controlled specific events in the cell cycle and that these events could be organized in pathways, much like metabolic pathways.[5] Eventually, all of these lines of investigation converged in the 1980s, leading to the discovery of cyclin-dependent kinases (CDKs).

Cyclin-Dependent Kinases

Arguably the most significant advance in understanding cell-cycle regulation was the discovery of CDKs.[6] These are binary, proline-directed, serine-threonine–specific protein kinases that consist of a catalytic subunit (the CDK) that has little if any intrinsic enzymatic activity and a requisite positive regulatory subunit known as a *cyclin*. In yeast, one CDK and numerous cyclins carry out cell-cycle regulatory functions, whereas in mammals, these same functions are carried out by a number of different CDKs and cyclins. In yeast, in which multiple cyclins activate the same CDK (CDK1, also known as Cdc28 or Cdc2, depending on the species) for distinct cell-cycle tasks, it is clear that most if not all substrate specificity beyond a rather degenerate primary structure target consensus lies in the cyclin subunit. In mammals, it is likely that substrate specificity is shared by CDK and cyclin subunits. Although not all pairwise combinations are permitted, there are enough combinatorial possibilities to create a significant level of substrate specificity.

CDKs have a structure similar to that of other protein kinases, consisting of two globular domains (the N-lobe and C-lobe) held together by a semiflexible hinge region. Protein substrates bound by the active enzyme are thought to fit into a cleft between the two domains. The N-lobe contains the adenosine triphosphate (ATP)–binding site. Studies comparing CDKs and CDK-cyclin complexes based on x-ray diffraction crystallography indicate that the primary role of the cyclin, in addition to substrate docking functions, is to realign critical active site residues into a catalytically permissive configuration and to open the catalytic cleft to accommodate substrates.[7] Once bound to a cyclin, the CDK active site is configured similarly to other protein kinases that do not require cyclin binding.

The known CDKs and cyclins and their presumptive intervals of function in the mammalian cell cycle are summarized in Figure 6.1. For the most part, the functional intervals of CDKs are determined by the accumulation and disappearance of cyclins. Whereas CDKs tend to be expressed at a constant level through the cell cycle, cyclin accumulation is usually dynamic, regulated at the level of biosynthesis and degradation (discussed in greater detail in "Cell-Cycle Machinery"). To summarize, three partially redundant D-type cyclins (D1, D2, and D3) activate two partially redundant CDKs (CDK4 and CDK6). Although, unlike most other cyclins, D-type cyclins do not appear to be expressed with high periodicity in cycling cells, the interval at which their primary activating function is thought to occur is from mid-to-late G_1 to direct phosphorylation of the cell-cycle inhibitor pRb and related proteins p107 and p130. Phosphorylation of these proteins by cyclin D–CDK4/6 inactivates their negative regulatory functions, allowing progression into S phase.[8,9]

Unlike D-type cyclins, E-type cyclins (E1 and E2) are expressed with high cell-cycle periodicity, accumulating in late G_1 and declining during S phase. E-type cyclins activate CDK2, and the fact that premature expression of cyclin E1 leads to accelerated entry into S phase[10,11] has suggested that the target(s) must be proteins responsible for initiation of DNA replication. However, the essentiality of cyclin E–CDK2 in this context has been put into question by the demonstration that cells from cyclin E1/E2 nullizygous mouse embryos can cycle with reasonably normal kinetics and can certainly initiate DNA replication.[12] The most likely explanation for the dispensability of E-type cyclins for S phase functions is redundancy with cyclin A, which also activates CDK2.

Cyclin A accumulates initially at the G_1/S-phase boundary and persists until prometaphase of mitosis. It has been best characterized as an activator of CDK2; however, it has also been reported to form complexes with CDK1. It is presumed that CDK2, activated by E-type cyclins and cyclin A, promotes cell-cycle progression from the G_1/S boundary through the G_2 interval.

At this time, B-type cyclins, in conjunction with CDK1, are responsible for getting cells into and through mitosis. Although mammalian cells express a number of B-type cyclins, only cyclin B1 appears to be essential. Cyclin B1 accumulates through S phase and G_2 and then is degraded at the metaphase-anaphase transition. It should be pointed out that the CDK family is extensive and that eukaryotes possess many additional CDKs that ostensibly have nothing to do with cell-cycle regulation.

The blueprint for CDK function through the mammalian cell cycle presented here is based on a large body of experimental evidence and most likely accounts for primary activities at each cell-cycle stage. However, this model does not account for potential redundancy of CDK function. Recently, however, it has been demonstrated that a *CDK2*-nullizygous mouse is viable, and furthermore, relatively normal.[13,14] Investigation of embryonic fibroblasts from these mice has suggested that in the absence of CDK2, CDK1 can carry out the functions normally attributed to CDK2.[15] However, the contribution of CDK1 to these functions in unperturbed cells remains to be determined.

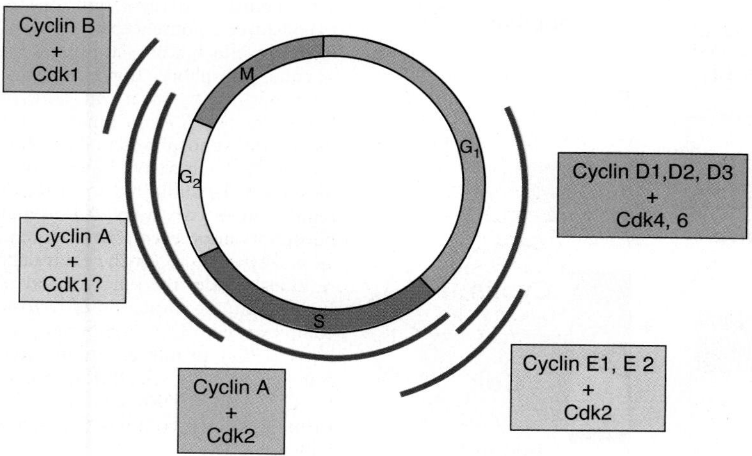

FIGURE 6.1 Windows of cyclin-dependent kinase (CDK) function in the cell cycle. D-type cyclins (cyclins D1, D2, and D3) activate CDK4 and CDK6 for functions extending from middle G_1 to the G_1/S-phase transition. E-type cyclins (cyclins E1 and E2) activate CDK2 for functions at the G_1/S-phase boundary, probably extending into early S phase. Cyclin A activates CDK2 for functions extending from the G_1/S-phase boundary and extending into G_2. Cyclin A is known to interact with CDK1 as well; however, no specific function for this complex has been identified. Finally, cyclin B activates CDK1 at the G_2/M-phase boundary with activity that lasts until cyclin B is degraded during anaphase.

Modes of Cyclin-Dependent Kinase Regulation

Because the activity of CDKs is central to cell survival, these enzymes are, of necessity, highly regulated.[6] As a result, a number of diverse regulatory mechanisms have evolved to allow for integration of environmental and internal signals (Fig. 6.2). A primary mode of CDK regulation is the availability of activating cyclins, as alluded to previously. For most cell-cycle regulatory CDKs, the relevant cyclins exhibit a distinct temporal program of accumulation and degradation, determining a precise window of CDK activation. Although D-type cyclins tend not to be highly regulated in cycling cells, they are strongly down-regulated as cells exit the cell cycle into a nonproliferative state and then resynthesized in response to mitogen stimulation and cell-cycle re-entry. The genes encoding cyclin E1 and E2 are transcribed periodically late in G_1 and up to the G_1-S phase transition. This, coupled with ubiquitin-mediated proteolysis of cyclin E in active cyclin E–CDK2 complexes, creates the observed window of cyclin E accumulation from late G_1 to mid-S phase.

Like cyclin E, the accumulation of cyclin A is determined by periodic transcription. However, unlike cyclin E, cyclin A remains stable in active CDK2 complexes. The timing of ubiquitin-mediated proteolysis of cyclin A is determined by activation of a protein-ubiquitin ligase known as the *anaphase-promoting complex/cyclosome* (APC/C) in prometaphase. Thus, the window of cyclin A accumulation is from the G_1-S transition until early in mitosis. Finally, B-type cyclin accumulation is also linked to periodic transcription. In this case, transcription begins in late S phase and persists through G_2. Similarly to cyclin A, B-type cyclins are targeted for ubiquitin-mediated proteolysis by the APC/C during mitosis, although their disappearance occurs slightly later in mitosis than that of cyclin A.

It is interesting to note that periodic transcription of cyclins E, A, and B mRNAs relies primarily on negative regulation. For cyclin E, an element known as *CERM* (cyclin E repressor module) binds a repressor complex containing the repressive member of the E2F family of transcription factors, E2F4, as well as the Rb-related protein p107 and a histone deacetylase.[16] Inactivation of the repressive complex in late G1 via phosphorylation of p107 by CDK4/6 allows the constitutive transcription factor, Sp1, to drive cyclin E transcription. Transcription of cyclin A and B mRNAs is similarly regulated. In this case, the repressor element is known as cell cycle genes homology region (CHR)[17] but the corresponding repressor complex has not yet been well characterized. However, once repression is relieved, transcription of both cyclin A and B mRNAs is driven the constitutive transcription factor, NF-Y.

A second important mode of CDK regulation is by phosphorylation. CDKs require an activating phosphorylation on a structural feature designated the *T loop*. Phosphorylation induces a movement of the T loop that has global effects on CDK structure, including an increase in CDK-cyclin contacts and changes in the substrate-binding site.[18] In most if not all instances, T-loop phosphorylation appears to constitute a housekeeping function that occurs concomitant with cyclin binding. However, negative regulatory phosphorylation of CDKs is a highly dynamic process. Proper cell-cycle regulation of CDK1, in particular, requires phosphorylation on two residues within the N-lobe, adjacent to the ATP-binding site: threonine 14 and tyrosine 15. During the normal course of the cell cycle, as cyclin B–CDK1 complexes accumulate, they are immediately phosphorylated at these sites and thereby kept inactive. This allows stockpiling of the large numbers of cyclin B–CDK1 complexes required for efficient entry into mitosis and maintaining them in an inactive state during late S phase and G_2. At the G_2/M-phase boundary, there is concerted dephosphorylation of these residues, causing cells to advance rapidly into mitosis. Although CDK2 and CDK4 have also been reported to undergo negative regulatory phosphorylation at the homologous residues, the function(s) of this regulation are not as clear-cut (but see "DNA Damage Checkpoints").

A third mode of CDK regulation is through the action of inhibitory proteins that can form either binary complexes with CDKs or ternary complexes with cyclin-CDK dimers. These exist in three major families. The INK4 family consists of four members (p15, p16, p18, and p19). All are composed of a series of conserved structural motifs known as *ankyrin repeats*

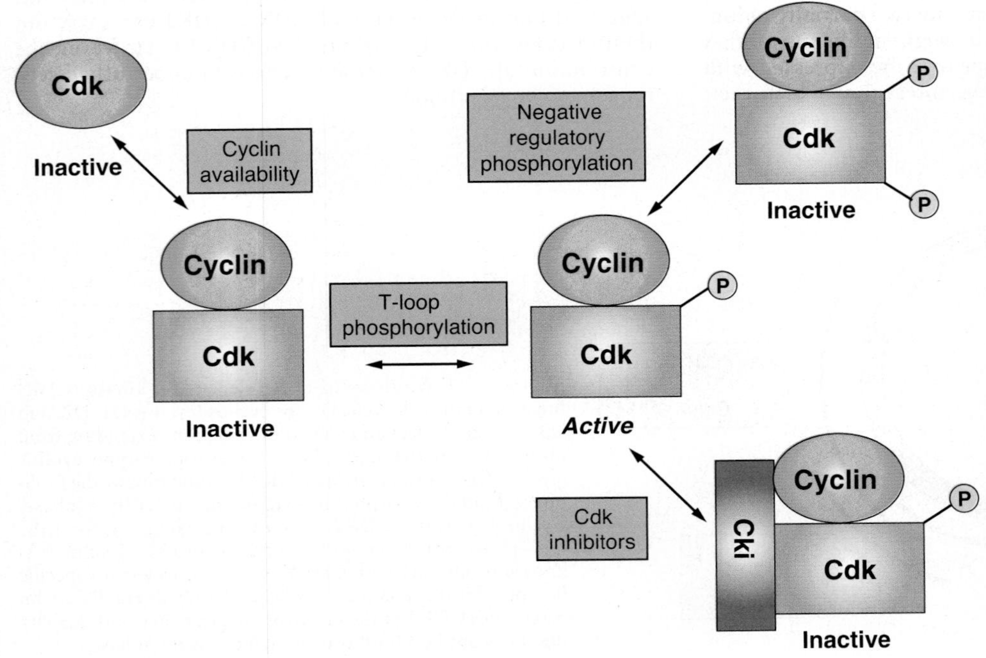

FIGURE 6.2 Principles of cyclin-dependent kinase (CDK) regulation. Because CDK catalytic subunits are inactive when unbound to cyclins, the first level of regulation is through the expression and availability of cyclins. The second level of regulation appears to constitute a housekeeping function in that cyclin binding stimulates an essential phosphorylation of a threonine within a structural feature known as the *T loop*. Binary complexes with phosphorylated T loops are active. Such active kinase complexes can be subjected to negative regulation in two ways. Additional phosphorylation events on threonine 14 and tyrosine 15 (or the equivalent residues) render the kinase inactive. In addition, the formation of ternary complexes with CDK inhibitory proteins (Ckis) promotes an inactive state. One class of Cki, INK4, specific for CDK4 and CDK6, can inhibit by forming binary complexes directly with the CDK.

and they specifically target CDK4 and CDK6. The mechanism of action of these inhibitors is to bind the CDK subunit and, by causing a rotation of the N-lobe relative to the C-lobe, constraining the kinase in an inactive conformation and, in addition, precluding cyclin binding.[19] The Cip/Kip family consists of three members in mammals: $p21^{Cip1}$, $p27^{Kip1}$, and $p57^{Kip2}$. All contain a conserved amino terminal cyclin-CDK–binding inhibitory domain and a divergent C-terminal domain possessing other less well-characterized functions. Although these have been characterized primarily as potent inhibitors of CDK2 and have more recently been shown to also be effective CDK1 inhibitors, the case for inhibition of CDK4 and CDK6 is less certain. Whereas Cip/Kip inhibitors are clearly capable of inhibiting CDK4 and CDK6 at high concentration, it is not clear that these conditions are met *in vivo*, and the situation is further complicated by the finding that Cip/Kip inhibitor binding is actually required to provide a chaperonin or assembly function for the efficient formation of active cyclin D–CDK4 complexes.[20] In the case of cyclin A–CDK2, where structural studies have been carried out, it appears that the Cip/Kip inhibitors first anchor via a high-affinity interaction with the cyclin.[21] This then allows the inhibitor polypeptide to invade and deform the N-lobe, thus interfering with ATP binding and catalysis.[16] The final class of inhibitors consists of two members of the pRb protein family, p107 and p130. Although these proteins have well-characterized functions as transcriptional inhibitors, they also are potent cyclin E/A–CDK2 inhibitors. p107 and p130 each contain cyclin-binding and CDK-binding sites that collaborate to confer inhibitory activity.

A final mode of CDK regulation is via control of nuclear import/export. This level of regulation is most obvious for cyclin B–CDK1 complexes, which are kept out of the nucleus via active nuclear export until late G_2, when phosphorylation inactivates *cis*-acting nuclear export signals allowing nuclear accumulation.[22] Sequestration of cyclin B–CDK1 in the cytoplasm is a redundant mechanism, along with negative regulatory phosphorylation of CDK1, for preventing premature phosphorylation of mitotic targets.

INDUCTION OF CELL-CYCLE PHASE TRANSITIONS

The cell cycle is composed of two action phases, S phase and M phase, in which the genetic material is duplicated and the components of a mother cell are divided into two daughter cells, respectively. The intervening phases, G_1 and G_2, are thought to exist primarily to allow time for cell growth and for regulatory inputs. Therefore, from the point of view of regulatory theory, cell proliferation is controlled operationally at two key transitions: that between G_1 and S phase and that between G_2 and M phase. The important characteristic of these two transitions is that, once initiated based on integration of regulatory signals, they must be executed decisively to maintain genetic and genomic integrity. This is accomplished by using a combination of positive and negative modulators to set up the equivalent of a molecular capacitor.

In cycling mammalian cells, the programmed accumulation of cyclins E and A via transcriptional induction provides the positive impetus for the G_1-S phase transition. However, these kinases are kept in check by the action of Cip/Kip family inhibitors. If the internal and external environments are permissive for proliferation, the continued accumulation of cyclins will eventually titrate the inhibitors, allowing the latter to be phosphorylated by free cyclin-CDK complexes. Phosphorylation then marks these inhibitors as targets of ubiquitin-mediated proteolysis. The concerted destruction of CDK inhibitors and concomitant activation of the entire pool of CDK complexes assure that the transition into S phase is rapid and irreversible.

Although the details of its regulation are somewhat different, the strategy underlying control of the G_2-M transition is similar. Cyclin B–CDK1 complexes accumulate starting near the end of S phase but are held in check not by CDK inhibitors but by negative regulatory phosphorylation of CDK1. This phosphorylation on threonine 14 and tyrosine 15 is carried out by kinases Wee1 and Myt1. Entry into M phase is signaled by the rapid dephosphorylation of T14 and Y15, resulting in activation of CDK1. This dephosphorylation is carried out by specialized protein phosphatases, CDC25B and CDC25C. The concerted dephosphorylation of CDK1 depends on activation of CDC25 isoforms by phosphorylation, as well as ubiquitin-mediated proteolysis of Wee1, also in response to phosphorylation. Although the initial activation of CDC25 isoforms is thought to be carried out by other protein kinases, such as Plk1, CDC25B and C are also activated by cyclin B–CDK1, establishing a positive feedback loop. These positive feedback dynamics leading to the simultaneous activation of a large accumulated pool of cyclin B–CDK1 assures that entry into mitosis is decisive. The turnover of Wee1 enforces irreversibility. Because entry into mitosis involves dismantling many of the cell's components and organelles, as well as construction and use of a complex apparatus for segregating the cell's genetic material, mitosis is a period of particular vulnerability, and therefore it is important that this transition and subsequent events be carried out rapidly and efficiently.

An important secondary transition that occurs within M phase is that between metaphase and anaphase (Fig. 6.3).[23] To preserve genomic integrity, all duplicated chromosomes must be aligned along the cell's equator and properly attached to microtubules of the mitotic spindle. The trigger for separation of sister chromatids and their movement to opposite poles of the cell is the activation of the protein-ubiquitin ligase APC/C. This is achieved via CDK1 activation, but more importantly by the binding of a key cofactor, CDC20, whose availability is linked to the proper attachment of chromosomes and the integrity of the spindle. The targets of the APC/C are a protein known as *securin* as well as cyclin B, both of which inhibit a specialized protease, separase. The key target of separase is a complex that binds sister chromatids together: cohesin. Cleavage of the Scc1 subunit of cohesin leads to a rapid execution of anaphase. It is the ability to stockpile a large pool of inactive securin-separase complexes that can be rapidly mobilized by irreversible proteolysis of securin and cyclin B that allows for a rapid irreversible metaphase-anaphase transition.

UBIQUITIN-MEDIATED PROTEOLYSIS

It is becoming increasingly evident that much of the regulation of cell-cycle phase transitions depends on ubiquitin-mediated proteolysis.[24] Ubiquitin is a 76-amino acid polypeptide that can be covalently linked to lysines of other proteins via the formation of an isopeptide bond with its C-terminal carboxylate. Additional ubiquitin molecules can then be attached to the lysines of already conjugated ubiquitin to form polyubiquitin chains. Polyubiquitylated proteins are usually targeted for rapid proteolysis by a large multisubunit protease known as the *proteasome*. The enzymes that transfer ubiquitin to target proteins are known as *protein-ubiquitin ligases*. From the perspective of cell-cycle control, two families of protein-ubiquitin ligases have predominant roles. The first family, SCF (Skp1-Cullin–F-box protein), specifically targets proteins that are marked for destruction by phosphorylation. This allows degradation of specific proteins to be regulated at a separate

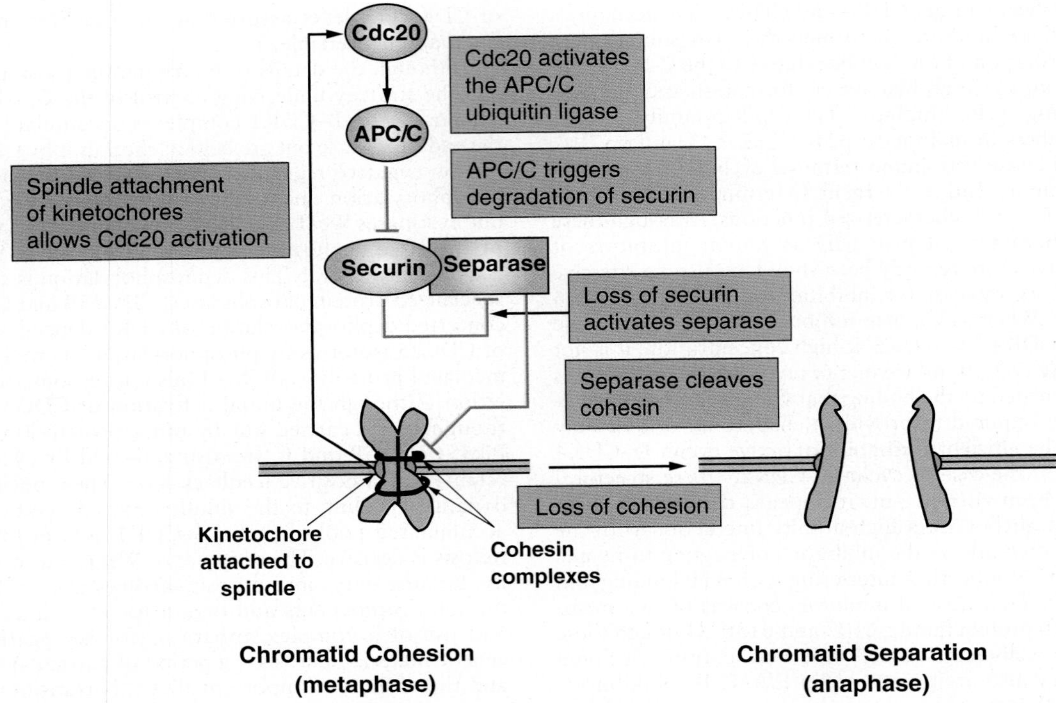

FIGURE 6.3 Regulation of the metaphase-anaphase transition. After replication, paired sister chromatids are held together by a complex of proteins, known collectively as *cohesin*, thus preventing anaphase. However, once paired chromatids have formed bivalent attachments to a functional mitotic spindle, inhibition of CDC20 mediated by the chromosome kinetochores is relieved. CDC20 is an essential cofactor of the protein-ubiquitin ligase anaphase-promoting complex/cyclosome (APC/C), which now becomes active. The primary initial target of the APC/C is securin, an inhibitor of the protease separase. Ubiquitin-mediated proteolysis of securin releases separase to cleave the cohesin subunit Scc1. This event releases paired chromatids from cohesion, thereby allowing anaphase to proceed.

level from the protein-ubiquitin ligase itself, which can be expressed constitutively and used to target a large number of substrates independently. SCF ligases consist of three invariant core components and one of a number of specificity factors (F-box proteins) that recognize phosphorylated substrates. A few notable examples of SCF protein-ubiquitin ligases are SCF^{Skp2} (containing the F-box protein Skp2), which targets p27[25] and p130,[26] and SCF^{CDC4} (containing the F-box protein CDC4, also known as FBXW7), which targets cyclin E.[27–29] The second family of protein-ubiquitin ligases that is critical for cell-cycle control is known collectively as the *APC/C*. The APC/C is a large complex consisting of 12 core subunits and 1 of 2 specificity factors, CDC20 and CDH1. Unlike SCF ubiquitin ligases, targeting of substrates by the APC/C is determined by ligase activation rather than substrate activation. APC^{CDC20} is active from metaphase until the end of mitosis as a result of periodic accumulation and degradation of CDC20 itself. APC^{CDH1}, on the other hand, which is negatively regulated by CDK-mediated phosphorylation, is activated on mitotic exit and during the subsequent G_1 interval when CDKs are inactive. In this manner, important mitotic targets, such as cyclin A, cyclin B, and securin (as well as many others), are degraded during mitosis and prevented from reaccumulating during the subsequent G_1 interval.

REGULATION OF THE CELL CYCLE

To preserve organismic function and integrity, the cell cycle must be regulated at a number of levels. These include entry into and exit from proliferation mode, coordination of cell-cycle events, and specialized responses that increase the probability of surviving a variety of environmental and internally generated insults.

Quiescence and Differentiation

The most fundamental aspect of cell-cycle control is the regulation of entry and exit. For mammalian cells, the decision to enter or exit the proliferative mode is based on environmental signals such as mitogens, growth factors, hormones, and cell-cell contact, as well as on internal differentiation programs. If the state of cell-cycle exit is reversible, it is referred to as *quiescence*. If it is in the context of terminal differentiation, cell-cycle exit may merely be one component of a differentiation program. Although cells entering quiescence and postmitotic differentiation vary from each other in many respects, from the perspective of cell-cycle control, they have much in common. First, cell-cycle exit is usually associated, at least initially, with an accumulation of G_1/S CDK inhibitors. Members of the INK4 family, targeting CDK4 and CDK6 and members of the Cip/Kip family, as well as the Rb-related protein p130, all targeting CDK2, are up-regulated. This causes accumulation of cells in G_1, from where cell-cycle exit can occur. Next, or simultaneously, the positive cell-cycle machinery is dismantled by down-regulation of CDKs and cyclins, primarily at the transcriptional level. In the case of quiescence, cell-cycle exit is paralleled by a reduced rate of protein synthesis, indicative that cells have entered a resting state.

Entry into and exit from quiescence are mediated largely by growth factors and mitogens that interact with cell surface receptors. These in turn are linked to intracellular signaling cascades that up-regulate the rate of protein synthesis as well as

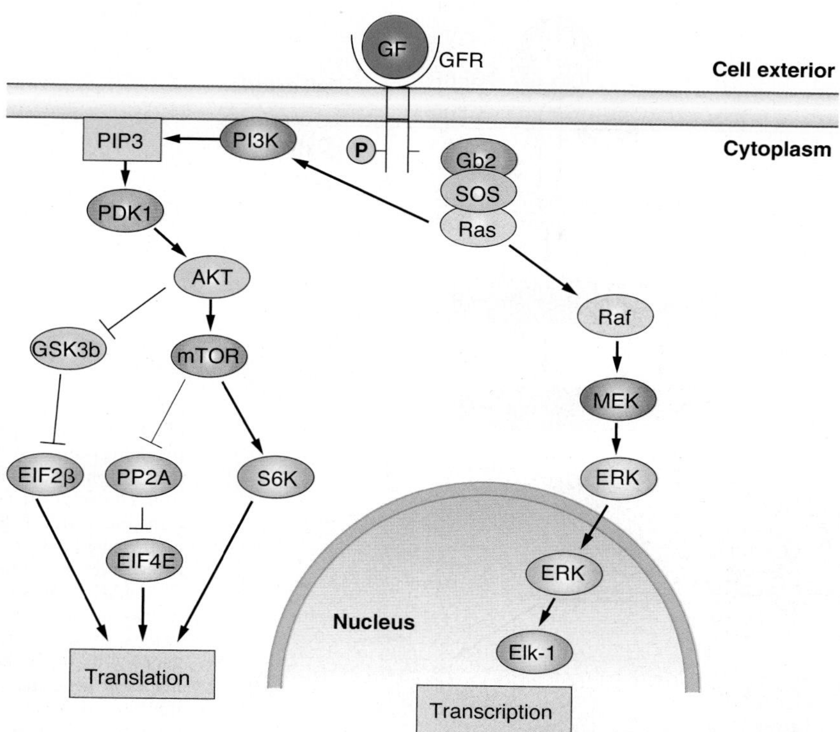

FIGURE 6.4 Growth factor (GF)/mitogen stimulator in response to occupancy of many GF receptors (GFRs) by ligand depends on the small guanosine triphosphatase transducer Ras. Receptor activation leads to phosphorylation of the receptor cytoplasmic domain. The phosphorylated receptor assembles a complex that includes Ras and its activated nucleotide exchange factor, son of sevenless (SOS), leading to activation of Ras. Activated Ras can then stimulate two important signal transduction pathways: the extracellular signaling–regulated kinase (ERK) pathway and the phosphoinositide 3 kinase (PI3K) pathway. Activated Ras stimulates the protein kinase activity of Raf, activating a protein kinase cascade consisting of Raf, MEK, and ERK. Activated ERK then translocates into the nucleus, where it phosphorylates and activates transcription factors, notably Elk-1. Genes important for growth and division are then transcribed. Activated Ras also stimulates PI3K activity, leading to the accumulation of phosphatidylinositol 3,4,5-triphosphate. This in turn stimulates the protein kinase activity of phosphoinositide-dependent kinase 1 (PDK1), activating a protein kinase cascade consisting of PDK1, AKT, and mTOR. Activation of this signal transduction pathway has the effect of stimulating translation and growth. AKT phosphorylates and inhibits the protein kinase glycogen synthase kinase 3 (GSK3β), thereby activating EIF2B required for translational initiation. mTOR phosphorylates and inhibits the protein phosphatase PP2A, thereby activating EIF4E, also required for translational initiation. Finally, mTOR phosphorylates and activates pp70S6 kinase, which in turn phosphorylates and activates ribosomal subunit S6.

the transcription of genes that promote proliferation, such as those encoding CDKs and cyclins. The two best-characterized signaling pathways in this context are the mitogen-activated protein kinase/extracellular signaling–regulated kinase pathway[30] and the phosphoinositide 3 (PI3) kinase/AKT pathway,[31] shown in Figure 6.4. Whereas the mitogen-activated protein kinase/extracellular signaling–regulated kinase pathway tends to stimulate expression of genes required for proliferation, the PI3-kinase/AKT pathway primarily stimulates protein synthesis and growth but also affects key cell-cycle regulatory proteins. Just as the presence of growth factors and mitogens stimulates these pathways, promoting cell-cycle entry, their removal shuts down these pathways, promoting quiescence. This is the basis for the reversibility of the quiescent state.

Antimitogenic Signals

An important aspect of control of cell division in mammals is antimitogenic signaling. Just as mitogens and growth factors bind to transmembrane receptors and use signal transduction pathways and downstream transcriptional programs to stimulate proliferation, parallel systems antagonize proliferation. The classic example of an antimitogenic signal is the effect of transforming growth factor-β (TGF-β) on epithelial cells (Fig. 6.5).[32] TGF-β, a cytokine, binds to a specific heterodimeric transmembrane receptor that, when occupied by ligand, phosphorylates a class of transcription factors, known as *SMADs*. These phosphorylated SMADs heterodimerize with non–receptor-interactive SMADs and translocate to the nucleus, where they complex with DNA-binding transcription factors and coactivators to transactivate specific genes. Relevant to cell-cycle regulation, stimulation of the TGF-β signaling pathway promotes transcription of the gene encoding p15. p15 is an INK4 class CDK inhibitor that specifically inactivates CDK4 and CDK6. However, the effects of p15 accumulation on cell-cycle regulators are more global than inhibition of CDK4/6.[33] INK4 inhibitors such as p15 have a secondary effect of displacing a pool of the Cip/Kip inhibitor p27 from cyclin D–CDK4/6 complexes, allowing it to then target and inactivate cyclin E–CDK2 and cyclin A–CDK2 (Fig. 6.5). Thus, exposure of epithelial cells to TGF-β has the effect of inhibiting G_1 and S phase CDK activities, thereby causing G_1 arrest.

Interestingly, in many cancers of epithelial origin, the response to TGF-β has been abrogated, suggesting that this and similar response pathways have an important role in maintaining control of proliferation. Interferons comprise another class of cytokines that have antiproliferative effects

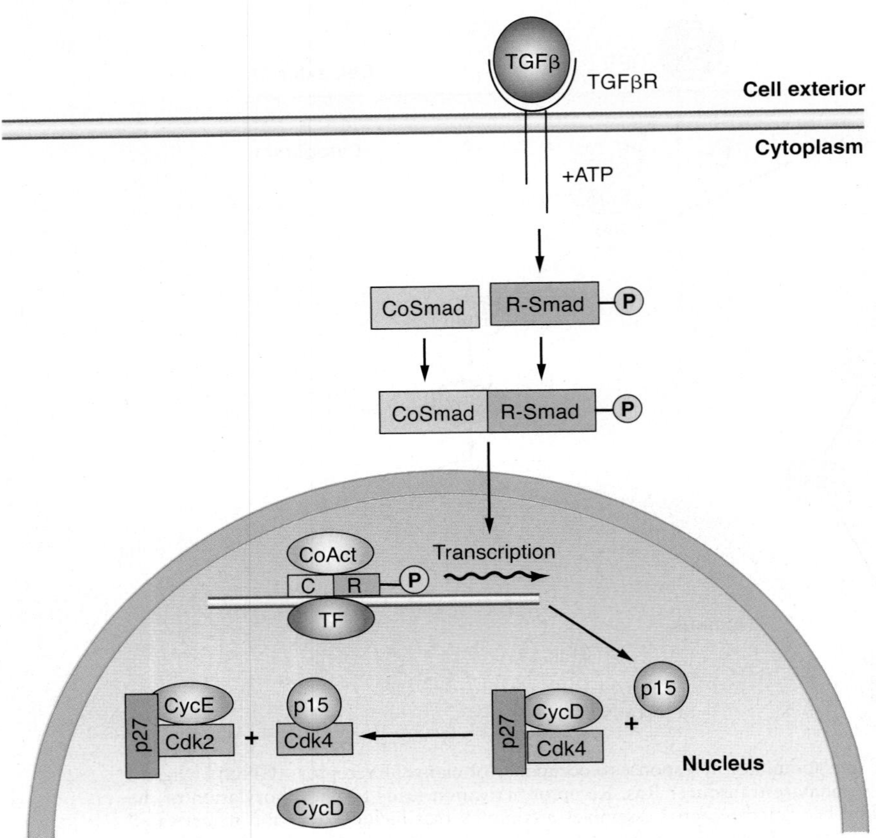

FIGURE 6.5 Transforming growth factor-β (TGF-β) antimitogenic pathway. Occupancy of the heterodimeric TGF-β receptor by ligand leads to phosphorylation of a class of transcription factor known collectively as *R-SMADs*. Phosphorylated R-SMADs then dimerize with nontargeted cofactors known as *CoSMADs* and translocate to the nucleus. There the R-SMAD/CoSMAD dimers complex with DNA-binding transcription factors and transcriptional coactivators to stimulate transcription of specific genes. One of the key targets of TGF-β signaling is the gene encoding p15/INK4b, a CDK4/6 inhibitor. p15, by binding to CDK4 and CDK6, inhibits these kinases and displaces a large pool of CDK4/6-bound p27, which is then free to inhibit CDK2 complexes. The result is G_1 arrest. ATP, adenosine triphosphate; TF, transcription factor; CoAct, coactivator.

on many cell types. Although the receptors used and signaling pathways are distinct from those used by TGF-β, the ultimate effects on the cell-cycle machinery are similar: up-regulation of CDK inhibitors and down-regulation of cyclins.

Checkpoints

Cells are constantly faced with insults, resulting in damage that can threaten their survival. These insults can be generated internally as chemically active by-products of metabolism or can originate in the external environment; for example, chemical agents or radiation. As a result, mechanisms have evolved to remove damaged molecules and make necessary repairs. In instances in which cell-cycle progression would be harmful or catastrophic before repair of damage, further mechanisms have evolved to delay progression pending repair. These are called *cell-cycle checkpoints*.[34] The necessity of checkpoints can be easily envisioned for genotoxic agents. Cells are particularly susceptible to the harmful effects of DNA damage at two points in the cell cycle: S phase and M phase. Unrepaired DNA damage poses a number of problems for cells undergoing DNA replication. Chromosomal lesions present physical barriers to replication forks. Replication that does traverse regions of unrepaired DNA damage is likely to be error-prone, resulting in accumulation of mutations. Likewise, segregation of severely damaged chromosomes at mitosis might lead to loss of genetic information, seriously threatening the survival or integrity of daughter cells. Therefore, cells possess mechanisms for preventing DNA replication and mitosis in response to genotoxic stress. Although the scope of this review does not permit a detailed description of all known checkpoints, those thought to be most basic to cell survival are characterized here.

DNA Damage Checkpoints

Although DNA damage exists in many forms, ranging from chemical adducts to double-strand breaks, they all pose similar problems for proliferating cells. As previously stated, impeded and error-prone DNA replication and loss of genetic material during mitosis are some of the likely consequences in the absence of DNA damage checkpoints. Therefore, cell-cycle progression is blocked at three points: before S phase entry (the G_1 DNA damage checkpoint), during S phase (the intra-S phase DNA damage checkpoint), and before M phase entry (the G_2 DNA damage checkpoint). Although the responses to different types of DNA damage are not identical, they are similar enough to generalize. DNA damage of various forms is first detected by DNA-bound protein complexes that serve as sensors. In mammalian cells, two related atypical protein kinases that share homology with lipid kinases, ATM and ATR,[35] are primary signal transducers that are activated by DNA damage at all points in the cell cycle. A key effector of the G_1 and G_2 checkpoint responses is a transcription factor known as *p53*.[36,37] In response to DNA damage, p53 is activated and stabilized leading to increased levels. The principal transcriptional target of p53 in the context of the G_1 checkpoint is the Cip/Kip inhibitor p21^{Cip1}. The resulting high levels of p21 block CDK2 activity and possibly CDK4 and CDK6 activity, leading to G_1 arrest. An additional transcriptional target of p53, GADD45, inhibits CDK1, thereby contributing to the G_2 DNA damage checkpoint. Another p53-dependent mechanism contributing to checkpoint-mediated G_2 arrest is through transcriptional repression of the genes encoding cyclin B1 and CDK1. This occurs via direct interaction p53 and NF-Y, the positive transcriptional activator of these genes. However, although p53-dependent mechanisms are required for long-term maintenance of arrest, the primary mechanism underlying the immediate G_2 DNA damage checkpoint is p53-independent. It involves one of two effector protein kinases known as *chk1* and *chk2* that have the effect of inhibiting CDC25C,[38] which carries out the activating dephosphorylation of CDK1. Therefore, in response to DNA damage, G_2 cells accumulate inhibited cyclin B–CDK1 complexes and are incapable of entering into mitosis. The intra-S phase DNA damage checkpoint response appears to be p53-independent but requires the chk1 or chk2 kinases, or both. A key target is CDC25A, responsible for activating CDK2 by dephosphorylation. In response to DNA damage, phosphorylation of CDC25A by chk1 or chk2 leads to its destabilization via ubiquitin-mediated proteolysis and thus the accumulation of inactive CDK2 complexes[39] phosphorylated on threonine 14 and tyrosine 15. Because ongoing DNA replication requires the activity of CDK2, DNA synthesis ceases until damage is repaired.

Replication Checkpoint

Under normal circumstances, DNA replication is complete well before the time when the accumulation and activation of cyclin B–CDK1 would drive cells into mitosis. However, through the action of toxins or the rare but finite probability that the duration of S phase will be excessively long, situations can be encountered in which completion of replication extends beyond the normal time of mitotic induction or replication is blocked entirely. Under such circumstances, it is necessary to delay or block entrance into M phase accordingly, as segregation of incompletely replicated chromosomes would be catastrophic, leading to chromosome breaks and/or nondisjunction events. Although the signaling pathways are somewhat different, the replication checkpoint ultimately functions like the G_2 DNA damage checkpoint in that mitotic entry is blocked by inhibiting CDC25C via the action of chk1, thus preventing activation of CDK1.

Spindle Integrity Checkpoint

The actual act of division is a dangerous time for a cell. It requires aligning duplicated chromosomes by attaching them via bipolar attachments to the spindle and then separating the chromatids so that each daughter cell gets a full complement. Errors result in aneuploidy, an extremely undesirable outcome. As a result, assembling a mitotic spindle and attaching chromosomes to it are extensively monitored processes. The mechanism of delay at prometaphase or metaphase in response to spindle defects or improper chromosome attachment is referred to as the *spindle integrity checkpoint*.[40] The sensor for this checkpoint consists of a number of proteins that reside at the chromosome kinetochores, sites of spindle microtubule attachment. The target is the essential APC/C cofactor, CDC20. Unattached or improperly attached kinetochores not experiencing an appropriate level of tension indicative of bipolar attachment inhibit CDC20 function. This in turn prevents the ubiquitylation and degradation of the anaphase inhibitors, securin and cyclin B. As a result, cells are prevented from initiating anaphase until all kinetochores are properly attached to a bipolar spindle (Fig. 6.3).

Restriction Point

Cells deprived of an essential nutrient or growth factor are blocked from cell-cycle progression at a point in mid-G_1.[41] Cells that have already passed this point, termed the *restriction point* or *R*, enter into S phase and complete the current cell cycle before arresting in the subsequent G_1 interval. In contrast, G_1 cells that have not reached the restriction point arrest immediately. The molecular basis for the restriction point has remained elusive. Initially it was thought that passage through the restriction point was a manifestation of G_1 CDK activation and/or phosphorylation the pRb family of transcriptional inhibitors. However, more recent work has indicated that CDK activation and pRb phosphorylation occur after passage through the restriction point.[42,43] Significantly, most malignant cells do not have a functional restriction point, which presumably helps them evade normal growth control signals.

Senescence

All normal mammalian cells have a finite proliferative lifespan. As cells approach the end of their proliferative capacity, they enter a state referred to as *replicative senescence*.[44,45] Although the reasons for programmed senescence are not known, it has been speculated that restricting cells to a finite number of divisions may be a protective mechanism against malignant growth. Although the rationale for senescence is not known, the mechanism has been largely elucidated, particularly for human cells. It is based on the requirement for a specialized replicase, telomerase, in the replication of the ends of chromosomes known as *telomeres*. Whereas germ line cells express telomerase, most if not all somatic cells do not. As a result, because of the topology of telomeres and the requirements of conventional DNA replication, progressive telomere shortening or attrition occurs with each cell cycle. Although linear chromosome ends create a discontinuity, which topologically is indistinguishable from a chromosome break, telomere-specific DNA sequences are shielded from the DNA damage checkpoints. However, when sufficient telomere attrition has removed these protected sequences, cells enter into a chronic checkpoint response, which is the molecular basis for senescence. Senescence is characterized by the accumulation of high levels of CDK inhibitors and ultimately permanent G_1 arrest. It should be noted that one of the requirements of malignant transformation of cells is to overcome the senescence barrier so as to provide tumor cells with unlimited proliferative capacity.

Regulation of DNA Replication

Entry into S phase is one of the key regulatory points of the cell cycle. The actual triggering of replication is attributed to the activation of CDK2 by cyclins E and A. However, the transcription of a large number of genes whose products are required for DNA replication requires the activity of CDK4 or CDK6, or both, driven by D-type cyclins. Mechanistically, this is based on the function of pRb and related proteins p130 and p107 serving as transcriptional repressors when bound to E2F family transcription factors (Fig. 6.6).[8] Phosphorylation by cyclin D–CDK4/6 relieves this repression. Once cells have synthesized all the necessary enzymes and initiated DNA replication, another serious regulatory problem is encountered. To maintain genomic integrity, cells must replicate all genomic sequences only once per cell cycle, necessitating that origins of replication, sites where DNA synthesis begins, are used once during each S phase. This is accomplished by requiring that replication origin preparation and firing are mediated, respectively, by distinct CDK environments.[46] Pre-replication complex assembly is triggered by low or absent CDK activity and therefore normally occurs as cells exit mitosis. This process requires the successive loading of proteins, CDC6, ctd1, and six MCM proteins (MCM2–7) to another complex of proteins, known as the *origin recognition complex*, which marks the origin site. Because of the requirement for low CDK activity, the permissive window for this process extends from the end of mitosis (telophase) until the point in G_1 when CDK activity begins to rise. The activation of CDK2 in late G_1 has

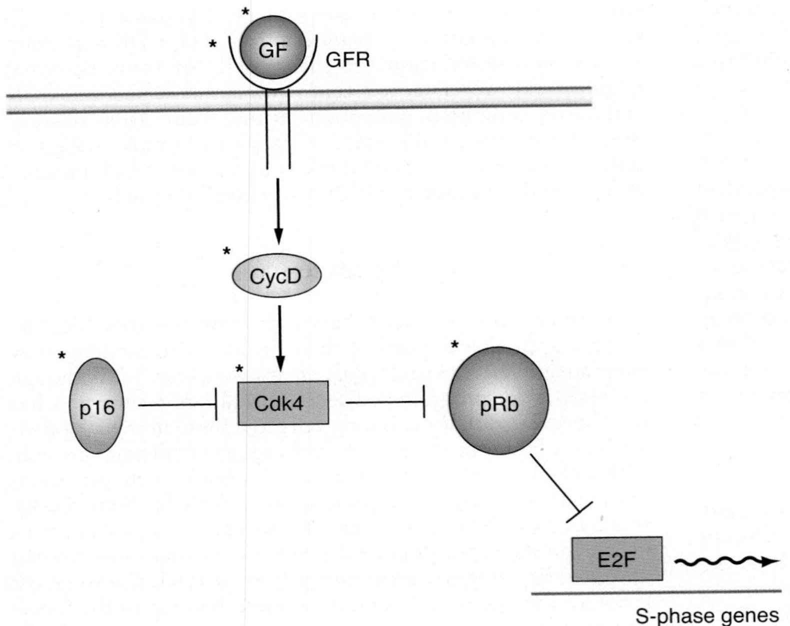

FIGURE 6.6 pRb pathway. pRb is a critical negative cell-cycle regulator that links growth factor (GF) signaling pathways to cell-cycle progression. One of the principal functions of pRb is to interact with E2F family transcription factors and, by recruitment of corepressors, to maintain many genes encoding proteins that are important for cell-cycle progression in a tightly repressed state. GF and mitogen-signaling pathways relieve this repression by stimulating accumulation of D-type cyclins on receptor occupancy. The resulting activation of CDK4 and CDK6 leads to phosphorylation of pRb and concomitant inactivation of its repressive functions. p16 is a CDK inhibitor of the INK4 family that down-regulates this pathway by inhibiting CDK4. It should be noted that all elements marked by an *asterisk* are found mutated or deregulated, or both, in human cancer. GFs, GF receptors (GFRs), and D-type cyclins are frequently overexpressed or deregulated. p16 is often not expressed or is underexpressed. Mutant versions of CDK4 that cannot bind p16 have been identified in human cancers. Finally, the gene encoding pRb is frequently mutated in cancer.

the dual effect of blocking further pre-replication complex assembly and causing DNA replication to initiate at primed origins. The maintenance of high levels of CDK activity (CDK2 followed by CDK1) for the remainder of the cell cycle assures that no new pre-replication complex assembly can occur until the end of mitosis, when CDK levels once again decline, and in doing so restricts origin function to once per cell cycle. Indeed, inhibiting CDK1 activity during G2 or early M phase is sufficient to promote a round of DNA replication without cell division.

CELL CYCLE AND CANCER

Cancer is partly a disease of uncontrolled proliferation. Because the proliferation of cells within an organism is normally tightly controlled by redundant regulatory pathways, it is not surprising that cell-cycle and checkpoint genes are often found misregulated or mutated in cancer. Genes in which mutations give rise to a gain of function or an enhanced level of function, leading to malignancy, are referred to as *protooncogenes*. Protooncogenes usually encode growth- or division-promoting proteins. Genes that give rise to loss of function mutations that lead to malignancy are referred to as *tumor suppressor genes*. Tumor suppressor genes usually encode negative regulators of growth and proliferation that protect cells from malignancy. Some cell-cycle genes commonly mutated or misregulated in cancer are listed in Table 6.1. Whereas mutations that create oncogenes tend to be dominant, mutations in tumor suppressor genes are usually recessive. This has led to the two-hit model of carcinogenesis (Fig. 6.7).[47] Briefly, recessive mutations occur in tumor suppressor genes but are latent because of the persistence of a wild type allele. The tumor suppressor phenotype, therefore, requires mutation or loss of the second allele, a process known as *loss of heterozygosity*. Alternatively, the second allele of a tumor suppressor gene can be silenced epigenetically without a direct genetic alteration. A number of genes encoding negative regulators of the cell cycle conform to this two-hit paradigm.

In theory, to achieve uncontrolled cell division, two basic requirements must be met. First, cells need a strong constitutive proliferation signal capable of overriding the environmental and internal restraints on division that normal cells experience. Second, the barrier of senescence needs to be dismantled to render tumor cells immortal. Mutations in a large variety of cell-cycle control and related genes are associated with malignancy, and most of these can be accommodated within this framework. This model of tumorigenesis has been confirmed in rodent tissue culture–based *in vitro* models. Transfection of primary rodent fibroblasts with individual plasmids programmed to express proteins that promote either growth or immortalization does not result in malignant transformation. However, cotransfection of two plasmids, one in each category, does promote transformation (Fig. 6.8). However, these results need to be interpreted cautiously in the context of human cancer because immortalization of rodent cells in culture most likely does not involve telomeres, which are much longer in rodents than in humans.[48] One idea that has emerged is that strong growth signals and other environmental pressures exerted on premalignant cells produce potent stress responses, leading to cell-cycle blockade or cell death.[49] Phenotypically, such stress-induced effects on fibroblasts closely resemble those associated with replicative senescence; therefore, this phenomenon has been termed *stress-induced senescence* (see following discussion). Therefore, genetic alterations are likely required to neutralize these stress responses to immortalize rodent cells. Transformation of human cells requires these same genetic alterations, but also telomere attrition must be reckoned with, requiring additional mutations.

Alterations in Pathways Affecting Growth and Proliferation

Mutations that regulate cell growth and proliferation can occur at many levels, ranging from cell surface receptor–mediated signaling pathways that control proliferation to elements of the core cell-cycle machinery itself.

TABLE 6.1

CELL-CYCLE GENES COMMONLY MUTATED OR ALTERED IN EXPRESSION IN HUMAN CANCER

Gene	Protein	Function	Alteration in Cancer
CCND1,2,3	D cyclins	Positive regulator of CDK4/6	Overexpressed
CCNE1	Cyclin E1	Positive regulator of CDK2	Overexpressed, deregulated
CDKN2A	p16, INK4a[a]	CDK4/6 inhibitor	Mutated, deleted, methylated
CDKN1B	$p27^{Kip1}$	CDK2 inhibitor	Underexpressed
CDKN1C	$p57^{Kip2}$	CDK2 inhibitor	Underexpressed, methylated
SKP2	Skp2	Turnover of p27	Overexpressed
CDK4	CDK4	Inactivates pRb	p16-resistant mutations
hCDC4	hCdc4	Turnover of cyclin E	Mutated, deleted
RB1	pRb	Represses E2F transcription	Mutated, deleted
RB2	p130	Inhibits CDKs, represses E2F	Mutated, deleted
CKS1,2	cks1, cks2	CDK-binding proteins	Overexpressed
AURKA	Aurora A	Mitotic kinase	Overexpressed
PLK	Plk1	Mitotic kinase	Overexpressed
PTTG1	Securin	Anaphase inhibitor	Overexpressed
TP53	p53	Checkpoints, apoptosis	Mutated, deleted
MTBP	MDM-2	Inhibitor of p53	Overexpressed
CDKN2A	$p14^{Arf}$[a]	Activator of p53	Mutated, deleted
ATM	ATM	Checkpoints, repair	Mutated, deleted
CHK2	chk2	Checkpoints	Mutated
NBS1	Nbs1	Checkpoints, repair	Mutated

[a] Interestingly, the $p16^{INK4A}$ and $p14^{Arf}$ are encoded by the same gene via alternative reading frames and different promoters.

Growth and Proliferation Signaling Pathways

Because a large number of receptors and pathways can influence cell proliferation, many mutations in elements of these pathways have been recovered in human malignancies. Only a few examples are cited here. One way to provide a strong constitutive proliferation signal is to overexpress or deregulate growth factor receptors. HER2/neu, a transmembrane tyrosine kinase receptor found on many epithelial cell types, is often overexpressed because of gene amplification in breast and other cancers.[50] Presumably the amplitude of proliferation signaling is abnormally high or completely deregulated in such tumors. Similarly, signaling elements downstream of mitogen receptors can be mutated to produce constitutive signaling. Perhaps the best-known example is the case of the Ras family

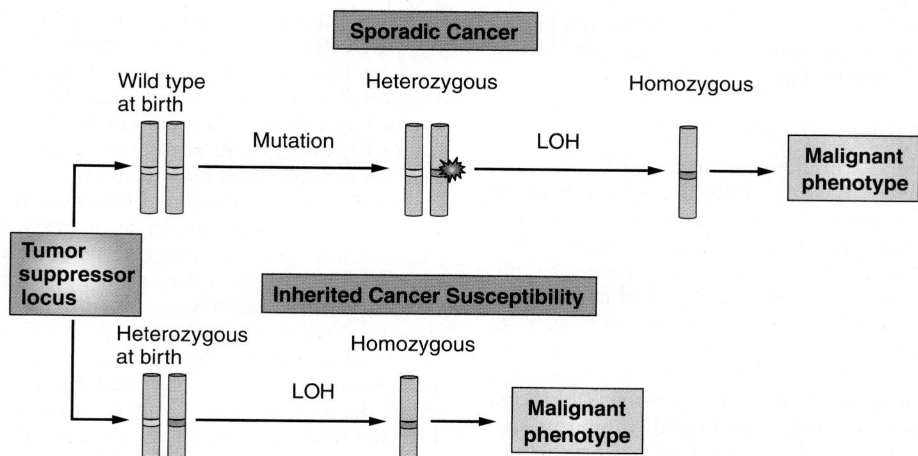

FIGURE 6.7 The two-hit model of tumor suppression. Tumor suppressors are proteins that are thought to provide protection from malignancy. Depicted is a chromosome carrying a tumor suppressor–encoding locus shown in white. At birth, normal individuals carry two wild type alleles (*yellow bands*) at tumor suppressor loci. Over time, however, spontaneous mutations occur at these loci (*red flash*) that render one allele nonfunctional (*orange band*). However, because such mutations are expected to be recessive to the wild type allele that is still present, there is no phenotypic consequence. Over time, additional events can lead to loss of the wild type allele, a phenomenon referred to as *loss of heterozygosity* (LOH). LOH then provides a tangible contribution to the malignant phenotype. However, because spontaneous mutations at specific loci and specific secondary allelic losses are rare events, malignancy usually develops only after a very long latency period. On the other hand, some individuals are born with inherited tumor suppressor mutations. Because only LOH is then required for expression of the tumor suppressor–null phenotype, cancer with decreased latency and higher penetrance develops in such individuals.

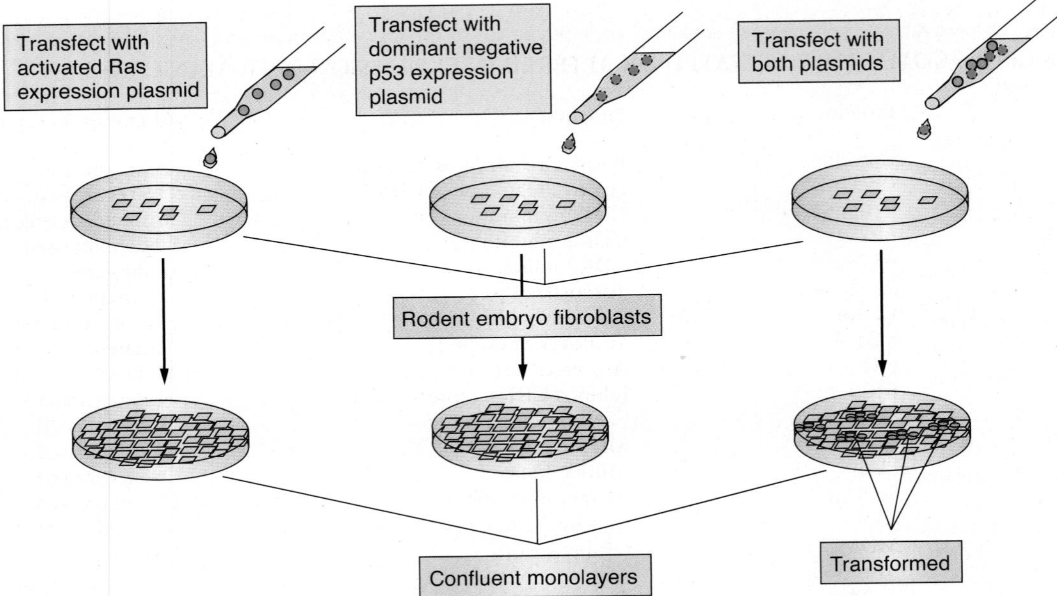

FIGURE 6.8 Malignant transformation requires multiple genetic alterations. Depicted is an *in vitro* experiment using primary rodent embryonic fibroblasts. Cells transfected with a plasmid programmed to express an activated Ras allele eventually grow to form a confluent monolayer, at which time proliferation ceases because of inhibition mediated by cell-cell contact. Similarly, cells transfected with a plasmid programmed to express a dominant-negative allele of p53 (encoding a protein that can complex with and inactivate endogenous wild type p53) from a confluent monolayer. However, cells transfected simultaneously with both plasmids from a confluent monolayer, out of which grow transformed foci. These piles of cells are no longer subject to the controls that restrict fibroblast proliferation and, as such, resemble cancer cells. The requirement for two perturbations in this system supports a mechanism whereby activated Ras stimulates growth and proliferation, and dominant negative p53 inactivates stress pathways that would cause these cells to have a limited proliferative lifespan.

guanosine triphosphatases, which serve as signal transducers for a number of key proliferation pathways. Dominant mutations in Ras isoforms that stabilize the activated state confer strong constitutive proliferation signaling. One of the pathways stimulated by Ras is the PI3-kinase pathway. A PI3 phosphatase, PTEN, normally reverses this phosphorylation, keeping the signal in check. Consistent with this, mutational loss of PTEN similarly to oncogenic mutations in Ras can lead to constitutive signaling contributing to carcinogenesis.

Cell-Cycle Machinery

Signaling pathways that stimulate proliferation impinge on the cell-cycle machinery by stimulating the biosynthesis of D-type cyclins and promoting the degradation of CDK inhibitors. Accumulation of D-type cyclins and concomitant activation of CDK4 and CDK6 have been shown to activate the cell-cycle program primarily by phosphorylation and inactivation of the retinoblastoma protein, pRb, and related proteins p107 and p130. These proteins form potent repression complexes with transcription factors that are critical for S-phase entry and progression, notably the E2F family, effectively blocking cell-cycle progression. In addition, INK4 family inhibitors specifically down-regulate CDK4 and CDK6, buffering their capacity to phosphorylate pRb and related proteins. Virtually all components of this pathway have been found to be misregulated or mutated in cancer to provide a constitutive proliferation signal (proteins with asterisks in Fig. 6.6).[51] The genes encoding D-type cyclins are found amplified in a broad spectrum of tumors. On the other hand, the gene encoding the INK4 inhibitor, p16, is mutated and lost in some types of cancer, whereas CDK4 has been found to be mutated so as not to bind p16. In many instances p16, although not genetically altered, is down-regulated at the epigenetic level. The p16 promoter contains a CpG island that is subject to repression via methylation. Finally, pRb is the tumor suppressor on which the so-called two-hit hypothesis was originally formulated. Inherited mutations in the *RB* gene and subsequent loss of heterozygosity invariably lead to childhood retinoblastoma and eventually other malignancies. However, somatic mutation of *RB1* and loss of heterozygosity are found in many sporadic noninherited cancers, underscoring the critical nature of negative cell-cycle regulation by pRb.

Like D-type cyclins, cyclin E is frequently found up-regulated in cancer. The fact that deregulated expression of cyclin E can drive cells prematurely into S phase suggests that cyclin E provides a growth/division stimulus during carcinogenesis. Furthermore, cells from cyclin E nullizygous mice are resistant to malignant transformation in tissue culture models.[12] However, other evidence suggests that deregulation of cyclin E may promote carcinogenesis principally by inducing genomic instability rather than by promoting growth (see "Mutations Causing Genetic and Genomic Instability"). Likewise, the CDK2 inhibitor $p27^{Kip1}$ is often found down-regulated in cancer, although never behaving as a classic tumor suppressor inactivated through mutation and allelic loss. However, as with cyclin E deregulation, it is not clear whether low p27 levels have an impact on carcinogenesis by promoting growth or genomic instability. While the CDK-inhibitory functions of p27 are restricted to the nucleus, hyperphosphorylation leads to cytoplasmic translocation, where non–CDK-bound p27 promotes cell migration. This may explain why p27 is rarely deleted in cancer, as cytoplasmic functions may be important for invasion and metastasis.[52]

Alterations in Pathways Affecting Senescence

In addition to a constitutive growth stimulus that overrides natural restraints, tumors need to have the capacity for unlimited proliferation. Normally, the limited lifespan of somatic cells imposed by the process of replicative senescence constitutes a natural barrier to tumorigenesis. Therefore, genes that mediate senescence are commonly mutated in cancer. However, the issue of senescence is complicated by functional overlap between senescence pathway genes and oncogenic stress pathway genes that also require inactivation.[48,49] Because senescence is a result of checkpoint responses to acute telomere attrition, genes that encode DNA checkpoint signaling elements and transducers are targeted. One of the most commonly mutated genes in human cancer encodes the checkpoint effector p53.[36] Inherited mutations in *TP53*, the gene encoding p53, confer a syndrome known as *Li-Fraumeni* characterized by early-onset cancer.[53] However, the majority of sporadic cancers are also mutated at the p53 locus. The role of p53 mutation in cancer as a promoter of immortalization is supported by the finding that cells from p53 nullizygous mice are immortal.[54] However, this conclusion is complicated by the fact that p53 is central to cellular stress responses that also require inactivation during malignant transformation, and as previously stated, telomere attrition is not likely to be a significant issue for immortalization in mice. Nevertheless, an observation supporting the idea that checkpoint genes likely to be triggered by telomere attrition are targeted to immortalize premalignant cells is that chk2, a signaling element of the DNA damage checkpoint response, is mutated in a subset of patients with Li-Fraumeni syndrome[53] rather than p53.

Mutation of the gene encoding Nbs1, required for activation of chk1 and chk2 kinases, is also associated with a hereditary cancer syndrome,[55] Nijmegen disease, as well as sporadic cancers, although the interpretation of this result is complicated by the fact that Nbs1 is also involved in DNA damage repair (see "Mutations Causing Genetic and Genomic Instability"). However, the most direct strategy to bypass senescence is to induce directly the expression of telomerase in somatic cells. c-Myc, a transcription factor linked to stimulation of proliferation, has also been shown to be a positive regulator of the gene encoding telomerase reverse transcriptase (hTERT), the catalytic subunit of telomerase.[56] This may explain the high frequency of human tumors exhibiting c-Myc amplification or overexpression, or both. However, there appear to be a number of different mutational targets that can lead to derepression of the *hTERT* gene.[57]

Mutations Neutralizing Stress Responses

Abnormally strong growth and proliferation signals provoke antagonistic stress responses leading to cell-cycle arrest or cell death. For example, it has been observed that expression of mutationally activated Ras alleles in nontransformed human fibroblasts leads to a cell-cycle arrest phenotype that closely resembles replicative senescence. As stated in "Alterations in Pathways Affecting Senescence," cellular stress responses are intimately related to checkpoint responses. Therefore, it is difficult to clearly categorize mutations that affect both. An example is p53, which is required for DNA damage checkpoint responses but also is a key effector of cellular stress responses.[37,48,49] In the case of activated Ras previously cited, the stress-activated MAP kinase pathway promotes phosphorylation and activation of p53 leading to cell-cycle arrest. Therefore, mutations that directly or indirectly inactivate p53 can promote oncogenesis by bypassing stress-dependent cell-cycle arrest or cell death. Murine double-minute gene-2, which is frequently amplified and overexpressed in human cancer, promotes turnover of p53, consistent with a role in neutralizing stress responses.[58] Conversely, p14^{Arf}, a protein that stabilizes p53 by antagonizing murine double-minute gene-2, is frequently found mutated or underexpressed in cancer.[58] Indeed, the p53 pathway is so frequently inactivated in human cancer most likely because loss of p53 function simultaneously antagonizes stress pathways and helps override cellular responses to telomere attrition. pRb may have a parallel function in maintenance of senescence, as loss of pRb has recently been shown to cause fibroblasts rendered senescent by expression of activated Ras to undergo DNA replication[59]. Thus, mutation of *RB* in cancer may contribute to escape from oncogene-induced senescence.

Mutations Causing Genetic and Genomic Instability

The pathway to malignancy minimally requires several mutations. In the case of tumor suppressor mutations, secondary genetic events mediating allelic loss are necessary. Therefore, any mutation that itself can confer genetic or genomic instability, or both, is likely to promote carcinogenesis.[60,61] Mutations in genes required for DNA repair result in a mutator phenotype linked to hyperaccumulation of secondary mutations. In this context, strong association between mutation of the gene encoding Nbs1, which is required for efficient DNA repair as well as checkpoint signaling, and carcinogenesis is easily understood.[55] Similarly, the association between mutation of components of the spindle integrity checkpoint, such as Bub1, and carcinogenesis can be rationalized.[62] Cells defective in this checkpoint experience deregulated mitosis, leading to chromosome instability and ultimately aneuploidy. In principle, aneuploidy potentiates amplification at oncogenic loci and allelic losses at tumor suppressor loci.

An interesting link between the core cell-cycle machinery and genomic instability is the case of cyclin E. Cyclin E is found overexpressed and deregulated in a broad spectrum of malignancies.[63] Although this correlation might be interpreted in the context of simply promoting proliferation, experiments on cells in culture have revealed that deregulation of cyclin E expression causes chromosome instability leading to aneuploidy and polyploidy.[64] This occurs because expression of cyclin E at inappropriate times in the cell cycle leads to impairment of DNA replication as well as of mitosis. Therefore, one possible role that cyclin E might play in promoting oncogenesis is to accelerate loss of heterozygosity at tumor suppressor loci. This was tested in a transgenic mouse mammary carcinogenesis model and, consistent with this idea, cyclin E deregulation led to accelerated loss of heterozygosity at the *TP53* locus (encoding p53), which correlated with higher tumor incidence.[65] Interestingly, an essential component of the ubiquitin ligase responsible for cell cycle–dependent targeting of cyclin E for proteolysis, hCDC4 (also known as FBXW7), is often found mutated in cancer,[27,29,66] and its deletion has been shown to also cause genomic instability in cultured cells.[67] Thus, genetic alterations that interfere with proper regulation of cell-cycle machinery have the potential of affecting not only the cell cycle itself, but also the genetic and genomic integrity of the cell.

MICRORNAs, THE CELL CYCLE, AND CANCER

Although discovered in the nematode *Caenorhabditis elegans* many years ago, the importance of microRNAs (miRs) in mammalian cells and human cancer has only recently begun to be appreciated.[68,69] These small RNAs target specific mRNAs via degradation or inhibition of translation. They confer unique regulatory possibilities in that they usually target several different mRNAs simultaneously, allowing for coordination of multiple pathways. At least five groups or clusters of miRs have been shown to target mRNAs encoding cell-cycle regulatory proteins. The miR-15a/16 cluster targets cyclin E1, cyclin D1, and cyclin D3, as well as CDK6. Not surprisingly, this miR cluster has been shown to have tumor suppressive functions in several different types of cancer. The miR-17/20 cluster, which targets cyclin D1 and E2F transcription factors, and let-7, which targets cyclin D1, cyclin D3 cyclin A, CDK4, and CDK6, have been also been shown to be tumor suppressive. Conversely, the miR-221-222 cluster and mir-21, which target a number of CDK inhibitors, has oncogenic properties. Understanding of the regulation and roles of miRs in normal cell function and cancer etiology is largely incomplete, and filling in the gaps poses a significant research challenge for the coming years.

THE CELL CYCLE AND CANCER THERAPY

Because cancer cells must proliferate, essential cell-cycle proteins have been suggested as targets for therapeutic exploitation. Notably, CDKs have been extensively screened for small-molecule inhibitors, some of which are in clinical trials. It is too early, however, to judge the efficacy of this approach beyond its success using *in vitro* models. An alternative approach being explored is to develop agents that undermine checkpoint responses. The presumption is that cancer cells, because of their highly proliferative state, might be more susceptible to loss of essential controls. This idea remains to be confirmed. However, it is noteworthy that many therapeutic approaches currently use compounds that normally trigger checkpoint responses, such as genotoxic agents or spindle poisons. It is assumed that these treatments are effective because tumor cells are actually impaired in their defensive checkpoint responses. An interesting approach that initially showed promise in model systems but has proven disappointing in clinical trials, uses the fact that a large percentage of malignancies are defective for p53 function in order to evade checkpoint and stress responses. A common human lytic virus known as *adenovirus,* expresses an essential gene, E1B p55K, specifically to down-regulate p53 in order to allow a productive infection. Oncolytic adenoviruses have therefore been engineered to not express E1B p55K.[70] These adenoviruses are harmless to normal cells but can productively infect and lyse p53-defective tumor cells in tissue culture and mouse xenograft models. However, technical issues such as low tumor infectivity, rapid viral clearance, and neutralizing immune responses in clinical trials have limited the efficacy of this approach.[70] On the other hand, if new generations of oncolytic viruses that circumvent these problems can be developed, this may constitute one of the more promising new therapeutic approaches.

Circadian rhythms may present another interesting link between cancer therapeutics and the cell cycle. Although circadian rhythms regulate virtually every aspect of human physiology, it is clear that cell-cycle regulatory gene expression and the cell cycle itself are entrained to the day-night cycle.[71] It has also been shown that tumor cells have largely lost this regulation. This difference, therefore, may be exploitable therapeutically. Indeed, the tolerance and efficacy of a variety of genotoxic chemotherapeutic agents varies with time of day, suggesting a possible link between the time of administration and the cell-cycle position of cells in healthy tissues. More detailed understanding of circadian regulation of the cell cycle may provide an avenue for optimization of current therapeutics.

Selected References

The full list of references for this chapter appears in the online version.

2. Johnson RT, Rao PN. Mammalian cell fusion: induction of premature chromosome condensation in interphase nuclei. *Nature* 1970;226:717.
3. Rao PN, Johnson RT. Mammalian cell fusion: studies on the regulation of DNA synthesis and mitosis. *Nature* 1970;225:159.
4. Masui Y, Markert CL. Cytoplasmic control of nuclear behavior during meiotic maturation of frog oocytes. *J Exp Zool* 1971;177:129.
5. Hartwell LH, Culotti J, Pringle JR, et al. Genetic control of the cell division cycle in yeast. *Science* 1974;183:46.
6. Harper JW, Adams PD. Cyclin-dependent kinases. *Chem Rev* 2001; 101:2511.
7. Jeffrey PD, Russo AA, Polyak K, et al. Mechanism of CDK activation revealed by the structure of a cyclinA-CDK2 complex. *Nature* 1995; 376:313.
8. Stevens C, La Thangue NB. E2F and cell cycle control: a double-edged sword. *Arch Biochem Biophys* 2003;412:157.
9. Stiegler P, Giordano A. The family of retinoblastoma proteins. *Crit Rev Eukaryot Gene Expr* 2001;11:59.
10. Ohtsubo M, Roberts JM. Cyclin-dependent regulation of G1 in mammalian fibroblasts. *Science* 1993;259:1908.
11. Resnitzky D, Gossen M, Bujard H, et al. Acceleration of the G1/S phase transition by expression of cyclins D1 and E with an inducible system. *Mol Cell Biol* 1994;14:1669.
12. Geng Y, Yu Q, Sicinska E, et al. Cyclin E ablation in the mouse. *Cell* 2003; 114:431.
13. Berthet C, Aleem E, Coppola V, et al. CDK2 knockout mice are viable. *Curr Biol* 2003;13:1775.
14. Ortega S, Prieto I, Odajima J, et al. Cyclin-dependent kinase 2 is essential for meiosis but not for mitotic cell division in mice. *Nat Genet* 2003; 35:25.
18. Russo AA, Jeffrey PD, Pavletich NP. Structural basis of cyclin-dependent kinase activation by phosphorylation. *Nat Struct Biol* 1996;3:696.
19. Russo AA, Tong L, Lee JO, et al. Structural basis for inhibition of the cyclin-dependent kinase CDK6 by the tumour suppressor p16INK4a. *Nature* 1998;395:237.
20. Cheng M, Olivier P, Diehl JA, et al. The p21(Cip1) and p27(Kip1) CDK inhibitors are essential activators of cyclin D-dependent kinases in murine fibroblasts. *EMBO J* 1999;18:1571.
24. Reed SI. Ratchets and clocks: the cell cycle, ubiquitylation and protein turnover. *Nat Rev Mol Cell Biol* 2003;4:855.
25. Carrano AC, Eytan E, Hershko A, et al. SKP2 is required for ubiquitin-mediated degradation of the CDK inhibitor p27. *Nat Cell Biol* 1999; 1:193.
26. Tedesco D, Lukas J, Reed SI. The pRb-related protein p130 is regulated by phosphorylation-dependent proteolysis via the protein-ubiquitin ligase SCF(Skp2). *Genes Dev* 2002;16:2946.
27. Strohmaier H, Spruck CH, Kaiser P, et al. Human F-box protein hCdc4 targets cyclin E for proteolysis and is mutated in a breast cancer cell line. *Nature* 2001;413:316.
28. Koepp DM, Schaefer LK, Ye X, et al. Phosphorylation-dependent ubiquitination of cyclin E by the SCFFbw7 ubiquitin ligase. *Science* 2001;294:173.
30. Davis RJ. Transcriptional regulation by MAP kinases. *Mol Reprod Dev* 1995;42:459.
31. Chang F, Lee JT, Navolanic PM, et al. Involvement of PI3K/Akt pathway in cell cycle progression, apoptosis, and neoplastic transformation: a target for cancer chemotherapy. *Leukemia* 2003;17:590.
32. Shi Y, Massague J. Mechanisms of TGF-beta signaling from cell membrane to the nucleus. *Cell* 2003;113:685.
34. Elledge SJ. Cell cycle checkpoints: preventing an identity crisis. *Science* 1996;274:1664.
35. Yang J, Yu Y, Hamrick HE. ATM, ATR, and DNA-PK: initiators of the cellular genotoxic stress responses. *Carcinogenesis* 2003;24:1571.
36. Vousden KH. Activation of the p53 tumor suppressor protein. *Biochim Biophys Acta* 2002;1602:47.
37. Taylor WR, Stark GR. Regulation of the G2/M transition by p53. *Oncogene* 2001;20:1803.
38. Bartek J, Lukas J. Chk1 and Chk2 kinases in checkpoint control and cancer. *Cancer Cell* 2003;3:421.
39. Sorensen CS, Syljuasen RG, Falck J, et al. Chk1 regulates the S phase checkpoint by coupling the physiological turnover and ionizing radiation-induced accelerated proteolysis of Cdc25A. *Cancer Cell* 2003;3:247.

40. Allshire RC. Centromeres, checkpoints and chromatid cohesion. *Curr Opin Genet Dev* 1997;7:264.
41. Blagosklonny MV, Pardee AB. The restriction point of the cell cycle. *Cell Cycle* 2002;1:103.
42. Ekholm SV, Zickert P, Reed SI, et al. Accumulation of cyclin E is not a prerequisite for passage through the restriction point. *Mol Cell Biol* 2001;21:3256.
43. Martinsson HS, Starborg M, Erlandsson F, et al. Single cell analysis of G1 check points—the relationship between the restriction point and phosphorylation of pRb. *Exp Cell Res* 2005;305:383.
44. Smith JR, Pereira-Smith OM. Replicative senescence: implications for in vivo aging and tumor suppression. *Science* 1996;273:63.
45. Harley CB, Sherwood SW. Telomerase, checkpoints and cancer. *Cancer Surv* 1997;29:263.
46. Woo RA, Poon RY. Cyclin-dependent kinases and S phase control in mammalian cells. *Cell Cycle* 2003;2:316.
47. Knudson AG Jr. Hereditary cancer. *JAMA* 1979;241:279.
49. Schmitt CA. Cellular senescence and cancer treatment. *Biochim Biophys Acta* 2007;1775:5.
51. Ortega S, Malumbres M, Barbacid M. Cyclin D-dependent kinases, INK4 inhibitors and cancer. *Biochim Biophys Acta* 2002;1602:73.
52. Lee J, Kim SS, The function of p27^{KIP1} during tumor development. *Ex. Mol Med* 2009; 41:765.
53. Varley J. TP53, hChk2, and the Li-Fraumeni syndrome. *Methods Mol Biol* 2003;222:117.
58. Zhang Y, Xiong Y. Control of p53 ubiquitination and nuclear export by MDM2 and ARF. *Cell Growth Differ* 2001;12:175.
60. Loeb KR, Loeb LA. Significance of multiple mutations in cancer. *Carcinogenesis* 2000;21:379.
61. Vessey CJ, Norbury CJ, Hickson ID. Genetic disorders associated with cancer predisposition and genomic instability. *Prog Nucleic Acid Res Mol Biol* 1999;63:189.
63. Donnellan R, Chetty R. Cyclin E in human cancers. *FASEB J* 1999;13: 773.
64. Spruck CH, Won KA, Reed SI. Deregulated cyclin E induces chromosome instability. *Nature* 1999;401:297.
68. Migliore C, Giordano S. MiRNAs as new master players. *Cell Cycle* 2009; 8:2185.
69. Yu Z, Baserga R, Chen L, et al. microRNA, cell cycle and human breast cancer. *Am J Pathol* 2010;176:1058.
71. Levi F, Alper O, Dulong S, et al. Circadian timing in cancer treatments. *Annu Rev Pharmacol. Toxicol* 2010; 50:377.

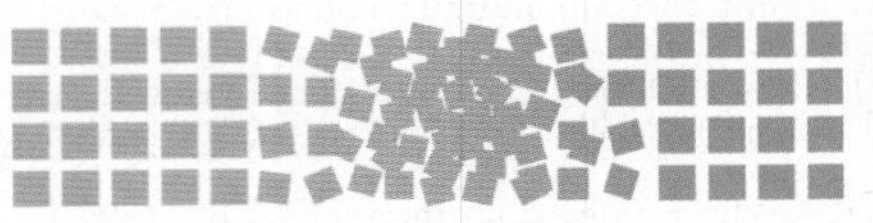

CHAPTER 7 MECHANISMS OF CELL DEATH

VASSILIKI KARANTZA AND EILEEN WHITE

Cell death has historically been subdivided into genetically controlled (or programmed) and unregulated mechanisms. Apoptosis has been recognized as a fundamental type of programmed cell death that is activated and repressed by specific genes and pathways. In contrast, necrosis has traditionally been considered an unregulated process and the result of cell death by acute physical trauma or overwhelming stress that is incompatible with cell survival. More recently, however, this strict classification of cell death mechanisms has been revisited, as mechanisms considered "programmed" were in certain instances shown to modulate necrosis and result in a regulated nonapoptotic cell death displaying necrotic morphology (necroptosis). It is also becoming apparent that disabling programmed cell death reveals novel survival mechanisms such as the catabolic autophagy pathway used by cancer cells to tolerate stress and starvation. Thus, cancer cells that acquire defects in programmed cell death are not merely "undead" but rather mobilize a novel physiologic state that actively enables survival. We review here the key aspects of the different cell death mechanisms and their regulation, and how they impact cancer development, progression, and treatment response.

APOPTOSIS

Apoptosis (or type I programmed cell death) is a genetic pathway for rapid and efficient killing of unnecessary or damaged cells that was initially described by Vogt (1842), and then Kerr et al.[1] and Wyllie et al.[2] They detailed a novel morphologic process for cell death that included swiftly executed cell shrinkage, blebbing of the plasma membrane, chromatin condensation, and intranucleosomal DNA fragmentation, after which cell corpses are engulfed by neighboring cells and professional phagocytes and degraded. Apoptosis (commonly pronounced ap-a-tow′-sis), a term coined from the Greek *apo* or from, and *ptosis* or falling, to make the analogy of leaves falling off a tree. Although underappreciated at the time, once the genes that controlled apoptosis were identified in model organisms and humans, and it was shown that perturbation of this program disturbed development and provoked disease, the importance of apoptosis was generally realized.

Cell death by apoptosis is involved in sculpting tissues in normal development. These developmental cell deaths span the removal of the interdigital webs and tadpole tails, to selection for and against specific B- and T-cell populations essential for controlling the immune response. Proper regulation of apoptosis is critical in that excessive apoptosis is associated with degenerative conditions, while deficient apoptosis promotes autoimmunity and cancer. Furthermore, apoptosis is required for eliminating damaged or pathogen-infected cells as a mechanism for limiting disease, especially cancer. In turn, tumors and pathogens have also evolved elegant mechanisms for disabling apoptosis to facilitate their persistence, often promoting disease progression. In human cancers, multiple mechanisms to disable apoptosis include loss of function of the apoptosis-promoting *p53* tumor suppressor and gain of function of the apoptosis-inhibitory and oncogenic B-cell chronic lymphocytic leukemia/lymphoma 2 (*BCL2*). It became apparent then that cancer progression was aided not only by increasing the rate of cell multiplication through activation of the *c-myc* oncogene, for example, but also by decreasing the rate of cell elimination through apoptosis, exemplified by gain of *BCL2* expression (Fig. 7.1). Indeed, activation of oncogenes such as *c-myc* or *E1A*,[3–5] or loss of tumor suppressor genes such as *Rb*,[6] can promote apoptosis, providing an explanation for the necessity for inactivation of the apoptotic pathway in many tumors. This may create a physiological state of cancer cells being "primed for death" where the necessity to up-regulate antiapoptotic mechanisms such as BCL2 to oppose oncogene activation poises cancer cells to reactivation of apoptosis providing a therapeutic window for cancer therapy.[7]

The effectiveness of many existing anticancer drugs involves or is facilitated by triggering the apoptotic response. Thus, a detailed understanding of the components, molecular signaling events, and control points in the apoptotic pathway has enabled rational approaches to chemotherapy aimed at restoring the capacity for apoptosis to tumor cells. Identification of the molecular means by which tumors inactivate apoptosis has led to cancer therapies directly targeting the apoptotic pathway. These drugs are now being used in the clinic to specifically reactivate apoptosis in tumor cells in which it is disabled to achieve tumor regression.

Model Organisms Provide Mechanistic Insight into Apoptosis Regulation

Key to elevating the field of programmed cell death from a descriptive to a mechanism-based process was the discovery of genes in the nematode *Ceanorhabditis elegans* that control cell death, the cell death defective or *ced* genes.[8] Genetic analysis revealed that *ced-4* and *ced-3* promote cell death, as worms with defective mutations in these genes possessed extra cells. In contrast, the *ced-9* gene inhibited the death-promoting function of *ced-4* and *ced-3*, thereby maintaining cell viability.[9] *ced-9* in turn was inhibited by *egl-1*, thereby promoting cell death. This creates a linear genetic pathway controlled upstream by cell-specific death specification regulators, and downstream by cell corpse engulfment and degradation mechanisms (Fig. 7.2).[10] These findings helped propel work in mammalian systems when it became apparent that Ced-9 was homologous to BCL2,[11] Ced-3 was homologous to interleukin1-β–converting enzyme, a cysteine protease that would later be classified as a member of the caspase family of aspartic acid proteases,[12] Egl-1 was a BH3-only protein homologue,[10] and that the

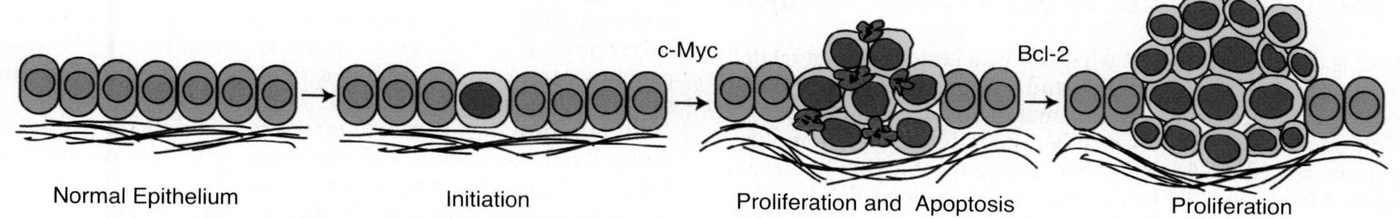

FIGURE 7.1 Tumor progression through cooperation of proliferative and antiapoptotic functions. In normal cells in epithelial tissues (*green cells*) initiating mutational events such as deregulation of *c-myc* expression deregulate cell growth control and promote abnormal cell proliferation (*yellow cells*) while triggering a proapoptotic tumor suppression (*red apoptotic cells*) mechanism that can restrict tumor expansion. Subsequent acquisition of mutations that disables the apoptotic response, exemplified by *Bcl-2* overexpression, prevents this effective means of culling emerging tumor cells, thereby favoring tumor expansion. Similar oncogenic events occur in lymphoid tissues.

proapoptotic factor apoptotic protease-activating factor (APAF-1)-1 identified in mammals was homologous to Ced-4.[13]

A similar cell death pathway in the fruit fly *Drosophila melanogaster* identified Reaper, Hid and Grim as inhibitors of the inhibitors of apoptosis proteins (IAPs) that negatively regulate caspase activation. This eventually led to the identification of their mammalian counterpart second mitochondrial-derived activator of caspase (SMAC), also known as direct IAP-binding protein with low pI (DIABLO).[14] These and other studies established the paradigm whereby proapoptotic BH3-only proteins inhibit antiapoptotic Bcl-2 proteins that prevent APAF-1-mediated caspase activation suppressed by IAPs, and the caspase-mediated proteolytic cellular destruction leads rapidly to cell death. It would later be realized that in mammals BH3-only proteins could also act as direct activators of the proapoptotic machinery (see later discussion).

Discovery of Bcl-2 and its Role as an Apoptosis Inhibitor in B-cell Lymphoma

To identify mechanisms of oncogenesis, the *bcl-2* gene was cloned from the site of frequent chromosome translocation t(14;18):(q32;q21) in human follicular lymphoma.[15–17] This chromosome rearrangement places *bcl-2* under the transcriptional control of the immunoglobulin heavy chain locus causing abnormally high levels of *bcl-2* expression. Distinct from other oncogenes at the time, instead of promoting cell proliferation, *bcl-2* promoted B-cell tumorigenesis by the novel concept of providing a survival advantage to cells stimulated to proliferate by *c-myc*.[18] Indeed, engineering high Bcl-2 expression in the lymphoid compartment in mutant mice promotes follicular hyperplasia that progresses to lymphoma upon *c-myc* translocation, and *bcl-2* synergizes with *c-myc* to produce lymphoid tumors, paralleling events in human follicular lymphoma.[19,20] Bcl-2 localizes to mitochondria where it has broad activity in promoting cell survival through suppression of apoptosis,[21] provoked by numerous events, including oncogene activation (*c-myc*, *E1A*), tumor suppressor activation (*p53*), growth factor and cytokine limitation, and cellular damage. It also became clear that inactivation of the retinoblastoma tumor suppressor (*Rb*) pathway promotes a *p53*-mediated apoptotic response, suggesting that apoptosis was part of a tumor suppression mechanism that responded to deregulation of cell growth.[6,22,23] Indeed, apoptotic defects acquired by a variety of means are a common event in human tumorigenesis.

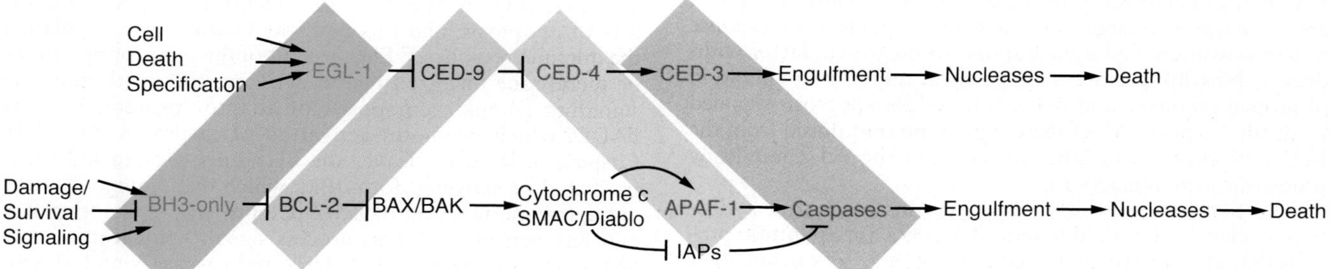

FIGURE 7.2 Analogous pathways regulate programmed cell death/apoptosis in metazoans. Regulation of programmed cell death in the nematode *Ceanorhabditis elegans* (**top**) and regulation of apoptosis in mammals (**bottom**). Shaded regions highlight corresponding homologous genes and protein families. In *C. elegans*, numerous cell death specification genes can up-regulate the transcription of the BH3-only protein Egl-1, which interacts with the antiapoptotic Bcl-2 homologue Ced-9 inhibiting is interaction with Ced-4. Ced-4, the Apaf-1 homologue, in turn, activates the caspase Ced-3, leading to cell death. A variety of engulfment gene products are then responsible for apoptotic corpse elimination and nucleases degrade the genome. In mammals, many survival, damage, and stress events impinge on the numerous members of the BH3-only class of proapoptotic proteins to either activate them to promote apoptosis or suppress their activation to enable cell survival. BH3-only proteins interact with and antagonize the numerous Bcl-2-related multidomain antiapoptotic proteins that serve to sequester proapoptotic Bax and Bak and may also contribute directly to Bax/Bak activation. Bax or Bak is essential for signaling apoptosis by permeabilizing the outer mitochondrial membrane to allow the release of cytochrome *c* and second mitochondrial-derived activator of caspase (SMAC). Cytochrome *c* acts as a cofactor for Apaf-1-mediated caspase activation in the apoptosome, and the SMAC amino-terminal four amino acids bind and antagonize the inhibitors of apoptosis proteins that interact with and suppress caspases, leading to their activation, widespread substrate cleavage, and cell death. Many engulfment gene products are responsible for corpse elimination and caspase-activated nucleases in the apoptotic cell itself, and additional nucleases within the engulfing cell are responsible for degradation of the genome.

Control of Apoptosis by Bcl-2 Family Members

Bcl-2 is the first member of what is now a large family of related proteins that regulate apoptosis and are conserved among metazoans including worms, flies, and mammals, and also viruses.[24–28] Multidomain Bcl-2 family members containing Bcl-2 homology regions 1-4 (BH1-4) are either antiapoptotic (Bcl-2, Bcl-x_L, Bcl-w, Mcl-1, and Bfl-1/A1, and virally encoded Bcl-2 homologues such as E1B 19K), or proapoptotic (Bax and Bak). Antiapoptotic proteins can block apoptosis by binding and sequestering Bax and Bak or by indirectly preventing Bax and Bak activation (Fig. 7.3).[25,29,30]

Bax and Bak are functionally redundant and required for signaling apoptosis through mitochondria, and deficiency in Bax and Bak produces a profound defect in apoptosis. Bax and Bak are considered the core apoptosis machinery controlled directly or indirectly by antiapoptotic Bcl-2-like proteins and proapoptotic BH3-only proteins. Remarkably, mice deficient in both Bax and Bak develop relatively normally, suggesting that other death mechanisms can compensate for loss of apoptosis in development.[31] In healthy cells, Bak is bound and sequestered by Mcl-1 and Bcl-x_L at cellular membranes, whereas Bax resides in the cytosol in a latent form and requires activation and translocation to membranes, where it is either sequestered by antiapoptotic Bcl-2-like proteins or otherwise induces apoptosis (Fig. 7.3).

Control of Multidomain Bcl-2 Family Proteins by the BH3-only Proteins

Bax and Bak deficiency abrogates the ability of BH3-only proteins to induce apoptosis, placing them upstream and dependent on the core apoptosis machinery.[32] BH3-only protein Bcl-2 family members (Bim, Bid, Nbk/Bik, Puma, Bmf, Bad, and Noxa) are proapoptotic and antagonize the survival activity of antiapoptotic Bcl-2-like proteins by binding and displacing Bax and Bak to allow apoptosis (BH3-only proteins as neutralizers of Bcl-2) (Fig. 7.4).[30] The different BH3-only proteins respond to specific stimuli to activate apoptosis (Fig. 7.3). For example, Bim induces apoptosis in response to taxanes, Puma and Noxa are transcriptional targets of and mediate apoptosis in response to *p53* activation, Bad signals apoptosis on growth factor withdrawal, Nbk/Bik promotes apoptosis in response to inhibition of protein synthesis, and Bid is required for apoptosis signaled by death receptors. All of these signals are transduced from the BH3-only proteins to other members of the Bcl-2 family by protein-protein interactions.

The BH3 region of BH3-only proteins binds to a hydrophobic cleft in the multidomain Bcl-2-like antiapoptotic proteins that also supports Bax and Bak binding,[33,34] causing their displacement (neutralization mode; Fig. 7.4).[30] Differential binding specificities among the BH3 regions of the different BH3-only proteins determine whether they bind one or more Bcl-2-like proteins and displace Bax or Bak or both.[35] Noxa binds and antagonizes Mcl-1, whereas Bad binds and antagonizes Bcl-2 and Bcl-x_L, necessitating cooperation between Noxa and Bad function for efficient apoptosis. In contrast, Bim, Bid, and Puma have broader binding specificity and antagonize Mcl-1, Bcl-2, and Bcl-x_L to release both Bax and Bak to induce apoptosis. Bim, the active form of Bid (truncated Bid or tBid) and possibly Puma can also be direct activators of Bax and Bak. For example, tBid can bind to latent, inactive Bax and promote its conformational change and translocation to the mitochondrial membrane that is required for apoptosis.[36] BH3-only proteins can inhibit Bcl-2-like proteins, releasing these direct activators of Bax and Bak to promote apoptosis in the de-repression mode (Fig. 7.4). BH3-only proteins that only interact with Bcl-2-like proteins can release activator BH3-only proteins to promote apoptosis in the sensitizer mode (Fig. 7.4). Thus, apoptosis induction by BH3-only proteins can occur through neutralization, de-repression and sensitizer functions.[28]

Importantly, it is this BH3 interaction with Bcl-2 that is the molecular basis for the BH3-mimetic class of proapoptotic, Bcl-2–antagonizing anticancer drugs (Fig. 7.5).[33,37–39] This detailed understanding of the Bcl-2 family member protein interactions and function is allowing rational, apoptosis-targeted therapy (see later discussion).

Role of Mitochondrial Membrane Permeabilization in Apoptosis

Once activated, Bax and Bak oligomerize in the mitochondrial outer membrane, rendering it permeable to proapoptotic mitochondrial proteins cytochrome *c* and SMAC.[40–44] How Bcl-2 family members permeabilize membranes is not entirely clear but it is likely related to a change in topology of the proteins in the membrane and formation of a channel or pore. Once released into the cytoplasm, cytochrome *c* interacts with the WD40 domains of APAF-1 in the apoptosome, a wheel-like particle with sevenfold symmetry that serves as a scaffold for caspase-9 activation.[45] SMAC functions to antagonize the caspase inhibitors, the IAP proteins, to facilitate caspase activation. The amino-terminus of SMAC binds to IAPs, neutralizing their caspase-inhibitor function. Subsequent effector caspase activation (e.g., caspase-3), leads to the rapid, orderly dismantling of the cell and cell death without activating the innate immune response.[46]

Control of Apoptosis by Death Receptors

One of the apoptotic pathways being modulated in cancer therapies is that belonging to the death receptors. Ligands related to tumor necrosis factor-α (TNF-α), including Fas/Apo1 (Fas) and tumor necrosis factor-related ligand (TRAIL) and their cognate receptors were identified as potent activators of apoptosis, and this pathway is critical for regulating the immune response.[47] Engagement of the receptor by soluble or membrane-localized ligand activates the death-inducing signaling complex composed of adaptor proteins such as FADD, which promotes activation of caspase-8 (Fig. 7.5). Caspase-8, in turn, cleaves the BH3-only protein Bid to its truncated or activated form tBid, which then antagonizes the antiapoptotic function of Bcl-2-like proteins, promoting Bax and Bak activation.[36] This process signals cytochrome *c* and SMAC release from mitochondria and caspase-9 and -3 activation and cell death. In some cell types that do not require this Bcl-2 family protein-regulated, mitochondrial amplification step, active caspase-8 can directly cleave and activate caspase-3 to cause cell death by apoptosis. Execution of apoptotic cell death is extremely rapid and efficient, resulting in cell death in less than 1 hour in mammalian cells.

Modulation of the Death Receptor Pathway in Cancer Therapy

The ability of soluble ligands to activate the apoptotic response has stimulated interest in using this pathway to therapeutically induce apoptosis preferentially in tumor cells. Although TNF-α and Fas proved highly toxic to both normal and tumor cells, tumor cells display preferential sensitivity to TRAIL,

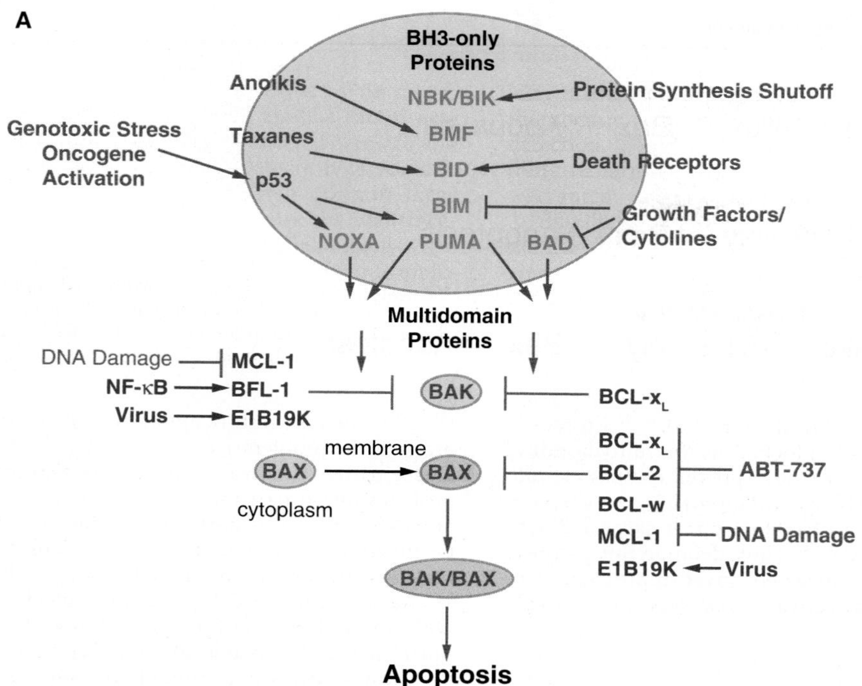

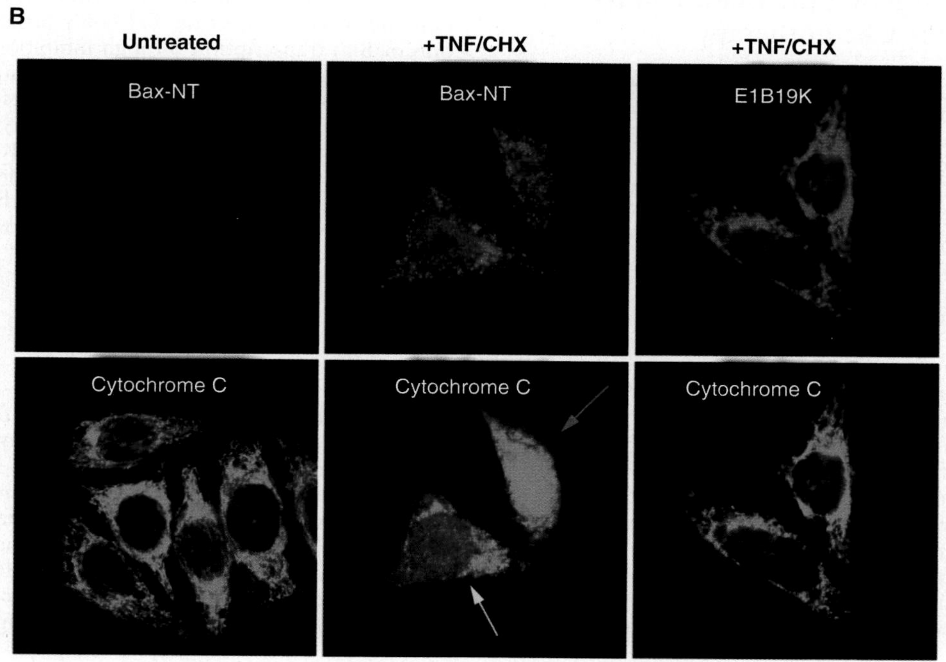

FIGURE 7.3 Regulation of apoptosis by the Bcl-2 family of proteins in mammals. **A:** Schematic of apoptosis regulation by the Bcl-2 family. Cytotoxic events activate, while survival signaling events suppress the activity of the BH3-only class of Bcl-2 family members (*orange*). BH3-only proteins are controlled at the transcription level and also by numerous posttranscriptional events that modulate phosphorylation, proteolysis, localization, sequestration, and protein stability. Once activated, BH3-only proteins disrupt functional sequestration of Bak and Bax by the multidomain antiapoptotic Bcl-2-like proteins (*blue*) and may also directly facilitate Bax/Bak activation. Although Bak is commonly membrane-associated in a complex with Mcl-1 and Bcl-x_L in healthy cells, Bax resides in the cytoplasm as an inactive monomer with its carboxy-terminus occluding the BH3-binding hydrophobic cleft.[138] Bax activation thereby additionally requires a change in protein conformation and membrane translocation by an unknown mechanism that may be facilitated by tBid binding. Binding specificity among BH3-only proteins for antiapoptotic Bcl-2-like proteins determines which complexes are disrupted, with some BH3-only proteins having broad specificity and others do not. Survival and death signaling events can also modulate apoptosis by targeting the multidomain antiapoptotic proteins either by antagonizing their function to promote apoptosis or induction their function to promote survival. ABT-737 is a rationally designed BAD BH3 mimetic that can bind Bcl-2, Bcl-x_L, and Bcl-w but not Mcl-1 that can promote apoptosis where survival does not depend on Mcl-1. Once activated, Bax or Bak oligomerization promotes apoptosis. **B:** Tumor necrosis factor-α (TNF-α) apoptotic signaling induces mitochondrial membrane translocation and a conformational change exposing the amino-terminus of Bax (visualized here by the Bax-NT antibody) and apoptosis, which is blocked by sequestration of Bax by the antiapoptotic viral Bcl-2 homologue E1B 19K. The human cancer cell line (HeLa cells) with or without E1B 19K expression, were then left untreated or treated with TNF/CHX. The localization of conformationally altered Bax (Bax-NT) and cytochrome *c* (**left and middle panels**), or E1B 19K and cytochrome *c* (**right panel**), are shown. The proapoptotic stimulus (TNF/CHX) induces Bax activation, mitochondrial translocation, and cytochrome *c* release from mitochondria that leads to caspase activation and apoptotic cell death, whereas expression of E1B 19K sequesters Bax thereby blocking cytochrome *c* release from mitochondria, caspase activation, and apoptotic cell death. The *yellow* and *red* arrows, respectively, mark cells with partial or complete cytochrome *c* release from mitochondria upon TNF/CHX treatment.

Neutralization Mode

BH3-only —| Bcl-2-like —| Bax → Apoptosis

De-repression Mode

Bcl-2-like —| BH3-only → Bax → Apoptosis

Sensitizer Mode

BH3-only —| Bcl-2-like —| BH3-only → Bax → Apoptosis

FIGURE 7.4 Modes of apoptosis activation by BH3-only proteins. The neutralization mode (**top**), de-repression mode (**middle**), and sensitizer mode (**bottom**). See text for explanation.

which has now entered clinical trials (Fig. 7.6).[48–52] Moreover, in cases in which apoptosis is blocked at the mitochondrial level in tumors, SMAC-mimetics have proved useful in stimulating the activity of TRAIL by antagonizing the caspase-inhibitory function of IAPs to facilitate direct caspase-3 activation by caspase-8 (Fig. 7.6).[53–56] Thus, defining this pathway to apoptosis regulation has revealed novel opportunities to rational therapy designed to activate apoptosis preferentially in tumor cells.

Drugs Targeting the Bcl-2 Family for Chemotherapy

In addition to Bcl-2 up-regulation in B-cell lymphoma as previously described, there are other mechanisms for directly or indirectly inactivating apoptosis in tumors that facilitate tumor progression and treatment resistance. Inactivation of the *p53* tumor suppressor, or the *p53* pathway through the gain of function of the *p53* inhibitor MDM-2, is a common occurrence in tumors that results in the loss of the proapoptotic and growth arrest functions of *p53*.[57,58] The BH3-only proteins Puma and Noxa are transcriptional targets of *p53*, the loss of which prevents induction of the *p53*-mediated response to genotoxic stress in tumors as a mechanism of tumor suppression. Various means for restoration of *p53* function in tumors are, therefore, an attractive therapeutic approach.[59–61]

Activation of the MAP kinase pathway is also common in tumors and results in stimulation of tumor cell proliferation, but also the phosphorylation and proteasome mediated degradation of the BH3-only protein Bim. This Bim inactivation promotes tumor growth, while also producing resistance to the taxane class of chemotherapeutic drugs. This loss of Bim function is rectified by blocking Bim degradation with a proteasome inhibitor (bortezomib) (Fig. 7.7).[62] Similarly, direct inhibition of MAP kinase pathway signaling with inhibitors (sorafenib, UO126) can also restore apoptotic function in addition to suppressing the proliferative response (Fig. 7.7). Receptor tyrosine kinase pathway activation in tumors also promotes tumor cell proliferation in part through MAP kinase pathway activation downstream and in part through Bim and thereby apoptosis inactivation. In chronic myelogenous leukemia in which chromosomal translocation and activation of the Bcr/Abl tyrosine kinase also leads to BIM inhibition, blocking kinase signaling with imatinib mesylate restores Bim and also Bad apoptotic function as a therapeutic strategy (Fig. 7.7).[63] Activation of the PI-3 kinase pathway commonly through loss of *PTEN* tumor suppressor function and AKT activation results in phosphorylation and inactivation of the BH3-only protein Bad and reduction of Bim transcription through inhibition of forkhead factors, resulting in down-regulation of apoptosis.[64] Thus, inhibitors of the PI-3 kinase pathway can restore apoptosis and facilitate tumor regression.[65] NF-κB, a cytokine-responsive transcription factor, also promotes tumor growth while turning on the expression of antiapoptotic regulators Bcl-x_L, Bfl-1 and IAPs (Fig. 7.3).[66] Strategies to inhibit NF-κB are likely to promote tumor regression in part through restoration of apoptotic function.[67]

Direct Modulation of Bcl-2 with BH3-mimetics

The observation that antiapoptotic Bcl-2 family members bound and sequestered BH3-regions in a hydrophobic cleft as a means to suppress apoptosis activation (Fig. 7.5) revealed the opportunity for the rational design of small molecules that occlude the cleft and disrupt this Bcl-2-like protein/proapoptotic protein interaction, thereby promoting apoptosis.[33] This was accomplished and resulted in ABT-737, which binds the BH3 binding pocket of Bcl-2, Bcl-x_L, and Bcl-w, but not Mcl-1, similarly to the Bcl-2 family protein binding by Bad (Fig. 7.5).

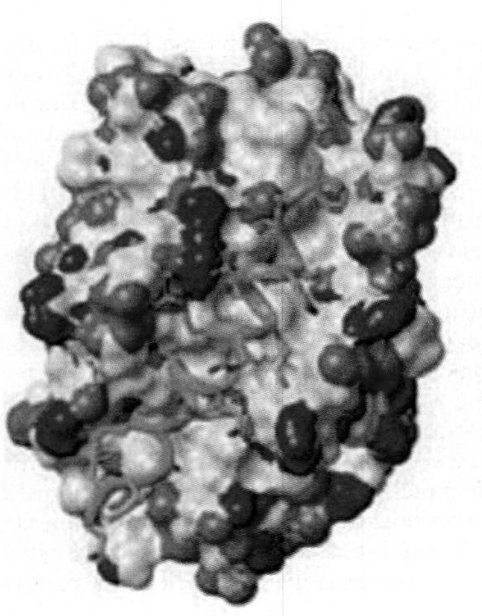

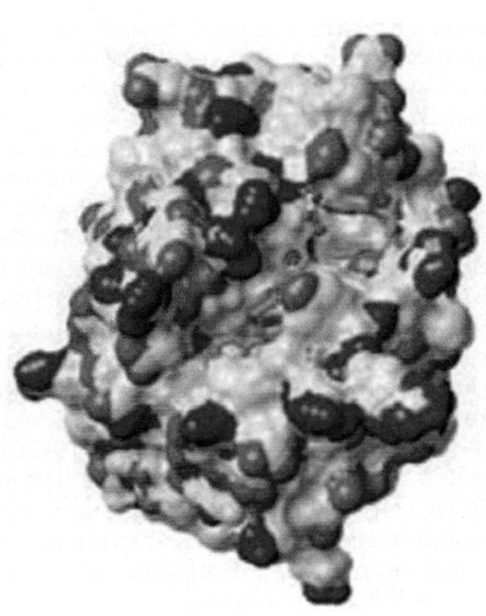

FIGURE 7.5 Three-dimensional structure of Bcl-x_L with bound Bad BH3 ligand and ABT-737. Space-filling model of Bcl-x_L illustrating the hydrophobic cleft binding the 25-mer peptide (*green helix*) of the Bad BH3 (**left**) or the rationally designed BH3-mimetic ABT-737 (**right**). (Reprinted from ref. 33, with permission.)

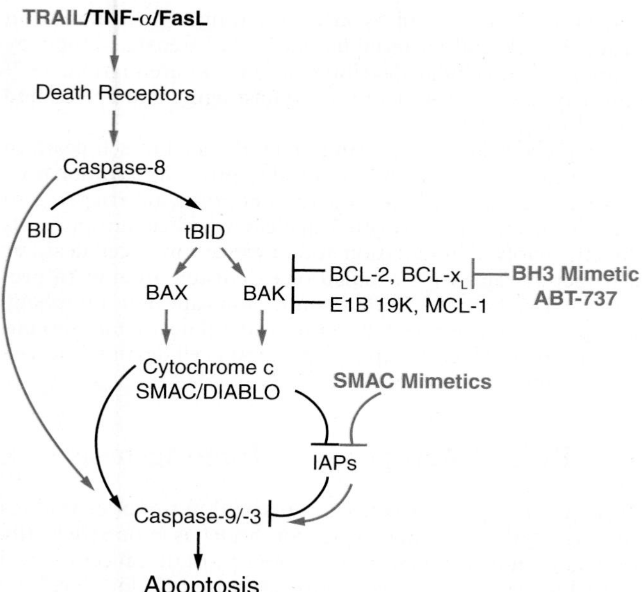

FIGURE 7.6 Therapeutic modulation of the apoptotic pathway downstream of death receptors. Tumor necrosis factor-related ligand (TRAIL) and related death-promoting ligands engage their cognate death receptors and activate caspase-8, which then cleaves Bid to active tBid. tBid can bind Bcl-2 and related antiapoptotic proteins to release Bax and Bak and may also directly promote their activation to permeabilize the mitochondrial outer membrane to release the APAF-1 cofactor cytochrome c, and the inhibitors of apoptosis protein antagonist second mitochondrial-derived activator of caspase (SMAC) for promote caspase-9 and -3 activation and cell death. BH3-mimetics such as ABT-737 can promote apoptosis-induction by TRAIL by relieving the protective capacity of the antiapoptotic Bcl-2-like proteins. In cells that do not depend on the mitochondrial apoptotic signal, TRAIL-mediated caspase-8 activation can directly promote downstream caspase activation and can synergize with SMAC mimetics in this case.

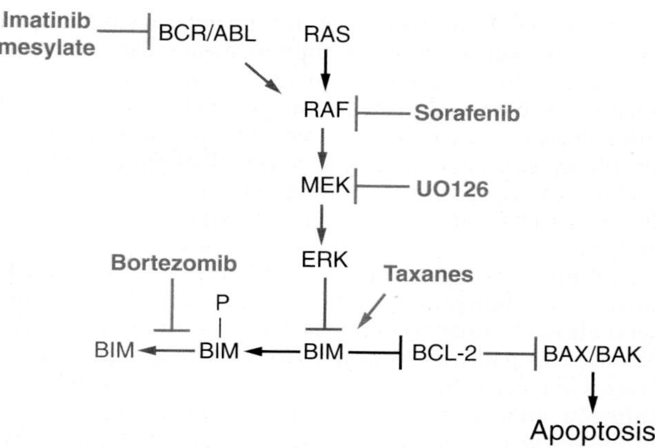

FIGURE 7.7 Therapeutic regulation of Bim and the MAP kinase pathway in cancer chemotherapy. Bim protein stability is regulated by Erk phosphorylation and proteasome-mediated degradation. Therapeutic modulation of the MAP kinase pathway (imatinib, sorafenib, and UO126) or proteasome function (bortezomib) can restore Bim protein levels and apoptosis function. Taxanes also stimulate Bim expression and promote Bim-mediated apoptosis, synergizing with the aforementioned inhibitors.

ABT-737 exhibited activity as a single agent against human lymphoma and small cell lung cancer cell lines *in vitro* and in mouse xenographs *in vivo*,[37] and in combination with various cytotoxic agents against acute myeloid leukemia,[68] multiple myeloma,[69] chronic lymphocytic leukemia,[70] and small cell lung cancer.[71] ABT-263, an orally bioavailable form of ABT-737, exhibited similar preclinical activity,[72] and has now entered clinical trials as a single agent or in combination with other anticancer drugs. Not surprisingly, given that ABT-737 does not bind to Mcl-1, resistance to ABT-737 has been associated with Mcl-1, as well as Bfl-1, up-regulation,[73] indicating that combinatorial treatment with anticancer agents that target Mcl-1[74] or Bfl-1 could be therapeutically beneficial. Alternate chemical approaches to generating BH3-mimetics to promote apoptosis in cancer cells are also producing encouraging results in the preclinical setting.[39] Thus, deciphering the mechanisms of apoptosis regulation in tumor cells is yielding novel opportunities for rational drug design and therapeutic intervention. These analyses can help predict which tumors have the potential to respond to apoptosis modulation and the types of drug combinations they may respond to.

Killing the Unkillable Cells: Alternate Approaches to Achieving Tumor Cell Death

An apoptotic response to therapy in tumors may not always be possible to achieve; therefore, it is important to determine alternate cell death processes and how to access them specifically in tumor cells. One intrinsic difference between normal and tumor cells is their altered metabolism and prevalence of aerobic glycolysis, which is an inefficient means for generation of adenosine triphosphate (ATP) required for sustaining homeostasis but an efficient means to generate synthetic precursors to support cell proliferation.[75,76] This tumor cell-specific altered metabolism can provide novel approaches to therapeutically target cancer but not normal cells.[75] Altered tumor cell metabolism is frequently coupled with high energy demand due to a rapid cell growth, with the potential to render tumor cells susceptible to cell death because of metabolic catastrophe where cellular energy consumption exceeds production.[77]

The means to specifically drive tumor cells toward metabolic catastrophe is through therapeutic nutrient deprivation that may be an additional consequence of the use of angiogenesis, growth factor, nutrient transporter, and metabolic pathway inhibitors. In addition, inhibition of the catabolic process of autophagy may similarly create metabolic deprivation and promote tumor cell death. Importantly, induction of cell death by interfering with metabolism can occur independently of an intact apoptotic response, suggesting that modulation of tumor cell metabolism may be therapeutically advantageous.

AUTOPHAGY

Role of Autophagy in Promoting Cell Survival to Metabolic Stress

Autophagy is an evolutionarily conserved, stress-activated catabolic lysosomal pathway that results in degradation of long-lived proteins and organelles. This process involves formation of the "autophagosome," a double-membrane vesicle in the cytosol that engulfs organelles and cytoplasm and then fuses with the lysosome to form the "autolysosome," where the sequestered contents are degraded and recycled to generate building blocks for macromolecular synthesis and maintenance of energy homeostasis.[78,79] Hence the name autophagy (commonly pronounced aw-tofʹə-je), a term coined from the Greek *auto* or oneself, and *phagy* or eating, accurately depicts the process. Although autophagy can potentially induce cell death through progressive cellular consumption (autophagy is sometime referred to as type II programmed cell death), physiologic conditions in mammals where this occurs have not yet been identified. In most settings, autophagy is a survival pathway that can delay apoptosis, support metabolism in nutrient stress, and mitigate cellular damage by preventing the accumulation of damaged proteins and organelles. In tumor cells with defects in apoptosis, it has recently become apparent that autophagy supports long-term survival of tumor cells,[80,81] newly revealing opportunities to target not only apoptosis, but also the mechanism by which cells survive once apoptosis is disabled.[82]

Autophagy is regulated by mTOR in the PI3-kinase/AKT pathway that functions to link nutrient availability to cellular metabolism.[83] Under conditions of nutrient limitation, normal cells use this pathway to turn down growth and protein synthesis while activating the catabolic process of autophagy to maintain energy and biosynthetic homeostasis.[79] Thus, autophagy is a temporary survival mechanism during starvation, as self-digestion provides an alternative energy source.[80,84–86]

On growth factor deprivation, hematopoietic cells activate autophagy, which is essential for maintenance of ATP production and cellular survival.[81] In normal mouse development, amino acid production by autophagic degradation of "self" proteins allows maintenance of energy homeostasis and survival during neonatal starvation.[87] Chronically ischemic myocardium induces autophagy, which inhibits apoptosis and may function as a cardioprotective mechanism.[88] These and other examples indicate that autophagy is essential for the maintenance of cellular energy homeostasis that enables survival particularly during stress and starvation.

Autophagy is not only involved in recycling of normal cellular constituents to support cellular metabolism, but is also essential for the removal of toxic-damaged proteins and organelles. The importance of this toxic garbage disposal mechanism is exemplified by the observation that defects in autophagy result in the accumulation of ubiquitin-positive and p62-positive protein aggregates, abnormal mitochondria, and deformed cellular structures associated with production of reactive oxygen species and cellular degeneration.[89–93] This protein and organelle quality control function of autophagy is important in preserving cellular health and viability in conjunction with metabolic support via catabolism.

Autophagy also contributes to innate immunity by protecting cells against infection with intracellular pathogens[94–97] and to acquired immunity by promoting T-lymphocyte survival and proliferation[98] and by affecting antigen presentation in dendritic cells and bacterial handling.[99] Moreover, autophagy is involved in cellular development and differentiation,[100,101] and may have a protective role against aging and age-related pathologies.[102,103]

Progressive autophagy can potentially lead to cell death in limited circumstances when allowed to proceed to completion, and when cells unable to undergo apoptosis are triggered to die. Unfortunately, it is often unclear whether autophagy is directly involved in initiation and/or execution of cell death or if it merely represents a failed or exhausted attempt to preserve cell viability.[104] Recent studies indicate that autophagy may play an active role in programmed cell death, but the conditions under which autophagy promotes cell death versus cell survival remain to be resolved.[105–108]

Role of Autophagy in Tumorigenesis

Defective autophagy has been implicated in tumorigenesis, as the essential autophagy regulator *becn1* is monoallelically deleted in human breast, ovarian, and prostate cancers[109] and some human breast cancers have decreased Beclin1 levels.[110] *Becn1* is the mammalian orthologue of the yeast *atg6/vps30* gene, which is required for autophagosome formation.[111] *Becn1* complements the autophagy defect present in *atg6/vps30*-disrupted yeast and in human MCF7 breast cancer cells, the latter in association with inhibition of MCF7-induced tumorigenesis in nude mice.[110] *Becn1*$^{-/-}$ mice die early in embryogenesis, whereas aging *Becn1*$^{+/-}$ mice have increased incidence of lymphoma and carcinomas of the lung and liver[112,113] In addition, mammary tissue from *Becn1*$^{+/-}$ mice shows hyperproliferative, preneoplastic changes.[113] Tumors forming in *Becn1*$^{+/-}$ mice express wild type Beclin1 mRNA and protein, indicating that *Becn1* is a haploinsufficient tumor suppressor.[112]

Recent studies revealed that autophagy enables tumor cell survival *in vitro* and *in vivo* that is particularly obvious in tumor cells when apoptosis is inactivated.[80,85,86] When angiogenesis is insufficient, autophagy localizes to the resulting hypoxic tumor regions where it supports tumor cell viability (Fig. 7.8).[80,85,86] This process of autophagy during nutrient deprivation allows recovery of growth and proliferative capacity with remarkably high fidelity when nutrients, oxygen, and

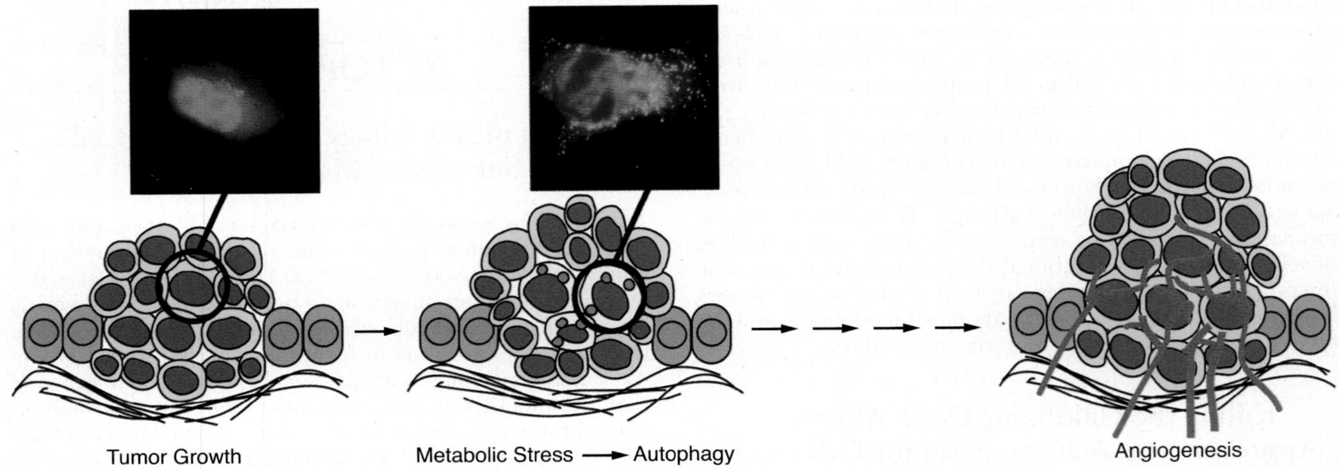

FIGURE 7.8 Role of autophagy in enabling survival of tumor cells to metabolic stress. As epithelial tumor cells proliferate and multiple cell layers accumulate, the initial absence of a blood supply produces metabolic stress in regions most distal to the supply of nutrients and oxygen often in the center of the tumor mass. In tumor cells with apoptosis defects, this allows tumor cells in these metabolically stressed tumor regions to survive through autophagy. Subsequent angiogenesis relieves metabolic stress, obviating the need for autophagy, fueling tumor growth.

growth factors are restored. Thus, autophagy may be a fundamental obstacle to tumor eradication.[80]

How inactivation of a survival pathway promotes tumorigenesis has been an intriguing question. The apparently conflicting pro-survival and pro-death functions of autophagy can, however, be reconciled if one considers autophagy a prolonged but interruptible pathway to cell death on stress and starvation, where nutrient restoration prior to its culmination can provide cellular salvation. This contrasts the death processes of apoptosis and necrosis, which are executed rapidly and are irreversible. As such, the identification of the precise mechanism by which autophagy supports survival is critical.

Autophagy not only provides an alternate means for energy generation during periods of starvation, but also has a role in cellular damage mitigation through promotion of protein and organelle quality control, especially under conditions of stress in which proteins and organelles become damaged. By degrading damaged proteins and organelles, autophagy prevents their accumulation, which can be toxic. This function of autophagy is particularly critical in stressed tissues and tumors, which are regularly subjected to metabolic stress by their dependence on the inefficient process of aerobic glycolysis and by their intermittently limited blood supply during rapid tumor growth or metastasis. Thus, autophagy defects in tissues and tumors reduce cellular fitness and render cells prone to DNA damage, mutation, and genomic instability,[85,86,92] which in turn contribute to tumor initiation and progression.[82,114,115]

In addition to these cell-autonomous mechanisms, defective autophagy can promote tumorigenesis in a non–cell-autonomous way by reducing tumor cell survival that causes chronic cell death and inflammation in tumors.[80,92,115] Autophagy can thereby be thought of as a double-edged sword. On the one hand, autophagy promotes tumor cell survival through maintaining energy homeostasis and mitigating oxidative damage by preventing the accumulation of aggregated proteins and abnormal organelles. On the other hand, defects in autophagy elevate oxidative stress, DNA damage, and mutation, and promote chronic cell death and inflammation, all of which are linked to promotion of cancer initiation and progression.[115] These observations have led to the notions that autophagy stimulation can prevent cancer, whereas inhibiting autophagy-mediated survival is an approach to treating established, aggressive cancers.[82,114]

Autophagy Modulation for Cancer Treatment

As autophagy can enable tumor cell survival to stress,[80,81] the means to block autophagy has the potential to promote cell death that may be therapeutically advantageous.[82,114] Moreover, both targeted and cytotoxic antineoplastic agents have been observed to induce autophagy in human cancer cell lines,[116,117] possibly as a survival mechanism in response to treatment-induced stress. Thus, autophagy inhibitors are expected to deprive cancer cells of an essential survival mechanism and consequently render them more susceptible to cell death. This novel paradigm in cancer therapy has been validated in several preclinical studies.[118–126] This approach is now under investigation in phase 1/2 clinical trials involving autophagy inhibition by the antimalarial drug hydroxychloroquine, which blocks lysosome degradation of the products of autophagy, in combination with standard chemotherapy.

NECROSIS

Recent evidence suggests that tumor cells in which apoptosis has been disabled can be diverted to necrosis, which has traditionally been considered an unregulated (and thus, not programmed) form of cell death implicated in pathologic states, such as ischemia, trauma, and infection.[127] Recent evidence is calling the unregulated nature of necrosis into question.

Necrosis is derived from the Greek word *nekros* for corpse, and it involves rapid swelling of the cell, loss of plasma membrane integrity, and release of the cellular contents into the extracellular environment, resulting in an acute inflammatory response. Necrosis is largely viewed as an accidental and unregulated cellular event triggered by cellular trauma (direct physical injury), acute energy depletion, or extreme stress.[128] Recently, a type of programmed necrotic cell death, called *necroptosis*,[129] has been identified as induced by interaction of death domain receptors with their respective ligands under conditions of defective or inhibited downstream apoptotic machinery.[130] Necroptosis depends on the serine/threonine kinase activity of the death domain receptor-associated adaptor Rip1 and its relative Rip3.[131–136] Necroptosis is potently inhibited by the Rip1 kinase inhibitors, the necrostatins.[133] In a genome-wide siRNA screen for necroptosis regulators, a set of 432 genes with enriched expression in the immune and nervous systems was identified and cellular sensitivity to necroptosis was found to depend on the same signaling network that mediates innate immunity.[131] Harnessing necroptosis to induce cell death in cancer is an exciting new prospect, the exploitation of which will require a deeper mechanistic insight into the process and its regulation.

Regarding necrosis as a therapeutic end point, tumor cell fate in response to treatment with DNA-damaging agents depends on the effect of the DNA repair protein poly(ADP-ribose) polymerase (PARP) on cellular metabolism. PARP activation by DNA-damaging alkylating agents causes PARP-mediated β-nicotinamide adenine dinucleotide (NAD) consumption, ATP depletion, and metabolic stress. The glycolytic state (Warburg effect) and inefficient mode of energy production in most cancer cells renders them sensitive to this ATP depletion in response to PARP activation, resulting in induction of necrotic cell death of apoptosis-defective tumor cells.[137] Tumor cells with defects in both apoptosis and autophagy may be particularly susceptible to death by necrosis as loss of autophagy potential deprives cells of an alternate energy source for maintenance of metabolism and viability in metabolic stress that is compounded by the Warburg effect.[80]

Manipulation of tumor cell metabolism is an appealing therapeutic approach, as it can be used to induce cancer cell death by metabolic catastrophe.[77] This is particularly relevant for tumors with increased proliferative capacity and high bioenergetic requirements, such as tumors with constitutive activation of the PI3-kinase/Akt pathway, which are unable to down-regulate metabolism and to activate autophagy in response to starvation. Thus, the very properties that confer cancer cells with the capacity for rapid growth may also render them susceptible to metabolic stress pharmacologically induced by a wide variety of means, including nutrient deprivation, angiogenesis inhibition, glycolysis inhibition, accelerated ATP consumption, or autophagy inhibition. Furthermore, necrotic cell death can be genetically determined indirectly through manipulation of cellular bioenergetics (decreased energy production through autophagy and catabolism inhibition, increased metabolic demand through elevated consumption, or decreased nutrient availability) or directly by activating Rip kinases or PARP. It will be of great interest to see if necrosis, like apoptosis, can be exploited for cancer therapy.

It is becoming clear that cells possess multiple death mechanism, and establishing how these are altered in tumors and can be activated with therapy is essential. Defining at the molecular level how apoptosis is regulated has led to the development of novel cancer therapies aimed at triggering or restoring apoptotic function in tumor cells, and this progress is likely to continue. Moreover, defining the mechanisms by which common mutations in human tumors inactivate apoptosis has yielded novel opportunities for tumor-genotype–specific rational chemotherapy targeting the apoptotic pathway. In tumor cells where apoptosis is disabled, it is apparent that alternate forms of cell death can be activated, including necrosis, the process by which remains poorly characterized. Finally, the catabolic process of autophagy can promote tumor cell survival to metabolic stress, providing new opportunities for therapeutic intervention, in part capitalizing on the altered metabolic state intrinsic to tumor cells.

Selected References

The full list of references for this chapter appears in the online version.

3. Rao L, Debbas M, Sabbatini P, Hockenbery D, Korsmeyer S, White E. The adenovirus E1A proteins induce apoptosis, which is inhibited by the E1B 19-kDa and Bcl-2 proteins. *Proc Natl Acad Sci U S A* 1992;89:7742.
4. Fanidi A, Harrington EA, Evan GI. Cooperative interaction between c-myc and bcl-2 proto-oncogenes. *Nature* 1992;359:554.
5. Evan GI, Wyllie AH, Gilbert CS, et al. Induction of apoptosis in fibroblasts by c-myc protein. *Cell* 1992;69:119.
6. Morgenbesser SD, Williams BO, Jacks T, DePinho RA. p53-dependent apoptosis produced by Rb-deficiency in the developing mouse lens. *Nature* 1994;371:72.
7. Certo M, Del Gaizo Moore V, Nishino M, et al. Mitochondria primed by death signals determine cellular addiction to antiapoptotic BCL-2 family members. *Cancer Cell* 2006;9:351.
9. Hengartner MO, Ellis RE, Horvitz HR. *Caenorhabditis elegans* gene ced-9 protects cells from programmed cell death. *Nature* 1992;356:494.
12. Yuan J, Shaham S, Ledoux S, Ellis HM, Horvitz HR. The *C. elegans* cell death gene ced-3 encodes a protein similar to mammalian interleukin-1 beta-converting enzyme. *Cell* 1993;75:641.
13. Zou H, Henzel WJ, Liu X, Lutschg A, Wang X. Apaf-1, a human protein homologous to C. elegans CED-4, participates in cytochrome c-dependent activation of caspase-3. *Cell* 1997;90:405.
15. Bakhshi A, Jensen JP, Goldman P, et al. Cloning the chromosomal breakpoint of t(14;18) human lymphomas: clustering around JH on chromosome 14 and near a transcriptional unit on 18. *Cell* 1985;41:899.
16. Cleary ML, Smith SD, Sklar J. Cloning and structural analysis of cDNAs for bcl-2 and a hybrid bcl-2/immunoglobulin transcript resulting from the t(14;18) translocation. *Cell* 1986;47:19.
17. Tsujimoto Y, Gorham J, Cossman J, Jaffe E, Croce CM. The t(14;18) chromosome translocations involved in B-cell neoplasms result from mistakes in VDJ joining. *Science* 1985;229:1390.
18. Vaux DL, Cory S, Adams JM. Bcl-2 gene promotes haemopoietic cell survival and cooperates with c-myc to immortalize pre-β cells. *Nature* 1988;335:440.
19. McDonnell TJ, Korsmeyer SJ. Progression from lymphoid hyperplasia to high-grade malignant lymphoma in mice transgenic for the t(14; 18). *Nature* 1991;349:254.
20. Strasser A, Harris AW, Bath ML, Cory S. Novel primitive lymphoid tumours induced in transgenic mice by cooperation between myc and bcl-2. *Nature* 1990;348:331.
22. Debbas M, White E. Wild-type p53 mediates apoptosis by E1A, which is inhibited by E1B. *Genes Dev* 1993;7:546.
23. Lowe SW, Ruley HE. Stabilization of the p53 tumor suppressor is induced by adenovirus 5 E1A and accompanies apoptosis. *Genes Dev* 1993;7:535.
31. Wei MC, Zong WX, Cheng EH, et al. Proapoptotic BAX and BAK: a requisite gateway to mitochondrial dysfunction and death. *Science* 2001;292:727.
32. Zong WX, Lindsten T, Ross AJ, MacGregor GR, Thompson CB. BH3-only proteins that bind pro-survival Bcl-2 family members fail to induce apoptosis in the absence of Bax and Bak. *Genes Dev* 2001;15:1481.
34. Muchmore SW, Sattler M, Liang H, et al. X-ray and NMR structure of human Bcl-xL, an inhibitor of programmed cell death. *Nature* 1996;381:335.
37. Oltersdorf T, Elmore SW, Shoemaker AR, et al. An inhibitor of Bcl-2 family proteins induces regression of solid tumours. *Nature* 2005;435:677.
40. Du C, Fang M, Li Y, Li L, Wang X. Smac, a mitochondrial protein that promotes cytochrome c-dependent caspase activation by eliminating IAP inhibition. *Cell* 2000;102:33.
42. Kluck RM, Bossy-Wetzel E, Green DR, Newmeyer DD. The release of cytochrome c from mitochondria: a primary site for Bcl-2 regulation of apoptosis. *Science* 1997;275:1132.
43. Verhagen AM, Ekert PG, Pakusch M, et al. Identification of DIABLO, a mammalian protein that promotes apoptosis by binding to and antagonizing IAP proteins. *Cell* 2000;102:43.
44. Yang J, Liu X, Bhalla K, et al. Prevention of apoptosis by Bcl-2: release of cytochrome c from mitochondria blocked. *Science* 1997;275:1129.
56. Fulda S, Wick W, Weller M, Debatin KM. Smac agonists sensitize for Apo2L/TRAIL- or anticancer drug-induced apoptosis and induce regression of malignant glioma in vivo. *Nat Med* 2002;8:808.
59. Xue W, Zender L, Miething C, et al. Senescence and tumour clearance is triggered by p53 restoration in murine liver carcinomas. *Nature* 2007;445:656.
60. Ventura A, Kirsch DG, McLaughlin ME, et al. Restoration of p53 function leads to tumour regression in vivo. *Nature* 2007;445:661.
62. Tan TT, Degenhardt K, Nelson DA, et al. Key roles of BIM-driven apoptosis in epithelial tumors and rational chemotherapy. *Cancer Cell* 2005;7:227.
68. Konopleva M, Contractor R, Tsao T, et al. Mechanisms of apoptosis sensitivity and resistance to the BH3 mimetic ABT-737 in acute myeloid leukemia. *Cancer Cell* 2006;10:375.
80. Degenhardt K, Mathew R, Beaudoin B, et al. Autophagy promotes tumor cell survival and restricts necrosis, inflammation, and tumorigenesis. *Cancer Cell* 2006;10:51.
81. Lum JJ, Bauer DE, Kong M, et al. Growth factor regulation of autophagy and cell survival in the absence of apoptosis. *Cell* 2005;120:237.
86. Mathew R, Kongara S, Beaudoin B, et al. Autophagy suppresses tumor progression by limiting chromosomal instability. *Genes Dev* 2007;21:1367.
87. Kuma A, Hatano M, Matsui M, et al. The role of autophagy during the early neonatal starvation period. *Nature* 2004;432:1032.
90. Komatsu M, Waguri S, Chiba T, et al. Loss of autophagy in the central nervous system causes neurodegeneration in mice. *Nature* 2006;441:880.
91. Hara T, Nakamura K, Matsui M, et al. Suppression of basal autophagy in neural cells causes neurodegenerative disease in mice. *Nature* 2006;441:885.
92. Mathew R, Karp CM, Beaudoin B, et al. Autophagy suppresses tumorigenesis through elimination of p62. *Cell* 2009;137:1062.
93. Komatsu M, Waguri S, Koike M, et al. Homeostatic levels of p62 control cytoplasmic inclusion body formation in autophagy-deficient mice. *Cell* 2007;131:1149.
102. Lee JH, Budanov AV, Park EJ, et al. Sestrin as a feedback inhibitor of TOR that prevents age-related pathologies. *Science* 2010;327:1223.
112. Yue Z, Jin S, Yang C, Levine AJ, Heintz N. Beclin 1, an autophagy gene essential for early embryonic development, is a haploinsufficient tumor suppressor. *Proc Natl Acad Sci U S A* 2003;100:15077.
113. Qu X, Yu J, Bhagat G, et al. Promotion of tumorigenesis by heterozygous disruption of the beclin 1 autophagy gene. *J Clin Invest* 2003;112:1809.
114. White E, DiPaola RS. The double-edged sword of autophagy modulation in cancer. *Clin Cancer Res* 2009;15:5308.
122. Degtyarev M, De Maziere A, Orr C, et al. Akt inhibition promotes autophagy and sensitizes PTEN-null tumors to lysosomotropic agents. *J Cell Biol* 2008;183:101.
123. Maclean KH, Dorsey FC, Cleveland JL, Kastan MB. Targeting lysosomal degradation induces p53-dependent cell death and prevents cancer in mouse models of lymphomagenesis. *J Clin Invest* 2008;118:79.
124. Carew JS, Nawrocki ST, Kahue CN, et al. Targeting autophagy augments the anticancer activity of the histone deacetylase inhibitor SAHA to overcome Bcr-Abl-mediated drug resistance. *Blood* 2007;110:313.
125. Amaravadi RK, Yu D, Lum JJ, et al. Autophagy inhibition enhances therapy-induced apoptosis in a Myc-induced model of lymphoma. *J Clin Invest* 2007;117:326.
130. Degterev A, Huang Z, Boyce M, et al. Chemical inhibitor of nonapoptotic cell death with therapeutic potential for ischemic brain injury. *Nat Chem Biol* 2005;1:112.
133. Degterev A, Hitomi J, Germscheid M, et al. Identification of RIP1 kinase as a specific cellular target of necrostatins. *Nat Chem Biol* 2008;4:313.
135. Cho YS, Challa S, Moquin D, et al. Phosphorylation-driven assembly of the RIP1-RIP3 complex regulates programmed necrosis and virus-induced inflammation. *Cell* 2009;137:1112.
136. He S, Wang L, Miao L, et al. Receptor interacting protein kinase-3 determines cellular necrotic response to TNF-alpha. *Cell* 2009;137:1100.
138. Suzuki M, Youle RJ, Tjandra N. Structure of Bax: coregulation of dimer formation and intracellular localization. *Cell* 2000;103:645.

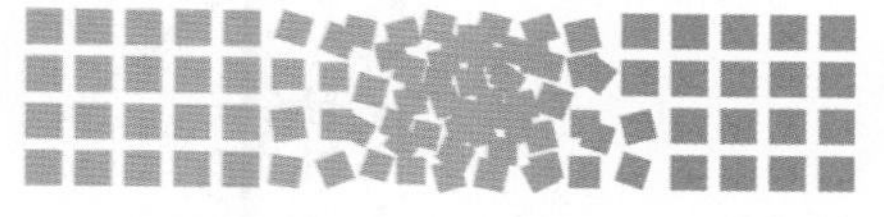

CHAPTER 8 CANCER METABOLISM

MATTHEW G. VANDER HEIDEN

One of the first distinctions noted between cancer tissues and normal tissues was a difference in metabolism. In the 1920s, the biochemist Otto Warburg observed that when provided with glucose, cancer tissues generate large amounts of lactate regardless of whether oxygen is present. This finding is in contrast to most normal tissues that only ferment glucose to lactate in the absence of oxygen. This metabolic difference between cancer cells and normal cells is referred to as the Warburg effect, and along with other metabolic alterations that characterize cancer cells, it remains an incompletely understood aspect of cancer biology. The metabolic phenotype of cancer cells has been exploited for cancer diagnostics and led to the development of some of the first successful chemotherapies. However, despite the fact that altered metabolism is shared across many different cancer types, few therapies exist that exploit differences in cellular metabolism. Efforts to understand cancer metabolism are currently an active area of investigation and hold great promise as a source of novel targets for cancer treatment.

ALTERED METABOLISM IN CANCER CELLS

The regulation of metabolic pathways in tumor tissues is different from that observed in most adult tissues.[1] Rapidly dividing cells must balance energy production with macromolecular synthesis, while most nonproliferating adult tissues utilize a greater fraction of nutrients for energy production and require less nutrient uptake. Cancer cells rely primarily on glycolysis for their metabolism, while the majority of normal cells in adult tissues utilize aerobic respiration to completely catabolize glucose and generate cellular energy.[2–5] Most differentiated cells primarily metabolize glucose to carbon dioxide in the presence of oxygen and only produce large amounts of lactate under anaerobic conditions. Warburg observed that cancer cells produce large amounts of lactate regardless of oxygen availability (Fig. 8.1).[6,7] Because cancer cells use glycolysis to make lactate from glucose in the presence of oxygen, this form of metabolism observed in cancer cells is also called aerobic glycolysis.

The primary energy source for cells in most tissues is glucose. The concentration of glucose in the blood remains relatively constant at around 4–6 mM (72–110 mg/dL). Glucose uptake into cells is controlled most proximally by the expression of glucose transport proteins on the cell surface (Fig. 8.2).[8] Insulin-responsive tissues rely on the regulated delivery of Glut4 transporters to the cell surface to increase glucose uptake. Noninsulin responsive tissues, including most cancers, do not use Glut4, but instead use the homologous Glut1, Glut2, or Glut3 proteins to transport glucose into cells. All of these glucose transporters allow the diffusion of glucose across the plasma membrane. The transporters differ in their affinity for glucose and capacity for transport. Glut1 is responsible for the basal level of glucose uptake in most normal cells and is thought to be the transporter responsible for glucose uptake in most tumor cells. Expression of Glut3 and other less well characterized glucose transporters have also been described in some cancers.[9,10] How these transporters differ from Glut1 and whether these differences are important for tumor biology and metabolism remain active areas of investigation.

Glucose is trapped in the cytoplasm of cells by the addition of a phosphate group to form glucose-6-phosphate (Fig. 8.2).[11] This reaction is catalyzed by the enzyme hexokinase, which also has several isoforms with different normal tissue distributions and enzymatic properties. The various isoforms of hexokinase can associate with the outer surface of mitochondria, and this proximity to a source of adenosine triphosphate (ATP) has been suggested to be important for the high rate of glucose uptake observed in many cancer cells.[12] The association of hexokinase with mitochondria has also been implicated in the regulation of apoptosis such that hexokinase may constitute a molecular link between glycolysis and the cell death machinery.[13]

Once trapped in cells, glucose can be metabolized via glycolysis to generate pyruvate in the cytosol.[11] The rate of glycolysis is controlled by glucose flux into cells, cofactor availability, and the activity of glycolytic enzymes (Fig. 8.3). Both the phosphofructokinase and pyruvate kinase steps of glycolysis are highly regulated and have been implicated in the control of tumor cell metabolism (Figs. 8.3 and 8.4).[14–16] Another major determinant of glucose metabolism by glycolysis is the availability of oxidized nicotinamide adenine dinucleotide (NAD) to serve as the electron acceptor for the conversion of glyceraldehyde-3-phosphate to 1,3-bisphosphoglycerate. This reaction, catalyzed by glyceraldehyde-3-phosphate dehydrogenase reduces NAD to NADH (reduced nicotinamide adenine dinucleotide). Because the size of the NAD/NADH cofactor pool in cells is small relative to the flux of glucose through glycolysis, continued cycling of NADH back to NAD is critical to permit continued glycolysis (Fig. 8.3). NADH can be reoxidized to NAD through a series of reactions that shuttle reducing equivalents into mitochondria for use in oxidative phosphorylation. This process is coupled to the further metabolism of pyruvate in the mitochondrial tricarboxylic acid (TCA) cycle and can result in the generation of large amounts of ATP. ATP is used as a source of free energy for cells to enable otherwise unfavorable biochemical processes. Mitochondrial oxidative phosphorylation requires the presence of oxygen (O_2) as the final acceptor of electrons from NADH and therefore is also referred to as aerobic respiration. Aerobic glycolysis also generates ATP; however, the ATP yield per molecule of glucose is much less than for aerobic respiration. The metabolism of glucose to pyruvate without mitochondrial respiration requires the enzyme lactate dehydrogenase (LDH) to produce lactate and regenerate NAD from NADH.

Several hypotheses for why aerobic glycolysis appears to be selected for in cancer cells have been proposed. Warburg

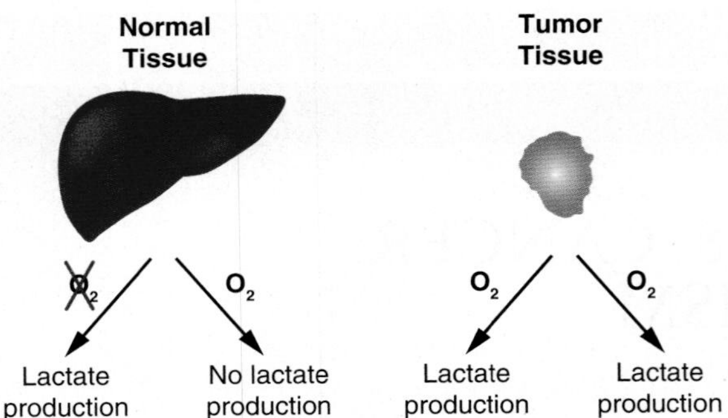

FIGURE 8.1 A graphic representation of Warburg's experiment is shown. Most normal tissues produce lactate in large quantities only when oxygen (O_2) is absent. In contrast, cancer cells tend to make lactate regardless of O_2 availability. This tendency of cancer cells to metabolize glucose to lactate (aerobic glycolysis) is often referred to as the Warburg effect.

hypothesized that cancer cells develop a defect in mitochondria that leads to impaired aerobic respiration and a subsequent reliance on glycolytic metabolism.[2] Although mutations in mitochondrial enzymes have been implicated in a subset of cancers (discussed in detail later in the chapter), subsequent studies demonstrated that mitochondrial function is not impaired in the majority of cancer cells.[17] Nevertheless, despite his hypothesis being incorrect, Warburg's original observation has held true with numerous reports describing that despite normally functioning mitochondria many cancer cells preferentially metabolize glucose via aerobic glycolysis.[4,18]

The growth of solid tumors is limited by the presence of an adequate blood supply to deliver oxygen and nutrients to support cell metabolism. Therefore, angiogenesis is an important process for tumor growth, and targeting this process has been successful for cancer therapy.[19] Because many tumors are characterized by inefficient angiogenesis, cells must survive periods of relative hypoxia and nutrient deprivation during tumorigenesis.[5] Therefore, it has been proposed that the relative hypoxia of tumors selects for glycolytic metabolism.[3] However, aerobic glycolysis is observed at the earliest stages of tumorigenesis. It is a characteristic feature of leukemia and lung cancers that arises under conditions of normal to high oxygen tensions and is found in normal rapidly proliferating tissues during embryogenesis and immune responses.[1] Therefore, it is likely that aerobic glycolysis provides another benefit to cancer cells that is selected for during tumorigenesis.[1] Aerobic glycolysis may still facilitate tumor survival during periods of hypoxia. The same pathways that regulate angiogenesis also promote aerobic glycolysis, suggesting that important connections between these two processes exist.[20,21]

The selective pressure for aerobic glycolysis in cancer cells may be related to the reprogramming of metabolism to accommodate rapid cell division. Cells metabolize glucose for purposes other than generating ATP.[1] Intermediates derived from the metabolism of glucose are used in other metabolic pathways

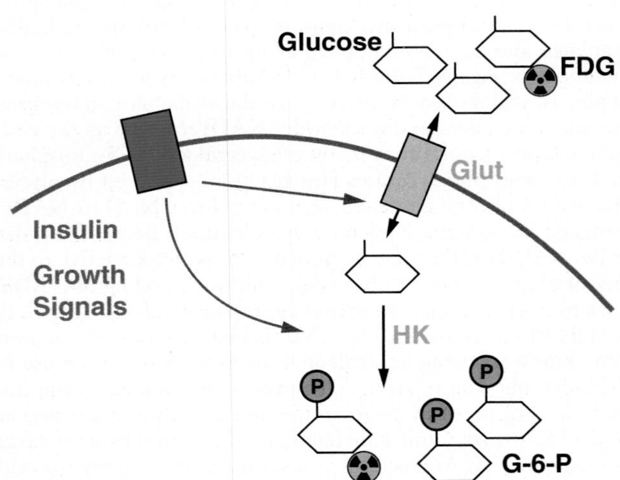

FIGURE 8.2 Glucose uptake is controlled in mammalian cells by the presence of glucose transporters on the cell surface (Glut). These transport proteins allow the diffusion of glucose across the plasma membrane where it is phosphorylated by the enzyme hexokinase (HK) and trapped in the cell. Glucose transporter expression is controlled by insulin signaling in insulin responsive tissues. Glucose uptake is also regulated by cell growth signals. A positron emission tomography (PET) scan can be used to monitor glucose uptake in the clinic. This assay uses the positron-emitting fluorine-18 (^{18}F)-conjugated glucose analogue fluoro-2-deoxyglucose (FDG), which can be phosphorylated by hexokinase and trapped in the cell but cannot be metabolized further.

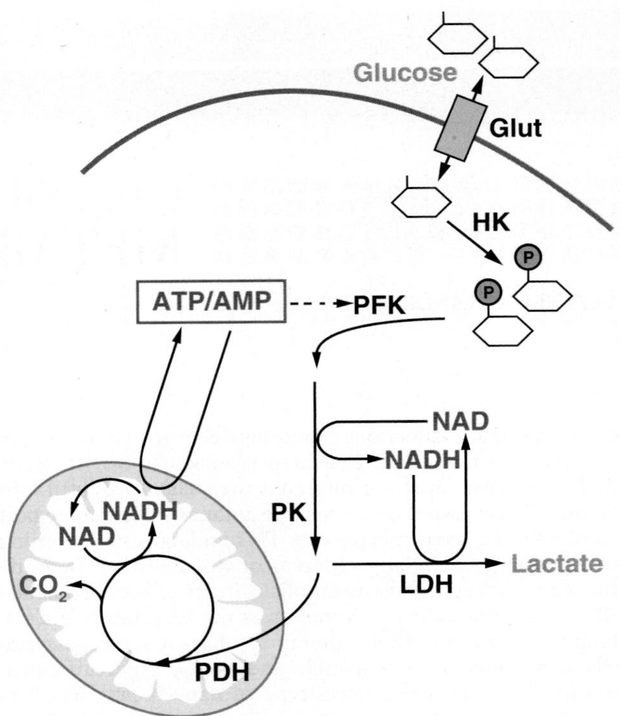

FIGURE 8.3 Cellular glucose metabolism is regulated at several steps. Uptake of glucose is regulated by glucose transporter expression (Glut). Glucose metabolism by glycolysis classically is considered to be regulated at three enzymatic steps: these include the reactions catalyzed by hexokinase (HK), phosphofructokinase (PFK) and pyruvate kinase (PK). The PFK step in glycolysis is a major point of regulation. One major allosteric input to PFK activity is the adenosine triphosphate: adenosine monophosphate (ATP:AMP) ratio. PFK activity and glycolysis are activated when the ATP:AMP ratio is low and inhibited when the ATP:AMP ratio is high. Glycolysis is also controlled by the availability of the cofactor nicotinamide adenine dinucleotide (NAD). NAD is reduced to NADH at the glyceraldehyde-3-phosphate dehydrogenase step of the pathway, and NADH must be recycled back to NAD to allow continued glycolysis. NADH can be converted to NAD by lactate dehydrogenase (LDH)-mediated conversion of pyruvate to lactate. NAD regeneration can also be coupled to the tricarboxylic acid (TCA) cycle and mitochondrial oxidative phosphorylation. Entry of pyruvate into the TCA cycle is controlled by pyruvate dehydrogenase (PDH) and allows the complete catabolism of glucose to carbon dioxide (CO_2) and maximum ATP production.

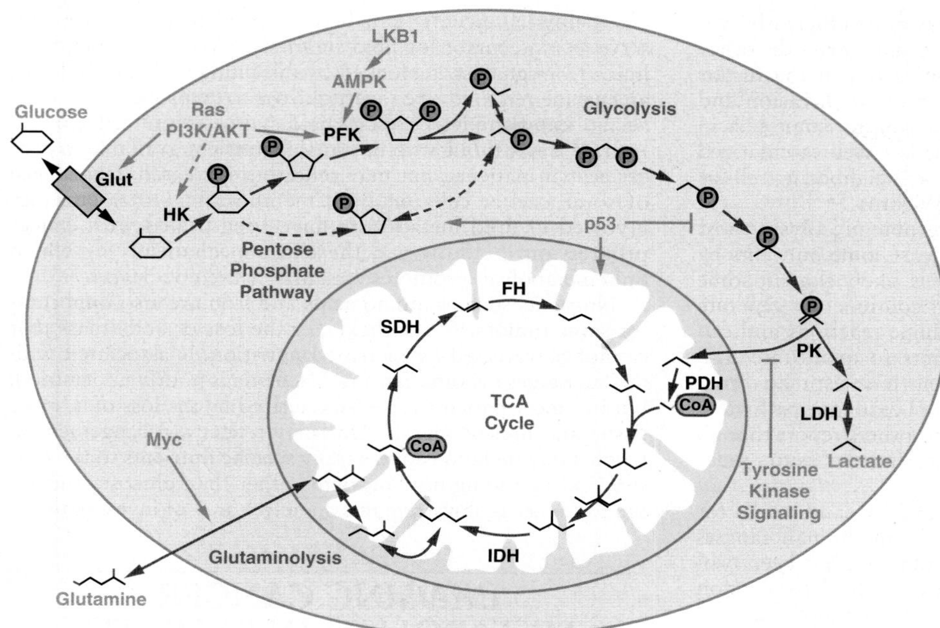

FIGURE 8.4 A schematic of central carbon metabolism is presented to show how glycolysis, the tricarboxylic acid (TCA) cycle, the pentose phosphate pathway, and glutamine metabolism are interconnected in cells. The major points of enzymatic regulation, along with the enzymes discussed in the text that have been demonstrated to be important in cancer, are shown for orientation within the pathways, Glut, glucose transporter; HK, hexokinase; PFK, phosphofructokinase; PK, pyruvate kinase; LDH, lactate dehydrogenase; PDH, pyruvate dehydrogenase; IDH, isocitrate dehydrogenase; SDH, succinate dehydrogenase; FH, fumarate hydratase. The site of regulation within these pathways by some of the major oncogenes and tumor suppressor genes is also shown.

in cells and ultimately provide much of the carbon necessary to produce biomass. The production of nucleic acids, amino acids, lipids, and carbohydrates needed to duplicate all the components of the dividing cell is the major metabolic requirement that distinguishes rapidly proliferating cancer cells from most normal cells. If glucose is completely catabolized to carbon dioxide (CO_2), as occurs during oxidative metabolism, there are no metabolic intermediates available for biosynthetic reactions. Thus, aerobic glycolysis may reflect how metabolism is altered to permit anabolic metabolism.[1] Indeed, many micro-organisms grow by fermentation when nutrients are abundant and display a metabolic phenotype analogous to aerobic glycolysis.[22]

ENERGETICS OF CELL PROLIFERATION

There is evidence that the rate of aerobic glycolysis, including the accompanying increased rate of glucose utilization, is not elevated in cancer cells solely to satisfy ATP demand. It has been suggested that glycolysis in tumors cells is limited by the rate of ATP consumption.[23,24] Cancer cells must balance the catabolism of nutrients to generate ATP with other metabolic needs to allow net biosynthesis and cell proliferation.[1] To produce a daughter cell, a proliferating cell must replicate the genome, duplicate the ribosomes and protein synthesis machinery, generate new organelles, and synthesize *de novo* enough lipids to duplicate cellular membranes. This imposes a large requirement of new nucleic acids, amino acids, and lipids for cell proliferation. While ATP hydrolysis provides free energy for many biosynthetic pathways, there are additional requirements to carry out these anabolic reactions. Synthesis of lipids and nucleic acids both require specific metabolite precursors and reducing equivalents provided by nicotinamide adenine dinucleotide phosphate (NADPH) (Fig. 8.5). In fact the need for NADPH and carbon skeletons on a molar basis exceeds the requirement for ATP in many biosynthetic reactions.[1] Aerobic glycolysis may allow cancer cells to balance the various metabolic requirements of proliferation.

Cancer Cells Can Metabolize Nutrients Other Than Glucose

Although tumor cell metabolism is adapted to facilitate anabolic metabolism for rapid proliferation, it is not clear why many cancer cells excrete lactate. Each lactate excreted wastes three carbons that might otherwise be recycled to fulfill some need in building a new cancer cell. It has been hypothesized that the excretion of lactate, which accompanies aerobic glycolysis, may enable faster proliferative metabolism.[1] In the early stages of tumorigenesis, cancer cells are not limited for nutrients. Cells

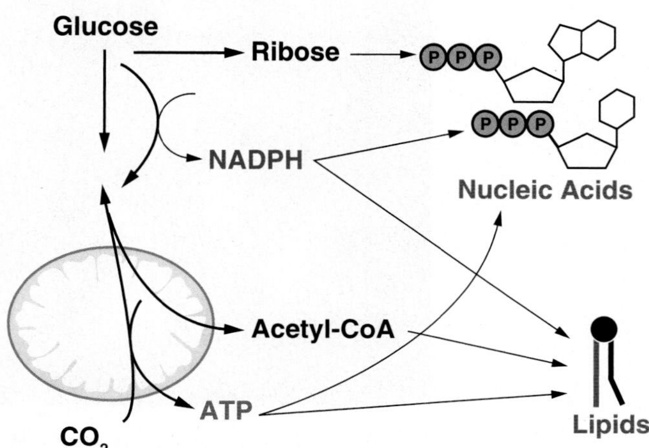

FIGURE 8.5 The generation of macromolecules requires several products of central carbon metabolism. In addition to adenosine triphosphate (ATP), the synthesis of nucleic acids and lipids both require reducing equivalents provided by nicotinamide adenine dinucleotide phosphate (NADPH) and carbon precursors that branch from different points of core metabolic pathways. Cancer cells must balance the production of specific macromolecular precursors such as ribose and acetyl-coA with the generation of enough NADPH and ATP to support proliferation.

that incorporate nutrients into biomass most efficiently will proliferate faster. Lactate production may provide other advantages to a tumor as well. Acidification of the tumor microenvironment has been shown to promote invasion and metastasis.[3] Lactate can also act as a nutrient for some cells in the tumor.[25] As tumors grow, cells in the less-well vascularized regions of a tumor can utilize lactate from neighboring cells as a carbon source to survive periods of cell stress.[26]

Despite an increased reliance on aerobic glycolysis, most tumor cells continue to metabolize at least some nutrients by oxidative phosphorylation. In fact, it is likely that in some cancer cells oxidative phosphorylation continues to generate much of the ATP required for biosynthetic reactions and cellular housekeeping functions.[4] Attempts to quantitate ATP production experimentally in cancer cells have estimated that 80% of the ATP generated is derived from oxidative pathways, while 20% comes from glycolysis,[27] and others report that up to 50% of the ATP in cancer cells can be derived from oxidative phosphorylation.[28]

Glucose is not the only substrate used by cancer cells for oxidative phosphorylation.[27,29] In fact, some human cancers do not demonstrate elevated glucose uptake. It has been proposed that at least some of these cancers may be dependent on the amino acid glutamine as a primary source of carbon. Glutamine can be metabolized via two transamination reactions to the TCA cycle intermediate α-ketoglutarate (Fig. 8.4), and glutamine is required for proliferation of many cancer cells.[30] In addition to glucose and glutamine, other nutrients have been shown to be important in some tumors. Several clinical studies have demonstrated that some human cancers show increased uptake of acetate by positron emission tomography (PET) scan using carbon-11 (^{11}C)-acetate as a tracer (see below).[31] Acetate can be converted to acetyl-coA and serve as a precursor for lipid synthesis.[32] When production of lipids from glucose is blocked by inhibiting ATP citrate lyase, an enzyme required to convert glucose to cytosolic acetyl-coA, acetate can completely rescue lipid synthesis and cell growth. Acetate is not thought to be a major nutrient available to cancer cells in patients, but may reflect an increased dependence of some cancer cells on lipid metabolism. Other enzymes involved in lipid metabolism have been linked with cancer progression,[33,34] however, the exact mechanisms by which lipid metabolism promotes malignancy are not clear.

Nutrients such as amino acids and iron are also important for some tumors.[35,36] Cachexia, or the loss of body mass that cannot be reversed by increased nutrition, is associated with the late stages of some cancers. Cachexia is poorly understood, but in cancer patients it is characterized by the loss of adipose tissue and muscle mass.[37] This may reflect a derangement in whole body metabolism to supply specific nutrients to the cancer. Understanding how nutrients other than glucose contribute to cancer biology remains an active area of investigation.

IMAGING CANCER METABOLISM IN PATIENTS

The characteristic increased glucose uptake of cancer cells has been exploited to image cancer in the clinic. The glucose analogue 2-deoxyglucose is permeable to glucose transporters and trapped in cells when phosphorylated by hexokinase (Fig. 8.2). The 2-deoxyglucose-6-phosphate is unable to be further metabolized,[38,38] and thus 2-deoxyglucose-6-phosphate

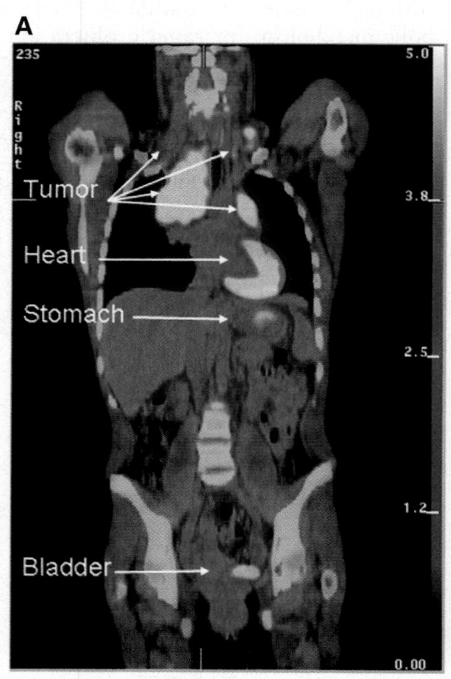

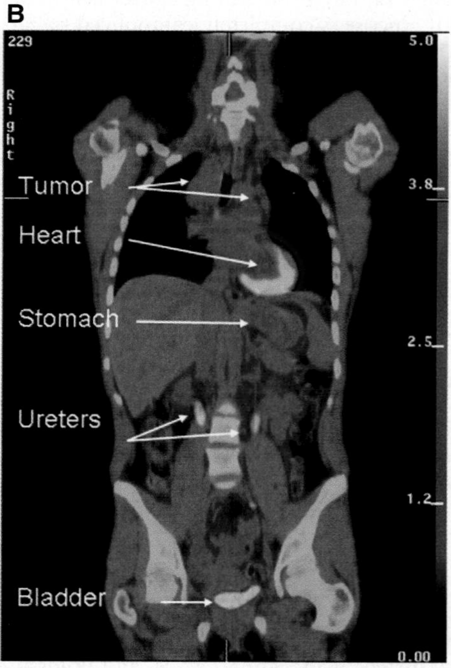

FIGURE 8.6 Early metabolic changes on ^{18}F-fluro-2-deoxyglucose position emission tomography/computed tomography (FDG-PET/CT) are highly predictive of final treatment response. Fused coronal FDG-PET/CT images in a 44-year-old woman with stage IIA Hodgkin's lymphoma at presentation (**A**) and after two cycles of ABVD (doxorubicin, bleomycin, vinblastine, dacarbazine) chemotherapy (**B**). The tumor seen in the mediastinum and bilateral neck shows intense avidity for the glucose analogue FDG prior to therapy consistent with increased glucose uptake in (**A**). Although a residual tumor mass is still seen on CT after two cycles of ABVD chemotherapy (**B**), it is no longer FDG-avid, and the patient has been in remission for over 2 years since completion of therapy. Normal FDG uptake and excretion is seen in the stomach, heart, and urinary tract, respectively. (Image courtesy of Tricia Locascio, Katherine Zukotynski, and Annick D. Van den Abbeele, Department of Imaging, Dana-Farber Cancer Institute.)

accumulation can be used to assess the rate of glucose uptake into cells. By conjugating the positron emitting isotope fluorine-18 (^{18}F) to 2-deoxyglucose, the uptake of glucose can be measured in patients using PET.[40] ^{18}F-fluro-2-deoxyglucose (FDG)-PET is used widely in the clinic to visualize tumors. The current use of FDG-PET is primarily as a staging tool for cancers, however, it is also sometimes used to characterize lesions observed by other imaging modalities. FDG-PET is also increasingly being used as a marker of response to therapy (Fig. 8.6). At least for some treatments, there is mounting evidence that decreased uptake of FDG by PET scan following therapy is a predictor of clinical efficacy.[41,42]

In the clinic, FDG-PET scan can be used to classify tumors. Although many tumors are visible by FDG-PET scan, some tumors do not display elevated FDG uptake. This illustrates that different tumors can display distinct metabolic phenotypes related to their genetic background or site of origin. As discussed above, some tumors rely on nutrients other than glucose. For instance increased ^{11}C-acetate uptake has been observed by PET in prostate tumors that do not demonstrate elevated signal on FDG-PET scan.[43] However, increased uptake of ^{11}C-acetate is also seen in some benign prostate conditions, so whether ^{11}C-acetate uptake defines a characteristic of some prostate cancers or reflects the underlying biology of the prostate gland remains to be determined.[44] New methods to image tumor metabolism by PET or magnetic resonance imaging (MRI) are being developed. If successful, such efforts will better define distinct metabolic phenotypes in patient tumors.

GENETIC EVENTS IMPORTANT FOR CANCER INFLUENCE METABOLISM

Human cancer occurs as a consequence of genetic events that promote the inappropriate proliferation of cells.[45] These events lead to the expression of oncogenes or the loss of tumor suppressor genes that contribute to tumor formation and progression. Although alterations involving specific oncogenes or tumor suppressor genes are hallmarks of specific malignant phenotypes, many of these genetic events are found in numerous types of cancer. These genetic changes occur in diverse cellular signaling and transcriptional pathways, and it is unclear how the various mutations converge to allow inappropriate cell growth and proliferation. One common downstream consequence of these genetic changes is altered cellular metabolism.

Efforts to understand the predisposition to malignancy displayed by von Hippel-Lindau (VHL) syndrome patients identified a link between cancer genetics and the regulation of cell metabolism.[46] VHL syndrome results when patients inherit one mutated copy of the *VHL* gene, leading to a spectrum of benign and malignant tumors including clear cell carcinoma of the kidney. In these patient's tumors, the normal *VHL* allele is lost, consistent with *VHL* acting as a tumor suppressor gene. Subsequent work demonstrated that the *VHL* gene product is also commonly lost in sporadic renal clear cell carcinomas. Although the exact mechanism by which *VHL* loss leads to renal cell carcinoma and other tumors is not known, loss of *VHL* has a profound impact on metabolic gene regulation, and these effects are thought to be important in the pathogenesis of these cancers.

The *VHL* gene encodes the substrate recognition component of a ubiquitin E3 ligase.[46] As an E3 ligase, the VHL protein-containing complex facilitates the transfer of ubiquitin to specific target proteins to effect their degradation. Among the targets of the VHL protein is the hypoxia-inducible transcription factor-1α (HIF-1α) (Fig. 8.7). HIF-1α levels are regulated by oxygen tension.[21,47] In the presence of oxygen HIF-1α is hydroxylated. The hydroxylated form of HIF-1α is recognized by VHL, leading to ubiquitination and degradation of the protein. When oxygen is absent, or when VHL is lost, HIF-1α protein accumulates, dimerizes with HIF-1α, and promotes the transcription of a number of hypoxia inducible genes. These genes include factors that promote angiogenesis to improve tissue blood supply as well as glucose transporters and most of the enzymes in glycolysis. Thus, inappropriate HIF-1α activation leads to the characteristic increased glucose uptake and glycolysis that is observed in cancer. HIF-1α accumulation is a direct consequence of VHL loss, providing a link between the loss of a tumor suppressor gene and the altered metabolic phenotype of malignant cells.

Increased expression of HIF-1α-regulated genes is found in many different types of cancer and correlates with poor patient prognosis.[48] Expression profiling of transformed cells demonstrates that metabolic genes are among the most strongly

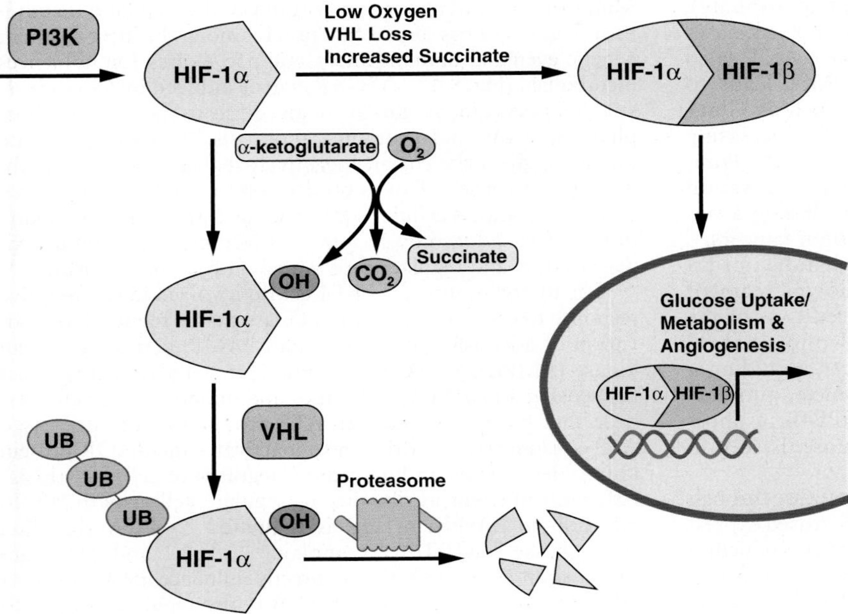

FIGURE 8.7 Transcription of many genes related to metabolism and angiogenesis is controlled by hypoxia-inducible transcription factor-1α (HIF-1α). HIF-1α levels are regulated by translational control downstream of phosphatidylinositol-3-kinase (PI3K) signaling and by the rate of proteosomal degradation. HIF-1α is marked for degradation by hydroxylation. This hydroxylation is sensitive to O_2, α-ketoglutarate, and succinate levels. The von Hippel-Lindau (VHL) protein facilitates ubiquitination and degradation of hydroxylated HIF-1α. Thus, PI3K signaling, hypoxia, succinate levels, and the presence of VHL all influence transcription of HIF-1a target genes. (Figure courtesy of Brooke J. Bevis, Whitehead Institute.)

up-regulated groups of genes.[49] Loss of expression of the HIF-1α target genes correlates with response to therapy in at least some models of cancer, suggesting that these genes are important for malignant cell proliferation and survival. Importantly, increased expression of glucose transporters and glycolytic enzymes under the control of HIF-1α are seen even in non-hypoxic tumors expressing VHL.[49,50] HIF-1α also drives expression of pyruvate dehydrogenase kinase, a negative regulator of the pyruvate dehydrogenase complex that catalyzes pyruvate entry into mitochondria.[51,52] Thus HIF-1α expression can promote aerobic glycolysis in cancer cells.

Transcription factors other than HIF-1α can promote the expression of metabolic enzymes. Expression of ChREBP-1, mondoA, and SREBP-1 has also been shown to be important in some cancers. ChREBP-1 is a key regulator of glycolytic enzyme expression and can promote anabolic metabolism.[53] MondoA is a key regulator of metabolic gene expression and coordinates glucose and glutamine metabolism.[54] Enzymes involved in cholesterol and lipid metabolism are controlled by the SREBP transcription factor,[55] and SREBP is induced as a result of oncogenic signaling.[56] Finally, increased HIF-1α–mediated gene transcription is observed in many cancers in the absence of hypoxia or VHL loss.[48] This has been attributed to increased production of HIF-1α that results from aberrant signaling downstream of phosphatidylinositol-3-kinase (PI3K), as discussed below.

Many Genetic Drivers of Cancer Increase Nutrient Uptake

Highlighting the central role that altered cellular metabolism plays in tumor biology, one shared consequence of many genetic events that promote cancer is increased glucose uptake and metabolism. Transformation is associated with elevated glucose uptake.[57,58] Activation of the PI3K signaling pathway is a common event in human cancer, and PI3K has a well-described role in glucose metabolism through its action as a proximal mediator of insulin signaling that leads to glucose uptake.[59] However, even in noninsulin dependent tissues, PI3K signaling can regulate glucose uptake and utilization and appears to drive this process in many cancers.

PI3K is activated downstream of receptor tyrosine kinases and transfers a phosphate to the membrane lipid phosphatidylinositol.[59,60] When phosphorylated on the 3-position (to generate phosphatidylinositol-3,4,5-triphosphate), the phosphorylated inositol species can recruit other kinases to the membrane, including the protein kinase AKT (also known as protein kinase B). Activation of AKT leads to increased expression of glucose transporters such as Glut1 and enhances the proximal steps in glycolysis by increasing hexokinase and phosphofructokinase activity (Fig. 8.4). Point mutations that result in growth-factor independent activation of PI3K are found in many human cancers, including a significant percentage of breast, ovarian, and colon cancers.[60] Loss of phosphatases that degrade the phosphatidylinositol species, leading to activation of signaling downstream of PI3K, are also common events in human cancer. Loss of the phosphatidylinositol-3,4,5-triphosphate-3-phosphatase PTEN is frequently observed in human cancer, including a sizable fraction of prostate cancer, breast cancer, glioblastoma, and melanoma.[60] Similarly, loss of INPP4B, a phosphatidylinsolitol-3,4-bisphosphate-4-phosphatase, is seen in breast and ovarian cancers.[61]

In addition to regulating glucose uptake and capture through activation of AKT, PI3K activation also leads to increased expression of enzymes in glucose metabolism via increased production of HIF-1α.[62] Activation of the mTOR kinase, an event downstream of PI3K signaling, induces expression of HIF-1α target genes at least in part through increased translation.[63–65] This activation of glucose metabolism results in the propensity for tumors with PI3K activation to be FDG-avid on PET scan. Small molecules that disrupt PI3K signaling lead to decreased glucose uptake by the tumors as measured by FDG-PET, and the ability to inhibit tumor FDG uptake correlates with tumor regression in PI3K-driven animal models of cancer.[66]

Increased glucose uptake and metabolism are also characteristic features of tumors with activated RAS signaling. RAS activation is frequently observed across human cancers. Glucose deprivation has been shown to drive the emergence of cells harboring an activating mutation in the *KRAS* gene.[67] This has led to the hypothesis that increased glucose uptake via Glut1 expression is a major downstream mediator of RAS signaling that contributes to tumorigenesis. In addition to increasing glucose transporter expression, RAS activation leads to increased phosphofructokinase activity and stimulates the proximal metabolism of glucose (Fig. 8.4).[14] Though less well studied, activating mutations in B-Raf, a kinase downstream of RAS, also result in increased nutrient uptake.[67] Mutations in receptor tyrosine kinases cause increased signaling through both the RAS and PI3K signaling pathways and also cause increased nutrient uptake.

Increased MYC expression is another frequent event in human cancer. MYC is a transcription factor, and many of the transcriptional targets of MYC include metabolic genes.[50] MYC regulates the transcription of enzymes involved in glucose uptake and metabolism, including LDH, the enzyme responsible for production of lactate. MYC-dependent tumors are sensitive to LDH inhibition.[68] MYC also directly and indirectly regulates the uptake of glutamine,[30,69] and MYC-dependent cancer cells are particularly sensitive to glutamine withdrawal.[70] Genetic alterations that lead to activation of MYC, PI3K, RAS, Raf, and receptor tyrosine kinases are among the best-understood driver events in human cancers. These seemingly disparate genetic alterations that promote cancer and occur across cancer types all lead to a converging metabolic phenotype characterized by enhanced cell autonomous nutrient uptake (Fig. 8.8).

Tumor Suppressor Gene Products Also Influence Cellular Metabolism

Many tumor suppressor gene products also regulate metabolism (Fig. 8.8). Loss of p53 function is among the most frequent genetic events in human cancer, and p53 expression influences metabolism (Fig. 8.4).[71] *TIGAR*, a gene induced by p53 expression, redirects glucose flux from glycolysis to the pentose phosphate pathway and promotes apoptosis.[72] Phosphoglycerate mutase, a glycolytic enzyme negatively regulated by p53, inhibits cell senescence.[73] Excess production of reactive oxygen species also promotes cellular senescence and apoptosis, and many of the genes induced by p53 are involved in adaptation to oxidative stress and regulation of mitochondrial metabolism.[74,75]

The tumor suppressor LKB1 is also involved in the adaptive response to cell stress. LKB1 is a kinase that is required for activation of adenosine monophosphate (AMP)-activated protein kinase (AMPK).[76–78] AMPK responds to cellular energy stress (by sensing a low ATP/AMP ratio) and initiates a signaling cascade that promotes increased ATP production and decreased ATP consumption.[79] AMPK also inactivates the mTOR protein kinase that acts as an important integrator of cell growth signals with nutrient availability to regulate cell growth.[80,81] In addition to AMPK, mTOR is regulated by PI3K signaling through the TSC1/TSC2 complex.[82,83] TSC1 and TSC2 are tumor suppressor genes that indirectly influence metabolism via effects on mTOR signaling.[84] mTOR is also regulated by amino

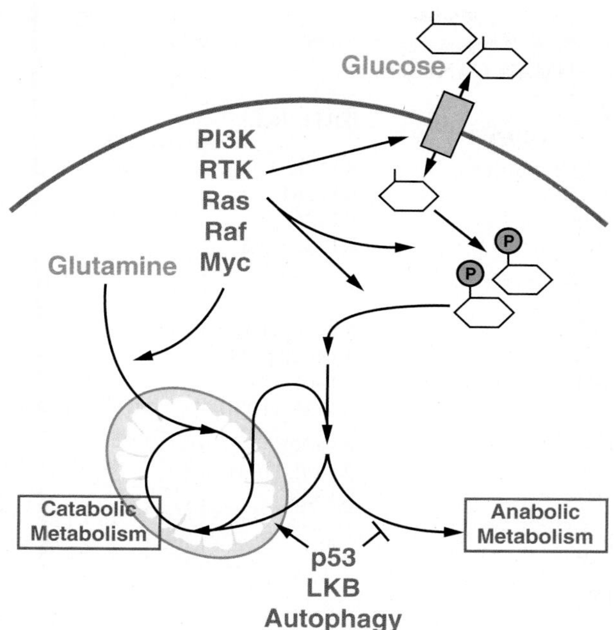

FIGURE 8.8 Many of the oncogenic events thought to drive cancer development influence metabolism by increasing glucose or glutamine uptake. Other genetic events and processes associated with cancer also influence metabolism but do not necessarily cause elevated nutrient uptake. Rather, these events appear to be involved in reprogramming of metabolism away from catabolic metabolism and promote the anabolic pathways necessary for cell growth and proliferation. Both the increase in nutrient uptake and the reprogramming of metabolism to support anabolism are required for cancer cells to proliferate. RTK, receptor tyrosine kinase.

acids such that the mTOR growth promoting activity is turned off under conditions of poor nutrient availability.[85] The response to cell stress also includes the induction of autophagy to catabolize existing cellular material for energy production and removal of damaged organelles.[86,87] Both mTOR signaling and nutrient stress regulate autophagy induction,[88] but the role of autophagy in cancer remains unclear. The use of mTOR inhibitors is gaining increasing use in the clinic to treat various cancers, yet the relationship between mTOR, autophagy, metabolic stress, and cancer is incompletely understood.

Other genetic changes may be important to promote anabolic metabolism in cancer cells. For instance, all cancer cells appear to express the M2 isoform of the glycolytic enzyme pyruvate kinase (PK-M2).[16,89] PK-M2 is normally expressed during embryonic development and is unique among the human pyruvate kinase isoforms in that it is regulated by tyrosine kinase signaling.[15] This regulation of PK-M2 by growth factor signaling promotes aerobic glycolysis in cells[89] and may constitute a molecular switch that allows cancer cells to metabolize glucose in a manner conducive to proliferation only when growth signals are present.

Mutations in Metabolic Enzymes Can Lead to Cancer

Altered cell metabolism can directly contribute to transformation as mutations in metabolic enzymes can promote cancer. Inherited loss of function mutations in genes that encode proteins involved in the proper assembly or function of the mitochondrial succinate dehydrogenase complex account for the subtypes of hereditary paraganglioma.[90–94] Succinate dehydrogenase (SDH) is an enzyme complex in the TCA cycle that catalyzes the oxidation of succinate to fumarate and supplies electrons to the mitochondrial electron transport chain.[11] These mutations lead to decreased activity of SDH and succinate accumulation. The enzymes that carry out the oxygen-dependent hydroxylation of HIF-1α also convert α-ketoglutarate to succinate as part of their catalytic mechanism.[95] Thus, accumulation of succinate leads to a decrease in HIF-1α hydroxylation, less HIF-1α degradation, and increased expression of HIF-1α target genes (Fig. 8.7). Loss-of-function SDH mutations that cause this "pseudohypoxia" account for some cases of renal cell carcinoma expressing normal amounts of VHL, supporting the notion that HIF-1α expression is an important event in some cancers.[93,95] Mutations in the TCA cycle enzyme fumarate hydratase (FH), which further metabolizes the fumarate produced by the succinate dehydrogenase complex, have also been described in renal cell carcinoma, leiomyomas, and other rare cancers.[95–97]

Isocitrate dehydrogenase (IDH) is another metabolic enzyme that is mutated in cancer.[98–100] All reported cases of IDH mutation occur in only one allele, with preservation of wild-type enzyme expression from the other allele (Fig. 8.9).[101] These mutations are frequent events in low-grade gliomas and secondary glioblastomas.[98,99,102] Interestingly, IDH-mutant gliomas appear to have a better prognosis,[98] suggesting that gliomas harboring these mutations represent a distinct subset of glioma with a different response to therapy or natural history. IDH mutations are also found in patients with acute myelogenous leukemia (AML) and myelodysplastic syndrome (MDS) and define a distinct clinical subset of these patients without other cytogenetic abnormalities.[100,103–105] IDH mutations have been proposed to be an early event in the pathogenesis of both AML and glioma.[101,105,106] Sporadic mutations in other cancers have also been reported. A summary of IDH mutations in human cancer is shown in Table 8.1, and the frequency of IDH1 or IDH2 mutations in specific cancer subsets is shown in Table 8.2.

The IDH mutations associated with cancer involve point mutations in the active site of either IDH1 or IDH2.[98–100,105] Other less frequent mutations involving residues in IDH1 have been reported in rare cases,[105,107–109] however, whether these represent driver mutations or polymorphisms remains unclear. IDH1 mutations involve R132, and mutations in the analogous active site residue (R172) are found in IDH2. This arginine (R132 in IDH1, R172 in IDH2) coordinates the CO_2 group that is lost during oxidative decarboxylation of isocitrate to α-ketoglutarate.[110] The other mutated residue in IDH2 (R140) makes contacts with the same CO_2 group in the IDH2 active

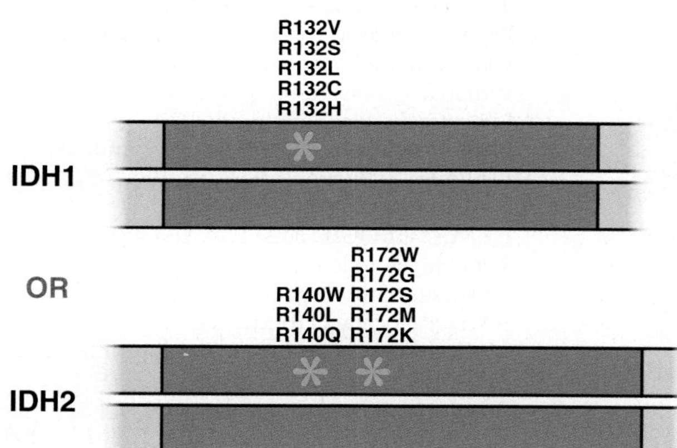

FIGURE 8.9 Mutations in isocitrate dehydrogenase-1 or -2 (IDH1 or IDH2) reported in human cancer are all monoallelic and involve a single residue in IDH1 or one of two residues in IDH2. (Figure adapted from Lenny Dang and Shengfang Jin, Agios Pharmaceuticals.)

TABLE 8.1

MUTATIONS IN IDH1 AND IDH2 REPORTED IN HUMAN CANCERS

Cancer Type	IDH1 (Ref.)	IDH2 (Ref.)
Glioma	R132H (98,102,150–153) R132C (98,154,155) R132S (98,99) R132G (99) R132L R132V (102)	R172K R172M (99) R172G R172S (155)
Acute myeloid leukemia (AML)	R132H (103) R132G (105) R132C (107)	R140Q (103,105) R140W (105) R140L R172K (107)
Myelodysplastic syndrome (MDS)	R132H (156) R132C R132L (104) R132G	R140Q) R140L (104) R172K
Acute lymphoblastic leukemia (ALL)	R132C (153)	
Prostate cancer	R132H (153) R132C	
Colorectal cancer	R132C (98)	
Paragangliomas	R132C (157)	
Thyroid cancer	R132H (109)	

Table provided by Lenny Dang and Shengfang Jin, Agios Pharmaceuticals. IDH, isocitrate dehydrogenase.

TABLE 8.2

FREQUENCY OF IDH1 AND IDH2 REPORTED IN HUMAN CANCERS

Tumor Classification	IDH1 Mutated (%)	IDH2 Mutated (%)
GLIOMA		
Secondary glioblastoma (grade IV)	73–88	—
Diffuse astrocytoma (grade II)	59–88	0.9
Oligodendroglioma (grade II)	68–82	2.3
Oligoastrocytoma (grade II)	50–94	1.3
Anaplastic astrocytoma (grade III)	52–78	0.9
Anaplastic oligodendroglioma (grade III)	60–86	3.4
Anaplastic oligoastrocytoma (grade III)	43–78	3.4
Primary glioblastoma (grade IV)	3–16	—
Primitive neuroectodermal tumor (grade IV)	6–33	—
Giant cell glioblastoma (grade IV)	*	—
Pediatric glioblastoma (grade IV)	*	—
Pilocytic astrocytoma (grade I)	*	—
Pleomorphic xanthoastrocytoma (grade II)	—	*
Compiled from references: (98, 99, 102, 106, 150, 153, 155, 158–161)		
HEMATOLOGIC MALIGNANCIES		
Acute myeloid leukemia (AML), all	4.4–9.1	15.4
AML, normal cytogenetics	7.1–16.2	19.3–19.4
AML, abnormal cytogenetics	0–5.4	—
Myelodysplastic syndrome/myeloproliferative neoplasm	1.1	5.8
B-acute lymphoblastic leukemia	2.0	—
Compiled from references: (100, 104, 105, 107, 108, 162–164)		

*,Less than 50 cases reported, too few to determine percentage mutated.
IDH, isocitrate dehydrogenase; — indicates no reported cases.
Table provided by Patrick S. Ward and Craig B. Thompson, University of Pennsylvania.

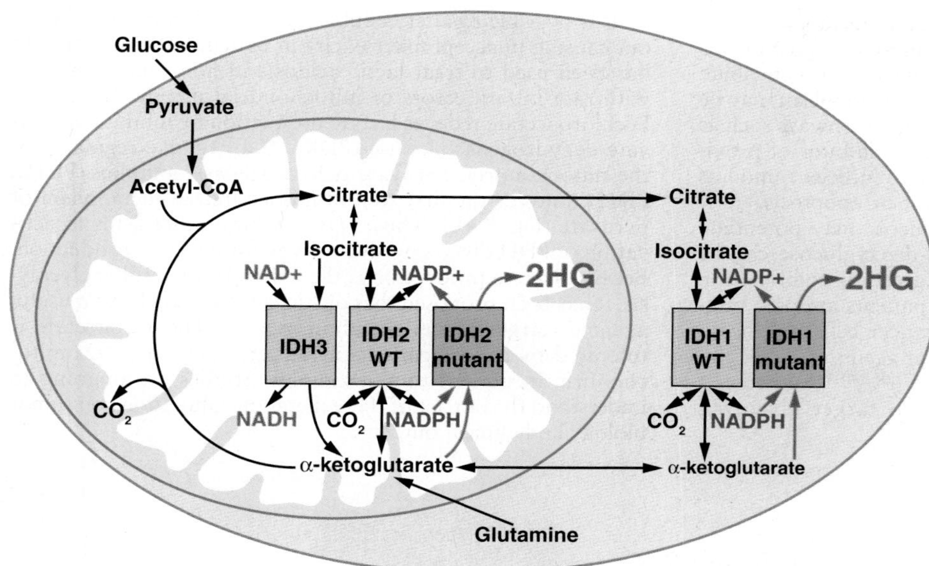

FIGURE 8.10 Human cancer associated mutations in isocitrate dehydrogenase-1 or -2 (IDH1 or IDH2) results in the neomorphic production of the metabolite 2-hydroxyglutarate (2HG). Because a wild-type version of both IDH1 and IDH2 remain even in IDH mutant cells, the normal activities of these enzymes persist despite the activity of the mutant enzyme to produce 2HG. The subcellular localization and enzymatic activities for all of the IDH isoforms is shown. (Figure courtesy of Patrick S. Ward and Craig B. Thompson, University of Pennsylvania.)

site.[105] All three mutations result in an alteration of enzyme activity that decreases the enzyme's ability to oxidatively decarboxylate isocitrate to α-ketoglutarate, but increases enzyme activity to reduce α-ketoglutarate. In the mutant enzymes, this reduction does not lead to incorporation of CO_2 to make isocitrate, but instead produces 2-hydroxyglutarate (2HG).[105,107,110] Because IDH mutations are monoallelic and the neomorphic activity acquired by the mutant enzyme is slow relative to the normal wild-type enzyme in these cells, the normal interconversion of isocitrate and α-ketoglutarate is not dramatically altered, and the main consequence of these mutations is 2HG production (Fig. 8.10).[105,107,110] The 2HG is produced in low levels in normal cells as an error product of various TCA cycle enzymes; however, in IDH mutant tumors 2HG accumulates to very high levels and has been linked with the pathogenesis of the disease.[110] Accumulation of 2HG has been demonstrated in rare patients with hereditary loss of the enzyme that degrades 2HG,[111] and gliomas have been described in a subset of these patients.[112] Mutations in IDH1 have been reported to result in HIF-1α accumulation,[113] however, the relationship among IDH mutation, 2HG accumulation, and HIF-1α accumulation remains unclear.

Recurrent mutations in yet another metabolic enzyme have recently been reported in colon cancer.[114] These are inactivating mutations of an enzyme involved in glucosamine metabolism, and signaling involving glucosamine-based protein modifications has been suggested to be important in cancer.[115] The exact mechanism by which the shunt from glucose to glucosamine impacts cellular metabolism and cancer remains to be determined.

TARGETING METABOLISM TO TREAT CANCER

The mechanisms by which cancer metabolism is regulated and how this regulation is impacted by genetic alterations known to be critical for cancer survival suggest cellular metabolic dependencies that could be exploited for cancer treatment. In fact, one of the first successful chemotherapies targeted folate metabolism. The observation that folate could enhance blood cell proliferation ultimately lead to the development of antifolates as chemotherapeutics.[116] Other active chemotherapeutics target purine metabolism. Although these agents are now thought of as "cytotoxic," they target metabolic dependencies of tumor cells and continue to play an important role in modern cancer therapy.

New therapies are being explored that directly or indirectly target cancer metabolism. A large fraction of human cancer is dependent on aberrant signaling through the PI3K/AKT pathway, and agents that target this pathway are being actively tested in the clinic.[117] The growing evidence that cancer cells depend on elevated glucose metabolism suggests that targeting key metabolic control points important for aerobic glycolysis might also be effective cancer therapies. Recent evidence suggests that drugs developed to treat metabolic diseases such as diabetes may provide a benefit to patients with cancer. A number of retrospective clinical studies have found a benefit to the widely used diabetic drug metformin (Glucophage) both in the primary prevention of cancer as well as improved outcomes when used with other cancer therapies.[118–120] The exact mechanism by which metformin lowers blood glucose levels is not completely understood; however, metformin decreases gluconeogenesis in the liver. Recently, metformin was discovered to be an activator of AMPK, and this effect was shown to be critical for inhibiting gluconeogenesis in the liver.[121] In addition, metformin has been shown to inhibit mitochondrial complex I and impair oxidative phosphorylation in cells.[122,123] Inhibition of oxidative phosphorylation and the subsequent decrease in energy charge (ATP:AMP ratio) is likely how metformin activates AMP kinase.

Recently, two separate clinical studies have shown a reduction in cancer-related mortality with metformin use.[118,119] This effect appears to be independent of blood glucose level as patients with similar glucose levels treated with insulin do not derive the same benefit as patients taking metformin. Another study reported that diabetic patients on metformin had a higher pathological complete response to neoadjuvant therapy for breast cancer than diabetic patients receiving other glucose lowering therapies.[120] Studies exploring metformin use for cancer therapy in numerous preclinical cancer models have suggested that these compounds may be selectively toxic to cancer cells with specific genetic backgrounds,[123–125] however, these compounds may also influence cancer therapy via their systemic effects on glucose metabolism. Increased insulin-like growth factor-1 (IGF1) levels, which accompany poor glucose control, may promote cancer growth.[126,127] Particularly in tumors with mutations that lead to activation of the PI3K pathway,[128] at least one effect of metformin may be to decrease the effect of IGF1 on cell growth.[129]

The success of FDG-PET scans as a diagnostic and predictive tool for treatment response in many cancers has lead some to suggest that targeting enzymes involved in metabolism may be an effective therapy.[130] Specific therapies may be possible for patients with mutations in metabolic enzymes that contribute directly to tumorigenesis.[130,131] In addition, metabolism may be sufficiently different in some cancers to target pathways such as glycolysis. 2-deoxyglucose is a competitive inhibitor of proximal glucose metabolism.[38,39] Cells exposed to sufficient amounts of 2-deoxyglucose undergo growth arrest or apoptosis,[132–134] and preclinical models show 2-deoxyglucose may potentiate standard cytotoxic chemotherapy.[135] 2-deoxyglucose can be administered to patients,[136] but when given in combination with radiation therapy to glioblastoma patients at doses sufficient to limit glucose metabolism in cancer cells significant toxicity is observed.[137–139] However, other agents to block glucose metabolism are being investigated. [67,130,140–146] Whether a sufficient therapeutic window exists to target glycolysis directly remains to be determined.

It is possible to alter cellular metabolism in a tumor without causing unacceptable toxicity in patients. Dichloroacetate has been used to treat lactic acidosis in non-cancer patients with rare inborn errors of mitochondrial metabolism. [147,148] Dichloroacetate reduces lactate production by inhibiting pyruvate dehydrogenase kinase (PDK),[149] a negative regulator of the mitochondrial pyruvate dehydrogenase complex (PDH). PDH catalyzes the first step in mitochondrial metabolism of pyruvate (Fig. 8.4).[11] Thus, PDK inhibition that leads to activation of PDH diverts pyruvate away from lactate production. Because lactate production is the hallmark of aerobic glycolysis, it has been proposed that dichloroacetate might be a useful agent to target cancer metabolism.[148,149] Dichloroacetate is tolerated by cancer patients at dosages that can alter mitochondria in patient tumor samples. Studies are ongoing to understand the impact of these metabolic alterations on tumor biology and clinical outcome.

Selected References

The full list of references for this chapter appears in the online version.

1. Vander Heiden MG, Cantley LC, Thompson CB. Understanding the Warburg effect: the metabolic requirements of cell proliferation. *Science* 2009;324:1029.
2. Warburg O. On the origin of cancer cells. *Science* 1956;123:309.
3. Gatenby RA, Gillies RJ. Why do cancers have high aerobic glycolysis? *Nat Rev Cancer* 2004;4:891.
4. Deberardinis RJ, Lum JJ, Hatzivassiliou G, et al. The biology of cancer: metabolic reprogramming fuels cell growth and proliferation. *Cell Metab* 2008;7:11.
5. Hsu PP, Sabatini DM. Cancer cell metabolism: Warburg and beyond. *Cell* 2008;134:703.
7. Warburg O, Posener K, Negelein E. Ueber den Stoffwechsel der Tumoren. *Biochemische Zeitschrift* 1924;152:319.
12. Mathupala SP, Ko YH, Pedersen PL. The pivotal roles of mitochondria in cancer: Warburg and beyond and encouraging prospects for effective therapies. *Biochim Biophys Acta* 2010;1797:1225.
17. Weinhouse S. The Warburg hypothesis fifty years later. *Z Krebsforsch Klin Onkol Cancer Res Clin Oncol* 1976;87:115.
19. Folkman J. Angiogenesis. *Annu Rev Med* 2006;57:1.
20. Bertout JA, Patel SA, Simon MC. The impact of O_2 availability on human cancer. *Nat Rev Cancer* 2008;8:967.
21. Semenza GL. Regulation of cancer cell metabolism by hypoxia-inducible factor 1. *Semin Cancer Biol* 2009;19:12.
24. Racker E. Why do tumor cells have a high aerobic glycolysis? *J Cell Physiol* 1976;89:697.
25. Sonveaux P, Vegran F, Schroeder T, et al. Targeting lactate-fueled respiration selectively kills hypoxic tumor cells in mice. *J Clin Invest* 2008;118:3930.
27. Guppy M, Leedman P, Zu X, et al. Contribution by different fuels and metabolic pathways to the total ATP turnover of proliferating MCF-7 breast cancer cells. *Biochem J* 2002;364:309.
29. DeBerardinis RJ, Mancuso A, Daikhin E, et al. Beyond aerobic glycolysis: transformed cells can engage in glutamine metabolism that exceeds the requirement for protein and nucleotide synthesis. *Proc Natl Acad Sci U S A* 2007;104:19345.
32. Hatzivassiliou G, Zhao F, Bauer DE, et al. ATP citrate lyase inhibition can suppress tumor cell growth. *Cancer Cell* 2005;8:311.
35. Lockart RZ Jr, Eagle H. Requirements for growth of single human cells. *Science* 1959;129:252.
37. Tisdale MJ. Mechanisms of cancer cachexia. *Physiol Rev* 2009;89:381.
40. Hawkins RA, Phelps ME. PET in clinical oncology. *Cancer Metastasis Rev* 1988;7:119.
41. Ben-Haim S, Ell P. 18F-FDG PET and PET/CT in the evaluation of cancer treatment response. *J Nucl Med* 2009;50:88.
46. Kaelin WG Jr. The von Hippel-Lindau tumour suppressor protein: O_2 sensing and cancer. *Nat Rev Cancer* 2008;8:865.
47. Kaelin WG Jr, Ratcliffe PJ. Oxygen sensing by metazoans: the central role of the HIF hydroxylase pathway. *Mol Cell* 2008;30:393.
48. Rankin EB, Giaccia AJ. The role of hypoxia-inducible factors in tumorigenesis. *Cell Death Differ* 2008;15:678.
49. Majumder PK, Febbo PG, Bikoff R, et al. mTOR inhibition reverses Akt-dependent prostate intraepithelial neoplasia through regulation of apoptotic and HIF-1-dependent pathways. *Nat Med* 2004;10:594.
50. Dang CV, Kim JW, Gao P, et al. The interplay between MYC and HIF in cancer. *Nat Rev Cancer* 2008;8:51.
57. Flier JS, Mueckler MM, Usher P, et al. Elevated levels of glucose transport and transporter messenger RNA are induced by ras or src oncogenes. *Science* 1987;235:1492.
58. Birnbaum MJ, Haspel HC, Rosen OM. Transformation of rat fibroblasts by FSV rapidly increases glucose transporter gene transcription. *Science* 1987;235:1495.
60. Engelman JA, Luo J, Cantley LC. The evolution of phosphatidylinositol 3-kinases as regulators of growth and metabolism. *Nat Rev Genet* 2006;7:606.
71. Cheung EC, Vousden KH. The role of p53 in glucose metabolism. *Curr Opin Cell Biol* 2010;22:186.
75. Matoba S, Kang JG, Patino WD, et al. p53 regulates mitochondrial respiration. *Science* 2006;312:1650.
79. Hardie DG. AMP-activated/SNF1 protein kinases: conserved guardians of cellular energy. *Nat Rev Mol Cell Biol* 2007;8:774.
82. Tee AR, Blenis J. mTOR, translational control and human disease. *Semin Cell Dev Biol* 2005;16:29.
83. Dann SG, Thomas G. The amino acid sensitive TOR pathway from yeast to mammals. *FEBS Lett* 2006;580:2821.
85. Shaw RJ, Cantley LC. Ras, PI(3)K and mTOR signalling controls tumour cell growth. *Nature* 2006;441:424.
86. Kundu M, Thompson CB. Autophagy: basic principles and relevance to disease. *Annu Rev Pathol* 2008;3:427.
87. Jin S, White E. Tumor suppression by autophagy through the management of metabolic stress. *Autophagy* 2008;4:563.
88. Wang RC, Levine B. Autophagy in cellular growth control. *FEBS Lett* 2010;584:1417.
90. Baysal BE, Ferrell RE, Willett-Brozick JE, et al. Mutations in SDHD, a mitochondrial complex II gene, in hereditary paraganglioma. *Science* 2000;287:848.
95. King A, Selak MA, Gottlieb E. Succinate dehydrogenase and fumarate hydratase: linking mitochondrial dysfunction and cancer. *Oncogene* 2006;25:4675.
98. Parsons DW, Jones S, Zhang X, et al. An integrated genomic analysis of human glioblastoma multiforme. *Science* 2008;321:1807.
100. Mardis ER, Ding L, Dooling DJ, et al. Recurring mutations found by sequencing an acute myeloid leukemia genome. *N Engl J Med* 2009;361:1058.
101. Thompson CB. Metabolic enzymes as oncogenes or tumor suppressors. *N Engl J Med* 2009;360:813.
110. Dang L, White DW, Gross S, et al. Cancer-associated IDH1 mutations produce 2-hydroxyglutarate. *Nature* 2009;462:739.
116. Farber S, Diamond LK. Temporary remissions in acute leukemia in children produced by folic acid antagonist, 4-aminopteroyl-glutamic acid. *N Engl J Med* 1948;238:787.
118. Evans JM, Donnelly LA, Emslie-Smith AM, et al. Metformin and reduced risk of cancer in diabetic patients. *BMJ* 2005;330:1304.
127. Pollak M. Insulin and insulin-like growth factor signalling in neoplasia. *Nat Rev Cancer* 2008;8:915.
128. Kalaany NY, Sabatini DM. Tumours with PI3K activation are resistant to dietary restriction. *Nature* 2009;458:725.
132. Laszlo J, Humphreys SR, Goldin A. Effects of glucose analogues (2-deoxy-D-glucose, 2-deoxy-D-galactose) on experimental tumors. *J Natl Cancer Inst* 1960;24:267.
141. Kroemer G, Pouyssegur J. Tumor cell metabolism: cancer's Achilles' heel. *Cancer Cell* 2008;13:472.
148. Michelakis ED, Sutendra G, Dromparis P, et al. Metabolic modulation of glioblastoma with dichloroacetate. *Sci Transl Med* 2010;2:31.

CHAPTER 9 ANGIOGENESIS

ROBERT S. KERBEL AND LEE M. ELLIS

INTRODUCTION: ORIGINS OF THE CONCEPT OF ANTIANGIOGENIC THERAPY FOR CANCER

Among the most significant advances in medical oncology over the last 6 years is the U.S. Food and Drug Administration (FDA) approval of several antiangiogenic drugs for the systemic treatment of a variety of metastatic malignancies. Prior to the first successful randomized phase 3 clinical trial involving an antiangiogenic agent[1] (bevacizumab, the humanized monoclonal antibody to vascular endothelial growth factor [VEGF]), enthusiasm in the field had waned by a combination of high expectations but little success in several pivotal phase 3 clinical trials. However, the initial success of bevacizumab, in combination with chemotherapy in the first-line treatment of metastatic colorectal cancer, initiated a resurgence in the field, in both the laboratory and the clinic, that has led to variable degrees of improvement in the therapy for advanced breast cancer, renal cell carcinoma (RCC), colorectal cancer, non–small cell lung cancer, glioblastoma, hepatocellular carcinoma, and ovarian cancer. However, despite these successes, clinical trials evaluating the use of these agents in some other malignancies has not yet led to similar success, and even where there is success, the clinical benefits are modest, as most notably in the case for breast cancer. Thus, it is essential to continue investigating basic mechanisms and mediators of angiogenesis with the aim of advancing the care of patients with malignant disease.

The era of antiangiogenic drug development began with the publication in 1971 of a landmark hypothesis article in the *New England Journal of Medicine* by M. Judah Folkman.[2] He hypothesized that inhibition of blood vessel growth within a tumor could prolong tumor dormancy and improve survival of patients with minimal toxicity. Following publication of his hypothesis, Folkman and colleagues reported a significant number of discoveries that were instrumental in advancing the field, including defining the nature of the angiogenic "switch" in tumors, raising awareness of the presence of both pro- and antiangiogenic factors that mediate both pathologic and physiologic processes.[3]

Although the hypothesis of the essential role of angiogenesis in tumor growth, and the proposed therapeutic benefit of antiangiogenic drugs for cancer treatment, have been partially validated, there have been many surprising twists and turns in the field over the ensuing decades necessitating some interesting modifications of the basic therapeutic concept.[4] These will be discussed in more detail later and include the following: (1) certain antiangiogenic drugs such as bevacizumab seem to have little or no clinical benefit when used as monotherapies to treat advanced disease of certain malignancies such as colorectal cancer, whereas they show clinical benefit only when used in combination treatments with other agents, particularly (thus far) chemotherapy[4–6]; (2) in addition to stimulators of angiogenesis, there are also a number of endogenous angiogenesis inhibitors, the expression of which may be down-regulated during tumor development, permitting a more robust angiogenic response[3]; (3) angiogenesis can also contribute to the growth of "liquid" hematologic malignancies, not just solid tumors[3,5,7]; (4) endothelial cells in developing blood vessels may be derived by incorporation and differentiation of systemically mobilized cells from the bone marrow, that is, circulating endothelial progenitor or precursor cells (CEPs) (Fig. 9.1.), not just by local division of pre-existing endothelial cells in resident vessels ("sprouting angiogenesis")[8,9]; and (5) there is not a single "TAF" but a large and diverse array of molecular mediators of angiogenesis.

SEQUENTIAL STEPS INVOLVED IN THE FORMATION OF BLOOD VESSEL CAPILLARIES IN TUMORS

There are a number of sequential and fairly well-defined steps involved in the development for new capillary blood vessels, and their subsequent formation into a functional network. The first step in the formation of a capillary sprout ("sprouting angiogenesis") from a pre-existing mature blood vessel is the localized degradation of the surrounding basement membrane of the parental postcapillary venule. This creates a break to allow the movement of differentiated endothelial cells toward the adjacent tumor cells and the stimuli produced by such cells. Localized degradation is likely the consequence of the ability of various proangiogenic growth factors secreted by the tumor cell population or reactive stromal cells to induce synthesis and export of a number of proteolytic enzymes such as matrix metalloproteinases, cathepsins, and urokinase plasminogen activator.

The next step involves the directed locomotion/migration of endothelial cells from the parental venule toward the angiogenic stimulus emanating from the tumor mass. This is followed by division of endothelial cells that, in concert with migration, lengthen the "stalk" of the endothelial cell sprout. Subsequently, lumen formation takes place with completion of capillary sprouts and loops, and the envelopment of nascent capillaries with new basement membrane structures along with recruitment of perivascular support cells, especially pericytes. Critical in this process are specialized endothelial cells at the ends of growing capillaries called *tip* cells, which fuse with other tip cells to create a fused (linked) network of new capillaries.[10] This sequence of events is thought to be quite similar to the formation of new blood vessel capillaries that occurs in developing embryos; however, the structure/morphology and function of

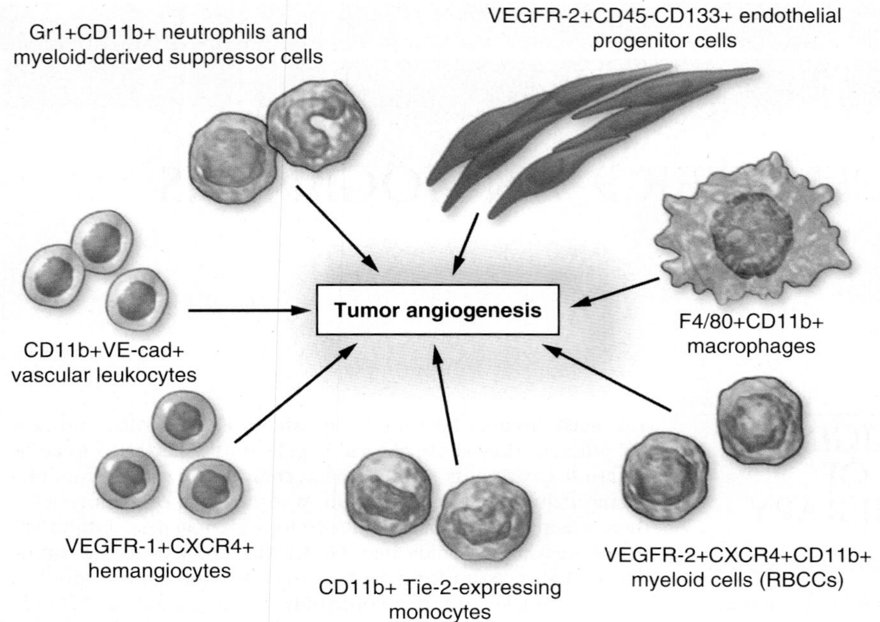

FIGURE 9.1 Circulating bone marrow–derived cell populations that stimulate or amplify tumor angiogenesis. The various hematopoietic (CD45-positive) cell types appear to have a perivascular location with respect to the tumor neovasculature, whereas the CD45-negative endothelial progenitor cells can become incorporated into the lumen of a growing blood vessel and differentiate into mature endothelial cells. In recent preclinical studies, neutrophils have also been shown to contribute to the induction of tumor angiogenesis. F4/80 is a pan macrophage cell-surface marker. CXCR4, CXC chemokine receptor 4; RBCCs, recruited bone marrow–derived circulating cells; VE-cad, vascular endothelial-cell cadherin (an adhesion molecule); VEGFR, vascular endothelial growth factor receptor. (From ref. 4, with permission.)

many tumor-associated blood vessels can be highly irregular, heterogeneous, and functionally abnormal.[6]

Although this abbreviated description of sprouting angiogenesis is the most common view of angiogenesis, over the past 5 to 10 years, modifications or alternative views of angiogenesis have emerged. The mechanisms of angiogenesis may be organ- and/or tumor-specific. For example, in vascular-rich organs such as the brain, co-option may play an important role in providing a nutrient blood supply to the growing tumor.[11] It has been hypothesized that parts of the vessel wall in tumors such as ocular melanoma or glioblastoma may be composed or melanoma cells, either in part (mosaic vessels)[12] or full[13] ("vascular mimicry"). Also noteworthy are the large number and diversity of molecular changes detected in endothelial cells in tumor blood vessels during angiogenesis, many of which suggest possible new targets for development of antiangiogenic drugs.[14,15] Some of these molecular changes might be related to the recently reported genetic and cytogenetic abnormalities detected in endothelial cells isolated from the tumor vasculature[16] or by endothelial cell uptake of tumor cell–derived membrane vesicles.[17]

PERICYTES

Pericytes (our definition of pericytes is a single layer of periendothelial smooth muscle cells) modulate endothelial cell function, and are critical for the development of a mature vascular network. Pericytes regulate vascular function, including vessel diameter (and thus blood flow) and vascular permeability.[18] Pericytes also provide mechanical support and stability to the vessel wall and maintain endothelial cell survival through direct cell-cell contact and paracrine circuits.[18,19]

The role of pericytes within the tumor vasculature is currently an intense area of study. The degree of pericyte coverage of endothelial cells in human tumors is controversial and discrepancies among studies may be because a single marker is not sufficient to examine pericyte presence and morphology. Markers such as alpha-smooth muscle actin, desmin, NG2, and RGS5 are commonly used, and confocal imaging is necessary to observe the true relationship of pericytes to endothelial cells.

Because of the role of pericytes in mediating endothelial cell survival,[19] these cells have emerged as an important therapeutic target for antiangiogenic therapy. Studies of antiangiogenic agents targeting endothelial cell survival have demonstrated that such drugs result in increased apoptosis in endothelial cells that are *not* associated with pericytes, leading to a relative increase in the proportion of vessels with pericyte coverage.[20] These data have led to the hypothesis that pericytes mediate resistance to antiangiogenic therapy. If this hypothesis is correct, targeting both endothelial cells and pericytes will increase the efficacy of antiangiogenic therapy, and there is some evidence in support of this hypothesis in preclinical studies.[21,22] However, there is currently some growing doubt about the clinical impact of targeting pericytes using drugs such as multitargeting tyrosine kinase inhibitors (TKIs), for example, sunitinib, sorafenib, and pazopanib, which target platelet-derived growth factor (PDGF) receptors (which are expressed by pericytes) in addition to vascular endothelial growth factor receptors (VEGFRs). Thus, the therapeutic impact of such drugs does not appear to be significantly greater compared with specific anti-VEGF antibodies with the exception, currently, of hepatocellular carcinoma. Moreover, there is some limited preclinical evidence that inhibition of pericyte function and attachment to endothelial cells may actually facilitate metastasis by allowing tumor cell intravasation and extravasation.[23] Still others have shown that inhibition of pericyte stimulatory factors may actually increase tumor growth, as pericytes may induce endothelial cell quiescence. Pericyte biology remains an important area of research that needs to be investigated more thoroughly.

DYSFUNCTIONAL NATURE OF THE TUMOR VASCULATURE

Although tumors possess the means to recruit and develop a new vascular network, this is not to suggest, as already mentioned, that such blood vessels are normal in either structure or function. Indeed, the characteristics of the vasculature in solid tumors are associated with a number of prominent abnormalities, the consequences of which have been hypothesized to have a significant impact on tumor growth, progression, and response to various anticancer therapies. For example, the structural and morphologic abnormalities include excessively dilated blood vessels, other vessels with areas containing absent or abnormal basement membranes, or having extreme corkscrewlike tortuosities, a relative lack of supporting perivascular cellular elements such as pericytes, or abnormalities in the pericyte population, and excessive vascular leakiness.[24,25] These abnormalities can be quite variable within a solid tumor mass, and such heterogeneity can also extend to the relative density of blood vessels, which can be quite high in certain areas, and low in others.

As a result of all of these features, blood flow and perfusion within tumors can be highly heterogeneous and often sluggish, with some areas therefore being deprived of oxygen and nutrients leading to adjacent areas of elevated hypoxia. This may account for slow growth of tumors in some regions and more rapid growth in others. In addition, the marked leakiness/hyperpermeability of the tumor vasculature can lead to a marked extravasation of high-molecular-weight plasma proteins and fluid into the extracellular microenvironment within tumors, which can lead to elevated interstitial fluid pressures.[24] It has been hypothesized that this can limit or retard the diffusion of anticancer drugs, especially antibodies or gene therapy vectors, and immune effector cells from the blood through the interstitium of the tumors.[24] Thus, given their nature, tumor blood vessels, while necessary for progressive tumor growth and hematogenous metastasis, may also actually limit the efficacy of a broad and diverse array of anticancer drugs and treatments, including chemotherapy, and oxygen required for optimal efficacy of radiation therapy.[24]

MOLECULAR MEDIATORS OF TUMOR ANGIOGENESIS: ANGIOGENIC STIMULATORS AND THEIR RECEPTORS

Several diverse families of growth factors (angiogenic factors) are now known to stimulate/mediate tumor angiogenesis. Some, like VEGF,[26] are primary, direct-acting factors that bind to cognate receptors that are primarily expressed on endothelial cells, especially when they are "activated." Other factors are likely secondary in nature, that is, indirect acting. In other words, they stimulate expression of one or more of the primary proangiogenic growth factors or recruit cells to sites of angiogenesis that amplify the angiogenic process. Included in this group are such molecules as transforming growth factor beta (TGF-β), TGF-α, hepatocyte growth factor, inflammatory cytokines such as interleukin-6 and interleukin-8, cytokines such as granulocyte-colony stimulating factor, chemokines such as stromal-derived factor-1, and sex hormones such as estrogens and androgens.[4] PDGFs have also been implicated as mediators of angiogenesis, for the most part through their effects on PDGF receptor-expressing pericytes, as previously mentioned. However, it is the primary, direct-acting factors, foremost among them VEGF,[26] that are considered to be the principal driving forces in stimulating both physiologic and pathologic angiogenesis, including tumor angiogenesis, in most cases.

Direct-acting, primary proangiogenic growth factors include the VEGF family and their cognate receptor tyrosine kinases,[26] the angiopoietins, especially angiopoietin-1 and -2 (ang-1/ang-2), and their cognate tyrosine kinase receptors, in particular tie-2 (see later discussion), and the Notch signaling receptor (specifically Notch 4) and its family of ligands, such as Deltalike ligand 4 (DLL4) and Jaggeds (see later discussion). All three systems have in common a high (but not absolute) degree of specificity for endothelial cells, and in particular activated endothelial cells associated with neovascularization. Another receptor tyrosine kinase-ligand system involved in angiogenesis is Eph receptor ephrin-B2.[27] Ephrin-B2 is a transmembrane ligand that is involved in "bidirectional signaling" whereby Eph receptors help regulate endothelial tip cell guidance in the sprouting and branching of new blood vessel capillaries. Ephrin-B2 mediates its effects, at least in part, by regulating VEGFR-2 function.[27]

Discovery of the VEGF family and their receptors (Fig. 9.2) represented a profound turning point in the field of tumor angiogenesis research and the development of antiangiogenic drugs.[26] Prior to the first published reports of VEGF, which was initially called vascular permeability factor,[28] basic fibroblast growth factor (bFG)F was considered to be the central mediator of angiogenesis, and was the first molecular mediator of angiogenesis to be identified.[3] However, bFGF lacks a signal sequence for cellular secretion, and therapeutic blockade of bFGF using antibodies did not cause consistent antitumor results, observations that raised doubts about a predominant role for bFGF in tumor angiogenesis.

VEGF was discovered in 1989 and reported to be a highly specific and potent mitogen for vascular endothelial cells.[26,29] When the genes for vascular permeability factor and VEGF were sequenced, it was realized they were the same molecule.[26] The vascular permeability function of VEGF is extremely potent (50,000-fold that of histamine) and probably accounts for much of the leakiness of the tumor vasculature. It is possible that enhanced permeability may be due to intercellular gaps between endothelial cells, decreased pericyte coverage (as a second barrier to permeability), and/or specialized endothelial cell organelles called *vesiculovacuolar organelles*,[30] transmembrane vacuoles that can form channels leading to extravasation of fluid and proteins. VEGF (VEGF-A) is the prototypical member of a family of ligands with ~40–80% homology: VEGF-A (also called simply VEGF), VEGF-B, VEGF-C, VEGF-D, and placental growth factor (PlGF) (Fig. 9.2). VEGF-A (hereafter called VEGF) actually exists in a number of variant isoforms based on RNA splicing. In humans, the most common splice variants are $VEGF_{121}$, $VEGF_{165}$, $VEGF_{189}$, and $VEGF_{206}$ (whereby the number denotes the number of amino acids in the mature protein). $VEGF_{121}$, the shortest isoform, is freely circulating, whereas $VEGF_{189}$ and $VEGF_{206}$ are strongly bound to heparin sulphate containing glycoproteins and thus remain cell-bound or sequestered in the extracellular matrix where they remain biologically inactive until mobilized by specific proteases. $VEGF_{165}$ has a heparin-binding sequence but can also freely circulate. Thus, $VEGF_{121}$ and $VEGF_{165}$ are generally considered to be the main VEGF family members that drive tumor angiogenesis. $VEGF_{121}$ and $VEGF_{165}$ bind to two tyrosine kinase receptors expressed by endothelial cells. These are known as VEGFR-1 (flt-1) and VEGFR-2 or KDR in humans (kinase insert domain receptor; with flk-1 being the KDR homolog in mice).[26] The major signaling receptor is VEGFR-2. In contrast, VEGFR-1 signals only weakly, after VEGF binding, despite the fact that it can bind VEGF with tenfold greater affinity compared with VEGFR-2. A naturally occurring soluble form of VEGFR-1 is thought to serve as a negative regulator in physiologic angiogenesis. In addition, neuropilins (e.g., neuropilin-1 and neuropilin-2), which can bind class 3 semaphorins involved in axon guidance, can also bind the larger VEGF isoforms, as $VEGF_{121}$ lacks the domain that binds to neuropilin.[31] Neuropilin likely contributes to angiogenesis by serving as a coreceptor to VEGF and enhancing binding of VEGF-A to VEGFR-2.[32] Antibodies that target both VEGF and neuropilin-1 yield better antiangiogenic responses than targeting a single protein.[33]

Binding of VEGF to up-regulated endothelial cell VEGFR-2 sets in motion a unique intracellular signaling cascade.[34] Various investigators have identified autophosphorylation on tyrosine

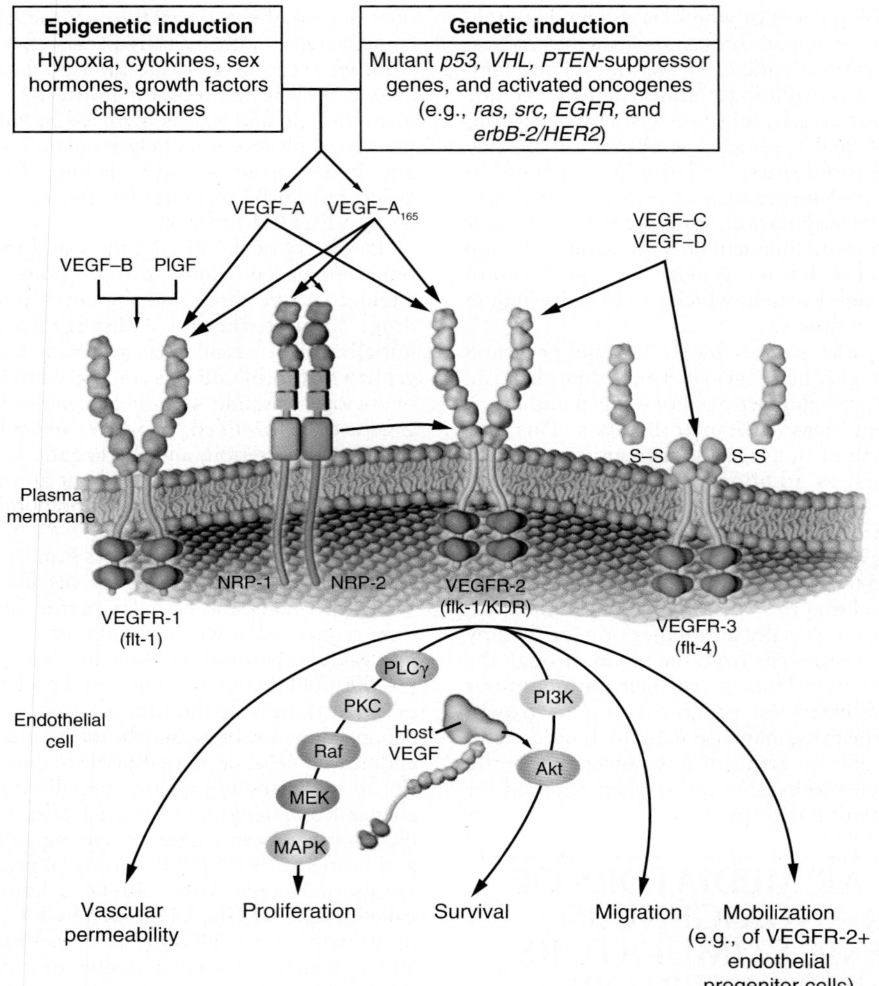

FIGURE 9.2 The family of vascular endothelial growth factor (VEGF) molecules and receptors. The major mediator of tumor angiogenesis is vascular endothelial growth factor A (VEGF-A, also called VEGF), specifically the circulating isoforms of VEGF, $VEGF_{121}$ and $VEGF_{165}$. These isoforms signal through VEGF receptor 2 (VEGFR-2), the major VEGF signaling receptor that mediates sprouting angiogenesis (called kinase-insert domain–containing receptor [KDR] in humans and fetal liver kinase 1 [flk-1] in mice). The role of VEGFR-1 in sprouting angiogenesis is much less clear. VEGF is expressed in most types of human cancer, and increased expression in tumors is often associated with a less favorable prognosis. Induction of or an increase in VEGF expression in tumors can be caused by numerous environmental (epigenetic) factors such as hypoxia, low pH, inflammatory cytokines (e.g., interleukin-6), growth factors (e.g., basic fibroblast growth factor), sex hormones (both androgens and estrogens), and chemokines (e.g., stromal cell–derived factor 1). Other causes include genetic inductive changes such as activation of numerous different oncogenes or loss or mutational inactivation of a variety of tumor suppressor genes. The binding of VEGF to VEGFR-2 leads to a cascade of different signaling pathways, two examples of which are shown, resulting in the up-regulation of genes involved in mediating the proliferation and migration of endothelial cells and promoting their survival and vascular permeability. For example, the binding of VEGF to VEGFR-2 leads to dimerization of the receptor, followed by intracellular activation of the phospholipase C gamma–protein kinase C–Raf kinase–MEK–mitogen-activated protein kinase (MAPK) pathway and subsequent initiation of DNA synthesis and cell growth, whereas activation of the phosphatidylinositol 3′–kinase (PI3K)–Akt pathway leads to increased endothelial cell survival. Activation of *src* can lead to actin cytoskeleton changes and induction of cell migration. VEGF receptors are located on the endothelial cell surface; however, intracellular ("intracrine")-signaling VEGF receptors (VEGFR-2) may be present as well, and they are involved in promoting the survival of endothelial cells. The detailed structure of the intracellular VEGFR-2 in endothelial cells is not yet known, but it is shown as the full-length receptor that is normally bound to the cell surface. Binding of VEGF-C to VEGFR-3 mediates lymphangiogenesis. $VEGF_{165}$ can bind to neuropilin (NRP) receptors, which can act as coreceptors with VEGFR-2 (*horizontal arrow*) to regulate angiogenesis. EGFR, epidermal growth factor receptor; flt-1, fms-like tyrosine kinase 1; PlGF, placental growth factor; PTEN, phosphatase and tensin homologue; S–S disulfide bond; VHL, von Hippel–Lindau. (From ref. 4, with permission.)

residues in VEGFR-2, including residues 951, 1054, 1059, 1175, and 1214. Phosphorylation of Y1175 leads to activation of phospholipase C gamma, that in turn stimulates the protein kinase C (PKC) pathway leading to inositol trisphosphate generation and calcium mobilization. In addition, this pathway, via PKCβ, stimulates the c-Raf-MEK-MAP-kinase cascade.

Another member of the VEGF family, PlGF, binds to VEGFR-1, but not VEGFR-2, and there may be circumstances where it contributes to tumor angiogenesis. Interestingly, heterodimers of VEGF-A/PlGF may prevent angiogenesis by limiting VEGF-A signaling.[35] VEGF appears to be a key mediator of embryonic angiogenesis, as well as both physiologic and pathologic forms of angiogenesis in the adult. A landmark discovery in this regard was the finding that disruption and inactivation of only one of the two VEGF alleles leads to embryonic lethality associated with marked developmental abnormalities of the vasculature ("haploininsufficiency").[36,37] Homozygous disruption of flk-1/VEGFR-2 or VEGFR-1 also leads to embryonic lethality accompanied by prominent vascular defects.[26]

There are at least four proposed roles by which VEGF is thought to promote tumor angiogenesis[26]: it can stimulate endothelial division, induce locomotion/migration, enhance endothelial cell survival[38] by up-regulating various inhibitors of apoptosis,[39] and mobilize endothelial progenitor cells from the bone marrow to sites of angiogenesis.[4] In addition, the permeability enhancing effects of VEGF might also stimulate tumor angiogenesis by causing extravasation of large molecular proteins such as fibrinogen, that can be crosslinked to form a fibrin gel in the extracellular milieu of tumors serving as a matrix for endothelial cell migration and blood vessel formation.[40] VEGF also has secondary effects including up-regulation of second messengers such as nitric oxide.

VEGF is expressed by most, if not all, human (and animal) cancers, often (but not always) at much higher levels than in corresponding normal tissues. Moreover, there are many reports showing elevated VEGF is an unfavorable prognostic marker.[26] The ubiquitous and elevated expression of VEGF in both human and animal tumors is likely the consequence of many factors that are commonly associated with tumors, as shown in Figure 9.2. Among the most important is hypoxia, a prominent feature associated with the Gompertzian growth of solid tumors. Hypoxia can stabilize and hence up-regulate the levels of the hypoxia-inducible transcription factor called HIF1α, which in turn regulates hundreds of genes, among the most important of which is VEGF.[41] In addition, a broad spectrum of oncogenes (e.g., *ras, src, Her* family members), and tumor suppressor genes, when they become mutated/inactivated or deleted, including *p53, PTEN*, and *VHL*, result in elevated VEGF expression.[4]

A second major growth factor signaling system that is known to be a major regulator of angiogenesis, especially for the later vessel maturation and stabilization stages, is the angiopoietin/tie-2 signaling pathway.[42] There are a number of members in the family including angiopoietins-1-4 (Ang) with Ang-1 and -2 being the best characterized.[43] Both of the latter bind to a highly specific endothelial cell-associated receptor tyrosine kinase, tie-2. Binding of Ang-1 to tie-2 causes an agonist effect whereas binding of Ang-2 is antagonistic. However, "pharmacologic levels" of Ang-2 may also serve as an agonist, which makes this system somewhat more complex and difficult to study.

Basic studies of this system suggest that Ang-1 is a stabilizing factor for endothelial cells; that is, it enhances endothelial cell survival and pericyte coverage. It is not truly a "proangiogenic" factor in the classic sense in that it does not promote endothelial cell proliferation. In fact, forced expression of Ang-1 in tumor cells leads to inhibited tumor growth from this "stabilizing" effect.[44] In contrast, Ang-2 is a destabilizing factor that, if present with VEGF, can promote angiogenesis. Hence, Ang-2 is a rationale for inhibiting tumor angiogenesis.[45] The tie-1 receptor remains an orphan receptor, with an undefined function. The Ang-1/tie-2 signaling pathway appears to be involved mainly in later stages of blood vessel formation, especially in the maturation and stabilization of vessels.[46]

Like VEGF and VEGF receptors, genetic disruption ("knockout") of either Ang-1 or tie-2 leads to embryonic lethality, although both alleles of Ang-1 (or tie-2) have to be silenced (homozygous disruption), unlike VEGF.[46] Studies of the role of Ang-1/tie-2 in tumor angiogenesis were hampered for many years by the inability to generate highly specific blocking antibodies or peptides. However, there are now a number of reports of the development not only of specific blocking peptides[47] ("peptibodies"), which have proceeded to clinical trial assessment,[45] but also monoclonal antibodies to Ang-2,[48] which cause robust antitumor activity; such reagents should help considerably in clarifying the role of this system in tumor angiogenesis.

There are a number of other factors implicated in the process of angiogenesis including interleukin-8, epidermal growth factor receptor ligands, basic and acidic FGF, PDGF, among many others. However, because of the need for brevity in this chapter, we have focused on a number of factors most relevant to clinical medicine, and perhaps the future of oncology. Some of the aforementioned factors may take on increasing importance as mediators of resistance to drugs that target the VEGF pathway of angiogenesis.[49,50]

ENDOGENOUS INHIBITORS OF TUMOR ANGIOGENESIS

In addition to the existence of multiple molecular stimulators of angiogenesis, there are a large number of endogenous and intrinsic inhibitors of angiogenesis. The existence of such inhibitors was first surmised by Folkman[3] on the basis of the observation that there are a number of tissues or organs that lack blood vessels and that also are rare sites of metastasis, such as cartilage or vitreous. It is also important to recognize the endogenous inhibitors are important in physiologic angiogenesis (wound healing, menstruation, luteal cycle) where a "stop" signal is necessary to prevent a pathologic condition.

A breakthrough in the field of endogenous inhibitors came with a series of reports by Dameron et al.[51] and Bouck et al.[52] beginning in 1989/1990. They reported a large glycoprotein that is a prominent member of the extracellular matrix, namely, thrombospondin-1 (TSP-1), which binds to CD36 receptors, and is a potent endogenous angiogenesis inhibitor. Moreover, the *p53* suppressor gene was found to up-regulate levels of TSP-1 in various cell types, and inactivation or loss of *p53* is associated with down-regulation of TSP-1 expression,[51] an observation that served to link the fields of cancer genetics—specifically the role of tumor suppressor genes and oncogenes in tumor development progression—with tumor angiogenesis.[3,4] Subsequently, a number of other proteins were identified as endogenous inhibitors of angiogenesis.[53–58] Many, if not most, are actually proteolytically cleaved fragments of larger proteins that are members of either the clotting/coagulation cascade family (e.g., angiostatin, which is a fragment of plasminogen[53]) or members of the extracellular matrix family of glycoproteins. Some examples of the latter category include endostatin,[54] tumstatin, and canstatin, fragments of type IV collagen.[55,56] Another endogenous inhibitor is known as vasostatin, which is a fragment of calreticulin.[57] Vasohibin is a secreted protein that is produced by endothelial cells on stimulation with an angiogenic stimulator such as VEGF. Vasohibin was the first example of an endogenous inhibitor that operates on the principles of a negative feedback mechanism.[58]

A theory that has emerged from this body of work is that tumor angiogenesis likely requires two broad functional events: the induction or elevated expression of one or more proangiogenic growth factors, such as VEGF, coinciding with the down-regulation with one or more endogenous inhibitors, such as TSP-1.[3,52,59]

A COOPERATIVE REGULATOR OF TUMOR ANGIOGENESIS: THE NOTCH RECEPTOR-DLL4 SIGNALING PATHWAY IN ENDOTHELIAL CELLS

During the last 5 years, the Notch/Notch ligand system has been shown to mediate embryonic and tumor angiogenesis.[60–65] Notch cell surface receptors (i.e., Notch 1, 2, 3, and 4) are expressed by a number of cell types and are involved in cell fate, differentiation, and proliferation. They interact with transmembrane-bound ligands (Jagged 1, Jagged 2, DLL 1, 3, and 4) on adjacent cells. The signaling aspects are unique: on ligand binding, the intracellular domain of Notch is cleaved by gamma secretase, where the Notch intracellular domain then translocates to the nuclear and acts as a transcription cofactor. It turns out that vascular endothelial cells express Notch 1 and Notch 4 receptors and Jagged 1, DLL1, and DLL4 ligands. Of these ligands, DLL4 is the only one that is selectively expressed by endothelial cells. It is expressed in small arteries and capillaries. Gene disruption experiments have shown that Notch/DLL4 signaling is absolutely essential for vascular development and arteriogenesis in embryos. Indeed, knockout of only one DLL4 allele (haploinsufficiency) is embryonic-lethal, similar to VEGF haploinsufficiency.[63] This would suggest that this system, like VEGF, would be a major stimulator of adult angiogenesis, including tumor angiogenesis. However, in some respects, Notch/DLL4 signaling is a *negative* regulator of tumor angiogenesis.[64] Thus, it turns out that DLL4 can be significantly up-regulated in the tumor vasculature in tumors, as a consequence of VEGF function. By using a combination of neutralizing antibodies to DLL4 or other types of approaches to block DLL4 function, blood vessel formation in tumors was found to be paradoxically increased, but these vessels are largely abnormal and functionally compromised such that blood flow and perfusion are impeded and tumor hypoxia increased.[60,64] This results in tumor growth inhibition. The impact of DLL4 signaling through Notch (Notch 1) is primarily restricted to tip cells at the leading edge of a growing vessel sprout or stalk, at least in the mouse retina.[61]

As a consequence of these biologic effects it appears that the Notch/DLL4 signaling pathway, though a "stimulator" of vasculogenesis and angiogenesis during early development, functions as an inhibitor of "productive" tumor angiogenesis in the adult. As such, it would seem that there is a sound therapeutic rationale for targeting the pathway to inhibit the growth of tumors, especially tumors that have become resistant to anti-VEGF therapies, by "converting" tumor blood vessels to a nonproductive or nonfunctional state.[60–64] It would appear that angiogenesis induced by VEGF can up-regulate DLL4 in endothelial cells of newly forming blood vessels and, in so doing, act as a negative feedback mechanism to prevent excessive functional angiogenesis.[62] Thus, vasohibin and DLL4 represent two negative feedback mechanisms to control/regulate tumor angiogenesis. However, the prospects of specifically targeting DLL4 received a setback recently when it was reported that chronic DLL4 blockade in mice using monoclonal antibodies caused the formation of subcutaneous vascular neoplasms and pathologic effects in organs such as the liver, thus raising critical safety concerns.[65] Hence, as always, one must carefully weigh the risk-benefit ratio of agents that may exhibit toxicities due to inhibition of pathways essential to homeostatic mechanisms.

STRATEGIES FOR DEVELOPMENT OF ANTIANGIOGENIC DRUGS

Given the aforementioned information, it can be appreciated that there are a number of possible strategies that have been developed to target tumor angiogenesis. These strategies have resulted in the discovery of an unusually large and diverse number of antiangiogenics.[25] The most obvious strategies would include developing drugs that neutralize proangiogenic growth factors such as VEGF, or block signaling from VEGFRs. In 1993, Kim et al.[66] reported that a highly specific neutralizing monoclonal antibody to human VEGF was capable of delaying the growth of VEGF expressing transplanted human tumor xenografts in immune-deficient mice, whereas it had no antiproliferative effect on the same tumor cells in cell culture, an observation consistent with an antiangiogenic mechanism of action. This was a seminal finding that opened the field of molecularly targeted antiangiogenic drugs for the treatment of cancer.

All of the currently approved antiangiogenic drugs either target VEGF or VEGFR tyrosine kinase receptors. For example, bevacizumab, as previously discussed, is a humanized derivative of a mouse monoclonal antibody that was developed to neutralize human VEGF.[26] There are also antibodies to VEGFR-2, which are in advanced clinical development,[67] a murine precursors of which has been studied extensively in preclinical studies.[68] Another antiangiogenic approach is the fusion of the extracellular binding domains of VEGFR-1 and -2 to an Fc backbone to create a "VEGF trap" molecule that primarily binds VEGF-A, but potentially binds other VEGFR-1 ligands as well such as PlGF.[69]

In addition to antibody/protein therapeutics a large number of small-molecule oral receptor tyrosine kinase inhibitors have been developed that block VEGF receptor phosphorylation. Such drugs, currently approved by the FDA, include sorafenib, sunitinib, and pazopanib.[70–72] These latter drugs are also known to affect other structurally similar receptor tyrosine kinases, including PDGF-α/β, c-kit, flt-3, CSF-1R, and the serine threonine (in the case of sorafenib), raf kinase. The antibody-based drugs, which clearly target a single pathway, rarely cause tumor regressions in preclinical models, whereas in contrast, there are instances where the small-molecule multikinase inhibitors can cause regressions of even large established tumors.[73] However, in such situations, the tumor responses induced may be a consequence of not only inhibition of angiogenesis, but also as a result of direct inhibition of tumor cell receptor tyrosine kinases involved in cell growth and survival. Furthermore, because they target PDGF receptors, the function of pericytes in stabilizing blood vessels may be compromised and this could conceivably also increase the initial efficacy of such drugs.[74]

It is important to note that at the present time it is not possible to determine which type of drug (antibody versus TKI) is optimal. With TKIs, multiple kinases may be affected, thus this class of drugs typically lead to many types of off-target toxicity and generally are more toxic than antibodies. In addition, it is more likely that there will be more patient-to-patient variation in drug exposure to small-molecule TKIs than antibodies (antibodies are dosed based on patient mass, whereas TKIs are dosed with a standard dose such as milligram per day and so forth).

A second broad approach to antiangiogenesis involves the administration of an endogenous angiogenesis inhibitor using recombinant genetically engineered protein. In this regard, there have been phase 1 clinical trials evaluating such drugs as endostatin, angiostatin, and TSP-1 peptide mimetics.[75] In general, this approach has not yet shown obvious clinical benefit in clinical trials.

Another important point about antiangiogenic drugs for the treatment of cancer is the concept of "accidental" angiogenesis inhibitors.[76] This refers to the idea that many anticancer drugs, both old and new, that were not developed with the intention of inhibiting angiogenesis, may in fact do so, which contributes to their overall antitumor effects. By way of example, chemotherapy drugs have been shown to have antiangiogenic effects.[77] There are at least two ways this can happen: either by directly targeting dividing endothelial cells present in growing tumor blood vessels,[78] or circulating bone marrow-derived endothelial progenitor cells and possibly other types of pro-angiogenic bone marrow derived circulating cells.[79] The nature of these different targets is important with respect to maximizing the antiangiogenic effects of chemotherapy. For example, there is limited preclinical evidence which shows that maximum tolerated doses of a chemotherapy drug can cause apoptosis of endothelial cells in the growing tumor vasculature of transplantable mouse tumors.[78] However, such a potential antiangiogenic effect is reversed during the subsequent drug-free break periods. This "repair" process may be mediated by a rapid mobilization and homing of endothelial progenitor cells to the drug-treated tumors.[5,80] By shortening the break periods or even eliminating them altogether, this process can be minimized or prevented. However, this requires giving relatively low doses of chemotherapy, that is, "metronomic chemotherapy," the antitumor effects of which can be markedly enhanced by combination with a targeted antiangiogenic drug.[81,82]

Metronomic chemotherapy has now been evaluated in phase 2 both randomized and nonrandomized clinical trials in a number of indications, with encouraging results, which will have to be validated in larger randomized phase 3 trials,[83–85] although there are examples of successful adjuvant metronomic chemotherapylike phase 3 trials, such as the daily oral administration of UFT, a 5-fluorouracil prodrug (comprising tegafur plus uracil) for 2 years with no breaks for non–small cell lung cancer[86] or breast cancer.[87]

ENHANCEMENT OF CHEMOTHERAPY EFFICACY AND OTHER THERAPEUTIC MODALITIES BY ANTIANGIOGENIC DRUGS

A concern in the early days of antiangiogenic drug development was that such drugs would not be useful for combination treatments involving chemotherapy or radiation therapy. By compromising blood flow/perfusion antiangiogenic drugs would "starve" tumors of oxygen, thus increasing levels of tumor hypoxia, a resistance factor to radiation and chemotherapy. However, in 1992 Teicher et al.[88] reported the first of a series of studies showing that the antitumor effects of chemotherapy on transplantable mouse tumors were actually enhanced by combination with a drug known to have antiangiogenic properties. The preclinical efficacy results were subsequently confirmed in many other studies, and foreshadowed the clinical benefit successes of bevacizumab in randomized phase 3 clinical trials in which the drug was combined with various chemotherapy regimens for the treatment of metastatic colorectal,[1] non–small cell lung[89] and breast cancers.[90] Consequently there has been considerable interest in unraveling the basis by which an antiangiogenic drug such as bevacizumab enhances the efficacy of chemotherapy. In addition, preclinical studies have shown that inclusion of an antiangiogenic drug with other therapeutic modalities—such as radiation,[91] signal transduction inhibitors,[92] oncolytic virus therapy,[93] and vascular disrupting agents[80]—can enhance the antitumor activity of all these aforementioned therapies as well as others.

With respect to the mechanistic basis by which antiangiogenic drugs enhance the efficacy of other types of anticancer therapy, most studies thus far have dealt with chemotherapy or dealing with radiation therapy, and a number of hypotheses have been proposed. One proposes that a proportion of the chaotic dysfunctional tumor-associated vasculature, which is responsible for heterogeneous and often sluggish blood flow within regions of tumors, and hence regional areas of hypoxia, can be transiently "normalized" by an antiangiogenic drug, in this case, a VEGF-targeted agent.[24] This can result in a paradoxical transient increase in regional blood flow, decreased hypoxia, and increased tumor cell proliferation.[24] If tumors are exposed to chemotherapy or radiation during the period of "vascular normalization," their efficacy will be increased. In addition, VEGF inhibition may decrease permeability, leading to a reduction in the high tumor interstitial fluid pressures, allowing better perfusion of tumor vessels.

The overall combined effect of all these changes would be transient episodes of increased tumor oxygenation and cell proliferation coinciding with an increased ability of the tumors to take up certain chemotherapy drugs during the "window" of vascular normalization, thus increasing the ability to affect a greater proportion of the tumor cell population than otherwise would be the case in the absence of the VEGF inhibition.[24,91] However aspects of this hypothesis have yet to be confirmed clinically. Thus, paradoxical increases in blood flow may not occur in all tumors, as single-agent anti-VEGF therapy for RCC is not associated with an increase in size prior to regression. Furthermore, clinical studies involving imaging (magnetic resonance imaging, computed tomographic scan) have not demonstrated an increase in blood flow with single-agent anti-VEGF therapy.

In addition, consistent evidence that the intratumoral delivery and distribution of conventional chemotherapy drugs is improved by normalization induced by antiangiogenic drugs is still lacking, especially with respect to clinical studies. A second theory is that the presence of an antiangiogenic drug during the extended drug-free break periods following each cycle of maximum tolerated dose chemotherapy will slow down the rate of tumor cell repopulation that inevitably follows tumor shrinkage, as repopulating tumor cells would require oxygen and nutrients normally supplied by the tumor vasculature.[94] In addition, there is some limited evidence that bolus injections of some cytotoxic chemotherapeutic drugs such as cyclophosphamide can cause a rapid mobilization of some of the bone marrow-derived cell populations shown in Figure 9.1 including CEPs.[79] Should some of these cells then home to sites of tumor angiogenesis in the drug-treated tumors, tumor cell repopulation would be accelerated.[5] There is some limited preclinical evidence that suggests this occurs after administration of a cytotoxiclike vascular disrupting agent or various chemotherapy drugs: tumor vascular disrupting agent (VDA)-induced CEPs home to the viable tumor rim that typically remains after VDA treatment and contributes to rapid tumor repopulation, a process that can be blocked by treatment with an antiangiogenic drug just before administration of the VDA.[80] Such systemic CEP responses constitute a form of "rebound vasculogenesis" and can occur after maximum tolerated dose chemotherapy as well.[95,96]

A third theory is that tumor stem or stemlike cells (self-renewing "tumor-initiating" cells) may reside in a vascular niche within tumors and depend on the vasculature for normal function and survival, as appears to be the case for glioma stem cells.[97] Disruption of the vascular niche can occur as a result of treatment with an antiangiogenic drug; the "compromised" tumor stem cell population might then be more sensitive to the chemotherapy than would otherwise be the case, provided chemotherapy retained access to the tumor.[98] This possibility also highlights an emerging area of research in tumor angiogenesis, namely the link between tumor stem cells and tumor angiogenesis, given the potent tumorigenic (tumor-initiating) property of the tumor stem cell subpopulation. There is growing interest in their proangiogenic phenotype in comparison to the bulk non tumor stem cell population.[97,99] On the contrary, there is also evidence in some systems that cancer stem cells may have an angiogenic-independent phenotype by adapting to hypoxic environments and using metabolic pathways that involve increased conversion of glycose to pyruvate and lactate.[100] This is an area of research that merits further analysis.

A fourth theory is that chemotherapy itself might be capable of causing direct damage to the dividing, activated endothelial cells of the tumor's growing vasculature, where the extent of such a vascular targeting effect is amplified by concurrent therapy with an antiangiogenic drug, such as an anti-VEGF antibody that would neutralize the prosurvival function of VEGF for endothelial cells, making endothelial cells more susceptible to the toxicity of chemotherapy.[81,101] However, even with single-agent anti-VEGF therapy, responses are noted in patients with metastatic RCC, providing indirect evidence that single-agent anti-VEGF therapy can lead to vascular regression.[102]

Finally, a fifth possibility is related to the fact that VEGF may act as a direct autocrine survival factor for certain tumor cell population by virtue of their expression of receptors that can bind VEGF, for example, VEGFR-1, VEGFR-2, or neuropilin-1.[103] Hence, blockade of VEGF signaling on tumor cells could conceivably directly render the cells more sensitive to chemotherapy in such cases.[103,104]

When considered together, these different theories serve to illustrate how difficult it is to dissect the mechanism of action of VEGF-targeted agents, despite its successes in the clinic. In addition, there are also clinical failures, and the successes observed in the clinic remain relatively modest as will be described later; thus there is a clear need to better understand mechanism(s) of action to improve efficacy and limit toxicity.

RESISTANCE TO ANTIANGIOGENIC DRUGS OR TREATMENTS

One of the theoretical advantages for antiangiogenic therapy of cancer hypothesized over 15 years ago was the possibility that this type of treatment strategy would be less susceptible to being rendered ineffective over time as a result of the development of acquired drug resistance.[105] However, preclinical experiments as well as clinical outcomes with angiogenesis inhibitors have shown that acquired resistance represents a significant problem, similar in nature to virtually every other anticancer drug or treatment modality. Intrinsic resistance is also a problem. In this regard, several investigators have shown that tumor endothelial cells from tumor neovasculature may not always be genetically stable, as was initially proposed. Klagsbrun and colleagues have shown that tumor endothelial cells are aneuploid, whereas others have actually reported similar genetic mutations in tumor cells and tumor associated endothelial cells.[106,107]

With respect to the clinical results, with rare exception, tumors of patients that initially show good responses to VEGF-targeted agents eventually stop responding. Preclinical investigations have revealed a number of mechanisms by which resistance to a drug such as bevacizumab or VEGF-targeted TKIs can develop when such drugs are administered as monotherapies, some of which are summarized in Figure 9.3.[108] Some of these resistance factors are discussed here.

(1) *Proangiogenic growth factor redundancy.* There are, as summarized earlier, many different growth factors that can stimulate angiogenesis, and moreover, the number and diversity of such growth factors expressed by tumors can increase with disease progression.[109] Thus, targeting a single proangiogenic pathway, especially in the context of advanced disease, by using a drug such as a monospecific antibody to VEGF or to VEGFR-2 can lead to the selection, and eventual overgrowth, of variants that can sustain angiogenesis despite persistence of VEGF/VEGFR-2 blockade.[50,110] By way of example, an alternative proangiogenic growth factor, such as bFGF, can assume control and begin to induce tumor angiogenesis during anti-VEGFR-2 antibody therapy, even though decreases in phosphorylated VEGFR-2 are detected in tumors that initially responded to the

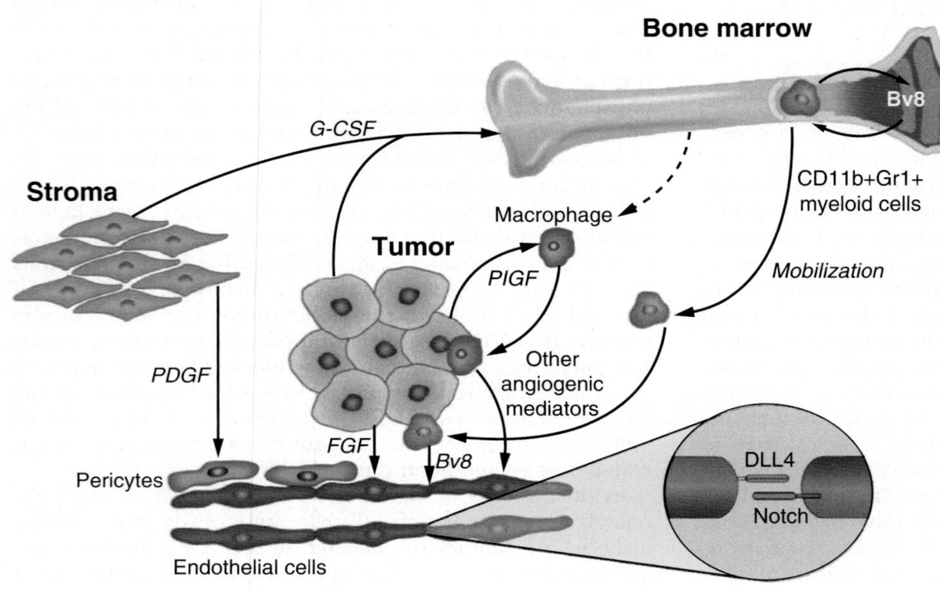

FIGURE 9.3 Some possible resistance pathways to vascular endothelial growth factor (VEGF)-targeted therapy. VEGF signaling plays a central role in tumor angiogenesis, but numerous compensatory angiogenic factors and cell types contribute to resistance to VEGF-targeted therapy. Mediators of resistance to VEGF-targeted therapy include soluble angiogenic factors such as fibroblast growth factor, placental growth factor, and Bv8; cell-bound Delta-like ligand 4 that can activate Notch on adjacent endothelial cells; pericytes that directly support endothelial cell survival; macrophages that secrete numerous angiogenic factors; and bone marrow–derived myeloid cells that also secrete soluble angiogenic factors. (From ref. 108, with permission.)

drug.[50,110] The bFGF was induced in the tumor cell population, probably as a consequence of elevated levels of hypoxia induced by drug treatment, and thus up-regulation of various growth factors known to be regulated by hypoxia.[50] Such findings would appear to support a theoretical advantage of using multitargeting TKI antiangiogenic drugs that block several proangiogenic pathways simultaneously as a means of significantly delaying or circumventing this type of acquired resistance. However, as previously mentioned, resistance to such drugs (e.g., sunitinib or sorafenib, as in RCC) eventually occurs in all patients who initially respond to treatment. One recent report implicated up-regulation of interleukin-8 as a mechanism for resistance to sunitinib in a model of RCC.[111] In some cases the source of a compensatory growth factor may be the tumor stroma, such as fibroblast-derived PDGF-C.[110] In addition, drugs such as sunitinib can induce elevated levels of multiple cytokines, chemokines, and growth factors such as granulocyte-colony stimulating factor, stromal-derived factor-1-1, PlGF, and VEGF in a tumor-independent fashion, and it is conceivable, but not yet proven, that these drug-induced changes could contribute to acquired resistance.[112]

(2) *Selection for hypoxia-resistant cells.* Cancer cells, as a result of certain genetic mutations (e.g., *p53* mutation/inactivation), can acquire an enhanced ability to survive under relatively hypoxic conditions, as would be expected to occur during an effective and long-term antiangiogenic therapy.[113] Thus, over time there could be a selection for mutant/variant subpopulations that depend less on tumor angiogenesis for survival, and possibly even cell growth.[113]

(3) *Co-option of normal organ vasculature.* It has been proposed that the ability of tumors to grow in certain vascular-rich organs such as the lung, brain, or liver might not be affected significantly by antiangiogenic drugs by virtue of the tumor cells exploiting ("co-opting") the existing mature normal vasculature to obtain the necessary oxygen and nutrients for robust growth[11]; this might also contribute to "mixed" responses in patients in whom tumors in one organ location respond to antiangiogenic treatment, but do not do so in a different organ.

(4) *Vascular remodeling.* Antiangiogenic drugs tend to preferentially target relatively immature growing neovasculature and have much reduced or even no efficacy on established/more mature vessels.[114] It has been reported that antiangiogenic therapy in preclinical tumor models can accelerate the maturation and remodeling of blood vessels, which become progressively less sensitive to the therapy.[114] The remodeled vasculature may be driven by increased expression of various factors that contribute to vessel stabilization and maturation (e.g., PDGF-BB and angiopoietin-1).[114]

With respect to development of new strategies that could have promise in dealing with tumors that are either intrinsically resistant to VEGF-targeted therapies, several strategies are being evaluated, such as sequential or salvage therapy with different antiangiogenic drugs (e.g., patients whose RCC stops responding to sunitinib may respond to sorafenib, or vice versa).[70] Combining VEGFR-2 pathway targeting drugs with other antiangiogenic drugs that block a different, complementary pathway (e.g., the tie-2/Ang2 pathway),[115] may be a promising strategy. Similarly, one might use drugs that target HIF-1α and the hypoxic tumor microenvironment, a consequence of VEGF-targeted therapies.

BIOMARKERS FOR TUMOR ANGIOGENESIS AND ANTIANGIOGENIC THERAPY

A challenge associated with the development and clinical use of antiangiogenic drugs, which is similar in nature to many other types of anticancer therapeutic modalities, especially "targeted" therapies, is the need for predictive and surrogate biomarkers to improve overall therapeutic benefit, including increasing efficacy, reducing toxicity, and improving cost-effectiveness.[116] It is important to make the distinction between predictive and surrogate markers. Predictive markers are identified prior to treatment to identify patients who may or may not benefit from therapy (predictive markers may also be used to identify patients who may develop toxicity). A surrogate marker is one that changes after initiation of therapy whereby the change may indicate target modulation and, hopefully, clinical benefit.[116]

Although there are a number of *in vivo* assays to monitor angiogenesis and hence inhibition of angiogenesis that are commonly used in mice, none of these are of practical use for use in humans.

Potential biomarkers for antiangiogenic therapies markers under investigation include circulating proteins, for example, VEGF or other proangiogenic growth factors, and soluble VEGF receptors.[116–118] In addition, circulating cells thought to be relevant to angiogenesis have been studied, including circulating endothelial cells and circulating endothelial progenitor cells.[4,9] Finally, another intensively studied approach is based on noninvasive imaging of blood flow or vascular permeability using such methods as dynamic contrast enhanced magnetic resonance imaging, computed tomographic scans incorporating flow parameters, or high-frequency microultrasound, among others.[103,116] Thus far, none of these approaches has yet been validated in prospective randomized clinical trials. However, recent studies have implicated the possibility that certain single nucleotide polymorphisms in angiogenesis-related genes (e.g., the *vegf* gene) may have promise as predictive markers for VEGF pathway targeting drugs such as bevacizumab, both for predicting clinical benefit as well as certain toxicities such as hypertension, a common side effect of VEGF inhibition.[119,120] Indeed, elevated hypertension is also currently being evaluated as a relatively simple and inexpensive surrogate biomarker, although this remains a point of controversy.[121]

To illustrate the nature of the considerable challenges involved in developing biomarkers for antiangiogenic drugs, attempts to exploit VEGF as a predictive marker for possible clinical benefit in patients receiving anti-VEGF monoclonal antibody (bevacizumab) therapy provides a compelling example. There is abundant literature reporting elevated levels of tumor VEGF are associated with a poor prognosis, so it might be anticipated that examining VEGF levels in tumors or in the circulation would be a relatively single predictive assay: the higher the levels of VEGF, the target of bevacizumab, the more likely a patient would benefit from bevacizumab therapy. However, neither VEGF expression in tumor tissue or circulating VEGF levels is predictive of clinical benefit for patients receiving either bevacizumab or other drugs that target the VEGF pathway.[122,123]

ANTIANGIOGENIC/ANTI-VEGF DRUG-BASED CLINICAL TRIALS

Research over the last two decades has shed a tremendous amount of light on the process of angiogenesis, which in turn has led the successful application of this knowledge to the care of patients with advanced-stage malignancies. All of the FDA-approved drugs considered to be antiangiogenic interfere with VEGF signaling, whereas the effectiveness of other agents remains to be determined. Because VEGF plays such diverse roles in regulating vascular development, function, and morphology, it is important at this stage in time to differentiate anti-VEGF therapy from other agents considered to be antiangiogenic. Anti-VEGF therapy can theoretically be of benefit to

TABLE 9.1

PHASE 3 TRIALS: CHEMOTHERAPY WITH OR WITHOUT VASCULAR ENDOTHELIAL GROWTH FACTOR (VEGF) TARGETED THERAPIES

Trial	Disease Site	Line of Rx	Total Patients on Trial	Primary End Point Met	ΔPFS
5-FU/LCV ± SU5416	mCRC	First	NA	No	NP
IFL ± BV	mCRC	First	923	Yes	4.4
FOLFOX ± PTK/ZK	mCRC	First	1168	No	0.2
XELOX/FOLFOX ± BV	mCRC	First	1400	Yes	1.4
FOLFOX ± BV	mCRC	Refractory	829	Yes	2.6
Capecitabine ± BV	mCRC	First	313	Yes	1.8
FOLFOX ± PTK/ZK	mCRC	Refractory	855	No	1.5
FOLFIRI ± sunitinib	mCRC	First	768	No	0.4–0.6
Chemo +/ cediranib vs chemo + BV[a]	mCRC	First	1,422	No	?
Chemo ± BV/BV	Stage II/III	Adjuvant	3,451	No	NA
FOLFOX ± BV/BV	Stage II/III CRC	Adjuvant	2,710	No	NA
5-FU/cisplatin ± BV	Gastric	First	774	No	1.4
Paclitaxel ± BV	mBreast Ca	First	715	Yes	5.9
Docetaxel ± BV	mBreast Ca	First	736	Yes	0.7–0.8
Capecitabine ± BV	mBreast Ca	Refractory	462	No	0.7
Chemo ± BV	mBreast Ca	First	1237	Yes	1.2–2.9
Chemo ± BV	M Breast Ca	First	684	Yes	1.3–2.2
Docetaxel ± sunitinib	mBreast Ca	First	?	No	?
Capecitabine ± sunitinib	mBreast Ca	Refractory	?	No	?
Carbo/Paclitaxel ± BV/ BV	Ovarian	First	1,873	No/yes	0.9/3.8
Carbo/Paclitaxel ± BV/BV	Ovarian	First	1,528	Yes	?
Carbo/Paclitaxel ± BV	Melanoma	First	?	No	1.4
Gem ± BV	Pancreatic Ca	First	602	No	0
Gem ± axitinib	Pancreatic Ca	First	597	No	2.3
Gem ± VEGF-Trap	Pancreatic Ca	First	?	No	?
Gemcitabine/erlotinib ± BV	Pancreatic Ca	First	301	No	1.0
Docetaxel ± BV	Prostate CA	Hormone-refractory	1050	No	2.4
Carbo/paclitaxel ± BV	NSCLC	First	878	Yes	1.9
Gem/Cis ± BV	NSCLC	First	1043	Yes	0.4–0.6
Carbo/paclitaxel ± sorafenib	NSCLC	First	926	No	–0.8

PFS, progression-free survival; 5-FU, 5-fluorouracil; LCV, mCRC, metastatic colorectal cancer; NP, not published at the time of writing; IFL, irinotecan, fluorouracil, leucovorin; FOLFOX, fluorouracil, leucovorin, oxaliplatin; BV, bevacizumab; PTK/ZK, PTK787/ZK222584; FOLFIRI, folinic acid, 5-FU, irinotecan, recently reported in press release but not yet presented at major meeting; NA, not available; Chemo, chemotherapy; Ca, cancer; Carbo, carboplatin; NSCLC, non–small cell lung cancer; Gem, gemcitabine; Cis, cisplatin.
[a]Head-to-head comparison.

patients by numerous mechanisms,[124] as discussed earlier in this chapter. Thus, it is appropriate to refer to agents that inhibit VEGF signaling as "anti-VEGF agents" or "VEGF-targeted therapies," providing a distinction from "generic" antiangiogenic agents that primarily target tumor endothelial cell proliferation.

Anti-VEGF therapy, despite all its high profile, does not always lead to patient benefit. A few principles derived from phase 3 clinical trial results deserve mention (Tables 9.1 and 9.2), with details of clinical trials being presented in other chapters in this text. First, for tumors other than RCC, anti-VEGF therapy is of benefit only to patients when combined with chemotherapy. The benefit to patients with RCC may be because there is a well-defined, dominant molecular alteration (loss of von Hippel–Lindau function) leading to tumors highly dependent on VEGF signaling. Second, despite the fact that anti-VEGF therapy appears to augment the effects of chemotherapy, this is not always the case. Tyrosine kinase inhibitors for patients with various types of metastatic cancer have so far failed to demonstrate improved efficacy over chemotherapy alone in multiple randomized phase 3 clinical trials, many of which have not yet been reported or published.[125,126] In addition, in trials in patients with metastatic breast cancer, bevacizumab augments the effects of paclitaxel in patients in the front-line setting, but in later lines of therapy the addition of bevacizumab provided no benefit when added to capecitabine. Lastly, anti-VEGF therapy leads to specific and sometimes unexpected toxicities, such as hypertension, proteinuria, bowel perforations, hemorrhage, arteriothrombotic events, and others. Some of these adverse effects may be due to our understanding of basic biology. For example, many investigators believe that hypertension associated with anti-VEGF therapy is due to inhibition of endothelial cell-derived nitric oxide, known pathway mediated by VEGFR-2 activation. However, the basis of other toxicities, such as bowel perforation, remain a mystery.[127]

It is important to point out that the benefits obtained with anti-VEGF/angiogenic therapy are incremental; cures are rare and tumor dormancy, if it occurs, is short-lived and rarely lasts beyond a year. The use of anti-VEGF therapy as "maintenance therapy" (after maximal tumor response with

TABLE 9.2

PHASE 3 TRIALS: VASCULAR ENDOTHELIAL GROWTH FACTOR-TARGETED THERAPIES (SINGLE AGENT OR WITH A BIOLOGIC)

Trial	Disease Site	Line of Rx	Total Patients on Trial	Primary End Point Met	ΔPFS
Sunitinib vs IFN-α	RCC	First	750	Yes	5.9
Sorafenib vs placebo	RCC	Refractory	903	Yes	2.7
IFN ± BV	RCC	First	641	Yes	4.8
Pazopanib vs placebo	RCC	Both	435	Yes	5.0
Sorafenib vs placebo	HCC	First	602	Yes	2.7
Sorafenib vs placebo	HCC	First	226	Yes	1.4
Sunitinib vs sorafenib	HCC	First	?	No	?
Sunitinib vs placebo	Pancreatic NET	First	170	Yes	5.9
Prednison ± Sunitinib	Prostate cancer	Hormone refractory	?	No	?

TPFS, progression-free survival; RCC, renal cell carcinoma; IFN, interferon; BV, bevacizumab; HCC, hepatocellular cancer; ?, recently reported in press release but not yet presented at major meeting; NET, neuroendocrine tumors.

chemotherapy) has only recently been tested in a clinical trial.[128] Furthermore, the use of anti-VEGF/angiogenic therapy in the adjuvant setting is under study, but with one exception (Table 9.1), results from most such trials will not be available for several years. The exception comes from the results of the first randomized phase 3 trial involving an antiangiogenic drug, which was recently announced.[129] The trial evaluated bevacizumab in combination with chemotherapy for 6 months followed by bevacizumab maintenance therapy for 6 additional months. The trial did not meet its primary end point of a progression-free survival benefit at 3 years despite prior interim analyses showing a transient benefit in the bevacizumab arm.[129] This benefit gradually disappeared over time, suggesting that there may be a change in the biological aggressiveness of tumor growth after the bevacizumab therapy has been completed.

Similarly, many recent phase 3 trials of bevacizumab plus chemotherapy have shown a benefit in progression-free survival but not overall survival. This has been reported for a number of trials in metastatic breast cancer, for example,[90] and also for trials in colorectal cancer,[130] gastric cancer,[131] and ovarian cancer.[128] The lack of overall survival benefit may be because of subsequent lines of therapy diluting the effect of front-line therapy. However, others have hypothesized that these findings suggest a possible change in the biology of tumor growth after an initial tumor response that reduces some of the initial clinical benefit. In this regard several recent preclinical studies have shown that there may be circumstances in which treatment with an antiangiogenic drug may accelerate tumor growth once treatment is stopped, and may also cause an increase in tumor cell invasion and/or metastasis.[112,132] With the possible exception of glioblastoma,[133,134] evidence for such increased malignant aggressiveness in the clinic has not yet been reported when drugs such as bevacizumab (plus chemotherapy) or single-agent antiangiogenic TKIs are used to treat various types of cancer. Moreover, if and when such increases in malignant aggressiveness occur, this does not mean that survival is decreased, but rather that the overall clinical benefits attained may be less than would otherwise be the case.[132] One theory to explain increases in malignant aggressiveness is that the elevated tumor hypoxia induced by antiangiogenic drug treatments will result in up-regulation of HIF-1α, which regulates numerous genes that contribute to tumor cell motility, invasion, and metastasis.[132,135,136]

LOOKING AHEAD: NEW TARGETS, NEW DRUGS, AND NEW STRATEGIES FOR ANTIANGIOGENIC THERAPY

We have stressed that, thus far, all approved antiangiogenic drugs involve the VEGF pathway as the only or primary target. Despite their successes, the limitations of such drugs highlight the need to develop alternative or complementary approaches to blocking tumor angiogenesis and improving the effects of existing drugs. With respect to new targets, there is currently considerable effort being put into defining molecular signatures of activated endothelial cells that may reveal new drivers of angiogenesis and/or promising molecular targets, especially those that are independent of the VEGF pathway. Some promising developments in this regard include the discovery and functional characterization of microRNAs—small noncoding RNA molecules that regulate gene expression at the posttranscriptional level—in vascular endothelial cells or tumor cells, and which thus can either stimulate or suppress angiogenesis.[137–139] For example, members of the microRNA-17-92 cluster have an antiangiogenic effect in endothelial cells[140] whereas *mir*-126, an endothelial-specific microRNA, can contribute to activation of VEGF signaling.[141]

Likewise, genomic and proteomic profiling of endothelial cells,[142] especially those isolated from the tumor vasculature, represents another approach being undertaken to uncover new molecular mediators of tumor angiogenesis.[15] With respect to new strategies, numerous possibilities exist, among them is the combining of antiangiogenic drugs with therapeutic modalities other than chemotherapy. For example, VEGF may have an impact on regulating components of the immune system, acting mainly as an immunosuppressive-regulating element.[143] Hence, VEGF inhibition may stimulate the immune system, making VEGF pathway targeting drugs ideal to combine with tumor vaccines or other immunotherapeutic methodologies. Many other types of combination treatment involving antiangiogenic drugs are currently under preclinical and clinical investigation.[93] Lastly, identifying patients likely to respond (or not respond) to current antiangiogenic therapies will lead to improvements in outcomes in those patients deemed likely to benefit from such therapies, while allowing other patients to be eligible for alternative antineoplastic approaches.

Selected References

The full list of references for this chapter appears in the online version.

1. Hurwitz H, Fehrenbacher L, Novotny W, et al. Bevacizumab plus irinotecan, fluorouracil, and leucovorin for metastatic colorectal cancer. *N Engl J Med* 2004;350:2335.
2. Folkman J. Tumor angiogenesis: therapeutic implications. *N Engl J Med* 1971;285:1182.
3. Folkman J. Angiogenesis: an organizing principle for drug discovery? *Nat Rev Drug Discov* 2007;6:273.
4. Kerbel RS. Tumor angiogenesis. *New Engl J Med* 2008;358:2039.
5. Kerbel RS. Antiangiogenic therapy: a universal chemosensitization strategy for cancer? *Science* 2006;312:1171.
6. Jain RK, Duda DG, Clark JW, Loeffler JS. Lessons from phase III clinical trials on anti-VEGF therapy for cancer. *Nat Clin Pract Oncol* 2006;3:24.
14. St. Croix B, Rago C, Velculescu V, et al. Genes expressed in human tumor endothelium. *Science* 2000;289:1197.
22. Bergers G, Song S, Meyer-Morse N, Bergsland E, Hanahan D. Benefits of targeting both pericytes and endothelial cells in the tumor vasculature with kinase inhibitors. *J Clin Invest* 2003;111:1287.
23. Xian X, Hakansson J, Stahlberg A, et al. Pericytes limit tumor cell metastasis. *J Clin Invest* 2006;116:642.
24. Jain RK. Normalization of tumor vasculature: an emerging concept in antiangiogenic therapy. *Science* 2005;307:58.
25. Kerbel RS, Folkman J. Clinical translation of angiogenesis inhibitors. *Nat Rev Cancer* 2002;2:727.
26. Ferrara N. Timeline: VEGF and the quest for tumour angiogenesis factors. *Nat Rev Cancer* 2002;2:795.
27. Sawamiphak S, Seidel S, Essmann CL, et al. Ephrin-B2 regulates VEGFR2 function in developmental and tumour angiogenesis. *Nature* 2010;465:487.
28. Senger DR, Galli S, Dvorak AM, Perruzzi CA, Harvey VS, Dvorak HF. Tumor cells secrete a vascular permeability factor that promotes accumulation of ascites fluid. *Science* 1983;219:983.
29. Leung DW, Cachianes G, Kuang W-J, Goeddel DV, Ferrara N. Vascular Endothelial Growth Factor is a secreted angiogenic molecule. *Science* 1989;246:1306.
32. Ellis LM. The role of neuropilins in cancer. *Mol Cancer Ther* 2006;5:1099.
34. Shibuya M, Claesson-Welsh L. Signal transduction by VEGF receptors in regulation of angiogenesis and lymphangiogenesis. *Exp Cell Res* 2006;312:549.
36. Ferrara N, Carver-Moore K, Chen H, et al. Heterozygous embryonic lethality induced by targeted inactivation of the VEGF gene. *Nature* 1996;380:439.
37. Carmeliet P, Ferreira V, Breier G, et al. Abnormal blood vessel development and lethality in embryos lacking a single VEGF allele. *Nature* 1996;380:435.
38. Alon T, Hemo I, Itin A, Pe'er J, Stone J, Keshet E. Vascular endothelial growth factor acts as a survival factor for newly formed retinal vessels and has implications for retinopathy of prematurity. *Nat Med* 1995;1(10):1024.
41. Semenza GL. Targeting HIF-1 for cancer therapy. *Nat Rev Cancer* 2003;3:721.
46. Hanahan D. Signaling vascular morphogenesis and maintenance. *Science* 1997;277:48.
47. Oliner J, Min H, Leal J, et al. Suppression of angiogenesis and tumor growth by selective inhibition of angiopoietin-2. *Cancer Cell* 2004;6:507.
48. Brown JL, Cao ZA, Pinzon-Ortiz M, et al. A human monoclonal anti-ANG2 antibody leads to broad antitumor activity in combination with VEGF inhibitors and chemotherapy agents in preclinical models. *Mol Cancer Ther* 2010;9:145.
49. Bergers G, Hanahan D. Modes of resistance to anti-angiogenic therapy. *Nat Rev Cancer* 2008;8:592.
50. Casanovas O, Hicklin D, Bergers G, Hanahan D. Drug resistance by evasion of antiangiogenic targeting of VEGF signaling in late stage pancreatic islet tumors. *Cancer Cell* 2005;8:299.
52. Bouck N, Stellmach V, Hsu SC. How tumors become angiogenic. *Adv Cancer Res* 1996;69:135.
60. Noguera-Troise I, Daly C, Papadopoulos NJ, et al. Blockade of Dll4 inhibits tumour growth by promoting non-productive angiogenesis. *Nature* 2006;444:1032.
61. Hellstrom M, Phng LK, Hofmann JJ, et al. Dll4 signalling through Notch1 regulates formation of tip cells during angiogenesis. *Nature* 2007;445:776.
66. Kim KJ, Li B, Winer J, et al. Inhibition of vascular endothelial growth factor-induced angiogenesis suppresses tumour growth *in vivo*. *Nature* 1993;362:841.
68. Prewett M, Huber J, Li Y, et al. Antivascular endothelial growth factor receptor (fetal liver kinase 1) monoclonal antibody inhibits tumor angiogenesis and growth of several mouse and human tumors. *Cancer Res* 1999;59:5209.
69. Lockhart AC, Rothenberg ML, Dupont J, et al. Phase I study of intravenous vascular endothelial growth factor trap, aflibercept, in patients with advanced solid tumors. *J Clin Oncol* 2010;28:207.
70. Rini BI, Atkins MB. Resistance to targeted therapy in renal-cell carcinoma. *Lancet Oncol* 2009;10:992.
78. Browder T, Butterfield CE, Kraling BM, Marshall B, O'Reilly MS, Folkman J. Antiangiogenic scheduling of chemotherapy improves efficacy against experimental drug-resistant cancer. *Cancer Res* 2000;60:1878.
80. Shaked Y, Ciarrocchi A, Franco M, et al. Therapy-induced acute recruitment of circulating endothelial progenitor cells to tumors. *Science* 2006;313:1785.
81. Klement G, Baruchel S, Rak J, et al. Continuous low-dose therapy with vinblastine and VEGF receptor-2 antibody induces sustained tumor regression without overt toxicity. *J Clin Invest* 2000;105:R15.
89. Sandler A, Gray R, Perry MC, et al. Paclitaxel-carboplatin alone or with bevacizumab for non-small-cell lung cancer. *N Engl J Med* 2006;355:2542.
90. Miller K, Wang M, Gralow J, et al. Paclitaxel plus bevacizumab versus paclitaxel alone for metastatic breast cancer. *N Engl J Med* 2007;357:2666.
97. Calabrese C, Poppleton H, Kocak M, et al. A perivascular niche for brain tumor stem cells. *Cancer Cell* 2007;11:69.
103. Hicklin DJ, Ellis LM. Role of the vascular endothelial growth factor pathway in tumor growth and angiogenesis. *J Clin Oncol* 2005;23:1011.
109. Relf M, LeJeune S, Scott PA, et al. Expression of the angiogenic factors vascular endothelial cell growth factor, acidic and basic fibroblast growth factor, tumor growth factor beta-1, platelet-derived endothelial cell growth factor, placenta growth factor, and pleiotrophin in human primary breast cancer and its relation to angiogenesis. *Cancer Res* 1997;57:963.
110. Ferrara N. Pathways mediating VEGF-independent tumor angiogenesis. *Cytokine Growth Factor Rev* 2010;21:21.
112. Ebos JML, Lee CR, Cruz-Munoz W, Bjarnason GA, Christensen JG, Kerbel RS. Accelerated metastasis after short-term treatment with a potent inhibitor of tumor angiogenesis. *Cancer Cell* 2009;15:232.
116. Murukesh N, Dive C, Jayson GC. Biomarkers of angiogenesis and their role in the development of VEGF inhibitors. *Br J Cancer* 2010;102:8.
120. Chen HX, Cleck JN. Adverse effects of anticancer agents that target the VEGF pathway. *Nat Rev Clin Oncol* 2009;6:465.
132. Paez-Ribes M, Allen E, Hudock J, et al. Antiangiogenic therapy elicits malignant progression of tumors to increased local invasion and distant metastasis. *Cancer Cell* 2009;15:220.
134. Norden AD, Young GS, Setayesh K, et al. Bevacizumab for recurrent malignant gliomas: efficacy, toxicity, and patterns of recurrence. *Neurology* 2008;70:779.
136. Pennacchietti S, Michieli P, Galluzzo M, Mazzone M, Giordano S, Comoglio PM. Hypoxia promotes invasive growth by transcriptional activation of the met protooncogene. *Cancer Cell* 2003;3:347.
137. Heusschen R, van GM, Griffioen AW, Thijssen VL. MicroRNAs in the tumor endothelium: novel controls on the angioregulatory switchboard. *Biochim Biophys Acta* 2010;1805:87.
139. Bonauer A, Boon RA, Dimmeler S. Vascular microRNAs. *Curr Drug Targets* 2010;11:943.

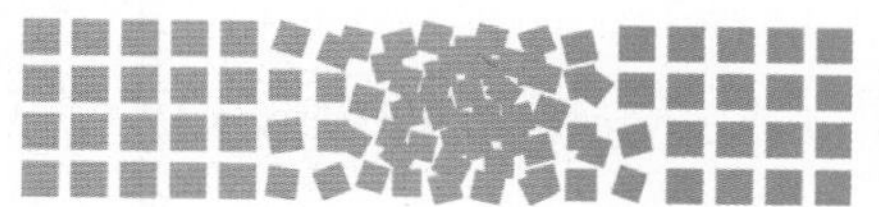

CHAPTER 10 INVASION AND METASTASIS

ANDY J. MINN AND JOAN MASSAGUÉ

Many of the gains in our understanding of the genetics and molecular mechanisms of cancer have been driven by the quest to understand characteristic anatomic and cellular traits of the disease. Pathologists have long observed that cancer seemingly can evolve from hyperplasia through a series of increasingly disorganized and invasive-appearing tumors that can then colonize distant organs in a nonrandom fashion. This spread of cancer from the organ of origin (primary site) to distant tissues is called *metastasis*. Much of the complex knowledge that has been acquired about cancer biology has been from a reductionistic approach that has focused on the inner workings of cancer cells with limited regard to interactions with the microenvironment and host biology. Although our understanding about cell proliferation, cell death, genomic instability, and signal transduction pathways has rapidly progressed, detailed understanding about the molecular mechanisms of metastasis has lagged considerably behind.

Inherent difficulties in studying metastasis have been due to technological limitations in analyzing a complex *in vivo* process rich with heterotypic interactions. Invasion, survival in the circulation, and growth in distant organs are not amenable to methods that primarily use *in vitro* models. Despite technical challenges, elegant experiments that started in the 1950s were done with mouse xenograft models and resulted in an important descriptive understanding of the biology of metastasis. With the accumulation of knowledge from studying cancer cells in isolation, subsequent advances in metastasis built on the classic studies. Unfortunately, metastasis remains responsible for the vast majority of cancer-related morbidity and mortality. Therefore, advancing our scientific and clinical understanding of metastasis is a high priority. In this chapter, we will first review the classic paradigm of cancer metastasis and then describe recent advances that are starting to better characterize metastasis on the molecular, cellular, and organismal level.

THE EVOLUTION AND PATHOGENESIS OF METASTASIS

Somatic Evolution of Cancer

Hyperplastic and dysplastic lesions need not always progress to cancer, but when they do, it can take years if not decades for this to occur. This protracted course to malignancy is consistent with epidemiologic studies that show an age-dependent increase in the incidence of cancer.[1] Mathematically, this precipitous rise can be explained by the accumulation of many stochastic events. These ideas have contributed to the widely accepted view that cancer requires several genetic alterations during a course of somatic evolution. However, the mutation frequency of human cells is thought to be too low to explain the high prevalence of the disease if so many stochastic genetic alterations are needed. To account for this disparity, cancer cells are widely believed to have a "mutator phenotype," a concept with much experimental support.[2]

Driven by increased mutability of the genome, the dynamics of tumor progression depend on mutation, selection, and tissue organization.[3] Mutations can result in activation of oncogenes or loss of tumor suppressor genes that increase fitness and cell autonomy. To oppose the accumulation of cells with tumorigenic mutations, tissue architecture often limits the spread of mutant cells that have reached fixation. For example, large compartments containing many cells accumulate advantageous mutations more rapidly than smaller compartments. Similarly, if there are only a limited number of precursor cells that have self-renewal capabilities (stem cells), this also has the effect of reducing the risk of enriching for tumorigenic mutations. However, despite the sequential mutations and steps predicted by the somatic evolution of cancer, the nature and/or sequence of genes that are altered during this evolution are mostly unknown.

Clinical, Pathologic, and Anatomic Correlations

Metastasis is often associated with several clinical and pathologic characteristics. Among these, tumor size and regional lymph node involvement are consistently associated with distant relapse. For tumor size, no clear threshold exists but trends are clear. For example, metastatic risk for breast cancer rises sharply after 2 cm,[4] while distant metastasis in sarcoma is more common for tumor sizes larger than 5 cm.[5] The involvement of regional lymph nodes is often, but not always, a harbinger for increased risk of distant metastasis. For head and neck cancer, the association between lymph node involvement and metastasis is predictable. Metastasis rarely occurs without prior involvement of cervical neck lymph nodes, and the lower down in the neck nodal involvement occurs, the more likely distant metastasis becomes.[6] For breast cancer, the presence of positive lymph nodes is the strongest clinicopathologic prognostic marker for distant relapse. Like head and neck cancer, the extent of nodal involvement is telling, as a precipitous rise in metastatic risk is observed for patients with more than four axillary lymph nodes.[4] However, lymph node metastasis does not always precede distant relapse. In sarcomas, for example, metastasis is often seen in the absence of nodal disease.[5]

When tumor cells appear to have aggressive traits on microscopic analysis, this often translates into increased risk for distant disease. Although many histopathologic traits for different cancer types have been reported to associate with poor prognosis, there are several that consistently appear to track with metastatic risk across various tumor types. These traits include: (1) *Tumor grade*. Tumors that are poorly differentiated, or retain few features of their normal tissue counterparts, are generally considered to be high grade. High-grade tumors often exhibit infiltrative rather than pushing borders and show signs of rapid cell division. Breast cancer and sarcomas are well recognized for displaying a markedly elevated risk of metastasis with higher tumor grade. (2) *Depth of invasion beyond normal tissue compartmental boundaries*. Some cancers like melanoma and gastrointestinal malignancies are staged by how deeply they extend beyond the basement membrane. Violation of deeper layers of the dermis, or invasion through the lamina propria, muscularis mucosa, and serosa, represent progressively more extensive invasion and higher risk of metastasis. (3) *Lymphovascular invasion*. Tumor emboli seen in the blood or lymphatic vessels generally carry a poorer prognosis than cancer without these features. Breast cancer and squamous cell cancers of the head and neck or female cervix are examples.

Tissue Tropism and the Seed and Soil Hypothesis

Despite apparent similarities in clinical and/or histologic features, different cancer types do not exhibit the same proclivity to metastasize to the same organs, and the same cancer type can preferentially metastasize to different organs (Table 10.1). This tissue tropism has long been recognized and has intrigued clinicians and pathologists to seek an explanation. In 1889, Stephen Paget proposed his "seed and soil" hypothesis (reviewed in ref. 7). This stated that the propensity of different cancers to form metastases in specific organs was due to the dependence of the seed (the cancer) on the soil (the distant organ). In contrast, James Ewing and others argued that tissue tropism could be accounted for based on mechanical factors and circulatory patterns of the primary tumor. For example, colorectal cancer can enter the hepatic-portal system, explaining its propensity for liver metastasis, and prostate cancer can traverse a presacral plexus that connects the periprostatic and vertebral veins, explaining its propensity for metastases to the lower spine and pelvis. Supporting the arguments for both views, current understanding would suggest that both seed and soil factors and anatomic ("plumbing") considerations contribute to metastatic tropism. A modern interpretation of the seed and soil hypothesis is an active area of investigation, with molecular definitions accumulating for both the cancer and the microenvironment.

Basic Steps in the Metastatic Cascade

From clinical, anatomic, and pathologic observations of metastasis, a picture of the steps involved in a metastatic cascade emerges. Numerous prerequisites and steps can be envisioned.

1. *Invasion and motility*. Normal tissue requires proper adhesions with basement membrane and/or neighboring cells to signal to each other that proper tissue compartment size and homeostasis is being maintained. Tumor cells display diminished cellular adhesion, allowing them to become motile, a fundamental property of metastatic cells. Tumor cells use their migratory and invasive properties in order to burrow through surrounding extracellular stroma and to gain entry into blood vessels and lymphatics.
2. *Intravasation and survival in the circulation*. Once tumor cells enter the circulation, or intravasate, they must be able to withstand the physical shear forces and the hostility of sentinel immune cells. Solid tumors are not accustomed to surviving as single cells without attachments and often interact with each other or blood elements to form intravascular tumor emboli.
3. *Arrest and extravasation*. Once arrested in the capillary system of distant organs, tumor cells must extravasate, or exit the circulation, into foreign parenchyma.
4. *Growth in distant organs*. Successful adaptation to the new microenvironment results in sustained growth. Of all the steps in the metastatic cascade, the ability to grow in distant organs has the greatest clinical impact and lies at the core of the seed and soil hypothesis. Accomplishing this step may be rate-limiting and may determine whether distant relapse occurs rapidly or dormancy ensues.

TABLE 10.1

STEREOTYPIC PATTERNS OF METASTASIS TO DISTANT ORGANS BY CANCER TYPE

Cancer Type	Site of Metastasis
Breast carcinomas	Primarily bone, lung, pleura and liver; less frequently brain and adrenal. ER-positive tumors preferentially spread to bone; ER-negative tumors metastasize more aggressively to visceral organs.
Lung cancers	The two most common types of lung cancer have different etiologies. SCLC disseminates rapidly to many organs including the liver, brain, adrenals, pancreas, contralateral lung, and bone. NSCLC often spreads to the contralateral lung and the brain, and also to adrenal glands, liver, and bones.
Prostate carcinoma	Almost exclusively to bone; forms osteoblastic lesions filling the marrow cavity with mineralized osseous matrix, unlike the osteolytic metastasis caused by breast cancer.
Pancreatic cancer	Aggressive spread to the liver, lungs, and surrounding viscera.
Colon cancer	The portal circulation pattern favors dissemination to the liver and peritoneal cavity, but metastasis also occurs in the lungs.
Ovarian carcinoma	Local spread in the peritoneal cavity.
Sarcomas	Various types of sarcoma; mesenchymal origin; mainly metastasize to the lungs.
Myeloma	Hematologic malignancy of the bone marrow that causes osteolytic bone lesions, sometimes spreading to other organs.
Glioma	These brain tumors display little propensity for distance organ metastasis, despite aggressively invading the central nervous system.
Neuroblastoma	Pediatric tumors arising from nervous tissue of the adrenal gland. Forms bone, liver, and lung metastases, which spontaneously regress in some cases.

ER, estrogen receptor; SCLC, small cell lung cancer; NSCLC, non–small cell lung carcinoma.

Heterogeneity in Cancer Metastasis and Rarity of Metastatic Cells

Because numerous sequential steps are needed for metastasis, multiple genetic changes are envisioned. A failure in any step would prevent metastasis altogether. Accordingly, tumor cells that can accumulate a full complement of needed alterations to endow them with metastatic ability should be rare. These ideas are supported by early experiments. Work by Fidler and colleagues[7] showed that subpopulations of tumor cells exist that display significant variation in their metastatic ability and metastatic lesions likely arose from single progenitor cells. Early cell fate studies revealed that less than 0.01% of tumor cells gave rise to metastases. More recent studies using *in vivo* video microscopy to visualize and quantitate cell fate confirmed that metastasis is an inefficient process (reviewed in ref. 8). Thus, important early studies helped to establish the idea that primary tumors are heterogeneous in their metastatic ability and that tumor cells that can successfully metastasize are exceedingly rare.

The Traditional Progression Model for Metastasis and its Implications

A synthesis of clinical observation, deduced steps in the metastatic cascade, and early studies of experimental metastasis in mice led to a traditional model for metastatic progression.[7] In this view, primary tumor cells undergo somatic evolution and accumulate genetic changes. Because numerous steps are required for metastasis, the number of genetic changes that are needed for full metastatic competency is large; hence, tumor cells that have acquired these changes are rare. Many clinicopathologic traits such as lymphovascular invasion and regional lymph node involvement represent successful completion of some of the steps in the metastatic cascade but not necessarily all. The clinical observation that metastatic risk increases with tumor size is explained by mathematical considerations predicting that genetic changes accumulate faster with increased population size. Larger tumors are more likely to contain rare cells that are metastatically competent, making metastasis a late event in tumorigenesis.

One of the primary objectives in the clinical management of cancer is to prevent or decrease the risk of metastasis. How this objective is approached is shaped by empiricism and perceptions about how metastasis proceeds. The idea that metastasis occurs as a late event in tumorigenesis argues that early detection and early eradication of the primary tumor will prevent metastasis and be sufficient for cure. Screening programs, radical versus more limited surgical excisions, and the use of adjuvant radiation to the surgical bed can be justified based on the idea that cancers caught early have not likely spread. Metastatic heterogeneity within the primary tumor and the rarity of tumor cells that can complete all the sequential steps in the metastatic cascade suggest that the detection of tumor cells caught in the act of undergoing an early step in the cascade may still represent an opportunity to stop metastasis in its tracks. This is a rationale for oncologic surgeries that include regional lymph node dissections and the use of regional radiation therapy. The likely emergence of rare metastatic cells late during tumorigenesis provides reason to add adjuvant systemic chemotherapy after local treatment of larger and more advanced primary tumors rather than smaller tumors with less aggressive features.

Alternative Models

Although the traditional model for metastasis has enjoyed favor, alternative models have been proposed. The clinical data for breast cancer has inspired a long-standing debate on whether metastasis follows a traditional progression model or a predetermination paradigm—also known as the Halsted model versus the Fisher model (discussed in ref. 9) for metastasis.[9] Both models seek to justify and explain clinical data looking at the benefit of aggressive local treatment of the primary tumor and draining lymph nodes versus the early use of adjuvant systemic chemotherapy. Although more anatomic than cellular in nature, the Halsted model looked at breast cancer from a traditional vantage point and imposed on it an orderly anatomic spread pattern from primary site, to regional lymph nodes, to distant organs. This orderly progression would make complete eradication of the primary and regional tumor burden sufficient to stop metastasis. In contrast, Fisher hypothesized that whether distant relapse occurs in breast cancer is predetermined from the onset of tumorigenesis (discussed in ref. 9). This view emphasizes breast cancer as a systemic disease for those tumors so fated and the importance of adjuvant systemic chemotherapy. The data from randomized trials for adjuvant treatment and from breast cancer screening programs do not clearly rule-out one model or the other.[10] To reconcile the clinical data, Hellman[9] proposed that breast cancer is best considered a spectrum of diseases bound by predetermination models and traditional progression models. Other models that conceptually differ from the traditional progression model include the clonal dominance model[11] and the dynamic heterogeneity model.[12]

Compatibility of Metastasis Models with Somatic Evolution

Both alternative and traditional progression models alike need to be compatible with the paradigm of somatic evolution, which presents a potential problem. Because it is not obvious why metastasis genes that promote growth at a distant site should have a fitness advantage for a primary tumor, the likelihood that multiple metastasis-specific genes will become fixed in a primary tumor would seem unlikely. To reconcile this, it has been suggested that the genes selected to drive primary tumor formation and progression are also the genes that mediate metastasis.[13] This notion would imply that metastasis is a predetermined property of primary tumors that principally depends on the history of oncogenes and tumor suppressor genes that the primary tumor acquires. Such early onset of metastatic ability could explain phenomenon like cancers of unknown primary and support earlier predetermination metastasis models for breast cancer. However, as previously mentioned, predetermination models are not always consistent with clinical data, in particular the ability of screening and early detection to decrease cancer mortality. Furthermore, the phenomenon of metastatic dormancy, whereby metastasis remains inactive and undetectable for years if not decades after treatment of the primary tumor, is difficult to explain unless further metastasis-promoting changes occur after the primary tumor has been removed.

AN INTEGRATED MODEL FOR METASTASIS

Different concepts on how metastasis progresses have individual merits and limitations. A clearer understanding of metastasis requires sophisticated insight on a molecular level. Recent advances in the field of metastasis research are beginning to bring together an integrated and more complex paradigm (Fig. 10.1) whereby elements from different models may be interconnected.[14] At the heart of this integrated paradigm are the principles of somatic evolution. Somatic evolution selects for functions and not directly for specific genes. Therefore,

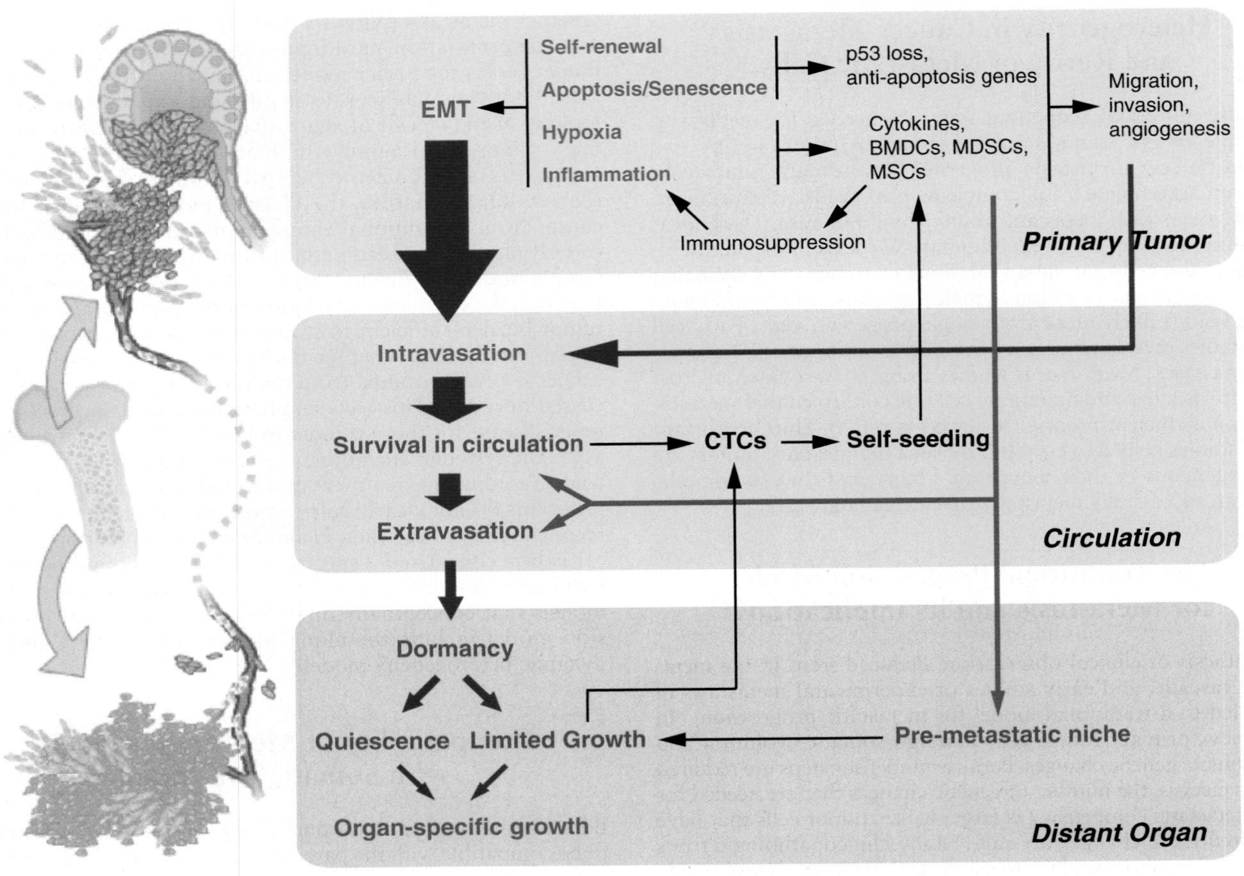

Metastasis Initiation Genes: **TWIST1, SNAI1, ZEB1, ZEB2, miR-10b, miR-200, miR-126**

Metastasis Progression Genes: **PTGS2, EREG, MMP1, LOX, ANGPTL4, CXCR4, CCL5/CCR5, VEGF, FSCN1, IL-6, IL-8, SRC, HBEGF**

Metastasis Virulence Genes: **IL11, SPARC, PTHRP, IL13RA2, IL-6, TNFα**

FIGURE 10.1 Selective pressures and steps from primary tumor growth to metastasis. Selective pressures at the primary tumor (labeled in *magenta*) can determine metastatic potential. Cancer is initiated by oncogenic changes. Of particular relevance to metastatic potential may be self-renewal pathways and the need to overcome apoptosis and senescence. Hypoxia and inflammation have important roles and lead to tumor cells co-opting bone marrow-derived cells (BMDCs), myeloid-derived suppressor cells (MDSCs), and mesenchymal stem cells (MSCs), to name a few. These cells and the cytokines that they produce enhance the ability of the tumor to migrate, invade, overcome hypoxia, and maintain an immunosuppressed environment. The ability of primary tumor cells to undergo an epithelial-to-mesenchymal transition (EMT) is also influenced by the selective pressures faced during primary tumor growth. EMT results in migration, invasion, and intravasation. Such functions (labeled in *red*) are examples of metastasis initiation functions. Although non–EMT-related migration and invasion can also lead to intravasation, EMT is likely a principle means by which circulating tumor cells (CTCs) are promoted. Further steps in the metastatic cascade are shown by *green arrows*, with the size of the arrow representing the likelihood that the step is successfully completed for many cancer types (e.g., breast cancer). Selective pressures encountered from the local microenvironment shape metastatic proclivity by selecting for tumorigenic functions that secondarily help cells navigate the metastatic cascade (metastasis-progression functions). Hypoxia and inflammation-related events contribute to metastasis-progression functions (labeled in *purple*) by enhancing the ability of CTCs to survive in the circulation, extravasate, and form a premetastatic niche. CTCs can either self-seed the primary tumor, which results in augmentation of tumor mass and further selection of metastatic traits, or extravasate into distant organs. Although a premetastatic niche facilitates adaptation to the foreign microenvironment of distant organs, further selection is needed for full colonization. This results in a period of dormancy whereby micrometastases remain quiescent or growth is counterbalanced by apoptosis and the lack of angiogenesis. Further somatic evolution within the distant organ can eventually result in selection of macrometastatic-colonization functions (labeled in *blue*) and organ-specific growth. On the bottom of the figure are examples of specific genes that play a role in metastasis initiation, metastasis progression, and macrometastatic colonization.

during primary tumor growth, the principal functions that are selected are *tumorigenic functions* that can be met by a large repertoire of oncogenic mutations. Examples of these tumorigenic functions include proliferative and metabolic autonomy, self-renewal ability, resistance to cell death, resistance to inhibitory signals, immune evasion, motility, invasion, and angiogenesis. Most of these traits were enumerated by Hanahan and Weinberg[15] as being hallmarks of cancer. Many of these tumorigenic functions allow transformed cells to attract supporting stroma and migrate and invade surrounding tissue, regardless of whether or not cells reside in the primary tumor. This subset of tumorigenic functions is a prerequisite for metastasis because such functions are needed for cells to invade, penetrate blood vessels, and give rise to circulating tumor cells. These functions are shared by primary tumors and metastasis and are defined as *metastasis initiation functions*. A prominent example includes epithelial-to-mesenchymal transition (EMT).

It is evident how genes with tumorigenic functions and genes with metastasis initiation functions can be selected for during primary tumor growth. However, how are metastasis-specific functions (i.e. functions that are not characteristic of general tumorigenesis) selected during growth at the primary site? Metastasis-specific functions include survival in the circulation, extravasation, survival in the microenvironment of distant organs, and organ-specific colonization. Recent experimental evidence reveals that some genes can mediate tumorigenic functions and secondarily serve metastasis-specific functions either in a general way or with particular organ selectivity.[16,17] These types of functions are called *metastasis-progression functions* and genes with this duality are defined as *metastasis-progression genes*. Metastasis-progression genes form the basis for predetermination models for metastasis. When metastasis-progression genes are selected for, their expression by the primary tumor will track with increased risk of metastasis. These genes will also mechanistically couple certain traits of primary tumor progression (e.g., rapid growth, invasiveness, resistance to hypoxia) with distant spread.

Cancer cells that have acquired metastasis-progression genes can undergo additional selective pressure during life away from the primary tumor. Functionally, genes selected by the pressures of a distant site are similar to metastasis-progression genes but they are not coupled to tumorigenic genes and so confer no advantage to a primary tumor. Therefore, altered expression of these genes would be rare or absent in the primary tumor and discernible only in the metastatic lesion. These genes are called *macrometastatic-colonization genes* and provide *macrometastatic-colonization functions*. Macrometastatic-colonization genes form the basis of traditional progression models for metastasis.

In this integrated view that stratifies genes into tumorigenic, metastasis initiation, metastasis progression, and macrometastatic colonization, the selection for tumorigenic functions during primary tumor growth provides essential prerequisites for future metastasis. Certain biases in the genes that are selected to fulfill particular tumorigenic functions may result in genes that can also fulfill specific metastatic functions, leading to an early proclivity toward distant spread. The further selection of metastasis-specific functions after infiltration of distant organs can continue to modify metastatic behavior through the acquisition of macrometastatic-colonization genes. Although the emerging evidence does not always allow clear delineation between genes that serve tumorigenic versus metastasis initiation versus metastasis-progression functions, recent molecular understanding and insight offer the underpinnings of this integrated view.

SELECTIVE PRESSURES AT THE PRIMARY TUMOR DRIVING ACQUISITION OF METASTASIS FUNCTIONS

Of all the tumorigenic functions required by aggressive primary cancers, several may additionally select for metastasis initiation or metastasis-progression genes (Fig. 10.1). Experimental and clinical evidence point toward the following factors.

Hypoxia

In order to disrupt tissue homeostasis during primary tumorigenesis, many barriers that can limit growth must be overcome. A near-universal need is for tumors to respond to hypoxia (reviewed in refs. 18 through 20). Normal tissue such as epithelium is separated from blood vessels by a basement membrane. When preinvasive tumor growth occurs, hypoxia can ensue because oxygen and glucose typically can only diffuse 100 to 150 microns, resulting in portions of the expanding mass becoming hypoxic. This can be seen in comedo-type ductal carcinoma *in situ* (DCIS) of the breast, whereby a necrotic center characterizes these preinvasive breast tumors. The fact that DCIS can take years to progress to invasive cancer, or never progresses to cancer, suggests that hypoxia can be a significant barrier.

Although there are multiple paths that cancer cells can take to adapt to hypoxia, the hypoxia-inducible factor (HIF) transcription factors have a central role. Under hypoxic conditions, HIF-1α and HIF-2α become stabilized, resulting in the transcription of over 100 HIF-α regulated genes. These target genes are involved in angiogenesis, glycolysis, and invasion, which together help hypoxic cells adapt. Up-regulated angiogenesis genes include vascular endothelial growth factor (VEGF) and platelet-derived growth factor (PDGF). These factors cause quiescent blood vessels to undergo remodeling, including the laying down of a matrix that activated endothelial cells use to form newly vascularized areas. Various glycolysis genes are expressed and their metabolic by-products lead to acidification of the extracellular space. This is normally toxic to cells and requires further adaptation either by up-regulation of H^+ transporters or acquired resistance to apoptosis. To assist in invasion toward newly vascularized areas, HIF-α up-regulates matrix metalloproteinase 1 and 2 (MMP1, MMP2), lysyl oxidase (LOX), and the chemokine receptor CXCR4. Degradation of the basement membrane by MMP2 and alteration of the extracellular matrix (ECM) by MMP1 and LOX clears away a barrier to migration. The activation of CXCR4 then stimulates cancer cells to migrate to regions of angiogenesis. Thus, if these series of events can be successfully completed, not only will preinvasive tumors successfully deal with hypoxia, but they will also likely invade through the basement membrane in the process. Invasion through the basement membrane defines invasive carcinomas.

Inflammation

When normal tissue homeostasis and architecture are disrupted, this can lead to vessel injury, hypoxic zones, extravasation of blood proteins, and the entry of foreign pathogens (reviewed in refs. 21 and 22). A rapid response is mounted by a front line composed of immune and bone marrow-derived cells (BMDCs) such as lymphocytes, neutrophils, macrophages, dendritic cells, eosinophils, and natural killer (NK) cells. The purpose is to restore homeostasis through several phases: inflammation, tissue formation, and tissue remodeling. In the initial phase, tissue breakdown attracts neutrophils to infiltrate the wounded area and release various proinflammatory cytokines such as interleukin (IL)-8), IL-1β, and tumor necrosis factor-α (TNF-α). In addition, reactive oxygen species and proteases such as urokinase-type plasminogen activator (uPA) are produced by neutrophils to fight pathogens and debride devitalized tissue. After a few days, neutrophils begin to undergo cell death and are replaced by macrophages that are either resident or recruited from circulating monocytes in response to proinflammatory cytokines and chemotactic gradients. Activated macrophages are thought to play an integral part in coordinating the wound response by providing matrix remodeling capabilities (uPA, MMP9), synthesis of growth factors (fibroblast growth factor [FGF], PDGF, transforming growth factor beta [TGF-β]), and production of angiogenesis factors (VEGF). These factors activate fibroblasts to synthesize new ECM and promote neovascularization in the formation of granulation tissue. Other cells that are important in wound healing include mesenchymal stem cells.[23] These fibroblastoid-like cells can be mobilized from the bone marrow or from niches within various tissues in order to aid wound healing by differentiating into different connective tissue cell types.

Cancer cells are often surrounded by activated fibroblasts and BMDCs. Because of the resemblances between primary tumors and normal tissue wound response, cancer has been described as a "wound that does not heal." Although Virchow hypothesized in the 1850s that inflammation was the cause of cancer, the presence of an inflammatory response has generally been interpreted as evidence that the immune system actively fights the cancer as it does with invading bacterial or viral pathogens. Under this scenario, the inflammatory response would apply significant selective pressure on the tumor to evade immune-mediated attack, and the nonhealing nature of the response suggests a back-and-forth struggle. Tumors that progress do so by orchestrating an immunosuppressive environment, a process known as *immunoediting*.[24]

To facilitate an immunosuppressive environment, the tumor microenvironment selects for cells that favor production of immunomodulatory factors like TGF-β, cycoloxygenase-2 (COX2), CSF-1 (macrophage growth factor, colony-stimulating factor-1), IL-10, and IL-6. These cytokines inhibit maturation of dendritic cells and promote tumor-associated macrophages (TAMs) that are immunosupressed.[25] Tumors also recruit BMDCs that have immunosuppressive properties such as myeloid-derived suppressor cells (MDSCs).[26] These cells are recruited through signaling events that involve stromal cell-derived factor-1 (SDF-1, also known as CXCL12) and its ligand CXCR4 and CXCL5/CXCR2, another chemokine/receptor pair. On arrival, the MDSCs increase local production of TGF-β, block T-lymphocyte function, and inhibit the activation of NK cells.[27] Thus, although the inflammatory response undoubtedly can help to limit cancer growth, cancers seem to select for cells that create immunosuppressive surroundings.

Rather than simply suppress the inflammatory response, cancer cells actually develop mechanisms to both co-opt and perpetuate it. For example, at the same time MDSCs are contributing to immunosuppression, these cells also facilitate tumor invasion by residing at the invasive front and secreting MMPs. The comingling of various stromal cells and other BMDCs with the cancer also actively contributes to tumor growth in a similar

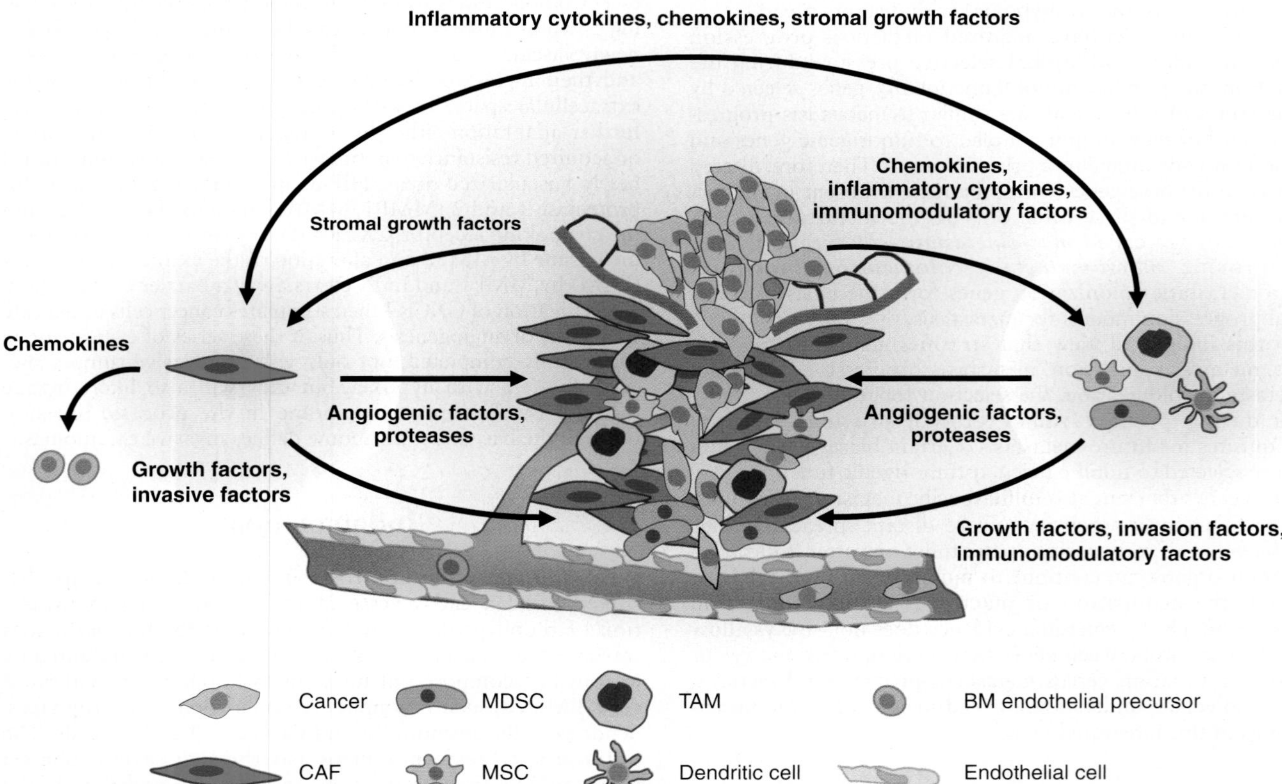

FIGURE 10.2 Interactions between cancer and stroma that promote invasion and metastasis. Cancerized stroma consists of fibroblasts, inflammatory cells, and other bone marrow-derived cells that have been conscripted to aid the tumor in overcoming hypoxia and in invasion and migration. Tissue breakdown, hypoxia, and inflammatory cytokines and chemokines secreted by the tumor cells result in recruitment of tumor-associated macrophages (TAMs), carcinoma-associated fibroblasts (CAFs), mesenchymal stem cells (MSCs), and myeloid-derived suppressor cells (MDSCs). TAMs and MDSCs can be found at points of basement membrane breakdown and at the invasive front of the tumor. These cells produce angiogenic factors to promote vascularization, proteases to degrade the extracellular matrix, and growth factors that stimulate tumor invasion and motility. CAFs also produce similar angiogenic factors, protease, and tumor growth factors. In addition, CAFs recruit bone marrow-derived endothelial precursors for angiogenesis. The cytokines and growth factors that TAMs and CAFs secrete are mutually beneficial to each other as part of an inflammatory/woundlike response. Cancers have been described as "wounds that do not heal." This chronic state is maintained by immunomodulatory cytokines that suppress immune functions to ensure a protumorigenic environment.

fashion. For example, TAMs are often found at points of basement membrane breakdown and, like MDSCs, end up at the invasive front to help tumors degrade extracellular proteins using uPA and MMPs or stimulate tumor growth and motility through EGF receptor ligands and PDGF. As in normal wound healing, growth factors secreted by the TAMs activate fibroblasts. These activated fibroblasts become carcinoma-associated fibroblasts (CAFs) and promote primary tumor growth by secreting CXCL12 to stimulate CXCR4 on tumor cells. Angiogenesis is also aided by the action of CAFs through recruitment of endothelial progenitor cells by CXCL12 and by the action of TAMs that are recruited to areas of hypoxia to produce VEGF. Figure 10.2 presents a summary of this interaction. Thus, although the question of whether the immune system is a friend or foe of malignancies is not a new one, it would seem that recent answers suggest that cancers actually find ways to turn an enemy into an accomplice.

Escaping Apoptosis and Senescence

A major mechanism to safeguard against a breakdown in tissue homeostasis due to cells that stray, become damaged, or spent, is to have these cells commit programmed cell death, or apoptosis.[28] This form of cell suicide is genetically regulated and can be triggered by a variety of signal transduction pathways linked to proteins that monitor environmental cues or act as damage sensors. Common cell intrinsic triggers for apoptosis include oncogene activation or tumor suppressor gene loss. For example, the inappropriate activation of c-MYC or the loss of Rb results in programmed cell death that must be countered by overexpression of antiapoptosis genes such as *Bcl-2* or loss of proapoptotic regulators like *p53*.[29] Extrinsic triggers for apoptosis include hypoxia, low pH, reactive oxygen species, loss of cell contact, and immune-mediated killing. Members of the TNF-receptor family can act as death receptors that mediate activation of proapoptotic proteases called *caspases* in response to loss of ECM adhesion[30] or after being engaged by immune cells for elimination. Cancer cells invariably ignore these cues, and their ability to resist cell death likely contributes to successful establishment of tumors.

In addition to apoptosis, senescence is another important barrier to cancer. This exit from the pool of proliferating cells results from telomere erosion, oncogene induction, and DNA damage. Similar to some forms of apoptosis, senescence is *p53*-dependent. Thus, pressure to escape senescence can result in the loss of *p53* or mutations in *p53*.

Self-Renewal Ability

Normal tissues result from the differentiation of precursor cells called *stem cells*, which are multipotent cells with self-renewal ability. In the adult, mature differentiated cells serve specialized tasks and have limited proliferative potential. However, adult tissue still undergoes turnover and is maintained through the self-renewal and multilineage differentiation of adult stem cells. Examples of this include skin, mucosa, and hematopoietic cells whereby a limited and spatially restricted pool of adult stem cells asymmetrically divides. One daughter cell maintains the stem cell pool by self-renewal, and the other daughter cell starts the process of terminal differentiation for tissue maintenance. The majority of cancers maintain some resemblance to their tissue of origin by virtue of persistent differentiation, albeit in an abnormal way. Thus, many cells in a tumor population may have limited proliferative potential and be incapable of sustained self-renewal, similar to their normal counterparts. The idea that only a limited subset of cells in a cancer is capable of self-renewal is called the *cancer stem cell hypothesis*.

The existence of cancer stem cells was first demonstrated in acute myeloid leukemia and recently shown in breast cancer, glioblastoma, and other cancer types.[31] These studies use cell surface markers to enrich for putative stem cell populations. In the case of breast cancer, $CD44^{high}/CD24^{low}$ cells were found to form tumors when injected into immunocompromised mice in low numbers and give rise to a diverse population that contained additional $CD44^{high}/CD24^{low}$ cells. In contrast, the injection of thousands of cells from other populations was nontumorigenic. Thus, the need for cancer cells to acquire self-renewal ability is paramount to the productive growth of the tumor. In principal, however, there is no advantage for cancer to keep this subpopulation of tumor-initiating cells small or fixed. Thus, tumors may contain a large proportion of cells with a tumor-perpetuating stem phenotype,[32] and this phenotype may be subject to back-and-forth reprogramming.

COUPLING TUMORIGENESIS WITH METASTASIS INITIATION

The selective pressures previously described that are encountered during primary tumor growth—hypoxia, inflammation, apoptosis, senescence, and need for proliferative, metabolic, and self-renewal sufficiency—drive primary tumors to acquire tumorigenic alterations that support aggressive growth. These same pressures collaterally support the initial stems of metastasis, and remain important throughout the subsequent malignant steps. One of the most striking types of metastasis initiation functions is EMT.

Selecting for Epithelial-to-Mesenchymal Transition

During development, the generation of many adult tissues and organs results from a series of EMT events and the reverse process, a mesenchymal-to-epithelial transition (MET).[33] For example, gastrulation and delamination of the neural crest are early developmental processes that layout the three germ layers (ectoderm, mesoderm, and endoderm) and give rise to diverse cell lineages (craniofacial cartilage and bone, smooth muscles, neurons, melanocytes), respectively. Both of these developmental events are characterized by epithelial cells loosening their cell-cell adhesion, losing cell polarity, and gaining the ability to invade and migrate under controlled cues. Important regulators include Notch and Wnt/β-catenin pathways, TGF-β family members, and FGF proteins that serve to set up regulatory networks involving EMT transcription factors such as Snail and Twist. These networks do not necessarily regulate cell fate, but rather drive morphogenetic movements by repression of the cell-cell adhesion protein E-cadherin, promoting cytoskeletal rearrangement, and increasing MMP activity. After cells complete EMT-mediated morphogenetic migration, they can then transiently differentiate into epithelial structures by repressing Snail and undergoing a MET. An example of cells that undergo a primary EMT that is followed by a MET includes neural crest cells giving rise to somites. These epithelial somites that have already experienced a primary EMT that is followed by a MET can then initiate a secondary EMT, which eventually results in development of muscle cells.

Growing evidence points toward EMT as an important characteristic of metastasis-prone cancers. EMT in cancer is not a concrete and tidy single process but rather a collection of cell reprogramming phenomena that share the property of down-regulating epithelial cell markers and, for convenience, the collective denomination of EMT. Hypoxia can induce Snail and Twist, a direct target of HIF-1α.[34] Low oxygen enhances β-catenin activity by inhibiting the activity of glycogen synthase kinase-3β, which normally induces the destruction of β-catenin. Accordingly, the presence of enhanced β-catenin signaling promotes Snail expression and subsequent EMT. Interestingly, the ability of hypoxia to liberate active β-catenin may set in place a feed-forward loop to help maintain EMT. Activation of Snail represses E-cadherin, which can then further enhance β-catenin and reinforce Snail expression.

Similar to hypoxia, the inflammatory microenvironment can also promote EMT. It has recently been demonstrated that TNF-α, which is an inflammatory mediator secreted by TAMs, sets into motion a signaling cascade that funnels through NF-κB and glycogen synthase kinase-3β to stabilize Snail and β-catenin, and thus, enhances cancer cell migration.[35] This ability of cancer cells to awaken an EMT program by co-opting an inflammatory microenvironment may be further reinforced by EMT itself. Snail-induced EMT is able to generate an environment of immunosuppressive T-regulatory cells and impaired dendritic cells partly through TGF-β and thrombospondin-1, helping to further perpetuate the inflammatory surroundings.[36]

Besides hypoxia and inflammation, the need for primary cancers to resist apoptosis and overcome senescence may be additional reasons to flip an EMT switch. Cells that have undergone EMT are associated with increased resistance to apoptosis, possibly through prosurvival activity conferred by Snail and Twist.[37,38] EMT can also help cancer overcome oncogene-induced senescence. Both Twist transcription factors and ZEB1 have been shown to suppress $p21^{cip1}$ and/or $p16^{ink4a}$, two p53-regulated cell cycle proteins that are critical in restraining oncogene-transformed cells via senescence.[39] These findings suggest that the pressure to resist apoptosis and bypass senescence can result in activation of EMT transcriptional regulators.

Acquiring the ability to sustain long-term self-renewal would provide an enormous advantage to cells in a growing tumor mass. Recent data suggest that selection for cells that are capable of undergoing EMT may provide a pool of cells with stemlike features.[40] Stem cell-enriched subpopulations with a $CD44^{high}/CD24^{low}$ cell surface marker profile have significantly higher levels of many EMT-related transcription factors, such as Snail and Twist, when compared with their $CD44^{low}/CD24^{high}$ counterparts. Furthermore, these EMT transcription factors are able to directly increase the number of cells with stemlike characteristics. Although it remains to be determined whether EMT is occurring in cancer stem cells or whether EMT occurs in non–self-renewing cells that then give them stemlike properties, these data argue for a another compelling reason for cancer cells to acquire EMT properties.

Epithelial-to-Mesenchymal Transition in Metastasis Initiation

Although the ability to awaken an EMT program would seem to offer numerous advantages for cells trying to expand within a primary tumor, it is not clear that primary tumor growth and invasion requires EMT. In fact, EMT-independent mechanisms have been shown to operate and allow carcinomas to invade and migrate at invasive fronts.[41] Despite this, mounting evidence suggests that for cancer cells that do satisfy tumorigenic functions with expression of EMT genes, these cells are also endowed with metastasis initiation functions. Early evidence that EMT genes can be dispensable for primary tumor growth but essential for metastasis has come from analyses of Twist.[42] In a breast cancer model, inhibition of Twist was shown to have no effect on primary tumor growth but potently reduced the number of metastatic lesions in the lung. Consistent with these findings, inhibiting Twist in either hypoxic cells or in cells overexpressing HIF-1α reversed both EMT and metastasis,[34] and inhibiting Snail decreased metastasis induced by inflammatory signals.[35] In total, these observations suggest that when imposing forces like hypoxia and inflammation select for cells capable of EMT, EMT genes become important in metastasis.

What makes EMT cells particularly adept at initiating early metastatic events? A careful analysis of the effect of Twist on metastasis revealed a role for Twist in establishing high levels of circulating tumor cells through enhancing intravasation and/or survival in the circulation.[42] The ability of cells undergoing EMT to intravasate is consistent with observations that EMT occurs at the invasive front of tumors whereby cells lose E-cadherin, detach, invade, and break down the basement membrane. Accordingly, experiments that directly analyzed EMT and non-EMT cells showed that only the EMT cells were able to penetrate surrounding stroma and intravasate.[43]

Another reason that EMT can make cells susceptible to distant spread may be related to the ability of EMT to confer stemlike properties. For the same reasons that primary tumors may rely on cancer stemlike cells for continued self-renewal, metastasis formation may also rely on cancer stemlike cells. Using pancreatic cancer models, it has been shown that a distinct subpopulation of $CD133^+/CXCR4^+$ cells localizes to the invasive edge of tumors and is more migratory than $CD133^+/CXCR4^-$ cells.[44] Interestingly, although both populations were equally capable of instigating primary tumor growth, only the $CD133^+/CXCR4^+$ cells could metastasize to the liver. Targeting CXCR4 either through depletion or pharmacologic targeting interfered with spontaneous metastasis formation. In breast cancer patients, $CD44^{high}/CD24^{low}$ cells, which are increased by EMT and express EMT markers, display stemlike properties and can be enriched both in the circulation and in the bone marrow.[45] Thus, EMT may play a role in metastasis initiation by ensuring that distant outgrowths are maintained with a pool of stemlike cells.

Prevalence of Primary Tumors with Metastasis-Initiation Functions and Early Dissemination

Considering that EMT can be selected by hypoxia and inflammation, resulting in invasive cancer cells that can intravasate and self-renew, one expectation might be that primary tumors can acquire metastasis-initiation functions early during tumorigenesis because EMT is acquired early. Indeed, recent evidence suggests that initial steps in metastasis can frequently occur far earlier than previously thought. By using transgenic mouse models of breast cancer, it has been shown that disseminated tumor cells (DTCs) can be found in bone marrow and lung tissue even before morphologic evidence of primary tumor invasion.[46,47] Closer inspection with electron microscopy reveals individual tumor cells from preinvasive atypical hyperplastic lesions breaching the basement membrane. Furthermore, preinvasive lesions also displayed high levels of Twist and MMP expression. These early DTCs progressed in parallel with the primary tumor and could give rise to metastatic lesions. Such experimental observations are consistent with clinical findings that patients with preinvasive DCIS also have cytokeratin-positive tumor cells in the bone marrow, as do a significant fraction of patients with early-stage breast cancers. However, despite these findings, patients with DCIS rarely develop metastasis, which highlights that metastasis-initiation functions are not sufficient to complete the metastatic cascade and indicates the need for metastasis-progression and macrometastatic-colonization genes.

COUPLING TUMORIGENESIS WITH METASTASIS PROGRESSION

The selection of genes that primarily fulfill tumorigenic functions may also result in genes that secondarily aid cancer cells after they have found their way into the circulation. In other words, when genes are selected to help the primary tumor grow, some of these genes have a collateral effect of benefiting the cancer after it disseminates by providing metastasis-specific tools. Such genes can be classified as metastasis-progression genes; however, a clear distinction with metastasis-initiation genes may not always be evident. In this section, we describe functions that can be classified as metastasis-progression functions.

Premetastatic Niche

Even before tumor cells colonize distant organs, they can help prepare foreign soil for the subsequent arrival of DTCs by remotely coordinating a "premetastatic niche" from the primary tumor.[48] These niches are often located within distant organs around terminal veins and are characterized by newly recruited hematopoietic progenitor cells of the myeloid lineage and by stromal cells. This niche provides an array of cytokines, growth factors, and adhesion molecules to help support metastatic cells on their arrival.

The remote coordination of the premetastatic niche by the primary tumor appears to be through cytokines and growth factors associated with the inflammatory and hypoxic microenvironment of the primary cancer. Through the secretion of cytokine profiles that include VEGF and placental growth factor, primary tumor cells can direct VEGFR1$^+$ myeloid cells to mobilize from the bone marrow and preferentially localize to areas in target organs with increased fibronectin.[49] If the primary tumor secretes VEGF, this promotes fibronectin deposition in the lung and directs the construction of the premetastatic niche there, while the combination of VEGF and placental growth factor leads to a more widespread pattern of niche assembly. Similarly, VEGF, TGF-β, and TNF-α produced at the primary tumor site can signal production of inflammatory proteins like S100A8 and S100A9 specifically within the lung parenchyma.[50,51] This results in the infiltration of myeloid cells into the lung and subsequent formation of the niche. Besides inflammatory signals from the primary tumor, LOX produced by a hypoxic primary tumor environment can also direct formation of a premetastatic niche.[52]

Once myeloid and activated stromal cells form the premetastatic niche, the local environment in the distant organ is altered by the production of inflammatory cytokines and MMPs, which begins bearing an evolving resemblance to the primary site. Consequently, when primary tumor cells start wandering in the circulation, the target organs with an established premetastatic niche become a better soil in which to attach, survive, and grow. Indeed, if the formation of the niche is disrupted, metastasis is inhibited. In this way, the shower of cytokines and growth factors that accompany inflammatory and hypoxic responses at the primary tumor not only selects for cancer cells that can flourish in the primary site but has the secondary effect of creating a more welcoming environment in distant organs after dissemination. Such a scenario would argue that the mechanism of premetastatic niche formation has properties consistent with metastasis-progression functions.

Survival in the Circulation

From experimental model systems, it has been estimated that approximately one million cancer cells per gram of tumor tissue can be introduced daily into the circulation.[53] Direct inoculation of tumor cells into mice demonstrates that metastasis can be an inefficient process because despite large numbers of circulating tumor cells (CTCs), relatively few metastases form.[8] In humans, the inefficiency of CTCs to give rise to detectable metastases was inadvertently demonstrated in ovarian cancer patients who received peritoneal-venous shunts for palliation of malignant ascites.[54] Despite the re-routing of millions of cancer cells from the peritoneum to the venous circulation, for years in some cases, the majority of the patients did not develop widespread metastases. Thus, even if cancer cells acquire metastasis-initiation functions like EMT, the ability to merely enter into the circulation often is not a rate-limiting step in metastasis. Other obstacles must be overcome.

After intravasation into the circulation from the primary tumor, tumor cells encounter significant physical stress due to shear forces or mechanical arrest in small-diameter vessels. The hepatic sinusoids can be activated by the mechanical restriction of tumor cells to secrete nitric oxide. Nitric oxide can cause apoptosis of arrested tumor cells and has been shown to be required for the massive cell death of experimentally injected melanoma cells.[55] Endothelial cells can also guard against wandering tumor cells through expression of DARC, a Duffy blood group glycoprotein.[56] DARC interacts with *KAI1* expressed on circulating tumor cells causing them to undergo senescence. *KAI1* was originally identified as a metastasis suppressor gene. The immune system can also actively attack circulating tumor cells.[57] For example, NK cells can engage and kill cancer cells via TNF-related molecules such as TRAIL or CD95L. In total, these mechanical and cell-mediated stresses can result in a short half-life for CTCs. Estimations derived from the enumeration of CTCs before and after removal of the primary tumor in patients with localized breast cancer demonstrate that the half-life can be as short as a few hours.[58]

How can CTCs evade cell death to enhance their metastatic potential? Growth at the primary tumor site will involve a selection for increased resistance to apoptosis. Antiapoptosis genes such as *BCL2* or $BCL\text{-}X_L$, or the loss of proapoptotic genes and genes downstream of the TNF-related receptor family, can result in increased metastasis.[59,60] Part of this may be the result of survival both in the circulation and shortly after extravasation. Both CTCs and platelets can also express the $\alpha v\beta 3$ integrin to promote aggregation of these cells to form tumor emoboli.[61] This aggregation not only facilitates arrest but can protect against shear forces and NK cell-mediated killing. Activation of $\alpha v\beta 3$ can result from CXCL12/CXCR4 signaling and has been shown to be required for formation of tumor emboli and metastasis.[62,63] Thus, the ability of a primary tumor to respond to apoptosis, senescence, and inflammatory signals can secondarily make cancer cells better able to survive in the circulation once metastasis has been initiated.

Extravasation and Colonization

After arresting in capillaries, tumor cells that are able to survive can grow intravascularly. This can lead to a physical disruption of the vessels.[64] However, more selective processes of extravasation exist. Cancer cells can mimic leukocytes and bind to endothelial E- and P-selectins.[65] Molecular mediators of extravasation include the cytoskeletal anchoring protein Ezrin, which links the cell membrane to the actin cytoskeleton and engages the cell with its microenvironment. Ezrin was discovered to promote metastasis in osteosarcoma by preventing cell death during migration into the lung.[66] VEGF expression by the tumor can also lead to disruptions in endothelial cell junctions and facilitate extravasation of cancer cells through enhanced vascular permeability. This is likely mediated by the activation of SRC family kinases in the endothelial cells, which is consistent with decreased lung metastasis in SRC nullizygous mice.[67] Expression of hypoxia-induced CXCR4 on CTCs allows for the selective extravasation into certain organs. This selectivity is due to the expression of its ligand CXCL12 by certain organs that include the lung, liver, bone, and lymph nodes.[68] Thus, the selection to successfully deal with hypoxia during primary tumor growth may bias the pattern of distant spread through the CXCR4-CXCL12 pathway.

The steps of extravasation and establishment of micrometastases help to illustrate a more concrete example of the concept of metastasis-progression genes. Using a mouse model system for breast cancer metastasis, a gene expression signature for aggressive lung metastasis was discovered that not only mediated experimental lung metastasis but was also expressed by primary human breast cancers with increased risk of metastasis selectively to the lung.[17] Four members of this lung metastasis gene expression signature (LMS), namely *EREG* (an EGF receptor ligand), *MMP1*, *MMP2*, and *COX2*, were selected during primary tumor growth and conferred a growth advantage by facilitating the assembly of new blood vessels.[16] The vascular remodeling program coordinated by these four genes was also critical to the extravasation of circulating breast cancer cells into the lung parenchyma, as its inhibition resulted in the intravascular entrapment of single cells. Another LMS gene that is a mediator of lung extravasation is the cytokine angiopoietin-like 4 (*ANGPTL4*).[69] *ANGPTL4* promotes the dissociation of endothelial cell-cell junctions and, consistent with it being a metastasis-progression gene, *ANGPTL4* is induced by TFG-β produced in the primary tumor microenvironment. The combined examples of VEGF, CXCR4, and several LMS genes illustrate how metastasis-progression genes can arise during primary tumor growth through the acquisition of genes that can cope with or respond to selective pressures at the primary site.

Cancer cells that have initiated the metastatic cascade can also epigenetically acquire metastasis-progression functions through paracrine factors secreted by the microenvironment of primary tumors. Mesenchymal stem cells recruited to the inflammatory stroma of a primary tumor have been shown in a xenograft model to produce CCL5 as a result of heterotypic interaction with neighboring breast cancer.[70] CCL5 can then act in a paracrine fashion to enhance motility, invasion, and extravasation into the lung. Accordingly, the prometastatic effects mediated by CCL5 were reversible when interactions with MSCs were removed. Thus, metastasis-progression functions acquired through events that occur in the primary tumor need not be accompanied by somatic changes in metastasis-progression genes.

Tumor Self-Seeding

As cancer cells selected by the inflammatory and hypoxic surroundings of the primary tumor wander through the circulation, might the most hospitable and likely destination for extravasation be the primary tumor from which they came? At least in theory, it would seem that compared with uncharted foreign environments or even premetastatic niches, the primary tumor would impose the least resistance to colonization.[71] Support for this concept of tumor self-seeding has recently been provided using mouse model systems and a variety of different cancer types by demonstrating that CTCs can seed the primary tumor and contribute to its mass.[72] The ability to self-seed is promoted by IL-6 and IL-8, common prometastatic cytokines found in the tumor microenvironment. The cancer cell expression of *MMP1* and Fascin-1, two previously identified lung metastasis genes, facilitates transendothelial migration and tumor self-seeding. In fact, metastatic cells in general are more efficient seeders, which may result from a direct cause and effect. Subpopulations of cancer cells selected to be efficient seeders can express an array of multiorgan metastasis genes. These observations suggest that disseminated cells capable of successfully navigating a round-trip rather than a one-way excursion help the primary tumor select for cells with metastatic functions.

FROM METASTASIS PROGRESSION TO MACROMETASTATIC COLONIZATION

Because metastasis-initiation functions and metastasis-progression functions are coupled to tumorigenic functions, the accumulating evidence that primary tumors can exhibit metastatic traits early on during primary tumorigenesis and with such high prevalence may not be surprising. However, despite the ability of EMT to drive invasion, intravasation, and self-renewal, and despite the remote influence the primary tumor has on survival in the circulation, extravasation, and premetastatic niche formation, the completion of the metastatic cascade is still relatively infrequent for many cancer types. This suggests an important requirement for macrometastatic colonization functions, or functions selected at distant sites for organ-specific colonization.

Dormancy

A major limiting step in metastasis is acquiring the ability to sustain growth within a distant site after extravasation. Many cancers such as breast and prostate will not give rise to metastasis until years or even decades after eradication of the primary tumor. Clinically, there is also a clear discrepancy between the proportion of patients with preinvasive or early-stage cancers that have cytokeratin-positive cells in the bone marrow and the proportion that develop overt metastasis. Experimentally, it has been shown that the vast majority of extravasated cancer cells do not form macrometastasis.[8] In aggregate, these observations of latency are referred to as *metastatic dormancy* and point toward the bottleneck that forms prior to outgrowth of macrometastasis.

A distinction has been made between tumor mass dormancy, which describes the process that inhibits expansion of a dividing tumor population, and cellular dormancy, which describes when cancer cells enter a state of growth arrest.[73] Tumor mass dormancy has been attributed to the existence of preangiogenic micrometastasis in which cell division is balanced by apoptosis.[74] Clinical evidence for this comes from one study whereby breast cancer patients with no evidence of disease years after mastectomy and considered candidates for having metastatic dormancy were shown to have detectable CTCs.[58] Later acquisition of angiogenic properties may allow such micrometastases to become vascularized and emerge from their occult state. Work with experimental models suggests that indolent metastasis may also be activated by coexisting with more aggressive metastasis secrete systemic factors like osteopontin (OPN).[75] Mechanisms that contribute to cellular dormancy may relate to the balance between the RAF-MEK-ERK pathway and the p38 MAPK pathway. Inhibition of the former and activation of the latter is associated with cellular quiescence in a G0-G1 state, and the exact balance between the two may depend on cross-talk between the tumor and the new microenvironment. Genes that may be important in blocking productive cross-talk between dormant metastasis and its microenvironment include metastasis suppressor genes such as *NME23*, *MKK4*, and *RKIP*, to name a few.[73,76] This functional class of genes specifically prevents growth of metastasis without influencing primary tumor growth.

Regardless of the nature of the dormancy, dormant cells must acquire genetic or epigenetic changes during residency at foreign sites in order to evolve into gross metastases. Tumor cells that are detected in the bone marrow and likely disseminated from the primary tumor at an early stage during tumorigenesis have been shown to undergo a separate evolution under separate selective pressures. Comparative genomic hybridizations of single breast cancer cells isolated from bone marrow were shown to be genetically heterogeneous in patients without overt metastasis.[77,78] These cells also showed few genetic features in common with matched primary tumors. In contrast, bone marrow-derived breast cancer cells from patients with overt metastatic disease displayed a marked reduction in genetic heterogeneity compared with patients with occult disease. These results are consistent with disseminated tumor cells departing from the primary tumor early on and being driven by different selective pressures found in the distant organ. Different metastatic sites that host dormant cells likely contribute unique selective pressures. This paves the way for the acquisition of macrometastatic colonization functions.

Organ Selective Growth

Bone

Homeostasis of the bone is maintained by a constant state of remodeling such that no net gain or loss of bone occurs. The mineralized bone matrix is reabsorbed by osteoclasts and filled in by osteoblasts. The differentiation of osteoclasts from bone marrow mononuclear cells is controlled by CSF-1 and the RANK receptor (reviewed in refs. 79 and 80). RANK interacts with its ligand RANKL produced by osteoblasts, leading to a tight coupling of these two cells with opposing actions. The activity of RANKL can also be controlled by osteoprotegerin (OPG). OPG is a secreted antagonist of RANKL and prevents interaction with RANK and resulting osteoclastogenesis. The differentiation of osteoblasts results from bone marrow mesenchymal stem cells under the control of a variety of regulators including insulin-like growth factor (IGF), endothelin-1, bone morphogenetic proteins, and WNT proteins.

The bone is one of the most common sites of distant spread. However, the latency period that precedes the development of gross osseous metastasis can be years, as illustrated by the high proportion of breast cancer patients with dormant cancer cells in the bone marrow. One factor that provides the ability to sustain this latency period is the SRC kinase, which is required for CXCL12- and IGF-mediated survival signals that protect indolent breast cancer cells in the bone marrow from TRAIL-mediated apoptosis.[81] Presumably, the sustained survival and dormancy afforded by SRC would allow time for the acquisition of bone-specific macrometastatic colonization genes.

When the dormancy period expires, gross osseous metastases are characterized by two basic types: osteoblastic and osteolytic. Many tumors such as lung, kidney, and breast carcinomas typically produce osteolytic lesions. Breast cancer cells achieve osteolytic metastasis competency by secreting factors including parathyroid hormone-related protein (PTHrP), TNF-α, IL-1, IL-6, IL-8, and IL-11 in order to orchestrate a vicious cycle of enhanced osteoclast activation, degradation of bone matrix, and the release of matrix-associated cytokines that stimulate the cancer cells[79,80] (Fig. 10.3). The secretion of PTHrP leads to the production of the membrane-bound RANKL on osteoblasts, resulting in RANK-mediated osteoclast activation. Other proinflammatory cytokines such as TNF-α, IL-1, IL-6, and IL-11 that are secreted by the tumor cell can lead to a synergistic effect on RANK-mediated signaling and may also inhibit production of OPG. Interestingly, RANK is also expressed on cancer cells and stimulates migratory activity.[82] On degradation of the bone matrix, embedded growth factors are released, including TGF-β and IGF. These liberated growth factors can further stimulate the tumor cells and enhance the entire vicious cycle.

A genomewide screen for genes involved in breast cancer bone metastasis uncovered IL-11, MMP1, ADAMTS1, CXCR4, connective tissue growth factor (CTGF), and OPN as mediators of osteolytic bone metastasis.[83] CXCR4 may enhance colonization of breast cancer cells to bone, MMP1 and ADAMTS1 proteolytically activate EGF receptor ligands,[84] and OPN and IL-11 may promote osteoclast differentiation. The expression of IL-11, CTGF, and PTHrP in breast cancer cells are targets for TGF-β, which is released by the bone matrix.[85] In total, these experimental data illustrate how tumor cells can survive and grow in the foreign environment of the bone by coercing resident cells to release secreted factors that are advantageous to the tumor. This cooperative situation between tumor cells and bone marrow cells is similar to that in the primary tumor whereby BMDCs and stromal cells act as accomplices.

Unlike osteolytic bone metastasis, osteoblastic metastasis is less common and typified by prostate cancer. Osteoblastic lesions result from the preferential stimulation of osteoblasts and/or the inhibition of osteoclasts. Like breast and other cancers that cause osteolytic lesions, prostate cancer also hijacks homeostatic regulation of bone remodeling to its advantage (reviewed in ref. 86). Various paracrine factors secreted by prostate cancer cells can regulate osteoblast proliferation or differentiation, including bone morphogenetic proteins, WNT, TGF-β, IGF, PDGF, FGF, and VEGF. Many of these signals converge on activation of RUNX2, a transcription factor that is essential for bone formation. In turn, the osteoblasts produce factors that stimulate the proliferation of prostate cancer as demonstrated by coculture experiments with either osteoblasts or their conditioned media. The exact factors that drive progression of prostate cancer metastasis have not been firmly established. Nonetheless, these results support the paradigm that a reciprocal relationship exists between the cancer cell and the cells of the microenvironment that contribute to bone-selective metastasis.

Lung

Lung is a common site of metastasis for many different cancers. Experimentally, colonization and growth in animal lungs has been used extensively to study metastasis and invasion by the direct inoculation of tumor cells into the venous circulation. With this method, the lung is the first organ encountered and may be the only organ encountered because of entrapment of tumor cells by the lung capillary bed. Although the list of genes that can contribute to enhanced experimental lung metastasis studied in this way is extensive, it can be difficult to know whether the genes are regulating a generic invasion pathway or contributing to organ-specific growth.

In a study seeking to gain insight into organ-selective metastasis genes, single cell-derived clones from a human breast cancer cell line were discovered to exhibit varying degrees of metastatic ability to the bone and to the lung.[87] Although there was no correlation between clones that metastasized well to the lung and those that metastasized effectively to the bone, metastatic tissue tropism did correlate with similarities in global gene expression patterns among the clones. These observations lead to the discovery of an LMS.[17] Several of these genes (some have already been discussed) were shown to cooperatively mediate experimental lung metastasis and consisted of secreted factors (*EREG, CXCL1, ANGPTL4,* and *SPARC*), cell surface receptors (*VCAM1* and *IL13R*α*2*), extracellular matrix protein (*TNC*) and proteases (*MMP1* and *MMP2*), and intracellular effectors (*ID1, Fascin-1,* and *COX2*). Although these genes mediated lung metastasis, they

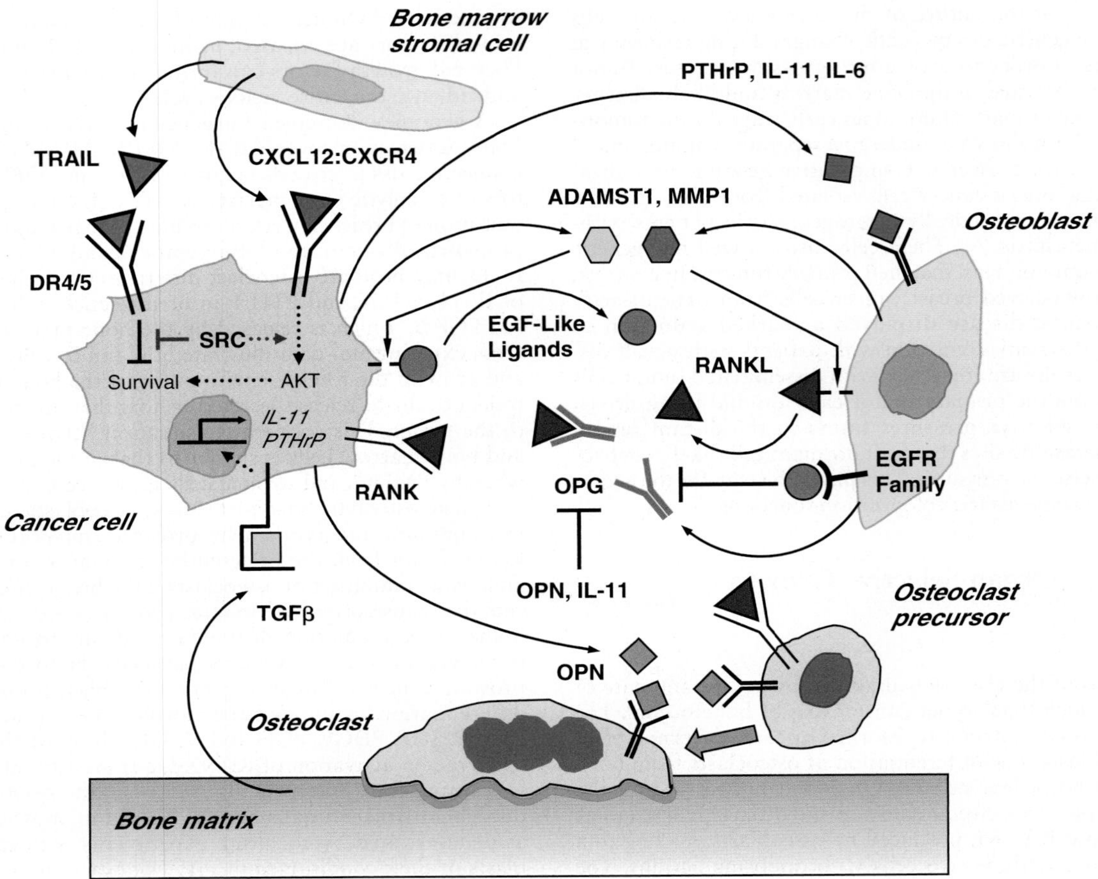

FIGURE 10.3 Interactions between cancer and the bone microenvironment lead to a "vicious cycle." Cancer cells can migrate to the bone microenvironment under the influence of CXCL12 (*blue triangle*), which also leads to cell activation and migration via its receptor CXCR4. The CXCL12:CXCR4 interaction promotes survival of metastatic cancer cells through AKT and SRC by counteracting proapoptotic stimuli directed by TRAIL (*red triangles*) and its receptor DR4/5. Survival can lead to dormancy, utilization of acquired metastasis-progression functions, and opportunities to accumulate additional macrometastatic-colonization genes. Surviving metastatic cells secretes factors such as PTHrP, IL-11, and IL-6 (*green squares*) that lead to production of membrane-bound RANKL (*brown triangles*) on osteoblasts. Tumor cell secretion of MMP1 (*red hexagon*) and ADAMST1 (*yellow hexagon*) can mobilize RANKL from osteoblasts and EGF-like ligands (*magenta circles*) from tumor cells. RANKL:RANK interaction stimulates tumor cells and promotes osteoclast differentiation and activation. RANKL can be antagonized by the decoy receptor osteoprotegerin, or OPG (*red-colored receptor*), that is normally produced by osteoblasts. Engagement of EGF receptor family members can inhibit OPG expression and thereby promote osteoclast activation and metastatic growth. Other tumor-derived factors like osteopontin, or OPN (*orange squares*), also promote osteoclast activation. Activation of osteoclasts leads to degradation of the bone matrix and release of TGF-β (*yellow square*). This further stimulates the tumor cells to transcriptionally activate genes such as *IL-11* and *PTHrP*, which contributes to the vicious cycle.

did not enhance bone metastasis and were largely distinct from a previously defined bone metastasis gene expression signature from the same cell line.

Many of the LMS genes are also expressed in a subset of primary human breast cancers. These patients with LMS-expressing tumors are at a higher risk for lung metastasis but not metastasis to bone or various other visceral sites.[17,88] In addition, LMS-expressing tumors are larger at the time of diagnosis compared with LMS-negative tumors, which is consistent with experimental data showing that LMS genes were selected for during growth in the mouse mammary gland. Mechanistically, the coupling of tumorigenic function and metastatic function is provided by the LMS genes *EREG, COX2, MMP1,* and *MMP2.* As described already, these genes are prototypical metastasis-progression genes in that they assist the primary tumor by promoting the assembly of new blood vessels.[16] However, as part of the metastatic cascade, these genes and other LMS genes enhance lung metastasis by promoting extravasation and by priming departing cancer cells for the lung parenchyma.[69,89] Some of the LMS genes such as *IL13Rα2* and *SPARC* do not enhance primary tumor growth and are not among the LMS genes expressed by primary tumors that track with lung metastasis; however, these genes do promote lung metastasis, making them macrometastatic-colonization genes that may be selected during residence away from the primary site.

Liver

The liver is supplied by both the portal and the systemic circulations. Metastasis to the liver is commonly seen with colorectal cancer and this bias is likely favored by the portal circulation for this organ. Metastasis from other cancers such as melanoma and breast and lung carcinomas generally occurs via the systemic circulation. Besides the bias for liver metastasis from the portal circulation, there is evidence that the microenvironment of the liver may be particularly favorable for metastasis from gastrointestinal tumors. Extracellular matrix extracted from primary rat hepatocytes was found to stimulate colorectal cancer cell lines better than ECM from fibroblasts.[90] Furthermore, CAFs isolated from metastatic colon cancer to the liver were found to secrete factors that enhance proliferation of colon cancer to a greater extent than the conditioned media from fibroblasts isolated from uninvolved liver or skin.[91] DNA microarray analysis demonstrated that the CAFs were more genetically similar than uninvolved fibroblasts and preferentially expressed genes associated in ECM remodeling (proteoglycan 1), proteases/protease inhibitors (tissue plasminogen activator, tissue plasminogen activator inhibitor type 1), growth factors (PDGF, FGF, CTGF, VEGF, TGF-β2), cytokines (IL-6, MCP-1), and intracellular mediators like COX2. This alteration in the microenvironment as a potential contributor to liver metastasis was also demonstrated for hepatocellular carcinoma, which tends to recur with intrahepatic metastasis. By comparing noninvolved hepatic tissue from patients with and without metastasis, genes associated with inflammation and/or immune responses were found to be associated with a "metastasis-inclined microenvironment." A major difference was noted in the cytokine profile of the metastasis-inclined tissue, which was strongly biases to a T_H2 rather than a T_H1 cytokine profile.[92] The latter is associated with cytotoxic T-cell activity and the former is associated with a humoral immune response. These different cytokine milieus may be driven in part by high levels of CSF-1.

Besides local microenvironmental influences on liver metastasis, contributing signaling molecules expressed by cancer cells have also been implicated. In a screen for genes associated with colon cancer metastasis to the liver, the *PRL-3* tyrosine phosphatase was identified.[93] Experimentally, *PRL-3* can trigger angiogenesis and enhance invasion. Clinically, its expression is found in primary colorectal tumors and correlates with metastasis. It is unclear whether *PRL-3* selectively mediates metastasis to the liver, as its expression is also found in other distant organs to which colorectal cancer relapses.[94]

Brain

The principal sources of brain metastasis are lung and breast carcinomas. Melanoma, colorectal, and renal cell carcinomas also can relapse in the brain, whereas some cancer types like prostate cancer rarely do. The microenvironment of the brain is unique in the sense that vascular access is more restricted because of the blood–brain barrier. This barrier is composed of tightly adjoined endothelial cells that are lined by basal lamina and astrocyte foot processes. The blood–brain barrier is a special consideration for pharmacologic intervention, but to what extent it uniquely deters circulating tumor cells from colonizing the brain is unclear. Once in the parenchyma, microenvironmental interactions occur with glial cells. Coculture experiments demonstrate enhanced adhesion and growth when astrocytes are partnered with cell lines from brain metastasis compared with lung metastasis.[95] This may involve IL-6, TGF-β, and IGF-1. Melanoma cells that metastasize to the brain have high STAT3 transcriptional activity compared with cutaneous metastases or primary melanoma specimens.[96] Manipulation of STAT3 activity was able to alter brain metastasis in animal models. Altered STAT3 affects expression of basic FGF, VEGF, and MMP2, and influences melanoma angiogenesis and invasion. Because of the dearth of cross-comparison studies with other organs, the selectivity of these effects for brain metastasis is unclear. Indeed, STAT3 has also been associated with metastasis to other visceral organs.[97]

In order to identify specific mediators of brain metastasis, a mouse model for breast cancer was used that incorporated both established cell lines and patient-derived samples.[98] Several genes were found to mediate metastasis to the brain, including *COX2*, the EGFR ligand *HBEGF*, and the α2,6-sialyltransferase, *ST6GALNAC5*. Notably, some of the newly identified brain metastasis genes overlapped with previously identified lung metastasis genes, a finding that is consistent with the known propensity for patients to develop synchronous or metachronous metastases to both organs. Accordingly, passage through the nonfenestrated capillaries of the brain and lungs could be promoted by *COX2* and *HBEGF*. In contrast, the specificity of the gene signature for the brain could be attributed to *ST6GALNAC5* and other associated genes that normally have a brain-restricted expression pattern. *ST6GALNAC5* enhances the ability of breast cancer cells to pass through the blood–brain barrier, although the exact mechanism remains unknown. Patients who express the genes in the brain metastasis signature also have a higher risk of succumbing to brain metastasis.

Lymphatics

The physiological function of the lymphatic system is to collect extravasated fluid, proteins, and immune cells from draining organs in order to return them for transport by the circulation. Lymphatics are low shear force vessels composed of a single layer of endothelial cells with little or no basement membrane and sparsely coated with pericytes. Lymphangiogenesis involves VEGF-C, VEGF-D, and their receptor VEGFR-3 (reviewed in ref. 99). In contrast to angiogenesis mediators like VEGF-A that responds to both inflammation and hypoxia, VEGF-C/D expression is induced by inflammation but not hypoxia. For example, macrophages that respond to inflammatory signals are a rich source of VEGF-C/D. Thus, angiogenesis can occur without lymphangiogenesis but under most circumstances lymphatic vessels grow concomitantly with blood vessels. Other non-VEGF family members can also induce lymphangiogenesis and include FGF2, PDGF, and angiopoietin proteins.

Unlike with angiogenesis, the functional advantage for tumors that induce lymphangiogenesis is a matter of debate. Possibilities include lowering interstitial fluid pressure in the tumor to facilitate blood perfusion and combat hypoxia, or the growth of new lymphatics may facilitate mechanisms that contribute to angiogenesis.[100] Alternatively, lymphangiogenesis may coincidentally result from induction of angiogenesis and/or the involvement of immune cells. Part of this uncertainty results from questions regarding the degree to which intratumoral lymphatics are functional. Lymphatics can be found in a peritumoral location or reside intratumorally. Although proliferating intratumoral lymphatic vessels are observed in animal models and cancers of the head and neck and melanoma, they may collapse under high intratumoral pressure. At least one study revealed that these intratumoral lymphatics were not important in conducting metastasis, rather peritumoral lymphatics were the main route.[101] Nonetheless, mouse models have revealed that inducing lymphangiogenesis does lead to lymph node metastasis.[102,103] Once in the lymph nodes, lymphatic stromal cells are a source for EGF, IGF-1, and various chemokines.[104] Like the lung parenchyma and the bone marrow, lymph nodes secrete CXCL12, which can interact with tumor-expressing CXCR4.[68] Other chemokine receptors such as CXCR3 also play a role in lymph node metatasis.[105]

Metastasis to the regional lymph nodes is considered one of the early signs of metastatic potential and/or distant spread. A long-standing question has been whether lymphatic metastasis selects cells that have enhanced metastatic ability but has not yet spread to distant organs or whether lymph node involvement is a marker for a tumor that may have already become metastatic in general. Reasons for the former include the idea that some tumors can only intravasate into lymphatics but not directly into blood vessels because they cannot overcome higher molecular or physical barriers. Explanations for the latter include underlying molecular mechanisms that couple angiogenesis, lymphangiogenesis, and metastatic ability, resulting in synchronous dispersal. To distinguish between these possibilities, lymphangiogenesis was inhibited in a mouse model for lung cancer metastasis using a soluble VEGFR-3-immunoglobulin fusion protein that traps VEGF-C/D and inhibits VEGFR-3 signaling. This approach blocked lymph node metastasis but had no effect on lung metastasis.[106] However, in another study, blocking VEGFR-3 signaling with mammary tumors suppressed metastases to both lymph nodes and the lungs.[107] Most likely, lymphatic-dependent and -independent metastasis are both possible and dictated by underlying biological mediators and selective pressures. This would also most fit clinical data. Markers for lymphatic-dependent and -independent spread would be useful to guide whether regional lymph nodes should be addressed therapeutically or less aggressively for prognostic staging.

Early, Multiorgan Metastasis

Most cancers such as breast, prostate, and sarcoma, to name a few, demonstrate appreciable latency periods. Depending on the onset of dissemination and colonization within distant organs, this provides varying and often lengthy periods for acquiring macrometastatic-colonization genes. In contrast, some cancers, like adenocarcinomas of the lung and pancreas, have short latency periods and exhibit early systemic metastasis often to multiple organs. One explanation for short versus long periods of latency is related to origin of the cell population initially targeted for transforming and tumorigenic events. The cancer stem cell hypothesis and the role of EMT in metastasis already suggest that early progenitor cells or cells that may have played a role in developmental processes can be predisposed to activate metastasis-progression mechanisms. An example of this has been demonstrated by introducing defined oncogenic alterations into different cell types.[108] When mammary epithelial cells or fibroblasts were transformed, these cells were tumorigenic but not metastatic. In contrast, oncogenic transformation of melanocytes resulted in aggressive metastasis. This difference was because of the expression of the EMT transcription factor Slug in the melanocytes but not the other tumor types. Thus, the transformation of certain unique cell types may predispose to early metastatic behavior and could explain certain phenomenon such as cancers of unknown primary.

Identification of genes that promote early metastasis in adenocarcinoma of the lung also supports the view that some carcinomas may not have an extensive requirement for macrometastatic-colonization functions. By using mouse models to dissect the molecular basis for lung metastasis, the existence of a WNT/TCF pathway was found capable of mediating rapid multiorgan metastasis through LEF1 and HOXB9.[109] A clinical predictor based on this pathway was associated with metastatic risk for patients with lung, but not breast, adenocarcinomas. This pathway is well characterized in stem cell and developmental biology, including EMT. Recent findings revealing that important drivers of aggressive metastasis can include developmental-related genes capable of causing genomewide changes[110,111] will likely help to uncover additional scenarios whereby macrometastatic-colonization functions play limited roles.

MICRO-RNAs AND METASTASIS

It was once thought that the effects of genes necessarily resulted from the proteins that they encode. However, as a result of developmental studies on the worm *Caenorhabditis elegans* that identified important roles for noncoding RNAs (ncRNAs), it is now appreciated that ncRNAs potentially influence cellular and organismal phenotypes on par with traditional protein-coding genes. In fact, microRNAs, which are approximately 22 nucleotide-long small ncRNAs, have been discovered to have important effects on metastasis.[112] MicroRNAs function by regulating the expression of hundreds of target genes through sequence-specific binding between the microRNA and the 3′ untranslated regions of mRNAs. This engagement results in either the degradation of the target mRNA or the inhibition of protein translation. Through this action, microRNAs can influence a large number of genes. In fact, it is predicted that microRNAs preferentially interact with genes that are central to highly connected networks.[113]

MicroRNAs can function both as metastasis activators and metastasis suppressors by influencing numerous genes involved in metastasis initiation, progression, and colonization. Several microRNAs, such as miR-10b, miR-9, and members of the miR-200 family, play critical roles in EMT or EMT-related events. For example, miR-10b influences cell migration, invasion, and metastasis by repressing HOXD10, a known inhibitor of a RHOC-mediated promotility program.[114] The expression of miR-10b is under the control of the EMT transcription factor Twist. In fact, miR-10b is essential for Twist-induced EMT and for metastasis, making miR-10b a metastasis activator. MiR-9 promotes metastasis by targeting E-cadherin, which results in β-catenin signaling and VEGF expression.[115] Accordingly, motility, invasion, angiogenesis, and metastasis ensue. MiR-200 family members also regulate EMT by inhibiting ZEB1 and ZEB2, which normally promote EMT through the suppression of E-cadherin.[116–118] Thus, in contrast to miR-10b, miR-200 family members act as metastasis suppressors. Other microRNAs such as miR-335, miR-126, miR-31, and let-7 also suppress distant spread. MiR-335 inhibits metastasis and invasion by targeting the LMS genes *SOX4* and *TNC*, while miR-125 suppresses overall tumor growth and proliferation.[119] MiR-31 represses multiple steps in the metastatic cascade, an effect that is related to its influence on multiple metastasis genes.[120] Let-7, which is one of the most extensively studied microRNAs, interferes with both self-renewal and distant colonization, and its expression can be controlled by metastasis suppressor genes.[76,121] Numerous other microRNAs that play a role in metastasis are being rapidly identified. Interestingly, even non-microRNA ncRNAs are being identified to influence aggressive distant spread.[110] The potential for microRNAs to serve as clinical markers and/or therapeutic targets is already starting to show promise.

Selected References

The full list of references for this chapter appears in the online version.

7. Fidler IJ. The pathogenesis of cancer metastasis: the 'seed and soil' hypothesis revisited. *Nat Rev Cancer* 2003;3:453.
8. Chambers AF, Groom AC, MacDonald IC. Dissemination and growth of cancer cells in metastatic sites. *Nat Rev Cancer* 2002;2:563.
9. Hellman S. Karnofsky memorial lecture: natural history of small breast cancers. *J Clin Oncol* 1994;12:2229.
13. Bernards R, Weinberg RA. A progression puzzle. *Nature* 2002;418:823.
14. Nguyen DX, Bos PD, Massague J. Metastasis: from dissemination to organ-specific colonization. *Nat Rev Cancer* 2009;9:274.
16. Gupta GP, Nguyen DX, Chiang AC, et al. Mediators of vascular remodelling co-opted for sequential steps in lung metastasis. *Nature* 2007;446:765.
17. Minn AJ, Gupta GP, Siegel PM, et al. Genes that mediate breast cancer metastasis to lung. *Nature* 2005;436:518.

25. Qian BZ, Pollard JW. Macrophage diversity enhances tumor progression and metastasis. *Cell* 2010;141:39.
26. Joyce JA, Pollard JW. Microenvironmental regulation of metastasis. *Nat Rev Cancer* 2009;9:239.
27. Yang L, Huang J, Ren X, et al. Abrogation of TGF beta signaling in mammary carcinomas recruits Gr-1+CD11b+ myeloid cells that promote metastasis. *Cancer Cell* 2008;13:23.
33. Thiery JP, Acloque H, Huang RY, Nieto MA. Epithelial-mesenchymal transitions in development and disease. *Cell* 2009;139:871.
34. Yang MH, Wu MZ, Chiou SH, et al. Direct regulation of TWIST by HIF-1alpha promotes metastasis. *Nat Cell Biol* 2008;10:295.
35. Wu Y, Deng J, Rychahou PG, Qiu S, Evers BM, Zhou BP. Stabilization of snail by NF-kappaB is required for inflammation-induced cell migration and invasion. *Cancer Cell* 2009;15:416.
36. Kudo-Saito C, Shirako H, Takeuchi T, Kawakami Y. Cancer metastasis is accelerated through immunosuppression during Snail-induced EMT of cancer cells. *Cancer Cell* 2009;15:195.
40. Mani SA, Guo W, Liao MJ, et al. The epithelial-mesenchymal transition generates cells with properties of stem cells. *Cell* 2008;133:704.
42. Yang J, Mani SA, Donaher JL, et al. Twist, a master regulator of morphogenesis, plays an essential role in tumor metastasis. *Cell* 2004;117:927.
44. Hermann PC, Huber SL, Herrler T, et al. Distinct populations of cancer stem cells determine tumor growth and metastatic activity in human pancreatic cancer. *Cell Stem Cell* 2007;1:313.
45. Pantel K, Brakenhoff RH, Brandt B. Detection, clinical relevance and specific biological properties of disseminating tumour cells. *Nat Rev Cancer* 2008;8:329.
46. Husemann Y, Geigl JB, Schubert F, et al. Systemic spread is an early step in breast cancer. *Cancer Cell* 2008;13:58.
47. Podsypanina K, Du YC, Jechlinger M, Beverly LJ, Hambardzumyan D, Varmus H. Seeding and propagation of untransformed mouse mammary cells in the lung. *Science* 2008;321:1841.
48. Psaila B, Lyden D. The metastatic niche: adapting the foreign soil. *Nat Rev Cancer* 2009;9:285.
49. Kaplan RN, Riba RD, Zacharoulis S, et al. VEGFR1-positive haematopoietic bone marrow progenitors initiate the pre-metastatic niche. *Nature* 2005;438:820.
51. Hiratsuka S, Watanabe A, Sakurai Y, et al. The S100A8-serum amyloid A3-TLR4 paracrine cascade establishes a pre-metastatic phase. *Nat Cell Biol* 2008;10:1349.
52. Erler JT, Bennewith KL, Cox TR, et al. Hypoxia-induced lysyl oxidase is a critical mediator of bone marrow cell recruitment to form the premetastatic niche. *Cancer Cell* 2009;15:35.
56. Bandyopadhyay S, Zhan R, Chaudhuri A, et al. Interaction of KAI1 on tumor cells with DARC on vascular endothelium leads to metastasis suppression. *Nat Med* 2006;12:933.
63. Felding-Habermann B, O'Toole TE, Smith JW, et al. Integrin activation controls metastasis in human breast cancer. *Proc Natl Acad Sci U S A* 2001;98:1853.
68. Muller A, Homey B, Soto H, et al. Involvement of chemokine receptors in breast cancer metastasis. *Nature* 2001;410:50.
70. Karnoub AE, Dash AB, Vo AP, et al. Mesenchymal stem cells within tumour stroma promote breast cancer metastasis. *Nature* 2007;449:557.
71. Norton L, Massague J. Is cancer a disease of self-seeding? *Nat Med* 2006;12:875.
72. Kim MY, Oskarsson T, Acharyya S, et al. Tumor self-seeding by circulating cancer cells. *Cell* 2009;139:1315.
73. Aguirre-Ghiso JA. Models, mechanisms and clinical evidence for cancer dormancy. *Nat Rev Cancer* 2007;7:834.
75. McAllister SS, Gifford AM, Greiner AL, et al. Systemic endocrine instigation of indolent tumor growth requires osteopontin. *Cell* 2008;133:994.
78. Schmidt-Kittler O, Ragg T, Daskalakis A, et al. From latent disseminated cells to overt metastasis: genetic analysis of systemic breast cancer progression. *Proc Natl Acad Sci U S A* 2003;100:7737.
81. Zhang XH, Wang Q, Gerald W, et al. Latent bone metastasis in breast cancer tied to Src-dependent survival signals. *Cancer Cell* 2009;16:67.
83. Kang Y, Siegel PM, Shu W, et al. A multigenic program mediating breast cancer metastasis to bone. *Cancer Cell* 2003;3:537.
87. Minn AJ, Kang Y, Serganova I, et al. Distinct organ-specific metastatic potential of individual breast cancer cells and primary tumors. *J Clin Invest* 2005;115:44.
88. Minn AJ, Gupta GP, Padua D, et al. Lung metastasis genes couple breast tumor size and metastatic spread. *Proc Natl Acad Sci U S A* 2007;104:6740.
89. Gupta GP, Perk J, Acharyya S, et al. ID genes mediate tumor reinitiation during breast cancer lung metastasis. *Proc Natl Acad Sci U S A* 2007;104:19506.
98. Bos PD, Zhang XH, Nadal C, et al. Genes that mediate breast cancer metastasis to the brain. *Nature* 2009;459:1005.
101. Wong SY, Haack H, Crowley D, Barry M, Bronson RT, Hynes RO. Tumor-secreted vascular endothelial growth factor-C is necessary for prostate cancer lymphangiogenesis, but lymphangiogenesis is unnecessary for lymph node metastasis. *Cancer Res* 2005;65:9789.
102. Skobe M, Hawighorst T, Jackson DG, et al. Induction of tumor lymphangiogenesis by VEGF-C promotes breast cancer metastasis. *Nat Med* 2001;7:192.
103. Stacker SA, Caesar C, Baldwin ME, et al. VEGF-D promotes the metastatic spread of tumor cells via the lymphatics. *Nat Med* 2001;7:186.
108. Gupta PB, Kuperwasser C, Brunet JP, et al. The melanocyte differentiation program predisposes to metastasis after neoplastic transformation. *Nat Genet* 2005;37:1047.
109. Nguyen DX, Chiang AC, Zhang XH, et al. WNT/TCF signaling through LEF1 and HOXB9 mediates lung adenocarcinoma metastasis. *Cell* 2009;138:51.
110. Gupta RA, Shah N, Wang KC, et al. Long non-coding RNA HOTAIR reprograms chromatin state to promote cancer metastasis. *Nature* 2010;464:1071.
114. Ma L, Teruya-Feldstein J, Weinberg RA. Tumour invasion and metastasis initiated by microRNA-10b in breast cancer. *Nature* 2007;449:682.
116. Gregory PA, Bert AG, Paterson EL, et al. The miR-200 family and miR-205 regulate epithelial to mesenchymal transition by targeting ZEB1 and SIP1. *Nat Cell Biol* 2008;10:593.
117. Korpal M, Lee ES, Hu G, Kang Y. The miR-200 family inhibits epithelial-mesenchymal transition and cancer cell migration by direct targeting of E-cadherin transcriptional repressors ZEB1 and ZEB2. *J Biol Chem* 2008;283:14910.
118. Park SM, Gaur AB, Lengyel E, Peter ME. The miR-200 family determines the epithelial phenotype of cancer cells by targeting the E-cadherin repressors ZEB1 and ZEB2. *Genes Dev* 2008;22:894.
119. Tavazoie SF, Alarcón C, Oskarsson T, et al. Endogenous human microRNAs that suppress breast cancer metastasis. *Nature* 2008;451:147.

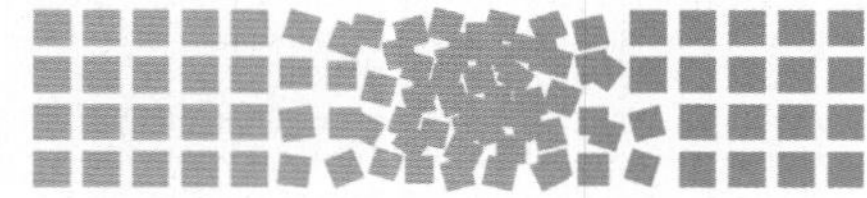

CHAPTER 11 CANCER STEM CELLS

JEAN C. Y. WANG AND JOHN E. DICK

A fundamental problem in cancer research is identification of the cell type capable of initiating and sustaining growth of the tumor—the cancer-initiating cell or cancer stem cell (CSC). Although it has long been known that only a fraction of cells within a tumor is capable of tumor generation upon transplantation, it has been unclear until recently whether this observed functional heterogeneity was attributable to stochastic influences or to intrinsic properties of the tumor cells. Evidence for the existence of biologically distinct CSCs, first demonstrated in a hematological malignancy and in the past 5 years in several solid tumors, has shaped a new paradigm of human cancer as a hierarchical disease whose growth is sustained by a population of CSCs. This conceptual shift has important implications not only for researchers seeking to understand mechanisms of tumor initiation and progression, but also for the development and evaluation of effective anticancer therapies.

TUMOR HETEROGENEITY

Our modern understanding of the origin of cancer can be traced to Rudolph Virchow, who in 1858 stated the heretical and revolutionary thesis "*omnis cellula e cellula*," that all cells come from cells. Out of his early theories grew the idea that cancer cells develop from normal cells that have undergone abnormal changes, a process now called somatic mutation. Nearly 150 years later, it is now well accepted that cancer is a genetic disease that arises from the clonal expansion of a single neoplastic cell. Simplistically, cancer has been viewed as the unregulated growth of abnormal cells, with the implication that all of the cells in the tumor are proliferating uncontrollably. However, this notion is incompatible with the observation made over four decades ago that only a fraction of cells within murine lymphomas were capable of clonogenic growth when transplanted into syngeneic mice.[1] Furthermore, autotransplants of cancer cell suspensions in humans demonstrated that tumor growth occurred only after inoculation of at least 10^4 to 10^5 cells.[2] These and similar observations demonstrated that there is functional heterogeneity in the proliferative ability of cells within a tumor.

Two contrasting theories have been proposed to explain this observed heterogeneity (Fig. 11.1).[3] One view is that extrinsic factors (e.g., host resistance, growth factor concentrations, niche availability) or intrinsic factors (e.g., timing of cell cycle entry) prevent every cell from behaving in the same way. In other words, the behavior of tumor cells is unpredictable and governed by probabilities that may be influenced by any or all of these factors. The end result is that cells will appear to be heterogeneous in their proliferative capacity when tested in a functional assay. The central tenet of this stochastic model is that every cell has equal potential to initiate and sustain tumor growth, but most cells do not proliferate extensively due to the low cumulative probability of permissive events.

The alternative model is based on the biology of normal somatic tissues, many of which are arranged as hierarchies comprising cell types with different growth properties. The nonproliferating mature cells that make up the majority of these normal tissues must be continuously replenished by a pool of rapidly proliferating progenitors, which in turn are replenished by rare stem cells at the apex of the hierarchy. A key property of stem cells that distinguishes them from progenitors and allows them to maintain tissue integrity is self-renewal, whereby at cell division one or both daughter cells retain the biological properties of the parent cell. According to this model, tumors retain features of normal tissue organization, in that they are made up of distinct classes of cells that are organized hierarchically and possess intrinsically different functional capacities. The tumor hierarchy is sustained at its apex by a population of CSCs that possess the capacity to self-renew (i.e., produce more CSCs) and to recapitulate tumor heterogeneity by generating all of the various nontumorigenic cell types that compose the bulk of tumor. The essential principle of this model is that CSCs are biologically distinct from the bulk cell population, which does not possess tumor-initiating activity.

Both the stochastic and CSC models predict that only a small number of cells within a tumor will have the capacity to initiate tumor growth (i.e., to behave as CSCs); however, their underlying biological principles are very different. According to the stochastic model, the oncogenic program is operative in all cells of the tumor, thus both research to understand neoplastic processes and drug development can be directed at the bulk cell population. In contrast, the CSC model implies that CSCs are biologically distinct from the majority of cells in the tumor due to irreversible epigenetic processes that influence cell function, layered onto the common genetic aberrations present in all cells of the tumor.[4] The biological consequence of a particular cancer pathway may be different in CSCs compared to cells without tumor-initiating capacity. Thus, research must be directed at the relevant cell populations as identified through functional assays, the ultimate goal being the rational development of therapies that interfere with the oncogenic program within CSCs.

In order to test these theories and address the fundamental question of how tumor heterogeneity arises, two things are required: first, the ability to purify subpopulations of tumor cells based on physical or functional properties such as surface antigen expression or dye exclusion, and second, a functional transplantation assay to test the ability of purified cell populations to generate tumors *in vivo*, as current *in vitro* culture techniques do not reproduce the necessary microenvironment for tumor development. According to the stochastic model, the behavior of tumor cells is random and cannot be predicted; therefore, tumor-initiating activity will appear in every isolated

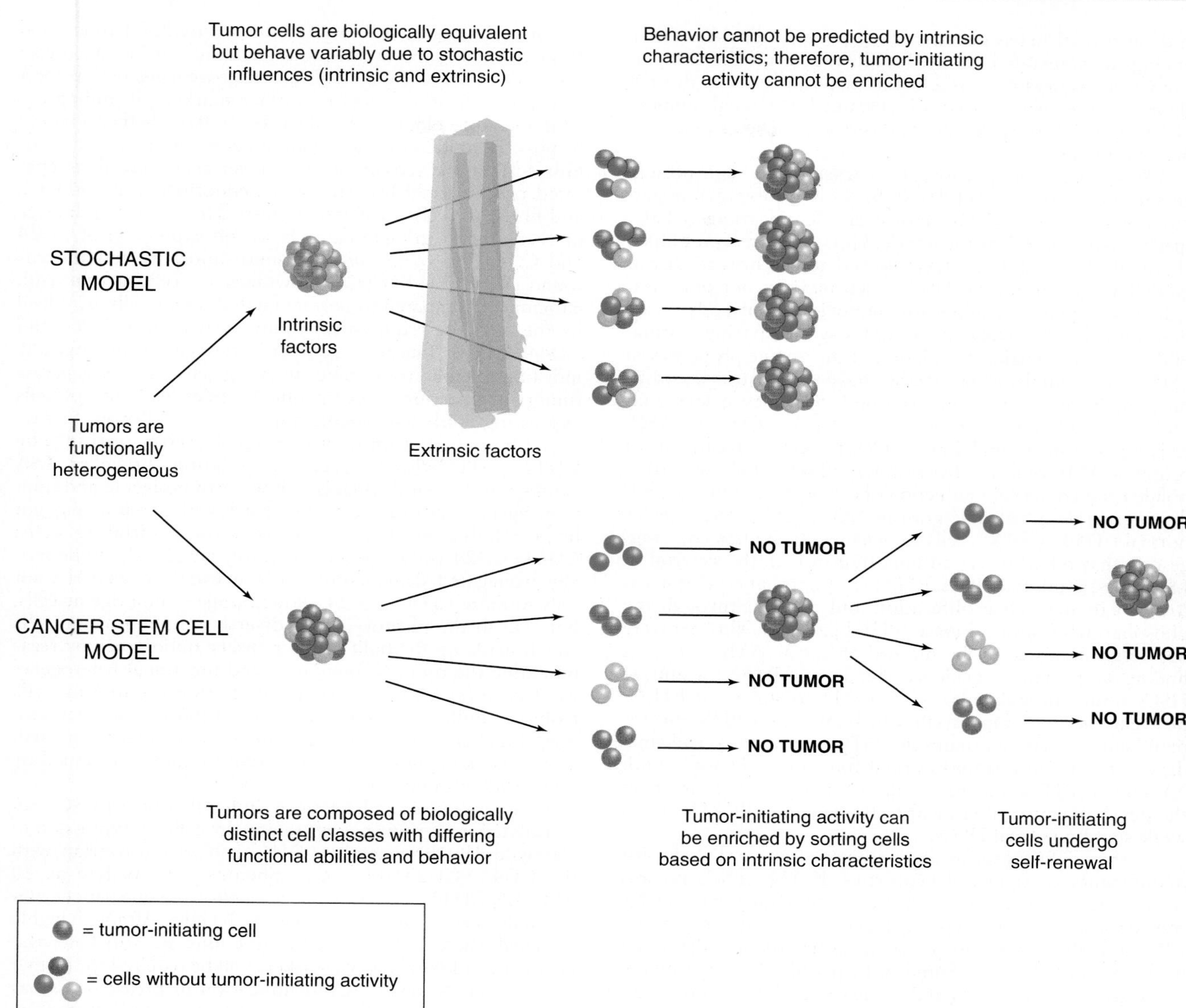
Tumor cells are biologically equivalent but behave variably due to stochastic influences (intrinsic and extrinsic)
Behavior cannot be predicted by intrinsic characteristics; therefore, tumor-initiating activity cannot be enriched
STOCHASTIC MODEL
Intrinsic factors
Extrinsic factors
Tumors are functionally heterogeneous
CANCER STEM CELL MODEL
NO TUMOR
NO TUMOR
NO TUMOR
NO TUMOR
NO TUMOR
NO TUMOR
Tumors are composed of biologically distinct cell classes with differing functional abilities and behavior
Tumor-initiating activity can be enriched by sorting cells based on intrinsic characteristics
Tumor-initiating cells undergo self-renewal
= tumor-initiating cell
= cells without tumor-initiating activity

FIGURE 11.1 Models of tumor heterogeneity. Tumors are composed of phenotypically and functionally heterogeneous cells. There are two theories as to how this heterogeneity arises. According to the stochastic model, tumor cells are biologically equivalent but their behavior is influenced by intrinsic and extrinsic factors and is therefore both variable and unpredictable. Thus, tumor-initiating activity cannot be enriched by sorting cells based on intrinsic characteristics. In contrast, the cancer stem cell model postulates the existence of biologically distinct classes of cells with differing functional abilities and behavior. Only a subset of cells has the ability to initiate tumor growth; these cancer stem cells possess self-renewal and give rise to nontumorigenic progeny that make up the bulk of the tumor. This model predicts that tumor-initiating cells can be identified and purified from the bulk non-tumorigenic population based on intrinsic characteristics. (Figure originally published in Dick JE. Stem cell concepts renew cancer research. *Blood* 2008;112:4793.) © The American Society of Hematology

cell fraction and cannot consistently be enriched. In contrast, the CSC model postulates that with an appropriate purification strategy, the CSCs with the capacity to initiate and sustain tumor growth *in vivo* can be identified and isolated from the bulk cells that do not have tumor-initiating activity (Fig. 11.1).

LEUKEMIA STEM CELLS

Based on the depth of knowledge gained from more than four decades of research in normal hematopoiesis, it is not surprising that identification of CSCs was first achieved in a hematological malignancy, acute myeloid leukemia (AML). This was made possible by prior detailed characterization of hematopoietic cell surface antigens and by the development of a xenotransplantation assay using severe combined immune-deficient (SCID) or nonobese diabetic (NOD)/SCID mice as recipients that allowed assessment of the ability of leukemic cells to initiate disease *in vivo*. When primary AML cells were fractionated based on expression of cell surface markers and transplanted into mice, only cells in the CD34+CD38− fraction composing less than 1% of the total blast population were able to initiate leukemic growth *in vivo*.[5,6] These leukemia stem cells (LSCs) possessed high self-renewal, as demonstrated by serial transplantation, and proliferated in the mice to produce large numbers of leukemic progenitors and nonproliferating blasts, generating a graft that recapitulated the phenotypic and functional heterogeneity of the patient's disease. These findings demonstrated that AML, like the normal hematopoietic system, is organized as a hierarchy of functionally distinct classes of cells whose growth is sustained by a small number of LSCs, which provides the first direct evidence supporting the CSC model.

LSCs share some phenotypic characteristics with normal hematopoietic stem cells (HSCs), for example expression patterns of CD34 and CD38. However, identification of LSC-specific markers such as the interleukin-3 (IL-3) receptor alpha chain (IL-3Rα, CD123)[7] has allowed researchers to distinguish LSCs from normal HSCs. Such markers not only provide a therapeutic window for monoclonal antibody-based therapies to selectively target LSCs while sparing normal HSCs,[8] but also enable elucidation of the unique properties of LSCs. For example, recent studies have demonstrated constitutive activation of the transcription factor nuclear factor κB (NF-κB) in quiescent primitive CD34+CD38−CD123+ AML cells but not in normal CD34+CD38− cells.[9] Treatment of primitive AML cells *in vitro* with the NF-κB inhibitor parthenolide resulted in rapid induction of cell death and loss of ability to generate a leukemic graft in NOD/SCID mice, whereas normal CD34+CD38− cells were generally unaffected,[10] suggesting that NF-κB plays an important role in the survival of LSCs but not normal HSCs. PTEN is a phosphatase that negatively regulates cell proliferation and survival through the phosphatidylinositol 3-kinase (PI3K) pathway. This pathway has been implicated in the survival of human AML LSCs,[11] a finding supported by evidence that loss of PTEN in murine HSCs results in leukemia.[12,13] Notably, treatment of PTEN-deficient mice with rapamycin, which targets the PI3K effector mammalian target of rapamycin (mTOR), prevented leukemia development and restored normal function to HSCs.[12] Both NF-κB and PTEN thus represent exciting potential targets in the development of therapeutic strategies to kill AML LSCs while sparing normal HSCs.

Normal HSCs require a microenvironmental niche for maintenance of stem cell properties. If AML LSCs possess unique requirements for interaction with a supportive niche, this association could represent another therapeutic target. CD44 is a ubiquitously expressed transmembrane protein that mediates cell adhesion. Some isoforms of CD44 are highly expressed on AML blasts and are associated with poor prognosis. Treatment of AML cells *in vitro* or *in vivo* with an activating monoclonal antibody (H90) directed against CD44 resulted in killing of LSCs, as demonstrated by loss of leukemic repopulation in NOD/SCID mice, while similarly treated normal cord blood and bone marrow cells were much less affected, if at all.[14] The mechanisms underlying eradication of LSCs included interference with homing to their microenvironmental niche, loss of engraftment ability, and induction of differentiation. These findings demonstrate that the leukemogenic process does not abrogate the niche dependence of LSCs and highlight a potential therapeutic target that may also be applicable to solid cancers.

CANCER STEM CELLS IN SOLID TUMORS

Breast Cancer Stem Cells

Investigations of mechanisms underlying solid tumor heterogeneity were first undertaken in human breast cancer. Al Hajj et al.[15] made single-cell suspensions of breast cancer specimens obtained from primary or metastatic sites in patients. Upon injection into the mammary fat pad of immune-deficient NOD/SCID mice, all samples studied were able to generate tumors. Thus, the NOD/SCID model provides a functional assay of the *in vivo* tumor-initiating ability of human breast cancer cells. Breast cancer cells are heterogeneous with respect to expression of a variety of surface markers, including the adhesion molecules CD24 and CD44. To test whether it would be possible to identify and isolate subpopulations enriched for tumor-initiating activity, breast cancer cells were first separated from normal hematopoietic, endothelial, mesothelial, and fibroblast cells by elimination of cells expressing lineage markers, then subfractionated based on expression of CD24 and CD44. All of the *in vivo* tumor-initiating activity was found in the CD44+CD24−/lowLineage− cell fraction, with enrichment compared to unfractionated tumor cells as judged by the cell dose required for tumor formation. CD44− and CD44+CD24+Lineage− cells, even though morphologically indistinguishable from tumor-initiating cells, did not generate tumors at injection sites. In some samples, isolation of cells expressing epithelial specific antigen (ESA) allowed further enrichment of tumor-initiating activity within the CD44+CD24−/lowLineage− population, however, ESA expression did not distinguish between tumorigenic and nontumorigenic cells in at least one sample, and therefore may not be a reliable marker for breast cancer-initiating cells. CD44+CD24−/lowLineage− tumorigenic cells could be serially propagated, demonstrating self-renewal, and gave rise not only to more CD44+CD24−/lowLineage− tumorigenic cells, but also to the phenotypically diverse nontumorigenic cells which made up the bulk of the primary tumor, thereby recapitulating the tumor's complexity and functional heterogeneity. This study was the first to isolate tumor-initiating cells from the bulk nontumorigenic population in a nonhematological malignancy, providing strong evidence that the growth of at least some types of human solid tumors is sustained by biologically distinct CSCs.

Other investigators have since shown that breast CSCs can be isolated from some patient tumors by cellular expression of aldehyde dehydrogenase (ALDH), with partial overlap with the CD44+CD24−Lineage− phenotype.[16] As few as 20 ALDH1+CD44+CD24−Lineage− cells from one patient cancer could generate tumors in NOD/SCID mice. Although highly enriched, these CSC-containing fractions are still heterogeneous, and additional CSC markers will be required for further purification. Nevertheless, identification of breast CSCs has moved cancer researchers away from studying bulk tumors and shifted their focus to understanding the biology of this subpopulation of cells. For example, Yu et al.[17] have shown that cell fractions enriched for breast CSCs have globally reduced microRNA expression compared to more differentiated cancer cells. In particular, the *let-7* family is not expressed and increases with differentiation. Lentiviral expression of *let-7* in Lineage−CD44+CD24− cells from patient breast cancers significantly reduced tumor formation in both primary and serially transplanted NOD/SCID mice. Insight into the biology of CSCs will be a crucial first step to develop an effective means to target them therapeutically.

Brain Cancer Stem Cells

Studies in several types of human brain cancers have clearly shown that the tumor cell population is functionally heterogeneous, in that only a fraction of cells have the ability to form tumor neurospheres when plated at low density in culture or generate tumors when transplanted *in vivo*.[18,19] As discussed above, demonstration that this heterogeneity arises from the existence of biologically distinct cell populations, rather than as a result of stochastic processes, requires isolation of tumor-initiating cells from the bulk nontumorigenic population. Singh et al.[20] reported that CD133+ cells in different types of human brain tumors possess extensive proliferative, differentiative, and self-renewal capacity *in vitro*. The development of a xenograft assay that involved injection of single-cell suspensions of human brain tumor samples into the NOD/SCID mouse brain enabled assessment of whether the CD133+ cells were capable of initiating tumor growth *in vivo*.[21] Tumors could be generated by as few as 100 CD133+ cells, while injection of up to 10^5 CD133− tumor cells did not result in tumor formation. Importantly, small numbers of viable CD133− tumor cells could be found at the injection site many weeks later, ruling out the possibility that CD133− cells did not form tumors simply because they died following transplantation. The tumors generated by CD133+ cells resembled the patient's original tumor by immunohistochemistry and consisted of a minority CD133+ and a majority CD133− cell population. CD133+ cells isolated from xenograft tumors could generate phenotypically similar tumors in secondary mice. Thus, CD133+ cells from human brain tumors possess the two key properties of CSCs: the ability to self-renew and to recapitulate tumor heterogeneity through differentiation. Interestingly, CD133 (also called prominin-1/AC133) has also been used as a marker to enrich normal human HSCs as well as stem cells in the human central nervous system, suggesting that it may be a marker of both normal and malignant stem cells.

Recently, there have been reports that CD133 may not be a universal marker of CSCs in brain cancer.[22–24] In addition, a study of neurosphere lines derived from *PTEN*-deficient human glioblastomas found that both CD133+ and CD133− cells could generate serially transplantable tumors in xenograft recipients and provided evidence that these tumors comprise a hierarchy of self-renewing CSC populations with variable tumorigenic capacity.[25] Unfortunately, these investigators were not able to study sorted cell populations directly isolated from patient tumors. Cell surface phenotype can change significantly during culture, without corresponding changes in stem cell function.[26] In addition, there is evidence that CD133 expression can vary as a function of cell cycle.[27] Thus, the results of these studies should be interpreted with caution. Nevertheless, it would not be surprising to find that the CSC phenotype is heterogeneous, even among tumors of the same histologic subtype, given the variety of genetic and epigenetic perturbations that can ultimately lead to tumor formation. These observations underscore the importance of characterizing candidate CSC populations through functional assays of their tumor-forming ability rather than relying solely on phenotypic identification.

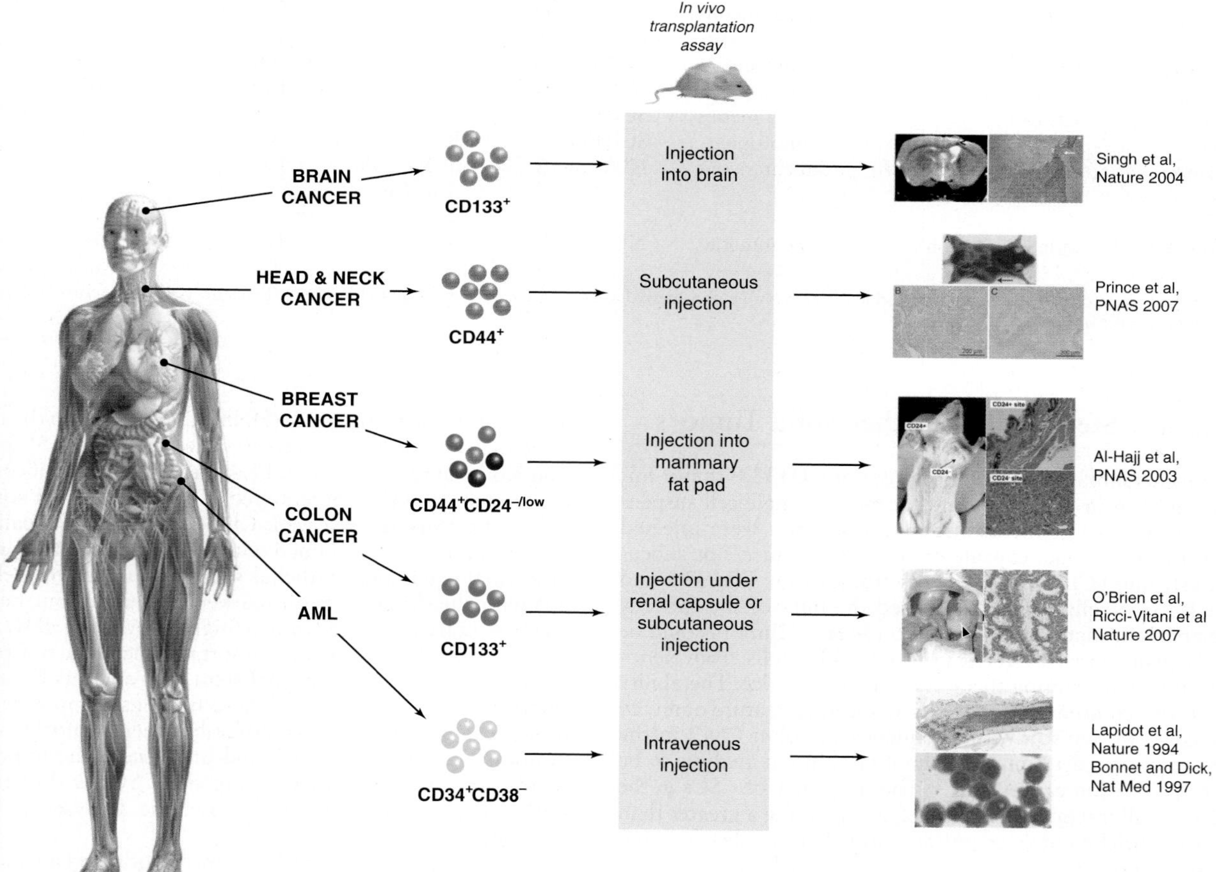

FIGURE 11.2 Identification of cancer stem cells (CSCs) in acute myeloid leukemia (AML) and solid tumors. Subfractions of tumor cells isolated from the bulk tumor population are assayed for their ability to initiate tumor growth *in vivo* using immune-deficient mice as recipients. CSCs are the only cells capable of initiating tumor growth, giving rise to more CSCs through self-renewal, and also to nontumorigenic differentiated progeny, thus recapitulating the functional heterogeneity of the original tumor. CSCs were first identified in AML and have now also been identified in several types of solid tumors (Table 11.1). (Brain cancer images adapted by permission from Macmillan Publishers Ltd: Nature (21), copyright 2004. Head and neck cancer and breast cancer images copyright 2007 (ref. 32) and 2003 (ref. 15), respectively, National Academy of Sciences, USA. Colon cancer images are from ref. 28.)

TABLE 11.1

PROSPECTIVE ISOLATION OF CANCER STEM CELLS FROM HUMAN LEUKEMIAS AND SOLID TUMORS

Tumor Type	CSC Marker	Transplantation Site	Mouse Strain	Frequency	Minimum Cell Dose for Tumor Formation	No. of Samples Engrafted	Ref.
AML	CD34+CD38−	Intravenous	SCID	1 in 2.5 × 10^5	2 × 10^5	1	5
AML	CD34+CD38−	Intravenous	NOD/SCID	0.2 to 100 per 10^6 bulk	5 × 10^3	7	6
Multiple myeloma	CD138−CD34−	Intravenous	NOD/SCID	NR	NA	1	114
Breast	CD44+CD24−/low	Orthotopic	NOD/SCID	5 in 10^5 bulk	10^3	8	15
Breast	CD44+CD24−	Orthotopic	NOD/SCID	NR	2 × 10^3	8	17
Breast	ALDH1+	Orthotopic	NOD/SCID	NR	500	4	16
Brain	CD133+	Orthotopic	NOD/SCID	NR	100	7	21
Brain	CD133+	Orthotopic	nu/nu	NR	500	2	101
Brain	A2B5+CD133±	Orthotopic	nu/nu	NR	1.5 × 10^4	5	24
Colon	CD133+	Kidney capsule	NOD/SCID	1 in 5.7 × 10^4 bulk; 1 in 262 CD133+	100	12	28
Colon	CD133+	Subcutaneous	SCID	NR	1.5 × 10^3	19	29
Colon	ESA+CD44+	Subcutaneous	NOD/SCID	NR	200	6	31
Colon	ESA+CD44+CD166+	Subcutaneous	NOD/SCID	NR	150	2	31
Colon	CD133+	Subcutaneous	nu/nu	NR	2.5 × 10^3	3	105
Head and neck	CD44+	Subcutaneous	NOD/SCID, Rag2$^{-/-}\gamma^{-/-}$	NR	5 × 10^3	9	32
Pancreas	CD133+	Orthotopic	NMRI-nu/nu	NR	500	7	37
Pancreas	CD44+CD24+ESA+	Orthotopic	NOD/SCID	NR	100	10	36
Lung	CD133+	Subcutaneous	SCID	NR	10^4	3	115
Liver	CD90+	Orthotopic	SCID/Beige	NR	10^3	NR	116
Melanoma	ABCB5+	Subcutaneous	NOD/SCID	1 in 10^6 bulk; 1 in 1.6 × 10^5 ABCB5+	10^4	4	39
Mesenchymal	Side population	Subcutaneous	NOD/SCID	NR	100	4	117

CSC, cancer stem cell; AML, acute myeloid leukemia; NOD, nonobese diabetic; SCID, severe combined immune-deficient; NR, not reported; ESA, epithelial specific antigen.

Cancer Stem Cells in Other Solid Tumors

Two groups initially reported isolation of CD133+ tumor-initiating cells from human colon cancers.[28,29] Single-cell suspensions of primary or metastatic tumor samples were injected either under the renal capsule of NOD/SCID mice[28] or subcutaneously into SCID mice.[29] In both studies, only CD133+ and not CD133− cells, which composed the bulk of the cancers, were able to initiate tumor formation *in vivo*. Tumors could be serially propagated by reisolating CD133+ cells from xenografts and transplanting them into secondary mice. The ability to perform quantitative analysis is an essential feature of any *in vivo* assay. In one study, the frequency of colon CSCs in the bulk tumor was determined by limiting dilution analysis to be 1 in 60,000 colon cancer cells.[28] The frequency of CSCs in the CD133+ cell fraction was 1 in 262, representing a greater than 200-fold enrichment over unfractionated cells. Clearly, however, the majority of CD133+ colon cancer cells are not CSCs. As has been shown in the CD34+ cell fraction of AML,[30] there may be a hierarchy of CSCs and progenitors in the CD133+ subpopulation of colon cancer cells. Another study identified colon CSCs in the EpCAMhighCD44+CD166+ cell fraction.[31] CD44+ cells generally constituted a minority subset of the CD133+ population, thus CD44 is a marker that could potentially be used to purify the CSC-containing fraction further.

Using methodology similar to that described above, CD44+ CSCs have recently been characterized in squamous cell carcinomas of the head and neck (HNSCC),[32] adding to the rapidly growing list of human cancers in which a distinct CSC population has been identified (Fig. 11.2, Table 11.1). Significantly, in moderately to well-differentiated HNSCC in which some tissue architecture is preserved, CD44+ cells were localized to the basal layer and costained with Cytokeratin 5/14, a marker of normal squamous epithelial stem and progenitor cells, but not with the differentiation marker involucrin. Furthermore, CD44+ cells expressed much higher levels of *BMI1* than CD44− cells. *BMI1* plays an important role in the self-renewal of hematopoietic and neuronal stem cells and has been implicated in tumorigenesis.[33–35] These findings demonstrate that biological pathways likely differ between tumorigenic and nontumorigenic populations and underscore the importance of identifying and characterizing the CSCs within tumors, both for gene expression and proteomic analyses as well as therapeutic targeting.

Expression of CD44 on CSCs from both breast cancer and HNSCC suggests that this adhesion molecule may also be a marker of CSCs in other tumors of epithelial origin. Recently, Li et al.[36] showed in pancreatic adenocarcinoma that cell fractions expressing CD44, CD24, epithelial specific antigen (ESA), or a combination of these markers were enriched for tumorigenic activity, as assessed by the frequency of tumor formation following subcutaneous or intrapancreatic injection into NOD/SCID mice. The most highly enriched fraction comprised cells that express all three of these markers, with tumor formation in half of mice receiving as few as 100 CD44+ CD24+ESA+ cells. However, injection of CD44−, CD24−, or ESA− cells also gave rise to tumors, albeit with lower frequency. Thus, none of the markers used in this study enabled clear separation of cells with tumor-initiating activity from the bulk nontumorigenic population. In contrast to these results, Hermann et al.[37] identified CSCs in pancreatic tumors by CD133 expression; as few as 500 freshly isolated CD133+ cells were able to generate tumors after orthotopic injection into immune-deficient mice, whereas as many as 1×10^6 CD133− cells could not.

The list of tumors in which CSC populations have been identified continues to grow (Table 11.1). There is frequent overlap in cell surface phenotype among CSCs from different tumor types, as evidenced in particular by expression of CD44 and CD133 on CSCs from epithelial tumors. Whether these are simply surrogate markers or play a functional role in CSC biology has yet to be determined.

Controversies and Future Directions

There have been a number of criticisms of the CSC model. As discussed above, characterization of CSC populations requires xenotransplantation into immune-deficient recipients. Some investigators have argued that inefficiencies of the xenotransplant system lead to underestimation of the frequency of cells with tumor-initiating ability.[38] In fact, when improvements have been made to these assay systems, for example through the use of more immune-deficient recipients such as NOD/SCID *Il2rg*$^{-/-}$ mice, the frequency of tumor initiating cells is sometimes dramatically increased, as seen recently for melanoma (greater than 4 log difference).[39,40] There are a number of issues to be considered here. First, such large increases in CSC frequency with the use of more immune-deficient recipients are not universal—for example, they have not been observed in AML[41,42,42a]—possibly reflecting variable sensitivity of tumor-initiating cells from different tumor types to residual host immune surveillance. Second, while human cell engraftment in xenotransplant assays is undoubtedly limited by residual elements of the recipient immune system, absence of cross-reactivity of cytokines, and other components of the host microenvironment, the low frequency of tumor-initiating cells seen in some cancers cannot be wholly explained by xenotransplantation barriers. For example, LSC frequency in two murine models of leukemia involving *MOZ-TIF* expression or *Pten* deletion was low (1 in 10^4 to 1 in 6×10^5) despite syngeneic bone marrow transplantation.[12,43] Furthermore, in contrast to the low frequency of LSCs generally seen when human AML cells are xenotransplanted, much higher LSC frequencies (on the order of 1%) have been observed in a genetically induced model of human B-cell acute lymphoblastic leukemia (ALL) that involves transplantation of human cord blood stem or progenitor cells expressing the *MLL-ENL* oncogene into immune-deficient mice.[42,44] This frequency was comparable to that reported for a murine model of *MLL-AF9*–induced AML (1 in 150).[45] These findings indicate that CSC frequencies can vary widely in different cancers, regardless of whether they are quantified using xeno- or syngeneic transplant assays, and likely relate at least in part to the specific underlying oncogenic pathways operating within the different tumors. Third, and perhaps most important, the CSC hypothesis does not address the absolute frequency of these cells: it is not required that CSCs be rare. The CSC model, at its most fundamental level, simply proposes that the basis of functional heterogeneity within tumors is the existence of cell populations that can be distinguished from other tumor cells by their ability to initiate malignant growth *in vivo*.

It is possible that some human cancers may not follow the CSC model. For example, the high frequency (one in four) and lack of a clear isolatable phenotype of tumor-initiating cells in melanoma suggest the absence of a hierarchical organization.[40] Regardless of whether a tumor contains a subpopulation of CSCs responsible for maintaining tumor growth or common tumorigenic cells with little evidence of a CSC hierarchy, all cancer cells with the ability to initiate disease must be identified and targeted therapeutically in order to achieve cure. Since the first published reports of CSCs in breast and brain cancers, there have been numerous studies of CSCs in other solid tumors, with varying degrees of robustness. When weighing evidence presented for or against the CSC hypothesis, one must consider not only the rigor of the xenotransplant assay but also experimental details such as whether cancer cells have been extensively cultured *in vitro* or passaged *in vivo*, both of which can lead to changes in function and phenotype, and whether freshly isolated cells from patients' tumors have been used versus cell lines that may not be representative of clinical disease.

Nevertheless, there is accumulating evidence that the growth of several types of human cancer is initiated and maintained by a subset of phenotypically and functionally distinct CSCs. Although the markers used to date to identify the CSC subset have enabled enrichment of this population compared to unsorted tumor cells, in all cases the enriched cell fractions are still functionally heterogeneous, containing both CSCs and their nontumorigenic progeny. One of the challenges of future research will be to obtain more purified populations of CSCs for use in molecular studies such as gene expression profiling. Novel protocols to purify cells with *in vivo* tumor-initiating capacity may combine cell surface markers with functional parameters such as Hoechst 33342 dye efflux, which identifies a "side population" of cells with high drug efflux capacity[46] or high aldehyde dehydrogenase activity.[47] Ultimately, rigorous proof for the existence of biologically distinct CSCs can only be obtained through demonstration that a single cell has the ability to self-renew and to recapitulate the entire tumor hierarchy. This will require either development of *in vivo* tumor models that support the growth of singly transplanted cells or clonal analysis techniques that enable tracking of the progeny of individually marked tumor cells *in vivo*, as demonstrated for AML LSCs.[30]

GENETIC DIVERSITY AND CLONAL EVOLUTION IN CANCER

Most of the initial studies identifying and characterizing CSCs in leukemia and solid tumors did not investigate the underlying genetic changes in cancer cells. Intratumor clonal heterogeneity has been described in many types of cancer[48] and may contribute to progression.[49] Investigators have proposed that intratumor heterogeneity arises through clonal evolution,[48] a long-standing concept in which cancer cells within a tumor acquire various mutations over time, leading to genetic drift and stepwise natural selection for the fittest, most aggressive cells, both of which drive tumor progression.[50] According to this model, the parallel growth and contraction of related but divergent subclones result in intratumor heterogeneity, and the genetic makeup of the tumor at any particular time reflects the activity of the dominant subclone(s). Recently, a number of studies have shown that phenotypically defined stem and progenitor populations in human breast cancers are clonally related but not identical.[51–53] There is now evidence from two studies in All[54,54a] that genetically distinct subclones that possess differing growth properties are present even at diagnosis. Examination of the genetic changes acquired by different subclones allowed reconstruction of their ancestry and provided evidence of a complex genetic architecture in ALL, with multiple subclones that are related in a branching rather than linear fashion. Importantly, the genetic diversity found in ALL patient samples was regenerated upon transplantation in immune-deficient mice, suggesting that leukemia-initiating cells are genetically diverse in this disease.

Although the existence of CSCs in most subtypes of human ALL is still under debate, based on these functional studies it may be reasonable to bring together the idea of clonal evolution driving intratumor genetic diversity and the existence of CSCs in a broader model of cancer progression, rather than viewing them as mutually exclusive concepts. Instead of being rigid, linear hierarchies that mirror normal tissue stem cell hierarchies, tumors should be thought of as genetically dynamic, comprising related but divergent subclones driven by CSCs, which are the units of evolutionary selection. On one hand, genetically distinct CSC clones may arise through changes acquired by existing CSCs. For example, the LSCs in an experimentally induced human leukemia can evolve through rearrangement of their immunoglobulin heavy chain genes.[44] On the other hand, CSCs may also arise through transformation of non-CSC populations, through acquisition of additional alterations or processes such as epithelial-mesenchymal transition (see below) (Fig. 11.3). Over time the genetic composition of the tumor may change, with different CSC-driven subclones becoming dominant or disappearing, either through natural selection based on cell-intrinsic or microenvironmental factors, or through selection by therapy. Indeed, clonal studies of matched diagnosis and relapse samples from pediatric patients with ALL have shown that relapse clones were often present as minor subpopulations at diagnosis.[55] Interestingly, therapy seemed to select for genetic abnormalities related to cell cycle regulation and B-cell development.

If found to be a property of cancer in general, genetic diversity of CSCs could have important implications for the development of anticancer therapies. Regardless of their origin, CSCs are the key cells that drive tumor growth and that must therefore be eliminated in order to achieve cure. If CSCs are genetically, and as a result functionally, diverse, they could represent a moving therapeutic target. Agents that target critical molecular pathways may fail if the selected targets are not present in some CSC subclones or if others have acquired changes that bypass their dependence on the targeted pathways. The development of successful therapeutic regimens will have to take into account the genetic and functional heterogeneity of CSCs.

THE ORIGINS OF CANCER STEM CELLS

A key focus of cancer research is elucidation of the molecular changes that underlie tumor initiation and progression. Tumorigenesis is a multistep process, and CSCs can be regarded as cells that have accumulated enough genetic or epigenetic changes to become fully transformed and that possess a stem cell program. However, little is known of the order or timing of such changes or of the cellular context in which they occur. Does cancer arise through the malignant transformation of normal stem cells or of committed downstream progenitors (or both)?[56] Unfortunately, the "stem" in "cancer stem

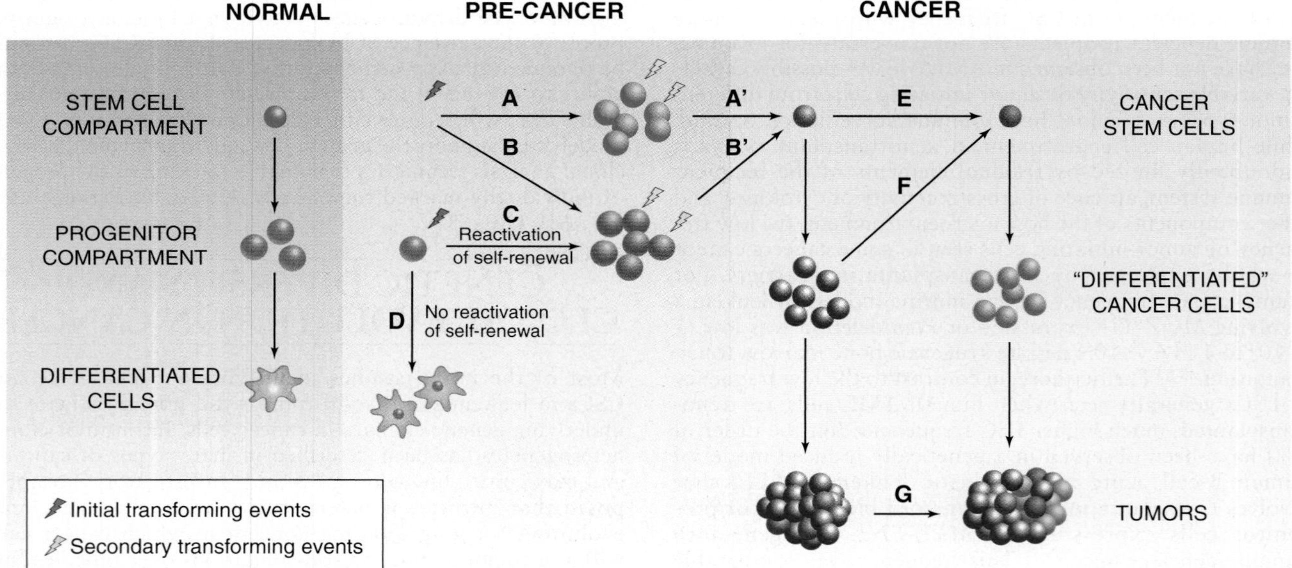

FIGURE 11.3 Models of tumor initiation and progression. Cancer stem cells (CSCs) might arise through neoplastic changes initiated in normal self-renewing stem cells, or downstream progenitors with limited or no self-renewal. Initial events in stem cells could cause (**A**) expansion of the stem cell pool and/or (**B**) expansion of downstream progenitors. Secondary events are more likely to occur in these expanded pools of target cells (A′, B′); thus, it is possible that transformation is initiated in a normal stem cell, but the final steps occur in downstream progenitors (B→B′). Reactivation of a self-renewal program is a central feature of oncogenic transformation of progenitors (**C**), as these short-lived cells will otherwise die or undergo terminal differentiation before enough mutations occur for full neoplastic transformation (**D**). CSCs themselves might acquire additional genetic or epigenetic changes during tumor progression (**E**), and non-CSCs can acquire CSC-like properties (**F**) through processes such as epithelial-mesenchymal transition (EMT), leading to evolution of tumor phenotype (**G**) and intratumor heterogeneity. Of note, the cell of origin debate centers around the cells and processes illustrated in the pink box, whereas CSC research focuses on characterization of cancer cell populations after they reach the green box. (Figure originally published in Wang JCY. Good cells gone bad: the cellular origins of cancer. *Trends Mol Med* 2010;16:145.)

cell" has led to the frequent misconception that CSCs always arise from stem cells.[57] On the contrary, emerging evidence suggests that although some cancers may originate in normal stem cells, committed progenitors can also be initial targets for transformation.

There has been a great deal of debate over the cellular origins of cancer. A number of conceptual arguments have been invoked to support stem cells as the cell of origin. One contention is that because self-renewal is a key property of CSCs, and stem cells already possess self-renewal capacity, they would theoretically require fewer neoplastic changes in order to become fully transformed. In contrast, despite their substantial proliferative ability, progenitors do not generally retain the self-renewal capacity of stem cells. Thus to become a CSC, a progenitor must acquire mutations that reactivate the cellular self-renewal machinery. In addition, there is greater opportunity for genetic changes to accumulate in individual, long-lived stem cells compared to more mature progenitors with a limited lifespan. If a short-lived progenitor acquires a genetic mutation that does not confer increased self-renewal, that cell is likely to die or undergo terminal differentiation before enough mutations occur for full neoplastic transformation.

On the other hand, stem cells are fewer in number and divide less frequently than progenitors; therefore, the probability that they will acquire the mutations needed for cancer development is correspondingly lower. Furthermore, some have argued that stem cells are the key to tissue regeneration and the only cells in adult tissues capable of self-renewal. Thus, they might have evolved sophisticated inhibitory machinery to keep self-renewal in check as an anticancer defense.[58] If this is true, stem cells could actually be less likely to acquire mutations that affect self-renewal and proliferation or to manifest biological changes as a result of such mutations, as compared to more committed progenitors. In other words, stem cells might be under evolutionary pressure to preserve genomic integrity over promoting survival in order to prevent oncogenic transformation.

Functional Studies in Leukemia

It is problematic to make inferences regarding the cellular origins of CSCs simply by studying their surface phenotype, as disruption of normal differentiation pathways by the neoplastic process can lead to aberrant expression of lineage-associated markers. Similarly, it is difficult to draw firm conclusions by studying the lineage involvement of the neoplastic clone. For example, in chronic myeloid leukemia (CML) patients, involvement of multiple hematopoietic lineages has been taken as evidence that CML originates from a multipotent HSC, whereas lineage restriction in some AML patients has been interpreted as disease origin from a committed progenitor. However, apparent lineage restriction of the leukemic clone in AML could also result from mutations that arise in a multipotent stem cell and suppress differentiation to one or more lineages.[59] The most direct way to determine whether CSCs arise from neoplastic transformation initiated in stem cells or progenitors is to test whether oncogene expression in directly isolated, functionally validated normal stem and progenitor cell populations is able to confer *in vivo* tumor-initiating ability.

This approach has been used to study leukemic initiation in the murine hematopoietic system, facilitated by previous detailed phenotypic and functional characterization of different classes of progenitors and HSCs. One focus of investigation has been the *mixed-lineage leukemia* (*MLL*) gene, which undergoes fusion with a wide variety of partner genes and is associated with myeloid, lymphoid, and biphenotypic acute leukemias in both children and adults. The fusion gene *MLL-GAS7* induces mixed-lineage leukemias when expressed in murine HSCs or multipotent progenitors, but not in lineage-restricted progenitors.[60] In contrast, *MLL-ENL* can initiate myeloid leukemias in both self-renewing HSCs and committed myeloid progenitors,[61] although much lower numbers of transformed HSCs compared to progenitors were required for tumor initiation *in vivo*. *MLL-AF9* is also able to generate LSCs from committed granulocyte macrophage progenitors (GMPs).[45] Interestingly, when *MLL-AF9* is expressed at lower, physiologic levels in a knock-in transgenic mouse model of leukemia, HSCs and CMPs, but not GMPs, from transgenic mice are able to initiate leukemia upon transplantation into wild type recipients.[62] Compared to retrovirally transduced GMPs, GMPs from knock-in mice had 170-fold lower expression of *MLL-AF9*. These findings imply that differences in experimental transformability of HSC and progenitor populations may be related to oncogene dosage. However, the nonequivalent transformation of HSCs and committed progenitors, even by supraphysiologic levels of retrovirally driven *MLL-ENL*,[61] points to the existence of inherent differences in susceptibility between these populations.

Taken together, these findings in the murine system indicate that MLL-expressing leukemias may be initiated in either HSCs or downstream progenitors, depending on the specific fusion partner involved. This likely depends on the ability of the fusion oncogene to reactivate a self-renewal program in committed progenitors. Indeed, the LSCs generated by *MLL-AF9* expression in GMPs possessed a surface immunophenotype and global gene expression profile similar to that of normal GMPs, but also demonstrated reactivation of a subset of genes highly expressed in HSCs and associated with self-renewal.[45,63] The capacity of *MLL* fusion genes to reactivate self-renewal machinery in progenitors confers a potent transforming ability to this group of oncogenes, as evidenced by the high frequency of leukemias in NOD/SCID mice transplanted with primitive human hematopoietic cells expressing an *MLL* fusion gene[44] and the infrequency of additional detectable genetic changes in human acute lymphoblastic leukemias with *MLL* rearrangements.[64]

Conclusions drawn from studies in *MLL* leukemias may not be generalizable, as *MLL* leukemia appears to be a unique disease distinct from other subtypes of acute leukemia.[65] However, there have been a few reports of the transforming ability of other leukemia-associated oncogenes. *MOZ-TIF* can initiate AML in HSCs as well as committed progenitors, while *BCR-ABL1* did not increase self-renewal *in vitro* or initiate disease when expressed in committed progenitors, despite the induction of myeloproliferative disease in mice transplanted with *BCR-ABL1*-transduced whole bone marrow.[43] These findings suggest that *BCR-ABL1* expression in more primitive HSCs is required for disease initiation, although this was not tested directly. Nevertheless, these results are consistent with data from studies of transgenic mouse models of CML, in which *BCR-ABL1* expression[66] or inactivation of *JunB*, a transcriptional regulator of myelopoiesis, in HSCs induces a transplantable myeloproliferative disorder, whereas *JunB* inactivation in more committed progenitors does not.[67] Interestingly, analysis of the *JunB*-deficient mice demonstrated expansion of the primitive HSC compartment as well as the GMP pool; however, the numbers of common myeloid progenitors and megakaryocytic-erythroid progenitors were similar to those of control animals, indicating that oncogenic changes in stem cells can have very specific effects in downstream progeny. Expansion or extended proliferation of progenitors may increase the risk of acquiring secondary cooperating events, resulting in progression to a fully transformed state. For example, transgenic mice that express reduced levels of the transcription factors PU.1[68] or GATA-1[69] are characterized by accumulation of an abnormal progenitor pool and a high propensity to develop acute leukemias, which in the PU.1 knockdown mice are frequently accompanied by additional chromosomal abnormalities. The mutant alleles in these engineered mice were expressed in every cell, thus it is impossible to determine whether reduced transcription factor levels would have equivalent transforming potential in the context of HSCs or progenitors. Patients with chronic phase CML have an expanded progenitor pool related at least in part to expression of *BCR-ABL*. Progression to blast crisis is associated with further expansion of GMPs that have activated β-catenin activity and increased self-renewal as demonstrated by *in vitro* replating assays.[70]

Overall, the accumulated evidence from studies in murine hematopoiesis indicates that the neoplastic changes that lead ultimately to generation of LSCs can be initiated in either normal HSCs or progenitors, depending on the ability of specific transforming events to overcome the inherent cellular barriers to transformation (Fig. 11.3). Potent oncogenes such as *MLL* that can reactivate self-renewal are able to transform committed progenitors, whereas less potent oncogenic changes must occur in self-renewing HSCs in order to initiate a tumorigenic program. Secondary neoplastic changes can occur within the stem cell compartment or within abnormally expanded downstream progenitor populations, ultimately resulting in the generation of LSCs. While the murine studies described above have provided significant insights, it will be important to carry out equivalent studies in the human hematopoietic system, as the processes underlying neoplastic transformation differ between mouse and man.[71]

Studies in Solid Tumors

Similar studies in solid tumors have been hampered by the lack of phenotypically and functionally defined stem and progenitor cell populations in most normal tissues. Recently, stem cells have been identified in murine[72,73] and human[74] mammary tissue and in murine prostate.[75–77] Lim et al.[78] proposed that luminal progenitors, rather than mammary stem cells, are the cell of origin for human basal breast cancers, which are associated with germline mutations in the tumor suppressor gene *BRCA1*, based on stronger similarity in gene expression profiles. Furthermore, the luminal progenitor population in premalignant breast tissue from *BRCA1* mutation carriers is expanded and has increased growth potential *in vitro*. However, analogous to targeting of HSCs in CML, it is also possible that *BRCA1* mutations target mammary stem cells and either drive development preferentially down the luminal lineage or have biological consequences only upon luminal differentiation. Transformation experiments of mammary cell subsets are needed to clarify this issue.

Despite the recent progress in characterizing normal cellular hierarchies in nonhematopoietic tissues, direct testing of the transformability of isolated stem and progenitor populations remains a challenge in most systems. Thus, researchers have turned to alternative methods to investigate the cell of origin in solid tumors. In brain cancer, genetic approaches have provided insights into the normal cell populations that might be targeted for transformation. Investigators used a transgenic mouse system that allows expression of oncogenes in a cell type-specific manner to show that selective expression of platelet-derived growth factor in nestin+ neural stem/progenitor cells generated oligodendrogliomas, whereas expression in GFAP+ astrocytes generated a mixture of oligodendrogliomas and oligoastrocytomas.[79] Similarly, the combined expression of activated Ras and Akt in nestin+ but not GFAP+ cells generated high-grade glioblastomas.[80] These findings suggest the existence of inherent differences in the transformability of neural cell populations but are confounded by the fact that GFAP marks neural stem cells as well as differentiated astrocytes.[81] In contrast, transduction of a constitutively active endothelial growth factor receptor mutant into either neural stem/progenitor cells or cortical astrocytes from *Ink4a/Arf−/−* mice gave rise to high-grade gliomas with similar latency, indicating that both cell compartments are permissive for transformation.[82] However, the isolated cell populations in this study were transduced only after a period of *in vitro* culture and were derived from age-mismatched animals, factors that can hamper direct comparisons of primitive and mature cell populations.

Using a different transgenic model, two groups found that activation of hedgehog (Hh) signaling, which is etiologically linked to medulloblastomas in mice and humans,[83] in both multipotent stem/progenitor cells and unilineage granule neuron precursors (GNPs), but not Purkinje neurons, generated transplantable medulloblastomas, but no tumors of other histological types.[84,85] Interestingly, Hh activation in stem/progenitor cells resulted in expansion and increased proliferation of these cells as well as committed GNPs, but caused no abnormalities in other downstream cell populations,[85] suggesting that Hh activation must occur in a lineage-specific context to manifest biological effects. The generation of medulloblastomas and no other histological tumor types is likely related to specific influences of Hh activation on target cell development, because conditional inactivation of tumor suppressor genes *p53*, *NF1*, and *Pten* (commonly mutated in human astrocytomas) in neural stem/progenitor cells generates high-grade astrocytomas.[86,87]

In the intestine, genetic lineage–tracing studies in mice have recently identified adult stem cell populations,[88–90] enabling studies of the cellular origin of intestinal tumors. Most human colorectal cancers are etiologically linked to mutations in the tumor suppressor gene *Apc*, with resultant activation of Wnt/β-catenin signaling.[91] In transgenic mouse models, rapid adenoma formation was consistently seen with conditional *Apc* deletion or expression of a stable β-catenin mutant in stem cell populations but not in more differentiated progenitors,[88,90,92] supporting a stem cell origin for intestinal tumors in the mouse. However, the findings from these transgenic models with full, constitutive β-catenin activation may not be fully applicable to human colorectal cancer, where studies have suggested that a specific degree or "dosage" of β-catenin signaling may be optimal for tumor formation,[93] as has been shown for leukemia stem/progenitor cells and *MLL* signaling. Clarification of these issues will require studies using human cells as target populations.

It is clear from these murine studies that cancers can originate in both stem cell and progenitor compartments, depending on the oncogene(s) involved, although stem and progenitor cells might differ in their inherent susceptibility to transformation. In addition, tumors generated by specific oncogenes are often phenotypically and functionally similar regardless of the cell of origin, suggesting that tumor heterogeneity in tissues is generated in large part by the differential effects of transforming events on the developmental program of the targeted cells, rather than by differences among target cells themselves. However, the results from murine studies must be confirmed in equivalent human studies using primary, functionally defined stem and progenitor cell populations. Insight into the cellular context in which the first steps of neoplastic transformation occur will be vital not only to understand how normal developmental processes become subverted during cancer initiation and progression, but also to advance our knowledge of CSC biology and facilitate the development of novel and effective therapies to eliminate these cancer-sustaining cells in patients.

EPITHELIAL-MESENCHYMAL TRANSITION

Epithelial-mesenchymal transition (EMT) is a complex molecular and cellular program involved in embryonic development whereby epithelial cells lose their differentiated characteristics and acquire a mesenchymal phenotype. There is recent evidence that EMT induction contributes to tumor progression by conferring properties such as invasiveness, the ability to metastasize, and resistance to therapy on epithelial cancer cells.[94,95] EMT induction of ras-transformed, SV40-immortalized human mammary epithelial cells (HMLEs) significantly increased their ability to generate tumors *in vivo* following subcutaneous injection into immune-deficient mice.[96] Notably, despite having undergone an EMT, transformed HMLEs did not exhibit *in vivo* tumor-initiating ability when EMT-inducing signals were removed, and the cells reverted to an epithelial phenotype when cultured further *in vitro*.[96] A number of groups have reported that EMT-inducing signals can originate from stromal cells in the tumor microenvironment.[97,98] Together, these observations suggest that in some epithelial tumors, acquisition and maintenance of CSC-like properties depend on continuous signals from the microenvironment, and support the notion that metastatic cancer cells revert to an epithelial state after dissemination and resultant loss of contact with a "tumor microenvironment." However, sustained induction of EMT might in some cases lead to irreversible, heritable epigenetic alterations that maintain the mesenchymal phenotype.[99] Such changes could have therapeutic implications, as breast cancer cells induced into EMT appear to be more resistant to standard chemotherapeutic drugs compared to control cells.[100] Furthermore, EMT of non-self-renewing cancer cell populations within a tumor could contribute to clonal evolution and intratumor heterogeneity of CSCs (Fig. 11.3). It should be noted, however, that the linkage between EMT and tumor initiation is still tenuous; a deeper understanding will require clonal assays, well-defined cell fractions, proof of self-renewal, and studies of primary tumors rather than cell lines.

CANCER STEM CELLS: TARGETED THERAPY

General Considerations

Implicit in the model of cancer as a hierarchical disease is the notion that CSCs are biologically distinct from the bulk cells in the tumor. Molecular pathways for survival and response to injury may be fundamentally different in these cells compared to nontumorigenic cells. Ultimately, to prevent disease relapse and achieve permanent cure, the CSCs that sustain tumor growth must be eradicated in addition to killing the bulk cells of the tumor. However, properties of CSCs, such as quiescence or expression of drug-resistance transporters, may make them difficult to eliminate using conventional cytotoxic drugs that kill the bulk tumor cells. It will be crucial to understand the unique biology of CSCs in order to develop novel treatments that effectively target these cells (Fig. 11.4).

There are several obstacles to be overcome in the development of effective CSC-targeted therapies. Such treatments must be selective for CSCs and spare normal stem cells. There is recent evidence in AML that the pathways that regulate self-renewal in normal stem cells are not completely abolished in LSCs.[30] In other words, CSCs, although transformed, likely retain aspects of normal developmental pathways. Thus, drugs that target critical processes in CSCs, such as survival or self-renewal, may prove intolerably harmful to their normal counterparts. Furthermore, normal stem or progenitor cells may in fact be more sensitive than CSCs to the effects of chemotherapy. CSCs will likely have acquired genetic or epigenetic changes that allow them to bypass normal tumor-suppressing processes such as senescence or apoptosis in response to DNA damage. Thus, treatment with agents that normally induce senescence or apoptosis may actually provide a growth advantage to CSCs.[101] Ideally, effective therapies will target pathways that are necessary for CSC survival but not for the survival of normal stem cells.

Clinical testing of CSC-targeted therapies must take into account the relative infrequency of these cells within some

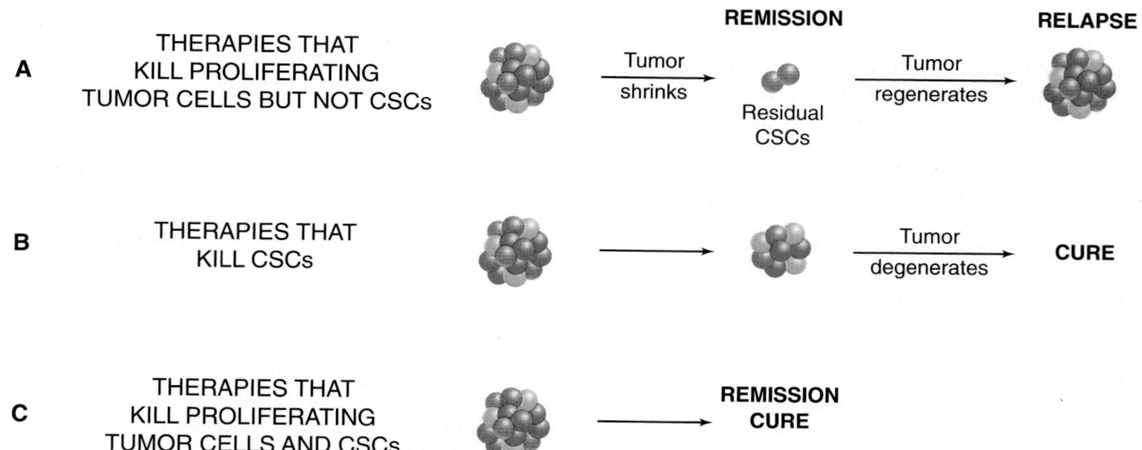

FIGURE 11.4 Development of effective anticancer therapies. **A:** Cancer stem cells (CSCs) are biologically distinct from bulk tumor cells and may not be effectively killed by conventional anticancer therapies due to properties such as quiescence or expression of drug-resistance transporters, leading to regrowth of the tumor and relapse after treatment. **B:** Ultimately, to prevent disease relapse and achieve permanent cure, the CSCs that sustain tumor growth must be eradicated. **C:** The most effective anticancer strategies will involve combination regimens that both reduce tumor bulk and kill CSCs, the latter likely best achieved through targeting of multiple critical pathways (see text). The development of new CSC-targeted therapies will require a greater understanding of the molecular pathways that drive tumor initiation and progression.

tumors. Treatments that eradicate CSCs may not have significant effects on proliferation or apoptosis of the bulk of tumor cells[102] and therefore may not cause rapid tumor regression or shrinkage.There is a significant risk that agents that selectively target CSCs will be overlooked in clinical trials if assessed simply on the basis of objective tumor response. In the evaluation of CSC-targeted therapies, delay in tumor progression would be a more relevant clinical end point. In the end, the ultimate test of the effectiveness of a CSC-targeted agent is whether relapse is prevented, an end point that requires long-term follow-up. A corollary to this concept is that evaluation of toxicity toward normal stem cells should also be measured in long-term studies, in order to properly assess effects on tissue maintenance. As tumor shrinkage is not an accurate measure of the efficacy of agents that selectively kill CSCs, clinical evaluation would be greatly aided by the development of sensitive real-time imaging modalities to detect and quantify residual CSCs in patients who undergo treatment. However, such technology is currently unavailable. As discussed above, current protocols for isolating tumor cell fractions enriched in CSCs do not yield pure populations, thus it is problematic simply to correlate therapeutic effectiveness with eradication of a phenotypically defined cell population. Ultimately, detection of residual CSCs with the ability to reinitiate tumor growth may depend on functional assays of tumorigenicity. However, such testing would be subject to the inherent limitations associated with *in vivo* detection of rare cells.

Resistance to Standard Therapy

The identification of CSCs in solid tumors and the development of *in vivo* assays to assess their tumorigenic properties have paved the way for studies to assess the impact of anticancer therapies on these cells. Radiation therapy for glioblastoma multiforme, an aggressive type of brain cancer, is transiently effective but is often followed by tumor recurrence or progression, implying that CSCs are not effectively eradicated. This notion is supported by recent evidence that ionizing-radiation treatment of glioblastoma grafts grown in mice leads to an increase in the proportion of CD133+ cells in the residual tumor population compared to unirradiated controls.[101] Irradiated CD133+ cells retain the ability to form heterogeneous tumors *in vivo* that can be serially propagated. *In vitro* experiments demonstrated that this radioresistance is likely due to increased activation of DNA damage checkpoint proteins and more efficient repair of DNA damage, resulting in a lower rate of apoptosis compared to CD133− cells. Intriguingly, treatment of CD133+ cells with an inhibitor of two checkpoint kinases disrupted their radioresistance, although the ability of treated cells to initiate tumor growth *in vivo* was not tested. A recent study that showed lower levels of pro-oxidants and higher expression of antioxidant genes in the CSC-enriched CD44+CD24−/lowLineage− cell population from primary human breast cancers compared to nontumorigenic cells suggests that lower levels of reactive oxygen species may also contribute to the relative radioresistance of CSCs.[103]

There have been a number of studies that indicated that CSCs may be resistant to standard chemotherapy. Following *in vitro* treatment of human pancreatic cancer cells with the nucleoside analogue gemcitabine, the CD133− population underwent apoptosis and was dramatically reduced, whereas most CD133+ cells survived, resulting in nearly 40-fold enrichment of the CD133+ fraction.[37] In addition, *in vivo* gemcitabine treatment of mice bearing pancreatic cancer cell line xenografts resulted in reduction of tumor bulk but approximately fourfold enrichment of the minority CD133+ population. These data suggest that the CSC-containing CD133+ cell population is relatively resistant to chemotherapy compared to non-CSCs. However, as discussed above, phenotypically defined populations enriched for CSCs are heterogeneous and contain non-CSCs as well. Thus, it is crucial to measure the effects of treatment on CSCs directly through functional assays. For example, Li et al.[104] showed that human breast cancer biopsy samples obtained from patients treated with standard chemotherapy had increased percentages of CD44+CD24−/low cells and increased clonogenic efficiency *in vitro*, implying enrichment of CSCs. Importantly, posttreatment samples were twice as efficient at generating tumor xenografts when implanted into the mammary fat pads of SCID/Beige mice, confirming a functional enrichment of CSCs surviving in the treated tumors.

CD133+ human colon cancer cells are more resistant to apoptosis induced by *in vitro* treatment with 5-fluorouracil or oxaliplatin compared to CD133− cells.[105] *In vivo* oxaliplatin treatment of mice bearing colon cancer xenografts led to a reduction in tumor size but an increase in the percentage of CD133+ cells, with associated resistance of CD133+ cells to apoptosis. Cotreatment of mice with oxaliplatin plus a neutralizing antibody against IL-4 resulted in delayed tumor growth that persisted after treatment was discontinued, as well as increased apoptosis of CD133+ cells, leading to enhanced killing of these cells. These findings suggest that chemoresistance of colon CSCs may be related at least in part to autocrine IL-4 signaling, possibly through up-regulation of an antiapoptotic program.[105] Similarly, *in vivo* treatment of early passage colon cancer xenografts with cyclophosphamide led to slowing of tumor growth but enrichment of cells with a CSC phenotype and a twofold increase in CSC number measured by limiting dilution serial transplantation assays.[106] ALDH1 activity catabolizes the cytotoxic metabolites of cyclophosphamide; short hairpin RNA–mediated knockdown of ALDH1 sensitized tumors to cyclophosphamide treatment *in vivo* and reduced the frequency of CSCs in residual tumors. Thus, identification of functional pathways such as ALDH1 that are important for CSC survival can provide not only markers for isolating these cells, but potential therapeutic targets as well. Future studies using primary human tumors tested in *in vivo* functional assays will be required to determine the clinical importance of CSCs in tumor response and relapse.

Targeting the Microenvironment

Angiogenesis is a critical factor in the early stages of tumor formation as well as in tumor progression and therefore represents a potential target for anticancer treatments. Regulation of angiogenesis involves a complex interplay between tumor cells and the neovasculature. Glioblastomas, for example, express high levels of vascular endothelial growth factor (VEGF).[107] A functional interaction between brain CSCs and endothelial cells is supported by the close association of CD133+ brain cancer cells with vascular endothelial cells *in vitro* and *in vivo*, and more importantly by the demonstration that coinjection of primary human endothelial cells enhances tumor formation by CD133+ medulloblastoma cells in immune-deficient mice.[102] Tumors initiated in mice by CD133+ cells from either primary glioblastoma biopsy specimens or xenograft cell lines are highly vascular.[107] Interestingly, treatment of xenograft tumors with bevacizumab, an antibody that neutralizes VEGF, not only potently inhibits tumor growth in mice[102,107] but also results in depletion of cells coexpressing CD133 and nestin, a marker of primitive neural cells, without directly affecting bulk tumor cell proliferation or death. Together, these results suggest that inhibition of brain tumor growth by antiangiogenic agents is mediated at least in part by disruption of a vascular niche required for maintenance of

CSCs. For the most part, these experiments were done using brain cancer cell lines rather than freshly isolated tumor cells, but they nevertheless make a compelling case for further characterization and therapeutic targeting of the unique microenvironment of CSCs.

Ginestier et al.[16,108] recently showed that human breast cancer cells expressing CXCR1, a receptor that binds the proinflammatory chemokine IL-8, are present almost exclusively within the CSC-containing ALDH1+ population. IL-8 has been implicated in tumor invasion, metastasis, and self-renewal.[109,110] Treatment of orthotopically transplanted tumors in NOD/SCID mice with the CXCR1/2 inhibitor repertaxin, the standard chemotherapeutic agent docetaxel, or a combination of both drugs all resulted in impaired tumor growth. However, tumors treated with docetaxel alone showed either unchanged or increased percentage of ALDH1+ cells compared with untreated controls, whereas repertaxin treatment alone or in combination with docetaxel significantly reduced the ALDH1+ population. Importantly, upon serial transplantation, tumor cells derived from control or docetaxel-treated primary animals were able to generate tumors in secondary mice with similar efficiency, while cells from repertaxin-treated animals showed a two- to fivefold reduction in tumor growth and were only able to generate tumors at the highest injected cell dose. These findings indicate that, contrary to standard chemotherapy with docetaxel, CXCR1 blockade with repertaxin directly targets and reduces the CSC population *in vivo* and underscore the importance of directly assaying effects on CSCs rather than relying on traditional measures of efficacy such as reduction of tumor bulk.

Differentiation Therapy

Another approach to anticancer therapy is induction of differentiation of CSCs, with consequent associated loss of self-renewal capacity. This strategy has been highly successful in acute promyelocytic leukemia (APL), where the addition of retinoic acid to conventional chemotherapy has significantly improved survival rates. The demonstration that the growth of solid tumors is sustained by CSCs with the capacity to generate tumor heterogeneity implies that it should be similarly possible to drive the differentiation of CSCs in these cancers. However, the clinical development of differentiation-inducing agents to treat solid tumors has been limited to date. Bone morphogenic proteins (BMPs) are soluble factors that induce normal neural precursor cells to differentiate. BMP treatment of CD133+ glioblastoma cells *in vitro* or in immune-deficient mice results in the formation of smaller, more differentiated, less invasive tumor grafts that cannot be serially propagated in mice,[111] demonstrating the therapeutic potential of differentiation-inducing agents in brain cancer. However, the differentiation response to BMP treatment may be impaired in a subset of glioblastoma CSCs due to epigenetic silencing of BMP receptor 1B (*BMPR1B*), a feature shared with early embryonic neural stem cells.[112] Indeed, in patient-derived glioblastoma cells with reduced *BMPR1B* expression, BMP2 induced proliferation rather than differentiation. Transgenic expression of a constitutively active BMPR1B mutant in these cells followed by orthotopic injection into neonatal SCID mice resulted in higher expression of GFAP by tumor cells, impaired tumor growth, and improved host survival compared to unmanipulated tumor cells. *BMPR1B* down-regulation was found in approximately 20% of primary human glioblastomas. This elegant study not only provides insight into the role of BMPs in brain CSC biology, but highlights the existence of intertumor CSC variability, even among tumors of the same histological class. As discussed above, tumor heterogeneity is likely related in large part to differences in the underlying oncogenic changes that drive tumor growth. Thus, therapeutic approaches such as induction of differentiation may require targeting of multiple pathways and will likely need to be tailored to some degree to the biology of individual tumors. A recent unbiased RNA interference screen identified several genes whose silencing induced a "differentiation phenotype" in glioblastoma cells derived from multiple patients' tumors.[113] The strongest and most reproducible of these was *TRRAP*, which encodes an adaptor protein found in multiprotein/chromatin complexes. Knockdown of TRRAP in three different patient-derived glioblastoma lines followed by orthotopic injection into SCID mice resulted in impaired tumor growth, a more differentiated xenograft phenotype, and improved host survival compared to control cells. Future studies are required to determine the applicability and efficacy of these treatment approaches in the clinic.

Selected References

The full list of references for this chapter appears in the online version.

1. Bruce WR, van der Gaag H. A quantitative assay for the number of murine lymphoma cells capable of proliferation in vivo. *Nature* 1963;199:79.
2. Southam CM, Brunschwig A, Dizon Q. Autologous and homologous transplantation of human cancer. In: Brennan MJ, Simpson WL, eds. *Biological interactions in normal and neoplastic growth. A contribution to the host-tumor problem.* Boston: Little, Brown, 1962:723.
5. Lapidot T, Sirard C, Vormoor J, et al. A cell initiating human acute myeloid leukemia after transplantation into SCID mice. *Nature* 1994;367:645.
6. Bonnet D, Dick JE. Human acute myeloid leukemia is organized as a hierarchy that originates from a primitive hematopoietic cell. *Nat Med* 1997;3:730.
7. Jordan CT, Upchurch D, Szilvassy SJ, et al. The interleukin-3 receptor alpha chain is a unique marker for human acute myelogenous leukemia stem cells. *Leukemia* 2000;14:1777.
8. Jin L, Lee EM, Ramshaw HS, et al. Monoclonal antibody-mediated targeting of CD123, IL-3 receptor alpha chain, eliminates human acute myeloid leukemic stem cells. *Cell Stem Cell* 2009;5:31.
10. Guzman ML, Rossi RM, Karnischky L, et al. The sesquiterpene lactone parthenolide induces apoptosis of human acute myelogenous leukemia stem and progenitor cells. *Blood* 2005;105:4163.
12. Yilmaz OH, Valdez R, Theisen BK, et al. Pten dependence distinguishes haematopoietic stem cells from leukaemia-initiating cells. *Nature* 2006;441:475.
14. Jin L, Hope KJ, Zhai Q, et al. Targeting of CD44 eradicates human acute myeloid leukemic stem cells. *Nat Med* 2006;12:1167.
15. Al Hajj M, Wicha MS, Benito-Hernandez A, et al. Prospective identification of tumorigenic breast cancer cells. *Proc Natl Acad Sci U S A* 2003;100:3983.
21. Singh SK, Hawkins C, Clarke ID, et al. Identification of human brain tumour initiating cells. *Nature* 2004;432:396.
25. Chen R, Nishimura MC, Bumbaca SM, et al. A hierarchy of self-renewing tumor-initiating cell types in glioblastoma. *Cancer Cell* 2010;17:362.
28. O'Brien CA, Pollett A, Gallinger S, et al. A human colon cancer cell capable of initiating tumour growth in immunodeficient mice. *Nature* 2007;445:106.
29. Ricci-Vitiani L, Lombardi DG, Pilozzi E, et al. Identification and expansion of human colon-cancer-initiating cells. *Nature* 2007;445:111.
30. Hope KJ, Jin L, Dick JE. Acute myeloid leukemia originates from a hierarchy of leukemic stem cell classes that differ in self-renewal capacity. *Nat Immunol* 2004;5:738.
37. Hermann PC, Huber SL, Herrler T, et al. Distinct populations of cancer stem cells determine tumor growth and metastatic activity in human pancreatic cancer. *Cell Stem Cell* 2007;1:313.
38. Kelly PN, Dakic A, Adams JM, et al. Tumor growth need not be driven by rare cancer stem cells. *Science* 2007;317:337.
40. Quintana E, Shackleton M, Sabel MS, et al. Efficient tumour formation by single human melanoma cells. *Nature* 2008;456:593.
42. Kennedy JA, Barabe F, Poeppl AG, et al. Comment on "Tumor growth need not be driven by rare cancer stem cells." *Science* 2007;318:1722.

42a. Ishizawa K, Rasheed ZA, Karisch R, et al. Tumor-initiating cells are rare in many human tumors. *Cell Stem Cell* 2010;7:279.
43. Huntly BJ, Shigematsu H, Deguchi K, et al. MOZ-TIF2, but not BCR-ABL, confers properties of leukemic stem cells to committed murine hematopoietic progenitors. *Cancer Cell* 2004;6:587.
44. Barabe F, Kennedy JA, Hope KJ, et al. Modeling the initiation and progression of human acute leukemia in mice. *Science* 2007;316:600.
45. Krivtsov AV, Twomey D, Feng Z, et al. Transformation from committed progenitor to leukaemia stem cell initiated by MLL-AF9. *Nature* 2006; 442:818.
48. Marusyk A, Polyak K. Tumor heterogeneity: causes and consequences. *Biochim Biophys Acta* 2010;1805:105.
54. Notta F, Mullighan CG, Wang JCY, et al. Evolution of human BCR-ALB1 lymphoblastic leukaemia-initiating cells. *Nature In Press.*
54a. Anderson K, Lutz C, van Delft FW, et al. Genetic variegation of clonal architecture and propagating cells in leukaemia. *Nature* 2010 doi:10.1038/nature09650.
60. So CW, Karsunky H, Passegue E, et al. MLL-GAS7 transforms multipotent hematopoietic progenitors and induces mixed lineage leukemias in mice. *Cancer Cell* 2003;3:161.
61. Cozzio A, Passegue E, Ayton PM, et al. Similar MLL-associated leukemias arising from self-renewing stem cells and short-lived myeloid progenitors. *Genes Dev* 2003;17:3029.
62. Chen W, Kumar AR, Hudson WA, et al. Malignant transformation initiated by Mll-AF9: gene dosage and critical target cells. *Cancer Cell* 2008;13:432.
63. Somervaille TC, Cleary ML. Identification and characterization of leukemia stem cells in murine MLL-AF9 acute myeloid leukemia. *Cancer Cell* 2006;10:257.
67. Passegue E, Wagner EF, Weissman IL. JunB deficiency leads to a myeloproliferative disorder arising from hematopoietic stem cells. *Cell* 2004;119:431.
70. Jamieson CH, Ailles LE, Dylla SJ, et al. Granulocyte-macrophage progenitors as candidate leukemic stem cells in blast-crisis CML. *N Engl J Med* 2004;351:657.
78. Lim E, Vaillant F, Wu D, et al. Aberrant luminal progenitors as the candidate target population for basal tumor development in BRCA1 mutation carriers. *Nat Med* 2009;15:907.
79. Dai C, Celestino JC, Okada Y, et al. PDGF autocrine stimulation dedifferentiates cultured astrocytes and induces oligodendrogliomas and oligoastrocytomas from neural progenitors and astrocytes in vivo. *Genes Dev* 2001;15:1913.
80. Holland EC, Celestino J, Dai C, et al. Combined activation of Ras and Akt in neural progenitors induces glioblastoma formation in mice. *Nat Genet* 2000;25:55.
82. Bruggeman SW, Hulsman D, Tanger E, et al. Bmi1 controls tumor development in an Ink4a/Arf-independent manner in a mouse model for glioma. *Cancer Cell* 2007;12:328.
84. Schuller U, Heine VM, Mao J, et al. Acquisition of granule neuron precursor identity is a critical determinant of progenitor cell competence to form Shh-induced medulloblastoma. *Cancer Cell* 2008;14:123.
85. Yang ZJ, Ellis T, Markant SL, et al. Medulloblastoma can be initiated by deletion of Patched in lineage-restricted progenitors or stem cells. *Cancer Cell* 2008;14:135.
90. Zhu L, Gibson P, Currle DS, et al. Prominin 1 marks intestinal stem cells that are susceptible to neoplastic transformation. *Nature* 2009;457:603.
92. Barker N, Ridgway RA, van Es JH, et al. Crypt stem cells as the cells-of-origin of intestinal cancer. *Nature* 2009;457:608.
96. Mani SA, Guo W, Liao MJ, et al. The epithelial-mesenchymal transition generates cells with properties of stem cells. *Cell* 2008;133:704.
100. Gupta PB, Onder TT, Jiang G, et al. Identification of selective inhibitors of cancer stem cells by high-throughput screening. *Cell* 2009;138:645.
101. Bao S, Wu Q, McLendon RE, et al. Glioma stem cells promote radioresistance by preferential activation of the DNA damage response. *Nature* 2006;444:756.
102. Calabrese C, Poppleton H, Kocak M, et al. A perivascular niche for brain tumor stem cells. *Cancer Cell* 2007;11:69.
104. Li X, Lewis MT, Huang J, et al. Intrinsic resistance of tumorigenic breast cancer cells to chemotherapy. *J Natl Cancer Inst* 2008;100:672.
105. Todaro M, Alea MP, Di Stefano AB, et al. Colon cancer stem cells dictate tumor growth and resist cell death by production of interleukin-4. *Cell Stem Cell* 2007;1:389.
106. Dylla SJ, Beviglia L, Park IK, et al. Colorectal cancer stem cells are enriched in xenogeneic tumors following chemotherapy. *PLoS One* 2008;3:e2428.
107. Bao S, Wu Q, Sathornsumetee S, et al. Stem cell-like glioma cells promote tumor angiogenesis through vascular endothelial growth factor. *Cancer Res* 2006;66:7843.
108. Ginestier C, Liu S, Diebel ME, et al. CXCR1 blockade selectively targets human breast cancer stem cells in vitro and in xenografts. *J Clin Invest* 2010;120:485.
111. Piccirillo SG, Reynolds BA, Zanetti N, et al. Bone morphogenetic proteins inhibit the tumorigenic potential of human brain tumour-initiating cells. *Nature* 2006;444:761.
112. Lee J, Son MJ, Woolard K, et al. Epigenetic-mediated dysfunction of the bone morphogenetic protein pathway inhibits differentiation of glioblastoma-initiating cells. *Cancer Cell* 2008;13:69.
113. Wurdak H, Zhu S, Romero A, et al. An RNAi screen identifies TRRAP as a regulator of brain tumor-initiating cell differentiation. *Cell Stem Cell* 2010;6:37.

CHAPTER 12 BIOLOGY OF PERSONALIZED CANCER MEDICINE

RAJU KUCHERLAPATI

It is well established that cancer is a genetic disease. At the genetic level cancer cells are different from their precursor cells. It is understood that a series of genetic changes are necessary for a normal cell to begin the process of transformation, eventually leading to cancer. Cancers can be generally classified into sporadic cancers and those that result from a genetic predisposition. Some individuals in the population inherit specific mutations in particular genes that predispose them to certain types of cancers. Although these individuals are born with a mutation in a predisposition gene, they do not develop tumors until later in life; and it is now well understood that, besides the inherited predisposition gene mutation, additional genetic changes are required for the cells in these individuals to become tumors. In sporadic cases a randomly acquired somatic mutation or another type of genetic change in a gene that is critical for the normal regulation of growth in the appropriate cell type might initiate a series of events that eventually leads to tumor formation. In addition to genetic mutations, changes in copy number of individual genes or subsets of genes; chromosomal aberrations including translocations, insertions, deletions and inversions; and changes in expression patterns of genes as well as epigenetic changes also play critical roles in tumor susceptibility, tumor initiation, and progression. Understanding all of the important genetic and genomic changes in each cancer type will help in accurate diagnosis and prognosis and increase the ability to stratify the patient populations to help assess the most optimal treatments for each patient. The use of such genetic and genomic information to determine treatment decisions is referred to as *personalized medicine*. Knowledge about the genetic and genomic changes that accompany cellular transformation and the events that are critical for initiation and maintenance of the cancerous state is increasing at a rapid pace. Because most cancers are clonal in origin and because it is possible to obtain an adequate amount of tumor material from tumor biopsies or resections, it is now possible to examine and document the genetic and genomic changes in tumor cells very accurately. As a result, understanding of the genetic and genomic changes in cancer is significantly greater than many other human diseases. This knowledge allows implementation of the principles of personalized medicine into clinical management of cancer patients. This chapter will consider examples of how cancer genetics and genomics are affecting the ability to manage cancer patients.

CANCER PREDISPOSITION

There is a large body of evidence that indicates that certain families have a higher incidence of a particular cancer. Epidemiological studies reveal that family members descendant from individuals who developed cancer, especially at a younger age, have a higher risk of developing cancer. This was followed by studies of families where the predisposition to develop cancer was found to be inherited. Another line of evidence that reveals the genetic basis for cancer came from studies of twins. Monozygotic twins have the same genetic composition, while dizygotic twins have a 50% probability of sharing an identical copy of any gene. The fact that there is a higher concordance of cancer incidence in monozygotic twins but not in dizygotic twins provides additional critical evidence for the genetic basis of cancer.[1] Studies during the past half century have established not only the familial predisposition of cancer but also to identified several genes that are involved in cancer predisposition. That knowledge, in turn, helps to explain the genetic processes and mechanisms that lead to cancer and to develop tests to identify individuals at risk for certain types of cancers.

There are several examples of gene mutations that are responsible for cancer predisposition. Cancers that show a familial predisposition include childhood retinoblastoma, colorectal cancer, early onset breast cancer, and several types of renal cancer, among many others. One cancer type where there is a large amount of information about familial predisposition is colorectal cancer (CRC).[2] CRC is one of the most common cancers, and it is estimated that as many 875,000 new cases of CRC are diagnosed every year in the world. The greater accessibility of the colon and rectum to detect or follow the cancer as well as the relative ease of obtaining biopsies facilitate study of this cancer.

CRC can be classified into familial cases and sporadic cases. Various estimates of the relative proportions of these two categories of CRC have been made and in some estimates the familial cases represent 10% of all CRCs, while other estimates place this number to be 25% or more.[3] Several genes that are involved in familial cases have been identified and are discussed in the sections that follow.

FAMILIAL ADENOMATOUS POLYPOSIS

Individuals with familiar adenomatous polyposis (FAP) are born normally and develop hundred to thousands of benign colonic polyps during their early adulthood. Unless these tumors are detected and treated (usually by surgery), one or more of them may develop into adenocarcinomas that can metastasize. Family studies revealed that this predisposition was inherited in an autosomal dominant fashion, and individuals who have inherited the susceptibility allele almost always exhibit the phenotype (near 100% penetrance). Linkage analysis revealed that the gene for FAP is located on human chromosome 5. Positional cloning has enabled the cloning of the gene that was designated as adenomatous polyposis coli (APC).[4,5] *APC* is a classic tumor suppressor gene, and inactivation or modification of both copies of the gene is necessary for the initiation of CRC development.

APC plays an important role not only in the relatively rare cases of FAP but also in a majority of sporadic CRC. Most of the sporadic colorectal tumors are also the result of the inactivation of both copies of the *APC* gene, but unlike FAP, where one copy is already mutated in the germline, in sporadic cases both copies are sequentially mutated in somatic colonic epithelial cells.[6] This observation explains the earlier onset of tumors and the abundance of tumors in FAP patients.

Since FAP is inherited in an autosomal dominant fashion and since individuals with FAP are born with a mutation in the *APC* gene, when an individual with FAP is identified it is recognized that all of the immediate family members are at risk to carry the mutant allele. The siblings of the affected individual are at 50% risk, and other relatives would also be at risk depending on the nature of familial relationship. Because the diagnosis of FAP is unambiguous, genetic testing is not always conducted. It is most desirable to sequence the germline DNA of the affected individual to identify the mutation, inform the relatives of their risk, and recommend the testing for the specific mutation as appropriate.

LYNCH SYNDROME

Another predisposition to CRC is Lynch syndrome (LS), named after Henry Lynch who first described this syndrome.[7] LS is also inherited as an autosomal dominant disorder, and individuals who inherit a disease allele develop CRC at an earlier age than sporadic CRC but later than FAP patients. The manifestation of colorectal neoplasms in individuals with this syndrome is less severe than in FAP patients, with the development of a few tumors later in life.

It was noted that the LS tumors have a unique feature in that they show genetic instability as revealed by expansion or contraction of the length of microsatellites.[8–10] Based on these observations these tumors are classified as microsatellite instable (MSI+). This knowledge of microsatellite instability plays an important role in discovering the genes important for LS. The first gene that was responsible for a subset of LS cases was found to be a human gene that has homology to a bacterial gene that is necessary for repairing single nucleotide mismatches and small insertions or deletions that result from errors in DNA replication.[11,12] This gene was designated Mut S homolog 2 (*MSH2*). *MSH2* encodes a protein that is required for recognition and repair of DNA mismatches. It was later discovered that mutations in other genes that encode members of the mismatch repair complex also cause LS. In addition to *MSH2* the genes that encode other members of this complex that are now known to be involved are Mut L homolog 1 (*MLH1*), Mut S homolog 6 (*MSH6*), postmeiotic segregation 2 (*PMS2*), and Mut L homolog 3 (*MLH3*). Mutations in all of these genes are now implicated in colon cancer susceptibility.[11,13–18]

Relatives of LS patients are also at increased risk to carry the mutant gene and, therefore, for CRC. As is the case for FAP it would be desirable to establish the specific mutation that causes LS and test the immediate relatives to establish or rule out the presence of the specific mutation in their germline. The presence or absence of mismatch repair proteins, especially *MLH1*, can also be detected by immunological methods, and individuals whose tumors do not have a detectable level of *MLH1* are excellent candidates for testing of their germline; if a germline mutation in the gene is detected, informing that patient's immediate relatives and testing them for the specific mutation may be warranted.

The precise incidence of LS in the population has been difficult to assess. Because individuals with LS develop fewer tumors and later in life than those with FAP, they are more difficult to distinguish from sporadic cases, and, therefore, testing for LS has not become routine. According to some studies the incidence of LS among patients with colorectal neoplasms is as high as 3%.[19] These results suggest that examination of all colorectal tumors for its MSI status and testing for mismatch repair gene mutations in individuals whose tumors are MSI+ may help identify individual at risk with a greater efficiency.[20,21]

OTHER POLYPOSIS SYNDROMES

There are other syndromes that are relatively rare that predispose individuals to CRC risk. These include Peutz-Jeghers syndrome, juvenile polyposis, and Cowden's disease. Genes that are involved in these syndromes have been identified and include *LKB1*, *SMAD4*, *BMPR1A*, and *PTEN*. Although all of the syndromes mentioned above are inherited in a dominant fashion, mutations in *MYH*, a homolog of an excision repair gene in *Escherichia coli*, cause a tumor predisposition but in a recessive fashion (de la Chapelle[22] gives a detailed review).

ASSOCIATION STUDIES

Most of the genetic mutations in genes described above result in CRC with high penetrance. This raises the question if there are other genes where mutations or variants cause a predisposition to CRC but with lower penetrance. Studies of sibling pairs that are concordant or discordant for CRC as well as association studies have identified regions of the genome or single nucleotide polymorphisms (SNP) that may be important in CRC susceptibility. One such polymorphism is that located on human chromosome 8. In an initial study Zanke et al.[23] examined a large cohort of individuals who had large bowel cancer and an equal number of controls for associations with genes or variants in the genome. In this study they identified SNPs at 8q24, which shows significant association with susceptibility to colon cancer. This region was also shown to be responsible for susceptibility to several other cancers.[24,25] Additional follow-up studies confirmed and extended these observations, implicating other regions of the genome in susceptibility to colon cancer among "sporadic" cancer cases.[26] Like several other SNP variants that have been shown to be associated with complex diseases, the SNPs at 8q24 also lie in a region that is not known to harbor any genes. However, Pomerantz et al.[27] were able to show that this variant is functionally important in regulating the expression of the cellular oncogene c-myc that is located a few hundred kilobases away from the variant. This group also showed that variants at 8q24 that are known to be involved in other solid tumors also act through their action on the myc oncogene.[28] These results suggest that it might be possible to identify individuals within the general population that show susceptibility to several different solid tumors. Identification of such susceptible individuals may, in turn, help in more careful monitoring or other interventions, which may lead to prevention of the cancers.

BREAST CANCER

Susceptibility to early onset breast cancer has been extensively studied. It was recognized that certain families have a high incidence of breast and ovarian cancers. Careful examination of these families revealed that the predisposition to these cancers is inherited in an autosomal dominant fashion. Genetic linkage analysis revealed that, at least in some families, this trait is linked to markers on human chromosome 17.[29] When positional cloning approaches became available, it was determined that mutations in a gene on this chromosome were found to be responsible for this predisposition.[30,31] That gene was designated *BRCA1* (BReast CAncer-1). In other families a second gene, *BRCA2*, located on chromosome 13, was found to be involved in the cancer predisposition. Women who inherit a mutation either in *BRCA1* or *BRCA2* are at high risk for development of breast or ovarian cancer. Mutations in these genes can be inherited or they could result from new mutational events. If an individual with mutations in either *BRCA1* or *BRCA2* has been identified, it would be important to assess if other members in their family are at risk. If inherited, since the mutations are dominant acting, each of the immediate relatives (siblings) would have a 50% risk of carrying the same mutation and therefore would also be at high risk for developing cancer. Individuals with known pathogenic mutations may elect prophylactic mastectomy and oophorectomy or careful surveillance to detect tumors at their earliest stage.

Testing individuals at high risk for breast cancer or colon cancer is a common practice. If an individual tests positive for a pathogenic mutation, it is prudent to test for the presence of the same mutation in that individual's immediate relatives and manage them based on the results.

It is estimated that only a fraction of women that carry a pathogenic mutation in *BRCA1* or *BRCA2* are detected. Detection of these mutations well in advance of the time at which they would develop their first breast or ovarian tumor would have significant positive implications for their health. A relatively simple way of identifying individuals at risk is through the use of family history. Several family history tools are available, and one that was developed by the surgeon general of the United States is easily accessible and free of charge on the U.S. Department of Health and Human Services Web site (search for "My Family Health Portrait Tool"). Algorithms that can assess relative risk have been developed, and depending on these risk predictions, appropriate individuals may be recommended to undergo genetic testing.

EARLY DETECTION

It is well established that the long-term survival of patients, whose tumors were diagnosed at early stages, are significantly greater than those whose tumors are detected at a later stage. For example, the long-term survival of patients whose colonic tumors were detected at stage I is 95%, while it is only 5% when the tumors are detected at stage IV.

There are different methods for early detection of cancers. For colon cancer detection, colonoscopies are recommended for all individuals over the age 50. Palpation of the prostate is a routine procedure during annual medical examinations. Mammograms are useful in detecting at least a significant portion of breast tumors. Some of these methods are expensive and patient compliance is not adequately high. Alternative strategies for detection of cancer at early stages are in development.

One approach to identify such markers was used by Faca et al.[32] In this study, a murine model for pancreatic cancer was used as a starting point. These mice reliably develop pancreatic tumors during specific periods of their life. Plasma samples from these mice at different stages of tumor development were sampled and analyzed for their protein composition using proteomic approaches. Several proteins that were found to be overexpressed during early stages of cancer were examined in the blood from 30 newly diagnosed patients with pancreatic cancer and an appropriate set of 30 controls. This approach enabled them to identify a panel of five proteins that was able to discriminate pancreatic cancer cases from matched controls in blood specimens obtained as much as 12 months prior to the diagnosis of pancreatic cancer. Similar approaches enabled identification of protein markers that are important for ovarian and colon cancers.[33,34]

The reason why tumor-specific markers can be detected in the circulating system prior to clinical diagnosis of disease is not well understood. It is possible that some tumor cells die, releasing their contents into circulation. Alternatively, some subsets of tumor cells escape their original site and are in circulation. Such cells are referred to as circulating tumor cells (CTC). Escape of tumor cells from their source of origin and entering the circulation is, of course, an important step in metastasis. Methods to detect CTC have advanced significantly in the past few years. It has been long known that tumor cells may express novel proteins on their cell surface. Although antibodies against many of these proteins are available, purification of circulating tumors cells proved to be difficult. However, many of the solid tumors are derived from epithelial cells, and such cells are not normally part of the circulation. Therefore, epithelial cell markers can be used as capture agents. This approach, together with the development of novel flow cells that allow for slow and gentle movement of cells through a substrate coated with the appropriate antibodies, is now shown to be a suitable method for capturing these rare circulating tumor cells.[35] The availability of intact cells will allow more detailed molecular examination of tumor cells, which could prove to be powerful in early diagnosis. It is important, however, to understand how well these circulating cells reflect the state of the tumor at its initial location. The ability to isolate circulating tumor cells has significant implications for our ability to understand the nature of the tumor and to devise appropriate interventions for the patients.

TUMOR CLASSIFICATION AND PATIENT STRATIFICATION

Assessment of the molecular origins of tumors and the molecular profiles of the tumors has important implications for accurate diagnosis, determination of the prognosis, and treatment decisions for a patient. Methodologies for assessing such features are rapidly evolving.

Early methods of tumor classification were based on cytogenetic methods in hematological malignancies. The first of chromosomal translocations that was identified as important in human cancer is the t(9;22)(q34;q11) associated with chronic myelogenous leukemia (CML).[36] Because the discovery was made from investigators from Philadelphia, this rearranged chromosome has been designated the Philadelphia chromosome. During the past 40 years hundreds of such translocations have been described in many different malignancies, and more than 300 different genes have been implicated in these abnormalities. For example, in acute myeloid leukemia 267 balanced rearrangements have been described.[37] These translocations sometimes result in inappropriate activation of genes or the creation of novel fusion genes, with novel functions resulting in cancer. The nature of these translocations is critical for accurate diagnosis and in several cases for targeted therapies. Although a majority of these translocations are described in hematological malignancies, several such translocations have been described in solid tumors, and it is now clear that such translocations are also common in most, if not all, solid tumors.[38,39] As is the case for hematological malignancies, specific translocations would not only help classify the tumors but also may provide novel targets for drug development. One such example is the EML-ALK4 translocation in lung cancer.[38]

Diagnosis of tumors can also be made on the basis of the gene expression profiles of the tumor. An example is the distinction between Burkitt's lymphoma and large B-cell lymphoma. These two disorders are treated differently, and, therefore, it is important to distinguish between them accurately. The diagnosis of Burkitt's lymphoma is largely based on morphologic findings, immunological data, and cytogenetic features. Diffuse large B-cell lymphoma and Burkitt's lymphoma have some overlapping clinical features. In addition, Burkitt's lymphoma has the t(8;14) translocation that results in the activation of the myc oncogene, but this translocation is also present in a subset of diffuse large B-cell lymphoma. Examination of Burkitt's lymphoma cases and large B-cell lymphoma samples by global gene expression profile analysis enabled the identification of a panel of genes whose expression profiles can distinguish the two categories with a very high level of accuracy.[40]

Some novel tests based on the patterns of gene expression profiling have been developed, and intensive efforts for additional tests are currently under way. An example of a type of test that was developed was one to predict the recurrence of cancer in women with tamoxifen-treated, node-negative breast cancer.[41] RNA extracted from paraffin-embedded sections of breast tumors from women who were enrolled in a clinical trial to study the effects of tamoxifen treatment were examined for expression of a panel of 21 genes. Based on the analysis of the data the investigators were able to translate the data into a recurrence score. It is likely that similar efforts with either gene expression profiles or protein expression profiles of tumors will result in identification of marker sets that can be used for accurate diagnosis and prognosis of many tumor types.

Efforts to use comprehensive genomic data for tumor diagnosis and stratification are proving to be extremely valuable. An example is the examination of human glioblastomas.[42] In this study several groups of investigators examined tumor samples from human glioblastomas and the corresponding normal DNA from the same patients for changes in gene and genomic copy number, gene expression profiles, and the mutational status of a large number of genes. Based on this comprehensive analysis this group of investigators was able to classify the tumors and assess the pathways that are deregulated in this cancer type. Similar types of efforts are under way for many other cancer types.

Other investigations have focused on a comprehensive examination of genetic changes in tumor cells and tumor tissue. These efforts have examined all of the coding regions of the tumor genome and in some cases the complete genomes of tumors.[43–46]

TREATMENT

As the understanding of the genetic and genomic changes that are responsible for tumor progression increases, it is becoming possible to understand the particular genetic changes and biochemical pathways that are modified in tumor cells. This knowledge, in turn, helps determine which patients are most likely to benefit from which drugs. There are several excellent examples of this feature and others are emerging rapidly. Some of these are briefly described below.

One of the first examples of a targeted therapy is for CML. In 1960 Nowell and Hungerford[47] described a marker chromosome in a human leukemia. In 1973 Rowley[48] defined this marker chromosome, designated the Philadelphia chromosome, to be the result of a translocation involving human chromosomes 9 and 22. It was later shown that this specific translocation results in a novel fusion gene product that involves a break point cluster region (BCR) and an oncogene that is homologous to the Abelson murine leukemia virus (ABL). The fusion product, designated BCR-ABL, is a tyrosine kinase and is expressed only in these tumor cells. It has been shown that the formation of this fusion gene is sufficient for the cells to become transformed. Mutational analysis of the fusion gene revealed that the loss of function of this protein leads to loss of its oncogenic activity. These observations led to the development of a specific inhibitor for this fusion protein. The drug, originally designated STI571, now imatinib, was found to be efficacious in preclinical studies. Clinical studies with this drug revealed that the drug that is orally administered is relatively safe and as many as 98% of the CML patients showed hematologic response in as little as 4 weeks of drug administration.[49,50] Additional studies showed that the drug's effects favorably compare with standard therapy for newly diagnosed CML patients. This is the current choice of drug for CML that is diagnosed to have the Philadelphia chromosome.

A second example of targeted therapy is for a subset of breast cancer patients. A subset of breast cancers (20% to 30%) are known to have amplification of a growth factor receptor gene, *ERBB2* (*HER2*). Women whose breast cancers have a high level of expression of this gene have a shortened survival. It has been shown that the amplification of the *HER2* gene is directly involved in the pathogenesis. Therefore, it was considered that development of inhibitors of this protein, which is expressed on the surface of the tumor cells, might provide an approach to treat these breast cancer patients. Several antibodies directed against this target were found to bind this target with high affinity and inhibit their proliferation. A humanized murine monoclonal antibody was developed as a therapeutic agent. This drug, trastuzumab, was found to be relatively safe, and its administration resulted in better disease-free progression and higher rates of overall response compared to chemotherapy alone. Combination of chemotherapy and trastuzumab improved the outcomes even more.[51,52] Based on these clinical trails the drug was approved and is currently the standard of therapy for patients whose breast tumors have amplification of HER2.

The role of genetic changes in drug response was well described in non–small cell lung cancer (NSCLC). Until the early part of this century the most widely used treatment for NSCLC has been chemotherapy, which results in a small increase in survival and is associated with several adverse effects. It was known that these lung cancer cells express higher levels of epidermal growth factor (EGFR) as compared to normal lung cells. EGFR is a member of a class of transmembrane signaling proteins. In the presence of its ligand, epidermal growth factor, the receptor dimerizes, resulting in phosphorylation of tyrosine in the intracellular domain and leading to a cascade of events that promote cell growth. One of the drugs that was developed to inhibit this tyrosine kinase activity is gefitinib. Treatment of patients with gefitinib resulted in variable responses among individuals with lung cancer. In early clinical trials individuals from Japan had better responses than those from the United States, and female never-smokers were better responders among both ethnic groups. In the United States the response rates were less than 20%, and the response did not correlate with EGFR levels as measured by immunohistochemistry. To understand the basis for this variable response, one group hypothesized that mutations in a receptor tyrosine kinase may be responsible for drug response.[53] To test this hypothesis they obtained tumor DNA samples from tumors prior to treatment and examined the DNA for mutations in the activation loops of 47 receptor kinase genes. A small number of tumors had heterozygous mutations in the *EGFR* gene. A more comprehensive examination revealed heterozygous missense and deletion mutations in a region corresponding to proximity of the adenosine triphosphate (ATP) binding cleft and the target of the drug gefitinib. Tumor DNA from patients who responded to the drug, obtained prior to initiation of treatment, had a mutation in *EGFR* in all responders, while only 1 of 61 nonselected patients had such a mutation. They were also able to show that lung caner cell lines that carried one of the mutations responded to low doses of gefitinib and also inhibited the autophosphorylation of the EGFR protein.

A second group of investigators reasoned that since the drug targets EGFR, mutations in that gene might be responsible for the differential effect of the drug.[54] To test this hypothesis they examined the biopsy samples from patients who later showed responses to gefitinib. These studies revealed that of the nine samples examined, eight had genetic changes in the region of the gene corresponding to the intracellular domain of the protein. The nature of the mutations detected were also point mutations, leading to a change in amino acid and deletions that resulted in loss of a few amino acids of the protein. No such mutations were detected in other tumor types, and the changes were found to be somatic. Using transient transfection of the mutant version of the gene into mammalian cells revealed that the mutations led to hyperactivation of the protein and to better responses to the drug at lower concentrations.

Both of these studies and another study published soon after[55] revealed that in NSCLC, the target of the drug gefitinib acquires certain somatic mutations, some of which result in activation of the protein. It is those patients whose EGFR has acquired one of these activation mutations who respond to the drug. These observations paved the way for the development of a molecular diagnostic test to identify patients who might be better responders to the tyrosine kinase inhibitors gefitinib and erlotinib.

To clinically assess if selection of patients whose lung tumors had an activation mutation would respond better to a tyrosine kinase inhibitor, several clinical trials were conducted. Although the trail designs and the number of patients in each trial varied, the general schema of several clinical trials was to examine the tumor DNA for *EGFR* mutations and assess their response rates and progression-free survival as well as long-term survival benefits of the drug.

In one study Mok et al.[56] compared the effectiveness of chemotherapy versus gefitinib treatment in patients with lung cancer. In a phase 3 study, they randomly assigned treatment-naive patients to receive gefitinib or chemotherapy. They observed that in the cohort who had *EGFR* mutations both the response rates as well as progression-free survival were better in the mutation-positive group. Interestingly, in the mutation-negative cohort chemotherapy yielded better response rates and better progression-free survival. These trial results suggest that patient stratification based on *EGFR* status and treatment with a tyrosine kinase inhibitor for mutation-positive patients and chemotherapy for mutation-negative patients would yield optimal response rates.

DEVELOPMENT OF RESISTANCE TO TYROSINE KINASE INHIBITORS

Despite the fact that individuals whose tumors have an activation mutation in EGFR respond better to tyrosine kinase inhibitors and such treatment leads to longer survival, all patients appear to relapse and tumor begins to grow again.

To understand the basis for this relapse Kobayashi et al.[57] obtained a biopsy sample from a relapsed patient and examined the status of the *EGFR* gene in the sample prior to treatment and the sample after relapse. Using direct DNA sequencing and sequencing of cDNA prepared from the tumor RNA sample, they observed that the relapsed tumor contained a novel mutation in the *EGFR* gene that resulted in a T790M mutation. Using molecular biological methods the investigators showed that the presence of this mutation in the background of an original responsive mutation rendered the EGFR protein 100 times more resistant to the drug. When they tested cells carrying the resistant allele with four commercial EGFR inhibitors, they found that an irreversible inhibitor of EGFR strongly inhibited EGFR function at relatively low concentrations. This observation suggested that periodic genetic monitoring of the tumor prior to treatment and at the time of relapse might help in the choice of the most appropriate drug or treatment for the patient.

ALTERNATIVE MECHANISMS OF RESISTANCE

It was observed that some individuals whose tumors have activating mutations in the *EGFR* gene do not respond to tyrosine kinase inhibitors. It is noted that some of these tumors have mutations in *KRAS*.[58–60] Activation of the EGFR-mediated signaling pathway involves the activation of the RAS-Map kinase pathway. Thus the product of RAS acts downstream of EGFR. Therefore, it is reasonable that independent activation of the downstream target renders the status of *EGFR* irrelevant to growth phenotype of these cells. These results form the basis for testing NSCLC for both *EGFR* and *KRAS* mutations. Patients who are most likely to respond to EGFR tyrosine kinase inhibitors would be those whose tumors have an activating mutation in *EGFR* and are wild type for *KRAS*.

Role of KRAS Mutations in Other Epidermal Growth Factor Receptor Inhibitors

Patients with colorectal cancer who failed chemotherapy were administered an antibody against EGFR, cetuximab. Although treatment with this monoclonal antibody resulted in improved overall survival, the disease progressed in more than 50% of the patients. Since a subset of colorectal tumors were known to have activating mutations in KRAS, a downstream component of EGFR signaling cascade, it is reasonable to assume that the *KRAS* mutations might render the treatment with cetuximab ineffective. This hypothesis was directly tested in a clinical trial. Patients who did not receive prior EGFR inhibitor treatment were randomized to receive cetuximab plus best supportive care or best supportive alone. Tumor samples, when available, were assessed for the status of *KRAS*. Approximately 40% of both groups had *KRAS* activation mutations. Patients with wild type *KRAS* tumors had better overall survival, better progression-free survival, and significantly better response rates than supportive care alone.[61] Similar results were obtained with the use of another monoclonal antibody against EGFR, panitumumab.[62] Based on these studies the U.S. Food and Drug Administration has changed the label for both drugs to require genetic testing of the *KRAS* prior to administration of either of these antibody drugs.

BRAF INHIBITORS

The RAS-Map kinase pathway is activated in a number of different tumor types. Efforts to identify small molecule inhibitors that can effectively inhibit this pathway have been under way for many years. There are different genetic changes that could result in the activation of this pathway.

EGFR amplification, mutations in the *EGFR* gene, mutations in a member of the *RAS* gene family, or certain mutations in *BRAF* are some of the examples of how this activation is accomplished. Efforts to target BRAF have been significantly successful.

Melanomas are capable of metastasis, and there are few effective therapies for metastatic melanoma. It was discovered that in melanomas as many as 40% to 60% may carry an activation mutation in *BRAF*. Interestingly, nearly 90% of the *RAF* mutations in this cancer involve codon 600, which results in a substitution of glutamic acid to valine (V600E). Two drugs, PLX4032 and PLX4720 (Plexxikon, Roche Pharmaceuticals, South San Francisco, California), effectively inhibit this modified protein in *in vitro* studies. Based on these encouraging data, clinical trials were conducted to assess the clinical efficacy of one of these drugs. In the initial dose escalation study the testing for the genetic status of *BRAF* was not a requirement, while in an extension study only those patients with an activation mutation in *BRAF* were included. In the dose escalation study a substantial number of patients were positive for the *BRAF* mutation. A substantial number (61%) of the patients responded to the drug, and all of the individuals whose tumors had *BRAF* mutations were among the responders, while patients without the mutation did not show a response.[63]

In the extension phase of the study only patients with the V600E mutation were treated with drug and remarkably 81% of them responded. The responses were durable and involved all metastatic sites of the tumor. The overall survival in this population is being assessed in a phase 3 trial. If these trials are successful it would benefit the patients to conduct testing for the status of *BRAF* and treat those who have the BRAF activation with this inhibitor. *BRAF* mutations are also detected in other tumor types, and the mutations detected in these tumors include V600E. Therefore, it is possible that this or other BRAF inhibitors will find widespread use in many tumor types.

The importance of genetic testing prior to treatment with BRAF inhibitors is underscored by studies that indicate that treatment of BRAF-negative melanoma patients with an RAF inhibitor may result in activation of the MAP kinase pathway and is therefore contraindicated.[64,65]

THE FUTURE

As the knowledge about the genetic changes that lead to the initiation and progression of cancer increases, so too the ability to choose the most appropriate drug to which the tumor will respond is also increasing. Understanding of the genetic and genomic changes in cancer has been fueled by new high-throughput technologies and large-scale approaches. During the past few years the ability to detect copy number changes, chromosomal aberrations, gene expression profile changes, global methylation changes, and DNA sequence changes has dramatically improved. More recently a significant reduction in the cost of DNA sequencing is also fueling efforts to sequence large sets of genes, whole exomes, and even whole genome sequencing from tumors and, when available, their corresponding normal samples. All of these results are increasing the understanding of the biology of cancer, but they are also increasing the ability to stratify patients and to choose the most appropriate drug or treatment based on the genetic composition of the tumor and the patient.

An illustrative example of the types of information that can be obtained from such large-scale studies can be found in the results on human glioblastomas published by two groups.[66,67] The Cancer Genome Atlas Research Network[42] analyzed copy number changes, expression profile changes, and methylation changes and sequenced a subset of genes in the genome in a large number of glioblastoma multiforme and compared them with normal samples obtained from the same patients. Parsons et al.[43] examined the coding sequence of more than 22,000 genes in 22 samples. They also examined copy number changes and expression profiles in these tumor samples. These studies identified a number of genes that were not previously implicated in gliomagenesis, most notably *NF1* and *IDH1*. The results also provided important clues about how glioblastoma multiforme acquire resistance to the alkylating agent temozolomide. Similar types of studies in other cancers have been published.

CHANGING FACE OF PERSONALIZED MEDICINE

As the information about critical genetic and genomic changes in many different cancers is accumulating, it is becoming possible to incorporate this information into patient treatment. The types of changes can be illustrated from the changes in treatment of lung cancer. The importance of *EGFR* and *KRAS* testing in making decisions about the suitability of tyrosine kinase inhibitors was described earlier in this chapter. A subset of lung tumors have mutations in the *BRAF* gene and, based on the results from clinical studies of melanoma patients, highly specific BRAF inhibitors might be the choice treatment for these patients. A subset of tumors have ErbB2 amplification, which is a common event in breast cancers, and patients whose breast tumors have this amplification respond well to trastuzumab. Clinical trials to evaluate the efficacy of using trastuzumab in lung cancer patients with ErbB2 amplification are under way. A subset of lung tumors also has activation mutations in one of several genes, leading to an activation of the PI3K pathway. There are several drugs, some of which are already approved for clinical use, that are effective inhibitors of this pathway, and these are excellent candidates with which to treat this group of patients. Another subset of patients has a unique translocation that involved the *EML* and *ALK4* genes. It has been shown that lung cancer patients with tumors that bear this translocation respond well to a new tyrosine kinase inhibitor crizotinib.[66]

Other NSCLC tumors have amplification in the oncogene *MET*. Inhibitors against this target and its ligand hepatocyte growth factor are in development, and some of them are being tested for their efficacy to treat lung cancer patients in clinical trials. Therefore, it is highly likely that in the near future tumors from patients diagnosed with NSCLC will be tested for the status of a battery of genes that include *EGFR*, *RAS*, *RAF*, *ErbB2*, *Met*, and the presence of the EML-ALK4 translocation to determine the most optimal treatment for each patient. Such efforts are already in place at several academic medical centers. A list of examples of genetic changes that could affect treatment decisions is presented in Table 12.1.

SUMMARY

The understanding of the genetic and genomic differences among individuals that affect cancer susceptibility and the

TABLE 12.1

EXAMPLES OF GENETIC CHANGES TO FACILITATE TREATMENT DECISIONS

Genetic Change	Indication
BCR-ABL translocation	Chronic myelogenous leukemia
ErbB2 amplification	Certain breast cancers
EGFR mutations	Sensitivity to tyrosine kinase inhibitors in NSCLC
EGFR mutations	Resistance to tyrosine kinase inhibitors in NSCLC
K-RAS	Resistance to tyrosine kinase inhibitors in NSCLC
K-RAS	Resistance to EGFR antibodies in colon cancer
B-RAF	Sensitivity to B-RAF inhibitors in melanoma
EML-ALK4 translocation	Sensitivity to ALK4 inhibitors
RAS-MAPK pathway members	Sensitivity to drugs that inhibit RAS-MAPK pathway
PTEN, AKT and PI3 kinase	Sensitivity to drugs that inhibit the AKT and PI kinase pathways
BRCA1 and BRCA2	Sensitivity to PARP inhibitors
HGF and MET mutations or amplification	Sensitivity to HGF and MET inhibitors
Mutations in genes in the angiogenesis pathway	Sensitivity to angiogenesis inhibitors

EGFR, epidermal growth factor receptor; NSCLC, non–small cell lung cancer; PARP, poly(adenosine diphosphate-ribose) polymerase; PI3, phosphatidylinositol 3; HGF, hepatocyte growth factor; MET, mesenchymal-to-epithelial transition.

genetic and genomic changes that are critical for the initiation and progression of cancer is increasing at a rapid pace. The rapid decrease in the cost of DNA sequencing and other genomic analysis is fueling this increase in knowledge. This new knowledge is helping in accurate prediction, early detection, and prognosis of cancer. Genetic differences among individuals and somatic changes during the development of cancer are also important in determining the appropriate treatment strategies for each patient. The use of genetic and genomic information is referred to as personalized medicine, which has the ability to transform the practice of oncology.

MOLECULAR BIOLOGY OF CANCER

Selected References

The full list of references for this chapter appears in the online version.

1. Lichtenstein P, Holm NV, Verkasalo PK, et al. Environmental and heritable factors in the causation of cancer—analyses of cohorts of twins from Sweden, Denmark, and Finland. *N Engl J Med* 2000;343:78.
2. Ashley DJ. Oesophageal cancer in Wales. *J Med Genet* 1969;6:70.
3. St. John DJ, McDermott FT, Hopper JL, et al. Cancer risk in relatives of patients with common colorectal cancer. *Ann Intern Med* 1993;118:785.
4. Nishisho I, Nakamura Y, Miyoshi Y, et al. Mutations of chromosome 5q21 genes in FAP and colorectal cancer patients. *Science* 1991;253:665.
5. Kinzler KW, Nilbert MC, Su LK, et al. Identification of FAP locus genes from chromosome 5q21. *Science* 1991;253(5020):661.
6. Nakamura Y, Nishisho I, Kinzler KW, et al. Mutations of the adenomatous polyposis coli gene in familial polyposis coli patients and sporadic colorectal tumors. *Princess Takamatsu Symp* 1991;22:285.
7. Lynch HT, Krush AJ. Heredity and adenocarcinoma of the colon. *Gastroenterology* 1967;53:517.
8. Parsons R, Li GM, Longley MJ, et al. Hypermutability and mismatch repair deficiency in RER+ tumor cells. *Cell* 1993;75:1227.
9. Aaltonen LA, Peltomäki P, Leach FS, et al. Clues to the pathogenesis of familial colorectal cancer. *Science* 1993;260:812.
10. Powell SM, Zilz N, Beazer-Barclay Y, et al. APC mutations occur early during colorectal tumorigenesis. *Nature* 1992;359:235.
11. Leach FS, Nicolaides NC, Papadopoulos N, et al. Mutations of a mutS homolog in hereditary nonpolyposis colorectal cancer. *Cell* 1993;75:1215.
12. Fishel R, Lescoe MK, Rao MR, et al. The human mutator gene homolog MSH2 and its association with hereditary nonpolyposis colon cancer. *Cell* 1993;75:1027.
13. Papadopoulos N, Nicolaides NC, Wei YF, et al. Mutation of a MutL homolog in hereditary colon cancer. *Science* 1994;263:1625.
14. Bronner CE, Baker SM, Morrison PT, et al. Mutation in the DNA mismatch repair gene homologue hMLH1 is associated with hereditary nonpolyposis colon cancer. *Nature* 1994;368:258.
15. Nicolaides NC, Papadopoulos N, Liu B, et al. Mutations of two PMS homologues in hereditary nonpolyposis colon cancer. *Nature* 1994;371:75.
16. Miyaki M, Konishi M, Tanaka K, et al. Germline mutation of MSH6 as the cause of hereditary nonpolyposis colorectal cancer. *Nat Genet* 1997;17:271.
17. Lipkin SM, Wang V, Jacoby R, et al. MLH3: a DNA mismatch repair gene associated with mammalian microsatellite instability. *Nat Genet* 2000;24:27.
18. Loukola A, Vilkki S, Singh J, Launonen V, Aaltonen LA. Germline and somatic mutation analysis of MLH3 in MSI-positive colorectal cancer. *Am J Pathol* 2000;157:347.
19. Aaltonen LA, Salovaara R, Kristo P, et al. Incidence of hereditary nonpolyposis colorectal cancer and the feasibility of molecular screening for the disease. *N Engl J Med* 1998;338:1481.
20. Loukola A, Salovaara R, Kristo P, et al. Microsatellite instability in adenomas as a marker for hereditary nonpolyposis colorectal cancer. *Am J Pathol* 1998;155:1849.
21. Salovaara R, Loukola A, Kristo P, et al. Population-based molecular detection of hereditary nonpolyposis colorectal cancer. *J Clin Oncol* 2000;18:2193.
22. de la Chapelle A. Genetic predisposition to colorectal cancer. *Nat Rev Cancer* 2004;4:769.
23. Zanke BW, Greenwood CM, Rangrej J, et al. Genome-wide association scan identifies a colorectal cancer susceptibility locus on chromosome 8q24. *Nat Genet* 2007;39:989.
24. Al Olama AA, Kote-Jarai Z, Giles GG, et al. Multiple loci on 8q24 associated with prostate cancer susceptibility. *Nat Genet* 2009;41:1058.
25. Gudmundsson J, Sulem P, Gudbjartsson DF, et al. Genome-wide association and replication studies identify four variants associated with prostate cancer susceptibility. *Nat Genet* 2009;41:1122.
26. Tenesa A, Farrington SM, Prendergast JG, et al. Genome-wide association scan identifies a colorectal cancer susceptibility locus on 11q23 and replicates risk loci at 8q24 and 18q21. *Nat Genet* 2008;40:631.
27. Pomerantz MM, Ahmadiyeh N, Jia L, et al. The 8q24 cancer risk variant rs6983267 shows long-range interaction with MYC in colorectal cancer. *Nat Genet* 2009;41:882.
28. Ahmadiyeh N, Pomerantz MM, Grisanzio C, et al. 8q24 prostate, breast, and colon cancer risk loci show tissue-specific long-range interaction with MYC. 2010 *Proc Natl Acad Sci U S A* 2010;107:9742.
29. Hall JM, Lee MK, Newman B, et al. Linkage of early-onset familial breast cancer to chromosome 17q21. *Science* 1990;250:1684.
30. Miki Y, Swensen J, Shattuck-Eidens D, et al. A strong candidate for the breast and ovarian cancer susceptibility gene BRCA1. *Science* 1994;266:66.

31. Futreal PA, Liu Q, Shattuck-Eidens D, et al. BRCA1 mutations in primary breast and ovarian carcinomas. *Science* 1994;266:120.
32. Faca VM, Song KS, Wang H, et al. A mouse to human search for plasma proteome changes associated with pancreatic tumor development. *PLoS Med* 2008;5:e123.
33. Pitteri SJ, JeBailey L, Faça VM, et al. Integrated proteomic analysis of human cancer cells and plasma from tumor bearing mice for ovarian cancer biomarker discovery. *PLoS One* 2009;4:e7916.
34. Hung KE, Faça V, Song K, et al. Comprehensive proteome analysis of an Apc mouse model uncovers proteins associated with intestinal tumorigenesis. *Cancer Prev Res* 2009;2:224.
35. Nagrath S, Sequist LV, Maheswaran S, et al. Isolation of rare circulating tumour cells in cancer patients by microchip technology. *Nature* 2007;450(7173):1235.
37. Mitelman F, Johansson B, Mertens F. The impact of translocations and gene fusions on cancer causation. *Nat Rev Cancer* 2007;7(4):233.
38. Soda M, Choi YL, Enomoto M, et al. Identification of the transforming EML4-ALK fusion gene in non-small-cell lung cancer. *Nature* 2007;448:561.
39. Tomlins SA, Laxman B, Dhanasekaran SM, et al. Distinct classes of chromosomal rearrangements create oncogenic ETS gene fusions in prostate cancer. *Nature* 2007;448:595.
40. Dave SS, Fu K, Wright GW, et al. Lymphoma/Leukemia Molecular Profiling Project. Molecular diagnosis of Burkitt's lymphoma. *N Engl J Med* 2006;354:2431.
41. Paik S, Shak S, Tang G, et al. A multigene assay to predict recurrence of tamoxifen-treated, node-negative breast cancer. *N Engl J Med* 2004;351(27):2817.
42. Cancer Genome Atlas Research Network. Comprehensive genomic characterization defines human glioblastoma genes and core pathways. *Nature* 2008;455:1061.
43. Parsons DW, Jones S, Zhang X, et al. An integrated genomic analysis of human glioblastoma multiforme. *Science* 2008;321:1807.
44. Jones S, Zhang X, Parsons DW, et al. Core signaling pathways in human pancreatic cancers revealed by global genomic analyses. *Science* 2008;321:1801.
45. Pleasance ED, Cheetham RK, Stephens PJ, et al. A comprehensive catalogue of somatic mutations from a human cancer genome. *Nature* 2010;463:191.
46. Mardis ER, Ding L, Dooling DJ, et al. Recurring mutations found by sequencing an acute myeloid leukemia genome. *N Engl J Med* 2009;361:1058.
47. Nowell P, Hungerford D. A minute chromosome in human chronic granulocytic leukemia *Science* 1960;132:1497.
48. Rowley JD. A new consistent chromosomal abnormality in chronic myelogenous leukemia. *Nature* 1973;243:290.
49. Druker BJ, Talpaz M, Resta DJ, et al. Efficacy and safety of a specific inhibitor of the BCR-ABL tyrosine kinase in chronic myeloid leukemia. *N Engl J Med* 2001;344:1031.
50. Druker BJ, Sawyers CL, Kantarjian H, et al. Activity of a specific inhibitor of the BCR-ABL tyrosine kinase in the blast crisis of chronic myeloid leukemia and acute lymphoblastic leukemia with the Philadelphia chromosome. *N Engl J Med* 2001;344:1038.
51. Slamon DJ, Leyland-Jones B, Shak S, et al. Use of chemotherapy plus a monoclonal antibody against HER2 for metastatic breast cancer that overexpresses HER2. *N Engl J Med* 2001;344:783.
52. Arteaga CL. ErbB-targeted therapeutic approaches in human cancer. *Exp Cell Res* 2003;284:122.
53. Paez JG, Jänne PA, Lee JC, et al. EGFR mutations in lung cancer: correlation with clinical response to gefitinib therapy. *Science* 2004;304:1497.
54. Lynch TJ, Bell DW, Sordella R, et al. activating mutations in the epidermal growth factor receptor underlying responsiveness of non-small-cell lung cancer to gefitinib. *N Engl J Med* 2004;350:2129.
56. Mok TS, Wu YL, Thongprasert S, et al. Gefitinib or carboplatin-paclitaxel in pulmonary adenocarcinoma. *N Engl J Med* 2009;361:947.
61. Karapetis CS, Khambata-Ford S, Jonker DJ, et al. K-ras mutations and benefit from cetuximab in advanced colorectal cancer. *N Engl J Med* 2008;359:1757.
63. Flaherty KT, Puzanov I, Kim KB, et al. Inhibition of mutated, activated BRAF in metastatic melanoma. *N Engl J Med* 2010;363:809.

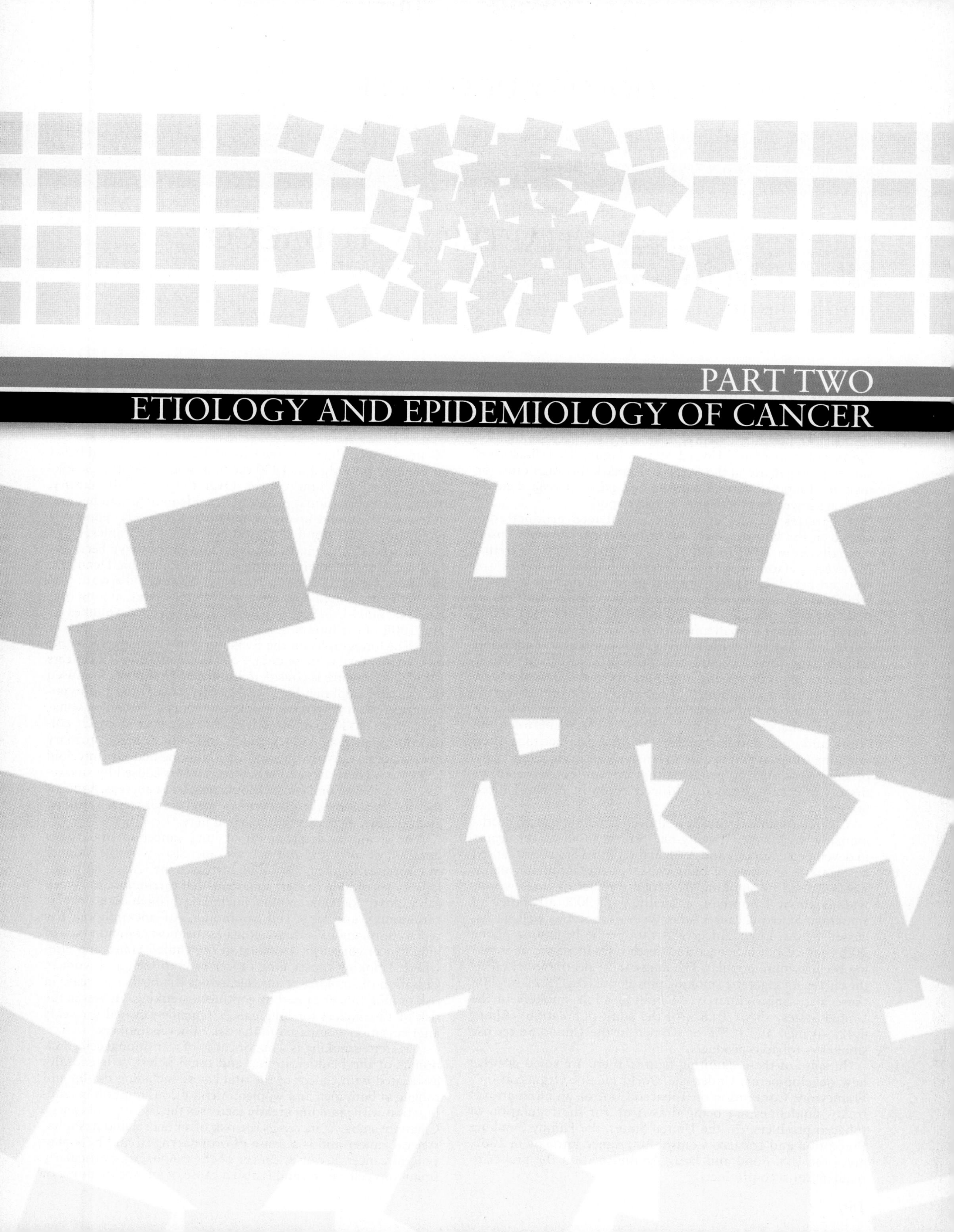

PART TWO
ETIOLOGY AND EPIDEMIOLOGY OF CANCER

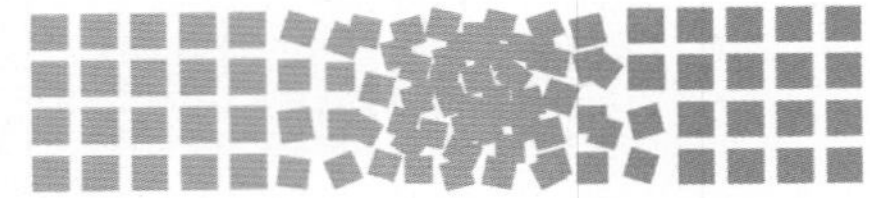

CHAPTER 13 TOBACCO

STEPHEN S. HECHT

The figures on worldwide tobacco use continue to be so large that they are numbing. There are about 1.2 billion smokers and hundreds of millions of smokeless tobacco users.[1,2] China alone has approximately 300 million male smokers, similar to the population of the United States. Figure 13.1 illustrates smoking prevalence in the world.[2,3] Remarkably high rates for men are found in eastern Europe and parts of Asia. Female rates are lower, but there are some hot spots.

Cigarettes are the main type of tobacco product consumed in the world. About 5.5 trillion cigarettes were used annually from 1990 to 2000; this is about 1,000 cigarettes for every person on Earth.[1] Over 15 billion cigarettes are smoked per day.[1] Other smoked products include *kreteks*, which are clove-flavored cigarettes popular in Indonesia, and "sticks," which are smoked in Papua New Guinea. *Bidis*, which consist of a small amount of tobacco wrapped in *temburni* leaf and tied with a string, are popular in India and neighboring areas. Cigars and pipes are still used. Water pipe smoking is increasing in popularity in the United States. And, a substantial amount of tobacco is consumed worldwide in the form of smokeless tobacco products, including chewing tobacco, moist snuff, which is placed between the cheek and gum, and *pan* or *betel quid*, a product that often contains tobacco and is used extensively in India. New types of smokeless tobacco products that are spitless, flavored, or dissolvable have been introduced recently in the United States.

Cigarette smoking causes well over 1 million cancer deaths annually worldwide.[2] Twenty-one percent of all cancer deaths in developed countries and 33% in the United States are caused by cigarette smoking.[4,5] Lung cancer is the dominant malignancy caused by smoking. The total number of cases worldwide is about 1.2 million annually, with 90% attributed to smoking.[6] Smoking causes other types of cancer as well, as discussed below. Lung cancer was rare at the beginning of the 20th century, but incidence and death rates increased as smoking became more popular. The lung cancer death rate parallels the curves for cigarette smoking prevalence (Fig. 13.2). In 2008 there were approximately 46 million adult smokers in the United States, about 20.6% of the adult population.[7] About 4.4% of men and 0.7% of women in the United States use smokeless tobacco products.[8]

In spite of these daunting figures, there are some positive new developments. Under the World Health Organization's Framework Convention on Tobacco Control, an international treaty, guidelines are being drawn up for the regulation of tobacco products.[9] In the United States, the Family Smoking Prevention and Tobacco Control Act, signed into law in 2009, gives the U.S. Food and Drug Administration the power to regulate tobacco products.

EPIDEMIOLOGY OF TOBACCO AND CANCER

Wynder and Graham[10] in the United States and Doll and Hill[11] in England published in 1950 the first large-scale studies linking smoking and lung cancer. Over the next half century, numerous international prospective epidemiologic studies and case-control studies involving millions of subjects repeatedly confirmed and extended these findings. As examples, large cohort studies of cigarette smoking and cancer have been carried out in the following countries: Canada, China, Denmark, Finland, Iceland, Japan, Norway, Sweden, Taiwan, the Netherlands, United Kingdom, and United States, among others.[6] The 2004 U.S. Surgeon General's Report and volumes 83 and 100E of the International Agency for Research on Cancer (IARC) Monographs on the Evaluation of Carcinogenic Risks to Humans review these data.[6,12,13] There are now 19 cancers for which evidence is considered sufficient that they are caused by cigarette smoking: lung, oral cavity, naso-, oro- and hypopharynx, nasal cavity and paranasal sinuses, larynx, esophagus (adeno- and squamous cell carcinoma), liver, stomach, colorectum, pancreas, kidney (body and pelvis), ureter, urinary bladder, cervix, ovary (mucinous), and bone marrow (myeloid leukemia). There are similarly three cancers caused by smokeless tobacco use: oral cavity, esophagus, and pancreas. Some of the important conclusions with respect to cigarette smoking and certain cancers are summarized here.[6]

The strongest determinant of lung cancer in smokers is duration of smoking, and risk also increases with the number of cigarettes smoked.[6] Smoking increases the risk of all histologic types of lung cancer: squamous cell carcinoma, small cell carcinoma, adenocarcinoma (including bronchiolar-alveolar carcinoma), and large cell carcinoma. Adenocarcinoma has replaced squamous cell carcinoma as the most common type of lung cancer caused by smoking in the United States and elsewhere. Smoking causes lung cancer in both men and women. Cessation of smoking at any age avoids the further increase in risk of lung cancer caused by continued smoking. However, the risk of ex-smokers for lung cancer remains elevated for years after cessation, compared to the risk of never smokers.

Cigarette smoking is a major cause of transitional cell carcinomas of the bladder, ureter, and renal pelvis. It is causally associated with cancer of the oral cavity including the lip and tongue in both men and women. Alcohol consumption in combination with smoking greatly increases the risk of oral cancer. Cigarette smoking increases the risk of sinonasal and nasopharyngeal cancer and is a cause of oropharyngeal and hypopharyngeal cancer. It causes cancer of the esophagus, particularly squamous cell cancer, and is also a cause of adenocarcinoma of

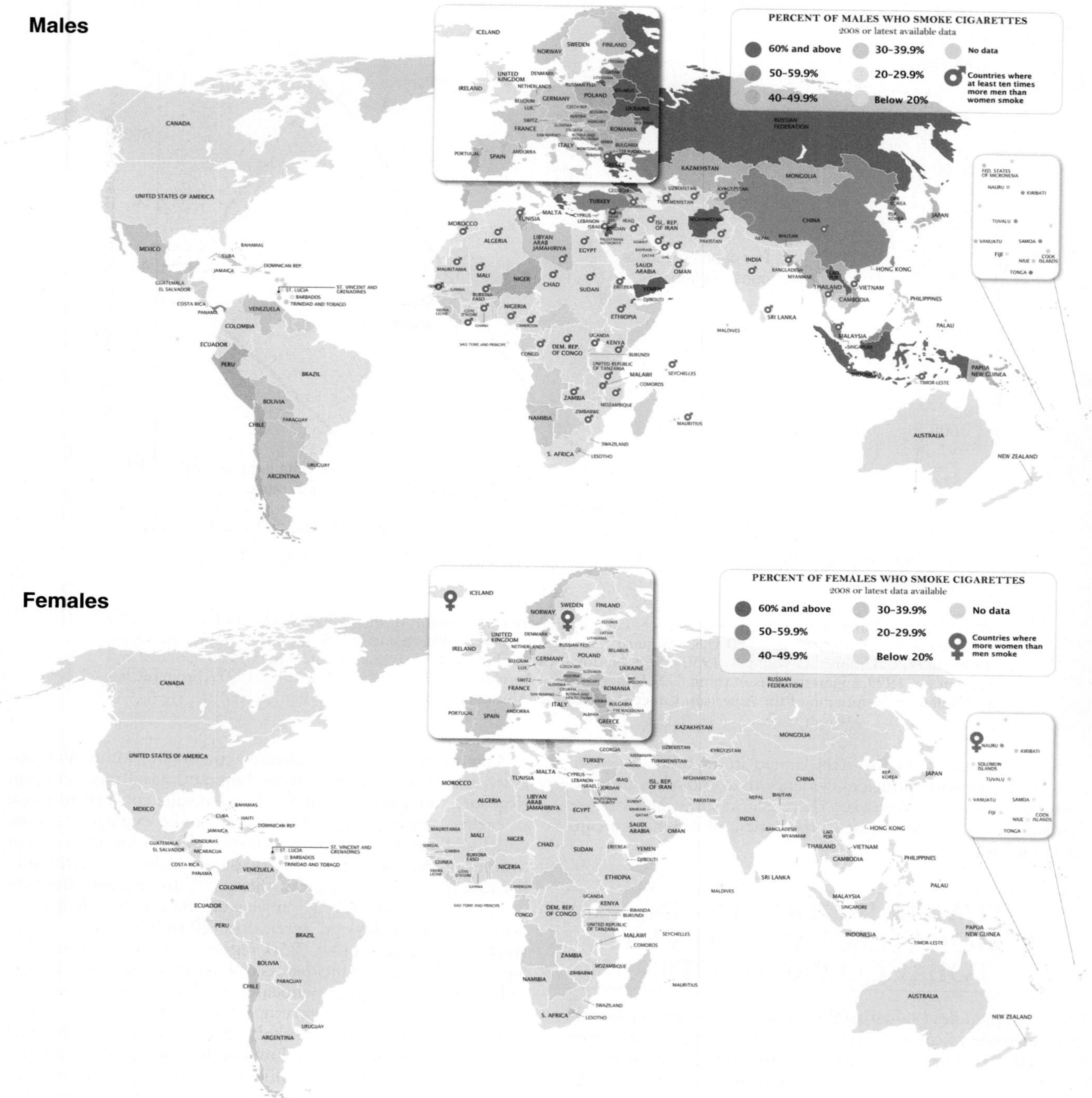

FIGURE 13.1 World smoking prevalence by gender (adapted from ref. 3).

the esophagus, which has been increasing in the United States. Laryngeal cancer is caused by cigarette smoking, and the risk is greatly enhanced by alcohol consumption. Similarly, pancreatic, stomach, and colon cancers are caused by cigarette smoking and are related to dosage.[6,13]

Cigarette smoking is a cause of liver cancer, independent of the effects of hepatitis B and C virus infection and alcohol consumption. It causes cervical squamous cell carcinoma, thus working in concert with or in addition to infection with human papilloma virus. Myeloid leukemia in adults is also causally related to cigarette smoking.[6]

Cigar and pipe smoking cause cancers of the oral cavity, oropharynx, hypopharynx, larynx, and esophagus, with the risk being similar to that of cigarette smoking. Dose–response relationships have been documented. Cigar or pipe smoking are causally associated with lung cancer and possibly with cancers of the pancreas, stomach, and urinary bladder.[6]

Secondhand smoke causes lung cancer in nonsmokers, although the risk is far less than that of a smoker. In spouses of smokers, the excess risk is about 20% in women and 30% in men. Workplace exposure to secondhand smoke also increases lung cancer risk in nonsmokers, by 12% to 19%.[6,14]

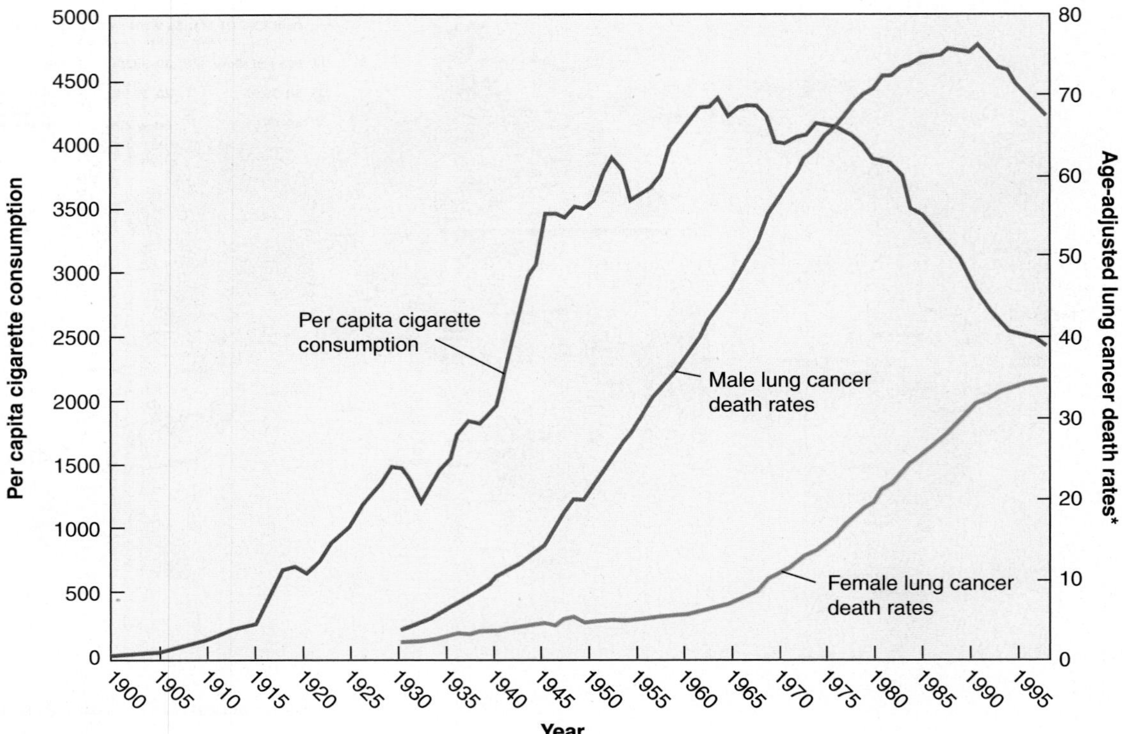

FIGURE 13.2 Lung cancer death rates and per capita cigarette consumption in the United States, 20th century. *Per 100,000 and age-adjusted to 1970 U.S. standard population. Sources: Death rates: U.S. mortality public use tapes, 1960–1997, U.S. mortality volumes, 1930–1959, National Center for Health Statistics, Centers for Disease Control and Prevention, 1999. Cigarette consumption: U.S. Department of Agriculture, 1900–1987, 1988, 1989–1997. (From ref. 95. Reprinted by permission of the American Cancer Society, Inc. All rights reserved.)

Epidemiologic studies from the United States, India, Pakistan, and Sweden provide sufficient evidence that smokeless tobacco causes oral cancer in humans.[8] There is also sufficient evidence that smokeless tobacco causes pancreatic and esophageal cancer in humans.[8,13]

TUMOR INDUCTION IN LABORATORY ANIMALS BY TOBACCO PRODUCTS

Laboratory studies evaluating the ability of cigarette smoke and its condensate to cause cancer in laboratory animals have been reviewed.[6,15,16] These works clearly demonstrate that inhalation of cigarette smoke and topical application of cigarette smoke condensate (CSC) cause cancer in animals.

Inhalation studies of cigarette smoke have been summarized.[6,15–21] Experiments have been carried out in hamsters, rats, mice, dogs, rabbits, nonhuman primates, and ferrets. Consistently, pronounced alterations of the larynx, including carcinoma, were induced by exposure of Syrian golden hamsters to cigarette smoke. In a study carried out by Dontenwill et al.[22] involving 4,440 hamsters, exposed nose only to the smoke of various cigarettes, the severity of alterations in the larynx depended on smoke dose and duration of treatment. These alterations were not observed in sham-exposed animals or in animals exposed only to the gas phase of smoke. The estimated concentration of smoke particles in the larynx was about 300 times greater than that in the lungs and bronchi under the conditions of these experiments, consistent with the observed tumor induction in the larynx rather than the lung.

One study in rats demonstrated convincing, although moderate, increases in tumors of the lung and nasal mucosa upon exposure to cigarette smoke.[23] These results contrast to those of earlier investigations of cigarette smoke exposure in rats, which did not consistently demonstrate significant increases in tumors of the lung, nasal cavity, or any other site, probably because the dosages were insufficient.[6,17] In another relatively recent study, female B6C3F$_1$ mice were exposed whole body, 6 hours per day, 5 days per week, for 920 to 930 days to mainstream cigarette smoke (250 mg/m^3) or sham exposed.[24] Significantly elevated incidences of lung adenoma, total benign pulmonary neoplasms, adenocarcinoma, and distal metastases were observed in the cigarette smoke–exposed mice. These results were even more remarkable because they were obtained in a strain of mouse with a low baseline incidence of pulmonary neoplasia.[25] Exposure of strain H neonatal mice to cigarette smoke for 120 consecutive days, starting at birth, resulted in a high incidence and multiplicity of benign lung tumors and significant increases in malignant lung tumors and other histopathological alterations.[26]

An A/J mouse model that is responsive to cigarette smoke has also been developed.[20] Benign lung tumors are induced in this highly susceptible strain by exposure to a mixture of 89% cigarette sidestream smoke (the main component of secondhand smoke) and 11% mainstream smoke. The animals are exposed for 5 months, then allowed a 4 month recovery period. In 18 individual studies reported by four different laboratories, a significant increase in lung tumor multiplicity was observed in 15 studies and a significant increase in lung tumor incidence in ten studies. The response is due to the gas phase constituents of smoke.

Smoke inhalation studies have been carried out with dogs trained to inhale cigarette smoke through tracheostomata and by nasal inhalation.[6,18] None of these studies provided convincing evidence of pulmonary tumor induction. Some studies have also been performed with rabbits and small numbers of nonhuman primates, all with negative results.[6,18]

Experiments in which CSC has been tested for tumor induction have been summarized.[6,15] CSC is roughly equivalent to cigarette smoke total particulate matter (TPM), the material collected on a glass fiber pad called a Cambridge filter, which has had smoke drawn through it. The term "tar," which has been used in official reports on cigarette brands, is equivalent to TPM but without nicotine and water.

CSC generation and collection techniques have been standardized.[21] The most widely used test system for carcinogenicity of CSC is mouse skin. Consistently, CSC induces benign and malignant skin tumors in mice. The carcinogenic activities of cigarettes of different designs as well as mechanisms of carcinogenesis have been investigated using the mouse skin assay. Mouse skin studies led to the identification of carcinogenic polycyclic aromatic hydrocarbons (PAH) in cigarette smoke as well as the demonstration that CSC has cocarcinogenic and tumor promoting activity.[27] The overall carcinogenic effect of CSC on mouse skin appears to depend on the composite interaction of the tumor initiators such as PAH, tumor promoters, and cocarcinogens. Tumors are not induced by the PAH alone, using dosages equivalent to their concentrations in CSC.[27]

CSC has also been tested by direct injection into the rodent lung, generally in a lipid vehicle. This caused squamous cell carcinomas of the lung in rats. Tumors were not observed in rats treated with the vehicle.[21]

An IARC working group concluded that there is sufficient evidence for the carcinogenicity of moist snuff in laboratory animals.[8] Squamous cell carcinomas and papillomas of the oral and nasal cavities and forestomach as well as other tumors developed in rats treated with snuff tobacco in a surgically created oral canal. However, other studies using this technique produced equivocal results, as has administration of extracts of snuff to laboratory animals. The combination of inoculation with human simplex virus-1 or -2 into the cheek pouches of hamsters, followed by repeated application of snuff tobacco to the cheek pouches, resulted in a high incidence of invasive squamous cell carcinoma in the cheek pouches. These tumors were not observed in cheek pouches treated with virus or snuff alone.

CARCINOGENS IN TOBACCO PRODUCTS

Table 13.1 summarizes carcinogens in cigarette smoke.[2] This table has been updated based on recently available analytical data, as cited in the table, and other comprehensive lists of tobacco smoke carcinogens.[28–30] The 72 compounds listed are only those that have been evaluated for carcinogenicity by IARC and placed in groups 1 (carcinogenic to humans), 2A (probably carcinogenic to humans), or 2B (possibly carcinogenic to humans). All of the compounds are carcinogenic in laboratory animals, and 15 are rated as carcinogenic to humans. There are other carcinogens in cigarette smoke that have not been evaluated by IARC. These include, for example, multiple PAH and aromatic amines with incompletely characterized occurrence levels and carcinogenic activities.[2,21]

PAH were first identified as carcinogenic constituents of coal tar.[31] They are products of incomplete combustion that occur as mixtures in tars, soots, broiled foods, automobile engine exhaust, and other materials. PAH are frequently locally acting carcinogens, and some, such as benzo[*a*]pyrene (BaP) have powerful carcinogenic activity. BaP is considered carcinogenic to humans by IARC.[32]

Other hydrocarbons include 1,3-butadiene, a powerful multiorgan carcinogen in the mouse, with weaker activity in the rat, and benzene, a known human leukemogen. Benzene and 1,3-butadiene are arguably the two most prevalent strong carcinogens in cigarette smoke.

N-Nitrosamines are a large class of carcinogens with demonstrated activity in at least 30 animal species.[33] *N*-Nitrosamines are potent systemic carcinogens that affect different tissues depending on their structures. Two of the most important *N*-nitrosamines in cigarette smoke are the tobacco-specific *N*-nitrosamines 4-(methylnitrosamino)-1-(3-pyridyl)-1-butanone (NNK) and *N*′-nitrosonornicotine (NNN).[34] NNK causes lung tumors in all species tested and has particularly high activity in the rat. NNK can also induce tumors of the pancreas, nasal cavity, and liver. NNN produces esophageal and nasal tumors in rats and respiratory tract tumors in mice and hamsters.[35] NNK and NNN are considered as carcinogenic to humans by IARC.[8]

Aromatic amines include the well-known human bladder carcinogens 2-naphthylamine and 4-aminobiphenyl, first identified as human carcinogens due to industrial exposures in the dye industry.[36] Heterocyclic aromatic amines are also combustion products and are best known for their occurrence in broiled foods.[37] Other heterocyclic compounds include nitrogen-containing analogues of PAH and simpler compounds such as furan, a liver carcinogen.

Aldehydes such as formaldehyde and acetaldehyde occur widely in the human environment and are also endogenous metabolites found in human blood. Phenolic compounds such as catechol are abundant in tobacco smoke, but have relatively weak carcinogenic activity. Catechol, however, is a potent cocarcinogen with PAH in mouse skin experiments.

Among the other carcinogenic organic compounds in cigarette smoke are the human carcinogens vinyl chloride, a liver carcinogen, and ethylene oxide, which is associated with malignancies of the lymphatic and hematopoietic system in both humans and experimental animals. Diverse metals and the radionuclide polonium-210 are also present in cigarette smoke.

Cigarette smoke also contains oxidants such as nitric oxide (up to 600 mcg per cigarette) and related species, and free radicals, which have been detected by electron spin resonance and spin trapping.[38] Other compounds may also be involved in oxidative damage produced by cigarette smoke. In addition, several studies demonstrate the presence in cigarette smoke of an as yet uncharacterized ethylating agent, which ethylates both DNA and hemoglobin.[39,40]

In summary, there are diverse carcinogens in cigarette smoke. Among the well characterized compounds listed in Table 13.2, the most important, based on their carcinogenic potency and established levels in cigarette smoke, are probably PAH, *N*-nitrosamines, aromatic amines, 1,3-butadiene, benzene, and aldehydes. The same carcinogens are also present in secondhand cigarette smoke, but human exposure is considerably less due to dilution with room air.

A variety of carcinogens have been detected in smokeless tobacco products.[8] The most abundant strong carcinogens are NNK and NNN, which are typically found in total amounts of 1 to 10 ppm in smokeless tobacco products, levels 10 to 1,000 times higher than *N*-nitrosamines in other products designed for human consumption. Considerable levels of PAH are also found in some products. Several other carcinogenic compounds such as formaldehyde, acetaldehyde, crotonaldehyde, cadmium, nickel, and polonium-210 are also present.[41,42]

Relationship of Carcinogens to Specific Cancers Caused by Tobacco Products

Data from carcinogenicity studies, product analyses, and biochemical and molecular biological investigations support a

TABLE 13.1

CONSTITUENTS OF CIGARETTE SMOKE CLASSIFIED BY THE INTERNATIONAL AGENCY FOR RESEARCH ON CANCER (IARC) AS CARCINOGENIC (UPDATED AND REVISED IN 2010)[a]

Carcinogen	Representative Amounts in Mainstream Cigarette Smoke, per Cigarette	*IARC Monographs* Evaluation of Carcinogenicity		IARC Group	IARC Monograph Volume, Year; and Additional References
		In Animals	In Humans		
POLYCYCLIC AROMATIC HYDROCARBONS (PAH)					
Benz[*j*]aceanthrylene[b]	Present	Limited		2B	(28,32); 92, 2010
Benz[*a*]anthracene	2.6–26.8 ng	Sufficient		2B	S7, 1987; (96,97); 92, 2010
Benzo[*b*]fluoranthene	1.3–17.0 ng	Sufficient		2B	S7, 1987; (96,97); 92, 2010
Benzo[*j*]fluoranthene	1.8–24.0 ng	Sufficient		2B	S7, 1987; (98); 92, 2010
Benzo[*k*]fluoranthene	0.5–3.3 ng	Sufficient		2B	S7, 1987; (96,97); 92, 2010
Benzo[*c*]phenanthrene[b]	Present	Limited		2B	(32)
Benzo[*a*]pyrene	1.0–15.2 ng	Sufficient	Limited	1	S7, 1987; (32,96,97,99,100); 92, 2010
Chrysene	2.6–24.7 ng	Sufficient		2B	(32,96); 92, 2010
Cyclopenta[*c,d*]pyrene[b]	Present	Sufficient		2A	(28,32); 92, 2010
Dibenz[*a,h*]anthracene	ND–6 ng	Sufficient		2A	S7, 1987; (97,98); 92, 2010
Dibenzo[*a,e*]pyrene	1.5–2.6 ng	Sufficient		2B	S7, 1987; (97,98); 92, 2010
Dibenzo[*a,i*]pyrene	0.7–1.2 ng	Sufficient		2B	S7, 1987; (97,98); 92, 2010
Dibenzo[*a,h*]pyrene[b]	5.0–9.5 ng	Sufficient		2B	(30,32); 92, 2010
Dibenzo[*a,l*]pyrene[b]	0.1 ng	Sufficient		2A	(32,101); 92, 2010
Indeno[1,2,3-*cd*]pyrene	0.65–11.2 ng	Sufficient		2B	S7, 1987; (97,98); 92, 2010
5-Methylchrysene[b]	ND–2 ng	Sufficient		2B	S7, 1987; (30); 92, 2010
OTHER HYDROCARBONS					
1,3-Butadiene	1.6–54.1 mcg	Sufficient	Sufficient	1	97, 2008; 71, 1999; (97,99,100)
Isoprene	42–586 mcg	Sufficient		2B	60, 1994; 71, 1999; (97,99,100)
Benzene	6.1–45.6 mcg	Sufficient	Sufficient	1	29, 1982; S7, 1987; (97,99,100)
Ethylbenzene[b]	Present	Sufficient	Inadequate	2B	77, 2000
Naphthalene	65–868 ng	Sufficient	Inadequate	2B	82, 2002; (102)
Styrene[b]	ND–48 mcg	Limited	Limited	2B	82, 2002; (96)
***N*-NITROSAMINES**					
N-Nitrosodimethylamine	ND–7.9 ng	Sufficient		2A	17, 1978; S7, 1987; (97)
N-Nitrosoethylmethylamine[b]	ND–0.2 ng	Sufficient		2B	17, 1978; S7, 1987; (30)
N-Nitrosodiethylamine[b]	ND–7.6 ng	Sufficient		2A	17, 1978; S7, 1987; (29)
N-Nitrosopyrrolidine	ND–19.7 ng	Sufficient		2B	17, 1978; S7, 1987; (97)
N-Nitrosopiperidine[b]	ND–231 ng	Sufficient		2B	17, 1978; S7, 1987; (30)
N-Nitrosodiethanolamine[b]	ND–290 ng	Sufficient		2B	17, 1978; 77, 2000; (30)
N′-Nitrosonornicotine	11–270 ng	Sufficient	Limited	1	S7, 1987; 89, 2004; (97,99,100)
4-(Methylnitrosamino)-1-(3-pyridyl)-1-butanone	13–223 ng	Sufficient	Limited	1	S7, 1987; 89, 2004; (97,99,100)
AROMATIC AMINES					
2-Toluidine	0.4–144 ng	Sufficient	Limited	2A	S7, 1987; 77, 2000; (97)
2,6-Dimethylaniline[b]	3.6–18.0 ng	Sufficient		2B	57, 1993; (30)
2-Naphthylamine	0.03–17.2 ng	Sufficient	Sufficient	1	4, 1974; S7, 1987; (97,99,100)
4-Aminobiphenyl	0.3–2.86 ng	Sufficient	Sufficient	1	1, 1972; S7, 1987; (97,99,100)
o-Anisidine[b]	Present	Inadequate	Sufficient	2B	73, 1999
HETEROCYCLIC AROMATIC AMINES[b]					
A-α-C	ND–260 ng	Sufficient		2B	40, 1986; S7, 1987; (30)
MeA-α-C	2–37 ng	Sufficient		2B	40, 1986; S7, 1987; (30)
IQ	0.3 ng	Sufficient		2A	S7, 1987; 56, 1993; (29)
Trp-P-1	0.2–0.3 ng	Sufficient		2B	31, 1983; S7, 1987; (30)
Trp-P-2	ND–0.2 ng	Sufficient		2B	31, 1983; S7, 1987; (30)
Glu-P-1	ND–0.89 ng	Sufficient		2B	40, 1986; S7, 1987; (30)
Glu-P-2	0.25–0.88 ng	Sufficient		2B	40, 1986; S7, 1987, (30)
PhIP	11–23 ng	Sufficient		2B	56, 1993; (30)

(*continued*)

TABLE 13.1

(CONTINUED)

Carcinogen	Representative Amounts in Mainstream Cigarette Smoke, per Cigarette	*IARC Monographs* Evaluation of Carcinogenicity: In Animals	In Humans	IARC Group	IARC Monograph Volume, Year; and Additional References
OTHER HETEROCYCLIC COMPOUNDS[b]					
Furan	18–65 mcg	Sufficient		2B	63, 1995; (30)
Dibenz[*a,h*]acridine	ND–0.1 ng	Sufficient		2B	32, 1983; S7, 1987; (30)
Dibenz[*a,j*]acridine	ND–10 ng	Sufficient		2B	32, 1983; S7, 1987; (30)
Dibenzo[*c,g*]carbazole	ND–0.7 ng	Sufficient		2B	32, 1983; S7, 1987; (30)
Benzo[*b*]furan	Present	Sufficient		2B	63, 1995; (30)
ALDEHYDES					
Formaldehyde	1.6–115.3 mcg	Sufficient	Sufficient	1	88, 2006; 62, 1995a; (97,99,100)
Acetaldehyde	32–828 mcg	Sufficient		2B	S7, 1987; 71, 1999; (97,99,100)
PHENOLIC COMPOUNDS					
Catechol	4.4–110 mcg	Sufficient		2B	S7, 1987; 71, 1999; (97,99,100)
Caffeic acid[b]	Present	Sufficient		2B	56, 1993; (30)
NITROHYDROCARBONS					
Nitromethane[b]	0.5–0.6 mcg	Sufficient		2B	77, 2000
2-Nitropropane	ND–18.7 ng	Sufficient		2B	S7, 1987; 71, 1999; (97)
Nitrobenzene[b]	25 ng	Sufficient		2B	65, 1996; (30)
MISCELLANEOUS ORGANIC COMPOUNDS					
Acetamide[b]	2.2–111 mcg	Sufficient		2B	S7, 1987; 71, 1999; (30)
Acrylamide[b]	2.3 mcg	Sufficient		2A	S7, 1987; 60, 1994; (30)
Acrylonitrile	0.5–19.6 mcg	Sufficient		2B	S7, 1987; 71, 1999; (97,99)
Vinyl chloride	ND–36.6 ng	Sufficient	Sufficient	1	97, 2008; S7, 1987; (97)
Ethylene oxide[b]	Present	Sufficient	Limited	1	97, 2008; 60, 1994
Propylene oxide[b]	Present	Sufficient		2B	60, 1994; S7, 1987
Urethane[b]	10–35 ng	Sufficient		2B	7, 1974; S7, 1987; (30)
Vinyl acetate[b]	1.6–4.0 mcg	Limited	Inadequate	2B	63, 1995
METALS AND INORGANIC COMPOUNDS					
Arsenic	ND–5.5 ng	Sufficient	Sufficient	1	84, 2004; (99)
Beryllium	ND–0.5 ng	Sufficient	Sufficient	1	S7, 1987; 58, 1993a; (103)
Nickel	ND–500 ng	Sufficient	Sufficient	1	S7, 1987; 49, 1990; (103)
Chromium (hexavalent)	ND–2.6 ng	Sufficient	Sufficient	1	S7, 1987; 49, 1990; (99,103)
Cadmium	1.6–101.0 ng	Sufficient	Sufficient	1	S7, 1987; 58, 1993a; (99,100)
Cobalt[b]	0.13–100.0 ng	Sufficient		2B	52, 1991; (30)
Lead (inorganic)	ND–39.2 ng	Sufficient	Limited	2A	23, 1980; S7,1987; 87, 2004b; (99)
Hydrazine[b]	24–57 ng	Sufficient		2B	S7, 1987; 71, 1999; (30)
Radio-isotope Polonium-210[b]	0.03–1.0 pCi	Sufficient		1	78, 2001

[a]This table (modified from [104] and IARC volume 83 [6] and updated in March 2010) shows compounds or elements in mainstream cigarette smoke, with representative amounts given per cigarette. Presence and amounts in cigarette smoke were assessed based on recent literature as cited and data given in references 28–30. Only constituents evaluated by IARC and included in groups 1 (15 constituents), 2A (10 constituents), or 2B (47 constituents) are listed. Virtually all these substances are known carcinogens in experimental animals. In combination with data on cancer in humans and—in some cases—other relevant data, *IARC Monographs* classifications for these agents have been established as Group 2B (possibly carcinogenic to humans), Group 2A (probably carcinogenic to humans), or Group 1 (carcinogenic to humans). When IARC evaluations were made more than twice, only the two most recent monographs are listed, with volume number and year of publication. No entry in the column "humans" indicates inadequate evidence or no data.

[b]Not commonly reported: values may be estimates or unreliable for the smoke of current cigarettes.

S7, Supplement 7 of the *IARC Monographs;* ND, not detected; A-α-C, 2-amino-9*H*-pyrido[2,3-*b*]indole; MeA-α-C, 2-amino-3-methyl-9*H*-pyrido[2,3-*b*]indole; IQ, 2-amino-3-methylimidazo[4,5-*f*]quinoline; Trp-P-1, 3-amino-l,4-dimethyl-5*H*-pyrido[4,3-*b*]indole; Trp-P-2, 3-amino-l-methyl-5*H*-pyrido[4,3-*b*]indole; Glu-P-1, 2-amino-6-methyl[1,2-*a*:3′,2′-*d*]imidazole; Glu-P-2, 2-aminodipyrido[1,2-*a*:3′,2′-*d*]imidazole; PhIP, 2-amino-l-methyl-6-phenylimidazo[4,5-*b*]pyridine; pCi, picoCurie.

TABLE 13.2

CARCINOGENS AND TOBACCO-INDUCED CANCERS

Cancer Type	Likely Carcinogen Involvement[a]
Lung	PAH, NNK (major) 1,3-butadiene, isoprene, ethylene oxide, ethyl carbamate, aldehydes, benzene, metals
Larynx	PAH
Nasal	NNK, NNN, other *N*-nitrosamines, aldehydes
Oral cavity	PAH, NNK, NNN
Esophagus	NNN, other *N*-nitrosamines
Liver	NNK, other *N*-nitrosamines, furan
Pancreas	NNK, NNAL
Cervix	PAH, NNK
Bladder	4-aminobiphenyl, other aromatic amines
Leukemia	Benzene
Colorectal	Heterocyclic aromatic amines

[a]Based on carcinogenicity studies in laboratory animals, biochemical evidence from human tissues and fluids, and epidemiological data, where available. NNAL, 4-(methylnitrosamino)-1-(3-pyridyl)-1-butanol; NNK, 4-(methylnitrosamino)-1-(3-pyridyl)-1-butanone; NNN, *N'*-nitrosonornicotine; PAH, polycyclic aromatic hydrocarbons. Adapted from Surgeon General's Report 2010, in press.

significant role for certain carcinogens in specific types of tobacco-induced cancer, but proof is difficult due to the complexity of tobacco smoke (Table 13.2).

Considerable evidence supports PAH and NNK as major causative factors in lung cancer. PAH can be potent locally acting carcinogens, and tobacco smoke fractions enriched in these compounds are carcinogenic.[43–45] PAH–DNA adducts have been detected in human lung, and the spectrum of mutations in the *p53* tumor suppressor gene isolated from lung tumors is similar to the spectrum of DNA damage produced *in vitro* by PAH diol epoxide metabolites and in cell culture by BaP, although similar changes are also produced by acrolein.[46–50]

NNK is a strong systemic lung carcinogen in rodents, inducing lung tumors independently of its route of administration.[35] The strength of NNK is particularly great in the rat, in which total doses as low as 6 mg/kg (and 1.8 mg/kg when considered as part of a dose–response trend) have induced a significant incidence of lung tumors.[51] This compares to an estimated 1.1 mg/kg dose of NNK in humans in 40 years of smoking.[35] DNA adducts derived from NNK or the related tobacco-specific nitrosamine NNN are present in lung tissue from smokers, and a metabolite of NNK, NNAL, is routinely found in the urine of smokers.[52,53] Levels of NNAL were related to lung cancer incidence in two prospective epidemiology studies.[54,55] Other compounds that could be involved in lung cancer include 1,3-butadiene, isoprene, ethylene oxide, ethyl carbamate, aldehydes, acrolein, benzene, and metals, but the collective evidence for each of these is not as strong as for PAH and NNK.[38,50]

The cigarette smoke particulate phase causes larynx tumors in hamsters. This could be attributed to PAH.[21] The *p53* gene mutations identified in tumors of the human larynx support a role for PAH in the development of this cancer.[46] *N*-Nitrosamines, as well as acetaldehyde and formaldehyde, induce nasal tumors in rodents and are likely candidates as causes of smoking-associated nasal tumors.[33] Levels of formaldehyde and acetaldehyde DNA adducts are higher in smokers than in nonsmokers or smokers who have stopped, respectively.[56,57] Based on animal studies, PAH, NNK, and NNN are the most likely causes of oral cancer in smokers, while NNK and NNN are the most probable in smokeless tobacco users.[58] *N*-Nitrosamines are the most effective esophageal carcinogens known, and NNN, which causes tumors of the esophagus in rats, is the most prevalent *N*-nitrosamine carcinogen in cigarette smoke and smokeless tobacco.

NNK and several other cigarette smoke *N*-nitrosamines are effective hepatocarcinogens in rats, as is furan.[33] NNK and its major metabolite NNAL are the only pancreatic carcinogens known to be present in tobacco products, and biochemical data from studies with human tissues provide some support for their role in smoking-related pancreatic cancer, although DNA adducts were not detected.[59–61] The link between smokeless tobacco use and pancreatic cancer is also plausibly due to NNK and its metabolite NNAL. Biochemical studies demonstrate that both NNK and PAH can reach the cervix in humans and are metabolically activated there.[62,63] DNA adducts derived from BaP and other hydrophobic compounds have been detected in cervical tissue from smokers.[48,63] Therefore, these compounds might contribute to the etiology of cervical cancer in smokers, in combination with human papilloma virus. The amines 4-aminobiphenyl and 2-naphthylamine are known human bladder carcinogens, and considerable data from human studies support the role of aromatic amines as the major cause of bladder cancer in smokers.[64,65] The most probable cause of leukemia in smokers is benzene, which occurs in large quantities in cigarette smoke and is a known cause of acute myelogenous leukemia in humans. Heterocyclic aromatic amines might be important in causing colon cancer in smokers.[13,66]

Cigarette smoke causes oxidative damage, probably because it contains free radicals such as nitric oxide and mixtures of hydroquinones, semiquinones, and quinones, which can induce redox cycling.[38,67] Smokers have lower levels of ascorbic acid, higher levels of oxidized lipids, and sometimes higher levels of oxidized DNA bases than nonsmokers, but the role of oxidative damage as a cause of specific tobacco-induced cancers remains unclear.[38]

OVERVIEW OF MECHANISMS OF TUMOR INDUCTION BY TOBACCO PRODUCTS

Figure 13.3 presents an overview of mechanisms by which cigarette smoke causes cancer[38,68]; a similar scheme would apply to smokeless tobacco products, but less is known. The major established pathway of cancer causation by cigarette smoke is presented in the central track of Figure 13.3. It involves exposure to carcinogens and the formation of covalent bonds between the carcinogens and DNA, thus producing DNA adducts. These adducts can cause miscoding, resulting in permanent mutations in critical genes of somatic cells.

Most people start smoking as teenagers, become addicted to nicotine, and then smoke habitually. While nicotine, the main known addictive agent in cigarette smoke, is not carcinogenic, it is accompanied in each puff by a mixture of the carcinogens listed in Table 13.1, along with thousands of other compounds. These carcinogens are mainly responsible for cancer induction by cigarette smoke. Extensive data in the literature demonstrate the uptake of these carcinogens by smokers and confirm the expected higher levels of their metabolites in urine of smokers than nonsmokers, as summarized later in this chapter.

Many cigarette smoke carcinogens are themselves unreactive and require a metabolic activation process, generally catalyzed by cytochrome P450 enzymes, to convert them to electrophilic entities that covalently bind to DNA, forming DNA adducts.[69,70] P450s 1A1 and 1B1, inducible by cigarette smoke via interactions of smoke compounds with the aryl hydrocarbon receptor, are particularly important in the metabolic activation of PAH.[71] The inducibility of these P450s may be a

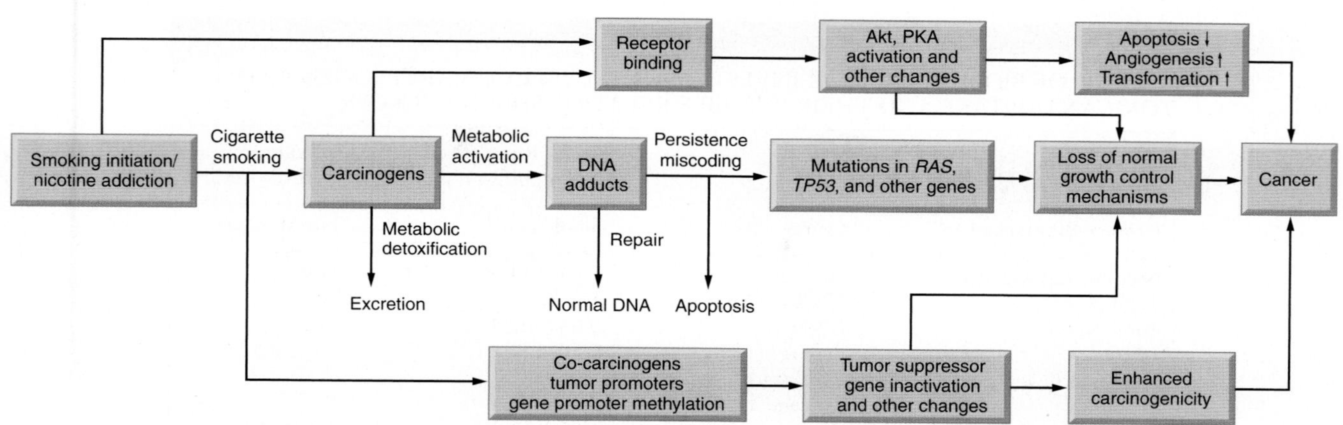

FIGURE 13.3 Conceptual model for understanding mechanisms of tobacco carcinogenesis.

critical aspect of cancer susceptibility in smokers. P450s 1A2, 2A13, 2E1, and 3A4 are also important in the activation of cigarette smoke carcinogens. Competing with metabolic activation is detoxification, which results in harmless excretion of carcinogen metabolites, and is catalyzed by a variety of enzymes including glutathione-*S*-transferases and UDP-glucuronosyl transferases.[72,73] The balance between carcinogen metabolic activation and detoxification varies among individuals and is very likely to affect cancer susceptibility with those having higher activation and lower detoxification capacity being at highest risk. Some support for this is found in the results of molecular epidemiologic studies of polymorphisms, or variants, in the genes coding for these enzymes, but there is also considerable negative data.[74,75]

Continuing along the central track of Figure 13.3, DNA adducts are absolutely central to the carcinogenic process. Extensive studies have examined the presence of DNA adducts in human tissues. There is massive evidence, especially from studies that use relatively nonspecific adduct measurement methods, that adduct levels in the lung and other tissues are higher in smokers than in nonsmokers, and some epidemiologic data link higher adduct levels with a higher cancer risk.[6]

Cellular repair systems can remove DNA adducts and return the structure of DNA to normal. These include direct base repair by alkyltransferases, excision of DNA damage by base and nucleotide excision repair, mismatch repair, and double strand repair. If these repair enzymes cannot efficiently perform, then adducts will persist, increasing the probability of cancer development. There are polymorphisms in genes coding for some DNA repair enzymes and the resulting deficient DNA repair could, in theory, increase the probability of cancer development.[76]

Persistent DNA adducts can cause miscoding during replication when DNA polymerase enzymes process them incorrectly. There is considerable specificity in the relationship between specific DNA adducts of cigarette smoke carcinogens and the types of mutations they cause. G-to-T and G-to-A mutations are frequently observed.[38] Mutations have been frequently observed in the *KRAS* oncogene in lung cancer and in the *TP53* tumor suppressor gene in a variety of cigarette smoke–induced cancers.[46,77,78] The cancer-causing role of these genes has been firmly established in animal studies.[79,80] In addition, numerous cytogenetic changes have been observed in lung cancer, and chromosome damage throughout the aerodigestive tract is strongly linked with cigarette smoke exposure. Gene mutations can cause loss of normal cellular growth control functions, via a complex process of signal transduction pathways, ultimately resulting in genomic instability, cellular proliferation, and cancer.[81,82] Apoptosis, or programmed cell death, is a protective process that can remove cells with DNA damage, and it serves as a counterbalance to these mutational events. The balance between mechanisms leading to apoptosis and those suppressing apoptosis will have a major impact on tumor growth.[82]

Although the central track of Figure 13.3 is clearly a major pathway by which cigarette smoke carcinogens cause cancer, epigenetic pathways also contribute, as indicated in the top and bottom tracks of Figure 13.3.[68,83] Nicotine and tobacco-specific nitrosamines bind to nicotinic and other cellular receptors, leading to activation of Akt (also known as protein kinase B), protein kinase A, and other changes, resulting in decreased apoptosis, increased angiogenesis, and increased transformation.[84,85] Cigarette smoke activates the epidermal growth factor receptor and cyclooxygenase-2.[86] The occurrence of cocarcinogens and tumor promoters in cigarette smoke is well established. Another important epigenetic pathway is enzymatic methylation of promoter regions of genes, resulting in gene silencing. If this occurs in tumor suppressor genes, the result can be unregulated proliferation.[87] Cigarette smoke also contains oxidants, inflammatory agents, and cilia-toxic compounds, all of which contribute to its carcinogenicity.

TOBACCO CARCINOGEN AND TOXICANT BIOMARKERS

The term "biomarker" has varied meanings. In the cancer research field in particular, this term is often associated with early detection of cancer. That is not the context here. *Merriam-Webster's Collegiate Dictionary* defines biomarker as "a distinctive biological or biologically derived indicator (as a metabolite) of a process, event, or condition." A biomarker in this chapter is any quantifiable substance, such as a metabolite, that can be specifically related to the uptake or effects of tobacco carcinogens or toxicants.

Tobacco carcinogen and toxicant biomarkers are currently recognized as critical in the study of tobacco and cancer.[88] It is likely that these biomarkers ultimately will play a significant role in the regulation of tobacco products and in increasing the understanding of susceptibility to tobacco-induced cancer. A panel of tobacco carcinogen and toxicant biomarkers is presented in Table 13.3.[53] All biomarkers have been validated analytically. Most have been used in multiple studies on hundreds or even thousands of smokers and nonsmokers. (The exceptions are HBMA, HEMA, N^6-hydroxymethyl-dAdo, and N^2-ethylidene-dGuo.) Some typical recent data are summarized

TABLE 13.3

A PANEL OF BIOMARKERS FOR INVESTIGATING TOBACCO CARCINOGEN AND TOXICANT UPTAKE AND THEIR POSSIBLE RELATIONSHIP TO CANCER

		Range of Recent Mean Values (nmol/24 h unless noted otherwise[a])	
Urinary Biomarkers	**Source**	**Smokers**	**Nonsmokers**
Nicotine equivalents	Nicotine	70.4–154 mcmol/24 h	NA[b]
Total NNAL	NNK	1.1–2.9	NA
Total NNN	NNN	0.049–0.24	NA
1-HOP	Pyrene	0.50–1.45	0.18–0.50
MHBMA	1,3-Butadiene	15.5–322	0.65–7.5
SPMA	Benzene	3.2–32.1	0.17–3.14
HPMA	Acrolein	5,869–11,190	1,131–1,847
HBMA	Crotonaldehyde	1,965–26,000	242–3,200
HEMA	Ethylene oxide	19.1–102	6.51–38.8
Cd	Cadmium	2.3–12.8	1.34–8.04
8-epi-$PGF_{2\alpha}$[c]	Oxidative damage	1.48–2.80	0.62–1.13
PGE-M	Inflammation	54–60	31.6–45.3
		Recent Data (pmol/g globin; mean ± S.D.)	
Hemoglobin Adducts	**Source**	**Smokers**	**Nonsmokers**
Cyanoethylvaline	Acrylonitrile	112 ± 81	6.5 ± 6.4
Carbamoylethylvaline	Acrylamide	84.1 ± 41.8	27.8 ± 7.1
Hydroxyethylvaline	Ethylene oxide	132 ± 92	21.1 ± 12.7
4-Aminobiphenyl-globin	4-Aminobiphenyl	0.26 ± 0.006[d]	0.067 ± 0.009[d]
		Recent Data (fmol/mcmol dN; mean ± S.D.)	
Leukocyte DNA Adducts	**Source**	**Smokers**	**Nonsmokers**
N^6-hydroxymethyl-dAdo	Formaldehyde	179 ± 205	15.5 ± 33.8
N^2-ethylidene-dGuo	Acetaldehyde	1,310 ± 1,720	705 ± 438
		Mean Concentrations	
Other	**Source**	**Smokers**	**Nonsmokers**
Exhaled CO	Carbon monoxide	17.4–34.4 ppm	2.6–6.5 ppm
Carboxyhemoglobin	Carbon monoxide	3.4–7.1%	0.35–1.45%

[a]Based on 1.3 g creatinine per 24 hours in smokers and 1.5 g creatinine per 24 hours in nonsmokers, or 1.5 L urine per 24 hours. Creatinine determinations were mainly by a modified Jaffe reaction using a certified automated clinical analyzer.
[b]NA, not applicable. These are not detected in the urine of nonsmokers unless they use other tobacco products, nicotine replacement products (for nicotine equivalents, and sometimes NNN or are exposed to secondhand smoke, in which case levels are usually less than 5% of smoker levels.
[c]Determined by mass spectrometry.
[d]Weighted mean ± S.D. (standard deviation).
nicotine equivalents, the sum of nicotine, cotinine, 3′-hydroxycotinine, and their glucuronides; total NNAL, 4-(methylnitrosamino)-1-(3-pyridyl)-1-butanol and its glucuronides; total NNN, *N*′-nitrosonornicotine and its glucuronides; 1-HOP, 1-hydroxypyrene and its glucuronides/sulfates; MHBMA, the sum of 1-hydroxy-2-(*N*-acetylcysteinyl)-3-butene and 1-(*N*-acetylcysteinyl)-2-hydroxy-3-butene; SPMA, *S*-phenyl mercapturic acid; HPMA, 3-hydroxypropyl mercapturic acid; HBMA, 4-hydroxybut-2-yl mercapturic acid; HEMA, 2-hydroxyethyl mercapturic acid; 8-epi-$PFG_{2\alpha}$, 9,11,15-trihydroxyprosta-5,13-dien-1-oic acid; PGE-M, 11α-hydroxy-9, 15-dioxo-2,3,4,5-tetranorprostane-1,20-dioic acid.
(From ref. 53, with permission.)

in Table 13.3. Although some of the ranges of values overlap between smokers and nonsmokers for certain biomarkers, biomarker levels are consistently higher in smokers compared to nonsmokers in individual studies.

The biomarkers in Table 13.3 represent a broad cross-section of carcinogens and toxicants in tobacco products. Among these compounds, NNK and NNN, BaP, 1,3-butadiene, benzene, ethylene oxide, cadmium, 4-aminobiphenyl, and formaldehyde are considered "carcinogenic to humans" by IARC.[32,89–93] Many of the compounds represented by the biomarkers in Table 13.3 also have considerable toxic effects. Although these constituents represent only a small percentage of the over 5,000 identified compounds in cigarette smoke,[28] they are collectively a powerful group and include all of those singled out by the World Health Organization for regulation under the Framework Convention on Tobacco Control: acetaldehyde, acrolein, benzene, BaP, 1,3-butadiene, carbon monoxide, formaldehyde, NNN, and NNK.[9] It is virtually inconceivable that a major reduction in their biomarker levels would not significantly impact cancer incidence in smokers. This is a significant goal pertinent to product regulation and cancer prevention.

Tobacco carcinogen biomarkers have proven critical in evaluating the exposure of nonsmokers to secondhand smoke. Total NNAL has been particularly effective in this respect because of its tobacco specificity.[94] The presence of NNAL in the urine of a nonsmoker confirms exposure to cigarette smoke, as this metabolite cannot come from the diet or other sources, only from NNK in tobacco smoke. Tobacco carcinogen biomarkers also have potential as measures of individual susceptibility to the effects of cigarette smoke. They could become part of an algorithm to predict which smoker will get cancer, information that is not presently available and could be very useful in cessation efforts.

Selected References

The full list of references for this chapter appears in the online version.

1. Mackay J, Eriksen M. *The tobacco atlas*. Geneva: World Health Organization, 2002.
2. International Agency for Research on Cancer. Tobacco smoke and involuntary smoking. In: *IARC monographs on the evaluation of carcinogenic risks to humans*, vol. 83. Lyon: IARC, 2004:53.
3. Shafey O, Eriksen MP, Ross H, et al. *The tobacco atlas*, 3rd ed. Atlanta: American Cancer Society and World Lung Foundation, 2009.
4. Peto R, Watt J, Boreham J. Deaths from smoking. World Wide Web URL: www. deathsfromsmoking.net, 2007.
5. Boyle P, Levin P. *World cancer report, 2008*. Lyon: IARC, 2008.
6. International Agency for Research on Cancer. Tobacco smoke and involuntary smoking. In: *IARC monographs on the evaluation of carcinogenic risks to humans*, vol. 83. Lyon: IARC, 2004:1179.
7. State-specific secondhand smoke exposure and current cigarette smoking among adults—United States, 2008. *MMWR Morb Mortal Wkly Rep* 2009;58;1232.
8. International Agency for Research on Cancer. Smokeless tobacco and tobacco-specific nitrosamines. In: *IARC monographs on the evaluation of carcinogenic risks to humans*, vol. 89. Lyon: IARC, 2007:57.
9. Burns DM, Dybing E, Gray N, et al. Mandated lowering of toxicants in cigarette smoke: a description of the World Health Organization tobacco regulation proposal. *Tobacco Control* 2008;17:132.
10. Wynder EL, Graham EA. Tobacco smoking as a possible etiologic factor in bronchiogenic carcinoma. A study of six hundred and eighty-four proved cases. *JAMA* 1950;143:329.
11. Doll R, Hill AB. Smoking and carcinoma of the lung. A preliminary report. *BMJ* 1950;2(4682):739.
12. U.S. Department of Health and Human Services. *The health consequences of smoking: a report of the surgeon general*. Atlanta: U.S. Department of Health and Human Services, Centers for Disease Control and Prevention, National Center for Chronic Disease Prevention and Health Promotion, Office on Smoking and Health, 2004.
13. Secretan B, Straif K, Baan R, et al. A review of human carcinogens—Part E: Tobacco, areca nut, alcohol, coal smoke, and salted fish. *Lancet Oncol* 2009;10:1033.
14. U.S. Department of Health and Human Services. *The health consequences of involuntary exposure to tobacco smoke: a report of the surgeon general*. Washington, DC: U.S. Dept. of Health and Human Services, Centers for Disease Control and Prevention, National Center for Chronic Disease Prevention and Health Promotion, Office on Smoking and Health, 2006.
20. Witschi H. A/J mouse as a model for lung tumorigenesis caused by tobacco smoke: strengths and weaknesses. *Exp Lung Res* 2005;31:3.
21. International Agency for Research on Cancer. Tobacco smoking. In: *IARC monographs on the evaluation of the carcinogenic risk of chemicals to humans*, vol. 38.Lyon: IARC, 1986:37.
23. Mauderly JL, Gigliotti AP, Barr EB, et al. Chronic inhalation exposure to mainstream cigarette smoke increases lung and nasal tumor incidence in rats. *Toxicol Sci* 2004;81:280.
24. Hutt JA, Vuillemenot BR, Barr EB, et al. Life-span inhalation exposure to mainstream cigarette smoke induces lung cancer in B6C3F$_1$ mice through genetic and epigenetic pathways. *Carcinogenesis* 2005;26:1999.
28. Rodgman A, Perfetti T. *The chemical components of tobacco and tobacco smoke*. Boca Raton, FL: CRC Press, 2009:1483.
32. Straif K, Baan R, Grosse Y, et al. Carcinogenicity of polycyclic aromatic hydrocarbons. *Lancet Oncol* 2005;6:931.
33. Preussmann R, Stewart BW. *N*-nitroso carcinogens. In: *Chemical carcinogens*, 2nd ed., ACS Monograph 182, vol. 2. CE Searle, ed. Washington, DC: American Chemical Society, 1984:643.
35. Hecht SS. Biochemistry, biology, and carcinogenicity of tobacco-specific *N*-nitrosamines. *Chem Res Toxicol* 1998;11:559.
36. Luch A. Nature and nurture—lessons from chemical carcinogenesis. *Nat Rev Cancer* 2005;5:113.
38. Hecht SS. Tobacco smoke carcinogens and lung cancer. *J Natl Cancer Inst* 1999;91:1194.
41. Stepanov I, Jensen J, Hatsukami D, et al. New and traditional smokeless tobacco: comparison of toxicant and carcinogen levels. *Nicotine Tobacco Res* 2008;10:1773.
42. Stepanov I, Villalta PW, Knezevich A, et al. Analysis of 23 polycyclic aromatic hydrocarbons in smokeless tobacco by gas chromatography-mass spectrometry. *Chem Res Toxicol* 2010;23:66.
52. Hecht SS. Human urinary carcinogen metabolites: biomarkers for investigating tobacco and cancer. *Carcinogenesis* 2002;23:907.
53. Hecht SS, Yuan J-M, Hatsukami DK. Applying tobacco carcinogen and toxicant biomarkers in product regulation and cancer prevention. *Chem Res Toxicol* 2010;23(6)1001.
54. Church TR, Anderson KE, Caporaso NE, et al. A prospectively measured serum biomarker for a tobacco-specific carcinogen and lung cancer in smokers. *Cancer Epidemiol Biomarkers Prev* 2009;18:260.
55. Yuan JM, Koh WP, Murphy SE, et al. Urinary levels of tobacco-specific nitrosamine metabolites in relation to lung cancer development in two prospective cohorts of cigarette smokers. *Cancer Res* 2009;69:2990.
56. Wang M, Cheng G, Balbo S, et al. Clear differences in levels of a formaldehyde-DNA adduct in leukocytes of smokers and non-smokers. *Cancer Res* 2009;69:7170.
57. Chen L, Wang M, Villalta PW, et al. Quantitation of an acetaldehyde adduct in human leukocyte DNA and the effect of smoking cessation. *Chem Res Toxicol* 2007;20:108.
68. Hecht SS. Tobacco carcinogens, their biomarkers, and tobacco-induced cancer. *Nature Rev Cancer* 2003;3:733.
70. Jalas J, Hecht SS, Murphy SE. Cytochrome P450 2A enzymes as catalysts of metabolism of 4-(methylnitrosamino)-1-(3-pyridyl)-1-butanone (NNK), a tobacco-specific carcinogen. *Chem Res Toxicol* 2005;18:95.
78. Ding L, Getz G, Wheeler DA, et al. Somatic mutations affect key pathways in lung adenocarcinoma. *Nature* 2008;455:1069.
82. Bode AM, Dong Z. Signal transduction pathways in cancer development and as targets for cancer prevention. *Prog Nucleic Acid Res Mol Biol* 2005;79:237.
88. Hatsukami DK, Benowitz NL, Rennard SI, et al. Biomarkers to assess the utility of potential reduced exposure tobacco products. *Nicotine Tobacco Res* 2006;8:169.
89. International Agency for Research on Cancer. Smokeless tobacco and tobacco-specific nitrosamines. In: *IARC monographs on the evaluation of carcinogenic risks to humans*, vol. 89. Lyon: IARC, 2007:421.
92. International Agency for Research on Cancer. Formaldehyde, 2-butoxyethanol and 1-*tert*-butoxypropan-2-ol. In: *IARC monographs on the evaluation of carcinogenic risks to humans*, vol. 88. Lyon: IARC, 2006:37.
93. International Agency for Research on Cancer. 1,3-Butadiene, ethylene oxide and vinyl halides (vinyl fluoride, vinyl chloride and vinyl bromide). In: *IARC monographs on the evaluation of carcinogenic risks to humans*, vol. 97. Lyon: IARC, 2008:45.
94. Hecht SS. Carcinogen derived biomarkers: applications in studies of human exposure to secondhand tobacco smoke. *Tobacco Control* 2003;13(Suppl 1):i48.

96. Ding YS, Trommel JS, Yan XJ, et al. Determination of 14 polycyclic aromatic hydrocarbons in mainstream smoke from domestic cigarettes. *Environ Sci Technol* 2005;39:471.
97. Roemer E, Stabbert R, Rustemeier K, et al. Chemical composition, cytotoxicity and mutagenicity of smoke from US commercial and reference cigarettes smoked under two sets of machine smoking conditions. *Toxicology* 2004;195:31.
98. Ding YS, Ashley DL, Watson CH. Determination of 10 carcinogenic polycyclic aromatic hydrocarbons in mainstream cigarette smoke. *J Agricul Food Chem* 2007;55:5966.
99. Counts ME, Hsu FS, Laffoon SW, et al. Mainstream smoke constituent yields and predicting relationships from a worldwide market sample of cigarette brands: ISO smoking conditions. *Regul Toxicol Pharmacol* 2004;39:111.
100. Hammond D, O'Connor RJ. Constituents in tobacco and smoke emissions from Canadian cigarettes. *Tobacco Control* 2008;17(Suppl 1):i24.
101. Seidel A, Frank H, Behnke A, et al. Determination of dibenzo[*a,l*]pyrene and other fjord-region PAH isomers with MW 302 in environmental samples. *Polycycl Aromat Comp* 2004;24:759.
102. Ding YS, Yan XJ, Jain RB, et al. Determination of 14 polycyclic aromatic hydrocarbons in mainstream smoke from U.S. brand and non-U.S. brand cigarettes. *Environ Sci Technol* 2006;40:1133.
104. Hoffmann D, Hoffmann I, El Bayoumy K. The less harmful cigarette: a controversial issue. A tribute to Ernst L. Wynder. *Chem Res Toxicol* 2001; 14:767.

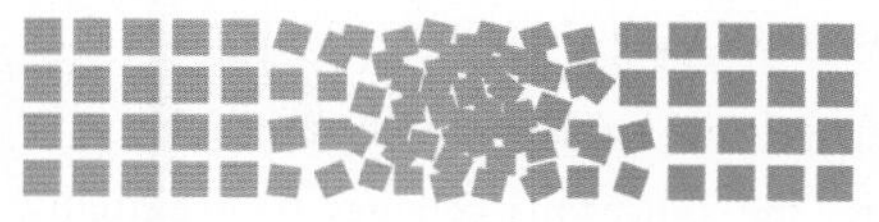

CHAPTER 14 CANCER SUSCEPTIBILITY SYNDROMES

ALICE HAWLEY BERGER AND PIER PAOLO PANDOLFI

Familial clustering of cancer susceptibility (CS) has been recognized for centuries, yet only 30 years ago scientists and geneticists were still actively debating whether cancer syndromes would indeed have a genetic inherited basis, in contrast to an environmental etiology. Importantly, whether built-in mechanisms to halt tumor initiation and progression would be operational in mammalian cells—a biological process that we now commonly refer to as *tumor suppression*—was also not clear. This sole fact testifies to the tremendous recent progress in defining biological concepts, progress that is being integrated into clinical practice and the way in which tumorigenesis, cancer prevention, and treatment are understood.

That such debate over the cause of cancer has persisted for so long probably reflects that, as it is now known, cancer is caused by both genetic and environmental factors. It has also become clear that the mechanism of cancer induction by these two factors is intricately intertwined—the primary mechanism of cancer development after exposure to environmental toxins is the development of mutations in the genome, some of which are favorable for tumor progression. Certainly some environmental factors can act at an epigenetic level as well, inducing modifications in gene expression through DNA methylation or other epigenetic mechanisms, but even these changes can be influenced by the landscape of genetic variations in a given individual. Further exemplifying the tight interplay between genetic and environmental factors in cancer development is the recent discovery that lung cancer susceptibility is influenced by genetic variation in a gene encoding for a nicotine receptor.[1–3] The association of this genetic variant with lung cancer may actually be mediated through its effect on smoking behavior; individuals with this variant generally smoked more cigarettes per day and showed more nicotine dependence than people without the variant. This finding suggests that the gene variant actually influences an individual's exposure to an environmental agent (tobacco smoke), and it is this higher exposure that is then responsible for the individual's increased risk of cancer.

Thus, in most settings, cancer development is due to complex interactions between gene and environment. However, some genetic mutations confer such pro-tumorigenic power that individuals who harbor these mutations are at extreme risk for cancer development in their lifetime. It is these mutations that are found in individuals with the highly penetrant CS syndromes that are discussed in this chapter.

The following sections will examine in detail the genetics of retinoblastoma, a paradigmatic CS syndrome that led to the formulation of the two-hit hypothesis by Alfred Knudson and the subsequent cloning of the *RB1* tumor suppressor gene. This hypothesis paved the way for two decades of dramatic advances and the generation of a detailed map of the molecular pathways, cellular functions, and the genes that are perturbed and mutated to trigger susceptibility in distinct tissues and cell types. The interplay between clinical and basic research, coupled with numerous technological advances, helped to accelerate this journey of discovery. A fluid communication from the bench to the clinic has been instrumental in identifying the syndromes and the affected families, and, with the identification of the aberrant gene, in determining the mechanistic functions of the genes and proteins involved in the observed phenotypes.

Currently, the ability to perturb the mouse genome and introduce the very same mutations and deletions observed in human syndromes offers additional insights in understanding the etiology of the syndrome, the function of the affected gene, and the way by which cancer can be prevented pharmacologically through testing of novel chemopreventative modalities in preclinical trials using transgenic or knockout models of CS syndromes. Conversely, mouse models are increasingly informing the search for new human cancer genes, as with the recent identification of *Dok* genes as lung tumor suppressors in the mouse and the subsequent recognition of human *DOK2* as a candidate human lung tumor suppressor in human lung adenocarcinoma.[4] This strategy will no doubt help in the identification of new cancer susceptibility genes, since some of these same genes may be mutated in familial cancer syndromes.

Whereas three decades ago the identification of families susceptible to specific cancer types unfortunately was accompanied by a limited array of diagnostic and therapeutic tools, today early genetic testing for some of these CS syndromes has proven critical because preventative approaches are possible (see the section "Genetic Testing"). Furthermore, the detailed knowledge of the pathways and cellular functions deregulated as a consequence of the various inherited genetic defects will allow for development of targeted chemopreventative therapies that might one day replace surgical-based preventive methods. For this reason, this chapter will summarize the common pathways mutated in CS syndromes, with a series of figures that accompany each section.

PRINCIPLES OF CANCER SUSCEPTIBILITY

This chapter will mainly focus on high-penetrance CS syndromes that can be classically inherited in an autosomal dominant or autosomal recessive fashion. However, high-penetrance susceptibility genes cannot account for most of the excess cancer risk seen in family members of patients with cancer compared with the general population. For example, high-penetrance alleles can account for only 20% of the cases of observed familial clustering of breast cancer.[5]

In addition, the fact that cancer is an epidemic disease expands the boundaries of the definition of "cancer susceptibility syndrome" to encompass the overall susceptibility of all individuals to develop cancer during their lifetimes. This susceptibility can be influenced by multiple somatic genetic and epigenetic changes as well as by a number of inherited mutations or variants in low-penetrance complex modifiers. The identification of such modifiers is aided by studies using mouse models[6] and could tremendously facilitate an accurate prediction of individual cancer risk. The recent advent of genome-wide association studies is further accelerating the identification of low-penetrance common genetic variants that can modestly affect an individual's cancer risk.[7–9] These studies will undoubtedly lead to a refinement in the understanding of cancer susceptibility and an expansion in the concept of cancer susceptibility to include both high-penetrance and low-penetrance genetic traits.

The RB Paradigm

More than 30 years ago, Alfred Knudson resolved a daunting genetic paradox regarding CS through the formulation of a revolutionary hypothesis: the "two-hit hypothesis."[10] At that time, it was already well established that CS could sometimes display a dominant inheritance modality (e.g., in the retinoblastoma syndrome). In contrast, data obtained in the laboratory through cell fusion experiments suggested that if cells had genes to oppose tumorigenesis, these genes should be recessive in their tumor suppressive function. Knudson postulated that the predisposition arises as a consequence of a heterozygous germline mutation in such a tumor suppressor, while a second acquired somatic mutation would be required for the tumor to develop. The model assumed that the second hit would take place in the remaining normal allele of this hypothetical tumor suppressor, hence resolving the paradox. In the two-hit hypothesis, because of the virtually 100% chance of eventually losing the second tumor suppressor allele, the cancer predisposition displays a dominant inheritance, while the activity of the tumor suppressor is recessive (Fig. 14.1, *left panel*).

Subsequently, Knudson's hypothesis was validated by the cloning of the *RB1* gene[11,12] and the realization that both alleles of the *RB1* gene are indeed frequently mutated in tumors from retinoblastoma patients.[13] The experimental generation and characterization of mice lacking *Rb1* in various tissues has further confirmed the *bona fide* role of *Rb1* in tumor suppression.[14–17] The pathogenesis and molecular basis of retinoblastoma are discussed in more detail later, in addition to detailed descriptions of four of the most prevalent CS syndromes and overviews of the remaining syndromes by function.

The RB paradigm represents a remarkable milestone in the understanding of the pathogenesis of human cancer, but a conceptual drift ensued that led to a dangerously unsubstantiated dogma in the following years; tumor suppressors are typically expected to be invariably recessive in their mode of action and thus their complete functional loss would be a prerequisite for a cellular phenotype to manifest and for cancer to develop. However, this is not always the case, as tumor suppressors can be haplo-insufficient in their mode of action in specific cell types or tissues, as discussed in the following sections.

What Is the Function of a Tumor Suppressor?

For cancer to initiate, the cancerous cell has to eventually acquire the ability to proliferate or to prolong its overall lifespan through the abrogation of programmed cell death. On this basis it was originally assumed that tumor suppressors would mostly regulate cell cycle progression (e.g., RB) and apoptosis (e.g., p53). It was subsequently recognized that two classes of tumor suppressors may cooperate in tumor formation: the ones that control proliferation and survival, the so-called gatekeepers, and the genes involved in the control of genomic integrity, the so-called caretakers.[18] Loss of DNA proofreading mechanisms (an example of loss of a caretaker) would, for instance, lead to the inactivation of gatekeeper tumor suppressors or the activation of proto-oncogenes.

It has become apparent in the past few years that this view needs to be further expanded on a number of levels. First, it is becoming clear that mammalian cells have evolved programs and checkpoints to ensure that an oncogenic cell is readily removed from the body. Such a professional tumor-suppressive response depends on cell type and the molecular trigger that elicits the response and includes apoptosis or cellular *senescence*, a permanent form of cell cycle arrest.[19] Second, additional processes, such as angiogenesis, when aberrantly regulated, could be critical driving forces of the oncogenic process[20] and, therefore, genes that oppose or regulate such processes could be potent tumor suppressors (e.g., *VHL*; see the section "Angiogenesis"). Lastly, in thinking about CS it is generally assumed that the cancer initiation process is strictly cell autonomous and that the germline mutation(s) should therefore be present and functionally relevant in cells from the tumor parenchyma. However, evidence is accumulating that certain tumor types could be driven in a non–cell autonomous manner through aberrant stromal–parenchymal interactions, and thus causative mutations could be found in the stromal cells instead.

Haplo-Insufficiency and the Effect of the Dose: The PTEN Paradigm

As discussed in the previous paragraphs, analysis of retinoblastoma and the *RB1* gene stimulated the development of fundamental concepts in tumor suppression. By contrast, the analysis of another critical tumor suppressor frequently mutated in human cancer and CS syndromes, *PTEN*, has allowed constructive revisitation of the Knudson two-hit hypothesis.

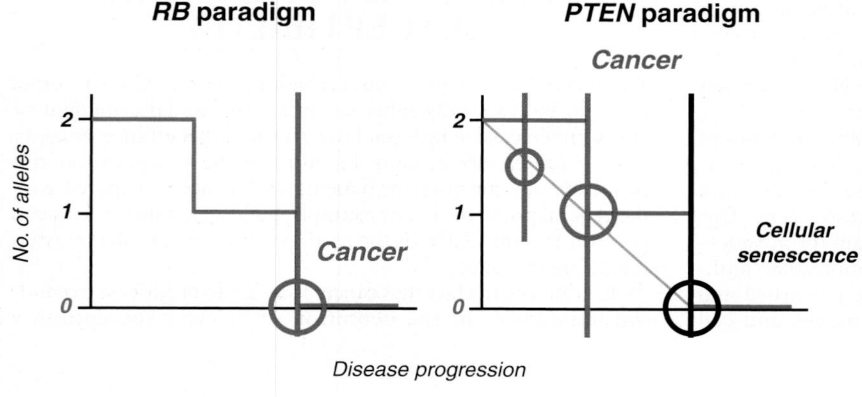

FIGURE 14.1 Revisiting the two-hit hypothesis. In Knudson's classic "two-hit" hypothesis of retinoblastoma (**left**), loss of both tumor suppressor alleles is required for tumor progression (*red circle/line*). In the PTEN paradigm (**right**), one hit is sufficient for cancer susceptibility, whereas a double hit actually opposes tumorigenesis through induction of irreversible growth arrest (senescence). Because *PTEN* is a dosage-sensitive gene, the relationship of PTEN function to gene dosage may be more appropriately depicted as a continuum (*gray line*). Certain types of cancer, such as breast cancer, can be induced with as little as a 20% reduction in *PTEN* gene expression (*small red circle/line*). (From ref. 23.)

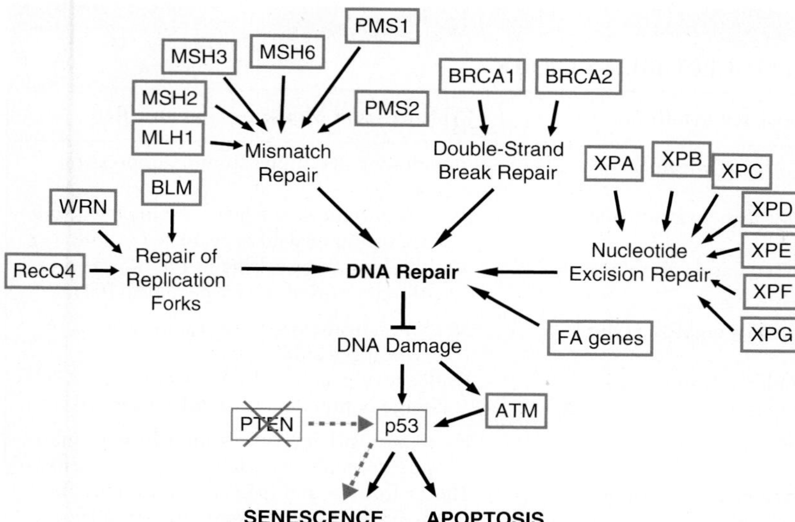

FIGURE 14.2 Genomic integrity and apoptosis pathways that are mutated in cancer susceptibility syndromes. A large number of proteins that regulate genomic integrity (caretakers) are mutated in cancer susceptibility syndromes. Tumor suppressor genes that underlie syndromes discussed in this chapter are boxed in green and include mismatch repair (MMR) genes frequently mutated in hereditary nonpolyposis colon cancer and the *BRCA1* and *BRCA2* tumor suppressors frequently mutated in human breast-ovarian cancer syndrome. The other genes and their respective syndromes are discussed in the section "Genomic Integrity and Apoptosis." Complete *PTEN* loss (*red cross*) can also lead to a p53-dependent cellular senescence response.

Contrary to the retinoblastoma paradigm, in which complete loss of the RB tumor suppressor is necessary for tumor progression in the eye, the case of *PTEN* in tumorigenesis establishes a novel paradigm. *PTEN* operates as a haplo-insufficient tumor suppressor to oppose tumor initiation in distinct tissues.[21,22] In the case of *PTEN*, cancer can develop in the absence of its complete genetic loss, because loss of one *PTEN* allele already has functional consequences, lending proliferation and survival advantages to the affected cell.[21,22] In fact, as little as a 20% reduction in *PTEN* expression can induce tumor formation (Fig. 14.1).[23] Additional loss of *PTEN* expression to 50% levels or below further enhances tumorigenesis.[24] In contrast to the RB paradigm, complete *PTEN* loss is actually antitumorigenic because it triggers a cellular senescence response that needs to be evaded for cancer to progress (Fig. 14.1, *right panel*, and Figs. 14.2 and 14.3).[25] Thus selective pressure may favor tumor cells with partial or heterozygous loss rather than complete loss of *PTEN*. These findings, in turn, open new venues for the development of a pro-senescence therapy for cancer, which aims to use the pharmacologic manipulation of the senescence response for cancer chemoprevention.[26]

The PTEN paradigm brings to light an important aspect in tumor suppressor biology with a profound impact on the requirements for tumorigenesis in CS patients; subtle incremental variations in the expression level or gene dosage can have devastating consequences, leading to distinct outcomes in distinct tissues.[23,24] The fact that even a subtle 20% reduction in *PTEN* level can initiate tumorigenesis in the mammary gland[23] provides a provocative example of how subtle variations in gene expression level may be responsible for dramatic pro-tumorigenic consequences. The unique sensitivity of cells to *PTEN* dosage further raises the possibility that epigenetic mechanisms that regulate *PTEN* expression could also significantly impact cancer risk and cancer development. These mechanisms could include cell-intrinsic mechanisms, such as expression of pseudogenes or long noncoding RNAs that act as competing endogenous RNAs (ceRNAs)[27] or alternatively could include environmental stimuli that alter gene expression, such as cigarette smoke.[28–30] These findings open a new frontier in the search for novel cancer susceptibility genes and the environmental stimuli that interact with such genetic conditions to induce cancer.

In addition to *PTEN*, numerous other tumor suppressor genes have been found to exhibit haplo-insufficiency (Table 14.1).[31] These tumor suppressors are not fully recessive in their modes of action, so heterozygosity for the tumor suppressor confers cancer susceptibility even with an absence of a second hit within the same gene.

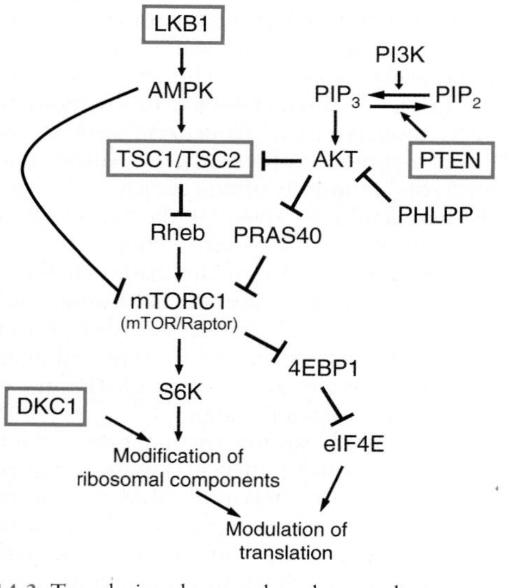

FIGURE 14.3 Translational control pathways that are mutated in cancer susceptibility (CS) syndromes. A number of critical tumor suppressors (*green boxes*) that can modulate translation are mutated in human CS syndromes.

GENETIC TESTING

An understanding of the genetic basis of CS syndromes has allowed for the development and implementation of genetic testing for CS syndromes. In fact, testing is now the standard of care for syndromes such as multiple endocrine neoplasia type 2, von Hippel-Lindau disease, and familial adenomatous polyposis.[32] However, testing should not be mistaken for a curative measure and is not recommended in all settings. Since 1996, the American Society of Clinical Oncology (ASCO) has maintained policy recommendations for genetic testing for CS, which were updated in 2010.[33] This updated report highlights the recent emergence of genetic tests for low-penetrance variants that confer moderate to weak cancer susceptibility.[33] In contrast to tests for high-penetrance susceptibility genes, no tests for low-penetrance genes have been shown to alter clinical

TABLE 14.1

EXAMPLES OF HAPLO-INSUFFICIENT CANCER SUSCEPTIBILITY GENES

Function	Gene	Associated Syndrome	Evidence from Mouse or Humans (Ref.)
Regulation of translation	*PTEN*	Cowden syndrome	*Pten* dosage determines tumor suppression (23, 24)
	LKB1	Peutz-Jeghers syndrome	Portion of tumors in *Lkb1* +/− mice without inactivation of wild-type allele (31, 68)
	PTCH1	Nevoid basal cell syndrome	Medulloblastomas arising in *Ptch1* +/− mice with retention of wild type allele (101)
Regulation of proliferation	*NF1*	Neurofibromatosis type 1	*Nf1*^{flox}/− stroma promotes tumorigenesis of *Nf1* null cells (68)
	APC	Familial adenomatous polyposis	Evidence of genetic selection of optimal APC dosage in human colorectal cancer (102)
Genomic integrity and apoptosis	*BLM*	Bloom's syndrome	Heterozygosity increases tumor formation in *Apc* +/− mice (31, 103)
	TP53	Li-Fraumeni syndrome	Tumor formation in *p53* +/− mice without loss-of-function of remaining *p53* allele (31, 104)

care. Even testing for high-penetrance genes is not yet warranted for the general (asymptomatic) population, but it can be beneficial to family members when a familial CS syndrome is suspected. Knowledge of a genetic lesion can cause significant distress to the patient and his or her family; therefore, the ASCO guidelines recommend genetic testing only if an individual is suspected of having a familial syndrome and if the genetic test can be adequately interpreted and will modify or aid the clinical strategy for patient care.[34]

If these criteria are met, genetic testing can offer significant advantages to the patient and the family, such as personalized consideration of the best methods for preventive and therapeutic care. In some cases, genetic testing can identify family members who do not carry the genomic alteration and are therefore predicted to be at lower or normal risk for the associated tumor type. In these instances, genetic testing can improve quality of life by reducing the patient's anxiety of developing cancer. ASCO has emphasized the importance of pre- and post-test genetic counseling to inform the patients of the complex benefits and risks of genetic testing. Informed consent of the patient must include education about the possible positive and negative consequences of obtaining such data, which can range from clinical consequences to psychological consequences to legal and insurance issues.[35]

In the clinic, how might a patient with a familial CS be identified? A cancer predisposition syndrome may be likely if a patient presents with a cancer at an unusually young age or exhibits multifocal or bilateral tumor development in the same organ or paired organs, respectively.[35,36] A high rate of cancer within the patient's family, particularly cancer of the same type as the patient, strongly suggests a hereditary CS.[36] More extensive guidelines for clinical diagnosis of specific syndromes have been described elsewhere for specific syndromes.

CANCER SUSCEPTIBILITY SYNDROMES

This section will describe in detail the inheritance and basis for retinoblastoma and, later, for four of the most prevalent CS syndromes. The section will also briefly examine a number of other CS syndromes and highlight their cellular function in signaling pathways controlling genomic integrity and apoptosis, proliferation, translation, and angiogenesis.

RB as the Paradigm

Incidence and Inheritance

Retinoblastoma is a tumor of the retinal photoreceptor precursor cells. Occurring in approximately 1 in 20,000 children, the tumors develop in affected individuals between birth and 8 years old.[37] Retinoblastoma occurs in both an inherited and sporadic fashion, which account for approximately 40% and 60% of total retinoblastoma cases, respectively.[36]

Genetic Basis

As discussed previously, Knudson's two-hit hypothesis for retinoblastoma postulated that retinoblastoma might be caused by the germline inheritance of an inactivated allele, followed by the "second hit" of a somatic mutation in the same allele. Indeed, familial retinoblastoma typically results from two distinct mutational events. The first clue to find the gene at the root of retinoblastoma came from karyotypic analysis of chromosomes in retinoblastoma tumor cells. In 1978, it was noticed that a fraction of chromosome 13q14 was sometimes missing in retinoblastoma cells.[37] This led to the cloning of the human *RB1* gene,[11,12] at which time it was demonstrated to be mutated in retinoblastoma.[13] Consistent with the hypothesis that *RB1* was a tumor suppressor gene whose function was lost in cancer, the mutations often consisted of large deletions of the gene and flanking DNA. Unlike the small clusters of gain-of-function mutations of oncogenes found in sporadic cancer, a remarkable variety of mutations in the *RB1* gene have now been documented. Hundreds of unique alleles have been reported, most of which are base substitutions or deletions. Mutations or variants have been reported in each of the exons and introns of the gene, although the most frequent mutations occur in exons 8 through 23.

In hereditary retinoblastoma, the function of the remaining wild type (i.e., normal) *RB1* allele is usually disrupted through a loss-of-heterozygosity (LOH) event. Rather than the creation of a novel loss-of-function mutation on the wild type allele, LOH refers to the loss of the wild type allele altogether, either through a chromosomal deletion event, whole chromosome loss (nondisjunction), or replacement of the wild type copy with another copy of the mutated germline allele through mitotic recombination.[37]

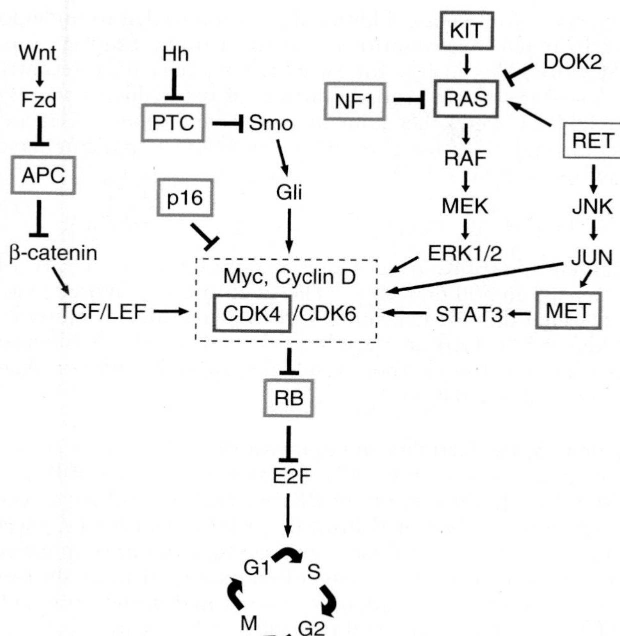

FIGURE 14.4 Regulation of proliferation is frequently perturbed in cancer susceptibility syndromes. Regulators of proliferation that are mutated in the syndromes discussed in this chapter include gatekeeper tumor suppressors (*green boxes*) and proto-oncogenes (*red boxes*; Table 14.2).

Molecular Mechanism

In the 20 years since the cloning of *RB1*, its function as a central regulator of the cell cycle has been elucidated. The *RB1* gene encodes a novel 105 kDa protein that undergoes phosphorylation at specific points in the cell cycle (Fig. 14.4).[37] In resting, noncycling G_0 cells, RB is unphosphorylated. On entrance into the cell cycle and G_1 growth phase, RB becomes weakly (but hypo-) phosphorylated on multiple serine and threonine amino acid residues.[37] When cells progress past the "restriction point" (considered the point of no return for cell cycle progression), RB phosphorylation is increased dramatically. The extensive phosphorylation persists until cells exit mitosis, when the PP1 phosphatase dephosphorylates RB, resetting the whole process. During G_0 and G_1, hypophosphorylated RB can bind to E2F transcription factors and prevent their activation of S phase-promoting proteins such as cyclin E. On entry into the cell cycle, the cyclin D-CDK4/6 complex can phosphorylate RB. Phosphorylated RB cannot bind E2F proteins, so phospho-RB dissociates from the complex.[38] Unbound E2F factors can then recruit transcriptional activators, and transcription of cyclin E and other cell-cycle genes is activated.[37] It should be mentioned that both RB and E2F are members of larger protein families. The differences and similarities between RB and its homologous genes p107 and p130 are beginning to be dissected but remain to be clarified, as discussed below.

Mouse Models

The cloning of the human *RB1* gene led to a race for a knockout mouse model of retinoblastoma. Given the clinical phenotype of human retinoblastoma, it was predicted that mice heterozygous for a null allele of *Rb1* would develop retinoblastoma at some frequency. Remarkably, back-to-back 1992 articles by three independent groups demonstrated that this was not the case.[14–16] Mice homozygous for inactivating *Rb1* mutations died between embryonic day 14 and 15. Surprisingly, heterozygotes did not display susceptibility to retinoblastoma at any measurable frequency, although they did exhibit susceptibility to pituitary tumors. It was hypothesized that *Rb1* heterozygote mice do not develop retinoblastoma because of compensation by RB family members p107 and p130 or because additional hits in other pathways are required. Generation of compound mouse mutants has addressed this hypothesis and illuminated the molecular requirements for retinoblastoma progression. Efforts by multiple groups culminated recently in the development of the St. Jude retinoblastoma (SJ-RBL) mouse, a conditional triple mutant for Rb, p107, and p53 in retinal progenitor cells.[17] These mice rapidly develop invasive retinoblastoma, exhibiting histological features of human retinoblastoma. These studies also highlighted the importance of p53 inactivation in retinoblastoma progression, a finding that has since been validated in human retinoblastoma cells.[39] This intriguing finding suggests additional "hits" may be a prerequisite for retinoblastoma progression. Other genetic aberrations in retinoblastoma tumors have been identified, such as *N-MYC* amplification.[40] Mouse models of retinoblastoma exhibit similar genetic aberrations, suggesting they may be of use to define the complete landscape of genetic changes in retinoblastoma.[41]

Clinical Features and Therapeutic Intervention

Children from families with retinoblastoma tend to present with multifocal or bilateral tumors, whereas sporadic cases of retinoblastoma are more likely unilateral.[36] Individuals with familial retinoblastoma are also at increased risk of osteosarcomas (usually occurring during adolescence) and other nonocular primary tumors.[37] Both the familial and the sporadic cases of retinoblastoma can be treated with surgery, chemotherapy, or radiation. With early detection, treatment can sometimes cure the patient with life and vision intact; however, treatment after late detection is less likely to prevent loss of vision quality for the patient.[42] Early detection and even prevention of retinoblastoma is now possible; both genetic testing and preimplantation diagnosis can now be performed to detect *RB* mutations.[42]

Most Prevalent Syndromes

Caretaker and gatekeeper genes cooperate in tumor suppression, so it is fitting that half of the four most prevalent CS syndromes result from mutations in caretaker genes and the other half from mutations in gatekeeper genes. Hereditary nonpolyposis colon cancer (HNPCC) and hereditary breast-ovarian cancer syndrome (HBOC) result from mutations in caretaker genes responsible for DNA repair and therefore genomic integrity (Fig. 14.2). Neurofibromatosis type 1 (NF1) and familial adenomatous polyposis (FAP), on the other hand, result from mutation of gatekeeper genes that restrain cellular proliferation (Fig. 14.4). These four syndromes are summarized below, followed by overviews of other syndromes categorized by the cellular functions frequently perturbed.

Hereditary Nonpolyposis Colon Cancer

Incidence. HNPCC, originally known as *Lynch syndrome*, is the most common CS disease and is responsible for at least 2% to 3% of total colon cancer cases.[37] HNPCC is distinct from the inherited polyposis colon cancer syndrome, familial adenomatous polyposis (FAP). FAP is another relatively common cancer syndrome that will be discussed in detail later. The overall incidence of HNPCC is estimated to be about 1 in 400.[43] HNPCC is inherited in an autosomal dominant fashion with a penetrance of about 90%. Males are affected at a higher penetrance, with females being less affected but at an additional risk of endometrial cancer.[43]

Genetic Basis. HNPCC can be caused by a germline mutation in one of six genes: *MLH1, MSH2, MSH3, MSH6, PMS1,* or *PMS2.*[35,43] All six genes function in DNA mismatch repair, so mutations in these genes affect genomic integrity (Fig. 14.2). More than 90% of HNPCC families exhibit mutations in *MLH1*, *MSH2*, or *MSH6*, with a minority exhibiting mutations in the *PMS* genes.[35,36] Approximately 70% of all mutations in the genes are predicted to yield a truncated protein. Similar to the retinoblastoma paradigm, patients generally inherit one inactivated (mutated) allele and the other, functional, allele is eventually lost through LOH.[44] Patients with mutations in mismatch repair genes exhibit microsatellite instability, a phenomenon in which errors in replication of highly repetitive sequences cannot be repaired, resulting in alterations of the length of the total repeat sequence.[37] Thus these genes are classified as caretakers. This type of instability often leads to mutation of other protein-coding genes, which can further promote tumorigenesis.[37] Surprisingly, somatic mutations of these genes in patients with sporadic colon cancer are very rare, even in cases with microsatellite instability[45] However, mismatch repair genes are undoubtedly important for sporadic tumor suppression, as evidenced by the fact that the expression of *MLH1* is frequently lost through methylation of its promoter.[45] This finding highlights the fact that other mechanisms besides mutation and chromosomal deletion can represent a "hit" in the progression of tumorigenesis. In fact, some hereditary cases of HNPCC are due to inherited hypermethylation of *MLH1*.[46]

Molecular Mechanism. The molecular mechanism of mismatch repair genes has been most extensively studied for the *Escherichia coli* homologs of MSH2 and MLH1, MutS and MutL. MutS recognizes errors that are introduced during DNA replication. The MutS:DNA complex is then recognized by MutL, which subsequently activates another protein, MutH. MutH introduces nicks in the DNA strand, resulting in excision of the mismatched base and subsequent resynthesis of the DNA fragment.[47]

Mouse Models. Mouse mutants of all six genes implicated in HNPCC have been generated. *Msh2* homozygous knockout mice are fertile and developmentally normal, but succumb to T-cell lymphomas by 1 year of age.[47] Consistent with the role of *MSH2* in human HNPCC, *Msh2* knockouts that survive past 6 months also develop gastrointestinal (GI) adenomas and carcinoma. Similarly, *Msh6* and *Mlh1* knockout mice develop T- and B-cell lymphomas and GI tumors. The phenotypes of the *Msh2* and *Msh6* knockout mice are slightly different, with the *Msh6* knockout mice exhibiting less or no microsatellite instability, whereas the *Msh2* knockouts exhibit extensive microsatellite instability.[47] *Msh3* knockout mice display CS at old age, and loss of *Msh3* cooperates with loss of *Msh6* to induce GI tumor formation as well as lymphomas and other cancers.[48] The phenotypes of *Pms1* and *Pms2* knockout mice are more dramatically different; *Pms1* knockout mice have no reported phenotype, whereas *Pms2* knockout mice develop lymphomas, are infertile, and do not develop GI tumors.[47]

Clinical Features and Therapeutic Intervention. HNPCC patients typically present with colon cancer at a younger average age than patients with sporadic colon cancer.[43] In contrast to other familial colon cancer syndromes, patients rarely exhibit polyps, making early detection difficult. Furthermore, colonic adenomas in HNPCC patients rapidly progress to carcinoma compared with the rate of progression in sporadic colon cancer patients. HNPCC patients also exhibit elevated risks for stomach, ovary, small intestine, ureter, and kidney cancers.[49] HNPCC family members should be screened annually by colonoscopy starting around age 20 to reduce both the incidence of and resultant mortality of colon cancer in HNPCC patients.[49] Women are additionally recommended to undergo yearly pelvic examinations and ultrasound examination. ASCO and the Society for Surgical Oncology have recently reviewed the recommended practices of risk-reducing surgery for HNPCC and other familial cancer syndromes.[50] General recommendations for clinical care of HNPCC patients have also been reviewed.[51–53]

Hereditary Breast-Ovarian Cancer Syndrome

Incidence. HBOC occurs in the population at a rate of between 1 in 500 or 1,000.[43] The syndrome is inherited in an autosomal dominant fashion with a penetrance of approximately 85%. Certain populations, such as the Ashkenazi Jewish population, harbor even higher rates of mutation than the general population.[35]

Genetic Basis. Germline mutations in *BRCA1* and *BRCA2* are estimated to cause up to 90% of cases of inherited HBOC.[43] More than 1,000 variants of *BRCA1* and *BRCA2* have been reported in the National Institute of Health's Breast Cancer Information Core Database.[54] Supporting a tumor suppressive role of these genes, mutations often consist of frameshift or nonsense mutations, leading to a truncated protein product. LOH of the remaining wild type allele is frequently observed. These genes are similarly important in somatic cancer, in which the function of at least one *BRCA1* or *BRCA2* allele is lost in 30% to 70% of sporadic breast and ovarian cancer cases.[55]

Molecular Mechanism. BRCA1 and BRCA2 function in DNA damage repair (Fig. 14.2). The localization of BRCA1 is altered in cells with stalled replication forks and double-stranded DNA breaks.[37] BRCA1 is recruited to these regions in concert with other proteins such as PCNA, Rad50, Rad51, and also BRCA2. These complexes function to repair the double-stranded break, although the precise role of BRCA1 and BRCA2 in these complexes remains unclear. BRCA1 and BRCA2 might also have non-DNA repair functions. For example, *BRCA1* mutant cells cannot silence one copy of the X chromosome, as typically occurs in female cells.[37]

Mouse Models. Conventional mouse knockouts of *Brca1*[56] and *Brca2*[57] are embryonic lethal, precluding analysis of breast cancer incidence in the adult animals. However, these models allowed for analysis of Brca-deficient cells and the realization that Brca proteins function to maintain genomic integrity, probably through double-strand break repair (Fig. 14.2). Conditional mouse mutants with mammary gland-specific deletion or mutation of either *Brca1*[58] or *Brca2*[59] develop mammary tumors after long latency. Interestingly, p53 loss cooperates with loss of either *Brca1* or *Brca2* to accelerate mammary tumorigenesis. In tumors arising in *Brca1* mutants on a *p53+/−* background, LOH of *p53* is usually observed, suggesting *p53* loss is required for tumor development induced by loss of *Brca1*.[58] Mutation of *p53* is present at a higher frequency in *BRCA1*- or *BRCA2*-associated human breast cancer compared with other breast cancer patients.[60] A wide variety of other conventional and conditional *Brca1* and *Brca2* mouse mutants have been constructed, and their characteristics and use in preclinical therapy trials have been recently reviewed.[61,62]

Clinical Features and Therapeutic Intervention. HBOC patients exhibit early onset breast cancer and an elevated risk for other cancers, including pancreatic cancer, stomach cancer, laryngeal cancer, fallopian tube cancer, and prostate cancer in male *BRCA* carriers.[43] Breast cancers arising in *BRCA1* mutant patients are typically high-grade invasive ductal carcinomas negative for estrogen receptor (ER) and HER2/neu,[61] which resemble certain types of sporadic breast cancer. This similarity is also supported by the strong overlap of gene expression profiles in comparisons between the familial *BRCA1* and sporadic subtypes. Tumors in *BRCA2* mutant carriers typically show a wider spectrum of histological features. Risk-reducing prophylactic breast surgery is an option for female patients who have tested positive for *BRCA1* or *BRCA2* mutations or have strong family histories of early onset breast cancer.[50] Genetic testing is available for HBOC, and recommendations for such testing and genetic counseling of patients have been issued by the National Society of Genetic Counselors.[63]

Neurofibromatosis Type 1

Incidence. NF1 affects, on average, approximately 1 in 3,500 people worldwide.[37] The trait is inherited in an autosomal dominant fashion, with a penetrance of 100% for neurofibromas. The spectrum of other phenotypes (described later) is variable and strongly influenced by the patient's genetic background.

Genetic Basis. Mutations in the *NF1* gene, cloned in 1990, are responsible for this syndrome. At least 70 different mutations have been reported, with approximately 70% leading to a truncated protein.[36] Neurofibromatosis type 2 results from inactivation of an unrelated gene, *NF2*, which occurs much less frequently than NF1[43] will not be discussed here because of space limitations. Similar to the other CS syndromes previously described, patients with NF1 inherit one mutant allele of *NF1*, with frequent LOH for the wild type allele in the malignant cells. Between 30% to 50% of the cases of NF1 occur because of *de novo* germline mutations in the *NF1* gene. The other cases occur in families with a history of neurofibromatosis and result from inherited germline alleles.[35] Recent reports also indicate that mutations in a different gene, *SPRED1*, can give rise to an NF1-like phenotype.[35,64]

Molecular Mechanism. NF1 encodes the neurofibromin protein, a 220 to 250 kDa guanosine triphosphate (GTPase) activating protein (GAP) for proteins of the Ras family,[37] RASGAP proteins stimulate the GTPase activity of Ras, converting the mitogenic Ras-GTP to Ras-GDP. Thus, loss of NF1 might mimic activation of Ras, a state that is frequently observed in sporadic cancer that results from oncogenic mutations in Ras that eliminate its catalytic activity and thereby increase the levels of Ras-GTP. In support of this function for NF1, hyperactive Ras signaling is observed in human and mouse NF1-deficient cells and inhibition of Ras activity can rescue the hyperproliferative phenotype of NF1-null cells.[65] Thus, the neurofibromatosis phenotype is presumed to result from hyperactive Ras signaling (Fig. 14.4).

Mouse Models. Homozygous *Nf1* knockout in mice results in embryonic lethality.[66] *Nf1* heterozygote mice are viable and, surprisingly, do not display a neurofibroma phenotype. These animals do display an increased incidence of pheochromocytomas and myeloid malignancies, reminiscent of the spectrum of tumor susceptibility seen in NF1 patients. Chimeric mice with both *Nf1−/−* and *Nf1+/+* cells develop plexiform neurofibromas that arise exclusively from the *Nf1−/−* cells,[67] demonstrating that biallelic loss of *Nf1* is required for tumor development and probably represents the rate-limiting step for tumorigenesis. Having *p53* heterozygosity can significantly accelerate the onset and lethality of tumors arising in *Nf1+/−* mice. Interestingly, data from mouse models indicate that *Nf1* may be haplo-insufficient in certain contexts (Table 14.1) because stromal *Nf1* heterozygosity enhances tumor formation of *Nf1* knockout cells compared with wild type stroma.[68] Recent preclinical trials in mouse models of NF1 have indicated that patients might benefit from treatment with the mTORC1 inhibitor, rapamycin[69] or the KIT inhibitor, imatinib.[70] In the latter study, the effectiveness of imatinib in the mouse model led the investigators to treat a patient with a large plexiform neurofibroma.[70] This patient showed a dramatic response, prompting ongoing full phase 2 and 3 clinical trials to examine the efficacy of imatinib for treatment of tumors in NF1 patients.

Clinical Features and Therapeutic Intervention. NF1 patients develop multiple benign neurofibromas, tumors formed from the cell sheaths of peripheral nervous system nerves.[37] A subset of these lesions will progress to neurofibrosarcomas. Patients are also at elevated risks for glioblastomas, pheochromocytomas, and myeloid leukemias. Café au lait macules are found in 100% of NF1 patients, and these increase in size and frequency with age.[36] A subset of patients may develop seizures and learning disabilities or mental retardation. Genetic testing is available but typically does not impact clinical management because the disorder is readily identified by phenotype.

Familial Adenomatous Polyposis

Incidence. FAP is a highly penetrant, autosomal dominant disorder with an incidence between 1 in 5,000 and 1 in 10,000.[43] This disorder is responsible for approximately 1% of all colon cancer cases.[43]

Genetic Basis. FAP is caused by germline mutations in the *APC* gene on chromosome 5q that are inherited in an autosomal dominant fashion. Mutations in this gene can be detected in 90% to 95% of FAP families.[35] Approximately 75% of cases are due to familial germline mutations, whereas the remainder are caused by first-generation *de novo* germline mutations.[35] Seventy percent to 80% of mutations result in truncation of the protein product.[35] Adenomatous polyposis coli (APC) is not only critical with regard to inherited colon cancer; more than 90% of sporadic colon carcinomas contain inactivating mutations in APC, and some of the remaining 10% of cases may inactivate the gene in other ways, including promoter hypermethylation.[37]

Molecular Mechanism. APC regulates Wnt signaling by promoting degradation of β-catenin (Fig. 14.4). APC functions in a cytoplasmic complex containing β-catenin, GSK3-β, and the scaffolding proteins axin and conductin.[37] When APC is present, the complex forms and GSK3-β phosphorylates β-catenin on several N-terminal residues. Phosphorylated β-catenin is targeted for degradation, preventing its translocation into the nucleus, where it acts as a transcriptional activator for Tcf/Lef family transcription factors. When APC expression is lost, β-catenin accumulates, resulting in persistent Wnt activation. In the normal intestinal epithelium, stem cells divide to give rise to one daughter cell that remains in the crypt and one daughter cell in which APC is expressed and functions to reduce levels of β-catenin.[37] This cell will proceed with differentiation and migration toward the distal end of the crypt. If APC expression is lost, both daughter cells are believed to remain stem cells and fail to migrate up the crypt toward the lumen of the colon.[71] On several successive cell divisions, a small area of dysplasia will develop, ultimately leading to the formation of an adenomatous polyp. Additional somatic genetic changes are then required for the transition from a polyp to a malignant lesion.

Mouse Models. The first model of FAP was actually generated prior to the identification of the *APC* gene as the site of the responsible genetic lesion in FAP. A mutant mouse was generated in an *N*-ethyl-*N*-nitrosourea (ENU) mutagenesis screen that exhibited multiple intestinal neoplasias,[72] so the responsible gene was termed *Min*. Shortly after the basis for human FAP was mapped to mutant *APC* in humans[73] the *Min* gene was mapped and discovered to be the murine homolog to human

APC[74]; the homologs are 90% identical at the amino acid level. Investigators identified a nonsense mutation in *Apc* as the responsible genetic culprit in the *Min* animals. Because nonsense mutations are frequently observed in FAP families, this mouse strain provided a model of intestinal neoplasia progression that closely mimicked FAP. One drawback of this, and other murine FAP models, is that murine tumors typically arise in the small intestine, not in the colon, as seen in human patients.

Many groups subsequently generated mice with mutations similar to those found in human FAP (these models have been reviewed in detail elsewhere[47,75]). Most models result in extensive adenomas and invasive cancer of the small intestine, with some variation in the number, latency, and lethality of the tumors. These models provide an experimental system in which to test the cooperation of environmental factors or other genes with *Apc* mutation, which led to the identification of *Mom1*, a gene that modifies the phenotype seen in *Apc* mutant animals by reducing the number of adenomas.[76] Evidence suggests that the syntenic chromosomal region in humans may act as a modifier of the FAP phenotype as well.[77] Finally, in yet another example of the power of mouse genetics, deletion of *myc* was demonstrated to rescue *Apc* deficiency in a conditional *Apc* knockout model of intestinal neoplasia.[78] Therefore, it is believed that the major functional consequence of *Apc* deletion is downstream activation of *myc* transcription by β-catenin (Fig. 14.4).

Clinical Features and Therapeutic Intervention. The hallmark of FAP is the presence of at least 100 (and often over 1,000) adenomatous polyps in the colorectum.[35] A subset of these polyps will progress to malignant colon cancer. The cancer risk for FAP patients is virtually 100% by age 40, but prophylactic colectomy is almost always performed to reduce this risk. Clinical genetic testing is increasingly common for this disorder. Patients with a positive genotype and significant polyp burden are recommended to undergo prophylactic colectomy. Nonsteroidal anti-inflammatory drugs can reduce the size and number of polyps, but are not recommended for FAP patients in place of surgery. FAP patients are also at elevated risk for upper GI tract neoplasms.[35] Other phenotypes observed in FAP patients include congenital hypertrophy of the retinal pigment epithelium, dental anomalies, epidermoid cysts, osteomas, desmoid tumors, and mesenteric fibrosis.[43]

Other Syndromes, by Function

In the past few decades, common themes have emerged regarding the biological functions necessary for cancer cell development and expansion. For example, six "hallmark" traits of cancer have been enumerated in the now-legendary "Hallmarks of Cancer" review by Hanahan and Weinberg.[20] Familial cancer syndromes exist as a result of mutations that confer at least one of these traits to the mutant cell. Additional somatic mutations are usually required for the progression to invasive cancer, even in familial cases. Because of space limitations here, the details of all of the well-established familial cancer syndromes will not be discussed (for an overview of the majority of syndromes, see Lindor et al.[35]). In the remainder of this chapter, additional familial cancer syndromes will be briefly summarized by the molecular function of the gene that is disrupted. To allow readers to quickly conceptualize the underlying molecular biology of these syndromes, the signaling pathways for each of the functions will be summarized and the genes that underlie the syndromes discussed in this chapter will be highlighted, as delineated in the figures. These pathways are in no way meant to be comprehensive or imply that there is no overlap in the distinct figures illustrated. For example, in addition to the function of the RAS/RAF/MEK/ERK pathway in proliferation (Fig. 14.4), this pathway is also intricately involved in regulation of translation (not shown in Fig. 14.3). ERK phosphorylates and inactivates the TSC1/TSC2 complex, thereby inhibiting mTORC1 activation. For simplicity, these interconnections have been omitted and the components have been restricted to those discussed in this chapter, separating the pathways based on the functional categorizations delineated in the section below.

Genomic Integrity and Apoptosis

Cancer is a genetic disease; thus, it may not come as a surprise that two of the four most common CS syndromes (HNPCC and HBOC) result from alterations in proteins that are important for maintenance of genomic integrity (i.e., caretakers). Human cancers are estimated to require two to seven mutations for cancer development. Based on the typical estimation of the average rate of mutations, random accumulation of mutations cannot explain the high rate of cancer in the human population. However, when the first mutations are acquired in genes that maintain genomic integrity, the mutation rate, and therefore the rate of cancer development, is greatly accelerated. CS syndromes resulting from mutation of genomic integrity genes include HNPCC and HBOC, as well as xeroderma pigmentosum (XP), ataxia telangiectasia, Werner syndrome, Rothmund-Thomson syndrome, Bloom syndrome, and Fanconi anemia (FA; Fig. 14.2).[37] XP is a rare autosomal recessive syndrome that results in sensitivity to sun damage and a 100% chance of developing skin cancer. XP results from mutation of any of eight genes that form the eight complementation groups of XP (*XPA*, *XPB*, *XPC*, *XPD*, *XPE*, *XPF*, *XPG*, and *XPV*). The first seven XP genes encode proteins that participate in a nucleotide excision repair (NER) complex. NER is a DNA repair process by which chemically altered nucleotides are first recognized by the alteration of the DNA double-helix structure and are then removed, along with many other nucleotides on either side of the lesion. Then DNA polymerases and ligases resynthesize a new strand. Ultraviolet light induces chemical changes in the DNA that can be recognized by the NER machinery. XP patients, unable to repair the mutations induced by ultraviolet light, quickly acquire multiple mutations, eventually in other important genes.

FA is another autosomal recessive syndrome caused by mutations in genes required for recognition or repair of DNA damage. FA is characterized by an increased risk of leukemias (mainly acute myelogenous) and cancers of the head and neck, esophagus, and vulva.[79] Interestingly, mutations in at least 13 different genes can manifest as FA. Biallelic mutations in *BRCA2* give rise to a form of FA, whereas monoallelic mutations result in HBOC.[79] Mutations in any of the 13 responsible genes (*FANCA*, *FANCB*, *FANCC*, *FANCD1/BRCA2*, *FANCD2*, *FANCE*, *FANCF*, *FANCG*, *FANCI*, *FANCJ/BRIP1*, *FANCL*, *FANCM/Hef*, and *FANCN*) result in a similar phenotype,[79] strongly suggesting that these genes function in the same pathway. Some of the FA proteins function at nuclear pores to allow monoubiquitination of FANCD2, which induces translocation of FANCD2 to sites of DNA damage.[79] The precise biochemical function of the proteins at the damage site and their role in its repair is not well understood and remains a hot area of investigation.

Bloom syndrome, Werner syndrome, and Rothmund-Thomson syndrome are all autosomal recessive syndromes caused by mutations of the human RecQ helicases BLM, WRN, and RECQ4, respectively.[80] These helicases are believed to repair damaged DNA replication forks, and they physically interact with many other proteins involved in DNA repair, including BRCA1 and MLH1 (in the case of BLM), and ATM (in the case of WRN; see also Fig. 14.2).[80] The phenotypes of these syndromes are all quite distinct, with some similarities. In Bloom syndrome, patients rapidly develop non-Hodgkin's lymphoma, leukemias, and breast, stomach, and skin cancers. In contrast, the onset and tumor spectrum of cancers is markedly different for Werner and Rothmund-Thomson syndromes.

If DNA damage is not repaired in a normal cell, the cell will undergo either senescence (irreversible arrest of proliferation) or more commonly apoptosis (cell death; Fig. 14.2). These mechanisms are cellular safeguards against the deleterious accumulation of mutations. Like all cellular pathways, the pathways that govern senescence and apoptosis rely on proteins that are themselves the product of genes. When these genes are mutated or lost, the cell can no longer transmit the signal from the DNA sensors to the apoptosis effectors, so the damage may persist and accumulate. One of the most important proteins with this function is p53. Mutations in p53 are found in the majority of sporadic cancers, and it is hypothesized that p53 function may be compromised in some way in all cancers. Missense mutations in p53 are the cause of Li-Fraumeni syndrome, a rare autosomal dominant familial cancer syndrome with a penetrance of 90% to 95%.[43] The most common cancers found in Li-Fraumeni patients are sarcomas, breast cancer, and brain tumors, but a wide spectrum of other tumor types may also occur.

The p53 protein is a labile DNA-binding transcription factor that is not expressed at high levels during normal cellular homeostasis.[37] It is regulated at the posttranslational level by, among other mechanisms, Mdm2-induced degradation of p53 protein. In response to cellular stress, including hypoxia and DNA damage, p53 protein is stabilized and activates transcription of growth arrest genes that halt the cell in phase G_1, DNA damage repair genes (including XP genes), and pro-apoptosis genes. The G_1 arrest halts the cell until damage can be repaired; if the damage persists, the cells remain in an irreversible G_1 arrest (senescence) or undergo apoptosis (Fig. 14.2). Sporadic and germline mutations typically abolish the DNA-binding capacity of p53. With no way to execute its transcriptional function, cells survive and may even continue in the cell cycle. Because of its critical role, p53 has been termed the *master guardian and executioner.*[37] Models of p53 nullizygosity and of specific p53 mutations have been generated and are too numerous to list here (but have been recently reviewed elsewhere[81,82]). Heterozygote *p53* mutant mice partially mimic aspects of Li-Fraumeni syndrome, including sarcomas and breast cancer, with variability depending on the strain background.

Regulation of Translation

Regulation of protein translation has been indirectly implicated in cancer progression because many proto-oncogenes and tumor suppressors can regulate or modulate ribosome function and translation.[83] Several genes with these functions are mutated in familial cancer syndromes, including the *DKC1* gene (dyskeratosis congenita), *PTEN* (Cowden syndrome), and *TSC1*, *TSC2* (tuberous sclerosis; Fig. 14.3). Proteins such as RB and p53 can also modulate translation, but the contribution of these functions to the overall phenotype of RB- or p53-mutant cells is not well understood.

Cowden syndrome is an autosomal dominant disorder in which patients develop numerous hamartomas of the skin, breast, thyroid, GI tract, and central nervous system. Patients develop malignant cancers in multiple tissues, and their elevated risk is most characterized for breast cancer (30% of females develop breast cancer).[36] The genetic basis of this disorder is germline mutations in the PTEN tumor suppressor, a lipid phosphatase that negatively regulates the proto-oncogene PI3K through modification of specific phosphoinositides at the plasma membrane (Fig. 14.3). PI3K can modulate translation through downstream activation of AKT, TOR, and the ribosomal protein S6. Phosphorylation of S6 is induced by multiple extracellular signals and results in increased translation of "TOP" mRNAs (mRNAs with a specific terminal oligopyrimidine tract in the 5′ untranslated region).[83] This class of mRNAs encodes proteins themselves that are involved in translation, including elongation factors, ribosomal proteins, and other ribosome biogenesis factors.[83] Therefore, PTEN, upstream of PI3K, can modulate translation. In mouse models of *Pten* deficiency, *Pten* heterozygote mice are susceptible to tumors of multiple origins (homozygote *Pten* deletion is lethal). In these models, inhibition of the mTORC1 complex by the drug rapamycin can reduce tumor-cell proliferation and tumor size, demonstrating that this pathway is critical for the tumor suppressive function of Pten.[83,84]

The tumor suppressors TSC1 and TSC2 can also modulate S6 phosphorylation and therefore can modulate translation and cell size.[83] The two proteins form a complex that acts as a GAP for the small GTPase, Rheb. *TSC1* and *TSC2* genes are inactivated in tuberous sclerosis, an autosomal dominant disorder also characterized by cortical tubers, hamartomas, multiple other benign lesions, and an increased risk of brain tumors and renal cancer. The majority of mutations found in tuberous sclerosis are truncating mutations, and LOH of the remaining allele has been reported.[44]

Dyskeratosis congenita (DC) is an X-linked recessive disorder caused by mutations in the *DKC1* gene,[83] although autosomal recessive and autosomal dominant forms of the disorder have also been reported (but represent less than 15% of all DC cases).[85] These rarer forms of DC result from mutations in the genes *TERC* or *TERT*, which encode for telomerase complex components.[35] Patients are susceptible to premature aging, anemia, hyperkeratosis of the skin, and possibly various malignancies, including myelodysplasia and carcinomas of the lung, larynx, esophagus, pancreas, and skin.[85] The *DKC1* gene, at Xq28, encodes dyskerin, a pseudouridine synthase responsible for posttranscriptional modification of ribosomal RNAs and TERC, a core RNA component of the telomerase complex.[85] Therefore, the DC phenotype is likely due to both defects in ribosomal RNA processing (leading to defects in translation)[83] and defective telomere maintenance.[86]

Finally, Peutz-Jeghers syndrome is another CS syndrome that might be caused by defects in translation. Peutz-Jeghers syndrome is an autosomal dominant disorder characterized by hamartomas of multiple tissues (in particular the GI tract) and a 20% to 50% chance of developing malignant tumors of the GI tract, pancreas, breast, or testis.[44] Mutations in *LKB1/STK11*, a serine threonine kinase, underlie the disorder, and a variety of loss-of-function mutations have been reported. The tumor suppressive function of LKB1 is believed to result from its upstream regulation of the AMP-activated protein kinase (AMPK), a key regulator of cellular metabolism (Fig. 14.3). AMPK can regulate mTORC1 signaling through phosphorylation of TSC1 and TSC2 and direct phosphorylation of the mTORC1 component Raptor.[87] In low-energy conditions, this phosphorylation leads to inhibition of mTORC1 activity and reduction in cell growth. In LKB1-deficient cells, the mTORC1 pathway remains activated, even in low-energy conditions, leading to unrestricted cell growth.[88]

Proliferation

Hyperproliferation is a common attribute of cancer cells, and, therefore, as expected, many CS syndromes result from mutations in proteins that regulate cellular proliferation (gatekeepers). These syndromes include NF1 and FAP, discussed in detail earlier, as well as familial renal cell carcinoma, familial malignant melanoma, multiple endocrine neoplasia type 2, and Gorlin syndrome. Gorlin syndrome, also known as nevoid basal cell carcinoma syndrome, is characterized by the early onset of numerous basal cell carcinomas of the skin. The syndrome is caused by mutations in the *Patched1* (*PTCH1*) gene, which encodes for a cell-surface protein that acts as a negative

TABLE 14.2

CANCER SUSCEPTIBILITY SYNDROMES CAUSED BY ACTIVATION OF PROTO-ONCOGENES

Syndrome	Gene	Protein Function
Costello Syndrome	*HRAS*	Small GTPase; positive regulator of proliferation
Hereditary papillary renal cancer	*MET*	Receptor tyrosine kinase; positive regulator of proliferation
Multiple endocrine neoplasia type 2	*RET*	
Hereditary gastrointestinal stromal tumors	*KIT*	
Familial melanoma	*CDK4*	Cell cycle regulator

regulator of pro-proliferative Sonic Hedgehog signaling (Fig. 14.4).[89] In a mouse model of nevoid basal cell carcinoma, heterozygous *Ptc1* mice are susceptible to basal cell carcinoma development following radiation exposure.[90]

Multiple endocrine neoplasia type 2 (MEN2) is similarly caused by mutation of a cell-surface regulator of proliferation, in this case the pro-proliferative receptor tyrosine kinase RET. Note that the RET mutations found in MEN2 are *activating* gain-of-function mutations, in contrast to the loss-of-function mutations that are most common in hereditary cancer syndromes. It is hypothesized that most oncogenic gain-of-function mutations are incompatible with embryonic development, explaining their rarity in hereditary cancer syndromes. However, a few other susceptibility syndromes are also caused by gain-of-function mutations (Table 14.2), including hereditary papillary renal cancer (caused by mutations in the *MET* gene) and familial gastrointestinal stromal tumors (caused by mutations in the *KIT* gene).[37] Both of these disorders are similar to MEN2 in that their genetic basis is oncogenic mutation of a receptor tyrosine kinase. Each of these syndromes results from mutation of cell-surface signaling receptors that regulate proliferation.

Of course mutation of downstream molecules in pro-proliferative signaling pathways can also result in CS (Fig. 14.4). Examples include FAP (discussed in detail earlier), which is caused by mutations in the cytoplasmic negative regulator of Wnt signaling, APC. NF1, also described in detail earlier, results from mutation of NF1, a cytoplasmic RASGAP that inhibits pro-proliferative Ras signaling. Similarly, another CS and developmental syndrome, Costello syndrome, is caused by activating HRAS mutations that prevent its regulation by RASGAP and therefore result in constitutive RAS signaling (another example of germline gain-of-function mutation).[91] Finally, familial malignant melanoma can result from loss-of-function mutations in the tumor suppressor gene *CDKN2A* (which encodes p16^{INK4A}, a CDK inhibitor for CDK4 or CDK6) or from gain-of-function mutations in the cell-cycle regulator CDK4 that abolish its ability to be bound by (and inhibited by) p16.[92] Thus, misregulation of cell-cycle regulators or their upstream signals can cause CS (summarized in Fig. 14.4).

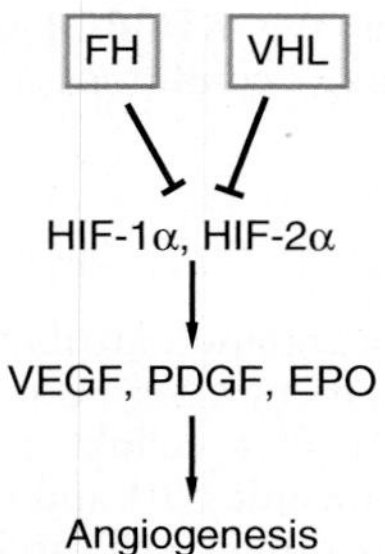

FIGURE 14.5 Angiogenic factors are also perturbed in human cancer susceptibility syndromes. Mutations in fumarate hydratase (FH) and von Hippel-Lindau (VHL) tumor suppressors cause up-regulation of pro-angiogenic factors that favor tumor survival. Green boxes indicate the genes or proteins in this diagram that are mutated in familial cancer syndromes.

Angiogenesis

Mutations in the *VHL* gene are the sole known cause of von Hippel-Lindau disease (VHL),[44] an autosomal dominant disorder characterized by a high incidence of renal cysts and clear cell renal carcinoma, benign pancreatic cysts, and hemangioblastomas of the central nervous system (Fig. 14.5).[36] Tumors and other neoplasms are often extensively vascularized. *VHL* encodes a 213 amino acid protein that acts as an ubiquitin ligase to target hypoxia-inducible factor (HIF)-1α and HIF-2α for degradation under normoxic conditions.[93] Without VHL binding, HIF-1α and HIF-2α accumulate and act as transcription factors to up-regulate the expression of pro-angiogenic genes, including *VEGF*, *PDGF*, and *EPO*.[93] VHL loss therefore results in accumulation of HIFs under normoxic conditions, stimulating enhanced angiogenesis. Consistently, *Vhl* heterozygote mice are susceptible to vascular neoplasms.[94] Finally, VHL is also a critical tumor suppressor for sporadic cancer; VHL function is disrupted in as many as 70% to 80% of sporadic clear cell renal carcinoma cases.[94]

Hereditary leiomyomatosis and renal cell cancer is another familial cancer syndrome that may be caused by alterations in angiogenesis. This syndrome was recognized in 2001 and subsequently shown to result from inactivating mutations in the fumarate hydratase (*FH*) gene.[93] FH is an enzyme that participates in the Krebs cycle to catalyze conversion of fumarate to malate. In multiple independent studies, FH-negative hereditary leiomyomatosis and renal cell cancer tumors are associated with strong HIF-1α overexpression.[93] The mechanism of such effect involves a buildup of fumarate in FH-deficient cells that then inhibits the prolyl hydroxylation of HIF-1α, preventing its degradation and resulting in increased cellular levels of HIF-1α.[95]

FUTURE DIRECTIONS

Although dramatic progress has been made in the past few years in determining the genetic basis of CS syndromes and, in general, of CS, it is clear that only the very tip of the iceberg of this phenomenon and only a few of the major determinants have been identified. With the human and mouse genomes in hand, coupled with technological advances, the identification of new tumor suppressor loci is proceeding at increasing speed. Furthermore, gene targeting in the mouse is unraveling a number of unexpected cancer phenotypes and a multitude of orphan tumor suppressors (i.e., demonstrated tumor suppressors with no as-yet-determined role in human CS syndromes). The role of these proteins in human tumorigenesis and in the pathogenesis of CS syndromes needs to be systematically assessed.

In the past few decades, the genetic basis for the most prevalent and penetrant CS syndromes has been identified. However, bulk of familial CS has just begun to be explained, and the understanding of CS is mainly limited to syndromes that obey a Mendelian pattern of dominant or recessive inheritance. Linkage mapping or association studies are not always sufficient to identify weaker modifiers, but might be revived because of the advent of single nucleotide polymorphism arrays that allow for rapid genome-wide genotyping (for a review of methods in human and mouse, see Balmain[6] and Pharoah et al.[96]). The identification of new weak modifiers along with the estimation of combinational effects (e.g., compound tumor suppressor haplo-insufficiency) will represent an important challenge in the years to come. Ultimately, these interactions must be defined to predict with increasing accuracy the CS risks in the population at large.

Additional challenges and exciting venues for research in the area of CS are also brought about by the realization that CS may be determined in part by epigenetic effects. In Beckwith-Wiedemann syndrome, a congenital syndrome of organ overgrowth and embryonal tumor CS, imprinting at the *IGF2* locus is frequently relaxed, resulting in an up-regulation of IGF2, a pro-proliferative growth factor.[97] In another example of germline "epimutation," multiple groups have reported heritable germline methylation of the HNPCC-susceptibility gene *MLH1*.[46] Moreover, mutations and variants that impact CS might be found in atypical regions of the genome, such as the loci coding for miRNAs, small RNAs that negatively regulate the translation of mRNA into proteins.[98] Importantly, miRNAs have already been found mutated both somatically in cancers of various histological origins and also in the germline of cancer patients. For example, germline mutations in *mir-16-1*, accompanied by LOH of the other allele, were found in 2 of 75 chronic lymphocytic leukemia patients compared with 0 of 160 controls.[99] Nonetheless, the prevalence of these mutations and the relative risk they incur remain to be determined.

A further and perhaps more provocative level of complexity has been introduced by the realization that CS is being firmly attributed to regions of the genome that do not seemingly encode for proteins or miRNA.[100] An understanding of the mechanisms by which these genetic variations could impact gene expression, cell behavior, chromosomal stability, and CS will require additional research. In this respect, a recent provocative finding demonstrates that noncoding RNAs or pseudogenes can act as ceRNAs to impact the expression of protein-coding genes.[27] The *PTEN* pseudogene *PTENP1*, which is expressed at the mRNA level but does not encode for a protein, is able to regulate the expression of *PTEN* through competitive binding of *PTEN*-regulating miRNAs.[27] Since PTEN function is particularly susceptible to subtle variations, mutation in *PTENP1* or changes in *PTENP1* expression could have significant consequences on PTEN function and ultimately cancer susceptibility. It is theoretically possible that germline changes in *PTENP1* could in fact induce a Cowden-like CS syndrome. Thus the realization that noncoding RNAs can dramatically impinge on coding RNA levels and function has important implications for the study of cancer and CS. Future work should be directed at questioning the effect of ceRNAs on cancer development and the analysis of the mechanisms by which noncoding areas of the genome confer CS.

Although all these aspects represent tremendous opportunities for understanding the rules underlying CS, the real challenge in future years will be to transform this wealth of novel information into concrete opportunities for cancer prevention that go beyond an early diagnosis and detection and effective surgical or chemical removal of the tumor lesion. Ultimately the principles of cancer susceptibility that are gleaned in these studies should be utilized to develop targeted therapeutic modalities for effective cancer chemoprevention commensurate to an accurate estimate of an individual's lifetime cancer risk.

Selected References

The full list of references for this chapter appears in the online version.

1. Hung RJ, McKay JD, Gaborieau V, et al. A susceptibility locus for lung cancer maps to nicotinic acetylcholine receptor subunit genes on 15q25. *Nature* 2008;452(7187):633.
2. Thorgeirsson TE, Geller F, Sulem P, et al. A variant associated with nicotine dependence, lung cancer and peripheral arterial disease. *Nature* 2008;452 (7187):638.
3. Amos CI, Wu X, Broderick P, et al. Genome-wide association scan of tag SNPs identifies a susceptibility locus for lung cancer at 15q25.1. *Nat Genet* 2008;40(5):616.
4. Berger AH, Niki M, Morotti A, et al. Identification of DOK genes as lung tumor suppressors. *Nat Genet* 2010;4(23):216.
5. Ponder BA. Cancer genetics. *Nature* 2001;411(6835):336.
6. Balmain A. Cancer as a complex genetic trait: tumor susceptibility in humans and mouse models. *Cell* 2002;108(2):145.
7. Stadler ZK, Thom P, Robson ME, et al. Genome-wide association studies of cancer. *J Clin Oncol* 2010;28(27):4255.
8. Easton DF, Eeles RA. Genome-wide association studies in cancer. *Hum Mol Genet* 2008;17(R2):R109.
9. Fletcher O, Houlston RS. Architecture of inherited susceptibility to common cancer. *Nat Rev Cancer* 2010;10(5):353.
10. Knudson AG Jr. Mutation and cancer: statistical study of retinoblastoma. *Proc Natl Acad Sci U S A* 1971;68(4):820.
11. Friend SH, Bernard R, Rogelj S, et al. A human DNA segment with properties of the gene that predisposes to retinoblastoma and osteosarcoma. *Nature* 1986;323(6089):643.
12. Lee WH, Hong F, Young LJ, Shew JY, Lee EY. Human retinoblastoma susceptibility gene: cloning, identification, and sequence. *Science* 1987;235(4794):1394.
13. Fung YK, Murphree AL, T'Ang A, Qian J, Hinrichs SH, Benedict WF. Structural evidence for the authenticity of the human retinoblastoma gene. *Science* 1987;236(4809):1657.
14. Jacks T, Fazeli A, Schmitt EM, Bronson RT, Goodell MA, Weinberg RA. Effects of an Rb mutation in the mouse. *Nature* 1992;359(6393):295.
15. Lee EY, Chang CY, Hu N, et al. Mice deficient for Rb are nonviable and show defects in neurogenesis and haematopoiesis. *Nature* 1992;359(6393):288.
16. Clarke AR, Maandag ER, van Roon M, et al. Requirement for a functional Rb-1 gene in murine development. *Nature* 1992;359(6393):328.
18. Kinzler KW, Vogelstein B. Cancer-susceptibility genes. Gatekeepers and caretakers. *Nature* 1997;386(6627):761.
19. Lowe SW, Cepero E, Evan G. Intrinsic tumour suppression. *Nature* 2004; 432(7015):307.
20. Hanahan D, Weinberg RA. The hallmarks of cancer. *Cell* 2000;100(1):57.
23. Alimonti A, Carracedo A, Clohessy JG, et al. Subtle variations in Pten dose determine cancer susceptibility. *Nat Genet* 2010;42(5):454.
24. Trotman LC, Niki M, Dotan ZA, et al. Pten dose dictates cancer progression in the prostate. *PLoS Biol* 2003;1(3):E59.
25. Chen Z, Trotman LC, Shaffer D, et al. Crucial role of p53-dependent cellular senescence in suppression of Pten-deficient tumorigenesis. *Nature* 2005;436(7051):725.
26. Alimonti A, Nardella C, Chen Z, et al. A novel type of cellular senescence that can be enhanced in mouse models and human tumor xenografts to suppress prostate tumorigenesis. *J Clin Invest* 2010;120(3):681.
27. Poliseno L, Salmena L, Zhang J, Carver B, Haveman WJ, Pandolfi PP. A coding-independent function of gene and pseudogene mRNAs regulates tumour biology. *Nature* 2010;465(7301):1033.
31. Fodde R, Smits R. Cancer biology. A matter of dosage. *Science* 2002;298 (5594):761.
32. Eng C, Hampel H, de la Chapelle A. Genetic testing for cancer predisposition. *Annu Rev Med* 2001;52:371.
33. Robson ME, Storm CD, Weitzel J, et al. American Society of Clinical Oncology policy statement update: genetic and genomic testing for cancer susceptibility. *J Clin Oncol* 2010;28(5):893.
35. Lindor NM, McMaster ML, Lindor CJ, et al. Concise handbook of familial cancer susceptibility syndromes, second edition. *J Natl Cancer Inst Monogr* 2008(38):1.
37. Weinberg RA. *The biology of cancer*. New York: Garland Science, 2007.
39. Laurie NA, Donovan SL, Chih C-S, et al. Inactivation of the p53 pathway in retinoblastoma. *Nature* 2006;444(7115):61.

43. Nagy R, Sweet K, Eng C. Highly penetrant hereditary cancer syndromes. *Oncogene* 2004;23(38):6445.
46. Suter CM, Martin DI, Ward RL. Germline epimutation of MLH1 in individuals with multiple cancers. *Nat Genet* 2004;36(5):497.
49. Garber JE, Offit K. Hereditary cancer predisposition syndromes. *J Clin Oncol* 2005;23(2):276.
50. Guillem JG, Wood WC, Moley JF, et al. ASCO/SSO review of current role of risk-reducing surgery in common hereditary cancer syndromes. *J Clin Oncol* 2006;24(28):4642.
64. Brems H, Chmara M, Sahbatou M, et al. Germline loss-of-function mutations in SPRED1 cause a neurofibromatosis 1-like phenotype. *Nat Genet* 2007;39(9):1120.
68. Santarosa M, Ashworth A. Haploinsufficiency for tumour suppressor genes: when you don't need to go all the way. *Biochim Biophys Acta* 2004;1654 (2):105.
70. Yang FC, Ingram DA, Chen S, et al. Nf1-dependent tumors require a microenvironment containing Nf1+/− and c-kit-dependent bone marrow. *Cell* 2008;135(3):437.
71. Radtke F, Clevers H. Self-renewal and cancer of the gut: two sides of a coin. *Science* 2005;307(5717):1904.
72. Moser AR, Pitot HC, Dove WF. A dominant mutation that predisposes to multiple intestinal neoplasia in the mouse. *Science* 1990;247(4940): 322.
73. Nishisho I, Nakamura Y, Miyoshi Y, et al. Mutations of chromosome 5q21 genes in FAP and colorectal cancer patients. *Science* 1991;253(5020):665.
74. Su LK, Kinzler KW, Vogelstein B, et al. Multiple intestinal neoplasia caused by a mutation in the murine homolog of the APC gene. *Science* 1992;256 (5057):668.
78. Sansom OJ, Meniel VS, Murcan V, et al. Myc deletion rescues Apc deficiency in the small intestine. *Nature* 2007;446(7136):676.
82. Donehower LA, Lozano G. 20 years studying p53 functions in genetically engineered mice. *Nat Rev Cancer* 2009;9(11):831.
83. Ruggero D, Pandolfi PP. Does the ribosome translate cancer? *Nat Rev Cancer* 2003;3(3):179.
91. Aoki Y, Niihori T, Kawame H, et al. Germline mutations in HRAS proto-oncogene cause Costello syndrome. *Nat Genet* 2005;37(10):1038.
92. Zuo L, Weger J, Yang Q, et al. Germline mutations in the p16INK4a binding domain of CDK4 in familial melanoma. *Nat Genet* 1996;12(1):97.
95. Linehan WM, Srinivasan R, Schmidt LS. The genetic basis of kidney cancer: a metabolic disease. *Nat Rev Urol* 2010;7(5):277.
96. Pharoah PD, Dunning Am, Ponder BA, Easton DF. Association studies for finding cancer-susceptibility genetic variants. *Nat Rev Cancer* 2004;4(11):850.
97. Rainier S, Johnson LA, Dobry CJ, Ping AJ, Grundy PE, Feinberg AP. Relaxation of imprinted genes in human cancer. *Nature* 1993;362(6422):747.
98. Esquela-Kerscher A, Slack FJ. Oncomirs—microRNAs with a role in cancer. *Nat Rev Cancer* 2006;6(4):259.

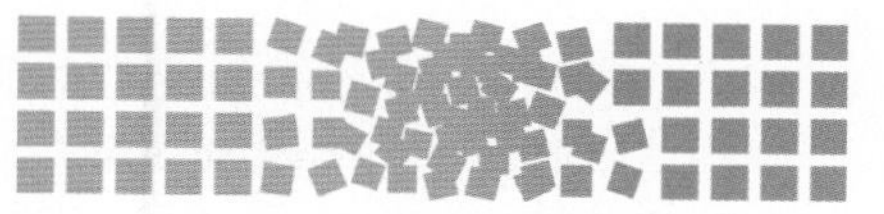

CHAPTER 15 DNA VIRUSES

PETER M. HOWLEY, DON GANEM, AND ELLIOTT KIEFF

HISTORY OF VIRAL ONCOLOGY

Viral oncology's foundation can be traced to scientific observations made at the turn of the century that defined the transmissibility of avian leukemia in Denmark in 1908 and avian sarcoma in chickens in 1911. These important discoveries were not appreciated at the time, and their impact on virology and medicine was not recognized for decades. The importance of the work of Peyton Rous,[1] showing that cell free extracts from a sarcoma in chickens could induce tumors in injected chickens within a few weeks, even when passed through filters that retained bacteria, was recognized with a Nobel Prize in 1968. Rous's original work pointed out that this infectious agent was not only capable of inducing tumors but also imprinting the phenotypic characteristics of the original tumor on the recipient cell. This early work, however, was at the time relegated to the rank of avian curiosities and its importance was not recognized for several decades.

In the 1930s Richard Shope published a series of papers demonstrating cell free transmission of tumors in rabbits. The first studies involved fibromatous tumors found in the footpads of wild cottontail rabbits that could be transmitted by injecting cell free extracts in either wild or domestic rabbits. Subsequent studies have shown that this virus, now referred to as the Shope fibroma virus, is a poxvirus. Additional studies carried out by Shope demonstrated that cutaneous papillomatosis in wild cottontail rabbits could also be transmitted by cell free extracts. In a number of cases, these benign papillomas would progress spontaneously into squamous cell carcinomas in infected domestic rabbits or in the infected cottontail rabbits.[2,3] In general, however, the field of viral oncology lay dormant until the early 1950s with the discovery of the murine leukemia viruses by Ludwig Gross and of the mouse polyoma virus by Gross, Stewart, and Eddy.[4–6] These findings of tumor viruses in mice led many cancer researchers and virologists to the field of viral oncology. These researchers had the hope that these initial observations in mammals could be extended to humans and that a fair proportion of human tumors might also be found to have a viral etiology.

The starting point of active research in human cancer viruses came in 1964 when Epstein et al. demonstrated herpes virus–like particles in human lymphoblasts derived from Burkitt's lymphoma: Epstein-Barr virus (EBV).[7,8] During the 1970s evidence accumulated for a role for hepatitis B virus (HBV) in primary hepatocellular carcinoma (HCC) in humans. Molecular biological analyses, however, revealed that only a portion of HCCs contained HBV nucleic acids, and subsequent studies have shown a role for hepatitis C virus in many of these HCCs.[9] In the 1970s specific human papillomaviruses were found by Orth et al.[10] to be associated with skin cancers in patients with a rare skin disease called epidermodysplasia verruciformis. In 1980, human T-lymphotropic virus 1 (HTLV-1) was isolated by the Gallo group and subsequently linked to adult T-cell leukemia.[11,12] In the mid-1980s specific human papillomaviruses (HPV) were identified in human cervical cancers by Boshart et al.[13] and Durst et al.[14] In the 1990s, a new herpes virus, Kaposi's sarcoma-associated herpesvirus (KSHV; also known as HHV-8) was identified by Yang Chang and Patrick Moore[15] and linked to Kaposi's sarcoma (KS). In 2008 using deep sequencing Chang and Moore[16] also identified a new candidate human tumor virus, a polyomavirus, from Merkel cell carcinomas (MCC), a rare tumor that is seen more frequently in immunosuppressed individuals. The details surrounding these discoveries are discussed in this chapter.

Because of the important role of retroviruses in murine tumors, much of the initial focus in the search for human tumor viruses was on the identification of human retroviruses in human cancers. However, with the exception of HTLV-1, no retrovirus has been directly linked as causative agent for human cancers. The human immunodeficiency virus (HIV), however, is an important cofactor in many human cancers, in part because it causes immunosuppression. General characteristics that have emerged for many human cancer viruses are: (1) the viruses that have been implicated in human carcinogenesis are frequently ubiquitous (e.g., EBV, HPV, hepatitis viruses); (2) cancer is a rare outcome of a virus infection and only a small percentage of infected individuals develops cancer; (3) the time intervals between the initial infection and cancer development is long (usually decades); (4) the cancers are usually clonal; and (5) chemical or physical agents are often implicated as playing cofactor roles.

Furthermore, many of the most important developments in modern molecular biology derive from studies in viral oncology through the decades from the 1960s. The discovery of reverse transcriptase, the development of recombinant DNA technology, the discovery of messenger RNA splicing, and the discovery of oncogenes and later tumor suppressor genes were all developments that derive directly from studies in viral oncology. Oncogenes were first recognized as cellular genes that had been acquired by retroviruses through recombinational processes to convert them into acute transforming RNA tumor viruses. Oncogenes are now known to participate in many different types of tumors and can be involved at different stages of tumorigenesis and have contributed significantly to our concepts in nonviral carcinogenesis. It is likely that the direct transforming, oncogene-transducing retroviruses do not play a major causative role in naturally occurring cancers in animals or in humans but rather represent laboratory generated recombinants. Similar to studies with the retroviruses, studies with DNA tumor viruses have also provided major insights into oncogenic mechanisms relevant to human cancer, including the discovery of tumor suppressor genes and p53.[17]

A list of human viruses with oncogenic properties is presented in Table 15.1. This list includes viruses such as the transforming adenoviruses, which are capable of transforming normal cells into malignant cells in the laboratory but have not

TABLE 15.1

HUMAN VIRUSES WITH ONCOGENIC PROPERTIES

Virus Family	Type	Associated Human Tumors	Cofactors
Adenovirus	Types 2, 5, 12	Not associated with human cancer	
Flaviviruses	Hepatitis C (HCV)	Hepatocellular carcinoma	—
Hepadnavirus	Hepatitis B (HBV)	Hepatocellular carcinoma	Aflatoxin, alcohol, smoking
Herpesviruses	EBV	Burkitt's lymphoma	Malaria
		Immunoblastic lymphoma	Immunodeficiency
		Nasopharyngeal carcinoma	Nitrosamines
		Hodgkin's lymphoma	—
		Leiomyosarcomas	—
		Gastric cancers	—
	KSHV (HSV8)	Kaposi's sarcoma	HIV infection
		Pulmonary effusion lymphoma	HIV infection
		Castleman's disease	HIV infection
Papillomaviruses	HPV-16, -18, -33, -39, others	Anogenital cancers and some upper airway cancers	Smoking, other factors
	HPV-5, -8, -17, others	? nonmelanoma skin cancer	EV, sunlight, immune suppression
Polyomavirus	Merkel cell virus	Merkel cell carcinomas	Immunosuppression
	SV40 (monkey virus)	? Brain tumors	—
		? Non-Hodgkin's lymphomas	—
		? Mesotheliomas	—
	JC virus	? Brain tumors	—
	BK virus	? Prostate cancer	—
Retroviruses	HTLV-1	Adult T-cell leukemia/lymphoma	Uncertain

KSHV, Kaposi's sarcoma–associated herpesvirus; HPV, human papillomavirus; HIV, human immunodeficiency virus; EV, epidermodysplasia verruciformis; HTLV, human T-lymphotropic virus.

been associated with any known human tumors. The list also includes viruses such as the papillomaviruses, which have been etiologically associated with specific human cancers and have been shown to encode transforming viral oncogenes. Finally, it includes viruses, such as the hepatitis B and hepatitis C, which have been closely linked with a specific human tumor, hepatocellular carcinoma, for which the evidence of a *bona fide* viral encoded oncogene is still unclear. This chapter focuses primarily on the DNA viruses that have been associated with specific human cancers and discusses the biology and pertinent molecular biology of these viruses. The preceding section of this chapter deals with the RNA viruses and in particular the human retroviruses. The evidence pertaining to the association of each of these viruses with specific types of human neoplasia is presented, and the mechanisms by which these viruses may contribute to malignant transformation are discussed.

HEPADNAVIRUSES AND HEPATOCELLULAR CARCINOMA

HCC is one of the world's most common malignancies. Though rare in the West, the disease is highly prevalent in Southeast Asia and Sub-Saharan Africa. In the 1970s, its distribution was recognized to mirror that of chronic HBV infection. This fact, along with the long-recognized histopathologic association between HCC and chronic hepatitis in the surrounding nontumorous liver, led to the strong presumption that chronic HBV infection predisposes to hepatic cancer. This presumption was then validated by large prospective epidemiologic studies in Taiwan, in which chronically infected individuals were followed for deaths due to HCC.[18] These studies established that chronic HBV infection is associated with a 100-fold increase in HCC risk over that of controls who are not chronically infected.

HBV is a small DNA virus classified as a member of the hepadnavirus family (for hepatotropic DNA viruses). HBV is the only human virus in this family, which also includes related viruses of woodchucks (woodchuck hepatitis virus, WHV), ground squirrels (ground squirrel hepatitis virus), and ducks (duck hepatitis B virus). Primary HBV infection produces either a subclinical infection or acute liver injury, but irrespective of their clinical manifestations 95% of such infections resolve, with clearance of virus from liver and blood and the induction of lasting immunity to reinfection.[19] However, 5% of patients go on to have persistent (usually lifelong) hepatic infection and viremia, and most of the demonstrated HCC risk falls within this subgroup of infections. In fact, patients with the highest levels of HBV viremia display the highest HCC risk.[20]

Another factor that adds to risk is the severity of chronic liver injury; asymptomatic carriers have lower HCC risk than those with chronic active hepatitis or cirrhosis. In chronic hepatitis B, hepatocyte injury is due to host immune responses triggered by recognition of viral antigens presented on the surface of infected cells.[19,21] The induction of immune-mediated hepatocellular injury is thought to be important in HCC pathogenesis because it triggers a stereotypic proliferative response in the liver. Such proliferation increases opportunities for replicative DNA errors (mutations) that over time can contribute to the loss of normal cellular growth control. Cells harboring such mutations would have a selective advantage that could further perpetuate this cell injury–proliferation cycle. As such, HBV serves indirectly as an agent of oncogenesis, chiefly by

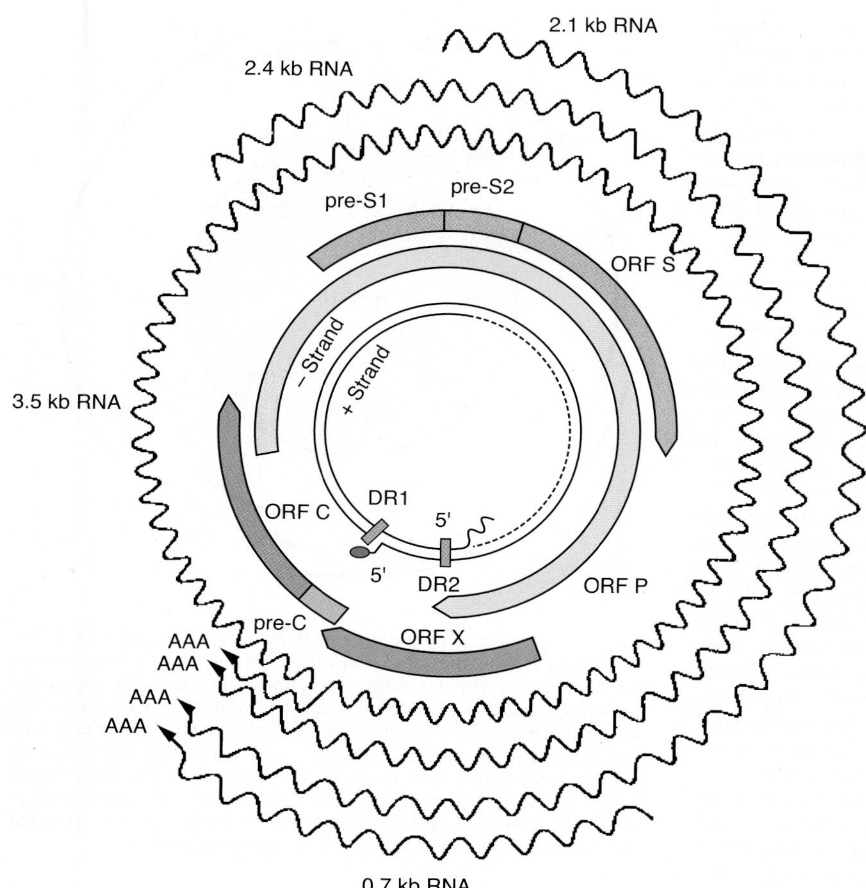

FIGURE 15.1 Genomic and transcriptional organization of the human hepatitis B virus. The inner circle represents the partially double stranded virion DNA, with dashes specifying the single-stranded genomic region. The locations of the direct repeat (DR1 and DR2) regions are indicated. The boxed arcs specify the viral coding regions and the arrows indicate the direction of translation. The outermost wavy lines depict the viral RNAs identified in infected cells with the arrows indicating the direction of transcription and the AAAs indicating the polyadenylated 3′ tails.

provoking cellular proliferation in response to immune-mediated injury; no direct genetic contribution is made by viral sequences acting *in cis* or viral gene products acting *in trans*. This view accords well with the fact that HCC risk is increased in every condition that provokes chronic liver injury and regeneration, including diseases as diverse as alcoholism, α1-antitrypsin deficiency, Wilson's disease, and hepatitis C virus infection.

Despite strong experimental support for the above pathogenetic scheme, there is reason to believe that hepadnaviruses may also make a more direct genetic contribution to HCC. Phylogenetic analyses of hepadnaviral genome organization reveal that the structure of the oncogenic mammalian viruses differs from that of the nononcogenic avian viruses in an important way—the mammalian viruses all harbor an additional coding region, termed ORF X (Fig. 15.1). This gene encodes a small regulatory protein (HBx) implicated possibly in a variety of signal transduction and transcriptional activation pathways. This open reading frame is absent in the avian viruses, which fail to induce HCC in their native hosts despite the regular induction of persistent infection. Interestingly, in several lines of transgenic mice that display constitutive hepatic expression of HBx hepatocellular carcinoma arises with increased frequency. Tumors in such mice do not begin until midlife, suggesting that additional genetic changes are necessary for loss of normal growth control. In addition, many HBV-related HCCs have deleted or inactivated the HBx coding region in their retained HBV DNA. Thus, if HBx expression is important in carcinogenesis *in vivo*, it must be involved at early stages and be dispensable during later tumor progression.

Another more direct genetic contribution that HBV might make to HCC derives from the activation or inactivation of cellular genes by the integrated copies of viral DNA in the tumor cells. Unlike retroviruses, hepadnaviruses do not specify genetic functions that direct genomic integration, and such integration is not essential for HBV replication. In fact, since every nucleotide of the viral genome is in a coding region, integration of HBV DNA generally disrupts essential genes and is incompatible with replication. Yet most hepatoma cells that arise in HBV-infected patients harbor multiple integrated HBV genomes, and in general active viral replication has been extinguished. The tumors are clonal with respect to these viral insertions: all cells of the tumor bear the same pattern of viral genome integrants, indicating that viral DNA integration preceded or accompanied the final transforming event. But close inspection of these integrants indicates that they are usually highly rearranged, with multiple deletions, inversions, reduplications, or other mutations typically present.[22] Although individual integrants may retain certain coding functions, no one viral coding region is invariably preserved, as are the *E6* and *E7* genes of the human papillomaviruses in human cervical cancer.

These facts have led to interest in the model that the viral sequences might be contributing *cis*-acting regulatory signals rather than transacting proteins to the host cell. Strong evidence that hepadnaviruses can mediate such activation events in *cis* has been proffered for WHV, which is strikingly oncogenic in its native host: virtually 100% of animals chronically infected from birth will develop HCC.[23] As in HBV-induced cancer, the tumors display multiple viral insertions, often highly rearranged, and in a clonal pattern. But here, remarkably, the vast majority of tumors can be shown to harbor at least one viral insertion in *cis* to the protooncogene N-*myc2*.[24] This gene, normally silent in adult liver, is strongly up-regulated by this insertion, and this activation can be seen early in the oncogenic sequence, even in premalignant lesions. Clearly, insertional activation of N-*myc* plays a major role in WHV oncogenesis. In contrast, in HCC there are only rare examples of integration within loci that might contribute to tumorigenesis as described (i.e., insertions near loci for retinoid receptors, *erb*-A or cyclin A).[25] Therefore, whereas insertional mutagenesis or specific oncogene activation may be important in individual cases of HCC, there is little evidence that it is of general mechanistic importance for HCC in humans.

PAPILLOMAVIRUSES

The papillomaviruses are nonenveloped DNA viruses that induce squamous epithelial and fibroepithelial tumors in their natural hosts. These viruses have a specific tropism for keratinocytes and express their full productive cycle only in squamous epithelial cells. The life cycle of the papillomaviruses, which leads to a productive infection, is linked to the differentiation state of the epithelial cell. In the squamous epithelium, the basal cell is the only cell normally capable of supporting cellular DNA synthesis and undergoing cellular division. The virus, therefore, must infect the basal cell in order to establish an infection. As the cells of an HPV infected lesion migrate upward within the epithelium into the granular layer, they undergo a program of differentiation. The control of papillomavirus late gene expression is tightly linked to the differentiation state of the squamous epithelial cells. Vegetative viral DNA synthesis and expression of the capsid proteins occur only in the most terminally differentiated epithelial cells.[26]

Over 140 different HPV types have now been recognized and each of them is associated with specific clinical lesions. All HPV types have a similar genomic organization. The DNA genomes of each of the HPVs sequenced as well as the other animal papillomaviruses are approximately 8,000 bp in size. All of the open reading frames (ORFs) that could serve to encode proteins for there viruses are located on only one of the two viral DNA strands. RNA studies have indicated that only one strand is transcribed. A more detailed description of the molecular biology of the papillomaviruses can be found in the recent edition of *Field's Virology*.[26]

The HPV genome can be divided into two distinct regions: an early region, which encodes the viral proteins involved in viral DNA replication, transcriptional regulation, and cellular transformation, and a late region, which encodes the viral capsid proteins. The genomic map of HPV-16 is shown in Figure 15.2. The genes located in the early region of the genes are designated as *E1*, *E2*, and so forth, and the two genes located in the late region that encode the capsid proteins are designated *L1* and *L2*. From studies with the HPVs, it is likely that *E4* encodes a late gene that is expressed only in productively infected keratinocytes. Thus although this gene is located within the so-called early region, its function may only be important in the later stages of vegetative replication of the virus. A listing of the functions assigned to the human papillomavirus ORFs is provided in Table 15.2.

The functions of the papillomavirus *E1* and *E2* genes appear to be highly conserved among different papillomavirus.[26] The papillomavirus *E2* gene has roles in the regulation of viral transcription, enhancing the activity of *E1* in initiating viral DNA replication and in ensuring the maintenance of the viral genome in persistently infected cells. E2 is a DNA-binding protein and can function as a transcriptional activator or a transcriptional repressor depending upon the context of its cognate sites in the promoter. In addition, E2 has a direct role in viral DNA replication. E2 forms a complex with the viral E1 protein to direct replication origin binding by E1 and to enhance E1-dependent replication. The *E1* gene encodes a protein necessary for initiating viral DNA replication. E1 has DNA binding, DNA helicase, and adenosine triphosphatase (ATPase) activities and binds components of the host cell replication machinery for recruitment to the viral DNA. Papillomaviruses do not encode a viral DNA polymerase and are dependent upon the host cell replication machinery to replicate the viral genomes.

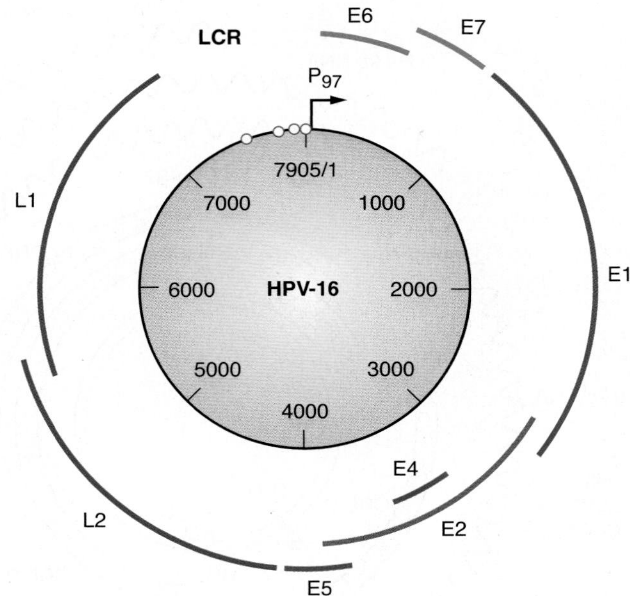

FIGURE 15.2 The genomic map of human papillomavirus 16 (HPV-16) deduced from the DNA sequence. The nucleotide numbers are noted within the circular maps, transcription proceeds clockwise, and the major open reading frames (E1 to E7, L1, and L2) are indicated. The only transcriptional promoter mapped to data for HPV-16 is designated (P_{97}). A_E and A_L represent the putative polyadenylation signals for the early and late transcripts, respectively. The viral long control region (LCR) containing the putative viral transcriptional and replication regulatory elements is noted. The closed circles on the genome represent the four E2 binding sites that have been noted in the LCR.

Because of their association with human cervical cancer, studies on the mechanisms of transformation have extensively focused on HPV-16 and HPV-18. The principal transforming genes for the cancer-associated HPVs are *E6* and *E7*.[26] *E7* is by

TABLE 15.2

HUMAN PAPILLOMAVIRUS GENE FUNCTIONS

ORF	FUNCTION
L1	L1 protein, major capsid protein (basis of current preventive VLP vaccines)
L2	L2 protein, minor capsid protein
E1	Initiation of viral DNA replication, helicase, ATPase
E2	Transcriptional regulatory protein, auxiliary role in viral DNA replication, genome maintenance
E4	Late protein; disrupts cytokeratins
E5	Membrane transforming protein; interacts with specific growth factor receptors
E6	Transformation; targets degradation of p53; activates telomerase
E7	Transformation; inactivates pRB and RB-related proteins, affects centrosome duplication

ORF, open reading frames; VLP, virus-like particles; ATPase, adenosine triphosphatase; pRB, product of the retinoblastoma tumor suppressor gene; RB, retinoblastoma.

itself sufficient for the transformation of established rodent cell lines such as 3T3 cells and can cooperate with an activated *ras* oncogene to transform primary rodent cells. Expression of *E6* and *E7* together are sufficient for the efficient immortalization of primary human cells, including keratinocytes,[27] the normal host cell for HPV. A number of cellular targets for the E6 and E7 oncoproteins have been identified and are discussed in detail below. HPV E5 may also have transforming activities and appears to function at least in part though interactions with the epidermal growth factor receptor. E5, however, is not required for HPV immortalization of keratinocytes and is generally not expressed in HPV-associated cancers.[26]

Papillomaviruses and Cancer

Only a subset of the papillomaviruses are associated lesions that are at risk for malignant progression. This is true for the human papillomaviruses as well as papillomaviruses in other animal species. The Shope papillomavirus (CRPV) that infects cotton-tailed rabbits was the first papillomavirus to be identified and is the etiologic agent of cutaneous papillomatosis in rabbits. CRPV has also been extensively studied as a model for papillomavirus-induced carcinogenesis. One of the features of carcinogenic progression with the papillomaviruses is the synergy between the virus and carcinogenic external factors. For instance, in the case of CRPV, carcinomas develop at an increased frequency in virus-induced papillomas that are painted with cool tar or methylcholanthrene.[28,29] CRPV-associated carcinomas contain viral DNA that is transcriptionally active, an observation that supports the hypothesis that these viruses play an active role in the cancers that develop.

Other animal papillomaviruses have also been associated with naturally occurring cancers. Of note is bovine papillomavirus 4 (BPV-4), which has been associated with esophageal papillomatosis in cattle and is also associated with squamous cell carcinomas of upper alimentary tract. Interestingly, however, only those cattle from the highlands of Scotland that are infected with BPV-4 that also feed on bracken fern (which is known to contain a radiomimetic substance) have a high incidence of squamous cell carcinomas of the esophagus and of the foregut. In contrast to the CRPV-associated carcinomas, in which the viral DNA can invariably be found, extensive analysis of the squamous cell carcinomas of the upper alimentary tract in these cattle infected with BPV-4 have failed to reveal a consistent pattern of viral DNA sequences within the malignant tumors. In the case of these alimentary tract tumors, it is possible that the continued presence of BPV-4 DNA sequences is not required for the maintenance of the cancer.[30]

Human Papillomaviruses and Anogenital Cancer

Cervical cancer is one of the most common cancers among women worldwide, with approximately 500,000 newly diagnosed cases each year, accounting for about 275,000 cancer deaths per year. Despite its worldwide distribution, the frequency of cervical cancer varies considerably.[31] Cervical cancer is the most common cancer of women in most developing countries. It occurs less frequently in developed countries because of effective screening programs. In the United States, there are about 12,000 newly diagnosed cases annually, and about one-third of these women will die of their malignant disease. The incidence of cervical cancer in the United States varies considerably between ethnic and socioeconomic groups, with the rate among black women being about twice that of white women.[32]

Epidemiologic studies had long implicated an infectious agent in the etiology of human cervical carcinoma.[33] Venereal transmission of a carcinogenic factor with a long latency had been suggested by epidemiologic studies. Sexual promiscuity, an early age of onset of sexual activity, and poor sexual hygienic conditions are known risk factors for cervical carcinoma. In the late 1960s and early 1970s genital infection by herpes simplex virus (HSV) type 2 was considered a possible etiologic candidate. Support for the notion that HSV might be a cancer-associated virus came from studies demonstrating the ability of HSV to transform certain rodent cells in the laboratory *in vitro* and from serologic studies, suggesting a higher frequency of antibodies to HSV-2 in patients with cervical carcinoma. However, subsequent carefully done molecular studies, which attempted to demonstrate HSV RNA or HSV DNA in cervical cancer tissues, did not provide convincing evidence for a role for HSV in cervical cancer.[34] Subsequent prospective epidemiologic studies have also failed to support the involvement of HSV infections as the major in etiologic agent in human cervical cancer.

In the mid-1970s, zur Hausen[35] suggested an association between papillomaviruses and genital cancers. The initial evidence that linked an HPV infection with cervical carcinoma came from the recognition that the morphologic changes previously interpreted on Papanicolaou (Pap) smears and tissue sections of the cervix as cervical dysplasia were due to a papillomavirus infection.[36] The association of an HPV with cervical dysplasia (also referred to as cervical intraepithelial neoplasia [CIN] or squamous epithelial lesions [SIL]) sparked an examination of cervical cancers for HPV sequences. The natural history linking CIN to carcinoma *in situ* and to invasive squamous cell carcinoma of the cervix had already been well established. Initial experiments from a number of laboratories revealed HPV sequences in occasional cases of cervical carcinoma and of anogenital carcinoma, but no consistent pattern of positivity emerged. Some initial studies focused on HPV-6 and HPV-11, which are related HPV types found in venereal warts (also known as condyloma acuminata). The majority of cervical carcinomas and other genital tract carcinomas, however, are negative for HPV-6 and HPV-11. Nonetheless, there are rare genital tract tumors that are positive for HPV-6 or HPV-11 in which there is malignant conversion of condyloma acuminata into squamous cell carcinoma. These lesions are referred to as Buschke-Lowenstein tumors and sometimes designated as giant condylomas. These tumors have characteristics similar to that of a locally invasive squamous cell carcinoma.

Using an HPV-11 DNA probe under low stringency hybridization conditions, Boshart et al.[13] and Durst et al.[14] identified two new papillomavirus DNAs, HPV-16 and HPV-18, in cellular DNA from human cervical cancers. Using these HPV DNAs as probes, HPV-16 and -18 could be demonstrated in approximately 70% of cervical carcinomas[37] and represent the two most frequent HPV types associated with the majority of human cervical cancers. The discovery of HPV-16 and HPV-18 and their association with cervical cancer led to zur Hausen receiving the Nobel Prize in Physiology or Medicine in 2008. The use of low stringency hybridization and polymerase chain reaction (PCR) with degenerative primers has led to the identification of over 20 different HPVs now associated with genital tract lesions, some of which are also associated with cervical cancer. These additional HPV types including HPV-31, HPV-33, HPV-39, HPV-42, among others that are each associated with a small percentage of cervical carcinomas. A causal role for HPV infections in cervical cancer has been documented beyond reasonable doubt and the association is present in virtually all cervical cancer cases worldwide.[38] Specific HPVs are also found in a lower percentage of other human genital tract carcinomas, including penile carcinomas, vulvar carcinomas, and perianal carcinomas.

Molecular studies of cervical cancers and derived cell lines have indicated that the HPV DNA is usually integrated, although there are some cases in which DNA is apparently also extrachromosomal. In those cases where the DNA is integrated, the pattern of integration is clonal, indicating that the association of the HPV preceded the clonal outgrowth of the tumor. Integration of the viral DNA is not at specific sites in the host chromosome, although in some cell lines the integration event has occurred in the vicinity of known oncogenes. For instance, in the HeLa cell lines (which is an HPV-18-positive cervical carcinoma cell line), the integration of the viral genome has occurred within approximately 50 kb of the c-*myc* locus on human chromosome 8. It seems quite plausible that in some individual cases of cervical cancer, the integration of the viral DNA could result in genetic changes that could contribute to carcinogenic progression by insertional mutagenesis.

In HPV-positive cancers there appears to be a selection for the integrity of the E6-E7 coding region and the upstream regulatory region in that *E6* and *E7* genes are regularly expressed in HPV-positive cervical cancers. Furthermore, integration of the HPV DNA into the host chromosome in the cancers is often associated with disruption of the viral *E1* or *E2* genes. HPV E2 is an important viral regulatory factor that can repress the promoter directing the *E6* and *E7* genes.[26] Disruption of the *E2* gene by the integration of the HPV genome releases the viral promoter of the *E6* and *E7* genes from the inhibitory activity of *E2*, resulting in the disregulated and increased expression of *E6* and *E7*.

The E6 and E7 proteins encoded by the high-risk HPVs are oncoproteins and contribute, at least in part, to cellular transformation by binding to the cell regulatory proteins p53 and RB, respectively (Fig. 15.3). The E7 proteins encoded by the high-risk HPVs share sequence similarity to adenovirus E1A and to SV40 large T antigen-transforming proteins.[39] In all three proteins, these regions of amino acid similarity are critical for their transformation properties. The regions of sequence similarity between E7 and adenovirus E1A that are shared with SV40 large T antigen are regions that participate in the binding to the product of the retinoblastoma tumor suppressor gene (pRB) and the related "pocket" proteins, p107 and p130.[40] One consequence of the interaction of E7 with pRB is the disruption of a complex between pRB and E2F transcription factors.[41] The E7-mediated release of E2F from these complexes activates the expression of genes required for cell cycle progression from G_1 into S. Mutational analyses with E7, however, indicate that there must be other cellular targets of E7, and that complex formation between E7 and the pocket proteins, including pRB, is not sufficient to account for the immortalization and transforming functions of this viral oncoprotein. A number of additional cellular targets have been proposed for HPV-16 E7.[42]

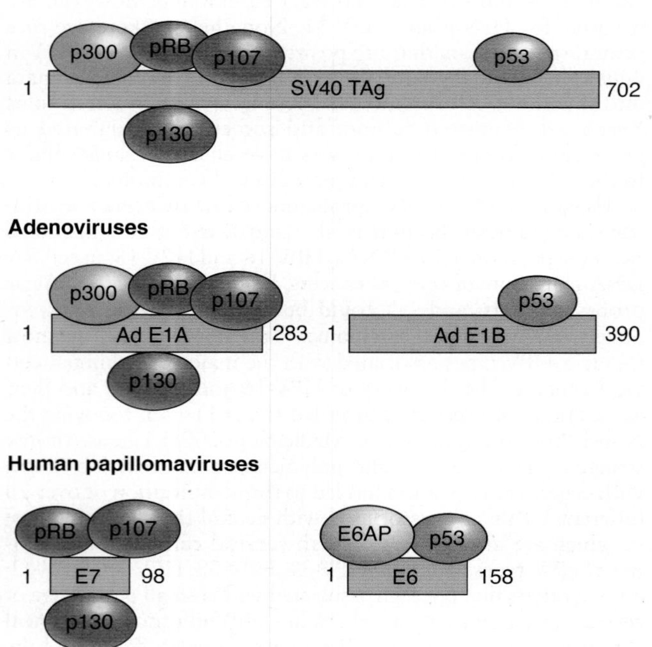

FIGURE 15.3 The transforming proteins encoded by three distinct groups of DNA tumor viruses target similar cellular proteins. The binding of human papillomavirus (HPV) E6 oncoproteins to p53 is mediated by a cellular protein called the E6-associated protein (E6AP). E6AP is an E3 ubiquitin protein ligase that targets the E6-dependent ubiquitylation of p53. (From refs. 169 and 49.)

In addition, the high-risk HPV E7 proteins cause genomic instability in normal human cells.[43] HPV-16 E7 induces G_1/S and mitotic cell cycle checkpoint defects and uncouples synthesis of centrosomes from the cell division cycle.[44] This causes formation of abnormal multipolar mitoses, leading to chromosome mis-segregation and aneuploidy.[45] This activity is not one that is not shared by the E7 proteins of the noncancer associated HPV types and therefore is likely to be functionally relevant to the contribution of high risk HPVs to malignant progression.

The transforming properties of the E6 protein were first revealed by studies using primary human cells, including keratinocytes.[27,46] Efficient immortalization of primary human cells requires both the *E6* and *E7* genes of the high-risk HPVs. The ability of the E6 and E7 proteins together to extend the lifespan of primary human keratinocytes is a characteristic of the high-risk HPVs, but not of the low-risk HPVs.[26] Like SV40 large T antigen and the 55 kd protein encoded by adenovirus E1B, the E6 proteins of the high-risk HPVs form a complex with the tumor suppressor protein p53.[47] The interaction of E6 with p53 is mediated by a cellular protein, called the E6-associated protein (E6AP), which promotes the ubiquitylation of p53, leading to its proteolysis.[48–50] E6 has other activities, and its immortalization and transformation properties cannot be fully explained through its interaction with p53.

Cells expressing E6 do not exhibit a functional p53 response. The p53 tumor suppressor is not required for normal cellular proliferation but rather functions as "guardian of the human genome" by integrating various signal transduction pathways that can sense cellular stress, including genotoxic and cytotoxic insults. The interaction of E6 with p53 appears to contribute to the chromosomal instability observed in cells infected by a high-risk HPV.[43] E6, however, has functions other than targeting the proteolysis of p53 that are important in cellular transformation and carcinogenesis. One important function that is p53 independent is that E6 causes the activation of the cellular telomerase in infected cells.[51]

Several additional cellular targets have also been identified for the high-risk E6 proteins in an attempt to define additional p53 independent activities.[26] One that may be of particular importance is the binding to cellular PDZ domain containing proteins. The high-risk E6 oncoprotein contains a X-(S/T)-X-(V/I/L)-COOH motif at the extreme C-terminus that can mediate the binding to cellular PDZ domain–containing proteins. This motif is unique in the high-risk HPV E6 proteins and is not present in the E6 proteins of the low-risk HPV types. E6 serves as a molecular bridge between these PDZ domain proteins and E6AP, facilitating their ubiquitylation and mediating their proteolysis. Among the PDZ domain proteins implicated as E6 targets are hDlg, the human homologue of the *Drosophila melanogaster* discs large tumor suppressor, and hScrib, the human homologue of the *Drosophila* Scribble tumor suppressor.[52,53] Other PDZ domain proteins have also been shown to be capable of binding to E6, and several PDZ-containing proteins have been shown to be involved in regulating cellular proliferation. Therefore, some of the p53 independent transforming activities of the high-risk E6 oncoproteins may be a consequence of the binding and degradation of specific PDZ motif–containing proteins.

HPV, while necessary, may not be sufficient for the development of cervical cancer. Only a small fraction of those individuals who are infected by a specific HPV will eventually develop cancer, and the time interval between infection and invasive cancer can be several decades. Thus E6 and E7 may initiate a process that can ultimately result in cancer. Other factors must therefore be involved in the progression to full cancers. Indeed epidemiologic studies have identified smoking as a risk factor for cervical carcinoma.[54]

Consistent with the multistep nature of tumorigenesis, cervical cancers have been shown to harbor cytogenetic alterations.[55] Certain cytogenetic changes have been found in a relatively high proportion of tumors.[56] Between one-quarter and one-half of cervical cancers show loss of heterozygosity in chromosome regions 3p14, 4p16, 4q21–35, 6p21–22, 11p15, 11q23, 17p13.3, and 18q12–22. Loss of heterozygosity in 3p has also been implicated in cervical dysplasias adjacent to cancers. This observation implies that inactivation of a putative tumor suppressor gene in this region may occur as an early event that could predispose to further progression, although the specific gene has not yet been identified.

Papillomaviruses and Head and Neck Cancer

The availability of specific HPV DNA probes has provided investigators the opportunity to carry out extensive screenings of a variety of human cancers for HPV sequences. Since HPVs infect squamous epithelial cells, cancers that arise from any squamous epithelium or an epithelium that has the potential to undergo squamous metaplasia would be potential candidates for an HPV association. Studies examining oral, upper airway, and tonsillar carcinomas have revealed that HPV is linked to some head and neck cancers, although not to the majority of the cancers in this region.[57–61] Most of these HPV-associated cancers are located in the oral pharynx, which includes the tonsils, tonsillar fossa, base of the tongue, and soft palette.

In the United Sates, the incidence of these cancers, but not those at other oral sites, has increased approximately 2% per year between 1973 and 1995, presumably because of the increase in sexually transmitted HPV infection.[62] Genital–oral sex may be a risk factor for these tumors, and the risk of HPV infection and cigarette smoking may be more than additive. HPV-positive tumors tend to have a characteristic basaloid morphology, are less likely to harbor mutations of p53 or pRb, and more likely to express p16. HPV positive head and neck cancers may also have improved disease-specific survival.

Papillomaviruses and Nonmelanoma Skin Cancer

The first evidence that HPVs might be associated with human cancer came from studies of skin cancers in patients with epidermodysplasia verruciformis (EV), a rare lifelong disease in humans that usually begins in infancy or childhood (reviewed in Jablonska et al.[63]). The disease is characterized by disseminated polymorphic cutaneous lesions that resemble flat warts and also as reddish macules sometimes referred to as pityriasis-like lesions. Approximately half of the patients with EV develop multiple skin cancers usually during the third of fourth decade of their lives. Papillomavirus can be detected within the benign lesions and not in the carcinomas. More than 20 different HPV types have now been demonstrated in individual lesions in patients with this rare disease. In approximately one-half of affected patients, EV occurs as an inherited disorder. Inheritance appears to have an autosomal recessive pattern in most affected families, although one family with apparent X-linked recessive inheritance has been reported. Cases with autosomal recessive inheritance appear to be genetically heterogeneous, as the condition in different families has been mapped to two distinct chromosomal loci[64] and two adjacent novel genes (*EVER1* and *EVER2*) have now been molecularly identified at one of these loci (17q25).[65] EV is a very rare disease, yet it has been under intense study by dermatologists and virologists.

The potential role of HPVs in cutaneous nonmelanoma skin cancers (NMSC) may extend beyond EV patients to other patients, both immunosuppressed and immunocompetent. Many HPV types distinct from those associated with genital tract lesions and comprising the beta genus of the phylogenetic branch of the human papillomaviruses have been found in NMSCs of immunosuppressed patients and in some of the same tumors in immunocompetent patients. The same HPV types that have been seen in skin cancers of patients with EV are also found in skin cancers seen in some immunosuppressed patients, such as renal transplant patients.

The relationship between the genus beta-HPVs and NMSC is important because NMSC is the most common form of malignancy among fair-skinned populations. Ultraviolet irradiation is the major risk factor for developing NMSC, but a pathogenic role for the beta-HPVs in NMSC has been proposed. Molecular studies reveal a likely role for HPV infection in skin carcinogenesis as a cofactor in NMSC.[66] The genus beta-HPV types are present in more than 90% of NMSCs in EV patients and are also detected at a high frequency in NMSC of immunosuppressed patients and of the general population. However, viral DNA cannot necessarily be found in every cell, and the viral DNA loads in the cancers is often low. This suggests that the role of the beta-HPVs in NMSC may be at the initiation stage of the tumor, and that it might not be required for maintenance. Furthermore, molecular studies on the beta-HPVs are limited compared to the high risk genital tact–associated genus alpha-HPVs. Several of the beta-HPV types have been shown to prevent apoptosis after ultraviolet radiation exposure, an activity that may be mediated by E6 targeting the degradation of the pro-apoptotic protein Bak.[67,68] Molecular analysis of this group of beta-HPVs is now an active area of research in the HPV field.

Papillomaviruses and Other Cancers

Esophageal carcinomas in humans have not yet been convincingly shown to be associated with an HPV. The esophagus is lined by a squamous epithelium, and squamous cell papillomas of the esophagus have been described in humans. Additional studies would seem warranted to investigate a possible role of HPV in human esophageal cancers. There are also sporadic reports associating occasional human tumors, including breast cancer, colon cancer, ovarian cancer, prostate cancer, and even melanomas, with the presence of HPV DNA in the literature. In general, it seems prudent to be skeptical of such reports until systematic and well carried out studies are confirmed in multiple laboratories.

Papillomavirus Prevention and Therapy

The development of a preventive vaccine for some of the major high-risk HPV types is one of the major advances in cancer prevention during this past decade. The expression in yeast and in insect cells of the major capsid protein L1, either alone or together with L2, leads to the assembly of virus-like particles

(VLPs), which are morphologically identical to native virion particles.[69] These VLPs present the conformational epitopes that are necessary for the development of a high-titer–neutralizing antisera. The L1 VLPs are highly immunogenic, inducing high titers of neutralizing antibodies that were conformationally dependent and type specific. Both Merck and GlaxoSmithKline have developed HPV VLP-based vaccines, both of which performed well in preclinical and proof of principle efficacy trials that reported almost complete protection in fully vaccinated women against persistent infection or dysplasia attributable to the HPV type(s) targeted by the vaccine.[70,71] High-level protection has now been shown to be durable for both vaccines, with serum antibody levels at least an order of magnitude higher than those seen following natural infection. Protection appears to be predominantly type specific. Gardasil, the U.S. Food and Drug Administration (FDA)–approved Merck vaccine is a quadrivalent vaccine containing VLPs from HPV-16, HPV-18, HPV-6, and HPV-11; and Cervarix, the FDA-approved GlaxoSmithKline commercial vaccine, is bivalent, composed of HPV-16 and HPV-18 VLPs in a proprietary adjuvant. Only 70% of cervical cancers are caused by HPV-16 or HPV-18, the remainder being caused by other high-risk HPV types. There will therefore likely be next generation VLP vaccines to protect against additional HPV infections by incorporating VLPs from additional HPV types. Gardasil has been shown to prevent genital warts in males, and its use in men and boys was approved by the FDA in 2009.

Despite the successes of the VLP vaccines, there are several important unresolved issues.[69] The immune response to the VLPs is very type specific and little if any cross-protection against HPV types not present in the vaccine has been seen. Furthermore, the VLP vaccine is expensive and is not heat stable, two characteristics that might impede its use in developing countries where the cervical cancer disease burden is the greatest.

The effect of the HPV vaccines on the reduction in the number of infections attributable to the HPV types in the vaccines will be seen much sooner than the impact on the incidence of cervical cancer, which may take decades. This plus the fact that there are still many oncogenic HPV types that can cause cervical cancer that are not affected by the vaccine; it will therefore be very important for vaccinated women to continue to undergo cervical cancer screening.

Additional approaches to improve the vaccine seem warranted. The use of L2 epitopes represents a potential alternate approach to develop a prophylactic vaccine against a broader spectrum of HPV types. Although they are not as immunogenic as the L1 neutralization epitopes, at least some of the L2 neutralization epitopes induce cross-neutralizing antibodies against papillomaviruses from different types.[72,73] In addition modifications of the L1 capsid protein allow the self-assembly of capsomeres, which are highly immunoprotective, can be produced in bacteria, and are more stable.[74] Finally, none of the preventive vaccines developed to date provide any therapeutic potential. The inclusion of antigens from some of the early gene products such as *E2*, *E6*, or *E7* might be expected to provide some therapeutic possibilities.

EPSTEIN-BARR VIRUS

Denis Burkitt, a British surgeon working in equatorial Africa, encountered and chronicled the high incidence of B-cell lymphomas among young children in malaria endemic regions. Because of the association with holoendemic malaria, Burkitt postulated an infectious etiology. His lectures in the United Kingdom about this unusual childhood lymphoma interested Anthony Epstein, an experimental pathologist studying virus infection of cells, in culture. Epstein succeeded in growing Burkitt's lymphoma (BL) cells in culture, which was soon identified as a new herpes virus that spontaneously replicated in an occasional BL cell (for review see Rickinson and Kieff[75]). Epstein-Barr virus (EBV) became the first candidate human cancer virus.[7]

The presence of a small fraction of cells permissive for EBV replication in BL cell cultures enabled researchers to test human sera for antibody to virus capsid antigens (VCA). This indirect immune fluorescence assay used fixed BL cells to detect immunoglobulin (Ig) M, IgG, or IgA human antibodies that react with the cytoplasm of the spontaneously reactivated infected BL cells grown in culture. Surprisingly, EBV is nearly ubiquitous and most humans have EBV VCA IgG. Henle et al.[76] discovered that adolescents or young adults with acute infectious mononucleosis (IM) seroconvert to first IgM and then IgG VCA antibodies. However, Africans with BL, Chinese with anaplastic nasopharyngeal carcinoma (NPC), and people from the United States, Europe, or South America with Hodgkin's lymphoma (HL) have significantly higher EBV antibody titers, consistent with Burkitt's hypothesis that EBV infection is a major risk factor for these malignancies.[77–79] An etiologic role for EBV in African BL, NPC, and HL was further supported by finding an EBV nuclear antigen, EBNA1, and EBV DNA in almost all African BL and NPC tumor cells and most Reed-Sternberg positive HL tumor cells.[80–83] The finding of EBV DNA by *in situ* hybridization in all tumor cells is strong evidence for an etiologic role in the above malignancies as well as in some gastric cancers, T or natural killer (NK) cell lymphomas, and in most lymphoproliferative diseases or lymphomas that occur in T-cell immune deficiency states, including posttransplantation, HIV infection, congenital immune deficiency states, and advanced aging (for review see Cohen et al.[84]).

The role of EBV in the pathogenesis of lymphoid malignancies was brought into focus by the discoveries that EBV efficiently converts human B lymphocytes into long-term lymphoblastoid cell lines (LCLs) and rapidly induces B-cell lymphomas following inoculation into nonhuman primates.[85,86] At the same time, Starzl et al.[87] observed that primary EBV infection after kidney transplantation and high doses of immune suppressants resulted in progression to acutely fatal polyclonal EBV infected B-lymphoproliferative disease (LPD). Children with X-linked, severe combined immunodeficiency (SCID) or sporadic immune deficiencies were also noted to develop EBV-positive multifocal malignant LPD, involving peripheral lymphoid organs or the brain.[88,89] LPDs in brain are typically similar in phenotype to LCLs, whereas peripheral LPDs can have a mixture of EBV and hyperexpression of c-*myc*, *BCL2*, or *BCL6* cell oncogenes. A decade later similar malignancies were noted in CD4-depleted HIV-infected AIDS patients.[90–93] Importantly, regular passive administration of immune serum globulin, which has antibody to EBV, has prevented serious EBV infection in children XLP-linked LPD, as initially envisaged.[94]

EBV latency III gene expression (Fig. 15.4) in LCLs, *in vitro*, and in human LPDs that are associated with severely T-cell immune compromised states, includes six nuclear proteins (EBNA-1, -2, LP, -3A, -3B, -3C), two integral membrane proteins (LMP-1, -2), two small RNAs (EBER1, 2), and multiple BHRF1 and BARF0 microRNAs.[95] Reverse genetic analyses indicate that EBNA2, EBNALP, EBNA3A, EBNA3C, and LMP1 are essential for the conversion of EBV infected peripheral blood B cells to LCLs, whereas LMP2 is also necessary for conversion of B-cell receptor negative cells and EBNA1 is necessary for efficient EBV episome persistence.[96–104] EBER RNAs remain of uncertain role in EBV infection, although modulation of interferon effects remains a possibility. EBV encodes more than 40 microRNAs, which are still mostly of uncertain function, except for a few that regulate EBV BHRF1, LMP1, and LMP2A RNAs levels.[105–107] EBV mir29b regulates TCL1A RNA and an EBV and KSHV conserved microRNAs target MICB mRNA, to down-regulate NK activity.[108,109] Recently, the putative targets

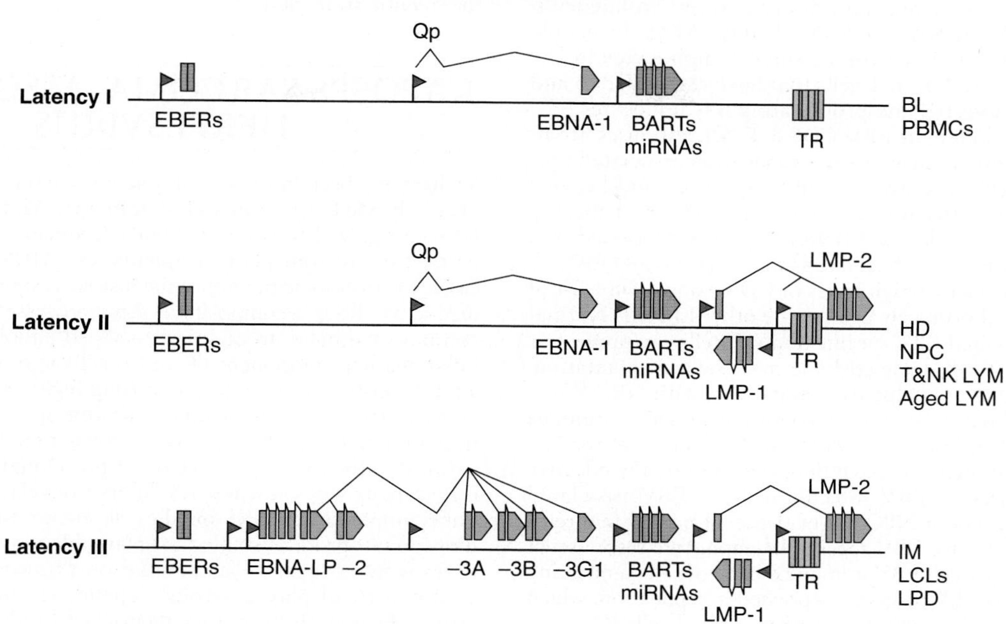

FIGURE 15.4 Epstein-Barr virus (EBV) RNAs expressed in latency I, II, or III infections *in vivo* or in cells in culture are shown projected on the linear virus genome. Protein-coding RNAs are black and BART microRNAs are white. BHRF1 microRNAs encoded by the EBNALP/-2 RNA are not shown. On the right are the normal or disease states that are characteristically associated with each form of latent infection.

of EBV and KSHV RNAs were identified by their association with Argonaut proteins.[110] Surprisingly, many of the EBV microRNA targets were up- rather than down-regulated.

Later onset posttransplant lymphomas, many of the peripheral lymphomas in HIV-infected people, and African BLs are usually composed of uniformly EBV-infected cells, but EBV gene expression is frequently restricted to latency I, characterized by expression of EBNA1, EBERs, and in some instances BARF0 mRNAs and microRNAs (Fig. 15.4). African BLs with latency I characteristically have a c-*myc*/Ig locus reciprocal translocation that results in c-*myc* overexpression and EBV latency III down-regulation, whereas HIV infection or late posttransplant LPDs may have c-*myc*, Bcl6, or Bcl2 translocations or other mutations that result in c-*myc*, Bcl-6, or Bcl-2 overexpression.[93,111] In contrast, EBV-associated HL and NPC are characteristically latency II infected, with EBNA1, LMP1, LMP2, EBERs, and BARF0 microRNA expression.[112–116]

When EBV infects a human B lymphocyte, the genome enters the nucleus and circularizes by joining the terminal direct repeats. *EBNA2* and *EBNALP* are the first EBV genes expressed in B lymphocytes. *EBNA2* and *EBNALP* act together to up-regulate virus and cell gene transcription.[117,118] *EBNA2* gets to specific promoters by direct interaction with the cell encoded, DNA sequence specific, transcription factors, RBP/CSL, PU.1, and AUF1.[119] *EBNA2* then activates transcription through its acidic activation domain, which binds basal and activation-related transcription factors. *EBNALP* removes repressors from promoters. *EBNA2* and *EBNA3A*, *EBNA3B*, and *EBNA3C* stably associate with RBP/CSL at high levels and coregulate overlapping sets of promoters. In targeting the cell transcription factor, RBP/CSL, and activating c-*myc*, EBNA2 imitates Notch receptors, which also activate transcription through RBP/CSL. Overexpressed Notch1 signaling is the usual cause of pediatric T-cell acute lymphoblastic leukemia (ALL),[120] consistent with the importance of RBP/CSL pathways in c-*myc* activation. *EBNA2*, *EBNALP*, *EBNA3A*, and *EBNA3C* jointly constitutively regulate the viral LMP1 promoter through RBP/CSL as well as the cell c-*myc* promoter, in large measure through RBP/CSL. *EBNA1* is essential for efficient conversion of lymphocytes to LCLs, because of its role in enabling EBV episome replication, persistence, and gene expression.

LMP1 is a key "transforming" component in EBV's constitutive proliferative and survival effects. LMP1 has six hydrophobic transmembrane domains that enable constitutive self-aggregation in cytoplasmic membranes, including the plasma membrane. LMP1 has two important C-terminal cytoplasmic signaling domains; one domain engages tumor necrosis factor (TNF) receptor cytoplasmic factors TRAF3, TRAF1, TRAF2, and TRAF5, and the other domain engages death domain proteins, including TRADD and RIP, without propagating a death signal.[121–123] Both domains activate nuclear factor kappa B (NF-κB), JNK and p38, although the TRAF interacting domain appears to be the principal IKKα activator and the TRADD interacting domain the principal activator of canonical NF-κB. The TRAF domain is also particularly important for LCL outgrowth, as well as for up-regulating TRAF1 and EGF receptor expression.[75] NF-κB activation is critical for LCL survival and may have a role in cell proliferation. Although, not important for LCL growth or survival, LMP2 mimics a constitutively active Ig receptor and desensitizes cells to Ig receptor signaling. LMP2 can also enhance cell survival as a result of low level forward signaling through PI3 kinase, particularly in pre- or pro-B-lymphocytes or epithelial cells.[124,125]

EBV is a remarkably unusual virus in potentially inducing malignant EBV infected B-lymphocyte proliferation in primary human infection.[75] Early in acute infection, latency III–infected B lymphocytes proliferate and may constitute up to 10% of peripheral blood B lymphocytes. These cells then seed into lymphatic organs. Normal humans have an unusually robust T-cell response to EBV latency III–infected cells. The high level of persistence of this response is evidence of ongoing latency III gene expression, although latency III proteins can also be expressed during replication.[126] Infected B-cell proliferation is dependent on EBNAs and LMPs, which cooperatively induce high level CD4+ and CD8+ T-lymphocyte responses. Latency III–infected cells exit from the cell cycle, revert to latency I, and express only EBNA1 or EBNA1 and LMP2. In people who develop IM, most of the dividing lymphocytes in the peripheral blood are NK or T cells that have responded to and eliminated EBV infected and proliferating B lymphocytes.[127]

Much of the dominant EBV CD8+ T cell responses are to EBNA3 or immediate early or early replication associated proteins. CD8+ T-cell responses are initially broad and become increasing focused after primary infection, but persist lifelong at readily measurable levels. EBNA1 is poorly processed into the class I pathway, and infected cells that express only EBNA1 can survive in the face of high levels of CD4+ and CD8+ T-cell immunity directed primarily against the other EBNAs. Normal or *in vitro* augmented EBV-specific donor T cells can prevent or treat LPD after T-cell depleted bone marrow transplantation. Similar approaches are being used in patients with NPC.[128,129]

EBV-infected B cells are the source of the almost continuous reactivated virus in human saliva.[130] In the context of the key role for CD4+ and CD8+ T lymphocytes in normally effective immune responses to EBV infected cells,[131] EBV-associated LPD, BL, HL, and even NPC are evidence of partial failure of the normally protective EBV specific T-lymphocyte response.[132] In part, transitory T-cell EBV immune escape of cells replicating EBV is enabled by EBV proteins, expressed in replication, which inhibit human T-cell recognition of EBV-infected cells.[133]

Overall, EBV is a substantial cause of LPD in heart, lung, liver, pancreas, or T-cell–depleted bone marrow transplant recipients, CD4 depleted HIV-infected patients, almost all African BLs, approximately 20% of non-African BLs, and approximately 50% of classical, Reed-Sternberg cell HL, particularly HL among postadolescents or Hispanics.[132] EBV latency 1 infection characterizes almost all NPCs worldwide and approximately 5% of gastric cancers (GCs), while unusual EBV-infected T-cell lymphomas and leiomyomas are more variable in latency type. Consistent latency III EBV infection is confined to LPD in severely T-cell immune deficient people, rare African BLs, and some T- or NK-cell lymphomas, whereas latency II, characterized by expression of EBNA1, LMP1, and LMP2, is evident in many NPCs and almost all EBV-associated HLs. Latency I is characteristic of most EBV-associated BLs. EBV is present at the onset of EBV-associated BL, HL, NPC, or GC since most tumor cells in these patients have EBV genomes with the same number of terminal repeats, whereas variability in terminal repeat number is a characteristic of independent EBV infection events.[134] Cell changes that accompany the presumed transformation from an EBV-infected cell or normal B cell to HL or BL have been partially characterized and include up regulation of c-*myc*, Bcl-6, or Rel expression.[135] EBV-infected HL tumor cells are similar to non-EBV infected HL cells in having nonproductive Ig mutations and up-regulated NF-κB and AP1 transcription.[136] EBV also causes oral hairy leukoplakia (OHL), a wart-like lesion on the tongue, caused by continuous EBV replication. OHL lesions have wild type and defective EBV genomes.[137] The lesions disappear in response to suppression of EBV replication with acyclovir.

Serology and peripheral blood EBV DNA levels have been useful for early detection of primary EBV NPC and recurrences.[138] The utility of serologic testing is dependent on ongoing clinical validation and intact patient immune responses. EBV LMP1 and LMP2 are likely to have important roles in the early survival of NPC cells. Loss of heterozygosity, chromosomal amplifications, and hypermethylations in NPC tumors likely have a role in tumor development or progression.[139] Among those from southern China, NPC is a very common malignancy. Families have been described with multiple affected members, enabling a familial genetic analysis and risk factor localization to 4p15.1–q12.[140] The expression of EBNA1 and of LMP1 and LMP2 in NPC and EBV-associated HL may render these cells susceptible to T-cell immune preventative and immune therapeutic strategies.[141–143]

KAPOSI'S SARCOMA–ASSOCIATED HERPESVIRUS

KS has long been known as an uncommon and indolent tumor of elderly Mediterranean and African men. More recently, it has been recognized to occur at higher frequency in immunosuppressed organ transplant recipients and AIDS patients. In all cases, the histologic picture of the disease is similar—and highly distinctive. KS is a composite of three processes: a proliferative component (made up of spindle-shaped endothelial cells), an inflammatory component (T and B cells and monocytes), and an angiogenic component (comprising highly aberrant, slit-like neovascular spaces). In advanced KS, the spindle cell proliferation dominates, resulting in nodule formation; but even in such cases, the disease is often oligo- or polyclonal.[144] This is only one of many ways in which KS differs from classical neoplasms. For example, cultured KS spindle cells are not fully tumorigenic: most do not produce stable transplantable tumors in nude mice or grow in soft agar. In fact, unlike most transformed cells they continue to display a strong dependence upon exogenous growth factors. (In turn, they themselves produce a large array of growth and angiogenic factors.) When transplanted into nude mice, they survive only transiently, but during their period of viability they recruit host inflammatory cells and neovascular structures very reminiscent of KS.[145] When the human spindle cells involute, the entire lesion disappears. This suggests a model for KS in which the entire process consists of paracrine signaling loops between its several components, not one of which is completely autonomous.[146,147]

KS had long been suspected to have a viral etiology. Early models attempted to relate spindle cell growth to HIV infection. Certainly, HIV infection is an enormous risk factor for KS development. However, spindle cells themselves are not targets of HIV infection, and KS epidemiology indicates that the lesion cannot depend solely upon HIV infection. First, of course, KS often arises in HIV-negative hosts, especially in the Mediterranean basin and Africa. More important, even within HIV-infected populations there are large differences in KS risk that must be attributed to factor s other than HIV.[148] KS risk is highest in homosexual men with untreated AIDS: 20% to 30% of such individuals will develop KS in the course of their HIV disease if no anti-HIV treatment is instituted. By contrast, less than 1% to 2% of AIDS cases related to blood product administration will be similarly afflicted, and KS is rarer still among pediatric AIDS cases in which HIV infection is acquired vertically from infected mothers. These and other data suggest the possibility of a sexually transmitted cofactor in KS etiology or pathogenesis. Chang et al.[15] used a PCR-based method to search for the putative causal virus by looking for DNA sequences that were present in DNA extracted from an AIDS-KS patient but absent in normal genomic DNA from the same patient. This search led to the discovery of the genome of the virus now known as KS-associated herpesvirus (KSHV), or human herpesvirus 8 (HHV-8).

Strong epidemiologic and molecular evidence indicates a pivotal role for this virus in KS development.[149] First, KSHV sequences are present in virtually all KS tumors, irrespective of their HIV status. And unlike HIV, in KS lesions KSHV DNA is found primarily in the spindle cells—the key cell type in KS pathogenesis. Most such cells display latent infection, though a small subpopulation is in the lytic cycle. In HIV-positive populations studied prospectively, KSHV infection precedes the development of KS, and prior infection with KSHV is strongly predictive of increased KS risk. Worldwide, there is a strong correlation between KSHV prevalence and KS risk: countries with high rates of classical KS display high rates of seropositivity for KSHV, and areas at low risk for KS typically have low prevalence of KSHV seropositivity. These data clearly indicate that KSHV is the agent predicted by KS epidemiology and strongly implicate KSHV in KS pathogenesis. KS is virtually never observed in the absence of documented KSHV infection, leading most experts in the field to conclude that KSHV is necessary for KS development. However, there is also strong consensus that it is not sufficient for this process. For example, 3% to 7% of the general population in the United States is infected by KSHV, yet this population has no significant KS risk. Clearly, therefore, some cofactor(s) in addition to KSHV is required to promote tumorigenesis. In the case of AIDS-KS, of course, that cofactor is HIV, although exactly what HIV contributes to pathogenesis is much debated. The nature of the cofactor(s) in the HIV-negative forms of KS remains unknown.

Studies of the global epidemiology of KSHV have yielded additional insights. First, the prevalence of KSHV in the general population is remarkably elevated in countries in which classical KS is common. For example, in southern Italy, Sicily and Sardinia, KSHV antibodies are found in over 20% of the general population; in many populations in Sub-Saharan Africa, where classical KS was common even in the pre-AIDS era, 60% to 80% of the population are seropositive. These numbers also reflect major epidemiologic differences between KSHV infection in Africa and the Mediterranean versus that in Western Europe and America. In the latter countries, homosexual men represent a major reservoir of infection, with much lower rates in women and very little infection in prepubertal children. By contrast, in Africa and the Mediterranean, seroconversions begin in childhood, and the seroprevalence rises nearly continuously throughout the first four or five decades of life. Moreover, seroprevalence is equal in males and females, in sharp contrast to Western Europe and the United States. The basis for this strikingly different epidemiology is not yet understood. The frequent occurrence of infection in young children in the Mediterranean and Africa suggests the existence of nonsexual routes of spread, and the equal infection rate in adult males and females also suggests different routes of spread from those observed in the United States. Exactly what these routes are remains conjectural, but the presence of virus in high titer in saliva of infected subjects suggests that a salivary route, as has been postulated for EBV transmission, is likely.

How does KSHV infection predispose to KS? Unlike EBV, in which the latency genes appear to be solely responsible for the oncogenic phenotypes, KS requires expression of both the KSHV latency genes and the lytic genes.[150] Much of what has been learned about the KSHV latency genes has come from the study of viral gene expression in cultured B cells from the KSHV-related primary effusion lymphomas (PEL). Most of the KSHV genes that are expressed in PEL have also been shown to be expressed in KS by *in situ* hybridization. There are seven latency genes known to be expressed in KS. One latency cluster expresses a set of three genes from a common promoter. Their products include *LANA*, an antigen that appears to function in KSHV genomic maintenance in latency, but also can impair p53 and Rb function as well as up-regulate the β-catenin pathway; expression of LANA in primary endothelial cells extends their survival, though it does not immortalize or transform them. Their products also include *V-cyclin*, a viral homologue of cellular cyclin D1 that can bind and activate cdk6, indicating that it is a functional cyclin. Its activity displays reduced sensitivity to the inhibitory effects of certain cdk inhibitors, suggesting that it might be refractory to normal regulatory controls imposed on its host counterparts. Their products include *V-FLIP*, a homologue of cellular inhibitors of caspase activation (Flice-inhibitory protein [FLIP]),which can also bind the inhibitor of κB (IκB) kinase complex and result in constitutive NF-κB activation.[151] The latter activity has been shown to be important in promoting cell survival and in inducing the cytoskeletal changes that give rise to the spindle cell morphology in infected endothelial cells. A second latent viral promoter directs production of transcripts encoding the kaposin family. These are transmembrane and soluble proteins that appear to be active in signal transduction. One of them, kaposin A, activates cytohesin-1, a protein involved in cell signaling cascades and regulating cell shape. Kaposins B and C appear to be involved in the regulation of signaling pathways that govern cytokine production.[150] This same promoter also engenders a series of microRNAs, most of which derive from an intron in the latent kaposin transcripts.[152] These small noncoding RNAs function by regulating the translation of other viral or host mRNAs, but the identities and functions of their putative targets are largely unknown. Deletion of most of the microRNAs promotes a modest increase in lytic reactivation, suggesting that one function of these small RNAs is to stabilize the latent state. A third latent promoter directs production of the K1 glycoprotein, a membrane protein that, when expressed in B cells, activates a signaling pathway similar to that of the B-cell antigen receptor. Its function in endothelial cells is unknown.

KS tumors also harbor smaller numbers of lytically infected cells that appear to be significant for the tumor phenotype. In patients with advanced AIDS, treatment with ganciclovir, a drug that blocks lytic but not latent KSHV infection, profoundly reduces the subsequent development of KS.[153] Although this result might mean simply that lytic reactivation from the lymphoid reservoir is necessary for spread to the endothelium to initiate latent infection there, it is also compatible with a requirement for ongoing KSHV replication in KS pathogenesis. The latter is an attractive notion because the virus contains numerous genes that are potent signaling molecules expressed principally during lytic growth.[154,155] Some of these are secreted factors (e.g., homologs of interleukin 6 [IL6], CC chemokines, and other factors), while others (e.g., the K1 protein and a virus-specific G protein–coupled receptor, v-GPCR) are transmembrane proteins that trigger deregulated signal transduction in the host, often leading to secretory products that can influence surrounding cells. For example, v-GPCR expression induces the release of vascular endothelial growth factor, a protein long speculated to play a role in the angiogenic phenotype of KS. Some of the viral chemokines can trigger angiogenesis as well; moreover, these molecules would be expected to contribute to the influx of inflammatory cells in the lesion—another hallmark of KS. Defining the relative contributions of latency and lytic growth to KS pathogenesis is an important area for KSHV research.

The homologies to EBV and HVS place KSHV/HHV-8 within the lymphotropic herpesvirus subfamily, an assignment supported by the finding of viral DNA in the B-cell compartment of the peripheral blood mononuclear cell population. KSHV is also associated with at least two lymphoproliferative conditions. The first is a rare B-cell lymphoma, PEL, which is largely limited to HIV-positive hosts.[156] These present as ascites tumors in the pleural and peritoneal cavities, often without clinically evident lymphadenopathy or bone marrow involvement. PEL cells are uniformly latently infected with KSHV; many (but not all) also bear latent EBV genomes as well. The other lymphoid lesion associated with KSHV is multicentric Castleman's disease (MCD), a complex and poorly understood lymphoproliferative syndrome that can occur in both HIV-positive and HIV-negative individuals. The HIV-positive form appears to be uniformly associated with KSHV, while only about half of the HIV-negative forms can be shown to harbor the virus.[157] Interestingly, KS and MCD can occur in the same individual; this provides an early epidemiologic clue suggesting the diseases have a common etiologic factor.

Study of viral gene expression in MCD has revealed some provocative surprises. Within the involved tissue, viral DNA is confined to B cells in the mantle zones surrounding the lymphoid follicles. There, both latently and lytically infected cells can be found, with a larger proportion of the infected cell population being in the lytic cycle than in KS.[158] Lytically infected cells produce large quantities of v-IL6, as well as host IL6, and it is thought that these factors drive the polyclonal expansion of B cells, which is the hallmark of this disorder. This is not to say that other viral gene products do not play a role in MCD; it seems likely that latency products are also involved, but the relative contributions of different viral gene products to pathogenesis is still being explored. Consistent with the importance of lytic infection in MCD, there is a report of transient remissions of fever and adenopathy in three patients with this condition who were treated with ganciclovir.[159] More robust therapeutic responses have been observed with rituximab, a monoclonal antibody to the B-cell antigen.[160] Interestingly, some patients with both KS and MCD have experienced worsening of their KS while on rituximab for treatment of MCD; the basis of this effect is unknown.

HUMAN POLYOMAVIRUSES

Merkel Cell Polyomavirus and Merkel Cell Carcinoma

Merkel cell carcinoma (MCC) is a highly lethal skin cancer that typically occurs in sun-exposed areas of elderly patients and in patients with HIV or chronic lymphocytic lymphoma. Because of the increased risk for MCC in immunocompromised individuals, Chang et al.[16] used next-generation sequencing of mRNA transcripts in MCC to search for viral sequences and found evidence for a novel human polyomavirus. Merkel cell polyomavirus (MCV) encodes a large T antigen (LT) and small T antigen (ST) highly similar to these oncoproteins encoded by the DNA tumor virus SV40. Several recent studies have found that approximately 70% of all MCC tumors contain chromosomally integrated copies of the MCV DNA. Furthermore, sequencing of the viral DNAs contained in MCC has revealed consistent evidence for mutations in the viral DNA that would retain expression of MCV ST and the N-terminal half of LT but delete the C-terminal half of MCV LT. The N-terminus of MCV LT, similar to other polyomavirus LT proteins, binds to Rb and Rb-related proteins to inactivate the Rb tumor suppressor pathway. Although 70% of all MCC contain integrated MCV viral DNA, there are no other features that have been found to distinguish between viral-positive and viral-negative cases of MCC.[161] Thus a causative role for this virus in MCC still needs to be established. Furthermore, MCV infection of skin turns out to be widespread, and over 80% of the population appears to be seropositive for this virus.[162]

SV40, the Human Polyomaviruses BK and JC and Human Cancer

There have been occasional reports for the past few decades suggesting the presence of SV40 DNA or antigens in a variety of different human cancers, including osteosarcomas, mesotheliomas, brain tumors, and non-Hodgkin's lymphomas. SV40 is a nonhuman primate virus that naturally infects Asian macaques. The major source of human exposure to SV40 was through contaminated poliovirus vaccines that were given between 1955 and 1963. SV40 is a highly oncogenic virus in rodent cells and has served as an extremely valuable model for determining the various mechanisms by which DNA tumor viruses transform cells and contribute to tumor formation. The possibility that SV40 might play an etiological role in specific human cancers has received some interest from the National Cancer Institute and from the Institute of Medicine.[163] These studies will not be summarized here, but the reader is referred to a number of recent reviews and on this subject.[164,165] There is, however, no epidemiologic evidence indicating a higher risk of cancers among the populations of individuals who received the SV40-contaminated vaccine.

There are no compelling data that the virus is circulating among human communities. Much of the data that claim an association of SV40 DNA with human tumors has been gathered by the use of the PCR assays, which are error prone, and has been difficult to confirm. In fact, the only double-blind study conducted thus far, involving nine different laboratories, was unable to confirm a correlation.[166] The possibility that SV40 (or any virus for that matter) is involved in the etiology of human cancer is strengthened when multiple lines of evidence (including epidemiology, as well as pathogenic and molecular mechanisms) converge. Thus it remains premature to consider SV40 a human cancer virus. Additional blind studies are ongoing to investigate the potential that SV40 may be associated with specific human cancers.

There have also been occasional reports implicating the human polyomaviruses BK and JC to specific human cancers. Both BK and JC are rather ubiquitous viruses, and over 80% of the population has antibodies to BK and JC. Like SV40, BK and JC are also highly oncogenic in rodents. JV can also cause glial tumors experimentally in inoculated nonhuman primates. Of potential interest is the finding of BK DNA in the epithelium of benign and proliferative inflammatory atrophy, suggesting that the virus may have some yet undefined role in early prostate cancer progression.[167] It should be noted, however, that a comprehensive blinded controlled analysis of human tumors for SV40, BK, or JC DNA sequences yielded no convincing evidence of any association.[168]

Selected References

The full list of references for this chapter appears in the online version.

1. Rous P. A sarcoma of the fowl transmissible by an agent separable from the tumor cells. *J Exp Med* 1911;13:397.
2. Shope RE, Hurst EW. Infectious papillomatosis of rabbits; with a note on the histopathology. *J Exp Med* 1933;58:607.
4. Gross L. Pathogenic properties, and "vertical" transmission of the mouse leukemia agent. *Proc Soc Exp Biol Med* 1951;62:523.
7. Epstein MA, Achong BG, Barr YM. Virus particles in cultured lymphoblasts from Burkitt's lymphoma. *Lancet* 1964;1:702.
10. Orth G, Favre M, Breitburd F, et al. Epidermodysplasia verruciformis: a model for the role of papillomaviruses in human cancer. *Cold Spring Harbor Conf Cell Prolif* 1980;7:259.
12. Poiesz BJ, Ruscetti FW, Reitz MS, Kalyanaraman VS, Gallo RC. Isolation of a new type C retrovirus (HTLV) in primary uncultured cells of a patient with Sezary T-cell leukemia. *Nature* 1981;294:268.
13. Boshart M, Gissman L, Ikenberg H, et al. A new type of papillomavirus DNA, its presence in genital cancer biopsies and in cell lines derived from cervical cancer. *EMBO J* 1984;3:1151.
14. Durst M, Gissmann L, Idenburg H, zur Hausen H. A papillomavirus DNA from a cervical carcinoma and its prevalence in cancer biopsy samples from different geographic regions. *Proc Natl Acad Sci U S A* 1983;80:3812.
15. Chang Y, Cesarman E, Pessin MS, et al. Identification of herpesvirus-like DNA sequences in AIDS-associated Kaposi's sarcoma. *Science* 1994;266:1865.
16. Feng H, Shuda M, Chang Y, Moore PS. Clonal integration of a polyomavirus in human Merkel cell carcinoma. *Science* 2008;319:1096.
18. Beasley RP. Hepatitis B virus—the major etiology of the hepatocellular carcinoma. *Cancer* 1988;61:1942.
19. Ganem D, Prince AM. Hepatitis B virus infection—natural history and clinical consequences. *N Engl J Med* 2004;350:1118.

21. Guidotti LG, Chisari FV. Immunobiology and pathogenesis of viral hepatitis. *Annu Rev Pathol* 2006;1:23.
25. Seeger C, Zoulim F, Mason WS. Hepadnaviruses. In: Knipe DM, Howley PM, eds. *Field's Virology*. Philadelphia: Lippincott Williams & Wilkins, 2007:2977.
26. Howley PM, Lowy DR. Papillomaviruses. In: Knipe DM, Howley PM, eds. *Field's Virology*. Philadelphia: Lippincott Williams & Wilkins, 2007:2299.
27. Münger K, Phelps WC, Bubb V, Howley PM, Schlegel R. The E6 and E7 genes of the human papillomavirus type 16 together are necessary and sufficient for transformation of primary human keratinocytes. *J Virol* 1989; 63:4417.
28. Rous P, Kidd JG. The carcinogenic effect of a virus upon tarred skin. *Science* 1936;83:468.
31. Parkin DM, Bray F, Ferlay J, Pisani P. Global cancer statistics, 2002. *CA Cancer J Clin* 2005;55:74.
36. Meisels A, Fortin R. Condylomatous lesions of the cervix and vagina. I. Cytologic patterns. *Acta Cytol* 1976;20:505.
40. Dyson N, Howley PM, Münger K, Harlow E. The human papillomavirus-16 E7 oncoprotein is able to bind the retinoblastoma gene product. *Science* 1989;243:934.
45. Duensing S, Lee LY, Duensing A, et al. The human papillomavirus type 16 E6 and E7 oncoproteins cooperate to induce mitotic defects and genomic instability by uncoupling centrosome duplication from the cell division cycle. *Proc Natl Acad Sci U S A* 2000;97:10002.
47. Werness BA, Levine AJ, Howley PM. Association of human papillomavirus types 16 and 18 E6 proteins with p53. *Science* 1990;248:76.
48. Huibregtse JM, Scheffner M, Howley PM. Cloning and expression of the cDNA for E6-AP: a protein that mediates the interaction of the human papillomavirus E6 oncoprotein with p53. *Mol Cell Biol* 1993;13:775.
49. Scheffner M, Huibregtse JM, Vierstra RD, Howley PM. The HPV-16 E6 and E6-AP complex functions as a ubiquitin-protein ligase in the ubiquination of p53. *Cell* 1993;75:495.
51. Klingelhutz AJ, Foster SA, McDougall JK. Telomerase activation by the E6 gene product of human papillomavirus type 16. *Nature* 1996;380:79.
52. Gardiol D, Kuhne C, Glaunsinger B, et al. Oncogenic human papillomavirus E6 proteins target the discs large tumour suppressor for proteasome-mediated degradation. *Oncogene* 1999;18:5487.
59. Gillison ML. Human papillomavirus-associated head and neck cancer is a distinct epidemiologic, clinical, and molecular entity. *Semin Oncol* 2004; 31:744.
67. Jackson S, Harwood C, Thomas M, Banks L, Storey A. Role of Bak in UV-induced apoptosis in skin cancer and abrogation by HPV E6 proteins. *Genes Dev* 2000;14:3065.
69. Lowy DR, Schiller JT. Prophylactic human papillomavirus vaccines. *J Clin Invest* 2006;116:1167.
72. Pastrana DV, Gambhira R, Buck CB, et al. Cross-neutralization of cutaneous and mucosal papillomavirus types with anti-sera to the amino terminus of L2. *Virology* 2005;337:365.
75. Rickinson AB, Kieff E. Epstein-Barr virus. In: Knipe DM, Howley PM, eds. *Field's virology*. Philadelphia: Lippincott Williams & Wilkins, 2007:2655.
79. Klein G, Giovanella BC, Lindahl T, et al. Direct evidence for the presence of Epstein-Barr virus DNA and nuclear antigen in malignant epithelial cells from patients with poorly differentiated carcinoma of the nasopharynx. *Proc Natl Acad Sci U S A* 1974;71:4737.
92. Pelicci PG, Knowles DM, Arlin ZA, et al. Multiple monoclonal B-cell expansions and c-myc oncogene rearrangements in acquired immunodefiency syndrome-related lymphoprolifeative disorders. *J Exp Med* 1986;164:2049.
94. Purtilo DT. Immune deficiency predisposing to Epstein-Barr virus-induced lymphoproliferative diseases: the X-linked lymphoproliferative syndrome as a model. *Adv Cancer Res* 1981;34:279.
95. Pfeffer S, Zavolan M, Grasser FA, et al. Identification of virus-encoded microRNAs. *Science* 2004;304:734.
109. Nachmani D, Stern-Ginossar N, Sarid R, Mandelboim O. Diverse herpesvirus microRNAs target the stress-induced immune ligand MICB to escape recognition by natural killer cells. *Cell Host Microbe* 2009;5:376.
110. Dolken L, Malterer G, Erhard F, et al. Systematic analysis of viral and cellular microRNA targets in cells latently infected with human gammaherpesviruses by RISC immunoprecipitation assay. *Cell Host Microbe* 2010;7:324.
114. Smuk G, Illes A, Keresztes K, et al. Pheno- and genotypic features of Epstein-Barr virus associated B-cell lymphoproliferations in peripheral T-cell lymphomas. *Pathol Oncol Res* 2010;16:377.
132. Kutok JL, Wang F. Spectrum of Epstein-Barr virus-associated diseases. *Annu Rev Pathol* 2006;1:375.
134. Raab-Traub N, Flynn K. The structure of the terminal of the Epstein-Barr virus as a marker of clonal cellular proliferation. *Cell* 1986;47:883.
135. Tinguely M, Rosenquist R, Sundstrom C, et al. Analysis of a clonally related mantle cell and Hodgkin lymphoma indicates Epstein-Barr virus infection of a Hodgkin/Reed-Sternberg cell precursor in a germinal center. *Am J Surg Pathol* 2003;27:1483.
137. Walling DM, Flaitz CM, Nichols CM. Epstein-Barr virus replication in oral hairy leukoplakia: response, persistence, and resistance to treatment with valacyclovir. *J Infect Dis* 2003;188:883.
146. Ensoli B, Sirianni MC. Kaposi's sarcoma pathogenesis: a link between immunology and tumor biology. *Crit Rev Oncog* 1998;9:107.
150. Ganem D. Kaposi's sarcoma-associated herpesvirus. In: Knipe DM, Howley PM., eds. *Field's Virology*. Philadelphia: Lippincott Williams & Wilkins, 2007:2847.
154. Moore PS, Boshoff C, Weiss RA, Chang Y. Molecular mimicry of human cytokine and cytokine response pathway genes by KSHV. *Science* 1996; 274:1739.
156. Cesarman E. The role of Kaposi's sarcoma-associated herpesvirus (KSHV/HHV-8) in lymphoproliferative diseases. *Recent Results Cancer Res* 2002; 159:27.
159. Casper C, Nichols WG, Huang ML, Corey L, Wald A. Remission of HHV-8 and HIV-associated multicentric Castleman disease with ganciclovir treatment. *Blood* 2004;103:1632.
161. Fischer N, Brandner J, Fuchs F, Moll I, Grundhoff A. Detection of Merkel cell polyomavirus (MCPyV) in Merkel cell carcinoma cell lines: cell morphology and growth phenotype do not reflect presence of the virus. *Int J Cancer* 2010;126:2133.
162. Pastrana DV, Tolstov YL, Becker JC, et al. Quantitation of human seroresponsiveness to Merkel cell polyomavirus. *PLoS Pathog* 2009;5:e1000578
164. Poulin DL, DeCaprio JA. Is there a role for SV40 in human cancer? *J Clin Oncol* 2006;24:4356.
168. Rollison DE, Utaipat U, Ryschkewitsch C, et al. Investigation of human brain tumors for the presence of polyomavirus genome sequences by two independent laboratories. *Int J Cancer* 2005;113:769.

CHAPTER 16 RNA VIRUSES

GARY L. BUCHSCHACHER, Jr. AND FLOSSIE WONG-STAAL

Viruses have long been hypothesized to cause some cancers. Although several DNA viruses are associated with the development of malignancy, members of only two RNA virus families—*Retroviridae* and *Flaviviridae*—have thus far been associated with development of neoplastic disease.[1,2] In humans, these viruses include the retroviruses human T-lymphotropic virus (HTLV) and human immunodeficiency virus (HIV), and the flavivirus hepatitis C virus (HCV). Human T-lymphotropic virus type 1 (HTLV-1) appears to contribute directly to the development of adult T-cell leukemia (ATL); HIV and HCV are associated with human malignancy, but likely contribute to its development in an indirect manner.

However, a number of animal retroviruses cause cancer in their natural hosts and have been important tools for understanding oncogenesis in both humans and animals. The discovery and characterization of oncogenes and the subsequent elucidation of protooncogene functions have been closely intertwined and made possible by the study of retroviruses. In this chapter, the discussion will focus on the molecular genetics and the characteristics of retroviruses relevant to oncogenesis, and will explore the roles of the retroviruses HTLV-1, HTLV-2, and HIV and of the flavivirus HCV in human cancers. In many examples, although these viruses may play key initiating or contributing roles to carcinogenesis, additional events are needed for infection to yield the full malignant phenotype.

RETROVIRUSES: BACKGROUND, REPLICATION CYCLE, AND MOLECULAR GENETICS

In the past, retroviruses had been classified on the basis of pathogenesis into the Oncoretrovirus (the retroviruses associated with tumor formation), Lentivirus, and Spumavirus groups, or on the basis of virus particle morphology (virus types A-D). Now, however, the retroviruses are organized into seven genera based on molecular genetic analysis: *Alpha-, Beta-, Gamma-, Delta-*, and *Epsilon-retroviruses, Lentiviruses,* and *Spumaviruses*. This taxonomic system divides the Oncoretroviruses into five genera. There are few known human retroviruses: the *Deltaretroviruses* HTLV-1 and HTLV-2 (additional *Deltavirus* isolates, termed *HTLV-3* and *HTLV-4* also have been reported[3–5]), and the *Lentiviruses* HIV-1 and HIV-2. The spumavirus formerly termed *human foamy virus* is, in fact, a simian retrovirus isolated from contaminated human cell cultures (it is now termed *chimpanzee foamy virus human isolate*). Human endogenous retroviruses are endogenous retroviral elements contained within the human genome but are not classified as retroviruses per se. Their possible roles in normal development and in disease pathogenesis, including development of cancer, are unclear at this time.[6–12] There also have been reports associating a *Gammaretrovirus,* xenotropic murine leukemia virus-related virus (XMRV), with prostate carcinoma, although confirmation and possible significance of this finding need further study.[13]

Retroviruses are unique among animal viruses in having an RNA genome that replicates through a DNA intermediate.[14] Retroviral virions contain two identical plus-sense RNA molecules. The RNA genome (Fig. 16.1) contains a 5′ untranslated region, the three genes common to all retroviruses—*gag, pol,* and *env*—and a 3′ untranslated region and polyadenylated tail. In general, the *gag* gene encodes viral structural proteins, *pol* encodes viral enzymatic proteins, and *env* encodes viral envelope glycoproteins.

The retroviral replication cycle is illustrated in Figure 16.2. Following entry into a cell, the single-stranded viral genome is converted to a double-stranded DNA copy (Fig. 16.1) by reverse transcriptase,[15] an RNA-dependent DNA polymerase. Then, the retroviral integrase protein inserts the double-stranded DNA viral genome into a host cell chromosome where it permanently resides as a provirus.[16] An integrated retroviral provirus resembles cellular genes in that it is duplicated along with the cell's genome, passed on to daughter cells during mitosis, and subsequently transcribed and processed into mRNA.

Reverse transcription is a complicated process that can use both viral RNA molecules as templates for DNA synthesis and involves RNA and DNA template strand-switching events during nucleotide polymerization. This process results in duplication of the 5′ and 3′ ends of the genome, thus forming the long terminal repeats (LTRs), which are composed of the U3, R, and U5 regions. The viral promoter and enhancer functions reside within the LTR. Transcription initiates in the 5′ LTR and proceeds to the polyadenylation (polyA) signal usually located in the 3′ LTR.

In summary, a number of features unique to the retroviral replication cycle demonstrate how retroviruses may be involved in the development of or used for the study of the molecular basis of cell transformation.[17] Integration of the provirus into the cellular genome can permanently introduce genes into a cell or can result in mutation or altered regulation of genes. In addition, the molecular mechanism by which reverse transcription occurs is a fertile environment in which alterations of genes or the creation of cancer-causing genes might take place.[18,19]

Mechanisms of Retroviral Oncogenesis

Infection by members of the *Alpha-, Beta-, Gamma-, Delta-*, and *Epsilon-retrovirus* genera may lead to the development of neoplastic disease in different ways (the genera are classified based on variations in genetic structure, not by shared mechanisms of pathogenesis), but, in general, individual members of each genus can be thought of as either acutely or slowly transforming

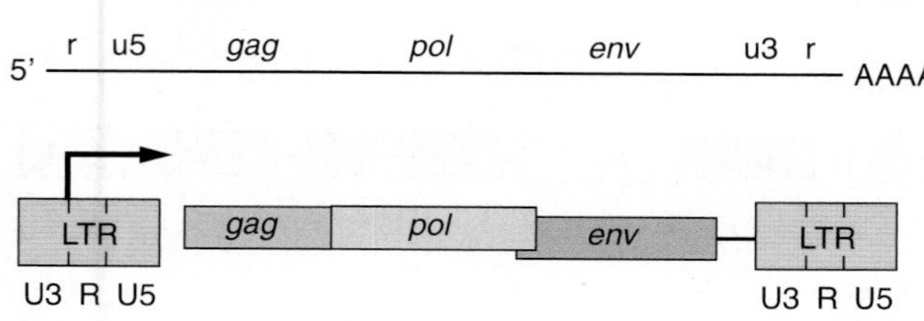

FIGURE 16.1 Retrovirus genetic organization. General genome structure of a typical replication competent oncoretrovirus. The structure of the double-stranded DNA copy (provirus) is shown below that of the genomic RNA. In the provirus, *gag* (encoding viral structural proteins), *pol* (viral replication enzymes), and *env* (viral envelope glycoproteins) genes are flanked on each end by the long terminal repeats (LTRs). The viral promoter/enhancer is located in the 5′ U3, with transcription termination and poly A signals located in the 3′ LTR. The *arrow* indicates point and direction of transcription initiation. U3, unique 3′ region; R, repeat; U5, unique 5′ region.

viruses. In the case of the acutely transforming retroviruses, virtually all infected cells are swiftly transformed, but for other retroviruses, transformation is an unusual and much delayed outcome that often depends on the cell's accrual of additional alteration of its DNA. This latter group includes the classic slowly transforming retroviruses and the *trans*-acting retroviruses. Reverse transcription and integration of the viral genome into the cell favors the three major mechanisms by which oncogenic retroviruses may participate in the malignant transformation process[20] (Fig. 16.3):

1. Slowly transforming viruses (e.g., avian leukosis virus, an *Alpharetrovirus*) alter cellular gene expression by random integration of a provirus within or adjacent to cellular protooncogenes (insertional mutagenesis). Direct physical disruption of a gene or effects of viral promoters and enhancers on cellular gene expression can lead to a malignant phenotype in infected cells.
2. Acutely transforming retroviruses (e.g., Rous sarcoma virus [RSV], an *Alpharetrovirus*) have incorporated into their genomes viral oncogenes derived from cellular protooncogenes (protooncogene capture) and subsequently transfer these altered or deregulated oncogenes into newly infected cells, thus leading to development of a malignant phenotype.
3. *Trans*-acting retroviruses (e.g., HTLV-1, a *Deltaretrovirus*) alter cellular gene expression and function and, consequently, the control of cell growth via viral protein(s) that act in *trans*.

Slowly Transforming Retroviruses: Insertional Mutagenesis

Simple integration of a provirus into the genome of a cell can, rarely, be tumorigenic by leading to aberrant activity of cellular genes. Retroviruses that act in this manner have been termed *chronic*, or slow-acting, tumor viruses: they do not transform cells in tissue culture and, *in vivo*, a long-latency period between infection and tumorigenesis is typical. In general, in addition to the mutagenesis caused by provirus integration, tumors caused by slowly transforming retroviruses require additional mutagenic events to take place in order that their transforming properties become apparent.

Most proviral integrations have no effect on the phenotype of the infected cell, but rarely can lead to phenotypically evident insertional mutagenesis in one of a number of ways. Proviral integration might disrupt a gene (typically a tumor suppressor gene) by integrating within the gene (in an exon or intron) or by disrupting the promoter of the gene, thereby preventing production of a functional protein. Alternatively, insertion upstream or within a gene can also result in aberrant production of a cellular protein if the retroviral promoters in either the 5′ or 3′ LTRs are active and, because of readthrough transcription, result in production of chimeric viral/cellular mRNAs. The protein derived from this mRNA may be wild type but produced in increased amounts, or may be a truncated or viral/cellular chimeric protein due to readthrough transcription and aberrant RNA splicing. The enhancers present in the retroviral LTRs also can affect expression of cellular genes either upstream or downstream of the provirus integration site and genes in either the sense or antisense orientation relative to the provirus.

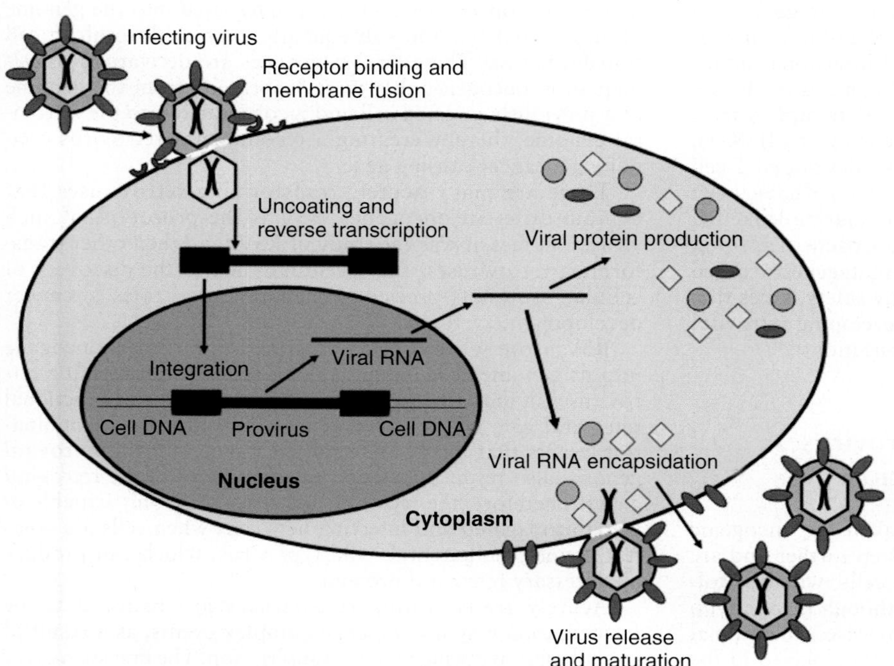

FIGURE 16.2 The retroviral replication cycle begins when retroviral envelope glycoproteins bind to specific cellular receptors and mediate fusion of viral and cellular membranes, resulting in release of the viral capsid into the cell. The retroviral RNA genome is then uncoated, reverse transcribed into a double-stranded DNA copy, and integrated into the host cell genome, where it resides as a provirus. Transcription of the provirus results in generation of viral RNA, which can be translated into viral proteins. These viral proteins then package viral genomic RNA into infectious virions that are released from the cell. (General features shared by retroviruses are illustrated; there are variations of these processes among different retroviruses.)

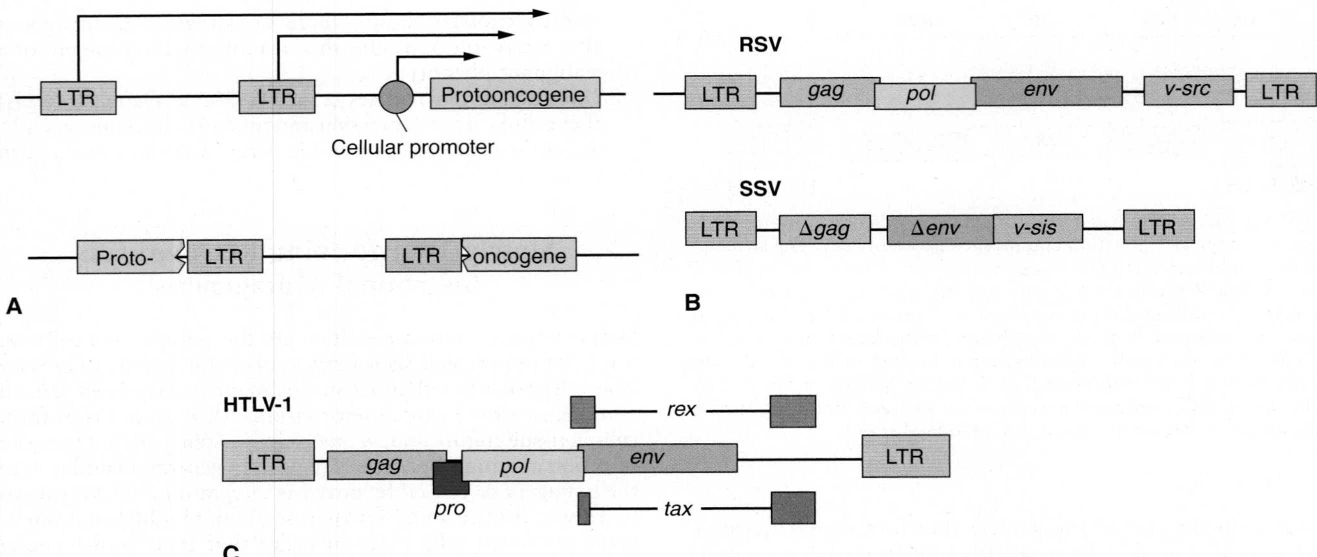

FIGURE 16.3 Three types of oncogenic retroviruses. **A:** Slowly transforming retroviruses. In the upper example, a provirus has integrated upstream of a cellular protooncogene. The viral promoters may alter protooncogene expression directly (via readthrough transcription originating from the 5′ long terminal repeat (LTR) or from transcripts aberrantly originating in the 3′ LTR or indirectly via the effect of viral enhancers increasing transcription from cellular promoters (the viral enhancer can also affect expression of cellular genes 5′ to and in the opposite orientation of the site of provirus integration). In the second example, insertional mutagenesis and consequent gene disruption is illustrated. This process may lead to inactivation of a tumor suppressor or to production of a mutant cellular protein that could lead to oncogenesis. In both cases, aberrant splicing could lead to production of chimeric viral-cellular proteins. *Arrows* indicate points of initiation and direction of transcription. **B:** Acutely transforming retroviruses. Rous sarcoma virus (RSV) and simian sarcoma virus (SSV), retroviruses that contain oncogenes, are shown. RSV is unique in that the oncogene, v-*src*, has been added to the viral genome without concomitant loss of replicative genes. SSV, an example of the more common oncogene-containing retroviruses, is not replication-competent; the recombination that led to v-*sis* insertion resulted in deletion of some viral sequences. **C:** *Trans*-acting retroviruses. In addition to *gag, pol,* and *env,* the human T-lymphotropic virus type 1 (HTLV-1) genome encodes the proteins Tax, Rev, $p12^{I}$, $p13^{I}$, and $p30^{II}$, derived from open reading frames I–IV located in the pX region. Tax (and possibly $p12^{I}$) is implicated in the genesis of adult T-cell leukemia through interactions with cellular transcription factors, resulting in alteration of expression of many T-cell growth regulation genes, including cytokines and cell cycle control elements.

With the exception of rare cases of T-cell malignancy that appears to involve a monoclonal expansion of an HIV-1–infected cell, naturally occurring retroviruses have not been shown to cause malignancy by insertional mutagenesis in humans. However, humans are clearly susceptible to malignancy associated with retroviral-mediated insertional mutagenesis. In a gene transfer clinical trial using a murine leukemia virus (a *Gammaretrovirus*) vector in an attempt to treat X-linked severe combined immunodeficiency (SCIDX-1), nearly half of the treated pediatric patients developed T-cell acute lymphoblastic leukemia that appears to have been caused, at least in part, by insertion of the murine leukemia virus vector provirus within or near protooncogenes (*LMO-2, BMI,1, CCND2*).[21–23] Possible insertional mutagenesis caused by retroviral vectors is just one of the many safety issues that must be taken into consideration when developing retroviral vectors for use in clinical gene transfer applications.[24]

Acutely Transforming Retroviruses: Oncogene Transduction

Acutely transforming retroviruses have taken the oncogenic potential of slow-acting retroviruses one step further and are capable of rapidly transforming infected cells, which is followed by subsequent tumor formation. Although there are no known acutely transforming human retroviruses, the animal viruses are important because of the roles they played in the discovery of oncogenes and in the continued study of the molecular mechanisms of tumor formation.

Acutely transforming retroviruses are mutant retroviruses that encode oncogenes that, when integrated into the genome of an infected cell and subsequently expressed, result in cell transformation. These viral oncogenes are derivatives of cellular protooncogenes that were "captured" from the genome of a previously infected cell and incorporated into the retroviral genome, thereby creating a recombinant retrovirus containing a cancer-causing gene.

There are many acutely transforming retroviruses that contain different oncogenes. RSV is the prototype of such viruses. In fact, it was the study of RSV (and then other transforming retroviruses) that eventually led to the discovery of cellular protooncogenes and their potential roles in cancer development.[25]

RSV arose when a retrovirus incorporated an oncogene into its genome; it is unique among acutely transforming retroviruses in that it encodes an oncogene (v-*src*) and functional retroviral *gag, pol,* and *env* genes. Typically, the recombination events that incorporate the oncogene into the retroviral genome also result in deletion of some or all of the retroviral genes. Therefore, the recombinant viruses are only capable of being propagated and infecting new cells when cells are coinfected with the parental, wild type virus, which can produce all necessary retroviral proteins.

Acutely transforming retroviruses are believed to be formed, following a number of complex events, as a result of recombination during reverse transcription. The first such event is the integration of a wild type retroviral provirus within or near a cellular protooncogene, as has been described for slowly transforming retroviruses. The next step involves formation of chimeric retroviral/cellular protooncogene mRNA, resulting from transcription from the 5′ LTR, with subsequent readthrough transcription into the cellular protooncogene. This chimeric viral/cellular mRNA can then be copackaged into a virion (which normally contain two identical copies of the viral genome) capable of infecting a new cell. Then, because reverse transcription of the retroviral genome involves template strand-switching events and also may lead to recombination events, nonhomologous recombination between wild type and chimeric molecules can occur, thereby resulting in a novel provirus with an oncogene incorporated into its genome.

A protooncogene generally is not transduced intact from the cell to the retroviral genome: deletion, frameshift, and point mutations are likely to occur during the process. In addition, the chimeric molecule can result in production of a viral/cellular fusion protein. Any or all of these alterations to the cellular protooncogene might contribute to altering the activity, level of expression, stability, function, or localization of the resulting protein, therefore resulting in the conversion of a cellular protooncogene with the *potential* to cause cancer into a viral oncogene *fully capable* of doing so.

Trans-Activating Retroviruses

A third manner of transformation involves *trans*-acting viral proteins that affect the expression or function of cellular growth and differentiation genes. This mechanism of oncogenesis is illustrated by HTLV-1, the only human retrovirus known to cause cancer directly.

HUMAN T-LYMPHOTROPIC VIRUS TYPE 1

The Viral Replication Cycle and Its Implications for Virus Spread

ATL is an aggressive malignancy of CD4+ T cells caused by HTLV-1.[26] Although HTLV-1 shares many features with other oncoretroviruses, it is considerably more complex genetically and biologically.[27] In addition to *gag, pol,* and *env,* the virus genome contains additional open reading frames (encoding Tax, Rex, p12^{I}, p13^{II}, p30^{II}) located in a region at the 3′ end of the genome termed pX.[28] HTLV-1 basic leucine zipper (HBZ) protein is transcribed from the complementary strand of the genome and may play a role in leukemogenesis.[29–31] The two best characterized of these accessory proteins are the *trans*-regulating proteins Tax and Rex. Both proteins are expressed early in the viral replication cycle and are important for expression of viral genes; as such, they are analogous to the HIV proteins Tat and Rev. Rex promotes the cytoplasmic accumulation of singly-spliced (*env*) and unspliced (genomic) mRNAs.[32] Tax activates transcription from the HTLV-1 LTR by associating with a number of cellular transcription factors. The precise roles in the viral replication cycle of the additional HTLV-1 proteins (p12^{I}, p13^{II}, p30^{II}) derived from translation of alternatively spliced RNA of the pX region are not entirely clear, but the proteins appear to be required for *in vivo* infectivity of the virus.

Although HTLV-1 shares a number of features with HIV—a complex genetic structure, tropism for CD4+ T lymphocytes, induction of syncytia in cultured T cells, and similar routes of transmission between individuals—HTLV-1 infection is not associated with marked cellular immunodeficiency unless ATL develops. In addition, although there are points during the course of HIV infection at which cell-to-cell transmission of the virus is important, infection by free virions is typical, with high levels of viremia detected in HIV-1–infected individuals. By contrast, in individuals infected with HTLV-1, significant viremia is not detected; it appears that both in culture and *in vivo,* virus spreads to uninfected cells by cell-to-cell transmission of the virus. This cell-to-cell spread of HTLV-1 appears to involve polarization of the cytoskeleton of infected cells to a cell-cell junction, promoting spread of virus to new cells.[33] In addition to cell-to-cell virus transmission, the number of HTLV-1–infected cells within an individual increases by simple mitosis of provirus-containing T cells, thereby amplifying the number of infected T cells. HTLV-1 infection in an individual patient can persist even in the presence of a strong immune response.[34,35]

Models for HTLV-1 Leukemogenesis

The most common outcome of HTLV-1 infection is an asymptomatic carrier state; HTLV-1 carriers have an estimated lifetime risk of developing ATL of around 3% to 5%, with a typical latency period from time of infection to development of malignancy of 30 to 50 years. Given these facts, it is apparent that factors other than simple viral infection must be necessary for leukemogenesis. The sites of proviral insertion are random from patient to patient, indicating that *cis*-acting insertional mutagenesis does not play a role in tumorigenesis. Nor does the virus appear to encode a host-derived oncogene: no homologies between human cellular genes and nonstructural HTLV-1 genes have been observed. A third genetic mechanism for tumorigenesis, which appears to be a multistep process, is thus implicated, with the Tax protein being central to transformation.[36–40]

Tax promotes viral gene expression by indirectly activating the viral promoter in the LTR via interaction with cellular transcription proteins. However, the interaction of Tax with various transcription factors also transactivates numerous cellular gene promoters.[41,42] The cellular transcription pathways activated by Tax include activating transcription factor/cyclic adenosine monophosphate-responsive element binding protein (ATF/CREB), nuclear factor-κB, and serum response factor. Tax is able to bind directly to the TATA-binding protein, a component of the transcriptional complex, and to p300 and CREB-binding protein, both of which are transcriptional coactivators.

Among the cellular genes transactivated by Tax, the most relevant are the interleukin (IL)-2 and IL-2 receptor α (IL-2Rα) genes. Unlike normal resting T cells, ATL cells and T cells transformed *in vitro* by HTLV-1 constitutively express the alpha chain of the IL-2 receptor at high levels, which can stimulate proliferation of infected cells. In addition, possible interactions between another HTLV-1 protein (p12^{I}) and the gamma subunit of IL-2R may contribute to ligand-independent activation of this receptor, potentially resulting in stimulation and expansion of the pool of infected cells.

Tax has also been shown to down-regulate expression of a cellular DNA repair enzyme, β-DNA polymerase, a potentially straightforward link to accelerated accumulation of mutations. In addition, expression of a large number of genes involved in cell proliferation is transactivated by Tax, including granulocyte-macrophage colony-stimulating factor, the protooncogenes *c-fos* and *c-sis,* HLA class I, vimentin, and tumor necrosis factor.

Tax also has been shown to interact with and presumably inactivate a number of cell cycle-related proteins,[43] including the cyclin-dependent kinase inhibitor p16^{INK4A} and the cell cycle checkpoint protein, MAD1. Tax activates the promoter of p21$^{waf1/cip1}$, also a cyclin-dependent kinase inhibitor, and, through the activation of the ATF/CREB pathway, suppresses

ETIOLOGY AND EPIDEMIOLOGY OF CANCER

the activity of p53, which can prevent p53-induced apoptosis. It also has been suggested that constitutive action of the IL-2 receptor pathway allows cells to avoid apoptosis through an unknown mechanism.

In summary, although the exact steps in HTLV-1-induced leukemogenesis are unclear, Tax (and probably p12^{I}) seems to play a critical role by direct interaction with cellular proteins involved in transcription, cell cycle regulation, cell proliferation, and apoptosis.[44] It appears that additional mutational events are necessary for the transition from cell immortalization to monoclonality and acute ATL. Immortalization and propagation of clones of infected cells probably allow alterations in the cell cycle and apoptosis pathways to accumulate, allowing a dominant transformed clone to emerge. Further work to determine the key events in the complex network of cell cycle/apoptosis pathways will help elucidate the fundamental cell biology leading to HTLV-1 leukemogenesis.

HUMAN T-LYMPHOTROPIC VIRUS TYPE 2

HTLV-2 is closely related to HTLV-1, sharing the same overall genetic organization and 70% homology at the amino acid level. The virus was isolated from a patient with atypical T-cell variant hairy cell leukemia and subsequently from two other individuals. Other disease associations have been reported; however, convincing epidemiologic data for an etiologic role for HTLV-2 in human disease are lacking.

HUMAN IMMUNODEFICIENCY VIRUS

HIV-1 and HIV-2 are members of the *Lentivirus* genus of retroviruses. Both viruses became human pathogens after zoonotic transmission to humans from primate reservoirs. Although HIV-2 can also cause AIDS in humans and monkeys, the majority of AIDS cases worldwide are the result of HIV-1 infection.[45] Therefore, this discussion will focus on HIV-1.

As with HTLV-1, the HIV genome (Fig. 16.4) and replication cycle are complex.[46–52] In sharp contrast to HTLV-1, however, HIV replicates actively following initial infection, which results in high levels of viremia. In addition, HIV, unlike HTLV-1, is highly cytopathic for CD4-positive T cells.

HIV encodes two *trans*-acting proteins, Tat and Rev, analogous in function to the HTLV-1 proteins Tax and Rex. Like HTLV-1 Tax, HIV Tat is necessary for efficient expression from the viral promoter in the 5′ LTR. At a molecular level, however, Tat and Tax act through different mechanisms. Instead of interacting indirectly with a region of the proviral LTR via interactions with cellular transcription factors, Tat interacts directly with a 5′ LTR region of HIV RNA known as the *trans*-activating region, and promotes processive transcription through further interactions with cellular factors that modify RNA polymerase II function. HTLV Rex and HIV Rev use similar mechanisms to promote expression of viral structural and enzymatic proteins by binding to their respective RNA response elements, *rxre* and *rre,* to mediate the export of full-length and singly spliced viral transcripts from the nucleus to the cytoplasm.[53]

In addition to Tat and Rev, HIV encodes a number of accessory proteins not found in other retroviruses. These proteins include Vpr, Vif, Vpu, and Nef, the functions of which are not yet fully elucidated, although each appears to play a role in allowing the virus to evade a variety of forms of cell restrictions on HIV replication. The protein Vpr also contributes to the ability of HIV to infect nondividing cells, a property unique to lentiviruses.[54] Although none of the accessory genes are absolutely necessary for generating infectious virions *in vitro,* growing evidence indicates they allow effective viral replication by counteracting cellular factors that would otherwise interfere with viral replication, thereby contributing to transmissibility, viral burden, and pathogenicity *in vivo.*[55–60]

The immunodeficiency resulting from HIV infection can contribute to the development of malignancies.[61] There is, however, no evidence to suggest that HIV is directly oncogenic. In HIV-infected persons, non-Hodgkin lymphoma (Burkitt, immunoblastic, and primary CNS), Kaposi sarcoma, and cervical cancer are all AIDS-defining illnesses. In addition, anal squamous cell carcinoma is commonly seen in AIDS patients. Many of the neoplasms common to AIDS patients are associated with infection by DNA viruses. These viruses include Kaposi sarcoma-associated herpesvirus/human herpes virus-8, Epstein-Barr virus, and human papilloma virus. These viruses and their associations with oncogenesis are discussed in detail elsewhere in this volume.

HEPATITIS C VIRUS

HCV infection is a well-established risk factor for the development of hepatocellular carcinoma (HCC).[62,63] However, its major role in oncogenesis is likely to be indirect. HCV belongs to the *Hepacivirus* genus of the *Flaviviridae* family of viruses. Virions consist of a single-stranded plus sense RNA molecule surrounded by a nucleocapsid and envelope. The viral genome (Fig. 16.5) has a single, large open reading frame encoding viral proteins (reviewed in ref. 64). The 5′ leader sequence of the viral genome is highly conserved among HCV isolates and contains stem-loop structures, one of which acts as an internal ribosome entry site. HCV encodes a polyprotein precursor that is proteolytically processed into viral structural and nonstructural proteins. The structural proteins include the capsid (C) protein and envelope (E1, E2) glycoproteins. Among the nonstructural proteins, NS2/NS3 is a metalloprotease that cleaves in *cis* at the NS2/3 junction; NS3 possesses serine protease and helicase activities; NS4A is a cofactor of the NS3 protease; NS4B may have various roles in HCV replication, one of which is the formation of a membranous web where replication occurs; NS5B encodes the RNA-dependent RNA polymerase responsible for viral nucleic acid replication. Additional proteins and peptides of undefined functions are also encoded by the open reading frame. The extreme 3′ end of the RNA genome contains a short untranslated region (composed of the VR, polyU/UC, and 3′X segments) important for viral nucleic acid replication.[65]

To gain entry into the hepatocyte, HCV first docks and attaches to the host cell surface, most likely via the interaction

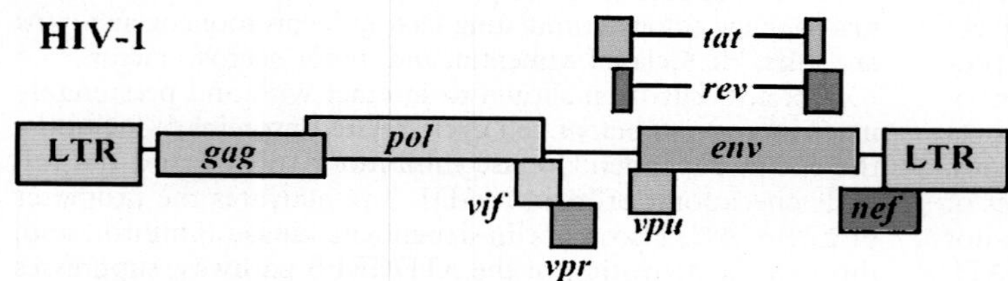

FIGURE 16.4 Human immunodeficiency virus (HIV) genome. Overall genomic organization of HIV is the same as for the simpler retroviruses, with *gag, pol,* and *env* genes flanked on each end by long terminal repeats (LTRs). HIV also encodes other proteins involved in the viral replication cycle.

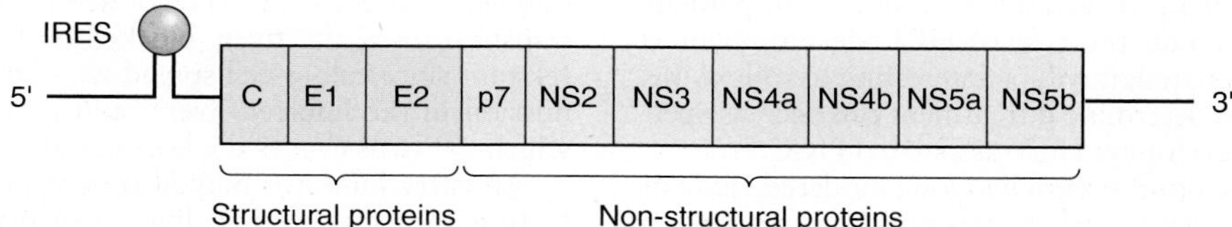

FIGURE 16.5 Hepatitis C virus (HCV) genome. The HCV genome consists of 5′ and 3′ untranslated regions and a single open reading frame encoding a protein precursor that is proteolytically processed into individual viral structural and enzymatic proteins. Structural proteins include the nucleocapsid (C) and envelope proteins (E1, E2). The NS2/3 metalloprotease and serine protease (NS3) perform most of the proteolytic processing of the polyprotein precursor. NS3 also possesses helicase activity. NS4A is a cofactor of the NS3 protease. NS4B is involved in membrane association of the replication complex. NS5B encodes the RNA-dependent RNA polymerase. The functions of NS1 (p7) and NS5A are still not known. Major protein domains are shown; further proteolytic processing also takes place. The 5′ untranslated region contains an internal ribosome binding site (IRES) that allows translation of the uncapped viral RNA.

with glycosaminoglycans. Attachment is followed by sequential specific interactions (direct or indirect) between the envelope glycoproteins with multiple HCV receptors, including CD81, the scavenger receptor B1 (SR-B1) and the tight junction proteins Claudin 1 and Occludin 1 (reviewed in ref. 66). After entry into cells, the viral genome is replicated by the viral-encoded RNA-dependent RNA polymerase via a minus-strand RNA intermediate; unlike the case with retroviruses, there is no DNA intermediate in the replication cycle.[67] Plus-strand viral RNA molecules lack the usual CAP modification at the 5′ end of mRNAs and are translated into a single polyprotein, using the internal ribosome entry site to initiate translation. The polyprotein produced is processed to yield all HCV enzymatic and structural proteins. Genomic RNA and structural proteins associate to form progeny virus particles, which are released from cells, most likely through the endoplasmic reticulum and host cell secretory pathways.

HCV is transmitted percutaneously in the majority of cases.[68] Prior to 1989, when screening for HCV began, use of contaminated blood products accounted for a significant fraction of new infections; spread via contaminated needles used by intravenous drug users continues to be a major problem. The virus also can be transmitted perinatally and via sexual routes; in about 10% of cases, known risk factors for transmission are not identified. It is estimated that around three million people in the United States are chronically infected with HCV.

HCV infection is strongly associated with the development of hepatic cirrhosis and HCC, although the regional prevalence of HCV infection in HCC varies. Following initial infection by HCV, about 25% of people develop acute clinical hepatitis while others are asymptomatic. HCV infection is chronic in 50% to 80% of cases. Of these cases, 60% to 70% will develop chronic hepatitis, with about 20% of this group progressing to cirrhosis. The estimated proportion of individuals chronically infected with HCV who develop HCC is estimated to be 1% to 5%. The rate of HCC development in those with cirrhosis is estimated to be 1% to 4% per year. Given the number of people infected with HCV (estimated to be approximately 170 million worldwide), such a percentage accounts for a large number of HCC cases per year. However, an individual patient's risk for progression to HCC development is difficult to assess because additional factors may affect the likelihood of HCC development. For example, alcohol consumption or coinfection with hepatitis B virus greatly increases the relative risk for developing HCC.

The role of HCV in HCC pathogenesis is not entirely clear.[69] It is unlikely that HCV itself is directly oncogenic, that is, capable on its own of fully transforming normal hepatocytes into neoplastic clones. After initial HCV infection, there is an approximately 10- to 20-year period prior to development of cirrhosis and a 20- to 30-year period prior to development of HCC. It appears likely that HCC largely develops indirectly as a result of the cellular turnover occurring during the inflammatory responses that lead to hepatocyte destruction, regeneration, and fibrosis characteristic of cirrhosis. It has been shown that reduction of viral burden will halt, or even reverse, the progression of cirrhosis.[70]

It has been postulated, however, that the virus may play a more direct role in neoplastic transformation of hepatocytes. For example, there have been results suggesting that the HCV core protein may contribute to tumor development: mice transgenic for the core gene developed tumors histologically similar to early HCV-associated HCC. The core protein also has been suggested to affect expression of genes that are ultimately involved in regulation of the cell cycle via the cyclin-dependent kinase pathway and to inhibit apoptosis. Further studies are required to determine the clinical significance of these observations. In addition, infection by different strains of HCV may also pose different levels of risk for HCC development. Many groups have reported that HCV genotype 1b confers an elevated risk for developing HCC. However, the observed effects were variable and not seen in all studies.

Because of the morbidity and mortality of associated cirrhosis and HCC, HCV is a major public health problem. Even though new infection rates have declined as the result of screening of blood donors, a large number of currently infected people are expected to progress to HCC. The incidence of HCC has increased during the last few decades.[71] An effective vaccine to prevent new HCV infections is still not available. For those infected with HCV, combined therapy with peg-interferon-α2a or -2b and ribavirin,[72–74] a synthetic guanosine analogue, has been the standard of care. However, this regimen is only effective in about 50% of patients infected with genotype 1 virus, the predominant genotype in the United States and Europe. Furthermore, there are serious side effects, including flulike symptoms, fever, fatigue, hemolytic anemia, and depression, resulting in low enrollment rates and patient compliance. Therefore, there is a great need for additional drugs that would synergize, and ultimately replace, this regimen. Like HIV, HCV exists as a quasispecies, and drug resistance is a major problem. It is likely that a combination of drugs that target both viral and host factors involved at different stages of the virus life cycle would be required for sustained viral response. So far, the majority of effort has been directed at development of antivirals directed at the HCV replication enzymes, namely the RNA polymerase and protease. Telaprevir,[75,76] an HCV 3/4A serine protease inhibitor, in conjunction with peg-interferon, can be effective in reducing viral load, with sustained response rates varying from around 50% to 80% (sustained response rates for genotype 1 are lower than for genotypes 2 and 3). In patients who respond to treatment, the risk of HCC development is decreased but not eliminated; it will be interesting to follow this subgroup of patients to determine if treatment can decrease permanently the risk of developing HCV-associated HCC.[77]

Lack of an *in vitro* culture system had long hindered study of the complete HCV life cycle,[78] and investigators have resorted to reporter systems that address specific steps of this process. For example, a replicon system allows studies of intracellular replication of the virus, and a pseudotyped virus system has allowed for studies of virus entry.[79] Use of these techniques has enabled screening for potential antiviral agents. The recent establishment of an infectious clone of HCV should open the door to greater understanding of the steps involved in the full HCV replication cycle, including virus maturation and release. Indeed, the pipeline of HCV therapies under development has greatly expanded in the last few years.[80] Most of these are directed against the HCV-encoded enzymes or proteins. A cyclosporine derivative (DEBIO-025) that inhibits HCV protein binding to cyclophilin, a cellular protein required for HCV replication, has recently garnered encouraging clinical results in early clinical trials.[81] Another interesting therapy under development is a small-molecule antagonist of the scavenger receptor B1 (SR-B1), an obligate cellular coreceptor for all HCV genotypes. This molecule, ITX5061, inhibits infection of HCV of diverse genotypes at nanomolar potency.[82] Furthermore, HCV can spread through cell-cell transmission even in the presence of neutralizing antibodies, but this transmission is effectively blocked by ITX5061.[83] This result is relevant since cell-to-cell spread may be a major route of transmission in the infected liver[84] and may be one mechanism by which the virus evades the host immune response.

An entry inhibitor may also be valuable in preventing reinfection in HCV-positive liver transplant patients. Although localized, directed therapies such as chemoembolization, radiofrequency ablation, or alcohol ablation can be useful in slowing tumor progression[85] and systemic treatment with the kinase inhibitor sorafenib may have limited impact on survival,[86] surgical resection of tumors or liver transplantation are the only two curative treatments for HCC. Unfortunately, the new graft is invariably reinfected.[87] An entry inhibitor may be able to forestall the reseeding of the infected cell reservoir.

In addition to hepatocytes, HCV may be able to infect other cell types. Recent evidence suggest that certain neuroepithelial cell lines can support HCV entry and replication,[88] raising the possibility that HCV can invade the CNS *in vivo*. It may also have an impact on hematopoietic cell disorders. Patients infected with HCV are suggested to be at increased risk for the development of B-cell non-Hodgkin lymphoma and other lymphoproliferative diseases,[89] although this association has not been observed in all infected patients.

Selected References

The full list of references for this chapter appears in the online version.

3. Gessain A. The human HTLV-3 and HTLV-4 retroviruses: new members of the HTLV family. *Pathol Biol* 2009;57:161.
8. Jern P, Coffin JM. Effects of retroviruses on host genome function. *Annu Rev Genet* 2008;42:709.
9. Ruprecht K, Mayer J, Sauter M, Roemer K, Mueller-Lantzsch. Endogenous retroviruses and cancer. *Cell Mol Life Sci* 2008;65:3366.
10. Cohen CJ, Lock WM, Mager, DL. Endogenous retroviral LTRs as promoters for human genes: a critical assessment. *Gene* 2009;448:105.
14. Buchschacher GL Jr. Introduction to retroviruses and retroviral vectors. *Somat Cell Mol Genet* 2001;26:1.
15. Temin HM, Mizutani S. RNA-dependent DNA polymerase in virions of RNA tumour viruses. *Nature* 1970;226:1211.
18. Zhang J, Temin HM. Rate and mechanism of nonhomologous recombination during a single cycle of retroviral replication. *Science* 1993;259:234.
20. Maeda N, Fan H, Yoshikai Y. Oncogenesis by retroviruses: old and new paradigms. *Rev Med Virol* 2008;18:387.
22. Hacein-Bey-Abina S, Garrigue A, Wang GP, et al. Insertional oncogenesis in 4 patients after retrovirus-mediated gene therapy for SCID-X1. *J Clin Invest* 2008;118:3132.
23. Howe SJ, Mansour MR, Schwarzwaelder K, et al. Insertional mutagenesis combined with acquired somatic mutations causes leukemogenesis following gene therapy of SCID-X1 patients. *J Clin Invest* 2008;118:3143.
24. Buchschacher GL Jr. Safety considerations associated with development and clinical application of lentiviral vector systems for gene transfer. *Curr Genom* 2004;5:19.
25. Parker RC, Varmus HE, Bishop JM. Expression of *v-src* and chicken *c-src* in rat cells demonstrates qualitative differences between pp60vsrc and pp60c-src. *Cell* 1984;37:131.
26. Poiesz BJ, Ruscetti FW, Reitz MS, et al. Isolation of a new type C retrovirus (HTLV) in primary uncultured cells of a patient with Sezary T-cell leukemia. *Nature* 1981;294:268.
28. Legros S, Boxus M, Dewulf JF, Dequiedt, Kettmann R, Twizere JC. Protein-protein interactions and gene expression regulation in HTLV-1 infected cells. *Front Biosci* 2009;14:4138.
31. Matsuoka M, Green PL. The HBZ gene, a key player in HTLV-I pathogenesis. *Retrovirology* 2009;6:71.
34. Boxus M, Willems L. Mechanisms of HTLV-1 persistence and transformation. *Br J Cancer* 2009;101:1497.
40. Taylor G. Molecular aspects of HTLV-I infection and adult T-cell leukaemia/lymphoma. *J Clin Pathol* 2007;60:1392.
44. Saggioro D, Silic-Benussi M, Biasiotto R, D'Agostino DM, Ciminale V. Control of cell death pathways by HTLV-1 proteins. *Front Biosci* 2009;14:3338.
46. Moore, MD, Hu WS. HIV-1 RNA dimerization: it takes two to tango. *AIDS Rev* 2009;11:91.
52. Martin Stoltzfus C. Regulation of HIV-1 alterntive RNA spicing and its role in virus replication. *Adv Virus Res* 2009;74:1.
55. Stevenson, M. Basic science summary. *Top HIV Med* 2009;17:30.
56. Malim MH, Emerman M. HIV-1 accessory proteins—ensuring viral survival in a hostile environment. *Cell Host Microbe* 2008;3:388.
60. Grambderg T, Sunseri N, Landau NR. Accessories to the crime: recent advances in HIV accessory protein biology. *Curr HIV/AIDS Rep* 2009; 6:36.
64. Lindenbach, BD, Rice CM. Molecular biology of flaviviruses. *Adv Virus Res* 2003;59:23–61.
68. Alter HJ, Purcell RH, Shih JW, et al. Detection of antibody to hepatitis C virus in prospectively followed transfusion recipients with acute and chronic non-A, non-B hepatitis. *N Engl J Med* 1989;321(22):1494.
71. Altekruse SF, McGlynn KA, Reichman ME. Hepatocellular carcinoma incidence, mortality, and survival trends in the United States from 1975 to 2005. *J Clin Oncol* 2009;27(9):1485.
75. Hezode C, Forestier N, Dusheiko G, et al. Telaprevir and perinterferon with or without ribavirin for chronic HCV infection. *N Engl J Med* 2009;360:1839.
79. Brass V, Moradpour D, Blum HE. Molecular biology of hepatitis C virus (HCV): 2006 update. *Int J Med Sci* 2006;3:29.
80. Lemon SM, McKeating JA, Pietschmann T, et al. Development of novel therapies for Hepatitis C. *Antiviral Res* 2010 86:79–92.
81. Coelmont L, Kaptein S, Paeshuyse J, et al. Debio 025, a cyclophilin binding molecule, is highly efficient in clearing hepatitis C virus (HCV) replicon-containing cells when used alone or in combination with specifically targeted antiviral therapy for HCV (STAT-C) inhibitors. *Antimicrob Agents Chemother* 2009;53:967–976.
82. Syder A, Lee H, Zeisel MJ, et al. Small molecule scavenger receptor BI antagonists are potent HCV entry inhibitors. *J Hepatology* 2011;54:46–53.
83. Grove J, Brimacombe C, Syder D, et al. Neutralising antibody resistant hepatitis C virus cell-to-cell transmission. *J Virol* 2010.
84. Liang Y, Shilagard T, Xiao S-Y, et al. Visualizing hepatitis C virus infections in human liver by two-photon microscopy. *Gastroenterology* 2009;137: 1448–1458.
85. Cheng BQ, Jia CQ, Liu CT, et al. Chemoembolization combined with radiofrequency ablation for patients with hepatocellular carcinoma larger than 3 cm. *JAMA* 2008;299:1669–1677.
86. Lovet JM, Rici S, Mazzaferro V, et al. Sorafenib in advanced hepatocellular carcinoma. *N Engl J Med* 2008;359:378–390.
87. Wright TL, Donegan E, Hsu HH, et al. Recurrent and acquired hepatitis C viral infection in liver transplant recipients. *Gastroenterology* 1992;103:317–322.
88. Fletcher NF, Yang JP, Farquhar MJ, et al. Hepatitis C virus infection of neuroepithelioma cell lines. *Gastroenterology* 2010;139:1365–1374.
89. Giordano TP, Henderson L, Landgren O, et al. Risk of non-Hodgkin lymphoma and lymphoproliferative precursor diseases in U.S. veterans with hepatitis C virus. *JAMA* 2007;297:2010.

CHAPTER 17 INFLAMMATION

GIORGIO TRINCHIERI

Inflammation is one of the predominant manifestations of innate resistance to pathogens, and it precedes, directs, and modulates the quality and strength of the adaptive immune response. The four classical symptoms of inflammation from Aulus Cornelius Celsus—*rubor*, *calor*, *tumor*, and *dolor*—and Virchow's *functio laesa* reflect the profound vascular, cellular, and humoral alterations that take place during the host's response to the alteration of tissue homeostasis upon a pathogen's invasion and the subsequent processes that lead to wound healing and tissue reconstitution. However, inflammatory responses may or may not be associated with infections, and they are not homogeneous. Different and often alternative inflammatory mechanisms are activated depending on the pathogen or cause of tissue damage, type and localization of the tissue involved, and the genotype of the host. In addition, like any action that induces a reaction, all proinflammatory responses are accompanied by anti-inflammatory responses. The optimal balance between proinflammatory and anti-inflammatory mechanisms determines the elimination of infection or damage with wound healing and re-establishment of tissue homeostasis but often also results in a state of equilibrium accompanied by chronic inflammation that may persist for a long time and may induce significant tissue damage.

Cancer is obviously one of the extreme consequences of alteration of tissue homeostasis and appropriately has been compared by Harvard pathologist Harold Dvorak[1] to a wound that does not heal. It is not surprising that the processes of inflammation may be closely related to the initiation, promotion, and progression as well as surveillance and control of the malignant disease (Fig. 17.1). Chronic inflammation induced by various pathologic conditions, associated or not with infections or altered response to the commensal flora, may create local conditions in which the early homeostatic, genetics, and epigenetics tissue and cellular alteration involved in tumor initiation are favored. Once intrinsic antitumor mechanisms are overcome and the initial tumor mass initiates expansion, a tumor-associated inflammation ensues, due to either intrinsic mechanisms in the transformed cells or the tissue of origin or to the extrinsic participation of inflammatory hematopoietic cells attracted and activated by chemotactic and proinflammatory factors produced by tumor cells and their associated stromal components. The tumor-associated inflammation promotes tumor growth as well as metastasis formation by favoring tissue remodeling and angiogenesis, providing growth factors and metabolic conditions that favor tumor cell expansion and chemotactic factors that affect migration of both tumor and inflammatory cells. Historically, the interaction of inflammation, innate resistance, and adaptive immunity with tumors was mostly interpreted as a defense response of the organism that attempts to eliminate the invading tumor and forms the basis of the tumor immune surveillance hypothesis, as discussed below. Although in many tumor types there is indeed evidence of an immune response against the tumors, this is quite ineffective because the tumor-associated microenvironment develops immunosuppressive mechanisms that are in part the same as those in the tumor-associated inflammatory response, which are responsible for promoting tumor growth and progression and are eventually responsible for tumor escape from immune surveillance. As depicted in Figure 17.1, different proinflammatory factors and cell types may have either an antitumor effect or a protumor effect, favoring tumor initiation and progression as well as immunoevasion. These different protumor effects of inflammation that act at different times during tumor initiation and progression may be in large part overlapping, and the characteristics of chronic inflammation that favor tumor initiation are likely quite similar, although not identical, to those observed in the progressing tumor or at metastatic sites.

TUMOR IMMUNE SURVEILLANCE

Over a century ago pioneering clinical studies of Fehleisen, Burns, and particularly of the New York surgeon William B. Coley, based on anecdotic historical reports of cancer remission in patients with acute infection, showed that artificial infection with inflammation-causing bacteria induced often dramatic regressions of otherwise incurable cancers.[2] More recently other proinflammatory therapies (e.g., the use of live bacille Calmette-Guérin [BCG] for local treatment of bladder carcinoma) have been based on the same principles.

Soon after, Paul Erlich proposed that the immune system may survey the appearance of new carcinomas and prevent the progression of most of them. The hypothesis of tumor immune surveillance was then formalized in the 1950s by MacFarlane Burnet and Lewis Thomas on the basis of the advanced understanding of the role of cellular immunity in elimination of allogeneic or altered cells, including cancer cells.[3] The theory of tumor immune surveillance, however, remained controversial and proved difficult to be demonstrated experimentally. In the past 10 years the availability of better genetic and immunological tools has allowed the investigators to obtain solid experimental evidence that both innate resistance and adaptive immunity control tumor development and progression. When a transformed cell escapes the intrinsic nonimmunologic tumor suppressor mechanisms, it may be recognized by the innate or adaptive immune system and eliminated (elimination phase).[4] If, however, the immune system fails to eliminate completely the growing tumor cells, a phase of equilibrium is established that applies selective pressure on the tumor cells, resulting in genetic instability, acquisition of new genetic mutations, and modulation of their immunogenicity (immune editing). This equilibrium phase is possibly responsible in part for the long phases of latency that are observed in clinical and experimental tumors.[5] In humans, the equilibrium phase may explain the appearance of tumors in

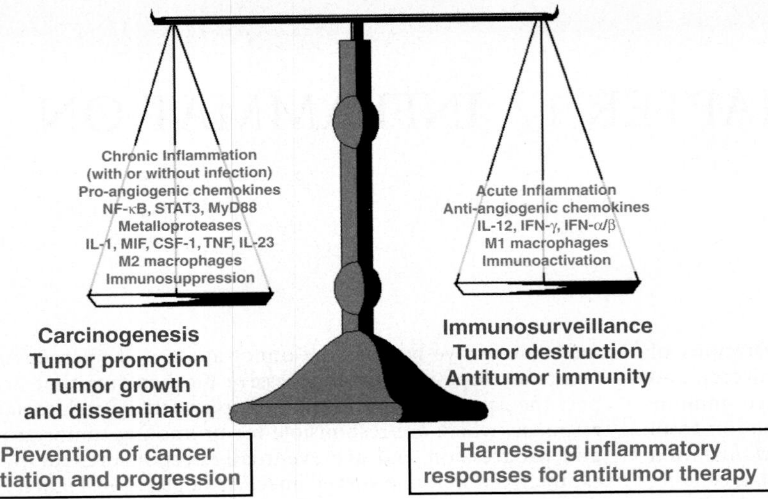

FIGURE 17.1 The contrasting effects of inflammation and immunity associated factors on cancer. Clinical observations and data from model of carcinogenesis in genetically modified experimental animals have allowed the investigators to identify inflammation-related factors that may be associated either with tumor initiation and progression or with resistance to tumor growth and antitumor effector mechanisms. Factors associated with chronic inflammation tend to be associated with protumor effects, whereas those associated with acute inflammation and immunity with an antitumor effect. However, this distinction is not absolute and, as discussed in the text, the same factors can have either a pro- or antitumor effect, depending on the tumor stage and the other factors present in the tumor microenvironment.

immunodepressed patients (see discussion below) or the development of donor-origin tumors such as melanomas in patients transplanted with tissues from donors who had survived a malignancy and had no evidence of disease for many years at the time of death.[6] If the growing tumor resists the suppressor effects of immunity (e.g., by eliciting immune suppressor mechanisms or becoming nonimmunogenic) and establishes favorable interactions with its microenvironment and stroma, then it will succeed to escape the surveillance mechanisms and tumor progression and dissemination will ensue.[4,7]

Overall, mice deficient in immune lymphocytes, T and B cells, as well as some of the effector molecules used in adaptive immunity (e.g., the pore-forming perforin involved in the lytic mechanisms of cell-mediated cytotoxicity) develop more tumors spontaneously or in response to chemical carcinogens such as methylcholanthrene (MCA). However, deficiency or activation of cells linked to innate immunity and of proinflammatory cytokines has also been found to affect tumor development.[4,8] These cell types include natural killer (NK) cells as well as natural killer T (NKT) cells and also T cells expressing γδT-cell receptors that are considered to mediate more innate rather than antigen-specific adaptive immune functions. Proinflammatory cytokines that negatively affect tumor development include type I interferon (IFN), interferon-γ (IFN-γ), and interleukin-12 (IL-12).

The experimental data that support a role of immune surveillance in controlling tumorigenicity have found strong support in epidemiologic studies of immunosuppressed transplantation patients in whom a significant increase in malignancies was observed.[9] However, as in immunodeficient experimental animals, not all types of tumors were increased in the patients. Whereas nonmelanoma skin cancers were increased more than 50-fold and oral, vaginal, and rectal cancers as well as non-Hodgkin's lymphoma were also significantly increased, the increase in other tumor types was modest and mostly nonsignificant.[9] Surprisingly, melanoma, a tumor type that is considered to be highly immunogenic, was among the tumor types that were only modestly affected by the immunosuppressive treatment.[9–11] In different studies increased risk of melanoma in immunodepressed patients ranged from not statistically significant to fivefold, but only in male patients.[9–11] Because the immune-suppressive regimen for transplantation was homogeneous in the cohorts of patients analyzed, it is possible that different types of tumors are controlled by different immunological mechanisms, and only some of these may have been suppressed in the patients. Conversely, it is possible that the deficit of immune surveillance in these patients is limited to tumors of viral origin or to those originating from tissues most exposed to both infectious and environmental inflammation-causing agents such as the skin and the mucosal surface open to the external environment. Significantly, however, the presence of tumor-infiltrating lymphocytes, particularly T cells with effector or memory characteristics, was found to be significantly associated with an improved prognosis in human tumors such as melanomas, colon carcinoma, ovarian cancers, and other carcinomas and hematopoietic cancers that have already progressed to clinically detectable levels or even to advanced stages of disease and thus escaped any mechanism of innate or immune surveillance.[12,13] The ability of the immune system to effectively control tumor progression is also clearly demonstrated by the presence of paraneoplastic neurological degenerations associated with cancer in certain patients. In these patients an immune response induced against neuronal antigens that are expressed in cancer cells effectively controls tumor growth but develops into an autoimmune neurodegenerative disease.[14] Thus, although the exact immunologic mechanisms of the antitumor effects remain to be fully investigated, the evidence in humans that the immune system may either prevent or control tumor growth is compelling.

INFLAMMATION AND TUMORIGENESIS

Unlike the evidence discussed above that suggests a tumor's protective role of innate resistance and immunity, an expanding number of observations are now linking inflammation with tumor initiation and promotion. Many types of tumors have been found to frequently originate on a background of prolonged chronic inflammation, and at least 15% of human tumors may have an infectious origin.[15] Table 17.1 shows examples of the association of cancer with chronic inflammation not known to be induced by pathogens, whereas Table 17.2 lists cancer types associated with chronic inflammation induced by infection. One of the early lines of evidence strongly linking cancer and inflammation has been the demonstration that the use of nonsteroidal anti-inflammatory drugs (NSAIDs)

TABLE 17.1

CHRONIC INFLAMMATORY CONDITIONS ASSOCIATED WITH TUMOR FORMATION

Pathologic Condition	Associated Tumor(s)	Etiologic Agent
Sunburned skin, burn scar	Basal cell carcinoma, squamous cell carcinoma (SCC), melanoma	Ultraviolet light
Severe thermal injury	Marjolin's ulcer (SCC)	—
Epidermolysis bullosa	SCC	Genetic, mechanical
Gingivitis, lichen planus	Oral SCC	—
Lichen sclerosus	Vulvar SCC	—
Sialadenitis	Salivary gland carcinoma	—
Sjögren syndrome, Hashimoto's thyroiditis	Mucosa-associated lymphoid tissue lymphomas	—
Asbestosis, silicosis	Mesothelioma, lung carcinoma	Asbestos fibers, silica particles
Bronchitis (nitrosamines, peroxides)	Lung carcinoma	Silica, asbestos, smoking
Reflux esophagitis, Barrett's esophagus	Esophageal carcinoma	Gastric acid, alcoholism, smoking
Hematochromatosis	Liver	Genetic
Liver cirrhosis	Hepatocellular carcinoma	Alcoholism
Chronic pancreatitis	Pancreatic carcinoma	Genetic (mutation in trypsinogen gene on chromosome 7), alcoholism, smoking
Inflammatory bowel disease, Crohn's disease, chronic ulcerative colitis	Colorectal carcinoma, small intestine carcinoma	—
Cystitis, bladder	Bladder carcinoma	Chronic indwelling, urinary inflammation catheters

decreases the incidence of tumors (e.g., colon carcinomas) in patients. Experimental models of chemical or transgenic carcinogenesis have now allowed the investigators to identify a series of proinflammatory products, including cytokines, chemokines, enzymes, and transcriptional factors, that are important or necessary for carcinogenesis. At first approximation, it could be concluded that an acute inflammatory or immune response tends to be associated with tumor prevention or an antitumor effect, whereas chronic, smoldering inflammation is rather associated with tumor initiation and progression. Various proinflammatory and anti-inflammatory factors have been studied and in part could be identified as either being associated with facilitation of tumor formation and progression or having an antitumor effect. Any of Hanahan's six hallmarks of cancer—self-sufficiency in growth signals, insensitivity to antigrowth signals, tissue invasion and metastasis, limitless replicative potential, and sustained angiogenesis—could be affected by innate and adaptive immune mechanisms.[16] In general, factors with antiapoptotic, proangiogenic, prometastatic, and immunosuppressive activity tend to favor tumor formation and progression, whereas those with proapoptotic, antiangiogenic, and immunostimulating activity tend to suppress tumor progression. Often factors and genes associated with the T helper-2 (Th-2) type of immune response and cytokines belong in the former group; whereas, Th-1 type factors are associated with an antitumor role. However, there are no fixed rules, and in some cases the same factors could be found associated with both tumor initiation and antitumor resistance. The best-known example is the cytokine tumor necrosis factor (TNF). As the name suggests, this cytokine was originally identified on the basis of its ability to induce hemorrhagic necrosis of several experimental tumors, and it has been clearly shown to play an important effector role in both innate and adaptive immune mechanisms primarily by its apoptotic

TABLE 17.2

CANCERS ASSOCIATED WITH INFLAMMATION CAUSED BY INFECTIOUS AGENTS

Pathologic Condition	Associated Tumor(s)	Pathogen(s)
Hepatitis	Hepatocellular carcinoma	Hepatitis B and C virus
Mononucleosis	B-cell non-Hodgkin's and Burkitts lymphoma	Epstein-Barr virus
AIDS	Non-Hodgkin's lymphoma, squamous cell carcinoma, Kaposi's sarcoma	Human immunodeficiency virus, human herpes virus type 8
Warts	Nonmelanoma skin cancer	Papillomaviruses
Pelvic inflammatory disease, chronic cervicitis	Ovarian carcinoma, cervical/anal carcinoma	*Neisseria gonorrhoeae, Chlamydia* spp., human papillomaviruses
Osteomyelitis	Skin carcinoma in draining sinuses	Bacteria
Chronic prostatitis	Prostate cancer	Gram(−) bacteria, others
Conjunctivitis	Ocular adnexal lymphoma	*Chlamydia psittaci*
Gastritis/ulcers	Gastric adenocarcinoma	*Helicobacter pylori*
Chronic cholecystitis	Gall bladder cancer	Bacteria, gall bladder stones
Opisthorchiasis, Cholangitis	Cholangiosarcoma, colon carcinoma	*Opisthorchis viverrini, O. sinensis* (liver flukes), bile acids
Chronic cystitis	Bladder, liver, rectal carcinoma, follicular lymphoma of the spleen	*Schistosoma hematobium, S. japonicum*, irradiation, carcinogens

effect on both tumor cells and endothelial cells.[17] However, it also induces activation of the nuclear factor κB (NF-κB) complex, and it has been shown to be required for tumor initiation in experimental models of carcinogenesis.[18] TNF, together with other cytokines, is expressed in many human tumors (e.g., ovarian, breast, and prostate cancers). Among the various possible mechanisms of the protumor effect of TNF is the induction of matrix metalloproteinase-9 (MMP-9) and of the chemokine monocyte chemotactic protein-1 (MCP-1) that regulates monocyte infiltration in the tumors.[18]

Although the full understanding of the role of inflammation in carcinogenesis is relatively recent, there were many historical observations already pointing in that direction. In 1828 Marjolin described a relatively uncommon ulcerative lesion associated with chronic inflammation following a skin thermal injury (Marjolin's ulcer) that progressed to malignant transformation.[19] Presently, many chronic skin inflammation or irritations are known to be associated with increased prevalence of squamous cell carcinoma.[20] In 1863, Rudolph Virchow for the first time proposed a link between inflammation and cancer by noting that inflammatory cells and factors were frequently present in the tumor stroma.[20] Overall, the strongest evidence in humans for a link between cancer and inflammation comes from the finding that NSAID therapy decreases the incidence of cancer and the observation of an association between chronic infectious or inflammatory lesions and cancer. Evidence supporting a link between chronic inflammation and colorectal cancer came from the epidemiologic observations that patients with long-term chronic inflammatory bowel disease often develop colorectal cancer. Specifically, colon carcinomas and particularly carcinomas of the small intestine were increased in Crohn's disease patients, whereas colon and rectal carcinomas were increased in patients with ulcerative colitis.[21] NSAIDs used in experimental animals and in humans were found to prevent colon cancer.[22] Cyclooxygenase-2 (COX-2) is expressed at increased levels in intestinal epithelial cells and colorectal tumors and, through its induction of prostaglandin E_2 (PGE_2), it controls inflammation, acting as a vasodilator, a regulator of angiogenesis, and an enhancer of hematopoietic cell homing. In addition it affects epithelial cell adhesion and apoptosis and regulates immune functions.[23] Chronic treatment with nonspecific cyclooxygenase inhibitors such as aspirin were found to decrease the risk of colon cancer by about 50%, although this cancer preventive action was associated with gastrointestinal site effects; specific COX-2 inhibitors were found to have less gastrointestinal site effects, but their use was mostly discontinued because of their reported cardiovascular toxicity.[22] COX-2-specific inhibitors increased overall and recurrence-free survival following surgical resection in the subset of patients with diagnosis of colorectal cancer that overexpressed COX-2 or presented mutated forms of its gene. Interestingly not only did COX-2 inhibitors prevent cancer formation, but they also decreased the number of already established polyps in patients with familial adenomatous polyposis.[22]

It has been estimated that approximately 15% of human cancers may have an infectious origin, although this may well be an underestimation. This proportion is significantly higher in developing countries, whereas it is lower in developed countries probably because of better prevention and lower exposure to infections.[15] Although some pathogens, viruses in particular, may directly induce cell transformation (e.g., Epstein-Barr virus and human papilloma viruses), other infections are more likely to give rise to cancer by establishing a chronic inflammatory microenvironment that would favor cell transformation and promote cancer progression. For example, hepatitis C infection in the liver predisposes to liver carcinoma, and *Schistosoma mansoni* infection induces inflammatory and mechanical damage in the bladder with increased incidence of both bladder and colon carcinomas.[24] *Helicobacter pylori* infects about 50% of the world's population, and it has been found to be responsible for chronic gastric inflammation that progresses to atrophy, metaplasia, dysplasia, and gastric cancer.[25] Notably, the risk of gastric cancer in patients with *H. pylori* infections was greatly enhanced by proinflammatory genetic polymorphisms at the IL-1B, IL-8, TNF, and IL-10 loci.[25] In mice, gastric atrophy in *Helicobacter* spp. infected animals was observed in mice that are prone to develop Th-1 immune responses (e.g., C57BL/6) rather than in those (e.g., BALB/c) that develop prevalently Th-2 responses.[25] Both in humans and in mice, coinfection with *Helicobacter* spp. and extracellular parasites that shift the immune responses to Th-2 was associated with decreased gastric atrophy and risk of cancer.[25] The commensal interaction of humans with *H. pylori* is of particular evolutionary interest. The presence of this pathogen in the stomach favored better immunological response against infection and better energy homeostasis, resulting in lean bodies but predisposed to gastric cancer at later ages. Its absence in modern populations due to decreased transmission and use of antibiotics protects against peptic ulcers and gastric cancer but may favor adiposity, type 2 diabetes, esophageal reflux, Barrett's esophagus, and adenocarcinoma.[26]

Unlike different chronic inflammatory conditions secondary to infections or to physical, chemical, or genetic causes, increased tumor incidence is in general not observed in autoimmunity probably because the antitissue immune response observed in autoimmune diseases is likely to have more of a protective rather than tumor-promoting effect. This is not the case in inflammatory bowel disease and either Crohn's disease or ulcerative colitis patients who have an approximately threefold increase in carcinoma frequency with a lifetime cumulative risk of 18%.[21] However, inflammatory bowel diseases are characterized by an altered immune response to the intestinal flora rather than an autoimmune response to the intestinal cells.

The association between inflammatory genes and carcinogenesis in experimental animals has been mostly based on experiments in which mice deficient for different inflammatory or immune genes were tested for tumor development in two-stage models of carcinogenesis in which treatment with a mutagen was followed by a tumor promoter (7,12-dimethylbenz[α]anthracene (DMBA)/12-O-tetradecanoylphorbol-13-acetate [TPA] for skin and azoxymethane [AOM]/dextran sulfate sodium [DSS] for colon carcinogenesis) or in different transgenic cancer models. In these experimental models the important role in carcinogenesis of inflammatory cytokines such as IL-1, TNF, colony-stimulating factor (CSF-1), macrophage-inhibiting factor (MIF), and IL-23 was determined. It should be noted that most of the studies on the role of immune surveillance were done using experimental models of systemic MCA-induced carcinogenesis or by studying spontaneous tumor formation in wild type or genetically altered mice. Because induction of inflammation is one of the modes of action of tumor promoters, the use of different models may perhaps explain some of the apparent contradictions between the results in the experiments of immune surveillance and those showing a link between cancer and inflammation.[27]

MECHANISMS OF CELL TRANSFORMATION AND CANCER INITIATION IN THE INFLAMMATORY ENVIRONMENT

Tumor initiation is a process in which normal cells mutate genes that regulate normal cell growth and homeostasis and eventually develop a growth advantage and survival mechanisms that allow them to expand at the expense of the surrounding normal cells and tissues. An inflammatory environment may create conditions of genetic instability and favor or induce the establishment of the initial gene mutation. A single mutation is, however, not sufficient in most cancers for successful tumor growth, and several successive inherited mutations must take place[16] Cancer can be initiated in tissues under conditions of chronic inflammation but also in tumors in which an initial inflammatory cause cannot be identified; cancer-associated inflammation is often observed that can be extrinsic and mediated by migration of inflammatory hematopoietic cells or intrinsic to the transformed cells that produce, often in response to mutation or activation of oncogenes, a cascade of proinflammatory factors, including cytokines, chemokines, and stroma-altering factors such as metalloproteases.[28] As a consequence of intrinsic inflammation, hematopoietic cells are attracted to the tumor microenvironment, with a feedback mechanism that augments the extrinsic inflammation and greatly contributes to the microenvironment, that promotes tumor growth and progression, but that could also induce genetic instability in the transformed cells with generation of successive gene mutation events.

Chronic inflammation can contribute with several possible mechanisms to increased DNA mutations and to genetic instability. Tissue damage and repair increase the proliferation rate in the affected tissue, increasing the probability of mutation or chromosomal translocation during mitosis. In addition, inflammation, reactive oxygen and nitrogen intermediates, and oxidative stress can reduce the expression and enzymatic activity of products of the mismatch DNA repair genes such as mutL homolog 1 (MLH1), mutS homolog (MSH) 2 and 6, resulting in an increased genetic instability and increased rate of DNA replication errors.[29,30] Particularly affected are genes, many of which control cell cycle or survival, that contain in their coding region unstable short repetitive DNA sequences known as microsatellites. Direct interaction of mucosal epithelial cells with microbial pathogens such as *H. pylori* and attaching and effacing enteropathogenic *Escherichia coli* rapidly results in decreased expression of MLH1 and MHS2.[31,32] In response to inflammation or interaction with bacterial pathogens, the expression of methyltransferases is increased with silencing of many genes, including the DNA repair genes and tumor suppressor genes, contributing to carcinogenesis.[33–35] Aberrant expression of activation-induced cytidine deaminase, an initiator of somatic hypermutation in B cells, in mucosal cells induced by inflammation, and in part mediated by TNF, IL-4, and IL-13, has been proposed to be linked to mutations in human colorectal cancer.[36] These mechanisms suggest that genomic instability, epigenetic changes, and functional protein modifications are involved in the early events of inflammation-induced cancer initiation.

Reactive oxygen and nitrogen species (ROS and RNS) contribute significantly to the pathological damage observed in inflamed tissues. Indeed it has been known that a pro-oxidant state could promote cancer initiation and growth.[37] ROS and RNS produced by inflammatory cells induce a series of cellular damage, including DNA strand breaks, single base DNA mutations, mutations in tumor suppressor genes, epigenetic modifications, and posttranslational modification of proteins that control apoptosis, survival, DNA repair, and cell cycle checkpoints.[37,38] Nitric oxide (NO) is one type of RNS that has complicated and apparently contradictory roles in cancer.[38] NO production is controlled by a family of nitric oxide synthases (NOS), of which NOS2 is expressed in inflammatory cells, and is inducible by various cytokines, including IFN-γ and TNF. The protumor role of NO includes its ability to induce DNA damage, to increase angiogenesis by inducing the production of vascular endothelial growth factor (VEGF), and to stimulate tumor cell proliferation and invasion. However, in different conditions and particularly when present at higher concentrations, NO can inhibit proliferation and induce apoptosis in cancer cells. These contrasting effects of NO have been in part explained by the status in the cancer cells of the *p53* tumor suppressor gene. NO stabilizes and activates p53, which then down-regulates NOS2. Activation of p53 results in induction of apoptosis, cell cycle arrest, and senescence in the exposed cancer cells. However, in the absence of p53, often mutated in many cancer types, NO is unable to induce apoptosis but instead stimulates cell growth and contributes to the genotoxic stress.[38]

Similar to the NOS family, the cyclooxygenase family comprises a constitutively expressed gene—*COX-1*—which contributes to maintaining the homeostasis of the gastrointestinal mucosa, and an inducible one—*COX-2*—that is regulated by various proinflammatory cytokines.[39] COXs are enzymes responsible for the production of prostaglandins from fatty acid, particularly prostaglandin E2 (PGE2). Although initially identified in colorectal cancer, COX-2 is highly expressed in almost every type of tumor from the very early stages of tumor formation. PGE2 can affect the DNA mutation rate and mediate tumor promotion by modulating angiogenesis, apoptosis, and formation of metastases.[39] Clinical trials with NSAID and particularly COX-2 selective inhibitors have shown a preventive effect on various types of cancer, particularly on the colon adenoma and adenocarcinoma, with a protective effect nearing 50%.[40] However, the significant cardiovascular side effects of these drugs, due to shunt of the COX-2 substrate—arachidonic acid—into the 5-cyclooxygenase pathway,[41] have resulted in the removal from distribution of many of these compounds and limited the indication for their prophylactic use in cancer.[39]

Several transcription factors activated in the inflammatory environment are instrumental in affecting cancer initiation and promotion, with NF-κB and STAT3 playing a particular central role. NF-κB target genes involves many genes that regulate the cell cycle, angiogenesis, and cell survival as well as genes encoding proinflammatory cytokines, chemokines, and proteases, including NOS2 and COX-2. Thus, NF-κB expression is required for cancer development, at least in the liver and in the colon, both in the tumor cells as well as in the infiltrating proinflammatory hematopoietic cells.[42,43] In most types of cancer, STAT3 is overexpressed and present in the nucleus in its phosphorylated form in tumor cells, stromal cells, and infiltrating hematopoietic cells. When overexpressed in tumor cells, STAT3 contributes to their survival, proliferation, and dissemination by controlling the expression of several cycle genes and of the protooncogene c-Myc. STAT3 activation also favors proliferation of malignant cells via an antiapoptotic effect, in part mediated by transcriptional down-regulation of p53 and by inducing factors that drive angiogenesis and metastasis, including VEGF and metalloproteases. Many factors released by the tumor and the tumor stroma, such as VEGF, IL-6, IL-10, and IL-11, contribute to STAT3 activation. Interestingly, several of these factors are themselves transcriptionally regulated by STAT3, thus creating a positive feedback regulation of their production.[44] Early expression of pSTAT3 in epithelial cells has been shown to be required for carcinogenesis, suggesting that activation of this transcriptional factor links inflammation with cancer initiation.[45] STAT3 in tumors also contributes to the recruiting of tumor-infiltrating hematopoietic cells by controlling production of chemotactic factors and the expression of their receptors on infiltrating cells. Although STAT3 activation induces recruitment of hematopoietic cells, STAT3 activation in tumor-associated macrophages and dendritic cells has a profound anti-inflammatory effect by preventing their complete maturation, inhibiting the production of proinflammatory cytokines such as IL-12 and favoring the maturation of alternatively activated macrophages.[44,46] These contrasting activities are well suited for tumor growth because proinflammatory cells provide factors for stromal development and angiogenesis but strong inflammatory responses with antitumor and antiangiogenic effects are prevented.

Epithelial cells can produce a variety of inflammatory cytokines and chemokines, metalloproteases, and angiogenic and growth factors that not only contribute to the migration and activation of infiltrating hematopoietic cells but could also act with an autocrine or paracrine feedback action favoring the continued production of these factors and affecting cell proliferation and differentiation. Oncogene products such as *RAS, RET, BRAF,* and *MYC* can induce this intrinsic pathway of inflammation in transformed epithelial cells, suggesting that this inflammatory feedback mechanism contributes both to the transforming phenotype of the epithelial cells as well as the proinflammatory environment that could promote tumor progression.[47] Continued activation or overexpression of oncogenes is not required for establishing this proinflammatory loop. It has been shown that transient activation of the *SRC* oncoprotein is sufficient to induce an epigenetic switch that through microRNA regulation, production of IL-6, and activation of its target transcription factors stably maintains the proinflammatory secretory loop even in the absence of the activated oncoprotein.[48] The proinflammatory secretory pattern observed in oncogene-transformed cells is very similar to that observed in senescent fibroblasts or epithelial cells.[49] Inflammation-dependent DNA damage favors cell senescence and through the activation of ataxia telangiectasia mutated (ATM) in response to double strand DNA breaks activates in a p53-independent way the secretion of proinflammatory factors that could than create conditions that promote the growth of cells with oncogene mutations and maintain their production of proinflammatory factors.[50]

Our understanding of the regulation of inflammation has been greatly enhanced in the past few years by the discovery and functional characterization of the receptors expressed in inflammatory cells that recognize shared structures (patterns) on microbes and pathogens (pattern recognition receptors, PRRs). The toll-like receptors (TLRs) represent the major class of PRRs, but in the past few years an increasing number of other cell surface or cytosolic receptors have also been identified.[51] In hematopoietic cells PRRs are very important for the induction of expression of the genes that encode proinflammatory factors and for the posttranslational regulation of their products, thus playing a central role in maintaining the inflammatory environment. These factors include cytokines, chemokines, proangiogenic and growth factors, as well as stroma-processing factors such as metalloproteases. However, PRRs such as TLRs are also expressed in nonhematopoietic cells, and their activation by way of infectious pathogens, commensal flora, or endogenous ligands induces a proinflammatory response that also affects cell proliferation, differentiation, and apoptosis.[52]

INFLAMMATORY CELLS AND STROMAL CELLS IN THE INITIATION OF NEOPLASIA AND IN THE TUMOR MICROENVIRONMENT

In order to better understand the complex interdependence between cancer and the mechanisms of inflammation it is important to look at the neoplastic lesion not as an extraneous structure growing within a normal tissue but as a complex interaction between the neoplastic cells, the tumor stroma, and the infiltrating hematopoietic cells. This is not unlike the infection by an efficient pathogen that, in order to expand in the host, needs to alter but not destroy tissue homeostasis and at the same time prevent an effective sterilizing immune response. This concept was already proposed in 1889 by Stephen Paget in his theory of seed and soil to explain the importance of the receiving tissue in metastasis formation, but it has been only in recent years that the mechanisms affecting the tumor–stroma interaction have started to be dissected and more thoroughly understood.[2,53] The initiating events in the development of carcinoma are likely to affect the epithelial cells as well as fibroblasts, endothelial cells, inflammatory cells, and other stromal cells. Only when the right equilibrium between the alterations in these different tissue components is established does the tumor find the conditions to establish itself, to progress, and eventually to disseminate.

An extreme example of the importance of the stromal and inflammatory components in regulating tumor initiation is provided by an experimental model of gastric cancer in *Helicobacter*-infected mice in which the tumor originated not from tissue epithelial or stem cells but from bone marrow–derived cells recruited to the site of inflammation.[54] A successful tumor survives a Darwinian microenvironment in which both the characteristics of the tumor cells and of the stroma and inflammatory cells are selected to allow tumor progression. Thus the immunogenicity of the tumor is apparently adapted to the environment (tumor immune editing), and the inflammatory response to a successful tumor favors angiogenesis, tumor growth, and dissemination, while the mechanisms potentially able to induce tumor destruction are blocked or attenuated.[3] The apparently paradoxical effects of the inflammatory and immune response to both favor and antagonize tumor initiation and progression can be better understood when viewed as elements of this delicate equilibrium that regulate tumor initiation. However, when a tumor is successfully established, it is difficult to change this equilibrium to induce tumor destruction both because of the multiple genetic and epigenetic mutations that have determined its fitness to survive and also because the inflammatory microenvironment polarization is maintained by positive and negative feedback mechanisms. Thus, it is possible to understand why immunotherapeutic approaches in cancer have proven more difficult than originally expected.

Both in acute and chronic inflammation lesions the most apparent histological trait is the infiltration with hematopoietic cells in which phagocytic cells, mostly neutrophils and macrophages, initially dominate but are then partially replaced by other cells, including lymphocytes, when the inflammation becomes chronic and polarized. In established tumors, the type and level of hematopoietic infiltration is variable but always present. Resident tissue cells, however, are the first to be exposed and respond to the proinflammatory insult such as infectious pathogens, and they coevolve with the transformed neoplastic cells to facilitate and allow tumor initiation and progression. Fibroblasts, endothelial cells, and adipocytes obviously have a major role in maintaining tissue homeostasis, whereas, among the tissue resident hematopoietic cells, tissue macrophages, mast cells, and dendritic cells represent the first line of reactivity and defense.[55] It is, however, very important to consider that in an inflamed tissue (or tumor microenvironment), not only the hematopoietic cells participate in the regulation of inflammation but every cell type in the tissue produces and responds to inflammation-regulating products, and this is instrumental in determining the ensuing type of inflammation. These cell types include not only tissue and cancer fibroblasts, discussed below, but also other stromal cells, including endothelial cells as well as epithelial cells and the tumor cell themselves.

Cancer-Associated Fibroblasts

Cancer-associated stromal fibroblasts (CAFs) acquire stable characteristics that make them better able to support tumor progression than fibroblasts from normal tissues.[56] In addition to expressing vimentin like other fibroblasts, CAFs express alpha-smooth muscle actin, and thus they have characteristics of myofibroblasts. Although the CAF phenotype can be maintained in culture and in adoptively transplanted cells, the CAFs are not immortalized and only in some studies genetic alterations, including loss of p53, have been found in the CAFs.[57] Thus, the CAF phenotype is likely to be due mostly to epigenetic modifications induced in tumor-promoting conditions associated with infection, inflammation, or irradiation. CAFs may differentiate from the pre-existing normal fibroblasts or from stem cells present in the tissues, or they may even possibly be derived from migrating bone marrow cells.[57] The protumor effect of CAFs is mediated mostly by their ability to secrete soluble factors able to induce angiogenesis, to attract inflammatory cells, and to directly support cancer cell growth and dissemination. Among the more relevant of these protumor factors produced by CAFs are the chemokine SDF-1/CXCL12, transforming growth factor beta (TGF-β), and other cytokines, growth factors, and MMPs.[58] The ability of SDF-1 to attract endothelial progenitor cells and to promote angiogenesis could be linked to its ability to activate MMP-9. Genetic alterations of tissue fibroblasts that block their responsiveness to TGF-β or induce them to overproduce growth factors, such as hepatocyte growth factor (HGF) endow them with the ability to induce tumor formation from epithelial cells in the absence of other carcinogenic stimuli.[35,38] Conversely, the malignant phenotype of tumor cells can be reversed by restoration of a normal microenvironment, even if the tumor cells retain all of their genetic mutations.[59] Thus, as suggested by Radisky et al.,[60] tumors may be seen as unique organs defined by abnormal signal and context, and tumorigenesis may be initiated by environmental (e.g., infections and inflammation) and inherited factors affecting the stromal cells.

Mast Cells

Mast cells with different characteristics are present in most tissues, and the ability of mast cells to affect angiogenesis has an important role in wound healing. In preneoplastic and neoplastic lesions, mast cells are present in increasing numbers associated with increased angiogenesis. Factors produced by mast cells are likely to affect tumor angiogenesis by recruiting and acting directly on endothelial cells and their precursors as well as other cells in the tumor stroma.[41,42] Many of the factors secreted by mast cells during inflammatory responses are preformed in the secretory granules, whereas others are formed *de novo*. Both heparin and histamine affect angiogenesis, but particularly important for the angiogenic effect of mast cells is the expression of MMP-2 and MMP-9 and serine proteases of the tryptase and chymase subclasses. The ability of these proteases to degrade the extracellular matrix may contribute both to angiogenesis and to tumor invasion and dissemination. In addition mast cells release several cytokines such as fibroblast growth factor-2 (FGF-2), VEGF, TGF-β, TNF, and IL-8, which not only affect angiogenesis but also have major effects on the recruitment and activation in the tumor of bone marrow–derived cells.

Dendritic Cells

Dendritic cells (DCs) are bone marrow–derived cells present in lymphoid tissues as well as in any other peripheral tissue. Several different subsets of DCs have been identified, but they can be classified into two major groups: the conventional DCs and the plasmacytoid DCs, also known as type I IFN-producing cells.

Conventional Dendritic Cells

Conventional DCs are characterized by an ability to rapidly respond to alteration of tissue homeostasis (e.g., by recognizing and uptaking pathogens or other microbial products due to their high expression of PRRs, including TLRs). They then rapidly undergo a process of activation or maturation characterized by secretion of proinflammatory cytokines, including IL-12, TNF, IL-6, IL-1, type I IFNs, and others. Activated or mature DCs rapidly migrate from the tissues to the T-cell area of lymph nodes through the draining lymphatic vessels. In the lymph nodes, they very efficiently present peptides derived from the antigens acquired in the tissues in the context of major histocompatibility complex (MHC) class I and II, to CD8+ and CD4+ T cells, respectively. Because of these specialized functions, DCs are considered the sentinels of the immune system, and they are among the firsts if not *the* first cells to initiate the inflammatory response and then to bridge innate resistance with adaptive immunity with their specialized activity of antigen presentation to both naive and memory T cells. Cytokines and chemokines produced during DC activation contribute to activate other tissue resident bone marrow–derived and stromal cells and to recruit inflammatory cells in the lesion. By their production of IL-12, type I IFNs, and other cytokines, they activate innate effector cells such as NK and NKT cells and in particular induce these cells to produce the proinflammatory and antiangiogenic cytokine IFN-γ. The ability of DCs to initiate an acute inflammatory response, resulting in the production of the group of cytokines associated with the Th-1 immune response, is often modulated by the characteristics of the stimulus or pathogen that activates them and also by their anatomical localization. For example, the ability of DC associated with mucosal surfaces to become fully activated and produce IL-12 is prevented in part by factors produced by epithelial cells or other tissue cell types, suppressing the Th-1 type inflammation and deviating it toward other types of responses, including Th-2 as well as immune tolerance. Similarly, in chronically infected tissues or in tumors, DCs are present, but their phenotype is altered by the interaction with other cells of the inflamed tissue or with the tumor cells, and in general they are hyporesponsive to stimuli that activate and induce maturation of the DCs from normal tissues. Among the factors either produced by tumor cells or by other stromal cells that contribute to this state of unresponsiveness in tumor associated DCs are the anti-inflammatory cytokines IL-10, TGF-β, IL-6, VEGF, and prostaglandins.[61] In human breast tumors, immature DCs are often observed in close contact and interspersed within the tumor cells, whereas mature DCs are present in the periphery of the tumors often in clusters of infiltrating cells and also containing T cells and other bone marrow–derived cells.[62] The prognostic significance of tumor infiltrating DCs has been studied in many human tumors and either shown to have positive prognostic relevance (e.g., in some studies in melanoma or in lung cancer) or to be irrelevant (e.g., in other studies in breast cancer).[63] The infiltration of activated T cells in primary human tumors has been in many studies considered a positive prognostic factor for tumor-free and overall survival, and this concept has been supported by recent studies in colorectal cancer that show that the type, activation state, density, and location of immune T cells provide a prognostic factor superior and independent to that of criteria related to the anatomic extent of the tumor.[13]

Plasmacytoid Dendritic Cells

The plasmacytoid DCs are cells with a very different biology and functions than the conventional DCs. They have a secretory morphology (plasmacytoid) with a smooth, round appearance, and only after activation *in vitro* or *in vivo* they acquire the dendritic morphology and some of the antigen-presenting functions of the conventional DCs.[64] Unlike conventional DCs, they migrate to the lymph nodes as well as to inflamed or infected tissues through the hematic rather than the lymphoid route.[46] They were originally described in the 1970s as interferon-producing cells (IPC), and they have now been confirmed to be a major *in vivo* producer cell of type I IFN during most virus infections and to play a central role in regulating virus resistance.[64] However, both *in vitro* and *in vivo* they have been shown to be able to induce immune tolerance with incompletely described mechanisms, which may include their ability to express the immunosuppressive enzyme indolamine 2,3-dioxygenase (IDO) and to activate IL-10–producing T cells by expressing inducible costimulator ligand (ICOS-L).[64,65] Plasmacytoid DCs (pDCs) able to induce immunosuppression have been isolated from human tumors, and, interestingly, the infiltration of a small percentage of primary human breast carcinoma with pDC have been shown to be an independent and dramatic negative prognostic factor for patient survival.[63]

Granulocytes

Neutrophilic granulocytes represent the early cells that infiltrate a site of infection or alteration of tissue integrity and precede the infiltration of macrophages and other inflammatory cell types. Neutrophils are also present in the tumor stroma, and they exert a strong angiogenic effect by expressing MMP-9 as well as a variety of cytokines.[19] In addition, neutrophils could link inflammation and carcinogenesis by inducing DNA damage through release of ROS and by metabolically activating carcinogenic compounds through secretion of myeloperoxidase (MPO).[66] In experimental cancer models it has been shown that expression of granulocyte colony-stimulating factor (G-CSF) increased malignancy and aggressiveness of transfected tumor cells, and that this effect was enhanced when granulocyte-macrophage CSF (GM-CSF) was also expressed in the cells.[67] This synergy between the two CSFs probably reflects the close cross-talk between neutrophils and macrophages; the characteristic functional phenotype of tumor-associated macrophages discussed below is probably significantly affected by the interaction with neutrophils and their products.[19]

Eosinophilic granulocytes have also been found to be associated with different types of human tumors.[68] In physiologic conditions, tissue eosinophils are mostly found in the gastrointestinal tract, and infiltration of eosinophils is observed in many mucosal inflammation states, particularly those dominated by Th-2 type responses. Peripheral blood eosinophilia and tumor-associated tissue eosinophilia are observed in certain human cancer patients and are also induced by cytokine immunotherapy (e.g., with IL-2 or GM-CSF). Within several tumor types, including gastrointestinal tumors, tumor-associated tissue eosinophilia has a favorable prognostic significance, whereas the opposite was observed in other tumor types such as oral squamous cell carcinoma. Tumor-associated eosinophils may have a cytotoxic effect on tumor cells, and they may also recruit and activate other hematopoietic cells. In addition they may alter the tumor microenvironment with suppression of the immune response and tumor promotion.[68] Indeed eosinophils are able to efficiently produce a large variety of cytokines, including those associated with Th-1 and Th-2 immune response as well as other immunoregulatory cytokines.[69] Together with the release of their secondary granules, containing the major basic proteins peroxidase and ribonuclease, eosinophils are also a source of ROS as well as leukotrienes and prostaglandins. They are, therefore, an important player in the regulation of the inflammatory response, participating in recruitment and activation of other inflammatory cells, tissue repair, and remodeling.[68]

Tumor-Associated Macrophages

Tumor-associated macrophages (TAMs) represent one of the major components of the infiltrating bone marrow–derived cells in the large majority of tumors. They originate from monocytes or monocyte precursors in the blood. They are attracted into the tumor by chemokines produced by the tumor or stromal cells. C-C chemokine ligand 2 (CCL2)/MCP-1 is the major chemokine responsible for the recruitment of TAMs, but other cytokines are also involved (e.g., macrophage-CSFs and VEGF). Activated macrophages can be cytotoxic for tumor cells and massive infiltration of tumor with activated macrophages, as observed in the presence of high production of CCL2, which results in tumor destruction; whereas the more balanced macrophage infiltration commonly observed in most progressing tumors promotes tumor formation.[70] These biphasic effects of the TAMs and of the chemokines that attract them have been incorporated in the "macrophage balance" hypothesis.[71]

The ability of TAMs to express different functional programs, either cytotoxic and antitumor or protumor and proangiogenic, is now considered to reflect the plasticity of macrophage activation in response to different inflammatory microenvironments. This is often simplified into a dichotomy between a classical type of activation—M1 macrophages—and an alternate one—M2 macrophages.[54,55] In general, intracellular pathogens induce type I polarized inflammation that is characterized by tissue infiltration by activated neutrophils and macrophages and often formation of granuloma, whereas type II inflammation is characteristic of infection with extracellular parasites and of allergic response, with eosinophilia, mastocytosis, alternate activated M2 macrophages, and tissue remodeling. Classical M1 macrophage activation is the phenotype displayed by macrophages activated by microbial products through PRRs such as TLRs and by IFN-γ. The classically activated or M1 macrophages produce high levels of proinflammatory cytokines and in particular IL-12, which favors a polarized type I response.[72] They also produce high levels of ROS and RNS. Thus, they are well poised to exert bactericidal and cytotoxic activity. The production of IFN-γ by innate lymphocytes such as NK and NKT cells and by the Th-1 cells under the influence of IL-12 and other proinflammatory cytokines such as TNF and IL-1 represents a potent, positive feedback for type I inflammation by maintaining macrophages and DC activation and boosting IL-12 production.[73] It should be noted that whereas IL-12 and IFN-γ at least in experimental animals have a protective effect in carcinogenesis experiments, other cytokines produced by M1 macrophages, in particular TNF, IL-1, and IL-23, are required for chemically induced carcinogenesis. Thus, although M1 macrophages may have a cytotoxic effect on established tumors, their products may still be players in the tumor promotion by acute or chronic inflammation.

In most established human and animal tumors, the TAMs have a functional phenotype of alternatively activated M2 macrophages. The dichotomy between M1 and M2 macrophages is, however, an oversimplification of the plasticity of macrophage activation, and phenotypes with subtle but important differences can be distinguished within the M2 population.[54,55,57] In general, M2 macrophages promote angiogenesis, tumor remodeling, and progression. M2 macrophages also produce much lower levels of IL-12 and proinflammatory cytokines than M1 macrophages. IL-4, IL-13, IL-10, and stimulation of TLR in the presence of immune complexes are all stimuli that induce alternatively activated macrophages. IL-4 and IL-13 induce M2a macrophages that are mostly involved in induction of Th-2 type responses and allergy, whereas IL-10 induces M2c macrophages that are mostly capable of immunosuppression, matrix deposition, and fibrosis.[52,54,55] It is of interest that, similar to IFN-γ, IL-4 and IL-13 are paradoxically potent up-regulators of IL-12 production, whereas IL-10 is a potent inhibitor, further complicating the understanding of the physiological role of M2a macrophages generated in the absence of IL-10.[73] M2b macrophages, activated by TLR ligands in the presence of immune complexes that trigger the receptors for the Fc fragment of immunoglobulin G (IgG), produce low levels of IL-12 but high levels of IL-10 and also of several proinflammatory cytokines including TNF.[74] The physiological role of M2b macrophages remains to be determined, but although they have a reduced ability to induce type I inflammation because of the reduced IL-12 production, they may not be immunosuppressive. Although Th-1 cells that produce IFN-γ would contribute to the maintenance of the M1 phenotype, in chronic infection extensively activated Th-1 cells become able to produce both IFN-γ and IL-10, thus down-regulating and controlling excessive type I immune response and inflammation.[75] In chronic infections and in tumors, IL-10 that favors the differentiation of M2 macrophages may also derive from Th-2 cells, T regulatory cells, as well as, in some cases, from the tumor cells themselves.

TAMs not only display many of the characteristics of M2 macrophages but also mediate protumor functions. Even when induced by potent M1 activating molecules such as TLR ligands, TAMs express low levels of proinflammatory cytokines, produce little NO or ROS, and have immunosuppressive functions by producing IL-10 and TGF-β. TAMs favor tumor growth and dissemination by inducing (1) angiogenesis through production of proangiogenic chemokines, VEGF, TNF, and FGF2; (2) tumor growth and survival through the production of growth factors and chemokines; and (3) matrix remodeling, tumor invasion, and metastasis formation through expression of MMPs, TGF-β, TNF, and chemokines.[70]

Although the anergic and immunosuppressive phenotype of macrophages and DCs that infiltrate the tumors is probably induced by several soluble factors and cellular interaction, their ability to respond to activating stimuli with induction of tumoricidal acute inflammation and induction of an antitumor immune response could surprisingly be re-established *in vivo* by neutralizing IL-10 alone.[76] Thus, tumor-infiltrating bone marrow–derived cells and in particular macrophages and DCs could be targets for immune therapeutic intervention with the goal of disrupting the symbiosis between the tumor and the microenvironment and preventing tumor progression.

Myeloid-Derived Suppressor Cells

A large number of recent studies have identified in mouse and human tumors a population of cells with myeloid characteristics and immune suppressive activity[77] that are now referred to as myeloid-derived suppressor cells (MDSC).[78] MDSC represent a heterogeneous population of immature myeloid cells (immature macrophages, granulocytes, DCs, and other immature myeloid cells) that in mice can be identified by the coexpression of the surface markers CD11b and Ly6G (Gr-1).[77] In humans these cells are characterized by the expression of CD34 and CD33 and also appear to be a heterogeneous population of immature myeloid cells. The ability of MDSC to form colonies in agar confirms that they are nonterminally differentiated cells. In healthy animals, cells with the characteristics of MDSC are found in bone marrow but are rare in blood or spleen. However, alteration of cytokine homeostasis during immune stress, infection, or tumor growth also alters the equilibrium of this population, inducing its accumulation in the periphery and within the tumors, and most important, its maturation to a suppressive phenotype.[77] Thus, the appearance of MDSC in the periphery seems to be a manifestation of the well-known early release of immature myeloid cells from bone marrow during stress responses, prompting leukocytosis (the clinical left shift response of granulocytes due to the appearance in circulation of immature forms of granulocytes with a lower average number of nuclear lobes). The profound immunoregulatory effect of these immature myeloid cells represents, however, a novel important functional aspect of this bone marrow response. Many of the tumor infiltrating hematopoietic cell populations (e.g., neutrophils, eosinophils, macrophages, DCs) with immunosuppressive or tumor promoting activity may indeed be comprised within the heterogeneous MDSC population. As expected in a population comprised of cells with different characteristics and functions, the immunoregulatory functions of MDSC appears to be mediated primarily by production of NO as well as arginase.[77] Because NO production is typical of M1 macrophages, whereas arginase is produced by M2 macrophages and prevents NO production by depleting the nitric oxide synthase substrate arginine, these findings appear to confirm the functional heterogeneity of the MDSC population.

B Lymphocytes

Although cancer patients often develop antibodies to their tumors, frequently they are not protective and paradoxically correlate with poor prognosis and decreased survival,[79] a phenomenon often referred to as antibody-mediated tumor enhancement. In an experimental model of skin carcinogenesis, it was recently demonstrated that B cells were necessary for tumor formation, and that their effect was reconstituted by transfer of serum antibodies; the antibodies promoted tumor progression by forming immune complexes that, by binding to receptors for the Fc fragment of IgG, modulated the inflammatory response and altered the tumor microenvironment.[79,80] B-cell–derived lymphotoxin was also shown to promote castration-resistant prostate cancer in an experimental mouse model.[81] Progression of prostate cancer in this model was shown to be associated with inflammatory infiltration and lymphotoxin-mediated IκB kinase α (IKKα) activation, which stimulates metastasis by an NF-κB–independent and cell autonomous mechanism. These studies open a new field of investigation by showing that antibodies, immune complexes, Fc receptors, and possibly complement factors may have an important role in tumor initiation and progression.

ETIOLOGY AND EPIDEMIOLOGY OF CANCER

Selected References

The full list of references for this chapter appears in the online version.

1. Dvorak HF. Tumors: wounds that do not heal. Similarities between tumor stroma generation and wound healing. *N Engl J Med* 1986;315:1650.
2. Philip M, Rowley DA, Schreiber H. Inflammation as a tumor promoter in cancer induction. *Semin Cancer Biol* 2004;14:433.
3. Dunn GP, Bruce AT, Ikeda H, et al. Cancer immunoediting: from immunosurveillance to tumor escape. *Nat Immunol* 2002;3:991.
5. Koebel CM, Vermi W, Swann JB, et al. Adaptive immunity maintains occult cancer in an equilibrium state. *Nature* 2007;450:903.
7. Dunn GP, Old LJ, Schreiber RD. The immunobiology of cancer immunosurveillance and immunoediting. *Immunity* 2004;21:137.
8. Dunn GP, Koebel CM, Schreiber RD. Interferons, immunity and cancer immunoediting. *Nat Rev Immunol* 2006;6:836.
9. Adami J, Gabel H, Lindelof B, et al. Cancer risk following organ transplantation: a nationwide cohort study in Sweden. *Br J Cancer* 2003;89:1221.

12. Bindea G, Mlecnik B, Fridman WH, et al. Natural immunity to cancer in humans. *Curr Opin Immunol* 2010;22:215.
13. Galon J, Costes A, Sanchez-Cabo F, et al. Type, density, and location of immune cells within human colorectal tumors predict clinical outcome. *Science* 2006;313:1960.
14. Albert ML, Darnell RB. Paraneoplastic neurological degenerations: keys to tumour immunity. *Nat Rev Cancer* 2004;4:36.
15. Pisani P, Parkin DM, Munoz N, et al. Cancer and infection: estimates of the attributable fraction in 1990. *Cancer Epidemiol Biomarkers Prev* 1997; 6:387.
16. Hanahan D, Weinberg RA. The hallmarks of cancer. *Cell* 2000;100:57.
18. Balkwill F. TNF-alpha in promotion and progression of cancer. *Cancer Metastasis Rev* 2006;25:409.
19. Balkwill F, Mantovani A. Inflammation and cancer: back to Virchow? *Lancet* 2001;357:539.
20. Mueller MM. Inflammation in epithelial skin tumours: old stories and new ideas. *Eur J Cancer* 2006;42:735.
21. Bernstein CN, Blanchard JF, Kliewer E, et al. Cancer risk in patients with inflammatory bowel disease: a population-based study. *Cancer* 2001;91:854.
23. Cha YI, DuBois RN. NSAIDs and cancer prevention: targets downstream of COX-2. *Annu Rev Med* 2007;58:239.
24. Coussens LM, Werb Z. Inflammation and cancer. *Nature* 2002;420:860.
25. Fox JG, Wang TC. Inflammation, atrophy, and gastric cancer. *J Clin Invest* 2007;117:60.
26. Blaser MJ, Falkow S. What are the consequences of the disappearing human microbiota? *Nat Rev Microbiol* 2009;7:887.
29. Colotta F, Allavena P, Sica A, et al. Cancer-related inflammation, the seventh hallmark of cancer: links to genetic instability. *Carcinogenesis* 2009;30: 1073.
30. Hakem R. DNA-damage repair; the good, the bad, and the ugly. *Embo J* 2008;27:589.
31. Maddocks OD, Short AJ, Donnenberg MS, et al. Attaching and effacing *Escherichia coli* downregulate DNA mismatch repair protein in vitro and are associated with colorectal adenocarcinomas in humans. *PLoS One* 2009;4:e5517.
32. Yao Y, Tao H, Park DI, et al. Demonstration and characterization of mutations induced by *Helicobacter pylori* organisms in gastric epithelial cells. *Helicobacter* 2006;11:272.
34. Das PM, Singal R. DNA methylation and cancer. *J Clin Oncol* 2004; 22:4632.
35. Fleisher AS, Esteller M, Harpaz N, et al. Microsatellite instability in inflammatory bowel disease-associated neoplastic lesions is associated with hypermethylation and diminished expression of the DNA mismatch repair gene, hMLH1. *Cancer Res* 2000;60:4864.
36. Endo Y, Marusawa H, Kou T, et al. Activation-induced cytidine deaminase links between inflammation and the development of colitis-associated colorectal cancers. *Gastroenterology* 2008;135:889.
37. Schetter AJ, Heegaard NH, Harris CC. Inflammation and cancer: interweaving microRNA, free radical, cytokine and p53 pathways. *Carcinogenesis* 2010;31:37.
40. Bertagnolli MM, Eagle CJ, Zauber AG, et al. Five-year efficacy and safety analysis of the Adenoma Prevention with Celecoxib Trial. *Cancer Prev Res (Phila)* 2009;2:310.
42. Karin M, Greten FR. NF-kappaB: linking inflammation and immunity to cancer development and progression. *Nat Rev Immunol* 2005;5:749.
43. Grivennikov SI, Greten FR, Karin M. Immunity, inflammation, and cancer. *Cell* 2010;140:883.
44. Yu H, Kortylewski M, Pardoll D. Crosstalk between cancer and immune cells: role of STAT3 in the tumour microenvironment. *Nat Rev Immunol* 2007;7:41.
45. Grivennikov SI, Karin M. Dangerous liaisons: STAT3 and NF-kappaB collaboration and crosstalk in cancer. *Cytokine Growth Factor Rev* 2010;21:11.
47. Borrello MG, Degl'Innocenti D, Pierotti MA. Inflammation and cancer: the oncogene-driven connection. *Cancer Lett* 2008;267:262.
48. Iliopoulos D, Hirsch HA, Struhl K. An epigenetic switch involving NF-kappaB, Lin28, Let-7 MicroRNA, and IL6 links inflammation to cell transformation. *Cell* 2009;139:693.
49. Coppe JP, Desprez PY, Krtolica A, et al. The senescence-associated secretory phenotype: the dark side of tumor suppression. *Annu Rev Pathol* 2010;5:99.
50. Rodier F, Coppe JP, Patil CK, et al. Persistent DNA damage signalling triggers senescence-associated inflammatory cytokine secretion. *Nat Cell Biol* 2009;11:973.
51. Takeuchi O, Akira S. Pattern recognition receptors and inflammation. *Cell* 2010;140:805.
52. Hasan UA, Caux C, Perrot I, et al. Cell proliferation and survival induced by toll-like receptors is antagonized by type I IFNs. *Proc Natl Acad Sci U S A* 2007;104:8047.
53. Mueller MM, Fusenig NE. Friends or foes—bipolar effects of the tumour stroma in cancer. *Nat Rev Cancer* 2004;4:839.
55. Littlepage LE, Egeblad M, Werb Z. Coevolution of cancer and stromal cellular responses. *Cancer Cell* 2005;7:499.
56. Bhowmick NA, Neilson EG, Moses HL. Stromal fibroblasts in cancer initiation and progression. *Nature* 2004;432:332.
59. Bissell MJ, Radisky D. Putting tumours in context. *Nat Rev Cancer* 2001; 1:46.
61. Zitvogel L, Tesniere A, Kroemer G. Cancer despite immunosurveillance: immunoselection and immunosubversion. *Nat Rev Immunol* 2006;6:715.
62. Bell D, Chomarat P, Broyles D, et al. In breast carcinoma tissue, immature dendritic cells reside within the tumor, whereas mature dendritic cells are located in peritumoral areas. *J Exp Med* 1999;190:1417.
64. Colonna M, Trinchieri G, Liu YJ. Plasmacytoid dendritic cells in immunity. *Nat Immunol* 2004;5:1219.
67. Obermueller E, Vosseler S, Fusenig NE, et al. Cooperative autocrine and paracrine functions of granulocyte colony-stimulating factor and granulocyte-macrophage colony-stimulating factor in the progression of skin carcinoma cells. *Cancer Res* 2004;64:7801.
70. Sica A, Schioppa T, Mantovani A, et al. Tumour-associated macrophages are a distinct M2 polarised population promoting tumour progression: potential targets of anti-cancer therapy. *Eur J Cancer* 2006;42:717.
71. Mantovani A, Sozzani S, Locati M, et al. Macrophage polarization: tumor-associated macrophages as a paradigm for polarized M2 mononuclear phagocytes. *Trends Immunol* 2002;23:549.
78. Gabrilovich DI, Bronte V, Chen SH, et al. The terminology issue for myeloid-derived suppressor cells. *Cancer Res* 2007;67:425.
79. Tan TT, Coussens LM. Humoral immunity, inflammation and cancer. *Curr Opin Immunol* 2007;19:209.

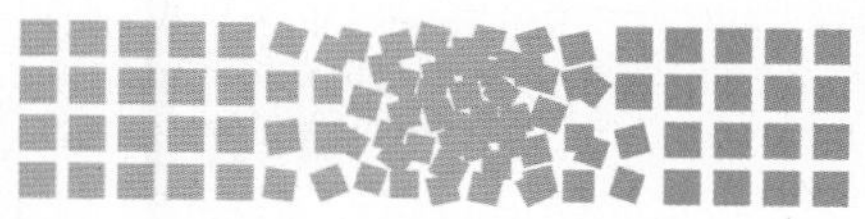

CHAPTER 18 CHEMICAL FACTORS

STUART H. YUSPA AND PETER G. SHIELDS

The chemical origin of human malignancies was recognized by observations of unusual cancer incidences in certain occupational groups. The capacity for chemicals to cause cancer was subsequently confirmed in numerous experimental animal studies. The extent to which chemical exposures contribute to cancer incidence was not fully appreciated until population-based studies documented differing organ-specific cancer rates of up to 300-fold among geographically distinct populations.[1,2] Changes in cancer frequency among migrating ethnic groups, high cancer rates associated with specific occupations, and the high risk of smoking-associated cancers confirmed that environmental and lifestyle exposures were major determinants of human cancer risk. For most common cancers, heritable factors also contribute to cancer risk, but twin studies show that for the common cancers, nongenetic risk factors are dominant, and the best associations for genetic risks of sporadic cancers indicate risks for specific genetic polymorphisms less than 1.5-fold.[3–5] Thus, for these common cancers, chemical exposures can be mechanistically linked to the carcinogenic process, and genetic susceptibilities modulate that risk, so studies of gene effects without considering gene-environment interactions only show small risks; genetics affect that risk through better or worse host defenses and other cellular mechanisms. Thus, most human cancer is not simply a genetically determined sequela of aging, but rather the manifestation of individual exposures (endogenous and exogenous), superimposed on an individually determined hereditary susceptibility. These factors have prompted the President's Cancer Panel Report to alert the cancer community of the urgent need to reduce environmental risk from contamination through industrial, agriculture, lifestyle, medical, military, and natural sources in their 2008–2009 report, although the magnitude of the risks asserted by the panel are not supported by current epidemiological studies (http://deainfo.nci.nih.gov/advisory/pcp/pcp08-09rpt/PCP_Report_08-09_508.pdf).

The experimental induction of tumors in animals and neoplastic transformation of cultured cells by chemicals, and the analysis of human tumors, have revealed important concepts regarding the pathogenesis of cancer and the consistency of pathways impacted for cancer development in rodent and human species (reviewed in refs. 3, 6–8). Chemical carcinogens usually affect specific organs, targeting the epithelial cells (or other susceptible cells within an organ) and causing genetic damage (genotoxic). The most commonly occurring exposures that increase cancer risk are tobacco, alcohol, ultraviolet light, diet, and reproductive factors (e.g., sexual behavior and hormones).[2,9] Chemically related DNA damage and consequent somatic mutations relevant to human cancer can occur either directly from exogenous exposures or indirectly by activation of endogenous mutagenic pathways (e.g., nitric oxide and oxyradicals).[10,11] The risk of developing a chemically induced tumor may be modified by nongenotoxic exogenous and endogenous exposures and factors (e.g., hormones, immunosuppression), and by accumulated exposure to the same or different genotoxic carcinogens.[3,6]

Analysis of how chemicals induce cancer in animal models and human populations has had a major impact on human health. Experimental studies have been instrumental in replicating hypotheses generated from human studies and identifying pathobiological mechanisms. For example, animal experiments confirmed the carcinogenic and cocarcinogenic properties of cigarette smoke and identified bioactive chemical and gaseous components.[9] Experimental animal studies are the mainstay of risk assessment as a screening tool to identify potential carcinogens in the workplace and the environment, although these studies do not prove chemical etiologies because of interspecies differences and the use of maximally tolerated doses that do not replicate human exposure. The transplacental carcinogenicity of diethylstilbestrol and the hazards of specific occupational carcinogens such as vinyl chloride, benzene, aromatic amines, and bis(chloromethyl) ether led to reduction of allowable exposures of suspected human carcinogens from the workplace and reduction of cancer rates. Dietary factors that enhance or inhibit cancer development and the contribution of obesity to specific organ sites have been identified in models of chemical carcinogenesis, and alterations in diet and obesity are expected to result in reduced cancer risk. The application of cancer chemoprevention strategies—particularly retinoids, rexinoids, deltanoids, antiestrogens, and inhibitors of the arachidonic acid cascade—are the direct result of studies conducted in models of chemical carcinogenesis,[12] and are reducing the tumor incidence in high-risk populations. However, the extrapolation of doses from experimental animal models for chemoprevention, timing of exposure, and the complexity of conducting such studies have been problematic for vitamins and other nutrients, and some trials in humans for vitamins and nutrients have been found to increase, rather than decrease cancer risk.[13,14]

THE NATURE OF CHEMICAL CARCINOGENS: CHEMISTRY AND METABOLISM

The National Toxicology Program lists over 200 chemical, physical and infectious agents as known or probable environmental carcinogens[15] (Table 18.1), and a small number are added with each quadrennial review (http://ntp.niehs.nih.gov). Experimental exposure to environmental carcinogens indicate that carcinogenic processes are very specific, and the great majority of the thousands of environmental chemicals are not known to be carcinogenic or have not been adequately tested (see President's Cancer Panel Report 2008–2009). Within chemical classes, stereoisomers may vary widely in carcinogenic potential. Most chemical carcinogens first undergo

TABLE 18.1

KNOWN OR SUSPECTED CHEMICAL CARCINOGENS IN HUMANS[a]

Target Organ	Agents	Industries	Tumor Type
Lung	Tobacco smoke, arsenic, asbestos, crystalline silica, benzo(a)pyrene, beryllium, bis(chloro)methyl ether, 1,3-butadiene, chromium VI compounds, coal tar and pitch, nickel compounds, soots, mustard gas, cobalt-tungsten carbide powders	Aluminum production, coal gasification, coke production, hematite mining, painters, grinding in oil and gas	Squamous, large cell, and small cell cancer and adenocarcinoma
Pleura	Asbestos, erionite	Insulation, mining	Mesothelioma
Oral cavity	Tobacco smoke, alcoholic beverages, nickel compounds	Boot and shoe production, furniture manufacturer, isopropyl alcohol production	Squamous cell cancer
Esophagus	Tobacco smoke, alcoholic beverages	—	Squamous cell cancer
Gastric	Smoked, salted and pickled foods	Rubber industry	Adenocarcinoma
Colon	Heterocyclic amines, asbestos	Pattern makers	Adenocarcinoma
Liver	Aflatoxin, vinyl chloride, tobacco smoke, alcoholic beverages, thorium dioxide	—	Hepatocellular carcinoma, hemangiosarcoma
Kidney	Tobacco smoke, phenacetin	—	Renal cell cancer
Bladder	Tobacco smoke, 4-aminobiphenyl, benzidine, 2-napthylamine, phenacetin	Magenta manufacture, auramine manufacture	Transitional cell cancer
Prostate	Cadmium	—	Adenocarcinoma
Skin	Arsenic, benzo(a)pyrene, coal tar and pitch, mineral oils, soots, cyclosporin A, PUVA	Coal gasification, coke production	Squamous cell cancer basal cell cancer
Bone marrow	Benzene, tobacco smoke, ethylene oxide, antineoplastic agents, cyclosporin A	Rubber workers	Leukemia, lymphoma

PUVA, psoralen-UV-A.
[a]These carcinogen designations are determined by regulatory or review agencies based on public health needs. They do not imply proof of carcinogenicity in individuals. This table is not all inclusive.
For additional information, the reader is referred to agency documents and publications.

metabolic activation by cytochrome P-450 or other metabolic pathways so that they react with DNA or alter epigenetic mechanisms.[8] This process, evolutionarily presumed to have been developed to rid the body of foreign chemicals, inadvertently generates reactive carcinogenic intermediates, and the metabolically activated carcinogens can bind cellular molecules, including DNA in the nucleus and mitochondria, and form covalent adducts or other alterations.[16] Because there is a good correlation between the ability to form DNA adducts and the potency to induce tumors in laboratory animals, DNA is considered the ultimate target for most carcinogens. However, the formation of DNA adducts is likely necessary, but not sufficient to cause cancer.

Genotoxic carcinogens may transfer simple alkyl or complexed (aryl) alkyl groups to specific sites on DNA bases.[11,16] These alkylating and aryl-alkylating agents include, but are not limited to, *N*-nitroso compounds, aliphatic epoxides, aflatoxins, mustards, polycyclic aromatic hydrocarbons, and other combustion products of fossil fuels and vegetable matter. Others transfer arylamine residues to DNA as exemplified by aryl aromatic amines, aminoazo dyes, and heterocyclic aromatic amines. For genotoxic carcinogens, the interaction with DNA is not random, and each class of agents reacts selectively with purine and pyrimidine targets.[3,11,16] Furthermore, targeting of carcinogens to particular sites in DNA is determined by nucleotide sequence, by host cell, and by selective DNA repair processes (see later discussion), making some genetic material at risk over others. As expected from this chemistry, genotoxic carcinogens are potent mutagens, particularly adept at causing base mispairing or small deletions, leading to missense or nonsense mutations. Others may cause macrogenetic damage such as chromosome breaks and large deletions. In all cases, mutations detected in tumors represent a combination of the effects of the mutagenic change on the function of the protein product and the functional alteration on the behavior of the specific host cell type. This is best typified by the signature mutations detected in the *p53* gene caused by ingested aflatoxin in human liver cancer[17] and by polycyclic aromatic hydrocarbons or acrolein in human lung cancer caused by inhalation of cigarette smoke.[6,18,19] Similarly, a distinct pattern of mutations is detected in pancreatic cancers from smokers when compared with pancreatic cancers from nonsmokers.[20]

Some chemicals that cause cancers in laboratory rodents are not demonstrably genotoxic. In general, these agents are carcinogenic in laboratory animals at high doses and require prolonged exposure. Synthetic pesticides and herbicides fall within this group, as do a number of natural products that are ingested. The mechanism of action by nongenotoxic carcinogens is controversial, and may be related in some cases to toxic cell death and regenerative hyperplasia. Induction of endogenous mutagenic mechanisms such as DNA oxyradical damage, depurination, and deamination of 5-methylcytosine by exposure to nongenotoxic carcinogens may contribute to carcinogenicity of these agents. In other cases, nongenotoxic carcinogens may have hormonal effects, influencing hormone-dependent tissues directly. Pesticides, herbicides, and fungicides are known to have endocrine-disrupting properties, although the relation to human cancer risk is unknown. Although the contribution of nongenotoxic carcinogens to human cancer causation is not certain, they may also serve as modifiers in concert with genotoxic agents, altering tissue homeostasis to provide an environment conducive for the selective expansion of a neoplastic clone. Both genotoxic and nongenotoxic carcinogens may alter gene expression through induction of DNA or histone methylation or by other nuclear mechanisms that influence the transcriptome.[21] Permanent epigenetic alterations in gene expression through chemical exposures is increasingly recognized as an important component of carcinogenesis.[22,23]

ANIMAL MODEL SYSTEMS AND CHEMICAL CARCINOGENESIS

Most forms of human cancer can be reproduced in experimental animals by exposure to specific chemical carcinogens, albeit in different organs, exposure pathways that do not exist for human exposure, or by chemicals that humans are not exposed to. In many cases the cell of origin, morphogenesis, phenotypic markers, and genetic alterations are qualitatively identical to corresponding human cancers. Furthermore, animal models have revealed the constancy of carcinogen-host interaction among mammalian species by reproducing organ-specific cancers in animals with chemicals identified as human carcinogens, such as coal tar and squamous cell carcinomas, vinyl chloride and hepatic angiosarcomas, aflatoxin and hepatocarcinoma, and aromatic amines and bladder cancer. The introduction of genetically modified mice designed to reproduce specific human cancer syndromes, and precancer models, has accelerated both the understanding of the contributions of chemicals to cancer causation and the identification of potential exogenous carcinogens.[24–27] Furthermore, construction of mouse strains genetically altered to express human drug-metabolizing enzymes has added both to the relevance of mouse studies for understanding human carcinogen metabolism and the prediction of genotoxicity from suspected human carcinogens and other chemical exposures.[28] Together, these studies have indicated that carcinogenic agents can directly activate oncogenes, inactivate tumor suppressor genes, and cause the genomic changes that are associated with autonomous growth, enhanced survival, and modified gene expression profiles that are required for the malignant phenotype.[29]

DNA REPAIR PROTECTS THE HOST FROM CHEMICAL CARCINOGENS

Protection of DNA integrity from chemical and physical damage is regulated by multiple endogenous repair systems linked to cancer proneness and presents compelling evidence for DNA as the ultimate target for carcinogenic stimuli and the importance of chemical damage to DNA for cancer initiation and progression. The capacity of cells to repair DNA damage is so dramatic that it prevents people from accumulating enough procarcinogenic mutations so that most cancer types are a disease of aging. Multiple DNA repair defects in diverse pathways have been identified in cancer-prone individuals, and repair-deficient mammalian cells are susceptible to transformation by chemical and physical carcinogens.[30,31] Nucleotide excision repair commonly removes carcinogen-DNA adducts or ultraviolet photoproducts by a complex process involving at least ten gene products, each potentially associated with mutations leading to human DNA repair defect syndromes and increased cancer rates. Nucleotide excision repair commonly favors adduct removal on the transcribed strand to protect protein synthesis. Genetically engineered mice deficient in genes involved in nucleotide excision repair are particularly sensitive to chemical and ultraviolet carcinogenesis at particular organ sites.

The highly mutagenic 0^6-methylguanine, a consequence of exposure to certain methylating agents, is repaired by 0^6-alkyldeoxyguanine-DNA alkyltransferase, an enzyme that protects the host from thymic lymphomas, colonic preneoplastic lesions, and colonic K-*ras* mutations after exposure of mice to methylating agents. Mutations in genes involved in nucleotide mismatch repair increase risk for colon cancer in humans, and engineered mice that are null for a gene in this pathway are predisposed to develop tumors.[31,32] The human cancer susceptibility genes *BRCA1/2* and *ATM* participate in repair of carcinogen-induced DNA double-strand breaks in pathways linked to homologous recombination.[33] Mutations in genes encoding a separate family of genes involved in homologous recombination, RecQ helicases, underlie two cancer-prone inherited diseases, Bloom and Werner syndromes, characterized by DNA rearrangements. Cells from these patients are particularly sensitive to genotoxic chemicals.[34]

GENETIC SUSCEPTIBILITY TO CHEMICAL CARCINOGENESIS

The identification and characterization of genes that modify risks for cancer development have been facilitated by substantial variation in susceptibility to chemically induced carcinogenesis at specific tissue sites among inbred strains of rodents and spontaneous or genetically modified mutant strains.[35–37] For a variety of tissue sites, including lung, liver, breast, and skin, pairs of inbred mice that differ by 100-fold in risk for tumor development after carcinogen exposure have been characterized. Genetically determined differences in the affinity for the aryl hydrocarbon hydroxylase (Ah) receptor or other differences in metabolic processing of carcinogens is one modifier that has a major impact on experimental and human cancer risk.[38,39] The development of mice reconstituted with components of the human carcinogen-metabolizing genome should facilitate the extrapolation of metabolic activity by human enzymes and cancer risk.[28] Other loci regulate the growth of premalignant foci, the response to tumor promoters, the immune response to metastatic cells, and the basal proliferation rate of target cells.[35] In mice susceptible to colon cancer due to a carcinogen-induced constitutive mutation in the *apc* gene, a locus on mouse chromosome 4 confers resistance to colon cancer.[36] The identification of the phospholipase A2 gene at this locus and subsequent functional testing in transgenic mice revealed an interesting paracrine protective influence on tumor development.[36] This gene, and several other genes mapped for susceptibility to chemically induced mouse tumors (*ptprj*, a receptor type tyrosine phosphatase, and *STK6/STK15*, an aurora kinase) have now been shown to influence susceptibility to organ-specific cancer induction in humans.[35,36] However, mouse studies have revealed the presence of multiple interacting loci that have powerful influences on susceptibility to chemically induced cancer at specific organ sites, making the interpretation of single nucleotide polymorphisms in the human genome extremely complex.[40,41]

In humans, the determination of genetic susceptibility can be assessed by phenotyping or genotyping methods. Phenotypes generally represent complex genotypes. Examples of phenotypes include the assessment of DNA repair capacity in cultured blood cells, mammographic breast density, or the quantitation of carcinogen-DNA adducts in a target organ.[7] New "omics" technologies, as discussed later, provide new phenotyping information implicating carcinogenic pathways.[42] The contribution of genetics to cancer risk from chemical carcinogens can range from small to large, depending on its penetrance. There are models for understanding how chemical exposures may be modulated by genetics in humans, the so-called gene-environment interactions, but the study of this can be complicated.[42–45] Highly penetrant cancer-susceptibility genes cause familial cancers, but account for less than 5% of all cancers. Low-penetrant genes cause common sporadic cancers, which have large public health consequences.

A genetic polymorphism (e.g., single nucleotide polymorphisms) is defined as a genetic variant present in at least 1% of the population. Because of the advent of improved genotyping methods that have reduced cost and increased high throughput, haplotyping and whole genome-wide association studies are ongoing.[5,46] Although haplotyping studies, facilitated through the International HapMap Project (www.hapmap.org) has not proven useful for predicting human cancers, high-density, whole genome-wide, single nucleotide polymorphism association studies have shown remarkable consistency for many gene loci, although the risk estimates are only 1.0–1.4.[5] For example, the contribution of genetic polymorphisms to cancer risk, at least for breast cancer, appears to improve risk modeling by only a few percent; known breast cancer risk factors account for about 58% of risk, and adding ten genetic variants increases risk only to 62%.[47]

Virtually any part of the carcinogenic process can be implicated as a heritable trait, given that single nucleotide polymorphisms are present in about every 300 base pairs. Genes under study are from pathways that affect behavior, activate and detoxify carcinogens, affect DNA repair, govern cell-cycle control, trigger apoptosis, effect cell signaling, and so forth.[48] Table 18.1 lists several investigated genetic polymorphisms and their possible associations with cancer risk, where biological hypotheses exist within the carcinogenic process. Virtually every cancer type has been examined for associations with genetic susceptibilities, and although there are many associations that have not been replicated, there is some consistency for cancers of the lung, breast, prostate, and colon.[46,49–54]

MOLECULAR EPIDEMIOLOGY, CHEMICAL CARCINOGENESIS, AND CANCER RISK IN HUMAN POPULATIONS

Molecular epidemiology is the application of biologically based hypotheses using molecular and epidemiologic methods and measures. New technologies continue to allow epidemiologic studies to improve testing of biologically based hypotheses. An important goal has been to identify cancer risk based on gene-environment interactions. Although experimental animal studies provide mechanistic models using modeled exposures with tumor initiation and promotion sequences, in humans, the best evidence that exists for how cancer develops is that of a genetic disease through multiple DNA-damaging events (e.g., mutations and alterations in gene expression through hypermethylation of promoter sequences), which have only loose temporal sequences, mostly occurring early.[21,55] More so, we remain challenged because cancer is a complex disease of diverse etiologies by multiple exposures causing damage in different genes, for example, $gene^N$-$environment^N$ interactions, for which how many "n" is not known.[56]

Two fundamental principles underlie current studies of molecular epidemiology. First, carcinogenesis is a multistage process, and behind each stage are numerous genetic events. Thus, characterizing a specific risk factor against a background of many risk factors is difficult and limits statistical power. Second, wide interindividual variation in response to carcinogen exposure and other carcinogenic processes indicate that the human response is not homogeneous, so that experimental models and epidemiology (e.g., the use of a single cell clone to study a gene's effect experimentally or the assumption that the population responds similarly to the mean in epidemiology studies), might not be representative of susceptible and resistant groups within a population.

Biomarkers of Cancer Risk

The evaluation of dose and risk estimates in epidemiologic studies can include four components, namely, external exposure measurements, internal exposure measurements, biomarkers estimating the biologically effective dose, and biomarkers of harm. The latter three measurements are biomarkers that improve on the first by quantifying exposure at the cellular level to characterize low-dose exposures in low-risk populations, providing a relative contribution of individual chemical carcinogens from complex mixtures, and/or estimating total burden of a particular exposure where there are many sources.[57]

Chemicals cause genetic damage in different ways, namely the formation of carcinogen-DNA adducts leading to base mutations, or gross chromosomal changes.[8,11] Adducts are formed when a mutagen, or part of it, irreversibly binds to DNA so that it can cause a base substitution, insertion, or deletion during DNA replication. Gross chromosomal mutations are chromosome breaks, gaps, or translocations. The level of DNA damage is the biologically effective dose in a target organ, and reflects the net result of carcinogen exposure, activation, lack of detoxification, lack of DNA repair, and lack of programmed cell death. A variety of assays have been used for determining carcinogen-macromolecular adducts in human tissues; for example, for assessing risk from tobacco smoking.[7,58,59] Important considerations for the assessment of biomarkers include sensitivity, specificity, reproducibility, accessibility for human use, and whether it represents a risk measured in a target organ or surrogate tissue. No single biomarker has been considered to be sufficiently validated for use as a cancer risk marker in an individual as it relates to chemical carcinogenesis.[59] However, there is some evidence that DNA adducts are cancer risk factors in both cohort and case-control studies[60,61] and possibly chromosomal aberrations.[57]

People are commonly exposed to *N*-nitrosamine and other *N*-nitroso compounds from dietary and tobacco exposures, which are associated with DNA adduct formation and cancer.[9,62] Exposure can occur through endogenous formation of *N*-nitrosamines from nitrates in food or directly from dietary sources, cosmetics, drugs, household commodities, and tobacco smoke. Endogenous formation occurs in the stomach from the reaction of nitrosatable amines and nitrate, used as a preservative, which is converted to nitrites by bacteria. The *N*-nitrosamines undergo metabolic activation by cytochrome P-450s (CYP2E1, CYP2A6, and CYP2D6) and form DNA adducts. Biomarkers are available to assess *N*-nitrosamine exposure from tobacco smoke (e.g., urinary tobacco-specific nitrosamine levels) or DNA, including in target organs such as the lungs.

Heterocyclic amines are formed from the overheating of food with creatine, such as meat, chicken, and fish.[63] Heterocyclic amines, estimated as consumption of well-done meat, have been associated with breast and colon cancer, presumably through metabolic activation mechanisms and DNA damage.[64,65] Aflatoxins, another food contaminant, are considered to be a major contributor to liver cancer in China and parts of Africa, especially interacting with hepatitis viruses,[7,66] Urinary aflatoxin adduct levels vary among regions of the world, depending on dietary exposures, which are predictors of liver cancer risk, especially as an interaction with hepatitis B infection.[61]

Aromatic amines are another class of human carcinogens. Aryl aromatic amines have been implicated in bladder carcinogenesis, especially in occupationally exposed cohorts (e.g., dye workers) and tobacco smokers.[67,68] These compounds are activated by cytochrome P-4501A2 and excreted via the *N*-acetyl transferase 2 gene. The quantitative assessment using biomarkers has been more difficult, but some persons have studied DNA adducts as well.[7]

Epidemiologic and experimental studies have linked benzene to hematologic toxicity including aplastic anemia, myelodysplastic syndrome, and acute myeloid leukemia. Benzene is metabolized by hepatic P-4502E1 (CYP2E1) yielding benzene oxide and hydroquinone, among other reactive metabolites. Circulating hydroquinones may be further metabolized to reactive benzoquinones by myeloperoxidase in bone marrow white blood cell precursors and stroma. Benzene metabolites are reported to have a variety of biological consequences on bone marrow cells including covalent binding to DNA and protein, alterations in gene expression, cytokine and chemokine abnormalities, and chromosomal aberrations.[69,70] In humans, functional polymorphisms in myeloperoxidase and the NAD(P):quinone oxidoreductase are associated with altered enzyme expression and benzene-related hematologic outcomes.[71] Similarly, functional polymorphisms in genes encoding proteins involved in maintaining genomic stability, including *p53*, *WRN*, and *BRCA2* that reduce their ability to contribute to double-strand DNA break repair, may increase hematotoxicity in occupationally exposed subjects.[72]

There are phenotyping assays that represent the lifetime response of a person's exposure to endogenous and exogenous chemical exposures. Examples of carcinogen-DNA adduct studies have been previously discussed. Other examples include measuring a person's capacity for DNA repair that has been extensively studied and found to predict cancer risk at multiple sites interacting with carcinogen exposure, and a genetic basis using twin study designs has been reported.[53] Another example is mammographic breast density, which carries as high as a sixfold risk of breast cancer and is related to exposures such as exogenous estrogens and alcohol drinking. The study of alterations in tumors can provide another type of phenotype suggesting the etiology of cancer risk in individuals. For example, researchers have linked the mutational spectra of the *p53* tumor suppressor gene[17] and hypermethylation of tumor suppressor genes.[73]

Emerging technologies using the omics approaches (genomics, measuring heritable variation, somatic mutations, and copy number; transcriptomics, measuring mRNA and microRNA expression; epigenomics; proteomics, measuring proteins; and metabolomics, measuring small metabolites) are increasingly being applied to chemical carcinogenesis and human cancer risk studies.[42] In the laboratory under experimental conditions, these methods are being used to characterize the pathways that respond to chemical exposure and how they contribute to their carcinogenic potential. In human studies, they are mostly used to identify pathways for future study (hypothesis generation) and to identify biomarkers that can be tested as risk markers. For example, in a small study of benzene-exposed workers, different pathways were shown to be affected depending on the omics being studied,[74] and smoking can induce different transcripts (microRNA and mRNA) in the same pathways.[75,76] The challenge, though, given that these mechanisms from transcripts to metabolism work concordantly in the cell, will be to integrate the data to determine how a specific chemical might affect the same pathway through different mechanisms.[42]

POLYCLIC AROMATIC HYDROCARBONS AS A MODEL FOR GENE-ENVIRONMENT INTERACTION

Polycyclic aromatic hydrocarbons (PAHs) are large aromatic (three or more fused benzene rings) compounds that are from a class of more than 200 chemicals. These compounds are ubiquitous in the environment and present in the ambient air. They are formed from overcooking foods, fireplaces, charcoal barbeques, burning of coal and crude oil, tobacco smoke, and in various occupational settings.[77–83] In order for PAHs to exert their toxic effect, they must undergo metabolic activation via cytochromes P-4501A1 and P-4503A4 to form DNA adducts, or are excreted via pathways involving the glutathione-S-transferase genes. It is important to note that different PAHs have different potential for carcinogenicity, depending on their chemical structure, and complex PAH mixtures, such as found in the aluminum and steel industry, cigarette smoke, coal tar, and diesel exhaust, have different types and ratios of PAHs so that these exposures have different cancer risks.[84] PAHs can be absorbed through the skin, inhaled, or ingested.

PAHs are associated with an increased risk of lung and skin cancer in the occupational setting.[84–86] Benzo(a)pyrene is among the most commonly studied PAH. It is classified as a known human carcinogen by the International Agency for Research on Cancer, and a suspected human carcinogen by the American Conference of Governmental Industrial Hygienists. It should be noted that other PAHs are considered as lesser classifications, and about 45 have not been shown to be carcinogenic or classified as group 3.[84,87,88] Benzo(a)pyrene (BaP) role in carcinogenesis serves as a model for chemical carcinogens. The bay region diol epoxide binds to DNA mostly as the N2-deoxyguanosine adduct. The evidence linking benzo(a)pyrene-deoxyguanosine adducts with a carcinogenic effect in lung cancer is very strong, including site-specific hotspot mutations in the *p53* tumor suppressor gene.[89–91] The experimentally obtained mutation spectra coincide with the spectra of mutations observed in lung cancer of smokers.[77,92] For dietary exposures, increased intake of charcoal-broiled meat was shown to increase PAH adducts in the DNA of white blood cells.[93] But the evidence for a clear association of dietary PAH, adducts, mutations, and cancer is lacking.

Workers with high PAH exposure have been extensively studied. PAH exposure is causally associated with lung cancer from inhalation exposures in the workplace, such as for aluminum, steel, coke oven, stokers, and asphalt workers.[84–86] Exposure to PAHs via other routes such as diet and skin absorption is not associated with lung cancer, even though the dietary contribution of PAHs to total body burden may be sizeable. A meta-analysis indicated that the unit relative risk for 100 mcg/m^3 years of PAH exposure to lung cancer was 1.2 (95% confidence interval, 1.11–1.29).[94] It is believed that PAHs in tobacco smoke are an important cause for the relationship of smoking to lung cancer. Skin cancer is the next most commonly associated cancer with PAH exposure.

Various biomarkers of exposure have been developed for assessing PAH exposure.[81,82,95–98] These include measuring DNA adducts, protein adducts, and urinary 1-hydroxypyrene; only the latter is a validated biomarker of exposure and no adducts have been validated as biomarkers of cancer risk. However, there are several case-control studies and a cohort study that indicates that PAH and other adducts are associated with cancer risk, and validating this further are adducts that are associated with *p53* mutations in lung tumors related to cigarette smoking.[99–101] There has been extensive research considering genetic susceptibility to PAH lung carcinogens, and although candidate polymorphisms plausibly increase risk, sufficient consistency to be considered a validated biomarker of cancer risk has not been achieved.[102] Examples include polymorphisms in the *CYP1A1*, *CYP3A4* glutathione transferase mu, and DNA repair genes.

Selected References

The full list of references for this chapter appears in the online version.

1. Parkin DM. International variation. *Oncogene* 2004;23:6329.
2. Colditz GA, Sellers TA, Trapido E. Epidemiology: identifying the causes and preventability of cancer? *Nat Rev Cancer* 2006;6(1):75.
3. Luch A. Nature and nurture: lessons from chemical carcinogenesis. *Nat Rev Cancer* 2005;5:113.
4. Lichtenstein P, Holm NV, Verkasalo PK, et al. Environmental and heritable factors in the causation of cancer: analyses of cohorts of twins from Sweden, Denmark, and Finland. *N Engl J Med* 2000;343:78.
5. Hunter DJ, Chanock SJ. Genome-wide association studies and "the art of the soluble." *J Natl Cancer Inst* 2010;102:836.
6. Wogan GN, Hecht SS, Felton JS, et al. Environmental and chemical carcinogenesis. *Semin Cancer Biol* 2004;14:473.
7. Poirier MC. Chemical-induced DNA damage and human cancer risk. *Nat Rev Cancer* 2004;4:630.
8. Irigaray P, Belpomme D. Basic properties and molecular mechanisms of exogenous chemical carcinogens. *Carcinogenesis* 2010;31:135.
9. Hecht SS. Tobacco carcinogens, their biomarkers and tobacco-induced cancer. *Nat Rev Cancer* 2003;3:733.
11. Shrivastav N, Li D, Essigmann JM. Chemical biology of mutagenesis and DNA repair: cellular responses to DNA alkylation. *Carcinogenesis* 2010;31:59.
12. Sporn MB, Liby KT. Cancer chemoprevention: scientific promise, clinical uncertainty. *Nat Clin Pract Oncol* 2005;2:518.
13. Omenn GS. Chemoprevention of lung cancers: lessons from CARET, the beta-carotene and retinol efficacy trial, and prospects for the future. *Eur J Cancer Prev* 2007;16:184.
14. Bresalier RS. Chemoprevention of colorectal cancer: why all the confusion? *Curr Opin Gastroenterol* 2008;24:48.
15. U.S. Department of Health and Human Services PHSNTP. *Report on Carcinogens*.11th ed. Washington, DC: U.S.Department of Health and Human Services; 2005.
16. Luch A. The mode of action of organic carcinogens on cellular structures. *EXS* 2006;(96):65.
17. Hussain SP, Schwank J, Staib F, et al. TP53 mutations and hepatocellular carcinoma: insights into the etiology and pathogenesis of liver cancer. *Oncogene* 2007;26:2166.
19. Porta M, Crous-Bou M, Wark PA, et al. Cigarette smoking and K-ras mutations in pancreas, lung and colorectal adenocarcinomas: etiopathogenic similarities, differences and paradoxes. *Mutat Res* 2009;682:83.
20. Blackford A, Parmigiani G, Kensler TW, et al. Genetic mutations associated with cigarette smoking in pancreatic cancer. *Cancer Res* 2009;69:3681.
21. Jones PA, Baylin SB. The epigenomics of cancer. *Cell* 2007;128:683.
22. Feinberg AP, Tycko B. The history of cancer epigenetics. *Nat Rev Cancer* 2004;4:143.
23. Fukushima S, Kinoshita A, Puatanachokchai R, et al. Hormesis and dose-response-mediated mechanisms in carcinogenesis: evidence for a threshold in carcinogenicity of non-genotoxic carcinogens. *Carcinogenesis* 2005;26:1835.
27. Cardiff RD, Anver MR, Boivin GP, et al. Precancer in mice: animal models used to understand, prevent, and treat human precancers. *Toxicol Pathol* 2006;34:699.
30. Cleaver JE. Cancer in xeroderma pigmentosum and related disorders of DNA repair. *Nat Rev Cancer* 2005;5:564.
31. Wijnhoven SW, Hoogervorst EM, de Waard H, et al. Tissue specific mutagenic and carcinogenic responses in NER defective mouse models. *Mutat Res* 2007;614:77.
32. Berndt SI, Platz EA, Fallin MD, et al. Genetic variation in the nucleotide excision repair pathway and colorectal cancer risk. *Cancer Epidemiol Biomarkers Prev* 2006;15:2263.
34. Reliene R, Bishop AJ, Schiestl RH. Involvement of homologous recombination in carcinogenesis. *Adv Genet* 2007;58:67.
35. Demant P. Cancer susceptibility in the mouse: genetics, biology and implications for human cancer. *Nat Rev Genet* 2003;4:721.
39. Di PG, Magno LA, Rios-Santos F. Glutathione S-transferases: an overview in cancer research. *Expert Opin Drug Metab Toxicol* 2010;6:153.
41. Fijneman RJ. Genetic predisposition to sporadic cancer: how to handle major effects of minor genes? *Cell Oncol* 2005;27:281.
42. Knox SS. From 'omics' to complex disease: a systems biology approach to gene-environment interactions in cancer. *Cancer Cell Int* 2010;10:11.
43. Vineis P, Berwick M. The population dynamics of cancer: a Darwinian perspective. *Int J Epidemiol* 2006;35:1151.
44. Hemminki K, Lorenzo BJ, Forsti A. The balance between heritable and environmental aetiology of human disease. *Nat Rev Genet* 2006; 7:958.
45. Hunter DJ. Gene-environment interactions in human diseases. *Nat Rev Genet* 2005;6:287.
46. Houlston RS, Peto J. The search for low-penetrance cancer susceptibility alleles. *Oncogene* 2004;23:6471.
47. Wacholder S, Hartge P, Prentice R, et al. Performance of common genetic variants in breast-cancer risk models. *N Engl J Med* 2010;362:986.
48. Spitz MR, Wu X, Mills G. Integrative epidemiology: from risk assessment to outcome prediction. *J Clin Oncol* 2005;23:267.
49. Liu G, Zhou W, Christiani DC. Molecular epidemiology of non-small cell lung cancer. *Semin Respir Crit Care Med* 2005;26:265.
50. Alberg AJ, Brock MV, Samet JM. Epidemiology of lung cancer: looking to the future. *J Clin Oncol* 2005;23:3175.
51. de La CA. Genetic predisposition to colorectal cancer. *Nat Rev Cancer* 2004;4:769.
52. Hsing AW, Chokkalingam AP. Prostate cancer epidemiology. *Front Biosci* 2006;11:1388.
53. Wu X, Gu J, Spitz MR. Mutagen sensitivity: a genetic predisposition factor for cancer. *Cancer Res* 2007;67:3493.
55. Vogelstein B, Kinzler KW. Cancer genes and the pathways they control. *Nat Med* 2004;10:789.
56. Shields PG, Harris CC. Cancer risk and low-penetrance susceptibility genes in gene-environment interactions. *J Clin Oncol* 2000;18:2309.
60. Veglia F, Loft S, Matullo G, et al. DNA adducts and cancer risk in prospective studies: a pooled analysis and a meta-analysis. *Carcinogenesis* 2008;29:932.
68. Neumann HG. Aromatic amines: mechanisms of carcinogenesis and implications for risk assessment. *Front Biosci* 2010;15:1119.
74. Zhang L, McHale CM, Rothman N, et al. Systems biology of human benzene exposure. *Chem Biol Interact* 2010;184:86.
84. International Agency for Research on Cancer (IARC). *Monographs on the Evaluation of Carcinogenic Risks to Humans: Some Non-Heterocyclic Polycyclic Aromatic Hydrocarbons and Some Related Exposures*. Vol 92. Lyon, France: IARC Press, 2010.
94. Armstrong B, Hutchinson E, Unwin J, Fletcher T. Lung cancer risk after exposure to polycyclic aromatic hydrocarbons: a review and meta-analysis. *Environ Health Perspect* 2004;112:970.
100. Boffetta P. Biomarkers in cancer epidemiology: an integrative approach. *Carcinogenesis* 2010;31:121.
101. Veglia F, Loft S, Matullo G, et al. DNA adducts and cancer risk in prospective studies: a pooled analysis and a meta-analysis. *Carcinogenesis* 2008;29:932.

CHAPTER 19 PHYSICAL FACTORS

MATS LJUNGMAN

Ionizing radiation (IR) and ultraviolet light (UV) have throughout time challenged the genetic integrity of all living organisms. By inducing DNA damage and subsequently mutations, these physical agents have promoted diversity through natural selection, and, as a result, organisms from all kingdoms of life carry genes that encode proteins that repair damaged DNA. In higher, multicellular organisms, many additional mechanisms of genome preservation have evolved such as cell cycle checkpoints and apoptosis. Despite the many sophisticated mechanisms to safeguard the human genome from the mutagenic actions of DNA-damaging agents, not all exposed cells successfully restore the integrity of their DNA and some cells may subsequently progress into malignant cancer cells. Furthermore, through man-made activities we are now exposed to many new physical agents, such as radiofrequency and microwave radiation, electromagnetic fields, asbestos, and nanoparticles, for which evolution has not yet had time to deliver genome-preserving response mechanisms. This chapter will highlight the molecular mechanisms by which these physical agents affect cells and how human exposure may lead to cancer.

IONIZING RADIATION

Ionizing radiation is defined as radiation that has sufficient energy to ionize molecules by displacing electrons from atoms. Ionizing radiation can be electromagnetic, such as x-rays and gamma rays, or consist of particles, such as electrons, protons, neutrons, alpha particles, or carbon ions. Natural sources of ionizing radiation make up about 80% of human exposure, while medical sources make up about 20%.[1] The increased medical use of diagnostic x-rays and computed tomography (CT) scanning procedures likely translates into higher incidences of cancer. Of the natural sources, radon exposure is the most significant exposure risk to humans. Importantly, with better and more comprehensive screening techniques, the human exposure to radon could be dramatically lowered.

Mechanisms of Damage Induction

Linear Energy Transfer

The biological effects of ionizing radiation are unique in that the induced damage is clustered due to the local deposition of energy in radiation tracks. The distance between the depositions of energy is biologically very relevant and unique to the energy and the type of radiation. The term linear energy transfer (LET) denotes the energy transferred per unit length of a track of radiation. Electromagnetic radiation, such as x-rays or gamma rays, are sparsely ionizing and therefore classified as low LET radiation, while particulate radiation, such as neutrons, protons, and alpha particles, are examples of high LET radiation.

Radiation Biochemistry

Radiation-induced damage to cellular target molecules, such as DNA, proteins, and lipids, can be either direct or indirect (Fig. 19.1). The *direct action* of radiation, which is the dominant mode of action of high LET radiation, is due to deposition of energy directly to the target molecule, resulting in one or more ionization events. The *indirect action* of radiation is due to the radiolysis of water molecules, which after initial absorption of radiation energy become excited and generate different types of radiolysis products where the reactive hydroxyl radical (•OH) can damage both DNA and proteins. About two-thirds of the damage induced by low LET radiation is due to the indirect action of radiation. Since the hydroxyl radical is very reactive (half-life is 10^{-9} seconds), it does not diffuse more than a few nanometers after it is formed before it reacts with other molecules, and, thus, only radicals formed in close proximity to the target molecule will contribute to the damage of that target.[2] However, by chemical recombination of the primary radiolysis products, hydrogen peroxide (H_2O_2) is formed, which in turn can produce hydroxyl radicals at a later time through the Fenton reaction. Since H_2O_2 is not very reactive, it can diffuse long distances away from the initial site of energy deposition.

Radical scavengers normally present in cells, such as glutathione, can protect target molecules by reacting with the hydroxyl radical (Fig. 19.1). Even after the target molecule has been hit and ionized, glutathione can contribute to cell protection by donating a hydrogen atom to the radical, allowing the unpaired electron present in the radical to pair up with the electron from the hydrogen atom. This is considered the simplest of all types of repair and is called *chemical repair.*[3] However, if oxygen molecules are present, they will compete with scavenger molecules for the ionized molecule, and if oxygen reacts with the ionized target molecule before the hydrogen donation occurs, the damage will be solidified as a peroxide not amendable to chemical repair. Instead, this lesion will require enzymatic repair for restoration. This augmenting biological effect of oxygen is called the *oxygen effect* and is considered an important factor for the effectiveness of radiation therapy.

Damage to DNA

The direct and indirect effects of radiation induce more or less identical types of lesions in DNA. However, the density of lesions induced in a stretch of DNA is higher for high LET radiation, and this increased complexity is thought to complicate the repair of these lesions. Radiation-induced lesions consist of more than 100 chemically distinct base lesions, such as the mutagenic lesions thymine glycol and 8-hydroxyguanine.[2,4,5] Furthermore, damage to the sugar moiety in the backbone of DNA and some types of base damage can result in single strand breaks (SSBs). Since the energy deposition of radiation is clustered even for low LET radiation, it is likely that two individual

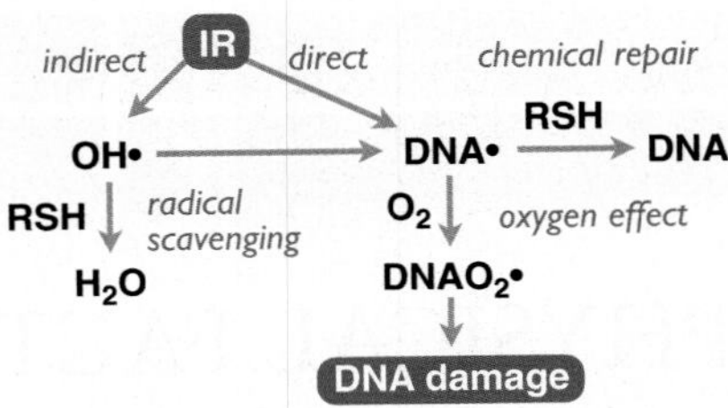

FIGURE 19.1 Factors affecting the induction DNA damage by ionizing radiation. Ionizing radiation can ionize DNA either by "direct action" or by "indirect action" in which radiation energy is absorbed by neighboring molecules, such as water, leading to the generation of hydroxyl radicals that attack DNA. Sulfur-containing cellular molecules (RSH), such as glutathione, can scavenge hydroxyl radicals by hydrogen atom donations and thereby protect the DNA from the indirect action of radiation. Glutathione can also donate hydrogen atoms to ionized DNA, thereby restoring the integrity of DNA in a process termed *chemical repair.* Oxygen can compete with chemical repair in a process termed the *oxygen effect,* resulting in the enhancement of the biological effect of ionizing radiation by the fixation of the initial DNA damage into DNA peroxides ($DNAO_2$•).

strand breaks are formed in close proximity on opposite strands, resulting in the formation of a double strand break (DSB). It has been estimated that 1 Gy of ionizing radiation gives rise to about 40 DSBs, 1,000 SSBs, 1,000 base lesions, and 150 DNA-protein cross-links per cell.[2] For a similarly lethal dose of UV light, about 400,000 lesions are required, demonstrating that the lesions induced by ionizing radiation are much more toxic than lesions induced by UV light. It is believed that DSBs are the critical lesions that lead to cell lethality following exposure to ionizing radiation.[6]

Damage to Proteins

Although proteins and lipids are subject to damage following exposure to ionizing radiation, the common belief is that DNA is the critical target for the biological effects of radiation. Indeed, abrogation of DNA damage surveillance or repair processes in cells results in enhanced induction of mutations and decreased cell survival following radiation.[5] However, studies of radiation-sensitive and -resistant bacteria imply that mechanisms that suppress protein damage may also play important roles in radiation resistance.[7] *Deinococcus radiodurans* is a bacterium that can survive radiation exposures of up to 17,000 Gy, and its extreme radioresistance has been linked to high intracellular levels of manganese that protect proteins from oxidation. The thought is that if a cell can limit protein oxidation, then its enzymes will remain active and cellular functions such as DNA repair will be able to restore the integrity of DNA even after severe DNA damage. It would be interesting to explore whether the concentration of manganese can be manipulated to sensitize tumor cells to radiation therapy. Furthermore, since protein damage due to reactive oxygen species (ROS) accumulate during the aging process, could supplements of manganese turn back the clock on aging?

Cellular Responses

DNA Repair

Ever since organisms started to utilize atmospheric oxygen for metabolic respiration many millions of years ago, they have been forced to deal with the cellular damage induced by ROS. Base excision repair (BER) (see Chapter 2) evolved to remove many of the different types of oxidative base lesions and DNA SSBs induced by ROS. However, ROS seldom induce DSBs unless the generation of hydroxyl radicals is clustered near the DNA molecule. A more important source of intracellular generation of DSBs may instead be the process of DNA replication, and it is possible that homologous recombination (HR) repair (see Chapter 2) primary evolved to overcome DSBs sporadically induced during the replication process. The other major pathway of DSB repair is the nonhomologous end-joining (NHEJ) pathway (see Chapter 2), which is utilized by immune cells in the process of antibody generation. Although the HR pathway has high fidelity due to the utilization of homologous sister chromatids to ensure that correct DNA ends are joined, the NHEJ pathway lacks this control mechanism and therefore occasionally rejoins ends incorrectly. Thus, the NHEJ pathway may contribute to the generation of mutations following radiation (Fig. 19.2). However, NHEJ is the only mechanism available for DSB repair in postmitotic cells and cells in the G_1 phase of the cell cycle since no sister chromatids are available in these cells to support HR repair.

Ataxia-Telangiectasia Mutated and Cell Cycle Checkpoints

Due to the enormous task of replicating the whole genome during the S phase and segregating the chromosomes during mitosis, proliferating cells are generally much more vulnerable to radiation than stationary cells. To prevent cells with damaged DNA to enter into these critical stages of the cell cycle, cells can activate cell cycle checkpoints (Fig. 19.2). The major sensor of radiation-induced damage in cells is the ataxia-telangiectasia mutated (ATM) kinase, which following activation can phosphorylate more than 700 proteins in cells.[8] Two

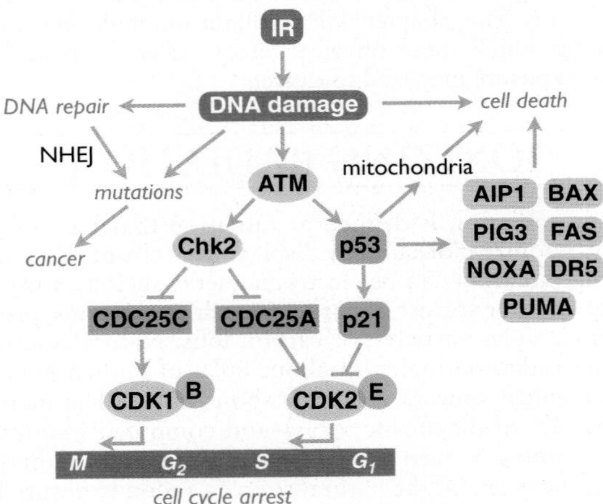

FIGURE 19.2 Cellular responses to ionizing radiation. Ionizing radiation induces predominantly base lesions, single and double strand breaks. Base lesions and single strand breaks are repaired by base excision repair (BER), while double strand breaks are repaired by nonhomologous end joining (NHEJ) and homologous recombination (HR). If DNA lesions are misrepaired by NHEJ or not repaired at all before cells enter S phase or mitosis, genomic instability is manifested as mutations or chromosome aberrations that promote carcinogenesis. In order for cells to assist DNA repair and safeguard against genetic instability and cancer, cells can induce cell cycle arrest or apoptosis. The ATM kinase is an early responder to DNA damage induced by ionizing radiation that activates the cell cycle checkpoint kinase Chk2 and the tumor suppressor p53. Chk2 inactivates the CDC25A and CDC25C phosphatases that are critical in promoting cell cycle progression by activating the cyclin-dependent kinases CDK2 or CDK1 and thereby arresting the cells at the G_1/S or G_2/M checkpoints. In addition, p53 can arrest cells at the G_1/S checkpoint by inducing the CDK inhibitor p21. P53 also plays a role in promoting apoptosis by inducing a number of pro-apoptotic proteins as well as translocating to mitochondria where it inhibits the actions of antiapoptotic factors.

ATM substrates, p53 and Chk2, are critical for the activation of cell cycle arrests at multiple sites in the cell cycle.[9,10] The kinase p53 regulates the gene expression of specific genes such as p21, which inhibits CDK2- and CDK4-mediated phosphorylation of the retinoblastoma protein, resulting in a block in the progression from the G_1 phase to the S phase of the cell cycle.[11,12] The Chk2 kinase promotes checkpoint activation in G_1 by targeting the CDC25A phosphatase[13] or in G_2/M by targeting the CDC25C phosphatase.[14] The activation of a cell cycle arrest following DNA damage provides the cell with additional time to repair the DNA before entering critical cell cycle stages and therefore promotes genetic stability. Loss or defects in the *ATM* or *p53* genes result in abrogation of radiation-induced cell cycle checkpoints, which manifests itself as the highly cancer-prone human syndromes ataxia telangiectasia[15] or Li-Fraumeni,[16] respectively.

Radiation-Induced Cell Death

Terminally differentiated and stationary cells, such as kidney, lung, brain, muscle, and liver cells, are in general more resistant to radiation-induced killing than are cells with a high turnover rate, such as different epithelial cells, spermatogonia, and hair follicles. However, the spleen and thymus, which consist of mostly nondividing cells, are among the most radiosensitive tissues, implying that the rate of cell proliferation is not the sole determinator of the radiation sensitivity of a tissue. An important factor regulating the induction of programmed cell death (apoptosis) in tissues is the tumor suppressor p53.[17] The p53 protein is activated in cells following exposure to IR by the ATM kinase (Fig. 19.2). When activated it regulates the expression of multiple genes that have roles in DNA repair, cell cycle arrest, and apoptosis. P53 can also localize to mitochondria following irradiation, where it triggers apoptosis through inactivation of antiapoptosis regulatory proteins.[18] Not all tissues induce the p53 response to the same degree after similar doses of IR, nor do they activate downstream pathways, such as DNA repair, cell cycle arrest, and apoptosis, in a similar way. For example, thymocytes have an intrinsic setting that favors apoptosis over cell cycle arrest following IR, while fibroblasts rarely induce apoptosis but instead activate a strong and lasting cell cycle arrest.[17]

Ionizing radiation can induce cell death in tissues by many different mechanisms. Apoptosis can occur rapidly in a p53-dependent manner and later in a p53-independent manner. This later wave of radiation-induced apoptosis is often initiated by mitotic catastrophe, which occurs as a result of complications during chromosome segregation. Cell death induced by ionizing radiation may in some cases be associated with autophagy, also called autophagocytosis, in which cells degrade cellular components via the lysosomal machinery. Whether autophagy is a programmed cell death or occurs in parallel with cell death is not clear. Interestingly, for some cell types, autophagy has been shown to actually protect the cells from radiation-induced death. Finally, tissue can undergo necrotic cell death following exposure to ionizing radiation. Necrosis is a clinical problem following radiation therapy that can occur in normal tissues many months after treatment and can contribute to the inflammatory response.

Cancer Risks

It is clear from epidemiologic studies of radiation workers and atomic bomb and Chernobyl victims that ionizing radiation can induce cancer.[19] Twenty years after the atomic bomb explosions in Japan during World War II, significant increases in the incidence of thyroid cancer and leukemia were observed. However, it took almost 50 years before solid tumors appeared in the population as a result of radiation exposure from the atomic bombs.[20] The incidences of solid tumors, such as breast, ovary, bladder, lung, and colon cancers, were estimated to have increased by a factor of 2 in the exposed group during this time period. The epidemiology studies following the nuclear power plant disaster in Chernobyl showed a clear increase in thyroid cancer as early as 4 years after the accident.[21] Young children were the most vulnerable to radiation exposure, with 1-year-old children being 237-fold more susceptible to thyroid cancer than the control group, while 10-year-old children were found to be sixfold more susceptible to thyroid cancer.[21] Many of the thyroid cancers that developed following the Chernobyl disaster could have been prevented if the population had not consumed locally produced milk that was contaminated with radioactive iodine.

The molecular signatures of radiation-induced tumors are complex but involve point mutations that could lead to the activation of the *RAS* oncogene or inactivation of the tumor suppressor gene *p53*. Furthermore, ionizing radiation induces DNA DSBs that may be unfaithfully repaired by the NHEJ pathway, leading to chromosome rearrangements. One such rearrangement found in 50% to 90% of the thyroid cancers examined following the Chernobyl accident involved the receptor tyrosine kinase c-RET, which when activated promotes cell growth.[21] Interestingly, no point mutations have been reported in the *RAS* or the *p53* genes in the thyroid tumors induced following the Chernobyl accident.[21]

The correlation between high exposure to ionizing radiation and cancer following the atomic bomb explosions and the Chernobyl accident is clear. What about the cancer risk following lower radiation exposures occurring in daily life? There are four theoretical risk models of radiation-induced cancer to consider. First, the *linear, no threshold* (LNT) *model* suggests that the induction of cancer is directly proportional to the dose of radiation, even at low doses of exposure. Second, the *sublinear* or *threshold model* suggests that below a certain threshold dose the risk of radiation-induced cancers is negligible. At these lower doses of radiation exposure, the DNA damage surveillance and repair mechanisms are thought to be fully capable of safeguarding the DNA to avoid the induction of mutations and cancer. Third, the *supralinear* or *stealth model* suggests that doses below a certain threshold or radiation with sufficiently low dose rates may not trigger the activation of DNA damage surveillance and repair mechanisms, resulting in suboptimal activation of cell cycle checkpoints and repair. This would be expected to lead to a higher rate of mutations and cancers than predicted by the LNT model but may be balanced by a higher incident of cell death. Fourth, the *linear-quadratic model* suggest that radiation effects at low doses are due to a single track of radiation hitting multiple targets, resulting in a linear induction rate, while at higher doses, multiple radiation tracks hit multiple cellular targets, resulting in a quadratic induction rate.

The BEIR VII report, released by the Committee on Biological Effects of Ionizing Radiation of the National Academy of Sciences and commissioned by the Environmental Protection Agency (EPA), is a review of published data regarding human health and cancer risks from exposure to low levels of ionizing radiation. Although this topic is controversial and not fully settled, the BIER VII report favored the LNT model.[1] Thus the "official" view is that no level of radiation is safe, and, therefore, careful consideration of risks versus benefits is necessary to ensure that the general population only receives radiation doses as low as reasonable achievable. Furthermore, the BIER VII committee concluded that the heritable effects of radiation were not evident in the published data, indicating that an individual is not likely to develop cancer due to radiation exposure of his or her parents.

The largest source of radiation exposure to the population is radon, which is a natural radioactive gas formed as a decay product of radium in the decay chain of uranium. Radon gas can accumulate to high levels in poorly ventilated basements in houses built on rock containing uranium. The major risk with radon is that some of its radioactive decay products can attach to dust particles that accumulate in lungs, leading to a continuous exposure of the lung tissues to high LET alpha particles. Due to this radiation exposure, the EPA claims that radon is the second leading cause of lung cancer in the United States. Another important source of human exposure to ionizing radiation is medical x-ray devices, and there is a growing concern about the dramatically increased use of whole body CT scans for diagnostic purposes. For a typical CT scan, a patient will receive about 100-fold more radiation than from a typical mammogram.[1] It is recommended that the use of whole body CT scans for children be very restricted due to the elevated risk of developing radiation-induced cancer for this age group.

Cancer patients who receive radiation therapy are at risk of developing secondary tumors induced by the radiation therapy treatment. This is particularly a concern for young patients since (1) children are more prone to radiation-induced cancer, (2) children have a relatively good chance of surviving the primary cancer and would have long life expectancies so a secondary tumor would have plenty of time to develop, and (3) many childhood cancers are promoted by genetic defects in DNA damage response pathways, making these patients highly prone to the geneotoxic effects of radiation and subsequent secondary cancers. The most sensitive tissues for the development of secondary cancer have been found to be the bone marrow (leukemia), thyroid, breast, and lung.

ULTRAVIOLET LIGHT

Depending on the wavelength, UV light is categorized into UVA (320 to 400 nm), UVB (290 to 320 nm), and UVC (240 to 290 nm) radiation. Most of the UVC light emitted from the sun is absorbed by the ozone layer in the atmosphere, and, thus, living organisms are mostly exposed to UVA and UVB irradiation.

Mechanisms of Damage Induction

UVC light is more damaging to DNA than UVA and UVB because the absorption maximum of DNA is around 260 nm. UVB and UVC induce predominantly pyrimidine dimers and 6-4 photoproducts, which consist of covalent ring structures that link two adjacent pyrimidines on the same DNA strand.[5] The formation of these lesions results in the bending of the DNA helix, resulting in the interference with both DNA and RNA synthesis. UVA light does not induce pyrimidine dimers or 6-4 photoproducts but can induce ROS, which in turn can form SSBs and base lesions in DNA of exposed cells.

Cellular Responses

DNA Repair

The nucleotide excision repair (NER) pathway removes pyrimidine dimers and 6-4 photoproducts from cellular DNA.[5] This pathway involves proteins that recognize the DNA lesions, nucleases that excise the DNA strand that contains the lesion, a DNA polymerase that synthesizes new DNA to fill the gap, and a DNA ligase that joins the backbone in the newly synthesized strand (see Chapter 2 for details). Genetic defects in the NER pathway result in the human syndrome xeroderma pigmentosum, with individuals more than 1,000-fold more prone to sun-induced skin cancer than normal individuals. In addition, human polymorphisms in certain NER genes are

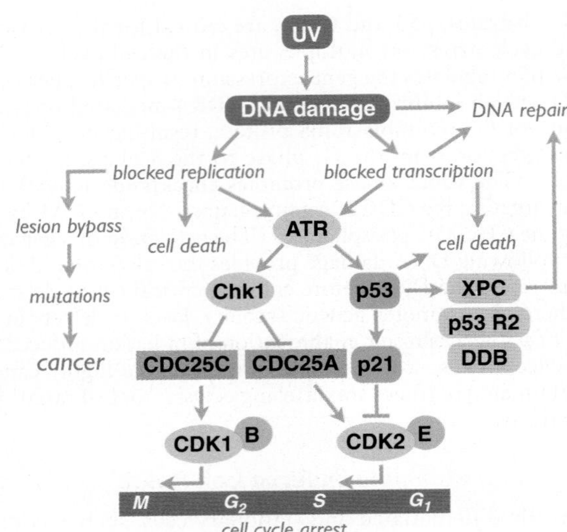

FIGURE 19.3 Cellular responses to ultraviolet (UV) light-induced DNA damage. UV light predominantly induces bulky DNA lesions that interfere with the processes of DNA replication and transcription. These lesions are removed from the global genome by global genomic nucleotide excision repair (GG-NER) and from transcribed DNA strands by transcription-coupled NER (TC-NER). Lesions blocking replication can be bypassed by exchanging processive DNA polymerases with less processive translesion DNA polymerases. While these polymerases allow cells to continue DNA synthesis and progress through the cell cycle, they have low fidelity, resulting in the potential induction of mutations promoting UV-induced carcinogenesis. To suppress mutations and support DNA repair efforts, the ataxia-telangiectasia and Rad3-related (ATR) kinase is activated in response to blocked replication or transcription. ATR activates the cell cycle checkpoint kinase Chk1, which, similar to Chk2, arrests cells in the G_1/S and G_2/M checkpoints by inhibiting CDC25A and CDC25C. ATR also activates p53, promoting G_1/S checkpoint activation via the induction of the Cdk-inhibitor p21. P53 also stimulates GG-NER by the transactivation of various NER genes and can promote apoptosis by induction of pro-apoptotic factors and translocation to mitochondria. Finally, apoptosis is induced if cells do not recover transcription in a certain time frame potentially due to the loss of survival factors or complications in S phase when replication encounters stalled transcription complexes.

thought to predispose individuals to cancers such as lung cancer, nonmelanoma skin cancer, head and neck cancer, and bladder cancer, indicating that NER is responsible for safeguarding the genome against many types of DNA adducts in addition to UV-induced lesions.[5]

UV-induced lesions formed in the transcribed strand of active genes block the elongation of RNA polymerase II, and if a cell does not restore transcription within a certain time frame, it may undergo apoptosis (Fig. 19.3).[22,23] To rapidly restore RNA synthesis and to avoid cell death, NER enzymes are recruited to the sites of blocked RNA polymerase II and the lesions are removed in a process called transcription-coupled repair (TCR).[24] Individuals with the Cockayne's syndrome (CS), tricothiodystrophy, or the UV-sensitive syndrome, are unable to utilize the TCR pathway following UV irradiation.[5] Cells from these individuals do not recover RNA synthesis following UV irradiation and are therefore very prone to UV-induced apoptosis. Interestingly, despite a clear DNA repair defect, these individuals are not predisposed to UV-induced skin cancer. It is thought that the inability of CS cells to remove the toxic lesions that block transcription following UV irradiation results in the suppression of tumorigenesis by the elimination of damaged cells by apoptosis. However, while protecting against tumorigenesis, the elevated level of apoptosis in these cells leads to increased cell loss, which in turn may lead to neurological degeneration.[22,25] Persistent transcription-blocking lesions in the genome has also been linked to aging.[26–28]

Translesion DNA Synthesis

Proliferating skin cells are very vulnerable to UV light because UV lesions block DNA replication (Fig. 19.3). Cells that have entered the S phase and initiated DNA synthesis have no choice but to finish replicating the whole genome or they will die. If DNA repair enzymes are not able to remove the blocking lesions from the template, the processive DNA polymerases may be exchanged for other, less processive DNA polymerases that can bypass the lesions. This is part of a "tolerance" mechanism, which allows cells to complete replication and eventually divide. However, the translesion DNA polymerases do not have the same fidelity as the processive DNA polymerases, and, thus, mutations may occur. This is thought to be a major pathway by which UV light induces mutagenesis and subsequently cancer (Fig. 19.3).

ATM and Rad3-Related Mediated Cell Cycle Checkpoints

In addition to utilizing the NER and BER pathways to repair UV-induced DNA damage, proliferating cells activate cell cycle checkpoints to allow more time for repair before entering critical parts of the cell cycle such as the S phase and mitosis. The ATM and Rad3-related (ATR) kinase is activated following UV irradiation by blocked replication or transcription (Fig. 19.3).[29] ATR phosphorylates a large number of proteins, many of which are the same as those phosphorylated by ATM after exposure to ionizing radiation.[8] Two important substrates of ATR are p53 and Chk1, which are critical in promoting cell cycle arrest. When induced by ATR, p53 transactivates the gene that encodes the cell cycle inhibitor p21, leading to the arrest of cells in the G_1 phase of the cell cycle, while Chk1 phosphorylates the CDK-activating phosphatases CDC25A and CDC25C, which targets them for degradation, resulting in an S-phase or G_2-phase arrest (Fig. 19.3).[30]

Activation of Cell Membrane Receptors

In addition to triggering cellular stress responses by inducing DNA damage, UV light can directly induce membrane receptor signaling by receptor phosphorylation. This is thought to be due to the direct UV-mediated inhibition of protein-tyrosine phosphatases that regulate the phosphorylation levels of various membrane receptors.[31] In addition, membrane receptors may physically aggregate following UV irradiation, leading to the activation of signal transduction pathways that regulate cell growth[32] or apoptosis.[33]

Cell Death

UV light effectively induces apoptosis in skin cells. The mechanism of how UV light induces cell death is not fully understood, but failure to adequately resume RNA synthesis following UV light exposure is strongly linked to apoptosis (Fig. 19.3).[22] Many potential mechanisms of how blocked transcription results in apoptosis have been suggested, such as a physical clash during S phase between elongating replication machineries and transcription complexes stalled at UV lesions. Another possible mechanism involves the preferential loss of survival factors coded by highly unstable mRNAs.[34] Induction of p53 may also contribute to UV-induced apoptosis,[35] although p53 appears to protect human fibroblasts[36] and keratinocytes[37] from UV-induced apoptosis. Although complications induced by DNA damage may be the predominant mechanism by which cells die following UV irradiation, UV light may in certain cell types induce apoptosis by directly promoting the physical aggregation of the death receptor Fas/APO1.[33]

Cancer Risks

The incidence of sun-induced skin cancer, especially melanoma, is on the increase due to higher sun exposure to the general population. The link between UV light exposure and skin cancer is very strong, but the role of UV light in the etiology of nonmelanoma and melanoma skin cancer differs. Although the risk of nonmelanoma cancer relates to the cumulative lifetime exposure to UV light, the risk of contracting melanoma appears to be linked to high sun light exposure during childhood.[38] What makes UV light such a potent carcinogen is that it can initiate carcinogenesis by inducing DNA lesions as well as suppressing the immune system, resulting in a greater probability that initiated cells will survive and grow into tumors.[39,40]

Nonmelanoma Skin Cancer

Basal cell carcinoma (BCC) and squamous cell carcinoma (SCC) are the two most common skin cancer types. BCC and SCC occur predominantly in sun-exposed areas of the skin, but there are examples of these cancers forming in nonexposed areas as well (see Chapter 117). The tumor suppressor genes *p53* and *p16* are frequently inactivated in BCC and SCC, while the hedgehog-signaling pathway is activated by mutations to the patched gene (PTCH). This scenario promotes proliferation without the opposition of the cell cycle inhibitors p53 and p16.

Melanoma

Melanoma arises from mutations in epidermal melanocytes and is the most dangerous form of skin cancer, since it has the highest propensity to metastasize (see Chapter 118). It is formed in both sun-exposed and shielded areas of the skin, and, therefore, the role of UV light as the major carcinogen in melanoma has been controversial.[38] Defects in the NER pathway do not seem to predispose development of melanoma, suggesting that pyrimidine dimers or 6-4 photoproducts induced by UVB are not the initiators of melanoma carcinogenesis. Instead, ROS induced by UVA may be responsible for the development of melanoma.[38] However, a study using next generation sequencing techniques to catalog all mutations in a melanoma cell line found a mutational spectrum of the over 33,000 mutations detected that strongly indicated that pyrimidine dimers and 6-4 photoproducts are the major mutagenic lesions in melanoma while a subset of mutations may be induced by ROS.[41] The incidence of mutations in the *p16* and *ARF* genes is high, while *p53* and *RAS* mutations are fairly uncommon in melanoma (see Chapter 118).

Photoimmunosuppression

Studies of transplantation of mouse skin cancers into syngeneic mice revealed that prior UVB irradiation of recipient mice promoted tumor growth, while transplantation into naïve unirradiated mice lead to rejection.[40] These studies established that UV light has local immunosuppressing ability, and subsequent studies found that UV light preferentially depletes Langerhans cells from irradiated skin.[39] Langerhans cells play an important role in the immune response by presenting antigens to the immune cells, and, thus, depletion of these cells leads to local immunosuppression. In addition to local immunosuppression, UV light has been shown to promote systemic immunosuppression.[42] This response is complex, but it is known that UV-induced DNA lesions in skin cells contribute to the systemic immunosuppression response.[43] Secretion of the immunosuppressing cytokine interleukin 10 (IL-10) from irradiated keratinocytes as well as UV-induced structural alteration of the epidermal chromophore urocanic acid may mediate the long-range immunosuppressive effects of UV light.[39,42]

RADIOFREQUENCY AND MICROWAVE RADIATION

Radiofrequency radiation (RFR) is electromagnetic radiation in the frequency range 3 kHz to 300 MHz, while microwave radiation (MR) is in the frequency range between 300 MHz to 300 GHz. RFR and MR do not have sufficient energies to cause ionizations in target tissues, rather the radiation energy is converted into heat as the radiation energy is absorbed. Sources of radiofrequency and microwave radiation include mobile phones, radio transmitters of wireless communication, radars, medical devices, and kitchen appliances.

Mechanism of Damage Induction

Since human exposure to RFR has increased dramatically in recent years, it is important to know whether this type of radiation give rise to genotoxic damage. Altough there are many studies showing that RFR can induce ROS, leading to genetic damage in cell culture systems, other studies have generated conflicting results.[44] One confounding factor when assessing the genotoxic effect of RFR, and especially MR, is the heating effect that occurs in the tissue when the radiation energy is absorbed. A recent study controlling for the potential heating effect of exposure found that RFR induces ROS and DNA damage in human spermatozoa *in vitro,* which is an alarming finding considering the potential hereditary implications.[45] It has been suggested that MR may affect the folding of proteins in cells that promote new protein synthesis.[46] Furthermore, exposure of cells to MR has been shown to lead to the phosphorylation of numerous cellular proteins largely through the activation of the p38/MAPK stress response pathway.[47] However, the biological consequences of these cellular changes are not clear. Epidemiology studies that monitored the genetic effects in individuals exposed to high levels of RF have revealed evidence of increased induction of chromosome aberrations in lymphocytes.[48] However, there is a level of uncertainty in these studies about exposure levels, making it difficult to come to meaningful conclusions.

Cancer Risks

Since the exposure of the population to radiofrequency and microwave radiation has dramatically increased in recent years, it is of great importance to assess the potential cancer risks of these types of radiation so that appropriate exposure limits could be implemented. A number of studies have focused on the potential cancer risks from mobile phone usage, and some of these studies indicate that long-term mobile phone usage may be associated with increased risks of developing brain tumors (see below). Other epidemiologic studies of cancer incidences in populations living near radio towers or mobile phone base stations are inconclusive. Some studies have shown a connection between proximity to mobile phone base stations and increased cancer incidence,[49] while another study found no association between exposure to RFR from mobile phone base stations and early childhood cancers.[50]

ELECTROMAGNETIC FIELDS

An electromagnetic field (EMF) is a physical field produced by electrically charged objects that can affect other charged objects in the field. Typical sources of EMF are electric power lines, electrical devices, and magnetic resonance imaging (MRI) machines.

Mechanisms of Damage Induction

A low frequency EMF does not transmit energy high enough to break chemical bonds, and, therefore, it is not thought to directly damage DNA or proteins in cells. The data obtained from studies to assess the potential genotoxic effects of EMF do not provide a clear conclusion. Some of the results obtained in cell culture studies suggest a harmful effect of EMF, but the concerns are that these effects may be related to heat production induced by EMF rather than from the magnetic field itself. A recent *in vitro* study detected DNA strand breaks in cells exposed to EMF, but this induction was thought to not be the result of ROS production but rather due to indirect effects through interference with DNA replication and induction of apoptosis in a subset of cells.[51] A study using an MRI found no evidence of induced formation of DNA DSBs in cell cultures.[52] EMF has been shown to induce nongenotoxic effects in cells, such as interference with cellular signaling pathways,[53] but the biological consequences of these effects are not fully understood.[54]

Cancer Risks

Studies with rodents have largely failed to detect an association between exposure to EMF and cancer. This is also true for numerous epidemiology studies, with the only exception being the association between EMF exposure and childhood leukemia where children exposed to doses of 0.4 mcT or above may have about a twofold increased risk of developing leukemia.[55,56] There is no strong link between EMF exposure and increased risks of contracting adult leukemia, brain tumors, or breast cancer.[57,58] Furthermore, a study investigating whether EMF exposure was associated with heritable effects found no correlation between parental exposure and childhood cancer.[59]

Potential Cancer Risks from Mobile Phone Usage

Mobile phones emit radiofrequency radiation (RFR) and generate EMFs. The biggest health concern with mobile phone usage is its potential role in the development of brain tumors. During mobile phone use, the brain tissue is exposed to doses, giving peak specific absorption rates (SAR) of 4 to 8 W/kg. At these intensities, induction of DNA damage has been detected in laboratory studies.[54] The current epidemiologic data are largely inconclusive on the association between mobile phone usage and brain tumor incidence. Meta-analysis studies of populations who had used mobile phones for more than 10 years concluded that mobile phone usage was associated with an elevated risk for brain tumors, such as acoustic neuroma and glioma cancer.[60–62] In contrast, another study that explored incidence trends of brain tumors in a population of 16 million adults over a period of 5 years found no evidence for increased brain tumor trends as a result of increased mobile phone usage.[63] It is important to point out that it generally takes 30 to 40 years for brain tumors to develop, and since mobile phones have only been in general use for about 15 years, there has not been sufficient time to fully evaluate the brain cancer risks of mobile phone usage.

ASBESTOS

Asbestos is a class of naturally occurring silicate minerals that have been widely used in building materials for its heat, sound, and electrical insulating qualities. Asbestos becomes a serious health hazard if the fibers are inhaled over a long period of time, and these health effects are increased dramatically if the exposed individual is a smoker. It was first reported in 1935 that asbestos might be an occupational health hazard that could induce cancer.[64,65] However, it was not until 1986 that the International Labor Organization recommended banning asbestos.[66] The use of asbestos products peaked in the 1970s but remains a major health hazard in many places around the world today.

Mechanisms of Damage Induction

Asbestos fibers can enter cells and induce ROS, especially if they contain high levels of iron.[67] In addition, ROS can be generated by "frustrated" phagocytosis, and this in turn can lead to the release of proinflammatory cytokines with subsequent inflammation of the tissue. ROS induce SSBs and base damage, such as 8-hydroxyguanine in DNA. Furthermore, if unsuccessfully repaired, asbestos-induced DNA damage has been shown to result in chromosome aberrations, micronuclei formation, and increased rates of sister chromatid exchanges.[68]

Cellular and Tissue Responses

Asbestos-induced ROS cause base lesions and DNA strand breaks, which require base excision repair for the restoration of DNA and for minimizing mutagenesis. In addition to DNA repair, a number of cellular signaling pathways are activated by asbestos. These include the epiderman growth factor (EGFR) and mitogen-activated protein kinase (MAPK) pathway, leading to the activation of nuclear factor κB (NF-κB) and transcription factor AP-1.[67,68] Activation of the NF-κB pathway leads to the induction of proinflammatory genes such as tumor necrosis factor (TNF), IL-6, and IL-8 and proliferation-promoting genes such as c-*Myc,* leading to inflammation and increased cell proliferation. Asbestos exposure also stimulates expression of the transforming growth factor beta (TGF-β), which in turn stimulates fibrogenesis in exposed tissues.[68]

Cancer Risks

Lung Cancer

Epidemiologic studies have found a strong link between asbestos exposure and lung cancer.[68] It has been estimated that about 5% to 7% of all lung cancers are attributable to asbestos exposure, and asbestos and tobacco smoking act in synergy to induce lung cancer. Mutational spectra due to 8-hydroxyguanine lesions formed by ROS can be linked to asbestos exposure, and point mutations in the tumor suppressor genes *p53* and *p16/INK4A* and in the *KRAS* oncogene have been found in tumors from asbestos-exposed individuals.

Mesothelioma

After being taken up by lung tissues, asbestos fibers can translocate into the pleurium, the body cavity that surrounds the lungs. The pleurium is covered with a protective lining, the mesothelia, consisting of squamous-like epithelial cells. Mesothelial cells can internalize asbestos fibers, resulting in induction of ROS and inflammatory responses subsequently leading to the initiation and progression of malignant mesothelioma.[69] Asbestos is considered one of the major causes of malignant mesothelioma, and frequent mutations are found in the *p16/INK4A* and *NF2* genes, while *p53* mutations are fairly rare.

NANOPARTICLES

Nanoparticles are defined as ultrafine particles of the size range 1 to 100 nm in diameter. Nanoparticle chemistry of a certain compound is different from bulk chemistry of that compound because of the high percentage of atoms at the surface of the particle. The production of nanoparticles has increased dramatically in recent years, and they are found in many industrial and consumer products such as paint, cosmetics, and sunscreens. They also have many potential medical applications, such as delivery vehicles for specific drugs to specific target tissues or tumors.

Mechanisms of DNA Damage Induction

Many of the cellular effects of nanoparticles are similar to the effects exerted by asbestos, such as the generation of ROS and inflammation.[67] Nanoparticles have been shown to induce oxidative DNA damage, such as DNA strand breaks and 8-hydroxyguanine lesions both directly and indirectly via the induction of inflammation.[70–73] Nanoparticle-induced DNA lesions are manifested as histone γ-H2AX nuclear foci, chromosome deletions, and micronuclei.

Cellular Responses

Nanoparticles induce ROS either directly or indirectly, resulting in DNA lesions, such as 8-hydroxyguanine-base damage and DNA strand breaks. These lesions are repaired by the base excision repair. Phosphorylation of histone H2AX has been shown to occur following exposure of cells to nanoparticles, suggesting that the DNA lesions trigger the activation of ATM or ATR stress kinases. Nanoparticles have also been found to affect the immune system[74] and can induce the release of the proinflammatory cytokine TNF-α from cells.

Cancer Risks

Some nanoparticles, such as titanium dioxide, which is used as pigments in paint, have been classified by the International Agency for Research on Cancer (IARC) as a group 2B carcinogen, "possible carcinogenic to humans." Although no epidemiologic evidence yet exists to link exposure of nanoparticles to cancer, it is likely that nanoparticles have the potential to induce lung cancer and mesothelioma in humans in a similar manner as asbestos.

ETIOLOGY AND EPIDEMIOLOGY OF CANCER

Selected References

The full list of references for this chapter appears in the online version.

1. Committee on Biological Effects of Ionizing Radiation of the National Academy of Sciences. *Health risks from exposure to low levels of ionizing radiation (BEIR VII)*. Washington, DC: National Academy Press, 2006.
2. Ward JF. DNA damage produced by ionizing radiation in mammalian cells: identities, mechanisms of formation, and repairability. *Prog Nucleic Acid Res Mol Biol* 1988;35:95.
4. Hutchinson F. Chemical changes induced in DNA by ionizing radiation. *Prog Nucleic Acid Res Mol Biol* 1985;32:115.

5. Friedberg E, Walker G, Siede W, Wood R, Schultz R, Ellenberger T. *DNA repair and mutagenesis*. Washington, DC: ASM Press, 2006.
7. Daly MJ. A new perspective on radiation resistance based on Deinococcus radiodurans. *Nat Rev Microbiol* 2009;7:237.
8. Matsuoka S, Ballif BA, Smogorzewska A, et al. ATM and ATR substrate analysis reveals extensive protein networks responsive to DNA damage. *Science* 2007;316:1160.
9. Kastan M, Onyekwere O, Sidransky D, Vogelstein B, Craig R. Participation of p53 protein in the cellular response to DNA damage. *Cancer Res* 1991; 51:6304.
10. Matsuoka S, Huang M, Elledge SJ. Linkage of ATM to cell cycle regulation by the Chk2 protein kinase. *Science* 1998;282:1893.
11. Harper J, Adami G, Wei N, Keyormarsi K, Elledge S. The p21 CDK-interacting protein Cip1 is a potent inhibitor of G1 cyclin-dependent kinases. *Cell* 1993;75:805.
12. El-Deiry W, Tokino T, Velculescu V, et al. WAF1, a potential mediator of p53 tumor suppression. *Cell* 1993;75:817.
13. Falck J, Mailand N, Syljuasen RG, Bartek J, Lukas J. The ATM-Chk2-Cdc25A checkpoint pathway guards against radioresistant DNA synthesis. *Nature* 2001;410:842.
14. Bartek J, Falck J, Lukas J. Chk2 kinase—a busy messenger [review]. *Nature Rev Mol Cell Biol* 2001;2:877.
15. Savitsky K, Bar-Shira A, Gilad S, et al. A single ataxia telangiectasia gene with a product similar to PI-3 kinase. *Science* 1995;268:1749.
16. Srivastava S, Zou ZQ, Pirollo K, Blattner W, Chang EH. Germ-line transmission of a mutated p53 gene in a cancer-prone family with Li-Fraumeni syndrome. *Nature* 1990;348:747.
17. Gudkov AV, Komarova EA. The role of p53 in determining sensitivity to radiotherapy. *Nat Rev Cancer* 2003;3:117.
18. Mihara M, Erster S, Zaika A, et al. p53 has a direct apoptogenic role at the mitochondria. *Mol Cell* 2003;11:577.
20. Thompson DE, Mabuchi K, Ron E, et al. Cancer incidence in atomic bomb survivors. Part II: solid tumors, 1958–1987. *Radiat Res* 1994;137:S17.
21. Williams D. Cancer after nuclear fallout: lessons from the Chernobyl accident. *Nat Rev Cancer* 2002;2:543.
22. Ljungman M, Zhang F. Blockage of RNA polymerase as a possible trigger for UV light-induced apoptosis. *Oncogene* 1996;13:823.
24. Hanawalt PC, Spivak G. Transcription-coupled DNA repair: two decades of progress and surprises. *Nat Rev Mol Cell Biol* 2008;9:958.
27. de Boer J, Andressoo JO, de Wit J, et al. Premature aging in mice deficient in DNA repair and transcription. *Science* 2002;296:1276.
28. Garinis GA, Uittenboogaard LM, Stachelscheid H, et al. Persistent transcription-blocking DNA lesions trigger somatic growth attenuation associated with longevity. *Nat Cell Biol* 2009;11:604.
29. Derheimer FA, O'Hagan H M, Krueger HM, et al. RPA and ATR link transcriptional stress to p53. *Proc Natl Acad Sci U S A* 2007;104:12778.
30. Kastan MB, Bartek J. Cell-cycle checkpoints and cancer. *Nature* 2004; 432:316.
31. Gross S, Knebel A, Tenev T, et al. Inactivation of protein-tyrosine phosphatases as mechanism of UV-induced signal transduction. *J Biol Chem* 1999;274:26378.
34. Ljungman M, Lane DP. Transcription—guarding the genome by sensing DNA damage. *Nat Rev Cancer* 2004;4:727.
39. Murphy GM. Ultraviolet radiation and immunosuppression. *Br J Dermatol* 2009;161(Suppl 3):90.
41. Pleasance ED, Cheetham RK, Stephens PJ, et al. A comprehensive catalogue of somatic mutations from a human cancer genome. *Nature* 2010;463:191.
42. Schwarz T. Photoimmunosuppression. *Photodermatol Photoimmunol Photomed* 2002;18:141.
43. Kripke ML, Cox PA, Alas LG, Yarosh DB. Pyrimidine dimers in DNA initiate systemic immunosuppression in UV-irradiated mice. *Proc Natl Acad Sci U S A* 1992;89:7516.
44. Vijayalaxmi, Prihoda TJ. Genetic damage in mammalian somatic cells exposed to radiofrequency radiation: a meta-analysis of data from 63 publications (1990–2005). *Radiat Res* 2008;169:561.
45. De Iuliis GN, Newey RJ, King BV, Aitken RJ. Mobile phone radiation induces reactive oxygen species production and DNA damage in human spermatozoa in vitro. *PLoS One* 2009;4:e6446.
48. Verschaeve L. Genetic damage in subjects exposed to radiofrequency radiation. *Mutat Res* 2009;681:259.
49. Khurana VG, Hardell L, Everaert J, et al. Epidemiological evidence for a health risk from mobile phone base stations. *Int J Occup Environ Health* 2010;16:263.
50. Elliott P, Toledano MB, Bennett J, et al. Mobile phone base stations and early childhood cancers: case-control study. *BMJ* 2010;340:c3077.
54. Hardell L, Sage C. Biological effects from electromagnetic field exposure and public exposure standards. *Biomed Pharmacother* 2008;62:104.
55. Ahlbom A, Day N, Feychting M, et al. A pooled analysis of magnetic fields and childhood leukaemia. *Br J Cancer* 2000;83:692.
57. Kheifets L, Monroe J, Vergara X, Mezei G, Afifi AA. Occupational electromagnetic fields and leukemia and brain cancer: an update to two meta-analyses. *J Occup Environ Med* 2008;50:677.
58. Chen C, Ma X, Zhong M, Yu Z. Extremely low-frequency electromagnetic fields exposure and female breast cancer risk: a meta-analysis based on 24,338 cases and 60,628 controls. *Breast Cancer Res Treat* 2010;123: 569.
60. Hardell L, Carlberg M, Hansson Mild K. Mobile phone use and the risk for malignant brain tumors: a case-control study on deceased cases and controls. *Neuroepidemiology* 2010;35:109.
61. Hardell L, Carlberg M, Soderqvist F, Hansson Mild K. Meta-analysis of long-term mobile phone use and the association with brain tumours. *Int J Oncol* 2008;32:1097.
62. Myung SK, Ju W, McDonnell DD, et al. Mobile phone use and risk of tumors: a meta-analysis. *J Clin Oncol* 2009;27:5565.
63. Deltour I, Johansen C, Auvinen A, et al. Time trends in brain tumor incidence rates in Denmark, Finland, Norway, and Sweden, 1974–2003. *J Natl Cancer Inst* 2009;101:1721.
64. Lynch K, Smith W. Pulmonary asbestosis. III Carcinoma of lung in asbestos-silicosis. *Am J Cancer* 1935;24:56.
66. LaDou J. The asbestos cancer epidemic. *Environ Health Perspect* 2004;112: 285.
67. Pacurari M, Castranova V, Vallyathan V. Single- and multi-wall carbon nanotubes versus asbestos: are the carbon nanotubes a new health risk to humans? *J Toxicol Environ Health A* 2010;73:378.
68. Nymark P, Wikman H, Hienonen-Kempas T, Anttila S. Molecular and genetic changes in asbestos-related lung cancer. *Cancer Lett* 2008; 265:1.
69. Jaurand MC, Renier A, Daubriac J. Mesothelioma: do asbestos and carbon nanotubes pose the same health risk? *Part Fibre Toxicol* 2009;6:16.
70. Bhabra G, Sood A, Fisher B, et al. Nanoparticles can cause DNA damage across a cellular barrier. *Nat Nanotechnol* 2009;4:876.
71. Trouiller B, Reliene R, Westbrook A, Solaimani P, Schiestl RH. Titanium dioxide nanoparticles induce DNA damage and genetic instability in vivo in mice. *Cancer Res* 2009;69:8784.

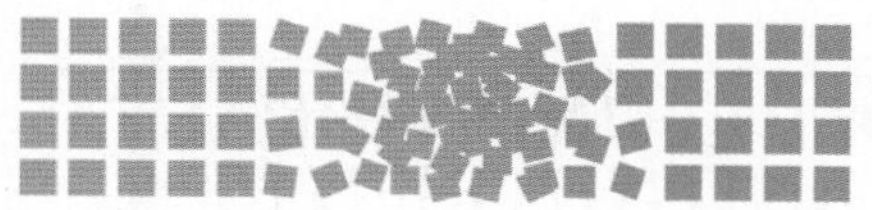

CHAPTER 20 DIETARY FACTORS

KARIN B. MICHELS AND WALTER C. WILLETT

Over two decades ago, Doll and Peto[1] speculated that 35% (range: 10% to 70%) of all cancer deaths in the United States may be preventable by alterations in diet. The magnitude of the estimate for diet exceeded that for tobacco (30%) and infections (10%).

Studies of cancer incidence among populations migrating to countries with different lifestyle factors have indicated that most cancers have a large environmental etiology. Although the contribution of environmental influences differs by cancer type, the incidence of many cancers changes by as much as five- to tenfold among migrants over time, approaching that of the host country. The age at migration affects the degree of adaptation among first-generation migrants for some cancers, suggesting that the susceptibility to environmental carcinogenic influences varies with age by cancer type. Identifying the specific environmental and lifestyle factors most important to cancer etiology, however, has proven difficult.

Environmental factors such as diet may influence the incidence of cancer through many different mechanisms and at different stages in the cancer process. Simple mutagens in foods, such as those produced by the heating of proteins, can cause damage to DNA, but dietary factors can also influence this process by inducing enzymes that activate or inactivate these mutagens, or by blocking the action of the mutagen. Dietary factors can also affect every pathway hypothesized to mediate cancer risk, for example, the rate of cell cycling through hormonal or antihormonal effects, aiding or inhibiting DNA repair, promoting or inhibiting apoptosis, and DNA methylation. Because of the complexity of these mechanisms, knowledge of dietary influences on risk of cancer will require an empirical basis with human cancer as the outcome.

METHODOLOGIC CHALLENGES

Study Types and Biases

The association between diet and the risk of cancer has been the subject of a number of epidemiologic studies. The most prevalent designs are the case-control study, the cohort study, and the randomized clinical trial. When the results from epidemiologic studies are interpreted, the potential for confounding must be considered. Individuals who maintain a healthy diet are likely to exhibit other indicators of a healthy lifestyle, including regular physical activity, lower body weight, use of multivitamin supplements, lower smoking rates, and lower alcohol consumption. Even if the influence of these confounding variables is analytically controlled, residual confounding remains possible.

Ecologic Studies

In ecologic studies or international correlation studies, variation in food disappearance data and the prevalence of a certain disease are correlated, generally across different countries. A linear association may provide preliminary data to inform future research but, due to the high probability of confounding, cannot provide strong evidence for a causal link. Food disappearance data also may not provide a good estimate for human consumption. The gross national product is correlated with many dietary factors such as fat intake.[2] Many other differences besides dietary fat exist between the countries with low fat consumption (less affluent) and high fat consumption (more affluent); reproductive behaviors, physical activity level, and body fatness are particularly notable and are strongly associated with specific cancers.

Migrant Studies

Studies of populations migrating from areas with low incidence of disease to areas with high incidence of disease (or vice versa) can help sort out the role of environmental factors versus genetics in the etiology of a cancer, depending on whether the migrating group adopts the cancer rates of the new environment. Specific dietary components linked to disease are difficult to identify in a migrant study.

Case-Control Studies

Case-control studies of diet may be affected by recall bias, control selection bias, and confounding. In a case-control study, participants affected by the disease under study (cases) and healthy controls are asked to recall their past dietary habits. Cases may overestimate their consumption of foods that are commonly considered "unhealthy" and underestimate their consumption of foods considered "healthy." Giovannucci et al.[3] have documented differential reporting of fat intake before and after disease occurrence. Thus, the possibility of recall bias in a case-control study poses a real threat to the validity of the observed associations. Even more importantly, in contemporary case-control studies using a population sample of controls, the participation rate of controls is usually far from complete, often 50% to 70%. Unfortunately, health-conscious individuals may be more likely to participate as controls and will thus be less overweight, consume fruits and vegetables more frequently, and less fat and red meat, which can substantially distort associations observed.

Cohort Studies

Prospective cohort studies of the effects of diet are likely to have a much higher validity than retrospective case-control studies because diet is recorded by participants before disease occurrence. Cohort studies are still affected by measurement error because diet consists of a large number of foods eaten in complex combinations. Confounding by other unmeasured or imperfectly measured lifestyle factors can remain a problem in cohort studies.

Now that the results of a substantial number of cohort studies have become available, their findings can be compared with those of case-control studies that have examined the same relations. In many cases, the findings of the case-control studies have not been confirmed; for example, the consistent finding of lower risk of many cancers with higher intake of fruits and vegetables in case-control studies has generally not been seen in cohort studies.[4] These findings suggest that the concerns about biases in case-control studies of diet, and probably many other lifestyle factors, are justified, and findings from such studies must be interpreted cautiously.

Randomized Clinical Trials

The gold standard in medical research is the randomized clinical trial (RCT). In a RCT on nutrition, participants are randomly assigned to one of two or more diets; hence, the association between diet and the cancer of interest should not be confounded by other factors. The problem with RCTs of diet is that maintaining the assigned diet strictly over many years, as would be necessary for diet to have an impact on cancer incidence, is difficult. For example, in the dietary fat reduction trial of the Women's Health Initiative (WHI), participants randomized to the intervention arm reduced their fat intake much less than planned.[5] The remaining limited contrast between the two groups left the lack of difference in disease outcomes difficult to interpret. Furthermore, the relevant time window for intervention and the necessary duration of intervention are unclear, especially with cancer outcomes. Hence, randomized trials are rarely used to examine the effect of diet on cancer but have better promise for the study of diet and outcomes that require considerably shorter follow-up time (e.g., adenoma recurrence). Also, the randomized design may lend itself better to the study of the effects of dietary supplements such as multivitamin or fiber supplements, although the control group may adopt the intervention behavior because nutritional supplements are widely available. For example, in the WHI trial of calcium and vitamin D supplementation, two-thirds of the study population used vitamin D or calcium supplements that they obtained outside of the trial, again rendering the lack of effect in the trial uninterpretable.

Diet Assessment Instruments

Observational studies depend on a reasonably valid assessment of dietary intake. Although, for some nutrients, biochemical measurements can be used to assess intake, for most dietary constituents a useful biochemical indicator does not exist. In population-based studies, diet is generally assessed with a self-administered instrument. Since 1980, considerable effort has been directed at the development of standardized questionnaires for measuring diet, and numerous studies have been conducted to assess the validity of these methods. The most widely used diet assessment instruments are the food frequency questionnaire, the 7-day diet record, and the 24-hour recall. Although the 7-day diet record may provide the most accurate documentation of intake during the week the participant keeps a diet diary, the burden of computerizing the information and extracting foods and nutrients has prohibited the use of the 7-day diet record in most large-scale studies. The 24-hour recall provides only a snapshot of diet on one day, which may or may not be representative of the participant's usual diet and is thus affected by both within-person variation and seasonal variation. The food frequency questionnaire, the most widely used instrument in large population-based studies, asks participants to report their average intake of a large number of foods during the previous year. Participants tend to substantially overreport their fruit and vegetable consumption on the food frequency questionnaire.[6] This tendency may reflect "social desirability bias," which leads to overreporting of healthy foods and underreporting of less healthy foods. Studies of validity using biomarkers or detailed measurements of diet as comparisons have suggested that carefully designed questionnaires can have sufficient validity to detect moderate to strong associations. Validity can be enhanced by using the average of repeated assessments over time.[7]

THE ROLE OF INDIVIDUAL FOOD AND NUTRIENTS IN CANCER ETIOLOGY

Energy

The most important impact of diet on the risk of cancer is mediated through body weight. Overweight, obesity, and inactivity are major contributors to cancer risk. (A more detailed discussion is provided in Chapter 21.) In the large American Cancer Society Cohort, obese individuals had substantially higher mortality from all cancers and in particular from colorectal cancer, postmenopausal breast cancer, uterine cancer, cervical cancer, pancreatic cancer, and gallbladder cancer than their normal-weight counterparts.[8] Adiposity and in particular waist circumference are predictors of colon cancer incidence among women and men.[9,10] Weight gain of 10 kg or more is associated with a significant increase in postmenopausal breast cancer incidence among women who never used hormone replacement therapy, while weight loss of comparable magnitude after menopause substantially decreases breast cancer risk.[11] Regular physical activity contributes to a lower prevalence of overweight and obesity and consequently reduces the burden of cancer through this pathway.

The mechanisms whereby adiposity increases risk of various cancers are probably multiple. Overweight is strongly associated with endogenous estrogen levels, which likely contribute to the excess risks of endometrial and breast cancers. The reasons for the association with other cancers are less clear, but excess body fat is also related to higher levels of insulin, lower levels of binding proteins for sex hormones and insulin-like growth factor-1(IGF1), and higher levels of various inflammatory factors, all of which have been hypothesized to be related to risks of various cancers.

Energy restriction is one of the most effective measures to prevent cancer in the animal model. While energy restriction is more difficult to study in humans, voluntary starvation among anorectics and situations of food rationing during famines provide related models. Breast cancer rates were substantially reduced among women with a history of severe anorexia.[12] Although breast cancer incidence was higher among women exposed to the Dutch famine during childhood or adolescence, such short-term involuntary food rationing for 9 months or less was often followed by overnutrition.[13] A more prolonged deficit in food availability during World War II in Norway, if it occurred during early adolescence, was associated with a reduction in adult risk of breast cancer.[14]

Alcohol

Besides body weight, alcohol consumption is the best established dietary risk factor for cancer. Alcohol is classified as a carcinogen by the International Agency for Research on Cancer. Consumption of alcohol increases the risk of numerous cancers, including those of the liver, esophagus, pharynx, oral cavity, larynx, breast, and colorectum in a dose-dependent fashion.[15] Evidence is convincing that excessive alcohol consumption increases the risk of primary liver cancer, probably through cirrhosis and alcoholic hepatitis. At least in the developed world about 75% of cancers of the esophagus, pharynx, oral cavity, and larynx are attributable to alcohol and tobacco, with a marked increase in risk among drinkers who also smoke, suggesting a multiplicative effect. Mechanisms may include direct damage to the cells in the upper gastrointestinal tract, modulation of DNA methylation, which affects susceptibility to DNA mutations, and an increase in acetaldehyde, the main metabolite of alcohol, which enhances proliferation of epithelial cells, forms DNA adducts, and is a recognized carcinogen. The association between alcohol consumption and breast cancer is notable because a small but significant risk has been found even with one drink per day. Mechanisms may include an interaction with folate, an increase in endogenous estrogen levels, and elevation of acetaldehyde. Some evidence suggests that the excess risk is mitigated by adequate folate intake possibly through an effect on DNA methylation.[16] Notably, for most cancer sites, no important difference in associations was found with the type of alcoholic beverage, suggesting a critical role of ethanol in carcinogenesis.

Dietary Fat

In recent years, reduction in dietary fat has been at the center of cancer prevention efforts. In the landmark 1982 National Academy of Sciences review of diet, nutrition, and cancer, reduction in fat intake to 30% of calories was the primary recommendation.

Interest in dietary fat as a cause of cancer began in the first half of the 20th century, when studies by Tannenbaum[17] indicated that diets high in fat could promote tumor growth in animal models. Dietary fat has a clear effect on tumor incidence in many models, although not in all; however, a central issue has been whether this is independent of the effect of energy intake. In the 1970s, the possible relation of dietary fat intake to cancer incidence gained greater attention as the large international differences in rates of many cancers were noted to be strongly correlated with apparent per capita fat consumption in ecologic studies.[2] Particularly strong associations were seen with cancers of the breast, colon, prostate, and endometrium, which include the most important cancers not due to smoking in affluent countries. These correlations were observed to be limited to animal, not vegetable, fat.

Dietary Fat and Breast Cancer

Breast cancer is the most common malignancy among women, and incidence has been increasing for decades, although a decline has been noted starting with the new millennium. Rates in most parts of Asia, South America, and Africa have been only approximately one-fifth that of the United States, but in almost all these areas rates of breast cancer are also increasing. Populations that migrate from low- to high-incidence countries develop breast cancer rates that approximate those of the new host country. However, rates do not approach those of the general U.S. population until the second or third generation.[18] This slower rate of change for immigrants may indicate delayed acculturation, although since a similar delay in rate increase is not observed for colon cancer, it may suggest an origin of breast cancer earlier in the life course.

The results from 12 smaller case-control studies that included 4,312 cases and 5,978 controls have been summarized in a meta-analysis.[19] The pooled relative risk (RR) was 1.35 ($P < .0001$) for a 100-g increase in daily total fat intake, although the risk was somewhat stronger for postmenopausal women (RR, 1.48; $P < .001$). This magnitude of association, however, could be compatible with biases due to recall of diet or the selection of controls.

Because of the prospective design of cohort studies, most of the methodologic biases of case-control studies are avoided. In an analysis of the Nurses' Health Study that included 121,700 U.S. female registered nurses, no association with total fat intake was observed, and there was no suggestion of any reduction in risk at intakes below 25% of energy.[20] Because repeated assessments of diet were obtained at 2- to 4-year intervals, this analysis provided a particularly detailed evaluation of fat intake over an extended period in relation to breast cancer risk. Similar observations were made in the National Institutes of Health (NIH)–American Association of Retired Persons (AARP) Diet and Health Study including 188,736 postmenopausal women[21] and in the European Prospective Investigation into Cancer and Nutrition (EPIC), which included 7,119 incident cases.[22] In a pooled analysis of seven prospective studies that included 337,000 women who developed 4,980 incident cases of breast cancer, no overall association was seen for fat intake over the range of less than 20% to more than 45% energy (reflecting the current range observed internationally).[23] A similar lack of association was seen for specific types of fat. This lack of association with total fat intake was confirmed in a subsequent analysis of the pooled prospective studies of diet and breast cancer that included over 7,000 cases.[24] These cohort findings therefore do not support the hypothesis that dietary fat is an important contributor to breast cancer incidence.

Endogenous estrogen levels have now been established as a risk factor for breast cancer. Thus, the effects of fat and other dietary factors on estrogen levels are of potential interest. Vegetarian women, who consume higher amounts of fiber and lower amounts of fat, have lower blood levels and reduced urinary excretion of estrogens, apparently due to increased fecal excretion. A meta-analysis has suggested that reduction in dietary fat reduces plasma estrogen levels,[25] but the studies included were plagued by the lack of concurrent controls, short duration, and confounding by negative energy balance. In a large, randomized trial among postmenopausal women with a previous diagnosis of breast cancer, reduction in dietary fat did not affect estradiol levels when the data were appropriately analyzed.[26]

The Women's Health Initiative Randomized Controlled Dietary Modification Trial similarly suggested no association between fat intake and breast cancer incidence,[5] but these results are difficult to interpret.[27] The data on biomarkers that reflect fat intake suggest little if any difference in fat intake between the intervention and control groups.[28] Even if dietary fat does truly have an effect on cancer incidence and other outcomes, this lack of adherence to the dietary intervention could explain the absence of an observed effect on total cancer incidence and total mortality.

Some prospective cohort studies suggest an inverse association between monounsaturated fat and breast cancer. This is an intriguing observation because of the relatively low rates of breast cancer in southern European countries with high intakes of monounsaturated fats due to the use of olive oil as the primary fat. In case-control studies in Spain, Greece, and Italy, women who used more olive oil had reduced risks of breast cancer.

In a report of findings from the Nurses' Health Study II cohort of premenopausal women, higher intake of animal fat was associated with an approximately 50% greater risk of breast cancer, but no association was seen with intake of vegetable fat.[29] This suggests that factors in foods containing animal fats, rather than fat *per se*, may account for the findings. In the same cohort, intake of red meat and total fat during adolescence was also associated with risk of premenopausal breast cancer.[30,31]

Dietary Fat and Colon Cancer

In comparisons among countries, rates of colon cancer are strongly correlated with national per capita disappearance of animal fat and meat, with correlation coefficients ranging

ETIOLOGY AND EPIDEMIOLOGY OF CANCER

between 0.8 and 0.9.[2] Rates of colon cancer rose sharply in Japan after World War II, paralleling a 2.5-fold increase in fat intake. Based on these epidemiologic investigations and on animal studies, a hypothesis has developed that higher dietary fat increases excretion of bile acids, which can be converted to carcinogens or act as promoters. However, evidence from many studies on obesity and low levels of physical activity increasing the risk of colon cancer suggests that at least part of the high rates in affluent countries previously attributed to fat intake is probably due to sedentary lifestyle.

The Nurses' Health Study suggested an approximately two-fold higher risk of colon cancer among women in the highest quintile of animal fat intake than in those in the lowest quintile.[32] In a multivariate analysis of these data, which included red meat intake and animal fat intake in the same model, red meat intake remained significantly predictive of risk of colon cancer, whereas the association with animal fat was eliminated. Other cohort studies have supported associations of colon cancer and consumption of red meat and processed meats but not other sources of fat or total fat.[33–35] Similar associations were also observed for colorectal adenomas. In a meta-analysis of prospective studies, red meat consumption was associated with risk of colon cancer (RR = 1.24; 95% CI [confidence interval], 1.09 to 1.41 for an increment of 120 g/d).[36] The association with consumption of processed meats was particularly strong (RR = 1.36; 95% CI, 1.15 to 1.61 for an increment of 30 g/d).

The apparently stronger association with red meat consumption than with fat intake in most large cohort studies needs further confirmation, but such an association could result if the fatty acids or nonfat components of meat (e.g., the heme iron or carcinogens created by cooking) were the primary etiologic factors. This issue has major practical implications because current dietary recommendations support the daily consumption of red meat as long as it is lean.[37]

Dietary Fat and Prostate Cancer

Although further data are desirable, the evidence from international correlations, case-control[38] and cohort studies[39–43] provides some support for an association between consumption of fat-containing animal products and prostate cancer incidence. This evidence does not generally support a relation with intake of vegetable fat, which suggests that either the type of fat or other components of animal products are responsible. Some evidence also indicates that animal fat consumption may be most strongly associated with the incidence of aggressive prostate cancer, which suggests an influence on the transition from the widespread indolent form to the more lethal form of this malignancy. Data are limited on the relation of fat intake to the probability of survival after the diagnosis of prostate cancer.

Dietary Fat and Other Cancers

Rates of other cancers that are common in affluent countries, including those of the endometrium and ovary, are also correlated with fat intake internationally. In prospective studies between Iowa and Canadian women, no evidence of a relation between fat intake and risk of endometrial cancer was found. Positive associations between dietary fat and lung cancer have been observed in many case-control studies. However, in a pooled analysis of large prospective studies that included over 3,000 incident cases, no association was observed.[44] These findings provide further evidence that the results of case-control studies of diet and cancer are likely to be misleading.

Summary

Largely on the basis of the results of animal studies, international correlations, and a few case-control studies, great enthusiasm developed in the 1980s that modest reductions in total fat intake would have a major impact on breast cancer incidence. As the findings from large prospective studies have become available, however, support for this relation has greatly weakened. Although evidence suggests that high intake of animal fat early in adult life may increase the risk of premenopausal breast cancer, this is not likely to be due to fat *per se* because vegetable fat intake was not related to risk. For colon cancer, the associations seen with animal fat intake internationally have been supported in numerous case-control and cohort studies, but this also appears to be explained by factors in red meat other than simply its fat content. Further, the importance of physical activity and leanness as protective factors against colon cancer indicates that international correlations probably overstate the contribution of diet to differences in colon cancer incidence. At present the available evidence most strongly suggests an association between animal fat consumption and risk of prostate cancer, particularly the aggressive form of this disease. As with colon cancer, the possibility remains that other factors in animal products contribute to risk.

Despite the large body of data on dietary fat and cancer that has accumulated since 1985, any conclusions should be regarded as tentative, because these are disease processes that are poorly understood and are likely to take many decades to develop. Because most of the reported literature from prospective studies is based on fewer than 20 years' follow-up, further evaluation of the effects of diet earlier in life and at longer intervals of observation are needed to fully understand these complex relations. Nevertheless, persons interested in reducing their risk of cancer could be advised, as a prudent measure, to minimize their intake of foods high in animal fat, particularly red meat. Such a dietary pattern is also likely to be beneficial for the risk of cardiovascular disease. On the other hand, unsaturated fats (with the exception of *transfatty* acids) reduce blood low-density lipoprotein cholesterol levels and the risk of cardiovascular disease, and little evidence suggests that they adversely affect cancer risk. Thus, efforts to reduce unsaturated fat intake are not warranted at this time and are likely to have adverse effects on cardiovascular disease risk. Because excess adiposity increases risks of several cancers and cardiovascular disease, balancing calories from any source with adequate physical activity is extremely important.

Fruits and Vegetables

General Properties

Fruits and vegetables have been hypothesized to be major dietary contributors to cancer prevention because they are rich in potential anticarcinogenic substances. Fruits and vegetables contain antioxidants and minerals and are good sources of fiber, potassium, carotenoids, vitamin C, folate, and other vitamins. Although fruits and vegetables supply less than 5% of total energy intake in most countries worldwide on a population basis, the concentration of micronutrients in these foods is greater than in most others.

The comprehensive report of the World Cancer Research Fund and the American Institute for Cancer Research published in 2007 and titled *Food, Nutrition, Physical Activity, and the Prevention of Cancer: A Global Perspective* reached the consensus based on the available evidence: "findings from cohort studies conducted since the mid-1990s have made the overall evidence, that vegetables or fruits protect against cancers, somewhat less impressive. In no case now is the evidence of protection judged to be convincing."[15]

Fruit and Vegetable Consumption and Colorectal Cancer

The association between fruit and vegetable consumption and the incidence of colon or rectal cancer has been examined prospectively in at least six studies. In some of these prospective cohorts, inverse associations were observed for individual foods or particular subgroups of fruits or vegetables, but no consistent pattern emerged and many comparisons revealed no such links. The results from the largest studies, the Nurses' Health Study and the Health Professionals' Follow-Up Study, suggested no important association between consumption of fruits and vegetables and incidence of cancers of the colon or rectum during 1,743,645 person-years of follow-up.[45] In these two large cohorts, diet was assessed repeatedly during follow-up with a detailed food frequency questionnaire. Similarly, in the Pooling Project of Prospective Studies of Diet and Cancer, including 14 studies, 756,217 participants, and 5,838 cases of colon cancer, no association with overall colon cancer risk was found.[46]

Fruit and Vegetable Consumption and Stomach Cancer

At least 12 prospective cohort studies have examined consumption of some fruits and vegetables and incidence of stomach cancer.[15] Seven of these studies considered total vegetable intake. Three found significant protection from stomach cancer, whereas three did not. All other comparisons were made for subgroups of vegetables and produced inconsistent results. Nine prospective cohort studies investigated the association between fruit consumption and stomach cancer risk. Four studies found an inverse association of borderline statistical significance.

Fruit and Vegetable Consumption and Breast Cancer

The most comprehensive evaluation of fruit and vegetable consumption and the incidence of breast cancer was provided by a pooled analysis of all cohort studies.[47] Data were pooled from eight prospective studies that included 351,825 women, 7,377 of whom developed incident invasive breast cancer during follow-up. The pooled relative risk adjusted for potential confounding variables was 0.93 (95% CI, 0.86 to 1.0; *P* for trend, .08) for the highest versus the lowest quartile of fruit consumption, 0.96 (95% CI, 0.89 to 1.04; *P* for trend, .54) for vegetable intake, and 0.93 (95% CI, 0.86 to 1.0; *P* for trend, .12) for total consumption of fruits and vegetables combined. The EPIC study confirmed this lack of association.[48] In a recent analysis within the Nurses' Health Study, an inverse association was seen between intake of vegetables and risk of estrogen receptor–negative breast cancer; this finding will need to be examined in other studies, as an inverse association could have been missed within this important subset of breast cancers.[49]

Fruit and Vegetable Consumption and Lung Cancer

The relation between fruit and vegetable consumption and the incidence of lung cancer was examined in the pooled analysis of cohort studies.[50] Overall, no association was observed, although a modest increase in lung cancer incidence was evident among participants with the lowest fruit and vegetable consumption.

Fruit and Vegetable Consumption and Total Cancer

An analysis of the Nurses' Health Study and the Health Professionals' Follow-Up Study, including over 9,000 incident cases of cancer, did not reveal a benefit of fruit and vegetable consumption for total cancer incidence.[51] Observations from the EPIC cohort were essentially consistent with these findings.[52] While there may be no or only a very weak protection conferred for cancer from consuming an abundance of fruits and vegetables, there is a substantial benefit for cardiovascular disease.

Summary

Consumption of fruits and vegetables and some of their main micronutrients appears to be less important in cancer prevention than previously assumed. With accumulation of data from prospective cohort studies and randomized trials, a lack of association of these foods and nutrients with cancer outcomes has become apparent. A modest association cannot be excluded because of imperfect measurement of diet, and it remains possible that a high consumption of fruits and vegetables during childhood and adolescence is more effective in reducing cancer risk than consumption in adult life due to the long latency of cancer manifestation.

Conversely, it is possible that, with the fortification of breakfast cereal, flour, and other staple foods, the frequent consumption of fruits and vegetables has become less essential for cancer prevention. Nevertheless, an abundance of fruits and vegetables as part of a healthy diet is recommended, because evidence consistently suggests that it lowers the incidence of hypertension, heart disease, and stroke.

Fiber

General Properties

Dietary fiber was defined in 1976 as "all plant polysaccharides and lignin which are resistant to hydrolysis by the digestive enzymes of men."[52a] Fiber, both soluble and insoluble, is fermented by the luminal bacteria of the colon. Among the properties of fiber that make it a candidate for cancer prevention are its "bulking" effect, which reduces colonic transit time, and the binding of potentially carcinogenic luminal chemicals. Fiber may also aid in producing short-chain fatty acids that may be directly anticarcinogenic, and fiber may induce apoptosis.

Dietary Fiber and Colorectal Cancer

In 1969, Dennis Burkitt hypothesized that dietary fiber is involved in colon carcinogenesis.[53] While working as a physician in Africa, Burkitt noticed the low incidence of colon cancer among African populations whose diet was high in fiber. Burkitt concluded that a link might exist between the fiber-rich diet and the low incidence of colon cancer. Burkitt's observations were followed by numerous case-control studies that seemed to confirm his theories. A combined analysis of 13 case-control studies[54] as well as a meta-analysis of 16 case-control studies[55] suggested an inverse association between fiber intake and the risk of colorectal cancer. Inclusion of studies was selective, however, and effect estimates unadjusted for potential confounders were used for most studies. Moreover, recall bias is a severe threat to the validity of retrospective case-control studies of fiber intake and any disease outcome.

Data from prospective cohort studies have largely failed to support an inverse association between dietary fiber and colorectal cancer incidence. Initial analyses from the Nurses' Health Study[56] and the Health Professionals' Follow-Up Study[35] found no important association between dietary fiber and colorectal cancer. A significant inverse association between fiber intake and incidence of colorectal cancer was reported from the EPIC study. The analysis presented on dietary fiber and colorectal cancer encompassed 434,209 women and men from eight European countries.[57] The analytic model used by the EPIC investigators included adjustments for age, height, weight, total caloric intake, sex, and center assessed at baseline and identified a significant inverse association between fiber intake and colorectal cancer. Applying the same analytic model used in EPIC to data from the Nurses' Health Study and the Health Professionals' Follow-Up Study encompassing 1.8 million person-years of follow-up and 1,572 cases of colorectal cancer revealed associations similar to those found in the EPIC study.[58] After more complete adjustment for confounding variables, however, the association vanished.[58] Results from the pooled analysis of 13 prospective cohort studies, including 8,081 colorectal cancer cases diagnosed during over 7 million person-years of follow-up, suggested an inverse relation between dietary fiber and colorectal cancer incidence in age-adjusted analyses, but this association disappeared after appropriate adjustment for confounding variables, particularly other dietary factors.[59] The NIH-AARP study, including 2,974 cases of colorectal cancer, confirmed the lack of association between total dietary fiber and colorectal cancer risk.[60]

The association between dietary fiber and colorectal cancer appears to be confounded by a number of other dietary and nondietary factors. These methodologic considerations must be taken into account when interpreting the evidence. It is possible that other dietary factors such as folate intake are more important for colorectal cancer pathogenesis than dietary fiber.

Dietary Fiber and Colorectal Adenomas

In a few prospective cohort studies, the primary occurrence of colorectal polyps was investigated, but no consistent relation was found.

The study of fiber intake and colorectal adenoma recurrence lends itself to a randomized clinical trial design because of the relatively short follow-up necessary and because fiber can be provided as a supplement. A number of RCTs have explored the effect of fiber supplementation on colorectal adenoma recurrence. Evidence has fairly consistently indicated no effect of fiber intake.[61–65] In one RCT, an increase in adenoma recurrence was observed among participants randomly assigned to use a fiber supplement, which was stronger among those with high dietary calcium.[66]

Dietary Fiber and Breast Cancer

Investigators have speculated that dietary fiber may reduce the risk of breast cancer through reduction in intestinal absorption of estrogens excreted via the biliary system.

Relatively few epidemiologic studies have examined the association between fiber intake and breast cancer. In a meta-analysis of ten case-control studies, a significant inverse association was observed. However, these retrospective studies were likely affected by the aforementioned biases—selection and recall bias, in particular. Results from at least six prospective cohort studies consistently suggested no association between fiber intake and breast cancer incidence.[67–72]

Dietary Fiber and Stomach Cancer

The results from retrospective case-control studies of fiber intake and gastric cancer risk are inconsistent. In the Netherlands Cohort Study, dietary fiber was not associated with incidence of gastric carcinoma.[73] Further investigation through prospective cohort studies must be completed before conclusions about the relation between fiber intake and stomach cancer incidence can be drawn.

Summary

The observational data presently available do not indicate an important role for dietary fiber in the prevention of cancer, although small effects cannot be excluded. The long-held perception that a high intake of fiber conveys protection originated largely from retrospectively conducted studies, which are affected by a number of biases, in particular, the potential for differential recall of diet, and from studies that were not well controlled for potential confounding variables.

OTHER FOODS AND NUTRIENTS

Red Meat

Regular consumption of red meat has been associated with an increased risk of colorectal cancer. In a recent meta-analysis the increase in risk associated with an increase in intake of 120 g/d was 24% (95% CI, 9% to 41%).[36] The association was strongest for processed meat; the relative risk of colorectal cancer was 1.36 (95% CI, 1.15 to 1.61) for a consumption of 30 g/d.[36] No overall association has been observed between red meat consumption and breast cancer in a pooled analysis of prospective cohorts.[74] However, among premenopausal women in the Nurses' Health Study II the risk for estrogen-receptor– and progesterone-receptor–positive breast cancer doubled with 1.5 servings of red meat per day compared to three or fewer servings per week.[75] No associations have been found in studies on poultry or fish.[15] Mechanisms through which red meat may increase cancer risk include anabolic hormones routinely used in meat production in the United States, heterocyclic amines, and polycyclic aromatic hydrocarbons formed during cooking at high temperatures, the high amounts of heme iron, and nitrates and related compounds in smoked, salted, and some processed meats that can convert to carcinogenic nitrosamines in the colon.

Milk, Dairy Products, and Calcium

The role of calcium in the prevention of colorectal cancer is not entirely clear,[76] but in the pooling project of prospective studies of diet and cancer, a modest inverse association was seen.[77] This finding is consistent with the results of a randomized trial in which calcium supplements reduced risk of colorectal adenomas.[78] Conversely, high intake of lactose from dairy products has been associated with a modestly higher risk of ovarian cancer.[79] In multiple studies high intake of calcium or dairy products has been associated with an increased risk of prostate cancer[80,81] or fatal prostate cancer.[82,83] Similar observations were made in the NIH-AARP study, although the increase in risk there did not reach statistical significance.[84] While the Multiethnic Cohort[85] and the Prostate, Lung, Colorectal, and Ovarian Cancer Screening Trial[86] did not find an important association between dairy consumption and prostate cancer, these cohort studies did not specifically include fatal prostate cancer cases. A meta-analysis of prospective studies generated an overall relative risk of advanced prostate cancer of 1.33 (95% CI, 1.00 to 1.78) for the highest versus the lowest intake categories of dairy products.[87] Thus, although the findings are not entirely consistent and are complicated by the widespread use of prostate-specific antigen (PSA) screening in the United States, the global evidence suggests an association between regular consumption of dairy products and the risk of fatal prostate cancer.

These observations are particularly important in the context of national dietary recommendations to drink three glasses of milk per day.[37] Possible mechanisms include an increase in endogenous IGF1 levels[88] and the fairly high steroid hormone content of cows' milk.

Vitamin D

Vitamin D is currently one of the most promising agents in cancer prevention research. In 1980, Garland and Garland[89] hypothesized that sunlight and vitamin D may reduce the risk of colon cancer. Since then, substantial research has been conducted in this area supporting an inverse association between circulating 25-hydroxyvitamin D [25(OH)D] levels and colorectal cancer risk.[90,91] A meta-analysis, including five nested case-control studies with prediagnostic serum, suggested a reduction of colorectal cancer risk by about half among individuals with serum 25(OH)D levels of more than 82 nmol/L compared to individuals with less than 30 nmol/L.[92] These observations are supported by similar findings for colorectal adenomas.[93] Vitamin D levels may particularly affect colorectal cancer prognosis; colorectal cancer mortality was 72% lower among individuals with 25(OH)D concentrations of 80 nmol/L or higher.[94] Although the data are not entirely consistent, high intake and high plasma levels of vitamin D have been associated with a decreased risk of several other cancers, including cancer of the breast,[95,96] prostate,[97] and pancreas.[98] Activation of vitamin D receptors by $1,25(OH)_2D$ induces cell differentiation and inhibits proliferation and angiogenesis.[99] Solar ultraviolet-B radiation is the major source of plasma vitamin D, and dietary vitamin D without supplementation has a minor effect on plasma vitamin D. To achieve sufficient plasma levels through sun exposure, at least 15 minutes of full-body exposure to bright sunlight is necessary. Sunscreen effectively blocks vitamin D production. Populations who live in geographic areas with limited or seasonal sun exposure may benefit from vitamin D supplementation of 1,000 IU/d.

Folate

Folate is a micronutrient commonly found in fruits and vegetables, particularly oranges, orange juice, asparagus, beets, and peas. Folate may affect carcinogenesis through various mechanisms: DNA methylation, DNA synthesis, and DNA repair. In the animal model, folate deficiency enhances intestinal carcinogenesis.[100] Folate deficiency is related to incorporation of uracil into human DNA and to an increased frequency of chromosomal breaks. A number of epidemiologic studies suggest that a diet rich in folate lowers the risk of colorectal adenomas and colorectal cancer.[15] Because folate content in foods is generally relatively low, is susceptible to oxidative destruction by cooking and food processing, and is not well absorbed, folic acid from supplements and fortification plays an important role. Pooled results from nine prospective studies suggests that intake of 400 to 500 mcg/d is required to minimize risk.[101]

Potential interactions among alcohol consumption, folic acid intake, and methionine intake have been described. Although alcohol consumption has been fairly consistently related to an increase in breast cancer incidence, the potential detrimental effect of alcohol seems to be eliminated in women with high folic acid intake.[16] A similar folic acid or methionine–alcohol interaction has been observed for colorectal cancer risk.[100]

Genetic susceptibility may also modify the relation between folate intake and cancer risk. A polymorphism of the *methylenetetrahydrofolate reductase (MTHFR)* gene (cytosine to thymine transition at position 677) may result in a relative deficiency of methionine. Homozygotes for the C677T mutation appear to experience the greatest protection from high folic acid or methionine intake and low alcohol consumption.[102] Although the interaction between this polymorphism and dietary factors needs to be investigated further, the consistently observed association between this polymorphism and risk of colorectal cancer suggests a role of folate in the etiology of colorectal cancer.

Conversely, evidence from animal and human studies suggests that a high folate status may promote progression of existing neoplasias.[103–105] Randomization of folic acid supplements among individuals with a history of colorectal adenoma resulted in either no effect on recurrent adenoma recurrence[106] or an increase in recurrence with over 6 to 8 years of follow-up.[107] The high proliferation rate of neoplastic cells requiring increased DNA synthesis is likely supported by folate, which is necessary for thymidine synthesis.[104] In addition, folate levels also affect availability of methyl groups via *S*-adenosylmethionine in the one-carbon metabolism.[105] The effects of folate on *de novo* methylation and subsequent gene silencing have been insufficiently studied. Whether the increase in colorectal cancer rates observed in the United States and Canada concurrent with the introduction of the folic acid fortification program is related to the high prevalence of colorectal adenomas in older individuals or an artifact of increase use of colonoscopy in the population remains to be evaluated.[108]

Soy Products

The role of soy products has been considered for breast carcinogenesis. In Asian countries, which traditionally have a high consumption of soy foods, breast cancer rates have been low until recently. In Western countries, soy consumption is generally low, and between-person variation may be insufficient to allow meaningful comparisons. Soybeans contain isoflavones, phytoestrogens that compete with estrogen for the estrogen receptor. Hence, soy consumption may affect estrogen concentrations differently depending on the endogenous baseline level. This mechanism may also contribute to the equivocal results of studies on soy foods and breast cancer risk. In a recent meta-analysis of 18 epidemiologic studies, including over 9,000 breast cancer cases, frequent soy intake was associated with a modest decrease in risk (odds ratio = 0.86; 95% CI, 0.75 to 0.99).[109] Wu et al.[110] observed that childhood intake of soy was more relevant to breast cancer prevention than adult consumption.

Carotenoids

Carotenoids, antioxidants prevalent in fruits and vegetables, enhance cell-to-cell communication, promote cell differentiation, and modulate immune response. In 1981, Doll and Peto[1] speculated that beta carotene may be a major player in cancer prevention and encouraged testing of its anticarcinogenic properties. Indeed, subsequent observational studies, mostly case-control investigations, suggested a reduced cancer risk—especially of lung cancer—with high intake of carotenoids. Clinical trials randomizing intake of beta carotene supplements, in contrast, have not revealed evidence of a protective effect of beta-carotene. In fact, beta carotene was found to increase the risk of lung cancer and total mortality among smokers in the Finnish Alpha-Tocopherol, Beta-Carotene Cancer Prevention Study.[111] However, these adverse affects disappeared during longer periods of follow-up.[112] In a detailed analysis of prospective studies, no association was seen between intake of beta carotene and risk of lung cancer.[113]

The particularly pronounced antioxidant properties of lycopene, a carotenoid mainly found in tomatoes, may explain the inverse associations with some cancers. Frequent consumption of tomato-based products has been associated with a decreased risk of prostate, lung, and stomach cancers.[114] Bioavailability of lycopene from cooked tomatoes is higher than from fresh tomatoes, making tomato soup and sauce excellent sources of the carotenoid.

DIETARY PATTERNS

Foods and nutrients are not consumed in isolation, and, when evaluating the role of diet in disease prevention and causation, it is sensible to consider the entire dietary pattern of individuals. Public health messages may be better framed in the context of a global diet than individual constituents.

During the past decade, dietary pattern analyses have gained popularity in observational studies. The most commonly employed methods are factor analyses and cluster analyses, which are largely data-driven methods, and investigator-determined methods such as dietary indices and scores. The search for associations between distinct patterns such as the "Western pattern"—characterized by high consumption of red and processed meats, high fat dairy products, including butter and eggs, and refined carbohydrates, such as sweets, desserts, and refined grains—and the "prudent pattern"—defined by frequent consumption of a variety of fruits and vegetables, whole grains, legumes, fish, and poultry—and the risk of cancer has been largely disappointing. Notable exceptions were the link between a Western dietary pattern and colon cancer incidence and an inverse relation between a prudent diet[115] and estrogen receptor–negative breast cancer,[116] but these findings have to be confirmed in additional studies. The apparent lack of association between global dietary habits and cancer supports a more modest role of nutrition during adult life in carcinogenesis than previously assumed.

DIET DURING EARLY PHASES OF LIFE

Some cancers may originate early in the course of life. A high birth weight is associated with an increase in the risk of childhood leukemia,[117] premenopausal breast cancer,[118] and testicular cancer.[119] Tall height is an indicator of the risk of many cancers and is in part determined by nutrition during childhood.[15] Until recently, most studies focused on the role of diet during adult life. However, the critical exposure period for nutrition to affect cancer risk may be earlier, and since the latent period for cancer may span several decades, diet during childhood and adolescence may be important. Relating dietary information during early life and cancer outcomes prospectively, however, is difficult, as nutrition records from the remote past are not available. Studies in which recalled diet during youth is used have to be interpreted cautiously due to misclassification, although recall has been found reasonably reproducible and consistent with recalls provided by participants' mothers.[120,121] The role of early life diet has been explored in only a few studies in relation to breast cancer risk. In a study nested in the Nurses' Health Study cohorts that used data recalled by mothers, frequent consumption of french fries was associated with an increased risk of breast cancer, while whole milk consumption was inversely related to risk.[122] Similarly, an inverse association with milk consumption during childhood was found among younger women (30 to 39 years), but not among older premenopausal women (40 to 49 years) in a Norwegian cohort.[123] Dietary habits during high school recalled by adult participants of the Nurses' Health Study and the Nurses' Health Study II suggested a positive association of total fat and red meat consumption.[30,31] More data are needed in this promising area of research.[124]

SUMMARY

A considerable proportion of cancers are potentially preventable through lifestyle changes. Besides curtailment of smoking, the most important strategies are maintaining a healthy body weight and regular physical activity, which contribute to a lower prevalence of overweight and obesity. Avoidance of a positive energy balance and becoming overweight are the most important nutritional factors in cancer prevention.

Although dietary patterns, including frequent fruit and vegetable consumption, appear to play a modest role in cancer prevention, knowledge gained about some specific foods and nutrients might inform a targeted approach. Vitamin D is a strong candidate to counter carcinogenesis, thus supplementation could be a feasible and safe route to avoid several types of cancer. Although the data on vitamin D and cancer incidence are not conclusive, the prevention of bone fractures is a sufficient reason to maintain good vitamin D status.

Limiting or avoiding red meat, processed meat, and alcohol reduces the risk of breast, colorectal, stomach, esophageal, and other cancers. Although the role of dairy products and milk remains to be more fully elucidated, current evidence suggests a potential increase in the risk of ovarian and prostate cancer with frequent milk consumption, which raises concern regarding current dietary recommendations of three glasses of milk per day. The relation of calcium intake to cancer is complex, as the evidence for reduction in risk of colorectal cancer is strong, but high intakes appear likely to increase the risk of fatal prostate cancer. Finally, consumption of tomato-based products may contribute to the prevention of prostate cancer.

LIMITATIONS

Studying the role of diet in health and disease requires overcoming a number of hurdles. Since biomarkers reflecting nutrient intake with sufficient accuracy are largely lacking, assessment of nutrition in a population-based study has to rely on self-reports of individuals, which inevitably leads to imprecision or error in diet assessment. Such misclassification may produce spurious associations in case-control studies or lead to underestimation of true associations in prospective cohort studies.

Most observational studies are conducted within populations or countries. Although reasonable variation in nutritional habits exists within populations, allowing the detection of substantial dietary risk factors for cardiovascular disease and diabetes, these contrasts may be too limited to detect small relative risks as they may exist for cancer. The pooled analysis of large prospective cohort studies across countries and continents attempts to overcome this limitation. Studies taking advantage of the large between-population variation in diet across developed and developing countries would appear to be advantageous, but would be plagued by confounding by other differences in lifestyle factors that might be difficult to assess and control adequately.

Few epidemiologic studies repeatedly capture dietary habits over time and thus account for potential changes in diet over time. Furthermore, the length of follow-up in prospective studies may not be sufficient to capture the impact of diet assessed at baseline. In case-control studies, recall of dietary habits prior to disease onset may be influenced by current disease status; moreover, the relevant time window for nutrition to act may be decades earlier, which is more difficult to remember.

Most epidemiologic studies of diet and cancer have assessed intake among adults. Due to greater susceptibility to genotoxic influences earlier in life, it is possible that data on diet during childhood or early adolescence are more relevant for carcinogenesis and cancer prevention. Studies that have collected dietary data during childhood and followed the subjects for cancer incidence would be most informative but are virtually nonexistent and will be challenging to conduct.

Finally, data on special diets including organic foods, whole foods, raw foods, and a vegan diet are limited.

FUTURE DIRECTIONS

Some of the most promising research at present is in the areas of vitamin D, milk consumption, and the effect of diet early in life on cancer incidence. Recent nutrition changes in countries previously maintaining a more traditional diet such as Japan and some developing countries have already been followed by increased cancer rates, providing a setting to study the effect of change over time. Additional insight may come from studies on gene–nutrient interaction and epigenetic changes induced by diet. To improve observational research methods, refined dietary assessment methods including identification of new biomarkers will be advantageous.

RECOMMENDATIONS

A wealth of data are available from observational studies on diet and cancer, and the current evidence supports suggestions made by Doll and Peto[1] that approximately 30% to 40% of cancer may be avoidable with changes in nutrition; however, much of this risk is related to being overweight and to inactivity. Excessive energy intake and lack of physical activity, marked by rapid growth in childhood and being overweight, have become growing threats to population health and are a major contributor to rising cancer rates.

Dietary recommendations must integrate the goal of overall avoidance of disease and maintenance of health and thus should not focus singularly on cancer prevention. The strength of the evidence and magnitude of the expected benefit should also be considered in recommendations. With these considerations in mind, the following recommendations are outlined, which are largely in agreement with the guidelines put forth by the American Cancer Society in 2006:[125]

1. *Engage in regular physical activity.* Physical activity is a primary method of weight control and it also reduces risk of several cancers, especially colon cancer, through independent mechanisms. Moderate to vigorous exercise for at least 30 minutes on most days is a minimum and more will provide additional benefits.
2. *Avoid overweight and weight gain in adulthood.* A positive energy balance that results in excess body fat is one of the most important contributors to cancer risk. Staying within 10 pounds of body weight at age 20 may be a simple guide, assuming no adolescent obesity.
3. *Limit alcohol consumption.* Alcohol consumption contributes to the risk of many cancers and increases the risk of accidents and addiction, but low to moderate consumption has benefits for coronary heart disease risk. The individual family history of disease as well as personal preferences should be considered.
4. *Consume lots of fruits and vegetables.* Frequent consumption of fruits and vegetables during adult life is not likely to have a major effect on cancer incidence, but will reduce the risk of cardiovascular disease.
5. *Consume whole grains and avoid refined carbohydrates and sugars.* Regular consumption of whole grain products instead of refined flour and low consumption of refined sugars lower the risk of cardiovascular disease and diabetes. The effect on cancer risk is less clear.
6. *Replace red meat and dairy products with fish, nuts, and legumes.* Red meat consumption increases the risk of colorectal cancer and coronary heart disease and should be largely avoided. Frequent dairy consumption may increase the risk of prostate cancer. Fish, nuts, and legumes are excellent sources of valuable mono- and polyunsaturated fats and vegetable proteins and may contribute to lower rates of cardiovascular disease and diabetes.
7. *Consider taking a vitamin D supplement.* A substantial proportion of the population, especially those living at higher latitudes, are vitamin D deficient. Most adults may benefit from taking 1,000 IU of vitamin D_3 per day during months of low sunlight intensity. Vitamin D supplementation will at a minimum reduce bone fracture rates, probably colorectal cancer incidence, and possibly other cancers.

Selected References

The full list of references for this chapter appears in the online version.

1. Doll R, Peto R. The causes of cancer: quantitative estimates of avoidable risks of cancer in the United States today. *J Natl Cancer Inst* 1981;66(6):1191.
2. Armstrong B, Doll R. Environmental factors and cancer incidence and mortality in different countries, with special reference to dietary practices. *Int J Cancer* 1975;15(4):617.
3. Giovannucci E, Stampfer MJ, Colditz GA, et al. A comparison of prospective and retrospective assessments of diet in the study of breast cancer. *Am J Epidemiol* 1993;137(5):502.
4. Riboli E, Norat T. Epidemiologic evidence of the protective effect of fruit and vegetables on cancer risk. *Am J Clin Nutr* 2003;78(3 Suppl):559S.
5. Prentice RL, Caan B, Chlebowski RT, et al. Low-fat dietary pattern and risk of invasive breast cancer: the Women's Health Initiative Randomized Controlled Dietary Modification Trial. *JAMA* 2006;295(6):629.
6. Michels KB, Bingham SA, Luben R, et al. The effect of correlated measurement error in multivariate models of diet. *Am J Epidemiol* 2004;160(1):59.
7. Willett W. *Nutritional epidemiology*, 2nd ed. New York: Oxford University Press, 1998.
11. Eliassen AH, Colditz GA, Rosner B, et al. Adult weight change and risk of postmenopausal breast cancer. *JAMA* 2006;296(2):193.
12. Michels KB, Ekbom A. Caloric restriction and incidence of breast cancer. *JAMA* 2004;291(10):1226.
13. Elias SG, Peeters PHM, Grobbee DE, et al. Breast cancer risk after caloric restriction during the 1944–1945 Dutch famine. *J Natl Cancer Inst* 2004;96(7):539.
15. World Cancer Research Fund. *Food, nutrition, physical activity, and the prevention of cancer: a global perspective. American Institute for Cancer Research.* Washington, DC: World Cancer Research Fund, 2007.
16. Zhang S, Hunter DJ, Hankinson SE, et al. A prospective study of folate intake and the risk of breast cancer. *JAMA* 1999;281(17):1632.
18. Kolonel L, Hinds M, Hankin J. Cancer patterns among migrant and native-born Japanese in Hawaii in relation to smoking, drinking, and dietary habits. In: Gelboin HV, Matsushima T, Sugimura T, et al., eds. *Genetics and environmental factors in experimental and human cancer.* Tokyo: Japan Scientific Societies Press, 1980.
23. Hunter DJ, Spiegelman D, Adami HO, et al. Cohort studies of fat intake and the risk of breast cancer—a pooled analysis. *N Engl J Med* 1996;334(6):356.
27. Michels KB. The Women's Health Initiative—curse or blessing? *Int J Epidemiol* 2006;35(4):814.
28. Michels KB, Willett WC. The Women's Health Initiative randomized controlled dietary modification trial: a post-mortem. *Breast Cancer Res Treat* 2009;114(1):1.
30. Linos E, Willett WC, Cho E, et al. Red meat consumption during adolescence among premenopausal women and risk of breast cancer. *Cancer Epidemiol Biomarkers Prev* 2008;17(8):2146.
31. Linos E, Willett WC, Cho E, et al. Adolescent diet in relation to breast cancer risk among premenopausal women. *Cancer Epidemiol Biomarkers Prev* 2010;19(3):689.
37. U.S. Department of Agriculture Food Pyramid. World Wide Web URL: www.mypyramid.gov/.
57. Bingham SA, Day NE, Luben R, et al. Dietary fibre in food and protection against colorectal cancer in the European Prospective Investigation into Cancer and Nutrition (EPIC): an observational study. *Lancet* 2003;361(9368):1496.
58. Michels KB, Fuchs CS, Giovannucci E, et al. Fiber intake and incidence of colorectal cancer among 76,947 women and 47,279 men. *Cancer Epidemiol Biomarkers Prev* 2005;14(4):842.

59. Park Y, Hunter DJ, Spiegelman D, et al. Dietary fiber intake and risk of colorectal cancer: a pooled analysis of prospective cohort studies. *JAMA* 2005;294(22):2849.
74. Missmer SA, Smith-Warner SA, Spiegelman D, et al. Meat and dairy food consumption and breast cancer: a pooled analysis of cohort studies. *Int J Epidemiol* 2002;31(1):78.
75. Cho E, Chen WY, Hunter DJ, et al. Red meat intake and risk of breast cancer among premenopausal women. *Arch Intern Med* 2006;166(20):2253.
77. Cho E, Smith-Warner SA, Spiegelman D, et al. Dairy foods, calcium, and colorectal cancer: a pooled analysis of 10 cohort studies. *J Natl Cancer Inst* 2004;96(13):1015.
78. Baron JA, Beach M, Mandel JS, et al. Calcium supplements for the prevention of colorectal adenomas. Calcium Polyp Prevention Study Group. *N Engl J Med* 1999;340(2):101.
82. Giovannucci E, Liu Y, Stampfer MJ, et al. A prospective study of calcium intake and incident and fatal prostate cancer. *Cancer Epidemiol Biomarkers Prev* 2006;15(2):203.
86. Ahn J, Albanes D, Peters U, et al. Dairy products, calcium intake, and risk of prostate cancer in the prostate, lung, colorectal, and ovarian cancer screening trial. *Cancer Epidemiol Biomarkers Prev* 2007;16(12):2623.
87. Gao X, LaValley MP, Tucker KL. Prospective studies of dairy product and calcium intakes and prostate cancer risk: a meta-analysis. *J Natl Cancer Inst* 2005;97(23):1768.
89. Garland CF, Garland FC. Do sunlight and vitamin D reduce the likelihood of colon cancer? *Int J Epidemiol* 1980;9(3):227.
92. Gorham ED, Garland CF, Garland FC, et al. Optimal vitamin D status for colorectal cancer prevention: a quantitative meta analysis. *Am J Prev Med* 2007;32(3):210.
95. Bertone-Johnson ER, Chen WY, Holick MF, et al. Plasma 25-hydroxyvitamin D and 1,25-dihydroxyvitamin D and risk of breast cancer. *Cancer Epidemiol Biomarkers Prev* 2005;14(8):1991.
101. Kim D, Smith-Warner S, Hunter D, et al. Pooled analysis of prospective cohort studies on folate and colorectal cancer. Pooling Project of Diet and Cancer Investigation. *Am J Epidemiol* 2001;153(Suppl):S118.
103. Kim YI. Folate: a magic bullet or a double edged sword for colorectal cancer prevention? *Gut* 2006;55(10):1387.
104. Mason JB. Folate, cancer risk, and the Greek god, Proteus: a tale of two chameleons. *Nutr Rev* 2009;67(4):206.
105. Osterhues A, Holzgreve W, Michels KB. Shall we put the world on folate? *Lancet* 2009;374(9694):959.
106. Wu K, Platz EA, Willett W, et al. A randomized trial on folic acid supplementation and risk of recurrent colorectal adenoma. *Am J Clin Nutr* 2009;90(6):1623.
107. Cole BF, Baron JA, Sandler RS, et al. Folic acid for the prevention of colorectal adenomas: a randomized clinical trial. *JAMA* 2007;297(21):2351.
108. Mason JB, Dickstein A, Jacques PF, et al. A temporal association between folic acid fortification and an increase in colorectal cancer rates may be illuminating important biological principles: a hypothesis. *Cancer Epidemiol Biomarkers Prev* 2007;16(7):1325.
111. The effect of vitamin E and beta carotene on the incidence of lung cancer and other cancers in male smokers. The Alpha-Tocopherol, Beta Carotene Cancer Prevention Study Group. *N Engl J Med* 1994;330(15):1029.
112. Virtamo J, Pietinen P, Huttunen JK, et al. Incidence of cancer and mortality following alpha-tocopherol and beta-carotene supplementation: a postintervention follow-up. *JAMA* 2003;290(4):476.
113. Mannisto S, Smith-Warner SA, Spiegelman D, et al. Dietary carotenoids and risk of lung cancer in a pooled analysis of seven cohort studies. *Cancer Epidemiol Biomarkers Prev* 2004;13(1):40.
114. Giovannucci E. Tomatoes, tomato-based products, lycopene, and cancer: review of the epidemiologic literature. *J Natl Cancer Inst* 1999;91(4):317.
117. Caughey RW, Michels KB. Birth weight and childhood leukemia: a meta-analysis and review of the current evidence. *Int J Cancer* 2009;124(11):2658.
118. Michels KB, Xue F. Role of birthweight in the etiology of breast cancer. *Int J Cancer* 2006;119(9):2007–25.
119. Michos A, Xue F, Michels KB. Birth weight and the risk of testicular cancer: a meta-analysis. *Int J Cancer* 2007;121(5):1123.
120. Chavarro JE, Rosner BA, Sampson L, et al. Validity of adolescent diet recall 48 years later. *Am J Epidemiol* 2009;170(12):1563.
122. Michels KB, Rosner BA, Chumlea WC, et al. Preschool diet and adult risk of breast cancer. *Int J Cancer* 2006;118(3):749.
124. Michels KB, Mohllajee AP, Roset-Bahmanyar E, et al. Diet and breast cancer: a review of the prospective observational studies. *Cancer* 2007;109(12 Suppl):2712.
125. Kushi LH, Byers T, Doyle C, et al. American Cancer Society Guidelines on Nutrition and Physical Activity for cancer prevention: reducing the risk of cancer with healthy food choices and physical activity. *CA Cancer J Clin* 2006;56(5):254.

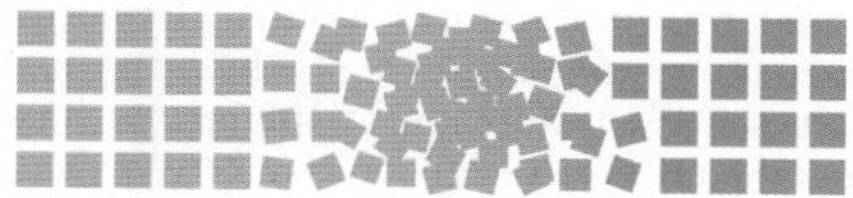

CHAPTER 21 OBESITY AND PHYSICAL ACTIVITY

KATHERINE D. HENDERSON, YANI LU, AND LESLIE BERNSTEIN

Evidence showing that physical activity is associated with decreased cancer risk and that obesity is associated with increased cancer risk at certain sites is rapidly accumulating. It is not yet known whether the action of these two factors is interrelated or independent. Physical activity may act to decrease cancer risk primarily by preventing weight gain and obesity. However, physical activity may also have independent effects on cancer risk. In this chapter, we present a summary of the current epidemiological literature on the possible associations between these exposures, physical activity and obesity, and risk of cancer at several organ sites.

Physical activity is defined as any movement of the body that results in energy expenditure. Here we focus on recreational physical activity, also called leisure-time physical activity or exercise, and occupational physical activity, including household activity. Occupational physical activity typically occurs over a longer period of time and generally requires less energy expenditure per hour than bouts of strenuous or moderate recreational physical activity.[1] The distinction between recreational and occupational activity is important because increasing mechanization and technological advances have led to decreased occupational physical activity in developed areas of the world, perhaps contributing to a decrease in overall physical activity. Obesity is defined as the condition of being extremely overweight. In epidemiological studies, the usual, but not necessarily the best measure of body mass in adults is Quetelet's Index, or body mass index (BMI), which is measured as weight in kilograms (kg) divided by the square of height in meters (m^2). The estimated proportion of the U.S. population that is obese, defined by having a BMI of 30 kg/m^2 or greater,[2] is 32.2% and 35.5% for adult men and women, respectively.[3] Physical inactivity has likely contributed to the high prevalence of obesity in the United States; data from the 2003–2004 National Health and Nutritional Examination Survey, a cross-sectional study of a sample of the civilian, noninstitutionalized population of the United States, has indicated that less than 5% of U.S. adults achieve 30 minutes per day of physical activity, and that men are more physically active than women.[4]

Epidemiological evidence on the association of physical activity and obesity with cancer comes from observational studies, including cohort studies, which follow populations forward in time after collecting exposure information, and case-control studies, which optimally identify a population-based series of newly diagnosed cases and healthy control subjects, collecting information retrospectively on exposures. In both study designs, physical activity information is usually self-reported and measures vary substantially with respect to timing and level of detail. Studies have measured lifetime or long-term physical activity, activity at defined ages or time points in life, and/or current or recent activity. Ideally, a study would capture activity by type (recreational, occupational, or other nonrecreational, such as activity related to transportation), duration (minutes per session), frequency (sessions per day), and intensity (low, moderate, or strenuous as defined by examples of activity types) across the lifetime. These studies have often measured height and weight by self-report at one time point, such as at the time of study entry. Some studies have collected other or more detailed anthropometric information, such as waist circumference, hip circumference, or weight at an additional time point like at age 18. Anthropometrics are directly measured by trained study personnel in only a few studies.

Epidemiological evidence for a role of physical activity or obesity in relation to cancer risk exists for cancers of the breast, colon, endometrium, esophagus, and kidney. Evidence is accumulating to link at least one of these "exposures" to incidence of pancreatic cancer, gallbladder cancer, non-Hodgkin lymphoma (NHL), and advanced prostate cancer. The evidence for an association between either physical activity or obesity and lung and ovarian cancer is inconclusive.

In addition to specific biological mechanisms pertinent to physical activity or to obesity at each specific organ site, several global mechanisms have been implicated in both relationships across a number of these organ sites. The steroid hormone and insulin/insulinlike growth factor (IGF) pathways are two such global mechanisms hypothesized to be involved in the links between physical activity or obesity and cancer.[2] The role of steroid hormones as a mediator in these relationships is perhaps best understood in the context of breast cancer and endometrial cancer, and will be discussed in those sections. The roles of the insulin and IGF pathways have been discussed in depth with respect to colon cancer and thus will be presented in that context. Although alterations in immune system function have been proposed as a global mechanism through which physical activity might influence cancer risk, little direct evidence for this currently exists.[5] Further, obesity has been shown to produce a proinflammatory state, and thus, inflammation may mediate the relationship between obesity and cancer risk.[6]

BREAST CANCER

Low level of physical activity is an established breast cancer risk factor among postmenopausal women and, to a lesser extent, premenopausal women.[2,7–9] This difference in the level of evidence may be partly related to the lower incidence of breast cancer in younger women; fewer studies have had sufficient numbers of premenopausal women to address the issue with confidence. Obesity appears to have a paradoxical relationship with breast cancer risk in that it is an established breast cancer risk factor among postmenopausal women, but may offer some protection for breast cancer among premenopausal women.[2]

The epidemiological literature has shown with relative consistency that breast cancer risk is reduced by increasing level of physical activity.[2,7–9] One of the earliest studies, a case-control study of women 40 years or younger, showed a dramatic reduction in risk of approximately 50% among women who averaged about 4 hours of activity per week during their reproductive years.[10] A meta-analysis of 29 case-control studies and 19 cohort studies published between 1994 and 2006 has provided strong evidence for an inverse association between physical activity and risk of breast cancer, citing that the evidence for an association between physical activity and premenopausal breast cancer was not as strong as that for postmenopausal breast cancer. The conclusion of the meta-analysis was that each additional hour of physical activity per week decreases breast cancer by approximately 6%.[8]

In the California Teachers Study (CTS), a prospective cohort study of over 133,000 female public school professionals, increasing levels of long-term strenuous recreational physical activity were associated with decreasing risk of *in situ* and invasive breast cancer; however, the decrease in risk reached statistical significance only among the most active women, who exercised, on average, 5 or more hours per week during their reproductive years.[11] In the CTS data, a variable combining strenuous and moderate long-term recreational physical activity was associated with reduced risk of estrogen receptor-negative but not estrogen receptor-positive invasive breast cancer, a result consistent with some[12] but not all[13–15] studies with receptor subtype available. A recent report from the Nurses' Health Study II has shown that recreational physical activity during youth, defined as between ages 12 and 22 years, may have a larger impact on premenopausal breast cancer risk than activity at older ages; these results did not differ by estrogen-receptor status.[16] Results from the National Institutes of Health-American Association of Retired Persons Diet and Health Study cohort showed that recent moderate-to-vigorous intensity recreational physical activity, and not activity at earlier age periods, was associated with decreased postmenopausal breast cancer risk, again with no apparent difference by tumor subtype. The European Prospective Investigation into Cancer and Nutrition (EPIC),[17] a study of over 200,000 premenopausal and postmenopausal women aged 20 to 80 years at cohort entry from nine European countries, captured data on occupational activity (which includes household activity) in addition to recreational physical activity. EPIC reported that increased physical activity in the form of household activity (highest vs. lowest quartile) was associated with a reduction in breast cancer risk of approximately 30% among premenopausal and 20% among postmenopausal women, but neither recreational activity nor occupational activity was significantly associated with risk.

In summary, epidemiological studies investigating the association between physical activity and breast cancer risk have produced relatively consistent results showing a reduction in breast cancer risk with increasing level of physical activity. The effect, most well established for recreational activity, has been observed in both premenopausal and postmenopausal women, and in women of different populations. Results to date suggest that moderate-to-strenuous activity may be required for the effect between physical activity and breast cancer risk to be clear; however, confirmation of this and clarification of other key details, such as the importance of timing and intensity of activity, or tumor characteristics, is pending.

Adult obesity and adult weight gain have both been associated with increased breast cancer risk among postmenopausal women.[2] Most studies among postmenopausal women have reported relative risks of 1.5 to 2.0 when comparing the most obese women or those with the largest weight gain to normal-weight women (BMI: 18.5–24.9 kg/m^2) or those with the least weight gain.[2] A pooled analysis of data from eight prospective studies indicated that breast cancer risk increased approximately 18% per 5 kg/m^2 increase in BMI.[18] Paradoxically, overweight or obese premenopausal women have an estimated 10% to 30% decreased risk of breast cancer compared with normal-weight or thinner women.[2]

Hormones are central in the discussion of biological mechanisms linking both physical activity and obesity with breast cancer risk. Physical activity can alter menstrual cycle patterns in premenopausal women, and hormone profiles in both premenopausal and postmenopausal women. Physical activity may lower body fat among children,[19] which in turn may delay age at menarche.[20] Later age at menarche has been associated with reduced breast cancer risk.[21] Physical activity may reduce the frequency of ovulatory cycles.[22] Having less frequent and therefore fewer cumulative ovulatory cycles is likely to reduce the lifetime exposure of the breast to endogenous ovarian hormones,[21] proven proliferative agents.[23] Physical activity also can have a direct impact on circulating estrogen levels among postmenopausal women.[24]

The defining biological event of the menopause is the cessation of ovarian hormone production. In the postmenopausal period adipose tissue is the primary source of endogenous hormones via aromatization of androstenedione to estrone.[25] Thus, heavier postmenopausal women have higher levels of circulating estrogen than women with less adipose tissue. The involvement of estrogen in the relationship between obesity and breast cancer risk is supported by the observation that obesity does not independently increase breast cancer risk among menopausal hormone therapy users[26]; the obesity-related increase in estrogen over that provided by exogenous estrogens is negligible. The breast tissue of overweight or obese perimenopausal and postmenopausal women with relatively high risk of breast cancer has been shown to have cytologic abnormalities and higher epithelial cell counts than that of normal-weight women.[27] In contrast, obese premenopausal women experience menstrual cycle disturbances, including anovulatory cycles and secondary amenorrhea, thereby lowering their cumulative exposure to estradiol and progesterone.[21]

Other likely mechanisms that may link physical activity[28,29] and obesity[30,31] with breast cancer risk include aspects of immune function, inflammatory mechanisms, oxidative stress and DNA repair capability, metabolic hormones, and growth factors.

COLON AND RECTAL CANCER

The epidemiological literature suggests that increased physical activity is protective for colon cancer.[2,32] In early studies, this effect was observed more consistently in men than in women. In cohort studies, a greater benefit among men is still observed, although results for case-control studies indicate that exercise benefits colon cancer similarly among men and women.[32] A meta-analysis of studies of physical activity and colon cancer showed a 31% reduction in colon cancer risk for case-control studies and a 17% reduction in risk for cohort studies when comparing individuals with the highest activity with those in the lowest activity group.[32] Among men, reductions in colon cancer risk associated with physical activity have been observed in studies of both occupational and recreational physical activity.[2]

One factor that might account for weaker results of studies of physical activity on colon cancer risk among older women is use of menopausal hormone therapy, which is associated with lower colon cancer risk.[33] This possibility has been investigated in the CTS. Mai et al.[34] reported that combined lifetime moderate and strenuous leisure-time physical activity was modestly associated with colon cancer risk in the CTS. The CTS participants who exercised at least 4 hours per week during their reproductive years had 25% lower risk of colon cancer relative to those who exercised no more than 30 minutes per week. Importantly, among postmenopausal CTS participants, those who had never used menopausal hormone therapy experienced a 46% decrease in colon cancer risk if they averaged at least 4 hours of exercise per week, whereas those who had used menopausal hormone therapy experienced no benefit from exercise, but retained a benefit from having used menopausal hormone therapy that was comparable to 4 hours of activity per week.

It has been argued that distal and proximal colon cancers have distinct etiologies.[35] Several studies of physical activity and colon cancer have examined risk by anatomic subsite, but results are inconsistent with regard to whether the association is stronger for distal tumors or for proximal tumors.[36–40]

In contrast to colon cancer, nearly all epidemiological studies have failed to show a relationship between physical activity and rectal cancer risk.[2] However, the National Institutes of Health-American Association of Retired Persons Diet and Health Study shows a modest reduction in rectal cancer risk for men but not for women after 6.9 years of follow-up.[40]

Obesity is an established risk factor for colon cancer in both men and women, although the relative risks for men have been marginally higher than those for women.[2] The adverse impact of overweight and obesity on colon cancer risk is stronger for cancers of the distal than for the proximal colon.[2] In addition, visceral adiposity appears to confer greater risk than abdominal adiposity or general overweight.[2] In the EPIC study, both high body weight and high BMI were statistically significantly associated with increased colon cancer risk in men, but not in women; however, other measures of adiposity including waist circumference and waist-to-hip ratio were associated with colon cancer risk in both men and women.[41] Again, no association between these adiposity measures and colon cancer risk was evident among postmenopausal women who had used menopausal hormone therapy, and no association was observed between any measure of adiposity and rectal cancer risk.[41]

The mechanisms explaining the relationship between physical activity and colon cancer are not clearly established, but include the impact on insulin sensitivity and IGF profiles, and inflammation, as well as some colon-specific mechanisms. Physical activity may stimulate stool transit in the colon, thereby decreasing the exposure of colonic mucosa to carcinogens in the stool.[5] Alternatively, physical activity-induced decreases in prostaglandin E_2 may decrease colonic cell proliferation rates and increase colonic motility.[5] In addition to steroid hormones, which have been clearly implicated as biological modifiers of the effect of physical activity and obesity on colon cancer risk, as previously discussed, the insulin and IGF pathways have been proposed as mediators of the associations between these exposures and colon cancer risk. In particular for obesity, the link can be inferred because obesity can lead to insulin resistance,[42] a syndrome characterized by high circulating insulin levels. High insulin levels appear to promote cell proliferation and tumor growth in the colon[6] and may also suppress expression of IGF binding proteins 1 and 2, leading to increased bioavailable IGF-1 levels.[43] In a recent nested colon cancer case-control study, Ma et al.[44] reported that men in the highest quintile of circulating IGF-1 concentration were at significantly higher risk for colon cancer. Another possible mechanistic pathway involves inflammation. Individuals with chronic colon conditions, such as inflammatory bowel disease, have higher colon cancer incidence than those without these conditions.[6] In addition, use of aspirin or other nonsteroidal anti-inflammatory drugs appears to reduce colon cancer risk.[6] Thus, obesity-induced inflammation may mediate the association between obesity and colon cancer by causing DNA damage in the colon and promoting the development of colon cancer, or more directly, by inducing insulin resistance.[6]

ENDOMETRIAL CANCER

The evidence for an association between physical activity and endometrial cancer risk is accumulating[2,45–49] but is not as definitive as that for the association between obesity and endometrial cancer or physical activity and postmenopausal breast cancer. The epidemiological literature to date has suggested that risk of endometrial cancer is decreased 20% to 40% in women who are in the highest versus lowest category of physical activity.[2,46] Adjustment for BMI minimally changes relative risk estimates, suggesting that physical activity is an independent protective factor for endometrial cancer. Although physical activity is associated with decreased risk of endometrial cancer in both normal-weight and obese women, two recent studies have suggested that this association is more pronounced for obese women.[45,49] Three recent studies have also reported an increased risk of endometrial cancer in sedentary women.[45,50,51]

Two meta-analyses of the association between physical activity and endometrial cancer have identified some inconsistencies in dose-response relationships, indicating the importance of differences in activity type and intensity.[46,47] Little evidence exists on how long-term or lifetime physical activity and activity patterns in different life periods might influence endometrial cancer risk; it has been suggested that recent or long-term activity might be more important than activity at early ages.[47]

In contrast, epidemiological studies have established the existence of a strong association between obesity and endometrial cancer risk.[2] Some studies have suggested a linear trend between increasing body weight and increasing endometrial cancer risk among postmenopausal women, whereas the association between body weight and endometrial cancer among premenopausal women may be present only among obese women.[2] Moreover, BMI appears to exert an effect on risk of endometrial that is independent of physical activity.[46]

Like breast and colon cancer, endometrial cancer is another hormone-dependent cancer; in fact, one of the best-established risk factors for endometrial cancer is menopausal hormone therapy in the form of unopposed estrogen.[52,53] Thus, physical activity and obesity are likely to influence endometrial cancer risk by altering endogenous hormone profiles.[21,43] As described earlier, heavier postmenopausal women have higher circulating levels of estrogen than do lighter postmenopausal women because of the aromatization of androstenedione in adipose tissue. This is pertinent to endometrial cancer risk because this aromatization occurs in the absence of progesterone, which counteracts the proliferative effects of estrogen on endometrial tissue. Physical activity may counter the proliferative effects of estrogen either directly or by restricting weight gain. Some evidence also links elevated insulin levels and diabetes to endometrial cancer risk.[54] Clearly, physical inactivity and obesity play a role in the development of insulin insensitivity and diabetes, providing another mechanism by which they may influence endometrial cancer risk.

ADENOCARCINOMA OF THE ESOPHAGUS

Several case-control studies[55–57] and one cohort study[58] have examined the association between physical activity and risk of adenocarcinoma of the esophagus. Zhang et al.[55] reported that participation in recreational physical activity more than once per week was associated with decreased risk of esophageal cancer in a non–statistically significant manner, although adenocarcinoma and squamous cell carcinoma were treated as a combined end point in this study. Lagergren et al.[56] reported no association between total, usual physical activity (recreational and occupational) and esophageal adenocarcinoma. Vigen et al.[57] showed that lifetime occupational physical activity (vigorous, moderate, or sedentary) was modestly related to decreased risk of adenocarcinoma of the esophagus, but average annual level of occupational physical activity before age 65 years was more strongly associated with risk with approximately a 40% reduction in risk of esophageal adenocarcinoma when the highest was compared with the lowest occupational physical activity category. Results from the cohort study also support the hypothesis that physical activity lowers risk of esophageal adenocarcinoma but not squamous cell esophageal cancer.[58]

High BMI has been implicated as a risk factor for adenocarcinoma of the esophagus in three population-based case-control studies conducted in the United States and Sweden; esophageal adenocarcinoma risk appears to increase directly with increasing level of usual or recent BMI.[56,59,60] Lagergren et al.[56] reported a 16-fold increased risk of esophageal adenocarcinoma when participants with a BMI in the obese range (>30 kg/m^2) were compared with the leanest participants (BMI <22 kg/m^2). With disease usually developing after age 60 years, the largest risks are observed among individuals who have been consistently heavy for an extended period of time.[56,60]

The possible biologic mechanisms linking increased physical activity to decreased esophageal adenocarcinoma risk include site-specific and general cancer mechanisms. It is possible that physical activity decreases digestive track transit time in a manner relevant to the stomach and esophagus. General cancer mechanisms include physical activity's impact on the immune system or steroid hormone pathways. It is likely that obesity impacts esophageal adenocarcinoma risk by influencing gastroesophageal reflux disease. Gastroesophageal reflux symptoms, which are more common among obese than normal-weight individuals and increase in prevalence as BMI increases, have been associated with risk of esophageal adenocarcinoma.[61] Gastroesophageal reflux may cause changes in the esophageal epithelium, leading to Barrett's esophagus, a precursor condition for esophageal adenocarcinoma.

KIDNEY/RENAL CELL CANCER

At least six cohort studies[2,62] and one case-control study[63] have investigated the association between kidney cancer and physical activity, with mixed results. In the Hawaii and Los Angeles Multiethnic Cohort Study, increased recreational physical activity was associated with increased kidney cancer risk among women but not among men.[62] Results from a large Canadian case-control study showed no effect of physical activity on kidney cancer risk among either sex.[63]

Obesity, in addition to high blood pressure and diabetes, is an established risk factor for kidney cancer.[2] Early studies showed that the association between obesity and renal cell cancer was stronger among women than men. Recent reports, however, have shown a more equal impact of BMI on kidney cancer risk among women and men, with an approximate 7% increase in risk per unit increase in BMI.[64]

PANCREATIC CANCER

Pancreatic cancer is relatively rare, is generally diagnosed at an advanced stage, and is associated with high mortality rates. Therefore case-control studies of pancreatic cancer are likely to exclude patients who die soon after diagnosis or who are too ill to participate. Prospective cohort studies require long duration of follow-up to accrue a sufficient number of pancreatic cancer cases to examine risk factors and to rule out confounding by changes in behavior due to subclinical prevalent disease. Despite these limitations, several prospective cohort studies have examined the association between physical activity and pancreatic cancer risk; no association between physical activity and pancreatic cancer risk has been established.[65] Evidence indicating that obesity is a risk factor for pancreatic cancer is growing. A meta-analysis of obesity and pancreatic cancer risk, based on 21 prospective cohort studies conducted throughout the United States, Europe, Japan, and Korea, and published between 1993 and 2006, concluded that for every 5 kg/m^2 increase in BMI, pancreatic cancer risk increased 12% overall.[66] The increase was greater for men (16%) than for women (10%). Results from the Hawaii and Los Angeles Multiethnic Cohort showed a 50% increase in pancreatic cancer risk among obese men, but in contrast to the findings in the meta-analysis, indicated that obese women experienced a 35% decrease in pancreatic cancer risk.[65]

GALLBLADDER CANCER

Gallbladder cancer occurs more frequently in women than in men, and the major risk factor is a history of gallstones,[67] which have been associated with use of exogenous estrogens.[68] To date, we have found no epidemiological literature investigating the possible association of physical activity and gallbladder cancer, although several studies have assessed the possible association between obesity and cancer of the gallbladder. Evidence from cohort and case-control studies has provided strong evidence that increased BMI is an independent risk factor for cancer of the gallbladder.[2,67,69] In a recent population-based case-control study conducted in Shanghai, higher BMI at all ages and a greater waist-to-hip ratio were associated with an increased risk of gallbladder cancer among subjects with and without a history of gallstones, suggesting that both overall and perhaps abdominal obesity may be important in the etiology of this disease.[69]

NON-HODGKIN LYMPHOMA

Studies addressing physical inactivity and obesity as potential risk factors for NHL have been mixed, in part because they have not had a sufficient number of cases to assess risk by NHL subtype. A large population-based case-control study in the United States reported that high BMI does not increase risk of NHL overall, but that extreme obesity (BMI ≥35 kg/m^2) was associated with 70% greater risk of diffuse NHL compared with individuals with normal BMI.[70] In this study, BMI was unrelated to risk of follicular NHL. Further, nonoccupational physical activity was associated with lower risk of NHL overall, but was strongest for diffuse NHL.[70] Physical activity also appeared to be associated with decreased risk of follicular NHL; however, when BMI and nonoccupational physical activity were included in a single model, only the association between high BMI and increased risk for diffuse NHL remained statistically significant. Prior studies of obesity and physical activity have reported similar results to those shown by Cerhan et al.,[70] with no overall association between high BMI or physical inactivity with NHL risk.[2] The observation that high BMI influences risk for diffuse NHL has been confirmed in two recent studies.[71,72] The prospective CTS cohort has shown that, among women, adiposity at age 18 was more important to overall B-cell NHL risk than adiposity later in life; no association was reported between long-term or recent recreational physical activity in this study.[73] At this time no definitive conclusions regarding physical activity can be drawn, and the results for BMI are suggestive of an impact, particularly for diffuse NHL.

PROSTATE CANCER

More than 20 studies have assessed the potential association between physical activity and prostate cancer.[2,74,75] Regardless of the varied approaches, population bases, or sample sizes used, the majority have suggested a modest reduction in risk with an increasing level of physical activity.[2]

In a review of the literature, Friedenreich and Orenstein[74] concluded that prostate cancer risk is reduced 10% to 30% when comparing the most active with the least active men and suggested that it may be high levels of physical activity earlier in life that are most relevant to this disease. In a Canadian population-based case-control study of advanced prostate cancer, defined as stage T2 or higher, in which lifetime histories of activity were assessed, physical activity during adolescence and overall lifetime strenuous activity were modestly related to lower prostate cancer risk.[75] Some[76–78] but not all[79] cohort studies have shown an association between adult physical activity and advanced prostate cancer. It is not yet clear whether these results reflect a true causal association or whether they are due to confounding by prostate-specific antigen testing,[77,78] which may be more common among physically active men.[77] The early epidemiological literature on the potential association between obesity and prostate cancer provided no consistent evidence of a relationship association.[2] In studies that excluded localized or low-grade prostate cancer, results have supported an association between obesity and advanced prostate cancer. Freedland et al.[80] have proposed that obesity may be protective for early-stage disease, but it may be a risk factor for aggressive prostate cancer. A cohort study conducted by the American Cancer Society in which obesity was associated with a 14% to 16% reduced risk for low-grade prostate cancer, but a 22% increased risk for nonmetastatic high-grade prostate cancer, and a 54% increased risk for metastatic or fatal prostate cancer[81] supports the explanation provided by Freedland et al.[80] Another possibility is that obesity may decrease the likelihood of diagnosis of less aggressive prostate cancer. Proposed mechanisms include paradoxical effects of testosterone on low-grade versus more advanced prostate cancer and alterations in insulin and circulating IGF-1 profiles.[81]

LUNG CANCER

The existence of relationships between physical activity or obesity and lung cancer risk is controversial. Physical activity may be protective for lung cancer, yet this effect is not considered well established.[2] A meta-analysis of nine studies published between 1966 and 2003 reported a 13% decreased risk for lung cancer associated with moderate recreational physical activity and a 30% decreased risk associated with strenuous activity.[51] The impact appeared to be slightly stronger among women than among men. Although these effects have been observed among smokers and after considering measures of pack-years smoked, it is still possible that control for confounding by smoking status and smoking intensity is insufficient to eliminate smoking effects or that the lower risk of lung cancer reflects unmeasured differences in smoking habits.

If a causal association exists between increased physical activity and decreased lung cancer risk, the effect should be apparent among never smokers, yet studies to date have not shown such an association. For example, in a large cohort study increased physical activity at cohort enrollment was associated with decreased lung cancer risk among former and current smokers, but not among those who never smoked.[82] Further, increasing physical activity was associated with decreasing risk of adenocarcinomas, but not other cell types. These results are consistent with those from two other studies in which results were stratified by smoking status.[83,84] These studies support the interpretation that the lower risk of lung cancer observed among smokers is due to residual confounding by cigarette smoking.

Several studies have suggested the existence of an inverse association between increasing BMI and lung cancer risk.[2] However, this inverse effect may have been due to weight loss caused by preclinical disease; this hypothesis is supported by the fact that the association disappears as length of follow-up increases. The inverse effect may also have arisen due to residual confounding by smoking; in fact, no association between BMI and lung cancer is seen in nonsmokers.[2]

OVARIAN CANCER

The literature on risk of ovarian cancer in relation to physical activity and obesity has been inconclusive. More than 18 studies have assessed the impact of physical activity on ovarian cancer risk. Risks of ovarian cancer with increasing physical activity range from no change to 67%.[2,85–87] A meta-analysis of 12 studies reported summary estimates for the decrease in ovarian cancer risk associated with physical activity in the highest category versus lowest category in the range of 20%.[87] Three cohort studies published after completion of the meta-analysis, one composed predominantly of premenopausal women[88] and two consisting predominantly of postmenopausal women,[89,90] have reported no association between physical activity and ovarian cancer risk. Results from a recent analysis of data from the American Cancer Society Cancer Prevention Study II cohort showed no evidence for an association between physical activity and ovarian cancer risk; however, an association between history of sedentary behavior (sitting ≥6 hours per day vs. <3 hours per day) was associated with more than a 50% increase in ovarian cancer risk.[85] The association with sedentary behavior is supported by subsequent results from one case-control study.[91]

The evidence for an association between obesity and increased ovarian cancer risk is weak, with few studies showing a statistically significant result.[2,92] A meta-analysis of 16 studies investigating the possible association between adult obesity and ovarian cancer risk indicated that adult obesity increases risk for ovarian cancer; the overall pooled effect estimate indicated that adult obesity was associated with a 30% increase in ovarian cancer risk; in addition, the suggestion of a dose-response effect was observed, and there was no evidence for heterogeneity of effect by histologic subtype.[92] The most likely pathways by which obesity may impact ovarian cancer risk are hormonal and include not only the impact of estrogens, but also the influence of BMI on androgens and insulin.

OVERVIEW

Table 21.1 illustrates the strength of evidence regarding increased physical activity as a protective factor and obesity as a risk factor for cancer. The strength of evidence for each exposure is classified as convincing (+++), probable (++), possible (+), or insufficient and inconclusive (?). Overall, for physical activity, convincing evidence exists for an association with postmenopausal breast cancer and colon cancer; for obesity, the evidence is convincing for breast, colon, endometrial, esophageal, and kidney/renal cell cancer. Evidence for associations between these exposures and several other cancer sites is accumulating. Despite some convincing evidence of the effects of physical activity and obesity on risk of certain cancers, it is difficult to make recommendations as to appropriate changes in lifestyle that will reduce a person's chances of developing cancer. We have no physical activity prescriptions to give at this time. Many questions remain to be answered. What are the ages at which physical activity will provide the most benefit? What types of activity should one do and at what intensity, frequency (times per week), and duration (hours per week)? Similarly, for BMI, is there some threshold below which the individual will not have excess cancer risk? Does purposeful weight loss during the adult years lower the risk associated with being overweight or obese? Finally, much necessary research is ongoing to identify the biological mechanisms that account for these effects, and to determine whether all persons are affected equally. For instance, it is possible that genetically defined subgroups of the population respond to physical activity or obesity differently. Understanding mechanisms and population variation in these effects will illuminate appropriate prescriptions for lifestyle change

TABLE 21.1

SUMMARY OF THE STRENGTH OF THE OBSERVATIONAL EPIDEMIOLOGIC EVIDENCE FOR PHYSICAL ACTIVITY AS A PROTECTIVE FACTOR AND OBESITY AS A RISK FACTOR FOR CANCER, BY TYPE OF CANCER

	Physical Activity	Overweight/ Obesity
Breast, postmenopausal	+++	+++
Breast, premenopausal	++	++ (protection)
Colon	+++	+++
Endometrium	+	+++
Esophagus, adenocarcinoma	?	+++
Kidney/renal cell	?	+++
Gallbladder	?	++
Pancreas	?	++
Non-Hodgkin lymphoma	?	+
Prostate, aggressive	+	+
Lung	+	?
Ovary	?	?

+++, evidence is convincing; ++, evidence is probable; +, evidence is possible; ?, evidence remains insufficient/inconclusive.

Selected References

The full list of references for this chapter appears in the online version.

1. Caspersen CJ, Powell KE, Christenson GM. Physical activity, exercise, and physical fitness: definitions and distinctions for health-related research. *Public Health Rep* 1985;100:126.
2. Vainio H, Bianchini F, eds. *Weight control and physical activity.* International Agency for Research on Cancer Vol 8.. Lyon, France: IARC Press; 2000.
3. Flegal KM, Carroll MD, Ogden CL, Johnson CL. Prevalence and trends in obesity among US adults, 1999–2000. *JAMA* 2002;288:1723.
5. Hardman AE. Physical activity and cancer risk. *Proc Nutr Soc* 2001;60:107.
6. Gunter MJ, Leitzmann MF. Obesity and colorectal cancer: epidemiology, mechanisms and candidate genes. *J Nutr Biochem* 2006;17:145.
7. Bull FC, Armstrong T, Dixon T, et al. Physical inactivity. In M. Ezzati, et al., eds. *Comparative Quantification of health risks: global and regional burden of disease due to selected major risk factors.* Geneva, Switzerland: World Health Organization; 2004:729.
8. Monninkhof EM, Elias SG, Vlems FA, et al. Physical activity and breast cancer: a systematic review. *Epidemiology* 2007;18:137.
9. World Cancer Research Fund / American Institute for Cancer Research: *Food, nutrition, physical activity, and the prevention of cancer: a global perspective.* Washington, DC: WCRF/AICR; 2007.
10. Bernstein L, Henderson BE, Hanisch R, Sullivan-Halley J, Ross RK. Physical exercise and reduced risk of breast cancer in young women. *J Natl Cancer Inst* 1994;86:1403.
21. Bernstein L. Epidemiology of endocrine-related risk factors for breast cancer. *J Mammary Gland Biol Neoplasia* 2002;7:3.
28. Bernstein L. Exercise and breast cancer prevention. *Curr Oncol Rep* 2009;11:490.
29. Neilson HK, Friedenreich CM, Brockton NT, Millikan RC. Physical activity and postmenopausal breast cancer: proposed biologic mechanisms and areas for future research. *Cancer Epidemiol Biomarkers Prev* 2009;18:11.
30. Cleary MP, Grossmann ME. Obesity and breast cancer: the estrogen connection. *Endocrinology* 2009;150:2537.
31. Brown KA, Simpson ER. Obesity and breast cancer: progress to understanding the relationship. *Cancer Res* 2010;70:4.
32. Wolin KY, Yan Y, Colditz GA, Lee IM. Physical activity and colon cancer prevention: a meta-analysis. *Br J Cancer* 2009;100:611.
35. Iacopetta B. Are there two sides to colorectal cancer? *Int J Cancer* 2002; 101:403.
43. Calle EE, Kaaks R. Overweight, obesity and cancer: epidemiological evidence and proposed mechanisms. *Nat Rev Cancer* 2004;4:579.
46. Voskuil DW, Monninkhof EM, Elias SG, et al. Physical activity and endometrial cancer risk, a systematic review of current evidence. *Cancer Epidemiol Biomarkers Prev* 2007;16:639.
47. Cust AE, Armstrong BK, Friedenreich CM, Slimani N, Bauman A. Physical activity and endometrial cancer risk: a review of the current evidence, biologic mechanisms and the quality of physical activity assessment methods. *Cancer Causes Control* 2007;18:243.
54. Kaaks R, Lukanova A, Kurzer MS. Obesity, endogenous hormones, and endometrial cancer risk: a synthetic review. *Cancer Epidemiol Biomarkers Prev* 2002;11:1531.
58. Leitzmann MF, Koebnick C, Freedman ND, et al. Physical activity and esophageal and gastric carcinoma in a large prospective study. *Am J Prev Med* 2009;36:112.
59. Chow WH, Blot WJ, Vaughan TL, et al. Body mass index and risk of adenocarcinomas of the esophagus and gastric cardia. *J Natl Cancer Inst* 1998;90:150.
62. Setiawan VW, Stram DO, Nomura AM, Kolonel LN, Henderson BE. Risk factors for renal cell cancer: the multiethnic cohort. *Am J Epidemiol* 2007;166:932.
64. Lipworth L, Tarone RE, McLaughlin JK. The epidemiology of renal cell carcinoma. *J Urol* 2006;176:2353.
65. Nothlings U, Wilkens LR, Murphy SP, et al. Body mass index and physical activity as risk factors for pancreatic cancer: the Multiethnic Cohort Study. *Cancer Causes Control* 2007;18:165.
66. Larsson SC, Orsini N, Wolk A. Body mass index and pancreatic cancer risk: A meta-analysis of prospective studies. *Int J Cancer* 2007;120: 1993.
67. Randi G, Franceschi S, La Vecchia C. Gallbladder cancer worldwide: geographical distribution and risk factors. *Int J Cancer* 2006;118:1591.
70. Cerhan JR, Bernstein L, Severson RK, et al. Anthropometrics, physical activity, related medical conditions, and the risk of non-Hodgkin lymphoma. *Cancer Causes Control* 2005;16:1203.
74. Friedenreich CM, Orenstein MR. Physical activity and cancer prevention: etiologic evidence and biological mechanisms. *J Nutr* 2002;132: 3456S.
80. Freedland SJ, Giovannucci E, Platz EA. Are findings from studies of obesity and prostate cancer really in conflict? *Cancer Causes Control* 2006;17:5.
82. Leitzmann MF, Koebnick C, Abnet CC, et al. Prospective study of physical activity and lung cancer by histologic type in current, former, and never smokers. *Am J Epidemiol* 2009;169:542.
87. Olsen CM, Bain CJ, Jordan SJ, et al. Recreational physical activity and epithelial ovarian cancer: a case-control study, systematic review, and meta-analysis. *Cancer Epidemiol Biomarkers Prev* 2007;16:2321.
92. Olsen CM, Green AC, Whiteman DC, et al. Obesity and the risk of epithelial ovarian cancer: a systematic review and meta-analysis. *Eur J Cancer* 2007;43:690.

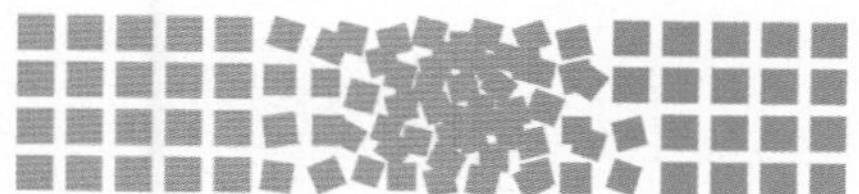

CHAPTER 22 EPIDEMIOLOGIC METHODS

XIAOMEI MA AND HERBERT YU

Epidemiology is the study of the distribution and determinants of health-related states or events in specified populations and the application of this study to control health problems.[1] Epidemiologic principles and methods have long been applied to cancer research, with the assumptions that cancer does not occur at random and the nonrandomness of carcinogenesis can be elucidated through systematic research. An example of such applications is the lung cancer study conducted by Doll and Hill[2] in the early 1950s, which linked tobacco smoking to an increased mortality of lung cancer in over 40,000 medical professionals in the United Kingdom. The observation from this study and many other studies, in conjunction with laboratory findings regarding the underlying biologic mechanisms for the effect of tobacco smoking, helped establish the role of tobacco smoking in the etiology of lung cancer. Epidemiologic methods are also used in clinical settings, where trials are conducted to evaluate the efficacy of new treatment protocols or preventive measures and observational studies of prognostic factors are done.

Epidemiologic studies can take different forms, but generally they can be classified into two broad categories: observational studies and experimental studies (Fig. 22.1). In experimental studies, an investigator allocates different study regimens to the subjects, usually with randomization (experimental studies without randomization are sometimes referred to as "quasi-experiments"[3]). Experimental studies can be individual based or community based. An experimental study most closely resembles laboratory experiments in that the investigator has control over the study condition. Experimental studies can be used to evaluate the efficacy of a treatment protocol (e.g., low-dose compared with standard-dose chemotherapy for non-Hodgkin's lymphoma[4]) or preventive measures (e.g., tamoxifen for women at an increased risk of breast cancer[5]). Although experimental studies are often considered the gold standard because of well-controlled study situations, they are only suitable for the evaluation of effects that are beneficial or at least not harmful due to ethical concerns. Experimental studies are discussed in detail in other chapters of this book. This section will focus on observational studies.

Observational studies do not involve artificial manipulation of study regimens. In an observational study, an investigator stands by to observe what happens or happened to the patients, in terms of exposure and outcome. Observational studies can be further divided into descriptive and analytical studies (Fig. 22.1). Descriptive studies focus on the *distribution* of diseases with respect to person, place, and time (i.e., who, where, and when), whereas analytical studies focus on the *determinants* of diseases. Descriptive studies are often used to *generate* hypotheses, while analytical studies are often used to *test* hypotheses. However, the two types of studies should not be considered mutually exclusive entities; rather, they are the opposite ends of a continuum. Descriptive studies are discussed in detail in the next section.

ANALYTICAL STUDIES

Ecologic Studies

As in experimental studies, the unit of analysis can be individuals or groups of people in observational studies. Studies that use groups of people as the unit of analysis are called ecologic studies, which are relatively easy to carry out when group level measures are available. However, a relationship observed between variables on a group level does not necessarily reflect the relationship that exists at an individual level. For example, the fraction of energy supply from animal products was founded to be positively correlated with breast cancer mortality in a recent ecologic study, which used preexisting data on both dietary supply and breast cancer mortality rates from 35 countries.[6] Since the data were country based, no reliable inference can be made at an individual level. Within each country, it could be that the people who had a low fraction of energy supply from animal products were actually dying from breast cancer. Results from ecologic studies are useful for inference at an individual level only when the within-group variability of the exposure is low so a group-level measure can reasonable reflect exposure at an individual level. Alternatively, if the implications for prevention or intervention are at a group level (e.g., taxation of cigarettes to reduce smoking), results from ecologic studies are very useful.

Cross-Sectional Studies

There are three main types of analytical studies in which the unit of analysis is individuals: cross-sectional, cohort, and case-control studies. In a cross-sectional study, the information on various factors is collected from the study population at a given point in time. From a public health perspective, data collected in cross-sectional studies can be of great value in assessing the general health status of a population and allocating resources. For example, the third National Health and Nutrition Examination Survey has provided valuable national estimates of health and nutritional status of the U.S. civilian, noninstitutionalized population.[7] Findings from cross-sectional studies can also help generate hypotheses that may be tested later in other types of studies. However, it should be noted that cross-sectional studies have serious methodological limitations if the research purpose is etiologic inference. Since exposures and disease status are evaluated simultaneously, it is usually not possible to know the temporality of events, unless the exposure cannot change over time (e.g., blood type, skin color, race, country of birth, etc.). If one observes that more brain cancer patients are depressed than people without brain cancer in a cross-sectional study, the correlation does not

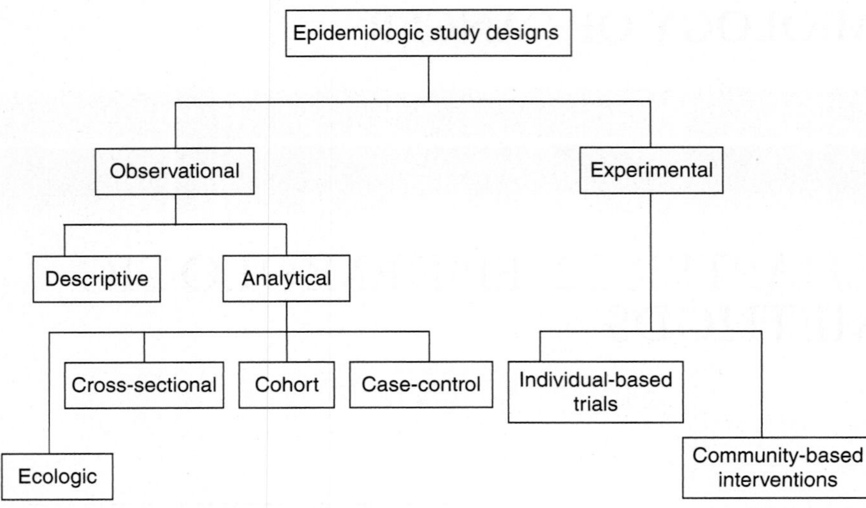

FIGURE 22.1 Classification of epidemiologic study designs.

necessarily mean that depression causes brain cancer. Depression may simply have resulted from the pathogenesis and diagnosis of brain cancer. Or, depression may have caused brain cancer in some patients and resulted from brain cancer in other patients. Without additional information on the timing of events, no conclusions can be made. Another concern in cross-sectional studies is the enrollment of prevalent cases, who survived different lengths of time after the incidence of disease. Factors then affect survival may also influence incidence. Prevalent cases may not be representative of incident cases, which makes etiologic inferences based on cross-sectional studies suspect at best.

Cohort Studies

In a cohort study, a study population free of a specific disease (or any other health-related condition) is grouped based on their exposure status and followed up for a certain period of time, and then the exposed and unexposed subjects are compared with respect to disease status at the end of the follow-up. The objective of a cohort study is usually to evaluate whether the incidence of a disease is associated with an exposure. The cohort design is fundamental in observational epidemiology and is considered "ideal" in that, if unbiased, cohort data reflect the real life cause–effect sequence of disease.[8] Subjects in cohort studies may be a sample of the general population in a geographic area, a group of workers who are exposed to certain occupational hazards in a specific industry, or people who are considered at a high risk for a specific disease. A cohort study is considered prospective or concurrent if the investigator starts following up the cohort from the present time into the future, and retrospective or historical if the cohort is established in the past based on existing records (e.g., an occupational cohort based on employment records) and the follow-up ends before or at the time of the study. Alternatively, a cohort study can be ambidirectional in that data collection goes both directions.[9] Whether a cohort study is prospective, retrospective, or ambidirectional, the key feature is that all the patients were free of the disease at the beginning of the follow-up and the study tracks the patients from exposure to disease. Follow-up time, ranging from days to decades, is an essential element in cohort studies.

In a cohort study, the incidence of disease in the exposed group and the unexposed group is compared. The incidence measure can be cumulative incidence or incidence density, depending on the availability of data. When comparing the incidence in the two groups, both relative differences and absolute differences can be assessed. In cohort studies, the relative risk of developing the disease is expressed as the ratio of the cumulative incidence in the exposed group to that in the unexposed group, which is also called cumulative incidence ratio or risk ratio. If we have data on the exact person-time of follow-up for every patient, we can also calculate an incidence density ratio (also called rate ratio) in a similar way. The numeric value of the risk or rate ratio reflects the magnitude of the association between an exposure and a disease. For example, a risk ratio of 2 would be interpreted as those exposed individuals have a doubled risk of developing a disease than unexposed individuals, while a risk ratio of 5 indicates that exposed individuals have a 5 times greater risk of developing a disease than unexposed individuals. Put in another way, a factor with a risk ratio of 5 has a stronger effect than another factor with a risk ratio of 2. In addition to risk ratio and rate ratio, another relative measure called the probability odds ratio can be calculated in cohort studies. The probability odds of disease is the number of individuals who developed a disease divided by the number of individuals who did not develop the disease, and the probability odds ratio is the probability odds in the exposed group divided by the probability odds in the unexposed group. Many investigators prefer risk ratio or rate ratio to probability odds ratio in cohort studies, since the ability to directly measure the risk of developing a disease is one of the most significant advantages in cohort studies. In practice, however, probability odds ratio is often used as an approximation for risk or rate ratio, especially when multivariate logistic regression models are employed to adjust for the effect of other factors that may influence the relationship between an exposure and a disease.

As for absolute differences, a commonly used measure is called attributable risk in the exposed, which is the incidence in the exposed group minus the incidence in the unexposed group. Attributable risk reflects the disease incidence that could be attributed to the exposure in exposed individuals and the reduction in incidence that we would expect if the exposure can be removed from the exposed individuals, provided there is a causal relationship between the exposure and the disease. Another absolute measure called population attributable risk extends this concept to the general population. It estimates the disease incidence that could be attributed to an exposure in the general population. Since both relative and absolute differences can be assessed in cohort studies, a natural question to ask is which measures to choose. In general, the relative differences are used more often if the main research objective is etiologic inference, and they can be used for the judgment of causality. Once causality is established or at least assumed, measures of absolute differences are more important from a public health perspective. This point can be illustrated using the following hypothetical example.

Assuming toxin X in the environment triples the risk of bladder cancer and toxin Y doubles the risk of bladder cancer, the effects of X and Y are entirely independent of each other, the prevalence of exposure to toxin Y in the general population is 20 times higher than the prevalence of exposure to toxin X, and there are only resources available to reduce the exposure to one toxin, it would be more effective to use the resources to reduce the exposure to toxin Y instead of toxin X. This is because the population attributable risk due to Y is higher than that due to X, although the risk ratio associated with toxin Y is smaller than that associated with toxin X.

Cohort studies have many advantages. A cohort design is the best way to study the natural history of a disease.[9] There is usually a clear temporal relationship between an exposure and a disease since all the individuals are free of the disease at the beginning of the follow-up (it can be a problem if an individual has a subclinical disease such as undetected prostate cancer). Furthermore, multiple diseases can be studied with respect to the same exposure. On the other hand, cohort studies, especially prospective cohort studies, are costly in terms of both time and money. A cohort design requires the follow-up of a large number of study participants over a sometimes extremely lengthy period of time and usually extensive data collection through questionnaires, physical measurements, and biological specimens at regular intervals. Participants may be "lost" during the follow-up because they became tired of the study, moved away from the study area, or died from causes other than the disease under study. If those who were lost during the follow-up are different from those who remained under observation with respect to exposure, disease, or other factors, that may influence the relationship between the exposure and the disease, and results from the study will be biased. To date, cohort studies have been used to study the etiology of a wide spectrum of diseases, including different types of cancer. If a cohort study is conducted to evaluate the etiology of cancer, usually the study sample size would need to be very large (such as the National Institutes of Health–American Association of Retired Persons Diet and Health Study, which included more than half a million subjects[10]) and the follow-up time would need to be long, unless the cohort selected is a high-risk population.

For simplicity, this chapter examines cohort studies in which the outcome of interest is the incidence of a specific disease and there are only two exposure groups. In practice, any health-related event can be the outcome of interest, and multiple exposure groups can be compared.

Case-Control Studies

Case-control design is an alternative to cohort design for the evaluation of the relationship between an exposure and a disease (or any other health condition). A case-control approach compares the odds of past exposure between cases and noncases (controls) and uses the exposure odds ratio as an estimate for relative risk. A primary goal in a case-control study is to reach the same conclusions as what would have been obtained from a cohort study, if one had been done.[11] If appropriately designed and conducted, a case-control study can optimize speed and efficiency as the need for follow-up is avoided.[8] The starting point of a case-control study is a source population from which the cases arise. Instead of obtaining the denominators for the calculation of risks or rates in a cohort study, a control group is sampled from the entire source population. After selecting control subjects, who ideally would have become cases had they developed the disease, an investigator collects data on past exposures from both the cases and the controls and then calculates an odds ratio, which is the odds of exposure in the cases divided by the odds of exposure in the controls.

There are two main types of case-control studies: case-based case-control studies and case-control studies within defined cohorts.[8] Some variations of the case-control design also exist. For instance, if the effect of an exposure is transient, sometimes a case can be used as his or her own control (case-crossover design). In case-based case-control studies, cases and controls are selected at a given point in time from a hypothetical cohort (i.e., at the end of follow-up). A cross-sectional ascertainment of cases will result in a case group that mostly contains prevalent cases, who may have survived for different lengths of time after disease incidence. Cases who died before an investigator began participant ascertainment would not be eligible to be included in the study. As a result, the cases finally included in the study may not be representative of all the cases from the entire hypothetical cohort. Another disadvantage of enrolling prevalent cases is that cases who were diagnosed a long time ago will likely have difficulties recalling exposures that occurred before disease incidence.

In case-control studies it is preferable to ascertain incident cases as soon as they are diagnosed and select controls as soon as cases are identified. Case-control studies that enroll only incident cases are sometimes called *prospective* case-control studies, in that the investigators need to wait for the incident cases to develop and be diagnosed. For cancer studies, the cases can be ascertained from population-based cancer registries or hospitals. A major advantage of using a cancer registry is the completeness of case ascertainment, but the reporting of cancer cases to registries is usually not instantaneous. There could be a lag time of several months or even over a year, and some case individuals could have died during the lag time. If the cancer under study has a poor survival or clinical specimens need to be obtained in a timely manner, it may be preferable to identify cases directly from hospitals using a rapid ascertainment protocol. As for the selection of controls, the key issue is that controls should be representative of the source population from which the cases arise, and theoretically the controls would have been ascertained as cases had they developed the disease. The most common types of controls include population-based controls (often selected through random digit dialing in case-control studies of cancer etiology), hospital controls, and friend controls. The advantages and disadvantages of different types of controls have been nicely summarized by Wacholder et al.[12] Since no follow-up is involved in case-based case-control studies, incidence risk or rate cannot be calculated directly for case and control groups. The odds ratio will be a good estimate of relative risk if the disease is uncommon.

In addition to case-based case-control studies, there are also case-control studies within defined cohorts (also known as hybrid or ambidirectional designs), including case-cohort studies and nested case-control studies. In case-cohort studies, cases are identified from a well-defined cohort after some follow-up time, and controls are selected from the baseline cohort. In nested case-control studies, cases are also identified from a cohort, but controls are selected from the individuals at risk at the time each case occurs (i.e., incidence density sampling).[8] In these types of designs, controls are a sample of the cohort, and the controls selected can theoretically become cases at some point. The possibility of selection bias in case-control studies within defined cohorts is lower than that in case-based case-control studies because the cases and the controls are selected from the same source population. Because of an increased awareness of the methodological issues inherent in the design of case-based case-control studies and the availability of a growing number of large cohorts, case-control studies within defined cohorts have become more common in recent years. The advantage of case-control studies within cohorts over traditional cohort studies is mainly the efficiency in additional data collection. For instance, a recent nested case-control study evaluated the relationship between endogenous sex hormones and prostate cancer risk.[13] Instead of measuring the serum hormone levels of the entire cohort (over 12,000 subjects), investigators chose to measure 300 cases and 300 controls selected from the cohort. Doing so not only significantly reduced the cost of measurements and the time it took to address the research question, but also helped preserve valuable serum samples for possible analyses in the future. In a case-cohort design, an odds ratio estimates risk ratio; in a nested case-control design, an odds ratio estimates rate ratio. In both designs, the disease under study does not have to be rare for the odds ratio to be a good estimate of the risk ratio or rate ratio.[8,14]

The biggest advantage of a case-control design is the speed and efficiency in obtaining data. It is claimed that investigators implement case-control studies more frequently than any other analytical epidemiologic study.[15] Since most types of cancer are uncommon and take a long time to develop, to date most epidemiologic studies of cancer have been case-control instead of cohort in design. A case-control study can be conducted to evaluate the relationship between many different exposures and a specific disease, but the study will have limited statistical power if the exposure is rare. In general, a case-control design tends to be more susceptible to biases than a cohort design. Such biases include but are not limited to selection bias when choosing and enrolling participants (especially controls) and recall bias when obtaining data from the participants. The status of the participants, that is, case or control, may affect how they recall and report previous exposures, some of which occurred years or even decades ago. It is important for investigators to explicitly define the diagnostic and eligibility criteria for cases, to select controls from the same population as the cases independent of the exposures of interest, to blind data collection staff to the case or control status of participants or the main hypothesis of the study, to ascertain exposure in a similar manner from cases and controls, and to take into account other factors that may influence the relationship between an exposure and a disease.[15]

INTERPRETATION OF EPIDEMIOLOGIC FINDINGS

This chapter has thus far discussed measures of effects in various study designs. However, a risk ratio of 3 from a cohort study or an odds ratio of 2.5 from a case-control study does not necessarily mean there is an association between an exposure and a disease. Several alternative explanations need to be assessed, including chance (random error), bias (systematic error), and confounding. Potential interaction also needs to be evaluated.

Statistical methods are required to evaluate the role of chance. The usual way is to calculate the upper and lower limits of a 95% confidence interval around a point estimate for relative risk (risk ratio, rate ratio, or odds ratio). If the confidence interval does not include one, one would say that the observed association is statistically significant; if the confidence interval includes one, one would say that the observed relationship is not statistically significant. The width of a confidence interval is directly related to the number of participants in a study, which is called sample size. A larger sample size leads to less variability in the data, a tighter confidence interval, and a higher possibility in finding a statistically significant relationship. A 95% confidence interval means that if the data collection and analysis could be replicated many times, the confidence interval should include the correct value of the measure 95% of the time.[16] It is better to consider a confidence interval to be a general guide to the amount of random error in the data but not necessarily a literal measure of statistical variability.[16]

Bias can be defined as any systematic error in an epidemiologic study that results in an incorrect estimate of the association between exposure and disease, and it can occur in every type of epidemiologic study design. There are two main types of bias: selection bias and information bias. Selection bias is present when individuals included in a study are systematically different from the target population. For example, if a study aimed to generate a sample representing all women in the United States, of the women contacted, more with a family history of breast cancer agreed to participate. This sample would be at a higher risk for breast cancer than the target population. Refusal to participate poses a constant challenge in epidemiologic studies. As individuals have become more concerned about privacy issues and as studies have become more demanding of time, biologic specimens, and other impositions, participation rates have dropped substantially in recent years. If nonparticipants are different from the participants with respect to study-related characteristics, the validity of the study is threatened. Information bias occurs when the data collected from the study subjects are erroneous. Information bias is also known as misclassification if the variable is measured on a categorical scale and the error causes a subject to be placed in a wrong category. Misclassification can happen to both exposure and disease. For example, in a case-control study of previous reproductive history and ovarian cancer, a woman who had an extremely early pregnancy loss may not even realize that she was ever pregnant and would mistakenly report no pregnancy, and another woman who has only subclinical presentations of ovarian cancer may be mistakenly selected as a control. Misclassification can be differential or nondifferential. An exposure misclassification is considered differential if it is related to disease status and nondifferential if not related to disease status. Similarly, a disease misclassification is considered differential if it is related to exposure status and nondifferential if not related to exposure status. If a binary exposure variable and a binary disease variable are analyzed, nondifferential misclassification will result in an underestimate of the true association. Differential misclassification can either exaggerate or underestimate a true effect. Usually not much can be done to control or correct bias at the data analysis stage, therefore, it is important to establish research protocols that are not prone to bias. The evaluation of potential bias is critical to the interpretation of study results. An invalid estimate is worse than no estimate.

Confounding refers to a situation in which the association between an exposure and a disease (or any health-related condition) is influenced by a third variable. This third variable is considered a confounding variable or confounder. A confounder must fulfill three criteria: (1) be associated with the exposure, (2) be associated with the disease independent of the exposure, and (3) not be an intermediate step between the exposure and the disease (i.e., not on the causal pathway). Unlike bias, which is primarily introduced by the investigator or study participants, confounding is a function of the complex interrelationship between various exposures and disease.[17] In a hypothetical case-control study of the effect of alcohol drinking on lung cancer, we may observe an odds ratio of 2.5 (usually called a "crude" odds ratio in the sense that no other variables were taken into account), which indicates that alcohol drinking increases the risk of lung cancer by 1.5-fold. However, if we classify all study subjects into two strata based on history of cigarette smoking and then calculate the odds ratio in the two strata (smokers and nonsmokers) separately, it is possible to have two stratum-specific odds ratios both equal to one, indicating that alcohol drinking is not associated with lung cancer risk. In this example, the crude odds ratio calculated to estimate the association between alcohol drinking and lung cancer without considering smoking is simply misleading. Being associated with both the exposure (i.e., alcohol drinking) and the disease (i.e., lung cancer), smoking acted as a confounder in this example. A stratified analysis is needed to evaluate the potential confounding effect of a third variable, whether it is done with pencil and paper or statistical modeling. Usually data are stratified based on the level of a third variable. If the stratum-specific effect measures are similar to one another but different from the crude effect measure, confounding is said to be present. This section has illustrated basic epidemiologic principles using an overly simplified scenario and only considers a single exposure. In practice, most, if not all diseases, cancer included, have a multifactorial etiology. Consequently, it is usually necessary to assess the potential confounding effect of a group of variables simultaneously using multivariate statistical models. The effect measure derived from a multivariate model will then be called an "adjusted" effect, in the sense that the effect of other factors was also adjusted for. Without controlling for the potential effect of other variables, an investigator cannot really judge whether an observed association between a given exposure and a specific disease is spurious.

If the effect of an exposure on the risk of a disease is not homogeneous in strata formed by a third variable, the third variable is considered an effect modifier, and the situation is called interaction or effect modification. Put in other words, interaction exists when the stratum-specific effect measures are different from one another. In the lung cancer example above, if the odds ratio for alcohol drinking is 1 in smokers but 3 in nonsmokers, then there is interaction and smoking is an effect modifier. The evaluation of interaction is essentially a stratified analysis, which is similar to the evaluation of confounding. Confounding and interaction can both be present in a given study. However, when interaction occurs, the stratum-specific effect measures should be reported. It is no longer appropriate to report a summary measure in the presence of interaction. Unlike confounding, a nuisance that an investigator hopes to remove, interaction is a more detailed description of the true relationship between an exposure and a disease.

MOLECULAR EPIDEMIOLOGY

Molecular epidemiology is transdisciplinary research that involves not only traditional epidemiology and biostatistics but also genetics, molecular biology, biochemistry, cellular biology, analytical chemistry, toxicology, pharmacology, and laboratory medicine. Unlike traditional epidemiology, research of cancer that focuses on exposures or risk factors ascertained through questionnaire-based interview or survey, molecular epidemiology studies expand the assessment of exposure to a much broader scope that includes analysis of biomarkers underlying internal exposure of exogenous and endogenous carcinogenic agents, molecular alterations in response to exposure, and genetic susceptibility to cancer. These include DNA, RNA, proteins, chromosomes, compound molecules (e.g., DNA and protein adducts), and various endogenous and exogenous substances that are related to cancer risk (e.g., steroids, nutrients, chemical or biological toxins, and phytochemicals). Molecular markers can reflect different aspects of the process of tumorigenesis, which include biomarkers of internal exposure, biomarkers of molecular or cellular changes in response to exposure, and biomarkers of precursor lesions or early diseases.[18,19] Depending on the source of molecules and location of diseases, surrogates are often used in epidemiologic studies. When using a surrogate marker or tissue, the relevance of a proxy to its underlying target needs to be established or justified.[19] This justification is especially important when conducting population-based epidemiologic studies that focus on organ-specific cancers, because assessing biomarkers in target tissue is difficult for controls—molecular markers from blood samples are often used as substitutes. If a biomarker in the blood does not travel to or act on the tissue or organ of interest, an association between the circulating marker and the cancer may not be relevant. Thus, establishing a close link between a surrogate and its target is crucial in molecular epidemiology research.

Gene–environment interaction plays an essential role in cancer development.[20] Common genetic variations are considered an important determinant of host susceptibility and are a major focus of molecular epidemiology research. Depending on the biologic mechanism involved, genetic variations can influence every aspect of the carcinogenic process, ranging from external and internal exposure to carcinogens or risk factors to molecular and cellular damage, alteration and response.[18,19] Currently, single nucleotide polymorphisms (SNPs) are the most studied genetic variations. It is believed that even if SNPs confer a small risk, they may still be important at the population level since these variations are common in the general population. It is also important that the impacts of SNPs on cancer are considered under the context of gene–gene and gene–environment interactions. As genotyping technology has advanced substantially with respect to its analytic quality, capacity, and cost, research of genetic polymorphisms has evolved rapidly from investigations of a single SNP to studies of haplotypes and tag SNPs, and from a pathway-based candidate gene approach to genome-wide association studies (GWAS).[21] A GWAS analyzes hundreds of thousands of SNPs simultaneously for hundreds or even thousands of study subjects. When these data are further combined with questionnaire information, such as environmental exposures, lifestyle factors, dietary habits, and medical history, enormous information is generated that requires a huge sample size to allow for reliable and complete assessment of these variables individually and jointly. A single epidemiologic study can no longer provide sufficient power for this type of investigation. Multicenter investigations or study consortia that pool study information and specimens together have emerged to address the sample size issue in recent years.[22] False-positive findings that result from multiple comparisons constitute a major challenge in epidemiologic studies of genetic associations with cancer.[23] A meta-analysis or pooled analysis can be used to address this problem if sufficient studies are already published and available for evaluation. To address this issue at the time of study design, one may adopt a two- or multiphase study design in which study subjects are divided into two or multiple groups for genotyping and data analysis. Selected or genome-wide SNPs are first screened in one group of the study participants (discovery phase), and then the significant findings determined by stringent statistical criteria (usually p values less than 1×10^{-5} or 1×10^{-7}) are reanalyzed in one or several other groups of participants for verification (validation phase). False-positive findings can also be addressed with various statistical methods, such as bootstrap, permutation test, estimate of false-positive report probability, prediction of false discovery rate, and the use of a much more stringent P value to accommodate multiple comparisons. For epidemiologic studies that are not population based or not conducted strictly following epidemiology principles, population stratification is a potential source of bias that may distort genetic associations.[24]

Since the previous edition of this book, a large number of GWAS have been completed in search for SNPs that influence host susceptibility to cancer. Considering that more than 5 million SNPs are present in the human genome, the numbers of SNPs that are found to be associated with cancer risk after rigorous validation are much fewer than what one would have anticipated. In addition, the risk associations detected are quite weak, with most of the odds ratios ranging from 1.1 to 1.5, and the functional relevance or biological implications are unclear for most of the SNPs. Furthermore, not many SNPs associated with cancer risk are located in protein-coding regions, and even fewer are in the loci of candidate genes suspected to be involved in tumorigenesis, such as oncogenes, tumor suppressor genes, DNA repair genes, and xenobiotic metabolizing or detoxification genes. Genes where SNPs are found to be linked to cancer by GWAS include *FGFR2*, *MAP3K1*, *MRPS30*, *LSP1*, *TNRC9*, *TOX3*, *STXBP1*, and *RAD51L1* for breast cancer,[25–27] *JAZF1*,

HNF1B, *MSMB*, *CTBP2*, and *KLK2/KLK3* for prostate cancer,[25,28] *SMAD7*, *CRAC1*, *EIF3H*, *BMP4*, *CDH1*, and *RHPN2* for colorectal cancer,[25,29] *CHRNA3* and *CHRNA5* for lung cancer,[30,31] *ABO* for pancreatic cancer,[32] *TACC3* and *PSCA* for bladder cancer,[33,34] and *KRT5* for basal cell carcinoma.[35] Among these genes identified by GWAS, two findings are considered especially interesting. One is the association of lung cancer with *CHRNA3* and *CHRNA5*, which encode neuronal nicotinic acetylcholine receptor subunits. Different genotypes of these receptor subunits appear to influence individual's addiction to tobacco, which further leads to different smoking exposure and lung cancer risk.[36,37] Another is the link of the *ABO* gene to pancreatic cancer. The association between pancreatic cancer risk and ABO blood type was observed 50 years ago. The GWAS finding not only confirms the relationship, but it also provides new clues for understanding the underlying biological mechanism.

Besides intragenic SNPs, GWAS also found many intergenic SNPs in association to cancer risk, which include those in the regions of 8q24, 5p15, 1p11, 1p36, 1q42, 2p15, 2q35, 3p12, 3p24, 3q28, 6p21, 6q25, 7q21, 7q32, 9p21, 9p22, 9p24, 9q22, 10p14, 11q13, 11q23, 14q13, 18q23, and 20p12.[25–27,29,35,38–44] Of these loci, SNPs in 8q24 are associated with several cancer sites, including prostate, breast, colon, and bladder.[25,27–29,43–45] Further analysis of 8q24 indicates that there are nine SNPs in five regions, and each region is independently related to different types of cancer, with SNPs in regions 1, 4, and 5 associated exclusively with prostate cancer, a SNP in region 2 related to breast cancer, and SNPs in region 3 linked to prostate, colon, and ovarian cancers.[46] No known genes are located within the region of 8q24, but an oncogene *c-MYC* resides about 330 kb downstream of the region.[47] Initial investigation found no evidence of the SNPs' influence on c-MYC expression,[43] but a recent study suggests that the SNPs in 8q24 may be distal enhancers of c-MYC, interacting with its promoter through a chromatin loop.[48] Another genomic region that is associated with the risk of multiple cancer sites is 5p15, a region involving TERT-CLPTM1L. Five types of cancer are found to be linked to this region, including basal cell carcinoma, lung, bladder, prostate, and cervical cancers.[49] TERT is a telomerase reverse transcriptase that extends the length of telomere and is associated with cell proliferation and abnormal telomere maintenance.[50] The risk alleles of TERT are associated with shorter telomere length among the elderly and with higher DNA adduct in the lung.[49,51]

GWAS has demonstrated its value in identifying disease-related SNPs in unknown regions of the genome, which provides new clues for investigators to interrogate and understand different regions of the human genome, especially in the gene-desert areas. Despite the strength, the low yield of significant findings from the GWAS has raised concerns in several areas, including the SNP coverage in the genome (rare SNPs and SNP representativeness in unknown regions), associations with low statistical significance (P value between 0.01 and 1×10^{-5}, the GWAS cutoff), other forms of genetic variations (copy number variation and other structural variations), cancer subtypes, and genetic interplay with environmental factors (gene–environment interaction).[52,53] To address these issues, investigators propose to perform fine mapping and resequencing to examine genetic regions more specifically and meticulously. Epidemiologists suggest that detailed environmental exposure and lifestyle factors should be included in the next wave of GWAS. Furthermore, to make the study more reliable and compelling, DNA specimens, instead of convenient samples, should come from well-designed and well-executed epidemiologic studies that pay close attention to the selection of study subjects and measurement of environmental and lifestyle factors to eliminate or minimize selection bias and measurement errors.

As described earlier, analytical epidemiology has two major study designs: case-control study and cohort study. It is important that investigators choose an appropriate study design to investigate molecular markers in epidemiologic studies. Two types of molecular markers, genotypic and phenotypic markers, can be considered. Genotypic markers refer to nucleotide sequences of genomic DNA, and all other molecules are considered phenotypic markers. The distinction between the two is a marker's status in relation to an outcome variable, usually a disease. Genotypic markers generally do not change over time and are not affected by the development of a disease, whereas phenotypic markers are likely to change over time or to be influenced by the presence of a disease, either itself or treatment associated with it. If measurements of a phenotypic marker are made from the specimens that are collected after or at the time of cancer diagnosis, investigators will have difficulties determining the status of the phenotypic marker before the cancer was diagnosed. A disease condition, however, does not affect genotypic markers such as SNPs, and therefore, a temporal relationship can be easily established even if the samples are collected after the disease is diagnosed. Based on this distinction, one can evaluate genotypic markers either in case-control or cohort studies, but a case-control study would be the design of choice because of efficiency and cost-effectiveness. A prospective cohort study design is ideal for phenotypic markers. Investigators, however, may use other study designs if they can demonstrate that the disease status does not influence the phenotypic markers of interest. To reduce study cost, investigators usually use nested case-control or case-cohort designs to avoid analysis of specimens from the entire cohort. The main reason to choose a cohort study design for molecular epidemiology investigation is to ensure that biospecimens are collected before the development of a disease so that a temporal relationship between a marker and disease development can be established.

The differences between molecular epidemiology and genetic epidemiology are the scope of molecular analysis and the emphasis on heredity. Sometimes molecular and genetic epidemiology both investigate genetic factors in association with cancer risk, but each has its own emphasis. The former assesses genetic involvement, but not necessarily inheritance, while the latter focuses mainly on heredity. Because of the difference in focus, study populations are different between the two types of investigation. Molecular epidemiology studies unrelated individuals, whereas genetic epidemiology investigates family members in the format of pedigrees, parent–child trios, or sibling pairs. Given different research focuses between genetic and molecular epidemiology, these investigations evaluate different genetic markers. Genetic epidemiology research is designed to identify genetic markers with high penetrance (strong association with an underlying disease) but low prevalence in the general populations, whereas molecular epidemiology investigation targets low penetrance markers that are commonly present in the general population. Given the difference in study design, analysis of a genetic marker's link to cancer is also different between the studies. Relative risks or odds ratios are calculated in molecular epidemiology studies since study participants are unrelated individuals, whereas linkage analysis is used in genetic epidemiology as individuals in the study are genetically related family members. Recently, both genetic and molecular epidemiology study designs have been considered in GWAS to improve study validity and to minimize false-positive findings. Another difference between genetic and molecular epidemiology research is that molecular epidemiology also studies nongenetic molecules. Thus, the scope of molecular analysis is much broader in molecular epidemiology research than in genetic epidemiology studies.

Laboratory analysis of molecular markers is another integral part of molecular epidemiology research, which has unique features that are different from basic laboratory research. Collection of biologic specimens is difficult and expensive in population-based epidemiologic studies. It not only results in additional cost, but also imposes constraints to multiple areas of epidemiology research. Specimen collection may adversely influence the response rate, potentially threatening study validity. For research of organ-specific cancer, investigating molecular markers in target tissue is difficult. Blood is the most common and versatile specimen used in molecular epidemiology research; other specimens used include urine, stool, nail, hair, sputum, buccal cells, and saliva. Tissue samples, either fresh frozen or chemically fixed, are also used, but the availability of these samples is highly limited to patients or selected subgroups of the overall study population. Comparability and generalizability are always problems in epidemiologic studies involving tissue specimens, except for those investigations that focus on cancer prognosis or treatment in which only cancer patients are involved. Attempts have been made to use a special body fluid for epidemiologic research, such as nipple aspirate and breast or pulmonary lavage, but the difficulty in specimen preparation and collection makes these samples impractical in large population-based studies.

Given the research value of biologic specimens and the difficulty in collecting them for population-based studies, technical issues related to specimen collection, processing, and storage become especially important in molecular epidemiology research. These include time and conditions for specimen transportation and processing, sample aliquot and labeling system, sample special treatment for storage and analysis, sample storage and tracking system, as well as backup plans and equipment for unexpected adverse events during long-term storage (e.g., power failure, earthquake, and flooding). Laboratory methods used to analyze biomarkers are also important in molecular epidemiology. Because large numbers of specimens are involved, laboratory methods are required to be robust, reproducible, high-throughput, low cost, and easy to use. These requirements are met in the analysis of nucleotide sequences that serve as genotypic markers. However, for phenotypic markers, many methods do not meet the requirements. Moreover, many phenotypic markers, such as proteins, require both qualitative and quantitative assessments. An ideal laboratory method should be quantitative (able to measure a wide range of values), sensitive (able to detect a small amount of analyte), specific (able to detect only the molecule of interest, no other molecules), reproducible (high precision and low variation), and versatile (easy to use). In addition, investigators need to implement appropriate quality assurance procedures during sample processing and testing as well as include appropriate quality control samples in specimen analysis.

Host–environment interaction is believed to play a key role in the etiology of most types of cancer. Genetic factors, including mutations and polymorphisms, are initially considered important host factors, but recent development in cancer research has indicated that epigenetic factors may also play a critical role in cancer as a host factor involved in host–environment interaction. Epigenetic factors that regulate the function of the human genome without altering the physical sequences of nucleotides include pretranscription regulation through nucleotide modification (e.g., cytosine methylation at CpG sites), chromosome modification (e.g., histone acetylation), and posttranscription regulation by noncoding small RNA (e.g., microRNAs). These epigenetic factors have two unique features that have captured the attention of cancer researchers, especially cancer epidemiologists who are interested in gene-environment interaction. It is known that epigenetic factors are heritable, but these inherited features are readily modifiable by environmental and lifestyle factors. Monozygotic twins have identical genome as well as epigenome at birth, but the latter undergo substantial changes over time, resulting in distinct epigenetic profiles that depend heavily on their environmental exposures.[54] Animal studies also indicated that maternal intake of dietary nutrients that involve one-carbon metabolism could influence the growth phenotypes of offspring that are regulated by DNA methylation.[55] As evidence mounts on epigenetic involvement in cancer, molecular epidemiologists start to look for clues in human populations that can link epigenetic factors to both lifestyle factors and cancer risk. Given that epigenetic regulation is tissue specific and time dependent, investigators face challenges in accurately assessing these phenotypic markers in etiologic studies. However, recent progress in the analysis of circulating methylation markers and microRNAs may provide an alternative to study epigenetic regulation in human cancer.

Selected References

The full list of references for this chapter appears in the online version.

1. Last J. *A dictionary of epidemiology*, 3rd ed. New York: Oxford University Press, 1995.
2. Doll R, Hill AB. Lung cancer and other causes of death in relation to smoking; a second report on the mortality of British doctors. *BMJ* 1956;12:1071.
3. Kleinbaum D, Kupper L, Morgenstern H. *Epidemiologic research*. New York: Van Nostrand Reinhold, 1982.
4. Kaplan LD, Straus DJ, Testa MA, et al. Low-dose compared with standard-dose m-BACOD chemotherapy for non-Hodgkin's lymphoma associated with human immunodeficiency virus infection. National Institute of Allergy and Infectious Diseases AIDS Clinical Trials Group. *N Engl J Med* 1997;336:1641.
5. Dunn BK, Kramer BS, Ford LG. Phase III, large-scale chemoprevention trials. Approach to chemoprevention clinical trials and phase III clinical trial of tamoxifen as a chemopreventive for breast cancer—the US National Cancer Institute experience. *Hematol Oncol Clin North Am* 1998;12:1019.
6. Grant WB. An ecologic study of dietary and solar ultraviolet-B links to breast carcinoma mortality rates. *Cancer* 2002;94:272.
7. NCHS. Third National Health and Nutrition Examination Survey, 1988–1994, Plan and Operations Procedures Manuals (CD-ROM). Hyattsville, MD: U.S. Department of Health and Human Services (DHHS). Centers for Disease Controls and Prevention, 1996.
8. Szklo M, Nieto F. *Epidemiology: beyond the basics*. Gaithersburg, MD: Aspen Publishers, 2000.
9. Grimes DA, Schulz KF. Cohort studies: marching towards outcomes. *Lancet* 2002;359:341.
10. Schatzkin A, Subar AF, Thompson FE, et al. Design and serendipity in establishing a large cohort with wide dietary intake distributions: the National Institutes of Health-American Association of Retired Persons Diet and Health Study. *Am J Epidemiol* 2001;154:1119.
11. Mantel N, Haenszel W. Statistical aspects of the analysis of data from retrospective studies of disease. *J Natl Cancer Inst* 1959;22:719.
12. Wacholder S, Silverman DT, McLaughlin JK, Mandel JS. Selection of controls in case-control studies. II. Types of controls. *Am J Epidemiol* 1992;135:1029.
13. Chen C, Weiss NS, Stanczyk FZ, et al. Endogenous sex hormones and prostate cancer risk: a case-control study nested within the Carotene and Retinol Efficacy Trial. *Cancer Epidemiol Biomarkers Prev* 2003;12:1410.
14. Pearce N. What does the odds ratio estimate in a case-control study? *Int J Epidemiol* 1993;22:1189.
15. Schulz KF, Grimes DA. Case-control studies: research in reverse. *Lancet* 2002;359:431.
16. Rothman K. *Epidemiology: an introduction*. New York: Oxford University Press, 2002.
17. Hennekens C, Buring J. *Epidemiology in medicine*. Boston: Little, Brown and Company, 1987.
18. Rundle A, Schwartz S. Issues in the epidemiological analysis and interpretation of intermediate biomarkers. *Cancer Epidemiol Biomarkers Prev* 2003;12:491.
19. Shields PG. Tobacco smoking, harm reduction, and biomarkers. *J Natl Cancer Inst* 2002;94:1435.
20. Hunter DJ. Gene-environment interactions in human diseases. *Nat Rev Genet* 2005;6:287.

21. Hirschhorn JN, Daly MJ. Genome-wide association studies for common diseases and complex traits. *Nat Rev Genet* 2005;6:95.
22. Breast Cancer Association C. Commonly studied single-nucleotide polymorphisms and breast cancer: results from the Breast Cancer Association Consortium. *J Natl Cancer Inst* 2006;98:1382.
23. Wacholder S, Chanock S, Garcia-Closas M, El Ghormli L, Rothman N. Assessing the probability that a positive report is false: an approach for molecular epidemiology studies. *J Natl Cancer Inst* 2004;96:434.
24. Clayton DG, Walker NM, Smyth DJ, et al. Population structure, differential bias and genomic control in a large-scale, case-control association study. *Nat Genet* 2005;37:1243.
25. Easton DF, Eeles RA. Genome-wide association studies in cancer. *Hum Mol Genet* 2008;17:R109.
26. Ahmed S, Thomas G, Ghoussaini M, et al. Newly discovered breast cancer susceptibility loci on 3p24 and 17q23.2. *Nat Genet* 2009;41:585.
27. Thomas G, Jacobs KB, Kraft P, et al. A multistage genome-wide association study in breast cancer identifies two new risk alleles at 1p11.2 and 14q24.1 (RAD51L1). *Nat Genet* 2009;41:579.
28. Thomas G, Jacobs KB, Yeager M, et al. Multiple loci identified in a genome-wide association study of prostate cancer. *Nat Genet* 2008;40:310.
29. Le Marchand L. Genome-wide association studies and colorectal cancer. *Surg Oncol Clin North Am* 2009;18:663.
30. Hung RJ, McKay JD, Gaborieau V, et al. A susceptibility locus for lung cancer maps to nicotinic acetylcholine receptor subunit genes on 15q25. *Nature* 2008;452:633.
31. Amos CI, Wu X, Broderick P, et al. Genome-wide association scan of tag SNPs identifies a susceptibility locus for lung cancer at 15q25.1. *Nat Genet* 2008;40:616.
32. Amundadottir L, Kraft P, Stolzenberg-Solomon RZ, et al. Genome-wide association study identifies variants in the ABO locus associated with susceptibility to pancreatic cancer. *Nat Genet* 2009;41:986.
33. Kiemeney LA, Sulem P, Besenbacher S, et al. A sequence variant at 4p16.3 confers susceptibility to urinary bladder cancer. *Nat Genet* 2010;42(5):415.
34. Wu X, Ye Y, Kiemeney LA, et al. Genetic variation in the prostate stem cell antigen gene PSCA confers susceptibility to urinary bladder cancer. *Nat Genet* 2009;41:991.
35. Stacey SN, Sulem P, Masson G, et al. New common variants affecting susceptibility to basal cell carcinoma. *Nat Genet* 2009;41:909.
36. Thorgeirsson TE, Geller F, Sulem P, et al. A variant associated with nicotine dependence, lung cancer and peripheral arterial disease. *Nature* 2008;452:638.
37. Spitz MR, Amos CI, Dong Q, Lin J, Wu X. The CHRNA5-A3 region on chromosome 15q24-25.1 is a risk factor both for nicotine dependence and for lung cancer. *J Natl Cancer Inst* 2008;100:1552.
38. Zheng W, Long J, Gao YT, et al. Genome-wide association study identifies a new breast cancer susceptibility locus at 6q25.1. *Nat Genet* 2009;41:324.
39. Gudmundsson J, Sulem P, Gudbjartsson DF, et al. Common variants on 9q22.33 and 14q13.3 predispose to thyroid cancer in European populations. *Nat Genet* 2009;41:460.
40. Gudmundsson J, Sulem P, Gudbjartsson DF, et al. Genome-wide association and replication studies identify four variants associated with prostate cancer susceptibility. *Nat Genet* 2009;41:1122.
41. Song H, Ramus SJ, Tyrer J, et al. A genome-wide association study identifies a new ovarian cancer susceptibility locus on 9p22.2. *Nat Genet* 2009;41:996.
42. Stacey SN, Gudbjartsson DF, Sulem P, et al. Common variants on 1p36 and 1q42 are associated with cutaneous basal cell carcinoma but not with melanoma or pigmentation traits. *Nat Genet* 2008;40:1313.
43. Zanke BW, Greenwood CM, Rangrej J, et al. Genome-wide association scan identifies a colorectal cancer susceptibility locus on chromosome 8q24. *Nat Genet* 2007;39:989.
44. Haiman CA, Patterson N, Freedman ML, et al. Multiple regions within 8q24 independently affect risk for prostate cancer. *Nat Genet* 2007;39:638.
45. Kiemeney LA, Thorlacius S, Sulem P, et al. Sequence variant on 8q24 confers susceptibility to urinary bladder cancer. *Nat Genet* 2008;40:1307.
46. Ghoussaini M, Song H, Koessler T, et al. Multiple loci with different cancer specificities within the 8q24 gene desert. *J Natl Cancer Inst* 2008;100:962.
47. Harismendy O, Frazer KA. Elucidating the role of 8q24 in colorectal cancer. *Nat Genet* 2009;41:868.
48. Wright JB, Brown SJ, Cole MD. Upregulation of c-MYC in cis through a large chromatin loop linked to a cancer risk-associated single-nucleotide polymorphism in colorectal cancer cells. *Mol Cell Biol* 2010;30(6):1411.
49. Rafnar T, Sulem P, Stacey SN, et al. Sequence variants at the TERT-CLPTM1L locus associate with many cancer types. *Nat Genet* 2009;41:221.
50. Fernandez-Garcia I, Ortiz-de-Solorzano C, Montuenga LM. Telomeres and telomerase in lung cancer. *J Thorac Oncol* 2008;3:1085.

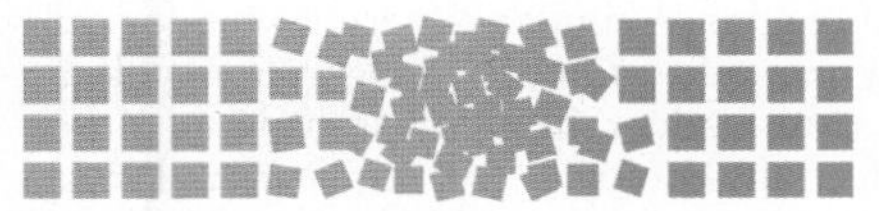

CHAPTER 23 GLOBAL CANCER INCIDENCE AND MORTALITY

MICHAEL J. THUN, AHMEDIN JEMAL, AND ELIZABETH WARD

The huge international variation in the occurrence of many types of cancer has historically provided important evidence that much of human cancer is avoidable.[1,2] For example, cancers of the breast and colon are rare among rural populations in Asia, but become progressively more common among migrants to urban cities in Asia and among those who move to western cities in North America and Europe. Conversely, the risk of stomach and liver cancer in first generation Chinese and Japanese migrants to California is lower than that in their country of origin, yet higher than that among long-term California residents.[3] The impact of migration on cancer rates is so large that it cannot be explained by differences in the accuracy or the completeness of diagnostic information in different countries, or by constitutional differences between migrants who venture abroad and their countrymen who stay at home. It can only be attributed to the changes in social, cultural, and behavioral factors that result from migration.

A second reason why a global perspective on cancer is critical is that the worldwide burden of cancer is no longer confined predominantly to the industrialized, wealthy countries but is rapidly shifting to low and medium resource countries.[4,5] This is partly because the population of low and medium resource countries accounts for 80% of the world population, partly because of increasing longevity in less developed countries due to reduction in infant mortality and deaths from infectious diseases, and partly because of the adoption of Western patterns of diet, physical inactivity, and tobacco use. In this chapter the authors describe global patterns of cancer incidence and mortality as these relate to changing risk factor profiles and the implications of these trends for health care systems.

DATA SOURCES AND MEASUREMENTS

Number of New Cancer Cases and Deaths

Counts of the number of newly diagnosed cases and deaths in a given year are the most basic measure of cancer burden. These are used to estimate the current and future health care and social services needs in a given geographic area. They also provide the numerator data for calculations of incidence and mortality rates (discussed below).

National mortality data are collected routinely in all industrialized countries and some less developed countries. Collectively, data on cancer mortality are available for approximately 30% of the world population. The quality of these data varies by country and by cause of death. Underlying cause of death is classified reasonably well in high-resource countries when data are abstracted from death certificates using systematic coding rules. In the United States, studies report approximately 90% agreement between death certificates and pathology reports on cancer diagnoses.[6] For countries with no death registration or limited information on cause of death, International Agency for Research on Cancer (IARC) estimates the number of deaths based on country- or region-specific incidence and survival data.[7]

Information on incident cases of cancer is collected nationally in only a few countries (Canada, Singapore, and all of the Nordic countries). Most cancer registries are regional rather than national, although these vary greatly in size. About 95% percent of the U.S. population is covered either by the Surveillance, Epidemiology, and End Results (SEER) program of the National Cancer Institute (NCI) or the National Program of Cancer Registries of the Centers for Disease Control. Information on cancer incidence in many less developed countries is collected through a network of regional registries coordinated by IARC. In countries with no registry, incidence rates are estimated based on mortality data or incidence rates in neighboring countries.[8] Types of cancer are coded according to the International Classification of Diseases for Oncology, which assigns an anatomic site and histologic code.[9]

Worldwide, the number of newly diagnosed cancer cases in 2008 was approximately 12.7 million, with 5.6 million in economically more developed countries and 7.1 million in less developed countries (Fig. 23.1).[10] The corresponding number of cancer deaths was approximately 7.6 million globally: 2.8 million in economically more developed and 4.8 million in economically less developed countries. These numbers are expected to grow rapidly because of growth and aging of the world population and the dissemination of Western lifestyles. By 2030, 21.4 million new cases and more than 13.2 million deaths are expected each year, based on current age-specific rates and census projections of population growth and aging. Barring unforeseen catastrophe, nearly two-thirds of these cases and deaths will occur in low and medium resource countries by 2030.

Actual data on the number of new cancer cases and deaths are always several years out of date due to the time required for collection and compilation of information on newly diagnosed cases and deaths by cancer registries or regional health departments.

Incidence and Mortality Rates

Crude incidence and mortality rates represent the average risk that individuals in a given population will develop or die from cancer in a single year. These rates are usually expressed per 100,000 people per year for adult cancers and per million per year for childhood cancers. Because the occurrence of most types of cancers increases rapidly with age, the rates are usually standardized for age or expressed within defined age strata. Age standardization simplifies comparisons among populations with different age compositions by summarizing the age-specific

Worldwide

Number of Cases: Male	Number of Cases: Female	Number of Deaths: Male	Number of Deaths: Female
Lung 1,095,186	Breast 1,383,523	Lung 951,023	Breast 458,367
Prostate 913,770	Cervix uteri 529,409	Liver 478,275	Lung 427,392
Colorectum 663,612	Colorectum 570,099	Stomach 464,435	Colorectum 288,049
Stomach 640,556	Lung 513,637	Colorectum 320,595	Corpus uteri 274,883
Liver 522,355	Stomach 349,042	Oesophagus 276,129	Stomach 273,634
Oesophagus 326,575	Corpus uteri 287,630	Prostate 258,381	Liver 217,568
Bladder 297,338	Ovary 225,484	Leukaemia 143,669	Ovary 140,153
Non-Hodgkin lymphoma 199,569	Liver 225,916	Pancreas 138,080	Oesophagus 130,677
Leukaemia 195,943	Thyroid 163,020	Bladder 112,255	Pancreas 127,949
Lip, oral cavity 170,903	Leukaemia 155,469	Non-Hodgkin lymphoma 109,465	Leukaemia 113,802
All sites but skin 6,639,430	All sites but skin 6,038,545	All sites but skin 4,225,662	All sites but skin 3,345,834

More Developed Regions

Number of Cases: Male	Number of Cases: Female	Number of Deaths: Male	Number of Deaths: Female
Prostate 658,751	Breast 1,383,523	Lung 411,988	Breast 189,488
Lung 482,642	Colorectum 337,747	Colorectum 166,159	Lung 188,379
Colorectum 389,667	Lung 241,683	Prostate 136,517	Colorectum 153,913
Bladder 177,793	Corpus uteri 142,196	Stomach 110,895	Pancreas 79,084
Stomach 173,697	Stomach 349,042	Pancreas 82,683	Stomach 70,765
Kidney 111,079	Ovary 100,254	Liver 75,413	Ovary 64,466
Non-Hodgkin lymphoma 95,742	Non-Hodgkin lymphoma 84,789	Bladder 55,006	Liver 39,871
Melanoma of skin 85,299	Melanoma of skin 81,561	Oesophagus 53,080	Leukaemia 38,689
Pancreas 84,154	Pancreas 80,938	Leukaemia 48,606	Non-Hodgkin lymphoma 33,452
Liver 81,701	Corpus uteri 76,507	Kidney 43,048	Cervix uteri 33,159
All sites but skin 2,985,477	All sites but skin 2,584,762	All sites but skin 1,528,197	All sites but skin 1,223,231

Less Developed Regions

Number of Cases: Male	Number of Cases: Female	Number of Deaths: Male	Number of Deaths: Female
Lung 612,544	Breast 691,281	Lung 539,035	Breast 268,879
Stomach 466,859	Cervix uteri 452,902	Liver 402,862	Cervix uteri 241,724
Liver 440,654	Lung 271,954	Stomach 353,540	Lung 239,013
Colorectum 273,945	Stomach 246,994	Oesophagus 223,049	Pancreas 79,084
Oesophagus 262,618	Colorectum 232,352	Colorectum 154,436	Stomach 202,869
Prostate 255,019	Liver 186,039	Prostate 121,864	Liver 177,697
Bladder 119,545	Corpus uteri 145,434	Leukaemia 95,063	Colorectum 134,136
Leukaemia 116,511	Oesophagus 137,889	Non-Hodgkin lymphoma 71,568	Ovary 75,687
Lip, oral cavity 107,736	Ovary 125,230	Brain, nervous system 63,652	Leukaemia 75,113
Non-Hodgkin lymphoma 103,827	Leukaemia 93,360	Lip, oral cavity 61,235	Brain, nervous system 50,282
All sites but skin 3,653,953	All sites but skin 3,453,783	All sites but skin 2,697,465	All sites but skin 2,122,603

FIGURE 23.1 Number of new cancer cases and deaths in 2008 for the ten leading cancer sites by sex, worldwide, and by level of economic development. (From ref. 10.)

rates into a single weighted average. The age-standardized incidence and death rates from selected types of cancer in relation to gender and regional level of economic development. As seen in Table 23.1, the incidence rates of cancers that are strongly related to screening, such as prostate and breast cancer, are considerably higher in regions with more economic development than in less developed regions. A similar pattern is seen for cancers that are strongly related to long-term cigarette smoking, such as lung, larynx, and bladder. In contrast, cancers caused predominantly by infectious etiologies (cervix, liver, and stomach) have much higher incidence rates in the less developed regions. The data in Table 23.1 are standardized to the age distribution of the 1960 world standard population, as is customary in international comparisons. In contrast, national statistics published by the United States, Europe, and certain other countries generally use the 2000 standard population from their own country or region to standardize incidence and mortality rates. Age-standardized rates can only be compared when the same age standard is applied to all of the populations of interest.[11]

The presentation of age-specific rather than age-standardized rates can sometimes reveal interesting differences that would otherwise be obscured. For example, Figure 23.2 shows the age-related increase in the incidence rate of all cancers combined among men (left panel) and women (right panel) in five populations in Asia and North America. The age-specific rates emphasize the much higher incidence rates in men than women and in the United States and Hong Kong than in China and India. They also reveal that men in Qidong County, China, have higher incidence of all cancers combined than the other populations shown in the age range 35 to 49 years. This results from very high incidence of liver cancer caused by endemic hepatitis B infection and exposure to aflatoxin contaminated grains in certain regions of China.[12] Liver cancer that results from vertical transmission of hepatitis B occurs at somewhat younger ages than most adult cancers.

Prevalence

Because it is currently impossible to distinguish between people who are still fighting their cancer and those who are cured, prevalent cancers are defined as the number (or proportion of the population) who are alive at some specified time point after being diagnosed with cancer. The NCI estimates that in 2006 in the United States, approximately 4 million cancer survivors had been diagnosed within the past 5 years (so-called partial prevalence), and 10.8 million survivors had at some time been diagnosed with an invasive cancer.[13]

Global estimates of the number of men and women alive 5 years after being diagnosed with cancer are shown in Figure 23.3, along with the proportionate distribution of prevalent cases by type of cancer.[7] An estimated 24.5 million people met the definition of a prevalent case in 2002. This number is expected to increase over time because of improvements in survival and the anticipated growth and aging of the world's population. Breast cancer accounted for 34% (n = 4,406,080) of all prevalent cases in women, followed by cervical cancer (11%, n = 1,432,491). In men, prostate cancer accounted for 21% (n = 2,424,967) of the total, followed by colon and rectum (13%, n = 1,501,170). Overall, there are more women than men who have survived cancer, by any definition, even though men have higher incidence rates for most cancers (Table 23.1).

Probability of Developing Cancer

The probability that an individual will develop or die from cancer by a given age or during a defined time period is another index of average risk in a population. Analyses of cumulative

TABLE 23.1

AGE-STANDARDIZED INCIDENCE AND MORTALITY RATES IN MORE AND LESS DEVELOPED REGIONS, 2008

	Males				Females			
	More Developed Regions		Less Developed Regions		More Developed Regions		Less Developed Regions	
Site	Incidence	Mortality	Incidence	Mortality	Incidence	Mortality	Incidence	Mortality
Bladder	16.6	4.6	5.4	2.6	3.6	1.0	1.4	0.7
Brain, nervous system	6.0	3.9	3.2	2.6	4.4	2.6	2.8	2.0
Breast					66.4	15.3	27.3	10.8
Cervix uteri					9.0	3.2	17.8	9.8
Colorectum	37.6	15.1	12.1	6.9	24.2	9.7	9.4	5.4
Corpus uteri					12.9	2.4	6.0	1.7
Gallbladder	2.4	1.6	1.4	1.1	2.1	1.5	2.2	1.7
Hodgkin lymphoma	2.2	0.4	0.9	0.6	1.9	0.3	0.5	0.3
Kidney	11.8	4.1	2.5	1.3	5.8	1.7	1.4	0.8
Larynx	5.5	2.4	3.5	2.1	0.6	0.2	0.6	0.4
Leukemia	9.1	4.8	4.5	3.7	6.0	2.9	3.6	2.9
Lip, oral cavity	6.9	2.3	4.6	2.7	2.4	0.6	2.6	1.5
Liver	8.1	7.2	18.9	17.4	2.7	2.5	7.6	7.2
Lung	47.4	39.4	27.8	24.6	18.6	13.6	11.1	9.7
Melanoma of skin	9.5	1.8	0.7	0.3	8.6	1.1	0.6	0.3
Multiple myeloma	3.3	1.9	0.9	0.8	2.2	1.3	0.7	0.6
Nasopharynx	0.6	0.3	2.1	1.4	0.2	0.1	1.0	0.6
Non-Hodgkin lymphoma	10.3	3.6	4.2	3.0	7.0	2.2	2.8	1.9
Oesophagus	6.5	5.3	11.8	10.1	1.2	1.0	5.7	4.7
Other pharynx	4.4	2.2	3.0	2.5	0.8	0.3	0.8	0.6
Ovary etc.					9.4	5.1	5.0	3.1
Pancreas	8.2	7.9	2.7	2.5	5.4	5.1	2.1	2.0
Prostate	63.0	10.6	12.0	5.6				
Stomach	16.7	10.4	21.1	16.0	7.3	4.7	10.0	8.1
Testis	4.6	0.3	0.8	0.3				
Thyroid	2.9	0.3	1.0	0.3	9.1	0.4	3.4	0.7
All sites but skin	**301.1**	**143.9**	**160.3**	**119.3**	**225.5**	**87.3**	**138.0**	**85.4**

Source: GLOBOCAN 2008.

risk are useful when comparing cancer risk in high and low resource countries, because they account for differences in longevity using an approach that is easier to understand than age-specific or age-standardized annual rates. Table 23.2 shows the average probability or cumulative risk of an individual being diagnosed with cancer by age 74 years for men and women in high and low resource countries. The cumulative risk of being diagnosed is nearly twice as high in economically more developed countries (30.1% in males and 22.0% in females) than in less developed countries (17.0% males and 14.0% females), yet the cumulative risk of dying from cancer by that age is similar, especially among women (9.1% in more developed countries, 9.0% in less developed countries). This reflects both the greater detection of potentially indolent cancers in high resource countries and the shorter survival in less developed countries, where many cancers are diagnosed at a late stage and treatment options are limited.

Survival

Relative survival represents the proportion of people alive at a specified point after diagnosis, usually 5 years, compared to that in a population of equivalent age without cancer. Thus, relative survival reflects the specific effects of cancer on shortened survival. For example, the 5-year relative survival for female breast cancers diagnosed in SEER areas of the United States in 2001 was 89.8%. This is equivalent to about 10% fewer female breast cancer patients surviving for 5 years compared to their peers in the general population. It is difficult to interpret changes in relative survival during time periods when screening is being widely introduced, because screening detects prevalent cancers at an earlier stage and may detect indolent tumors that might not otherwise be diagnosed. Because of so-called lead time bias, the increase in relative survival from screening may overestimate the extent to which screening prolongs life.

Survival data have been compared across a number of countries in the CONCORD project[14] (Fig. 23.4). The observed variations in survival reflect differences in the use of screening tests as well as in the availability of effective and timely treatment.[15] For countries with no survival data, 5-year relative survival is approximated by computing the ratio of the mortality rate to the incidence rate.[7]

OVERALL CANCER RISK

In addition to the effects of age on the overall risk of developing or dying from cancer, risk varies by gender, socioeconomic status, race or ethnicity, and geographic location.

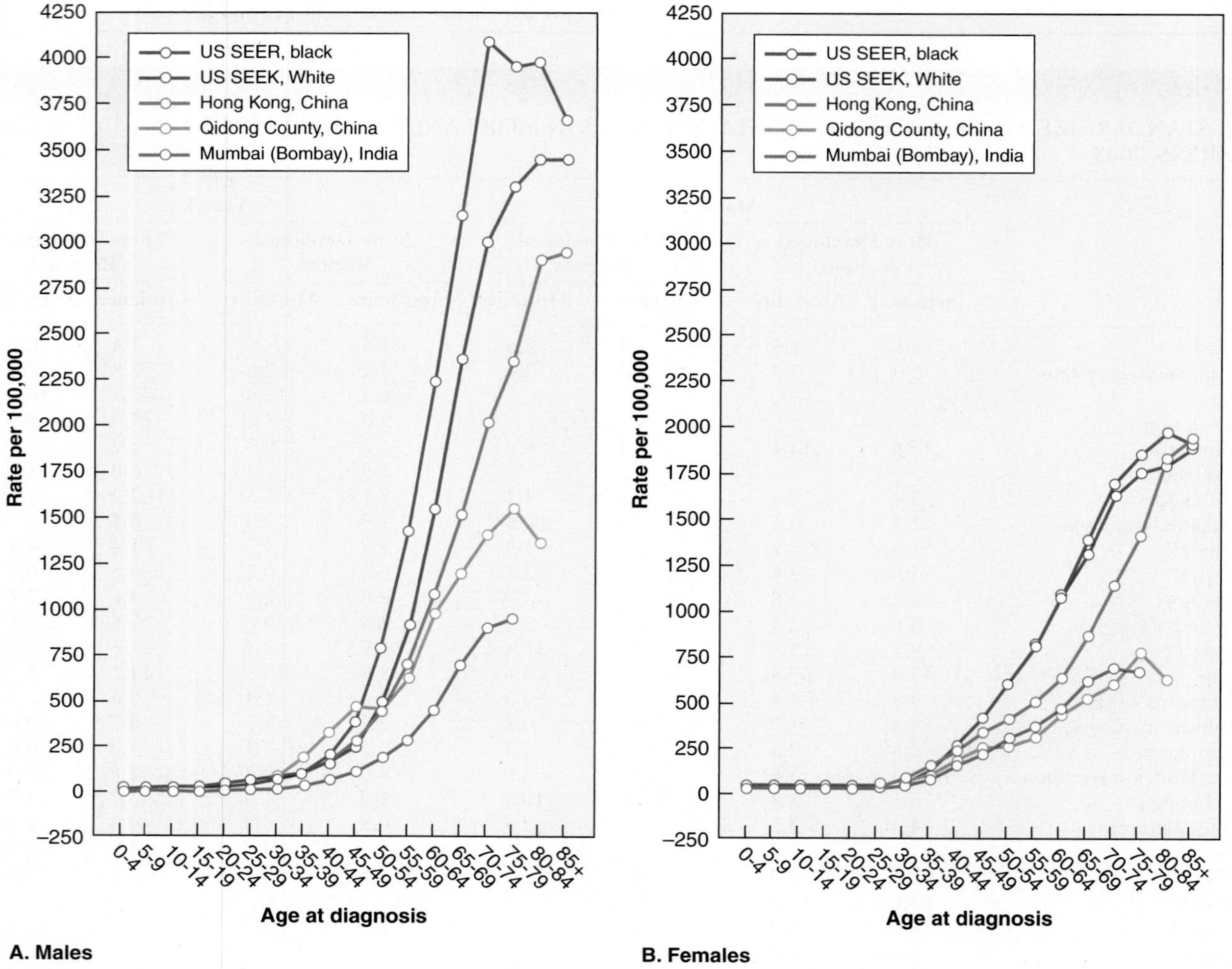

US SEER, black
US SEEK, White
Hong Kong, China
Qidong County, China
Mumbai (Bombay), India

Rate per 100,000

Age at diagnosis

A. Males

B. Females

FIGURE 23.2 Age- and sex-specific incidence rates for all cancers combined from selected populations in North America and Asia, 1993–1997. (From Cancer Incidence in Five Continents, Volume VIII (http://www.dep.iarc.fr/) accessed on February 20, 2007. Surveillance, Epidemiology, and End Results (SEER) Program (www.seer.cancer.gov) SEER*Stat Database: Incidence-SEER 9 Regs Limited-Use, Nov 2006 Sub (1973–2004)–Linked to County Attributes–Total U.S., 1969–2004 Counties, National Cancer Institute, DCCPS, Surveillance Research Program, Cancer Statistics Branch, released April 2007, based on the November 2006 submission.)

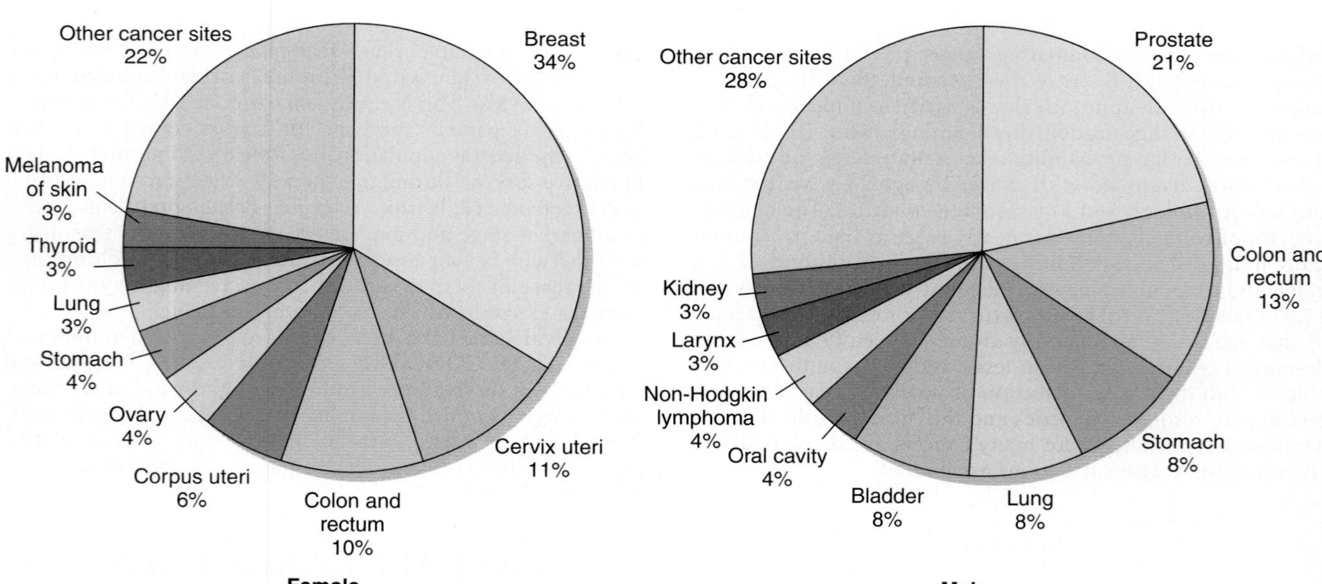

FIGURE 23.3 Percentage distribution of the types of cancer among all prevalent cancers diagnosed in the past 5 years, global estimates by sex, 2002. (From Ferlay J, Bray F, Pisani P, Parkin DM, eds. *Globocan 2002: Cancer Incidence, Mortality and Prevalence Worldwide*. Lyon, France: IARC Press, 2004.)

TABLE 23.2

CUMULATIVE RISK (%) OF DEVELOPING OR DYING FROM CANCER FROM BIRTH TO AGE 74 BY SEX, CANCER SITE, AND LEVEL OF ECONOMIC DEVELOPMENT, 2008

	Males				Females			
	More Developed Regions		Less Developed Regions		More Developed Regions		Less Developed Regions	
Site	Incidence	Mortality	Incidence	Mortality	Incidence	Mortality	Incidence	Mortality
Bladder	1.90	0.46	0.63	0.28	0.41	0.09	0.16	0.07
Brain, nervous system	0.59	0.42	0.33	0.27	0.43	0.28	0.28	0.21
Breast					7.14	1.69	2.83	1.16
Cervix uteri					0.85	0.33	1.86	1.10
Colorectum	4.44	1.69	1.42	0.76	2.74	1.01	1.08	0.58
Corpus uteri					1.56	0.28	0.68	0.20
Gallbladder	0.26	0.17	0.17	0.13	0.23	0.16	0.26	0.19
Hodgkin lymphoma	0.18	0.04	0.08	0.06	0.15	0.03	0.05	0.03
Kidney etc.	1.39	0.47	0.29	0.14	0.67	0.19	0.16	0.08
Larynx	0.68	0.30	0.44	0.26	0.08	0.02	0.07	0.04
Leukemia	0.89	0.48	0.41	0.34	0.56	0.28	0.32	0.26
Lip, oral cavity	0.80	0.28	0.54	0.31	0.26	0.06	0.31	0.17
Liver	0.97	0.85	2.15	1.98	0.30	0.27	0.86	0.82
Lung	5.72	4.66	3.34	2.91	2.25	1.61	1.30	1.11
Melanoma of skin	1.01	0.20	0.07	0.04	0.85	0.12	0.06	0.03
Multiple myeloma	0.38	0.21	0.11	0.09	0.26	0.14	0.09	0.07
Nasopharynx	0.06	0.03	0.23	0.16	0.02	0.01	0.10	0.06
Non-Hodgkin lymphoma	1.10	0.38	0.45	0.31	0.76	0.22	0.30	0.20
Oesophagus	0.81	0.64	1.43	1.21	0.14	0.11	0.67	0.54
Other pharynx	0.53	0.27	0.37	0.29	0.09	0.04	0.09	0.07
Ovary etc.					1.04	0.59	0.53	0.35
Pancreas	0.98	0.93	0.32	0.30	0.62	0.57	0.25	0.23
Prostate	7.90	0.89	1.38	0.52				
Stomach	1.99	1.20	2.54	1.87	0.82	0.50	1.13	0.88
Testis	0.35	0.03	0.07	0.02				
Thyroid	0.29	0.04	0.11	0.04	0.85	0.04	0.35	0.09
All cancers excl. nonmelanoma skin cancer	**30.14**	**14.97**	**16.97**	**12.69**	**22.00**	**9.11**	**14.01**	**9.01**

Source: GLOBOCAN 2008.

Sex

The incidence rates of most cancers that affect both men and women are higher in men than women (Table 23.3). An extreme example is cancer of the larynx, for which the incidence rate is seven times higher in men than women. The few exceptions in which cancers that affect both sexes are more common in women than men are breast, thyroid, and gallbladder.[4] For breast cancer, the incidence rate is more than 100 times higher in women than men in the United States (data not shown).

Socioeconomic Status

The incidence and death rates from most diseases are inversely related to socioeconomic status (SES). This is true for many types of cancer, although the relationships are changing over time and depend upon the level of economic development of the country. In wealthy countries, incidence rates of smoking-related cancers were historically higher in affluent men, who began smoking first. This socioeconomic gradient reversed over time, however, so that most of the major risk factors for cancer and other chronic diseases are currently more common in low rather than in average or high SES groups. The opposite is true for cancers that have screening tests. Currently, the incidence of prostate cancer is higher in high and middle SES groups than in the poor, simply because of greater detection. However, the death rate from all cancers combined is inversely related to SES (educational attainment) as shown for whites in the United States in Figure 23.5. Compared to their contemporaries who have completed college, white males aged 25 to 64 with less than 12 years of education have more than three times the overall death rate for cancer. White women with less than 12 years of education have twice the death rate from all cancers combined as college graduates.[16]

In many economically less developed countries, major cancer risk factors such as cigarette smoking, obesity, and physical inactivity continue to be more common among the educated, higher SES groups than the poor.[17] For example, 36% of female Turkish doctors are current cigarette smokers compared to 15% for women in the general population.[18,19]

Race and Ethnicity

In general, the large disparities in cancer incidence and death rates associated with race and ethnicity are thought to reflect social, economic, and cultural factors rather than differences in inherited genetic susceptibility. Inherited genetic susceptibility

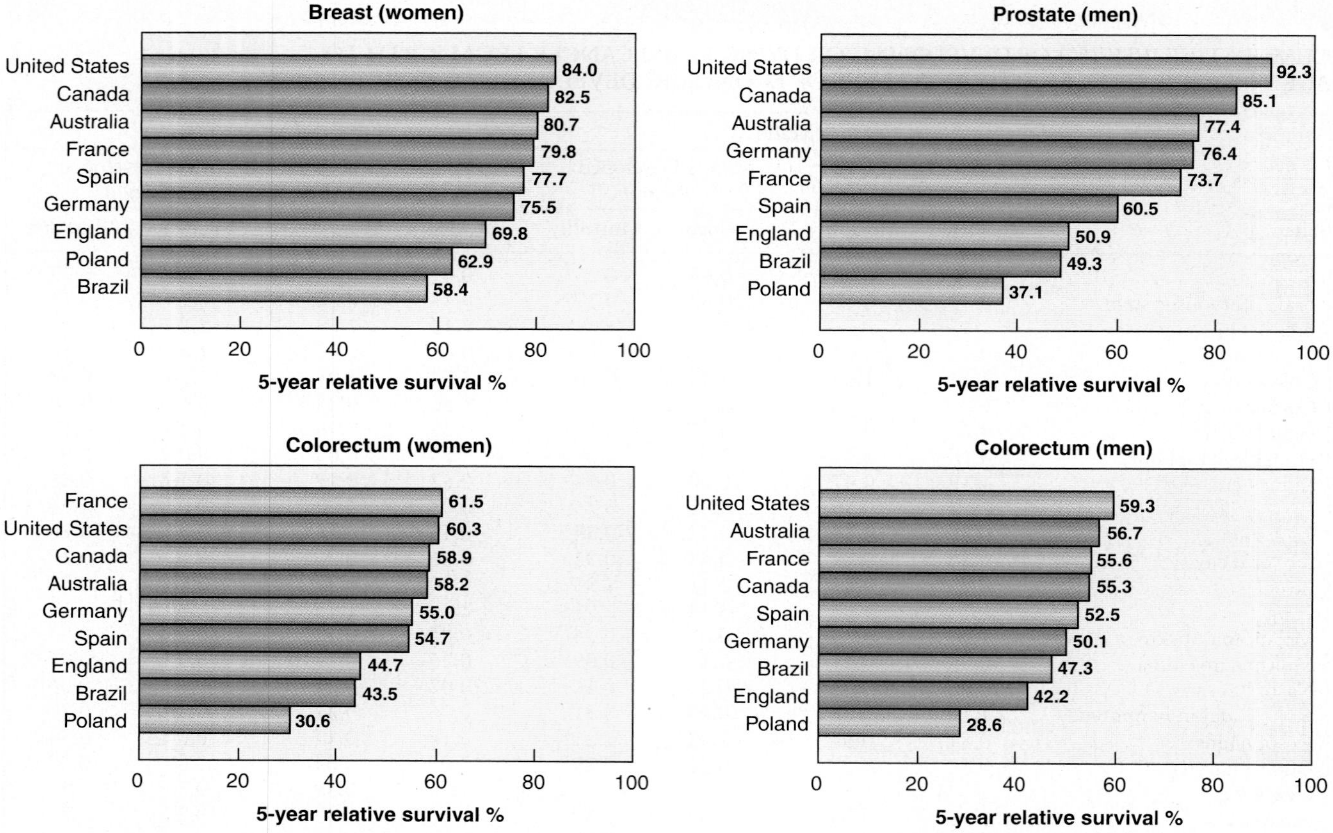

Breast (women)

	5-year relative survival %
United States	84.0
Canada	82.5
Australia	80.7
France	79.8
Spain	77.7
Germany	75.5
England	69.8
Poland	62.9
Brazil	58.4

Prostate (men)

	5-year relative survival %
United States	92.3
Canada	85.1
Australia	77.4
Germany	76.4
France	73.7
Spain	60.5
England	50.9
Brazil	49.3
Poland	37.1

Colorectum (women)

	5-year relative survival %
France	61.5
United States	60.3
Canada	58.9
Australia	58.2
Germany	55.0
Spain	54.7
England	44.7
Brazil	43.5
Poland	30.6

Colorectum (men)

	5-year relative survival %
United States	59.3
Australia	56.7
France	55.6
Canada	55.3
Spain	52.5
Germany	50.1
Brazil	47.3
England	42.2
Poland	28.6

FIGURE 23.4 Relative five-year survival for breast, prostate, and colorectal cancer in selected countries. (From ref 14.)

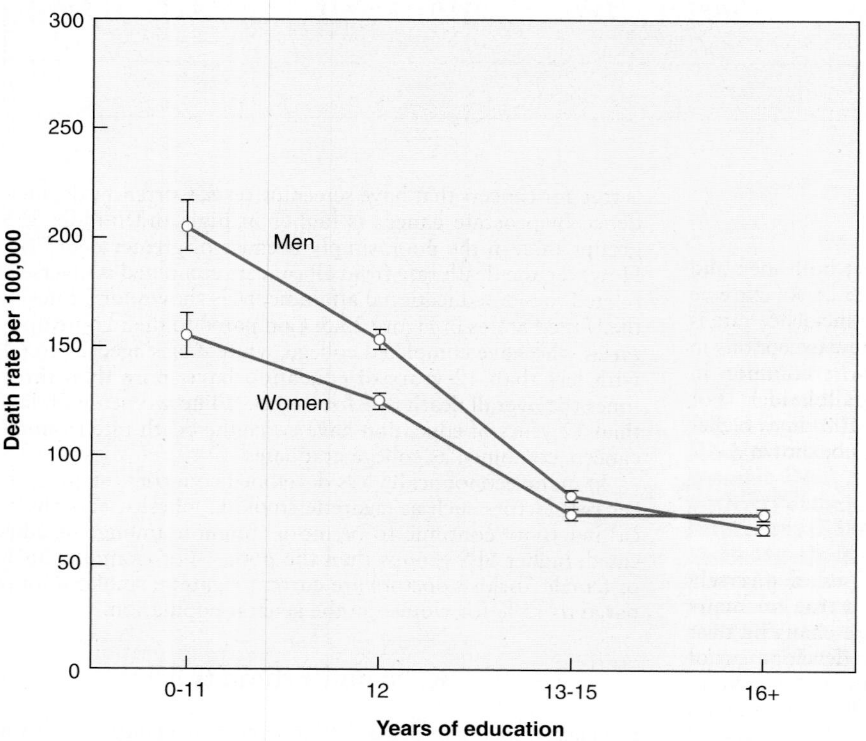

FIGURE 23.5 Age-standardized death rates from all cancers combined in non-Hispanic white men and women aged 25 to 64 years by years of education, United States in 2001. Mortality data were obtained from the National Center for Health Statistics (NCHS). The denominators used to calculate rates (populations of men and women aged 25 to 64 within strata of education, attained age, and race) were obtained from the Current Population Survey (CPS) of the U.S. Bureau of the Census for the year 2001 (data provided by NCHS). The analyses exclude three states with more than 20% of education data missing on the death certificates (Georgia, Rhode Island, and South Dakota). (From Jemal A, Thun MJ, Ward EE, et al. 2008. Mortality from leading causes by education and race in the United States, 2001. *Am J Prev Med* 2008;34:1–8.)

TABLE 23.3

AGE-STANDARDIZED INCIDENCE AND MORTALITY RATES FROM CANCER (PER 100,000) BY SEX WORLDWIDE, 2008

	Incidence			Mortality		
	Males	Females	Rate Ratio M/F	Males	Females	Rate Ratio M/F
Bladder	9.1	2.2	4.1	3.3	0.9	3.7
Brain, nervous system	3.9	3.1	1.3	3.0	2.2	1.4
Breast		39.0			12.5	
Cervix uteri		15.2			7.8	
Colorectum	20.4	14.6	1.4	9.7	7.0	1.4
Corpus uteri		8.2			2.0	
Gallbladder	1.8	2.2	0.8	1.3	1.7	0.8
Hodgkin lymphoma	1.2	0.8	1.5	0.5	0.3	1.7
Kidney	5.2	2.8	1.9	2.2	1.1	2.0
Larynx	4.1	0.6	6.8	2.2	0.3	7.3
Leukemia	5.9	4.3	1.4	4.3	3.1	1.4
Lip, oral cavity	5.3	2.6	2.0	2.6	1.2	2.2
Liver	16.0	6.0	2.7	14.6	5.7	2.6
Lung	34.0	13.5	2.5	29.4	11.0	2.7
Melanoma of skin	3.1	2.6	1.2	0.8	0.5	1.6
Multiple myeloma	1.7	1.2	1.4	1.2	0.9	1.3
Nasopharynx	1.7	0.8	2.1	1.1	0.4	2.8
Non-Hodgkin lymphoma	6.0	4.2	1.4	3.3	2.1	1.6
Oesophagus	10.2	4.2	2.4	8.6	3.4	2.5
Other pharynx	3.4	0.8	4.3	2.4	0.5	4.8
Ovary etc.		6.3			3.8	
Pancreas	4.4	3.3	1.3	4.2	3.1	1.4
Prostate	28.5			7.5		
Stomach	19.8	9.1	2.2	14.3	6.9	2.1
Testis	1.5			0.3		
Thyroid	1.5	4.7	0.3	0.3	0.6	0.5
All sites but skin	204.4	164.9	1.2	128.8	87.6	1.5

Source: GLOBOCAN 2008.

alone is estimated to account for less than 5% of all cancers,[7] whereas the interaction of inherited genes with environmental factors account for the great majority of cancer.

Migrant studies have helped to differentiate whether variations in cancer rates across countries and among racial and ethnic groups are due to environmental factors or to inherited genetic factors.[20] Table 23.4 shows the difference in death rates from selected cancers comparing Japanese in Japan with first- and second-generation Japanese in California, and with native California whites.[3] Death rates from cancers of the stomach and liver were much higher among Japanese in Japan than in California whites between 1950 and 1960. The risk of these infection-related cancers was substantially lower among first-generation Japanese men who migrated to California than in Japan, although still higher than that of California whites. The risk among Japanese migrants and whites became more similar by the second generation. In contrast, the risk of death from colon cancer increased rapidly after migration from Japan to California, approximately doubling in the first-generation Japanese who moved to California and approaching the rates of

TABLE 23.4

DEATH RATES FROM STOMACH, COLON, AND LIVER CANCER RISKS IN JAPANESE MEN IN JAPAN, MIGRANTS TO CALIFORNIA AND CALIFORNIA WHITES AGE 45–64, 1956–1962

		Japanese		
Cancer Site	Whites California	2nd Generation in California	1st Generation in California	Japan
Stomach	1.0	2.8	3.8	8.4
Colon	1.0	0.9	0.4	0.2
Liver	1.0	2.2	2.7	4.1

Source: Adapted with permission, from Buell et al., 1965.

TABLE 23.5

AGE-STANDARDIZED INCIDENCE AND DEATH RATES[a] FOR SELECTED CANCERS BY RACE AND ETHNICITY, US, 1999 TO 2003

	All Races	White	African American	Asian American/Pacific Islander	American Indian/Alaska Native[b]	Hispanic-Latino[c]
Incidence Rates						
All sites						
Male	562.1	555.0	639.8	385.5	359.9	444.1
Female	415.3	421.1	383.8	303.3	305.0	327.2
Breast (female)	128.2	130.8	111.5	91.2	74.4	92.6
Colon & rectum						
Male	64.2	63.7	70.2	52.6	52.7	52.4
Female	46.7	45.9	53.5	38.0	41.9	37.3
Kidney & renal pelvis						
Male	17.9	18.0	18.5	9.8	20.9	16.9
Female	9.2	9.3	9.5	4.9	10.0	9.4
Liver & bile duct						
Male	8.2	7.2	11.1	22.1	14.5	14.8
Female	3.0	2.7	3.6	8.3	6.5	5.8
Lung & bronchus						
Male	89.6	88.8	110.6	56.6	55.5	52.7
Female	54.7	56.2	50.3	28.7	33.8	26.7
Prostate	165.0	156.0	243.0	104.2	70.7	141.1
Stomach						
Male	10.7	9.7	17.4	20.0	21.6	16.1
Female	5.1	4.4	9.0	11.4	12.3	9.1
Uterine cervix	9.1	8.6	13.0	9.3	7.2	14.7
Death Rates						
All sites						
Male	243.7	239.2	331.0	144.9	153.4	166.4
Female	164.3	163.4	192.4	98.8	111.6	108.8
Breast (female)	26.0	25.4	34.4	12.6	13.8	16.3
Colon & rectum						
Male	24.3	23.7	33.6	15.3	15.9	17.5
Female	17.0	16.4	23.7	10.5	11.1	11.4
Kidney & renal pelvis						
Male	6.1	6.2	6.1	2.6	6.8	5.3
Female	2.8	2.8	2.8	1.2	3.3	2.4
Liver & bile duct						
Male	7.0	6.3	9.6	15.5	7.8	10.7
Female	3.0	2.8	3.8	6.7	4.0	5.0
Lung & bronchus						
Male	74.8	73.8	98.4	38.8	42.9	37.2
Female	41.0	42.0	39.8	18.8	27.0	14.7
Prostate	29.1	26.7	65.1	11.8	18.0	22.1
Stomach						
Male	6.1	5.4	12.4	11.0	7.1	9.2
Female	3.1	2.7	6.0	6.7	3.7	5.2
Uterine cervix	2.7	2.4	5.1	2.5	2.6	3.4

[a]Rates are per 100,000 and age adjusted to the 2000 US standard population.
[b]Incidence rates are for diagnosis years 1999-2002.
[c]Persons of Hispanic/Latino origin may be of any race.
Source: Incidence (except American Indian and Alaska Native): Howe HL, Wu X, Ries LAG, et al. Annual report to the nation on the status of cancer 1975–2003, featuring cancer among US Hispanic/Latino populations. *Cancer* 2006;107:1643–1658.
Incidence (American Indian and Alaska Native) and Mortality: Ries LAG, Harkins D, Krapcho M, et al.

California white men by the second generation. Currently, colorectal cancer death rates among Japanese in both the United States and Japan are higher than rates in whites, presumably reflecting changing dietary and physical activity patterns in Asia as well as among migrants to the United States.

Table 23.5 illustrates the large difference in the incidence and death rates between black and white Americans in the time period 2002 to 2006. The incidence of all cancers combined was 25% higher in black than white men and the mortality rate was 43% higher. Similarly, the death rate from all cancers combined was nearly 20% higher in black than white women, despite lower incidence rates. Disparities of the same magnitude have been reported in cancer incidence and death rates between the indigenous aboriginal and white populations in Australia.[21] These differences reflect a combination of disparities that affect prevention, early detection, and treatment. The extent to which inherited differences in cancer susceptibility contribute to the observed differences is not yet clear, but is likely to be very small. In contrast, other major racial and ethnic groups have lower incidence and mortality for all sites combined and for the four most common cancer sites (lung and bronchus, colon and rectum, prostate, and female breast). For certain cancer sites, the incidence in Hispanic and Asian migrants remains higher than that in whites. This is particularly true for cancers of the stomach, liver, cervix uteri, and intrahepatic bile duct. All of these cancers are affected by specific infectious agents that are more prevalent in the countries of origin than in the United States.

Geographic Location

As noted above, the incidence and death rates from many specific types of cancer and from all cancers combined vary widely by geographic location. The large observed geographic variability in cancer occurrence, together with migrant studies and surveillance data on cancer trends, has stimulated important hypotheses about the etiology and potential preventability of many cancers. The geographic variability is larger for some cancers than for others, but even the incidence of all cancers combined varies by more than fourfold in men, and three- to four-fold in women, comparing the World Health Organization (WHO) region with the highest incidence rate (North America) with the regions that have the lowest rates (Northern and Western Africa).

Large geographic variations in the incidence rate of specific cancers may reflect a combination of differences in the prevalence of underlying risk factors, differences in host susceptibility, or variations in detection, completeness of reporting, treatment, and classification of disease. For example, the approximately 100-fold variations in the incidence of Kaposi sarcoma reflect differences in both risk factor prevalence and treatment. Kaposi sarcoma remains the second most commonly diagnosed cancer in Eastern Africa (Table 23.6). This reflects the high prevalence of combined infection with human immunodeficiency virus (HIV) and human herpes virus 8 (HHV-8) and the lack of widespread availability of intensive antiretroviral therapy. Similarly, the more than 44-fold variation in the incidence rate of prostate cancer comparing the United States (83.8/100,000) and Bangladesh (1.9/100,000) reflects both a true difference in incidence and much more aggressive screening for prostate cancer in the United States than in Bangladesh.

Most of the cancers related to tobacco smoking or infectious etiologies have a three- to 10-fold variation in incidence between the WHO region with the highest rate and that with the lowest. The incidence rate of tobacco-related cancers—oral cavity, larynx, lung (Fig. 23.6), esophagus, urinary bladder, and (in men) pancreas and kidney—varies by at least

TABLE 23.6

FOUR MOST COMMONLY DIAGNOSED CANCERS (% OF TOTAL) BY WHO REGION, BOTH SEXES COMBINED, 2008

WHO Region	Cancer Sites			
Eastern Africa	Cervix uteri (14.2%)	Kaposi sarcoma (11.3%)	Breast (8.1%)	Oesophagus (7.2%)
Middle Africa	Liver (16.2%)	Breast (12.4%)	Cervix uteri (12.3%)	Prostate (6.2%)
Northern Africa	Breast (17.0%)	Lung (7.3%)	Bladder (7.3%)	Non-Hodgkin lymphoma (6.7%)
Southern Africa	Breast (11.4%)	Prostate (9.8%)	Oesophagus (8.5%)	Cervix uteri (8.2%)
Western Africa	Breast (16.0%)	Cervix uteri (15.7%)	Liver (11.2%)	Prostate (7.2%)
Caribbean	Prostate (20.1%)	Breast (11.3%)	Lung (10.7%)	Colorectum (8.5%)
Central America	Prostate (11.6%)	Breast (9.9%)	Cervix uteri (8.8%)	Stomach (8.0%)
South America	Breast (13.6%)	Prostate (12.9%)	Lung (7.8%)	Colorectum (7.4%)
Northern America	Lung (14.8%)	Prostate (13.3%)	Breast (12.8%)	Colorectum (11.0%)
Eastern Asia	Lung (17.4%)	Stomach (16.2%)	Liver (12.7%)	Colorectum (9.7%)
South-Eastern Asia	Lung (13.5%)	Breast (12.0%)	Liver (10.3%)	Colorectum (9.5%)
South Central Asia	Cervix uteri (12.2%)	Breast (12.1%)	Lung (7.2%)	Lip, oral cavity (6.9%)
Western Asia	Breast (12.7%)	Lung (12.2%)	Colon and rectum (8.3%)	Stomach (6.7%)
Eastern Europe	Lung (14.0%)	Colorectum (13.2%)	Breast (11.6%)	Stomach (7.5%)
Northern Europe	Prostate (15.9%)	Breast (14.2%)	Colorectum (12.3%)	Lung (12.0%)
Southern Europe	Colorectum (14.4%)	Breast (12.8%)	Lung (11.9%)	Prostate (11.2%)
Western Europe	Prostate (16.4%)	Breast (14.4%)	Colorectum (13.4%)	Lung (10.4%)
Australia/ New Zealand	Prostate (16.5%)	Colorectum (13.7%)	Breast (12.8%)	Melanoma of skin (10.8%)
Melanesia	Lip, oral cavity (12.0%)	Cervix uteri (10.3%)	Breast (9.1%)	Liver (6.9%)
Micronesia	Breast (19.7%)	Lung (18.9)	Colorectum (13.4%)	Prostate (7.2%)
Polynesia	Breast (14.6%)	Lung (13.6%)	Prostate (10.1%)	Thyroid (6.7%)

Source: GLOBOCAN 2008.

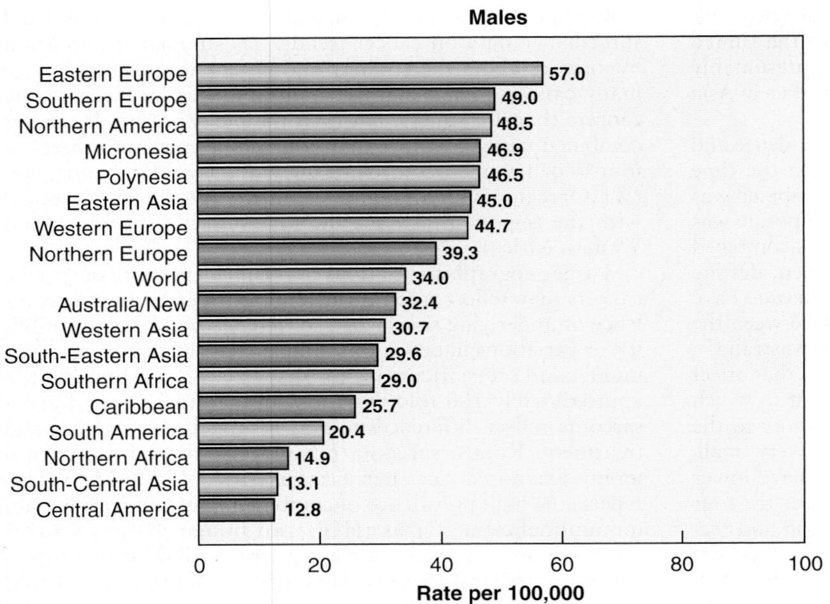

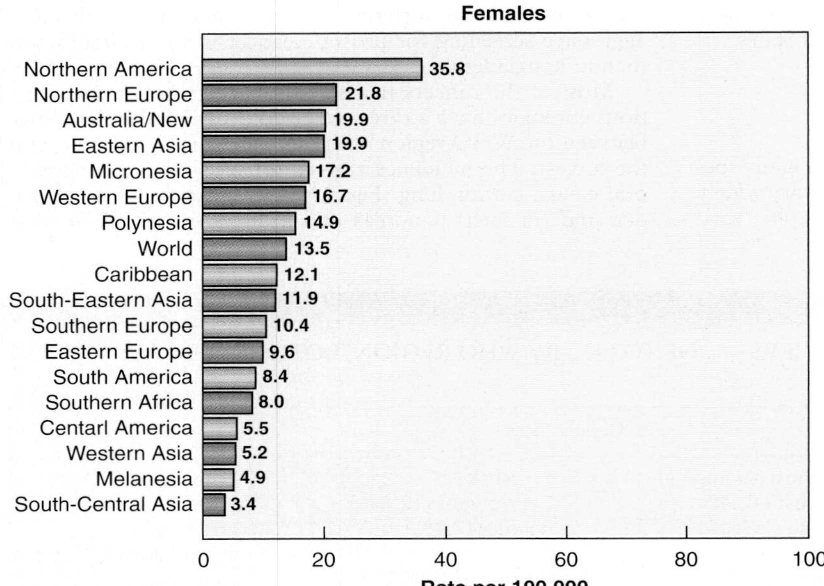

FIGURE 23.6 Age-standardized lung cancer incidence rates by World Health Organization region and sex, 2008. (From ref. 10.)

20-fold among countries. Cancer sites for which incidence rates vary by approximately fivefold across the WHO regions include female breast (3.6-fold, Fig. 23.7), ovary (5.1-fold), non-Hodgkin's lymphoma (5.0-fold males, 5.8-fold females), and thyroid (6.5-fold males, 5.8-fold females). More extreme variations are seen when cancer incidence rates are examined by country than by WHO region.

High-risk areas for specific cancers may or may not be well characterized by official administrative boundaries, such as county, state, or national borders. For example, the very high incidence and death rates from esophageal cancer around the Caspian Sea are highest in areas that are most remote from towns and where access to fresh fruits and vegetables is nonexistent for much of the year.[22] In the United States, the area with the highest death rates from cervical cancer spanned much of Appalachia,[23] where women in the past lacked access to regular Pap testing or treatment. This observation motivated the U.S. Congress to create the National Breast and Cervical Cancer Early Detection Program (NBCCEDP) to improve access to breast and cervical cancer screening and diagnostic services for low-income women.[24] While this program currently serves only 14.3% of eligible women aged 40 to 64 and 7.3% of those aged 18 to 64 because of insufficient funding for NBCCEDP, it illustrates how a national or multinational approach may be needed for public health problems that extend across state or national borders.

Geographic information system (GIS) analysis is a relatively new tool for describing cancer patterns by place of residence, using the address at diagnosis or death. It is a powerful automated system for the capture, storage, retrieval, analysis, and display of spatial data. Examples of GIS application in

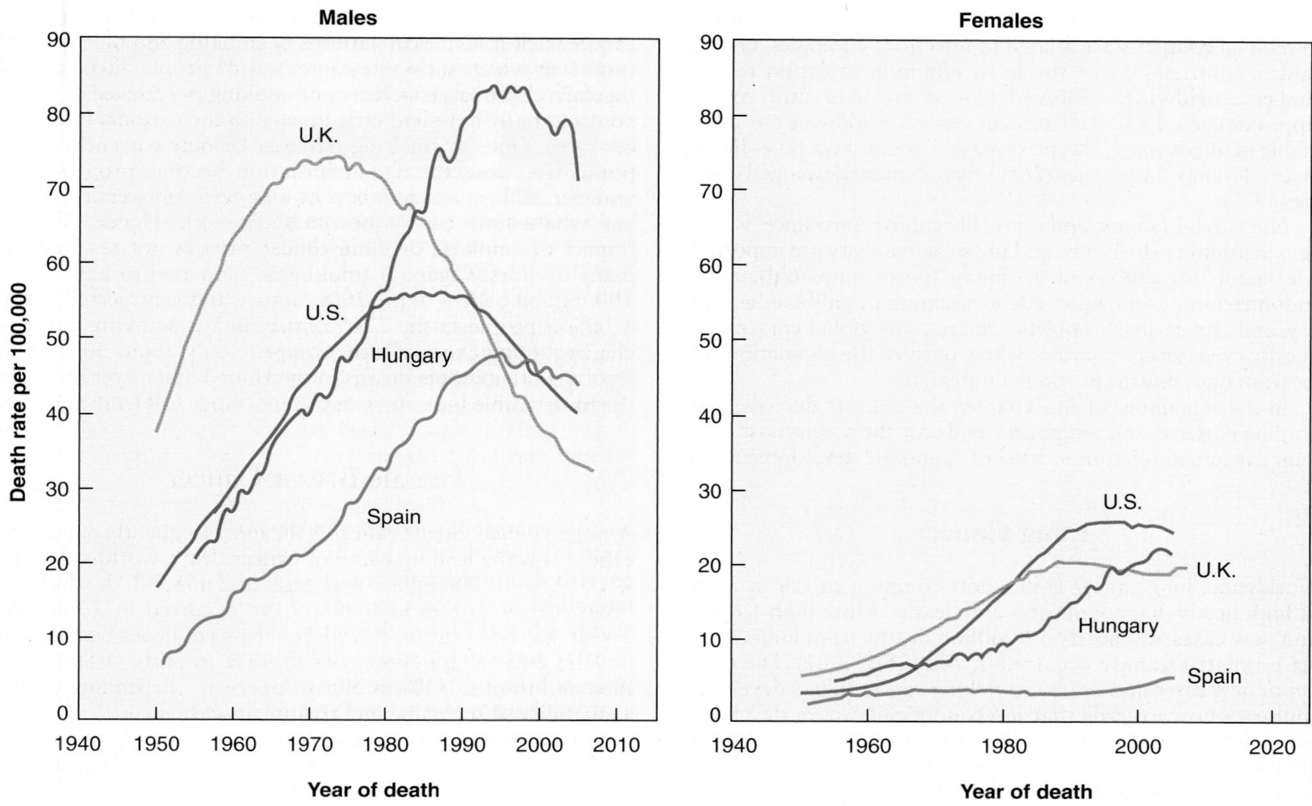

FIGURE 23.7 Age-standardized female breast cancer incidence and death rates by World Health Organization region for 2008. (From ref. 10.)

cancer epidemiology include identification of geographic areas with a high proportion of distant stage breast cancers in New Jersey[25] and finding an inverse relationship between travel distance to the nearest radiation therapy facility and receipt of radiotherapy after breast-conserving surgery in New Mexico.[26]

Temporal Trends

Two broad patterns are seen in the temporal trends in cancer incidence and mortality rates worldwide. First, cancers that are strongly related to infectious etiologies, for example, stomach, liver, and uterine cervix, are, in general, decreasing globally, although these tumors remain common regionally in less developed countries. A notable exception to this general pattern is Kaposi sarcoma, which is increasing only in low and middle income countries where access to and acceptance of antiretroviral treatment is limited. A second global trend is the rapid increase in the occurrence of malignancies that were historically common only in wealthy countries, but that now are increasing in middle and low resource countries. These include cancers of the lung, breast, prostate, and colon or rectum. The global spread of these cancers is a direct consequence of international and national tobacco marketing and of the adoption of Western patterns of diet and physical inactivity. The temporal trends in a number of specific cancer sites and in all cancers combined are discussed in greater detail below.

INCIDENCE AND MORTALITY PATTERNS FOR COMMON CANCERS

Cancer incidence and mortality rates for all cancers combined and several specific cancers are shown in Table 23.1. The ten most common types of cancer in 2008 are listed for economically more and less developed countries in Figure 23.1. In economically more developed countries, the three most commonly diagnosed cancers are prostate, lung, and colorectum among men, and breast, colorectum, and lung in women. In contrast, in economically less developed countries, the three most commonly diagnosed cancers are lung, stomach, and liver cancers in men, and breast, cervix uteri, and lung cancers in women. In both economically more and less developed countries, these same cancer sites are also the three leading causes of cancer death. As the global use of tobacco (especially manufactured cigarettes) has increased, so has the number and proportion of all cancers related to tobacco use. Cigarette smoking and other forms of tobacco use accounted for an estimated 21% of all cancer deaths worldwide in the year 2000.[27] Approximately 60% of these deaths were from lung cancer, and 21% were from upper aerodigestive tract cancers. The number of cancers attributable to tobacco continues to increase globally, even as smoking prevalence decreases in wealthy countries, because of expansion of the world's population and an increase in long-term cigarette consumption in economically less developed countries.

Currently three of the five most common cancers in less developed countries are related to infectious etiologies. Gastric cancer continues to be the most common infection-related cancer worldwide, followed closely by liver and cervix. Approximately 15% of all incident cancers worldwide are attributable to infections.[28] This percentage is about three times higher in less developed countries (26%) than in more developed countries (8%).

Nutritional factors, and especially caloric imbalance, weight gain in adulthood, obesity, and physical inactivity are important risk factors for cancers of the breast (postmenopausal), colon, endometrium, esophagus (adenocarcinoma), gallbladder, kidney, and certain hematopoietic cancers. The global epidemic of obesity even affects countries where parts of the population suffer from undernutrition and malnutrition.

In the remainder of this chapter, the authors describe geographic patterns and temporal trends for the seven most common cancers in relation to level of economic development.

Lung Cancer

Worldwide, lung cancer is the most common cancer in terms of both newly diagnosed cases and deaths. More than 1.6 million new cases and nearly 1.4 million deaths from lung cancer are estimated to have occurred in 2008 (Fig. 23.1). The number of new cases and deaths from lung cancer in less developed countries now exceeds that in economically more developed countries, even though the proportion of all cancer deaths attributable to lung cancer is higher in more developed (21%) than in less developed (16.1%) countries.

Lung cancer is more strongly associated with cigarette smoking than any other cancer site.[29] Globally, an estimated 85% of lung cancers in men and 47% in women are attributable to tobacco smoking.[30] This percentage is higher (90% to 95%) among men in Europe and North America, where cigarette smoking has been entrenched for many decades.

The lung cancer incidence rates vary by nearly fivefold in men and over 10-fold in women across the WHO regions (Fig. 23.6), reflecting differences in historical patterns of smoking. The highest rates are among men in Eastern Europe, Southern Europe, and North America, whereas the lowest rates are observed in Central America and South Central Asia. Lung cancer incidence and death rates among men have begun to fall in North America, Northern Europe, Australia, and New Zealand but continue to rise in many other countries (Fig. 23.8).

Lung cancer patterns in women differ from those in men because the uptake of widespread cigarette smoking among women lagged behind that in men by approximately 25 years, even in industrialized countries. The prevalence of cigarette smoking is still low among women in much of Asia and Africa, but in Europe and parts of South America, teenage girls are now smoking more than teenage boys.[4] The highest lung cancer rates among women are currently in North America, Northern Europe (especially Scandinavia), and Australia and New Zealand. Lung cancer rates among women have leveled off but not yet declined in the United States.

Factors other than cigarette smoking contribute to the relatively high background rate of lung cancer among women in parts of China. The lung cancer incidence rate per 100,000 for 2008 among Chinese women (21.3/100,000) is higher than that among women in Germany (16.4) and France (14.7), despite their lower prevalence of smoking. Factors thought to contribute to the high lung cancer rate among Chinese women in certain regions of China include indoor exposure to coal smoke,[31] indoor emissions from burning other fuels,[32] exposure to fumes from frying foods at high temperatures,[33] and to secondhand smoke.[34]

Temporal trends in lung cancer and other tobacco-related cancers reflect historical patterns of smoking and the length of time over which substantial numbers of people have smoked regularly. Even large increases in smoking prevalence in young adults initially have had little impact on the national lung cancer rates. Only as smoking patterns become entrenched in a population does the age at initiation become progressively younger, and greater numbers of long-term smokers reach the age where lung cancer becomes common. Hence, the full impact of smoking on lung cancer rates is not reached for many decades. Cigarette smoking is estimated to have killed 100 million people in the 20th century and is projected to kill 1 billion people in the 21st century unless smoking patterns change.[4] Lung cancer deaths comprise only about 30% of all smoking-attributable deaths in the United States, yet these are the most visible indicators of the enormous toll from tobacco.

Female Breast Cancer

Among women, breast cancer is the most frequently diagnosed cancer and the leading cause of cancer death worldwide (Fig. 23.1). About 1.38 million new cases and 458,000 deaths from breast cancer are estimated to have occurred in 2008. The 5-year survival rates vary widely across countries from about 30% in Sub-Saharan countries to 45% in parts of Southeast Asia and to over 80% in North America,[28] depending on the availability of screening and treatment services.

Female breast cancer incidence rates are highest in the economically more developed countries in Western and Northern Europe and North America (Fig. 23.7). Low rates are found in most of Africa, Asia, and Central America. Factors that contribute to the striking international variation include historical differences in reproductive factors (age at menarche and menopause, first live birth, number of children, and duration of breastfeeding), use of hormone replacement therapy, obesity after menopause, alcohol intake, and screening practices. Women in affluent countries are more likely to delay childbearing, have fewer children, and use hormone replacement therapy after menopause. Early detection of breast cancer through mammography screening contributes to higher incidence rates but lower mortality. Inherited genetic mutations with high penetrance, such as *BRCA1* and *BRCA2*, that are more common in women of Ashkenazi Jewish descent, increase risk of breast cancer[35] in affected individuals but have little impact on global geographic differences or temporal trends.[36]

Although historical data are limited, the incidence of breast cancer is thought to have increased over most of the 20th century in more developed countries, first because of changes in reproductive patterns and more recently because of increased screening.[37]

In the past 50 years, breast cancer incidence rates have also been rising in many less developed countries, with the most notable increases in traditionally low-incidence African countries.[37] The reasons for these trends are not completely understood but likely reflect changes in reproductive patterns, nutrition, and physical inactivity.

During the past decade, female breast cancer death rates have decreased in the United States and certain European countries (the United Kingdom, Netherlands, Denmark, etc.) In the United States, this decline has been attributed to a combination of increased mammography and improvements in treatment.[38] Changes in breast cancer treatment may account for most of the decrease in mortality rates in Europe, where mammography is less prevalent.

In contrast to the trends in the United States and United Kingdom, female breast cancer death rates in Asian countries, such as Japan and Singapore, are increasing. The increase

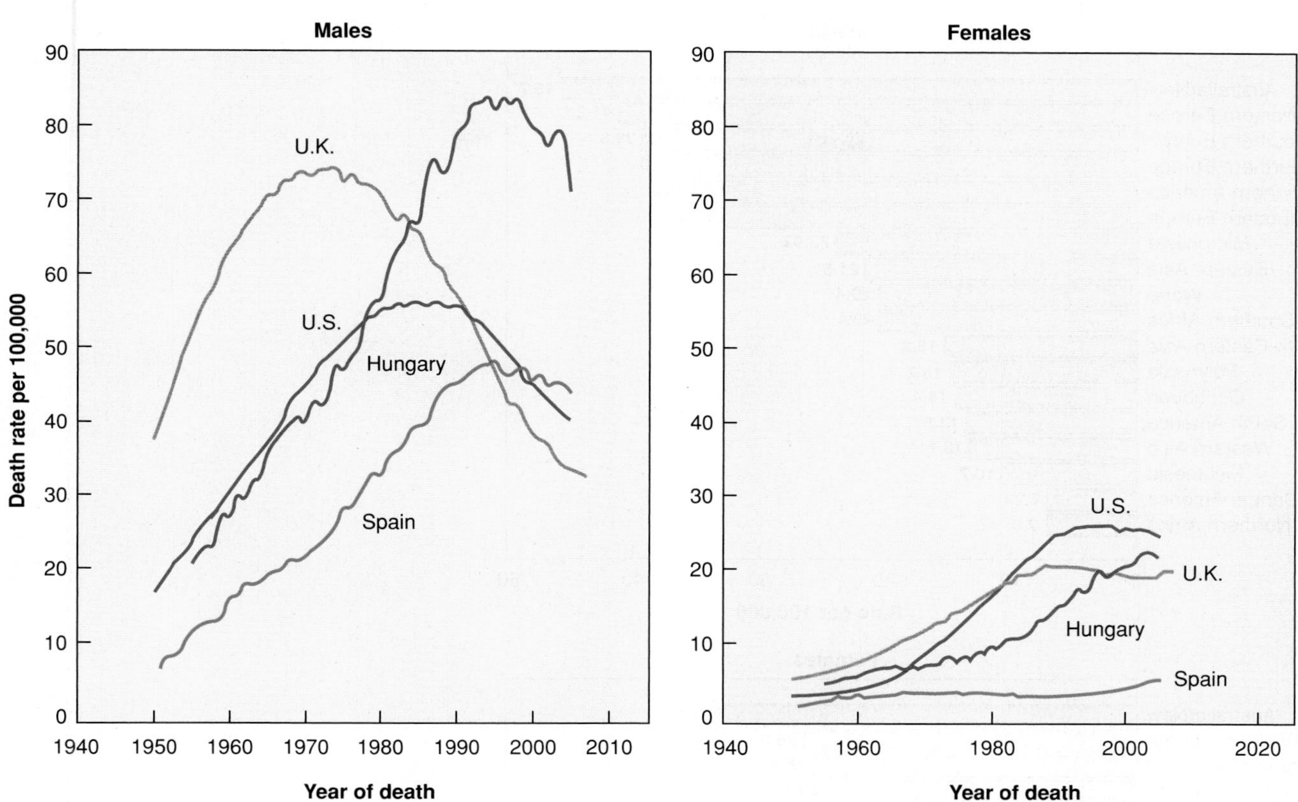

FIGURE 23.8 Trends in age-standardized lung cancer death rates in males and females in four countries. (From World Health Organization. Mortality database. Available at www.who.int/whosis/whosis. Accessed March 5, 2010.)

follows Westernization of reproductive and nutritional patterns, including younger age at menarche and increased use of hormone replacement therapy.

Colon and Rectum Cancer

Cancers of the colon and rectum (colorectal cancer) are the third most common cancer diagnosed in men and women. Worldwide, over 1.2 million new cases and 608,000 deaths are estimated to have occurred in 2008 (Fig. 23.1). Over half (59%) of these cases occur in economically more developed countries. The 5-year survival rate for colorectal cancer varies from less than 15% in Sub-Saharan Africa to 65% in United States.[39]

The incidence rate of colorectal cancer varies by more than 20-fold across countries and six- to sevenfold among WHO regions (Fig. 23.9). Historically the highest incidence rates were in North America, Europe, New Zealand, and Australia. Rates remain low in Africa, Central America, and much of Asia. However, the incidence of colorectal cancer has increased dramatically in Japan since World War II.

Migrant studies have shown that the incidence of colorectal cancer rises rapidly among populations who move from a low- to a high-risk country. This increase occurs within the first generation, implying that potentially modifiable exposures in adulthood profoundly affect risk.

Recent trends in colorectal cancer incidence and death rates are also affected by international differences in colorectal cancer screening. Both incidence and death rates are rapidly decreasing in the United States, coincident with increases in screening that can detect and remove precancerous polyps and identify early stage cancers.[40–42]

Stomach Cancer

About 737,000 people die from stomach cancer each year (Fig. 23.1), making it the third leading cause of cancer death in men and the fifth in women, despite a global decrease in incidence and death rates over the past 50 years.[10] Generally, incidence rates are about twice as high in men as in women. In the United States, the median age at diagnosis is 70 years in men and 74 years in women. Survival in most countries is poor, although 5-year survival rates as high as 50% are reported in Japan where screening for stomach cancer is common.[43]

Stomach cancer incidence rates are highest in Eastern Asia and Central and Eastern Europe (Fig. 23.10). Among countries the incidence rates (per 100,000) range from 62.2 in Korea to 2.4 cases in Gabon for men and from 25.9 in Guatemala to 1.3 in the Central African Republic. Factors that contribute to the geographic patterns include variation in prevalence of chronic *Helicobacter pylori* infection and diets high in salt and processed foods and low in fresh vegetables and fruit.[44] *H. pylori* infection accounts for an estimated 64% of the stomach cancer cases in less developed countries and 61% in more developed countries.[8] The prevalence of *H. pylori* infection is reportedly as high as 80% among adults in Eastern European countries.[28]

Mortality rates from stomach cancer have decreased by more than 80% in most industrialized countries over the past 50 years. Similar trends have been noted in some less developed countries, including China, although the decrease is smaller and the rates remain high regionally. Factors that have contributed to these remarkable decreases are thought to include increased availability of fresh fruits and vegetables, decreased reliance on salted and preserved foods, reduction in

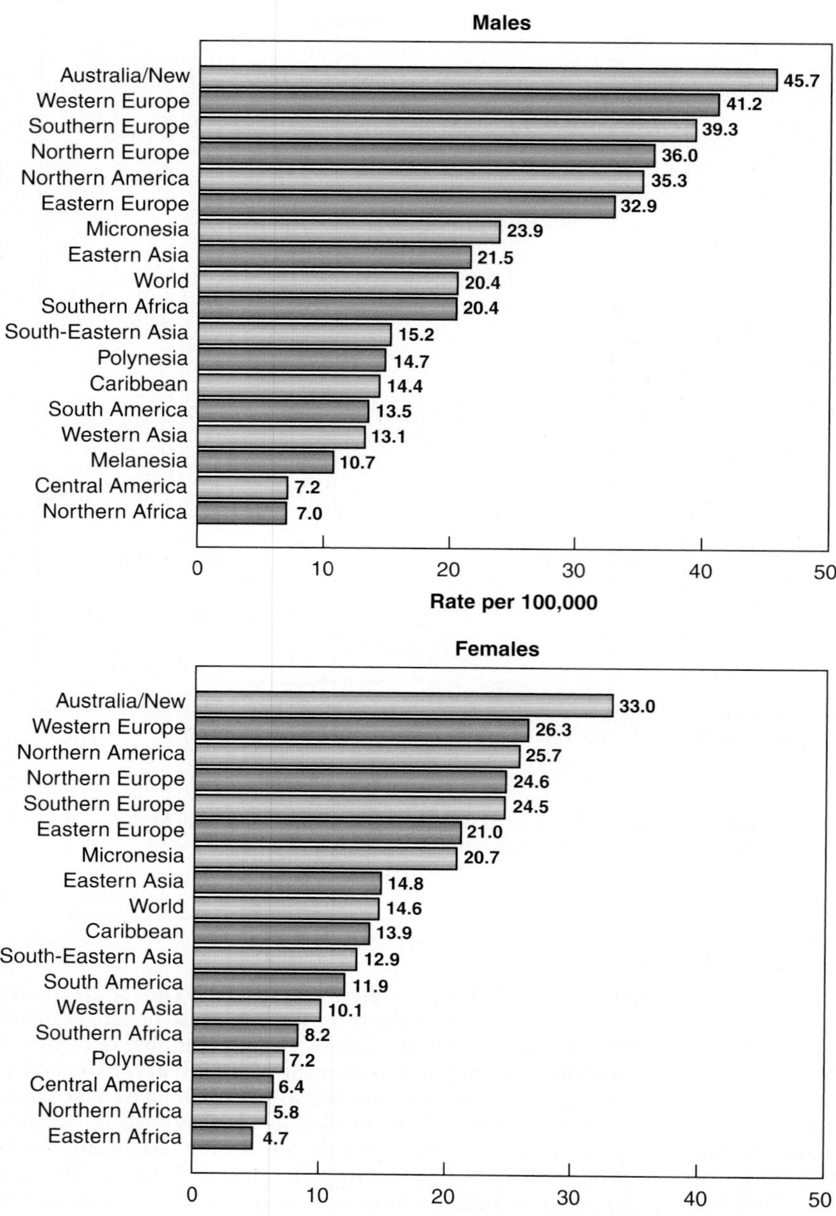

FIGURE 23.9 Age-standardized colorectal cancer incidence rates by World Health Organization region and sex for 2008. (From ref. 10.)

chronic *H. pylori* infection due to sanitation and antibiotics,[27] and (in Japan) increased screening.[45]

Prostate Cancer

Prostate cancer is the second most frequently diagnosed cancer and the sixth most common fatal cancer among men worldwide. Nearly three quarters (72%) of the more than 913,000 cases estimated to have been diagnosed in 2008 were in economically more developed countries (Fig. 23.1). The only well-established risk factors for prostate cancer are age, race or ethnicity, and family history of the disease. Prostate cancer incidence rates are strongly affected by screening with the prostate-specific antigen (PSA) blood test. Screening facilitates the detection of prevalent cases, including indolent cancers that might otherwise go undetected.[46]

The incidence rates of prostate cancer vary by nearly eightfold across WHO regions (Fig. 23.11). The highest rates are recorded in Australia and New Zealand and the lowest rates in parts of Africa and Asia. International variation in testing for PSA accounts for much of the variation in incidence.

Variation in the age-standardized mortality rate from prostate cancer is substantially smaller than that observed for incidence (Fig. 23.11), largely because most aggressive tumors would ultimately be diagnosed, albeit at a later stage, even without PSA testing. In the United States, the death rate per 100,000 from prostate cancer decreased by 40% from 39.3 in 1991 to 23.6 in 2006. Smaller decreases were observed in Europe over the same time period, but the age-standardized death rate in Western Europe remains higher than that in North America (Fig. 23.11).

Men in Western Africa and their descendants in North America and Jamaica have the highest prostate cancer

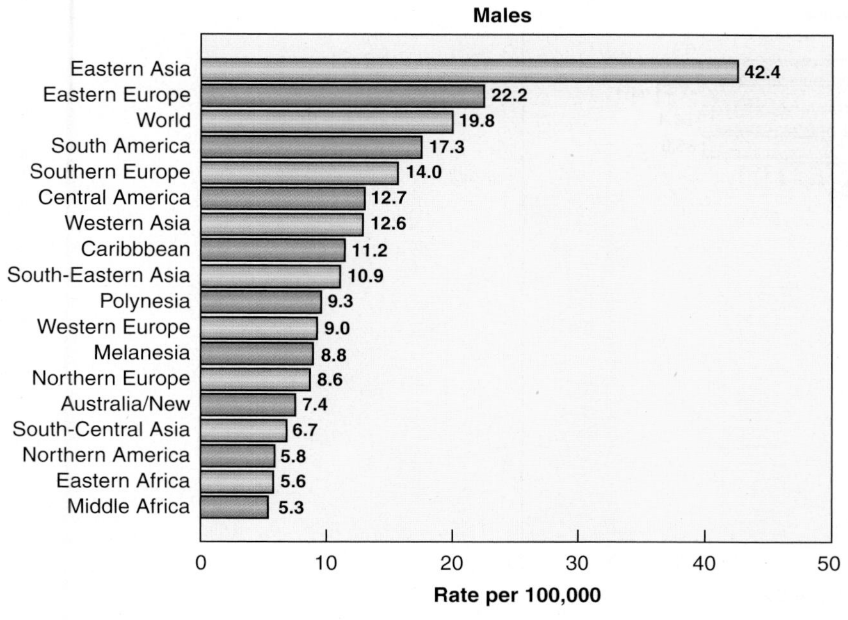

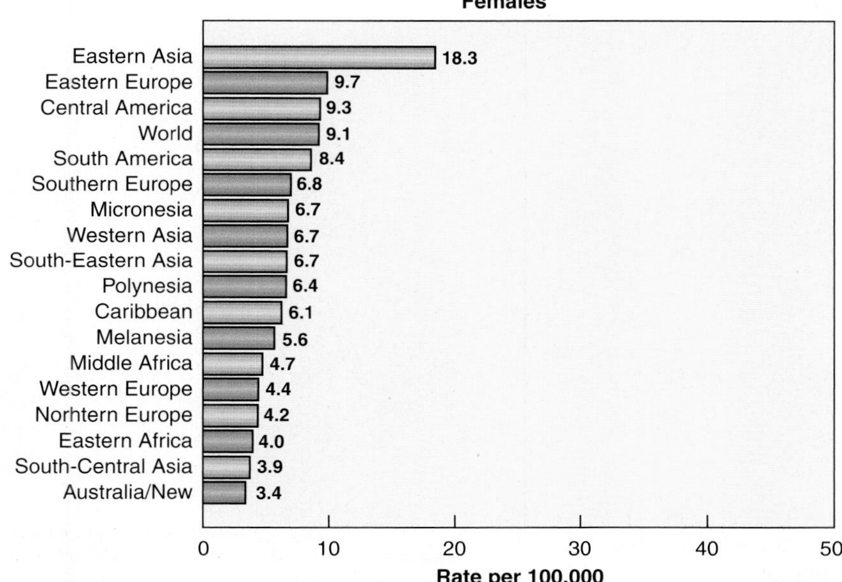

FIGURE 23.10 Age-standardized stomach cancer incidence rates by World Health Organization region and sex for 2008. (From ref. 10.)

mortality rates in the world. This accounts for the higher overall rates among men in the Caribbean WHO, which are almost three times the age-standardized mortality rate from prostate cancer than the overall male population in North America and more than ten times the rate of men in Eastern Asia (Fig. 23.11). The reason why men in Western Africa and black men in the Caribbean and North America have high prostate cancer risk is still poorly understood.

Australia and New Zealand and Western Europe have the highest prostate cancer incidence rates, whereas Asia, Eastern Africa, and Northern Africa have the lowest (Fig. 23.11). As noted, regional differences in PSA testing account for much of this variation. The geographic variation may also reflect biological differences in susceptibility. This may contribute to the moderately high incidence rates in Caribbean (Trinidad and Tobago and Jamaica), where PSA testing is less frequent, and to the 60% higher incidence rates among blacks than white males in the United States, despite lower prevalence of PSA testing.[47]

Liver Cancer

Liver cancer is the fifth most common cancer in men and the eighth in women, but is the second leading cause of cancer death in men and the sixth in women. It is among the most fatal cancers, with 5-year relative survival rates less than 10% even in more developed nations. Over 83% of the approximately 747,000 cases estimated to have occurred in 2008 will be in less developed countries (Fig. 23.1). China alone accounts for 53.4% of all cases. Hepatocellular carcinoma (HCC) is the most common subtype of primary liver cancers, comprising an estimated 70% to 85% of cases worldwide.[48] Rates are more than twice as high in men as in women.

Liver cancer incidence rates are highest in Eastern Asia and much of Africa (Fig. 23.12) and are lowest in India, Europe, and Australia and New Zealand. Globally, the geographic patterns largely mirror the prevalence of hepatitis B virus (HBV)

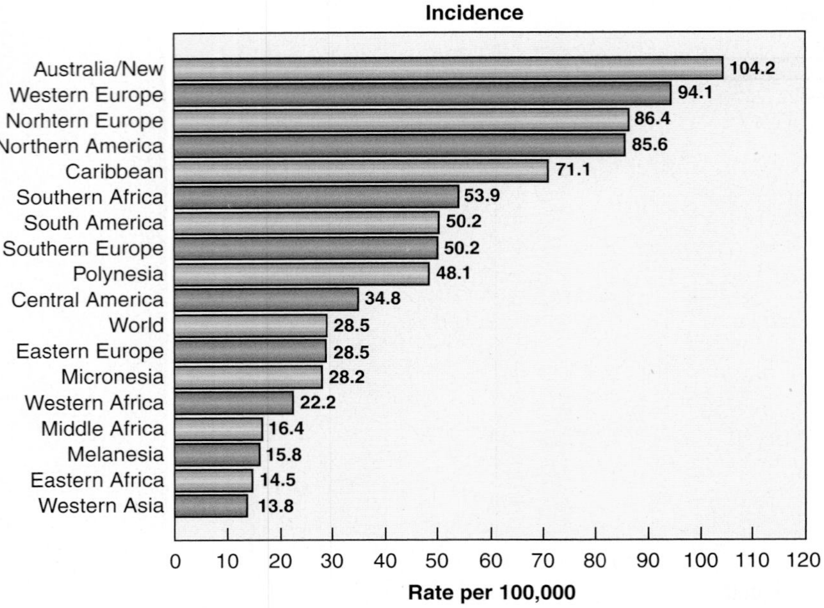

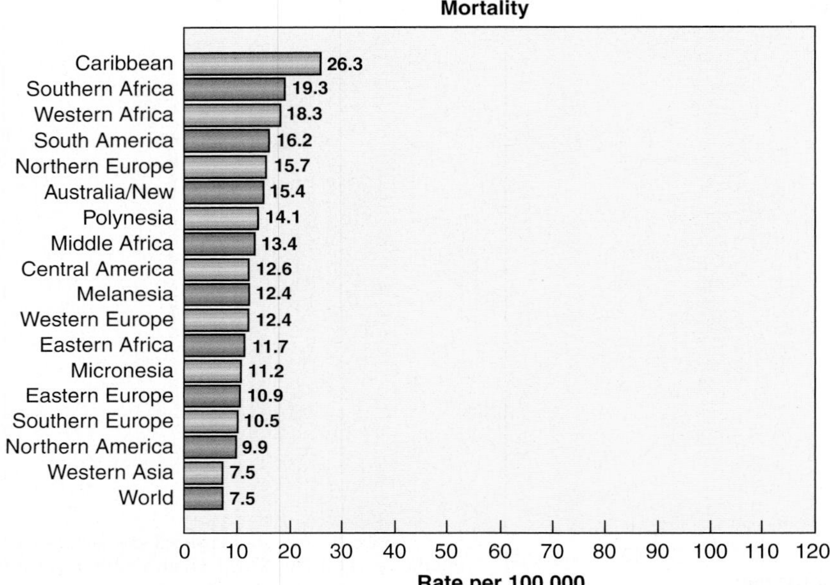

FIGURE 23.11 Age-standardized prostate cancer incidence and death rates by World Health Organization region for 2008. (From ref. 10.)

infection, which accounts for about 55% cases worldwide.[28] Chronic infection with HBV affects up to 18% of adults in China, Southeast Asia, and Sub-Saharan Africa. In low-risk areas of northern Europe and North America, the prevalence of HBV is as low as 0.5%. Large variations in the incidence of liver cancer are observed within as well as among countries. In San Francisco, the incidence of liver cancer (per 100,000) among racial and ethnic subgroups from 2000 to 2004 ranged from 6.6 cases in non-Hispanic white, to 24.1 in Chinese, and to 33.6 in Korean men.[49]

Ingestion of aflatoxin-contaminated grain has been hypothesized to be an important cofactor in HCC risk for persons chronically infected with HBV.[51] Heavy alcohol consumption and tobacco smoking also increase risk. Chronic infection with hepatitis C Virus (HCV) causes liver disease, cirrhosis, and HCC, especially when combined with alcohol consumption.[50] Although chronic HCV is an established cause of primary liver cancer, the global distribution of HCV infection is substantially different from that of either HBV or HCC.[50]

During the past two decades, the incidence rate of liver cancer has declined in Chinese populations in Singapore and Shanghai, coincident with reductions in the prevalence of HBV infection.[50,52] In contrast, rates have continued to increase in the United States, Japan, and several other Western countries. Possible explanations for the increase in HCC in the United States include chronic liver disease from obesity and HCV infections from intravenous drug use.[53]

Cervical Cancer

Cancer of the uterine cervix is the second most commonly diagnosed cancer and the fourth leading cause of cancer death among women worldwide. Approximately 529,000 cases and 274,000 deaths from cervical cancer are estimated to have

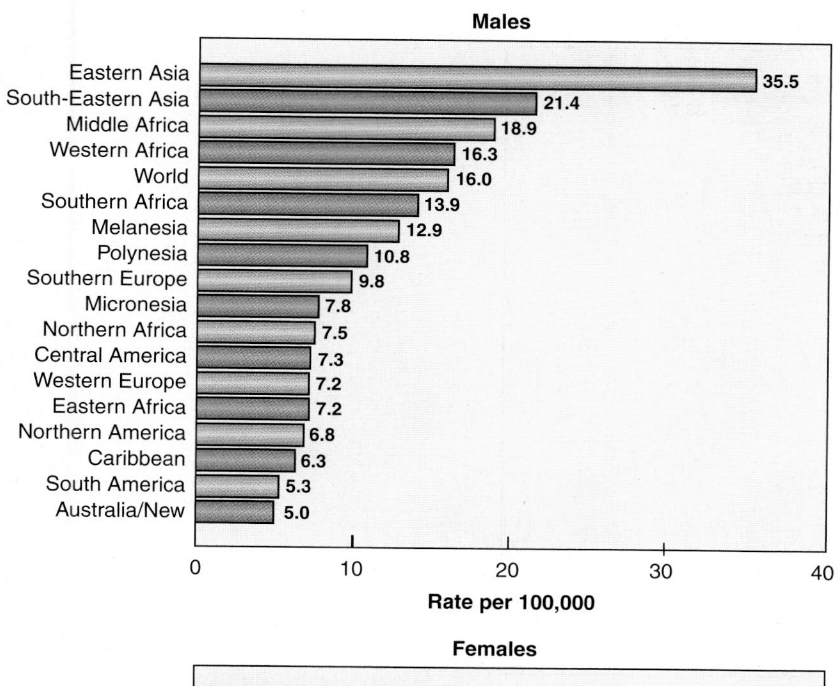

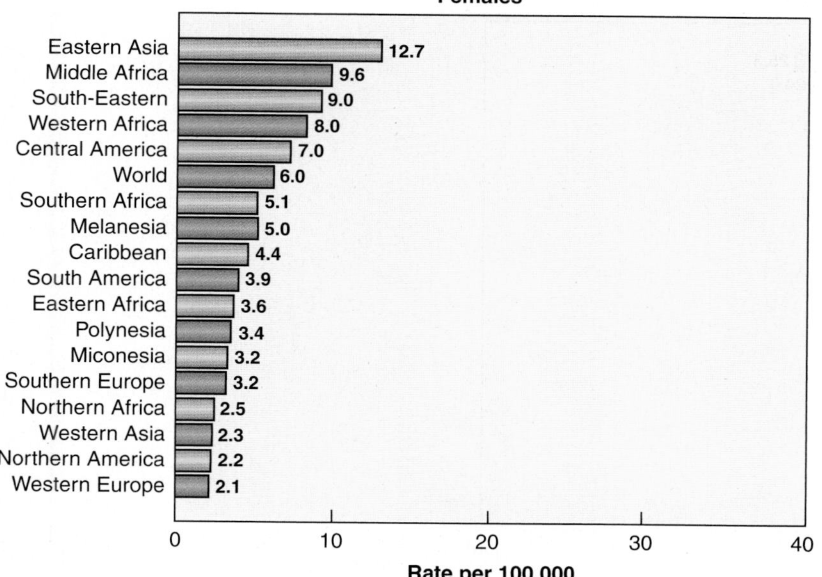

FIGURE 23.12 Age-standardized liver cancer incidence rates by World Health Organization region and sex for 2008. (From ref. 10.)

occurred in 2008 (Fig. 23.1). More than 85% of all new cases and deaths occur in less developed countries. India, the second most populous country in the world, accounts for 25% of the total cases. The 5-year relative survival rate varies widely, from less than 30% in Africa to 70% in North America and Northern Europe.[13,15,54]

Worldwide, cervical cancer incidence rates are the highest in Africa, Melanesia, and Central America (Fig. 23.13), with rates as high as 56.3 per 100,000 in Guinea. Rates are lowest in Western Asia, Northern America, and Australia and New Zealand. Historically, cervical cancer was as common in the United States and Europe as it is today in parts of Africa and Asia.

Cervical cancer incidence and mortality have been declining since the 1960s in many more developed countries where screening has been in place for a number of years (Fig. 23.14). It is estimated that up to 80% of cervical cancer can be prevented if comprehensive screening programs are made available.[55] However, many less developed countries lack the infrastructure or financial resources to conduct comprehensive screening. Persistent infection with one of several strains of human papillomavirus (HPV) is the major environmental cause of cervical cancer. The prevalence of oncogenic HPV types correlates with the incidence rates of cervical cancer in populations without effective screening programs.[56] The development of vaccines to prevent HPV infection offer great hope for curbing the epidemic in less developed countries, although cost will limit population-wide vaccination programs, at least in the near term.

Historically, the death rate from cervical cancer among women in affluent countries was as high as is seen today in parts of Africa and Asia. The introduction of Pap smear screening led to a dramatic decrease in the incidence and mortality rates from squamous cell carcinoma of the cervix. However, even in wealthy countries screening and appropriate treatment does not reach all women. Over 11,069 new cases and 3,869 deaths from cervical cancer are estimated to have occurred among U.S. women in 2008.

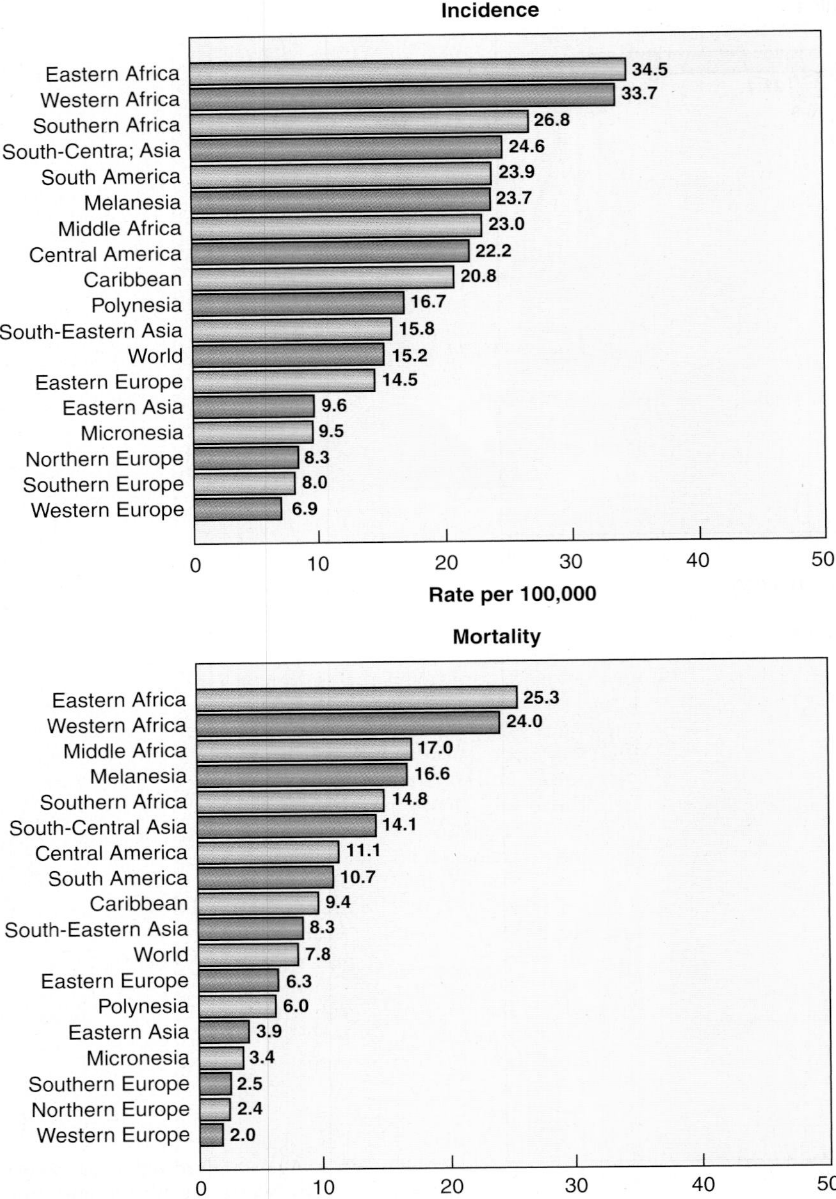

FIGURE 23.13 Age-standardized cervical cancer incidence and death rates by World Health Organization region for 2008. (From ref. 10.)

ISSUES IN INTERPRETING TEMPORAL TRENDS

A challenge in interpreting temporal trends in cancer incidence rates is to distinguish actual changes in disease occurrence from artifacts due to changes in disease detection or classification, delayed reporting of newly diagnosed cases to registries, or revisions in the estimated population at risk. Increases in incidence rates may signal increased exposure to risk factors or increased detection due to the introduction of screening or more sensitive diagnostic tests. Alternatively, decreases in incidence rates may represent progress in primary prevention, saturation or withdrawal of a screening test, or incomplete registration due to delayed reporting of cases in the most recent years.

Trends in cancer mortality rates are easier to interpret and less susceptible to artifact than are trends in incidence and survival. This is particularly true for cancers with a high prevalence of undetected indolent disease, such as prostate cancer.

The current decrease in death rates from breast and prostate cancers that can be observed in many of the more developed countries reflects genuine progress in reducing the lethality of these diseases. Death rates are not susceptible to the problems of lead time bias that complicate the interpretation of trends in relative survival. However, even mortality rates can be affected by revisions of population estimates and by changes in diagnosis and disease classification.

In describing temporal trends, epidemiologists often refer to period and cohort effects. A period effect results from medical advances (the introduction of a new screening technique or improved treatment) or from changes in disease classification that increase or decrease the incidence rate across all age groups in the same calendar period. A striking contemporary example of a period effect is the sharp increase and subsequent decrease in prostate cancer incidence rates in almost all age groups between the late 1980s and early 1990s in the United States, reflecting the introduction and dissemination of PSA testing in the late 1980s.[57]

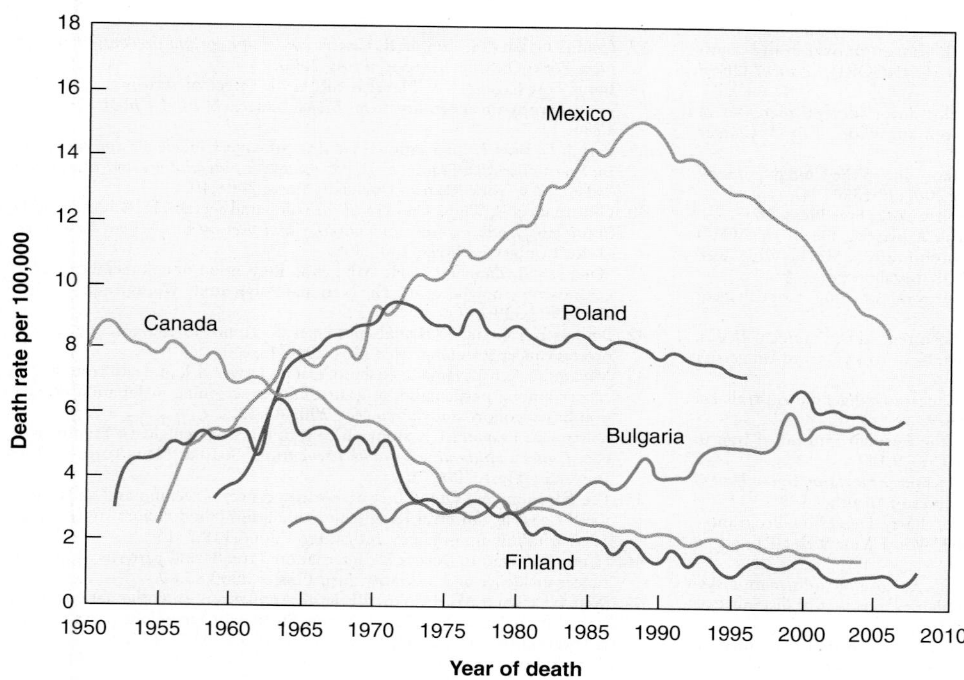

FIGURE 23.14 Trends in age-standardized death rates from cervical cancer in selected countries. (From World Health Organization. Mortality database. Available at www.who.int/whosis/whosis. Accessed March 5, 2010.)

In contrast, a birth cohort effect typically results from the introduction (or increased prevalence) of a risk factor that becomes established at a young age in people born during the same time period. Birth cohort patterns reflect the disease consequences from exposures that begin early in life but affect cancer incidence later in life, as birth cohorts age.

CONCLUSION

The burden of cancer worldwide varies across countries according to differences in risk factors, detection practices, treatment availability, age structure, and completeness of reporting. Cancers related to infections account for about 28% of the cases in less developed countries and less than 8% of the cases in more developed countries. Cancers in less developed countries more often result in death largely because they are generally diagnosed at a late stage and the resources for early detection and treatment are limited. Overall, the number of people dying from cancer worldwide is projected to grow from 7.6 million in 2007 to more than 13.2 million in 2030 due to increased life expectancy and as people in less developed countries adopt Western lifestyles, including cigarette smoking, higher consumption of saturated fat and calorie-dense foods, and reduced physical activity at work and during leisure time.

The exact percentage of cancer deaths that could, in principle, be avoided is a matter of some uncertainty, but has been estimated to be as high as 75% to 80%.[2] Population-based surveillance of cancer and risk factors for cancer is an essential tool for measuring progress against these diseases. Surveillance data can be used to convince legislators and policymakers of the importance of cancer prevention, early detection, and treatment. While cancer registration is now well accepted as a public health priority in the more developed world, including the United States, less emphasis is given to it in the developing world. According to the International Associations of Cancer Registries, about 21% of the world population (most of whom live in more affluent countries) is covered by population-based cancer registries,[58] with high quality incidence data for only 9%. Therefore, expansions of registries in geographic coverage, quality, and scope will be a necessary step in promoting cancer control programs worldwide.

Selected References

1. Doll R. Epidemiological evidence of the effects of behaviour and the environment on the risk of human cancer. *Recent Results Cancer Res* 1998; 154:3.
2. Doll R, Peto R. The causes of cancer: quantitative estimates of avoidable risks of cancer in the United States today. *J Natl Cancer Inst* 1981;66:1191.
3. Buell P, Dunn J. Cancer mortality among Japanese Issei and Nisei of California. *Cancer* 1965;18:656.
4. Mackay J, Lee N, Parkin D. *The cancer atlas*. Atlanta: American Cancer Society, 2006.
5. Thun MJ, DeLancey JO, Center MM, et al. The global burden of cancer: priorities for prevention. *Carcinogenesis* 2009;31:100.
6. Kircher T, Nelson J, Burdo H. The autopsy as a measure of accuracy of the death certificate. *N Engl J Med* 1985;313:1263.
7. Parkin DM, Bray F, Ferlay J, et al. Global cancer statistics, 2002. *CA Cancer J Clin* 2005;55:74.
8. Parkin DM, Bray F, Ferlay J, et al. Estimating the world cancer burden: GLOBOCAN 2000. *Int J Cancer* 2001;94:153.
9. Fritz A, Percy C, Jack A, et al. *International classification of diseases for oncology*, 3rd ed. Geneva: World Health Organization, 2000.
10. Ferlay J, Shin H, Bray F, et al. *GLOBOCAN 2008: cancer incidence, mortality, and prevalence worldwide*. Lyon: International Agency for Research on Cancer, 2010.
11. Anderson RN, Rosenberg HM. Age standardization of death rates: implementation of the year 2000 standard. *Natl Vital Stat Rep* 1998; 47:1.
12. Groopman JD, Johnson D, Kensler TW. Aflatoxin and hepatitis B virus biomarkers: a paradigm for complex environmental exposures and cancer risk. *Cancer Biomark* 2005;1:5.
13. Horner MJ, Ries L, Krapcho M, et al. *SEER cancer statistics review, 1975–2006*. Bethesda, MD: National Cancer Institute, 2009.

14. Coleman MP, Quaresma M, Berrino F, et al. Cancer survival in five continents: a worldwide population-based study (CONCORD). *Lancet Oncol* 2008;9:730.
15. Sant M, Capocaccia R, Coleman MP, et al. Cancer survival increases in Europe, but international differences remain wide. *Eur J Cancer* 2001;37:1659.
16. Albano JD, Ward E, Jemal A, et al. Cancer mortality in the United States by education level and race. *J Natl Cancer Inst* 2007;99:1384–94.
17. Rogers E. *Diffusion of innovation*, 5th ed. New York: Free Press, 2003.
18. Health Professionals and Tobacco Control. A briefing file of the WHO European Region. World Health Organization, 2005. World Wide Web URL: http://www.euro.int/document/tob/TOB_factsheet.pdf.
19. WHO Europe. *The European tobacco control report 2007*. Copenhagen: WHO Regional Office for Europe, 2007.
20. Kolonel L, Wilkens L. Migrant studies. In: Schottenfeld D, Fraumeni JJ, eds. *Cancer epidemiology and prevention*, 3rd ed. New York: Oxford University Press, 2006:189.
21. Condon JR, Armstrong BK, Barnes A, et al. Cancer in indigenous Australians: a review. *Cancer Causes Control* 2003;14:109.
22. Ghadirian P. Food habits of the people of the Caspian Littoral of Iran in relation to esophageal cancer. *Nutr Cancer* 1987;9:147.
23. Devesa SS, Grauman D, Blot W, et al. *Atlas of cancer mortality in the United States 1950–1994*. Bethesda: National Institutes of Health, 1999.
24. The National Breast and Cervical Cancer Early Detection Program—Reducing mortality through screening, 2003. World Wide Web URL: http://www.cdc.gov/cancer/nbccedp/about.htm.
25. Roche LM, Skinner R, Weinstein RB. Use of a geographic information system to identify and characterize areas with high proportions of distant stage breast cancer. *J Public Health Manag Pract* 2002;8:26.
26. Athas WF, Adams-Cameron M, Hunt WC, et al. Travel distance to radiation therapy and receipt of radiotherapy following breast-conserving surgery. *J Natl Cancer Inst* 2000;92:269.
27. Ezzati M, Henley SJ, Lopez AD, et al. Role of smoking in global and regional cancer epidemiology: current patterns and data needs. *Int J Cancer* 2005;116:963.
28. Parkin DM. The global health burden of infection-associated cancers in the year 2002. *Int J Cancer* 2006;118:3030.
29. Thun M, Henley S. Tobacco. In: Schottenfeld D, Fraumeni JJ, eds. *Cancer epidemiology and prevention*, 3rd ed. New York: Oxford University Press, 2006:217.
30. Peto R. Smoking and death: the past 40 years and the next 40. *BMJ* 1994;309:937.
31. Lan Q, He X. Molecular epidemiological studies on the relationship between indoor coal burning and lung cancer in Xuan Wei, China. *Toxicology* 2004;198:301.
32. Chen BH, Hong CJ, Pandey MR, et al. Indoor air pollution in developing countries. *World Health Stat Q* 1990;43:127.
33. Yu IT, Chiu YL, Au JS, et al. Dose-response relationship between cooking fumes exposures and lung cancer among Chinese nonsmoking women. *Cancer Res* 2006;66:4961.
34. Wen W, Shu XO, Gao YT, et al. Environmental tobacco smoke and mortality in Chinese women who have never smoked: prospective cohort study. *BMJ* 2006;333:376.
35. Ford D, Easton DF, Bishop DT, et al. Risks of cancer in BRCA1-mutation carriers. Breast Cancer Linkage Consortium. *Lancet* 1994;343:692.
36. Struewing JP, Hartge P, Wacholder S, et al. The risk of cancer associated with specific mutations of BRCA1 and BRCA2 among Ashkenazi Jews. *N Engl J Med* 1997;336:1401.
37. Colditz G, Baer H, Tamimi R. *Cancer epidemiology and prevention*, 3rd ed. New York: Oxford University Press, 2006.
38. Berry DA, Cronin KA, Plevritis SK, et al. Effect of screening and adjuvant therapy on mortality from breast cancer. *N Engl J Med* 2005;353:1784.
39. Parkin D, Bray F. International patterns of cancer incidence and mortality. In: Schottenfeld D, Fraumeni JJ, eds. *Cancer Epidemiology and prevention*, 3rd ed. New York: Oxford University Press, 2006:101.
40. Giovannucci E, Wu K. Cancers of the colon and rectum. In: Schottenfeld D, Fraumeni JJ, eds. *Cancer epidemiology and prevention*, 3rd ed. New York: Oxford University Press, 2006:809.
41. Winawer SJ, Zauber AG, Ho MN, et al. Prevention of colorectal cancer by colonoscopic polypectomy. The National Polyp Study Workgroup. *N Engl J Med* 1993;329:1977.
42. Phillips KA, Liang SY, Ladabaum U, et al. Trends in colonoscopy for colorectal cancer screening. *Med Care* 2007;45:160.
43. Miyamoto A, Kuriyama S, Nishino Y, et al. Lower risk of death from gastric cancer among participants of gastric cancer screening in Japan: a population-based cohort study. *Prev Med* 2007;44:12.
44. Shibata A, Parsonnet J. Stomach cancer. In: Schottenfeld D, Fraumeni JJ, eds. *Cancer epidemiology and prevention*, 3rd ed. New York: Oxford University Press, 2006:707.
45. Lee KJ, Inoue M, Otani T, et al. Gastric cancer screening and subsequent risk of gastric cancer: a large-scale population-based cohort study, with a 13-year follow-up in Japan. *Int J Cancer* 2006;118:2315.
46. Hsing AW, Tsao L, Devesa SS. International trends and patterns of prostate cancer incidence and mortality. *Int J Cancer* 2000;85:60.
47. Weir HK, Thun MJ, Hankey BF, et al. Annual report to the nation on the status of cancer, 1975–2000, featuring the uses of surveillance data for cancer prevention and control. *J Natl Cancer Inst* 2003;95:1276.
48. Perz JF, Armstrong GL, Farrington LA, et al. The contributions of hepatitis B virus and hepatitis C virus infections to cirrhosis and primary liver cancer worldwide. *J Hepatol* 2006;45:529.
49. Chang ET, Keegan TH, Gomez SL, et al. The burden of liver cancer in Asians and Pacific Islanders in the Greater San Francisco Bay Area, 1990 through 2004. *Cancer* 2007;109:2100.
50. Bosch FX, Ribes J, Diaz M, et al. Primary liver cancer: worldwide incidence and trends. *Gastroenterology* 2004;127:S5.
51. London W, McGlynn K. Liver cancer. In: Schottenfeld D, Fraumeni JJ, eds. *Cancer epidemiology and prevention*, 3rd ed. New York: Oxford University Press, 2006:763.
52. McGlynn KA, Tsao L, Hsing AW, et al. International trends and patterns of primary liver cancer. *Int J Cancer* 2001;94:290.
53. El-Serag HB. Hepatocellular carcinoma: recent trends in the United States. *Gastroenterology* 2004;127:S27.
54. Sankaranarayanan R, Black R, Parkin DM. *Cancer survival in developing countries*. Publication No. 145. Lyon: IARC Scientific Publications, 1999.
55. International Agency for Research on Cancer (IARC). *Cervix cancer screening*. Lyon: IARC Press, 2005.
56. Schiffman M, Hildesheim A. Cervical cancer. In: Schottenfeld D, Fraumeni JJ, eds. *Cancer epidemiology and prevention*, 3rd ed. New York: Oxford University Press, 2006:1044.
57. Potosky AL, Miller BA, Albertsen PC, et al. The role of increasing detection in the rising incidence of prostate cancer. *JAMA* 1995;273:548.
58. Parkin DM. The evolution of the population-based cancer registry. *Nat Rev Cancer* 2006;6:603.

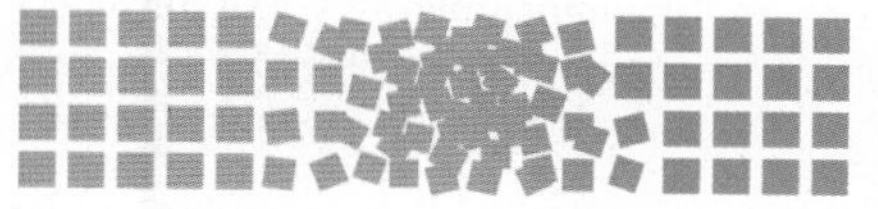

CHAPTER 24 TRENDS IN CANCER MORTALITY

TIM E. BYERS

Cancer surveillance is now a well-established part of the public health system in the United States. Cancer incidence registries now cover nearly all of the population, both state-based vital records systems and aggregate national systems regularly report trends in both cancer incidence and mortality, and various surveys routinely monitor cancer-related risk factors in the population. These surveillance systems have documented substantial changes in both risk factors for cancer and in cancer incidence and mortality rates in the United States over the past two decades.

In 1996 the American Cancer Society (ACS) set an ambitious challenge goal for the United States: to reduce cancer mortality from its apparent peak in 1990 by 50% in the 25-year period ending in 2015.[1] In 1998 the ACS then also challenged the United States to reduce cancer incidence rates from their peak in 1992 by 25% by the year 2015.[2] In this chapter, we will examine trends and projections in cancer risk factors as well as cancer incidence and mortality rates over the 25-year period between 1990 and 2015. To do this we will need to consider not only past trends, but also how historic and projected changes in risk factors are likely to affect cancer trends in the coming decade.

CANCER SURVEILLANCE SYSTEMS

The National Cancer Institute has supported high-quality cancer incidence and outcomes registration in selected states and cities since 1973 within the Surveillance, Epidemiology, and End Results (SEER) system.[3] The most precise measures of trends in cancer incidence come from SEER-9, a set of nine SEER registries that together include about 10% of the United States population. The populations included in the SEER-9 registries have the longest history of highly standardized cancer case ascertainment, staging, treatment, and outcomes. Despite this national resource, cancer incidence is largely a state-based activity in the United States, as cancer incidence rates are ascertained and reported annually by state cancer registries. The Centers for Disease Control and Prevention (CDC) organizes these state-based cancer registries within the National Program of Cancer Registries, which now reports on the collective data on cancer incidence from over 40 different state-based registries providing data that meets strict quality standards.[4] Deaths from cancer are well ascertained in all states via state-based vital records systems, which are aggregated into national mortality reports by the CDC National Center for Health Statistics. Each year, the ACS, the National Cancer Institute, and the CDC publish a "Report to the Nation" on trends in cancer incidence and mortality in the United States.[5] Trends in the prevalence of behavioral risk factors that are tied to cancer and other chronic diseases are tracked by the Health Interview Survey, an in-person interview of a nationally representative sample of adults every 2 years, and by the Behavioral Risk Factor Surveillance System, a telephone-based survey operated by state departments of health and organized by CDC, reported annually.[6]

MAKING SENSE OF CANCER TRENDS

Understanding the reasons for cancer trends requires understanding trends in cancer-related risk factors. Relating risk factor trends to cancer trends can be difficult, however, as in many instances quantifying relationships is complicated by incomplete understandings about latency periods between exposures and cancer incidence. In most situations, all that is possible is to infer crude qualitative relationships between temporal trends in risk factors for cancer and subsequent trends in cancer rates. Statistical methods such as linear regression join point analysis can tell us when inflections in cancer trends occur, but accounting for the precise reasons for changing rates is often impaired by our incomplete knowledge about the impacts of variations in cancer screening, diagnosis, and treatment, and by uncertainties about latencies between interventions and outcomes.[7]

TRENDS IN CANCER RISK FACTORS

Trends in major cancer risk factors have been mixed (Table 24.1). Downward trends in tobacco smoking among adults that began in the 1960s slowed after 1990, but there has been a continuing downward trend in the number of cigarettes smoked per day by continuing smokers.[8] Obesity trends have been adverse among both men and women, with a doubling of the prevalence of obesity since 1990.[9] Long-term trends in the use of hormone replacement therapy (HRT) are not routinely monitored, but HRT use increased substantially in the last two decades of the 20th century. Then, following the 2002 publication of the Women's Health Initiative trial, which showed clear adverse effects of HRT, there was a rapid and substantial drop in HRT use.[10,11] The use of endoscopic screening for colorectal cancer (sigmoidoscopy or colonoscopy) has increased substantially in recent years, approximately doubling since the mid-1990s, although about a third of adults aged 50 and older report never having had an endoscopic examination. Mammography use increased progressively through the 1990s, but mammogram usage then leveled off after 2000.[12,13] Widespread prostate-specific antigen (PSA) testing began in the middle to late 1980s, then increased substantially during the 1990s. By 2002 the majority of U.S. men aged 50 and older reported having been tested.

TABLE 24.1

TRENDS IN RISK FACTORS AND CANCER SCREENING PRACTICES IN THE UNITED STATES, 1990 TO 2009[a]

Year	Smoking		Obesity	CRC Screening	Mammography	PSA Testing
	Men	Women				
1990	24.9	21.3	11.6	—	58.3	—
1991	25.1	21.3	12.6	—	62.2	—
1992	24.2	21.0	12.6	—	63.1	—
1993	24.0	21.1	13.7	—	66.5	—
1994	23.9	21.6	14.4	—	66.6	—
1995	24.8	20.9	15.8	29.4	68.6	—
1996	25.5	21.9	16.8	—	69.2	—
1997	25.4	21.1	16.6	32.4	70.3	—
1998	25.3	20.9	18.3	—	72.3	—
1999	24.2	20.8	19.7	43.7	72.8	—
2000	24.4	21.2	20.1	—	76.1	—
2001	25.4	21.2	21.0	—	—	—
2002	25.7	20.8	22.1	48.1	75.9	53.9
2003	24.8	20.2	—	—	—	—
2004	23.0	19.0	23.2	53.0	74.7	52.1
2005	22.1	19.2	24.4	—	—	—
2006	22.2	18.4	25.1	57.1	76.5	53.8
2007	21.2	18.4	26.3	—	—	—
2008	20.3	16.7	26.6	61.8	76.0	54.8
2009	19.5	16.7	27.1	—	—	—

CRC, colorectal cancer; PSA, prostate-specific antigen.
[a]Median percent of the population across all states in the Behavioral Risk Factor Surveillance System. Survey covered such areas as body mass index was based on self-reported height and weight. Are you a regular cigarette smoker? Have you ever had a proctoscopic examination (1995)? Have you ever had a sigmoidoscopy or proctoscopic examination (1999 and after) among adults aged 50 and older. Have you had a mammogram in the past 2 years, among women aged 40 and older. Have you ever had a PSA test, among men aged 50 and older.
(From ref. 6.)

TABLE 24.2

TRENDS IN AGE-ADJUSTED CANCER INCIDENCE RATES IN THE UNITED STATES BY CANCER SITE, 1990 TO 2007[a]

Year	Lung		Colorectal	Breast	Prostate	All Sites
	Men	Women				
1990	96.9	47.7	60.7	131.7	170.9	481.7
1991	97.2	49.6	59.5	133.7	214.8	502.8
1992	97.1	49.8	58.0	131.9	237.2	510.3
1993	93.9	49.1	56.8	129.1	209.4	493.1
1994	90.9	50.5	55.6	130.9	180.1	483.1
1995	89.8	50.4	54.0	132.5	168.9	476.4
1996	87.9	51.2	54.7	133.5	169.1	478.6
1997	86.2	52.6	56.4	137.8	173.2	485.8
1998	87.9	52.9	56.7	141.1	170.3	487.3
1999	84.5	52.4	55.4	141.2	183.0	489.6
2000	81.9	51.2	54.1	136.3	182.2	484.7
2001	81.0	51.6	53.3	138.0	183.7	487.1
2002	79.9	52.2	52.8	134.7	180.7	483.6
2003	80.3	52.6	50.3	125.6	167.8	470.1
2004	75.4	51.5	49.3	126.3	163.2	469.3
2005	74.5	53.0	46.9	124.4	153.2	462.6
2006	72.4	52.4	45.7	123.6	165.7	462.1
2007	69.9	51.6	44.6	124.7	165.8	461.0
Annual % change	−2.2	+0.3	−1.5	0	−1.1	−0.4

[a]Data source is the Surveillance, Epidemiology, and End Results-9 populations for cancer incidence. Rates are age-adjusted to the Year 2000 population standard. Annual percent change is the mean percent change per year across the 17-year period, 1990 to 2007.
(From ref. 3.)

CANCER TRENDS

In this chapter we will assess cancer trends using cancer mortality data from the National Center for Health Statistics and cancer incidence data from the SEER-9 registry.[3,14] All rates were age-adjusted to the U.S. 2000 standard population by the direct method, using 10-year age intervals. Cancer death rates for the years 1999 to 2006 were further adjusted to account for cancer site-specific coding changes between the International Classification of Diseases, ninth and tenth revisions, coding rules.[15] Over the period 1990 to 2007, all-site cancer incidence rates in the United States declined by about 0.4% per year (Table 24.2). Increases in incidence in the early 1990s were due principally to a surge in prostate cancer diagnoses resulting from the use of PSA screening (Fig. 24.1).[16] Both lung cancer incidence and death rates increased among women between 1990 and 1998, then stabilized through 2007. Reductions in cancer incidence have also been observed for cancers of the prostate, lung (men), and colorectum. A downward incidence trend began to be apparent for breast cancer after 1999 and was particularly steep after 2002. Between 1990 and 2006, the all-site cancer death rates declined in the United States by about 1% per year (Table 24.3). Declines in mortality have been particularly steep for breast cancer, prostate cancer, colorectal cancer, and for lung cancer among men.

Lung Cancer

The lung is the second leading site for cancer incidence and the leading cause of cancer death among both men and women in the United States.[17] Trends in lung cancer incidence and mortality have been nearly identical because there are few effective treatments for lung cancer and survival time remains short. Lung cancer trends follow historical declines in tobacco use, lagged by about 20 years.[18] Between 1965 and 1985, tobacco use among U.S. adults dropped substantially, more in men than in women.[19] Lung cancer mortality rates began to decline among men in 1990, but rates increased among women throughout the 1990s. The stabilization of lung cancer incidence trends among women since 2000 foretells a coming decline in their lung cancer mortality rates as well.

The effectiveness of annual examination by use of chest radiographs in reducing lung cancer mortality is now being studied as part of the Prostate, Lung, Colorectal, Ovary (PLCO) trial, and the effectiveness of screening by computed tomography of the lung fields is being examined in the National Lung Screening Trial (NLST).[20,21] Neither the PLCO nor the NLST are likely to produce results until after 2011, but if either of these trials shows lung cancer mortality reductions, predicting effects of new efforts to screen for lung cancer on future lung cancer incidence and mortality will be possible. If a useful

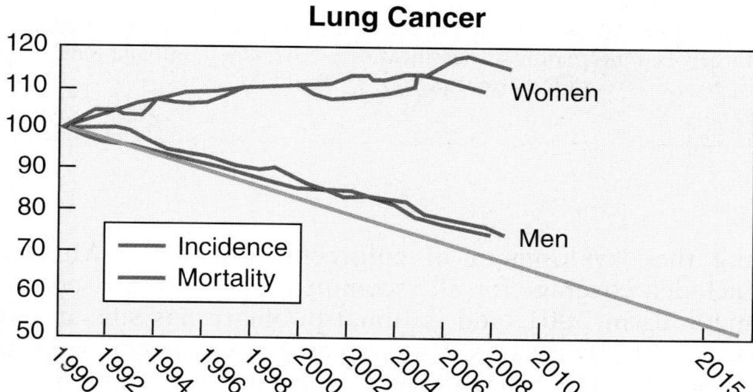

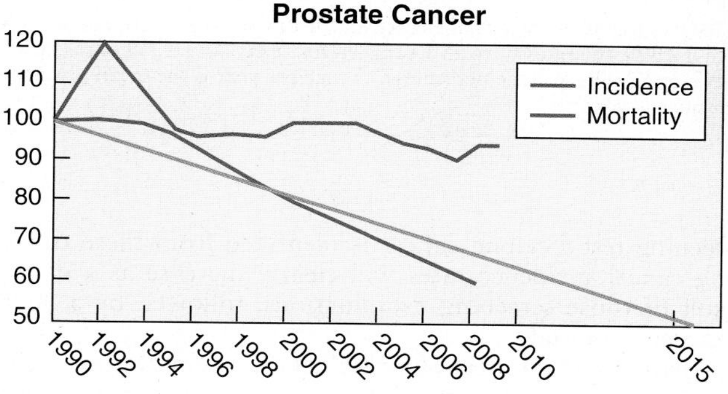

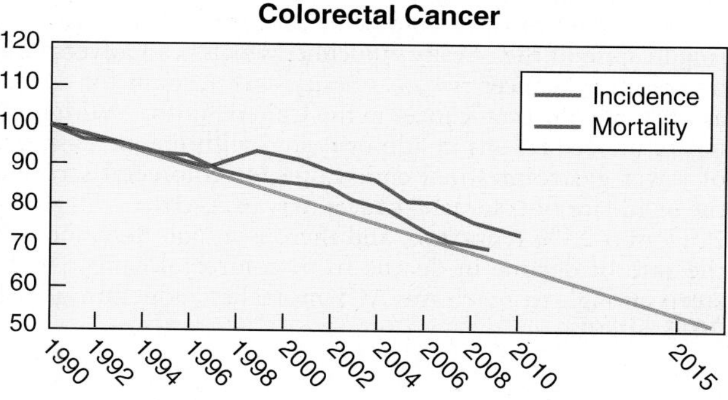

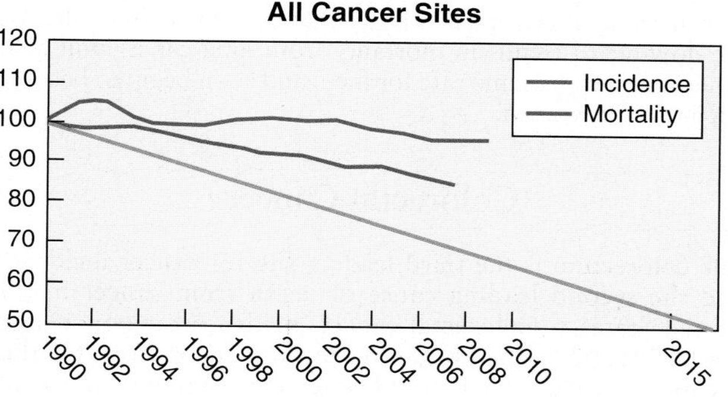

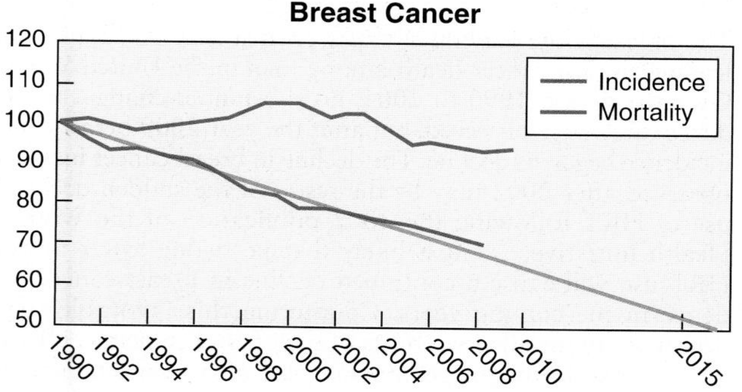

FIGURE 24.1 Trends in cancer incidence and mortality between 1990 and 2007. Incidence rates are for the populations in the Surveillance, Epidemiology, and End Results—registries, and mortality rates are for the entire United States. Rates are age-adjusted to the year 2000 standard. The y-axis rates are expressed as a percentage of the 1990 incidence rates. The *dotted lines* represent incidence rates and the *solid lines* represent mortality rates. The *straight line* is the linear trend that would need to be followed to achieve a 50% mortality reduction between 1990 and 2015. (Data from refs. 3 and 14.)

TABLE 24.3

TRENDS IN AGE-ADJUSTED CANCER MORTALITY RATES IN THE UNITED STATES BY CANCER SITE, 1990 TO 2006[a]

	Lung					
Year	Men	Women	Colorectal	Breast	Prostate	All Sites
1990	91.9	37.1	24.5	33.3	38.4	216.0
1991	90.0	37.8	23.7	32.7	38.9	215.2
1992	88.1	38.8	23.4	31.6	38.9	213.5
1993	87.6	39.4	23.1	31.4	39.0	213.5
1994	85.6	39.7	22.7	30.9	38.2	211.7
1995	84.2	40.3	22.4	30.5	37.0	209.8
1996	82.6	40.4	21.7	29.5	35.7	216.7
1997	81.2	40.9	21.4	28.2	33.9	203.5
1998	79.7	41.1	21.1	27.6	32.4	200.7
1999	78.2	40.9	20.7	26.5	30.9	204.2
2000	78.0	42.0	20.6	26.7	30.0	203.1
2001	76.3	41.7	20.0	25.9	28.7	199.5
2002	74.4	42.3	19.5	25.5	27.5	198.8
2003	72.9	42.0	18.9	25.1	26.1	193.4
2004	71.3	41.6	17.8	24.4	25.1	189.1
2005	70.1	41.2	17.3	24.0	24.2	187.0
2006	68.2	40.7	17.0	23.4	23.2	184.0
Annual % change	−2.0	+0.6	−2.2	−2.1	−3.0	−1.1

[a]Data source is the National Center for Health Statistics national mortality data set. Rates are age-adjusted to the Year 2000 population standard. After 1999, the rates were also adjusted for the coding changes in cause of death between International Classification of Diseases, ninth and tenth revisions.[16] The average percentage change per year is the mean percent change per year across the 16-year period, 1990 to 2006.
(From ref. 14.)

screening test for lung cancer is identified from these trials, lung cancer incidence rates will clearly increase as a direct result of those screening examinations, followed by a later decrease in mortality.

Apart from this effect of possible increases in future screening, the major factor that will determine lung cancer incidence in the coming decade is the past history of tobacco use. Considering all factors, it is likely that over the coming decade the downward trends in mortality from lung cancer will continue at about the same rate for men, and soon begin to become apparent for women.

Colorectal Cancer

The colorectum is the third leading site for cancer incidence and the second leading cause of death from cancer in the United States.[17] Colorectal cancer incidence rates increased until 1985, when they began to decline. The reasons for this decline are not clear, but could be related to downward trends in cigarette smoking, increasing use of nonsteroidal anti-inflammatory drugs (NSAIDs), and increasing HRT use.[23] The recent decline in HRT use following publication of the Women's Health Initiative trial results may adversely affect colorectal trends among women in the coming years, as HRT reduces risk for colorectal cancer among women.[10] Recent trials have demonstrated the potential for NSAIDs to reduce colorectal neoplasia, but adverse effects from these agents will limit their widespread use for that purpose. Nonetheless, even the sporadic use of NSAIDs for other indications will contribute to continuing declines in colorectal cancer incidence in the coming years.

Screening with either sigmoidoscopy or colonoscopy leads to the identification and removal of adenomas, thus preventing the development of colorectal cancer.[24,25] Medicare included coverage for all recommended colorectal screening methods in 2001, and national publicity has substantially increased public interest in screening.[26] Colorectal screening rates have been increasing over time, now with about 62% of adults over age 50 reporting having ever been screened by lower gastrointestinal endoscopy (Table 24.1).

Decreasing rates of colorectal cancer incidence are occurring in spite of the obesity epidemic, which is an adverse force on colorectal cancer risk, as obesity may account for as much as 20% of colorectal cancer in the United States.[27] With potential future reductions in adiposity and with the increasing use of lower gastrointestinal endoscopy for colorectal screening, the incidence of colorectal cancer may exceed the ACS goal for 2015 of a 25% reduction, and there is a high likelihood that the rate of decline in deaths from colorectal cancer will be steep enough to reach the ACS mortality reduction goal for 2015 of 50%.

Breast Cancer

The breast is the leading site cancer incidence and the second leading site for cancer death among men in the United States.[17] Over the period 1990 to 2001, no substantial changes in incidence rates were observed, but after the year 2000 breast cancer incidence began to decline. The decline in breast cancer incidence observed after 2002 may be the result of the sudden decline in use of HRT following the 2002 publication of the Women's Health Initiative.[10–12] It is likely that persisting lower rates of HRT use will cause a continued decline in breast cancer incidence in the coming years. Countering this favorable trend, however, are the adverse effects of the obesity epidemic. Obesity, a major risk factor for postmenopausal breast cancer, increased substantially between 1990 and 2005, now with over 27% of U.S. women being obese.[27,28] It is important to note that the rate of increase in obesity has slowed noticeably since 2005, which may foretell coming decreases in obesity as a result of recent publicity and interventions. If the obesity epidemic can be slowed and reversed in the coming decade, this could have substantial beneficial effects on the future trends in breast cancer incidence.

After persistent increases in the use of mammography over a 20-year period, mammography rates declined modestly between 2000 and 2004, then leveled off.[13] Recent downgrading of the evidence recommendations by the U.S. Preventive Services Task Force for mammography for women aged 40 to 49 and recommendations for every-other-year mammography for women aged 50 and older will likely result in lower mammogram utilization in the coming decade. This trend will have an adverse effect on breast cancer mortality, but will tend to reduce breast cancer incidence somewhat because of lack of detection of very early stage cancers. The antiestrogens tamoxifen and raloxifene have both been shown to reduce the risk of incident breast cancer.[29] The safety profile for tamoxifen discourages its widespread use, but the more favorable risk-benefit balance of raloxifene may make it more commonly used, thus reducing future breast cancer incidence rates.

The average decline in breast cancer death rates of over 2% per year since 1990 is the combined result of earlier diagnosis and better treatment.[30] Progress in breast cancer treatment is continuing, especially in the development and application of hormone-targeted therapies. Aromatase inhibitors have largely replaced tamoxifen therapy for breast cancer treatment for postmenopausal women. Both of these antiestrogens, tamoxifen and raloxifene, substantially reduce the incidence of second primary cancers in the contralateral breast. In the coming decade, the longer term effects of decreased HRT use, increased antiestrogen use, reversal of the obesity trends, and continued improvements in therapies will likely lead to continued decreases in both the incidence and mortality rates from breast cancer.

Prostate Cancer

The prostate is the leading site for cancer incidence and the second leading site for cancer death among men in the United States.[17] The incidence of prostate cancer has been extremely variable over the period 1990 to 2003. The sharp increase in incidence observed in the early 1990s actually began in the late 1980s, coincident with the advent of PSA testing.[16] The reasons for the approximately 3% per year downward trend in prostate cancer mortality since 1990 are uncertain, as the ongoing PSA screening trials have not yet demonstrated a mortality benefit as great as that observed since 1990.[31,32] In fact, the interim trial findings to date suggest that there was virtually no mortality benefit within the first decade following the initiation of screening. It is therefore not possible to know how much of this favorable trend was related to early diagnosis, how much was related to improvements in treatment, or how much might have been related to other factors, such as changes in the way cause of death is listed on death certificates.

The Prostate Cancer Prevention Trial provided an important proof of principle that antiandrogen therapies can reduce prostate cancer risk.[33] Although the net benefits of finasteride for prevention are not clearly demonstrated from this trial, other agents that interfere with androgen effects on prostate cancer growth could prove to be useful for prostate cancer chemoprevention in the future. Prostate cancer incidence trends will likely continue to be driven largely by rates of PSA screening in the coming decade. In the coming years, final results of a benefit to mortality from either the PLCO trial in the United States or the European PSA trial would help to better specify screening recommendations.[31,32]

Other Cancers

Even though mortality rates have been declining by about 2% per year from the four most common causes of cancer death (lung, colorectal, breast, and prostate), very little progress has been made in reducing death rates from the other half of all adult cancers in the United States. Continuing progress in tobacco control will have beneficial effects on many other types of cancer linked to tobacco (e.g., oral, esophageal, bladder), and stopping the obesity epidemic will have favorable effects on many obesity-related cancers that have been increasing in recent years, such as adenocarcinoma of the esophagus and renal cancer.[27] Melanoma rates have been increasing substantially in recent years, likely the result of the combined effects of previous sun exposure and increased awareness and surveillance for pigmented lesions. Declining rates of stomach cancer incidence and mortality over several decades may be related to the combined effects of historic improvements in nutrition and the declining prevalence of chronic infection with *Helicobacter pylori*. Liver cancer incidence has been substantially increasing in the past decades, likely resulting from historical trends in chronic infection with hepatitis B and C viruses. As a result, liver cancer will likely continue to rise in the United States over the coming decade.

The incidence of thyroid cancer has been increasing in the United States for the past several decades, but the mortality rates have been stable, a pattern most likely due to increased detection from improved diagnostic techniques. Invasive cervical cancer is uncommon in the United States because of widespread screening using Pap smears. The newly approved vaccine for the human papillomavirus has been shown to be highly effective in protecting against the serotypes that together account for 70% of cervical cancer cases, but so far coverage has been poor among young women in the United States. For many of the other cancers—such as cancers of the pancreas, brain, ovary, and the hematopoietic malignancies—risk factors are poorly understood and there are no effective early detection methods. For these cancers, current hope for improvement resides in the development of better methods for early cancer detection and treatment.

PREDICTING FUTURE CANCER TRENDS

In the United States, cancer is the leading cause of death under age 85 years.[18] Over the first half of the ACS 25-year challenge period, overall cancer incidence rates have declined by about 0.4% per year, and mortality rates have declined by about 1% per year. Using simple linear extrapolation, it therefore seems that the ACS challenge goals of reducing cancer incidence by 25% and mortality by 50% over 25 years may be only half achieved.[34,35] Clearly, though, estimating future trends only by linear extrapolation is a crude way to foretell future events. There has been considerable statistical work done on the challenge of predicting cancer incidence at the onset of each year.[36] These methods use various statistical models to predict cancer by lagging cancer incidence and mortality data by 2 to 3 years. Projecting cancer trends into the more distant future is more difficult, though, as many past trends have been nonlinear. Nonetheless, knowledge about changes in major cancer risk factors can lead to reasonable predictions about the direction and approximate slope of future trends.

One method to incorporate knowledge about trends in risk factors into estimates of future cancer trends is to estimate the impact of changes in the attributable risk (also called the "preventable fraction") in the population for each risk factor.[37] By making assumptions about latency period, then tying changes in factors to changes in cancer incidence and mortality, cancer trends resulting from risk factor changes can be predicted. For example, if there were a factor that explained 30% of a particular cancer, then cutting that exposure in half would eventually lead to a projected 15% reduction in rates (50% of 30%). This method was used to project cancer mortality trends to 2015, and seems to have projected trends that are quite similar to those observed in recent years.[34,35,37] However, it is important to remember that any predictions are only best guesses based on past events and reasonable judgments.

Progress in cancer prevention, early detection, and treatment since 1990 has been persistent, and there are many reasons to be optimistic about the future. Just how much steeper the future downward slope in cancer death rates can be driven will depend on the extent to which we can discover new factors causing cancer, and effectively enact efforts to better act on our current knowledge about how to prevent and control cancer.[38,39] Especially important will be progress in reversing the epidemics of tobacco use and obesity, and assuring that the coming improvements to health care access will lead to access for all to state-of-the-art cancer screening and therapy.

Selected References

1. American Cancer Society Board of Directors. ACS Challenge goals for U.S. Cancer Mortality for the Year 2015. *Proceedings of the Board of Directors.* Atlanta, GA: American Cancer Society, 1996.
2. American Cancer Society Board of Directors. ACS Challenge goals for U.S. Cancer Incidence for the Year 2015. *Proceedings of the Board of Directors.* Atlanta, GA: American Cancer Society, 1998.
3. Surveillance, Epidemiology, and End Results. SEER program information. http://seer.cancer.gov.
4. National Program of Cancer Registries. http://cdc.gov/cancer/npcr.
5. Edwards B, Ward E, Kohler B, et al. Annual Report to the Nation on the Status of Cancer, 1975-2006, featuring colorectal cancer trends and impact of interventions (risk factors, screening, and treatment) to reduce future rates. *Cancer* 2010;116:544-73.
6. Behavioral Risk Factor Surveillance System. http://cdc.gov/brfss.
7. Ward E, Thun M, Hannan L, Jemal A. Interpreting cancer trends. *Ann NY Acad Sci* 2006;1076:29.
8. Centers for Disease Control. http://cdc.gov/tobacco.
9. Mokdad A, Bowman B, Ford E, et al. The continuing epidemic of obesity and diabetes in the United States. *JAMA* 2001;286:1195.
10. Writing group for the Women's Health Initiative Investigators. Risks and benefits of estrogen plus progestin in healthy postmenopausal women: principal results from the Womens Health Initiative randomized controlled trial. *JAMA* 2002;288:321.
11. Hersh A, Stefanick M, Stafford R. National use of postmenopausal hormone therapy. *JAMA* 2004;291;47.
12. Kondro W. Decline in breast cancer since HRT study. *CMAJ* 2007;176(2):160.
13. Ryerson AB, Miller J, Eheman CR, White MC. Use of mammograms among women aged ≥40 years—United States, 2000–2005. *MMWR* 2007;56:49.
14. Centers for Disease Control. U.S. mortality data. http://wonder.cdc.gov.
15. Anderson R, Minino A, Hoyert D, Rosenberg H. Comparability of cause of death between ICD-9 and ICD-10: preliminary estimates. *National Vital Statistics Reports* 2001;49(2), May.
16. Potosky A, Feuer E, Levin D. Impact of screening on incidence and mortality of prostate cancer in the United States. *Epidemiol Rev* 2001;23(1):181.
17. Jemal A, Siegel R, Ward E, Hao Y, Xu J, Thun M. Cancer statistics, 2009. *CA Cancer J Clin* 2009;59:225.
18. Giovino GA. Epidemiology of tobacco use in the United States. *Oncogene* 2002;21:7326.
19. Wingo P, Ries L, Giovino G, et al. Annual report to the nation on the state of cancer, 1973-1996, with a special section on lung cancer and tobacco smoking. *J Natl Cancer Inst* 1999;91:675.
20. Gohagan J, Prorok P, Hayes R, et al. The Prostate, Lung, Colorectal and Ovarian (PLCO) Cancer Screening Trial of the National Cancer Institute: history, organization, and status. *Control Clin Trials* 2000;21(6 Suppl):251S.
21. Warner E, Mulshine J. Lung cancer screening with spiral CT: toward a working strategy. *Oncology* 2004;18(5):564.
22. Anonymous. Low-dose CT shows clear mortality benefit for lung cancer screening in heavy smokers. NCI cancer Bulletin. Nov 16, 2010. http://www.cancer.gov/ncicancerbulletin/111610/page 4.
23. Martinez ME. Primary prevention of colorectal cancer: lifestyle, nutrition, exercise. *Recent Results Cancer Res* 2005;166:177.
24. Winawer S, Zauber A, Ho M, et al. Prevention of colorectal cancer by colonoscopic polypectomy: the National Polyp Study Workgroup. *N Engl J Med* 1993;329:1977.
25. Atkin W, Edwards R, Kralj-Hans I, et al. Once-only flexible sigmoidoscopy screening in prevention of colorectal cancer: a multi-centre randomized controlled trial. *Lancet* 2010;375:1624.
26. Cram P, Fendrick A, Inadomi J, et al. The impact of celebrity promotional campaign on the use of colon cancer screening: the Katie Couric effect. *Arch Intern Med* 2003;163(13):1601.
27. International Agency for Cancer Research. *Weight control and physical activity.* Handbook 6. Lyon, France: IARC Press, 2002.
28. Ogden CL, Carroll MD, Curtin LR, McDowell MA, Tabak CJ, Flegal KM. Prevalence of overweight and obesity in the United States, 1999–2004. *JAMA* 2006;295:1549.
29. Vogel V, Constantino J, Wickerham D, et al. Effects of tamoxifen vs raloxifene on the risks of developing invasive breast cancer and other disease outcomes: the NSABP Study of Tamoxifen and Raloxifene (STAR) P-2 trial. *JAMA* 2006;295:2727–41.
30. Berry D, Cronin K, Plevritis S, et al. Effect of screening and adjuvant therapy on mortality from breast cancer. *N Engl J Med* 2005;353:1784.
31. Andriole GL, Crawford ED, Grubb RL 3rd, et al. 2009. Mortality results from a randomized prostate-cancer screening trial. *N Engl J Med* 360(13): 1310.
32. Schröder FH, Hugosson J, Roobol MJ, et al. 2009. Screening and prostate-cancer mortality in a randomized European study. *N Engl J Med* 360(13): 1320.
33. Thompson I, Goodman P, Tengen C, et al. The influence of finasteride on the development of prostate cancer. *N Engl J Med* 2003;349:215.
34. Byers T, Barrera E, Fontham E, et al. A midpoint assessment of the American Cancer society challenge goal to halve the U.S. cancer mortality rates between the years 1990 and 2015. *Cancer* 2006;107:396.
35. Sedjo R, Byers T, Barrera E, et al. A midpoint assessment of the American Cancer Society challenge goal to decrease cancer incidence by 25% between 1992 and 2015. *CA Cancer J Clin* 2007;57:326.
36. Pickle L, Hao Y, Zhaohui Z, et al. A new method of estimating United States and state-level cancer incidence counts for the current calendar year. *CA Cancer J Clin* 2007;57:30.
37. Byers T, Mouchawar J, Marks J, et al. The American Cancer Society challenge goals: how far can cancer rates decline in the U.S. by the year 2015? *Cancer* 1999;86:715.
38. Curry S, Byers T, Hewitt M, eds. *Fulfilling the potential of cancer prevention and early detection.* National Cancer Policy Board, Institute of Medicine, The National Academies Press, Washington, DC; 2003.
39. World Cancer Research Fund/American Institute for Cancer Prevention. Policy and Action for Cancer Prevention. *Food, nutrition, and physical activity: a global perspective.* Washington, DC: AICR, 2009.

PART THREE
PRINCIPLES OF CANCER TREATMENT

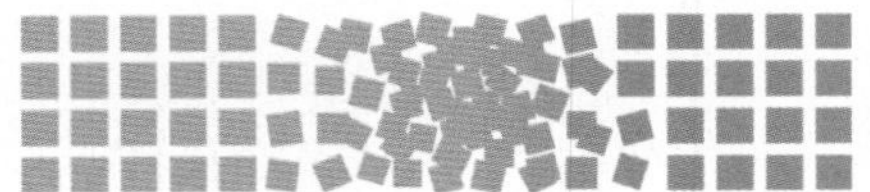

CHAPTER 25 SURGICAL ONCOLOGY: GENERAL ISSUES

STEVEN A. ROSENBERG

Surgery is the oldest treatment for cancer and, until recently, was the only treatment that could cure patients with cancer. The surgical treatment of cancer has changed dramatically over the past several decades. Advances in surgical techniques and a better understanding of the patterns of spread of individual cancers have allowed surgeons to perform successful resections for an increased number of patients. Improvements in radiation therapy and the development of systemic treatments that can control microscopic disease have prompted surgeons to reassess the magnitude of surgery necessary. The surgeon has a central role in the prevention, diagnosis, treatment, palliation, and rehabilitation of the cancer patient. The principles underlying each of these roles of the surgical oncologist are discussed in this chapter.

HISTORICAL PERSPECTIVE

Although the earliest discussions of the surgical treatment of tumors are found in the Edwin Smith papyrus from the Egyptian Middle Kingdom (circa 1600 BC), the modern era of elective surgery for visceral tumors began in frontier America in 1809.[1,2] Ephraim McDowell removed a 22-pound ovarian tumor from a patient, Mrs. Jane Todd Crawford, who survived for 30 years after the operation. This procedure, the first of 13 ovarian resections performed by McDowell, was the first elective abdominal operation and provided a stimulus to the development of elective surgery.

The surgical treatment of increasing numbers of cancer patients depended on two subsequent developments in surgery. The first of these was the introduction of general anesthesia by two dentists, Dr. William Morton and Dr. Crawford Long. The first major operation using general ether anesthesia was the excision of the submaxillary gland and part of the tongue, performed by Dr. John Collins Warren on October 16, 1846, at the Massachusetts General Hospital. The second major development resulted from the introduction of the principles of antisepsis by Joseph Lister in 1867. Based on the concepts of Pasteur, Lister introduced carbolic acid in 1867 and described the principles of antisepsis in an article in the *Lancet* that same year.

These developments freed surgery from pain and sepsis and greatly increased its use for the treatment of cancer. In the decade before the introduction of ether, only 385 operations were performed at the Massachusetts General Hospital. By the last decade of the 19th century, more than 20,000 operations per year were performed at that hospital.[3]

Table 25.1 lists selected milestones in the history of surgical oncology. Although this list does not include all the important developments, it indicates the tempo of the application of surgery to cancer treatment.[4] Major figures in the evolution of surgical oncology included Albert Theodore Billroth, who, in addition to developing meticulous surgical techniques, performed the first gastrectomy, laryngectomy, and esophagectomy. In the 1890s, William Stewart Halsted elucidated the principles of *en bloc* resections for cancer, exemplified by the radical mastectomy. Examples of radical resections for cancers of individual organs include the radical prostatectomy performed by Hugh Young in 1904, the radical hysterectomy performed by Ernest Wertheim in 1906, the abdominoperineal resection for cancer of the rectum performed by W. Ernest Miles in 1908, and the first successful pneumonectomy performed for cancer by Evarts Graham in 1933. Modern technical innovations continue to extend the surgeon's capabilities. Recent examples include the development of microsurgical techniques that enable the performance of free graft procedures for reconstruction, automatic stapling devices, sophisticated equipment that allows for a wide variety of endoscopic surgery, and major improvements in postoperative management and critical care of patients that have improved the safety of major surgical therapy.

Critics who believe that the application of surgery has reached a plateau beyond which it will not progress should remember the words of a famous British surgeon Sir John Erichsen, who, in his introductory address to the medical institutions at University College, said: "There must be a final limit to the development of manipulative surgery, the knife cannot always have fresh fields for conquest and although methods of practice may be modified and varied and even improved to some extent, it must be within a certain limit. That this limit has nearly, if not quite, been reached will appear evident if we reflect on the great achievements of modern operative surgery. Very little remains for the boldest to devise or the most dextrous to perform." These comments, published in *Lancet* in 1873, preceded most important developments in modern surgical oncology.

ANESTHESIA FOR ONCOLOGIC SURGERY

Modern anesthetic techniques have greatly increased the safety of major oncologic surgery. Regional and general anesthesia play important roles in a wide variety of diagnostic techniques, in local therapeutic maneuvers, and in major surgery.

Anesthetic techniques may be divided into those for regional and those for general anesthesia.[5] *Topical anesthesia* refers to the application of local anesthetics to the skin or mucous membranes. Local anesthesia involves injection of anesthetic agents directly into the operative field. *Field block* refers to injection of local anesthetic by circumscribing the operative field with a continuous wall of anesthetic agent. Lidocaine (Xylocaine) in concentrations from 0.5% to 1.0%

TABLE 25.1

SELECTED HISTORICAL MILESTONES IN SURGICAL ONCOLOGY

Year	Surgeon	Event
1809	Ephraim McDowell	Elective abdominal surgery (excised ovarian tumor)
1846	John Collins Warren	Use of ether anesthesia (excised submaxillary gland)
1867	Joseph Lister	Introduction of antisepsis
1860–1890	Albert Theodore Billroth	First gastrectomy, laryngectomy, and esophagectomy
1878	Richard von Volkmann	Excision of cancerous rectum
1880s	Theodore Kocher	Development of thyroid surgery
1890	William Stewart Halsted	Radical mastectomy
1896	G. T. Beatson	Oophorectomy for breast cancer
1904	Hugh H. Young	Radical prostatectomy
1906	Ernest Wertheim	Radical hysterectomy
1908	W. Ernest Miles	Abdominoperineal resection for rectal cancer
1912	E. Martin	Cordotomy for the treatment of pain
1910–1930	Harvey Cushing	Development of surgery for brain tumors
1913	Franz Torek	Successful resection of cancer of the thoracic esophagus
1927	G. Divis	Successful resection of pulmonary metastases
1933	Evarts Graham	Pneumonectomy
1935	A. O. Whipple	Pancreaticoduodenectomy
1945	Charles B. Huggins	Adrenalectomy for prostate cancer
1958	Bernard Fisher	Organization of NSABP to conduct prospective randomized trials

NSABP, National Surgical Adjuvant Breast and Bowel Project.

is the most common anesthetic agent used for this purpose. Peripheral nerve block results from the deposition of a local anesthetic surrounding major nerve trunks. It can provide local anesthesia to entire anatomic areas.

Major surgical procedures in the lower portion of the body can be performed using epidural or spinal anesthesia. Epidural anesthesia results from the deposition of a local anesthetic agent into the extradural space within the vertebral canal. Catheters can be left in place in the epidural space, allowing the intermittent injection of local anesthetics for prolonged operations and for postoperative pain control. The major advantage of epidural over spinal anesthesia is that it does not involve puncturing the dura, and the injection of foreign substances directly into the cerebrospinal fluid is avoided.

Spinal anesthesia involves the direct injection of a local anesthetic into the cerebrospinal fluid. Puncture of the dural sac generally is performed between the L2 and L4 vertebrae. Spinal anesthesia provides excellent anesthesia for intra-abdominal operations, operations on the pelvis, or procedures involving the lower extremities. Because the patient can be awake during spinal anesthesia and is breathing spontaneously, it is often thought that spinal anesthesia is safer than general anesthesia. There is no difference in the incidence of intraoperative hypotension with spinal anesthesia and with general anesthesia, and there is no clear benefit in using spinal anesthesia for patients with ischemic heart disease.[6] Because patients are awake during spinal anesthesia and can become agitated during the surgical procedure, spinal anesthesia actually can cause more myocardial stress than general anesthesia. The health status of patients with preoperative evidence of congestive heart failure is more likely to be worsened by general anesthesia than by spinal anesthesia. Because of the local irritating effects of general anesthesia on the lung, it has been suggested that spinal anesthesia may be safer for patients with severe pulmonary disease.

General anesthesia refers to the reversible state of loss of consciousness produced by chemical agents that act directly on the brain. Most major oncologic procedures are performed using general anesthesia, which can be induced using intravenous or inhalational agents. The advantages of intravenous anesthesia are the extremely rapid onset of unconsciousness and improved patient comfort and acceptance.

A variety of inhalational anesthetic agents are in clinical use. Nitrous oxide is popular, usually in combination with narcotics and muscle relaxants. This technique provides a safe form of general anesthesia with the use of nonexplosive agents. Fluorinated hydrocarbons were introduced in the mid-1950s and represented a major improvement over other inhalational agents such as ether or chloroform because they facilitated more rapid induction and emergence than other inhalational agents. Halothane was widely used but had several significant side effects; It has been replaced by other agents. Isoflurane, approved in 1979, rapidly replaced halothane as the most commonly used inhalational agent. Isoflurane induces less reduction of cardiac output and less sensitization to the arrhythmia-inducing effects of catecholamines, although isoflurane-induced tachycardia continues to represent a clinical problem. Sevoflurane and desflurane are other inhalational agents in common use.

Intravenous agents are often used to induce anesthesia, although they are rarely used to provide total anesthesia for surgical procedures. Intravenous induction is rapid, pleasant, and safe and is usually preferred over inhalational induction. The five most common intravenous agents used in the United States for induction of anesthesia are sodium thiopental, ketamine, propofol, etomidate, and midazolam.

Virtually all general anesthetics affect biochemical mechanisms, with actions including depression of bone marrow, alteration of the phagocytic activity of macrophages, and immunosuppression. General anesthetic agents such as cyclopropane and diethyl ether rarely are used because of their explosive potential.

Intravenous neuromuscular blocking agents, called *muscle relaxants*, are commonly used during general anesthesia. These agents either are nondepolarizing (e.g., rocuronium and *cis*-atracuronium), preventing access of acetylcholine to the receptor site of the myoneural junction, or are depolarizing (e.g., succinylcholine), acting in a manner similar to that of acetylcholine by depolarizing the motor endplate. These agents induce profound muscle relaxation during surgical procedures but have the disadvantage of inhibiting spontaneous respiration because of paralysis of respiratory muscles. Succinylcholine is short acting (3 to 5 minutes) with a rapid recovery phase, whereas nondepolarizing agents can cause more prolonged paralysis (30 to 40 minutes).

DETERMINATION OF OPERATIVE RISK

As with any treatment, the potential benefits of surgical intervention in cancer patients must be weighed against the risks of surgery. The incidence of operative mortality is of major importance in formulating therapeutic decisions and is a complex function of the basic disease process that involves surgical factors, anesthetic technique, operative complications, and, most importantly, the general health status of patients and their ability to withstand operative trauma.

In an attempt to classify the physical status of patients and their surgical risks, the American Society of Anesthesiologists (ASA) has formulated a general classification of physical status that appears to correlate well with operative mortality.[7] Patients are classified into five groups depending on their general health status, as shown in Table 25.2.

Operative mortality usually is defined as mortality that occurs within 30 days of a major operative procedure. In oncologic patients, the basic disease process is a major determinant of operative mortality. Patients undergoing palliative surgery for widely metastatic disease have a high operative mortality rate even if the surgical procedure can alleviate the symptomatic problem. Examples of these situations include surgery for intestinal obstruction in patients with widespread ovarian cancer and surgery for gastric outlet obstruction in patients with cancer of the head of the pancreas. These simple palliative procedures are associated with mortality rates up to 20% because of the debilitated state of the patient and the rapid progression of the underlying disease.

Anesthesia-related mortality has decreased in the past four decades, largely because of the development of rigid practice standards and improved intraoperative monitoring techniques.[8–12] A study of 485,850 instances of anesthetic administration in 1986 in the United Kingdom revealed the risk of death from anesthesia alone to be approximately 1 in 185,000.[9] In a retrospective review encompassing cases from 1976 through 1988, Eichhorn[10] estimated anesthetic mortality in ASA class I and II patients to be 1 in 200,200. These are probably underestimates because underreporting of anesthetic-related deaths is a problem in all studies. Most cancer patients undergoing elective surgery fall between physical status classes I and II; thus, an anesthetic mortality rate of 0.01% to 0.001% is a realistic estimate for this group.

TABLE 25.2

AMERICAN SOCIETY OF ANESTHESIOLOGISTS CLASSIFICATION OF PHYSICAL STATUS

CLASS I
A normal healthy patient with no organic, physiologic, biochemical, or psychiatric disturbance. The abnormal process for which operation is to be performed is localized and does not entail a systemic disturbance (i.e., a fit patient with inguinal hernia or a fibroid uterus in an otherwise healthy woman).

CLASS II
A patient with mild to moderate systemic disturbance caused either by the condition to be treated surgically or by other pathophysiologic processes (i.e., nonorganic or only slightly limiting organic heart disease, mild diabetes, essential hypertension, or anemia). Some might list the neonate or the octogenarian, even if no discernible systemic disease is present. Extreme obesity and chronic bronchitis may be included in this category.

CLASS III
A patient with severe systemic disease that limits activity but is not incapacitating, even though it may not be possible to define the degree of disability with finality (i.e., severely limiting organic heart disease; severe diabetes with vascular complications; moderate to severe degrees of pulmonary insufficiency; and angina pectoris or healed myocardial infarction).

CLASS IV
A patient with an incapacitating systemic disease that is a constant threat to life and not always correctable by operation (i.e., patients with organic heart disease showing marked signs of cardiac insufficiency, persistent anginal syndrome, or active myocarditis; and advanced degrees of pulmonary, hepatic, renal, or endocrine insufficiency).

CLASS V
A moribund patient who is not expected to survive 24 hours without operation or who has little chance of survival but is submitted to operation in desperation (i.e., the burst abdominal aneurysm with profound shock, major cerebral trauma with rapidly increasing intracranial pressure, and massive pulmonary embolus). Most of these patients require operation as a resuscitative measure with little, if any, anesthesia.

STATUS E
In the event of emergency operation, precede the number with an E. Any patient in one of the classes listed previously who is operated on as an emergency is considered to be in poorer physical condition. The letter E is placed beside the numeric classification. Thus, the patient with a hitherto uncomplicated hernia now incarcerated and associated with nausea and vomiting is classified as IE. By definition, class V always constitutes an emergency.

(From ref. 7, with permission.)

TABLE 25.3

RISK FACTORS ASSOCIATED WITH 7-DAY OPERATIVE MORTALITY

Variable	Description	Relative Odds of Dying
Patient factors		
Age	>80 y vs. <60 y	3.29
Gender	Female vs. male	0.77
Physical status	ASA III–V vs. ASA I–II	10.65
Surgical factors		
Operation type	Major vs. minor	3.82
Length	>2 h vs. <2 h	1.08
Urgency	Emergency vs. elective	4.44
Anesthesia factors		
Techniques	Inhalation + narcotic vs. inhalation alone	0.76
	Narcotic alone vs. inhalation alone	1.41
	Narcotic + inhalation vs. inhalation alone	0.79
	Spinal vs. inhalation alone	0.53
	Number of anesthetic drugs: 1–2 vs. >3	2.94
Experience of anesthetist	>600 procedures/y for 8+ y vs.<600 procedures/y for <8 y	1.06

ASA, American Society of Anesthesiologists.
(From ref. 13, with permission.)

Anesthesia-related mortality is rare, and factors related to the patient's pre-existing general health status and disease are far more important indicators of surgical outcome. A study of the factors contributing to the risk of 7-day operative mortality after 100,000 surgical procedures yielded the findings shown in Table 25.3.[13] The 7-day perioperative mortality in this study was 71.4 deaths per 10,000 cases, and the major determinants of death were the physical status of the patient, the emergent nature of the procedure, and the magnitude of the operation.

The five most common causes of death after surgery are bronchopneumonia, congestive heart failure, myocardial infarction, pulmonary embolism, and respiratory failure. Perioperative pulmonary complications, therefore, are a major threat, and the major patient-related risk factors associated with postoperative pulmonary complications are smoking, age over 70, obesity, and chronic obstructive pulmonary disease (Table 25.4). Patients with a recent myocardial infarction have a significantly higher incidence of reinfarction and cardiac death associated with surgery. Significant improvements have occurred as new techniques

TABLE 25.4

PATIENT-RELATED RISK FACTORS ASSOCIATED WITH POSTOPERATIVE PULMONARY COMPLICATIONS

Potential Risk Factor	Type of Surgery	Relative Risk Associated with Factor
Smoking	Coronary bypass	3.4
	Abdominal	1.4–4.3
ASA class higher than II	Unselected	1.7
	Thoracic or abdominal	1.5–3.2
Age older than 70 y	Unselected	1.9–2.4
	Thoracic or abdominal	0.9–1.9
Obesity	Unselected	1.3
	Thoracic or abdominal	0.8–1.7
Chronic obstructive pulmonary disease	Unselected	2.7–3.6
	Thoracic or abdominal	4.7

ASA, American Society of Anesthesiologists.
(From ref. 8, with permission.)

TABLE 25.5

LIFE EXPECTANCY AS A FUNCTION OF AGE

Male		Female	
Age (y)	Life Expectancy (years)	Age (y)	Life Expectancy (years)
62	19.2	62	23.6
63	18.4	63	22.7
64	17.6	64	21.9
65	16.9	65	21.0
66	16.1	66	20.2
67	15.4	67	19.4
68	14.7	68	18.6
69	14.0	69	17.9
70	13.3	70	17.1
71	12.7	71	16.4
72	12.1	72	15.6
73	11.5	73	14.9
74	10.9	74	14.3
75	10.4	75	13.6
76	9.9	76	12.9
77	9.4	77	12.3
78	8.9	78	11.7
79	8.4	79	11.1
80	8.0	80	10.5
81	7.5	81	10.0
82	7.1	82	9.5
83	6.8	83	9.0
84	6.4	84	8.5
85	6.1	85	8.0
86	5.8	86	7.6
87	5.5	87	7.1
88	5.2	88	6.7
89	4.9	89	6.4
90	4.7	90	6.0
91	4.4	91	5.6
92	4.2	92	5.3
93	4.0	93	5.0
94	3.8	94	4.7
95	3.6	95	4.4
96	3.4	96	4.4
97	3.2	97	4.1
98	3.0	98	3.8
99	2.8	99	3.5
100	2.6	100	3.3
101	2.4	101	3.0
102	2.2	102	2.8
103	2.0	103	2.6
104	1.9	104	2.4

of anesthetic monitoring and hemodynamic support have been developed.[14–16]

The impact of general health status on operative mortality is seen when operative mortality as a function of age is analyzed. In a study of the postoperative mortality of 17,199 patients undergoing general surgical procedures, the overall mortality rate for patients younger than age 70 was 0.25%, compared with 9.2% for patients older than age 70.[17] In these elderly patients, the operative mortality rate for emergency operations was 36.8%, compared with 7.8% for elective surgical procedures. The four leading causes of operative mortality that accounted for approximately 75% of all postoperative deaths in this age group were pulmonary embolism, pneumonia, cardiovascular collapse, and the primary illness itself.

Hoskings et al.[18] reviewed the outcome of surgery performed on 795 patients aged 90 years or older. Surgery was generally well tolerated. As with younger patients, the ASA classification was an important predictor of outcome.

Cancer is often a disease of the elderly, and there is sometimes a tendency to avoid even curative major surgery for cancer in patients of advanced age. In the United States and in most Western countries, life expectancies for the elderly have increased substantially. The life expectancy in years of patients between the ages of 62 and 104 in the United States is shown in Table 25.5. The average life expectancies for 80-year-old men and women in the United States are 8 and 10.5 years, respectively. The expected survival of 90-year-old men and women is 4.7 and 6.0 years, respectively. Thus, even in the very old cancer patient, aggressive curative surgery can be warranted.[19]

ROLES FOR SURGERY

Prevention of Cancer

All surgical oncologists should be aware of the high-risk situations that require surgery to prevent subsequent malignant disease. Some underlying conditions or congenital or genetic traits are associated with an extremely high incidence of subsequent cancer. When these cancers are likely to occur in nonvital organs, it is necessary to remove the potentially involved organ to prevent subsequent malignancy.[20] Examples of diseases associated with a high incidence of cancer that can be prevented by prophylactic surgery are presented in Table 25.6 and are considered in more detail in Chapter 52. An excellent illustration is presented by patients with the genetic trait for multiple polyposis of the colon. If colectomy is not performed in these patients, approximately half will develop colon cancer by the age of 40. By age 70, virtually all patients with multiple polyposis will develop colon cancer.[20] It is therefore advisable for all patients containing the mutant gene for multiple polyposis to undergo prophylactic colectomy before age 20 to prevent these cancers. Approximately 40% of patients with ulcerative colitis who have total colonic involvement ultimately die of colon cancer if they survive the ulcerative colitis.[21] Three percent of children with ulcerative colitis develop cancer of the colon by the age of 10, and 20% develop cancer during each ensuing decade.[22] Colectomy is indicated for patients with ulcerative colitis if the chronicity of this disease is well established. Patients with multiple endocrine neoplasia type 2A can be screened using polymerase chain reaction–based direct DNA testing for mutations in the *RET* protooncogene. This is the preferred method for screening kindred with multiple endocrine neoplasia type 2A to identify individuals in whom total thyroidectomy is indicated, regardless of the plasma calcitonin levels.[23] A more complex example of the role of surgery in cancer prevention involves women at high risk for breast cancer. Because the risk of cancer in some women is increased substantially over the normal risk (but does not approach 100%), counseling that explains the benefits and risks of prophylactic mastectomy is an important part of the care of these patients. Genetic tests for the presence of *BRCA1* and *BRCA2* mutations provide valuable information. Statistical techniques can provide approximations of the risk for patients, depending on the frequency of disease in the family history, the age at the first pregnancy, and the presence of fibrocystic disease.

TABLE 25.6

CONDITIONS IN WHICH PROPHYLACTIC SURGERY CAN PREVENT CANCER

Underlying Condition	Associated Cancer	Prophylactic Surgery
Cryptorchidism	Testicular	Orchiopexy
Polyposis coli	Colon	Colectomy
Familial colon cancer	Colon	Colectomy
Ulcerative colitis	Colon	Colectomy
Multiple endocrine neoplasia types 2 and 3	Medullary cancer of the thyroid	Thyroidectomy
Familial breast cancer	Breast	Mastectomy
Familial ovarian cancer	Ovary	Oophorectomy

Diagnosis of Cancer

The major role of surgery in the diagnosis of cancer lies in the acquisition of tissue for exact histologic diagnosis. The principles underlying the biopsy of malignant lesions vary, depending on the natural history of the tumor under consideration. Various techniques exist for obtaining tissues suspected of malignancy, including aspiration biopsy, needle biopsy, incisional biopsy, and excisional biopsy.

Aspiration biopsy involves the aspiration of cells and tissue fragments through a needle that has been guided into the suspect tissue. In *needle biopsy*, a core of tissue is obtained through a specially designed needle introduced into the suspect tissue. The core of tissue provided by needle biopsy is sufficient for the diagnosis of most tumor types. *Incisional biopsy* refers to removal of a small wedge of tissue from a larger tumor mass. Incisional biopsies often are necessary for diagnosis of large masses that require major surgical procedures for even local excision. *Excisional biopsy* refers to excision of the entire suspected tumor tissue with little or no margin of surrounding normal tissue. Care should be taken to avoid contaminating new tissue planes or further compromising the ultimate surgical procedure.

The following principles guide the performance of all surgical biopsies:

1. Needle tracks or scars should be placed so that they can be conveniently removed as part of the subsequent definitive surgical procedure. Placement of biopsy incisions is extremely important, and misplacement often can compromise subsequent care. Incisions on the extremity generally should be placed longitudinally so as to make the removal of underlying tissue and subsequent closure easier.
2. Care should be taken to avoid contaminating new tissue planes during the biopsy procedure. The development of large hematomas after biopsy can lead to tumor spread and

must be scrupulously avoided by securing excellent hemostasis during the biopsy. For biopsies on extremities, the use of a tourniquet may help to control bleeding. Instruments used in a biopsy procedure are another potential source of contamination of new tissue planes. It is not uncommon to take biopsy samples from several suspected lesions at one time. Care should be taken to avoid using instruments that may have come in contact with a tumor when obtaining tissue from a potentially uncontaminated area.

3. Adequate tissue samples must be obtained to meet the needs of the pathologist. For the diagnosis of selected tumors, electron microscopy, tissue culture, or other techniques may be necessary. Sufficient tissue must be obtained for these purposes if diagnostic difficulties are anticipated.
4. When knowledge of the orientation of the biopsy specimen is important for subsequent treatment, it is important to mark distinctive areas of the tumor to facilitate subsequent orientation of the specimen by the pathologist. Certain fixatives are best suited to specific types or sizes of tissue. If all biopsy specimens are placed in formalin immediately, the opportunity to perform valuable diagnostic tests may be lost. The handling of excised tissue is the surgeon's responsibility.
5. Placement of radiopaque clips during biopsy and staging procedures is sometimes important to delineate areas of known tumor and to guide the subsequent delivery of radiation therapy to these areas.

Treatment of Cancer

Surgery can be a simple, safe method to cure patients with solid tumors when the tumor is confined to the anatomic site of origin. The extension of the surgical resection to include areas of regional spread can cure some patients, although regional spread often is an indication of undetectable distant micrometastases.

The role of surgery in the treatment of cancer patients can be divided into six areas: (1) definitive surgical treatment for primary cancer, selection of appropriate local therapy, and integration of surgery with other adjuvant modalities; (2) surgery to reduce the bulk of disease (e.g., ovarian cancer); (3) surgical resection of metastatic disease with curative intent (e.g., pulmonary metastases in sarcoma patients, hepatic metastases from colorectal cancer); (4) surgery for the treatment of oncologic emergencies; (5) surgery for palliation; and (6) surgery for reconstruction and rehabilitation. In each area, integration with other treatment modalities can be essential for a successful outcome.

Resection of the Primary Cancer

Three major challenges confront the surgical oncologist in the definitive treatment of solid tumors: accurate identification of patients who can be cured by local treatment alone; development and selection of local treatments that provide the best balance between local cure and the impact of treatment morbidity on the quality of life; and development and application of adjuvant treatments that can improve the control of locally invasive and distant metastatic disease. The selection of the appropriate local therapy to be used in cancer treatment varies with the individual cancer type and the site of involvement. In many instances, definitive surgical therapy that encompasses a sufficient margin of normal tissue is sufficient local therapy. The treatment of many solid tumors falls into this category, including the wide excision of primary melanomas in the skin, which can be cured locally by surgery alone in approximately 90% of cases. The resection of colon cancers with a 5-cm margin from the tumor results in anastomotic recurrences in fewer than 5% of cases.

In other instances, surgery is used to obtain histologic confirmation of diagnosis, but primary local therapy is achieved through the use of a nonsurgical modality, such as radiation therapy. Examples include the treatment of Ewing sarcoma in long bones and the treatment of selected primary malignancies in the head and neck. In each instance, selection of the definitive local treatment involves careful consideration of the likelihood of cure balanced against the morbidity of the treatment modality.

The magnitude of surgical resection is modified in the treatment of many cancers by the use of adjuvant treatment modalities. Rationally integrating surgery with other treatments requires a careful consideration of all effective treatment options. It is knowledge of this rapidly changing field that most distinctly separates the surgical oncologist from the general surgeon.

In some instances, the availability of effective adjuvant modalities has led to a decrease in the magnitude of surgery. The evolution of treatment for childhood rhabdomyosarcoma is a striking example of the successful integration of adjuvant therapies with surgery in the treatment of cancer.[24,25] Childhood rhabdomyosarcoma is the most common soft-tissue sarcoma in infants and children. Before 1970, surgery alone was used almost exclusively, and 5-year survival rates of 10% to 20% were commonly reported. Local surgery alone failed in patients with rhabdomyosarcomas of the prostate and extremities because of extensive invasion of surrounding tissues and the early development of metastatic disease. The failure of surgery alone to control local disease in patients with childhood rhabdomyosarcoma led to the introduction of adjuvant radiation therapy. This resulted in a marked improvement in local control rates that was further improved dramatically by the introduction of combination chemotherapy. Long-term cure rates are now in the range of 80%. Many other examples of the integration of surgery with other treatment modalities appear throughout this text.

Cytoreductive Surgery

In some instances, the extensive local spread of cancer precludes the removal of all gross disease by surgery. The partial surgical resection of bulk disease in the treatment of selected cancers improves the ability of other treatment modalities to control residual gross disease that has not been resected.[26,27] Studies that suggest the merit of this approach are discussed in Chapter 104 dealing with ovarian cancer.

Enthusiasm for cytoreductive surgery has led to the inappropriate use of surgery to reduce the bulk of tumor in some cases. Clearly, cytoreductive surgery is of benefit only when other effective treatments are available to control the residual disease that is unresectable. Except in rare palliative settings, there is no role for cytoreductive surgery in patients for whom little other effective therapy exists.

Metastatic Disease

The value of surgery in the cure of patients with metastatic disease tends to be overlooked and is often underused. As a general principle, patients with a single site of metastatic disease that can be resected without major morbidity should undergo resection of that metastatic cancer. Some patients with limited metastases to lung or liver or brain can be cured by surgical resection. This approach is especially appropriate for cancers that do not respond well to systemic chemotherapy. The resection of pulmonary metastases from soft-tissue and bony sarcomas can be curative in as many as 30% of patients. As effective systemic therapy is developed for the treatment of these diseases, cure rates may increase. Studies have shown that similar cure rates occur in patients with adenocarcinomas when resected metastatic disease in the lung is the sole clinical site of metastases. Small numbers of pulmonary metastases often are the only clinically apparent metastatic disease in patients with sarcomas. However, this is rare in the natural history of most adenocarcinomas. If solitary metastases to the lung do occur in patients with carcinoma of the colon or other adenocarcinomas, surgical resection is indicated.

Similarly, resection of hepatic metastases, especially from colorectal cancer, in patients in whom the liver is the only site of known metastatic disease can lead to long-term cure in approximately 25% of patients. This far exceeds the cure rates of any other available treatment.

Resection for cure of solitary brain metastases should also be considered when the brain is the only site of known metastatic disease. The exact location and functional sequelae of resection should be considered when making this treatment decision.

Oncologic Emergencies

As for all patients, emergencies arise for oncologic patients that require surgical intervention. These generally involve the treatment of exsanguinating hemorrhage, perforation, drainage of abscesses, or impending destruction of vital organs. Each category of surgical emergency is unique and requires an individual approach.

The oncologic patient often is neutropenic and thrombocytopenic and has a high risk of hemorrhage or sepsis. Perforations of an abdominal viscus can be caused by direct tumor invasion or by tumor lysis resulting from effective systemic treatments. Perforation of the gastrointestinal tract after effective treatment for lymphoma involving the intestine is not uncommon. Surgery to decompress cancer invading the central nervous system represents another emergency surgical procedure that can lead to preservation of function.

Palliation

Surgical resection often is required for the relief of pain or functional abnormalities. The appropriate use of surgery in these settings can improve the quality of life for cancer patients. Palliative surgery may include procedures to relieve mechanical problems, such as intestinal obstruction, or the removal of masses that are causing severe pain or disfigurement. A study by Krouse et al.[28] has emphasized the role of surgery in the palliative treatment of cancer patients.

Reconstruction and Rehabilitation

Surgical techniques are being refined that aid in the reconstruction and rehabilitation of cancer patients after definitive therapy. The ability to reconstruct anatomic defects can substantially improve function and cosmetic appearance. The development of free flaps using microvascular anastomotic techniques is having a profound impact on the ability to bring fresh tissue to resected or heavily irradiated areas. Lost function (especially of extremities) often can be restored by surgical approaches. This includes lysis of contractures or muscle transposition to restore muscular function that has been damaged by previous surgery or radiation therapy.

SURGICAL ONCOLOGIST

In the past decade, a substantial increase has been seen in the creation of separate sections of surgical oncology in departments of surgery within universities. This enthusiasm derives from the recognition that modern oncologic management requires levels of expertise in cancer surgery, chemotherapy, and radiation therapy that are not common in most general surgeons and from a desire to effectively use the resources being committed to cancer care and research by hospitals, private foundations, and the federal government. A sense of urgency has existed because some surgical leaders believe that the surgeon is experiencing a declining intellectual role in modern cancer treatment and research, and that steps must be taken to reassert the surgeon's role in modern oncology.

Within the next several decades, the United States will experience a dramatic growth in the number of older individuals. The 2000 Nationwide Inpatient Sample and the 1996 National Survey of Ambulatory Surgery estimated that by 2020 the number of patients undergoing oncologic procedures will increase by 24%, and that these will include both outpatient and inpatient procedures.[29] The increase in the number of surgical oncology fellowships available is playing a valuable role in ensuring the supply of surgical oncologic specialists. In one study, 69% of all surgical oncology fellows trained at a major cancer center held "academic full-time" positions.

Further fueling the need for specialists in surgical oncology is a vast body of accumulating data that indicate that the number of difficult surgical procedures for cancer performed by the surgeon is directly related to patient outcome. Many studies have shown that increasing hospital volume for major cancer surgery also has positive impact on patient survival. In one study of 5,013 patients in the Surveillance, Epidemiology, and End Results registry of patients aged 65 years or older, high hospital volume was linked with lower mortality for patients undergoing pancreatectomy ($P = .004$), esophagectomy ($P < .001$), liver resection ($P = .04$), and pelvic exenteration ($P = .04$). In patients undergoing esophagectomy, for example, operative mortality was 17.3% in low-volume hospitals compared with 3.4% in high-volume hospitals. For patients undergoing pancreatectomy, the corresponding rates were 12.9% versus 5.8%.[30] In another study of 474,108 patients who underwent one of eight cardiovascular procedures or cancer resections, a highly significant inverse relationship was seen between surgeon volume and operative mortality for lung resection ($P = .003$) and for bladder cystectomy, esophagectomy, and pancreatic resection ($P < .001$). These differences could not be attributed to differences in the rates of use of adjuvant therapy.[31,32] A recent study emphasized the learning curve involved in the performance of extensive surgical procedures such as pancreaticoduodenectomy. Comparing the first 60 cases per surgeon to the second 60 cases per surgeon, there were statistically significant drops in median blood loss ($P < .001$), operative time ($P < .001$), lengths of stay ($P = .004$), and the incidence of positive or suspicious margins ($P < .001$).[33]

Surgical oncology is increasingly becoming an acknowledged specialty within surgery. The creation of a World Federation of Surgical Oncology societies is helping to increase information exchange. Another positive development in this area was the creation of the American College of Surgeons Oncology Group to bring surgeons together in the performance of clinical trials in surgical oncology. This program has initiated multiple trials exploring the role of surgery in treatment of a variety of cancer types.[34]

The development of surgical oncology as a specialty area of surgery depends on a clear delineation of its role. The Society of Surgical Oncology in the United States has formalized training guidelines for surgeons intending to specialize in surgical oncology that fall in four broad areas, presented in Table 25.7.

TABLE 25.7

TRAINING REQUIREMENTS FOR SPECIALISTS IN SURGICAL ONCOLOGY

Knowledge, Skills, and Clinical Experiences

Clinical and technical skills for providing comprehensive care to cancer patients. An essential component of the fellowship is training in new techniques to produce surgeons capable of providing state-of-the-art surgical care to cancer patients.

Skills in performing special and unusual operations for patients with complex or recurrent neoplasms.

Expertise in diagnosis and management of rare or unusual tumors, based on knowledge of the natural history of such cancers.

Knowledge and experience to determine disease stage and treatment options for individual cancer patients, at the time of diagnosis and throughout the disease course.

Broad knowledge of other cancer treatment modalities (including radiotherapy, chemotherapy, immunotherapy, and endocrine therapy). This requires an understanding of the fundamental biology of cancer, clinical pharmacology, tumor immunology, and endocrinology as well as an understanding of potential complications of multimodality therapy.

Expertise in the selection of patients for surgical therapy in combination with other forms of cancer treatment, as well as knowledge of the benefits and risks associated with a multidisciplinary approach.

Expertise in palliative techniques, including proper selection of patients, proper performance of appropriate palliative surgical procedures, and knowledge of nonsurgical palliative treatments.

Knowledge of tumor biology, carcinogenesis, epidemiology, tumor markers, and tumor pathology.

Cancer Research

Knowledge to design and implement a prospective database and to conduct clinical cancer research, especially prospective clinical trials.

Sufficient familiarity with statistical methods to properly evaluate results of published research studies.

Knowledge to guide a trainee or other personnel in laboratory or clinical oncology research.

Knowledge of the interface of basic science with clinical cancer care, to facilitate translational research.

Cancer Education

Educational knowledge and skills to train students and physicians in the multimodal management of cancer patients.

Knowledge and skills to train nonphysicians (e.g., physician assistants, oncology nurses, enterostomal therapists) in specialized cancer care.

Skills to organize and conduct cancer-related public education programs.

Leadership in Oncology

Skills to develop and support the following:

- Institutional programs relating to cancer, including a tumor registry
- Institutional policies regarding cancer programs and problems
- Interdisciplinary meetings and discussions on cancer topics, patient care, and oncology research program
- Psychosocial and rehabilitative programs for cancer patients and their families

References

1. Brested JH. *The Edwin Smith surgical papyrus*. Chicago: University of Chicago Press; 1930.
2. Thorwald J. *Science and the secrets of early medicine*. New York: Harcourt, Brace, and World; 1962.
3. Wangensteen OH. Has medical history importance for surgeons? *Surg Gynecol Obstet* 1975;140:434.
4. Hill GJ. Historic milestones in cancer surgery. *Semin Oncol* 1979;6:409.
5. Strichartz GR, Berde CB. Local anesthetics. In: Miller RD, ed. *Anesthesia*. New York: Churchill Livingstone; 1994.
6. Goldman L, Caldera DL, Nussbaum SR, et al. Multifactorial index of cardiac risk in noncardiac surgical procedures. *N Engl J Med* 1977;297:845.
7. Dripps RD, Eckenhoff JE, Vandam LD. *Introduction to anesthesia*, 2nd ed. Philadelphia: WB Saunders; 1988.
8. Miller, RD, ed. *Anesthesia*, 5th ed. Philadelphia: Churchill Livingstone; 2000.
9. Buck N, Devlin HB, Lunn JN. *Report on the confidential enquiry into perioperative deaths*. London: Nuffield Provincial Hospitals Trust, The Kings Fund Publishing House; 1987.
10. Eichhorn JH. Prevention of intraoperative anesthesia accidents and related severe injury through safety monitoring. *Anesthesiology* 1989;70:572.
11. Eichhorn JH. Documenting improved anesthesia outcome. *J Clin Anesth* 1991;3:351.
12. Ross AF, Tinker JH. Anesthesia risk. In: Miller RD, ed. *Anesthesia*. New York: Churchill Livingstone; 1994.
13. Cohen MM, Duncan PG, Tate RB. Does anaesthesia contribute to operative mortality? *JAMA* 1988;260:2859.
14. Topkins MJ, Artusio JF. Myocardial infarction and surgery: a five year study. *Anesth Analg* 1964;43:715.
15. Tarhan S, Moffitt EA, Taylor WF, et al. Myocardial infarction after general anesthesia. *JAMA* 1972;199:318.
16. Rao TLK, Jacobs KH, El-Etr AA. Reinfarction following anesthesia in patients with myocardial infarction. *Anesthesiology* 1983;59:499.
17. Palmberg S, Hirsjarvi E. Mortality in geriatric surgery. *Gerontology* 1979;25:103.
18. Hoskings MP, Warner MA, Lobdell EM, et al. Outcomes of surgery in patients 90 years of age and older. *JAMA* 1989;261:1909.
19. Manton KC, Vaupel JW. Survival after the age of 80 in the United States, Sweden, France, England, and Japan. *N Engl J Med* 1995;333:1232.
20. Mulvihill JJ. Cancer control through genetics. In: Arrighi FE, Rao PN, Stubblefield E, eds. *Genes, chromosomes, and neoplasia*. New York: Raven Press; 1980.
21. MacDougall IPM. The cancer risk in ulcerative colitis. *Lancet* 1964;2:655.
22. Devroede GJ, Taylor WF, Sauer WG. Cancer risk and life expectancy of children with ulcerative colitis. *N Engl J Med* 1971;285:17.
23. Wells SA, Chi DD, Toshima K, et al. Predictive DNA testing and prophylactic thyroidectomy in patients at risk for multiple endocrine neoplasia type 2A. *Ann Surg* 1994;220:237.
24. Kilman JW, Clatworthy HW Jr, Newton WA, et al. Reasonable surgery for rhabdomyosarcoma: a study of 67 cases. *Ann Surg* 1973;3:346.
25. Heyn RM, Holland R, Newton WA, et al. The role of combined chemotherapy in the treatment of rhabdomyosarcoma in children. *Cancer* 1974;34:2128.
26. McCarter MD, Fong Y. Role for surgical cytoreduction in multimodality treatments for cancer. *Ann Surg Oncol* 2001;8:38.
27. Wong RJ, De Cosse JJ. Cytoreductive surgery. *Surg Gynecol Obstet* 1990;170:276.

28. Krouse RS, Nelson RA, Farrell BR, et al. Surgical palliation at a cancer center. *Arch Surg* 2001;136:773.
29. Etzioni DA, Liu JH, Maggard MA, et al. Workload projections for surgical oncology: will we need more surgeons? *Ann Surg Oncol* 2003;10:1112.
30. Begg CB, Cramer LD, Hoskins WJ, et al. Impact of hospital volume on operative mortality for major cancer surgery. *JAMA* 1998;280:1747.
31. Birkmeyer JD, Stukel TA, Siewers AE, et al. Surgeon volume and operative mortality in the United States. *N Engl J Med* 2003;349:2117.
32. Birkmeyer JD, Sun Y, Wong SL, Stukel TA. Hospital volume and late survival after cancer surgery. *Ann Surg* 2007;245:777.
33. Tseng JF, Pisters, PWT, Lee JE, et al. The learning curve in pancreatic surgery. *Surgery* 2007;141:456.
34. Wells SA. The American College of Surgeons Oncology Group: its genesis and future directions. *Bull Am Coll Surg* 1998;83:13.

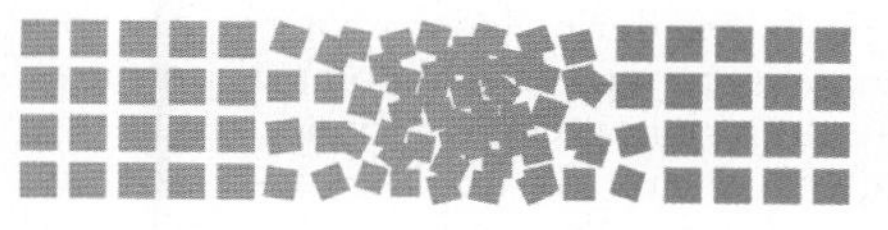

CHAPTER 26 SURGICAL ONCOLOGY: LAPAROSCOPIC SURGERY

YOSHINORI HOSOYA AND ALAN T. LEFOR

Laparoscopy is a valuable tool in the diagnosis and management of many diseases, and is the worldwide standard of care for cholecystectomy, resulting in a dramatically decreased length of hospital stay, increased patient comfort, and rapid return to employment compared to open surgery. Laparoscopy has become an important tool in the care of patients with cancer as well.

The development of laparoscopy spans over a century, and much of the early work is credited to Georg Kelling.[1] In 1901, in a canine model, Kelling insufflated the abdomen via a puncture and then placed a hollow tube through which a viewing laparoscope was inserted. Laparoscopy has a role in the diagnosis, staging, treatment, and palliation of many types of malignancies. The development of new instrumentation was essential for the advancement of laparoscopic surgery, enabling procedures to be performed through air-tight ports inserted into the abdominal cavity (Fig. 26.1). The invention of laparoscopic biopsy instruments has allowed the verification of malignancy by providing tissue specimens, and ultrasound guided biopsy allows the biopsy of masses deep within solid organs. Laparoscopic staging can identify unresectable disease, which often dramatically alters therapy. For resectable disease, a wide range of curative laparoscopic resections have been described. After resection, tumor surveillance can be performed by direct observation, with carcinomatosis identified in second-look operations. In the case of unresectable disease or complications of advanced disease, laparoscopic procedures can provide palliation.

NEW TECHNOLOGY

Innovative techniques to benefit patients are being developed to further refine existing laparoscopic surgical techniques. Recent efforts have included ways to reduce invasiveness of procedures, to improve imaging techniques, and to improve technical results.

Single-Port Access Laparoscopy and Natural Orifice Transluminal Endoscopic Surgery

In attempts to reduce the invasiveness of surgery, recent efforts have focused on single-port access (SPA) laparoscopy as well as natural orifice transluminal endoscopic surgery (NOTES). These techniques have potential importance in laparoscopic diagnosis and staging of malignancies. SPA surgery is being used in a variety of procedures. At a single center, investigators reported having successfully performed cholecystectomy, colon resection, small bowel resection, liver biopsy, splenectomy, and adrenalectomy.[2] Two port access has also been reported for the staging of gynecologic cancers.[3] The clinical application of NOTES has been appropriately restrained but is being applied to cholecystectomy and appendectomy in the context of closely monitored clinical trials at a limited number of institutions.[4] This deserves close monitoring because it may become more important in the future use of laparoscopy in the care of patients with cancer.

Imaging Systems

Attempts are also being made to improve the results of laparoscopic surgery by improving the imaging systems used. In a study of high definition (HD) video versus conventional definition video, participants not only preferred the HD image but also had significantly improved knot-tying performance.[5] Face-mounted binocular displays have also been tested in laparoscopic surgery. In one study, they were found to reduce neck and back strain with improvement of both visualization and overall satisfaction.[6] More recently, the head-mounted display was compared with a conventional wall-mounted display.[7] These authors found improved performance and concluded that the greatest promise may be in combination with other advances in imaging technology.

Robotic Surgery

The use of surgical robots allows surgeons to have several degrees of freedom in the motion of an instrument without tremor. Further randomized prospective trials are needed to define the benefits and limitations of robotic-assisted laparoscopic surgery in the care of the cancer patient. The robotic-assisted radical prostatectomy (RARP) has become the preferred approach at many centers in the United States. The procedure is associated with a steep learning curve and demands careful case selection early in the surgeon's experience as well as an appropriate discussion with the patient regarding surgical margins.[8] Robot-assisted tumor specific rectal surgery (RTSRS) has also been reported. In an analysis of 112 patients from three centers, investigators found a conversion rate of 4.9%, a mean of 14.1 lymph nodes harvested, and margin status comparable to that reported in open surgery series.[9] Further clinical studies will be needed to establish the benefits of this procedure. Robot-assisted gastrectomy (RAG) has also been reported in a series of 100 consecutive patients from the same institution.[10] Investigators reported 33 total gastrectomies and 67 subtotal gastrectomies with D1 + β or D2 lymph node resections. The mean total operative time was 230 minutes. This study establishes the feasibility of this complex procedure. A consensus statement on robotic surgery serves as a resource to the surgical community.[11]

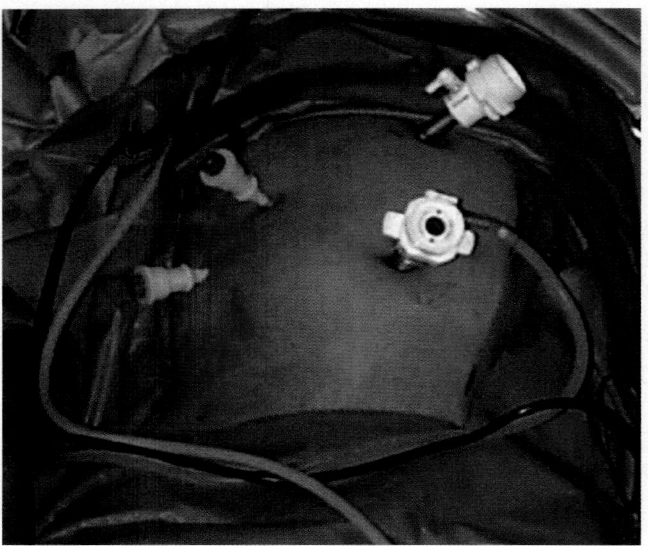

FIGURE 26.1 The placement of operating ports in the insufflated abdomen provides access to the abdominal cavity for laparoscopic surgery.

PHYSIOLOGY OF LAPAROSCOPY

Immunologic Effects

Systemic immunocompetence is better preserved after laparoscopic surgery than after open procedures. Some studies have shown significant decreases in the CD4 and CD8 cell counts in patients undergoing open cholecystectomy, and others have shown a derangement in the ratios of the T-cell subsets.[12] Vallina and Velasco[13] studied peripheral lymphocyte populations in 11 patients undergoing laparoscopic cholecystectomy and found a transient decrease in the CD4 to CD8 ratio, with no difference in absolute CD4 and CD8 cell counts, followed by a return to the preoperative ratio within 1 week of surgery.

Cardiac Effects

In a hemodynamic study carried out during laparoscopic colectomy for carcinoma, patients were monitored with arterial and pulmonary artery catheters along with transesophageal echocardiography.[14] The mean arterial pressure, central venous pressure, mean pulmonary artery pressure, pulmonary capillary wedge pressure, and systemic vascular resistance all increased significantly. Cardiac index and ejection fraction decreased significantly, whereas heart rate remained relatively unchanged. It is likely that the decrease in cardiac function is the direct result of an interaction between decreased venous return and increased transmitted intrathoracic pressure.

Pulmonary Effects

To understand the effects of laparoscopy on an injured lung, a porcine adult respiratory distress syndrome (ARDS) model was used.[15] After ARDS was induced, animals were divided into two groups; one underwent laparoscopy and the other underwent conventional laparotomy. The laparoscopic group demonstrated significantly decreased pulmonary compliance compared with the laparotomy group, had a higher pCO_2, and was more acidotic. Despite the increase in pulmonary derangements caused by laparoscopy in animals with adult respiratory distress syndrome, overall cardiopulmonary function was preserved.

Effects on Malignant Cells

A common physiologic change during laparoscopy is the exposure of abdominal contents to high intraabdominal pressures. Gutt et al.[16] exposed cultures of two human tumor cell lines to 0-mm Hg, 6-mm Hg, and 12-mm Hg CO_2 pressures. The proliferation of colon carcinoma cells increased significantly as pressure increased, whereas pancreatic carcinoma cells proliferated with CO_2 exposure independently of ambient pressure. In a rat model, 36 anesthetized rats underwent laparoscopy and a 1-mL suspension of a moderately differentiated colon adenocarcinoma line was injected intraperitoneally and pneumoperitoneum was held for 60 minutes.[17] Rats that underwent higher pressure laparoscopy had a greater volume of tumor.

Port-Site Metastases

Case reports of port-site metastases in the early 1990s increased in frequency and led to restraint by many surgeons in the application of laparoscopic techniques to patients with cancer. *Port-site metastasis*, broadly defined, is the recurrence of tumor at the small wounds created for the transabdominal placement of ports used to pass instruments or retrieve specimens. Early series reported the incidence of port-site metastases in up to 21% of patients.[18] Hughes et al.[19] reviewed data for 1,603 patients with colon carcinoma treated with conventional laparotomy and found a total recurrence rate of 0.8%. Recurrences included 11 cases in the laparotomy scar and five in the stoma or drain site. Based on large retrospective studies, the wound recurrence in open cases is estimated to be less than 1%. Later reports showed such port-site recurrences to be an uncommon phenomenon. Results for a series of 480 patients in the American Society of Colon and Rectal Surgeons laparoscopic registry showed a port-site recurrence rate of 1.1%.[20] In 2001, Zmora and Weiss[21] performed a meta-analysis of laparoscopic colorectal resections for carcinoma. Of 1,737 patients, they identified 17 (0.6%) with port-site metastases.

More recently, concerns about port-site metastases have waned somewhat after the results of numerous prospective trials, especially in the laparoscopic resection of colorectal tumors, showing that the incidence of this complication is very low. Table 26.1 briefly outlines some of the factors that have

TABLE 26.1

POSSIBLE CAUSES OF TUMOR CELL DISSEMINATION IN LAPAROSCOPIC SURGERY FOR CANCER

Possible Cause	Intervention to Potentially Minimize This Cause
Adverse effects of CO_2 gas	Use helium, nitrogen, or ambient room air.
Dispersion of cells by insufflation gas	Avoid sudden loss of pneumoperitoneum.
Tumor spillage from manipulation and instrumentation	Avoid excessive manipultion of the tumor.
Tumor spillage at extraction site	Use protected tumor extraction (plastic bag).
Immunosuppressive effect of pneumoperitoneum	Irrigate the abdomen with tumoricidal solutions.

been suggested to be responsible for port-site metastases and interventions to minimize the effects of these factors.

LAPAROSCOPY IN THE DIAGNOSIS OF MALIGNANCY

Although it is rare that the diagnosis of malignancy is unknown before surgical intervention, in certain situations, such as retroperitoneal adenopathy, imaging and material gained from core biopsy may not reliably diagnose a lymphoma. Since this information determines which radiotherapeutic or chemotherapeutic regimen will be instituted, diagnostic laparoscopy, which is less invasive and may allow earlier definitive therapy, becomes an important tool. Similarly, a tumor in the mesentery is often not amenable to image-guided biopsy but is accessible to laparoscopic biopsy and extirpation. In this situation, laparoscopy provides a diagnosis, stages the intra-abdominal disease, and provides treatment in a single procedure. Figure 26.2*A* shows a large tumor in the left upper quadrant, with a liver metastasis as shown in Figure 26.2*B*. The liver lesion was considered difficult to safely biopsy percutaneously but was easily and safely approached laparoscopically.

In addition to direct biopsy of visualized masses, laparoscopy allows for cytologic evaluation via washings. In a prospective study, laparoscopic peritoneal lavage was performed in patients without ascites with upper gastrointestinal malignancy; 100% of those patients with cytologic findings positive for malignancy died.[22] Similar results have been reported in patients with other gastrointestinal malignancies such as pancreatic cancer.[23]

The introduction of laparoscopic intracorporeal ultrasonography (LICU) has permitted the detection and biopsy of masses deep in solid organs such as the liver, which was not previously possible. The 1-cm size limitation for detection of malignancy by routine computed tomography (CT) scanning does not apply to LICU, in which lesions smaller than 1 cm can be identified, subjected to biopsy, and even treated by adjunctive laparoscopic ablation techniques. Also, LICU permits real-time retroperitoneal examination and focused exploration. The addition of Doppler ultrasound allows identification of vascular structures to be avoided intraoperatively. The acoustic interference from bowel gas and distance that limits transabdominal ultrasound is eliminated by the use of LICU and a clearer picture is obtained.

LAPAROSCOPY IN THE STAGING OF MALIGNANCY

One of the most important benefits of laparoscopic staging is the ability to exclude patients from undergoing a major operation by identifying metastatic disease or unresectable disease. One very clear advantage is the ability to identify peritoneal carcinomatosis, which is easily missed on imaging studies, and perform biopsy of the lesions. Lesions deeper than the peritoneal surfaces can also be identified using intraoperative ultrasound, and biopsy can then be safely performed. With increased accuracy in staging, many patients can be spared the pain of and hospitalization for a nontherapeutic laparotomy. Laparoscopy may be most useful in the diagnosis of malignancy where other modalities have not demonstrated disease, as a supplement to noninvasive pretherapeutic staging methods. Figures 26.3*A* and 26.3*B* show an example of a patient with a large lesion at the esophagogastric junction but no other findings on CT scan. Laparoscopic exploration showed disseminated carcinomatosis that was proven to be adenocarcinoma on biopsy.

Esophagus Cancer

Because of the inaccuracies of noninvasive staging methods, the use of laparoscopy for staging has generated interest. Krasna et al.[24] reviewed results for 111 patients who underwent thoracoscopic/laparoscopic (Ts/Ls) staging along with CT, magnetic resonance imaging (MRI), and endoscopic ultrasound (EUS). The staging accuracy for mediastinal and abdominal metastases was 58% and 68%, respectively, for imaging staging and 91% and 96% for Ts/Ls staging. In a study of Ts/Ls staging, of 137 patients, 73% met the requirement for Ts/Ls staging.[25] Among those for which both imaging and Ts/Ls staging were performed, 53% of patients were found to have positive lymph nodes. Based on prospective data, it appears that Ts/Ls staging is more accurate than imaging staging alone for patients with esophageal cancer. More important, noninvasive staging may incorrectly overstage disease and thus prevent an attempt at curative resection.

Stomach Cancer

To reduce unnecessary operations in patients with gastric cancer, laparoscopic staging has been advocated to improve staging

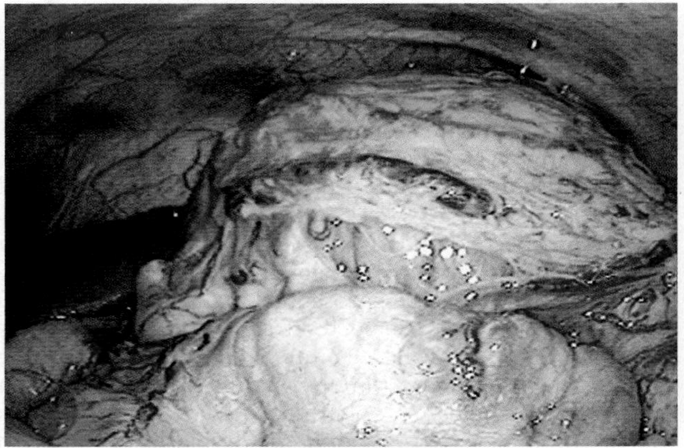

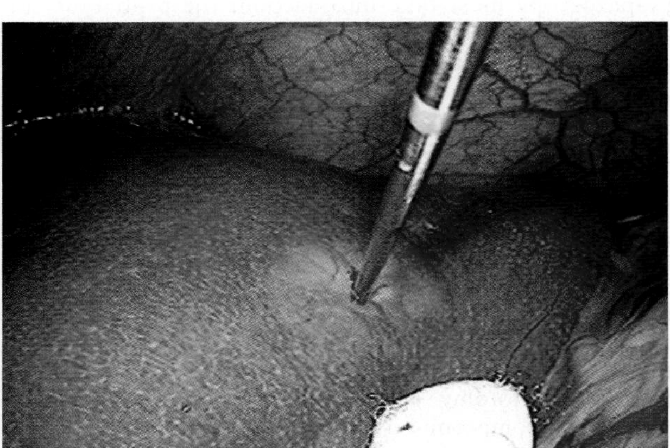

FIGURE 26.2 **A:** A 53-year-old man presented with a large left upper quadrant tumor, shown laparoscopically. **B:** Preoperative computed tomography scan suggested a liver lesion that was not amenable to percutaneous biopsy. Laparoscopic biopsy was performed (Fig. 26.3*B*), establishing the diagnosis of a metastatic neuroendocrine tumor of the pancreas.

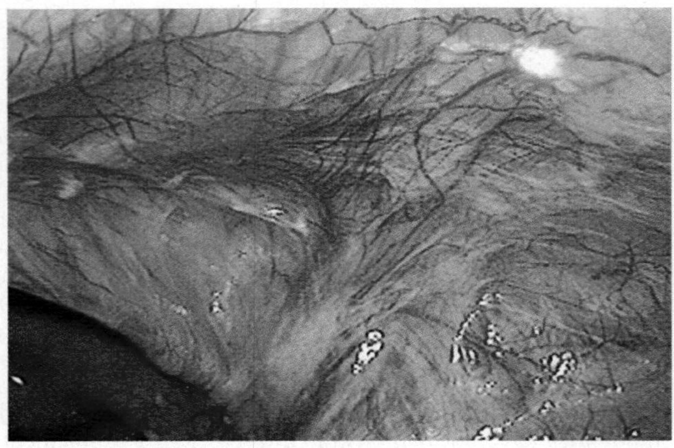

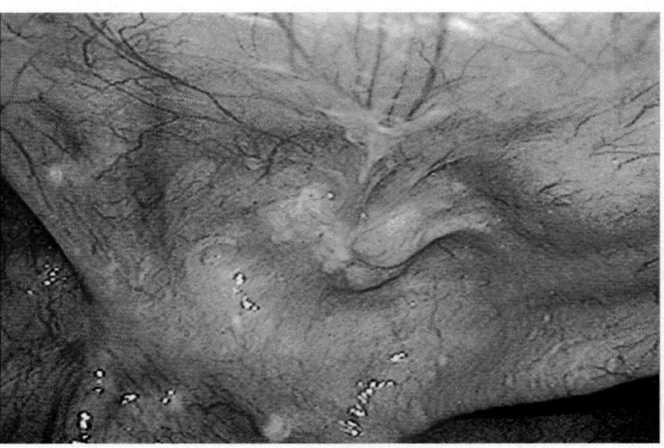

FIGURE 26.3 **A:** A 65-year-old man presented with a computed tomography (CT) scan showing a large tumor at the esophagogastric junction, and CT suggested broad serosal invasion. **B:** Staging laparoscopy showed multiple disseminated nodules (shown in A and B), but not suggested on CT scan. Peritoneal washings for cytology were also obtained at laparoscopy and were positive for malignancy.

and resection rates. Positive cytologic findings are rare for T1 to T2, M0 cases, whereas the rate of positive findings approaches 10% for T3 to T4 disease and is much higher for M1 disease.[26] Cytologic washings should be taken as part of the laparoscopic staging of patients with gastric cancer. The value of lavage cytology, especially in patients receiving neoadjuvant chemotherapy, was shown by Nakagawa et al.[27] They found that 22% of patients were able to avoid unnecessary laparotomy following staging laparoscopy. In the case of smaller asymptomatic lesions, for which laparoscopy might have the greatest impact, the likelihood of finding metastatic disease diminishes rapidly.

Laparoscopic staging can be performed as an outpatient before definitive resection is scheduled or during diagnostic laparoscopy immediately preceding laparotomy. In a detailed review, undetected metastatic disease was found in 13% to 57% of patients initially staged as having no metastatic disease using conventional imaging, such as that illustrated in Figure 26.3.[26] The discovery of unexpected metastatic disease obviated the need for exploratory laparotomy in over 20% of the cases. Prospective studies have shown accuracy rates of more than 90% for laparoscopy in detection of metastatic disease and carcinomatosis, whereas detection accuracy for imaging was between 70% and 80%.

In a study of 24 patients with advanced disease (T3/T4), Song et al.[28] found unsuspected peritoneal carcinomatosis in 62.5% of cases. They conclude that patient selection for staging laparoscopy must take into account the probability of peritoneal lesions. Laparoscopy altered the treatment plan in one-third of the patients.

Pancreatic Cancer

The goal of laparoscopy in the staging of carcinoma of the pancreas is to avoid the need for laparotomy in those patients who, despite being deemed to have resectable disease by preoperative imaging studies, have distant disease. About 25% of patients who are considered resectable after preoperative imaging studies are found to have metastases or advanced unresectable lesions at surgery in groups evaluated by laparoscopy or by laparotomy. Those patients who underwent laparotomy had a compromised quality of life and a delay in the start of appropriate therapy, while the laparoscopic group avoided unnecessary laparotomy.[29]

Early studies that compared conventional imaging to a combination of laparoscopy and LICU reported an approximately 20% rate of detection of M1 or unresectable disease that resulted in a change in the operative plan to either no resection or a palliative procedure by the use of laparoscopy. However, the role of laparoscopic staging for tumors of the pancreas continues to be redefined. In a study of 1,045 patients with radiographically resectable pancreatic or peripancreatic lesions, laparoscopy identified unresectable disease in 145 (14%).[30] Furthermore, the yield of laparoscopy showed a marked downward trend from 19% in 1999 to just 3% in 2005. They conclude that "when high-quality cross-sectional imaging reveals no evidence of unresectable disease, routine staging laparoscopy may not be warranted for pancreatic or peri-pancreatic tumors other than presumed pancreatic adenocarcinoma."

With the use of combined imaging modalities such as high-quality helical CT, MRI, and EUS, the intraoperative detection of occult unresectability has declined to 4% to 13% of cases.[31] Careful patient selection is essential to use laparoscopy appropriately in patients with pancreatic lesions. In a study of 198 patients with no signs of disseminated disease, Mortensen et al.[32] found that patient management was altered in 27.3% by using laparoscopic ultrasonography. The liver and pancreas were the main targets of the biopsies, and the procedure was shown to be safe and have an impact on the management of a significant fraction of patients.

Liver Tumors

Staging for primary hepatic cancer such as hepatocellular cancer (HCC) and cholangiocarcinoma remains very important, because there is no role for palliative hepatic resection in the event that the tumor is found to be unresectable or M1 disease is discovered. A nontherapeutic laparotomy adds cost, creates patient discomfort, and delays therapy until healing has occurred.

In a prospective study from 1998 to 2000, 68 consecutively treated patients with HCC lesions suggested to be resectable by imaging underwent laparoscopic staging using LICU.[33] The preoperative workup included ultrasound with either lipiodol contrast CT or dual-phase spiral CT. At the time of laparoscopy, 63 of 68 primary tumors were histologically proven to be HCC; the remainder included two cases of cholangiocarcinoma and three cases of high-grade dysplastic nodules. Thus, diagnosis was changed in five cases (7%). In 14 cases (22%), new malignant HCC nodules were identified as well as a case of adrenal metastasis. The sizes of the new lesions were small, averaging 14 mm, and many were below the 10-mm limit of detection of CT. Laparoscopic staging changed the operative procedure in 12 of the 15 patients with additional tumor nodules. This particular study highlights the issues with laparoscopic staging of HCC. When additional tumor nodules are identified, numerous treatment modalities are available; some are treatable by laparoscopy as a stand-alone procedure or in combination with conventional resection.

The staging of secondary hepatic malignancies has been studied extensively, particularly in patients with colorectal metastases to the liver. In a large prospective study, D'Angelica et al.[34] analyzed data for 401 patients who underwent staging laparoscopy for hepatobiliary malignancy. There were 199 colorectal metastases (49.6%), 59 hilar cholangiocarcinomas (14.7%), 50 gallbladder carcinomas (12.5%), and 33 hepatocellular carcinomas (8.2%). Two hundred sixty-six patients (66.3%) had previously undergone a laparotomy. Eighty-four patients (20.9%) were found to have unresectable disease. Laparoscopy and LICU had the least yield in determining unresectability in metastatic colorectal carcinoma, detecting 10% of the total of 20% unresectable colorectal cases. Preoperatively, the surgeon's impression of resectability was statistically significant in determining outcomes. The authors of the study pointed out that in their experience, as time progressed, the ability to exclude laparotomy by laparoscopic staging decreased from approximately one-third in prior studies to the current level of 10% through the use of modern imaging methods.

Prostate Cancer

There is still some debate in the urologic oncology community about the extent of pelvic lymph node dissection needed in patients with prostate cancer. In a study comparing limited lymphadenectomy (N = 381) with extended lymphadenectomy (N = 163), complication rates and conversion rates were similar in both groups.[35] Furthermore, in the extended lymphadenectomy group, in 38% of the cases, metastases were found in lymph nodes outside those dissected in the limited lymphadenectomy procedure. Laparoscopic staging is often combined with laparoscopic prostatectomy, which reduces morbidity, lowers costs, shortens hospital stays, and reduces the number of blood transfusions.

In another study, the role of laparoscopic sentinel lymph node biopsy in the staging of prostate cancer was evaluated.[36] A series of 28 patients with prostate cancer underwent laparoscopic pelvic lymphadenectomy, with identification of the sentinel node using a gamma probe. All sentinel nodes were removed successfully without intra- or postoperative complications. This study shows that laparoscopic sentinel lymph node dissection in patients with prostate cancer is feasible.

Testicular Cancer

Current management options after radical orchiectomy for low-stage mixed malignant germ cell tumors include observation, chemotherapy, or lymph node dissection. Open lymph node dissection is considered the standard approach, but laparoscopic lymph node dissection also is performed. In a retrospective study of 26 patients, Skolarus et al.[37] found excellent oncologic results with the laparoscopic procedure, and no increase in surgical complications. Laparoscopic staging is an excellent option for this malignancy, which has a generally favorable prognosis.

Gynecologic Cancer

To reduce the morbidity of the procedure, laparoscopic staging has been advocated because of its theorized lower rate of adhesion formation. One prospective randomized controlled trial compared laparotomy staging, laparoscopic staging, and clinical staging in locally advanced cervical cancer.[38] For those patients undergoing surgical staging, no difference was seen in operating time, blood loss, lymph node yield, or survival with laparoscopic staging versus staging at laparotomy. Twenty-five percent of patients had lymph node metastases. It appears that open and laparoscopic staging are both effective in detecting unresectable disease. Several studies have shown acceptable rates of recurrence, but guidelines have not yet been universally established in determining eligibility for these procedures.[39] It has also been suggested that laparoscopic pelvic lymphadenectomy can help identify patients who are the best candidates for pelvic exenteration.[40] However, the exact role of laparoscopic surgery in the evaluation of patients with locally advanced cervical cancer remains undefined.

Sentinel node techniques have recently been evaluated in the staging of cervical cancer.[41] In a study of 33 patients with locally advanced or early stage disease, laparoscopic sentinel node biopsy was performed. These investigators found that the sentinel node technique was less accurate in locally advanced disease than in early stage cervical cancer. Further applications of laparoscopic surgery await more data from prospective trials.

The use of laparoscopy in the comprehensive surgical staging of uterine cancer was recently reported in the results of a large multicenter study.[42] Patients with clinical stage I to IIA were randomized to undergo laparoscopic (N = 1,696) or open laparotomy, including hysterectomy, salpingo-oophorectomy, pelvic cytology, and lymphadenectomy. The conversion rate was 26%, and the laparoscopic group had a significantly longer operating time (204 minutes vs. 130 minutes). Hospital stay was shorter in the laparoscopy group, and there was no difference in the detection rate of advanced disease. This study establishes the feasibility and safety of this procedure in patients with uterine cancer.

Lymphoma

This diverse group of malignancies is categorized by histologic findings into Hodgkin's lymphoma (HL) and non-HL (NHL). To secure the diagnosis, a lymph node biopsy is usually required because of the high false-negative and false-positive rates with fine-needle aspiration. Treatment for HL in the past was based on the stage of the disease, and the procedures have been described using laparoscopic approaches. However, the importance of surgical staging has greatly diminished with the use of high-quality imaging techniques and the administration of chemotherapeutic agents, even in patients with relatively early stage disease, resulting in improved survival. Thus, the role of laparoscopy is limited to obtaining diagnostic material when it is not available from more superficial sites.

For NHL, differences in histologic characteristics and prognosis make it difficult to evaluate the efficacy of a particular therapy. Despite the wide variation in disease behavior, the staging of NHL typically does not require a laparotomy.[43] In cases in which NHL is suspected to reside in the spleen and a tissue diagnosis is required, laparoscopic splenectomy is indicated for diagnostic purposes.

LAPAROSCOPY IN THE TREATMENT OF MALIGNANCY

The three major concerns regarding laparoscopic surgery for the treatment of cancer are (1) maintenance of the integrity of the oncologic resection (e.g., margins of resection, lymph node harvest), (2) demonstration of improved outcome parameters for the resection (e.g., decreased hospital stay, decreased pain, decreased cost, more rapid return to work), and (3) absence of any negative impact on survival (e.g., induction of carcinomatosis or metastasis by laparoscopy, port-site recurrences).

Esophagus Cancer

Minimally invasive resection of esophageal tumors is performed throughout the world. In a report from the University of Pittsburgh, investigators described a series of 222 patients who underwent minimally invasive esophagectomy using both laparoscopy and thoracoscopy, and a cervical esophagogastric anastomosis.[44] This series showed a mortality of 1.4%, an anastomotic leak rate of 11%, and an incidence of pneumonia of 7.7%. Some have observed that this operation (whether performed open or laparoscopically) has a higher incidence of strictures and anastomotic leaks, as well as recurrent laryngeal nerve injury due to extensive neck dissection. Some surgeons therefore prefer the Ivor-Lewis approach, utilizing an intrathoracic anastomosis. The same group from the University of Pittsburgh reported a series of 50 patients who underwent a minimally invasive Ivor-Lewis esophagectomy.[45] There was a 6% operative mortality and a 6% postoperative leak rate, with 8% developing postoperative pneumonia, and no incidence of recurrent laryngeal nerve injuries. This report shows that the technique is feasible with good initial results in the hands of very experienced, minimally invasive surgeons.

There are few randomized trials of laparoscopy in the treatment of esophageal cancer. A prospective study of 104 consecutive minimally invasive esophagectomies was recently reported.[46] The majority of these were performed for esophageal cancer and most were performed using a thoracoscopic or laparoscopic esophagectomy with a cervical anastomosis or a minimally invasive Ivor-Lewis esophagectomy. The conversion rate was 2.9%. Leaks occurred in 9.6% and anastomotic strictures occurred in 26%. The authors conclude that this is a feasible approach with low conversion rate, acceptable morbidity, and low mortality.

Patient positioning for these procedures remains an area of interest, with most surgeons using the left lateral position. Recently, excellent results with prone positioning have been reported.[47] The authors felt that this position led to improved ergonomics, lower operative time, and fewer respiratory complications.

Stomach Cancer

In countries with well-established mass-screening programs that identify patients with early stage gastric cancer, laparoscopic gastric resection with lymphadenectomy is commonly performed, which includes T1/T2, N0, M0 cases. Better short-term outcome following laparoscopic procedures has been reported; recovery is faster, hospital stay shorter, there is less pain, and cosmesis is better. Long-term results have been reported, showing 5-year disease-free survival rates of 99.8% (stage IA), 98.7% (stage IB), and 85.7% (stage II).[48] A randomized controlled trial of subtotal gastrectomy was also reported from Italy.[49] This study showed that 5-year overall and disease-free survival rates are not significantly different for the two operative approaches.

In the Western world, acceptance of laparoscopic resection of gastric cancer has been somewhat delayed, in part because of the lower incidence of early disease amenable to resection. In a review of the technical feasibility and oncologic efficacy of this procedure, Strong et al.[50] found that laparoscopic gastric resection is safe, with improved short-term outcomes, including decreased length of stay, decreased use of narcotics, and fewer complications.

A prospective randomized trial of laparoscopic distal gastrectomy versus open distal gastrectomy was recently reported by Kim et al.[51] This study specifically examined the impact of the procedure on quality of life (QOL) and randomized 164 patients to the two groups, with 82 patients each. These authors found that the laparoscopic group had improved QOL compared to the open group with regard to physical functioning, appetite loss, sleep disturbance, anxiety, and body image. Other outcomes including intraoperative blood loss, postoperative narcotic use, and hospital stay were all improved in the laparoscopic group. Based on these results, laparoscopic gastric resection is well accepted for patients with early gastric cancer.

Gastrointestinal Stromal Tumor

Gastrointestinal stromal tumor (GIST) is the most common sarcoma of the GI tract. Sixty percent to 70% of GIST tumors occur in the stomach, followed by small intestine (25%), the rectum (5%), the esophagus (2%), and a variety of other locations. The role of surgery in the treatment of a GIST tumor is to resect the tumor with adequate margins and an intact pseudocapsule. Lymph node involvement is rare with GIST tumors, and, thus, no effort is made to perform an extended lymph node dissection. Based on this concept, a laparoscopic resection is a useful operation for patients with GIST tumors. A recent study showed that laparoscopic surgery is oncologically safe. Recent guidelines suggest that laparoscopic resection should be limited to tumors less than 2 cm in size.[52,53] A comparison of various resection techniques was recently reported by Pisters et al.[54] Adjuvant imatinib is recommended after surgical resection in some patients. The tumor must be handled with care to prevent intra-abdominal rupture and port-site metastasis by using a specimen bag for extraction. In particular, delivery of a posterior gastric tumor through an anterior gastrotomy can be problematic. A new technique to manage such lesions while minimizing the risk of rupture has been described.[55]

Pancreatic Cancer

Laparoscopic performance of a variety of pancreatic resections has been reported. Widespread application of laparoscopy to surgery of the pancreas is limited by the technically demanding nature of these operations.[56] The laparoscopic pancreaticoduodenectomy was first reported in 1994 by Gagner.[57] A recent study reported a retrospective study of 42 patients from a single center who underwent laparoscopic pancreatoduodenectomy.[58] The reconstructive phase of the operation is particularly demanding, and there have been no established techniques to makes this more generally applicable. Therefore, the laparoscopic resection of pancreatic lesions requiring pancreatoduodenectomy remains an investigative procedure.

Laparoscopy has been applied successfully to the resection of pancreatic neuroendocrine tumors, with good results. In a review of 176 patients from multiple reports over 8 years, successful laparoscopic resection of neuroendocrine tumors was reported in 84% of patients.[59] Conversion to open surgery was performed in 16% of cases, with hemorrhage being the most common reason. Further, the use of hand-assisted laparoscopic technology seems to have decreased the conversion rate. Complications occurred in 15% of patients with a pancreatic leak rate of 8.5%. Although long-term data regarding oncologic outcome in these series remain to be reported, it may be a promising approach in selected patients with neuroendocrine tumors of the pancreas.

Another application of laparoscopy to pancreatic lesions is the resection of tumors of the distal pancreas. This was first reported in 1993 and remains a potentially useful technique when performed on the appropriate patient by an experienced surgeon. A number of series have been published, showing reasonable length of stay, conversion rates ranging from 0% to 29%, and complication rates similar to those seen in open surgery. In a review of 212 patients who underwent laparoscopic distal pancreatectomy at nine academic medical centers, the authors concluded that the laparoscopic procedure has similar short- and long-term oncologic outcomes compared with the open procedure.[60] The laparoscopic operation is an acceptable approach for resection of selected pancreatic lesions. The relative rarity of these lesions will make prospective trials difficult to perform.

Liver Tumors

Laparoscopic liver wedge resections have been performed for some time with low morbidity. With no laparotomy incision, pain is substantially reduced, which permits rapid recovery and early hospital discharge. In addition, for liver malignancies, laparoscopic ablative techniques under laparoscopic ultrasonographic guidance allow detection and treatment of small metastases that would be missed by conventional imaging. Figure 26.4 shows the CT scan of a patient with significant comorbidities and a colon cancer metastasis at the confluence of the hepatic veins who was treated by laparoscopic radiofrequency ablation. The development of new approaches has revolutionized the application of minimally invasive techniques to solid organ resections. The rapid advances in technology, including the use of electrical energy, ultrasonic energy, and radio frequency energy in devices to divide the liver parenchyma, has made these rapid advances possible.[14] Major liver resections are now carried out laparoscopically at many centers around the world. The techniques for these technically demanding procedures are becoming standardized and promulgated through available courses.

A review of the world literature on laparoscopic liver resection was conducted by Nguyen et al.[61] The range of procedures being performed laparoscopically continues to expand. Of the 2,804 patients reviewed, 50% were for malignant lesions, 45% were for benign lesions, and the remainder for a variety of other reasons, including living-related donor partial hepatectomy. Of the procedures, 75% were done completely laparoscopically. Procedures included a wedge resection (45%), left lateral segmentectomy (20%), right hepatectomy (9%), and left hepatectomy (7%). The conversion rate was 4.1%. Overall mortality was 0.3%. The authors conclude that laparoscopic hepatic resection is safe with acceptable morbidity and mortality as well as oncologic outcomes similar to open surgery in this selected group of patients.

Laparoscopic radiofrequency ablation (RFA) has also been widely applied to malignant lesions of the liver. Buell et al.[62] confirmed that laparoscopic RFA serves as a useful bridge to transplantation in patients with HCC with a low recurrence rate. This review also conforms the safety of laparoscopic

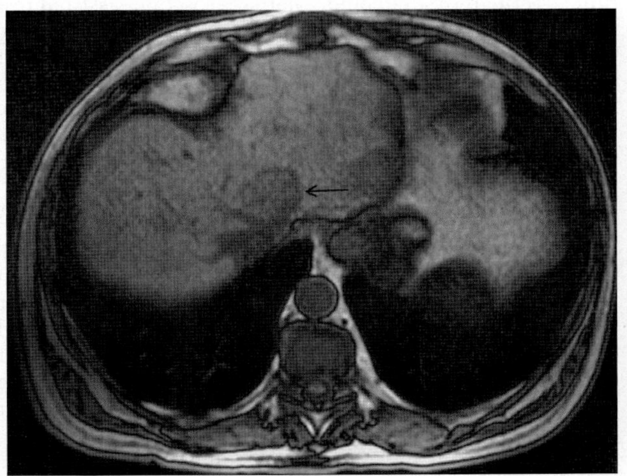

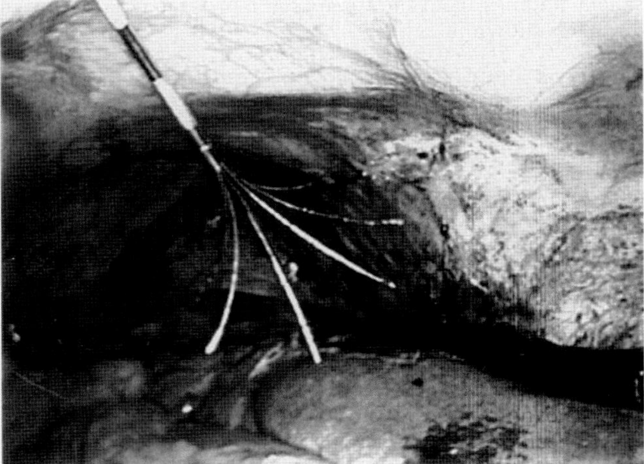

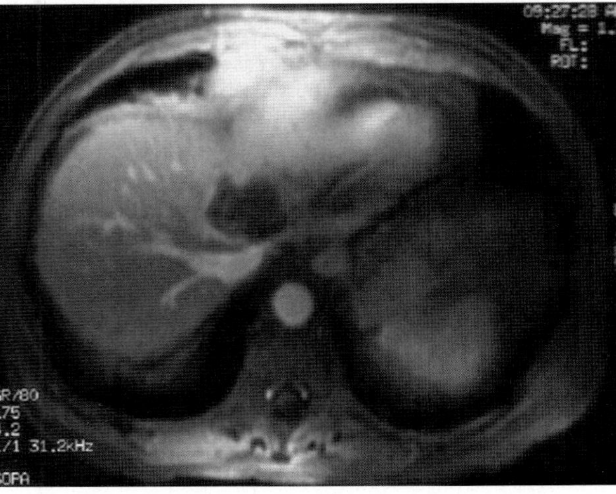

FIGURE 26.4 A 79-year-old man presented for treatment with colon cancer metastatic to the liver at the hepatic vein confluence. The lesion was treated by laparoscopic radiofrequency ablation. **A:** Preoperative magnetic resonance image (MRI) of the lesion. **B:** The radiofrequency probe. **C:** Postoperative MRI of the lesion.

TABLE 26.2

SUMMARY OF FINDINGS FROM PROSPECTIVE RANDOMIZED TRIALS FOR COLON CANCER RESECTION

			Open Resection			Laparoscopic Resection		
Study (Ref.)	No. of Patients	Conversion Rate (%)	Patients	Operating Room Time (min)	Time to Discharge (days)	Patients	Operating Room Time (min)[a]	Time to Discharge (days)[a]
COST Trial (54)	865	21	432	95	5	433	150	6
COLOR Trial (57)	1,248	17	621	115	9.3	627	145	8.2
CLASICC Trial (56)	794	29	268	135	11	526	180	9

[a]Indicates statistically significant difference between open surgery group and laparoscopic group ($P < .05$).

hepatic resection for a variety of malignant lesions. Santambrogio et al.[63] evaluated laparoscopic RFA compared to surgical resection in the management of patients with HCC and cirrhosis and found similar survival rates.

Colon Cancer

Laparoscopic colon resection for malignancy is a natural extension of previously developed procedures. Early reports showing a high incidence of port-site metastases quickly diminished enthusiasm for this procedure and led to restraint by many, awaiting the results of prospective trials. A summary of salient findings from the three major prospective randomized trials is shown in Table 26.2.

Clinical Outcomes of Surgical Therapy Trial

The National Cancer Institute funded the large randomized controlled Clinical Outcomes of Surgical Therapy (COST) study to evaluate (1) disease-free survival, (2) overall survival, and (3) QOL with colon cancer.[64] The QOL component measures included symptoms distress scale, QOL Index, and single item global rating scale at 2 days, 2 weeks, and 2 months postoperatively and showed that there were *no* significant differences in QOL between the two groups.[65]

The final results of this study were published in 2004 and included the "oncologic outcomes."[64] There were no significant differences in the 30-day mortality, readmission rate, or overall rate of complications. The cumulative incidence of recurrence in patients who underwent laparoscopic resection was not significantly different from those who underwent open resection ($P = .32$). Overall survival was also similar in the two groups. The authors concluded that there were no significant differences between the two treatment groups in regard to time to recurrence, disease-free survival, or overall survival for any stage.

This well-designed multicenter prospective randomized trial supports the safety of laparoscopic colon resection for patients with colon cancer, in regard to rate of complications, time to recurrence, disease-free survival, and overall survival. Factors relating to the technical conduct of the procedure such as number of lymph nodes resected, length of bowel and mesentery resected, and bowel margins also showed no differences in the two treatment groups. Furthermore, the authors point out that the study was not designed to show whether laparoscopic resection is superior to open resection, only that it is not inferior to open resection. The authors concluded that laparoscopic colon resection is an acceptable alternative to open colon resection for patients with carcinoma of the colon.

CLASICC Trial

The Conventional versus Laparoscopic ASsited Surgery in patients with Colorectal Cancer (CLASSICC) trial was conducted at 27 centers in the United Kingdom.[66] This study was somewhat different from others in that patients with carcinoma of the rectum were included. Overall, in terms of tumor status, nodal status, quality of life, and the defined short-term end points, these authors found no significant differences between laparoscopic resection and open surgery for patients with carcinoma of the colon and rectum. Surgical resection margins were similar in both groups except for patients who had laparoscopic anterior resection for carcinoma of the rectum. Although they conclude that laparoscopic-assisted resection of colon cancer is reasonable and should have no long-term differences in outcome compared to open surgery, they state that due to impaired short-term outcomes and pathologic features after laparoscopic anterior resection, these results do not justify routine use of laparoscopic-assisted resection in patients with carcinoma of the rectum.

Colon Cancer Laparoscopic or Open Resection Trial

The colon cancer laparoscopic or open resection (COLOR) trial was conducted in Europe as a multicenter, prospective, randomized trial to assess the safety and benefit of laparoscopic resection compared to open resection for patients with carcinoma of the right or left colon.[67] Analysis of short-term outcomes show that although the duration of surgery is longer for laparoscopic resection, patients undergoing laparoscopic resection have less blood loss, tolerate fluid intake earlier, and spend less time in the hospital. Oncologic outcomes such as positive margins, tumor size, and number of lymph nodes resected were equivalent in the two groups. Although long-term follow-up is pending, these results suggest that laparoscopic resection of the colon is a reasonable procedure and the equivalent oncologic short-term outcomes suggest that the two procedures will result in similar long-term results.

Meta-Analyses

In one meta-analysis, the authors analyzed a number of factors, including the time until return of bowel function, quality of life, and length of hospitalization as short-term variables.[68] These authors concluded that laparoscopy is superior in reducing pain during the same length of the postoperative period when compared to open surgery. Regarding hospital stay, the authors conclude that there is adequate level I evidence to show that laparoscopy for malignancy is associated with more rapid discharge from the hospital compared to open surgery for colon cancer. Reviewing long-term outcome, the authors evaluated recurrence rates and survival. A review of survival reported in the studies reviewed demonstrated that case-controlled and cohort studies have not demonstrated any differences in 5-year survival between patients undergoing open resection of colon cancer and those undergoing laparoscopic resection. Overall, the authors conclude that there are no significant differences in survival for patients undergoing laparoscopic resection of colon cancer compared to those undergoing open resection, with high-level evidence.

In a well-designed meta-analysis, investigators looked at 10 published randomized controlled trials of laparoscopic colon resection for cancer published from 1997 through 2005.[69] Overall, they found no significant differences in cancer-related mortality, cancer recurrence, or number of lymph nodes retrieved when comparing laparoscopic resection to conventional open surgery. They also found a trend toward improved cancer-related survival and fewer recurrences in the laparoscopic groups, although there was no significant difference observed. There were no significant differences observed in end points for the two groups of patients, laparoscopic versus open surgical resection. They conclude that laparoscopic resection for patients with colorectal cancer is oncologically sound and may offer distinct advantages.

In a meta-analysis of the Barcelona trial as well as the COST, COLOR, and CLASICC trials, authors reviewed 796 patients who underwent laparoscopic resection and 740 patients who underwent open resection.[70] They found that 3-year disease-free and overall survival rates were similar in the two groups. When evaluated separately, disease-free and overall survival rates for stages I, II, and III did not differ between the two treatments. These authors conclude that laparoscopically assisted colectomy for cancer is oncologically safe.

Hand-Assisted Laparoscopic Colon Resection

Hand-assisted laparoscopic surgery (HALS) allows the surgeon to use a gloved hand to facilitate laparoscopic surgery. Using the HALS technique, a hand is inserted into the abdomen through a seal that allows maintenance of the pneumoperitoneum. Thus, the excellent vision afforded by the laparoscope is maintained, while the surgeon can also have tactile feedback, which facilitates exposure, retraction, and dissection as well as the rapid control of bleeding. However, this technique necessitates the creation of a relatively large incision, and this may obviate some of the patient benefits of "minimally invasive" surgery.

A randomized prospective trial was carried out to evaluate results with HALS compared to routine laparoscopic-assisted colectomy.[71] A total of 54 patients were enrolled in this study, with 27 in the laparoscopic group and 27 in the HALS group. These authors conclude that the hand-assist device is helpful in difficult intraoperative situations and should be considered as an adjunct to conventional laparoscopic procedures when needed.

Lymph Node Harvest

In a study of 729 patients undergoing colorectal cancer resections (243 laparoscopic and 486 open), El-Gazzaz et al.[72] showed that the number of lymph nodes retrieved did not differ between laparoscopic and open surgery ($P = .4$). Numbers of lymph nodes harvested did depend on the site of resection (right vs. left). Number of lymph nodes remains an important oncologic outcome in these procedures.

The caution with which surgeons approached laparoscopic resection of colon cancer was in large part due to the early experience with port-site metastases, and the resulting hesitation to perform the procedure without results from well-designed trials may be a model for future careful application of some new technologies. The large body of high-level evidence has led to joint endorsement of the technique by the American Society of Colon and Rectal Surgeons (ASCRS) and the Society of American Gastrointestinal Endoscopic Surgeons (SAGES). In part, this endorsement states "Laparoscopic colectomy for curable cancer results in equivalent cancer related survival compared to open colectomy when performed by experienced surgeons."[68] Many patients prefer minimally invasive techniques, and these data support that it is safe to offer this approach to our patients.

Rectal Cancer

At this time, routine laparoscopic resection of rectal cancer is not justified by some of the available data.[66] The different results in the CLASICC trial for colon and rectal cancer underscores the need to consider these diseases separately when evaluating the use of laparoscopic surgery. Many clinicians are skeptical about the use of laparoscopic surgery in the treatment of rectal cancer. Poon et al.[73] conducted a meta-analysis of laparoscopic resection for rectal cancer. They concluded that laparoscopic resection of rectal cancer does benefit patients, with reduced blood loss, earlier return of bowel function, and shorter hospital stay. Caution, however, is warranted due to the paucity of randomized controlled trials. This procedure should only be performed by expert, trained surgeons who are evaluating outcomes carefully and in the setting of a controlled trial. There are currently two ongoing multicenter trials, and these data are eagerly awaited.

In the past 20 years, the treatment of rectal cancer has changed greatly, in part because of the growing support for total mesorectal excision (TME), which has led to higher incidences of sphincter and nerve preservation, reduced recurrence rates, and improved overall survival.[74] The literature is not yet conclusive about the method of performing laparoscopic total mesorectal excision (LTME), however. There are currently ongoing prospective trials, including COLOR II, designed to answer these questions. In a recent survey study, Cheung et al.[74] found a high level of agreement among surgeons for some practices such as medial-to-lateral dissection, ultrasonic hemostasis, high ligation of the inferior mesenteric artery, and pelvic drainage. There was less agreement regarding other practices such as identification of the right ureter, location of the mini-laparotomy, and construction of a colonic pouch.

Spleen Tumors

Laparoscopic splenectomy was first reported in 1991 and is the standard treatment for benign lesions of the spleen. Benefits to the patient for laparoscopic resection of the spleen are similar to those observed in the laparoscopic resection of other organs, with shortened hospital stay and decreased postoperative pain. Indications for laparoscopic splenectomy include lymphoproliferative disorders, myeloproliferative disorders, vascular tumors, metastatic tumors, and other lesions such as sarcomas. Most of these patients are older, many have anemia, coagulation disorders, or thrombocytopenia. In a review of three series containing 327 patients combined, 95 of whom had malignant lesions, morbidity, mortality, and postoperative complication are all improved in patients undergoing laparoscopic surgery compared to historical data for those having open surgery.[75] Patients who need a splenectomy in the management of their malignant disease should undergo laparoscopic splenectomy using well-described techniques when technically feasible. To ensure the acquisition of ideal pathologic information, the spleen should usually be removed intact. Morselization of the spleen may be acceptable in some cases, and discussion with pathology colleagues may be helpful in this decision-making process.

The management of splenomegaly deserves special attention. For most surgeons, patients with splenomegaly should undergo traditional open splenectomy. In some cases, laparoscopic splenectomy may be a reasonable alternative. Another alternative is HALS splenectomy. In a recent review comparing hand-assisted laparoscopic splenectomy with open splenectomy in patients with splenomegaly, the hand-assisted laparoscopic splenectomy technique resulted in less postoperative pain, shorter hospital stay, and a shorter incision.[76] Laparoscopy is also useful in treating recurrent hematologic diseases of splenic origin, such as immune thrombocytopenia purpura, but preoperative imaging studies are essential.[77]

Adrenal Cancer

Open adrenalectomy generally requires a generous incision, resulting in pain for the patient and, despite the incision size, often results in a poor visual field for the surgeon. However, laparoscopic adrenalectomy changed the situation for both surgeon and patient and was first described in 1991. Laparoscopic resection reduced postoperative pain, reduced hospital stay, and improved morbidity, while the laparoscope provides excellent visualization of the operative field. Laparoscopic adrenalectomy is considered the standard approach for most lesions, although open adrenalectomy must remain a viable option when indicated.

A wide array of lesions including adrenal metastases, malignant pheochromocytoma, and adrenocortical carcinoma have been treated by laparoscopic resection. In a review of 232 adrenalectomies from one institution, there was a 2% conversion rate, a 0.4% mortality rate, and a 6% postoperative complication rate. Relative contraindications for laparoscopic adrenalectomy include invasive adrenocortical lesions and very large tumors, greater than 12 cm.[78] The incidence of adrenocortical lesions increases with size, as does the technical difficulty of the procedure. In a review of laparoscopic resection of lesions greater than 5 cm, Sharma et al.[79] reported on 29 patients with adrenal lesions having a mean size of 7 cm. Operative time was greater in larger lesions, but they concluded that laparoscopic adrenalectomy is safe when performed by experienced surgeons.

In addition, laparoscopy has emerged as the method of choice for the resection of incidentally identified adrenal lesions (also called an incidentaloma). The patients should undergo appropriate preoperative testing with functional biochemical testing, adrenal imaging, as well as appropriate cancer screening. The most common laparoscopic approach to the adrenal gland is transabdominal. In a review of 255 consecutive adrenalectomies from 13 centers, Conzo et al.[80] found that the indications for adrenalectomy may have changed with the availability of laparoscopic adrenalectomy. In a review of 42 patients who underwent laparoscopic adrenalectomy for incidentaloma, 30% of patients with borderline elevated urine or plasma metanephrine levels had a pheochromocytoma.[81] Routine alpha-blockade is recommended in these patients.

Prostate Cancer

Laparoscopic approaches to surgery of the kidney and prostate have been reported widely. In 2003 results of a series of more than 1,000 patients in Germany were reported; procedures included 450 radical prostatectomies, 558 nodal dissections, 45 radical nephrectomies, 22 radical nephroureterectomies, 12 partial nephrectomies, and 11 adrenalectomies.[82] At a median follow-up of 58 months, there were only eight local recurrences (0.73%) and two port-site metastases (0.18%). In the hands of these surgeons, the laparoscopic approach to surgery for urologic malignancy appears to be safe and feasible; however, no randomized trials have confirmed these data.

There are now three different surgical approaches to prostatectomy, including open surgery, conventional laparoscopic resection, and robotic resection. In North America, prostatectomy is increasingly performed using robotic surgery techniques. The prostate is an ideal organ for robotic surgery because the operative field is limited and meticulous dissection is required to avoid complications, including incontinence. With the improved visualization provided by high-quality optics, the operating time using robotic surgery techniques has been reported to be shorter than that for conventional laparoscopic surgery.[83] Postoperative urinary function and sexual function have been reported to be improved in patients undergoing robotic surgery.[83] Although robotic-assisted prostatectomy is widely performed, there remains an absence of randomized studies in the literature to allow valid comparisons.[84] In one meta-analysis, investigators report no clear differences between the techniques regarding operative time, complication rates, and hospital stay.[84] Other studies have shown that short-term data, including functional outcomes, urinary continence, and sexual function, are similar using the various approaches.[85] However, cost considerations favor open surgery, with the robotic laparoscopic approach having the highest cost.[85] Data from long-term prospective trials, which currently do not exist, are necessary to objectively evaluate these techniques.

Renal Cancer

The incidence of renal cortical tumors, the most common of which is renal cell carcinoma, has significantly increased with the increased use of abdominal imaging techniques. This early detection has also resulted in the identification of more lesions in early stages compared with historical data. This has also led to the increased use of minimally invasive surgical techniques for resection of these tumors.[69] Laparoscopic radical nephrectomy is now widely accepted for the treatment of both benign and malignant lesions, and can be done by either a transperitoneal or retroperitoneal approach. The retroperitoneal approach has a benefit in the patient who has had previous surgery where adhesions may be present. Laparoscopic resection of renal tumors has a definitely established role at this time and is generally considered to be the standard approach to these tumors.[86]

More recently, laparoscopic partial nephrectomy has continued to evolve. Over the past 5 years, there has been a considerable reduction in warm ischemia time and complication rates. In a review of 184 patients who underwent laparoscopic partial nephrectomy at a single center, investigators found that while there were some differences over the course of the study, the mean tumor size was about 3 cm and the warm ischemia time was 30 minutes.[87] At a median follow-up of 18 months, there were no local or distant tumor recurrences reported. Over time, these investigators feel that the laparoscopic procedure is appropriate in larger and more complex tumors. Brandina and Aron[88] report that the morbidity and oncologic outcomes of laparoscopic partial nephrectomy are comparable to the open procedure. It is considered an established procedure for the resection of T1a renal tumors as well as some T1b and more complex tumors.

Gynecologic Cancer

In general, all of the procedures required to treat a variety of gynecologic malignancies have been described using the laparoscopic approach.[89] Unlike colorectal and urologic cancers, the role of laparoscopic surgery for gynecologic malignancies remains somewhat undefined in part due to early experience with ovarian carcinoma, where results seemed poor and were attributed to the surgical approach chosen. Laparoscopic surgery is considered the standard approach in the diagnosis of adnexal masses, but the mass should be removed intact, avoiding accidental puncture of the wall.[89] In a randomized prospective trial comparing open transperitoneal, open extraperitoneal, and laparoscopic pelvic lymphadenectomy in the management of patients undergoing radical hysterectomy for cervical cancer, 168 patients were evaluated.[90] This study established that laparoscopic lymphadenectomy is safe and feasible with a shorter hospital stay, although with longer operating times and significantly fewer lymph nodes retrieved using the laparoscopic approach compared to the open approach. These authors point out that standard treatment for early stage cervical cancer remains radical hysterectomy and pelvic lymphadenectomy, and that laparotomy is still considered the standard approach. The laparoscopic hysterectomy remains a procedure for which there are no universally accepted standards.

The surgical treatment of invasive ovarian cancer does not include laparoscopy in most patients, although it may be useful in second-look procedures in patients originally thought to have benign masses.[89] Laparoscopy can be useful in confirming the diagnosis and determining respectability. Further studies are under way, particularly in patients with early stage ovarian cancer.

A recent study directly compared operative results for patients with endometrial cancer, comparing 210 patients who underwent laparoscopic surgery to historic controls.[91] The conversion rate was less than 5%, and there was no influence of body mass index, age, or previous surgery on the conversion rate. Operative time was similar and the mean number of lymph nodes retrieved was greater in the laparoscopic group. In another series, 159 women with early stage endometrial cancer were randomized to undergo total laparoscopic hysterectomy or abdominal hysterectomy with lymphadenectomy.[92] Mean operating time was slightly longer in the laparoscopic group (136 minutes vs. 123 minutes), and length of hospital stay was significantly less in the laparoscopic group (2.1 days vs. 5.1 days). The results of further multicenter randomized trials are awaited to evaluate long-term oncologic outcomes.

LAPAROSCOPY IN THE PALLIATION OF MALIGNANCY

The role of laparoscopy extends beyond diagnosis and treatment. At times patients need palliation of the complications from their malignancy or from the therapy for their malignancy. A common scenario is gastric outlet obstruction or intestinal obstruction. When the gastric outlet is obstructed by a tumor such as an incurable gastric or pancreatic cancer, a laparoscopic stapled gastrojejunostomy can be performed quickly to provide pain relief and allow resumption of eating. Intestinal stomas can also be created when bowel loops are involved with tumor and intestinal bypass is not feasible. The ideal method of palliation remains unclear, although laparoscopic gastrojejunostomy is considered by some to be the standard approach. In a meta-analysis comparing open gastrojejunostomy to endoscopic stenting and laparoscopic gastrojejunostomy, the endoscopic stenting showed superior results to open surgery, although there are still an insufficient number of studies to compare endoscopic stenting to laparoscopic bypass procedures.[93]

When small bowel loops are matted in the pelvis after radiation therapy for cervical cancer, an intestinal bypass procedure can relieve the symptoms resulting from treatment of the malignancy. The aforementioned palliative bypass or intestinal stoma creation procedures can be done as stand-alone procedures for a known malignancy or can be performed during the diagnostic laparoscopic phase when a cancer is first diagnosed and found to be unresectable. Other adjunct laparoscopic procedures for therapy and palliation include the placement of feeding tubes for alimentary nutrition or for decompression of obstruction.

Selected References

The full list of references for this chapter appears in the online version.

2. Podolsky ER, Curcillo PG. Single port access surgery—a 24-month experience. *J Gastrointest Surg* 2010;14:759.
4. Horgan S, Cullen JP, Talamini M, et al. Natural orifice surgery: initial clinical experience. *Surg Endosc* 2009;23:1512.
5. Hagiike M, Phillips EH, Berci G. Performance differences in laparoscopic surgical skills between true high-definition and three chip CCD video systems. *Surg Endosc* 2007;21:1849.
9. Pigazzi A, Luca F, Patriti A, et al. Multicentric study on robotic tumor specific mesorectal excision for the treatment of rectal cancer. *Ann Surg Oncol* 2010;17:1614.
10. Song J, Oh SJ, Kang WH, et al. Robot-assisted gastrectomy with lymph node dissection for gastric cancer. *Ann Surg* 2009;249:927.
11. Herron DM, Marohn M, SAGES-MIRA Robotic Surgery Consensus Group. A consensus document on robotic surgery. *Surg Endosc* 2008; 22:313.
16. Gutt NC, Kim ZG, Hollander D, et al. CO2 environment influences the growth of cultured human cancer cells dependent on insufflation pressure. *Surg Endosc* 2001;15:314.
20. Vukasin P, Ortega AE, Greene FL, et al. Wound recurrence following laparoscopic colon cancer resection: results of the American Society of Colon and Rectal Surgeons laparoscopic registry. *Dis Colon Rectum* 1996;39:S20.
25. Krasna MJ, Reed CE, Nedzwiecki D, et al. CALGB 9380: a prospective trial of the feasibility of thoracoscopy/laparoscopy in staging esophageal cancer. *Ann Thorac Surg* 2001;71:1073.
27. Nakagawa S, Nashimoto A, Yabusaki H. Role of staging laparoscopy with peritoneal lavage cytology in the treatment of locally advanced gastric cancer. *Gastric Cancer* 2007;10:29.
28. Song KY, Kim JJ, Kim SN, et al. Staging laparoscopy for advanced gastric cancer: is it also useful for the group which has an aggressive surgical strategy? *World J Surg* 2007;31:1228.
30. White R, Winston C, Gonen M, et al. Current utility of staging laparoscopy for pancreatic and peripancreatic neoplasms. *J Am Coll Surg* 2008;206: 445.
32. Mortensen MB, Fristrup C, Ainsworth A, et al. Laparoscopic ultrasound-guided biopsy in upper gastrointestinal tract cancer patients. *Surg Endosc* 2009;23:2738.
36. Corvin S, Schilling D, Eichhorn K et al. Laparoscopic sentinel lymph node dissection—a novel technique for the staging of prostate cancer. *Eur Urol* 2006;49:280.
42. Walker JL, Piedmonte MR, Spirtos NM, et al. Laparoscopy compared with laparotomy for comprehensive surgical staging of uterine cancer: Gynecologic Oncology Group Study LAP2. *J Clin Oncol* 2009;27:5332.
43. Lefor AT. Laparoscopic interventions in lymphoma management. *Semin Laparosc Surg* 2000;7:129.
44. Luketich JD, Alvelo-Rivera M, Buenaventura PO, et al. Minimally invasive esophagectomy outcomes in 222 patients. *Ann Surg* 2003;238:486.
46. Nguyen NT, Hinojosa MW, Smith BR, et al. Minimally invasive esophagectomy: lessons learned from 104 operations. *Ann Surg* 2008;248:1081.
48. Kitano S, Shiraishi N, Uyama I, et al. A multicenter study on oncologic outcome of laparoscopic gastrectomy for early gastric cancer in Japan. *Ann Surg* 2007;245:68.
50. Strong VE, Devaud N, Karpeh M. The role of laparoscopy for gastric surgery in the West. *Gastric Cancer* 2009;12:127.
51. Kim YW, Baik YH, Yun YH, et al. Improved quality of life outcomes after laparoscopy-assisted distal gastrectomy for early gastric cancer: results of a prospective randomized clinical trial. *Ann Surg* 2008;248:721.

53. Blay JY, Bonvalot S, Casali P, et al. Consensus meeting for the management of gastrointestinal stromal tumors. Report of the GIST Consensus Conference of 20–21 March 2004, under the auspices of ESMO. *Ann Oncol* 2005;16:566.
54. Pisters PW, Patel SR. Gastrointestinal stromal tumors: current management. *J Surg Oncol* 2010;102:530.
55. Warsi AA, Peyser PM. Laparoscopic resection of gastric GIST and benign gastric tumours: evolution of a new technique. *Surg Endosc* 2010; 24:72.
56. Takaori K, Tanigawa N. Laparoscopic pancreatic resection: the past, present, and future. *Surg Today* 2007;37:535.
58. Palanivelu C, Jani K, Senthilnathan P, et al. Laparoscopic pancreaticoduodenectomy: technique and outcomes. *J Am Coll Surg* 2007;205: 222.
60. Kooby DA, Hawkins WG, Schmidt CM, et al. A multicenter analysis of distal pancreatectomy for adenocarcinoma: is laparoscopic resection appropriate? *J Am Coll Surg* 2010;210:779.
61. Nguyen KT, Gamblin C, Geller D. World review of laparoscopic liver resection—2804 patients. *Ann Surg* 2009;250:831.
62. Buell JF, Thomas MT, Rudich S, et al. Experience with more than 500 minimally invasive hepatic procedures. *Ann Surg* 2008;248:475.
64. Weeks JC, Nelson H, Gelber S, et al. Short term quality of life outcomes following laparoscopic-assisted colectomy vs open colectomy for colon cancer: a randomized trial. *JAMA* 2002;287:321.
65. COST Study Group. A comparison of laparoscopically assisted and open colectomy for colon cancer. *N Engl J Med* 2004;350:2050.
66. Guillou PJ, Quirke P, Thorpe H, et al. Short term endpoints of conventional versus laparoscopic assisted surgery in patients with colorectal cancer (MRC CLASSIC trial): muticentre randomized controlled trial. *Lancet* 2005;365:1718.
67. COLOR Study Group. Laparoscopic surgery versus open surgery for colon cancer: short-term outcomes of a randomized trial. *Lancet Oncol* 2005; 6:477.
68. Cera S, Wexner SD. Minimally invasive treatment of colon cancer. *Cancer J* 2005;11:26.
69. Jackson TD, Kaplan GG, Arena G, et al. Laparoscopic versus open resection for colorectal cancer: a meta-analysis of oncologic outcomes. *J Am Coll Surg* 2007;204:439.
72. El-Gazzaz G, Hull T, Hammel J, Geisler D. Does a laparoscopic approach affect the number of lymph nodes harvested during curative surgery for colorectal cancer? *Surg Endosc* 2010;24:113.
73. Poon JTC, Law WL. Laparoscopic resection for rectal cancer: a review. *Surg Endosc* 2009;16:3038.
75. Burch M, Monali M, Phillips EH. Splenic malignancy: a minimally invasive approach. *Cancer J* 2005;11:36
76. Barbaros U, Dinccag A, Sumer A, et al. Prospective randomized comparison of clinical results between hand-assisted laparoscopic and open splenectomies. *Surg Endosc* 2010;24:25.
78. Ogilvie JB, Duh QY. New approaches to the minimally invasive treatment of adrenal lesions. *Cancer J* 2005;11:64.
79. Sharma R, Ganpule A, Veeramani M, et al. Laparoscopic management of adrenal lesions larger than 5 cm in diameter. *Urol J* 2009;6:254.
81. Lee JA, Zarnegar R, Shen WT, et al. Adrenal incidentaloma, borderline elevations of urine or plasma metanephrine levels and the subclinical pheochromocytoma. *Arch Surg* 2007;142:870.
82. Rassweiller Jens, Tsivian A, Ravi Kumar AV, et al. Oncologic safety of laparoscopic surgery for urological malignancy: experience with more than 1,000 operations. *J Urol* 2003;169:2072.
83. Menon M, Shrivastava A, Tewari A. Laparoscopic radical prostatectomy: conventional and robotic. *Urology* 2005;66(Suppl 5A):101.
86. Trabulsi EJ, Kalra P, Gomella LG. New approaches to the minimally invasive treatment of kidney tumors. *Cancer J* 2005;11:57.
88. Brandina R, Aron M. Laparoscopic partial nephrectomy: advances since 2005. *Curr Opin Urol* 2010;20:111.
90. Panici PB, Plotti F, Zullo MA, et al. Pelvic lymphadenectomy for cervical carcinoma: Laparotomy extraperitioneal, transperitoneal or laparoscopic approach? A randomized study. *Gyn Oncol* 2006;103:859.
91. Eisenkop SM. Total laparoscopic hysterectomy with pelvic/aortic lymph node dissection for endometrial cancer—a consecutive series without case selection and comparison to laparotomy. *Gynecol Oncol* 2010;117:216.
92. Malzoni M, Tinelli R, Cosentino F, et al. Total laparoscopic hysterectomy versus abdominal hysterectomy with lymphadenectomy for early-stage endometrial cancer: a prospective randomized study. *Gynecol Oncol* 2009;112:126.
93. Ly J, O'Grady G, Mittal A, et al. A systematic review of methods to palliate malignant gastric outlet obstruction. *Surg Endosc* 2010;24:290.

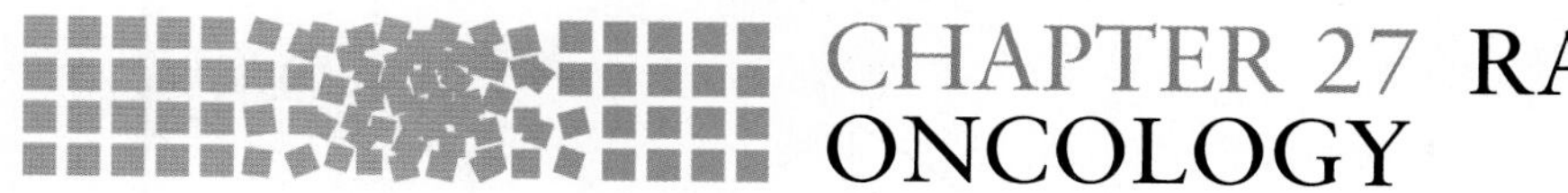

CHAPTER 27 RADIATION ONCOLOGY

MEREDITH A. MORGAN, RANDALL K. TEN HAKEN, AND THEODORE S. LAWRENCE

People have been exposed to radiation throughout the millennium, but it is only in the past approximately 100 years that the potential diagnostic and therapeutic use of radiation has been harnessed. This beneficial use was launched by the experiments of Wilhelm Roentgen, who in 1895 found that x-rays could pass through materials that were impenetrable to light. Emil Grubbe provided one of the early examples of the therapeutic use of radiation by treating an advanced ulcerated breast cancer with x-rays in January 1896. We have made great progress from these early days when rudimentary applications of radioactivity were used to treat tumors. This progress has been strongly influenced by research in radiation chemistry, biology, and physics, which are described here. This chapter will conclude with the clinical application of radiation therapy.

BIOLOGIC ASPECTS OF RADIATION ONCOLOGY

Radiation-Induced DNA Damage

Radiation is administered to cells either in the form of photons (i.e., x-rays and gamma rays) or particles (protons, neutrons, and electrons). When photons or particles interact with biological material, they cause ionizations that can either directly interact with subcellular structures or they can interact with water, the major constituent of cells, and generate free radicals that can then interact with subcellular structures (Fig. 27.1).

The direct effects of radiation result in the consequence of the DNA in chromosomes absorbing energy, which leads to ionizations. This is the major mechanism of DNA damage induced by charged nuclei (such as a carbon nucleus) and neutrons and is termed *high linear energy transfer* (Fig. 27.2). In contrast, the interaction of photons with other molecules such as water results in the production of free radicals, some of which possess a lifetime long enough to be able to diffuse to the nucleus and interact with DNA in the chromosomes. This is the major mechanism of DNA damage induced by x-rays and has been termed *low linear energy transfer*.[1]

A free radical generated through the interaction of photons with other molecules that possess an unpaired electron in their outermost shell (e.g., hydroxyl radicals) can abstract a hydrogen molecule from a macromolecule such as DNA to generate damage. Cells that have increased levels of free radical scavengers such as glutathione would have less DNA damage induced by x-rays, but have similar levels of DNA damage induced by a carbon nucleus that is directly absorbed by chromosomal DNA. Furthermore, a low oxygen environment would also protect cells from x-ray–induced damage as there would be fewer radicals available to induce DNA damage in the absence of oxygen; but this environment would have little impact on DNA damage induced by carbon nuclei.[2]

Cellular Responses to Radiation-Induced DNA Damage

Checkpoint Pathways

The cell cycle must progress in a specific order; checkpoint genes ensure that the initiation of late events is delayed until earlier events are complete. There are three principal places in the cell cycle at which checkpoints induced by DNA damage function: the border between G_1 phase and S phase, intra-S phase, and the border between G_2 phase and mitosis (Fig. 27.3). Cells with intact checkpoint function that have sustained DNA damage stop progressing through the cycle and become arrested at the next checkpoint in the cell cycle. For example, cells with damaged DNA in G_1 phase avoid replicating that damage by arresting at the G_1/S interface. If irradiated cells have already passed the restriction point, a position in G_1 phase that is regulated by the phosphorylation of the retinoblastoma tumor suppressor gene (*Rb*) and its dissociation from the E2F family of transcription factors, they will transiently arrest in the S phase. The G_1 or S and intra-S phase checkpoints inhibit the replication of damaged DNA and work in a coordinated manner with the DNA repair machinery to allow the restitution of DNA integrity, thereby increasing cell survival.

The earliest response to radiation is activation of ataxia-telangiectasia mutated (ATM), which involves a conformational change that results in activation of its kinase domain and phosphorylation of serine 1981 (Fig. 27.3).[3] This phosphorylation causes the ATM homodimer to dissociate into active monomers that phosphorylate a wide range of proteins such as p53BP1,[4] the histone variant H2AX,[5] Nbs1 (Nijmegen breakage syndrome; a member of the *MRN complex*, composed of Mre11, Rad50, and Nbs1),[6] BRCA1,[7] and SMC1 (structural maintenance of chromosomes),[6] and these proteins coordinate repair with the cell cycle. In response to DNA damage, H2AX is rapidly phosphorylated by ATM and localizes to sites of DNA double-strand breaks in multiprotein complexes described as foci (Fig. 27.4). Phosphorylation of H2AX by ATM results in the direct recruitment of Mdc1 and forms a complex with H2AX to recruit additional ATM molecules, forming a positive feedback loop.[8]

The G_1/S phase checkpoint is the best understood. In response to DNA damage, activated ATM can directly phosphorylate p53 and mdm2, the ubiquitin ligase that targets p53 for degradation. These phosphorylations are important in increasing the stability of p53 protein. In addition to ATM, the checkpoint kinases (Chk) also phosphorylate p53 and mdm2 and can enhance p53 stability. Activated p53 transcriptionally increases the expression of the $p21^{WAF1/CIP1}$ gene, which results in a sustained inhibition of G_1 cyclin/Cdk's and prevents phosphorylation of pRb and progression from G_1 into the S phase.[9] Mutations in p53 that are commonly found in solid tumors

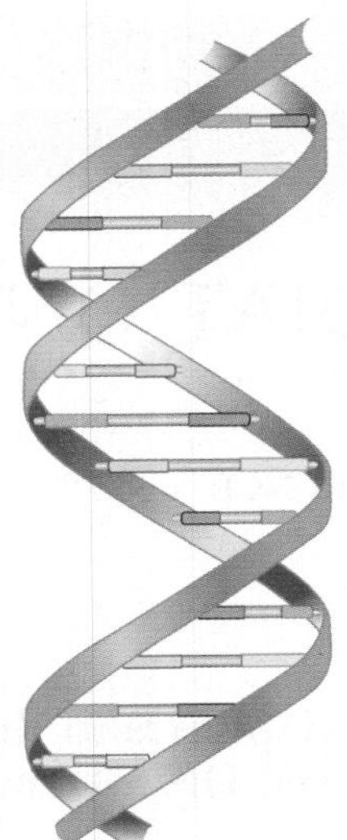

FIGURE 27.1 The direct and indirect effects of ionizing radiation on DNA. Incident photons transfer part of their energy to free electrons (Compton scattering). These electrons can directly interact with DNA to induce DNA damage or they can first interact with water to produce hydroxyl radicals that can then induce damage.

result in loss of transcriptional activity and compromised checkpoint function. A second more rapid, but transient G_1- to S-phase checkpoint is activated by DNA damage and mediated through Chk1 phosphorylation of the Cdc25A phosphatase.[10] Cdc25A activation produces rapid inhibition of cyclin E/Cdk2 and cyclin A/Cdk2 complex activity and cell-cycle arrest. This Chk1-Cdc25A checkpoint works independently of p53, but results in only a short-lived checkpoint response unless p53 is induced.

Control of the S-phase checkpoint is also in part mediated by the Cdc25A phosphatase inhibiting Cdk2 activity and the loading of Cdc45 onto chromatin. If Cdc45 fails to bind to chromatin, DNA polymerase-α is not recruited to replication

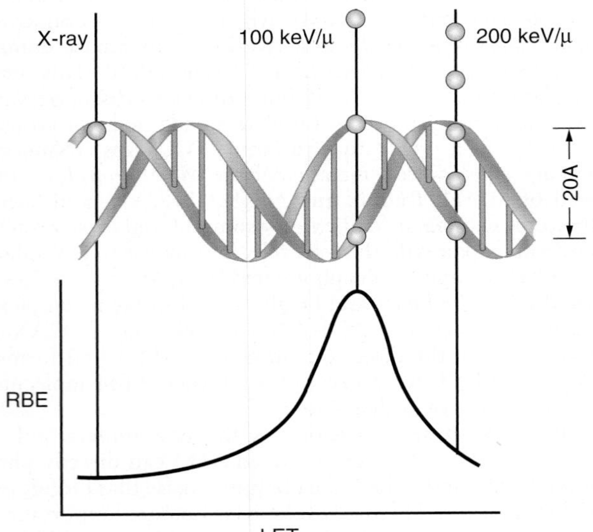

FIGURE 27.2 Linear energy transfer and DNA damage. Ionizing radiation deposits energy along track (linear energy transfer [LET]) that causes DNA damage and cell killing. The most biologically potent (highest relative biological effectiveness [RBE]) LET is 100 keV/mcm because the separation between ionizing events is the same as the diameter of the DNA double helix (2 nm). (From ref. 1, with permission.)

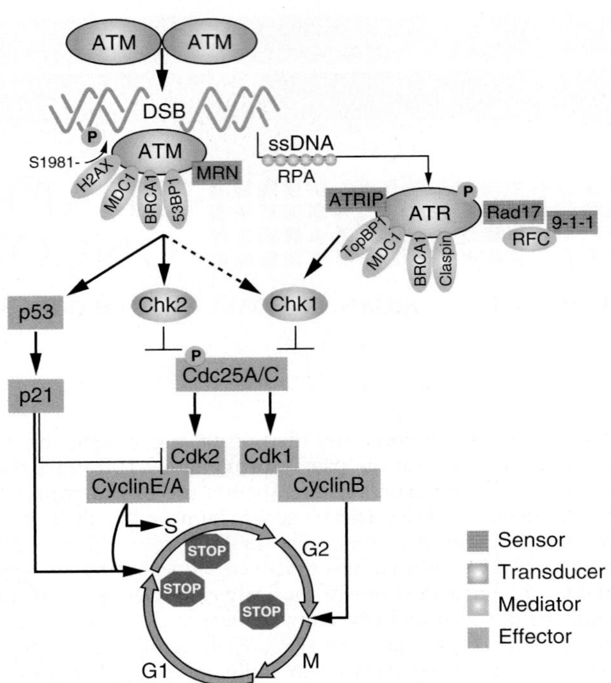

FIGURE 27.3 In response to DNA damage the MRN complex, composed of MRE11, Rad50, and NBS1, together with ATM (ataxia-telangiectasia mutation) and H2AX are the earliest proteins recruited to the site of the break. ATM is released from its homodimer complex, activated by transautophosphorylation and in turn, phosphorylates H2AX. Other members are recruited to the complex such as BRCA1 and 53BP1. As the DNA at the double-strand break (DSB) is resected, single-stranded DNA is formed and bound by replication protein A (RPA), resulting in activation of the ataxia-telangiectasia and Rad3-related (ATR) pathway. The net result of ATM/ATR activation is downstream activation of p53, leading to transcription of the Cdk inhibitor, p21, and activation of Chk1/Chk2, resulting in degradation of Cdc25 phosphatases, Cdk-cyclin complex inactivation, and cell cycle arrest at phase G_1, intra-S, or G_2. Note that in other models ATM is thought to be a sensor of changes in chromatin structure induced by DNA breaks.

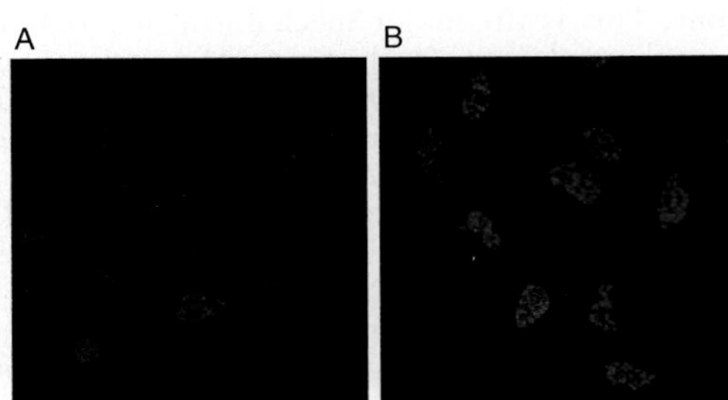

FIGURE 27.4 Phosphorylated histone variant H2AX as a marker of DNA damage. Phosphorylated histone variant H2AX (also called gamma H2AX) localizes to sites of DNA double strand breaks, so that its appearance and disappearance correspond with induction and repair of breaks. The cells in panels A and B have been stained with DAPI (4′,6-diamidino-2-phenylindole) (*blue*), in order to visualize cell nuclei, and stained with an antibody which recognizes *gamma* H2AX (*red*). The cells in A are untreated and exhibit little to no gamma H2AX staining, while the cells in B are treated with 7.5 Gy radiation and exhibit strong gamma H2AX staining at punctate foci in the nuclei which are thought to correlate with sites of DNA double strand breaks. (Image provided by Dr. Leslie Parsels, University of Michigan.)

origins and replicon initiation fails to occur.[10] A more prominent mechanism for S-phase arrest is signaled through the MRN complex and the cohesin protein SMC1 by ATM.[6] Loss of ATM, MRN components, or SMC1 leads to loss of intra-S phase checkpoint function and increased radiosensitivity.[6] Both the CDC45 and ATM pathways represent parallel, but seemingly independent, pathways to protect replication forks from trying to replicate through DNA strand breaks. Although ATM has received the lion's share of attention in signaling checkpoint activation in response to ionizing radiation, its family member ATR (ataxia telangiectasia and rad3-related) also plays a role in S-phase checkpoint responses.[11] ATM kinase activity is inducible by radiation, whereas ATR kinase activity is constitutive and does not significantly change with irradiation. In contrast to Cdc45 and ATM, ATR is probably more important in monitoring perturbations in replications that are the result of stalled replication forks to prevent the formation of DNA double-strand breaks.

The arrest of cells in G_2 phase following DNA damage is one of the most conserved evolutionary responses to ionizing radiation. It makes sense to have a final checkpoint in G_2 phase to prevent cells from entering into mitosis with damaged DNA that could be transmitted to their progeny. It follows that cells lacking the G_2 checkpoint are radiosensitive because they try to divide with damaged chromosomes that cannot be aligned at metaphase to be properly apportioned to daughter cells. At the biochemical level, the regulation of the mitosis-promoting factor cyclin B/Cdk1 is the critical step in the activation of this checkpoint. At the molecular level, ATM and Chk are activated by DNA damage in G_2 phase and inhibit the activation of Cdc25C phosphatases, which are essential for the activation of cyclin B/Cdk1.[12,13] The polo-like kinase family (Plk1 and Plk3) also responds to DNA damage and can inhibit Cdc25C activation.[14] A great deal of effort has been focused on the development of small molecules to inhibit checkpoint response proteins, such as Chk1, with the idea that they would inhibit radiation-induced G_2 arrest and perhaps repair and thus be used as radiation sensitizers.[15]

DNA Repair

Ionizing radiation causes base damage, single-strand breaks, double-strand breaks, and sugar damage, as well as DNA-DNA, and DNA-protein crosslinks. The critical target for ionizing radiation-induced cell inactivation and cell killing is the DNA double-strand break.[16,17] In eukaryotic cells, DNA double-strand breaks can be repaired by two processes: homologous recombination repair (HRR), which requires an undamaged DNA strand as a participant in the repair, and nonhomologous end joining (NHEJ), which mediates end-to-end joining.[18] In lower eukaryotes such as yeast, homologous recombination repair is the predominant pathway used for repairing DNA double-strand breaks, whereas mammalian cells use both homologous and nonhomologous recombination to repair their DNA. In mammalian cells, the choice of repair is biased by the phase of the cell cycle and by the abundance of repetitive DNA. HRR is used primarily in the late S to G_2 phases of the cell cycle, and NHEJ predominates in the G_1 phase of the cell cycle (Fig. 27.5). NHEJ and HRR are not mutually exclusive, and both have been found to be active in the late S to G_2 phase of the cell cycle, indicating that factors in addition to cell-cycle phase are important in determining which mechanism will be used to repair DNA strand breaks.

Nonhomologous End Joining. In the G_1 phase of the cell cycle, the ligation of DNA double-strand breaks is primarily through NHEJ, as a sister chromatid does not exist to provide a template for repair. The damaged ends of DNA double-strand breaks must first be modified before rejoining. The process of NHEJ can be divided into at least four steps: synapsis, end processing, fill-in synthesis, and ligation (Fig. 27.6).[19] Synapsis is the critical initial step where the Ku heterodimer and the DNA-dependent protein kinase catalytic subunit DNA-PKcs bind to the ends of the DNA double-strand break. Ku recruits not only DNA-PKcs to the DNA ends, but also artemis, a protein that possesses endonuclease activity for 5′ and 3′ overhangs as well as hairpins.[20] DNA-PKcs that is bound to the broken DNA ends phosphorylates artemis and activates its endonuclease activity for end processing. This role of artemis's endonuclease in NHEJ may not necessarily be required for the ligation of blunt ends or ends with compatible termini. DNA polymerase-μ is associated with the Ku/DNA/XRCC4/DNA ligase IV complex and is probably the polymerase that is used in the fill-in reaction. The actual rejoining of DNA ends is mediated by a XRCC4/DNA ligase IV complex, which is also probably recruited by the Ku heterodimer.[21,22] Although NHEJ is effective in rejoining DNA double-strand breaks, it is highly error prone. In fact, the main physiologic role of NHEJ is to generate antibodies through V(D)J rejoining, and the error-prone nature of NHEJ is essential for generating antibody diversity.

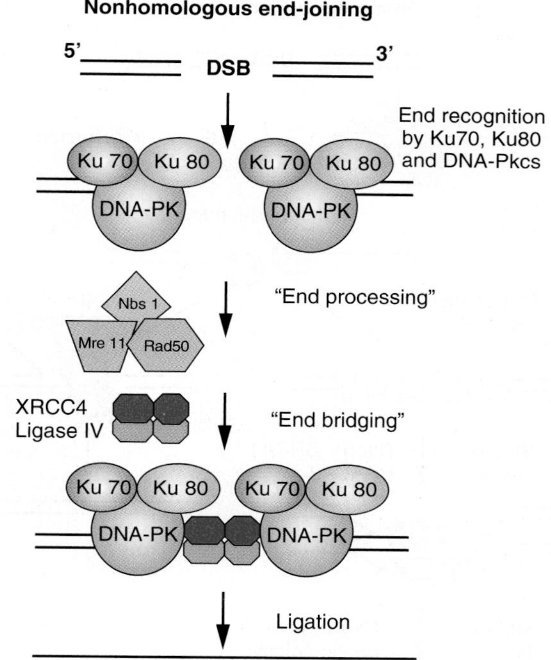

FIGURE 27.5 Schematic of the critical steps and proteins involved in nonhomologous end joining (NHEJ). The process of NHEJ can be divided into at least four steps: synapsis, end processing, fill-in synthesis, and ligation. DSB, double-strand break.

Homologous Recombination. HRR provides the mammalian genome a high-fidelity pathway of repairing DNA double-strand breaks. In contrast to NHEJ, HRR requires physical contact with an undamaged DNA template such as a sister chromatid for repair to occur. In response to a double-strand break, ATM as well as the complex of Mre11, Rad50, and Nbs1 proteins (MRN complex) are recruited to sites of DNA double-strand breaks[23] (Fig. 27.6). In lower eukaryotes, the MRN complex facilitates nucleosome displacement and histone variant H2A phosphorylation near sites of DNA strand breaks.[23] The MRN complex is also involved in the recruitment of the breast cancer tumor suppressor gene *BRCA1* to the site of the break.[24] In addition to recruiting *BRCA1* to the site of the DNA strand break, Mre11 and as yet unidentified

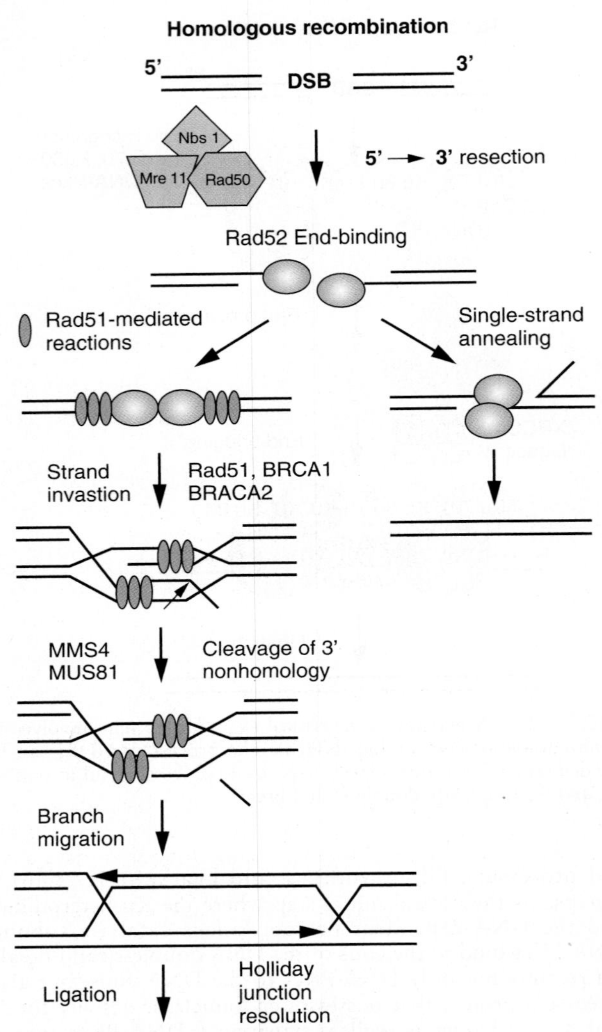

FIGURE 27.6 Schematic of the critical steps and proteins involved in homologous recombination repair (HRR). The process of HRR can be divided into the following steps: double-strand break (DSB) targeting by H2AX and the MRN complex, recruitment of the ATM (ataxia-telangiectasia mutation) kinase, end processing and protection, strand exchange, single-strand gap filling, and resolution into unique double stranded molecules.

endonucleases resect the DNA, resulting in a 3′ single-strand DNA that serves as a binding site for Rad51. *BRCA2*, which is recruited to the double-strand break by BRCA1, facilitates the loading of the Rad51 protein onto replication-protein A (RPA)-coated single-strand overhangs that are produced by endonuclease resection.[25] The Rad51 protein is a homologue of the *Escherichia coli* recombinase RecA, and it possesses the ability to form nucleofilaments and catalyze strand exchange with the complementary strand of the undamaged chromosome, an essential step in HRR. Five additional paralogs of Rad51 also bind to the RPA-coated single-stranded region and recruit Rad52, which binds DNA and protects against exonucleolytic degradation.[26] To facilitate repair, the Rad54 protein uses its ATPase activity to unwind the double-stranded molecule. The two invading ends serve as primers for DNA synthesis, resulting in structures known as Holliday junctions. These Holliday junctions are resolved either by noncrossing over, in which case the Holliday junctions disengage and DNA strands align followed by gap filling, or by crossing over of the Holliday junctions and gap filling. Because inactivation of most of the HRR genes discussed previously results in radiosensitivity and genomic instability, these genes provide a critical link between HRR and chromosome stability.

Chromosome Aberrations Result from Faulty DNA Double-Strand Break Repair

Unfaithful restitution of DNA strand breaks can lead to chromosome aberrations such as acentric fragments (no centromeres) or terminal deletions (uncapped chromosome ends). Radiation-induced DNA double-strand breaks also induce exchange-type aberrations that are the consequence of symmetric translocations between two DNA double-strand breaks in two different chromosomes (Fig. 27.7). Symmetrical chromosome translocations often do not lead to lethality, as genetic information is not lost in subsequent cell divisions. In contrast, when two DNA double-strand breaks in two different chromosomes recombine to form one chromosome with two centromeres and two fragments of chromosomes without centromeres or telomeres, cell death is inevitable. These types of chromosome aberrations are the consequence of asymmetrical chromosome translocations where the genetic material is

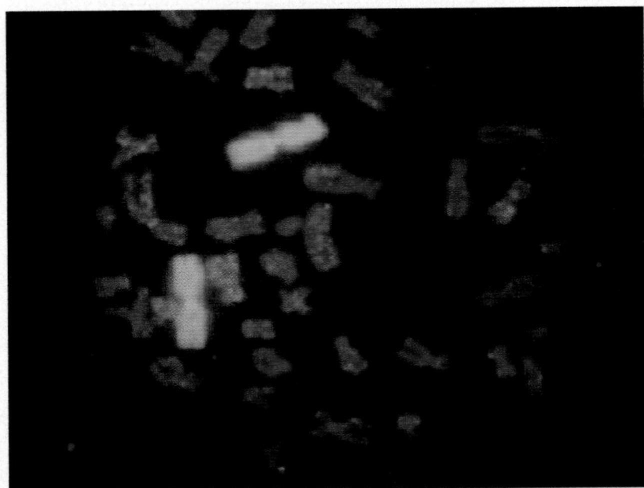

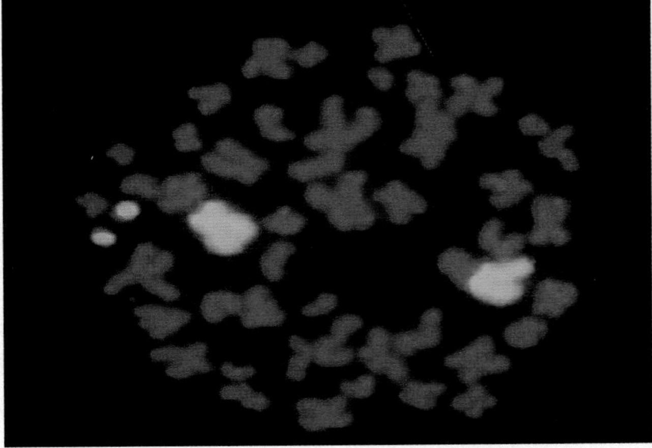

FIGURE 27.7 Fluorescent *in situ* hybridization of DNA probes that specifically recognize chromosome 4. In unirradiated cells (**top**), two chromosome 4s are visualized. In irradiated cells (**bottom**), one chromosome 4 illegitimately recombined with another chromosome to produce an asymmetrical chromosome aberration, with resulting acentric fragments that will be lost in subsequent cell divisions.

recombined in what has been termed an *illegitimate* manner (e.g., a chromosome containing an extra centromere).

During mitosis when a cell divides, aberrant chromosomes that have two centromeres or lack a centromere or are in the shape of a ring have difficulty in separating, resulting in daughter cells with unequal or asymmetric distribution of the parental genetic material. The quantification of asymmetric chromosome aberrations induced by radiation is difficult and has to be performed by the first cell division, as these aberrations will be lost during subsequent cell divisions. For this reason, symmetrical chromosome aberrations have been used to assess radiation-induced damage many generations after exposure as they are not lost from the population of exposed cells. In fact, symmetrical chromosome aberrations can be detected in the descendants of survivors of Hiroshima and Nagasaki, indicating that they are stable biomarkers of radiation exposure.[27]

The Effect of Radiation on Cell Survival

The potential consequences of cells exposed to ionizing radiation are normal cell division, DNA damage-induced senescence (reproductively inactive but metabolically active), DNA damage-induced apoptosis, or mitotic-linked cell death (Fig. 27.8). These manifestations of DNA damage can occur within one or two cell divisions or can manifest at later times after many cell divisions.[28] Effects that occur at later times have been termed *delayed reproductive cell death* and may also be influenced by secreted factors that are induced in response to radiation exposure.[29]

The ability to culture cells derived from both normal and tumor tissue has provided insight into how radiosensitivity varies between tissues by analyzing the shape of survival curves. Survival curves of tumor cells often possess a shouldered region at low doses that becomes shallower as the dose increases and eventually becomes exponential. A shoulder on a survival means that these low doses of radiation are less efficient in cell killing, presumably because cells are efficient in repairing DNA strand breaks.[16,17] Killing at low doses of radiation can be described in the form of a linear quadratic equation: $S = e^{-\alpha D - \beta D^2}$ (Fig. 27.9).[30] In this equation, S is the fraction of cells that survive a dose (D) of radiation, whereas α and β are constants. Cell killing by the linear and quadratic components are equal when $\alpha D = \beta D^2$ or $D = \alpha/\beta$. Over a larger dose range, the relationship between cell killing and dose is

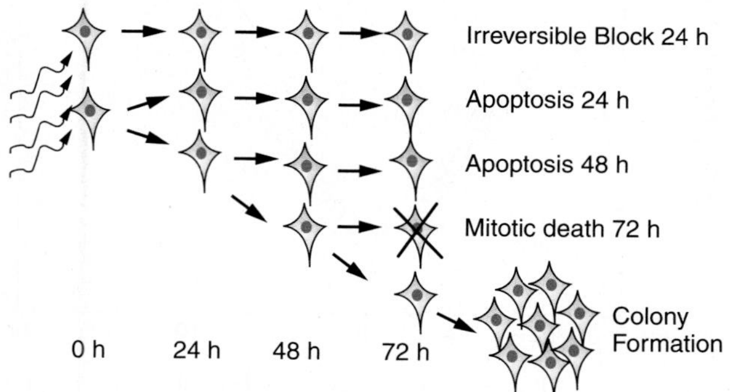

FIGURE 27.8 Consequences of exposure to ionizing radiation at the cellular level. Cells exposed to ionizing radiation can enter a state of senescence where they are unable to divide, but are still able to secrete growth factors. Alternatively, cells can die through apoptosis, mitotic linked cell death, or they can repair their DNA damage and produce viable progeny.

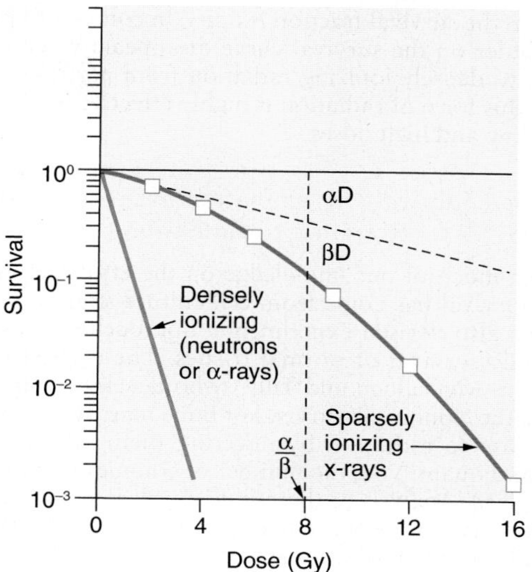

FIGURE 27.9 Analysis of survival curves for mammalian cells exposed to radiation by the linear quadratic model. The probability of hitting a critical target is proportional to dose (αD): the alpha component. The probability of hitting two critical targets will be the product of those probabilities; therefore, it will be proportional to dose^2 (βD^2): the beta component. The dose at which killing by both the alpha and beta components is equal is defined as D = α/β. (From ref. 1, with permission.)

more complex and is described by three different components: an initial slope (D_1), a final slope (D_0), and the width of the shoulder (n, the extrapolation number) or D_q, the quasi-threshold dose (Fig. 27.10). The extrapolation number, n, defines the place where the shoulder intersects the ordinate when the dose is extrapolated to zero, and the quasi-threshold dose D_q defines the width of the shoulder by cutting the dose

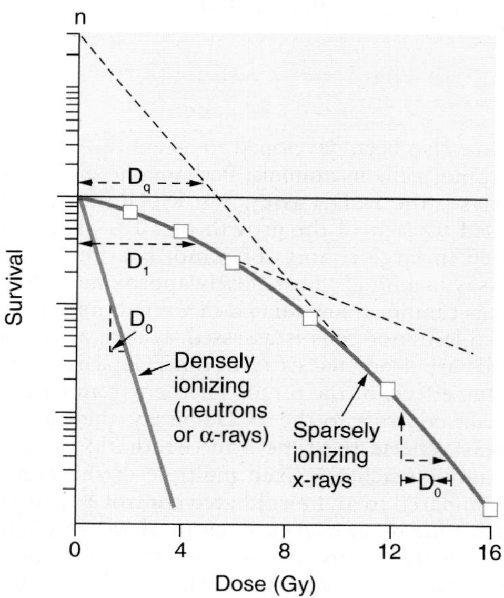

FIGURE 27.10 Analysis of survival curves for mammalian cells exposed to radiation by the multitarget model. This survival is described by an initial slope (D_1; dose to decreased survival to 37% on initial portion of the curve), a final slope (D_0; dose to decrease survival from starting point to 37% of that point on straight line portion of the curve), an extrapolation number (n; an estimate of the width of the shoulder), and a quasi-threshold (D_q; a type of threshold dose below which radiation has no effect). (From ref. 1, with permission.)

axis when the survival fraction is unity. In contrast to photons, the shoulder on the survival curve disappears when cells are exposed to densely ionizing radiation from particles, indicating that this form of radiation is highly effective in killing cells at both low and high doses.

In Vivo Survival Determination of Normal Tissue Response to Radiation

Although much of our knowledge on the effects of radiation on cell survival has come from cell culture studies, investigators have also devised experimental approaches to assess the clonogenic survival of normal tissues. The earliest example came from McCulloch and Till,[31] who developed an assay to measure the clonogenic survival of bone marrow–derived cells in response to radiation by injecting them into a recipient mouse and quantifying the number of colonies that developed in the spleen. Analysis of these *in vivo* spleen assays indicated that bone marrow cells are highly radiosensitive (perhaps the most radiosensitive of all mammalian cells) in that their cell survival curve lacked a shoulder. These experiments represent two important firsts in the radiation sciences: they described the first development of an *in vivo* assay to assess normal tissue survival to radiation and they demonstrated the first existence of normal tissue stem cells. Soon after, Withers[32,33] developed an assay to assess the survival of skin stem cells, and Withers and Elkind[34] developed an assay to quantify the viability of small intestinal clonogens.

Because these ingenious approaches cannot be applied to all normal tissues, loss of tissue function instead of clonogenic survival has been used as an end point to assess radiation effects. Effects on tissue function can be grouped into the acute or late variety. Desquamation of skin by radiation is an example of an acute loss of function, whereas loss of spinal cord function is an example of a late functional effect. Acutely sensitive tissues such as skin, bone marrow, and intestinal mucosa possess a significant component of tissue cell division, whereas delayed sensitive tissues such as spinal cord, breast, and bone do not possess a significant amount of cell division or turnover and manifest radiation effects at later times.

In Vivo Determination of Tumor Response to Radiation

Assays have also been developed to assess the clonogenic survival of tumor cells in animals. Perhaps the most relevant of these assays is the TCD_{50} assay,[35] in which the dose of radiation needed to control the growth of 50% of the tumors is determined in large cohorts of tumor-bearing animals. The TCD_{50} assay in animals most closely approximates the clinical situation as tumors are irradiated in animals and the ability to kill all viable tumor cells is assessed. Unlike assays in which tumor cells are irradiated *ex vivo*, the TCD_{50} assay takes into account the effects of the tumor microenvironment on tumor response. In contrast to the TCD_{50} assay, the tumor growth delay assay reflects the time after irradiation that a transplanted tumor reaches a fixed multiple of the pretreatment volume compared to an unirradiated control.[36] This end point can be achieved by measuring tumor volume through the use of calipers or by noninvasive measurement of tumor volume using bioluminescent molecules such as luciferase or fluorescent proteins. In the latter approach, all the tumor cells are stably transfected with a bioluminescent marker before implantation, and tumor growth is measured by bioluminescent activity.[37] The advantage of this approach is that tumor cells can be assessed even if they are orthotopically transplanted into their tissue of origin. In another approach, tumors or cells are first irradiated *in vivo*, the tumor is excised and made into a single-cell suspension, and these cells are then injected into a non–tumor-bearing animal. If the cells are injected subcutaneously under the skin, the end point is tumor formation.[38] If the tumor cells are injected in the tail vein of the mouse, the end point is colony formation in the lungs.[39] The major advantage of these assays is that the actual number of viable cells can be determined.

FACTORS THAT AFFECT RADIATION RESPONSE

The Fundamental Principles of Radiobiology

Studies on split dose repair (SDR) by Elkind et al.[40] uncovered three of what we now recognize as the most fundamental principles of fractionated radiotherapy: repair, reassortment, and repopulation (Fig. 27.11). (Reoxygenation, described below, is the fourth.) SDR describes the increased survival or tumor growth delay found if a dose of radiation is split into two fractions compared to the same dose administered in one fraction. This repair is likely due to DNA double-strand break rejoining. Elkind et al. found that the survival of cells increased with increasing time between doses for up to a maximum of about 6 hours. This finding is consistent with the clinical observation that separation of radiation treatments by 6 hours produces similar normal tissue injury as a 24-hour separation. The shoulder of a survival curve is strongly influenced by SDR: the broader the shoulder the more SDR and the smaller α/β ratio.

Similar to repair, reassortment and repopulation are also dependent on the interval of time between radiation fractions. If cells are given short time intervals between doses, they can progress from a resistant portion of the cell cycle (e.g., S phase) to a sensitive portion of the cell cycle (e.g., G_2 phase). This transit between resistant and sensitive phases of the cell cycle is termed *reassortment*. If irradiated cells are provided even

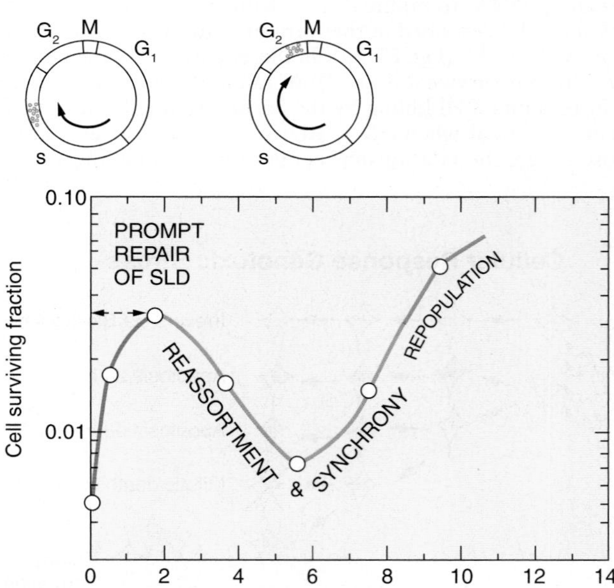

FIGURE 27.11 Idealized survival curve of rodent cells exposed to two fractions of x-rays. This figure illustrates how the time interval between doses alters the sensitivity of cells when exposed to multiple fractions. In this case, cells move from a resistant phase of the cell cycle (late S phase) to a sensitive phase of the cell cycle (G_2 phase). This is known as *reassortment*. If longer periods of time occur between fractions of radiation, cells will undergo division. This latter process is called *repopulation*. SLD, sublethal damage. (From ref. 1, with permission.)

longer intervals of time between doses, the survival of the population of irradiated cells will increase. This increase in split-dose survival after longer periods of time is the result of cell division and has been termed *repopulation*. Reassortment and repopulation appear to have more protracted kinetics in normal tissues than rapidly proliferating tumor cells and thereby enhance the tumor response to fractionated radiotherapy compared to normal tissues.

Dose-Rate Effects

For sparsely ionizing radiation, dose rate plays a critical factor in cell killing. Lowering the dose rate, and thereby increasing exposure time, reduces the effectiveness of killing by x-rays because of increased SDR. Further reduction in dose rate results in more SDR and reduces the shoulder of the survival curve. Thus, if one plots the survival for individual doses in a multifraction experiment so that there is sufficient time for SDR to occur, the resulting survival curve would have little shoulder and appear almost linear.[41] In some cell types, there is a threshold to the lowering of dose rate, and in fact one paradoxically finds an increase, instead of a decrease, in cell killing. This increase in cell killing under these conditions of protracted dose rate is due to accumulation of cells in a radiosensitive portion of the cell cycle. In summary, the magnitude of the dose-rate effect varies between cell types because of SDR, the redistribution of cells through the cell cycle, and time for cell division to occur.

Cell Cycle

The phase of the cell cycle at the time of radiation influences the cell's inherent sensitivity to radiation. Cells synchronized in late-G_1 to early-S and G_2 or M phases are most sensitive while cells in G_1 and mid- to late-S phases are more resistant to radiation.[1] These differences in sensitivity during the cell cycle are exploited by the concept of reassortment during fractioned radiotherapy as well by the use of chemotherapeutic agents that reassort cells into more sensitive phases of the cell cycle in combination with radiation.

Tumor Oxygenation

The major microenvironmental influence on tumor response to radiation is molecular oxygen.[42] Decreased levels of oxygen (hypoxia) in tissue culture result in decreased killing after radiation, which can be expressed as an oxygen enhancement ratio (OER).[36] Operationally, OER is defined as the ratio of doses to give the same killing under hypoxic and normoxic conditions. At high doses of radiation, the OER is approximately 3, whereas at low doses it is closer to 2.[43] Oxygen must be present within 10 μsec of irradiation to achieve its radiosensitizing effect. Under hypoxic conditions, damage to DNA can be repaired more readily than under oxic conditions where damage to DNA is "fixed" because of the interaction of oxygen with free radicals generated by radiation. These changes in radiation sensitivity are detectable at oxygen ranges below 30 mm Hg. Most tumor cells exhibit a survival difference halfway between fully aerobic and fully anoxic cells when exposed to a partial pressure of oxygen between 3 and 10 mm Hg.[1] The presence of hypoxia has greater significance for single-dose fractions used in the treatment of certain primary tumors and metastases and is less important for fractionated radiotherapy where reoxygenation occurs between fractions. Furthermore, most hypoxic cells are not actively undergoing cell division, thus impeding the efficacy of conventional chemotherapeutic agents that are targeted to actively dividing cells.

Although normal tissue and tumors vary in their oxygen concentrations, only tumors possess levels of oxygen low enough to influence the effectiveness of radiation killing. Although the variations in normal tissue oxygenation are in large part due to physiology governing acute changes in oxygen consumption, the variations in tumor oxygen can be directly attributed to abnormal vasculature that results in a more chronic condition. Thomlinson and Gray[44] observed that variations in tumor oxygen occur because there is insufficient vasculature to provide oxygen to all tumor cells. They hypothesized that oxygen is unable to reach tumor cells beyond 10 to 12 cell diameters from the lumen of a tumor blood vessel because of metabolic consumption by respiring tumor cells. This form of hypoxia caused by metabolic consumption of oxygen has been termed *chronic* or *diffusion-mediated hypoxia*. In contrast, changes in blood flow, due either to interstitial pressure changes in tumor blood vessels that lack a smooth muscle component or red blood cell fluxes, can cause transient occlusion of blood vessels, resulting in *acute* or *transient hypoxia*. Chronically hypoxic cells will only become reoxygenated when their distance from the lumen of a blood vessel decreases, such as during fractionated radiotherapy when tumor cords shrink. In contrast, tumor cells that are acutely hypoxic because of changes in blood flow or interstitial pressure often cycle in an unpredictable manner between oxic and hypoxic states as blood flow changes.

Based on studies demonstrating that hypoxia can alter radiation sensitivity and decrease tumor control by radiotherapy, strategies have been developed to increase tumor oxygenation. Most important, it appears that tumor oxygen levels increase during a course of fractionated radiation. This may be one of the most important benefits of fractionated radiation and is termed *reoxygenation*. Tumor reoxygentation during a course of fractionated radiation may also offer an explanation for the general lack of clinical efficacy of hypoxic cell sensitizers, despite the clear evidence that hypoxia causes radioresistance.

Aside from using fractionated radiation, the most direct approach to increasing tumor oxygenation is to expose patients who receive radiotherapy to hyperbaric oxygen therapy. The underlying concept is that increasing the amount of oxygen in the bloodstream should result in more oxygen available for diffusion to the hypoxic regions of tumors. Experimentally, hyperbaric oxygen therapy increases the sensitivity of transplanted tumors to radiation. The results of clinical studies with hyperbaric oxygen therapy when combined with radiotherapy showed improvement for two sites—head and neck and cervix cancers—but failed to show an improvement with other sites, thus calling into question its general usefulness in radiotherapy.[45] In a related approach, erythropoietin (EPO), a hormone released by the kidney that increases red blood cell production, should also increase tumor oxygenation by increasing the delivery of hemoglobin-bound oxygen molecules. EPO has been effective in correcting anemia but has not been successful in combination with radiation to control head and neck cancer and may, in fact, stimulate tumor growth.[46,47]

Another strategy to increase tumor oxygenation has been the combined use of nicotinamide, which increases tissue perfusion and carbogen (95% O_2 and 5% CO_2) breathing (arcon therapy). Clinical studies in head and neck cancer suggest that this combination may increase the effectiveness of radiotherapy in head and neck cancer.[48] Biologics such as anti–vascular endothelial growth factor (VEGF) therapy have also been demonstrated to increase tumor oxygenation.[49] Anti-VEGF therapy may increase tumor oxygenation by eliminating abnormal vessels that are inadequate in perfusing tumor cells, the so-called vascular normalization hypothesis. Although there is solid experimental evidence to support this hypothesis, there appears to be only a short window of time in which it could be effectively combined with radiotherapy.

Because the presence of hypoxia has both prognostic and potential therapeutic implications, substantial effort has been invested in trying to image hypoxia.[50,51] The goal of using imaging to "paint" radiation doses to different regions of tumors, although technically possible (as described in the next section "Radiation Physics"), faces the problem that changes in oxygenation are dynamic.[52] In the future, hypoxia-directed treatment may evolve from the use of cytotoxics that are activated under hypoxic conditions to targeted drugs that exploit the genomic and proteomic changes induced by hypoxia such as hypoxia-inducible factor-1α (HIF-1α) or those involved in translational control and the unfolded protein response. However, despite the strong rationale supporting their use, at this time there are no agents used in the clinic that target hypoxia.

DRUGS THAT AFFECT RADIATION SENSITIVITY

For over 30 years now, chemotherapy and radiotherapy have been administered concurrently. In order to maximize the efficacy of radiochemotherapy it is necessary to understand the biological mechanisms underlying radiosensitization by chemotherapeutic agents. The several classes of standard chemotherapeutic agents as well as novel molecularly targeted agents that possess radiosensitizing properties will be discussed in this section.

Antimetabolites

The chemotherapeutic radiation sensitizer 5-fluorouracil is among the most commonly used. Given in combination with radiation, it has led to clinical improvements in a variety of cancers, including those of the head and neck, esophagus, stomach, pancreas, rectum, anus, and cervix. The combination of 5-fluorouracil with radiation is now a standard therapy for cancers of the stomach (adjuvant), pancreas (unresectable), and rectum. For other cancers such as head and neck, esophagus, or anal, 5-fluorouracil and radiation are combined with cisplatin or mitomycin C, respectively. Being an analogue of uracil, 5-flourouracil is misincorporated into RNA and DNA. However, the ability of 5-fluorouracil to radiosensitize is related to its ability to inhibit thymidylate synthase, which leads to depletion of dTTP and inhibition of DNA synthesis. This slowed, inappropriate progression through the S phase in response to 5-fluorouracil is thought to be the mechanism underlying radiosensitization.[53] Similarly to 5-fluorouracil, the oral thymidylate synthase inhibitor capecitabine is also being increasingly used in combination with radiation.

Gemcitabine (2′,2′-deoxyfluorocytdine [dFdCyd]) is another potent antimetabolite radiosensitizer. Preclinical studies have demonstrated that radiosensitization by gemcitabine involves depletion of dATP (related to the ability of dFdCDP to inhibit ribonucleotide reductase) as well as redistribution of cells into the early S phase of the cell cycle.[54] The combination of gemcitabine with radiation in clinical trials has suggested improved clinical outcomes for patients with cancers of the lung, pancreas, and bladder. Gemcitabine-based chemoradiation has developed into a standard therapy for locally advanced pancreatic cancer. However, in some clinical trials, such as those in lung and head and neck cancers, the combination of gemcitabine with radiation has led to increased mucositis and esophagitis.[55] Thus it should be emphasized that in the presence of gemcitabine, radiation fields must be defined with great caution. Such is the case in pancreatic cancer, where the combination of full-dose gemcitabine with radiation to the gross tumor can be safely administered if clinically uninvolved lymph nodes are excluded.[56] Conversely, inclusion of the regional lymphatics in the treatment field in combination with full-dose gemcitabine produces unacceptable toxicities.[57]

Platinums

Cisplatin is likely the most commonly used chemotherapeutic agent in combination with radiation. While cisplatin was the prototype for several other platinum analogues, carboplatin is also frequently used in combination with radiation. Cisplatin in combination with radiation, and sometimes in conjunction with a second chemotherapeutic agent, is indicated for cancers of the head and neck, esophagus (with 5-fluorouracil), lung, cervix, and anus.

Radiosensitization by cisplatin is related to its ability to cause inter- and intrastrand DNA crosslinks. Removal of these crosslinks during the repair process results in DNA strand breaks. Although there are multiple theories to explain the mechanism(s) of radiosensitization by cisplatin, two plausible explanations are that cisplatin inhibits the repair (both homologous and nonhomologous) of radiation-induced DNA double-strand breaks or increases the number of lethal radiation-induced double-strand breaks.[58]

Taxanes

The taxanes, paclitaxel and docetaxel, act to stabilize microtubules, resulting in accumulation of cells in the G_2 or M phase, the most radiation sensitive phase of the cell cycle. The radiosensitizing properties of the taxanes are thought to be attributable to redistribution of cells into G_2 or M phase. Paclitaxel in combination with radiation (with cis- or carboplatin) has demonstrated clinical benefit in the treatment of unresectable lung carcinoma.[59,60]

Molecularly Targeted Agents

Molecularly targeted agents are especially appealing in the context of radiosensitization as they are generally less toxic than standard chemotherapeutic agents and need to be given in multimodality regimens (given their often inadequate efficacy as single agents). The epidermal growth factor receptor (EGFR) has been intensely pursued as a target, thus both antibody and small molecule EGFR inhibitors, such as cetuximab and erlotinib, respectively, have been developed. Head and neck seems to be the most promising tumor site for the combination of EGFR inhibitors with radiation therapy. Preclinical data have demonstrated that the schedule of administration of EGFR inhibitors with radiation is important; EGFR inhibition before chemoradiation may produce antagonism.[61,62] In a randomized phase 3 trial, cetuximab plus radiation produced a significant survival advantage over radiation alone in patients with locally advanced head and neck cancer.[63] Subsequent trials are under way to test the efficacy of cetuximab in combination with concurrent, cisplatin-based chemoradiation in head and neck cancer as well.

Although EGFR inhibition concurrent with radiation is by far the best established combination of a molecularly targeted agent with radiation, other exciting molecularly targeted agents are being developed as radiation sensitizers. Targeting DNA damage response pathways is one approach to radiosensitization. Recently, Chk1 inhibitors have been shown to radiosensitize tumor cells and are currently in clinical development in combination with chemotherapy, with clinical trials in combination with radiation planned.[64] In addition, poly(adenosine diphosphate-ribose) polymerase (PARP) inhibitors have been demonstrated to induce radiosensitization preclinically, and at least one clinical trial to test a PARP inhibitor with whole-brain radiation is under way, with others likely to follow.[65]

Other Agents

While the most common clinically used agents in combination with radiation that have been shown to produce significant clinical benefit are described above, other agents with different mechanisms of action have been used as radiation sensitizers as well as radiation protectors. The vinca alkaloids, such as vincristine, possess radiosensitizing properties due to their ability to block mitotic spindle assembly and thus arrest cells in the M phase. Although, vincristine is used in combination with radiation to treat medulloblastoma, rhabdomyosarcoma, and brainstem glioma, its use is principally based on its lack of myelosuppressive side effects, which are dose limiting for radiation in these types of tumors, rather than its potential radiosensitizing properties.

Also worth mention in a discussion of modulators of radiation sensitivity are agents designed to radioprotect normal tissues. One such type of drug, amifostine is a free radical scavenger with some selectivity toward normal tissues, which express more alkaline phosphatase than tumor cells, the enzyme which converts amifostine to a free thiol metabolite. Clinical trials in head and neck as well as lung cancers have shown a reduction in radiation-related toxicities such as xerostomia, mucositis, esophagitis, and pneumonitis, respectively.[66,67] However, further clinical investigation is necessary to conclusively demonstrate a lack of tumor protection and safety in combination with chemoradiotherapy regimens.

RADIATION PHYSICS

Physics of Photon Interactions

Tumors requiring radiation can be found at depths ranging from zero to tens of centimeters below the skin. The goal of treatment is to delivery sufficient radiation to the tumor site, which can result in absorbed dose. This involves both the availability of treatment beams and delivery techniques, together with methods to plan the treatments and ensure their safe delivery. This section will establish the general physical basis for the use of ionizing radiation in the treatment of tumors, briefly describe some of the treatment equipment, indicate physical qualities of the treatment beams themselves, and summarize the treatment planning process. Those who desire more in-depth detail are referred to textbooks dedicated to medical physics and the technological aspects of radiation oncology.[68–74]

Most patients who are treated with radiation receive high-energy external-beam photon therapy. Here, "external" indicates that the treatment beam is generated and delivered from outside the body. High-energy (6 to 20 MeV) photon beams (electromagnetic radiation) penetrate tissue, enabling the treatment of deep-seated tumors. Modern equipment generates these beams with sufficient fluence to ensure delivery of therapeutic fractions of dose in short treatment sessions. Other types of particles and beams also exist for use in treating tumors both externally and internally. They are mentioned briefly later. However, as external photon beams dominate the scene (and as common basic physics principles related to delivered dose exist among the modalities), the focus here will be on photon beam generation and interactions in tissue.

As mentioned earlier, ionizing radiation kills cells via both direct and indirect mechanisms. Radiation therapy aims to instigate those ionizations and events in the tumor cells. Photons are massless, uncharged packets of energy that interact with matter via electromagnetic processes. As a consequence of those interactions, the incident photons become either entirely absorbed (giving up their energy to the ejection of an atomic electrons [photoelectric effect] or create an energetic electron-positron pairs [pair production]) or scatter (reduction in energy and change in direction of incident photons with subsequent transfer of parts of their energy to a free electrons [Compton scattering]). The secondary electrons generated as a consequence of these interactions have residual energy, mass, and, most important, electric charge. They slow down in matter through multiple interactions with (primarily) the electrons of atoms, leading to excitation and ionization of those atoms. These ionizations (hence the term *ionizing radiation*) lead to local absorption of energy (i.e., dose, energy absorbed per unit mass) and the direct and indirect cell-killing effects necessary to treat tumors.

Thus, the use of external photon beams for cancer therapy involves a two-step process; interaction (scattering) of the photons, with subsequent dose deposition via the secondary electrons. The probability of photon interactions is energy dependent. Photoelectric interactions dominate at lower photon energies. Whereas these beams are ideal for diagnostic procedures (for their preferential absorption by tissues of differing atomic number, leading to good subject contrast), they are attenuated too quickly in tissue to supply enough interactions to be useful for therapy for any but the most superficial tumors. Pair production interactions dominate at higher photon energies; however, the probability of interacting in tissue for those high-energy photons is so low as to preclude them from general use as well. In the 10s to 100s of kiloelectron volt to the few megaelectron volt photon energy range, Compton scattering dominates. As will be shown, these beams have sufficient penetration and can be generated with sufficient intensity to be useful for tumor treatments, especially when combined in treatment plans that comprise multiple beams entering the patient from different directions but overlapping at the tumor.

It is useful to point out physical scales of reference for external photon beam therapy. A typical megavoltage photon beam may have an average photon energy near 2 MeV. Those photons primarily undergo Compton scattering with a mean free path of approximately 20 cm for a 2-MeV photon in tissue. An average Compton interaction results in a secondary electron with a mean energy near 0.5 MeV (and a Compton scattered photon near 1.5 MeV, that likely escapes or scatters elsewhere in the patient). A typical secondary electron of approximately 0.5 MeV will cause excitations and ionizations of atoms as it dissipates its energy over a path length of approximately 2 mm. This could be expected to lead to approximately 10,000 ionizations, or about 5 ionizations per micron of tissue. As can be seen, therapeutic killing of cancer cells will require many Compton scatterings with statistical interaction among the ionizations because of the resulting slow down of the secondary electrons.

Photon Beam Generation and Treatment Delivery

As previously mentioned, effective external-beam photon treatments require higher energy beams capable of reaching deep-seated tumors with sufficient fluence to make it likely that the dose deposition will kill tumor cells. To spare normal tissues and maximize targeting, beams are arranged to enter the patient from several directions and to intersect at the center of the tumor (treatment isocenter). Although machines containing collimated beams from high-intensity radioactive sources (primarily ^{60}Co) are still in use, today's modern treatment machine accelerates electrons to high (million electron volt) energy and impinges them onto an x-ray production target, leading to the generation of intense beams of Bremsstrahlung x-rays. A typical photon beam treatment machine[75,76] (Fig. 27.12) consists of a high-energy (6 to 20 MeV) linear

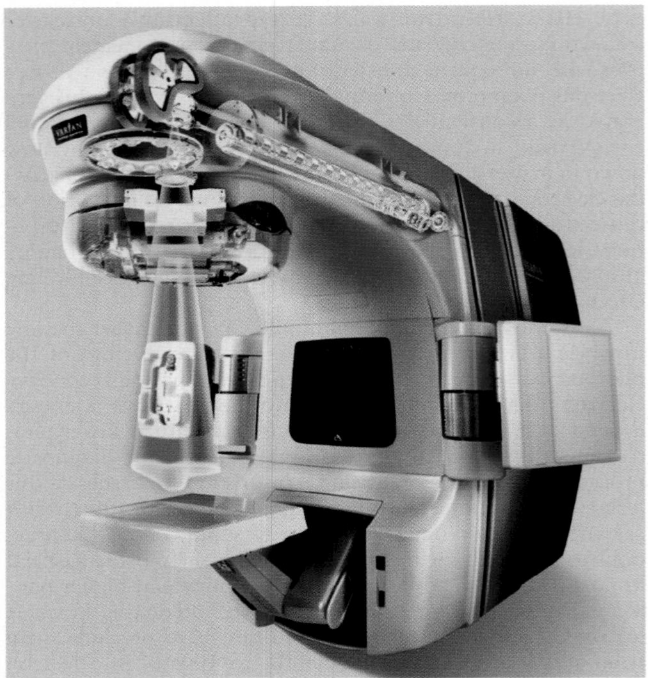

FIGURE 27.12 Shadow view of C-arm linear accelerator. Electron beam (originating at upper right) is accelerated through a linear accelerator wave guide, selected for correct energy in a bending magnet and then impinges on an x-ray production target. The x-ray beam (originating at target upper left) is flattened and collimated before leaving the treatment head. Also illustrated (downstream from the beam) is an electric portal imager that is used to measure (image) the beam exiting a patient. (From Varian Medical Systems, Palo Alto, CA, with permission.)

electron accelerator, electromagnetic beam steering and monitoring systems, x-ray generation targets, high-density treatment field-shaping devices (collimators), and up to a ton of radiation shielding on a mechanical C-arm gantry that can rotate precisely around a treatment couch (Fig. 27.13). These treatment-delivery machines routinely maintain mechanical isocenters for patient treatments to within a sphere of 1 mm radius. The development of "stereotactic radiotherapy," which will be described in the section "Clinical Application of Types of Radiation," depends on this level of machine precision.

X-ray production by monoenergetic high-energy electrons results in an x-ray (photon) beam that contains a continuous spectrum of energies with maximum photon energy near that of the incident electron beam. Lower energy photons appear with a much greater probability than do the highest energy ones, but they also become preferentially filtered out of the beam through absorption in the target and attenuation in the flattening filter. This generally results in a treatment beam energy spectrum with mean photon energy of approximately one-third of the initial electron beam energy. In this energy range the resulting photon beam exits the production target with a narrow angular spread focused primarily in the forward direction. These forward-peaked intensity distributions generally need to be modulated (flattened) to produce a large (up to 40 cm diameter) photon beam with uniform intensity across the beam. All modern treatment units extensively take advantage of computer control, monitoring, and feedback. Thus, these machines produce highly stable and reproducible treatment beams.

The resulting photon beam requires beam shaping for conformal dose delivery. Some combination of primary high-density field blocks (collimators) together with additional edge blocks generally provide the required shaping and shielding (producing beams that project in size up to 40 cm by 40 cm at the patient). Modern machines use computer-controlled multileaf collimators (Fig. 27.14) for the edge sculpting subsequent to setting the primary collimators for maximal shielding. This computer control provides high precision and reproducibility in the definition of field edges. Additionally, automation allows precise reshaping of the treatment beam for each angle of incidence, allowing not only conformation of irradiation to target volumes but also modulation of the beam intensity patterns across the field (intensity-modulated radiation therapy [IMRT]).

Variations on the standard linear accelerator (linac) plus C-arm scenario that are being used for external-beam radiation treatments throughout the body include helical tomotherapy and nonisocentric miniature linac robotic delivery systems.[77] In helical tomotherapy, the accelerator, photon-production target and collimation system are mounted on a ring gantry (similar to those found on diagnostic computed tomography [CT] scanners) (Fig. 27.15). It produces a fan-beam of photons, the intensity of each part of the fan modulated by a binary collimator. As the gantry rotates, the patient simultaneously slides through the bore of the machine (again analogous to modern x-ray-CT imagers), which allows the continuous delivery of intensity-modulated radiation in a helical pattern from all angles around a patient. Another delivery system uses an industrial robot to hold a miniature accelerator plus photon beam-production system (Fig. 27.16). The bulk of the system is reduced by keeping the field sizes small (spot-like). However, computer control of the robot provides flexibility in irradiating tumors from nearly any position external to the patient. The same control allows the selection and use of many differing beam angles to build up dose at the tumor location.

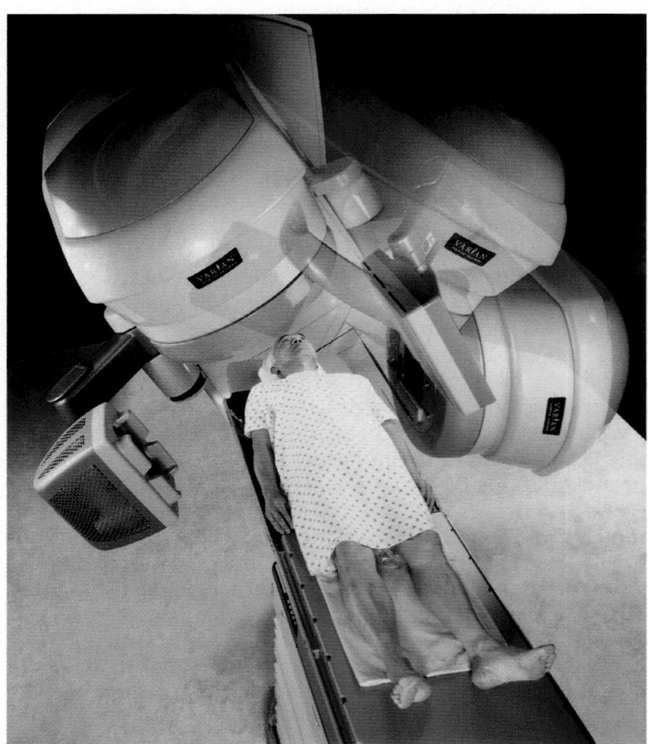

FIGURE 27.13 Model in treatment position on patient support table. The treatment delivery head on the gantry's C-arm rotates about the patient, enabling the delivery of beams throughout 360 degrees of rotation. (From Varian Medical Systems, Palo Alto, CA, with permission.)

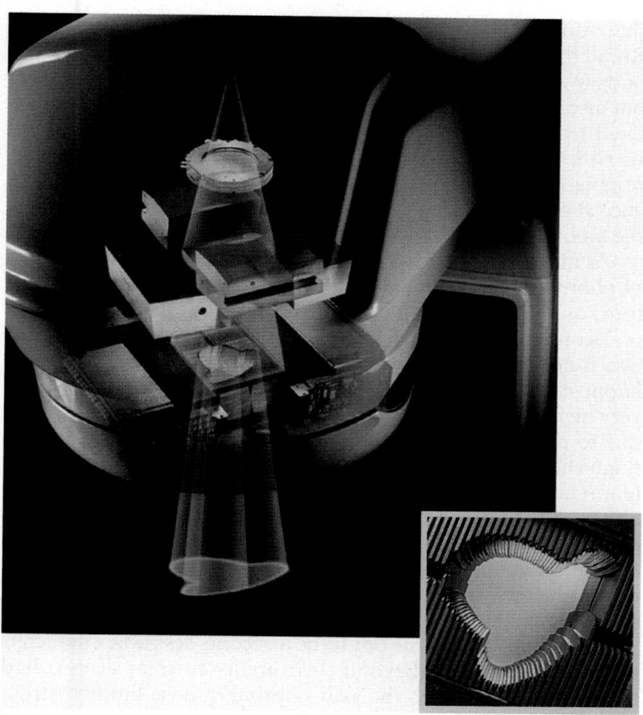

FIGURE 27.14 Multileaf collimator shaping of x-ray treatment beam from a linear accelerator. Inset shows view of multileaf collimator. (From Varian Medical Systems, Palo Alto, CA, with permission.)

To take advantage of the precision of modern beam delivery, it is crucial to localize the patient's tumor and normal tissue.[78] This process can be divided into patient immobilization (i.e., limiting the motion of the patient) and localization (i.e., knowing the tumor and normal tissue location precisely in space). Although these concepts of immobilization and localization are related, they are not identical. Patients can be held reasonably comfortably in their treatment pose with the aid of foam molds and meshes (immobilization devices). Traditionally,

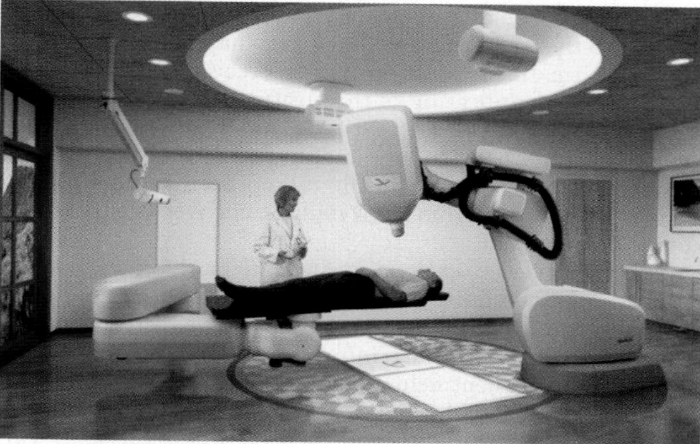

FIGURE 27.16 Miniature accelerator plus x-ray production system on a robotic delivery arm. Both treatment table and treatment head set by computer for multiple arbitrary angles of incidence. (From Accuray, Sunnyvale, CA, with permission.)

localization has been achieved by indexing the immobilization device to the computer-controlled treatment couch and by using low-power laser beams aligned to skin marks. These techniques make it possible to reproducibly couple the surface of each patient with the treatment machine isocenter.

However, what is truly needed is to localize the tumor and normal tissues. The development of in-room, online x-ray, ultrasound, and infrared imaging equipment can now be used to ensure that the intended portions of each patient's internal anatomy are correctly positioned at the time of treatment. In particular, the development of rugged, low-profile, active matrix flat-panel imaging devices, either attached to the treatment gantry or placed in the vicinity of the treatment couch, together with diagnostic x-ray generators or the patient treatment beam (Fig. 27.13), allows the digital capture of projection x-ray images of patient anatomy with respect to the isocenter and treatment field borders. These digitized electronic images are immediately available for analysis. Software tools allow comparison to reference images and the generation of

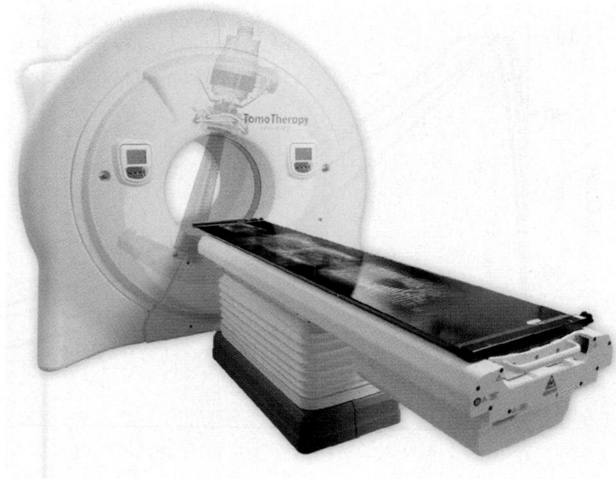

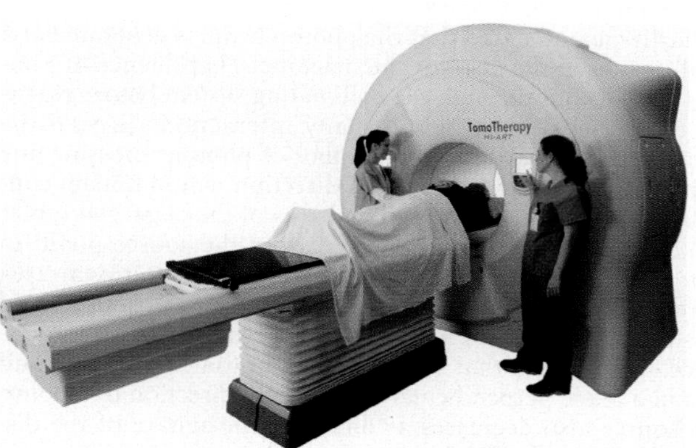

FIGURE 27.15 **A:** Shadow view of linear accelerator, x-ray beam production system, and x-ray fan beam for helical tomotherapy treatment delivery. The beam production system rotates within its enclosed gantry. **B:** Model patient on treatment table slides into treatment unit. During treatment the table moves as the collimated fan beam rotates about the patient, creating a modulated helical dose delivery pattern. (From TomoTherapy, Inc., Madison, WI, with permission.)

correction coordinates, which are in turn available for downloading to the treatment couch for automated fine adjustment of patient treatment position. Other precise localization systems rely on identification of the positions of small, implanted radiopaque markers or other types of "smart" position-reporting devices. Careful use of these image-guided radiation therapy (IGRT) systems[78–80] can result in repeated reducibility of patient position to within a few millimeters over a 5- to 8-week course of treatment.

The final part of external-beam patient treatment is dose delivery. All modern treatment units have computer monitoring (and often control) of all mechanical and dose-delivery components. Treatment-planning information (treatment machine parameters, treatment field configurations, dose per treatment field segment) is downloaded to a work station at the treatment unit that first assists with and then records treatment. This information, together with the readbacks from the treatment machine, are used to reproducibly set up and then verify each patient's treatment parameters, which prevents many of the variations that used to occur when all treatment was performed simply by following instructions written in a treatment chart.

Treatment Beam Characteristics and Dose-Calculation Algorithms

Beyond a basic understanding of the interactions of ionizing radiation with matter lies the requirement of being able to characterize the treatment beams for purposes of planning and verifying treatments. By virtue of a couple of underlying principles, this generally can be accomplished via a two-step process of absolute calibration of the dose at some reference point in a phantom (measurement media representative of a patient's tissues), with relative scaling of dose values in other parts of the beam or phantom with respect to that point.

As mentioned earlier, the predominant mode of interaction for therapeutic energy photon beams in tissue-like materials is through Compton scattering. The probability of Compton scattering events is primarily proportional to the relative electron density of the media with which they interact. As many body tissues are "water-like" in composition, it has been possible to make photon beam dosimetric measurements in phantoms consisting mostly of water (water tanks) or tissue-equivalent plastic and to then scale the interactions via relative electron density values (as can be derived from computed x-ray-CT, for example) to other water-like materials. Thus, the relative fluence of photons in a therapeutic treatment beam is attenuated as it passes through a phantom, primarily via Compton scattering.

Earlier it was stated that the photon beam is generated at a small region in the head of the machine. That fluence of photons spreads out through the collimating system before reaching the patient. Thus, without any interactions (e.g., if the beam were in a vacuum) the number of photons crossing any plane perpendicular to the beam direction would remain constant. However, the cross-sectional area of the plane gets larger and larger the farther it is located from the source point. In fact, both the width and length of the cross-sectional area increase in proportion to the distance from the source, and thus the area increases in proportion to the square of the distance. This means that the primary photon fluence per unit area in a plane perpendicular to the beam direction of a point-like source also decreases as one over the square of the distance, the so-called $1/r^2$ reduction in fluence as a function of distance, r, from the source.

Thus, we have two processes, attenuation and $1/r^2$ reduction, that reduce the photon fluence from an external therapeutic beam as a function of depth in a patient. There is also a process that can increase the photon fluence at a point downstream. Recall that Compton scattering interactions lead not only to secondary electrons (which are responsible for deposition of dose) but also to Compton scattered photons. These photons are scattered from the interaction sites in multiple, predominantly forward-looking directions. Thus, Compton-scattered photons originating from many other places can add to the photon fluence at another point. As the irradiated area (field size) increases, the amount of scattered radiation also increases.

As mentioned earlier, dose "deposition" is a two-step process of photon interaction (proportional to the local fluence of photons) and energy transfer to the medium via the slowing down of secondary electrons. Thus, the point where a photon interacts is not the place where the dose is actually deposited, which happens over the track of the secondary electron. Dose has a very strict definition of energy "absorbed" per unit mass (i.e., due to the slowing down charged particles) and should be distinguished from the energy released at a point, defined as kerma (e.g., energy transfer from the scattering incident photon). Thus, although the photon beam fluence will always be greatest at the entrance to a patient or phantom, the actual "absorbed dose" for a megavoltage photon beam builds up over the first couple of centimeters, reaching a maximum (d-max) at a depth corresponding to the range of the higher energy Compton electrons set in motion. This turns out to be a second desirable characteristic of these beams (beyond their ability to treat deep-seated lesions), as the dose to the skin (a primary dose-limiting structure in earlier times) is greatly reduced.

The relative distributions of dose, normalized to an absolute dose measurement (using a small thimble-like air ionization chamber at a standard depth and for a standard field size according to nationally and internationally accepted protocols), are the major inputs into treatment-planning systems. The major features of these distributions are (1) the initial dose buildup up to a depth of d-max, with a more gradual drop off in dose as a function of depth into the phantom due to the attenuation and $1/r^2$ factors at deeper depths (relative depth dose), and (2) the shape of the dose in the plane perpendicular to the direction of the beams; both as a function of field size. Typical central axis depth dose curves for typical external photon beams are shown in Figure 27.17 for two beam energies and for both a large and smaller field size.

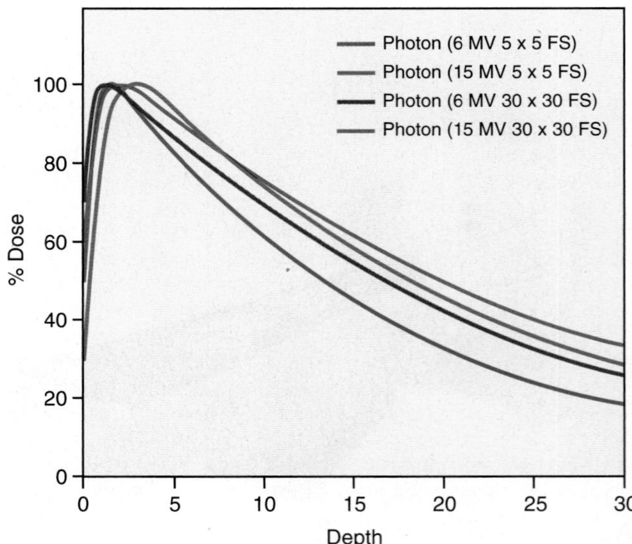

FIGURE 27.17 Sample depth-dose curves (change in delivered dose as a function of depth) along the central axis of some typical photon treatment beams for low (6 MV) and intermediate (15 MV) energy beams and large (30 × 30 cm²) and smaller (5 × 5 cm²) field sizes (FS).

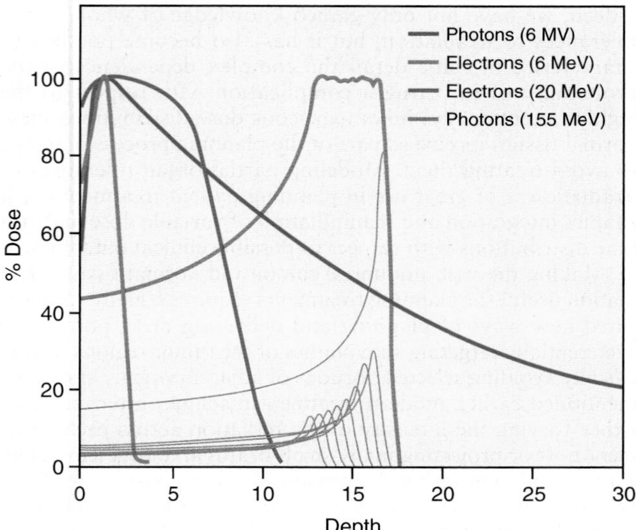

FIGURE 27.18 Sample depth-dose curves along the central axis of some typical charged particle treatment beams compared with that of a 6-MV proton beam. The spread out Bragg peak at the end of the 155-MeV proton beam (*thick pink curve*) is a composite dose deposition pattern from addition of the multiple range-shifted proton curves (*thinner pink curves*).

Notice both the expected increase in penetration with increasing beam energy and the increase in dose at a particular depth with increasing field size; the latter effect due to increased numbers of secondary Compton-scattered photons for larger irradiated areas. The change in dose perpendicular to the central axis is less remarkable, as the beams are designed to be uniform dose across a field as a function of depth.

It is useful to also point out the depth dose characteristics of clinical external treatment beams produced using ionizing radiations other than photons, primarily through the direct use of charged particles. Those beams (Fig. 27.18) illustrate interesting characteristics, which, when added to the options available for treatment planning (or used by themselves), can produce advantageous results. The authors notice that (relative to the photon beam) direct use of electron beams leads to deposition of dose over a more localized range, but at the expense of a relative lack of penetration. Thus, electron beams are most widely used for treating, or boosting the treatment of, more superficial tumors and regions (see the section "Clinical Application of Types of Radiation"). The heavier charged particle beams (protons and carbon ions) appear to exhibit even more interesting "depth-dose" characteristics, with the advantage of being both (when necessary) highly penetrating but also lacking significant dose beyond a certain depth (a depth that can be controlled and purposefully placed, for example, at the distal edge of a target volume).

The results of these measurements have been modeled so as to develop dose-calculation algorithms used in treatment-planning systems. These models all use measured beam data to set or adjust parameters used by those algorithms in their dose-distribution computations. As most of the input data used for beam fitting come from measurements in water (or water-like plastic) phantoms, patient specific adjustments are needed to the water phantom data to account for both geometry and tissue properties. It is the task of the dose-calculation algorithms to take those changes into account. The accuracy and precision actually realized for all dose-calculation algorithms generally need to be traded off against the time required to complete the calculation. Although the availability of ever more powerful computers has made calculation time less of a concern for broad open-beam treatment planning, issues still remain for more specialized planning exercises that use many small beams or parts of beams such as IMRT, discussed later. Typically, relative dose distributions can be computed within patients on the scale of a few millimeters with a precision of better than a few percentage points.

An important area of research is the development of treatment-planning systems that calculate dose based on the principles of how radiation interacts with tissues, rather than simply by fitting data. These approaches use Monte Carlo techniques,[79] which build a dose distribution by summing the calculated paths of thousands of photons and scattered electrons. This approach is more accurate than beam-fitting algorithms in regions of differing tissue densities, such as the lung, and therefore will ultimately replace the current generation of treatment-planning systems, particularly for complex conditions. However, the time to perform these calculations is still prohibitive for a clinic, and it is anticipated that Monte Carlo calculations will be introduced over a period of years by balancing the need for accuracy in a particular clinical situation with the need to initiate patient treatment.

TREATMENT PLANNING

As discussed in the previous section, single-treatment beams usually deposit more dose closer to where they enter the patient than they do at depths corresponding to where a deep-seated tumor might be located. The use of multiple beams entering the patient from different directions that overlap at the target produces more dose per unit volume throughout the tumor volume than is received by normal tissues. In fact, as noticed earlier, the treatment-delivery machines are designed to make this easy to accomplish. Planning patient treatments under these circumstances should be a somewhat trivial matter of first selecting a sufficient number of beam angles to realize the desired buildup of dose in the overlap region relative to the doses in the upstream parts of each beam, and then second, designing beam apertures that shape the edges of the beams to match the target. However, often, dose-limiting normal tissues also lie in the paths of one or more of the beams; normal tissues are often more sensitive to radiation damage than the tumor, to which it is best to minimize the dose in any case as a general principle. Computerized treatment-planning systems function to develop patient-specific anatomic or geometric models and then use these models together with the beam-specific dose deposition properties (derived from phantom measurements, as previously described) to select beam angles, shapes, and intensities that meet an overall prescribed objective. That is, modern radiation oncology dose prescriptions contain both tumor and normal tissue objectives, and the modern computerized treatment-planning systems make it possible to design treatments that meet these objectives.

The development and use of three-dimensional (3D) models of each patient's anatomy, treatment geometry, and dose distribution led to a paradigm shift in radiation therapy treatment planning. Computerized radiation treatment planning began in the 1980s as a mainly x-ray-CT–based reconstruction of 3D geometries from information manually contoured on multiple 2D transverse CT images. Today these models often incorporate imaging data from multiple sources. Geometrically accurate anatomic information from x-ray-CT still anchors these studies (as well as provides tissue density information necessary for dose calculations). However, it is now quite common to also register the CT data set with other studies such as magnetic resonance imaging (MRI), which may add anatomic detail for soft tissues, or functional MRI or positron emission tomography (PET) studies,[81,82] which provide physiological or molecular information about tumors and normal tissues. Once

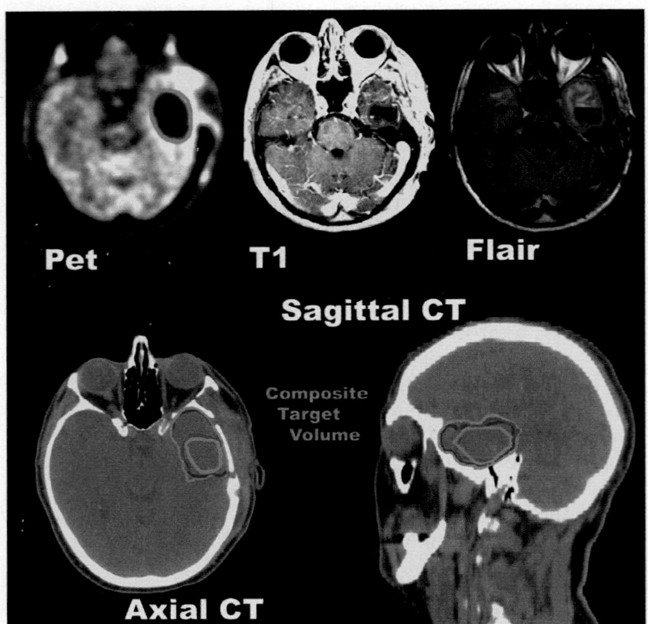

FIGURE 27.19 Illustration of brain tumor target volume delineated on coregistered nuclear medicine and magnetic resonance imaging studies fused with computed tomography (CT) data for treatment planning. PET, positron emission tomography.

registered with each other, the unique or complementary information from each data set can be fused for inspection and incorporated into the design of each patient's target and normal tissue volumes (Fig. 27.19). Beyond the ability to more fully define the extent of the primary target volume (for instance, as the encompassing envelope of disease appreciated on all the imaging studies) lies the ability to define subvolumes of the tumor volume that might be appropriate for simultaneous treatment to higher dose. For example, it should soon become possible to define different biological components of the tumor that could potentially be targeted and then monitored for response using these same imaging techniques.[83]

Current treatment planning makes the tacit assumption that the planning image yields "the truth" about the location and condition of tumors and normal tissues throughout the course of treatment. However, this ignores the complexity inherent in attempting to build accurate 3D models from multimodality imaging for purposes of planning patient treatments. First, patients breathe and undergo other physiological processes during a single treatment, changes that require dynamic modeling or other methods of accounting for the changes. Furthermore, the patient's condition may change over time (and hence their model). Thus, a complete design and assessment of a patient undergoing high-precision treatment requires the construction of 4D patient models. Indeed, the recent ready availability of multidetector CT scanners with subsecond gantry rotations, and even more recently the availability of cone-beam CT capabilities on the radiation therapy treatment simulators and treatment machines themselves, now makes it possible to construct 4D patient models.[84] A very active area of physics research deals with 4D patient models (including distortions and changes in anatomy) of the motion over time and the determination of the accumulated dose received by a moving tumor as well as the surrounding normal tissues such as uninvolved lung.

Complementary to the availability of these patient and dose models has come a much better understanding of the doses safely tolerated by normal tissues adjacent to a tumor volume (e.g., spinal cord) or surrounding it (e.g., brain, lung, liver).[85] Indeed, we have not only gained knowledge of whole organ tolerances to irradiation, but it has also become possible to characterize in some detail the complex dependence of the probability of incurring a complication with respect to the highly (intentionally) inhomogeneous dose distributions these normal tissues receive as part of the planning process designed to avoid treating them. Modeling partial organ tolerances to irradiation is of great use in planning patient treatments as it enables integration and manipulation of variable dose and volume distributions with respect to possible clinical outcomes.

Making the vast amount of tumor and normal tissue information useful for planning treatments requires equally sophisticated new ways of planning and delivering dose, potentially preferentially targeting subvolumes of the tumor regions or specifically avoiding selected portions of adjacent organs at risk. As mentioned earlier, modern treatment machines are capable of either varying the intensity of the radiation across each treatment port or projecting many small beams at a targeted region. This modulation of beam intensities from a given beam direction, together with the use of multiple beams (or parts of beams) from different directions, gives many degrees of freedom to create highly sculpted dose distributions, given that a system for designing the intensity modulation is available. Much computer programming and computational analysis has gone into the design of treatment-planning optimization systems to perform these functions are readily available.[86,87]

In IMRT as most often applied, each treatment beam portal is broken down into simple basic components called beamlets, typically 0.5 to 1 cm by 1 cm in size, evenly distributed on a grid over the cross-section of each beam. Optimization begins with precomputation of the relative dose contribution that each of these beamlets gives to every subportion of tumor and normal tissue that the beamlet traverses as it goes through the patient model. Sophisticated optimization engines and search routines then iteratively alter the relative intensities of each beamlet in all the beams to minimize a cost function associated with target and normal tissue treatment goals. These often hundreds of beamlets (each with its own intensity) (Fig. 27.20)

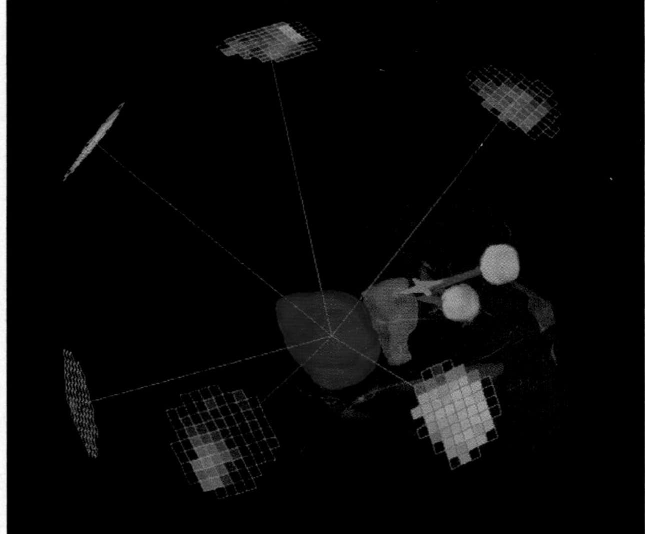

FIGURE 27.20 Six intensity modulated treatment ports planned for treatment of a brain tumor (*large object in red*). Differing intensities of the 5 × 5 mm "beamlets" in each port illustrated by gray scale (brighter beamlet = higher intensity). Computer optimization of the beamlet intensities designed to generate a delivered dose distribution that will conform to the tumor region, yet avoid critical normal tissues such as the brainstem (*dark pink*), optic chiasm (*green*), and optic nerves (*red tubular structures*).

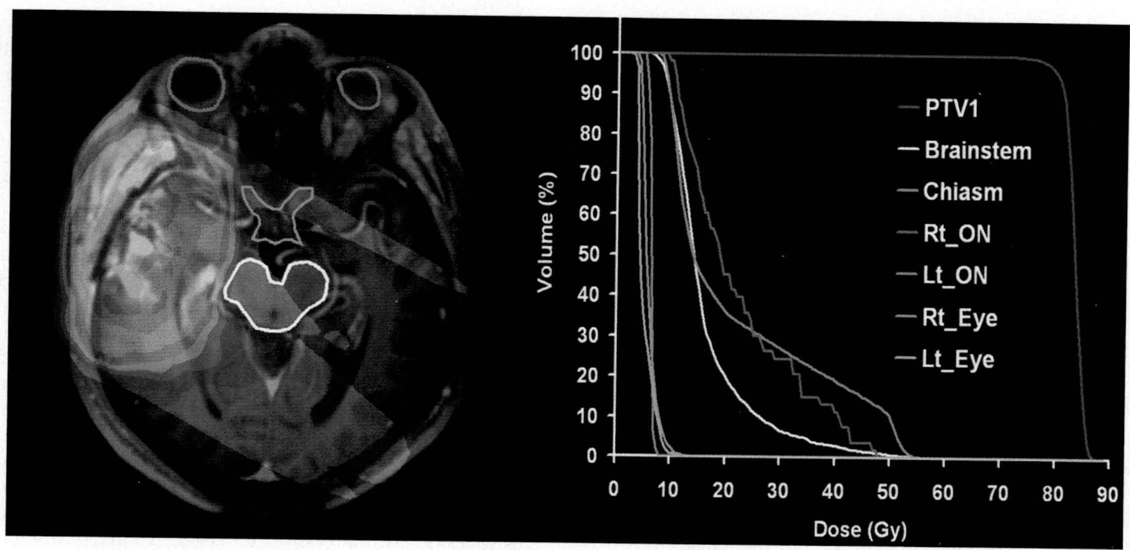

FIGURE 27.21 Resulting isodose distribution for an optimized intensity-modulated brain treatment. Dose-intensity pattern in the left panel is overlaid on the patient's magnetic resonance images used in planning. Also contoured are the optic chiasm (*green*), brain brainstem (*white*), and eyes (*orange*). In the right panel, the dose distribution throughout all slices of the patient's anatomy is summarized via cumulative dose-volume histograms for the various tissues and volumes that have been previously segmented. Each location on each curve represents the fraction of the volume of that tissue (%) that receives greater than or equal to the corresponding dose level.

provide the necessary flexibility and degrees of freedom to create dose distributions that can preferentially irradiate subportions of targets and also produce sharp dose gradients to avoid nearby organs at risk (Fig. 27.21). The cost-function approach also facilitates the ability to include factors such as the normal tissue and tumor-response models, mentioned previously in the optimization process, thus integrating the overall effects of the complex dose distributions across whole organ systems or target volumes within the planning process.

OTHER TREATMENT MODALITIES

Other types of external-beam radiation treatments use atomic or nuclear particles rather than photons. Beams of fast neutrons have been used for some cancers,[88] primarily because of the dense ionization patterns they produce as they slow down in tissue (making cell killing less dependent on the indirect effect previously discussed). Being uncharged particles, neutron beams of therapeutic energy penetrate in tissue (have depth-dose characteristics) similar to photon beams, but with denser dose deposition in the cellular scale. Most other external-beam treatments use charged particles, primarily either electrons[89] (produced on the same machines used for photon beam treatments) or protons or heavier particles such as carbon ions.[73,90] The latter beams have desirable dose-deposition properties (Fig. 27.18), as they can spare tissues downstream from the target volume and generally give less overall dose to normal tissue. There can also be some radiobiological advantage to the heavier charged particle beams, similar to neutrons. Generation and delivery of proton and heavier charged particle beams generally requires an accelerator (in its own vault) plus a beam transport system and some sort of treatment nozzle, often located on an isocentric gantry. The cost of the accelerator is generally leveraged by having it supply beams to multiple treatment rooms, but these units still cost many times that of a standard linear accelerator.

Brachytherapy is a form of treatment that uses direct placement of radioactive sources or materials within tumors (interstitial brachytherapy) or within body or surgical cavities (intracavitary brachytherapy), either permanently (allowing for full decay of short-lived radioactive materials) or temporarily (either in one extended application or over several shorter-term applications). The ability to irradiate tumors from close range (even from the inside out) can lead to conformal treatments with low normal tissue doses. The radioactive isotopes most generally used for these treatments are contained within small, tube- or seed-like sealed source enclosures (preventing direct contamination). They emit photons (gamma and x-rays) during their decay, which penetrate the source cover and interact with tissue via the same physical processes as described for external-beam treatments. The treatments have the advantage of providing a high fluence (and dose) very near each source that drops in intensity as 1 over the square of the distance from the source ($1/r^2$). Radioactive sources decay in an exponential fashion characterized by their individual half-lives. After each half-life ($T_{1/2}$), only one half of the radioactive parent isotope present at the beginning of that period remains. Thus, the strength of each source decreases by half each $T_{1/2}$. Brachytherapy treatments are further generally classified into the two broad categories of low-dose-rate and high-dose-rate treatments. Low-dose-rate treatments attempt to deliver tumoricidal doses via continuous irradiation from implanted sources over a period of several days. High-dose-rate treatments use one or more higher activity sources (stored external to the patient) together with a remote applicator or source transfer system to give one or more higher-dose treatments on time scales and schedules more like external-beam treatments.

Isotopes for brachytherapy treatments are selected on the basis of a combination of specific activity (how much activity can be achieved per unit mass; i.e., to keep the source sizes small), penetrating ability of the decay photons (together with the $1/r^2$ falloff determines how many sources or source location will be required for treatment), and the half-life of the radioactive material (must be accounted for in computation of dose, but also determines how often reusable sources will need to be replaced). Table 27.1 lists those isotopes most commonly used, along with some of their primary applications.

TABLE 27.1

COMMON ISOTOPES FOR BRACHYTHERAPY TREATMENT

Isotope	Form	Primary Applications
^{125}I	Implantable sealed seed	LDR: Permanent prostate implants, brain implants, tumor bed implants, eye plaques
^{192}Ir	Implantable sealed seed	LDR: Interstitial solid tumor treatments
^{192}Ir	High activity sealed source on a remote transfer wire	HDR: Intracavatory GYN treatments, intraluminal irradiations
^{137}Cs	Sealed source tubes	LDR: Intracavatory GYN treatments

LDR, low-dose rate; HDR, high-dose rate; GYN, gynecologic.

The dose-deposition patterns surrounding each type of source can be measured or computed. These data (or the parameterization of same) can be stored within a computerized treatment-planning system. Planning a brachytherapy treatment-delivery scheme (desirable source strengths and arrangements) proceeds within the planning system by distributing the sources throughout the treatment area and having the computer add up the contributions of each source to designated tumor and normal tissue locations (e.g., obtained from a CT scan). Source strengths or spacing can be adjusted until an acceptable result is obtained. Indeed, optimization systems are now routinely used to fine-tune this process.

Other types of therapeutic treatments with internal sources of ionizing radiation, generally classified as systemic targeted radionuclide therapy (STaRT), use antibodies or other conjugates or carriers such as microspheres to selectively deliver radionuclides to cancer cells.[91,92] Computing the effective dose to tumors and normal tissues via these techniques requires information on how much of the injected activity reaches the targets (biodistribution) as well as the energy and decay properties of the radionuclide being delivered. Imaging techniques and computer models are aiding in these computations.

CLINICAL APPLICATIONS OF RADIATION THERAPY

In contrast to surgical oncology and medical oncology, which focus on early- or late-stage disease, respectively, the field of radiation oncology encompasses the entire spectrum of oncology. Board certification requires 5 years of postdoctoral training, typically beginning with an internship in internal medicine or surgery, followed by 4 years of radiation oncology residency. Education, as defined by leaders in the field,[93] begins with a thorough knowledge of the biology, physics, and clinical applications of radiation. It also includes training in the theoretical and practical aspects of the administration of radiation protectors and anticancer agents used as radiation sensitizers and the management of toxicities that result from those treatments. In addition, residents receive education in palliative care, supportive care, and symptom and pain management. This training is in preparation for a practice that, in a given week, might include patients with a 2-mm vocal cord lesion or a 20-cm soft tissue sarcoma, both of whom can be treated with curative intent, as well as a patient with widely metastatic disease who needs palliative radiation, medical care for pain and depression, and discussion of end-of-life issues. More than 50% of (nonskin) cancer patients receive radiation therapy during the course of their illnesses.[94]

Clinical Application of Types of Radiation

Electrons are now the most widely used form of radiation for superficial tumors. Electrons that are produced by a standard linear accelerator can penetrate into about 6 cm of tissue and thus are very effective for superficial treatments, such as of skin cancer, the lumpectomy cavity (after whole-breast photon radiation in the treatment of breast cancer), or superficial lymph nodes (e.g., cervical lymph nodes in squamous cell carcinoma of the head and neck, or inguinal lymph nodes for anal or vulvar cancer). Because the depth of penetration can be well controlled by the energy of the beam, it is possible to treat, for instance, a small part of the breast while sparing the underlying lung, or the cervical lymph nodes but not the spinal cord, which lies several centimeters more deeply. A variety of electron energies can be produced by a standard linear accelerator. Superficial tumors such as those of skin cancers can also be treated very effectively with low-energy (kilovoltage) photons, but their use has decreased because a separate machine is required for their production.

The main form of treatment for deep tumors is photons. As described in the "Radiation Physics" section, photons spare the skin and deposit dose along their entire path until the beam leaves the body. The use of multiple beams that intersect on the tumor allows high doses to be delivered to the tumor with relatively sparing normal tissue. During the past 20 years, this concept has been exploited in progressive steps, from 2D, to 3D, to IMRT, with dramatic improvements that resulted from the use of intersecting beams that more accurately target the tumor. IMRT uses hundreds of beams, which allows the treatment of concave shapes with relative sparing of the central region (Figs. 27.20 and 27.21). However, as each beam continues on its path beyond the tumor, this use of multiple beams means that a significant volume of normal tissue receives a low dose. There has been considerable debate concerning the magnitude of the risk of second cancers produced by radiating large volumes with low doses of radiation.[95]

Charged particle beams (proton and carbon, in this discussion) differ from photons in that they interact only modestly with tissue until they reach the end of their path, where they then deposit the majority of their energy and stop (the Bragg peak; Fig. 27.18). This ability to stop at a chosen depth gives them the potential advantage of treating tumors that are close to critical structures. The chief form of charged particle used today is the proton. Their main application has been in the treatment uveal melanomas, base-of-skull chondrosarcomas, and chordomas.[96] In the 2D-3D era, proton therapy could deliver higher doses of radiation to the target than photon therapy because protons could produce a more rapid falloff of dose between the target and the critical normal tissue (e.g., tumor and brainstem). In the modern era of IMRT photons, it is difficult to determine whether protons will allow a higher target dose to be delivered. If the tumor abuts the critical normal structure, the residual uncertainties in beam physics and the geometry of patient setup (in the range of 2 to 3 mm) will limit the final dose for both IMRT photons and protons.

Although the majority of patients who have received proton therapy have prostate cancer, there is as yet no evidence that higher dose of radiation can be delivered with protons[97] than with 3D or IMRT planned photons.[98,99] However, in contrast to these issues of target dose, protons have the potential to decrease regions of low dose, which may decrease the chance of second malignancies. This would be of particular importance in the treatment of pediatric malignancies. There is considerable controversy about whether the current generation of proton machines, which use scattering foils, produce a neutron bath that would subject patients to a higher dose of radiation outside the treatment field than was previously recognized.[95] Newer forms of protons generation should overcome this potential disadvantage. A carbon ion beam has an additional potential biological advantage over protons. As discussed in the section "Biologic Aspects of Radiation Oncology," hypoxic cells, which are found in many tumors, are up to three times more resistant to photon or proton radiation than well-oxygenated cells. In contrast, hypoxia does not cause resistance to a carbon beam. Whether hypoxia is a cause of clinical resistance to fractionated radiation is still debated.[100] A carbon beam is available at a few sites in Europe and Japan.[96]

Whereas there is general agreement that charged particle beams have superior dose-deposition characteristics compared with photons, two major issues affect their widespread acceptance. The most widely recognized is cost. Proton (approximately $120 million) and carbon-beam facilities (in excess of $200 million) are substantially more expensive than a similar-sized photon facility (approximately $25 million). The operating costs appear to be significantly higher as well. The magnitude of these costs makes the determination of the appropriate applications and number of charged particles of societal importance.[101] Although less-expensive single-gantry proton units are under construction, there are no functioning units at the time of this writing. A second, less well-appreciated issue concerns the need to develop full integration of charged particle beams with IGRT, as has already been accomplished with photons.

As one contemplates these expenses, it is worth stepping back and asking the question of whether giving doses higher than can be safely achieved by 2D therapy improves clinical outcome. The answer is yes. The best modern example comes from prostate cancer, for which three randomized trials now show that biochemical relapse from patients receiving the higher dose (in the range of 78 Gy) is decreased compared with lower doses (in the range of 70 Gy).[97,102,103] If one looks across multiple studies, it can be estimated that the 5-year survival rate of biologically having no evidence of disease for patients with prostate cancer increases by 1% to 2%/Gy above 70 Gy within the tested range.[98] Similarly, 3D planning and now IMRT have allowed the safe delivery of higher doses of radiation to lung[104] and liver[105] cancers, which appears to have improved local control and, possibly, survival. Conversely, these advanced techniques can preserve the target dose and local control produced by 2D treatment in the treatment of head and neck cancer while, at the same time, decreasing xerostomia (by sparing the parotid gland) and dysphagia or aspiration (by sparing the constrictor muscles).[106] Thus, the increased dose to the target (or normal tissue-sparing) allowed by the advance from 2D treatment to 3D and IMRT has produced a remarkable increase in tumor control (or a decrease in toxicity); it will be of great interest to determine if charged particle therapy can produce similar gains.

Neutron therapy attracted significant interest in the 1980s, based on the principle that it would be more effective than photons against hypoxic cells that some have thought are responsible for radiation resistance of tumors. The effectiveness of neutron therapy has been limited by initial difficulties with collimation and targeting, although there is evidence that they have a role in the treatment of refractory parotid gland tumors.[107]

Brachytherapy refers to the placement of radioactive sources next to or inside the tumor. The chief sites where brachytherapy plays a role are in prostate and cervix cancer, although it has applications in head and neck cancers, soft tissue sarcomas, and other sites. In the case of prostate cancer, most experience is with low-dose-rate permanent implants using ^{125}I or, more recently, ^{103}Pd. Over the past 5 years there has been an increased emphasis on improving the accuracy of seed placement, guided by ultrasound and confirmed by CT or MRI,[108] and, in skilled hands, outstanding results can be achieved. In the case of cervix cancer, high-dose-rate treatment, which can be performed on an outpatient basis, has essentially replaced low-dose-rate treatment, which typically requires general anesthesia and a 2-day hospital stay. The results from both techniques appear to be approximately equivalent.

Yttrium microspheres represent a distinct form of brachytherapy. These spheres carry ^{90}Y, a pure beta emitter with a range of about 1 cm. These have been used to treat both primary hepatocellular cancer and colorectal cancer metastatic to the liver (hepatic arterial or systemic chemotherapy) by administration through the hepatic artery.

TREATMENT INTENT

Radiation doses are chosen so as to maximize the chance of tumor control without producing unacceptable toxicity. The dose of radiation required depends on the tumor type, the volume of disease (number of tumor cells), and the use of radiation-modifying agents (such as chemotherapeutic drugs used as radiation sensitizers). Except for a subset of tumors that are exquisitely sensitive to radiation (e.g., seminoma and lymphoma), doses that are required are often close to the tolerance of the normal tissue. A key fact driving the choice of dose is that a 1 cm^3 tumor contains approximately 1 billion cells. It follows that the reduction of a tumor that is 3 cm in diameter to 3 mm, which would be called a complete response by CT scan, would still leave 1 million tumor cells. Because each radiation fraction appears to kill a fixed fraction of the tumor, the dose to cure occult disease needs to be more similar to the dose for gross disease than one might otherwise expect. Thus, radiation doses (using standard fractionation) of 45 to 54 Gy are typically used in the adjuvant setting when there is moderate suspicion for occult disease, 60 to 65 Gy for positive margins or high suspicion for occult disease, and 70 Gy or more for gross disease.

It is common during a course of radiation to give higher doses of radiation to regions that have a higher tumor burden. For example, regions that are suspected of harboring occult disease may be targeted to receive (in once-daily 2-Gy fractions) 54 Gy, whereas, to control the gross tumor, the goal may be to administer a total dose of 70 Gy. As the gross tumor will invariably reside within the region at risk for occult disease, it has become standard practice to deliver 50 Gy to the entire region, and then an additional "boost" dose of 20 Gy to the tumor. This sequence is called the *shrinking field technique*. With the development of IMRT, it has become possible to treat both regions with different doses each day and achieve both goals simultaneously. For example, on each of 35 days of treatment, the gross tumor might receive 2 Gy, and the region of occult disease 1.7 Gy (total dose, 59.5 Gy, which is of approximately equal biological effectiveness to 54 Gy in 1.8-Gy fractions because of the lower dose per fraction; see the section "Biologic Aspects of Radiation Oncology").

Radiation therapy alone is often used with curative intent for localized tumors. The decision to use surgery or radiation therapy involves factors determined by the tumor (Is it resectable without a serious compromise in function?) and the patient (Is the patient a good operative candidate?). The most common tumor in this group is prostate cancer, but patients with early stage larynx cancer often receive radiation for voice preservation, and there are many patients with early stage lung cancer who are not operative candidates. Control rates for these early stage lesions are in excess of 70% (and as high as 90% for early stage larynx cancer) and are usually a function of tumor size. Stereotactic body radiation may provide an improved method of curing early stage lung cancer. This approach uses precise localization and image guidance to deliver a small number (less than five) of high doses of radiation, with the concept of ablating the tumor, rather than using fractionation to achieve a therapeutic index (see the section "Fractionation"). Although early results are encouraging,[109] there are as yet no randomized trials between standard fractionated radiation and stereotactic treatment.

Locally advanced or aggressive cancers can be cured with radiation alone or with the combination of radiation and chemotherapy or a molecularly targeted therapy. The most common examples are locally advanced lung cancer, head and neck, esophageal, and cervix cancers, with cure rates in the 15% to 40% range, and these are discussed in detail in their own chapters in this book. A general principle that has emerged during the past decade is that combination chemoradiation has increased the cure rates of locally advanced cancers by 5% to 10% at the cost of increased toxicity.

An important consideration in the use of radiation (with or without chemotherapy) with curative intent is the concept of organ preservation. Perhaps the best example of achieving organ preservation in the face of gross disease involves the use of chemotherapy and radiation to replace laryngectomy in the treatment of advanced larynx cancer. Combined radiation and chemotherapy does not improve overall survival compared with radical surgery; however, the organ-conservation approach allows voice preservation in approximately two-thirds of patients with advanced larynx cancer.[110] The treatment of anal cancer with chemoradiation can also be viewed in this light, with chemoradiotherapy producing organ conservation and cure rates superior to radical surgery used decades ago.[111] Multiple randomized trials have demonstrated that lumpectomy plus radiation for breast cancer produces survival rates equal to that of modified radical mastectomy, while allowing preservation of the breast.

In the past decade, it has become clear that some patients with metastatic disease can be cured with radiation (with or without chemotherapy). The concept underlying this approach was established by the surgical practice of resecting a limited number of liver or lung metastases. A significant fraction of patients have a limited number of liver metastases that cannot be resected because of location, but they are able to undergo high-dose radiation (often combined with chemotherapy). This radical approach to oligometastases[112] can produce 5-year survival rates in the range of 20% in selected patients.[105,113] Patients with a limited number of lung metastases from colorectal cancer or soft tissue sarcomas are now being approached with stereotactic body radiation with a similar concept as has been used to justify surgical resection.[109]

Radiation therapy can also contribute to the cure of patients when used in an adjuvant setting. If the risk of recurrence after surgery is low or if a recurrence could be easily addressed by a second resection, adjuvant radiation therapy is not usually given. However, when a gross total resection of the tumor is still associated with a high risk of residual occult disease or if local recurrence is morbid, adjuvant treatment is often recommended. A general finding across many disease sites is that adjuvant radiation can reduce local failure rates to below 10%, even in high-risk patients, if a gross total resection is achieved. If gross disease or positive margins remain, higher doses or larger volumes may be required, which may be less well tolerated and are less successful in achieving tumor control.

Adjuvant therapy can be delivered before or after definitive surgery. There are some advantages to giving radiation therapy after surgery. The details of the tumor location are known and, with the surgeon's cooperation, clips can be placed in the tumor bed, allowing increased treatment accuracy. In addition, compared with preoperative therapy, postoperative therapy is associated with fewer wound complications. However, in some cases it is preferable to deliver preoperative radiation. Radiation can shrink the tumor, diminishing the extent of the resection or making an unresectable tumor resectable. In the case of rectal cancer, the response to treatment may carry more prognostic information than the initial TNM (tumor, necrosis, metastasis) staging.[114] In patients who will undergo significant surgeries (particularly a Whipple's procedure or an esophageal resection), preoperative (sometimes called neoadjuvant) therapy can be more reliably administered than postoperative therapy. Most important, after resection of abdominal or pelvic tumors (such as rectal cancers or retroperitoneal sarcomas), the small bowel may become fixed by adhesions in the region that requires treatment, increasing the morbidity of postoperative treatment. A randomized trial has shown that preoperative therapy produces fewer gastrointestinal side effects and at least as good efficacy as postoperative adjuvant therapy for locally advanced rectal cancer.[115] Taken together, there appears to be a trend toward preoperative or neoadjuvant therapy in cancers of the gastrointestinal track (esophagus, stomach, pancreas, rectum), and postoperative radiation seems to be favored in head and neck, lung, and breast cancer, and soft tissue sarcoma seems equally split.

The effectiveness of adjuvant therapy in decreasing local recurrence has been demonstrated in randomized trials in lung, rectal, and breast cancers. More recently, randomized trials have shown that postmastectomy radiation improved the survival for women with breast cancer and four or more positive lymph nodes, all of whom also received adjuvant chemotherapy. A fascinating analysis has revealed that, across many treatment conditions, each 4% increase in 5-year local control is associated with a 1% increase in 5-year survival.[116] It has been proposed that the long-term survival benefit of radiation in these more recent studies was revealed by the introduction of effective chemotherapy, which prevented a high fraction of women from dying early with metastatic disease.[117] This concept has been developed into a hypothesis that the effect of adjuvant radiation on survival will depend importantly on the effectiveness of adjuvant chemotherapy. If chemotherapy is either ineffective or very effective, adjuvant radiation may have little influence on the survival in a disease in which systemic relapse dominates survival. Radiation will have its greatest impact on survival when chemotherapy is moderately effective.[118]

In addition to these curative roles, radiation plays an important part in palliative treatment. Perhaps most important, emergency irradiation can begin to reverse the devastating effects of spinal cord compression and of superior vena cava syndrome. A single 8-Gy fraction is highly effective for many patients with bone pain from a metastatic lesion. Some have advocated the use of body stereotactic radiation to treat vertebral body metastases in patients who have a long projected survival or who need retreatment after previous radiation,[119] but the role of stereotactic body radiotherapy is still being defined in this setting. Stereotactic treatment can relieve symptoms from a small number of brain metastasis, and fractionated whole-brain radiation can mitigate the effects of multiple metastases. Bronchial obstruction can often be relieved by a brief course of treatment, as can duodenal obstruction from pancreatic cancer. Palliative treatment is usually delivered in a smaller number of larger radiation fractions (see the section "Fractionation") because the desire to simplify the treatment for a patient with limited life expectancy outweighs the somewhat increased potential for late side effects.

FRACTIONATION

Two crucial features that influence the effectiveness of a physical dose of radiation are the dose given in each radiation treatment (fraction) and the total amount of time required to complete the course of radiation. Standard fractionation for radiation therapy is defined as the delivery of one treatment of 1.8 to 2.25 Gy/d. This approach produces a fairly well understood chance of tumor control and risk of normal tissue damage (as a function of volume). By altering the fractionation schemes, one may be able to improve the outcome for patients undergoing curative treatment or simplify the treatment for patients receiving palliative therapy.

Two forms of altered fractionation have been tested for patients undergoing curative treatment: accelerated fractionation and hyperfractionation. Accelerated fractionation emerged from analyses of the control of head and neck cancer as a function of dose administered and total treatment time. It was found that with increasing dose there was increasing local control, but that protraction of treatment was associated with a loss of local control that was equivalent to about 0.75 Gy/d.[120] The data were best modeled by assuming that, approximately 2 weeks into treatment, tumor cells began to proliferate more rapidly than they were proliferating early in treatment (called *accelerated repopulation*).[121] In accelerated fractionation, the goal is to complete radiation before the accelerated tumor cell proliferation occurs. The most common method of achieving accelerated fractionation is to give a standard fraction to the entire field in the morning and to give a second treatment to the boost field in the afternoon (called *concomitant boost*). As in standard radiation, the boost would be given by extending the length of the treatment course; this concomitant boost approach can shorten treatment from 7 weeks to 5 weeks in head and neck cancer.

The second approach to altering fractionation is called *hyperfractionation*. Hyperfractionation is defined as the use of more than one fraction per day separated by more than 6 hours (see the section "Biologic Aspects of Radiation Oncology" above), with a dose per fraction that is less than standard. Hyperfractionation is expected to produce fewer late complications for the same acute effects against both rapidly dividing normal tissues and tumors. Pure hyperfractionation might give 1 Gy twice a day, so that the total dose per day would be 2 Gy, and thus be equal to standard fractionation. In practice, hyperfractionated treatments are usually in the range of 1.2 Gy, which means that, compared with standard fractionation, a somewhat higher dose is administered during the same period of time (so that most hyperfractionation also includes modest acceleration). The overall effect is to increase the acute toxicity (which resolves) and tumor response, while not increasing the (dose-limiting) late toxicity, which can improve the cure rate. Both accelerated fractionation and hyperfractionation have been demonstrated in a meta-analysis to be superior to standard fractionation in the treatment of head and neck cancer with radiation alone.[122]

Hypofractionation refers to the administration of a smaller number of larger fractions than is standard. Hypofractionation might be expected to cause more late toxicity for the same antitumor effect than standard or hyperfractionation. In the past, this approach was reserved for palliative cases, with the sense that a modest potential for increased late toxicity was not a major concern in patients with limited life expectancy. However, more recently, it has been proposed that the ability to better exclude normal tissue by using IGRT may allow hypofractionation to be used safely, and that in the specific case of prostate cancer, hypofractionation may have beneficial effects.[123] There are now several clinical trials of hypofractionation using IGRT, although it is too early to tell if important late toxicities will be seen.

Although optimization of fractionation has been shown to have a significant impact on the effectiveness of radiation alone, its role is unclear when radiation is combined with chemotherapy. Chemotherapy may prevent repopulation during a course of treatment and therefore make accelerated fractionation unnecessary. It is clear that combining hyperfractionated or accelerated radiation with chemotherapy increases treatment toxicity substantially.

ADVERSE EFFECTS

Radiation produces adverse effects in normal tissues. Although these are discussed in detail in other chapters of this book as part of comprehensive discussions of organ toxicity, it is worth making some general comments here from the perspective of how radiation biology relates to the clinical toxicities. The term *radiation toxicity* is used to describe the adverse effects caused by radiation alone and radiation plus chemotherapy. Although this latter toxicity would be better labeled as *combined modality toxicity*, the pattern typically resembles a more severe form of the toxicity produced by radiation alone. Adverse effects from radiation can be divided into acute, subacute, and chronic (or late) effects. Acute effects are common, rarely serious, and usually self-limiting. Acute effects tend to occur in organs that depend on rapid self-renewal, most commonly the skin or mucosal surfaces (oropharynx, esophagus, small intestine, rectum, and bladder). This is due to radiation-induced cell death that occurs during mitosis, so that cells that divide rapidly show the most rapid cell loss. In the treatment of head and neck cancer, mucositis becomes worse during the first 3 to 4 weeks of therapy, but then will often stabilize as the normal mucosa cell proliferation increases in response to mucosal cell loss. It seems likely that normal tissue stem cells are relatively resistant to radiation compared with the more differentiated cells, as these stem cells survive to allow the normal mucosa to re-epithelialize. Acute side effects typically resolve within 1 to 2 weeks of treatment completion, although occasionally these effects are so severe that they lead to consequential late effects, as described later.

As lymphocytes are exquisitely sensitive to radiation, there has been considerable investigation into the effects of radiation on immune function. In contrast to mucosal cell killing, which requires mitosis, radiation kills lymphocytes in all phases of the cell cycle by apoptosis, so that lymphocyte counts decrease within days of initiating treatment. These effects do not tend to put patients at risk for infection, as granulocytes, which are chiefly responsible for combating infections, are relatively unaffected.

Two acute side effects of radiation do not fit neatly into these models that relate to cell kill: nausea[124,125] and fatigue.[126,127] The origin of radiation-induced nausea is not related to acute cell loss, as it can occur within hours of the first treatment. Nausea is usually associated with radiation of the stomach but can sometimes occur during brain irradiation or as a result of large-volume irradiation that involves neither the brain nor the stomach. Irradiation typically produces fatigue, even if relatively small volumes are irradiated. It seems likely that origins of both of these "abscopal" effects of radiation (effects that occur systemically or at a distance for the site of irradiation) are related to the release of cytokines, but little is known for certain.

Radiation can also produce subacute toxicities in the form of radiation pneumonitis and radiation-induced liver disease. These typically occur 2 weeks to 3 months after radiation has been completed. The risk of radiation pneumonitis and radiation-induced liver disease is proportional to the mean dose delivered.[128,129] Thus, the 3D tools that allow the calculation of dose-volume histograms described above are currently used to determine the maximum safe treatment that can be delivered in terms of dose and volume. These toxicities appear to be initiated subclinically during the course of radiation as a cascade of cytokines in which transforming growth factor-beta (TGF-β), tumor necrosis factor-α, interleukin 6, and other cytokines play a role.[130] High TGF-β plasma levels during a course of treatment have been found to be associated with a greater risk of

TABLE 27.2

RADIATION TOLERANCE DOSES FOR NORMAL TISSUES

	TD 5/5 (Gy)[a]			TD 50/5 (Gy)[b]			
	Portion of Organ Irradiated			Portion of Organ Irradiated			
Site	1/3	2/3	3/3	1/3	2/3	3/3	Complication End Point(s)
Kidney	50	30	23	—	40	28	Nephritis
Brain	60	50	45	75	65	60	Necrosis, infarct
Brainstem	60	53	50	—	—	65	Necrosis, infarct
Spinal cord	50 (5–10 cm)	—	47 (20 cm)	70 (5–10 cm)	—	—	Myelitis, necrosis
Lung	45	30	17.5	65	40	24.5	Radiation pneumonitis
Heart	60	45	40	70	55	50	Pericarditis
Esophagus	60	58	55	72	70	68	Stricture, perforation
Stomach	60	55	50	70	67	65	Ulceration, perforation
Small intestine	50	—	40	60	—	55	Obstruction, perforation, fistula
Colon	55	—	45	65	—	55	Obstruction, perforation, fistula, ulceration
Rectum	(100 cm³ volume)		60	(100 cm³ volume)		80	Severe proctitis, necrosis, fistula
Liver	50	35	30	55	45	40	Liver failure

[a]TD 5/5, the average dose that results in a 5% complication risk within 5 years.
[b]TD 50/5, the average dose that results in a 50% complication risk within 5 years.
(Adapted from ref. 145.)

radiation pneumonitis.[131] Thus, in the future, researchers might look toward a combination of physical dose delivery, measured by the dose-volume histogram, functional imaging of normal tissue damage, and the detection of biomarkers of toxicity, such as TGF-β, to improve the ability to individualize therapy.

Late effects, which are typically seen 6 months or more after a course of radiation, include fibrosis, fistula formation, or long-term organ damage. Two theories for the origin of late effects have been put forth: late damage to the microvasculature and direct damage to the parenchyma. Although the vascular damage theory is attractive, it does not account for the differing sensitivities of organs to radiation. Perhaps the microvasculature is unique in each organ.[132] Regardless of the mechanism of toxicity, the tolerance of whole-organ radiation is now fairly well established (Table 27.2). Late complications can also be divided into two categories: consequential and true late effects. The best example of a consequential late effect is fibrosis and dysphagia after high-dose chemoradiation for head and neck cancer. Here, late fibrosis or ulceration appears to be the result of the mucosa becoming denuded for a prolonged time period. Late effects consequential are distinct from true late effects, which can follow a normal treatment course of self-limited toxicity and a 6-month or more symptom-free period. Examples of true late effects are radiation myelitis, radiation brain necrosis, and radiation-induced bowel obstruction. In the past, radiation fibrosis was thought to be an irreversible condition. Therefore, an exciting recent development is that severe radiation-induced breast fibrosis is an active process that can be reversed by drug therapy (pentoxifylline and vitamin E).[133] Radiation therapy also causes second cancers.

PRINCIPLES OF COMBINING ANTICANCER AGENTS WITH RADIATION THERAPY

Combining chemotherapy with radiation therapy has produced important improvements in treatment outcome. Randomized clinical trials show improved local control and survival through the use of concurrent chemotherapy and radiation therapy for patients with high-grade gliomas and locally advanced cancers of the head and neck, lung, esophagus, stomach, rectum, and anus. There are least two proposed reasons why chemoradiotherapy might be successful. The first is radiosensitization. In the laboratory, radiosensitization is defined as a synergistic relationship, using mathematical approaches such as isobologram or median effect analysis.[134,135] The underlying concept is that the observed effect of using chemotherapy and radiation concurrently is greater than simply adding the two together. A second proposed reason to combine radiation and chemotherapy is to realize the benefit of improved local control radiation along with the systemic effect of chemotherapy, a concept called *spatial additivity*.[136]

Clinical results show that both radiosensitization and spatial additivity contribute to varying extents in different clinical settings. In the case of head and neck cancer, radiosensitization predominates. This conclusion is supported by the meta-analysis of head and neck cancer: sequential chemotherapy and radiotherapy produce little if any improvement in survival, whereas concurrent chemoradiation produces a significant increase in survival.[137] Furthermore, in the early positive studies using concurrent chemoradiation, systemic metastases were unaffected, although survival was improved. Radiosensitization may also predominate in the success of chemoradiotherapy for locally advanced lung cancer. For instance, although initial studies indicate that sequential chemotherapy and radiation had some benefit for lung cancer,[138] more recent work indicates that concurrent therapy is superior, and it is now the standard treatment.[139] However, there are also examples of spatial additivity. For example, both radiosensitization and spatial additivity are provided by the use of chemoradiation for locally advanced cervix cancer, in that both local and systemic relapse are decreased by combined therapy.[140]

By targeting aberrant growth factor or pro-angiogenic pathways that are specific to cancer cells, rather than all rapidly proliferating cells, molecularly targeted therapies offer the potential to improve outcome without increasing toxicity. Even a selective cytostatic effect against the tumor

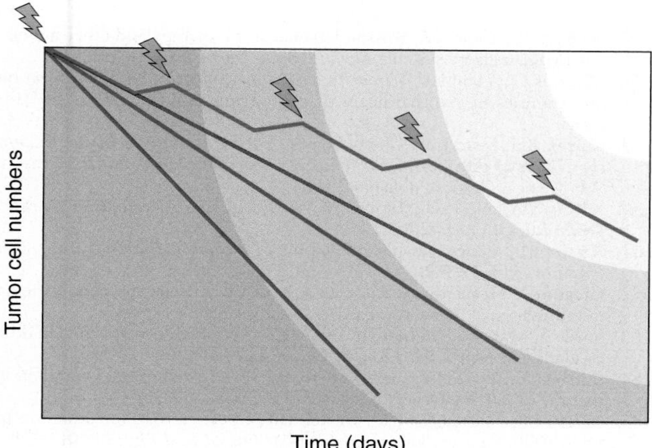

FIGURE 27.22 Potential mechanisms of synergy between epidermal growth factor receptor (EGFR) inhibitors and radiation. Although each daily radiation treatment kills a fraction of the cells, some cells grow back by the next day, which attenuates the effectiveness of radiation. If an EGFR inhibitor has only a selective cytostatic effect and blocks regrowth between fractions, the result would be a dramatic increase in radiation efficacy. The benefit of the inhibitor would be even greater if it caused tumor cell cytotoxicity or radiosensitization.

would be predicted to act synergistically with radiation (Fig. 27.22). Although preclinical studies (summarized earlier) have highlighted the potential therapeutic gains that could be achieved by adding EGFR inhibitors to radiation, the best validation of this combination has been from the results of clinical trials in head and neck cancer. A phase 3 clinical trial demonstrated that, in a cohort of 424 patients with locoregionally advanced squamous cell carcinoma of the head and neck, the addition of cetuximab nearly doubled the median survival of patients (compared to radiotherapy alone), from 28 to 54 months. This study represents the first major success achieved by the addition of an EGFR antagonist to radiotherapy. This improvement was achieved without enhanced toxicity. Notably, the rates of pharyngitis and weight loss were identical in the two arms.[63] Local control was improved rather than the development of metastases, suggesting synergy rather than spatial additivity. Thus, the principle that can be derived from this study is that in tumors that express high EGFR levels and are likely to depend on aberrant EGF signaling, a combination of a true cytotoxic agent such as radiation with a cytostatic agent such as cetuximab has considerable promise.

Because of the success of chemoradiotherapy, the natural tendency has not been to substitute molecularly targeted agents such as cetuximab for chemotherapy but to add cetuximab to chemoradiotherapy. Thus, the combination of cisplatin, cetuximab, and radiation is now being tested against cisplatin and radiation for patients with locally advanced head and neck cancer in the Radiation Therapy Oncology Group's trial RTOG 0522. The best method of combining all three is unknown. However, it has been shown preclinically that when EGFR inhibitors are given prior to chemotherapy, they can produce antagonism,[141] and it has been speculated[142] that scheduling may have played a role in the negative INTACT (Iressa Non–Small Cell Lung Cancer Trial Assessing Combination Treatment) 1 and 2 trials.[143,144] Thus, it is possible, for instance, that if a patient is receiving cisplatin, cetuximab, and radiation, cisplatin should be given, for example, on Monday, cetuximab on Tuesday, and radiation Monday through Friday. The principles of adding molecularly targeted therapy to chemoradiation are still evolving.

Selected References

The full list of references for this chapter appears in the online version.

1. Hall EJ, Giaccia AJ. *Radiobiology for the radiologist*. Philadelphia: Lippincott Williams & Williams, 2006.
2. Fowler JF. Developing aspects of radiation oncology. *Med Phys* 1981;8: 427.
3. Lavin MF. Ataxia-telangiectasia: from a rare disorder to a paradigm for cell signalling and cancer. *Nat Rev Mol Cell Biol* 2008;9:759.
7. Cortez D, Wang Y, Qin J, Elledge SJ. Requirement of ATM-dependent phosphorylation of brca1 in the DNA damage response to double-strand breaks. *Science* 1999;286:1162.
9. Sherr CJ, McCormick F. The RB and p53 pathways in cancer. *Cancer Cell* 2002;2:103.
10. Bartek J, Lukas J. Chk1 and Chk2 kinases in checkpoint control and cancer. *Cancer Cell* 2003;3:421.
11. Abraham RT. Cell cycle checkpoint signaling through the ATM and ATR kinases. *Genes Dev* 2001;15:2177.
13. Donzelli M, Draetta GF. Regulating mammalian checkpoints through Cdc25 inactivation. *EMBO Rep* 2003;4:671.
15. Dai Y, Grant S. New insights into checkpoint kinase 1 in the DNA damage response signaling network. *Clin Cancer Res* 2010;16:376.
16. Giaccia A, Weinstein R, Hu J, Stamato TD. Cell cycle-dependent repair of double-strand DNA breaks in a gamma-ray-sensitive Chinese hamster cell. *Somat Cell Mol Genet* 1985;11:485.
18. Helleday T, Lo J, van Gent DC, Engelward BP. DNA double-strand break repair: from mechanistic understanding to cancer treatment. *DNA Repair (Amst)* 2007;6:923.
19. Hefferin ML, Tomkinson AE. Mechanism of DNA double-strand break repair by non-homologous end joining. *DNA Repair (Amst)* 2005;4:639.
23. Tsukuda T, Fleming AB, Nickoloff JA, Osley MA. Chromatin remodelling at a DNA double-strand break site in Saccharomyces cerevisiae. *Nature* 2005;438:379.
26. Sleeth KM, Sorensen CS, Issaeva N, et al. RPA mediates recombination repair during replication stress and is displaced from DNA by checkpoint signalling in human cells. *J Mol Biol* 2007;373:38.
27. Littlefield LG, Kleinerman RA, Sayer AM, Tarone R, Boice JD Jr. Chromosome aberrations in lymphocytes—biomonitors of radiation exposure. *Prog Clin Biol Res* 1991;372:387.
29. Sowa Resat MB, Morgan WF. Radiation-induced genomic instability: a role for secreted soluble factors in communicating the radiation response to non-irradiated cells. *J Cell Biochem* 2004;92:1013.
30. Elkind MM. The initial part of the survival curve: does it predict the outcome of fractionated radiotherapy? *Radiat Res* 1988;114:425.
31. McCulloch EA, Till JE. The sensitivity of cells from normal mouse bone marrow to gamma radiation in vitro and in vivo. *Radiat Res* 1962;16:822.
32. Withers HR. The dose-survival relationship for irradiation of epithelial cells of mouse skin. *Br J Radiol* 1967;40:187.
33. Withers HR. Recovery and repopulation in vivo by mouse skin epithelial cells during fractionated irradiation. *Radiat Res* 1967;32:227.
34. Withers HR, Elkind MM. Microcolony survival assay for cells of mouse intestinal mucosa exposed to radiation. *Int J Radiat Biol Relat Stud Phys Chem Med* 1970;17:261.
35. Suit H, Wette R. Radiation dose fractionation and tumor control probability. *Radiat Res* 1966;29:267.
39. Hill RP, Bush RS. A lung-colony assay to determine the radiosensitivity of cells of a solid tumour. *Int J Radiat Biol Relat Stud Phys Chem Med* 1969;15:435.
41. Elkind MM, Whitmore GF. *Radiobiology of cultured mammalian cells*. New York: Gordon and Breach, 1967.
44. Thomlinson RH, Gray LH. The histological structure of some human lung cancers and the possible implications for radiotherapy. *Br J Cancer* 1955;9:539.
45. Overgaard J, Horsman MR. Modification of hypoxia-induced radioresistance in tumors by the use of oxygen and sensitizers. *Semin Radiat Oncol* 1996;6:10.

46. Machtay M, Pajak TF, Suntharalingam M, et al. Radiotherapy with or without erythropoietin for anemic patients with head and neck cancer: a randomized trial of the Radiation Therapy Oncology Group (RTOG 99-03). *Int J Radiat Oncol Biol Phys* 2007;69:1008.
49. Willett CG, Boucher Y, di Tomaso E, et al. Direct evidence that the VEGF-specific antibody bevacizumab has antivascular effects in human rectal cancer. *Nat Med* 2004;10:145.
51. Rischin D, Hicks RJ, Fisher R, et al. Prognostic significance of [18F]-misonidazole positron emission tomography-detected tumor hypoxia in patients with advanced head and neck cancer randomly assigned to chemoradiation with or without tirapazamine: a substudy of Trans-Tasman Radiation Oncology Group Study 98.02. *J Clin Oncol* 2006; 24:2098.
52. Lee NY, Mechalakos JG, Nehmeh S, et al. Fluorine-18-labeled fluoromisonidazole positron emission and computed tomography-guided intensity-modulated radiotherapy for head and neck cancer: a feasibility study. *Int J Radiat Oncol Biol Phys* 2008;70:2.
53. Lawrence TS, Davis MA, Tang HY, Maybaum J. Fluorodeoxyuridine-mediated cytotoxicity and radiosensitization require S phase progression. *Int J Radiat Biol* 1996;70:273.
54. Lawrence TS, Chang EY, Hahn TM, Hertel LW, Shewach DS. Radiosensitization of pancreatic cancer cells by 2′,2′-difluoro-2′-deoxycytidine. *Int J Radiat Oncol Biol Phys* 1996;34:867.
55. Eisbruch A, Shewach DS, Bradford CR, et al. Radiation concurrent with gemcitabine for locally advanced head and neck cancer: a phase I trial and intracellular drug incorporation study. *J Clin Oncol* 2001;19:792.
56. McGinn CJ, Zalupski MM, Shureiqi I, et al. Phase I trial of radiation dose escalation with concurrent weekly full-dose gemcitabine in patients with advanced pancreatic cancer. *J Clin Oncol* 2001;19:4202.
57. Wolff RA, Evans DB, Gravel DM, et al. Phase I trial of gemcitabine combined with radiation for the treatment of locally advanced pancreatic adenocarcinoma. *Clin Cancer Res* 2001;7:2246.
58. Wilson GD, Bentzen SM, Harari PM. Biologic basis for combining drugs with radiation. *Semin Radiat Oncol* 2006;16:2.
59. Lau D, Leigh B, Gandara D, et al. Twice-weekly paclitaxel and weekly carboplatin with concurrent thoracic radiation followed by carboplatin/paclitaxel consolidation for stage III non-small-cell lung cancer: a California Cancer Consortium phase II trial. *J Clin Oncol* 2001; 19:442.
60. Bradley JD, Bae K, Graham MV, et al. Primary analysis of the phase II component of a phase I/II dose intensification study using three-dimensional conformal radiation therapy and concurrent chemotherapy for patients with inoperable non–small-cell lung cancer: RTOG 0117. *J Clin Oncol* 2010;28:2475.
61. Nyati MK, Morgan MA, Feng FY, Lawrence TS. Integration of EGFR inhibitors with radiochemotherapy. *Nat Rev Cancer* 2006;6:876.
62. Debucquoy A, Machiels JP, McBride WH, Haustermans K. Integration of epidermal growth factor receptor inhibitors with preoperative chemoradiation. *Clin Cancer Res* 2010;16:2709.
63. Bonner JA, Harari PM, Giralt J, et al. Radiotherapy plus cetuximab for locoregionally advanced head and neck cancer: 5-year survival data from a phase 3 randomised trial, and relation between cetuximab-induced rash and survival. *Lancet Oncol* 2010;11:21.
64. Morgan MA, Parsels LA, Zhao L, et al. Mechanism of radiosensitization by the Chk1/2 inhibitor AZD7762 involves abrogation of the G2 checkpoint and inhibition of homologous recombinational DNA repair. *Cancer Res* 2010;70:4972.
65. Bolderson E, Richard DJ, Zhou BB, Khanna KK. Recent advances in cancer therapy targeting proteins involved in DNA double-strand break repair. *Clin Cancer Res* 2009;15:6314.
66. Brizel DM, Wasserman TH, Henke M, et al. Phase III randomized trial of amifostine as a radioprotector in head and neck cancer. *J Clin Oncol* 2000;18:3339.
67. Winczura P, Jassem J. Combined treatment with cytoprotective agents and radiotherapy. *Cancer Treat Rev* 2010;36:268.
68. Hendee WR, Ibbott GS, Hendee EG. *Radiation therapy physics*, 3rd ed. Philadelphia: Wiley, 2004.
69. Khan FM. *The physics of radiation therapy*, 4th ed. Philadelphia: Lippincott Williams & Wilkins, 2010.
70. Levitt SH, Purdy JA, Perez CA, et al., ed. *Technical basis of radiation therapy*. Philadelphia: Springer, 2006.
71. Mayles P, Nahum A, Rosenwald J-C. *Handbook of radiotherapy physics: theory and practice*. Boca Raton, FL: Taylor and Francis Group, 2007.
72. Podgorsak EB. *Radiation physics for medical physicists*. Berlin Heidelberg: Springer-Verlag, 2010.
73. Schlegel W, Bortfeld T, Grosu AL, ed. *New technologies in radiation oncology*. Berlin Heidelberg: Springer-Verlag, 2006.
74. Van Dyk J, ed. *The modern technology of radiation oncology*, Vol. 2. Madison, WI: Medical Physics Publishing, 2005.
75. Karzmark CJ, Nunan CS, Tanabe E. *Medical electron accelerators*. New York.: McGraw-Hill, 1993.
76. Greene D, Williams PC. *Linear accelerators for radiation therapy*, 2nd ed. New York: Taylor and Francis Group, 1997.
77. Fenwick JD, Tome WA, Soisson ET, et al. Tomotherapy and other innovative IMRT delivery systems. *Semin Radiat Oncol* 2006;16:199.
78. Mageras GS, guest ed., Tepper JE, ed. Management of target localization uncertainties in external-beam therapy. *Semin Radiat Oncol* 2005;15: 133.
79. Curran BH, Balter JM, Chetty IJ, eds. *Integrating new technologies into the clinic: Monte Carlo and image-guided radiation therapy*. Madison, WI: Medical Physics Publishing, 2006.
80. Jaffray DA, guest ed., Tepper JE, ed. Image-guided radiation therapy. *Semin Radiat Oncol* 2007;17:243.
81. Kessler ML. Image registration and data fusion in radiation therapy. *Brit J Radiol* 2006;79:S99.
82. Gregoire V, Haustermans K, Geets X, et al. PET-based treatment planning in radiotherapy: a new standard? *J Nucl Med* 2007;48:68S.
83. Søvik Å, Malinen E, Olsen DR. Strategies for biologic image-guided dose escalation: a review. *Int J Radiat Oncol Biol Phys* 2009;73:650.
84. Bortfeld T, Chen GTY, guest eds., Tepper JE, ed. High-precision radiation therapy of moving targets. *Semin Radiat Oncol* 2004;14:1.
85. Marks LB, Ten Haken RK, Martel MK. Guest editor's introduction to QUANTEC: a users guide. *Int J Radiat Oncol Biol Phys* 2010;76:S1.
86. Bortfeld T. IMRT: a review and preview. *Phys Med Biol* 2006;51:R363.
87. Webb S. *Contemporary IMRT developing physics and clinical implementation*. London: IOP Publishing, 2005.
88. Maughan RL, Yudelev M. Neutron therapy. In: Van Dyk J, ed. *The modern technology of radiation oncology*. Madison, WI: Medical Physics Publishing, 1999:871.
89. Hogstrom KR, Almond PR. Review of electron beam therapy physics. *Phys Med Biol* 2006;51:R455.
90. Webb S, Evans PM, guest eds., Tepper JE, ed. Innovative techniques in radiation therapy. *Semin Radiat Oncol* 2006;16:193.
91. Knox SJ, guest ed., Tepper JE, ed. Systemic radiation therapy. *Semin Radiat Oncol* 2000;11:71.
92. Meredith RF. Systemic targeted radionuclide therapy (STaRT). *Int J Radiat Oncol Biol Phys* 2006;66(2)S2.
93. Tripuraneni P, Watson RL, Ang KK, et al. Intersociety Radiation Oncology Summit—SCOPE II. *Int J Radiat Oncol Biol Phys* 2008;72:323.
94. Delaney G, Jacob S, Featherstone C, et al. The role of radiotherapy in cancer treatment: estimating optimal utilization from a review of evidence-based clinical guidelines. *Cancer* 2005;104:1129 [erratum appears in *Cancer* 2006;107(3):660].
96. Schulz-Ertner D, Tsujii H. Particle radiation therapy using proton and heavier ion beams. *J Clin Oncol* 2007;25:953.
97. Zietman AL, Bae K, Slater JD, et al. Randomized trial comparing conventional-dose with high-dose conformal radiation therapy in early-stage adenocarcinoma of the prostate: long-term results from Proton Radiation Oncology Group/American College of Radiology 95-09. *J Clin Oncol* 2010;28:1106.
98. Symon Z, Griffith KA, McLaughlin PW, et al. Dose escalation for localized prostate cancer: substantial benefit observed with 3D conformal therapy. *Int J Radiat Oncol Biol Phys* 2003;57:384.
99. Zelefsky MJ, Chan H, Hunt M, et al. Long-term outcome of high dose intensity modulated radiation therapy for patients with clinically localized prostate cancer. *J Urol* 2006;176:1415.
100. Overgaard J. Hypoxic radiosensitisation—adored and ignored. *J Clin Oncol* 2007;25:4066.
101. Brada M, Pijls-Johannesma M, De Ruysscher D. Proton therapy in clinical practice: current clinical evidence. *J Clin Oncol* 2007;25:965.
102. Al-Mamgani A, van Putten WL, Heemsbergen WD, et al. Update of Dutch multicenter dose-escalation trial of radiotherapy for localized prostate cancer. *Int J Radiat Oncol Biol Phys* 2008;72:980.
103. Kuban DA, Tucker SL, Dong L, et al. Long-term results of the M. D. Anderson randomized dose-escalation trial for prostate cancer. *Int J Radiat Oncol Biol Phys* 2008;70:67.
104. Kong F-M, Ten Haken RK, Schipper MJ, et al. High-dose radiation improved local tumor control and overall survival in patients with inoperable/unresectable non-small-cell lung cancer: long-term results of a radiation dose escalation study. *Int J Radiat Oncol Biol Phys* 2005;63:324.
105. Ben-Josef E, Normolle D, Ensminger WD, et al. Phase II trial of high-dose conformal radiation therapy with concurrent hepatic artery floxuridine for unresectable intrahepatic malignancies. *J Clin Oncol* 2005;23:8739.
106. Feng FY, Kim HM, Lyden TH, et al. Intensity-modulated chemoradiotherapy aiming to reduce dysphagia in patients with oropharyngeal cancer: clinical and functional results. *J Clin Oncol* 2010;28:2732.
108. Merrick GS, Butler WM, Wallner KE, et al. Variability of prostate brachytherapy pre-implant dosimetry: a multi-institutional analysis. *Brachytherapy* 2005;4:241.
109. Lo SS, Fakiris AJ, Chang EL, et al. Stereotactic body radiation therapy: a novel treatment modality. *Nat Rev Clin Oncol* 2010;7:44.
110. Urba S, Wolf G, Eisbruch A, et al. Single-cycle induction chemotherapy selects patients with advanced laryngeal cancer for combined chemoradiation: a new treatment paradigm. *J Clin Oncol* 2006;24:593.

111. Bartelink H, Roelofsen F, Eschwege F, et al. Concomitant radiotherapy and chemotherapy is superior to radiotherapy alone in the treatment of locally advanced anal cancer: results of a phase III randomized trial of the European Organization for Research and Treatment of Cancer Radiotherapy and Gastrointestinal Cooperative Groups. *J Clin Oncol* 1997;15:2040.
112. Hellman S, Weichselbaum RR. Oligometastases. *J Clin Oncol* 1995;13:8.
115. Sauer R, Becker H, Hohenberger W, et al. Preoperative versus postoperative chemoradiotherapy for rectal cancer. *N Engl J Med* 2004;351:1731.
116. Clarke M, Collins R, Darby S, et al. Effects of radiotherapy and of differences in the extent of surgery for early breast cancer on local recurrence and 15-year survival: an overview of the randomised trials. *Lancet* 2005;366:2087.
119. Jin J-Y, Chen Q, Jin R, et al. Technical and clinical experience with spine radiosurgery: a new technology for management of localized spine metastases. *Technol Cancer Res Treat* 2007;6:127.
120. Tarnawski R, Fowler J, Skladowski K, et al. How fast is repopulation of tumor cells during the treatment gap? *Int J Radiat Oncol Biol Phys* 2002;54:229.
122. Bourhis J, Overgaard J, Audry H, et al. Hyperfractionated or accelerated radiotherapy in head and neck cancer: a meta-analysis. *Lancet* 2006;368:843.
123. Fowler JF, Ritter MA, Chappell RJ, et al. What hypofractionated protocols should be tested for prostate cancer? *Int J Radiat Oncol Biol Phys* 2003;56:1093.
128. Dawson LA, Ten Haken RK. Partial volume tolerance of the liver to radiation. *Semin Radiat Oncol* 2005;15:279.
129. Kong F-M, Hayman JA, Griffith KA, et al. Final toxicity results of a radiation-dose escalation study in patients with non-small-cell lung cancer (NSCLC): predictors for radiation pneumonitis and fibrosis. *Int J Radiat Oncol Biol Phys* 2006;65:1075.
131. Hart JP, Broadwater G, Rabbani Z, et al. Cytokine profiling for prediction of symptomatic radiation-induced lung injury. *Int J Radiat Oncol Biol Phys* 2005;63:1448.
137. Pignon JP, Bourhis J, Domenge C, et al. Chemotherapy added to locoregional treatment for head and neck squamous-cell carcinoma: three meta-analyses of updated individual data. MACH-NC Collaborative Group. Meta-Analysis of Chemotherapy on Head and Neck Cancer. *Lancet* 2000;355:949.
139. Vokes EE. Optimal therapy for unresectable stage III non–small-cell lung cancer. *J Clin Oncol* 2005;23:5853.
142. Baselga J. Combining the anti-EGFR agent gefitinib with chemotherapy in non–small-cell lung cancer: how do we go from INTACT to impact? *J Clin Oncol* 2004;22:759.

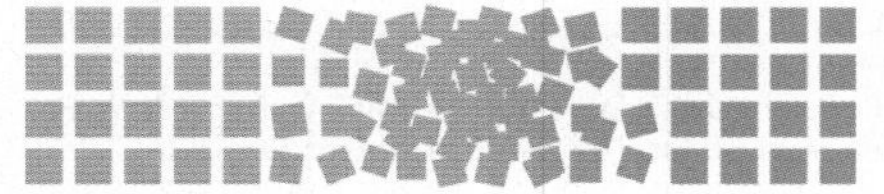

CHAPTER 28 MEDICAL ONCOLOGY

VINCENT T. DEVITA, Jr. AND EDWARD CHU

INTRODUCTION

Chemotherapy, which includes newly developed targeted treatments, is the principle tool of the medical oncologist. The development of effective combination chemotherapy programs for childhood leukemia, advanced Hodgkin's lymphoma, and diffuse large B-cell lymphomas in the 1960s provided curative therapeutic strategies for patients with advanced malignancies of all types. These advances confirmed the principle that chemotherapy could indeed cure advanced cancer and provided the rationale for using chemotherapy in the adjuvant setting following surgical resection and for integrating chemotherapy into combined modality programs with surgery and radiation therapy in locally advanced disease. The principal obstacles to the clinical efficacy of chemotherapy have been toxicity to the normal tissues of the body and the development of cellular drug resistance. The advances in molecular technology have also provided insights into the molecular and genetic events within cancer cells that confer chemosensitivity to drug treatment. This enhanced understanding of the molecular pathways by which chemotherapy exerts its cytotoxic activity and by which genetic instability results in resistance to drug therapy has provided the rational basis for the development of innovative therapeutic strategies to directly attack these novel targets. As such, chemotherapy has now evolved into more specific targeted treatment and is moving from empiric delivery to a more individually tailored approach. The implementation of such novel treatment approaches provides an important paradigm shift as to how chemotherapy is administered. The long-term goal of these research efforts is to enhance the clinical outcome for cancer patients undergoing treatment, especially those with cancers that traditionally have been resistant to conventional chemotherapy.

Historical Perspective

The systemic treatment of cancer has its roots in the initial work of Paul Ehrlich, who coined the term *chemotherapy*. The use of *in vivo* rodent model systems to develop antibiotics for treating infectious diseases led Clowes and colleagues at Roswell Park Memorial Institute, in the early 1900s, to develop inbred rodent lines bearing transplanted tumors to screen potential anticancer drugs. This *in vivo* system provided the foundation for mass screening of novel compounds.[1] Alkylating agents represent the first class of chemotherapeutic drugs to be used in the clinical setting. Of note, application of this class of compounds was a direct product of the secret gas program of the United States during both World Wars, and was based on the astute observation that exposure to mustard gas resulted in bone marrow and lymphoid hypoplasia. This experience led to the first clinical use of nitrogen mustard in a patient with non–Hodgkin's lymphoma in 1942. Subsequent treatment with this alkylating agent resulted in dramatic regressions in advanced lymphomas and thereby generated significant excitement in the field of cancer pharmacology.

In the late 1940s, Sidney Farber reported that folic acid had a significant proliferative effect on leukemic cell growth in children with lymphoblastic leukemia. These observations led to the development of folic acid analogs as cancer drugs to inhibit cellular folate metabolism. This work initiated the era of cancer chemotherapy. In fact, the entire class of antimetabolites, including antifolates, fluoropyrimidines, deoxycytidine analogs, and the purine analogs were all designed with the expectation that they would target critical biochemical pathways involved in *de novo* pyrimidine and purine metabolism, respectively, and thereby inhibit cancer cell proliferation and growth. Indeed, these compounds represent the first examples of targeted anticancer agents to be developed for clinical application. Current targeted treatments, in contrast, focus on key elements of the cellular signaling apparatus uncovered since then.

Clinical Application of Chemotherapy

Presently, chemotherapy is used in four main clinical settings: (1) primary induction treatment for advanced disease or for cancers for which there are no other effective treatment approaches (Tables 28.1 and 28.2); (2) as the primary or neoadjuvant treatment for patients with localized disease for which local forms of therapy, such as surgery, radiation, or both, are ineffective by themselves (Table 28.3); (3) adjuvant treatment for early-stage disease following local methods of treatment, including surgery, radiation therapy, or both (Table 28.4); and (4) direct instillation into sanctuary sites or site-directed perfusion of specific regions of the body directly affected by the cancer.

Primary induction chemotherapy refers to drug therapy administered as the first treatment for patients who present with advanced cancer for which no alternative treatment exists.[2,3] This approach applies for patients with advanced, metastatic disease. Studies involving a wide range of solid tumor types have shown that chemotherapy confers survival benefit when compared with only supportive care in patients with advanced disease, which provides sound rationale for the early initiation of drug treatment. Cancer chemotherapy can be curative in a small but significant subset of patients who present with advanced disease. In adults, these curable cancers include Hodgkin's and non–Hodgkin's lymphoma, acute lymphoblastic and myelogenous leukemia, germ cell cancer, ovarian cancer, limited-stage small cell lung cancer, and choriocarcinoma. In pediatric patients, the major curable cancers include the acute leukemias, Burkitt lymphoma, Wilms tumor, and embryonal rhabdomyosarcoma.

TABLE 28.1

PRIMARY CHEMOTHERAPY: CANCERS FOR WHICH CHEMOTHERAPY IS A PRIMARY TREATMENT MODALITY

Acute leukemias
Non-Hodgkin lymphoma
Myeloma
Hodgkin lymphoma
Germ cell cancer
Primary central nervous system lymphoma
Ovarian cancer
Small cell lung cancer
Wilms tumor
Embryonal rhabdomyosarcoma

Neoadjuvant chemotherapy refers to the use of chemotherapy as the primary treatment in patients who present with localized cancer for which local therapies, such as surgery and/or radiation, exist but are less than completely effective.[4] For chemotherapy to be used as the initial treatment for a cancer that would be partially curable by either surgery or radiation therapy, there is usually documented evidence for its efficacy in the advanced disease setting. At present, neoadjuvant therapy is used to treat locally advanced anal cancer, bladder cancer, breast cancer, gastroesophageal cancer, head and neck cancer, non–small cell lung cancer (NSCLC), rectal cancer, and osteogenic sarcoma. Clinical benefit can be optimized when chemotherapy is administered in combination with radiation therapy, either concurrently or sequentially. One potential advantage of neoadjuvant therapy is to reduce the size of the primary tumor such that it allows for higher rates of surgical resection while reducing the potential spread of micrometastatic spread. Moreover, neoadjuvant chemotherapy may allow for preservation of vital organs such as the larynx, anal sphincter, limbs, and bladder.

One of the most important roles for cancer chemotherapy is as an adjuvant to local treatment modalities such as surgery and radiation therapy, and this approach has been termed *adjuvant chemotherapy*.[5] The development of disease recurrence, either locally or systemically, after surgery, radiation, or both, is mainly due to the spread of occult micrometastases. Thus, the goal of adjuvant therapy is to eradicate micrometastases, thereby reducing the incidence of both local and systemic recurrence and improving the overall survival of patients. In general, chemotherapy regimens with clinical activity against advanced disease are used in the adjuvant setting and may have curative potential after surgical resection of the primary tumor, provided the appropriate dose and schedule are used. The efficacy of adjuvant chemotherapy in prolonging disease-free and overall survival is now well established in a wide range of tumors, including breast cancer, colon cancer, gastric cancer, NSCLC, ovarian cancer, head and neck cancer, and cervical cancer, Wilms tumor, and osteogenic sarcoma. There is also evidence to support the use of adjuvant chemotherapy in patients with anaplastic astrocytomas. Patients with primary malignant melanoma at high risk of metastases derive clinical benefit from adjuvant treatment with the biologic agent interferon-α, although this treatment must be given for 1 year. Finally, the antiestrogens tamoxifen, anastrozole, and letrozole are effective agents in the adjuvant therapy of postmenopausal women whose breast tumors express the estrogen receptor. Because these agents are cytostatic as opposed to cytocidal in their action, they must be administered on a prolonged basis, and the standard recommended treatment length for adjuvant endocrine therapy is for a total of 5 years.

TABLE 28.2

PRIMARY CHEMOTHERAPY: CANCERS FOR WHICH THERE IS AN EXPANDING ROLE FOR PRIMARY CHEMOTHERAPY OF ADVANCED DISEASE

Bladder	Head and neck
Breast	Nasopharyngeal
Cervical	Non–small cell lung
Colorectal	Pancreatic
Esophageal	Prostate
Gastric	

TABLE 28.3

NEOADJUVANT CHEMOTHERAPY: CANCERS FOR WHICH NEOADJUVANT CHEMOTHERAPY IS INDICATED FOR LOCALLY ADVANCED DISEASE

Anal cancer	Head and neck cancer
Bladder cancer	Ovarian cancer
Breast cancer	Osteogenic sarcoma
Cervical cancer	Rectal cancer
Gastroesophageal cancer	Soft tissue sarcoma
Non–small cell lung cancer	

Principles of Cancer Cell Kinetics

The key principles of chemotherapy were initially defined by Skipper et al.[6] and Skipper[7] using the murine leukemia L1210 cells as their experimental model system. However, drug treatment of human cancers requires a clear understanding of the differences between the growth characteristics of this rodent leukemia and those of human cancers, as well as an understanding of the differences in growth rates of normal target tissues in mice and in humans. For example, L1210 is a rapidly growing leukemia with a high percentage of cells synthesizing DNA. In fact, this system has a growth fraction of 100% (i.e., all its cells are actively progressing through the cell cycle) and, as such, its life cycle is consistent and predictable.

Based on the experimental findings with the murine L1210 model, the cytotoxic effects of anticancer drugs are predicted to follow logarithmic cell-kill kinetics, and a given agent or treatment regimen is predicted to kill a constant fraction of cells as opposed to a constant number. Thus, if an individual drug leads

TABLE 28.4

ADJUVANT CHEMOTHERAPY: CANCERS FOR WHICH ADJUVANT THERAPY IS INDICATED AFTER SURGERY

Anaplastic astrocytoma
Breast cancer
Colorectal cancer
Gastric cancer
Melanoma
Non–small cell lung cancer
Osteogenic sarcoma
Pancreatic cancer

to a 3 log kill of cancer cells and reduces the tumor burden from 10^{10} to 10^7 cells, the same dose used at a tumor burden of 10^5 cells reduces the tumor mass to 10^2. Cell kill is therefore proportional, regardless of tumor burden. When treatment failed in sensitive cell lines, it was because the initial tumor burden was too high for even potentially curative doses of chemotherapy to eradicate the very last leukemia cell. The cardinal rule of chemotherapy—the invariable inverse relation between cell number and curability—was established with this model system, and this relationship has been applied to other model systems, including both hematologic malignancies and solid tumors.

Although growth of murine leukemias simulates exponential cell kinetics, mathematical modeling data suggest that most human solid tumors do not grow in such a manner. Taken together, the experimental data for human solid cancers support a Gompertzian model of tumor growth and regression. The critical distinction between Gompertzian and exponential growth is that in Gompertzian kinetics, the growth fraction of the tumor is not constant but decreases exponentially with time. The Gompertzian model predicts that the growth fraction peaks when the tumor is approximately 37% of its maximum size. In general, when patients with advanced solid tumors are treated, the tumor mass is larger, its growth fraction is low, and the fraction of cells killed is therefore small. An important feature of Gompertzian growth is that response to chemotherapy in drug-sensitive tumors depends largely on where the tumor is in its particular growth phase.

Predictions can be made about the behavior of small tumors, such as microscopic tumors present after primary surgical therapy. When the tumor is clinically undetectable, its growth fraction is at its highest level, and although the numerical reduction in cell number is small, the fractional cell kill from a known-to-be-effective therapeutic dose of a chemotherapy agent would be significantly higher than later in the tumor course. This observation was initially used to justify dose reductions at lower tumor volumes. However, such an unnecessary dose reduction may account for some of the disappointments in the outcomes of studies of adjuvant chemotherapy in early-stage breast cancer. The Gompertzian model for tumor growth is important because it predicts patterns of regrowth of residual tumor cells. Norton[8] analyzed the clinical data from multiple adjuvant studies for primary breast cancer and from available studies of untreated patients with localized disease. In each clinical study, the Gompertzian model precisely fit the growth curves of these tumors. In the adjuvant setting, the model predicted that relapse-free survival and overall survival curves would be unable to discriminate between a residual cell population of only one cell and a residual population of one million cells, because the regrowth of residual cell populations would be faster for smaller volumes than for larger volumes, and identical results would be produced sometimes at 5 years after diagnosis and treatment. Unless total eradication of micrometastases (cure) was achieved, varying residual volumes would produce similar 5-year relapse-free survival rates and obscure the major differences in tumor reduction by different programs. This mathematical modeling has been especially useful in the design of new adjuvant treatment protocols for early-stage breast cancer, as well as in the design of dose-dense regimens for metastatic breast and colorectal cancer, which have now been shown to produce results superior to conventional doses and schedules.

Principles Governing the Use of Chemotherapy

With rare exceptions (e.g., choriocarcinoma and Burkitt lymphoma), single drugs at clinically tolerable dosages are unable to cure cancer. In the 1960s and early 1970s, drug combination regimens were initially developed based on known biochemical actions of available anticancer drugs rather than on their clinical efficacy. Perhaps not surprisingly, these initial drug regimens were largely ineffective. The era of effective combination chemotherapy was ushered in when a number of active drugs representing different classes became available for use in combination in the treatment of acute leukemias and lymphomas. After this initial success with hematologic malignancies, combination chemotherapy was extended to the treatment of solid tumors.

Combination chemotherapy using conventional cytotoxic agents accomplishes several important objectives not possible with single-agent monotherapy. First, it provides maximal cell kill within the range of toxicity tolerated by the host for each drug as long as dosing is not compromised; that is, each agent used in combination is given at full doses. Second, it provides a broader range of interaction between drugs and tumor cells with different genetic abnormalities in a heterogeneous tumor population. Finally, it may prevent and/or slow the subsequent development of cellular drug resistance.

Certain principles have been useful in guiding the selection of drugs in the most effective drug combinations, and they provide a paradigm for the development of new drug programs. First, only drugs known to be partially effective against the same tumor when used alone should be selected for use in combination. If available, drugs that produce some fraction of complete remission are preferred to those that produce only partial responses. Second, when several drugs of a class are available and are equally effective, a drug should be selected that has toxicity that does not overlap with the toxicity of other drugs to be used in the combination. Although such selection leads to a wider range of side effects, it minimizes the risk of a lethal effect caused by multiple insults to the same organ system by different drugs and allows dose intensity to be maximized. In addition, drugs should be used at their optimal dose and schedule, and drug combinations should be given at consistent intervals. Because long intervals between cycles negatively affect dose intensity, the treatment-free interval between cycles should be the shortest possible time necessary for recovery of the most sensitive normal target tissue, which is usually the bone marrow.

Finally, there should be a clear understanding of the biochemical, molecular, and pharmacokinetic mechanisms of interaction between individual drugs in a given combination, to allow for maximal effect. Omission of a drug from a combination may allow overgrowth by a tumor clone sensitive to that drug alone and resistant to other drugs in the combination. Finally, arbitrary reduction in the dosage of an effective drug to incorporate other less-effective drugs may dramatically reduce the dosage of the most effective agent below the threshold of effectiveness and destroy the capacity of the combination to cure disease in a given patient.

Most standard treatment programs were designed around the kinetics of recovery of the bone marrow in response to chemotherapy exposure. The introduction of the colony-stimulating factors, such as filgrastim and the long-acting molecule pegfilgrastim, has been a significant advance for cancer therapy as these growth factors help to accelerate bone marrow recovery and prevent the onset of severe myelosuppression. Their use has played a pivotal role in facilitating the delivery of dose-intense chemotherapy by reducing the incidence of infections and the need for hospitalizations.

Norton and Day[9] developed a mathematical model to aid in the design and scheduling of combination regimens in cancer chemotherapy. Based on their work, the sequential use of drug combinations was predicted to outperform alternating cycles. This approach was based on the fact that no two combinations were likely to have equal cell-killing capacity or be strictly non–cross-resistant. There is now a growing list of clinical examples in which scheduled sequential therapies have outperformed alternating cyclic use of the same drugs used concurrently, when the dose intensity of the two regimens is carefully controlled.[10,11]

One final issue relating to chemotherapy relates to the optimal duration of drug administration. Several randomized trials of the adjuvant treatment of breast and colorectal cancer have shown that short-course treatment on the order of 6 months is as effective as long-course therapy (12 months).[12,13] One study from the United Kingdom has shown that 3 months adjuvant therapy with 5-fluorouracil (5-FU)-based chemotherapy is equivalent to 6 months of therapy. As a result, a large international effort is currently underway to definitively compare the clinical efficacy of 3 months versus 6 months of adjuvant oxaliplatin-based chemotherapy (FOLFOX or XELOX) in the treatment of stage III colon cancer.

With respect to the advanced disease setting, progressive disease during chemotherapy is a clear indication to stop treatment. However, the optimal duration of chemotherapy for patients without evidence of disease progression has not been well defined. With the development of more potent drug regimens, the potential risk of cumulative adverse events, such as cardiotoxicity secondary to the anthracyclines and neurotoxicity secondary to the taxanes and the platinum analogs, must also be factored into the decision-making process. There is, however, no evidence of clinical benefit in continuing therapy indefinitely until disease progression. Several randomized studies have been performed in advanced colorectal cancer comparing continuous and intermittent chemotherapy, and they showed that a policy of stopping and rechallenging with the same chemotherapy provides a reasonable treatment option for patients.[14–16] In particular, patients with good prognostic features may derive greater benefit from a chemotherapy-free interval than those patients whose tumors have a more aggressive phenotype.

Similar observations have been made in the treatment of metastatic disease, including NSCLC, breast cancer, germ cell cancer, ovarian cancer, and small cell lung cancer. Several requirements must be met, however, for such an intermittent treatment approach to be adopted into clinical practice. First, the induction chemotherapy regimen must be of sufficient clinical efficacy and duration to ensure that the majority of responses are achieved during the treatment period. Second, a good response must be shown to reinitiation of the same chemotherapy and/or to administration of an effective salvage chemotherapy regimen. Third, there should be a sufficient time interval between the termination of primary induction chemotherapy and the onset of progressive disease. Finally, patients whose active chemotherapy regimen is stopped must continue to be closely followed to ensure that treatment can be reinstituted at the first sign of disease progression and the onset of tumor-related symptoms.

Dose Intensity and Combination Chemotherapy

One of the main factors limiting the ability of chemotherapy and radiation therapy to achieve cure is effective dosing. The dose-response curve in biologic systems is usually sigmoidal, with a threshold, a lag phase, a linear phase, and a plateau phase. For chemotherapy and radiation therapy, therapeutic selectivity is significantly dependent on the differential between the dose-response curves of normal tissues and tumor tissues. In experimental *in vivo* models, the dose-response curve is usually steep in the linear phase, and a reduction in dose when the tumor is in the linear phase of the dose-response curve almost always results in a loss in the capacity to cure the tumor effectively, even before a reduction in the antitumor activity is observed. Thus, although complete remissions continue to be observed with dose reductions in the range of 20%, residual tumor cells may not be entirely eliminated, which thereby allows for eventual relapse to occur. In experimental systems, a dose reduction of 20% results in a reduction of cure rate by 50% without a change in the complete response rate. Because anticancer drugs are associated with toxicity, it is often appealing for clinicians to avoid acute toxicity by simply reducing the dose or by increasing the time interval between each cycle of treatment. Such empiric modifications in dose may represent a major reason for treatment failure in patients with drug-sensitive tumors who are receiving chemotherapy in either the adjuvant or advanced disease setting.

As noted earlier, a major issue facing clinicians is the ability to deliver effective doses of chemotherapy in a dose-intense manner. The concept of dose intensity was first put forth by Hryniuk[17] and Hryniuk and Goodyear,[18] who defined *dose intensity* as the amount of drug delivered per unit of time. Specifically, this was expressed as milligrams per square meter per week, regardless of the schedule or route of administration. The dose intensity of each drug regimen is then determined based on the time period in which the treatment program is administered. Specific calculations can be made of the intended dose intensity, which is the dose intensity originally proposed in the treatment regimen, or of the received dose intensity. However, it is the received dose intensity, rather than the intended dose intensity, that is the more clinically relevant issue, as it reflects the direct impact of dose reductions and treatment delays imposed in actual clinical practice. A positive relationship between dose intensity and response rate has been nicely documented in several solid tumors, including advanced ovarian, breast, lung, and colon cancers, as well as in hematologic malignancies, including the lymphomas.

The term *summation dose intensity* has also been developed to reflect the close relationship between dose and combination chemotherapy.[19] As part of this concept, the final outcome of a combination treatment must be related in some manner to the sum of the dose intensities of all the agents used in that treatment. For nearly all treatable malignancies, a combination regimen incorporating at least three active drugs is necessary for cure. In the case of childhood leukemia, the cure rate increases linearly when the number of active drugs increases from three to seven. The critical issue for this concept is that all active agents must be used at their full therapeutic doses. Although the concept of summation dose intensity is not new, it offers a unified approach for the careful design and interpretation of clinical trials.

Calculations of the impact of dose intensity on outcome are particularly important in estimating the efficacy of adjuvant chemotherapy. The steep dose-response curve for most anticancer drugs indicates that dose reductions in adjuvant chemotherapy programs are likely to be associated with significantly less therapeutic effect. Historically, dose reduction was incorporated in the design of adjuvant chemotherapy trials. One example is the standard CMF (cyclophosphamide, methotrexate, and 5-FU) regimen for breast cancer. The initial reports for this regimen revealed an impressive complete remission rate of approximately 30% in the advanced disease setting, albeit at the expense of considerable toxicity. When this regimen was advanced for use in Italy at the Istituto Nazionale Tumori by Bonadonna and Zambetti[11] and in the cooperative group setting, doses of the respective agents were arbitrarily reduced without first testing the potential impact of such reductions on clinical outcome. In addition, further reduction was empirically made for patients older than 60 years, on the assumption that such a dose reduction would be required for age. Careful analysis of the data suggests that such dose reductions have had a negative impact on clinical outcome. In premenopausal women, the differences in relapse-free survival at low and high doses of

CMF are statistically significant. The importance of dose effect was further confirmed by a large study in which a survival benefit was observed as a result of increasing dose intensity in the adjuvant chemotherapy for women with stage II node-positive breast cancer.[20]

At present, there are three main approaches to delivery of chemotherapy in a dose-intense fashion. The first approach is through dose escalation in which doses of a given anticancer agent are increased. The second strategy is to administer anticancer agents in a dose-dense manner by reducing the interval between treatment cycles.[20] The third approach involves sequential scheduling of either single agents, which is, in effect, combination chemotherapy in sequence.

The growth of most solid tumors follows a pattern of Gompertzian kinetics. In this setting, the growth of cells is significantly faster in the early part of the growth curve than at any other stage in the growth kinetics. The log cell kill generated by chemotherapy would, therefore, be higher in tumors of small volume than in those of large volume. In such cases, the regrowth of cancer cells between chemotherapy cycles is more rapid. Thus, the more frequent administration of cytotoxic chemotherapy represents an attractive strategy to minimize residual tumor burden and prevent regrowth. In computer simulations, this relatively simple maneuver has indeed achieved significantly higher benefit by minimizing the regrowth of cancer cells between cycles of treatment. The clinical relevance of dose density was supported by a landmark randomized phase 3 trial comparing dose-dense versus conventionally scheduled chemotherapy in the adjuvant treatment of node-positive primary breast cancer (INT C9741). In this study, a dose-dense schedule in which the anticancer agents doxorubicin, cyclophosphamide, and paclitaxel were administered every 2 weeks rather than at the conventional 3-week intervals resulted in significantly improved clinical outcomes with respect to disease-free survival and overall survival.[21] Of note, with the concomitant use of the colony-stimulating factor filgrastim (granulocyte colony-stimulating factor), dose-dense therapy was not accompanied by an increase in toxicity.

Although a dose-dense approach may have its greatest application in the adjuvant setting, there is now growing evidence for the potential efficacy of this strategy in the treatment of metastatic disease. Dose-dense regimens have shown superior clinical activity compared with standard chemotherapy in metastatic colorectal cancer, extensive-stage small cell lung cancer, and poor-prognosis germ cell cancer. A phase 1 study of biweekly capecitabine for patients with metastatic breast cancer, based on the Norton-Simon mathematical model, showed that such a dose-dense approach is well tolerated and allows for safe delivery of higher daily doses of capecitabine than those routinely used in clinical practice even in heavily pretreated patients.[22]

One of the potential limitations of modern combination chemotherapy is that dose levels of individual drugs are generally reduced in an effort to limit toxicity when the drugs are used in combination. To address this issue, investigators have administered drug combinations in an alternating sequence to deliver a greater number of different drugs per unit of time. This strategy may not allow for enhanced dose intensity, however; in fact, it may actually compromise clinical benefit. A randomized clinical trial conducted by Bonadonna and Zambetti[11] observed that four 3-week cycles of doxorubicin followed by eight 3-week cycles of CMF in women with high-risk primary breast cancer (four or more positive lymph nodes) resulted in improved clinical efficacy in terms of disease-free and overall survival than an alternating schedule of doxorubicin and CMF at the same dose intensity. Sledge et al.[23] addressed the issue of sequential versus combination therapy in the Eastern Cooperative Oncology Group E1193 randomized phase 3 trial of combination chemotherapy in sequence, with doxorubicin and paclitaxel versus a combination of the two agents as the first-line treatment for metastatic breast cancer. Combination therapy yielded a superior response rate and time to disease progression but has not yet translated into a survival benefit when compared with sequential single-agent therapy. Such sequential strategies are being tested for treatment of other solid tumors, including colorectal cancer and ovarian cancer.

BIOLOGY OF DRUG RESISTANCE

The main obstacle to the clinical efficacy of chemotherapy is the development of cellular drug resistance. In 1979, Goldie and Coldman[24] proposed that the development of resistance to anticancer drugs by cancer cells could arise without prior exposure to these drugs. They suggested that the nonrandom cytogenetic changes associated with the development of most human cancers were tightly associated with the development of the capacity to resist the action of certain types of anticancer drugs. They developed a mathematical model that highlighted the tight linkage between the rate at which tumor cells mutate to drug resistance and the inherent genetic instability of a particular tumor. Their model predicted that such events would begin to occur at population sizes between 10^3 and 10^6 tumor cells (1,000 to 1 million cells), much lower than the mass of cells considered to be clinically detectable (10^9, or 1 billion cells). The probability that a given tumor contains resistant clones at the time of initial diagnosis was a function of both tumor size and the inherent mutation rate. If the mutation rate was as low as 10^{-6}, a tumor composed of 10^9 cells (a 1-cm mass) would be predicted to have at least one drug-resistant clone; however, the absolute number of resistant cells in a tumor composed of 10^9 cells would be relatively small. Therefore, in the clinical setting, such tumors should initially respond to treatment with a partial or complete remission but would recur as the resistant tumor clone(s) expands to repopulate the tumor mass. Such a pattern is commonly seen in the clinical setting with the use of chemotherapy, even in drug-responsive tumors.

In addition, there is what is best described as *physiologic resistance*, a term that applies to most normal cells. A prime example of this type of resistance is human breast tissue. Neoadjuvant chemotherapy programs in breast cancer patients are focused on cytoreduction of the invasive tumor, but biopsies of the breast always shows normal breast tissue to be intact. In this context, the normal tissue was relatively more resistant than the cancer, implying that the sensitivity to chemotherapy of the invasive cancer was an acquired characteristic. If so, this finding may provide an explanation as to why cancers in their earlier stages are not always as responsive to chemotherapy as would be predicted based on cell kinetic data alone.

In other cancers, such as the lymphomas, where the cell of origin has easy access to apoptotic mechanisms during development, the tumor cells are much more sensitive to cytotoxic insults at the outset but, as with follicular lymphomas, rarely is it possible to eradicate them completely, presumably because of the presence of intact mechanisms for repairing DNA damage (see later discussion). When these lymphomas transform to the more aggressive diffuse large B-cell lymphomas, they can then be cured by chemotherapy, again suggesting that the exquisite sensitivity to chemotherapy is an acquired characteristic. Finally, tumors that were once sensitive to chemotherapy but grow resistant with repeated exposure to drugs develop an acquired form of drug resistance, a commonly observed phenomenon in the clinic.

One of the most challenging areas of research is in identifying relevant molecular profiles associated with chemosensitivity in drug-curable advanced cancers. For more than 40 years, the classic view of anticancer drug action has involved the specific interaction between a given drug and its respective target. Cell death arises as a direct consequence of this drug-receptor interaction. However, the critical signaling events involved, from facilitation of the initial coupling of the stimulus to the final response of the cell, were never clearly elucidated. Given our enhanced understanding of the molecular mechanisms underlying the control of the cell cycle and the process of programmed cell death (apoptosis), it is clear that this model is overly simplistic and insufficient to explain the cytotoxic effects of anticancer agents and more modern views of cellular drug resistance. It is now well established that the drug-receptor interaction acts as the initial stimulus that then sets off a cascade of downstream cellular signaling events that eventually results in apoptosis. This process is exceedingly complex and typically involves a sensor that detects a death-inducing signal, a signal transduction network, and execution machinery that facilitates the process of cell death. Moreover, this process is highly dependent on the cell of origin of a specific tumor type, and its access to these mechanisms during normal development, the specific anticancer agent and/or regimen being tested, and the particular cellular context and environment in which the drug-target interaction takes place.

The ability of certain cancers to resist the cytotoxic effects of cancer chemotherapy appears to be more closely connected with the underlying genetic instability of tumor cells and/or to alterations in key pathways involved in cell-cycle checkpoint control and apoptosis than to the specific biochemical mechanisms of resistance that have been characterized for each agent. This observation is underscored by the general failure to overcome resistance to chemotherapy in the clinic with approaches that attack only the classic biochemical or molecular mechanisms of resistance (or both).

As previously noted, one of the remarkable features of both radiation therapy and chemotherapy is that their cytotoxic effects initially appears to be greater in tumor cells than in normal host tissues, such as the bone marrow and the gastrointestinal (GI) tract. Doses that eradicate chemosensitive tumors will not ablate the bone marrow or destroy the capacity of the GI mucosa to regenerate. Molecular genetic studies have revealed that, in contrast to malignant cells, normal cells, such as those derived from the bone marrow and gut, express an intact genetic machinery. As a result, the normal mechanisms for apoptosis and cell-cycle arrest after exposure to genotoxic and cytotoxic stresses remain present. Thus, normal bone marrow and GI precursor cells are able to effectively monitor and repair DNA damage after exposure to a genotoxic stress, as well as destroy cells with irreparable DNA, rather than allowing damaged cells to progress through the normal cell cycle and potentially replicate their damaged DNA. Because normal cells express an intact genetic machinery, they are able to recover from exposure to DNA-damaging anticancer agents. The exception to this is high-dose chemotherapy as observed with stem cell transplantation. In the transplant setting, high doses of chemotherapy are able to overwhelm these protective mechanisms, thereby resulting in direct cellular necrosis.

p53 As a Mediator of Chemosensitivity

The p53 protein is a tumor suppressor protein and critical transcriptional activator that plays a key role in mediating G_1 and G_2 arrest of the cell cycle after exposure to DNA-damaging agents and other genotoxic stress.[25,26] This function is thought to be essential in preserving the integrity of the cellular genome in response to treatment with a cytotoxic agent. In addition to playing a role in preserving the cell-cycle checkpoint, p53 is a potent inducer of programmed cell death (apoptosis) in response to DNA damage. The basis for the cell's decision to undergo growth arrest with subsequent repair of DNA damage or to induce apoptosis remains unclear. Significant research efforts have focused on elucidating the critical factors that determine the eventual cellular function of p53. This is a complex issue that involves the extent of DNA damage, the stage of the cell cycle at which the DNA damage occurs, the presence of other genetic abnormalities in either the cell-cycle regulatory apparatus or the signaling machinery, the specific cellular environment within the cell, and exogenous factors within the cellular matrix.

Mutations in the *p53* gene are among the most common genetic alterations observed in human tumor samples, occurring in at least 50% of all human tumors. In addition to point mutations in the *p53* gene, there are other mechanisms by which the function of p53 can be inactivated. Posttranslational inactivation of p53 through binding to other cellular protein partners (e.g., murine double-minute 2 [MDM2]) or enhancement of degradation (e.g., the E6 protein of the human papillomavirus), as well as translational repression by binding of the folate-dependent enzyme thymidylate synthase to wild type p53 messenger RNA result in an impaired ability of the cell to undergo cell-cycle arrest or apoptosis in response to DNA damage. The initial studies documenting a tight association between loss of *p53* function and resistance to chemotherapy and radiotherapy came from *in vivo* model systems using *p53* knockout mice. Subsequent studies confirmed that various malignant cell lines and tumors expressing mutant or deleted *p53* were chemoresistant to a wide range of anticancer agents. However, loss of p53 function is not always associated with chemoresistance. Some studies suggest that cells with impaired p53 function may become sensitized to various anticancer agents. Thus, the relationship between p53 status and chemosensitivity is complex and is presumably dependent on a number of factors, including the specific cytotoxic insult, tissue-specific differences, and the specific cellular context that incorporates the overall genetic machinery and the various intracellular signaling pathways.

Role of Bcl-2 Family Members in Mediating Chemosensitivity

Because apoptosis is a genetically programmed event, inactivation of genes that induce the apoptotic program or activation of antiapoptotic genes can result in the development of cellular drug resistance. Bcl-2 is a potent suppressor of apoptotic cell death, and a number of studies have shown that its expression leads to repression of cell death triggered by either γ-irradiation or a variety of anticancer agents.[27] In addition, the Bcl-2 protein is overexpressed in several human cancers, including non–Hodgkin's lymphoma, prostate cancer, melanoma, breast cancer, and NSCLC. In further support of the pivotal role of Bcl-2 as an inhibitor of cell death are preclinical *in vitro* and *in vivo* studies demonstrating that treatment of certain human leukemia or non–Hodgkin's lymphoma cell lines with an antisense strategy directed against Bcl-2 and/or with small molecule inhibitors leads to the reversal of chemoresistance.

The phosphorylation status of Bcl-2 plays an important role in determining chemosensitivity. There is growing evidence that the phosphorylated form of Bcl-2 interacts less efficiently with its heterodimer protein partner bax, which results in cell death. Bcl-x_L, a functional and structural homologue of Bcl-2, is also able to confer protection against radiation-induced apoptosis as well as against a wide number of anticancer agents, including bleomycin, cisplatin, etoposide, and vincristine. Recently, the antiapoptotic effects of Bcl-2 and Bcl-x_L were compared using FL5.12 lymphoid cells. These two proteins have a differential ability to protect against chemotherapy-induced cell death. This differential effect depends more on the molecular mechanism targeted than on the cell-cycle specificity of an individual drug. In contrast to Bcl-2 and Bcl-x_L, other family members, including Bax, Bcl-x_s, and Bak, have been shown to promote apoptosis in response to either radiation or various anticancer drugs (or both).

The underlying mechanisms through which these Bcl-2 family members control apoptosis are complex, and this field remains an active area of investigation. Given the pivotal role of Bcl-2 as a mediator of apoptosis and its increased expression in a number of human solid tumors and hematologic malignancies, significant efforts have focused on Bcl-2 as a potential target for drug development.[28] Specifically, antisense phosphorothioate oligonucleotides targeting the first 18 nucleotides of the human Bcl-2 protein-coding region as well as small molecules that target the BH3-domain-binding site of Bcl-2 have been tested in the preclinical and clinical settings either alone or in combination with chemotherapy. These molecules have now been studied in a broad range of tumor types, and in particular, in non–Hodgkin's lymphoma and chronic lymphocytic leukemia where inhibition of Bcl-2 expression and function appears to be a potentially effective anticancer strategy.

Death Executioner Pathway

The molecular mechanisms and intracellular signal transduction pathways initiated by a given cytotoxic or genotoxic stress may differ significantly. However, the final stage of these various death pathways is mediated through the activation of caspases,[29] which represent a highly conserved family of cysteine proteases. The specific caspases involved in apoptosis include 3, 6, 7, 8, and 9, and they exert their effects through cleavage of protein kinases and other signal transduction proteins, cytoskeletal proteins, chromatin-modifying protein, and DNA repair proteins.

The activation of caspases is determined by the intrinsic and extrinsic pathways of apoptosis. The intrinsic pathway is a mitochondrial-dependent pathway mediated by the Bcl-2 family of proteins. Exposure to cytotoxic stress results in disruption of the mitochondrial membrane, which then leads to release of cytochrome *c* and other protease activators. Cytochrome *c* binds with Apaf-1, which allows for interaction with procaspase 9 and other proteases. Caspase 9 is subsequently activated, setting off a cascade of events that commits the cell to undergo apoptosis. The extrinsic pathway is mediated by ligand binding to the tumor necrosis factor (TNF) family of receptors, which includes TNF receptor-1, Fas, DR3, DR4 (TNF-related apoptosis-inducing ligand [TRAIL] R1), DR5 (TRAILR2), or DR6, coupled with an intracytoplasmic death domain protein and certain essential adaptor proteins. These adaptor proteins recruit various proteases and then cleave the N-terminal domain of caspase 8, which leads to activation of the caspase cascade. There are important links between the intrinsic and extrinsic pathways, and caspase 3 plays the key role in this regard. Studies of several knockout mouse models expressing germ line disruptions of Apaf-1, caspase 3, or caspase 9 have shown that these genetically engineered mice are resistant to chemotherapy and δ-irradiation.

NFκB Signaling

The presence of several external stimuli, including various cytokines, TNF-α-, chemotherapy, and radiation, leads to activation of the transcription factor nuclear factor κB (NFκB).[30] Paradoxically, activation of NFκB results in potent suppression of the apoptotic potential of these stimuli. Several studies have demonstrated that inhibition of NFκB *in vitro* leads to enhanced apoptosis in response to different stimuli. These findings suggest that activation of NFκB expression in response to chemotherapy may represent an important mechanism of inducible tumor chemoresistance. They also suggest that strategies to inhibit NFκB may represent a rational approach to enhance and/or restore chemosensitivity to antitumor therapy through increased apoptosis.

Bortezomib is a modified dipeptidyl boronic acid that functions as a reversible inhibitor of the chymotrypsin-like activity of the 26S proteasome in mammalian cells.[31] The 26S proteasome is a large adenosine triphosphate (ATP)-dependent multicatalytic protein complex that degrades ubiquitinated proteins. The ubiquitin-proteasome degrades several short-lived intracellular regulatory proteins that govern certain critical signaling pathways involved in cell cycle, transcription factor activation, apoptosis, angiogenesis, cell trafficking, invasion, and metastasis. Specifically, this system mediates proteolysis of IκB, the endogenous inhibitor of NFκB. Degradation of IκB by the proteasome leads to activation of NFκB, which then results in stimulation of cell growth, inhibition of apoptosis, and induction of cellular drug resistance. Inhibition of the proteasome multienzyme complex by bortezomib results in inhibition of targeted proteolysis of multiple critical cellular proteins, with the end effect being cell-cycle arrest, induction of apoptosis, and restoration of chemosensitivity.

In preclinical models of multiple myeloma, bortezomib was shown to induce apoptosis, reduce adherence of myeloma cells to bone marrow stromal cells, and block production and intracellular signaling of interleukin-6. This work was subsequently extended into the clinical setting, where this agent has shown promising clinical activity initially in patients with refractory multiple myeloma but also in the front-line treatment of multiple myeloma.

Resistance to Targeted Therapy

Over the past 10 years, significant advances have been made in the development of novel targeted therapies for the treatment of human cancers. In large part, these advances came about as a result of an enhanced understanding of the genetic alterations and key signaling pathways in human cancer. As with traditional cytotoxic chemotherapy, one of the major challenges to targeted cancer therapy is the development of intrinsic and/or acquired resistance mechanisms.[32] An enhanced understanding of the molecular pathways that mediate drug resistance may identify the subset of patients who may not be appropriate candidates for targeted therapy. Moreover, these studies may lead to the development of certain predictive biomarkers that could then allow for improved patient selection. Finally, this work may have relevance with respect to drug development as it may provide the rational basis for developing novel strategies that can prevent and/or circumvent cellular drug resistance that can be directly translated into patient care.

Resistance to HER2 and EGFR-Targeted Therapy

Trastuzumab is an IgG1 monoclonal antibody targeted against the human epidermal growth factor receptor (HER)2 tyrosine kinase, which is overexpressed in up to 25% to 35% of invasive breast cancers. Although a significant number of patients exhibit an initial response to trastuzumab-based regimens, disease progression is usually observed within 1 year of treatment initiation. Several potential mechanisms of resistance have now been identified,[33,34] albeit mainly in preclinical models, and they include: (1) prevention of trastuzumab binding to HER2 through epitope masking by the membrane-associated glycoprotein MUC4; (2) up-regulation of alternative signaling pathways downstream of HER2, such as loss of function of PTEN or mutations in PI3K and/or Akt that lead to constitutive PI3K/Akt activation; (3) up-regulation of alternative growth factor receptor signaling pathways and, specifically, overexpression of the insulinlike growth factor-1 receptor (IGF-1R) and/or the c-Met receptor; and (4) inhibition of immunologic-mediated mechanisms. In addition, a fifth mechanism has been identified that results from the presence of a constitutively active, truncated form of the HER2 receptor, p95HER2.[34] This protein has kinase activity but in contrast to the intact HER2 receptor, it lacks the extracellular domain and binding site of trastuzumab. In one study, this truncated p95HER2 was present in 60% of breast tumors that were strongly positive for the intact HER2, and a recent retrospective clinical study identified a strong association between the presence of p95HER2 and clinical resistance to trastuzumab therapy.

Epidermal growth factor receptor (EGFR) is an important target for several different solid tumor types, including colorectal cancer (CRC), NSCLC, and head and neck cancer. Two main strategies have been taken to inhibit this pathway. One approach was to develop small molecule inhibitors that target the tyrosine kinase domain, while the second strategy was to develop monoclonal antibodies that targeted the external cell surface domain of the receptor. In the case of small molecule TKIs, gefitinib and erlotinib were approved by the U.S. Food and Drug Administration in 2003 and 2004, respectively, for the treatment of relapsed NSCLC. Somatic mutations in EGFR have been identified in up to 40% of patients with NSCLC, and in patients with sensitizing mutations, treatment with the EGFR TKIs is associated with initial response rates in the 60% to 80% range. The efficacy of these agents, however, is limited by the development of either primary or acquired resistance.[35]

A well-described primary resistance mechanism is the presence of an insertion mutation in exon 20 of *EGFR*. Although such insertion mutations in exon 20 occur in less than 5% of all documented *EGFR* gene mutations, studies have shown that tumor cells with these mutations have activated EGFR signaling. As such, the TKIs are ineffective at inhibiting EGFR signaling. Interestingly, exon 20 insertion mutations in *HER2* are also associated with the presence of intrinsic TKI resistance. In addition to mutations in *EGFR* and *HER2,* mutations in *KRAS* confer resistance to TKIs. *KRAS* mutations have been observed in 20% to 30% of patients with NSCLC and are seen more frequently in smokers (30%–45%) as opposed to nonsmokers (5%–7%). The presence of *BRAF* mutations, loss of expression of the tumor suppressor *PTEN*, and activation of alternative signaling pathways, such as IGF-1R, have also been identified as potential primary resistance mechanisms, although their exact clinical relevance remains to be defined.

In the setting of sensitizing somatic *EGFR* mutations, the initial response to TKI therapy is quite high. Unfortunately, disease progression invariably develops, in large part due to acquired resistance. Perhaps the best characterized resistance mechanism identified to date is the T790M mutation in exon 20 of the EGFR kinase domain. This mutation is found in up to 50% of patients who develop resistance to TKIs. Three other EGFR mutations have been identified involving amino acid substitutions at D761Y, L747S, and T854A, but each of these mutations occur at a much lower frequency than the T790M mutation. A second important mechanism of acquired resistance involves activation of parallel signaling pathways in which the critical downstream mediators of EGFR are activated independently of EGFR. The best examples identified to date are activation of MET signaling through *MET* amplification, which has been identified in up to 20% of patients who develop resistance to TKIs, and activation of IGF-1R signaling. Activation of either of these key pathways can then lead to activation of PI3K, thereby resulting in enhanced survival. Finally, there may be other mechanisms that lead to activation of the PI3K/Akt axis, including loss of *PTEN* expression as well as mutations in either *PI3K* or *Akt*.

Cetuximab and panitumumab are monoclonal antibodies that are currently active as monotherapy or in combination with cytotoxic chemotherapy in the treatment of metastatic CRC. However, only at most 20% to 30% of patients will derive clinical benefit when treated with antibody therapy. In contrast to NSCLC, somatic mutations in the *EGFR* are extremely rare in CRC, and when present, they do not appear to impact on clinical activity. Over the past 2 to 3 years, a significant body of evidence has demonstrated that *KRAS* mutations confer resistance to anti-EGFR antibody therapy.[36] *KRAS* mutations occur in approximately 30% to 40% of patients with CRC, regardless of tumor stage, and they typically reside in codons 12, 13, and 61. These mutations lead to constitutive activation of RAS-RAK-MAPK signaling, which then circumvents the effects of antibody therapy. In Europe and the United States, the use of anti-EGFR antibody therapy is presently restricted to mCRC patients whose tumors express wild type *KRAS*. However, it should be noted that there is recent evidence suggesting that there may be differences in response to antibody therapy depending on the location of the specific *KRAS* mutation.[37] Even though this situation occurs in probably less than 1% of the mutant *KRAS* population, this finding may explain why a small number of patients treated with cetuximab and panitumumab may still derive some level of clinical benefit.

KRAS is a highly specific negative predictive biomarker with a specificity of over 90%. However, it a relatively poor sensitive biomarker, with a sensitivity of only 45%. Thus, even in the presence of wild type *KRAS*, the large majority of patients will continue to be resistant to anti-EGFR antibody therapy. BRAF is a serine/threonine protein kinase that plays a key role as a member of the RAS-RAF-MAPK pathway downstream of EGFR. Mutations in *BRAF* have been identified in codon 600 (V600E), and they have been found in up to 10% of patients with CRC. Of note, mutations in *BRAF* occur exclusive of *KRAS* mutations, and previous studies have shown that these mutations are associated with a worse overall prognosis. Based on retrospective analyses, patients who experienced a clinical response to cetuximab or panitumumab therapy did not have *BRAF* mutations. Perhaps of greater significance was the fact that the presence of a *BRAF* mutation was a negative predictor for response to antibody treatment.[37]

Oncogenic activation of the *PI3K/Akt* signaling pathway is another acquired resistance mechanism. This pathway can be dysregulated through activating mutations in *PI3K*, mutations in *Akt*, or by inactivation of PTEN. *PI3K* mutations have been implicated in drug resistance, but the data are not as clean as they are for *KRAS* or *BRAF* mutations. Recent work suggests that the particular location of the mutation, whether in the exon 9 or exon 20 hotspots, may play a crucial role in determining whether resistance to antibody therapy develops. Finally, activation of parallel signaling pathways, such as IGF-1R, may provide an alternative route for tumor cells to circumvent and/or overcome the effects of cetuximab and panitumumab.

Resistance to Antiangiogenic Therapy

Bevacizumab, sunitinib, and sorafenib are antiangiogenic agents that target the vascular endothelial growth factor (VEGF) signaling pathway. These agents have been approved for the treatment of a number of solid tumors, including CRC, NSCLC, breast cancer, renal cell cancer, hepatocellular cancer, gastrointestinal stromal tumors (GIST), and glioblastoma multiforme. The long-held view was that resistance to antiangiogenic agents could not develop in the clinical setting as these agents were targeting genetically stable endothelial cells and not tumor cells. However, both preclinical and clinical studies have now shown that this original concept was incorrect and that resistance can indeed develop to this class of agents.

There appear to be at least five distinct mechanisms by which resistance to antiangiogenic therapies can develop.[38,39] The specific resistance mechanism most likely depends on the particular tumor type as well as the specific antiangiogenic therapy. The first resistance mechanism involves activation and/or up-regulation of alternative proangiogenic signaling pathways within the tumor. The proangiogenic factors that have been typically up-regulated include members of the fibroblast growth factor, ephrin A1 and ephrin A2, angiopoietin 1, and the chemokine interleukin-8 (IL-8). A second mechanism involves tumor hypoxia-driven up-regulation of hypoxia-induced factor-1-α, which then leads to increased circulating levels of VEGF and platelet-derived growth factor (PDGF). The increased levels of these ligands might then be sufficient to circumvent and/or overcome the inhibitory effects on VEGF signaling exerted by either antibodies targeting VEGF or small molecules targeting VEGFR-TKs. Recruitment of bone marrow-derived myeloid cells into tumor tissue with production of proangiogenic cytokines, including IL-6 and IL-8, has also been shown to induce tumor angiogenesis. In addition, tumor-associated macrophages and monocytes may express certain key cytokines and growth factors that are able to circumvent anti-VEGF therapy. A fourth mechanism involves increased pericyte coverage of the tumor vasculature, which serves to mediate endothelial cell survival, thereby protecting a core of pre-existing blood vessels. In the presence of anti-VEGF therapy, blood vessels that are heavily covered by pericytes would be much better able to survive inhibitor therapy and would allow the tumor to continue to grow, albeit at a potentially slower rate.

Finally, several studies have recently shown that activation of mechanisms involved in invasion and metastasis can occur in the setting of antiangiogenic therapy. With this scenario, tumor cells migrate along the outside of normal blood vessels and use them as conduits to migrate into normal tissue and/or infiltrate through the extracellular matrix.

Resistance to Bcr-Abl Targeted Therapy

Chronic myeloid leukemia (CML) arises from the translocation of *c-ABL* from chromosome 9 and *BCR* on chromosome 22, which then leads to the formation of the BCR-ABL1 fusion oncoprotein with constitutive tyrosine kinase (TK) activity. Imatinib is a phenylaminopyrimidine compound, and it was the first small molecule TK inhibitor (TKI) approved for the treatment of CML. This molecule binds almost exclusively to the BCR-ABL1 tyrosine kinase, but has inhibitory effects against only a limited number of other tyrosine kinases, including KIT, ARG, and PDGFR. Despite the dramatic success with imatinib in the treatment of CML, resistance mechanisms have been identified.[40] Mutations in the kinase domain of BCR-ABL1 represent the main mechanism by which acquired resistance can develop. Specifically, various mutations have been observed in the context of clinical resistance to imatinib, and they reside within four distinct locations: (1) imatinib binding site, (2) P-loop ATP binding site, (3) catalytic domain, and (4) activation loop. Mutations within the ATP binding domain account for nearly 50% of the mutations identified with imatinib resistance. The T315I mutation has been termed the *gatekeeper* mutation, and it is located in the imatinib binding site and occurs in 5% to 20% of resistant cases. This mutation is of particular importance as it confers resistance to imatinib as well as to the next generation of TKI inhibitors, including dasatinib and nilotinib. Although mutations have been observed in at least 25 amino acids throughout the kinase domain, substitutions at only 7 residues account for up to 85% of the resistance-associated mutations.

In addition to mutations in the BCR-ABL kinase domain, other resistance mechanisms have been identified.[40] Amplification of the *BCR-ABL* fusion gene results in overexpression of BCR-ABL1 TK, which leads to drug resistance. In contrast to mutations in the TK domain, however, this resistance mechanism is a relatively uncommon event as one clinical study of 66 imatinib-resistant patients showed that *BCR-ABL* gene amplification was present in only two patients. An association between activation of BCR-ABL1–independent signaling pathways and imatinib resistance has been identified in both the preclinical and clinical settings. Specifically, up-regulation of two members of the SRC-family of tyrosine kinases, HCK and LYN, results in imatinib resistance. Finally, overexpression of the multidrug efflux transporters of the ATP-binding cassette (ABC) transporter family, which include the multidrug-resistant gene product P-glycoprotein (P-gp and ABCB1) and the breast cancer-resistant protein (ABCG2), has been identified in imatinib-resistant CML patients in blast phase.

Because imatinib also inhibits the KIT tyrosine kinase, this agent is active in the treatment of unresectable and/or metastatic GIST as well as in the adjuvant therapy of GIST following resection of localized disease. In about 10% of patients, primary resistance to imatinib has been observed, usually in the setting of wild type *KIT* and *PDGFRA*, mutations in exon 9 of *KIT*, or in the setting of a D842V substitution of *PDGFRA*.[41] In addition, gene amplification of *KIT* and *PDGFRA* has been observed in the setting of primary resistance. In the absence of gene amplification or mutations in either *PDGFRA* or *KIT*, activation of the BRAF signaling pathway resulting from activation mutations in the *BRAF* gene has been observed in resistant patients.

As observed with imatinib resistance in CML, the development of acquired resistance in GIST is most often associated with the presence of secondary mutations in *KIT* or *PDGFRA*.[41] These mutations reside within the ATP binding site of the kinase domain located in exons 13 and 14 or the kinase activation loop in exons 17 and 18. Of note, there is a "gatekeeper" mutation involving threonine residue 670 (T670I) homologous to the threonine 315 residue (T315I) in the BCR-ABL TK that directly inhibits imatinib binding, thereby leading to imatinib resistance. Other resistance mechanisms have recently been identified, including gene amplification of *KIT* and *PDGFRA* and activation of alternate signaling pathways, such as IGF-1R, focal adhesion kinase, and Axl.

References

1. Marshall EK Jr. Historical perspectives in chemotherapy. *Adv Chemother* 1964;1:1.
2. DeVita VT. The evolution of therapeutic research in cancer. *N Engl J Med* 1978;298:907.
3. Muggia FM. Primary chemotherapy: concepts and issues. In: *Primary Chemotherapy in Cancer Medicine*. New York: Alan R. Liss; 1985:377.
4. Frei A 3rd, Clark JR, Miller D. The concept of neoadjuvant chemotherapy. In: Salmon SE, ed. *Adjuvant Therapy of Cancer*, 5th ed. Orlando, FL: Grune and Stratton; 1987:67.
5. Goldie JH. Scientific basis for adjuvant and primary (neoadjuvant) chemotherapy. *Semin Oncol* 1987;14:1.
6. Skipper HE, Schabel FM Jr, Mellet LB, et al. Implications of biochemical, cytokinetic, pharmacologic and toxicologic relationships in the design of optimal therapeutic schedules. *Cancer Chemother Rep* 1950;54:431.
7. Skipper HE. Kinetics of mammary tumor cell growth and implications for therapy. *Cancer* 1971;28:1479.
8. Norton LA. A Gompertzian model of human breast cancer growth. *Cancer Res* 1988;48:7067.

9. Norton L, Day RS. Potential innovations in scheduling in cancer chemotherapy. In: DeVita VT Jr, Hellman S, Rosenberg SA, eds. *Important Advances in Oncology 1991*. Philadelphia: Lippincott-Raven Publishers; 1991:57.
10. Buzzoni R, Bonadonna G, Valagussa P, et al. Adjuvant chemotherapy with doxorubicin plus cyclophosphamide, methotrexate, and fluorouracil in the treatment of resectable breast cancer with more than three positive axillary nodes. *J Clin Oncol* 1991;9:2134.
11. Bonadonna G, Zambetti M. Sequential or alternating doxorubicin and CMF regimens in breast cancer with more than three positive nodes. *JAMA* 1995;273:542.
12. McArthur HL, Hudis CA. Adjuvant chemotherapy for early-stage breast cancer. *Hematol Oncol Clin North Am* 2007;21:207.
13. Wolpin BM, Mayer RJ. Systemic treatment of colorectal cancer. *Gastroenterology* 2008;134:1296.
14. Maughan TS, James RD, Kerr DJ, et al. Comparison of intermittent and continuous palliative chemotherapy for advanced colorectal cancer: a multicenter randomized trial. *Lancet* 2003;361:457.
15. Tournigand C, Cervantes A, Figer A, et al. OPTIMOX1: a randomized study of FOLFOX4 or FOLFOX7 with oxaliplatin in a stop-and-go fashion in advanced colorectal cancer—a GERCOR study. *J Clin Oncol* 2006; 20:394.
16. Chibaudel B, Maindrault-Goebel F, Lledo G, et al. Can chemotherapy be discontinued in unresectable metastatic colorectal cancer? The GERCOR OPTIMOX2 Study. *J Clin Oncol* 2009; 27:5727.
17. Hryniuk WM. Average relative dose intensity and the impact on design of clinical trials. *Semin Oncol* 1987;14:65.
18. Hryniuk W, Goodyear M. The calculation of received dose intensity. *J Clin Oncol* 1990;8:1935.
19. Hryniuk W, Frei E 3rd, Wright FA. A single scale for comparing dose-intensity of all chemotherapy regimens in breast cancer: summation dose-intensity. *J Clin Oncol* 1998;16:3137.
20. Wood W, Korzan AH, Cooper R, et al. Dose and dose intensity of adjuvant chemotherapy for stage II node positive breast cancer. *N Engl J Med* 1994;330:1253.
21. Citron ML, Berry DA, Cirrincione C, et al. Randomized trial of dose-dense versus conventionally scheduled and sequential versus concurrent combination chemotherapy as postoperative adjuvant treatment of node-positive primary breast cancer: first report of intergroup trial C9741/Cancer and Leukemia Group B Trial 9741. *J Clin Oncol* 2003;12:1431.
22. Traina TA, Theodoulou M, Felgin K, et al. Phase I study of a novel capecitabine scheduled based on the Norton-Simon mathematical model in patients with metastatic breast cancer. *J Clin Oncol* 2008;26:1797.
23. Sledge GW, Neuberg D, Bernardo P, et al. Phase III trial of doxorubicin, paclitaxel, and the combination of doxorubicin and paclitaxel as front-line chemotherapy for metastatic breast cancer: an intergroup trial (E1193). *J Clin Oncol* 2003;21:588.
24. Goldie JH, Coldman AJ. A mathematical model for relating the drug sensitivity of tumors to the spontaneous mutation rate. *Cancer Treat Rep* 1979;63:1727.
25. El-Deiry WS. The role of p53 in chemosensitivity and radiosensitivity. *Oncogene* 2003;22:7486.
26. Lowe SW, Bodis S, McClatchey A, et al. p53 status and the efficacy of cancer therapy in vivo. *Science* 1994;266:807.
27. Adams JM, Cory S. The BCL-2 apoptotic switch in cancer development and therapy. *Oncogene* 2007;26:1324.
28. Chanan-Khan A. Bcl-2 antisense therapy in hematologic malignancies. *Curr Opin Oncol* 2004;16:581.
29. Meng XW, Lee SH, Kaufmann SH. Apoptosis in the treatment of cancer: a promise kept? *Curr Opin Cell Biol* 2006;18:668.
30. Melisi D, Chiao PJ. NF-kappaB as a target for cancer therapy. *Expert Opin Ther Targets* 2007;11:133.
31. Jackson G, Einsele H, Moreau P, Miguel JS. Bortezomib, a novel proteasome inhibitor, in the treatment of hematologic malignancies. *Cancer Treat Rev* 2005;31:591.
32. Ellis L, Hicklin D. Resistance to targeted therapies: refining anticancer therapy in the era of molecular oncology. *Clin Cancer Res* 2009;15(24):7471.
33. Pohlmann P, Mayer I. Resistance to trastuzumab in breast cancer. *Clin Cancer Res* 2009;15:7479.
34. Nahta R, Yu D, Hung M. Mechanisms of disease: understanding resistance to HER2-targeted therapy in human breast cancer. *Nat Clin Pract Oncol* 2006;3:269.
35. Hammerman P, Janne P, Johnson B. Resistance to epidermal growth factor receptor tyrosine kinase inhibitors in non-small cell lung cancer. *Clin Cancer Res* 2009;15:7502.
36. Bardelli A, Siena S. Molecular mechanisms of resistance to cetuximab and panitumumab in colorectal cancer. *J Clin Oncol* 2010;28:1254.
37. Banck M, Grothey A. Biomarkers of resistance to epidermal growth factor receptor monoclonal antibodies in patients with metastatic colorectal cancer. *Clin Cancer Res* 2009;15:7492.
38. Bergers G, Hanahan D. Modes of resistance to anti-angiogenic therapy. *Nat Rev Cancer* 2008;8:592.
39. Cao Y, Zhong W, Sun Y. Improvement of antiangiogenic cancer therapy by understanding the mechanisms of angiogenic factor interplay and drug resistance. *Sem Cancer Biol* 2009;29:338-343,
40. Milojkovic D, Apperley J. Mechanisms of resistance to imatinib and second-generation tyrosine inhibitors in chronic myeloid leukemia. *Clin Cancer Res* 2009;15:7519.
41. Gramza A, Corless C, Heinrich M. Resistance to tyrosine kinase inhibitors in gastrointestinal stromal tumors. *Clin Cancer Res* 2009;15:7510.

CHAPTER 29 ASSESSMENT OF CLINICAL RESPONSE

ANTONIO TITO FOJO AND SUSAN ELAINE BATES

The "modern era" of drug development began in 1976 when 16 experienced oncologists who treated lymphoma gathered to decide what would be considered a reliable measure of response to a therapy.[1] Each oncologist measured 12 "simulated tumor masses" employing "usual clinical methods"—calipers or rulers. A principal goal was to identify the amount of shrinkage that *could not* be ascribed to operator error and that *would not* be found if a placebo was administered. Unknown to the participants two pairs of these "tumors" were identical in size. The results showed that when measuring two identical sized spheres a single investigator incorrectly concluded there was a difference of *50% in the product of the perpendicular diameters* 6.8% of the time. If two investigators measured the same sphere and compared sizes, then 7.8% of the time their calculations of the *product of the perpendicular diameters* that ideally would have been the same in fact differed by 50%. Because differences of *25% in the product of the perpendicular diameters* were found in an unacceptably high 19% and 24.9% of measurements, Moertel and Hanley[1] concluded: "In the clinical setting it is recommended that the 50% reduction criterion be employed and that the investigator should anticipate an objective response rate of 5 to 10% due to human error in tumor measurement." It was from this auspicious beginning that our current methodologies of response assessment evolved. The important point to note is that the decision to use a 50% reduction in tumor as a measure of response was made to reduce error and *not because it represented a value that conferred clinical benefit.*

This medical science progressed from calipers and rulers in lymphoma to diagnostic imaging and the bidimensional World Health Organization (WHO) criteria and on to one-dimensional Response Evaluation Criteria in Solid Tumors (RECIST). In 1981, 5 years after the rationale for accepting a 50% decrease as a measure of response was published, Miller et al.[2] reported the recommendations from a WHO initiative to develop standardized approaches for the "reporting of response, recurrence and disease-free interval." In concordance with the 1976 recommendations, the WHO criteria recommended malignant disease be "measured in two dimensions by ruler or caliper with *surface area* determined by multiplying the longest diameter by the greatest perpendicular diameter." Furthermore, complete response (CR) was defined as the disappearance of all known disease, determined by two observations not less than 4 weeks apart; while a designation of a partial response (PR) was assigned if there was a "50% or more decrease in *total tumor load* of the lesions that have been measured to determine the effect of therapy by two observations not less than four weeks apart," and with multiple lesions, a "*50% decrease in the sum of the products of the perpendicular diameters of the multiple lesions*" was needed. Thus the 50% reduction initially chosen as an "operationally" optimal value became institutionalized as the threshold for declaring efficacy in the majority of cancers. This measure of efficacy was perpetuated when in 2000 a recommendation was made to replace the WHO criteria with the now widely used RECIST criteria.[3] The authors noted "the definition of a partial response, in particular, is an arbitrary convention—there is no inherent meaning for an individual patient of a 50% decrease in overall tumor load." Nevertheless, the threshold chosen, a 30% reduction in one dimension, was comparable to the 50% decrease in the sum of the products of the perpendicular diameters and thus perpetuated the 1976 standard. Table 29.1 compares the WHO criteria with those of RECIST 1.0 and RECIST 1.1,[2–5] while Figure 29.1 provides a visual presentation of the differences and underscores the higher threshold required to qualify as PD when using RECIST.[6]

OVERALL RESPONSE RATE AND STABLE DISEASE

Overall response rate (ORR) is the portion of patients with a tumor size reduction of a predefined amount for a minimum time period. The U.S. Food and Drug Administration (FDA) has generally defined ORR as the sum of PR plus CR. Although overall survival (OS) remains the gold standard, ORR has been used both in drug development and in clinical practice to indicate antitumor efficacy of a given agent or regimen. Table 29.2 summarizes the attributes and drawbacks of using ORR as a method of assessment. Using the standardized definitions of response that evolved from the original exercise on tumor measurements, it has been shown that ORR (often) correlates with OS. For example a meta-analysis of 3,791 patients enrolled in 25 randomized trials of first-line treatment of colorectal cancer found that an increase in ORR translated into an increase in OS,[7] although ORR explained less than half of the variability of the survival benefits in the 25 trials. Similarly, a meta-analysis on individual data from 2,126 metastatic breast cancer patients enrolled in ten randomized trials to compare standard versus intensified epirubicin-containing chemotherapy found that the achievement of a response to chemotherapy was associated with a true OS benefit.[8] Finally, an examination of over 7,000 patients reported in 143 phase 2 trials found a strong correlation ($P < .0001$) of ORR with progression-free survival (PFS) and OS.[9] Equally important, however, is the duration of response, a value that is measured from the time of initial response until documented tumor progression.

The FDA has generally not been willing to include stable disease (SD), defined as shrinkage that qualifies as neither response nor progression, as part of the ORR as it is often indicative of the underlying disease biology rather than attributed to the drug's therapeutic effect.[10,11] Nevertheless, investigators are increasingly using the term *clinical benefit rate* (CBR) to include CR + PR + SD. This represents a misuse of the term clinical benefit since CR, PR, and SD are objective tumor findings that do not address the true clinical

TABLE 29.1

KEY FEATURES OF DIFFERENT EVALUATION CRITERIA

	WHO	RECIST 1.0	RECIST 1.1
Measurable lesion definition	Uni- and bidimensional[a]	Unidimensional, longest diameter, ≥10 mm (spiral CT); ≥20 mm other modalities	Unidimensional, longest diameter tumor lesions ≥10 mm (CT; skin by calipers); ≥20 mm if CXR
Measurable node definition	Not defined	Not defined	≥15 mm short axis
Disease burden to be assessed at baseline	All (not specified)	Measurable target lesions up to ten total (five per organ); other lesions nontarget	Measurable target lesions up to five total (two per organ); other lesions nontarget
Baseline sum	Sum of products of bidimensional diameters or Sum of linear unidimensional diameters	Sum of longest diameters all measurable lesions	Sum of diameters target lesions, short axis nodes, longest diameter others
CR	Disappearance of all known disease	Disappearance of all known disease	Disappearance of all known disease; malignant nodes must be <10 mm
PR	Bidimensional disease, 50% decrease in sum of products of diameters[b]	Measurable target lesions, 30% decrease in sum of longest diameters; all other disease, no evidence of progression	Measurable target lesions, 30% decrease in sum of longest diameters; all other disease, no evidence of progression
Response confirmation?	Yes, 4 weeks	Yes, 4 weeks	Yes, 4 weeks (if response primary end point) No, if secondary end point
Progression	Measurable disease, ≥25% increase in size of one or more measurable lesions[c] or appearance of new lesions	Measurable disease, 20% increase in sum longest diameters, taking as reference smallest sum in study; or appearance of new lesions	20% increase in sum of diameters, with minimum absolute increase of 5 mm, taking as reference smallest sum in study; or appearance of new lesions
	Nonmeasurable disease, estimated increase of ≥25%	Nonmeasurable disease, unequivocal progression	Nonmeasurable disease, unequivocal progression
Stable disease	Stable disease or non-PR and non-PD for 4 weeks	Non-PR, non-PD; minimum time defined by protocol	Non-PR, non-PD; minimum time defined by protocol

WHO, World Health Organization; RECIST, Response Evaluation Criteria in Solid Tumors; CT, computed tomography; CXR, chest x-ray; PR, partial remission; CR, complete remission; PD, progressive disease.
[a]By convention, bidimensional measurement is generally used in trials assessing response using the WHO criteria.
[b]Unidimensional measurable and estimated nonmeasurable disease, 50% decrease also allowed by WHO criteria.
[c]In practice, some groups changed this to 25% increase in sum of products of diameter.
(Adapted from ref. 4.)

benefit of a therapy. Although it is tempting to assign a clinical benefit to a reduction in tumor size or SD, in fact there is no evidence of such. CB was originally delineated to assess the benefit of gemcitabine in pancreatic cancer.[12] The primary efficacy measure was *clinical benefit response*, a composite of measurements of pain (analgesic consumption and pain intensity), Karnofsky performance status, and weight. CB required a sustained (4 weeks or longer) improvement in at least one parameter without worsening in any others.[12] Using CBR to include tumors scored as SD as meaningful responses is unlikely to generate data that are comparable across institutions and disease types. The latter is due in part to the fact that in the majority of trials SD is not defined, and a value that is not defined has limited utility. In an analysis of over 140 phase 2 clinical trials, SD rates did not correlate with either PFS or OS in trials with either cytotoxic or targeted therapies.[9] And SD was not defined in nearly 80% of these trials. Failing the "clear communication between investigators" test for clinical trial end points,[13] SD should not be used as a response end point in the absence of standardized definitions that are shown to effect meaningful changes in clinical outcome.

ALTERNATE RESPONSE CRITERIA

Despite the value of ORR, not every tumor type has been amenable to standardized definitions. Examples include bony disease in prostate cancer, pleural and peritoneal surface disease in mesothelioma and ovarian cancer, and gastrointestinal stroma tumors (GIST), which often remain the same size as the center of the tumor mass undergoes necrosis. Different strategies have emerged to quantify these diseases, including biomarkers and positron emission tomography (PET) criteria, as discussed below.

International Working Group Criteria for Lymphoma

Because lymph nodes represent special challenges in disease assessment, an International Working Group (IWG) was convened in 1999 to develop recommendations for assessment of response in malignant lymphoma. These guidelines were

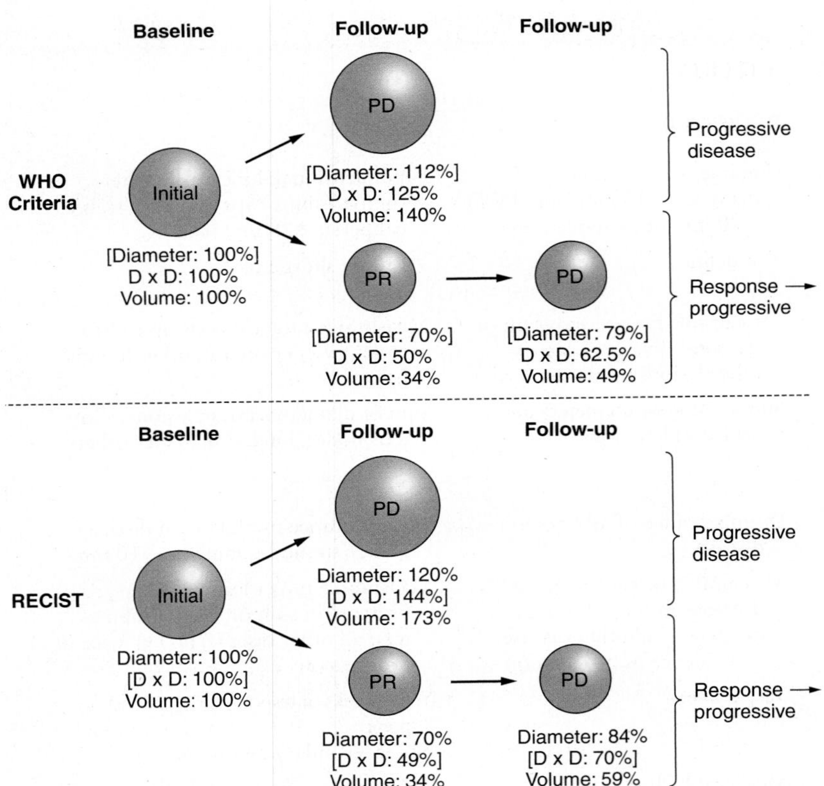

FIGURE 29.1 Comparison of World Health Organization (WHO) and Response Evaluation Criteria in Solid Tumors (RECIST) thresholds in three parameters: diameter, product of diameters, and volume. In the figure, spheres meeting WHO and RECIST criteria for progressive disease (PD) and for partial response (PR) are shown with percentage relative to baseline calculated for each parameter. According to WHO criteria, PD was scored when the product of the perpendicular diameters exceeded 125%. In a sphere this represents a 112% increase in diameter and a 140% increase in volume. By comparison RECIST allows the longest diameter to increase to 120%, equivalent to a 144% increase in the product of the perpendicular diameters and a 173% increase in volume in a sphere. Because of the 33% higher threshold to meet PD (and comparable increase in stable disease [SD] classification), studies that used the WHO criteria cannot be compared directly to studies in the RECIST era (from ref. 6). In contrast, PR definitions are almost identical. Brackets identify the measure *not used* in the criteria portrayed.

TABLE 29.2

ATTRIBUTES AND DRAWBACKS OF USING RESPONSE RATE AS A CRITERIUM

Attributes	Drawbacks
Standardized: WHO, RECIST, IWG/Cheson, Prostate Cancer Working Groups	Requires prospective, consistent definition. Meaningful response durations not standardized. One-size-fits-all approach not ideal.
Because spontaneous regressions rare, tumor regression after treatment indicates treatment effect	Short-lived responses rarely clinically meaningful.
Response rate is a surrogate for clinical benefit	Uncertain correlation between ORR and clinical benefit.
Early end point, often reached within months of initiating treatment	Requires confirmation. May require validation by independent review for credibility.
Definition of progressive disease (PD) identifies uniform time to end treatment and data capture	Definition of PD is arbitrary without evidence it actually represents end of benefit period Some tumors difficult to measure (e.g., ovarian cancer, mesothelioma, or gastrointestinal stromal tumor following imatinib)

WHO, World Health Organization; RECIST, Response Evaluation Criteria in Solid Tumors; IWG, International Working Group; ORR, overall response rate.

subsequently updated to incorporate ^{18}F-fluorodeoxyglucose (FDG)-PET assessments of disease metabolic activity.[14] The definition of CR requires complete disappearance of detectable disease, but a posttreatment residual mass is allowed if it is PET-negative. For lymphomas that are not consistently FDG avid, or FDG avidity is unknown, a CR can only be scored if nodes that were greater than 1.5 cm before therapy regress to less than 1.5 cm, and nodes that were 1.1 to 1.5 cm in their long axis and more than 1.0 cm in their short axis shrink to 1.0 cm or less in their short axis. The definition of PR resembles the WHO criteria, in that a greater than 50% decrease in the sum of the product of the diameters in up to six nodal masses or in hepatic or splenic nodules must be documented. The IWG criteria, sometimes called the Cheson criteria, address in detail the response assessment in the different manifestations and varied histopathologies of malignant lymphoma.[14]

Serial Biomarker Levels

Biomarkers have been developed for multiple purposes: for screening, for early detection of recurrent disease, and for monitoring response to systemic therapy (Table 29.3). Only the latter indication will be discussed here. Predictive biomarkers, scoring the likelihood of response to specific treatments, require extensive validation, specifically large randomized clinical trials and meta-analyses.

The use of serum biomarkers to monitor treatment in oncology has been slow to crystallize, and consequently there are few clinically validated biomarkers.[15] In addition to issues regarding sensitivity and specificity, their use and development has also been hindered by the modest efficacy of our therapies—biomarkers are of little value without highly effective primary and salvage therapies. For example, a recent clinical trial indicates that in *asymptomatic patients* with ovarian cancer, whose only evidence of disease progression is an isolated rising CA 125, nothing is gained by instituting treatment

TABLE 29.3

RESPONSE CRITERIA FOR BIOMARKERS

Type (Ref.)	Baseline	Response	Progression
CA 125 in ovarian cancer (GCIG criteria) (15)	Two pretreatment samples >2 × ULN	CA 125 decline ≥50% confirmed at 28 days	2 × nadir OR 2 × ULN if normalized on therapy
PSA in prostate caanser (PSA WG 1)[a] (20, 21)	≥5 ng/mL and documentation of two consecutive increases in PSA over a previous reference value	PSA decline of 50% from baseline (measured twice 3 to 4 weeks apart)	PSA increase by 25%[2] above nadir or entry value (50% increase if response achieved) AND >5 ng/mL, or back to baseline, whichever is lower
PSA in prostate cancer (PCWG2)[a] (22)	Minimum starting value: ≥2.0 ng/mL Estimate pretherapy PSA-DT: Need ≥3 values ≥4 weeks apart	Report percentage change from baseline (rise or fall) at 12 weeks, and separately, the maximal change (rise or fall) at any time using a waterfall plot	PSA increase ≥25% and ≥2 ng/mL above the nadir, confirmed by a second value ≥3 weeks later (i.e., a confirmed rising trend) OR ≥25% and ≥2 ng/mL >12 weeks
hCG and AFP in testicular cancer (23–26)		Long half-life of decay(>3.5 days for hCG, >7 days for AFP) is indicative of a poor response	
Choi Criteria for GIST			
Choi criteria for CT images in GIST (27)		≥10% decrease in tumor size OR ≥15% reduction in tumor density	
EORTC Criteria for PET			
EORTC criteria for response when using a PET scan (30)	ROI should be drawn, SUV calculated	CMR: Complete resolution of uptake PMR: SUV reduction ≥25% after more than one treatment cycle SMD: <25% increase and <15% decrease in SUV	PMD: SUV increase of >25% in regions defined on baseline, or appearance of new FDG avid lesions

GCIG, Gynecologic Cancer Inter Group; ULN, Upper limit of normal; PSA, prostate-specific antigen; PSA WG 1, PSA Working Group 1; PCWG2: Prostate Cancer Working Group 2; PSA-DT, PSA-doubling time; hCG, human chorionic gonadotropin; AFP, alpha-fetoprotein; CT, computed tomography; GIST, gastrointestinal stromal tumor; EORTC, European Organisation for the Research and Treatment of Cancer; PET, positron emission tomography; ROI, region of interest; SUV, standardized uptake value; CMR, complete metabolic response; PMR, partial metabolic response; SMD, stable metabolic disease; PMD, progressive metabolic disease.

[a]Guidelines for PSA assessment have evolved from those of the PSA WG 1 (refs. 20, 21), where responses were dichotomized based on the percentage decline, to those in the PCWG2 (ref. 22), where PSA response is considered a continuous variable. Recently, emphasis has shifted to assessing PSA doubling time.

before there is other evidence of progression.[12] As noted by the authors, the results highlight "the need for improved salvage therapies for recurrent ovarian cancer."[16]

- **Cancer antigen (CA) 125:** Despite its recognized limitations, CA 125 is used widely. For example, the Gynaecologic Cancer InterGroup (GCIG) criteria have evolved to help determine whether a patient's tumor has responded to therapy.[18–20] Consistently, the fraction of patients scored as having a tumor response using CA 125 criteria is higher than the response defined by RECIST. Whether this is more or less accurate is the subject of some controversy.[16]
- **Prostate-specific antigen (PSA):** Similar issues have confronted those who care for patients with prostate cancer. The PSA Working Group 1 guidelines, first published in 1999, established PSA criteria, particularly for use in patients with disease that was difficult to quantify.[22,23] There followed a second working group (PCWG2) that recommended plotting the percentage of PSA change for each patient in a waterfall plot so as to avoid creating a dichotomous variable from the changes in PSA.[24] PCWG2 also recommended keeping patients on trial until evidence of a change in clinical status, either symptomatic or radiographic progression. The latter addressed concerns with patients in whom PSA changes did not reflect clinical status, particularly those with transient increases in the first 12 weeks of a new therapy.
- **Human chorionic gonadotropin (hCG) and alpha-fetoprotein (AFP):** Because testicular cancer is a highly curable disease with validated biomarkers, outcome assessment has focused on the rapid detection of patients whose tumors have a poor response to therapy. Since both markers have relatively short half-lives—1 to 2 days for hCG and 5 to 7 days for serum AFP—the rate of decline can be determined. Various methods have demonstrated that a rapid decline or early normalization of marker levels is indicative of a good outcome, without any one method achieving

widespread acceptance.[25–27] Nonetheless, the 2010 American Society of Clinical Oncology (ASCO) guidelines on serum tumor markers concluded there was still insufficient evidence to recommend changing therapy solely on the basis of a slow marker decline.[28] Rising levels after two cycles of therapy (outside the first week of treatment when rises can be due to tumor lysis) can be considered an indication to change treatment plan.

Computed Tomography–Based Tumor Density

One approach that has gained some support advocates assessing tumor response in GIST based on density on computed tomography (CT) (Table 29.3). This variation was prompted by the evident response to treatment with imatinib but with minimal tumor shrinkage.[29] Confirmation of this approach by other investigators is awaited.

Fluorodeoxyglucose-Positron Emission Tomography

Regulatory approval of new agents has focused on response assessments by WHO, RECIST, or IWG criteria, with FDG-PET utilized at most as an adjunct to those standardized criteria (Table 29.3). Although FDG uptake is a powerful diagnostic tool that strongly correlates with tumor activity, it has some limitations: there are tumors with variable FDG avidity; there is variation due to patient activity, carbohydrate intake, blood glucose, and timing; and there are several benign sources of uptake, including inflammatory and postsurgical sites. Numerous methods to quantitate FDG-PET and assess response have been proposed,[30] but to date there is no consensus. Standardized uptake values (SUV), the most commonly used method of PET measurement, should be corrected for lean body mass (SUL).[30,31] The European Organisation for Research and Treatment of Cancer (EORTC) criteria, with its four response categories, are commonly used, but are in need of updating.[32] Other approaches are also under study.

Several of the examples above represent approaches for specific diseases. There are other diseases where specific strategies for response assessment are required, such as in cutaneous T-cell lymphoma, where skin lesions coexist with blood and nodal involvement; acute leukemia, where bone marrow criteria have been defined; mesothelioma, where volumetric measurement is needed since tumors are not spherical; and pancreatic cancer, where clinical benefit has been defined, as noted above. In every case, response assessment requires an active agent. But the greatest need is for clinicians to work together with regulatory agencies to define a common language of response. This requires establishing criteria that are then revisited periodically and refined over time.

WATERFALL PLOTS

The arbitrary nature of the initial 50% cutoff, discussed above, and its evolution to the current RECIST threshold of 30% reduction in the size of the maximum diameter raise valid queries as to why 30% is valuable and not 29% or 25%. For this reason waterfall plots, such as the one shown in Figure 29.2, have become increasingly popular, because they depict the benefit or lack thereof in all patients as a continuum of response, rather than a dichotomized response rate.[33] The correlations that have been observed between ORR and PFS and OS[7–9] would most likely be higher if the threshold for response required an even greater magnitude than 30% shrinkage. Similarly one could envision that if SD were more narrowly defined, such as responses covering the range from 20% to 29%, then SD might be seen to correlate with PFS and OS. The reason this value was chosen as an operational optimum in lymphoma over 30 years ago and has endured is that 30% shrinkage in one dimension (RECIST definition of response) represents a volumetric decrease of over 65%, a magnitude of tumor regression that not surprisingly impacts OS in the majority of cancers. Because a 20% decrease represents a 50% decrease in volume, it would not be surprising to find that some responses that are currently scored as SD could nevertheless impact PFS and OS.

PROGRESSION FREE SURVIVAL AND TIME TO PROGRESSION

In cancer drug development one usually finds ORR assessed as an indicator of activity in phase 2 trials, while randomized phase 3 trials rely on other end points, including PFS and time to progression (TTP) (Table 29.4). While PFS and TTP attempt to assess efficacy in close proximity to a therapy, they score responses differently and should not be seen as interchangeable. TTP is defined as the time from randomization to the *time of disease progression.*[10] In TTP analyses, deaths are censored either at the time of death or at an earlier visit. In contrast, PFS is defined from the *time of randomization to the time of disease progression or death.* Although patients who come off a trial because of adverse events might be censored in both analyses, patients who die while in a study are censored

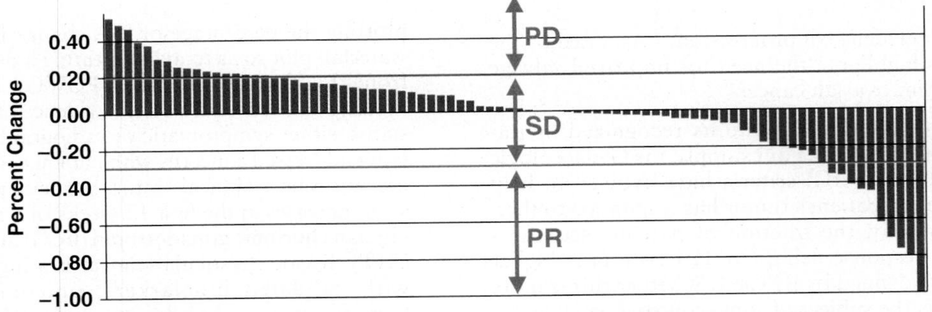

FIGURE 29.2 Example of a waterfall plot demonstrating for each patient the maximum benefit obtained with the study therapy. Those on the left represent patients whose tumors increased, while those on the right represent patients whose tumors regressed. The vertical red lines at +20% and −30% define the boundaries of stable disease according to Response Evaluation Criteria in Solid Tumors (RECIST). Ideally all responses should be confirmed after a period of at least 4 weeks. The example shown is of patients with renal cell carcinoma treated with the microtubule targeting agent ixabepilone. PD, progressive disease; SD, stable disease; PR, partial response. (From ref. 33.)

TABLE 29.4

PROGRESSION-FREE SURVIVAL VERSUS TIME TO TUMOR PROGRESSION

			Off-Study Reason			
Scheduled Assessment	No. Alive	Continuing Treatment	No. of Progressive Disease	No. Dead[a]	PFS (%)	TTP (%)
Enrollment	10	10	0	0	100	100
1st	10	9	1	0	90 (9/10)	90 (9/10)
2nd	10	8	2	0	80 (8/10)	80 (8/10)
3rd	9	6	3	1	60 (6/10)	66 (3/9)
4th	9	5	4	1	50 (5/10)	55 (5/9)
5th	8	4	4	2	40 (4/10)	50 (4/8)
6th	8	3	5	2	30 (3/10)	37.5 (3/8)
7th	8	2	6	2	20 (2/10)	25 (2/8)
8th	7	1	6	3	10 (1/10)	14 (1/7)
9th	7	0	7	3	0 (0/10)	0 (0/7)

PFS, progression-free survival; TTP, time to tumor progression.
[a]Dead, whether due to adverse event or unrelated event, but without documented progressive disease prior to death.

only in the TTP analysis. Those who favor TTP analyses argue that if a patient dies but the tumor has not meet criteria for progression, one cannot accurately estimate when progression might have occurred, so the data should be censored. However, those who favor PFS argue that in some cases death might be an adverse effect of the therapy. High-dose therapies represent an example of why PFS might be a preferable (regulatory) end point. If in a given tumor there is evidence of a dose–response relationship for an active drug, then high doses may have a greater response. However, such high doses may also be responsible for a greater number of deaths. Assessing only those who survive the high-dose therapy and ignoring those who die (TTP) may lead to the conclusion the high-dose therapy is more effective. The balance sheet that includes death (PFS) would clearly demonstrate this efficacy came at too great a price. Table 29.4 shows an example of how TTP, by censoring deaths, can result in a longer time to "progression." In the example, if assessments were being conducted at 3-month intervals, the median PFS would be 12 months, whereas the median TTP would be 15 months.

Although some have argued PFS and TTP should be acceptable end points for cancer clinical trials, in the majority of tumors there is no convincing evidence PFS is a surrogate for OS, and in those where there is some evidence, its value is arguable.[34] Table 29.5 presents the attributes and drawbacks of PFS and TTP. Note that the definition of progression is often difficult, particularly in some tumor types, and that investigator bias can thus influence PFS and TTP. For example, an investigator convinced of the efficacy of an experimental drug may leave patients in a study an additional restaging interval and thereby improve PFS or TTP by the length of that interval. Precise definitions of disease progression can help with this problem, but these may have the problem of being too stringent in clinical practice. Conversely, *ascertainment bias* can lead to earlier diagnosis of progression, especially if evaluation (*ascertainment*) occurs before a scheduled interval to a greater extent in the control arm compared to the experimental arm.

TABLE 29.5

ATTRIBUTES AND DRAWBACKS OF USING PROGRESSION-FREE SURVIVAL AND TIME TO TUMOR PROGRESSION AS OVERALL CRITERIA

Attributes	Drawbacks
All patients are included in efficacy analysis	Requires randomized clinical trial design to provide control group.
Earlier trial end point than overall survival	Disease progression definition is difficult—requires precision.
Not confounded by crossover effects or use of second-line therapies	Little agreement on magnitude of PFS or TTP that constitutes clinical benefit. Statistically significant improvement in TTP or PFS may not translate into improved OS nor represent clinical benefit.
Patients who suffer complications of disease (PFS/TTP), or adverse effects (PFS/TTP), and are removed from study; or who suffer death while on study (TTP) are censored at time of event and still included in analysis	Subject to investigator bias, particularly in unblinded clinical trials. External review committees or blinded trials can reduce investigator bias.
	Requires uniform, frequent, and consistent disease measurement to avoid "ascertainment bias."[a]
Less expensive than an OS end point	More expensive than other clinical trial end points.

PFS, progression-free survival; TTP, time to tumor progression; OS, overall survival.
[a]"Ascertainment bias" occurs when patients in one arm of the study are evaluated (ascertained) more frequently before a planned assessment. Because disease progression can occur between scheduled observations—particularly if assessments occur infrequently—"ascertainment bias" can lead to a greater likelihood of "looking" for progression in one arm of the study.

OVERALL SURVIVAL

Table 29.6 summarizes the attributes and drawbacks of OS as an end point. Defined as the time from randomization to death, OS has been considered the gold standard of clinical trial end points. In part, this is because OS is unambiguous and does not suffer from interpretation bias. An additional advantage of the survival end point is that it can balance the

TABLE 29.6

ATTRIBUTES AND DRAWBACKS TO USING OVERALL SURVIVAL AS A CRITERIUM

Attributes	Drawbacks
Unambiguous	Requires a large sample size
Direct clinical benefit	May require long follow-up
Not dependent on assessment intervals	Posttrial therapies may confound end point
Includes treatment-related mortality that can obscure benefit in a subset	Crossover to the experimental arm at disease progression can obscure survival advantage in the experimental arm
Patient benefit can be described as superior survival or noninferior survival if the trial is prospectively designed as a noninferiority trial	Requires randomized, controlled trials

effect of therapies with high treatment-related mortality even if tumor control is substantially better with the new treatment. However, some worry that because patients may receive multiple lines of therapy following the clinical trial, the results may be confounded by those subsequent therapies. The latter concern is often cited as the reason for why an advantage in PFS or TTP disappears when one looks to OS. But as a review of clinical trials confirms,[35] the magnitude of the difference does not disappear, only the statistical validity (see examples in Reck et al.[36] and Hortobagyi et al.[37]) as illustrated in Figure 29.3.[38]

When evaluating a randomized controlled trial, it is important that the OS as well as the PFS are always analyzed by intention to treat (ITT). In an ITT analysis, often described as "once randomized, always analyzed,"[39] all patients assigned to a group at the time of randomization are analyzed regardless of what occurred subsequently. An ITT analysis avoids the bias introduced by omitting dropouts and noncompliant patients who can negate randomization and overestimate clinical effectiveness.

KAPLAN-MEIER PLOTS

In a typical clinical trial, data are represented as a Kaplan-Meier plot. In discrete time intervals, the number of patients in each group who are progression free and alive (PFS analysis) or alive (OS analysis) at the end of the interval are counted and divided by the total number of patients in that group at the beginning of the time interval. One excludes from this calculation patients censored for a reason other than progressive disease or death during the same interval. This has the advantage that it allows one to include censored patients in estimates of the probability of PFS or OS up to the point when they were censored; they are excluded only beyond the point of censoring. In most clinical trials, a fraction of patients are typically censored.

In constructing the Kaplan-Meier plot, probabilities are calculated for each interval of time. The probability of surviving

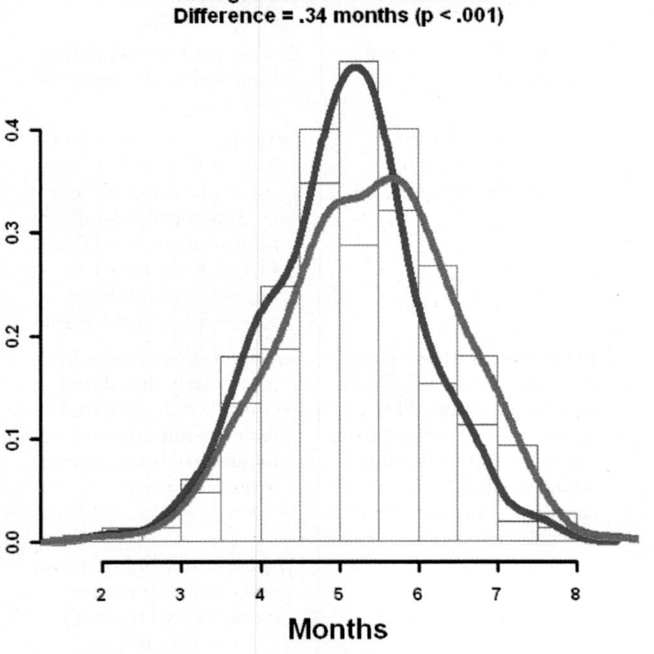

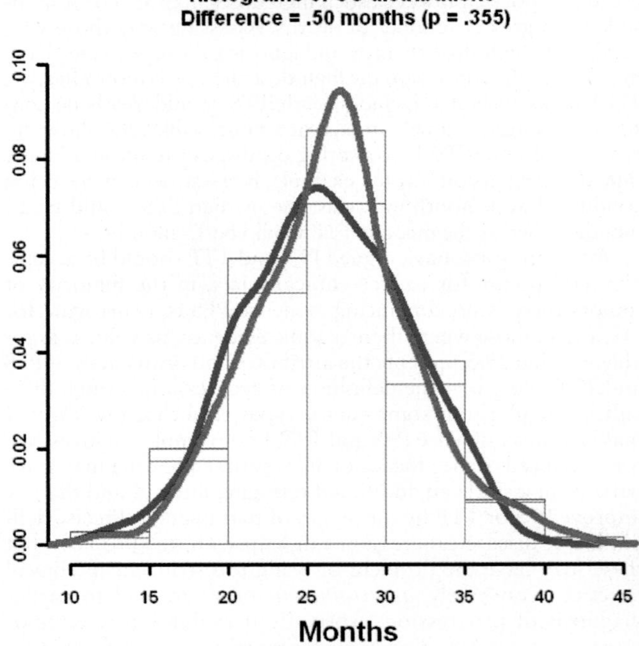

FIGURE 29.3 Hypothetical distribution of progression-free survival (PFS) and overall survival (OS) data demonstrating "disappearance of PFS benefit." Because chemotherapy does not exert a lasting effect on underlying tumor biology, and because PFS is a shorter interval, measured in increments—not daily as is OS—PFS differences often "disappear." The hypothetical example shown illustrates this phenomenon. The panel on the left shows a histogram of PFS distributions with a difference of 0.34 months that nevertheless achieves statistical significance over the short interval when PFS is measured. The panel on the right depicts similar histograms for OS, captured over a longer time period. Despite a larger absolute difference of 0.5 months, the OS difference does not reach statistical significance. For these hypothetical curves random number generated data sets (with normal distribution), histograms, and density plots were generated using R Development Core's R version 2.11.1 (2010-05-31). (from ref. 38). The differences were deliberately chosen to be small, but a similar "disappearance" can also occur with larger differences. As can be seen what disappears is not the absolute benefit, but rather the statistical validity.

progression free or being counted as a "survivor" to the end of an interval of assessment is the product of the probabilities of surviving in all the preceding assessment intervals multiplied by the probability for the interval of interest. As might be expected, with different rates of death and progression, together with differences in the number of patients censored, Kaplan-Meier plots vary greatly. One might ask to what extent the two curves in each study differ. One measure that is of value is the median PFS or OS—a value calculated in most studies from a Kaplan-Meier plot.

HAZARD RATIOS

Increasingly, however, hazard ratios are incorrectly cited in preference to the more traditional measures of efficacy such as the median PFS and median OS. *Because a hazard ratio is a value that has no dimension, it has very limited value, informing the reader only with regard to the reliability and uniformity of the data.* It does not quantify the magnitude of the benefit. A physician and especially a patient want to know the magnitude of the benefit—the extent to which a life will be prolonged—not what a dimensionless hazard ratio is. By definition, the hazard ratio is a ratio of the hazard rates. The hazard rate quantifies the likelihood that a patient will experience a hazardous event or a hazard during a defined interval of observation expressed as a rate (or percentage). Specifically the hazard rate represents the conditional probability that a patient will continue to be alive without progression of disease or death in the upcoming period of time. The hazard rate can be easily obtained from the data used to generate a Kaplan-Meier plot. As commonly presented, the lower the hazard ratio, the better the experimental therapy. To determine whether the hazard ratio has statistical significance, one can (1) use a log-rank test to show the null hypothesis that the two treatments lead to the same survival probabilities is wrong or (2) use a parametric approach writing a regression model and fitting the data to the model so that one can establish the hazard ratio for the whole trial and its statistical significance. In many cases, the Cox proportional hazard model is used. Although the ideal hazard ratio would capture the differential benefit throughout the period of study, in practice the entire time depicted in a Kaplan-Meier plot may not be analyzed. As time progresses, the number of patients who have not yet died or experienced progression of their disease declines, and any such event generates a disproportionate effect on the hazard rate and in turn the hazard ratio. Consequently, these areas of the Kaplan-Meier plot are often not used in calculating the overall hazard ratio. While intuitively reasonable, this has the effect of ignoring portions of the Kaplan-Meier curve that are less beneficial for the superior arm of the study, and this enhances the hazard ratio.

FOREST PLOTS

As therapies have become more "targeted" and as benefits have become increasingly marginal, there is greater interest in determining whether there is heterogeneity in a treatment effect, such that a treatment works better in some subgroups than others. While simple in concept, these attempts can be subject to error since subgroups are composed of smaller numbers and the confidence intervals are therefore wider than those for the entire group. Forest plots are increasingly used to display treatment effects across subgroups. The most common presentation includes a vertical line at the "no effect point" (e.g., a hazard ratio of 1.0), with symbols of varying size representing the subgroups, each with its confidence interval depicted by a line that stretches from the symbol to both sides (the symbol size is usually proportional to the size of the subgroup). If the confidence interval for a subgroup crosses the no effect point, this is commonly interpreted, not necessarily correctly, as a lack of effect in the subgroup. The information one seeks from a forest plot is whether the effect size for different subgroups varies significantly from the main effect and this is determined by a test for heterogeneity.[40]

META-ANALYSES

Meta-analysis is the statistical process of combining information from several trials that address the same question.[34] The most common type of meta-analysis uses data culled from published reports. Such meta-analyses can be flawed because of publication bias or exclusion bias; further, the data provided in the publications may be inadequate to perform meaningful calculations. A second type of meta-analysis uses summary data obtained directly from investigators, whether published or unpublished, and avoids publication and exclusion biases. Moreover, simple but unbiased summary statistics can be obtained even for outcomes that are time related. The best approach is a meta-analysis based on individual patient data. Such meta-analyses have contributed to therapeutic progress, and they have recently been used to discern which early end points can serve as surrogates for later end points.

QUALITY OF LIFE

The assessment of cancer patients enrolled on a clinical trial can be said to consist of two sets of end points: cancer outcomes and patient outcomes. Cancer outcomes measure the response of the tumor to treatment, the duration of the response, the symptom-free period, and the early recognition of relapse. In contrast, patient outcomes assess the benefit achieved with a given therapy by measuring the increase in survival, and the quality of life (QOL) before and after therapy. Unfortunately, physicians tend to concentrate on cancer-related outcomes, often neglecting assessments of QOL.

Several instruments to assess QOL have been developed and refined in the past two decades. Early studies equated QOL with functional status as measured by performance status scales. However, functional status and QOL have shown weak correlations, suggesting that although QOL and functional status are related, QOL encompasses more—symptoms, side effects, and social, psychologic, spiritual, family, and financial dimensions. Although QOL assessment in clinical settings is possible with currently available instruments, there must be continued development and refinement of these instruments. Such development must focus not only on extracting valuable information in an unbiased manner, but also, equally importantly, on developing an instrument that is user friendly and will be completed in a high percentage of encounters. Poor compliance is common, as seen in a recent multinational randomized phase 3 study that noted "these results might have been affected by the low return rate of the questionnaires, which decreased from about 70% at baseline to less than 15% at the end of study."[41]

NOVEL END POINTS

Randomized Discontinuation Trial

The randomized discontinued trial (RDT) phase 2 design is especially suited for agents likely to benefit only a selected, yet to be identified patient population. Initially a broad patient population is enrolled. Those with tumor shrinkage deemed of

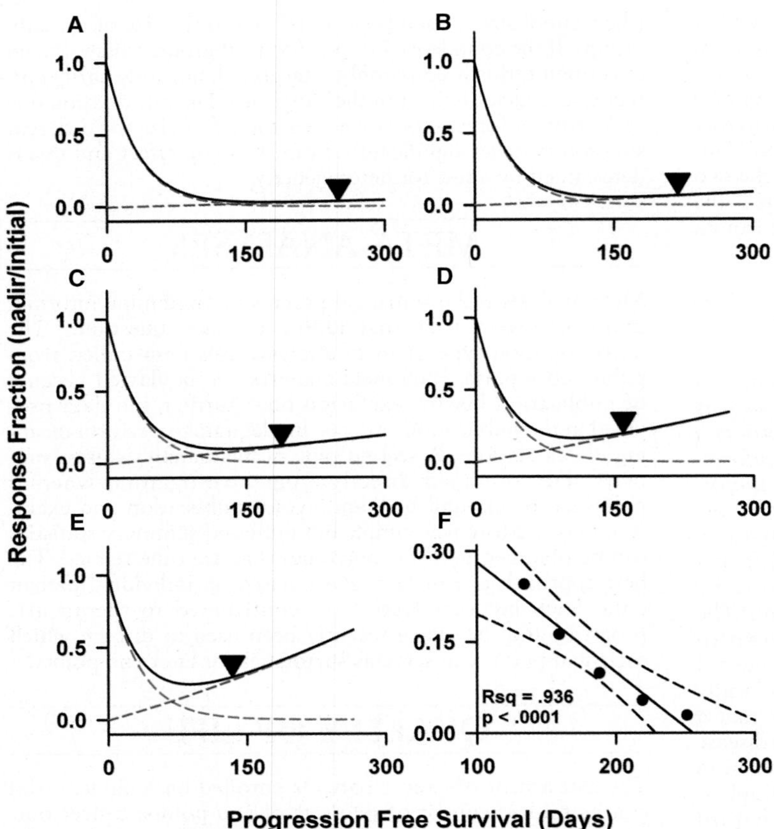

FIGURE 29.4 The effect of the growth rate constant and two commonly reported clinical values: the extent of tumor shrinkage and progression-free survival (PFS). The black line in panels (A) thru (E) depicts the tumor quantity measured as patients receive chemotherapy. This clinical measurement (*solid black line*) can be described by fitting the data to concurrent tumor regression (*dashed red line*) and growth (*dashed blue line*) curves that can be described by a rate constant and a first order kinetic equation (from ref. 43). To demonstrate the correlation between the growth rate constant, tumor shrinkage, and PFS, the same regression rate has been "modeled" in panels (A) thru (E). In contrast, the growth rate constant of each successive panel is greater (faster). Each plot has an arrow where the tumor size (*black line*) has reached a point 20% above the nadir (Response Evaluation Criteria in Solid Tumors [RECIST] definition of progressive disease). As the growth rate constant increases (faster tumor growth) from panels (A) to (E), the nadir is reached sooner, and the depth of the nadir is less. So too is the point at which PFS is scored (illustrated in each panel by an *arrow*). The correlation between PFS and extent of tumor shrinkage (nadir) is shown in panel (F), plotting the correlation between PFS and response fraction, defined as the ratio of nadir to initial value, clinically the number reported as a percentage of tumor remaining. Although the examples shown were chosen with the same regression rate constant so as to illustrate the effect of the growth rate constant, the curves are based firmly on data obtained from patients enrolled on clinical trials.

clinical significance continue treatment, while those with progressive disease or toxicity discontinue the therapy. The remaining patients with SD are randomized in a double-blind manner to continue or discontinue therapy. The primary end point is the fraction of patients progression free after an additional period or the time to progression after randomization. By identifying those with SD and thus enriching for a possible sensitive population, the RDT can confidently assesses if SD was a consequence of the investigational agent while minimizing the number of patients exposed to placebo.[42]

Growth Rate Constant

Using data gathered while a patient is receiving therapy and a novel, but simple two-phase mathematical equation, one can estimate the concomitant rates of tumor regression and growth (and derive regression and growth rate constants). A high correlation has been observed between OS and the growth rate constant, although not the regression rate constant. Other implications can be derived from calculation of the growth rate constant. As shown in Figure 29.4, the response of a tumor to a therapy is exemplified by the nadir, the time to the nadir, and the PFS and thse values are all surrogates of the growth rate constant. Besides providing a measure that is highly correlated with OS, calculating the growth rate constant allows one to (1) compare efficacy across trials; (2) predict the outcome if therapy is continued longer; and (3) provide accurate measures of efficacy that are not subject to ascertainment bias or bias that repeatedly delays evaluation of patients enrolled in one arm of a study. The utility of this approach awaits further validation.[43]

References

1. Moertel CG, Hanley JA. The effect of measuring error on the results of therapeutic trials in advanced cancer. *Cancer* 1976;38:388.
2. Miller AB, Hoogstraten B, Staquet M, Winkler A. Reporting results of cancer treatment. *Cancer* 1981;47:207.
3. Therasse P, Arbuck SG, Eisenhauer EA, et al. New guidelines to evaluate the response to treatment in solid tumors. European Organization for Research and Treatment of Cancer, National Cancer Institute of the United States, National Cancer Institute of Canada. *J Natl Cancer Inst* 2000;92:205.
4. Adjei AA, Christian M, Ivy P. Novel designs and end points for phase II clinical trials. *Clin Cancer Res* 2009;15:1866.
5. Eisenhauer EA, Therasse P, Bogaerts J, et al. New response evaluation criteria in solid tumours: revised RECIST guideline (version 1.1). *Eur J Cancer* 2009;45:228.
6. Mazumdar M, Smith A, Schwartz LH. A statistical simulation study finds discordance between WHO criteria and RECIST guideline. *J Clin Epidemiol* 2004;57:358.
7. Buyse M, Thirion P, Carlson RW, et al. Relation between tumour response to first-line chemotherapy and survival in advanced colorectal cancer: a meta-analysis. Meta-Analysis Group in Cancer. *Lancet* 2000;356:373.
8. Bruzzi P, Del ML, Sormani MP, et al. Objective response to chemotherapy as a potential surrogate end point of survival in metastatic breast cancer patients. *J Clin Oncol* 2005;23:5117.
9. Vidaurre T, Wilkerson J, Simon R, Bates SE, Fojo T. Stable disease is not preferentially observed with targeted therapies and as currently defined has limited value in drug development. *Cancer J* 2009;15:366.
10. Pazdur R. Endpoints for assessing drug activity in clinical trials. *Oncologist* 2008;13(Suppl 2):19.

11. McKee AE, Farrell AT, Pazdur R, Woodcock J. The role of the U.S. Food and Drug Administration review process: clinical trial endpoints in oncology. *Oncologist* 2010;15(Suppl 1):13.
12. Burris HA 3rd, Moore MJ, Andersen J, et al. Improvements in survival and clinical benefit with gemcitabine as first-line therapy for patients with advanced pancreas cancer: a randomized trial. *J Clin Oncol* 1997;15:2403.
13. Ohorodnyk P, Eisenhauer EA, Booth CM. Clinical benefit in oncology trials: is this a patient-centred or tumour-centred end-point? *Eur J Cancer* 2009;45:2249.
14. Cheson BD, Pfistner B, Juweid ME, et al. International Harmonization Project on Lymphoma. Revised response criteria for malignant lymphoma. *J Clin Oncol* 2007;25:579.
15. Buyse M, Sargent DJ, Grothey A, Matheson A, de Gramont A. Biomarkers and surrogate end points—the challenge of statistical validation. *Nat Rev Clin Oncol* 2010;7:309.
16. Karam AK, Karlan BY. Ovarian cancer: the duplicity of CA125 measurement. *Nat Rev Clin Oncol* 2010;7:335.
17. Ferrandina G, Ludovisi M, Corrado G, et al. Prognostic role of Ca125 response criteria and RECIST criteria: analysis of results from the MITO-3 phase III trial of gemcitabine versus pegylated liposomal doxorubicin in recurrent ovarian cancer. *Gynecol Oncol* 2008;109:187.
18. Vergote I, Rustin GJ, Eisenhauer EA, et al. Re: new guidelines to evaluate the response to treatment in solid tumors [ovarian cancer]. Gynecologic Cancer Intergroup. *J Natl Cancer Inst* 2000;92:1534.
19. Guppy AE, Rustin GJ. CA125 response: can it replace the traditional response criteria in ovarian cancer? *Oncologist* 2002;7:437.
20. Rustin GJ, Quinn M, Thigpen T, et al. Re: new guidelines to evaluate the response to treatment in solid tumors (ovarian cancer). *J Natl Cancer Inst* 2004;96:487.
21. Gronlund B, Hansen HH, Høgdall C, Høgdall EV, Engelholm SA. Do CA125 response criteria overestimate tumour response in second-line treatment of epithelial ovarian carcinoma? *Br J Cancer* 2004;90:377.
22. Bubley GJ, Carducci M, Dahut W, et al. Eligibility and response guidelines for phase II clinical trials in androgen-independent prostate cancer: recommendations from the Prostate-Specific Antigen Working Group. *J Clin Oncol* 1999;17:3461. [Erratum in *J Clin Oncol* 2007;25:1154. *J Clin Oncol* 2000;18:2644].
23. Bubley GJ, Carducci M, Dahut W, et al. Update: eligibility and response guidelines for phase II clinical trials in androgen-independent prostate cancer. *Classic Papers Curr Comments* 2001;6:311.
24. Scher HI, Halabi S, Tannock I, et al. Prostate Cancer Clinical Trials Working Group. Design and end points of clinical trials for patients with progressive prostate cancer and castrate levels of testosterone: recommendations of the Prostate Cancer Clinical Trials Working Group. *J Clin Oncol* 2008;26:1148.
25. Mazumdar M, Bajorin DF, Bacik J, et al. Predicting outcome to chemotherapy in patients with germ cell tumors: the value of the rate of decline of human chorionic gonadotrophin and alpha-fetoprotein during therapy. *J Clin Oncol* 2001;19:2534.
26. Fizazi K, Culine S, Kramar A, et al. Early predicted time to normalization of tumor markers predicts outcome in poor-prognosis nonseminomatous germ cell tumors. *J Clin Oncol* 2004;22:3868.
27. Toner GC. Early identification of therapeutic failure in nonseminomatous germ cell tumors by assessing serum tumor marker decline during chemotherapy: still not ready for routine clinical use. *J Clin Oncol* 2004;22:3842.
28. Gilligan TD, Seidenfeld J, Basch EM, et al. American Society of Clinical Oncology Clinical Practice Guideline on uses of serum tumor markers in adult males with germ cell tumors. *J Clin Oncol* 2010;28:3388.
29. Choi H, Charnsangavej C, Faria SC, et al. Correlation of computed tomography and positron emission tomography in patients with metastatic gastrointestinal stromal tumor treated at a single institution with imatinib mesylate: proposal of new computed tomography response criteria. *J Clin Oncol* 2007;25:1753.
30. Wahl RL, Jacene H, Kasamon Y, Lodge MA. From RECIST to PERCIST: evolving considerations for PET response criteria in solid tumors. *J Nucl Med* 2009;50(Suppl 1):122S.
31. Shankar LK, Hoffman JM, Bacharach S, et al. Consensus recommendations for the use of 18F-FDG PET as an indicator of therapeutic response in patients in National Cancer Institute Trials. *J Nucl Med* 2006;47:1059.
32. Young H, Baum R, Cremerius U, et al. Measurement of clinical and subclinical tumour response using [18F]-fluorodeoxyglucose and positron emission tomography: review and 1999 EORTC recommendations. European Organization for Research and Treatment of Cancer (EORTC) PET Study Group. *Eur J Cancer* 1999;35:1773.
33. Huang H, Menefee M, Edgerly M, et al. A phase II clinical trial of ixabepilone (Ixempra; BMS-247550; NSC 710428), an epothilone B analog, in patients with metastatic renal cell carcinoma. *Clin Cancer Res* 2010;16:1634.
34. Buyse M. Use of meta-analysis for the validation of surrogate endpoints and biomarkers in cancer trials. *Cancer J* 2009;15:421.
35. Wilkerson J, Fojo T. Progression-free survival is simply a measure of a drug's effect while administered and is not a surrogate for overall survival. *Cancer J* 2009;15:379.
36. Reck M, von Pawel J, Zatloukal P, et al. Overall survival with cisplatin-gemcitabine and bevacizumab or placebo as first-line therapy for non-squamous non-small-cell lung cancer: results from a randomised phase III trial (AVAiL). *Ann Oncol* 2010;21:1804.
37. Hortobagyi GN, Gomez HL, Li RK, et al. Analysis of overall survival from a phase III study of ixabepilone plus capecitabine versus capecitabine in patients with MBC resistant to anthracyclines and taxanes. *Breast Cancer Res Treat* 2010;122:409.
38. R Development Core Team. R: a language and environment for statistical computing. R Foundation for Statistical Computing, Vienna, Austria. 2010. World Wide Web URL: http://www.R-project.org.
39. Hennekens CH, Buring JE, Mayrent SL. *Epidemiology in medicine*. Boston: Little, Brown, 1987:207.
40. Cuzick J. Forest plots and the interpretation of subgroups. *Lancet* 2005;365:1308.
41. Pirker R, Pereira JR, Szczesna A, et al. Cetuximab plus chemotherapy in patients with advanced non-small-cell lung cancer (FLEX): an open-label randomised phase III trial. *Lancet* 2009;373:1525.
42. Stadler W. Other paradigms: randomized discontinuation trial design. *Cancer J* 2009;15:431.
43. Stein WD, Huang H, Menefee M, et al. Other paradigms: growth rate constants and tumor burden determined using computed tomography data correlate strongly with the overall survival of patients with renal cell carcinoma. *Cancer J* 2009;15:441.

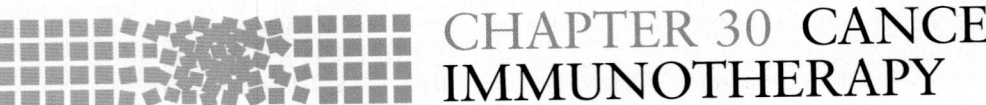

CHAPTER 30 CANCER IMMUNOTHERAPY

STEVEN A. ROSENBERG, PAUL F. ROBBINS, AND NICHOLAS P. RESTIFO

Recent progress in understanding basic aspects of cellular immunology and tumor–host immune interactions have led to the development of effective immune-based therapies capable of mediating the rejection of metastatic cancer in humans. Early studies of allografts and transplanted syngeneic tumors in mice demonstrated that it was the cellular arm of the immune response rather than the action of antibodies (humoral immunity) that was responsible for tissue rejection. Thus most modern studies of the immunotherapy of solid tumors have emphasized attempts to increase levels of immune lymphocytes capable of recognizing cancer antigens and destroying established cancers. Although antibodies that recognize growth factors on the surface of tumors can contribute to tumor regression, these antibodies appear to act primarily by interfering with growth signals rather than by the direct destruction of tumor cells, and this will be considered in Chapter 48.

Evidence for specific tumor recognition by cells of the immune system was obtained in experiments first conducted in the 1940s using murine tumors generated or induced by the mutagen methylcholanthrene (MCA). Mice that received a surgical resection of previously inoculated tumors could be protected against a subsequent tumor challenge; however, while these mice were protected against challenge with the immunizing tumor, either no or limited protection was observed against challenge with additional MCA tumors. Subsequent observations indicated that CD8+ cytotoxic T cells were the cells that were primarily responsible for mediating the rejection of MCA-induced tumors in mice. These studies led to the identification of genes that encoded tumor rejection antigens expressed on murine tumors as well as the subsequent identification of antigens recognized by human tumor-reactive T cells. The observation that many human tumor antigens represented shared, nonmutated gene products led to the expectation that effective vaccine therapies could be developed for the treatment of cancer patients. The results of vaccination therapies that boost the antitumor immune response of individuals with cancer have, however, to this point been disappointing, although the recent success of a cell-based vaccine that prolonged the life of patients with metastatic prostate cancer has stimulated renewed interest in this field. Vaccination with viruslike particles expressing human papilloma virus (HPV) proteins are successful in preventing the establishment of cervical cancer; however, this vaccine works by preventing viral infection (see Chapter 50). In spite of the presence of highly immunogenic HPV epitopes on cervical cancers, vaccination appears to be ineffective for the treatment of patients with existing disease that results from infection with this highly immunogenic virus. However, immune-based therapies have been developed that are capable of resulting in the regression of large, established tumor metastases in the human. Nonspecific immune stimulation with interleukin-2 (IL-2) administration or inhibition of regulatory pathways with an antibody that blocks the CTLA-4 cell surface molecule on lymphocytes can mediate objective regressions in about 15% of patients with metastatic melanoma. The adoptive transfer of melanoma reactive T cells can mediate objective clinical responses in 50% to 70% of patients with melanoma, and the ability to genetically modify antitumor lymphocytes is expanding this cell transfer therapy approach to the treatment of patients with other cancer histologies. Intensive studies are under way to better understand the basic mechanisms that regulate immune responses to cancer in order to design more effective immunotherapies for patients with cancer.

APPROACHES TO THE IDENTIFICATION OF HUMAN TUMOR ANTIGENS

Three major approaches have been used to identify the molecular nature of antigens that are naturally processed and presented on tumor cells, which to date comprise more than 100 antigenic proteins or epitopes (examples in Table 30.1). Most antigens have been identified using T cells with the ability to recognize intact cancer cells, as assessed by either specific cytokine release or lysis when T cells and cancer cells are cocultured. These T cells can be derived by repeated *in vitro* sensitization with tumor cells or by the culture of tumor infiltrating lymphocytes (TIL). The antitumor T cells can be used to screen tumor cDNA libraries transfected into target cells containing the appropriate major histocompatibility complex (MHC) restriction element. Alternatively, peptides can be eluted from cancer cells and used to pulse histocompatibility leukocyte antigen (HLA) matched target cells that are then tested for recognition by the antitumor T cells. To identify HLA class II–restricted tumor antigens, cellular proteins can be fractionated and fed to antigen presenting cells (APCs) until a single protein species is identified.

A second approach to identify cancer antigens uses a "reverse immunology" method in which putative antigens are used to generate tumor reactive T cells by repeated *in vitro* sensitization with candidate peptides or proteins.[1] The *in vitro*-generated tumor reactive T cells are then tested for the ability to recognize intact cancer cells to determine whether the putative antigens are naturally processed and presented on the surface of cancer cells. Alternatively, mice transgenic for human MHC molecules can be immunized with candidate antigens, and the murine T cells are used to test for cancer cell recognition. Only a small percentage of the potential epitopes are naturally presented on the cell surface at sufficient levels to allow detection by T cells. Peptides that are presented on the cell surface in association with class I molecules appear to be processed in the proteasome, a multisubunit catalytic complex that is responsible for generating the carboxy terminus of processed peptides (Fig. 30.1).[2] Thus, although it has been surprisingly easy to use these techniques to generate T cells against

TABLE 30.1

REPRESENTATIVE HLA CLASS I AND CLASS II RESTRICTED T-CELL EPITOPES

Category	Tumor Expression Pattern	Epitope	HLA Restriction Amino Acid Element		Ref.
CANCER TESTIS					
MAGE-A1	Many	EADPTGHSY	161–169	A1	319
MAGE-A3	Many	EVDPIGHLY	168–176	A1	25
NY-ESO-1	Many	SLLMWITQC	157–165	A2	30
NY-ESO-1	Many	SLLMWITQCFLPVF	157–170	DPβ1*0401/2	35
MELANOCYTE DIFFERENTIATION ANTIGEN					
MART-1	Melanoma	AAGIGILTV	27–35	A2	40
gp100	Melanoma	ITDQVPSFV	209–217	A2	47
gp100	Melanoma	YLEPGPVTA	280–288	A2	48
Tyrosinase	Melanoma	YMDGTMSQV	369–377	A2	135
Tyrosinase	Melanoma	QNILLSNAPLGPQFP	56–70	DRβ1*0401	57
Tyrosinase	Melanoma	SYLQDSDPDSFQD	450–462	DRβ1*0401	57
gp100	Melanoma	TTEWVETTARELPIPEPE	420–437	DRβ1*0701	61
OVEREXPRESSED GENE PRODUCT					
PRAME	Melanoma	LYVDSLFFL	301–309	A24	63
FGF-5	Renal carcinoma	NTYASPRFK	172–176 and 204–207	A3	136
MUTATED ANTIGEN					
CDK4	Melanoma	ACDPHSGHFV	23–32	HLA-A2	83
p14ARF:125–133,	Many	AVCPWTWLR	125–133	HLA-A*1101	87
p16INK4a:111–119	Many	AVCPWTWLR	111–119	HLA-A*1101	87
HLA-A*1101	Melanoma	—	—	HLA-A*1101	87

HLA, histocompatibility leukocyte antigen.

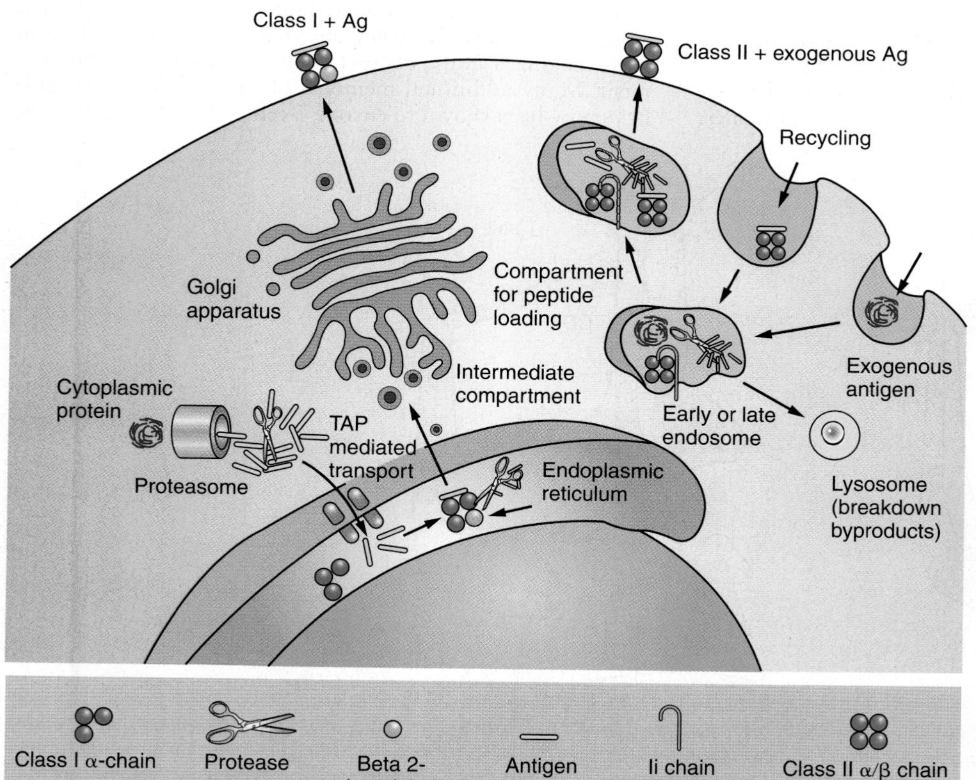

FIGURE 30.1 Intracellular trafficking pathways in the presentation of endogenous and exogenous antigen. Cytoplasmic proteins are digested by proteases in the proteasome molecular complex, trimmed, and transported into the endoplasmic reticulum by TAP (transporter associated with antigen-processing) molecules. Accessory proteins facilitate assembly of the peptide–major histocompatibility complex (MHC) class I complex. The complexes pass through the Golgi apparatus to the cell surface for presentation of antigen to CD8+ T cells. Exogenous antigen (Ag) uptake occurs by endocytosis in immature dendritic cells, macrophages, and B lymphocytes. Acid-dependent proteases digest antigens in acidified lysosomes, where peptides form complexes with MHC class II molecules. The assembled complexes move to the cell surface for presentation of antigen to CD4+ T cells. (Illustration by Emily Green Shaw.)

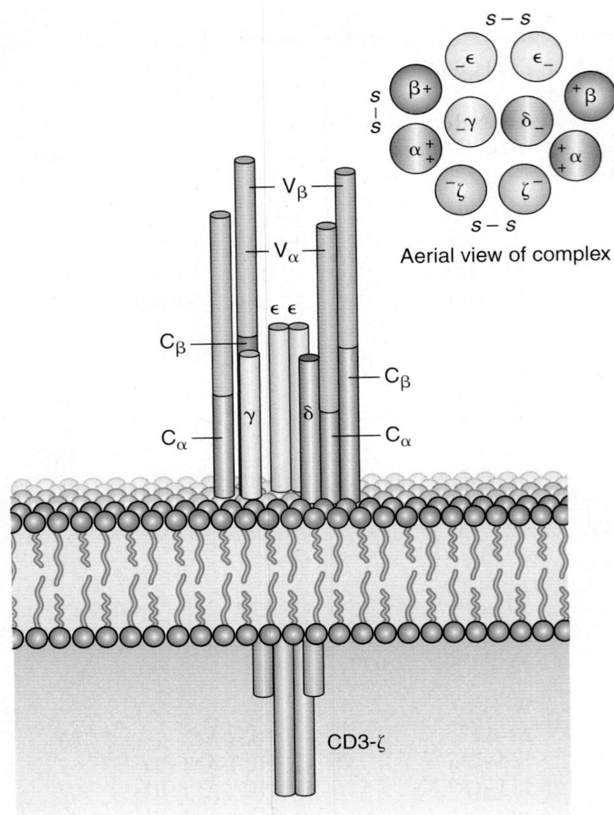

FIGURE 30.2 T-cell receptor (TCR) complex. α, α chain of the TCR; β, β chain of the TCR; V, polypeptide variable region; C, polypeptide constant region; ε, γ, δ, and ζ, chains that constitute the CD3 complex. (An alternative nomenclature includes only ε, γ, and δ chains in the CD3 complex.) (Illustration by Emily Green Shaw.)

individual peptides, only a limited number of these peptides are naturally presented on the surface of tumor cells.

All tumor antigens are recognized by T-cell receptors that recognize peptides presented on cell surface MHC molecules. CD8+ T cells recognize peptides on class I MHC and CD4+ T cells recognize peptides on class II MHC molecules (Fig. 30.2). CD8 and CD4 cells use different molecules that interact with MHC class I and II molecules, respectively, on the cell surface and serve to potentiate immune reactions (Fig. 30.3).

A third approach to the identification of tumor antigens is a method that has been termed SEREX (serological analysis of recombinant cDNA expression) libraries.[3] This method, which utilizes antisera from cancer patients to screen cDNA libraries constructed from tumor cells, has resulted in the identification of thousands of target molecules.[4] Although some of the proteins identified using this technique are expressed in a tumor-specific manner, many of the proteins identified using this technique are expressed in normal tissues but appear to be overexpressed in tumor cells. Normal proteins released from large masses of necrotic and apoptotic tumor cells may also be processed by dendritic cells (DC), which may also lead to the generation of antibodies against intracellular products that are normally sequestered from the immune system.

CATEGORIES OF TUMOR ANTIGENS CAN BE DEFINED BY EXPRESSION PATTERNS

Nonmutated Self-Antigens Recognized by CD8+ and CD4+ T Cells

Cancer/Testis Antigens

The first antigen shown to be recognized by human tumor reactive T cells, termed MAGE-1, was isolated by screening a melanoma genomic DNA library derived from the MZ2-MEL cell line with a cytotoxic T lymphocyte (CTL) clone that recognized MZ2-MEL cells.[5] The gene that was isolated, termed *MAGE-1*, was found to be a nonmutated gene that was a member of a large, previously unidentified gene family. The T-cell epitope identified using the MAGE-1 reactive CTL clone was recognized in the context of the HLA-A1 restriction element. Many additional members of the MAGE gene family have now been shown to encode T-cell epitopes recognized by

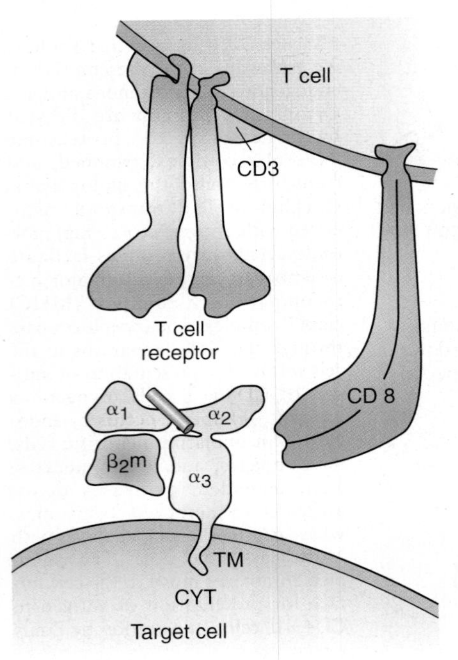

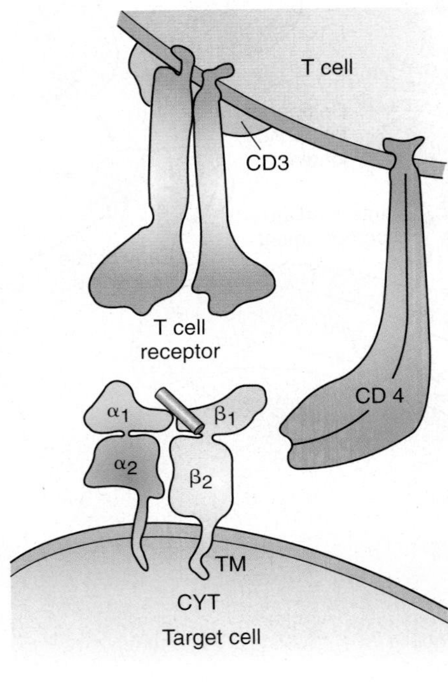

FIGURE 30.3 CD8 and CD4 cells use different molecules that interact with major histocompatibility complex (MHC) class I and II molecules respectively on the cell surface and serve to potentiate immune reactions.

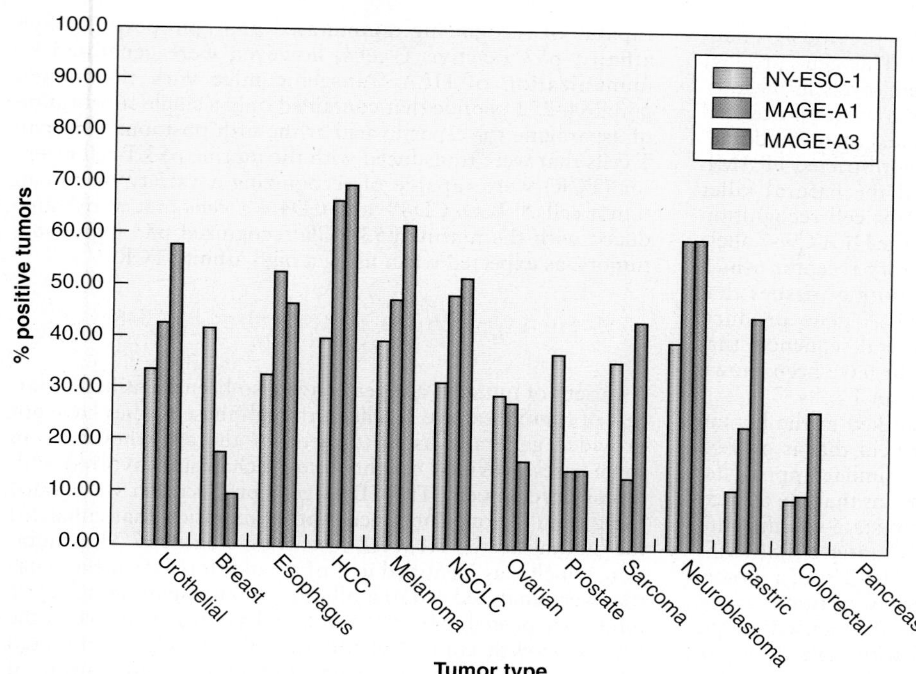

FIGURE 30.4 Expression of three different cancer/testes antigens in many different tumor types is shown. These data reflect reverse transcription-polymerase chain reaction measurements and is more sensitive than results obtained by immunohistochemistry. (Data compiled by Dr. J. Wargo. Massachusetts General Hospital.)

tumor reactive T cells.[6] These genes are expressed exclusively either in the testes or in placenta but not in other normal tissues and have been termed cancer/testis antigens. The testes and placenta fail to express HLA molecules and thus are not recognized by T cells reactive with members of this gene family. Members of the MAGE gene family are expressed in a variety of tumor types including melanoma, breast, prostate, and esophageal cancers. Although variable levels of expression were observed in these tumor types, methylation was found to play a predominant role in regulating expression of MAGE family genes. Methylation of the MAGE-1 promoter correlated with gene expression, and treatment of cultured cells with the demethylating agent 5-aza-2′-deoxycytidine upregulated gene expression in tumor cells as well as normal cultured fibroblasts.[7] Expression of three different cancer/testes antigens in many different tumor types is shown in Figure 30.4.

The NY-ESO-1 antigen, which was initially identified using the SEREX technique,[8] represents a cancer/testis antigen that is unrelated to the MAGE family of genes. The peripheral blood of a melanoma patient with a high serum titer of anti-NY-ESO-1 antibodies was found to contain HLA class I–restricted T cells directed against this antigen, and further studies resulted in the identification of the NY-ESO-1:157–165 peptide as a dominant epitope recognized by HLA-A2–restricted, NY-ESO-1 reactive T cells.[9,10] The NY-ESO-1 molecule is expressed in approximately 30% of breast, prostate, as well as melanoma tumors. In contrast to other antigens such as tyrosinase and MAGE-1, for which infrequent antibody responses have been observed, many patients with NY-ESO-1 positive tumors generate antibodies against this antigen.[11] Tumor burden was associated with the titer of anti-NY-ESO-1 antibodies.

Melanocyte Differentiation Antigens

The gene encoding the melanoma antigen designated MART-1[12] or Melan-A[13] was isolated following the screening of melanoma cDNA libraries with an HLA-A2–restricted tumor reactive TIL and a CTL clone derived by *in vitro* sensitization, respectively. The *MART-1* gene encoded a 118 amino acid protein that is expressed in 80% to 90% of fresh melanomas and cultured melanoma cell lines.[14] The majority of melanoma reactive, HLA-A2–restricted TIL were shown to recognize MART-1, indicating that this is a highly immunodominant antigen.[15,16]

The MART-1 antigen is representative of a set of gene products, termed *melanocyte differentiation antigens* (MDAs), that are expressed in melanoma as well as in normal melanocytes and are present in the skin as well as in the eye and ear. Tumors arising from glial cells have also been shown to express MDAs, and low levels of expression of these products have been detected in normal brain tissue.[17] Expression of these gene products results from the activity of tissue specific promoters, an observation that is consistent with the fact that normal melanocytes as well as glial cells are derived from neuroectodermal tissue. The results of peptide screening assays demonstrated that HLA-A2–restricted, MART-1 reactive T cells recognized a single nonamer peptide AAGIGILTV (MART-1:27-35). Several proteins were initially shown to be involved in the synthesis of melanin but were subsequently found to represent MDAs, including the gp100, tyrosinase, TRP-1, and TRP-2 gene products.[18,19]

Several of the MDAs initially identified as the targets of class I–restricted T cells have also been shown to be recognized by class II–restricted CD4+ T cells. Two epitopes of tyrosinase were found to be recognized in the context of HLA-DRβ1*0401.[20] Additional shared class II–restricted epitopes that have been described, including an epitope that is shared between TRP-1 and TRP-2,[21] as well as multiples epitopes derived from the gp100 glycoprotein.[22–24]

Overexpressed Gene Products

Gene products that are expressed at low levels in normal tissues but are overexpressed in a variety of tumor types have also been shown to be recognized by T cells. Screening of an autologous renal carcinoma cDNA library with a tumor reactive, HLA-A3–restricted T-cell clone resulted in the isolation of FGF5,[25] a protein that was expressed only at low levels in normal tissues but up-regulated in multiple renal carcinomas as well as prostate and breast carcinomas. Use of a similar approach with an HLA-A24–restricted melanoma reactive

T-cell clone resulted in the isolation of a previously undescribed gene that was termed *PRAME*.[26] This gene product appeared to be expressed in relatively high levels in melanomas as well as in additional tumor types, but was also detected in a variety of normal tissues that included testis, endometrium, ovary, and adrenals. The HLA-A24–restricted PRAME reactive T-cell clone, however, expressed the natural killer (NK) inhibitory receptor p58.2, and tumor cell recognition was dependent upon loss of expression of the HLA Cw-7 allele that represented the ligand for the inhibitory receptor, which may explain the lack of recognition of normal tissues that express relatively high levels of this HLA gene product. Products derived from endogenous retroviral sequences that are overexpressed specifically in tumor cells have been shown to be recognized by murine as well as human T cells.[27]

Immunogenic peptides have been identified in the human carcinoembryonic antigen (CEA),[28] a protein that is overexpressed in colon and breast carcinomas. Similar approaches have been used to identify epitopes in proteins that are overexpressed in prostate carcinomas, such as prostate-specific antigen (PSA)[29] and prostate-specific membrane antigen (PSMA).[30] Attempts to generate T cells reactive with Her-2/neu, a protein that is frequently overexpressed in a variety of tumor types, including breast carcinomas, have primarily focused on the Her-2/neu:369-377, a peptide that binds with high affinity to HLA-A2. Initial studies indicated that T cells generated with this peptide recognized the appropriate tumor targets.[31] Subsequently, immunization of patients with the same peptide in Freund's incomplete adjuvant was found to result in the generation of peptide reactive T cells following two *in vitro* stimulations of postvaccination peripheral blood mononuclear cell (PBMC) from three of the four patients who were tested.[32] Although these T cells recognized target cells that were pulsed with relatively low concentrations of the Her-2/neu:369-377 peptide, they failed to recognize HLA-A2+/Her-2/neu+ tumor cells, and objective clinical responses were not observed in this trial.

A peptide corresponding to amino acids 540-548 of the human telomerase reverse transcriptase (hTERT) catalytic subunit was initially reported to generate tumor-reactive T cells.[33] The results reported by additional investigators, however, failed to provide evidence that T cells generated using this peptide recognized tumor targets.[34,35] Inefficient processing may be responsible for these findings, as the incubation of a long peptide corresponding to amino acids 534 to 554 of the telomerase protein with purified proteosomes resulted in the production of multiple cleavage products but did not result in the generation of peptides containing the appropriate carboxy terminus,[34] in contrast to results observed with T-cell epitopes that are naturally processed and presented.[36]

Another method that has been used to identify naturally processed epitopes is the use of mass spectrometry to sequence peptides that have been eluted from MHC molecules isolated from the surface of human tumor cells. Use of this technique, coupled with microarray gene expression profiling, resulted in the identification of peptides that were derived from proteins that were overexpressed in tumor cells.[37] Peptides identified using this approach may in many cases not be immunogenic, as the expression of these proteins at some level in normal tissues may lead to self-tolerance; however, one of the peptides that was identified in this study also appeared to be recognized by human tumor reactive T cells.

Transgenic mice that express human HLA molecules have also been immunized in an attempt to identify T-cell epitopes that are naturally processed and presented on tumor cells. Missense mutations have been shown to result in overexpression of p53 in a wide variety of tumor types; however, self-tolerance due to the wide expression of p53 in normal cells appears to be responsible for the difficulty in generating T cells capable of recognizing nonmutated p53 epitopes.[38,39] High affinity, p53 reactive T cells, however, were generated by immunization of HLA transgenic mice with the human p53:264–272 peptide that contained only a single substitution of asparagine for aspartic acid at the fifth position.[40] Human T cells that were transduced with the murine p53 T-cell receptor (TCR) were capable of recognizing a variety of human tumor cells.[41] Both CD8+ and CD4+ T cells that were transduced with the murine p53 TCR recognized p53 expressing tumors, as expected when using a high affinity TCR.

Mutated Gene Products Recognized by CD8+ and CD4+ T Cells

A variety of mutated antigens have also been identified as targets of tumor reactive T cells. Although these studies have not provided generally useful targets for therapy, they have in some cases provided insights into mechanisms involved with tumor development. The CDK4 gene product that was cloned using a CTL clone contained a point mutation that enhanced the binding to the HLA-A2 restriction element.[42] This mutation, which was identified in 1 of an additional 28 melanomas that were analyzed, led to inhibition of binding to the cell cycle inhibitory protein $p16^{INK4a}$ and may have played a role in the loss of growth control in this tumor cell. A point-mutated product of the β-catenin gene, containing a substitution of phenylalanine for serine at position 37, was isolated by screening a cDNA library with an HLA-24–restricted, melanoma reactive TIL line.[43] The peptide epitope corresponded to amino acids 27-35 of the mutated β-catenin gene product, and the phenylalanine substitution appeared to have generated an optimal peptide for binding to HLA-A24. This mutation was found to stabilize the β-catenin gene product by altering a critical serine phosphorylation site, and 2 of 24 additional melanoma cell lines were found to express transcripts with identical mutations.[44] Previous studies demonstrating that β-catenin functions as a transcriptional activator are consistent with the hypothesis that the mutated gene products may have played a role in the development of these tumors. Additional mutated gene products identified as the targets of tumor reactive T cells, such as the mutated caspase-8 transcript identified using T cells reactive with a head and neck carcinoma[45] as well as an epitope derived from frame-shifted p14ARF and p16INK4a gene products,[46] may also play a role in tumorigenesis. A variety of mutated gene products have also been identified following screening carried out with class II–restricted, tumor reactive T cells.[47]

The observations made in murine studies that indicate that immunization against an individual tumor does not generally result in cross-protection against multiple tumors have led to the suggestion that mutant T-cell epitopes represent the dominant antigens responsible for tumor rejection.[48] Nevertheless, the studies described below suggest that normal self-proteins can represent tumor rejection antigens, as the adoptive transfer of cells whose predominant reactivity is directed against MDAs such as MART-1 and gp100 can lead to the regression of even bulky tumor deposits.

Attempts have been made to generate tumor reactive T cells using epitopes that result from mutational hot spots that are present in some oncogenes. This approach has been used to generate responses against p21ras, which is frequently mutated at positions 12 and 61, as well as peptides that result from junctional sequences present in bcr-abl fusion products that are frequently expressed in cancers such as acute lymphoblastic leukemia, as reviewed in Cheever et al.[49] and Plautz et al.[50] Although caution is needed in evaluating the reactivity of T cells generated using candidate epitope approaches, antigen presentation of class II–restricted epitopes may not result in direct recognition of tumor cells. Constitutive expression of

HLA class II has been observed in some tumor types, in particular melanoma, but is not generally observed in other tumor histologies. Antigen-presenting cells such as dendritic cells and monocytes, however, can process and present exogenous proteins derived from tumor cells to class II–restricted T cells.

Antigens in Viral-Associated Cancers

Although the expression of viral oncogenes has been shown in experimental systems to lead to the development of a wide variety of cancers, viruses have not been shown to play a role in the development of the majority of human cancers. Nevertheless, it is now clear that viruses play an important role in the etiology of cancers such as genital and hepatic carcinomas. Infection with papilloma viruses, a group of double-stranded DNA viruses that infect squamous epithelium, is highly associated with the development of a variety of genital lesions that range from warts to carcinoma. Nearly 100 HPV genotypes have been identified, and infection with HPV-16 and -18 as well as several additional genotypes is highly associated with the development of genital cancers.[51] The viral proteins E6 and E7 have been shown to lead to cellular transformation *in vitro*[52] and appear to be responsible for the induction of tumorigenesis following *in vivo* infection with HPV. Kenter et al.[53] reported on the use of a synthetic long peptide vaccine in women with HPV-16-positive high-grade vulvar intraepithelial neoplasia. Fifteen of 19 patients had clinical responses including 9 patients with complete regression of all lesions. Recombinant vaccines have been produced by the generation of viruslike particles (VLP), self-assembling particles that form following the expression of the HPV L1 protein in recombinant viral and yeast systems, that were initially found to be protective in animal models.[54,55] The results of a phase 2 trial in which 2,392 women between 16 and 23 years of age were immunized with HPV-16 VLPs indicated that 100% of those who were vaccinated were protected against infection with HPV-16.[56,57] Chapter 50 presents a detailed discussion of these preventive cancer vaccines based on immunization against viral antigens. Although vaccination with VLP does not lead to the regression of established disease, a variety of therapeutic vaccination strategies are also being tested.

A role for both hepatitis B virus (HBV) and hepatitis C virus (HCV) infection in the development of cirrhosis as well as hepatocellular carcinoma has been clearly demonstrated. Hepatitis is a noncytopathic virus, and infection of normal healthy individuals is generally controlled as a result of immune responses directed against HBV; however, in about 3% of individuals, chronic infection leads to cirrhosis and hepatocellular carcinoma. Damage to the liver appears to result in part from immune responses directed against HBV-infected cells and nonspecific inflammatory responses.[58] In contrast to HPV, studies have failed to provide evidence that oncogenic proteins derived from HBV or HCV result in transformation. The increased cell turnover that results from chronic hepatitis infection may lead to carcinoma development by increasing the number of somatic mutations generated in normal hepatocytes.[59] Vaccination with HBV has been found to be effective at reducing the rate of development of hepatoma.[60]

Immunosuppression in the Tumor Microenvironment

Peripheral T cells isolated from the majority of cancer patients do not, however, appear to exhibit a state of either generalized immunosuppression or suppression of specific tumor antigen responses, as demonstrated by the ability of patients with progressive disease to respond to vaccination with tumor antigen peptides.[61–65] In addition, many of the tumor antigen epitopes that have been studied represent self-antigens that bind MHC molecules with relatively low affinities and may not efficiently activate peripheral T cells, which are generally in a resting state. Considerable evidence exists, however, for the functional impairment of T cells present within the tumor microenvironment. The analysis of T cells present within melanomas as well as tumor-invaded lymph nodes has provided evidence for the functional impairment of T cells present at these sites, whereas T cells present in the peripheral blood analyzed simultaneously show little evidence for impairment.[66] Myeloid cells present in the tumor microenvironment have also been shown to express arginase, resulting in down-regulation of TCR zeta chain expression and impaired T-cell function in a mouse tumor model, and has been observed in human renal cancer patients.[67] Expression of arginase as well as nitric oxide synthase, which also plays a role in arginine metabolism, has been observed in human prostate carcinomas.[68] Expression of the inhibitory molecule indolamine 2,3 dioxygenase, which is involved with degradation of tryptophan, was also observed in plasmacytoid dendritic cells within tumor-draining lymph nodes.[69] Mouse studies have provided evidence that a subpopulation of monocytes that express the Gr-1 molecule can down-regulate T-cell responses.[70,71] The ability of tumors to secrete granulocyte-macrophage colony-stimulating factor (GM-CSF) has been associated with the accumulation of a population of CD34+ suppressor cells that may correspond in humans to a recent described population of cells termed myeloid suppressor cells.[72] Myeloid-derived suppressor cells have been identified in mice and humans and appear to play an important role in suppressing antitumor immune reactions.[73] Further discussion of these regulatory cell types is also considered in Chapter 17.

The identification of T regulatory (Treg) cells as potent modulators of immune responses has led to an examination of their potential role in modulating antitumor responses. Recent analyses carried out using antibodies directed against the FoxP3 protein, which serves as a marker for T regulatory cells, indicate that relatively high numbers of regulatory T cells may be present in the microenvironment of both human and murine tumors,[74,75] which may act to limit anticancer immune responses. These FoxP3+CD4+ cells infiltrating into the tumor were unable to secrete IL-2 or interferon-gamma upon *ex vivo* stimulation and were three to five times more prevalent in tumors than in peripheral blood of the same patients.[76] The majority of tumor infiltrating lymphocytes in melanomas including MART-1 antigen reactive lymphocytes expressed the PD-1 molecule and exhibited impaired cytokine secretion as well.[77] The expansion of Treg cells may result in part from expression of transforming growth factor beta (TGF-β) in the tumor environment.

Additional data have suggested that the levels of T-cell subsets detected within tumors can be associated with enhanced or decreased survival of patients with a variety of tumor types, including ovarian cancer,[78] melanoma,[79] and colon cancer.[80,81] Conflicting data concerning the exact phenotypic properties associated with prognosis have led to considerable confusion in this area. These findings may reflect the presence of an ongoing antitumor immune response that may act to limit the growth of malignant cells. The cross-presentation of tumor antigens by DC, which can be influenced by many factors, may also be important for priming effective immune responses. Thus, the balance between factors that act to promote effective antitumor immune responses and suppressive factors that act to limit those responses may be responsible for determining progression of tumor growth.

CANCER IMMUNOTHERAPIES

A wide variety of therapies have been evaluated in model systems and are now being developed for the treatment of patients

TABLE 30.2

THREE MAIN APPROACHES TO CANCER IMMUNOTHERAPY

1. Nonspecific stimulation of immune reactions
   a. Stimulate effector cells
   b. Inhibit regulatory cells
2. Active immunization to enhance antitumor reactions (cancer vaccines)
3. Passively transfer activated immune cells with antitumor activity (adoptive immunotherapy)

with cancer. These include nonspecific approaches, those that involve direct immunization of patients with a variety of immunogens, and approaches that involve the adoptive transfer of activated effector cells (Table 30.2). Much confusion related to the effectiveness of cancer immunotherapy has resulted from the lack of proper evaluation of the results of therapy using standard, accepted oncologic criteria such as the World Health Organization or the Response Evaluation Criteria in Solid Tumors (RECIST). Many clinical trials reported a positive use of "soft" criteria such as lymphoid infiltration or tumor necrosis that can occur in the natural course of cancer growth. Because of the delayed responses seen with some immunotherapy approaches, including tumor regression after initial tumor growth, guidelines have been published suggesting the use of an alternate set of immune-related response criteria for the evaluation of immune-based cancer treatments.[82,83] Other confusion has arisen from the use of inappropriate animal models. Although animal model systems have provided important clues that may lead to improved therapies, model systems that employ artificially introduced foreign antigens or that evaluate protection from tumor challenge do not appear to be relevant to the treatment of patients with bulky metastases. Short-term lung metastasis models involve the treatment of relatively small, nonvascularized tumors and also may not be directly relevant to the majority of tumors that are the targets of current clinical trials.

TABLE 30.3

RESPONSE OF PATIENTS WITH METASTATIC CANCER TREATED USING HIGH-DOSE BOLUS INTERLEUKIN-2

Diagnosis	Total[a]	CR	PR	CR + PR
		No. of Patients		
Melanoma	305	12 (4%)	27 (9%)	39 (13%)
Renal cell cancer	264	21 (8%)	32 (12%)	53 (20%)
Total	569	33 (6%)	59 (10%)	92 (16%)

CR, complete response; PR, partial response.
[a]Patients accrued between September 1985 and December 2005. Follow-up as of March 15, 2007 (median follow-up 14.3 years).

Nonantigen Specific Therapies

Interleukin-2 Therapy

The first clear evidence that immunologic manipulations could mediate the regression of large, vascularized metastatic cancers in humans comes from studies of the administration of recombinant IL-2. Early tumor treatment studies in mice demonstrated that the administration of high-dose IL-2 could result in substantial tumor regression.[84] Subsequently, clinical trials that employed treatment with high-dose IL-2 resulted in objective tumor regression in 10% to 20% of patients with metastatic melanoma and renal cancer (Table 30.3 and Fig. 30.5).[85] Almost half of the responses are complete, and over 80% of these complete responses are ongoing beyond 10 years. Thus, although the frequency of response is relatively low, response durations can be substantial and in many cases curative. These results led to the approval of IL-2 by the U.S. Food and Drug Administration for the treatment of patients with metastatic melanoma and renal cancer. The factors that are responsible for these responses are not clear. Recent

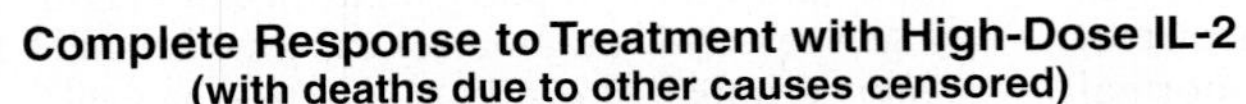

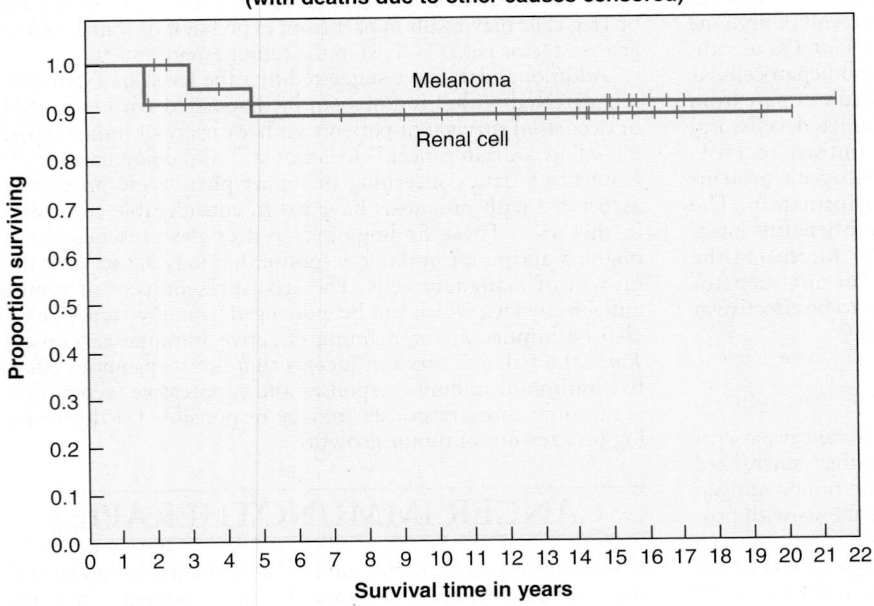

FIGURE 30.5 Actuarial survival of patients with metastatic melanoma or renal cancer who achieve a complete response.

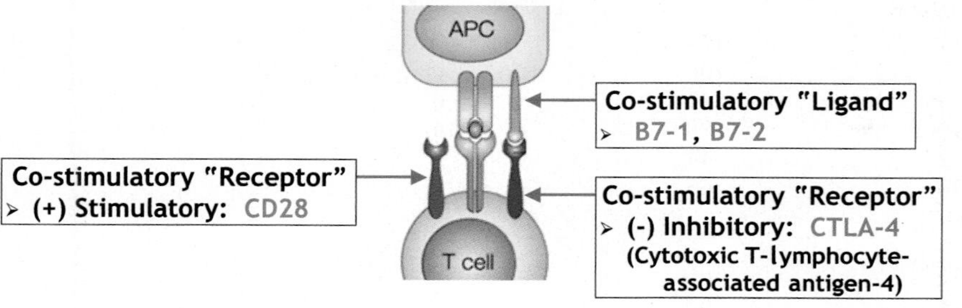

FIGURE 30.6 Mechanism of action of cytotoxic T lymphocyte–associated antigen 4 (CTLA-4). When CD28 is engaged on the T cell, reactivity of the T cell is enhanced. When CTLA-4 is engaged on the T cell, reactivity of the T cell is inhibited. Blocking of CTLA-4 with a monoclonal antibody can elicit antitumor immunity but also autoimmunity.

findings demonstrate that IL-2 administration can also lead to the expansion of peripheral Treg cells.[86,87] As many tumors have been shown to contain relatively high frequencies of Treg cells, these clinical responses may reflect the relative balance between Treg and effector T cells. At the present time the administration of high-dose IL-2 represents the best chance for the curative treatment of patients with metastatic melanoma and renal cell cancer since many of the new targeted therapies often produce few complete responses.

Anticytotoxic T Lymphocyte–Associated Antigen-4 Antibody Therapy

Cytotoxic T lymphocyte–associated antigen 4 (CTLA-4) is an immunomodulatory molecule, expressed on both CD8+ and CD4+ T cells, that maintains peripheral tolerance by suppressing T-cell activation and proliferation (Fig. 30.6). Triggering through CTLA-4 results in a decrease in T-cell responsiveness and raises the threshold for T-cell activation.[88] Mice genetically deficient in the expression of CTLA-4 develop profound autoimmunity and die of a lymphoproliferative disease at 4 weeks of age. Similarly, in humans, CTLA-4 gene polymorphisms have been linked to the development of various autoimmune diseases, including autoimmune hypothyroidism and type 1 diabetes.

Blockade of CTLA-4 function provides a means of enhancing antitumor immunity since tumors primarily express nonmutated, self-antigens. Administration of an anti-CTLA-4 blocking antibody has been shown to result in enhanced regression in murine tumor model systems when administered in combination with tumor vaccination[89] or with antibodies directed against activating molecules such as 4-1BB.[90] Translation of these findings in clinical trials demonstrated that the administration of an anti-CTLA-4 blocking antibody mediated objective responses in approximately 15% of patients with metastatic melanoma.[91] Objective responses correlated with grade 3 or 4 autoimmune manifestations, including dermatitis, enterocolitis, hepatitis, and hypophysitis. A prospective randomized trial of an anti-CTLA4 monoclonal antibody, ipilimumab, in patients with metastatic melanoma demonstrated an improvement in median survival from 6.4 months to 10.1 months in patients previously treated with other systemic approaches.[92] Grade 3 or 4 immune-related adverse events occurred in 10% to 15% of patients. Complete responses occurred in only 3 of 406 patients who received ipilimumab, suggesting that the significant improvement in survival resulted from prolonged partial responses or stabilization of disease in many patients.

The programmed death-1 (PD-1) molecule is an inhibitory receptor expressed on the surface of activated T cells and can lead to the suppression of antitumor immune responses. Phase 1 studies of an anti-PD-1 monoclonal antibody (MDX-1106) in 39 patients with advanced cancer resulted in an objective response in one patient each with colorectal cancer, melanoma, and renal cancer.[93] Objective responses were also reported by Sznol et al. in an abstract presented at the 2010 American Society of Clinical Oncology. Further evaluation of this approach is ongoing.

Active Immunization Approaches to Cancer Therapy

The molecular characterization of multiple cancer antigens led to a large number of clinical trials that attempted to actively immunize against these antigens with the expectation that cellular immune reactions would be generated capable of inhibiting the growth of established cancers. There is a paucity of murine tumor models that suggests that active vaccine approaches can mediate the regression of established vascularized tumors, so it is not surprising that these approaches have, with a few exceptions, shown little efficacy in humans. Enthusiasm about the effectiveness of cancer vaccines has often been grounded in surrogate and subjective end points, rather than reliable objective cancer regressions using standard oncologic criteria. In a review of 1,306 published vaccine treatments, including those conducted in the Surgery Branch at the National Cancer Institute (NCI), a 3.3% overall objective response rate was observed[94] (Table 30.4). In many cases relatively soft criteria such as stable disease or the regression of individual metastases in the presence of progressive disease at other sites have been reported. A variety of immunizing vectors have been used, including tumor-derived peptides, proteins, whole tumor cells, recombinant viruses, dendritic cells, and heat-shock proteins.[94–106] Although many of these approaches can lead to the development of circulating T cells that can recognize the immunizing tumor antigen, these T cells rarely cause the inhibition of established tumors, a point that has led to much confusion in the field of tumor immunology. The generation of antitumor T cells *in vivo* is likely a necessary, but certainly not a sufficient criteria for the development of a clinically active immunotherapy. Often T cells with weak avidity for tumor recognition are generated and the tolerizing and inhibitory influences that exist *in vivo* must be overcome for an effective immune response to cause tumor destruction.

Peptide Vaccines

Vaccines based on the administration of tumor-derived peptides administered in a variety of adjuvants have been extensively explored. Immunization was shown to result in the expansion of T cells reactive with peptides from melanoma-melanocyte antigens such as gp100, MART-1, and tyrosinase as well as against many of the cancer-testes antigens such as

TABLE 30.4

REVIEW OF CLINICAL VACCINE STUDIES IN PATIENTS WITH METASTATIC CANCER

Published	No. of Trials	Total (No. of Patients)	Objective Responders	Percent
Peptide	11	175	7	4.0
Pox virus	7	200	0	0
Tumor cells	5	142	6	4.2
Dendritic cells	10	198	14	7.1
Heat shock proteins	2	44	2	4.5
Total	33	765	29	4.0
SURGERY BRANCH				
Peptide	15	366	9	2.9
Virus or DNA	8	160	3	1.9
Dendritic cells	2	15	2	13.3
Total	25	541	14	2.6
Overall:	58	1,306	43	3.3

NY-ESO-1, MAGE A1, and MAGE A3. Although the expansion of T cells directed against the immunizing peptide was observed in many of these trials, generally less than 3% of the treated patients demonstrated clinical responses. Additional findings demonstrate that tumor progression can occur even in the presence of relatively high frequencies of tumor antigen reactive T cells. In an adjuvant trial of patients with no evidence of disease at the start of the course of vaccination, multiple courses of peptide immunization were carried out over a course of 48 weeks, using the modified gp100:209–217 2M peptide, and resulted in the induction of high levels of peptide and tumor reactive T cells.[64] Analysis of reactivity of PBMC obtained following multiple tests using enzyme-linked immunospot (ELISPOT) assays indicated that in 44% of the immunized patients between 1% and 10% of all peripheral CD8+ T cells recognized the immunogen, and in 17% of patients more than 10% of peripheral CD8+ T cells recognized this peptide. Although immunoselection for loss of antigen or HLA-A2 expression could have been partially responsible for some of the recurrences, patients did recur in the presence of tumors that clearly expressed both antigen and HLA-A2.

In a phase 2 study a heteroclitic peptide vaccine derived from the gp100 melanoma/melanocyte tumor antigen administered along with IL-2 to patients with metastatic melanoma was reported to increase the objective response rate compared to the administration of IL-2 alone.[63] At the 2009 annual meeting of the American Society of Clinical Oncology Schwartzentruber et al.[107] reported a prospective randomized study in 185 patients confirming that the addition of this peptide vaccine doubled the response rate to IL-2 ($P = .022$) and improved progression-free survival ($P = .010$) but only a trend to improved survival was seen ($P = .096$). In a prospective randomized trial the addition of this peptide vaccine did not improve the results when added to the administration of an anti-CTLA4 monoclonal antibody, ipilimumab.[92]

Whole Cell Vaccines

Clinical trials employing whole tumor cells as a vaccine represents an attractive immunization approach since one could theoretically immunize against multiple antigens at the same time.[108] Despite many attempts, no whole cell vaccines have been shown to be clinically effective in humans. In historically controlled analyses treatment with a combination of three irradiated allogeneic melanoma cells with BCG (Canvaxin trial) resulted in an overall survival rate of 49%, as opposed to a rate of 37% in patients who did not receive the vaccine.[109] Patients in the treatment group appeared to have all of the same tumor and demographic characteristics as the vaccine patients. Further evaluation of this approach in phase 3 trials, however, showed no significant difference in survival of stage III or IV melanoma patients receiving this treatment compared to controls receiving BCG, and this approach is no longer being used.[110]

Gene-modified cells have been evaluated for their effectiveness in cancer therapy protocols. In a murine model system, mice that were immunized with B16 melanoma cells transduced individually with genes encoding ten cytokines were examined for their resistance to a subsequent inoculation of the wild type B16 tumor.[111] The results indicated that tumors transduced with the GM-CSF gene provided significant protection against B16 tumor challenge. In a clinical trial to study immunization of patients with autologous renal carcinoma cells that had been transduced with the GM-CSF gene, immune responses against the parental renal carcinomas were observed, as measured by delayed-type hypersensitivity (DTH) responses, and an objective clinical response was observed in 1 of the 16 fully evaluable patients.[112]

Two recent trials have pointed to a possible danger of using GM-CSF as an immune adjuvant to a cancer vaccine.[113] A recent study that randomized 121 patients with completely resected stage IIB to IV melanoma to receive a multiple peptide vaccine alone or with GM-CSF showed a significant decrease in CD8+ T cell responses when GM-CSF was added ($P<.001$) and a significant decrease in CD4+ tetanus responses as well ($P = .005$).[114] Overall and progression-free survivals were lower with GM-CSF, but this was not statistically significant. Similarly, another prospective randomized trial that added GM-CSF to a whole cell vaccine in patients with resected stage IIB to IV melanoma resulted in a decrease in immune parameters and a significant decrease in survival at 2 years in the GM-CSF group ($P = .002$).[115]

Vaccines Using Antigen Presenting Cells

Other approaches have utilized immunization with professional antigen-presenting cells such as autologous DC. In one trial, patients were vaccinated with autologous DC that was pulsed either with peptide or melanoma lysates, which resulted in objective clinical responses in 5 of 16 treated patients[116]; however, follow-up studies that involved treatment of larger numbers of patients using this approach have not been reported by this group. Another approach has employed immunization of patients with DCs that have been transfected either with mRNA encoding individual tumor antigens or bulk mRNA isolated from tumor cells.[117,118]

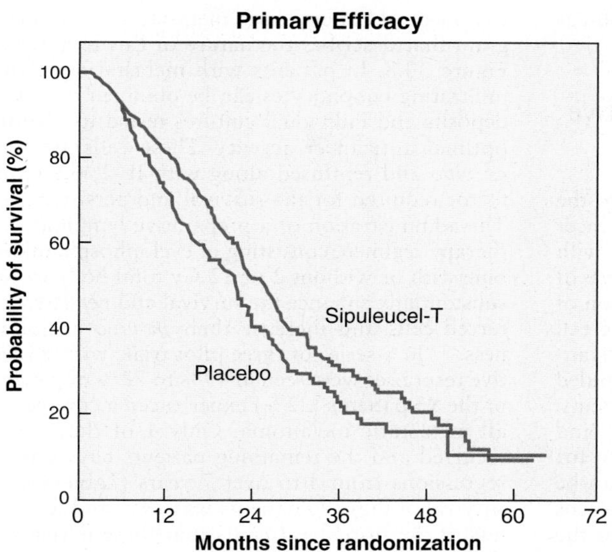

Number at risk

Sipuleucel-T	341	274	129	49	14	1
Placebo	171	123	55	19	4	1

FIGURE 30.7 Kaplan-Meier estimate of the overall survival in patients with metastatic castration-resistant prostate cancer treated with Sipuleucel-T antigen–presenting cell immunotherapy. A modest but statistically significant improvement in survival was seen ($P = .03$).

Although expansion of tumor-reactive T cells following these treatments has been reported, only sporadic cases of tumor regression were observed in these trials. Additional trials are also being carried out using dendritic cells pulsed with either tumor lysates or using hybrids of dendritic cells and cancer cells. Recently, however, a prospective randomized trial that showed a clinical benefit of immunization with antigen-presenting cells was carried out by the Dendreon Corporation (Seattle, Washington). This trial used an antigen-presenting cell vaccine loaded with prostatic acid phosphatase linked to GM-CSF compared to placebo in men with hormone-refractory prostate cancer.[119] Of 330 patients who received the vaccine treatment, 1 objective partial response was seen. Eight patients experienced a PSA drop of at least 50%. There was no difference in the time to disease progression; however, the vaccine group had a median survival of 25.8 months compared to 21.7 months in the placebo group, and based on this statistically significant survival improvement, this treatment was approved by the U.S. Food and Drug Administration (Fig. 30.7).

Other Vaccine Approaches

Multiple trials have been carried out using either recombinant viral constructs or naked DNA encoding particular tumor antigens. In these trials, recombinants that contained either full-length gene products or minigenes containing individual or multiple T-cell epitopes were evaluated. The failure in general to detect enhanced precursor frequencies directed against the tumor antigens may have resulted from the dominance of viral epitopes. Attempts have also been made to enhance the potency of vaccination protocols through the provisions of costimulatory signals. In studies carried out in a mouse model system, evidence for enhanced immunity was obtained following immunization with a recombinant virus that contain the genes encoding the candidate tumor antigen CEA along with genes encoding LFA-3, ICAM-1, and B7-1, termed TRICOM.[120,121] One objective response was also observed in 58 patients with advanced CEA-expressing cancers that were treated with TRICOM-CEA.[122] No improvement in survival was seen in a randomized trial using TRICOM MUC-1/CEA in patients with pancreatic cancer. Larger randomized patient studies will be needed to test the efficacy of this approach. A randomized phase 2 trial was performed of a poxviral-based vaccine (TRICOM/PSA) targeting PSA administered with GM-CSF. Although the primary end point of progression-free survival showed no difference between the vaccine and the control group, there was a significant survival improvement in patients treated with the vaccine. This trial is now being repeated with survival as the primary end point.[120]

The first autologous heat shock protein (HSP) vaccine introduced in clinical trials was Oncophage or, HSPPC-96 (heat-shock protein-peptide complex 96) (Antigenics Inc, Woburn, Massachusetts), produced from surgically resected cancer tissue and formulated for intradermal or subcutaneous injection. Numerous HSP vaccine trials have been carried out in a variety of patients, including those with resected pancreatic adenocarcinoma, renal cell carcinoma, melanoma, colorectal cancer, non-Hodgkin's lymphoma, and gastric cancer. However, prospective randomized trials in patients with renal cancer and with melanoma failed to demonstrate a survival advantage using these HSP-based vaccines.[123]

The presence of idiotypic determinants on the immunoglobulin molecules expressed by B-cell lymphomas has presented investigators with unique targets for vaccine trials of patients with hematopoietic malignancies. Immunization with idiotypic proteins that have been coupled to carrier proteins has been shown to result in long-term tumor regression in some patients. These responses were associated with serological anti-idiotypic responses as well as FcγRIIIa polymorphisms, suggesting that humoral immunity may play a significant role in these responses. Immunization with DCs that have been pulsed with idiotype protein was also shown to result in tumor regression in four of ten vaccinated patients.[124] Two randomized trials using an idiotype–keyhole limpet hemocyanin (KLH) vaccine in patients with non-Hodgkin's lymphoma failed to demonstrate an improvement in progression-free survival. However a report by Schuster et al.[125] at the 2009 meeting of the American Association of Clinical Oncology reported a prospective randomized trial of an idiotype-KLH/GM-CSF vaccine that showed an improvement in the time to relapse in patients with follicular lymphoma.[125]

Passive Immunological Treatments: Adoptive Cell Transfer

Adoptive cellular immunotherapy refers to the transfer to the tumor-bearing host of immune lymphocytes with anticancer activity. Studies that used cell transfer therapy in patients with metastatic melanoma have provided the clearest evidence of the power of the immune system to mediate the regression of advanced metastatic cancers in humans.[126–131] Adoptive cell therapy has several theoretical as well as practical advantages.[129] Lymphocytes with antitumor activity can be expanded to very large numbers *ex vivo* for infusion into cancer patients. These cells can be tested *in vitro* for antitumor activity, and cells with appropriate properties such as high avidity for tumor recognition and a high proliferative potential can be identified and selectively expanded for treatment. These cells can be activated *in vitro* and thus are not subjected to the tolerizing influences that exist *in vivo*. Perhaps most important, the host can be manipulated prior to the transfer of the anticancer cells to provide an optimal tumor microenvironment free of *in vivo* suppressive factors.[129] Studies have shown that the transfer of cultured lymphocytes with antiviral activity can prevent Epstein-Barr virus infections as well as the subsequent development of posttransplant lymphoproliferative diseases. Cultured lymphocytes have been used for the treatment of patients with established Epstein-Barr virus (EBV)–induced lymphomas.[132–134]

The best evidence for the ability of adoptive cell transfer to successfully treat patients with solid tumors comes from the treatment of patients with metastatic melanoma.[128–131] A diagram that describes the nature of this treatment is shown in Figure 30.8. In patients with metastatic melanoma, tumor-infiltrating lymphocytes can be obtained from resected tumor deposits and individual cultures tested to identify those with optimal anticancer activity. These cells are then expanded *ex vivo* and reinfused along with IL-2, the requisite growth factor required for the survival and persistence of these cells. The administration of a preparative lymphodepleting chemotherapy regimen, consisting of cyclophosphamide and fludarabine with or without 2 or 12 Gy total body irradiation, could substantially enhance the survival and persistence of the transferred cells and increase their *in vivo* antitumor effectiveness.[130] In a series of three pilot trials with 93 patients objective responses were seen in 49% to 72% of patients.[131] Twenty of the 93 patients (22%) experienced a complete regression of all metastatic melanoma. Only 1 of these 20 patients has recurred and the remaining patients have ongoing complete regressions from 3 to over 7 years (Table 30.5). The 5-year survival of these 93 patients was 29% and was similar regardless of the prior treatments that these patients had received (Fig. 30.9).

Tumor-infiltrating lymphocytes with antitumor activity can only be reproducibly obtained from patients with metastatic melanoma but not from other tumors. To more widely apply adoptive cell therapy, techniques have been developed to genetically modify lymphocytes using retroviral transduction to insert antitumor T-cell receptors into the normal lymphocytes of patients.[135] In early trials the infusion of transduced circulating autologous lymphocytes with genes encoding T-cell receptors reactive with either the MART-1 or the gp100 melanoma/melanocyte tumor antigens has resulted in objective responses in 30% of patients.[136] The targeting of these normal

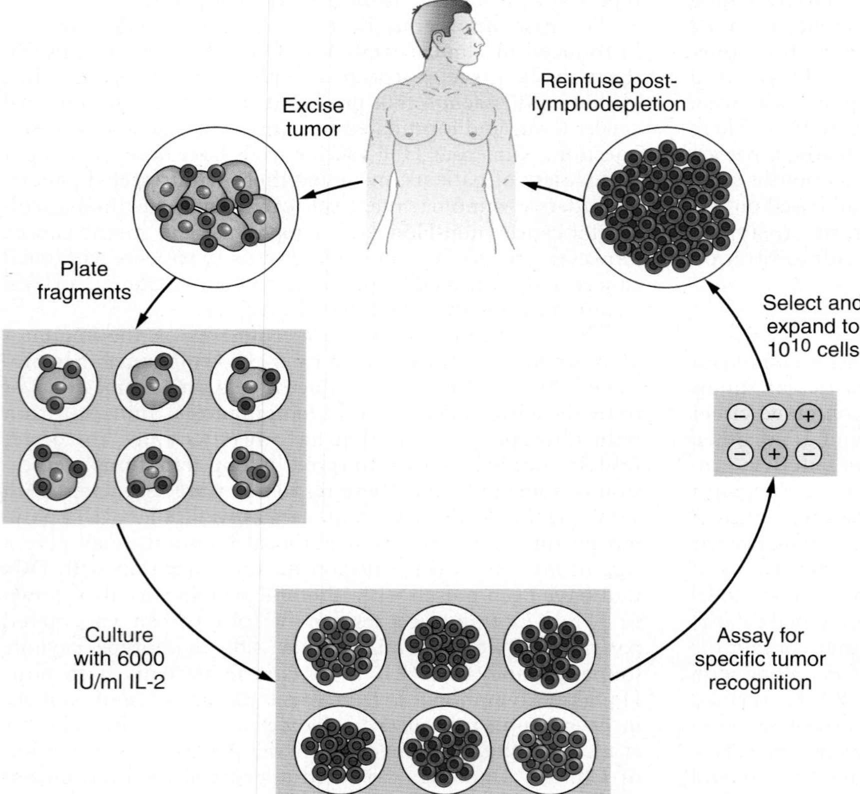

FIGURE 30.8 Diagram of the adoptive cell therapy of patients with metastatic melanoma. Tumors are resected and individual cultures are grown and tested for antitumor reactivity. Optimal cultures are expanded *in vitro* and reinfused into the autologous patient who had received a preparative lymphodepleting chemotherapy.

TABLE 30.5

CELL TRANSFER THERAPY IN PATIENTS WITH METASTATIC MELANOMA

Treatment	Total	PR	CR	OR (%)
		Number of Patients (duration in months)		
No TBI	43	16(37%) (84, 36, 29, 28, 14, 12, 11, 7, 7, 7, 7, 4, 4, 2, 2, 2)	5(12%) (82+, 81+, 79+, 78+, 64+)	21 (49%)
200 TBI	25	8(32%) (14, 9, 6, 6, 5, 4, 3, 3)	5(20%) (68+, 64+, 60+, 57+, 54+)	13 (52%)
1,200 TBI	25	8 (32%) (21, 13, 7, 6, 6, 5, 3, 2)	10 (40%) (48+, 45+, 44+, 44+, 39+, 38+, 38+, 38+, 37+, 19)	18 (72%)
TOTAL	93	32 (34%)	20 (22%)	52 (56%)

antigens caused mild uveitis and auditory problems that could be overcome by the application of topical steroids. Similar studies that utilized the transduction of autologous lymphocytes with genes encoding T-cell receptors reactive with the NY-ESO-1 cancer antigen have also shown objective responses in patients with metastatic synovial cell sarcoma (in press). Approaches using chrimeric antigen receptors that utilize the combining site of monoclonal antibodies genetically fused to intracellular signaling chains have resulted in the *in vitro* generation of T cells capable of recognizing cell surface antigens based on recognition by antibodies instead of T-cell receptors.[137] Utilization of this approach has shown evidence of *in vivo* clinical effect in patients with neuroblastoma and in patients with B-cell lymphomas.

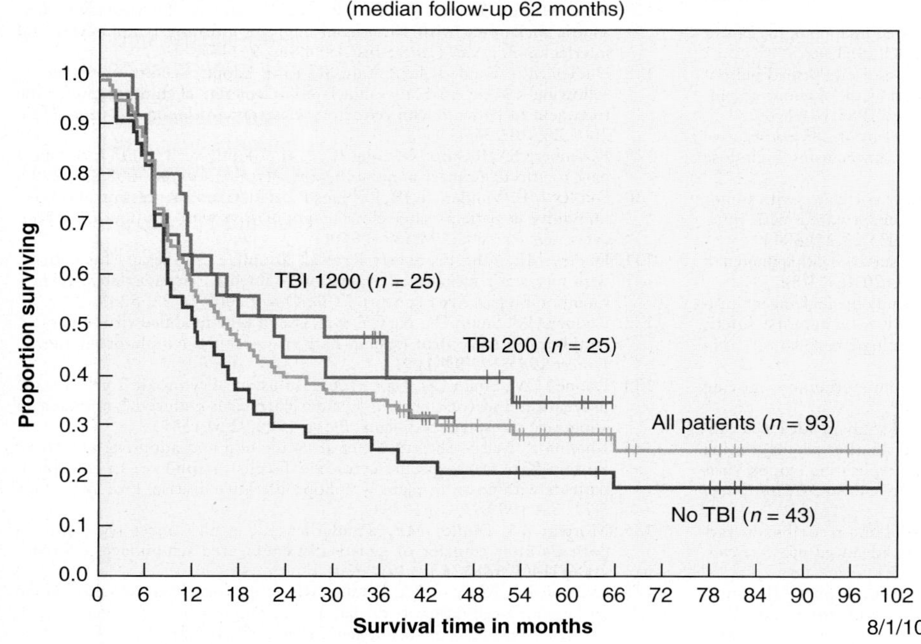

FIGURE 30.9 Kaplan-Meier estimate of the overall survival in patients with metastatic melanoma treated with adoptive cell therapy after receiving a preparative lymphodepleting regimen of cyclophosphamide/fludarabine alone or with 2 or 12 Gy total body irradiation.

Selected References

The full list of references for this chapter appears in the online version.

5. van der Bruggen P, Traversari C, Chomez P, et al. A gene encoding an antigen recognized by cytolytic T lymphocytes on a human melanoma. *Science* 1991;254(5038):1643.
8. Chen YT, Scanlan MJ, Sahin U, et al. A testicular antigen aberrantly expressed in human cancers detected by autologous antibody screening. *Proc Natl Acad Sci U S A* 1997;94(5):1914.
12. Kawakami Y, Eliyahu S, Delgado CH, et al. Cloning of the gene coding for a shared human melanoma antigen recognized by autologous T cells infiltrating into tumor. *Proc Natl Acad Sci U S A* 1994;91(9):3515.
24. Parkhurst MR, Riley JP, Robbins PF, et al. Induction of CD4+ Th1 lymphocytes that recognize known and novel class II MHC restricted epitopes from the melanoma antigen gp100 by stimulation with recombinant protein. *J Immunother* 2004;27(2):79.
53. Kenter GG, Welters MJP, Valentijn AR, et al. Vaccination against HPV-16 oncoproteins for vulvar intraepithelial neoplasia. *N Engl J Med* 2009;361(19):1838.
56. Koutsky LA, Ault KA, Wheeler CM, et al. A controlled trial of a human papillomavirus type 16 vaccine. *N Engl J Med* 2002;347(21):1645.
57. Villa LL, Costa RL, Petta CA, et al. Prophylactic quadrivalent human papillomavirus (types 6, 11, 16, and 18) L1 virus-like particle vaccine in young women: a randomised double-blind placebo-controlled multicentre phase II efficacy trial. *Lancet Oncol* 2005;6(5):271.
63. Rosenberg SA, Yang JC, Schwartzentruber DJ, et al. Immunologic and therapeutic evaluation of a synthetic peptide vaccine for the treatment of patients with metastatic melanoma. *Nat Med* 1998;4(3):321.
64. Rosenberg SA, Sherry RM, Morton KE, et al. Tumor progression can occur despite the induction of very high levels of self/tumor antigen-specific CD8+ T cells in patients with melanoma. *J Immunol* 2005;175(9):6169.
73. Gabrilovich DI, Nagaraj S. Myeloid-derived suppressor cells as regulators of the immune system. *Nat Rev Immunol* 2009;9(3):162.
76. Ahmadzadeh M, Felipe-Silva A, Heemskerk B, et al. FOXP3 expression accurately defines the population of intratumoral regulatory T cells that selectively accumulate in metastatic melanoma lesions. *Blood* 2008; 112(13):4953.
77. Ahmadzadeh M, Johnson LA, Heemskerk B, et al. Tumor antigen-specific CD8 T cells infiltrating the tumor express high levels of PD-1 and are functionally impaired. *Blood* 2009;114(8):1537.
80. Galon J, Costes A, Sanchez-Cabo F, et al. Type, density, and location of immune cells within human colorectal tumors predict clinical outcome. *Science* 2006;313(5795):1960.
82. Wolchok JD, Hoos A, O'Day S, et al. Guidelines for the evaluation of immune therapy activity in solid tumors: immune-related response criteria. *Clin Cancer Res* 2009;15(23):7412.
83. Hoos A, Eggermont AM, Janetzki S, et al. Improved endpoints for cancer immunotherapy trials. *J Natl Cancer Inst* 2010;102(18):1388.
84. Rosenberg SA, Mule JJ, Spiess PJ, et al. Regression of established pulmonary metastases and subcutaneous tumor mediated by the systemic administration of high dose recombinant IL-2. *J Exp Med* 1985;161:1169.
85. Rosenberg SA, Yang JC, Topalian SL, et al. Treatment of 283 consecutive patients with metastatic melanoma or renal cell cancer using high-dose bolus interleukin-2. *JAMA* 1994;271:907.
91. Attia P, Phan GQ, Maker AV, et al. Autoimmunity correlates with tumor regression in patients with metastatic melanoma treated with anti-cytotoxic T-lymphocyte antigen-4. *J Clin Oncol* 2005;23(25):6043.
92. Hodi FS, O'Day SJ, McDermott DF, et al. Improved survival with ipilimumab in patients with metastatic melanoma. *N Engl J Med* 2010;363(8):711.
93. Brahmer JR, Drake CG, Wollner I, et al. Phase I study of single-agent anti-programmed death-1 (MDX-1106) in refractory solid tumors: safety, clinical activity, pharmacodynamics, and immunologic correlates. *J Clin Oncol* 2010;28(19):3167.
94. Rosenberg SA, Yang JC, Restifo NP. Cancer immunotherapy: moving beyond current vaccines. *Nat Med* 2004;10(9):909.
97. Marshall JL, Hoyer RJ, Toomey MA, et al. Phase I study in advanced cancer patients of a diversified prime-and-boost vaccination protocol using recombinant vaccinia virus and recombinant nonreplicating avipox virus to elicit anti-carcinoembryonic antigen immune responses. *J Clin Oncol* 2000;18(23):3964.
98. Eder JP, Kantoff PW, Roper K, et al. A phase I trial of a recombinant vaccinia virus expressing prostate-specific antigen in advanced prostate cancer. *Clin Cancer Res* 2000;6(5):1632.
107. Schwartzentruber DJ, Lawson D, Richards J, et al. A phase III multi-institutional randomized study of immunization with the gp100:209–217(210M) peptide followed by high dose IL-2 alone in patients with metastatic melanoma. *J Clin Oncol* 2009;27:18s (abst CRA9011).
110. Faries MB, Morton DL. Therapeutic vaccines for melanoma: current status. *BioDrugs* 2005;19(4):247.
111. Dranoff G, Jaffee E, Lazenby A, et al. Vaccination with irradiated tumor cells engineered to secrete murine granulocyte-macrophage colony-stimulating factor stimulates potent, specific, and long-lasting anti-tumor immunity. *Proc Natl Acad Sci U S A* 1993;90(8):3539.
112. Simons JW, Jaffee EM, Weber CE, et al. Bioactivity of autologous irradiated renal cell carcinoma vaccines generated by ex vivo granulocyte-macrophage colony-stimulating factor gene transfer. *Cancer Res* 1997;57(8):1537.
113. Eggermont AM. Immunostimulation versus immunosuppression after multiple vaccinations: the woes of therapeutic vaccine development. *Clin Cancer Res* 2009;15(22):6745.
114. Slingluff CL, Petroni GR, Olson WC, et al. Effect of granulocyte/macrophage colony-stimulating factor on circulating CD8+ T-cell responses to a multipeptide melanoma vaccine: Outcome of a multicenter randomized trial. *Clin Cancer Res* 2009;15(22):7036.
115. Faries MB, Hsueh EC, Ye X, et al. Effect of granulocyte/macrophage colony-stimulating factor on vaccination with an allogeneic whole-cell melanoma vaccine. *Clin Cancer Res* 2009;15(22):7029.
116. Nestle FO, Alijagic S, Gilliet M, et al. Vaccination of melanoma patients with peptide- or tumor lysate-pulsed dendritic cells. *Nat Med* 1998; 4(3):328.
119. Kantoff PW, Higano CS, Shore ND, et al. Sipuleucel-T immunotherapy for castration-resistant prostate cancer. *N Engl J Med* 2010;363(5):411.
120. Kantoff PW, Schuetz TJ, Blumenstein BA, et al. Overall survival analysis of a phase II randomized controlled trial of a poxviral-based PSA-targeted immunotherapy in metastatic castration-resistant prostate cancer. *J Clin Oncol* 2010;28(7):1099.
121. Hodge JW, Sabzevari H, Yafal AG, et al. A triad of costimulatory molecules synergize to amplify T-cell activation. *Cancer Res* 1999;59(22):5800.
122. Marshall JL, Gulley JL, Arlen PM, et al. Phase I study of sequential vaccinations with fowlpox-CEA(6D)-TRICOM alone and sequentially with vaccinia-CEA(6D)-TRICOM, with and without granulocyte-macrophage colony-stimulating factor, in patients with carcinoembryonic antigen-expressing carcinomas. *J Clin Oncol* 2005;23(4):720.
123. Wang HH, Mao CY, Teng LS, Cao J. Recent advances in heat shock protein-based cancer vaccines. *Hepatobiliary Pancreat Dis Int* 2006;5(1):22.
124. Weng WK, Czerwinski D, Timmerman J, et al. Clinical outcome of lymphoma patients after idiotype vaccination is correlated with humoral immune response and immunoglobulin G Fc receptor genotype. *J Clin Oncol* 2004;22(23):4717.
125. Schuster SJ, Neelapu SS, Gause BL, et al. Idiotype vaccine therapy (BiovaxID) in follicular lymphoma in first complete remission: phase III clinical trial results. *J Clin Oncol* 2009;27(18S):2.
126. Rosenberg SA, Spiess P, Lafreniere R. A new approach to the adoptive immunotherapy of cancer with tumor-infiltrating lymphocytes. *Science* 1986;233(4770):1318.
127. Rosenberg SA, Yannelli JR, Yang JC, et al. Treatment of patients with metastatic melanoma with autologous tumor-infiltrating lymphocytes and interleukin 2. *J Natl Cancer Inst* 1994;86(15):1159.
128. Dudley ME, Wunderlich JR, Yang JC, et al. Adoptive cell transfer therapy following non-myeloablative but lymphodepleting chemotherapy for the treatment of patients with refractory metastatic melanoma. *J Clin Oncol* 2005;23(10):2346.
129. Rosenberg SA, Restifo NP, Yang JC, et al. Adoptive cell transfer: a clinical path to effective cancer immunotherapy. *Nat Rev Cancer* 2008;8(4):299.
130. Dudley ME, Wunderlich JR, Robbins PF, et al. Cancer regression and autoimmunity in patients after clonal repopulation with antitumor lymphocytes. *Science* 2002:298(5594):850.
131. Dudley ME, Yang JC, Sherry R, et al. Adoptive cell therapy for patients with metastatic melanoma: evaluation of intensive myeloablative chemoradiation preparative regimens. *J Clin Oncol* 2008;26(32):5233.
132. Rooney CM, Smith CA, Ng CY, et al. Use of gene-modified virus-specific T lymphocytes to control Epstein-Barr-virus–related lymphoproliferation. *Lancet* 1995;345(8941):9.
133. Rooney CM, Smith CA, Ng CY, et al. Infusion of cytotoxic T cells for the prevention and treatment of Epstein-Barr virus–induced lymphoma in allogeneic transplant recipients. *Blood* 1998;92(5):1549.
134. Khanna R, Bell S, Sherritt M, et al. Activation and adoptive transfer of Epstein-Barr virus–specific cytotoxic T cells in solid organ transplant patients with posttransplant lymphoproliferative disease. *Proc Natl Acad Sci U S A* 1999;96(18):10391.
135. Morgan RA, Dudley ME, Wunderlich JR, et al. Cancer regression in patients after transfer of genetically engineered lymphocytes. *Science* 2006;314(5796):126.
136. Johnson LA, Morgan RA, Dudley ME, et al. Gene therapy with human and mouse T-cell receptors mediates cancer regression and targets normal tissues expressing cognate antigen. *Blood* 2009;114(3):535.
137. Eshhar Z, Waks T, Gross G, Schindler DG, et al. Specific activation and targeting of cytotoxic lymphocytes through chimeric single chains consisting of antibody-binding domains and the gamma or zeta subunits of the immunoglobulin and T-cell receptors. *Proc Natl Acad Sci U S A* 1993; 90(2):720.

CHAPTER 31 HEALTH SERVICES RESEARCH AND ECONOMICS OF CANCER CARE

CRAIG C. EARLE AND DEBORAH SCHRAG

Cancer-related health services research is a field of study that focuses primarily on how cancer care is delivered in the "real world." Its central questions consider how research discoveries made in the laboratory and in experimental settings such as clinical trials are translated into practice and the outcomes realized within the broader context of communities and populations. In cancer medicine, clinical trials establish the theoretic *efficacy* of health care interventions under controlled, ideal conditions. Indeed, most chapters in this book focus on delineating the incremental body of knowledge gained as a consequence of basic science, translational studies, and clinical trials that determine efficacy. Health services research investigates the *effectiveness* of these interventions as they are rolled out into diverse settings. It considers the differences between efficacy and effectiveness and explores the underlying reasons for variation in practice and effectiveness across settings.

The impetus for health services research emerged in response to societal concerns regarding access to care and variation in the outcomes, quality, and costs of care both within the United States and between the United States and other countries. In 1979, the Institute of Medicine (IOM)[1] defined health services research as "inquiry to produce knowledge about the structure, processes, and effects of personal health services." A 1995 update[2] defined it as a "multidisciplinary field of inquiry, both basic and applied, that examines the use, costs, quality, accessibility, delivery, organization, financing, and outcomes of health care services to increase knowledge and understanding of the structure, processes, and effects of health services for individuals and populations." The most recent definition adopted by the Board of Directors of the Association for Health Services Research[3] in 2000 broadens the scope of health services research even further to include personal behaviors (e.g., smoking, diet, and exercise) and social factors (e.g., income, educational attainment, occupation, residential neighborhood) recognized as having important influences on the need for services and on the potential benefit or impact of health services on outcomes. A key feature of health services research is that it is inherently multidisciplinary and inevitably draws on methods from a variety of science and social science disciplines. The term is sometimes used synonymously with health outcomes research to signify research that focuses on nontraditional end points in health care such as quality of life, satisfaction with care and with health care decisions, and the economic consequences of care.[4]

This chapter provides overviews of four broad themes in health services:

1. Studies of health service delivery in cancer medicine,
2. Patient reported outcomes assessment,
3. The economics of cancer care,
4. Comparative effectiveness research.

STUDIES OF HEALTH SERVICE DELIVERY IN CANCER MEDICINE

Methodologic Issues

Because health services research so often involves analysis of real-world observational data that are not subject to controlled settings, baseline differences in the groups of patients being compared introduce *selection bias* that is not easily overcome. For example, consider a study that seeks to determine whether patients in small medical oncology practices versus hospital-affiliated multidisciplinary clinics are more likely to complete their prescribed breast cancer adjuvant chemotherapy regimens. The patients who seek care from hospital-affiliated clinics may well differ from those who obtain care in private medical oncology practices in important ways. Unless it is possible to capture and measure all of those, it is likely that this selection bias will influence any observed associations between the primary predictor (the type of clinic) and the outcome (completion of a course of adjuvant chemotherapy). Strategies to mitigate the effects of selection bias are essential to the design of health services research studies and must be considered in the conceptual model and the analytic plan.

In epidemiologic terms, selection bias often plagues health services research because of *confounders*, factors that are associated both with the outcome of interest and the primary predictor. In our hypothetical example, residence in a rural area may be associated with both receipt of chemotherapy in a small medical oncology practice and noncompletion of adjuvant breast cancer treatment because of the distance patients are required to travel rather than the type of clinic. In the process of considering what variables influence relationships of interest, it is often helpful to distinguish between observable and unobservable parameters. For example, clinical performance status, patient address (from which travel distance can be calculated), and bone marrow reserve would be potentially important parameters in a study seeking to determine the association between site of care and adjuvant chemotherapy completion rates. Clinical performance status and travel distance are observable and could be controlled for in statistical analysis; however, in most cases bone marrow reserve is not. If there was, for some reason, a predominance of patients with poor bone marrow reserve in one group, it would confound the results. Unobservable parameters can really only be controlled for with a randomized design. If too many important parameters are either unobservable or observable but not easily measured, the model or the analytic strategy needs to be revised.

Planning the analytic strategy for a health services research study may rely on classic clinical trial designs, involve secondary collection of data within the context of a clinical trial, require opportunistic analyses of data collected for nonresearch purposes in the context of routine care delivery, or demand *de novo* data collection specific to the research question. A critical step is to distinguish between descriptive methods and those that seek to formally test hypotheses. Randomized designs may be used. For example, breast cancer survivors have been randomized to receive follow-up surveillance from their primary care physicians or from their oncologist to compare clinical outcomes and patient satisfaction.[5]

Health services researchers use a variety of multivariable statistical techniques to attempt to control for selection bias and confounding in observational studies. These include focus on patient subgroups, stratification, multivariable modeling to adjust for known confounders, and use of propensity scores. Each of these strategies can help minimize the potential for confounding by adjusting for known factors that can be measured. Instrumental variable analysis is a statistical approach adopted from econometrics that uses an "instrument" that is associated with the probability of assignment to a particular treatment but independent of the outcome of treatment. An example of a common instrument is geographic variation in the utilization of an intervention. Patients in different regions are assumed to be similar (known covariates can still be controlled for) and to derive similar benefits from a treatment if they receive it. Therefore, the outcomes of patients in areas of low versus high utilization of the intervention can be compared to infer the effectiveness of the intervention.[6] In randomized trials, randomization is the instrument. In this way, instrumental variable analysis attempts to simulate randomization. Notwithstanding use of these techniques, none are able to completely eliminate the potential for selection bias.

Common Data Sources for Cancer-Related Health Services Research

In order to understand real-world care, access to sources of data that provide information about large groups of patients and not simply those select few who participate in clinical research studies is of paramount importance. Data collected in highly controlled and monitored studies are rich in clinical detail. Unfortunately, because data collection is laborious and resource intensive, this level of detail is typically not available for large groups of patients on a population basis. In contrast, data collected in routine care delivery generates very large sample sizes. However, extensive detail is usually not documented consistently or in a way that facilitates subsequent research, so it is very expensive to assemble and codify. This sets up an important conundrum for all health services research: the tradeoff between generalizability and detailed information.

Health services researchers must be resourceful and often leverage different approaches to address a question. For example, population-based data from the Surveillance, Epidemiology, and End Results (SEER) program of high-quality tumor registries provides sufficient data for a health services researcher to determine the use of breast-conserving surgery versus mastectomy for age-, race-, and clinical stage–specific cohorts of women with breast cancer. However, this data set lacks information about access to providers, the types of providers women see, personal risk factors, comorbidity, and baseline performance status. Alternatively, assessment of the factors associated with breast-conserving surgery versus mastectomy in women who participated in an adjuvant chemotherapy trial would likely provide more information about potentially important determinants of the type of surgery chosen, but would lack the generalizability available from the SEER sample.

Combining multiple sources of existing data to create resources that have richer detail is often necessary in order to obtain useful insights about health care delivery. The most important example of this in cancer health services research is the linkage of SEER registry data with Medicare claims.[7] Registries collect detailed information about cancer site, stage at diagnosis, histology, and initial surgery and radiation. However, important information like chemotherapy use, disease recurrence, and later treatment is not collected. In contrast, administrative claims (billing records) that itemize the diagnostic and procedure codes submitted by health care providers to the Centers for Medicare and Medicaid Services (CMS) for reimbursement can be scrutinized to characterize downstream care, including hospitalizations, use of surgery, chemotherapy, radiation, and management of comorbid illnesses. The claims allow identification of health care providers, including physicians and hospitals, as well as the costs associated with care. Because cancer predominates among persons older than age 65, and because most persons age 65 and older in the United States are insured by Medicare, the SEER-Medicare–linked data approximate a population-based data source for persons with cancer. The reliability of using claims to capture major cancer treatment such as chemotherapy and radiation has been validated by comparing claims histories to medical record review.[8,9] This linkage has created fertile soil for health services researchers, and many hundreds of publications using this resource have now been published.

Linkage efforts may also relate large-scale surveys of patients or providers to patient-based data such as health insurance claims. Many studies have linked physician attributes recorded by the American Medical Association or hospital attributes recorded by the American Hospital Association to administrative claims in order to understand health care delivery in light of providers' training, experience, and access to specialized facilities. Linkage of health care data to census information helps to characterize neighborhoods and communities where patients reside and provides ecologic measures of socioeconomic status at the level of the census tract. These linkages have identified substantial variation across geographic regions and even within regions based on community attributes and infrastructure.[10] Table 31.1 displays some important data sources used by cancer-related health services researchers.

Patterns of Care

Patterns of care studies are typically descriptive analyses that examine how health care interventions, spanning the spectrum from cancer prevention and screening to treatment, surveillance, and end-of-life care, are disseminated into community practice subsequent to demonstration of efficacy in experimental settings. Because clinical trials often involve strict criteria for eligibility and typically exclude patients with impaired functional status or substantial comorbidity, it is important to assess how health care interventions are adopted into the broader community and whether the efficacy observed in clinical trails translates into effectiveness in the population.[6,11]

A great deal of oncology care is delivered in the outpatient setting, often in private practice medical oncology clinics that do not have data collection systems amenable to research. This complicates reliable ascertainment of utilization rates—for example, of chemotherapy and hormonal therapy—and makes data collection laborious and expensive. To address this problem, patterns of care data are collected under a congressional mandate to the National Cancer Institute that recognizes the importance of ensuring that progress in cancer research is translated into general practice. Such analyses use the population-based SEER program as a platform. Special supplemental studies are routinely carried out that involve medical record

TABLE 31.1

IMPORTANT DATA SOURCES FOR HEALTH SERVICES RESEARCH STUDIES IN CANCER

Data Source	Examples	Advantages	Limitations
Cancer registry data	SEER registries	Population-based Inexpensive, public use Reliably tracks incidence, mortality, histology, and stage at diagnosis	No longitudinal follow-up other than vital status. Minimal detail on treatment
Administrative (billing) claims	Medicare claims Medicaid claims Commercial insurance claims	Inexpensive to obtain and analyze Permits longitudinal tracking Large sample sizes	Patients may switch insurance Stage information missing Billing records not designed for research and may not reliably capture important aspects of care
Linked registry-administrative claims	SEER-Medicare	Mitigate drawbacks of each source when used alone	No source of claims covers the whole population
Hospital discharge registries	Nationwide inpatient sample and state-specific data collected by the Health Care Cost and Utilization Project (HCUP)	Detailed information about reasons for hospitalizations, length of stay, secular trends in hospitalization, and inpatient cancer care delivery across many states	Lack information about cancer stage and histology that limits the ability to evaluate appropriateness of care Unable to follow patients into outpatient care settings or subsequent hospitalizations
Patient surveys	National Health Interview Survey (NHIS) National Health and Nutrition Examination Survey (NHANES)	Longitudinal large-scale surveys of patient risk factors including smoking and cancer screening specific to geographic region, age, race, and gender	Not easily linked to other data sources such as tumor registries
Provider surveys	AMA physician surveys AHA hospital surveys	Characterize providers in terms of age, practice site and type, specialty, experience, and credentialing	Incomplete responses; not current; minimal detail
Large-scale care delivery networks	Cancer Research Network (CRN) affiliation of HMOs	Systematic collection of comparable data elements in the context of routine primary and specialty care permits assessment of care patterns before and after cancer diagnosis. Includes longitudinal detail about medication use, inpatient and outpatient records	HMO populations are typically less heterogeneous than the population at large and underrepresent the very ill, the very old, and the very poor Because enrollment is often employer-based, patients may disenroll
Specialty care networks	National Comprehensive Cancer Network (NCCN) Outcomes Database Projects (breast, non-Hodgkin's lymphoma, and colorectal cancers)	Abstraction of medical records yields detailed information about care delivery at specialty centers Linkage to practice guidelines permits assessment of the extent to which practice conforms to standards	Information about patients' care prior to diagnosis not always accessible Patients may not be representative of general cancer population
Large-scale prospective cohort studies	Prostate Cancer Outcomes Study (PCOS) Cancer Care Outcomes and Research Surveillance Consortium (CanCORS)	Includes record review and patient interviews to create comprehensive portrait of care delivery and outcomes in real-world contexts	Federally funded multicenter studies that are extremely expensive to conduct and implement Difficult to sustain and thereby difficult to use for ongoing quality assessment, intervention, and reassessment
Clinical trial data	Cooperative Group Cancer Control and Health Outcomes Studies (e.g., CALGB, NSABP)	Efficient to supplement collection of clinical trial data with data elements that permit evaluation of research questions that evaluate care delivery systems and sources of variation	Small, select patient groups

SEER, Surveillance, Epidemiology, and End Results; AMA, American Medical Association; AHA, American Hospital Association; HMO, health maintenance organization; CALGB, Cancer and Leukemia Group B; NSABP, National Surgical Adjuvant Breast and Bowel Project.

reviews, and in some cases patient interviews have helped determine the extent to which important therapeutic interventions such as adjuvant treatments penetrate into community practice.[12] By linking these data collection efforts to SEER registries, population-based estimates of the dissemination of new treatments are obtained.

SEER-Medicare–linked data have also become a widely used source to document patterns of care in population-based samples. Numerous studies have documented the inverse relationship between treatment rates and age in situations in which evidence exists that the elderly derive benefits similar to younger patients. For example, in SEER-Medicare cohorts aged 65 and older diagnosed with colon cancer in the late 1990s, 78% of patients aged 65 to 69 received recommended adjuvant treatment, while only 52% of those aged 75 to 79 and 34% of those 80 to 84 did so.[13] Several studies have demonstrated that patients who reside in more affluent neighborhoods are more likely to receive recommended care. Moreover, a woefully large body of literature repeatedly documents lower rates of treatment with standard therapies among nonwhite populations. Lower rates of cancer care are especially predominant for black Americans and are evident, although less consistently so, among Hispanic Americans. For example, black Americans are less likely to undergo thorough staging for lung cancer and less likely to undergo potentially curative resection when diagnosed with early stage disease.[14] Blacks are less likely to receive adjuvant chemotherapy and radiation for breast and colorectal cancers and less likely to receive palliative treatment for advanced lung, esophageal, and pancreas cancers.[15]

Patterns of care studies also evaluate variation based on physician and hospital characteristics. For example, Hawley et al.[16] surveyed breast cancer surgeons about their use of mastectomy versus breast cancer surgery and of breast cancer reconstruction for women with early stage breast cancer. By measuring patient characteristics, surgeon characteristics, and referral patterns, they were able to determine that surgeons' characteristics are strongly associated with the type of surgery a woman receives and that surgeons have varying propensity to refer patients to plastic surgeons. Another study compared postoperative mortality for whites and blacks and determined that a substantial proportion of observed racial disparity (higher mortality for blacks) could be attributed to the characteristics of the hospitals where blacks and whites tend to have cancer surgery.[17]

Volume–Outcome Associations

Volume–outcome relationships in health care were described by Luft et al.[18] in 1979, and since then there has been a persistent debate about whether complex, elective care such as cancer surgery should be restricted to high-volume centers. Although regional specialization is accepted practice in organ transplantation, it has penetrated less completely into cancer surgery. Numerous studies have shown that higher hospital volume is associated with lower postoperative mortality and morbidity rates after a great number of different surgical procedures. Dudley et al.[19] found lower hospital mortality at high-volume hospitals in 123 of 128 analyses involving 40 different procedures. Using Medicare data, Birkmeyer et al.[20] found that higher volume hospitals had lower operative mortality for eight major cancer operations, including colectomy, gastrectomy, esophagectomy, pancreatectomy, cystectomy, nephrectomy, and lung lobectomy or pneumonectomy and hepatectomy. The evidence in support of these associations is greatest for those procedures with the highest risk such as pancreatectomy and esophagectomy[21]; and indeed, for those procedures the IOM, payors, and consumer organizations such as the Leapfrog group have advocated regionalization to centers of excellence.[22] In these high-risk procedures the difference in 30-day mortality between hospitals with low- and high-case volume can approach 5% to 10%.[23] In contrast, for lower-risk operations such as colectomy and prostatectomy, where surgical mortality is less frequent, the magnitude of these differences is in the realm of 0.5% to 2%.[19,21]

The volume–outcome literature has been extended to include the association between case volume and long-term survival[24] and has focused on individual surgeon volume as well as hospital volume.[25] In general, the findings of these studies all suggest that volume–outcome relationships exist. However, interpretation of this large body of literature requires considerable caution. First, there are no clear or consistent volume thresholds or standards for what counts as high volume. Second, most analyses rely on observational data, typically administrative databases such as discharge abstract registries. The information collected is typically insufficient to characterize comorbidity, making it difficult, if not impossible, to discern whether the observed variation in outcomes is attributable to "case mix," namely that patients who travel to receive care from higher-volume providers are somehow healthier than those who remain in their local communities. The small studies that have relied on detailed clinical records to examine volume–outcome relationships have not demonstrated strong associations.[26] From both a statistical and a policy perspective, it is also important to consider whether volume–outcome associations represent a consistent pattern among low-volume providers or whether they can be attributed to a select subset of outliers who obtain especially poor results.

Quality of Care Studies

Since the late 1990s, the perception that cancer care delivery systems are suboptimal as well as the desire for greater accountability have stimulated efforts to develop strategies to track and benchmark the quality of care. A series of influential reports released by the IOM documented the extent to which health care delivery in general and cancer care in particular falls well short of what could be achieved given existing knowledge, resources, technology, and levels of investment. The 1999 IOM Report *Ensuring Quality Cancer Care* documented shortcomings in cancer care delivery as well as in the infrastructure and knowledge available to translate the fruits of biomedical research into practice. It found that "there is a wide gulf between ideal cancer care and the reality experienced by many Americans".[27] The 2001 IOM Report *Crossing the Quality Chasm* noted "the health care system is for many, particularly for patients with cancer, a nightmare to navigate".[28] As a result of these influential syntheses and the variation observed by patterns of care studies, efforts to define, measure, and ultimately improve the quality of cancer care delivery have become a major focus of health services research in oncology.

The IOM defines quality of care as "the degree to which health care services for individuals and populations increase the likelihood of desired health outcomes and are consistent with current professional knowledge".[29] This definition has been extended to emphasize the importance of patients' experiences by considering "care that incorporates respect for patients' values and preferences".[27]

Specific criteria for what constitutes high-quality care usually come from accepted guidelines. In cancer medicine, these have been developed primarily by provider organizations like the American Society of Clinical Oncology (ASCO), Cancer Care Ontario, and the National Comprehensive Cancer Network (NCCN). Practice guidelines seek to develop and codify standards for management of a particular cancer or cancer-related complications. Comparative effectiveness research will increasingly inform these efforts. Technology assessment is a related endeavor that evaluates evidence in favor of a particular health care intervention, often one for which clinical trial data are incomplete. Guidelines from ASCO and Cancer Care Ontario are strictly evidence based. They begin with systematic reviews of the primary literature and consideration of other efforts to increase the evidence base by pooling many studies.[30] For example, the Cochrane Collaborative in the United Kingdom conducts exhaustive literature reviews and performs meta-analyses to review the basis for recommending specific interventions. The NCCN practice guidelines, on the other hand, are developed through an explicit consensus process that is informed by evidence. In this way, they have been able to provide guidance on the management of most malignancies across disease stages and phases of illness. The National Guideline Clearinghouse is a federally sponsored effort to make evidenced-based practice guidelines readily available, and a user-friendly Web interface facilitates searches for guidelines pertinent to hundreds of scenarios in clinical medicine.

Once quality care is defined, measuring it is an involved and complicated process that requires development of specific criteria. Donabedian,[31] a leader in the health care quality movement, noted that the reason to measure quality is to "create an environment of watchful concern that motivates everyone to perform better." The simple act of measuring quality may itself catalyze change in behavior and practice patterns. Donabedian also developed a conceptual framework for thinking about health care quality and developing measures that are still widely used. He distinguished between the *structure* of care (the contexts in which care is rendered), the *process* of care (what we do to patients), and the *outcomes* of care (what ultimately happens to patients) (Table 31.2).

The growing demand for accountability and transparency in cancer care delivery has stimulated enormous effort to develop quality metrics, often termed *quality indicators*. A quality indicator represents an aspect of health care delivery, usually an intervention, that when performed is known to lead to superior outcomes. Because outcomes typically reflect the cumulative effect of many interrelated factors, including both care delivery and patient factors, process measures most easily identify specific areas of care for targeting improvement initiatives. Consequently, most quality metrics focus on implementation of specific care processes, for example, delivery of adjuvant hormonal therapy to women with hormone receptor–positive breast cancer.

Assessment of process measures of quality typically focuses on determination of *underuse*, *overuse*, or *misuse* of a particular intervention. Underuse measures (e.g., failure to administer adjuvant therapy) are usually easier to define than overuse measures (e.g., numerous surveillance imaging scans). Misuse refers to applying an intervention incorrectly (e.g., inadequate radiation fields). Quality metrics are typically represented as a series of "if . . . then" statements. The "if" defines the group of patients in the denominator and the "then" defines the numerator. For example, *if* patients undergo curative resection of stage III colon cancer, *then* they should receive adjuvant chemotherapy within 16 weeks of surgery. The resulting proportion yields a measure for evaluating quality. The inclusion and exclusion criteria for both the numerator and denominator can clearly have a profound impact on results of measurement and the feasibility of assessment. For example, if the denominator excludes patients with a host of comorbidities and complications, then assessment requires record review to determine whether any such conditions pertain. Table 31.3 illustrates some of the important dimensions for quality metrics.

Quality metrics also consider structural aspects of health care. For example, the availability of emergency resuscitation equipment and expertise in practice settings where chemotherapy with potential for anaphylaxis is administered represents a structural aspect of quality. Accreditation assessments usually focus on such structural aspects of quality. Relatively fewer quality metrics focus directly on outcomes such as achieving a specific benchmark for complication rates or mortality after major cancer operations. Increasingly, mortality outcomes and patient satisfaction ratings are being voluntarily reported by hospitals and made publicly available. Although lower mortality rates may be presented as emblematic of hospital quality, interpretation of these results is challenging because of the need to consider risk adjustment and baseline differences in patient characteristics when interpreting variation in outcomes.

It is important to recognize that quality measures may be used for somewhat different purposes by different target audiences. Increasingly, providers supply report cards displaying clinical performance measurements for consumers to make decisions based on quality. These may be externally posted or submitted to intermediary organizations like the National Committee for Quality Assurance or the Joint Commission for Accreditation of Healthcare Organizations. Purchasers and consumers are often thought to be the key audience for these reports. Health care purchasers' primary interest is in using accountability data to guide the selection of providers or set financial rewards to providers for performance. This allows comparison of providers in terms of efficiency and enables payors to steer patients toward desirable providers. In contrast, health care providers may be motivated to measure and report quality both to improve their own level of care (internal quality improvement) as well as to market their own expertise in comparison to competitors.

TABLE 31.2

TYPES OF QUALITY MEASURES USED TO ASSESS CANCER CARE DELIVERY

Quality Domain	Definition	Examples
Structure	Features of an organization or clinician relevant to the capacity to provide health care.	Training, credentials, and experience of providers. Availability of an experienced chemotherapy pharmacist in outpatient practice settings.
Process	Evaluates a health care service provided to a patient. Process measures are often used to assess adherence to recommendations for clinical practice based on evidence or consensus.	Delivery of adjuvant hormonal therapy for women with hormone receptor–positive breast cancer. Removal of at least 12 lymph nodes in colorectal cancer surgery. Patient involvement in decision-making. Radiation after breast conserving surgery.
Outcome	A health state of a patient resulting from health care delivery.	Disease-free survival. Quality of life. Satisfaction with care. Costs of care.

TABLE 31.3

IMPORTANT DIMENSIONS OF QUALITY MEASURE

Dimension	Definition
MEASURE IMPORTANCE	
Relevance to stakeholders	The measure is of significant interest to multiple stakeholders preferably to patients, providers, and payors.
Impact on health	The measure addresses an aspect of health that is clinically important as defined by high prevalence or incidence and a significant effect on the burden of illness.
Relevance for measuring equitable distribution of health care	The measure can be analyzed by subgroups to examine whether disparities in care exist among a population of patients.
Evidence of need for improvement	There is evidence indicating that there is substantial variation or overall poor quality so as to justify the need for targeted measurement and improvement initiatives in a particular area.
Potential for change	Measures should focus on aspects of health care where there is leverage and the potential to bring about meaningful change based on findings. Evidence of poor or uneven quality if identified can be translated and operationalized into action plans leading to improvements in care delivery.
SCIENTIFIC SOUNDNESS	
Strength of evidence	The topic area of the measure should be supported by a robust evidence base.
Comprehensible	Measure results should be understood to a broad array of stakeholders.
MEASURE PROPERTIES	
Reliability	Results of the measure should be reproducible and reflect results of interventions when implemented over time.
Validity	Measure should be associated with the construct it purports to measure and generalizable across settings and time periods.
FEASIBILITY	
Explicit specification	A measure should have straightforward specification for both numerator and denominators that is the criteria for considering both that a quality measure has been achieved and for inclusion in the population of subjects considered eligible for inclusion in the analytic sample.
Data availability	Data sources needed to implement a quality measure should be readily available, accessible, and amenable to expeditious efficient data collection. The data sources to be used for measurement should be explicitly stated.
Burden of measurement	The effort required to perform measurement and the time and costs required to access, abstract, and analyze data should be considered in relation to the importance of the knowledge to be gained.

Health services researchers have focused on the development of systems to integrate quality measurement and improvement into clinical workflow and culture. Developing quality measurement initiatives that are sustainable over time and that involve a manageable burden of data collection is a major challenge. Cancer centers, health care systems, payors, and increasingly individual providers are becoming actively engaged in systems designed to facilitate this goal. For example, ASCO has developed a provider-driven program, the Quality Oncology Practice Initiative, in which community medical oncology practices assess their practice patterns and submit data to a central database. They receive back reports showing their performance relative to other participating practices and have the opportunity to apply for special certification through the program. Additionally, the National Quality Forum has developed preliminary quality measure sets for colorectal cancer end-of-life cancer care, and ASCO and NCCN have developed a quality toolbox with a common agreed-on measure set for colorectal and breast cancers.

PATIENT-REPORTED OUTCOMES ASSESSMENT

Traditional outcomes in oncology have included overall survival, disease-specific survival, disease-free survival, objective response, and time to progression. However, given that most cancer treatments have relatively modest effects on these outcomes and are often accompanied by considerable toxicity, monitoring the symptoms of disease and toxicity from treatment is appropriate as well. This section will define and consider patient-reported outcomes (PROs), ranging from limited measures of specific symptoms or toxicities experienced and reported by patients, through the broader multidimensional evaluation of health-related quality of life (HRQOL), to preference-based measurement of the value or utility placed on the health effects of a disease and its treatment.

There is little consensus about how to measure PROs. Early instruments had health care providers or family members respond to questions about patients' symptoms, but such assessments have not been found to be as accurate as patient reports. This is particularly true of nonobservable outcomes such as pain, nausea, or depression. Consequently, many competing *instruments* (e.g., questionnaires, rating scales) have been developed to measure PROs.

Development of a new instrument should be undertaken only if there is no existing instrument to be used or adapted. The first step in creating an instrument is to identify the relevant *domains* (concepts, such as dyspnea or psychological distress) to measure. This can be based on clinical experience, literature review, patient interviews, or focus groups. Then a draft instrument composed of *items* (questions) that try to characterize these domains can be made. This involves many choices. How many items will be required to characterize each domain? Which response categories should be used? These can range from simple yes-no checklists, to Likert scales with ordered response options (e.g., excellent, very good, good, fair, poor) and numerical analog scales (e.g., 1 to 10), to visual analog scales in which respondents mark a line along a continuous scale. How long should the recall period be? Shorter instruments with only a few types of response options, a short recall period, and that do not frame all items in a positive or negative light are preferred. Should it be self-administered, either without supervision such as a mailed or Internet survey, or with supervision, such as in a waiting room with a research assistant? Or should an interviewer administer it in person or by the telephone? It is essential that use of the instrument be as consistent as possible, that is, clear and explicit instructions to the respondent for self-administered instruments or standardized training for interviewers if they are being used. Each of these choices may influence response rate and the results obtained.

Once there is a draft instrument, what ensues is an iterative cycle of performance evaluation, modification of the instrument, followed by repeat evaluation. The first step is to do pilot testing and in-depth cognitive debriefing interviews with a small number of respondents to make sure the instructions and items are clear and understood in the way they were intended, and then to revise the instrument to correct any problems. Larger and more formal studies are required to assess other properties. *Reliability* is assessment of whether the instrument produces similar results among similar or even the same patient on repeat administration (e.g., "test-retest reliability"). *Internal consistency* is assessment of whether items meant to measure the same domain produce correlated results. For interviewer-administered instruments, *inter-interviewer reproducibility* examines whether the results are similar when different interviewers administer the instrument. There should be sufficient *variability* in responses among the target population, ideally using the entire response range, in order to be able to discriminate between patients with different health states. It is important to know both what a *minimal clinically important difference* (MCID) is, and that the instrument can detect such differences or changes. Studies can evaluate this, for example, by asking patients to complete the instrument at two different times and rating whether there has been no, a small, medium, or large change in their health status in the interim or comparing the results to another objective clinical measure. The change in the instrument's score that corresponds to a small but appreciable change in health status represents the MCID. It has been observed as a rule of thumb that the MCID often approximates one-half of one standard deviation. For utilities (described later), the MCID is approximately 0.05 on a scale ranging from 0 to 1.

Investigators often describe instruments as "validated," but it is important to recognize that validation is an ongoing process and that there are several aspects of validity. *Content validity* usually involves surveys or interviews with patients and clinicians to ensure that all of the relevant items and domains necessary to describe a particular outcome such as depression or pain are included in the instrument. *Construct validity* testing involves relating the results of the instrument to some external standard so as to ensure that the intended concept is indeed the one being captured. Examples include correlating results to those of another simultaneously administered validated instrument that has some overlap in domains, or showing that the results discriminate between patients with different objective clinical situations, such as different stages of cancer or those responding versus progressing on treatment. If the expected relationships are observed, it adds support to the instrument's construct validity.

Data from different methods of administration or from any alteration in an instrument, such as omission or reordering of questions, change in the response options, altered format or mode of administration, or altered recall period are not necessarily interchangeable and would ideally require empirical evidence of validation. Similarly, translation into different languages is challenging because there are also cultural concerns to attend to. Ideally, independent "back-translation" from the new language into the original language is done to ensure that the meaning was accurately conveyed in translation.

Analytic Considerations

Missing data is a common problem with patient-reported outcomes. In fact, a review of HRQOL studies in lung cancer found that only about half of the patients had more than a baseline evaluation,[32] making it difficult to determine repeated measures analyses and even comparisons of the proportions of patients who improved versus worsened. If the data are missing for some random reason (e.g., the patient missed an appointment because of a snowstorm), it is referred to as *missing completely at random*. In such a case it is thought to be "uninformative" in the sense that the fact that the data from the visit are missing does not imply anything about the outcome being measured. If, on the other hand, they did not come in because they were feeling too sick, then the fact of the missing data is "informative," as it is missing because the patient is experiencing a poor outcome. Similarly, patients may be too sick to even fill out a mailed questionnaire or may skip sections. Such informative missing data can introduce bias into the results of a study.

As an example of the analytic problems presented by missing data, imagine a trial in a cancer with a progressive natural history, in which patients are receiving a toxic therapy. If PROs are measured at baseline and then repeatedly over time, the outcomes would be expected to worsen. If, however, patients become too ill to fill out the instrument or the patient died, average outcomes calculated at each time point will appear to improve as the sickest patients drop out, when in fact they generally worsen for most patients. If outcomes are calculated only on those with complete data, then the subgroup analyzed will tend to be those with the least disease burden, most indolent course, or the best response to treatment and consequently may not be representative of the broader population. The commonly used last observation carry forward approach to handling missing data assumes that the missing data point is the same as the prior measurement. Imputation approaches involve attempting to predict—for example, through regression analyses of characteristics of similar patients without missing data—what the missing value would likely be. In general, it is usually best to also consider worst and best case scenarios, for example, by assuming that all patients with missing data had extreme negative outcomes and assess the effect of that assumption on the study results. In the end, the best way to handle missing data is to minimize it by avoiding overly long and burdensome instruments, pilot testing data collection procedures in order to identify problems before embarking on a study, and supervising study staff to ensure maximal data capture.

Analytically, items can either stand on their own as a *battery* or *profile*, or be combined, sometimes with a weighting scheme, into a summary score or *index* across all or part of the instrument. There are statistical procedures such as factor analysis that can help determine the most appropriate scoring scheme and suggest unnecessary items that can be eliminated from an instrument. The primary end point(s) in an analysis of PROs must be prespecified because each domain, and even item, has the potential to serve as an end point. Multiple analyses of such end points would substantially increase the risk of finding spurious associations (type I error). On the other hand, if more than one component of an instrument is being evaluated, they are probably correlated to some extent and so common adjustments (e.g., the Bonferroni correction) for multiple testing may be too conservative. If one chooses to have a summary score as the primary end point, there is a risk of losing sensitivity to change because it will probably include domains that are less likely to be affected by a disease or intervention (e.g., incorporating social role function in a composite score that measures HRQOL in groups of patients who receive different chemotherapy drugs for an advanced cancer). If the goal is to show that an intervention affects overall HRQOL, then it is necessary to provide evidence that the disease impairs all measured domains and that the treatment improves all domains. Domains such as family support and spirituality are important but may not be differentially affected by alternative chemotherapy drugs. This is one of the reasons why the U.S. Food and Drug Administration (FDA) is reluctant to consider claims about HRQOL improvement in approval decisions, preferring to look instead at measures of clinical benefit that focus on particular domains or symptoms.[33] An example of this was the clinical benefit response outcome devised by the FDA for evaluation of gemcitabine in pancreatic cancer.[34] It consisted of a composite end point that looked for changes in pain, performance status, and weight. In a randomized trial, gemcitabine was found to meet the definition of conferring clinical benefit to patients, although its approval was eventually based on a somewhat unexpected observation of survival benefit.

Commonly Used Health-Related Quality of Life Instruments

HRQOL is a particular type of PRO that tries to incorporate a number of domains. The broadest definition of quality of life includes such things as economic prosperity, personal security, and social support. The domains commonly considered to be encompassed by HRQOL instruments are impact of an illness and its treatment on physical, psychological, and social function. They can either be generic or specific to particular diseases, populations, or treatments. A common strategy is to combine a generic instrument with a disease-specific instrument in order to be able to compare results across conditions while still capturing the important unique issues related to the disease.

There are several high-quality HRQOL instruments in existence but no single commonly agreed on measure or even core set of instruments. One of the most commonly used generic instruments is the SF-36, which is a 36-item short form of the battery of measures used in the Medical Outcomes Study.[35] Because it is not cancer specific, it is a good choice for studies related to screening or survivorship. Other generic measures commonly encountered in the literature include the Hospital Anxiety and Depression Scale, the Profile of Mood States, the Spitzer Quality of Life Index, the Sickness Impact Profile, the Brief Symptom Inventory, and the Nottingham Health Profile.

There are several general cancer measures, but the current most commonly used ones are the European Organisation for Research and Treatment of Cancer Quality of Life Cancer Questionnaire (EORTC QLQ-C30) and, in the United States, the Functional Assessment of Cancer Therapy, General (FACT-G) scale. Both are core instruments that allow comparison across studies in different cancer populations, being designed to be supplemented by modules to more specifically detect relevant changes in outcomes related to a specific cancer or symptom. Both use a combination of Likert and numerical analog scale format questions[36] to characterize HRQOL in the week leading up to its administration. Other commonly used general cancer measures include the Rotterdam Symptom Checklist, the Cancer Rehabilitation Evaluation System, and the Functional Living Index–Cancer. Several of these also have shorter versions (e.g., the SF-12) to reduce patient burden.

The EORTC QLQ-C30 consists of 30 questions. Because it was developed primarily for use in clinical trials, the EORTC scale focuses on cancer-related symptoms and treatment-related toxicity. As a result, its psychometric properties are thought to be especially good in situations in which patients are relatively ill and receiving anticancer therapy. It is sometimes limited in this application, though, by its length and complexity, which may make it difficult to administer to the sickest patients.

The FACT-G[37] consists of 34 questions. It was developed using patient input as well as that of medical professionals for item generation and review, providing it with content validity. With patient input from the outset, it emphasizes social and emotional well-being. It does not have as comprehensive an assessment of symptoms, however, and so it may be most successfully used in monitoring patients who are not as ill or those receiving supportive care rather than aggressive anticancer treatment.

An example of a disease-specific instrument is the Lung Cancer Symptom Scale.[38] It focuses exclusively on the symptoms of lung cancer (e.g., dyspnea and cough, but not sexual dysfunction or urinary symptoms) and does not attempt to assess the toxicity of treatment. It is very simple, consisting only of nine visual analog scales and six optional items for an observer to fill out and asks about HRQOL in the previous 24 hours. It is responsive to changes in the symptoms of lung cancer, but it is difficult to put the results in context for patients with other diseases.

A new approach in health outcomes research is borrowed from educational testing: rather than using a fixed instrument, select specific items whose performance have been extensively characterized from an *item bank* using computer-adaptive methods and *item response theory*. Such an approach creates a highly tailored battery that can characterize PROs very precisely with the minimum number of questions. If it is known where responses to various items lie along the continuum of severity for a domain, the response to an initial question aimed at the middle of the domain can direct the next question toward either the more or less severe part of the severity scale. In this way, problem areas and the severity of the respondent's symptoms can be determined very efficiently. This may also decrease respondent burden, thereby increasing response rates and minimizing missing data. Such an approach is logistically more complex and expensive than using a traditional battery of instruments, however. The NIH is sponsoring a Patient-Reported Outcomes Measurement Information System (PROMIS) network that has as one of its goals to develop a set of publically available computerized adaptive tests for the research community.

Preference-Based Measures

Although PROs and HRQOL instruments can indicate the severity of a symptom or side effect, they do not incorporate a relative valuation of how much that symptom affects overall perception of health. For example, perhaps severe nausea is worse than severe pain for a particular respondent. The *utility* is a measure of preference for a given health state rated on a scale from 0 (the worst imaginable health state) to 1 (perfect health). In this way, it attaches a value to the health effects: rather than just rating the amount of, for example, dyspnea and depression a patient is experiencing, the utility considers the value attached to these symptoms (Table 31.4). The terms utilities, values, and preferences are used interchangeably. The main application of preference-based methods is in economic analysis, as described later.

There are two ways to measure utilities: directly and indirectly. The most commonly used direct methods are the standard gamble (SG), the time trade-off, and visual analog scales. According to expected utility theory, a utility is derived most accurately by SG.[39] SG exercises ask patients to decide on a risk of death they would accept to be returned to perfect health (conceptually similar to undergoing a risky surgical procedure

TABLE 31.4

SELECTED UTILITIES FOR CANCER-RELATED HEALTH STATES

Health State	Utility Range
Death	0.00
Last month of life with acute leukemia	0.00
Extensive SCLC with progressive disease	0.31
Progressive metastatic breast cancer (depending on toxicity from treatment)	0.41–0.69
Stable metastatic breast cancer (depending on toxicity from treatment)	0.50–0.80
Metastatic NSCLC	0.69
Early progressive prostate cancer (moderate pain/fatigue)	0.83
Induction interferon for stage II and III melanoma	0.94
Maintenance interferon for stage II and III melanoma	0.97
Extensive SCLC in complete remission	0.99
Perfect health	1.00

SCLC, small-cell lung cancer; NSCLC, non–small cell lung cancer.
(From ref. 71, with permission.)

that could cure a morbid illness). Time trade-off involves finding the balance between a shorter survival in perfect health and a longer time in a particular health state affected by disease or treatment (such as chemotherapy). There is controversy around whether these utilities should be derived from patients, their families, health care workers, or lay societal "jurors" who are given detailed scenarios describing the health state. Recent guidelines favor the latter as being most consistent with a societal perspective.[40] However, there is concern that people without relevant disease experience may not properly understand the health state. Indeed, utilities derived from the general population are generally lower than those derived from actual patients, demonstrating the phenomenon of adaptation to the disease state by persons with chronic illness such as cancer.

Alternatively, indirect approaches use multiattribute instruments such as the Health Utilities Index, Quality of Well Being Scale, or the EQ-5D that are specifically designed to be able to estimate utilities. These instruments are associated with preexisting utility functions usually derived by relating answers of a population-based sample to concurrent direct utility estimation. Subjects complete these instruments and their responses are mapped on to the utility function to impute their utility. Completing these questionnaires is a less complex cognitive task than performing the standard gamble or time trade-off exercises. Furthermore, they can be self-administered, making them easier to use than the direct measures. There have been attempts to create cross walks between common HRQOL instruments and utilities, but most standard quality of life instruments have not undergone the testing required to accurately convert their scores into utilities.

Satisfaction with Care

Another outcome of interest in certain situations is patients' satisfaction with care. Evaluation of satisfaction has some challenges. Patients are usually quite satisfied with care so there is a "ceiling effect" whereby the majority of responses cluster at the top of a satisfaction scale, resulting in little variability and consequently little ability to differentiate between groups. Moreover, patients can be very satisfied with poor-quality care. Things such as waiting times, parking, physical comfort, amenities, and food quality often drive satisfaction. All of these things may be present while a patient receives incorrect treatment recommendations. Satisfaction measurement must also ensure that patients are not concerned that their feedback can be relayed to their providers in an identifiable manner. Commonly used general instruments include the Picker Survey of satisfaction with hospital care or the Consumer Assessment of Health Plans, while examples of cancer-specific scales are the FAMCARE measure of family satisfaction with palliative care and the Princess Margaret Hospital Patient Satisfaction with Doctor Questionnaire.

Value Added

Does measurement of PROs provide additional information beyond that of the traditional biomedical outcomes like response, survival, toxicity, and performance status? If an intervention is curative, it is unlikely that HRQOL effects will affect decision making, so it is probably not necessary to monitor anything beyond treatment toxicity on a clinical trial. On the other hand, for a palliative, noncurative intervention, HRQOL is often an important secondary end point used to determine the balance between symptom improvement and treatment toxicity. For example, a randomized trial comparing continuous versus intermittent chemotherapy in metastatic breast cancer showed improved overall quality of life with continuous treatment.[41] A treatment judged to be without important tumor activity can still improve HRQOL, and in cases wherein a survival difference is not found, HRQOL effects could be the determining factor when choosing a course of treatment. One of the best-known examples of this was the approval of mitoxantrone added to prednisone for the treatment of metastatic prostate cancer.[42] In a randomized trial in which survival was not expected to differ, the primary end point was a 2-point decrease in pain on a 6-point scale without increase in analgesic medication. Such a symptomatic response was observed in 29% of patients treated with the combination compared with only 12% of patients on prednisone alone. As the array of cancer treatment options expands, the importance of PROs in oncology is expected to increase.

THE ECONOMICS OF CANCER CARE

Health care costs in the United States are approximately $2 trillion annually, or around $7,000 per person.[43] It was just 5% of the gross domestic product (GDP) in 1965 but is projected to be 20% by 2014.[44] Approximately 30% of costs are incurred in the last year of life, with more than half of those costs in the last 60 days.[45] The inability to stem the rising cost of medical care has led to insurance premiums rising faster than inflation, which in turn has resulted in a decline in employer-provided health insurance.[46]

The current cost of cancer care has been estimated to be about $100 billion in the United States in 2007, accounting for approximately 5% of overall medical spending, and, in the older population, 10% of total Medicare expenditures.[43] The costs of care related to cancer are rising faster than other health care costs from the development of many new and effective but costly treatments,[47] demographic changes leading to an aging population with more people in the age groups at highest risk of cancer, and a more informed and activist patient population demanding access to new and even experimental therapies.[48] Lung cancer is the site accounting for the largest

TABLE 31.5

THE RISING COST OF SYSTEMIC TREATMENT FOR METASTATIC COLON CANCER

Chemotherapy Regimen	Era	Approximate 8-week Drug Cost ($)	Approximate Median Survival (months)
FU + FA	1960s	<300	10–12
FU + FA + (IRI or OX)	Late 1990s	10,000	14–16
FU + FA + (IRI or OX) + BEV	2004+	20,000	20–24
FU + FA + (IRI or OX) + CET		30,000	

FU, 5-fluorouracil; FA, folinic acid; IRI, irinotecan; OX, oxaliplatin; BEV, bevacizumab; CET, cetuximab.
(From ref. 47, with permission.)

proportion, 13.3% of total expenditures, followed by breast cancer at 11.2%.

Cancer drugs account for more than 40% of Medicare drug spending.[44] The high prices of drugs under 20-year patent protection reflect the estimated approximately $1 billion it costs to take a new drug to market, as well as profit, which is argued to be necessary to stimulate innovation.[49] The prices of the newer so-called targeted drugs are generally even higher than conventional compounds because of their greater costs of development and manufacture (Table 31.5). Moreover, neither the FDA in its approval decisions nor Medicare in its coverage decisions explicitly considers cost. Current studies are investigating the use of multiple targeted agents in combination, moving them up to earlier treatment phases and continuing them beyond primary therapy into periods of disease stability or quiescence. Consequently, if we realize the goal of turning cancer into a chronic disease, some patients may remain on these drugs for many years, with significant economic implications.

In the 1990s, managed care organizations were transiently successful in stemming the rise in health care costs by implementing criteria under which procedures of marginal or questionable effectiveness could be used and requiring preauthorization on a case-by-case basis.[50] However, because of adverse publicity and high-profile lawsuits, insurers have become increasingly reluctant to interfere with cancer care. More recent approaches have focused on cost sharing, with lower priced high-deductible plans, higher copayments and coinsurance, and health savings accounts. The idea is that if patients are responsible for more of their health care costs, they will be better consumers than when they are effectively insulated from prices through traditional fee-for-service or indemnity insurance. However, patients often have little choice but to accept treatment for illness, and when sick, particularly with life-threatening illness, are unlikely to shop around for lowest prices. Oncologists are also uncomfortable discussing economic issues with patients[51] and are reluctant to mention options that they do not think patients can reasonably obtain.[52] A recent national survey found that 84% of medical oncologists say that patients' out of pocket expenses influence treatment recommendations.[53] This raises the potential for patients missing out on useful therapies for economic reasons.

As cancer is a disease of the elderly, more than half of U.S. cancer patients are eligible for Medicare. Consequently, CMS is interested in payment schemes that will control costs while maintaining quality. For example, the prospective payment system for inpatient care, based on diagnosis-related grouping that reimburses at a fixed level for management of a specific problem, thereby providing an incentive to the hospital to provide care as efficiently as possible, was associated with a decline in the lengths of stay related to cancer operations.[54] For outpatient cancer care, there is evidence that chemotherapy reimbursement incentives lead providers to choose more expensive management options.[55,56] The Medicare Modernization Act tried to change this by pegging reimbursement to the average sales price instead of the average wholesale price, but this still gives providers more money when they prescribe more expensive drugs. Another tack is the *competitive acquisition program* in which physicians receive drugs from contractors and only receive payments from Medicare for administration costs. However, uptake of this has been low. Also being explored are the previously described pay-for-performance programs in which reimbursement rates are tied to the provision of guideline concordant care or measures on sets of quality of care indicators.[50] Indeed, "bending the cost curve" is one of the goals of health care reform, although the path to achieving this is far from clear.

Economic Analysis

Given these increasing and widespread economic ramifications of cancer care, economic analysis has emerged as a research technique to assess whether an intervention represents value for money in order to inform medical policy decisions. The question in an economic study is not how much something costs, but how much more it costs and how much benefit is gained compared to the most appropriate alternative strategy (e.g., the current standard, or a "do nothing" alternative). There are four types of commonly used economic evaluations. Each involves a comparison of both the costs and consequences of alternative interventions. The main differences between them are the methods used to measure their consequences.

Cost-minimization or *cost-analysis* assumes that the outcomes or effectiveness of the interventions are equal. Resource utilization is the only significant difference between the options. The direct costs associated with each intervention are compared, and the least costly strategy is the preferred choice. These studies are not common because cancer treatments rarely produce equivalent survival or quality of life.

If the interventions being assessed are not of equal effectiveness, *cost-effectiveness analysis* includes a comparison of outcomes such as cases diagnosed, cases averted, or life years gained. These outcomes are then related to the direct costs of the procedure by calculating ratios of incremental cost per unit of incremental effectiveness, such as cost per life year gained. As such, they are relatively easy to understand.

A *cost-utility analysis* is similar to a cost-effectiveness analysis, except that the denominator is the quality-adjusted life year (QALY).[57] The QALY is a measure of the quantity of life gained by a treatment weighted by the utility (described previously). For example, consider a treatment that prolongs survival by an average of 6 months, but because of toxicity and disease morbidity, the average utility experienced by patients during that time is 0.8. The treatment provides 0.5 years × 0.8 utility = 0.4 QALYs. Because the QALY is not disease specific, it allows comparison of the relative efficiency of health care interventions for different conditions. Consequently, the U.S. Preventive Health Service Panel on Cost-Effectiveness recommended the use of QALYs as the best way to estimate outcomes in cost-effectiveness analysis.[58] However, an evaluation of 110 interventions for cancer showed that the incorporation of utilities would only affect decision making in no more than 5% of cases.[59] Therefore, it could be argued that in cases in which the treatment is not expected to have dramatic effects on quality of life in one direction or the other, expensive and time-consuming attempts to precisely measure utilities for a study may not be justified. An alternative analytic approach in such situations would be to estimate the utility *ad hoc* and vary it over a wide range of plausible values in sensitivity analysis (described later) to see whether it would materially change the interpretation of the results.

Cost-benefit analysis is in theory the gold standard of the different forms of economic evaluation. The QALYs in the denominator are valued in monetary terms to arrive at the absolute benefit of the intervention. An intervention is cost-beneficial if the benefits (measured in currency) are greater than the costs. Because these analyses always produce a monetary outcome, it is relatively easy to compare different potential uses of resources, even those beyond health care. However, placing a monetary value on the often-intangible outcomes of health care, in particular the value of a life, is problematic. As a result, true cost-benefit analyses are rare.

Identification and Assessment of Costs

An economic analysis can consider several types of costs. *Direct treatment costs* are the resources used by the health care system to provide treatment, like health care provider fees, drugs, and hospitalization. There are *fixed costs* incurred by each patient regardless of the total number of patients, such as the cost of chemotherapy drugs used. On the other hand, *variable* or *marginal costs* depend on volume and are subject to economies of scale. For example, the cost of doing one extra screening in an established screening program is not the same as the cost of doing the first screening in that program.

Charges are often a poor measure of cost because they are influenced by market forces and reflect profit and cost shifting and the effects of government health care regulations and taxation.[60] Thus, they may bear little resemblance to the resources required to provide a service.[61] Most hospital accounting systems are able to provide departmental cost-to-charge ratios that can be used to estimate costs from charges. Alternatively, reimbursements are sometimes used as a reasonable proxy for cost.[62] In other cases, it is necessary to collect primary data using "microcosting" approaches, such as time and motion studies in which the different components of care are observed, tabulated, and timed.

Direct nontreatment costs are those costs incurred by patients and family to participate in treatment, such as travel, parking, and accommodations near a cancer treatment center. These often are measured by having patients complete diaries or questionnaires about out-of-pocket expenses and time spent. However, these measurements may suffer from missing data and inaccuracies with recall.

Indirect costs include the time patients or informal caregivers spend related to care. This includes time spent traveling to and from clinics, waiting for appointments, or in hospital. It is important to point out that in accounting practice indirect cost refers to overhead, but in health economics overhead is usually considered a direct cost. The value of patient time is often measured as the median wage for all ages (approximately $15 per hour currently in the United States), whether the specific patient is employed or not, in this way recognizing loss of leisure time to be an important consideration as well. Other approaches, however, try to more directly quantify the measurable productivity effects for the specific people affected.[63]

Indirect costs can be nontrivial. For example, it has been estimated in colorectal cancer that these are equivalent to 19% of the direct medical costs of treatment in the first year after diagnosis, rising to 37% in the last year of life.[63] Translated, they can range from a few hundred dollars in the first year after diagnosis of an early stage cancer, to more than $7,000 for metastatic solid tumors in the United States in the last year of life. Overall, in the United States in 2005 it was estimated that patient time costs for the initial phase of cancer care were $2.3 billion for 11 common tumor sites.[64]

The *perspective* of an analysis will affect the range of costs and benefits estimated and, ultimately, the conclusions of the evaluation. Commonly relevant perspectives are those of the providers or purchasers of health care. For example, a program of early discharge after major surgery might save a hospital money, but by shifting costs to home care and outpatient services it becomes relatively cost neutral from the payor's perspective. On the other hand, family members may lose wages staying home to provide additional care and thereby incur more cost from their perspective.[65] It is recommended that a full economic evaluation consider the costs and benefits to all sectors of society affected by the interventions, but also to present the costs and benefits broken down into the component relevant perspectives.[58]

The choice of *time horizon* is also important to ensure that the analysis has considered all the health care resources that may be used. Usually, clinical care is thought of in terms of a new intervention with "upfront" costs such as physician visits, diagnostic tests, procedures, hospitalization, and drugs and dispensing fees. It would also include management of any toxicity or morbidity. These upfront costs could be balanced by "downstream costs," however, like savings from averting the need for treatment of recurrent disease and terminal care. Optimally, a lifetime time horizon is chosen, which would also include estimation of the cost of treating diseases that would not have occurred had the patient died earlier.

Economic Modeling

Some degree of modeling is usually required in order to estimate economic outcomes. Prospectively captured economic data, such as that gathered as part of a clinical trial, is expensive to collect and so may not be available. Even if they are available, long-term outcomes such as survival often need to be estimated from the shorter-term outcomes, such as progression-free survival, that are usually measured in clinical trials. Furthermore, in clinical trials there are usually concerns about patient selection and representativeness, which could affect toxicity and effectiveness estimates for the usually older general cancer population with more comorbidity. Additionally, there are protocol effects that may dictate more visits and tests than would be done in routine practice. Modeling is used to extrapolate to a lifetime time horizon, to adjust the data to be relevant to the general cancer population, and to account for protocol effects.

Costs and benefits that occur in the future should be adjusted, or *discounted*, to their present value. This is because of time preference. It is generally preferred to incur benefits sooner rather than later and costs later rather than sooner. Thus, future costs and benefits have less weight than current costs and benefits and are usually accounted for by applying a constant discount rate, usually in the range of 3% to 6% per year.[40,66] Some recommend discounting benefits as well as costs. Such adjustment favors therapeutic procedures that provide immediate benefit while rendering preventive and screening programs, which require immediate expenditure for future benefits, less attractive.

Because there are so many variables in economic analyses that an investigator can choose to include or exclude in a study, there is always the possibility of bias. Readers of economic analyses have to be especially critical of studies sponsored by pharmaceutical companies, as this industry has a strong interest in seeing these studies come out in favor of their product, and such studies do indeed tend to show favorable results.[67,68] It is possible that publication bias may contribute to this finding. Still, transparency about assumptions and how resource consumption, cost valuations, and benefits were derived are important, and data should be presented in a disaggregated form so readers can make their own judgments about it.

Detailed *sensitivity analyses* should be conducted in any economic study. Such analyses assess how the study results change in response to varying the estimates of resource use, cost, effectiveness, discount rate, and others over a range of plausible possibilities. If altering the value of key parameters changes the conclusion of the study, it is "sensitive" to those parameters and not "robust." The question becomes not whether all estimates of resource use and survival were accurate, but whether any errors would have a meaningful impact on the results.

Economic evaluation itself is not a costless activity.[69] Not every medical technology requires an economic analysis. The more modest the difference in therapeutic effectiveness between two interventions, the more likely it is that economic issues may influence decision making. On the other hand, if the cost of an effective treatment is large but only applicable to a small proportion of the population, an economic evaluation is unlikely to be influential, as the overall cost to the health care system would be small. Lastly, political and cultural considerations must be taken into account. If a treatment is already so ingrained in day-to-day practice that physicians are unlikely to change their practice regardless of the economic data, such a study may not be worth undertaking.

Assessing Cost-Effectiveness

The cost-effectiveness ratio is the *incremental* cost of an intervention divided by its *incremental* benefits, as given by the formula:

$$\text{Cost Effectiveness} = \frac{Cost_1 - Cost_2}{Effectiveness_1 - Effectiveness_2}$$

What constitutes a cost-effective intervention? The value of a consumer product is usually determined by how much people are willing to pay for it. However, this willingness to pay approach can be problematic in health economics because medical care is generally not a discretionary purchase. A patient cannot reasonably decide to refuse life-saving surgery because he or she does not think it is a good bargain. Moreover, whether something represents value for money greatly depends on the income and wealth of the person being asked.

Another approach is to have a threshold for determining acceptable interventions. In the United States, a commonly cited threshold is that interventions costing less than $50,000 per QALY are considered cost-effective,[60] similar to the cost-effectiveness of hemodialysis. The rationale for this is that because Congress debated its funding when it was first introduced, the decision to fund hemodialysis is held up as a precedent for the willingness of society to fund similarly cost-effective programs. An affluent country may be able to support interventions with cost-effectiveness analyses much greater than $50,000/QALY, whereas a poor country may have a lower threshold. To account for this, in international public health the threshold is often set at up to three times a nation's per capita GDP. The current per capita GDP of the United States is approximately $40,000 in 2010, and indeed, many cancer interventions covered by Medicare have estimated cost-effectiveness ratio thresholds exceeding $100,000.

Using Cost-Effectiveness Information in Decision Making

In many countries, cost-effectiveness analysis is explicitly used to decide which health services are essential and consequently covered as part of a universal health insurance package to all citizens. For example, both Australia and the Province of Ontario (Canada) require economic analyses to be part of new drug approval submissions.[70] In contrast, in the United States, policy makers have been slow to use economic studies when setting policy. In fact, the statute that established the Medicare program explicitly prohibits consideration of economic factors in decisions about coverage. However, this is starting to change. The decision to have Medicare pay for pneumococcal vaccination is thought to have been based on the results of a cost-effectiveness analysis.[58]

Why have decision makers not embraced economic analyses? One reason is that the data presented do not always address their immediate needs. Advances in the methodology have brought about routine inclusion of societal costs, which sometimes drive the analysis' conclusion. However, the typical decision maker is usually more concerned with the immediate effects of an intervention on the budget he or she controls. An insurer, for example, is unlikely to realize financial rewards from shifting resources away from treatment for a condition toward a long-term prevention strategy that will have a payoff many years in the future. They are going to be more influenced by arguments that an intervention can be cost neutral or cost savings in the short term. A public health policy maker, on the other hand, may be able to advocate for resources for the preventive program using societal funds. Both perspectives are important but not always clearly presented in published studies.

Another challenge to incorporation of economic information in allocation decisions is that relying on willingness to pay or simple thresholds as described previously could bankrupt a health care system if there is a proliferation of cost-effective interventions. A commonly discussed decision rule to address this is to rank interventions based on their cost-effectiveness in a "league table" and then sequentially fund the most cost-effective until funds are exhausted (Table 31.6).[71] This should theoretically maximize the health gained from limited resources. Perhaps the most prominent example of this was the attempt by the state of Oregon to prioritize medical reimbursements on the basis of cost-effectiveness. A problem with this approach, however, is that comparing studies of varying quality that used different methodologies makes the exercise not as valid as it might seem. Additionally, there are other considerations like social justice and providing treatment preferentially to the young or those with no other options that are important in allocation decisions.[72] In the end, cost-effectiveness analysis can only inform decisions and should not be solely used to make them.

COMPARATIVE EFFECTIVENESS RESEARCH

The American Recovery and Reinvestment Act of 2009 created the Federal Coordinating Council for Comparative Effectiveness Research (CER) to administer a $1.1 billion allocation for studies comparing the benefits and harms of established treatments and strategies for specific conditions. It is

TABLE 31.6

AN ONCOLOGY COST-UTILITY "LEAGUE TABLE"

Description of Intervention, Alternative, and Target Population	Cost ($)/QALY
One-time Pap smear screening program versus no screening program for a low-income 70-year-old black woman seeking medical care from a municipal hospital outpatient clinic	<0[a]
Biennial breast cancer screening in age group 50–70 versus triennial breast cancer screening in age group 50–65	6,900
Adjuvant chemotherapy following surgery, assuming a 15% gain in life expectancy, versus surgery alone for stage II or III colorectal cancer patients	8,100
Adjuvant high-dose interferon alfa-2b therapy versus no interferon treatment for newly diagnosed resectable primary cutaneous melanoma patients	16,000
Chemotherapy versus no chemotherapy for 60-year-old premenopausal women who have undergone surgery for node-negative, ER-negative stage I or IIa breast cancer	25,000
Biennial breast cancer screening in age group 40–70 versus biennial breast cancer screening in age group 50–70	70,000
Breast cancer screening every 2 years versus no breast cancer screening past age 75	80,000
CXR screen versus no testing to follow patients with resected intermediate thickness, local cutaneous melanoma	220,000
IV immune globulin versus no IV immune globulin for chronic lymphocytic leukemia and hypogammaglobulinemia	7,900,000
Follow-up of various intensities versus no follow-up for colorectal cancer patients previously treated by surgery	D

QALY, quality-adjusted life year; ER, estrogen receptor; CXR, chest x-ray; IV, intravenous; D, dominated (more costly but not more effective).
[a]<0, cost-saving.
(From ref. 71, with permission.)

important to note that consideration of cost is not included in the definition of CER. The IOM convened a committee that was asked to prioritize topics across all of health care and produced a list of 100 for initial attention, grouped into quartiles of priority.[73] Although many of the suggestions cut across more than one disease, several are specific to cancer. Examples from the highest priority quartile include comparison of the effectiveness of different management strategies for localized prostate cancer and ductal carcinoma *in situ* and the effectiveness of genetic and biomarker testing in the management of common cancers. Other recommendations are to compare the effectiveness of newer technologies for breast and colorectal cancer screening, management options for liver metastases, and models of end-of-life and palliative care.

Efficacy research addresses the question as to how well this intervention can work. In contrast, effectiveness research addresses the question of how well this intervention actually works in real world contexts. The IOM committee has defined CER as "the generation and synthesis of evidence that compares the benefits and harms of alternative methods to prevent, diagnose, treat, and monitor a clinical condition or to improve the delivery of care. The purpose of CER is to assist consumers, clinicians, purchasers, and policy makers to make informed decisions that will improve health care at both the individual and population levels".[74] The core questions of CER are to determine which treatment works best, for whom, and under what circumstances. Engaging stakeholders, who confront decisions about what treatments to use when, in prioritizing research questions, and thus the consumers of the knowledge gained from this research, is a tenet of CER.[75]

CER often uses the PICO framework to crystallize an analysis. (PICO stands for *P*opulation, *I*ntervention, *C*omparison, and *O*utcome.) By defining each of these attributes of an analysis, the comparison is made explicit. The PICO framework is sometimes expanded to PICOTT, adding information about the *T*ype of question being asked (therapy, diagnosis, prognosis, toxicity) and the *T*ype of study design most appropriate to address the particular question. Using this framework helps to make CER analyses explicit and facilitates communication about study results.

CER involves a variety of research methods. First is the use of existing data resources about the outcomes of care in routine clinical settings. As with all observational research, access to sufficient clinical information and detail to minimize the impact of selection bias and confounding is essential and a perpetual challenge. The dissemination of electronic medical records and strategies for encryption of confidential data has facilitated the potential to leverage observational data sets to compare outcomes of different treatment approaches. In addition, the use of statistical techniques, such as propensity score analyses and instrumental variable analyses, is important to mitigate confounding that may arise when observational data are used to compare outcomes. CER also extends to include prospective data collection, including the concept of the pragmatic clinical trial, sometimes referred to as large simple trials. In contrast to the typical efficacy trial, these studies have few exclusion criteria, are performed in everyday community practice settings, and involve simple measurements of covariates and outcome variables. A particular subtype of pragmatic trial is the cluster randomized trial. In this design, individual patients are not randomized; instead, providers, or more often clinic sites, are randomized to adopt one strategy or another. Then, the outcomes of patients treated at centers who adopt strategy A versus B are compared.[76,77]

Finally, in order to derive benefit from research it must be communicated to practitioners and policy makers and actually put into use. Consistent application of the knowledge already known have would have an impact on the prevention and treatment of cancer on par with many of the largest scientific advances. It is apparent from the variations in care quality described previously that presentation of research results in scientific meetings and publication in journals is insufficient to alter practice in many cases. Common strategies to better implement research include the creation of guidelines for providers and decision aids for patients. Newer approaches include involvement of policy makers in applied research early on and direct attempts to provide summaries to them in written or presentation formats. Identification of strategies to translate research into practice is a key element of CER.

Selected References

The full list of references for this chapter appears in the online version.

4. Lee SJ, Earle CC, Weeks JC. Outcomes research in oncology: history, conceptual framework, and trends in the literature. *J Natl Cancer Inst* 2000; 92:195.
5. Grunfeld E, Levine MN, Julian JA, et al. Randomized trial of long-term follow-up for early-stage breast cancer: a comparison of family physician versus specialist care. *J Clin Oncol* 2006;24:848.
6. Earle CC, Tsai JS, Gelber RD, et al. Effectiveness of palliative chemotherapy for advanced lung cancer: instrumental variable and propensity analysis. *J Clin Oncol* 2001;19:1064.
7. Warren JLJ, Klabunde CNC, Schrag DD, Bach PBP, Riley GFG. Overview of the SEER-Medicare data: content, research applications, and generalizability to the United States elderly population. *Med Care* 2002;40:3.
8. Lamont EB, Herndon JE, Weeks JC, et al. Measuring disease-free survival and cancer relapse using Medicare claims from CALGB breast cancer trial participants (companion to 9344). *J Natl Cancer Inst* 2006; 98:1335.
9. Lamont EB, Herndon JE, Weeks JC, et al. Criterion validity of Medicare chemotherapy claims in Cancer and Leukemia Group B breast and lung cancer trial participants. *J Natl Cancer Inst* 2005;97:1080.
13. Schrag D, Cramer LD, Bach PB, Begg CB. Age and adjuvant chemotherapy use after surgery for stage III colon cancer. *J Natl Cancer Inst* 2001; 93:850.
14. Bach PB, Cramer LD, Warren JL, Begg CB. Racial differences in the treatment of early-stage lung cancer. *N Eng J Med* 1999;341:1198.
15. Krzyzanowska MK, Weeks JC, Earle CC. Treatment of locally advanced pancreatic cancer in the real world: population-based practices and effectiveness. *J Clin Oncol* 2003;21:3009.
16. Hawley ST, Hofer TP, Janz NK, et al. Correlates of between-surgeon variation in breast cancer treatments. *Med Care* 2006;44:609.
19. Dudley RA, Johansen KL, Brand R, Rennie DJ, Milstein A. Selective referral to high-volume hospitals: estimating potentially avoidable deaths [comments]. *JAMA* 2000;283:1159.
20. Birkmeyer JDJ, Siewers AEA, Finlayson EVE, et al. Hospital volume and surgical mortality in the United States. *N Eng J Med* 2002;346:1128.
21. Halm EA, Lee C, Chassin MR. Is volume related to outcome in health care? A systematic review and methodologic critique of the literature. *Ann Intern Med* 2002;137:511.
22. Birkmeyer JD, Finlayson EV, Birkmeyer CM. Volume standards for high-risk surgical procedures: potential benefits of the Leapfrog initiative. *Surgery* 2001;130:415.
23. Begg CB, Cramer LD, Hoskins WJ, Brennan MF. Impact of hospital volume on operative mortality for major cancer surgery. *JAMA* 1998;280:1747.
24. Bach PB, Cramer LD, Schrag D, et al. The influence of hospital volume on survival after resection for lung cancer. *N Engl J Med* 2001;19(345):181.
25. Schrag D, Panageas KS, Riedel E, et al. Hospital and surgeon procedure volume as predictors of outcome following rectal cancer resection. *Ann Surg* 2002;236:583.
31. Donabedian A. Evaluating the quality of medical care. *Milbank Mem Fund Q* 1966;44:166.
32. Earle CC. Outcomes research in lung cancer. *J Natl Cancer Inst Monogr* 2004;33:56.
33. Bradley C. Feedback on the FDA's February 2006 draft guidance on patient reported outcome (PRO) measures from a developer of PRO measures. *Health Qual Life Outcomes* 2006;4:78.
35. Tarlov AR, Ware JE Jr, Greenfield S, et al. The Medical Outcomes Study. An application of methods for monitoring the results of medical care. *JAMA* 1989;262:925.
36. Aaronson NK, Ahmedzai S, Bergman B, et al. The European Organization for Research and Treatment of Cancer QLQ-C30: a quality-of-life instrument for use in international clinical trails in oncology. *J Natl Cancer Inst* 1993;85:365.
37. Cella DF, Tulsky DS, Gray G, et al. The functional assessment of Cancer Therapy Scale: development and validation of the general measure. *J Clin Oncol* 1993;11:570.
38. Hollen PJ, Gralla RJ, Kris MG, Eberly SW, Cox C. Normative data and trends in quality of life from the Lung Cancer Symptom Scale (LCSS). *Support Care Cancer* 1999;7:140.
39. Torrance GW, Feeny D. Utilities and quality-adjusted life years. *Int J Tech Assess Health Care* 1989;5:559.
40. Siegel JE, Weinstein MC, Russell LB, Gold MR. Recommendations for reporting cost-effectiveness analyses. *JAMA* 1996;276:1339.
42. Tannock IF, Osoba D, Stockler MR, et al. Chemotherapy with mitoxantrone plus prednisone or prednisone alone for symptomatic hormone-resistant prostate cancer: a Canadian randomized trial with palliative end points. *J Clin Oncol* 1996;14:1756.
43. Pauly MV. Is high and growing spending on cancer treatment and prevention harmful to the United States economy? *J Clin Oncol* 2007;25:171.
44. Meropol NJ, Schulman KA. Cost of cancer care: issues and implications. *J Clin Oncol* 2007;25:180.
45. Lubitz JD, Riley GF. Trends in Medicare payments in the last year of life. *N Engl J Med* 1993;328:1092.
47. Schrag D. The price tag on progress—chemotherapy for colorectal cancer. *N Engl J Med* 2004;351:317.
51. Schrag D, Hanger M. Medical oncologists' views on communicating with patients about chemotherapy costs: a pilot survey. *J Clin Oncol* 2007;25:233.
55. Hadley J, Mandelblatt JS, Mitchell JM, et al. Medicare breast surgery fees and treatment received by older women with localized breast cancer. *Health Serv Res* 2003;38:553.
56. Jacobson M, O'Malley AJ, Earle CC, et al. Does reimbursement influence chemotherapy treatment for cancer patients? *Health Aff (Millwood)* 2006;25:437.
57. Greenberg D, Earle C, Fang CH, Eldar-Lissai A, Neumann PJ. When is cancer care cost-effective? A systematic overview of cost-utility analyses in oncology. *J Natl Cancer Inst* 2010;102:82.
58. Gold MR, Siegel JE, Russell LB, Weinstein MC, eds. *Cost-effectiveness in health and medicine*. New York: Oxford University Press, 1996.
59. Tengs TO. Cost-effectiveness versus cost-utility analysis of interventions for cancer: does adjusting for health-related quality of life really matter? *Value Health* 2004;7:70.
60. Hayman J, Weeks J, Mauch P. Economic analyses in health care: an introduction to the methodology with an emphasis on radiation therapy. *Int J Rad Oncol Biol Phys* 1996;35:827.
61. Finkler SA. The distinction between costs and charges. *Ann Intern Med* 1982;96:102.
62. Brown ML, Riley GF, Schussler N, Etzioni R. Estimating health care costs related to cancer treatment from SEER-Medicare data. *Med Care* 2002;40(Suppl):IV-104.
63. Yabroff KR, Warren JL, Knopf K, Davis WW, Brown ML. Estimating patient time costs associated with colorectal cancer care. *Med Care* 2005;43:640.
64. Yabroff KR, Davis WW, Lamont EB, et al. Patient time costs associated with cancer care. *J Natl Cancer Inst* 2007;99:14.
65. Grunfeld E, Glossop R, McDowell I, Danbrook C. Caring for elderly people at home: the consequences to caregivers. *Can Med Assoc J* 1997;157:1101.
66. Torrance GW, Blaker D, Detsky A, et al. Canadian guidelines for economic evaluation of pharmaceuticals. *Pharmacoeconomics* 1996;9:535.
67. Friedberg M, Saffran B, Stinson TJ, Nelson W, Bennett CL. Evaluation of conflict of interest in economic analyses of new drugs used in oncology. *JAMA* 1999;282:1453.
69. Drummond MF, Coyle D. The role of pilot studies in the economic evaluation of health technologies. *Int J Tech Assess Health Care* 1998;14:405.
71. Earle CC, Chapman RH, Bell CM, et al. A systematic overview of cost-utility assessments in oncology. *J Clin Oncol* 2000;18:3302.
72. Drummond MF, Mason AR. European perspective on the costs and cost-effectiveness of cancer therapies. *J Clin Oncol* 2007;25:191.
76. Murray DM, Pals SL, Blitstein JL, Alfano CM, Lehman J. Design and analysis of group-randomized trials in cancer: a review of current practices. *J Natl Cancer Inst* 2008;100:483–491.
77. Zwarenstein M, Treweek S, Gagnier JJ, et al. Improving the reporting of pragmatic trials: an extension of the CONSORT statement. *BMJ*. 2008;337:a2390.

PART FOUR

PHARMACOLOGY OF CANCER THERAPEUTICS

SECTION 1: CHEMOTHERAPY AGENTS

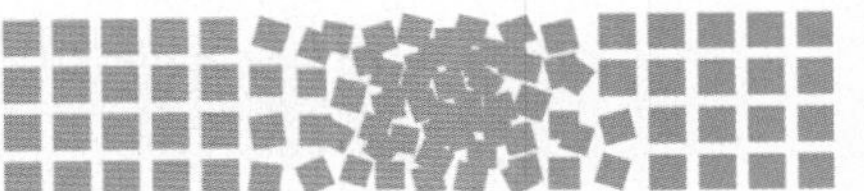

CHAPTER 32 PHARMACOKINETICS AND PHARMACODYNAMICS

CHRIS H. TAKIMOTO, CHEE M. NG, AND THOMAS PUCHALSKI

The pharmacologic treatment of human malignancies involves the clinical use of some of the most challenging therapeutic agents in all of medicine. The practicing medical oncologist must manage the risk of serious toxicities, optimize therapies with relatively narrow efficacy profiles, and adjust on a routine basis the administration of various therapeutic regimens to heterogeneous patient populations. In this chapter, the use of the term *drug* will apply equally to small molecules and to biologically derived therapeutics. Because the science of clinical pharmacology attempts to rationally explain and predict the sources of variability of drug action, it has great relevance for the field of medical oncology. Clinical pharmacology can be broadly defined as the study of drugs in humans, and it can be subdivided into two major disciplines: *pharmacokinetics* and *pharmacodynamics*.[1] Atkinson[1] defined pharmacokinetics as "the quantitative analysis of the process of drug absorption, distribution and elimination that determine the time course of drug action." Ratain and Mick[2] have paraphrased this definition of pharmacokinetics as "what the body does to the drug." Classically, pharmacokinetics involves the characterization of an agent's absorption, distribution, metabolism, and excretion through the measurement of drug concentrations in an accessible compartment over time. In contrast, *pharmacodynamics* relates drug dose and kinetics to clinical drug effects, such as efficacy or toxicity. In simplified terms, pharmacodynamics can be defined as "what the drug does to the body."[2]

WHY STUDY PHARMACOKINETICS AND PHARMACODYNAMICS?

The clinical importance of pharmacokinetics and pharmacodynamics is predicated on the principle that concentration–response relationships are less variable than dose–response relationships for any specific agent.[1] Drug receptor theory predicts that drug concentrations in measurable compartments at equilibrium are directly proportional to the concentrations at the effective site of action. Understanding interpatient variability in drug kinetics allows for the implementation of strategies to reduce this variability and thereby achieve more consistent clinical results. The ultimate goal of the medical oncologist is to use pharmacokinetic and pharmacodynamic knowledge to maximize therapeutic benefits for individual patients. Typically, the clinical pharmacology of a new anticancer agent is characterized during integrated pharmacokinetic and pharmacodynamic studies initiated early in the drug development process. Data obtained from these analyses, when rationally applied to general clinical practice, allow the practicing oncologist to optimize treatment regimens for patients even before the first dose is administered. It also provides valuable information on how to adjust treatment doses and schedules when the initial treatment is unsatisfactory because of excessive toxicities or other complications.

Understanding a drug's kinetic properties provides the medical oncologist and drug development scientist with clinically useful descriptive, explanatory, and predictive information.[3] The descriptive power of pharmacokinetics is easily illustrated by summarizing a drug's behavior in a defined population using a specific pharmacokinetic model. For example, the characterization of a one-compartment, open, linear pharmacokinetic model with first-order elimination and mean values for the volume of distribution and the elimination rate constant can succinctly describe an extensive amount of concentration versus time data for a group of cancer patients (Fig. 32.1). Furthermore, the relative standard deviations of the population estimates of the volume of distribution and elimination rate constant can provide insight into the degree of interpatient variability in drug kinetics in the study population.[3]

Pharmacokinetic analyses can also provide substantial explanatory information about the underlying physiologic processes affecting drug behavior.[3] This can lead to specific hypotheses about the underlying mechanisms responsible for the distribution, elimination, or metabolism of a specific agent. For example, if a correlation is observed between drug clearance and creatinine clearance, then renal excretion may be hypothesized to be an important route of drug elimination (Fig. 32.2). Such findings suggest that caution is warranted if the drug is administered to patients with renal impairment. Furthermore, a correlation between renal function and drug clearance may serve as a basis for individualized dosing algorithms using pretreatment estimations of the glomerular filtration rate (GFR). A widely employed clinical example is the Calvert formula used to dose carboplatin to achieve a target area under the concentration curve (AUC).[4] Variability in pharmacokinetic parameters may also be affected by other important covariates, including age, gender, hepatic dysfunction, body surface area, concomitant medications, or pharmacogenetic polymorphisms in key drug-metabolizing enzymes. These covariate relationships may explain a substantial portion of the pharmacokinetic variability present within the study population. The reduction of interpatient variability by the *a priori* adjustment of individual treatment regimens is a major goal of applied clinical pharmacology.

Finally, understanding drug kinetics allows for specific predictions to be made when different doses and schedules of administration are used.[3] For example, pharmacokinetic parameter estimates obtained after a single intravenous drug

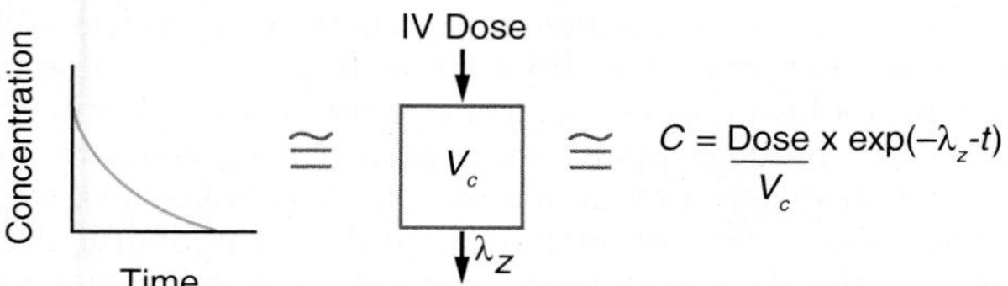

FIGURE 32.1 One-compartment, open pharmacokinetic model with intravenous bolus input is defined by two pharmacokinetic parameters: the apparent volume of distribution, V_c, and the elimination rate constant, λ_z. The raw pharmacokinetic concentration versus time data can be represented by a schematic box diagram or by a monoexponential mathematical formula with two unknown parameters, V_c and λ_z. In the mathematical representation of these data, time (t) is the independent variable, concentration (C) is the dependent variable, and *dose* is a known constant.

bolus can be used to calculate the steady-state concentration profile during a prolonged continuous infusion. This predictive function is clinically important for making rational dose adjustments during an ongoing treatment course. However, for agents with saturable pharmacokinetics, it may be difficult to predict exact drug concentrations following dose adjustment. For example, paclitaxel is a commonly used antitumor agent with well-characterized nonlinear pharmacokinetic behavior.[5]

Pharmacodynamic studies are directly relevant to the practice of medical oncology because of their focus on clinical end points.[6] Drug kinetics may account for only a portion of the variability seen in treatment outcomes. Patients with identical systemic exposures may experience very different responses to drug therapy in terms of efficacy and toxicity. For example, a patient with a history of extensive prior chemotherapy or radiation therapy may experience more myelosuppressive toxicity than a minimally pretreated patient at the same dose and exposure. A well-defined pharmacodynamic model minimizes the contribution of pharmacokinetic variability and allows the investigator to focus on inherent differences in target tissue susceptibility. Our understanding of pharmacodynamic variability in malignant tissues is still quite limited; however, molecular profiling of tumors is likely to improve our understanding of cancer sensitivity and resistance. The integration of molecular pharmacodynamics into early clinical trials of newer targeted anticancer agents is now a standard in oncology drug development. An example of molecularly defined pharmacodynamic differences occurs in advanced colorectal cancer patient with *K-ras* mutations. These patients are highly resistant to treatment with anti–epidermal growth factor receptor (EGFR) antibodies.[7]

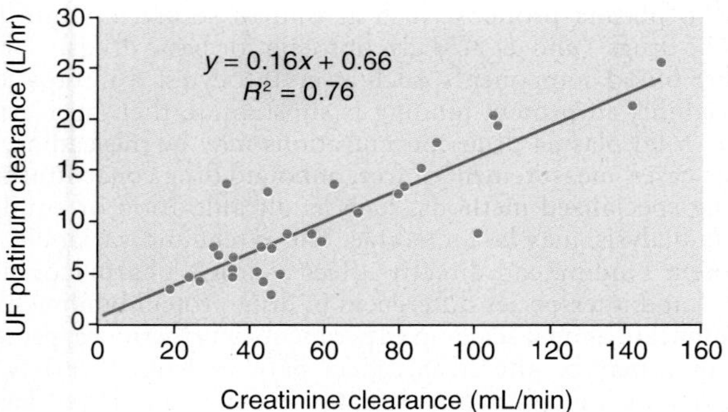

FIGURE 32.2 Correlation between the clearance of platinum species from plasma ultrafiltrates (UF) and the measured 24-hour urinary creatinine clearance in adult solid-tumor patients with varying degrees of renal dysfunction after treatment with oxaliplatin. (Data taken from a clinical trial described in ref. 56.)

CANCER PATIENTS PRESENT UNIQUE CHALLENGES

The design of rational, pharmacologically sound treatment strategies for cancer patients presents some unique challenges to the medical oncologist. The therapeutic index of any cancer therapy is defined as the ratio between the systemic exposure associated with unacceptable toxicity and the exposure that maximizes the likelihood of the intended treatment response. The therapeutic index of cancer therapies is probably the narrowest of any class of agents in common use. Furthermore, pharmacokinetic variability in cancer patients may be enhanced by a variety of factors, including prior gastrointestinal surgery, poor nutritional status, hypoalbuminemia, polypharmacy, advanced age, and altered renal or hepatic function. Factors that may alter pharmacodynamic drug effects include prior chemotherapy or radiation therapy, poor performance status, comorbid disease states, and bone marrow involvement by the underlying tumor. Finally, the pharmacodynamics of most anticancer agents are complex because of the long lag time between drug exposure and clinically relevant outcomes, such as myelosuppressive toxicity or tumor response. All of these factors must be accounted for when designing pharmacologic strategies for treating patients with cancer. Despite these obstacles, the number of new, molecularly targeted agents with activity in the treatment of human malignancies continues to grow. The challenge for the practicing oncologist is to apply knowledge about the clinical pharmacology of these new therapies in the most expeditious way possible to maximize therapeutic benefit.

PHARMACOKINETIC CONCEPTS

A drug's pharmacokinetic properties in a specific patient population can be defined by a relatively small set of pharmacokinetic parameters. These parameters are related to fundamental processes affecting drug behavior over time, such as drug absorption, distribution, and elimination. In the following sections, some basic pharmacokinetic and pharmacodynamic parameters are described, with an emphasis on their clinical relevance.

Bioavailability

Historically, most anticancer therapies have been administered intravenously; however, the use of orally administered agents is growing with the development of many small-molecule targeted cancer therapeutics, such as imatinib, erlotinib, sunitinib, sorafenib, lapatinib, dasatinib, and others. The pharmacokinetic parameter most closely associated with oral absorption is bioavailability (F), defined as the dose fraction that reaches the systemic circulation relative to a reference method of administration, which is most commonly intravenous delivery. For an oral agent, bioavailability is defined as the AUC achieved following oral administration divided by the AUC observed after intravenous administration. Oral bioavailability can range from 0 to 1.0 and is defined by the following formula[8]:

$$F = dose(IV) \times AUC(oral)/[dose(oral) \times AUC(IV)], \quad \text{(Eq. 1)}$$

where *dose(IV)* and *dose(oral)* are the intravenous and oral doses, respectively, and *AUC(oral)* and *AUC(IV)* are the resulting oral and intravenous AUC values, respectively. The actual extent of absorption from the gut into the systemic circulation can only be determined if both an oral and an intravenous formulation are available. In oncology, intravenous formulations of oral treatment agents are not always tested clinically; however, clearance and volume of distribution can still be assessed using standard methods if the results are corrected for bioavailability.[8] Thus, apparent volume of distribution can be reported as *V/F* and clearance (*CL*) as *CL/F*, even when bioavailability, *F*, is not determined explicitly.

Bioavailability is directly related to absorption processes that dictate how an agent enters the systemic circulation. For an oral agent, this complex series of events begins with ingestion followed by drug disintegration, dissolution, diffusion through gastrointestinal fluids, membrane permeation, portal circulation uptake, passage through the liver, and, finally, entry into the systemic circulation.[9] Extensive drug metabolism in the gut and liver or avid biliary excretion can limit the entry into the systemic circulation of an oral drug, a process called the *first-pass effect.*[10] Oral bioavailability may be altered in cancer patients by the simultaneous consumption of food, nausea and vomiting, changes in product formulation, or by altered integrity of the gastrointestinal tract arising from surgery, chemotherapy side effects, or radiation therapy. For biological therapies such as monoclonal antibodies, intravenous administration is typical, but bioavailability may be calculated for nonintravenous routes of administration such as subcutaneous injections.[11]

Volumes of Distribution

The volume of distribution relates the amount of drug in the body to the concentration observed in the measured compartment; thus, it represents a constant of proportionality. The volume of distribution may or may not correspond to an actual physiologic compartment. Several volume of distribution terms are in common clinical use, and not all volume terms are directly representative of drug distribution processes. In oncology studies, commonly reported parameters include the apparent volume of distribution at steady state (V_{ss}), volume of distribution of the central compartment (V_c), and volume of distribution during the terminal elimination phase (V_z or V_{area}).

The apparent volume of distribution at steady state (V_{ss}) is the constant of proportionality relating the amount of drug in the body to the steady-state concentration.[12] This volume term has high clinical relevance because it is heavily influenced by the anatomic space occupied by the drug and by the amount of deep tissue penetration at equilibrium.[10] The V_{ss} is independent of drug clearance and half-life, and its estimation does not require steady-state drug administration. In a multicompartment model, V_{ss} is defined by

$$V_{ss} = V_1 + V_2 + \cdots + V_n, \qquad \text{(Eq. 2)}$$

where *n* is the number of compartments in the model. Using noncompartmental analysis methods based on statistical moment theory, the V_{ss} can be calculated after a single intravenous bolus dose as follows[12]:

$$V_{ss} = dose(AUMC)/(AUC)^2 \qquad \text{(Eq. 3)}$$

where *AUMC* is the area under the first moment curve (concentration multiplied by time plotted versus time) and *AUC* is the area under the concentration versus time curve. After an infusion, V_{ss} can be calculated from the following[12]:

$$V_{ss} = dose(AUMC)/(AUC)^2 - [R_0T^2/2(AUC)], \qquad \text{(Eq. 4)}$$

where *T* is the duration of the infusion and R_0 is the dose rate of infusion. For protein-based therapeutics, slightly modified approaches are recommended.[13] In general, larger V_{ss} values suggest more widespread tissue distribution, whereas a V_{ss} approximating the plasma volume is consistent with an agent confined to the intravascular space.

The volume of distribution of the central compartment (V_c) is the constant of proportionality relating drug dose and the immediate postbolus infusion drug concentration. This parameter is useful for the determining the maximal drug concentration (C_{max}) immediately after an intravenous drug bolus; however, it provides little or no information about the extent of drug distribution or tissue binding, making it a less useful volume term for clinical use.[10]

The terminal disposition volume of distribution (V_z or V_{area}) is the constant of proportionality associated with the amount of drug in the measured compartment during the terminal elimination phase. This volume term is useful for calculating the loading dose necessary to ensure that average drug concentrations never fall below the targeted steady-state concentration. This volume term can be estimated from the following formula:

$$V_z = V_{area} = CL/\lambda_z = dose/(\lambda_z \times AUC), \qquad \text{(Eq. 5)}$$

where λ_z is the elimination rate constant and *CL* is clearance. The clinical utility of this parameter may vary because V_z does not always reflect changes in the drug distribution process.[10] Although V_z may approximate V_{ss} in some situations, for drugs with high clearance rates, V_z will exceed V_{ss} values independent of any distribution processes.[10]

The rate and extent to which a drug distributes into various tissues depend on a number of factors, including the drug lipophilicity, tissue permeability, tissue-binding constants, and local organ blood flow. Large apparent volumes of distribution are common for agents with high tissue binding or high lipid solubility. Distribution into specific body compartments may be limited by physiological processes, such as the blood–brain barrier protecting the central nervous system, or the blood–testes barrier. Poor drug penetration into these compartments may have clinical relevance. For example, the treatment of carcinomatous meningitis or acute leukemia in the central nervous system typically requires direct intrathecal chemotherapy administration.[14]

Protein Binding and Free Drug Concentrations

Bioanalytical drug assays typically measure total plasma concentrations and do not distinguish between the free and protein-bound drug fractions. Although at equilibrium free and bound drug vary in parallel, only the free fraction directly equilibrates with extravascular compartments, making it the most relevant for predicting pharmacodynamic drug effects. Most small-molecule therapeutics show some degree of binding to plasma proteins, such as human serum albumin for acidic drugs[13] and α_1-acid glycoprotein for basic drugs,[15] or to other blood components, such as erythrocytes. If intrapatient variability in protein binding is substantial, then measuring only total plasma drug concentrations may be misleading. In such cases, measurement of free, unbound drug concentrations using specialized methods, such as ultrafiltration or equilibrium dialysis, may be preferable. The extent and variability of protein binding can directly affect a drug's pharmacokinetics,[15] and interspecies differences in drug protein binding may complicate animal scale-up experiments. Furthermore, protein binding may be altered in cancer patients from a variety of factors, including renal or hepatic dysfunction, altered levels of the acute-phase reactant α_1-acid glycoprotein, or hypoalbuminemia caused by malnutrition, poor biosynthetic reserve in the liver, or paraneoplastic nephrotic syndrome. Thus, protein binding may be an important source of interpatient variability in drug kinetics.

Drug Clearance

Of all the parameters in clinical pharmacology, clearance has the most clinical relevance because it reflects all processes in the body that contribute to the elimination of a drug over time. These can include metabolism in the liver, urinary excretion, or excretion through the biliary system. Clearance is not a rate; instead, it is a unit of volume that is cleared of drug per time. For a drug with dose-proportional kinetics, clearance is independent of concentration and dose, which underscores its fundamental clinical importance. Total systemic drug clearance (CL) is the sum of all individual clearance processes occurring throughout the body and can be defined by the following equation:

$$CL = CL_{renal} + CL_{hepatic} + CL_{other}, \quad \text{(Eq. 6)}$$

where CL_{renal} is renal clearance, $CL_{hepatic}$ is hepatic clearance, and CL_{other} is all other clearance processes in the body.

Drug clearance is relevant because it defines the key relationship between drug dose as prescribed by the practicing clinician and systemic drug exposure or AUC as measured by the pharmacokineticist. The AUC is directly calculated from concentration versus time data using simple mathematical integration methods (Fig. 32.3).[8] If $AUC_{0\text{-}INF}$ is the area under the concentration versus time curve extrapolated to infinity after a single dose of drug, then

$$CL = dose/AUC_{0\text{-}INF}, \quad \text{(Eq. 7a)}$$

or, rearranging,

$$AUC_{0\text{-}INF} = dose/CL. \quad \text{(Eq. 7b)}$$

As seen in Equation 7b, clearance is the sole determinant of systemic drug exposure for any given dose. Interpatient variability in drug clearance can be described by the coefficient of variation ($CV\%$), which is the relative standard deviation expressed as a percentage of the mean clearance. Many anticancer agents have $CV\%$ in clearance in the range of 20% to 40%. Clearance also defines the steady-state concentrations (C_{ss}) observed during continuous, prolonged drug infusions, as defined by the formula:

$$CL = infusion\ rate/C_{ss}. \quad \text{(Eq. 8)}$$

Whether recognized or not, the practicing medical oncologist estimates an individual's drug clearance every time cancer chemotherapy is prescribed on a milligram per square meter basis. Dosing of cancer chemotherapy using body surface area (BSA) inherently assumes that CL is directly related to body size (Eq. 7b). However, this CL and BSA correlation is often weak and may not justify the uncritical widespread implementation of this practice.[16] The routine use of BSA-based dosing for small-molecule therapeutics has been heavily criticized. In some situations, alternative dosing regimens based on lean body mass,[17] or even the use of flat, fixed doses for patients of different sizes may be a more rational approach.[18,19]

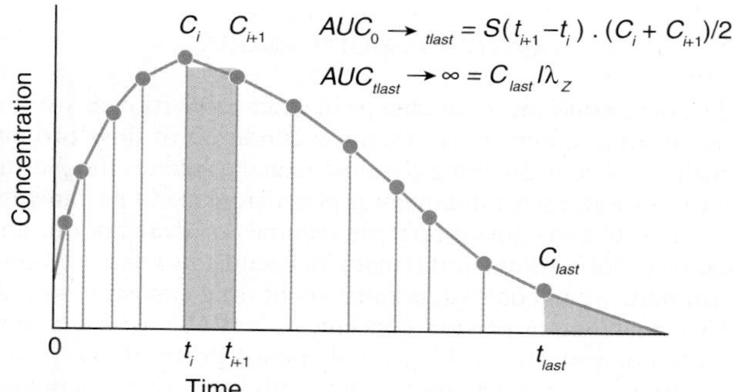

FIGURE 32.3 Estimation of the area under the concentration versus time curve (AUC) using the log-linear trapezoidal rule. The area under the curve from time zero to t_{last} is defined by $AUC_{0 \rightarrow tlast} = S(t_{i+1} - t_i) \times (C_i + C_{i+1})/2$, and the area under the curve from time t_{last} extrapolated to infinity is defined by $AUC_{tlast} \rightarrow \infty = C_{last}/\lambda_z$, where λ_z is the elimination rate constant. The total AUC extrapolated to infinity, $AUC_0 \rightarrow \infty$, is the sum of these two AUC terms.

For most small-molecule therapeutics, drug metabolism is a major route of systemic clearance. The liver is the predominant site for most drug-metabolizing reactions, although biotransformation can also occur in the gut, lung, kidneys, blood, tumors, and virtually anywhere else in the body. Traditionally, drug-metabolizing reactions have been divided into phase I and II reactions, both of which typically generate more polar, biologically inactive metabolites. Phase I reactions add a functional group through enzymatic oxidation or reduction, often converting the molecule into a substrate for subsequent phase II conjugation reactions. The cytochrome P-450 mono-oxygenase system is the best characterized family of phase I drug-metabolizing enzymes. These enzymes are grouped into 17 families with numerous subgroups identified based on amino acid sequence homology. In humans, CYP1, CYP2, and CYP3 families are involved in most drug-metabolizing reactions, with two isoforms, CYP3A4 and CYP3A5, being responsible for approximately 50% of human drug metabolism. Individual cytochrome P-450 isoforms have characteristic induction and inhibition profiles, and their substrate specificity is typically well defined, although overlap between different isoforms is common. These enzymes are involved in the endogenous biosynthesis of fatty acids and steroids, and they were presumed to have an evolutionary role in protecting against xenobiotic toxins. In most circumstances, these phase I metabolic pathways are detoxifying reactions; however, activation of drugs and carcinogens by the action of cytochrome P-450 can also occur.[20] Clinically significant drug interactions due to the inhibition of CYP3A4-medicated drug metabolism by agents such as ketoconazole, ritonavir, erythromycin, and clarithromycin are well documented.[20]

Phase II reactions involve drug conjugation to glucuronic acid, amino acids, glutathione, or sulfate groups. The resulting water-soluble polar metabolites are usually substrates for subsequent drug excretion in urine or bile. Glucuronidation is mediated through uridine diphosphate glucuronosyltransferases found in the liver, intestines, kidney, and skin. Glucuronidation followed by biliary excretion is important for the elimination of endogenous compounds such as steroids, bile acids, and bilirubin, and it is a major rate-limiting pathway for the excretion of anticancer agents such as SN-38, the active metabolite of irinotecan. *N*-acetyltransferases and sulfotransferases found in the liver and other tissues are also responsible for drug transformation to more water-soluble species. Genetic polymorphisms in all types of drug-metabolizing enzymes are increasingly being recognized as an important source of variability in drug-metabolizing pathways.[21] The impact of hepatic dysfunction on liver drug-metabolizing pathways can be difficult to assess. Liver dysfunction can affect glucuronidation, and cirrhosis can reduce drug-metabolizing capacity by 30% to 50%.[22] Malnutrition has also been implicated in alterations in hepatic clearance of drugs.[23]

Drug clearance may also be mediated by excretion processes occurring in either the kidneys or the biliary system. The importance of assessing renal function before dosing renally excreted agents is well recognized.[4] Agents such as topotecan, etoposide, and carboplatin require dose adjustments in patients with impaired renal function. Usually, dosing decisions are based on estimations of the GFR; however, renal drug excretion may be influenced by other processes such as tubular secretion and reabsorption. In the proximal tubules, drugs are actively excreted via the action of adenosine triphosphate (ATP)-binding cassette (ABC) drug efflux pumps such as ABCB1 (P-glycoprotein) and ABCC2 (MRP2/cMOAT).[24] In distal tubules and collecting ducts, passive reabsorption dominates, and these processes are often greatly affected by urinary pH. The excretion of weak acids is often enhanced by urinary alkalinization. Finally, because body size affects GFR, individual estimates of GFR should be scaled to BSA and expressed in term of milliliters per minute per 1.73 m^2 whenever BSA-adjusted drug dosing schemes are used.[25]

The ABC transporters in the biliary canaliculi are important in mediating biliary drug excretion pathways. The ABCB1 and ABCC2 transport proteins can interact with organic cations and conjugated metabolites, such as drug glucuronides and sulfates. Biliary excretion is an important route of drug clearance for anticancer agents such as the irinotecan metabolite SN-38 and the anthracycline doxorubicin. The inducible activity of these biliary transport enzymes can lead to clinically significant changes in drug clearance. Cancer patients treated with enzyme-inducing antiepileptic drugs, such as phenytoin and carbamazepine, may have twofold to threefold higher drug clearance than control patients.[26] Biliary excretion pathways are also involved in enterohepatic circulation of some anticancer agents. Cleavage of glucuronidated metabolites of irinotecan by endogenous gut flora can lead to enterohepatic circulation and prolonged retention within the gastrointestinal tract.[27]

The relevance of renal and hepatic clearance mechanisms in medical oncology is highlighted by the treatment of patients with end-organ dysfunction. Alterations in hepatic function are quite common in patients with hepatic metastases from colorectal cancer and can lead to significant diminutions in drug clearance. Although not the most sensitive measure of hepatic function, baseline bilirubin and alanine aminotransferase/aspartate aminotransferase are often used to select a dose for drugs that principally undergo hepatic metabolism. In other cancer patients, administration of nephrotoxic chemotherapeutic agents, such as cisplatin, or tumor-induced obstructive nephropathies may result in chronic renal impairment that complicates the use of renally excreted agents. Increasingly, formal pharmacokinetic studies in cancer patients with abnormal renal and hepatic function are being conducted during the later stages of the drug development process to provide important dosing guidelines for these unique patient populations.[28,29]

Elimination Half-Life

The elimination half-life is the amount of time required for 50% of an administered drug to be eliminated.[1] The terminal elimination half-life ($t_{1/2}$) can be readily calculated from the elimination rate constant, λ_z, using the following formula:

$$t_{1/2} = ln(2)/\lambda_z, = 0.693/\lambda_z. \quad \text{(Eq. 9)}$$

The terminal elimination rate constant, λ_z, is expressed in units of time^{-1} and can be estimated by unweighted regression of the log-linear terminal elimination phase of the concentration versus time curve (Fig. 32.4).[8] The relationship between clearance, volume of distribution, and λ_z is defined by the following formula:

$$CL = V_c \times \lambda_z. \quad \text{(Eq. 10)}$$

The terminal elimination half-life is not considered a fundamental pharmacokinetic parameter because it is derived from clearance and the apparent volume of distribution (Eq. 10) and it is the inverse of the elimination rate constant.[1] The time to reach steady state on a multidose schedule or during a continuous intravenous drug infusion is directly related to the terminal elimination half-life for a drug with dose-proportional kinetics. After an infusion period of four half-lives, the drug concentrations will be 94% of the steady-state value.

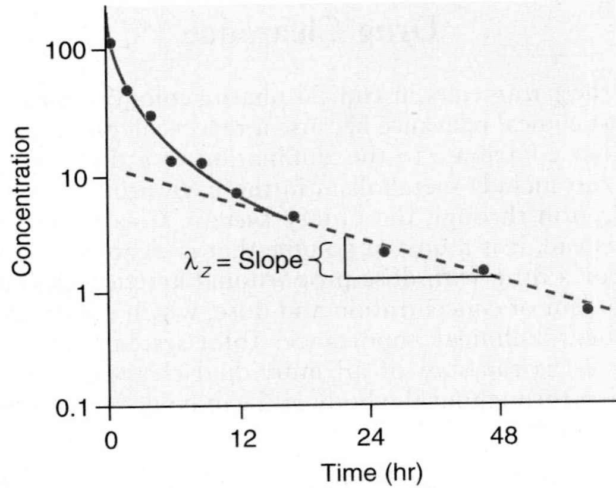

FIGURE 32.4 Estimation of the terminal elimination rate constant, λ_z, by regression analysis of the terminal portion of the log-linear concentration versus time plot.

Because half-life is an easily visualized pharmacokinetic parameter, its clinical utility is often overemphasized. In actual practice, the terminal elimination half-life may not be relevant for determining the proper time interval for repeated drug dosing. For example, if an agent is converted into active metabolites, the biologically effective half-life may be much longer than the measured half-life. Furthermore, drugs with multicompartmental pharmacokinetic behavior may demonstrate several different half-lives, depending on the sensitivity of the analytical method used. For example, if a highly sensitive mass spectroscopic assay is used to measure plasma 5-fluorouracil concentrations, then extremely low plasma concentrations of this agent can be detected for an unusually long period after drug administration.[30] This previously unrecognized long terminal 5-fluorouracil elimination half-life is attributed to the slow efflux of drug from deep tissue compartments. However, these low plasma drug concentrations do not relate to any clinical drug effects and, thus, are of limited biological relevance. In other situations, prolonged terminal drug elimination half-life may have profound clinical consequences. For example, after distribution of methotrexate into large third-space fluid compartments, such as ascites or pleural effusions, the drug is slowly released back into the systemic circulation over time. The resulting prolongation of the terminal half-life can induce substantial drug toxicity.[31] Thus, the clinical relevance of the terminal elimination half-life varies depending on the specific agent and the clinical situation.

Dose Proportionality

When drug concentrations change in strict proportionality to the dose of drug administered, then the condition of dose proportionality holds. If doubling the dose exactly doubles the plasma concentration, then fundamental pharmacokinetic parameters, such as rate constants, apparent volumes of distribution, and clearance, are constant and remain independent of dose and concentration.[32,33] In contrast, parameters of drug exposure, such as *AUC*, steady-state plasma concentrations (C_{ss}), or maximum plasma concentrations (C_{max}), will change proportionally with drug dose. By strict definition, drugs with linear pharmacokinetics are dose-proportional. Linear pharmacokinetics means that a drug's pharmacologic behavior can be described by a series of linear differential equations, such as those used to describe a multicompartmental model with first-order rate constants.

Dose proportionality is clinically important because it means that dose adjustments will generate predictable changes in systemic drug exposure. For drugs that lack dose proportionality, parameters such as clearance will demonstrate concentration, time dependence, or both, making it difficult to predict the effect of dose adjustments on plasma drug concentrations. Such drugs may also demonstrate high degrees of pharmacokinetic variability. Factors that can contribute to non–dose proportional kinetics include metabolism by enzymes with Michaelis-Menten kinetics, saturable oral absorption, capacity-limited distribution, saturable protein binding, or autoinduction of drug-metabolizing enzymes.

There are a number of different techniques available to test for dose proportionality.[32,33] The most robust study design to test for dose proportionality is a crossover pharmacokinetic study in which each patient receives a series of low, moderate, and high doses over time. However, such studies are rare in oncology because of the required use of low, ineffective doses, which may raise ethical issues for cancer patients. More often, dose proportionality is assessed in phase 1 dose-escalation trials in which small groups of patients are treated at a single dose level using a parallel study design. The statistical power of such studies to detect deviations from dose proportionality is poor; however, these phase 1 dose-escalation trials are often the only opportunity to examine drug kinetics over a wide dose range. In these studies, dose proportionality can be assessed by plotting the weighted regression of the *AUC* or C_{max} against dose level to see if the resulting line passes through the origin (the intercept test).[8] If the 95% confidence interval of the regression line includes the origin, then these data are consistent with dose-proportional pharmacokinetics (doubling the dose doubles the *AUC*). More rigorous tests of dose proportionality include the application of the power model[32] or analysis of variance testing of the log-transformed *CL* or log-transformed dose-normalized *AUC* (*AUC*/dose) values examined across various dose levels.[8,32]

PHARMACODYNAMIC CONCEPTS

Pharmacodynamic models relate clinical drug effects with drug dose, concentrations, or other pharmacokinetic parameters indicative of drug exposures.[2] In oncology, pharmacodynamic variability may account for substantial differences in clinical outcomes, even when systemic exposures are uniform. Variability in pharmacodynamic response may be heavily influenced by clinical covariates such as age, gender, prior chemotherapy, prior radiotherapy, concomitant medications, or other variables.[34] The kinetic parameters that are most often correlated with drug effects are markers of drug exposure, such as *AUC*, or plasma drug concentrations, such as C_{max} or C_{ss}. Other parameters may also have pharmacodynamic utility. For example, the toxic effects of highly schedule-dependent agents may be better explained by the duration that drug concentrations remain above a particular threshold value than by using the standard *AUC*. This approach has been successfully applied to pharmacodynamic studies of paclitaxel.[35] In general, the specific parameter used as the independent variable in a pharmacodynamic analysis depends on the particular characteristics of the study drug.

In oncology, pharmacodynamic studies of drug effects have most often focused on toxicity end points. Continuous response variables, such as the percentage fall in the absolute blood count from baseline, are easily analyzed using nonlinear regression methods. Dose-limiting neutropenia has been frequently analyzed using a sigmoid maximum effect model described by the modified Hill equation (Fig. 32.5)[36]:

$$\text{Percentage fall in blood counts} = 100\% \times C^h/[C^h + (EC_{50})^h], \quad \text{(Eq. 11)}$$

where C is the input parameter of drug exposure (often *AUC* or C_{ss}), EC_{50} is the value of C that produces a 50% fall in blood counts, and *h* is the Hill constant that is related to the

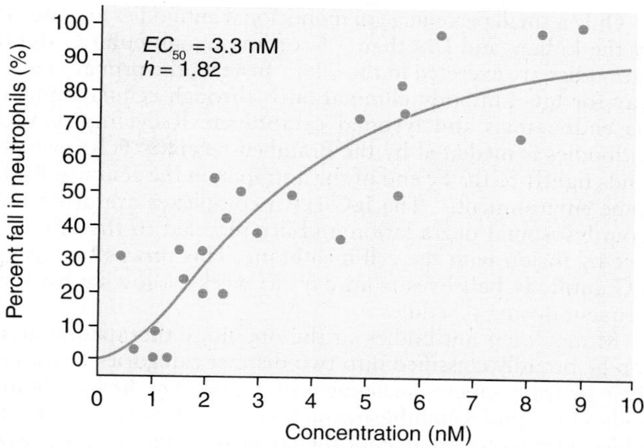

FIGURE 32.5 Pharmacodynamic sigmoid E_{max} model. The percentage fall in the absolute neutrophil count from baseline in adult solid-tumor patients treated with a 72-hour infusion of 9-aminocamptothecin (9-AC) is graphed as a function of the steady-state plasma drug concentration. The EC_{50} is the plasma concentration of 9-AC lactone associated with a 50% fall in neutrophil counts from baseline, and *h* is the Hill coefficient. (Data taken from a clinical trial described in ref. 55.)

degree of sigmoidicity of the exposure-effect curve. The pharmacodynamic analysis of subjectively graded clinical end points, such as common toxicity criteria scores that assess drug-related adverse events as mild (grade 1), moderate (grade 2), severe (grade 3), or life-threatening (grade 4), may require more sophisticated statistical methods. Logistical regression methods have been used to model these types of categorical (ordinal) response or outcome variables.[2]

Physiological pharmacodynamic models describing the severity and time course of drug-related myelosuppression induced by paclitaxel[35,37] and pemetrexed[38] have been derived using population mixed-effect methods. The ability of these models to predict both the severity and duration of drug-induced neutropenia substantially enhances their clinical usefulness. In contrast to small-molecule therapeutics, biological therapies such as monoclonal antibodies may not demonstrate toxicities directly related to dose levels. For these large-molecule therapeutics, a thorough understanding of the pharmacokinetic/pharmacodynamic relationships using a modeling approach may be critical for optimal dose selection.

SPECIAL TOPICS IN PHARMACOKINETICS AND PHARMACODYNAMICS

Pharmacokinetic Concepts for Biological Agents

The number of approved biologic agents for the treatment of human malignancies has increased substantially in the modern era. These powerful therapeutics have unique pharmacokinetic characteristics, distinct from small-molecule agents or classic chemotherapies.

Because of their large molecular weight and susceptibility to protein degradation, monoclonal antibodies cannot be absorbed from the gastrointestinal tract and require direct systemic administration, most often via short-term intravenous infusions. Typically, monoclonal antibodies are not bound to plasma proteins and their tissue distribution is independent of lipophilicity, tissue permeability, tissue-binding constants, or local organ blood flow. Convection is the principal mechanism for antibody distribution and this process is well characterized.[39]

Only a small percentage of monoclonal antibodies are filtered by the kidney and less than 1% of immunoglobulin G (IgG) antibodies are excreted in the bile.[40] Instead, the primary pathway for IgG antibody elimination is through cellular uptake via endocytosis and lysomal catabolism. Recycling of IgG antibodies is mediated by the Brambell receptor, FcRn, which binds tightly to the Fc end of the antibody in the acidified lysosome environment.[41] The IgG-FcRn complexes are protected from lysosomal degradation and are recycled to the cell surface by fusion with the cell membrane. This process prolongs IgG antibody half-lives from days to weeks, allowing for less frequent dosing schedules.

Monoclonal antibodies in the oncology therapeutic area can be broadly classified into two distinct categories based on their pharmacologic mechanism of action. The first are antibodies that bind to soluble ligand targets, such as bevacizumab, which targets vascular endothelial growth factor. For these agents, the antibody concentrations at clinically relevant doses are in large molar excess compared with the soluble ligand target. Consequently, binding to the ligand does not affect antibody clearance, resulting in dose-proportional pharmacokinetics. The second class of antibodies involves those that bind to membrane-bound receptors, such as cetuximab or trastuzumab, which target EGFR and ErbB2, respectively. Binding to cell surface receptors can lead to antibody internalization, which may contribute to overall drug clearance when the receptor target is relatively abundant in tissues.[42] This process, known as *target-mediated disposition*, can result in non–dose-proportional pharmacokinetics. For example, cetuximab at lower doses is rapidly removed from the central compartment because of target binding and clearance in tissues expressing EGFR receptors.[43] However, once binding is saturated, target-mediated disposition is minimized, and the pharmacokinetics become dose-proportional. Because of these phenomena, cetuximab is typically administered using a loading dose followed by a lower maintenance dose level.

Any exogenously administered protein can be viewed as foreign and trigger an immune response, resulting in the generation of endogenous antidrug antibodies. All currently marketed monoclonal antibodies exhibit some level of immunogenicity.[44] In general, murine antibodies are more immunogenic than chimeric, humanized, or fully human monoclonal antibodies.[45] Prolonged treatment with a monoclonal antibody may result in an increased probability of developing antidrug antibodies. This type of immune response can alter pharmacokinetics and increase clearance rates by forming immune complexes, which may impair efficacy. In addition, these immune complexes can alter the safety profile and increase adverse events.[46]

POPULATION PHARMACOKINETICS/ PHARMACODYNAMICS

Ultimately, the goal of a pharmacokinetic/pharmacodynamic study is to define a drug's pharmacokinetic and pharmacodynamic behavior in a population of patients.[45] Traditionally, this was performed using a classic "two-stage" analysis in which parameter estimates for individual patients are pooled and characterized using summary statistics, such as means, variances, or covariances. In this approach, the relative standard deviation or coefficient of variation (*CV*%) for each pharmacokinetic/pharmacodynamic parameter reflects the degree of interpatient variability within the population.[2] However, this approach has substantial limitations because the estimations of interindividual variability are confounded by the presence of random residual error. In addition, numerous blood samples were needed to obtain individual parameter estimates, which raises ethical concerns when patients are critically ill, extremely young, or elderly and frail. Population pharmacokinetics takes a more sophisticated approach by using a one-step, nonlinear, mixed-effect model to estimate both interindividual and random residual variability simultaneously. Implementation of this approach using powerful software programs such as NONMEM (Icon, Ellicott City, Maryland)[47] can evaluate the impact of individual patient covariates on pharmacokinetic variability. Such population approaches are clinically useful because of their ability to provide insights into the nature of pharmacokinetic/pharmacodynamic variation within a heterogeneous population. Population analyses using Bayesian estimation techniques can also provide accurate estimates of pharmacokinetic parameters for individual patients using relatively few blood samples (sparse sampling strategies). Finally, an exciting area of drug development is the use of pharmacokinetic-pharmacodynamic population models as a tool for detailed simulations of phase 3 studies to help design more innovative and efficient clinical studies. Such an approach has great potential for improving the design and efficacy of large-scale randomized clinical trials.[48]

PHARMACOKINETICS AND PHARMACODYNAMICS IN ONCOLOGY DRUG DEVELOPMENT

Carefully designed clinical pharmacology studies should be fully integrated into the overall drug development plan. Ideally, the collection of pharmacokinetic and pharmacodynamic information should begin at the earliest stages of drug development. Preclinical laboratory studies can characterize potential risk of serious drug interactions by identifying important drug-metabolizing enzymes, such as CYP3A4, using *in vitro* test systems.[49] These studies can also suggest important pathways of drug clearance. At this stage, analytical assays can be developed and validated with sufficient sensitivity and reliability to perform pharmacokinetic studies. Efforts should also be directed toward validating measurements of pharmacodynamic end points by characterizing suitable biomarkers for informing about an agent's mechanism of action. Application of these assays to animal models provides the first information about pharmacokinetic-pharmacodynamic relationships in intact organisms. These experiments can provide valuable information for the design of first-time-in-human studies and the pharmacokinetic exposure needed for optimal pharmacodynamic effect.

The first-time-in-human phase 1 trial is the initial opportunity to obtain detailed clinical pharmacokinetic information about a new molecular entity. Summary descriptive pharmacokinetics allows an assessment of the degree of intrapatient and interpatient pharmacokinetic variability, and covariate analyses can highlight the important factors that underlie this variability. A comparison of the pharmacokinetic parameters at the recommended phase 2 dose to the pharmacokinetic exposure needed in preclinical models provides valuable criteria for dose selection. Because dose escalation is a hallmark of traditional phase 1 oncologic studies, an analysis of dose proportionality over the dose range studied can be implemented. For monoclonal antibodies, the immunogenicity data collected in early trials can be used to determine the immunogenicity risk profile. Toxicity assessments are also important end points in phase 1 studies; thus, pharmacodynamic correlations between drug exposure and drug toxicity can also be initiated at this phase of drug development. Increasingly, with the development of molecularly targeted therapies, an early examination of drug efficacy can occur at the end of phase 1 by the addition of expansion cohorts of molecularly defined patients subsets, selected for treatment based on testing for the presence of potential predictive biomarkers. Finally, the information obtained in these early intensive pharmacokinetic studies can be used to develop optimal and limited sampling strategies that can readily be applied to pharmacokinetic monitoring in clinical studies during later stages of development.

A new type of first-in-human study that is being explored in the drug development process is the phase 0 trial.[50,51] These are novel early clinical trials conducted in patients or volunteers that are of limited duration and have no therapeutic intent. Using the U.S. Food and Drug Administration's Exploratory Investigational New Drug mechanism,[52] phase 0 trials reduce the requirement for preclinical testing prior to entry into human clinical trials. Although not designed to supplant traditional phase 1 and 2 trials, this new pathway provides a means to accelerate the entry of novel therapeutics into clinical testing. Such studies may range from microdose pharmacokinetic or imaging studies to mechanism of action or pharmacodynamic biomarker studies. Although the full impact of this new type of early clinical trial must still be defined, it represents an attempt to enhance innovation in oncology drug development.

In phase 2 studies, clinical efficacy trials are typically conducted at multiple institutions in multiple disease types. Thus, the total number of patients treated increases substantially from this point forward. Often, fiscal and logistical difficulties prohibit extensive pharmacokinetic sampling at this stage. However, the implementation of formal limited or sparse pharmacokinetic sampling strategies may allow for further expansion of the pharmacokinetic database. Pooled data from all the pharmacokinetic studies performed can be analyzed in population pharmacokinetic studies. Nonlinear mixed-effect modeling can further characterize the magnitude of kinetic variation within the population and can identify important covariates that may be used in selecting special subpopulations for further study. Finally, comprehensive population pharmacokinetic-pharmacodynamic models developed at this stage can serve as the basis for early clinical trial forecasting and simulations that assist in the design of larger, more resource-intense randomized phase 3 trials.[48]

Simultaneously with expanded single-agent phase 2 testing, combination phase 1 studies may be initiated at this stage. Coadministration of a new agent with standard anticancer therapies can be rationally planned based on synergistic antitumor activity or because the agent is being targeted for use in a specific disease type such as lung, colon, or breast cancer. A phase 1 trial of any new drug combination should always include pharmacokinetic monitoring to define potential drug interactions. However, in most instances these studies are not formally statistically powered to examine the drug interaction. Other specialized clinical trials include formal mass balance studies that define the total excretion of an experimental agent in urine and feces and other bodily fluids over time. Typically, these studies are performed in carefully controlled settings with radioactively labeled drug. The results of mass balance studies combined with information obtained from other early pharmacokinetic trials can precisely define the major routes of drug elimination and may highlight the need to perform additional specialized studies. For example, a drug that is largely excreted unchanged in the urine will need to be carefully examined in pharmacokinetic studies in patients with renal dysfunction. In contrast, a hepatically metabolized drug or one that undergoes biliary excretion should be examined in formal studies in patients with liver dysfunction. Finally, if the growing body of clinical information identifies potential drug interactions, then a formal statistically rigorous drug interaction study can be performed with the compound of interest. Other pharmacokinetic studies of potential importance include phase 1 trials in special populations such as pediatric cancer patients, patients with acute leukemia, or geriatric patients. This phase of drug development may temporally overlap with other phases of drug development and may even stretch into the postmarketing period.

The final and most resource-intense phase of drug development is the randomized phase 3 trial. Consequently, the growing field of clinical trial forecasting and simulation based on pharmacokinetic-pharmacodynamic modeling may offer the greatest benefit immediately before this stage of drug development.[48] Ideally, this involves the maximal use of all pharmacologic information collected up to that time. Formalized simulations of various study designs and possible outcomes can then be explored in detail. If the results are favorable, then this stage culminates in the initiation of a randomized phase 3 clinical trial, most often the final step in a successful registration program.

Drug development is a very time-consuming and expensive process. A new drug requires an average of 13.5 years and over 1.5 billion dollars in research and development costs to reach a market today.[53] In comparison with other therapeutic areas, new oncology drugs have lower success rates and higher incidences of late-stage failure in large phase 3 studies, resulting in substantial development costs.[53] Ironically, at a time when genomics and molecular biology have created exponentially increasing therapeutic opportunities, translation of scientific discoveries into innovative safe and effective cancer therapies is now rate-limiting. The U.S. Food and Drug Administration recently established a new approach to assess the efficacy and safety of investigational drugs through its Critical Path Initiative in order to overcome these problems associated with drug development.[54] One aspect of this initiative is to transition from empirical to model-based drug development. This new approach emphasizes the use of modeling and simulation technologies to integrate drug-specific pharmacokinetic and pharmacodynamic information into the overall drug development process. This strategy uses our growing understanding of pharmacology and the underlying disease process to improve the efficiency of drug development. Ultimately, this approach holds great promise for lowering costs and shortening development times for novel therapeutics.

References

1. Atkinson AJ. Introduction to clinical pharmacology. In: Atkinson AJ, Abernethy DR, Daniels CE, et al., eds. *Principles of Clinical Pharmacology*. 2nd ed. Amsterdam: Academic Press, 2007:1.
2. Ratain MJ, Mick R. Principles of pharmacokinetics and pharmacodynamics. In: Schilsky RL, Milano GA, Ratain MJ, eds. *Principles of Antineoplastic Drug Development and Pharmcology. Basic and Clinical Oncology.* New York: Marcel Dekker, 1996:123.
3. Bourne DWA. *Mathematical Modeling of Pharmacokinetic Data*. Lancaster: Technomic, 1995:95.
4. Calvert AH. Dose optimisation of carboplatin in adults. *Anticancer Res* 1994;14:2273.
5. Gianni L, Kearns CM, Giani A, et al. Nonlinear pharmacokinetics and metabolism of paclitaxel and its pharmacokinetic/pharmacodynamic relationships in humans. *J Clin Oncol* 1995;13:180.

6. Ratain MJ, Schilsky RL, Conley BA, et al. Pharmacodynamics in cancer therapy. *J Clin Oncol* 1990;8:1739.
7. Khambata-Ford S, Garrett CR, Meropol NJ, et al. Expression of epiregulin and amphiregulin and K-*ras* mutation status predict disease control in metastatic colorectal cancer patients treated with cetuximab. *J Clin Oncol* 2007;25:3230.
8. Noe DA. Noncompartmental pharmacokinetic analysis. In: Grochow LB, Ames MM, eds. *A Clinician's Guide to Chemotherapy: Pharmacokinetics and Pharmacodynamics*. Baltimore: Williams & Wilkins, 1998:515.
9. Martinez MN, Amidon GL. A mechanistic approach to understanding the factors affecting drug absorption: a review of fundamentals. *J Clin Pharmacol* 2002;42:620.
10. Gibaldi M, Perrier D. *Pharmacokinetics*. 2nd ed. New York: Marcel Dekker, 1982.
11. Lundin J, Kimby E, Bjorkholm M, et al. Phase II trial of subcutaneous anti-CD52 monoclonal antibody alemtuzumab (Campath-1H) as first-line treatment for patients with B-cell chronic lymphocytic leukemia (B-CLL). *Blood* 2002;100:768.
12. Perrier D, Mayersohn M. Noncompartmental determination of the steady-state volume of distribution for any mode of administration. *J Pharm Sci* 1982;71:372.
13. Mordenti J, Rescigno A. Estimation of permanence time, exit time, dilution factor, and steady-state volume of distribution. *Pharm Res* 1992;9:17.
14. Blaney SM, Balis FM, Poplack DG. Current pharmacological treatment approaches to central nervous system leukaemia. *Drugs* 1991;41:702.
15. Stewart CF, Zamboni WC. Plasma protein binding of chemotherapeutic agents. In: Grochow LB, Ames MM, eds. *A Clinician's Guide to Chemotherapy: Pharmacokinetics and Pharmacodynamics*. Baltimore: Williams & Wilkins, 1998:55.
16. Sawyer M, Ratain MJ. Body surface area as a determinant of pharmacokinetics and drug dosing. *Invest New Drugs* 2001;19:171.
17. Prado CM, Baracos VE, McCargar LJ, et al. Body composition as an independent determinant of 5-fluorouracil-based chemotherapy toxicity. *Clin Cancer Res* 2007;13:3264.
18. Grochow LB, Baraldi C, Noe D. Is dose normalization to weight or body surface area useful in adults? *J Natl Cancer Inst* 1990;82:323.
19. Ng CM, Lum BL, Gimenez V, et al. Rationale for fixed dosing of pertuzumab in cancer patients based on population pharmacokinetic analysis. *Pharm Res* 2006;23:1275.
20. Hasler JA. Pharmacogenetics of cytochromes P450. *Mol Aspects Med* 1999;20:12.
21. McLeod HL, Evans WE. Pharmacogenomics: unlocking the human genome for better drug therapy. *Annu Rev Pharmacol Toxicol* 2001;41:101.
22. Hoyumpa AM, Schenker S. Is glucuronidation truly preserved in patients with liver disease? *Hepatology* 1991;13:786.
23. Murry DJ, Riva L, Poplack DG. Impact of nutrition on pharmacokinetics of anti-neoplastic agents. *Int J Cancer Suppl* 1998;11:48.
24. Cascorbi I. Role of pharmacogenetics of ATP-binding cassette transporters in the pharmacokinetics of drugs. *Pharmacol Ther* 2006;112:457.
25. Ratain MJ. Dear doctor: we really are not sure what dose of capecitabine you should prescribe for your patient. *J Clin Oncol* 2002;20:1434.
26. Relling MV, Pui CH, Sandlund JT, et al. Adverse effect of anticonvulsants on efficacy of chemotherapy for acute lymphoblastic leukaemia. *Lancet* 2000;356:285.
27. Gupta E, Lestingi TM, Mick R, et al. Metabolic fate of irinotecan in humans: correlation of glucuronidation with diarrhea. *Cancer Res* 1994;54:3723.
28. Gibbons J, Egorin MJ, Ramanathan RK, et al. Phase I and pharmacokinetic study of imatinib mesylate in patients with advanced malignancies and varying degrees of renal dysfunction: a study by the National Cancer Institute Organ Dysfunction Working Group. *J Clin Oncol* 2008;26: 570.
29. Ramanathan RK, Egorin MJ, Takimoto CH, et al. Phase I and pharmacokinetic study of imatinib mesylate in patients with advanced malignancies and varying degrees of liver dysfunction: a study by the National Cancer Institute Organ Dysfunction Working Group. *J Clin Oncol* 2008; 26:563.
30. van Groeningen CJ, Pinedo HM, Heddes J, et al. Pharmacokinetics of 5-fluorouracil assessed with a sensitive mass spectrometric method in patients on a dose escalation schedule. *Cancer Res* 1988;48:6956.
31. Chabner BA, Stoller RG, Hande K, et al. Methotrexate disposition in humans: case studies in ovarian cancer and following high-dose infusion. *Drug Metab Rev* 1978;8:107.
32. Gough K, Hutchison M, Keene O, et al. Assessment of dose proportionality: Report from the statisticians in the pharmaceutical industry/pharmacokinetics UK joint working party. *Drug Inform J* 1995;29:1039.
33. Smith BP, Vandenhende FR, DeSante KA, et al. Confidence interval criteria for assessment of dose proportionality. *Pharm Res* 2000;17:1278.
34. Karlsson MO, Molnar V, Bergh J, et al. A general model for time-dissociated pharmacokinetic-pharmacodynamic relationship exemplified by paclitaxel myelosuppression. *Clin Pharmacol Ther* 1998;63:11.
35. Kearns CM, Gianni L, Egorin MJ. Paclitaxel pharmacokinetics and pharmacodynamics. *Semin Oncol* 1995;22:16.
36. Gabrielsson J, Weiner D. *Pharmacokinetic and Pharmacodynamic Data Analysis, Concepts and Applications*. 2nd ed. Stockholm, Swedish Pharmaceutical Press, 1997.
37. Minami H, Sasaki Y, Saijo N, et al. Indirect-response model for the time course of leukopenia with anticancer drugs. *Clin Pharmacol Ther* 1998;64:511.
38. Latz JE, Schneck KL, Nakagawa K, et al. Population pharmacokinetic/pharmacodynamic analyses of pemetrexed and neutropenia: effect of vitamin supplementation and differences between Japanese and Western patients. *Clin Cancer Res* 2009;15:346.
39. Wang W, Wang EQ, Balthasar JP. Monoclonal antibody pharmacokinetics and pharmacodynamics. *Clin Pharmacol Ther* 2008;84:548.
40. Delacroix DL, Hodgson HJ, McPherson A, et al. Selective transport of polymeric immunoglobulin A in bile: quantitative relationships of monomeric and polymeric immunoglobulin A, immunoglobulin M, and other proteins in serum, bile, and saliva. *J Clin Invest* 1982;70:230.
41. Brambell FW, Hemmings WA, Morris IG. A theoretical model of gamma-globulin catabolism. *Nature* 1964;203:1352.
42. Mager DE, Jusko WJ. General pharmacokinetic model for drugs exhibiting target-mediated drug disposition. *J Pharmacokinet Pharmacodyn* 2001; 28:507.
43. Baselga J, Pfister D, Cooper MR, et al. Phase I studies of anti-epidermal growth factor receptor chimeric antibody C225 alone and in combination with cisplatin. *J Clin Oncol* 2000;18:904.
44. Tabrizi MA, Tseng CM, Roskos LK. Elimination mechanisms of therapeutic monoclonal antibodies. *Drug Discov Today* 2006;11:81.
45. Hwang WY, Foote J. Immunogenicity of engineered antibodies. *Methods* 2005;36:3.
46. Roskos L, Kellermann S, Foon K. Human antiglobulin responses. In: Lotze M, Thomson A, eds. *Measuring Immunity: Basic Science and Clinical Practice*. London, Elsevier Ltd, 2005:172.
47. Beal SL, Sheiner LB. *NONMEM User's Guides*. San Francisco, University of California, 1989.
48. Holford NH, Kimko HC, Monteleone JP, et al. Simulation of clinical trials. *Annu Rev Pharmacol Toxicol* 2000;40:209.
49. Obach RS, Walsky RL, Venkatakrishnan K, et al. In vitro cytochrome P450 inhibition data and the prediction of drug-drug interactions: qualitative relationships, quantitative predictions, and the rank-order approach. *Clin Pharmacol Ther* 2005;78:582.
50. Kummar S, Kinders R, Gutierrez ME, et al. Phase 0 clinical trial of the poly (ADP-ribose) polymerase inhibitor ABT-888 in patients with advanced malignancies. *J Clin Oncol* 2009;27:2705.
51. Kummar S, Kinders R, Rubinstein L, et al. Compressing drug development timelines in oncology using phase '0' trials. *Nat Rev Cancer* 2007;7:131.
52. U.S. Food and Drug Administration. *Guidance for Industry, Investigators, and Reviewers: Exploratory IND Studies*. Washington, DC: U.S. Food and Drug Administration, 2006.
53. Paul SM, Mytelka DS, Dunwiddie CT, et al. How to improve R&D productivity: the pharmaceutical industry's grand challenge. *Nat Rev Drug Discov* 2010;9:203.
54. U.S. Food and Drug Administration. *Innovation Stagnation Critical Path Opportuities Report*. Washington, DC: U.S. Food and Drug Administration, 2006.
55. Takimoto CH, Dahut W, Marino MT, et al. Pharmacodynamics and pharmacokinetics of a 72-hour infusion of 9-aminocamptothecin in adult cancer patients. *J Clin Oncol* 1997;15:1492.
56. Takimoto CH, Remick SC, Sharma S, et al. Dose-escalating and pharmacological study of oxaliplatin in adult cancer patients with impaired renal function: A National Cancer Institute Organ Dysfunction Working Group Study. *J Clin Oncol* 2003;21(14):2664.

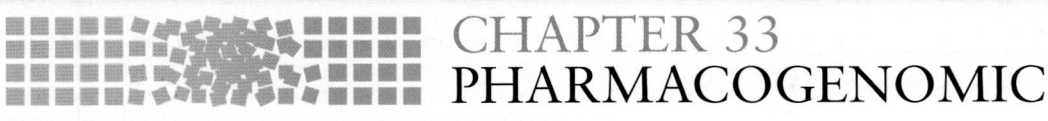

CHAPTER 33 PHARMACOGENOMICS

ANTHONY EL-KHOUEIRY AND HEINZ JOSEF LENZ

If it were not for the great variability among individuals, medicine might as well be a science and not an art.

—Sir William Osler, 1892

Genetic variability among patients leads to variable responses to therapies and drugs, which compels the treating physician to attempt to tailor the treatment to the patient. This need to individualize the treatment approach to a specific patient has been a central theme in the "art of medicine." However, the evolution of scientific knowledge about genetic variability and the advancement of technology have brought art closer to science through the field of pharmacogenomics. Rather than trying to individualize therapy based on broad clinical and environmental characteristics, pharmacogenomics uses novel genomic technologies to elucidate the influence of a patient's genetic makeup on the variability in individual responses to drugs. One of the main goals of pharmacogenomics is to elucidate a genetic signature or profile that can be used to tailor therapy to the individual patient and move away from the "one size fits all" approach. In the field of cancer therapy, being able to individualize the treatment could revolutionize cancer care by contributing to improved survival and reduced toxicity. This chapter contains a brief overview of the field of pharmacogenomics in cancer care while highlighting the limitations and challenges that need to be addressed prior to a broader clinical application of pharmacogenomics in the treatment of cancer patients.

DEFINITIONS: TERMS AND CONCEPTS

In this review of the field of pharmacogenomics, it is important to define several terms that are essential to the understanding of the field and to the accurate interpretation of the data presented.

Pharmacogenomics is the science of incorporating information on inherited genetic variability into predicting treatment response. Pharmacogenomics includes studies of germline polymorphisms, somatic mutations, and variations in RNA expression.[1] Germline polymorphisms are inherited genetic variants that are present in all cells of the body and can therefore be assayed at the DNA level, which is extracted from readily available normal tissue cells, most commonly peripheral blood mononuclear cells. The examination of variations in RNA expression (gene expression analysis) is intended to evaluate the association between specific genes and distinct phenotypes, such as the resistance to a chemotherapeutic drug. Gene expression analysis depends on access to tumor tissue and the utilization of molecular biology techniques such as real-time polymerase chain reaction or high-throughput methods such as arrays and gene chips. The discussion about pharmacogenomics and cancer in this chapter will focus on germline polymorphisms with occasional reference to gene expression data. Genome-wide arrays will not be discussed in detail.

The initial studies that evaluated the impact of pharmacogenomic alterations on the efficacy or toxicity of a specific treatment were retrospective in nature and limited by the small sample sizes. Over the past few years, pharmacogenomic analyses have been incorporated into prospective clinical trials with the goal of validating previously observed associations.

A *polymorphism* (Fig. 33.1) is a variation within a gene in which two or more alleles exist at a frequency of at least 1% in the general population. Different types of polymorphisms exist, including microsatellites (e.g., dinucleotide repeats), insertions, deletions, and single nucleotide changes. A variation at a single nucleotide is referred to as a *single nucleotide polymorphism* (SNP). The human genome contains approximately 1.4 million SNPs with 60,000 SNPs being in exons. There are two exonic SNPs per gene, with 93% of genetic loci containing one or more SNPs.[2] An SNP can have a functional consequence if it exists within a coding or regulatory region of a gene. Alternatively, an SNP may be silent if it results in a synonymous amino acid substitution or if it resides in a noncoding region of the DNA, except in rare occasions.

A *predictive marker* is a genetic or molecular variation that would help predetermine the likelihood of response and toxicity to a specific drug. The concept of a predictive marker is usually applied to individual patients with the goal of tailoring therapy to maximize efficacy and minimize toxicity. In more specific and practical terms, a predictive marker could assist a clinician in deciding "what to treat with and how much to give."

A *prognostic marker* is a genetic or molecular variation that would influence clinical outcome by affecting the natural history of the disease. This concept is generally applied to populations with the aim of determining the need for a therapeutic intervention. For example, a prognostic marker could assist a clinician in deciding "whom and when to treat" with adjuvant chemotherapy.

PHARMACOGENOMICS AND PREDICTIVE MOLECULAR MARKERS

Single Nucleotide Polymorphisms in Single Genes as Predictors of Response and Survival

Single nucleotide polymorphisms have been associated with changes in drug disposition by affecting genes involved in drug transport and metabolism as well as changes in drug targets such as receptors and enzymes. These changes have been correlated with the probability of response or survival following treatment with a specific drug. Presented here are examples of

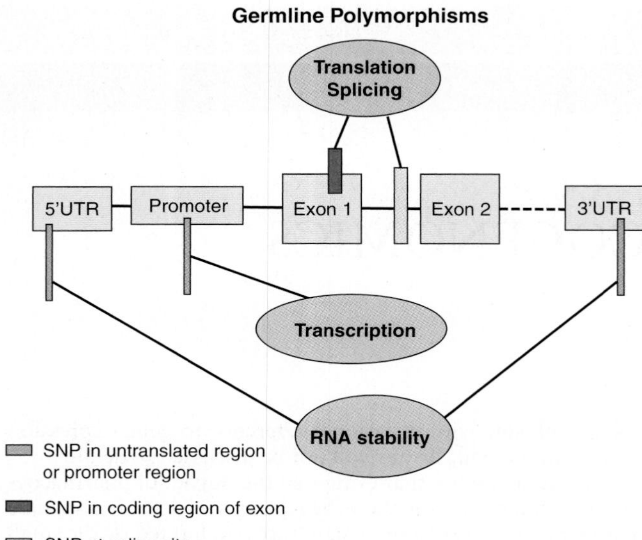

FIGURE 33.1 This figure illustrates the impact that germline polymorphisms can have on the transcription or translation of a gene. The location of such polymorphisms tends to correlate with specific functional alterations. If a polymorphism affects the activity of a protein critical for the efficacy or toxicity of a chemotherapy drug, it may be associated with clinical outcome or tolerance of the drug. SNP, single nucleotide polymorphism.

single variations in single genes that have been shown to be possible predictors of outcome to treatment with a drug.

Thymidylate Synthase

Thymidylate synthase (TS) is the main target of the 5-fluorouracil (5-FU) metabolite, fluorodeoxyuridine monophosphate (FdUMP), which forms a ternary complex with TS and folic acid and inhibits the conversion of deoxyuridine monophosphate to deoxythymidine monophosphate.[3] Several studies have shown an inverse relationship between the level of TS gene expression and the likelihood of response or survival in patients with colorectal or gastric cancer treated with 5-FU.[4,5] The 5′-untranslated region functions as a *cis*-acting transcriptional enhancer element and contains polymorphic 28-base pair (bp) tandem repeats. The presence of three tandem repeats (3R) has been associated with approximately two- to fourfold greater gene expression compared with double repeats (2R).[6] In a retrospective study of 52 patients with metastatic colorectal cancer (CRC), TS gene expression levels were 3.6 times higher in patients who were homozygous for the triple repeat (3R/3R) 28-bp sequence compared with those homozygous for the double repeat variant (2R/2R) ($P = .004$). Patients homozygous for the double repeats (2R/2R) showed a significantly better response rate to 5-FU compared with those homozygous for the triple repeats (3R/3R) (50% vs. 9%; $P = .04$).[7] Kawakami et al.[8] reported higher TS protein expression levels with the 3R/3R genotype, which suggested improved translational efficiency as a potential mechanistic explanation for the genotype-dependent difference in expression. A prospective study of 102 patients with metastatic CRC treated with 5-FU revealed that the 2R/2R genotype conferred the longest survival (median survival of 19 months for 2R/2R, 10 months for 2R/3R, and 14 months for 3R/3R; $P = .025$). All three groups had similar objective response rates.[9]

CYP2D6 Polymorphisms and Outcome in Women Treated with Adjuvant Tamoxifen. The activity of tamoxifen, which is used as adjuvant therapy in women with early hormone receptor positive breast cancer, is dependent on its metabolites, 4-hydroxytamoxifen and endoxifen. Variations in the polymorphic cytochrome P450 2D6 (CYP2D6) enzyme have been associated with significant differences in survival among women with early breast cancer who are treated with tamoxifen.[10] Patients were classified as having extensive, heterozygous/intermediate, or poor CYP2D6 metabolism based on genotype for variants associated with reduced (*10, *41) or absent (*3, *4, *5) enzyme activity. Compared with extensive metabolizers, those with decreased CYP2D6 activity (heterozygous extensive/intermediate and poor metabolism) had worse event-free survival (HR,1.33; 95% CI [confidence interval], 1.06 to 1.68) and disease-free survival (HR [hazard ratio], 1.29; 95% CI, 1.03 to 1.61), but there was no significant difference in overall survival (HR, 1.15; 95% CI, 0.88 to 1.51).

Vascular Endothelial Growth Factor and Vascular Endothelial Growth Factor Receptor

In a large multicenter prospective randomized trial (E2100) of metastatic breast cancer patients treated with paclitaxel versus paclitaxel and bevacizumab (a monoclonal antibody against vascular endothelial growth factor [VEGF]), two polymorphisms of VEGF (VEGF 2578 C/A and VEGF 1154 G/A) were associated with improved overall survival, but had no impact on response rate or progression-free survival. These findings await further validation.[11]

Epidermal Growth Factor Receptor

Another example of SNPs in one gene serving as predictors of response can be found in the association between epidermal growth factor receptor (EGFR) mutations and the likelihood of response to gefitinib in patients with advanced non–small cell lung cancer. Two independent reports found associations between somatic mutations in the tyrosine kinase domain of the *EGFR* gene and sensitivity to gefitinib in patients with non–small cell lung cancer.[12,13] These mutations consisted of small in-frame deletions or amino acid substitutions clustered around the adenosine triphosphate (ATP)-binding pocket of the tyrosine kinase domain. The functional significance of these mutations was further studied *in vitro* where they were linked to enhanced tyrosine kinase activity in response to epidermal growth factor.

Multiple other examples of SNPs in single genes serving as predictors of clinical efficacy of a drug exist (Table 33.1). However, the activity of a drug is more likely to depend on more than one single nucleotide variation in one gene or more than one gene in one pathway.

Multiple Genes in One Pathway as Predictors of Response or Survival

The Example of 5-Fluorouracil Metabolism: Multiple Genes in One Pathway

Elevated TS gene expression has been helpful in identifying patients who are unlikely to respond to 5-FU–based therapy, as mentioned earlier. However, low TS expression levels do not necessarily predict response to 5-FU. The lack of response in patients with low TS levels may be explained by the influence of other genes in the 5-FU metabolism pathway, such as dihydropyrimidine dehydrogenase (DPD) and thymidine phosphorylase (TP). DPD is a crucial enzyme in the catabolism of 5-FU as it degrades more than 80% of 5-FU in the liver. TP is involved in the conversion of 5-FU to fluorodeoxyuridine, which is then converted to FdUMP, the active metabolite of 5-FU.[3] Salonga et al.[14] evaluated the combined role of TS, TP, and DPD in predicting response to 5-FU. Patients who

TABLE 33.1

EXAMPLES OF GENETIC POLYMORPHISMS THAT HAVE AN IMPACT ON DRUG METABOLISM AND THEIR CLINICAL CONSEQUENCES[a]

Gene	Type of Genetic Variation	Functional Significance	Clinical Impact	Disease Type
TS	Number of 28 bp tandem repeats in 5′ region (2 vs. 3)	Increased gene expression with the 3R variant	Lower response and survival rates to 5-FU in 3R/3R patients in comparison with 2R/2R patients Increased risk of grade 2 or more adverse events in 2R/2R patients	Colorectal cancer
TS	6-bp deletion in 3′ region	May increase mRNA degradation	Clinical impact noted only in combination analysis with polymorphisms in ERCC1, XPD, and GSTP-1 (see text)	Colorectal cancer
EGFR	Small in-frame deletions in the tyrosine kinase domain	Enhanced tyrosine kinase activity in response to EGF	Increased likelihood of response to treatment with gefitinib	Non–small cell lung cancer
ERCC1	C to T single nucleotide change at position 118	Unknown but possible trend toward higher *ERCC1* expression with higher number of T alleles	T/T group had a 1.86 increased risk of dying compared to the C/C group when treated with 5-FU, leucovorin, and oxaliplatin	Colorectal cancer
XPD	Polymorphism in exon 23 causing a Lys751 to Gln substitution	Unknown but possibly decreased nucleotide excision repair efficacy with Lys allele	Gln/Gln group had a 2.55-fold increased risk of dying compared with Lys/Lys group when treated with 5-FU, leucovorin, and oxaliplatin	Colorectal cancer
GSTP-1	Polymorphism at position 313 causing an isoleucine to valine substitution	Diminished enzymatic activity of GSTP-1-105Val, a detoxifying enzyme involved in platinum resistance	Ile/Ile group had a 2.96-fold increased risk of dying compared with the Val/Val group when treated with 5-FU, leucovorin, and oxaliplatin	Colorectal cancer
*UGT1A1*28*	2-bp (TA) insertion in promoter region leading to 7 TA repeats instead of 6	Decreased protein expression of UGT1A1	Increased risk of neutropenia with irinotecan therapy in patients homozygous for the 7 TA repeats	Colorectal cancer
*SLCO1B1*5*	A T to C single nucleotide change at position 521	Reduced transport function of SN-38 from blood to liver	CT and CC genotypes have a higher irinotecan AUC compared with TT genotype	Colorectal cancer
DPD	A G to C single nucleotide change in exon 14	Decreased enzymatic activity of DPD responsible for 5-FU breakdown	Severe toxicity when treated with 5-FU	Colorectal cancer
OPRT	A G to A single nucleotide change at position 213	Increased enzymatic activity of OPRT involved in the activation of 5-FU	Increased risk of grade 2 or more diarrhea or leucopenia when treated with 5-FU	Colorectal cancer

bp, base pair; 3R, three tandem repeats; 5-FU, 5-fluorouracil; 2R, two tandem repeats; XPD, xeroderma pigmentosum group; GSTP-1, glutathione-S-transferase P1; EGF, epidermal growth factor; AUC, area under the curve; DPD, dihydropyrimidine dehydrogenase; OPRT, orotate phosphoribosyltransferase.

[a]All examples listed are discussed in the text. This table is not meant to give a comprehensive overview of all relevant polymorphisms for the genes mentioned or of all relevant genes involved in a specific drug metabolism.

responded to 5-FU had low expression levels of all three genes. Nonresponders had at least one gene with high expression values. These data highlight the importance of assessing several markers simultaneously because the response to a drug does not depend on a single gene in a single pathway.

The Example of Combined Chemotherapy: Multiple Polymorphisms in Related Pathways

The combination of 5-FU, leucovorin, and oxaliplatin (FOLFOX) is commonly used in the treatment of metastatic colorectal cancer, which means that the response depends on more than one drug. Furthermore, the metabolism and efficacy of each drug is influenced by more than one enzyme. An increased ability to repair DNA damage through the nucleotide excision repair (NER) pathway is thought to lead to increased resistance to platinum drugs. The excision repair cross-complementation group 1 enzyme (ERCC-1), XRCC-1, and the xeroderma pigmentosum group (XPD) are all members of the NER pathway and harbor functional polymorphisms.[15] Glutathione-S-transferase P1 (GSTP-1) belongs to a superfamily of enzymes that catalyze the conjugation of reduced glutathione, thereby protecting cellular macromolecules from damage caused by carcinogenic and chemotherapeutic agents. An SNP at position 313 results in an isoleucine to valine substitution. The GSTP-1-105 Val is thought to have diminished enzymatic detoxification activity.[16] In a retrospective study of 106 patients with metastatic CRC who were treated with FOLFOX, Stoehlmacher et al.[17] performed a combinational analysis of polymorphisms in XPD-751, ERCC1-118, GSTP1-105, and TS-3′-untranslated region that revealed that patients who possessed two or more favorable genotypes survived a median of 17.4 months compared to 10.2 months in patients with one favorable genotype and 5.4 months in patients with no favorable genotype ($P < .001$). Two of these polymorphisms as well as other previously reported ones from single institution series were evaluated in a prospective multi-institutional clinical trial (N9741) that compared FOLFOX to IFL (bolus 5-FU, leucovorin, and irinotecan) and IROX (irinotecan and oxaliplatin) in patients with metastatic colon cancer. In this trial, there was no association between any single polymorphism and outcome and no combinational analysis was performed.[18] Despite the absence of any association with outcome, this prospective analysis established the feasibility of pharmacogenetic studies being successfully performed in large multicenter trials. It also served as a reminder that associations of polymorphisms with outcome made in small single institution studies may be false positives and that careful validation is needed.

Molecular Predictors of Toxicity

Pharmacogenomics may represent an important tool in predicting excessive or preventable toxicities to chemotherapy. Such predictions may influence the choice of a single drug or combination regimen for an individual patient when alternatives are available. They may also result in the adoption of aggressive supportive care measures or dose modification for a known toxicity. The examples of 5-FU, irinotecan, and oxaliplatin will be discussed to highlight specific and relevant concepts related to the role of pharmacogenomics in predicting toxicity. Irinotecan plays a central role in the treatment of metastatic CRC and can result in dose-limiting neutropenia and diarrhea. The active metabolite of irinotecan, SN38, is metabolized in human liver by UGT1A1 to an inactive compound, SN-38G. A 2-bp (TA) insertion in the TATA box in the promoter region of UGT1A1 leads to seven TA repeats instead of six and results in the variant allele UGT1A1*28.[19] UGT1A1*28 leads to decreased protein expression of UGT1A1 and increased risk of neutropenia with irinotecan in patients homozygous for the seven TA repeats.[20] These data resulted in a label change for irinotecan that incorporated the UGT1A1 molecular assay information. The label change states: "a reduction in the starting dose by at least one level should be considered for patients known to be homozygous for the UGT1A1*28 allele." The clinical impact of this label change has been limited for practical and molecular reasons. On the practical level, the test identifies the patients who are at high risk of neutropenia only, and not the patients who are at risk of another common toxicity of irinotecan, which is diarrhea. Furthermore, because of the low frequency of the UGT1A1*28 homozygous genotype (7/7 genotype), testing for this polymorphism only reduced the risk of grade 4 neutropenia from 18% to 17%. When evaluated prospectively, the same polymorphism did not predict the risk of toxicity in patients who received bolus 5IFL in clinical trial N9741.[21] Statistically significant associations were found between the 7/7 genotype and the risk of grade 4 neutropenia in the patients treated with IROX (55% vs. 15%; $P = .002$) or when all three arms were pooled for analysis ($P = .003$).[18] Given the complexity of irinotecan metabolism, a more comprehensive and clinically applicable toxicity algorithm needs to account for the effect of other genes involved in the metabolism and transport of irinotecan and SN-38. Innocenti et al.[22] examined the role of several transporters involved in the metabolism of irinotecan along with UGT1A1. Twelve haplotypes of ABCC2 were identified and haplotype 4 was correlated with SN-38G/SN-38 area under the curve (AUC) ratio ($P < .0001$). SLCO1B1*5 (521T >C) CT and CC genotypes had a higher irinotecan AUC compared with TT genotype ($P = .0001$). Using a multivariate model, SLCO1B1, ABCC2, and UGT1A1 gene variants along with total bilirubin were associated with the risk of neutropenia in this retrospective study of 65 patients. Once again, such data highlight the importance of the interplay among several genetic variations in determining toxicity to a drug. In the case of 5-FU, associations between polymorphisms in several genes involved in 5-FU metabolism and side effects have been identified. A G to C mutation in the invariant GT splice donor site flanking exon 14 results in decreased DPD enzymatic activity, which is responsible for about 80% of the catabolism of 5-FU. This mutation has been associated with severe, potentially lethal toxicity with 5-FU therapy.[23] Other SNPs in orotate phosphoribosyltransferase (OPRT), which is involved in one of the activation pathways of 5-FU, and 5'UTR region of TS have been associated in adverse events to 5-FU based therapy.[24] Oxaliplatin frequently results in sensory neurotoxicity that results in treatment interruption or dose reduction, and that has significant morbidity on the patient. When evaluated prospectively in the clinical trial N9741, GSTP1 I105V genotype TT was associated with a higher risk of treatment discontinuation with FOLFOX secondary to neurotoxicity and a higher risk of grade 3 neurotoxicity in patients treated with IROX.[18]

PHARMACOGENOMICS AND PROGNOSTIC MARKERS

A Single Gene as a Prognostic Marker: Gene Expression Data

Although a detailed comprehensive discussion of current data about prognostic molecular markers is beyond the scope of this chapter, it is important to note that prognostic molecular markers that help predict tumor behavior as well as host–tumor interactions can be helpful in risk stratification and in restriction of treatment to patients who would derive the most benefit from it. For instance, the prognostic role of ERCC1, a member of the NER family involved in DNA repair, as discussed previously, was documented through the evaluation of intratumoral *ERCC1* gene expression in a series of 51 patients with non–small cell lung cancer who underwent surgical resection of their primary tumor. Multivariate analysis revealed that high *ERCC1* expression independently predicted for longer survival.[25] In addition to its prognostic role, *ERCC1* was also found to have a predictive role in regard to benefit from adjuvant cisplatin-based chemotherapy in patients with stages I to III non–small-cell lung cancer. Using immunohistochemistry to assess *ERCC1* gene expression at the protein level in 761 patient tumor samples, adjuvant chemotherapy resulted in significantly prolonged survival among patients with ERCC1-negative tumors, but not among patients with ERCC1-positive tumors.[26]

A Comprehensive Molecular Profile: Genome-Wide Arrays

Genome wide arrays have become technically feasible over the past few years and have been used in genome-wide association studies with the goal of establishing a comprehensive risk profile for a specific cancer or identifying an accurate prognostic signature. This approach holds significant promise given the acceptance that a patient's risk or prognosis generally depends on more than one gene in one pathway. The arrays were originally designed to identify thousands of SNPs across the genome simultaneously. The technology has since then expanded to investigate copy number variations and loss of heterozygosity in cancer cells.[27] Numerous examples of susceptibility alleles identified through genome-wide association studies exist in the literature. For instance, Turnbull et al.[28] genotyped 582,886 SNPs in 3,659 patients with a family history of breast cancer and 4,897 controls. Promising associations were then evaluated in a second stage comprising over 12,000 controls and cases. Five susceptibility loci and three SNPs were identified to have associations with risk. Similar examples of such associations have been published for other cancers such as lung, testicular, and colon.[29–32] In addition to identifying subgroups of patients at higher risk for specific cancers, the concept of a multigene signature is the subject of intense investigation in an attempt to better stratify patients regarding risk of cancer recurrence and overall prognosis. These prognostic signatures are based on technologies that measure gene expression using real-time reverse transcriptase quantitative polymerase chain reaction (qPCR) or DNA microarray profiling. We will not discuss this approach in detail in this chapter since it extends beyond the field of pharmacogenomics. However, it is important to note that it has begun to influence clinical practice as illustrated by the example of breast cancer recurrence score based on a 21-gene profile (Onctoype DX™) or the 70-gene oligonucleotide microassay (MammaPrint).[33,34]

Population Pharmacogenomics and Cancer

Variations in toxicity and efficacy of specific therapies have been observed among specific ethnic groups or geographic regions of the world. Genetic diversity affecting drug metabolism and the expression of drug targets, combined with other biologic and environmental factors, may offer a potential explanation for such variability.[35] In lung cancer, similar treatment regimens were observed to have a different outcome in Japan and the United States. To further investigate this issue, investigators of the Southwest Oncology Group and their counterparts from Japan designed and conducted three phase 3 trials with similar eligibility and a common arm of carboplatin and paclitaxel. The outcome was similar in the two Japanese trials but significantly different from the U.S. trial regarding survival and neutropenia. Pharmacogenomic analysis of genes involved in the metabolism of paclitaxel and in DNA damage repair was conducted. There was a significant difference between Japanese and U.S. patients in genotypic distribution for *CYP3A4*1B* (P = .01), *CYP3A5*3C* (P = .03), *ERCC1* 118 (P <.0001), *ERCC2* K751Q (P <.001), and *CYP2C8* R139K (P = .01). Genotypic associations were observed between *CYP3A4*1B* for progression-free survival (HR, 0.36; 95% CI, 0.14 to 0.94; P = .04) and ERCC2 K751Q for response (HR, 0.33; 95% CI, 0.13 to 0.83; P = .02). For grade 4 neutropenia, the HR for ABCB1 3425C3T was 1.84 (95% CI, 0.77 to 4.48; P = .19).[36] The genotype-related associations with patient outcomes were exploratory in nature and need to be confirmed. Nonetheless, this study provided proof of feasibility and a model for further exploring population-related pharmacogenomics as a potential basis for differences in outcome and side-effect profile to similar therapies across different ethnic populations.

PHARMACOLOGY OF CANCER THERAPEUTICS

CURRENT CHALLENGES AND FUTURE DIRECTIONS

The overview of the field of pharmacogenomics as it relates to cancer treatment presented in this chapter highlights its great promise in the quest for personalized medicine. The recent incorporation of pharmacogenomic assessments into prospective clinical trials represents an important step toward the goal of validating or disproving associations with clinical outcome previously made in small retrospective studies. In addition to the emphasis on prospective data collection, the validation of pharmacogenomic associations can be achieved through careful statistical designs that allow for replication of these associations in independent cohorts and through the assessment of the functional role of the associated polymorphisms or genes. Understanding the functionality of single gene variations or multigene signatures that are associated with outcome, prognosis, or risk of developing a cancer is an essential step toward being able to harness their potential as new therapeutic targets.

References

1. Ulrich CM, Robien K, McLeod HL. Cancer pharmacogenomics: polymorphisms, pathways and beyond. *Nat Rev Cancer* 2003;3:912.
2. The International SNP Map Working Group. A map of human genome sequence variation containing 1.42 million single nucleotide polymorphisms. *Nature* 2001;409:928.
3. Longley D, Harkin P, Johnston P. 5-Fluorouacil: mechanisms of action and clinical strategies. *Nature Rev* 2003;3:330.
4. Leichman CG, Lenz HJ, Leichman L, et al. Quantitation of intratumoral thymidylate synthase expression predicts for disseminated colorectal cancer response and resistance to protracted infusion fluorouracil and leucovorin. *J Clin Oncol* 1997;15:3223.
5. Lenz HJ, Leichman CG, Danenberg KD, et al. Thymidylate synthase mRNA level in adenocarcinoma of the stomach: a predictor for primary tumor response and overall survival. *J Clin Oncol* 1996;14:176.
6. Horie N, Aiba H, Oguro K, et al. Functional analysis and DNA polymorphism of the tandemly repeated sequences in the 5′ terminal regulatory region of the human gene for thymidylate synthase. *Cell Struct Funct* 1995;20:191.
7. Pullarkat ST, Stoehlmacher J, Ghaderi V, et al. Thymidylate synthase gene polymorphism determines response and toxicity of 5-FU based chemotherapy. *Pharmacogenomics J* 2001;1:65.
8. Kawakami K, Salonga D, Park JM, et al. Different lengths of a polymorphic repeat sequence in the thymidylate synthase gene affect translational efficiency but not its gene expression. *Clin Cancer Res* 2001;7:4096.
9. Etienne MC, Chazal M, Laurent-Puig P, et al. Prognostic value of tumoral thymidylate synthase and p53 in metastatic colorectal cancer patients receiving fluorouracil-based chemotherapy: phenotypic and genotypic analyses. *J Clin Oncol* 2002;20:2832.
10. Scroth W, Goetz M, Hamman U, et al. Association between CYP2D6 polymorphisms and outcomes among women with early stage breast cancer treated with tamoxifen. *JAMA* 2009;302(13):1429.
11. Schneider BP, Wang M, Radovich M, et al. Association of vascular endothelial growth factor and vascular endothelial growth factor receptor 2 genetic polymorphisms with outcome in a trial of paclitaxel compared with paclitaxel and bevacizumab in advanced breast cancer: ECOG 2100. *J Clin Oncol* 2008;26:4672.

12. Paez JC, Jänne PA, Lee JC, et al. Clinical response to gefitinib therapy mutations in lung cancer: correlation with EGFR. *Science* 2004;304:1497.
13. Lynch TJ, Bell DW, Sordella R, et al. Activating mutations in the epidermal growth factor receptor underlying responsiveness of non–small-cell lung cancer to gefitinib. *N Engl J Med* 2004;350:2129.
14. Salonga D, Danenberg KD, Johnson M, et al. Colorectal tumors responding to 5-fluorouracil have low gene expression levels of dihydropyrimidine dehydrogenase, thymidylate synthase, and thymidine phosphorylase. *Clin Cancer Res* 2000;6:1322.
15. Kweekel DM, Gelderblom H, Guchelaar HJ. Pharmacology of oxaliplatin and the use of pharmacogenomics to individualize therapy. *Cancer Treat Rev* 2005;31:90.
16. Srivastava S, Singhal S, Hu X, et al. Differential catalytic efficiency of allelic variants of human glutathione S-transferase Pi in catalyzing the glutathione conjugation of thiotepa. *Arch Biochem Biophys* 1999;366:89.
17. Stoehlmacher J, Park DJ, Zhang W, et al. A multivariate analysis of genomic polymorphisms: prediction of clinical outcome to 5FU/oxaliplatin combination chemotherapy in refractory colorectal cancer. *Br J Cancer* 2004;91:344.
18. Mcleoad HL, Sargent DJ, Marsh S, et al. Pharmacogenetic predictors of adverse events and response to chemotherapy in metastatic colorectal cancer: results from North American Gastrointestinal Intergroup Trial N9741. *J Clin Oncol* 2010;28(20):3227.
19. Iyer L, Das S, Janisch L, et al. UGT1A1*28 polymorphism as a determinant of irinotecan disposition and toxicity. *Pharmacogenomics J* 2002;2:43.
20. Innocenti F, Undevia SD, Iyer L, et al. Genetic variants in the UDP-glucuronosyltransferase 1A1 gene predict the risk of severe neutropenia of irinotecan. *J Clin Oncol* 2004;22:1382.
21. McLeod HL, Parodi L, Sargent DJ, et al. UGT1A1*28, toxicity and outcome in advanced colorectal cancer: results from Trial N9741. ASCO Annual Meeting Proceedings Part I. *J Clin Oncol* 2006;24(18S):3520.
22. Innocenti F, Undevia SD, Rosner GL, et al. Irinotecan (CPT-11) pharmacokinetics (PK) and neutropenia: interaction among UGT1A1 and transporter genes. *Proc Am Soc Clin Oncol* 2005;23(16S): (abstr 2006).
23. van Kuilenburg ABP, Muller EW, Haasjes J, et al. Lethal outcome of a patient with a complete dihydropyrimidine dehydrogenase (DPD) deficiency after administration of 5-fluorouracil: frequency of the common IVS14+1G: a mutation causing DPD deficiency. *Clin Cancer Res* 2001;7:1149.
24. Ichikawa W, Takahashi T, Nihei Z, et al. Polymorphisms of orotate phosphoribosyl transferase (OPRT) gene and thymidylate synthase tandem repeat (TSTR) predict adverse events (AE) in colorectal cancer (CRC) patients treated with 5-fluorouracil (FU) plus leucovorin (LV). *Proc Am Soc Clin Oncol* 2003;22(265): (abstr 1063).
25. Simon G, Sharma S, Cantor A, et al. ERCC1 expression is a predictor of survival in resected patients with non–small-cell lung cancer. *Chest* 2005;127:978.
26. Olaussen KA, Dunant A, Fouret P, et al. DNA repair by ERCC1 in non–small-cell lung cancer and cisplatin-based adjuvant chemotherapy. *N Engl J Med* 2006;355:983.
27. LaFramboise T. Single nucleotide polymorphism arrays: a decade of biological, computational and technological advances. *Nucleic Acids Res* 2009;37(13):4181.
28. Turnbull C, Ahmed S, Morrison J, et al. Genome-wide association study identifies five new breast cancer susceptibility loci. *Nature Genetics* 2010; 42:504.
29. Truong T, Hung RJ, Amos CI, et al. Replication of lung cancer susceptibility loci at chromosomes 15q25, 5p15, and 6p21: a pooled analysis from the International Lung Cancer Consortium. *J Natl Cancer Inst* 2010;102(13): 959.
30. Li Y, Sheu CC, Ye Y, et al. Genetic variants and risk of lung cancer in never smokers: a genome-wide association study. *Lancet Oncol* 2010;11:321.
31. Turnbull C, Rapley EA, Seal S, et al. Variants near DMRT1, TERT and ATF7IP are associated with testicular germ cell cancer. *Nat Genet* 2010; 42:604.
32. Tenesa A, Farrington SM, Prendergast JG, et al. Genome-wide association scan identifies a colorectal cancer susceptibility locus on 11q23 and replicates risk loci at 8q24 and 18q21. *Nat Genet* 2008;40:631.
33. Goldstein LJ, Gray R, Badve S, et al. Prognostic utility of utility of the 21-gene assay in hormone receptor positive operable breast cancer compared with classical clinicopathologic features. *J Clin Oncol* 2008;26: 4063.
34. van deVijver MJ, He YD, van'tVeer LJ, et al. A gene expression signature as a predictor of survival in breast cancer. *N Engl J Med* 2002;347:1999.
35. Ma BB, Hui EP, Mok TS. Population-based differences in treatment outcome following anticancer drug therapies. *Lancet Oncol* 2010;11:75.
36. Gandara DR, Kawagushi T, Crowley J, et al. Japanese-US common-arm analysis of paclitaxel plus carboplatin in advanced non–small-cell lung cancer: a model for assessing population-related pharmacogenomics. *J Clin Oncol* 2009;27:3540.

CHAPTER 34 ALKYLATING AGENTS

KENNETH D. TEW

PERSPECTIVES

Alkylating agents were the first anticancer molecules developed, and they are still used today. After more than 50 years of use, the basic chemistry and pharmacology of this drug family is well understood and has not changed substantially. The family contains six major classes: nitrogen mustards, aziridines, alkyl sulfonates, epoxides, nitrosoureas, and triazene compounds, although a few nonstandard agents have recently been developed. Most epoxides tend to be quite nonspecific with respect to their reactivity and, as such, few have useful clinical characteristics. This chapter provides perspective on how the limited varieties of alkylating agents continue to be useful in the therapeutic management of cancer patients.

The alkylating agents are a diverse group of anticancer agents with the commonality that they react in a manner such that an electrophilic alkyl group or a substituted alkyl group can covalently bind to cellular nucleophilic sites. Electrophilicity is achieved through the formation of carbonium ion intermediates and can result in transition complexes with target molecules. Ultimately, reactions result in the formation of covalent linkages by alkylation with a broad range of nucleophilic groups, including bases in DNA, and these are believed responsible for ultimate cytotoxicity and therapeutic effect. Although the alkylating agents react with cells in all phases of the cell cycle, their efficacy and toxicity result from interference with rapidly proliferating tissues. From a historical perspective, the vesicant properties of mustard gas used during World War I were shown to be accompanied by suppression of lymphoid and hematologic functions in experimental animals[1] and led to the development of mechlorethamine as the first alkylating agent used in the management of human cancer.[2] Subsequently, a number of related drugs have been developed, and these have roles in the treatment of a range of leukemias, lymphomas, and solid tumors. Most of the alkylating agents cause dose-limiting toxicities to the bone marrow and, to a lesser degree, the intestinal mucosa, with other organ systems also affected contingent on the individual drug, dosage, and duration of therapy. Despite the present trend toward targeted therapies, this class of "nonspecific" drugs maintains an essential role in cancer chemotherapy.

CHEMISTRY

Alkylating reactions are generally classified through their kinetic properties as S_N1 (nucleophilic substitution, first order) or S_N2 (nucleophilic substitution, second order) (Fig. 34.1). The first-order kinetics of the S_N1 reactions depend on the concentration of the original alkylating agent. The rate-limiting step is the initial formation of the reactive intermediate, and the rate is essentially independent of the concentration of the substrate. The S_N2 alkylation reaction is a bimolecular nucleophilic displacement with second-order kinetics, where the rate depends on the concentration of both alkylating agent and target nucleophile. Reactivity of electrophiles[3] suggests that the rates of alkylation of cellular nucleophiles (including thiols, phosphates, amino and imidazole groups of amino acids, and various reactive sites in nucleic acid bases) are most dependent on their potential energy states, which can be defined as "hard" or "soft," based on the polarizability of their reactive centers.[4] Although the metabolism and metabolites of nitrogen mustards and nitrosoureas differ, the active alkylating species of each is the alkyl carbonium ion (Fig. 34.1), a highly polarized hard electrophile as a consequence of its highly positive charge density at the electrophilic center. Alkyl carbonium ions will react most readily with hard nucleophiles (possessing a highly polarized negative charge density), where the high-energy transition state (a potential energy barrier to the reaction) is most favorable. In specific terms, an active alkylating species from a nitrogen mustard will demonstrate selectivity for cellular nucleophiles in the following order: (1) oxygen in phosphate groups of RNA and DNA, (2) oxygens of purines and pyrimidines, (3) amino groups of purine bases, (4) primary and secondary amino groups of proteins, (5) sulfur atoms of methionine, and (6) thiol groups of cysteinyl residues of protein and glutathione.[3] The least favored reactions will still occur but at much slower rates unless they are catalyzed.

Alkylation through highly reactive intermediates (e.g., mechlorethamine) would be expected to be less selective in their targets than the less reactive S_N2 reagents (e.g., busulfan). However, the therapeutic and toxic effects of alkylating agents do not correlate directly with their chemical reactivity. Clinically useful agents include drugs with S_N1 or S_N2 characteristics, and some with both.[5] These differ in their toxicity profiles and antitumor activity, but more as a consequence of differences in pharmacokinetics, lipid solubility, penetration of the CNS, membrane transport, metabolism and detoxification, and specific enzymatic reactions capable of repairing alkylation sites on DNA.

CLASSIFICATION

The major classes of clinically useful alkylating agents are illustrated in Table 34.1 and summarized in the following sections. Doses and schedules of the various agents are shown in Table 34.2.

Alkyl Sulfonates

Busulfan is used for the treatment of chronic myelogenous leukemia. It exhibits S_N2 alkylation kinetics and shows nucleophilic selectivity for thiol groups, suggesting that it may exert cytotoxicity through protein alkylation rather than through

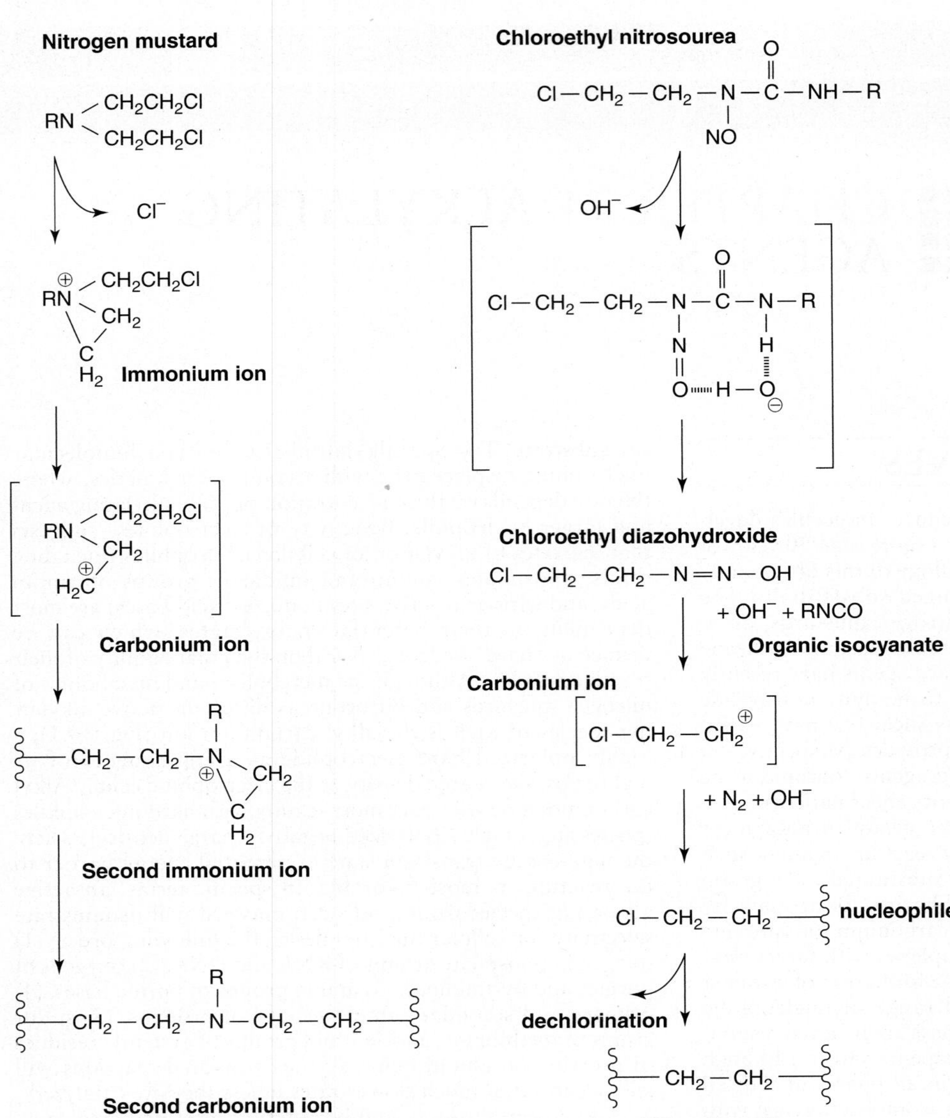

FIGURE 34.1 Comparative decomposition and metabolism of a typical nitrogen mustard compared to a nitrosourea. Although intermediate metabolites are distinct, the active alkylating species is a carbonium ion in each case. This electrophilic moiety reacts with target cellular nucleophiles.

DNA. In contrast to the nitrogen mustards and nitrosoureas, busulfan has a greater effect on myeloid cells than lymphoid cells, thus its use against chronic myelogenous leukemia.[6]

Aziridines

Aziridines are analogs of ring-closed intermediates of nitrogen mustards and are less chemically reactive, but they have equivalent therapeutic properties. Thiotepa has been used in the treatment of carcinoma of the breast, ovary, for a variety of CNS diseases, and with increasing frequency as a component of high-dose chemotherapy regimens.[7] Thiotepa and its primary desulfurated metabolite TEPA (triethylenethiophosphoramide) alkylate through aziridine ring openings, a mechanism similar to the nitrogen mustards.

Triazines

Perhaps the newest clinical development in the alkylating agent field is the emergence of temozolomide (TMZ). This agent acts as a prodrug and is an imidazotetrazine analog that undergoes spontaneous activation in solution to produce 5-(3-methyltriazen-1-yl) imidazole-4-carboxamide (MTIC), a triazine derivative. It crosses the blood–brain barrier with concentrations in the CNS approximating 30% of plasma concentrations.[8] Resistance to the methylating agent occurs quite frequently and has adversely affected the rate and durability of the clinical responses of patients. However, because of its favorable toxicity and pharmacokinetics, TMZ is being combined with numerous other classes of anticancer drug in an effort to improve response rates in diseases such as malignant melanomas, gliomas, brain metastasis from solid tumors, and refractory leukemias. Many of these trials are currently underway.[9]

Nitrogen Mustards

Bischloroethylamines or nitrogen mustards are extensively administered in the clinic. As an initial step in alkylation, chlorine acts as a leaving group and the β-carbon reacts with the nucleophilic nitrogen atom to form the cyclic, positively charged, reactive aziridinium moiety. Reaction of the aziridinium ring with an electron-rich nucleophile creates an initial alkylation product. The remaining chloroethyl group achieves bifunctionality through formation of a second aziridinium.

TABLE 34.1

MAJOR CLASSES OF CLINICALLY USEFUL ALKYLATING AGENTS

Drug	Main Therapeutic Uses	Clinical Pharmacology	Major Toxicities	Notes
ALKYL SULFONATES				
Busulfan	Bone marrow transplantation, especially in chronic myelogenous leukemia	Bioavailability, 80%; protein bound, 33%; $t_{1/2}$, 2.5 h	Pulmonary fibrosis, hyperpigmentation thrombocytopenia, lowered blood platelet count and activity	Oral or parenteral; high dose causes hepatic veno-occlusive disease
ETHYLENEIMINES/METHYLMELAMINES				
Altretamine		Protein bound, 94%; $t_{1/2}$, 5–10 h	Nausea, vomiting, diarrhea, and neurotoxicity	Not widely used
Thio TEPA	Breast cancer, ovarian cancer, and bladder cancer; also bone marrow transplant	$t_{1/2}$, 2.5 h; urinary excretion at 24 h, 25%; substrate for CYP2B6 and CYP2C11	Myelosuppression	Nadirs of leukopenia, occur 2 wk; thrombocytopenia, 3 wk (correlates with AUC of parent drug)
NITROGEN MUSTARDS				
Mechlorethamine	Hodgkin's lymphoma		Nausea, vomiting, myelosuppression	Precursor for other clinical mustards
Melphalan (L-phenylalanine mustard)	Multiple myeloma and ovarian cancer, and occasionally malignant melanoma	Bioavailability 25%–90%; $t_{1/2}$, 1.5 h; urinary excretion at 24 h, 13%; clearance, 9 mL/min/kg	Nausea, vomiting, myelosuppression	Causes less mucosal damage than others in class
Chlorambucil	Chronic lymphocytic leukemia	$t_{1/2}$, 1.5 h; urinary excretion at 24 h, 50%	Myelosuppression, gastrointestinal distress, CNS, skin reactions, hepatotoxicity	Oral
Cyclophosphamide	Variety of lymphomas, leukemias and solid tumors	Bioavailability, >75%; protein bound, >60%; $t_{1/2}$, 3–12 h; urinary excretion at 24 h, <15%	Nausea and vomiting, bone marrow suppression, diarrhea, darkening of the skin/nails, alopecia (hair loss), lethargy, hemorrhagic cystitis	IV; primary excretion route is urine
Ifosfamide	Testicular cancer; breast cancer; lymphoma (non–Hodgkin's); soft tissue sarcoma; osteogenic sarcoma; lung cancer; cervical cancer; ovarian cancer; bone cancer	$t_{1/2}$, 15 h; urinary excretion at 24 h, 15%	As for cyclophosphamide	Ifosfamide is often used in conjunction with mesna to avoid cystinuria
NITROSOUREAS				
Carmustine	Glioma, glioblastoma multiforme, medulloblastoma and astrocytoma, multiple myeloma and lymphoma (Hodgkin's and non–Hodgkin's)	Bioavailability, 25%; protein bound, 80%; $t_{1/2}$, 30 min	Bone marrow and pulmonary toxicities are a function of lifetime cumulative dose	Clinically, nitrosoureas do not share cross-resistance with nitrogen mustards in lymphoma treatment

(*Continued*)

PHARMACOLOGY OF CANCER THERAPEUTICS

TABLE 34.1

CONTINUED

Drug	Main Therapeutic Uses	Clinical Pharmacology	Major Toxicities	Notes
Streptozotocin	Cancers of the islets of Langerhans	$t_{1/2}$, 35 min; excreted in the urine (15%), feces (<1%), and in the expired air	Nausea and vomiting; nephrotoxicity can range from transient protein urea and azotemia to permanent tubular damage; can also cause aberrations of glucose metabolism	A natural product from *Streptomyces achromogenes*
TRIAZENES				
Dacarbazine	Malignant melanoma and Hodgkin's lymphoma	$t_{1/2}$, 5 h; protein bound, 5% hepatic metabolism	Nausea, vomiting, myelosuppression	IV or IM
Temozolomide	Glioblastoma; astrocytoma; metastatic melanoma	Protein bound, 15%; $t_{1/2}$, 1.8 h; clearance, 5.5 l/h/m^2	Nausea, vomiting, myelosuppression	Oral; derivative of imidazotetrazine, prodrug of dacarbazine; rapidly absorbed

$t_{1/2}$, half-life; TEPA, triethylenethiophosphoramide; AUC, area under curve; IV, intravenous; IM, intramuscular.

Melphalan (L-phenylalanine mustard), chlorambucil, cyclophosphamide, and ifosfamide (Table 34.1) replaced mechlorethamine as primary therapeutic agents. These derivatives have electron-withdrawing groups substituted on the nitrogen atom, reducing the nucleophilicity of the nitrogen and rendering them less reactive, but enhancing their antitumor efficacy.

One distinguishing feature of melphalan is that an amino acid transporter responsible for uptake influences its efficacy across cell membranes.[10] Although a number of glutathione (GSH) conjugates of alkylating agents are effluxed through adenosine triphosphate–dependent membrane transporters,[11] specific uptake mechanisms are generally rare for cancer drugs. Cyclophosphamide and ifosfamide are prodrugs that require cytochrome P-450 metabolism to release active alkylating species. Cyclophosphamide continues to be the most widely used alkylating agent and has activity against a variety of tumors.[12]

Nitrosoureas

The nitrosoureas form a diverse class of alkylating agents that has distinct metabolism and pharmacology that separates it from others.[13] Under physiological conditions, proton abstraction by a hydroxyl ion initiates spontaneous decomposition of the molecule to yield a diazonium hydroxide and an isocyanate (Fig. 34.1). The chloroethyl carbonium ion generated is the active alkylating species. Through a subsequent dehalogenation step, a second electrophilic site imparts bifunctionality.[14] Thus, while cross-linking similar to those lesions caused by nitrogen mustards may occur, the chemistry leading to the end point is distinct. The isocyanate species generated are also electrophilic, showing nucleophilic selectivity toward sulfhydryl and amino groups that can inhibit a number of enzymes involved in nucleic acid synthesis and thiol balance.[15] Because carbamoylation is considered of minor importance to the therapeutic efficacy of clinically used nitrosoureas, chlorozotocin and streptozotocin were designed to undergo internal carbamoylation at the 1- or 3-OH group of the glucose ring, with the consequence that no carbamoylating species are produced.[16,17] Streptozotocin is also unusual in that most methylnitrosoureas have only modest therapeutic value. However, its lack of bone marrow toxicity and strong diabetogenic effect in animals led to its use in cancer of the pancreas[18] (Table 34.1). The dose-limiting toxicities in humans are gastrointestinal and renal, but the drug has considerably less hematopoietic toxicity than the other nitrosoureas. Because of their lipophilicity and capacity to cross the blood–brain barrier, the chloroethylnitrosoureas were found to be effective against intracranially inoculated murine tumors. Indeed, early preclinical studies showed that many mouse tumors were quite responsive to nitrosoureas. The same extent of efficacy was not found in humans. Subsequent analyses demonstrated that an enzyme responsible for repair of O6 alkyl guanine (O^6-methylguanine-DNA methyltransferase [MGMT] or the Mer/Mex phenotype[19]) was expressed at low levels in mice, but high levels in humans, a contributory factor in the reduced clinical efficacy of nitrosoureas in humans. Particularly in the 1980s a number of new nitrosoureas were tested in patients in Europe and Japan, but none established a regular role in standard cancer treatment regimens.

O^6-methylguanine-DNA methyltransferase promoter methylation is crucial in MGMT gene silencing and can predict a favorable outcome in glioblastoma patients receiving alkylating agents.[20] This biomarker is on the verge of entering clinical decision making and is currently used to stratify or even select glioblastoma patients for clinical trials. In other subtypes of glioma, such as anaplastic gliomas, the relevance of MGMT promoter methylation might extend beyond the prediction of chemosensitivity, and could reflect a distinct molecular profile.

TABLE 34.2

DOSE AND SCHEDULES OF CLINICALLY USEFUL ALKYLATING AGENTS

Alkylating Agent	Disease Sites and Dose Ranges Used Clinically	Notes
BCNU (Carmustine)	General antineoplastic	Infusion 1–2 h; in combination, dose usually reduced by 25%–50%
	150–200 mg/m² (IV, every 6 weeks)	
	Cutaneous T-cell lymphoma	Side effects include irritant dermatitis, telangiectasia, erythema, and bone marrow suppression
	200–600 mg (topical solution)	
	Adjunct to surgical resection of brain tumor	Up to 8 wafers (7.7 mg of carmustine) implanted
	61.6 mg (implant)	
Busulfan	Chronic myelogenous leukemia and myeloproliferative disorders	Dispensed over 3–4 days, with cyclophosphamide
	4–8 mg (daily PO)	
	1.8 mg/m² (daily PO)	
	Bone marrow transplant	
	640 mg/m² (daily PO)	
Carboplatin	Advanced ovarian cancer—monotherapy	With cyclophosphamide
	360 mg/m² (IV, every 4 weeks)	Patients usually receive marrow transplantation or peripheral stem cell support
	Ovarian cancer—combination	
	300 mg/m² (IV, every 4 weeks for 6 cycles)	
	Ovarian cancer—intraperitoneal	
	200–500 mg/m² (IP, 2 L dialysis fluid)	
	Ovarian and other sites phase 1/2 setting—high-dose therapy	
	800–1,600 mg/m² (IV)	
Cisplatin	Metastatic testicular cancer:	With other antineoplastic agents
	20 mg/m²/day for 5 days of each cycle (IV)	With cyclophosphamide (600 mg/m² once every 4 weeks)
	Metastatic ovarian cancer:	
	75–100 mg/m² (IV, once every 4 weeks)	With vincristine, bleomycin, and fluorouracil
	Head and neck cancer:	With methotrexate and fluorouracil
	100 mg/m² (IV)	MVAC regimen (methotrexate, vinblastine, doxorubicin, and cisplatin) used for cervical cancer
	Bladder cancer:	
	(combination prior to cystectomy)	
	50–70; initiate dosing at 50 mg/m² (IV, once every 3–4 weeks)	Administration preceded by paclitaxel 135 mg/m² every 3 weeks
	Metastatic breast cancer:	With radiation therapy
	20 mg/m² (IV, days 1–5 every 3 weeks)	
	Cervical cancer:	
	70 mg/m² (IV, dosing cycled every 4 weeks)	
	Non–small cell lung cancer:	
	75 mg/m² (IV, every 3 weeks)	
	Esophageal cancer:	
	75 mg/m² on day 1 of weeks 1, 5, 8, and 11 (IV)	
Cyclophosphamide	General antineoplastic	Dose used as monotherapy for patients with no hematologic toxicity
	1–5 mg/kg (daily PO)	
	40–50 mg/kg (IV, in divided doses over 2–5 days)	
	40–50 mg/kg (IV, in divided doses over 2–5 days)	
	10–15 mg/kg (IV, every 7–10 days)	
	10–15 mg/kg (IV, every 7–10 days)	
	3–5 mg/kg (IV twice per week)	
	High-dose regimen in bone marrow transplantation and for other autoimmune disorders	
	200 mg/kg (IV)	
	1–2.5 mg/kg (daily PO 7–14 days/mo)	
Dacarbazine	General antineoplastic	Administered for 10 days, may be repeated at 4-week intervals
	2–4.5 mg/kg/day (IV)	
	150 mg/m²/day (IV)	With other anticancer agents; treatment lasts 5 days, may be repeated every 4 weeks

(*Continued*)

TABLE 34.2

CONTINUED

Alkylating Agent	Disease Sites and Dose Ranges Used Clinically	Notes
Etoposide	Testicular cancer 50–100 mg/m²/day (IV, slow infusion over 30–60+ min for 5 days) Small cell lung cancer 35–50 mg/m²/day (IV, slow infusion over 30–60+ min for 4–5 days)	Alternatively, 100 mg/m²/day on days 1, 3, and 5 may be used. Doses for combination therapy and are repeated at 3- to 4-wk intervals after recovery from hematologic toxicity Doses are for combination therapy and repeated at 3- to 4-week intervals after recovery from hematologic toxicity. Oral dose is twice the IV, rounded to the nearest 50 mg
Ifosfamide	General antineoplastic 1.2 g/m²/day (IV, for 5 consecutive days)	Repeat every 3 weeks
Melphalan	Multiple myeloma: 16 mg/m² (IV, infusion over 15–20 min) 6 mg (daily PO) Epithelial ovarian cancer: 0.2 mg/kg (daily PO)	2-week intervals for 4 doses, 4-week intervals thereafter After 2–3 weeks treatment, should be discontinued for up to 4 weeks, then reinstituted at 2–4 mg/day Daily dose for a 5-day course, repeated every 4–5 weeks
Streptozotocin	Pancreatic tumors 500 mg/m²/day; 1,000 mg/m²/day (IV; IV)	500 mg for 5 consecutive days every 6 weeks, 1,000 mg is for 2 weeks, followed by an increase in weekly dose not to exceed 1,500 mg/m²/wk
Temozolomide	Brain tumors 150 mg/m² (daily PO)	Dose adjusted on the basis of blood counts
Thiotepa	General antineoplastic: 0.3–0.4 mg/kg (IV) Papillary carcinoma of the bladder: 60 mg/wk for 4 weeks (bladder catheter) Control of serous effusions: 0.6–0.8 mg/kg (intracavitary)	Rapid administration given at 1- to 4-week intervals 30 or 60 mL should be retained for 2 h, so the patient is usually dehydrated prior to administration of the drug

IV, intravenously; PO, by mouth.

At this time, standardization of MGMT assays will be critical in establishing prospective prognostic or predictive effects. In addition, eventual clinical trials will need to determine, for each subtype of glioma, the extent to which methylation patterns are predictive or prognostic and whether such assays could be incorporated into an individualized approach to clinical practice.[20]

CLINICAL PHARMACOKINETICS/ PHARMACODYNAMICS

The pharmacokinetics of the alkylating agents are highly variable, depending on the individual agent. Nevertheless, they are generally characterized by high reactivity and short half-lives. Although detailed studies on clinical pharmacology are available,[21] Table 34.1 summarizes some of the primary kinetic characteristics of the major clinically useful drugs. Mechlorethamine is unstable and is administered rapidly in a running intravenous infusion to avoid its rapid breakdown to inactive metabolites. In contrast, chlorambucil and cyclophosphamide are sufficiently stable to be given orally, and are rapidly and completely absorbed from the gastrointestinal tract, while others like melphalan have poor and variable oral absorption. Cyclophosphamide,[22] ifosfamide, and dacarbazine are unusual in that they require activation by cytochrome P-450 in the liver before they can alkylate cellular constituents. The nitrosoureas also require activation, albeit nonenzymatic. The major route of metabolism of most alkylating agents is spontaneous hydrolysis, although many can also undergo some degree of enzymatic metabolism. This is particularly pertinent for phase II metabolic conversions where reactivity with nucleophilic thiols precedes conversion to mercapturates, with the result that most of the alkylating agents are excreted in the urine. One example of complex multistep metabolism is provided by cyclophosphamide (Fig. 34.2). Activation by CYP2B6 is followed by conversion of aldehyde dehydrogenase to reactive alkylating species or possible detoxification through GSH conjugation reactions. The latter is particularly important for acrolein because it is believed to contribute to the bladder toxicities associated with the drug.

The alkylating agents form covalent bonds with a number of nucleophilic groups present in proteins, RNA, and DNA (e.g., amino, carboxyl, sulfhydryl, imidazole, phosphate). Under physiological conditions, the chloroethyl group of the nitrogen mustards undergoes cyclization, with the chloride acting as a leaving group forming an intermediate carbonium ion that attacks nucleophilic sites (Fig. 34.1). Bifunctional alkylating agents (with two chloroethyl side chains) can undergo a subsequent cyclization to form a covalent bond with an adjacent nucleophilic group, resulting in DNA:DNA or DNA:protein cross-links. The N7 or O6 positions of guanine are particularly susceptible and may represent primary targets that determine both the cytotoxic and mutagenic consequences of therapy.[23] The nitrosoureas have a similar, but distinct, mechanism of action, spontaneously forming both alkylating and carbamoylating agents in aqueous media (Fig. 34.1). The carbamoylating moieties are generally believed to be inconsequential to the therapeutic properties of the nitrosoureas.

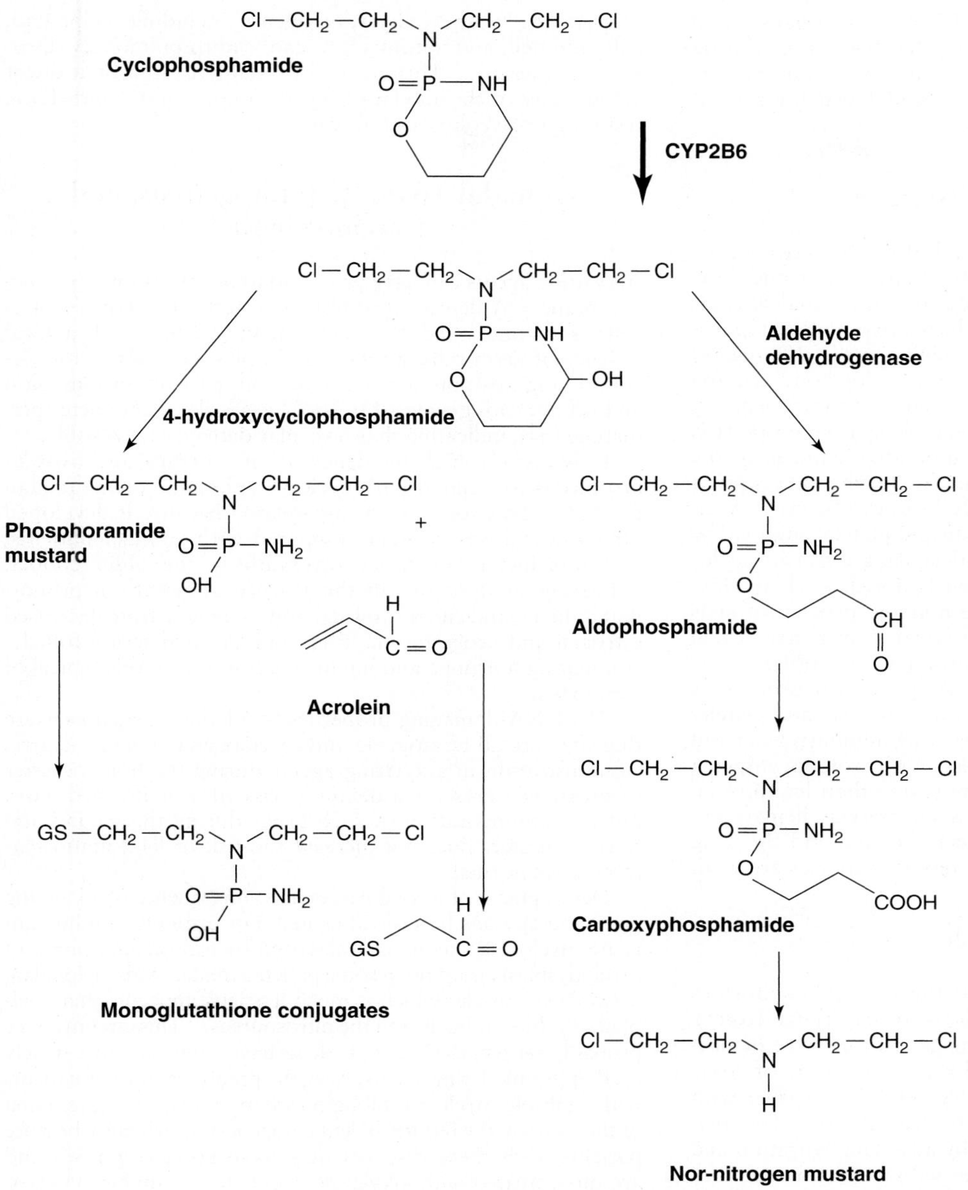

Cyclophosphamide

CYP2B6

4-hydroxycyclophosphamide

Aldehyde dehydrogenase

Phosphoramide mustard

Acrolein

Aldophosphamide

Carboxyphosphamide

Monoglutathione conjugates

Nor-nitrogen mustard

FIGURE 34.2 Activation and detoxification routes of metabolism for cyclophosphamide.

THERAPEUTIC USES

The alkylating agents are frequently used in combination therapy to treat a variety of types of cancer. Perhaps the most versatile is cyclophosphamide, while the other alkylating agents are of more restricted clinical use. Because of early successes, many disease states are managed with drug combinations that contain several alkylating agents. Cyclophosphamide is employed to treat a variety of immune-related diseases and to purge bone marrow in autologous marrow transplant situations.[24] A general summary of the clinical uses of the primary alkylating agents is shown in Table 34.1.

TOXICITIES

The alkylating agents show significant qualitative and quantitative variability in the sites and severities of their toxicities. The primary dose-limiting toxicity is suppression of bone marrow function, with secondary limiting effects on the proliferating cells of the intestinal mucosa.

Contraindications to the use of alkylating agents would identify patients with severely depressed bone marrow function and patients with hypersensitivity to these drugs. Other listed precautions to these drugs include carcinogenic and mutagenic effects and impairment of fertility. Precaution is also advised in patients with (1) leukopenia or thrombocytopenia, (2) previous exposure to chemotherapy or radiotherapy, (3) tumor cell infiltration of the bone marrow, and (4) impaired renal or hepatic function. These drugs can also increase toxicity in adrenalectomized patients and interfere with wound healing. A brief summary of dose-limiting toxicities is shown in Table 34.1, and a narrative of each follows here.

Nausea and Vomiting

Nausea and vomiting are frequent side effects of alkylating agent therapy and are not well controlled by conventional antiemetics.[23] They are a major source of patient discomfort and a significant cause of lack of drug compliance and even discontinuation of therapy. Frequency and extent are highly variable among patients. The overall frequency of nausea and vomiting is directly proportional to the dose of alkylating agent. Onset of nausea may occur within a few minutes of the administration of the drug or may be delayed for several hours.

Bone Marrow Toxicity

Bone marrow toxicity can involve all of the blood elements, leukocytes, platelets, and red cells.[25] The extent and time course of suppression show marked interindividual fluctuation. Relative platelet sparing is a characteristic of cyclophosphamide treatment. Even at the very high doses (<200 mg/kg) of cyclophosphamide (used in preparation for bone marrow transplantation), some recovery of hematopoietic elements occurs within 21 to 28 days. This stem cell–sparing property is further reflected by the fact that cumulative damage to the bone marrow is rarely seen when cyclophosphamide is given as a single agent, and repeated high doses can be given without progressive lowering of leukocyte and platelet counts. The biochemical basis for the stem cell–sparing effect of cyclophosphamide is related to the presence of high levels of aldehyde dehydrogenase in early bone marrow progenitor cells (Fig. 34.2). Busulfan is particularly toxic to bone marrow stem cells,[25] and treatment can lead to prolonged hypoplasia. The hematopoietic depression produced by the nitrosoureas is characteristically delayed. The onset of leukocyte and platelet depression occurs 3 to 4 weeks after drug administration and may last an additional 2 to 3 weeks.[21,25] Thrombocytopenia appears earlier and usually is more severe than leukopenia. Even if the nitrosourea is given at 6-week intervals, hematopoietic recovery may not occur between courses, and the drug dose often must be decreased when repeated courses are used.

Renal and Bladder Toxicity

Hemorrhagic cystitis is unique to the oxazaphosphorines (cyclophosphamide and ifosfamide) and may range from a mild cystitis to severe bladder damage with massive hemorrhage.[26] This toxicity is caused by the excretion of toxic metabolites (particularly acrolein) (Fig. 34.2) in the urine, with subsequent direct irritation of the bladder mucosa. The incidence and severity can be lessened by adequate hydration and continuous irrigation of the bladder with a solution containing 2-mercaptoethane sulfonate (MESNA) and frequent bladder emptying.[27] MESNA is given in divided doses every 4 hours in dosages of 60% of those of the alkylating agent.

At high cumulative doses, all commonly used nitrosoureas can produce a dose-related renal toxicity that can result in renal failure and death.[28] In patients developing clinical evidence of toxicity, increases in serum creatinine usually appear after the completion of therapy and may be first detected up to 2 years after treatment.

Interstitial Pneumonitis and Pulmonary Fibrosis

Long-term busulfan therapy can lead to the gradual onset of fever, a nonproductive cough, and dyspnea, followed by tachypnea and cyanosis, progressing to severe pulmonary insufficiency and death.[29] If busulfan is stopped before the onset of clinical symptoms, pulmonary function may stabilize, but if clinical symptoms are manifest, the condition may be rapidly fatal. Cyclophosphamide, bischloroethylnitrosourea and methyl-1-(2-chloroethyl)-3-cyclohexyl-1-nitrosourea in cumulative doses exceeding 1,000 mg/m^2 may also lead to similar side effects.[30] Other alkylating agents, including melphalan, chlorambucil, and mitomycin C can lead to pulmonary fibrosis after therapy.[31] This effect is probably caused by a direct cytotoxicity of the alkylating agent to pulmonary epithelium, resulting in alveolitis and fibrosis.

Gonadal Toxicity, Teratogenesis, and Carcinogenesis

Alkylating agents can have profound toxic effects on reproductive tissue.[32] A depletion of testicular germ (but not Sertoli's) cells is accompanied by aspermia. In patients with a total absence of germ cells, an increase in plasma levels of follicle-stimulating hormone occurs. However, patients in remission and off alkylating agents for 2 to 7 years show complete spermatogenesis, indicating that testicular damage is reversible.

In women, a high incidence of amenorrhea and ovarian atrophy is associated with cyclophosphamide or melphalan therapy.[33] This seems to be age-related because it developed after lower doses in older compared with younger patients, and was less likely to be reversible in the older cohort. Pathologic analysis reveals the absence of mature or primordial follicles, and endocrinology studies demonstrate decreased estrogen and progesterone levels and elevated serum follicle-stimulating hormone and luteinizing hormone levels typical of menopause.

The DNA-damaging properties of alkylating agents ensure that they are all teratogenic and carcinogenic to some degree. Administration of alkylating agents during the first trimester of pregnancy presents a definitive risk of a malformed fetus, but the administration of such drugs during the second and third trimesters does not increase the risk of fetal malformation above normal.[34]

Development of second cancer as a consequence of alkylating agent therapy has been documented. For example, a fulminant acute myeloid leukemia characterized by a preceding phase of myelodysplasia is found in some patients treated with melphalan, cyclophosphamide (which is much less leukemogenic than melphalan), chlorambucil, and the nitrosoureas.[32] This circumstance probably reflects the fact that these have been the most widely used of the alkylating agents. Also, the preponderance of patients with multiple myeloma, Hodgkin's lymphoma, and carcinoma of the ovary in the reports of leukemogenesis is probably because patients with these diseases may have good responses and are often treated with alkylating agents for a number of years. The rate of occurrence of acute leukemia in patients with ovarian cancer who survive for 10 years after treatment with alkylating agents might be as high as 10%. Acute leukemia has been the most frequently described second malignancy, and it usually develops 1 to 4 years after drug exposure.[35] Other malignancies, including solid tumors, also have been reported to develop in patients treated with alkylating agents.[36]

The last four decades have yielded significant improvement in survival of children diagnosed with cancer (5-year survival is approximately 80%). As many as two-thirds of the survivors of childhood malignancies can experience delayed drug toxicities that may be severe or even life-threatening. Such complications include impairment in growth and development, neurocognitive dysfunction, cardiopulmonary compromise, endocrine dysfunction, renal impairment, gastrointestinal dysfunction, musculoskeletal sequelae, and second cancers.[37]

Alopecia

The degree of alopecia after cyclophosphamide administration may be quite severe, especially when this drug is used in combination with vincristine sulfate or doxorubicin hydrochloride.[38] Regrowth of hair inevitably occurs after cessation of therapy but may be associated with a change in the color and greater curl. Use of a tourniquet or ice pack applied to the scalp during and for a short period after cyclophosphamide administration reduces the impact.

Allergic Reactions

Alkylating agents covalently bind to proteins, and these conjugates can act as haptens and produce allergic reactions.[39] An increasing number of reports of skin eruption, angioneurotic edema, urticaria, and anaphylactic reactions after systemic administration of alkylating agents have appeared.

Immunosuppression

Alkylating agents suppress both humoral and cellular immunity in a variety of experimental systems.[40] The most immunosuppressive is cyclophosphamide, reported to cause (1) selective suppression of B-lymphocyte function, (2) depletion of B-lymphocytes, and (3) suppression of lymphocyte functions that are mediated by T cells, such as the graft-versus-host response and delayed hypersensitivity. Most intermittent antitumor regimens do not uniformly produce profound immunosuppression, and recovery is usually prompt. Sustained drug treatments can lead to severe lymphocyte depletion and profound immunosuppression and may be accompanied by an increase of viral, fungal, and protozoal infections.[40]

COMPLICATIONS WITH HIGH-DOSE ALKYLATING AGENT THERAPY

At standard doses, alkylating agents produce myelosuppression as their dose-limiting toxicity. Less severe effects on gastrointestinal epithelium, lung, bladder, and kidney may become problems with long-term treatment, but rarely limit initial therapy. For this reason, and because of their steep dose response to tumor-killing curves, the alkylating agents have become a logical tool, either alone or in combination, for high-dose chemotherapy regimens in which bone marrow toxicity is expected, and is accommodated by bone marrow transplantation, stem cell reconstitution from peripheral blood monocytes, and growth factor rescue. In this high-dose setting, toxicities that affect the gut, lung, liver, and CNS become dose-limiting and life-threatening.[41] The highly lipid-soluble alkylators, especially ifosfamide, busulfan, the nitrosoureas, and thiotepa, cause CNS dysfunction, including seizures, altered mental status, cerebellar dysfunction, cranial nerve palsies, and coma.[42] High-dose ifosfamide is most frequently the cause of neurotoxicity.[43] Clinical manifestations of grade 4 neurotoxicities were reported in approximately one-fourth of those patients receiving ifosfamide. The side-chain *N*-linked chloroethyl moiety of ifosfamide (Table 34.1) is more likely than the bischloroethyl group of cyclophosphamide to undergo oxidation and subsequent *N*-deethylation and lead to the formation of chloroacetaldehyde. High-dose busulfan is also frequently used in a variety of conditioning regimens for hematopoietic cell transplantation. In this setting, busulfan causes neurotoxicity manifesting in seizures that generally are tonic-clonic in character. Phenytoin has been the preferred drug to treat busulfan-induced seizures although some emerging clinical data support the use of benzodiazepines, most notably clonazepam and lorazepam, to prevent busulfan-induced seizures. Moreover, the second-generation antiepileptic drug levetiracetam possesses the characteristics of optimal prophylaxis for busulfan-induced seizures.[44]

Cyclophosphamide at doses exceeding 100 mg/kg during a 48-hour period (preparatory to bone marrow transplantation) can cause cardiac toxicity.[45] No evidence exists for cumulative damage to the heart after repeated moderate or low doses of the drug. Cardiac toxicity occurs with greatest frequency in patients older than 50 years or in those previously treated with anthracyclines.[45]

ALKYLATING AGENT–STEROID CONJUGATES

Adapting the rationale that steroid receptors may function to localize and concentrate attached drug species intracellularly in hormone-responsive cancers, a number of synthetic conjugates of nitrogen mustards and steroids have been developed. Of these, two made the transition into clinical use.

Prednimustine is an ester-linked conjugate of chlorambucil and prednisolone designed to function as a prodrug for chlorambucil. Release of the alkylating agent occurs after cleavage by serum esterases[46] that can release the ester link of prednimustine, producing the hormone and active alkylating drug. The elimination phase of chlorambucil in patient plasma is significantly longer after administration of prednimustine than after chlorambucil. Estramustine is a carbamate ester-linked conjugate of nor-nitrogen mustard and estradiol. Unlike prednimustine, the pharmacology of estramustine is governed by the presence of the carbamate group in the steroid-mustard linkage. The relative resistance of the carbamate bond to enzymatic cleavage eliminates the alkylating activity of the molecule and conveys an entirely new pharmacology.[47] Crystal structural and mechanism of action studies showed that estramustine has antimitotic activity, an activity shared by some other steroids.[48] Estramustine has found a clinical niche used in combination with other antimitotic drugs in the management of hormone refractory prostate cancer.[49]

DRUG RESISTANCE AND MODULATION

As with all drugs, intrinsic or acquired resistance to alkylating agents occurs and limits the therapeutic utility of this class of anticancer drugs.[50] A plethora of preclinical studies have characterized mechanisms by which cells develop resistance and, to a lesser degree, these have been shown to occur clinically. Because alkylating agents have a narrow therapeutic index, the emergence of resistance can have a significant impact on clinical success. Some of the factors that can contribute to the expression of resistance to alkylating agents include (1) alterations in drug uptake or transport; (2) increased repair of drug-induced nucleic acid damage; (3) failure to activate alkylating agent prodrugs; (4) increased scavenging of drug species by nonessential cellular nucleophiles; (5) increased enzymatic detoxification of drug species; and (6) altered expression of genes coding for cellular commitment to apoptosis.

RECENT DEVELOPMENTS

In the era of directed targeted therapies, the lack of specificity of alkylating agents would seem to limit the likelihood that novel drugs will be forthcoming. High toxicities, narrow therapeutic indices, and chemical instabilities are all properties that consign this drug class to the lower echelons of popularity in drug-discovery platforms. Although covalent bonding to specific target sites is one approach to direct targeting, the random electrophilic attraction toward nucleic acids and proteins is not an optimal property by today's standards. Nevertheless, the relative success of the alkylating agents in gaining therapeutic responses to diseases that are difficult to treat continues to serve as an impetus to use alkylating moieties as a means to kill cells. Some novel agents are presently in development. Cyclophosphamide and ifosfamide were prodrugs synthesized in the hope that high levels of phosphoamidase in epithelial tumors would selectively activate the drugs.[26] Other efforts to improve selectivity have centered on the synthesis of antibody-enzyme conjugates that bind to tumor-specific surface antigens. Enzymes frequently associated with the cell surface include peptidases, nitroreductases, and γ-glutamyl transpeptidase; to some degree, each has been targeted to cleave circulating alkylating prodrugs, thereby in a localized fashion releasing active alkylating species. Antibody-directed enzyme prodrug therapy is exemplified by the use of an antibody linked to the peptidase carboxypeptidase G-2, which releases an active alkylator from an inactive γ-glutamyl conjugate.[51] Linkage of the peptidase to any antibody that localizes selectively to a tumor cell membrane is a viable option. Expression of the peptidase on the cell surface then leads to prodrug activation and cell kill. Such approaches have had limited clinical impact to this time; however, their development does continue.

A further rationale for enhancing tumor-specific delivery takes advantage of the observation that glutathione-*S*- transferase *pi* (GSTP1-1) is preferentially expressed in a number of solid tumors and some lymphomas. In this case, the prodrug consists of an unusual alkylating agent conjugated to a substituted glutathione peptidomimetic. GSTP initiates the cleavage thereby creating a cytotoxic alkylating species.[52] The initial canfosfamide design strategy relied on the principle that proton-abstracting sites at the active site of GST could initiate a cleavage reaction that would convert an inactive prodrug into a cytotoxic species. The presence of a histidine residue in proximity to the G binding site was integral to the removal of the sulfhydryl proton from the GSH cosubstrate, resulting in the generation of a nucleophilic sulfide anion. This moiety would be more reactive with electrophiles in the absence of GSH. Unlike other standard nitrogen mustard drugs, canfosfamide contains a tetrakis (chloroethyl) phosphorodiamidate moiety. Other compounds bearing this structure have been shown to be more cytotoxic than a similar structure with a single bis-(chloroethyl) amine group.[53]

As in other nitrogen mustards, the chlorines can act as leaving groups, thus creating aziridinium ions with electrophilic characteristics. Although the exact temporal or sequential formation of the four possible chlorine leaving events is not known, the assumption is that these species possess cytotoxic properties through their capacity to alkylate target nucleophiles such as DNA bases. Tetrafunctionality could result in the formation of cross-links with bonding distances greater than for bifunctional agents. However, a number of caveats apply to this interpretation. For example, alkylating agents, whether mono-, bi-, or putatively tetrafunctional, generally lead to some form of myelosuppression. A number of clinical trials with canfosfamide have now been completed. These include, phase 1,[54] phase 1/2a,[55] phase 2,[56] and phase 3.[57] The phase 3 study was in platinum refractory ovarian cancer patients and proved negative for enhanced survival. Nevertheless, additional trials are still in progress.

Another targeting approach delivers the gene for a cytochrome P-450 isoenzyme to tumors by viral vector, thereby enhancing specific tumor cell activation of cyclophosphamide.[58] Because this therapy has its base in gene delivery technologies, successful development in humans will await further advances in this arena.

Laromustine is in the sulfonylhydrazine class of alkylating agents. It is presently in clinical development for the treatment of malignancies such as acute myelogenous leukemia (AML).[59] Similar to nitrosoureas, laromustine is a prodrug that yields a chloroethylating and a carbamoylating (methyl isocyanate) species. As with nitrosoureas, the cytotoxicity of laromustine is attributed primarily to the chloroethylating mediated alkylation of DNA and subsequent interstrand cross-links.[60] The carbamoylating species can inhibit DNA repair and other cellular enzyme systems. Phase 1 trials in patients with solid tumors indicated the expected myelosuppression, although few extramedullary toxicities were observed, indicating potential efficacy in the treatment of hematologic malignancies. Phase 2 trials have been completed in patients with untreated AML, high-risk myelodysplastic syndrome, and relapsed AML. The most encouraging results have been found in patients older than 60 years with poor-risk, *de novo* AML for which no standard treatment exists. Laromustine is currently in phase 2/3 trials for AML and phase 2 trials for myelodysplastic syndrome and solid tumors.[61] Laromustine appears to be a promising agent in elderly patients who do not respond to or are not fit for intensive chemotherapy.

Although not a new drug, bendamustine is a unique cytotoxic agent with structural similarities to alkylating agents and antimetabolites, but lacking cross-resistance with other established alkylating agents both *in vitro* and in the clinic.[62] Its mechanism of action is similar to other mustards in causing DNA intra- and interstrand cross-links. In comparison with other more commonly used alkylating agents, such as cyclophosphamide or phenylalanine mustard, more DNA double-strand breaks are formed at equitoxic dosages. Treatment with bendamustine induces a concentration-dependent apoptosis as evidenced by changes in Bcl-2 and Bax expression profiles in chronic B-cell lymphocytic leukemia.[63] DNA damage produced by bendamustine is repaired via base-excision repair mechanisms, implicating an unusual mode of action, which was recently confirmed through gene expression profiling analyses. This also provided an explanation for the lack of cross-resistance with other alkylating agents, as observed *in vitro* with anthracycline-resistant breast cancer and cisplatin-resistant ovarian cancer.[63,64]

Clinical studies conducted in Germany more than 30 years ago suggested activity in indolent non–Hodgkin's lymphoma. Subsequent American trials showed responses in more than 70% of patients with drug refractory disease, with the implication that bendamustine may be the most effective drug in this patient population. Combinations of bendamustine and rituximab elicited response rates of 90% to 92%, with complete remission in 55% to 60% in follicular and mantle cell lymphoma. Superiority over chlorambucil in previously untreated patients with chronic lymphocytic leukemia (CLL) led to its recent approval for this disease in the United States. Bendamustine is approved in Germany for the treatment of patients with indolent non–Hodgkin's lymphoma, CLL, and multiple myeloma. Activity has also been noted in patients with breast cancer and non–small cell lung cancer.

Bendamustine has been used both as a single agent and in combination with other agents including etoposide, fludarabine, mitoxantrone, methotrexate, prednisone, rituximab, and vincristine. A multicenter phase 2 trial in lymphomas had an overall response rate of 89%; (35% complete response and 54% partial response). In previously treated patients the overall response rate was 76% (38% complete response and 38% partial response). The estimated median progression-free survival was 19 months.[64] In CLL patients, the drug is administered at 100 mg/m^2 intravenously over 30 minutes on days 1 and 2 of a 28-day cycle, for up to six cycles. Efficacy relative to first-line therapies other than chlorambucil has not been established. It is also indicated for the treatment of patients with indolent B-cell non–Hodgkin's lymphoma that has progressed during, or within, 6 months of treatment with rituximab or rituximab-containing regimens. As with most alkylating agents, the primary dose-limiting toxicity is myelosuppression; nonhematologic toxicities were mild and included fatigue, nausea, loss of appetite, and vomiting. At this stage of development, optimization of dose and schedule, response relative to other drugs, and management of toxicities remain to be optimized. However, the availability of bendamustine provides another effective treatment option for patients with lymphoid malignancies.[65]

Selected References

The full list of references for this chapter appears in the online version.

1. Adair FE, Bagg HJ. Experimental and clinical studies on the treatment of cancer by dichlorethylsulphide (mustard gas). *Ann Surg* 1931;93(1):190.
2. Rhoads C. Nitrogen mustards in treatment of neoplastic disease. *JAMA* 1946;131:6568.
3. Coles B. Effects of modifying structure on electrophilic reactions with biological nucleophiles. *Drug Metab Rev* 1985;15:1307.
4. Pearson R, Songstad J. Application of the principle of hard and soft acids and bases to organic chemistry. *J Am Chem Soc* 1967;89:1827.
8. Agarwala SS, Kirkwood JM. Temozolomide, a novel alkylating agent with activity in the central nervous system, may improve the treatment of advanced metastatic melanoma. *Oncologist* 2000;5(2):144.
9. Tentori L, Graziani G. Recent approaches to improve the antitumor efficacy of temozolomide. *Curr Med Chem* 2009;16(2):245.
10. Vistica DT. Cytotoxicity as an indicator for transport mechanism: evidence that murine bone marrow progenitor cells lack a high-affinity leucine carrier that transports melphalan in murine L1210 leukemia cells. *Blood* 1980;56(3):427.
11. Dean M, Rzhetsky A, Allikmets R. The human ATP-binding cassette (ABC) transporter superfamily. *Genome Res* 2001;11(7):1156.
12. Sensenbrenner LL, Marini JJ, Colvin M. Comparative effects of cyclophosphamide, isophosphamide, 4-methylcyclophosphamide, and phosphoramide mustard on murine hematopoietic and immunocompetent cells. *J Natl Cancer Inst* 1979;62(4):975.
13. Montgomery JA, James R, McCaleb GS, Johnston TP. The modes of decomposition of 1,3-bis(2-chloroethyl)-1-nitrosourea and related compounds. *J Med Chem* 1967;10(4):668.
14. Brundrett RB, Cowens JW, Colvin M. Chemistry of nitrosoureas: decomposition of Deuterated 1,3-bis(2-chloroethyl)-1-nitrosourea. *J Med Chem* 1976;19(7):958.
15. Tew KD, Kyle G, Johnson A, Wang AL. Carbamoylation of glutathione reductase and changes in cellular and chromosome morphology in a rat cell line resistant to nitrogen mustards but collaterally sensitive to nitrosoureas. *Cancer Res* 1985;45(5):2326.
17. Anderson T, McMenamin MG, Schein PS. Chlorozotocin, 2-(3-(2-chloroethyl)-3-nitrosoureido)-D-glucopyranose, an antitumor agent with modified bone marrow toxicity. *Cancer Res* 1975;35(3):761.
19. Pieper RO. Understanding and manipulating O6-methylguanine-DNA methyltransferase expression. *Pharmacol Ther* 1997;74(3):285.
20. Weller M, Stupp R, Reifenberger G, et al. MGMT promoter methylation in malignant gliomas: ready for personalized medicine? *Nat Rev Neurol* 2010;6(1):39.
21. Tew K, Colvin OM, Jones RB. Clinical and high dose alkylating agents. In: Chabner BA, Longo DL, eds. *Cancer: Chemotherapy and Biotherapy: Principles and Practice.* Philadelphia: Lippincott-Raven, 2005:283.
22. Brookes P, Lawley PD. The reaction of mono- and di-functional alkylating agents with nucleic acids. *Biochem J* 1961;80(3):496.
23. Penta JS, Poster DS, Bruno S, Macdonald JS. Clinical trials with antiemetic agents in cancer patients receiving chemotherapy. *J Clin Pharmacol* 1981;21(8-9 Suppl):11S.
25. Elson L. Hematological effects of the alkylating agents. *Ann N Y Acad Sci* 1958;68:826.
26. Cox PJ. Cyclophosphamide cystitis—identification of acrolein as the causative agent. *Biochem Pharmacol* 1979;28(13):2045.
27. Andriole GL, Sandlund JT, Miser JS, Arasi V, Linehan M, Magrath IT.The efficacy of mesna (2-mercaptoethane sodium sulfonate) as a uroprotectant in patients with hemorrhagic cystitis receiving further oxazaphosphorine chemotherapy. *J Clin Oncol* 1987;5(5):799.
31. Kreisman H, Wolkove N. Pulmonary toxicity of antineoplastic therapy. *Semin Oncol* 1992;19(5):508.
32. Kumar R, Biggart JD, McEvoy J, McGeown MG. Cyclophosphamide and reproductive function. *Lancet* 1972;1(7762):1212.
33. Miller JJ 3rd, Williams GF, Leissring JC. Multiple late complications of therapy with cyclophosphamide, including ovarian destruction. *Am J Med* 1971;50(4):530.
34. Nicholson HO. Cytotoxic drugs in pregnancy: review of reported cases. *J Obstet Gynaecol Br Commonw* 1968;75(3):307.
35. Reimer RR, Hoover R, Fraumeni JF Jr, Young RC. Acute leukemia after alkylating-agent therapy of ovarian cancer. *N Engl J Med* 1977;297(4):177.
36. Penn I. Second malignant neoplasms associated with immunosuppressive medications. *Cancer* 1976;37(2 Suppl):1024.
37. Bhatia S, Constine LS. Late morbidity after successful treatment of children with cancer. *Cancer J* 2009;15(3):174.
38. Calvert W. Alopecia and cytotoxic drugs. *Br Med J* 1966;2(5517):831.
39. Weiss RB, Bruno S. Hypersensitivity reactions to cancer chemotherapeutic agents. *Ann Intern Med* 1981;94(1):66.
40. Santos GW, Sensenbrenner LL, Burke PJ, et al. Marrow transplanation in man following cyclophosphamide. *Transplant Proc* 1971;3(1):400.
43. Pratt CB, Goren MP, Meyer WH, Singh B, Dodge RK. Ifosfamide neurotoxicity is related to previous cisplatin treatment for pediatric solid tumors. *J Clin Oncol* 1990;8(8):1399.
45. Steinherz LJ, Steinherz PG, Mangiacasale D, et al. Cardiac changes with cyclophosphamide. *Med Pediatr Oncol* 1981;9(5):417.
46. Bastholt L, Johansson CJ, Pfeiffer P,et al. A pharmacokinetic study of prednimustine as compared with prednisolone plus chlorambucil in cancer patients. *Cancer Chemother Pharmacol* 1991;28(3):205.
47. Tew KD, Glusker JP, Hartley-Asp B, Hudes G, Speicher LA. Preclinical and clinical perspectives on the use of estramustine as an antimitotic drug. *Pharmacol Ther* 1992;56(3):323.
48. Punzi JS, Duax WL, Strong P, et al. Molecular conformation of estramustine and two analogues. *Mol Pharmacol* 1992;41(3):569.
49. Hudes GR, Greenberg R, Krigel RL, et al. Phase II study of estramustine and vinblastine, two microtubule inhibitors, in hormone-refractory prostate cancer. *J Clin Oncol* 1992;10(11):1754.
50. Tew K, Houghton JA, Houghton PJ. *Preclinical and Clinical Modulation of Anticancer Drugs*. Boca Raton, FL: CRC Press, 1993.
52. Tew KD. TLK-286: a novel glutathione S-transferase-activated prodrug. *Expert Opin Investig Drugs* 2005;14(8):1047.
53. Borch RF, Valente RR. Synthesis, activation, and cytotoxicity of aldophosphamide analogues. *J Med Chem* 1991;34(10):3052.
56. Kavanagh JJ, Gershenson DM, Choi H, et al. Multi-institutional phase 2 study of TLK286 (TELCYTA, a glutathione S-transferase P1-1 activated glutathione analog prodrug) in patients with platinum and paclitaxel refractory or resistant ovarian cancer. *Int J Gynecol Cancer* 2005;15(4):593.
57. Vergote I, Finkler N, del Campo J, et al. Phase 3 randomised study of canfosfamide (Telcyta, TLK286) versus pegylated liposomal doxorubicin or topotecan as third-line therapy in patients with platinum-refractory or -resistant ovarian cancer. *Eur J Cancer* 2009;45(13):2324.
58. Chase M, Chung RY, Chiocca EA. An oncolytic viral mutant that delivers the CYP2B1 transgene and augments cyclophosphamide chemotherapy. *Nat Biotechnol* 1998;16(5):444.
59. Vey N, Giles F. Laromustine (cloretazine). *Expert Opin Pharmacother* 2010;11(4):657.
60. Pigneux A. Laromustine, a sulfonyl hydrolyzing alkylating prodrug for cancer therapy. *IDrugs* 2009;12(1):39.
61. Schiller GJ, O'Brien SM, Pigneux A, et al. Single-agent laromustine, a novel alkylating agent, has significant activity in older patients with previously untreated poor-risk acute myeloid leukemia. *J Clin Oncol* 2010;28(5):815.
62. Eichbaum M, Bischofs E, Nehls K, Schneeweiss A, Sohn C.Bendamustine hydrochloride—a renaissance of alkylating strategies in anticancer medicine. *Drugs Today (Barc)* 2009;45(6):431.
63. Rasschaert M, Schrijvers D, Van den Brande J, et al. A phase I study of bendamustine hydrochloride administered day 1+2 every 3 weeks in patients with solid tumours. *Br J Cancer* 2007;96(11):1692.

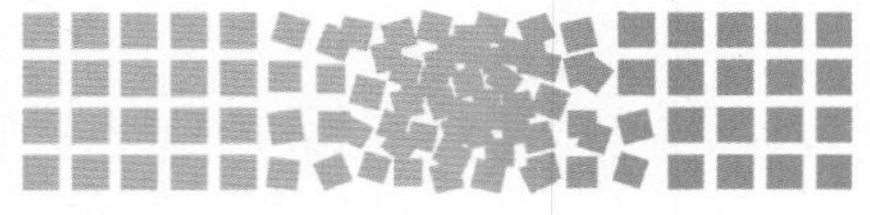

CHAPTER 35 PLATINUM ANALOGS

EDDIE REED

Since the introduction of cisplatin in the 1970s, three agents have come to constitute the most broadly used class of anticancer agents, the platinum compounds.[1,2] Either alone or in combination with other drugs, cisplatin, carboplatin, and oxaliplatin are the current mainstays of systemic therapy for non–small cell lung cancer, small cell lung cancer, aerodigestive malignancies, lower gastrointestinal malignancies, gynecologic malignancies, and genitourinary malignancies. In addition, they are key to the treatment of important subsets of breast cancer, non–Hodgkin's lymphoma, childhood malignancies, and others tumors.

Table 35.1 is a summary of how the platinum analogues are currently used in the treatment of several major cancers. Extensive reviews of the relevant data are given in the respective chapters of this text. Generally, in most circumstances in which cisplatin and carboplatin have been tested in phase 3 trials, cisplatin is clearly the more toxic agent. Cisplatin commonly causes renal toxicity, neurotoxicity, auditory toxicity, and a range of other side effects. That said, there are several diseases in which cisplatin remains the mainstay of therapy because of strong evidence of an advantage in clinical efficacy. Those diseases include testicular cancer, bladder cancer, small cell lung cancer, esophageal cancer, gastric cancer, and cervix cancer. In several of these malignancies, the utility of cisplatin is partly due to its role as a radiation sensitizer.

In ovarian cancer, cisplatin and carboplatin are viewed as having equivalent clinical efficacy, with carboplatin associated with a much lower rate of observed toxicities. For this reason, carboplatin has supplanted cisplatin in this disease. In colorectal cancer, the level of efficacy seen for oxaliplatin in phase 2 clinical trials far exceeded the historical phase 2 data for cisplatin and carboplatin. Oxaliplatin is therefore considered much more efficacious in this disease than the other two compounds, even though direct comparisons are mostly lacking.

Cisplatin, *cis*-diammine-dichloroplatinum (II), is the prototype of this family of agents, having the broadest range of clinical activity and the most substantial toxicity profile. Clinical dosing is in milligrams per squared meter per dose. The most common dosing schedule is one dose, given intravenously (IV), every 3 to 4 weeks. Intraperitoneal (IP) dosing was once popular in the treatment of ovarian cancer and has been reinvigorated, as discussed later.

Chemically, the platinum core of cisplatin has two ammine groups in the *cis*-configuration, which are opposite the two chloride leaving groups also in the *cis*- configuration. The majority of work on platinum chemistry has been done using cisplatin. This is also true for work done on subcellular mechanisms of cellular sensitivity and cellular resistance. In this chapter, reference to these topics will refer mainly to work done with cisplatin, unless specifically stated otherwise.

Carboplatin, *cis*-diammine(cyclobutanedicarboxylato)-platinum (II), has the same range of clinical activity as cisplatin but is less nephrotoxic and less emetogenic. In some diseases, such as testicular cancer, cisplatin is more clinically effective; therefore, cisplatin remains the drug of choice in that disease. Carboplatin is more toxic to bone marrow than cisplatin. Carboplatin dosing is usually given in milligrams per squared meter × minute, or area under the drug exposure curve (AUC). AUC dosing is associated with more predictable myelosuppression. Carboplatin may be given every 3 to 4 weeks. Chemically, the carboplatin core has two ammine groups in the *cis*- configuration, which are opposite the cyclobutane- dicarboxylato leaving group. The difference between the cisplatin and carboplatin molecules is in the leaving groups. Once the leaving groups are dissociated from the respective parent compounds, the resulting moieties for cisplatin and carboplatin are the same.

Oxaliplatin, 1,2-diamminocyclohexaneoxalato-platinum (II), is approved by the United States Food and Drug Administration for the treatment of colorectal cancer. In combination with other anticancer agents, oxaliplatin is currently the standard of care for initial systemic therapy when such therapy is needed. Whereas cisplatin is effective in upper gastrointestinal malignancies such as esophageal cancer and stomach cancer, oxaliplatin is much more effective in colorectal cancer. The reason for this clinical difference is not known, but is suspected to be related to the 1,2-diamminocyclohexane carrier ligand. This ligand inhibits replicative bypass of platinum-DNA adducts, which is a mechanism of cellular resistance to platinum compounds.[3] The platinum core of the oxaliplatin molecule behaves similarly to cisplatin in its physical chemistry characteristics.[4] The leaving group for oxaliplatin is the oxalato moiety, which results in the parent platinum molecule with two reactive *cis*- bonds, similar to cisplatin and carboplatin. The carrier ligand remains covalently bound to the parent platinum core. This carrier ligand probably also contributes to differences in the clinical pharmacology of the compound.

A potentially promising new analogue of cisplatin is satraplatin (bis-aceto-ammine-dichloro-cyclohexylamine platinum IV, or JM216).[5–8] Satraplatin is an orally active platinum analogue that has preclinical activity in tumor cell lines resistant to cisplatin, taxanes, and/or anthracyclines. This drug appears to be particularly active in prostate cancer.[6] A recent phase 3 randomized trial compared satraplatin plus prednisone to prednisone plus placebo in castrate-resistant prostate cancer. Satraplatin was orally administered at 80 mg/m^2, as a single daily dose, on days 1 to 5 of a 35-day treatment cycle. All study participants received prednisone at 5 mg orally, twice daily.

When the satraplatin group was compared with the placebo-treated group, the satraplatin-treated group showed statistically significant improvement in progression-free survival, time to progression, prostate-specific antigen responses, and pain responses. However, there was similar overall survival comparing satraplatin to placebo. One subset analysis of this study was an assessment of satraplatin performance in patients who had previously received docetaxel chemotherapy. In this subgroup it was observed that satraplatin treatment was

TABLE 35.1

DISEASE COMPARISONS OF PLATINUM ANALOGUES

Ovarian cancer	Prospective randomized trials showed clinical equivalency for cisplatin and carboplatin. Cisplatin was more toxic.
Testicular cancer	Prospective randomized trials showed clinical superiority for cisplatin combinations over carboplatin combinations.
Non–small cell lung cancer	Meta-analyses suggest that cisplatin-based regimens *may* offer improved efficacy over carboplatin-based regimens.
Small cell lung cancer	Recent randomized trials suggest that carboplatin-based regimens may have equal efficacy and less toxicity.
Colorectal cancer	Phase 2 data for oxaliplatin are strongly superior over historical phase 2 data for cisplatin or carboplatin.
Bladder cancer	Prospective randomized trials showed clinical superiority for cisplatin combinations over carboplatin combinations.
Cervix cancer	Cisplatin is optimal radiosensitizer. Carboplatin is active. Oxaliplatin is much less active than cisplatin or carboplatin.
Gastric cancer	Cisplatin-based regimens appear superior. Oxaliplatin-based regimens may be equivalent to cisplatin-based regimens. Carboplatin is less active.
Esophageal cancer	Cisplatin is optimal radiosensitizer. Carboplatin is active. Generally, cisplatin/5- fluorouracil is used concurrent with radiation.
Head and neck cancers	Cisplatin is optimal radiosensitizer. Carboplatin is active.

associated with prolonged progression-free survival and a trend toward improved overall survival ($P = .06$). Further studies are indicated.

Satraplatin is the first platinum IV compound to demonstrate clinical effectiveness. Also, it is the first platinum compound to achieve clinical effectiveness by the oral route of administration. *In vitro* studies show that the DNA lesions generated by satraplatin are similar to those of cisplatin, carboplatin, and oxaliplatin and that they are repaired with similar kinetics within cells by the nucleotide excision repair pathway.[8] A brief overview of cisplatin, carboplatin, oxaliplatin, and satraplatin is given in Table 35.2.

COMMON FEATURES OF PLATINUM CHEMISTRY

Platinum is the core element of the four compounds previously listed, giving each of these compounds some commonalities of chemistry[1,2,4,5] Each of these compounds induces its cell-killing effects through the development of covalent bifunctional DNA adducts with cellular DNA. Covalent binding to other subcellular components occur as well, including proteins, lipids, RNA, and mitochondrial DNA. However, the scientific consensus is that the primary mode of cell killing is through damage to cellular DNA.

The platinum (II) molecules exist in a planar structure. For cisplatin the core platinum element, the two amine groups, and the two chloride leaving groups all exist in the same two dimensional plane. For carboplatin and for oxaliplatin, the core elements of the platinum molecule also exist in a planar structure. For platinum (IV) compounds, such as satraplatin, there are also two potentially reactive groups in the Z plane. In the case of satraplatin, these are aceto- groups, which are perpendicular to the chloride leaving moieties.

Platination of cellular DNA is different from alkylation of cellular DNA. With the bifunctional alkylating agents, carbon is the pivot atom. Thus, the reactive arms of the bifunctional alkylating agents are movable about the central carbon core. Therefore, when alkylating agents form bifunctional adducts with cellular DNA, that DNA has spatial flexibility relative to the covalently bound drug, and vice versa. For platinum compounds,

TABLE 35.2

KEY FEATURES OF PLATINUM ANALOGUES

Cisplatin
- Administered IV in normal saline. Dosing is in mg/m^2.
- Usual dose: 50–75 mg/m^2, in 250 mL NS, every 3–4 weeks.
- Infusion time: 1 h, but can be up to 4 h.
- Very effective in a wide range of epithelial malignancies.
- Toxicity is problematic, particularly renal toxicity, neurotoxicity, and nausea.
- Use mannitol to protect against renal toxicity; avoid furosemide.

Carboplatin
- Administered IV in normal saline. Dosing is in $mg/m^2 \times$ minute (AUC).
- Usual dose: 4, 5, or 6 $mg/m^2 \times$ minute, in 250 mL NS, every 3–4 weeks.
- Infusion time: 1 h, but can be up to 4 h.
- Range of effectiveness is similar to cisplatin, but not exactly the same.
- Less toxic than cisplatin, but more myelosuppressive than cisplatin.
- Renal toxicity is often underestimated.
- A new method for measuring serum creatinine, will affect AUC dosing.

Oxaliplatin
- Administered IV in 5% dextrose. Dosing is in mg/m^2.
- Usual dose: 85 to 130 mg/m^2 every 2–3 weeks, depending on regimen.
- Infusion time: 6 h, but 2 h and 4 h sometimes used.
- Primarily used in colorectal cancer.
- Toxicities similar to those of cisplatin and carboplatin.

Satraplatin
- Administered orally, daily times five. Dosing is in mg/m^2.
- Prostate cancer dose: 80 mg/m^2/day for 5 consecutive days with prednisone.
- Other doses and dose schedules are being studied.
- Early studies show effectiveness in prostate cancer.
- Toxicities similar to those of cisplatin and carboplatin.

IV, intravenously; NS, normal saline; AUC, area under the curve.

the bifunctional reactive groups are fixed in space relative to the platinum core, with an average distance of 3.3 nanometers between binding sites. As a consequence, the DNA that is covalently bound to the platinum compound is also fixed in space, relative to the platinum core. This platinum-DNA adduct is repaired by the nucleotide excision repair (NER) pathway. DNA repair studies suggest that the types of DNA lesions formed by cisplatin, carboplatin, oxaliplatin, and satraplatin are all very similar,[3,8] with cisplatin studied most extensively.

The N7-d(GpG)-intrastrand platinum-DNA adduct accounts for about 60% of total platinum binding to DNA. The N7-d(ApG)-intrastrand adduct accounts for about 30% of total platinum binding to DNA. The N7-d(GpXpG)-intrastrand adduct represents about 10% of total platinum binding to DNA. And the N7-d(X)-d(X)-interstrand cross-link accounts for less than 2% of total platinum binding to DNA. There has been debate over the question of which lesion may be the most lethal to the cells, or which lesion may be the most mutagenic. The definitive answers to these questions have been elusive. What has been consistently observed is that the level of platinum-DNA damage is directly related to the level of cell killing, regardless of the lesion measured.

Two very important features of the platinum compounds include the nature of the leaving groups and the nature of the carrier ligands. Although important, it has not been possible to predict how a specific leaving group, or a specific carrier ligand, will affect the behavior of a particular platinum analogue.

Oxaliplatin has a leaving group and a carrier ligand. The diaminocyclohexane carrier ligand of oxaliplatin gives the compound unique intracellular characteristics once the drug is covalently bound to DNA. This carrier ligand has influence on DNA repair activities within the cell, as well as inhibiting replicative bypass of platinum-DNA adduct within the cell. Satraplatin is a platinum (IV) analogue, with potentially four leaving groups, as well as a carrier ligand. Although not as well studied as the previous three platinum analogues, we do know that the platinum-DNA damage caused by satraplatin is repaired by NER, similar to other platinum compounds.[8] This suggests the possibility that, practically, the chloride leaving groups of satraplatin drive the intracellular behavior of the drug with respect to DNA damage. Important summary points for platinum analogue chemistry are given in Table 35.3.

Among the most exciting of new developments in the chemistry of platinum analogues is the preclinical development of cisplatin nanocapsules and carboplatin nanocapsules.[9–12] Cisplatin nanocapsules were discovered during work to develop better methods for enclosing cisplatin in liposomes. For cisplatin, such nanoparticles have approximate bidimensional measurements of 50 to 120 nm. The cisplatin-to-lipid molar ratio is about ten. The solid core of the nanoparticle is 90% the dichloride species of cisplatin, and the outer lipid bilayer is very different from that of liposomes. A slight modification of the method used for cisplatin is used to develop carboplatin nanocapsules. There are slight, but measurable, differences in molar ratios and other specific values when comparing cisplatin nanocapsules to carboplatin nanocapsules. Most importantly, when comparing the IC_{50} values of cisplatin nanocapsules to cisplatin, and that of carboplatin nanocapsules to carboplatin, in both cases the nanocapsules are two orders of magnitude more cytotoxic than their parent drug, against IGROV-1 human ovarian cancer cells.

TABLE 35.3

KEY FEATURES OF THE CHEMISTRY OF PLATINUM ANALOGUES

DNA lesions are similar for all four clinically active platinum agents.
- N7-d(GpG)-intrastrand adducts: ~60% of total DNA binding
- N7-d(ApG)-intrastrand adducts: ~30% of total DNA binding
- N7-d(GpXpG)-intrastrand adducts: ~10% of total DNA binding
- N7-d((X)-d(X)-interstrand crosslinks: <2% of total DNA binding

The nature of the DNA lesion is different from that formed by alkylating agents.
- Platinum core is planar, and fixed.
- Clinically active agents have reactive species in the *cis*-configuration.
- DNA bends to conform to the platinum core of the compound.
- The DNA adducts formed, are similar for all four analogues.
- NER is the DNA repair pathway that repairs DNA lesions for all four drugs.

Additional characteristics impact on the subcellular behavior of the compound.
- Platinum (II) versus platinum (IV).
- The nature of the leaving groups.
- The nature of the carrier ligand.
- Satraplatin is the only platinum-IV to date, with clinical efficacy.

NER, nucleotide excision repair.

CLINICAL PHARMACOLOGY

Cisplatin

When given as a single agent or in combination with other drugs, cisplatin is usually administered as a single IV dose of 50 to 75 mg/m^2 every 3 to 4 weeks. Drug is usually given in 250 mL of normal saline, as a 1- to 4-hour infusion. The 1-hour time frame is the most common. Shorter infusion times are associated with greater clinical toxicity. It is important that the patient is prehydrated and posthydrated with at least 2 liters of IV fluid to maintain good urine flow. Mannitol, 125 mg, may be mixed with drug in the 250 mL, 1-hour cisplatin infusion. Furosemide and other renal tubule inhibitors should be avoided. When cisplatin is administered IV or IP, it is usually given in normal saline, without cations (e.g., Mg^{2+}, Ca^{2+}) of any type in the IV solution, as these may partially inactivate the drug. Bicarbonate solutions should be avoided as well. Details of pharmacokinetics and pharmacodynamics of each of the platinum analogues are given in previous editions of this text.

The IP route of delivery is associated with increased efficacy in some subsets of patients with advanced-stage ovarian cancer.[13–16] Hess et al.[13] performed a meta-analysis for 1,716 ovarian cancer patients treated from January 1990 through January 2006. In this report, the pooled hazard ratios favored IP therapy for progression-free survival (hazard ratio, 0.792, $P = .001$) and for overall survival (hazard ratio, 0.799, $P = .0007$. For cisplatin, the IP route is associated with an increased pharmacologic advantage for exposure to intraperitoneal tumors.[14]

However, careful analyses suggest that the improved pharmacologic advantage is only part of the story. The IP route of administration is associated with increased ovarian tumor exposure to drug from the systemic circulation for a prolonged period of time.[14] When drug is administered IP, IV use of thiosulfates is recommended to minimize renal toxicity from drug. Long-term follow-up of patients demonstrate that long-term survival does occur from IP therapy.[15,16]

Common toxicities from cisplatin, given IV or IP, include renal insufficiency with cation wasting, nausea and vomiting, peripheral neuropathy, auditory impairment, and myelosuppression with thrombocytopenia prominent. Catheter complications are common when using the IP route. Less common but serious side effects include hypersensitivity, visual impairment, seizures, and late leukemia as a secondary treatment-related condition. Renal damage can be minimized by ensuring vigorous hydration during therapy. Vigorous premedication for nausea and vomiting should be routinely administered as well. Myelosuppression can be addressed by the use of appropriate bone marrow cytokines.

Aggressive pre-emption of nausea and vomiting is critically important for successful cisplatin therapy and for all platinum compounds. Adequate prevention of nausea and vomiting can be ensured by following the guidelines of the 2004 Perugia International Antiemesis Consensus Conference, recently reviewed by Hesketh.[17] Generally, level 4 antiemesis regimens should always be used for cisplatin-based regimens. Level 4 antiemesis regimens consist of a defined combination before chemotherapy and a defined combination after chemotherapy. Before chemotherapy, one should administer a serotonin 5-hydroxy tryptamine type 3 (5-HT3) receptor antagonist, dexamethasone, and aprepitant. After chemotherapy, one should administer dexamethasone on days 2, 3, and 4, and aprepitant on days 2 and 3.

For carboplatin or for oxaliplatin, level 3 antiemesis can be administered. In level 3 antiemesis treatment, one should administer a 5-HT3 receptor antagonist and dexamethasone before chemotherapy. After chemotherapy, one should administer a 5-HT3 receptor antagonist and dexamethasone on days 2 and 3. However, for some patients, level 4 antiemesis therapy will be needed, even for carboplatin and for oxaliplatin. Remember, the goal is patient safety and avoidance of unnecessary side effects.

Carboplatin

Carboplatin is usually dosed by AUC in an effort to attain predictable myelosuppression. This approach for this drug was initially developed by Jodrell et al.[18] and refined and simplified by Calvert and Egorin[19] and Calvert et al.[20] The Calvert formula, which is now commonly used to calculate dose, is: AUC (carboplatin) = dose/(creatinine clearance + 25). The usual administered dose is an AUC of 4, 5, or 6 mg/m^2 × minute. Prior to common adoption of AUC dosing, carboplatin was assumed to be equivalent to cisplatin at a ratio of 4 mg to 1 mg; that is, 400 mg of carboplatin was clinically equivalent to 100 mg of cisplatin.

Controversy has arisen on the topic of carboplatin dosing with respect to the AUC approach. The calculation of AUC is generally based on the Calvert formula[19,20] using a serum creatinine measured by an approach that has been in use for a number of years.[19,20] From the first reports of AUC dosing it was clear that this approach was imperfect, with substantial variability.[21,22]

Recently, the National Institute of Standards and Technology (NIST) has developed a more accurate method for measuring serum creatinine.[23] The clinical problem is that when the NIST measurement is used to calculate the carboplatin AUC, the carboplatin milligram dose may be substantially larger than it would have been using the older serum creatinine measurement.[24] This has resulted in an increase in the development of adverse treatment-related events.

Further complicating this issue is that, with increasing cumulative dose of cisplatin or carboplatin, there develops a moderate type of heavy metal renal toxicity that is commonly seen with exposures to substances such as lead, mercury, and cadmium.[25,26] That is, there develops a disassociation between the serum creatinine and the glomerular filtration rate.[25,26] In this setting, the serum creatinine may possibly not be a reliable measure of glomerular filtration rate, whatever method might be used for measuring creatinine.

In a practical sense, the National Cancer Institute Cancer Therapy Evaluation Program is in the process of developing specific guidance on how to handle this problem. In the meantime, this is an issue that the oncology clinician should be aware of, with emphasis on the need to closely monitor renal function when using platinum compounds in any setting.

Like cisplatin, carboplatin is given as a single IV dose per cycle every 3 to 4 weeks. Like cisplatin, carboplatin should be given in a normal saline solution. Carboplatin should be given as a 1- to 4-hour infusion. The 1-hour time frame is the most common.

Carboplatin excretion is more dependent on good kidney function than cisplatin. Further, if patients are not adequately hydrated, carboplatin administration can result in loss of kidney function by more than 50%, as measured by creatinine clearance.[24,25] The toxicity profile is similar to that of cisplatin, but with notable differences. Carboplatin is much less emetogenic, but more myelosuppressive. The potential for kidney damage should not be underestimated and should be monitored in a fashion as one would for cisplatin.

Oxaliplatin

Unlike cisplatin and carboplatin, oxaliplatin should be administered in a 5% dextrose chloride-free IV solution. The common dose range is 85 up to 130 mg/m^2 every 2 to 3 weeks, depending on the other agents used and the specific disease treated. In addition to colorectal cancer, oxaliplatin is a recommended treatment option in recurrent ovarian cancer. Oxaliplatin is usually given as a 2-hour IV infusion, but 4- and 6-hour infusions may be used. Oxaliplatin pharmacokinetics have not been as extensively characterized as those of cisplatin or carboplatin.

A substantial fraction of oxaliplatin is retained in red blood cells after a drug dose. However, oxaliplatin does not accumulate to any significant levels after multiple drug exposures. This is in stark contrast to cisplatin, which accumulates to a substantial degree. When given in combination with 5-fluorouracil, the most important toxicities are myelosuppression with neutropenia predominant, diarrhea and stomatitis, peripheral neuropathy, and mild to moderate nausea and vomiting. Unusual but serious toxicities include anaphylaxis, hemolytic anemia, and laryngopharyngeal dysesthesias.

Satraplatin

Several different oral dosing regimens for satraplatin have been published. The dosing regimen associated with the most impressive clinical results is 80 mg/m^2/day for 5 consecutive days, with prednisone 5 mg orally twice daily.[6] As with other platinum compounds, the treating physician should be particularly mindful of vigorous hydration for the patient. Myelosuppression is prominent, and the maximum concentration after the first drug dose is directly related to neutropenia and to thrombocytopenia. The platelet nadir is also directly related to the cumulative dose of satraplatin, and to the AUC of total drug administered, but not to the AUC of the ultrafiltrable drug.

DETERMINANTS OF CELLULAR SENSITIVITY AND RESISTANCE TO PLATINUM AGENTS

On the subcellular level, there are more than ten putative general mechanisms through which cells may become sensitive or resistant to platinum compounds. These are listed in Table 35.4.

TABLE 35.4

MECHANISMS OF CELLULAR RESISTANCE TO PLATINUM COMPOUNDS

Mechanisms acting before DNA damage occurs
Decreased cellular uptake of drug
Increased cellular efflux of drug
Detoxification of drug intracellularly
Mechanisms directly related to DNA damage
Decreased binding of drug to DNA
Altered DNA repair
Increased tolerance to DNA damage
Mechanisms acting after DNA damage
Decreased apoptosis
Inhibition of apoptosis
Increased levels of chaperone proteins
Altered cell-signaling pathways
Altered cell-cycle regulation

In the context of these listed molecular mechanisms, there are more than 60 specific genes that have been reported to show alterations of some type, in platinum-sensitive or platinum-resistant cells. This range of potential molecular mechanisms and of various genes may be partly due to the range of cell lines studied and the range of systems studied.

As indicated in Table 35.4, one can separate the various mechanisms of cellular sensitivity and resistance into three categories: mechanisms acting before DNA damage occurs, mechanisms directly related to DNA damage and its repair, and mechanisms acting after DNA damage occurs. This is a simplified version of a very complex view of platinum drug resistance. Interestingly, there is linkage between very early work in platinum drug resistance and recent clinical observations from molecular correlative studies.

Prior to the current wave of gene discovery, three groups conducted studies to assess the relative importance of three different types of mechanisms of cellular resistance to platinum compounds. Eastman et al.,[27] Parker et al.,[28] Godwin et al.[29] and Calvert et al.[30] assessed the relative contributions of cellular accumulation of drug, cytosolic inactivation of drug, and repair of DNA-bound drug. Eastman et al. worked in *Escherichia coli* cell lines, with varying levels of *in vitro*-induced resistance to cisplatin. Parker et al., Godwin et al., and Calvert et al. worked with human ovarian cancer cells of varying levels of induced cisplatin resistance.

All of these groups reached similar conclusions. For what was termed *low levels of cisplatin resistance,* up to 10- to 15-fold over baseline, the two major contributors to platinum resistance were altered cellular accumulation of drug and altered DNA repair. For levels of cisplatin resistance above 15-fold over baseline, cytosolic inactivation of drug appeared predominant. Recent studies by Fokkema et al.[31] and Cullen et al.[32] suggest that these high levels of resistance may be clinically relevant.

CELLULAR ACCUMULATION AND CYTOSOLIC INACTIVATION OF DRUG

We now know that cellular accumulation of cisplatin is a combined function of cellular uptake of drug and cellular efflux of drug.[33] Cellular uptake of drug may be influenced by the extracellular pH, the copper transporter *CTR1*, characteristics of the cell membrane, and a range of genes that regulate endocytosis and transmembrane transport of naturally occurring compounds. Cellular efflux of drug may be modulated by the copper transporters *ATP7A* and *ATP7B*, along with other genes that may influence the efflux of compounds that occur naturally.

There is evidence that *CTR1*, a normal copper transporter in the cell membrane, may be a major contributor to the active uptake of all three major platinum drugs by cells, including cisplatin, carboplatin, and oxaliplatin.[34,35] Also, there is good evidence that *ATP7A* and *ATP7B*, normal copper efflux proteins in the cell membrane, are major contributors to the efflux of platinum drugs in cancer cells.[36] In addition, the human organic cation transporters 1, 2, and 3, have been implicated in modulating the cellular uptake of platinum compounds, specifically as it may relate to human renal toxicity.[37,38]

Cytosolic inactivation of drug, which occurs at high levels of resistance, is mediated through the glutathione detoxification pathways,[29,30] and by metallothioneins.[39,40] It is not clear whether the proximity of histones to cellular DNA or the proximity of other DNA-related proteins may in some cases serve as a sink for platinum agents that can transverse the cytosol.

DNA DAMAGE AND REPAIR

The importance of DNA repair to cellular and clinical resistance to platinum compounds has been confirmed by a large number of laboratory and clinical studies. The repair of platinum-DNA adduct is executed by the NER pathway.[41–45] When NER is up-regulated, platinum-DNA adduct repair is increased, which leads to increased cellular resistance.[46,47] When NER is down-regulated, platinum-DNA adduct repair is reduced, which leads to increased cellular sensitivity. There are several good markers for the activity of the NER process. One such marker is the gene *ERCC1*, which can be followed using mRNA, protein, or specific polymorphisms of the gene.[46,47]

There are between 10 and 13 currently known separable DNA repair pathways.[48] For each, there are reports in the literature of some association with cellular resistance to platinum compounds, in an *in vitro* system. Table 35.5 lists the currently recognized separable DNA repair pathways. Of

TABLE 35.5

TEN TO THIRTEEN DIFFERENT DNA REPAIR PATHWAYS, EACH OF WHICH MAY HAVE IMPACT ON PLATINUM DRUG RESISTANCE

Nucleotide excision repair (two subtypes)
Global genomic repair
Transcription coupled repair
Base excision repair (two subtypes)
Short patch repair
Long patch repair
Double-strand break repair (two subtypes)
Homologous recombination
Nonhomologous end-joining
Mismatch repair
Direct reversal
Translesional synthesis
Template switching
Fanconi anemia (FANC) pathway
ATM-mediated DNA damage repair signaling
ATR-mediated DNA damage repair signaling

ATM, ataxia-telangiectasia mutated; ATR, ATM- and Rad3-related.

these, there are two pathways with unequivocal evidence of clinical relevance. One is the NER pathway, with *ERCC1* being a critical gene in that pathway, and an important clinical biomarker. The other is the base excision repair pathway, with *PARP1* being an important gene. The proposed *PARP1* relationship of clinical resistance to carboplatin is complex and involves the theoretical importance of double-strand breaks in cellular resistance to platinum compounds.[48]

The *in vitro* evidence to support the role of NER in the platinum-resistant phenotype is quite substantial. In paired Chinese hamster ovary cells, the absence of a functional *ERCC1* renders cells hypersensitive to cisplatin, and those cells are not able to repair platinum-DNA damage.[49] In the paired *ERCC1*-competent Chinese hamster ovary cells there is restored resistance to cisplatin and restored ability to repair platinum-DNA damage. Following this seminal observation, cellular expression of *ERCC1* was observed to be directly related to platinum resistance in every cell line studied. This includes such cancers as germ cell, ovary, bladder, cervix, lung, and colon.[50] *In vitro* studies led to a series of clinical molecular correlative studies to address this question, in that setting.

The molecular biology of NER has been the collective accomplishment of the work of many groups.[41–45] Whereas the complete NER process involves more than three dozen genes, there are about 17 genes that are critical to the steps of DNA damage recognition and excision. DNA damage excision is rate-limiting to NER, with the repairosome complex executing this function. Among the genes of this complex are *ERCC1, XPA, XPB, XPD, XPF,* and *CSB*, with *ERCC1* as a key gene.[46–50]

Clinically, several of the major genes in the repairosome appear to be up-regulated together or down-regulated together in human ovarian cancer tissues. This appears to be related to common regulatory elements in the 5′ untranslated regions (5′UTR) of these genes,[51] as well as common responses to known transcriptional regulatory proteins. Genes previously listed in the NER repairosome appear to be up-regulated by *AP1*,[52] through the jun kinase pathway or the ERK pathway.[53,54] These genes appear to be down-regulated by *MZF1*[55] and possibly by *RFX1*.[56]

Of the many features of *ERCC1*, one that may have clinical relevance is the silent polymorphism at codon 118, which results in the same amino acid but is associated with a 50% reduction in codon usage. This codon 118 polymorphism is associated with reduced ERCC1 mRNA and protein, reduced platinum-DNA adduct repair, and enhanced sensitivity to platinum compounds. This was first reported by Yu et al.[57,58] in human ovarian cancer cells and appears to be relevant in colon cancer, ovarian cancer, and other malignancies.[46–48]

PARP1 inhibition induces enhanced sensitivity to platinum compounds *in vitro*[59–61] and this has translated into improved clinical efficacy in human breast cancer when using carboplatin combinations in *BRCA*-positive breast cancer.[59–61] There appears to be a good fit between the *in vitro* data and the clinical trials observations in terms of *PARP1* inhibition and clinical efficacy of platinum compounds. However, useful biomarkers that are proven to track the process have yet to be fully developed.

The first observations regarding the association of high expression of *ERCC1* with clinical resistance to platinum-based therapy were made in human ovarian cancer. In a study of 26 patients who received platinum-based chemotherapy, *ERCC1* mRNA levels were found to be 2.6-fold higher in tumor tissues of patients who did not respond to chemotherapy[62,63]; mRNA levels for *ERCC1* and *XPA* were high in nonresponders and low in responders (*ERCC1*, $P = .026$; *XPA*, $P = .011$). Alternatively, spliced species of *ERCC1* mRNA were noted in material extracted from platinum-sensitive and platinum-resistant tumors.

Subsequent to these initial reports, there have been numerous observations in a wide range of malignancies validating the use of *ERCC1* as a clinical biomarker for cisplatin sensitivity and resistance.[46–48] This area is best developed in non–small cell lung cancer.[64,65] Redon et al.[66] have reported on the possible use of gamma-*H2AX* as a biomarker for the effective inhibition of *PARP1* in clinical specimens. The definitive clinical trials are currently in progress.[66]

Selected References

The full list of references for this chapter appears in the online version.

3. Chaney SG, Vaisman A. Specificity of platinum-DNA adduct repair. *J Inorg Biochem* 1999;77:71.
4. Spingler B, Whittington DA, Lippard SJ. 2.4 A crystal structure of an oxaliplatin 1,2-d(GpG) intrastrand cross-link in a DNA dodecamer duplex. *Inorg Chem* 2001;40:5596.
5. Carr JL, Tingle MD, McKeage MJ. Satraplatin activation by haemoglobin, cytochrome C and liver microsomes in vitro. *Cancer Chemother Pharmacol* 2006;57:483.
6. Sternberg CN, Petrylak DP, Sartor O, et al. Multinational, double-blind, phase III study of prednisone and either satraplatin or placebo in patients with castrate-refractory prostate cancer progressing after prior chemotherapy: the SPARC trial. *J Clin Oncol* 2009;27:5431.
8. Reardon JT, Vaisman A, Chaney SG, Sancar A. Efficient nucleotide excision repair of cisplatin, oxaliplatin, and bis-aceto-ammine-dichloro-cyclohexylamine-platinum(IV) (JM216) platinum intrastrand DNA diadducts. *Cancer Res* 1999;59:3968.
9. Burger KN, Staffhorst RW, Vijlder HC, et al. Nanocapsules: lipid coated aggregates of cisplatin with high toxicity. *Nat Med* 2002;8:81.
10. Chupin V, de Kroon AI, de Kruijff B, Molecular architecture of nanocapsules, bilayer enclosed solid particles of cisplatin. *J Am Chem Soc* 2004; 126:13816.
11. Hamelers IH, de Kroon AI. Nanocapsules: a novel formulation technology for platinum-based anticancer drugs. *Future Lipidol* 2007;2:445.
12. Hamelers IH, van Loenen E, Staffhorst RW, de Kruijff B, de Kroon AI. Carboplatin nanocapsules: a highly cytotoxic, phospholipid-based formulation of carboplatin. *Mol Cancer Ther* 2006;5:2007.
15. Barakat RR, Sabbatini P, Bhaskaran D, et al. Intraperitoneal chemotherapy for ovarian carcinoma: results of long-term follow-up. *J Clin Oncol* 2002; 20:694.
16. Fujiwara K, Armstrong D, Morgan M, Markman M. Principles and practice of intraperitoneal chemotherapy for ovarian cancer. *Int J Gynecol Cancer* 2007;17:1.
17. Hesketh PJ. Chemotherapy induced nausea and vomiting. *N Engl J Med* 2008;358:2482.
19. Calvert AH, Egorin MJ. Carboplatin dosing formulae: gender bias and the use of creatinine-based methodologies. *Eur J Cancer* 2002;38:11.
20. Calvert AH, Newell DR, Gumbrell LA, et al. Carboplatin dosage: prospective evaluation of a simple formula based on renal function. *J Clin Oncol* 1989;7:1748.
25. Reed E, Jacob J. Carboplatin and renal dysfunction [letter]. *Ann Intern Med* 1989;110: 409.
26. Reed E, Jacob J, Brawley, O. Measures of renal function in cisplatin-related chronic renal disease. *J Natl Med Assoc* 1991;83:522.
28. Parker RJ, Eastman A, Bostick-Bruton F, et al. Acquired cisplatin resistance in human ovarian cancer cells is associated with enhanced repair of cisplatin-DNA lesions and reduced drug accumulation. *J Clin Invest* 1991;87:772.
29. Godwin AK, Meister A, O'Dwyer PJ, Huang CS, Hamilton TC, Anderson ME. High resistance to cisplatin in human ovarian cancer cell lines is associated with marked increase of glutathione synthesis. *Proc Natl Acad Sci U S A* 1992;89:3070.
32. Cullen KJ, Newkirk KA, Schumaker LM, Aldosari N, Rone JD, Haddad BR. Glutathione S-transferase pi amplification is associated with cisplatin resistance in head and neck squamous cell carcinoma cell lines and primary tumors. *Cancer Res* 2003;63:8097.

34. Zhou B, Gitschier J. hCTR1: a human gene for copper uptake identified by complementation in yeast. *Proc Natl Acad Sci U S A* 1997;94:7481.
35. Holzer AK, Manorek GH, Howell SB. Contribution of the major copper influx transporter CRT1 to the cellular accumulation of cisplatin, carboplatin, and oxaliplatin. *Mol Pharmacol* 2006;70:1390.
36. Samini G, Katano K, Holzer AK, Safaei R, Howell SB, Modulation of the cellular pharmacology of cisplatin and its analogs by the copper exporters ATP7A and ATP7B. *Mol Pharmacol* 2004;66:25.
38. Ciarimboli G, Ludwig T, Lang D, et al. Cisplatin nephrotoxicity is critically mediated via the human organic cation transporter 2. *Am J Pathol* 2005; 167:1477.
40. Smith DJ, Jaggi M, Zhang W, et al. Metallothioneins and resistance to cisplatin and radiation in prostate cancer. *Urology* 2006;67:1341.
44. De Laat WL, Jaspers NG, Hoeijmakers JH. Molecular mechanism of nucleotide excision repair. *Gene Dev* 1999;13:768
45. Wood RD, Mitchell M, Lindahl T. Human DNA repair genes, 2005. *Mutat Res* 2005;577:275.
47. Reed E. ERCC1 measurements in clinical oncology. *N Engl J Med* 2006; 355:1054.
48. Reed E. DNA damage and repair in translational oncology: an overview. *Clin Cancer Res* 2010;16:4511.
49. Lee KB, Parker RJ, Bohr VA, Cornelison TC, Reed E. Cisplatin sensitivity/resistance in UV-repair deficient Chinese hamster ovary cells of complementation groups 1 and 3. *Carcinogenesis* 1003;14:2177.
51. Zhong Z, Thornton K, Reed E. Computer based analyses of the 5′-flanking regions of selected genes involved in the nucleotide excision repair excision complex. Int J Oncol 2000;17:375.
52. Li Q, Gardner K, Zhang L, Tsang B, Bostick-Bruton F, Reed E. Cisplatin induction of ERCC1 mRNA expression in A2780/CP70 human ovarian cancer cells. *J Biol Chem* 1998;273:23419.
55. Yan QW, Reed E, Zhong XS, Thornton K, Guo Y, Yu JJ. MZF1 possesses a repressively regulatory function in ERCC1 expression. *Biochem Pharmacol* 2006;71:761.
56. Yu JJ, Thornton K, Guo Y, Kotz H, Reed E. An ERCC1 splicing variant involving the 5'UTR of the mRNA may have a transcriptional modulatory function. *Oncogene* 2001;20:7694.
57. Yu JJ, Mu C, Lee KB, et al. A nucleotide polymorphism in ERCC1 gene in human ovarian cancer cell lines and tumor tissues. *Mutat Res Genom* 1997;382:13.
58. Yu JJ, Lee KB, Mu C, Li Q, Abernathy TV, Bostick-Bruton F, Reed E. Comparison of two human ovarian carcinoma cell lines (A2780/CP70 and MCAS) that are equally resistant to platinum, but differ at codon 118 of the ERCC1 gene. *Int J Oncol* 2000;16:555.
59. Annunziata CM, O'Shaughnessy J. Poly(ADP-Ribose) Polymerase as a novel therapeutic target in cancer. *Clin Cancer Res* 2010;16;4517.
60. Fong PC, Boss DS, Yap TA, et al. Inhibition of poly(ADP-ribose) polymerase in tumors from BRCA mutation carriers. *N Engl J Med* 20099; 361(2):123.
61. Tutt A, Robson M, Garber JE, et al. Oral poly(ADP-ribose) polymerase inhibitor olaparib in patients with BRCA1 or BRCA2 mutations and advanced breast cancer: a proof-of-concept trial. *Lancet* 2010;376(9737): 235.
62. Dabholkar M, Bostick-Bruton F, Weber C, Bohr VA, Egwuagu C., Reed E. ERCC1 and ERCC2 expression in malignant tissues from ovarian cancer patients. *J Natl Cancer Inst* 1992;84:1512.
63. Dabholkar M, Vionnet JA, Bostick-Bruton F, Yu JJ, Reed E. mRNA Levels of XPAC and ERCC1 in ovarian tumor tissue correlates with response to platinum containing chemotherapy. *J Clin Invest* 1994;94:703.
64. Vilmar A, Sorensen JB. Excison repair cross-complementation group 1 (ERCC1) in platinum-based treatment of non-small cell lung cancer with special emphasis on carboplatin: a review of the current literature. *Lung Cancer* 2009;64(2):131.
65. Olaussen KA, Mountzios G, Soria JC. ERCC1 as a risk stratifier in platinum-based chemotherapy for non-small cell lung cancer. *Curr Opin Pulm Med* 2007;13(4):284.

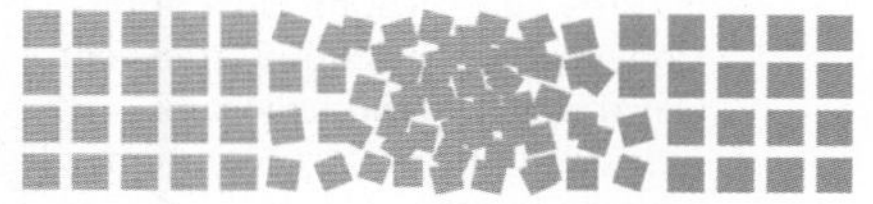

CHAPTER 36 ANTIMETABOLITES

M. WASIF SAIF AND EDWARD CHU

ANTIFOLATES

Aminopterin was the first antimetabolite to demonstrate clinical activity in the treatment of children with acute leukemia in the 1940s. This antifolate analogue was subsequently replaced by methotrexate (MTX), the 4-amino, 10-methyl analogue of folic acid, which remains the most widely used antifolate analogue, with activity against a wide range of cancers (Table 36.1), including hematologic malignancies (acute lymphoblastic leukemia and non-Hodgkin's lymphoma) and many solid tumors (breast cancer, head and neck cancer, osteogenic sarcoma, bladder cancer, and gestational trophoblastic cancer). Pemetrexed is a pyrrolopyrimidine, multitargeted antifolate analogue that targets multiple enzymes involved in folate metabolism, including thymidylate synthase (TS), dihydrofolate reductase (DHFR), glycinamide ribonucleotide (GAR) formyltransferase, and aminoimidazole carboxamide (AICAR) formyltransferase.[1,2] This agent has broad-spectrum activity against solid tumors, including malignant mesothelioma and breast, pancreatic, head and neck, non–small cell lung, colon, gastric, cervical, and bladder cancers.[3–5] The third antifolate compound to have entered clinical practice is pralatrexate (10-propargyl-10-deazaaminopterin), a 10-deazaaminopterin antifolate compound that was rationally designed to bind with higher affinity to the reduced folate carrier (RFC)-1 transport protein, when compared with MTX, leading to enhanced membrane transport into tumor cells. It is also an improved substrate for the enzyme folylpolyglutamyl synthetase (FPGS), resulting in enhanced formation of the cytotoxic polyglutamate metabolites.[6,7] When compared with MTX, this analogue is a more potent inhibitor of multiple enzymes involved in folate metabolism, including TS, DHFR, GAR formyltransferase, and AICAR formyltransferase. This agent is presently approved for the treatment of relapsed or refractory peripheral T-cell lymphomas.[8]

Mechanism of Action

The antifolate compounds are tight-binding inhibitors of DHFR, a key enzyme in folate metabolism.[1] DHFR plays a pivotal role in maintaining the intracellular folate pools in their fully reduced form as tetrahydrofolates, and these compounds serve as one-carbon carriers required for the synthesis of thymidylate, purine nucleotides, and certain amino acids.

The cytotoxic effects of MTX, pemetrexed, and pralatrexate are mediated by their respective polyglutamate metabolites, which are formed by the enzyme FPGS, adding up to five to seven glutamyl groups in a γ-peptide linkage. These polyglutamate metabolites exhibit prolonged intracellular half-lives, thereby allowing for prolonged drug action in tumor cells. Moreover, these polyglutamate metabolites are potent, direct inhibitors of several folate-dependent enzymes, including DHFR, TS, AICAR formyltransferase, and GAR formyltransferase.[1]

Mechanisms of Resistance

The development of cellular resistance to antifolates remains a major obstacle to its clinical efficacy.[9,10] In experimental systems, resistance to antifolates arises from several mechanisms, including an alteration in antifolate transport because of either a defect in the reduced folate carrier or folate receptor systems, decreased capacity to polyglutamate the antifolate parent compound through either decreased expression of FPGS, or increased expression of the catabolic enzyme γ-glutamyl hydrolase, and alterations in the target enzymes DHFR and/or TS through increased expression of wild type protein or overexpression of a mutant protein with reduced binding affinity for the antifolate. Gene amplification is a common resistance mechanism observed in various experimental systems, including tumor samples from patients. In *in vitro* and *in vivo* experimental model systems, the levels of DHFR and/or TS protein acutely increase after exposure to MTX and other antifolate compounds. This acute induction of target protein in response to drug exposure is mediated, in part, by a translational regulatory mechanism, which may represent a clinically relevant mechanism for the acute development of cellular drug resistance.

Clinical Pharmacology

The oral bioavailability of MTX is saturable and erratic at doses greater than 25 mg/m^2. MTX is completely absorbed from parenteral routes of administration, and peak serum levels are achieved within 30 to 60 minutes of administration. The distribution of MTX into third-space fluid collections, such as pleural effusions and ascitic fluid, can substantially alter MTX pharmacokinetics. The slow release of accumulated MTX from these third spaces over time prolongs the terminal half-life of the drug, leading to potentially increased clinical toxicity. It is advisable to evacuate these fluid collections before treatment and monitor plasma drug concentrations closely.

Renal excretion is the main route of elimination of MTX, and this process is mediated by glomerular filtration and tubular secretion. About 80% to 90% of an administered dose is eliminated unchanged in the urine. Doses of MTX, therefore, should be reduced in proportion to reductions in creatinine clearance. Renal excretion of MTX is inhibited by probenecid, penicillins, cephalosporins, aspirin, and nonsteroidal anti-inflammatory drugs.

TABLE 36.1

Drug	Main Therapeutic Uses	Main Doses and Schedule	Major Toxicities
Methotrexate	Non-Hodgkin's lymphoma Primary CNS lymphoma Acute lymphoblastic leukemia Breast cancer Bladder cancer Osteogenic sarcoma Gestational trophoblastic cancer	Low dose: 10–50 mg/m² IV every 3–4 weeks. Low dose weekly: 25 mg/m² IV weekly. Moderate dose: 100–500 m/m² IV every 2–3 weeks. High dose: 1–12 gm/m² IV over a 3- to 24-hour period every 1–3 weeks. Intrathecal (IT): 10–15 mg IT 2 times weekly until CSF is clear, then weekly dose for 2–6 weeks, followed by monthly dose.	Mucositis, diarrhea, myelosuppression, acute renal failure, transient elevations in serum transaminases and bilirubin, pneumonitis, neurologic toxicity
Pemetrexed	Mesothelioma Non–small cell lung cancer	500 mg/m² IV, every 3 weeks	Myelosuppression, skin rash, mucositis, diarrhea, fatigue
Pralatrexate	Peripheral T-cell lymphoma	30 mg/m² IV, weekly for 6 weeks. Cycles repeated every 7 weeks	Myelosuppression, skin rash, mucositis, diarrhea, elevation of serum transaminases and bilirubin, mild nausea/vomiting
5-Fluorouracil	Breast cancer Colorectal cancer Anal cancer Gastroesophageal cancer Hepatocellular cancer Pancreatic cancer Head and neck cancer	Bolus monthly schedule: 425–450 mg/m² IV on days 1–5 every 28 days. Bolus weekly schedule: 500–600 mg/m² IV every week for 6 weeks every 8 weeks. Infusion schedule: 2,400–3,000 mg/m² IV over 46 hours every 2 weeks. 120-hour infusion: 1,000 mg/m²/day IV on days 1–5 every 21–28 day Protracted continuous infusion: 200–400 mg/m²/day IV	Nausea/vomiting, diarrhea, mucositis, myelosuppression, neurotoxicity, coronary artery vasospasm, conjunctivitis
Capecitabine	Breast cancer Colorectal cancer Gastroesophageal cancer Hepatocellular cancer Pancreatic cancer	Recommended dose for monotherapy is 1,250 mg/m² PO bid for 2 weeks with 1 week rest. May decrease dose of capecitabine to 850–1,000 mg/m² bid on days 1–14 to reduce risk of toxicity without compromising efficacy. An alternative dosing schedule for monotherapy is 1,250–1,500 mg/m² PO bid for 1 week on and 1 week off. This schedule appears to be well tolerated, with no compromise in clinical efficacy. Capecitabine should be used at lower doses (850–1,000 mg/m² bid on days 1–14) when used in combination with other cytotoxic agents, such as oxaliplatin and lapatinib.	Diarrhea, hand-foot syndrome, myelosuppression, mucositis, nausea/vomiting, neurologic toxicity, coronary artery vasospasm
Cytarabine	Hodgkin's lymphoma Non-Hodgkin's lymphoma Acute myelogenous leukemia Acute lymphoblastic leukemia	Standard dose: 100 mg/m² /day IV on days 1–7 as a continuous IV infusion, in combination with an anthracycline as induction chemotherapy for acute myelogenous leukemia. High-dose: 1.5–3.0 g/m² IV q 12 hours for 3 days as a high-dose, intensification regimen for acute myelogenous leukemia. SC: 20 mg/m² SC for 10 days per month for 6 months, associated with IFN-α for treatment of chronic myelogenous leukemia. IT: 10–30 mg IT up to 3 times weekly in the treatment of leptomeningeal carcinomatosis secondary to leukemia or lymphoma.	Nausea/vomiting, myelosuppression, cerebellar ataxia, lethargy, confusion, acute pancreatitis, drug infusion reaction, hand-foot syndrome, High-dose therapy: noncardiogenic pulmonary edema, acute respiratory distress and *Streptococcus viridans* pneumonia, conjunctivitis and keratitis

(continued)

TABLE 36.1
(CONTINUED)

Drug	Main Therapeutic Uses	Main Doses and Schedule	Major Toxicities
Gemcitabine	Pancreatic cancer Non–small cell lung cancer Breast cancer Bladder cancer Hodgkin's lymphoma Ovarian cancer Soft tissue sarcoma	Pancreatic cancer: 1,000 mg/m² IV every week for 7 weeks with 1 week rest. Treatment then continues weekly for 3 weeks followed by 1 week off. Bladder cancer: 1,000 mg/m² IV on days 1, 8, and 15 every 28 days. Non–small cell lung cancer: 1,000-1,200 mg/m² IV on days 1 and 8 every 21 days.	Nausea/vomiting, myelosuppression, flulike syndrome, elevation of serum transaminases and bilirubin, pneumonitis, infusion reaction, mild proteinuria and rarely hemolytic-uremic syndrome and thrombotic thrombocytopenic purpura
6-Mercaptopurine	Acute lymphoblastic leukemia	Induction therapy: 2.5 mg/kg PO daily. Maintenance therapy: 1.5–2.5 mg/kg PO daily.	Myelosuppression, nausea/vomiting, mucositis and diarrhea, hepatotoxicity, immunosuppression
6-Thioguanine	Acute myelogenous leukemia Acute lymphoblastic leukemia	Induction: 100 mg/m² PO every 12 hours on days 1–5, usually in combination with cytarabine. Maintenance: 100 mg/m² PO every 12 hours on days 1–5, every 4 weeks, usually in combination with other agents. Single agent: 1–3 mg/kg PO daily.	Myelosuppression, nausea/vomiting, mucositis and diarrhea, hepatotoxicity, immunosuppression
Fludarabine	Chronic lymphocytic leukemia Non-Hodgkin's lymphoma	25 mg/m² IV on days 1–5 every 28 days. For oral usage, the recommended dose is 40 mg/m² PO on days 1–5 every 28 days.	Myelosuppression, immunosuppression with increased risk of opportunistic infections, mild nausea/vomiting, hypersensitivity reaction
Cladribine	Hairy cell leukemia Chronic lymphocytic leukemia Non-Hodgkin's lymphoma	Usual dose is 0.09 mg/kg/day IV via continuous infusion for 7 days. One course is usually administered	Myelosuppression, immunosuppression, mild nausea/vomiting, fever
Clofarabine	Acute lymphoblastic leukemia	52 mg/m² IV daily for 5 days every 2–6 weeks	Myelosuppression nausea/vomiting, diarrhea, systemic inflammatory response syndrome, increased risk of opportunistic infections, renal toxicity

IV, intravenously; CSF, cerebrospinal fluid; PO, by mouth; bid, twice daily; SC, subcutaneously.

Pemetrexed enters the cell via the RFC system and, to a lesser extent, by the folate receptor protein. As with MTX, it undergoes polyglutamation by FPGS within the cell to the pentaglutamate form, which is at least 60-fold more potent than the parent compound. This agent is primarily cleared by renal excretion, and in the setting of renal dysfunction, the terminal half-life of the drug is significantly prolonged to up to 20 hours. Pemetrexed, therefore, should be used with caution in patients with renal dysfunction. In addition, renal excretion is inhibited in the presence of other agents including probenecid, penicillins, cephalosporins, aspirin, and nonsteroidal anti-inflammatory drugs.

As with other antifolate analogues, pralatrexate is taken up into the cell by the RFC carrier protein and then metabolized by FPGS to form longer-chain polyglutamates, with up to four additional glutamate residues attached to the parent molecule. About 34% of parent drug is cleared in the urine during the first 24 hours after drug administration, and as such, caution is advised when using pralatrexate in patients with renal dysfunction. As with MTX and pemetrexed, the concomitant administration of other agents such as probenecid, penicillins, cephalosporins, aspirin, and nonsteroidal anti-inflammatory drugs, may inhibit renal clearance.

Toxicity

The main side effects of MTX are myelosuppression and gastrointestinal (GI) toxicity, which are usually completely reversed within 14 days, unless drug-elimination mechanisms are impaired. In patients with compromised renal function, even small doses of MTX may result in serious toxicity. MTX-induced nephrotoxicity is thought to result from the intratubular precipitation of MTX and its metabolites in acidic urine. Antifolates may also exert a direct toxic effect on the renal tubules. Vigorous hydration and urinary alkalinization have greatly reduced the incidence of renal failure in patients on high-dose regimens. Acute elevations in hepatic enzyme levels and hyperbilirubinemia are often observed during high-dose therapy, but these levels usually return to normal within 10 days.

The main toxicities of pemetrexed include dose-limiting myelosuppression, mucositis, and skin rash, usually in the form of the hand-foot syndrome. Other toxicities include reversible transaminasemia, anorexia and fatigue syndrome, and GI toxicity. These side effects are reduced by supplementation with folic acid (350 μg orally daily) and vitamin B_{12} (1,000 μg subcutaneously given at least 1 week before starting

PHARMACOLOGY OF CANCER THERAPEUTICS

therapy, and then repeated every three cycles). To date, there is no evidence to suggest that vitamin supplementation adversely affects the clinical efficacy of pemetrexed.

The main toxicities of pralatrexate include dose-limiting mucositis and myelosuppression. Other side effects include reversible transaminasemia, anorexia, and fatigue. As with pemetrexed, these toxicities are reduced by supplementation with folic acid (1–1.25 mg orally daily) starting at least 10 days before initiation of therapy and vitamin B_{12} (1 mg intramuscularly given no more than 10 weeks before starting therapy, and then repeated every 8-10 weeks thereafter).

5-FLUOROPYRIMIDINES

The fluoropyrimidine 5-fluorouracil (5-FU) was synthesized in the mid-1950s, and to this day, it remains one of the most widely used anticancer agents, showing activity in a broad range of solid tumors (Table 36.1), including GI malignancies (esophageal, gastric, pancreatic, colorectal, anal, and hepatocellular cancers), and breast, head and neck, and ovarian carcinomas.[11] It continues to serve as the main backbone for combination regimens used to treat advanced colorectal cancer (CRC) and as adjuvant therapy of early-stage colon cancer.

Mechanism of Action

5-FU enters cells via the facilitated uracil transport mechanism and is then anabolized to various cytotoxic nucleotide forms by several biochemical pathways. It is thought that 5-FU exerts its cytotoxic effects through various mechanisms, including (1) inhibition of TS, (2) incorporation into RNA, and (3) incorporation into DNA. In addition to these mechanisms, the genotoxic stress resulting from TS inhibition may also activate programmed cell-death pathways in susceptible cells, which leads to induction of parental DNA fragmentation.

Mechanisms of Resistance

Several resistance mechanisms have been identified in experimental and clinical settings. Alterations in the target enzyme TS represent the most commonly described mechanism of resistance. *In vitro, in vivo,* and clinical studies have documented a strong correlation between the levels of TS enzyme activity/TS protein and chemosensitivity to 5-FU. In this regard, cell lines and tumors with higher levels of TS are relatively more resistant to 5-FU. Mutations in TS protein have been identified that result in reduced binding affinity of the 5-FU metabolite FdUMP to the TS protein. Reduced expression and/or diminished activity of key activating enzymes may interfere with formation of cytotoxic 5-FU metabolites. Decreased expression of mismatch repair enzymes, such as hMLH1 and hMSH2, and increased expression of the catabolic enzyme dihydropyrimidine dehydrogenase (DPD) are associated with fluoropyrimidine resistance. At this time, the relative contribution of each of these mechanisms in the development of cellular resistance to 5-FU in the actual clinical setting remains unclear.

Clinical Pharmacology

5-FU is not orally administered, given its erratic bioavailability resulting from high levels of the catabolic enzyme DPD present in the gut mucosa. After intravenous bolus doses, metabolic elimination is rapid, with a half-life of 8 to 14 minutes. More than 85% of an administered dose of 5-FU is enzymatically inactivated by DPD. A pharmacogenetic syndrome has been identified in which partial or compete deficiency in the DPD enzyme is present in 3% to 5% and 0.1% of the general population, respectively. In this setting, patients experience excessive, severe toxicity in the form of myelosuppression, diarrhea and mucositis, and neurotoxicity.[12] It is now increasingly appreciated that DPD mutations are unable to account for all of the observed cases of excessive 5-FU toxicity because up to 50% of patients who experience 5-FU toxicity will have no documented alterations in the *DPD* gene. Moreover, individuals with normal DPD enzyme activity may be diagnosed with high plasma levels of 5-FU, resulting in increased toxicity.

Biomodulation of 5-FU

Significant efforts have focused on enhancing the antitumor activity of 5-FU through the process of biochemical modulation in which 5-FU is combined with various agents, including leucovorin, MTX, *N*-phosphonoacetyl-L-aspartic acid, interferon-α, interferon-γ, and a whole host of other agents.[13,14] For the past 20 to 25 years, the reduced folate LV has been used as the main biochemical modulator of 5-FU. An alternative approach has been to alter the schedule of 5-FU administration. Given the S phase specificity of this agent, prolonged exposure of tumor cells to 5-FU would increase the fraction of cells being exposed to drug. Overall response rates are significantly higher in patients treated with infusional schedules of 5-FU than in those treated with bolus 5-FU, and this improvement in response rate has translated into a survival benefit, albeit of only 1 month. However, the overall safety profile is improved with infusional regimens. A hybrid schedule of bolus and infusional 5-FU was originally developed in France, and this regimen has shown superior clinical activity compared with bolus 5-FU schedules. This hybrid schedule has now been simplified by using only the 46-hour infusion of 5-FU and completely eliminating the 5-FU bolus doses.

Toxicity

The spectrum of 5-FU toxicity is dose- and schedule-dependent. The main side effects are diarrhea, mucositis, and myelosuppression. The hand-foot syndrome is more commonly observed with infusional 5-FU therapy. Acute neurologic symptoms have also been reported, and they include somnolence, cerebellar ataxia, and upper motor signs. Treatment with 5-FU can, on rare occasions, cause coronary vasospasm, resulting in a syndrome of chest pain, cardiac enzyme elevations, and electrocardiographic changes.

CAPECITABINE

Capecitabine is an oral fluoropyrimidine carbamate that was rationally designed to allow for selective 5-FU activation in tumor tissue.[15] This oral agent was initially approved in anthracycline- and taxane-resistant breast cancer and subsequently approved for use in combination with docetaxel as second-line therapy in metastatic breast cancer and in combination with lapatinib, a tyrosine kinase inhibitor of human epidermal growth factor receptor type 2 (HER2) and epidermal growth factor receptor (EGFR) in women with HER2-positive metastatic breast cancer following progression on trastuzumab-based therapy.[16] This agent is also approved by the U.S. Food and Drug Administration for the first-line treatment of metastatic CRC (mCRC) and as adjuvant therapy for stage III colon cancer when fluoropyrimidine therapy alone is preferred.[17] In Europe and throughout much of the world, the combination of capecitabine plus oxaliplatin (XELOX) is approved for the treatment of mCRC as well as for the adjuvant therapy of stage III colon cancer.[18]

Clinical Pharmacology

Capecitabine is rapidly and extensively absorbed by the gut mucosa, with nearly 80% oral bioavailability. It is inactive in its parent form and undergoes enzymatic conversion via three successive steps. Of note, the third and final step occurs in tumor tissue and involves the conversion of 5′-deoxy-5-fluorouridine to 5-FU by the enzyme thymidine phosphorylase, which is expressed at much higher levels in tumors when compared with corresponding normal tissue. Capecitabine and capecitabine metabolites are primarily excreted by the kidneys, and in contrast to 5-FU, caution must be taken in the presence of renal dysfunction, with appropriate dose reduction. The use of capecitabine is absolutely contraindicated in patients whose creatinine clearance is less than 30 mL/min.

Toxicity

The main side effects of capecitabine include diarrhea and hand-foot syndrome. The incidence of myelosuppression, neutropenic fever, mucositis, alopecia, and nausea/vomiting is lower with capecitabine when compared with 5-FU. Elevations in indirect serum bilirubin can be observed, but are usually transient and clinically asymptomatic. Patients in the United States appear to be unable to tolerate as high doses of capecitabine as European patients, either as monotherapy or in combination with other cytotoxic chemotherapy.[19] Although the underlying reasons for this discrepancy are not known, it may in part be related to the increased fortification of the U.S. diet with folate and the increased focus on vitamin and folic acid supplementation.

CYTARABINE

Cytarabine (ara-C) is one of several arabinose nucleosides isolated from the sponge *Cryptothethya crypta*, differing from its physiologic counterpart by virtue of a stereotypic inversion of the 2′-hydroxyl group of the sugar moiety.[20] A regimen of ara-C combined with an anthracycline, given as a 5- or 7-day continuous infusion, is considered the standard induction treatment for acute myeloid leukemia (AML). Ara-C is active against other hematologic malignancies, such as non-Hodgkin's lymphoma, chronic myelogenous leukemia, and acute lymphocytic leukemia (Table 36.1). However, this agent has absolutely no activity against solid tumors.

Mechanism of Action

Ara-C enters cells via nucleoside transport proteins, the most important one being the equilibrative inhibitor-sensitive (es) receptor. Once inside the cell, ara-C requires activation for its cytotoxic effects.[20,21] The first metabolic step is the conversion of ara-C to ara-C monophosphate (ara-CMP) by the enzyme deoxycytidine kinase (dCK) with subsequent phosphorylation to the di- and tri-phosphate metabolites, respectively. Ara-CTP is a potent inhibitor of DNA polymerases α, β, and γ, which, in turn, interferes with DNA chain elongation, DNA synthesis, and DNA repair. Ara-CTP is also incorporated directly into DNA and functions as a DNA chain terminator, interfering with chain elongation. Catabolism of ara-C involves two key enzymes, cytidine deaminase and deoxycytidylate deaminase. These breakdown enzymes convert ara-C and ara-CMP into the inactive metabolites, ara-U and ara-UMP, respectively. The balance between intracellular activation and degradation is critical in determining the amount of drug that is ultimately converted to ara-CTP and, thus, its subsequent cytotoxic and antitumor activity.

Mechanisms of Resistance

Several mechanisms of resistance to ara-C have been described. Impaired transmembrane transport, decreased rate of anabolism, and increased rate of catabolism may result in the development of ara-C resistance.[20,22,23] The level of cytidine deaminase enzyme activity has been shown to correlate with clinical response in patients with AML undergoing induction chemotherapy with ara-C–containing regimens.

Clinical Pharmacology

Ara-C has poor oral bioavailability given its extensive deamination within the GI tract. As a result, ara-C is administered intravenously via continuous infusion. After administration, ara-C undergoes extensive metabolism in the liver, plasma, and peripheral tissues. Within 24 hours, up to 80% of drug is recovered in the urine as the ara-U metabolite. Ara-C crosses the blood–brain barrier when used at high doses, with cerebrospinal fluid levels between 7% and 14% of plasma levels and reaching peak levels of up to 10 μM.

PHARMACOLOGY OF CANCER THERAPEUTICS

Toxicity

The toxicity profile of ara-C is highly dependent on the dose and schedule of administration. Myelosuppression is dose-limiting with a standard 7-day regimen. Leukopenia and thrombocytopenia are observed most frequently, with nadirs occurring between days 7 and 14 after drug administration. GI toxicity commonly manifests as a mild-to-moderate degree of anorexia, nausea, and vomiting along with mucositis, diarrhea, and abdominal pain. In rare cases, acute pancreatitis has been observed. The ara-C syndrome has been described in pediatric patients with hematologic malignancies, usually begins within 12 hours after start of drug infusion, and is characterized by fever, myalgia, bone pain, maculopapular rash, conjunctivitis, malaise, and occasional chest pain.

Administration of ara-C at high doses (2 to 3 g/m^2 with each dose) is associated with profound myelosuppression.[24] Severe GI toxicity in the form of mucositisand/or diarrhea is also observed. Neurologic toxicity is significantly more common with high-dose ara-C than with standard doses, and presents with seizures, cerebral and cerebellar dysfunction, and peripheral neuropathy. Clinical signs of cerebellar dysfunction occur in up to 15% of patients and include dysarthria, dysmetria, and ataxia. Change in alertness and cognitive ability, memory loss, and frontal lobe release signs reflect cerebral toxicity. Despite discontinuation of therapy, clinical recovery is incomplete in up to 30% of affected patients. Pulmonary complications may include noncardiogenic pulmonary edema, acute respiratory distress, and pneumonia, resulting from *Streptococcus viridans* infection. Other side effects associated with high-dose ara-C include conjunctivitis (often responsive to topical corticosteroids), a painful hand-foot syndrome, and, rarely, anaphylactic reactions.

GEMCITABINE

Gemcitabine (2′,2′-difluorodeoxycytidine) is a difluorinated deoxycytidine analogue. Despite its similarity in structure, metabolism, and mechanism of action to ara-C, the spectrum of antitumor activity of gemcitabine is much broader.[20,25] This compound has significant clinical activity against several human solid tumors, including pancreatic, small cell and non–small cell lung, bladder, ovary, and breast cancers as well as hematologic malignancies, namely Hodgkin's and non-Hodgkin's lymphoma (Table 36.1).

Mechanism of Action

Transport of gemcitabine into cells requires the nucleoside transporter system. Gemcitabine is inactive in its parent form and requires intracellular activation for its cytotoxic effects. The steps involved in the metabolic activation of gemcitabine are similar to those observed with ara-C, with both drugs being activated by the same enzymatic machinery to the active triphosphate metabolite. Gemcitabine triphosphate is then incorporated into DNA, resulting in chain termination and inhibition of DNA synthesis and function, or the triphosphate form can directly inhibit DNA polymerases α, β, and γ, which, in turn, interferes with DNA chain elongation, DNA synthesis, and DNA repair. The triphosphate metabolite is also a potent inhibitor of ribonucleotide reductase, which further mediates inhibition of DNA biosynthesis, by reducing the levels of key deoxynucleotide pools.

Mechanisms of Resistance

Several mechanisms of resistance to gemcitabine have been described in various preclinical experimental models.[26,27] Nucleoside transport–deficient cells are highly resistant to gemcitabine. Furthermore, the efficiency of gemcitabine uptake can vary significantly according to the specific nucleoside transporter expressed on the cell surface. Several enzymes involved in the intracellular metabolism of gemcitabine have been implicated in the development of cellular drug resistance, including reduced expression and/or deficiency in dCK enzyme activity as well as increased expression and/or activity of the catabolic enzymes cytidine deaminase and dCMP deaminase. Recent studies have also identified a subset of CD44-positive cancer stem cells within pancreatic tumors that sustain tumor formation and growth, and are resistant to gemcitabine therapy.[28]

Clinical Pharmacology

Gemcitabine is administered via the intravenous route, typically over a 30-minute intravenous infusion, and it undergoes extensive metabolism by deamination to the catabolic metabolite, difluorodeoxyuridine (dFdU), with more than 90% of metabolized drug being recovered in urine. Plasma clearance is about 30% lower in women and in elderly patients, and this pharmacokinetic difference may result in an increased risk of toxicity in these respective patient populations.

Toxicity

Gemcitabine is a relatively well-tolerated drug when used as a single agent. The main dose-limiting toxicity is myelosuppression, with neutropenia more commonly experienced than thrombocytopenia. Toxicity is schedule-dependent, with longer infusions producing greater hematologic toxicity. Transient flu-like symptoms including fever, headache, arthralgias, and myalgias occur in 45% of patients. Asthenia and transient transaminasemia may occur. Renal microangiopathy syndromes, including hemolytic-uremic syndrome and thrombotic thrombocytopenic purpura, have been reported rarely.

6-THIOPURINES

The development of the purine analogues in cancer chemotherapy began in the early 1950s with the synthesis of the thiopurines, 6-mercaptopurine (6-MP) and 6-thioguanine (6-TG). 6-MP has an important role in maintenance therapy for acute lymphoblastic leukemia, whereas 6-TG is active in remission induction and in maintenance therapy for AML (Table 36.1).

Mechanism of Action

The thiopurines, 6-MP and 6-TG, act similarly with respect to their cellular biochemistry.[29] In their respective monophosphate nucleotide forms, they inhibit enzymes involved in *de novo* purine synthesis and purine interconversion reactions. The triphosphate nucleotide forms can get directly incorporated into either cellular RNA or DNA, leading to inhibition of RNA and DNA synthesis and function, respectively.

Mechanisms of Resistance

The development of cellular resistance to 6-thiopurines results from a decreased level of key cytotoxic nucleotide metabolites, either through decreased formation or increased breakdown. Resistant cells have been identified that express either complete or partial deficiency of the activating enzyme HGPRT. In clinical samples derived from patients with AML, drug resistance has been associated with increased concentrations of a membrane-bound alkaline phosphatase or a conjugating enzyme, 6-thiopurine methyltransferase (TPMT), the end-result being reduced formation of cytotoxic thiopurine nucleotides. Finally, decreased expression of mismatch repair enzymes, including hMLH1 and hMSH2, has been associated with cellular drug resistance.

Clinical Pharmacology

Oral absorption of 6-MP is highly erratic, with only 16% to 50% of an administered dose reaching the systemic circulation. This effect is mainly related to rapid first-pass metabolism in the liver. The major route of drug elimination is via metabolism by several enzymatic pathways. 6-MP is oxidized to the inactive metabolite 6-thiouric acid by xanthine oxidase. Enhanced 6-MP toxicity may result from the concomitant administration of 6-MP and the xanthine oxidase inhibitor allopurinol. In patients receiving both 6-MP and allopurinol, the 6-MP dose must be reduced by at least 50% to 75%. 6-MP also undergoes S-methylation by the enzyme TPMT to yield 6-methylmercaptopurine.[30]

6-TG is administered orally in the treatment of AML. Its oral bioavailability is erratic, with peak plasma levels occurring 2 to 4 hours after ingestion. The catabolism of 6-TG differs from 6-MP in that it is not a direct substrate for xanthine oxidase.

TPMT enzyme activity may vary considerably among patients as a result of point mutations or loss of alleles of TPMT.[31] Approximately 0.3% of the white population expresses either a homozygous deletion or mutation of both alleles of the *TPMT* gene. In these patients, grossly elevated TGN concentrations, profound myelotoxicity with pancytopenia, and extensive GI symptoms are observed after only a brief course of thiopurine treatment. An estimated 10% of patients may be at increased risk for toxicity because of heterozygous loss of the gene or a mutant allele coding for a less enzymatically active TPMT.

Toxicity

The major dose-related toxicities of the thiopurines are myelosuppression and GI toxicity in the form of nausea/vomiting, anorexia, diarrhea, and stomatitis.[32] In TPMT-deficient patients, dosage reduction to 5% to 25% of the standard dosage is necessary to prevent severe excessive toxicity. Thiopurine hepatotoxicity occurs in up to 30% of adult patients and presents mainly as cholestatic jaundice, although elevations of hepatic transaminases may also be seen. Combinations of thiopurines with other known hepatotoxic agents should be avoided, and liver function should be closely monitored. The thiopurines are also potent suppressors of cell-mediated immunity, and prolonged therapy results in an increased predisposition to bacterial and parasitic infections.

FLUDARABINE

Fludarabine (9-β-D-arabinosyl-2-fluoroadenine monophosphate, F-ara-AMP) is an active agent in the treatment of chronic lymphocytic leukemia (CLL) (Table 36.1).[33,34] It is also active against indolent non-Hodgkin's lymphoma, prolymphocytic leukemia, cutaneous T-cell lymphoma, and Waldenstrom macroglobulinemia. This agent has also shown promising activity in mantle cell lymphoma. In contrast to its activity in hematologic malignancies, this compound has virtually no activity against solid tumors.

Mechanism of Action

The active cytotoxic metabolite is the triphosphate metabolite F-ara-ATP, which competes with deoxyadenosine triphosphate (dATP) for incorporation into DNA and serves as a highly effective chain terminator. In addition, F-ara-ATP directly inhibits enzymes involved in DNA replication, including DNA polymerases, DNA primase, DNA ligase I, and ribonucleotide reductase.[35] F-ara-ATP is also incorporated into RNA, causing inhibition of RNA function, processing, and mRNA translation. In contrast to other antimetabolites, fludarabine is active against nondividing cells. In fact, the primary effect of fludarabine may result from activation of apoptosis, through an as yet ill-defined mechanisms.[36] This finding may explain the activity of fludarabine in indolent lymphoproliferative diseases with relatively low growth fractions.

Mechanisms of Resistance

Decreased expression of the activating enzyme dCK resulting in diminished intracellular formation of F-ara-AMP is one of the main resistance mechanisms identified in preclinical models.[37] A high degree of cross-resistance develops to multiple nucleoside analogues requiring activation by dCK, including cytarabine, gemcitabine, cladribine, and clofarabine. Reduced cellular transport of drug has also been identified as a resistance mechanism.

Clinical Pharmacology

Peak concentrations of F-ara-A are reached 3 to 4 hours after intravenous administration.[38] The main route of elimination is via the kidneys, with about 25% of a given dose of drug being excreted unchanged in the urine.

Toxicity

Myelosuppression and immunosuppression are the major side effects of fludarabine as highlighted by dose-limiting and possibly cumulative lymphopenia and thrombocytopenia. Suppression of the immune system affects T-cell more than B-cell function. Fevers, often in the setting of neutropenia, occur in 20% to 30% of patients. Lymphocyte counts, specifically CD4-positive cells, decrease rapidly after initiation of therapy, and recovery of CD4-positive cells to normal levels may take longer than 1 year. Common opportunistic pathogens include varicella-zoster virus, *Candida*, and *Pneumocystis carinii*. In general, patients are empirically placed on sulfamethoxazole trimethoprim prophylaxis to prevent the development of *P. carinii* infection. Other uncommon toxicities include skin rash, nausea, vomiting, diarrhea, stomatitis, anorexia, increased salivation, abdominal cramps, a metallic taste, transient elevations in levels of hepatic enzymes, and renal dysfunction.

CLADRIBINE

Cladribine (2-CdA) is a purine deoxyadenosine analogue, and it is the drug of choice for hairy cell leukemia with activity in low-grade lymphoproliferative disorders (Table 36.1).[39,40] Salvage treatment of patients previously treated with interferon-α or splenectomy is as effective as first-line treatment. Retreatment with cladribine results in complete response in up to 60% of relapsing patients. In addition, this agent has promising activity in patients with CLL and non-Hodgkin's lymphoma.

Mechanism of Action

On entry into the cell, 2-CdA undergoes initial conversion to cladribine-monophosphate (Cd-AMP) via the reaction catalyzed by dCK, and Cd-AMP is subsequently metabolized to the active metabolite, cladribine-triphosphate. The triphosphate metabolite competitively inhibits incorporation of the normal dATP nucleotide into DNA, a process that results in termination of chain elongation.[41] Progressive accumulation of the triphosphate metabolite leads to an imbalance in deoxyribonucleotide pools, thereby inhibiting further DNA synthesis and repair. Finally, the triphosphate metabolite is a potent inhibitor of ribonucleotide reductase, which further facilitates inhibition of DNA biosynthesis.

Mechanisms of Resistance

Resistance to 2-CdA has been attributed to altered intracellular drug metabolism. A reduction in the activity of dCK, the enzyme responsible for generating cytotoxic nucleotide metabolites, is a major determinant of acquired resistance. The monophosphate and triphosphate metabolites are dephosphorylated by the cytoplasmic enzyme 5′-nucleotidase. Interestingly, resistant cells derived from a patient with CLL exhibited both low levels of dCK expression and high-levels of 5′-nucleotidase.

Clinical Pharmacology

2-CdA is orally bioavailable, with 50% of an administered dose orally absorbed. Approximately 50% of an administered dose of drug is cleared by the kidneys, and 20% to 35% of the drug is excreted unchanged in the urine. Of note, this nucleoside can cross the blood–brain barrier with penetration into the cerebrospinal fluid.

Toxicity

At conventional doses, myelosuppression is dose-limiting. After a single course of drug, recovery from thrombocytopenia usually occurs within 2 to 4 weeks, while recovery from neutropenia takes place in 3 to 5 weeks. GI toxicities are generally mild, with nausea/vomiting and diarrhea. Mild-to-moderate neurotoxicity occurs in 15% of patients and is at least partly reversible with discontinuation of the drug. Immunosuppression accounts for the late morbidity observed in 2-CdA–treated patients. Lymphocyte counts, particularly CD4-positive cells, decrease within 1 to 4 weeks of drug administration and may remain depressed for several years. After discontinuation of 2-CdA, a median time of up to 40 months may be required for complete recovery of normal CD4-positive counts. Although opportunistic infections occur, they do so less frequently than with fludarabine therapy. Infectious complications correlate with decreases in CD4-positive count, and they include herpes zoster, *Candida*, *Pneumocystis*, *Pseudomonas aeruginosa*, *Listeria monocytogenes*, *Cryptococcus neoformans*, *Aspergillus*, *P. carinii,* and cytomegalovirus.

CLOFARABINE

Clofarabine is a purine deoxyadenosine nucleoside analogue, and it is approved for the treatment of pediatric patients with relapsed or refractory acute lymphoblastic leukemia (Table 36.1).[42] Ongoing studies are exploring the benefit of clofarabine alone and in combination with other agents in less heavily pretreated patients and in the use of different dose schedules for other hematologic malignancies.[43]

Mechanism of Action

Clofarabine is inactive in its parent form and, like other purine analogues, it requires intracellular activation by dCK to form the monophosphate nucleotide, which undergoes further metabolism to the cytotoxic triphosphate metabolite. Clofarabine triphosphate is then incorporated into DNA, resulting in chain termination, and inhibition of DNA synthesis and function or the triphosphate form can directly inhibit DNA polymerases α, β, and γ, which in turn interferes with DNA chain elongation, DNA synthesis, and DNA repair. The triphosphate metabolite is also a potent inhibitor of ribonucleotide reductase, further mediating inhibition of DNA biosynthesis by reducing the levels of key deoxyribonucleotide pools.

Mechanisms of Resistance

Several resistance mechanisms have been identified in various preclinical systems, and they include decreased activation of drug through reduced expression of the anabolic enzyme deoxycytidine kinase, decreased transport of drug into cells via the nucleoside transporter protein, and increased expression of CTP synthetase activity resulting in increased concentrations of competing physiologic nucleotide substrate dCTP. To date, the precise resistance mechanism(s) that are relevant in the clinical setting remain to be determined.

Clinical Pharmacology

Approximately 50% to 60% of an administered dose of drug is excreted unchanged in the urine, and the terminal half-life is on the order of 5 hours. To date, the pathways for nonrenal elimination have not been well defined. Caution should be exercised in patients with abnormal renal function, and concomitant use of medications known to cause renal toxicity should be avoided during drug treatment.

Toxicity

Myelosuppression is dose-limiting with neutropenia, anemia, and thrombocytopenia. The capillary leak syndrome (systemic inflammatory response syndrome) presents with tachypnea, tachycardia, pulmonary edema, and hypotension. In essence, this adverse event is part of the tumor lysis syndrome and results from rapid cytoreduction of peripheral leukemic cells following treatment. Other side effects may include nausea/vomiting, reversible liver dysfunction (hyperbilirubinemia and elevated serum transaminases), renal dysfunction (approximately 10%), and cardiac toxicity in the form of tachycardia and acute pump dysfunction.

References

1. Monahan BP, Allegra CJ. Antifolates. In: Chabner BA, Longo DL, eds. *Cancer Chemotherapy and Biotherapy: Principles and Practice,* 4th ed. Philadelphia: Lippincott–Raven, 2006:91.
2. Chattopadhyay S, Moran RG, Goldman ID. Pemetrexed: biochemical and cellular pharmacology, mechanisms, and clinical applications. *Mol Cancer Ther* 2007;6:404.
3. Vogelzang NJ, Rusthoven JJ, Symanowski J, et al. Phase III study of pemetrexed in combination with cisplatin versus cisplatin alone in patients with malignant pleural mesothelioma. *J Clin Oncol* 2003;21:2636.
4. Kindler HL. Sysemic treatments for mesothelioma: standard and novel. *Curr Treat Options Oncol* 2008;9:171.
5. Joerger M, Omlin A, Cerny T, Fruh M. The role of pemetrexed in advanced non small-cell lung cancer: special focus on pharmacology and mechanism of action. *Curr Drug Targets* 2010;11:37.
6. Sirotnak FM, DeGraw JI, Moccio DM, et al. New folate analogs of the 10-deaza-aminopterin series. *Cancer Chemother Pharmacol* 1984;12:18.
7. Krug LM, Ng KK, Kris MG, et al. Phase I and pharmacokinetic study of 10-propargyl-10-deazaaminopterin, a new antifolate. *Clin Cancer Res* 2000;6:3493.
8. O'Connor OA. Pralatrexate: an emerging new agent with activity in T-cell lymphomas. *Curr Opin Oncol* 2006;18:591.
9. Bertino JR, Goker E, Gorlick R, Li WW, Banerjee D. Resistance mechanisms to methotrexate in tumors. *Oncologist* 1996;1:223.
10. Zhao R, Goldman ID. Resistance to antifolates. *Oncogene* 2003;22:7431.
11. Grem JL. 5-Fluorouracil: forty-plus and still ticking. A review of its preclinical and clinical development. *Invest New Drugs* 2000;18:299.
12. Zhang X, Diasio RB. Regulation of human dihydropyrimidine dehydrogenase: implications in the pharmacogenetics of 5-FU-based chemotherapy. *Pharmacogenomics* 2007;8:257.
13. Grem JL. Biochemical modulation of 5-FU in systemic treatment of advanced colorectal cancer. *Oncology (Williston Park)* 2001;15(1 Suppl 2):13.
14. The Meta-Analysis Group in Cancer. Modulation of fluorouracil by leucovorin in patients with advanced colorectal cancer: an updated meta-analysis. *J Clin Oncol* 2004;22:3766.
15. Shimma N, Umeda I, Arasaki M, et al. The design and synthesis of a new tumor-selective fluoropyrimidine carbamate, capecitabine. *Bioorg Med Chem* 2000;8:1697.
16. Geyer CE, Forster J, Lindquist D, et al. Lapatinib plus capecitabine for *HER2*-positive advanced breast cancer. *N Engl J Med* 2006;355:2733.
17. Chu E. Efficacy and safety of capecitabine therapy for colorectal cancer. *Am J Oncol Rev* 2003;2(Suppl 3):4.
18. Van Custem E, Verslype C, Tejpar S. Oral capecitabine: bridging the Atlantic divide in colon cancer treatment. *Semin Oncol* 2005;32:43.
19. Haller DG, Cassidy J, Clarke SJ, et al. Potential regional differences for the tolerability profiles of fluoropyrimidines. *J Clin Oncol* 2008;26:2118.
20. Ryan DP, Garcia-Carbonero R, Chabner BA. Cytidine analogs. In: Chabner BA, Longo DL, eds. *Cancer Chemotherapy and Biotherapy: Principles and Practice,* 4th ed. Philadelphia: Lippincott–Raven, 2006:183.

21. Braess J, Wegendt C, Feuring-Buske M, et al. Leukemic blasts differ from normal bone marrow mononuclear cells and CD34+ hematopoietic stem cells in their metabolism of cytosine arabinoside. *Br J Haematol* 1999;105:388.
22. Momparler RL, Laliberte J, Eliopoulos N, et al. Transfection of murine fibroblast cells with human cytidine deaminase cDNA confers resistance to cytosine arabinoside. *Anticancer Drugs* 1996;7:266.
23. Cai J, Damaraju VL, Groulx N, et al. Two distinct molecular mechanisms underlying cytarabine resistance in human leukemic cells. *Cancer Res* 2008;68:2349.
24. Kern W, Estey EH. High-dose cytosine arabinoside in the treatment of acute myeloid leukemia: review of three randomized trials. *Cancer* 2006;107:116.
25. Mini E, Nobili S, Caciagli B, Landini I, Mazzei T. Cellular pharmacology of gemcitabine. *Ann Oncol* 2006;17(Suppl 5):v7:7.
26. Bergman AM, Pinedo HM, Peters GJ. Determinants of resistance to 2′,2′-difluorodeoxycytidine (gemcitabine). *Drug Resist Update* 2002;5:19.
27. El Maalouf G, Le Tourneau C, Batty GN, et al. Markers involved in resistance to cytotoxic and targetd therapeutics in pancreatic cancer. *Cancer Treat Rev* 2009;35:167.
28. Hong SP, Wen J, Bang S, et al. CD44-positive cells are responsible for gemcitabine resistance in pancreatic cancer cells. *Int J Cancer* 2009;125:2323.
29. Hande KR. Purine antimetabolites. In: Chabner BA, Longo DL, eds. *Cancer Chemotherapy and Biotherapy: Principles and Practice,* 4th ed. Philadelphia: Lippincott–Raven, 2006:212.
30. Evans WE. Pharmacogenetics of thiopurine S-methyltransferase and thiopurine therapy. *Ther Drug Monitor* 2004;26:186.
31. Wang L, Weinshilboum R. Thiopurine S-methyltransferase pharmacogenetics: insights, challenges, and future directions. *Oncogene* 2006;25:1629.
32. Vora A, Mitchell CD, Lennard L, et al. Medical Research Council; National Cancer Research Network Childhood Leukaemia Working Party. Toxicity and efficacy of 6-thioguanine versus 6-mercaptopurine in childhood lymphoblastic leukaemia: a randomised trial. *Lancet* 2006;368:1339.
33. Gandhi V, Plunkett W. Cellular and clinical pharmacology of fludarabine. *Clin Pharmacokinet* 2002;41:93.
34. Montillo M, Ricci F, Tedeschi A. Role of fludarabine in hematological malignancies. *Expert Rev Anticancer Ther* 2006;6:1141.
35. Van den Neste E, Cardoen S, Offner F, Bontemps F. Old and new insights into the mechanism of action of two nucleoside analogs active in lymphoid malignancies: fludarabine and cladribine. *Int J Oncol* 2005;27:1113.
36. Huang P, Robertson LE, Wright S, et al. High molecular weight DNA fragmentation: a critical event in nucleoside analog-induced apoptosis in leukemia cells. *Clin Cancer Res* 1995;1:1005.
37. Dumontet C, Fabianowska-Majewska K, Mantincic D, et al. Common resistance mechanisms to deoxynucleoside analogs in variants of the human erythroleukemic line K562. *Br J Haematol* 1999;106:78.
38. Malspeis L, Grever MR, Staubus AE, et al. Pharmacokinetics of 2-F-ara-A (9-b-D-arabinofuranosyl-2-fluoroadenine) in cancer patients during the phase I clinical investigation of fludarabine phosphate. *Semin Oncol* 1990;17(Suppl 8):18.
39. Grevz N, Saven A. Cladribine: from the bench to the bedside: focus on hairy cell leukemia. *Expert Rev Anticancer Ther* 2004;4:745.
40. Gidron A, Tallman MS. 2-CdA in the treatment of hairy cell leukemia: a review of long-term follow-up. *Leuk Lymphoma* 2006;47:2301.
41. Seto S, Carrera CJ, Kubota M, et al. Mechanism of deoxyadenosine and 2-chlorodeoxyadenosine toxicity to nondividing human lymphocytes. *J Clin Invest* 1985;75:377.
42. Bonate PL, Arthaud L, Cantrell WR Jr, et al. Discovery and development of clofarabine: a nucleoside analogue for treating cancer. *Nat Rev Drug Discov* 2006;5:855-863.
43. Faderi S, Gandhi V, Keating MJ, et al. The role of clofarabine in hematologic and solid malignancies: development of a next generation nucleoside analog. *Cancer* 2005;102:1985.

CHAPTER 37 TOPOISOMERASE-INTERACTING AGENTS

ZESHAAN A. RASHEED AND ERIC H. RUBIN

TOPOISOMERASE BIOLOGY

DNA topoisomerases are a general class of enzymes that alter the topology of DNA and are found in all organisms, including Archaebacteria, viruses, yeast, *Drosophila*, and humans.[1] The importance of and fundamental need for DNA topoisomerases in all cells are related to the double-helical structure of DNA. Access to DNA during processes such as replication, transcription, and recombination requires double-helical DNA to be separated, which results in torsional stress that is resolved by DNA topoisomerases. There are two general classes of topoisomerases, type I and type II, distinguished by the number of DNA strand breaks they make during catalysis.[1] Mammalian cells contain one type IB topoisomerase, topoisomerase I (Top1), and two type IA topoisomerases, topoisomerase IIIα (Top3α) and topoisomerase IIIβ (Top3β). Additionally, mammalian cells contain two type II topoisomerases, topoisomerase IIα (Top2α) and topoisomerase IIβ (Top2β). In mammalian cells Top1, Top2α, and Top2β are essential, as disruption of any of these topoisomerase genes leads to lethality during embryogenesis or at birth.[2] In mammalian cells Top1 is important in supporting replication fork movement during DNA replication and to relax super coils generated during transcription[1] Top2α is responsible for unlinking intertwined daughter duplexes during DNA replication, contributes to DNA relaxation during transcription, and facilitates remodeling of chromatin structure.[1]

Type I topoisomerases cleave a single strand of DNA and change the linking number of DNA by one per cycle of activity, and type II topoisomerases cleave both strands of DNA and change the linking number of DNA by two (Figs. 37.1 and 37.2). The mechanism of action of Top1 involves an initial noncovalent interaction with DNA. Top1 then cleaves a single strand of DNA and forms a covalent intermediate via a phosphodiester linkage between tyrosine-723 of Top1 and the 3′-phosphate group of the scissile strand of DNA. The intact DNA strand is then passed through the break and then Top1 relegates the DNA and releases from the complex.[1,2] In contrast, type II topoisomerase enzymes function as homo- or heterodimers and require adenosine triphosphate for catalysis. A topoisomerase dimer binds to DNA, forming a double-strand DNA break in which the proteins are covalently bound to the 5′ end of broken DNA strands to form the Top2 cleavable complex. In this state the protein dimer is stabilized, forming a gate in the DNA through which a second DNA double-helix strand can pass in an energy-dependent fashion.

As described below, several U.S. Food ad Drug Administration (FDA)-approved anticancer drugs target either Top1 or Top2 isozymes. Additional topoisomerase-targeting compounds are under investigation in the clinic. Some of these target both Top1 and Top2 enzymes. Top3-targeting anticancer drugs have not yet been identified.

CAMPTOTHECINS

Camptothecin is a naturally occurring alkaloid that was identified in the 1960s by Wall and Wani[3] in a screen of plant extracts for antineoplastic drugs. Early trials with the sodium salt of camptothecin produced modest responses, which were complicated by unexpected severe myelosuppression and hemorrhagic cystitis, and the drug was deemed too toxic for clinical use. Subsequently, it was discovered that the carboxylic acid form of camptothecin in the sodium salt that was used in earlier trials is much less active than the form containing a lactone ring at position 20.[4] Further development of camptothecin led to two water-soluble derivatives that can be delivered as the more active lactone forms: topotecan and irinotecan. These are currently approved for the treatment of several cancer types. In addition, several topoisomerase I-targeting drugs are under clinical investigation, including various camptothecin derivatives and formulations (including high-molecular weight conjugates or liposomal formulations), as well as non-camptothecin compounds that exhibit greater potency or noncross resistance to irinotecan and topotecan in preclinical cancer models.

Mechanism of Action

Camptothecins are called topoisomerase "poisons" since they kill cells not by inhibiting topoisomerase catalysis, but by stabilizing the normally transient reaction intermediate in which the enzyme is covalently linked to DNA (Fig. 37.1).[5] A crystal structure of the topotecan-Top1-DNA ternary complex is available and has helped elucidate this mode of action[6] In the complex, topotecan stacks into the DNA duplex at the Top1 cleavage site, thereby preventing relegation of DNA at the site of the single-strand nick. The formation of the ternary complex and formation of DNA nicks alone do not account for camptothecin-mediated cell death, since these lesions are reversible and disappear with removal of the drug. According to the replication fork collision model, a replication fork encounters the ternary complex, leading to lethal double-strand DNA breaks,[5] which may also account for the S-phase specificity of the cell cycle of camptothecin cell toxicity.[7]

Mechanisms of Resistance

The mechanisms underlying *de novo* and acquired clinical resistance to camptothecins are not completely understood. However, based on preclinical studies, it is likely that clinical resistance to these drugs might be the result of inadequate accumulation of drug in the tumor, impaired metabolism of the prodrug (as in the case of irinotecan), alterations in the

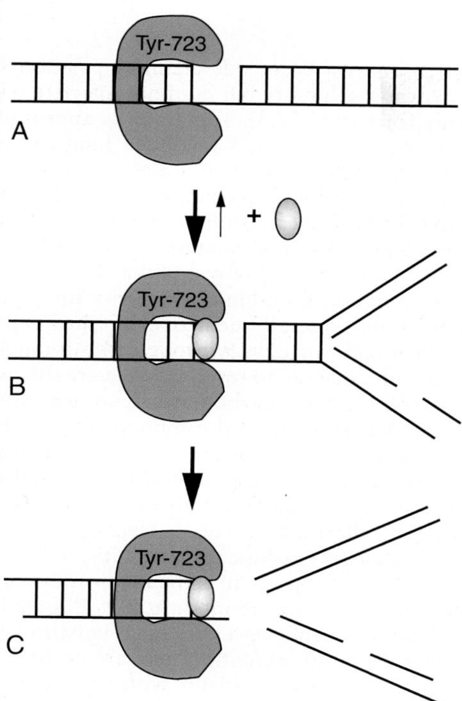

FIGURE 37.1 Topoisomerase I (Top1) mechanism of action and replication fork collision model for camptothecin cytotoxicity. **A:** Top1 (*blue*) normally relaxes super coiled DNA by forming a covalent interaction between tyrosine-723 and the 3′ end of the nicked DNA. **B:** Addition of camptothecin (*yellow*) results in the formation of the ternary complex and prevents relegation of DNA. **C:** Collision of the advancing replication fork with the ternary complex leads to DNA damage and cell death.

target (Top1), or alterations in the cellular response to the Top1-camptothecin interaction.[8]

Both active and passive transport mechanisms are implicated in intestinal cell uptake of camptothecin,[9] and ovarian cancer cells contain active transporters that are required for the influx of topotecan and SN-38 (the active metabolite of irinotecan).[10] Additionally, efflux mechanisms may play a role in resistance. MDR1 (P-glycoprotein) overexpression confers resistance to camptothecin derivatives, albeit to a lesser degree than to other substrates of P-glycoprotein, such as the anthracyclines.[11] Antisense oligonucleotides directed against the *ABCC2* MRP2 gene can increase cellular sensitivity to irinotecan.[12] Additionally, multidrug resistance secondary to BCRP gene overexpression has been implicated in resistance in some but not all camptothecins.[13–15]

Cellular metabolism may be particularly important for irinotecan as it is a prodrug that is converted to its active form, SN-38, by cellular carboxylesterases,[16–19] and increased levels of this enzyme correlate with increased cellular sensitivity to the drug.[16,20] Furthermore, SN-38 is also conjugated and detoxified by UDP-glucuronosyltransferase (UGT) to yield an SN-38-glucuronide.[21] Glucuronidation of SN-38 is associated with increased efflux of the drug from colon cancer cells,[22] and glucuronidation of the camptothecins has been associated with altered chemosensitivity of breast cancer cells and lung cancer cells.[23,24]

Camptothecin specifically targets Top1, therefore, it is not surprising that Top1 mutations that confer resistance to camptothecin have been identified in various mammalian and yeast cells and, more recently, in tumor tissue from a patient treated with irinotecan.[25] Most of the point mutations can be found clustered in three regions of the protein, one of which is near the catalytic tyrosine at position 723 and in other regions that participate in interactions with minor and major grooves of DNA and the intercalated drug.[6,8,26]

Interactions between Top1 and other proteins may affect cellular sensitivity to camptothecins. The Top1-binding protein nucleolin may recruit Top1 to the nucleolus as a result of the high rate of transcription in this region,[27] and yeast lacking the orthologue of nucleolin are resistant to camptothecin.[28] Studies in yeast and cell culture models have implicated the response of several DNA replication, DNA damage checkpoint, and DNA repair proteins to the formation of the cleavable complex, which also plays a role in camptothecin resistance. Loss of function of the checkpoint proteins, Chk1 or ATR, is associated with increased cellular sensitivity to camptothecin.[29,30] Additionally, loss of RAD9, a checkpoint protein that is activated by DNA damage and induces G2 arrest in yeast, was shown to enhance Top1-induced cell death.[31,32] Studies in murine cells implicate the loss of the Werner syndrome protein, a helicase that interacts with Top1, in camptothecin hypersensitivity.[33] Deletion of multiple proteins involved in DNA repair have been implicated in camptothecin hypersensitivity, including MSH2, a mismatch repair protein[34]; Pnk1, a eukaryotic polynucleotide kinase that plays a role in camptothecin-induced DNA damage repair[35]; and a tyrosine-DNA phosphodiesterase that specifically cleaves Top1 and is covalently linked to DNA.[36,37] Notably, overexpression of the DNA repair protein, x-ray repair cross-complementing gene I protein (XRCC), leads to camptothecin resistance in cells.[38]

Cellular processes downstream from induction and repair of DNA damage may also be important in the resistance to

PHARMACOLOGY OF CANCER THERAPEUTICS

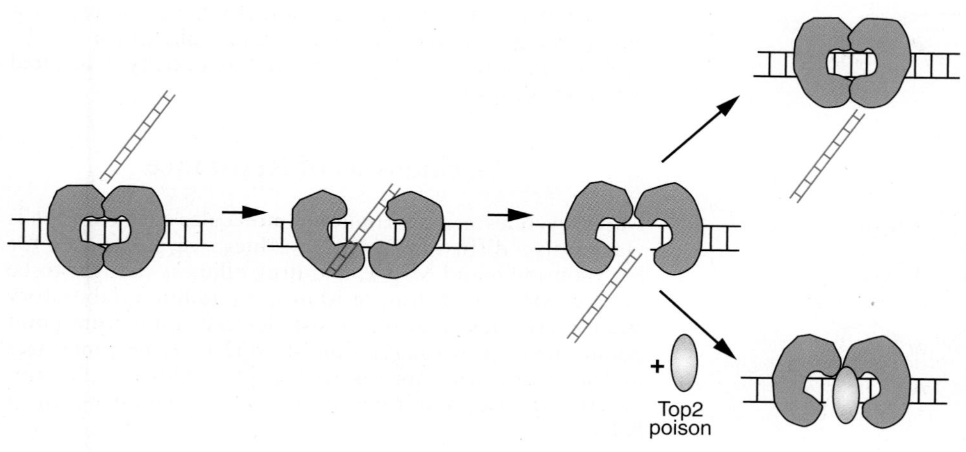

FIGURE 37.2 Topoisomerase II (Top2) mechanism of action and model for drug cytotoxicity. A Top2 (*blue*) homodimer binds to DNA, forming a double-strand DNA break in which the proteins are covalently bound to the 5′ end of broken DNA strands to form the Top2 cleavable complex. A second DNA double-helix strand (*red*) can then pass through this "gate" in an energy-dependent fashion. Finally, the broken DNA is relegated. In the presence of Top2 poisons (*yellow*) DNA is unable to relegate, leading to double-strand DNA breaks and cell death.

camptothecin. Overexpression of bcl-2 and p21$^{Waf1/Cip1}$ has been associated with relative resistance to camptothecin.[39–41] Tumor cells deficient in camptothecin-induced Top1 down-regulation were found to be more sensitive to camptothecin,[42] and pretreatment of cells with bortezomib (a dipeptide proteasome inhibitor) enhanced SN-38-mediated cellular cytotoxicity,[43] implicating ubiquitination of Top1 as an important determinant of cellular sensitivity.

Retrospective gene expression profiling has also been used to identify a gene expression "signature" in cell lines and tumor biopsy specimens that predicts for resistance to topotecan.[44] Prospective studies are needed to validate this exciting finding.

Irinotecan

Irinotecan is a prodrug containing a bulky dipiperidino side chain at C-10 (Fig. 37.3) that must be cleaved by a carboxylesterase-converting enzyme in the liver and other tissues to generate the active metabolite, SN-38. Irinotecan is FDA approved for the treatment of colorectal cancer[45,46] but is also active in the treatment of small-cell and non–small-cell lung cancers, gastric cancer, and cervical cancer (Table 37.1). Irinotecan is usually administered intravenously as a weekly infusion of 125 mg/m^2 for 4 weeks with a 2-week rest period or, alternatively, 240 to 350 mg/m^2 every 3 weeks (Table 37.2).

The most common toxicities associated with irinotecan are diarrhea and myelosuppression. Two mechanisms are involved in irinotecan-induced diarrhea. Acute cholinergic effects produced by inhibition of acetylcholinesterase by the prodrug can cause abdominal cramping and diarrhea in less than 24 hours, which can be treated with administration of atropine. Mucosal cytotoxicity that leads to diarrhea observed after 24 hours can be treated with administration of loperamide. Renal excretion of irinotecan accounts for up to 25% of the administered dose, with the remainder being eliminated by hepatic metabolism and biliary excretion. SN-38 is glucuronidated in the liver by UGT1A1, and deficiencies in this pathway may increase the risk of diarrhea and myelosuppression. Dose reductions are recommended for patients who are homozygous for the UGT1A1*28 allele,[47] for which an FDA-approved test for detection of the UGT1A1*28 allele in patients is available.[48] Additionally, dose reductions in irinotecan are also recommended for patients with hepatic dysfunction.[49]

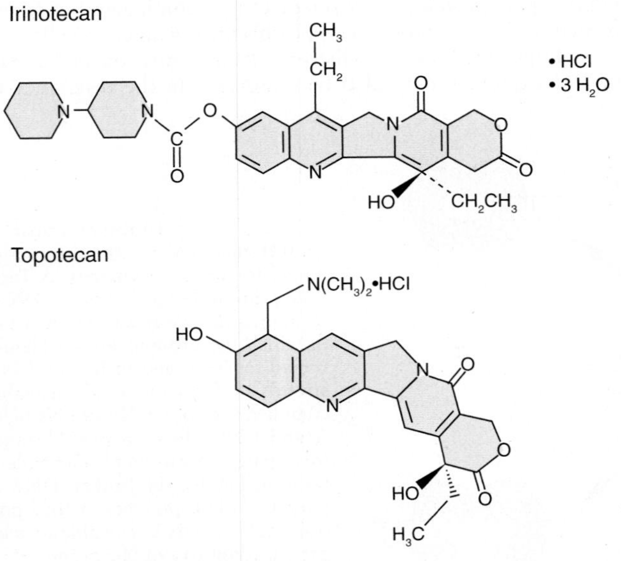

FIGURE 37.3 Camptothecin structures.

Topotecan

Topotecan contains a basic side chain at position C-9 that enhances its water solubility but does not interfere with interactions with Top1 (Fig. 37.3). Topotecan is approved for the treatment of ovarian cancer,[50] small-cell lung cancer,[51] and cervical cancer.[52] Additionally, it is active in non–small-cell lung cancer, acute myeloid leukemia, and myelodysplastic syndrome (Table 37.1). Typically, it is administered intravenously at a dose of 1.5 mg/m^2 as a 30-minute infusion daily for 5 days, followed by a 2-week period of rest (Table 37.2).

The most common dose-limiting toxicity for topotecan is myelosuppression, especially neutropenia when counts typically reach their nadir on days 9 through 14. Although thrombocytopenia and moderate to severe anemia are somewhat less common, extensive prior carboplatin treatment specifically increases the risk of subsequent thrombocytopenia.[53] Extensive prior radiation or previous bone marrow–suppressive chemotherapy increases the risk of topotecan-induced myelosuppression. Other less frequent and typically milder toxicities include nausea, vomiting, diarrhea, low-grade fevers, fatigue, alopecia, skin rash, and transient hepatic transaminitis.

Renal clearance of topotecan is the major route of elimination of the drug and its metabolites. A 50% dose reduction is recommended for patients with mild renal impairment (creatinine clearance 40 to 60 mL/min). There are no formal guidelines for dose reductions in patients with hepatic dysfunction (serum bilirubin less than10 mg/dL). Topotecan penetration into the central nervous system is greater than that of other camptothecins, resulting in cerebrospinal fluid drug concentrations that are approximately 30% of plasma levels.[54]

ANTHRACYCLINES

Anthracyclines are natural products derived from *Streptomyces peucetius* variation *caesius*. Daunorubicin and doxorubicin were discovered in the 1960s and 1970s and in the 1980s were found to target Top2.[55] They have an extremely broad range of therapeutic activity and clinical use. Subsequent searches for less toxic drugs and formulations led to the approval of liposomal doxorubicin, idarubicin, and epirubicin (Fig. 37.4).

Mechanism of Action

The anthracyclines are flat, planar molecules that are relatively hydrophobic (Fig. 37.4). They poison Top2 by intercalating DNA with high affinity and stabilize the DNA-Top2 cleavable complexes, leading to DNA double-strand breaks (Fig. 37.2).[56] Additionally, the quinone structure of anthracyclines enhances the catalysis of oxidation-reduction reactions, thereby promoting the generation of oxygen free radicals, which may be involved in antitumor effects as well as toxicity associated with these drugs.[57]

Mechanisms of Resistance

Anthracyclines are hydrophobic molecules that enter cells via passive diffusion. Anthracyclines are substrates for P-glycoprotein and Mrp-1, and drug efflux is thought to be a major affecter of drug resistance. In addition, laboratory studies have indicated that resistance can result from point mutations or down-regulation of Top2 isozymes; increases in drug-neutralizing species, such as glutathione or glutathione transferase; mutations in p53; and overexpression of Bcl-2.[58]

TABLE 37.1

MAJOR CLASSES OF CLINICALLY USEFUL TOPOISOMERASE TARGETING AGENTS

Drug	Main Therapeutic Uses	Clinical Pharmacology	Major Toxicities	Notes
CAMPTOTHECINS				
Irinotecan	FDA approved: colorectal cancer Other uses: small cell lung cancer, non–small cell lung cancer, gastric cancer, cervical cancer	50% protein bound; $t_{1/2}$ of SN-38 (active metabolite) 10–20 h; renal (25%) and biliary excretion	Diarrhea, myelosuppression	Dose reductions recommended for patients homozygous for UGT1A1*28 allele or hepatic dysfunction
Topotecan	FDA approved: ovarian cancer, cervical cancer, small cell lung cancer Other uses: non–small cell lung cancer, AML, MDS	30% protein bound; 40% oral bioavailability; $t_{1/2}$ 2–3 h (IV) or 3–6 h (oral); 33% fecal excretion (oral) and renal excretion (30% IV and 20% oral)	Myelosuppression	CSF drug levels reach 30% of plasma levels; dose reductions for renal dysfunction
ANTHRACYCLINES				
Doxorubicin and liposomal doxorubicin	FDA approved: ALL, AML, CLL, mantle cell lymphoma, non-Hodgkin's lymphoma, Hodgkin's lymphoma, Kaposi's sarcoma, mycosis fungoides, thyroid cancer, prostate cancer, breast cancer, gastric cancer, Ewing's sarcoma, non–small cell lung caner, nephroblastoma, neuroblastoma, ovarian cancer, transitional cell bladder cancer, cervical cancer, Langerhans cell cancer, multiple myeloma Other uses: soft tissue sarcoma, carcinoid, osteosarcoma, liver cancer	75% protein bound; $t_{1/2}$ 20–48 h; 40% biliary and 10% renal excretion	Myelosuppression, congestive heart failure, cardiac dysrhythmia, "radiation recall" (pericarditis, pleural effusion), secondary leukemia, mucositis	Dose reductions for hepatic dysfunction; extravasation can lead to severe skin and tissue necrosis
Daunorubicin	FDA approved: ALL, AML Other uses: Ewing's sarcoma, nephroblastoma, chronic myeloid leukemia, and non-Hodgkin's lymphoma	$T_{1/2}$ 18.5 h; 40% fecal and 25% renal excretion	Myelosuppression, congestive heart failure, cardiac dysrhythmia, secondary leukemia	Dose reductions for hepatic or renal dysfunction
Epirubicin	FDA approved: breast cancer Other uses: esophageal cancer, gastric cancer, ovarian cancer, small cell carcinoma, soft tissue sarcoma, and Hodgkin's lymphoma	77% protein bound; $t_{1/2}$ 30–36 h; 34% fecal and 27% renal excretion	Myelosuppression, congestive heart failure, cardiac dysrhythmia, secondary leukemia	Dose reductions for hepatic or renal dysfunction; extravasation can lead to severe skin and tissue necrosis

(continued)

TABLE 37.1

(CONTINUED)

Drug	Main Therapeutic Uses	Clinical Pharmacology	Major Toxicities	Notes
Idarubicin	FDA approved: AML Other uses: ALL		Myelosuppression, congestive heart failure, cardiac dysrhythmia, secondary leukemia	Dose reductions for hepatic dysfunction; extravasation can lead to severe skin and tissue necrosis
ANTHRACENEDIONES				
Mitoxantrone	FDA approved: prostate, AML Other uses: breast cancer, liver cancer, non-Hodgkin's lymphoma, ALL	78% protein bound; $t_{1/2}$ 75 h; 25% fecal and 10% renal excretion	Myelosuppression, secondary leukemia, hepatoxicity	Dose reductions for hepatic dysfunction
ACTINOMYCINS				
Dactinomycin	FDA approved: Ewing's sarcoma, gestational trophoblastic cancer, testicular cancer, nephroblastoma, rhabdomyosarcoma	$T_{1/2}$ 36 h; 50% fecal and 10% renal excretion	Myelosuppression, hepatotoxicity, veno-occlusive disease of the liver, "radiation recall"	Dose adjustments for obesity or edema; extravasation can lead to severe skin and tissue necrosis
EPIPODOPHYLLOTOXINS				
Etoposide	FDA approved: small-cell lung cancer, testicular cancer Other uses: ALL, AML, Hodgkin's lymphoma, non-Hodgkin's lymphoma, primary cutaneous T-cell lymphoma, MDS, multiple myeloma, endometrial cancer, ovarian germ cell tumor, gestational trophoblastic caner, non–small cell lung cancer, gastric cancer, osteosarcoma, retinoblastoma	25%–75% bioavailability (IV); $t_{1/2}$ 3–12 h; 40%–60% renal excretion	Myelosuppression, mucositis, secondary leukemia	Dose reductions for renal dysfunction
Teniposide	FDA approved: pediatric ALL Other uses: non-Hodgkin's lymphoma, neuroblastoma	99% protein bound; $t_{1/2}$ 5 h; 40% renal excretion	Myelosuppression, secondary leukemia, hypersensitivity reactions	Dose reductions for hepatic or renal dysfunction

FDA, U.S. Food and Drug Administration; ALL, acute lymphocytic leukemia; AML, acute myeloid leukemia; CLL, chronic lymphocytic leukemia; MDS, myelodysplastic syndrome.

Cardiac Toxicity

Anthracyclines are associated with cardiac toxicities, and special considerations are necessary from the perspective of this side effect. Acute doxorubicin cardiotoxicity is reversible, and clinical signs include tachycardia, hypotension, electrocardiogram changes, and arrhythmias. Acute toxicity develops during or within days of anthracycline infusion, the incidence of which has been significantly reduced by slowing doxorubicin infusion rates. Chronic cardiotoxicity is the most common type of anthracycline damage and is irreversible. Chronic cardiotoxicity peaks at 1 to 3 months but can occur even years after therapy. Congestive heart failure from congestive cardiomyopathy is more common and of greater clinical significance than are the acute cardiac effects associated with anthracyclines. Myocardial damage occurs by several mechanisms, the most important of which is generation of reactive oxygen species during electron transfer from the semiquinone to quinone moieties of the anthracycline.[57] The generation of hydrogen peroxide and the

TABLE 37.2

COMMON DOSES FOR THE CAMPTOTHECINS

Drug	FDA Indication	Usual Dose	Dose Adjustments
Irinotecan	Colorectal	125 mg/m^2 weekly for 4 weeks with a 2-week rest or 350 mg/m^2 every 3 weeks or 180 mg/m^2 every 2 weeks	Homozygous UGT1A1*28 or Hepatic dysfunction
Topotecan	Small-cell lung Ovarian Cervical	1.5 mg/m^2 daily for 5 days every 3 weeks 0.75 mg/m^2 daily for 3 days every 3 weeks	Renal dysfunction

FDA, U.S. Food and Drug Administration.

peroxidation of myocardial lipids contribute to myocardial damage. Endomyocardial biopsy is characterized by a predominant finding of multifocal areas of patchy and interstitial fibrosis (stellate scars) and occasional vacuolated myocardial cells (Adria cells). Myocyte hypertrophy and degeneration, loss of cross-striations, and absence of myocarditis are also characteristic of this diagnosis.[59] The incidence of cardiomyopathy is related to both cumulative dose and schedule of administration, and predisposition to cardiac damage includes a previous history of heart disease, hypertension, radiation to the mediastinum, age younger than 4 years, prior use of anthracyclines or other cardiac toxins, and coadministration of other chemotherapy agents (e.g., paclitaxel, cyclophosphamide, or trastuzumab).[60,61] Sequential administration of paclitaxel followed by doxorubicin in breast cancer patients is associated with cardiomyopathy at total doxorubicin doses above 340 to 380 mg/m^2, whereas the reverse sequence of drug administration did not yield the same systemic toxicities.[62] Table 37.2 lists the incidence of clinically detectable congestive heart failure when doxorubicin is given at doses of 40 to 75 mg/m^2 as a bolus injection every 3 to 4 weeks. When doxorubicin is given by a low-dose weekly regimen (10 to 20 mg/m^2/wk) or by slow continuous infusion over 96 hours, cumulative doses of more than 500 mg/m^2 can be given. Doses of epirubicin below 1,000 mg/m^2 and daunorubicin below 550 mg/m^2 are considered safe. Additionally, liposomal doxorubicin is associated with less cardiac toxicity.

Cardiac function can be monitored during treatment with anthracyclines by electrocardiography, echocardiography, or radionuclide scans. Numerous studies demonstrate the danger of embarking on anthracycline therapy in patients with underlying cardiac disease (e.g., a baseline left ventricular ejection fraction of less than 50%) and of continuing therapy after a documented decrease in ejection fraction by more than 10% (if this decrease falls below the lower limit of normal). Dexrazoxane is a metal chelator that decreases the myocardial toxicity of doxorubicin in breast cancer patients and is approved for that use by the FDA.[62] Dexrazoxane chelates iron and copper, thereby interfering with the redox reactions that generate free radicals and damage myocardial lipids.

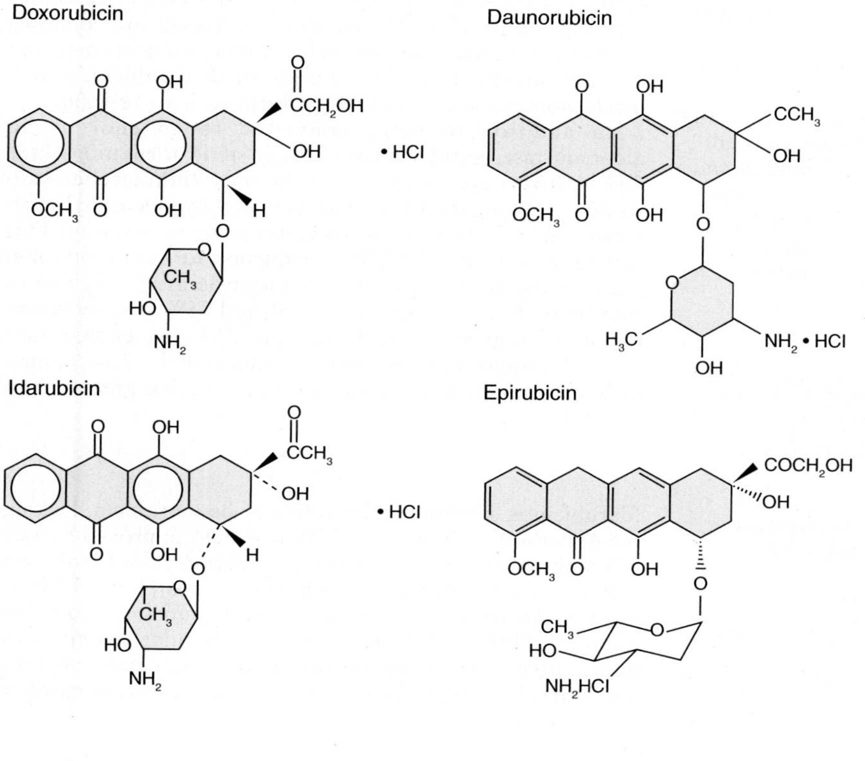

Doxorubicin

Daunorubicin

Idarubicin

Epirubicin

FIGURE 37.4 Anthracycline structures.

Doxorubicin

Doxorubicin differs from daunorubicin by a single hydroxyl group at C14 (Fig. 37.4). It is available in a standard salt form and as a liposomal formulation. FDA-labeled indications for standard doxorubicin include acute lymphoid leukemia, acute myeloid leukemia, chronic lymphoid leukemia, Hodgkin's lymphoma, non-Hodgkin's lymphoma, mantle cell lymphoma, multiple myeloma, mycosis fungoides, Kaposi's sarcoma, breast cancer (adjuvant therapy and advanced), advanced prostate cancer, advanced gastric cancer, Ewing's sarcoma, thyroid cancer, advanced nephroblastoma, advanced neuroblastoma, advanced non–small-cell lung cancer, advanced ovarian cancer, advanced transitional cell bladder cancer, cervical cancer, and Langerhans cell tumors. Doxorubicin has activity in other malignancies as well, including soft tissue sarcoma, osteosarcoma, carcinoid, and liver cancer (Table 37.1). Liposomal doxorubicin is FDA-approved for Kaposi's sarcoma and advanced ovarian cancer[63] (Table 37.1). Doxorubicin is typically administered at a recommended dose of 30 to 75 mg/m^2 every 3 weeks intravenously, and liposomal doxorubicin doses range from 20 to 60 mg/m^2 every 3 weeks intravenously (Table 37.3).

Major acute toxicities of doxorubicin include myelosuppression, mucositis, alopecia, nausea, and vomiting. Myelosuppression is the acute dose-limiting toxicity and the white blood cell count typically reaches a nadir at 10 to 14 days. Diarrhea, nausea, vomiting, mucositis, and alopecia are dose- and schedule-related toxicities. Prophylactic antiemetics are routinely given with bolus doses of doxorubicin and longer infusions are associated with less nausea. Doxorubicin is a potent vesicant, and extravasation can lead to severe necrosis of skin and local tissues, requiring surgical debridement and skin grafts. Care must be taken to avoid extravasation, and longer infusions are recommended via a central venous catheter. Acute treatment with ice and dimethyl sulfoxide may minimize extravasation-induced tissue damage. In contrast, a "flare reaction" of erythema around the infusion site is a benign reaction. Patients should also be warned to expect their urine to redden after drug administration. Liposomal doxorubicin is associated with less nausea and vomiting and relatively mild myelosuppression. Liposomal doxorubicin can also cause hand-foot syndrome and an acute infusion reaction manifested by flushing, dyspnea, edema, fever, chills, rash, bronchospasm, and hypertension. These infusion-related events appear to be related to the rate of drug infusion.

Other toxicities of doxorubicin are "radiation recall" and the risk of developing secondary leukemia. "Radiation recall" is an inflammatory reaction at sites of previous radiation and can lead to pericarditis, pleural effusion, and skin rash. Secondary leukemias are thought to be a result of balanced translocations that result from Top2 poisoning by the anthracyclines, albeit to lesser degree than other Top2 poisons, such as the epipodophyllotoxins.[64]

TABLE 37.3

INCIDENCE OF CONGESTIVE HEART FAILURE AS A FUNCTION OF CUMULATIVE DOSE OF DOXORUBICIN

Cumulative Dose of Doxorubicin (mg/m^2)	Incidence of Congestive Heart Failure (%)
300	1–2
400	3–5
450	5–8
500	6–20

Anthracyclines are metabolized in the liver and excreted in the bile. Dose reductions should be made in patients with elevated plasma bilirubin. Doxorubicin may be dose reduced by 50% for plasma bilirubin concentrations ranging from 1.2 to 3.0 mg/dL, by 75% for values of 3.1 to 5.0 mg/dL, and withheld for values greater than 5 mg/dL. Additionally, anthracyclines are reduced to enols at the 13-keto group by aldoreductases, which are found in most tissues. The enols are active, however, slightly less than the parental compounds because of reduced lipophilicity and decreased cellular penetration. Doxorubicin is less avidly metabolized by this route. Finally, urinary excretion of doxorubicin and other anthracyclines is low, comprising less than 10% of the administered dose.

Daunorubicin

Daunorubicin is similar in structure to doxorubicin (Fig. 37.4). It is FDA approved for the treatment of acute lymphoid leukemia and acute myeloid leukemia. Additionally, it has activity in Ewing's sarcoma, nephroblastoma, chronic myeloid leukemia, and non-Hodgkin's lymphoma (Table 37.1). Daunorubicin is typically administered intravenously 30 to 45 mg/m^2 on 3 consecutive days in combination chemotherapy (Table 37.4). Daunorubicin has similar toxicities to doxorubicin, including myelosuppression, cardiac toxicity, nausea, vomiting, and alopecia. Similar to doxorubicin, care should be taken to prevent extravasation. Daunorubicin is metabolized by the liver and also undergoes substantial elimination by the kidneys. Therefore, 50% dose reductions are recommended for serum creatinine greater than 3 mg/dL. Dose reductions of 25% are recommended for plasma bilirubin concentrations ranging from 1.2 to 3.0 mg/dL, and 50% for values of greater than 3 mg/dL.

Epirubicin

Epirubicin is an epimer of doxorubicin with increased lipophilicity (Fig. 37.4). It is FDA approved for adjuvant therapy of breast cancer but is also active in esophageal cancer, gastric cancer, ovarian cancer, small-cell carcinoma, soft tissue sarcoma, and Hodgkin's lymphoma (Table 37.1). Typical doses of epirubicin are 60 to 120 mg/m^2 every 3 to 4 weeks given intravenously (Table 37.4). The incidence of nausea and vomiting, alopecia, and cardiac toxicity is less with epirubicin compared to doxorubicin. However, similar to doxorubicin, severe myelosuppression can occur. Epirubicin is also a vesicant.

In addition to being converted to an enol by an aldoreductase, epirubicin has a unique steric orientation of the C-4 hydroxyl group, making it the only anthracycline substrate for conjugation reactions mediated by glucuronyltransferases and sulfatases. Dose adjustments are recommended for hepatic dysfunction: 50% dose reduction for serum bilirubin 1.2 to 3 mg/dL or aspartate aminotransferase (AST) two to four times the upper limit of normal, and 75% dose reduction for bilirubin greater than 3 mg/dL or AST greater than four times the upper limit of normal. Additionally, dose adjustments are recommended for serum creatinine greater than 5 mg/dL.

Idarubicin

Idarubicin is a synthetic derivative of daunorubicin, lacking the 4-methoxy group (Fig. 37.4). It is FDA approved as part of combination chemotherapy for acute myeloid leukemia and is also active in acute lymphoid leukemia (Table 37.1). It is given intravenously at a dose of 12 mg/m^2 for 3 consecutive days (Table 37.4). Idarubicin has similar toxicities as daunorubicin, including myelosuppression, nausea, vomiting, alopecia, cardiac toxicity, and tissue necrosis in cases of

TABLE 37.4

COMMON DOSES FOR THE ANTHRACYCLINES

Drug	FDA Indication	Usual Dose	Dose Adjustments
Doxorubicin	ALL AML CLL Kaposi's sarcoma Non-Hodgkin's lymphoma Mantle cell lymphoma Mycosis fungoides Hodgkin's lymphoma Breast Gastric Ewing's sarcoma Prostate Thyroid Nephroblastoma Neuroblastoma Non–small cell lung Ovarian Transitional cell bladder	40–60 mg/m² every 3–4 weeks or 60–75 mg/m² every 3 weeks	Hepatic dysfunction
	Cervical	30 mg/m²	
	Langerhans cell	50 mg on days 1 and 22 every 42 days	
	Multiple myeloma	9 mg/m² continuous infusion days 1 to 4	
Liposomal doxorubicin	Kaposi's sarcoma Ovarian	20 mg/m² every 3 weeks 50 mg/m² every 4 weeks	Hepatic dysfunction
Daunorubicin	ALL AML	30–45 mg/m² daily for 3 days	Renal or hepatic dysfunction
Epirubicin	Breast	100–120 mg/m² every 3–4 weeks or 60 mg/m² weekly for 2 weeks followed by 1–2 weeks rest	Hepatic or renal dysfunction
Idarubicin	AML	10–12 mg/m² daily for 2–3 days	Hepatic or renal dysfunction

FDA, U.S. Food and Drug Administration; ALL, acute lymphocytic leukemia; AML, acute myeloid leukemia; CLL, chronic lymphocytic leukemia.

extravasation. Aldoreductases convert idarubicin to idarubicinol, which is more lipophilic than the enols of other anthracyclines. Fifty percent dose reductions are recommended for serum bilirubin of 2.6 to 5 mg/dL and it should not be given if the bilirubin is greater than 5 mg/dL. Additionally, dose reductions in renal impairment are advised, but specific guidelines are not available.

ANTHRACENEDIONES

Mitoxantrone

Mitoxantrone is the only anthracenedione that is FDA approved (Fig. 37.5). It was originally synthesized in the 1970s in a search for anthracycline analogs with less cardiac toxicity. Mitoxantrone is a DNA intercalator and stabilizes the Top2-DNA complex, leading to double-strand DNA breaks.[65] Relative to anthracyclines, mitoxantrone is less likely to undergo oxidation-reduction reactions and form free radicals, thereby decreasing its cardiac toxicity. Mechanisms of resistance to mitoxantrone include drug efflux by BCRP,[66] mutant Top2α,[67–69] and loss of DNA mismatch repair proteins, MSH2 and MLH1.[70]

Mitoxantrone is FDA approved for treatment of advanced hormone-refractory prostate cancer[71] and acute myeloid leukemia.[72] It also has activity in metastatic breast cancer, liver cancer, non-Hodgkin's lymphoma, and acute lymphoid leukemia (Table 37.1). This drug is typically administered intravenously at a dose of 12 mg/m² for 3 days in the treatment of acute myeloid leukemia (typically in combination with cytosine arabinoside), and 12 to 14 mg/m² every 3 weeks in the treatment of prostate cancer (Table 37.5).

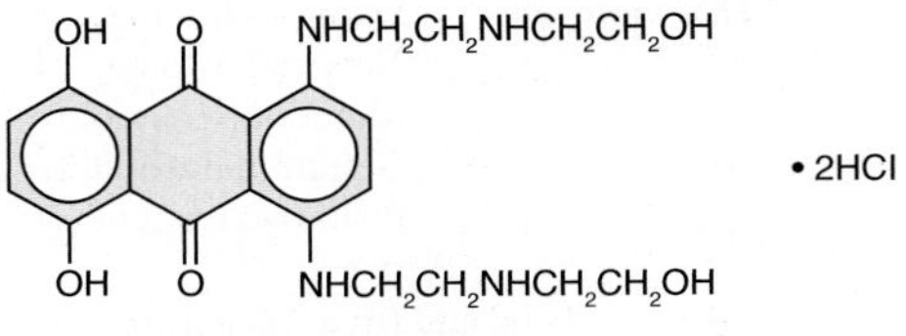

FIGURE 37.5 Mitoxantrone structure.

TABLE 37.5

COMMON DOSES FOR MITOXANTRONE

Drug	FDA Indication	Usual Dose	Dose Adjustments
Mitoxantrone	Prostate	12–14 mg/m² every 3 weeks	Hepatic dysfunction
	AML	12 mg/m² daily for 3 days	

FDA, U.S. Food and Drug Administration; AML, acute myeloid leukemia.

Dose-limiting toxicities involve myelosuppression. Nausea, vomiting, alopecia, and mucositis are less common compared to doxorubicin. Cardiac toxicity is generally seen at cumulative doses greater than 160 mg/m².[73] Mitoxantrone is rapidly cleared from the plasma and is highly concentrated in tissues. A small amount is cleared via the kidney and most of the drug is excreted in the feces. Dose adjustments for hepatic dysfunction are recommended, but formal guidelines are not available.

Dactinomycin

Actinomycins were the first anticancer antibiotics isolated from the culture broth of *Streptomyces* in the 1940s. The derivative presently in use is dactinomycin. Structurally, dactinomycin is a "chromopeptide," consisting of a planar phenoxazone ring (which produces the yellow-red color of the drug), attached to two peptide side chains (Fig. 37.6). Dactinomycin can intercalate into DNA between adjacent guanine-cytosine bases, thereby poisoning Top2 and leading to lethal double-strand DNA breaks. Dactinomycin was one of the first drugs shown to be transported by P-glycoprotein, which represents the major mechanism of cellular resistance.[74]

Dactinomycin is FDA approved for Ewing's sarcoma, gestational trophoblastic neoplasm, metastatic testicular cancer, nephroblastoma, and rhabdomyosarcoma (Table 37.1). Typically it is administered intravenously at doses of 12 to 15 mcg/kg for 5 days (Table 37.6). Toxicities include myelosuppression, veno-occlusive disease of the liver, nausea, vomiting, alopecia, erythema, and acne. Additionally, similar to doxorubicin, dactinomycin can cause "radiation recall" and severe tissue necrosis in cases of extravasation. Dactinomycin is largely excreted unchanged in the feces and urine. Guidelines for dosing in patients with impaired renal or liver function are not available.

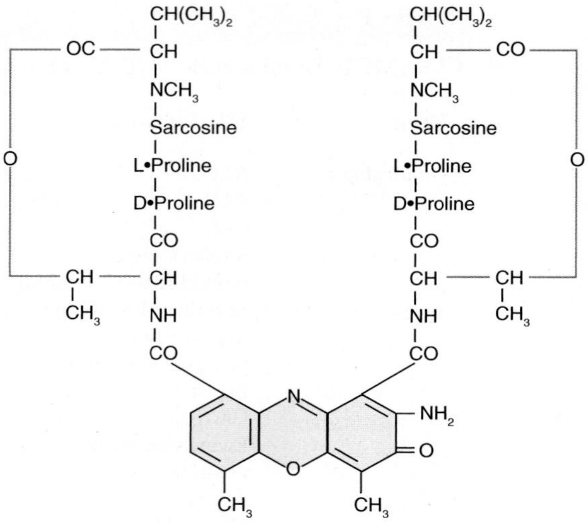

FIGURE 37.6 Dactinomycin structure.

EPIPODOPHYLLOTOXINS

Epipodophyllotoxins are glycoside derivatives of podophyllotoxin, an antimicrotubule agent extracted from the mandrake plant (Fig. 37.7). Interestingly, rather than having antimicrotubule activity, two derivatives, etoposide and teniposide, function as Top2 poisons.

Mechanism of Action

Although epipodophyllotoxins were shown to poison Top2 isozymes, they are not DNA intercalators and, therefore, poison Top2 by a mechanism that is distinct from that of the anthracyclines and other DNA intercalators.[75]

Mechanisms of Resistance

Similar to other natural product-derived Top2-targeting agents, epipodophyllotoxins are substrates for P-glycoprotein.[76] Additionally, altered localization of Top2α decreased cellular expression of Top2α[77] and impaired phosphorylation of Top2 have been implicated in resistance to etoposide.[78]

Etoposide

Etoposide (Fig. 37.7) is available in intravenous and oral forms. It is FDA approved for treatment of small-cell lung cancer and

TABLE 37.6

COMMON DOSES FOR DACTINOMYCIN

Drug	FDA Indication	Usual Dose	Dose Adjustments
Dactinomycin	Ewing's sarcoma Nephroblastoma Rhabdomyosarcoma Gestational trophoblastic	12–15 mcg/kg daily for 5 days	Obesity or edema
	Pediatric testicular	1,000 mcg/m²	

FDA, U.S. Food and Drug Administration.

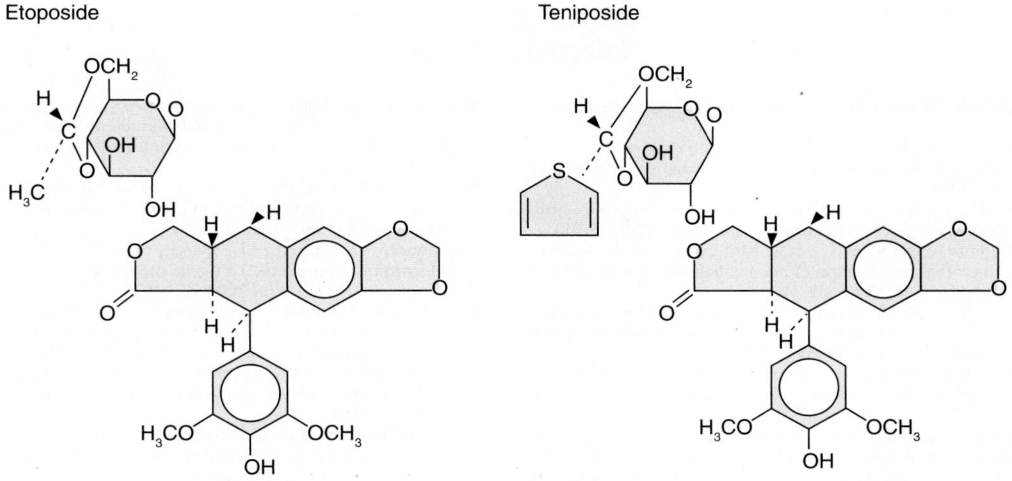

Etoposide

Teniposide

FIGURE 37.7 Epipodophyllotoxin structures.

refractory testicular cancer. It also has activity in acute lymphoid leukemia, acute myeloid leukemia, Hodgkin's and non-Hodgkin's lymphoma, primary cutaneous T-cell lymphoma, myelodysplastic syndrome, multiple myeloma, endometrial cancer, gastric cancer, ovarian germ cell tumor, gestational trophoblastic neoplasm, non–small cell lung cancer, osteosarcoma, and retinoblastoma (Table 37.1). The intravenous form is generally administered at doses of 35 to 50 mg/m^2 for 4 to 5 days every 3 to 4 weeks in combination therapy for small cell lung cancer and 50 to 100 mg/m^2 for 5 days every 3 to 4 weeks in combination therapy for refractory testicular cancer (Table 37.7). The dose of oral etoposide is usually twice the intravenous dose.

The dose-limiting toxicity for etoposide is myelosuppression, with white blood cell count nadirs typically occurring on days 10 to 14. Thrombocytopenia is less common than leukopenia. Additionally, mild to moderate nausea, vomiting, diarrhea, mucositis, and alopecia are associated with etoposide. Among the Top2 poisons, epipodophyllotoxins are associated with the greatest risk for development of secondary malignancies, with a 4% 6-year cumulative risk.[79] Myelomonocytic (FAB M4) and monoblastic (FAB M5) variants of acute myeloid leukemia are the most common presentations of epipodophyllotoxin-related leukemia resulting from balanced translocations affecting the breakpoint cluster region of the *MLL* gene at chromosome 11q23.[64]

The oral bioavailability of etoposide is dependent on intestinal P-glycoprotein and is highly variable, with an average value of about 50%.[80] The majority of etoposide is cleared unchanged by the kidneys and a 25% dose reduction is recommended in patients with a creatinine clearance of 15 to 50 mL/min. A 50% dose reduction is recommended in patients with a creatinine clearance less than 15 mL/min. Given that the unbound fraction of etoposide is dependent on albumin and bilirubin concentrations, dose adjustments for hepatic dysfunction are advised, but consensus guidelines are not available.

Teniposide

Teniposide contains a thiophene group in place of the methyl group on the glucose moiety of etoposide (Fig. 37.7). Teniposide is FDA approved for refractory pediatric acute lymphoid leukemia and is also used in adult neuroblastoma and non-Hodgkin's lymphoma (Table 37.1). The typical dose in adults ranges from 30 to 100 mg/m^2 intravenously, used either alone or in combination chemotherapy (Table 37.7). Similar to etoposide, the dose-limiting toxicity of teniposide is myelosuppression. Additional toxicities include mild to moderate nausea, vomiting, diarrhea, alopecia, and secondary leukemia. Teniposide is associated with greater frequency of hypersensitivity reactions compared to etoposide.

Teniposide is 99% bound to albumin and compared to etoposide is more hepatically metabolized and less renally cleared. No specific guidelines are available on dose adjustments for renal or hepatic dysfunction.

TABLE 37.7

COMMON DOSES FOR THE EPIPODOPHYLLOTOXINS

Drug	FDA Indication	Usual Dose	Dose Adjustments
Etoposide	Small-cell lung	35–50 mg/m^2 intravenously for 4–5 days repeated every 3–4 weeks (oral dose is twice the intravenous dose)	Renal dysfunction
	Testicular	50–100 mg/m^2 intravenously daily for 5 days every 3–4 weeks	
Teniposide	Pediatric ALL	165–250 mg/m^2 weekly or twice weekly	Hepatic or renal dysfunction

FDA, U.S. Food and Drug Administration; ALL, acute lymphocytic leukemia.

Selected References

The full list of references for this chapter appears in the online version.

1. Wang JC. DNA topoisomerases. *Annu Rev Biochem* 1996;65:635.
2. Champoux JJ. DNA topoisomerases: structure, function, and mechanism. *Annu Rev Biochem* 2001;70:369.
3. Wall ME, Wani MC. Camptothecin and taxol: discovery to clinic—thirteenth Bruce F. Cain Memorial Award Lecture. *Cancer Res* 1995;55:753.
4. Hertzberg RP, Caranfa MJ, Holden KG, et al. Modification of the hydroxy lactone ring of camptothecin: inhibition of mammalian topoisomerase I and biological activity. *J Med Chem* 1989;32:715.
5. Hsiang YH, Lihou MG, Liu LF. Arrest of replication forks by drug-stabilized topoisomerase I-DNA cleavable complexes as a mechanism of cell killing by camptothecin. *Cancer Res* 1989;49:5077.
6. Staker BL, Hjerrild K, Feese MD, et al. The mechanism of topoisomerase I poisoning by a camptothecin analog. *Proc Natl Acad Sci U S A* 2002;99:15387.
7. D'Arpa P, Beardmore C, Liu LF. Involvement of nucleic acid synthesis in cell killing mechanisms of topoisomerase poisons. *Cancer Res* 1990;50:6919.
8. Rasheed ZA, Rubin EH. Mechanisms of resistance to topoisomerase I-targeting drugs. *Oncogene* 2003;22:7296.
9. Gupta E, Luo F, Lallo A, et al. The intestinal absorption of camptothecin, a highly lipophilic drug, across Caco-2 cells is mediated by active transporter(s). *Anticancer Res* 2000;20:1013.
10. Ma J, Maliepaard M, Nooter K, et al. Reduced cellular accumulation of topotecan: a novel mechanism of resistance in a human ovarian cancer cell line. *Br J Cancer* 1998;77:1645.
14. Honjo Y, Hrycyna CA, Yan QW, et al. Acquired mutations in the MXR/BCRP/ABCP gene alter substrate specificity in MXR/BCRP/ABCP-overexpressing cells. *Cancer Res* 2001;61:6635.
16. Danks MK, Morton CL, Pawlik CA, Potter PM. Overexpression of a rabbit liver carboxylesterase sensitizes human tumor cells to CPT-11. *Cancer Res* 1998;58:20.
17. Ahmed F, Vyas V, Cornfield A, et al. In vitro activation of irinotecan to SN-38 by human liver and intestine. *Anticancer Res* 1999;19:2067.
21. Ciotti M, Basu N, Brangi M, Owens IS. Glucuronidation of 7-ethyl-10-hydroxycamptothecin (SN-38) by the human UDP-glucuronosyltransferases encoded at the UGT1 locus. *Biochem Biophys Res Commun* 1999;260:199.
23. Brangi M, Litman T, Ciotti M, et al. Camptothecin resistance: role of the ATP-binding cassette (ABC), mitoxantrone-resistance half-transporter (MXR), and potential for glucuronidation in MXR-expressing cells. *Cancer Res* 1999;59:5938.
25. Tsurutani J, Nitta T, Hirashima T, et al. Point mutations in the topoisomerase I gene in patients with non-small cell lung cancer treated with irinotecan. *Lung Cancer* 2002;35:299.
26. Kerrigan JE, Pilch DS. A structural model for the ternary cleavable complex formed between human topoisomerase I, DNA, and camptothecin. *Biochemistry* 2001;40:9792.
27. Bharti AK, Olson MO, Kufe DW, Rubin EH. Identification of a nucleolin binding site in human topoisomerase I. *J Biol Chem* 1996;271:1993.
30. Cliby WA, Lewis KA, Lilly KK, Kaufmann SH. S phase and G2 arrests induced by topoisomerase I poisons are dependent on ATR kinase function. *J Biol Chem* 2002;277:1599.
33. Lebel M, Leder P. A deletion within the murine Werner syndrome helicase induces sensitivity to inhibitors of topoisomerase and loss of cellular proliferative capacity. *Proc Natl Acad Sci U S A* 1998;95:13097.
34. Pichierri P, Franchitto A, Piergentili R, Colussi C, Palitti F. Hypersensitivity to camptothecin in MSH2 deficient cells is correlated with a role for MSH2 protein in recombinational repair. *Carcinogenesis* 2001;22:1781.
37. Barthelmes HU, Habermeyer M, Christensen MO, et al. TDP1 overexpression in human cells counteracts DNA damage mediated by topoisomerases I and II. *J Biol Chem* 2004;279:55618.
38. Park SY, Lam W, Cheng YC. X-ray repair cross-complementing gene I protein plays an important role in camptothecin resistance. *Cancer Res* 2002;62:459.
40. Walton MI, Whysong D, O'Connor PM, et al. Constitutive expression of human Bcl-2 modulates nitrogen mustard and camptothecin induced apoptosis. *Cancer Res* 1993;53:1853.
41. Zhang Y, Fujita N, Tsuruo T. p21Waf1/Cip1 acts in synergy with bcl-2 to confer multidrug resistance in a camptothecin-selected human lung-cancer cell line. *Int J Cancer* 1999;83:790.
42. Desai SD, Li TK, Rodriguez-Bauman A, Rubin EH, Liu LF. Ubiquitin/26S proteasome-mediated degradation of topoisomerase I as a resistance mechanism to camptothecin in tumor cells. *Cancer Res* 2001;61:5926.
43. Cusack JC Jr, Liu R, Houston M, et al. Enhanced chemosensitivity to CPT-11 with proteasome inhibitor PS-341: implications for systemic nuclear factor-kappaB inhibition. *Cancer Res* 2001;61:3535.
45. Douillard JY, Cunningham D, Roth AD, et al. Irinotecan combined with fluorouracil compared with fluorouracil alone as first-line treatment for metastatic colorectal cancer: a multicentre randomised trial. *Lancet* 2000;355:1041.
46. Saltz LB, Cox JV, Blanke C, et al. Irinotecan plus fluorouracil and leucovorin for metastatic colorectal cancer. Irinotecan Study Group. *N Engl J Med* 2000;343:905.
48. Innocenti F, Undevia SD, Iyer L, et al. Genetic variants in the UDP-glucuronosyltransferase 1A1 gene predict the risk of severe neutropenia of irinotecan. *J Clin Oncol* 2004;22:1382.
49. Schaaf LJ, Hammond LA, Tipping SJ, et al. Phase 1 and pharmacokinetic study of intravenous irinotecan in refractory solid tumor patients with hepatic dysfunction. *Clin Cancer Res* 2006;12:3782.
50. ten Bokkel Huinink W, Gore M, Carmichael J, et al. Topotecan versus paclitaxel for the treatment of recurrent epithelial ovarian cancer. *J Clin Oncol* 1997;15:2183.
51. Ardizzoni A, Hansen H, Dombernowsky P, et al. Topotecan, a new active drug in the second-line treatment of small-cell lung cancer: a phase II study in patients with refractory and sensitive disease. The European Organization for Research and Treatment of Cancer Early Clinical Studies Group and New Drug Development Office, and the Lung Cancer Cooperative Group. *J Clin Oncol* 1997;15:2090.
54. Baker SD, Heideman RL, Crom WR, et al. Cerebrospinal fluid pharmacokinetics and penetration of continuous infusion topotecan in children with central nervous system tumors. *Cancer Chemother Pharmacol* 1996;37:195.
56. Tewey KM, Rowe TC, Yang L, Halligan BD, Liu LF. Adriamycin-induced DNA damage mediated by mammalian DNA topoisomerase II. *Science (New York)* 1984;226:466.
58. Rubin EH, Li TK, Duann P, Liu LF. Cellular resistance to topoisomerase poisons. *Cancer Treat Res* 1996;87:243.
62. Shan K, Lincoff AM, Young JB. Anthracycline-induced cardiotoxicity. *Ann Intern Med* 1996;125:47.
63. Harrison M, Tomlinson D, Stewart S. Liposomal-entrapped doxorubicin: an active agent in AIDS-related Kaposi's sarcoma. *J Clin Oncol* 1995;13:914.
64. Felix CA, Kolaris CP, Osheroff N. Topoisomerase II and the etiology of chromosomal translocations. *DNA Repair* 2006;5:1093.
65. Crespi MD, Ivanier SE, Genovese J, Baldi A. Mitoxantrone affects topoisomerase activities in human breast cancer cells. *Biochem Biophys Res Commun* 1986;136:521.
67. Mirski SE, Cole SP. Cytoplasmic localization of a mutant M(r) 160,000 topoisomerase II alpha is associated with the loss of putative bipartite nuclear localization signals in a drug-resistant human lung cancer cell line. *Cancer Res* 1995;55:2129.
68. Harker WG, Slade DL, Parr RL, et al. Alterations in the topoisomerase II alpha gene, messenger RNA, and subcellular protein distribution as well as reduced expression of the DNA topoisomerase II beta enzyme in a mitoxantrone-resistant HL-60 human leukemia cell line. *Cancer Res* 1995;55:1707.
69. Wessel I, Jensen PB, Falck J, et al. Loss of amino acids 1490Lys-Ser-Lys1492 in the COOH-terminal region of topoisomerase IIalpha in human small cell lung cancer cells selected for resistance to etoposide results in an extranuclear enzyme localization. *Cancer Res* 1997;57:4451.
70. Fedier A, Schwarz VA, Walt H, et al. Resistance to topoisomerase poisons due to loss of DNA mismatch repair. *Int J Cancer* 2001;93:571.
71. Tannock IF, Osoba D, Stockler MR, et al. Chemotherapy with mitoxantrone plus prednisone or prednisone alone for symptomatic hormone-resistant prostate cancer: a Canadian randomized trial with palliative end points. *J Clin Oncol* 1996;14:1756.
72. Reece DE, Elmongy MB, Barnett MJ, et al. Chemotherapy with high-dose cytosine arabinoside and mitoxantrone for poor-prognosis myeloid leukemias. *Cancer Invest* 1993;11:509.
75. Ross W, Rowe T, Glisson B, Yalowich J, Liu L. Role of topoisomerase II in mediating epipodophyllotoxin-induced DNA cleavage. *Cancer Res* 1984;44:5857.
77. Valkov NI, Gump JL, Engel R, Sullivan DM. Cell density-dependent VP-16 sensitivity of leukaemic cells is accompanied by the translocation of topoisomerase IIalpha from the nucleus to the cytoplasm. *Br J Haematol* 2000;108:331.
78. Takano H, Kohno K, Ono M, Uchida Y, Kuwano M. Increased phosphorylation of DNA topoisomerase II in etoposide-resistant mutants of human cancer KB cells. *Cancer Res* 1991;51:3951.
79. Smith MA, Rubinstein L, Anderson JR, et al. Secondary leukemia or myelodysplastic syndrome after treatment with epipodophyllotoxins. *J Clin Oncol* 1999;17:569.

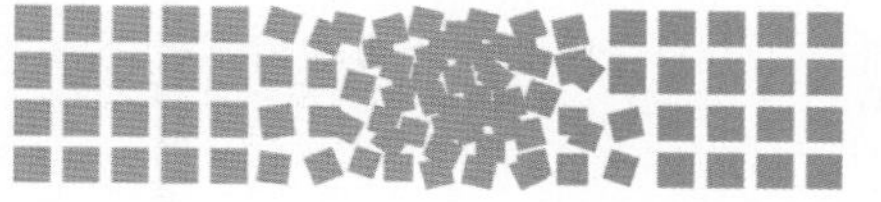

CHAPTER 38 ANTIMICROTUBULE AGENTS

MAYSA M. ABU-KHALAF AND LYNDSAY N. HARRIS

MICROTUBULES

Microtubules are vital and dynamic cellular organelles that play a critical role in cell division, directional transport of vesicles and organelles, signaling, cell shape, and polarity.[1] Microtubules are composed of 13 linear protofilaments of polymerized $\alpha\beta$-tubulin heterodimers arranged in parallel around a cylindrical axis.[2] The specific biologic functions of microtubules are due to their unique polymerization dynamics. Tubulin polymerization is mediated by a nucleation-elongation mechanism. One end of the microtubule, termed the *plus end*, is kinetically more dynamic than the other end, termed the *minus end*. Microtubule dynamics are governed by two principal processes. The first, known as *treadmilling*, is the net growth at one end of the microtubule and the net shortening at the opposite end.[2] The second dynamic behavior, termed *dynamic instability*, is a process in which the microtubule ends switch spontaneously between states of slow sustained growth and rapid shortening.

TAXANES

The unique chemical structure and mechanism of action of the taxanes, coupled with their broad antitumor activities, has rendered the taxanes one of the most important classes of anticancer agents. Interest in the taxanes began in 1963, when a crude extract of the bark of the Pacific yew tree, *Taxus brevifolia*, was shown to have impressive activity in preclinical tumor models. In 1971, paclitaxel was identified as the active constituent of the bark extract.[3] The initial development of paclitaxel was hampered by the limited supply of its source as a natural product and its poor aqueous solubility, however, its novel mechanism of action encouraged its evaluation in preclinical and clinical settings. The early search for taxanes derived from more abundant and renewable resources led to the development of docetaxel, which is synthesized by the addition of a side chain to 10-deacetylbaccatin III, an inactive taxane precursor found in the needles and other components of more abundant yew species.[3] The structures of paclitaxel and docetaxel are shown in Figure 38.1. The taxane rings of paclitaxel and docetaxel are linked to an ester side chain attached to the C13 position of the ring, which is essential for antimicrotubule and antitumor activity. Their respective structures differ with respect to substitutions at position C10 of the taxane ring position and on the ester side chain attached at position C13.

Paclitaxel initially received regulatory approval in the United States in 1992 for the treatment of patients with ovarian cancer after failure of first-line or subsequent chemotherapy (Table 38.1).[3] Subsequently, it has been approved for several other indications, including advanced breast cancer after failure of combination chemotherapy or at relapse within 6 months of adjuvant chemotherapy[4]; advanced ovarian cancer in combination with a platinum compound; adjuvant combination chemotherapy of lymph node–positive breast cancer sequentially after standard doxorubicin-based chemotherapy[5]; second-line treatment of AIDS-related Kaposi's sarcoma S; and first-line treatment of non–small cell lung cancer in combination with cisplatin (Table 38.1).[6] In addition to the U.S. Food and Drug Administration (FDA) on-label indications, paclitaxel is widely used for several other tumor types, such as cancer of unknown origin, bladder, esophagus, gastric, head and neck, and cervical cancers. The U.S. patent for paclitaxel expired in 2002, and a generic form of paclitaxel is now available.

Docetaxel was first approved for use in the United States in 1996 for patients with metastatic breast cancer that progressed or relapsed after anthracycline-based chemotherapy, which was later broadened to a general second-line indication (Table 38.1).[3,4] Subsequently, it received regulatory approval for several other indications: adjuvant chemotherapy of lymph node–positive breast cancer in combination with adriamycin-based chemotherapy (TAC)[7]; first-line chemotherapy for locally advanced or metastatic breast cancer[8]; nonresectable, locally advanced, or metastatic non–small cell lung cancer after failure of cisplatin-based therapy, first-line treatment of nonresectable, locally advanced, or metastatic non–small cell lung cancer in combination with cisplatin[9]; androgen-independent (hormone-refractory) metastatic prostate cancer in combination with prednisone[10]; first-line treatment of gastric adenocarcinoma, including gastroesophageal junction adenocarcinoma in combination with cisplatin and 5-fluorouracil (5-FU)[11]; inoperable locally advanced squamous cell cancer of the head and neck in combination with cisplatin and 5-FU (Table 38.1). Docetaxel is currently manufactured by Sanofi-Aventis; however, it is expected to come off patent in November 2010.

Mechanisms of Action

The unique mechanism of action for paclitaxel was initially defined by Schiff et al.[12] in 1979, who showed that it bound to the interior surface of the microtubule lumen at binding sites completely distinct from those of exchangeable guanosine 5′-triphosphate (GTP), colchicine, podophyllotoxin, and the vinca alkaloids.[2] Docetaxel, which is slightly more water soluble than paclitaxel, appears to share the same tubulin-binding site as paclitaxel. The taxanes profoundly alter the tubulin dissociation rate constants at both ends of the microtubule, suppressing treadmilling and dynamic instability. However, in sharp contrast to the vinca alkaloids, they do not alter the association rate constants and the process of tubulin polymerization. The ability of the taxanes to induce mitotic arrest is associated with stoichiometric drug binding to microtubules, which occurs at submicromolar concentrations that are readily achieved in the clinic.

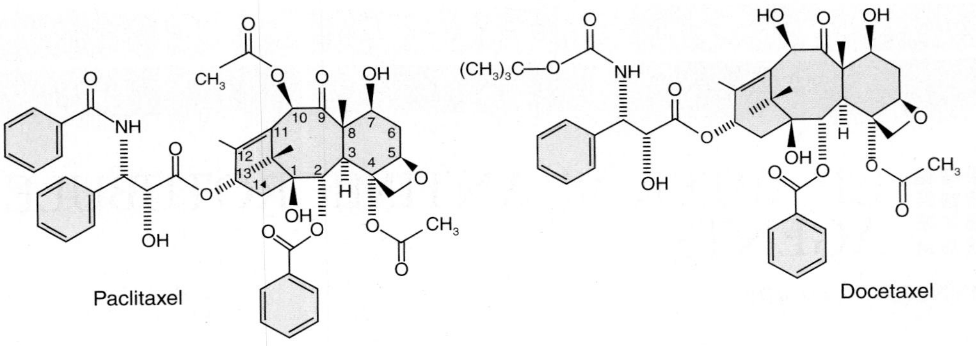

FIGURE 38.1 Structures of paclitaxel and docetaxel.

TABLE 38.1

ANTIMICROTUBULE AGENTS: DOSAGES AND TOXICITIES

Chemotherapeutic Agent	Dosage	Indications	Common Toxicities
Paclitaxel	135 to 200 mg/m² IV over 3 h or 135 mg/m² IV over 24 h every 3 wk; or 80 mg/m² IV over 1 h weekly	Adjuvant therapy of node-positive breast cancer; metastatic breast, ovarian, non–small cell lung, bladder, esophagus, cervical, gastric, and head and neck cancer; AIDS-related Kaposi's sarcoma; cancer of unknown origin	Myelosuppression, nausea and, vomiting, alopecia, arthralgia, myalgia, peripheral neuropathy
Docetaxel	60 to 100 mg/m² IV over 1 h every 3 wk	Adjuvant therapy of node-positive breast cancer; metastatic breast, gastric, head and neck, prostate, non–small cell lung, and ovarian cancer	Myelosuppression, edema, alopecia, nail damage, rash, diarrhea, nausea, vomiting, asthenia, neuropathy
Cabazitaxel	25 mg/m² IV every 3 weeks over 1 h	Patients with hormone-refractory metastatic prostate cancer previously treated	Neutropenia, infections, myelosuppression, diarrhea, nausea, vomiting, constipation, abdominal pain, asthenia
Albumin-bound paclitaxel	260 mg/m² IV over 30 min every 3 wk; or 125 mg/m² IV weekly on days 1, 8, and 15 every 28 days	Metastatic breast cancer	Myelosuppression, nausea, vomiting, alopecia, myalgia, peripheral neuropathy
Ixabepilone	40 mg/m² IV over 3 hours every 3 weeks.	Metastatic and locally advanced breast cancer	Myelosuppression, fatigue/asthenia, myalgia/arthralgia, alopecia, nausea, vomiting, stomatitis/mucositis, diarrhea, musculoskeletal pain
Vincristine	0.5 to 1.4 mg/m²/wk IV (maximum 2 mg per dose); or 0.4 mg/d continuous infusion for 4 days	Lymphoma, acute leukemia, neuroblastoma, rhabdomyosarcoma, AIDS-related Kaposi's sarcoma, multiple myeloma, testicular cancer	Constipation, nausea, vomiting, alopecia, diplopia, myelosuppression
Vinblastine	6 mg/m² IV on days 1 and 15 as part of the ABVD regimen; or 0.15 mg/kg IV on days 1 and 2 as part of the PVB regimen	Hodgkin's and non-Hodgkin's lymphoma; Kaposi's sarcoma; breast, testicular, bladder, prostate, and renal cell cancer	Myelosuppression, constipation, alopecia, malaise, bone pain
Vinorelbine	25 to 30 mg/m² IV weekly	Non–small cell lung, breast, cervical, and ovarian cancer	Alopecia, diarrhea, nausea, vomiting, asthenia, neuromyopathy
Estramustine	14 mg/kg PO daily in 3 or 4 divided doses	Metastatic prostate cancer	Nausea, vomiting, gynecomastia, fluid retention

ABVD, doxorubicin (Adriamycin), bleomycin, vinblastine, dacarbazine; PVB, cisplatin, vinblastine, bleomycin; IV, intravenous; PO, by mouth.

Clinical Pharmacology

Paclitaxel

With prolonged infusion schedules (6- and 24-hour), drug disposition is a biphasic process with values for alpha and beta half-lives averaging approximately 20 minutes and 6 hours, respectively.[3] When administered via shorter infusion schedules, most notably as a 3-hour infusion, its pharmacokinetic behavior is nonlinear. True nonlinear pharmacokinetics may have important clinical implications, particularly regarding dose modifications, because a small increase in dose may result in a disproportionate increase in drug exposure and hence toxicity. In contrast, a small dose reduction may result in a disproportionate decrease in drug exposure, thereby decreasing antitumor activity. Approximately 71% of an administered dose of paclitaxel is excreted in stool via the enterohepatic circulation over 5 days as either parent compound or metabolites in humans. Renal clearance of paclitaxel and metabolites is minimal, accounting for 14% of the administered dose. In humans, the bulk of drug disposition is metabolized by cytochrome P-450 mixed-function oxidases, specifically the isoenzymes CYP2C8 and CYP3A4, which metabolize paclitaxel to hydroxylated 3′p-hydroxypaclitaxel (minor) and 6α-hydroxypaclitaxel (major), as well as dihydroxylated metabolites.

Docetaxel

The pharmacokinetics of docetaxel on a 1-hour schedule are triexponential and linear at doses of 115 mg/m^2 or less.[3] Terminal half-lives ranging from 11.1 to 18.5 hours have been reported. The most important determinants of docetaxel clearance were the body surface area (BSA), hepatic function, and plasma α_1-acid glycoprotein concentration. Plasma protein binding is high (greater than 80%), and binding is primarily to α_1-acid glycoprotein, albumin, and lipoproteins. The hepatic cytochrome P-450 mixed-function oxidases, particularly isoforms CYP3A4 and CYP3A5, are principally involved in biotransformation. The principal pharmacokinetic determinants of toxicity, particularly neutropenia, are drug exposure and the time that plasma concentrations exceed biologically relevant concentrations. The baseline level of α_1-acid glycoprotein may be an independent predictor of response and a major objective prognostic factor of survival in patients with non–small cell lung cancer treated with docetaxel chemotherapy.

Drug Interactions

Sequence-dependent pharmacokinetic and toxicologic interactions between paclitaxel and several other chemotherapy agents have been noted.[13] The sequence of cisplatin followed by paclitaxel (24-hour schedule) induces more profound neutropenia than the reverse sequence, which is explained by a 33% reduction in the clearance of paclitaxel after cisplatin.[13] Treatment with paclitaxel on either a 3- or 24-hour schedule followed by carboplatin has been demonstrated to produce equivalent neutropenia and less thrombocytopenia as compared to carboplatin as a single agent, which is not explained by pharmacokinetic interactions. Neutropenia and mucositis are more severe when paclitaxel is administered on a 24-hour schedule before doxorubicin, compared to the reverse sequence, which is most likely due to an approximately 32% reduction in the clearance rates of doxorubicin and doxorubicinol when doxorubicin is administered after paclitaxel. Several agents that inhibit cytochrome P-450 mixed-function oxidases interfere with the metabolism of paclitaxel and docetaxel in human microsomes *in vitro*; however, the clinical relevance of these findings is not known.[13]

Toxicity

Paclitaxel

Neutropenia is the principal toxicity of paclitaxel. The onset is usually on days 8 to 10, and recovery is generally complete by days 15 to 21 with an every-3-week dosing regimen. Neutropenia is noncumulative, and the duration of severe neutropenia, even in heavily pretreated patients, is usually brief. The most important pharmacologic determinant of the severity of neutropenia is the duration that plasma concentrations are maintained above biologically relevant levels (0.05 to 0.10 mcmol). Major hypersensitivity reactions occur in 3% of patients with effective prophylaxis. Major hypersensitivity reactions usually occur within the first 10 minutes after the first treatment and resolve completely after stopping treatment. Patients who have major reactions have been rechallenged successfully after receiving high doses of corticosteroids. Hypersensitivity reactions are probably caused by a nonimmunologically mediated release of histamine-like substances, most likely due to its polyoxyethylated castor oil vehicle.

Paclitaxel induces a peripheral neuropathy that presents in a symmetric stocking glove distribution.[14] Neurologic examination reveals sensory loss and loss of deep tendon reflexes, and neurophysiologic studies reveal axonal degeneration and demyelination.[14] Severe neurotoxicity is uncommon when paclitaxel is given alone at doses below 200 mg/m^2 on a 3- or 24-hour schedule every 3 weeks or below 100 mg/m^2 on a continuous weekly schedule. There is no convincing evidence that any specific measure is effective at ameliorating existing manifestations or preventing the development or worsening of neurotoxicity.[14] The most common cardiac rhythm disturbance, a transient sinus bradycardia, can be observed in up to 30% of patients. Routine cardiac monitoring during paclitaxel therapy is not necessary but is advisable for patients who may not be able to tolerate bradyarrhythmias. Drug-related gastrointestinal effects, such as vomiting and diarrhea, are uncommon. Severe hepatotoxicity and pancreatitis have also been noted rarely. Pulmonary toxicities, including acute bilateral pneumonitis, have been reported. Extravasation of large volumes can cause moderate soft tissue injury. Paclitaxel also induces reversible alopecia of the scalp in a dose-related fashion. Nail disorders have also been reported with paclitaxel use and include ridging, nail bed pigmentation, onychorrhexis, and onycholysis.[15,16] These side effects have been reported more commonly with dose-intensified paclitaxel regimens.

Cytochrome P-450 polymorphisms (2C8, 3A4) have been shown to alter paclitaxel metabolism *in vitro* and *in vivo*.[17,18] Rodriguez-Antona et al.[18] reported that CYP2C8 haplotypes, named B and C with frequencies of 24% and 22% in whites, respectively, caused a significant increased and reduced paclitaxel 6 α-hydroxylation in 49 human liver samples. Speed et al.[19] evaluated the global frequency distributions of ten single nucleotide polymorphisms across 132 kb of CYP2C8 and CYP2C9 in 2,500 individuals, representing 45 populations. There was considerable geographic variation in haplotype frequencies, which may have pharmacogenomic implications for drug interactions. These polymorphisms have been suggested to modify paclitaxel-related toxicity. Leskala et al.[20] reported an association between polymorphisms in cytochrome P-450 2C8 and 3A5 with neurotoxicity in 118 patients treated with paclitaxel. CYP2C8 haplotype C and CYP3A5*3 was associated with less toxicity and CYP2C8 with increased toxicity. This suggests an important role for metabolism and hydroxylated paclitaxel metabolites in the development of paclitaxel-related neurotoxicity.

In addition, recent studies have suggested a role for ABC transporter polymorphisms in the development of neuropathy.

Sissung et al.[21] reported that patients carrying two reference alleles for the *ABCB1* (P-glycoprotein, MDR1) 3435C greater than T polymorphism had a reduced risk to develop neuropathy as compared to patients carrying at least one variant allele ($P = .09$). Additionally, patients who were homozygous variant at the 2677 and 3435 loci had a significantly greater percentage decrease in absolute neutrophil count at nadir ($P = .02$). This suggests that paclitaxel-induced neuropathy and neutropenia might be linked to inherited variants of *ABCB1*. However, data from a large controlled trial to evaluate these and other candidate polymorphisms failed to detect a significant association between genotype and outcome or toxicity for any of the genes analyzed (*ABCB1*, *ABCC1*, *ABCC2*, *ABCG2*, *CDKN1A*, *CYP1B1*, *CYP2C8*, *CYP3A4*, *CYP3A5*, *MAPT*, and *TP53*) in 914 ovarian cancer patients from the Scottish Randomised Trial in Ovarian Cancer phase 3 trial who were treated at presentation with carboplatin and taxane regimen.[22] Further studies are required to adequately assess the role of these variants in predicting toxicity from taxane therapy.

Docetaxel

Neutropenia is the main toxicity of docetaxel.[3,23] When docetaxel is administered on an every-3-week schedule, the onset of neutropenia is usually noted on day 8 with complete resolution by days 15 to 21. Neutropenia is significantly less when low doses are administered weekly. Docetaxel induces a unique fluid retention syndrome characterized by edema, weight gain, and third-space fluid collection.[3] Fluid retention is cumulative and is due to increased capillary permeability. Prophylactic treatment with corticosteroids has been demonstrated to reduce the incidence of fluid retention. Aggressive and early treatment with diuretics has been successfully used to manage fluid retention. Hypersensitivity reactions were noted in approximately 31% of patients who received the drug without premedications in early studies.[3] Symptoms include flushing, rash (with or without pruritus), chest tightness, back pain, dyspnea, and fever or chills. Severe hypotension, bronchospasm, generalized rash, and erythema may also occur.[24] Major reactions usually occur during the first two courses and within minutes after the start of treatment. Signs and symptoms generally resolve within 15 minutes after cessation of treatment, and docetaxel can usually be reinstituted without sequelae after treatment with an H1-receptor antagonist. Skin toxicity may occur in as many as 50% to 75% of patients[3]; however, premedication may reduce the overall incidence of this effect. Recent evidence suggests a shorter duration of premedication may provide adequate protection from fluid retention.[24] Other cutaneous effects include palmar-plantar erythrodysesthesia and onychodystrophy. Docetaxel produces neurotoxicity, which is qualitatively similar to that of paclitaxel; however, neurosensory and neuromuscular effects are generally less frequent and less severe than with paclitaxel.[14] Mild to moderate peripheral neurotoxicity occurs in approximately 40% of untreated patients.[14] Asthenia has been a prominent complaint in patients who have been treated with large cumulative doses.[3] Stomatitis appears to occur more frequently with docetaxel than with paclitaxel.

NEW TAXANE FORMULATIONS

Albumin-Bound Paclitaxel

Albumin-bound paclitaxel (ABI-007) is a solvent-free formulation of paclitaxel and is a colloidal suspension with nanoparticle albumin (Table 38.1). It received regulatory approval in the United States in 2005 for treatment of patients with metastatic breast cancer on the basis of a randomized, trial versus paclitaxel that enrolled 460 women with metastatic breast cancer, and two single-arm, open-label studies with a total of 106 participants.[25] Early clinical trials evaluated two different schedules of albumin-bound paclitaxel administration: an every-3-week schedule and a weekly schedule. The maximum tolerated dose (MTD) for the every-3-week schedule was 300 mg/m^2, while the MTD for the weekly schedule was 150 mg/m^2. Noticeably, severe hypersensitivity reactions have not been observed during the infusion period, which represents a potential advantage of the albumin-bound formulation over the traditional cremophor-based paclitaxel. The main toxicities observed with either of these schedules were neutropenia and sensory neuropathy. Other toxicities include alopecia, diarrhea, nausea and vomiting, elevations in liver enzymes, arthralgia, myalgia, and asthenia. In breast cancer, albumin-bound paclitaxel was evaluated extensively and showed significantly higher tumor response rates compared to cremophor-based paclitaxel and significantly longer time to tumor progression.[25] The incidence of severe neutropenia was significantly lower in albumin-bound paclitaxel arm, and severe sensory neuropathy was more frequent in the albumin-bound paclitaxel arm. A randomized, multicenter study phase 2 study examined the antitumor activity and safety of weekly and every-3-week nab-paclitaxel compared with docetaxel as first-line treatment in patients with metastatic breast cancer. Nab-paclitaxel 150 mg/m^2 weekly demonstrated significantly longer progression-free survival (PFS) than docetaxel 100 mg/m^2 every 3 weeks by both independent radiologist assessment (12.9 vs. 7.5 months, respectively; $P = .0065$) and investigator assessment (14.6 vs. 7.8 months, respectively; $P = .012$). Grade 3 or 4 fatigue, neutropenia, and febrile neutropenia were less frequent in all nab-paclitaxel arms.[26]

In addition to the ongoing clinical trials to evaluate albumin-bound paclitaxel as adjuvant and neoadjuvant therapy for breast cancer patients, it is actively being tested in clinical trials for other solid cancers. A phase 2 trial evaluated the combination of nab-paclitaxel, carboplatin, and bevacizumab in 48 advanced (stage IIIB/IV) nonsquamous non–small cell lung cancer, which resulted in a 31% response rate. Median PFS was 9.8 months and median survival was 16.8 months.[27] A phase 2 clinical trial to evaluate the use of nab-paclitaxel in 47 patients with histologically or cytologically confirmed epithelial cancer of the ovary, fallopian tube, or peritoneum resulted in a 64% objective response rate (ORR) and estimated median PFS of 8.5 months.[29] In addition, a phase 2 clinical trial to evaluate the activity of nab-paclitaxel and gemcitabine (in 44 patients with pancreatic cancer) resulted in a median overall survival time of 12.2 months, a doubling of survival compared to historic control of gemcitabine administered alone.[29] A phase 3 study that evaluated 1,052 patients with stage IIIB or IV non–small cell lung cancer showed that the nab-paclitaxel and carboplatin combination resulted in a superior response compared to a carboplatin and paclitaxel combination, which is considered the current standard of care.[30]

The superior response seen with nab-paclitaxel has been attributed to targeting an albumin-specific receptor (gp60), thereby activating transcytosis through the proliferating blood vessel wall and allowing the administered drugs to reach the tumor cells in higher concentration.[31] This hypothesis is the subject of ongoing preclinical and clinical research. The significant activity and favorable toxicity profile from these trials provides a basis for further evaluation in phase 3 trials in early stage breast cancer and in other solid tumors in combination with other chemotherapeutic and targeted agents.

Cabazitaxel

Cabazitaxel is a semisynthetic derivative of the natural taxoid 10-deacetylbaccatin III. It binds to and stabilizes tubulin, resulting in the inhibition of microtubule depolymerization and cell division, cell cycle arrest in the G_2/M phase, and the inhibition of tumor cell proliferation. Cabazitaxel is a poor substrate for the membrane-associated, multidrug resistance (MDR), P-glycoprotein (P-gp) efflux pump and therefore may be useful for treating multidrug-resistant tumors. In addition, it penetrates the blood–brain barrier.[32,33] A phase 3 multi-institutional study enrolled 755 men with metastatic hormone refractory metastatic prostate cancer who had failed a docetaxel-containing regimen. Patients were randomized to treatment with cabazitaxel or mitoxantrone. Median survival was 15.1 months for patients receiving cabazitaxel versus 12.7 months for patients receiving mitoxantrone. Cabazitaxel also improved PFS and was associated with higher response rates compared with mitoxantrone. Cabazitaxel was associated with more grade 3 or 4 neutropenia (82%) than mitoxantrone (58%). Cabazitaxel was approved by the FDA in June 2010 to be used with prednisone to treat hormone-refractory metastatic prostate cancer in those who had received prior chemotherapy. Side effects reported in more than 20% of patients treated with cabazitaxel included myelosuppression, diarrhea, nausea, vomiting, constipation, abdominal pain, or asthenia. Fatal infectious adverse events (sepsis or septic shock) in setting of grade 4 neutropenia occurred in five patients.[34]

VINCA ALKALOIDS

The vinca alkaloids have been some of the most active agents in cancer chemotherapy since their introduction 40 years ago. The naturally occurring members of the family, vinblastine (VBL) and vincristine (VCR), were isolated from the leaves of the periwinkle plant *Catharanthus roseus G. Don*. In the late 1950s, their antimitotic and, therefore, cancer chemotherapeutic potential was discovered by groups both at Eli Lilly Research Laboratories and at the University of Western Ontario, and they came into widespread use for the single-agent treatment of childhood hematologic and solid malignancies and, shortly after, for adult hematologic malignancies (Table 38.1).[1] Their clinical efficacy in several combination therapies has led to the development of various novel semisynthetic analogues, including vinorelbine (VRL), vindesine (VDS), and vinflunine (VFL) (Fig. 38.2).

Mechanism of Action

In contrast to the taxanes, the vinca alkaloids depolymerize microtubules and destroy mitotic spindles.[1] At low but clinically relevant concentrations, vinblastine does not depolymerize spindle microtubules, yet it powerfully blocks mitosis, and this has been suggested to occur as a result of suppression of microtubule dynamics rather than microtubule depolymerization. This group of compounds binds to the beta subunit of tubulin dimers at a distinct region called the vinca-binding domain. Importantly, binding of vinblastine induces a conformational change in tubulin in connection with tubulin self-association. In mitotic spindles, slowing of the growth and shortening or treadmilling dynamics of the microtubules block mitotic progression. This suppression of dynamics has at least two downstream effects on the spindle: it prevents the mitotic spindle from assembling normally, and it reduces the tension at the kinetochores of the chromosomes. Mitotic progress is delayed in a metaphase-like state, with chromosomes often stuck at the spindle poles, unable to congress to the spindle equator. The cell cycle signal to the anaphase-promoting complex to pass from metaphase into anaphase is blocked, and tumor cells eventually die by apoptosis. The naturally occurring vinca alkaloids VCR and VBL, the semisynthetic analogue VRL, and a novel bifluorinated analogue vinflunine have similar mechanisms of action.

Tissue and tumor sensitivities to the vinca alkaloids, which relate in part to differences in drug transport and accumulation, also vary. Intracellular or extracellular concentration ratios range from five- to 500-fold depending on the individual cell type.[35] Although the vinca alkaloids are retained in cells for long periods of time and thus may have prolonged cellular effects, intracellular retention is markedly different among the various vinca alkaloids. The results of early studies suggested that the vinca alkaloids entered cells by energy- and temperature-dependent transport processes, but it now appears that temperature-independent, nonsaturable mechanisms, analogous to simple diffusion, account for the majority of drug transport, and temperature-dependent saturable processes are less important.[1] Another important determinant of drug accumulation and retention is lipophilicity. In this regard, VBL appears to be retained to a much greater degree than either VCR or VDS.[35,36] Drug uptake and retention are also influenced by tissue-specific factors, as illustrated by studies that demonstrate that the accumulation and retention of VRL in neurons are less than those of other vinca alkaloids. One important tissue-specific factor is tubulin isotype composition, which may influence the intracellular accumulation of the vinca alkaloids and other antimicrotubule agents that avidly bind tubulin.[37] Tubulin isotypes confer variable drug-binding characteristics, involve different drug uptake and efflux pump mechanisms, and determine the magnitude of the intracellular reservoir for drug accumulation. In addition, differences in the type and quantity of microtubule-associated proteins (MAPs) and GTP, which may influence drug interactions with tubulin, and variability in cellular permeation and retention may influence the formation and stability of complexes formed between the vinca alkaloids and tubulin.[1] Newer theories of mechanism of action of antimicrotubule agents have emerged, suggesting that the more important target of these drugs may be the tumor vasculature, as reviewed in the next section.

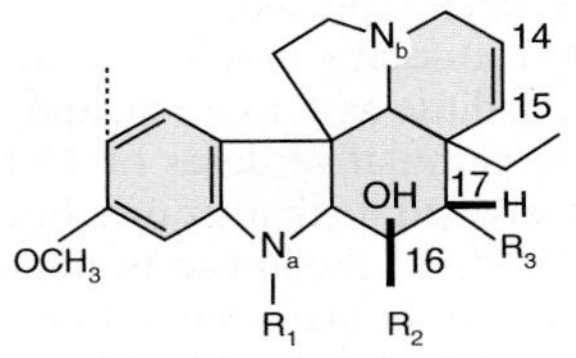

Vindoline nucleus

	R_1	R_2	R_3
Vindesine	CH_3	$CONH_2$	OH
Vincristine	CHO	CO_2CH_3	$OCOCH_3$
Vinblastine	CH_3	CO_2CH_3	$OCOCH_3$
Vinorelbine	CH_3	CO_2CH_3	$OCOCH_3$

FIGURE 38.2 Structural modifications of the vindoline ring in various vinca alkaloids.

Clinical Pharmacology

The vinca alkaloids are usually administered intravenously as a brief infusion, and their pharmacokinetic behavior in plasma has generally been explained by a three-compartment model. The vinca alkaloids share many pharmacokinetic properties, including large volumes of distribution, high clearance rates, and long terminal half-lives that reflect the high magnitude and avidity of drug binding in peripheral tissues. Large inter- and intraindividual variability is present in their pharmacologic behavior, which has been attributed to differences in protein and tissue binding, hepatic metabolism, and biliary clearance.[38]

Although prolonged infusion schedules may avoid excessively toxic peak concentrations and increase the duration of drug exposure in plasma above biologically relevant threshold concentrations for any given tumor, there is little, if any, evidence to support the notion that prolonged infusion schedules are more effective than bolus schedules. VCR had the longest terminal half-life and the lowest clearance rate, VBL had the shortest terminal half-life and the highest clearance rate, and VDS had intermediate characteristics. Comparable values for VLR overlap with those of VDS and VBL. The longest half-life and lowest clearance rate of VCR may account for its greater propensity to induce neurotoxicity, but there are many other nonpharmacokinetic determinants of tissue sensitivity, as discussed earlier.

Vincristine

After conventional doses of VCR (1.4 mg/m^2) given as brief infusions, peak plasma levels approach 0.4 mcmol. Plasma clearance is slow, and terminal half-lives that range from 23 to 85 hours have been reported. VCR is metabolized and excreted primarily by the hepatobiliary system. Seventy-two hours after the administration of radiolabeled VCR, approximately 12% of the radiolabel is excreted in the urine (at least 50% of which consists of metabolites), and approximately 70% to 80% is excreted in the feces (40% of which consists of metabolites).[39] The nature of the VCR metabolites identified to date, as well as the results of metabolic studies *in vitro*, indicate that VCR metabolism is mediated principally by hepatic cytochrome P-450 CYP3A5.

Vinblastine

The clinical pharmacology of VBL is similar to that of VCR. Binding of VBL to plasma proteins and formed elements of blood is extensive.[40,41] Peak plasma drug concentrations are approximately 0.4 mcmol after rapid intravenous injections of VBL at standard doses. Distribution is rapid, and terminal half-lives range from 20 to 24 hours. Like VCR, VBL disposition is principally through the hepatobiliary system with excretion in feces (approximately 95%); however, fecal excretion of the parent compound is low, indicating that hepatic metabolism is extensive.[34]

Vinorelbine

The pharmacologic behavior of VRL is similar to that of the other vinca alkaloids, and plasma concentrations after rapid intravenous administration have been reported to decline in either a biexponential or triexponential manner.[35,42] After intravenous administration, there is a rapid decay of VRL concentrations followed by a much slower elimination phase (terminal half-life, 18 to 49 hours). Plasma protein binding, principally to α_1-acid glycoprotein, albumin, and lipoproteins, has been reported to range from 80% to 91%, and drug binding to platelets is extensive.[35] VRL is widely distributed, and high concentrations are found in virtually all tissues, except the central nervous system.[35] The wide distribution of VRL reflects its lipophilicity, which is among the highest of the vinca alkaloids. As with other vinca alkaloids, the liver is the principal excretory organ, and up to 80% of VRL is excreted in the feces, whereas urinary excretion represents only 16% to 30% of total drug disposition, the bulk of which is unmetabolized VRL. Studies in humans indicate that 4-O-deacetyl-VRL and 3,6-epoxy-VRL are the principal metabolites, and several minor hydroxy-VRL isomer metabolites have been identified. Although most metabolites are inactive, the deacetyl-VRL metabolite may be as active as VRL. The cytochrome P-450 CYP3A isoenzyme appears to be principally involved in biotransformation.

Drug Interactions

Methotrexate accumulation in tumor cells is enhanced *in vitro* by the presence of VCR or VBL, an effect mediated by a vinca alkaloid–induced blockade of drug efflux; however, the minimal concentrations of VCR required to achieve this effect occur only transiently *in vivo*.[43] The vinca alkaloids also inhibit the cellular influx of the epipodophyllotoxins *in vitro*, resulting in less cytotoxicity, but the clinical implications of this potential interaction are unknown. L-asparaginase may reduce the hepatic clearance of the vinca alkaloids, which may result in increased toxicity. To minimize the possibility of this interaction, the vinca alkaloids should be given 12 to 24 hours before L-asparaginase. The combined use of mitomycin C and the vinca alkaloids has been associated with acute dyspnea and bronchospasm. The onset of these pulmonary toxicities has ranged from within minutes to hours after treatment with the vinca alkaloids or up to 2 weeks after mitomycin C.

Treatment with the vinca alkaloids has precipitated seizures associated with subtherapeutic plasma phenytoin concentrations.[43] Reduced plasma phenytoin levels have been noted from 24 hours to 10 days after treatment with VCR and VBL. Because of the importance of the cytochrome P-450 CYP3A isoenzyme in vinca alkaloid metabolism, administration of the vinca alkaloids with erythromycin and other inhibitors of CYP3A may lead to severe toxicity.[44] Concomitantly administered drugs, such as pentobarbital and H_2-receptor antagonists, may also influence VCR clearance by modulating hepatic cytochrome P-450 metabolic processes.[43]

Toxicity

Despite close similarities in structure, the vinca alkaloids differ significantly in their safety profiles. VCR principally induces neurotoxicity characterized by a peripheral, symmetric mixed sensory-motor and autonomic polyneuropathy.[45,46] Its primary neuropathologic effects are axonal degeneration and decreased axonal transport due to interference with axonal microtubule function. Initially, only symmetric sensory impairment and paresthesias are usually experienced. Neuritic pain and loss of deep tendon reflexes may develop with continued treatment, which may be followed by foot drop, wrist drop, motor dysfunction, ataxia, and paralysis. Nerve conduction velocities are usually normal, although diminished amplitude of sensory and motor nerve action potentials and prolonged distal latencies, suggesting axonal degeneration, may be noted. Cranial nerves may be affected rarely, and the uptake of VCR into the central nervous system is low. Toxic manifestations include constipation, abdominal cramps, paralytic ileus, urinary retention, orthostatic hypotension, and hypertension. Laryngeal paralysis has also been reported.

In adults, neurotoxicity may occur after treatment with cumulative doses as little as 5 to 6 mg, and manifestations may be profound after cumulative doses of 15 to 20 mg. Children appear to be less susceptible than adults, but the elderly are particularly prone. However, the apparent influence of age may, in fact, be due to previously inadequate dose calculation by body weight in children and adults and by BSA in infants. In infants, VCR doses are now calculated according to body weight. Patients with antecedent neurologic disorders, such as Charcot-Marie-Tooth disease, hereditary and sensory neuropathy type 1, and Guillain-Barré, are highly predisposed. Impaired drug metabolism and delayed biliary excretion in patients with hepatic dysfunction or obstructive liver disease are associated with increased risk of neurotoxicity. The manifestations of neurotoxicity are similar for the other vinca alkaloids; however, they are typically less common and severe.[47] Severe neurotoxicity is observed infrequently with VBL and VDS. VRL has been shown to have a lower affinity for axonal microtubules than either VCR or VBL, which seems to be confirmed by clinical observations.[48] Mild to moderate peripheral neuropathy, principally characterized by sensory effects, occurs in 7% to 31% of patients, and constipation and other autonomic effects are noted in 30% of subjects, whereas severe toxicity occurs in 2% to 3%. Muscle weakness, jaw pain, and discomfort at tumor sites may also occur.

Neutropenia is the principal dose-limiting toxicity of VBL and VRL. Thrombocytopenia and anemia occur less commonly. The onset of neutropenia is usually 7 to 11 days after treatment, and recovery is generally by days 14 to 21. Myelosuppression is not typically cumulative. Clinically relevant hematologic effects are uncommon after VCR treatment, but may be observed after inadvertent administration of high doses or in the presence of hepatic dysfunction. Gastrointestinal effects, aside from those caused by autonomic dysfunction, may be caused by all vinca alkaloids.[25,33–38] Gastrointestinal autonomic dysfunction, as manifested by bloating, constipation, ileus, and abdominal pain, occur most commonly with VCR or high doses of the other vinca alkaloids. Mucositis occurs more frequently with VBL than with VRL and is least common with VCR. Nausea, vomiting, and diarrhea may also occur to a lesser extent. Pancreatitis has been reported with VRL.[49]

The vinca alkaloids are potent vesicants and may cause tissue damage if extravasation occurs. If extravasation is suspected, treatment should be discontinued, and aspiration of any residual drug remaining in the tissues should be attempted.[50] In animal models, cold appears to increase toxicity, whereas heat limits tissue damage. Therefore, the immediate application of heat for 1 hour four times daily for 3 to 5 days and the injection of hyaluronidase, 150 to 1,500 U (15 U/mL in 6 mL 0.9% sodium chloride solution) subcutaneously, through six clockwise injections in a circumferential manner using a 25-gauge needle (changing the needle with each new injection) into the surrounding tissues, is the treatment of choice for minimizing discomfort and latent cellulitis. A surgical consultation to consider early debridement is also recommended. Discomfort, signs of phlebitis, and latent sclerosis may also occur along the course of an injected vein. The risk of phlebitis is increased if the vein is not adequately flushed after treatment.

Mild and reversible alopecia occurs in approximately 10% and 20% of patients treated with VLR and VCR, respectively. Acute cardiac ischemia, chest pains without evidence of ischemia, fever without an obvious source, Raynaud's syndrome, hand-foot syndrome, and pulmonary and liver toxicity (transaminitis and hyperbilirubinemia, to a lesser extent) have also been reported with use of the vinca alkaloids. All of the vinca alkaloids can cause syndrome of inappropriate secretion of antidiuretic hormone (SIADH), and patients who are receiving intensive hydration are particularly prone to severe hyponatremia secondary to SIADH. Hyponatremia generally responds to fluid restriction, as with hyponatremia associated with SIADH due to other causes, but in some cases, treatment with demeclocycline is warranted.

Mechanism of Resistance to Microtubule Inhibitors

The development of cellular drug resistance is one of the main factors that limits the clinical efficacy of taxanes and vinca alkaloids. Drug resistance is often complex and multifaceted and can involve diverse mechanisms such as (1) factors that reduce the ability of drugs to reach their cellular target (e.g., activation of detoxification pathways and decreased drug accumulation); (2) modifications in the drug target; and (3) events downstream of the target (e.g., decreased sensitivity to, or defective, apoptotic signals). Many tubulin binding agents are substrates for multidrug transporters such as P-glycoprotein (Pgp) and the multidrug resistance gene (*MDR1*).[51,52]

The *MDR1*-encoded gene product MDR1 (ABC subfamily B1; ABCB1) and MDR2 (ABC subfamily ABCB4) are the best-characterized adenosine triphosphate binding cassette (ABC) transporters thought to confer drug resistance to taxanes.[51,53] MDR-related taxane resistance can be reversed by many classes of drugs, including the calcium channel blockers, cyclosporin A, and antiarrhythmic agents.[51,53] However, the clinical utility of this approach has never been proven, despite several clinical trials. Hence, the role of ABC transporters in resistance to microtubule inhibitors appears doubtful at this time.[54]

An increasing number of studies suggest that the expression of individual tubulin isotypes are altered in cells resistant to antimicrotubule drugs and may confer drug resistance.[52,55] Inherent differences in microtubule dynamics and drug interactions have been observed with some isotypes *in vitro* and *in vivo*.[56] Several taxane-resistant mutant cell lines that have structurally altered α- and β-tubulin proteins and an impaired ability to polymerize into microtubules have also been identified.[57] Mutations of tubulin isotype genes, gene amplifications, and isotype switching have also been reported in taxane-resistant cell lines.[57] Higher levels of class III β-tubulin RNA levels have also been reported in non–small cell lung cancers of patients who did not respond to taxane treatment, consistent with *in vitro* findings. Monzo et al.[58] reported that 16 of 41 patients with stage IIIB or IV non–small cell lung cancer with β-tubulin mutations in exons 1 or 4 showed no response to treatment with a 3- or 24-hour infusion of paclitaxel. In another study, expression of class III β-tubulin was examined immunohistochemically in 91 baseline tumor samples from stage III and IV non–small cell lung cancer patients, including 47 who received paclitaxel-based regimens and 44 who received regimens without tubulin-binding agents. The authors reported that low levels of class III β-tubulin isotype is predictive of response to therapy and outcome in patients receiving paclitaxel-based chemotherapy, whereas this variable was not found to be predictive in patients receiving regimens without tubulin-binding agents.[59] While tubulin mutations for the ubiquitous α-tubulin and β-tubulin genes were not detected in both resistant and sensitive cases in a cohort of 41 patients with advanced ovarian, the authors reported that overexpression of class III β-tubulin was associated with paclitaxel resistance.[54] In opposition to taxanes, resistance to vinca alkaloids has been associated with decreased class II β-tubulin expression.[55,56]

Microtubule-associated proteins (MAPs) are important structural and regulatory components of microtubules. Alterations in the activity and expression of MAPs can profoundly affect microtubule function, and altered expression of MAPs has also been associated with the development of drug resistance.[57] The overexpression of stathmin, a regulatory protein that destabilizes microtubules in breast cancer cells, has been reported to decrease sensitivity to paclitaxel and vinblastine.[52,60] Higher levels of MAP4 in multiple cancer cell lines increased sensitivity to paclitaxel but decreased sensitivity to vinca alkaloids.[42,44,52,61,62] MAP4 promotes the polymerization of microtubules, which could explain the disparate response to taxanes (stabilizing agents) and vinca alkaloids (destabilizing agents). An analysis of predictive or prognostic factors in a large phase 3 study (National Surgical Adjuvant Breast and Bowel Project NSABP-B 28) in patients with node-positive breast cancer showed that tau was a prognostic factor, however, it did not show an association between tau expression levels and benefit from paclitaxel-based chemotherapy.[52,63]

ESTRAMUSTINE PHOSPHATE

Estramustine is a conjugate of nor-nitrogen mustard linked to 17β-estradiol by a carbamate ester bridge. Estramustine phosphate received regulatory approval in the United States in 1981 for treating patients with hormone-refractory prostate cancer (HRPC). Although the recommended daily dose of estramustine phosphate is 14 mg/kg/d, patients are usually treated in the daily dosing range of 10 to 16 mg/kg in three to four divided daily doses (Table 38.1). Estramustine has significant activity in HRPC and is generally used in combination with vinblastine or docetaxel. A recent phase 3 study in patients with HRPC showed a significant improvement in median survival with docetaxel and estramustine, as compared with mitoxantrone and prednisone.[64]

Estramustine binds to β-tubulin at a site distinct from the colchicine and vinca alkaloid binding sites. This agent depolymerizes microtubules and microfilaments, binds to and disrupts MAPs, and inhibits cell growth at high concentrations, resulting in mitotic arrest and apoptosis in tumor cells. The selective accumulation and actions of estramustine and its metabolite, estromustine, in specific tissues appear to be dependent on the expression of the estramustine-binding protein (EMBP). The disposition of estramustine is principally by rapid oxidative metabolism of the parent compound to estromustine. Estromustine concentrations in plasma are maximal within 2 to 4 hours after oral administration, and the mean elimination half-life of estromustine is 14 hours. Estromustine and estramustine are principally excreted in the feces, with only small amounts of conjugated estrone and estradiol detected in the urine (less than 1%).

In general, this agent has a manageable safety profile. Nausea and vomiting are the principal toxicities encountered. In contrast to the taxanes and the vinca alkaloids, myelosuppression is rarely clinically relevant. Common estrogenic side effects include gynecomastia, nipple tenderness, and fluid retention. Thromboembolic complications may occur in up to 10% of patients.

EPOTHILONES

The success with the taxanes provided the rationale to develop novel agents with similar mechanisms of action yet with improved properties relating to safety profile, convenience, and clinical pharmacology. Moreover, significant focus has been placed on developing new molecules that did not display cross-resistance to the taxanes and the vinca alkaloids. Several classes of natural products, including the epothilones, eleutherobins, discodermolides, sarcodictyins, and laulimalides, all of which promote tubulin polymerization, have been identified.[65] The epothilones are macrolide compounds that were initially isolated from the mycobacterium *Sorangium cellulosum.* They exert their cytotoxic effects by promoting tubulin polymerization and inducing mitotic arrest.[66] In general, the epothilones are more potent than the taxanes. In contrast to the taxanes and vinca alkaloids, overexpression of the efflux protein P-glycoprotein minimally affects the cytotoxicity of epothilones. Epothilone B (patupilone; EPO906), aza-epothilone B (BMS-247550), a water-soluble semisynthetic analogue of epothilone B (BMS-310705), epothilone D (deoxyepothilone B, KOS-862), and a synthetic analogue, ZK-EPO, are currently undergoing clinical testing.[66]

BMS-247550 (ixabepilone) is aza-epothilone B, which has been evaluated in several schedules using a cremophor-based formulation.[66] It is active in breast cancer previously treated with paclitaxel or docetaxel. Ixabepilone has been approved by the FDA for the treatment of patients with breast cancer. The principal toxicities observed to date include neutropenia and peripheral neuropathy.[14,66] It also has been evaluated in other solid tumors such as ovarian, prostate, and renal cell carcinoma. The Gynecologic Oncology Group phase 2 evaluation of the efficacy and safety of ixabepilone in patients with recurrent or persistent platinum- and taxane-resistant primary ovarian or peritoneal carcinoma resulted in a 14.3% ORR, with three complete and four partial responses. The median time to progression was 4.4 months and median survival was 14.8 months (95% confidence interval [CI], 0.8 to 50.0). Adverse effects included peripheral neuropathy, neutropenia fatigue nausea or emesis, and diarrhea (4%).[67] A randomized, noncomparative, multicenter, clinical trial evaluated ixabepilone or mitoxantrone/prednisone (MP) as second-line chemotherapy in 41 patients with taxane-refractory, hormone-refractory, prostate cancer, which resulted in 10.4 months median survival with ixabepilone and 9.8 months with MP.[68] A phase 2 study to evaluate the efficacy and safety of ixabepilone in 87 patients with metastatic renal cell carcinoma reported one patient had a complete response, 10 patients had partial responses, and the median duration of response was 5.5 months.[69] Ixabepilone appears to have promising phase 2 activity in various solid tumors, and additional evaluation in a large phase 3 setting is needed to confirm these results.

EPO906 is an epothilone B that is active in breast and ovarian cancers and is undergoing evaluation in clinical trials. The toxicity profile of EPO906 is different from that of BMS-247550, and diarrhea is the dose-limiting toxicity of EPO906.

NOVEL COMPOUNDS TARGETING MICROTUBULES AND MITOTIC MOTOR PROTEINS

LY355703 is a synthetic analogue of cryptophycin depsipeptides with potent inhibitory effects on microtubule polymerization in tumor xenografts displaying the MDR phenotype. The dolastatins noncompetitively inhibit the binding of the vinca alkaloids to tubulin, inhibit tubulin polymerization, and possess cytotoxic activity in the picomolar to low nanomolar range. A multicenter phase 2 trial evaluated LY355703 in 26 previously treated stage IIIB (pleural effusion) or stage IV non–small cell lung cancer. After dose reduction for toxicity, LY355703 failed to produce measurable responses utilizing this schedule.[70] LY355703 has modest activity in patients with platinum-resistant advanced ovarian cancer. As reported in a phase 2 study that enrolled 26 patients, LY355703 (1.5 mg/m^2) was administered intravenously on days 1 and 8, every 3 weeks, infused over 2 hours. From 24 patients evaluable for response, three partial responses and seven disease stabilizations were reported, for an overall clinical benefit of 41.7%. Fourteen patients experienced a progression of the disease during treatment. Among the 25 patients evaluable for toxicity, two episodes of grade 3 anemia; one episode of grade 3 thrombocytopenia; one episode of grade 4 elevation of creatinine; and one episode of grade 3 hyperbilirubinemia were reported.[71]

Dolastatin-10 and -15, and semisynthetic analogues, TZT-1027 (soblidotin) and ILX651 (synthadotin), are undergoing active clinical development. Halichondrin B and synthetic macrocyclic ketone analogues (ER-076349 and ER-086526) inhibit tubulin polymerization and are undergoing clinical development.

Kinesin spindle protein (KSP; also known as EG5) is a kinesin motor protein required to establish mitotic-spindle bipolarity.[64] Several KSP inhibitors have been evaluated in early phase clinical trials. SB-715992 (ispinesib) is a small-molecule inhibitor of KSP adenosine triphosphatase (ATPase) and has been evaluated in two different schedules.[65] The dose-limiting toxicity is neutropenia. Ispinesib was found to be inactive in phase 2 studies evaluating efficacy in patients with androgen-independent and largely docetaxel-resistant prostate cancer, advanced renal cancer, and head and neck cancer.[72–74] SB-743921 and MK-0731 are KSP inhibitors in early clinical development.[65]

Aurora kinases are mitotic kinases crucial for mitosis. MK-0457 (or VX-680) and AZD1152 are aurora kinase inhibitors currently in clinical development. The main dose-limiting toxicity of these agents is neutropenia. Phase 2 trials in non–small cell lung cancer and acute myeloid leukemia are ongoing. Polo-like kinases (PLKs) are serine or threonine kinases crucial for cell cycle process. Overexpression of PLKs has been shown to be related to histologic grading and poor prognosis in several types of cancer. BI-2536 and ON01910 are PLK inhibitors in early clinical development.[65]

Selected References

The full list of references for this chapter appears in the online version.

1. Jordan MA, Wilson L. Microtubules as a target for anticancer drugs. *Nat Rev Cancer* 2004;4(4):253.
2. Nogales E. Structural insight into microtubule function. *Annu Rev Biophys Biomol Struct* 2001;30:397.
3. Rowinsky EK. Antimicrotubule agents. In: Chabner BA, Longo DL, eds. *Cancer chemotherapy and biotherapy: principles and practice*, 4th ed. Philadelphia: Lippincott Williams & Wilkins, 2005:237.
5. Mamounas EP, Bryant J, Lembersky B, et al. Paclitaxel after doxorubicin plus cyclophosphamide as adjuvant chemotherapy for node-positive breast cancer: results from NSABP B-28. *J Clin Oncol* 2005;23(16):3686.
7. Martin M, Pienkowski T, Mackey J, et al. Adjuvant docetaxel for node-positive breast cancer. *N Engl J Med* 2005;352(22):2302.
8. Jones SE, Erban J, Overmoyer B, et al. Randomized phase III study of docetaxel compared with paclitaxel in metastatic breast cancer. *J Clin Oncol* 2005;23(24):5542.
10. Tannock IF, de Wit R, Berry WR, et al. Docetaxel plus prednisone or mitoxantrone plus prednisone for advanced prostate cancer. *N Engl J Med* 2004;351(15):1502.
11. Van Cutsem E, Moiseyenko VM, Tjulandin S, et al. Phase III study of docetaxel and cisplatin plus fluorouracil compared with cisplatin and fluorouracil as first-line therapy for advanced gastric cancer: a report of the V325 Study Group. *J Clin Oncol* 2006;24(31):4991.
14. Lee JJ, Swain SM. Peripheral neuropathy induced by microtubule-stabilizing agents. *J Clin Oncol* 2006;24(10):1633.
15. Hussein S, Anderson D, Salvatti ME, et al. Oncholysis as a complication of systemic chemotherapy. *Cancer* 2000;88:2367.
17. Dai D, Zeldin DC, Blaisdell JA, et al. Polymorphisms in human CYP2C8 decrease metabolism of the anticancer drug paclitaxel and arachidomic acid. *Pharmacogenetics* 2001;11:597.
18. Rodriguez-Antona C, Niemi M, Backman JT, et al. Characterization of novel CYP2C8 haplotypes and their contribution to paclitaxel and repalinide metabolism. *Pharmacogenomics J* 2008;8:268.
19. Speed W, Kang PK, Tuck D, Harris L, Kidd K. Global variation in CYP2C8-CYP2C9 functional haplotypes. *Pharmacogenomics J* 2009;9:283.
20. Leskala S, Jara C, Leandro-Garcia LJ, et al. Polymorphisms in cytochromes P450 2C8 and 3A5 are associated with paclitaxel neurotoxicity. *Pharmacogenomics J* 2010. Doi 10.1038/tpj.2010.13.
21. Sissung T, Mross K, Steinberg S, et al. Association of *ABCB1* genotypes with paclitaxel-mediated peripheral neuropathy and neutropenia. *Eur J Cancer* 2006;42:2893.
24. Baker J, Ajani J, Scotté F, et al. Docetaxel-related side effects and their management. *Eur J Oncol Nurs* 2009;13(1):49.
25. Gradishar WJ, Tjulandin S, Davidson N, et al. Phase III trial of nanoparticle albumin-bound paclitaxel compared with polyethylated castor oil-based paclitaxel in women with breast cancer. *J Clin Oncol* 2005;23(31): 7794.
26. Gradishar WJ, Krasnojon D, Cheporov S, et al. Significantly longer progression-free survival with nab-paclitaxel compared with docetaxel as first-line therapy for metastatic breast cancer. *J Clin Oncol* 2009;27(22):3611.
29. Von Hoff D. Epithelium and stroma: double trouble. Presented at the "Progress in Pancreatic Cancer" session on April 18 at the 101st annual meeting of the American Association for Cancer Research (AACR), Washington, DC.
30. Socinski R, Bondarenko IN, Karaseva NA, et al. Results of a randomized, phase III trial of nab-paclitaxel (nab-P) and carboplatin (C) compared with cremophor-based paclitaxel (P) and carboplatin as first-line therapy in advanced non-small cell lung cancer (NSCLC). Presented at the 46th annual meeting of the American Society of Clinical Oncology (ASCO), Chicago. *J Clin Oncol* 2010;28(Suppl 18s): (abstr LBA7511).
31. Desai N, Trieu V, Yao Z, et al. Increased antitumor activity, intratumor paclitaxel concentrations, and endothelial cell transport of cremophor-free, albumin-bound paclitaxel, ABI-007, compared with cremophor-based paclitaxel. *Clin Cancer Res* 2006;12(4):1317.
33. Mita AC, Denis LJ, Rowinsky EK, et al. Phase I and pharmacokinetic study of XRP6258 (RPR 116258A), a novel taxane, administered as a 1-hour infusion every 3 weeks in patients with advanced solid tumors. *Clin Cancer Res* 2009;15(2):723.
35. Rahmani R, Zhou XJ. Pharmacokinetics and metabolism of vinca alkaloids. In: Workman P, Graham M, eds. *Cancer surveys*, vol. 17: *Pharmacokinetics and cancer chemotherapy*. Plainview, NY: Cold Spring Harbor Laboratory Press, 1993:269.
37. Zhou J, Giannakakou P. Targeting microtubules for cancer chemotherapy. *Curr Med Chem Anticancer Agents* 2005;5(1):65.
38. Jackson DV Jr. The periwinkle alkaloids. In: Lokich JJ, ed. *Cancer chemotherapy by infusion*. Chicago: Precept Press, 1990:155.
42. Rowinsky EK, Noe DA, Trump DL, et al. Pharmacokinetic, bioavailability, and feasibility study of oral vinorelbine in patients with solid tumors. *J Clin Oncol* 1994;12(9):1754.
45. Quasthoff S, Hartung HP. Chemotherapy-induced peripheral neuropathy. *J Neurol* 2002;249(1):9.
46. Peltier AC, Russell JW. Recent advances in drug-induced neuropathies. *Curr Opin Neurol* 2002;15(5):633.
51. Gottesman MM, Fojo T, Bates SE. Multidrug resistance in cancer: role of ATP-dependent transporters. *Nat Rev Cancer* 2002;2(1):48.
52. Perez EA. Microtubule inhibitors: differentiating tubulin-inhibiting agents based on mechanisms of action, clinical activity, and resistance. *Mol Cancer Ther* 2009;8(8):2086.
53. Fojo AT, Menefee M. Microtubule targeting agents: basic mechanisms of multidrug resistance (MDR). *Semin Oncol* 2005;32(6 Suppl 7):S3.
54. Mozzetti S, Ferlini C, Concolino P, et al. Class III β-tubulin overexpression is a prominent mechanism of paclitaxel resistance in ovarian cancer patients. *Clin Cancer Res* 2005;11:298
55. Drukman S, Kavallaris M. Microtubule alterations and resistance to tubulin-binding agents [review]. *Int J Oncol* 2002;21(3):621.
56. Verrills NM, Kavallaris M. Improving the targeting of tubulin-binding agents: lessons from drug resistance studies. *Curr Pharm Des* 2005;11(13): 1719.
57. Orr GA, Verdier-Pinard P, McDaid H, Horwitz SB. Mechanisms of taxol resistance related to microtubules. *Oncogene* 2003;22(47):7280.
59. Sève P, Mackey J, Isaac S, et al. Class III β-tubulin expression in tumor cells predicts response and outcome in patients with non–small cell lung cancer receiving paclitaxel. *Mol Cancer Ther* 2005;4(12):2001.
60. Alli E, Bash-Babula J, Yang JM, Hait WN. Effect of stathmin on the sensitivity to antimicrotubule drugs in human breast cancer. *Cancer Res* 2002;62: 6864.
61. Zhang CC, Yang JM, White E, et al. The role of MAP4 expression in the sensitivity to paclitaxel and resistance to vinca alkaloids in p53 mutant cells. *Oncogene* 1998;16:1617.
62. Zhang CC, Yang JM, Bash-Babula J, et al. DNA damage increases sensitivity to vinca alkaloids and decreases sensitivity to taxanes through p53-dependent repression of microtubule-associated protein 4. *Cancer Res* 1999;59:3663.
63. Pusztai L, Jeong J, Gong Y, et al. Evaluation of microtubule associated protein τ expression as prognostic and predictive marker in the NSABP-B 28 randomized clinical trial. Presented at the 31st annual SABCS Meeting. 2008: (abst 54).
65. Jackson JR, Patrick DR, Dar MM, Huang PS. Targeted anti-mitotic therapies: can we improve on tubulin agents? *Nat Rev Cancer* 2007;7(2):107.
66. Goodin S, Kane MP, Rubin EH. Epothilones: mechanism of action and biologic activity. *J Clin Oncol* 2004;22(10):2015.
67. De Geest K, Blessing JA, Morris RT, et al. Phase II clinical trial of ixabepilone in patients with recurrent or persistent platinum- and taxane-resistant ovarian or primary peritoneal cancer: a Gynecologic Oncology Group study. *J Clin Oncol* 2010;28(1):149.
68. Rosenberg JE, Weinberg VK, Kelly WK, et al. Activity of second-line chemotherapy in docetaxel-refractory hormone-refractory prostate cancer patients : randomized phase 2 study of ixabepilone or mitoxantrone and prednisone. *Cancer* 2007;110(3):556.
69. Huang H, Menefee M, Edgerly M, et al. A phase II clinical trial of ixabepilone (Ixempra; BMS-247550; NSC 710428), an epothilone B analog, in patients with metastatic renal cell carcinoma. *Clin Cancer Res* 2010;16(5)1634–1641.

CHAPTER 39 TARGETED THERAPY WITH SMALL MOLECULE KINASE INHIBITORS

CHARLES L. SAWYERS

In 2001 the first tyrosine kinase inhibitor, imatinib, was approved for clinical use in chronic myeloid leukemia (CML). The spectacular success of this first-in-class agent ushered in a transformation in cancer drug discovery from efforts that were largely based on novel cytotoxic chemotherapy agents to an almost exclusive focus on molecularly targeted agents across the pharmaceutical and biotechnology industry and academia. This chapter summarizes this remarkable decade of progress with the focus on the concepts underlying this paradigm shift as well as the considerable challenges that remain (Tables 39.1 and 39.2). Readers in search of more specific details on individual drugs and their indications should consult the relevant disease-specific chapters elsewhere in this volume as well as references cited within this chapter. Readers should also note that the epidermal growth factor receptor (EGFR) and human epidermal growth factor receptor 2 (HER2) tyrosine kinases covered here have also been successfully targeted by monoclonal antibodies that engage these proteins at the cell surface. These drugs, often referred to as biologics rather than small molecule inhibitors, are covered in other chapters. The chapter is organized around kinase targets rather than diseases and, intentionally, has a historical flow to make certain thematic points and illustrate the broad lessons that have been and continue to be learned through the clinical development of these exciting agents.

Perhaps the most stunning discovery from the clinical trials of the ABL kinase inhibitor imatinib was the recognition that tumor cells acquire exquisite dependence on the BCR-ABL fusion oncogene, created by the Philadelphia chromosome translocation.[1] Although this may seem intuitive at first glance, consider the fact that the translocation arises in an otherwise normal hematopoietic stem cell whose survival is regulated by a complex array of growth factors and interactions with the bone marrow microenvironment. While BCR-ABL clearly gives this cell a growth advantage that, over years, results in the clinical phenotype of CML, there was no reason to expect that these cells would depend on BCR-ABL for their survival when confronted with an inhibitor. In the absence of BCR-ABL, these tumor cells could presumably rely on the marrow microenvironment for their survival, just like their normal nontransformed neighbors. Thus, it seemed more likely that by shutting down the driver oncogene, BCR-ABL inhibitors would halt the progression of CML but not eliminate the preexisting tumor cells. But in fact, CML progenitors are eliminated after just a few months of anti-BCR-ABL therapy, indicating they are dependent on the driver oncogene for their survival and have "forgotten" how to return to normal. This phenomenon, subsequently documented in a variety of human malignancies, is colloquially termed "oncogene addiction."[2] Although the molecular basis for this addiction remains to be defined, the notion of finding an Achilles' heel for each cancer has captivated the cancer research community, spawning a broad array of efforts to elucidate the molecular identity of these targets and discover relevant inhibitors.

EARLY SUCCESSES: TARGETING CANCERS WITH WELL-KNOWN KINASE MUTATIONS

From the beginning, clinical trials of imatinib were restricted to patients with Philadelphia chromosome–positive CML. For what seem like obvious reasons, there was never any serious discussion about treating patients with Philadelphia chromosome–negative leukemia because the assumption was that only patients with the BCR-ABL fusion gene would have a chance of responding. This was clearly a wise decision because hematologic response rates approached 90% and cytogenetic remissions were seen in nearly half of the patient in the early phase studies.[3] It was obvious the drug worked and imatinib was approved in record time. Unwittingly, the power of genome-based patient selection was demonstrated in the clinical development of the very first kinase inhibitor. It has taken a decade for this lesson to be fully learned. Today the much larger clinical experience with an array of different kinase inhibitors across many tumor types has led to a much better understanding of the principles that dictate oncogene addiction that, in retrospect, were staring researchers in the face. Foremost among them is the notion that tumors with somatic mutation or amplification of a kinase drug target are much more likely to be dependent on that target for survival. Hence, a patient whose tumor has such a mutation is much more likely to respond to treatment with the appropriate inhibitor.

After CML, the next example to illustrate this principle was gastrointestinal stromal tumor (GIST), which is associated with mutations in the KIT tyrosine kinase receptor or, more rarely, in the platelet-derived growth factor receptor (PDGFR).[4,5] Serendipitously, imatinib inhibits both KIT and PDGFR; therefore, the clinical test of KIT inhibition in GIST followed quickly on the heels of the success in CML.[6] In retrospect, the rapid progress made in these two diseases was based, in part, on the fact that the driver molecular lesion (BCR-ABL or KIT mutation, respectively) is present in nearly all patients who are diagnosed with these two diseases. The molecular analysis merely confirmed the diagnosis that was made using standard clinical and histological criteria. Consequently, clinicians could identify the patients most likely to respond based on clinical criteria rather than rely on an elaborate molecular profiling infrastructure to prescreen patients. Consequently, clinical trials evaluating kinase inhibitors in CML and GIST accrued quickly and the therapeutic benefit became clear almost immediately.

TABLE 39.1

APPROVED KINASE INHIBITORS

Target	Drug	Approved Indications	Anticipated Future Indications[a]
BCR-ABL	Imatinib Dasatinib Nilotinib	Chronic myeloid leukemia Philadelphia chromosome positive acute lymphoid leukemia	
KIT	Imatinib Sunitinib	Gastrointestinal stromal tumor	
PDGFRα/β	Imatinib	Chronic myelomonocytic leukemia (with TEL-PDGFRβ fusion) Hypereosinophilic syndrome (with PDGFRβ fusion) Dermatofibrosarcoma protuberans	
HER2	Lapatinib	Her2+breast cancer	
EGFR	Gefitinib Erlotinib	Lung adenocarcinoma (with EGFR mutation, although not required for initial approval)	
VEGFR	Sorafenib Sunitinib	Kidney cancer Hepatocellular carcinoma (sorafenib only)	Hepatocellular carcinoma (sunitinib) Pancreatic neuroendocrine tumors (sunitinib) Thyroid cancer (sorafenib)
TORC1 (mTOR)	Sirolimus (rapamycin) Everolimus Temsirolimus	Kidney cancer	Mantle cell lymphoma Endometrial cancer

[a]Indications are considered "anticipated" based on data from randomized phase 2 trials that led to initiation of phase 3 registration studies.

TABLE 39.2

UNAPPROVED KINASE INHIBITORS WITH CLEAR EVIDENCE OF CLINICAL ACTIVITY

Target	Drug	Clinical Development Path	Clinical Trial Stage	Other Potential Indications
BRAF	PLX4032 GSK2118436	BRAF mutant melanoma	Phase 3 Phase 1	Thyroid cancer Colon cancer
ALK	PF02341066	ALK mutant lung cancer	Phase 3	ALK-positive anaplastic lymphoma ALK-mutant neuroblastoma
JAK2	INCB018424 TG101348	Myelofibrosis	Phase 3 Phase 2	Polycythemia vera Essential thrombocytosis
FLT3	Midostaurin (PKC412) AC220	FLT3 mutant acute myeloid leukemia	Phase 1 Phase 2	FLT3 mutant acute lymphoid leukemia
MEK	AZD6244 GSK1120212	BRAF mutant melanoma	Phase 2 Phase 1	Combination therapy with PI3K pathway inhibitors (many tumor types) or RAF inhibitors (BRAF mutant melanoma)
RET	Vandetanib (AZD6474) Sorafenib XL184 motesanib (AMG706)	Thyroid cancer	Phase 3 Phase 3 Phase 3 Phase 2	Combination with chemotherapy (lung cancer, motesanib phase 3 trial)[a]
VEGFR	Axitinib (AG013736) Tivozanib (AV951) Pazopanib (GW786034)	Kidney cancer	Phase 3 Phase 3 Phase 3	Combination therapy with TORC1 inhibitors (in kidney cancer) Hepatocellular carcinoma

[a]Based on the success of chemotherapy in combination with the VEGF antibody bevacizumab in several tumor types, several VEGFR inhibitors and RET inhibitors (which have activity against VEGFR) have been evaluated in chemotherapy combinations in lung cancer and colon cancer. Most trials have failed in the phase 3 setting.

The notion that molecular alteration of a driver kinase determines sensitivity to a cognate kinase inhibitor was further validated during the development of the dual EGFR/HER2 kinase inhibitor lapatinib. Clinical trials of this kinase inhibitor were conducted in women with advanced HER2-positive breast cancer based on earlier success in these same patients with the monoclonal antibody trastuzumab that targets the extracellular domain of the HER2 kinase. Lapatinib was initially approved in combination with the cytotoxic agent capecitabine for women with resistance to trastuzumab,[7] then was subsequently approved for frontline use in metastatic breast cancer in combination with chemotherapy or hormonal therapy, depending on estrogen-receptor status. A key ingredient that enabled the clinical development of lapatinib was the routine use of HER2 gene amplification testing in the diagnosis of breast cancer, pioneered during the development of trastuzumab several years earlier. This widespread clinical practice allowed rapid identification of those patients most likely to benefit. If lapatinib trials had been conducted in unselected patients, the clinical signal in breast cancer would likely have been missed.

The Serendipity of Unexpected Clinical Responses

In contrast to the logical development of imatinib and lapatinib in molecularly defined patient populations, the EGFR kinase inhibitors gefitinib and erlotinib entered the clinic without the benefit of such a focused clinical development plan. Although considerable preclinical data implicated EGFR as a cancer drug target, there was little insight into which patients were most likely to benefit. The first clue that EGFR inhibitors would have a role in lung cancer came from the recognition, by several astute clinicians, of remarkable responses in a small fraction of patients with lung adenocarcinoma.[8] Further studies revealed the curious clinical circumstance that those patients most likely to benefit tended to be never smokers, women, and those of Asian ethnicity.[9] Clearly there was a strong clinical signal in a subgroup of patients who could perhaps be enriched based on these clinical features, but it seemed that a unifying molecular lesion must be present. Three academic groups simultaneously converged on the answer. Mutations in the *EGFR* gene were detected in the 10% to 15% of patients with lung adenocarcinoma who had radiographic responses.[10–12] It may seem surprising that mutations in a gene as highly visible as *EGFR* and in such a prevalent cancer had not been detected earlier. But the motivation to search aggressively for *EGFR* mutations was not there until the clinical responses were seen. Perhaps even more surprising was the failure of the pharmaceutical company sponsors of the two most advanced compounds, gefitinib and erlotinib, to embrace this important discovery and refocus future clinical development plans on patients with *EGFR* mutant lung adenocarcinoma.

Clinical development of cytotoxic agents has always proceeded empirically. Typically, small numbers of patients with different cancers are treated in "all comer" phase 1 studies (no enrichment for subgroups) with the goal of eliciting a clinical signal in at least one tumor type. A single agent response rate of 20% to 30% in a disease-specific phase 2 trial can justify a randomized phase 3 registration trial where the typical end point for drug approval is time to progression or survival. Cytotoxics are also typically evaluated in combination with existing standard of care treatment (typically approved chemotherapy agents) with the goal of increasing the response rate or enhancing the duration of response.

The clinical development of gefitinib and erlotinib followed the cytotoxic model. Both drugs had similarly low but convincing single agent response rates (10% to 15%) in chemotherapy-refractory advanced lung cancer. Indeed, gefitinib was originally granted accelerated approval by the U.S. Food and Drug Administration (FDA) in 2003 based on the impressive nature of these responses, contingent on the completion of formal phase 3 studies with survival end points.[13] The sponsors of both drugs therefore conducted phase 3 registration studies in patients with chemotherapy-refractory advanced stage lung cancer but without prescreening patients for EGFR mutation status. (In fairness, these trials were initiated prior to the discovery of EGFR mutations in lung cancer.) Erlotinib was approved in 2004 on the basis of a modest survival advantage over placebo (the BR.21 trial); however, gefitinib failed to demonstrate a survival advantage in essentially the same patient population.[14,15] This difference in outcome was surprising since the two drugs have highly similar chemical structures and biological properties. Perhaps the most important difference in the two trials was drug dose. Erlotinib was given at the maximum tolerated dose, which produces a high frequency of rash and diarrhea. Both side effects are presumed "on target" consequences of EGFR inhibition since EGFR is highly expressed in skin and gastrointestinal epithelial cells. In contrast, gefitinib was dosed slightly lower to mitigate these toxicities, with the rationale that responses should not be compromised since clinical responses were clearly documented at lower doses.

In parallel with the single agent phase 3 trials in chemotherapy-refractory patients, both gefitinib and erlotinib were studied as upfront therapy for advanced lung cancer to determine if either would improve the efficacy of standard "doublet" (carboplatin/paclitaxel or gemcitabine/cisplatin) chemotherapy when all three drugs were given in combination. These trials, termed INTACT-1 and INTACT-2 (gefitinib with either gemcitabine/cisplatin or with carboplatin/paclitaxel) and TRIBUTE (erlotinib with carboplatin/paclitaxel) collectively enrolled over 3,000 patients.[16–18] Excitement in the oncology community was high based on the clear single agent activity of both EGFR inhibitors. But both trials were spectacular failures—neither drug showed any benefit over chemotherapy alone. The emerging data on *EGFR* mutations in the 10% to 15% of patients who responded to single agent *EGFR* inhibitor therapy provided a logical explanation. Only a small fraction of patients enrolled in these phase 3 trials had a chance of benefit since the clinical signal from those whose tumors had *EGFR* mutations was diluted by all the patients whose tumors had no *EGFR* alterations, many of whom benefited from chemotherapy.

The convergence of the *EGFR* mutation discovery with these clinical trial results will be remembered as a remarkable time in the history of targeted cancer therapies, not just for the important role of these agents as lung cancer therapies but for the delays in studying whether *EGFR* genotype should drive treatment selection. Perhaps the most egregious error came from a retrospective analysis of tumors from patients treated in the BR.21 trial that concluded that *EGFR* mutations did *not* predict for a survival advantage.[19] (*EGFR* gene amplification *was* associated with survival but only in univariate analysis.) This conclusion was concerning because less than 30% of patients on the trial had tissue available for EGFR mutation analysis, raising questions about the adequacy of the sample size. Furthermore, the *EGFR* mutation assay used by the authors was subsequently criticized because a significant number of the *EGFR* mutations reported in these patients were in residues not previously found by others who had sequenced thousands of tumors. Many of these mutations were suspected to be an artifact of working from formalin-fixed biopsies. (Formalin fixed, paraffin-embedded tissue samples present special challenges for nucleic acid analysis that can be avoided if the tissue is fresh frozen at the time of acquisition or can be overcome with additional controls.)

More recently, clinical investigators in Asia, where a greater fraction of lung cancers (roughly 30%) are positive for *EGFR* mutations, addressed the question of whether mutations predict for clinical benefit in a prospective trial. In this study known as IPASS, gefitinib was clearly superior to standard doublet chemotherapy as frontline therapy for patients with advanced *EGFR* mutation–positive lung adenocarcinoma.[20] Conversely, *EGFR* mutation–negative patients fared much worse with gefitinib and benefited from chemotherapy. In addition, *EGFR* mutation–positive patients had a more favorable overall prognosis regardless of treatment, indicating that *EGFR* mutation is also a prognostic biomarker. The IPASS trial serves as a compelling example of a properly designed (and executed) biomarker-driven clinical trial. Although the rationale for this clinical development strategy had been demonstrated years earlier with BCR-ABL in leukemia, KIT in GIST, and HER2 in breast cancer, it was difficult to derail the empiric approach that had been used for decades in developing cytotoxic agents.

Platelet-Driven Growth Factor Receptor Leukemias and Sarcoma

The discovery of *EGFR* mutations in lung cancer (motivated by dramatic clinical responses in a subset of patients treated with EGFR kinase inhibitors) is the most visible example of the power of bedside-to-bench science, but it is not the only (or the first) such example from the kinase inhibitor era. Shortly after the approval of imatinib for CML in 2001, two case reports documented dramatic remissions in patients with hypereosinophilic syndrome (HES), a blood disorder characterized by prolonged elevation of eosinophil counts and subsequent organ dysfunction from eosinophil infiltration, when treated with imatinib.[21,22] Although HES resembles myeloproliferative diseases such as chronic myeloid leukemia, the molecular pathogenesis of HES was completely unknown at the time. Reasoning that these clinical responses must be explained by inhibition of a driver kinase, a team of laboratory-based physician scientists quickly searched for mutations in the three kinases known to be inhibited by imatinib (ABL, KIT, and PDGFR). ABL and KIT were quickly excluded, but the *PDGFRα* gene was targeted by an interstitial deletion that fused the upstream FIP1L1 gene to PDGFRα.[23] FIP1L1-PDGFRα is a constitutively active tyrosine kinase, analogous to BCR-ABL, and also inhibited by imatinib. As with *EGFR*-mutant lung cancer, the molecular pathophysiology of HES was discovered by dissecting the mechanism of response to the drug used to treat it.

The HES/FIP1L1-PDGFRα story serves as a nice bookend to an earlier discovery that the t(5,12) chromosome translocation, found rarely in patients with chronic myelomonocytic leukemia, creates the TEL-PDGFRβ fusion tyrosine kinase.[24] Similar to HES, treatment of patients with t(5,12) translocation-positive leukemias with imatinib has also proven successful.[25] A third example comes from dermatofibrosarcoma protuberans, a sarcoma characterized by a t(17,22) translocation that fuses the *COL1A* gene to the gene for *PDGFB ligand* (not the receptor). COL1A-PDGFB is oncogenic through autocrine stimulation of the normal PDGFR in these tumor cells. Patients with dermatofibrosarcoma protuberans respond to imatinib therapy because it targets the PDGFR, just one step downstream from the oncogenic lesion.[26]

Exploiting the New Paradigm: Searching for Other Kinase-Driven Cancers

The benefits of serendipity notwithstanding, the growing number of examples of successful kinase inhibitor therapy in tumors with mutation or amplification of the drug target begged for a more rational approach to drug discovery and development. In 2002, the list of human tumors known to have mutations in kinases was quite small. Due to advances in automated gene sequencing, it became possible to ask whether a much larger fraction of human cancers might also have such mutations through a brute force approach. To address this question comprehensively, one would have to sequence all of the kinases in the genome in hundreds of samples of each tumor type. Several early pilot studies demonstrated the potential of this approach by revealing important new targets for drug development. Perhaps the most spectacular was the discovery of mutations in the BRAF kinase in over half of patients with melanoma, as well as in a smaller fraction of colon and thyroid cancers[27] Another was the discovery of mutations in the Janus-associated tyrosine kinase 2 (*JAK2*) in nearly all patients with polycythemia vera, as well as a significant fraction of patients with myelofibrosis and essential thrombocytosis.[28–30] A third example was the identification of *PIK3CA* mutations in a variety of tumors, with the greatest frequencies in breast, endometrial, and colorectal cancers.[31] *PIK3CA* encodes a lipid kinase that generates the second messenger phosphatidyl inositol 3-phosphate (PIP3). PIP3 activates growth and survival signaling through the AKT family of kinases as well as other downstream effectors. Coupled with the well-established role of the PTEN (phosphatase and tensin homologue) lipid phosphatase in dephosphorylating PIP3, the discovery of *PIK3CA* mutations focused tremendous attention on developing inhibitors at multiple levels of this pathway, as discussed further below.

Each of these important discoveries—BRAF, JAK2, PIK3CA—came from relatively small efforts (less than 100 tumors) generally focused on resequencing only those exons that coded for regions of kinases where mutations had been found in other kinases (typically the juxtamembrane and kinase domains). These restricted searches were largely driven by cost. In 2006, a comprehensive effort to sequence all of the exons in all kinases in 100 tumors could easily exceed several million dollars. Financial support for such projects could not be obtained easily through traditional funding agencies as the risk/reward ratio was considered too high. Furthermore, substantial infrastructure for sample acquisition, microdissection of tumor from normal tissue, nucleic acid preparation, high throughput automated sequencing, and computational analysis of the resulting data were essential. Few institutions were equipped to address these challenges. In response, the National Cancer Institute in the United States (in partnership with the National Human Genome Research Institute) and an international group known as the International Cancer Genome Consortium (ICGC) launched large-scale efforts to sequence the complete genomes of thousands of cancers. By 2010 the U.S. effort (called The Cancer Genome Atlas [TCGA]) had completed an analysis of glioblastoma[32] and ovarian cancer and had launched efforts in lung, kidney, endometrial, and other cancers. The international consortium had committed to sequencing 25,000 tumors representing 50 different cancer subtypes.[33] Both groups stipulated immediate release of all sequence information to the research community free of charge so that the entire scientific community could learn from the data. These grand-scale projects were possible due to a dramatic decline in sequencing costs. Discussions just a few years earlier about which genes (or regions of genes) to include in such projects were no longer necessary. The cost of complete exome (all exons from all genes in the human genome—not just kinases) and complete genome (all DNA) resequencing had fallen to about $5,000 per sample.

Rounding Out the Treatment of Myeloproliferative Disorders: JAK2 and Myelofibrosis

Taken together with the BCR-ABL translocation in chronic myeloid leukemia and FIP1L1-PDGFRα in HES, the discovery of *JAK2* mutations in polycythemia, essential thrombocytosis, and myelofibrosis provided a unifying understanding of myeloproliferative disorders as diseases of abnormal kinase activation. JAK family kinases are the primary effectors of signaling through inflammatory cytokine receptors and had therefore been considered compelling targets for anti-inflammatory drugs. But the JAK2 mutation discovery immediately shifted these efforts toward developing JAK2 inhibitors for myeloproliferative disorders. Since most patients have a common JAK2 V617F mutation, these efforts could rapidly focus on screening for activity against a single genotype. Progress has been rapid. Two compounds (INCB018424 and TG101348) were active in phase 2 studies in myelofibrosis, one of which has already progressed to a randomized phase 3 trial.[34,35] Myelofibrosis was selected as the initial indication (instead of essential thrombocytosis or polycythemia vera) because the time to registration is expected to be shortest. Currently there are no approved treatments for myelofibrosis and shrinkage in spleen size can be used as an end point for drug approval. Successful trials in myelofibrosis will likely lead to studies in essential thrombocytosis and polycythemia vera.

BRAF Mutant Melanoma: Several Missteps before Finding the Right Inhibitor

As with JAK2 mutations in myeloproliferative disorders, the discovery of *BRAF* mutations in patients with melanoma launched widespread efforts to find potent BRAF inhibitors. One early candidate was the drug sorafenib, which had been optimized during drug discovery to inhibit RAF kinases. (Sorafenib also inhibits vascular endothelial growth factor receptor [VEGFR], which led to its approval in kidney cancer as discussed later in this chapter.) Despite the compelling molecular rationale for targeting BRAF, clinical results of sorafenib in melanoma were extremely disappointing and reduced enthusiasm for pursuing BRAF as a drug target.[36] In hindsight, this concern was completely misguided. Sorafenib dosing is limited by toxicities that preclude achieving serum levels in patients that potently inhibit RAF (but are sufficient to inhibit VEGFR). In addition, patients were enrolled without screening for *BRAF* mutations in their tumors. Although the frequency of *BRAF* mutations in melanoma is high, the inclusion of patients without *BRAF* mutation diluted the chance of seeing any clinical signal. In short, the clinical evaluation of sorafenib in melanoma was poorly designed to test the hypothesis that BRAF is a therapeutic target. The danger is that negative data from such clinical experiments can slow subsequent progress. It is critical to know the pharmacodynamic properties of the drug and the molecular phenotype of the patients being studied when interpreting the results of a negative study.

The fact that RAF kinases are intermediate components of the well-characterized RAS/MAP kinase pathway (transducing signals from RAS to RAF to MEK to ERK) raised the possibility that tumors with BRAF mutations might respond to inhibitors of one of these downstream kinases (Fig. 39.1). Preclinical studies revealed that tumor cell lines with BRAF mutation were exquisitely sensitive to inhibitors of the

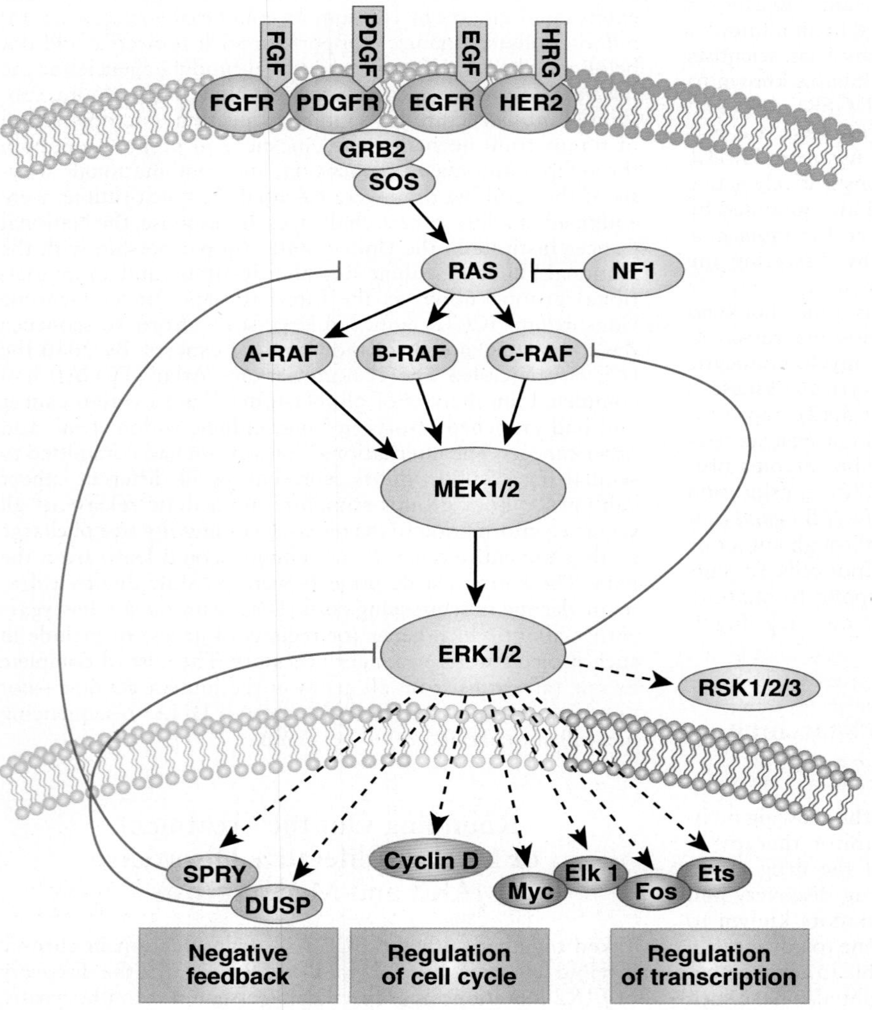

FIGURE 39.1 The RAS-RAF-MEK-ERK signaling pathway. The classical mitogen-activated protein kinase (MAPK) pathway is activated in human tumors by several mechanisms, including the binding of ligand to receptor tyrosine kinases (RTK), mutational activation of an RTK, by loss of the tumor suppressor NF1, or by mutations in RAS, BRAF, and MEK1. Phosphorylation and thus activation of ERK regulates transcription of target genes that promote cell cycle progression and tumor survival. The ERK pathway contains a classical feedback loop in which the expression of feedback elements such as SPRY and DUSP family proteins are regulated by the level of ERK activity. Loss of expression of SPRY and DUSP family members due to promoter methylation or deletion is thus permissive for persistently elevated pathway output. In the case of tumors with mutant BRAF, pathway output is enhanced by impaired upstream feedback regulation. (From ref. 114, with permission.)

downstream kinase MEK.[37] Sorafenib, in contrast, does not show this profile of activity.[38] Thus, proper preclinical screening would have revealed the shortcomings of sorafenib as a BRAF inhibitor. Curiously, cell lines with mutation or amplification of *EGFR* or *HER2*, which function upstream in the pathway, were insensitive to MEK inhibition. Even tumor lines with RAS mutations were variably sensitive. In short, the preclinical data made a strong case that MEK inhibitors should be effective in *BRAF* mutant melanoma but not in other subtypes. The reason that *HER2, EGFR*, and *RAS* mutant tumors were not sensitive to MEK inhibitors is explained, at least in part, by the existence of negative feedback loops that modulate the flux of signal transduction through MEK.[39]

In parallel with the generation of these preclinical findings, clinical trials of several MEK inhibitors were initiated. Patients with various cancers were enrolled in the early studies but there was a strong bias to include melanoma patients. Significant efforts were made to demonstrate MEK inhibition in tumor cells by measuring the phosphorylation status of the direct downstream substrate ERK using immunohistochemical analysis of biopsies from patients with metastatic disease. Phase 1 studies of the two earliest compounds in clinical development (PD325901 and AZD6244) documented reduced phospho-ERK staining at multiple dose levels in several patients on whom baseline and treatment biopsies were obtained.[40,41] These pharmacodynamic studies, while well intentioned, were not quantitative enough to document the magnitude of MEK inhibition in these patients. Furthermore, clinical responses were observed in a few patients with BRAF mutant melanoma. Armed with this confidence, a randomized phase 2 clinical trial of AZD6244 was conducted in advanced melanoma, with the chemotherapeutic agent temozolomide (approved for glioblastoma) as the comparator arm. Clinical development of PD325901 was discontinued because of safety concerns about ocular and neurologic toxicity. Disappointingly, patients receiving AZD6244 had no benefit in progression-free survival when compared to temozolomide-treated patients, raising further concerns about the viability of BRAF as a drug target.[42] Closer examination of the data revealed that clinical responses were, indeed, seen in patients receiving AZD6244. The fact that *BRAF* mutation status was not required for study entry likely diminished the clinical signal in the AZD6244 arm, a lesson learned from the EGFR inhibitor trials in lung cancer. In addition, the results in the control group were better than expected and reflect greater activity of temozolomide in melanoma than previously believed.

All doubts about BRAF as a target vanished in 2009 to 2010 when dramatic clinical responses were observed with a novel BRAF inhibitor PLX4032. Like sorafenib, this compound was optimized to inhibit RAF but with an additional focus on mutant BRAF. PLX4032 differs dramatically from sorafenib because it potently inhibits BRAF without the additional broad range of activities that sorafenib has against other kinases like VEGFR.[43] The greater selectivity of PLX4032 relative to sorafenib resulted in much greater tolerability such that it could be given at high doses while avoiding significant toxicity. The early days of PLX4032 clinical development were plagued by challenges in maximizing the oral bioavailability of the drug.[44] Consequently, the initial phase 1 clinical trial was temporarily halted to develop a novel formulation (the coingredients in the drug capsule or tablet that improve solubility and absorption through the gastrointestinal tract). Much higher serum levels were obtained in patients who received the new PLX4032 formation and, shortly thereafter, complete and partial responses were observed in about 80% of the melanoma patients with *BRAF* mutant tumors. Strikingly, no activity was observed in patients whose tumors were wild type for *BRAF*.[45,46] The data were so compelling that PLX4032 was immediately advanced to a phase 3 registration trial. Similarly impressive responses in *BRAF* mutant melanoma patients were observed in a phase 1 trial of another, even more potent RAF inhibitor GSK2118436,[47] providing further proof that BRAF is an important cancer target.

The PLX4032 and GSK2118436 data also provide insight into why sorafenib and the early MEK inhibitor trials failed to demonstrate activity. One lesson is the critical importance of achieving adequate target inhibition. Clinical responses with PLX4032 were observed only after the drug was reformulated to achieve substantially higher serum levels. Reductions in phospho-ERK staining (as documented by immunohistochemistry) were documented in the earlier trials but, in retrospect, the assays were not sensitive enough to distinguish between modest (approximately 50%) kinase inhibition versus more complete BRAF or MEK inhibition. Efficacy in preclinical models is significantly improved using doses that give greater than 80% inhibition, and the human trial data suggest that this degree of pathway blockade is also required for a high clinical response rate.[46] Interestingly, investigators conducting a phase 1 clinical trial with a third MEK inhibitor, GSK1120212, have reported a high response rate (approximately 40%) in BRAF-mutant melanoma patients. These data appear to be substantially better than those observed with the earlier MEK inhibitors, although not as impressive as with PLX4032.[48] There is speculation that this newer MEK inhibitor inhibits MEK more completely that the earlier generation compounds, but this remains to be demonstrated in patients. Collectively, these experiences illustrate the critical need for quantitative pharmacodynamic assays to measure target inhibition early in clinical development. A second lesson is the importance of genotyping all patients for mutation or amplification of the relevant drug target. Not only does this ensure that a sufficient number of patients with the biomarker of interest are included in the study, the results also provide compelling evidence early in clinical development in support (or not) of the preclinical hypothesis.

Getting It Right: ALK and Lung Cancer

The development of the ALK inhibitor crizotinib (PF02341066), which is currently under evaluation in a phase 3 registration trial in lung cancer, illustrates how an unexpected signal obtained in a small number of patients can quickly shift a program in an entirely new direction with a high probability of success. The key ingredient is this story is a familiar one—a strong molecular hypothesis backed up by clinical response data in a small number of carefully selected patients. Crizotinib emerged from a drug discovery program at Pfizer focused on finding inhibitors of the MET receptor tyrosine kinase and entered the clinic with this target as its lead indication.[49] As discussed above with imatinib, essentially all kinase inhibitors have activity against other targets (so-called off target activities), which can sometimes prove to be advantageous. Off target activities are typically discovered by screening compounds against a large panel of kinases to establish profiles of relative selectivity against the intended target. Off target activity, potency, and pharmaceutical properties (bioavailability, half-life) are all factors that influence the decision of which compound to advance to clinical development. The primary off target activity of crizotinib is against the ALK tyrosine kinase.

ALK was first identified as a candidate driver oncogene in 1994 through the cloning of the t(2,5) chromosomal translocation associated with anaplastic large cell lymphoma, which creates the NPM-ALK fusion gene.[50] This discovery, together with the demonstration that NPM-ALK causes lymphoma in mice, made a compelling case for ALK as a drug target in this disease. But there was limited interest in developing ALK inhibitors because this particular lymphoma subtype is rare and most commonly found in children. Companies are generally reluctant to develop drugs solely for pediatric indications because of complexities related to dose selection and additional regulatory guidelines. Efforts to streamline this development process are under way.

In 2007, another ALK fusion gene called *EML4-ALK* was discovered in a small fraction of patients with lung adenocarcinoma, with an estimated frequency of 1% to 5%.[51] This discovery did not immediately capture the attention of drug developers, but several academic groups that had already begun testing lung cancer patients seen at their institutions for *EGFR* mutations simply added an *EML4-ALK* fusion test to the screening panel. Astute clinical investigators participating in the phase 1 trial of crizotinib, which was designed to include patients with a broad array of advanced cancers, were aware of the off target ALK activity and enrolled several lung cancer patients with *EML4-ALK* fusions in the study. These patients had remarkably dramatic responses.[52] This serendipitous finding in a few *ALK*-positive patients was confirmed in a larger cohort, resulting in the initiation of a phase 3 study in *ALK*-positive lung cancer, just 2 years after the discovery of the *EML4-ALK* fusion. Crizotinib is also being evaluated in other diseases associated with genomic alterations in *ALK*, including large cell anaplastic lymphoma, neuroblastoma,[53] and inflammatory myofibroblastic sarcoma.[54]

Extending the Model to RET Mutations in Thyroid Cancer

Subsets of patients with papillary or medullary thyroid cancer have activating mutations or translocations targeting the RET tyrosine kinase receptor, raising the question of whether RET inhibitors might have a role in this disease.[55] Although no drugs specifically designed to inhibit RET have entered the clinic, four compounds with off target activity against RET (vandetanib, sorafenib, motesanib, and XL184) have all shown single agent activity in phase 2 thyroid cancer studies.[56–60] Three are currently under evaluation in phase 3 registration trials, one of which (vandetanib) has recently reported improved progression-free survival. Because all four compounds also inhibit VEGFR, it is unclear whether the clinical benefit observed in these studies is explained by inhibition of RET, VEGFR, or both. Unlike the crizotinib trials in *ALK*-positive lung cancer, enrollment in these registration studies was not restricted to patients with *RET* mutations. In addition to the fact that thyroid cancer patients are not routinely screened for these mutations, the primary reason for including all comers in these studies is that clinical responses are observed in a larger fraction of patients than can be accounted for based on the suspected frequency of *RET* mutation. Responses in patients without *RET* mutation (if they occur) might be explained by mutations in other genes in the RAS-MAP kinase pathway such as *BRAF* or *HRAS*, which are found in a substantial fraction of patients and are typically nonoverlapping with *RET* alterations.[55] Clearly, detailed genotype–response correlations, as demonstrated in lung cancer and melanoma, will clarify the role of these mutations in predicting response to these drugs. Thyroid cancer is also a compelling indication for the BRAF and MEK inhibitors discussed above in melanoma.

FLT3 Inhibitors in Acute Myeloid Leukemia

Shortly after the success of imatinib, the receptor tyrosine kinase FLT3 emerged as a compelling drug candidate based on the presence of activating mutations in about one-third of patients with acute myeloid leukemia (AML).[61] Laboratory studies documented that FLT3 alleles bearing these mutations, which occur as internal tandem duplications (ITDs) of the juxtamembrane domain or point mutation in the kinase domain, function as driver oncogenes in mouse models, giving phenotypes analogous to BCR-ABL.[62] As with RET in thyroid cancer, no compounds had been specifically optimized to target FLT3, but several drugs with off target FLT3 activity were redirected to AML. Disappointingly, the first three of the compounds tested (midostaurin, lestaurtinib, sunitinib) showed only marginal single agent activity in relapsed AML patients, even in those with *FLT3* mutations.[63–65] Despite the strong molecular rationale for FLT3 as a driver lesion, questions were raised about the viability of FLT3 as a drug target. Pharmacodynamic studies showed evidence of FLT3 kinase inhibition in tumor cells, but the magnitude and duration of these effects were difficult to quantify, raising the possibility of inadequate target inhibition.[63] Indeed, the dose of all three compounds was limited by toxicities believed to be independent of FLT3. A more pessimistic interpretation was that FLT3, although presumably important for initiation of AML, was no longer required for tumor maintenance due to the accumulation of additional driver genomic alterations. If true, even complete FLT3 blockade with a highly selective inhibitor would be expected to fail. But this view was not supported by the fact that clinical responses were observed in the somewhat analogous situation of single agent ABL kinase inhibitor treatment of chronic myeloid leukemia in blast crisis, where BCR-ABL is just one of many additional genomic alterations that contributes to disease progression yet complete remissions are observed in many patients.

Despite this pessimism about FLT3 as a viable drug target, two drugs are now advancing toward drug registration trials. Midostaurin, one of the early compounds that showed disappointing single agent activity in relapsed AML, is being evaluated in a randomized phase 3 trial for newly diagnosed AML combined with standard induction chemotherapy. A single arm phase 2 study showed higher and more durable remission rates in FLT3 mutant patients when compared to historical controls.[66] The second compound, AC220, is a next generation FLT3 inhibitor with greater potency and specificity and with impressive single agent activity in *FLT3*-mutant relapsed AML—precisely the population where midostaurin and others failed.[67,68] It is not clear if this success is due to more potent FLT3 inhibition in patients since detailed pharmacodynamic studies are not yet available. Assuming these compounds prove successful in AML, it will be important to examine their activity in the rare cases of pediatric acute lymphoid leukemia associated with *FLT3* mutation. Although testing is still inconclusive on FLT3 inhibitors, the failure of early compounds in AML is reminiscent of the failures of early RAF and MEK inhibitors in melanoma. Collectively, these examples emphasize the importance of using optimized compounds to test a molecularly based hypothesis in patients and to focus enrollment on those patients with the relevant molecular lesion.

Kidney Cancer: Targeting the Tumor and the Host

A recurring theme in this chapter is the critical role of driver kinase mutations in guiding the development of kinase inhibitors. Ironically, four kinase inhibitors have been approved for kidney cancer over the past 5 years in a tumor type with no known kinase mutations. The most common molecular alteration in kidney cancer is loss of function in the Von Hippel-Lindau (*VHL*) tumor suppressor gene, resulting in activation of the hypoxia inducible factor[66] pathway.[69] As a consequence of *VHL* loss, which normally targets hypoxia-induced factor

(HIF) proteins for proteosomal degradation, HIF1α and HIF2α are constitutively active transcription factors that function as oncogenes through activation of an array of downstream target genes. Among these is the angiogenesis factor VEGF, which is secreted by HIF-expressing cells and promotes the development and maintenance of tumor neovasculature. HIF-mediated secretion of VEGF by tumor cells likely explains the highly vascular histopathology of clear cell renal carcinoma. All three currently approved angiogenesis inhibitors (the monoclonal antibody bevacizumab targeting VEGF and the kinase inhibitors sorafenib and sunitinib targeting its receptor VEGFR) have single agent clinical activity in clear cell carcinoma.[70–72] The high specificity of bevacizumab for VEGF leaves little doubt that the activity of this drug is explained by antiangiogenic effects. In contrast, the off target activities of sorafenib and sunitinib include several kinases expressed in kidney tumor cells, stroma, and inflammatory cells (PDGFR, RAF, RET, FLT3, and others). Interestingly, the primary effect of bevacizumab in kidney cancer is disease stabilization, whereas sorafenib and sunitinib have substantial partial response rates. This raises the question of whether the superior antitumor activity of the VEGFR kinase inhibitors is due to concurrent inhibition of other kinases. However, partial responses rates with next generation VEGFR inhibitors (axitinib, pazopanib, and tivozanib), all of which have greater potency and selectivity for VEGFR, are similarly high and reinforce the importance of VEGFR as the critical target in kidney cancer.[73–75] Molecular characterization of tumors from these patients should clarify the mechanism by which each of these inhibitors exerts antitumor activity, particularly if drug-resistant kinase domain mutations are found in any of the targets at relapse.

Two inhibitors of the mammalian target of rapamycin (mTOR) kinase (temsirolimus and everolimus) are also approved for advanced renal cell carcinoma.[76,77] Both temsirolimus and everolimus are known as rapalogs since both are chemical derivatives of the natural product sirolimus (rapamycin). Sirolimus was approved more than 10 years ago to prevent graft rejection in transplant recipients based on its immunosuppressive properties against T cells. Sirolimus also has potent antiproliferative effects against vascular endothelial cells and, on that basis, is incorporated into drug eluting cardiac stents to prevent coronary artery restenosis following angioplasty.[78] Rapalogs differ from other kinase inhibitors discussed in this chapter in that they inhibit the kinase through an allosteric mechanism rather than by targeting the mTOR kinase domain. Because rapalogs also inhibit the growth of cancer cell lines from different tissues of origin, clinical trials were initiated to study their potential role as anticancer agents in a broad range of tumor types. Based on responses in a few phase 1 patients with different tumor types (including kidney cancer), exploratory phase 2 studies were conducted in several diseases. Single agent activity of temsirolimus was observed in a phase 2 kidney cancer study[79] then confirmed in a phase 3 registration trial.[76] The phase 3 everolimus trial, which was initiated after temsirolimus, was noteworthy because clinical benefit was demonstrated in patients who had progressed on the VEGFR inhibitors sorafenib or sunitinib.[77]

In parallel with the empirical clinical development of rapalogs, various laboratories explored the molecular basis for mTOR dependence in cancer cells. mTOR functions at the center of a complex network that integrates signals from growth factor receptors and nutrient sensors to regulate cell growth and size (Fig. 39.2). It does so, in part, by controlling the translation of various mRNAs with complex 5′ untranslated regions into protein. mTOR exists in two distinct complexes known as TORC1 and TORC2. Rapalogs only inhibit the TORC1 complex, which is largely responsible for downstream phosphorylation of targets such as S6K1/2 and 4EBP1/2, which regulate protein translation.[80] The TORC2 complex contributes to activation of AKT by phosphorylating the important regulatory serine residue S473 and is unaffected by rapalogs.

Two hypotheses have emerged to explain the clinical activity of rapalogs in kidney cancer. The antiproliferative activity of these compounds against endothelial cells suggests an antiangiogenic mechanism and is consistent with the clinical activity of the VEGFR inhibitors. But rapalogs also inhibit the growth of kidney cancer cell lines in laboratory models where the effects on tumor angiogenesis have been eliminated. Interestingly, mRNAs for HIF1/2 are among those whose translation is impaired by rapalogs, and this effect has been implicated as the primary mechanism of rapalog activity in kidney cancer xenograft models.[81] As with the VEGFR inhibitors, detailed molecular annotation of tumors from responders and nonresponders will shed light on these issues.

Other Potential Indications for Mammalian Target of Rapamycin Inhibitors

The fact that rapalogs inhibit the growth of cancer cell lines and xenografts from different tumor types raised hopes for a broad role in cancer, but clinical trials of rapalogs outside of kidney cancer have generally been disappointing. Two exceptions are mantle cell lymphoma and endometrial cancer, where convincing single agent activity has led to ongoing drug registration trials.[82–85] Mantle cell lymphoma is characterized by a chromosome translocation that results in constitutive expression of the cell cycle regulatory protein cyclin D1, which functions as a driver oncogene in this disease. Rapalogs inhibit translation of cyclin D1 mRNA in laboratory models, analogous to the inhibition of HIF1/2 translation by rapalogs observed in *VHL*-mutant kidney cancer models. Endometrial cancers often have mutations in one of several genes in the PI3K pathway (*PTEN, PIK3CA, PIK3R1*), any one of which causes pathway activation. Because mTOR functions downstream of PI3K, tumors with these mutations should, in theory, respond to rapalogs. Many studies of cell lines, xenografts, and genetically engineered mouse models have linked PI3K pathway activation to increased sensitivity to rapalogs.[86,87] In fact, endometrial hyperplasia in mice with heterozygous loss of *Pten* is completely reversible by temsirolimus treatment.[88] As with kidney cancer, molecular annotation of the tumors from the mantle cell lymphoma and endometrial cancer patients on these trials is essential to address these questions.

It is unclear why rapalogs have failed in other tumor types. One likely explanation is the concurrence of PI3K pathway mutations with alterations in other pathways that mitigate sensitivity to rapalogs. Another possibility is the disruption of negative feedback loops regulated by mTOR that inhibit signaling from upstream receptor tyrosine kinases. Rapalogs paradoxically *increase* signaling through PI3K due to loss of this negative feedback. A primary consequence is *increased* AKT activation, which signals to an array of downstream substrates that can enhance cell proliferation and survival (other than TORC1, which remains inhibited by rapalog) (Fig. 39.2). This problem might be overcome by combining rapalogs with an inhibitor of an upstream kinase in the feedback loop, such as the insulin-like growth factor receptor (IGFR), to block this undesired effect of rapalogs on PI3K activation.[89] Alternatively, this feedback-mediated activation could, in theory, prevent use of inhibitors of PI3K itself or of the TORC2 complex that activates AKT.

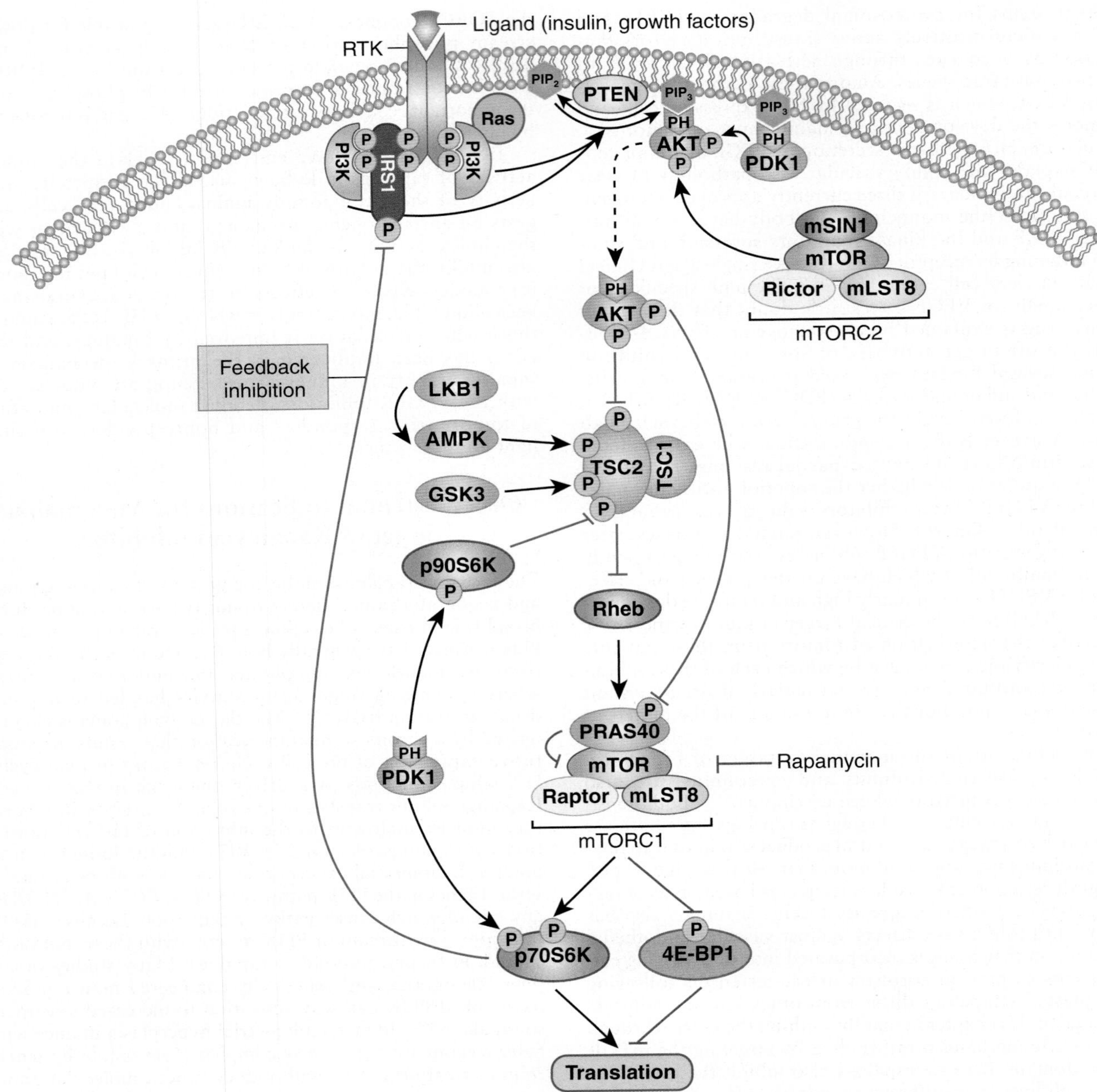

FIGURE 39.2 Feedback inhibition of the phosphatidylinositol 3-kinase (PI3K) pathway. Activated AKT regulates cellular growth through mammalian target of rapamycin (mTOR), a key player in protein synthesis and translation. mTOR forms part of two distinct complexes known as mTORC1 (which contains mTOR, Raptor, mLST8, and PRAS40) and mTORC2 (which contains mTOR, Rictor, mLST8, and mSIN1). mTORC1 is sensitive to rapamycin and controls protein synthesis and translation, at least in part, through p70S6K and eukaryotic translation initiation factor 4E–binding protein 1 (4E-BP1). AKT phosphorylates and inhibits tuberous sclerosis complex 2 (TSC2), resulting in increased mTORC1 activity. AKT also phosphorylates PRAS40, thus relieving the PRAS40 inhibitory effect on mTOR and the mTORC1 complex. mTORC2 and 3-phosphoinositide-dependent kinase (PDK1) phosphorylate AKT on Ser473 and Thr308, respectively, rendering it fully active. mTORC1-activated p70S6K can phosphorylate insulin receptor substrate 1 (IRS1), resulting in inhibition of PI3K activity. In addition, PDK1 phosphorylates and activates p70S6K and p90S6K. The latter has been shown to inhibit TSC2 activity through direct phosphorylation. Conversely, LKB1-activated AMP-activated protein kinase (AMPK) and glycogen synthase kinase 3 (GSK3) activate the TSC1/TSC2 complex through direct phosphorylation of TSC2. Thus, signals through PI3K as well as through LKB1 and AMPK converge on mTORC1. Inhibition of mTORC1 can lead to increased insulin receptor–mediated signaling, and inhibition of PDK1 may lead to activation of mTORC1 and may, paradoxically, promote tumor growth. (From ref. 115, with permission.)

TARGETING THE PI3K PATHWAY DIRECTLY

Mutations or copy number alterations (amplification or deletion of oncogenes or tumor suppressor genes) in PI3K pathway genes (*PIK3CA, PIK3R1, PTEN, AKT1*, and others) are among the most common abnormalities in cancer. Consequently, intensive efforts at many pharmaceutical companies have been devoted to the discovery of small molecule inhibitors targeting kinases in the PI3K pathway. Inhibitors of PI3K-, AKT-, and ATP-competitive (rather than allosteric) inhibitors of mTOR that target both the TORC1 and TORC2 complex are all in clinical development (Table 39.3). Phase 1 clinical trials have, in general, established that the pathway can be efficiently targeted without serious toxicity other than easily manageable effects on glucose metabolism (anticipated based on the importance of PI3K signaling in insulin signaling). Unfortunately, there has been no evidence to date of dramatic single agent clinical activity with any of these agents. To be fair, most compounds are still in a very early clinical development stage and have been evaluated without enriching for patients with PI3K pathway mutations.

Conducting a PI3K pathway mutation-enriched trial is challenging because no single tumor type has such a high frequency of mutations that it becomes the obvious disease for early clinical development (in contrast to BRAF in melanoma). A compelling case can be made for PIK3CA mutant breast or endometrial cancer, but these trials are not straightforward because PIK3CA mutations in breast cancer are associated with good prognosis disease that is often cured by standard therapy.[90] A further complication is the fact that mutations in the PI3K pathway can occur in one of many different genes in the pathway (*PIK3CA, PIK3R1, PTEN, AKT1*, etc.) and sometimes in combination.[91] Treatment response may vary depending on the type of mutation; therefore, lumping patients with different PI3K pathway mutations into the same trial may complicate data interpretation. Indeed, tumor cell lines with PIK3CA mutation respond differently to a PI3K pathway inhibitor compared to those with PTEN loss.[92] There are also technical challenges in developing an assay to determine mutation status for genes like *PTEN*, which can be inactivated by point mutation, deletion, or transcriptional silencing. The success or failure of these drugs as single agents should become clear in the next few years based on the outcome of many phase 2 studies that are currently under way.

COMBINATIONS OF KINASE INHIBITORS

Preclinical studies indicate that combinations of kinase inhibitors are required to realize their full potential as anticancer agents. The most common rationale is to address the problem of concurrent mutations in different pathways that alleviate dependence on a single driver oncogene. The best examples are cancers with mutations in both the RAS/MAP kinase pathway (*RAS* or *BRAF*) and the PI3K pathway (*PIK3CA* or *PTEN*). In mouse models, such doubly mutant tumors fail to respond to single agent treatment with either an AKT inhibitor or a MEK inhibitor. However, combination treatment can give dramatic regressions.[93] Similarly, genetically engineered mice that develop KRAS-driven lung cancer respond only to combination therapy with a PI3K inhibitor and a MEK inhibitor.[94] Several combination therapy trials combining different PI3K pathway and RAS/MAP kinase pathway inhibitors have recently been initiated.

Many of the tumor types discussed in this chapter *do* respond to treatment with a single agent kinase but relapse despite continued inhibitor therapy. Research into the causes of "acquired" kinase inhibitor resistance has revealed two primary mechanisms: novel mutations in the kinase domain of the drug target that preclude inhibition, or "bypass" of the driver kinase signal by activation of a parallel kinase pathway. In both cases, the solution is combination therapy to prevent the emergence of resistance. An elegant demonstration of this approach comes from CML where resistance to imatinib is primarily caused by mutations in the BCR-ABL kinase domain.[95,96] The second-generation ABL inhibitors dasatinib and nilotinib are effective against most imatinib-resistant BCR-ABL mutants and were initially approved as single agent therapy for imatinib-resistant chronic myeloid leukemia.[97,98] Very recently, both drugs have proven superior to imatinib in upfront treatment of chronic myeloid leukemia, due to

TABLE 39.3

COMPOUNDS IN CLINICAL DEVELOPMENT THAT TARGET THE PI3K PATHWAY

Compound	Target	Company	Clinical Trial Stage
BEZ235	PI3K & mTOR	Novartis	Phase 2
BKM120	PI3K	Novartis	Phase 1
SF1126	PI3K family	Semafore	Phase 1
GSK1059615B	PI3K & mTOR	GSK	Phase 1
XL765	PI3K & mTOR	Exelixis	Phase 2
XL147	PI3K	Exelixis	Phase 2
GDC0941	PI3K alpha	Genentech	Phase 1
PX-866	PI3K	Oncothyreon	Phase 1
VQD-002 (triciribine)	pan-AKT	VioQuest	Phase 1
GSK690693	pan-AKT	GSK	Phase 1
MK-2206	AKT	Merck	Phase 2
Perifosine (KRX-0401)	pan-AKT	Keryx	Phase 2
Everolimus (RAD001)	TORC1 (mTOR)	Novartis	Approved
Temsirolimus (CCI779)	TORC1 (mTOR)	Wyeth	Approved
Rapamycin (Rapamune)	TORC1 (mTOR)	Wyeth	Approved
AZD8055	TORC1/2 (mTOR)	AstraZeneca	Phase 1
OSI-027	TORC1/2 (mTOR)	OSI	Phase 1
INK-128	TORC1/2 (mTOR)	Intellikine	Phase 1

increased potency and fewer mechanisms of acquired resistance.[99–101] However, one BCR-ABL mutation called T315I is resistant to all three drugs. A novel ABL kinase inhibitor AP24534 that blocks T315I has shown promising activity in a phase 1 clinical trial that included CML patients with the T315I mutation.[102,103] If AP24534 proves successful, a two drug combination of AP24534 with either dasatinib or nilotinib would likely shut off all mechanisms of relapse, analogous to triple drug highly active antiretroviral therapy (HAART) for human immunodeficiency virus (HIV). Analogous approaches should also be successful in other diseases such as EGFR-mutant lung cancer and KIT-mutant GIST where acquired resistance to the front-line kinase inhibitor is also associated with mutations in the target kinase.[104,105]

The clinical development of kinase inhibitor combinations to prevent acquired resistance is straightforward. Since the frontline drug is already approved, success would be determined by an improvement in response duration using the combination. The situation is more complex when two experimental compounds (e.g., a PI3K pathway inhibitor and a MEK inhibitor) are combined, neither of which shows significant single agent activity. Current regulatory guidelines require a four arm study that compares each single agent to the combination and to a control group in order to obtain approval of the combination. This design can discourage drug developers as well as patients from moving forward because it requires a large sample size, and it requires that 75% of the patients be assigned to treatment arms that are expected to be inactive. In response to growing preclinical evidence supporting the unique activity of certain combinations, these guidelines are now under revision. A more challenging issue may be optimization of the dose and schedule needed to safely combine two investigational drugs. Much like the development of combination chemotherapy several decades ago, it may be important to select compounds with nonoverlapping toxicities to allow sufficient doses of each drug to be achieved. Investigators may also need to adopt higher toxicity thresholds.

SPECULATIONS ON THE FUTURE ROLE OF KINASE INHIBITORS IN CANCER MEDICINE

The role of genomics in predicting response to kinase inhibitor therapy is now irrefutable. As the number of kinase driver mutations continues to grow, the field is likely to move away from the current strategy of a "companion diagnostic" for each drug. Rather, comprehensive mutational profiling platforms that query each tumor for hundreds of potential cancer mutations are more likely to emerge as the diagnostic platform. Only a small number of mutations are "actionable" in 2010 (meaning the presence of a mutation defines a treatment decision), but this number will undoubtedly grow. In addition, the presence or absence of concurrent mutations will guide decisions about combination therapies.

More effort must be devoted to manipulating the dose and schedule of kinase inhibitor therapy to maximize efficacy and minimize toxicity. To date all kinase inhibitors have been developed based on the assumption that 24/7 coverage of the target is required for efficacy. Consequently, most compounds are optimized to have a long serum half-life (12 to 24 hours). Phase 2 doses are then selected based on the maximum tolerated dose determined with daily administration. But a recent clinical trial of the ABL inhibitor dasatinib in CML indicates that equivalent antitumor activity can be achieved with intermittent therapy.[106] By giving larger doses intermittently, higher peak drug concentrations were achieved that resulted in equivalent and possibly superior efficacy.[107] Similar results were observed in laboratory studies of EGFR inhibitors in EGFR-mutant lung cancer. Clinically robust, quantitative assays of target inhibition are needed to hasten progress in this area.

Although the focus of this chapter is kinase inhibitors, the themes developed here should apply broadly to inhibitors of other cancer targets. Early clinical results with inhibitors of the G-protein coupled receptor smoothened (SMO) in patients with metastatic basal cell carcinoma or medulloblastoma establish that the driver mutation hypothesis extends beyond kinase inhibitors. SMO is a component in the hedgehog pathway that is constitutively activated in subsets of patients with basal cell carcinoma and medulloblastoma due to mutations in the hedgehog ligand binding receptor Patched-1. Treatment with the SMO inhibitor GDC-0449 led to impressive responses in basal cell carcinoma and medulloblastoma patients whose tumors had Patched-1 mutations.[108,109] Other novel cancer targets are emerging from cancer genome sequencing projects. Somatic mutations in the Krebs cycle enzyme isocitrate dehydrogenase (*IDH1/2*) were found in subsets of patients with glioblastoma and acute myeloid leukemia.[110–112] Mutations in enzymes involved in chromatin remodeling were recently found in kidney cancer.[113] Drug discovery programs are already under way to find inhibitors of several of these mutant enzymes. Kinase inhibitors are just the first wave of molecularly targeted drugs ushered in through understanding of the molecular underpinnings of cancer cells. There is much more to follow.

Selected References

The full list of references for this chapter appears in the online version.

1. Sawyers CL. Shifting paradigms: the seeds of oncogene addiction. *Nat Med* 2009;15(10):1158.
2. Weinstein IB. Cancer. Addiction to oncogenes—the Achilles heal of cancer. *Science* 2002;297(5578):63.
3. Druker BJ, Talpaz M, Resta DJ, et al. Efficacy and safety of a specific inhibitor of the BCR-ABL tyrosine kinase in chronic myeloid leukemia. *N Engl J Med* 2001;344(14):1031.
4. Hirota S, Isozaki K, Moriyama Y, et al. Gain-of-function mutations of c-kit in human gastrointestinal stromal tumors. *Science* 1998; 279(5350):577.
6. Demetri GD, von Mehren M, Blanke CD, et al. Efficacy and safety of imatinib mesylate in advanced gastrointestinal stromal tumors. *N Engl J Med* 2002;347(7):472.
7. Geyer CE, Forster J, Lindquist D, et al. Lapatinib plus capecitabine for HER2-positive advanced breast cancer. *N Engl J Med* 2006;355 (26):2733.
8. Kris MG, Natale RB, Herbst RS, et al. Efficacy of gefitinib, an inhibitor of the epidermal growth factor receptor tyrosine kinase, in symptomatic patients with non-small cell lung cancer: a randomized trial. *JAMA* 2003;290(16):2149.
10. Paez JG, Jänne PA, Lee JC, et al. EGFR mutations in lung cancer: correlation with clinical response to gefitinib therapy. *Science* 2004; 304(5676):1497.
11. Lynch TJ, Bell DW, Sordella R, et al. Activating mutations in the epidermal growth factor receptor underlying responsiveness of non–small-cell lung cancer to gefitinib. *N Engl J Med* 2004;350(21):2129.
12. Pao W, Miller V, Zakowski M, et al. EGF receptor gene mutations are common in lung cancers from "never smokers" and are associated with sensitivity of tumors to gefitinib and erlotinib. *Proc Natl Acad Sci U S A* 2004;101(36):13306.
14. Shepherd FA, Rodrigues Pereira J, Ciuleanu T, et al. Erlotinib in previously treated non-small-cell lung cancer. *N Engl J Med* 2005;353(2):123.
19. Tsao MS, Sakurada A, Cutz JC, et al. Erlotinib in lung cancer—molecular and clinical predictors of outcome. *N Engl J Med* 2005;353(2):133.

20. Mok TS, Wu YL, Thongprasert S, et al. Gefitinib or carboplatin-paclitaxel in pulmonary adenocarcinoma. *N Engl J Med* 2009;361(10):947.
23. Cools J, DeAngelo DJ, Gotlib J, et al. A tyrosine kinase created by fusion of the PDGFRA and FIP1L1 genes as a therapeutic target of imatinib in idiopathic hypereosinophilic syndrome. *N Engl J Med* 2003;348(13):1201.
27. Davies H, Bignell GR, Cox C, et al. Mutations of the BRAF gene in human cancer. *Nature* 2002;417(6892):949.
28. Baxter EJ, Scott LM, Campbell PJ, et al. Acquired mutation of the tyrosine kinase JAK2 in human myeloproliferative disorders. *Lancet* 2005;365(9464):1054.
29. James C, Ugo V, Le Couédic JP, et al. A unique clonal JAK2 mutation leading to constitutive signalling causes polycythaemia vera. *Nature* 2005;434(7037):1144.
30. Levine RL, Wadleigh M, Cools J, et al. Activating mutation in the tyrosine kinase JAK2 in polycythemia vera, essential thrombocythemia, and myeloid metaplasia with myelofibrosis. *Cancer Cell* 2005;7(4):387.
31. Samuels Y, Wang Z, Bardelli A, et al. High frequency of mutations of the PIK3CA gene in human cancers. *Science* 2004;304(5670):554.
37. Solit DB, Garraway LA, Pratilas CA, et al. BRAF mutation predicts sensitivity to MEK inhibition. *Nature* 2006;439(7074):358.
45. Flaherty KT, Puzanov I, Kim KB, et al. Inhibition of mutated, activated BRAF in metastatic melanoma. *N Engl J Med* 2010;363(9):809.
46. Bollag G, Hirth P, Tsai J, et al. Clinical efficacy of a RAF inhibitor needs broad target blockade in BRAF-mutant melanoma. *Nature* 2010;467:596.
51. Soda M, Choi YL, Enomoto M, et al. Identification of the transforming EML4-ALK fusion gene in non-small-cell lung cancer. *Nature* 2007; 448(7153):561.
61. Sawyers CL. Finding the next Gleevec: FLT3 targeted kinase inhibitor therapy for acute myeloid leukemia. *Cancer Cell* 2002;1(5):413.
67. Zarrinkar PP, Gunawardane RN, Cramer MD, et al. AC220 is a uniquely potent and selective inhibitor of FLT3 for the treatment of acute myeloid leukemia (AML). *Blood* 2009;114(14):2984.
70. Yang JC, Haworth L, Sherry RM, et al. A randomized trial of bevacizumab, an anti-vascular endothelial growth factor antibody, for metastatic renal cancer. *N Engl J Med* 2003;349(5):427.
71. Escudier B, Eisen T, Stadler WM, et al. Sorafenib in advanced clear-cell renal-cell carcinoma. *N Engl J Med* 2007;356(2):125.
72. Motzer RJ, Hutson TE, Tomczak P, et al. Sunitinib versus interferon alfa in metastatic renal-cell carcinoma. *N Engl J Med* 2007;356(2):115.
76. Hudes G, Carducci M, Tomczak P, et al. Temsirolimus, interferon alfa, or both for advanced renal-cell carcinoma. *N Engl J Med* 2007;356(22):2271.
77. Motzer RJ, Escudier B, Oudard S, et al. Efficacy of everolimus in advanced renal cell carcinoma: a double-blind, randomised, placebo-controlled phase III trial. *Lancet* 2008;372(9637):449.
81. Thomas GV, Tran C, Mellinghoff IK, et al. Hypoxia-inducible factor determines sensitivity to inhibitors of mTOR in kidney cancer. *Nat Med* 2006;12(1):122.
82. Hess G, Herbrecht R, Romaguera J, et al. Phase III study to evaluate temsirolimus compared with investigator,s choice therapy for the treatment of relapsed or refractory mantle cell lymphoma. *J Clin Oncol* 2009; 27(23):3822.
86. Neshat MS, Mellinghoff IK, Tran C, et al. Enhanced sensitivity of PTEN-deficient tumors to inhibition of FRAP/mTOR. *Proc Natl Acad Sci U S A* 2001;98(18):10314.
87. Majumder PK, Febbo PG, Bikoff R, et al. mTOR inhibition reverses Akt-dependent prostate intraepithelial neoplasia through regulation of apoptotic and HIF-1-dependent pathways. *Nat Med* 2004;10(6):594.
88. Podsypanina K, Lee RT, Politis C, et al. An inhibitor of mTOR reduces neoplasia and normalizes p70/S6 kinase activity in Pten+/– mice. *Proc Natl Acad Sci U S A* 2001;98(18):10320.
89. O,Reilly KE, Rojo F, She QB, et al. mTOR inhibition induces upstream receptor tyrosine kinase signaling and activates Akt. *Cancer Res* 2006;66 (3):1500.
93. She QB, Halilovic E, Ye Q, et al. 4E-BP1 is a key effector of the oncogenic activation of the AKT and ERK signaling pathways that integrates their function in tumors. *Cancer Cell* 2010;18(1):39.
94. Engelman JA, Chen L, Tan X, et al. Effective use of PI3K and MEK inhibitors to treat mutant Kras G12D and PIK3CA H1047R murine lung cancers. *Nat Med* 2008;14(12):1351.
95. Gorre ME, Mohammed M, Ellwood K, et al. Clinical resistance to STI-571 cancer therapy caused by BCR-ABL gene mutation or amplification. *Science* 2001;293(5531):876.
96. Shah NP, Nicoll JM, Nagar B, et al. Multiple BCR-ABL kinase domain mutations confer polyclonal resistance to the tyrosine kinase inhibitor imatinib (STI571) in chronic phase and blast crisis chronic myeloid leukemia. *Cancer Cell* 2002;2(2):117.
97. Shah NP, Tran C, Lee FY, et al. Overriding imatinib resistance with a novel ABL kinase inhibitor. *Science* 2004;305(5682):399.
98. Talpaz M, Shah NP, Kantarjian H, et al. Dasatinib in imatinib-resistant Philadelphia chromosome-positive leukemias. *N Engl J Med* 2006; 354(24):2531.
99. Kantarjian H, Shah NP, Hochhaus A, et al. Dasatinib versus imatinib in newly diagnosed chronic-phase chronic myeloid leukemia. *N Engl J Med* 2010;362(24):2260.
100. Sawyers CL. Even better kinase inhibitors for chronic myeloid leukemia. *N Engl J Med* 2010;362(24):2314.
101. Saglio G, Kim DW, Issaragrisil S, et al. Nilotinib versus imatinib for newly diagnosed chronic myeloid leukemia. *N Engl J Med* 2010;362(24): 2251.
104. Pao W, Miller VA, Politi KA, et al. Acquired resistance of lung adenocarcinomas to gefitinib or erlotinib is associated with a second mutation in the EGFR kinase domain. *PLoS Med* 2005;2(3):e73.
105. Antonescu CR, Besmer P, Guo T, et al. Acquired resistance to imatinib in gastrointestinal stromal tumor occurs through secondary gene mutation. *Clin Cancer Res* 2005;11(11):4182.
106. Shah NP, et al. Intermittent target inhibition with dasatinib 100 mg once daily preserves efficacy and improves tolerability in imatinib-resistant and -intolerant chronic-phase chronic myeloid leukemia. *J Clin Oncol* 2008;26(19):3204.
107. Shah NP, Kasap C, Weier C, et al. Transient potent BCR-ABL inhibition is sufficient to commit chronic myeloid leukemia cells irreversibly to apoptosis. *Cancer Cell* 2008;14(6):485.

CHAPTER 40 HISTONE DEACETYLASE INHIBITORS AND DEMETHYLATING AGENTS

STEVEN D. GORE, STEPHEN B. BAYLIN, AND JAMES G. HERMAN

The past decade has seen remarkable progress toward an understanding of the role of chromatin in the control of gene expression.[1] The role of epigenetic abnormalities in the progression of cancer[2,3] and the possibility of epigenetically targeted therapies in cancer have been increasingly recognized and explored.[2–4] Of these epigenetic abnormalities, the most thoroughly examined is the occurrence of abnormal cytosine guanine (CpG) promoter region DNA methylation and associated altered chromatin, resulting from histone modifications, in the transcriptional silencing of genes, including many tumor suppressor genes.[2–4] This chapter describes the basis of epigenetic changes in cancer and discusses approaches that target reexpression of silenced genes for cancer therapy. The two approaches most mature in development are the inhibition of DNA methyltransferases, which mediate the abnormal promoter DNA methylation, and the inhibition of histone deactylases, which remove histone modifications associated with active chromatin that alone, or in association with DNA methylation, are associated with transcriptional repression.[2–4]

Aberrant gene function and altered patterns of gene expression are key features of cancer.[2] Although genetic alterations remain the best characterized in the development and progression of cancer, increasingly it is appreciated that epigenetic abnormalities cooperate with genetic alterations to cause dysfunction of key regulatory pathways. This chapter will outline the understanding of how epigenetic alterations contribute to cancer and how this abnormality has led to novel therapeutic approaches that target the most well-characterized epigenetic changes, using inhibitors of DNA methylation and histone deacetylases.

EPIGENETICS AND GENE SILENCING

Epigenetic changes are defined as alterations in gene expression that are heritable but are not accompanied by changes in DNA sequence. This definition clearly delineates the two key features of epigenetic regulation important for an understanding of therapies described in this chapter. Specifically, the distinction from genetic alterations (point mutations, deletions, or translocations) implies that the coding sequence of targeted genes remains intact. Thus, reversal of changes in gene expression can restore the normal function of that gene or protein. Second, the heritable nature of epigenetic changes, that is the ability of a cell to pass on regulation of gene expression through DNA replication, suggests that such changes are relatively stable, if not permanent. Thus, reprogramming of patterns of gene expression could result in a long-term change in the cancer cell phenotype, even after the therapeutic agent used to alter gene expression is removed.

Gene silencing at the level of chromatin is necessary for the life of multicellular eukaryotic organisms and is critical for regulating important biological processes, including differentiation, imprinting, and silencing of large chromosomal domains, including the X chromosome of female mammals. For example, the diversity of structure and function of cells derived from epithelial or mesenchymal origin, ultimately differentiating into cells lining the intestine or lung or forming mature granulocytes and myocytes, result from heritable changes in gene expression that are not the result of a change in DNA sequence. While in many species silencing can be initiated and maintained solely by processes involving the covalent modifications of histones and other chromatin components, vertebrates utilize an additional layer of gene regulation. This process involves the only natural covalent modification of DNA in humans and is characterized by DNA cytosine methylation that occurs nearly exclusively at the fifth position of the cytosine ring in cytosines preceding guanine, the so-called CpG dinucleotide.

Gene Silencing and Cancer

Like most biological processes, the normal patterns of silencing can be altered, resulting in the development of disease states. Thus, activation of genes normally not expressed, or silencing of a gene that should be expressed, can contribute to the dysregulation of gene function that characterizes cancer and, when stably present, represent epigenetic alterations.[2] Most studies have focused on the silencing of normally expressed genes. For the purposes of understanding the rationale behind epigenetic therapy it is important to understand the mechanisms through which gene silencing occurs. Alterations in gene expression associated with epigenetic changes that give rise to a growth advantage would be expected to be selected for in the host tissue, leading to progressive dysregulated growth of the tumor. Such dysregulation is commonly associated with increases in promoter region DNA methylation and is associated with repressive chromatin changes.

CHANGES IN DNA METHYLATION

The importance of promoter cytosine methylation in CpG islands and gene silencing has been clearly established in the past decade and been shown convincingly to be involved in cancer development.[2] The CpG dinucleotide, usually underrepresented in the genome, is clustered in the promoter regions of many human genes. These promoter regions have been termed *CpG islands*, which are largely protected from methylation in normal cells, with the exception of genes on the inactive X chromosome and imprinted genes.[5] This protection is critical, since methylation of promoter region CpG islands is associated with loss of gene expression. This change serves as an alternative mechanism for loss of tumor suppressor gene function. Recent studies have also suggested that adjacent regions, termed *CpG island shores*, are abnormally methylated in cancers[6] and may be altered in stem cell populations.[7] The relative cancer specificity of changes in CpG island methylation makes reversal of these changes by targeting DNA methyltransferase logical for cancer therapeutics. As an example, the most studied tumor suppressor gene for promoter hypermethylation is the *p16* gene, currently designated *CDKN2A*, a cyclin-dependent kinase inhibitor that functions in the regulation of the phosphorylation of the Rb protein. Hypermethylation associated with loss of expression of the *CDKN2A* gene has been found to be one of the most frequent alterations in neoplasia. Methylation of the *p16* gene is common in lung, head and neck, gliomas, colorectal, and breast carcinomas,[8,9] indeed in most types of cancer. A member of the same gene family, *p15* or *CDKN2B*, also regulates Rb and is silenced in association with promoter methylation in many forms of leukemia and in myelodysplastic syndrome,[10] of relevance for the clinical uses of epigenetic therapies discussed below.

Many hundreds of genes may be inactivated in a single cancer by promoter methylation,[11] providing potential targets for gene reactivation using epigenetic therapies.[12] This represents one of the potential ways in which epigenetic therapy may be effective: multiple genes and gene pathways, all repressed by changes in DNA methylation and chromatin modification, can be reactivated by demethylating agents and histone deacetylase (HDAC) inhibitors, thereby restoring normal cell cycle control, differentiation, and apoptotic signaling. In general, methylated CpG islands are not capable of the initiation of transcription unless the methylation signal can be overridden by alterations in factors that modulate chromatin, such as removal of methylated cytosine-binding proteins. However, reversal of DNA methylation with secondary changes in histone modification or directed reversal of repressive histone modifications represents a target for epigenetic therapies.

Most studies of DNA methylation, particularly in the study of cancer, have focused on CpG island promoter methylation. However, about 40% of human genes do not contain *bona fide* CpG islands in their promoters.[13] The primary focus on CpG islands has resulted from the clear demonstration that CpG-island promoter methylation permanently silences genes both physiologically and pathologically in mammalian cells. However, recent work has shown correlations between tissue-specific expression and methylation of non-CpG islands, including, for example, the maspin gene,[14] and as mentioned above, regions near CpG islands,[6,7] suggesting that many additional genes could be regulated, either normally or abnormally, by changes in DNA methylation.

Chromatin in Gene Regulation

Heritable gene silencing involves the interplay between DNA methylation, histone covalent modifications, and nucleosomal remodeling. The histone code refers to the posttranslational modifications that occur on certain amino acid residues of the tails of histone proteins. Acetylation, deacetylation, methylation, phosphorylation, and other modifications all modify chromatin structure and thereby alter gene expression. Some of the enzymes that catalyze these modifications include DNA methyltransferase (DNMTs), HDACs, histone methyltransferases (HMTs), and most recently histone demethylases. These modifications establish a heritable repressive state at the start site of genes, resulting in gene silencing through repression of gene transcription.

A link between covalent histone modifications and DNA methylation has been clearly established[15,16] whereby cytosine methylation attracts methylated DNA-binding proteins and HDACs to methylated CpG sites during chromatin compaction and gene silencing. In addition, the DNA methylation binding protein (MBD2) interacts with the nucleosomal remodeling complex (NuRD) and directs the complex to methylated DNA.[17] Thus, the three processes of DNA cytosine methylation, histone modification, and nucleosomal remodeling are intimately linked, and alterations in these processes result in the permanent silencing of cancer-relevant genes.

Enzymes Regulating DNA Methylation and Histone Acetylation

DNA methylation involves the covalent addition of a methyl group to the 5′ position of cytosine. In mammals, three enzymes have been shown to catalyze this transfer of a methyl group from the methyl donor S-adenosylmethionine. Most of the methyltransferase activity present in differentiated cells is derived from the expression of DNMT1.[18] This enzyme is thought to be most important in maintaining DNA methylation patterns following DNA replication and thus is referred to as a maintenance methyltransferase. However, the enzyme does possess the ability to methylate previously unmethylated DNA sequences (*de novo* activity).[19] In contrast, the other enzymes, DNMT3a and DNMT3b, are efficient at methylating previously unmethylated DNA and thus are considered *de novo* methyltransferases. Each of these enzymes possesses a similar catalytic site, a fact important for the inhibition of DNMT enzymes by nucleoside analogues, discussed later in this chapter.

DNA methylation is closely associated with changes in the histone modifications. Histone proteins are the central components of the nucleosome, and modifications of the histone tails of core histones are associated with active or repressed chromatin, sometimes referred to as the histone code.[20] Although it is beyond the scope of this chapter to fully discuss the complex series of modifications to the histone tails of histone H3 and H4, a few well characterized modifications should be mentioned that are relevant to therapies targeted to modifying the histone code. In reference to currently investigated epigenetic therapies, changes in histone acetylation are of importance.[20] Acetylation of histones H3 and H4 at key amino acids is associated with the active chromatin present at the promoters of transcribed genes, while the absence of histone acetylation is associated with repressed, silenced genes. Histone acetyltransferases (HATs) HDACs have opposing functions to maintain the proper level of histone acetylation for gene expression.

HDACs specifically deacetylate the lysine residues of the histone tails, which then is associated with condensation and closed chromatin formation, leading to transcriptional repression. There are four classes of HDACs.[21] Class I HDACs are characterized by their similarity to the yeast Rpd3 HDAC. In humans, this class of enzymes includes HDAC1, -2, -3, and -8. These HDACs are thought to be ubiquitously expressed in tissue throughout the body. In contrast, class II HDACs are similar to yeast Hda1 and include HDAC4, -5, -6, -7, -9, and -10, and they have a greater degree of tissue specificity. Class III HDACs are similar to yeast Sir2 and are set apart from the other classes by their dependence on nicotinamide adenine dinucleotide (NAD+) as a cofactor. Finally, class IV includes HDAC11.[21]

Reversal of Layers of Gene Silencing

The interaction between DNA methylation and HDAC activity and repressive chromatin marks in maintaining aberrant

TABLE 40.1

SMALL MOLECULES TARGETING EPIGENETIC ABNORMALITIES IN CLINICAL DEVELOPMENT

Drug	Class	Target	Dose Range	Schedule	Route of Administration
5-Azacitidine	Nucleoside	DNA methyltransferase	30–75 mg/m²/d	Daily × 7–14 days/ 28 days	Subcutaneous or intravenous
2′-Deoxy-5-azacytidine	Nucleoside	DNA methyltransferase	10–45 mg/m²/d	Daily × 3–5 days/ 4–6 weeks	Intravenous
Valproic acid	Small chain fatty acid	Histone deacetylase (class I and II)	25–50 mg/kg/d	Daily	Oral or intravenous
Vorinostat	Hydroxamic acid	Histone deacetylase (class I and II)	400–600 mg/d	Divided doses	Oral
SNDX-275	Benzamide	Histone deacetylase (class I)	2–8 mg/m²	Weekly	Oral
Belinostat	Hydroxamic acid	Histone deacetylase (class I and II)	600–1,000 mg/m²	Daily × 5/28 days	Intravenous
Romidepsin	Cyclic tetrapeptide	Histone deacetylase (class I and II)	13–18 mg/m²	Weekly	Intravenous
LBH-589	Hydroxamic acid	Histone deacetylase (class I and II)	5–11 mg/m²	Daily × 3	Intravenous
MGCD-0103	Benzamide	Histone deacetylase (class I)	40–125 mg/m²	Twice weekly	Oral
CI-994	Benzamide	Histone deacetylase (class I)	5–8 mg/m²	Daily	Oral

silencing of hypermethylated genes in cancer has therapeutic implications for epigenetic therapies. Experimental evidence suggests that DNA methylation functions as a dominant event that locks in complete transcriptional repression. Inhibition of HDAC activity alone, by potent and specific drugs such as trichostatin (TSA), does not result in the reactivation of aberrantly silenced and hypermethylated genes in tumor cells.[22] In contrast, treatment with HDAC inhibitors can reactivate densely silenced genes if the cells are first treated with demethylating drugs, such as 5-aza-cytidine.[22] The clinical implications of this observation are discussed in more detail below (Table 40.1).

DNA Methyltransferase Inhibitors

Originally synthesized as cytotoxic antimetabolite drugs in the 1960s,[23] azacytosine nucleosides were recognized as inhibitors of DNA methylation in the early 1980s. The inhibitors 5-azacitidine (5AC) and 2′-deoxy-5-azacitidine induced muscle, fat, and chondrocyte differentiation in mouse embryo cells, in association with reversal of DNA methylation.[24,25] Incorporation of azacytosine nucleosides into DNA in lieu of cytosine residues was shown to be associated with inhibition of DNMT activity.[26,27] DNMT inhibition requires incorporation of decitabine triphosphate into DNA. The incorporated azacytosine nucleoside forms an irreversible inactive adduct with DNMT. Sequential reversal of DNA methylation results when DNA replication proceeds in the absence of active DNMT.[28] The inhibitor 5AC must be phosphorylated and converted to decitabine diphosphate by ribonucleotide reductase before it can be activated through triphosphorylation; decitabine does not require ribonucleotide reductase. The inhibitor 5AC can also be incorporated into RNA. DNMT2, a misnamed protein that is actually an RNA specific methyltransferase,[29] becomes inhibited, leading to depletion of methylated tRNA.[27] This may contribute to inhibition of protein synthesis and is a potential difference between azacytidine and decitabine.[30]

The azacytosine nucleosides exhibit complex dose–response characteristics. At low concentrations (0.2 to 1 mcM), the "epigenetic" activities of these drugs predominate, with dose-dependent reversal of DNA methylation[31] and induction of terminal differentiation in some systems. As concentrations are increased, DNA damage and apoptosis become more prominent.[31] Cell lines with 30-fold resistance to the cytotoxic effects of decitabine continue to reverse methylation in response to this nucleoside, suggesting that the methylation reversing and cytotoxic activities of this compound can be separated.[32] The ability of these drugs to inhibit the cell cycle, at least in part through induction of $p21^{WAF1/CIP1}$ expression, complicates the goal of reversing DNA methylation, since the latter requires DNA replication with the azacytosine nucleoside incorporated into the DNA.

The two azacytosine nucleosides in clinical use are highly unstable in aqueous solution. In aqueous solutions, the drugs readily hydrolyzed and inactivated.[33] In clinical practice, the drugs must be administered shortly after reconstitution. The drugs are also metabolized by cytidine deaminase,[34] leading to a short half-life in plasma. When injected subcutaneously, 5AC reaches a maximal plasma concentration at 30 minutes, with a terminal half-life of 1.5 to 2.3 hours.[12,35] At the U.S. Food and Drug Administration (FDA) approved dose of 5AC (75 mg/m² administered subcutaneously daily for 7 days), peak plasma concentrations were 3 to 5 mcM, which is well within the range of DNMT inhibitory concentrations.[12,35] Intravenous (IV) administration of the same dose has led to higher peak plasma concentrations (11 mcM) with a shorter half-life (approximately 22 minutes).[35] Decitabine given over 1 hour IV at 15 to 20mg/m² produced plasma concentrations of 1.1 to 1.6 mcM during the infusion,[36] while in a phase 1 study in patients with thoracic malignancies, patients were treated with escalating doses of decitabine for 72-hour IV infusions for two 35-day cycles. The maximum tolerated total dose was 60 to 75 mg/m² with neutropenia as the dose-limiting toxicity. Steady-state plasma concentrations ranged from 25 to 40 nM, which is less than those usually used to induce expression of methylated genes in tissue culture models.[37] These differences in drug concentration, according to schedule of administration, will be discussed later concerning therapeutic activity.

The less-than-ideal pharmacologic characteristics of the azacytosine nucleosides have led investigators to explore alternative means of DNMT inhibition and methylation reversal. Procainamide has been shown to inhibit DNMT1 with a Ki of 7 mcM; it does not appear to inhibit DNMT3a or DNMT3b.[38] Considerably higher concentrations (200 mcM) have been required to reverse methylation in some cell lines.[39] Hydralazine and the green tea polyphenol(−)-epigallocatechin-3-gallate, also previously reported to inhibit DNMT, appear to have low potency.[39] The cytidine analogue zebularine appears more stable in aqueous solution and is a potent inhibitor of DNMT.[40,41] Unfortunately, this drug appears to have limited bioavailability in primates,[42] and the ability of this drug to reverse methylation is somewhat limited.[43] MG-98 is a phosphorothioate antisense oligodeoxynucleotide directed at DNMT1. In a phase 1 study, administration of this antisense molecule was not associated with consistent inhibition of DNMT mRNA.[44] Finally, 5-fluoro-2′-deoxycytidine has been investigated as a clinical DNMT inhibitor in conjunction with the cytidine deaminase inhibitor tetrahydrouridine.[45] However, at present, only 5AC and decitabine appear to be potent demethylating agents that are clinically active.

HISTONE DEACETYLASE INHIBITORS

The increasing recognition of the critical importance of histone modifications in regulating the transcriptional permissivity of chromatin has led to intense interest in compounds that can inhibit the activity of HDAC proteins, facilitating acetylation of lysines associated with transcriptional activation of genes. The first generation of HDAC inhibitors were small chain fatty acids, including sodium butyrate, arginine butyrate, sodium phenylbutyrate, and valproic acid. These agents require submillimolar to millimolar concentrations to inhibit HDACs.[46–48] Like the DNMT inhibitors, these compounds have complex pharmacodynamic properties. At the lowest concentrations associated with HDAC inhibitory activity, these compounds may increase cellular proliferation.[49,50] At high concentrations, cell cycle arrest occurs, associated with induction of $p21^{WAF1/CIP1}$ and evidence of differentiation. At concentrations exceeding 1 mM, apoptosis is induced.[49,51]

Second generation HDAC inhibitors include hydroxamic acids, cyclic depsipeptides, and benzamides. The hydroxamic acid HDAC inhibitors include vorinostat (suberoylanilide hydroxamic acid [SAHA]), which was synthesized as a derivative of the differentiation inducer hexamethylene bisacetamide.[52] Other hydroxamic acid HDAC inhibitors under clinical investigation include belinostat (PXD1010)[53] and panobinostat (LBH589).[54] Hydroxamic HDAC inhibitors fit into and interact with the catalytic core of HDACs.[55] Hydoxamic acids inhibit class I and II HDACs.[56] Romidepsin is a depsipeptide with potent HDAC inhibitory activity that requires reduction for optimal activity and appears to specifically inhibit class I HDACs.[57] The benzamide HDAC inhibitors include entinostat (SNDX 275, MS 275),[58] CI 994[59], and MGCD 0103 and are selective for class I HDACs.[56]

Many proteins in addition to histones serve as substrates for protein acetylases and can thus be impacted by HDAC inhibitors. These include transcription factors such as p53, E2F1, and GATA1.[60–62] DNA binding proteins such as HMG1[63] and tubulin can also be acetylated by acetyltransferases.[64] Protein acetylation can result in increased DNA binding, impact protein–protein interactions, and increase protein stability, as reviewed by Fuks et al.[61]

Given that a wide variety of proteins can undergo acetylation in the presence of HDAC inhibitors, it is not surprising that administration of HDAC inhibitors has been associated with broad effects on cellular physiology. As predicted, administration of HDAC inhibitors induces alterations in gene expression. This includes both up- and down-regulation. Expression profiling has suggested that between 2% and 10% of genes studied may have their expression altered by exposure to HDAC inhibitors; however, the number of genes whose expression is reliably altered in a number of different cancer cell lines in response to a variety of HDAC inhibitors is few.[65] Expression of $p21^{WAF1/CIP1}$ is uniformly increased by treatment with HDAC inhibitors; not surprisingly, this is often associated with cell cycle arrest. Induction of p21 expression occurs even in cells in which p53 is mutant or null.[66]

Inhibitors in the Treatment of Hematologic Malignancies

The successful development of 5AC for the treatment of myelodysplastic syndrome can be credited largely to Silverman et al. in the Cancer and Leukemia Group B (CALGB). The inhibitor 5AC had successfully induced the expression of hemoglobin F in patients with sickle cell anemia.[12,67] Viewing this compound as a potential inducer of terminal differentiation, Silverman et al. conducted a series of phase 2 trials of 5AC administered as a continuous intravenous infusion or as subcutaneous injections for the treatment of myelodysplastic syndrome (MDS).[68,69] Based on significant hematologic responses, the group performed a phase 2 trial (CALGB 9221) in which patients with low- and high-risk MDS with significant hematopoietic compromise were randomly assigned to receive subcutaneous 5AC (75 mg/m^2/day daily for 7 days, repeated on a 28-day cycle) or observation. Patients on the observation arm with progressive disease could cross over to receive 5AC. This study firmly established the ability of 5AC to induce hematologic improvement, and, less frequently, complete and partial responses.[69,70] The median time to development of acute myeloid leukemia (defined by 30% bone marrow blast cells) or death was greater in the 5AC arm by 9 months (21 vs. 12 months); of note, the observation arm included patients who subsequently crossed over to 5AC treatment.

In a subsequent phase 3 trial (AZA001),[71] patients with higher risk myelodysplastic syndromes were randomly assigned one-to-one to receive azacitidine (75 mg/m^2 per day for 7 days every 28 days) or conventional care (best supportive care, low-dose cytarabine, or intensive chemotherapy as selected by investigators before randomization). Three hundred fifty-eight patients were randomly assigned to receive azacitidine (n = 179) or conventional care regimens (n = 179). After a median follow-up of 21.1 months (interquartile range [IQR] 15.1 to 26.9), median overall survival was 24.5 months (9.9 not reached) for the azacitidine group versus 15.0 months (5.6 to 24.1) for the conventional care group (hazard ratio [HR] 0.58; 95% confidence interval [CI], 0.43 to 0.77; P = .0001). At 2 years, on the basis of Kaplan-Meier estimates, 50.8% (95% CI, 42.1 to 58.8) of patients in the azacytidine group were alive compared with 26.2% (95% CI, 18.7 to 34.3) in the conventional care group (P <.0001). Median time to acute myeloid leukaemia transformation was 17.8 months (IQR 8.6 to 36.8; 95% CI, 13.6 to 23.6) in the azacitidine group compared with 11.5 months (4.9 not reached; 8.3 to 14.5) in the conventional care group (HR 0.50; 95% CI, 0.35 to 0.70; P <.0001).

The early development of decitabine in MDS took place primarily in Europe under the leadership of Wijermans et al.[72,73] These investigators pursued intravenous scheduling of decitabine administered three times daily for 3 days (45 mg/m^2/d total dose). This cycle was repeated every 6 weeks. Phase 2 studies suggested a response rate of approximately 50% in MDS patients. In a randomized trial of decitabine versus observation, patients with International Prognostic Score risk categories intermediate 1 to high received the above schedule of decitabine or observation. No cross-over was allowed in this trial. Response rates reported were: complete response 9%, partial response 8%, hematologic improvement 13%.[74] A 10% induction death rate occurred, suggesting that this schedule of decitabine may be more toxic than the CALGB schedule of 5AC (1% induction mortality). Decitabine has also been investigated in low-dose daily intravenous dosing[75] and in daily-times-five schedules. The latter appears convenient and well tolerated. A very high response rate has been reported in response to a 20 mg/m^2/d daily times five phase 2 trial; however, this trial used response criteria designed for acute myeloid leukemia (AML) studies, which do not require demonstration of stability of hematologic response. These criteria included a category of "marrow complete response" in which hematologic improvement is not required; additionally, response duration was not reported in this study.[74] However, additional studies have explored this daily times five dosing of decitabine. Ninety-nine patients with MDS (*de novo* or secondary) of any French-American-British (FAB) subtype and an International Prognostic Scoring System (IPSS) score equal to or greater than 0.5 were treated, with an overall response rate of 32% (17 complete responses [CR] plus 15 marrow CRs [mCRs]).[76] Among patients who improved, 82% demonstrated responses by the end of cycle two. This well-tolerated regimen allows outpatient administration, and as noted above, provides plasma levels of decitabine that inhibit DNMTs. The 3-day intravenous schedule of decitabine has been studied in two randomized trials compared to supportive care in patients with higher risk MDS. The first trial confirmed the hematologic activity of decitabine in this patient population but failed to show an improvement in survival in the decitabine-treated patients.[77] Survival was also not increased in the subsequent trial, performed by the European Organisation for Research and Treatment of Cancer (EORTC), thus far published only in abstract form.[78] The failure of the randomized decitabine trials to show a survival benefit may be due to study design. Both randomized trials of 5AC continued treatment until disease progression for patients who did not achieve complete remission; in fact, this meant that most patients received maintenance therapy. In contrast, both randomized trials of decitabine allowed a maximum of eight cycles of treatment. The need for maintenance therapy in patients treated with DNMT inhibitors has not been tested in prospective randomized trials.

An additional difference in the conduct of the two sets of DNMT inhibitor trials involves the duration of therapy administered. The median number of cycles of treatment administered in the two randomized trials of decitabine was three, compared to nine in the azacytidine trials. This may reflect greater toxicity of the FDA-approved schedule of decitabine compared to that of 5AC. The impact of the alternative 5-day schedule of decitabine on survival has not been studied. While the differences in survival may reflect differences in trial design and trial conduct, emerging data suggests that despite similarities in methylation reversal, the two drugs differ in other potentially important biological parameters, which may contribute to clinical outcomes.[29,30,43]

The azacytosine nucleosides require prolonged administration to demonstrate hematologic improvement in MDS. Median time to development of first clinical response in the CALGB studies of 5AC was three cycles; 90% of responses developed by cycle six.[69] In the phase 3 trial of decitabine, median time to response was two cycles,[77] as also seen in the alternative regimen of decitabine.[76] It is therefore extremely important when treating patients with azacytosine nucleosides to commit to administering between four and six cycles of therapy before determining whether a patient is responding to treatment. Furthermore, survival benefit is seen even in patients not showing bone marrow improvement for 5AC, perhaps related to decreased transfusion requirements or delayed progression to AML.[71]

Since AML in the context of MDS is somewhat arbitrarily defined based on marrow blast count, activity of the azanucleoside analogues in AML should not be surprising. In CALGB 9221, 20 patients were reclassified upon central pathology review as meeting criteria for AML (greater than 30% blasts). Their outcomes were comparable to the overall population in the study.[70] In all three CALGB studies among patients meeting current World Health Organization (WHO) criteria for AML (greater than 20% blasts), complete response was achieved in 9% and hematologic improvement in 26%.[69] A retrospective review of 20 patients with AML, including eight patients with bone marrow blasts greater than 29% treated with 5AC, reported complete remission in four patients, partial response in five, and hematologic improvement in three. Median duration of response was 8 months (range 3 to 33).[79] Decitabine induced complete hematologic response in 2 or 20 patients treated who had the blastic phase of chronic myeloid leukemia.[80] These studies suggest activity of the azacytosine nucleosides in the treatment of a subset of AML patients. Current studies do not allow determination of whether this subset is limited to MDS-associated AML (AML with trilineage dysplasia), which tends to have low white blood cell counts and have a low proliferative rate, or whether these compounds are also active for those with AML without a history of antecedent hematologic disorder. Several reports describe the azanucleoside's sensitivity for MDS and AML, characterized by abnormalities of chromosome 7 and associated with poor outcome in response to cytarabine-based therapy. In one nonrandomized retrospective study, survival of such patients following administration of DNMT inhibitors surpassed survival in response to conventional cytotoxic chemotherapy, similar to the outcomes of AZA001.[81–83]

Whether the clinical activity of azacytosine analogues requires reversal of gene methylation remains uncertain. Administration of decitabine has been shown to induce transient decrements of methylation in noncoding regions, including LINE and ALU elements.[84] Although this finding indicates that clinical administration of the compounds inhibits DNMT, reversal of methylation of noncoding elements is not associated with clinical response. Early studies that examined methylation reversal of the target gene p15^{INK4B} in response to decitabine showed no correlation between methylation reversal and clinical response.[75,85] Clinical responders to decitabine developed significantly higher expression of this gene following treatment, but the biological impact of the low levels of p15 expression induced by the drug remain uncertain. However, clinical response was closely associated with reversal of methylation of p15 or CDH-1 during the first cycle of treatment with 5AC followed by the HDAC inhibitor sodium phenylbutyrate.[12] In that study, it was noteworthy that administration of 5AC prior to the addition of an HDAC inhibitor was associated with induction of histone acetylation. Although the mechanism underlying this activity is unknown, histone acetylation has been observed following DNA damage due to gamma irradiation.[86] Subsequent studies have found demethylation following treatment with either decitabine or 5AC,[87–90] but not consistently associated with response.[87,88,90] More work will be required to answer the important mechanistic question underpinning the clinical activity of azacytosine analogues.

A variety of HDAC inhibitors have been explored for the treatment of a variety of hematopoietic neoplasms. These will be discussed according to the chemical class of the inhibitor.

Small Chain Fatty Acids

The earliest report of the use of an HDAC inhibitor to treat leukemia described the treatment of a child with refractory

AML with intravenous sodium butyrate, with a concomitant clearance of peripheral blood blast cells and a decrement in bone marrow blasts.[91] No responses developed in a subsequent study of nine AML patients who were treated with intravenous butyrate.[92] Phase 1 studies of sodium phenylbutyrate (NaPB) in MDS and AML explored 7-day continuous infusions administered monthly or biweekly, and 21-day continuous infusions administered monthly.[93,94] At the maximum tolerated dose (375 mg/kg/d), the mean steady-state plasma concentration was 0.3 mM, within the range of HDAC inhibition.[49,93,94] Isolated patients developed hematologic improvement in response to sodium phenylbutyrate.

Similar to NaPB, valproic acid (VPA) requires near millimolar concentrations to effectively inhibit HDACs. Of 18 patients with MDS or AML with trilineage dysplasia treated with VPA to target plasma concentrations of 0.3 to 0.7 mM, six patients developed hematologic improvement.[95] Of 20 elderly patients with AML treated with VPA, only 11 could remain in control long enough to be considered evaluable for response. Five had improvement in platelet counts.[96] VPA induced hematologic improvement in combination with all transretinoic acid in two of eight patients treated with AML; fluorescence *in situ* hybridization analysis showed definitive evidence of terminal differentiation of the malignant cells.[97] A larger study of this combination induced hematologic response in only 2 of 26 elderly patients with AML.[50] It appears unlikely that the short chain fatty acids will develop an important role in the treatment of malignancy, given the availability of HDAC inhibitors with vastly greater potency.

Hydroxamic Acids

The FDA approved vorinostat as the first commercially available HDAC inhibitor. The approval was based on activity of this agent in cutaneous T-cell lymphoma (CTCL). Thirty-three patients with a median number of five prior systemic therapy regimens received one of three dose schedules of vorinostat in a single institution study.[98] Eight patients achieved a partial response, with a median time to response of 12 weeks and a median duration of response of 15 weeks. Overall 45% of patients had relief of pruritus. Fatigue, diarrhea, nausea, and thrombocytopenia were common toxicities. In a multicenter phase 2 trial, 74 patients with relapsed or refractory CTCL were treated with 400 mg daily.[99] Similar to the prior study, 29% of patients responded, consisting almost entirely of partial responses. Median time to response was 56 days, and median duration of response was greater than 6 months. In phase 1 trials, responses to vorinostat have developed in other non-Hodgkin's and Hodgkin's lymphoma.[100]

Panobinostat (LBH589), a cinnamic hydroxamic acid HDAC inhibitor, reduced peripheral blood blast percentage but did not induce remissions in a phase 1 trial of daily times seven oral dosing in patients with a variety of relapsed hematologic malignancies.[74] Asymptomatic changes in electrocardiographic T waves developed in 80% of treated patients. Gastrointestinal symptoms and thrombocytopenia were common.

Cyclic Tetrapeptides

Romidepsin has recently been FDA approved for the treatment of CTCL[101] and is undergoing phase 2 studies in peripheral T-cell lymphoma.[102,103] Antitumor activity, including tumor lysis syndrome, was demonstrated in a phase 1 study that enrolled patients with chronic lymphocytic leukemia and AML, but no complete or partial remissions were seen.[35] Administration of romidepsin induces electrocardiographic changes, including T-wave flattening and ST-T wave depression in greater than half of the posttreatment tracings; however, no changes in serum cardiac troponin levels or left ventricular ejection fraction have been reported.[104]

Benzamides

Entinostat, formerly known as MS-275, was administered weekly times four to patients with relapsed and refractory AML in a phase 1 study. Infections, unsteady gate, and somnolence were dose-limiting toxicities. No clinical responses developed, although improvement in neutrophil counts were observed.[105]

PHARMACODYNAMIC OBSERVATIONS

Administration of oral vorinostat was associated with a transient increase in acetylation of histone H3 in peripheral blood lymphocytes, which peaked at 2 hours postdosing and reverted to baseline by 8 hours; similar changes were observed in the lymph node of a treated patient with lymphoma.[100] Treatment with vorinostat was associated with translocation of phosphorylated STAT-3 from nucleus to cytoplasm in responding patients and with reduced microvessel density.[98]

Similar changes in acetylation of histones 2B and 3 were observed in peripheral blood cells from patients treated with LBH589.[74] Romidepsin induced acetylation of H3 and H4 in peripheral blood tumor cells within 4 hours of dosing[35]; of interest, $p21^{WAF1/CIP1}$ protein levels also increased, associated with an increase in acetylation of H4 at the p21 promoter (using chromatin immunoprecipitation).

Treatment with entinostat led to increased acetylation of H3 and H4 in both peripheral blood and bone marrow. This increase was detectable within 8 hours and remained above baseline throughout the treatment cycle. Thus, this compound may provide the most prolonged inhibition of protein deacetylation of HDAC inhibitors under current investigation.[105] Increases in $p21^{WAF1/CIP1}$ and activation of caspase 3 were also demonstrated in these samples.

No clinical studies to date have examined other potentially important pharmacodynamic parameters in patients receiving HDAC inhibitors. The apparent sensitivity of CTCL to HDAC inhibitors as a class has not yet been explained.

Combining Inhibitors in the Treatment of Hematologic Malignancies

Methyl binding proteins recruit HDACs as part of transcriptional corepression complexes to areas of cytosine methylation. Optimal reexpression of transcriptionally silenced genes with promoter methylation *in vitro* can be achieved by the sequential application of DNMT inhibitors followed by HDAC inhibitors.[22] This *in vitro* treatment paradigm has led to a variety of clinical studies that have attempted to apply this concept to the treatment of hematologic malignancies. The first study of sequential DNMT/HDAC inhibitors administered a variety of doses of 5AC for 5 to 14 days followed by 7 days of NaPB by continuous infusion at its maximum tolerated dose to patients with MDS and AML.[12] The combination was well tolerated, and clinical responses were frequent in patients receiving 5AC at 50 mg/m²/d daily for 10 days and 25 mg/m²/da daily for 14 days, with 5 of 14 patients at those dose schedules achieving complete or partial response.

In a pilot study, ten patients with MDS or AML were treated with 5AC at 75 mg/m²/d daily times seven followed by 5 days of NaPB given at 200 mg/kg/d as a 1- to 2-hour infusion. Three patients developed a partial response.[106]

In a similar study, investigators at M. D. Anderson Cancer Center treated leukemic patients with decitabine (15 mg/m²/d IV daily times ten) and concomitant VPA at a variety of doses. Twelve of 54 patients achieved complete remission or complete remission with incomplete platelet recovery.[107] The inhibitors 5AC, VPA, and all transretinoic acid have been administered to patients with AML and MDS. Fourteen of 33 previously untreated patients over the age of 60 developed a complete remission or a complete remission with inadequate platelet recovery.[108] A subsequent study of 5AC and VPA suggests increased efficacy of this combination in high-risk MDS.[109]

Entinostat has been successfully combined with azacytidine in patients with myeloid malignancies[90]; the U.S. Leukemia Intergroup has recently completed a randomized phase 2 trial of this combination compared with azacytidine alone. Other current studies combine DNMT inhibitors with vorinostat and belinostat. It remains to be established whether combination therapies are more effective than single-agent demethylating therapies.

Epigenetically Targeted Therapy in Nonhematologic Malignancies

The intense interest in the application of epigenetically targeted drugs to hematologic malignancies derives from the empiric observation of the activity of 5AC for the treatment of MDS and the ability to easily sample tumor cells for pharmacodynamic measurements. Nonetheless, these approaches are being appropriately studied in epithelial malignancies that are known to have very abnormal epigenomes. NaPB was investigated in phase 1 studies of continuous intravenous infusions, twice daily infusions, and oral administration. Stable disease was observed in some patients.[110–112] Partial responses were observed in patients with papillary thyroid cancer, mesothelioma, and laryngeal cancer who were treated on a phase 1 study of oral vorinostat.[113]

In addition to its activity in lymphoma, romidepsin induced clinical responses in renal cell carcinoma in a phase 1 study[114]; however, few responses were seen in a phase 2 study in that disease.[115] No objective responses occurred in a phase 1 trial in refractory pediatric solid tumors.[116] Entinostat administration was associated with stable disease in a phase 1 study at the National Cancer Institute.[117]

Although it appears unlikely that HDAC inhibitors will have marked activity as monotherapy in solid tumors, their widespread effects on numerous important cellular pathways make them attractive compounds for development in therapeutic combinations.

The recent identification of other regulatory enzymes involved in histone modifications, including histone methyltransferases and histone demethylases (i.e., LSD1), provides novel targets for epigenetically targeted drugs. It is expected that these agents will be further developed and tested in the coming years, with anticipated activity either alone or strategically combined with other epigenetic agents.

Selected References

The full list of references for this chapter appears in the online version.

2. Herman JG, Baylin SB. Gene silencing in cancer in association with promoter hypermethylation. *N Engl J Med* 2003;349:2042.
3. Jones PA, Baylin SB. The epigenomics of cancer. *Cell* 2007;128:683.
12. Gore SD, Baylin S, Sugar E, et al. Combined DNA methyltransferase and histone deacetylase inhibition in the treatment of myeloid neoplasms. *Cancer Res* 2006;66:6361.
22. Cameron EE, Bachman KE, Myohanen S, Herman JG, Baylin SB. Synergy of demethylation and histone deacetylase inhibition in the re-expression of genes silenced in cancer. *Nat Genet* 1999;21:103.
29. Schaefer M, Hagemann S, Hanna K, Lyko F. Azacytidine inhibits RNA methylation at DNMT2 target sites in human cancer cell lines. *Cancer Res* 2009;69:8127.
30. Hollenbach PW, Nguyen AN, Brady H, et al. A comparison of azacitidine and decitabine activities in acute myeloid leukemia cell lines. *PLoS One* 2010;5:e9001.
36. Blum W, Klisovic RB, Hackanson B, et al. Phase I study of decitabine alone or in combination with valproic acid in acute myeloid leukemia. *J Clin Oncol* 2007;25:3884.
37. Schrump DS, Fischette MR, Nguyen DM, et al. Phase I study of decitabine-mediated gene expression in patients with cancers involving the lungs, esophagus, or pleura. *Clin Cancer Res* 2006;12:5777.
43. Flotho C, Claus R, Batz C, et al. The DNA methyltransferase inhibitors azacitidine, decitabine and zebularine exert differential effects on cancer gene expression in acute myeloid leukemia cells. *Leukemia* 2009;23:1019.
52. Richon VM, Emiliani S, Verdin E, et al. A class of hybrid polar inducers of transformed cell differentiation inhibits histone deacetylases. *Proc Natl Acad Sci U S A* 1998;95:3003.
69. Silverman LR, McKenzie DR, Peterson BL, et al. Further analysis of trials with azacitidine in patients with myelodysplastic syndrome: studies 8421, 8921, and 9221 by the Cancer and Leukemia Group B. *J Clin Oncol* 2006; 24:3895.
70. Silverman LR, Demakos EP, Peterson BL, et al. Randomized controlled trial of azacitidine in patients with the myelodysplastic syndrome: a study of the Cancer and Leukemia Group B. *J Clin Oncol* 2002;20:2429.
71. Fenaux P, Mufti GJ, Hellstrom-Lindberg E, et al. Efficacy of azacitidine compared with that of conventional care regimens in the treatment of higher-risk myelodysplastic syndromes: a randomised, open-label, phase III study. *Lancet Oncol* 2009;10:223.
72. Wijermans P, Lubbert M, Verhoef G, et al. Low-dose 5-aza-2′-deoxycytidine, a DNA hypomethylating agent, for the treatment of high-risk myelodysplastic syndrome: a multicenter phase II study in elderly patients. *J Clin Oncol* 2000;18:956.
74. Kantarjian H, Oki Y, Garcia-Manero G, et al. Results of a randomized study of 3 schedules of low-dose decitabine in higher-risk myelodysplastic syndrome and chronic myelomonocytic leukemia. *Blood* 2007; 109:52.
76. Steensma DP, Baer MR, Slack JL, et al. Multicenter study of decitabine administered daily for 5 days every 4 weeks to adults with myelodysplastic syndromes: the alternative dosing for outpatient treatment (ADOPT) trial. *J Clin Oncol* 2009;27:3842.
84. Yang AS, Doshi KD, Choi SW, et al. DNA methylation changes after 5-aza-2′-deoxycytidine therapy in patients with leukemia. *Cancer Res* 2006;66: 5495.
85. Daskalakis M, Nguyen TT, Nguyen C, et al. Demethylation of a hypermethylated P15/INK4B gene in patients with myelodysplastic syndrome by 5-Aza-2′-deoxycytidine (decitabine) treatment. *Blood* 2002;100:2957.
90. Fandy TE, Herman JG, Kerns P, et al. Early epigenetic changes and DNA damage do not predict clinical response in an overlapping schedule of 5-azacytidine and entinostat in patients with myeloid malignancies. *Blood* 2009;114:2764.
98. Duvic M, Talpur R, Ni X, et al. Phase 2 trial of oral vorinostat (suberoylanilide hydroxamic acid, SAHA) for refractory cutaneous T-cell lymphoma (CTCL). *Blood* 2007;109:31.
100. O'Connor OA, Heaney ML, Schwartz L, et al. Clinical experience with intravenous and oral formulations of the novel histone deacetylase inhibitor suberoylanilide hydroxamic acid in patients with advanced hematologic malignancies. *J Clin Oncol* 2006;24:166.
103. Piekarz RL, Frye R, Turner M, et al. Phase II multi-institutional trial of the histone deacetylase inhibitor romidepsin as monotherapy for patients with cutaneous T-cell lymphoma. *J Clin Oncol* 2009;27:5410.
105. Gojo I, Jiemjit A, Trepel JB, et al. Phase 1 and pharmacologic study of MS-275, a histone deacetylase inhibitor, in adults with refractory and relapsed acute leukemias. *Blood* 2007;109:2781.
106. Maslak P, Chanel S, Camacho LH, et al. Pilot study of combination transcriptional modulation therapy with sodium phenylbutyrate and 5-azacytidine in patients with acute myeloid leukemia or myelodysplastic syndrome. *Leukemia* 2006;20:212.
107. Garcia-Manero G, Kantarjian HM, Sanchez-Gonzalez B, et al. Phase 1/2 study of the combination of 5-aza-2′-deoxycytidine with valproic acid in patients with leukemia. *Blood* 2006;108:3271.
108. Soriano AO, Yang H, Faderl S, et al. Safety and clinical activity of the combination of 5-azacytidine, valproic acid, and all-trans retinoic acid in acute myeloid leukemia and myelodysplastic syndrome. *Blood* 2007;110: 2302.
109. Voso MT, Santini V, Finelli C, et al. Valproic acid at therapeutic plasma levels may increase 5-azacytidine efficacy in higher risk myelodysplastic syndromes. *Clin Cancer Res* 2009;15:5002.
117. Ryan QC, Headlee D, Acharya M, et al. Phase I and pharmacokinetic study of MS-275, a histone deacetylase inhibitor, in patients with advanced and refractory solid tumors or lymphoma. *J Clin Oncol* 2005;23:3912.

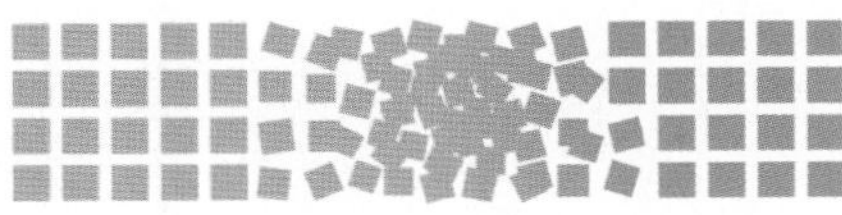

CHAPTER 41 PROTEASOME INHIBITORS

MICHAEL G. KAUFFMAN, CHRISTOPHER J. MOLINEAUX, CHRISTOPHER J. KIRK, AND CRAIG M. CREWS

BIOCHEMISTRY OF THE UBIQUITIN-PROTEASOME PATHWAY

The vast majority of intracellular proteins are degraded via the ubiquitin-proteasome pathway. A key step in this process is "tagging" of proteins targeted for degradation with multiple copies of ubiquitin, a 76-amino acid protein whose primary sequence and structure is highly conserved in organisms ranging from yeast to mammals.[12,13] Once polyubiquitinated, proteins targeted for degradation bind to the 26S proteasome, a holoenzyme composed of two 19S regulatory complexes capping a central 20S proteolytic core. The 20S core is a hollow "barrel" consisting of four stacked heptameric rings. The subunits are classified as either α-subunits (outer two rings) or β-subunits (inner two rings). The 19S regulatory complex consists of a lid that recognizes ubiquitinated protein substrates with high fidelity, and a base that contains six adenosine triphosphatases, unfolds protein substrates, removes the polyubiquitin tag, and threads them into the catalytic chamber of the 20S particle in an adenosine triphosphate-dependent manner.[14,15]

Unlike typical proteases, the 20S proteasome in eukaryotic cells contains multiple proteolytic activities resulting in cleavage of protein targets at multiple sites. For example, the proteasome hydrolyzes peptide bonds after bulky hydrophobic amino acid residues, reminiscent of chymotrypsin. Similarly, it also cleaves peptide bonds after basic residues, analogous to trypsin, and those after acidic residues, analogous to caspases. Hence, these activities are referred to as the chymotrypsin-like (CT-L), the trypsin-like (T-L), and the caspase-like (C-L) activities, respectively. These activities are encoded by the genes *PSMB5* (β5), *PSMB2* (β2), and *PSMB1* (β1), respectively.[16] A systematic study of the individual proteolytic sites within the 26S proteasome revealed that all three types of activities contribute significantly to proteolysis, although their relative importance varies widely according to the specific primary amino acid sequence of the substrate.[17]

PROTEASOME INHIBITORS

Natural Product Proteasome Inhibitors

Mode of action studies have revealed several natural products to be selective, potent PIs including lactacystin[18,19] and the peptide α', β'-epoxyketone epoxomicin.[20] Epoxomicin targets the 20S proteasome[9] but unlike other classes of PIs (e.g., boronates) that inhibit serine proteases and other enzymes, epoxomicin and its derivatives are highly specific for the active sites of the proteasome, which are the major *N*-terminal Thr proteases in the cell.[21] Other natural product inhibitors of the proteasome include TMC-95A, fellutamide B, and NPI-0052, a β-lactone member of the lactacystin class of inhibitors. NPI-0052 (salinosporamide A) is an orally bioavailable PI isolated from *Salinispora tropica* currently being developed by Nereus Pharmaceuticals, Inc. (San Diego, California).[22]

Disclosure

C.M.C. was a founder of Proteolix, Inc., the initial developer of carfilzomib. C.J.M. is a former employee of Proteolix, Inc., and Onyx Pharmaceuticals, Inc.

The ubiquitin proteasome system is involved in the degradation of more than 80% of cellular proteins, including those that control cell-cycle progression, apoptosis, DNA repair, and the stress response.[1] Given its key role in maintaining cellular homeostasis, the ubiquitin proteasome system appeared to be an unlikely target for pharmaceutical intervention; however, a variety of studies suggested that inhibitors of proteasome function might prove to be viable therapeutic agents.[2]

Initial studies used substrate-related peptide aldehydes to investigate the proteolytic functions and specificity of the proteasome.[3] *In vitro* and *in vivo* studies with these inhibitors demonstrated their ability to induce apoptosis as well as inhibit tumor growth.[4–7] The subsequent discovery that several natural products with antitumor activity exert their action via proteasome inhibition[8,9] provided additional rationale for the development of selective proteasome inhibitors (PIs).

The first PI clinically validated for use in cancer was the boronate-based dipeptide, bortezomib. Initially approved in 2003 for treatment of patients with relapsed/refractory multiple myeloma (R/R MM), bortezomib is currently approved for two indications by the U.S. Food and Drug Administration (FDA): for patients with MM, and for patients with mantle cell lymphoma (MCL) who have received at least one prior therapy.[10] A separate class of synthetic, peptide-based epoxyketone inhibitors related to the natural product epoxomicin include carfilzomib, which is now entering phase 3 clinical trials for the treatment of MM, and ONX 0912 (formerly PR-047), which will be among the first orally active PIs to be evaluated in clinical studies. In addition, three other Pis, which are orally active in animals, include the boronate-based PIs CEP-18770 and MLN9708, and the lactacystin analogue NPI-0052. All three compounds have entered phase 1 clinical studies using intravenous (IV) administration protocols, and MLN9708 has also entered clinical studies using oral dosing regimen.[11] A comprehensive summary of the drugs described in this chapter is provided in Table 41.1.

TABLE 41.1

NATURAL PRODUCT AND SYNTHETIC PROTEASOME INHIBITORS

Drug	Other Names	Structure[11]	Route(s) of Administration	Therapeutic Use(s)[a]	In vivo Biochemistry	
					IC$_{50}$ $\beta_5/\beta_2/\beta_1$ (nM)	Dissociation $t_{1/2}$ (min)[b]
Lactacystin			N/A	Preclinical investigation only	N/A	N/A
Epoxomicin			N/A	Preclinical investigation only	N/A	N/A
Eponemycin			N/A	Preclinical investigation only	N/A	N/A
TMC-95A			N/A	Preclinical investigation only	N/A	N/A

Fellutamide B		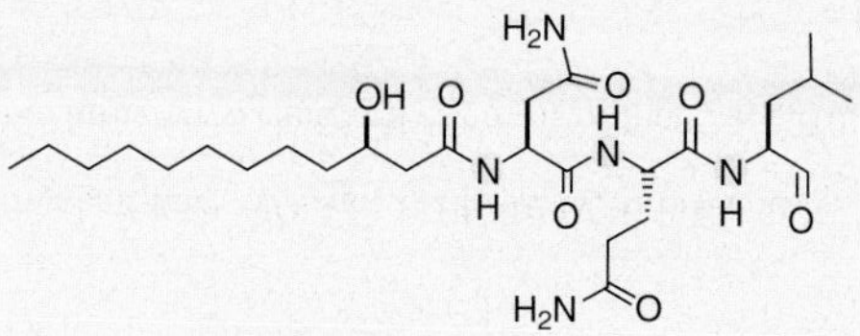	N/A	Preclinical investigation only	N/A	N/A
Salinosporamide A	NPI-0052; marizomib	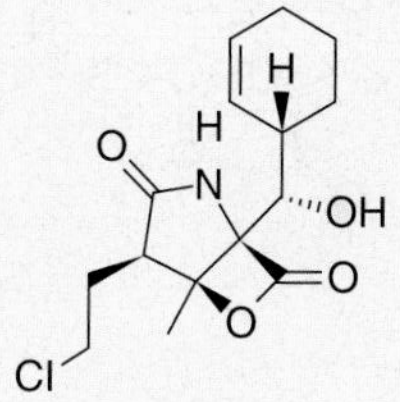	IV, oral	Under clinical investigation for treatment of relapsed and/or refractory multiple myeloma, refractory lymphoma, and advanced solid tumors (including NSCLC, pancreatic cancer, and melanoma)	3.5/28/430	Irreversible
Bortezomib	Velcade	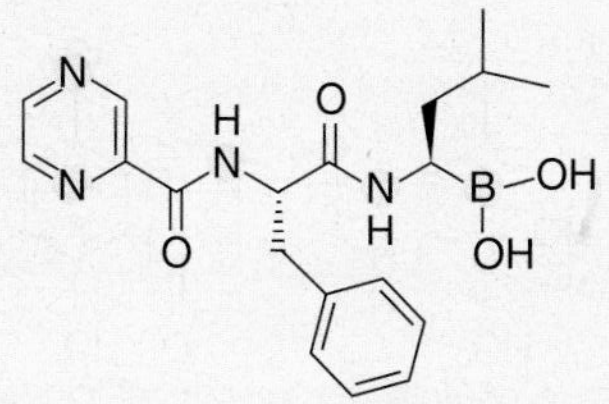	IV	Approved by FDA and EMEA for treatment of multiple myeloma and mantle cell lymphoma[c]	2.4–7.9/590–4200/24–74	110
Carfilzomib	PR-171	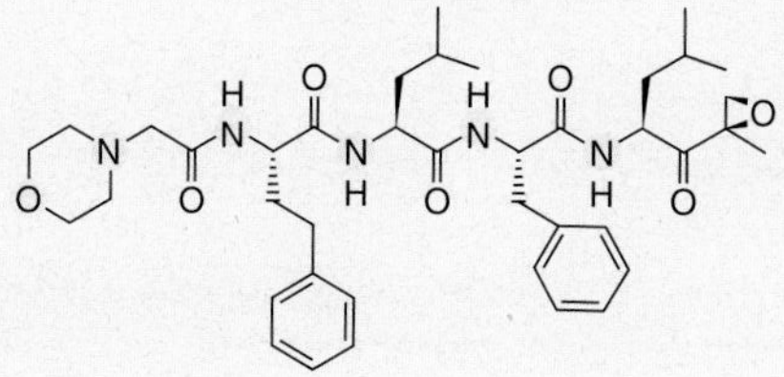	IV	Under clinical investigation for treatment of primary and relapsed or refractory multiple myeloma, and advanced solid tumors (including NSCLC, SCLC, renal, and ovarian cancers)	6/3600/2400	Irreversible
CEP-18770		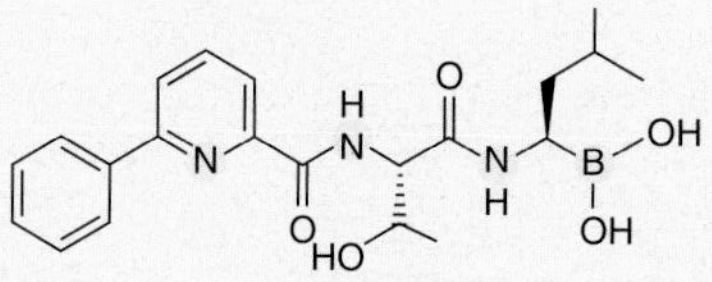	IV, oral	Under clinical investigation for treatment of relapsed multiple myeloma, refractory solid tumors, and non-Hodgkin's lymphoma	3.8/>100/<100	NR—slowly reversible

(continued)

TABLE 41.1

(CONTINUED)

Drug	Other Names	Structure[1]	Route(s) of Administration	Therapeutic Use(s)[a]	*In vivo* Biochemistry: IC_{50} $\beta_5/\beta_2/\beta_1$ (nM)	*In vivo* Biochemistry: Dissociation $t_{1/2}$ (min)[b]
MLN9708			IV, oral	Under clinical investigation for treatment of relapsed and refractory multiple myeloma, lymphoma (including Hodgkin's lymphoma), and advanced nonhematologic malignancies for which standard treatment is no longer effective (including NSCLC, head and neck cancer [squamous cell cancer], soft tissue sarcoma, or prostate cancer)	3.4/3500/31	18
ONX-0912	PR-047		Oral	Under clinical investigation for treatment of advanced refractory or recurrent solid tumors	36/NR/NR	Irreversible

IC_{50}, half maximal inhibitory concentration; $t_{1/2}$, half-time; N/A, not available; IV, intravenously; NSCLC, non–small cell lung cancer; FDA, U.S. Food and Drug Administration; EMEA, European Medicines Agency; NR, not reported.

[a]Information on therapeutic uses obtained from http://www.clinicaltrials.gov as of June 24, 2010.

[b]Data from ref. 11. [c]Data from ref. 10.

Synthetic Proteasome Inhibitors: Preclinical Development

Bortezomib (PS-341, Velcade), developed by Millennium Pharmaceuticals (Cambridge, Massachusetts), was the first PI approved for clinical use.[10,23] Unlike lactacystin and the epoxyketones, the boronic acid inhibitors do not produce covalent adducts with the proteasome, instead forming stable, slowly reversible tetrahedral intermediates. Recovery of proteasome activity following bortezomib inhibition *in vitro* and *in vivo* likely takes place primarily because of *de novo* synthesis of new proteasomal proteins, rather than by reversibility of the boronate tetrahedral complex.[24] Like NPI-0052, bortezomib is a time-dependent inhibitor of proteasome activity and predominantly targets the CT-L activities of both the constitutive proteasome (β5) and the immunoproteasome (LMP7).

Carfilzomib (PR-171), a tetrapeptide epoxyketone derivative of epoxomicin,[25] is currently in development by Onyx Pharmaceuticals, Inc. (Emeryville, California, which acquired Proteolix Inc., in November 2009). Like NPI-0052, carfilzomib is an irreversible PI. Carfilzomib displays 300-fold selectivity for the CT-L active sites of both the constitutive proteasome and the immunoproteasome,[25] and is in late-stage clinical trials for treatment of MM. Although both carfilzomib and bortezomib potently inhibit the CT-L activity of the proteasome, bortezomib exhibits off-target activity toward several additional serine proteases with a preference for Leu/Phe/Tyr in the P1 position.[26] The extent to which off-target inhibition contributes to the toxicities of bortezomib, especially peripheral neuropathy (PN), remains to be determined. Carfilzomib, on the other hand, displays minimal off-target activity because it only binds to N-terminal Thr proteases. The greater specificity/selectivity that carfilzomib exhibits toward the CT-L activity of the proteasome may explain the increased *in vivo* potency of carfilzomib relative to bortezomib and its ability to overcome bortezomib resistance both *in vitro* and *in vivo*.[25,27] Moreover, unlike bortezomib, carfilzomib is well tolerated when given to animals and humans in daily IV doses for up to 5 days (maximum number of daily doses tested) resulting in an extremely high degree (>80%) of prolonged proteasome inhibition.[27]

CEP-18770, a dipeptide boronate derivative, is an orally active PI in animals[28] and also inhibits the proteasome CT-L, with similar potency to bortezomib. This inhibitor suppresses NF-κB-mediated signaling pathways and induces tumor cell death *in vitro* and in mouse models of MM following oral administration.[29] CEP-18770 appears to exhibit a more favorable cytotoxicity profile toward nontransformed cells when compared with bortezomib. It has recently entered human clinical trials in R/R MM, non-Hodgkin's lymphoma (NHL), and advanced-stage solid tumors.

PRECLINICAL PHARMACOLOGY OF PIS

In vitro and *in vivo* Antitumor Activity of PIs

In vitro, both naturally derived and synthetic PIs display potent, concentration-dependent cytotoxic activity against transformed cells of hematologic and nonhematologic origins.[27,30–32] Prolonged incubation of PIs with cells in culture results in extensive concentration-dependent cytotoxicity, including in nontransformed cells. In contrast, brief (1 hour) incubation of PIs followed by washout, which likely reflects the exposure seen *in vivo* (see later discussion), results in preferential cytotoxic activity against hematologic tumor cell lines but minimal to no cell death in nontransformed cells.[27]

Development of subunit-specific inhibitors of the proteasome has demonstrated that inhibition of the CT-L activity is sufficient to induce apoptosis[33,34] through caspase-mediated events. In addition, PIs have been shown to affect the half-life of the "BH3-only" members of the Bcl-2 family, specifically BH3-interacting-domain death agonist (Bid) and Bcl-2 interacting killer (Bik).[35] Proteasome inhibition also up-regulates the expression of several key cell-cycle checkpoint proteins that include p53 (an inducer of G_0/G_1 cell-cycle arrest through accumulation of the cyclin-dependent kinase [CDK] inhibitor p27), the CDK inhibitor p21, mammalian cyclins A, B, D, and E, and transcription factors E2F and Rb.[36,37] The transcription factor NF-κB, an important regulator of cell survival and cytokine/growth factor production,[38] is also affected by proteasome inhibition in multiple ways. However, the net effect on NF-κB signaling is not consistent across various assays and cell lines, and its relative importance in the antitumor effects of PIs remains unclear.

PIs are active in mouse models of human cancer. Preclinical studies with bortezomib have been published extensively (reviewed in ref. 30), and a detailed description of these studies is beyond the scope of this chapter. For carfilzomib, *in vivo* antitumor activity was demonstrated to depend on the schedule of administration, with intensive dose schedules (e.g., daily dosing) showing excellent responses in tumor xenograft models, resistant to the twice-weekly, days 1 and 4, schedule of bortezomib.[27] NPI-0052 has shown antitumor activity as a single agent and in combination with several approved chemotherapeutics in models of leukemia and in human MM xenografts. In a number of studies, NPI-0052 overcame resistance to conventional treatments and to bortezomib.[31,39]

Pharmacokinetics and Pharmacodynamics of Proteasome Inhibitors in Animals

Following IV administration to rodents and other animals, proteasome activity is inhibited in a dose-dependent fashion within minutes; however, PIs such as bortezomib and carfilzomib are also rapidly cleared from circulation.[27,32,40,41] Recovery of proteasome activity in animals occurs in tissues with a half-life of approximately 24 hours, mirroring the recovery time of cells exposed to sublethal concentrations of PIs *in vitro*[27] and likely reflects new protein synthesis. In safety studies both in animals and in humans, carfilzomib was well tolerated using highly intensive daily dosing schedules (2–5 consecutive days) that are not possible with bortezomib because of severe morbidity and mortality.[42,43]

PROTEASOME INHIBITORS IN CANCER

Clinical Activity of Bortezomib

Bortezomib is typically administered on days 1, 4, 8, and 11 of a 3-week cycle. Increasing doses of bortezomib inhibit proteasome activity in blood in a dose-dependent fashion, reaching a maximum of 74% inhibition at a dose of 1.38 mg/m^2. Daily dosing schedules in animal studies have been associated with severe toxicity and have not been attempted in humans. In clinical trials, thrombocytopenia and PN were common adverse events.[10] Bortezomib has shown remarkable single-agent antitumor activity in a wide range of hematologic malignancies, including MM, NHL, Waldenström macroglobulinemia, and other diseases. In 2003, bortezomib was approved by the FDA for use as a single agent for the treatment of patients with MM following two prior therapies and who demonstrated disease progression with their most recent therapy.[44] The CREST trial in R/R MM yielded a 50% overall response rate (ORR), defined as patients having more than 25% drop in circulating myeloma M-protein levels, for patients receiving bortezomib at 1.3 mg/m^2 for up to eight cycles.[45] Long-term follow-up from the CREST study revealed a median survival of 60 months.[46] Improved response rates have been observed with bortezomib in earlier-stage MM patient populations. A single-agent ORR of 38% (6% complete response [CR] rate) was seen in the phase 3 APEX study in early relapsed MM, with a time to progression (TTP) of 6.2 months and a median duration of response of 8 months.[47–50] In the frontline setting, bortezomib demonstrated a single-agent response rate of 41% (5% CR rate).[51] In APEX, the major grade 3 and 4 toxicities were PN, 12%; dysesthesia and related symptoms, 8% to 10%; anemia, 8%; diarrhea, 8%; neutropenia, 14%; and fatigue, 12%.

Bortezomib is also approved for newly diagnosed MM in combination with melphalan and prednisone (VMP). The phase 3 VISTA trial evaluated VMP in patients with untreated MM who were ineligible for high-dose therapy.[52] The addition of bortezomib significantly improved response rates in this setting with an ORR of 71% for VMP (including 30% CR) versus 35% (with only 4% CR) for MP.[52] VMP was associated with a TTP of ~24 months, compared with ~16.6 months with MP. For VMP versus MP, the median overall survival was not estimable versus 43.1 months, and the 3-year overall survival rate was 68.5% versus 54.0%, respectively, with improvements across all patient subgroups.[53]

Bortezomib has also shown promise when combined with other agents in R/R MM patients. The combination of bortezomib with pegylated doxorubicin (Doxil, Centocor Ortho Biotech Products, L.P., Horsham, PA) resulted in an ORR of 79% in relapsed patients, and toxicities were similar to those observed with each agent administered separately.[54] A phase 3 study in 646 patients with R/R MM compared this treatment with bortezomib alone, with the combination only producing a 44% ORR. Treatment with doxorubicin extended the TTP from 6 to 9.3 months.[55,56] This combination received FDA approval in 2007 for use in bortezomib-naïve patients with MM following one prior therapy.[57] Other agents being tested in combination include vorinostat, the anti-CS1 mAb, elotuzumab, the Hsp90 inhibitor tanespimycin, and the Akt inhibitor perifosine.[58–62]

Frontline combinations with bortezomib in MM patients have shown high ORRs with a notable improvement in CR rates. In longer-term studies, CR rates with bortezomib-based combinations have been shown to be associated with improved clinical outcomes.[63,64] A community-based phase 3b study evaluating bortezomib + dexamethasone (VD) versus bortezomib + thalidomide + dexamethasone (VTD) versus VMP found similar ORR (60%, 70%, and 52%, respectively) and CR rates (13%, 18%, and 15%, respectively).[63] Bortezomib + melphalan + prednisone + thalidomide (VMPT) followed by bortezomib + thalidomide (VT) maintenance resulted in a superior CR rate compared with VMP with no maintenance (34% versus 21%) and improved 2-year progression-free survival (70% vs. 58.2%).[64] A protocol modification changing from twice weekly to weekly bortezomib administration yielded similar TTP but reduced the incidence (21% vs. 43%) and severity of PN (2% grade 3/4 vs. 14%).[64] There are as yet no complete data on responses rates or overall survival using weekly administration of bortezomib in combination with other agents.

Bortezomib has also shown activity in other hematologic cancers, most notably MCL. As a single agent in 155 R/R MCL patients, bortezomib yielded an ORR of 33% (8% CR), a median duration of response of 9.2 months, and a TTP of 6.2 months.[65] Toxicities observed were similar to those seen in patients with MM and included thrombocytopenia, PN, and fatigue. When bortezomib was used to treat both newly diagnosed and refractory MCL, a response rate of 46% was observed in both populations,[66] leading to FDA approval late in 2006. Encouraging data with other lymphomas, notably follicular lymphoma, have led to investigations of additional combinations.

Bortezomib has been tested in a variety of solid tumors in phase 1 and 2 studies.[67] Partial responses (PRs) were reported in 8% of patients with refractory non–small cell lung cancer (NSCLC), although the TTP was 1.5 months.[68] Exacerbation of PN was common. Bortezomib was subsequently tested in combination with paclitaxel, irinotecan, and gemcitabine/carboplatin; however, results have not been encouraging. Bortezomib continues to be tested in combination with other agents in a variety of tumor types.[69,70]

Development of Other Proteasome Inhibitors

Carfilzomib

Parallel phase 1 studies of carfilzomib have been conducted in patients with multiple tumor types, and two phase 1 dose-finding studies targeting B-cell malignancies have been completed. The first study used daily IV bolus dosing with doses up to 20 mg/m^2 for 5 consecutive days followed by 9 days of rest and resulted in substantial inhibition of proteasome activity.[43] In the second study, carfilzomib was administered daily for 2 days for 3 consecutive weeks (days 1, 2, 8, 9, 15, and 16), followed by 12 days of recovery.[71,72] This dosing regimen provides three periods of proteasome inhibition per cycle, with each lasting for 48 hours or more. Despite a high rate of baseline neuropathy (~30% in the second phase 1 study), new-onset PN was infrequent and no grade 3/4 PN was reported. Hematologic toxicities were the most frequent adverse events, observed along with transient, noncumulative elevations in serum creatinine, usually with increases in serum urea nitrogen, and consistent with a "prerenal" etiology. Among 20 evaluable patients (including bortezomib-refractory patients), four PRs and one minor response were seen. Responses were also durable, lasting more than 1 year in some cases. Although the maximum tolerated dose of carfilzomib was not established in this study, a dose of 20 mg/m^2 was initially selected for the phase 2 studies.

Based on the phase 1 studies, two open-label, single-arm, phase 2 studies of single-agent carfilzomib in MM were initiated in 2007. The first, PX-171-003, was conducted in heavily pretreated patients with R/R MM.[73] The second, PX-171-004, is in earlier-stage MM patients with one to three prior therapies.[74] In PX-171-003, patients must have previously received bortezomib and either thalidomide or lenalidomide, must have relapsed after two or more therapies that had to include "standard" agents (e.g., glucocorticoids and alkylating agents), and their disease must have been refractory to the most recently received therapy. Carfilzomib was administered as an IV bolus on the twice-weekly dose schedule. Patients enrolled in the initial phase of the study (003-A0) had received a median of five prior therapies and 78% of patients had grade 1/2 PN at entry.[73] Among 39 evaluable patients in 003-A0, 10 (26%) achieved a minor response or better, including 5 PRs, and 16 additional patients with stable disease.[75] Four patients completed all 12 cycles of dosing and most have continued therapy. As safety information accumulated from continued phase 1 studies and patients were given oral and IV hydration to reduce any prerenal effects, the protocol was amended and the carfilzomib dose was escalated to 27 mg/m^2 after the first cycle (003-A1) in July 2008. In addition, the trial was increased to 250 patients and overall survival was added as an end point. Interim safety data from the first 141 patients receiving 003-A1 have been reported.[73] Major adverse events (grade 3/4) included 3.5% neutropenia, 13.5% anemia, and 4.3% fatigue;

grade 3/4 PN was reported in one patient (0.7%) and grade 3/4 gastrointestinal complaints occurred in less than 1% of patients (antidiarrheal prophylaxis was not routinely given).[73]

The parallel PX-171-004 trial enrolled patients with relapsed MM following one to three prior treatments and who may have been refractory to one or more of these therapies. Approximately 150 evaluable patients are planned for enrollment into 2 groups: bortezomib-naïve and bortezomib-treated. Thirty-five patients have been enrolled in the bortezomib-treated arm and 120 in the bortezomib-naïve cohorts. In patients with relapsed disease, nonhematologic and hematologic toxicity profiles were similar.[76] Despite high rates of baseline PN, reports of worsening neuropathic symptoms were infrequent (2% incidence of grade 3 and no grade 4 events).[77] In PX-171-004, carfilzomib demonstrated considerable activity in bortezomib-naïve patients, inducing PR or better in 46% of 54 evaluable patients at 20 mg/m^2 and 53% of patients at 27 mg/m^2.[74] These represent some of the highest single-agent activities of currently available antimyeloma agents.[74] The response rate in patients previously exposed to bortezomib was lower (18%).[74] Responses across groups are durable, typically 8 to 9 months.[74]

In both the PX-171-003 and -004 studies, tumor lysis syndrome (TLS) was initially observed or suspected in 4 of 77 patients treated at the 20 mg/m^2 dose prior to the implementation of TLS prophylaxis guidelines. Since these measures were implemented, including oral and IV hydration with 4 mg dexamethasone premedication during the first cycle, no documented cases of symptomatic TLS have been observed, with more than 350 patients treated in phase 2 trials (Onyx Pharmaceuticals, Inc., data on file). To date, no clinically significant, cumulative toxicities have been noted with carfilzomib, allowing an indefinite duration of dosing to patients with good disease control.

Trials of carfilzomib in combination with other agents in MM have been initiated, including a phase 1b/2 safety and efficacy study of carfilzomib in combination with lenalidomide and low-dose dexamethasone (CRd). The dose-escalation phase (1b) of this study has completed enrollment and carfilzomib has been safely combined at the doses used in the 003 and 004 trials with the maximum recommended dose of lenalidomide (25 mg once daily days 1–21 of a 28-day cycle). CRd has been well tolerated to date and no dose-limiting toxicities have been observed up to the maximum protocol-specified dose. Based on this excellent tolerability, the phase 2 portion of the study enrolled 44 additional patients.[78] High levels of disease control have been noted in preliminary evaluations despite the fact that most patients were previously treated with bortezomib and lenalidomide (and/or thalidomide). The CRd combination is now being tested in an international, multicenter, randomized, open-label phase 3 study in comparison with lenalidomide and low-dose dexamethasone (Rd) in approximately 700 patients with relapsed MM following one to three prior therapies.

An ongoing phase 1b/2 study with carfilzomib in patients with advanced-stage solid tumors and MM is exploring carfilzomib administered as a 30-minute infusion and includes planned dose escalations to 88 mg/m^2.[79] Interestingly, the prerenal effects of carfilzomib were found to be associated with C_{max} in animals (Onyx Pharmaceuticals, Inc., data on file), and phase 1 clinical studies of carfilzomib have now been modified to administer the drug over 30 minutes (rather than 2–5 minutes as in the original studies). This has allowed the administration of carfilzomib at doses up to 56 mg/m^2 with generally good tolerability.[79] When carfilzomib was administered as an IV bolus (20 mg/m^2 on days 1 and 2 followed by 36 mg/m^2 on subsequent days), responses based on RECIST criteria were seen in small cell lung cancer and in renal (clear cell) carcinoma, with several patients (including patients with refractory small cell lung cancer and NSCLC) continuing to receive single-agent carfilzomib for more than 18 cycles.[80] Nonhematologic adverse events in the solid tumor study are similar to those seen in the phase 2 hematologic studies; however, the rate of hematologic toxicities appears to be substantially lower than that observed in patients with MM, perhaps because of improved bone marrow reserves in patients with solid tumors.

NPI-0052

NPI-0052 (marizomib) has been studied as a single agent in several phase 1 trials in patients with advanced solid tumors or refractory lymphomas[81] and MM.[82] A separate study is evaluating NPI-0052 with vorinostat in patients with advanced NSCLC.[83] In a phase 1 trial in MM, patients were treated with NPI-0052 IV weekly for 3 weeks in 4-week cycles at doses ranging from 0.025 mg/m^2 to 0.7 mg/m^2. At the maximum dose of 0.7 mg/m^2, inhibition of CT-L activity in whole blood was 73% and 99% at days 1 and 15, respectively. Because NPI-0052 is an irreversible PI, the increased inhibition seen at day 15 is likely due to cumulative inhibition in enucleated erythrocytes. One patient with IgA$^+$ MM had a 71% decrease in M-protein (unconfirmed PR; off study after three cycles). A second patient with nonsecretory disease had a ~50% reduction in involved light chain and remained on study 5+ months. In addition, eight patients with R/R MM remained on study for 6 to 15 months (including three patients for >1 year) with stable disease and no significant toxicity. Two patients in this latter group had bortezomib-refractory disease.[82,84] Toxicities were comparable with those of bortezomib but notable for an apparent lack of PN. One patient, however, did develop reversible renal insufficiency. Stable disease was seen as the best response in several patients with previously progressing MM, and further studies are underway. Dose escalation of NPI-0052 was halted at 0.8 mg/m^2, as dose-limiting toxicities of transient "hallucinations" (visual imprints when eyes closed) and dizziness/unsteady gait were observed at 0.9 mg/m^2.[85] Distinguishing NPI-0052 from other PIs (e.g., bortezomib, carfilzomib, CEP-18770) is its ability to penetrate the blood–brain barrier.[27,29,32] NPI-0052 inhibits brain proteasome CT-L activity by more than 90%,[32] indicating possible utility in the treatment of CNS tumors, but raising potential safety concerns around long-term treatment because of the link between abnormalities in the ubiquitin proteasome system and neurodegenerative diseases.[86,87]

MLN9708 (MLN2238)

MLN9708 is an orally bioavailable peptide boronic acid analogue of bortezomib currently being developed by Millennium Pharmaceuticals. When exposed to aqueous solutions or plasma, the compound spontaneously hydrolyzes to produce the active drug, MLN2238.[88] *In vivo* studies have demonstrated efficacy of MLN2238 in several tumor models, including prostate, diffuse large B-cell lymphoma, colon, and lymphoma models.[89] Interestingly, 14 mg of MLN2238 resulted in proteasome inhibition in bone marrow that was stronger and more sustained that that seen in blood, along with increased reversibility compared with bortezomib.[89,90] Associated with this finding, statistically significant tumor growth inhibition was seen in an intratibial MDA-MB-231 breast cancer xenograft model.[89] Additionally, greater proteasome inhibition was seen in both tumor and bone marrow than in blood,[91] indicating substantial distribution of MLN2238 into these tissues. MLN9708 is currently being investigated, using both IV and oral dosing, in phase 1 studies in lymphoma and solid tumors. The schedules of administration are the same as those for bortezomib (weekly and twice weekly).

ONX 0912 (formerly PR-047)

Data from *in vitro* models of Waldenström macroglobulinemia and in mouse xenograft models of NHL and colorectal cancer demonstrated that ONX 0912, the orally bioavailable epoxyketone analogue of carfilzomib, appears to have antitumor activity equivalent to that of carfilzomib.[92,93] Absolute oral bioavailability of up to 39% was seen in rodents and dogs.[94] Following oral administration of ONX 0912 in mice, rapid absorption, tissue distribution, and proteasome inactivation were reported.[93] Like carfilzomib, ONX 0912 has demonstrated synergistic activity with a CDK4/6 inhibitor in chemoresistant MM cells.[95] ONX 0912 has entered phase 1 clinical testing as an orally administered agent delivered on a dose-intensive (5 times a day) schedule.

Selected References

The full list of references for this chapter appears in the online version.

2. Rolfe M, Chiu MI, Pagano M. The ubiquitin-mediated proteolytic pathway as a therapeutic area. *J Mol Med* 1997;75(1):5.
3. Vinitsky A, Michaud C, Powers JC, Orlowski M. Inhibition of the chymotrypsin-like activity of the pituitary multicatalytic proteinase complex. *Biochemistry* 1992;31(39):9421.
6. Orlowski RZ, Eswara JR, Lafond-Walker A, Grever MR, Orlowski M, Dang CV. Tumor growth inhibition induced in a murine model of human Burkitt's lymphoma by a proteasome inhibitor. *Cancer Res* 1998;58(19):4342.
7. Delic J, Masdehors P, Omura S, et al. The proteasome inhibitor lactacystin induces apoptosis and sensitizes chemo- and radioresistant human chronic lymphocytic leukaemia lymphocytes to TNF-alpha-initiated apoptosis. *Br J Cancer* 1998;77(7):1103.
8. Meng L, Kwok BH, Sin N, Crews CM. Eponemycin exerts its antitumor effect through the inhibition of proteasome function. *Cancer Res* 1999;59(12):2798.
9. Meng L, Mohan R, Kwok BH, Elofsson M, Sin N, Crews CM. Epoxomicin, a potent and selective proteasome inhibitor, exhibits in vivo antiinflammatory activity. *Proc Natl Acad Sci U S A* 1999;96(18):10403.
11. Dick LR, Fleming PE. Building on bortezomib: second-generation proteasome inhibitors as anti-cancer therapy. *Drug Discov Today* 2010;15(5-6):243.
12. Wilkinson KD. Ubiquitination and deubiquitination: targeting of proteins for degradation by the proteasome. *Semin Cell Dev Biol* 2000;11(3):141.
13. Kopp F, Hendil KB, Dahlmann B, Kristensen P, Sobek A, Uerkvitz W. Subunit arrangement in the human 20S proteasome. *Proc Natl Acad Sci U S A* 1997;94(7):2939.
15. Groll M, Ditzel L, Lowe J, et al. Structure of 20S proteasome from yeast at 2.4 A resolution. *Nature* 1997;386(6624):463.
16. Orlowski M, Wilk S. Catalytic activities of the 20 S proteasome, a multicatalytic proteinase complex. *Arch Biochem Biophys* 2000;383(1):1.
17. Kisselev AF, Callard A, Goldberg AL. Importance of the different proteolytic sites of the proteasome and the efficacy of inhibitors varies with the protein substrate. *J Biol Chem* 2006;281(13):8582.
21. Groll M, Bajorek M, Kohler A, et al. A gated channel into the proteasome core particle. *Nat Struct Biol* 2000;7(11):1062.
22. Feling RH, Buchanan GO, Mincer TJ, Kauffman CA, Jensen PR, Fenical W. Salinosporamide A: a highly cytotoxic proteasome inhibitor from a novel microbial source, a marine bacterium of the new genus salinospora. *Angew Chem Int Ed Engl* 2003;42(3):355.
23. Adams J, Palombella VJ, Sausville EA, et al. Proteasome inhibitors: a novel class of potent and effective antitumor agents. *Cancer Res* 1999;59(11):2615.
25. Kuhn DJ, Chen Q, Voorhees PM, et al. Potent activity of carfilzomib, a novel, irreversible inhibitor of the ubiquitin-proteasome pathway, against preclinical models of multiple myeloma. *Blood* 2007;110(9):3281.
26. Arastu-Kapur S, Shenk K, Parlati F, Bennett MK. Non-proteasomal targets of proteasome inhibitors bortezomib and carfilzomib [abstract presented at the 50th Annual Meeting of the American Society of Hematology, San Francisco, CA, December 6–9]. *Blood*. 2008;112(11):Abstract 2657.
27. Demo SD, Kirk CJ, Aujay MA, et al. Antitumor activity of PR-171, a novel irreversible inhibitor of the proteasome. *Cancer Res* 2007;67(13):6383.
28. Dorsey BD, Iqbal M, Chatterjee S, et al. Discovery of a potent, selective, and orally active proteasome inhibitor for the treatment of cancer. *J Med Chem* 2008;51(4):1068.
29. Piva R, Ruggeri B, Williams M, et al. CEP-18770: A novel, orally active proteasome inhibitor with a tumor-selective pharmacologic profile competitive with bortezomib. *Blood* 2008;111(5):2765.
31. Chauhan D, Hideshima T, Anderson KC. A novel proteasome inhibitor NPI-0052 as an anticancer therapy. *Br J Cancer* 2006;95(8):961.
33. Parlati F, Lee SJ, Aujay M, et al. Carfilzomib can induce tumor cell death through selective inhibition of the chymotrypsin-like activity of the proteasome. *Blood* 2009;114(16):3439.
34. Myung J, Kim KB, Lindsten K, Dantuma NP, Crews CM. Lack of proteasome active site allostery as revealed by subunit-specific inhibitors. *Mol Cell* 2001;7(2):411.
35. Zhang HG, Wang J, Yang X, Hsu HC, Mountz JD. Regulation of apoptosis proteins in cancer cells by ubiquitin. *Oncogene* 2004;23(11):2009.
36. Pagano M, Tam SW, Theodoras AM, et al. Role of the ubiquitin-proteasome pathway in regulating abundance of the cyclin-dependent kinase inhibitor p27. *Science* 1995;269(5224):682.
39. Chauhan D, Catley L, Li G, et al. A novel orally active proteasome inhibitor induces apoptosis in multiple myeloma cells with mechanisms distinct from Bortezomib. *Cancer Cell* 2005;8(5):407.
41. Orlowski RZ, Stinchcombe TE, Mitchell BS, et al. Phase I trial of the proteasome inhibitor PS-341 in patients with refractory hematologic malignancies. *J Clin Oncol* 2002;20(22):4420.
42. Kirk CJ, Jiang J, Muchamuel T, et al. The selective proteasome inhibitor carfilzomib is well tolerated in experimental animals with dose intensive administration [abstract presented at the 50th Annual Meeting of the American Society of Hematology, San Francisco, CA, December 6–9]. *Blood*. 2008;112(11):Abstract 2765.
43. O'Connor OA, Stewart AK, Vallone M, et al. A phase 1 dose escalation study of the safety and pharmacokinetics of the novel proteasome inhibitor carfilzomib (PR-171) in patients with hematologic malignancies. *Clin Cancer Res* 2009;15(22):7085.
46. Jagannath S, Barlogie B, Berenson JR, et al. Updated survival analyses after prolonged follow-up of the phase 2, multicenter CREST study of bortezomib in relapsed or refractory multiple myeloma. *Br J Haematol* 2008;143(4):537.
47. Richardson PG, Sonneveld P, Schuster M, et al. Extended follow-up of a phase 3 trial in relapsed multiple myeloma: final time-to-event results of the APEX trial. *Blood* 2007;110(10):3557.
48. Richardson PG, Barlogie B, Berenson J, et al. A phase 2 study of bortezomib in relapsed, refractory myeloma. *N Engl J Med* 2003;348(26):2609.
49. Richardson PG, Sonneveld P, Schuster MW, et al. Bortezomib or high-dose dexamethasone for relapsed multiple myeloma. *N Engl J Med* 2005;352(24):2487.
50. Richardson PG, Barlogie B, Berenson J, et al. Extended follow-up of a phase II trial in relapsed, refractory multiple myeloma: final time-to-event results from the SUMMIT trial. *Cancer* 2006;106(6):1316.
51. Richardson PG, Chanan-Khan A, Schlossman RL, et al. Phase II trial of single-agent bortezomib (VELCADE(R)) in patients with previously untreated multiple myeloma (MM) [abstract presented at the 46th Annual Meeting of the American Society of Hematology, San Diego, CA, December 4–7]. *Blood*. 2004;104(11):Abstract 336.
52. San Miguel JF, Schlag R, Khuageva NK, et al. Bortezomib plus melphalan and prednisone for initial treatment of multiple myeloma. *N Engl J Med* 2008;359(9):906.
53. Mateos M-V, Richardson PG, Schlag R, et al. Bortezomib plus melphalan-prednisone continues to demonstrate a survival benefit vs melphalan-prednisone in the phase III VISTA trial in previously untreated multiple myeloma after 3 years' follow-up and extensive subsequent therapy use [abstract presented at the 51st Annual Meeting of the American Society of Hematology, New Orleans, LA, December 5–8]. *Blood*. 2009;114(22): Abstract 3859.
56. Orlowski RZ, Nagler A, Sonneveld P, et al. Randomized phase III study of pegylated liposomal doxorubicin plus bortezomib compared with bortezomib alone in relapsed or refractory multiple myeloma: combination therapy improves time to progression. *J Clin Oncol* 2007;25(25):3892.
58. Richardson P, Wolf JL, Jakubowiak A, Zonder JA, Lonial S, Irwin DH, et al. Perifosine in combination with bortezomib and dexamethasone extends progression-free survival and overall survival in relapsed/refractory multiple myeloma patients previously treated with bortezomib: updated phase I/II trial results [abstract presented at the 51st Annual Meeting of the American Society of Hematology, New Orleans, LA, December 5–8]. *Blood*. 2009;114(22):Abstract 1869.
64. Palumbo A, Bringhen S, Rossi D, Ria R, Offidani M, Patriarca F, et al. Bortezomib, melphalan, prednisone and thalidomide (VMPT) followed by maintenance with bortezomib and thalidomide for initial treatment of elderly multiple myeloma patients [abstract presented at the 51st Annual Meeting of the American Society of Hematology, New Orleans, LA, December 5–8]. *Blood*. 2009;114(22):Abstract 128.
71. Alsina M, Trudel S, Vallone M, Molineaux C, Kunkel L, Goy A. Phase 1 single agent antitumor activity of twice weekly consecutive day dosing of the proteasome inhibitor carfilzomib (PR-171) in hematologic malignancies [abstract presented at the 49th Annual Meeting of the American Society of Hematology, Atlanta, GA, December 8–11]. *Blood*. 2007;110(11):Abstract 411.
73. Jagannath S, Vij R, Stewart K, Somlo G, Jakubowiak A, Trudel S, et al. Final results of PX-171-003-A0, part 1 of an open-label, single-arm, phase II

study of carfilzomib (CFZ) in patients (pts) with relapsed and refractory multiple myeloma (MM) [abstract presented at the 2009 Annual Meeting of the American Society of Clinical Oncology, Orlando, FL, May 29–June 2]. *J Clin Oncol.* 2009;27(15S):Abstract 8504.

74. Vij R, Siegel DS, Kaufman JL, et al. Results of an ongoing open-label, phase II study of carfilzomib in patients with relapsed and/or refractory multiple myeloma (R/R MM) [abstract presented at the 2010 Annual Meeting of the American Society of Clinical Oncology, Chicago, IL, June 4–8]. *J Clin Oncol.* 2010;28(7s):Abstract 8000.
77. Vij R, Wang L, Orlowski RZ, et al. Carfilzomib (CFZ), a novel proteasome inhibitor for relapsed or refractory multiple myeloma, is associated with minimal peripheral neuropathic effects [abstract presented at the 51st Annual Meeting of the American Society of Hematology, New Orleans, LA, December 5–8]. *Blood.* 2009;114(22):Abstract 430.
78. Niesvizky R, Wang L, Orlowski RZ, et al. Phase Ib multicenter dose escalation study of carfilzomib plus lenalidomide and low dose dexamethasone (CRd) in relapsed and refractory multiple myeloma (MM). Blood (ASH Annual Meeting Abstracts). 2009 November 20, 2009;114(22): 304.
79. Lee P, Burris H, Papadopoulos KP, et al. Updated results of a phase 1b/2 study of carfilzomib (CFZ) in patients (pts) with relapsed malignancies. American Society of Clinical Oncology Meeting Abstracts. 2010 May 21, 2010;28.
80. Rosen PJ, Gordon M, Lee PN, et al. Phase II results of Study PX-171-007: A phase Ib/II study of carfilzomib (CFZ), a selective proteasome inhibitor, in patients with selected advanced metastatic solid tumors [abstract]. *J Clin Oncol* 2009;27(15s):A3515.
84. Richardson P, Hofmeister C, Jakubowiak A, et al. Phase 1 clinical trial of the novel structure proteasome inhibitor NPI-0052 in patients with relapsed and relapsed/refractory multiple myeloma (MM). ASH Annual Meeting Abstracts. 2009 November 20, 2009;114(22):431.
93. Zhou HJ, Aujay MA, Bennett MK, et al. Design and synthesis of an orally bioavailable and selective peptide epoxyketone proteasome inhibitor (PR-047). *J Med Chem* 2009;52(9):3028.
94. Muchamuel T, Aujay M, Bennett MK, et al. Preclinical pharmacology and in vitro characterization of PR-047, an oral inhibitor of the 20S proteasome. ASH Annual Meeting Abstracts. 2008 November 16, 2008;112 (11):3671.

PHARMACOLOGY OF CANCER THERAPEUTICS

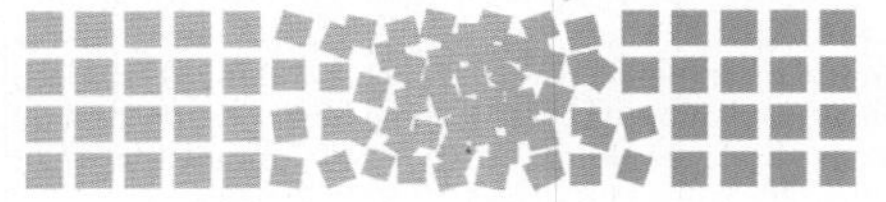

CHAPTER 42 POLY(ADP-RIBOSE) POLYMERASE INHIBITORS

ALAN ASHWORTH

Cancer cells frequently harbor defects in DNA repair pathways leading to genomic instability. This can foster tumorigenesis but also provides a weakness that can be exploited therapeutically. Tumors with compromised ability to repair double-strand DNA breaks by homologous recombination, including those with defects in the *BRCA1* and *BRCA2* genes, are highly sensitive to blockade of the repair of DNA single-strand breaks, via the inhibition of the enzyme PARP. This provides the basis for a "synthetic lethal" approach to cancer therapy, which is showing considerable promise in the clinic.

CELLULAR DNA REPAIR PATHWAYS

DNA is continually damaged by environmental exposures and endogenous activities, such as DNA replication and cellular free radical generation, which cause diverse lesions including base modifications, double-strand breaks (DSBs), single-strand breaks (SSBs), and intrastrand and interstrand cross-links.[1] These aberrations are repaired by distinct repair pathways, which are coordinated to maintain the stability and integrity of the genome. This faithful repair of DNA damage is an essential prerequisite for the maintenance of genomic integrity and cellular and organismal viability. Where one DNA strand is affected and the intact complementary strand is available as a template, the base-excision repair (BER), nucleotide-excision repair, or mismatch repair pathways are used and these pathways are highly efficient at repairing damage. DSBs, more problematic than SSBs as the complementary strand is not available as a template, are repaired by the homologous recombination (HR) or nonhomologous end-joining (NHEJ) pathways.[1]

Endogenous base damage, including SSBs, is the most common DNA aberration and it has been estimated that the average cell may repair 10,000 such lesions every day. BER is an important pathway for the repair of SSBs and involves the sensing of the lesion followed by the recruitment of a number of other proteins. PARP-1 (poly[ADP]ribose polymerase) is a critical component of the major "short-patch" BER pathway. PARP is an enzyme, discovered over 40 years ago,[2] that produces large branched chains of poly(ADP) ribose (PAR) from NAD^+. In humans, there are 17 members of the PARP gene family but most of these are poorly characterized.[3,4] The abundant nuclear protein PARP-1 senses and binds to DNA nicks and breaks, resulting in activation of catalytic activity causing poly(ADP)ribosylation of PARP-1 itself as well as other acceptor proteins including histones. This modification may signal the recruitment of other components of DNA repair pathways as well as modify their activity. The highly negatively charged PAR that is produced around the site of damage may also serve as an antirecombinogenic factor. In addition to the BER pathway PARP enzymes have been implicated in numerous cellular pathways.[3,4]

Two main DSB repair pathways are available within eukaryotic cells: NHEJ and HR.[5,6] HR can be further subdivided into the gene conversion (GC) and single-strand annealing (SSA) subpathways.[1] Both GC and SSA rely on sequence homology for repair whereas NHEJ uses no, or little, homology.[2,3] NHEJ is the most important pathway for the repair of DSBs during G_0, G_1, and early S phases of the cell cycle, although it is likely active throughout the cell cycle.[7,8] This form of DSB repair usually results in changes in DNA sequence at the break site and, occasionally, in the joining of previously unlinked DNA molecules, potentially resulting in gross chromosomal rearrangements such as translocations.[9] GC uses a homologous sequence, preferably the sister chromatid, as a template to resynthesize the DNA surrounding the DSB, and therefore generally results in accurate repair of the break. Repair by GC is critically dependent on the recombinase function of RAD51 and is facilitated by a number of other proteins. SSA also involves the use of homologous sequences for the repair of DSBs, but unlike GC, SSA is RAD51-independent and involves the annealing of DNA strands formed after resection at the DSB. The detailed mechanism of SSA is still obscure but it frequently results in the loss of one of the homologous sequences and deletion of the intervening sequence.[9] SSA is a potentially important pathway of mutagenesis because a significant fraction of mammalian genomes consist of repetitive elements. GC and SSA are cell-cycle regulated and are most active in S-G_2 phases of the cell cycle.[10]

THE DEVELOPMENT OF PARP INHIBITORS

PARP inhibitors were originally developed as chemopotentiators, which are agents that enhance the effects of DNA damage—a common mechanism of action of drugs used to treat cancer. The rationale is that inhibition of the repair of chemotherapy-induced DNA damage might give greater efficacy. Early studies using relatively nonspecific PARP inhibitors such a 3–aminobenzamide, demonstrated potential synergy with alkylating agents.[11] Subsequent studies with more potent PARP inhibitors demonstrated synergy with temozolomide, an observation that was taken into a clinical trial with AG014699, a PARP inhibitor developed by Pfizer.[12] Although the major focus of this chapter is the use of PARP inhibitors in synthetic lethal therapeutic strategies, their use in chemopotentiation in combination with chemotherapy remains under active investigation, as described later.

BRCA1 AND *BRCA2* MUTATIONS AND DNA REPAIR

Heterozygous germ line mutations in the *BRCA1* and *BRCA2* genes confer a high risk of breast (up to 85% lifetime risk) and ovarian (10% to 40%) cancer in addition to a significantly increased risk of pancreatic, prostate, and male breast cancer.[13] The genes have been classified as tumor suppressors, as the wild type *BRCA* allele is frequently lost in tumors, a phenomenon that occurs by a variety of mechanisms. The *BRCA1* and *BRCA2* genes encode large proteins that likely function in multiple cellular pathways including transcription, cell-cycle regulation, and the maintenance of genome integrity. However, it is the roles of BRCA1 and BRCA2 in DNA repair that have been best documented.[14]

BRCA1- and BRCA2-deficient cells are highly sensitive to ionizing radiation and display chromosomal instability, which is likely to be a direct consequence of unrepaired DNA damage.[14] The similar genomic instability in BRCA1- and BRCA2-deficient cells and the interaction of both BRCA1 and BRCA2 with RAD51 suggested a functional link between the three proteins in the RAD51-mediated DNA damage repair process. However, although BRCA2 is directly involved in RAD51-mediated repair, affecting the choice between GC and SSA, BRCA1 acts upstream of these pathways[15]; both GC and SSA are reduced in BRCA1-deficient cells, placing BRCA1 before the branch point of GC and SSA.[15]

BRCA1 has a role in signaling DNA damage and cell-cycle checkpoint regulation,[14,15] whereas BRCA2 has a more direct role in DNA repair itself. BRCA2 is thought to promote genomic stability through a role in the error-free repair of DSBs by GC via association with RAD51. Aberrations in *BRCA2*-deficient cells arise at least in part by the use of the SSA pathway. NHEJ, however, is apparently unaffected in BRCA2-deficient cells.[14,15] Loss of BRCA2, therefore, results in the repair of DSBs by preferential utilization of error-prone mechanism potentially explaining the apparent chromosome instability associated with *BRCA2* deficiency.[15]

The physical interaction between BRCA2 and RAD51 is essential for error-free DSB repair. BRCA2 is required for the localization of RAD51 to sites of DNA damage, where RAD51 forms the nucleoprotein filament required for recombination. Foci of RAD51 protein are apparent in the nucleus after certain forms of DNA damage and these likely represent sites of repair by HR; BRCA2-deficient cells do not form RAD51 foci in response to DNA damage.[15] Two different domains within BRCA2 interact with RAD51, the eight BRC repeats in the central part of the protein and a distinct domain, TR2, at the C-terminus.[16]

PARP1 INHIBITION AS A SYNTHETIC LETHAL THERAPEUTIC STRATEGY FOR THE TREATMENT OF BRCA-DEFICIENT CANCERS

Synthetic lethality is defined as the situation when mutation in either of two genes individually has no effect but combining the mutations leads to death.[17] This effect was first described and studied in genetically tractable organisms such as *Drosophila* and yeast.[17,18] This effect can arise because of a number of different gene-gene interactions. Examples include two genes in separate semiredundant or cooperating pathways, and two genes acting in the same pathway where loss of both critically affects flux through the pathway. The implication is that targeting one of these genes in a cancer where the other is defective should be selectively lethal to the tumor cells but not toxic to the normal cells. In principle, this should lead to a large therapeutic window.[19] The original suggestion that the concept of synthetic lethality could be used in the selection or development of cancer therapeutics came from Hartwell et al.[18] and from experiments performed in yeast. Comprehensive synthetic lethal screens have now been performed in a number of model organisms[20] and to a certain extent in human cells.[21] These have revealed multiple potential gene-gene interactions, some of which could be exploited clinically. However, synthetic lethal therapies have not been clinically used until recently, when evidence has been provided for PARP1 inhibition as a potential synthetic lethal approach for the treatment of *BRCA*-mutation associated cancers.

PARP-1 inhibition causes failure of the repair of SSB lesions but does not affect DSB repair.[22] However, a persistent DNA SSB encountered by a DNA replication fork will cause stalling of the fork and may result in either fork collapse or the formation of a DSB.[23] Therefore, loss of PARP-1 increases the formation of DNA lesions that might be repaired by GC. As loss of function of either BRCA1 or BRCA2 impairs GC,[14,15] loss of PARP-1 function in a BRCA1 or BRCA2 defective background could result in the generation of replication-associated DNA lesions normally repaired by sister chromatid exchange. If so, this might lead to cell-cycle arrest and/or cell death. Therefore, PARP inhibitors could be selectively lethal to cells lacking functional BRCA1 or BRCA2 but might be minimally toxic to normal cells. This would indicate a synthetic lethal interaction between PARP and BRCA1 or BRCA2.

Exemplifying this principle, decreasing PARP-1 expression levels using RNA interference causes a reduction in the clonogenic survival of BRCA1- and BRCA2-deficient cells compared with wild type cells.[24] This suggests that chemical inhibitors of PARP activity might have similar effects. Potent inhibitors of PARP were used to probe test the sensitivity of cells deficient in either BRCA1 or BRCA2. Cell survival assays showed that cell lines lacking wild type BRCA1 or BRCA2 were extremely sensitive to the potent PARP inhibitors KU0058684 and KU0058948 compared with heterozygous mutant or wild type cells.[24] Similar results were obtained with nonembryonic cells such as Chinese hamster ovary cells deficient in Brca2,[10] which showed a greater than 1,000-fold enhanced sensitivity compared with a Brca2-complemented derivative.[24] Depletion of *BRCA1* mRNA in MCF7 human breast cancer cells or of *BRCA2* mRNA in MCF7 or MDA-MB-231 cells also induced hypersensitivity to PARP inhibition.[24,25] No selective effect on cells heterozygous for *BRCA1* or *BRCA2* mutations was apparent; this is important as the normal tissue in *BRCA* patients carries only one copy of the relevant wild type *BRCA* gene. Potent PARP inhibitors seem to be required, as relatively ineffective PARP inhibitors do not cause this effect.[26,27]

To explain these observations, a model was proposed whereby persistent single-strand gaps in DNA caused by PARP inhibition when encountered by a replication fork, might trigger fork arrest, collapse, and/or a DSB.[28] Normally, these DSBs would be repaired by RAD51-dependent GC.[14,15] However, in the absence of BRCA1 or BRCA2, the replication fork cannot be restarted and collapses, causing persistent chromatid breaks. When repaired by the alternative error-prone DSB repair mechanisms of SSA or NHEJ, large numbers of chromatid aberrations would be induced, leading to cell lethality.[28] That it is the defect in GC that is being targeted in BRCA-deficient cells is supported by the demonstration that deficiency in other genes implicated in HR also confers sensitivity to PARP inhibitors.[29] This further suggests that this approach may be more widely applicable in the treatment of sporadic cancers with impairments of the HR pathway or "BRCAness"[30] (and see below).

MECHANISMS OF RESISTANCE TO PARP INHIBITORS

Resistance to targeted therapy frequently occurs, but it is unclear how resistance might arise to a synthetic lethal therapy. No studies have yet reported mechanisms of resistance in patients treated with PARP inhibitors. Potential mechanisms of resistance to PARP inhibitors have, however, been elucidated both directly *in vitro* and in mouse models, and indirectly in the clinic by studying platinum resistance in *BRCA* mutation carriers.[31] An *in vitro* model for resistance was developed by producing cells from the highly PARP inhibitor sensitive BRCA2-deficient cell line CAPAN1, which carries a c.6174delT *BRCA2* frameshift mutation. CAPAN1 cells cannot form damage-induced RAD51 foci, are defective for HR, and are extremely sensitive to treatment with PARP inhibitors.[29] PARP inhibitor resistant clones were highly resistant (over 1,000-fold) to the drug and were also cross-resistant to the DNA cross-linking agent cisplatin, but not to the microtubule-stabilizing drug docetaxel. PARP inhibitors and cisplatin both exert their effects on BRCA-deficient cells by increasing the frequency of misrepaired DSBs in the absence of effective HR. Therefore, this observation indicates that the resistance of PARP inhibitor resistant clones to PARP inhibitors might be because of restored HR. This contention was supported by the acquisition in PARP inhibitor resistant clones cells of the ability to form RAD51 foci after PARP inhibitor treatment or exposure to irradiation.[31]

DNA sequencing of PARP inhibitor-resistant clones revealed the unexpected presence of novel *BRCA2* alleles that resulted in elimination of the c.6174delT mutation and restoration of an open reading frame.[31] Resistance in this case, therefore, arises because of gain of function mutations in the synthetic lethal partner (BRCA2) rather than the direct drug target (PARP). An alternative mechanism of PARP inhibitor resistance has been described. A mouse model of *BRCA1*-associated mammary gland cancer demonstrated the efficacy of olaparib *in vivo* and was used to study mechanisms of resistance.[32] Resistance seemed to be caused by up-regulation of *ABCB1a/b*, which encode P-glycoprotein pumps; this effect could be reversed with the P-glycoprotein inhibitor tariquidar.

Mechanisms of resistance to PARP inhibitors in patient material have not yet been assessed because clinical trials are still at an early stage. However, cisplatin and carboplatin are part of the standard of care for the treatment of ovarian cancer, including individuals with *BRCA1* or *BRCA2* mutations. Platinum salts are thought to exert their BRCA-selective effects by a similar mechanism to PARP inhibitors.[15] Clinical observations suggest that *BRCA* mutation carriers with ovarian cancer usually respond better to these agents than patients without *BRCA* mutations[33,34]; however, resistance does eventually occur. To investigate this effect, *BRCA1* and *BRCA2* have been sequenced in tumor material from mutation carriers.[31,35] These studies revealed mutations in *BRCA1* or *BRCA2* that restored the open reading frame and likely contributed to platinum resistance. These observations suggest that specific mutations in *BRCA1* or *BRCA2* and sensitivity to therapeutics in cell lines and patients can be suppressed by intragenic deletion. Presumably these mutations occur randomly and are then selected for by differential drug sensitivity. Therefore, the best use of these agents is likely to be earlier in the disease process when the disease burden is smaller, which will reduce the probability of resistance based on stochastic genetic reversion.

INITIAL CLINICAL RESULTS TESTING SYNTHETIC LETHALITY

The profound sensitivity of BRCA mutant cells to PARP inhibition has led to the development of a number of clinical trials to test the efficiency of the synthetic lethal approach. A phase 1 clinical trial of olaparib (AstraZeneca, London, UK; formerly KU-0059436, KuDOS Pharmaceuticals, Cambridge, UK) and AZD2281 (AstraZeneca, London, UK) was performed in patients with refractory solid tumors.[36] This study was designed to enrich for patients with a mutation in *BRCA1* or *BRCA2*. Olaparib at doses of 60 mg or higher twice daily was associated with greater than 90% inhibition of PARP. Dose-limiting toxic effects were observed at 400 mg and 600 mg (twice daily); therefore, the dose-expansion cohort of *BRCA1/2* mutation carriers received 200 mg twice daily. Adverse effects were minimal (predominantly gastrointestinal and fatigue) and, strikingly, partial responses in 63% of patients (12 of 19) were documented, including 8 patients with ovarian cancer. This strong suggestion of clinical activity is preliminary vindication of the synthetic lethal therapeutic strategy.[36]

This trial has now reported an expanded cohort of patients with advanced *BRCA1/2* mutation associated ovarian, primary peritoneal, and fallopian tube cancers.[37] Of 50 patients treated with olaparib, the clinical benefit that was evaluated by radiologically and/or CA 125 response was 46% (relative risk, 40%; stable disease for more than 4 months, 6%) and the median duration of response was 28 weeks (range, 10–86 weeks). Importantly, the overall clinical benefit rate decreased significantly with platinum insensitivity (platinum sensitive, 69%; platinum resistant, 46%; platinum refractory, 23%). Furthermore, there was a positive association between the overall platinum-free interval and response to olaparib (P = .002). Although the clinical efficacy of olaparib diminished with decreasing platinum-free interval, it is noteworthy that the antitumor activity was substantial in both platinum-resistant disease and platinum-refractory disease states compared with other known agents.[37]

These promising results led to phase 2 multicenter single-arm, open-label sequential dosing cohort studies of *BRCA1/BRCA2* mutation carriers with either advanced chemorefractory ovarian cancer or metastatic breast cancer; these trials provided formal proof-of-concept of synthetic lethality.[38,39] Other PARP inhibitors, AG014699/PF-01367338 (Pfizer, New York, New York) and BSI-201 (BiPAR/Sanofi-Aventis, Paris, France) are undergoing evaluation in phase 2 trials of patients with *BRCA*-associated advanced ovarian cancer (Table 42.1).

THE USE OF PARP INHIBITORS IN SPORADIC CANCERS WITH "BRCANESS"

Germ line mutations in *BRCA1* or *BRCA2* are relatively common in hereditary breast and ovarian cancer. However, inactivation of *BRCA* genes by mutation in sporadic cancers is rare at least in breast cancer, which may seem to limit the application of PARP inhibitors to a wider range of patients. However, many tumors display features in common with BRCA-deficient tumors including similar defects in DNA repair due to either epigenetic mutation of *BRCA1*, such as promoter methylation, or mutation of other components of BRCA-associated pathways.[30] This "BRCAness" may make these tumors also susceptible to PARP inhibition.[30] For example, *PTEN* mutations, which occur with a frequency estimated at 50% to 80% in sporadic tumors,[40] may cause PARP inhibitor sensitivity in preclinical models, most likely because PTEN null cells display BRCAness phenotypes

TABLE 42.1

PARP INHIBITORS IN CLINICAL DEVELOPMENT FOR CANCER

Drug	Company	Indication	Status (Phase)
Olaparib (AZD2281)	KuDOS/AstraZeneca	*BRCA*-related breast cancer *BRCA*-related ovarian cancer Various other malignancies	2 2 2
Iniparib (BS1-201)	BiPAR/Sanofi-Aventis	Triple-negative breast cancer Various other malignancies	3
Veliparib (ABT-888)	Abbot	Various malignancies	2
AG014699 (PF-01367338)	Pfizer	Various malignancies	2
MK 4827	Merck	*BRCA*-related ovarian cancer and other malignancies	1
CEP-9722	Cephalon	Various malignancies	1

such as the inability to efficiently repair certain forms of DNA damage.[41]

Traditional histopathologic methods and, more recently, gene expression profiling approaches have shown the phenotypic overlap between triple-negative breast cancers, basal-like breast cancers, and *BRCA1* familial breast cancers.[42,43] In gene expression profiling studies it has been observed that *BRCA1* familial cancers strongly segregate with basal-like tumors and share features such as high-grade and pushing margins.[30,42,43] Although the overlap is not absolute, it leads to the hypothesis that there may be a subset of sporadic breast cancers that exhibits features of BRCAness, including deficiencies in HR and may be susceptible to treatment with drugs such as PARP inhibitors.[28,30]

On the basis of these shared characteristics, O'Shaughnessy et al.[44] performed a randomized phase 2 study comparing gemcitabine and carboplatin with or without the BiPAR PARP inhibitor BSI-201 in triple-negative breast cancer patients. Gemcitabine (1,000 mg/m^2 intravenously [IV]) and carboplatin (area under the curve = 2; IV) were given on days 1 and 8, and BSI-201 (5.6 mg/kg, IV) on days 1, 4, 8, and 11 every 21 days. The trial showed an objective response rate of 48% versus 16% (P = .002) in those treated with the PARP inhibitor and a difference in overall survival of 9.2 versus 5.7 months, respectively.[44] No excess toxicity was noted in the BSI-201 arm. A phase 3 study has now completed accrual and results are awaited. As previously discussed, PARP inhibitors were originally proposed as anticancer agents given their ability to sensitize cells to chemo- and radiotherapy. Therefore, it is possible that the effects observed in the BSI-201 triple-negative trial represent, in part at least, a chemosensitization effect perhaps combined with synthetic lethality, with an HR defect in the triple-negative subgroup.

PROSPECTS

Currently, the treatments for cancers arising in carriers of *BRCA1* or *BRCA2* mutations are the same as those occurring sporadically matched for tumor pathology and age of onset. However, tumors in *BRCA1* or *BRCA2* mutation carriers lack wild type *BRCA1* or *BRCA2* but normal tissues retain a single wild type copy of the relevant gene. This is a potentially targetable alteration that provides the basis for new mechanism-based approaches to the treatment of cancer. The biochemical difference in capacity to carry out HR between the tumor and normal tissues, in a *BRCA1* or *BRCA2* carrier, provides the rationale for this approach. Inhibiting the DNA repair protein PARP results in the generation of specific DNA lesions that require *BRCA1* and *BRCA2* specialized repair function(s) for

TABLE 42.2

PARP INHIBITORS: DOSAGES AND TOXICITIES

PARP Inhibitor	Dosage	Indications	Common Toxicities
Olaparib (AZD2281)	100–400 mg bid continuous	*BRCA1* or *BRCA2* defective breast ovarian and prostate cancer	Nausea, fatigue
Iniparib (BSI–201)	5.6 mg/kg (IV) days 1, 4, 8 and 11 every 21 days. Given with gemcitabine (1,000 mg/m^2, IV) and carboplatin (AUC = 2; IV)	Triple-negative breast cancer	No reported additional toxicities compared with chemotherapy alone
AG014699	12 mg/m^2 with 200 mg/m^2 temozolomide	Melanoma, various malignancies	No additional toxicity compared with temozolomide

IV, intravenously; AUC, area under the curve.

their removal. Preclinical data indicate that tumors defective in wild type *BRCA1* or *BRCA2* could be much more sensitive to PARP inhibition than unaffected heterozygous tissues, providing a potentially large therapeutic window. The safety and efficacy of this approach is currently being tested in clinical trials. Early indications are that these therapies show low toxicity with some preliminary indications of activity (Table 42.2).

Synthetic lethality by combinatorial targeting of DNA repair pathways may have usefulness as a therapeutic approach beyond familial cancers. The majority of solid tumors also exhibit genomic instability and aneuploidy. This suggests that pathways involved in the maintenance of genomic stability are dysfunctional in a significant proportion of neoplastic disorders.[45] Understanding which specialized DNA damage response and repair pathways are abrogated in sporadic tumor subtypes may allow the development of therapies that target the residual repair pathways on which the cancer, but not normal tissue, is now completely dependent. These potential therapies may significantly improve response rates while causing fewer treatment-related toxicities. However, these approaches may be associated with mechanism-associated resistance, and careful consideration of their optimal use will be required.

References

1. Hoeijmakers JH. Genome maintenance mechanisms for preventing cancer. *Nature* 2001;411:366.
2. Chambon P, Weill JD, Mandel P. Nicotinamide mononucleotide activation of new DNA-dependent polyadenylic acid synthesizing nuclear enzyme. *Biochem Biophys Res Commun* 1963;11:39.
3. Ame JC, Spenlehauer C, de Murcia G. The PARP superfamily. *Bioessays* 2004;26:882.
4. Otto H, Reche PA, Bazan F, et al. In silico characterization of the family of PARP-like poly(ADP-ribosyl)transferases (pARTs). *BMC Genomics* 2005; 6:139.
5. van Gent DC, Hoeijmakers JH, Kanaar R. Chromosomal stability and the DNA double-stranded break connection. *Nat Rev Genet* 2001;2:196.
6. Shin DS, Chahwan C, Huffman JL, et al. Structure and function of the double-strand break repair machinery. *DNA Repair (Amst)* 2004;3:863.
7. Takata M, Sasaki MS, Sonoda E, et al. Homologous recombination and non-homologous end-joining pathways of DNA double-strand break repair have overlapping roles in the maintenance of chromosomal integrity in vertebrate cells. *Embo J* 1998;17:5497.
8. Rothkamm K, Kruger I, Thompson LH, et al. Pathways of DNA double-strand break repair during the mammalian cell cycle. *Mol Cell Biol* 2003;23: 5706.
9. Stark JM, Pierce AJ, Oh J, et al. Genetic steps of mammalian homologous repair with distinct mutagenic consequences. *Mol Cell Biol* 2004;24:9305.
10. Elliott B, Richardson C, Jasin M. Chromosomal translocation mechanisms at intronic alu elements in mammalian cells. *Mol Cell* 2005;17:885.
11. Durkacz BW, Omidiji O, Gray DA, Shall S. (ADP ribose)n participates in DNA excision repair. *Nature* 1980;283(5747):593.
12. Tertoli L, Graziani G. Chemosensitisation by PARP inhibitors in cancer therapy. *Pharmacol Res* 2005;52:25.
13. Wooster R, Weber BL. Breast and ovarian cancer. *N Engl J Med* 2003;348: 2339.
14. Gudmundsdottir K, Ashworth A. The roles of BRCA1 and BRCA2 and associated proteins in the maintenance of genomic stability. *Oncogene* 2006;25: 5864.
15. Tutt AN, Lord CJ, McCabe N, et al. Exploiting the DNA repair defect in BRCA mutant cells in the design of new therapeutic strategies for cancer. *Cold Spring Harb Symp Quant Biol* 2005;70:139.
16. Lord CJ, Ashworth A. RAD51, BRCA2 and DNA repair: a partial resolution. *Nat Struct Mol Biol* 2007;14:461.
17. Dobzhansky T. Genetics of natural populations: Xiii. Recombination and variability in populations of *Drosophila pseudoobscura*. *Genetics* 1946;31: 269.
18. Hartwell LH, Szankasi P, Roberts CJ, et al. Integrating genetic approaches into the discovery of anticancer drugs. *Science* 1997;278:1064.
19. Kaelin WG Jr. The concept of synthetic lethality in the context of anticancer therapy. *Nat Rev Cancer* 2005;5:689.
20. Ooi SL, Pan X, Peyser BD, et al. Global synthetic-lethality analysis and yeast functional profiling. *Trends Genet* 2006;22:56.
21. Iorns E, Lord CJ, Turner N, et al. Utilizing RNA interference to enhance cancer drug discovery. *Nat Rev Drug Discov* 2007;6:556.
22. Noel G, Giocanti N, Fernet M, et al. Poly(ADP-ribose) polymerase (PARP-1) is not involved in DNA double-strand break recovery. *BMC Cell Biol* 2003;4:7.
23. Haber JE. DNA recombination: the replication connection. *Trends Biochem Sci* 1999;24:271.
24. Farmer H, McCabe N, Lord CJ, et al. Targeting the DNA repair defect in BRCA mutant cells as a therapeutic strategy. *Nature* 2005;434:917.
25. Bryant HE, Schultz N, Thomas HD, et al. Specific killing of *BRCA2*-deficient tumours with inhibitors of poly(ADP-ribose) polymerase. *Nature* 2005; 434:913.
26. McCabe N, Lord CJ, Tutt AN, et al. *BRCA2*-deficient CAPAN-1 cells are extremely sensitive to the inhibition of poly (ADP-ribose) polymerase: an issue of potency. *Cancer Biol Ther* 2005;4:934.
27. Gallmeier E, Kern SE. Absence of specific cell killing of the *BRCA2*-deficient human cancer cell line CAPAN1 by poly(ADP-ribose) polymerase inhibition. *Cancer Biol Ther* 2005;4:703.
28. Ashworth A. A synthetic lethal therapeutic approach: PARP inhibitors for the treatment of cancers deficient in double-strand break repair. *J Clin Oncol* 2008;26:3785.
29. McCabe N, Turner NC, Lord CJ, et al. Deficiency in the repair of DNA damage by homologous recombination and sensitivity to poly(ADP-ribose) polymerase inhibition. *Cancer Res* 2006;66:8109.
30. Turner N, Tutt A, Ashworth A. Hallmarks of 'BRCAness' in sporadic cancers. *Nat Rev Cancer* 2004;4:814.
31. Edwards S, Brough R, Lord CJ, et al. Resistance to therapy caused by intragenic deletion in *BRCA2*. *Nature* 2008;451(7182):1111.
32. Rottenberg S, Jaspers JE, Kersbergen A, et al. High sensitivity of *BRCA1*-deficient mammary tumors to the PARP inhibitor AZD2281 alone and in combination with platinum drugs. *Proc Natl Acad Sci U S A* 2008;105:17079.
33. Cass I, Baldwin RL, Varkey T, et al. Improved survival in women with BRCA-associated ovarian carcinoma. *Cancer* 2003;97:2187.
34. Pal T, Permuth-Wey J, Kapoor R, et al. Improved survival in BRCA2 carriers with ovarian cancer. *Fam Cancer* 2007;6:113.
35. Sakai W, Swisher EM, Karlan BY, et al. Secondary mutations as a mechanism of cisplatin resistance in *BRCA2*-mutated cancers. *Nature* 2008;451:1116.
36. Fong PC, Boss DS, Yap TA, et al. Inhibition of poly(ADP-ribose) polymerase in tumors from BRCA mutation carriers. *N Engl J Med* 2009;361:123.
37. Fong PC, Yap TA, Boss DS, et al. Poly(ADP)-ribose polymerase (PARP) inhibition: frequent durable responses in BRCA carrier ovarian cancer correlating with platinum-free interval. *J Clin Oncol* 2010;28:2512.
38. Audeh MW, Carmichael J, Penson RT, et al. Oral poly(ADP-ribose) polymerase inhibitor olaparib in patients with *BRCA1* or *BRCA2* mutations and recurrent ovarian cancer: a proof-of-concept trial. *Lancet* 2010;376:245.
39. Tutt A, Robson M, Garber JE, et al. Oral poly(ADP-ribose) polymerase inhibitor olaparib in patients with *BRCA1* or *BRCA2* mutations and advanced breast cancer: a proof-of-concept trial. *Lancet* 2010;376:235.
40. Salmena L, Carracedo A, Pandolfi PP. Tenets of PTEN tumor suppression. *Cell* 2008;133:403.
41. Mendes-Pereira AM, Martin SA, Brough R, et al. Synthetic lethal targeting of PTEN mutant cells with PARP inhibitors. *EMBO Mol Med* 2009;1:315.
42. Foulkes WD, Stefansson IM, Chappuis PO, et al. Germline BRCA1 mutations and a basal epithelial phenotype in breast cancer. *J Natl Cancer Inst* 2003;95:1482.
43. Turner NC, Reis-Filho JS. Basal-like breast cancer and the BRCA1 phenotype. *Oncogene* 2006;25:5846.
44. O'Shaughnessy J, Osborne C, Pippen J, et al. Iniparib plus chemotherapy in metastic triple-negative breast cancer. *N Engl J Med* 2011;3:205–214.
45. Lengauer C, Kinzler KW, Vogelstein B. Genetic instabilities in human cancers. *Nature* 1998;396:643.

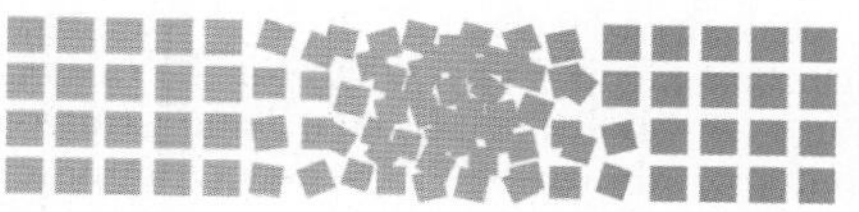

CHAPTER 43 MISCELLANEOUS CHEMOTHERAPEUTIC AGENTS

M. SITKI COPUR, MICHAL ROSE, AND SCOTT GETTINGER

SIROLIMUS AND TEMSIROLIMUS

Sirolimus (rapamycin) was isolated from the soil bacteria *Streptomyces hygroscopicus,* which was isolated from the South Pacific in the mid-1970s.[1] This bacterial macrolide later became the preferred immunosuppressant for kidney transplantation, as it was mildly immunosuppressive but, in contrast to cyclosporine A, it did not enhance tumor incidence.[2] Sirolimus is the prototypic inhibitor of the mammalian target of rapamycin (mTOR), a serine/threonine protein kinase that is a highly conserved regulatory protein involved in cell-cycle progression, proliferation, and angiogenesis.[3] Signaling pathways both upstream and downstream of mTOR have been shown to be commonly dysregulated in cancer. mTOR functions through two main mechanisms, depending on the presence and activity of the mTOR-associated protein complexes, mTORC1 and mTORC2. Of note, sirolimus and its analog compounds temsirolimus and everolimus form a complex with the FK binding protein (FKBP) and inhibit activation of a subset of mTOR proteins, residing within mTORC1. In contrast, mTORC2 holds mTOR in a form that is not as readily inhibited by these rapamycin analogs, and it appears that up-regulation of mTORC2 may represent a mechanism by which resistance can develop to this class of compounds.

Temsirolimus (CCI-779), a novel functional ester of sirolimus, is a water-soluble dihydroxymethyl propionic acid ester that rapidly undergoes hydrolysis to sirolimus after intravenous (IV) administration, reaching peak concentrations within 0.5 to 2.0 hours.[4] This drug is widely distributed in tissues, and steady-state drug levels are reached in 7 to 8 days. Temsirolimus is metabolized primarily in the liver by CYP3A4 microsomal enzymes to yield sirolimus as the main metabolite. The terminal half-life of temsirolimus is 17 hours, while that of sirolimus is approximately 55 hours. When bound to temsirolimus, mTOR is unable to phosphorylate the key protein translation factors, such as 4E-BP1 and S6K1, which then leads to translational inhibition of several critical regulatory proteins involved in cell-cycle control. Several other cellular proteins involved in regulation of angiogenesis, such as hypoxia-inducible factor-1α and vascular endothelial growth factor, are suppressed through mTOR inhibition by temsirolimus.

Phase 1 studies of temsirolimus have investigated various schedules and doses, ranging from 7.5 to 220 mg given as a weekly 30-minute infusions.[4] A phase 2 study in patients with cytokine-refractory renal cell cancer (RCC) investigated the efficacy and safety of three different dose levels (25, 75, and 250 mg, respectively) administered on a weekly schedule. This study showed promising antitumor activity for all three dose levels with no significant difference in efficacy or toxicity.[5] As a result, the 25-mg dose was eventually selected as the monotherapy dose for further study. The phase 3 randomized advanced RCC trial compared interferon, temsirolimus, and the combination of the two agents in previously untreated patients with advanced RCC who had at least three of six poor-prognostic features.[6] Once-weekly IV temsirolimus, 25 mg, prolonged the median overall survival of patients with poor prognostic features by 49% from 7.3 months (95% confidence interval [CI], 6.1 to 8.8 months) in the interferon arm to 10.9 months (95% CI, 8.6 to 12.7 months) in the single-agent temsirolimus arm, $P = .008$. Single-agent temsirolimus also extended median progression free survival by 77%, from 3.1 months in the interferon arm to 5.5 months in the temsirolimus arm, $P < .001$. Moreover, temsirolimus was effective for both clear cell and nonclear cell histologies.[7]

Mantle cell lymphoma was the first hematologic malignancy in which mTOR inhibition was explored as a treatment strategy. The rationale for this approach was that mantle cell lymphoma is characterized by overexpression of cyclin D1, which is a cyclin whose expression appears to be tightly regulated by mTOR signaling. In a phase 3 trial, once-weekly temsirolimus, 175 mg IV for 3 weeks followed by 75 mg once-weekly schedule, improved progression-free survival and overall response rate.[8] The early-phase clinical trials of temsirolimus showed promising activity against non–Hodgkin's lymphomas, multiple myeloma, and myeloid leukemias, and further studies are underway to confirm the activity of this drug in these various hematologic malignancies.[9]

In terms of safety profile, the most common adverse events associated with temsirolimus were asthenia and fatigue, dry skin with acneiform skin rash, nausea/vomiting, mucositis, and anorexia. Hyperlipidemia with increased serum triglycerides and/or cholesterol as well as hyperglycemia occur in up to 90% of patients. Allergic, hypersensitivity reactions have been observed in about 10% of patients, and pulmonary toxicity, presenting as increased cough, dyspnea, fever, and pulmonary infiltrates, is a relatively rare event, occurring in less than 1% of patients. However, the risk of pulmonary toxicity increases in patients with underlying pulmonary disease.[10]

EVEROLIMUS

Everolimus (RAD001) is an orally active hydroxyethyl ether analog of rapamycin containing a 2-hydroxyethyl chain substitution at position 40:40-O-(2-hydroxyethyl)-rapamycin. Thus, this molecule is significantly more water-soluble than sirolimus. As with sirolimus and temsirolimus, everolimus targets mTOR by forming a complex with mTOR and FKBP, resulting in inhibition of mTOR activity. Few data are available regarding the actual differences in the ability of temsirolimus and everolimus to inhibit mTOR. One preclinical *in vitro* study showed that the binding of everolimus to FKBP was approximately threefold weaker than that of sirolimus.[11] *In vivo* studies, however, have documented similar efficacy of the two agents in terms of immunosuppressive activity as well as antitumor activity. In preclinical models, administration of everolimus results in inhibition of mTOR, similar to what has been observed with the other rapamycin analogs.[12,13] In terms of clinical pharmacology, peak drug levels are achieved within 1 to 2 hours after oral administration, and food with a high fat content reduces oral bioavailability by up to 20%. This compound is metabolized in the liver, mainly by the CYP3A4 system, and six main metabolites have been identified. In general, these metabolites are less active than the parent compound. Elimination is mainly hepatic with excretion in feces, and caution should be used in patients with moderate liver impairment (Child-Pugh class B).[14,15] In this setting, the daily dose of drug should be reduced to 5 mg. In patients with severe liver dysfunction (Child-Pugh class C), the use of this drug is contraindicated.

Encouraging clinical activity was initially observed in phase 1/2 trials in patients with non–small cell lung, gastric, and esophageal cancers, sarcomas and pancreatic neuroendocrine tumors as well as hematologic malignancies.[16-20] Presently, everolimus is indicated and approved for the prophylaxis of organ rejection in adult patients at low to moderate immunologic risk following kidney transplantation and for the treatment of adults with advanced RCC after failure with sunitinib or sorafenib.[21] Based on these pivotal trials, the recommended dose of everolimus for the treatment of advanced RCC is 10 mg, to be taken once daily.

The safety profile of everolimus is similar to what has been observed with temsirolimus. The most common adverse events include asthenia and fatigue, dry skin with acneiform skin rash, nausea/vomiting, mucositis, and anorexia. Hyperlipidemia with increased serum triglycerides and/or cholesterol as well as hyperglycemia occur in up to 90% of patients. Allergic, hypersensitivity reactions have been observed in about 10% of patients, and pulmonary toxicity, presenting as increased cough, dyspnea, fever, and pulmonary infiltrates, are a relatively rare event, occurring in less than 1% of patients. However, the risk of pulmonary toxicity increases in patients with underlying pulmonary disease.

L-ASPARAGINASE

L-Asparaginase (L-asparagine aminohydrolase, EC 3.5.1.1) is a naturally occurring enzyme found in a variety of plants and microorganisms.[22,23] It catalyzes the hydrolysis of the essential amino acid L-asparagine to L-aspartic acid and ammonia depleting circulating pools of L-asparagine. Cancer cells depend on an exogenous source of L-asparagine for survival. Normal cells, however, are able to synthesize asparagine and are less affected by the effects of L-asparaginase. In addition to depletion of L-asparagine, L-asparaginase may exert its antitumor activity through a glutaminase effect, whereby depletion of essential glutamine stores leads to inhibition of DNA biosynthesis. L-Asparaginase is available in three preparations, two of which are native forms purified from bacterial sources. These include *Escherichia coli* and *Erwinia carotovora*, respectively. A third preparation, PEG-L-asparaginase, is a chemically modified form of the enzyme in which native *E. coli* L-asparaginase has been covalently conjugated to polyethylene glycol.[24]

After IV administration, plasma levels correlate closely with a given dose. After intramuscular (IM) injection, peak plasma levels are reached within 14 to 24 hours, and they are approximately one-half of those achieved with IV administration. Plasma protein binding is on the order of 30%. The pharmacokinetics of L-asparaginase vary depending on the particular source of the enzyme.[25] Pharmacokinetic studies in newly diagnosed children with acute lymphocytic leukemia (ALL) have shown peak serum concentrations in the range of 1 to 10 IU/mL, which are observed 24 to 48 hours after a single injection of 2,500 to 25,000 IU/m² of the enzyme derived from *E. coli*. After a dose of 25,000 IU/m² of the enzyme derived from *Erwinia* species, peak serum levels are achieved within 24 hours; however, the half-life is significantly shorter (15 hours) than that observed for *E. coli* L-asparaginase (40 to 50 hours). In contrast, PEG–L-asparaginase, when administered at a dose of 2,500 IU/m², achieves peak drug levels at 72 to 96 hours and has a significantly longer half-life (5.7 days) than for the *E. coli* L-asparaginase preparation.[25] Clinical trials have demonstrated the efficacy, safety, and tolerability of PEG- L-asparaginase administered intramuscularly, subcutaneously, or intravenously as part of multiagent chemotherapy regimens in the management of newly diagnosed and relapsed pediatric and adult ALL.

L-Asparaginase has been shown to antagonize the antineoplastic effects of methotrexate when administered either together or when given immediately before. Thus, these two drugs should be administered sequentially at least 24 hours apart. L-Asparaginase has also been shown to inhibit the metabolic clearance of vincristine, and can result in increased neurotoxicity. Toxicity is less pronounced when L-asparaginase is administered after vincristine, and for this reason, vincristine is normally administered at least 12 to 24 hours before L-asparaginase.

Hypersensitivity reactions occur in up to 25% of patients, manifested as skin rash and urticaria, or with life-threatening anaphylactic reactions such as facial edema, hypotension, bronchospasm, and respiratory distress. The risk is increased with repeated exposure, and when L-asparaginase is used as a single agent without the concurrent use of steroids. Although PEG–L-asparaginase is less immunogenic than the native nonpegylated forms of the enzyme, hypersensitivity reactions can still occur. A number of other side effects are observed that are secondary to the inhibitory effects of L-asparaginase on cellular protein synthesis. Decreased serum levels of insulin, key lipoproteins, and albumin have been reported. L-Asparaginase can cause alterations in thyroid function tests as early as 2 days after an administered dose, and this effect is believed to be secondary to a reduction in the serum levels of thyroxine-binding globulin. Alterations in coagulation parameters with prolonged thrombin time, prothrombin time, and partial thromboplastin time have been observed. In addition, decreased levels of vitamin K–dependent clotting factors, including factors V, VII, VIII, and IX, and a reduction in fibrinogen levels have been observed. Reductions in serum antithrombin III, protein C, protein S, plasminogen, and α_2-antiplasmin can also be caused by treatment. Patients treated with L-asparaginase are, therefore, at increased risk for bleeding and for thromboembolic events.[26] L-Asparaginase is contraindicated in patients with a prior history of pancreatitis, as there is a 10% incidence of acute pancreatitis. Neurologic toxicity includes lethargy, confusion, agitation, hallucinations, and/or coma, and in many instances, the severe form of neurotoxicity resembles ammonia toxicity. In contrast to the other anticancer agents used to treat ALL, myelosuppression is rarely seen with L-asparaginase therapy.

BLEOMYCIN

Of the 13 identifiable fractions, the main component is bleomycin A2. The drug's primary cytotoxic action is probably related to its excising effect on free bases after binding to DNA, resulting in single-strand breaks.[27] Bleomycin-mediated DNA damage requires the presence of Fe^{2+} metal ion in the presence of oxygen to generate the activated free radical species. Moreover, bleomycin mediates the oxidative degradation of all major classes of cellular RNAs. The effects of bleomycin are cell cycle-specific, as its main effects are mediated in the G_2 and M phases of the cell cycle.[28] Presently, bleomycin is primarily used as part of combination regimens for the treatment of Hodgkin's and non–Hodgkin's lymphoma, germ cell tumors, squamous cell cancer of the head and neck, and squamous cell carcinomas of the skin, cervix, vulva, and penis. It has also been used as a sclerosing agent to control malignant pleural effusions and ascites, as well as an intralesional agent with electrochemotherapy in the management of cutaneous malignancies.[29]

The oral bioavailability of bleomycin is poor, and it must be administered via the IV or IM routes. The initial distribution half-life is on the order of 10 to 20 minutes, whereas the terminal half-life is in the range of 3 hours. Bleomycin is absorbed rapidly after IM injection, and peak blood levels approximately one-third to one-half those achieved after an IV dose are usually reached in 30 to 60 minutes. In contrast to nearly all other anticancer agents, bleomycin can also be administered via the intracavitary route to control malignant pleural effusions or ascites, or both. Approximately 45% to 55% of an administered intracavitary dose of bleomycin is absorbed into the systemic circulation. Elimination is primarily via the kidneys, and approximately 60% to 70% of an administered dose is excreted unchanged in the urine. In patients with a creatinine clearance of less than 25 to 35 mL/min, dose reductions are required.

The dose-limiting toxicity of bleomycin is the development of pulmonary toxicity.[30] Bleomycin-induced pneumonitis occurs in approximately 10% of patients, and this side effect is related to the cumulative dose of drug received. The risk is increased in patients older than 70 years and in those who receive a total cumulative dose greater than 400 units. In addition, patients with underlying lung disease, prior irradiation to the chest or mediastinum, and exposure to high concentrations of inspired oxygen are also at increased risk for development of pulmonary toxicity. An increased use of granulocyte colony-stimulating factor (G-CSF) has been paralleled by an increased incidence of bleomycin-induced pulmonary toxicity. The exacerbating effects of G-CSFs seem to be associated with a marked infiltration of activated neutrophils along with the lung injury caused by the direct effects of bleomycin.[31,32] In a retrospective review, 18% of a total of 141 patients with Hodgkin's lymphoma treated with a bleomycin-containing regimen developed pulmonary toxicity. G-CSF use was one of the key factors associated with the development of this complication, and omission of bleomycin had no impact on clinical outcome.[33]

Patients with bleomycin-induced pulmonary toxicity may present with cough, dyspnea, dry inspiratory crackles, and infiltrates on chest radiograph. Pulmonary function testing is the most sensitive approach to monitor patients, and pulmonary function tests should be obtained at baseline before the start of therapy and before each cycle of therapy, with specific focus on the carbon monoxide diffusion capacity in the lung and vital capacity. A decrease of greater than 15% in either diffusion capacity of carbon monoxide or vital capacity should mandate immediate discontinuation of bleomycin. Early clinical trials and isolated case reports suggest that bleomycin-induced acute hypersensitivity reactions occur in 1% of patients with lymphoma and less than 0.5% of those with solid tumors. The reactions are mainly characterized by high-grade fever, chills, hypotension, and in a few cases, cardiovascular collapse, which can lead to death. The exact mechanism of these reactions is unclear, but is thought to be related to the release of endogenous pyrogens from the host cells. Supportive care, including hydration, steroids, antipyretics, and antihistamines, may resolve the symptoms. Clinicians should monitor their patients for any signs and symptoms of acute hyperpyrexic reactions during bleomycin administration. Because the onset of the reactions can occur with any dose of bleomycin and at any time, routine test dosing does not seem to predict when drug reactions may occur.[34] Mucocutaneous toxicity presents as mucositis, erythema, hyperpigmentation, induration, hyperkeratosis, and skin peeling that may progress to ulceration, usually developing in the second and third week of treatment and after a cumulative dose of 150 to 200 units of the drug. Of note, levels of bleomycin hydrolase are relatively low in lung and skin tissue, perhaps offering an explanation as to why these normal tissues are more adversely affected by bleomycin. Myelosuppression and immunosuppression are relatively mild. In rare cases, vascular events, including myocardial infarction, stroke, and Raynaud phenomenon, have been reported.

PROCARBAZINE

Procarbazine is a 1-methyl-2-benzyl derivative of hydrazine, and this agent was originally developed as a monoamine oxidase inhibitor. In its parent form, it is inactive, and it must be converted to its cytotoxic metabolites. This activation process may occur either spontaneously or by an enzymatic reaction mediated by the cytochrome P-450 system.[35,36] After conversion, the precise mechanism of action is uncertain. Proposed mechanisms involve inhibition of protein synthesis by inhibiting or damaging the action of DNA, RNA, or transfer RNA. Procarbazine is a cell-cycle phase, nonspecific antineoplastic agent, and the precise mechanism by which it exerts its antitumor activity is not entirely clear. However, it seems that procarbazine metabolites may function in a similar way as alkylating agents, although there is cross-resistance between procarbazine and classical alkylators.[37] This agent was initially approved by the Food and Drug Administration (FDA) in 1969 as part of the MOPP (mechlorethamine, vincristine, procarbazine, and prednisone) regimen for the treatment of Hodgkin's lymphoma. Since then it has also demonstrated clinical activity in non–Hodgkin's lymphoma, cutaneous T-cell lymphoma, and brain tumors.

Procarbazine is rapidly and completely absorbed from the gastrointestinal tract. Following oral administration, peak drug levels are reached within 10 to 15 minutes. Moreover, procarbazine crosses the blood–brain barrier and rapidly equilibrates between plasma and cerebrospinal fluid after oral administration. Peak cerebrospinal fluid drug levels are reached within 30 to 90 minutes after drug administration. The biological half-life of procarbazine hydrochloride in both plasma and cerebrospinal fluid is approximately 1 hour. Procarbazine is metabolized to active and inactive metabolites by two main pathways, chemical breakdown in aqueous solution and liver microsomal P-450 system. Approximately 70% of procarbazine is excreted in urine within 24 hours, and less than 5% to 10% of drug is eliminated in an unchanged form.[38,39]

A careful food and drug history is required before starting a patient on procarbazine therapy, as there are several potential drug-drug and drug-food interactions that may occur. Patients should avoid tyramine-containing foods, such as dark beer, wine, cheese, yogurt, bananas, and smoked foods as they may lead to increased nausea/vomiting, visual disturbances, headache, and elevations in blood pressure. Procarbazine produces a disulfiram-like reaction with concurrent use of alcohol. Acute hypertensive reactions may occur with coadministration of tricyclic antidepressants and sympathomimetic drugs. Finally, concurrent use of procarbazine with antihistamines and other CNS depressants can result in CNS and/or respiratory depression.

Dose-limiting toxicity is myelosuppression. Thrombocytopenia is more commonly observed than neutropenia, and the nadir in platelet count is generally observed at 4 weeks with return of platelet counts to normal in 4 to 6 weeks. Patients with glucose-6-phosphate dehydrogenase deficiency can develop hemolytic anemia while receiving procarbazine therapy. Mild nausea and vomiting develop shortly after administration, usually within the first days of therapy, but improves with continued therapy. Diarrhea may also be observed. Stepwise dose increments over the first few days of drug administration may minimize gastrointestinal intolerance. A flulike syndrome in the form of fever, chills, sweating, myalgias, and arthralgias usually occurs with initial therapy. Paresthesias and peripheral neuropathies, myalgias, arthralgias, and altered mental status have also been reported, including psychotic reactions, which may be related to its underlying monoamine oxidase inhibitory activity. Hypersensitivity reactions with pruritus, urticaria, maculopapular skin rash, flushing, eosinophilia, and pulmonary infiltrates can occur. Skin rash responds to steroid therapy, and the treatment may be continued. On rare occasions, procarbazine may induce interstitial pneumonitis, which mandates discontinuation of therapy. Azospermia and infertility after treatment with MOPP can be attributed, in part, to procarbazine. In addition, this agent is associated with an increased risk of secondary malignancies, especially acute leukemia.

THALIDOMIDE

Thalidomide (α-N-phthalimidoglutarimide; Thalomid) is a synthetic glutamic acid derivative that was initially synthesized in 1953. It was used widely in Europe between 1956 and 1962 as a sleeping aid and antiemetic for pregnant women, before it was discovered to cause severe congenital malformations. Initial reports of its efficacy in multiple myeloma were published in 1999 and it was approved by the FDA for the indication in 2006.

Thalidomide and its derivatives are designated immunomodulatory drug but their exact mechanism of action is not fully understood. It likely involves immunomodulatory, anti-inflammatory, and antiangiogenic effects. Thalidomide inhibits tumor necrosis factor-α production by activated monocytes, and causes T cell and natural killer cell costimulation. Its antiangiogenesis effects occur through modulation of chemotactic factors involved in endothelial cell migration. Thalidomide and/or its metabolites appear to have direct antiproliferative and proapoptotic effects. These properties are believed to be in part mediated by inhibition of the transcriptional activity of NFKB in multiple myeloma cells, with resultant decrease in the production of antiapoptotic molecules in tumor cells. Thalidomide also interferes with the adhesion of multiple myeloma cells to bone marrow stromal cells and inhibits the production and release of various growth factors (e.g., vascular endothelial growth factor, basic fibroblast growth factor, tumor necrosis factor-α, and interleukin-6) that regulate angiogenesis and tumor cell proliferation. Finally, thalidomide possesses potent immunomodulatory effects including enhanced natural killer cell-mediated cytotoxicity.[40]

Thalidomide is poorly soluble, and it is absorbed slowly from the gastrointestinal tract, reaching peak plasma concentration in 3 to 6 hours, with 55% to 66% bound to plasma proteins. The exact metabolic route and fate of thalidomide is not known. Thalidomide does not appear to be hepatically metabolized, but rather undergoes spontaneous nonenzymatic hydrolysis in plasma to multiple metabolites, with a half-life of elimination ranging from 5 to 7 hours. These metabolites are believed to be responsible for the antitumor effects of thalidomide. Less than 1% is excreted into the urine as unchanged drug.[41]

Thalidomide frequently causes drowsiness, constipation, and fatigue. Peripheral neuropathy is a common, potentially severe, and irreversible side effect occurring in up to 30% of patients. An increased incidence of venous thromboembolic events, such as deep venous thrombosis and pulmonary embolus, has also been observed with thalidomide, particularly when used in combination with dexamethasone or anthracycline-based chemotherapy. Patients who are appropriate candidates may benefit from concurrent prophylactic anticoagulation or aspirin treatment.[42] Other side effects of thalidomide include rash, nausea, dizziness, orthostatic hypotension, bradycardia, and mood changes.

Thalidomide received FDA approval in May 2006 for use with dexamethasone in newly diagnosed multiple myeloma based on a result of a phase 3 clinical trial randomizing 207 such patients to therapy with pulse dexamethasone therapy versus the same regimen of dexamethasone with 200 mg of thalidomide given daily.[43] With the addition of thalidomide, response rates were 63% compared with 41% with dexamethasone alone (P = .0017), and these results were confirmed in a similar larger-scale trial.[44] Two trials have also demonstrated that the addition of daily thalidomide to a combination of melphalan and prednisone in elderly patients with newly diagnosed multiple myeloma results in a higher response rate and progression-free survival in the thalidomide-treated patients.[45,46] However, the use of thalidomide has dropped precipitously in the United States with the FDA approval of more efficacious and less toxic therapies for myeloma.

LENALIDOMIDE

Lenalidomide (3-(4-amino-1-oxo 1,3-dihydro-2*H*-isoindol-2-yl) piperidine-2,6-dione; Revlimid) is a thalidomide derivative that shares the immunomodulatory and antineoplastic properties of its parent compound. However, lenalidomide appears to be more potent *in vitro* with less nonhematologic toxicities in clinical studies. It has well-established clinical activity in the treatment of both multiple myeloma and the myelodysplastic syndromes associated with a deletion of 5q cytogenetic abnormality with or without additional cytogenetic abnormalities.

The mechanism of action of lenalidomide remains incompletely understood. Its antineoplastic and immunomodulatory properties appear to be more potent than those of thalidomide.[40] It is associated with CD4+ and CD8+ T-cell costimulation, resulting in an increased Th1 cytokine production, natural killer cell expansion, secretion of cytokines including interferon γ, and enhanced natural killer cell antibody-dependent cellular cytotoxicity. Like its parent compound it possesses antiangiogenic properties. Multiple myeloma cells appear to be particularly sensitive to lenalidomide, with inhibition of malignant cell growth in the MM.1S human multiple myeloma cell line by inducing cell-cycle arrest and apoptosis.

Lenalidomide is administered orally and is rapidly absorbed from the gastrointestinal tract. Maximum plasma concentration is reached in 0.625 to 1.5 hours after dosing, with approximately 30% bound to plasma proteins. The half-life of elimination is approximately 3 hours, with little information currently available concerning metabolism. Approximately 70% of an administered dose is excreted unchanged by the kidneys.[47]

Compared with thalidomide, lenalidomide is associated with less sedation, constipation, and peripheral neuropathy. However, myelosuppression in the form of neutropenia and thrombocytopenia can be dose-limiting. As with thalidomide, the incidence of thromboembolic events is significant with the combination of dexamethasone and lenalidomide. A pooled analysis of 691 patients enrolled in two randomized studies reported a 12% incidence of thrombotic or thromboembolic events with the combination, compared with 4% with dexamethasone alone.[48]

Lenalidomide initially received FDA approval in December 2005 for the treatment of patients with transfusion-dependent anemia secondary to low or intermediate-risk myelodysplastic syndromes associated with a deletion 5q cytogenetic abnormality, with or without additional cytogenetic abnormalities. Approval was based on a phase 2 multicenter trial of 148 such patients who were treated with lenalidomide, 10 mg, either daily for 21 days every 4 weeks or with continuous daily dosing.[49] Transfusion independence was achieved in 67% of patients (95% CI, 59 to 74) with a median response duration of 116 weeks. An additional 10% benefited with less frequent need for blood transfusion. Major cytogenetic responses were observed in 44% of the evaluable patients. Grade 3/4 thrombocytopenia and neutropenia were observed in 44% and 55%, respectively, and response rates were higher in patients with more severe treatment-related cytopenias. [50]

Two randomized, multinational phase 3 studies evaluated the efficacy and safety of lenalidomide as salvage therapy in multiple myeloma.[51,52] These double-blind, placebo-controlled studies compared lenalidomide plus oral pulse high-dose dexamethasone therapy with dexamethasone therapy alone. Both trials were unblinded after preplanned interim analyses revealed a significant benefit in time to progression, the primary end point of the study, with the combination. With median follow-up of 17.1 months and 16.5 months, respectively, time to progression was 11.1 versus 4.7 months ($P < .001$)[51] and 11.3 versus 4.7 months ($P < .001$),[52] favoring the addition of lenalidomide to high-dose dexamethasone in each study. Grade 3/4 neutropenia was more common with dexamethasone/lenalidomide: 16.5% versus 1.2% in the former trial, and 36.2% versus 4.5% in the latter. The incidence of thromboembolic events was also higher with the lenalidomide combination: 8.5 versus 4.5%, and 15 versus 3.5%, respectively. In June 2006, lenalidomide in combination with dexamethasone was approved by the FDA for the treatment of patients with multiple myeloma who had received at least one prior therapy.[48] A pivotal study comparing lenalidomide plus high-dose dexamethasone versus lenalidomide plus low-dose dexamethasone in newly diagnosed patients with multiple myeloma has demonstrated better survival in the group treated with low-dose dexamethasone.[53] Based on this trial, lenalidomide, 25 mg on days 1 through 21, plus oral dexamethasone, 40 mg on days 1, 8, 15, and 22 of a 28-day cycle, has become a very popular, well-tolerated, and efficacious regimen in newly diagnosed patients. Preliminary promising results combining lenalidomide with bortezomib and dexamethasone in patients with newly diagnosed myeloma have been also been reported, with 100% response rates in a phase 2 trial.[54] A summary of characteristics of miscellaneous drugs mentioned in this chapter is provided in Table 43.1.

TABLE 43.1

MISCELLANEOUS CHEMOTHERAPEUTIC AGENTS

	Main Therapeutic Uses	Clinical Pharmacology	Major Toxicities	Notes
Temsirolimus	Advanced renal cancer	Peak concentration 0.5–2 h, widely distributed in tissues, steady-state levels reached in 7–8 days, $t_{1/2}$ 17 h	Asthenia, fatigue, dry skin, acneiform skin rash, mucositis, anorexia, hyperlipdemia, hyperglycemia	Efficacy shown for both clear cell and non-clear cell histologies. Efficacy in hematologic malignancies (mantle cell lymphoma, non–Hodgkin's lymphoma, multiple myeloma
Everolimus	Advanced renal cell carcinoma	Peak concentration 1–2 h, reduced bioavailability with high fat content food, metabolized by CYP3A4 system, mainly hepatic excretion	Asthenia, fatigue, dry skin, nausea, vomiting, mucositis, hyperlipidemia, hyperglycemia, allergic hypersensitivity reactions, pulmonary toxicity	Contraindicated in Child-Pugh class C patients, encouraging activity in gastric, non–small cell lung, esophageal cancers, sarcomas, approved for organ rejection prophylaxis
L-Asparaginase	Pediatric and adult acute lymphocytic leukemia	Peak concentration 7–12 h after IV administration, 30% plasma protein binding, pegylated form has longer half-life 5.7 days, antagonize effects of methotrexate if given before or concurrently	Hypersensitivity reactions, alterations in thyroid function, prolonged PT/PTT, decreased levels of vitamin K–dependent factors, acute pancreatitis.	Myelosupression is rare, hypersensitivity reaction risk increases with repeated exposure and when used as single agent, pegylated form is less immunogenic
Bleomycin	Hodgkin's disease, neoplastic pleural effusion, non–Hodgkin's lymphoma, squamous cell carcinoma of cervix, squamous cell carcinoma of nasopharynx, squamous cell carcinoma of penis, squamous cell carcinoma of the head and neck, squamous cell carcinoma of vulva, testicular cancer	Terminal $t_{1/2}$ 3 h, peak concentration 3 h, can be given intracavitary, 45%–55% of intracavitary dose absorbed systemically, elimination via kidneys if Cr Cl <25–35 mL/min dose reduction required	Pulmonary toxicity dose-limiting, more if age >70 y, cumulative dose >400 units, acute hypersensitivity reactions, rare (1%), mucositis, erythema, hyperpigmentation	Not myelosupressive immunosuppressive, metabolizing enzyme, bleomycine hydrolase enzyme low in lung and skin tissue, G-CSF use seems to exacerbate pulmonary toxicity

(*Continued*)

TABLE 43.1

(CONTINUED)

	Main Therapeutic Uses	Clinical Pharmacology	Major Toxicities	Notes
Procarbazine	Hodgkin's lymphoma	Rapid complete oral absorbtion, peak concentration, 10–15 min, crosses blood–brain barrier, $t_{1/2}$ 1 h, several drug-drug and food-drug interactions, metabolized by hepatic microsomal P-450 system 70% excreted in urine	Dose-limiting toxicity is myelosuppression more commonly thrombocytopenia nadir at 4 weeks, G-6PD-deficient patients can develop hemolytic anemia, nausea, vomiting, diarrhea, flulike symptoms, peripheral neuropathy, hypersensitivity reactions	Avoid tyramin-containing foods, disulfiram-like reaction with concurrent alcohol use, hypertensive reaction with concurrent tricylic antidepressant use, increased risk for azospermia/infertility and secondary malignancy
Thalidomide	Multiple myeloma, erythema nodosum leprosum	Oral absorbtion slow, peak concentration 3–6 h, 55%–66% bound to plasma proteins, $t_{1/2}$ 5–7 h, spontaneous nonenzymatic hydrolysis in plasma	Drowsiness, constipation, fatigue, skin rash, increased risk for thromboembolic complications	Pregnancy category X, may be present in semen, serious skin reactions including Stevens-Johnson syndrome
Lenalidomide	Low-intermediate risk myelodysplastic syndrome associated with 5q deletion, multiple myeloma	Rapid oral absorbtion, peak concentration in 0.6–1.5 h, $t_{1/2}$ 3 h, 70% excreted unchanged by kidneys	Less sedation, drowsiness, constipation than thalidomide, myelosupression, thromboembolic events, peripheral neuropathy	Pregnancy category X, caution in patients with renal function impairment, neutropenia, thrombocytopenia may be dose-limiting

$t_{1/2}$, half-life; IV, intravenous; PT, prothrombin time; PTT, partial thromboplastin time; Cr Cl, creatinine clearance; G-CSF, granulocyte colony-stimulating factor; G-6PD, glucose-6-phosphate dehydrogenase.

Selected References

The full list of references for this chapter appears in the online version.

1. Sehgal SN, Baker H, Vezina C. Rapamycin (AY-22,989), a new antifungal antibiotic: II. fermentation, isolation and characterization. *J Antibiot (Tokyo)* 1975;28:727.
3. Wullschleger S, Loewith R, Hall MN. TOR signaling in growth and metabolism. *Cell* 2006;124:471.
4. Raymond E, Alexandre J, Faivre S, et al. Safety and pharmacokinetics of escalated doses of weekly intravenous infusion of CCI-779, a novel mTOR inhibitor in patients with cancer. *J Clin Oncol* 2004;22:2336.
6. Hudes G, Carducci M, Tomczak P, et al. Temsirolimus, interferon alfa, or both for advanced renal-cell carcinoma. *N Engl J Med* 2007;356:2271.
8. Hess G, Herbecht R, Romaguera J, et al. Phase III study to evaluate temsirolimus compared with investigator's choice therapy for the treatment of relapsed or refractory mantle cell lymphoma. *J Clin Oncol* 2009;27:3822.
11. Schuler W, Sedrani R, Cottens S, et al. SDZ RAD, a new rapamycin derivative: pharmacological properties in vitro and in vivo. *Transplantation* 1997;64:36.
12. Dudkin L, Dilling MB, Cheshire PJ, et al. Biochemical correlates of mTOR inhibition by the rapamycin ester CCI-779 and tumor growth inhibition. *Clin Cancer Res* 2001;7:1758.
14. Kirchner GI, Meier-Wiedenbach I, Manns MP. Clinical pharmacokinetics of everolimus. *Clin Pharmacokinet* 2004;43:83.
15. Jacobsen W, Serkova N, Hausen B, Morris RE, Benet LZ, Christians U. Comparison of the in vitro metabolism of the macrolide immunosuppressants sirolimus and RAD. *Transplant Proc* 2001;70:425.
16. O'Donnell A, Faivre S, Burris HA, et al. Phase I pharmacokinetic and pharmacodynamic study of the oral mammalian target of rapamycin inhibitor everolimus in patients with advanced solid tumors. *J Clin Oncol* 2008;26:1588.
21. Motzer R, Escudier B, Oudard S, et al. Efficacy of everolimus in advanced renal cell carcinoma: a double-blind, randomized, placebo-controlled phase III trial. *Lancet* 2008;372:449.
23. Verma N, Kumar K, Kaur G, Anand S. L-Asparaginase: a promising chemotherapeutic agent. *Crit Rev Biotechnol* 2007;27:45.
24. Zeidan A, Wang ES, Wetzler M, et al. Pegasparaginase: where do we stand? *Expert Opin Biol Ther* 2009;9:111.
27. Evans WE, Yee GC, Crom WR, et al. Clinical pharmacology of bleomycin and cisplatin. *Head Neck Surg* 1981; 4:98.
28. Chen J, Stubbe J. Bleomycins: towards better therapeutics. *Nat Rev Cancer* 2005;2:102.
31. Azulay E, Herigault S, Levame M, et al. Effect of granulocyte colony-stimulating factor on bleomycin-induced acute lung injury and pulmonary fibrosis. *Crit Care Med* 2003;31:21.
35. Swaffar DS, Horstman MG, Jaw JY, et al. Methylazoxyprocarbazine, the active metabolite responsible for the anticancer activity of procarbazine against L1210 leukemia. *Cancer Res* 1989;49:2442.
40. Quach H, Ritchie D, Stewart AK, et al. Mechanism of action of immunomodulatory drugs (IMiDs) in multiple myeloma. *Leukemia* 2010;24:22.
42. Bennett CL, Angelotta C, Yarnold PR. Thalidomide and lenalidomide associated thromboembolism among patients with cancer. *JAMA* 2006;296:2558.
45. Palumbo A, Bringhen S, Liberati AM, et al. Oral melphalan, prednisone, and thalidomide in elderly patients with multiple myeloma: updated results of a randomized controlled trial. *Blood* 2008;112:3107.
52. Dimopoulos M, Spencer A, Attal M, et al. Lenalidomide plus dexamethasone for relapsed or refractory multiple myeloma. *N Engl J Med* 2007;357:2123.

CHAPTER 44 INTERFERONS

VERNON K. SONDAK, JÜRGEN C. BECKER, AND AXEL HAUSCHILD

The interferons are immunomodulatory proteins with a variety of oncologic and nononcologic clinical applications. Interferons belong to a family of secreted proteins that stimulate intracellular and intercellular networks and regulate resistance to viral infections, enhance innate and acquired immune responses, and modulate normal and tumor cell survival and death. Both the desired and the adverse effects of interferons can vary dramatically based on the dose, schedule, and route of administration, as well as based on pharmacologic manipulations of the interferon molecule. This chapter will examine the biologic properties of interferons, discuss the dose-, schedule-, and route dependencies of their effects, and provide examples of how the interferons are used therapeutically.

Interferons were initially discovered as secreted proteins that "interfered" with the ability of viruses to infect cells.[1] These initial reports lead to the eventual isolation, characterization, and ultimate cloning of the interferon genes. In humans, the interferons are made up of three classes: type I, II, and III interferons, with type I interferons being the most diverse and clinically relevant class.[2,3] Production of all types of interferons, both *in vitro* and *in vivo*, is transient and requires stimulation by viruses, microbial products, or chemical inducers. Interferons induce a state in which viral replication is impaired by the synthesis of a number of proteins that interfere with cellular and viral processes. Interferons are also critical factors in shaping the immune response to cancer. In addition, these proteins have potent antiproliferative and antiangiogenic activities. These additional activities induced by interferons can be viewed as an extension or enhancement of their antiviral activities. It was these additional functions induced by interferons that resulted in their evaluation as anticancer agents.

The type I interferon (IFN) family is composed of α (by convention, the recombinant forms of interferon-α are referred to as *interferon alfa*), β, δ, ε, κ, τ, and ω subtypes. The number of functional genes identified that encode type I IFNs is even higher: 17 nonallelic genes have been described in humans. All lack introns and cluster on chromosome 9. Of the type I interferons, there are 13 interferons-α genes, whereas to date only one gene has been discovered for each of the others.[4] Although type I interferons have qualitative and quantitative differences in their antiviral and other actions, the reasons behind the origin and maintenance of this diversity through evolution are as yet unknown.[5] The type I interferons all belong to the helical cytokine superfamily with secondary structures of a five α-helix bundle held in position by two disulfide bonds. The type II interferon family has only one member, interferon-γ. The type III interferon family has three subtypes of IFN-λ.[3] The various types and subtypes are further subdivided for pharmaceutical preparations (e.g., interferon-α2a, interferon-γ1b).

The interferon families are quite distinct. Type I interferons are induced primarily in response to viral or microbial infection, although they also play a profound role in modeling both the adaptive and innate immune response to cancer. Interferon-α and interferon-ω are produced predominantly from leukocytes, but interferon-β can be produced by most cell types, especially fibroblasts. Type I interferons act through a cell surface receptor composed of two ubiquitously expressed transmembrane proteins, interferon-α receptor (IFNAR) 1 and 2. Formation of the interferon receptor complex is initiated by binding of the interferon protein interacting with IFNAR2; the binding affinity is in the nanomolar range. Subsequently, IFNAR1 binds interferons with an affinity 1,000-fold weaker than that of IFNAR2. Binding studies are consistent with the ternary complex between the two receptors and interferons having a 1:1:1 stoichiometry. The assembly of the ternary complex is a two-step process; the interferons binds first to either of the receptors and then recruit the second with no identified interaction between the two interferon-α receptors. The genes for the IFNAR are clustered on chromosome 21. Since type I interferons bind to the receptor with relatively low affinity, efforts to increase binding of modified interferons to the receptor could ultimately result in enhanced therapeutic activity.[6]

Interferon-γ is produced predominantly by T lymphocytes, natural killer (NK), and natural killer T (NKT) cells in response to immune or inflammatory stimuli. Interferon-γ binds to its own unique multisubunit receptor, which is composed of IFNGR1 and IFNGR2 subunits. The type III interferons are coproduced with IFN-α and activate the same main signaling pathway as type I interferons, but have evolved a completely different receptor structure.[3]

INTERFERON SIGNALING PATHWAYS

The binding of an interferon to its receptor initiates a signaling cascade through the Janus-associated tyrosine kinase (Jak)—signal transducers and activators of transcription (STAT) pathway that culminates in the expression of hundreds of proteins in a distinctive cell- and interferon subtype–specific program that profoundly alters cellular function.[7] The ternary complex composed of type I interferons and the IFNAR1 and IFNAR2 subunits associates with the Janus kinases Jak1 and Tyk2 (Fig. 44.1).[8,9] The binding of any type I interferon to this receptor results in the activation of Jak1 and Tyk2, which leads to the tyrosine phosphorylation of STAT1, STAT2, STAT3, and STAT5.[10] The phosphorylation of STATs results in homo- or heterodimerization, dissociation from the interferon receptor, and translocation to the nucleus. In the nucleus, the STAT1 or STAT2 dimer associates with the protein IRF9. This complex,

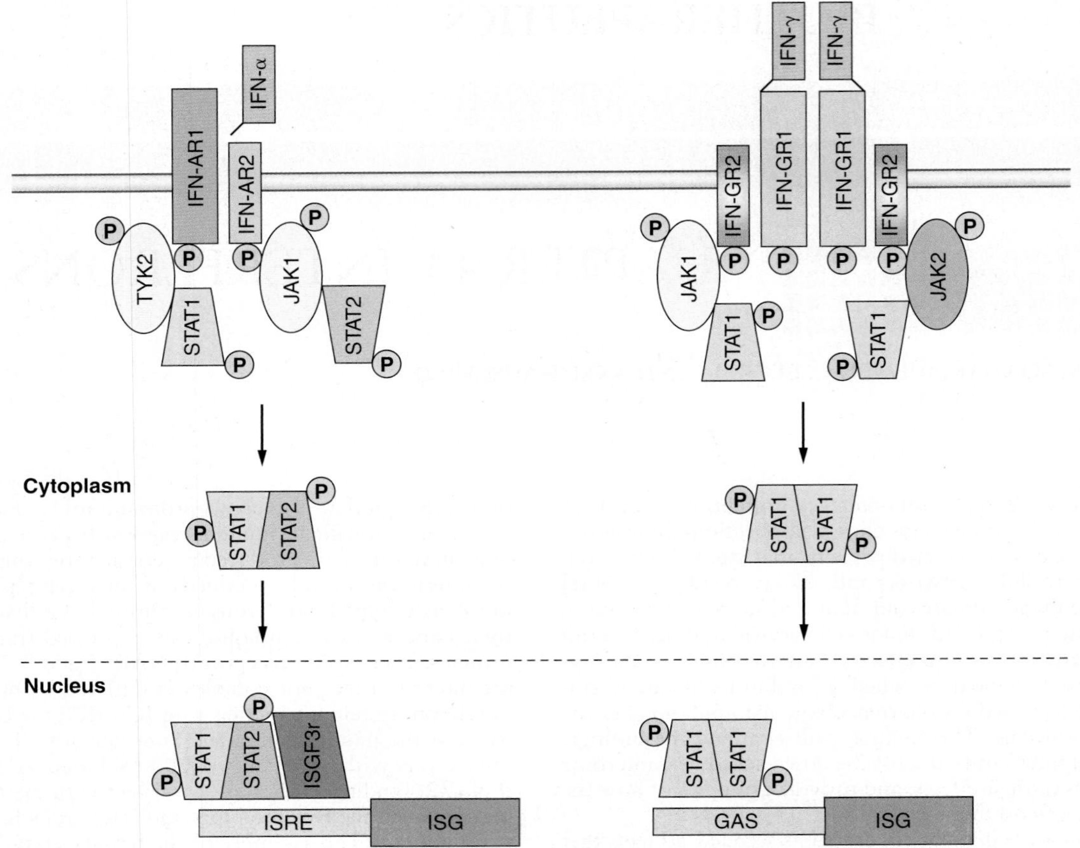

FIGURE 44.1 The effects of interferon (IFN) are mediated by receptors on the cell surface. Different receptors bind type I interferons (e.g., α, *left side of figure*) and type II interferons (γ, *right side of figure*). For both types of interferon, binding to their respective receptor initiates phosphorylation of cytoplasmic proteins, which result in nuclear translocation and binding to interferon-stimulated response elements (ISRE) or γ-activating sequences (GAS), which lead to regulation of interferon-stimulated genes (ISG). IFN-AR, interferon-α receptor; IFN-GR, interferon-γ receptor; ISGF, interferon-stimulated gene factor; JAK, Janus kinase; P, phosphorylation site; STAT, signal transducers and activators of transcription; TYK, tyrosine kinase. (From ref. 58, with permission.)

called *interferon-stimulated gene factor 3* (ISGF3), binds to the interferon-stimulated response element (ISRE) of the so-called interferon-stimulated genes (ISG). Binding to the ISRE results in the induction of interferon target genes, which are ultimately responsible for the biologic effects of the type I interferons. Other STAT homo- and heterodimer complexes are also stimulated by the type I interferons; these bind to the interferon-γ activated sites (GAS) that are present in the promoter regions of ISG. Of the numerous ISG, some have ISRE elements, some have GAS elements, and some have both in their promoters.

Although initial studies were carried out primarily in human fibroblasts, recent studies have identified additional complexity that allows individual cell types to respond by activating different STATs in response to the same interferons.[11] Upon activation of receptors, the Jaks undergo autophosphorylation and transphosphorylation to increase their activity, and then phosphorylate the interferon receptors and finally STATs. However, these mechanisms are not sufficient to explain all nuances of signaling. Tissue-specific differences in activating additional protein kinases probably contribute to the differential responses of various cells. In at least some cell types, the p85 subunit of phosphatidylinositol 3-kinase (PI3K), extracellular response kinases (ERKs), and p38 are associated with IFNAR1.[12] IFN-dependent activation of these stimulates the phosphorylation of NFκ and AP-1. These activated transcription factors may then either drive gene expression independently of activated STATs or cooperate with activated STATs on certain promoters.

In contrast to the type I interferons, interferon-γ only activates GAS elements since it does not induce the formation of ISGF3 complexes and therefore does not induce binding at ISRE sites. Distinct ensembles of STATs are activated depending on the subtype of interferon and cell type involved.[13] This mechanism may help to customize the cellular response. For example, interferon-α–induced STAT4 induces interferon-γ during viral infection, but interferon-α–induced STAT1 can actually suppress interferon-γ production during a viral infection.[14]

Interferon-γ binds as a homodimer to the interferon-γ receptor. The interferon-γ receptor is also a multisubunit complex, consisting of IFNGR1 and IFNGR2 (Fig. 44.1). Dimerization of the receptor activates Jak1 and Jak2, which ultimately results in the tyrosine phosphorylation of STAT1, leading to a conformational change and homodimerization. The STAT1 homodimer then translocates to the nucleus and binds to GAS elements of interferon-stimulated genes. Interferon-γ does not induce ISGF3 and thus cannot activate genes containing only ISRE elements in their promoters. Interestingly, a single nucleotide polymorphism in the interferon-γ promoter, 764G/C, appears to code for a markedly improved probability of viral clearance of hepatitis C with interferon-α therapy, arguing for an important role for interferon-γ in interferon-α antiviral activity.[15] Perhaps even more significantly, it implies that there may be identifiable host factors that can predict the likelihood of therapeutic benefit from interferon therapy.

In addition to the tyrosine phosphorylation needed for STAT activity, serine phosphorylation of the serine 727 residue on STAT1 and STAT2 molecules is also induced by type I and II interferons, via the protein kinase C (PKC) family (which is itself also induced by interferons).[16] STAT complexes interact with numerous other proteins, which they recruit to help modify chromatin to maximize the transcriptional response. These proteins include p300 and core binding protein (CBP), which have histone acetyltransferase activity, and the transcriptional coactivator GCN5.[10] Additionally, and somewhat surprisingly, it has been shown that histone deacetylase activity is also essential for STAT transcription.[17]

Although the Jak-STAT system is necessary for interferon signaling, it is not sufficient to reproduce the entire repertoire of interferon effects. The mitogen-activated protein kinase (MAPK) p38α is phosphorylated in a type I interferon–dependent manner in interferon-sensitive cell lines.[18] The PI3K signaling pathway is also induced by interferon. It appears that PI3K activation by type I or II interferons causes activation of PKC-δ, which in turn phosphorylates serine 727 on STAT1 and STAT2, making them transcriptionally competent.[16]

Although these potent signaling systems are recruited by interferon, there are also negative feedback signals that inhibit interferon stimulated signal transduction and gene transcription programs. The suppressor of cytokine signaling (SOCS) proteins suppress Jak-STAT signaling and appear to be a check on uncontrolled interferon-induced signal transduction.[19] Currently, there are eight members of this family, SOCS1 through SOCS7 and the related cytokine-inducible SH2 (CIS) protein. Specifically, the SOCS1 and SOCS3 proteins are known to inhibit interferon-α–induced antiviral and antiproliferative activity,[20,21] SOCS1 deficient mice are much more sensitive to the antitumor effects of interferon-α than SOCS-competent mice, and SOCS proteins are transiently induced by interferon-α in humans undergoing interferon treatment.[22]

Prior cytokine exposure can condition how a cell will respond to interferons. Conversely, interferons condition responses to other cytokines (e.g., exposure of human macrophages to interferon changes their response to interleukin-10 [IL-10] from activation of STAT3 to activation of STAT1).[23] As STAT1 and STAT3 drive essentially opposite biological responses, signal-dependent changes in their concentrations will affect their relative activation by a further signal. Indeed, an increase in the ratio of STAT1 to STAT3 after interferon-α treatment of patients with melanoma correlated with improved survival.[24]

TABLE 44.1

IMMUNOLOGIC AND NONIMMUNOLOGIC EFFECTS OF INTERFERONS

IMMUNOLOGIC EFFECTS
Innate Immunity
Stimulatory effects on natural killer (NK) cells:
  Increased proliferation, trafficking, secretion of IFN-γ, cytolytic activity
Increased lymphokine-activated killer (LAK) cell activity
Adaptive Immunity
Effects on macrophages and antigen-presenting cells:
  Activation, increased MHC class II antigen expression, increased differentiation
Effects on B lymphocytes:
Increased trafficking, increased IgG secretion, decreased IgE secretion
Effects on T lymphocytes:
Increased trafficking, shift to Th1 phenotype, increased cytolytic activity
Regulatory and immunomodulatory effects on cytokine/chemokine secretion
Direct Effects on Tumor Cells
Increased MHC class I antigen expression, increased expression of tumor-associated antigens, increased expression of adhesion molecules

NONIMMUNOLOGIC EFFECTS
Antiangiogenesis Effects
Direct cytostatic and cytotoxic effects on tumor cells
Antimetastatic effects on tumor cells

IFN, interferon; MHC, major histocompatibility complex; Ig, immunoglobulin.
(Data from refs. 25 and 31.)

IMMUNOLOGIC EFFECTS OF INTERFERON

The biologic effects of interferons on the immune system are profound and involve both innate and adaptive responses (Table 44.1).[25] The interferons can enhance the activity of the cellular components of the innate immune response, which is composed of NK cells, NKT cells, and macrophages. In addition, interferon-γ induces the production of chemokines that are selective for the recruitment of lymphocytes and macrophages. These chemokines include inducible protein-10 (IP-10) and macrophage inhibitory protein-1 alpha (MIP-1α).[26] Both type I and type II interferons enhance the major histocompatibility complex (MHC) class I antigen presentation pathway. They do this by increasing the expression of MHC class I and β_2-microglobulin, as well as by increasing essential elements of the class I antigen-processing pathway. Essential proteins in this pathway that are up-regulated include transporters associated with antigen processing 1 and 2 (TAP1, TAP2) and low molecular mass polypeptide 2 (LMP-2).[27]

Interferons also interact with the adaptive immune response through their effects on dendritic cells. Dendritic cells are unique antigen-presenting cells that are able to stimulate a naïve T-cell response to antigen. In their immature state dendritic cells take up antigen, while after maturation they are able to present antigen to T cells. Type I and II interferons can induce the *in vitro* maturation of dendritic cells.[28] In the presence of granulocyte macrophage colony stimulating factor (GM-CSF), type I interferons can up-regulate the expression of the chemokine receptor CCR7, which is integral to dendritic cell trafficking to lymph nodes.[29] In this regard, interferons are one of several molecules that regulate the relationship between the innate and the adaptive immune responses. Interferon-γ also reduces the activity of the immunoinhibitory CD4+ CD25+ T cells (Tregs), which are now thought to be an important mechanism of tumor immune escape.[30]

Much of our insight into the immunomodulatory effects of interferon comes from studies on transplanted or chemically induced tumors in mice. Interferon-γ insensitive mice develop chemically induced sarcomas three- to fivefold more frequently than controls.[31] Mice deficient in STAT1 also have increased tumor formation. It appears that $\gamma\delta$ T cells are an important source of interferon-γ in the process of rejecting tumors.[32] The potent cytokine IL-12, which is known to cause tumor regression of established chemically induced tumors in several mouse models, appears to cause tumor rejection through the production of interferon-γ.[33] In addition, interferon-γ causes up-regulation of tumor antigens, causing tumors to be more visible to the immune system.[31]

The type I interferons can also cause potent immune rejection in syngeneic tumor models.[34] Mice that are treated with a type I interferon receptor–blocking antibody fail to reject immunogenic tumors that are rejected by control mice.[32] Escape from tumor surveillance mechanisms is an important requirement for tumor growth. Since the interferons play a major role in immunosurveillance, tumors can escape through defects in interferon signaling. Specifically, melanoma, squamous cell cancers, prostate cancer, and lung cancer are often insensitive to interferon and display defects in the Jak-STAT pathway or overexpression of SOCS1, a negative regulator of interferon signaling.[35] Although type II interferon signaling defects in tumors appear to be an important mechanism of escape, by contrast type I interferon signaling defects are more important for the host immune system.[22,36]

Interferon-γ also up-regulates the MHC class II antigen processing pathway, which is constitutively expressed on dendritic cells and B lymphocytes. This pathway is regulated by a single interferon-γ–inducible master transcription factor called class II transactivator.[37,38] MHC class II proteins are selectively up-regulated by interferon-γ, but not by type I interferons due to the STAT2-dependent induction of SOCS1.[39] Another specific effect of interferon-γ is the ability to inhibit the expression of IL-4. By inhibiting IL-4, interferon-γ plays an integral role in the skewing of the immune response to a T helper 1 (cellular) response and away from a T helper 2 (antibody-mediated) response.[26]

Interferons also promote accumulation of leukocytes at sites of inflammation by induction of the expression of vascular adhesion molecules, including intracellular adhesion molecule 1 (ICAM1). Furthermore, interferons induce the production of chemokines that participate in leukocyte recruitment (e.g., CXCL9, also known as MIG, monokine induced by interferon-γ, CXCL10, also known as IP-10, interferon-γ 10 kD inducible protein, and CXCL11, also known as I-TAC, interferon-inducible T cell α-chemoattractant). As implied by their names, these chemokines are not expressed in the absence of interferon signaling.

NONIMMUNOLOGIC ANTIANGIOGENIC EFFECTS OF INTERFERON

Interferons, either directly or indirectly, exhibit antiangiogenic properties by altering the stimulatory factors produced by tumor cells and by directly inhibiting endothelial cells.[40] Endothelial cells exhibit inhibited motility and undergo coagulation necrosis in response to interferons. Type I interferons inhibit the synthesis of basic fibroblast growth factor, IL-8, and collagenase type IV, which are proangiogenic factors.[41] Interferons also inhibit vascular endothelial growth factor (VEGF) mRNA and protein expression by regulating its promoter.[42] These effects have been exploited in the therapy of infantile hemangiomas,[43] hemangioblastomas,[44] and giant cell tumors of the mandible.[45] Interferon-α has shown activity in Kaposi's sarcoma, a neoplastic virally induced endothelial tumor.[46] In addition, as discussed above, interferon-γ induces the chemokines CXCL9, CXCL10, and CXCL11, which are strong angiogenesis inhibitory molecules. Conflicting angiogenic signals are also possible from proteins induced by type I interferons. The gene for hypoxia-inducible factor (HIF) 1α is induced by interferon-α, which in turn activates transcription of vascular endothelial growth factor. However, interferon-α treatment fails to induce transcription of several prototypic HIF-responsive genes (VEGF-A, PPARγ, and prostacyclin synthase) due to an insufficient increase in HIF-1α protein levels.[47] Moreover, knockdown of HIF-1α significantly reduces the capacity of interferon-α to inhibit endothelial cell proliferation.

DIRECT ANTITUMOR EFFECTS OF INTERFERONS

Interferons can induce pro-apoptotic proteins and cause cell cycle arrest or death directly or when combined with other therapies. They can shift the balance toward apoptosis by activating a number of pathways. Induction of apoptosis by Apo2 ligand, also called tumor necrosis factor-related apoptosis-inducing ligand (APO2L/TRAIL) and Fas has been identified in many malignant cell types, as has induction of APO2L/TRAIL on immune effector cell surfaces, thus sensitizing tumor cells to T-cell, NK-cell, and macrophage-mediated cytotoxicity.[48] The cyclin-dependent kinase inhibitor $p21^{waf}$ is induced by interferon-α in lymphoma cell lines.[49] In chronic myelogenous leukemia (CML) and myeloma cells, interferon caused cell death through recruitment of the death receptor Fas-associated protein with death domain (FADD) and activation of caspase 8.[50,51] Similarly, basal cell carcinoma, melanoma, and cholangiocarcinoma can be sensitized to Fas ligand–mediated apoptosis. Through interactions with p53 and the inhibitor of apoptosis, X-linked inhibitor of apoptosis prein (XIAP), the interferon-stimulated gene product XIAP-associated factor 1 (XAF1) may allow APO2L/TRAIL to fully activate downstream caspases.[52] Similarly, IRF1 can suppress another antiapoptotic protein, survivin. Interferons can also increase the expression of caspases in breast cancer,[53] colon cancer,[54] and melanoma.[55] Another mechanism that has been postulated to cause interferon-induced cell cytotoxicity is via the death-associated protein kinases, which are caspase independent and activated by interferon and can have reduced expression in some malignancies.[56]

CLINICAL TOXICITY OF INTERFERON ADMINISTRATION

Constitutional Toxicities

The most extensive toxicity analysis of interferon in an oncology patient population is from trials of recombinant interferon-α in the adjuvant treatment of high-risk melanoma.[57,58] There is also an extensive literature on the toxicity profile of interferon-α in the treatment of hepatitis C.[59] Clinical trials with recombinant interferon-γ have also been reported.[60] The clinical toxicities associated with interferon administration are schedule and dose dependent as well as highly variable in type and degree between individuals. The most common toxicities seen with all interferons are constitutional. Acute administration can result in fever, chills, myalgias, arthralgias, headache, nausea, vomiting, and fatigue. With repetitive dosing, tachyphylaxis occurs in relation to fever and chills. Rigors can occur with interferon but are not common. Fatigue usually increases with repetitive dosing until a baseline level of fatigue is reached at a stable dose of interferon. For many patients, appropriate timing of interferon administration (e.g., at or just before bedtime) can limit the impact of symptoms. Anorexia and weight loss are commonly seen with higher dose regimens and can be related to nausea or can occur independent of any gastrointestinal symptoms.

Hematologic Toxicities

Hematologic toxicities associated with interferon administration are anemia, neutropenia, and thrombocytopenia and appear to be dose related, as they are rarely reported in lower-dose regimens. Neutropenia requiring dosage reduction is reported to occur in 26% to 60% of patients receiving high-dose interferon-α for the adjuvant treatment of high-risk melanoma.[57] However, neutropenic fevers or infections that require antibiotic administration or hospitalization are quite rare. Thrombocytopenia is rarely severe enough to warrant dose reductions.

Organ Toxicities

Interferon administration has direct effects on several organ systems. Interferon can cause supraventricular tachydysrhythmias, most notably atrial fibrillation. The risk of cardiac toxicity is increased in elderly patients and those with pre-existing cardiac disease. Rare cases of reversible cardiomyopathy associated with interferon have been reported.[61,62] Hypotension may be seen both acutely, within 2 hours of administration, or chronically due to diminished fluid intake and increased fluid losses. Acute hypotension generally responds to fluid resuscitation but may rarely require the administration of vasopressors. Interferon effects on the kidneys have included reversible proteinuria and rarely nephrotic syndrome or interstitial nephritis. Proteinuria occurs in 15% to 20% of patients. Rarely, interferon has been associated with thrombotic microangiopathy in chronic myelogenous leukemia patients treated for several years.[63] This is in contrast to other nephropathies associated with interferon, which usually manifest after only several months of treatment. The skin can also be a target of interferon toxicity with occasional macular rashes and reports of psoriatic type skin reactions, which require treatment and resolve with discontinuation of therapy.[64,65]

High-dose interferon regimens can cause acute hepatic toxicity. This toxicity manifests itself as an increase in serum alanine aminotransferase/aspartate aminotransferase (ALT/AST) levels and can result in fatal hepatic failure.[57] This serious complication was identified in the initial trial of high-dose interferon-α for adjuvant therapy of melanoma. Once careful monitoring was instituted with requirements for dose reduction tied to serum transaminases elevations, there were no further cases of fatal hepatotoxicity on this trial or subsequent cooperative group trials using the same dose and schedule. Hence, with careful monitoring and appropriate dosage modification, fatal complications can be avoided and therapy can generally continue for patients who develop transaminase elevations during high-dose therapy.

Type I interferon administration has been associated with retinopathy.[66] The retinopathy includes retinal hemorrhages and cotton wool spots, either alone or together. The retinopathy can be unilateral or bilateral. The retinal hemorrhages occur mainly around the optic disc and can be linear or patchy. The incidence of interferon retinopathy has been reported to occur from 18% to 86% in different series. The different rates may reflect a dosage effect, may be related to the surveillance intensity, or both. Diabetes mellitus may be an associated risk factor for the development as well as the progression of interferon retinopathy. The retinopathy rarely results in any visual disturbance and disappears spontaneously during treatment or resolves after interferon is discontinued.

Neuropsychiatric Toxicities

The neuropsychiatric toxicities associated with interferon therapy can manifest as subtle changes that are detected only by formal testing or can be overt with depression, hypomania, or suicidal ideation, requiring discontinuation of interferon and active intervention.[67–69] Acute neurocognitive changes include impaired memory, difficulty in concentration, and decreased initiative. With the continued administration of interferon, subacute and chronic changes are manifest. These consist of behavioral (personality), mood, and affect changes. The prophylactic use of the selective serotonin reuptake inhibitor (SSRI) paroxetine (Paxil) has been suggested to ameliorate depressive symptoms in a small, placebo-controlled trial involving patients receiving adjuvant high-dose interferon for melanoma.[70] Changes in tryptophan metabolism were observed in untreated depressed patients, and it appeared that paroxetine attenuated the consequences of these changes.[71] In the randomized study, however, the placebo group had a higher rate of discontinuation of interferon therapy due to depression (35%) than previously reported. In previous trials of adjuvant interferon for high-risk melanoma, less than 10% of patients were reported as having grade 3 or 4 depression.[57,58] In patients with a past history of clinical depression or psychiatric disorders, the benefits and risks of interferon use should be considered carefully. Whether SSRIs such as paroxetine should be used routinely or selectively in patients receiving high-dose interferon-α remains an unresolved issue. Other strategies for ameliorating the constitutional and neuropsychiatric effects of high-dose interferon, such as the use of methylphenidate or exercise, remain the subject of investigation.[72,73]

Endocrine and Metabolic Toxicities

Thyroid abnormalities have been reported in 5% to 31% of patients receiving interferon therapy.[68,74] Although up to 70% to 80% of patients exhibiting thyroid disorders while on interferon have detectable thyroid autoantibodies, the exact mechanism of thyroid toxicity is unknown. It may be a direct effect of interferon on the thyroid gland or an indirect effect due to suppressing thyroid-stimulating hormone (TSH) release. Autoimmune thyroiditis may be a manifestation of an increase risk of autoimmune disorders in general that has been seen in patients on interferon. Interestingly, as further described below, the development of clinical or serologic evidence of autoimmunity has been associated with improved outcomes for melanoma patients treated with interferon-α2b in the adjuvant setting in some, but not all, studies.[75,76] Nevertheless, a high degree of clinical suspicion for thyroid dysfunction needs to be maintained because of the similarities between hypothyroidism and the clinical spectrum of fatigue and hair loss that can be seen from interferon administration in the euthyroid patient.

Metabolic alterations in the blood lipid profile associated with interferon include hypertriglyceridemia and elevated low-density lipoprotein, secondary to inhibition of lipoprotein lipase.[77] Interferon may depress the plasma cholesterol in 15% to 40% of patients.

Autoimmunity

As noted above, interferon treatment is associated with autoimmune effects. In addition to thyroid disorders, other autoimmune alterations that have been reported include rheumatoid arthritis and Raynaud's and Sjögren's syndromes.[78–80] Associations between female gender and longer duration of therapy with interferon have been reported for autoimmune disorders. Gogas et al.[75] reported on a study of 200 patients treated with adjuvant high-dose interferon-α2b for high-risk melanoma where patients were assessed for clinical and serologic markers of autoimmunity. Autoantibodies or clinical manifestations of autoimmunity were detected in 52 patients (26%); evidence of autoimmunity was associated with a statistically significantly superior outcome. The median relapse-free survival was 16 months among patients without autoimmunity (108 of 148 had a relapse) and was not reached (more than 45 months) among patients with autoimmunity (7 of 52 had a relapse). The median survival was 37.6 months among patients without autoimmunity (80 of 148 died) and was not reached (greater than 45 months) among patients with autoimmunity (2 of 52 died). Multivariate regression analyses showed that autoimmunity was an independent marker for improved relapse-free survival and overall survival ($P < .001$). A subsequent analysis of patients treated with pegylated interferon called into question whether the association between autoimmunity and outcome, also seen to an extent with that agent, was real or a manifestation of lead-time bias built into the analytical model used.[76]

Other Reported Toxicities Associated with Interferon Therapy

Rhabdomyolysis has been reported with high-dose interferon.[81] Another unusual but potentially serious association is the occurrence of sarcoidosis in patients receiving interferon.[82,83] Both pulmonary and cutaneous manifestations of sarcoidosis have been reported. If symptomatic, the manifestations of sarcoid usually regress after the discontinuation of interferon. The pulmonary manifestations of sarcoid can be misinterpreted to represent progressive cancer. A diagnosis of sarcoid is a contraindication to interferon administration, as is pre-existing active autoimmune disease.

POTENTIAL DRUG INTERACTIONS

Potential interactions between interferons and other drugs have not been extensively studied, particularly for the high-dose interferon-α2b regimen used for adjuvant therapy. In a study of 17 patients, treatment with high-dose interferon-α resulted in inhibition of the activity of cytochrome P450 isozymes CYP1A2 and CYP2D within 24 hours of the first intravenous dose.[84] After 26 days of treatment, significant inhibition of CYP2C19 was found. The implication of these findings is that drugs metabolized by these enzymes would be expected to be diminished after interferon therapy; examples of such drugs include tricyclic antidepressants, SSRIs, theophylline, phenytoin, and many others. To date, no clinically significant drug–interferon interactions have been proven, but at least two cases of hepatotoxicity associated with gemfibrozil therapy for interferon-α–induced hypertriglyceridemia have been reported. These cases could represent a drug interaction on the basis of cytochrome P450 inhibition.[85]

ONCOLOGIC APPLICATIONS OF INTERFERONS

Pharmacology and Dosage

Interferons are available for clinical usage in both natural and recombinant forms, with the latter used most commonly for oncologic applications.[86] Commercially available type I interferon formulations include human leukocyte-derived interferon-αn3 (Alferon N), multisubtype human interferon-α (Multiferon), recombinant "consensus" interferon alfacon-1, produced from a 166 amino acid sequence derived by sequencing several natural interferon-α subtypes and assigning the most frequent amino acid in each corresponding position (Infergen), recombinant interferon-α2a (Roferon-A), recombinant interferon-α2b (Intron-A), recombinant interferon-β1a (Rebif), recombinant interferon-β1b (Betaseron), and recombinant interferon-γ1b (Actimmune). Most of the oncologic experience has been accumulated with interferon-α2a and -α2b, which are approved by the U.S. Food and Drug Administration for use in hairy cell leukemia, AIDS-related Kaposi's sarcoma, and Philadelphia chromosome–positive CML (interferon-α2a), and hairy cell leukemia, acquired immunodeficiency syndrome-related Kaposi's sarcoma, follicular lymphoma, and melanoma (interferon-α2b). Experience has been accumulated with interferons of various types in a host of other tumor types as well.

The half-life of recombinant interferon-α2 in the blood varies between 2 hours and 8 hours after subcutaneous or intramuscular administration and is probably somewhat shorter after intravenous administration. Oral delivery is impractical due to proteolytic degradation. Peak plasma concentrations are highest after intravenous administration.[84] Generally speaking, intravenous administration of interferon-α is performed daily (5 days per week in the most commonly used regimen for adjuvant therapy of interferon), while subcutaneous or intramuscular administration is performed three times weekly. Other dose schedules have been explored in the hope of maximizing certain properties of interferons while minimizing toxicities (e.g., low-dose, twice daily schedules of subcutaneous interferon-α for "antiangiogenesis" trials).

Neutralizing Antibodies

The development of neutralizing antibodies can alter the pharmacology and efficacy of recombinant cytokines after repeated administration. Neutralizing antibodies have been observed in 25% to 30% of patients treated with interferon-α2a, but less than 3% of patients treated with interferon-α2b.[87,88] Neutralizing antibodies are also frequently encountered after administration of interferon-β.[89] The development of neutralizing antibodies has been associated with a loss of clinical efficacy. Some patients who have developed neutralizing antibodies to recombinant interferon preparations have been successfully treated with natural interferon.[90,91]

Effects of Dose and Schedule on Efficacy and Toxicity

A great variety of doses, schedules, and routes of administration of interferon have been tested in clinical trials, particularly in the setting of adjuvant therapy for melanoma patients at risk of recurrence after complete surgical resection. Interferon-α has been shown to have detectable but low levels of antitumor activity in melanoma patients with metastatic disease, resulting in objective regressions in approximately 10% of patients treated with any of several dose and schedule regimens.[92] There has been no consistent observation that responses are linked to a specific dose or schedule of administration. Responses are more common in patients with small, generally soft tissue or lung nodules. Interferon-γ in immunologically active doses has failed to demonstrate more than minimal activity in metastatic melanoma[93] and was likewise ineffective in two randomized trials evaluating similar doses in the adjuvant setting.[60,94]

The remarkable variety of doses, schedules, and routes of administration of interferon-α that have been tested in clinical trials is, in part, due to a lack of knowledge regarding the specific mechanisms responsible for interferon's antitumor activity. To date, surrogate markers of immunologic or other parameters have not been informative in determining what constitutes a sufficient dose and route of delivery.[95–97] Clinical trials have clearly established a greater incidence of grade 3 and 4 toxicity for high-dose regimens than for lower doses.[98–100] The results of the E1690 trial, a three-arm U.S. Intergroup trial that compared high-dose and low-dose interferon-α2b to observation after surgery for high-risk stage II and stage III (thick node-negative or node-positive) melanoma are representative.[98]

The effect of dose and schedule of adjuvant interferon therapy on overall survival has been more controversial.[101,102] When all three randomized phase 3 trials of high-dose interferon-α2b in melanoma were included in a meta-analysis, there was a 15% ± 8% reduction in deaths associated with high-dose interferon treatment, more of an impact than was seen in the low-dose trials, but this did not reach statistical significance (P = .06).[103] Another meta-analysis, evaluating overall survival at 2 years as the primary end point, did demonstrate a statistically significant benefit for 1 year of high-dose interferon-α.[104] Most recently, a new meta-analysis of all adjuvant interferon studies showed a statistically significant 11% reduction in the risk of death associated with adjuvant interferon treatment (hazard ratio 0.89; 95% confidence interval, 0.83 to 0.96; P = .002) but could demonstrate no dose-related heterogeneity between trials and no significant difference in survival between the interferon-α treatment arms in trials that used high-dose versus low-dose interferon.[105]

Interferon-α2a versus -α2b

No direct comparative data exist to allow any conclusions regarding the relative efficacy of equitoxic doses or the relative toxicity of equally effective doses of recombinant interferon-α2a and -α2b. All adjuvant therapy trials to date involving intravenous administration have used interferon-α2b. Because of uncertainty regarding the equivalent dosing for intravenous administration of interferon-α2a, its substitution for interferon-α2b in high-dose adjuvant therapy cannot be recommended.[106]

Pharmacologic Modification of Interferons

As is the case with many cytokines, the relatively short half-life of interferons requires repetitive dosing to maintain exposure to biologically effective concentrations. Toxicity may well be related to peak plasma concentrations, while efficacy may be more closely linked to binding efficacy and duration of exposure (area under the curve). The possibility of engineering a mutant recombinant interferon-α with improved binding affinity for the type I interferon receptor has already been mentioned.[6] A pharmacologic approach to improving interferon efficacy or decreasing toxicity has been to couple the recombinant interferon molecule with a polyethylene glycol moiety (pegylation). This slows metabolism of the interferon, providing more sustained levels of exposure, but also diminishes the specific activity of the interferon due to steric interference, decreasing binding affinity with its receptor. Two commercial pegylated interferons are available, each utilizing a different form of polyethylene glycol: branched-chain pegylated interferon-α2a (peginterferon-α2a [Pegasys]) and succinimidyl carbonate-polyethylene glycol 12,000 (straight-chain pegylated) interferon-α2b (peginterferon-α2b [PegIntron]). When utilized in comparable concentrations, each pegylated interferon formulation appears to have identical biologic activity to the unmodified recombinant molecule.[107,108]

The pharmacodynamics properties of pegylated interferon have been studied and provide a framework for comparison to the peak and sustained concentrations obtained with weekly administration of pegylated interferon compared to daily intravenous or thrice weekly subcutaneous administration of recombinant interferon.[109,110]

There have been no direct comparative studies evaluating pegylated versus unmodified interferon in oncologic applications to date, but their efficacy in hepatitis C appears to be as good or better than standard recombinant interferon when used at equitoxic doses.[59,111,112] In a phase 1 and 2 trial involving 35 patients with advanced solid tumors of a variety of histologies, the maximum tolerated dose (MTD) of pegylated interferon-α2b for long-term treatment was found to be 6 mcg/kg/wk.[113] Similar results were obtained in a phase 1 trial in patients with Philadelphia chromosome–positive chronic myelogenous leukemia.[114] In the CML study, a complete hematologic or improved cytogenetic response was observed in 48% of patients who were intolerant to or did not respond to prior interferon-α therapy. In the solid tumor trial, 9 of 69 patients (13%) experienced objective remissions, including four complete responses, with responses predominantly seen at or above 6.0 mcg/kg/wk. Responses were seen in both visceral and nonvisceral sites. Results in previously untreated patients with renal cell carcinoma were encouraging; objective responses were seen in 6 of 14 patients (44%), including 2 complete responders. Two of six melanoma patients also had complete responses. A randomized phase 2 trial evaluated three different doses of pegylated interferon-α2a in 150 patients with metastatic melanoma.[115] Objective responses were seen in 6% of the lowest dose cohort, and 8% and 12% in the higher dose cohorts. In total, five patients (3%) had complete responses. These clinical results certainly appear to be at least comparable to those achieved with nonpegylated recombinant interferon-α, with equal or less toxicity. Moreover, pegylated interferons seem better suited to chronic administration as they allow once-a-week dosing, which has prompted a randomized trial of very long-term (5 years) pegylated interferon-α versus observation for patients with stage III melanoma. In this 1,256-patient trial, relapse-free survival was significantly higher in the pegylated interferon–treated patients, especially in those with microscopic nodal disease, compared to those in the observation arm (hazard ratio 0.82; 95% confidence interval, 0.71 to 0.96; P = .01). Overall survival was not significantly different in either arm, although the median follow-up of 3.8 years is relatively short.[116] Pegylated interferons may also be better choices for investigating the antiangiogenesis properties of interferon therapy.

Combinations of Interferon and Other Agents

The activity and toxicity profiles of interferons make them logical candidates for combination with other immunologic and cytotoxic therapies. To date, combination therapy including interferon has been evaluated in a multitude of clinical trials, but no studies have established a definitive role for combination regimens. Randomized trials have established that high-dose interferon does not diminish the ability to respond to a ganglioside vaccine[117] and may augment or maintain the immune response to vaccines.[118,119] Nonetheless, specific evidence for synergy between interferon and immunologic or cytotoxic therapy is lacking.[120]

Selected References

The full list of reference for this chapter appears in the online version.

1. Isaacs A, Lindenmann J. Virus interference. The interferons. *Proc R Soc London* 1957;147:258.
8. Der SD, Zhou A, Williams BRG, Silverman RH. Identification of genes differentially regulated by interferon α, β, or γ using oligonucleotide arrays. *Proc Natl Acad Sci U S A* 1998;95:15623.
9. Holko M, Williams BRG. Functional annotation of IFN-α-stimulated gene expression profiles from sensitive and resistant renal cell carcinoma cell lines. *J Interferon Cytokine Res* 2006;26:534.
10. Platanias LC. Mechanisms of type-I- and type-II-interferon-mediated signalling. *Nat Rev Immunol* 2005;5:375.
14. Nguyen KB, Watford WT, Salomon R, et al. Critical role for STAT4 activation by type 1 interferons in the interferon-γ response to viral infections. *Science* 2002;297:2063.
22. Zimmerer J, Lesinski GB, Kondadasula SV, et al. IFN-α–induced signal transduction, gene expression, and antitumor activity of immune effector cells are negatively regulated by suppressor of cytokine signaling proteins. *J Immunol* 2007;178:4832.
24. Wang W, Edington HD, Rao UNM, et al. Modulation of signal transducers and activators of transcription 1 and 3 signaling in melanoma by high-dose IFNα2b. *Clin Cancer Res* 2007;13:1523.
25. Brassard DL, Grace MJ, Bordens RW. Interferon-α as an immunotherapeutic protein. *J Leukoc Biol* 2002;71:565.
31. Kaplan DH, Shankaran V, Dighe AS, et al. Demonstration of an interferon γ-dependent tumor surveillance system in immunocompetent mice. *Proc Natl Acad Sci U S A* 1998;95:7556.
32. Dunn GP, Koebel CM, Schreiber RD. Interferons, immunity and cancer immunoediting. *Nat Rev Immunol* 2006;6:836.
36. Lesinski GB, Valentino D, Hade EM, et al. Expression of STAT1 and STAT2 in malignant melanoma does not correlate with response to interferon-alpha adjuvant therapy. *Cancer Immunol Immunother* 2005;54:815.
41. Fidler IJ. Regulation of neoplastic angiogenesis. *J Natl Cancer Inst Monogr* 2001;28:10.
42. von Marschall Z, Scholz A, Cramer T, et al. Effects of interferon alpha on vascular endothelial growth factor gene transcription and tumor angiogenesis. *J Natl Cancer Inst* 2003;95:437.
46. Krown SE, Li P, Von Roenn JH, et al. Efficacy of low-dose interferon with antiretroviral therapy in Kaposi's sarcoma: a randomized phase II AIDS Clinical Trials Group study. *J Interferon Cytokine Res* 2002;22:295.
48. Chawla-Sarkar M, Lindner DJ, Liu Y-F, et al. Apoptosis and interferons: role of interferon-stimulated genes as mediators of apoptosis. *Apoptosis* 2003;8:237.
57. Kirkwood JM, Bender C, Agarwala S, et al. Mechanisms and management of toxicities associated with high-dose interferon alfa-2b therapy. *J Clin Oncol* 2002;20:3703.
60. Sondak VK, Kopecky KJ, Smith JW II, et al. Is interferon-γ detrimental? Results of a Southwest Oncology Group randomized trial of adjuvant human interferon-γ versus observation in malignant melanoma. In: Salmon SE, ed. *Adjuvant therapy of cancer VIII*. Philadelphia: Lippincott-Raven, 1997:259.
62. Cohen MC, Huberman MS, Nesto RW. Recombinant alpha 2 interferon-related cardiomyopathy. *Am J Med* 1988;85:549.
65. Funk J, Langeland T, Schrumpf E, Hanssen LE. Psoriasis induced by interferon-alpha. *Br J Dermatol* 1991;125:463.
66. Hayasaka S, Nagaki Y, Matsumoto M, Sato S. Interferon associated retinopathy. *Br J Ophthalmol* 1998;82:323.
67. Trask PC, Esper P, Riba M, Redman B. Psychiatric side effects of interferon therapy: prevalence, proposed mechanisms, and future directions. *J Clin Oncol* 2000;18:2316.
70. Musselman DL, Lawson DH, Gumnick JF, et al. Paroxetine for the prevention of depression induced by high-dose interferon alfa. *N Engl J Med* 2001;344:961.
72. Schwartz AL, Thompson JA, Masood N. Interferon-induced fatigue in patients with melanoma: a pilot study of exercise and methylphenidate. *Oncol Nurs Forum* 2002;29:E85.
74. Monzani F, Caraccio N, Dardano A, Ferrannini E. Thyroid autoimmunity and dysfunction associated with type I interferon therapy. *Clin Exp Med* 2004;3:199.
75. Gogas H, Ioannovich J, Dafni U, et al. Prognostic significance of autoimmunity during treatment of melanoma with interferon. *N Engl J Med* 2006;354:709.
76. Bowhuis MG, Suciu S, Testori A, et al. Phase III trial comparing adjuvant treatment with pegylated interferon alfa-2b versus observation: prognostic significance of autoantibodies—EORTC 18991. *J Clin Oncol* 2010;28:2460.
77. Wong S-F, Jakowatz JG, Taheri R. Management of hypertriglyceridemia in patients receiving interferon for malignant melanoma. *Ann Pharmacother* 2004;38:1655.
79. Schapira D, Nahir AM, Hadad N. Interferon-induced Raynaud's syndrome. *Semin Arthritis Rheum* 2002;32:157.
81. Reinhold U, Hartl C, Hering R, et al. Fatal rhabdomyolysis and multiple organ failure associated with adjuvant high-dose interferon alfa in malignant melanoma. *Lancet* 1997;349(9051):540.
82. Li SD, Yong S, Srinivas D, Van Thiel DH. Reactivation of sarcoidosis during interferon therapy. *J Gastroenterol* 2002;37:50.
84. Islam M, Frye RF, Richards TJ, et al.. Differential effect of IFNα-2b on the cytochrome P450 enzyme system: a potential basis of IFN toxicity and its modulation by other drugs. *Clin Cancer Res* 2002;8:2480.
86. Jonasch E, Haluska FG. Interferon in oncological practice: review of interferon biology, clinical applications, and toxicities. *Oncologist* 2001;6:34.
93. Schiller JH, Pugh M, Kirkwood JM, et al. Eastern Cooperative Group trial of interferon gamma in metastatic melanoma: an innovative study design. *Clin Cancer Res* 1996;2:29.
94. Kleeberg UR, Suciu S, Bröcker EB, et al. Final results of EORTC 18871/DKG 80-1 randomised phase III trial. rIFN-α2b versus rIFN- γ gamma versus ISCADOR M® versus observation after surgery in melanoma patients with either high-risk primary (thickness >3 mm) or regional lymph node metastasis. *Eur J Cancer* 2004;40:390.
95. Kirkwood JM, Bryant J, Schiller JH, et al. Immunomodulatory function of interferon-gamma in patients with metastatic melanoma: results of a phase II-B trial in subjects with metastatic melanoma, ECOG study E 4987. Eastern Cooperative Oncology Group. *J Immunother* 1997;20:146.
96. Kirkwood JM, Richards T, Zarour HM, et al. Immunomodulatory effects of high-dose and low-dose interferon α2b in patients with high-risk resected melanoma: the E2690 laboratory corollary of Intergroup adjuvant trial E1690. *Cancer* 2002;95:1101.
97. Sondak VK. How does interferon work? Does it even matter? *Cancer* 2002;95:947.
98. Kirkwood JM, Ibrahim JG, Sondak VK, et al. High- and low-dose interferon alfa-2b in high-risk melanoma: first analysis of Intergroup trial E1690/S9111/C9190. *J Clin Oncol* 2000;18:2444.
99. Cascinelli N, Belli F, Mackie RM, et al. Effect of long-term adjuvant therapy with interferon alpha-2a in patients with regional node metastases from cutaneous melanoma: a randomised trial. *Lancet* 2001;358(9285):866.
100. Hancock BW, Wheatley K, Harris S, et al. Adjuvant interferon in high-risk melanoma: the AIM HIGH study—United Kingdom Coordinating Committee on Cancer Research randomized study of adjuvant low-dose extended-duration interferon alfa-2a in high-risk resected malignant melanoma. *J Clin Oncol* 2004;22:53.
103. Wheatley KM, Ives N, Hancock B, et al. Does adjuvant interferon-α for high-risk melanoma provide a worthwhile benefit? A meta-analysis of the randomised trials. *Cancer Treat Rev* 2003;29:241.
104. Verma S, Quirt I, McCready D, et al. Systematic review of systemic adjuvant therapy for patients at high risk for recurrent melanoma. *Cancer* 2006;106:1431.
105. Mocelli S, Pasquali S, Rossi CR, Nitti D. Interferon alpha adjuvant therapy in patients with high-risk melanoma: a systematic review and meta-analysis. *J Natl Cancer Inst* 2010;102:493.
109. Eggermont AMM, Bouwhuis MG, Kruit WH, et al. Serum concentrations of pegylated interferon α-2b in patients with resected stage III melanoma receiving adjuvant pegylated interferon α-2b in a randomized phase III trial (EORTC 18991). *Cancer Chemother Pharmacol* 2010;65:671.
110. Daud AI, Xu C, Hwu W-J, et al. Pharmacokinetic/pharmacodynamic analysis of adjuvant pegylated interferon α-2b in patients with resected high-risk melanoma. *Cancer Chemother Pharmacol* 2010; available online.
113. Bukowski R, Ernstoff MS, Gore ME, et al. Pegylated interferon alfa-2b treatment for patients with solid tumors: a phase I/II study. *J Clin Oncol* 2002;20:3841.
115. Dummer R, Garbe C, Thompson JA, et al. Randomized dose-escalation study evaluating peginterferon alfa-2a in patients with metastatic malignant melanoma. *J Clin Oncol* 2006;24:1188.
116. Eggermont AMM, Suciu S, Santinami M, et al. Adjuvant therapy with pegylated interferon alfa-2b versus observation alone in resected stage III melanoma: final results of EORTC 18991, a randomised phase III trial. *Lancet* 2008;372(9633):117.
117. Kirkwood JM, Ibrahim J, Lawson DH, et al. High-dose interferon alfa-2b does not diminish antibody response to GM2 vaccination in patients with resected melanoma: results of the multicenter Eastern Cooperative Oncology Group phase II trial E2696. *J Clin Oncol* 2001;19:1430.
120. Falkson CI, Ibrahim J, Kirkwood JM, et al. Phase III trial of dacarbazine versus dacarbazine with interferon alpha-2b versus dacarbazine with tamoxifen versus dacarbazine with interferon alpha-2b and tamoxifen in patients with metastatic malignant melanoma: an Eastern Cooperative Oncology Group study. *J Clin Oncol* 1998;16:1743.

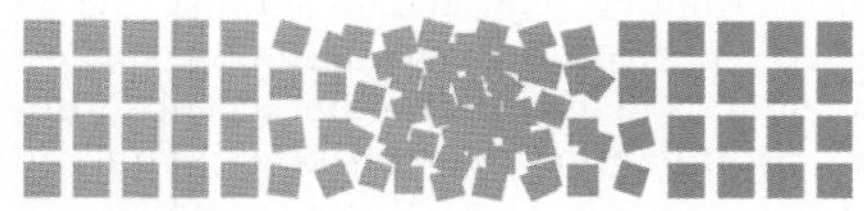

CHAPTER 45 INTERLEUKIN THERAPY

MICHAEL T. LOTZE

INTERLEUKINS AS THERAPEUTICS

Purified recombinant cytokines are proven agents, useful for patients with cancer, and include the cytokines erythropoietin, interferon alpha (IFN-α), and interleukin 2 (IL-2). It is now clear that most adult tumors arise in the setting of chronic inflammation and many of the other cytokine therapies were ineffective for most patients with cancer. However, the notable successes of IFN-α (see Chapter 44) and of IL-2 (see following discussion) in small numbers of patients with renal cell carcinoma, melanoma, and lymphoma provided an impetus for development of interleukins alone and in combination with other more conventional cancer therapeutics. Currently the novel γc receptor binding cytokines, IL-7, IL-15, and IL-21 are in active clinical trials.

The nomenclature for individuals just entering the field is formidable[1]; modern compendiums of cytokines extend over thousands of pages and, in our summation, two volumes. As a way to gain understanding of the literally hundreds of cytokines now apparent in biology, in part revealed from the sequencing of the human genome, there are a couple of brief pointers. The first is that all cytokines—factors literally "moving cells" to grow, move, or exert effector function—can be considered in two categories. The first are the hematopoietins (factors working predominantly within the hematopoietic system and sharing structural disulfide-linked immunoglobulin-domainlike structures) and similar secreted, leader sequence, conventional cytokines that are synthesized in the rough endoplasmic reticulum, and exported through the Golgi stack to the cell membrane and/or secreted. Thus, these are the "leader" cytokines, including most of the interleukins, interferons, chemokines, and tumor necrosis family (TNF) members. The second category, which includes so-called *leaderless* secreted proteins, use alternative means to gain access to the extracellular space to mediate their biologic function, and include the IL-1 family (now numbering 11 family members), the fibroblast growth factors, and oxidoreductases such as thioredoxin and migration inhibitory factor, as well as an emergent family of molecules collectively referred to as *damage-associated molecular pattern* (DAMP) molecules.[2] These are released or secreted by damaged or injured cells and include the S100 family of molecules, the heat shock proteins, and the nuclear protein, HMGB1, high mobility group B1. Although within the interleukins, a collective originally designed to signify production by one white cell and acting on another, one can find leaderless cytokines such as members of the IL-1 family (IL-1α and IL-1β, IL1 receptor antagonist, IL-18, IL-33, IL37, and IL38),[3] and leadered cytokines including members of the IL-2R family (IL-2, IL-4, IL-7, IL-9, IL-13, IL-15, and IL-21), the IL-17 family (IL-17 and IL-25), the colony-stimulating factors IL-3, IL-11, and IL-36, the chemokine family with 50 members (IL-8 is a member important in angiogenesis), the extended IL-6 family (IL-6 itself, IL-12, IL-23, and IL-27), and the IL-10–related members of the interferon family (IL-10, IL-19, IL-20, IL-22, and IL-24).

Although representing diverse family members with distinct biologic and possibly clinical roles as "replacement" or inductive active immunotherapies or as targets for inhibition, the current collection serves as a means to illustrate some of their roles in the clinic, and future editions of this text may group them more appropriately along family lines! Here we briefly review the status of the major subclasses of interleukins that have been introduced into therapy.

INTERLEUKIN-1 FAMILY

The IL-1 extended family (IL-1Fx) of beta trefoil cytokines now includes a total of 11 members. Their major role in immunity remains not fully explored. They are important for the initial critical events in recruiting and activating myeloid and lymphoid cells, serving as DAMPs or pathogen-associated molecular pattern molecules (PAMPs), the so-called signal 0s alerting the host to damage or injury. Subsequent delivery of antigen/major histocompatibility complex (signal 1) and B7/CD28 (signal 2) during polarization (signal 3) of the immune response prompts the adaptive immune response. During the effector phase they serve as signal 4s associated with tissue-specific signaling and homing, driving either inflammation or healing and the fibroblastic response, mediated by IL-1β during the effector phase of the immune response as signal 5s.[3,4] They also deliver activation signals across the immunologic synapse to T and natural killer (NK)-cells.[5,6]

The β trefoil IL-1 family now totals 11 members. The function of the new members (IL-1F5–IL-1F10, IL-33, and IL-37) and what their role might be in the initiation or maintenance of the immune response remains unclear. The IL-1 family members are proinflammatory cytokines that initiate the innate immune response by activating a set of transcription factors including NF-κB and AP-1.[7] The better-studied members of the IL-1 familyIL-1F1(IL-1α), IL-1F2 (IL-1β), IL-1F3 (IL-1RA), and IL-1F4 (IL-18)—as well as the fibroblast growth factors are structurally related as β trefoil cytokines[8] that are secreted without signal peptides and do not follow the typical secretion pathways. Both apoptotic cells producing IL-1 and IL-18 as well as activated cells can release these cytokines into the local milieu[9] but this appears only to be associated with caspase-1 activation. Recently, secretion of IL-1β, IL-18, and likely other family members in the form of rapidly shed microvesicles budding off of the plasma membrane has been identified as a method for secretion, and this appears to be true for other members of the IL-1 family including IL-18 as well as the novel factor HMGB1 released during necrotic cell death and secreted by activated monocytes.[2]

Interleukin-1F1 and Interleukin-1F2

IL-1α and IL-1β bind the type I IL-1 receptor with subsequent recruitment of a signaling component, the IL-1R accessory protein (IL-1Racp[10,11]). Both are potently secreted by dendritic cells (DCs).[12] IL-1β increases CD40L-induced cytokine secretion by monocyte-derived DC, CD34(+)-derived DC, and peripheral blood DC. Neither has been effective in cancer clinical trials alone or in combination with IL-2 for patients seeking either antitumor effects or restorative hematologic effects warranting the toxicity of hypotension, fever, rigors, and myalgia. Some increase in platelet counts have been observed.[13–39]

Interleukin-1F3

IL-1F3 (IL-1RA) also binds the type I receptor but does not recruit IL-1Racp, thereby preventing signaling by IL-1F1 (IL-1α) or IL-1F2 (IL-1β). The type II IL-1 receptor is a molecular decoy of IL-1 activity, binding IL-1 without signaling, and has been approved for the treatment of patients with rheumatoid arthritis. Recent studies suggest activity in type II diabetes mellitus,[14] juvenile rheumatoid arthritis,[15] familial cold autoinflammatory syndrome,[16,17] posterior uveitis,[18] hyperimmunoglobulinemia D,[19] panniculitis,[20] and likely other IL-1–associated inflammatory diseases.

Interleukin-1F4/Interleukin-18

IL-1F4 (IL-18) is a family member promoting IFN-γ production from T cells, B cells, and NK cells, especially in synergy with IL-12.[21] IL-18 has a similar signaling pathway to IL-1α and IL-1β but uses the IL-1R–related protein (IL-1Rrp) and a nonbinding chain, IL-1R accessory proteinlike (IL1RAcPL) and IL-1RAcPL. An IL-18 binding protein located on the same chromosome and produced largely by the same cells with several pox virus homologues has also been identified.[22] Our studies suggested that the antitumor effects of IL-18 are mediated by T cells, NK cells, and DCs.[23]

Enhanced serum levels of IL-18BP in patients[24] treated with IL-12 were observed in melanoma patients at presentation, with the levels up to 22 ng/mL rising to 95 ng/mL following treatment with IL-12. IL-18 and IL-18BP circulate in normal and cancer patients. Phase 1/2 trials of IL-18 have been performed and recently reported.[24,25] Patients given rhIL-18 ranging from 3 to 1,000 mcg/kg had chills, fever, nausea, headache, and hypotension along with neutropenia, thrombocytopenia, anemia, hypoalbuminemia, hyponatremia, and elevations in liver transaminases, but with limited, unconfirmed responses. Ongoing trials in combination with therapeutic monoclonal antibodies are still ongoing (Z. Jonak, personal communication, 2011).

Interleukin 33 (Interleukin-1F11)

HMGB1[2] and the recently described IL-33 are abundant chromatin-associated nuclear factors with potent proinflammatory cytokine activities. ST2 is an IL-1 receptor family member, a mechanically induced cardiomyocyte protein, found in patients with acute myocardial infarction or chronic heart failure. Recently, IL-33 was identified as a functional ligand of ST2L, allowing exploration of the role of ST2 in the myocardium. Recombinant IL-33 treatment reduced hypertrophy and fibrosis and improved survival in animal models. Thus, it is a cardioprotective cytokine and may have potential in cardiac patients[26] for beneficially regulating the myocardial response.

Interleukin 37 (Interleukin-1F7b)

Sadly, the human cytokine, initially called IL-1H4 or IL-1F7b, has been found to be spliced out in the mouse genome, limiting our ability to discern function. Antitumor effects of placing the human gene in murine tumors suggested an agonist role on nominally, still-expressed receptors, but new findings[27] suggest that its expression in macrophages or epithelial cells suppresses production of proinflammatory cytokines. Thus, in humans it may play a possible role as a natural suppressor of innate inflammatory and immune responses.

INTERLEUKIN 3, INTERLEUKIN 11, AND INTERLEUKIN 34

These cytokines are grouped together because their primary established role is in promoting hematopoiesis, broadly in the case of IL-3,[28] like the IL-1 family members and granulocyte-macrophage colony-stimulating factor (GM-CSF), and more narrowly supporting megakaryopoiesis and thrombopoiesis, like IL-11. IL-11 use shortens the duration of chemotherapy-induced thrombocytopenia; it is approved by the U.S. Food and Drug Administration (FDA).[29]

Interleukin 3

Two versions of IL-3 have been tested in the clinic. This includes the recombinant molecule[30–32] as well as a fusion product with GM-CSF, termed *PIXY-321*.[32,33] Neither has been approved for use, although IL-3 had prominent pluripoietinlike effects in patients treated. Following treatment with rhIL-3, bone marrow erythroid (burst forming units-erythroid) and multilineage (multipotential colony-forming cells) progenitors increased, as did total leukocyte, neutrophil, platelet, and eosinophil counts. Although rhIL-3 induced a multilineage response stimulating proliferation of multipotential and lineage-restricted progenitors, randomized studies[34] failed to show sufficient benefit to warrant approval.

Interleukin 11

IL-11 supports megakaryopoiesis and promotes small bowel mucosal integrity. Randomized clinical trials[35,36] of IL-11 demonstrated decreased need for platelet support and decreased evidence of infection, presumably because of its activities on the small bowel integrity, It has been approved for clinical use in the setting of thrombocytopenia. New indications exploring other activities of the cytokine are being explored, including a role in autoimmunity and in the response to mechanical stress in osteoblasts.[37]

Interleukin 34

IL-34 is a recently identified cytokine, without homology to other known cytokines or other genes, acting to promote myeloid proliferation and survival, acting on the macrophage colony-stimulating factor receptor, CSF-1. It binds to primary human monocytes and activates ERK1/2 phosphorylation as well as the human monocytic cell line, THP-1.

INTERLEUKIN-2 FAMILY

IL-2 was the first agent available for the treatment of metastatic cancer that functions solely through the activation of the immune system. Originally described as a growth factor for activated T cells, IL-2 was later found to exert multiple effects on cellular immune function and to induce tumor regression in mice. Subsequent clinical trials involving patients with renal cell carcinoma and malignant melanoma have demonstrated sufficient efficacy to establish IL-2 as an FDA-approved treatment for both of these malignancies.

Isolation, Characterization, and Cloning of Interleukin 2

In 1976, Morgan et al.[38] demonstrated the existence of a growth factor present in the conditioned medium of lectin-stimulated human peripheral blood mononuclear cells that could sustain indefinitely the *ex vivo* proliferation of human T cells. This initial report was followed in short order by the isolation, biochemical characterization, and ultimately, the cloning of what was then termed the *T-cell growth factor*.[39] Subsequently designated IL-2, this factor was shown to be a 15-kD polypeptide made up of 153 amino acids, the first 20 of which form a signal sequence that is proteolytically cleaved during secretion. Natural IL-2 is glycosylated, although the attachment of sugar moieties is not essential for biologic activity. The molecule has cysteine residues at positions 58, 105, and 125, the first two of which form an intramolecular disulfide bridge. The third cysteine is not essential for biologic activity and can be replaced with alternative amino acids to minimize polymerization and increase shelf life; commercially available IL-2 has a serine for cysteine substitution at this position and is provided lyophilized in mannitol and a weak detergent, SDS. Crystallographic analysis indicates that IL-2 is a spherical molecule comprised of six α-helical regions. Production and response to IL-2, like many other immune products, appears to be regulated by miRNA.[40,41]

Interleukin 2 Receptor

The biologic effects of IL-2 are the result of the binding of the lymphokine to specific surface receptors. As with IL-2 itself, the expression of high-affinity IL-2 receptors is induced as a result of signaling through the T-cell antigen receptor. With the exception of a minor population of memory T cells that presumably were activated *in vivo* by a prior antigen exposure, freshly isolated peripheral blood T cells do not constitutively express high-affinity IL-2 receptors.

The high-affinity IL-2 receptor consists of three distinct subunits designated the α, β, and γ chains (Fig. 45.1). The α chain is a 251–amino acid polypeptide with a large extracellular domain, a transmembrane span, and a short 13-residue cytoplasmic tail. The extracellular domain of this protein binds IL-2 with low affinity. The cytoplasmic domain of this receptor has no known biologic function and is dispensable for IL-2–induced signaling.

The IL-2 receptor β chain has a 214–amino acid extracellular domain, a transmembrane motif, and a large 286-residue cytoplasmic tail.[42] In contrast to the cytoplasmic domain of the α chain, that of the β chain is essential for IL-2 signaling. The IL-2 receptor γ chain has paired cysteines at two sites within the extracellular domain and a perimembrane WSXWS motif characteristic of the members of an enlarging cytokine receptor superfamily that includes the receptors for IL-3, IL-4, IL-6, IL-7, GM-CSF, prolactin, erythropoietin, and growth hormone. This activity[43] is possibly related to binding abundant molecules such as HMGB1,[44] which could facilitate cytokine/cytokine receptor interactions.

The γ chain is a novel 64-kD protein that physically associates with the β chain. Like the β chain, the γ chain is a member of the cytokine receptor superfamily.[45] These two together

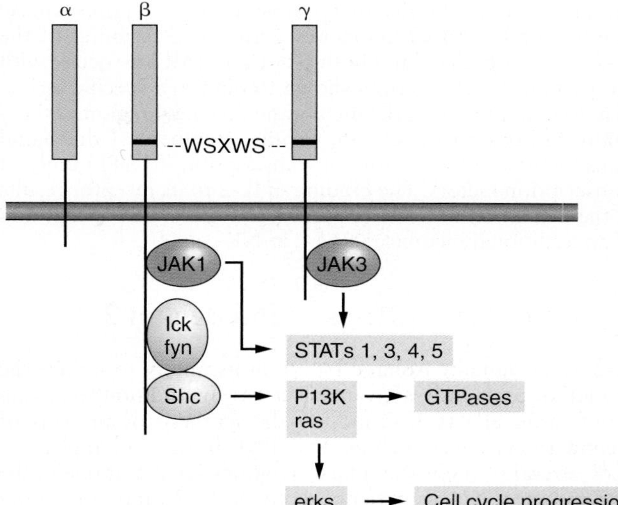

FIGURE 45.1 The high-affinity interleukin-2 receptor and associated signaling pathways. The cytoplasmic domains of the β and γ chains contain several tyrosines that, when phosphorylated, provide docking and activation sites for numerous downstream kinases that affect cell proliferation, gene expression, and cell motility. GTPases, guanosine triphosphatases; JAK, janus kinase; PI3K, phosphoinositide 3 kinase; STAT, signal transduction and activators of transcription.

bind IL-2 with intermediate affinity. When cotransfected along with the complementary DNAs of the α and β chains, the complementary DNA encoding the γ chain yields a high-affinity IL-2 receptor that transduces signals and is internalized in response to IL-2 binding. More recent studies have demonstrated that this receptor chain is shared by the receptors for several lymphokines, including IL-4, IL-7, IL-9, IL-15, and IL-21 as well as IL-2.[46] Mutations in the gene encoding this receptor chain account for most, if not all, cases of X-linked severe combined immunodeficiency.[47] When antibodies against these receptor chains were used, resting T cells were found to constitutively express low levels of the IL-2 receptor α chain but not the β or γ chains. All three chains are up-regulated as a result of antigenic stimulation. Resting NK cells constitutively express the β chain, and both the α and γ chains are induced in these cells by exposure to IL-2 or IL-12.[48]

Signaling Pathways

The binding of IL-2 to its receptor induces the tyrosine phosphorylation of numerous cellular proteins, including the IL-2 receptor β and γ chains. Because all three chains of the IL-2 receptor lack intrinsic tyrosine kinase activity, these events must be transduced through kinases that physically associate with the cytoplasmic domains of the receptor subunits (Fig. 45.1). IL-2 also induces the recruitment and subsequent tyrosine phosphorylation of the adaptor protein Shc to the IL-2 receptor β chain. This particular association is thought to be largely responsible for the activation of $p21^{ras}$ and the downstream mitogen-activated protein kinases erk-1 and erk-2 in response to IL-2.[49] The IL-2 receptor-γ chain is also essential for IL-2–induced signaling, because mutant T-cell lines expressing the α and β chains and a mutant version of the γ chain lacking the C-terminal 68 residues failed to express the protooncogenes *c-fos*, *c-jun*, and *c-myc* when stimulated with IL-2.[50]

In addition to associating with src family tyrosine kinases, both the β and γ receptor chains associate with members of

PHARMACOLOGY OF CANCER THERAPEUTICS

the Janus kinase family of tyrosine kinases.[51] Janus kinase family member JAK3 associates with the C-terminal of the IL-2 receptor β chain and both JAK1 and JAK2 associate with the γ chain. JAK1 has been shown to bind to a specific serine-rich domain present in the membrane proximal region of the γ chain. Janus kinases activate various members of the signal transduction and activators of transcription (STAT) family of transcription factors. The binding of IL-2 to its receptor results in the activation of STAT1, STAT3, and STAT5 in T cells and of an additional member, STAT4, in NK cells.[52]

In Vitro Effects of Interleukin 2

IL-2 was originally isolated based on its ability to induce the growth of previously activated T cells.[38] In addition to having proliferative effects, IL-2 induces the synthesis of an array of secondary cytokines such as IL-1, TNF, IL-6, and lymphotoxin.[49] Several of these secondary cytokines are detectable in the circulation of cancer patients receiving IL-2 immunotherapy and are thought by many investigators to contribute to the side effects of IL-2 therapy.[53]

The biologic effect of IL-2 arguably most pertinent to its use as an antitumor agent is its ability to enhance the cytolytic activity of antigen-specific cytotoxic T lymphocytes and NK cells.[54] The biochemical basis for this enhanced cytolytic function is currently unclear, but it is thought to be due in part to the increased expression of genes encoding the lytic components of cytotoxic granules (e.g., perforin, granzymes) as well as adhesion molecules (LFA-1) that facilitate the binding of activated leukocytes to tumor endothelium and the tumor cells themselves. In addition to increasing the HLA-restricted cytolytic activity of cytotoxic T lymphocytes for cells expressing a particular antigen and that of NK cells for susceptible tumor cell targets, IL-2 markedly diversifies the range of target cells susceptible to killing by these effectors. Indeed, human peripheral blood lymphocytes exposed only to high concentrations of IL-2 without prior exposure to tumor cells are able to kill virtually all tumor cell lines and most freshly isolated tumor cells *in vitro* regardless of the particular HLA class I alleles expressed by the target cell. Some nontransformed cells, in particular cultured endothelial cells, are similarly susceptible to IL-2–primed peripheral blood lymphocytes in isotope release assays. The cells responsible for this HLA-unrestricted killing in response to IL-2 have been termed *lymphokine-activated killer* (LAK) cells.[55] LAK cells appear to be a mixture of activated NK cells and CD3+/CD8+ cytotoxic T cells, the relative contributions of which depend on the duration of culture in IL-2 and whether human peripheral blood lymphocytes or murine spleen suspensions are used as an LAK cell source. As described in clinical investigations involving high-dose IL-2, these *ex vivo*–activated LAK cells featured prominently in the early clinical trials carried out with IL-2 in cancer patients.

Role of Interleukin 2 in Driving T-Regulatory Cells

Subsequent to the approval of IL-2 as a therapeutic agent, it was found to be an important component of expansion of so-called T-regulatory cells (Tregs). IL-2R signaling delivers signals for thymic development of Tregs and promotes their function, even with limited IL-2. Although an important marker for Tregs, neither IL-2 nor CD25 appear to be essential for their maintenance. Although Tregs appear to increase following IL-2 administration, there is no clear relationship with response to treatment. Prophylactic depletion of Tregs using monoclonal antibodies in mice stimulates antitumor immune responses and can prevent tumor development, but clinical trials have so far been disappointing.

Preclinical Studies with Interleukin 2 in Tumor-Bearing Mice

The results of the *in vitro* studies cited earlier in *in vitro* effects of IL-2 demonstrating that IL-2 could enhance the cytolytic activity of NK cells and tumor-specific cytotoxic T lymphocytes suggested that systemically administered IL-2 might induce tumor regression in tumor-bearing mice. IL-2 has since undergone extensive evaluation as an antitumor agent in a variety of murine tumor models. IL-2 has been used alone, in combination with other cytokines, and in conjunction with the adoptive transfer of various *ex vivo*–activated lymphoid preparations to eradicate a wide range of local and metastatic tumors. Early studies demonstrated that IL-2 used alone could reduce or eliminate pulmonary metastases from methylcholanthrene-induced sarcoma and melanoma cell lines and that this antitumor effect was strictly dependent on the dose of IL-2 administered.[56] In some animal models, tumor eradication by IL-2 administration resulted in immunization against the tumor. In other studies in which mice were immunized with dendritic cells pulsed with tumor lysates, the concurrent systemic administration of IL-2 was shown to enhance the efficacy of the vaccine.[57]

In several studies, the effects of IL-2 could be enhanced by the concurrent administration of LAK cells generated by culturing splenocytes *ex vivo* in IL-2–containing media.[58] Mice bearing hepatic micrometastases from poorly immunogenic MCA-105 or MCA-102 sarcomas or MCA-38 adenocarcinoma cells, for example, were highly responsive to treatment with the combination of IL-2 and LAK cells but unresponsive to LAK cells alone and only partially responsive to IL-2.

Lymphocytes present within tumor infiltrates are often enriched for effector cells capable of killing tumor cells. When isolated and tested *in vitro* for cytolytic activity against autologous tumor cells, these tumor-infiltrating lymphocytes (TILs) are 50- to 100-fold more potent than IL-2–activated splenocytes (LAK cells). This apparent superiority was also evident *in vivo*. The infusion of 2×10^6 TILs with IL-2, for example, completely eradicated the pulmonary metastases of mice previously inoculated with MCA-105 sarcoma cells.[59] As many as 2×10^8 LAK cells were required for a comparable antitumor effect.

Clinical Applications of Interleukin 2

The potent immunomodulatory and antitumor effects of IL-2 in the *in vitro* experiments and preclinical animal tumor models described earlier prompted the rapid movement of IL-2 into the clinical setting. Early clinical trials involving the brief administration of modest doses of purified, cell-derived IL-2 produced only transient fever and lymphopenia, but no sustained ill effects or tumor responses. Because preclinical trials had shown that tumor responses were dose-dependent and maximal when IL-2 was combined with LAK cells, the advent of recombinant IL-2 led quickly to a series of trials using higher doses of IL-2 with and without LAK cells.

Clinical Investigations Involving High-Dose Interleukin 2

We at the National Cancer Institute (NCI) Surgery Branch developed a regimen that involved the administration of high-dose intravenous (IV) bolus IL-2.[60] In this regimen, IL-2 was administered at 600,000 to 720,000 IU/kg IV every 8 hours on days 1 to 5 and 15 to 19 of a treatment course. A maximum of 28 to 30 doses per course was administered; however, doses were frequently withheld because of excessive toxicity. Treatment courses were repeated at 8- to 12-week intervals in responding patients. During initial studies, patients underwent daily leukapheresis on days 8 to 12 during which large numbers of lymphocytes were obtained to be cultured in IL-2 for 3 or 4 days to generate LAK cells; these LAK cells were then reinfused into the patient during the second 5-day period of IL-2 administration.

This high-dose IL-2 regimen with or without LAK cells produced overall tumor responses in 15% to 20% of patients with metastatic melanoma or renal cell cancer in clinical trials conducted at either the NCI Surgery Branch or within the Cytokine Working Group (formerly the Extramural IL-2 and LAK Working Group).[61] Complete responses were noted in 4% to 6% of patients with each disease and were frequently durable. Rare responses, usually partial and of shorter duration, were also noted in patients with either Hodgkin's or non–Hodgkin's lymphoma, or non–small cell lung, colorectal, or ovarian carcinoma.[62] Randomized and sequential clinical trials comparing IL-2 plus LAK cells with high-dose IL-2 alone failed to show sufficient benefit for the addition of LAK cells to justify their continued use.[63] Because of the quality and durability of tumor responses to this high-dose IL-2 regimen, IL-2 received FDA approval for the treatment of metastatic renal cell carcinoma in 1992 and for treatment of metastatic melanoma in 1998.[64,65] Long-term follow-up data for patients with melanoma and renal cell cancer treated in the initial high-dose bolus IL-2 trials presented to the FDA[66,67] have confirmed the earlier findings of response durability, with median duration for complete responses yet to be reached and few, if any, relapses observed in patients free of disease for longer than 30 months. In fact, several patients have remained free of disease in excess of 20 years since initiating treatment. These data suggest that high-dose IL-2 treatment may actually have led to the cure of some patients with these advanced malignancies previously considered incurable.

Toxicity of High-Dose Interleukin 2

The usefulness of high-dose IL-2 therapy has been limited by toxicity, many features of which resemble bacterial sepsis. Side effects are dose-dependent and, fortunately, largely predictable and rapidly reversible. Common side effects or findings include fever, chills, lethargy, diarrhea, nausea, anemia, thrombocytopenia, eosinophilia, diffuse erythroderma, hepatic dysfunction, and confusion.[68] Myocarditis also occurs in approximately 5% of patients. IL-2 therapy also commonly produces a "capillary leak syndrome," leading to fluid retention, hypotension, early adult respiratory distress syndrome, prerenal azotemia, and occasionally myocardial infarction. As a consequence of these side effects, few patients are able to receive all of the proposed therapy. IL-2 has produces a neutrophil chemotactic defect that predisposes patients to infection with Gram-positive and occasionally Gram-negative bacteria.[69] Early high-dose IL-2 studies were associated with 2% to 4% mortality, largely related to infection or cardiac toxicity.[65,68] The routine use of antibiotic prophylaxis, more extensive cardiac screening, and more judicious IL-2 administration have greatly enhanced the safety of this therapy; since 1990 the mortality rates at experienced treatment centers have been less than 1%[70] (Table 45.1). Nonetheless, the considerable toxicity of the high-dose IL-2 regimen has continued to limit its application to highly selected patients with excellent performance status and adequate organ function treated at medical centers with considerable experience with this approach.

Laboratory studies have suggested that the toxicity of IL-2 is in part mediated by the release of secondary cytokines such

TABLE 45.1

SAFETY OF HIGH-DOSE INTRAVENOUS BOLUS RECOMBINANT INTERLEUKIN-2 THERAPY: THE NATIONAL CANCER INSTITUTE EXPERIENCE[a]

Adverse Event	1985 Incidence (%)	1997 Incidence (%)
Hypotension	81	31
Diarrhea	92	12
Neuropsychiatric toxicity	19	8
Line sepsis	18	4
Pulmonary complications	12	3

[a]Dose: 720,000 IU/kg every 8 hours. With patient selection and experience in managing side effects, high-dose recombinant interleukin-2 is safe. There were no treatment-related deaths in 809 consecutive patients. Incidence of grade 3–4 adverse events has been greatly reduced. (Adapted from ref. 70.)

as angiopoietin-2, TNF-α, IL-1, and IL-6.[53] Nonetheless, attempts to block the toxicity of IL-2 by the coadministration of soluble receptors of IL-1 or TNF, or CNI-1493, an inhibitor of IL-1 and TNF signaling, have yielded only a modest reduction in the hypotension, vascular leak, and other serious side effects routinely observed in patients receiving high-dose IL-2.[71–73] The hypotension associated with IL-2 is partly due to the overproduction of the vasodilator nitric oxide. This diffusible gas is generated from the deamination of the amino acid arginine, and its production can be inhibited with various arginine analogues. Kilbourn et al.[74] were able to demonstrate that the administration of NG-monomethyl-L-arginine to patients with renal cell carcinoma reversed the hypotension associated with IL-2 treatment. The concurrent administration of M40403, a superoxide dismutase mimetic, has also been shown to reduce IL-2–associated hypotension in tumor-bearing mice.[75] This particular agent also appeared to enhance the antitumor activity of IL-2, presumably through the inhibition of superoxide production by macrophages. Clinical trials of human protein tyrosine phosphatase β inhibitors, which stabilize Tie2 phosphorylation and limit the vascular leak, have shown promise in murine models and are entering the clinic in conjunction with IL-2 soon.

Management of Patients Receiving High-Dose Interleukin 2

The safe administration of high-dose IL-2 requires, first of all, a careful selection of patients capable of tolerating the fever, hypotension, and edema that often develop during treatment. Because of this, high-dose IL-2 should be considered a reasonable treatment option only in patients without significant cardiac disease (i.e., angina, congestive heart failure, arrhythmia, or prior myocardial infarction). Patients older than 40 years should undergo stress testing, and those found to have exercise-induced ischemia should be excluded. Patients should be specifically screened for central nervous system metastases, and those with positive findings on head computed tomographic scan or magnetic resonance image should only cautiously be given high-dose IL-2. Anecdotal responses to IL-2 have been observed in patients with brain metastases receiving IL-2 alone or in combination with other agents. Patients should also have adequate renal, hepatic, and pulmonary function with a serum creatinine level of less than 1.6 mg/dL, bilirubin level of less than 1.5 mg/dL, and a forced expiratory volume in 1 second of more than 2 liters. They should also have a performance score on the Eastern Cooperative Oncology Group scale of less than 2.

Once a decision is made to offer high-dose IL-2 to a patient, the various treatment-associated side effects[68] can be ameliorated by the concomitant administration of acetaminophen and indomethacin to reduce fever and chills, H_2 blockers to prevent gastritis, and prophylactic antibiotics to prevent central line–associated infections. Patients should receive antiemetics and antidiarrheals as needed. IL-2–induced pruritus and dermatitis can be minimized with diphenhydramine and various skin creams. Steroids should be avoided because they antagonize the immunostimulatory properties of IL-2. Hypotension is best managed initially with fluid replacement, but many patients require IV dopamine and, in some instances, both dopamine and phenylephrine. Most patients require supplemental IV sodium bicarbonate to prevent acidosis. In the event of life-threatening toxicity (e.g., hypotension refractory to pressors), the IL-2 is discontinued but may be resumed after the resolution of the problem. Generally, doses of IL-2 withheld because of toxicity are not made up at the end of a treatment cycle. With careful patient selection and the appropriate use of concurrent medications, most patients can safely receive high-dose IL-2; however, the unusual array and severity of treatment side effects mandate that this form of immunotherapy be administered by a team of physicians and nurses experienced in the use of this agent.

Lower-Dose or Alternative Interleukin 2 Regimens

Because of the significant toxicity associated with the high-dose IV bolus IL-2 regimen and the expense involved with the necessary hospitalization and intensive monitoring, various investigators have attempted to establish active regimens using lower doses of IL-2. In these regimens, IL-2 was administered either by lower-dose IV bolus, continuous IV infusion, or subcutaneous injection in an effort to reduce toxicity without compromising antitumor efficacy. The more commonly used lower-dose regimens are listed in Table 45.2.

The maximum tolerated dose of IL-2 when administered by a 5-day (120-hour) continuous infusion was shown to be 18 MIU/m²/d or approximately one-fifth the total amount of IL-2 tolerated by IV bolus IL-2 regimens.[76] Although continuous-infusion IL-2 regimens were shown to produce response rates similar to those of the high-dose IV bolus IL-2 regimen, the toxicity was also generally comparable. Other regimens, such as those using lower doses of IL-2 administered either by IV bolus or subcutaneous injections, are better tolerated and enable patients to be treated on a conventional inpatient hospital ward or even as outpatients. Side effects associated with these regimens are generally limited to flulike or constitutional symptoms, which allows even patients with limited cardiopulmonary reserve to receive this agent. However, it remains to be seen whether or not a less toxic, lower-dose regimen can be devised that duplicates the benefits of high-dose IL-2.

The question of whether high-dose regimens are more effective than those using lower doses remains controversial. In the case of metastatic melanoma, low-dose regimens consistently yield response rates below 5% and are regarded as clearly inferior to high-dose IL-2.[77] In contrast, studies of low-dose IL-2 in treatment of patients with renal cancer have consistently shown tumor regression in 10% to 20% of patients, comparable to the rate achieved with high-dose IL-2 in some studies. However, a phase 3 randomized trial assigning patients with renal cancer to either high-dose IL-2 or one of two lower-dose regimens (one IV and one subcutaneous) yielded a 21% response rate in the high-dose limb,[78] but only 13% and 10% response rates for the low-dose IV and subcutaneous regimens, respectively. Although no survival difference between the treatment groups was discernible, more durable responses were seen in patients receiving high-dose IL-2, which suggests an advantage to the high-dose regimens.

As part of this trial, investigators examined the pharmacokinetics of IL-2 in an effort to explain differences in biologic and clinical effects of the various administration schedules.[79] Peak concentrations of 4,680 ± 1,188 IU/mL were achieved after the first injection of high-dose IL-2. Subsequent clearance was biphasic with an initial half-life of 12.6 ± 5.4 minutes and a terminal half-life of 1.6 ± 0.4 hours. Patients receiving IV low-dose IL-2 had peak serum levels of 486 ± 198 IU/mL with a similar clearance pattern and rate. Those receiving IL-2 by subcutaneous injection had peak levels of 61 ± 34 IU/mL 2 to 3 hours after the injection with a half-life of 5.3 ± 1.9 hours. Levels in excess of 18 IU/mL were maintained in those treated with either the high-dose IV or subcutaneous regimen. The inability of lower-dose regimens to produce sustained blood levels above the K_d of the low-affinity IL-2 receptor has been proposed as a potential explanation for their apparent diminished efficacy.

In addition to simply lowering the IL-2 dose, there have been several other attempts at improving the therapeutic index of IL-2. One example is the use of BAY 50-4798, a selective IL-2 receptor agonist engineered to bind preferentially to the high-affinity IL-2 receptor on T cells and less well to the lower-affinity IL-2 receptor present on NK cells. The rationale for the development of this agent rested on the unproven assumption that cytotoxic T cells expressing high-affinity IL-2 receptors were responsible for IL-2–induced tumor regression, whereas NK cells expressing only the β- and γ-receptor chains were

TABLE 45.2

COMMONLY USED TREATMENT REGIMENS OF INTERLEUKIN-2 (IL-2)

Regimen	IL-2	IL-2	Clinical Setting
High-dose bolus	600,000–720,000 IU/kg	IV q8h d 1–5, 15–19	ICU-like
Continuous infusion	18 MIU/m²/d	CIV infusion d 1–5, 15–19	ICU-like
Low-dose IV bolus	72,000 IU/kg	IV q8h d 1–5, 15–19	Ward
Subcutaneous	250,000 IU/kg/d	SC d 1–5, wk 1	Outpatient
	125,000 IU/kg/d	SC d 1–5, wk 2–6	
Decrescendo	18 MIU/m²/6 h	CIV infusion 1 d	Ward
	18 MIU/m²/12 h	CIV infusion 1 d	
	18 MIU/m²/24 h	CIV infusion 1 d	
	4.5 MIU/m²/24 h	CIV infusion 3 d	
Ultra-low-dose	<1 MIU/d	CIV infusion 14–42 d	Outpatient

IV, intravenous; ICU-like, intensive care unit or specialized unit capable of providing blood pressure support; CIV, continuous intravenous.

responsible for the production of pyrogenic cytokines and much of the toxicity of IL-2. This novel version of IL-2 was expected to enhance T-cell–mediated tumor killing while minimizing toxicity. Although clinical investigations with this agent appeared to show some reduction in toxicity, the antitumor activity of the cytokine has not yet been shown to be comparable to that of conventional IL-2.[80] Other approaches including the formulation of IL-2 into liposomes and the direct intratumoral administration of a plasmid DNA–lipid complex containing the IL-2 gene have been abandoned in large part.[81,82]

At the present time the high-dose bolus IL-2 regimen remains the treatment of choice for appropriate patients with access to such treatment and is the gold standard to which other IL-2–based regimens should be compared. The addition of tumor-infiltrating lymphocytes, other cytokines, or chemotherapeutics have failed to improve on the durable partial and complete responses observed with high-dose IL-2 treatment. Recently, administration of the antibody to CTLA-4 (ipilimumab), enabling the increased burst size of responsive clones of T cells, has apparently added to IL-2 response rates in randomized, prospective clinical trials. Ipilimumab, at a dose of 3 mg/kg of body weight, is administered every 3 weeks for up to four treatments (induction). The median overall survival with ipilimumab alone was 10.1 months (hazard ratio for death in the comparison with the gp100 vaccine alone, 0.66; $P = .003$). Grade 3 or 4 immune-related adverse events occurred in 10% to 15% of patients treated with ipilimumab. It will likely be approved by the regulatory agencies in 2010[83] and be available for combination studies with IL-2.

Predictors of Response to Interleukin 2-Based Therapy

Because of the toxicity and expense of high-dose IL-2 treatment, considerable effort has been expended to identify patient populations most likely to benefit from this therapy. In the initial experience with high-dose IL-2 in melanoma patients, tumor responses were more likely in those with a good performance status (score of 0 on the Eastern Cooperative Oncology Group scale) and those who had not received prior systemic therapy.[64,65] Other factors associated with treatment include the development of systemic autophagy,[84] various autoimmune phenomena[85,86] such as thyroiditis and vitiligo and the presence of metastases restricted to the skin and soft tissues.[86] In addition, even in patients receiving high-dose IL-2, the likelihood of response appeared to correlate with the amount of IL-2 administered.[87] Analysis of tumors during IL-2 therapy for the presence of RNA transcripts of various immunoregulatory genes correlated tumor response to the pattern of gene expression.[88] Although these investigations have enhanced the understanding of the mechanisms underlying the antitumor effects of IL-2 activity, they have generally dealt with events that occur during and after treatment, and although these data are not without interest, they do not serve as a guide to clinicians in the selection of patients for IL-2–based therapy.

In the case of renal carcinoma, tumor response has been variably associated with performance status on the Eastern Cooperative Oncology Group scale, the number of metastatic sites, absence of bone metastases, prior nephrectomy, presence of tumor carbonic anhydrase IX, favorable (clear cell) histology, the degree of treatment-related thrombocytopenia, thyroid dysfunction, the extent of rebound lymphocytosis after treatment, erythropoietin production, low pretreatment plasma IL-6 levels, and high posttreatment levels of TNF-α and IL-1.[89] Data from a Cytokine Working Group phase 3 trial comparing high-dose IL-2 administered in hospital with IL-2 and IFN given on an outpatient basis (see "Combination IL-2–Based Therapy") suggested that in those receiving outpatient treatment, disease site factors such as an unresected primary tumor or the presence of hepatic or skeletal metastases correlated with poor treatment outcome.[90] These factors were less predictive of response in patients receiving high-dose IL-2. Additional retrospective studies suggested that the histologic pattern of the renal cancer also correlates with the probability of response to IL-2.[91] Response rates as high as 40% have been seen in patients whose primary tumors possessed favorable histologic features, such as clear cell histologic type with alveolar but no papillary or granular cell components. Conversely, those whose tumors displayed papillary or more than 50% granular features were unlikely to show a response. These correlations have been independently confirmed for metastatic lesions. The SELECT trial conducted by the Cytokine Working Group failed to demonstrate an ability to predict response, which still was remarkably good with a 25% response rate in patients with clear cell carcinoma. Immunohistochemical studies have suggested that the expression of the G250 antigen (carbonic anhydrase IX) on a large percentage of renal cancer cells is also associated with an increased likelihood of benefit from IL-2 treatment.[92,93]

Combination Interleukin 2-Based Therapy

A number of agents have been combined with IL-2 in an effort to improve the activity of IL-2–based therapy. These agents are listed in Table 45.3. Although preclinical laboratory and animal studies

TABLE 45.3

APPROACHES TO IMPROVE THE ACTIVITY OF INTERLEUKIN-2 (IL-2)

NOVEL PREPARATIONS
Liposomal IL-2
IL-2–based gene therapy
IL-2 selective agonists

COMBINATION WITH OTHER CYTOKINES
Interferon-α
Interferon-γ
Tumor necrosis factor
IL-4, IL-12, IL-18
Granulocyte-macrophage colony-stimulating factor

COMBINATION WITH MONOCLONAL ANTIBODIES
Tumor antigen target
T-cell activation antigen target

COMBINATION WITH VACCINES
Nonspecific tumor derived
HLA-restricted peptide
Dendritic cell based

COMBINATION WITH ADAPTIVE IMMUNOTHERAPY
Lymphokine-activated killer cell
Tumor-infiltrating lymphocytes (TILs) or T-cells transfected TCR
CD8+ selected TILs
Tumor antigen–specific CD8+ TILs

IL-2–BASED BIOCHEMOTHERAPY
5-Fluorouracil based
Cisplatin-dacarbazine based

DIMINUTION OF IMMUNE SUPPRESSION
Histamine
Lymphodepletion
CTLA-4 Antibody

may have provided a strong rationale for these combinations, for the most part, the subsequent clinical trials with the exception of CTLA4 antibody have failed to demonstrate any advantage of these combinations over high-dose IL-2 monotherapy.[94]

A major focus of this line of investigation has involved combinations of IL-2 and IFN-α. Despite promising laboratory studies suggesting synergy, early clinical studies with high-dose IL-2 and IFN have not demonstrated any benefit over high-dose IL-2 alone.[95,96] On the other hand, a number of regimens involving combinations of low-dose IL-2 and IFN appeared promising. These regimens can be administered safely in an outpatient setting and appear to possess sufficient antitumor activity to be considered by many as an alternative to high-dose IL-2.[97,98] In addition, these low-dose IL-2 and IFN combinations can be modified to include other potentially active agents such as chemotherapeutic drugs.

Phase 3 investigations of low-dose IL-2 and IFN combinations have, however, prompted a reconsideration of these apparent advantages. For example, the Cytokine Working Group completed a phase 3 trial comparing high-dose IL-2 therapy with IL-2 and IFN therapy given in an outpatient setting in patients with metastatic renal cancer. This study demonstrated a higher response rate in those randomly selected to receive the high-dose bolus IL-2 regimen (23% vs. 9%), with more patients progression-free at 3 years (10 vs. 3).[99] In addition, despite the greater acute toxicity associated with high-dose IL-2, the overall quality of life appeared to be at least equivalent to that of patients receiving the more protracted lower-dose regimen.[100]

Low-dose IL-2 regimens are generally ineffective in melanoma,[77] and it remains to be seen whether the addition of IFN and other agents (e.g., chemotherapeutic drugs) appreciably extends the survival of patients with advanced metastatic disease. Despite promising phase 2 data, several phase 3 studies have failed to show any advantage for biochemotherapy (the addition of cisplatin and dacarbazine–based chemotherapy to IL-2 and IFN) relative to chemotherapy or immunotherapy alone.[101–103] Preliminary data suggest that the addition of maintenance low-dose IL-2 after an initial course of biochemotherapy may improve overall responses. If this proves true in large prospective studies, a modified form of biochemotherapy featuring long-term low-dose IL-2 administration may yet revive the interest of clinicians in complicated multiagent regimens of this sort.

Efforts to combine IL-2 with other potentially active cytokines such as IFN-α TNF, IL-4, and GM-CSF were largely unsuccessful and have been abandoned.[94] One study has suggested that IL-2 can restore and maintain the biologic activity of IL-12 when it is administered chronically and that such restoration may enhance the clinical efficacy of this agent; however, overall response rates for this combination were still modest at best.[104] Combinations of IL-2 with a variety of monoclonal antibodies directed either against tumor antigens (GD2 or GD3 gangliosides or CD20) or T-cell activation antigens (CD3) have also been disappointing.[78,105,106] Histamine has been administered in association with IL-2 in an effort to block immune dysfunction associated with superoxide production by macrophages. Although a randomized phase 3 trial comparing low-dose IL-2 plus histamine with low-dose IL-2 alone in patients with metastatic melanoma produced few tumor responses, improved survival was noted for those receiving the combination, particularly in the subset of patients with hepatic metastases.[107] A confirmatory trial restricted to patients with hepatic metastases has recently been completed and results should be available shortly. We have demonstrated that the antimalarial agent, chloroquine, used as an autophagy inhibitor has activity in combination with IL-2 therapy, and a randomized phase 2 Cytokine Working Group trial will be initiated soon.

Investigators have also continued to pursue the use of IL-2 together with cellular therapy approaches. IL-2 and TIL combinations were extremely promising in animal tumor models,[108] and preliminary studies involving administration of IL-2 and TILs to patients with melanoma or IL-2 plus IFN and selected CD8+ TILs to patients with renal cell carcinoma yielded encouraging results; however, selection bias could not be excluded as an explanation for the unusually high response rates reported.[109] A subsequent randomized trial of low-dose IL-2 with or without CD8+ TILs in patients with metastatic renal cell carcinoma produced such a disappointingly low response rate for both treatment arms[110] that no definite conclusion could be drawn regarding the potential role of TILs in the treatment of this disease. Interest in adoptive immunotherapy has been revived by an NCI Surgery Branch study involving the administration of clonally expanded, tumor antigen–specific CD8+ lymphocytes and IL-2 after fludarabine-induced lymphodepletion that showed encouraging antitumor activity in patients with refractory melanoma.[111] This has been extended to include the use of T-cell receptors recognizing melanoma and transfected into autologous lymphocytes administered in conjunction with nonmyeloablative chemotherapy, and most recently radiotherapy with impressive responses in patients with advanced melanoma.[112–114]

TILs have also proven to be a valuable tool for identifying melanoma-associated tumor regression antigens.[115] Extensive research at the NCI Surgery Branch and elsewhere has identified HLA-restricted melanocyte lineage–specific antigens that are recognized by the cellular immune system in patients exhibiting a response to IL-2–based therapy. Active immunization trials with immunodominant peptides derived from these tumor regression antigens have produced some encouraging results.[116] For example, vaccination with a mutated version of the gp100 peptide antigen together with high-dose IL-2 produced tumor responses in more than 40% of patients.[117] Although the Cytokine Working Group found that only 10% of patients exhibited tumor responses,[118] a randomized multicenter trial of high-dose IL-2 with or without the gp100 peptide vaccine were reported at the 2009 meeting of the American Society of Clinical Oncology with statistically significant increases in response to treatment with the combination when compared with IL-2 alone; this study has now been submitted for publication (Schwartzentruber D, Lawson D, Richards J, et al., unpublished data, 2009).

Although the clinical application of IL-2 has benefited only a small portion of patients with either melanoma or renal cancer to date, it remains the only treatment that can produce durable benefit in more than an occasional patient with one of these diseases. Unfortunately, efforts to build on the successes seen with high-dose IL-2 alone have been largely disappointing. However, as more information is gained about the mechanism of action of IL-2 and the workings of the immune system in general, it is likely that IL-2–based treatment regimens will be refined and the appropriate patient populations to receive IL-2 will be better defined, which will lead ultimately to improved therapeutic results. Recently, the ability of IL-2 to modify Tregs, a concern in preclinical studies, has failed to show dramatic effects on circulating functional activities.[119,120]

Interleukin 4

IL-4 has also been successfully administered to patients with malignancy alone and in combination with IL-2. We initiated studies in 1988[121–123] based on evidence that it enhanced expansion of tumor infiltrating lymphocytes from melanomas.[124] We demonstrated rhinitis, acute gastric mucosal injury, and hypotension in these studies without apparent increased efficacy. Subsequent clinical trials[125–132] have demonstrated similar flulike illnesses and little evidence of clinical responses alone or as a gene therapy (Lotze MT, unpublished data, 1999). IL-4 administration caused degranulation of eosinophils with release of major basic protein and enhanced eosinophil number and survival,[133] although previous studies had suggested that the IL-2–induced hypereosinophilia to extraordinary levels was mediated likely by IL-5 induced by this treatment.[134]

Interleukin 7

We initially suggested that IL-7 might be useful for cancer therapy based on results suggesting its role as a lymphopoietin, enhancing lymphokine-activated killer cell activity and promoting the growth of tumor-infiltrating lymphocytes.[135–137] We also showed subsequently that it could be used to expand T cells recognizing tumor cells of epithelial origin[138–140] consistent with its role in immunity. Although reports of IL-7 gene therapy soon followed,[141,142] it was not until the last couple of years that rIL-7 in sufficient quantities was available for clinical testing.[143,144] These studies suggested that IL-7 might be useful in the treatment of patients with lymphopenia, enhancing cell number without increasing Tregs. When rhIL-7 was given subcutaneously every other day for 2 weeks in a dose-escalation study, only mild to moderate constitutional symptoms, reversible spleen and lymph node enlargement, and marked increase in peripheral CD3(+), CD4(+), and CD8(+) lymphocytes were observed in a dose-dependent and age-independent manner.[144]

Interleukin 9

IL-9, originally described as a factor capable of enhancing T-helper 2 (Th2) activity, has not been given to patients. Its inhibition is suggested by intriguing studies in allogeneic skin transplants in which it appears to be critical for maintenance of Tregs through a mast cell–dependent process.[145]

Interleukin 15

Discovered almost 2 decades ago, IL-15 has just entered clinical trials at the National Institutes of Health. It shares both the β and γ signaling chains of IL-2, and yet in many studies it has been demonstrated to have substantial ability to increase T cells specific for tumor without impacting on Tregs and to be required for NK expansion, recently with targeted inhibition of IL-15 in the setting of NK leukemias.[146] In primate models, IL-15 administration expands memory CD8(+) and CD4(+) T cells, and NK cells in the peripheral blood, with minimal increases in CD4(+)CD25(+)Foxp3(+) regulatory T cells, boding well for the ongoing clinical trials.[147]

Interleukin 21

IL-21 shares a common γ chain receptor with other members of the extended IL-2 family and has recently entered clinical trials in patients with renal cell carcinoma and melanoma; it is associated with cytokinelike effects. Complete and partial responses have been observed in patients with melanoma and renal cell carcinoma.[148,149] Increases in serum-soluble CD25, frequencies of CD25(+) NK and CD8(+) T cells, and mRNA for IFN-γ, perforin, and granzyme B in CD8(+) T and NK cells, consistent with known biologic effects of this cytokine were observed. rIL-21 administered at 30 mcg/kg/d in 5-day cycles every second week is biologically active and well tolerated in patients with metastatic melanoma.

INTERLEUKIN 6 FAMILY

Interleukin 6

IL-6 is increased in the serum of patients with acute trauma, burns, and infections and is found in the serum of patients with chronic disease states including autoimmunity, chronic viral infection, and cancer. As such, it serves as a suitable surrogate for disease progression in many states. The rationale for its application clinically was based on activity in murine models, although a more modern sense is that its inhibition, largely in autoimmune settings, might be useful.[150] Clinical trials of IL-6 have shown essentially no clinical antitumor activity with a variety of constitutional, hematologic, and neurologic effects.[151–153] Recently, clinical trials of anti-IL6R antibodies (Tocilizumab) in patients with rheumatoid arthritis[154] have shown great promise as have chimeric anti-IL6 (siltuximab) antibodies in patients with the atypical lymphoproliferative disorder Castleman disease,[155] most of whom had complete eradication of apparent disease.

Interleukin-12

IL-12 is a dendrikine, identified and cloned from Epstein-Barr virus–transformed B-cell lines. Although originally defined as an NK-stimulating factor and a cytolytic lymphocyte maturation factor, it became clear that IL12 acted early in immunity to polarize and promote T-helper 1 (Th1) development. Enhancing IFN-γ production, proliferation and cytolytic activity of NK and T cells, IL-12 primarily promotes cellular immunity, In the absence of IFNγ or with immature immune cells such as those derived from cord blood, IL-12 can actually promote a Th2 response. Although we demonstrated substantial antitumor activity of IL-12 in several preclinical studies, our clinical trials with either recombinant IL-12 or its application as a gene therapy demonstrated limited efficacy. More recently identified IL-12 family members (IL-23 and IL-27) are now available to be considered for either administration or blocking in the setting of cancer.

Our animal[156,157] and human clinical studies that attribute improved clinical outcome[158] and mechanisms of IL-12–based therapy[159] to strong type 1 responses *in situ*. IL-12 is produced as a heterodimeric cytokine composed of two covalently linked p35 and p40 subunits[160] by activated macrophages, neutrophils, and DCs, acting as adaptors/regulators of cell-mediated responses. The biological functions of IL-12 are mediated by the IL-12 receptor[161] composed of two chains (β1 and β2). Engaging these receptors activates JAK2/Tyk2 and in turn causes phosphorylation of STAT4.[161] More recent studies support its critical role as a third signal for $CD8^+$ T cell differentiation,[162,163] and its ability to serve as an important factor in the reactivation and survival of memory $CD4^+$ T cells.[164]

PHARMACOLOGY OF CANCER THERAPEUTICS

Innate and Adaptive Immunity Promoted by Interleukin 12

IL-12 enhances generation and survival of cytotoxic T cells by promoting transcription expression of perforin and granzyme.[165] Production of the IL-12 heterodimer (IL-12p70) occurs when bacterial products, so-called (PAMPs) or DAMPs, and cytokines such as IFN-γ or CD40L-CD40 ligand receptor interactions act in concert for production of both p35 and p40 subunits.[166] Conversely, IL-10 and TGF-β1 negatively regulate IL-12 production by suppressing transcription of the IL-12 p40 subunit.[167,168] We[169,170] as well as others[171] demonstrated that IL-12 had potent antitumor activity at very low doses against established murine tumors requiring both $CD4^+$ and $CD8^+$ T cells. The efficacy of IL-12 was diminished in nude mice and this activity was mediated by NK cells. We also demonstrated that combinations of IL-12 with IL-18[172] in preclinical models profoundly synergized engaging NK, NKT, $CD4^+$ and $CD8^+$ T cells.[171,173]

Clinical Studies with Interleukin 12

IL-12 has been evaluated in patients with solid and hematologic tumors,[104,174–179] most frequently in patients with melanoma or renal cell carcinomas. It has been applied as either monotherapy (Table 45.4) or in combination with other therapies

TABLE 45.4

CLINICAL STUDIES OF SYSTEMIC INTERLEUKIN 12 (IL-12) ALONE

Tumors	Route of Administration	No. of Patients	OR (%)	Immune Modulation	Angiogenesis-Related Effects	Refs.
Individual solid tumors[a]	IV	40	5	■ Dose-dependent ↑ sIFN-γ; peak at 24–48 h after IL-12 ■ ↓ CD4+/CD8+ and CD16+ cells; nadir at 24 h after IL-12 ■ ↑ of NK cell adhesion molecules (CD2, LFA-1)	ND	174, 200
Melanoma[a]	SC	10	0 3 MRs	■ ↑ sIFN-γ within 24 h after the 1st IL-12 injection; ■ ↑ IL-10 during the second cycle; ■ Lymphopenia and CD4/CD8 ratio inversion. ■ ↓ CD16+cells 24 h after the 1st injection; ■ ↑ Frequency of antitumor CTL precursors; ■ Tumor infiltration by CD8+ memory T cells.	■ ↓ Urine bFGF in 2 of 3 patients with MR	179, 180
Renal cell carcinoma[a]	SC	51	2	■ ↑ sIFN-γ with peak level at 24 h after the first maintenance dose	ND	201
Cutaneous T-cell lymphoma[a]	SC or intralesionally	10	56	■ ↑ CD8+ and/or TIA-1+ T cells in skin biopsy from regressing lesions	ND	175
Melanoma, renal cell carcinoma[a]	IV	28	3	■ Induction of IFN-γ, IL-15 and IL-18, maintained in patients with tumor regression or prolonged disease stabilization	ND	181
Renal cell carcinoma[b]	SC	30	7	■ ↑ sIFN-γ, IL-10 and neopterin, maintained in cycle 2	ND	202
Abdominal tumors[a]	IP	29	7	■ ↑ peritoneal CD3+ and ↓ CD14+ cells	■ ↓ bFGF and VEGF in tumor; ■ ↑IFN-γ and IP-10 transcripts in peritoneal exudate cells	183
Bladder cancer[a]	Intravesically	15	0	No urine/serum IFN-γ induction	ND	182
Renal cell carcinoma[a]	SC	26	NA	■ Dose-dependent ↑ sIFN-γ, TNF-α, IL-10, IL-6 and IL-8 at first injection. ■ Lymphopenia; ■ Further ↑ IL-10 during treatment	ND	203
Cervical carcinoma[b]	IV	34	3	■ ↑ lymphoproliferative responses to HPV 16 E4, E6 and E7 peptides.	ND	204
Head-neck carcinoma[a]	Intratumorally	10	ND	■ ↑ CD56+ NK cells in the primary tumor; ■ high IFN-γ mRNA expression at lymph node level	ND	205
AIDS-related Kaposi sarcoma[a]	SC	34	50 (71 at highest doses)	■ ↑ sIFN-γ after 1st dose, persisting after week 4	↑ sIP-10 after the 1st dose, persisting after week 4	177
Mycosis fungoides[b]	SC	23	43	ND	ND	206

OR, overall response; IV, intravenously; IFN, interferon; ND, not done; NK, natural killer; MR, minor response; ↓, decrease; ↑, increase; SC, subcutaneously; s, serum; bFGF, basic fibroblastic growth factor; CTL, cytotoxic T-lymphocyte; VEGF, vascular endothelial growth factor; IP, intraperitoneally; NA, not available.

[a]Pilot/phase 1 trial.

[b]Phase 2 trial.

(Modified from Del Vecchio M, Bajetta E, Canova S, et al. Interleukin-12: biological properties and clinical application. *Clin Cancer Res* 2007;13:4677–4685.)

TABLE 45.5

CLINICAL STUDIES OF SYSTEMIC INTERLEUKIN 12 (IL-12) IN COMBINATION WITH VACCINES, OTHER CYTOKINES, OR ANTITUMOR MONOCLONAL ANTIBODIES

Tumors	Combined Treatment	No. of Patients	OR (%)	Immune Modulation	Angiogenesis-Related Effects	Refs
Melanoma[a]	gp100 and tyrosinase peptides	48	ND.	■ Ag-specific immune response against the peptide vaccine, as shown by ↑IFN-γ release in most patients	ND	176
Melanoma[a]	Melan-A/Mart-1 and influenza peptides	28	8	■ ↑ sIFN-γ within 24 h after the 1st IL-12 injection.	ND	207
Melanoma[b]	Melan-A/Mart-1 peptide-pulsed PBMC	20	10	■ ↑ IFN-γ-producing T cells directed to Melan-A/Mart-1 after vaccination	ND	208
Melanoma, renal cell carcinoma[a]	IL-2	28	11	■ ↑ IFN-γ production and expansion of NK cells	↑ IP-10 production	104
Melanoma, renal cell carcinoma*	IFN-α2b	26	11	■ CD80 and IFN-γ induction in PBMCs of selected patients by RT-PCR.	RT-PCR on PBMCs showed induction of IP-10 and IFN-γ in selected patients	185
HER2+ tumors[a]	Trastuzumab	15	6	■ ↑ IFN-γ production by NK cells in responsive or stable patients; associated with IFN-γ gene polymorphism.	■ ↑ sMIP-1α, TNF-α and IP-10	186
B-cell NHL (previously treated patients)[b]	Rituximab	58	41	■ In a few patients ↑ expression of IL-12-related genes as IFN-γ, CXCL10, IFIT2, IFIT4, Il-8 and CXCL2; ■ Greater variability in TCR repertoire from concurrent rituximab-treated patients	ND	178

OR, overall response; ND, not done; ↑, increase; IFN, interferon; NK, natural killer; PBMCs, peripheral blood mononuclear cells; RT-PCR, reverse transcription polymerase chain reaction; TNF, tumor necrosis factor; NHL, non–Hodgkin's lymphoma; TCR, T-cell receptor.
[a]Pilot/phase 1 trial.
[b]Phase 2 trial.
(Modified from Del Vecchio M, Bajetta E, Canova S, et al. Interleukin-12: biological properties and clinical application. *Clin Cancer Res* 2007;13:4677–4685.)

(Table 45.5). Efficacy in patients with cutaneous T-cell lymphoma,[175,176] AIDS-related Kaposi sarcoma,[177] and B-cell non–Hodgkin's lymphoma,[178] was noted. In the first published trial, we[174] enrolled 40 patients, including 20 with renal cancer and 12 with melanoma, in a phase 1 dose-escalation study of IV-administered recombinant human IL-12 (rHuIL-12). The maximum-tolerated dose was 500 ng/kg, and dose-limiting toxicities included liver function test abnormalities and stomatitis. A transient complete response (at pleural and cervical lymph node level; duration, 4 weeks) in a melanoma patient and one partial response in a patient with renal cell cancer were documented. Both responses were observed in previously untreated patients. Toxicity was mild and included fever, fatigue, nausea, vomiting, and headache. Bajetta et al.[179] enrolled ten pretreated patients with advanced melanoma in a pilot study. The patients received a fixed dose of rHuIL-12 (0.5 mcg/kg) on days 1, 8, and 15 for two sequential 28-day cycles. No partial or complete responses were documented, but tumor shrinkage involving subcutaneous metastases, superficial adenopathy (duration up to 14 weeks), and hepatic metastases was observed. IL-12[180] administration induced a striking burst, in the periphery, of HLA-restricted cytotoxic T-lymphocyte precursors (CTLp) directed to autologous tumor and to an immunogenic tumor-associated antigen (Melan-A/Mart-1_{26-35} peptide). Interestingly, infiltration of neoplastic tissue by CD8+ T cells with a memory and cytolytic phenotype identified by immunohistochemistry in eight of eight posttreatment metastatic lesions, but not in five of five pretreatment metastatic lesions from three patients.[180]

Using twice-weekly injection[181] increased serum levels of IFN-γ, IL-15, and IL-18 were noted in treated patients. Interestingly, although IFN-γ and IL-15 induction were attenuated during the first cycle in patients with disease progression, patients with tumor regression or stable disease showed constant higher levels of IFN-γ, IL-15 and IL-18.[181] Intravesical IL-12[182] in patients with recurrent superficial transitional cell carcinoma of the bladder was evaluated giving intravesical IL-12 weekly for 6 weeks. No objective responses were observed. Intraperitoneal administration[183] of IL-12 to patients with peritoneal carcinomatosis through an indwelling peritoneal catheter had essentially no responses. When applied as an adjuvant to vaccination[176] in patients with melanoma, enhanced delayed type hypersensitivity reactivity and IFNγ reactivity to the gp100 antigen was noted in most patients. Subsequent studies[176] with rHuIL-12 administered with melanoma peptides intradermally demonstrated mixed clinical responses Although profound antitumor responses were observed in our murine tumor models, the reasons for the limited clinical efficacy of IL-12 in patients is poorly understood. Our studies[184] showed tachyphylaxis to IL-12 following initial administration. A strategy of slowly increasing the dose of IL-12 (*crescendo ma non troppo*) that we proposed was never tested. Use of IL-12 in combination with other cytokines or tumor-specific monoclonal antibodies were likewise of limited efficacy.[185,186]

Evaluation of Interleukin 12 Gene Therapy

We have treated over 30 patients with direct injection of IL-12–transfected fibroblasts without response, publishing our results in Korean studies[187] with only transient reduction of tumor size. Similar studies using tumors transduced or direct injection of plasmid DNA–encoding IL-12 were ineffective.[187–190]

Interleukin 23

IL-23 shares the p40 chain with IL-12, associating with the p19 chain.[191] IL-23 serves to promote TH4/TH_{17} cells producing the cytokines IL-6, IL-17, IL-22, and IL-25. These cytokines appear to play roles in the priming and reactivation of polarized T-cell responses. Both IL-12p70 and IL-27 can exert effects in the priming of Th1 $CD4^+$ T cell responses,[192,193] with recent data suggesting a critical role for Treg survival. IL-12 and IL-23 enhance responses of memory T cells,[194] while IL-27 engagement with its receptor appears to limit inflammatory T-cell responses.[195] A further promising area of investigation, with potentially relevant clinical applications, stems from the emerging knowledge on newly discovered IL-12 family members. For example, in murine models, both IL-23 and IL-27 have been used to effectively treat tumors.[196,197] Comparison of ustekinumab (an IL-12 and IL-23 blocker targeting the p40 chain of IL-12) and etanercept (an inhibitor of TNF-α), showed superiority for p40 blockade for the treatment of patients with psoriasis.[198] Antibodies to both IL-23 and IL-23R are in clinical testing.

Interleukin 27 and Interleukin 35

IL-27 is also an heterodimeric cytokine composed of the EBI3 (Epstein-Barr virus–induced molecule 3) that associates with the IL-27 p28 chain.[191] These three proteins, IL-12, IL-23 and IL-27, show overlapping and distinct properties on the regulation of innate and adaptive immune responses. Similarly to IL-12, IL-23 and IL-27 are produced predominantly by macrophages and DCs and affect IFN-γ production by T and NK cells.[191] IL-27 suppresses development of TH4/TH_{17} cells,[199] promoting Th1 development with expression of T-bet and IL-12Rβ2. The Epstein-Barr-virus–induced gene 3 (*Ebi3*, which encodes IL-27β) and IL-12α are expressed by mouse Tregs but not by CD4+ T cells. An *Ebi3*-IL-12α heterodimer is secreted by Tregs. This novel *Ebi3*-IL-12α heterodimeric cytokine has been designated IL-35. IL-35 confers regulatory activity on naive T cells, whereas recombinant IL-35 suppresses T-cell proliferation.[191] No clinical trials of either IL-27 or IL-35 have been conducted.

INTERLEUKIN 10 FAMILY

The IL-10 family members are closely related to the type I (IFNα and IFNβ and type II (IFNγ) interferons. Nominally, IL-10 exerts anti-inflammatory actions by counteracting many biological effects of IFN-γ, but we showed that systemic administration or delivery by retroviral vectors was associated with substantial antitumor effects.[209,210] To our knowledge, IL-10 has never been tested in patients with cancer but it has been given to patients with inflammatory bowel disease,[211–213] with only minimal improvement in patients treated in a number of clinical trials. Interestingly, in treated patients, significant increases in serum neopterin and phytohemagglutinin-induced IFN-γ production, possibly important for the lack of amelioration.[214] The newer IL-10 family members, IL-19, IL-20, IL-22, IL-24, IL-28, and IL-29, have yet to be tested in the clinic or to have demonstrable antitumor activity.[215–218] IL-28A, IL-28B, and IL-29 (also designated type III interferons) are a new subfamily within the IL-10 family, produced primarily by DCs after viral infection with antiviral and cytostatic activities. They could be interesting agents for patients with viral infections or tumors.[219] Tolerence is regulated by the IL-10 family and downstream effects of the IL2α chain.[220,221]

Selected References

The full list of references for this chapter appears in the online version.

1. Thomson AW, Lotze MT. *The Cytokine Handbook*. 4th ed. London: Academic Press, 2003.
2. Rubartelli A, Lotze MT. Inside, outside, upside-down: damage associated molecular pattern molecules and Redox. *Trends Immunol* 2007;28(10):429.
7. Sims JE, March CJ, Cosman D, et al. cDNA expression cloning of the IL-1 receptor, a member of the immunoglobulin superfamily. *Science* 1988;241(4865):585–589.
8. Schreuder H, Tardif C, Trump-Kallmeyer S, et al. A new cytokine-receptor binding mode revealed by the crystal structure of the IL-1 receptor with an antagonist. *Nature* 1997;386(6621):194.
22. Xiang Y, Moss B. Correspondence of the functional epitopes of poxvirus and human interleukin-18-binding proteins. *J Virol* 2001;75(20):9947–9954.
24. Robertson MJ, Mier JW, Logan T, et al. Clinical and biological effects of recombinant human interleukin-18 administered by intravenous infusion to patients with advanced cancer. *Clin Cancer Res* 2006;12(14 Pt 1):4265.
34. Hofstra LS, Kristensen GB, Willemse PH, et al. Randomized trial of recombinant human interleukin-3 versus placebo in prevention of bone marrow depression during first-line chemotherapy for ovarian carcinoma. *J Clin Oncol* 1998;16(10):3335–3344.
37. Kido S, Kuriwaka-Kido R, Umino-Miyatani Y, et al. Mechanical stress activates Smad pathway through PKCδ to enhance interleukin-11 gene transcription in osteoblasts. *PLoS One* 2010;5(9). pii:e13090.
38. Morgan DA, Ruscetti FW, Gallo R. Selective in vitro growth of T lymphocytes from normal human bone marrows. *Science* 1976;193(4257):1007.
39. Taniguchi T, Matsui H, Fujita T, et al. Structure and expression of a cloned cDNA for human interleukin-2. *Nature* 1983;302(5906):305.
47. Noguchi M, Yi H, Rosenblatt HM, et al. Interleukin-2 receptor gamma chain mutation results in X-linked severe combined immunodeficiency in humans. *Cell* 1993;73(1):147.
51. Russell SM, Johnston JA, Noguchi M, et al. Interaction of IL-2R beta and gamma c chains with Jak1 and Jak3: implications for XSCID and XCID. *Science* 1994;266(5187):1042–1045.

54. Lotze MT, Grimm EA, Mazumder A, Strausser JL, Rosenberg SA. Lysis of fresh and cultured autologous tumor by human lymphocytes cultured in T-cell growth factor. *Cancer Res* 1981;41(11 Pt 1):4420.
60. Rosenberg SA, Lotze MT, Muul LM, et al. Observations on the systemic administration of autologous lymphokine-activated killer cells and recombinant interleukin-2 to patients with metastatic cancer. *N Engl J Med* 1985;313(23):1485.
63. Rosenberg SA, Lotze MT, Yang JC, et al. Prospective randomized trial of high-dose interleukin-2 alone or in conjunction with lymphokine-activated killer cells for the treatment of patients with advanced cancer. *J Natl Cancer Inst* 1993;85(8):622.
65. Atkins MB, Lotze MT, Dutcher JP, et al. High-dose recombinant interleukin 2 therapy for patients with metastatic melanoma: analysis of 270 patients treated between 1985 and 1993. *J Clin Oncol* 1999;17(7):2105–2116.
78. Yang JC, Sherry RM, Steinberg SM, et al. Randomized study of high-dose and low-dose interleukin-2 in patients with metastatic renal cancer. *J Clin Oncol* 2003;21(16):3127–3132.
111. Dudley ME, Wunderlich JR, Robbins PF, et al. Cancer regression and autoimmunity in patients after clonal repopulation with antitumor lymphocytes. *Science* 2002;298(5594):850–854.
114. Morgan RA, Dudley ME, Wunderlich JR, et al. Cancer regression in patients after transfer of genetically engineered lymphocytes. *Science* 2006;314(5796):126.
124. Kawakami Y, Haas GP, Lotze MT. Expansion of tumor-infiltrating lymphocytes from human tumors using the T-cell growth factors interleukin-2 and interleukin-4. *J Immunother Emphasis Tumor Immunol* 1993;14(4):336–347.
128. Atkins MB, Vachino G, Tilg HJ, et al. Phase I evaluation of thrice-daily intravenous bolus interleukin-4 in patients with refractory malignancy. *J Clin Oncol* 1992;10(11):1802.
138. Maeurer MJ, Martin D, Walter W, et al. Human intestinal Vdelta1+ lymphocytes recognize tumor cells of epithelial origin. *J Exp Med* 1996;183(4):1681.
146. Morris JC, Janik JE, White JD, et al. Preclinical and phase I clinical trial of blockade of IL-15 using Mikbeta1 monoclonal antibody in T cell large granular lymphocyte leukemia. *Proc Natl Acad Sci U S A* 2006;103(2):401.
151. Weber J, Yang JC, Topalian SL, et al. Phase I trial of subcutaneous interleukin-6 in patients with advanced malignancies. *J Clin Oncol* 1993;11(3):499.
160. Kobayashi M, Fitz L, Ryan M, et al. Identification and purification of natural killer cell stimulatory factor (NKSF), a cytokine with multiple biologic effects on human lymphocytes. *J Exp Med* 1989;170(3):827.
169. Nastala CL, Edington HD, McKinney TG, et al. Recombinant IL-12 administration induces tumor regression in association with IFN-gamma production. *J Immunol* 1994;153(4):1697–1706.
170. Tahara H, Zeh HJ III, Storkus WJ, et al. Fibroblasts genetically engineered to secrete interleukin 12 can suppress tumor growth and induce antitumor immunity to a murine melanoma in vivo. *Cancer Res* 1994;54(1):182–189.
174. Atkins MB, Robertson MJ, Gordon M, et al. Phase I evaluation of intravenous recombinant human interleukin 12 in patients with advanced malignancies. *Clin Cancer Res* 1997;3(3):409.
187. Kang WK, Park C, Yoon HL, et al. Interleukin 12 gene therapy of cancer by peritumoral injection of transduced autologous fibroblasts: outcome of a phase I study. *Hum Gene Ther* 2001;12(6):671.
192. Pflanz S, Timans JC, Cheung J, et al. IL-27, a heterodimeric cytokine composed of EBI3 and p28 protein, induces proliferation of naive CD4(+) T cells. *Immunity* 2002;16(6):779.
209. Berman RM, Suzuki T, Tahara H, et al. Systemic administration of cellular IL-10 induces an effective, specific, and long-lived immune response against established tumors in mice. *J Immunol* 1996;157(1):231–238.
210. Suzuki T, Tahara H, Narula S, et al. Viral interleukin 10 (IL-10), the human herpes virus 4 cellular IL-10 homologue, induces local anergy to allogeneic and syngeneic tumors. *J Exp Med* 1995;182(2):477.
213. Colombel JF, Rutgeerts P, Malchow H, et al. Interleukin 10 (Tenovil) in the prevention of postoperative recurrence of Crohn's disease. *Gut* 2001;49(1):42–46.

CHAPTER 46 ANTISENSE AGENTS

CY A. STEIN AND HARRIS S. SOIFER

How can the specificity of chemotherapy be increased and the nonspecific toxicity decreased? One of the more conceptually elegant ways to accomplish this is to target the messenger RNA (mRNA) that encodes the nucleic acid sequence and will be translated by the ribosome into a specific protein. If that protein is responsible for the growth or viability of a tumor cell, then a knockdown in its expression may lead to either sensitization of the cell to cytotoxic chemotherapy or to cellular death. The targeting of the Bcl-2 mRNA, which will be discussed below, is an example of such a strategy that has found clinical application.

In targeting the mRNA that encodes the protein, advantage can be taken of the exquisite specificity of the Watson-Crick base pair interaction that should, at least in theory, produce a highly specific therapy. All that is required is to know the sequence of the mRNA and a small piece of DNA, or siRNA, can be chemically synthesized complementary to it. A simple calculation demonstrates that an oligodeoxynucleotide of 15 to 17 mer in length is sufficiently long so that its sequence is represented only once in the entire human genome.[1] Because the mRNA sequence is defined as "sense," the complementary oligodeoxyribonucleotide is the "antisense." The binding of the antisense oligodeoxyribonucleotide (oligonucleotide) to its target mRNA forms a hybrid mRNA-DNA duplex species. The formation of this duplex leads, as will be described, to the inhibition of translation of that mRNA into protein.

In theory, antisense biotechnology provides a highly specific way of eliminating the activity of a protein because of the specificity of the Watson-Crick base pair interaction. In practice, however, it has been far more difficult to obtain clinical successes with antisense oligonucleotides than was ever considered at the time extensive research on this method began more than 25 years ago.[2]

OLIGONUCLEOTIDE STABILITY AND EFFICACY: THE ROLE OF PHOSPHOROTHIOATES

Normal DNA, which contains phosphodiester linkages bridging the deoxyribose sugars in the oligonucleotide chain, cannot be used as antisense molecules. This is because they are digested rapidly in human plasma, mostly by exonuclease activity.[3] The class of oligonucleotide that is currently used in the clinic is the phosphorothioate. In a phosphorothioate oligonucleotide, a sulfur atom, replaces an oxygen atom at a nonbridging position at each phosphorus in the chain, but the charge, and thus the property of aqueous solubility, is retained. Phosphorothioate oligonucleotides are also much more nuclease resistant than phosphodiesters,[4] but they are not nuclease proof. It is also possible that the nonantisense, nonspecific properties of phosphorothioates can synergize with their sequence specific functions. This may produce the types of overall anticancer effects that have been commonly observed both *in vitro* and *in vivo*, which invariably appear to be the result of a combination of antisense plus nonantisense effects.

Mechanism of Action of the Antisense Effect

The binding of a charged oligonucleotide to its complementary mRNA elicits the activity of a ubiquitous intranuclear enzyme known as RNase H. This enzyme cleaves the mRNA strand of the mRNA-oligonucleotide duplex.[5] This renders the antisense oligonucleotide "pseudocatalytic," as it can then dissociate from the cleaved mRNA and bind to another identical mRNA. The cleaved mRNA is then very rapidly degraded. Due to the activity of RNase H, one can employ phosphorothioate oligonucleotides at submicromolar concentrations to produce antisense effects. Essentially, the only classes of oligonucleotide that can elicit RNase H activity are phosphodiesters and phosphorothioates. All other classes of oligonucleotide, including peptide nucleic acids and morpholino oligonucleotides, cannot. Although the activity of RNase H is important for the submicromolar efficacy of antisense phosphorothioate oligonucleotides, a problem arises because the enzyme is not stringent. For example, although G3139, the anti-Bcl-2 phosphorothioate oligonucleotide that has completed several phase 3 clinical trials, is 18 mer in length, RNAse H does not require an intact 18 mer mRNA-G3139 duplex to cleave the Bcl-2 mRNA. Rather, it may require a duplex region of only 6 to 10 mer in length in order to cleave the target.[6] However, in any 18 mer, there are a relatively large number of nested 6- to 10-mer sequences, although these short sequences are not unique to the Bcl-2 mRNA. In fact, these short sequences may be scattered throughout the entire human transciptome, although many of these sites on nontargeted mRNAs will not be accessible either to the oligonucleotide, or to RNase H, or both. In theory, this lack of stringency can result in the RNase H cleavage of nontargeted mRNAs.[7] Despite the questions of nonsequence specificity, irrelevant cleavage, and myriad other issues, one phosphorothioate oligonucleotide has emerged, as of this writing, as the lead candidate to be the first anticancer antisense oligonucleotide, the anti-Bcl-2 molecule G3139.

Delivery of Oligonucleotides into Cells

For 20 years, it was universally accepted that gene silencing by oligonucleotides (oligos) cannot be accomplished to any significant extent *in vitro* unless the oligos are transfected into the cells,[8,9] usually by a lipid-based transfection reagent. Such reagents are usually cationic lipids, which form complexes with charged (but not uncharged) oligonucleotides, after which the lipid–oligo complex adsorbs to the cell surface and undergoes endocytosis into endosomes.[10] Within the endosome, the cationic lipid dissociates from the oligonucleotide[11] and inserts into the endosomal membrane, altering the lipid phase of the membrane and increasing the rate of endosomal rupture.[12] Once in the cytoplasm, oligonucleotides delivered by cationic lipids undergo transport to the nucleus by an unknown mechanism where the antisense effect is believed to occur.

The requirement for cationic lipids was born in part from the notion that the polarity of charged or uncharged oligonucleotides renders them impermeable to the hydrophobic lipid bilayer of the plasma membrane. However, even in the absence of cationic lipids, charged oligonucleotides such as phosphorothioates adsorb to the heparin-binding domains in plasma membrane proteins and undergo adsorptive endocytosis with the cell membrane to become localized within intracellular endosomal vesicles. Uncharged oligonucleotides, on the other hand, exhibit very low affinity for heparin-binding domains and thus can only be internalized from the bulk, or fluid, phase by the process of pinocytosis, and they too localize in endosomes.[8] The pinocytotic process is inefficient compared to adsorptive endocytosis, which is another reason that uncharged oligonucleotides are difficult to employ as antisense molecules. Even after adsorptive endocytosis of charged oligonucleotides in tissue culture, the slow rate of spontaneous endosomal rupture (endosomolysis) in the absence of cationic lipids was considered a significant barrier given that high levels of oligonucleotide in the nucleus were believed to be critical for antisense efficacy.

While endosomolysis and nuclear delivery may be important to the antisense effect when cationic lipids are employed to deliver oligonucleotides to cells in culture, recent evidence indicates that phosphorothioate oligonucleotides can promote efficient sequence-specific gene silencing in the absence of transfection reagents in tissue culture systems. This method of antisense silencing, in which the oligos were delivered "naked" (*gymnos* in Greek), that is, without conjugates or transfectants, has been named gymnotic delivery.

Gymnotic Delivery of Oligonucleotides in Tissue Culture

Gymnotic delivery, defined as the ability to achieve antisense effects in cells by oligonucleotide delivery in the absence of any carrier whatsoever,[13] represents a dramatic change in the oligo delivery paradigm that challenges the current proposed mechanism of gene silencing by antisense DNA. The long-held notion that high nuclear levels of oligo are required for gene silencing has now been demonstrated to be untrue, as oligos delivered by gymnosis are active in the cytoplasm. Further, endosome escape may not be necessary for productive gene silencing to occur, as gymnosis delivers oligo to cytoplasmic foci that interact with the RNA silencing machinery. In addition, gymnotic delivery can define optimum oligo chemistry for *in vivo* applications, as *in vitro* gymnosis appears to correlate with productive *in vivo* gene silencing.[13]

Gymnotic delivery does not require the use of any transfection reagent or any serum additives to serum whatsoever to promote gene silencing. Unmodified phosphorothioate oligos are not gymnotically active, with the exception of G3139. Optimum results were obtained with locked nucleic acid (LNA) phosphorothioate gapmers. The two LNA moieties at the 5′ and one base upstream from the 3′ molecular termini increase the T_m of the mRNA-DNA duplex by approximately 4 to 6°C/base modification, as well as virtually eliminate 3, 5 exonuclease digestion.[14] In a typical gymnotic silencing experiment, adherent cells are seeded at low plating density so that they would just attain confluence on the final day of the experiment. The day after plating, oligos are added directly to the culture media (typical concentrations were 1 to 5 mcM). Measurement of the antisense effect through RNA or protein analysis is conducted 6 to 10 days following PS-LNA gapmer treatment. Long-term gene silencing (more than 180 days) could be achieved through serial passage of cells at low density and oligo retreatment. Efficient gymnotic silencing has been observed in a wide variety of human cancer cell lines, and *in vivo* as well.

CLINICAL TRIALS OF G3139 (OBLIMERSEN) IN CHRONIC LYMPHOCYTIC LEUKEMIA

Increasing evidence suggests that the pathogenesis of chronic lymphocytic leukemia is linked to Bcl-2 overexpression.[15] High levels of Bcl-2 expression have been correlated with resistance to chemotherapy, and in the case of chronic lymphocytic leukemia (CLL), seem to directly influence tumor aggressiveness.[16,17] Preclinical studies demonstrated that oblimersen had significant single-agent activity against CLL cell lines and enhanced the cytotoxicity of several agents commonly used to treat this cancer, including fludarabine.[18,19] Phase 1 and 2 clinical data confirmed the modest single-agent activity of oblimersen in the treatment of relapsed or refractory CLL.[20]

Two hundred forty-one patients with relapsed or refractory CLL were randomized to receive treatment with chemotherapy alone (fludarabine $mg/m^2/d$ intravenous [IV] for 3 days plus cyclophosphamide 250 $mg/m^2/d$ IV for 3 days every 28 days) with or without oblimersen (3 mg/kg/d administered on days 1 through 7 by continuous intravenous infusion, plus fludarabine and cyclophosphamide administered at the same doses on days 5, 6, and 7).[21] Patients were stratified according to response to prior fludarabine therapy (responsive vs. refractory), number of prior treatment regimens (one or two vs. three or more), and duration of response to last prior therapy (6 months vs. 6 months). Patients were considered refractory if they failed to achieve at least a partial response (PR) or if disease recurred within 6 months of last prior treatment and were considered relapsed if disease recurred after achievement of at least a PR lasting more than 6 months. Responses were evaluated according to the National Cancer Institute Working Group Guidelines.[22] One hundred twenty patients received treatment with chemotherapy and oblimersen, and 121 patients received chemotherapy alone. Twenty patients (17%) in the oblimersen group achieved a complete remission (CR) or nodular partial response (nPR) compared with 8 patients (7%, considerably lower than anticipated) in the chemotherapy alone group ($P = .025$). Eleven patients (9%) in the oblimersen group and 3 patients (2%) in the chemotherapy-alone group achieved CR ($P = .03$).

Although there was no overall significant difference in time to progression (TTP) between the two treatment groups, TTP was closely correlated with response ($P < .001$). Among patients who achieved a CR or nPR, TTP was 2 years or greater in 70% of patients who received oblimersen, in comparison to 50% for those in the chemotherapy-alone group. Patients in both groups who achieved CR or nPR appeared to have substantial clinical benefit, with documented resolution of CLL related symptoms, including fever, night sweats, fatigue, and abdominal discomfort.

Although the overall estimated median survival did not differ significantly between the two treatment groups (33.8 months for the oblimersen group vs. 32.9 months in the chemotherapy-alone group) (Fig. 46.1), survival was closely correlated with

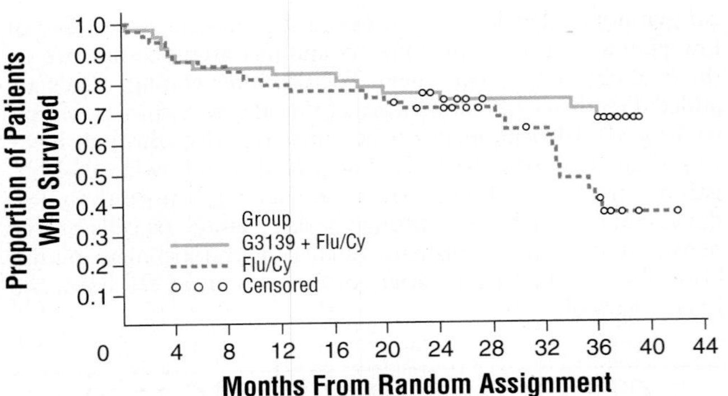

FIGURE 46.1 Oblimersen in chronic lymphocytic leukemia. Kaplan-Meier survival curves by treatment group. Fludarabine-sensitive patients median overall survival, not reached at 36 months for the oblimersen group and 33.2 months for chemotherapy-only (fludarabine and cyclophosphamide [Flu/Cy]) group (hazard ratio 0.53; P = .05). (Reprinted with permission © 2007 American Society of Clinical Oncology. All rights reserved.)

response (P <.001). The 5-year survival rate[23] among patients who achieved CR or nPR was 47% of the oblimersen group and 24% for those who received fludarabine and cyclophosphamide chemotherapy alone and was statistically significant (hazard ratio [HR] 0.60; P = .038). Increases in survival were observed in both CR and nPR patients. Most important, the greatest benefit was observed in patients who were fludarabine sensitive; the reduction in the risk of death at 5 years was 50% (P = .004), a marked improvement over data obtained at 3 years (HR 0.53; P = .05).

Nausea was the major non-hematologic adverse event observed in both treatment groups (72% for the oblimersen group versus 48% for patients treated with chemotherapy alone) (Table 46.1). However, this did not translate into a difference in antiemetic use between the two treatment groups. Catheter-related complications occurred more frequently among patients who received oblimersen (16% vs. 3%). Hematological toxicity, including thrombocytopenia and febrile neutropenia, occurred more often in the oblimersen group than in the chemotherapy-alone group. The oblimersen group experienced more bleeding events (all grades) than did the chemotherapy-alone group (19% vs. 8%), but the grade 3 to 4 bleeding events were low for both groups (4% and 2%, respectively). Five patients in the oblimersen group (4%) experienced a treatment-related adverse event with an outcome of death (septic shock, cytokine release syndrome, acute renal failure) versus two patients (2%) in the chemotherapy-alone arm (neutropenic sepsis and pseudomonal pneumonia).

CLINICAL TRIALS IN ADVANCED MELANOMA

The data obtained from a relatively small phase 1/2 trial led to the initiation of the largest phase 3 trial in advanced melanoma.[24] Between July 2000 and February 2003, 771 chemotherapy naïve patients with advanced malignant melanoma were randomly assigned to receive treatment with dacarbazine alone (1,000 mg/m^2/d intravenously for 60 minutes) or with oblimersen (7 mg/kg/d by continuous infusion for 5 days) followed by the same dacarbazine dose. Patients were stratified according to Eastern Cooperative Oncology Group (ECOG) performance status (0 vs. 1–2), presence or absence of liver metastasis, and disease site or serum lactate dehydrogenase (LDH) level. This latter category included two groups, patients with nonvisceral disease (skin, subcutaneous tissue, or lymph node disease) *and* normal LDH, and those with visceral disease (excluding liver) *or* elevated LDH (baseline serum level at least 1.1 times the upper limit of normal [ULN]).

With a minimum follow-up of 24 months, the median overall survival in the oblimersen-dacarbazine cohort was 9.0 months, compared with 7.8 months observed in the dacarbazine alone group (HR 0.87; 95% CI, 0.75 to 1.01; P = .077) (Fig. 46.2). Overall response rates (complete plus partial response) were 13.5% for patients treated with oblimersen plus dacarbazine and 7.5% for patients receiving dacarbazine alone (P = .007). Durable responses (>6 months) were also increased for the oblimersen-dacarbazine group (7.3% vs. 3.6%; P = .03). Eleven patients (2.3%) in the combination treatment arm achieved CR in comparison to three patients

TABLE 46.1

OBLIMERSEN IN CHRONIC LYMPHOCYTIC LEUKEMIA: NONHEMATOLOGIC ADVERSE EVENTS BY TREATMENT GROUP (OBLIMERSEN + FLUDARABINE/CYCLOPHOSPHAMIDE VS. FLUDARABINE/CYCLOPHOSPHAMIDE ALONE)

Frequently Reported Nonhematologic Adverse Events by Treatment Group: Treated Patients

	Grade 1 + Grade 2 (%)		Grade 3 + Grade 4 (%)	
Adverse Event[a]	Oblimersen Group	Chemotherapy-Only	Oblimersen Group	Chemotherapy-Only
Nausea	64.3	46.1	7.8	1.7
Pyrexia	44.3	26.1	3.5	2.6
Fatigue	38.3	27.0	6.1	4.3
Vomiting	24.3	22.6	6.1	0.9
Cough	27.0	21.7	0.9	0.0
Constipation	24.3	18.3	1.7	0.9
Headache	22.6	11.3	0.9	2.6
Diarrhea	20.9	13.0	0.9	0.9
Dyspnea	15.7	14.8	5.2	1.7

[a]Includes events reported in ≥ 20% of patients in either treatment group.
(From ref 23. Reprinted with permission © 2007 American Society of Clinical Oncology. All rights reserved.)

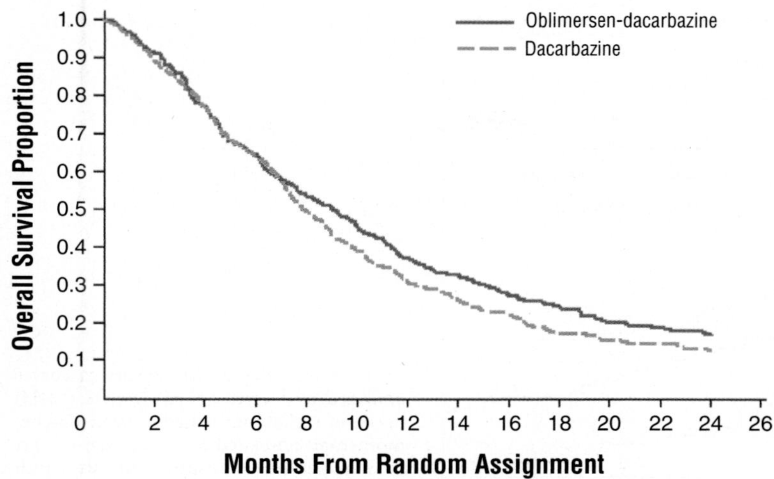

FIGURE 46.2 Oblimersen in melanoma. Kaplan-Meier estimates of overall survival. Median overall survival 9.0 months for oblimersen-dacarbazine versus 7.8 months for dacarbazine (P = .077; hazard ratio 0.87; 95% confidence interval [CI], 0.75 to 1.01). (From ref 24. Reprinted with permission © 2006 American Society of Clinical Oncology. All rights reserved.)

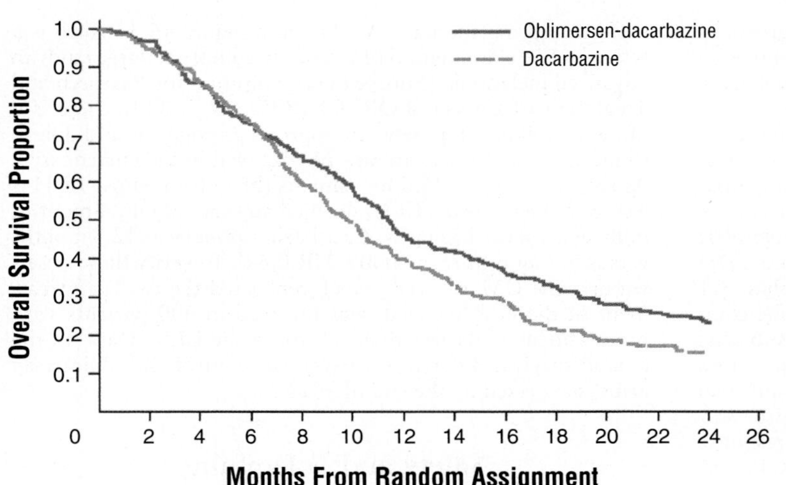

FIGURE 46.3 Oblimersen in melanoma. Kaplan-Meier estimates of overall survival in patients with normal (less than 1.1 time the upper limit of normal [ULN]) baseline serum lactate dehydrogenase (LDH) (n = 508). Median overall survival, 11.4 months for oblimersen-dacarbazine versus 9.7 months for dacarbazine (P = .02; hazard ratio 0.79; 95% confidence interval [CI], 0.65 to 0.96). (From ref 24. Reprinted with permission © 2006 American Society of Clinical Oncology. All rights reserved.)

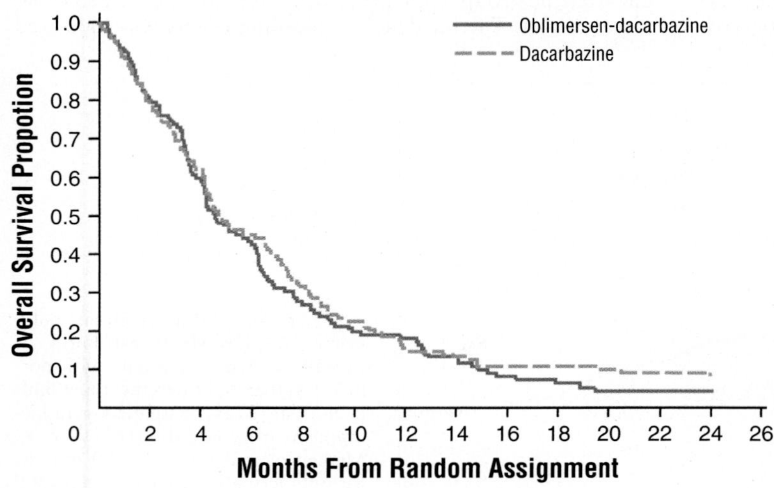

FIGURE 46.4 Oblimersen in melanoma. Kaplan-Meier estimates of overall survival of patients with elevated (greater than 1.1 times the upper limit of normal [ULN]) baseline serum lactate dehydrogenase (LDH) (n = 252). Median overall survival, 4.6 months for oblimersen-dacarbazine versus 4.7 months for dacarbazine (P = .41). (From ref 24. Reprinted with permission © 2006 American Society of Clinical Oncology. All rights reserved.)

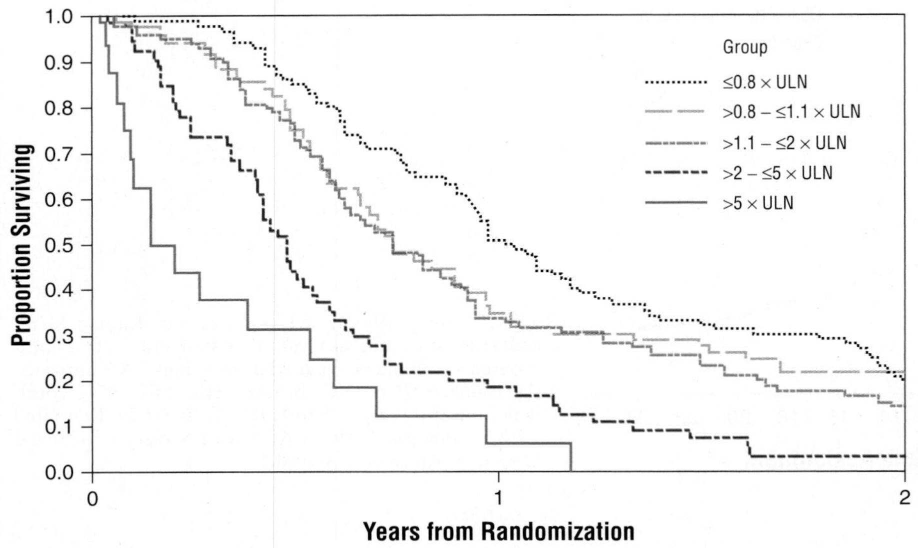

FIGURE 46.5 Kaplan-Meyer survival curves analyzed by lactate dehydrogenase (LDH) decile in melanoma patients receiving chemotherapy unrelated to oblimersen as part of European Organisation for Research and Treatment of Cancer (EORTC) 18951. (From ref 25. Reprinted with permission from Elsevier.)

(0.8%) in the dacarbazine alone group. Median progression-free survival was also significantly longer among patients who received oblimersen than in those treated with dacarbazine alone (2.6 vs. 1.6 months, HR 0.75; $P < .001$).[24]

Outcome data was analyzed according to the LDH stratification category. It should be noted that LDH has long been recognized as an important independent biomarker of poor prognosis in malignant melanoma.[25] In this trial, multivariate analyses that accounted for differences in baseline prognostic factors revealed an interaction between treatment and LDH activity level. Study patients with LDH values less than 1.1 times the ULN who received the oblimersen-dacarbazine combination (approximately two-thirds, 508 of the 771 subjects) were observed to have significantly better treatment outcomes for all efficacy end points. These included overall survival (median, 11.4 vs. 9.7 months; $P = .02$), progression-free survival (median, 3.1 vs. 1.6 months; $P < .001$), overall response (17.2% vs. 9.3%; $P = .009$), complete response (3.4% vs. 0.8%), and durable response (9.6% vs. 4.0%; $P = .01$) (Figs. 46.3 and 46.4). In sharp contrast, significant differences between treatment groups were not observed for patients with elevated (greater than 1.1 times the ULN) baseline LDH levels. New data have revealed the dramatic extent to which LDH stratification, *even within the "normal" range*, is predictive of prognosis in advanced melanoma.[26] As shown in Figure 46.5, which is a retrospective examination of a recently completed large study in advanced melanoma (European Organisation for Research and Treatment of Cancer [EORTC] 18951, N = 330), there is a dramatic relationship between improving prognosis and diminishing LDH levels, as can also be observed in the current trial. As shown in Figure 46.6 for patients (N = 108) whose LDH is less than 0.8 times the ULN, the median survival (at 24 months, oblimersen-dacarbazine vs. dacarbazine alone) was 12.3 months versus 9.9 months ($P = .0009$; HR 0.64). To verify these observations, the GM307 trial, which replicated the two-arm treatment of the GM301 trial, was initiated in 300 patients with pretreatment LDH less than 0.8 times the ULN. Data on the overall survival difference between the control and oblimersen arms is expected by the end of 2010.

Safety and Tolerability

The most significant adverse events were neutropenia and thrombocytopenia (Table 46.2). Grade 3 to 4 neutropenia with infection occurred at a rate of 4.3% for the oblimersen-dacarbazine group, compared with 2.8% for the dacarbazine-alone cohort. The incidence of bleeding events was increased

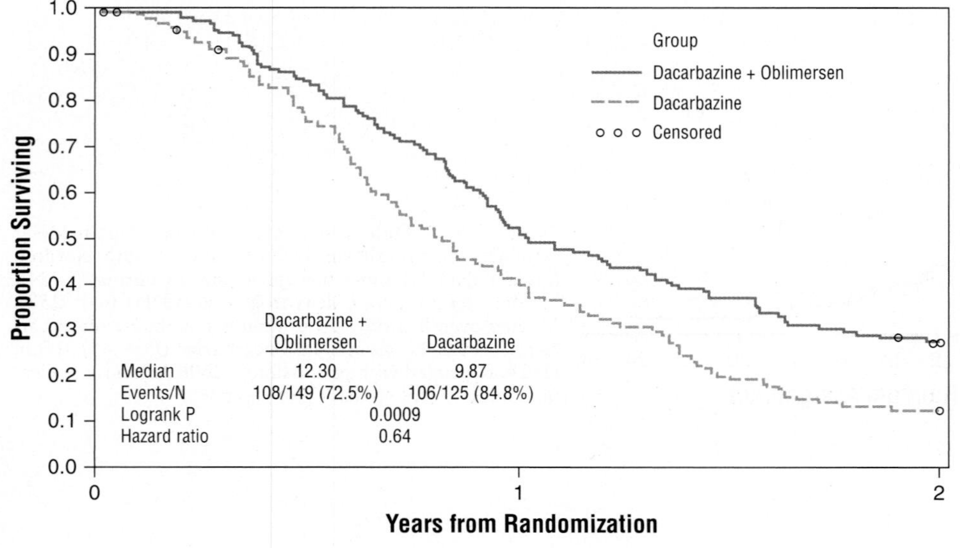

FIGURE 46.6 Oblimersen in melanoma. Kaplan-Meier estimates of overall survival in patients with normal (less than 0.8 times the upper limit of normal [ULN]) baseline serum lactate dehydrogenase (LDH) ($n = 274$). Median overall survival, 12.3 months for oblimersen-dacarbazine versus 9.9 months for dacarbazine ($P = .0009$; hazard ratio 0.64; 95% confidence interval [CI], 0.49 to 0.83). (From ref 26. Reprinted with permission from Elsevier.)

TABLE 46.2

OBLIMERSEN IN MELANOMA

	Adverse Events Occurring in ≥15% of Patient											
	Any Grade				Grade 3				Grade 4			
	Oblimersen-Dacarbazine (*n* = 371)		Dacarbazine (*n* = 360)		Oblimersen-Dacarbazine (*n* = 371)		Dacarbazine (*n* = 360)		Oblimersen-Dacarbazine (*n* = 371)		Dacarbazine (*n* = 360)	
Adverse Event	No.	%	No.	%	No.	%	No.	%	No.	%	No.	%
Gastrointestinal												
Nausea[a]	231	62.3	169	46.9	25	6.7	8	2.2	0	0	1	0.3
Vomiting[b]	139	37.5	75	20.8	16	4.3	6	1.7	0	0	1	0.3
Constipation	103	27.8	93	25.8	8	2.2	3	0.8	0	0	0	0
Diarrhea[b]	100	27.0	63	17.5	6	1.6	2	0.6	0	0	1	0.3
Hematologic/lymphatic												
Thrombocytopenia[a]	107	28.8	40	11.1	49	13.2	19	5.3	10	2.7	4	1.1
Neutropenia[a]	103	27.8	56	15.6	40	10.8	30	8.3	39	10.5	15	4.2
Anemia[b]	86	23.2	61	16.9	24	6.5	14	3.9	3	0.8	3	0.8
Leukopenia[a]	62	16.7	31	8.6	23	6.2	13	3.6	5	1.3	1	0.3
Infection (any)[a]	123	33.2	65	18.1	35	9.4	11	3.1	7	1.9	2	0.6
Other												
Pyrexia[b]	197	53.1	63	17.5	16	4.3	6	1.7	0	0	1	0.3
Fatigue	171	46.1	142	39.4	16	4.3	9	2.5	1	0.3	2	0.6
Anorexia[a]	114	30.7	56	15.6	9	2.4	1	0.3	0	0	0	0
Headache[a]	97	26.1	47	13.1	10	2.7	1	0.3	0	0	0	0
Rigors[b]	76	20.5	16	4.4	3	0.8	0	0	0	0	0	0
Dizziness (excluding vertigo)[b]	56	15.1	22	6.1	1	0.3	0	0	1	0.3	0	0
Pain[b]	56	15.1	32	8.9	13	3.5	6	1.7	1	0.3	0	0

NOTE. In the event that a patient had both grade 3 and grade 4 occurrences of an event that patient was included in the grade 4 column.
[a]Denotes a statistically significant difference between treatment groups in the number of patients with any grade of the event as well as in the number of patiens with grade 3 or grade 4 occurrences of the event
[b]Denotes a statistically significant difference between tretment in the number of patients with any grade of the event.
Adverse events occurring in ≥15% by treatment group.
(From ref 24. Reprinted with permission © 2006 American Society of Clinical Oncology. All rights reserved.)

in the oblimersen-dacarbazine group at 13.7%, an increase from 9.2% observed for the dacarbazine-alone group. However, these were events primarily in grade 1 to 2 epistaxis or hematuria. In fact, more grade 3 to 4 bleeding events (mostly gastrointestinal events) occurred in the dacarbazine-alone group (3.1% vs. 2.2%). Also of note was an apparent increased rate of catheter-related events (venous thrombosis, infection, occlusion) observed for the combination oblimersen-dacarbazine group (19.1%), in comparison to the dacarbazine-alone group (8.6%). Patients without elevated baseline LDH values appeared to fare better with respect to safety findings and had lower rates of adverse events that resulted in treatment discontinuation or death.

Although treatment with oblimersen was associated with an increased incidence of grade 3 to 4 neutropenia (21%) and thrombocytopenia (16%), these rates are still substantially lower than those associated with other drugs and drug regimens used for the treatment of advanced melanoma.[27,28] Moreover, the rates of serious bleeding events and the incidence of neutropenic infections were both low for patient who received oblimersen. On the other hand, catheter-related problems remain an issue, which might be expected given that the treatment was provided via continuous intravenous infusion.

At this point there is no question that oblimersen has substantial clinical activity. But does this activity validate the antisense approach to cancer therapeutics? This is an extremely controversial point, as data exist both for and against the idea that the effects of oblimersen in melanoma cells are in any way related to the down-regulation of Bcl-2 expression. Nevertheless, this scientific discourse should not vitiate acceptance of the clinical benefits of agents like oblimersen for the cancer patient population.

References

1. Stein CA, Cheng YC. Antisense oligonucleotides as therapeutic agents—is the bullet really magical? *Science* 1993;261:1004.
2. Stephenson ML, Zamecnik PC. Inhibition of Rous sarcoma viral RNA translation by a specific oligodeoxyribonucleotide. *Proc Natl Acad Sci U S A* 1978;75:285.
3. Eder PS, De Vine RJ, Dagle JM, et al. Substrate specificity and kinetics of degradation of antisense oligonucleotides by a 3′ exonuclease in plasma. *Antisense Res* 1991;1:141.
4. Stein CA, Subasinghe C, Shinozuka K, et al. Physicochemical properties of phosphorothioate oligodeoxynucleotides. *Nucl Acids Res* 1988;16:3209.
5. Walder RY, Walder JA. Role of RNase H in hybrid-arrested translation by antisense oligonucleotides. *Proc Natl Acad Sci U S A* 1988;14:6433.
6. Monia BP, Lesnik EA, Gonzalez C, et al. Evaluation of 2′-modified oligonucleotides containing 2′-deoxy gaps as antisense inhibitors of gene expression. *J Biol Chem* 1993;268:14514.

7. Stein CA. Is irrelevant cleavage the price of antisense efficacy? *Pharmacol Ther* 2000;85:231.
8. Akhtar S, Basu S, Wickstrom W, et al. Interactions of antisense DNA oligonucleotide analogs with phospholipid membranes (liposomes). *Nucl Acids Res* 1991;19:5551.
9. Lebedeva I, Benimetskaya L, Stein CA, et al. Cellular delivery of antisense oligonucleotides. *Eur J Pharm Biopharm* 2000;50:101.
10. Zabner J, Fasbender AJ, Moninger T, et al. Cellular and molecular barriers to gene transfer by a cationic lipid. *J Biol Chem* 1995;270:18997.
11. Benimetskaya L, Takle GB, Vilenchik M, et al. Cationic porphyrins: novel delivery vehicles for antisense oligodeoxynucleotides. *Nucl Acids Res* 1998; 26:5310.
12. Zelphati O, Szoka FC Jr. Mechanism of oligonucleotide release from cationic liposomes. *Proc Natl Acad Sci U S A* 1996;93:11493.
13. Stein CA, Rode Hansen B, Lai J, et al. Efficient gene silencing by delivery of locked nucleic acid antisense oligonucleotides, unassisted by transfected reagents. *Nucl Acids Res* 2010;38:e3.
14. Koch T, Rosenbohm C, Hansen H, et al. Locked nucleic acid: properties and therapeutic aspects. In: Kurreck J, ed. *Therapeutic oligonucleotides*. Cambridge: RSC Publishing, 2008:103.
15. Schena M, Larsson L-G, Cottardi D, et al. Growth- and differentiation-associated expression of Bcl-2 in B-chronic lymphocytic leukemia cells. *Blood* 1992;79:2981.
16. Reed JC, Kitada S, Takayama S, et al. Regulation of chemoresistance by the Bcl-2 oncoprotein in non-Hodgkin's lymphoma and lymphocytic leukemia cell lines. *Ann Oncol* 1994;5:61.
17. Meijerink JP, Van Lieshout EM, Beverloo HB, et al. Novel murine B-cell lymphoma/leukemia model to study Bcl-2-driven oncogenesis. *Int J Cancer* 2005;114:917.
18. Auer RL, Corbo M, Fegan CD, et al. Bcl-2 antisense (Genasense) induces apoptosis and potentiates activity of both cytotoxic chemotherapy and rituximab in primary CLL cells. *Blood* 2001;98: (abst 3358).
19. Castro JE, Kitada S, Mota M, et al. Phosphorothioate oligodeoxynucleotides can induce apoptosis of chronic lymphocytic leukemia B cells via a mechanism that does not depend upon specific interference of Bcl-2 gene expression. *Blood* 2002;100: (abst 1470).
20. O'Brien SM, Cunningham CC, Golenkov AK, et al. Phase I to II multicenter study of oblimersen sodium, a Bcl-2 antisense oligonucleotide, in patients with advanced chronic lymphocytic leukemia. *J Clin Oncol* 2005;23:7697.
21. O'Brien S, Moore JO, Boyd TE, et al. Randomized phase III trial of fludarabine plus cyclophosphamide with or without oblimersen sodium (Bcl-2 antisense) in patients with relapsed or refractory chronic lymphocytic leukemia. *J Clin Oncol* 2007;25:1114.
22. Cheson BD, Bennett JM, Grever M, et al. National Cancer Institute–sponsored Working Group guidelines for chronic lymphocytic leukemia: revised guidelines for diagnosis and treatment. *Blood* 1996;87:4990.
23. O'Brien S, Moore J, Boyd T, et al. 5-Year survival in patients with relapsed or refractory chronic lymphocytic leukemia in a randomized, phase III trial of fludarabine plus cyclophosphamide with or without oblimersen. *J Clin Oncol* 2009;27:5208.
24. Bedikian A, Millward M, Pehamberger H, et al. Bcl-2 antisense (oblimersen sodium) plus dacarbazine in patients with advanced melanoma: the Oblimersen Melanoma Study Group. *J Clin Oncol* 2006;24:4738.
25. Manola J, Atkins M, Ibrahim J, et al. Prognostic factors in metastatic melanoma: a pooled analysis of Eastern Cooperative Oncology Group trials. *J Clin Oncol* 2000;18:3782.
26. Agarwala S, Keilholz U, Gilles E, et al. LDH correlation with survival in advanced melanoma from two large, randomized trials: oblimersen (GM301) and EORTC 18951. *Eur J Cancer* 2009;45:1807.
27. Avril MF, Aamdal S, Grob J, et al. Fotemustine compared with dacarbazine in patients with disseminated malignant melanoma: a phase III study. *J Clin Oncol* 2004;22:1118.
28. Chapman PB, Einhorn LH, Meyers ML, et al. Phase III multicenter randomized trial of the Dartmouth regimen versus dacarbazine in patients with metastatic melanoma. *J Clin Oncol* 1999;17:2745.

CHAPTER 47 ANTIANGIOGENESIS AGENTS

CINDY H. CHAU AND WILLIAM D. FIGG

The spread of cancer occurs through metastasis whereby cancer cells penetrate into lymphatic and blood vessels, and circulate through the bloodstream to invade and grow in the normal tissues elsewhere. Characterization of the growth and invasion of solid tumors to understand this metastatic process is the subject of intense research for over a century that stemmed from the "seed-and-soil" hypothesis of Dr. Stephen Paget.[1] Through observations made by the study of autopsy data, Paget proposed that specific tumors had a predictable pattern of metastasis such that the seeds of tumor cells form metastatic deposits only if they land in appropriate soils.

Early cancer researchers investigating the conditions necessary for cancer metastasis observed that one of the critical events required for tumor growth is an increased vascularization and the formation of a new network of blood vessels called *angiogenesis*. Indeed it was nearly 70 years ago that the existence of tumor-derived factors responsible for promoting new vessel growth was postulated[2] and that tumor growth is essentially dependent on vascular induction and the development of a neovascular supply.[3] By the late 1960s, Dr. Judah Folkman and colleagues[4] had begun the search for a tumor angiogenesis factor. In the 1971 landmark report, Folkman[5] proposed that inhibition of angiogenesis by means of holding tumors in a nonvascularized dormant state would be an effective strategy to treat human cancer, and hence laid the groundwork for the concept behind the development of "antiangiogenic" drugs. This fostered the search for angiogenic factors, regulators of angiogenesis, and antiangiogenic molecules over the next three decades and shed light on angiogenesis as an important therapeutic target for the treatment of cancer and other diseases.

Successful development and clinical translation of antiangiogenesis agents depends on the complete understanding of the biology of angiogenesis and the regulatory proteins that govern this angiogenic process, topics that have been covered in greater detail in another section of this textbook. This chapter will briefly review the mechanisms behind angiogenesis followed by an in-depth discussion of antiangiogenic therapy.

UNDERSTANDING THE ANGIOGENIC PROCESS

Angiogenic Switch and Regulatory Proteins

Tumor development and progression depend on angiogenesis. Recruitment of new blood vessels to the tumor site is required for delivery of nutrients and oxygen to the cancerous growths and for the removal of waste products.[6] Cancer cells promote angiogenesis at an early stage of tumorigenesis beginning with the release of molecules that send signals to the surrounding normal host tissue and stimulating the migration of microvascular endothelial cells (ECs) in the direction of the angiogenic stimulus. These angiogenic factors not only mediate EC migration, but also EC proliferation and microvessel formation in tumors undergoing the switch to the angiogenic phenotype.[7] Experimental evidence for this "angiogenic switch" was observed when hyperplastic islets in transgenic mice (RIP-Tag model) switch from small (<1 mm), white microscopic dormant tumors to red, rapidly growing tumors.[7]

Dormant tumors have been discovered during autopsies of individuals who died of causes other than cancer.[8] These autopsy studies suggest that the vast majority of microscopic, *in situ* cancers never switch to the angiogenic phenotype during a normal lifetime. Such incipient tumors are usually not neovascularized and can remain harmless to the host for long periods of time as microscopic lesions that are in a state of dormancy.[9,10] These nonangiogenic tumors cannot expand beyond the initial microscopic size and become clinically detectable, lethal tumors until they have switched to the angiogenic phenotype[11–13] through neovascularization and/or blood vessel cooption.[14] Depending on the tumor type and the environment, this switch can occur at different stages of the tumor progression pathway and ultimately depends on a net balance of positive and negative regulators. Thus, the angiogenic phenotype may result from the production of growth factors by tumor cells and/or the down-regulation of negative modulators.

Changes in this angiogenic balance affecting the levels of activator and inhibitor molecules dictate whether an EC will be in a quiescent or an angiogenic state. Normally, the inhibitors predominate, thereby blocking growth. Should a need for new blood vessels arise, the balance will shift in favor of the angiogenic state with an increase in the amount of activators and a decrease in inhibitors. This prompts the activation, growth, and division of vascular ECs resulting in the formation of new blood vessels. The activated ECs produce and release matrix metalloproteinases (MMPs) into the surrounding tissue. These degradative enzymes break down the extracellular matrix to allow the ECs to migrate into the surrounding tissues and organize themselves into hollow tubes that eventually evolve into a mature network of blood vessels.

Proangiogenic factors or positive regulators of angiogenesis include vascular endothelial growth factor (VEGF), basic fibroblast growth factor, platelet-derived growth factor (PDGF), placental growth factor, transforming growth factor-β, pleiotrophins, and others.[15] Activation of the hypoxia-inducible factor-1 (HIF-1) via tumor-associated hypoxic conditions is also involved in the up-regulation of several angiogenic factors.[16] The angiogenic switch also involves down-regulation of angiogenesis suppressor proteins that include endostatin, angiostatin, thrombospondin, and others (reviewed in refs. and 17 and 18). Most notably, however, is the link between many oncogenes and angiogenesis and the significant role oncogenes play in driving the angiogenic switch. These proangiogenic oncogenes not only induce the expression of stimulators but may also down-regulate inhibitors of angiogenesis (reviewed in ref. 19).

Endogenous Inhibitors of Angiogenesis

The infrequency of microscopic *in situ* tumors that actually undergo the angiogenic switch (<1%) suggests that naturally occurring endogenous inhibitors exist in the body to defend against the angiogenic switch in pathologic conditions and limit physiological angiogenesis.[9] These circulating endogenous inhibitors could also prevent microscopic metastases from growing into visible tumors. Early studies by Langer et al.[20,21] demonstrated the possible existence of such inhibitors through the extraction of a functional inhibitor from cartilage, a tissue that is poorly vascularized. Since then, dozens of endogenous angiogenesis inhibitors have been identified, and some of these are listed in Table 47.1.[17,18] Many of the endogenous inhibitors of angiogenesis that have been discovered to date are proteolytically cleaved fragments of larger proteins that are members of either the clotting/coagulation system or members of the extracellular matrix family of glycoproteins. The discovery of angiostatin, an internal fragment of plasminogen, first revealed that an angiogenesis inhibitory peptide could be enzymatically released from a parent protein that lacked this inhibitory property.[22] Soon thereafter endostatin, an internal fragment of collagen XVIII, demonstrated for the first time that a basement-membrane collagen contained an antiangiogenic peptide.[23] Endostatin is the most well-studied endogenous angiogenesis inhibitor (reviewed in ref. 24). Other potent endogenous angiogenesis inhibitors include thrombospondin-1[25] and tumstatin, a 232-amino acid antiangiogenic peptide in the α-3 chain of collagen type IV.[26] The discovery of vasohibin, an endogenous inhibitor that is selectively induced in ECs by proangiogenic stimulatory growth factors such as VEGF, demonstrated the existence of some kind of intrinsic and EC-specific feedback inhibitor control mechanism.[27] More recently, a second endothelium-produced negative regulator of angiogenesis has been discovered, the notch 4/DLL4 signaling system.[28,29] Both intrinsic factors have since been shown to control tumor angiogenesis by an autoregulatory or negative-feedback mechanism.

Perhaps the most compelling genetic evidence that endogenous inhibitors suppress pathologic angiogenesis was observed in studies using mice deficient in tumstatin, endostatin, or thrombospondin-1 (TSP-1).[30] These experiments demonstrate that normal physiological levels of the inhibitors can retard the tumor growth, and that their absence leads to enhanced angiogenesis and increased tumor growth by two- to threefold. Tumors grow twofold faster in the tumstatin/TSP-1 double-knockout mice, compared with either the tumstatin- or the TSP-1–deficient mice. Additionally, tumor growth in transgenic mice overexpressing endostatin specifically in the ECs (a 1.6-fold increase in the circulating levels) is threefold slower than the tumor growth in wild type mice. Collectively, these results strongly suggest that endogenous inhibitors of angiogenesis can act as endothelium-specific tumor suppressors.

The connection between a tumor suppressor protein and angiogenesis is best illustrated by the classic tumor suppressor *p53*. *p53* is known to link the biology of the cell cycle to tumorigenesis and for its role in regulating tumor cell proliferation. However, *p53* can also inhibit angiogenesis by increasing the expression of thrombospondin-1,[31] by repressing VEGF[32] and basic fibroblast growth factor binding protein,[33] and by degrading HIF-1,[34] which blocks downstream induction of VEGF expression. Furthermore, a recent study revealed that *p53*-mediated inhibition of angiogenesis occurs in part via the antiangiogenic activity of endostatin and tumstatin.[35] This landmark finding clearly demonstrates that *p53* not only controls cell proliferation but can also repress tumor angiogenesis through enzymatic mobilization of these endogenous angiogenesis inhibitor proteins to prevent ECs from being recruited into the dormant, microscopic tumors and thereby preventing the switch to the angiogenic phenotype.[36] It remains to be established whether other angiogenesis inhibitors are regulated by *p53* or by other tumor suppressor genes. Nevertheless, the discovery that these endogenous angiogenesis inhibitors can suppress the growth of primary tumors raises the possibility that such inhibitors might also be able to slow tumor metastasis. Indeed, inhibition of angiogenesis by angiostatin significantly reduced the rate of metastatic spread.

TABLE 47.1

EXAMPLES OF ENDOGENOUS INHIBITORS OF ANGIOGENESIS

Alphastatin
Angiostatin
Antithrombin III (cleaved)
Arrestin
Canstatin
Endostatin
Interferon alpha/beta
2-Methoxyestradiol (2-ME)
Pigment epithelial-derived factor (PEDF)
Platelet factor-4 (PF4)
Tetrahydrocortisol-S
Thrombospondin-1
TIMP-2
Tumstatin
Vasohibin

DRUG DEVELOPMENT OF ANGIOGENESIS INHIBITORS

The first angiogenesis inhibitor was reported in 1980 and involved low-dose administration of interferon-α.[37–39] Over the next decade several compounds were discovered to have potent antiangiogenic activity, which included protamine and platelet-factor 4,[40] trahydrocortisol,[41] and the fumagillin analogue TNP-470.[42] The proof of concept that targeting angiogenesis is an effective strategy for treating cancer came with the approval of the first angiogenesis inhibitor, bevacizumab, by the U.S. Food and Drug Administration (FDA) following a phase 3 study showing a survival benefit. Since then, several antiangiogenic agents have received FDA approval for cancer treatment (Table 47.2) and two additional agents (pegaptanib and ranibizumab) are approved for the treatment of wet age-related macular degeneration. There are numerous investigational angiogenesis inhibitors currently being tested in clinical trials (Table 47.3).

Rationale for Antiangiogenic Therapy

Antiangiogenic therapy stems from the fundamental concept that tumor growth, invasion, and metastasis are angiogenesis-dependent. The microvascular EC recruited by a tumor has become an important second target in cancer therapy. Unlike the cancer cell (the primary target of cytotoxic chemotherapy) that is genetically unstable with unpredictable mutations, the genetic stability of ECs may make them less susceptible to

TABLE 47.2

ANTIANGIOGENIC AGENTS THAT HAVE RECEIVED U.S. FOOD AND DRUG ADMINISTRATION APPROVAL FOR CANCER TREATMENT

Drug	Class	Mechanism (Cellular Targets)	Year of Approval	Indications	Dosages
Bevacizumab (Avastin)	Anti-VEGF mAB	VEGF	2004	1st-line and 2nd-line metastatic CRC	5 mg/kg IV q2wk + bolus-IFL; 10 mg/kg IV q2wk + FOLFOX4
			2006	1st-line NSCLC	15 mg/kg IV q3wk + carboplatin/paclitaxel
			2009	GBM that has progressed after prior treatment	10 mg/kg IV q2wk
			2009	Metastatic RCC	10 mg/kg IV q2wk + IFN
Sorafenib (Nexavar, BAY439006)	Small-molecule RTKI	VEGFR2, VEGFR3, PDGFR, FLT3, c-Kit	2005	Advanced RCC	400 mg PO bid (w/o food)
			2007	Unresectable HCC	400 mg PO bid (w/o food)
Sunitinib (Sutent, SU11248)	Small-molecule RTKI	VEGFR1, VEGFR2, VEGFR3, PDGFR, FLT3, c-Kit, RET	2006	Imatinib-resistant or -intolerant GIST	50 mg PO qd, 4 wk on / 2 wk off
			2006	Advanced RCC	50 mg PO qd, 4 wk on / 2 wk off
Pazopanib (Votrient)	Small-molecule RTKI	VEGFR1, VEGFR2, VEGFR3, PDGFR, Itk, Lck, c-Fms	2009	Advanced RCC	800 mg PO qd (w/o food)
Thalidomide (Thalomid)	Immunomodulatory agent	Unknown	2006	Newly diagnosed MM	200 mg PO qd + dex
Lenalidomide (Revlimid, CC-5013)	Immunomodulatory agent	Unknown	2005	Deletion 5q MDS	10 mg PO qd
			2006	Previously treated MM	25 mg PO qd on days 1–21 of repeated 28-day cycles + dex
Temsirolimus (Torisel)	mTOR inhibitor	mTOR	2007	Advanced RCC	25 mg IV qwk (infused over 30–60 min)
Everolimus (Afinitor, RAD-001)	mTOR inhibitor	mTOR	2009	2nd-line advanced RCC after VEGFR-TKI failure	10 mg PO qd

mAB, monoclonal antibody; VEGF, vascular endothelial growth factor; CRC, colorectal cancer; IV, intravenous; IFL, irinotecan, 5-fluorouracil, and leucovorin; NSCLC, non–small cell lung cancer; *HER2*, human epidermal receptor-2; BC, breast cancer; GBM, glioblastoma multiforme; RCC, renal cell carcinoma; IFN, interferon-alfa; RTKI, receptor tyrosine kinase inhibitor; VEGFR, VEGF receptor; PDGFR, platelet-derived growth factor receptor; PO, orally; bid, twice daily; FLT, Fms-like tyrosine kinase; c-Kit, stem cell factor receptor; HCC, hepatocellular carcinoma; RET, glial cell line-derived neurotrophic factor receptor; GIST, gastrointestinal stromal tumor; Itk, interleukin-2 receptor inducible T-cell kinase; Lck, leukocyte-specific protein tyrosine kinase; c-Fms, transmembrane glycoprotein receptor tyrosine kinase; MM, multiple myeloma; MDS, myelodysplastic syndrome; dex, dexamethasone; mTOR, mammalian target of rapamycin.

acquired drug resistance.[43] Moreover, ECs in the microvascular bed of a tumor may support 50 to 100 tumor cells. Coupling this amplification potential together with the lower toxicity of most angiogenesis inhibitors results in the use of antiangiogenic therapy that should be significantly less toxic than conventional chemotherapy. Therefore, treating both the cancer cell and the EC in a tumor may be more effective than treating the cancer cell alone.

Classification of Antiangiogenic Agents

Various strategies for the development of antiangiogenic dugs have been investigated over the years, with these agents being classified into several different categories depending on their mechanism of action. Some inhibit ECs directly, while others inhibit the angiogenesis signaling cascade or block the ability of ECs to break down the extracellular matrix. Some antiangiogenic agents may target either VEGF directly through neutralizing the protein, blocking the tumor expression of the angiogenic factor, or blocking the receptor for the angiogenic factor on the ECs. Finally, these inhibitors may also be characterized by the degree of their blocking potential: drugs that block one main angiogenic protein, drugs that block two or three main angiogenic proteins, or drugs that have a broad-spectrum effect, blocking a range of angiogenic regulators.[44] These broad-spectrum inhibitors may target the angiogenic regulators and/or signaling pathways in both the tumor and ECs.

TABLE 47.3

EXAMPLES OF INVESTIGATIONAL ANTIANGIOGENESIS AGENTS AND THEIR CELLULAR TARGETS IN CLINICAL TRIALS

Drug	Cellular Targets
Anti-VEGF agents	
VEGF-AS (antisense oligonucleotide)	VEGF, VEGF-C, VEGF-D
VEGF Trap	VEGF, PlGF
(Multi)targeted agents that interfere with growth factor receptor signaling pathways	
Axitinib (AG13736)	VEGFR1, VEGFR2, PDGFR
Cediranib (AZD2171)	VEGFR1, VEGFR2, VEGFR3, PDGFR, c-Kit
BMS582664	VEGFR2, FGFR
Motesanib (AMG706)	VEGFR1, VEGFR2, VEGFR3, PDGFR, c-Kit
OSI930	VEGFR2, c-Kit
RPI.4610 (Angiozyme)	mRNA for VEGFR1
Tandutinib (MLN518/CT53518)	FLT3, PDGFR, c-Kit
Vatalanib (PTK787/ZK222584)	VEGFR1, VEGFR2, VEGFR3, PDGFR, c-Kit
Vandetanib (ZD6474)	VEGFR1, VEGFR2, VEGFR3
XL184	VEGFR2, MET, FLT3, Tie2
XL999	VEGFRs, FGFR, PDGFR, FLT3, c-Kit
Agents that target other proteins or pathways	
AMG386	Angiopoietins
AMG479	Insulin-like growth factor-1 receptor
CP751871	Insulin-like growth factor-1 receptor
TNP-470	Methionine animopeptidase-2
TRC105	Endoglin (CD105)
Volociximab (M200)	$\alpha 5\beta 1$ integrin receptor

VEGF, vascular endothelial growth factor; PlGF, platelet growth factor; VEGFR, VEGF receptor; PDGFR, platelet-derived growth factor receptor; FGFR, fibroblast growth factor receptor; c-Kit, stem cell factor receptor; FLT3, Fms-like tyrosine kinase 3; MET, hepatocyte growth factor receptor; Tie2, angiopoietin receptor.

Angiogenesis inhibitors may also be referred to as either being *exclusive* or *inclusive*. Drugs that are *exclusively* antiangiogenic only have one known function, which is to exhibit antiangiogenic activity. Examples of these drugs include bevacizumab or VEGF-Trap and treatment with these agents is known as anti-VEGF therapy. For other angiogenesis inhibitors, the antiangiogenic activity is *included* with other functions of the drug. Among them are certain cancer agents that exhibit dual roles. In many cases, the antiangiogenic activity is discovered as a secondary function after the drug has received FDA approval for a different primary function. For example, bortezomib is a proteasome inhibitor that is approved for multiple myeloma and later found to possess antiangiogenic activity via inhibiting VEGF. Certain orally available small-molecule drugs display their antiangiogenic activity through inducing the expression of endogenous angiogenesis inhibitors such as celecoxib, a cyclooxygenase-2 inhibitor, which inhibits angiogenesis by increasing levels of endostatin.[24] Examples of these inclusive angiogenesis inhibitors are highlighted in Table 47.4.

Drugs with antiangiogenic activity may also be classified as either *direct* or *indirect* angiogenesis inhibitors (Fig. 47.1). A direct angiogenesis inhibitor blocks vascular ECs from proliferating, migrating, or increasing their survival in response to proangiogenic proteins. They target the activated endothelium directly and inhibit multiple angiogenic proteins. Direct angiogenesis inhibitors are presumed to be less likely to induce acquired drug resistance because they target the genetically stable ECs. Examples of direct angiogenesis inhibitors include many of the endogenous inhibitors of angiogenesis such as endostatin, angiostatin, and thrombospondin-1. ABT-510 is synthetic peptide that mimics the antiangiogenic activity of the endogenous protein thrombospondin-1. Results from phase 1/2 trials of ABT-510 in patients with advanced malignancies,[45,46] advanced soft tissue sarcoma,[47] and renal cell carcinoma[48] demonstrated a favorable toxicity profile but failed to yield compelling evidence of strong single-agent activity in these patient populations. Given the favorable toxicity profile, studies may still consider the evaluation of ABT-510 in combination therapy.

TABLE 47.4

EXAMPLES OF DRUGS THAT POSSESS ANTIANGIOGENIC ACTIVITY OR INHIBIT ANGIOGENESIS AS A SECONDARY FUNCTION

Drug	Class
Cetuximab Panitumumab Trastuzumab	EGFR/HER monoclonal antibodies
Gefitinib Erlotinib	EGFR small-molecule tyrosine kinase receptor inhibitors
Belinostat (PXD101) LBH589 Vorinostat (SAHA)	HDAC inhibitors
Celecoxib	COX-2 inhibitors
Bortezomib	Proteasome inhibitors
Zoledronic acid	Bisphosphonates
Rosiglitazone	PPAR-gamma agonists
Doxycycline	Antibiotic

EGFR, epidermal growth factor receptor; HDAC, histone deacetylase; COX-2, cyclooxygenase-2; PPAR, peroxisome-proliferator-activated-receptor.

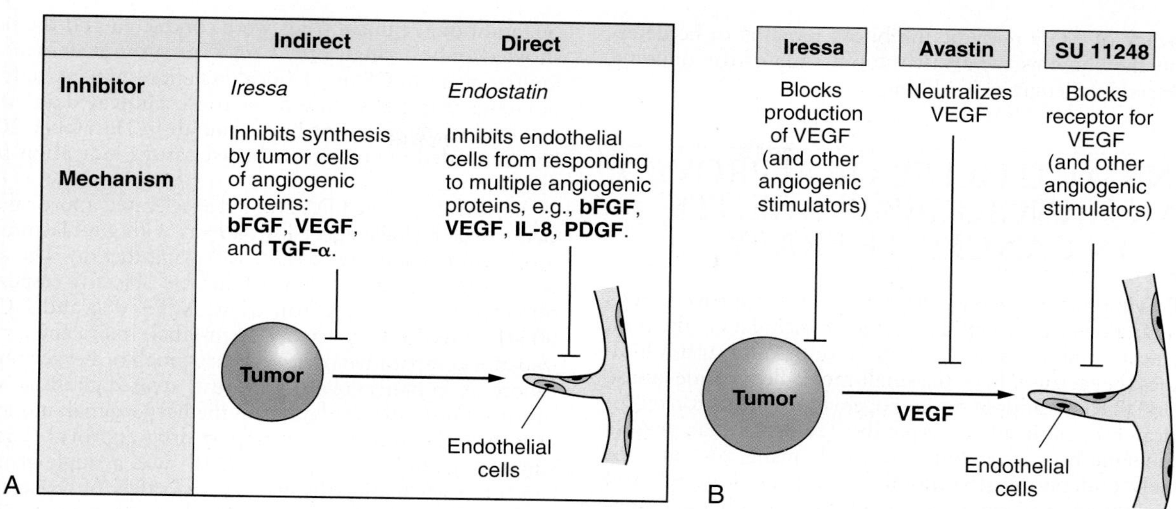

FIGURE 47.1 **A:** An "indirect" angiogenesis inhibitor blocks synthesis of an angiogenic protein by a tumor cell, neutralizes the angiogenic protein, or blocks the endothelial receptor for that protein. Several drugs have been designed to block oncogene expression or to block the signal transduction pathway of an oncogene block expression of the angiogenic proteins that were induced by the oncogene (e.g., Iressa blocks the epidermal growth factor receptor tyrosine kinase). A "direct" angiogenesis inhibitor prevents endothelial cells from responding to a wide spectrum of angiogenic stimuli (e.g., endostatin). (From ref. 137, with permission.) **B:** Three examples of "indirect" angiogenesis inhibitors. (From ref. 136, with permission.) bFGF, basic fibroblast growth factor; IL, interleukin; PDGF, platelet-derived growth factor; TGF, transforming growth factor; VEGF, vascular endothelial growth factor.

Indirect angiogenesis inhibitors decrease or block expression of a tumor cell product, neutralize the tumor product itself, or block its receptor on ECs. Examples of drugs that interfere with the angiogenesis signaling pathway include bevacizumab, sorafenib, and sunitinib (as described later). These drugs target the major signaling pathways in tumor angiogenesis: VEGF, PDGF, and their respective receptors as well as other growth factors and/or signaling pathways. VEGF (also known as vascular permeability factor) is a potent proangiogenic growth factor and its expression is up-regulated by most cancer cell types. It stimulates EC proliferation, migration, and survival as well as induces increased vascular permeability. The different forms of VEGF bind to transmembrane tyrosine kinase receptors (RTKs) on ECs: VEGFR1 (Flt-1), VEGFR2 (KDR/Flk-1), or VEGFR3 (Flt-4).[49] This results in receptor dimerization, activation, and autophosphorylation of the tyrosine kinase domain, thereby triggering downstream signaling pathways. Other signaling molecules that may represent attractive therapeutic targets include PDGF and angiopoietin-2. PDGF-B/PDGF receptor (R)-β plays an important role in the recruitment of pericytes and maturation of the microvasculature.[50] Angiopoietin-2 (which binds the Tie-2 receptor) is mostly expressed in tumor-induced neovasculature, whereby its selective inhibition results in reduced EC proliferation.[51] Most indirect angiogenesis inhibitors are designed to target these signaling pathways and can block the activity of one, two, or a broad spectrum of proangiogenic proteins and/or their receptors. The limitation to indirect inhibitors is that over time tumor cells may acquire mutations that lead to increased expression of other proangiogenic proteins that are not blocked by the indirect inhibitor. This may give the appearance of drug resistance and warrants the addition of a second antiangiogenic agent, one that would target the expression of these up-regulated proangiogenic proteins.

Another group of angiogenesis inhibitors is directed against the MMPs, enzymes that catalyze the breakdown of the extracellular matrix. Because breakdown of the matrix is required to allow ECs to migrate into surrounding tissues and proliferate into new blood vessels, drugs that target MMPs also can inhibit angiogenesis. Although inhibiting the activity of MMPs has been considered for potential therapeutic targets, clinical development of MMP inhibitors (MMPIs) has yielded disappointing results. Incyclinide (COL-3) showed biological activity in AIDS-related Kaposi sarcoma[52] but no activity in advanced soft tissue sarcomas.[53] A broad-spectrum MMPI, BMS-275291, demonstrated inadequate efficacy in patients with advanced or metastatic cancer,[54] castrate-resistant prostate cancer with bone metastases,[55] and patients with human immunodeficiency virus-associated Kaposi sarcoma.[56] Other MMPIs, such as BAY-129566 or BB-2516, have failed to show therapeutic efficacy in human malignancies despite preclinical antimetastatic and antiangiogenic activity. The challenges of anti-MMP therapy are complex and the reasons for the disappointing trial results observed with MMPIs in cancer therapy remain to be established.[57,58] These negative results of MMPIs have definitely raised serious concerns and doubts about pursuing future developments of MMPIs as a therapeutic target.

Integrins are cell surface adhesion molecules that play an essential role in cell–cell and cell–matrix adhesion. They are responsible for transmitting signals important for cell migration, invasion, proliferation, and survival. One member of the integrin family, $\alpha 5$-β_3 integrin, is expressed on tumor and ECs. The involvement of integrin in tumor angiogenesis was demonstrated in studies that show the β-4 subunit of integrin promoting endothelial migration and invasion.[59] Therefore, agents that target integrins (inhibitors of $\alpha_v\beta_3$ and $\alpha_v\beta_5$) have been evaluated as potential therapeutic options and include etaracizumab (Abegrin, MEDI-522), a monoclonal antibody, and cilengitide (EMD-121974), the RGD (arginine-glycine-aspartic acid)-mimetic cyclic peptide. Integrin inhibitors have proven to be largely ineffective in various cancer trials[60–62] with the exception of cilengitide in the glioblastoma patient population, which has shown promising activity in phase 2 studies.[63,64] The poorer than expected efficacy of integrin inhibitors in clinical trials may be due to insufficient levels of drug in the body. Recent *in vivo* studies demonstrated that low concentrations of RGD-mimetic integrin inhibitors can paradoxically enhance VEGF-mediated angiogenesis and stimulate tumor growth.[65]

The efficacy of RGD-mimetic inhibitors remains to be determined in the clinic as we await the outcome of the ongoing phase 3 trial of cilengitide in glioblastoma.

CLINICAL UTILITY OF APPROVED ANTIANGIOGENIC AGENTS IN CANCER THERAPY

The following section reviews the current FDA-approved drugs with antiangiogenic activity. These agents include: (1) the pure angiogenesis inhibitors such as the monoclonal anti-VEGF antibodies (bevacizumab) or the small-molecule tyrosine kinase inhibitors' (TKIs) multiple proangiogenic growth factor receptors (sorafenib, sunitinib, pazopanib); (2) drugs that possess antiangiogenic properties but with mechanisms that are not completely understood (thalidomide and lenalidomide); and (3) drugs that are antiangiogenic in addition to other activities such as inhibition of cell proliferation (inhibitors of the mammalian target of rapamycin—temsirolimus, everolimus).

Bevacizumab

Bevacizumab is a recombinant humanized anti-VEGF-A monoclonal antibody that received FDA approval in February 2004 for use in combination therapy with fluorouracil-based regimens for metastatic colorectal cancer. Bevacizumab binds VEGF and prevents the interaction of VEGF to its receptors (Flt-1 and KDR) on the surface of ECs. It is the first antiangiogenic agent clinically proven to extend survival following a large, randomized, double-blind, phase 3 study in which bevacizumab was administered in combination with bolus irinotecan, 5-fluorouracil, and leucovorin (IFL) as first-line therapy for metastatic colorectal cancer.[66] In 2006, its approval extended to first- or second-line treatment of patients with metastatic carcinoma of the colon or rectum. This recommendation is based on the demonstration of a statistically significant improvement in overall survival (OS) in patients receiving bevacizumab plus FOLFOX4 (5-flourouracil, leucovorin, and oxaliplatin) when compared to those receiving FOLFOX4 alone. In 2006, it received an additional approval for use in combination with carboplatin and paclitaxel, and is indicated for first-line treatment of patients with unresectable, locally advanced, recurrent, or metastatic nonsquamous, non–small cell lung cancer. This recommendation is based on the demonstration of a statistically significant improvement in OS in patients receiving bevacizumab with carboplatin and paclitaxel compared to those receiving chemotherapy alone.[67]

In February 2008, the FDA granted a conditional, accelerated approval for bevacizumab to be used in combination with paclitaxel for the treatment of patients who have not received chemotherapy for metastatic human epidermal growth factor receptor-2 (*HER2*)-negative breast cancer. The approval was based on the demonstration of an improvement in progression-free survival (PFS) in patients receiving bevacizumab with paclitaxel compared to those receiving paclitaxel alone as a first-line treatment for metastatic breast cancer (E2100 trial).[68] Additionally, the product labeling specifies that bevacizumab is not indicated for patients with breast cancer that has progressed following anthracycline and taxane chemotherapy administered for metastatic disease following the failure of a randomized phase 3 trial of bevacizumab and capecitabine used as second- or third-line treatment of refractory metastatic breast cancer patients (AVF2119 trial).[69] No data are currently available that demonstrate an improvement in disease-related symptoms or increased OS with bevacizumab in breast cancer. After the accelerated approval of bevacizumab for breast cancer, additional clinical trials were conducted and the new data showed only a small effect on PFS without evidence of an improvement in OS or a clinical benefit to patients sufficient to outweigh the risks. Based on these clinical data, the FDA recinded its approval of bevacizumab in December 2010 and recommended removing the breast cancer indication from the drug's label.[69a–69c]

In May 2009, the FDA granted accelerated approval to bevacizumab as a single agent for patients with glioblastoma multiforme with progressive disease following therapy. The approval was based on demonstration of durable objective response rates observed in two single-arm trials, AVF3708g and NCI 06-C-0064E.[70] AVF3708g was an open-label, multicenter, randomized, noncomparative trial of bevacizumab or bevacizumab plus irinotecan in patients with previously treated glioblastoma multiforme. Only efficacy data from the bevacizumab monotherapy arm (N = 85) was used to support drug approval. The second supporting study (NCI 06-C-0064E) was a single-arm, single-center trial evaluating the efficacy and safety of bevacizumab in patients (N = 56) with recurrent high-grade gliomas. Finally, in July 2009, bevacizumab was approved for use in combination with interferon-α (IFN-α) for the treatment of patients with metastatic renal cell carcinoma (RCC). The approval was based on results from the BO17705 (or AVOREN) trial, a multinational study evaluating the combination of bevacizumab plus IFN-α-2a to IFN-α-2a plus placebo in patients with metastatic RCC, which demonstrated a 5-month improvement in median PFS in patients treated with bevacizumab.[71] Another phase 3 trial of bevacizumab plus IFN-α versus IFN-α monotherapy was conducted in patients with previously untreated, metastatic clear cell RCC (Cancer and Lymphoma Group B [CALGB] 90206). The median PFS times were 8.4 months versus 4.9 months in favor of the bevacizumab combination.[72] Both studies did not demonstrate a statistically significant advantage in OS.[73,74]

Clinical studies of bevacizumab in combination with oxaliplatin-containing and 5-fluorouracil-based regimens have shown that combination therapy is well tolerated with its toxicity being not substantially greater than that of the chemotherapy alone.[75] Its side effects include grade 3 hypertension, grade 1 or 2 proteinuria, a slight increase (less than two percentage points) in grade 3 or 4 bleeding, and impaired surgical wound healing in patients who undergo surgery during treatment with bevacizumab. However, potentially life-threatening events (arterial thrombotic events, gastrointestinal perforation, hemoptysis) have occurred in a small number of patients, thus requiring close patient monitoring in individuals who are at greater risk of adverse events (reviewed in ref. 76). At the time of writing, there are currently ~490 actively recruiting, ongoing trials investigating the clinical benefits of bevacizumab in combination with chemotherapeutic regimens or as adjuvant therapy in various stages of breast cancer, RCC, pancreatic cancer, ovarian cancer, and castrate-resistant prostate cancer as well as other solid tumors (http://clinicaltrial.gov and reviewed in ref. 77).

Sorafenib

Sorafenib is a small-molecule Raf kinase and VEGF receptor kinase (VEGFR2 and VEGFR3) inhibitor. It has been shown to exhibit broad-spectrum effects on multiple targets (PDGFR, c-KIT, p38) that affect the maintenance of the tumor vasculature and angiogenesis.[78] In December 2005 the FDA granted approval for sorafenib, considered the first multikinase inhibitor, for the treatment of patients with advanced RCC. The efficacy and safety of sorafenib was proven in the largest phase 3, multicenter, randomized, double-blind, placebo-controlled study conducted in advanced RCC. Treatment with sorafenib was shown to prolong PFS as compared with placebo.[79] The final OS analysis demonstrated that although an OS benefit was not seen on a primary intent-to-treat analysis, results of a secondary OS analysis censoring placebo patients demonstrated a survival advantage for those receiving sorafenib, suggesting an important cross-over effect.[80] In November 2007, sorafenib was approved for the treatment of patients with unresectable hepatocellular carcinoma (HCC) based on the results of an international, multicenter, randomized, double-blind, placebo-controlled trial in patients with advanced HCC who had not received previous systemic treatment. Median survival and the time to radiologic progression were nearly 3 months longer for patients treated with sorafenib than for those given placebo.[81]

Sorafenib was generally well tolerated with a predictable safety profile. The most common adverse events include diarrhea, rash/desquamation, fatigue, hand-foot skin reaction, alopecia, and nausea/vomiting. Grade 3/4 adverse events were 38% for sorafenib versus 28% for placebo. Sorafenib induced hypertension in patients with metastatic RCC. The treatment-related hypertension was noted to be a class effect observed not only with VEGFR inhibitors but also with the VEGF monoclonal antibody as well (reviewed in ref. 76). No significant relationship between previously described mediators of blood pressure and the magnitude of increase was found in a study evaluating the mechanism of sorafenib-induced hypertension in patients.[82]

One therapeutic combination of particular interest involves simultaneous blockade of VEGFRs with depletion of secreted VEGF. The rationale behind this approach is based on the observation that serum VEGF levels increase following administration of VEGFR inhibitors, including sorafenib. There are currently over 200 actively recruiting, ongoing clinical trials investigating the clinical benefit of sorafenib alone or in combination with chemotherapy or other targeted agents (such as bevacizumab) in patients with various solid tumors (http://clinicaltrial.gov).

Sunitinib

Sunitinib (SU11248) is a novel, oral, small-molecule, multitargeted RTK inhibitor of angiogenesis. It exhibits potent antitumor and antiangiogenic activity. Sunitinib is an inhibitor of multiple RTKs, including VEGFR-1, -2, -3; stem cell factor receptor (c-KIT); PDGF receptors; Fms-like tyrosine kinase 3 (FLT-3); colony stimulating factor receptor type 1 receptor; and the glial cell line–derived neurotrophic factor receptor. Previous TKIs such as SU6668 and SU5416 (semaxanib) had little success in the clinic because of poor pharmacologic properties and limited efficacy. Therefore, sunitinib was rationally designed and chosen for its high bioavailability and its nanomolar-range potency against the antiangiogenic RTKs.

In January 2006, sunitinib was granted approval by the FDA for the treatment of gastrointestinal stromal tumor after disease progression on, or intolerance to, imatinib and accelerated approval for the treatment of advanced RCC.[83] The accelerated approval for RCC was based on durable partial responses, with a response rate of 26% to 37%, and a median duration of response of 54 weeks from two phase 2, single-arm, multicenter trials of patients with cytokine-refractory RCC.[84] In February 2007, the FDA converted the accelerated approval of sunitinib for advanced RCC to regular approval following confirmation of an improvement in PFS. Efficacy data, based on an interim PFS analysis, was determined in a phase 3, multicenter, international randomized trial enrolling 750 patients with treatment-naive metastatic RCC to receive either sunitinib or IFN-α.[85] Final OS analysis of this trial showed that sunitinib demonstrated longer OS compared with IFN-α plus improvement in response and PFS in the first-line treatment of patients with metastatic RCC.[86]

Sunitinib demonstrated significant efficacy (prolonged median time to progression) in imatinib-resistant or -intolerant gastrointestinal stromal tumor in a randomized, double-blind, placebo-controlled phase 3 trial.[87] Adverse effects (grade 1 or 2 in severity) including diarrhea, mucositis, asthenia, skin abnormalities, and altered taste were more common in patients receiving sunitinib. In addition, a decrease in left ventricular ejection fraction and severe hypertension were also more commonly reported in the sunitinib arm. Grade 3 or 4 treatment-emergent adverse events were reported in 56% versus 51% of patients on sunitinib versus placebo, respectively.

Sunitinib has demonstrated robust antitumor activity in preclinical studies, resulting not only in tumor growth inhibition, but tumor regression in models of colon cancer, non–small cell lung cancer, melanoma, renal carcinoma, and squamous cell carcinoma, which were associated with inhibition of VEGFR and PDGFR phosphorylation. Clinical activity was evaluated in neuroendocrine, colon, and breast cancers in phase 2 studies. Studies investigating sunitinib alone in various tumor types and in combination with chemotherapy are ongoing.

Pazopanib

Pazopanib is an oral, second-generation, multitargeted, TKI that binds to VEGFR-1, -2, -3, PDGFR-α and -β, c-KIT, and several other key proteins responsible for angiogenesis, tumor growth, and cell survival. Pazopanib exhibited *in vivo* and *in vitro* activity against tumor growth and early clinical trials demonstrated potent antitumor and antiangiogenic activity.[88] A phase 3 clinical trial in treatment-naive and cytokine-pretreated patients with advanced and/or metastatic RCC showed a significant improvement in PFS and tumor response compared with placebo,[89] leading to the approval of pazopanib in the United States in October 2009. The drug is generally well tolerated in this population, with the most common adverse events being diarrhea, fatigue, anorexia, hypertension, and hair depigmentation as well as laboratory abnormalities in elevated aspartate aminotransferase and alanine aminotransferase. Pazopanib has shown clinical activity in a variety of tumors including breast cancer, soft tissue sarcoma, thyroid cancer, HCC, and cervical cancer.[90] Ongoing phase 2 and 3 trials are further evaluating pazopanib in these malignancies.

Thalidomide and Its Analogue Lenalidomide

Another antiangiogenic drug used in human malignancies is thalidomide, although its exact mechanism of action is still unclear. Thalidomide analogues, referred to as *immunomodulatory drugs,* were developed to enhance the immunomodulatory effects while minimizing the toxic effects of the parent drug. Thalidomide was originally prescribed outside the United States as a sedative and antiemetic for morning sickness and was subsequently marketed worldwide in the late 1950s. It was once notorious for producing severe limb abnormalities and other congenital defects in newborn babies whose mothers were given the drug during pregnancy. This resulted in the birth of over 10,000 infants worldwide with severe malformations and led to the withdrawal of the drug in the early 1960s. The drug was subsequently found to be effective in the treatment of erythema nodosum leprosum lesions, a painful inflammatory dermatologic reaction of lepromatous leprosy (also known as Hansen disease) and was granted approval by the FDA in 1998 for this indication. Off the market for several decades, thalidomide re-emerged in recent years as a somewhat effective treatment for various cancers, neurologic, and inflammatory diseases.[91]

Thalidomide was originally shown to inhibit angiogenesis by D'Amato et al.[92] in 1994 and this was subsequently confirmed in several different *in vitro* and *ex vivo* assays.[93–96] Interestingly, unlike other mechanisms of action, the antiangiogenic activity of thalidomide is believed to require enzymatic activation. The extent to which the antiangiogenic properties of thalidomide and its analogues play a role in its antimyeloma activity is not clearly understood. However, several mechanisms have been proposed that involve down-regulation of cytokines in EC, inhibition of EC proliferation, decrease in the level of circulating ECs, or modulation of adhesion molecules between the multiple myeloma cells and the endogenous bone marrow stromal cells, thereby decreasing the production of VEGF and interleukin-6.[97–100] In addition to its antiangiogenic activity, thalidomide and its immunomodulatory drugs also display anti-inflammatory and immunomodulatory properties.

In May 2006, thalidomide was granted accelerated approval for use in combination with dexamethasone for the treatment of newly diagnosed multiple myeloma patients. The effectiveness of thalidomide is based on objective improved response rates and shorter time to response in a phase 3 trial of 207 diagnosed patients randomly assigned to receive thalidomide plus dexamethasone or dexamethasone alone.[101] The response rate with thalidomide plus dexamethasone was significantly higher than with dexamethasone alone (63% vs. 41%, respectively; P = .0017). There are no controlled trials thus far demonstrating a clinical benefit. Because of thalidomide's known teratogenicity, the FDA is controlling thalidomide's marketing in the United States via the System for Thalidomide Education and Prescribing Safety (S.T.E.P.S.) program. This mandatory registry includes authorized patients, prescribers, and pharmacies, extensive patient education regarding thalidomide's safety, and is designed to prevent fetal exposure to thalidomide during pregnancy. The most common toxicities associated with thalidomide were grade 3 or higher venous thromboembolism, neuropathy, somnolence, constipation, and rash.

Lenalidomide has undergone rapid clinical development for the treatment of multiple myeloma.[102] It received fast-track designation from the FDA and was designated an orphan drug by the European Commission for Multiple Myeloma. In June 2006, the FDA approved lenalidomide for use in combination with dexamethasone in patients with multiple myeloma who have received one prior therapy. Lenalidomide is also available under a special restricted distribution program called RevAssist. Efficacy and safety were demonstrated in two randomized, double-blind, multicenter, multinational, placebo-controlled phase 3 studies comparing the combination of lenalidomide plus oral pulse dexamethasone versus dexamethasone alone in multiple myeloma patients who had received at least one prior therapy. In December 2005, lenalidomide was also granted FDA approval for patients with myelodysplastic syndromes associated with a deletion 5q cytogenetic abnormality with or without additional chromosomal abnormalities.

Thalidomide and its immunomodulatory analogues are being investigated in several phase 2/3 trials for treating various tumors including RCC,[103] prostate cancer, and HCC. Because both the docetaxel/thalidomide and the docetaxel/bevacizumab combinations exhibit significant activity in castrate-resistant prostate cancer,[96] presumably through targeting different angiogenic factors, a phase 2 trial of a four-drug combination consisting of docetaxel, prednisone, thalidomide, and bevacizumab was conducted in men with chemotherapy-naive, progressive castrate-resistant prostate cancer. Results from this study demonstrated the addition of bevacizumab and thalidomide to docetaxel is a highly active combination with manageable toxicities with an estimated median survival that is encouraging, given the generally poor prognosis of this patient population.[104] Phase 2 trials have shown promising results with thalidomide in combination with cytotoxic chemotherapy, but conducting randomized phase 3 trials is essential in order to validate these findings.

Temsirolimus and Everolimus

The mammalian target of rapamycin (mTOR) pathway is a central component of the PI3K/Akt signaling pathway and a regulator of many biological processes that are essential for angiogenesis, cell proliferation, and metabolism.[105] Inhibition of the mTOR kinase prevents downstream signaling via the Akt pathway, resulting in inhibition of protein translation and cell growth. mTOR plays a key role in angiogenesis and specifically regulates the expression of HIF-1, which is upregulated by the loss of the von Hippel Lindau gene in RCC. In May 2007, temsirolimus was approved for the treatment of advanced RCC. Efficacy and safety were demonstrated at a second interim analysis of a phase 3, multicenter, international, randomized, open-label study in previously untreated patients (N = 626) with poor risk features of metastatic RCC assigned to one of three treatment arms: IFN-α alone, temsirolimus 25 mg alone, or the combination of temsirolimus (15 mg) and IFN-α.[106] Single-agent temsirolimus was associated with a statistically significant improvement in OS when compared with IFN; the addition of temsirolimus to IFN did not improve OS. The most common adverse reactions that occurred were rash, asthenia, mucositis, nausea, edema, and anorexia. Rare serious adverse reactions associated with temsirolimus included interstitial lung disease, bowel perforation, and acute renal failure.

Everolimus (RAD001) was approved in March 2009 for patients with advanced RCC after failure of treatment with sunitinib or sorafenib, based on a longer PFS time than with placebo. Efficacy was demonstrated in a phase 3 trial of everolimus in patients with mRCC whose disease had progressed on VEGFR-targeted therapy (sunitinib or sorafenib).[107] The primary end point was PFS with the median PFS of 4.9 and 1.9 months in the everolimus and placebo arms, respectively (hazard ratio = 0.33; P <.0001). The most common adverse reactions were stomatitis, infections, asthenia, fatigue, cough, and diarrhea. The most common grade 3/4 adverse reactions were infections, dyspnea, fatigue, stomatitis, dehydration, pneumonitis, abdominal pain, and asthenia. Both temsirolimus and everolimus are currently being evaluated in phase 2 studies of various cancer types. By down-regulating HIF-1 in the tumor cell, mTOR inhibitors may complement the effects of TKIs at the level of the EC; thus, the combination of mTOR inhibitors with other targeted agents such as bevacizumab or sorafenib/sunitinib are also being investigated.

COMBINATION THERAPIES

Tumor angiogenesis is a highly complex process involving multiple growth factors and their receptor signaling pathways. Based on current evidence, with a few exceptions, effective therapy will probably rely on a combinatorial approach that involves targeting multiple pathways simultaneously. However, a recent study has demonstrated that simultaneous inhibition of the VEGF and EGF pathways in combination with chemotherapy shortens rather than prolongs PFS as compared to inhibition of the VEGF pathway alone in combination with chemotherapy.[108] Whether other targeted agents exhibit beneficial effects when combined with VEGF inhibitors remains to be investigated. Moreover, a number of studies have shown that antiangiogenic agents in combination with chemotherapy or radiotherapy result in additive or synergistic effects. Several models have been proposed to explain the mechanism responsible for this potentiation, keying in on the chemosensitizing effects of antiangiogenic therapy.[109] One hypothesis is that antiangiogenic therapy may normalize the tumor vasculature, thus resulting in improved oxygenation, better blood perfusion, and, consequently, improved delivery of chemotherapeutic drugs.[110] A second model suggests that chemotherapy delivered at low doses and at close, regular intervals with no extended drug-free break periods preferentially damages ECs in the tumor neovasculature[111,112] and suppresses circulating endothelial progenitor cells.[113,114] This regimen, also called *metronomic chemotherapy,* sustains antiangiogenic activity and reduces acute toxicity.[115] Thus, the efficacy of metronomic chemotherapy may increase when administered in combination with specific antiangiogenic drugs.

Finally, the third model addresses the use of antiangiogenic drugs to slow down tumor cell repopulation between successive cycles of cytotoxic chemotherapy.[116] This model underscores the importance of timing and sequence in achieving the maximal therapeutic benefit from combination therapies. Nevertheless, it remains a challenge to determine why bevacizumab has proved largely ineffective as a single agent whereas VEGF RTKIs have repeatedly failed in randomized phase 3 trials when used in combination with chemotherapy. Ongoing studies are continuing to evaluate the most effective combination of antiangiogenic agents with other targeted therapies and conventional therapies in order to improve clinical outcomes and to address what role drug combinations play in the efficacy of antiangiogenic agents.

SURROGATE MARKERS OF ANTIANGIOGENIC THERAPY

Antiangiogenic therapy has created a need to develop effective biomarkers to assess the activity of these inhibitors. Surrogate markers of tumor angiogenesis activity are important to guide clinical development of these agents and to select patients most likely to benefit from this approach. Although there are currently no validated biomarkers for clinically assessing the efficacy of or selecting patients who will respond to antiangiogenic therapies, a number of candidate markers including tissue, imaging, and circulating biomarkers are emerging that need to be prospectively validated.[117,118] Several avenues are currently being investigated and include tumor biopsy analysis, microvessel density, noninvasive vascular imaging modalities (positron emission tomography, dynamic contrast-enhanced magnetic resonance imaging), and measuring circulating biomarkers (levels of angiogenic factors in serum, plasma, urine or circulating ECs and their precursors).[119] Recent research efforts have focused on identifying genetic and toxicity biomarkers to predict which patients will benefit from anti-VEGF/VEGFR therapy and identify patients at risk of adverse events. The existence of VEGF single nucleotide polymorphisms and their association with clinical outcome may be predictive of patient response to bevacizumab. When patients with metastatic breast cancer were treated with paclitaxel and bevacizumab (E2100 trial), single nucleotide polymorphism analysis demonstrated that the VEGF-2578 AA and VEGF-1154 AA genotypes predicted an improved median OS, whereas the VEGF-634 CC and VEGF-1498 TT genotypes predicted protection from grade 3/4 hypertension in the combination treatment arm.[120]

Another candidate biomarker of response for antiangiogenic therapy is hypertension, one of the most common toxicities in patients taking VEGF inhibitors. The degree of hypertension can serve as a predictive biomarker of survival in patients after bevacizumab or TKI treatment. In the same E2100 trial, patients who experienced grade 3 or 4 hypertension survived significantly longer, although hypertension was seen in patients with the VEGF634 CC and VEGF1498 TT variants.[120] Other pharmacodynamic biomarkers of response to antiangiogenic therapy include elevated VEGF and placental growth factor levels,[117] while biomarkers of resistance include circulating basic fibroblast growth factor, stromal cell-derived factor 1α, and viable circulating endothelial cells increased when tumors escaped treatment.[121] If validated, these findings could help identify which subgroup of patients should receive antiangiogenic therapy and lead the way to possible future tailoring of individualized antiangiogenic therapy.

RESISTANCE TO ANTIANGIOGENIC THERAPY

Clinical experience with angiogenesis inhibitors reveals that VEGF-targeted therapy often prolongs survival of cancer patients by only months because tumors elicit evasive resistance.[122] Resistance to VEGF inhibitors may be observed in late-stage tumors when tumors regrow during treatment, after an initial period of growth suppression from these antiangiogenic agents. This resistance involves reactivation of tumor angiogenesis and increased expression of other proangiogenic factors. As the disease progresses, it is possible that redundant pathways might be implicated, with VEGF being replaced by other angiogenic pathways, warranting the addition of a second angiogenesis inhibitor that would target these secondary growth factors and/or their activated receptor pathways or the use of a multitargeted TKI antiangiogenic drug (e.g., sunitinib, sorafenib). However, resistance to these drugs eventually occurs, implicating the existence of additional pathways mediating resistance to antiangiogenic therapies. Whether the administration of angiogenic drugs at earlier stages of the disease may be a more effective and beneficial approach remains to be determined. Moreover, tumor cells bearing genetic alterations of the *p53* gene may display a lower apoptosis rate under hypoxic conditions, which might reduce their reliance on vascular supply and thereby their responsiveness to antiangiogenic therapy.[123] Therefore, the selection and overgrowth of tumor-variant cells that are hypoxia-resistant and thus less dependent[123] on angiogenesis and vasculature remodeling resulting in vessel stabilization[124] could also explain the resistance to antiangiogenic drugs. Other possible mechanisms for acquired resistance to antiangiogenic drugs include tumor vessels becoming less sensitive to antiangiogenic agents, tumor regrowth via rebound revascularization, and vessel cooption.[125–130] Perhaps one of the most intriguing finding is that although ECs are assumed to be genetically stable, they may under some circumstances harbor genetic abnormalities and thus acquire resistance as well.[131,132]

Recent studies report that VEGF-targeted therapies induce primary tumor shrinkage and inhibit tumor progression but can also initiate mechanisms that increase malignancy to promote tumor invasiveness and metastasis.[133–135] These mechanisms of resistance to antiangiogenic therapy involve tumor and host-mediated pathways and may allow for differential efficacy in different stages of disease progression.[130] Specifically, antiangiogenic drug resistance mechanisms involve pathways mediated by the tumor, whether intrinsic or acquired in response to therapy or by the host, which is either responding directly to therapy or indirectly to tumoral cues. Taken together, antiangiogenic therapy can enhance tumor invasiveness and metastasis to facilitate and/or accelerate disease in microscopic tumors and hence reduce OS benefit. Understanding the mechanisms of resistance, whether intrinsic or acquired, after exposure to antiangiogenic drug treatment is essential for developing strategies that will allow for optimal exploitation of the potential of VEGF inhibitors to block primary tumor growth while at the same time suppressing prometastatic effects. It is equally important to identify biomarkers of drug resistance and the factors mediating this resistance as the development of reliable biomarkers can be valuable to monitor the development of evasive resistance to angiogenesis inhibitors, thereby rendering this therapy more effective in the future.

Selected References

The full list of references for this chapter appears in the online version.

5. Folkman J. Tumor angiogenesis: therapeutic implications. *N Engl J Med* 1971;285:1182.
7. Hanahan D, Folkman J. Patterns and emerging mechanisms of the angiogenic switch during tumorigenesis. *Cell* 1996;86:353.
9. Folkman J, Kalluri R. Cancer without disease. *Nature* 2004;427:787.
10. Weidner N, Semple JP, Welch WR, Folkman J. Tumor angiogenesis and metastasis—correlation in invasive breast carcinoma. *N Engl J Med* 1991;324:1.
12. Naumov GN, Bender E, Zurakowski D, et al. A model of human tumor dormancy: an angiogenic switch from the nonangiogenic phenotype. *J Natl Cancer Inst* 2006;98:316.
13. Holmgren L, O'Reilly MS, Folkman J. Dormancy of micrometastases: balanced proliferation and apoptosis in the presence of angiogenesis suppression. *Nat Med* 1995;1:149.
14. Holash J, Maisonpierre PC, Compton D, et al. Vessel cooption, regression, and growth in tumors mediated by angiopoietins and VEGF. *Science* 1999;284:1994.
16. Carmeliet P, Dor Y, Herbert JM, et al. Role of HIF-1alpha in hypoxia-mediated apoptosis, cell proliferation and tumour angiogenesis. *Nature* 1998;394:485.
23. O'Reilly MS, Boehm T, Shing Y, et al. Endostatin: an endogenous inhibitor of angiogenesis and tumor growth. *Cell* 1997;88:277.
27. Kerbel RS. Vasohibin: the feedback on a new inhibitor of angiogenesis. *J Clin Invest* 2004;114:884.
28. Noguera-Troise I, Daly C, Papadopoulos NJ, et al. Blockade of Dll4 inhibits tumour growth by promoting non-productive angiogenesis. *Nature* 2006;444:1032.
29. Ridgway J, Zhang G, Wu Y, et al. Inhibition of Dll4 signalling inhibits tumour growth by deregulating angiogenesis. *Nature* 2006;444:1083.
31. Dameron KM, Volpert OV, Tainsky MA, Bouck N. Control of angiogenesis in fibroblasts by p53 regulation of thrombospondin-1. *Science* 1994;265:1582.
35. Teodoro JG, Parker AE, Zhu X, Green MR. p53-mediated inhibition of angiogenesis through up-regulation of a collagen prolyl hydroxylase. *Science* 2006;313:968.
36. Folkman J. Tumor suppression by p53 is mediated in part by the antiangiogenic activity of endostatin and tumstatin. *Sci STKE* 2006;2006:e35.
44. Folkman J. Angiogenesis: an organizing principle for drug discovery? *Nat Rev Drug Discov* 2007;6:273.
49. Ferrara N, Gerber HP, LeCouter J. The biology of VEGF and its receptors. *Nat Med* 2003;9:669.
50. Lindahl P, Johansson BR, Leveen P, Betsholtz C. Pericyte loss and microaneurysm formation in PDGF-B-deficient mice. *Science* 1997;277:242.
62. Desgrosellier JS, Cheresh DA. Integrins in cancer: biological implications and therapeutic opportunities. *Nat Rev Cancer* 2010;10:9.
65. Reynolds AR, Hart IR, Watson AR, et al. Stimulation of tumor growth and angiogenesis by low concentrations of RGD-mimetic integrin inhibitors. *Nat Med* 2009;15:392.
66. Hurwitz H, Fehrenbacher L, Novotny W, et al. Bevacizumab plus irinotecan, fluorouracil, and leucovorin for metastatic colorectal cancer. *N Engl J Med* 2004;350:2335.
67. Sandler A, Gray R, Perry MC, et al. Paclitaxel-carboplatin alone or with bevacizumab for non-small-cell lung cancer. *N Engl J Med* 2006;355:2542.
68. Miller K, Wang M, Gralow J, et al. Paclitaxel plus bevacizumab versus paclitaxel alone for metastatic breast cancer. *N Engl J Med* 2007;357:2666.
69a. Miles DW, Chan A, Dirix LY, et al. Phase III study of bevacizumab plus docetaxel compared with placebo plus docetaxel for the first-line treatment of human epidermal growth factor receptor 2-negative metastatic breast cancer. *J Clin Oncol* 2010;28:3239–3247.
69b. Robert NJ, Dieras V, Glaspy J, et al. RIBBON-1: Randomized, double-blind, placebo-controlled, phase III trial of chemotherapy with or without bevacizumab (B) for first-line treatment of HER2-negative locally recurrent or metastatic breast cancer (MBC). *J Clin Oncol* 2009;27(suppl):1005.
69c. Brufsky A, Rivera AA, Hurvitz SA, et al. Progression-free survival (PFS) in patient subgroups in RIBBON-2, a phase III trial of chemotherapy (chemo) plus or minus bevacizumab (BV) for second-line treatment of HER2-negative, locally recurrent or metastatic breast cancer (MBC). *J Clin Oncol* 2010;28 (suppl):1021.
71. Escudier B, Pluzanska A, Koralewski P, et al. Bevacizumab plus interferon alfa-2a for treatment of metastatic renal cell carcinoma: a randomised, double-blind phase III trial. *Lancet* 2007;370:2103.
72. Rini BI, Halabi S, Rosenberg JE, et al. Bevacizumab plus interferon alfa compared with interferon alfa monotherapy in patients with metastatic renal cell carcinoma: CALGB 90206. *J Clin Oncol* 2008;26:5422.
76. Chen HX, Cleck JN. Adverse effects of anticancer agents that target the VEGF pathway. *Nat Rev Clin Oncol* 2009;6:465.
77. Grothey A, Galanis E. Targeting angiogenesis: progress with anti-VEGF treatment with large molecules. *Nat Rev Clin Oncol* 2009;6:507.
79. Escudier B, Eisen T, Stadler WM, et al. Sorafenib in advanced clear-cell renal-cell carcinoma. *N Engl J Med* 2007;356:125.
81. Llovet JM, Ricci S, Mazzaferro V, et al. Sorafenib in advanced hepatocellular carcinoma. *N Engl J Med* 2008;359:378.
85. Motzer RJ, Hutson TE, Tomczak P, et al. Sunitinib versus interferon alfa in metastatic renal-cell carcinoma. *N Engl J Med* 2007;356:115.
87. Demetri GD, van Oosterom AT, Garrett CR, et al. Efficacy and safety of sunitinib in patients with advanced gastrointestinal stromal tumour after failure of imatinib: a randomised controlled trial. *Lancet* 2006;368:1329.
89. Sternberg CN, Davis ID, Mardiak J, et al. Pazopanib in locally advanced or metastatic renal cell carcinoma: results of a randomized phase III trial. *J Clin Oncol* 2010;28:1061.
92. D'Amato RJ, Loughnan MS, Flynn E, Folkman J. Thalidomide is an inhibitor of angiogenesis. *Proc Natl Acad Sci U S A* 1994;91:4082.
106. Hudes G, Carducci M, Tomczak P, et al. Temsirolimus, interferon alfa, or both for advanced renal-cell carcinoma. *N Engl J Med* 2007;356:2271.
107. Motzer RJ, Escudier B, Oudard S, et al. Efficacy of everolimus in advanced renal cell carcinoma: a double-blind, randomised, placebo-controlled phase III trial. *Lancet* 2008;372:449.
108. Tol J, Koopman M, Cats A, et al. Chemotherapy, bevacizumab, and cetuximab in metastatic colorectal cancer. *N Engl J Med* 2009;360:563.
109. Kerbel RS. Antiangiogenic therapy: a universal chemosensitization strategy for cancer? *Science* 2006;312:1171.
110. Jain RK. Normalization of tumor vasculature: an emerging concept in antiangiogenic therapy. *Science* 2005;307:58.
115. Kerbel RS, Kamen BA. The anti-angiogenic basis of metronomic chemotherapy. *Nat Rev Cancer* 2004;4:423.
117. Jain RK, Duda DG, Willett CG, et al. Biomarkers of response and resistance to antiangiogenic therapy. *Nat Rev Clin Oncol* 2009;6:327.
120. Schneider BP, Wang M, Radovich M, et al. Association of vascular endothelial growth factor and vascular endothelial growth factor receptor-2 genetic polymorphisms with outcome in a trial of paclitaxel compared with paclitaxel plus bevacizumab in advanced breast cancer: ECOG 2100. *J Clin Oncol* 2008;26:4672.
121. Batchelor TT, Sorensen AG, di Tomaso E, et al. AZD2171, a pan-VEGF receptor tyrosine kinase inhibitor, normalizes tumor vasculature and alleviates edema in glioblastoma patients. *Cancer Cell* 2007;11:83.
122. Kerbel RS. Tumor angiogenesis. *N Engl J Med* 2008;358:2039.
123. Yu JL, Rak JW, Coomber BL, Hicklin DJ, Kerbel RS. Effect of p53 status on tumor response to antiangiogenic therapy. *Science* 2002;295:1526.
128. Bergers G, Hanahan D. Modes of resistance to anti-angiogenic therapy. *Nat Rev Cancer* 2008;8:592.
130. Ebos JM, Lee CR, Kerbel RS. Tumor and host-mediated pathways of resistance and disease progression in response to antiangiogenic therapy. *Clin Cancer Res* 2009;15:5020.
131. Streubel B, Chott A, Huber D, et al. Lymphoma-specific genetic aberrations in microvascular endothelial cells in B-cell lymphomas. *N Engl J Med* 2004;351:250.
133. Loges S, Mazzone M, Hohensinner P, Carmeliet P. Silencing or fueling metastasis with VEGF inhibitors: antiangiogenesis revisited. *Cancer Cell* 2009;15:167.
134. Ebos JM, Lee CR, Cruz-Munoz W, et al. Accelerated metastasis after short-term treatment with a potent inhibitor of tumor angiogenesis. *Cancer Cell* 2009;15:232.
135. Paez-Ribes M, Allen E, Hudock J, et al. Antiangiogenic therapy elicits malignant progression of tumors to increased local invasion and distant metastasis. *Cancer Cell* 2009;15:220.
136. Folkman J, Kalluri N. Medicine. Tumor angiogenesis. In: Kufe DW, Pollock RE, Weichselbaum RR, et al. eds. *Cancer Medicine*, 6th ed. Hamilton, Ontario: BC Decker; 2003:161.
137. Kerbel R, Folkman J. Clinical translation of angiognesis inhibitors. *Nat Rev Cancer* 2002;2:727.

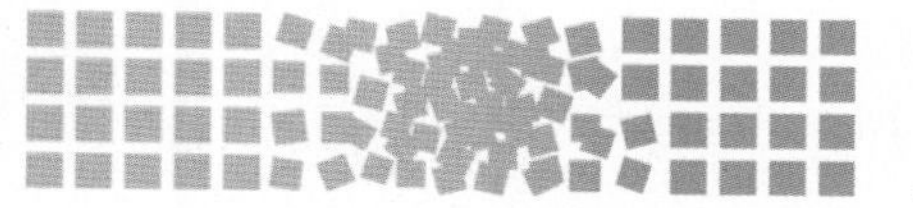

CHAPTER 48 MONOCLONAL ANTIBODIES

MATTHEW K. ROBINSON, HOSSEIN BORGHAEI, GREGORY P. ADAMS, AND LOUIS M. WEINER

Antibody-based therapeutics have become important components of the cancer therapeutic armamentarium. Early antibody therapy studies attempted to explicitly target cancers based on the structural and biologic properties that distinguish neoplastic cells from their normal counterparts. The first generation of monoclonal antibodies (MAbs) that were evaluated in clinical trials demonstrated a limited effectiveness. To a large degree, this was because of their immunogenicity and inefficient effector functions.[1–3] Initial MAbs used in clinical trials were murine in origin and patients developed human antimouse antibody responses against the therapeutic agents that limited both efficacy of the MAb by rapidly clearing it from the body and the number of times the therapy could be administered. More recently, work with engineered chimeric, humanized, and fully human MAbs has identified a number of important and useful applications for antibody-based cancer therapy. Currently, the U.S. Food and Drug Administration (FDA) has approved ten antibodies for the treatment of cancer (Table 48.1) and many more are under evaluation in late-stage clinical trials.[4] Antibodies provide an important means by which to exploit the immune system by specifically recognizing and directing antitumor responses.

Antibodies are produced by B cells and arise in response to exposures to a variety of structures, termed *antigens,* as a result of a series of recombinations of V, D, and J germ line genes. Immunoglobulin-G (IgG) molecules are most commonly employed as the working backbones of current therapeutic MAbs, although various other isotypes of antibodies have specialized functions (e.g., IgA molecules play important roles in mucosal immunity and IgE molecules are involved in anaphylaxis). The advent of hybridoma technology by Kohler and Milstein[5] made it possible to produce large quantities of antibodies with high purity and monospecificity for a single binding region (epitope) on an antigen.

The mechanisms that antibody-based therapeutics employ to elicit antitumor effects include focusing components of the patient's immune system to attack tumor cells[6,7] and methods to alter signal transduction pathways that drive tumor progression.[8,9] Antibody-based conjugates employ the targeting specificity of antibodies to deliver toxic compounds, such as radionuclides or chemotherapeutics, specifically to the tumor sites.

IMMUNOGLOBULIN STRUCTURE

Structural and Functional Domains

An IgG molecule is typically divided into three domains consisting of two identical antigen-binding (Fab) domains connected to an effector or Fc domain by a flexible hinge sequence. Figure 48.1 shows the structure of an IgG molecule, as well as enzymatically derived or recombinantly prepared antibody fragments. The IgG antibodies are composed of two identical light chains and two identical heavy chains, with the chains joined by disulfide bonds, resulting in a bilaterally symmetrical complex. The Fab domains mediate the binding of IgG molecules to their cognate antigens and are composed of an intact light chain and half of a heavy chain. Each chain in the Fab domain is further divided into variable and constant regions, with the variable region containing hypervariable, or complementarity determining regions (CDRs) in which the antigen-contact residues reside. The light and heavy chain variable regions each contain three CDRs (CDR1, CDR2, and CDR3). All six CDRs combine to form the antigen-binding pocket and are collectively defined in immunologic terms as the idiotype of the antibody. Although each of the six CDRs contribute to the binding process, in the majority of cases the variable heavy chain CDR3 plays a dominant role.[10]

The different isotypes of immunoglobulins are defined by the structure and function of their Fc domains. The Fc domain, composed of the CH2 and CH3 regions of the antibody's heavy chains, is the critical determinant of how an antibody mediates effector functions, transports across cellular barriers, and persists in circulation.[7,11]

MODIFIED ANTIBODY-BASED MOLECULES

Advances in antibody engineering and molecular biology have facilitated the development of many novel antibody-based structures with unique physical and pharmacokinetic properties (Fig. 48.1). These include chimeric human-murine antibodies with human-constant regions and murine-variable regions,[12] humanized antibodies in which murine CDR sequences have been grafted into human IgG molecules, and entirely human antibodies derived from human hybridomas and more recently from transgenic mice expressing human immunoglobulin genes.[13] Accepted product source identifiers and oncologic indicators are listed in Table 48.2. If the MAb is used as an immunoconjugate, a second word identifies the conjugated moiety. Engineering has also facilitated development of antibody-based fragments. In addition to the classic, enzymatically derived, Fab and $F(ab')_2$ molecules, a plethora of promising IgG derivatives have been developed that retain antigen-binding properties of intact antibodies (Fig. 48.1) (reviewed in ref. 14). The basic building block for these molecules is the 25-kDa, monovalent single-chain Fv (scFv) that is composed of the variable domains (V_H and V_L) of an antibody derived from either murine hybridomas[15] or phage-display libraries[16] and fused together with a short peptide linker. Examining the behavior of these engineered molecules has allowed the identification of many critical properties that impact the uptake of the antibodies into solid tumors.

TABLE 48.1

FOOD AND DRUG ADMINISTRATION–APPROVED ANTIBODIES FOR THE TREATMENT OF CANCER

Generic Name (Trade Name)	Origin	Isotype and Format	Indication	Target	Dose	Year Approved
UNCONJUGATED MAbs						
Rituximab (Rituxan)	Chimeric	Human IgG1	NHL, CLL	CD20	NHL, 375 mg/m^2 QWK; CLL, 375 mg/m^2 (1st cycle) and 500 mg/m^2 in cycle 2–6 (Q 28 days)	1997
Trastuzumab (Herceptin)	Humanized	Human IgG1	Breast	HER2	4 mg/kg loading, 2 mg/kg maintenance QWK	1998
Alemtuzumab (Campath-1H)	Humanized	Human IgG1	CLL	CD52	Escalate on defined schedule to 30 mg/day, 3 × per week on alternate days for 12 wk	2001
Cetuximab (Erbitux)	Chimeric	Human IgG1	Colorectal, head and neck	EGFR	400 mg/m^2 loading, 250 mg/m^2 maintenance QWK	2004
Bevacizumab (Avastin)	Humanized	Human IgG1	Colorectal, lung, renal cell, GBM, breast	VEGF	CRC, 5 mg/kg (10 mg/kg) Q2 wk with bolus-IFL (FOLFOX4); BrCa, GBM, RCCC: 10 mg/kg Q2 wk; NSCLC, 15 mg/kg Q3 weeks	2004
Panitumumab (Vectibix)	Human (XenoMouse)	Human IgG2	Colorectal cancer	EGFR	6 mg/kg Q2 wk	2006
Ofatumumab (Arzerra)	Human (XenoMouse)	Human IgG1	CLL	CD20	300 mg initial dose followed 1 wk later by 2,000 mg QWK × 7, followed 4 wk later by 2,000 mg Q4 wk for 4 doses	2009
IMMUNOCONJUGATES						
Gemtuzumab Ozogamicin (Mylotarg)	Humanized	Human IgG4 (calicheamicin conjugate)	Acute myelogenous leukemia	CD33	9 mg/m^2 Q 2 wk for 2 doses	2000
Ibritumomab Tiuxetan (Zevalin)	Murine	Murine IgG1 (^{90}Y-conjugate)	NHL	CD20	Day 1, 250 mg/m^2 Rituximab + 5 mCi ^{111}In-Zevalin; Day 3 or 4, imaging scan; Day 7, 8, or 9, 250 mg/m^2 Rituximab + 0.3–0.4 mCi/kg ^{90}Y-Zevalin (<32 mCi)	2002
Tositumomab (Bexxar)	Murine	Murine IgG2A (^{131}I-conjugate)	NHL	CD20	Day 1, 450 mg Tositumomab + 5 mCi ^{131}I-Tositumomab; day 3–8, two imaging scans; day 8, 450 mg Tositumomab + 0.655 Gy (35 mg) ^{131}I-Tositumomab	2003

MAb, monoclonal antibody; NHL, non–Hodgkin's lymphoma; CLL, chronic lymphocytic lymphoma; IgG, immunoglobulin-G; GBM, glioblastoma multiforme; RCCC, renal clear cell carcinoma; NSCLC, non–small cell lung cancer.

FACTORS REGULATING ANTIBODY-BASED TUMOR TARGETING

A number of obstacles to treatment efficacy have been identified in preclinical studies and in clinical trials and are summarized in Table 48.3.

Antibody Size

Nonuniform distribution of systemically administered antibody is generally observed in biopsied specimens of solid tumors. Heterogeneous tumor blood supply limits uniform antibody delivery to tumors, and elevated interstitial pressures in the center of tumors oppose inward diffusion.[17] This high interstitial pressure leads to a net outward gradient from the tumor center and is predicted to slow the diffusion of molecules from their vascular extravasation site in a size-dependent manner.[18,19] The relatively large transport distances in the tumor interstitium also substantially increase the time required for large IgG macromolecules to reach target cells.[20]

To the first approximation, the pharmacokinetic behavior of a protein correlates with its size relative to the renal threshold; proteins less than approximately 65 kDa are small enough to pass through the glomeruli of the kidney and undergo rapid,

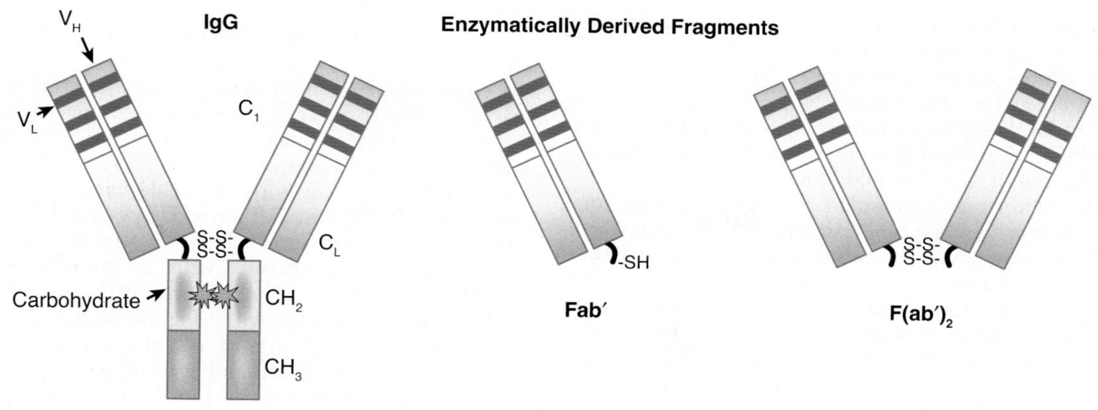

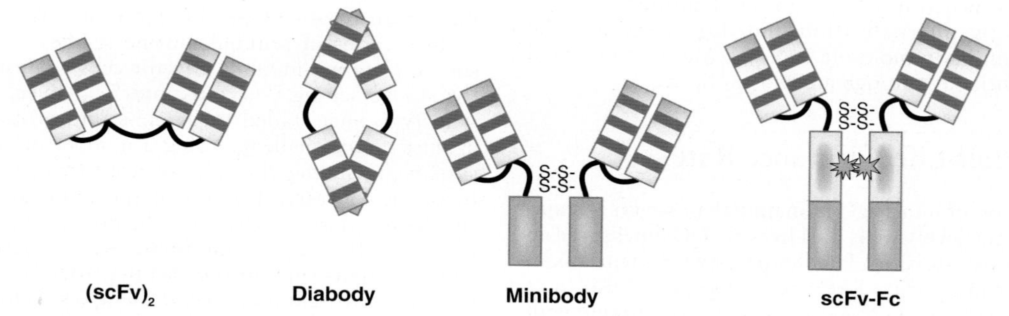

FIGURE 48.1 Antibody-based targeting proteins. C, constant; V, variable; H, heavy chain; L, light chain; IgG, immunoglobulin-G; Fab, fragment of IgG; F(ab′)$_2$, fragment of IgG after pepsin digestion; scFv, single-chain Fv; (scFv)$_2$, dimeric scFv.

first-pass renal clearance.[21] In the case of the antibody-based molecules described in Figure 48.1, only the scFv, (scFv′)$_2$, and diabody are small enough to be eliminated in this manner. The more rapid tumor penetration exhibited by these molecules is therefore coupled with a rapid clearance from the tumor-bearing host.[22]

TABLE 48.2

RULES FOR NAMING MONOCLONAL ANTIBODIES FOR THE TREATMENT OF CANCER

PRODUCT SOURCE IDENTIFIERS	
-e-	Hamster
-a-	Rat
-i-	Primate
-o-	Mouse
-xi-	Chimeric
-zu-	Humanized
-u-	Human
ONCOLOGIC INDICATION	
-col-	Colorectal
-mel-	Melanoma
-mar-	Breast
-got-	Testis
-gov-	Ovarian
-pr(o)-	Prostate
-tu(m)-	Miscellaneous

Tumor Antigens

Access to the target antigen is undoubtedly a critical determinant of therapeutic effect of antibody-based applications. The heterogeneity of antigen expression by tumor cells can contribute to this phenomenon. Moreover, shed antigen in the serum, tumor microenvironment, or both may saturate the antibody's binding sites and prevent binding to the cell surface. Alternatively, a rapid internalization of an antibody/antigen complex may deplete the quantity of cell surface MAb capable of initiating antibody-dependent cellular cytotoxicity (ADCC) or cytotoxic signal transduction events. Finally, target antigens are normally *tumor-associated* rather than *tumor-specific*. Tumor-specific antigens that exhibit high levels of expression limited to malignant tissue are both highly desirable and rare. Typically these antigens arise as a result of unique genetic recombinations that are the cause or consequence of oncogenic

TABLE 48.3

OBSTACLES TO SUCCESSFUL MONOCLONAL ANTIBODY THERAPY

Impaired antibody distribution and delivery to tumor sites
Inadequate trafficking of effector cells to tumor
Intratumoral and intertumoral antigenic heterogeneity
Shed or internalized targets
Insufficient tumor specificity of target antigens
Human antimouse antibody responses

transformation, such as clonal immunoglobulin idiotypes expressed on the surface of B-cell lymphomas.[23]

Antibody affinity for its target antigen has complex effects on tumor targeting. The "binding-site barrier" hypothesis postulates that antibodies with extremely high affinity for target antigen would bind irreversibly to the first antigen encountered on entering the tumor, which would limit the diffusion of antibody into the tumor and accumulate instead in regions surrounding the tumor vasculature.[24] Adams et al.[25,26] described the effect of antibody affinity on tumor retention and penetration in more detail in a set of experiments using a series of anti-HER2/neu scFv with affinities ranging from 1.6×10^{-6} M to 1.5×10^{-11} M. In direct support of the binding site barrier hypothesis, a low-affinity scFv distributed diffusely throughout the vascularized regions of the tumors within 24 hours postinjection, whereas an scFv with 10,000-fold higher affinity was only detected within several cell diameters of the blood vessels. These results may be explained by tumor cell internalization and degradation of high-affinity antibodies. In tumor spheroids, the *in vitro* penetration of engineered antibodies is primarily limited by internalization and degradation.[27] The valence of an antibody molecule can increase the functional affinity of the antibody through an avidity effect.[28–30]

Half-Life/Clearance Rate

The concentration of intact IgG in mammalian serum is maintained at constant levels with half-lives of IgGs measured in days. This homeostasis is regulated in part by the major histocompatibility complex class I–related Fc receptor, FcRn (n = neonatal). FcRn is a dimer composed of a 50-kDa protein with homology to the major histocompatibility complex α-chains and the 15-kDa nonpolymorphic β_2-microglobulin, an invariant component of major histocompatibility complex class I. FcRn is expressed in endothelial cells, the predominant cell type in the body and one with close proximity to the vasculature. Mutations in the Fc domain of IgGs that alter the affinity for FcRn modify IgG half-life in serum.[31,32] The IgG mutations that increase serum half-life in a wild type mouse fail to do so in C57BL/6 mice that lack a functional FcRn.[11]

Multiple strategies have been developed to increase the serum persistence of antibody-based fragments and other classes of protein therapeutics (reviewed in ref. 14). For example, MM-111, a bispecific anti-HER2/HER3 scFv-albumin fusion protein that is currently in clinical trials, was developed using this approach.[33]

Glycosylation

Immunoglobulin-Gs undergo N-linked glycosylation at the conserved Asn residue at position 297 within the C_H2 domain of the constant region. Glycosylation status of the residue has long been known to impact the ability of IgGs to bind effector ligands such as FcγR and C1q and in turn affect their ability to participate in Fc-mediated functions such as ADCC and complement-dependent cytotoxicity (CDC).[34–36] The glycosylation of MAbs can be altered to increase ADCC by producing them in a Chinese hamster ovary cell line engineered to express the β(1,4)-*N*-acetylglucosaminyltransferase III (GnTIII), the enzyme required to add the bisecting GlcNAc residues.[35]

UNCONJUGATED ANTIBODIES

The majority of MAbs approved for clinical use display intrinsic antitumor effects that are mediated by one or more of the following mechanisms.

Cell-Mediated Cytotoxicity

As components of the immune system, effector cells such as natural killer (NK) cells and monocytes/macrophages represent a natural line of defense against oncologically transformed cells. Effector cells express Fcγ receptors (FcγR) on their cell surfaces that interact with the Fc domain of IgG molecules. This family is composed of three classes (type I, II, and III) that are further divided into subclasses (IIa/IIb and IIIa/IIIb).[37] Recognition of transformed cells by immune effector cells leads to cell-mediated killing through processes such as ADCC and phagocytosis, as shown in Figure 48.2, and can be mediated by FcγRI, a high-affinity receptor capable of binding to monomeric IgG, or FcγRII and FcγRIII, which are low-affinity receptors that preferentially bind multimeric complexes of IgG. Signaling through type I, IIa, and IIIa receptors results in activation of effector cells due to associated immunoreceptor tyrosine-based activation motifs, whereas engagement of type IIb receptors inhibits cells activation through associated immunoreceptor tyrosine-based inhibitory motifs.[37]

In a series of seminal murine studies[38] antibodies were shown to target immune effector cells against cancer cells in the *in vivo* setting.[39,40] Fc receptor $\gamma^{-/-}$ mice, unlike congenic wild type mice, failed to demonstrate protective immunity against tumor challenge using a number of antibody/antigen systems, including clinically relevant trastuzumab and rituximab. In contrast, deletion of the inhibitory type II FcγR (FcγRIIb) led to an increase in the protective effect, suggesting that FcγRIIB acts to modulate ADCC activity *in vivo*.[40] Clinical results support the idea that ADCC can play a role in the efficacy of antibody-based therapies. Naturally occurring polymorphisms in FcγRs alter their affinity for human IgG1 and have been linked to clinical response.[41,42] A polymorphism in the *FCGR3A* gene results in either a valine or phenylalanine at position 158 of FcγRIIIa. Human IgG1 binds more strongly to FcγRIIIa-158V than FcγRIIIa-158F, and likewise to NK cells from individuals that are either homozygous for 158F or heterozygous for this polymorphism.[43] The FcγRIIIa-158v was a predictor of early response and was associated with progression free survival (PFS). Patients homozygous for 158V had a 2-year PFS of 45%, compared with 14% for F carriers. A second polymorphism, FcγRIIa-131H/R, did not predict early response but was an independent predictor of TTP.[42]

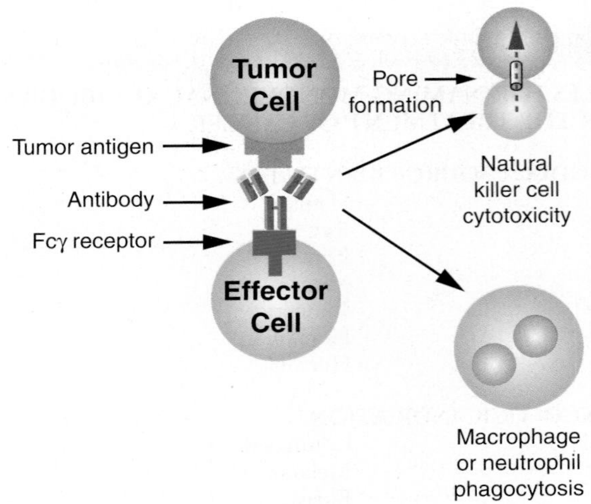

FIGURE 48.2 Antibody-dependent cellular cytotoxicity. The antibody engages the tumor antigen and the Fc domain binds to cellular Fc receptors to bridge effector and target cells. This bridging induces effector cell activation, resulting in natural killer cell cytotoxicity or phagocytosis by neutrophils, monocytes, or macrophages.

Taken together, these data suggest that modulating the affinity of MAbs for FcγRIIIa, FcγRIIa, or both, may increase the efficacy of therapeutic MAbs.

Each class of FcγR exhibits a characteristic specificity for IgG subclasses.[44] For example, the activating FcγRIII binds preferentially to IgG1 and IgG3, whereas the inhibitory FcγRIIb binds with somewhat less affinity for IgG1, suggesting that IgG1 may be the best backbone to elicit effector function. Many groups have focused on modifying the Fc domain of IgGs to optimize engagement of subclasses of FcγR and induction of ADCC. This work is based in large part on the findings of Shields et al.,[31] who performed a series of mutagenesis experiments to map the residues required for IgG1-FcγR interaction.

Ocrelizumab, a humanized version of rituximab, has been engineered for increased binding to low-affinity FcγRIIIa variants. In a phase 1/2 trial in patients with rituximab-relapsed/refractory non–Hodgkin's lymphoma (NHL), ocrelizumab had a 36% relative risk. A third-generation anti-CD20 antibody, PRO131921, is an engineered form of ocrelizumab. It binds with higher affinity to CD20, and the Fc domain of this humanized antibody has been engineered to increase binding affinity for both FcγRIIIa and C1q as compared with rituximab and ocrelizumab. In recent phase 1 trials, PRO131921 has demonstrated clinical activity in the setting of rituximab-relapsed/refractory NHL patients.[45] Responses seen with these and other engineered anti-CD20 antibodies in these heavily pretreated patient populations warrant further study of these novel agents.

An alternative to modifying the Fc region of MAbs is to create bispecific antibodies that recognize both a tumor-associated antigen and a "trigger antigen" present on the surface of an immune effector cell.[43] Simultaneous engagement of both antigens can redirect the cytotoxic potential of the effector cell against the tumor.[46–48] Such antibodies are capable of eliciting effector function against tumor cell lines *in vitro* and in animal models. Two HER2-directed bispecific antibodies, 2B1 and MDX-H210, have been tested in phase 1 clinical trials.[49,50]

Bispecific antibodies have a number of possible advantages over IgG molecules, including flexible choices of cytotoxic trigger molecules,[51] recruitment of effector function in the presence of excess IgG,[47] and custom tailoring of the affinity of the bispecific antibody to match effector cell characteristics. These advantages have been associated with improved methods of bispecific antibodyproduction.[52] BiTE (bispecfic T-cell engager) antibodies represent a novel class of bispecific single-chain Fv antibodies that have the benefits of the classic bispecific antibodies previously described, but overcome the production issues associated with those molecules.[53] Promising results have been seen in early-phase clinical trials with at least two BiTE antibodies. In phase 1 trials in the setting of relapsed NHL, doses as low as 0.005 mg/m^3 of the anti-CD19/anti-CD3 blinatumomab led to clearance of CD19+ tumor cells in blood. All patients (7 of 7) treated at the 0.06 mg/m^3 dose level experienced tumor regression.[54] Promising phase 1 trial results have also been reported in interim analysis of the anti-EpCAM/anti-CD3 MT110 BiTE in the setting of advanced lung and gastrointestinal tumors.[55]

Complement-Dependent Cytotoxicity

In addition to cell-mediated killing (see previous discussion), MAbs can recruit the complement cascade to kill cells via CDC. Although IgM is the most effective isotype for complement activation, it is not widely used in clinical oncology. Similar to ADCC, the human IgG subclass used to construct a therapeutic MAb dictates its ability to elicit CDC; in contrast to IgG2 and IgG4, IgG1 is extremely efficient at fixing the complement.[56] Antibodies activate complement through the classic pathway, by engaging multiple C1q to trigger activation of a cascade of serum proteases, which kill the antibody-bound cells.[57,58] The anti-CD20 MAb rituximab has been found to depend in part on CDC for its *in vivo* efficacy.[59] Antibody engineering approaches have identified residues in the C_H2 domain of the Fc region that either suppress or enhance the ability of rituximab to bind C1q and activate CDC.[60] The ability to manipulate complement fixation through engineering approaches warrants *in vivo* testing to determine the impact of these changes on the efficacy and toxicity of MAbs.

Immunomodulation

Cytotoxic T-lymphocyte associated antigen 4 (CTLA-4) is a critical inhibitory receptor of T-cell activation. Antibodies directed against CTLA-4 have been shown to increase CD8+ and CD4+ immune response and induce tumor regression in a number of experimental systems.[61,62] Two such antibodies are undergoing phase 3 clinical trials in the setting of metastatic melanoma and have shown clinical therapeutic responses according to the response evaluation criteria in solid tumors (RECIST).[63] Adverse events observed in the clinical trials are consistent with antibody-based induction of autoimmune responses through interference with CTLA-4 engagement of its cognate ligands. Induction of these autoimmune responses in melanoma patients correlates with tumor regression.[64] These results suggest that combinatorial therapeutic strategies that incorporate anti-CTLA-4 antibodies with other antibodies that induce ADCC, with vaccines or with cytotoxic chemotherapy or radiotherapy, offer the potential of enhancing tumor antigen-specific immune responses. Other costimulatory molecules that are the target of antibodies in clinical development include CD40 and CD137.[65] More recently, additional regulators of costimulation through CD137 have been identified and offer new avenues to expand and direct tumor antigen-specific immune responses.[66]

ALTERING SIGNAL TRANSDUCTION

Growth factor receptors represent a well-established class of targets for therapeutic intervention. Normal signaling through these receptors often leads to mitogenic and prosurvival responses. Unregulated signaling, as seen in a number of common cancers due to receptor overexpression, promotes tumor cell growth and insensitivity to chemotherapeutic agents. Clinically relevant MAbs can modulate signaling through their target receptors to normalize cell growth rates and sensitize tumor cells to cytotoxic agents. Binding of cetuximab or panitumumab to the epidermal growth factor receptor (EGFR) physically blocks ligand binding[67] and prevents the receptor from assuming the extended conformation required for dimerization.[68] Pertuzumab binds to the dimerization domain of HER2, thereby sterically inhibiting subsequent receptor heterodimerization with other ligand-bound family members.[69] Alternatively, signaling through growth factor receptors can be indirectly modified by MAbs that bind to activating ligands, as is seen with the anti–vascular endothelial growth factor (VEGF) MAb bevacizumab.[70]

Activation of the proapoptotic TRAIL-R1 and TRAIL-R2 through use of agonistic antibodies represents a potential therapeutic modality. HGS-ETR1 (mapatumumab), a fully human agonistic monoclonal antibody specific for TRAIL-R1, induces cell death in tumor cell lines by activating both the extrinsic and intrinsic arms of the apoptotic pathway. The intrinsic

TABLE 48.4

ADVANTAGES OF DIFFERENT IMMUNOCONJUGATE STRATEGIES

IMMUNOTOXINS
Exceedingly potent
Catalytic action
Well-defined biology and chemistry
DRUG IMMUNOCONJUGATES
Proven efficacy of antineoplastic components in cancer medicine
Well-defined spectra of efficacy and toxicity
Possibility of bystander effect
Internalization of immunoconjugate not required
RADIOIMMUNOCONJUGATES
Multiple available isotopes permit customized approaches
Multiple cell radius of action to address antigenic heterogeneity
Internalization not usually required
Predictable toxicity based on dosimetry

activity of HGS-ETR1 suppresses the growth of colon, lung, and renal tumors in xenograft models in athymic mice[71] and led to phase 1 clinical trials of HGS-ETR1, alone and in combination with either gemcitabine or cisplatin. Preliminary results from these trials have confirmed the pharmacokinetics, safety of the agent, with hints of clinical activity.

IMMUNOCONJUGATES

MAbs that are not capable of directly eliciting antitumor effects, either by altering signal transduction or directing immune system cells, can still be effective against tumors by delivering cytotoxic payloads (Table 48.4). MAbs have been employed to deliver a wide variety of agents including chemotherapy, toxins, radioisotopes, and cytokines (reviewed in ref. 4). In theory, the appropriate combination of toxic agent and MAb could lead to a synergistic effect. For example, delivery of a therapeutic radioisotope by a MAb would be significantly enhanced if by binding to its target antigen the MAb also activated a signaling event that increased the target cell's sensitivity to ionizing radiation.

Immunodrug Conjugates

Gemtuzumab ozogamicin (Mylotarg), approved by the FDA in 2000 for the treatment of patients with relapsed CD33-positive acute myeloid leukemia, represents the only FDA-approved immunodrug conjugate to date. Gemtuzumab ozogamicin is composed of a humanized IgG4 anti-CD33 antibody conjugated to the cytotoxic antibiotic calicheamicin. Binding of gemtuzumab to CD33, which is expressed on the surface of 85% to 90% of leukemia progenitor cells but not mature granulocytes or nonhematopoietic cells,[72] focuses the DNA-damaging activity of calicheamicin to leukemia cells as compared with normal tissue. Gemtuzumab ozogamicin has exhibited a combined overall response rate of 26% (71 of 277), with age and duration of first remission being the two most critical determinants of response.[73]

Successful development of immunodrug conjugates requires that attention be paid not only to effective tumor targeting of the antibody but also to efficient delivery of active drug once the conjugate is bound to the tumor cell surface. Strategies to overcome difficulties associated with delivery of active drug to tumor cells are well illustrated by the development of cantuzumab mertansine and its subsequent derivatives[74,75] as well as trastuzumab-DM1.[76] Cantuzumab has had limited success in clinical trials.[75,77] Linker structure and subsequent drug metabolites can affect the efficacy of immunoconjugates *in vivo* in a manner that would not necessarily be predicted from *in vitro* toxicity data.[74,78]

Coupling DM1 to trastuzumab (T-DM1) through a nonreducible thioether linkage offered improved pharmacokinetics, efficacy, and therapeutic window as compared with disulfide-based cleavable linkers.[76] Phase 2 clinical trials demonstrate that T-DM1 has robust single-agent activity. Overall response and clinical benefit rates of 33% and 44.5%, respectively, were achieved in heavily pretreated HER2-positive metastatic breast cancer patients who had progressed after both trastuzumab and lapatinib-based therapies.[79,80] Advances in the engineering of immunodrug conjugates and clinical successes with agents such as T-DM1 have led to an increased focus on development of immunodrug conjugates. A wide variety of immunodrug conjugates are currently undergoing clinical testing. Examples include, but are not limited to, the anti-PSMA MLN2704 in castration-resistant prostate cancer,[81] the anti-GPNMB CR011-vcMMAE in melanoma,[82,83] as well as a number of immunodrug conjugates (SGN-35, CMC-544, and SAR3419) in various lymphomas.[84–87]

Antibodies also can be used to target liposome-encapsulated drugs[88] and other cytotoxic agents such as antisense RNA[89] or radionuclides to tumors.

Immunotoxins

Catalytic toxins derived from plants (e.g., ricin) and microorganisms (e.g., pseudomonas) represent another class of cytotoxic agents being investigated for their utility in immunoconjugate strategies.[90] Immunotoxins have demonstrated significant antitumor effects in preclinical models. For example, Kreitman et al.[91] have reported complete regressions of human Burkitt lymphoma xenografts in mice that were treated with BL22, a recombinant anti-CD22 immunotoxin composed of the RFB4(dsFv) and a truncated form of *Pseudomonas exotoxin,* at relevant doses based on those tolerated by cynomolgus monkeys. This led to a phase 1 clinical trial in hairy cell leukemia patients who were resistant to cladribine.[92] Eleven of 16 patients exhibited complete remissions and the observance of minimal side effects. Clinical trials with other immunotoxins have been associated with unacceptable neurotoxicity[93] and life-threatening vascular leak syndrome.[94]

Superantigens, such as staphylococcal enterotoxin E superantigen (SEA/E-120) incorporated into Naptumomab estafenatox, have been fused to antibodies as well. Decoration of tumor cells with superantigen-based immunotoxins results in a potent, localized T cell–dependent killing of the tumor cells as well as induction of inflammatory and tumoricidal cytokine responses that can induce a bystander effect (reviewed in ref. 95).

Immunocytokine Conjugates

Immunocytokine fusions have been investigated as an approach to direct the patient's immune response to his or her own tumor.[96] A number of cytokines have been incorporated into antibody-based constructs, including interleukin-2 (IL-2),[97,98] γ-interferon,[99] tumor necrosis factor-α,[99] VEGF,[100] and IL-12.[101] Because immunocytokine conjugates based on intact IgG molecules often suffer from accelerated systemic clearance, site-directed mutagenesis of the FcRn site on the Fc domain has been employed to prolong their retention in circulation.[102]

Radioimmunoconjugates

Two anti-CD20 radioimmunoconjugates are FDA approved for radioimmunotherapy of NHL. Ibritumomab (Zevalin) and tositumomab (Bexxar) are murine MAbs labeled with yttrium-90 (^{90}Y) and iodine-131 (^{131}I), respectively. Both are associated with impressive clinical efficacy.[103] Treatment with ibritumomab leads to an overall response rate of 67%, with low-grade disease exhibiting an even better overall response rate of 82%.[104] Significantly, therapeutic efficacy was seen even in the presence of bulky disease and splenomegaly. Although these MAbs are of murine origin, human antimouse antibody responses (described earlier) are not frequently observed with these two radioimmunoconjugates.[105] Despite significant preclinical evidence supporting the use of radioimmunotherapy for solid malignancies, clinical results have not demonstrated consistent antitumor activity.[4]

UNCONJUGATED ANTIBODIES APPROVED FOR USE AGAINST SOLID TUMORS

Trastuzumab

RhuMAb HER2,[106] also known as trastuzumab (Herceptin), is a humanized antibody derived from 4D5, a murine monoclonal antibody that recognizes HER2/neu. HER2/neu (c-erbB-2), a member of the EGFR family, has been targeted for antibody therapy as it is overexpressed by gene amplification in 25% of breast cancers. In a phase 2 trial in women with metastatic breast cancer, Baselga et al.[107] reported an objective response rate of 11.6%, with responses seen in the liver, mediastinum, lymph nodes, and chest wall metastases, and Cobleigh et al.[108] treated 222 women with metastatic breast cancer, finding an objective response rate of 16%. Thus, trastuzumab clearly has single-agent activity in breast cancer patients who overexpress *HER2/neu* and was the first FDA-approved therapeutic antibody targeting solid tumors. Furthermore, trastuzumab in combination with cytotoxic chemotherapy demonstrates improved response rates compared with chemotherapy alone, from 25.0% to 57.3% with a taxane regimen.[109] Use of trastuzumab in the adjuvant setting has been associated with approximately a 50% reduction in recurrence after 1 year in multiple phase 3 trials.[110,111] Subsequent follow-up at a median time point of 2 years showed both better disease-free survival and overall survival rates in patients randomized to adjuvant trastuzumab therapy as compared with observation alone.[112] Myocardial dysfunction seen with anthracycline therapy was observed with increased frequency in patients receiving antibody alone[113] or with doxorubicin or epirubicin.

Cetuximab

Cetuximab (Erbitux) targets the EGFR. This chimeric IgG1 binds to domain III of the EGFR with roughly a tenfold higher affinity than either EGF or transforming growth factor (TGF)-α ligands and thereby inhibits ligand-induced activation of this tyrosine kinase receptor. Cetuximab may also function to down-regulate EGFR-dependent signaling by stimulating EGFR internalization.[114] Cetuximab is approved for the treatment of colorectal cancer and more recently for the treatment of squamous cell cancer of the head and neck.

The efficacy and safety of cetuximab against colorectal cancer was demonstrated alone and in combination with irinotecan in a phase 2, multicenter, randomized, controlled trial of 329 patients.[102] The combination of irinotecan plus cetuximab provided an increase in both overall response and median duration of response as compared with cetuximab alone. Additionally, patients with irinotecan refractory disease responded to treatment with the combination regimen. Recent studies in patients with colorectal cancers have indicated that patients with KRAS mutations in codon 12 or 13 should not receive anti-EGFR therapy.[115,116]

An international, multicenter, phase 3 trial comparing definitive radiotherapy with radiotherapy plus cetuximab in squamous cell carcinoma of the head and neck demonstrated that EGFR blockade with radiotherapy significantly reduced the risk of locoregional failure by 32% and the risk of death by 26%. In advanced-stage non–small cell lung cancer expressing EGFR, the combination of cetuximab and standard doublet chemotherapy (cisplatin plus vinorelbine) was studied in a prospective randomized phase 3 trial.[117] Addition of cetuximab was associated with a slight, but statistically significant, benefit in overall survival over chemotherapy alone (median overall survival, 10.1 vs. 11.3 months). A similar study using the carboplatin plus paclitaxel backbone in combination with cetuximab did not meet its primary end point of improved PFS, although cetuximab-treated patients exhibited higher objective response rates.[118] Therefore, the benefit of adding cetuximab to standard chemotherapy for patients with advanced non–small cell lung cancer is unclear.

Panitumumab

Panitumumab (Vectibix) is a fully human IgG2 monoclonal antibody that binds to EGFR. Similar to cetuximab, panitumumab inhibits EGFR activation by blocking binding of EGF and TGF-α. However, it does so by binding to EGFR with a higher affinity than cetuximab (5×10^{-11} M vs. 1×10^{-10} M). As previously mentioned, the IgG2 class of antibodies does not induce activation of immune system cells via Fc-receptor mechanism, so the primary action of panitumumab appears to be interference with EGFR-ligand interactions.

A phase 3 trial of 463 patients with metastatic colorectal cancer compared panitumumab plus best supportive care with best supportive care alone.[119] A partial response rate of 8% and a stable-disease rate of 28% were reported for the panitumumab arm compared with a 10% stable disease rate in the best supportive care arm of the study. As with cetuximab, patients with metastatic colorectal cancers who have KRAS mutations in codons 12 or 13 are not routinely offered therapy with panitumumab.[120]

Bevacizumab

Bevacizumab (Avastin or rhuMab VEGF) is a humanized monoclonal antibody targeting VEGF. VEGF is a critical determinant of tumor angiogenesis, a process that is a necessary component of tumor invasion, growth, and metastasis. VEGF expression by invasive tumors has been shown to correlate with vascularity and cellular proliferation and is prognostic for several human cancers.[121–123] Interestingly, inhibition of VEGF signaling via bevacizumab treatment may normalize tumor vasculature, promoting more effective delivery of chemotherapy agents.[124] Bevacizumab is approved for use as a first-line therapy for metastatic colorectal cancer and non–small cell lung cancer when given in combination with appropriate cytotoxic chemotherapy regimens. Phase 3 clinical trials leading to the approval of bevacizumab for the treatment of colorectal cancer demonstrated improved response rates from 35% to 45% compared with 5-fluorouracil–based chemotherapy alone. Enhanced response durations and improved patient survival were seen in patients treated with chemotherapy plus bevacizumab as compared with patients receiving chemotherapy alone.[125] A survival benefit was also seen in the setting of non–small cell lung cancer. A randomized phase 3 trial (ECOG 4599) of paclitaxel and carboplatin with or without bevacizumab in patients with advanced nonsquamous non–small cell lung cancer led to a significant improvement in median survival (12.5 vs. 10.2 months; P = .0075) for patients in the bevacizumab arm,[126] with significantly higher response rates. A higher incidence of bleeding was associated with bevacizumab (4.5% vs. 0.7%). Five of ten treatment-related deaths occurred as a result of hemoptysis, all in the bevacizumab arm.

A phase 3 trial randomized 722 patients with metastatic breast cancer with no prior chemotherapy for advanced disease to either paclitaxel or paclitaxel and bevacizumab.[127] Progression-free survival was significantly better in the paclitaxel plus bevacizumab arm (median, 11.8 vs. 5.9 months; hazard ratio for progression, 0.60; P <.001) with an increased response rate (36.9% vs. 21.2%; P <.001). Overall survival, however, was similar.

In contrast,[128] in a randomized phase 3 trial capecitabine/bevacizumab increased response rates compared with capecitabine alone in 462 anthracycline and taxane pretreated metastatic breast cancer patients but did not meet its primary end point of improved progression-free survival. Overall survival and time to deterioration in quality of life were comparable in both treatment groups.

Bevacizumab has not demonstrated activity in the adjuvant colorectal cancer setting.[129] In breast cancer, several trials are evaluating the efficacy of bevacizumab in the adjuvant setting as well. As an example, the BEATRICE trial (clinicaltrial.gov identifier: NCT00528567) is investigating the potential utility of the addition of bevacizumab to standard chemotherapy in patients with triple-negative breast cancer. No formal analysis of this trial is available at this point.

ANTIBODIES USED IN HEMATOLOGIC MALIGNANCIES

Rituximab

Rituximab (Rituxan) is a chimeric anti-CD20 monoclonal antibody that was the first MAb to be approved by the FDA for use in human malignancy.[130,131] Studies have shown that multiple doses can be safely administered, and *in vitro* studies have demonstrated multiple mechanisms by which anti-CD20 antibodies can lead to cell death.[132] Efficacy of rituximab monotherapy was established in phase 2 trials in patients with previously treated low-grade, or follicular, B-cell lymphoma. Response rates approaching 50% were seen with minimal toxicities. A separate phase 2 trial evaluated rituximab in relapsing or refractory diffuse large B-cell lymphoma, mantle cell lymphoma, or other intermediate or high-grade B-cell NHLs,[133] with an overall response rate of 31%. Patients with refractory disease and those with histologies other than diffuse large B-cell lymphoma appeared to have lower response rates.

Rituximab has also been tested in conjunction with chemotherapy based on supportive preclinical data.[134,135] The combination of rituximab with cylcophosphamide, doxorubicin, vincristine, and prednisolone (CHOP) resulted in a 95% overall response rate (55% complete response, 40% partial response) among 40 patients with low-grade or follicular B-cell NHL. Seven of eight patients who had initially been positive for the bcl-2 translocation became negative for the translocation by polymerase chain reaction assay after therapy.[136] A long-term study of elderly patients with previously untreated diffuse large-cell lymphoma randomized to either CHOP chemotherapy plus rituximab (R-CHOP) or CHOP alone demonstrated a significant improvement in outcome for the combination arm.[137] At a median follow-up of 5 years, event-free survival, progression-free survival, disease-free survival, and overall survival were all statistically improved with R-CHOP. No significant differences in long-term toxicity were noted.

Low-grade B-cell lymphoma patients possessing the (158 v/v) polymorphism in FcγRIII experience superior response rates and outcomes when treated with rituximab.[41,42] These findings signify that antibody Fc domain::Fc receptor interactions underlie at least some of the clinical benefit of rituximab, and indicate a possible role for ADCC that depends on such interactions.

Combination of active agents (such as lenalidomide and thalidomide) that are also immune modulating may be additive with rituximab,[138] and perhaps synergize by increasing ADCC.[139] Cytokines such as IL-2, -12, or -15 and myeloid growth factors may also enhance therapeutic antibody activity, as suggested by preclinical data demonstrating that IL-2 can promote NK cell proliferation and activation and enhance rituximab activity[140] and clinical efficacy.[141,142] Myeloid growth factors in combination with rituximab may also activate ADCC.[143] Alternative approaches to induce effector cell activity by combining toll-like receptor agonists, such as CpG oligonucleotides, are also being investigated.[144] Altering the balance of pro- and antiapoptotic signals could generate more rituximab-induced cytotoxicity. Bcl-2 down-regulation by antisense oligonucleotides was found to enhance rituximab efficacy in preclinical testing.[145,146] However, small molecules that bind to the BH-3 domain common to many members of the bcl-2 family of proteins may be better therapeutic agents.[147–149]

Ofatumumab

The anti-CD20 ofatumumab[150] binds an epitope on CD20 distinct from that bound by rituximab and is engineered for better complement activation, although it induces less ADCC. It is a fully human antibody and therefore may reduce infusion-related reactions and antibody responses associated with the chimeric rituximab. Ofatumumab has received regulatory approval for treatment of patients with fludarabine-refractory chronic lymphocytic leukemia. In a recently reported, planned interim analysis that included 138 chronic lymphocytic leukemia patients with treatment-refractory disease or bulky (>5 cm) lymphadenopathy, treatment with ofatumumab led to an overall response rate (primary end point) of 47% in patients with bulky disease and 5% in patients refractory to both alemtuzumab and fludarabine.[151] Additional humanized anti-CD20 antibodies (veltuzumab[152] and ocrelizumab) are under development.

Alemtuzumab

Alemtuzumab (Campath-1H) targets the CD52 glycopeptide, which is highly expressed on T and B lymphocytes. It has been tested as a therapeutic agent for chronic lymphocytic leukemia and promyelocytic leukemias, as well as other NHLs.

Selected References

The full list of references for this chapter appears in the online version.

4. Adams GP, Weiner LM. Monoclonal antibody therapy of cancer. *Nat Biotechnol* 2005;23:1147.
5. Kohler G, Milstein C. Continuous cultures of fused cells secreting antibody of predefined specificity. *Nature* 1975;256:495.
10. Komissarov AA, Calcutt MJ, Marchbank MT, et al. Equilibrium binding studies of recombinant anti-single-stranded DNA Fab. Role of heavy chain complementarity-determining regions. *J Biol Chem* 1996;271:12241.
11. Ghetie V, Popov S, Borvak J, et al. Increasing the serum persistence of an IgG fragment by random mutagenesis. *Nat Biotechnol* 1997;15:637.
13. Kudo T, Saeki H, Tachibana T. A simple and improved method to generate human hybridomas. *J Immunol Methods* 1991;145:119.
15. Huston JS, Levinson D, Mudgett-Hunter M, Tai M-S, Novotny J. Protein engineering of antibody binding sites: recovery of specific activity in an anti-digoxin single-chain Fv analogue produced in E coli. *Proc Natl Acad Sci U S A* 1988;85:5879.
16. Clackson T, Hoogenboom HR, Griffiths AD, et al. Making antibody fragments using phage display libraries. *Nature* 1991;352:624.
18. Jain RK. Physiological barriers to delivery of monoclonal antibodies and other macromolecules in tumors. *Cancer Res* 1990;50:814S.
24. Fujimori K, Covell DG, Fletcher JE, et al. A modeling analysis of monoclonal antibody percolation through tumors: a binding site barrier. *J Nucl Med* 1990;31:1191.
26. Adams GP, Schier R, McCall AM, et al. High affinity restricts the localization and tumor penetration of single-chain fv antibody molecules. *Cancer Res* 2001;61:4750.
28. Adams GP, Tai MS, McCartney JE, et al. Avidity-mediated enhancement of in vivo tumor targeting by single-chain Fv dimers. *Clin Cancer Res* 2006;12:1599.
31. Shields RL, Namenuk AK, Hong K, et al. High resolution mapping of the binding site on human IgG1 for Fc gamma RI, Fc gamma RII, Fc gamma RIII, and FcRn and design of IgG1 variants with improved binding to the Fc gamma R. *J Biol Chem* 2001;276:6591.
35. Umana P, Jean-Mairet J, Moudry R, et al. Engineered glycoforms of an antineuroblastoma IgG1 with optimized antibody-dependent cellular cytotoxic activity. *Nat Biotechnol* 1999;17:176.
37. Raghavan M, Bjorkman PJ. Fc receptors and their interactions with immunoglobulins. *Annu Rev Cell Dev Biol* 1996;12:181.
40. Clynes RA, Towers TL, Presta LG, et al. Inhibitory Fc receptors modulate in vivo cytoxicity against tumor targets. *Nat Med* 2000;6:443.
41. Cartron G, Dacheux L, Salles G, et al. Therapeutic activity of humanized anti-CD20 monoclonal antibody and polymorphism in IgG Fc receptor FcgammaRIIIa gene. *Blood* 2002;99:754.
42. Weng WK, Levy R. Two immunoglobulin G fragment C receptor polymorphisms independently predict response to rituximab in patients with follicular lymphoma. *J Clin Oncol* 2003;21:3940.
47. Weiner LM, Holmes M, Richeson A, et al. Binding and cytotoxicity characteristics of the bispecific murine monoclonal antibody 2B1. *J Immunol* 1993;151:2877.
50. Weiner LM, Clark JI, Davey M, et al. Phase I trial of 2B1, a bispecific monoclonal antibody targeting c-erbB-2 and FcgammaRIII. *Cancer Res* 1995;55:4586.
51. Liu MA, Kranz DM, Kurnick JT, et al. Heteroantibody duplexes target cells for lysis by cytotoxic T lymphocytes. *Proc Natl Acad Sci U S A* 1985; 82:8648.
54. Bargou R, Leo E, Zugmaier G, et al. Tumor regression in cancer patients by very low doses of a T cell-engaging antibody. *Science* 2008;321:974.
59. Di Gaetano N, Cittera E, Nota R, et al. Complement activation determines the therapeutic activity of rituximab in vivo. *J Immunol* 2003;171:1581.
64. Attia P, Phan GQ, Maker AV, et al. Autoimmunity correlates with tumor regression in patients with metastatic melanoma treated with anti-cytotoxic T-lymphocyte antigen-4. *J Clin Oncol* 2005;23:6043.
68. Li S, Schmitz KR, Jeffrey PD, et al. Structural basis for inhibition of the epidermal growth factor receptor by cetuximab. *Cancer Cell* 2005;7:301.
70. Presta LG, Chen H, O'Connor SJ, et al. Humanization of an anti-vascular endothelial growth factor monoclonal antibody for the therapy of solid tumors and other disorders. *Cancer Res* 1997;57:4593.
71. Pukac L, Kanakaraj P, Humphreys R, et al. HGS ETR1, a fully human TRAIL-receptor 1 monoclonal antibody, induces cell death in multiple tumour types in vitro and in vivo. *Br J Cancer* 2005;92:1430.
73. Bross PF, Beitz J, Chen G, et al. Approval summary: gemtuzumab ozogamicin in relapsed acute myeloid leukemia. *Clin Cancer Res* 2001;7:1490.
76. Lewis Phillips GD, Li G, Dugger DL, et al. Targeting HER2-positive breast cancer with trastuzumab-DM1, an antibody-cytotoxic drug conjugate. *Cancer Res* 2008;68:9280.
79. Krop I, LoRusso P, Miller KD, et al. A phase II study of trastuzumab-DM1 (T-DM1), a novel HER2 antibody-drug conjugate, in patients with HER2+ metastatic breast cancer who were previously treated with an anthracyline, a taxane, capecitabine, lapatinib, and trastuzumab, San Antonio Breast Cancer Symposium. San Antonio, TX, 2009, pp 710.
80. Vogel CL, Burris HA, Limentani S, et al. A phase II study of trastuzumab-DM1 (T-DM1), a HER2 antibody-drug conjugate (ADC), in patients (pts) with HER2+ metastatic breast cancer (MBC): final results. *J Clin Oncol* 2009;27:1017.
92. Kreitman RJ, Wilson WH, Bergeron K, et al. Efficacy of the anti-CD22 recombinant immunotoxin BL22 in chemotherapy-resistant hairy-cell leukemia. *N Engl J Med* 2001;345:241.
96. Lode HN, Xiang R, Becker JC, et al. Immunocytokines: a promising approach to cancer immunotherapy. *Pharmacol Ther* 1998;80:277.
103. Juweid ME. Radioimmunotherapy of B-cell non-Hodgkin's lymphoma: from clinical trials to clinical practice. *J Nucl Med* 2002;43:1507.
104. Witzig TE, White CA, Wiseman GA, et al. Phase I/II trial of IDEC-Y2B8 radioimmunotherapy for treatment of relapsed or refractory CD20(+) B-cell non-Hodgkin's lymphoma. *J Clin Oncol* 1999;17:3793.
106. Carter P, Presta L, Gorman CM, et al. Humanization of an anti-p185HER2 antibody for human cancer therapy. *Proc Natl Acad Sci U S A* 1992; 89:4285.
110. Piccart-Gebhart MJ, Procter M, Leyland-Jones B, et al. Trastuzumab after adjuvant chemotherapy in HER2-positive breast cancer. *N Engl J Med* 2005;353:1659.
111. Romond EH, Perez EA, Bryant J, et al. Trastuzumab plus adjuvant chemotherapy for operable HER2-positive breast cancer. *N Engl J Med* 2005; 353:1673.
112. Smith I, Procter M, Gelber RD, et al. 2-Year follow-up of trastuzumab after adjuvant chemotherapy in HER2-positive breast cancer: a randomised controlled trial. *Lancet* 2007;369:29.
116. Van Cutsem ELI, D'haens G. KRAS status and efficacy in the first-line treatment of patients with metastatic colorectal cancer (metastatic CRC) treated with FOLFIRI with or without cetuximab: the CRYSTAL experience. Abstract 2. *J Clin Oncol* 2008;26:5s.
117. Pirker R, Pereira JR, Szczesna A, et al. Cetuximab plus chemotherapy in patients with advanced non-small-cell lung cancer (FLEX): an open-label randomised phase III trial. *Lancet* 2009;373:1525.
119. Gibson TB, Ranganathan A, Grothey A. Randomized phase III trial of panitumumab, a fully human anti-epidermal growth factor receptor monoclonal antibody, in metastatic colorectal cancer. *Clin Colorectal Cancer* 2006;6:29.
120. Amado RG, Wolf M, Peeters M, et al. Wild-type KRAS is required for panitumumab efficacy in patients with metastatic colorectal cancer. *J Clin Oncol* 2008;26:1626.
125. Hurwitz H, Fehrenbacher L, Novotny W, et al. Bevacizumab plus irinotecan, fluorouracil, and leucovorin for metastatic colorectal cancer. *N Engl J Med* 2004;350:2335.
126. Sandler A, Gray R, Perry MC, et al. Paclitaxel-carboplatin alone or with bevacizumab for non-small-cell lung cancer. *N Engl J Med* 2006; 355:2542.
127. Miller K, Wang M, Gralow J, et al. Paclitaxel plus bevacizumab versus paclitaxel alone for metastatic breast cancer. *N Engl J Med* 2007;357:2666.
130. Maloney D, Grillo-Lopez A, Bodkin D, et al. IDEC-C2B8: results of a phase I multiple-dose trial in patients with relapsed non-Hodgkin's lymphoma. *J Clin Oncol* 1997;3266.
133. Coiffier B, Haioun C, Ketterer N, et al. Rituximab (anti-CD20 monoclonal antibody) for the treatment of patients with relapsing or refractory aggressive lymphoma: a multicenter phase II study. *Blood* 1998;92:1927.
137. Feugier P, Van Hoof A, Sebban C, et al. Long-term results of the R-CHOP study in the treatment of elderly patients with diffuse large B-cell lymphoma: a study by the groupe d'Etude des lymphomes de l'Adulte. *J Clin Oncol* 2005;23:4117.
142. Khan KD, Emmanouilides C, Benson DM Jr, et al. A phase 2 study of rituximab in combination with recombinant interleukin-2 for rituximab-refractory indolent non-Hodgkin's lymphoma. *Clin Cancer Res* 2006;12:7046.
151. Wierda WG, Kipps TJ, Mayer J, et al. Ofatumumab as single-agent CD20 immunotherapy in fludarabine-refractory chronic lymphocytic leukemia. *J Clin Oncol* 2010;28:1749.

CHAPTER 49 ENDOCRINE MANIPULATION

MATTHEW P. GOETZ, CHARLES ERLICHMAN, MANISH KOHLI, AND CHARLES L. LOPRINZI

Hormonal agents are commonly used as a treatment of hormonally responsive cancers, such as breast, prostate, or endometrial carcinomas. Other uses for some hormonal therapies include the treatment of paraneoplastic syndromes, such as carcinoid syndrome, and symptoms caused by cancer, including anorexia. This chapter discusses the major hormonal agents for such therapy, first with a general overview of their use in practice, then with more detailed pharmacologic information regarding them (Table 49.1).

SELECTIVE ESTROGEN RECEPTOR MODULATORS

Tamoxifen

Tamoxifen continues to be a very important hormonal therapy for the treatment of breast cancer worldwide. The continued importance of tamoxifen is reflected in that it is the only hormonal agent approved by the U.S. Food and Drug Administration (FDA) for the prevention of premenopausal breast cancer,[1] the treatment of ductal carcinoma *in situ*,[2] and the treatment of surgically resected premenopausal estrogen receptor (ER)–positive breast cancer.[3] In these settings, there is a general consensus, at present, that tamoxifen use should be continued for 5 years.

The standard daily dose of tamoxifen is 20 mg. The most common toxicity from tamoxifen is hot flashes, affecting approximately 50% of treated women. These hot flashes are of varying intensity and duration. Tamoxifen-induced hot flashes appear to increase over the first 3 months of therapy and then plateau. They appear to be more prominent in women with a history of hot flashes or estrogen replacement use. Although tamoxifen-induced hot flashes can be ameliorated by a number of different pharmacotherapies including low doses of megestrol,[4] antidepressants such as venlafaxine, paroxetine, or fluoxetine,[5–7] and the anticonvulsant drug gabapentin,[8] a growing body of evidence suggests that some of these drugs (e.g., paroxetine and fluoxetine) potently inhibit CYP2D6 and thus alter the metabolic activation of tamoxifen to endoxifen.

The estrogenic properties of tamoxifen are responsible for both beneficial and deleterious side effects. Although the incidence of endometrial cancer in patients who receive tamoxifen is increased, the absolute risk is small and primarily appears to involve only postmenopausal women. For women who receive tamoxifen, the increase in the annual incidence of endometrial cancer is approximately 2.58 (ratio of incidence rates).[9] The incidence of a rarer form of uterine cancer, uterine sarcoma, is also increased after tamoxifen use.[10] This form of endometrial cancer comprises approximately 15% of all uterine malignancies that develop after tamoxifen use.[10] Beneficial estrogenic effects from tamoxifen include a decrease in total cholesterol[11] and the preservation of bone density in postmenopausal women.[12] In premenopausal women, however, tamoxifen has a negative effect on bone density.[13] Although most patients do not complain of vaginal symptoms, a few complain of vaginal dryness, whereas others have increased vaginal secretions and discharge, the latter an indication of the estrogenic activity on tamoxifen on the vagina. In the Arimidex, Tamoxifen, Alone or in Combination (ATAC) trial that compared tamoxifen to anastrozole, a commonly observed tamoxifen side effect was vaginal bleeding, leading to a higher hysterectomy rate for patients randomized to tamoxifen (5%) compared to anastrozole (1%).[14] An uncommon effect from tamoxifen is retinal toxicity. This drug can also increase the risk of cataracts. However, no difference in the rate of vision-threatening ocular toxicity has been seen among prospectively treated tamoxifen patients.[15] Tamoxifen predisposes patients to thromboembolic phenomena, especially if used with concomitant chemotherapy. Depression has also been described, but this association with tamoxifen is not clear. Although liver cancers have been noted in laboratory animals, there is no established association between tamoxifen and liver cancers in humans.

Pharmacology

Tamoxifen acts by blocking estrogen stimulation of breast cancer cells, inhibiting both translocation and nuclear binding of the ER. This alters transcriptional and posttranscriptional events mediated by this receptor.[16] Tamoxifen has agonistic, partial agonistic, or antagonistic effects, depending on the species, tissue, or end points that have been assessed. Additionally, there are marked differences between the antiproliferative properties of tamoxifen and its metabolites.[17]

Resistance to tamoxifen can be intrinsic or acquired, and the potential mechanisms for this resistance are reviewed below. At each step of the signal transduction pathway with which tamoxifen or its metabolites interferes, there is potential for an alteration in response. The most important factor appears to be the level of ER, which is highly predictive for response to tamoxifen. Tamoxifen is ineffective in ER-negative breast cancer. Although decreased or absent expression of the progesterone receptor (PR) is associated with a worse prognosis, the relative risk reduction in tamoxifen-treated patients is the same regardless of the presence or absence of the PR.

Following binding to the ER, subsequent translocation of the tamoxifen/ER complex to the nucleus and binding to an estrogen-response element may occur. This binding prevents transcriptional activation of estrogen-responsive genes. Laboratory and clinical data have demonstrated that ER-positive breast cancers that overexpress HER2 may be less responsive to tamoxifen and to hormonal therapy in general.[18–21] In these tumors, ligand-independent activation of the ER by mitogen-activated protein kinase (MAPK) pathways may contribute to resistance.[22–24] In addition, expression of AIB1, an estrogen-receptor coactivator, has been associated with

TABLE 49.1

OVERVIEW OF MAJOR HORMONAL AGENTS USED IN CANCER

Class of Drug	Individual Drug	Dose	Route of Delivery	Frequency of Delivery
Selective estrogen receptor modulator	Tamoxifen	20 mg	Oral	Once daily
	Toremifene	60 mg	Oral	Once daily
	Raloxifene	60 mg	Oral	Once daily
Aromatase inhibitor	Anastrozole	1 mg	Oral	Once daily
	Letrozole	2.5 mg	Oral	Once daily
	Exemestane	25 mg	Oral	Once daily
Estrogen receptor down-regulator	Fulvestrant	500 mg	IM	Once monthly
Luteinizing hormone releasing hormone agonist	Goserelin	7.5	IM	Once monthly[a]
	Leuprolide	3.6	IM	Once monthly[a]
GnRH antagonist	Degarelix	240 mg loading dose	SC	80 mg SC monthly maintenance dose
Antiandrogen	Flutamide	250 mg	Oral	Three times daily
	Bicalutamide	50 mg	Oral	Once daily
	Nilutamide	300 mg for 30 days then 150 mg	Oral	Once daily
CYP17 lyase inhibitors	Abiraterone Acetate	1,000 mg (four 250 mg capsules)	Oral	Once Daily
AR "super antagonists"	MDV3100	160–240 mg	Oral	Daily
Androgen	Fluoxymesterone	10 mg	Oral	Twice daily
Estrogen	Estradiol	10 mg	Oral	Up to three times daily
Somatostatin analogue	Octreotide	Varies	Subcu or intravenous	Up to three times daily[b]
Progestational agents	Megestrol	Varies	Oral	Once daily
	Medroxyprogesterone acetate	Varies	Oral or IM	Varies

IM, intramuscular; SC, subcutaneous; GnRH, gonadotropin-releasing hormone; CYP, cytochrome P-450; AR, androgen receptor.
[a]Longer acting depot preparations (every 3 months) are available.
[b]Depot formulations are available.

tamoxifen resistance in patients whose breast cancers overexpress HER2.[25] Recent data suggest that PAX2, a tamoxifen-recruited transcriptional repressor of the *ERBB2* gene, and AIB1 compete for binding and regulation of ERBB2 transcription, and that elevated levels of PAX2 are associated with improved recurrence-free survival compared to PAX2-negative tumors.[26]

In some cases resistance may result from decrease or loss of ER expression.[27,28] Although ER mutation has been suggested as a mechanism of resistance, little evidence for such changes in the ER has been demonstrated.[29] Phosphorylation of the ER can mediate the hormone binding, DNA binding, and ultimately transcriptional activation. Alterations in this phosphorylation, mediated by changes in protein kinases A and C, could lead to resistance. Finally, modifications of the estrogen-response element, such as sequence alteration and element duplication, may lead to binding of the tamoxifen–ER complex with increased transcription of the estrogen-response genes.

The carcinogenic potential of tamoxifen has been recognized in rat studies[30–32] and in humans (endometrial cancer).[33] Although the mechanism of these carcinogenic effects is not understood, it has been proposed that generation of reactive intermediates that bind covalently to macromolecules underlies the process. Such reactive intermediates have been demonstrated *in vitro*.[33–36] In addition, induction of covalent DNA adducts in rat livers treated with tamoxifen has been reported.[37] Both constitutive and inducible cytochrome P-450 (CYP) enzymes have been implicated in the formation of metabolites with tamoxifen,[38,39] and the flavone-containing mono-oxygenase has been implicated in the formation of the *N*-oxide of tamoxifen. Reactive intermediates from such metabolic steps are being evaluated for their carcinogenic potential *in vitro* and *in vivo*.

Multiple studies to evaluate tumor gene-expression profiling have identified gene expression patterns or specific genes associated with resistance to tamoxifen therapy. A commonly utilized gene expression assay, Oncotype DX 21 gene assay (Genomic Health, Redwood City, California), measures the expression of genes known to be involved in estrogen signaling (e.g., ER, PR), HER2, proliferation (e.g., Ki-67), and others. In multiple different data sets, the recurrence score has been associated with a higher risk of breast cancer recurrence in patients treated with hormonal therapy (e.g., tamoxifen or aromatase inhibitors) without concomitant chemotherapy.[40–42]

The pharmacokinetics of tamoxifen is complex. The chemical structure and metabolic pathway of tamoxifen are shown in Figure 49.1. Tamoxifen is a prodrug, and metabolic activation is associated with greater pharmacological activity. The two most active tamoxifen metabolites are 4-hydroxytamoxifen (4-OH tamoxifen) and 4-OH-N-desmethyltamoxifen (endoxifen). A series of studies carried out to characterize endoxifen pharmacology have demonstrated that it has equivalent potency *in vitro* to 4-hydroxytamoxifen in estrogen receptor-alpha (ERα) and -beta (ERβ) binding,[43] for suppression of ER-dependent human breast cancer cell line proliferation,[17,43] and in global ER-responsive gene expression.[44] A recent study suggests that endoxifen's effect on the ER may differ from 4-hydroxytamxoifen, given its ability to degrade ERα.[45]

PHARMACOLOGY OF CANCER THERAPEUTICS

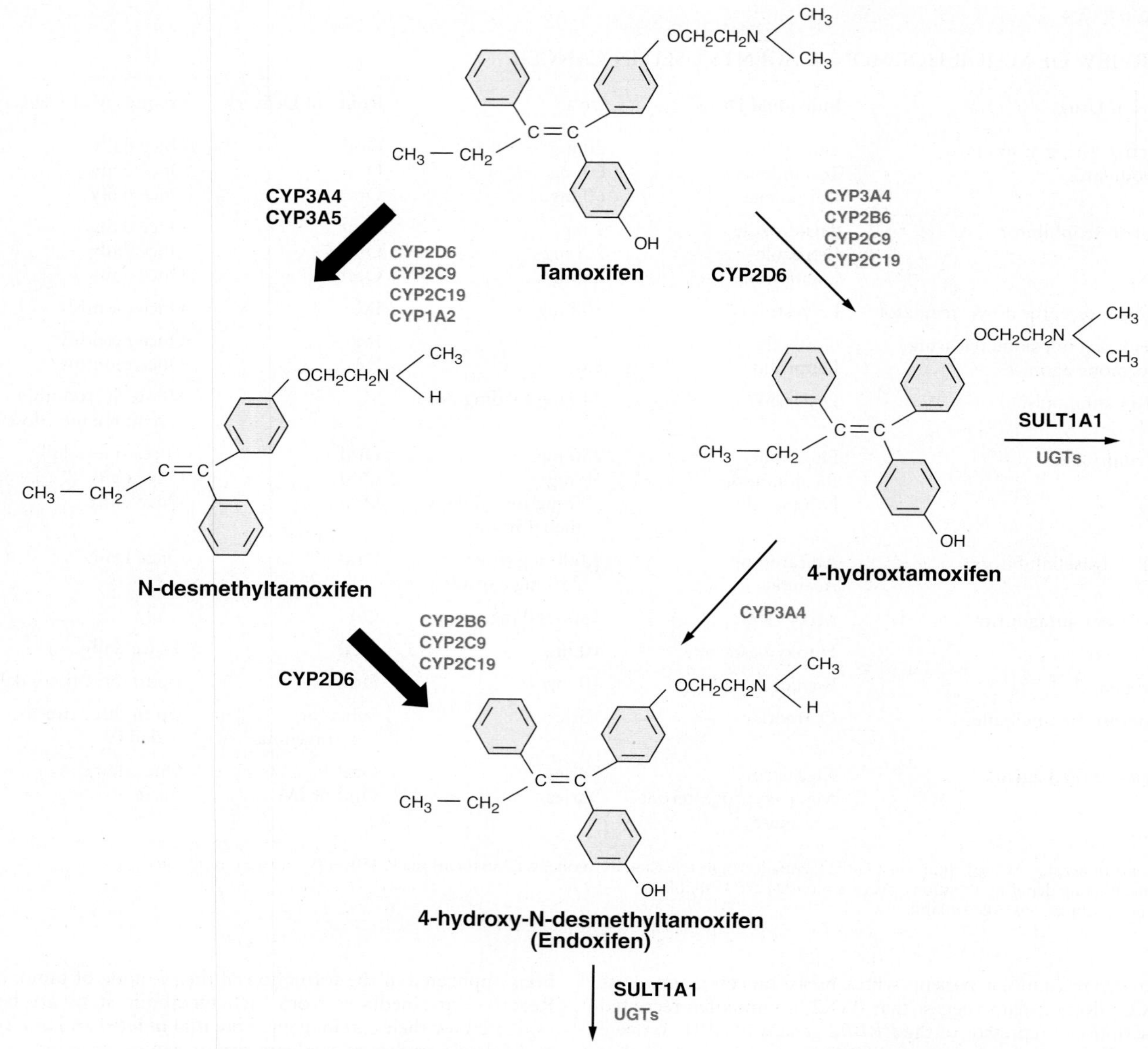

FIGURE 49.1 Metabolic pathway of tamoxifen biotransformation. (Modified in part from ref. 46.)

In women who receive tamoxifen at a dose of 20 mg/d, plasma endoxifen steady-state concentrations are generally six to ten times higher than 4-hydroxytamoxifen.[46] Although the metabolism of tamoxifen to 4-OH-tamoxifen is catalyzed by multiple enzymes, endoxifen is formed predominantly by the CYP2D6-mediated oxidation of *N*-desmethyltamoxifen, the most abundant tamoxifen metabolite (Fig. 49.1).[47] Recent clinical studies have demonstrated that common *CYP2D6* genetic variation (leading to low or absent CYP2D6 activity) or drug-induced inhibition of CYP2D6 significantly lowers endoxifen concentrations.[46,48] The *CYP2D6* gene is highly polymorphic, with more than 70 major alleles with four well-defined phenotypes: poor metabolizers (PM), intermediate metabolizers (IM), extensive metabolizers (EM), and ultrarapid metabolizers (UM).

The clinical studies to evaluate the association between *CYP2D6* polymorphisms and tamoxifen outcome have yielded conflicting results. Although initial[49] and follow-up data[50,51] demonstrate that CYP2D6 PM had an approximately two- to threefold higher risk of breast cancer recurrence (compared to CYP2D6 EM), other studies have not demonstrated this association.[52–54] An FDA Advisory Committee initially recommended a change to the label of tamoxifen to include a warning related to an increased risk of breast cancer recurrence for women who are deficient in CYP2D6 metabolism. However, a formal label change has yet to occur.

Many drugs are known to inhibit CYP2D6 activity. In tamoxifen-treated women, the coadministration of fluoxetine or paroxetine converts a patient with normal CYP2D6 metabolism to a phenotypic PM.[55] Venlafaxine appears to have little or no CYP2D6 inhibition.[55] Many other clinically important drugs have been reported to inhibit the CYP2D6 enzyme system, but their effects on tamoxifen metabolism have not been studied. As with the data regarding CYP2D6 genotype, the data regarding CYP2D6 inhibitors has additionally been controversial. Two recently published "pharmacy" database studies reported opposite findings with regard to CYP2D6 inhibitor use and breast cancer recurrence or death.[56,57] Although these data remain controversial, caution should be exercised when prescribing drugs that inhibit CYP2D6 enzyme, with the greatest caution related to drugs that are potent inhibitors of the enzyme system.

Following the metabolic activation of tamoxifen, the hydroxylated metabolites undergo conjugation, with both glucuronidation and sulfation. Peak plasma levels of tamoxifen (C_{max}) are seen 3 to 7 hours after oral administration. Assuming an oral bioavailability of 30%, the volume of distribution has been calculated to be 20 L/kg, and plasma clearance ranges from 1.2 to 5.1 L/h.[58] The terminal half-life of tamoxifen has been reported to range between 4 and 11 days.[59,60] The elimination half-life of tamoxifen increases with successive doses, consistent with saturable kinetics.[59,61] The drug's distribution in tissues is extensive. Levels of the parent drug and metabolites have been reported to be higher in tissue than in plasma in animal studies.[62,63] Reports of tamoxifen concentrations 10- to 60-fold higher than plasma concentrations in liver, lung, brain, pancreas, skin, and bone have appeared.[64,65] Concentrations of tamoxifen in pleural, pericardial, and peritoneal effusions approach those in plasma, with effusion to serum ratios ranging between 0.2 and 1.0. These findings are consistent with the large calculated volume of distribution. Elevated levels of tamoxifen with biliary obstruction have been reported.[66]

Tamoxifen has been reported to interact with warfarin,[61,67–69] digitoxin, phenytoin,[70] and medroxyprogesterone.[61] Tamoxifen-induced activation of hPXR, resulting in induction of CYP3A4, may increase elimination of concomitantly administered CYP3A substrates[71] such as anastrozole.[72]

Toremifene

Toremifene is an agent similar to tamoxifen. It is available in the United States for the treatment of patients with metastatic breast cancer but is approved in other countries for the adjuvant treatment of ER-positive breast cancer. A recent pooled analysis by the International Breast Cancer Study Group demonstrated no difference in either disease-free or overall survival when toremifene was compared with tamoxifen for the treatment of ER-positive breast cancer.[73] Additionally, a randomized comparison of toremifene and tamoxifen in metastatic breast cancer suggested that these two medications are equivalent.[74] Clinical trials in postmenopausal women with metastatic breast cancer concluded that there is major cross-resistance between tamoxifen and toremifene.[75,76]

Pharmacology

Toremifene is an antiestrogen with a chemical structure that differs from that of tamoxifen by the substitution of a chlorine for a hydrogen atom that is retained when toremifene undergoes metabolism.[77] Like tamoxifen, toremifene is metabolized by CYP3A,[78] with secondary metabolism to form hydroxylated metabolites that appear to have similar binding affinities to 4-OH tamoxifen.[77,79] The importance of these metabolites or the role of metabolism to the hydroxylated metabolites is unknown, but may play a role, given the structural similarity of toremifene to tamoxifen. Although the oral bioavailability has not been defined, toremifene's oral absorption appears to be good. The time to peak plasma concentrations after oral administration ranges from 1.5 to 6.0 hours,[80] with the terminal half-lives for toremifene and one metabolite, 4-hydroxytoremifene, being 5 to 6 days.[81,82] The apparent clearance is 5.1 L/h. The terminal half-life for the major metabolite, *N*-desmethyltoremifene, is 21 days.[83] The time to reach plasma steady-state concentrations is 1 to 5 weeks. Plasma protein binding is more than 99%. As with tamoxifen, toremifene tissue distribution in rats has been studied and found to be extensive and in high concentrations. Consistent with this is the high apparent volume of distribution, 958 L. Seventy percent of the drug is excreted in feces as metabolites. Studies in patients with impaired liver function secondary to alcoholic cirrhosis and in patients on anticonvulsants known to induce CYP3A have demonstrated that hepatic dysfunction decreases the clearance of toremifene and *N*-desmethyltoremifene,[83] whereas those patients on anticonvulsants had an increased clearance. Although toremifene appeared to be less carcinogenic than tamoxifen in preclinical models,[36,84,85] the adjuvant studies comparing tamoxifen to toremifene demonstrated similar rates of endometrial cancer.[73]

Raloxifene

Raloxifene is an estrogen agonist and antagonist that was developed as an agent to treat osteoporosis. Large placebo-controlled randomized trials demonstrated reduced rates of osteoporosis and a reduction in new breast cancers in treated women, leading to the development of a second-generation breast cancer chemoprevention trial (National Surgical Adjuvant Breast and Bowel Project, NSAPB P2) in which raloxifene was compared with tamoxifen in high-risk postmenopausal women. In the most recent analysis of the NSABP study, tamoxifen was superior to raloxifene in terms of both invasive and noninvasive cancer events. However, tamoxifen use is associated with a significantly higher risk of thromboembolic events and endometrial cancer.[86]

Pharmacology

Raloxifene is partially estrogenic in bone[87] and lowers cholesterol.[88] It is antiestrogenic in mammary tissue[89,90] and uterine tissue.[91]

The pharmacokinetics of raloxifene have been studied principally in postmenopausal women.[92–94] Pharmacokinetic parameters of raloxifene show considerable interindividual variation. Limited information is available on the pharmacokinetics of raloxifene in individuals with hepatic impairment, renal impairment, or both.

Raloxifene is rapidly absorbed from the gastrointestinal tract. Because raloxifene undergoes extensive first-pass glucuronidation, oral bioavailability of unchanged drug is low. Although approximately 60% of an oral dose is absorbed, the absolute bioavailability as unchanged raloxifene is only 2%. However, systemic availability of raloxifene may be greater than that indicated in bioavailability studies, because circulating glucuronide conjugates are converted back to the parent drug in various tissues.

After oral administration of a single 120- or 150-mg dose of raloxifene hydrochloride, peak plasma concentrations of raloxifene and its glucuronide conjugates are achieved at 6 hours and 1 hour, respectively. Plasma concentrations of raloxifene's glucuronide conjugates exceed those of the parent drug, and the time to achieve maximum concentrations of the drug and glucuronide metabolites depends on the extent and rate of systemic interconversion and enterohepatic circulation. After oral administration of radiolabeled raloxifene, less than 1% of total circulating radiolabeled material in plasma represents parent drug.

The area under the curve (AUC) for plasma concentration and time after a single dose of raloxifene is the same as the AUC after multiple doses of the drug. Increasing the dose of raloxifene hydrochloride over a range of 30 to 150 mg results in a slightly less than proportional increase in the AUC of raloxifene. Administration of raloxifene with a standardized high-fat meal increases the raloxifene peak plasma concentration by 28% and the AUC by 16% when compared with administration on an empty stomach but does not result in clinically important changes in systemic exposure.

Results of a single-dose study in patients with cirrhosis of the liver (Child-Pugh class A) and total serum bilirubin concentrations of 0.6 to 2.0 mg/dL indicate that plasma raloxifene concentrations correlate with serum bilirubin concentrations and are 2.5 times higher in such individuals than in those with normal hepatic function. In postmenopausal women who received raloxifene in clinical trials, plasma concentrations of raloxifene and the glucuronide conjugates in those with renal impairment (i.e., estimated creatinine clearance values as low as 23 mL/min) were similar to values in women with normal renal function.

Distribution of raloxifene into body tissues and fluids has not been fully characterized. Raloxifene and raloxifene 4′-glucuronide have been detected in saliva after oral administration of radiolabeled drug. In studies in rats given radiolabeled raloxifene 6-glucuronide, the liver contained the highest concentration of radioactivity, followed by serum, lung, and kidney. Although bone and the uterus contained relatively low concentrations of radiolabeled metabolite, 24% of the radioactivity in bone, 14% in the uterus, and 23% in the liver represented raloxifene. Results of this study indicate that the conversion of metabolite to parent drug occurs readily in a variety of tissues, including the liver, lung, spleen, kidney, bone, and uterus. The apparent volume of distribution after oral administration of single doses of raloxifene hydrochloride, 30 to 150 mg, is 2,348 L/kg, suggesting extensive tissue distribution. The volume of distribution is not dose dependent over a dosage range of 30 to 150 mg daily.

Raloxifene and its monoglucuronide conjugates are more than 95% bound to plasma proteins. Raloxifene binds to albumin and α_1-acid glycoprotein. Raloxifene undergoes extensive first-pass metabolism to the glucuronide conjugates raloxifene 4′-glucuronide, 6-glucuronide, and 6,4′-diglucuronide. UGT1A1 and -1A8 have been found to catalyze the formation of both the 6-β-and 4′-β-glucuronides, whereas UGT1A10 formed only the 4′-β-glucuronide.[95] Metabolism of raloxifene does not appear to be mediated by CYP enzymes (such as CYP2D6), as metabolites other than glucuronide conjugates have not been identified.

The plasma elimination half-life of raloxifene at steady state averages 32.5 hours (range, 15.8 to 86.6 hours). Raloxifene is excreted principally in feces as unabsorbed drug and via biliary elimination as glucuronide conjugates, which, subsequently, are metabolized by bacteria in the gastrointestinal tract to the parent drug. After oral administration, less than 0.2% of a raloxifene dose is excreted as parent compound and less than 6% as glucuronide conjugates in urine.

Fulvestrant

An alternative endocrine treatment to tamoxifen is fulvestrant. Fulvestrant is an ER antagonist that has no known agonist activity and results in ER down-regulation.[96–99] Like tamoxifen, fulvestrant competitively binds to the ER but with a higher affinity—approximately 100 times greater than that of tamoxifen[96,100–102]—thus preventing endogenous estrogen from exerting its effect in target cells.

Results from two phase 3 clinical trials have shown fulvestrant to be as effective as anastrozole in the treatment of postmenopausal women with advanced hormone receptor–positive breast cancer previously treated with antiestrogen therapy (mainly tamoxifen).[100–104] Based on these data, fulvestrant has been approved in the United States for the treatment of postmenopausal women with hormone receptor–positive metastatic breast cancer after progression on antiestrogen therapy. In the setting of first-line hormone-responsive metastatic breast cancer, a randomized phase 3 clinical trial to compare tamoxifen to fulvestrant (250 mg/mo) demonstrated no differences in response or time to progression.[105] However, a randomized phase 2 of high dose fulvestrant (500 mg/mo) compared to anastrozole (1 mg/d) in the first-line metastatic setting demonstrated similar clinical benefit rates and response rates, but longer time to progression for fulvestrant.[106]

Fulvestrant is well tolerated. The most common drug-related events (greater than 10% incidence) from the randomized phase 3 studies were injection-site reactions and hot flashes. Common events (1% to 10% incidence) included asthenia, headache, and gastrointestinal disturbances such as nausea, vomiting, and diarrhea, with minor gastrointestinal disturbances being the most commonly described adverse event.

Pharmacology

Fulvestrant is a steroidal molecule derived from E_2 with an alkylsulphonyl side chain in the 7-α position (Fig. 49.2). Because fulvestrant is poorly soluble and has low and unpredictable oral bioavailability, a parenteral formulation of fulvestrant was developed in an attempt to maximize delivery of the drug.[99] The intramuscular formulation provides prolonged release of the drug over several weeks. The pharmacokinetics of three different single doses of fulvestrant (50, 125, and 250 mg) have been published.[99] In this phase 1 and 2 multicenter study, postmenopausal women with primary breast cancer who were awaiting curative surgery received either fulvestrant, tamoxifen, or placebo. After single intramuscular injections of fulvestrant, the time of maximal concentration (t_{max}) ranged from 2 to 19 days, with the median being 7 days for each dose group. At the interval of 28 days, C_{min} values were two- to fivefold lower than the C_{max} values. For most patients in the 125- and 250-mg dose groups, significant levels of fulvestrant were still measurable 84 days after administration. Pharmacokinetic modeling of the pooled data from the 250-mg cohort was best described by a two-compartment model in which a longer terminal phase began approximately 3 weeks after administration. Because of the long time needed to reach steady state, concern was raised that the unimpressive clinical findings to date may partly reflect the long time needed to reach steady state plasma concentrations. Prospective studies using a loading dose[107] or simply a higher dose (500 mg/mo) have demonstrated equivalence compared to the aromatase inhibitors exemestane and anastrozole in the metastatic setting. Furthermore, pharmacokinetic data testing the loading dose regimen (500 followed by 250 mg day 14) confirm that steady state concentrations are achieved within 1 month.[108]

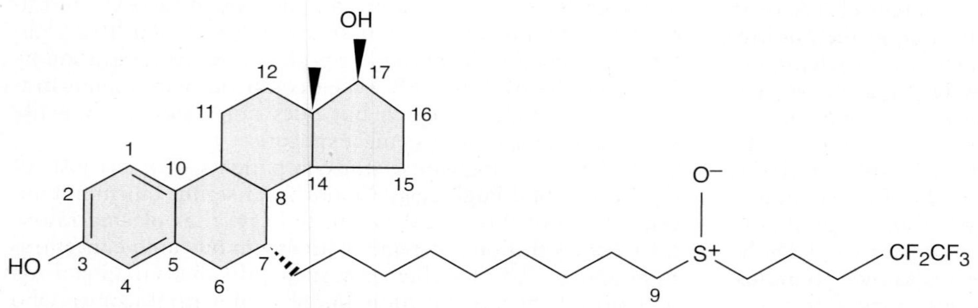

FIGURE 49.2 Structure of fulvestrant.

AROMATASE INHIBITORS

At menopause, the synthesis of ovarian hormones ceases. However, estrogen continues to be converted from androgens (produced by the adrenal glands) by aromatase, an enzyme of the CYP superfamily. Aromatase is the enzyme complex responsible for the final step in estrogen synthesis via the conversion of the androgens androstenedione and testosterone to the estrogens estrone (E_1) and E_2. This biologic pathway served as the basis for the development of the antiaromatase class of compounds. Alterations in aromatase expression have been implicated in the pathogenesis of estrogen-dependent disease, including breast cancer, endometrial cancer, and endometriosis. The importance of this enzyme is also highlighted by the fact that selective aromatase inhibitors are commonly used as first-line therapy for the treatment of postmenopausal women with estrogen-responsive breast cancer. Aminoglutethimide was the first clinically used aromatase inhibitor. When it became available, it was used to cause a *medical adrenalectomy*. Because of the lack of selectivity for aromatase and the resultant suppression of aldosterone and cortisol, aminoglutethimide is no longer recommended for treating metastatic breast cancer. Aminoglutethimide has also occasionally been used to try to reverse excess hormone production by adrenocortical cancers.[109]

Aromatase (cytochrome P-450 19 [CYP19]) is encoded by the *CYP19* gene. Recent sequencing of the aromatase gene led to the identification of multiple novel single-nucleotide polymorphisms, some of which appear to be functionally important.[110] Some early studies suggest that some of these polymorphisms may have clinical significance.[111,112]

Aromatase inhibitors have been classified in a number of different ways, including first, second, and third generation; steroidal and nonsteroidal; and reversible (ionic binding) and irreversible (suicide inhibitor, covalent binding).[113] The nonsteroidal aromatase inhibitors include aminoglutethimide (first generation), rogletimide and fadrozole (second generation), and anastrozole, letrozole, and vorozole (third generation). The steroidal aromatase inhibitors include formestane (second generation) and exemestane (third generation).

Steroidal and nonsteroidal aromatase inhibitors differ in their modes of interaction with, and their inactivation of, the aromatase enzyme. Steroidal inhibitors compete with the endogenous substrates androstenedione and testosterone for the active site of the enzyme and are processed into intermediates that bind irreversibly to the active site, causing irreversible enzyme inhibition.[14] Nonsteroidal inhibitors also compete with the endogenous substrates for access to the active site, where they then form a reversible bond to the heme iron atom so that enzyme activity can recover if the inhibitor is removed; however, inhibition is sustained whenever the inhibitor is present.[14] It is unclear whether the type of inhibition (i.e., reversible or irreversible) has clinical implications.

Letrozole and Anastrozole

Both letrozole and anastrozole have been extensively studied in the metastatic and adjuvant settings. When compared to tamoxifen, both letrozole and anastrozole have demonstrated superior response rates and progression-free survival in the metastatic setting.[114,115] In the adjuvant setting, two trials have been performed and demonstrated superiority in terms of relapse-free survivals of both anastrozole (ATAC)[116] and letrozole (BIG 1-98).[117] Additionally, anastrozole has been studied in a sequential approach, and the sequence of tamoxifen followed by anastrozole is superior to 5 years of tamoxifen alone.[118]

The side effects of both anastrozole and letrozole are similar and include arthralgias and myalgias in up to 50% of patients. Both letrozole and anastrozole are associated with a higher rate of bone fracture, compared with the tamoxifen.[119] At the present time, minimal long-term (longer than 5 years) clinical data regarding the effect of aromatase inhibitors on bones are available. When offering anastrozole for extended periods of time to patients with early breast cancer, attention to bone health is paramount, and bone density should be monitored carefully on all patients. Data presented at the 2006 American Society for Clinical Oncology meeting, however, report that it is extremely uncommon for patients with normal bone mineral density (no osteopenia) to develop osteoporosis with 5 years of anastrozole.[14] Those patients with documented development of substantial bone loss should be offered bisphosphonate therapy. Prospective studies have demonstrated that bisphosphonates prevent aromatase-inhibitor–induced bone loss and should be considered in patients with a high risk of fracture.[120]

No impact has been seen with anastrozole on adrenal steroidogenesis at up to ten times the clinically recommended dose.[121] Although letrozole may decrease basal and adrenocorticotropic hormone–stimulated cortisol synthesis,[122,123] the clinical effect appears to be minimal. Aromatase inhibitors appear to have differential effects on lipids. In a study of over 900 patients with metastatic disease, anastrozole showed no marked effect on lipid profiles, compared with baseline.[124] Conversely, administration of letrozole in women with advanced breast cancer resulted in a significant increase in total cholesterol and low-density lipoprotein from baseline after 8 and 16 weeks of therapy.[125] In the Breast International Group 1-98 trial, more women who received letrozole experienced grade 1 hypercholesterolemia compared to women who received tamoxifen.[117]

Letrozole is a nonsteroidal aromatase inhibitor with a high specificity for the inhibition of estrogen production (Fig. 49.3). Letrozole is 180 times more potent than aminoglutethimide as an inhibitor of aromatase *in vitro*. Aldosterone production *in vitro* is inhibited by concentrations 10,000 times higher than those required for inhibition of estrogen synthesis.[126,127] In a normal male volunteer study, letrozole was shown to decrease E_2 and serum E_1 levels to 10% of baseline with a single 3-mg dose. In phase 1 studies, letrozole caused a significant decline in plasma E_1 and E_2 within 24 hours of a single oral dose of 0.1 mg.[128,129] After 2 weeks of treatment, the blood levels of E_2, E_1, and estrone sulfate were suppressed 95% or more from baseline. This continued over the 12 weeks of therapy. There was no apparent alteration in plasma levels of cortisol and aldosterone with letrozole or after corticotropin stimulation.[128] In postmenopausal women with advanced breast cancer, the drug did not have any effect on follicle-stimulating hormone (FSH), luteinizing hormone (LH), thyrotropin (previously thyroid-stimulating hormone), cortisol, 17-α-hydroxyprogesterone, androstenedione, or aldosterone blood levels.[130,131]

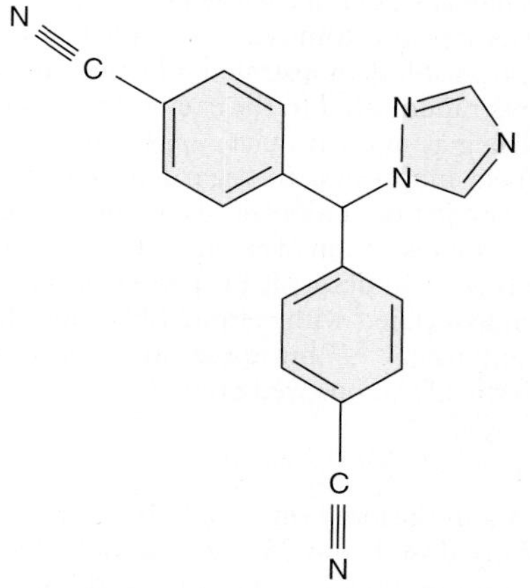

FIGURE 49.3 Structure of letrozole.

Anastrozole is a nonsteroidal aromatase inhibitor that is 200-fold more potent than aminoglutethimide.[132] No effect on the adrenal glands has been detected. In human studies, the t_{max} is 2 to 3 hours after oral ingestion.[133] Elimination is primarily via hepatic metabolism, with 85% excreted by that route and only 10% excreted unchanged in urine. The main circulating metabolite is triazole after cleavage of the two rings in anastrozole by *N*-dealkylation. Linear pharmacokinetics have been observed in the dose range of 1 to 20 mg and do not change with repeat dosing. The terminal half-life is approximately 50 hours, and steady-state concentrations are achieved in approximately 10 days with once-a-day dosing and are three to four times higher than peak concentrations after a single dose. Plasma protein binding is approximately 40%.[134] In one study, anastrozole, 1 mg and 10 mg daily, inhibited *in vivo* aromatization by 96.7% and 98.1%, respectively, and plasma E_1 and E_2 levels were suppressed 86.5% and 83.5%, respectively, regardless of dose.[135] Thus, 1 mg of anastrozole achieves near maximal aromatase inhibition and plasma estrogen suppression in breast cancer patients.

A recent prospective study to evaluate the pharmacokinetics of anastrozole (1 mg/d) demonstrated large interindividual variations in plasma anastrozole and anastrozole metabolite concentrations, as well as pretreatment and postdrug plasma E_1, E_2, and E_1 conjugate and estrogen precursor (androstenedione and testosterone) concentrations.[136] Further research is needed to determine the basis for the wide variability in the pharmacokinetics of anastrozole and whether these findings are clinically relevant.

Exemestane

Exemestane has been compared to tamoxifen in both the metastatic and adjuvant settings. In the setting of tamoxifen-refractory metastatic breast cancer, exemestane is superior to megestrol acetate, as demonstrated in a phase 3 trial in which improvements in both median time to tumor progression and median survival were observed.[137] In the adjuvant setting, the international exemestane study compared 2 to 3 years of tamoxifen with 2 to 3 years of exemestane in women who had previously competed 2 to 3 years of adjuvant tamoxifen. In this trial, a switch to exemestane resulted in superior disease-free and overall survival in the hormone receptor–positive subtype.

Exemestane has a steroidal structure and is classified as a type 1 aromatase inhibitor, also known as an *aromatase inactivator*, because it irreversibly binds with and permanently inactivates the enzyme.[123]

Side Effects of Exemestane

Although preclinical studies have suggested that exemestane prevented bone loss in ovariectomized rats,[138] the Intergroup exemestane adjuvant trial still demonstrated a higher rate of bone fracture for patients randomized to the exemestane arm. Side effects, including arthralgias and myalgias, appear to be similar to the other aromatase inhibitors. In regard to steroidogenesis, no impact on either cortisol or aldosterone levels was seen in a small study after the administration of exemestane for 7 days.[139] Finally, exemestane has weak androgenic properties, and its use at higher doses has been associated with steroidal-like side effects, such as weight gain and acne,[140,141] but these side effects have not been observed with the FDA-approved dose (25 mg/d).[142]

Pharmacology

Exemestane is administered once daily by mouth, with the recommended daily dose being 25 mg. The time needed to reach maximal E_2 suppression is 7 days,[143] and its half-life is 27 hours.[144] At daily doses of 10 to 25 mg, exemestane suppresses estrogen concentrations to 6% to 15% of pretreatment levels. This activity is more pronounced than that produced by formestane and comparable to that produced by the nonsteroidal aromatase inhibitors anastrozole and letrozole.[145–147] Exemestane does not appear to affect cortisol or aldosterone levels when evaluated after 7 days of treatment, based on dose-ranging studies including doses from 0.5 to 800 mg.[139] Exemestane is metabolized by CYP3A4.[123] Although drug–drug interactions have not been formally reported for exemestane, there is the potential for interactions with drugs that affect CYP3A4.[123]

GONADOTROPIN-RELEASING HORMONE ANALOGUES

Gonadotropin-releasing hormone (GnRH) analogues result in a *medical orchiectomy* in men and are used as a means of providing androgen ablation for metastatic prostate cancer.[148] Because the initial agonist activity of GnRH analogues can cause a *tumor flare* from temporarily increased androgen levels, concomitant use of the antiandrogen flutamide has been used to prevent this effect. GnRH analogues can also cause tumor regressions in hormonally responsive breast cancers[149] and have received FDA approval for the treatment of metastatic breast cancer in premenopausal women. Data suggest that these drugs may be useful as adjuvant therapy of premenopausal women with resected breast cancer.[150] The use of these drugs in combination with tamoxifen or exemestane in premenopausal women with primary breast cancer is the subject of large, ongoing, international clinical trials. The primary toxicities of GnRH analogues are secondary to the ablation of sex steroid concentrations and include hot flashes, sweating, and nausea.[151] These symptoms can be reversed with low doses of progestational analogues.[4] In males treated with GnRH analogues for prostate cancer, an alternate strategy of intermittent schedule of GnRH administration has resulted in improved tolerability and quality of life, with comparable efficacy compared with continuous GnRH analogue administration.[152]

GnRH analogues available for clinical use include goserelin[153,154] and leuprolide.[155] Both are available in depot intramuscular preparations to be given at monthly intervals. The recommended monthly dose of leuprolide is 7.5 mg and of goserelin is 3.6 mg. There are also longer-acting depot preparations to be administered every 3 months and even every 6 months (triptorelin).[156]

Pharmacology

Analogues of the decapeptide GnRH[153,155,157] have been synthesized by modifications of position 6 in which the L-glycine has been exchanged for a D-amino acid and the C-terminal amino acid has been either replaced by an ethylamide or substituted for a modified amino acid. These changes increase the affinity of the analogue for the GnRH receptor and decrease the susceptibility to enzymatic degradation. There is an amino acid structure of GnRH with the substitutions for leuprolide and goserelin. Initial administration of these compounds results in stimulation of gonadotropin release. However, prolonged administration has led to profound inhibition of the pituitary–gonadal axis.[157] Plasma E_2 and progesterone are consistently suppressed to postmenopausal or castrate levels after 2 to 4 weeks of treatment with goserelin or leuprolide.[151,158] These drugs are administered intramuscularly or subcutaneously in a parenteral sustained-release microcapsule preparation, because parenteral administration of the parent drug otherwise is associated with rapid clearance. The GnRH analogues are metabolized in the liver, kidney, hypothalamus, and pituitary gland by neutral peptidase cleavage of the peptide bond between the tyrosine in the 5 position and the amino acid in the position 6 and by a postproline-cleaving enzyme that cleaves the peptide bond between proline in the 9 position and the glycine-NH_2 in the 10 position. Substitutions at the glycine 6 position and modification of the C-terminal make these analogues more resistant to this enzymatic cleavage.

Leuprolide is approximately 80 to 100 times more potent than endogenous GnRH. It induces castrate levels of testosterone in men with prostate cancer within 3 to 4 weeks of drug administration after an initial sharp increase in LH and FSH. The mechanisms of action include pituitary desensitization after reduction in pituitary GnRH receptor binding sites and possibly a direct antitumor effect in ER-positive human breast cancer cells.[155] The depot form results in a dose rate of 210 mcg/d of leuprolide. Peak concentrations of the depot form, achieved approximately 3 hours after drug administration, have been reported to range between 13.1 and 54.5 mcg/L. There appears to be a linear increase in the AUC for doses of 3.75, 7.5, and 15.0 mg in the depot form. The parenteral bioavailability of subcutaneously injected leuprolide is 94%. The volume of distribution ranges from 27.4 to 37.1 L. In human studies, leuprolide urinary excretion as a metabolite was the primary route of clearance.

Goserelin is approximately 100 times more potent than the naturally occurring GnRH. Like leuprolide, it causes stimulation of LH and FSH acutely, and with subsequent administration, GnRH receptor numbers decrease, and the pituitary becomes desensitized with decreasing LH and FSH levels. Castrate levels of testosterone are achieved within 1 month. In women, goserelin inhibits ovarian androgen production, but serum levels of dehydroepiandrosterone sulfate and, to a lesser extent, androstenedione, are preserved. *In vitro*, goserelin has demonstrated antitumor activity in estrogen-dependent MCF7 human breast cancer cells and LNCaP2 prostate cancer cells. The drug is released at a continuous mean rate of 120 mcg/d in the depo form, with peak concentrations in the range of 2 to 3 mcg/L achieved. The mean volume of distribution in six patients has been reported to be 13.7 L,[159] consistent with extracellular fluid volume. Goserelin is principally excreted in the urine, with a mean total body clearance of 8 L/h in patients with normal renal function. The total body clearance is reduced by approximately 75%, with renal dysfunction and the elimination half-life increased two- or threefold. However, dose adjustment for renal insufficiency does not appear to be necessary. The 5 to 10 hexapeptide and the 4 to 10 hexapeptide were detected in urine in animal studies.[160] The terminal half-life of goserelin is approximately 5 hours after subcutaneous injection. Protein binding is low, and no known drug interactions have been documented.

GONADOTROPIN-RELEASING HORMONE ANTAGONISTS

Modification to the structure of GnRH has resulted in the development of GnRH antagonist compounds that are currently being used in the treatment of prostate cancer. Abarelix was initially approved by the FDA in 2003 as the first depot injectable GnRH antagonist but was subsequently withdrawn in 2005 for economic reasons. Degarelix is a synthetically modified compound with GnRH antagonist activity that was approved for use by the FDA in 2008 for the management of prostate cancer.[161] Its effect in prostate cancer treatment is to block the GnRH receptor, thereby preventing the trigger for production of LH, which mediates androgen synthesis. In contrast to GnRH analogues, degarelix does not cause *tumor flare* symptoms secondary to a temporary increased androgen production. A large randomized clinical trial demonstrated that degarelix was associated with a rapid and sustained reduction in serum testosterone, prostate-specific antigen (PSA), FSH and LH levels with a loading dose of 240 mg subcutaneously followed by a monthly maintenance dose of 80 mg[162] and comparable efficacy to leuprolide.[163] The most common side effects (greater than 10%) with degarelix include hot flashes and pain at injection site in this trial[163] when patients were provided degarelix for a 12-month period. It is unknown as of yet if degarelix will have a similar chronic side effect profile as is associated with long-term use of GnRH analogues, which includes metabolic syndrome, osteoporosis, and higher incidence of type 2 diabetes.

Pharmacology

The recommended loading dose of degarelix is 240 mg, administered as two injections of 120 mg each subcutaneously. Monthly maintenance doses of 80 mg as a 20 mg/mL solution is started 28 days after the loading dose. In an analysis of pharmacokinetic/pharmacodynamic (PK/PD) properties of degarelix in 60 healthy males, after a single subcutaneous dose, a terminal $t_{1/2}$ of 47 days was observed.[164] The K_i of degarelix with endogenous GnRH at its receptor was 0.082 ng/mL, indicating a prolonged antagonism that resulted in reduction of the GnRH receptors available for LH and testosterone synthesis. The mean time of blockade was estimated to be 4.5 days. PK properties of degarelix have been evaluated when administered as a subcutaneous depot of drug as a gel in six different doses to 48 healthy males and with intravenous administration. Using data from several clinical trials, the rate of drug diffusion from subcutaneous administration results in detectable drug up to 60 days after a single dose compared to less than 4 days when the drug is injected intravenously.

Due to a lack of available data, no dose reduction is recommended in renal insufficiency, despite the observation that 20% to 30% of degarelix is excreted unchanged in urine. Likewise no change in dose is recommended in hepatic impairment.

ANTIANDROGENS

Flutamide

The antiandrogen flutamide is used in men with metastatic prostate cancer either as initial therapy, combined with GnRH analogue administration, or when the metastatic prostate cancer is unresponsive, despite androgen ablation therapy. The recommended dose is 250 mg by mouth three times a day. In patients whose prostate cancer is growing despite flutamide use, stopping flutamide can clearly cause a flutamide-withdrawal response.

The most common toxicity seen with flutamide is diarrhea, with or without abdominal discomfort. Gynecomastia, which can be tender, frequently occurs in men who are not receiving concomitant androgen ablation therapy.[165] Flutamide can rarely cause hepatotoxicity, a condition that is reversible if detected early, but this toxicity can also be fatal.[166] There is no accepted, clinically recommended testing schedule to screen for flutamide-induced hepatotoxicity other than being aware of this phenomenon and testing for liver function if hepatic symptoms develop.

Pharmacology

Flutamide is a pure antiandrogen with no intrinsic steroidal activity.[167] Flutamide's mechanism of action is as an androgen-receptor antagonist. This binding prevents the dihydrotestosterone binding and subsequent translocation of the androgen-receptor complex into the nuclei of cells. Because it is a pure antiandrogen, it acts only at the cellular level, with no progestational effects. Administration of flutamide alone leads to increased LH and FSH production and a concomitant increase in plasma testosterone and E_2 levels. Plasma protein binding ranges between 94% and 96% for flutamide and between 92% and 94% for 2-hydroxyflutamide, its major metabolite. When the drug is administered three times a day, steady-state levels are achieved by day 6. The steady-state C_{max} is 112.7 ng/L and occurs at approximately 1.13 hours after drug administration. The steady-state C_{max} is between three and five times higher than after the first dose. The elimination half-life at steady state is 7.8 hours, and 2-hydroxyflutamide achieves concentrations 50 times higher than the parent drug at steady state and has a potency equal to or greater than that of flutamide.[167] The mean C_{max} averaged 1,719 ng/mL at steady state and was achieved 1.9 hours after drug administration. The elimination half-life for the metabolite is 9.6 hours. The high plasma concentrations of 2-hydroxyflutamide, as compared with flutamide, suggest that the therapeutic benefits of flutamide are mediated primarily through its active metabolite.[168]

Bicalutamide

Bicalutamide is another nonsteroidal antiandrogen that has been approved by the FDA for use in the United States. The recommended dose is one 50-mg tablet per day. One randomized trial reported that bicalutamide compared favorably with flutamide in patients with advanced prostate cancer.[169] Bicalutamide appears to be relatively well tolerated and is associated with a lower incidence of diarrhea than is flutamide.

Pharmacology

Bicalutamide has a binding affinity to the androgen receptor in the rat prostate that is four times greater than that of 2-hydroxyflutamide.[170,171] *In vivo*, bicalutamide caused marked inhibition of growth of accessory sex organs in rats, with a potency five to ten times greater than that of flutamide. Unlike flutamide, bicalutamide did not cause a significant increase in LH or testosterone in rats. Bicalutamide bioavailability in humans has not been defined. The drug has a long plasma half-life of 5 to 7 days, so the drug may be administered on a weekly schedule. Pharmacokinetics of the drug showed a dose-dependent increase in mean peak plasma concentrations, and the AUC increased linearly with dose. The half-life of bicalutamide in humans was approximately 6 days, and the drug clearance was not saturable at plasma concentrations up to 1,000 ng/mL. Daily dosing of the drug led to an approximately tenfold accumulation after 12 weeks of administration. In contrast to results in rats, serum concentrations of testosterone and LH increased significantly from baseline at all dose levels tested in humans. Whereas serum FSH concentrations remained essentially unchanged, the median serum E_2 concentrations increased significantly.[172]

Nilutamide

Nilutamide represents the third variation of an antiandrogen available for use in patients with prostate cancer. The observation of unique toxicities, night blindness, and pulmonary toxicity has limited its use.

NOVEL ANTIANDROGENS

Although testosterone depletion remains an unchallenged standard for advanced stage hormone sensitive disease, evidence has emerged that "castration-recurrent" prostate cancer remains androgen receptor (AR) dependent and is neither "hormone refractory" nor "androgen-independent," which were commonly used terms to define progression of advanced stage disease following androgen deprivation therapy. Recognition of AR functioning despite the paucity of circulating androgens is evidenced by the elevation of AR messenger RNA in castration-recurrent tumor tissue relative to androgen-dependent tumors and re-expression of some androgen-regulated genes during clinical castration resistance. Recently the AR axis has been the focus of therapeutic targeting.

Abiraterone Acetate

After the failure of initial androgen manipulation with GnRH analogues and peripheral antiandrogens, prostate cancer continues to respond to a variety of second- and third-line hormonal interventions. Based on this observation, CYP17, a key enzyme in androgen and estrogen synthesis, was targeted using ketoconazole, which is a weak, reversible and nonspecific inhibitor of CYP17 resulting in modest antitumor activity of short durability. More recently, abiraterone, a more potent (20 times more than ketoconazole), selective, and irreversible inhibitor of CYP17, has been investigated in castration recurrent prostate cancer and significant objective responses have been observed.[173] Chemically, it is a 3-pyridyl steroid pregnenolone–derived compound available in a oral prodrug form of abiraterone acetate. Its main toxicity is from symptoms of mineralocorticoid excess (including hypokalemia, hypertension, and fluid overload), since continuous CYP17 blockade results in raising adrenocorticotrophic hormone (ACTH) levels that increase steroid levels upstream of CYP17, including corticosterone and deoxycorticosterone. These adverse effects are best avoided by the coadministration of steroids. PK studies support a once daily oral dose of four capsules (250 mg each).

MDV3100

For inhibiting the testosterone-AR axis at the receptor levels, novel AR inhibitors like MDV3100 have been developed. MDV3100 is a new diarylthiohydantoin compound targeting AR by binding overexpressed AR in advanced stage disease with an affinity that is several-fold greater than previously obtained with antiandrogens (bicalutamide and flutamide). This class of novel AR inhibitor drugs also disrupts the nuclear translocation of AR and impairs DNA binding to androgen response elements and recruitment of coactivators and thus have multifunctional antitumor capabilities.[174] In early clinical trials, promising results have been observed despite adequate castration and subsequent chemotherapy failure. Since the oral bioavailability is excellent, doses ranging from 30 to 600 mg daily have been evaluated with unacceptable toxicity of fatigue, seizure, asthenia, anemia, and arthralgia observed with increasing dose levels.

OTHER SEX STEROID THERAPIES

Fluoxymesterone

Fluoxymesterone is an androgen that has been used in women with metastatic breast cancer who have hormonally responsive cancers and who have progressed on other hormonal therapies such as tamoxifen, an aromatase inhibitor, or megestrol acetate. The usual dose is 10 mg given twice daily. Although the overall response rate is low for fluoxymesterone used in this clinical situation,[175] there are some patients who have substantial antitumor responses lasting for months or even years.

Toxicities associated with fluoxymesterone are those that would be expected with an androgen: hirsutism, male-pattern baldness, voice lowering (hoarseness), acne, enhanced libido, and erythrocytosis. Fluoxymesterone can also cause elevated liver function test results in some patients and, rarely, has been associated with hepatic neoplasms.

Pharmacology

Fluoxymesterone is a chlorinated synthetic analogue of testosterone with potent androgenic and anabolic activity in humans. Limited pharmacologic information is available on this agent. Colburn,[176] using a radioimmunoassay, studied two patients after a single oral administration of a 50-mg dose. Peak serum concentrations were achieved between 1 and 3 hours after administration, with the average peak concentrations being 335 ng/mL. By 5 hours after drug administration, serum levels had declined to approximately 50% of the peak concentration. Urinary excretion of a 10-mg dose can be detected for 24 hours, and at least 6-hydroxy, 4-ene, 3-β, and 11-hydroxy metabolites of fluoxymesterone have been detected.[177]

Estrogens: Diethylstilbestrol and Estradiol

Diethylstilbestrol (DES) used to be the primary hormonal therapy for postmenopausal metastatic breast cancer. Randomized comparative trials demonstrated it had a similar response rate to that of tamoxifen.[178,179] However, based on these trials, DES use was supplanted by tamoxifen primarily because DES has more toxicity. DES is occasionally used in metastatic breast cancer patients who have hormonally sensitive cancers that have failed to respond to multiple other hormonal therapies. The usual dose in this situation is 15 mg/d (either as a single dose or as divided doses). DES was also used as androgen ablation therapy in men with metastatic prostate cancer.[180] Doses of approximately 3 mg/d result in testosterone levels that are seen in an anorchid state.

DES toxicities include nausea and vomiting, breast tenderness, and a darkening of the nipple–areolar complex. DES increases the risk of thromboembolic phenomenon, and this may result in life-threatening complications. Although DES is not clinically available in the United States, similar antitumor effects and toxicities are seen with estradiol, with a target dose of 10 mg by mouth three times a day. The pharmacology of E_2 has been extensively described elsewhere.[181]

Medroxyprogesterone and Megestrol

Medroxyprogesterone and megestrol are 17-OH-progesterone derivatives differing in a double bond between C6 and C7 positions in megestrol. Megestrol historically was used as a hormonal agent for patients with advanced breast cancer, usually at a total daily dose of 160 mg. Additionally, it is still used for the treatment of hormonally responsive metastatic endometrial cancer, at a dose of 320 mg/d. In addition, doses of 160 mg/d are occasionally used as a hormonal therapy for prostate cancer.[182] Megestrol has also been extensively evaluated for the treatment of anorexia/cachexia related to cancer or AIDS.[183–186] Various dosages ranging from 160 to 1,600 mg/d have been used. A prospective study has demonstrated a dose–response relationship with doses up to 800 mg/d.[187] Low dosages of megestrol (20 to 40 mg/d) have been shown to be an effective means of reducing hot flashes in women with breast cancer and in men who have undergone androgen ablation therapy.[4] Although megestrol has historically been commonly administered four times per day, the long terminal half-life supports that once-per-day dosing is reasonable.

Megestrol is a relatively well-tolerated medication, with its most prominent side effects being appetite stimulation and resultant weight gain. Although these may be beneficial effects in patients with anorexia/cachexia, they can be important problems in patients with breast or endometrial cancers. Another side effect of megestrol acetate is the marked suppression of adrenal steroid production by suppression of the pituitary–adrenal axis.[188] Although this appears to be asymptomatic in the majority of patients, reports suggest that this adrenal suppression can cause clinical problems in some patients.[189] This drug has been abruptly stopped for decades without the recognition of untoward sequelae in patients, and it seems reasonable to continue this practice. Nonetheless, if Addisonian signs or symptoms develop after drug discontinuation, corticosteroids should be administered. Furthermore, if patients who receive megestrol have a significant infection, experience trauma, or undergo surgery, then corticosteroid coverage should be administered. There appears to be a slightly increased incidence of thromboembolic phenomena in patients receiving megestrol alone.[187] This risk appears to be higher if megestrol is administered with concomitant cytotoxic therapy.[190] There are conflicting reports regarding megestrol causing edema.[191] If it does, the edema is generally minimal and easily handled with a mild diuretic. Megestrol may cause impotence in some men.[192] The incidence of this is controversial, although it is generally agreed that this is a reversible situation. Megestrol can cause menstrual irregularities, the most prominent of which is withdrawal menstrual bleeding within a few weeks of drug discontinuation.[4] Although nausea and vomiting have sometimes been attributed as a toxicity of this drug, there are data to demonstrate that this drug has antiemetic properties.[185,186,190] In terms of magnitude, megestrol appears to decrease both nausea and vomiting in advanced-stage cancer patients by approximately two-thirds.

Medroxyprogesterone has many of the same properties, clinical uses, and toxicities as megestrol acetate. It has never been used commonly in the United States for the treatment of breast cancer but has been used more in Europe. Medroxyprogesterone is available in 2.5- and 10-mg tablets and in injectable formulations of 100 and 400 mg/L. Dosing for the treatment of metastatic breast or prostate cancer has commonly been 400 mg/wk or more and 1,000 mg/wk or more for metastatic endometrial cancer. Injectable or daily oral doses have been used for controlling hot flashes.

Pharmacology

The exact mechanism of antitumor effect of medroxyprogesterone and megestrol is unclear. These drugs have been reported to suppress adrenal steroid synthesis,[193] suppress ER levels,[194] alter tumor hormone metabolism,[195] enhance steroid metabolism,[196] and directly kill tumor cells.[197] In addition, progestins may influence some growth factors,[198] suppress plasma estrone sulfate formation, and, at high concentrations, inhibit P-glycoprotein.

The oral bioavailability of these progestational agents is unknown, although absorption appears to be poor for medroxyprogesterone, relative to megestrol.

The terminal half-life for megestrol is approximately 14 hours,[199,200] with a t_{max} of 2 to 5 hours after oral ingestion.[201] The AUC for a single megestrol dose of 160 mg is between 2.5- and 8-fold higher than that for single-dose medroxyprogesterone at 1,000 mg with a radioactive dose of megestrol; 50% to 78% is found in the urine after oral administration, and 8% to 30% is found in the feces.

Metabolism and excretion of medroxyprogesterone have been incompletely characterized. In humans, 20% to 50% of a [^{3}H]medroxyprogesterone dose is excreted in the urine and 5% to 10% in the stool after intravenous administration.[202–204] Metabolism of medroxyprogesterone occurs via hydroxylation, reduction, demethylation, and combinations of these reactions.[205] The major urinary metabolite is a glucuronide. Less than 3% of the dose is excreted as unconjugated medroxyprogesterone in humans. Clearance of medroxyprogesterone has been reported to range between 27 and 70 L/h.[204] The initial volume of distribution is between 4 and 8 L in humans. The mean terminal half-life is 60 hours. The t_{max} for medroxyprogesterone occurs 2 to 5 hours after oral administration. Medroxyprogesterone appears to be concentrated in small intestine, colon, and adipose tissue in human autopsy studies.[206] Drug interactions of medroxyprogesterone have been reported with aminoglutethimide, which decreases plasma medroxyprogesterone levels.[207] Medroxyprogesterone may reduce the concentration of the *N*-desmethyltamoxifen metabolite concentration. Progestational agents also may increase plasma warfarin levels.[208] These reports are consistent with CYP3A being the site of interaction.

OTHER HORMONAL THERAPIES

Octreotide

Octreotide is a somatostatin analogue that is administered for the treatment of carcinoid syndrome and other hormonal excess syndromes associated with some pancreatic islet cell cancers and acromegaly. Response rates (measured in terms of reduction in diarrhea and flushing) are high and, on average, last for several months, sometimes for years. Occasionally, antitumor responses temporarily related to octreotide are seen with these tumors. Octreotide may be useful to alleviate 5-fluorouracil–associated diarrhea.[209–212]

Octreotide can be administered intravenously or subcutaneously. Initial doses of 50 mcg are given two to three times on the first day. The dose is titrated upward, with a usual daily dose of 300 to 450 mcg/d for most patients. A depot preparation is available, allowing doses to be administered at monthly intervals. Octreotide is generally well tolerated overall. It appears to cause more toxicity in acromegalic patients, with such problems as bradycardia, diarrhea, hypoglycemia, hyperglycemia, hypothyroidism, and cholelithiasis.

Pharmacology

Octreotide is an 8-amino acid synthetic analogue of the 14-amino acid peptide somatostatin.[213] Octreotide has a similar high affinity for somatostatin receptors, as does its parent compound, with a concentration that inhibits the receptor by 50% in the subnanomolar range. Octreotide inhibits insulin, glucagon, pancreatic polypeptide, gastric inhibitory polypeptide, and gastrin secretion. It has a much longer duration of action than the parent compound because of its greater resistance to enzymatic degradation. Its absorption after subcutaneous administration is rapid, and bioavailability is 100% after subcutaneous injection. Peak concentrations of 4 mcg/L after a 100-mcg dose occur within 20 to 30 minutes of subcutaneous injection and are 20% to 40% of the corresponding intravenous injection. Both peak concentration and AUC for octreotide increase linearly with dose. The total body clearance in healthy volunteers is 9.6 L/h. Hepatic metabolism of octreotide accounts for 30% to 40% of the drug's disposition, and 11% to 20% is excreted unchanged in the urine. The volume of distribution ranges between 18 and 30 L, and the terminal half-life is reported to be between 72 and 98 minutes. Sixty-five percent of the drug is protein bound primarily to the lipoprotein fraction.[213,214] Because of the short half-life, classic octreotide is administered subcutaneously two or three times per day.[215] A slow-release form of octreotide, designed for once-per-month administration, controls the symptoms of carcinoid syndrome at least as well as three-times-per-day octreotide.[216]

Selected References

The full list of references for this chapter appears in the online version.

1. Fisher B, Costantino JP, Wickerham DL, et al. Tamoxifen for the prevention of breast cancer: current status of the National Surgical Adjuvant Breast and Bowel Project P-1 study. *J Natl Cancer Inst* 2005;97:1652.
2. Fisher B, Dignam J, Wolmark N, et al. Tamoxifen in treatment of intraductal breast cancer: National Surgical Adjuvant Breast and Bowel Project B-24 randomised controlled trial. *Lancet* 1999;353:1993.
3. Colleoni M, Gelber S, Goldhirsch A, et al. Tamoxifen after adjuvant chemotherapy for premenopausal women with lymph node-positive breast cancer: International Breast Cancer Study Group Trial 13-93. *J Clin Oncol* 2006;24:1332.
4. Loprinzi CL, Michalak JC, Quella SK, et al. Megestrol acetate for the prevention of hot flashes. *N Engl J Med* 1994;331:347.
5. Loprinzi CL, Kugler JW, Sloan JA, et al. Venlafaxine in management of hot flashes in survivors of breast cancer: a randomised controlled trial. *Lancet* 2000;356:2059.
6. Loprinzi CL, Sloan JA, Perez EA, et al. Phase III evaluation of fluoxetine for treatment of hot flashes. *J Clin Oncol* 2002;20:1578.
7. Stearns V, Beebe KL, Iyengar M, et al. Paroxetine controlled release in the treatment of menopausal hot flashes: a randomized controlled trial. *JAMA* 2003;289:2827.
8. Pandya KJ, Morrow GR, Roscoe JA, et al. Gobapentin for hot flashes in 420 women with breast cancer: a randomised double-blind placebo-controlled trial. *Lancet* 2005;366(9488):818–824.
9. Tamoxifen for early breast cancer: an overview of the randomised trials. Early Breast Cancer Trialists' Collaborative Group. *Lancet* 1998;351:1451.
10. Wickerham DL, Fisher B, Wolmark N, et al. Association of tamoxifen and uterine sarcoma. *J Clin Oncol* 2002;20:2758.
17. Lim YC, Desta Z, Flockhart DA, et al. Endoxifen (4-hydroxy-*N*-desmethyl-tamoxifen) has anti-estrogenic effects in breast cancer cells with potency similar to 4-hydroxy-tamoxifen. *Cancer Chemother Pharmacol* 2005;55:471.
19. Borg A, Baldetorp B, Ferno M, et al. ERBB2 amplification is associated with tamoxifen resistance in steroid-receptor positive breast cancer. *Cancer Lett* 1994;81:137.
25. Osborne CK, Bardou V, Hopp TA, et al. Role of the estrogen receptor coactivator AIB1 (SRC-3) and HER-2/neu in tamoxifen resistance in breast cancer. *J Natl Cancer Inst* 2003;95:353.
26. Hurtado A, Holmes KA, Geistlinger TR, et al. Regulation of ERBB2 by oestrogen receptor-PAX2 determines response to tamoxifen. *Nature* 2008;456:663.
32. Williams GM, Iatropoulos MJ, Djordjevic MV, et al. The triphenylethylene drug tamoxifen is a strong liver carcinogen in the rat. *Carcinogenesis* 1993;14:315.
33. Rutqvist LE, Johansson H, Signomklao T, et al. Adjuvant tamoxifen therapy for early stage breast cancer and second primary malignancies. Stockholm Breast Cancer Study Group. *J Natl Cancer Inst* 1995;87:645.
42. Paik S, Shak S, Tang G, et al. A multigene assay to predict recurrence of tamoxifen-treated, node-negative breast cancer. *N Engl J Med* 2004;351:2817.
43. Johnson MD, Zuo H, Lee KH, et al. Pharmacological characterization of 4-hydroxy-*N*-desmethyl tamoxifen, a novel active metabolite of tamoxifen. *Breast Cancer Res Treat* 2004;85:151.
45. Wu X, Hawse JR, Subramaniam M, et al. The tamoxifen metabolite, endoxifen, is a potent antiestrogen that targets estrogen receptor alpha for degradation in breast cancer cells. *Cancer Res* 2009;69:1722.
46. Jin Y, Desta Z, Stearns V, et al. CYP2D6 genotype, antidepressant use, and tamoxifen metabolism during adjuvant breast cancer treatment. *J Natl Cancer Inst* 2005;97:30.
47. Desta Z, Ward BA, Soukhova NV, et al. Comprehensive evaluation of tamoxifen sequential biotransformation by the human cytochrome P450 system in vitro: prominent roles for CYP3A and CYP2D6. *J Pharmacol Exp Ther* 2004;310:1062.
48. Stearns V, Johnson MD, Rae JM, et al. Active tamoxifen metabolite plasma concentrations after coadministration of tamoxifen and the selective serotonin reuptake inhibitor paroxetine. *J Natl Cancer Inst* 2003;95:1758.
49. Goetz MP, Rae JM, Suman VJ, et al. Pharmacogenetics of tamoxifen biotransformation is associated with clinical outcomes of efficacy and hot flashes. *J Clin Oncol* 2005;23:9312.

56. Dezentjé VO, van Blijderveen NJ, Gelderblom H, et al. Effect of concomitant CYP2D6 inhibitor use and tamoxifen adherence on breast cancer recurrence in early-stage breast cancer. *J Clin Oncol* 2010;28(14):2423.
57. Kelly CM, Juurlink DN, Gomes T, et al. Selective serotonin reuptake inhibitors and breast cancer mortality in women receiving tamoxifen: a population based cohort study. *BMJ* 2010;340:c693.
73. Pagani O, Gelber S, Price K, et al. Toremifene and tamoxifen are equally effective for early-stage breast cancer: first results of International Breast Cancer Study Group Trials 12-93 and 14-93. *Ann Oncol* 2004;15:1749.
74. Hayes DF, Van Zyl JA, Hacking A, et al. Randomized comparison of tamoxifen and two separate doses of toremifene in postmenopausal patients with metastatic breast cancer. *J Clin Oncol* 1995;13:2556.
89. Anzano MA, Peer CW, Smith JM, et al. Chemoprevention of mammary carcinogenesis in the rat: combined use of raloxifene and 9-cis-retinoic acid. *J Natl Cancer Inst* 1996;88:123.
92. Allerheiligen S, Geiser J, Knadler M. Raloxifen (RAL) pharmacokinetics and the associated endocrine effects in premenopausal women treated during the follicular, ovulatory, and luteal phases of the menstrual cycle. *Pharmaceut Res* 1996;13:S430.
96. Coopman P, Garcia M, Brunner N, et al. Anti-proliferative and anti-estrogenic effects of ICI 164,384 and ICI 182,780 in 4-OH-tamoxifen-resistant human breast-cancer cells. *Int J Cancer* 1994;56:295.
97. Howell A, DeFriend DJ, Robertson JF, et al. Pharmacokinetics, pharmacological and anti-tumour effects of the specific anti-oestrogen ICI 182780 in women with advanced breast cancer. *Br J Cancer* 1996;74:300.
103. Howell A, Robertson JF, Quaresma Albano J, et al. Fulvestrant, formerly ICI 182,780, is as effective as anastrozole in postmenopausal women with advanced breast cancer progressing after prior endocrine treatment. *J Clin Oncol* 2002;20:3396.
105. Howell A, Robertson JF, Abram P, et al. Comparison of fulvestrant versus tamoxifen for the treatment of advanced breast cancer in postmenopausal women previously untreated with endocrine therapy: a multinational, double-blind, randomized trial. *J Clin Oncol* 2004;22:1605.
106. Robertson JF, Llombart-Cussac A, Rolski J, et al. Activity of fulvestrant 500 mg versus anastrozole 1 mg as first-line treatment for advanced breast cancer: results from the FIRST study. *J Clin Oncol* 2009;27:4530.
107. Chia S, Gradishar W, Mauriac L, et al. Double-blind, randomized placebo controlled trial of fulvestrant compared with exemestane after prior nonsteroidal aromatase inhibitor therapy in postmenopausal women with hormone receptor-positive, advanced breast cancer: results from EFECT. *J Clin Oncol* 2008;26:1664.
110. Ma CX, Adjei AA, Salavaggione OE, et al. Human aromatase: gene resequencing and functional genomics. *Cancer Res* 2005;65:11071.
114. Mouridsen H, Gershanovich M, Sun Y, et al. Phase III study of letrozole versus tamoxifen as first-line therapy of advanced breast cancer in postmenopausal women: analysis of survival and update of efficacy from the International Letrozole Breast Cancer Group. *J Clin Oncol* 2003;21:2101.
115. Goss PE, Ingle JN, Martino S, et al. A randomized trial of letrozole in postmenopausal women after five years of tamoxifen therapy for early-stage breast cancer. *N Engl J Med* 2003;349:1793.
116. Howell A, Cuzick J, Baum M, et al. Results of the ATAC (Arimidex, Tamoxifen, Alone or in Combination) trial after completion of 5 years' adjuvant treatment for breast cancer. *Lancet* 2005;365:60.
117. Thurlimann B, Keshaviah A, Coates AS, et al. A comparison of letrozole and tamoxifen in postmenopausal women with early breast cancer. *N Engl J Med* 2005;353:2747.
118. Jakesz R, Jonat W, Gnant M, et al. Switching of postmenopausal women with endocrine-responsive early breast cancer to anastrozole after 2 years' adjuvant tamoxifen: combined results of ABCSG trial 8 and ARNO 95 trial. *Lancet* 2005;366:455.
120. Gnant M, Mlineritsch B, Schippinger W, et al. Endocrine therapy plus zoledronic acid in premenopausal breast cancer. *N Engl J Med* 2009;360: 679.
132. Dukes M, Edwards PN, Large M, et al. The preclinical pharmacology of "Arimidex" (anastrozole; ZD1033)—a potent, selective aromatase inhibitor. *J Steroid Biochem Mol Biol* 1996;58:439.
135. Geisler J, King N, Dowsett M, et al. Influence of anastrozole (Arimidex), a selective, non-steroidal aromatase inhibitor, on in vivo aromatisation and plasma oestrogen levels in postmenopausal women with breast cancer. *Br J Cancer* 1996;74:1286.
136. Ingle JN, Buzdar AU, Schaid DJ, et al. Variation in anastrozole metabolism and pharmacodynamics in women with early breast cancer. *Cancer Res* 2010;70(8):3278.
140. Bajetta E, Zilembo N, Noberasco C, et al. The minimal effective exemestane dose for endocrine activity in advanced breast cancer. *Eur J Cancer* 1997;33:587.
142. Coombes RC, Hall E, Gibson LJ, et al. A randomized trial of exemestane after two to three years of tamoxifen therapy in postmenopausal women with primary breast cancer. *N Engl J Med* 2004;350:1081.
148. Ahmann FR, Citrin DL, deHaan HA, et al. Zoladex: a sustained-release, monthly luteinizing hormone-releasing hormone analogue for the treatment of advanced prostate cancer. *J Clin Oncol* 1987;5:912.
150. Kaufmann M, Jonat W, Blamey R, et al. Survival analyses from the ZEBRA study. goserelin (Zoladex) versus CMF in premenopausal women with node-positive breast cancer. *Eur J Cancer* 2003;39:1711.
154. Vogelzang NJ, Chodak GW, Soloway MS, et al. Goserelin versus orchiectomy in the treatment of advanced prostate cancer: final results of a randomized trial. Zoladex Prostate Study Group. *Urology* 1995;46:220.
166. Wysowski DK, Freiman JP, Tourtelot JB, et al. Fatal and nonfatal hepatotoxicity associated with flutamide. *Ann Intern Med* 1993;118:860.
168. Radwanski E, Perentesis G, Symchowicz S, et al. Single and multiple dose pharmacokinetic evaluation of flutamide in normal geriatric volunteers. *J Clin Pharmacol* 1989;29:554.
173. Attard G, Reid AH, A'Hern R, et al. Selective inhibition of CYP17 with abiraterone acetate is highly active in the treatment of castration-resistant prostate cancer. *J Clin Oncol* 2009;27(23):3742.
174. Tran C, Ouk S, Clegg NJ, et al. Development of a second-generation antiandrogen for treatment of advanced prostate cancer. *Science* 2009;324:787.
178. Ingle JN, Ahmann DL, Green SJ, et al. Randomized clinical trial of diethylstilbestrol versus tamoxifen in postmenopausal women with advanced breast cancer. *N Engl J Med* 1981;304:16.
185. Loprinzi CL, Ellison NM, Schaid DJ, et al. Controlled trial of megestrol acetate for the treatment of cancer anorexia and cachexia. *J Natl Cancer Inst* 1990;82:1127.
187. Loprinzi CL, Michalak JC, Schaid DJ, et al. Phase III evaluation of four doses of megestrol acetate as therapy for patients with cancer anorexia and/or cachexia. *J Clin Oncol* 1993;11:762.
204. Utaaker E, Lundgren S, Kvinnsland S, et al. Pharmacokinetics and metabolism of medroxyprogesterone acetate in patients with advanced breast cancer. *J Steroid Biochem* 1988;31:437.
210. Cascinu S, Fedeli A, Fedeli SL, et al. Octreotide versus loperamide in the treatment of fluorouracil-induced diarrhea: a randomized trial. *J Clin Oncol* 1993;11:148.
216. Rubin J, Ajani J, Schirmer W, et al. Octreotide acetate long-acting formulation versus open-label subcutaneous octreotide acetate in malignant carcinoid syndrome. *J Clin Oncol* 1999;17:600.

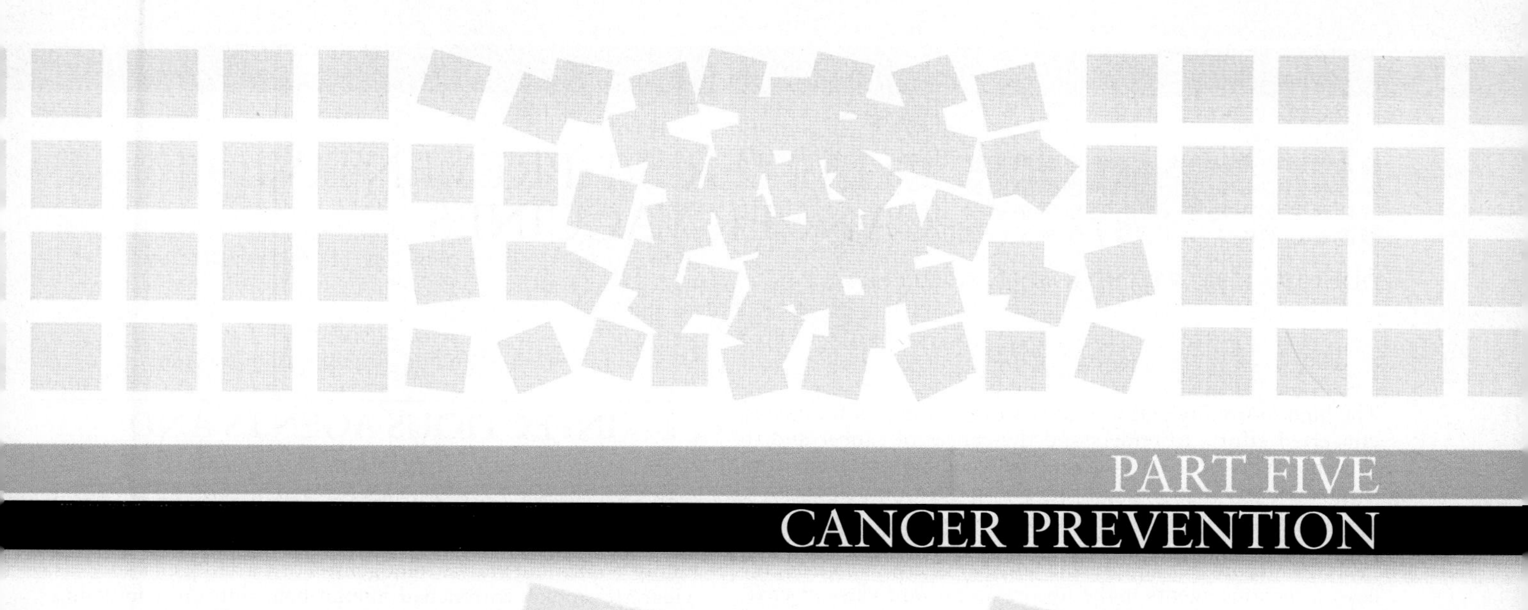

PART FIVE
CANCER PREVENTION

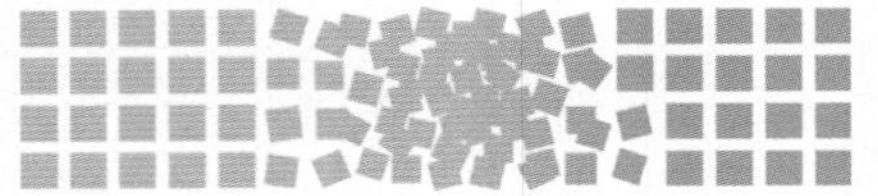

CHAPTER 50 PREVENTIVE CANCER VACCINES

DOUGLAS R. LOWY AND JOHN T. SCHILLER

The high morbidity and mortality from cancer has stimulated concerted efforts to understand the causes of cancer and to prevent cancer from developing. The recognition that environmental factors may account for the majority of cancers has encouraged researchers to identify the exogenous factors that trigger the carcinogenic process, define their role in tumorigenesis, and develop approaches that interfere with this process. Infectious agents make up one important class of environmental factors implicated in tumor development, and prophylactic vaccines have a long history of success in preventing nonmalignant diseases induced by infectious agents.[1,2] This chapter discusses the efforts to use this approach to prevent malignant disease induced by infectious agents implicated in cancer etiology and pathogenesis. It highlights the two cancer-causing viruses for which preventive vaccines are now available, hepatitis B virus (HBV) and human papillomavirus (HPV), and ongoing efforts to develop a vaccine against a bacterial pathogen, *Helicobacter pylori*, which worldwide is responsible for more cancers than any other infectious agent.

BACKGROUND

Although the oncogenic potential of some infectious agents, such as EBV and HBV, was recognized in the 1970s, many of the infectious agents now believed to be oncogenic were discovered since then (Table 50.1).[2,3] The latter include the oncogenic HPVs, hepatitis C virus, herpesvirus type 8, Merkel cell polyoma virus, and *H. pylori*. It seems likely that further research will result in additional forms of cancer being attributed to infectious agents. The expanded list will arise by demonstrating that infectious agents already recognized as oncogenic may be causally involved with additional forms of cancer or by attributing these additional cancers to other infectious agents not yet recognized as oncogenic.

Identification of an infectious agent in the etiology of a malignant process implies that timely interference with the infection could prevent the tumor from arising. The development of effective vaccines against infectious carcinogenic agents represents a potentially powerful form of intervention. The prototype for this approach is the HBV vaccine, which can protect immunized individuals against both acute disease and the malignant consequences attributable to the virus.[4,5] More recently, papillomavirus vaccines have been shown to prevent HPV infection and HPV-associated premalignant neoplastic disease.[6,7]

This chapter briefly considers how infectious oncogenic agents lead to cancer, discusses general issues related to developing vaccines against these agents, and presents individual portions devoted to the three agents that account for the most cancers worldwide: *H. pylori*, HBV, and HPV. Together they represent about 78% of the tumors attributable to infectious agents. Hepatitis C virus accounts for another 10%.[8,9]

INFECTIOUS AGENTS AND CANCER

Reducing exposure to an identified carcinogen represents the principal approach to decreasing the carcinogenic effects of many environmental carcinogens. For carcinogens such as cigarette smoke, entrenched human behavior and conflicting economic interests may present considerable obstacles to reducing or eliminating exposure. By contrast, a vaccine against an infectious carcinogen does not require modification of the behavior that leads to exposure because the vaccine attenuates the oncogenic activity of the infectious agent by reducing or preventing infection of target tissue.[10] Furthermore, the induction of herd immunity via the widespread use of an effective vaccine offers the possibility of reducing the risk of nonimmunized individuals to exposure to the infectious agent, as well as the long-term possibility of eliminating the agent from the environment.

Before considering vaccination itself, it is worthwhile reviewing some features of oncogenic infectious agents, as their characteristics may have implications for vaccine development, testing, and implementation. Viruses, bacteria, and parasites have been implicated in the pathogenesis of human cancer (Table 50.1). It is estimated that approximately 18% of cancers worldwide may be attributed to infectious agents (Tables 50.1 and 50.2).[2] In the United States and other developed countries, a smaller proportion of cancers (approximately 8%) are associated with these agents, while they account for a higher proportion (approximately 26%) in developing countries.

Several factors contribute to these regional differences. Some of the infectious agents, such as parasites with oncogenic potential, are extremely uncommon in the United States, or the rate of infection may vary greatly, as with HBV.[11,12] For others, such as HPV, infection in the United States is common, but Papanicolaou (Pap) smear screening for premalignant lesions in the cervix leads to effective treatment before carcinomas develop.[13] In still other instances, as with HPV, HPV, and *H. pylori*, strain differences or the interaction between the infectious agent and environmental factors, host factors, or both, might help determine the rate of carcinogenic progression.[14–16]

The identified oncogenic infectious agents share at least three characteristics: the ability to establish chronic infection, the establishment of chronic infection for many years before the development of malignancy, and a benign (i.e., nonmalignant) outcome for most infected individuals. These characteristics imply that cancer attributable to infectious agents develops only after prolonged infection, that a malignant outcome arises only after the development of infection-dependent changes in the host, and that induction of cancer is not part of the normal life cycle of the infectious agent.

TABLE 50.1

ONCOGENIC INFECTIOUS AGENTS

Agent	Tumor Types	Annual Cases Worldwide (Estimate)
BACTERIA		
Helicobacter pylori	Stomach cancer, gastric lymphoma	603,000
VIRUSES		
Human papillomavirus	Cervical, anal, vaginal, other cancers	561,000
Hepatitis B virus	Liver cancer	330,000
Hepatitis C virus	Liver cancer	195,000
Human immunodeficiency virus	Kaposi's sarcoma, non-Hodgkin's lymphoma	102,000[a]
Human herpes type 8	Kaposi's sarcoma	66,000[a]
Epstein-Barr virus	Nasopharyngeal carcinoma, Lymphomas (Hodgkin's, non- Hodgkin's, Burkitt)	113,000[a]
Human T-cell lymphotropic virus-1	Adult T-cell leukemia	3,000
PARASITES		
Schistosomes	Bladder cancer	11,000
Liver flukes	Cholangiocarcinoma	2,000

[a]The human immunodeficiency virus (HIV) cases include the 66,000 cases of Kaposi's sarcoma included under human herpes type 8, plus 36,000 cases of non-Hodgkin's lymphoma. The Epstein-Barr virus cases do not include the estimated 24,000 cases of HIV-associated non-Hodgkin's lymphoma that contain Epstein-Barr virus.
(Adapted from ref. 2.)

CANCER PREVENTION

Consistent with current concepts of the multistep nature of carcinogenesis, the changes in the host probably involve genetic alterations in potential target cells, impairment of the immune system, or both. Because not all infectious agents that establish a chronic infection are carcinogenic, chronic infection with agents not implicated in carcinogenesis must be much less efficient in inducing the types of changes that lead to cancer than are those agents that are implicated in carcinogenesis.

Infection seems to induce tumors by three main mechanisms, either singly or in combination, depending on the agent. In some instances, such as with HPV, the agent infects the potential target cell population and induces a series of changes from within those cells that lead to cancer.[13,17] The viral genes that continue to be expressed in tumors contribute directly to the tumorigenic phenotype by, for example, inactivating the activity of tumor suppressor genes. In a second scenario, as

TABLE 50.2

CANCERS ATTRIBUTABLE TO INFECTION: ESTIMATE OF WORLDWIDE DISTRIBUTION ACCORDING TO TYPE (ANNUAL NUMBER OF CASES IN THOUSANDS)[a]

Tumor Type	Developed Countries	Developing Countries	World	Percentage of Tumor Type Attributable to Infection
Stomach cancer	192	400	592	63
Liver cancer	50	475	525	85
Cervical cancer	83	409	493	100
Nasopharyngeal cancer	6	72	78	97
Kaposi's sarcoma in acquired immunodeficiency syndrome	4	62	66	100
Non-Hodgkin's lymphoma in acquired immunodeficiency syndrome	9	27	36	67
Hodgkin's lymphoma	12	17	29	45
Anal cancer	13	14	27	90
Vulvar/vaginal cancer	7	9	16	40
Bladder cancer	0	11	11	3
Gastric lymphoma	6	6	12	77
Burkitt's lymphoma	0	7	7	83
Leukemias	1	2	3	
Cholangiocarcinoma	0	2	2	

[a]Figures in each column represent the estimated number of cases of that tumor type attributed to infection, except for the column on the right, which represents the percentage of all cancers of that type worldwide attributed to an infectious cause.
(Adapted from ref. 2.)

with *H. pylori*, the infectious agent is present in the target tissue and induces cancer by local effects, usually chronic inflammation, but the agent remains outside the tumor cells.[16] By the time the tumor is capable of distant metastasis, if not sooner, its growth may be independent of the infectious agent. The third mechanism, which is more indirect, results in increased tumor risk secondary to suppression of the host immune system, as with human immunodeficiency virus infection. These tumors are often associated with coinfection by an oncogenic virus.[2,18]

PROPHYLACTIC VERSUS THERAPEUTIC VACCINATION

Vaccination against an infectious oncogenic agent can be contemplated in three possible clinical settings: as a prophylactic vaccine to prevent infection or acute disease, a therapeutic vaccine to treat an established infection before a malignancy has been induced, and a therapeutic vaccine to treat the infection after the malignant tumor has developed, as long as the tumor still depends on the presence of the infectious agent. The use of vaccines in the treatment of cancer is covered in Chapter 45.

An ideal vaccine would be effective both in preventing and treating premalignant disease, as well as in reducing the likelihood of transmitting the agent to uninfected individuals. The long interval between the initial infection and cancer development means there is a relatively long opportunity to identify and treat the infected population. In addition, it is usually easier to carry out therapeutic clinical trials that determine efficacy, compared with prophylactic trials. A therapeutic vaccine trial can limit its enrollment to infected individuals at a particular stage of disease, and the response to vaccine can be evaluated, usually within a short period, by suppression of infection and of the disease. A vaccine with therapeutic efficacy would also have the advantage of reducing the incidence of malignant disease much sooner than a prophylactic vaccine because the ability to target people with active infection intervenes much later in the infectious process than a purely prophylactic vaccine, which must be given prior to exposure to the agent. These considerations underscore the potential utility of determining whether successes with therapeutic vaccines in experimental animal systems, such as *H. pylori*[19,20] and papillomaviruses,[21,22] can be achieved in people.

Despite these theoretical advantages of vaccines with therapeutic efficacy, the challenge to develop such vaccines remains formidable. It has proven easier to develop prophylactic vaccines against infectious agents than therapeutic ones. Of the more than 20 approved vaccines in the United States, all are approved for prevention, rather than treatment, of established infection.[10] The comparative ease with which prophylactic vaccines can be developed and the fact that worldwide public health vaccine efforts are designed primarily for the administration of prophylactic vaccines support this approach. Safety is especially important for a prophylactic cancer vaccine, as malignancy develops in only a small minority of individuals.

The long interval between infection and tumor development implies that it requires many years to determine whether a candidate prophylactic vaccine can prevent cancer. Thus, while many studies have shown that HBV vaccination is highly effective in preventing acute disease (hepatitis), there is less documentation that this vaccine actually reduces the frequency of hepatocellular carcinoma.[4,5]

Although cancer prevention might appear to be a necessary end point for establishing the efficacy of a cancer vaccine, there can be serious ethical and practical obstacles to using this clinical end point. For those clinical situations in which the standard of care involves the treatment of premalignant lesions to prevent the development of malignancy, as with cervical abnormalities related to Pap smear screening, it may be unethical to delay treatment until cancer develops. Premalignant end points were used in licensing the HPV vaccine.[13] For those oncogenic infectious agents that induce nonmalignant diseases that carry significant morbidity and economic cost long before they cause cancer, it may be more practical to use a nonmalignant end point in efforts to demonstrate efficacy, with the effect on cancer being determined, directly or indirectly, by follow-up studies.[23] This was the approach taken with the HBV vaccine.

The most critical information for vaccine development lies in determining which antigens can induce protective immunity. For HBV and HPV, many aspects of their immunology and their role in carcinogenesis remain incompletely understood, but identification of a protective viral antigen was able to lead to development of an effective vaccine for both viruses.[11,13]

It appears to be easier to develop vaccines against agents such as HBV and HPV whose natural history in most individuals is characterized by self-limited infection and long-term resistance to reinfection. A successful vaccine can induce protective immunity against these agents by mimicking key aspects of the effective immune response to natural infection. By contrast, it is much more challenging to develop vaccines against agents such as *H. pylori*[19,20] and hepatitis C virus,[8,9] where infection is commonly lifelong and resolution of the infection may not be associated with long-term resistance to reinfection. Therefore, a successful vaccine against these agents has the added burden of inducing an immune response that is substantially more effective than the response to natural infection.

In natural infection, the cellular and humoral arms of the adaptive immune system generally function together to interfere either with the initial phases of infection or the eradication of established infection. Antibodies capable of neutralizing the infectious agent appear to be the prime effectors in preventing infection, while CD8+ T cells usually serve more critical roles in the resolution of established infection.[10,24] The success of prophylactic vaccines in inducing long-term protection against infection probably lies primarily in their ability to induce neutralizing antibodies, although other immune components may also contribute to their overall effectiveness.

HEPATITIS B VIRUS

The identification of HBV in the 1960s led to epidemiologic studies that clarified its worldwide role in hepatocellular cancer.[11,25,26] Although infection with this DNA virus can cause acute hepatitis, its most serious global consequences are chronic hepatitis, cirrhosis, and hepatocellular carcinoma, all of which are associated with chronic HBV infection.[27] It is estimated that there are more than 1 million chronic HBV carriers in the United States and approximately 350 million carriers throughout the world. The virus is believed to account for approximately 1 million deaths per year worldwide, approximately one-third of them secondary to hepatocellular carcinoma.

In highly endemic areas, the lifetime risk of exposure may exceed 50%, with most infections occurring perinatally or in early childhood. In areas of low endemicity, HBV transmission occurs mainly in adults, often via sexual exposure or parenteral exposure from infected shared needles used with illicit drugs. The risk of medical exposure to infected blood products has been greatly reduced by systematic screening of these materials for HBV.

The HBV carrier state, which is a measure of persistent infection, is a critical determinant of the long-term risk for hepatocellular carcinoma. HBV carrier rates vary dramatically in different populations, being less than 0.5% in the United States and many other countries with high standards of living, to rates of 10% to 20% in parts of Africa, Asia, and the South Pacific. The relative incidence of cancer attributable to HBV follows a similar geographic distribution.

The frequency with which persistent HBV infection is established varies inversely with the age of exposure. The highest risk by far occurs during the perinatal period and the first year of life. More than 70% of exposed neonates born to infected mothers become chronic carriers, compared with around 8% of those exposed at 3 years of age and an even lower proportion in immunocompetent adults. HBV is much more likely to induce acute hepatitis in older age groups, while acute infection is usually asymptomatic when exposure occurs in the perinatal period. The relative immunoincompetence of infants probably accounts for their lack of symptoms, which result from acute inflammation, and for the high frequency with which the virus establishes persistent infection in this age group. Thus, infants and children are the main target population for preventing HBV-associated cancer, although adult vaccination may be useful for preventing acute morbidity and developing herd immunity.[4,28,29]

The precise role of the virus in the development of hepatocellular carcinoma has not been fully determined.[11,26] Persistent infection appears to lead to cancer mainly as the result of chronic inflammation and repeated cellular regeneration. Most cases of liver cancer associated with HBV infection arise after chronic hepatitis has led to cirrhosis. Hepatocellular carcinoma may develop in as little as 5 to 10 years of infection, but it does not usually occur until an individual has been infected for at least 20 to 30 years. Ongoing infection continues to be a risk factor for carcinoma, with an estimated cumulative risk of 15% for an individual who has had persistent infection for 50 years. The rate of hepatocellular carcinoma attributable to HBV is at least three times higher in males than in females, in part because of the higher frequency with which the HBV carrier state is established in male subjects (close to two to one) and the greater likelihood of female subjects to eliminate the carrier state. An effective therapeutic vaccine would have great utility, but does not yet exist.

The HBV vaccine is the prototype prophylactic vaccine against an oncogenic infectious agent. A key to HBV vaccine development was the recognition that the neutralizing antibodies were directed against the hepatitis B surface antigen (HBsAg), and that there is only one HBV serotype. The HBsAg is expressed in relatively pure form as circulating enveloped lipid membrane-based viruslike particles (VLPs) in the blood of infected HBV carriers. The HBsAg particles do not carry the viral genome and are not infectious. It was possible to purify the particles, inactivate possibly contaminating infectious virus with formalin (which should also have inactivated other viruses), and to test the particles as a subunit vaccine in human clinical trials, which were initiated in 1975.

The systemically administered HBsAg vaccine was well tolerated, induced an immune response in almost all vaccinees, and reduced the infection rate in adults by at least 95% and in neonates by at least 85%. The protection rates in neonates may be further increased by giving hepatitis B immune globulin in addition to the vaccine. The vaccine was licensed in the United States in 1981.

An analogous HBsAg particle vaccine produced in yeast by recombinant DNA technology was licensed in the United States in 1986. The recombinant vaccine has replaced the blood-derived vaccine, following efficacy trials showing that the recombinant vaccine confers a similar rate of protection against HBV.[11,15] In addition, the recombinant vaccine is less expensive to manufacture and does not have the theoretical concern of contaminating infectious material.

The initial series of immunizations, with either vaccine preparation, confers protection against infection for at least several years. In instances in which breakthrough infection has occurred, it has not been associated with development of a chronic carrier state. Routine revaccination is not recommended at this time by vaccine advisory groups in the United States.[28]

The long interval between HBV infection and the development of hepatocellular carcinoma means that relatively limited data thus far indicate directly that vaccination can actually decrease the incidence of cancer attributable to HBV. Data from an HBV vaccination program in Taiwan, an area with high HBV endemicity where universal vaccination was instituted in 1984, show the incidence of hepatocellular carcinoma in vaccinees 6 to 19 years of age is about one-third the rate before implementing vaccination, with the current cases more likely to occur in individuals who received fewer than the recommended three doses of vaccine or whose mothers were chronic carriers.[5] These results indicate that HBV vaccination can achieve the long-term goal of cancer reduction. However, such a reduction will occur only if the populations most at risk are given the vaccine in a timely manner. To this end, considerable effort has been required to increase HBV vaccine coverage to developing nations with a high prevalence of chronic HBV infection.[15,30]

HUMAN PAPILLOMAVIRUS

Papillomaviruses are epitheliotropic agents that induce benign papillomas of the skin and mucous membranes.[13,17] In contrast to HBV, there are more than 100 HPV genotypes (types).[31] A subset of HPV types that are almost always transmitted sexually are the main cause of cervical cancer. Infection with these HPV types is a strong risk factor for cervical cancer, and HPV DNA from one or more of these types is found in virtually all cervical tumors.[32,33] The virus encodes oncoproteins that appear to be required both for the induction and the maintenance of the cancer. HPV infection has also been linked to the majority of anal cancers, in which the molecular pathogenesis seems to be similar to that of the cervix, as well as to other anogenital malignancies and to tumors of the upper aerodigestive tract.[2,13]

As with HBV, cancer attributable to HPV develops only after many years of persistent HPV infection and is an infrequent outcome of infection.[14,34] Cervical HPV infection is remarkably common; it is estimated that in the United States a woman has at least a 75% chance of having at least one genital HPV infection during her lifetime, with the highest prevalence occurring in the first few years after becoming sexually active. Most infections are self-limited, and clinical cures are associated with at least partial resistance to reinfection. The antigenic divergence between HPV types is such that protection appears to be largely type specific. Genital HPV infection in the male has been studied less intensively, but appears to share many features with that in females. Worldwide, only about 10% of cancers attributable to HPV infection occur in males because cervical cancer accounts for most cases of HPV-induced cancer. In the United States, by contrast, about one-third of HPV-associated cancers occur in males, mainly because of the reduction in the incidence of cervical cancer from cervical cancer screening together with an increase in HPV-associated oropharynx cancer, mainly among males.[35]

The HPVs associated with cervical and anal cancer are usually designated as high-risk types, as contrasted with the low-risk types, which also participate in anogenital infection but are almost never found in cervical or anal cancers. Although there are several high-risk HPV types, HPV-16 is the most common type, being present in more than one-half of cervical cancers worldwide, with HPV-18 being second in frequency. Together they account for about 70% of cervical cancer and an even higher proportion of the other HPV-associated cancers. The viral *E6* and *E7* genes of the high-risk types are preferentially retained and expressed in the tumors, where they contribute to tumorigenesis by inactivating the p53 and Rb tumor suppressor proteins, respectively, in addition to altering the activity of other endogenous proteins.

In principle, cervical cancer is already a largely preventable disease.[14] In countries in which Pap smear screening reaches most women, the incidence of cervical cancer has decreased markedly. In the United States, for example, the rate of cervical cancer has decreased several-fold since the 1950s, from more than 50 in 100,000 to less than 10 in 100,000. This decrease in cancer rates is even more impressive because it has occurred during a period in which increased sexual promiscuity has been associated with an increased frequency of genital HPV infection.

However, the cost of Pap smear screening and follow-up is high (estimated to be more than $6 billion annually in the United States), and Pap smear screening is not routinely available in many less well-developed countries. This situation has made cervical cancer the leading cancer among women in many developing countries, and it remains the third most common female cancer worldwide.[13,14]

Establishing the etiologic link between HPV infection and cervical cancer (and other tumors) focused interest on developing an HPV vaccine. The main goal would be to reduce the incidence of cervical cancer, which accounts for approximately 75% of the cancers worldwide attributable to HPV infection, although such a vaccine should also reduce the other HPV-associated cancers. Because cervical cancer is especially prevalent in developing countries, an HPV vaccine would potentially have its greatest public health impact in these populations. In the United States, an effective HPV vaccine might reduce the incidence of cervical cancer below its current level by reaching populations that do not receive adequate Pap screening. In addition, widespread vaccine use in the United States would be expected to decrease the frequency of genital HPV infection, thereby reducing the number of cervical dysplasias that require treatment and the overall cost of cervical cancer screening programs. Thus, fewer women would need to deal with the personal, social, medical, and economic issues associated with a diagnosis of genital HPV infection and the conditions it causes.

As papillomaviruses contain oncogenes and prophylactic vaccines are directed toward healthy young individuals, HPV vaccine efforts have emphasized a subunit approach, analogous to that used for HBV.[13,23] The current prophylactic HPV vaccines are based on the observation that high-level expression of the L1 major structural viral protein, even in nonmammalian cells, will lead to its efficient self-assembly into nonenveloped icosahedral VLPs that resemble authentic viral capsids structurally and antigenically. Preparative amounts of VLPs can be synthesized in eukaryotic cells and are suitable immunogens that, as is true of authentic virions, possess the immunodominant conformational epitopes capable of raising high-titer neutralizing antibodies.

It was unclear whether intramuscular administration of this subunit vaccine would induce protection against a local mucosal infection. However, successful proof of principle efficacy trials of VLP-based HPV vaccines undertaken by two pharmaceutical companies (Merck and GlaxoSmithKline) led both of them to initiate and complete large international 4-year phase 3 trials of commercial versions of their respective vaccines.[6,7] One is a bivalent HPV-16/18 VLP vaccine (manufactured by GlaxoSmithKline) that is produced in insect cells and uses a proprietary adjuvant, AS04. Together these two HPV types are responsible for about 70% of cervical cancer. The other is a quadrivalent vaccine (manufactured by Merck) produced in yeast and composed of VLPs from HPV-6, -11, -16, and -18. As HPV-6 and -11 together account for about 90% of genital warts, this latter vaccine also targets this condition. In fully vaccinated women, the phase 3 trials from both manufacturers found close to complete protection against moderate-grade cervical dysplasia or worse pathology (CIN2+) attributable to incident infection by HPV-16 and -18 (Table 50.3).[6,7] The Merck vaccine was found in addition to confer virtually complete protection against the development of moderate-grade dysplasia or worse of the vulva and vagina, as well as against genital warts, attributable to the HPV types targeted by the vaccine.

As noted earlier, cervical cancer could not be used as an end point for the trials, as it is unethical to allow cervical lesions that arise in women in a vaccine study population to progress to malignancy. A cancer end point would also require more than 10 years to establish, given the long interval between infection and cancer. Fortunately, the surrogate end points of persistent HPV infection and high-grade cervical dysplasia have been shown to be tightly linked to the risk of progression to invasive cancer.[14,34]

Thus far, protection has been shown to last at least 6 years for the vaccines from both companies used in the proof of principle studies. However, it seems likely that protection

TABLE 50.3

HUMAN PAPILLOMAVIRUS (HPV) VACCINE EFFICACY TRIAL OUTCOMES[a]

Study (Ref.)	Vaccine[b]	Number of Subjects: Vaccine	Number of Subjects: Control	End Point	Vaccine Efficacy: Percent (95% confidence limits)
Munoz et al. 2010 (7)	6/11/16/18	4,616	4,680	CIN 2/3 (AIS)	100 (90–100)
		4,689	4,735	VIN 2/3, VAIN 2/3, GW	95 (70–100)
Paavonen et al. 2009 (6)	16/18	7,344	7,312	CIN 2/3	98 (88–100)

CIN, cervical intraepithelial neoplasia; 2, intermediate, 3, severe; AIS, adenocarcinoma *in situ*; GW, genital warts; VIN, vulvar intraepithelial neoplasia; VAIN, vaginal intraepithelial neoplasia.

[a]Efficacy measured as prevention in fully vaccinated women of incident (new) infection and disease caused by the HPV types in each vaccine.

[b]HPV-6/11/16/18, Merck vaccine (Gardasil); HPV-16/18, GlaxoSmith Kline vaccine (Cervarix).

will last longer, as serum antibody levels in vaccines reach a plateau within the first 2 years after vaccination, and protection was seen for the duration of the phase 3 trials. Protection for both vaccines is predominantly type specific, although both display some cross-protection against closely related high-risk HPV types. However, partial cross-protection from the GlaxoSmithKline vaccine, which is even more immunogenic than the Merck vaccine,[36] extends to HPV-31, -33, and -45, while that of the Merck vaccine extends only to HPV-31. It is unclear whether this difference is attributable to differences in the production of the VLPs, the adjuvant used, or both.

The U.S. Food and Drug Administration licensed the Merck vaccine in 2006 for females and in 2009 for males and the GlaxoSmithKline vaccine for females in 2009. The vaccines have also been licensed in the European Union and other countries. These are the first vaccines whose principal goal is to reduce the incidence of cancer and the first subunit vaccines that successfully target a local sexually transmitted infection.

It will be important to develop public health policies for the appropriate age for vaccination of women and the degree to which men should also be vaccinated. The VLP vaccines will be most cost-effective if given prior to initiating sexual activity, and the highest priority target population are young adolescent females.[13] There should also be benefit to catch-up vaccination for older adolescents. However, it is unclear how much serious disease will be prevented by the vaccines when they are given to women who have been sexually active for more than 5 to 10 years.[37]

The type-restricted nature of protection means that even vaccinated women should follow the same cervical cancer screening as nonvaccinated women, as the current vaccines are not expected to prevent about 30% of serious infections. In principle, the vaccine could have the largest public health impact in the developing world, but its high cost and the logistical difficulty in this setting of giving multiple injections to adolescents will probably prevent its widespread implementation there for the foreseeable future.

These considerations make it attractive to develop second-generation HPV vaccines, and it is likely that some will be developed.[23,38] The current vaccine manufacturers will probably broaden the HPV coverage of their respective vaccine by adding VLPs from more HPV types, providing that such additions do not impair the immunogenicity of the types in the current vaccine. Other approaches, such as those that reduce the number of immunizations or use an approach that does not require injection, might be easier to deliver as a prophylactic vaccine in a developing-world setting. The presence of epitopes in the L2 minor capsid protein that induce broadly cross-neutralizing antibodies might result in a broadly protective vaccine that was easier to produce, if the lower immunogenicity of these epitopes can be overcome. It should also be noted that the current candidate prophylactic vaccines are not expected to benefit the approximately 5 million women with prevalent HPV infection who are destined over the next 20 years to develop cervical cancers from which they will die. For these women, it is possible to develop and implement cost-effective screening programs.[39] In addition, an effective therapeutic vaccine, ideally one that might also have prophylactic capabilities, would also be highly desirable.[21,22]

HELICOBACTER PYLORI

H. pylori, which was discovered in 1982, induces chronic gastric infection of almost one-half the world population. Infection with *H. pylori* is associated with a variable proportion of several disorders, including duodenal ulcer, gastric ulcer, gastric carcinoma, which is the second most common cancer worldwide, and the much less-common gastric mucosa-associated lymphoid tissue lymphomas.[16,40]

H. pylori is usually acquired in childhood. It disproportionately affects people of lower socioeconomic status, and the majority of adults from developing countries are infected. The bacterium is found less frequently among individuals in developed countries such as the United States, and the low rate of infection in children from developed countries suggests the proportion in adults will continue to fall.

Most *H. pylori* infections are asymptomatic and have a benign outcome. When infection does lead to stomach cancer, it usually takes decades. In this process, bacterially induced chronic gastritis is believed to progress to atrophic gastritis and metaplasia, and then to cancer. The bacterium appears to be required only until atrophic gastritis develops. Experimental *H. pylori* infection of Mongolian gerbils can induce these sequential pathologic changes, including gastric adenocarcinoma.[41]

Gastric mucosa-associated lymphoid tissue lymphoma is much less common than gastric carcinoma and has a distinct pathogenesis.[42] This B-cell lymphoma arises from *H. pylori*–dependent chronic stimulation of the Peyer's patches in the gastric mucosa. Localized mucosa-associated lymphoid tissue tumors often remain dependent on continued stimulation by bacterial antigens, and eradication of the bacteria with antibiotic treatment may frequently be associated with lymphoma regression at this stage. However, the growth of more invasive tumors, which may become widely disseminated, is usually autonomous, and these tumors typically do not respond to antibacterial therapy.

Several bacterial virulence factors account for the ability of *H. pylori* to colonize and persist in the gastric mucosa.[16,40] Although different isolates of *H. pylori* are closely related antigenically, those that are associated with carcinoma contain a cassette of genes that are designated a pathogenicity-associated island whose marker is a cytotoxic-associated antigen (CagA).

In principle, *H. pylori* infection can be eradicated by combined treatment with several antimicrobial agents plus proton pump inhibitors. However, the high cost and the emergence of antibiotic resistance make this approach poorly suited for bacterial eradication from whole populations.[43] These limitations have fostered efforts to develop *H. pylori* vaccines.[20,44]

However, although humoral and cellular immune responses develop in most infected individuals, it is uncommon for these infections to disappear spontaneously, and reinfection may occur after successful antibiotic treatment. These characteristics of *H. pylori* infection, combined with imperfect animal models, pose a challenge to successful vaccine development. However, responses in preclinical vaccine studies have been obtained with animal models. Mucosal immunization with bacterial lysates, purified bacterial antigens, or with attenuated salmonellae encoding *H. pylori* antigen can all prevent experimental infection. Some of these vaccines have also had some success in eradicating established infection in the animal models. It remains to be determined which of these approaches will prove efficacious in human vaccine trials. Thus far, clinical trials with single antigens have been disappointing, and efforts are under way to test vaccines that consist of several antigens. The most desirable outcome would be a cost-effective vaccine that could eradicate established infection while also protecting against new infections. Such a vaccine would have the long-term benefits of a purely prophylactic vaccine while reducing the incidence of gastric cancer after a much shorter interval.

References

1. Ehreth J. The economics of vaccination from a global perspective: present and future. 2–3 December, 2004, Vaccines: all things considered, San Francisco, CA, USA. *Expert Rev Vaccines* 2005;4:19.
2. Parkin DM. The global health burden of infection-associated cancers in the year 2002. *Int J Cancer* 2006;118:3030.
3. Feng H, Shuda M, Chang Y, Moore PS. Clonal integration of a polyomavirus in human Merkel cell carcinoma. *Science* 2008;319:1096.
4. Chang MH. Cancer prevention by vaccination against hepatitis B. *Recent Results Cancer Res* 2009;181:85.
5. Chang MH, You SL, Chen CJ, et al. Decreased incidence of hepatocellular carcinoma in hepatitis B vaccinees: a 20-year follow-up study. *J Natl Cancer Inst* 2009;101:1348.
6. Paavonen J, Naud P, Salmeron J, et al. Efficacy of human papillomavirus (HPV)-16/18 AS04-adjuvanted vaccine against cervical infection and precancer caused by oncogenic HPV types (PATRICIA): final analysis of a double-blind, randomised study in young women. *Lancet* 2009;374:301.
7. Munoz N, Kjaer SK, Sigurdsson K, et al. Impact of human papillomavirus (HPV)-6/11/16/18 vaccine on all HPV-associated genital diseases in young women. *J Natl Cancer Inst* 2010;102:325.
8. Strickland GT, El-Kamary SS, Klenerman P, Nicosia A. Hepatitis C vaccine: supply and demand. *Lancet Infect Dis* 2008;8:379.
9. Stoll-Keller F, Barth H, Fafi-Kremer S, Zeisel MB, Baumert TF. Development of hepatitis C virus vaccines: challenges and progress. *Expert Rev Vaccines* 2009;8(3):333.
10. Graham BS, Crowe JE Jr. Immunization against viral diseases. In: Knipe DM, Howley PH, eds. *Fields virology.* Vol. 1. 5th ed. Philadelphia: Lippincott Williams & Wilkins, 2007:487.
11. Hollinger FB, Liang TJ. Hepatitis B viruses. In: Knipe DM, Howley PH, eds. *Fields virology.* Vol. 2. 4th ed. Philadelphia: Lippincott Williams & Wilkins, 2001:2971.
12. Marcellin P. Hepatitis B and hepatitis C in 2009. *Liver Int* 2009;29(Suppl 1):1.
13. Lowy DR, Solomon D, Hildesheim A, Schiller JT, Schiffman M. Human papillomavirus infection and the primary and secondary prevention of cervical cancer. *Cancer* 2008;113(7 Suppl):1980.
14. Schiffman M, Castle PE, Jeronimo J, Rodriguez AC, Wacholder S. Human papillomavirus and cervical cancer. *Lancet* 2007;370:890.
15. Zanetti AR, Van Damme P, Shouval D. The global impact of vaccination against hepatitis B: a historical overview. *Vaccine* 2008;26:6266.
16. Herrera V, Parsonnet J. *Helicobacter pylori* and gastric adenocarcinoma. *Clin Microbiol Infect* 2009;15:971.
17. Howley PM, Lowy DR. Papillomaviruses. In: Knipe DM, Howley PH, eds. *Fields virology.* Vol. 2. 5th ed. Philadelphia: Lippincott Williams & Wilkins, 2007:2299.
18. Engels EA, Biggar RJ, Hall HI, et al. Cancer risk in people infected with human immunodeficiency virus in the United States. *Int J Cancer* 2008;123:187.
19. Agarwal K, Agarwal S. *Helicobacter pylori* vaccine: from past to future. *Mayo Clin Proc* 2008;83:169.
20. Del Giudice G, Malfertheiner P, Rappuoli R. Development of vaccines against *Helicobacter pylori. Expert Rev Vaccines* 2009;8:1037.
21. Kanodia S, Da Silva DM, Kast WM. Recent advances in strategies for immunotherapy of human papillomavirus-induced lesions. *Int J Cancer* 2008;122:247.
22. Kenter GG, Welters MJ, Valentijn AR, et al. Vaccination against HPV-16 oncoproteins for vulvar intraepithelial neoplasia. *N Engl J Med* 2009;361:1838.
23. Schiller JT, Lowy DR. Vaccines to prevent infections by oncoviruses. *Annu Rev Microbiol* 2010;64:23.
24. Ha SJ, West EE, Araki K, Smith KA, Ahmed R. Manipulating both the inhibitory and stimulatory immune system towards the success of therapeutic vaccination against chronic viral infections. *Immunol Rev* 2008;223:317.
25. Beasley RP. Hepatitis B virus. The major etiology of hepatocellular carcinoma. *Cancer* 1988;61:1942.
26. Seeger C, Zoulim F, Mason WS. Hepadnaviruses. In: Knipe DM, Howley PH, eds. *Fields virology.* Vol. 2. 5th ed. Philadelphia: Lippincott Williams & Wilkins, 2007:2977.
27. Goldstein ST, Zhou F, Hadler SC, et al. A mathematical model to estimate global hepatitis B disease burden and vaccination impact. *Int J Epidemiol* 2005;34:1329.
28. Mast EE, Weinbaum CM, Fiore AE, et al. A comprehensive immunization strategy to eliminate transmission of hepatitis B virus infection in the United States: recommendations of the Advisory Committee on Immunization Practices (ACIP). Part II: immunization of adults. *MMWR Recomm Rep* 2006;55:1.
29. Chen DS. Hepatitis B vaccination: the key towards elimination and eradication of hepatitis B. *J Hepatol* 2009;50:805.
30. Kane MA, Brooks A. New immunization initiatives and progress toward the global control of hepatitis B. *Curr Opin Infect Dis* 2002;15:465.
31. Bernard HU, Burk RD, Chen Z, et al. Classification of papillomaviruses (PVs) based on 189 PV types and proposal of taxonomic amendments. *Virology* 2010;401:70.
32. Munoz N, Bosch FX, de Sanjose S, et al. Epidemiologic classification of human papillomavirus types associated with cervical cancer. *N Engl J Med* 2003;348:518.
33. Schiffman M, Rodriguez AC, Chen Z, et al. A population-based prospective study of carcinogenic human papillomavirus variant lineages, viral persistence, and cervical neoplasia. *Cancer Res* 2010;70:3159.
34. Koutsky L. The epidemiology behind the HPV vaccine discovery. *Ann Epidemiol* 2009;19:239.
35. Chaturvedi AK. Beyond cervical cancer: burden of other HPV-related cancers among men and women. *J Adolesc Health* 2010;46:S20.
36. Einstein MH, Baron M, Levin MJ, et al. Comparison of the immunogenicity and safety of Cervarix and Gardasil human papillomavirus (HPV) cervical cancer vaccines in healthy women aged 18–45 years. *Hum Vaccin* 2009;5:705.
37. Rodriguez AC, Schiffman M, Herrero R, et al. Longitudinal study of human papillomavirus persistence and cervical intraepithelial neoplasia grade 2/3: critical role of duration of infection. *J Natl Cancer Inst* 2010;102:315.
38. Schiller JT, Nardelli-Haefliger D. Chapter 17: Second generation HPV vaccines to prevent cervical cancer. *Vaccine* 2006;24:S147.
39. Sankaranarayanan R, Nene BM, Shastri SS, et al. HPV screening for cervical cancer in rural India. *N Engl J Med* 2009;360:1385.
40. Wroblewski LE, Peek RM Jr, Wilson KT. *Helicobacter pylori* and gastric cancer: factors that modulate disease risk. *Clin Microbiol Rev* 2010;23:713.
41. Kabir S. Effect of *Helicobacter pylori* eradication on incidence of gastric cancer in human and animal models: underlying biochemical and molecular events. *Helicobacter* 2009;14:159.
42. Sagaert X, Van Cutsem E, De Hertogh G, Geboes K, Tousseyn T. Gastric MALT lymphoma: a model of chronic inflammation-induced tumor development. *Nat Rev Gastroenterol Hepatol* 2010;7:336.
43. Suzuki H, Nishizawa T, Hibi T. *Helicobacter pylori* eradication therapy. *Future Microbiol* 2010;5:639.
44. Hernandez-Hernandez Ldel C, Lazcano-Ponce EC, Lopez-Vidal Y, Aguilar-Gutierrez GR. Relevance of *Helicobacter pylori* virulence factors for vaccine development. *Salud Publica Mex* 2009;51:S447.

CHAPTER 51 TOBACCO DEPENDENCE AND ITS TREATMENT

ELLEN R. GRITZ, CHO Y. LAM, DAMON J. VIDRINE, AND MICHELLE CORORVE FINGERET

Tobacco use and its relation to cancer have been studied extensively for over 50 years. The 1964 U.S. Surgeon General's Report on Smoking and Health was the first definitive document in the United States to establish the causal relationship of smoking to lung cancer.[1] In 1988, the Surgeon General's Report firmly established nicotine as the addictive agent in tobacco.[2] Understanding the biobehavioral and social aspects of smoking remains critical to reducing smoking initiation in youth and promoting smoking cessation in adults. The pharmacologic treatment of smoking cessation has been expanding over decades as our understanding of the complex actions of nicotine in the brain deepens. We have now entered the era of research aimed at tailored treatments based on genetics, phenotypes of nicotine addiction, and comorbidities. Policy, regulation, taxation, and outreach to disadvantaged and vulnerable populations where tobacco use is most entrenched are critical aspects of tobacco control today. The National Institutes of Health State of the Science Conference held in June 2006 resulted in a panel statement and a series of expert presentations summarized in a recent publication that will be of substantial interest to the reader.[3] However, relatively little attention has been focused on the cancer patient and smoking in the oncology setting. There is a growing body of evidence that establishes the connection between smoking and adverse outcomes on cancer treatment, recurrence, second primary tumors, survival, and quality of life. This chapter will provide an overview of the area for the oncologic audience, summarizing scientific evidence, providing a clinical framework for behavioral and pharmacologic treatment, and outlining important areas of future research.

NICOTINE AND THE NEUROBIOLOGICAL BASIS OF SMOKING

Nicotine stimulates the mesolimbic dopaminergic system, an important reward circuitry in the brain targeted by many psychostimulant drugs of abuse.[4] Specifically, nicotine increases extracellular concentrations of dopamine in the nucleus accumbens.[5,6] Although the exact mechanism by which the activation of the mesolimbic dopaminergic system controls smoking remains unclear, researchers have suggested that this activation is involved in the experience of nicotine's rewarding effect.[4] Others have hypothesized that the increase in extracellular dopamine in the nucleus accumbens enhances the incentive value of the smoking behaviors, making them more likely to be repeated.[7] It is also suggested that dopaminergic neurotransmission is involved in the assignment of incentive salience to environmental cues associated with smoking.[8] As a result, these environmental cues may become conditioned reinforcers that serve to maintain smoking behaviors. Furthermore, the nucleus accumbens has been implicated in drug reinstatement or relapse.[9] A comprehensive discussion on neurobiology of nicotine addiction is beyond the scope of the present chapter. Interested readers are referred to reviews prepared by Balfour[7] and Di Chiara.[10]

SMOKING PREVALENCE AND QUIT RATES

Data from the 2009 National Health Interview Survey (NHIS) indicate that the prevalence of smoking among adults in the United States is 20.6%, approximately 46.0 million individuals. This represents a significant decrease in smoking prevalence over the past 10 years. However, smoking prevalence has remained essentially unchanged over the 5 most recent NHIS survey years.[11]

Based on these trends, it is not anticipated that the *Healthy People 2010* objective to reduce the prevalence of cigarette smoking to 12% will be met. As noted by the Centers for Disease Control and Prevention, the lack of progress in reducing tobacco use among U.S. adults highlights the need for improving efforts to establish sustained, comprehensive, evidence-based tobacco-control programs.[11] A population in particular need of such efforts is oncology patients. Increased attention must be given to prioritize cessation in the oncology setting due to elevated rates of smoking in certain cancer patient populations and the critical relevance of continued smoking to cancer treatment outcomes. Despite high interest and motivation to quit smoking documented among cancer patients, the opportunity to intervene is often missed by health care professionals.

Across different studies, rates of current smoking among patients with head and neck or lung tumors at diagnosis have ranged from 40% to 60%.[12–15] Further research indicates that patients with smoking-related tumors may be quite receptive to smoking cessation interventions even as they continue to smoke. One study found that among head and neck patients who underwent surgical treatment and continued to smoke postoperatively, 92% reported an interest in quitting, 84% made at least one quit attempt, and 69% made multiple quit attempts.[15] These figures contrast with general population estimates of 70% of smokers who want to quit completely[16] and 42.5% of smokers who attempt to quit within the preceding 12 months.[17] Elevated interest and motivation to quit smoking following cancer diagnosis can be used as a window of opportunity to intervene and provide assistance in the quitting process. A continuum of potential teachable moments to promote smoking cessation in the oncology setting have been described by McBride et al.,[18] beginning with screening and diagnostic testing and extending into the period of cancer survivorship.

Although the strongest predictor of quitting following cancer diagnosis has been disease site, limited data are available on the smoking behaviors of patients with non–smoking-related tumors. In a population of stage I non–small cell lung cancer patients, 83.2% of smokers made a quit attempt in the first year following surgery, with 53% achieving continuous abstinence at the end of the first year.[19] Walker et al.[12] reported quit rates of 73.2% at 3 months, 69.9% at 6 months, and 63.1% at 12 months following surgery for non–small cell lung cancer. Ostroff et al.[15] found a 65% cessation rate among head and neck cancer patients following surgical intervention. In contrast, studies of patients with cancers less strongly associated with smoking typically find moderate to high quit rates but lower continuous abstinence rates (e.g., 31% among bladder cancer patients).[20]

It is likely that a more explicit connection between diagnosis and smoking status facilitates smoking cessation. A number of additional factors such as prognosis, length and number of hospitalizations, and treatment side effects may also differentially influence smoking behaviors. For example, patients with higher cure rates and improved prognosis may minimize the risks of continued smoking. Alternatively, patients with long or multiple hospitalizations (where smoking is not permitted) or those whose illness and treatment interfere with smoking behaviors are more likely to have higher sustained cessation rates.

Despite elevated cessation rates in certain cancer groups, 30% to 50% of individuals who smoked at diagnosis do not quit or relapse following initial quit attempts. As cancer survivors recover from their treatment, particular attention must be given to promoting sustained abstinence and relapse prevention. Although relapses in the general population usually occur within the first week after cessation, relapses in cancer patients are often delayed because of surgical and other posttreatment healing. In one study with head and neck cancer patients, the majority of relapses did not occur until 1 to 6 months after surgery.[21] Other findings indicate that rates of smoking relapse are relatively high among lung cancer patients who had quit a year or more prior to cancer diagnosis.[22] It is thus recommended that oncology health care providers be vigilant in addressing smoking behaviors with their patients well into the period of cancer survivorship.

Similar to the trends observed in the general population, data from the *Cancer Trends Progress Report—2009/2010 Update* suggest that the prevalence of current smoking among long-term adult cancer survivors (all sites combined) has significantly declined from 1992 to 2008. While the smoking prevalence among long-term survivors aged 45 years or older is approximately the same as the prevalence in the general population, the prevalence among the younger long-term survivors is significantly higher. Specifically, the prevalence of smoking among long-term survivors 18 to 44 years is 40.4% compared to 24.7% among the same age group in the general population.[23] Findings from other national surveys have documented similar trends (i.e., elevated rates of smoking among younger long-term survivors).[24,25] An important caveat to these findings is that many smoking-related tumors have high mortality rates (lung, head and neck, pancreas), so that these individuals are not represented among long-term survivors. Indeed, survivors of cervical cancer, a smoking-related tumor with a low mortality rate, were among those in the under-40 group in the Bellizzi et al.[24] study.

EFFECTS OF CONTINUED SMOKING ON CANCER TREATMENT OUTCOMES

An ever-growing body of evidence indicates that smoking represents an important variable affecting both the treatment course and survivorship experience for individuals diagnosed with smoking-related and non–smoking-related cancers.[26,27] Continued smoking following a cancer diagnosis results in reduced treatment effectiveness and an increased risk of treatment-related complications. Cigarette smoking can adversely affect outcomes associated with each of the major cancer treatment modalities (i.e., surgery, radiation therapy, and chemotherapy). Continued smoking is also an important predictor of cancer recurrence, risk of second cancers, disease-specific survival, and overall survival. Finally, cigarette smoking after a cancer diagnosis is associated with poor performance status and health-related quality of life.

Surgery

Several published reports suggest that cancer patients who undergo surgical procedures have an increased risk of complications. This increased risk has been observed among patients who undergo thoracotomy for suspected lung cancer, in which current smokers were twice as likely to experience a respiratory complication.[28] Similarly, cigarette smoking has been identified as the most important predictor of pulmonary complications among patients who undergo head and neck surgery.[29]

In addition to surgical procedures for smoking-related cancers, current smoking has been linked to adverse outcomes among women who receive reconstructive surgery for breast cancer. Chang et al.[30] observed significantly more adverse outcomes among current smokers who received free pedicled transverse rectus abdominis myocutaneous (TRAM) flap procedures for breast reconstruction compared to former and never smokers. Specifically, current smokers were more likely to experience mastectomy flap necrosis, abdominal flap necrosis, and hernia. Of interest, these authors also found that women who successfully quit smoking at least 4 weeks prior to reconstructive procedures experienced a significant reduction in risk compared to women who continued to smoke.

Several mechanisms have been identified that may explain the increased risk of complications experienced in smokers who undergo surgical procedures. First, smokers who received general anesthesia have higher levels of sputum production compared to nonsmokers, which can lead to respiratory complications.[31] Second, smokers are more likely than nonsmokers to experience tissue hypoxia. This may be caused by both increased levels of carboxyhemoglobin levels, limiting the oxygen carrying capacity of the blood, and by compromised capillary blood flow due to nicotine-induced vasoconstriction.[1] The result of these conditions is an increased risk of infection and poorer wound healing.[32,33]

Radiation Therapy

Cigarette smoking may also have an adverse effect on patients who undergo radiation therapy. Work by Browman et al.[34] indicates that head and neck cancer patients who received radiation treatment and yet continued to smoke were significantly less likely to a have a complete response to treatment. Smoking among individuals who receive radiation therapy for head and neck cancer is also associated with an elevated risk of treatment-related adverse events, such as mucositis, xerostomia, poor voice quality, and disfigurement.[35,36] In a more recent study Zevallos et al.[37] confirmed an elevated rate of treatment-related complications in patients who were being irradiated for laryngopharyngeal cancer and continued to smoke from diagnosis through treatment compared to those who quit smoking and abstained throughout treatment. Complications were more common in those who continued to smoke versus quitters, and included mucositis, feeding tube placement and duration, and pharyngeal stricture. Two complications reached statistical significance (need for hospitalization for reasons related to dehydration, airway management, pneumonia, and pain control [$P = .04$] and osteiradionecrosis [$P = .03$]). Similarly, lung cancer patients who receive radiation therapy and continue to smoke are more likely to experience adverse events, such as clinical radiation pneumonitis.[38]

Persistent smoking while undergoing radiation therapy can also increase the risk of adverse outcomes for patients with non–smoking-related cancers. For example, Jagsi et al.[39] found that among women who received radiation therapy for early stage breast cancer, those who continued to smoke during treatment were significantly more likely to experience a myocardial infarction or coronary artery disease. Smoking has a negative impact on treatment effectiveness in men who receive radiation therapy for localized prostate cancer. Specifically, patients who were current smokers at the time they received a course of external beam radiotherapy were significantly more likely to develop metastatic disease. This relationship remained significant even after controlling for T stage, Gleason score, and prostate-specific antigen (PSA) level.[40]

Although the exact biological mechanisms that explain the association between smoking during radiation treatment and health outcomes are not fully understood, several possibilities have been identified. For example, Grau et al.[41] hypothesize that hypoxia caused by high carbohemoglobin levels in smokers may modulate tumor response to radiation. Another hypothesis to explain the poorer outcomes among current smokers is that smoking results in aberrant methylation of gene promoter sequences. Consistent with this, Enokida et al.[42] found that the methylation status of prostate cancer tumor tissue was significantly associated with smoking status. Methylation status was also significantly correlated with markers of disease progression, such as Gleason scores and PSA levels.

Chemotherapy

Patients who receive chemotherapy frequently experience adverse side effects, such as immune suppression, weight loss, fatigue, and cardiac or pulmonary toxicities. Because cigarette smoking is also associated with these events, patients who smoke during treatment may experience more severe treatment-related toxicities.[43] Emerging evidence also indicates that smoking may reduce the effectiveness of certain anticancer or cancer preventive agents. For example, results from a phase 3 trial designed to assess the efficacy of isotretinoin to prevent second primary tumors among stage I non–small cell lung cancer patients indicated the presence of a smoking status by treatment interaction. More specifically, results indicated that isotretinoin increased the risk of lung cancer recurrence and mortality among current smokers compared to those who never smoked.[14]

Findings from another trial also indicate that those who never smoked have better treatment outcomes compared to smokers. In this retrospective study of a large sample of advanced-stage lung cancer patients treated with chemotherapy, patients who were never smokers had significantly better responses to treatment and lower rates of progressive disease compared to former and current smokers.[44] In another study, van der Bol et al.[45] found that smokers being treated with irinotecan experienced less neutropenia compared with nonsmokers. Although lower toxicity may appear, on the surface, to be a positive occurrence, it more likely indicates that cigarette smoking increased the metabolic rate of irinotecan. This accelerated metabolism may ultimately reduce the therapeutic effectiveness of irinotecan in smokers.[45,46] In fact, cigarette smoking is well known to interact with numerous drugs through a variety of mechanisms. In the case of irinotecan, smoking may induce drug metabolizing enzymes. This may also be true for erlotinib, the epidermal growth factor receptor (EGFR) tyrosine kinase inhibitor.[47] Waller et al.[48] conducted a dose escalation study and established a recommended phase 2 dose in patients who continue to smoke (300 mg daily vs. 150 mg daily for nonsmokers). These findings need to be further explored in pharmacokinetic research and via clinical trials. However, with other drugs, smoking may inhibit metabolizing enzymes.[46]

Intriguing *in vitro* findings indicate that nicotine can interfere with chemotherapeutic efficacy via cellular functions. In lung cancer cell lines, nicotine induces resistance to chemotherapy-induced apoptosis (cisplatin, etoposide) by modulating mitochondrial signaling.[49] Nicotine improves cell survival and causes modest increases in DNA synthesis. Nicotine decreases apoptosis via nuclear factor κB (NF-κB)–dependent survival and Akt-dependent proliferation.[50] Similarly, nicotine has been shown to inhibit apoptosis-induced cisplatin in human oral cancer cell lines.[51] The effect of nicotine is, at least in part, mediated by up-regulation of surviving protein in a time- and dose-dependent manner. The authors suggest that elucidating the signaling pathways underlying the antiapoptotic effects of nicotine may facilitate the development of therapeutic strategies for oral cancers in patients who continue to smoke.

In recent years, more attention has been focused on developing treatments designed to target cancer cells based on their molecular phenotypes. Agents that target specific epigenetic abnormalities and restore normal cell regulation could not only improve cancer treatment, but may potentially lead to preventive approaches as well.[52] Because of the role that EGFR plays in disease progression, tyrosine kinase inhibitors (TKIs) designed to inhibit EGFR (e.g., erlotinib and gefitinib) have been developed. The effectiveness of the TKIs depends on the mutation status of the tumor, rather than on the clinical characteristics of the patient. In the Iressa Pan-Asia Study (IPASS) trial, patients with EGFR mutations responded to gefitinib with prolonged progression-free survival, while those without mutations benefited more from carboplatin-paclitaxel chemotherapy.[53] These patients were Asian never-smokers or light ex-smokers with adenocarcinoma histology. In the United States, less than 30% of lung cancer patients carry these mutations, but those who do have a 70% chance of responding. The likelihood of having EGFR abnormalities decreases as exposure to tobacco increases.[54,55] Tobacco-related adenocarcinomas are associated with other mutations, such as k-*ras*.[56]

Survival

Given the evidence that smoking after a cancer diagnosis negatively affects surgical, radiation, and medical treatment, it is not surprising that smoking is also an independent predictor of disease-free and overall survival. Findings from several large studies, both cohort and tumor registry, clearly indicate that current smoking or a history of smoking is associated with poorer survival for patients with lung, liver, head and neck, pancreatic, breast, and prostate cancers.[57,58] Other studies that have focused only on the effects of continued smoking after a cancer diagnosis have reported similar findings. For example,

Browman et al.[59] found that patients receiving radiation therapy for head and neck cancer who continued to smoke during the treatment period had poorer 2-year survival rates compared to patients who did not smoke. A large, multicenter chemoprevention trial designed to assess the efficacy of isotretinoin in stage I and II head and neck cancer patients yielded similar results. In this trial, current smokers were significantly more likely to be diagnosed with a second primary tumor and have a shorter survival time compared to former and never smokers.[60] Similar findings were also reported by Videtic et al.[61] who observed poorer survival rates among patients who received chemoradiotherapy for non–small cell lung cancer and continued to smoke compared to former smokers. Research findings also indicate that continued smoking negatively affects cause-specific survival among patients with operable colorectal cancer. As with the aerodigestive cancer patients, colorectal cancer patients who continued to smoke after surgical resection had poorer survival as compared to never smokers and former smokers.[62] Thus, cancer patients who smoke during their treatment period frequently have poorer survival rates compared to those who do not smoke. A further finding of interest concerns the role of tobacco use on disease outcomes among patients with human papillomavirus (HPV)–positive squamous cell carcinomas of the oropharynx (SCCOP). HPV-positive patients have a more favorable outcome than HPV-negative patients. Tobacco use (current) and history (20 or more pack-years) negatively affect further disease and overall survival in both HPV-positive and HPV-negative patients.[63,64] Never users of tobacco who have HPV-positive SCCOP have the best outcomes of all.[65] Further research is indicated to determine whether targeted therapy with respect to tobacco history will improve survival and quality of life and whether HPV-positive nonsmoking SCCOP patients may receive less intensive treatment without affecting outcome.[64]

Health-Related Quality of Life

In addition to the adverse clinical outcomes associated with continued smoking among individuals with cancer, continued smoking also appears to negatively affect health-related quality of life (HRQOL) outcomes, both short term and long term. For example, several studies of head and neck cancer patients indicate that continued smoking is a significant predictor of several HRQOL domains, such as vitality, physical functioning, social functioning, emotional functioning, and general health perceptions 12 months following treatment.[66,67] In addition to these more general domains, several head and neck specific domains (e.g., head and neck pain, swallowing, weight loss, and social eating) are also negatively affected by continued smoking.[68] Research conducted with lung cancer patients has yielded similar findings. Results from a study by Baser et al.[69] indicated that patients treated for non–small cell lung cancer who continued to smoke had significantly lower performance status at both 6 and 12 months postdiagnosis compared to patients who quit smoking at diagnosis. In another study with lung cancer patients, Garces et al.[70] found that compared to never smokers, patients who continued to smoke had significantly poorer overall quality of life. In addition, the current smokers had poorer functioning in several lung cancer–specific domains, such as appetite, fatigue, cough, and shortness of breath. A cross-sectional survey of 893 lung cancer patients (mostly late stages IIIb and IV), 17% of whom were classified as persistent smokers, showed that the continuing smokers reported significantly higher levels of usual pain than former or nonsmokers, even after adjusting for other demographic factors and lung cancer symptoms.[71] The area of pain and smoking is an important one to explore in future research. Additional findings from studies conducted with cancers not typically associated with smoking—stomach cancer[72] and hematologic cancers[73]—also indicate that patients who continue to smoke experience poorer HRQOL compared to never smokers and former smokers. Although the evidence linking continued smoking among cancer patients with poor quality of life is not as extensive as the evidence linking continued smoking with other adverse health outcomes, the implications for cancer survivorship appear clear.

In sum, the existing literature strongly demonstrates that smoking not only increases the risk of numerous types of cancer, but can also significantly impact the effectiveness of cancer treatment. Promoting cessation in the oncology setting has the potential to significantly enhance medical management and improve the cancer survivorship experience of patients diagnosed with both smoking- and non–smoking-related cancers.

CESSATION TREATMENT AND RESEARCH

Delivering smoking cessation interventions within the context of cancer diagnosis and treatment presents unique challenges for the clinician. Effective tailoring of treatment to the individual needs of cancer patients requires sensitivity to limitations imposed by disease and treatment, knowledge of medical contraindications to certain types of pharmacologic treatment, and attention to comorbid conditions (e.g., depression, alcohol dependence).[27] Smoking following cancer diagnosis may be reflective of particularly high levels of nicotine dependence in individuals with long histories of heavy tobacco use. Patients are likely to be particularly sensitive to any perceived blame for their illness, especially when diagnosed with a smoking-related cancer.[26,27] Urgency of cessation is another unique treatment issue for this patient group, considering the critical relevance of continued smoking to cancer treatment outcomes.[74]

Thus far, treatment of the tobacco-dependent cancer patient has been largely informed by interventions evaluated in the general population. Although literature in the area of empirically based smoking cessation interventions for cancer patients is slowly growing, more work is clearly needed to determine effective treatment strategies for this group and the optimal timing, duration, and mode of intervention delivery relative to cancer diagnosis. Following a description of clinical practice guidelines for treating tobacco use and dependence in the general population and detailed information on pharmacotherapy and pharmacogenetic approaches to treatment, this chapter presents an overview of cessation research conducted with cancer patients. It then highlights a unique program providing state-of-the-art tobacco treatment services to all current tobacco users or recent quitters at a comprehensive cancer center in the United States.

Clinical Practice Guideline

Treating Tobacco Use and Dependence is a Public Health Service–sponsored clinical practice guideline designed to assist health care providers in delivering and supporting effective smoking cessation treatment.[75] This guideline urges clinicians and health care delivery systems to institutionalize the consistent identification, documentation, and treatment of every tobacco user seen in a health care setting. Effective treatment strategies, ranging from brief (requiring 5 minutes or fewer of direct clinician time) to more intensive, are discussed and a detailed approach to promote cessation at each patient visit is outlined. It is important to note that the benefits of providing brief physician advice have been well documented, with physician-delivered interventions significantly increasing long-term abstinence rates.[75]

Because of considerable new data emerging in the area of tobacco research and clinical practice, this guideline was updated in 2008.[76] The updated version highlights additional effective medication options and provides strong support for counseling and use of quit lines as effective intervention strategies. The core of the guideline remains to outline clear strategies to assist clinicians in delivering and supporting effective treatments for tobacco use and dependence. The five major steps in conducting smoking cessation interventions in a primary care setting as outlined by the clinical practice guideline include: (1) documenting tobacco use for every patient, (2) strongly urging every tobacco user to quit, (3) determining the willingness of the user to attempt quitting, (4) using counseling and pharmacotherapy to aid in quitting, and (5) scheduling follow-up contact, preferably within the first week after the quit date. These steps are referred to as the five A's: Ask, Advise, Assess, Assist, and Arrange.

A convenient algorithm is provided to guide clinicians in implementing the five A's (Fig. 51.1). The first step (Ask) to delivering effective smoking cessation treatment is to inquire about and document smoking behaviors for every patient at every visit. Routine evaluation for tobacco use at subsequent clinic visits is considered necessary for all patients who currently use tobacco, have recently quit, or have a history of multiple quit attempts with subsequent relapse. Several ideas have been suggested to develop a more universal and systematic method for documenting tobacco use status. Fiore et al.[77] recommend including smoking as "the fifth vital sign." With a simple institutional intervention consisting of including smoking status as part of the vital sign assessment, these authors not only found dramatic increases in the rate of identifying patients who smoked but also increases in the rates of advising and intervening in patients who smoked. Alternatives to expanding the vital signs are placing tobacco-use status stickers on patient charts or using an electronic record reminder system.

A standard way to evaluate smoking history is to inquire whether patients have smoked at least 100 cigarettes in their lifetime and whether they currently smoke. This provides a minimum of information about smoking status (i.e., current, former, or never smoker) and conforms to national standards of assessment (e.g., National Health Interview Survey). In order to conduct a thorough evaluation of tobacco use, additional information such as dose (number of cigarettes smoked per day) at initial assessment, age of smoking initiation, duration of smoking, general patterns of use, and previous quit attempts should be included. Table 51.1 provides a list of recommended items to consider asking during an initial patient visit to obtain relevant detailed information about smoking behavior. The items listed in Table 51.1 have also been suggested for inclusion in oncology clinical trials to refine the understanding of the effects of smoking on treatment efficacy and outcome.[26] Of particular value to clinicians is the item "How soon after waking do you smoke your first cigarette?" Level of nicotine dependence can be quickly assessed by determining whether a patient smokes during the first 30 minutes of waking.[78] Nicotine dependence is a good indicator of the intensity of cessation treatment needed and can further guide recommendations for pharmacologic treatment.

The second step in promoting cessation (Advise) involves giving clear, strong, and personalized advice to quit. This advice should indicate the importance of quitting smoking, not just cutting down. Personalized advice optimally links tobacco use to current health or illness and can also include a discussion of social and economic costs as well as the impact of tobacco use on children and others in the household. For all oncology patients, this includes providing explicit information on the risks of continued smoking and benefits of cessation for cancer treatment outcomes and overall health regardless of cancer diagnosis. For oncology patients with smoking-related cancers, discussing the link between their diagnosis and

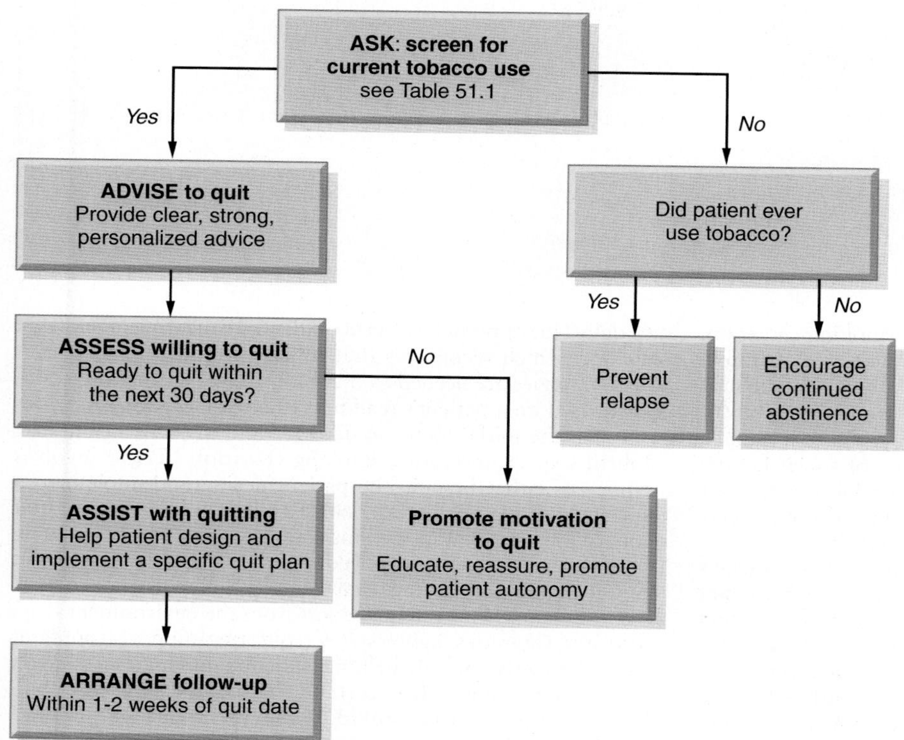

FIGURE 51.1 Algorithm to guide implementation of the five A's (Ask, Advise, Assess, Assist, Arrange).

TABLE 51.1

EVALUATION OF TOBACCO USE AND RELATED BEHAVIORS

All individuals	Have you smoked at least 100 cigarettes in your entire life? (5 packs = 100 cigarettes) *If no—code as never smoker Have you ever used other forms of tobacco? (identify all that apply) a. Pipe b. Cigar c. Chew tobacco d. Snuff e. Others *If never smoker, and no history of other forms of tobacco—end interview	
Ever-tobacco users	Do you NOW smoke cigarettes? a. Everyday b. Some days c. Not at all *If a or b, code as current smoker *If c, code as former smoker	Do you use other forms of tobacco NOW? a. Everyday b. Some days c. Not at all
Current smokers	On average, how many cigarettes per day do you smoke? *reflects dose (1 pack = 20 cigarettes) How soon after you wake up do you smoke your first cigarette? a. Within 5 minutes b. Within 6–30 minutes c. After 30 minutes *Responses a or b reflect high level of nicotine dependence Are you seriously thinking about quitting smoking in the next 30 days? *If yes, consider helping patient implement a quit plan, If no, consider motivational enhancement interventions How many times in the last 12 months have you tried to quit smoking and stayed off for at least 24 hours? Do people in your household smoke? (If so, who)	
Current and former smokers	At what age did you begin smoking regularly? *age of initiation (Duration for current smokers = current age minus age of initiation) For how many years have you smoked regularly? *duration of smoking for former smokers	
Former smokers	How long has it been since you last smoked regularly? a. Within the past month b. Within the past 3 months c. Within the past 6 months d. Within the past year e. Within the past 5 years f. Within the past 15 years g. More than 15 years ago h. Never smoked regularly *a–d = recent quitter, e–g = long-term former smoker	

smoking behaviors is believed to facilitate smoking cessation. As further discussed in the American Society of Clinical Oncology (ASCO) Cancer Prevention Curriculum on Tobacco Control in the Oncology Setting,[79] clinicians must be particularly sensitive to avoid contributing to any perceived blame for the patient's illness. Reminding patients of social factors that contributed to nicotine dependence in adolescence prior to full knowledge or showing understanding of the adverse effects of smoking might be useful in this context.

In the third step (Assess), it is recommended that clinicians evaluate whether the patient is willing to make a quit attempt within the next 30 days. Determining the patient's motivation and interest in quitting is a critical element of smoking cessation treatment and influences the types of intervention strategies to be employed. Different strategies are outlined in the clinical practice guideline for helping the patient willing to quit (i.e., ready to quit within 30 days) and for the patient unwilling to quit. This approach is based on the transtheoretical model of change, which recognizes that unique intervention messages and strategies are needed to optimally promote smoking cessation based on a patient's readiness to quit smoking.[80,81]

With the initial focus on delivering brief interventions, the fourth step in promoting smoking cessation (Assist) involves clinicians either helping the patient design and implement a specific quit plan or broadly enhancing the motivation to quit tobacco. For the patient willing to quit smoking, the following brief strategies can be employed to assist with the development of a quit plan: (1) setting a quit date (ideally within 2 weeks), (2) removing all tobacco products from the environment (e.g., ashtrays, cigarettes, lighters), (3) requesting support from family and friends, and (4) helping patients anticipate challenges to the quit attempt. It is further recommended that supplementary materials be provided to patients (see Table 51.2 for suggested references). Except in the presence of special

TABLE 51.2

SUGGESTED REFERENCES/RESOURCES TO SUPPLEMENT CESSATION ADVICE

You Can Quit Smoking: Consumer Guide (based on the Clinical Practice Guideline), available in English and Spanish: www.surgeongeneral.gov/tobacco/conspack.html
American Cancer Society (www.cancer.org): brochures and fact sheets on the importance of smoking cessation
Centers for Disease Control and Prevention (www.cdc.gov/tobacco/how2quit.htm): a collection of online resources, information, and materials about quitting tobacco use
American Legacy Foundation (www.americanlegacy.org): a national independent public health foundation offering programs to help people quit and resources about the health effects of tobacco use
Tobacco Free Nurses (www.tobaccofreenurses.org): an organization aimed at engaging nurses in tobacco cessation efforts
Smoking Cessation Leadership Center Toolkit and Resources: http://smokingcessationleadership.ucsf.edu/Resources.html
North American Quitline Consortium (http://www.naquitline.org): information on local and national cessation quitlines, 1-800-QUITNOW

circumstances, physicians are urged to encourage the use of pharmacotherapies to assist with quitting. A comprehensive overview of pharmacologic approaches to smoking cessation is offered in the next section.

For patients unwilling to make a quit attempt, primary emphasis is placed on enhancing motivation to quit smoking. Such patients are believed to respond best when the clinician educates, reassures, and gently encourages them to consider changing their smoking behaviors. Specific strategies include discussing the personal relevance of smoking and benefits to cessation, providing support and acknowledging the difficulty of quitting, and educating patients about the negative consequences of smoking and available pharmacologic methods to assist quitting. Primary emphasis must be placed on promoting patient autonomy to quit. Additional information on motivational strategies for patients unwilling to quit has been published elsewhere.[75,79,81]

The final step (Arrange) in a clinician-delivered smoking cessation intervention involves scheduling follow-up contact with the patient, preferably within 1 to 2 weeks after the identified quit date. Additional contacts are to be scheduled as needed, either via phone or in person. During the follow-up period, clinicians can briefly discuss accomplishments and setbacks regarding remaining abstinent and assess pharmacotherapy use and problems. It is critical to create a supportive environment for patients to feel comfortable acknowledging whether they have returned to smoking. Framing lapses as a learning experience can be helpful. It is further recommended that a patient's recommitment to quit be encouraged by setting another quit date. Referrals to a psychologist or professionally trained smoking cessation counselor should be considered for patients with numerous unsuccessful quit attempts, comorbid depression, anxiety, additional substance abuse disorders, or inadequate social support.

Pharmacologic Treatment for Smoking Cessation

The latest edition of the clinical practice guideline identifies five nicotine- (nicotine gum, vapor inhaler, nasal spray, lozenge and transdermal patch) and two non–nicotine-based (bupropion and varenicline) agents as effective first-line pharmacotherapies for smoking cessation.[76] This guideline further recommends that certain combinations of first-line medications can be effective in treating tobacco use and dependence (see Table 51.3 for a brief summary of both nicotine-, non–nicotine-based, and combination treatment).

Nicotine is the key addictive substance in tobacco. Nicotine replacement therapy (NRT) replaces nicotine from cigarettes. As such, NRT facilitates smoking cessation by reducing craving and withdrawal that smokers experience during abstinence. NRT also weans smokers off nicotine by providing a lower level and in some cases slower infusion of nicotine than smoking.[82] There is strong evidence that all commercially available forms of NRT are effective treatments for smoking cessation. For instance, a meta-analysis of over 100 randomized clinical trials found that, compared to placebo, NRT increased the odds of quitting long term by as much as twofold, with no overall significant difference among different agents.[83] When trials of all forms of NRT were pooled, results showed that 17% of smokers receiving NRT were able to quit compared to 10% of those given placebo, representing a 74% increase in the odds of abstinence after at least 6 months.[83]

Since NRT delivers nicotine without exposing users to carcinogens found in cigarette smoke, it may be especially suited for treating cancer patients who are unable to abstain from nicotine but want to reduce immediately their carcinogenic exposure. However, for certain neoplastic illness, like head and neck cancer, surgeons would not treat smokers with oral forms of NRT (gum, lozenge, or inhaler). Furthermore, nicotine increases peripheral vasoconstriction. As such, there are concerns that NRT may compromise postsurgical wound healing among patients who have received surgical treatments or reconstructive procedures. Thus, under these circumstances, other pharmacologic agents may be preferable.

Another class of agents, antidepressant medications, has been widely studied as nonnicotine-based pharmacotherapy for smoking cessation. The hypothesis that nicotine suppresses depressive affect in humans and the strong association between smoking and depression may have prompted researchers to promote antidepressants for smoking cessation. Currently, bupropion is the only antidepressant approved by the U.S. Food and Drug Administration (FDA) for the treatment of tobacco dependence. Bupropion inhibits the reuptake of both dopamine and norepinephrine and has been shown to increase the dopamine and norepinephrine concentrations in the mesolimbic dopaminergic and the noradrenergic systems, respectively.[7,84] Another study suggests that bupropion is a nicotinic acetylcholine receptor antagonist that blocks the stimulation of nicotinic receptors, thereby lowering the rewarding effects of nicotine.[85] Should an abstinent smoker lapse, bupropion may function to reduce the pleasure of cigarette smoking experienced by the smoker[86] and help to prevent further lapse and relapse. Bupropion is an effective treatment for smoking cessation. A meta-analysis found that smokers who received bupropion were twice as likely as those who received placebo to have achieved long-term abstinence at either 6- or 12-month follow-ups (odds ratio [OR] 2.06; 95% confidence interval [CI], 1.77 to 2.40).[87]

Varenicline received FDA approval for treating tobacco dependence in 2006. It is a partial agonist of the $\alpha 4\beta 2$ nicotinic acetylcholine receptor that combines both agonist and antagonist properties. As a partial agonist, varenicline produces a sustained dopamine release in the mesolimbic system. This sustained release maintains a normal systemic level of the neurotransmitter, which helps to reduce craving and withdrawal during abstinence.[88] In addition, by blocking nicotinic receptors (antagonist effect), varenicline dampens nicotine's rewarding effects. Since varenicline attenuates the pleasure smokers experience from smoking, it may decrease motivation to smoke and protect them from relapse. A randomized clinical

TABLE 51.3

PHARMACOLOGIC AGENTS USED IN TREATMENT OF NICOTINE DEPENDENCE

Generic Name	Trade Name	Dosage	Drug Type	Drug Function
FIRST-LINE AGENTS[a]				
Nicotine gum, patch, inhaler, nasal spray, lozenge	Nicorette, Habitrol, Nicoderm, Nicotrol, Commit	Gum: smokers smoking less than 24 cigarettes/day use 2 mg (max 24 pieces/day); smokers smoking more then 24/day use 4 mg (max 24 pieces/day) Patch: 21 mg (one/day for 4 weeks), 14 mg (one/day for 2 weeks), 7 mg (one/day for 2 weeks) Inhaler: 6–16 cartridges/day Nasal spray: 0.5 mg (8–40 doses/day) Lozenge: 2–4 mg (max 24 pieces/day)	NRT	FDA-approved smoking cessation treatment. Nicotine-based treatments replace nicotine obtained from cigarettes. NRT helps smokers by reducing craving and withdrawal symptoms.
Bupropion	Wellbutrin, Zyban	150 mg every day for 3 days, then 150 mg twice a day	Atypical antidepressant	FDA-approved smoking cessation treatment. Bupropion increases the level of dopamine in the brain through the blockade of reuptake. It may also act as a nicotine antagonist and reduces the pleasure smokers may experience from smoking by blocking nicotine from nicotinic receptors.
Varenicline	Chantix	0.5 mg every day for 3 days, 0.5 mg twice a day for 4 days, then 1 mg twice a day	$\alpha 4\beta 2$ partial agonist and antagonist	FDA-approved smoking cessation treatment. As a partial agonist, varenicline reduces the withdrawal symptoms by maintaining dopaminergic tone at the nucleus accumbens. As an antagonist, varenicline reduces the pleasure smokers may experience from smoking by blocking nicotine from nicotinic receptors.
SECOND-LINE AGENTS				
Clonidine		0.15–0.75 mg every day	$\alpha 2$ agonist	Clonidine is an antihypertensive agent.
Nortriptyline		75–100 mg every day	Tricyclic antidepressant	The mechanism of action of tricyclics is believed to be mediated primarily through the noradrenergic system. It increases the synaptic concentration of norepinephrine by blocking the reuptake of the neurotransmitters.
OTHER AGENTS				
Rimonabant			Cannabinoid (CB1) receptor antagonist	Completed phase 3 clinical trials. Rimonabant was initially developed for weight reduction. However, in several animal models, rimonabant has also been shown to reduce both the nicotine additive effects and nicotine-seeking behavior via its antagonist activity on CB1 receptors. Thus, rimonabant may help smokers to both quit smoking and prevent weight gain.
TA-NIC, Nic VAX			Nicotine vaccine	Completed phase 1 trials. Nicotine vaccine stimulates the production of nicotine-specific antibodies. These antibodies sequester nicotine in the blood, preventing nicotine from entering the central nervous system.

NRT, nicotine replacement therapy; FDA, U.S. Food and Drug Administration.
[a]Combinations of first-line agents recommended for use by the clinical practice guideline include: (1) patch + ad libitum NRT (gum or nasal spray), (2) patch + inhaler, (3) patch + bupropion SR.

trial that compared varenicline (2 mg), bupropion (300 mg), and placebo showed overall continuous abstinence rates between 9 to 52 weeks postquit of 23%, 15%, and 10%, respectively.[89] Varenicline more than doubled the odds of quitting over placebo (OR 2.66; 95% CI, 1.72 to 4.11) and performed significantly better than bupropion (OR 1.77; 95% CI, 1.19 to 2.63). Furthermore, compared to smokers who received placebo, those who received varenicline reported significantly less craving and withdrawal symptoms throughout the trial. Additional data suggest that a 1-mg dose per day of varenicline can be effective for treatment of tobacco use and dependence. The effectiveness of the standard dose (2 mg/d) and the 1 mg/d was addressed by a recent meta-analysis.[76] Results indicated that the 1 mg daily dose approximately doubled while the 2 mg daily dose approximately tripled the likelihood of long-term abstinence (6 months) compared to placebo. As a result, the 1 mg daily dose can be considered as an alternative should the patient experience significant dose-related side effects.

In February 2008, the FDA issued a warning after reports that some patients attempting to quit smoking while using varenicline experienced exacerbations of psychiatric illnesses, which involved depressed mood, agitation, changes in behavior, suicide ideation, as well as suicide. This has prompted recommendations that health care providers elicit information about a patient's psychiatric history prior to prescribing varenicline and to closely monitor changes in mood and behavior during the course of treatment.

The clinical practice guideline also identifies two non–nicotine-based medications—clonidine and nortriptyline—as second-line pharmacotherapies for tobacco dependence. According to the guideline, a second-line agent is used when a smoker cannot use first-line medications due to either contraindications or lack of effectiveness. Both clonidine, an antihypertensive, and nortriptyline, a tricyclic antidepressant, have been shown to effectively assist smokers to achieve abstinence.[87,90] Researchers are also working on identifying novel agents for the treatment of tobacco dependence. For instance, a new compound emerging on the horizon is rimonabant, a selective cannabinoid receptor blocker. Randomized clinical trials showed that smokers who took a 20-mg dose of rimonabant were more likely than those who took placebo to abstain from smoking continuously at 1-year follow-up (OR 2.21; $P < .01$).[91] Smokers on active medication also experienced significantly less postcessation weight gain.[92] Nicotine vaccine, another product under development, offers smokers the convenience of a treatment that does not require daily administration. Vaccine sequesters nicotine in the blood by binding nicotine to nicotine-specific antibodies and prevents nicotine from crossing the blood–brain barrier to reach nicotinic receptors in the brain.[93,94] Findings from phase 1 studies indicate that nicotine vaccine is safe and well-tolerated by smokers.[95,96] Preliminary data from phase 1 studies also suggest that nicotine vaccine may increase smoking abstinence.[95,97] A recent phase 2 randomized controlled trial failed to find a significant treatment effect for vaccination against nicotine.[98] That is, participants assigned to the vaccine group did not achieve a higher rate of continuous abstinence than those assigned to the placebo group. Nevertheless, the results from this trial showed that a subgroup of vaccinated smokers with high antibody levels were significantly more likely than those who received placebo to report continuous abstinence 6 months after vaccine injection (OR 2.9; 95% CI, 1.4 to 5.9). The findings suggest that smokers respond differently to a nicotine vaccine and that only the high antibody responders may benefit from the vaccine's treatment effect.

Despite the many efficacious pharmacotherapies that are now available to smokers who desire to quit, many who quit will eventually relapse, and their long-term abstinence rate remains low. Since smoking poses enormous health risks to individuals and their families, even modest improvement in smoking reduction may translate into a significant impact on public health.[85] Thus, to facilitate smokers' success in achieving abstinence, many tobacco researchers have begun to use genetic information to (1) better tailor existing treatment agents to smokers and (2) discover new compounds for treating tobacco dependence. These nascent efforts to develop pharmacogenetic treatments are discussed in the next section.

Pharmacogenetic Approach to Smoking Cessation Treatment

Tobacco use is a heritable trait. Classic twin studies have shown that genetic factors account for substantial variability in smoking initiation,[99] progression from initiation to nicotine depenence,[100] and smoking persistence.[101] To examine how heredity influences the risk of smoking, tobacco researchers have largely focused on examining genes that regulate neurotransmitters involved in the experience of nicotine reward as well as genes that regulate nicotine and medication metabolism.

One of the more commonly studied variants is the *Taq*1 (A1) restriction fragment length polymorphism, previously thought to be in the dopamine D2 receptor gene (*DRD2*). One study indicates that the *Taq*1A polymorphism actually lies in the neighboring *ANKK1* gene.[102] The A1 allele is associated with a decrease in dopamine receptor density[103,104] and may reflect an innate reward deficiency that may increase nicotine use in an effort to offset the deficit. A meta-analysis reported mixed results regarding the association between the *DRD2 Taq*1A polymorphism and smoking.[105] Using a fixed-effects model, the analysis revealed that individuals with the A1 variant (i.e., carrier of either A1/A1 or A1/A2 genotype) were more likely than those with homozygous A2/A2 genotype to initiate, adopt, and persist with smoking. Those with the A1 variant also reported a higher cigarette consumption rate. However, these effects were no longer significant when a random-effects model was used to analyze the data. Furthermore, regardless of the models used, Munafo et al.[105] did not find significant effect for *DRD2* A1 variant on smoking cessation.

Nevertheless, two pharmacogenetic studies found that smokers with different *DRD2 Taq*1A polymorphisms might benefit differentially from NRT.[106,107] The studies examined 755 British smokers and found that among smokers with the A1 allele, those who received the nicotine patch were significantly more likely than those who received a placebo to achieve abstinence. No treatment effect was found for carriers of the homozygous A2/A2 genotype.

Several studies examined the association between the *DRD2 Taq*1A polymorphism and bupropion treatment and found that smokers with homozygous A2/A2 genotype might be more apt to benefit from the medication. Specifically, David et al.[108] found a significant genotype X bupropion treatment effect and showed that at 6 months postquit, smokers with the A2/A2 allele showed significantly better treatment response (i.e., higher abstinence rates among those who received bupropion than those who received placebo) than smokers with the A1 allele. *Taq*1A variant may also influence cessation outcome via an interaction among genotype, treatment, and postcessation side effects. For instance, the *Taq*1A polymorphism has been found to influence adherence to bupropion treatment.[109] In this study, female smokers with the A1 allele were more likely than their counterparts with the homozygous A2/A2 genotype to experience bupropion's side effects and to discontinue medication, resulting in a trend toward higher abstinence rate for the A2/A2 smokers. No such difference was found in men.

Besides the *Taq*1A polymorphism, two other functional variants of the *DRD2* gene, the –141C *Ins/Del* and the *C957T* variants, have also received attention from tobacco researchers. The *InsC* variant is associated with increased transcriptional efficiency,[110,111] possibly increasing receptor expression and sensitivity to dopamine. The *C957T* variant is associated with decreased mRNA stability and protein synthesis.[112] Lerman et al.[113] have shown that smokers who carry the *DelC* allele or the T allele of *C957T* are more likely to quit smoking when given NRT, whereas those who carry the *InsC* allele benefit more from bupropion.

The studies reviewed thus far have focused on examining the *DRD2* gene, which regulates dopamine neurotransmission, in an effort to better pair existing treatments to smokers with a different genotype. Although it is premature to consider putting any of the pharmacogenetic findings into practice, the results on the *DRD2* gene have several implications. First, smokers who carry the A1 allele at *Taq*1A, the *DelC* allele at –141C *Ins/Del*, or the T allele of the *C957T* are likely to benefit from NRT. Second, smokers with A2/A2 genotype showed superior response to bupropion than those with the A1 allele. Third, female smokers with the A1 allele may have difficulty tolerating the side effects of bupropion and therefore may stop taking their medication and abort their quit efforts prematurely.

In addition to the investigation of genes that regulate neurotransmitters involved in the experience of nicotine reward, researchers also study genes that regulate nicotine and medications metabolism. The hepatic enzyme CYP2A6 mediates the process of converting nicotine into cotinine, a primary metabolite of nicotine.[114] The activity of the CYP2A6 enzyme is controlled by the *CYP2A6* gene. Several studies have found that four genetically deficient variants of the *CYP2A6* gene (*CYP2A6*2*, *CYP2A6*4*, *CYP2A6*9*, and *CYP2A6*12*) are associated with impaired CYP2A6 enzyme activity that inhibits its nicotine metabolism.[115,116] Since it takes longer for individuals with the defective *CYP2A6* variants to eliminate nicotine from their systems, these slow metabolizers consumed significantly fewer cigarettes per day and were less likely to become nicotine dependent.[117–119] Compared to normal metabolizers, slow metabolizers smoke for a shorter duration and are more successful at quitting.[119,120]

In a recent placebo-controlled clinical trial that compared the efficacy between a standard (8 weeks) and an extended (6 months) regimen of nicotine replacement therapy, participants were classified, based on their CYP2A6 genotype, as either reduced metabolizers (RMs) or normal metabolizers (NMs).[121] The study found that RMs who were assigned to the extended therapy were significantly more likely to achieve abstinence than RMs who were assigned to the standard therapy. NMs did not differ in their responses to either the standard or the extended therapies. The results suggest that smokers with reduced nicotine metabolism benefited from an extended NRT regimen more than their normal metabolism counterparts.

Encouraged by findings that genetically deficient *CYP2A6* variants are associated with smoking abstinence, some tobacco researchers set out to identify compounds that mimic these variants' metabolic inhibitory effects.[122,123] They hypothesized that concurrent use of such compounds and NRT may enhance smoking cessation. That is, by coadministering a CYP2A6 inhibitor with NRT, one may reduce the CYP2A6 enzyme's nicotine metabolic activity and help smokers to maintain a higher plasma nicotine level. A higher systemic nicotine tone may in turn decrease smokers' motivation to smoke, resulting in higher abstinence rates. Three studies that paired methoxsalen, a CYP2A6 inhibitor, with NRT (nicotine gum or transdermal patch) have found that smokers who received methoxsalen and NRT showed significantly higher plasma nicotine levels than those who received placebo and NRT.[124–126] These preliminary results suggest that methoxsalen may have the potential to become a supplemental treatment for smoking cessation.

CYP2B6 is an enzyme that metabolizes bupropion into hydroxybupropion.[127] Among the variant alleles that had been identified for the *CYP2B6* gene, *CYP2B6*6* was shown to be associated with reduced activity in bupropion metabolism.[128] It is hypothesized that a slow bupropion metabolizer may experience higher levels of bupropion plasma levels, possibly increasing the medication's therapeutic effects for these smokers. In a clinical trial that examined bupropion versus placebo for smoking cessation, Lee et al.[129] found that slow bupropion metabolizers (i.e., participants with *6 allele) who received bupropion achieved a significantly higher rate of abstinence than slow metabolizers who received placebo. Bupropion did not increase abstinence rates over placebo for normal metabolizers (i.e., participants with *1 allele).

Thus, there are preliminary indications that the efficacy of various smoking cessation treatments may vary as a function of genetic predisposition. Research in the development of pharmacogenetic treatments of tobacco dependence is still in its infancy. One of the biggest challenges confronted by pharmacogenetic researchers is the failure to replicate earlier findings.[130] Although findings from early pharmacogenetic investigations are promising, more studies will be needed prior to assessing the utility of using genetic information to improve current smoking cessation treatments. This research may ultimately benefit not only smokers in the general population but also those who have been diagnosed with and treated for cancer, including long-term survivors.

Empirically Tested Cessation Interventions with Cancer Patients

Cessation research with cancer patients has been conducted in various settings, ranging in intensity, methodologic rigor, and sample characteristics, and has shown mixed results. Twelve intervention studies have been identified that target smoking behaviors among cancer patients. Gritz et al.[131] conducted the first randomized cessation intervention in this area and tested the efficacy of a surgeon- or dentist-delivered treatment for 186 newly diagnosed patients with head and neck cancer. The intervention consisted of strong personalized advice to stop smoking, a contracted quit date, tailored written materials, and booster advice sessions and was compared to a minimal advice control condition. For this study, usual care advice was standardized and physician training was provided as advice-giving practices among providers varied widely from none at all to inquiries and warnings about smoking behavior at every visit.

Although no significant differences were found between the enhanced and minimal advice control conditions, a 70.2% continuous abstention rate was found at 12-month follow-up regardless of treatment condition. These high sustained quit rates were quite promising and suggest that many cancer patients can benefit from even brief physician-delivered advice. The authors suggested that a "stepped care" approach may be the most useful, with brief advice incorporated into usual care and more intensive treatment offered for patients with continued difficulty in quitting.

A later study by Schnoll et al.[132] also failed to find significant differences in quit rates for cancer patients randomized to a more intensive cognitive-behavioral treatment compared to standardized health education advice on smoking cessation. All patients received NRT. Quit rates in both groups approached 50% at 1-month follow-up and 40% at 3-month follow-up, perhaps lower than the rates of Gritz et al.[131] because there was a mixed sample of head and neck and lung cancer patients with greater variation in time since diagnosis. Timing of intervention may be a key factor, with the Gritz et al. study capitalizing on the "teachable moment" of cancer diagnosis. Further, head and neck cancer patients may exhibit higher quit rates due to oral complications from diagnosis and treatment. Nevertheless, the quit rates found by Schnoll et al. support the benefits of even brief advice on smoking outcomes. Clearly, further work is needed to develop intensive cessation interventions to target cancer patients with particular difficulty quitting.

Four smaller studies examined nurse-delivered cessation interventions for cancer patients. These studies included patients with varying cancer diagnoses and contained sample sizes ranging from 15 to 80 patients. The lowest cessation rates were found with a single session intervention (21% cessation rate in intervention group vs. 14% in usual care group 6 weeks postintervention).[133] Higher cessation rates were found with a more intensive intervention, consisting of three inpatient visits, supplementary materials, and five postdischarge follow-up contacts. This multisession intervention was conducted in three separate studies. Wewers et al.[134] found a 64.3% abstinence rate among intervention participants (vs. 50% among usual-care control participants), Stanislaw and Wewers[135] reported a 75% abstinent rate among intervention participants (vs. 43% among usual-care control participants), and Wewers et al.[136] found a 40% abstinence rate among intervention participants (no control group) at 6 weeks postdischarge. Differences in sample composition are noteworthy as the first two studies included large numbers of head and neck cancer patients, while the third study was comprised of lung cancer patients. Although larger, more rigorous studies are clearly needed to demonstrate the effectiveness of nurse-delivered hospital interventions for cancer patients, these findings are promising.

Larger-scale smoking cessation studies conducted with cancer patients reinforce the benefits of cessation treatment for patients with smoking-related tumors and emphasize the need for early intervention. In a trial coordinated by the Eastern Cooperative Oncology Group, cancer patients ($n = 432$) were randomly assigned to a brief physician-delivered intervention (comprised of cessation advice, optional NRT, and written materials) or usual care (unstructured advice from physicians).[137] Both 6- and 12-month posttreatment abstinence rates ranged from 12% to 15% across groups. Although there were no significant intervention effects and generally low abstinence rates, cancer diagnosis emerged as a significant predictor of abstinence. Specifically, patients with head and neck or lung cancer were significantly more likely to have quit smoking compared to patients with tumors that were not smoking related. Two additional retrospective studies were conducted to analyze tobacco treatment outcomes for specific cancer groups compared to matched controls at the Mayo Clinic Nicotine Dependence Center. Sanderson Cox et al.[138] found that although lung cancer patients were more likely to achieve 6-month tobacco abstinence than controls (22% vs. 14%), significant differences were not found after adjusting for covariates. Garces et al.[70] also found no significant differences in abstinence rates between head and neck cancer patients and controls (33% vs. 26%). However, both studies found that duration of time between cancer diagnosis and treatment significantly affected treatment outcome. Significantly higher abstinence rates were found for both head and neck and lung cancer patients treated within 3 months of diagnosis compared to those treated more than 3 months after diagnosis. It is likely that the patients referred to the nicotine dependence program were the most heavily addicted, and that other patients were able to quit upon the advice of their oncologic treating physicians.

Another study considered the importance of addressing smoking, depression, and alcohol use among head and neck cancer patients. Duffy et al.[139] randomized head and neck cancer patients with at least one of these conditions to usual care or 9 to 11 sessions of a nurse-administered intervention consisting of cognitive-behavioral therapy and medications. Targeting comorbid smoking, problem drinking, and depression resulted in significantly increased quit rates at 6-month follow-up for the intervention group compared to the usual control group (47% vs. 31%; $P < .05$). Alcohol and depression rates were found to improve in both conditions, with no significant group differences in these outcomes at 6-month follow-up.

The most recent study of oncology patients was a double-blind placebo-controlled trial, in which 246 cancer patients were randomized to 9 weeks of placebo or bupropion, stratified by pretreatment depression symptoms.[140] All patients received transdermal nicotine and behavioral counseling. Major efforts over 5.5 years were required to identify and enroll patients, including telephone screening of over 7,500 potential patients. Barriers to enrollment included low eligibility, which was mostly related to current smoking status and rate, distance from treatment, multiple languages, medical contraindications, and comorbidities (depression, alcohol use).[141] Results showed no main effect of bupropion versus placebo on abstinence rates at 12- or 27-week follow-up. Patients with depression symptoms had significantly lower cessation rates that patients without depression symptoms; bupropion selectively increased abstinence rates, lowered withdrawal, and increased quality of life in this group of patients. Patients without depression symptoms did equally well when treated with bupropion versus transdermal nicotine and counseling alone.[140] This study indicates the importance of affect comorbidity in guiding smoking cessation treatment. The patient mix (multiple tumor sites, 32% tobacco related), treatment status (awaiting treatment to completed treatment), variation in stage of disease (29% late stage disease), and the relatively low percentage of patients with symptoms of depression (22% and patients with major depression excluded) reflect the difficulty of conducting research in the oncology setting and the need to explore these key variables in future studies with larger sample sizes.

As cessation research with cancer patients continues to expand, studies have begun that include patients with a broader range of disease sites. Emmons et al.[142] conducted a randomized controlled trial of a peer-based counseling intervention versus self-help intervention for young adult survivors of pediatric cancer ($n = 796$). The intervention was delivered by a trained childhood cancer survivor and included six calls, tailored and targeted written materials, and optional NRT. Significantly higher quit rates were found in the counseling group compared to the self-help group at all reported follow-up time points, including 12 months (15% vs. 9%; $P < .01$). Low rates of smoking cessation were found in another intervention study conducted with a mixed group of cancer patients. Wakefield et al.[143] conducted a randomized controlled trial of a motivational interviewing-based smoking cessation intervention in a south Australian hospital. The intervention, delivered over a 3-month period, consisted of multiple contacts with a trained counselor, provision of supplementary material tailored to cancer patients, and NRT. The control group received brief advice to quit and generic supplementary material. Quit rates did not differ by treatment group (5% to 6% at 3-month follow-up); however, the intervention group was significantly more likely to report attempts to quit smoking.

Many of the intervention components described above have been drawn from extensive research on smoking cessation in the general population. Previous research has clearly identified the benefits of brief physician-delivered cessation advice for cancer patients and the responsiveness of patients with smoking-related tumors (especially head and neck cancer patients) to cessation treatment. Much additional work is needed to effectively target patients with non–smoking-related cancers and to develop intensive interventions for cancer patients with particular difficulty quitting.

A Model Tobacco Treatment Program

The Tobacco Treatment Program, first made available to patients at the University of Texas M. D. Anderson Cancer Center on January 17, 2006, was designed to evaluate and treat all M. D. Anderson patients who self-report as current tobacco users or recent quitters.[144] The program has since expanded to offer smoking cessation treatment to the institution's employees. An allocation of funds from the State of Texas Tobacco Settlement has been made available to support this program and ensure that patients and employees can quickly access state-of-the-art tobacco cessation services. This program provides an empirically based therapeutic intervention centered around the clinical practice guideline,[75] tailored to meet the needs of cancer patients. Each year, the program serves over 700 new cancer patients who are referred from over 50 departments across the authors' institution.

Tobacco cessation services are provided within the context of the patient's overall cancer treatment plan, in cooperation with the patient's attending physician. Physicians and providers throughout the institution are able to make direct referrals using an electronic Consult On-Line system. Identification and referral of eligible patients are facilitated by including the assessment of smoking status as an additional vital sign during all clinic visits. Additionally, a Tobacco Registry is being developed to electronically identify all tobacco users at new patient registration for the purpose of providing proactive treatment. Pilot programs for the proactive identification of smokers have been successfully carried out in several treatment centers within the institution, with future plans for an institution-wide roll out of this system.

The program is staffed by a multidisciplinary treatment team comprised of psychologists, social workers, tobacco counselors, a research nurse, a physician assistant, and an addiction psychiatrist. Treatment includes behavioral counseling conducted in person, via telephone, or via Web-cam, and tobacco cessation pharmacologic intervention, including various nicotine replacement therapies, bupropion, varenicline, and other medications. The general treatment model consists of 12 counseling sessions (30 to 45 minutes each) with particular consideration given to the level of nicotine dependence, impending cancer treatment, presence of comorbid disorders (e.g., depression, alcohol or substance abuse), spouse's tobacco use and involvement in treatment, and frequency, duration, and timing of previous quit attempts. Telephone follow-ups are provided as needed, and long-term follow-up is available for 3 to 12 months. More extensive counseling and ancillary therapy are provided when needed. Table 51.4 provides a list of potential intervention strategies used in the Tobacco Treatment Program, which are delivered as indicated.

The Tobacco Treatment Program is functioning well within the operations of M. D. Anderson Cancer Center, and physicians and patients have consistently expressed positive feedback regarding the service of the program. Although this is primarily a clinical service, the data from these patients will provide hypothesis-generating material for future research and descriptive data on a population and treatment that has yet to be fully appreciated in the cancer care literature. The scope and magnitude of this program is believed to be truly unique and unlike any other offered in cancer centers in this country.

TABLE 51.4

A SELECTION OF TREATMENT STRATEGIES USED IN THE TOBACCO TREATMENT PROGRAM (DELIVERED AS INDICATED)

Provide and monitor the use of nicotine replacement therapies
Provide education regarding the health effects of tobacco use and its addictive and relapsing nature
Identify environmental and psychological cues for tobacco use
Generate alternative behaviors for tobacco use
Use stimulus control principles to generate changes in routine and environment to support cessation efforts
Assist in optimization of social support for cessation efforts
Relapse prevention, including the identification of future high-risk situations and plans for specific behaviors in those situations, as well as the interpretation of and response to potential future lapse
Motivation interventions as needed throughout treatment
Relaxation techniques such as guided imagery and progressive muscle relaxation
Behavioral strategies to address depressed mood (e.g., increasing pleasurable activities)
Crisis intervention including appropriate referrals and emergency intervention if indicated

FUTURE RESEARCH AND CLINICAL OPPORTUNITIES

Treatment Research

Intervention studies must be targeted and tailored to cancer patients and survivors. Studies conducted up to now are generally evidence-based (clinical practice guideline), but it is not known how much these interventions would benefit from more specific personalization by organ or cancer site, including smoking-related and non–smoking-related malignancies and oncologic treatment, pharmacologic or pharmacogenetic tailoring, and timing of intervention. The treatment of underserved cancer patients, high-risk patients, and those with medical or substance use or psychiatric comorbidities have not been addressed in research. Clinically, many of these factors are likely taken into account, but systematic research has yet to be conducted to evaluate the efficacy of such interventions. Sustained or ongoing cessation treatment, potentially for longer than 1 year, as well as relapse prevention and retreatment of lapsed quitters are also very important. The goal is to help patients become permanently abstinent.

Provider Awareness and Skill Training

There are relatively few opportunities for oncology professionals to learn and practice smoking cessation intervention skills. Few oncology meetings offer such educational workshops or talks,[145,146] and they are often poorly attended when they are offered. More in-person talks as well as written and Web-based training should be made available. Toward this end, the ASCO Prevention Curriculum has a chapter devoted to educating oncology health care professionals on the evaluation and treatment of tobacco use.[147] Innovative curricula, such as the Texas Tobacco Outreach Education Program (TOEP), are available and can facilitate program development in other states. The TOEP is a Web-based course on tobacco prevention or cessation, which provides online continuing medical education credits in ethics or professional responsibility to Texas physicians at no cost.[148]

Finally, specialty programs in tobacco cessation treatment that are based in cancer centers and other medical centers are valuable resources that needs to be further developed. The Tobacco Treatment Program at M. D. Anderson Cancer Center, highlighted earlier in the chapter, represents a comprehensive approach to providing cessation services in a cancer center.[144] Examples of highly reputed cessation programs in other medical settings include the Mayo Clinic Nicotine Dependence Centers and the ACT Center for Tobacco Treatment, Education, and Research located in Mississippi.

Systems Issues: Reimbursement, Systematic Integration of Tobacco Treatment

Not only should providers be aware of the need for tobacco cessation and available interventions, but health care institutions must build such treatment into their overall system of care. Thus, identification of patients who smoke, referral or direct treatment by providers, billing and reimbursement for treatment provided, and national pressure from professional oncology organizations are critically important.[145] A recent survey of the 58 NCI-designated cancer centers indicated that about 80% of respondents had a tobacco use program available to their patients (59% in the cancer center and 21% in the university or health care system), but less than 50% of centers had a designated individual who provided services; about 60% routinely offered educational smoking cessation materials.[149] As further research identifies biologic effects of continued smoking that adversely affect oncology treatment outcome, produce harmful interactions with cancer treatment agents, increase recurrence and second primary tumors, and reduce survival and quality of life, there will be an increasing evidence base to justify systematic identification and treatment of smokers and reimbursement for services provided.[26,46,145]

It may be particularly useful to consider the benefits of routine cotinine screening for smoking, which would provide unequivocal and objective evidence of smoke exposure. Cotinine, the major proximate metabolite of nicotine, can be measured in various biological specimens such as blood, saliva, or urine. A recent study by Benowitz et al.[150] found that self-report of smoking behaviors substantially underestimated the true prevalence of smoke exposure among 948 patients admitted to an urban public hospital in San Francisco. Among patients who denied smoking, 15% were biochemically determined to be active smokers and 17% were found to be recent smokers or heavily exposed to secondhand smoke. Biochemical verification of tobacco use has important advantages to be considered. Further information on biochemical markers most useful for assessing tobacco use and optimal cut-points for biomarker values are discussed in a publication by the Society for Research on Nicotine and Tobacco (SRNT) Subcommittee on Biochemical Verification.[151]

Leadership Roles by Oncologic Professional Societies

Increasingly, medical and oncology professional societies are taking leadership roles in recognizing the need to learn more about the effects of tobacco in medical treatment and the critical role of tobacco cessation. The American Medical Association passed a resolution supporting the documentation of smoking behavior in clinical trials, from trial registration through treatment, follow-up, and to end of study or death,[152] and the Oncology Nursing Society has also been very active in this area.[153,154] In conjunction with its 2010 annual meeting, the American Association for Cancer Research (AACR) published a strong white paper on the medical and public health evidence against tobacco use and urged the need for action by scientists, policy makers, and other advocates to prevent further suffering and death and to improve public health, worldwide.[155] Most recently, the American Society of Clinical Oncology (ASCO) has joined forces with the American Legacy Foundation to produce a Tobacco Cessation Toolkit for the oncology setting (personal communication, Jon Larsen, ASCO, April 7, 2010).

Policy Implications

The tremendous public health burden from tobacco-related disability and death, particularly in cancer, has not been countered by a proportional level of funding in tobacco control, cancer treatment research, or public advocacy. Researchers, clinicians, and advocates must come together to persuade policy makers to increase funding in tobacco-related research, treatment, and policy initiatives on behalf of healthy individuals and patients. Traditionally, these forces have battled over resources. A united front is critically needed in support of a common agenda that includes both increased tobacco control efforts and additional funding for disease-related research and treatment.[145]

Selected References

The full list of references for this chapter appears in the online version.

1. U.S. Department of Health and Human Services. *The health consequences of smoking: a report of the surgeon general.* Atlanta: U.S. Department of Health and Human Services, Centers for Disease Control and Prevention, National Center for Chronic Disease Prevention and Health Promotion, Office on Smoking and Health, 2004.
2. U.S. Department of Health and Human Services. *The health consequences of smoking for women: nicotine addiction. A report of the surgeon general, 1998.* Washington, DC: U.S. Department of Health and Human Services, 1998.
3. National Institutes of Health. NIH State-of-the-Science Conference statement on tobacco use: prevention, cessation, and control. *Ann Intern Med* 2006;145:839.
6. Pontieri FE, Tanda G, Orzi F, et al. Effects of nicotine on the nucleus accumbens and similarity to those of addictive drugs. *Nature* 1996;382:255.
7. Balfour DJ. The neurobiology of tobacco dependence: a preclinical perspective on the role of the dopamine projections to the nucleus accumbens. *Nicotine Tob Res* 2004;6:899.
8. Berridge KC, Robinson TE. What is the role of dopamine in reward: hedonic impact, reward learning, or incentive salience? *Brain Res Brain Res Rev* 1998;28:309.
10. Di Chiara G. Role of dopamine in the behavioural actions of nicotine related to addiction. *Eur J Pharmacol* 2000;393:295.
11. Centers for Disease Control and Prevention. Vital Signs: current cigarette smoking among adults aged-18 years—United States, 2009. *MMWR Morb Mortal Wkly Rep* 2010;59(35):1135–1140.
12. Walker MS, Vidrine DJ, Gritz ER, et al. Smoking relapse during the first year after treatment for early-stage non-small-cell lung cancer. *Cancer Epidemiol Biomarkers Prev* 2006;15(12):2370.
13. Gritz ER. Smoking and smoking cessation in cancer patients. *Br J Addict* 1991;86:549.

14. Lippman SM, Lee JJ, Karp DD, et al. Randomized phase III intergroup trial of isotretinoin to prevent second primary tumors in stage I non-small-cell lung cancer. *J Natl Cancer Inst* 2001;93(8):605.
15. Ostroff JS, Jacobsen PB, Moadel AB, et al. Prevalence and predictors of continued tobacco use after treatment of patients with head and neck cancer. *Cancer* 1995;75(2):569.
18. McBride CM, Emmons KM, Lipkus IM. Understanding the potential of teachable moments: the case of smoking cessation. *Health Educ Res* 2003;18(2):156.
19. Gritz ER, Nisenbaum R, Elashoff RE, et al. Smoking behavior following diagnosis in patients with stage I non-small cell lung cancer. *Cancer Causes Control* 1991;2(2):105.
20. Ostroff J, Garland J, and Moadel A, et al. Cigarette smoking patterns in patients after treatment of bladder cancer. *J Cancer Educ* 2000;15:86.
26. Gritz ER, Dresler C, Sarna L. Smoking, the missing drug interaction in clinical trials: ignoring the obvious. *Cancer Epidemiol Biomarkers Prev* 2005;14(10):2287.
27. Gritz ER, Fingeret MC, Vidrine DJ, et al. Successes and failures of the teachable moment: smoking cessation in cancer patients. *Cancer* 2006;106(1):17.
34. Browman GP, Wong G, Hodson I, et al. Influence of cigarette smoking on the efficacy of radiation therapy in head and neck cancer. *N Engl J Med* 1993;328(3):159.
46. Benowitz NL. Cigarette smoking and the personalization of irinotecan therapy. *J Clin Oncol* 2007;25(19):2646.
47. Hughes AN, O'Brien MER, Petty WJ, et al. Overcoming CYP1A1/1A2 mediated induction of metabolism by escalating erlotinib dose in current smokers. *J Clin Oncol* 2009; 27(8):1220.
57. Park SM, Lim MK, Shin SA, et al. Impact of prediagnosis smoking, alcohol, obesity, and insulin resistance on survival in male cancer patients: National Health Insurance Corporation Study. *J Clin Oncol* 2006;24(31):5017.
59. Browman GP, Mohide EA, Willan A, et al. Association between smoking during radiotherapy and prognosis in head and neck cancer: a follow-up study. *Head Neck* 2002;24(12):1031.
60. Khuri FR, Lee JJ, Lippman SM, et al. Randomized phase III trial of low-dose isotretinoin for prevention of second primary tumors in stage I and II head and neck cancer patients. *J Natl Cancer Inst* 2006;98(7):441.
61. Videtic GM, Stitt LW, Dar AR, et al. Continued cigarette smoking by patients receiving concurrent chemoradiotherapy for limited-stage small-cell lung cancer is associated with decreased survival. *J Clin Oncol* 2003;21(8):1544.
66. Duffy SA, Terrell JE, Valenstein M, et al. Effect of smoking, alcohol, and depression on the quality of life of head and neck cancer patients. *Gen Hosp Psychiatry* 2002;24(3):140.
76. Fiore MC, Jaén CR, Baker TB, et al. *Treating tobacco use and dependence: 2008 update.* Clinical Practice Guideline. Rockville, MD: U.S. Department of Health and Human Services, Public Health Service, 2008.
79. Gritz ER, Fingeret MC, Vidrine DJ. Tobacco control in the oncology setting. In: Brawley OW, Khuri FR, Rock CL, eds. *ASCO cancer prevention curriculum.* Alexandria, VA: American Society of Clinical Oncology, 2007.
82. Henningfield JE, Keenan RM. Nicotine delivery kinetics and abuse liability. *J Consult Clin Psychol* 1993;61:743.
83. Silagy C, Lancaster T, Stead L, et al. Nicotine replacement therapy for smoking cessation. *Cochrane Database Syst Rev* 2004;1: CD000146.
84. Ascher JA, Cole JO, Colin JN, et al. Bupropion: a review of its mechanism of antidepressant activity. *J Clin Psychiatry* 1995;56(9):595.
87. Hughes JR, Stead LF, Lancaster T. Antidepressants for smoking cessation. *Cochrane Database Syst Rev* 2003;1: CD000031.
88. Coe JW, Brooks PR, Vetelino MG, et al. Varenicline: an alpha4beta2 nicotinic receptor partial agonist for smoking cessation. *J Med Chem* 2005;48(10):3474.
89. Jorenby DE, Hays JT, Rigotti NA, et al. Efficacy of varenicline, an alpha4-beta2 nicotinic acetylcholine receptor partial agonist, vs placebo or sustained-release bupropion for smoking cessation: a randomized controlled trial. *JAMA* 2006;296(11):1355.
95. Hatsukami D, Rennard S, Jorenby D, et al. Safety and immunogenicity of a nicotine conjugate vaccine in current smokers. *Clin Pharmacol Ther* 2005;78:456.
99. Heath AC, Cates R, Martin NG, et al. Genetic contribution to risk of smoking initiation: comparisons across birth cohorts and across cultures. *J Subst Abuse* 1993;5:221.
100. Kendler KS, Neale MC, Sullivan P, et al. A population-based twin study in women of smoking initiation and nicotine dependence. *Psychol Med* 1999;29:299.
101. Heath AC, Martin NG. Genetic models for the natural history of smoking: evidence for a genetic influence on smoking persistence. *Addict Behav* 1993;18:19.
105. Munafo M, Clark T, Johnstone E, et al. The genetic basis for smoking behavior: a systematic review and meta-analysis. *Nicotine Tob Res* 2004;6:583.
106. Johnstone EC, Yudkin PL, Hey K, et al. Genetic variation in dopaminergic pathways and short-term effectiveness of the nicotine patch. *Pharmacogenetics* 2004;14:83.
107. Yudkin P, Munafo M, Hey K. Effectiveness of nicotine patches in relation to genotype in women versus men: randomised controlled trial. *BMJ* 2004;328:989.
113. Lerman C, Jepson C, Wileyto EP, et al. Role of functional genetic variation in the dopamine D2 receptor (DRD2) in response to bupropion and nicotine replacement therapy for tobacco dependence: results of two randomized clinical trials. *Neuropsychopharmacology* 2006;31:231.
121. Lerman C, Jepson C, Wileyto EP, et al. Genetic variation in nicotine metabolism predicts the efficacy of extended-duration transdermal nicotine therapy. *Clin Pharmacol Ther* 2010;87(5):553.
122. Lee AM, Tyndale RF. Drugs and genotypes: how pharmacogenetic information could improve smoking cessation treatment. *J Psychopharmacol* 2006;20:7.
125. Tyndale RF, Li Y, Kaplan HL, et al. Inhibition of nicotine's metabolism: a potential new treatment for tobacco dependence. *Clin Pharmacol Ther* 1999;65:145.
131. Gritz ER, Carr CR, Rapkin D, et al. Predictors of long-term smoking cessation in head and neck cancer patients. *Cancer Epidemiol Biomarkers Prev* 1993;2(3):261.
132. Schnoll RA, Rothman RL, Wielt DB, et al. A randomized pilot study of cognitive-behavioral therapy versus basic health education for smoking cessation among cancer patients. *Ann Behav Med* 2005;30:1.
137. Schnoll RA, Zhang B, Rue M, et al. Brief physician-initiated quit-smoking strategies for clinical oncology settings: a trial coordinated by the Eastern Cooperative Oncology Group. *J Clin Oncol* 2003;21(2):355.
139. Duffy SA, Ronis DL, Valenstein M, et al. A tailored smoking, alcohol, and depression intervention for head and neck cancer patients. *Cancer Epidemiol Biomarkers Prev* 2006;15:2203.
142. Emmons KM, Puleo E, Park E, et al. Peer-delivered smoking counseling for childhood cancer survivors increases rate of cessation: the partnership for health study. *J Clin Oncol* 2005;23:6516.
147. Gritz ER, Fingeret MC, Vidrine DJ. Tobacco control in the oncology setting. In: *Cancer Prevention.* An ASCO Curriculum, Chapter 4. Alexandria, VA: American Society of Clinical Oncology; 2007.
148. Stancic N, Mullen PD, Prokhorov AV, et al. Continuing medical education: what delivery format do physicians prefer? *J Contin Educ Health Prof* 2003;23:162.

CHAPTER 52 ROLE OF SURGERY IN CANCER PREVENTION

JOSÉ G. GUILLEM, ANDREW BERCHUCK, JEFFREY F. MOLEY, JEFFREY NORTON, AND SHERYL G. A. GABRAM

Since the heritable component of some cancer predispositions has been linked to mutations in specific genes, clinical interventions have been formulated for mutation carriers within affected families. The primary interventions for mutation carriers for highly penetrant syndromes, such as multiple endocrine neoplasia, familial adenomatous polyposis, hereditary nonpolyposis colon cancer, and hereditary breast and ovarian cancer syndromes, are primarily surgical. This chapter is divided into five sections addressing breast (Gabram), gastric (Norton), ovarian and endometrial (Berchuck), and multiple endocrine neoplasias (Moley) and colorectal (Guillem). For each, the clinical and genetic indications and timing of prophylactic surgery and its efficacy, when known, are provided.

Prophylactic surgery in hereditary cancer is a complex process, requiring a clear understanding of the natural history of the disease and variance of penetrance, a realistic appreciation of the potential benefit and risk of a risk-reducing procedure in an otherwise potentially healthy individual, and the long-term sequelae of such surgical intervention, as well as the individual patient's and family's perception of surgical risk and anticipated benefit.

PATIENTS AT HIGH RISK FOR BREAST CANCER

Identification of Patients at Risk

The American Society of Clinical Oncology (ASCO) updated their policy on genetic and genomic testing for cancer susceptibility and it includes information on genetic tests of uncertain clinical utility and direct-to-consumer (DTC) marketing, both of which impact the practice of oncology and preventive medicine.[1] Historically genetic counseling and testing were offered by health care providers, but with the advent of DTC, individuals may obtain tests and receive results directly from a company. ASCO still endorses pre- and posttest counseling for thorough disclosure of the impact of testing. Before any woman considers risk-reduction surgery such as bilateral mastectomy or salpingo-oophorectomy, referral to a high-risk or genetic screening program is desirable since women often overestimate actual risk for breast cancer.[2]

The most common cancer syndromes that place women at risk for breast cancer are BRCA1[3] and BRCA2[4] gene mutations. Other less common syndromes are listed in Table 52.1.[5,6]

Following referral for genetic assessment, three groups of patients emerge.[7] The first consists of those women who have undergone genetic testing and have been found to harbor a mutated gene associated with high penetrance for breast cancer. Given that the possibility of developing breast cancer in this group may be as high as 90%, there is a role for enhanced surveillance or prophylactic surgery. The American Cancer Society has published guidelines for magnetic resonance imaging (MRI) screening as a method for enhanced surveillance.[8] Women in this first group qualify for such screening, which can be offered annually but staggered at 6-month intervals with screening mammography to increase the rate of identifying interval cancers. Alternatively, simultaneous screening with MRI and mammography to compare one modality with the other on an annual basis may also be offered. Another choice for this group of women is to pursue bilateral prophylactic mastectomy with an option for immediate reconstruction. Bilateral salpingo-oophorectomy for BRCA1 and BRCA2 mutation carriers may also be considered, as this procedure has been shown to reduce breast cancer risk by almost 50%.[7,9] This is especially true for BRCA2 mutation carriers, who tend to develop hormone-positive breast cancers.

The second group consists of women with strong family histories suggestive of hereditary breast cancer who test negative for either the BRCA1/2 mutations or other described syndromes. In this group, there may not have been a family member with cancer who was tested for the mutation. Therefore, a negative test does not necessarily indicate that a woman's risk is equivalent to that of the general population. There may also be an undetected mutation in such a family, indicating the possibility of higher-than-average risk for that particular woman. Given the current limitations of testing, however, it may be impossible to accurately define the risk. These women may or may not qualify for enhanced surveillance with MRI screening,[8] and accurate assessment of their risk thus depends on the use of other tools,[2] evaluating for the presence of lobular carcinoma *in situ*, atypical lobular hyperplasia (ALH), or atypical ductal hyperplasia (ADH), and a more intensive surveillance regimen for those whose breasts are heterogeneously or extremely dense on mammography.

The third group consists of women with a strong family history of breast cancer who, for various reasons, have chosen not to pursue genetic testing. These individuals may have other health-related problems, psychological concerns, or cost issues, or they may fear perceived medical insurance discrimination. Women in all groups can be educated that with passage of the Genetic Information Nondiscrimination Act in 2008, significant protections have been established to protect patients from discrimination by employers and health insurers.[10]

Women in the second and third groups may still qualify for bilateral prophylactic mastectomy and immediate reconstruction.

TABLE 52.1

HEREDITARY CARCINOMA SYNDROMES INCLUDING BREAST CANCER

Syndrome	Chromosome/Gene	Primary Carcinoma	Secondary Carcinoma	Breast Cancer Penetrance
Familial breast cancer/ ovarian cancer syndrome	17g21; *BRCA1* Autosomal dominant	Breast cancer, ovarian cancer	Colon, prostate	60%–80%
Familial breast cancer/ ovarian cancer syndrome	13q12; *BRCA2* Autosomal dominant	Breast cancer, ovarian cancer	Male breast cancer, endometrial, prostate, oropharyngeal, pancreatic	60%–80%
Li-Fraumeni syndrome	17p13.1 and 22q12.1; *TP53* and *CHEK2* Autosomal dominant	Soft tissue cancers (including breast)	Soft tissue sarcoma, leukemia, osteosarcoma, melanoma, colon, pancreas, adrenal syndrome, cortex, and brain tumors	50%–85% (for all types of cancers in this syndrome)
PTEN Hamartoma syndrome (Cowden's)	10q23.31; *PTEN* mutation Autosomal dominant	Breast cancer	Thyroid (follicular) and endometrial carcinoma	25%–50%
Peutz-Jeghers syndrome	19p13.3; *STK11* Autosomal dominant	Gastrointestinal cancers	Esophagus, stomach, small intestine, large bowel, pancreas, lung, ovary, endometrial	29%
Diffuse gastric cancer	16q22.1; *CDH1* Autosomal dominant	Diffuse gastric cancer	Colorectal, lobular breast cancer	39% Lobular breast cancer
Louis-Bar syndrome	11q22.3; *ATM* Autosomal recessive	Leukemia and lymphoma	Ovarian, breast, gastric, melanoma, leiomyomas, sarcomas	38% (for all types of cancers in the syndrome)

From refs. 5 and 6.

Often, women who elect this path are influenced by their family history or by witnessing breast or ovarian cancer deaths in close family members, giving them a significant fear of diagnosis. For women in all three groups, the decision to pursue or not pursue risk-reducing surgery is difficult. Often the expertise of a cancer clinical psychologist or psychiatrist is enlisted, as prophylactic mastectomy does involve an irreversible procedure with body image and sexual implications.

In 1993 the Society of Surgical Oncology published a statement on the role of prophylactic mastectomy for patients at high risk for breast cancer, as well as those patients recently diagnosed with breast cancer who are considering contralateral prophylactic breast surgery.[11] For women at high risk, indications fall into three broad categories: presence of BRCA mutations or other genetic susceptibility genes; strong family history with no demonstrable mutation; and histologic risk factors (biopsy-proven atypical ductal hyperplasia, lobular hyperplasia, or lobular carcinoma *in situ*). Recommendations for patients with recently diagnosed breast cancer are similar in that they include the risk-reduction indications for high-risk individuals noted above, as well as future surveillance challenges for the opposite breast (clinically and mammographically dense breast tissue or diffuse, indeterminate microcalcifications in the contralateral breast). Another important consideration is the need for symmetry in patients with large, ptotic, or disproportionately sized contralateral breasts. These regularly updated guidelines can be easily accessed on the Web site for the Society of Surgical Oncology.[11]

Surgical Issues and Technique

In a single institution's experience over 33 years,[12] the risk for breast cancer in both moderate- and high-risk groups of women based on family history was reduced by at least 89% if they had a bilateral prophylactic mastectomy. Patients underwent either subcutaneous mastectomy (removal of the majority of breast tissue with sparing of the nipple–areola complex) or total mastectomy (removal of the entire breast through the nipple–areolar complex). Most of the recurrences occurred in women undergoing a subcutaneous mastectomy. However, this may have resulted from the fact that this was the most frequent procedure performed at that time.[1] In a large series[13] of women with known BRCA1 or BRCA2 mutations, bilateral prophylactic mastectomy reduced the risk of breast cancer by 95% in those undergoing previous or concurrent prophylactic bilateral oophorectomy and by approximately 90% in women with intact ovaries. Since it is doubtful that a randomized trial will ever be feasible for these very high-risk patients, prospective observational studies, such as described above, provide the best available information for counseling patients.

Another surgical option for high-risk women is prophylactic bilateral salpingo-oophorectomy. This is currently reserved for patients with BRCA1 or BRCA2 mutations in order to reduce ovarian cancer risk.[7,9] As an additional benefit, however, this procedure also decreases the risk of breast cancer for BRCA1 and BRCA2 mutation carriers, likely through the mechanism of decreasing hormonal exposure at a younger age.[7]

Contemporary surgical procedures for risk-reducing bilateral mastectomy include total mastectomy; skin-sparing mastectomy (preservation of the skin envelope by removal of the entire breast through a circumareolar incision around the nipple–areolar complex); subcutaneous mastectomy; areola-sparing mastectomy (removal of the nipple while sparing the areola), and nipple-sparing mastectomy (removal of entire breast and nipple core tissue but preservation of nipple–areolar skin).[14] Given advances in reconstructive nipple–areolar techniques, it appears that total mastectomy with or without skin-sparing methods reduces the risk of breast cancer to the greatest extent with reasonable cosmesis. More limited and long-term follow-up data are available on areola- and nipple-sparing techniques. The potential downside to these procedures are distortion of the nipple–areolar complex and lack of sensitivity after breast tissue has been completely removed.[7]

Immediate reconstruction is offered to patients and performed in the vast majority of patients. Choices of procedure include bilateral transverse rectus abdominis muscle (TRAM) flap; bilateral latissimus flap with or without implant or expanders; or bilateral implant or expander placement alone. Although tissue flap transfer gives a more natural appearance and texture to the reconstructed site, individual body contour drives the ultimate plan for reconstruction. This important decision should be made by the plastic surgeon with input from the surgical oncologist.

Although the risk reduction is dramatic for bilateral mastectomies, residual breast tissue may be left behind especially with skin-sparing procedures. Patients should be educated that careful chest wall surveillance is therefore encouraged after such a procedure. Local recurrences after bilateral implant reconstruction are reliably detected by clinical examination. Recurrences after reconstruction with autologous tissue present most commonly on the skin, 50% to 72% of the time and detectable by physician examination.[15] Nonpalpable deeper recurrences in this setting are less common, and use of mammography image surveillance may be indicated especially if significant breast tissue has been left behind unintentionally during the bilateral mastectomy procedure. Often an initial "screening" mammogram performed well after all healing has taken place can delineate the amount of visible breast tissue on imaging. This drives future decisions of whether to follow a patient with imaging. Finally, all patients should be instructed to return for clinical breast examination with the health provider if *any* changes are noted on the reconstructed breasts, regardless of imaging plan.

Although prophylactic mastectomy may be exceedingly beneficial for high-risk women, especially for those testing positive for BRCA1, BRCA2, or other deleterious mutations or belonging to a family afflicted with a cancer syndrome, it is an option among those outlined above. Along with prophylactic bilateral salpingo-oophorectomy, prophylactic mastectomy resides at the far end of the spectrum of individual choices.[16] It should be offered only after a woman's risk has been accurately assessed, appropriate counseling has been given, and in-depth consideration of this irreversible procedure has taken place.

HEREDITARY DIFFUSE GASTRIC CANCER

Gastric cancer is the fourth most common cause of cancer worldwide, and by 2030 deaths from gastric cancer globally are predicted to rise to the tenth leading cause of cancer mortality.[17] Although environmental agents, including *Helicobacter pylori* and diet, are the primary risk factors for this disease, approximately 1% to 3% of gastric cancers are a result of an inherited gastric cancer predisposition syndrome.[18,19]

Histologically, gastric cancers may be classified as either diffuse type or intestinal type. The intestinal type histopathology is linked to environmental factors and advanced age. The diffuse type occurs in younger patients and is associated with a familial predisposition. Because of a decrease in intestinal type gastric cancers, the overall incidence of gastric cancer has declined significantly in the past 50 years. However, the incidence of diffuse gastric cancer (DGC), which is also called signet ring cell or linitis plastica, has remained stable, and by some reports may be increasing.

Hereditary diffuse gastric cancer (HDGC) is a genetic cancer susceptibility syndrome defined by one of the following:

1. Two or more documented cases of DGC in first- or second-degree relatives, with at least one diagnosed before the age of 50;
2. Three or more cases of documented DGC in first- or second-degree relatives, independent of age of onset.

The average age of onset of HDGC is 38, and the pattern of inheritance is autosomal dominant.[20] Figure 52.1 shows a pedigree with HDGC.

In 1998 inactivating germline mutations in the E-cadherin gene *CDH1* were identified in three Maori families, each with multiple cases of poorly differentiated DGC.[21] The CDH1 mutations in these families were inherited in an autosomal dominant pattern, with incomplete but high penetrance. Onset of clinically apparent cancer was early, with the youngest affected individual dying of DGC at the age of 14.[21] Since then, germline mutations of CDH1 have been identified in 30% to 50% of all patients with HDGC.[19,22] More than 50 mutations have been recognized across diverse ethnic backgrounds, including European, African American, Pakistani, Japanese, Korean, and others.[19] In addition to gastric cancers, germline CDH1 mutations are associated with increased risk of lobular carcinoma of the breast and possibly with increased risk of signet ring cell colorectal cancer and prostate cancer as well.[23] CDH1 is, to date, the only gene implicated in HDGC. Penetrance of DGC in patients carrying a CDH1 mutation is

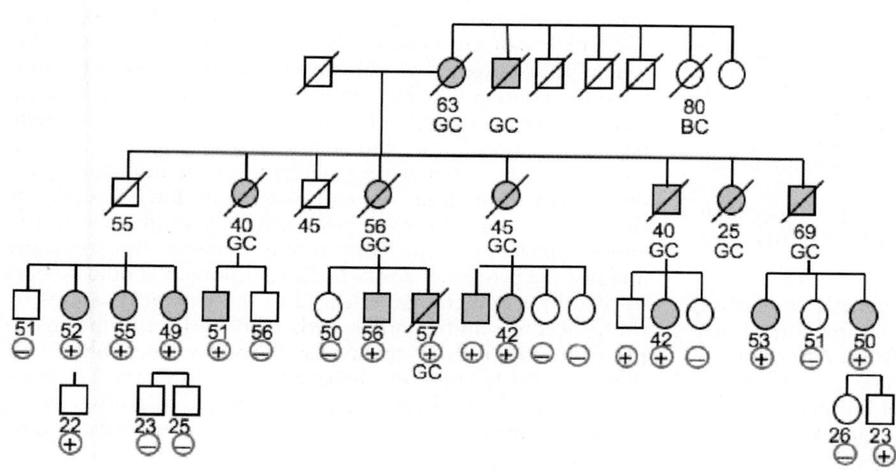

FIGURE 52.1 A family pedigree showing autosomal dominant inheritance of gastric cancer (GC). Individual mutation testing results for the codon 1003 CDH1 mutation are indicated by + or −. Individuals affected with gastric cancer are shaded. The six who underwent prophylactic gastrectomy on the current study are numbered 1–6. Four other individuals who have had prophylactic gastrectomies are labeled a–d. (From ref. 19.)

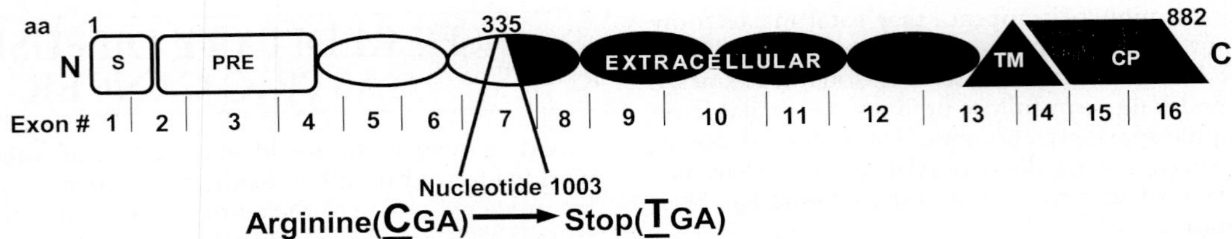

FIGURE 52.2 The mutation in this kindred is located in the central region of the E-cadherin gene that codes for the extracellular cadherin domains of the protein containing calcium-binding motifs important in the adhesion process. The C → T transition in exon 7 of nucleotide 1003 results in a premature stop codon (R335X), producing truncated peptides lacking the transmembrane and cytoplasmic β-catenin binding domains essential for tight cell-cell adhesion. Black area indicates truncated portion of peptide. N, N-terminus; C, C-terminus; S, signal peptide; PRE, precursor sequence; TM, transmembrane domain; CP, cytoplasmic domain. (From ref. 19.)

estimated at 70% to 80%, but may be higher. The need for a systematic study of specimens is supported by recent work by Gaya et al.[24] in which initial total gastrectomy specimens were reported as negative but detailed sectioning and analysis showed invasive carcinoma.

CDH1 is localized on chromosome 16q22.1 and encodes the calcium-dependent cell adhesion glycoprotein E-cadherin. Functionally, E-cadherin impacts maintenance of normal tissue morphology and cellular differentiation. It is hypothesized that CDH1 acts as a tumor suppressor gene in HDGC, with loss of function leading to loss of cell adhesion and subsequently to proliferation, invasion, and metastases. Figure 52.2 shows the CDH1 mutation for the pedigree depicted in Figure 52.1.

The germline CDH1 mutation is most frequently a truncating mutation. Germline missense mutations are causative in a few HDGC kindreds but are more often clinically insignificant. *In vitro* assays for cellular invasion and aggregation may predict the functional impact of missense mutations to aid in this distinction.[22] Within the gastric mucosa, the "second hit" leading to complete loss of E-cadherin function results from CDH1 promoter methylation or an inactivating point mutation.[25]

It remains unclear whether specific CDH1 mutations are associated with distinctive phenotypic characteristics or rates of penetrance, although this may become apparent as more recurrent mutations are recognized. To date, most identified mutations have been novel and distributed throughout CDH1. Recognition of recurrent mutations has usually resulted from independent events; however, there is evidence for the role of founder effects in certain kindreds.[22] At present it is also unclear whether HDGC patients without detectable CDH1 mutations have mutation of a different gene or merely a CDH1 mutation that has gone unrecognized.

New recommended screening criteria for CDH1 mutations are as follows:

1. Families with one or more cases of diffuse gastric cancer.
2. Individuals with diffuse gastric cancer before the age of 40 years without a family history.
3. Families or individuals with cases of diffuse gastric cancer (one case below the age of 50 years) and lobular breast cancer.
4. Cases where pathologists detect *in situ* signet ring cells or pagetoid spread of signet ring cells adjacent to diffuse type gastric cancer.[18,26]

As in other familial cancer syndromes, genetic counseling should take place prior to genetic testing so that the family understands the potential impact of the results. After obtaining informed consent, a team comprising a geneticist, gastroenterologist, surgeon, and oncologist should discuss the possible outcomes of testing and the management options associated with each. Genetic testing should first be performed on a family member with HDGC or on a tissue sample if no affected relative is living. In addition to direct sequencing, multiplex ligation-dependent probe amplification (MLPA) is recommended to test for large genomic rearrangements. If a CDH1 mutation is identified, asymptomatic family members may proceed with genetic testing, preferably by the age of 20.[19] If no mutation is identified in the family member with DGC, the value of testing asymptomatic relatives is low.

Among individuals found to carry a germline CDH1 mutation, clinical screening is problematic. Histologically, DGC is characterized by multiple infiltrates of malignant signet ring cells, which may underlie normal mucosa.[27] Because these malignant foci are small in size and widely distributed, they are difficult to identify via random endoscopic biopsy. Chromoendoscopy and positron emission tomography (PET) have reportedly been used, but the clinical utility of these tools in early detection remains unproven. Lack of a sensitive screening test for HDGC makes early diagnosis extremely challenging. By the time patients are symptomatic and present for treatment, many have diffuse involvement of the stomach or linitis plastica, and rates of mortality are high. Published case reports describe patients who have presented with extensive DGC despite recent normal endoscopy and negative biopsies.[28] The 5-year survival rate for individuals who develop clinically apparent DGC is only 10%, with the majority dying before age 40.

Because of high cancer penetrance, poor outcome, and inadequacy of clinical screening tools for HDGC, prophylactic total gastrectomy is recommended as a management option in asymptomatic carriers of CDH1 mutations.[18] Although total gastrectomy is performed with prophylactic intent in these cases, most specimens have been found to contain foci of diffuse signet ring cell cancer.[19,28,29] Foci of DGC have been identified even in patients who have undergone extensive negative screening, including high-resolution computed tomography (CT), PET scan, chromoendoscopy-guided biopsies, and endoscopic ultrasonography.[19] However, HGDC in asymptomatic CDH1 carriers is usually completely resected by prophylactic gastrectomy, as pathological analysis of resected specimens have shown only T1N0 disease.

Because these signet ring cell cancers are multifocal and distributed throughout the entire stomach, but especially in the cardia,[30] prophylactic gastrectomy should include the entire stomach, and the surgeon must transect the esophagus and not the proximal stomach. Furthermore, it should be performed by a surgeon experienced in the technical aspects of the procedure and familiar with HDGC. In asymptomatic patients, lymph node metastases have not been observed; therefore, D2 lymph node resection is not necessary. The optimal timing of prophylactic gastrectomy in individuals with CDH1 mutations is unknown, but recent consensus recommendations indicate that age 20 is reasonable.[18]

Although it is a potentially lifesaving procedure, prophylactic gastrectomy for CDH1 mutation carries significant risks that must be considered. Overall mortality for total gastrectomy is estimated to be as high as 2% to 4%, although it is estimated that it should be 1% when performed prophylactically. Patients must also be aware that there is a nearly 100% risk of long-term morbidity associated with this procedure, including diarrhea, dumping, weight loss, and difficulty eating.[19] Because of these complications and the fact that lymph node spread has not been observed, some recommend vagus-preserving gastrectomy done either open or laparoscopically. In addition, because the penetrance of CDH1 mutations is incomplete, some patients who undergo prophylactic gastrectomy would never have gone on to develop clinically significant gastric cancer. Prophylactic gastrectomy has, in fact, been performed on several patients reported to show no evidence of gastric cancer on pathology.[29,31]

Some individuals with CDH1 mutations choose not to pursue prophylactic gastrectomy. These individuals should undergo careful surveillance, including biannual chromoendoscopy with biopsies, beginning when they are at least 10 years younger than the youngest family member with DGC was at time of diagnosis. It is recommended that any endoscopically visible lesion is targeted and that six random biopsies are taken from the following regions: antrum, transitional zone, body, fundus, and cardia. Additionally, because women with CDH1 mutations have a nearly 40% lifetime risk of developing lobular breast carcinoma, they should be carefully screened with annual mammography and breast MRI starting at age 35.[23] They should also do monthly self-examinations and every 6 months have a breast examination by a physician. The same surveillance recommendations are probably appropriate for HDGC families without identifiable CDH1 mutations, although no current guidelines for this exist.

The emergence of gene-directed gastrectomy as a treatment strategy for patients with HDGC represents the culmination of a successful collaboration between molecular biologists, geneticists, oncologists, gastroenterologists, and surgeons. It is anticipated that the recognition of similar molecular markers in other familial cancer syndromes will transform the approach to the early diagnosis and treatment of a variety of tumors.

SURGICAL PROPHYLAXIS OF HEREDITARY OVARIAN AND ENDOMETRIAL CANCER

Hereditary Ovarian Cancer (BRCA1, BRCA2)

Inherited mutations in BRCA1 and BRCA2 strongly predispose women to breast and ovarian cancer.[32] The incidence of fallopian tube cancer also appears to be increased, but many of these cancers present at an advanced stage and it is often difficult to determine whether the cancer arose in the ovary, the fallopian tube, or in the peritoneal cavity. About two-thirds of hereditary ovarian cancers are due to BRCA1 mutations and one-third of BRCA2 mutations and hereditary cases account for about 10% of all invasive epithelial ovarian cancers and 15% of high-grade serous cases. The lifetime risk of ovarian cancer increases from a baseline of 1.5% to about 15% to 25% in BRCA2 carriers and 25% to 40% in BRCA1 carriers.[33,34] BRCA mutations are rare in most populations (less than 1 in 500 individuals); one notable exception is the Ashkenazi Jewish population, in which the carrier frequency is 1 in 40. The median age of sporadic epithelial ovarian cancer is around 60, compared to the mid-40s for BRCA1-associated cases. BRCA2-associated ovarian cancers occur later, with a median age in the mid-50s or early 60s.[35]

Genetic testing for inherited mutations in the *BRCA1/2* genes should be discussed with women who have a significant family history of early onset breast cancer or cancers of the ovary, fallopian tube, or peritoneum. Involvement of a genetic counselor prior to testing is helpful, as they have expertise in managing the inherent clinical and social issues. *BRCA1* is mutated more often than *BRCA2* in women with hereditary ovarian cancer. Most BRCA1/2 mutations involve deletions or insertions, encoding truncated protein products that are clearly dysfunctional. Less frequently, disease causing point mutations may occur that alter a single amino acid, but most of these missense variants represent innocent polymorphisms. The clinical significance of point mutations can sometimes be elucidated by determining whether they track with cancer in other family members. In addition, genomic rearrangements may occur that inactivate *BRCA1* or *BRCA2*, and identification of such alterations requires molecular testing beyond sequencing.

Risk-reducing bilateral salpingo-oophorectomy (RRSO) is strongly recommended in women who carry BRCA1/2 mutations because of the high mortality rate of ovarian cancer and the lack of effective screening and prevention approaches. The past practice of performing prophylactic surgery based solely on family history should largely be abandoned. Clinical management of women with a strong family history in whom a mutation is not found or those with variants of uncertain significance are resolved on a case-by-case basis. Fortunately, the risk of hereditary ovarian cancer does not rise dramatically until the late 30s in women with BRCA1 mutations, and the 40s for women with BRCA2 mutations, so women have the opportunity to complete their family prior to undergoing RRSO.[35] The age at which RRSO should be performed is not clearly established, but typically is done by the mid-30s to 40 for BRCA1 carriers. BRCA2 carriers may choose to delay surgery a bit longer due to their lower risk, but there is little to be gained. If a mutation carrier chooses to pursue fertility into her 40s, particularly a BRCA1 carrier, she should be counseled that she is at high risk of developing a life-threatening ovarian cancer. Removal of the ovaries usually has little effect on body image and self-esteem and most BRCA1/2 mutation carriers elect to undergo RRSO. The ovaries are internal organs, and most women experience only modest feelings of altered body image and self-esteem after surgery, in contrast to the more profound effects experienced after mastectomy. Insurance companies will almost always pay for prophylactic RRSO in proven mutation carriers.

Several retrospective studies have provided evidence of the efficacy of RRSO. In one study of BRCA1/2 carriers, women who underwent surgery had a 75% lower rate of breast and ovarian cancers over several years of follow-up compared to those who did not undergo the procedure.[9] A separate study examined outcome in 551 BRCA1/2 carriers from various registries.[36] Among 259 women who had undergone RRSO, 6 (2.3%) were found to have stage I ovarian cancer at the time of the procedure and 2 women (0.8%) subsequently developed serous peritoneal carcinoma. Among the controls, 58 women (20%) developed ovarian cancer after a mean follow-up of 8.8 years. With the exclusion of the six women whose cancer was diagnosed at surgery, RRSO reduced ovarian cancer risk by 96%. Finally, an international registry study of over 1,800 subjects with median follow-up of 3.5 years found that RRSO reduced ovarian, tubal, and peritoneal cancer risk by 80% due to incident cancers and an estimated 6% residual life-time risk of primary peritoneal cancer.[37]

The pros and cons of surgical prophylaxis for hereditary ovarian cancer are summarized in Table 52.2. RRSO can be performed laparoscopically (or robotically) in most women, with discharge home in less than 24 hours. If a laparoscopic approach is problematic due to obesity or adhesions, the

TABLE 52.2

PROS AND CONS OF PROPHYLACTIC SALPINGO-OOPHORECTOMY IN *BRCA1/2* CARRIERS

PROS
Strikingly decreased ovarian and fallopian tube cancer incidence and mortality
Can be delayed to allow completion of childbearing
Can be performed laparoscopically in most cases
Impact on body image and self-esteem acceptable
Estrogen replacement can ameliorate consequences of menopause
Decreases breast cancer risk

CONS
Cost
Potential operative morbidity and mortality
Residual risk of primary peritoneal carcinoma
Surgical menopause in women who elect not to take hormone replacement

surgery can be performed through a small lower abdominal incision. Morbidity, including bleeding, infection, and damage to the urinary or gastrointestinal tracts, can occur, but the incidence of serious complications is very low. Since the fallopian tubes and ovaries are small, discrete organs, they are relatively easy to remove completely. Attention should be paid to transecting the ovarian artery and vein proximal to the ovary so that remnants are not left behind. This involves opening the pelvic sidewall peritoneum, visualizing the ureter, and then isolation of the infundibular pelvic ligament that contains the ovarian blood supply. If there are adhesions between the adnexa and adjacent structures, careful dissection should be performed to ensure complete removal of the ovaries and fallopian tubes. If the uterus is not removed, care should be taken to remove the entire fallopian tube. A small portion of the tube inevitably will be left in the cornu of the uterus, but thus far there are no case reports of fallopian tube cancer developing in such remnants.

Although there is not strong evidence that BRCA1/2 mutations increase uterine cancer risk, many women elect to have the uterus removed as part of the surgical procedure because they have completed their family or have other gynecologic indications. Hysterectomy somewhat increases operative time, blood loss, surgical complications, and hospital stay, but usually can be performed laparoscopically and serious adverse outcomes are infrequent. Furthermore, the likelihood of future exposure to tamoxifen in the context of breast cancer prevention or treatment, which increases endometrial cancer risk two- to threefold, also supports concomitant hysterectomy. Women who receive hormone replacement therapy after surgery will require a progestin along with estrogen to protect against the development of endometrial cancer if the uterus is not removed.

In younger women, surgical menopause after RRSO is associated with vasomotor symptoms, vaginal atrophy, decreased libido, and an accelerated onset and incidence of osteoporosis and cardiovascular disease. In premenopausal women who do not have a personal history of breast cancer, estrogen replacement can be administered to ameliorate many of the deleterious effects of premature menopause. Systemic estrogen levels are lower in oophorectomized premenopausal women taking hormone replacement than if the ovaries had been left in place. The therapeutic benefit of oophorectomy in women with breast cancer has long been appreciated, and more recent studies support the contention that RRSO is protective against breast cancer in BRCA1/2 carriers. Many carriers are identified after developing early onset breast cancer, and this group represents the most difficult in which to balance the potential risks and benefits of estrogen replacement therapy.

Early cancers of the fallopian tube and ovary have been identified in some RRSO specimens. The frequency of occult malignancies has varied between reports but appears to be about 3%.[38] In view of this, the pelvis and peritoneal cavity should be examined carefully during surgery. Malignant cells also have been found in pelvic peritoneal cytologic specimens, and washings of the pelvis should be obtained when performing RRSO. The pathologist should be informed of the indication for surgery, and multiple sections of the ovaries and fallopian tubes should be examined to exclude the presence of occult carcinoma. There is now strong evidence to suggest that most high-grade serous cancers that are found in the ovary, tube, and peritoneum are derived from cells of the tubal fimbria.[39] Most early cancers discovered at RRSO in BRCA1/2 carriers appear to originate in the fallopian tube fimbria, and *in situ* carcinomas that overexpress mutant TP53 also are frequently found.

Cases of peritoneal serous carcinoma indistinguishable from ovarian cancer have been observed after RRSO, but the origin of these cancers is unclear. Some peritoneal cancers that occur years later may represent recurrences of occult ovarian or tubal cancers. In this regard, retrospective examination of the ovaries and fallopian tubes sometimes has revealed cancers that were not originally recognized. Some of these cancers likely arise directly from epithelial cells that have implanted on the peritoneum. In view of this, patients who undergo RRSO should be made aware of their residual risk of cancer.

In summary, surgical prophylaxis with RRSO represents the best approach for decreasing ovarian and fallopian tube cancer mortality in BRCA1/2 carriers. For younger women who wish to maintain fertility, periodic screening with the cancer antigen 125 (CA 125) serum marker and transvaginal sonography, although of unproven benefit, is often advised. Prevention by using oral contraceptives may also be of benefit during the reproductive years, but RRSO is the standard of care and should be strongly recommended to women who carry BRCA1/2 mutations.

HEREDITARY ENDOMETRIAL CANCER (LYNCH SYNDROME)

Although Lynch syndrome (previously referred to as hereditary nonpolyposis colorectal cancer) typically manifests as familial clustering of early onset colon cancer,[40] there is also an increased incidence of several other types of cancers—most notably endometrial cancer in women. About 3% to 5% of endometrial cancers are attributable to inherited mutations in the DNA mismatch repair (MMR) genes that cause Lynch syndrome. Most often *MSH2* and *MLH1* are implicated, but mutations in *MSH6*, *PMS1*, and *PMS2* also occur. The risk of ovarian cancer is also significantly increased in Lynch syndrome but to a lesser degree, and this accounts for only about 1% of all ovarian cancers.

Cells in which one of the MMR genes has been inactivated exhibit a phenomenon called microsatellite instability (MSI). This occurs as DNA mismatches cause shortening or lengthening of repetitive DNA sequences, and these mismatches go unrepaired. This results in generation of alleles in the cancer that contain a greater or lesser number of repeats than are present in normal cells from that individual. MSI occurs in most Lynch syndrome–associated colon and endometrial cancers.[40] However, MSI is found in about 20% of sporadic cancers that arise in these organs, and in most cases is caused by silencing of the *MLH1* gene due to promoter methylation.

Screening strategies for identification of mismatch repair gene alterations in families with Lynch syndrome–associated cancers include analysis of tumor tissue for MSI or loss of DNA mismatch repair gene expression using immunohistochemisty.[41] In cancers with MSI or loss of expression of one of the mismatch repair genes or in families with pedigrees suggestive of Lynch syndrome, these genes can be sequenced to identify disease-causing mutations, most of which cause truncated protein products.

The risk of a woman who carries an MMR mutation developing endometrial cancer ranges from 20% to 60% in various reports.[42,43] The risk of ovarian cancer is increased to about 5% to 12%. Whereas the mean age of women with sporadic endometrial cancers is the early 60s, cancers that arise in association with the Lynch syndrome are often diagnosed before menopause, with an average age for women in their 40s. The clinical features of Lynch syndrome–associated endometrial cancers are similar to those of most sporadic cases (well-differentiated, endometrioid, early stage), and survival is about 90%.[42] The mean age of onset of ovarian cancer in Lynch syndrome families is the early 40s, and the clinical features of these cancers are generally more favorable than in sporadic cases. They usually are identified at an early stage, are well or moderately differentiated, and about 20% occur in the setting of a synchronous endometrial cancer.

Recommendations for screening and risk-reducing surgery in Lynch syndrome are better established for colorectal cancer than for extracolonic malignancies.[44] Transvaginal ultrasound has been proposed as a screening test for endometrial cancer (and ovarian cancer) in Lynch syndrome families, but its efficacy is unproven.[45] Endometrial biopsy is the most sensitive means of diagnosing endometrial cancer, and it has been suggested that this should be employed periodically beginning around age 30 to 35. However, there are no published data that demonstrate that this approach is superior to simply performing a biopsy if abnormal uterine bleeding occurs.

Most experts believe that risk-reducing hysterectomy has a role in the management of some women with Lynch syndrome because of the high incidence of endometrial cancer and because the uterus does not serve a vital function once childbearing has been completed (Table 52.3). One study demonstrated that there were no cases of endometrial cancer in 61 Lynch syndrome carriers who underwent risk-reducing hysterectomy, while endometrial cancer developed in 69 of 210 (33%) who did not undergo surgery.[46] However, since most endometrial cancers are diagnosed early and cured, it is conceivable that prophylactic hysterectomy may not appreciably decrease mortality. In view of the increased risk of ovarian cancer in Lynch syndrome, concomitant bilateral salpingo-oophorectomy should be strongly considered. Estrogen replacement therapy after removal of the ovaries is not contraindicated in women with Lynch syndrome, as there is no evidence that this adversely affects the incidence of other cancers.

Many women who belong to Lynch syndrome families elect to undergo risk-reducing colectomy, which provides an opportunity to perform concomitant hysterectomy. Hysterectomy in concert with colectomy, either via laparoscopy or laparotomy, does not greatly increase operative time or surgical complications. If an endometrial biopsy has not been performed preoperatively, an intraoperative inspection of the uterine cavity and possibly frozen section should be performed to exclude the presence of cancer. If cancer is found in the uterus, surgical staging—including sampling of the regional lymph nodes—should be considered in addition to hysterectomy. It is also appropriate to discuss risk-reducing hysterectomy with Lynch syndrome carriers who do not elect to undergo prophylactic colectomy. In such cases, the operative approach (vaginal vs. laparotomy vs. laparoscopy) can be determined based on the presence or absence of uterine pathology (e.g., myomas), whether or not the patient has had prior abdominal surgery, and whether the ovaries are also to be removed.

TABLE 52.3

PROS AND CONS OF PROPHYLACTIC HYSTERECTOMY IN HEREDITARY NONPOLYPOSIS COLORECTAL CANCER

PROS
Can be performed in concert with prophylactic colectomy
Decreases uterine cancer incidence
Can be delayed to allow completion of childbearing
Can be performed laparoscopically in most cases
Impact on body image and self-esteem acceptable
CONS
Cost
Potential operative morbidity and mortality
Unproven to decrease endometrial cancer mortality

MULTIPLE ENDOCRINE NEOPLASIA TYPE 2

Gene Carriers

The multiple endocrine neoplasia (MEN) type 2 syndromes include MEN-2A, MEN-2B, and familial (non-MEN) medullary thyroid carcinoma (FMTC).[47] These are autosomal dominant–inherited syndromes caused by germline mutations in the *RET* protooncogene. Their hallmark is the development of multifocal, bilateral medullary thyroid carcinoma (MTC) associated with C-cell hyperplasia. MTCs arise from the thyroid C cells, also called parafollicular cells. C cells secrete the hormone calcitonin, a specific tumor marker for MTC. A slow-growing tumor in most cases, MTC causes significant morbidity and death in patients with uncontrolled local or metastatic spread. Large tumor burden is associated with diarrhea and flushing. In the MEN-2 syndromes, there is almost complete penetrance of MTC. Other features are variably expressed, with incomplete penetrance (Table 52.4).

In MEN-2A, all patients develop MTC. Approximately 42% of affected patients also develop pheochromocytomas, associated with adrenal medullary hyperplasia, and hyperparathyroidism develops in 10% to 35%. Cutaneous lichen amyloidosis and Hirschsprung's disease are infrequently associated with MEN-2A.[48–50]

MEN-2B appears to be the most aggressive form of hereditary MTC. In MEN-2B, MTC develops in all patients at a very young age (infancy). All affected individuals develop neural gangliomas, particularly in the mucosa of the digestive tract, conjunctiva, lips, and tongue; 40% to 50% develop pheochromocytomas. MEN-2B patients may also have megacolon, skeletal abnormalities, and markedly enlarged peripheral nerves. They do not develop hyperparathyroidism.

Familial, non-MEN medullary thyroid carcinoma is characterized by development of MTC in the absence of any other endocrinopathies. MTC in these patients has a more indolent clinical course. Some individuals with FMTC never manifest clinical evidence (i.e., symptoms or a lump in the neck), although biochemical testing and histologic evaluation of the thyroid demonstrates MTC.

TABLE 52.4

CLINICAL FEATURES OF SPORADIC MEDULLARY THYROID CARCINOMA, MULTIPLE ENDOCRINE NEOPLASIA 2A, MULTIPLE ENDOCRINE NEOPLASIA 2B, AND FAMILIAL MEDULLARY THYROID CARCINOMA

Clinical Setting	Features of MTC	Inheritance Pattern	Associated Abnormalities	Genetic Defect
Sporadic MTC	Unifocal	None	None	Somatic *RET* mutations in greater than 20% of tumors
MEN-2A	Multifocal, bilateral	Autosomal dominant	Pheochromocytomas, hyperparathyroidism	Germline missense mutations in extracellular cysteine codons of *RET*
MEN-2B	Multifocal, bilateral	Autosomal dominant	Pheochromocytomas, mucosal neuromas, megacolon, skeletal abnormalities	Germline missense mutation in tyrosine kinase domain of *RET*
FMTC	Multifocal, bilateral	Autosomal dominant	None	Germline missense mutations in extracellular or intracellular cysteine codons of *RET*

MTC, medullary thyroid carcinoma; MEN, multiple endocrine neoplasia; FMTC, familial medullary thyroid carcinoma.

RET Genotype-Phenotype Correlations

Mutations in the *RET* protooncogene are responsible for MEN-2A, MEN-2B, and FMTC. This gene encodes a transmembrane protein tyrosine kinase.[48,51] The mutations that cause the MEN-2 syndromes are activating, gain-of-function mutations affecting constitutive activation of the protein. This is unusual among hereditary cancer syndromes, which are usually caused by loss-of-function mutations in the predisposition gene (e.g., familial polyposis, *BRCA1* and *BRCA2*, von Hippel-Lindau, and MEN-1). More than 30 missense mutations have been described in patients affected by the MEN-2 syndromes (Table 52.5).

There is a relationship between the type of inherited *RET* mutation and presentation of MTC. The most virulent form is seen in patients with MEN-2B. These patients most commonly have a germline mutation in codon 918 of *RET* (ATG→ACG), although other mutations have been described (codon 883 and 922). As noted above, MTC in MEN-2B has an extremely early age of onset (infancy). Despite its distinctive clinical appearance and associated gastrointestinal difficulties, however, the disease is often not detected until the patient evidences a neck mass. Metastatic spread is usually present at the time of initial treatment, and calcitonin levels often remain elevated postoperatively.

MTC has a variable course in patients with MEN-2A, similar to that of sporadic MTC. Codon 634 and 618 mutations are the most common *RET* mutations associated with MEN-2A, although mutations at other codons are also observed (Table 52.5). Some patients do extremely well for many years, even with distant metastases, while others develop inanition; symptomatic liver, lung, or skeletal metastases; and disabling diarrhea. Recurrence in the central neck, with invasion of the airway or great vessels, may cause death.

In patients with FMTC, MTC is usually indolent. These individuals most commonly have mutations of codons 609, 611, 618, 620, 768, 804, or 891, although mutations of other codons have been identified (Table 52.5). Many patients with FMTC are cured by thyroidectomy alone, and even those with persistent elevation of calcitonin levels do well for many years. Occasionally FMTC patients survive into the seventh or eighth decade without clinical signs of disease, although pathologic examination of the thyroid will reveal MTC or C-cell hyperplasia.[52]

TABLE 52.5

***RET* MUTATIONS IN HEREDITARY MEDULLARY THYROID CARCINOMA**

	Missense Germline Mutations in the RET Protooncogene	
Syndrome	**Exon**	**Codon**
MEN-2A, FMTC	10	609
		611
		618
		620
11	631[a]	634
13	790	791
15	891	
FMTC	8	533
11	630	
13	768	
14	804	844[a]
15	913	918
MEN-2B	16	883

MEN, multiple endocrine neoplasia; FMTC, familial medullary thyroid carcinoma.
[a]Clinical features not yet characterized.

Risk-Reducing Thyroidectomy in RET Mutation Carriers

Genetic counseling and informed consent should be obtained prior to genetic testing. In RET mutation testing, DNA is extracted from the peripheral blood or other tissue source. Regions of the *RET* protooncogene are then amplified by polymerase chain reaction, and mutations are detected by one of several techniques. These include direct DNA sequencing; analysis of restriction sites introduced or deleted by a mutation; or gel shift analysis (denaturing gradient gel electrophoresis or single-strand conformation polymorphism analysis).

It has been shown that RET mutation carriers may harbor foci of MTC in the thyroid gland even when calcitonin levels are normal.[53] Although the age of onset and rate of disease

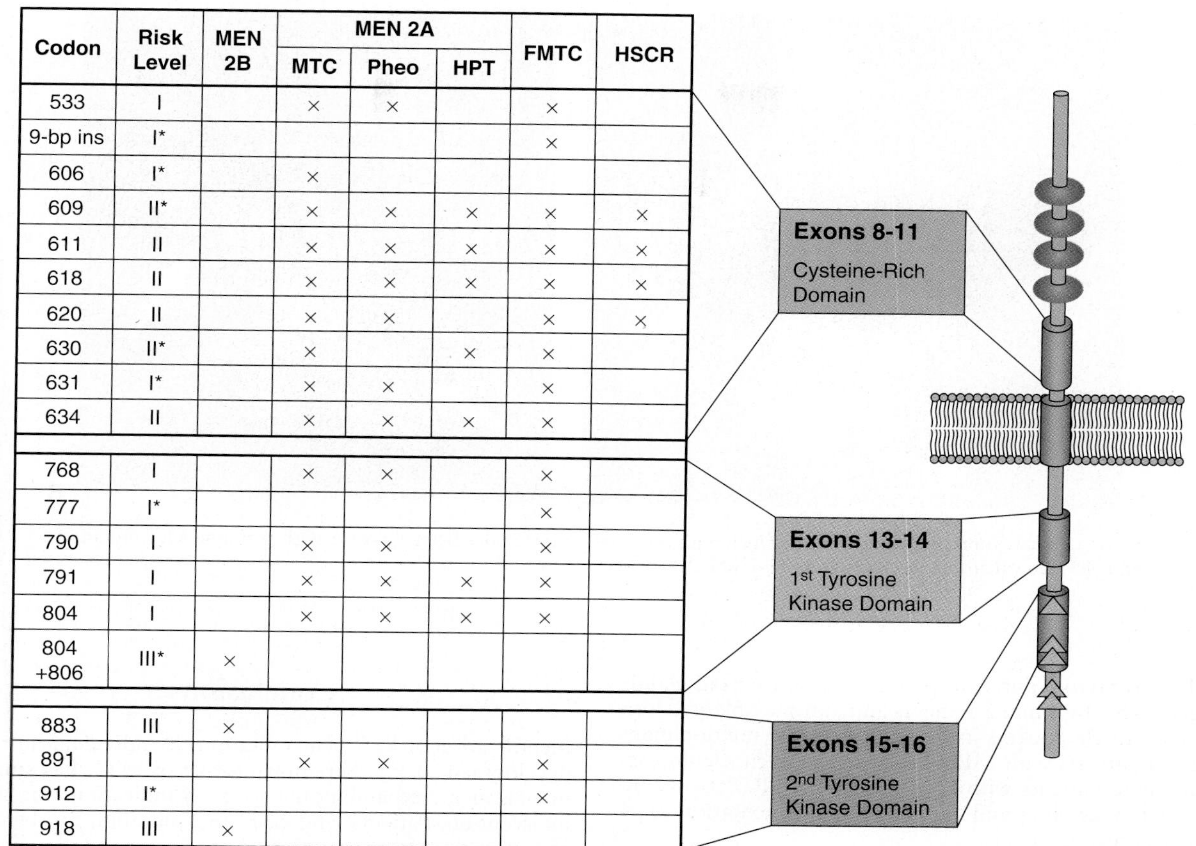

Codon	Risk Level	MEN 2B	MEN 2A			FMTC	HSCR
			MTC	Pheo	HPT		
533	I		×	×		×	
9-bp ins	I*					×	
606	I*		×				
609	II*		×	×	×	×	×
611	II		×	×	×	×	×
618	II		×	×	×	×	×
620	II		×	×		×	×
630	II*		×		×	×	
631	I*		×	×		×	
634	II		×	×	×	×	
768	I		×	×		×	
777	I*					×	
790	I		×	×		×	
791	I		×	×	×	×	
804	I		×	×	×	×	
804 +806	III*	×					
883	III	×					
891	I		×	×		×	
912	I*					×	
918	III	×					

FIGURE 52.3 RET mutation sites associated with multiple endocrine neoplasia 2 (MEN-2) syndromes. Codons previously reported in association with MEN-2 syndromes are listed by structural domain within the RET protein. Risk level is based on consensus guidelines or more recent clinical reports. Previously reported phenotypes for each codon are shown. MTC, medullary thyroid carcinoma; Pheo, pheochromocytoma; HPT, hyperparathyroidism; FMTC, familial medullary thyroid carcinoma; HSCR, Hirschsprung's disease. * indicates risk level based on recent clinical reports, not available at publication of the consensus guidelines. (From ref. 51, with permission.)

progression may differ, the lifetime penetrance of MTC is near 100% in carriers of RET mutations associated with MEN-2 syndromes. At-risk individuals who are found to have inherited a *RET* gene mutation are therefore candidates for thyroidectomy, regardless of their plasma calcitonin levels.

The best option for prevention of MTC in RET mutation carriers is complete surgical resection prior to malignant transformation. Preventative thyroidectomy is the goal in these patients, prior to the development of MTC. A number of studies have demonstrated improved biochemical cure rates or decreased recurrence rates from early thyroidectomy, performed after positive screening by calcitonin testing or RET mutation testing.[54–56]

MEN-2B mutations are the highest risk level, designated level III (Fig. 52.3).[57,58] Patients with MEN-2B have the most aggressive form of MTC, with invasive disease reported in patients less than 1 year of age. These patients should have preventative surgery early in the first year of life if possible. Identification and preservation of parathyroid glands can be extremely difficult in these infants due to their small size, translucent appearance, and the presence of exuberant thymic and perithyroidal nodal tissue. These procedures should be performed by surgeons experienced in parathyroid operations and pediatric thyroidectomy.

MEN-2A patients with mutations in codons 634, 620, 618, and 611 are considered high risk (level II).[57,58] Patients with level II mutations should undergo a total thyroidectomy at 5 to 6 years of age. There is evidence that the risk of lymph node metastasis is very low in MEN-2A patients under the age of 8, with normal calcitonin levels. Central lymph node dissection is associated with higher risk of hypoparathyroidism and recurrent laryngeal nerve injury and should be reserved for patients with elevated calcitonin levels.

A larger subset of RET mutations, associated with MEN-2A or FMTC, are considered lowest risk (level I).[57,58] These include mutations at codons 768, 790, 791, 804, and 891. For patients with low-risk, level I mutations, total thyroidectomy is recommended, and surgery before age 5 to 10 years is appropriate. As with the level II mutations, the need for central lymph node dissection should be guided by calcitonin levels and clinical features of the patient and kindred.

Until recently, some groups recommended total thyroidectomy with central neck lymph node dissection and total parathyroidectomy with autotransplantation for RET mutation carriers. Recent studies and personal experience, however, have demonstrated an extremely low likelihood of nodal metastases in MEN-2A or FMTC patients younger than 8 and in patients with a normal calcitonin level.[56] The current strategy is to leave the parathyroid *in situ* in these patients if possible.[59] Often, however, the desired complete removal of thyroid tissue results in compromise of parathyroid blood supply. In these situations, autotransplantation of devascularized parathyroid is required. The authors routinely remove and autotransplant the parathyroid if a central node dissection is

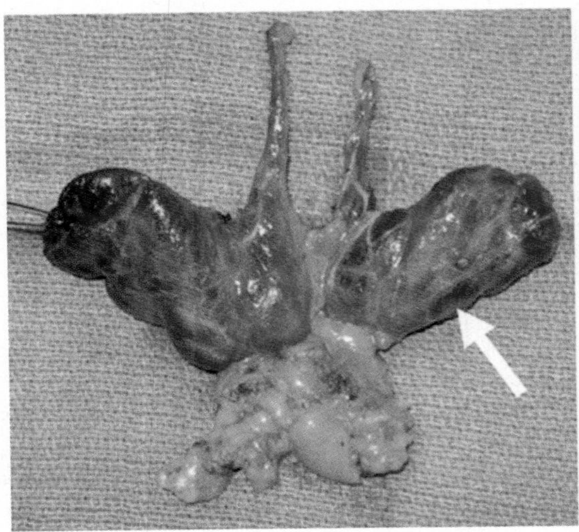

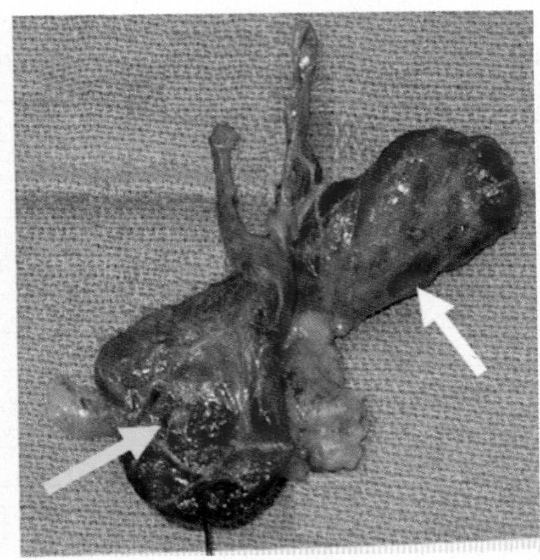

FIGURE 52.4 Total thyroidectomy specimen with attached central nodes from a patient with germline *RET* mutation and elevated calcitonin levels. Note small visible foci of MTC (*arrows*).

done. In parathyroid autotransplantation, parathyroid glands are sliced into 1 by 3 mm fragments and autotransplanted into individual muscle pockets in the muscle of the nondominant forearm in patients with MEN-2A or in the sternocleidomastoid muscle in patients with FMTC or MEN-2B. Patients are maintained on calcium and vitamin D supplementation for 4 to 8 weeks postoperatively.

In a series of thyroidectomies performed in 50 individuals with MEN-2A (identified by genetic screening), total thyroidectomy and central node dissection with parathyroidectomy and parathyroid autografting were performed in all patients (Fig. 52.4).[56] All autografts functioned, but three patients required supplemental calcium. The percentage of individuals requiring calcium supplementation following parathyroidectomy with parathyroid autografting reportedly ranges from 0% to 18%. Parathyroidectomy should be done in all patients showing gross parathyroid enlargement or biochemical evidence of parathyroid disease at time of surgery. The operating surgeon should have expertise in preservation of parathyroid function. It is important that the surgeon who performs an operative procedure for MTC be familiar with the techniques described here. If not, the patient should be referred to a center where these procedures are routinely done.

Follow-Up

Following thyroidectomy, thyroid hormone replacement is required for life. Patients may need several weeks of oral calcium and vitamin D until parathyroid function recovers. Intermittent calcitonin testing may be done to monitor for persistent or recurrent MTC.

The term *biochemical cure* is used to refer to patients with normal calcitonin levels after surgery for MTC. Complete postoperative normalization of calcitonin has been associated with decreased long-term risk of MTC recurrence, though the evidence is less clear for a survival benefit. A persistent or recurrent elevation in calcitonin indicates residual or recurrent MTC and warrants additional investigation by imaging, at a minimum. However, as most MTC has a fairly indolent course, patients with biochemical evidence of recurrent disease may not have corollary imaging findings for some time.

Conclusions

Identification of *RET* gene mutations in individuals at risk for development of the hereditary forms of MTC has simplified management, expanding the scope of indications for surgical intervention. Patients who carry this mutation can be offered operative treatment at a very young age, hopefully before the cancer has developed or spread; and those identified as not having the mutation are spared further genetic and biochemical screening. This achievement marks a new paradigm in surgery: the indication that an operation be performed based on the results of a genetic test. As in the decision to perform any surgical procedure, meticulous preparation and detailed discussion with patient and family must precede the final recommendation. It is also important that the patient and family be involved in preoperative discussion with genetic counselors.

FAMILIAL ADENOMATOUS POLYPOSIS, *MYH*-ASSOCIATED POLYPOSIS, AND LYNCH SYNDROME

Inherited colorectal cancer syndromes with adenomatous polyps are comprised primarily of two syndromes that predispose to disease by germline mutations transmitted in an autosomal dominant fashion. Familial adenomatous polyposis (FAP), accounting for less than 1% of the annual colorectal cancer burden, is caused by mutations in the tumor-suppressor adenomatous polyposis coli (*APC*) gene. It is characterized by the presence of 100 or more adenomatous polyps in the colorectum, nearly 100% penetrance, and an inevitable risk of colorectal cancer at the average age of 40 if prophylactic colectomy is not performed.[7,60] In the less severe form, attenuated FAP (AFAP), patients can present with fewer than 100 colorectal adenomas, which tend to be proximally located. Biallelic germline mutations in the base-excision-repair gene *MYH* may account for 7.5% of patients with a classical FAP phenotype who have no demonstrable APC mutation.[61] *MYH*-associated polyposis (MAP) shows an autosomal recessive pattern of inheritance and often presents as attenuated polyposis.

Lynch syndrome, also called hereditary nonpolyposis colorectal cancer, accounts for 2% to 3% of all colorectal cancer and is attributable to a germline mutation in one of the DNA MMR genes (*hMLH1*, *hMSH2*, *hMSH6*, and *PMS2*). Recent studies suggest that germline deletions in cell adhesion molecule (*EpCAM*) also known as *TACSTD1*, may account for 6.3% of Lynch syndrome cases.[62] Lynch syndrome is characterized by early age-of-onset colorectal cancer, predominance (70%) of lesions proximal to the splenic flexure, an increased rate of metachronous colorectal tumors, and a unique spectrum of benign and malignant extracolonic tumors. Lifetime risk of colorectal cancer in Lynch syndrome patients is approximately 80%. MSI, reflecting a deficiency in DNA repair secondary to the mutation in the MMR genes, is a common feature of Lynch syndrome–related tumors.[63]

Differences in penetrance, phenotypic expression, and certainty of disease development mandate distinctly different surgical approaches in the three most common adenomatous polyp syndromes, namely FAP, MAP, and Lynch syndrome.[64] This includes the type and timing of risk-reducing colon and rectal surgery.

Familial Adenomatous Polyposis

Surveillance (based on genetic testing or annual flexible sigmoidoscopy) of at-risk family members should begin around puberty (10 to 12 years). At-risk individuals who belong to families with an AFAP phenotype should undergo colonoscopic screening. In families with a demonstrated *APC* mutation, informative genetic testing is possible and mutations are detected in 90% to 95% of FAP pedigrees. Patients with either a positive genotype or with adenomatous polyps identified on sigmoidoscopy should undergo full colonoscopy to establish the severity of their polyposis. Timing of surgery depends to some degree on the extent of polyposis, because the risk of colorectal cancer development is partially associated with colon and rectal polyp burden. Patients with mild polyposis and a correspondingly lower cancer risk can undergo surgery in their late teens. Patients with severe polyposis, high degree of dysplasia, multiple adenomas larger than 5 mm in size, and symptoms (bleeding, persistent diarrhea, anemia, failure to thrive, psychosocial stress, etc.) should undergo risk-reducing colorectal surgery as soon as is practical after diagnosis.[60,65] However, in carefully selected, fully asymptomatic patients who have small adenomas but a strong family history of aggressive abdominal desmoid disease, consideration can be given to delaying prophylactic colectomy, as the risk of desmoid-related complication may be greater than the risk of developing colorectal cancer.

The three current surgical options for patients with FAP are total proctocolectomy with permanent ileostomy (TPC), total colectomy with ileorectal anastomosis (IRA), and proctocolectomy with ileal pouch-anal anastomosis (IPAA). IPAA can be a double-stapled, end-of-pouch-to-anus anastomosis, which may leave behind approximately 1 cm of anal transition zone. An alternative approach, which is preferred when there is carpeting of the anal transition zone with adenomas, is to perform a mucosal stripping of the anal transition zone down to the dentate line followed by a hand-sewn per anal anastomosis of pouch to the dentate line. Selection of the optimal procedure for an individual patient is based on several factors, including characteristics of the FAP syndrome within the patient and family, differences in likely postoperative functional outcome, preoperative anal sphincter status, and patient preference.[7]

TPC with permanent ileostomy, although rarely chosen as a primary procedure, is used in patients with unacceptably poor baseline sphincter function, patients with invasive cancer involving the sphincters or levator complex, or patients for whom an IPAA is not technically feasible (secondary to desmoid disease and foreshortening of the small bowel mesentery, making it surgically impossible to bring the ileal pouch to the anus) nor likely to lead to good function such as massive obesity or weak anal sphincters. However, TPC is occasionally chosen as a primary procedure by patients who perceive that their lifestyle would be compromised by the frequent bowel movements (five to six per day) sometimes associated with the IPAA procedure.

In addition to the issues mentioned above, the key in deciding between an IPAA and an IRA is based primarily on the risk of rectal cancer development if the rectum is left *in situ*. The risk of rectal cancer following IRA may be as high as 4% to 8% at 10 years and 26% to 32% after 25 years.[66,67] The magnitude of risk in an individual patient is, however, related to the overall extent of colorectal polyposis. IRA may be considered for patients with less than 1,000 colorectal polyps (including those with attenuated FAP) and less than 20 rectal adenomas, as these individuals have a relatively low risk of developing rectal cancer.[60,65,66] Patients with severe rectal (greater than 20 adenomas) or colonic (greater than 1,000 adenomas) polyposis, an adenoma larger than 3 cm, or an adenoma with severe dysplasia should ideally undergo proctectomy.[60,65,66]

The risk of secondary rectal excision, due to uncontrollable rectal polyposis or rectal cancer, may be estimated by identifying the specific location of the causative APC mutation. Patients with a mutation located between codons 1250 and 1464 have been shown to have a 6.2-fold increased risk of rectal cancer compared to those with a mutation prior to codon 1250 or after codon 1464 (mean number of rectal polyps 42 vs. 22, respectively).[7] Although the concept of using genotype-phenotype relations to help guide the management of a specific patient is appealing and results from multiregistry studies show promise for this approach,[68] it is important to recognize the variability of phenotypic expression that exists even among members of the same family. This suggests that at the current time, the choice between an IRA and an IPAA should be based primarily on clinical (rather than genetic) grounds.[60]

The risk of polyp and cancer development following primary surgery is not limited to patients undergoing IRA. In patients undergoing IPAA, neoplasia may occur at the site of ileal pouch anastomosis; the frequency appears to be greater after stapled anastomosis (28% to 31%) than after mucosectomy and hand-sewn anastomosis (10% to 14%).[69] In the case of neoplasia developing at the anal transition zone after a stapled anastomosis, transanal mucosectomy can often be performed, followed by advancement of the pouch to the dentate line. Of additional concern is the development of adenomatous polyps in the ileal pouch, which occurs in 35% to 45% of patients by 7 to 10 years of follow-up.[70] Consequently, lifetime surveillance of the rectal remnant (after IRA) or the ileal pouch (after IPAA) is required following either procedure.

Another important consideration in choosing between IPAA and IRA is postoperative bowel function and quality of life. Some studies have associated IPAA with higher frequency of both daytime and nocturnal bowel movements, higher incidence of passive incontinence and incidental soiling, and greater postoperative morbidity.[71] However, long-term follow-up studies have shown that the IPAA results in a good quality of life when compared to the general population.[72] Therefore, although the choice of procedure must be carefully individualized, because of the risk of rectal cancer associated with IRA the authors favor IPAA for most FAP patients whenever feasible. However, an IRA should be considered in specific circumstances, such as when there is mild rectal polyposis (as in attenuated FAP), or a young patient with rectal sparing who is not interested in undergoing the multiple procedures that accompany an IPAA and diverting loop ileostomy, or a young woman interested in having children and trying to avoid the decreased fecundity associated with an IPAA procedure. Although the authors attempt to perform a diverting loop ileostomy in all IPAA procedures, it is not always feasible due to a number of anatomical factors, including body habitus.

Endoscopic surveillance of the rectal segment at 6- to 12-month intervals after the index surgery is recommended. With increasing numbers of adenomas, frequency of surveillance should be increased. Although small (less than 5 mm) scattered adenomas can be safely observed or removed with a biopsy forceps, polyps greater than 5 mm should be removed with a snare. However, repeated fulguration and polypectomy over many years can lead to difficulty with subsequent polypectomy, reduced rectal compliance, and difficulty identifying flat cancers within a background of scar tissue. The development of severe dysplasia, or villous adenomas not amenable to endoscopic removal, is indication for proctectomy.

Long-Term Considerations from Extracolonic Manifestations

Despite the reduced risk of colorectal cancer–related death following prophylactic colectomy, FAP patients are still at increased risk of mortality from both rectal cancer and other causes relative to the general population. The three main causes of death following IRA are progression of desmoid disease, upper gastrointestinal malignancy, and perioperative mortality.

Desmoids

Desmoids may occur in up to 30% of patients with FAP[65] and, unlike those found in the general population, tend to be intra-abdominal (up to 80%) and to arise after prior abdominal surgery. Although conflicting reports exist, it appears that female patients, those with extracolonic manifestations of FAP, a positive family history of desmoids, and APC mutations located at 3′ of codon 1440 are at increased risk of developing desmoids.[73–75] These tumors often involve the small bowel mesentery (greater than 50%), making complete resection difficult or impossible; they may also involve the ureters. Morbidity following attempted resection—which often involves removal of a variable length of small bowel—is significant. Furthermore, the rate of recurrence is high following attempted resection, with recurrent disease often more aggressive than the initial desmoid. Therefore, resection is usually not recommended.

Intra-abdominal desmoids may be more common and severe after IRA than after IPAA. Desmoids that involve the small bowel mesentery may preclude the formation of an IPAA secondary to foreshortening of the small bowel mesentery, especially in patients undergoing proctectomy after an initial IRA. Surgery for abdominal wall desmoids should be reserved for small, well-defined tumors with clear margins.

MYH-Associated Polyposis

MAP should be suspected in patients with more than ten colorectal adenomas, a weak history of colorectal cancer, and no family history of FAP. The diagnosis is confirmed by *MYH* gene testing.[76]

Depending on the polyp burden, the management of the colon and rectum of a patient with a biallelic *MUTYH* mutation can be endoscopic or surgical. If the polyp burden is limited and an endoscopic approach is pursued, colonoscopy should be performed at least annually in order to ensure that polyps larger than 5 mm are removed. If, at diagnosis, the polyp burden is not amenable to an endoscopic approach, a resection is indicated at that time. In most cases in which surgery is deemed necessary, an IRA is sufficient. However, if rectal polyposis is severe, an IPAA may be indicated. Indications for surgery following an initial endoscopic surveillance program include increasing polyp size or number or worsening histology.

Because of the increased risk of duodenal cancer, MAP patients should also undergo upper gastrointestinal endoscopy starting between 18 and 20 years of age.[60]

Lynch Syndrome

Due to ambiguity, the term hereditary nonpolyposis colorectal cancer has been abandoned and replaced by Lynch syndrome, which refers to individuals with a predisposition to colorectal cancer and other malignancies as a result of a germline MMR mutation.[77] Overall, colorectal cancer occurs in 78% to 80% of Lynch syndrome patients at a mean age of 46 years.[7] Endometrial cancer occurs in 43%, gastric cancer in 19%, urinary tract cancer in 18%, and ovarian cancer in 9% of affected individuals. The Amsterdam Criteria, which led to the identification of the Lynch syndrome-associated MMR gene mutations, require that there be three relatives (one a first-degree relative of the other two) with colorectal, endometrial, small bowel, ureteral, or renal pelvis cancer, in two or more successive generations, with at least one case of diagnosed colorectal cancer at less than 50 years of age and FAP excluded.[78] Although useful for determining whom to test for Lynch syndrome, only 60% of families that meet the Amsterdam Criteria will have a mutation in an MMR gene.[79] Families meeting Amsterdam Criteria and lacking an MMR mutation are referred to as having "familial colorectal cancer type X" and appear to have a lower incidence of colorectal and extracolonic cancers than those with Lynch syndrome (Fig. 52.5). Of note, they have an increased incidence of left-sided tumors and nonmucinous MSS tumors.[80,81]

The Amsterdam Criteria and revised Bethesda Criteria[82] (Table 52.6) are used in clinical practice to identify patients at risk for Lynch syndrome and who require further testing. Patients with colorectal cancer who belong to pedigrees suspicious for Lynch syndrome should be offered screening by immunohistochemistry (IHC) for loss of MMR protein expression or by MSI analysis. Since the sensitivity of IHC testing for loss of MMR protein expression is comparable to MSI testing, either approach can be pursued. However, IHC testing is less expensive and can also identify a specific MMR protein loss, which can help target subsequent germline testing. Routine IHC testing for loss of MMR protein in individuals younger than 50 at the time of colorectal cancer diagnosis is feasible and has led to the identification of patients with Lynch syndrome who might otherwise have been missed.[83] Patients with MSI-high tumors should undergo testing for germline MMR mutations in *hMSH2*, *hMLH1*, *MSH6*, and *PMS2*. In families for which tumor tissue is not available, initial germline testing may be considered. As in FAP, a mutation in an affected individual must be established for testing in at-risk individuals to be conclusive.

Although development of colorectal cancer in Lynch syndrome is not a certainty, the 80% lifetime risk,[7] the 45% rate of metachronous colorectal neoplasms, and the possibly accelerated adenoma-to-carcinoma sequence[84] mandate consideration of prophylactic surgical options. Patients with Lynch syndrome, with a colon cancer, or more than one advanced adenoma should be offered the options of prophylactic total

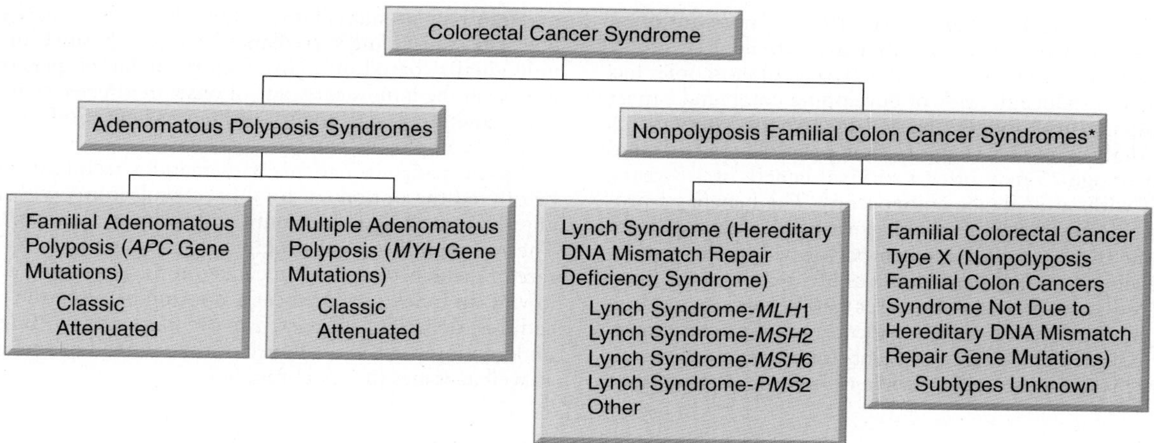

FIGURE 52.5 Schematic showing the two categories of colorectal cancer syndromes, illustrating that nonpolyposis disorders are heterogeneous but based on tumor biology and can be distinguished as those having defective mismatch repair (Lynch syndrome; group A) and those with proficient mismatch repair (group B in this study, called here familial colorectal cancer type X). Diagram excludes syndromes characterized by hamartomatous/hyperplastic polyposis. *Defined by any number of pedigree or laboratory criteria, including but not limited to the Amsterdam criteria. Hereditary nonpolyposis colon cancer syndrome is the term that has traditionally been used in this context, encompassing those entities that have emerged as distinguishable clinical entities (i.e., Lynch syndrome and familial colorectal cancer type X). (From ref. 92, Copyright © 2005 American Medical Association. All rights reserved.)

colectomy with IRA or segmental colectomy with annual postoperative surveillance colonoscopy.[84,85] Careful surveillance is also necessary after total colectomy and IRA, as the risk of cancer in the retained rectum is approximately 12% at 10 to 12 years.[86] Although there has been no trial demonstrating an improved survival for Lynch syndrome patients undergoing total colectomy and IRA versus segmental colectomy, mathematical models suggest a benefit for total colectomy and IRA, especially in younger individuals with early-stage cancers.[87] In addition, because of increased rates of metachronous polyp development and abdominal surgeries in those undergoing a segmental resection, a total colectomy and IRA has emerged as the procedure of choice for the index cancer.[88,89] Recently, targeted genetic testing approaches—such as the single amplicon MSH2 A636P mutation test in Ashkenazi Jewish patients with colorectal cancer—have demonstrated how a rapid and inexpensive preoperative genetic test can help direct the extent of colon resection.[90]

Mismatch repair mutation-positive patients with a normal colon may also be offered prophylactic colectomy in highly selected situations. One rationale for this approach is the similarity of lifetime cancer risk between patients with *APC* and *MMR* gene mutations, and the fact that total abdominal colectomy with IRA produces less functional disturbance than the prophylactic procedure recommended for FAP (total proctocolectomy with IPAA). However, an alternate strategy for these individuals is surveillance by colonoscopy, which is cost-effective and greatly reduces the rate of colorectal cancer development and overall mortality.[91] There is a risk of colorectal cancer development in the interval between colonoscopies,

TABLE 52.6

THE REVISED BETHESDA GUIDELINES FOR TESTING COLORECTAL TUMORS FOR MICROSATELLITE INSTABILITY

Tumors from individuals should be tested for MSI in the following situations:

1. Colorectal cancer diagnosed in a patient who is less than 50 years of age.
2. Presence of synchronous, metachronous colorectal, or other HNPCC-associated tumors,[a] regardless of age.
3. Colorectal cancer with the MSI-H[b] histology[c] diagnosed in a patient who is less than 60 years of age.[d]
4. Colorectal cancer diagnosed in one or more first-degree relatives with an HNPCC-related tumor, with one of the cancers being diagnosed under age 50 years.
5. Colorectal cancer diagnosed in two or more first- or second-degree relatives with HNPCC-related tumors, regardless of age.

MSI, microsatellite instability; HNPCC, hereditary nonpolyposis colorectal cancer; MSI-H, microsatellite instability–high.
[a]HNPCC-related tumors include colorectal, endometrial, stomach, ovarian, pancreas, ureter and renal pelvis, biliary tract, and brain (usually glioblastoma as seen in Turcot syndrome) tumors, sebaceous gland adenomas and keratoacanthomas in Muir-Torre syndrome, and carcinoma of the small bowel.
[b]MSI-H in tumors refers to changes in two or more of the five National Cancer Institute–recommended panels of microsatellite markers.
[c]Presence of tumor infiltrating lymphocytes, Crohn's-like lymphocytic reaction, mucinous/signet ring differentiation, or medullary growth pattern.
[d]There was no consensus among the workshop participants on whether to include the age criteria in guideline 3 above; participants voted to keep less than 60 years of age in the guidelines.
(From ref. 82.)

but if the interval is less than 2 years these tumors are often identified at an early stage, when they are curable. Recently, a shorter (every 1 to 2 years) interval between colonoscopies has been shown to reduce the risk of developing colorectal cancer when compared to a longer (every 2 to 3 years) interval.[84] A decision analysis model suggests that prophylactic subtotal colectomy at age 25 may offer a survival benefit of 1.8 years, compared with surveillance colonoscopy. The benefit of prophylactic colectomy decreases when surgery is delayed until later in life and is negligible when performed at the time of cancer development.[87] When quality of life is considered, however, surveillance provides the greatest benefit in quality-adjusted life years. Based on this evidence, prophylactic surgery is clearly indicated only in those patients for whom colonoscopic surveillance is not technically possible or in those who refuse to undergo regular surveillance. Thus, the decision between prophylactic surgery and surveillance for a gene-positive, unaffected individual is based on many factors, including penetrance of disease in the family, early age of onset in affected family members, functional and quality-of-life considerations, and likelihood of compliance with surveillance.

Lynch syndrome patients with an index rectal cancer should be offered the options of total proctocolectomy with IPAA or anterior proctosigmoidectomy with primary reconstruction.[85] The rationale for total proctocolectomy is the 17% to 45% rate of metachronous colon cancer in the remaining colon following an index rectal cancer. Choosing between the two procedures depends, in part, on the patient's willingness to undergo intensive surveillance of the retained proximal colon, as well as issues of bowel function.

Selected References

The full list of references for this chapter appears in the online version.

1. Robson ME, Storm CD, Weitzel J, Wollins DS, Offit K. American Society of Clinical Oncology policy statement update: genetic and genomic testing for cancer susceptibility. *J Clin Oncol* 2010;28:893.
2. Amir E, Freedman OC, Seruga B, Evans DG. Assessing women at high risk of breast cancer: a review of risk assessment models. *J Natl Cancer Inst* 2010;102:680.
7. Guillem JG, Wood WC, Moley JF, et al. ASCO/SSO review of current role of risk-reducing surgery in common hereditary cancer syndromes. *J Clin Oncol* 2006;24:4642.
8. Saslow D, Boetes C, Burke W, et al. American Cancer Society guidelines for breast screening with MRI as an adjunct to mammography. *CA Cancer J Clin* 2007;57:75.
9. Kauff ND, Satagopan JM, Robson ME, et al. Risk-reducing salpingo-oophorectomy in women with a BRCA1 or BRCA2 mutation. *N Engl J Med* 2002;346:1609.
10. Genetic Information Non-Discrimination Act of 2008 (GINA). Public Law No.110-233.
11. Society for Surgical Oncology: position statement on prophylactic mastectomy. World Wide Web URL: http://www.surgonc.org/default.aspx?id=179. Accessed May 7, 2010.
13. Meijers-Heijboer H, van Geel B, van Putten WL, et al. Breast cancer after prophylactic bilateral mastectomy in women with a BRCA1 or BRCA2 mutation. *N Engl J Med* 2001;345:159.
14. Eldor L, Spiegel A. Breast reconstruction after bilateral prophylactic mastectomy in women at high risk for breast cancer. *Breast J* 2009;15(Suppl 1):S81.
15. Zakhireh J, Fowble B, Esserman LJ. Application of screening principles to the reconstructed breast. *J Clin Oncol* 2010;28:173.
16. Gabram SG, Dougherty T, Albain KS, et al. Assessing breast cancer risk and providing treatment recommendations: immediate impact of an educational session. *Breast J* 2009;15(Suppl 1):S39.
18. Fitzgerald RC, Hardwick R, Huntsman D, et al. Hereditary diffuse gastric cancer: updated consensus guidelines for clinical management and directions for future research. *J Med Genet* 2010;47:436.
19. Norton JA, Ham CM, Van Dam J, et al. CDH1 truncating mutations in the E-cadherin gene: an indication for total gastrectomy to treat hereditary diffuse gastric cancer. *Ann Surg* 2007;245:873.
21. Guilford P, Hopkins J, Harraway J, et al. E-cadherin germline mutations in familial gastric cancer. *Nature* 1998;392:402.
22. Kaurah P, MacMillan A, Boyd N, et al. Founder and recurrent CDH1 mutations in families with hereditary diffuse gastric cancer. *JAMA* 2007;297:2360.
28. Huntsman DG, Carneiro F, Lewis FR, et al. Early gastric cancer in young, asymptomatic carriers of germ-line E-cadherin mutations. *N Engl J Med* 2001;344:1904.
30. Rogers WM, Dobo E, Norton JA, et al. Risk-reducing total gastrectomy for germline mutations in E-cadherin (CDH1): pathologic findings with clinical implications. *Am J Surg Pathol* 2008;32:799.
33. Struewing JP, Hartge P, Wacholder S, et al. The risk of cancer associated with specific mutations of BRCA1 and BRCA2 among Ashkenazi Jews. *N Engl J Med* 1997;336:1401.
34. Risch HA, McLaughlin JR, Cole DE, et al. Prevalence and penetrance of germline BRCA1 and BRCA2 mutations in a population series of 649 women with ovarian cancer. *Am J Hum Genet* 2001;68:700.
35. King MC, Marks JH, Mandell JB. Breast and ovarian cancer risks due to inherited mutations in BRCA1 and BRCA2. *Science* 2003;302:643.
36. Rebbeck TR, Lynch HT, Neuhausen SL, et al. Prophylactic oophorectomy in carriers of BRCA1 or BRCA2 mutations. *N Engl J Med* 2002;346:1616.
37. Finch A, Beiner M, Lubinski J, et al. Salpingo-oophorectomy and the risk of ovarian, fallopian tube, and peritoneal cancers in women with a BRCA1 or BRCA2 mutation. *JAMA* 2006;296:185.
41. Hampel H, Frankel W, Panescu J, et al. Screening for Lynch syndrome (hereditary nonpolyposis colorectal cancer) among endometrial cancer patients. *Cancer Res* 2006;66:7810.
42. Watson P, Vasen HF, Mecklin JP, Jarvinen H, Lynch HT. The risk of endometrial cancer in hereditary nonpolyposis colorectal cancer. *Am J Med* 1994; 96:516.
44. Koornstra JJ, Mourits MJ, Sijmons RH, et al. Management of extracolonic tumours in patients with Lynch syndrome. *Lancet Oncol* 2009;10:400.
46. Schmeler KM, Lynch HT, Chen LM, et al. Prophylactic surgery to reduce the risk of gynecologic cancers in the Lynch syndrome. *N Engl J Med* 2006; 354:261.
47. Traugott AL, Moley JF. Multiple endocrine neoplasia type 2: clinical manifestations and management. *Cancer Treat Res* 2009;153:321.
48. Eng C, Clayton D, Schuffenecker I, et al. The relationship between specific RET proto-oncogene mutations and disease phenotype in multiple endocrine neoplasia type 2. International RET mutation consortium analysis. *JAMA* 1996;276:1575.
56. Skinner MA, Moley JA, Dilley WG, et al. Prophylactic thyroidectomy in multiple endocrine neoplasia type 2A. *N Engl J Med* 2005;353:1105.
57. Brandi ML, Gagel RF, Angeli A, et al. Guidelines for diagnosis and therapy of MEN type 1 and type 2. *J Clin Endocrinol Metabo* 2001;86(12): 5658.
58. Kloos RT, Eng C, Evans DB, et al. Medullary thyroid cancer: management guidelines of the American Thyroid Association. *Thyroid* 2009;19:565.
59. Moley JF. Medullary thyroid carcinoma: management of lymph node metastases. *J Natl Compr Canc Netw* 2010;8:549.
60. Vasen HF, Moslein G, Alonso A, et al. Guidelines for the clinical management of familial adenomatous polyposis (FAP). *Gut* 2008;57:704.
61. Sieber OM, Lipton L, Crabtree M, et al. Multiple colorectal adenomas, classic adenomatous polyposis, and germ-line mutations in MYH. *N Engl J Med* 2003;348:791.
64. Steinhagen E, Markowitz AJ, Guillem JG. How to manage a patient with multiple adenomatous polyps. *Surg Oncol Clin North Am* 2010;19:711.
65. Church J. Familial adenomatous polyposis. *Surg Oncol Clin North Am* 2009;18:585.
66. Sinha A, Tekkis PP, Rashid S, Phillips RKS, Clark SK. Risk factors for secondary proctectomy in patients with familial adenomatous polyposis. *Br J Surg* 2010;97:1710.
68. Nieuwenhuis M, Blow S, Bjrk J, et al. Genotype predicting phenotype in familial adenomatous polyposis: a practical application to the choice of surgery. *Dis Colon Rectum* 2009;52:1259.
71. Aziz O, Athanasiou T, Fazio VW, et al. Meta-analysis of observational studies of ileorectal versus ileal pouch-anal anastomosis for familial adenomatous polyposis. *Br J Surg* 2006;93:407.
72. Ganschow P, Pfeiffer U, Hinz U, et al. Quality of life ten and more years after restorative proctocolectomy for patients with familial adenomatous polyposis coli. *Dis Colon Rectum* 2010;53:1381.

74. Nieuwenhuis MH, De Vos Tot Nederveen Cappel W, Botma A, et al. Desmoid tumors in a Dutch cohort of patients with familial adenomatous polyposis. *Clin Gastroenterol Hepatol* 2008;6:215.
77. Palomaki G, McClain M, Melillo S, Hampel H, Thibodeau S. EGAPP supplementary evidence review: DNA testing strategies aimed at reducing morbidity and mortality from Lynch syndrome. *Gen Med* 2009;11:42.
80. Valle L, Perea J, Carbonell P, et al. Clinicopathologic and pedigree differences in amsterdam I-positive hereditary nonpolyposis colorectal cancer families according to tumor microsatellite instability status. *J Clin Oncol* 2007;25:781.
82. Umar A, Boland CR, Terdiman JP, et al. Revised Bethesda Guidelines for hereditary nonpolyposis colorectal cancer (Lynch syndrome) and microsatellite instability. *J Natl Cancer Inst* 2004;96:261.
83. Lee-Kong SA, Markowitz AJ, Glogowski E, et al. Prospective immunohistochemical analysis of primary colorectal cancers for loss of mismatch repair protein expression. *Clin Colorectal Cancer* 2010;9:255.
84. Vasen HF, Abdirahman M, Brohet R, et al. One to 2-year surveillance intervals reduce risk of colorectal cancer in families with Lynch syndrome. *Gastroenterology* 2010;138:2300.
86. Rodriguez-Bigas MA, Vasen HF, Pekka-Mecklin J, et al. Rectal cancer risk in hereditary nonpolyposis colorectal cancer after abdominal colectomy. International Collaborative Group on HNPCC. *Ann Surg* 1997;225:202.
89. Kalady MF, McGannon E, Vogel JD, et al. Risk of colorectal adenoma and carcinoma after colectomy for colorectal cancer in patients meeting Amsterdam Criteria. *Ann Surg* 2010;252:507.
90. Guillem JG, Glogowski E, Moore HG, et al. Single-amplicon MSH2 A636P mutation testing in Ashkenazi Jewish patients with colorectal cancer: role in presurgical management. *Ann Surg* 2007;245:560.
91. de Jong AE, Hendriks YM, Kleibeuker JH, et al. Decrease in mortality in Lynch syndrome families because of surveillance. *Gastroenterology* 2006;130:665.

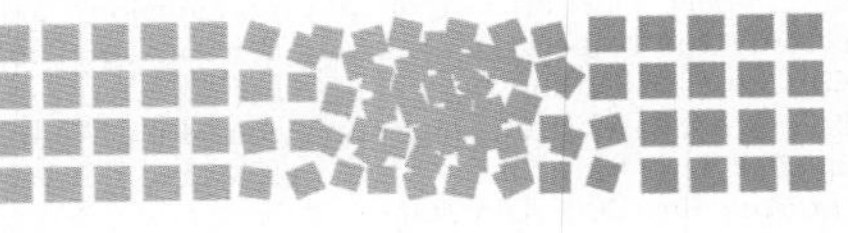

CHAPTER 53 PRINCIPLES OF CANCER RISK REDUCTIVE INTERVENTION

DEAN E. BRENNER

WHY CANCER PREVENTION AS A CLINICAL ONCOLOGY DISCIPLINE?

Until recently, clinical oncology has been defined as a medical specialty that attempts to intervene in order to slow or reverse the final stage of the cancer process—the clonally derived, genomically damaged, invasive cell mass. A stepwise carcinogenesis process that includes critical molecular events and loss of cellular control functions occurs prior to and during the morphologic changes that define neoplasia. Morphologic changes, such as subtle increases in cellular proliferation that progress to early and late precancerous lesions containing dysplastic cells, characterize the carcinogenesis process (Fig. 53.1).[1,2] Opportunities for intervention in this process can include diverse, nonpharmacologic approaches (e.g., obesity management via nutritional diet based interventions, exercise) or pharmacologic interventions (e.g., drugs, purified nutritional extracts, standardized nutritional component mixtures) aimed at delaying or reversing the carcinogenesis process prior to or following the appearance of early morphologic changes. Cancer screening and early detection strategies (e.g., surveillance endoscopy, fecal occult blood testing, mammography) identify not only those individuals with early stage, curable malignant transformations but also those individuals with noninvasive neoplasias that identify those at higher risk than the general population for progression to transformed invasive malignancies.

Historically, many cancer preventive interventions have been considered standards of practice of nononcologic specialists. Nevertheless, oncologists remain community resources in cancer, called on to address broad cancer-related questions that encompass prevention as well as treatment of advanced malignancy. The understanding, use, and management of interventions designed to delay or reverse the carcinogenesis process have become integral components of the oncologist's role as community experts and leaders in cancer care.[19]

DEFINING CANCER RISK REDUCTIVE INTERVENTION (CHEMOPREVENTION)

Cancer risk reductive intervention, commonly referred to as chemoprevention, is the use of a range of interventions from purified drugs to purified dietary extracts to dietary modulation to block, reverse, or prevent the development of invasive cancer.[20,21] Human cancer risk reductive intervention asserts that one can intervene at many steps in the carcinogenesis process, which occurs over many years. This prolonged latency provides opportunities to intervene at many time points and at multiple events in the carcinogenesis process but risks intervention-associated toxicity in otherwise healthy populations. Successful deployment of cancer risk–reductive interventions will reduce cancer-associated mortality or delay the age of mortality.

IDENTIFYING POTENTIAL CANCER RISK REDUCTIVE INTERVENTIONS

Cancer risk reductive interventions (CRRIs) result from the synthesis of data from population, basic, translational, and clinical sciences. Data sets from all of these disciplines are combined to contribute to identification of products with potential to delay or reverse the carcinogenesis process (Fig. 53.1).

Cellular Transformation Mechanism–Based Development of Cancer Risk Reductive Interventions

During the past three decades, signaling pathway intermediate molecules controlling the following cellular functions have been identified to play critical regulatory roles in neoplastic cellular development: self-sufficiency in growth signals, insensitivity to growth-inhibitory signals, evasion of apoptosis, limitless replication potential, sustained angiogenesis, and tissue invasion and metastasis.[22] These alterations can be triggered by a large array of genetic and environmental stressors such as chronic inflammation, oxidation, inherited genetic mutations, and exogenous environmental exposures. Many such signaling intermediates have a common function in multiple organ sites (Fig. 53.1). For example, growth factor receptors or their ligands that regulate cellular proliferation processes have been primary targets for cancer therapeutic interventions (erlotinib and cetuximab [epidermal growth factor receptor], trastuzumab [human epidermal growth factor receptor 2]).[18] The complexity and overlap of signal transduction pathways suggest that single targets may not always be effective. Interventions at multiple pathways or targets may be required to arrest or reverse cellular carcinogenesis.

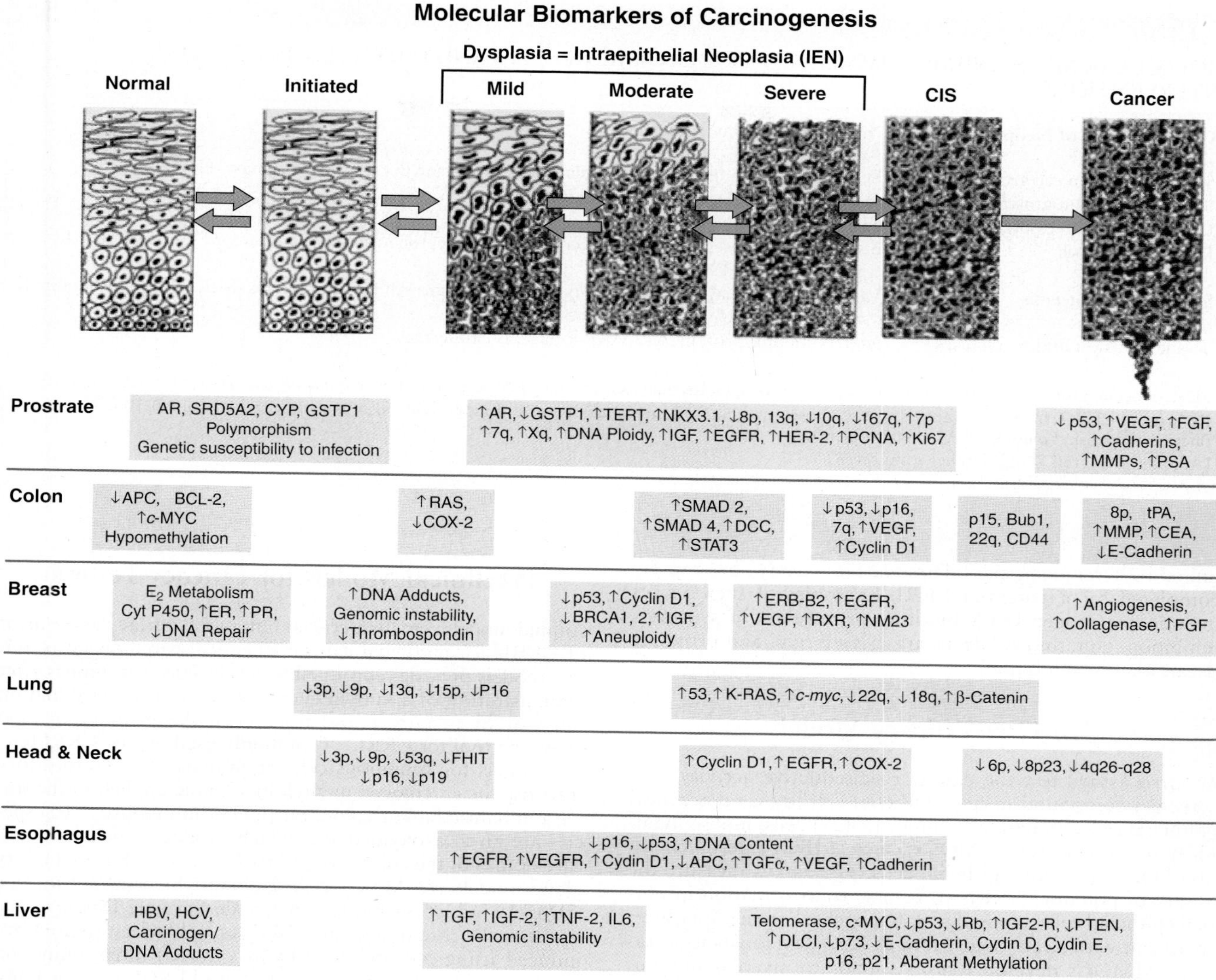

FIGURE 53.1 Genetic progression in major cancers. Carcinogenesis is driven by genetic progression. This progression is marked by the appearance of molecular biomarkers in distinctive patterns representing accumulating changes in gene expression and correlating with changes in histologic phenotype as cells move from normal through the early stages of clonal expansion to dysplasia and finally to early invasive, locally advanced, and metastatic cancer. The figure shows candidate molecular biomarkers of genetic progression in seven target organs: prostate (refs. 3–5) colon (refs. 1, 6), breast (refs. 7, 8), lung (refs. 9–11), head and neck (refs. 12–15), esophagus (refs. 6, 16), and liver (ref. 17). (Figure and revised caption from ref. 18, published with permission from the American Association for Cancer Research.)

Prominent interventions and their modulator targets are listed in Table 53.1.

PRECLINICAL DEVELOPMENT OF CANCER RISK REDUCTIVE INTERVENTIONS

Similar to the development of therapeutic interventions, assessment of efficacy and toxicity of single chemically synthesized entities, agents designed *in silico*, botanicals, purified nutritional extracts, and nutritional supplements for cancer risk reductive efficacy proceeds through a translational paradigm that identifies efficacy in cell culture models, in live animal models, and in humans. Models that simulate the carcinogenesis process in target epithelia identify molecular biomarker events for modulation by interventions. These models can be used to assess toxicity of interventions and to assess the effect of interventions on the development and progression of neoplasia or on preinvasive lesions or intraepithelial neoplasms.[23]

The U.S. National Cancer Institute's preclinical CRRI (chemoprevention) drug screening program is a prime example of a rational strategy to select promising agents for clinical trials through a stepwise approach of preclinical *in vitro* testing followed by *in vivo* screening.[23] This system involves several phases: biochemical prescreening assays, *in vitro* efficacy models, *in vivo* short-term screening, and animal efficacy testing.

Biochemical Prescreening Assays

Prescreening assays are a series of short-term, mechanistic assays developed to evaluate the ability of a test compound to modulate biochemical events presumed to be mechanistically

TABLE 53.1

MOLECULAR MECHANISMS COMMON TO TRANSFORMING CELLS AND POTENTIAL PREVENTIVE INTERVENTIONS

Characteristics of Neoplasia	Possible Molecular Targets
Self-sufficiency in cell growth	Epidermal growth factor receptor, platelet-derived growth factor, MAP-kinase, PI3K
Insensitivity to antigrowth signals	SMADs, pRb, cyclin-dependent kinases, myc
Limitless replicative potential	hTERT, pRb, p53
Evading apoptosis	Bcl-2, BAX, caspases, Fas, tumor necrosis factor receptor, insulin growth factor/PI3K/AKT, mTOR p53, NF-κB, PTEN, *Ras*
Sustained angiogenesis	Vascular endothelial growth factor, basic fibroblast growth factor, integrins ($\alpha_v\beta_3$), thrombospondin-1, hypoxia-inducible factor-1α
Tissue invasion and metastases	Matrix metalloproteinases, MAP-kinase, E-cadherin

PI3K, phosphoinositol-3-kinase; SMAD, drosophila protein, mothers against decapentaplegic gene and the *elegans* protein SMA; pRb, phosphorylate Rb protein; hTERT, human telomerase reverse transcriptase; mTOR, mammalian target of rapamycin; NF-κB, nuclear factor kappa B; PTEN, phosphatase and tensin homolog; MAP, mitogen-activated protein.
(Adapted from ref. 7 and derived from ref. 6.)

linked to carcinogenesis.[23] These *in vitro* assays are rapidly completed for a potential CRRI. Examples of such assays include carcinogen-DNA binding, prostaglandin synthesis inhibition, glutathione-S-transferase inhibition, and ornithine decarboxylase inhibition.

In Vitro Efficacy Models

In vitro assays test the cancer risk reductive activity of a screened compound in five epithelial cell lines: rat tracheal epithelial cells, human lung tumor (A427) cells, mouse mammary organ cultures (MMOCs), mouse JB6 epidermal cells, and human foreskin epithelial cells. The assays measure the ability of potential CRRIs to reverse transformation in normal epithelial cells exposed to carcinogens. For example, after treatment with a carcinogen such as 7,12-demethylbenzathracene, MMOCs develop lesions similar to alveolar nodules that are considered precancerous in mouse mammary glands *in vivo*.[24] Protocols pretreating organ cultures or treating after carcinogen exposures measure the effect of cancer risk reductive agents in the initiation or promotion stages of carcinogenesis. Three of these assays (using rat tracheal epithelial, A427, and MMOC cells) have shown predictive values of 76% to 83% for cancer risk reductive efficacy for *in vivo* models.[23]

In Vivo Short-Term Screening

Short-term screening evaluates the effectiveness of a test agent in early phases of carcinogenesis. For example, two experimental models commonly used include aberrant crypt foci (ACF) assays in rat and mouse colon and the rat mammary gland ductal carcinoma *in situ* (DCIS) assay.[23] For ACF assays, F344 rats are injected with azoxymethane and sacrificed 6 weeks later. ACF lesions consist of large, thick crypts seen in methylene-blue–stained specimens of colon.[25] The occurrence patterns of ACF and their response to CRRIs prior to or following azoxymethane injection parallel those of adenomas and carcinomas in rodent carcinogenesis models.[26] The DCIS carcinogenesis protocol consists of injecting weanling Sprague-Dawley rats with 1-methyl-1-nitrosourea (MNU). CRRIs are administered in the diet continuously starting 1 week after carcinogen administration. Forty-five to 50 days later, the mammary glands are excised and the number of DCIS lesions counted.[27]

Preclinical Models for Efficacy Testing

Animal models remain a crucial link in the efficacy assessment of CRRIs for epithelial cancer. Chemical carcinogenesis animal models provide reproducible development of tumors after administration of a known chemical initiator or combination initiator or promoter and have been the primary *in vivo* screening tool for CRRI.[28] Commonly used *in vivo* CRRI testing models for squamous cell carcinomas of the respiratory tract use the carcinogen methylnitrosamine applied to the trachea in hamsters. For colon, rat (F344) and mouse (CF1) species are given azoxymethane, which produces adenomas and carcinomas of the colon over 36 to 40 weeks.[29] Rat mammary gland models use MNU or 7,12-dimethylbenz(a)-anthracene (DMBA) induction models in female Sprague-Dawley rats, resulting in carcinomas at 120 days.[27] Bladder tumors are induced using *N*-butyl-*N*-(4-hydroxybutyl) nitrosamine via intragastric administration in 50-day-old BDF mice or F344 rats. Bladder tumors occur at 180 days posttreatment.[30] Skin carcinogenesis can be mimicked using DMBA and 12-O-tetradecanoylphorbol-13-acetate in a two-stage protocol, topically to SENCAR or CD-1 mice. Squamous cell carcinomas occur by 18 weeks.[28]

Carcinogenesis models that employ genetically engineered mouse models are a promising alternative to chemical carcinogenesis models. Transgenic models that express a viral or cellular oncogene (e.g., mice overexpressing *Ras*) have not found acceptance as models for CRRI efficacy. Subsequent efforts to manipulate the endogenous genome to create mutations that mimic those found in human tumors have yielded useful data. For example, the mice with manipulated adenomatous polyposis coli, such as Min+ mice, spontaneously develop gut tumors.[31,32] Nonsteroidal anti-inflammatory drugs reduce adenomas and prolong survival in these models.[33,34] Knockout or genetic mutational models create accelerated neoplastic progression that does not accurately recapitulate the more complex, stepwise human carcinogenesis process and, with many genes, can result in embryonic lethality. Conditional alleles allow controlled deletion, reactivation, or mutation of endogenous genes at specific epithelial sites. Recombinant alleles can be driven by the addition of drug-sensitive regulatory elements, such as tetracycline or tamoxifen analogs, to achieve temporal control over specific gene expression. Such mouse models may more accurately recapitulate human carcinogenesis and may be useful for future CRRI efficacy testing.[29,35,36]

TABLE 53.2

CLINICAL DEVELOPMENT OF CANCER RISK REDUCTIVE INTERVENTIONS: RESEARCH PHASES AND END POINTS COMPARED WITH CLINICAL DEVELOPMENT OF CANCER TREATMENT INTERVENTIONS

Phase	Cancer Risk Reductive Clinical Trial Phase	Cancer Treatment Clinical Trial Phase
1	Dose-intervention biomarker trial. Search for lowest dose to modulate biomarker of drug delivery and carcinogenesis biology. End point = biomarker change without toxicity.	Dose-response trial designed to search maximum tolerated dose. Primary end point = toxicity. Secondary end points may be biomarker for targeted therapeutics.
2	2a: Short-term, multiple dose to define lowest safe dose to modulate biomarker(s) associated with carcinogenesis of an epithelial target. 2b: Intermediate (6–12 months) to long duration (3 years +), randomized clinical trial with a validated biomarker end point that may be used as a surrogate for a cancer incidence at an epithelial target.	Preliminary efficacy testing. Trials designed to define biological response through the use of an imaged view of an invasive neoplasm at a primary or metastatic site or biomarker end point related to mechanism of action of a targeted agent. End point usually reduction in size of the imaged invasive neoplasm.
3	Randomized, controlled clinical trial in a high-risk population. Cancer incidence the primary end point.	Randomized, controlled clinical trial with a survival, disease-free survival, or time to progression end point.

CLINICAL DEVELOPMENT OF CANCER RISK REDUCTIVE INTERVENTIONS

Special Features of Cancer Risk Reductive Intervention Development

Clinical efficacy assessment of chemopreventive agents employs phased testing (phase 1 to 3) models used for development of drugs,[37] but with crucial differences in study design and end points (Table 53.2). Special features for the clinical development of CRRIs create the following challenges to be overcome:

1. Large therapeutic index. The potential toxicity of an intervention aimed at delaying or reversing transformation should be acceptable to individuals who are asymptomatic yet may benefit from an extended (years) treatment course.
2. Long latency to malignant transformation. Assessment of effectiveness based on the reduction in cancer incidence requires studies lasting for years and involving thousands of participants.
3. Adherence. Once-daily dosing regimens using interventions that have sufficiently prolonged half-lives may minimize the impact of a dropped dose yet maintain the biological impact on the physiologic target. Minimal toxicity and strong psychological commitment to preventive goals also enhance adherence.[38]
4. Complex risk assessment for cancer. Individuals with highly penetrant but infrequent germ line genetic mutations predict for cancer risk for breast and colon cancers[39,40] are candidates for CRRIs and will accept some toxicity for reduced cancer risk. For individuals at lower risk than germ line mutation carriers but who are at higher risk than normal based upon epidemiologic associations, such as environmental exposures, lifestyle variables (e.g., diet, exercise, smoking), quantitative risk assessment algorithms may be useful in the future to identify optimal CRRI.

Biomarkers as Cancer Risk Reductive Intervention Targets and Efficacy End Points

A biomarker is a characteristic that is measured and evaluated as an indicator of normal biologic processes, pathogenic processes, or pharmacologic responses to therapeutic interventions.[41] A surrogate end point for cancer prevention assumes that a measured biological feature will predict the presence or future development of a cancer outcome.[42] The primary motivation for development of such surrogate end points concerns the ability to diagnose cancer at an early stage, to identify individuals at high risk for cellular transformation, and to enable reduction in the size and duration of an intervention trial by replacing a rare or distal end point with a more frequent, proximate end point.[43] Intraepithelial neoplasia (IEN) has served as and continues to serve as a biomarker for invasive malignancy (Table 53.3). Although many advocate the use of IEN-based biomarkers as regulatory surrogate end points, others caution that IEN may not serve as a sufficiently robust surrogate biomarkers for cancer incidence or mortality.[44]

In order to be useful as end points for cancer risk reductive efficacy testing as regulatory end points, any biomarker must have statistical accuracy, precision, and effectiveness of results[44] that demonstrates prediction of a "hard" disease end point—cancer incidence or mortality. The validation data set must address defined standards of validation, avoiding and accounting for overfitting and bias. The biomarker must be generalizable to the specific clinical or screening population (Table 53.4). Future progress in linking the genetic changes in neoplastic progression with biologically important functional consequences will provide improved biomarkers, interventional targets, and strategies.

TABLE 53.3

COMMON INTRAEPITHELIAL NEOPLASIAS

Epithelium	Intraepithelial Neoplasia	Reference
Colon and rectum	Adenoma	45
Lower esophagus	Barrett's esophagus	46
Upper esophagus	Squamous dysplasia	47, 48
Skin-squamous/ basal cell	Actinic keratosis	49
Skin-pigmented	Dysplastic nevus	50
Cervix	Cervical intraepithelial neoplasia	51
Head and neck	Leukoplakia	52
Lung	Bronchial dysplasia	53

TABLE 53.4

CHARACTERISTICS OF BIOMARKERS FOR USE AS ENDPOINTS IN CANCER RISK REDUCTIVE EFFICACY ASSESSMENT

- Variability of expression between phases of the carcinogenesis process
- Detected early in the carcinogenesis process
- Genetic progression or protein pathway based
- Target of modulation by preventive interventions
- Changes in biomarker linked to reduction in incident cancer of epithelial target
- Changes in biomarker linked to clinical benefit
- Can be quantified directly or via closely related activity such as a downstream target or upstream kinase
- Measurable in an accessible biosample (preferably urine, serum, saliva, stool, or breath)
- High throughput, technically feasible, analytical procedure with strong quality assurance or quality control procedures
- Cost-effective

Phases of Cancer Risk Reductive Intervention Development

Phase 1 cancer risk reductive trials define an optimal cancer risk reductive dose (Table 53.2). An optimal cancer risk reductive dose is one that is usually nontoxic, scheduled once daily, and modulates a tissue, cellular, or serum surrogate of drug activity (e.g., the dose of aspirin that inhibits prostaglandin production in a target tissue site). Definition of a maximal tolerable dose is not an essential end point of phase 1 cancer risk reductive trials. Higher, yet nontoxic doses may reduce cancer risk reductive efficacy. For example, beta carotene at high doses has pro-oxidant activity and may enhance the carcinogenesis process, while at low doses it is a potent antioxidant and differentiating agent.[54]

Phase 2 cancer risk reductive trials begin to define cancer risk reduction efficacy. These short-term (6 months to 1 year) treatment periods gather evidence of risk reduction by assessing drug effect on tissue, cellular, or blood surrogates of carcinogenesis. Phase 2a trials are nonrandomized, biomarker modulation trials. Phase 2b trials are randomized, placebo-controlled trials of several hundred subjects with changes in recurrence of a pathologic, usually IEN, cellular dynamic (e.g., proliferation, apoptotic index), biochemical or molecular (e.g., p53, cyclin D, microsatellite expression) end point(s). For example, trials of aspirin,[55] calcium,[56] or a combination of sulindac and difluoromethylornithine[57] reduce the recurrence of sporadic adenomatous polyps in humans, strongly suggesting colorectal cancer risk reduction efficacy for these interventions.

Phase 3 cancer risk reductive trials define reduction in a hard cancer end point such as cancer incidence or mortality. Such trials use large, high-risk populations in a randomized, double-blinded intervention and are designed to identify a standard of preventive care for a given risk population. For example, trials of tamoxifen for the reduction of breast cancer incidence,[58,59] finasteride for the reduction of prostate cancer incidence,[60] and beta carotene for the reduction of lung cancer incidence serve as examples of well-conducted, definitive phase 3 cancer risk reductive clinical trials.[61]

Some investigators consider randomized, controlled clinical trials with an end point sufficient for regulatory review as phase 3. Using such a definition, a clinical trial with an end point of reduction in adenoma recurrence is considered a phase 3 trial. Other investigators define phase 3 cancer risk reductive trials as randomized, controlled clinical trials with a cancer incidence or mortality end point. This controversy causes confusion in the literature. For the purpose of clarity in this chapter, the later definition of phase 3 trial is used—a prospective, randomized, controlled clinical trial with a cancer incidence or mortality end point. Randomized, controlled clinical trials with a surrogate biomarker end point such as an IEN (e.g., adenoma) are defined as phase 2b cancer risk reductive trials.

IMPLEMENTATION OF CANCER RISK REDUCTIVE INTERVENTIONS IN THE COMMUNITY

A systemic approach to identification, preclinical, and clinical testing of potential cancer risk reductives ultimately results in interventions for individuals, families, and populations at varying degrees of risk for the development of future cancers. CRRIs for the prevention of colorectal adenocarcinoma[55,56] and breast cancer[58] have shown efficacy, yet uptake into community practice has been limited. A personalized CRRI strategy based on specific biomarker profiles defining increased risk for cancer at a given organ matched with activity or toxicity profiles of currently available CRRIs promises to improve generalization to community use. Future strategies aim to improve the therapeutic index of CRRIs by identification of dietary components and extracts with strong cancer risk reductive mechanisms and combining CRRIs at lower, less toxic doses. The inclusion of CRRIs into daily medical practice will be based on evidence of individual cancer risk and CRRI-demonstrated reduction in cancer incidence and mortality.

Selected References

The full list of references for this chapter appears in the online version.

1. Fearon ER, Vogelstein B. A genetic model for colorectal tumorigenesis. *Cell* 1990;61:759.
2. Sidransky D. Emerging molecular markers of cancer. *Nat Rev Cancer* 2002;2:210.
3. Nelson WG, De Marzo AM, Isaacs WB. Prostate cancer. *N Engl J Med* 2003;349:366.
6. Barrett MT, Sanchez CA, Prevo LJ, et al. Evolution of neoplastic cell lineages in Barrett oesophagus. *Nat Genet* 1999;22:106.
7. Dontu G, Liu S, Wicha MS. Stem cells in mammary development and carcinogenesis: implications for prevention and treatment. *Stem Cell Rev* 2005;1:207.
10. Massion PP, Carbone DP. The molecular basis of lung cancer: molecular abnormalities and therapeutic implications. *Respir Res* 2003;4:12.
11. Mao L, Lee JS, Kurie JM, et al. Clonal genetic alterations in the lungs of current and former smokers. *J Natl Cancer Inst* 1997;89:857.
14. Califano J, van der Riet P, Westra W, et al. Genetic progression model for head and neck cancer: implications for field cancerization. *Cancer Res* 1996;56:2488.
15. Braakhuis BJ, Tabor MP, Kummer JA, et al. A genetic explanation of Slaughter's concept of field cancerization: evidence and clinical implications. *Cancer Res* 2003;63:1727.
16. Reid BJ, Levine DS, Longton G, et al. Predictors of progression to cancer in Barrett's esophagus: baseline histology and flow cytometry identify low- and high-risk patient subsets. *Am J Gastroenterol* 2000;95:1669.
18. Kelloff GJ, Lippman SM, Dannenberg AJ, et al. Progress in chemoprevention drug development: the promise of molecular biomarkers for prevention of intraepithelial neoplasia and cancer—a plan to move forward. *Clin Cancer Res* 2006;12:3661.

19. Lippman SM, Levin B, Brenner DE, et al. Cancer prevention and the American Society of Clinical Oncology. *J Clin Oncol* 2004;22:3848.
20. Wattenberg L. Chemoprevention of cancer. *Cancer Res* 1985;45:1.
21. Greenwald P, Kelloff G. The role of chemoprevention in cancer control. *IARC Sci Publ (Lyon)* 1996;139:13.
22. Hanahan D, Weinberg RA. The hallmarks of cancer. *Cell* 2000;100:57.
23. Steele VE, Boone CW, Lubet RA, et al. Preclinical drug development paradigms for chemopreventives. *Hematol Oncol Clin North Am* 1998;12:943.
24. Mehta RG, Naithani R, Huma L, et al. Efficacy of chemopreventive agents in mouse mammary gland organ culture (MMOC) model: a comprehensive review. *Curr Med Chem* 2008;15:2785.
26. Khare S, Chaudhary K, Bissonnette M, et al. Aberrant crypt foci in colon cancer epidemiology. *Methods Mol Biol* 2009;472:373.
27. Medina D. Chemical carcinogenesis of rat and mouse mammary glands. *Breast Dis* 2007;28:63.
28. Hoenerhoff MJ, Hong HH, Ton TV, et al. A review of the molecular mechanisms of chemically induced neoplasia in rat and mouse models in National Toxicology Program bioassays and their relevance to human cancer. *Toxicol Pathol* 2009;37:835.
29. Rosenberg DW, Giardina C, Tanaka T. Mouse models for the study of colon carcinogenesis. *Carcinogenesis* 2009;30:183.
31. Moser AR, Pitot HC, Dove WF. A dominant mutation that predisposes to multiple intestinal neoplasia in the mouse. *Science* 1990;247:322.
32. Corpet DE, Pierre F. Point: From animal models to prevention of colon cancer. Systematic review of chemoprevention in min mice and choice of the model system. *Cancer Epidemiol Biomarkers Prev* 2003;12:391.
35. Olive KP, Tuveson DA. The use of targeted mouse models for preclinical testing of novel cancer therapeutics. *Clin Cancer Res* 2006;12:5277.
36. Jeet V, Russell PJ, Khatri A. Modeling prostate cancer: a perspective on transgenic mouse models [Review]. *Cancer Metastasis Rev* 2010;29:123.
37. Shureiqi I, Reddy P, Brenner DE. Chemoprevention: general perspective. *Crit Rev Oncol Hematol* 2000;33:157.
38. Becker M. Adherence to prescribed therapies. *Med Care* 1985;23:539.
39. Miki Y, Swensen J, Shattuck-Eidens D, et al. A strong candidate for the breast and ovarian cancer susceptibility gene BRCA1. *Science* 1994;266:66.
40. Powell SM, Petersen GM, Krush AJ, et al. Molecular diagnosis of familial adenomatous polyposis. *N Engl J Med* 1993;329:1982.
41. Definitions Working Group. *Biomarkers and surrogate endpoints*. Bethesda, MD: National Institutes of Health, Food and Drug Administration, 1999.
42. Schatzkin A, Freedman LS, Schiffman MH, et al. Validation of intermediate end points in cancer research. *J Natl Cancer Inst* 1990;82:1746.
43. Prentice R. Surrogate endpoints in clinical trials: definition and operational criteria. *Stat Med* 1989;8:431.
44. Ransohoff DF. Rules of evidence for cancer molecular-marker discovery and validation. *Nat Rev Cancer* 2004;4:309.
45. Winawer SJ, Zauber AG, Ho MN, et al. Prevention of colorectal cancer by colonoscopic polypectomy. The National Polyp Study Workgroup. *N Engl J Med* 1993;329:1977.
48. Taylor P, Li B, Dawsey S, et al. Prevention of esophageal cancer: the nutrition intervention trials in Linxian, China. Linxian Nutrition Intervention Trials Study Group. *Cancer Res* 1994;54:2029s.
49. Sober A, Burstein J. Precursors to skin cancer. *Cancer* 1995;75(Suppl):645.
50. Tucker M, Halpern A, Holly E, et al. Clinically recognized dysplastic nevi. A central risk factor for cutaneous melanoma. *JAMA* 1997;277:1439.
51. Gustafsson L, Adami H-O. Natural history of cervical neoplasia: consistent results obtained by an identification technique. *Br J Cancer* 1989;60:132.
52. Cawson R. Premalignant lesions in the mouth. *Br Med Bull* 1975;31:164.
53. Saccomanno G, Archer VE, Auerbach O, et al. Development of carcinoma of the lung as reflected in exfoliated cells. *Cancer* 1974;33:256.
55. Baron JA, Cole BF, Sandler RS, et al. A randomized trial of aspirin to prevent colorectal adenomas. *N Engl J Med* 2003;348:891.
56. Baron JA, Beach M, Mandel JS, et al. Calcium supplements for the prevention of colorectal adenomas. Calcium Polyp Prevention Study Group. *N Engl J Med* 1999;340:101.
57. Meyskens FL Jr, McLaren CE, Pelot D, et al. Difluoromethylornithine plus sulindac for the prevention of sporadic colorectal adenomas: a randomized placebo-controlled, double-blind trial. *Cancer Prev Res (Phila Pa)* 2008;1:32.
58. Fisher B, Costantino J, Wickerham D, et al. Tamoxifen for prevention of breast cancer: report of the National Surgical Adjuvant Breast and Bowel Project P-1 study. *J Natl Cancer Inst* 1998;90:1371.
59. Vogel VG, Costantino JP, Wickerham DL, et al. Update of the National Surgical Adjuvant Breast and Bowel Project study of tamoxifen and raloxifene (STAR) P-2 Trial: preventing breast cancer. *Cancer Prev Res (Phila Pa)* 2010;3:696.
60. Thompson IM, Goodman PJ, Tangen CM, et al. The influence of finasteride on the development of prostate cancer. *N Engl J Med* 2003;349:215.
61. Omenn G, Goodman G, Thornquist M, et al. Effects of a combination of beta carotene and vitamin A on lung cancer and cardiovascular disease. *N Engl J Med* 1996;334:1150.

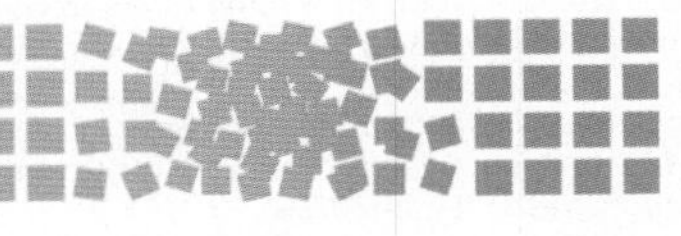

CHAPTER 54 RETINOIDS, CAROTENOIDS, AND OTHER MICRONUTRIENTS IN CANCER PREVENTION

SUSAN T. MAYNE, EDWARD GIOVANNUCCI, AND SCOTT M. LIPPMAN

Cancer chemoprevention can be defined as pharmacologic intervention with specific nutrients or other chemicals to suppress or reverse carcinogenesis and to prevent the development of invasive cancer.[1] Two basic concepts support this cancer control strategy: multistep and field carcinogenesis. Carcinogenesis is a chronic, multistep process characterized by the accumulation of specific genetic, epigenetic, and phenotypic alterations that can evolve over a 10- to 20-plus-year period from the first initiating event. The premise of human chemoprevention is that one can intervene (and suppress) at many steps in the carcinogenic process and over a period of many years. A wave of new technology (e.g., high-resolution endoscopy, laser-capture microdissection, multiplex gene/expression/protein arrays, and small interfering RNA) is rapidly increasing our understanding of neoplastic evolution. It is now understood that this process can involve mutations in key tumor suppressor genes and/or oncogenes, epigenetic changes via aberrations of histone acetylation or DNA methylation, genetic instability, and defects in signal transduction, with clonal expansion and, remarkably, intraepithelial spread/metastasis of premalignant cells.[2] Certain micronutrients can modulate microRNA expression in tobacco smoke-exposed rat lungs,[3] and recent data showing smoking-dependent changes in microRNA expression in human-airway epithelium suggest that these changes may be important in the early pathogenesis of certain lung cancers.[4,5] Field carcinogenesis was first described in the early 1950s as "field cancerization" in the head and neck, and subsequently was ascribed to many epithelial sites. The field concept is that patients have a wide surface area of carcinogenic tissue change that can be detected at the gross (oral premalignant lesions, polyps), microscopic (metaplasia, dysplasia), and/or molecular (gene loss or amplification) levels. Recent molecular studies detecting profound genetic alterations in histologically normal tissue from high-risk individuals have provided strong support for the field carcinogenesis concept. The implication of the field effect is that multifocal, genetically distinct, and clonally related premalignant lesions can progress over a broad tissue region. The essence of chemoprevention, then, is intervention within the multistep carcinogenic process and throughout a wide field.

To date, retinoids (the natural derivatives and synthetic analogs of vitamin A) and β-β-carotene (a member of the carotenoid class) are among the best-studied agents in human chemoprevention, for which their record includes several completed phase 3 efficacy trials. As will be discussed in detail later, whereas some trials have demonstrated chemopreventive efficacy for retinoids and carotenoids, adverse effects have also been noted, particularly in some patient populations. The "antioxidant" nutrient vitamin E and the trace mineral selenium have also been evaluated in phase 3 randomized cancer prevention trials, as will be discussed in this chapter. Other micronutrients such as folate, calcium, and vitamin D also have been of interest for chemoprevention, with some completed trials to date, as will also be discussed. Because of space limitations, this chapter will emphasize these compounds, with brief mention of other selected micronutrients in human cancer chemoprevention. The structure of this chapter is based on organ sites for the benefit of clinicians interested in preventive interventions for specific tumor sites.

HEAD AND NECK CANCER CHEMOPREVENTION

Squamous cell carcinomas of the head and neck have been a model for chemoprevention research involving micronutrients for decades. This particular organ site has many advantages for prevention research purposes: intermediate markers (e.g., oral premalignant lesions) and easily visualized target tissue are available, it is a well-characterized risk model and classic model of field carcinogenesis, and it is frequently a site of the important clinical problem of recurrences and second primary tumors (SPTs) in curatively treated cancer patients.

Risk Considerations

Early risk assessments focused on the histology of oral premalignant lesions, which include leukoplakias and erythroplakias. Small hyperplastic leukoplakia lesions have a 30% to 40% spontaneous regression rate and less than a 5% risk of malignant transformation; in contrast, erythroleukoplakia and dysplastic leukoplakia lesions have a low rate of spontaneous regression and a 30% to 40% long-term risk of oral cancer.[2,6] In more recent work, 3-year oral cancer risks associated with various microsatellite marker profiles (of loss of heterozygosity or microsatellite instability) in oral leukoplakia patients range from 25% to 70%.[7,8] The ability of markers such as these to predict future risk of malignancy may be important in targeting chemopreventive agents toward individuals most likely to benefit from preventive interventions, and could minimize the number of trial participants who will be exposed to chemopreventive agents that may have unknown adverse effects (improved risk-benefit profile). Therefore, risk prediction is an important part of chemoprevention development for all organ sites, but is only briefly mentioned here to illustrate the point.

Head And Neck Trials: Premalignancy

Some of the first evidence supporting micronutrient-based chemoprevention came from studies in the 1980s in populations at a relatively high risk of oral cancer (tobacco chewers, betel quid chewers). Early trials demonstrated that supplemental β-carotene and retinol significantly reduced the frequency of oral micronuclei; this supported further evaluation of β-carotene/retinol/retinoids in oral premalignant lesions. As summarized in a meta-analysis,[9] treatment with β-carotene, lycopene, and vitamin A was associated with significant rates of clinical resolution, compared with placebo or absence of treatment.

Retinoids also have been studied extensively in the reversal of oral premalignant lesions.[2,6] An important early randomized placebo-controlled study (reported in 1986) found that high-dose 13-*cis*-retinoic acid (13cRA; 2 mg/kg/d) was highly active but intolerable and ceased working after drug was stopped.[10] A subsequent trial found that low-dose 13cRA (0.5 mg/kg/d) (following high-dose 13cRA induction) was more effective in preventing progression of oral premalignant lesions than was β-carotene (30 mg/d)—progression rates of 8% (13cRA) versus 55% (β-carotene) ($P < .001$), although toxicity results favored the β-carotene arm.[11] Other randomized trials of retinoids showing significant preventive activity in oral premalignancy include one of *N*-(4-hydroxyphenyl) retinamide (4HPR, or fenretinide) versus control,[12] two involving retinol,[13,14] and one involving *N*-4-(hydroxycarbophenyl) retinamide (4HCR)[15]—all indicating significant retinoid chemopreventive activity. In a nonrandomized phase 2 trial, 4HPR (200 mg/d for 3 months) produced 12 (34.3%) partial clinical responses (95% confidence interval [CI], 19.2%–52.4%) in 35 oral leukoplakia patients who had not responded (*de novo* resistance) or who had responded and then relapsed (acquired resistance) to previous treatment with natural retinoids.[16]

Evidence of chemopreventive efficacy in the oral premalignancy model is necessary but not sufficient for recommending clinical use of a putative chemopreventive agent. Trials in premalignancy generally lack the sample size needed to fully characterize benefits and risks associated with the long-term use of an agent (e.g., effects on cancer-specific and all-cause mortality). As will be discussed later, results of phase 3 trials of retinoids and the carotenoid β-carotene have greatly limited the clinical development of these agents, despite consistent evidence of efficacy in the oral premalignancy model.

Head and Neck Trials: Malignancy

There have been three completed phase 3 adjuvant chemoprevention trials of retinoids and three involving β-carotene in head and neck cancer. Conducted by Hong et al.,[17] the first retinoid trial is historic because it provided the first proof of the principle of cancer chemoprevention. High-dose 13cRA (50-100 mg/m²/d) produced no significant differences in primary disease recurrence (local, regional, or distant) or survival but significantly lowered the rate of SPTs (vs. placebo) ($P = .005$) in 103 head and neck cancer patients followed for a median of 32 months. Reanalyzed after a median follow-up of 55 months, the reduction in SPTs in the aerodigestive tract persisted in the treated group (vs. placebo) ($P = .008$).[18] Substantial retinoid toxicity, however, including skin dryness and peeling, cheilitis, conjunctivitis, and hypertriglyceridemia, necessitated dose reductions in 30% of the retinoid-treated patients and prevented 18% from completing the intervention (12 months).

A follow-up phase 3 trial of low-dose, long-term 13cRA was conducted in 1,190 randomized patients who had been curatively treated for stage I or II head and neck squamous cell carcinoma. These patients were randomized to receive either 13cRA or placebo for 3 years and were followed for 4 more years. There was no significant difference between the treatment and placebo arms in overall survival or SPT- or recurrence-free survival.[19] In the third randomized trial (conducted in France), the synthetic retinoid etretinate (50 mg/d for 1 month, then 25 mg/d for 2 years) was well tolerated but did not significantly reduce SPTs (vs. placebo) at a median follow-up of 41 months in 316 patients following definitive therapy of stage I to III (T1,2N0,1) squamous cell carcinoma of the oral cavity and oropharynx.[20]

Supplemental β-carotene has been studied as a single agent and in combination with other agents for prevention of SPTs of the mouth and throat. After definitive local therapy, 264 patients with stage I or II head and neck cancer were randomized to either supplemental β-carotene (50 mg/d) or identical placebo.[21] The median follow-up was 51.1 months from the date of randomization. There was no significant benefit for risk of second head and neck cancer (relative risk [RR] = 0.69; 95% CI 0.39-1.25) or lung cancer (RR = 1.44; 95% CI, 0.62-3.39). Another secondary prevention trial involving β-carotene (30 mg/d) and alpha tocopherol (400 IU/d) was initiated in 540 head and neck cancer patients. β-Carotene was discontinued during the trial, based on adverse effects on lung cancer observed in other trials (see the section "Lung Trials: Malignancy"), but the trial continued with alpha tocopherol intervention. After a median 6.5 years of follow-up, all-cause mortality was significantly increased in the supplemented group.[22] A smaller Italian trial of β-carotene only (75 mg/d for 3 months with 1-month drug holiday) observed no significant harm or benefit in comparison to no treatment.[23] Another adjuvant chemoprevention study, the European Study on Chemoprevention with Vitamin A and *N*-Acetylcysteine (EUROSCAN), included both head and neck and lung cancer patients and is discussed in the section "Lung Trials: Malignancy."

In summary, both retinoids and β-carotene appear to have chemopreventive efficacy in oral premalignancy, but the trials with cancer end points have either failed to demonstrate significant efficacy or have raised serious concerns over side effects (further discussed in the section "Lung Trials: Malignancy"). For these reasons, retinoids and β carotene are not in current clinical use in head and neck cancer chemoprevention. Further interest in retinoids combined with other agents continues, however. For example, a pharmacogenomic study showed that a retinoic acid-based regimen significantly decreased head and neck cancer development in high-risk patients who had a certain cyclin D1 genotype[24]; this work may lead to future study of retinoid combinations in head and neck and lung cancer chemoprevention in targeted patient populations.[25]

LUNG CANCER CHEMOPREVENTION

Lung Trials: Premalignancy

The Tyler (Texas) Chemoprevention Trial randomized 755 asbestos workers to receive β-carotene (50 mg/d) and retinol (25,000 IU every other day) versus placebo to see if the nutrient combination could reduce the prevalence of atypical cells in sputum. After a mean intervention period of 58 months, there was no significant difference in the two groups in the prevalence of sputum atypia.[26]

In a French trial, chronic smokers with squamous metaplasia of the bronchial epithelium detected in initial bronchoscopy specimens were treated with etretinate (25 mg/d) for 6 months.[27] In this uncontrolled trial, a decline in the extent of squamous metaplasia was observed in most treated patients. The positive result of this French study led to three randomized trials—one of etretinate in Canada, and one of 13cRA and another of fenretinide in the United States. The Canadian study evaluated the ability of 25 mg of etretinate per day for 6 months to reverse sputum atypia in chronic smokers.[28] Toxicity was mild and the number of subjects requiring dose reductions or dropping out was very small and similar in both arms. No difference in the degree of atypia occurred between the etretinate and placebo groups. In the U.S. 13cRA study, chronic smokers underwent bronchoscopy with endobronchial biopsies taken from six specific anatomic sites within the proximal lung field,[29] as reported in the earlier single-arm French study.[27] Ninety-three of the 152 chronic smokers who underwent bronchoscopic biopsies had squamous metaplasia or dysplasia. Eligible smokers with metaplasia or dysplasia were randomized to 6 months of 13cRA or placebo. The extent of metaplasia decreased similarly (in approximately 50% of subjects) in both study arms. Only smoking cessation was associated significantly with a reduction in the metaplasia index during the 6-month intervention. Fenretinide was studied in the most recent trial.[30] This study was similar to the earlier 13cRA study with respect to overall design and lack of treatment effect.[29] Retinoid studies have also focused on high-risk former smokers, with preliminary promising results involving intermediate end points that led to chemoprevention studies with other agents in former smokers.[31] Clinical trial results and correlative *in vitro* studies indicated that phosphatidylinositol 3-kinase (PI3K) may be an important target of natural agents for lung cancer chemoprevention.[32]

Lung Trials: Malignancy

Two large trials of β-carotene plus other micronutrients for primary prevention of lung cancer have been completed. The first, known as the Alpha-Tocopherol, Beta-Carotene (ATBC) Trial, involved 29,133 men aged 50 to 69 years old from Finland, who were heavy cigarette smokers at entry.[33] The study design was a 2 × 2 factorial with participants randomized to receive either supplemental alpha tocopherol (50 mg/d), β-carotene (20 mg/d), the combination, or placebo for 5 to 8 years. Unexpectedly, participants receiving β-carotene (alone or in combination with alpha tocopherol) had a statistically significant 18% increase in lung cancer incidence (RR = 1.18; 95% CI, 1.03-1.36) and 8% increase in total mortality (RR =1.08; 95% CI, 1.01-1.16) relative to participants receiving placebo. Supplemental β-carotene did not appear to affect the incidence of other major cancers occurring in this population. Although not the primary outcome of this trial, an interesting observation was made with regard to vitamin E and prostate cancer. That is, men randomized to receive alpha tocopherol had a 32% decrease in prostate cancer incidence and a 41% decrease in prostate cancer mortality.[34] This finding led to a large follow-up phase 3 trial, the Selenium and Vitamin E Chemoprevention Trial (SELECT; see the section "Prostate Cancer Chemoprevention").

The finding of an increased incidence of lung cancer in β-carotene–supplemented smokers was replicated in another major trial. The Carotene and Retinol Efficacy Trial (CARET) was a multicenter lung cancer prevention trial of supplemental β-carotene (30 mg/d) plus retinol (25,000 IU/d) versus placebo in asbestos workers and smokers.[35] CARET was terminated early because interim analyses of the data indicated that should the trial have continued for its planned duration, it is highly unlikely that the intervention would have been found to be beneficial. Furthermore, the interim results indicated that the supplemented group was developing more lung cancer, not less, consistent with the results of the ATBC trial. Overall, lung cancer incidence was increased by 28% in the supplemented subjects (RR = 1.28; 95% CI, 1.04-1.57) and total mortality was also increased (RR = 1.17; 95% CI, 1.03-1.33). The increase in lung cancer following supplementation with β-carotene and retinol was observed for current but not former smokers. In contrast, the Physicians' Health Study (PHS) of supplemental β-carotene versus placebo in 22,071 male U.S. physicians reported no significant effect—positive or negative—of 12 years of supplementation of β-carotene (50 mg every other day) on total cancer, lung cancer, or cardiovascular disease.[36] The relative risk for lung cancer in current smokers randomized to β-carotene was 0.90 (95% CI, 0.58-1.40). Among nonsmokers, the relative risk was 0.78 (95% CI, 0.34-1.79). A similar lack of effect of supplemental β-carotene on overall cancer incidence was seen in the Women's Health Study, although the duration of intervention was short (median, 2.1 years),[37] and in the Medical Research Council/British Heart Foundation Heart Protection Study of antioxidant vitamin supplementation, although a combination intervention was used (600 mg of vitamin E, 250 mg of vitamin C, and 20 mg of β-carotene daily).[38]

A clear mechanism to explain the apparent enhancement of lung carcinogenesis by supplemental β-carotene, alone or in combination with retinol, in smokers has yet to emerge, although several theories have been suggested. As detailed elsewhere,[39] it should be noted that the two trials that observed this enhancing effect had higher median plasma β-carotene concentrations in their intervention groups than did the trials that did not observe an enhancing effect. High tissue concentrations of β-carotene in the presence of strongly oxidative tobacco smoke appear to interact to promote carcinogenesis. Wang et al.[40] have used the ferret to model β-carotene/tobacco interactions in lung and noted a relative lack of both retinoic acid and RARß expression in the lung of smoke-exposed ferrets given high-dose β-carotene. The authors suggested that oxidative metabolites of β-carotene might cause diminished retinoid signaling and thus increase tumorigenesis. In contrast with a pharmacologic dose of β-carotene, a physiological dose of β-carotene in smoke-exposed ferrets had no potentially detrimental effects and may have afforded weak protection against lung damage induced by cigarette smoke.[41] Characterization of the complex array of oxidation products of β-carotene is under way, along with mechanistic studies to evaluate the effects of such products. Although mechanistic studies continue, it is recommended that heavy smokers avoid high-dose supplements of β-carotene.

Early data suggesting that retinoid chemoprevention may help control SPTs, recurrence, and mortality of stage I non–small cell lung cancer patients led to two large-scale phase 3 retinoid trials in the setting of SPT prevention. One of these was a European trial called EUROSCAN,[42] which was an open-label multicenter trial employing a 2 × 2 factorial design to test 2 years of retinyl palmitate and *N*-acetylcysteine in preventing SPTs in 2,592 patients. Patients had completed definitive therapy of early-stage head and neck cancer (larynx: Tis, T1-3, and N0-1; oral cavity: T1-2 and N0-1) and non–small cell lung cancer (T1-2, N0-1, and T3N0). Retinyl palmitate and/or *N*-acetylcysteine produced no improvement in event-free survival, survival, or incidence of SPTs.

The other large SPT trial, called the Lung Intergroup Trial, was a multicenter U.S. National Cancer Institute Intergroup phase 3 trial involving 1,166 patients with pathologic stage I non–small cell lung cancer (6 weeks to 3 years from definitive resection and no prior radiotherapy or chemotherapy), who were randomly assigned to receive placebo or 13cRA

(30 mg/d) for 3 years in a double-blind fashion. The primary end point was time to SPT, and the secondary end points were times to recurrence and death. After a median follow-up of 3.5 years, there were no statistically significant differences between the placebo and 13cRA arms with respect to the time to SPTs, recurrences, or mortality.[43] Whereas this trial had null results overall, a different picture emerged on stratification of patient smoking status. In this subgroup analysis, 13cRA was apparently harmful in current smokers yet beneficial in former smokers, with a statistically significant interaction between treatment and smoking status (mortality was highest in current smokers randomized to 13cRA). Overall, the carotenoid and retinoid trials indicate that chemoprevention in current smokers may be particularly challenging.[44]

BREAST CANCER CHEMOPREVENTION

Moon et al.[45] first showed that fenretinide was a promising cancer chemopreventive agent for the breast, having a high therapeutic index and synergistic interaction with tamoxifen in mammary carcinogenesis model studies. This laboratory work led to a large-scale randomized trial of fenretinide (vs. no treatment) for 5 years to prevent contralateral breast cancer in women aged 30 to 70 years with a history of resected early breast cancer and no prior adjuvant therapy.[46] The intervention produced no significant overall effect. Subset analyses suggested that fenretinide reduced contralateral and ipsilateral breast cancer rates in premenopausal women, with an opposite (adverse) trend observed in postmenopausal women. The reduced incidence of second breast cancer in premenopausal patients was subsequently confirmed in a 15-year follow-up report.[47] Secondary analyses also indicated a fenretinide-related decrease in ovarian cancer.[48]

Promising preclinical data on retinoid X receptor (RXR)-selective retinoids show the potential of this retinoid class for preventing estrogen receptor (ER)–negative breast cancer,[49] and RXR-selective bexarotene currently is in a clinical trial in high-risk women.[50] The preclinical data include (1) a study showing that an RXR-selective retinoid combined with a selective estrogen receptor modulator (SERM) produced striking preventive results in an ER-negative, neu-positive animal mammary tumor model,[51] and (2) recent data showing the potent efficacy of a combination of a rexinoid and triterpenoid in preventing ER-negative mammary carcinogenesis in mice.[52] The ability of SERMs to reduce breast cancer risk is firmly established (the SERMs tamoxifen and raloxifene are approved by the U.S. Food and Drug Administration for this indication), but they prevent only ER-positive tumors.[53] Therefore, the data on retinoid potential in preventing ER-negative breast tumors could have important clinical implications for managing breast cancer.

Vitamin D is another agent that has received considerable attention for a possible role in the prevention of breast[54] and other cancers. Technically, vitamin D is not a vitamin as adequate levels of vitamin D can be made through skin exposure to solar UVB radiation. However, many individuals are at risk for vitamin D deficiency because they avoid solar radiation or do not make adequate vitamin D following solar radiation. The main known role of vitamin D has been for calcium homeostasis and bone health. Although some observational studies have reported that higher serum vitamin D is associated with lower breast cancer risk, the association is inconsistent.[55,56] With regard to randomized trials, no trials have yet investigated vitamin D as a single agent for prevention of breast cancers. The large Women's Health Initiative (WHI) gave a combination of calcium and vitamin D (1,000 mg calcium and 400 IU vitamin D/day); there was no significant effect of this combination on breast cancer risk (hazard ratio [HR], 0.96; 95% CI, 0.85-1.09).[57] Lappe et al.[58] conducted a trial that examined the relation between calcium plus vitamin D (1,100 IU/d) supplementation (vs. calcium alone or placebo) in 1,179 healthy postmenopausal women in Nebraska. Although fracture was the primary outcome of the trial, total cancer incidence was reportedly lower in the calcium plus vitamin D group, although the number of end points was very small (n = 50 total cancers observed during the follow-up). A new randomized trial of vitamin D and omega-3 fatty acids has been initiated (the *VIT*amin D and Omeg*A*-3 Tria*L* [VITAL]). The aims are to evaluate the role of vitamin D and long-chain marine omega-3 polyunsaturated fatty acid (eicosapentaenoic acid plus docosahexaenoic acid) supplements in the primary prevention of cancer and cardiovascular disease. The dose of vitamin D is 2,000 IU/d, and 20,000 participants are expected to be randomized for a treatment period of 5 years. This trial is expected to provide more definitive data on a possible role of vitamin D in chemoprevention of breast and other cancers.

SKIN CANCER CHEMOPREVENTION

Data suggest that topical all-*trans*-retinoic acid (ATRA) has significant dose-related activity in reversing premalignant skin lesions (e.g., actinic keratoses, which undergo a malignant transformation rate of 5%).[59] Systemic retinoid therapy has produced significant activity in the two reported randomized trials.[60,61] Several small, single-arm studies have found that systemic retinoids can reduce skin cancer incidence significantly in very high-risk patients with xeroderma pigmentosum (XP)[62] and in renal and heart transplant recipients.[63,64]

Published in 1988, the XP trial was a landmark trial for the field of chemoprevention.[62] Although including only five XP patients, the extremely high rate of skin cancer development and rigorous documentation of skin tumor rates before, during, and after the 2-year high-dose (2 mg/kg/d) 13cRA intervention provided statistically valid results. The overall average reduction in skin cancer incidence during therapy was 63% ($P = .019$). As was the case with high-dose retinoid trials in head and neck cancer, this trial revealed severe, acute mucocutaneous toxicity with the 13cRA. Also, the preventive effect of the retinoid was lost after stopping retinoid therapy, as indicated by a mean 8.5-fold increase in the annual rate of skin tumor development ($P = .007$). The retinoid chemopreventive effect in this study was greatest in the XP patients with the highest frequency of *de novo* skin tumor development, and, in subsequent studies, was found to be dose-related.

A randomized, placebo-controlled trial of the retinoid acitretin (30 mg/d for 6 months) was conducted in 38 renal transplant recipients.[65] The retinoid group had significant reductions in (1) premalignant lesions ($P = .008$), (2) the number of patients with skin cancer ($P = .01$), and (3) the cumulative number of skin cancers ($P = .009$). Nine of the 19 placebo patients developed a total of 18 skin cancers, and two of the 19 retinoid patients developed skin cancer, one cancer each. After completing the intervention, the rate of skin cancer development in the retinoid arm increased and became similar to that of the placebo arm. Toxicity in the retinoid group was frequent but mild in degree, and the retinoid had no adverse effect on renal function. There have been two other randomized acitretin trials in this setting, one significantly reducing skin squamous cell carcinoma[66] and one significantly reducing actinic keratoses.[67]

Three large-scale randomized phase 3 trials of retinoids and skin cancer have been reported. A trial of very low-dose

13cRA (10 mg/d)[68] and one of retinol (25,000 IU) or 13cRA (5-10 mg/d) versus placebo in patients with prior skin cancers had negative findings.[69] The third trial, involving retinol in patients with prior actinic keratoses, did see a significant reduction of squamous but not basal skin cancers in the retinoid arm.[70]

A phase 3 adjuvant trial of a retinoid combination, 13cRA (1 mg/kg/d orally) plus interferon-α (3×10^6 U subcutaneously 3 times per week), taken for 6 months did not improve time to tumor recurrence and/or SPTs (vs. the control of no adjuvant therapy) in 66 patients with aggressive skin squamous cell carcinoma.[71] The treatment hazard ratio of time to recurrence and SPT was 1.13 (95% CI, 0.53-2.41), of time to recurrence was 1.08 (95% CI, 0.43-2.72), and of time to SPT was 0.89 (95% CI, 0.27-2.93). The regimen was moderately tolerable, with dose reductions for grade 3 or 4 toxicities required in 29% of patients in the treatment arm.

Greenberg et al.[72] conducted a large randomized clinical trial of supplemental β-carotene (50 mg/d for 5 years) in 1,805 people with a previous nonmelanoma skin cancer. There was no difference between the two groups in the rate of occurrence of the first new nonmelanoma skin cancer (RR =1.05; 95% CI, 0.91-1.22). Subgroup analyses revealed a significant interaction (P = .04) between the treatment assignment and smoking status: the relative risk for new nonmelanoma skin cancer was 1.44 (95% CI, 0.99-2.09) in current smokers randomized to β-carotene, versus a relative risk of 0.97 (95% CI, 0.82-1.15) for never smokers randomized to β-carotene (as compared with placebo). Supplemental β-carotene (30 mg/d) also did not prevent either basal cell carcinoma or squamous cell carcinoma of the skin in an Australian trial.[73]

Selenium is another nutrient that has been evaluated for efficacy in the prevention of second skin cancers. As initially reported in 1996, Clark et al.[74] randomized a total of 1,312 patients with a history of nonmelanoma skin cancer to 200 mcg/d selenium or placebo. Selenium did not affect the incidence of second skin cancers (RR = 1.10 for basal cell carcinoma and RR = 1.14 for squamous cell carcinoma). However, there was a significant reduction in total cancer mortality (RR = 0.50; 95% CI, 0.31-0.80), mainly because of reductions in incident lung, colorectal, and prostate cancers. A further report of this trial in 2003 after longer follow-up indicated that there was a significant increase in total nonmelanoma skin cancer (HR = 1.17; 95% CI, 1.02-1.34) and squamous cell skin cancer (HR = 1.25; 95% CI, 1.03-1.51).[75] As these cancers have excellent prognoses, the possible benefit for prostate cancer and all-cause mortality supported a follow-up phase 3 trial involving selenium for prostate cancer prevention (SELECT, discussed in the section "Prostate Cancer Chemoprevention").

BLADDER CANCER CHEMOPREVENTION

Three randomized clinical trials have tested the retinoid etretinate in patients following resection of their superficial (noninvasive) bladder tumors, which recur in 40% to 90% of cases. All three studies observed substantial mucocutaneous toxicity in the retinoid arms.[76–77] In two of the three trials, prolonged (>1 year) low-dose etretinate (25 mg/d) was significantly better than placebo in reducing recurrences. These positive results require a cautious reading, however, because of small patient numbers and short-term follow-up.

A multicenter phase 3 trial of 4HPR (200 mg/d orally for 12 months) versus placebo was conducted for preventing tumor recurrence in patients with nonmuscle-invasive bladder transitional cell carcinoma (stages Ta, Tis, or T1) after transurethral resection with or without adjuvant intravesical bacillus Calmette-Guerin.[79] A total of 149 patients were enrolled, and 137 were evaluable for recurrence. The 1-year recurrence rates by Kaplan-Meier estimate were similar in the two groups: 32.3% (placebo) versus 31.5% (4HPR) (P = .88 log-rank test). 4HPR was well tolerated. Another chemoprevention trial randomized 65 patients with biopsy-confirmed transitional cell carcinoma of the bladder to a multivitamin (recommended dietary allowance [RDA] levels) alone or supplemented with 40,000 IU of retinol, 100 mg of pyridoxine, 2,000 mg of ascorbic acid, 400 units of alpha tocopherol, and 90 mg of zinc.[80] The 5-year estimate of tumor recurrence was 91% in the RDA arm versus 41% in the megadose arm (P = .0014). These results are promising in that the intervention was essentially nontoxic, with only one patient (3%) requiring dose reduction for mild stomach upset. Further research is needed to replicate this finding and to identify which vitamin(s) were responsible for chemopreventive efficacy.

CERVICAL CANCER CHEMOPREVENTION

Many randomized and nonrandomized chemoprevention studies have been conducted in cervical dysplasia. Randomized trials include two studies of folic acid, four of interferons, four of β-carotene, and five of retinoids. Only one of these trials, using topical ATRA,[81] found a significant treatment effect. Three hundred one patients with moderate (cervical intraepithelial neoplasia 2) and severe (cervical intraepithelial neoplasia 3) dysplasia were randomly assigned to topical ATRA versus placebo. This trial administered a 0.372% β-ATRA solution by collagen sponge in a cervical cap delivery system for 4 days initially, then for 2 days at months 3 and 6. The major finding was a higher complete response rate in the ATRA group (43%) than the placebo group (27%; P = .041) among the 141 patients with moderate dysplasia. No significant differences in dysplasia regression rates between the two study arms were detected in patients with severe dysplasia. Acute toxicity was infrequent, mild, and reversible, consisting primarily of local (vaginal and vulvar) irritation occurring in less than 5% of treated subjects. Major problems with compliance (e.g., 52 patients were lost to follow-up) suggest a cautious interpretation of this trial. More recent randomized retinoid studies involving topical ATRA[82] and oral fenretinide,[83] 13cRA,[84] and 9cRA[85] have all had negative findings.

Four randomized trials involving β-carotene have been published. The first was a trial from the Netherlands that randomized women with a histologic diagnosis of cervical dysplasia to either 10 mg/d of β-carotene for 3 months or placebo. After 3 months of intervention, there was no detectable effect of supplemental β-carotene on the regression and progression of cervical dysplasia.[86] Romney et al.[87] randomized women with cervical dysplasia to 30 mg/d of β-carotene (n = 39) or placebo (n = 30). After 9 months of intervention, there was no beneficial effect of β-carotene supplementation. An Australian trial used a factorial design to investigate the effects of supplemental β-carotene (30 mg/d) or vitamin C (500 mg/d) in 141 women with minor cervical abnormalities.[88] There was no significant effect of either agent in this trial. The most recently reported trial randomized 101 women with high-grade cervical intraepithelial neoplasia to β-carotene (30 mg/d) or placebo; regression rates were similar in both arms when stratified by cervical intraepithelial neoplasia grade.[89]

ESOPHAGEAL/GASTRIC CANCER CHEMOPREVENTION

Certain regions of China (Huixian and Linxian) have strikingly high incidence rates of esophageal and gastric cancers; moreover, intake and blood levels of various micronutrients are consistently low in these populations. These observations have led to several esophageal and/or gastric cancer prevention trials in China.[90-92] The first was in high-risk Chinese subjects from Huixian that tested the combination of retinol, riboflavin, and zinc for 13.5 months. After the intervention, there was no overall difference between the two arms in the occurrence of premalignant lesions or the prevalence or severity of dysplasia.[90]

Two trials were done in Linxian County. The first trial was conducted in residents from the general population.[91] Nearly 30,000 men and women aged 40 to 69 years took part in the study, which tested the efficacy of four different nutrient combinations at inhibiting the development of esophageal and gastric cancers. The nutrient combinations included retinol plus zinc, riboflavin plus niacin, ascorbic acid plus molybdenum, and the combination of β-carotene, selenium, and vitamin E. After a 5-year intervention period, those who were given the combination of β-carotene, vitamin E, and selenium had a 13% reduction in total cancer deaths (RR = 0.87; 95% CI, 0.75-1.00), a 4% reduction in esophageal cancer deaths (RR = 0.96; 95% CI, 0.78-1.18), and a 21% reduction in gastric cancer deaths (RR = 0.79; 95% CI, 0.64-0.99). None of the other nutrient combinations reduced gastric or esophageal cancer deaths significantly in this trial. The treatment benefit has now been shown to persist for 10 years after intervention, with new data indicating greater benefits in parti pants under age 55 years.[93] The finding that vitamin supplements reduced cancer deaths in this population provides compelling data supporting the concept of cancer prevention via nutrients; however, the applicability of these results for populations with adequate nutritional status and for other tumor sites may be limited. Also, it is unclear which nutrient(s) (β-carotene, vitamin E, or selenium) was responsible for the observed protection in this population.

The other Linxian trial was done to determine whether a multivitamin/multimineral preparation plus β-carotene (15 mg) reduced esophageal and gastric cardia cancers in 3,318 residents with esophageal dysplasia.[92] Cumulative esophageal/gastric cardia death rates after the 6-year intervention period were 8% lower (RR = 0.92; 95% CI, 0.67-1.28), esophageal cancer mortality was 16% lower (RR = 0.84; 95% CI, 0.54-1.29), and total cancer mortality was 4% lower (RR = 0.96; 95% CI, 0.71-1.29) in the supplemented group. Surprisingly, stomach cancer mortality was 18% higher (RR = 1.18; 95% CI, 0.76-1.85) in the supplemented group. None of the results was statistically significant.

A large, randomized trial from China tested the effects of one-time *Helicobacter pylori* treatment and long-term vitamin or garlic supplements in reducing the prevalence of advanced precancerous gastric lesions. The "vitamin" arm in this 3 × 3 × 3 factorial trial included 500 mg of vitamin C, 200 IU of vitamin E, and 75 mcg of selenium (from yeast) given daily. Although *H. pylori* treatment reduced the prevalence of precancerous gastric lesions, there were no beneficial effects from the vitamin intervention, despite the long duration (7.3 years) and high compliance.[94]

Intermediate end point trials have also been done in other parts of the world. A trial from Uzbekistan used a factorial design to study the combination of β-carotene, retinol, and alpha tocopherol, with and without riboflavin, in subjects with chronic esophagitis.[95] The risk of progression or no change versus regression was nonsignificantly decreased by 34% in those receiving retinol, β-carotene, and alpha tocopherol (odds ratio = 0.66; 95% CI, 0.37-1.16) versus those who did not receive these agents. Correa et al.[96] conducted a trial of supplemental antioxidant nutrients (β-carotene, vitamin C) and anti–*H. pylori* therapy in participants with gastric dysplasia in Colombia. In contrast to the results from the most recent Chinese trial,[94] all three basic interventions resulted in statistically significant increases in the rates of regression.

COLORECTAL CANCER CHEMOPREVENTION

Several randomized trials aimed at the prevention of recurrent colorectal adenomas with micronutrients have been completed. Beginning with supplemental β-carotene, the Australian Polyp Prevention Project evaluated the efficacy of reducing dietary fat to 25% of total calories, and supplementing the diet with 25 g of wheat bran and/or 20 mg of β-carotene daily, in a factorial design.[97] Beta carotene did not reduce the incidence of adenomas in this trial. Another trial (n = 291) using a lower dose of 15 mg/d of β-carotene also failed to see a reduction in adenomas with supplementation.[98] The largest trial studied 751 patients who had had an adenoma diagnosed and removed within the previous 3 months.[99] Participants were randomized using a 2 × 2 factorial design, with the active treatments being β-carotene (25 mg/d), and the combination of 1 g of vitamin C plus 400 mg of vitamin E. There was no evidence that either β-carotene or vitamins C and E reduced the incidence of adenomas in this 4-year trial. The relative risk for β-carotene was 1.01 (95% CI, 0.85-1.20); for vitamins C and E it was 1.08 (95% CI, 0.91-1.29). A subsequent report from this trial noted that alcohol intake and cigarette smoking modified the efficacy of β-carotene.[100] Among nonsmokers and nondrinkers, β-carotene was associated with a significant decrease in the risk of one or more recurrent adenomas (RR = 0.56); however, among persons who smoked and also drank more than one alcoholic drink per day, β-carotene significantly increased the risk of recurrent adenoma (RR = 2.07).

Observational epidemiological studies have shown a relatively consistent inverse association between low calcium intake, including that from supplements, and increased colorectal and colon cancer risk.[101,102] A role of calcium on colorectal carcinogenesis has also been supported by randomized intervention trials with recurrent colorectal adenomas as the outcome. In a trial by Baron et al.,[103] 930 subjects with a recent history of colorectal adenomas were randomly assigned to receive either calcium carbonate (1,200 mg/d of elemental calcium) or placebo. Follow-up colonoscopies were performed 1 and 4 years after the qualifying colonoscopy. The main analysis was based on the 832 subjects (409 in the calcium group and 423 in the placebo group) who completed both follow-up examinations. At least one adenoma was diagnosed between the first and second follow-up endoscopies in 127 subjects in the calcium group (31%) and 159 subjects in the placebo group (38%). The adjusted risk ratio was 0.81 (95% CI, 0.67-0.99; P = .04), and the adjusted ratio of the average number of adenomas in the calcium group to that in the placebo group was 0.76 (95% CI, 0.60-0.96; P = .02). A further analysis indicated that the effect of calcium was only evident in participants with higher levels of 25-OH vitamin D, suggesting that calcium and vitamin D may interact.[104]

A smaller, similar study of calcium gluconolactate and carbonate (2 g of elemental calcium daily) was conducted in Europe on 665 patients with a history of colorectal adenomas, of whom 552 participants completed the follow-up examination.[105] The adjusted odds ratio for adenoma recurrence was

CANCER PREVENTION

0.66 (95% CI, 0.38-1.17; $P = .16$) for calcium treatment. The findings were similar to those of Baron et al.,[103] but with the smaller sample size, the results were not statistically significant. The optimal dose and form of calcium that may be most protective cannot be determined by the randomized trials. Observational epidemiological studies suggest that benefits of calcium may plateau at 1,000 mg/d or less.[101,102]

As noted earlier, some evidence suggests that vitamin D may be important as an agent for cancer prevention, especially for colorectal cancer.[106] As systematically reviewed by the Agency for Healthcare Research and Quality,[55] a number of studies show that individuals with lower blood vitamin D levels have a higher risk of colorectal cancer or adenoma.

Only one adequately powered phase 3 trial, the WHI, has examined calcium and vitamin D intake in relation to risk of colorectal cancer. The WHI, a randomized, placebo-controlled trial of 400 IU of vitamin D plus 1,000 mg/d of calcium in 36,282 postmenopausal women did not confirm a protective role of calcium and vitamin D over a period of 7 years, with 332 colorectal cancer cases diagnosed.[107] The null findings for calcium plus vitamin D in this trial should be interpreted cautiously for the following reasons: (1) the vitamin D dose was relatively low (400 IU/d), (2) compliance was suboptimal, (3) a high percentage of women took nonstudy supplements, and (4) mean baseline intake of calcium was already high (>1,151 mg/d). With regard to vitamin D as a single agent, there was also no suggestion of benefit for colon cancer incidence in a 5-year British trial of vitamin D (100,000 IU every 4 months) that reported colon cancer incidence, although this was not a primary end point.[108] An ongoing randomized trial (NCT00153816) is examining 1,000 IU/d of vitamin D on risk of recurrent colorectal adenoma.

The B vitamins, including folate, vitamin B_6 (pyridoxine), and vitamin B_{12}, may be important for risk reduction for colon and perhaps certain other cancers (e.g., breast, pancreas). Folate is a water-soluble B vitamin found in foods, whereas folic acid is the synthetic form found in supplements and fortified foods. Adequate folate is critical for DNA methylation, repair, and synthesis.[109,110] It is now recognized that the methylation status of genes can play a key role in gene silencing/gene expression, lending plausibility to the idea that folate could be a key nutrient in regulating cell growth/proliferation. Epidemiological studies have linked low folate intake with higher risk of several cancers, most notably colorectal cancer.[111] Long-term use of multivitamin supplements, which are a major source of folate and other B vitamins, has been associated with a 20% to 70% reduction in risk of colon cancer in some studies.[112-114] Supporting an anticancer role of folate is that genotypes for methylene tetrahydrofolate reductase, an enzyme known to be involved in folate metabolism, predict risk of colon cancer dependent on folate intake or status.[115] Vitamin B_6 has been less studied in relation to cancer than folate, but recent studies suggest that vitamin B_6 may be an important preventive factor for colorectal cancer.[116,117] These effects could be related to one-carbon metabolism as for folate, but vitamin B_6 participates in more than 100 enzymatic reactions, and a number of mechanisms have been proposed for anticancer benefits.[118] A higher risk of cancer related to deficiencies of these vitamins has been proposed for alcohol drinkers.

Data from five randomized clinical trials of folic acid supplementation for the prevention of colorectal adenomas in patients with prior adenomas ("recurrent adenomas") have been reported. Two of these trials were quite small, and reported at least suggestions of benefit of folic acid supplementation.[119,120] However, benefits were not observed in two much larger trials, the Aspirin/Folate Polyp Prevention Study (AFPPS) (dose 1,000 mcg of folic acid daily) and the United Kingdom Colorectal Adenoma Prevention (ukCAP) trial (dose 500 mcg of folic acid daily).[121,122] In fact, the AFPPS trial found indications of an increased risk for advanced lesions and multiple adenomas with prolonged treatment and follow-up.[121] A third large trial, the NHS/HPFS folic acid polyp prevention trial, showed no overall risk reduction, although there were suggestions of decreased risks among those with higher alcohol intake and lower folate levels at baseline.[123] Other trials involving folic acid for various disease end points are ongoing, including a trial examining folic acid, vitamin B_{12}, and vitamin B_6 in relation to colorectal adenoma in women. The lack of efficacy for supplemental folic acid observed in recent large trials suggests a greater emphasis on food sources of folate (foods naturally rich in folate include leafy green vegetables, fruits, and dried beans and peas); a recent meta-analysis showed that folate from foods alone but not total folate (from foods and supplements) was associated with a lower risk of colorectal cancer.[124]

PROSTATE CANCER CHEMOPREVENTION

Recent evidence suggests that oxidative stress may play a role in the etiology of prostate cancer, and several antioxidant nutrients including lycopene, vitamin E, and selenium have been of interest for preventing prostate cancer. As described earlier, provocative secondary analyses of prior phase 3 National Cancer Institute–supported trials of selenium to prevent skin cancer[74] and vitamin E to prevent lung cancer[34] indicated that men randomized to vitamin E or selenium experienced fewer incidents of prostate cancer. In response, the National Cancer Institute supported the initiation of SELECT, a phase 3 trial testing selenium and vitamin E in a 2×2 factorial design.[125] SELECT is translational, with prospectively collected data and a biorepository for ancillary molecular epidemiological and other biological studies of prostate carcinogenesis and agent effects. SELECT recruited 35,534 randomized men, including 21% minority men overall and 15% black men, the highest percentage of blacks recruited to a large chemoprevention trial to date.[126]

Primary results of SELECT were reported in 2009[125] and included the following hazard ratios for prostate cancer (99% CIs) after a median overall follow-up of 5.46 years: vitamin E HR = 1.13 (99% CI, 0.95-1.35; n = 473), selenium HR = 1.04 (99% CI, 0.87-1.24; n = 432), and vitamin E plus selenium HR = 1.05 (99% CI, 0.88-1.25; n = 437) versus placebo (HR = 1.00; n = 416). No arm significantly reduced the risk of any other prespecified cancer end point as well. The risks of prostate cancer in the vitamin E arm and of type 2 diabetes mellitus in the selenium arm were increased nonsignificantly, although these increases did not occur in the selenium plus vitamin E arm. Negative/neutral findings also were reported for vitamins E and C and prostate and total cancer in the PHS II randomized controlled trial.[127]

Recent selenium pharmacogenetic research from cohort data has suggested that selenium may prevent poorer prognosis prostate cancer and its progression, but only in men with genetic backgrounds that influence selenium requirements[128,129] (notwithstanding the overall negative effect of selenium in SELECT). This finding is intriguing, but replication (e.g., in SELECT) is needed.

Carotenoids are a group of at least 600 compounds manufactured by plants and account for many of the bright colors in the plant kingdom. Only about 14 carotenoids are found in appreciable levels in human tissues, and the most common in the human diet and plasma are β-carotene, α-carotene, lycopene, lutein, and β-cryptoxanthin.[130] In recent years, lycopene, which comes primarily from tomatoes and tomato-based products, has generated much interest in regard to prostate cancer risk. This carotenoid does not contribute to vitamin A, but is a strong antioxidant and is the most commonly consumed carotenoid in most populations evaluated to date. In a number of epidemiological studies, although not all, both high consumers of tomato products and men with high serum or plasma levels of lycopene have been at lower risk of prostate cancer.[131] A meta-analysis of all the relevant observational studies published up to March 2003 found statistically significant moderate risk reductions for intake of tomatoes, cooked tomatoes and lycopene, and for circulating lycopene levels.[132] Several intervention trials have been conducted based on lycopene supplements, but these studies have been small, short term, based on intermediate end points, and have not had adequate control groups. The specific use of lycopene-concentrated pills for prostate chemoprevention needs to be evaluated in clinical trials before recommendations for these can be made, as the data available thus far have been from observational studies and have dealt only with tomato intake, or lycopene intake or levels, which are essentially markers of tomato products in the diet. The use of a tomato sauce-based intervention is supported by recent animal data indicating that tomato powder (which includes lycopene along with other phytochemicals), but not lycopene alone, was effective at inhibiting prostate carcinogenesis.[133]

CONCLUSIONS

This chapter has highlighted selected high-impact studies of retinoids, carotenoids, folic acid, calcium/vitamin D, vitamin E, and selenium in human cancer prevention. As reviewed herein, many trials of these agents for cancer prevention have been completed. Some of the trials have observed statistically significant reductions in risk of the primary end point (e.g., retinoids and β-carotene in oral premalignancy, retinoids in skin carcinogenesis models, calcium in colorectal adenomas, antioxidant nutrients in Linxian, China, for gastric cancer prevention), whereas others have observed statistically significant increases in the risk of the primary end point (β-carotene lung cancer prevention trials in smokers and selenium prevention trials in patients at risk of nonmelanoma skin cancer). Considering the completed trials, there is clear evidence against the general use of nutrient supplements for cancer prevention, which is the conclusion also reached by the World Cancer Research Fund/American Institute for Cancer Research,[134] which concluded that nutrient supplements are not recommended for cancer prevention.

Having said that, there are other themes emerging from this growing body of research. One such theme is that nutrient supplementation may be of benefit to some but not all. One such population that may benefit includes persons who are low in the nutrient of interest at baseline. This was suggested in the Linxian Country trial (done in a micronutrient-deficient population) and in subgroup analyses of several completed trials, but this hypothesis has not been formally tested in intervention trials to date.

Another consistent theme is that lifestyle factors (e.g., smoking) and also genetics (polymorphisms) may determine who is most likely to benefit from supplementation. Trial data will likely be increasingly mined to identify single nucleotide polymorphism profiles associated with both better outcomes (risk prediction) and response to intervention.[135,136] Ultimately a more personalized approach to cancer prevention may emerge, consistent with the movement toward a more personalized approach for cancer treatment. In the meantime and while the research continues, the most prudent recommendation for cancer prevention with regard to these agents is to follow the cancer prevention recommendations of the World Cancer Research Fund/American Institute for Cancer Research,[134] which emphasizes consumption of micronutrient-dense foods of plant origin, including nonstarchy vegetables, fruits, and whole grains, and the avoidance of nutrient supplements for cancer prevention.

Suggested Readings

The full list of references for this chapter appears in the online version.

1. Lippman SM, Benner SE, Hong WK. Cancer chemoprevention. *J Clin Oncol* 1994;12:851.
2. Lippman SM, Hong WK. Cancer prevention science and practice. *Cancer Res* 2002(62):5119–5125.
9. Lodi G, Sardella A, Bez C, et al. Interventions for treating oral leukoplakia. *Cochrane Database Syst Rev* 2006(4):CD001829 [update of *Cochrane Database Syst Rev* 2004;(3):CD001829].
10. Hong W, Endicott J, Itri LM, et al. 13-cis retinoic acid in the treatment of oral leukoplakia. *N Engl J Med* 1986;315:1501–1505.
11. Lippman SM, Batsakis JG, Toth BB, et al. Comparison of low-dose isotretinoin with beta carotene to prevent oral carcinogenesis. *N Engl J Med* 1993;328:15–20.
17. Hong WK, Lippman SM, Itri LM, et al. Prevention of second primary tumors with 13cRA in squamous-cell carcinoma of the head and neck. *N Engl J Med* 1990;323:795–801.
19. Khuri FR, Lee JJ, Lippman SM, et al. Randomized phase III trial of low-dose isotretinoin for prevention of second primary tumors in stage I and II head and neck cancer patients. *J Natl Cancer Inst* 2006;98:441–450.
20. Bolla M, Lefur R, Ton Van J, et al. Prevention of second primary tumours with etretinate in squamous cell carcinoma of the oral cavity and oropharynx. Results of a multicentric double-blind randomised study. *Eur J Cancer* 1994;30A:767–772.
21. Mayne ST, Cartmel B, Baum M, et al. Randomized trial of supplemental beta-carotene to prevent second head and neck cancer. *Cancer Res* 2001(61):1457–1463.
28. Arnold AM, Browman GP, Levine MN, et al. The effect of the synthetic retinoid etretinate on sputum cytology: results from a randomized trial. *Br J Cancer* 1992;65:737.
29. Lee JS, Lippman SM, Benner SE, et al. Randomized placebo-controlled trial of isotretinoin in chemoprevention of bronchial squamous metaplasia. *J Clin Oncol* 1994;12:937–945.
30. Kurie JM, Lee JS, Khuri FR, et al. N(4-hydroxyphenyl) retinamide in the chemoprevention of squamous metaplasia and dysplasia of the bronchial epithelium. *Clin Cancer Res* 2000;6:2973–2979.
33. The Alpha-Tocopherol, Beta Carotene Cancer Prevention Study Group. The effect of vitamin E and beta carotene on the incidence of lung cancer and other cancers in male smokers. *N Engl J Med* 1994;330:1029–1035.
35. Omenn GS, Goodman GE, Thornquist MD, et al. Effects of a combination of beta carotene and vitamin A on lung cancer and cardiovascular disease. *N Engl J Med* 1996;334:1150–1155.
36. Hennekens CH, Buring JE, Manson JE, et al. Lack of effect of long-term supplementation with beta carotene on the incidence of malignant neoplasms and cardiovascular disease. *N Engl J Med* 1996;334:1145–1149.
38. Heart Protection Study Collaborative Group. MRC/BHF Heart Protection Study of antioxidant vitamin supplementation in 20,536 high-risk individuals: a randomized placebo-controlled trial. *Lancet* 2002;360(9326):23–33.
42. van Zandwijk N, Dalesio O, Pastorino U, et al. EUROSCAN, a randomized trial of vitamin A and N-acetylcysteine in patients with head and neck cancer or lung cancer. For the European Organization for Research and Treatment of Cancer Head and Neck and Lung Cancer Cooperative Groups. *J Natl Cancer Inst* 2000;92:977–986.
43. Lippman SM, Lee JJ, Karp DD, et al. Randomized phase III intergroup trial of isotretinoin to prevent second primary tumors in stage I non-small-cell lung cancer. *J Natl Cancer Inst* 2001;93:605–618.
44. Mayne ST, Lippman SM. Cigarettes: a smoking gun in cancer chemoprevention. *J Natl Cancer Inst* 2005;97:1319–1321.
46. Veronesi U, De Palo G, Marubini E, et al. Randomized trial of fenretinide to prevent second breast malignancy in women with early breast cancer. *J Natl Cancer Inst* 1999;91:1847–1856.
55. Chung M, Balk EM, Brendel M, et al. *Vitamin D and Calcium: A Systematic Review of Health Outcomes*. Evidence Report No. 183. (prepared by the Tufts Evidence-based Practice Center under Contract No. HHSA 290-2007-10055-1). Rockville, MD:AHRQ;2009. AHRQ Publication No 09-E015.

56. IARC. Vitamin D and Cancer. *IARC Working Group Reports*. Vol. 5. Lyon, France: International Agency for research on Cancer; 2008.
57. Chlebowski RT, Johnson KC, Kooperberg C, et al. Calcium plus vitamin D supplementation and the risk of breast cancer. *J Natl Cancer Inst* 2008;100:1581–1591.
62. Kraemer KH, DiGiovanna JJ, Moshell AN, et al. Prevention of skin cancer in xeroderma pigmentosum with the use of oral isotretinoin. *N Engl J Med* 1988;318:1633–1637.
68. Tangrea JA, Edwards BK, Taylor PR, et al. Long-term therapy with low-dose isotretinoin for prevention of basal cell carcinoma: a multicenter clinical trial. *J Natl Cancer Inst* 1992;84:328.
69. Levine N, Moon TE, Cartmel B, et al. Trial of retinol and isotretinoin in skin cancer prevention: a randomized, double-blind, controlled trial. Southwest Skin Cancer Prevention Study Group. *Cancer Epidemiol Biomarkers Prev* 1997;6:957–961.
70. Moon TE, Levine N, Cartmel B, et al. Effect of retinol in preventing squamous cell skin cancer in moderate-risk subjects: a randomized, double-blind, controlled trial. *Cancer Epidemiol Biomarkers Prev* 1997;6:949–956.
71. Brewster AM, Lee JJ, Clayman GL, et al. Randomized trial of adjuvant 13-cis-retinoic acid and interferon alfa for patients with aggressive skin squamous cell carcinoma. *J Clin Oncol* 2007;25:1974–1978.
72. Greenberg ER, Baron JA, Stukel TA, et al. and the Skin Cancer Prevention Study Group. A clinical trial of beta carotene to prevent basal cell and squamous cell cancers of the skin. *N Engl J Med* 1990;323:789–795.
74. Clark LC, Combs GF Jr, Turnbull BW, et al. Effects of selenium supplementation for cancer prevention in patients with carcinoma of the skin. A randomized controlled trial. Nutritional Prevention of Cancer Study Group. *JAMA* 1996;276:1957–1963.
79. Sabichi AL, Lerner SP, Atkinson EN, et al. Phase III prevention trial of fenretinide in patients with resected non-muscle-invasive bladder cancer. *Clin Cancer Res* 2008;14:224.
81. Meyskens FL, Surwit E, Moon TE, et al. Enhancement of regression of cervical intraepithelial neoplasia II (moderate dysplasia) with topically applied all-trans-retinoic acid: a randomized trial. *J Natl Cancer Inst* 1994;86:539–543.
91. Blot WJ, Li J-Y, Taylor PR, et al. Nutrition intervention trials in Linxian, China: supplementation with specific vitamin/mineral combinations, cancer incidence, and disease-specific mortality in the general population. *J Natl Cancer Inst* 1993;85:1483–1492.
94. You WC, Brown LM, Zhang L, et al. Randomized double-blind factorial trial of three treatments to reduce the prevalence of precancerous gastric lesions. *J Natl Cancer Inst* 2006;98(14):974–983.
96. Correa P, Fontham ET, Bravo JC, et al. Chemoprevention of gastric dysplasia: randomized trial of antioxidant supplements and anti-helicobacter pylori therapy. *J Natl Cancer Inst* 2000;92(23):1881–1888.
99. Greenberg ER, Baron JA, Tosteson TD, et al. and the Polyp Prevention Study Group. A clinical trial of antioxidant vitamins to prevent colorectal adenoma. *N Engl J Med* 1994;331:141–147.
103. Baron JA, Beach M, Mandel JS, et al. Calcium supplements for the prevention of colorectal adenomas. The Calcium Polyp Prevention Study Group. *N Engl J Med* 1999;340:101–107.
105. Bonithon-Kopp C, Kronborg O, Giacosa A, et al. Calcium and fibre supplementation in prevention of colorectal adenoma recurrence: a randomized intervention trial. *Lancet* 2000;356:1300.
107. Wactawski-Wende J, Kotchen JM, Anderson GL, et al. Calcium plus vitamin D supplementation and the risk of colorectal cancer. *N Engl J Med* 2006;354:684–696.
111. Giovannucci E. Epidemiologic studies of folate and colorectal neoplasia: a review. *J Nutr* 2002;132:2350S–2355S.
117. Wei EK, Giovannucci E, Selhub J, et al. Plasma vitamin B6 and the risk of colorectal cancer and adenoma in women. *J Natl Cancer Inst* 2005;97:684–692.
121. Cole BF, Baron JA, Sandler RS, et al. Folic acid for the prevention of colorectal adenomas: a randomized clinical trial. *JAMA* 2007;297:2351–2359.
122. Logan RF, Grainge MJ, Shepherd VC, Armitage NC, Muir KR. Aspirin and folic acid for the prevention of recurrent colorectal adenomas. *Gastroenterology* 2008;134:29–38.
123. Wu K, Platz EA, Willett WC, et al. A randomized trial on folic acid supplementation and risk of recurrent colorectal adenoma. *Am J Clin Nutr* 2009;90:1623–1631.
125. Lippman SM, Klein EA, Goodman PJ, et al. Effect of selenium and vitamin E on risk of prostate cancer and other cancers: the Selenium and Vitamin E Cancer Prevention Trial (SELECT). *JAMA* 2009;301:39–51.
129. Penney KL, Schumacher FR, Li H, et al. A large prospective study of SEP15 genetic variation, interaction with plasma selenium levels, and prostate cancer risk and survival. *Cancer Prev Res (Phila Pa)* 2010;3:604–610.
131. Giovannucci E. Tomatoes, tomato-based products, lycopene, and cancer: review of the epidemiologic literature. *J Natl Cancer Inst* 1999;91:317–331.
132. Etminan M, Takkouche B, Caamano-Isorna F. The role of tomato products and lycopene in the prevention of prostate cancer: a meta-analysis of observational studies. *Cancer Epidemiol Biomarkers Prev* 2004;13:340–345.
134. World Cancer Research Fund, American Institute for Cancer Research. *Food, Nutrition, Physical Activity, and the Prevention of Cancer: a Global Perspective*. The Second Expert Report. Washington D.C.; 2007.
136. Wu X, Spitz MR, Lee JJ, et al. Novel susceptibility loci for second primary tumors/recurrence in head and neck cancer patients: large-scale evaluation of genetic variants. *Cancer Prev Res (Phila Pa)* 2009;2:617–624.

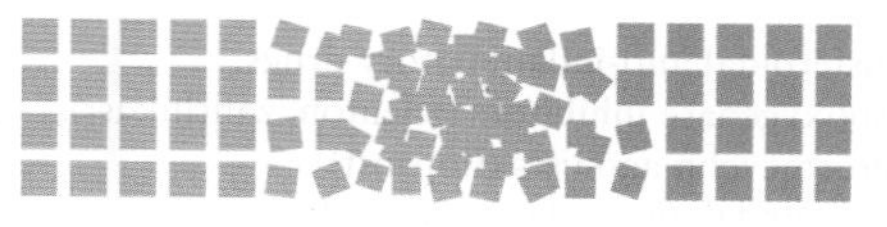

CHAPTER 55 DRUGS AND NUTRITIONAL EXTRACTS FOR CANCER RISK REDUCTION (CHEMOPREVENTION)

MADHURI KAKARALA AND DEAN E. BRENNER

The genetic events associated with cellular progression from differentiated function to neoplastic transformation present opportunities for intervention in order to delay or reverse these processes. The agents with potential capacity to inhibit the carcinogenesis process have traditionally been called *chemopreventive drugs*; however, this term invokes the negative connotations of the toxicities of cytotoxics used in cancer treatment. It also does not encompass the broad range of interventions to reduce risk of transformation, including behavioral change such as smoking cessation or increased exercise, dietary interventions, nutritional extracts such as curcumin or resveratrol, and drugs. Therefore, this chapter will refer to the field of study of these interventions as *cancer risk reduction* and the agents or interventions studied as *cancer risk reductive interventions* (CRRIs) rather than chemopreventive drugs.

Drugs or nutritional extracts with demonstrated efficacy or potential efficacy to delay or reverse the carcinogenesis process at common epithelial sites target key internal or external homeostatic processes associated with neoplastic transformation—inflammation with enhanced cellular oxidative stress, over- or underexpression of intracellular signal transduction pathways that control cellular proliferation, apoptotic events, and epigenetic modulation (Table 55.1).[1]

Despite the identification of critical targets and demonstrated success in translating preclinical data to reduction in cancer incidence at important epithelial targets (breast, colon, prostate), safety concerns have limited CRRI entry into clinical practice. Long-term administration of drugs to healthy populations imposes more stringent safety thresholds than treatments of clinical conditions that cause symptomatic reduction of quality of life. The risk-benefit ratio varies based on the long-term risk of developing cancer. For example, an individual with an 80% lifetime risk of developing breast cancer may be willing to tolerate more toxicity than an individual with a 3% lifetime risk.

This chapter reviews prominent drugs and nutritional extracts that delay or reverse transformation of common epithelial cancers. Selected new drugs or nutritional extracts with promising preliminary data are also discussed.

ANTI-INFLAMMATORY DRUGS

Nonsteroidal Anti-Inflammatory Agents

Mechanism

Nonsteroidal anti-inflammatory drugs (NSAIDs) represent a class of drugs that reduce cellular inflammation through modulation of eicosanoid metabolism.[2,3] Eicosanoids are metabolites of dietary fatty acids, primarily linoleic acid. Linoleic acid is metabolized to arachidonic acid, which is stored in the lipid membrane, and once mobilized from the membrane is further metabolized by prostaglandin-H synthases (PGHS) 1 and 2 to PGD_2, PGE_2, $PGF_{2\alpha}$, PGI_2, or thromboxane A_2 by specific synthases (Fig. 55.1). Leukotriene pathways involve conversion of arachidonic acid to leukotriene A_4 by 5-lipoxygenase and subsequent hydrolysis of leukotriene A_4 to other downstream leukotrienes. Newly formed prostaglandins and leukotrienes exit cells and function primarily through binding to EP receptors, releasing coupled G-proteins to elicit responses in the same or neighboring cells.[4]

NSAIDs vary in their binding and ultimately their inhibition of the cyclooxygenase (Cox) domain of the PGHS protein.[5] Although no drug can completely selectively inhibit one Cox isoform over the other, selective inhibitors of the Cox domain of PGHS-2 (Cox-2 inhibitor) were developed as less gastric toxic alternatives to nonselective NSAIDs. Prostaglandins play crucial roles in controlling cellular proliferation, apoptosis, cellular invasiveness, angiogenesis, and modulating immunosuppression.[4] Because PGE_2 is the most abundant PG in tumors, reducing local concentrations of PGE_2 may be a pivotal colorectal cancer preventive maneuver.[4] The role of leukotrienes in the carcinogenesis process is not known.

PGHS-independent mechanisms of NSAID action, such as inhibition of stem cell proliferation via Cox products,[6,7] may, at least in part, explain NSAID preventive efficacy.[2–4] Selective Cox-2 inhibitors also inhibit Akt signaling and induce apoptosis of human colorectal and prostate cancer cells *in vitro* in a Cox-2-independent manner via inhibition of phosphoinositide-dependent kinase-1. NSAIDs inhibit nuclear factor (NF)-κB at pharmacologic concentrations and key cellular proliferation signaling intermediates such as activator protein and other intermediates of the mitogen-activated protein (MAP)-kinase pathway. The impact of NSAIDs on carcinogenesis events driven by these upstream pathways remains unclear.

Epidemiology

The majority of population-based case-control studies found that aspirin taken at least 16 times per month confers a 50% reduction in risk of occurrence of colorectal cancer.[8] However, in a 12-year follow-up study, the Physician's Health Study reported that random assignment to a 325-mg daily aspirin dose was associated with a relative risk (RR) for colorectal cancer of 1.03 (95% confidence interval [CI], 0.83–1.28).[9] The Nurse's Health study suggests that frequent ingestion of aspirin is required for more than 10 years in order to detect colorectal cancer risk reduction (RR, 0.62; CI, 0.44–0.8]).[10] An inverse relationship with NSAID use is seen consistently with esophageal squamous (RR, 0.58; 95% CI, 0.43–0.78), esophageal

TABLE 55.2

CHEMOPREVENTION CLINICAL TRIALS OF NONSTEROIDAL ANTI-INFLAMMATORY DRUGS AND ADENOMATOUS COLORECTAL POLYPS

Population	Drug (Dose), Duration	Phase	End Point	Outcome	Ref.
GENE-ASSOCIATED					
Familial adenomatous polyposis	Sulindac (100 mg tid), 4 mo	2b	Polyp regression	Polyps regressed in 6 patients, partly in 3	126
Familial adenomatous polyposis	Sulindac (150 mg bid), 9 mo	2b	Polyp regression	Number of polyps decreased by 56% and size by 65%	21
Familial adenomatous polyposis	Sulindac (400 mg), 6 mo	2b`	Polyp regression	Duodenal polyps regressed in 11 treated patients	127
Familial adenomatous polyposis	Celecoxib (100 mg bid or 400 mg), 6 mo	2a	Polyp regression	Celecoxib significantly decreased number of colon polyps	20
Apc mutation carriers	Sulindac (75 or 150 mg bid), 48 mo	2b	Polyp regression	Sulindac did not prevent the development of adenomas	22
SPORADIC RISK					
Previous adenomatous polyps	Sulindac (300 mg), 4 mo	2b	Polyp regression	Sulindac did not significantly decrease the number or size of polyps	24
Previous adenomatous polyps	Piroxicam (7.5 mg), 2 y	2b	Polyp recurrence	Colorectal mucosal PGE_2 reduced in piroxicam-treated arm, unacceptable toxicity	25
Previous adenomatous polyps, healthy subjects	Aspirin (40, 81, 325, 650 mg qd), 1 day, 4 wk	1, 2a	Dose-biomarker	Aspirin dose of 81 mg daily sufficient to suppress colorectal mucosal prostaglandin E_2	128–130
Prior colorectal cancer	Aspirin (325 mg qd), 3 y	2b	Polyp recurrence	Aspirin use associated with delayed development of adenomatous polyps	131
Previous adenomatous polyps	Aspirin (81 mg qd or 325 mg qd) and/or folate, 3 y	2b	Polyp recurrence	Low-dose aspirin reduced the recurrence of adenomatous polyps	132
Previous adenomatous polyps	Celecoxib	2b	Polyp recurrence	Celecoxib reduced the recurrence of adenomatous polyps, unacceptable toxicity	27
Previous adenomatous polyps	Celecoxib	2b	Polyp recurrence	Celecoxib reduced the recurrence of adenomatous polyps, unacceptable toxicity	26
Previous adenomatous polyps	Rofecoxib	2b	Polyp recurrence	Rofecoxib reduced the recurrence of adenomatous polyps, unacceptable toxicity	28
POPULATION-BASED					
Healthy Women (Women's Health Study)	Aspirin (100 mg qod) 10 y	3	Colorectal cancer	Aspirin does not reduce risk of colorectal cancer	29
Healthy male physicians (Physicians Health Study)	Aspirin (325 mg qod) 5 y	3	Colorectal cancer	Aspirin does not reduce the risk of colorectal cancer	30

the incidence of contralateral second primary breast cancers during adjuvant treatment regimens catalyzed the push for its development as a CRRI.[45–47]

Table 55.3 summarizes the phase 3 data for SERM-based breast cancer risk reduction. In the updated analysis at 8-year median follow-up of Cuzick et al.,[48] 142 breast cancers (invasive and ductal carcinoma *in situ* [DCIS]) were diagnosed in the 3,579 women in the tamoxifen group versus 195 breast cancers in the 3,575 women in the placebo group (risk ratio, 0.73; 95% CI, 0.58–0.91). The incidence of invasive, ER-positive breast cancer was 26% lower in the tamoxifen arm. There is no effect on ER-negative breast cancers (risk ratio, 1.00; 95% CI, 0.61–1.65). The reduction in cancer and DCIS incidence persists even at 13-year follow-up after the discontinuation of tamoxifen.[48,49] In all trials, tamoxifen causes an approximately twofold increase in risk of endometrial adenocarcinoma.[50] These cancers are low-grade, early-stage cancers without related deaths. Tamoxifen also causes a two- to threefold increased risk of venous

TABLE 55.3

PHASE 3 RANDOMIZED, CONTROLLED CLINICAL TRIALS OF SELECTIVE ESTROGEN RECEPTOR MODULATORS FOR THE PREVENTION OF BREAST CANCER

Study	Drug	Dose/Day (mg)	*N*	Treatment Duration (y)	Entry Criteria	Outcome	Ref.
NSABP P-1	Tamoxifen	20	13,388	5	Gail model: 5 y predicted risk of ≥1.66%	RR = 0.51 (95% CI, 0.39–0.66)	51
IBIS-1	Tamoxifen	20	7,139	5	>2-fold relative risk	OR = 0.73 (95% CI, 0.58–0.91)	48
Royal Marsden	Tamoxifen	20	2,471	8	Family history	HR = 0.78 (95% CI, 0.58–1.04)	49
Italian	Tamoxifen	20	5,408	5	Normal risk, hysterectomy	RR = 0.84 (95% CI, 0.60–1.17)	133
NSABP P-2	Raloxifene	60	19,747	5	Gail model: 5 y predicted risk of ≥1.66%	Vs. tamofen RR = 1.02 (95% CI, 0.81–1.28)	134

NSABP, National Surgical Adjuvant Breast and Bowel Project; RR, relative risk; CI, confidence interval; IBIS, International Breast Cancer Intervention Study; OR, odds ratio; HR, hazard ratio.

thromboembolism[48,51] with reported excess deaths from this toxicity.[51] Tamoxifen nonsignificantly reduces the incidence of skeletal fractures but has no effect on the incidence of coronary artery disease.

The U.S. Food and Drug Administration approved tamoxifen for the prevention of breast cancer, yet only 3% to 20% of eligible high-risk women agree to take tamoxifen for primary prevention. The low willingness of eligible women to take tamoxifen for 5 years demonstrates the issue of risk:benefit for CRRIs. Women with high short-term risk (5-year Gail risk of >5%)—for example, those with ER-positive atypical hyperplasia, lobular carcinoma *in situ,* and the majority of non–high-grade DCIS lesions—may be most likely to respond to SERMs with an acceptable risk:benefit ratio. In the National Surgical Adjuvant Breast and Bowel Project, tamoxifen-treated women with a *BRCA2* mutation but not a *BRCA1* mutation had reduced cancer incidence,[52] but subsequent data from another group have found reduced cancer risk in both *BRCA* mutations.[53]

The dose of tamoxifen tested in the large prevention trials, 20 mg per day, was derived from doses used for breast cancer treatment rather than for a prevention indication. Tamoxifen, 1 or 5 mg daily, had no difference in biomarker effects (Ki-67 proliferative index)[54] and reduced concentrations of C-reactive protein, fibrinogen, and antithrombin III compared with the standard, 20-mg daily dose. These data suggest that low doses of tamoxifen might be an effective estrogen antagonist in the breast yet a less potent estrogen agonist at other organ targets. This work emphasizes the importance of careful early-phase study of CRRIs defining dose response for cancer risk reductive efficacy using biomarker and toxicity end points.

Raloxifene

The benzothiophene structure of raloxifene confers a different tissue-specific ER binding profile than the triphenylethylene tamoxifen. Raloxifene has greater estrogen agonist activity in bone but reduced estrogen agonist activity in the uterus. Raloxifene was studied for treatment and prevention of osteoporosis in a large, pivotal trial (Multiple Outcomes of Raloxifene Evaluation, or MORE) and found to reduce the rate of vertebral fracture as compared with placebo in postmenopausal women.[55] In addition, a significant reduction occurred in breast cancer incidence in the raloxifene-treated group (62% reduction in all breast cancers, 72% reduction in all invasive breast cancers, and 84% reduction in ER-positive breast cancers but no reduction in ER-negative tumors), with no increased risk of thromboembolism or endometrial adenocarcinoma.[40,41,56]

In a phase 3 chemoprevention trial comparing tamoxifen with raloxifene (Table 55.3), the invasive breast cancer preventive efficacy of raloxifene was found to be equivalent to that of tamoxifen, but with an improved safety profile (reduced thromboembolic events, cataracts, and lower risk of endometrial cancer).[50] However, there was more DCIS and mixed *in situ* disease in the raloxifene arm (111 in tamoxifen vs. 137 in the raloxifene group; RR, 1.22; 95% CI, 0.95–1.59), with nearly equal rates in lobular carcinoma *in situ*.[50] Raloxifene does not differ from tamoxifen in risk of fractures, other cancers, or cardiovascular events.[50] The lower risk of raloxifene for endometrial adenocarcinomas compared with tamoxifen needs to be weighed against the increased risk of stroke seen in a cardiovascular prevention trial.[57] Its impact on the risk of thromboembolism is unclear. The effectiveness of raloxifene in the community may also be compromised by its poor bioavailability (2%) due to rapid phase 2 enzyme metabolism in the gut and liver,[58] whereas tamoxifen is more bioavailable and has active metabolites that permit prolonged drug effect. Missed raloxifene doses may potentially compromise efficacy and prevention outcomes in widespread community use.

Aromatase Inhibitors

In adjuvant clinical trials for breast cancer, aromatase inhibitors (anastrozole, exemestane, letrozole) given after 5 years of tamoxifen enhance reduction of breast cancer recurrence in the contralateral breast compared with tamoxifen alone.[59] In a phase 1 chemoprevention trial, letrozole reduces the Ki-67 proliferation index of breast epithelial cells aspirated from high-risk women.[60] Aromatase inhibitors are associated with increased risk of fractures, hot flashes, and very commonly increased joint and muscle pains; therefore, they were deemed too toxic for phase 3 study as CRRIs in the United States.[61,62] Ongoing trials in the United Kingdom (anastrozole) and Canada (exemestane) will define the role and toxicity profiles of aromatase inhibitors as breast cancer risk reductives.

Finasteride

Mechanism

Prostate cancers require androgens to proliferate and to evade apoptosis. The primary nuclear androgen responsible for maintenance of epithelial function is dihydrotestosterone. The testes and adrenal gland synthesize dihydrotestosterone by the conversion of testosterone by 5α-steroid reductase types 1 and 2 isozymes. Dihydrotestosterone binds to intracellular androgen receptors to form a complex that binds to DNA hormone response elements controlling cellular proliferation and apoptosis. Finasteride, a selective, competitive inhibitor of type 2 5α-steroid reductase,[63] inhibits proliferation in the transformed prostate cell. In the 3,2′-dimethyl-4-aminobiphenyl (DMAB), methylnitrosourea (MNU), and testosterone chemical carcinogenesis models in rats, finasteride reduces prostate tumor incidence by nearly sixfold. Finasteride appears to be more effective in the promotion phase of prostate carcinogenesis.[64]

Cancer Preventive Activity

A randomized, placebo-controlled cancer incidence end point risk reductive clinical trial demonstrated that finasteride reduced the incidence of prostate cancer by 24.8%.[65] The initial analysis suggested that tumors of high Gleason's grade (7–10) were higher in the finasteride arm (37%) compared with the placebo arm (22%). Sexual function side effects (erectile dysfunction, loss of libido, gynecomastia) were more common in the finasteride treatment arm.[65,66] Dutasteride inhibits both 5α-steroid reductase inhibitor types 1 and 2 isoforms, whereas finasteride inhibits only the type 2 isoform. In a cancer incidence, randomized, placebo-controlled prostate cancer risk reduction trial, dutasteride reduced the relative risk of prostate cancer by 22% and the absolute risk reduction was 5.1%. Similar to the finasteride study, in the final 2 years of observation, more high-grade (Gleason's grade 8–10) tumors were observed in the dutasteride-treated arm than in the placebo arm.[67]

Although these data support a conclusion that finasteride prevents prostate cancer or delays the progression of prostate cancer from microscopic to macroscopic size as demonstrated in the preclinical data, the concerns over the apparent selection by finasteride of high-grade Gleason's score tumors and the accompanying drug-associated toxicities have reduced enthusiasm for generalized use of finasteride in population-based prevention. The ability of finasteride to reduce prostate-specific antigen, reduce gland size, and alter the prostate histology through increased apoptosis and reduced proliferation of glandular epithelium may have confounded the grading of biopsies after treatment.[66,68]

SIGNAL TRANSDUCTION MODIFIERS

Both cancer therapy and cancer prevention have investigated drugs that modify specific targets in signal transduction pathways. Even though the emphasis in drug development has focused on cancer treatment, interventions aimed at modulating signal transduction pathways promise new approaches to interventions in the carcinogenesis process. Because of the complexity of signaling systems, inhibition of single targets may not be effective or may cause unacceptable toxicity.

Difluoromethylornithine

Polyamines (spermidine, spermine, and the diamine, putrescine) are required to maintain cellular growth and function.[69] In mammalian cells, polyamine inhibition by genetic mutation or pharmaceutical agents is associated with virtual cessation in cellular growth. Difluoromethylornithine (DFMO) is an enzyme-activated irreversible inhibitor of ornithine decarboxylase (which is transactivated by the *c-myc* oncogene and cooperates with the *ras* oncogene in malignant transformation).[70] Extensive preclinical data have found that DFMO prevents tumor promotion in a variety of systems—skin, mammary, colon, cervical, and bladder carcinogenesis models.[69] Synergistic or additive activity with retinoids, butylated hydroxyanisole, tamoxifen, piroxicam, and fish oil has been demonstrated with low concentrations of DFMO.[69]

In phase 1 prevention trials, DFMO at a dose of 0.5 mg/m^2 per day reduces tissue polyamines in colon and skin,[71,72] causes regression of cervical IEN when used topically,[73] but does not reduce cellular proliferation of tissue polyamines or other biomarkers in the human breast.[74] The major preventive dose-limiting toxicity is reduction in hearing acuity. The bulk of clinical data suggest that doses below 0.5 g/m^2 per day cause changes in pure tone-only hearing, which are rapidly reversible.

Growth Factor Receptor Modulators

Growth factor receptors and their ligands are primarily targets for a new generation of drugs developed for cancer treatment. Antibodies that bind to the receptor protein (e.g., cetuximab) are unlikely to be useful as CRRIs because of the potential for immune reactions to the antibody molecule. Agents that primarily target the intracellular kinase portion of the receptor (gefitinib, erlotinib) appear to have a superior safety profile for use as cancer risk reductives.

Early clinical trials of these agents in patients with intraepithelial neoplasms have shown mixed results. Treatment of 65 patients with intermediate- or high-grade DCIS with gefitinib during the interval from biopsy to surgical removal reduced the Ki-67 proliferation index and nuclear MAP kinase. The treatment-associated rash may be dose-limiting for cancer risk reductive interventions.[75] Similar data have been reported for erlotinib in the same patient population.[76] These early trials intended for treatment of cancer suggest promise for prevention indications if dose and toxicity can be managed.

Statins

Statins or hydroxyl-3-methylglutaryl coenzyme A (*HMG-CoA*) reductase inhibitors are the second most prescribed drug in the United States.[77] Statins have been suggested to decrease risk of cancer in preclinical studies by inhibiting *Ras-* and *Rho*-mediated cell proliferation, up-regulation of cell-cycle inhibitors (e.g., p21 and p27), induction of apoptosis of transformed cells, and inhibition of angiogenesis.[78,79]

Although several large trials of statins on cardiovascular disease risk with cancer as secondary end points have shown no benefit to cancer risk with follow-ups between 18 months to 4 years, these trials were not adequately powered to examine cancer end points. Several case-control studies that have examined the effect of statins on colorectal adenocarcinoma have shown a decrease in odds ratios ranging from 0.53 to 0.91, all statistically significant,[77,80] while secondary analysis of a celecoxib prevention trial demonstrated no protection against colorectal neoplasms.[81] Prospective longitudinal studies have shown mixed results with the Physician's Health Study, suggesting statin protection for prostate cancer (adjusted RR, 0.51),[82] while the Nurse's Health Study showed no decrease in risk of breast cancer.[83] Statins may be effective CRRIs in individuals with the A/A genotype variant of the predominant T/T genotype of rs12654264 of the *HMG-CoA* reductase gene.[84]

Metformin

Metformin, an oral antidiabetic drug in the biguanide class,[85] is the first-line drug of choice for the treatment of type 2 diabetes.[86]

Cancers are more common in diabetics and obese individuals than their normal-weight and normoglycemic counterparts, leading to the hypothesis that elevated serum insulin concentrations promote cancer risk.[87] Insulin and insulinlike growth factors (IGF1 and 2) stimulate cellular DNA synthesis, proliferation, and tumor growth through PI3-kinase, mTOR, and the *Ras*-MAPK signaling pathways.[88] Case-control studies have shown that metformin therapy reduces risk of cancers of the pancreas and breast in treated individuals.[87,89] Metformin causes few adverse effects (e.g., gastrointestinal upset) and does not cause hypoglycemia.

Multiagent Chemoprevention

In the transition to molecular-targeted interventions, combinations of targets that logically address critical carcinogenesis pathways may have greater efficacy than single agents. For example, interactive signaling of epidermal growth factor receptors and Cox-2, experiments in Min$^+$ mice[90] demonstrate chemopreventive synergism. Attacking the eicosanoid synthesis pathway through substrate presentation and enzyme inhibition also enhances cancer risk reductive effect while reducing toxicity.[91] Combining atorvastatin with selective or nonselective Cox inhibitors enhanced the inhibition of azoxymethane-induced colon carcinogenesis in F344 rats and reduced the dose of the combined drugs required to achieve reduction of colon carcinogenesis.[92]

DFMO plus sulindac inhibited adenoma formation in a phase 2b trial of 375 patients with prior history of adenomas followed for 36 months.[93] Cardiovascular adverse outcomes were higher in DFMO/sulindac-treated patients who had preexisting high baseline cardiovascular risk; however, the cardiovascular adverse events were similar to placebo-treated in moderate or low cardiovascular risk patients.[94] Using insulin growth factor-1 as a biomarker, Guerrieri-Gonzaga et al.[95] showed that the combination of low-dose tamoxifen with low-dose fenretinide is safe but not synergistic. As more data accumulate from *in vivo* models, combined drugs aimed at specific targets in coordinated signaling pathways will enter clinical biomarker-based trials. Optimal doses, toxicity, and biomarker modulation data will select those combinations useful for risk reduction trials and, ultimately, generalized use in at-risk populations.

Nutritional Extracts as CRRIs

Polyphenol nutritional extracts such as curcumin, resveratrol, epigallocatechin gallate, genistein, quercetin, and others are attractive as CRRIs for their low toxicity and multimechanistic cancer-preventive properties. One polyphenol, curcumin, the major yellow pigment extracted from turmeric, a commonly used spice, has long been used as a treatment for inflammation, skin wounds, and tumors[96] in India and the Far East. Curcumin suppresses Cox and lipoxygenase, protein kinases, and scavenges reactive oxygen species, inducing Cox-2 gene expression. The pleiotropic effects of curcumin have been explained through its inhibition of NF-κB[97]; however, recent work demonstrates that curcumin down regulates *Wnt* and *Notch* signaling pathways.[98] Curcumin is a potent anticarcinogen in rodent models of breast, skin, and colon carcinogenesis.[96,99] Curcumin, like other polyphenols, is extensively metabolized and poorly absorbed in the gastrointestinal tract and is largely converted to glucuronidated and sulfated forms.[100,101] *In vivo* studies demonstrating biomarker effect with no detectable curcumin parent compound raise the possibility of biologically active conjugates or deconjugation at the target site.[100–102]

Resveratrol (3,5,4′-trihydroxy-*trans*-stilbene) is a phytoalexin found in grapes, mulberries, peanuts, and *Cassia quinquangulata* plants that may help to protect against cancer[103] via inhibition of a variety anti-inflammatory (Cox, lipoxygenase inhibition) and protein kinase signal transduction pathways (e.g., STAT-3, HER2/neu, MAP kinases, and Akt). Resveratrol given to mice reduces high caloric diet-induced body weight, increases lifespan, and decreases IGF-1 concentrations.[104] Resveratrol inhibits carcinogenesis in rodent models (colon, breast).[105–107] Data in humans to date are limited, suggesting poor bioavailability when measured in human plasma,[108] similar to other nutritional polyphenols.[102,109] Tenfold higher concentrations in human colon tissue as compared with plasma tissue suggests that resveratrol has sufficient bioavailability in human tissue to be considered for further CRRI investigators.[110]

ANTI-INFECTIVES

Major infective carcinogens include the human hepatitis viruses, hepatitis B virus and hepatitis C virus for hepatocellular carcinoma,[111] *Helicobacter pylori* for gastric adenocarcinoma,[112] human papillomaviruses for cervical, anal, vulva, penis, and oral cavity and pharynx,[113] herpes virus-8 for Kaposi sarcoma,[114] and schistosomes for bladder carcinoma.[115] The success of human papillomavirus vaccine in reducing the incidence of epithelial intraepithelial neoplasia of the cervix (reviewed in Chapter 50) is one example that demonstrates the potential of immunochemoprevention for epithelial targets for which an etiologic agent can be identified.

Helicobacter pylori

Intestinal-type gastric adenocarcinoma arises through a multistep process, known as the Correa cascade that begins with chronic gastritis, progressing through gastric mucosal atrophy, intestinal metaplasia to dysplasia, and ultimately to adenocarcinoma.[116] The cascade is commonly initiated by *H. pylori*, which infects 50% of the world's population.[112] Infection occurs early in life and remains quiescent and may be associated with chronic gastritis of variable intensity but with minimal symptoms. Although the majority of *H. pylori* organisms remain in the gastric mucous layer, 10% adhere to the gastric mucosa through adhesion *BabA*, an outer membrane protein that binds to the histo-blood group antigen Le^b.[112] Progression to atrophic gastritis and peptic ulcer disease (occurs in 10%–15% of infected individuals) requires other bacterial and host cofactors.[112,116] Infection with *H. pylori* is associated with an odds ratio of 2.7 to 6.0 for gastric cancer; *CagA* virulence protein increases this risk by 20- to 40-fold. The risk of developing gastric adenocarcinoma with *H. pylori* infection is estimated to be 1% to 3%.[112,116]

Eradication of *H. pylori* with antibiotics and anti-inflammatory agents (e.g., amoxicillin, metronidazole, and bismuth subsalicylate) increases the rate of regression of nonmetaplastic gastric atrophy and intestinal metaplasia[117] but may not reduce the progression to gastric cancers.[118,119] Long-term therapy with proton pump inhibitors, producing achlorhydria, may increase the risk of atrophic gastritis in individuals infected with *H. pylori*,[120] but this point remains controversial.[121] Some clinical data support eradicating *H. pylori* with antibiotics prior to long-term treatment with proton pump inhibitors as a method to reduce the risk of progression to gastric cancer,[122,123] although no study to date has observed an increased risk of gastric cancer in proton pump inhibitor–treated patients.

Selected References

The full list of references for this chapter appears in the online version.

1. Kelloff GJ, Lippman SM, Dannenberg AJ, et al. Progress in chemoprevention drug development: the promise of molecular biomarkers for prevention of intraepithelial neoplasia and cancer—a plan to move forward. *Clin Cancer Res* 2006;12:3661.
2. Thun MJ, Henley SJ, Patrono C. Nonsteroidal anti-inflammatory drugs as anticancer agents: mechanistic, pharmacologic, and clinical issues. *J Natl Cancer Inst* 2002;94:252.
4. Wang D, Mann JR, DuBois RN. The role of prostaglandins and other eicosanoids in the gastrointestinal tract. *Gastroenterology* 2005;128:1445.
8. Thun MJ, Namboodiri MM, Heath C Jr. Aspirin use and reduced risk of fatal colon cancer. *N Engl J Med* 1991;325:1593.
10. Chan AT, Giovannucci EL, Meyerhardt JA, et al. Long-term use of aspirin and nonsteroidal anti-inflammatory drugs and risk of colorectal cancer. *JAMA* 2005;294:914.
12. Wang WH, Huang JQ, Zheng GF, et al. Non-steroidal anti-inflammatory drug use and the risk of gastric cancer: a systematic review and meta-analysis. *J Natl Cancer Inst* 2003;95:1784.
14. Eliassen A, Chen W, Spiegelman D, et al. Use of aspirin, other NSAIDs, and acetaminophen and risk of breast cancer among premenopausal women in the Nurses Health Study II. *Arch Intern Med* 2008;169:115–121.
17. Kawamori T, Rao C, Seibert K, et al. Chemopreventive effect of celecoxib, a specific cyclooxygenase-2 inhibitor on colon carcinogenesis. *Cancer Res* 1998;58:409.
21. Giardiello FM, Hamilton SR, Krush AJ, et al. Treatment of colonic and rectal adenomas with sulindac in familial adenomatous polyposis. *N Engl J Med* 1993;328:1313.
22. Giardiello FM, Yang VW, Hylind LM, et al. Primary chemoprevention of familial adenomatous polyposis with sulindac. *N Engl J Med* 2002;346:1054.
26. Arber N, Eagle CJ, Spicak J, et al. Celecoxib for the prevention of colorectal adenomatous polyps. *N Engl J Med* 2006;355:885.
27. Bertagnolli MM, Eagle CJ, Zauber AG, et al. Celecoxib for the prevention of sporadic colorectal adenomas. *N Engl J Med* 2006;355:873.
29. Cook NR, Lee IM, Gaziano JM, et al. Low-dose aspirin in the primary prevention of cancer: the Women's Health Study: a randomized controlled trial. *JAMA* 2005;294:47.
31. Grosser T, Fries S, FitzGerald GA. Biological basis for the cardiovascular consequences of COX-2 inhibition: therapeutic challenges and opportunities. *J Clin Invest* 2006;116:4.
32. Bresalier RS, Sandler RS, Quan H, et al. Cardiovascular events associated with rofecoxib in a colorectal adenoma chemoprevention trial. *N Engl J Med* 2005;352:1092.
35. Routine aspirin or nonsteroidal anti-inflammatory drugs for the primary prevention of colorectal cancer: U.S. Preventive Services Task Force recommendation statement. *Ann Intern Med* 2007;146:361.
40. Fabian CJ, Kimler BF. Selective estrogen-receptor modulators for primary prevention of breast cancer. *J Clin Oncol* 2005;23:1644.
41. Jordan VC. Chemoprevention of breast cancer with selective oestrogen-receptor modulators. *Nat Rev Cancer* 2007;7:46.
46. Rutqvist LE, Cedermark B, Glas U, et al. Contralateral primary tumors in breast cancer patients in a randomized trial of adjuvant tamoxifen therapy. *J Natl Cancer Inst* 1991;83:1299.
47. Fisher B, Redmond C. New perspective on cancer of the contralateral breast: a marker for assessing tamoxifen as a preventive agent. *J Natl Cancer Inst* 1991;83:1278.
48. Cuzick J, Forbes JF, Sestak I, et al. Long-term results of tamoxifen prophylaxis for breast cancer—96-month follow-up of the randomized IBIS-I trial. *J Natl Cancer Inst* 2007;99:272.
49. Powles TJ, Ashley S, Tidy A, et al. Twenty-year follow-up of the Royal Marsden randomized, double-blinded tamoxifen breast cancer prevention trial. *J Natl Cancer Inst* 2007;99:283.
50. Vogel VG, Costantino JP, Wickerham DL, et al. Update of the National Surgical Adjuvant Breast and Bowel Project Study of Tamoxifen and Raloxifene (STAR) P-2 Trial: preventing breast cancer. *Cancer Prev Res* 2010;3:696.
52. King MC, Wieand S, Hale K, et al. Tamoxifen and breast cancer incidence among women with inherited mutations in BRCA1 and BRCA2: National Surgical Adjuvant Breast and Bowel Project (NSABP-P1) Breast Cancer Prevention Trial. *JAMA* 2001;286:2251.
54. Decensi A, Robertson C, Viale G, et al. A randomized trial of low-dose tamoxifen on breast cancer proliferation and blood estrogenic biomarkers. *J Natl Cancer Inst* 2003;95:779.
65. Thompson IM, Goodman PJ, Tangen CM, et al. The influence of finasteride on the development of prostate cancer. *N Engl J Med* 2003;349:215.
66. Thompson IM, Tangen CM, Goodman PJ, et al. Chemoprevention of prostate cancer. *J Urol* 2009;182:499; discussion 8.
67. Andriole GL, Bostwick DG, Brawley OW, et al. Effect of dutasteride on the risk of prostate cancer. *N Engl J Med* 2010;362:1192.
68. Thompson IM, Chi C, Ankerst DP, et al. Effect of finasteride on the sensitivity of PSA for detecting prostate cancer. *J Natl Cancer Inst* 2006;98:1128.
69. Gerner EW, Meyskens FL Jr. Polyamines and cancer: old molecules, new understanding. *Nat Rev Cancer* 2004;4:781.
72. Alberts DS, Dorr RT, Einspahr JG, et al. Chemoprevention of human actinic keratoses by topical 2-(difluoromethyl)-dl-ornithine. *Cancer Epidemiol Biomarkers Prev* 2000;9:1281.
73. Meyskens FL Jr, Surwit E, Moon TE, et al. Enhancement of regression of cervical intraepithelial neoplasia II (moderate dysplasia) with topically applied all-trans-retinoic acid: randomized trial. *J Natl Cancer Instit* 1994;86:539.
74. Fabian CJ, Kimler BF, Brady DA, et al. A phase II breast cancer chemoprevention trial of oral alpha-difluoromethylornithine: breast tissue, imaging, and serum and urine biomarkers. *Clin Cancer Res* 2002;8:3105.
77. Gonyeau MJ, Yuen DW. A clinical review of statins and cancer: helpful or harmful? *Pharmacotherapy* 2010;30:177.
80. Poynter JN, Gruber SB, Higgins PD, et al. Statins and the risk of colorectal cancer. *N Engl J Med* 2005;352:2184.
81. Bertagnolli MM, Hsu M, Hawk ET, et al. Statin use and colorectal adenoma risk: results from the adenoma prevention with celecoxib trial. *Cancer Prev Res* 2010;3:588.
84. Lipkin SM, Chao EC, Moreno V, et al. Genetic variation in 3-hydroxy-3-methylglutaryl CoA reductase modifies the chemopreventive activity of statins for colorectal cancer. *Cancer Prev Res* 2010;3:597.
87. Evans JM, Donnelly LA, Emslie-Smith AM, et al. Metformin and reduced risk of cancer in diabetic patients. *BMJ* 2005;330:1304.
88. Pollack MN. Insulin, insulin-like growth factors, insulin resistance, and neoplasia. *Am J Clin Nutr* 2007;86:s820.
90. Torrance CJ, Jackson PE, Montgomery E, et al. Combinatorial chemoprevention of intestinal neoplasia. *Nat Med* 2000;6:1024.
92. Reddy BS, Wang CX, Kong AN, et al. Prevention of azoxymethane-induced colon cancer by combination of low doses of atorvastatin, aspirin, and celecoxib in F 344 rats. *Cancer Res* 2006;66:4542.
93. Meyskens FL Jr, McLaren CE, Pelot D, et al. Difluoromethylornithine plus sulindac for the prevention of sporadic colorectal adenomas: a randomized placebo-controlled, double-blind trial. *Cancer Prev Res* 2008;1:32.
94. Zell JA, Pelot D, Chen WP, et al. Risk of cardiovascular events in a randomized placebo-controlled, double-blind trial of difluoromethylornithine plus sulindac for the prevention of sporadic colorectal adenomas. *Cancer Prev Res* 2009;2:209.
96. Sharma RA, Gescher AJ, Steward WP. Curcumin: the story so far. *Eur J Cancer* 2005;41:1955.
99. Aggarwal BB, Sung B. Pharmacological basis for the role of curcumin in chronic diseases: an age-old spice with modern targets. *Trends Pharmacol Sci* 2009;30:85.
103. Jang M, Cai L, Udeani GO, et al. Cancer chemopreventive activity of resveratrol, a natural product derived from grapes. *Science* 1997;275:218.
104. Pirola L, Frojdo S. Resveratrol: one molecule, many targets. *IUBMB Life* 2008;60:323.
112. Fox JG, Wang TC. Inflammation, atrophy, and gastric cancer. *J Clin Invest* 2007;117:60.
113. Saslow D, Castle PE, Cox JT, et al. American Cancer Society Guideline for human papillomavirus (HPV) vaccine use to prevent cervical cancer and its precursors. *CA Cancer J Clin* 2007;57:7.
117. Correa P, Fontham ET, Bravo JC, et al. Chemoprevention of gastric dysplasia: randomized trial of antioxidant supplements and anti-*Helicobacter pylori* therapy. *J Natl Cancer Inst* 2000;92:1881.
122. Ohkusa T, Fujiki K, Takashimizu I, et al. Improvement in atrophic gastritis and intestinal metaplasia in patients in whom *Helicobacter pylori* was eradicated. *Ann Intern Med* 2001;134:380.

PART SIX
CANCER SCREENING

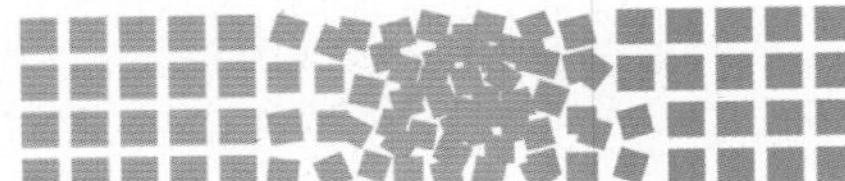

CHAPTER 56 PRINCIPLES OF CANCER SCREENING

JACK S. MANDEL AND ROBERT SMITH

Cancer screening (hereafter referred to as *screening*) is synonymous with secondary prevention, in which earlier therapeutic intervention is possible through screening an asymptomatic population to identify cancer at an earlier stage than it would have been diagnosed in the absence of screening.[1] Screening is distinguished from case detection or case finding, which occurs when the patient presents to a physician with symptoms or suspicion of a condition. The goal of screening is to reduce mortality from the disease and/or reduce the severity of the disease through early diagnosis and treatment.

Screening is the application of a test to an asymptomatic population to determine who is *likely* to have the disease and who is *not likely* to have the disease. Thus, screening tests are not generally diagnostic tests. The detection of occult disease through screening is a two-phase process because those who have positive results from a screening test must undergo diagnostic procedures to determine if they actually have the disease.

There are circumstances in which screening can contribute to primary prevention. for example, when colorectal cancer screening leads to the identification and removal of an adenoma, which subsequently reduces the incidence of colorectal cancer.[2,3]

Screening for cancer began with the Pap smear, a test developed by George Papanicolaou, who in 1941 published his seminal article: "The diagnostic value of vaginal smears in carcinoma of the uterus" in the *American Journal of Obstetrics and Gynecology.*[4] He initially presented his research at the Third Race Betterment Conference in Battle Creek, Michigan, in 1928, but his colleagues were sufficiently discouraging of his ideas about detecting cancer through exfoliative cytology that Papanicolaou abandoned the work for many years. He returned to it more than a decade later and eventually established the correlation between cells scraped from the surface of the cervix and the detection of cervical carcinoma, which he published in 1941. In 1942, he published "Diagnosis of uterine cancer by the vaginal smear."[4] The first widespread use of this technology may have been as early as 1937 when Dr. Elise L'Esperance established a cancer detection center in New York and began using the Pap smear to test women for cervical cancer. Cervical cytology followed by biopsy of a positive test is still the principal method for cervical cancer screening in the world.[5]

Breast cancer screening started in the 1960s when mammography became available. To determine if mammography screening would reduce breast cancer mortality, the Health Insurance Plan of New York study was initiated in 1963.[6] This landmark study of 62,000 women aged 40 to 64 years lasted 25 years and provided the first experimental evidence of the efficacy of breast cancer screening. This study also increased awareness of two important concepts in cancer screening: lead time bias and length bias sampling, which are discussed later.

A number of other cancer screening trials followed the Health Insurance Plan study, including additional breast cancer screening trials in Europe and Canada. Lung cancer screening trials using chest radiograph and sputum cytology were conducted in the 1970s, and the first colorectal cancer screening trial was initiated in 1975. Three other colorectal cancer trials followed. Subsequently, trials evaluating tests for prostate and ovarian cancers were initiated in the 1990s. Today the only proven cancer screening tests are for cervical, breast, and colorectal cancers, although trials have been underway for prostate, lung, and ovarian cancers. Results recently published for prostate cancer screening using the prostate-specific antigen (PSA) test were not consistent.[7,8]

PRINCIPLES OF SCREENING

Although most cancers have a better prognosis if diagnosed earlier in their natural history, this basic observation is not in itself sufficient to justify screening an asymptomatic population for cancer. A number of criteria should be met before initiating cancer screening, these having been first outlined by Wilson and Junger[9] in 1968 for the World Health Organization. These principles of cancer screening along with some additional considerations are as follows:

- The disease should be an important public health problem in terms of its frequency and/or severity. Historically, the development of this principle was in the general context of screening for infectious and chronic diseases and not related specifically to cancer. Today some of the cancer sites considered for screening are not particularly common diseases; nevertheless, early detection and subsequent reduction of mortality can result in a significant benefit in life-years saved.
- The natural history of the disease presents a window of opportunity for early detection. For cancer this generally refers to a detectable preclinical phase (DPCP), and it represents the interface between characteristics of the disease and the screening technology. It is during this period that screening is considered optimal to detect the disease early and prior to the development of symptoms. For screening to be effective, the recommended screening interval must be shorter than the estimate of the DPCP.
- An effective treatment should be available that favorably alters the natural history of the disease. Usually for cancer this means a reduction in cause-specific mortality.
- The treatment should be more effective if initiated during the presymptomatic (or earlier) stage than during the symptomatic (or later) stage; that is, if treating early (presymptomatic) stage has no advantage over treating late

(symptomatic) stage, then the cost and the risk of screening cannot be justified.

- A suitable screening test should be available, that is, one that is accurate, acceptable to the population, fairly easy to administer, safe, and relatively inexpensive.
- There should be an appropriate screening strategy for the target population (i.e., an age to begin screening and a screening interval).

The screening guidelines should be based on good scientific evidence (usually based on results of a randomized controlled clinical trial) and economically feasible:

- Screening programs should have high rates of participation from the eligible population.
- Screening programs for a particular geographic area should take into account specific resources available for screening, diagnosis, and treatment so that countries can focus on optimal recommendations based on available resources.
- Screening programs should be sensitive to patient and provider concerns.
- Screening programs should ensure prompt follow-up of positive tests with a diagnostic examination and prompt treatment of cases.
- Screening programs should be cost-effective.
- Screening programs should be monitored and regularly evaluated.

Most of these principles are fairly straightforward, but a few warrant further discussion.

EVALUATING SCREENING TESTS

Test Validity

The accuracy or validity of a screening test, that is, its ability to distinguish between diseased and nondiseased people, is measured by sensitivity and specificity (Table 56.1). Sensitivity refers to the ability of the screening test to correctly identify people with the disease among the screened population and is defined as the number of people screened with a positive test divided by those who actually have the disease. Specificity refers to the ability of the test to correctly identify people without the disease among the screened population and is defined as the number of people with a negative test divided by the number of people who do not have the disease. Ideally, sensitivity and specificity would be 100% accurate, but unfortunately there is no cancer screening test that performs this well. Hence, although a majority of people undergoing screening will have accurate test results, some will be labeled by the screening test as positive but eventually will be found not to have the disease following the diagnostic workup (false-positives), and some with the disease will be labeled negative by the screening test and thus are missed cases or false-negatives. Sensitivity and specificity are inversely related, ultimately increasing one results in a decrease in the other after a certain threshold of accuracy is reached.

For a quantitative test (e.g., a quantitative immunochemical test for colorectal cancer), the cutoff level to designate a test positive can be adjusted to the extent that all potential cases can be identified (sensitivity equals 100%). However, to do so would sacrifice specificity, resulting in a large number of individuals who would be unnecessarily subjected to a costly and sometimes risky diagnostic procedure. Thus, balancing sensitivity and specificity (when possible) is important in determining the outcome of a screening program.

Measuring Test Performance

Evaluating the sensitivity and specificity of cancer screening tests in community practice poses unique challenges. Specificity is more easily measured as false-positive outcomes are identified in the near term because of the workup of individuals with positive tests. Measuring sensitivity is a greater challenge. Although identifying true positives, like false-positives, occurs at the conclusion of the diagnostic evaluation, those with cancer who test negative are not subjected to a diagnostic evaluation. Hence, immediate ascertainment of the false-negative rate generally is not possible. In practice, estimates of test sensitivity rely on long-term follow-up through cancer registries to determine which individuals were diagnosed with cancer within a fixed interval after a negative screening test. This is the most common method, and it measures cases diagnosed between screenings (interval cancers) as the criterion for a false-negative test result. This method assumes that these cases were detectable at the screening but were missed.

In research settings, test performance may be measured by applying definitive diagnostic tests to all individuals with normal and abnormal screening test results, although this methodology is uncommon because the prevalence of detectable cancer is low and the costs associated with this study design are very high. Alternatively, test performance may be measured by applying the screening test to a group of symptomatic patients. However, this method does not measure screening performance accurately as the results from this approach are not applicable to an asymptomatic population that ultimately will be screened. Regardless of the complexity of screening technology under evaluation, the test may have much better performance in a symptomatic population than in an asymptomatic population.

The proportion of the population with detectable preclinical disease is an important factor in determining the success of screening. If the proportion is low, then relatively few cases will be detected and the yield may be considered too low

TABLE 56.1

OUTCOMES OF A SCREENING AND DIAGNOSTIC PROGRAM[a]

	Diseased	Not Diseased	Total
Positive screening test	True positives (a)	False-positives (b)	Test positives (a + b)
Negative screening test	False-negatives (c)	True negatives (d)	Test negatives (c + d)
Total	Total with disease (a + c)	Total without disease (b + d)	Total screened (a + b + c + d)

Sensitivity = a/(a + c).
Specificity = d/(b + d).
Positive predictive value = a/(a + b).
Negative predictive value = d/(c + d).

CANCER SCREENING

relative to the cost. The length of the DPCP will also influence the frequency of screening. A screening test that can detect a lesion very early in its development will generally be associated with a longer DPCP than a test that more commonly detects a lesion that is more advanced. However, if a screening program is detecting a high percentage of advanced cases, this suggests either the screening interval is too long, allowing considerable tumor progression during the DPCP, or that the test has low test sensitivity perhaps resulting from poor quality assurance. More commonly, host characteristics limit optimal performance of screening tests in same subpopulations.

Positive Predictive Value

An important parameter in evaluating a screening program is positive predictive value (PPV), which is the proportion of individuals with a positive screening test who actually have the disease. The PPV can be computed only after the diagnostic examinations of those who test positive had been completed. A PPV of 10% means that only one in ten of the patients with positive test results truly had the disease. The other nine received the diagnostic examination and incurred cost and risks that are commonly described as "unnecessary." Actually, it is not reasonable to label all false-positives as unnecessary because additional tests and invasive procedures often are necessary in the presence of a positive screening test in order to confirm the presence or absence of cancer. As previously noted, screening tests are not diagnostic tests. Thus, it is important to distinguish, at least conceptually, between what might be labeled as unavoidable versus avoidable follow-up tests. If poor quality results in an excess rate of false-positives, the workups prompted by this fraction of positive test results truly can be labeled as unnecessary and avoidable.

The PPV is influenced by three factors: sensitivity and specificity of the test and the prevalence of disease. Specificity has a bigger effect on PPV because most people who are screened for cancer do not have the disease. If the specificity is increased to improve PPV, at some point the sensitivity will likely decrease (as sensitivity and specificity ultimately are inversely related) and the number of false-negative findings will increase. If the rate of disease increases with increasing age, the PPV also will improve in the higher age groups, even if sensitivity and specificity do not change at all. Alternatively, focusing the screening on a population with a higher prevalence of disease can be accomplished by restricting the screening program to higher-risk individuals who are more likely to have the disease.

Although the PPV is regarded as a measure of effectiveness, a proper interpretation of it requires data on the tumor characteristics of the cancers detected and the cancer detection rate. A program with a very high PPV, but mostly very large tumors, will achieve less than a program with a lower PPV, but a greater cancer detection rate, and a more favorable distribution of tumor characteristics.

Test Sensitivity Versus Program Sensitivity

There is a difference between the performance of a screening test applied once (test sensitivity) and the performance of a screening test applied multiple times to the same population (program sensitivity). If a population is highly adherent with screening recommendations, program sensitivity will generally be higher than test sensitivity because of the greater chance of detecting a cancer on the second round of screening that was missed on the first round of screening. If the screening interval is considerably shorter than the DPCP, then the limitations of a test with lower sensitivity can be overcome with dependable, successive opportunities for detection. However, under circumstances with the same test sensitivity, if adherence with the screening interval is poor, then program sensitivity will be lower because the screening program may be dominated by both missed cancers and cancers detected symptomatically out of interval.

Test sensitivity and program sensitivity also will vary based on the proportion of the population that has undergone screening. When evaluating a test applied to a population, there generally will be different outcomes from the initial screening that detects prevalent cases than from the subsequent screenings that detect incident cases (usually prevalence is greater than incidence). This observation applies to the program overall, but also to the subpopulations that enter the ongoing screening program for the first time. The initial screening will generally detect more cases, and more advanced cases, than subsequent screenings because the pool of prevalent cancers has been reduced after the initial round of screening.

In evaluating program performance over time, the underlying prevalence of disease overall and in subpopulations will influence PPV. Thus, a screening program administered to a lower-risk population will have a different outcome than one administered to a higher-risk population. Variability in PPV can be seen in screening for the same cancer where the underlying prevalence of disease is lower in the younger population undergoing screening than the older population, even if test sensitivity is the same. The quality of the screening and the quality of the diagnostic workup will also influence the outcome of the program.

Threats to Validity

Because of various biases that can affect survival in screening-detected versus nonscreening-detected cancers, such as lead time and length bias sampling (described later), survival alone (case fatality) cannot be used to determine the efficacy of screening. The most informative evaluation of a screening test is a randomized controlled clinical trial (RCT) comparing cause-specific mortality among individuals randomly allocated to screening and individuals randomly allocated to usual care. Overall mortality (i.e., all-cause mortality) is not a sensitive indicator if the number of deaths from the disease of interest represents a relatively small proportion of the total number of deaths, as is the case with most cancers. Further, the goal of screening for a particular cancer is not to prevent an individual from dying of any cause, but rather to avoid a premature death or significant morbidity for a particular cancer.

Generally RCTs for cancer screening tests are expensive and take considerable time to complete. A large number of participants are usually needed, and they must be engaged in the study for many years to be able to detect a difference in cause-specific mortality if in fact the test is effective. For example, in evaluating fecal occult blood testing for colorectal cancer there have been four major RCTs involving a total of more than 300,000 people. The duration of the trials was at least 15 years. Following the successful completion of trials for one screening test such as Hemoccult (Beckman Coulter Inc., Fullerton, California) for colorectal cancer, is it necessary to conduct a full-scale RCT for another similar test such as an immunochemical fecal occult blood test? Because there are a number of similar fecal occult blood tests, each would have to be evaluated using thousands of people studied over a 15-year period. Clearly, such trials are not needed for every test, and a study could be designed to evaluate the performance of a new fecal occult blood test against the proven one using many fewer people over a shorter period of time.

Case-control studies, which can be conducted with fewer people and in a relatively short period of time, have been used to evaluate screening tests, but because of potential selection bias these studies are not sufficient to provide definitive evidence of effectiveness. The U.S. Preventive Services Task Force, which develops recommendations for screening tests, including cancer screening tests, relies primarily on RCTs for proof that a test is effective in reducing deaths.

Lead Time Bias

In the evaluation of cancer screening tests, it is important to distinguish between the survival rate and the mortality rate, which principally is the reason there is a distinction between lead time and lead-time bias. Because screening advances the time of diagnosis, the duration of time between when a cancer is detected by screening and when it would have been detected because of symptoms is referred to as the *lead time,* and achieving lead time is a fundamental goal of screening. The lead time gained nearly always is less than the DPCP, as there will be few individuals who have perfect concordance between the date of screening and the date that their cancer entered the DPCP. As previously noted, the recommended screening interval must be shorter than the estimated DPCP in order to have the greatest probability of detecting most cancers through regular screening.

The survival rate is the percentage of people diagnosed with a particular cancer who are alive after a specific duration of time. In the absence of screening, survival is measured from the time of diagnosis associated with symptomatic disease and the proportion dying or surviving over a particular duration. In a screening program, survival time is measured by the average time between the date of diagnosis as a result of a screening that detected occult tumor and the proportion surviving or dying over a particular duration. However, if screening results in earlier detection of disease, but death occurs at the same time as it would in the absence of screening, then there will appear to be an increase in mean survival associated with screening when in fact there is not. This is referred to as *lead-time bias* and is represented by the interval of time between detection by screening and the time when the diagnosis would have been made in the absence of screening, that is, generally when the patient is symptomatic. It represents the amount of time by which treatment is advanced because of earlier detection, but there is no survival advantage for the patient. However, the proportion of cases that survive for some time after diagnosis will be higher, thus giving the impression that screening is effective.

The goal of screening is to reduce the incidence rate of advanced disease, and that is achieved by advancing the lead time before a cancer becomes symptomatic. Prospective RCTs avoid lead-time bias because the end point of interest is mortality. Studies that show higher survival in screening-detected cancers compared with symptom-detected cancers, however encouraging, do not provide sufficient evidence to endorse a policy of offering screening to the population because lead-time bias cannot be ruled out.

Although lead-time bias can increase survival in screening-detected cases, its true influence is limited by the duration of the detectable preclinical phase. Thus, the effect of lead-time bias on survival occurs in the near term, whereas long-term differences in survival are more likely to be influenced by length bias, which is discussed next.

Length-Bias Sampling

Length-bias sampling refers to the tendency for screening to be more successful at detecting slow-growing, less aggressive disease, and to be less successful at detecting more aggressive, faster-growing disease. *Length bias* simply refers to the greater likelihood of screening-detected cancers having a longer DPCP, and hence a greater likelihood of being detected.

Length-bias sampling is a function of the variability in cancer progression rates. For any given screening interval, there is a greater probability of detecting a slower-growing cancer than a faster-growing cancer. If the slower-growing cancers have better prognosis, the screening will selectively identify cases at a lower risk of death, and this "length-bias sampling" will create the impression that screening is more effective than it actually is, when in fact the increased survival is simply the result of the detection of slower-growing cancers with a more favorable prognosis. Overdiagnosis is an extreme case of length-bias sampling, but it is difficult to estimate the rate of overdiagnosis as there is no way to prove that a given tumor would remain subclinical indefinitely.

Overdiagnosis

A consequence of screening can be overdiagnosis, which is the detection of a cancer that would not have progressed to become symptomatic in the person's lifetime. Such lesions, when detected, are currently indistinguishable from lesions that are, or evolve, to become clinically significant. The example generally cited to illustrate overdiagnosis bias resulting from screening is the detection of prostate cancer using the PSA test. Because of the high prevalence of latent prostatic cancer in older men, a screening test such as PSA will detect some cancers that, in the absence of screening, would have remained asymptomatic during the remainder of the person's lifetime. As a result of the testing they are identified and subsequently treated in the same manner and perhaps with the same urgency as all other prostate cancers. However, there may be the same serious consequences for patients undergoing treatment of these latent cancers, including short-term disability, unnecessary costs, and long-term treatment-related side effects as experienced by those who needed to be treated to avoid premature death. Further, in reality the screening has produced no true benefit for these patients because they did not have a life-threatening cancer, although there may appear to be a benefit in that the patient's outcome in terms of survival is favorable.

Overdiagnosis is largely a theoretical and statistical concept. It is very difficult to measure, and where experimental evidence has shown that screening is associated with a reduction in deaths from cancer, overdiagnosis likely represents a small contribution to the harms in comparison to a larger benefit from screening.

Selection Bias

Individuals who participate in cancer screening are usually different from those who do not participate, and these differences could have an affect on disease outcomes. For example, compared with the population who does not undergo screening, those who do generally will be more health conscious and healthier, more aware of the signs and symptoms of disease, have access to better health care, and be more adherent to treatment.

DEVELOPING AND EVALUATING A CANCER SCREENING PROGRAM

Cancer screening programs are generally designed to administer tests multiple times on a recommended schedule (e.g., annual mammograms). Current cancer screening tests are generally not designed for a one-time application, although one test, colonoscopy for colorectal cancer (the diagnostic examination), has been considered as a screening test that could be applied periodically (every 10 years) or even once in a lifetime. Continued screening of a population will lessen the consequences of false-negative results because these cancers may be detected in subsequent screenings. If disease progression is not too rapid, as for example in most colorectal cancers, then a false-negative finding on a single screen may not have serious long-term consequences if the cancer is detected on a follow-up screen. An effective screening test may not significantly reduce disease-specific morbidity and mortality in the population if the participation rate with the screening and/or the diagnostic evaluation in the program is low. Thus, adherence to the screening and subsequent diagnostic program is essential to ensure that the benefit accrues to the population. A good health education program is important to ensure that the population understands the disease and the importance of screening, the screening method to be used, the diagnostic procedures, potential risks, and treatment options. Some countries are able to rely on population registers to remind individuals that screening tests are due, whereas in the United States, the referring physician plays a key role.

Once screening has been introduced in a population, how soon should benefits be evident in population trends of disease rates? The answer to this question is not easily answered, and depends on the duration of the rollout period, the rate of uptake, nonscreening influences on incidence and mortality (e.g., behavioral changes, improvements in therapy), the lag in surveillance data, and the ability to isolate screened and nonscreened cohorts in an analysis. In 2009, several publications on cancer screening argued that the benefits of screening were lower and harms higher than commonly perceived[10,11] and challenged the value of screening for breast and prostate cancer as trends in incidence and mortality were not more favorable in the presence of significant screening rates.[11] They stated that optimal screening should have produced a rise in incidence rates, followed by a fall in rates, and then a return to prescreening rates, which should have a more favorable stage distribution. This theoretical scenario would result from a rise in incidence during screening related to lead time, followed by the decline in incidence from cancers already having been detected, and then a return to prescreening incidence rates. They observed that in the United States, breast and prostate cancer screening has not produced that trend, but instead has led to an increase in localized disease, without a decline in advanced disease. Despite contrary results from RCTs, these studies concluded that screening is not very effective at altering the natural history of aggressive disease, and mostly detects less aggressive and indolent (i.e., overdiagnosed) cases.

However, this scenario is not very realistic because the entire population is different from the potentially screened population, the actually screened population, and the occasionally and regularly screened populations. Incidence rates include cancers detected in adults who are not eligible for screening, have no access to screening, are eligible but refuse screening, are irregularly screened, screened but did not have their early-stage disease detected, and those who entered the screening cohort for the first time, of which the latter group will generally manifest the characteristics of a prevalent screening round. The conclusion that much of the excess of disease represented significant overdiagnosis may be explained by the short period of observation, a trend in rising incidence rates, and the expected effect of lead time. Even though overdiagnosis is a significant problem in prostate cancer screening,[12] it is likely a small problem in breast cancer screening, and mostly limited to ductal carcinoma *in situ*.[13,14] Short-term evaluations of population surveillance data are not a sound basis for judging the effectiveness of screening.[15]

Beyond population adherence, it is important to continuously evaluate screening programs to measure performance and apply corrective action where appropriate. Screening must be appreciated as a continuum of interrelated steps. Compromises in the quality at any one step can significantly reduce the benefit of a screening program.

References

1. Morrison A. *Screening in Chronic Disease*. New York: Oxford University Press, 1992.
2. Mandel JS, Church TR, Bond JH, et al. The effect of fecal occult-blood screening on the incidence of colorectal cancer. *N Engl J Med* 2000; 343:1603.
3. Winawer SJ, Zauber AG, Ho MN, et al. Prevention of colorectal cancer by colonoscopic polypectomy. The National Polyp Study Workgroup. *N Engl J Med* 1993;329:1977.
4. Michalas SP. The Pap test: George N. Papanicolaou (1883–1962). A screening test for the prevention of cancer of uterine cervix. *Eur J Obstet Gynecol Reprod Biol* 2000;90:135.
5. Ngoma T. World Health Organization cancer priorities in developing countries. *Ann Oncol* 2006;17(Suppl 8):viii9.
6. Shapiro S, Venet W, Strax P, Venet L. *Periodic Screening for Breast Cancer: the Health Insurance Plan Project and its Sequelae*. Baltimore: Johns Hopkins University Press, 1988.
7. Schroder FH, Hugosson J, Roobol MJ, et al. ERSPC Investigators Screening and prostate-cancer mortality in a randomized European study. *N Engl J Med* 2009;360(13):1320.
8. Andriole GL, Crawford ED, Grubb RL, et al, for the PLCO Project Team. Mortality results from a randomized prostate-cancer screening trial. *N Engl J Med* 2009;360(13):1310.
9. Wilson JMG, Junger G. *Principles and Practice of Screening for Disease*. Geneva, Switzerland: World Health Organization, 1968.
10. Screening for breast cancer: U.S. Preventive Services Task Force recommendation statement. *Ann Intern Med* 2009;151:716.
11. Esserman L, Shieh Y, Thompson I. Rethinking screening for breast cancer and prostate cancer. *JAMA* 2009;302:1685.
12. Etzioni R, Penson DF, Legler JM, et al. Overdiagnosis due to prostate-specific antigen screening: lessons from U.S. prostate cancer incidence trends. *J Natl Cancer Inst* 2002;94:981.
13. Duffy SW, Lynge E, Jonsson H, Ayyaz S, Olsen AH. Complexities in the estimation of overdiagnosis in breast cancer screening. *Br J Cancer* 2008;99:1176.
14. Yen MF, Tabar L, Vitak B, Smith RA, Chen HH, Duffy SW. Quantifying the potential problem of overdiagnosis of ductal carcinoma in situ in breast cancer screening. *Eur J Cancer* 2003;39:1746.
15. Etzioni R, Feuer E. Studies of prostate-cancer mortality: caution advised. *Lancet Oncol* 2008;9:407.

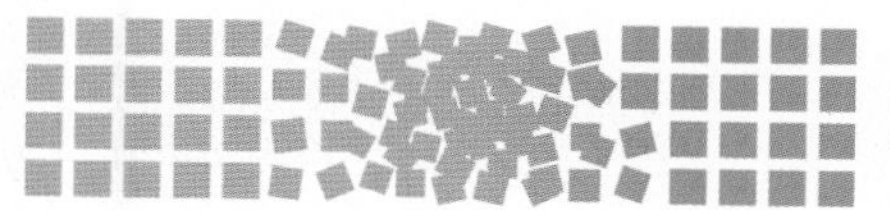

CHAPTER 57 EARLY DETECTION USING PROTEOMICS

VIRGINIA ESPINA, CLAUDIO BELLUCO, EMANUEL F. PETRICOIN III, AND LANCE A. LIOTTA

CELLULAR PROTEOMICS

Essential Information for the Individualized Therapy of Cancer

Advances in cancer molecular targeted therapies have created a tremendous need to more precisely define patients who will derive the most benefit from molecular targeted agents.[1] Staging parameters such as tumor size, degree of tumor cell differentiation, presence or absence of metastases, cytogenetic analysis, and immunohistochemical scoring all play an important role in therapeutic decision making. Nevertheless, these parameters fail to address the complexity and tumor-specific molecular alterations that determine success or failure of a targeted therapeutic agent. Completion of the human genome sequence[2,3] was just the beginning of what promises to be a new era in medicine.[4] The new and current challenge is to generate a comprehensive understanding of the cellular "software and the hardware." Full penetration of the causal mechanisms driving carcinogenesis and cancer progression requires analytical tools ranging from direct DNA sequencing, to microRNA expression monitoring, to protein sequencing, and finally, metabolic profiling to develop molecular network maps. In response to this need, the rapidly emerging field of cellular proteomics has the potential to generate essential information for individualized therapy.

The final functional network state of cancer cells is a product of the individual genetic derangement of that cancer cell within the context of the tissue microenvironment. Cellular metabolism associated with disease may be due to posttranslational processes regulated by the cellular environment, and these disease-associated changes cannot be inferred from DNA or RNA profiles. Signal network proteins coalesce into pathways following a stimulus. Once the stimulus is removed the interconnected proteins disperse and the network organization dissolves.

As we are learning more about how signaling networks are continually remodeling under the influence of the tissue microenvironment, the diagnostic report of the future will be an individualized network map, or the equivalent of a different street map, for each patient. Moreover, the most meaningful measurements may be the strength of connections between nodes in the network, not just the amount of each node, or protein, in the network.[5] Accordingly, elucidation of the human proteome requires an understanding of the corresponding repertoire of potential posttranslational modifications and matching functional correlations. Thus, a complete understanding of the molecular basis of cancer depends on a multidisciplinary approach combining genetics, pathology, proteomics, cell biology, bioinformatics, and clinical medicine.

New Technology to Realize the Promise of Individualized Therapy Profiling

Realizing the potential of tissue proteomics for individualized therapy is not possible unless appropriate new technology is available to overcome the key challenges to tissue proteomic profiling. Laser capture microdissection (LCM) has solved the first challenge, procuring enriched cell populations from heterogeneous tissue samples.[6,7] The second challenge, measuring the functional states of cellular signaling pathways, has been solved by protein microarrays.[8–11] The third challenge is preservation of the labile tissue protein antigen. This last challenge is being solved with new classes of tissue-preservative chemistries.[12,13] With all these technologies in place, tissue proteomics has graduated from basic science to clinical trial implementation.[5] This chapter will review all three classes of technology and show how they are currently in use in clinical research trials based on individualized molecular targeted therapy.

Laser Capture Microdissection

Solving the Challenge of Tissue Heterogeneity

LCM enables researchers to isolate specific cells of interest, under direct microscopic visualization, without contamination from surrounding cells (Fig. 57.1).[7,14–17] Heterogeneous tissue may confound molecular analysis because it is currently impossible to discern which cells contribute which cellular constituents to a given tissue lysate. A twofold signal difference is considered highly significant for gene arrays and protein analytes, but there may be greater than twofold differences in cell population numbers between different tissue sections from the same tumor, making molecular profile comparisons invalid for heterogeneous, nonmicrodissected samples.[16,17] Tumor-stromal interactions are now regarded as important communications for tumor development,[18–22] embryonic development,[23,24] and wound healing.[25] Thus, molecular profiling of microdissected tissue cell populations, which is reflective of the cell population's *in vivo* genomic and proteomic state, is essential for correlating molecular signatures in diseased and disease-free cells.[11,15,26,27]

Laser Microdissection Systems

Prior to 1996 investigators used manual scraping with tools such as needles, or had attempted laser ablation, of all unwanted cells in a tissue field, so as to leave behind the desired cells.[28,29] LCM, launched by a publication in *Science*,[7] was developed as a means for directly procuring and physically capturing the

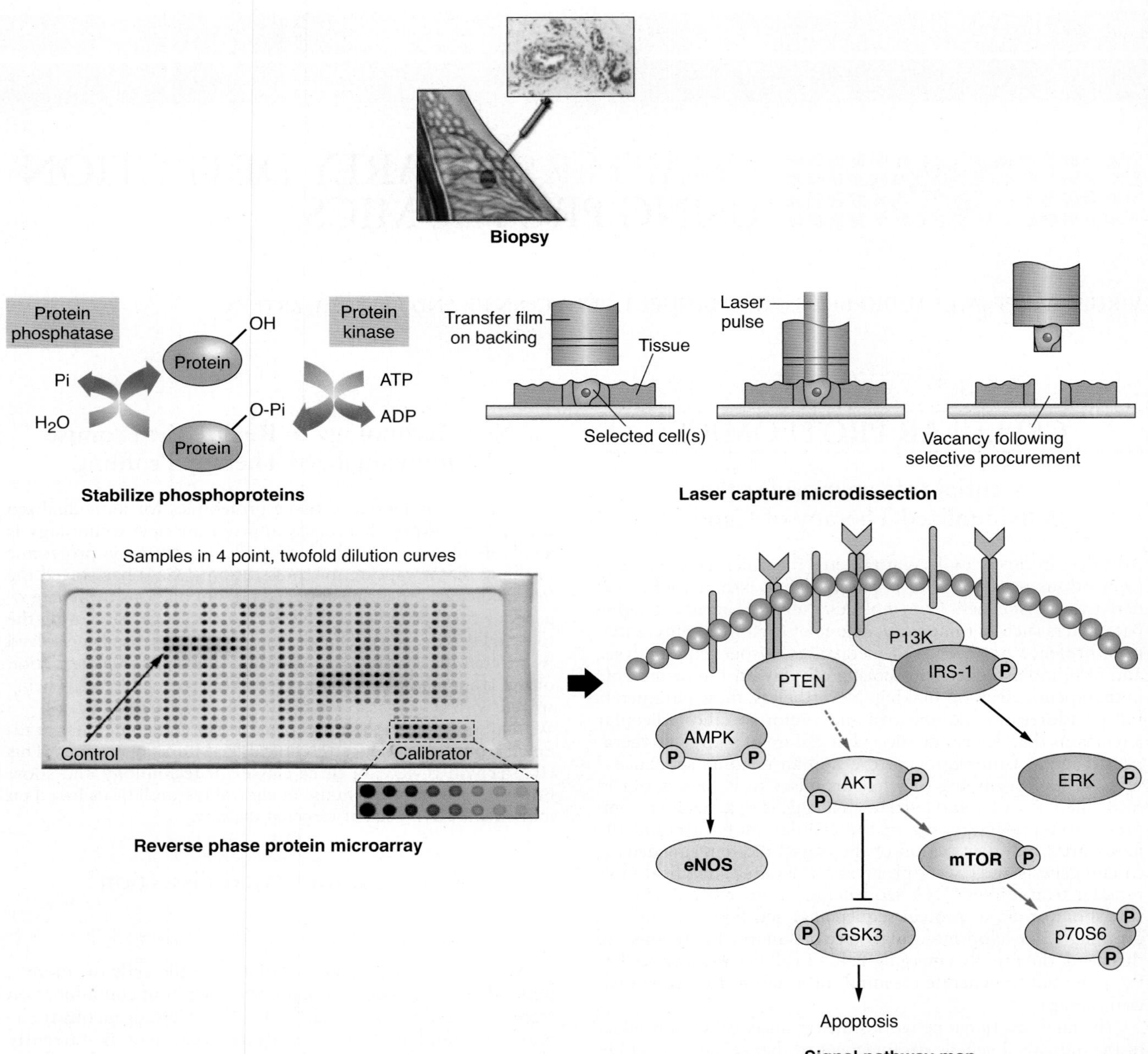

FIGURE 57.1 Proteomics workflow for mapping cell signaling kinase activity. Biopsy samples are divided into aliquots for diagnosis or translational research. Protein conformation and enzymatic activity are retained if the tissue is frozen or fixed in a solution that blocks both phosphatase and kinase activity. Tissues contain heterogeneous cellular populations (e.g., epithelium, cancer cells, fibroblasts, endothelium, and immune cells). Laser capture microdissection (LCM), using a stained tissue section under direct microscopic visualization, is used to procure pure cell populations. LCM directly procures the subpopulation of cells selected for study, while leaving behind all of the contaminating cells. A stained section of the heterogeneous tissue is mounted on a glass microscope slide and viewed under high magnification. The experimenter selects the individual cell(s) to be studied via a computer screen. A stationary near-IR (infrared) laser mounted in the optical axis of the microscope stage is used for melting a thermolabile polymer film, which is mounted on the bottom surface of an optical-quality plastic cap. The polymer melts only in the vicinity of the laser pulse, forming a polymer-cell composite. When the polymer cap is lifted from the tissue section, only the desired cells for study are excised from the heterogeneous cellular population. Using appropriate buffers, the cellular constituents are solubilized and printed in a multiplexed, reverse phase protein microarray format. Proteins from all subcellular locations can be mapped based on activity level, thus generating a cell-signaling profile of a specific cellular population. (Adapted from Mueller C, Liotta LA, Espina V. Reverse phase protein microarrays advance to use in clinical trials. *Mol Oncol* 2010;4(6):461–481.)

desired cells in one step. The principal components of laser microdissection technology are (1) visualization of the cells of interest via microscopy, (2) transfer of laser energy to a thermolabile polymer with formation of a polymer-cell composite (infrared [IR] system), or photo volatilization of cells surrounding a selected area (ultraviolet [UV] system), and (3) removal of the cells of interest from the heterogeneous tissue section (Fig. 57.1). Using LCM, frozen or fixed tissues, or live cells, can be successfully dissected and recovered cells can be used for DNA, RNA, and protein analysis (Fig. 57.2).[14,30–38]

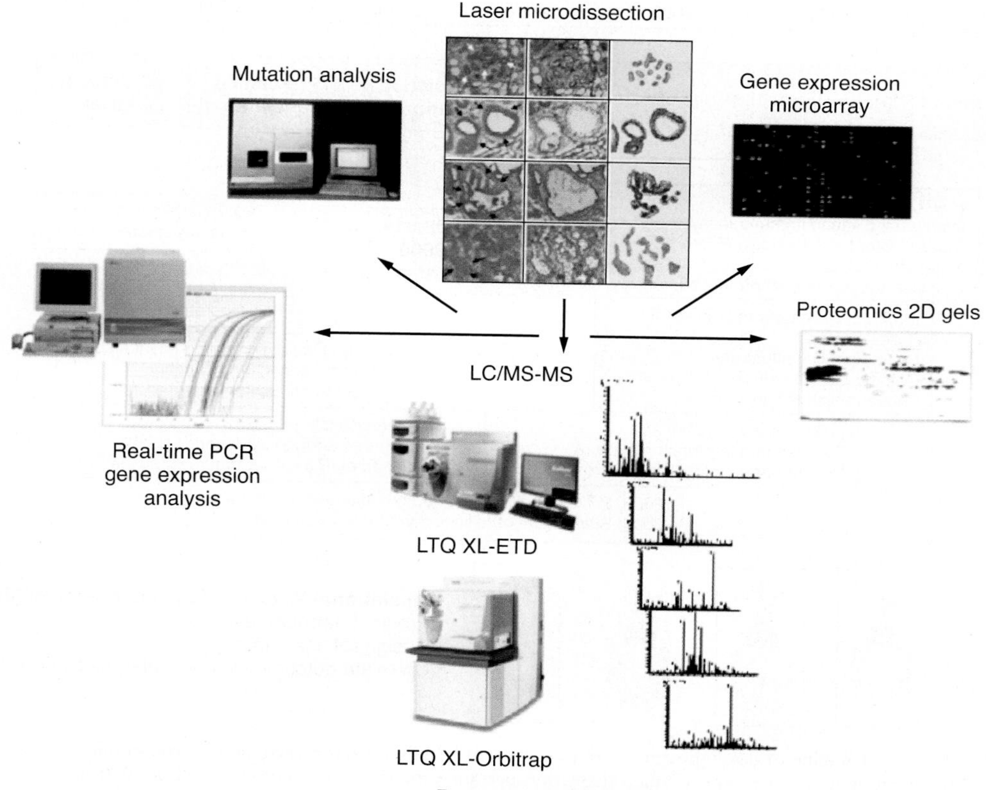

FIGURE 57.2 Applications of laser capture microdissection to genomic and proteomic discovery and analysis of cell type-specific molecular changes. The extracted proteins, DNA, or RNA can be analyzed by any method that has sufficient sensitivity. Examples include gene-associated somatic mutation analysis of tumor etiology and progression (*upper left*), gene expression measurement by real-time polymerase chain reaction (PCR) (*middle left*), or transcript arrays (*upper right*), proteomic fractionization of proteins by two-dimensional (2D) gels (*middle right*), and protein sequencing by mass spectrometry (MS) (*lower*) such as LC/MS-MS, liquid chromatography/mass spectrometry or LTQ-XL-ETD, electron transfer dissociation.

Protein Array Technology

Multiplex Analysis of Cellular Signaling Proteins

Protein microarrays represent an emerging technology that is quickly becoming a powerful tool for drug discovery, biomarker identification, and signal transduction profiling of cellular material (Fig. 57.3). The advantage of protein microarrays lies in their ability to provide a "map" of known cellular signaling proteins that can reflect, in general, the state of information flow through protein networks in individual specimens in a manner that is not possible with gene arrays. Identification of critical nodes, or interactions, within the network is a potential starting point for drug development and/or the design of individual therapy regimens.[11,15,17,27,39–42] Protein microarrays may be used to monitor changes in protein phosphorylation over time, before and after treatment, or between disease and nondisease states, allowing one to infer protein activity levels in a particular pathway to tailor treatment to each patient's cellular "circuitry" (Fig. 57.1).[11,15,17,27,39–42]

Protein microarray formats fall into two major classes, forward phase arrays (FPA) and reverse phase arrays (RPMA), depending on whether the analyte(s) of interest is captured from the solution phase or bound to the solid phase.[10,43–52] In an FPA format (antibody array), capture molecules, such as antibodies, are immobilized onto the substratum and act as the bait molecule. Each FPA is incubated with one test sample (e.g., a cellular lysate from one treatment condition or serum sample from disease/control patients), and multiple analytes are measured at once. A number of excellent reviews summarize recent applications, obstacles, and new advances in FPA technology.[53–56]

Reverse Phase Protein Microarray Technology

RPMAs are a direct descendant of miniaturized immunoassays (Fig. 57.3).[8,9] The introduction of gene expression microarray technology in 1995 provided researchers with technology needed to fabricate high-throughput protein microarrays.[57] The term *reverse phase* refers to the fact that the analyte (antigen) is immobilized as a capture molecule, rather than immobilizing an antibody as the capture molecule (Fig. 57.1).[10] RPMAs were originally developed to quantitatively measure numerous proteins extracted from a small number of cells obtained from tissue microdissection,[15–17,19,27,39,58–60] but the technology has been used in preclinical stuides of human cell lysates,[61–64] cell lines,[65–69] and serum/plasma.[70–74] RPMA makes it possible to evaluate the state of entire portions of a signaling pathway or cascade, even though the cell is lysed, by quantifying posttranslationally modified or total cellular proteins from multiple samples printed on a series of identical arrays (Fig. 57.1) with high sensitivity (femtogram-attogram range) and good precision (<15% coefficient of variation).[10,11,27,75–78]

Protein Stability and Preanalytical Variability

The promise of tissue protein biomarkers to provide revolutionary diagnostic and therapeutic information will never be

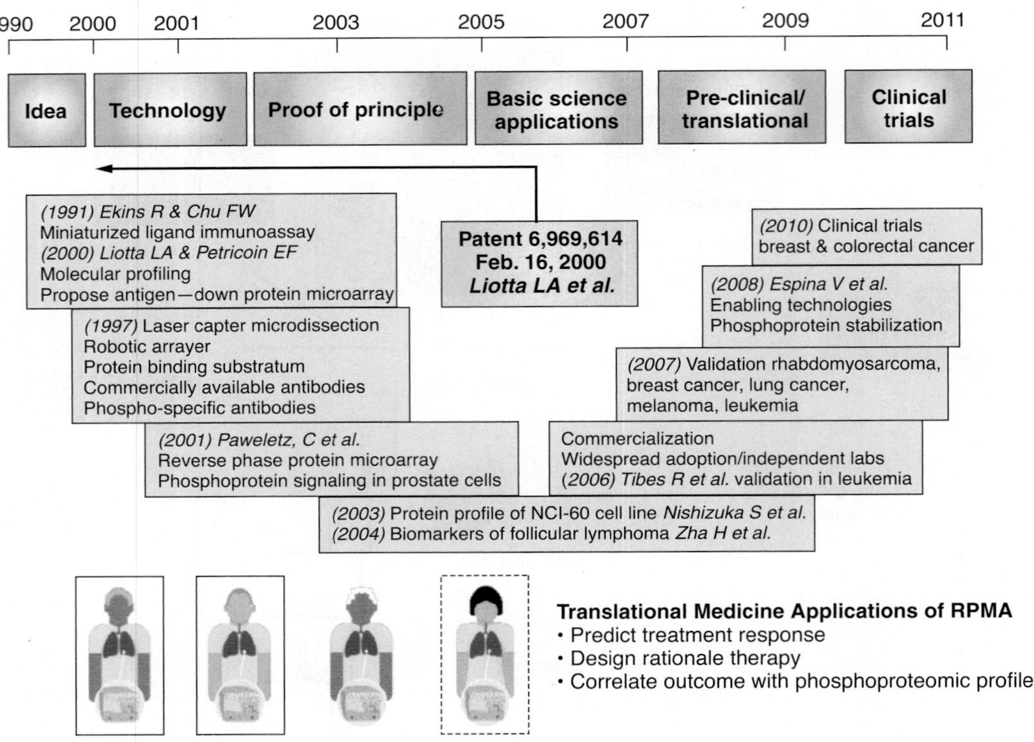

FIGURE 57.3 Timeline of development for laser capture microdissection, reverse phase protein microarrays, and enabling technologies. Laser capture microdissection permits procurement of enriched cell populations for DNA, RNA, or protein analysis. Reverse phase protein microarray technology allows specific proteomic posttranslational modifications to be quantified in a multiplex format. Validation of these technologies in independent laboratories, and commercialization of the platforms, coupled with emerging technologies for specimen preservation, have supported translational medicine applications such as designing rationale therapy and predicting treatment response. (Adapted from Mueller C, Liotta LA, Espina V. Reverse phase protein microarrays advance to use in clinical trials *Mol Oncol* 2010;4(6);461–481.)

realized unless the problem of tissue protein biomarker instability is recognized and solved. Cells within a tissue biopsy react and adapt to the trauma of excision, ischemia, hypoxia, acidosis, accumulation of cellular waste, absence of electrolytes, and temperature changes.[12,79] A large surge of stress, hypoxia, and wound repair–related protein signal pathway proteins and transcription factors are induced in the tissue immediately following procurement.[80,81] Investigators have worried about the effects of vascular clamping and anesthesia prior to excision on the fidelity of molecular data in tissues.[82] A much more significant and underappreciated issue is the fact that excised tissue is alive and reacting to *ex vivo* stress.[12,83–85] Without stabilization, imbalances of kinases/phosphatases will significantly distort the tissue's molecular signature compared to the state of *in vivo* markers.

At any point in time within the tissue cellular microenvironment, the phosphorylated state of a protein is a function of the local stoichiometry of associated kinases and phosphatases specific for the phosphorylated residue. Thus, in the absence of kinase activity, proteins may be dephosphorylated by phosphatases, reducing the level of a phosphoprotein analyte causing a false-negative result. This can be prevented by a variety of chemical- and protein-based phosphatase inhibitors.[86,87] However if the kinase remains active, then the addition of a phosphatase inhibitor alone will result in an augmentation of the phosphoepitope, generating a false-positive result. Consequently, cellular samples for kinase network analysis require stabilization of the kinases and phosphoproteins immediately after tissue procurement, and these stabilizing solutions (preservatives) are currently being evaluated in clinical research trials.[12,88]

Guidelines for Reducing Tissue Preanalytical Variability

Based on the emerging published data revealing that excised tissue is reactive and can introduce sources of variability for diagnostic molecular end points, the following guidelines can be proposed for the reduction of preanalytical variables.[12,83–85,89,90] (1) Tissue should be stabilized within 20 minutes of excision. (2) Stabilization methods should block both sides of the kinase/phosphatase kinetic reaction. (3) Tissue-preservation methods should be compatible with the intended downstream analysis while maintaining histology and morphology. (4) Sample excision/collection time, elapsed time to stabilization, and length of fixation time are critical data elements for sample quality assessment.

Nonformalin Fixation Chemistries for Molecular Analysis

Although it is now possible to extract proteins from formalin-fixed tissue,[91–93] formalin penetrates tissue at a variable rate, reported within the range of millimeters per hour.[94–96] During this permeation period the portion of the living tissue deeper than a few millimeters would be expected to undergo significant fluctuations in regard to phosphoprotein analytes.[91,94,97] Because the dimensions of the tissue and the depth of the block from which samples are prepared are unknown variables, formalin fixation would be expected to cause significant variability in protein and phosphoprotein stability for molecular diagnostics.[94,98,99]

Although new fixatives have been developed for preservation and/or extraction of RNA from formalin-fixed tissue, there is an awakening recognition that new chemistries are needed for preserving proteins as well.[100–102] Rapid-fixation chemistries and formalin alternatives are being developed but as yet have not been thoroughly evaluated in a time course analysis of fluctuating posttranslationally modified proteins.[97,100,101,103–106] Thermal/pressure inactivation of proteins has been developed as an effective, rapid protein stabilization/inactivation method,[107] but fails to maintain tissue morphology. Ultrasound rapid fixation[97,103,104,106,108] and non–formalin-based fixatives[100,105] processed with or without microwave assistance are technologies designed to preserve diagnostic macromolecules for subsequent histopathologic analysis. Espina et al.[12] have described an ethanol-based fixative chemistry that contains phosphatase and kinase inhibitors to successfully arrest the reactive kinase pathways activated *ex vivo* following procurement while maintaining tissue histomorphology for frozen-section preparation and paraffin embedding.

LCM and RPMA in the Molecular Oncology Clinic

LCM and RPMA have been successfully combined to analyze the functional state of signaling pathways within microdissected human malignant lesions, including comparisons to adjacent normal epithelium, invasive carcinoma, or host stroma.[11,12,15,17,27,39,58,59,109,110] Preclinical data generated from RPMA performed following professional (College of American Pathologists) and federal laboratory standards (Clinical Laboratory Improvement Amendments) have propelled the technology into several clinical research trials.[13,15,17]

I-SPY 1 and I-SPY 2 Breast Cancer Clinical Trials

I-SPY 1 and I-SPY 2 (Investigation of Serial Studies to Predict Your Therapeutic Response with Imaging and Molecular Analysis) are a series of national clinical trials for patients with stage II/III breast cancer.[111] A primary objective of I-SPY 1 was to establish a research infrastructure for combining imaging, comparative genomic hybridization, gene expression, fluorescent *in situ* hybridization, immunohistochemistry, and RPMA data that were generated at independent research centers. I-SPY 1 was the first clinical trial in which RPMA analysis of frozen core needle biopsies was reduced to practice in a College of American Pathologists/Clinical Laboratory Improvement Amendments compliant laboratory. I-SPY 2 is an adaptive trial design that will be used to correlate response and outcome with molecular targeted inhibitors (figitumumab/neratinib/ABT-888).[5]

Individualized Therapy for Metastatic Colorectal Cancer (NITMEC) Trial

An urgent clinical need exists to identify new drug targets for metastatic lesions because the metastasis cell signaling network is different from the primary tumor.[20,112] The extent of cell signaling changes associated with colorectal metastasis, compared to the primary tumor, was the basis for developing a score to stratify patients for a phase 1/2 study (NITMEC) of imatinib alone or in combination with panitumumab. The score was developed based on RPMA, which indicated that a high percentage of liver metastasis with wild type *K-ras* had high levels of phosphorylated c-KIT and PDGF; thus implying that the liver metastasis may be sensitive to imatinib. Investigators in the NITMEC trial are profiling cells procured by LCM from hepatic metastasis samples to evaluate the feasibility of a predefined proteomic score to predict which patient may be responsive to imatinib treatment.[58]

Individualized Therapy for Metastatic or Locally Recurrent Breast Cancer

Molecular profiling to individualize therapy for patients with refractory, metastatic breast cancer is the basis for a trial sponsored by TGen Drug Development Services and Side Out Foundation. In order to assess whether individualized therapy can change the clinical course of disease a growth modulation index will be calculated for each patient. The growth modulation index is the ratio of progression-free survival under the individualized therapy to the time to progression for the most recent regimen on which the patient has progressed. Biopsies of the metastatic disease are analyzed using immunohistochemistry, transcript arrays, and RPMA. For the RPMA, biopsies are subjected to LCM prior to RPMA analysis, and the activated state of selected signal pathways is scored. Data from all three assays are used to select a therapy for each patient.

Prevention of Invasive Breast Neoplasia by Chloroquine Trial

Prevention of Invasive breast Neoplasia by Chloroquine (PINC) is a neoadjuvant therapy trial for patients with breast ductal carcinoma *in situ* (DCIS) sponsored by Inova Health Systems (USA). The therapeutic target is the autophagy pathway and the proposed treatment is oral Aralen (chloroquine phosphate). The therapeutic strategy is based on data that support the hypothesis that cellular autophagy is necessary for the survival and propagation of DCIS neoplastic cells.[13] Patients with estrogen receptor (ER)-positive high-grade DCIS will receive standard of care tamoxifen, plus Aralen. Patients with low-grade, ER-positive DCIS will receive tamoxifen only. Patients who are ER-negative will receive Aralen only. The activated state of 100 signal pathway proteins associated with autophagy, hypoxia, adhesion apoptosis, and p53-mediated cell survival will be measured by RPMA before and after therapy within the microdissected epithelial and stromal compartments.[13]

Phase 2 Trial of Trastuzumab and/or Lapatinib Plus Chemotherapy for *HER2*-Positive Breast Cancer

Lapatinib and trastuzumab have different modes of action on the *HER2/EGFR* signaling cascade. Lapatinib, a small-molecule inhibitor, is a dual tyrosine kinase inhibitor that blocks both EGFR (ErbB1) and *HER2* (ErbB2) by binding to the adenosine triphosphate pocket. Lapatinib can also inhibit truncated forms of the receptor,[113] while trastuzumab, a monoclonal antibody, binds directly to the *HER2* extracellular domain.[114] RPMAs are providing quantitative cell signaling data related to the *in vivo* effects of these molecular targeted therapies before and after treatment (US Oncology 05–074 /GlaxoSmithKline LPT109096 sponsored trial). This multisite trial recently completed patient accrual (N = 100) and has established a proteomic workflow for breast core needle biopsy preservation and shipping without the need for dry ice or frozen samples.[12] Two important questions are being addressed in this clinical trial: (1) Does mono or combination *HER2* inhibition therapy improve complete patient response? (2) Can we prospectively identify responders to *HER2* targeted therapy?

Phase 2 Trial of Radiation, Cisplatin, and Panitumumab in Head and Neck Cancer

The University of Pittsburgh–sponsored trial (NCT00798655) for squamous cell carcinoma of the head and neck will evaluate progression-free survival of patients undergoing postoperative chemoradiotherapy plus panitumumab.[5] Patient inclusion criteria include stage III/IVa tumors, without any prior chemotherapy or EGFR pathway inhibitor therapy. RPMAs are being used in baseline archival paraffin-embedded tumor tissue samples to correlate potential efficacy parameters with EGFR, angiogenesis, and downstream pathway activation for at least 17 total or phosphorylated cell-signaling proteins, as well as with genetic polymorphisms.

BIOMARKER PROTEOMICS

Opportunities, Challenges, and New Technology

Biomarker discovery is moving away from the idealized single cancer-specific biomarker. Despite decades of effort, single biomarkers have not been found that can reach an acceptable level of specificity and sensitivity required for routine clinical use for detection or monitoring of the most common cancers. Most investigators believe that this is because of patient-to-patient tumor molecular heterogeneity, tumor location, size, histology, grade, and stage. Moreover, an individual patient's organ may harbor tumor cells coexisting at multiple stages in the same tissue (e.g., *in situ* and invasive cancer). Epidemiologic heterogeneity, including differences in age, sex, and genetic background, is a third level of patient-to-patient variability that can reduce cancer biomarker specificity. Taking a cue from gene arrays, the hope is that panels of tens to hundreds of protein and peptide markers may transcend the heterogeneity to generate a higher level of diagnostic specificity.

Serum/Plasma Proteomics: An Expanding Diagnostic Window

The recognition that cancer is a product of the proteomic tissue microenvironment and involves communication networks shifts the emphasis away from therapeutic targets being directed solely against individual molecules within pathways and focuses the effort on targeting "nodes" in multiple pathways inside and outside the cancer cell that cooperate to orchestrate the malignant phenotype. Second, the tumor-host communication system may involve unique enzymatic events and sharing of growth factors. Consequently, the microenvironment of the tumor-host interaction could be a source for biomarkers that could ultimately be shed into the serum proteome (Fig. 57.4).[20,115–117] Although normal cellular processes (and the peptide content generated by these processes) are also a manifestation of the tissue microenvironment, the tumor microenvironment, through the process of aberrant cell growth, cellular invasion, and altered immune system function, represents a unique constellation of enzymatic (e.g., kinases, phosphatases) and protease activity (e.g., matrix metalloproteases). This results in changed stoichiometry of molecules within the peptidome itself (low-molecular-weight range of the serum proteome, peptides <50,000 Da) compared with the "normal" milieu.

The peptidome hypothesis states that a large variety of proteins and peptides are shed into the local circulation from the tumor microenvironment. This includes whole functional proteins, such as degradative enzymes, and many classes of cleaved proteins. Shedding of protein and peptides into the circulation is facilitated by the leaky nature of newly formed blood vessels and the increased hydrostatic pressure within tumors.[116] This pathologic physiology would tend to push molecules from the tumor interstitium into the circulation. As cells die within the microenvironment, they will shed the degraded products. The mode of death, apoptosis versus necrosis, would be expected to generate different classes of degraded cellular constituents.

Although some dismissed the peptidome as biologically irrelevant "noise,"[118,119] others have proposed that just the opposite is the case: it may contain a rich, untapped source of disease-specific diagnostic information.[41,120–129] This dichotomy is partly due to tissue proteins that are normally too large to passively diffuse through the endothelium but may enter the circulation as fragments of the parent molecule (Fig. 57.4). The information in the peptidome resides in multiple dimensions: (1) identity of the parent protein (i.e., isoform); (2) peptide fragment size and cleavage ends, and posttranslational glycosylation,[130,131] phosphorylation sites,[132,133] or cleavage sites[121,122,128,134]; (3) specific size of the peptide; (4) quantity of the peptide itself; and (5) nature of the carrier protein to which it is bound.[123,131,135]

Combinations of peptidome markers representing specific interactions of the tumor tissue microenvironment at the enzymatic level can achieve a higher specificity and a higher sensitivity for early-stage cancers.[72,122,123,125,126,128,129,136–143] This optimism is partly based on the concept that biomarkers derived from a population of cells comprise a volume that is greater than from the small precancerous lesion itself. In this way the peptidome can potentially supersede individual single biomarkers and transcend the issues of tumor and population heterogeneity. The implication is that measuring panels of peptidome markers can potentially overcome the failures of previous biomarkers to achieve adequate clinical sensitivity and specificity.[41,120–129]

Biomarker Discovery and Analysis

Biomarkers Hitch a Ride on Albumin

Candidate biomarkers are expected to exist in very low concentration, have the potential to be rapidly excreted, and must be separated from high-abundance blood proteins such as albumin, that exists in a billion-fold excess. Consequently, the greatest challenge to biomarker discovery is the isolation of very rare candidate proteins within a highly concentrated complex mixture of blood proteins massively dominated by seemingly nonrelevant proteins. Peptidome biomarkers are sequestered in the circulation because they accumulate on high-concentration resident proteins such as albumin and then acquire albumin's longer half-life, thereby protecting the bound species from kidney clearance.[41,123,127,129,144]

The starting point for rigorous biomarker discovery and analysis is the development of a discovery study set consisting of a population of serum or plasma samples from patients who have (1) histologically verified cancer, (2) benign or inflammatory nonneoplastic disease, and (3) unaffected and apparently healthy controls or hospital controls, depending on the intended use. The issue of including specimens for initial discovery from patients with no evidence of cancer but with inflammatory conditions, reactive disease, and benign disorders is of critical importance to ensure that specific markers are enriched for from the outset. This issue is critical for cancer research especially as the disease almost always occurs in the background of inflammatory processes that are part of the disease pathogenesis itself.[41,120–129] However, as has already

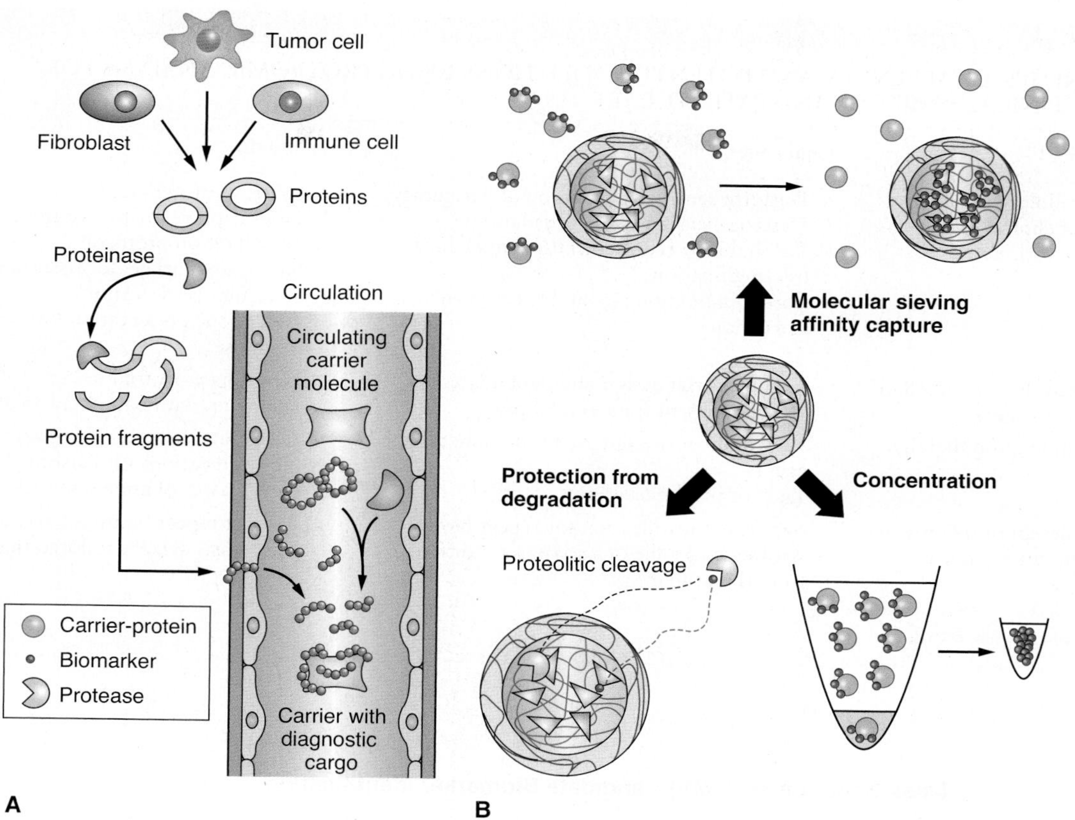

FIGURE 57.4 Emerging technology for harvesting low-abundance peptides and low-molecular proteins. **A:** Potential biomarker proteins, including secreted and intracellular molecules, are shed from living or dying tumor cells, stromal cells, vascular cells, and immune cells interacting in the tissue microenvironment. Proteolytic cascades within the tissue generate peptides and protein fragments that diffuse into the circulation where they associate with high-abundance carrier molecules such as albumin. The association with carrier molecules protects the biomarkers from renal clearance and lengthens their half-life so that they increase in concentration in the blood. The extracellular proteins are further modified by proteinases derived from any of the cell types. **B:** Hydrogel nanoparticles offer a method of protein harvesting and concentration from blood and body fluids. Hydrogel nanoparticles sequester proteins based on molecular weight (size sieving), protect the protein from degradation by trapping it within the nanoparticle three-dimensional structure, and concentrate the protein of interest to a level within the limit of detection of current mass spectrometers or enzyme-linked immunosorbent assay.

happened,[122] care must also be taken not to immediately overreach and dismiss peptide fragment markers that may be construed as nonspecific simply because their parental forms are known to be part of "normal" or inflammatory physiological processes.

The most critical stage of research clinical validation is blinded testing of the biomarker panel using an independent (not used in discovery), large clinical study set that is ideally drawn from at least three geographically separate locations. Employing previously verified controls and calibrators, under standard clinical chemistry guidelines for immunoassays,[145] the sensitivity and specificity can be determined for a test population. Sensitivity and specificity in an experimental test population do not translate to the positive predictive value that would be seen if the putative test is used routinely in the clinic. The true positive predictive value is a function of the indicated use and the prevalence of the disease. For example, the percentage of expected cancer cases in a population of patients at high genetic risk for cancer is higher than the general population. Consequently, the probability of false-positive results in the latter population would be much higher. For this reason the ultimate adoption of a peptidome-based test will be strongly dependent on the clinical context of its use.

Solving Remaining Hurdles for Clinical Implementation and the Future of Clinical Proteomics

New proteomic technology has been developed to overcome all of these fundamental challenges to biomarker discovery. A new class of nanoparticle has been created that performs three independent functions within minutes, in one step, in solution (serum, plasma, or urine): (1) molecular size sieving, (2) affinity capture of all solution phase low abundance target analyte molecules, and (3) complete protection of harvested proteins from degradation (Fig. 57.4).[72,146] This technology can concentrate a biomarker many hundred-fold, and fully prevent biomarker degradation. Multiple reaction monitoring mass spectrometry is a new class of quantitative mass spectrometry that can be used to specifically identify a known protein, without the requirement for a specific antibody (Fig. 57.5).[147–149] These tandem technologies offer a new level of optimism for the biomarker discovery.

Clinical proteomics can have important direct "bedside" applications. The pathologist of the future will detect early manifestations of disease using proteomic patterns of body-fluid

TABLE 57.1

OPPORTUNITIES, CHALLENGES, AND POTENTIAL SOLUTIONS USING PROTEOMIC ANALYSIS FOR ROUTINE CLINICAL PRACTICE AND PATIENT CARE

Opportunities	Challenges	Solutions
Proteomic cellular circuit analysis of clinical biopsy specimens	■ Platform sensitivity precision and accuracy ■ Heterogeneity of tissue populations ■ Perishability: requirement for immediate freezing/fixation ■ Formalin fixation unsuitable for protein extraction	■ Sensitive protein microarrays ■ Laser capture microdissection ■ New fixation protocols ■ Surrogate markers for tissue and blood molecular preservation ■ New tissue preservation kits for operating room use
Individualized therapy based on molecular profiling	■ Complex trial design and data analysis ■ Patient consent for serial biopsies	■ New classes of trial design ■ Dialogues with patient advocates and IRB
Tailored combination therapy	■ Low number of approved candidate targeted agents ■ Lack of preclinical data	■ Accelerate discovery of novel agents ■ New indications for existing drugs ■ New classes of animal models
Rational redesign of therapy in the setting of recurrence	■ Safety and justification for repeat biopsy ■ Molecular profile of metastasis is different from the primary	■ Restrict repeat biopsy to accessible sites ■ Metastasis-specific tailored therapy

IRB, institutional review board.

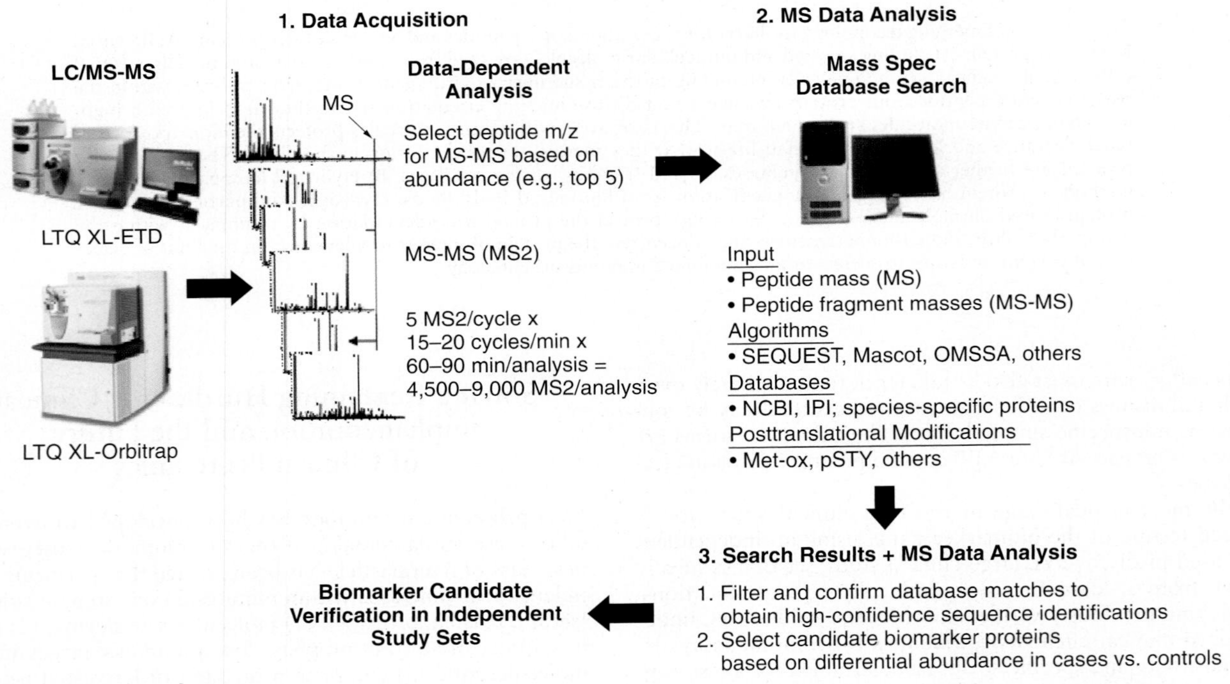

FIGURE 57.5 Workflow for mass spectrometry (MS) sequencing and confirmation of candidate protein biomarkers. 1. Spectra from the mass spectrometric analysis are generated based on mass/charge (m/z) ratios of the trypsin-digested proteins. 2. MS data analysis relies on search algorithms that compare species, protein modifications, cleavage fragment sites, and m/z ratios for protein sequencing. Results from the sequencing algorithms are compared to known protein databases for protein identification. 3. Results are filtered and annotated to obtain high-confidence sequence protein identifications. Candidate biomarkers are selected based on confirmation of differential abundance in cases versus controls.

samples and will provide the primary physician a diagnosis based on proteomic signatures as a complement to histopathology. Based on this knowledge, recommendations will be made for an individualized selection of therapeutic combinations of agents that target the entire disease-specific protein network. The pathologist and the diagnostic imaging physician will assist the clinical team to perform real-time assessment of therapeutic efficacy and toxicity. Proteomic and genomic analysis of recurrent tumor lesions could be the basis for rational redirection of therapy because it could reveal changes in the diseased protein network that are associated with drug resistance. The paradigm shift will directly affect clinical practice because it has an impact on all of the crucial elements of patient care and management (Table 57.1).

Selected References

The full list of references for this chapter appears in the online version.

2. Lander ES, Linton LM, Birren B, et al. Initial sequencing and analysis of the human genome. *Nature* 2001;409:860.
4. Collins FS, Green ED, Guttmacher AE, et al. A vision for the future of genomics research. *Nature* 2003;422:835.
7. Emmert-Buck MR, Bonner RF, Smith PD, et al. Laser capture microdissection. *Science* 1996;274:998.
9. Ekins RP, Chu FW. Multianalyte microspot immunoassay–microanalytical "compact disk" of the future. *Clin Chem* 1991;37:1955.
10. Liotta LA, Espina V, Mehta AI, et al. Protein microarrays: meeting analytical challenges for clinical applications. *Cancer Cell* 2003;3:317.
11. Paweletz CP, Charboneau L, Bichsel VE, et al. Reverse phase protein microarrays which capture disease progression show activation of pro-survival pathways at the cancer invasion front. *Oncogene* 2001;20:1981.
12. Espina V, Edmiston KH, Heiby M, et al. A portrait of tissue phosphoprotein stability in the clinical tissue procurement process. *Mol Cell Proteomics* 2008;7:1998.
13. Espina V, Mariani BD, Gallagher RI, et al. Malignant precursor cells pre-exist in human breast dcis and require autophagy for survival. *PloS One* 2010;5:e10240.
15. Petricoin EF 3rd, Espina V, Araujo RP, et al. Phosphoprotein pathway mapping: Akt/mammalian target of rapamycin activation is negatively associated with childhood rhabdomyosarcoma survival. *Cancer Res* 2007;67:3431.
17. Wulfkuhle JD, Speer R, Pierobon M, et al. Multiplexed cell signaling analysis of human breast cancer applications for personalized therapy. *J Proteome Res* 2008;7:1508.
18. Geho DH, Bandle RW, Clair T, et al. Physiological mechanisms of tumor-cell invasion and migration. *Physiology (Bethesda)* 2005;20:194.
20. Liotta LA, Kohn EC. The microenvironment of the tumour-host interface. *Nature* 2001;411:375.
21. Liotta LA, Stracke ML. Tumor invasion and metastases: biochemical mechanisms. *Cancer Treat Res* 1988;40:223.
22. Stracke ML, Murata J, Aznavoorian S, et al. The role of the extracellular matrix in tumor cell metastasis. *In Vivo* 1994;8:49.
29. Noguchi S, Motomura K, Inaji H, et al. Clonal analysis of predominantly intraductal carcinoma and precancerous lesions of the breast by means of polymerase chain reaction. *Cancer Res* 1994;54:1849.
32. Espina V, Wulfkuhle JD, Calvert VS, et al. Laser-capture microdissection. *Nat Protoc* 2006;1:586.
33. Kolble K. The LEICA microdissection system: design and applications. *J Mol Med* 2000;78:B24.
34. Micke P, Ostman A, Lundeberg J, et al. Laser-assisted cell microdissection using the PALM system. *Methods Mol Biol* 2005;293:151.
40. Liotta L, Petricoin E. Molecular profiling of human cancer. *Nat Rev Genet* 2000;1:48.
41. Liotta LA, Ferrari M, Petricoin E. Clinical proteomics: written in blood. *Nature* 2003;425:905.
46. Haab BB. Antibody arrays in cancer research. *Mol Cell Proteomics* 2005;4:377.
48. MacBeath G, Schreiber SL. Printing proteins as microarrays for high-throughput function determination. *Science* 2000;289:1760.
57. Schena M, Shalon D, Davis RW, et al. Quantitative monitoring of gene expression patterns with a complementary DNA microarray. *Science* 1995;270:467.
65. Mazzone M, Selfors LM, Albeck J, et al. Dose-dependent induction of distinct phenotypic responses to Notch pathway activation in mammary epithelial cells. *Proc Natl Acad Sci U S A* 2010;107:5012.
72. Longo C, Patanarut A, George T, et al. Core-shell hydrogel particles harvest, concentrate and preserve labile low abundance biomarkers. *PloS One* 2009;4:e4763.
79. Spruessel A, Steimann G, Jung M, et al. Tissue ischemia time affects gene and protein expression patterns within minutes following surgical tumor excision. *Biotechniques* 2004;36:1030.
81. Li X, Friedman AB, Roh MS, et al. Anesthesia and post-mortem interval profoundly influence the regulatory serine phosphorylation of glycogen synthase kinase-3 in mouse brain. *J Neurochem* 2005;92:701.
88. Espina V, Mueller C, Edmiston KH, et al. Tissue is alive: New technologies are needed to address the problems of protein biomaker pre-analytical variability. *Proteomics Clin Appl* 2009;3:874.
92. Ronci M, Bonanno E, Colantoni A, et al. Protein unlocking procedures of formalin-fixed paraffin-embedded tissues: application to MALDI-TOF imaging MS investigations. *Proteomics* 2008;8:3702.
94. Fox CH, Johnson FB, Whiting J, et al. Formaldehyde fixation. *J Histochem Cytochem* 1985;33:845.
103. Nadji M, Nassiri M, Vincek V, et al. Immunohistochemistry of tissue prepared by a molecular-friendly fixation and processing system. *Appl Immunohistochem Mol Morphol* 2005;13:277.
111. Barker AD, Sigman CC, Kelloff GJ, et al. I-SPY 2: an adaptive breast cancer trial design in the setting of neoadjuvant chemotherapy. *Clin Pharmacol Ther* 2009;86:97.
112. Mendoza M, Khanna C. Revisiting the seed and soil in cancer metastasis. *Int J Biochem Cell Biol* 2009;41:1452.
121. Lopez MF, Mikulskis A, Kuzdzal S, et al. High-resolution serum proteomic profiling of Alzheimer disease samples reveals disease-specific, carrier-protein-bound mass signatures. *Clin Chem* 2005;51:1946.
122. Lopez MF, Mikulskis A, Kuzdzal S, et al. A novel, high-throughput workflow for discovery and identification of serum carrier protein-bound peptide biomarker candidates in ovarian cancer samples. *Clin Chem* 2007;53:1067.
123. Lowenthal MS, Mehta AI, Frogale K, et al. Analysis of albumin-associated peptides and proteins from ovarian cancer patients. *Clin Chem* 2005;51:1933.
127. Tirumalai RS, Chan KC, Prieto DA, et al. Characterization of the low molecular weight human serum proteome. *Mol Cell Proteomics* 2003;2:1096.
135. Schulz-Knappe P, Schrader M, Zucht HD. The peptidomics concept. *Comb Chem High Throughput Screen* 2005;8:697.
136. Adam BL, Qu Y, Davis JW, et al. Serum protein fingerprinting coupled with a pattern-matching algorithm distinguishes prostate cancer from benign prostate hyperplasia and healthy men. *Cancer Res* 2002;62:3609.
141. Villanueva J, Philip J, Entenberg D, et al. Serum peptide profiling by magnetic particle-assisted, automated sample processing and MALDI-TOF mass spectrometry. *Anal Chem* 2004;76:1560.
144. Mehta AI, Ross S, Lowenthal MS, et al. Biomarker amplification by serum carrier protein binding. *Dis Markers* 2003;19:1.
146. Luchini A, Geho DH, Bishop B, et al. Smart hydrogel particles: biomarker harvesting: one-step affinity purification, size exclusion, and protection against degradation. *Nano Lett* 2008;8:350.
147. Baker M. Mass spectrometry. *Nature Methods* 2010;7:157.
148. Choudhary C, Mann M. Decoding signalling networks by mass spectrometry-based proteomics. *Nat Rev Mol Cell Biol* 2010;11:427.
149. Mueller C, Liotta LA, Espina V. Reverse phase protein microarrays advance use in clinical trials. *Mol Oncol* 2010;4:461.

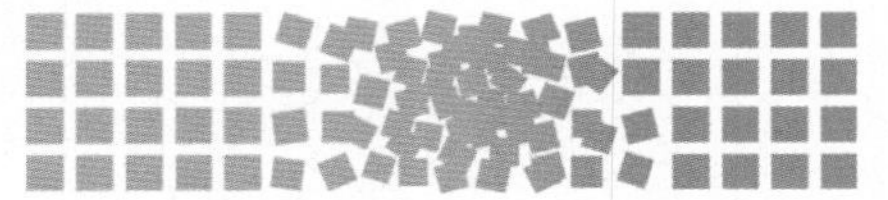

CHAPTER 58 SCREENING FOR GASTROINTESTINAL CANCERS

TIMOTHY R. CHURCH AND JACK S. MANDEL

HISTORY OF COLORECTAL CANCER SCREENING

Jemal et al.[1] report that among U.S. men, cancer death rates decreased by 21.0% between 1990 and 2006, and among women, cancer death rates decreased by 12.3% between 1991 and 2006. Much of the decrease came from lower mortality from colorectal cancer. In addition, the authors report that cancer incidence rates also decreased annually for both men and women in the last 6 to 8 years, also partly related to decreases in newly diagnosed cases of colorectal cancer. In the United States, colorectal cancer accounts for 9% of cancer incidence and 9% of cancer deaths in men, and 10% of cancer incidence and 9% of cancer mortality in women. Of the decrease in colorectal cancer incidence and mortality, the authors say, "The accelerated decrease in colorectal cancer incidence rates from 1998 to 2006 largely reflects increases in screening that can detect and remove precancerous polyps."[1]

The idea of detecting colorectal cancer early enough to improve survival came from combining the observation that Dukes stage A cancers[2] were frequently successfully treated by excision with the increasing availability of endoscopes that could visualize the colon and rectum. The earliest demonstrations of the potential for colorectal cancer screening used observational methods to evaluate the rigid proctoscope or sigmoidoscope.[3–6] Subsequently, work extended to flexible sigmoidoscopy[7–9] and, ultimately, colonoscopy.[10,11] The early development of the fecal occult blood test resulted from the perceived failure of sigmoidoscopy. In 1967, Greegor[12] noted that only one malignant polyp was detected in 2,500 sigmoidoscopic examinations, whereas he would have expected one carcinoma in every 300 to 500 examinations. In a review of all large bowel carcinomas, he found that all patients but one had a positive reaction for occult blood in at least one of three stool specimens submitted at the initial visit. He concluded that testing one portion of one specimen would be inadequate but using the commercially available Hemoccult test (Beckman Coulter, Inc., Brea, California) on at least two or three portions of three stools would be preferable. In a subsequent article, Greegor[13] presented an argument for multiple guaiac tests. Because of the number of false-positive findings (27 of 29 test positives), Greegor added a step to the process, which was the requirement for a meat-free diet during the collection of the specimens. In responding to the assertion that early cancers do not bleed, he presented data that showed that most of the cases in his series were detected at a curable stage. Thus, testing for stool blood became a plausible screening method early on.[14]

Imaging by radiograph with barium contrast has long been a way to noninvasively examine the colon and to diagnose polyps and cancer there, so it was natural to think of such means for early detection.[15–18] As x-ray techniques become more sophisticated, incorporating computed tomography (CT)[19] and mathematical reconstruction of three-dimensional structures, the sensitivity and specificity of such methods improve commensurately. "Virtual" colonoscopy using CT allows a physician to visually reproduce the endoscopic examination on a computer screen. Recent evidence suggests a growing role for this newest technology, and some guidelines have incorporated colonography as screening test.[20] However, challenges in the implementation include not only inconvenience of preparation and the discomfort of the procedure, but also the lack of reimbursement by most payors.[21]

Publication of the results of the Health Insurance Plan study of breast cancer screening by mammography[22] demonstrated that large-scale, randomized clinical trials could be used to assess the efficacy of cancer screening. Taking a similar approach to evaluating fecal occult blood testing, Gilbertsen et al.[14] randomized 46,551 adults in Minnesota with equal probability to one of annual screening, biennial screening, or usual care. Screening was largely performed with a rehydrated guaiac test. In 1993, after 13 years of follow-up, the study participants who were offered annual screens showed a 33% reduction in colorectal cancer mortality compared to the usual-care participants.[23] This result was the evidence used by the U.S. Preventive Services Task Force to make the first recommendation for colorectal cancer screening.[24] The screening effect persisted through 18 years of follow-up, at which time the participants who were offered biennial screens showed a 21% reduction in colorectal cancer mortality.[25] In addition, relative to the usual-care participants, both screening arms showed significant reductions through 18 years in colorectal cancer incidence: 18% for biennial screening and 21% for annual screening.[26] This study was the first to definitively demonstrate that screening for colorectal cancer could reduce both mortality and incidence from the disease.

In 1996 two additional randomized trials published findings of significant reductions of 15% to 18% in colorectal cancer mortality from biennial screening with guaiac-based fecal occult blood testing.[27,28] With these confirming results, colorectal cancer screening began to be accepted to a greater degree by the medical community in the United States and Europe.

A Cochrane Review evaluated the results from all the fecal occult blood test trials and concluded that the overall mortality reduction was 16%, and adjusting for screening attendance increased that reduction to 25%.[29] Current recommendations for screening in the United States include fecal occult blood testing on an annual basis, based on the consistent results of randomized trials showing mortality reductions and the larger reduction for annual screening as well as the reduction in incidence shown in the Minnesota trial.[25,26]

POLYP REMOVAL AND COLORECTAL CANCER PREVENTION

Most colorectal cancers are believed to begin as adenomas that undergo additional mutations to become invasive adenocarcinoma. Based on this hypothesis, the endoscopic removal of polyps has long been advocated as a method to prevent colorectal cancer. Indeed, the earliest attempts at endoscopic screening focused on adenoma removal to prevent cancer.[3] Two randomized trials have demonstrated that endoscopic removal of polyps does in fact reduce the incidence of colorectal cancer by about 20% in a population screened either by rehydrated fecal occult blood testing[26] or by flexible sigmoidoscopy.[30] Two notable attempts to estimate the effect of polyp removal specifically in those patients with polyps came from the National Polyp Study, which estimated a 78% to 95% reduction,[31] and from the Polyp Prevention Study group, which found no effect.[32] As the latter authors point out, neither estimate comes from comparing equivalent groups and, thus, the estimates may be biased. However, there is sufficient evidence to believe that polyp detection and removal is important to reduce colorectal cancer incidence.

METHODS OF SCREENING FOR COLORECTAL CANCER

Colorectal cancer screening is unique in that there are at least five different screening methods that are recommended in existing guidelines. This variety reflects the multiple ways that colorectal cancer screening developed as a concept and the ways it continues to develop. The bleeding often associated with colorectal cancer and large adenomas gave rise to fecal tests (guaiac, immunochemical, and genetic), the presence of precancerous lesions, and the ability to remove them endoscopically gave rise to visualization methods, including barium-enema x-rays, flexible sigmoidoscopy, optical colonoscopy, and virtual colonoscopy. In this chapter, the state of the various screening methods are described and summarized.

Fecal Occult Blood Testing

Although it remains the only method to have been proven effective in replicated randomized trials against usual care, after years of increasing, the rates of screening by fecal occult blood testing have been declining in general.[33] An exception is the Veterans Administration population, in which a study of the Veterans Administration database showed that colorectal cancer screening has dramatically increased, with fecal occult blood testing as the dominant method of screening.[34] Newer fecal occult blood testing methods are gaining acceptance. The guaiac method has the drawback of being nonspecific to cancer or adenomas. Guaiac tests detect the pseudoperoxidase activity of heme, and fecal excretion of heme is an indicator of gastrointestinal pathology. Any source of blood, including dietary, can lead to a positive test. Shortcomings in guaiac-based fecal occult blood testing[35] have led to the development of immunochemical testing methods.[36] These tests are more specific because they are designed to react only to human blood, rather than any animal blood. This also gives them the added advantage that they can be used without dietary restrictions because they do not react with nonhuman hemoglobin or with uncooked fruits and vegetables that may contain peroxidase activity.[37] These immunochemical tests have been studied in case-control studies, particularly in Japan, and by comparing them with the older guaiac-based tests in general have shown themselves to have lower rates of false positivity and equal or greater sensitivity for polyps.[38]

Mass screening with a 1-day immunochemical hemagglutination test (Immudia-Hem Sp or HemSelect: Fujirebio, Tokyo, Japan) was introduced in Japan in 1986 and evaluated through case-control studies.[39,40] The studies evaluating immunochemical tests in Japan have provided consistent results showing the benefit of screening, with odds ratios as low as 0.19, suggesting an 81% reduction in colorectal cancer mortality. Overall in Japan, six million people (about 17% of the eligible population) have been screened with immunochemical tests.[40] The overall positivity rate was 7.1% (N = 430,000); 60% of the positive test results complied with the diagnostic protocol, which consisted of colonoscopy or flexible sigmoidoscopy with double-contrast barium enema. The colorectal cancer detection rate was 1.6 per 1,000 population with 69% Dukes A and 14% Dukes B stages, suggesting to the authors that the program was working well.

Other immunochemical tests have been evaluated by comparing their performance with that of Hemoccult or Hemoccult Sensa and they generally performed better and resulted in greater compliance.[41–44] Particularly noteworthy was the performance of a relatively new immunochemical test, Insure (Quest Diagnostics, Edison, New Jersey), which uses a brush-based sampling technique and a test result that is quantifiable in terms of the amount of blood present in the sample.[37] For this test, the participant samples toilet bowl water from the surface of the stool by swishing the brush in the bowl and then wiping the brush onto the test card. In a direct comparison with Hemoccult Sensa and another immunochemical test, called FlexSure OBT (Beckman Coulter, Inc.), the participation rate was highest for Insure, which, according to the authors, was because of the simplified sampling technique and lack of dietary restrictions.[45]

The Scottish Bowel Screening Programme adopted a two-tiered screening program using both guaiac and immunochemical tests. This strategy, using an immunochemical test on guaiac-positive patients, appears to reduce the number of colonoscopies and the overall cost of the screening program.[46]

Stool and Blood DNA Testing

Most recently, researchers are examining molecular methods in both stool[47] and blood.[48] Although promising, the challenges of acceptance of collecting whole-stool samples for the former and of confirming adequate sensitivity and specificity for both the former and the latter need to be addressed. Finding the right molecular markers in both is key to the effective implementation of these strategies, and doing so will require fairly large samples of cancer patients and controls. Eventually, such methods will need to be evaluated in large populations to determine efficacy relative to already accepted methods of screening.

Endoscopy

Rigid Proctoscopy/Sigmoidoscopy

One of the earliest proponents of colorectal cancer screening, Victor Gilbertsen, was a surgeon who sought to use the rigid proctoscope to detect and remove early cancers and precancerous adenomas from asymptomatic men and women.[3] He screened and followed 20,000 patients from his clinic and reported an observed rectal-cancer mortality reduction of 100%. Although this was an uncontrolled study with a selected population and incomplete follow-up, these results encouraged the further study of endoscopic screening.

A study by Selby et al.[6] evaluated the program of screening by rigid sigmoidoscope that Kaiser-Permanente had had in place for many years. The study estimated a reduction in mortality from cancers of the rectum and sigmoid colon of 59%. Although later publications estimated smaller reductions from the same study,[49] this study directly led to the inclusion of flexible sigmoidoscopy in screening guidelines.[24]

Flexible Sigmoidoscopy

Flexible sigmoidoscopy allows a more thorough examination of the rectum and sigmoid colon, up to the descending colon, and has replaced rigid sigmoidoscopy. It is estimated that flexible sigmoidoscopy will find 60% to 83% of cancers and polyps found by colonoscopy.[50] In addition to the Kaiser-Permanente study previously cited, there have been numerous other observational studies of flexible sigmoidoscopy that have estimated sizable reductions in mortality and incidence from screening asymptomatic individuals. However, observational studies may not be able to control for the biases inherent in screening evaluation.[49] One large-scale randomized trial in the United Kingdom recently reported that a one-time flexible sigmoidoscopy reduced colorectal cancer mortality by 31% and reduced incidence by 23%,[30]– results very similar to those from annual rehydrated fecal occult blood screening that showed 33% and 20% reductions, respectively.[25,26] A U.S. randomized trial of two flexible sigmoidoscopy screens 3 to 5 years apart is currently ongoing and is expected to report results by 2015.[51] These studies will provide more reliable estimates of flexible sigmoidoscopy efficacy as a one-time or repeated screening tool.

Colonoscopy

Colonoscopy, which allows a complete examination of the rectum and colon to the cecum, has become the screening method for colorectal cancer preferred by gastroenterologists and many other physicians and public health experts. In spite of a lack of direct evidence, the enthusiasm rests on inference from other, indirect evidence. The 15% to 33% reductions in mortality from fecal occult blood screening are attributable to the colonoscopies that almost universally followed positive test results. Not only were cancers found and initially treated using colonoscopy in those studies, but precancerous adenomas that were found during the examinations were removed and mostly likely led to the reduction in incidence seen in at least one of the studies.[26] The recently published study of one-time flexible sigmoidoscopy showing a 31% mortality reduction and a 23% incidence reduction[30] further supports the use of colonoscopy under the assumption that the colonoscope can examine the right colon as well as the left colon and rectum reached by the sigmoidoscope. In addition, the positive observational studies of both sigmoidoscopy and colonoscopy support the efficacy of colonoscopy as a screening method. However, because the actual effect on mortality and incidence is unknown, cost-effectiveness analyses comparing the different screening methods have depended on unreliable estimates.

The results of the studies on flexible sigmoidoscopy compared with recent large observational analyses examining the impact of colonoscopy on mortality and incidence have led to rethinking the superiority of colonoscopy to other methods of screening. In two large case-control studies and one very large cohort study, no statistically significant effect of colonoscopy on incidence or mortality involving cancer in the proximal colon was found, and the reduction in the distal colon and rectum was only slightly larger than that estimated for sigmoidoscopy.[52] Clearly, more research in this area is needed to determine the relative value of the different screening methods.

In current U.S. guidelines, colonoscopy is recommended every 10 years in those at average risk.[17,18] The reasoning is based on evidence from observational studies because the efficacy of colonoscopy has not been studied directly. It is generally believed that the average time from development of a polyp to development of invasive malignancy is at least 10 years. Because the sensitivity of colonoscopy for cancer and significant polyps is very high, by screening every 10 years, nearly all polyps will be detected before they become malignant, and those few that do will be found in the early stages.[17,18]

Interestingly, colonoscopy, the diagnostic test for colorectal cancer, is not without problems. In a recent review of studies in which tandem or back-to-back colonoscopies were performed, Van Rijn et al.[53] showed that 21% of adenomas were missed; 26% of adenomas 1 to 5 mm and 2% of adenomas 10 mm or more. Rex[54] addressed the issue of the wide variability in performance of screening colonoscopy among gastroenterologists, arguing that improvements in technology (e.g., chromoendoscopy, autofluorescence, Third Eye Retroscope, wide-angle colonoscopy, Avantis Medical Systems, Sunnyvale, CA) would help, but the time and costs for the procedures would increase. He suggests that the best colonoscopist achieves effective and safe bowel preparation, is sufficiently slow and careful during withdrawal, and identifies all adenomas. Trecca et al.[55] evaluated chromoendoscopy in addition to conventional colonoscopy for the detection of flat neoplasms and showed that chromoendoscopy, particularly for nonpolypoid lesions, detected lesions with advanced histology that were missed by conventional colonoscopy.

Imaging CT Colonography (Virtual Colonoscopy)

CT imaging for detecting colorectal cancer was proposed in 1980.[56] Helical CT provides a noninvasive way to create a three-dimensional image of the colon and rectum that can be examined for the presence of polyps and cancers. By use of contrast agents such as barium, and bowel preparation to minimize fecal artifact, radiologists have achieved detection performance similar to that of optical colonoscopy in moderately large trials.[20] The main findings are presented in Table 58.1.[20]

Even larger, multicenter trials are currently being conducted to further evaluate virtual colonoscopy as a viable screening method. Its main value is that it is less invasive and potentially could have higher compliance than colonoscopy. Several issues remain to be addressed. One issue is that the patients who exhibit significant lesions must undergo optical colonoscopy to remove them for pathologic examination. Because cathartic bowel preparation for both virtual and optical colonoscopy can be bothersome and painful for patients, it would be best to only require it once per screen. Some researchers are studying preparation methods for virtual colonoscopy that tag the bowel and thereby identify fecal artifact more easily. Perfection of such methods would only require patients with positive findings on virtual colonoscopy to undergo cathartic preparation for the follow-up optical colonoscopy. An alternative would be to develop centers that permit immediate optical colonoscopy following a positive virtual colonoscopy, so that the same preparation would be used for both procedures. A related issue is determining a criterion for optical colonoscopy based on the size or number of lesions found in virtual colonoscopy. In spite of these issues, the consensus for routine

TABLE 58.1

PERFORMANCE CHARACTERISTICS OF VIRTUAL COLONOSCOPY AND OPTICAL COLONOSCOPY FOR THE DETECTION OF ADENOMAS

Variable	Size Category (mm)				
	≥6	≥7	≥8 (no./total no.) (% [95% CI])	≥9	≥10
Analysis according to patient[a]					
Virtual colonoscopy					
Sensitivity	149/168 (88.7 [82.9–93.1])	100/110 (90.9 [83.9–95.6])	77/82 (93.9 [86.3–98.0])	53/57 (93.0 [83.0–98.1])	45/48 (93.8 [82.8–98.7])
Specificity	848/1065 (79.6 [77.0–82.0])	981/1123 (87.4 [85.3–89.2])	1061/1151 (92.2 [90.5–93.7])	1116/1176 (94.9 [93.5–96.1])	1138/1185 (96.0 [94.8–97.1])
Accuracy	997/1233 (80.9 [78.6–83.0])	1081/1233 (87.7 [85.7–89.5])	1138/1233 (92.3 [90.7–93.7])	1169/1233 (94.8 [93.4–96.0])	1183/1233 (95.9 [94.7–97.0])
Test-positive rate[b]	366/1233 (29.7 [27.1–32.3])	242/1233 (19.6 [17.4–22.0])	167/1233 (13.5 [11.7–15.6])	113/1233 (9.2 [7.6–10.9])	92/1233 (7.5 [6.1–9.1])
Sensitivity of optical colonoscopy[c]	155/168 (92.3 [87.1–95.8])	100/110 (90.9 [83.9–95.6])	75/82 (91.5 [83.2–96.5])	51/57 (89.5 [78.5–96.0])	42/48 (87.5 [74.8–95.3])
Analysis according to polyp[d]					
Sensitivity of virtual colonoscopy	180/210 (85.7 [80.2–90.1])	119/133 (89.5 [83.0–94.1])	88/95 (92.6 [85.4–97.0])	56/61 (91.8 [81.2–97.3])	47/51 (92.2 [81.1–97.8])
Sensitivity of optical colonoscopy	189/210 (90.0 [85.1–93.7])	120/133 (90.2 [83.9–94.7])	85/95 (89.5 [81.5–94.8])	55/61 (90.2 [79.8–96.3])	45/51 (88.2 [76.1–95.6])

CI, confidence interval.
[a]For analyses according to patient:
Sensitivity: percentage of all examinations in individuals with at least one polyp in the size category that were reported as having at least one by the examination; for example, the sensitivity of virtual colonoscopy for polyps ≥6 mm indicates that 88.7% of all polyps that size were detected in the virtual colonoscopic examination.
Specificity: percentage of all examinations of individuals with no polyps in the size category that report none in that category; for example, the specificity of virtual colonoscopy for polyps ≥6 mm indicates that 79.6% of all examinations in individuals with no polyps reported no polyps ≥6 mm.
Accuracy: the percentage of all examinations that gave the accurate result according to the polyp size category; for example, the accuracy of virtual colonoscopy for polyps ≥6 mm indicates that 80.9% of all examinations reported accurately that there was a polyp ≥6 mm or that there was no polyp ≥6 mm.
Test-positive rate: percentage of all examinations that reported at least one polyp in the size category; for example, the test-positive rate for polyps ≥6 mm indicates that 29.7% of all examinations found a polyp ≥6 mm.
[b]Data are for the virtual colonoscopic studies that were deemed to be positive each size category.
[c]The data for optical colonoscopy are for the initial optical colonoscopy performed before the results on virtual colonoscopy were revealed.
[d]For analyses according to polyp:
Sensitivity: percentage of all polyps in the size category that are reported by the examination; for example, the sensitivity of virtual colonoscopy indicates that 85.7% of all polyps ≥6 mm were reported by the examination.
(From ref. 20, with permission.)

use of virtual colonoscopy is growing, especially in cases in which optical colonoscopy might be difficult because of frailty or reluctance of the patient.

Rosman and Korsten[57] conducted a meta-analysis of 30 CT colonography studies and found that sensitivity was higher for larger than smaller polyps, two-dimensional and three-dimensional CT colonography performed about equally as well, CT colonography was superior to air-contrast barium enema, and that optical colonoscopy performed better than CT colonography for smaller polyps. To overcome the extensive bowel preparation and radiation exposure associated with CT colonography, Florie et al.[58] evaluated magnetic resonance colonography in high-risk patients (those with personal or family history of colorectal cancer or polyps) scheduled for optical colonoscopy. A minimal bowel preparation was used that consisted largely of a low-fiber diet and ingestion of 12 g of lactulose powder in 6-g packets dissolved in water once per day. An oral contrast agent was added to all major meals. For polyps over 6 mm, sensitivity and specificity were 65% and 67%, respectively, and for polyps over 10 mm, sensitivity and specificity were 75% and 93%, respectively. The authors concluded that the results were modest and use of screening magnetic resonance colonography should await further technical developments.

Vijan et al.[59] found that CT colonography was cost-effective compared to no screen, was more expensive and less effective than optical colonoscopy, and that further improvements will need to be made for it to be a cost-effective screening option.

Other Imaging Technology

Capsule endoscopy (CE), a simple, noninvasive, wireless capsule containing a miniaturized camera, a light source, and a wireless circuit for acquiring and transmitting signals, is well tolerated by patients. It has the potential for the detection of lesions in the small bowel.[60] The commonest use for CE is for

TABLE 58.2

COLON CANCER SCREENING RECOMMENDATIONS FOR PEOPLE WITH FAMILIAL OR INHERITED RISK

Familial Risk Category	Screening Recommendation
First-degree relative affected with colorectal cancer or an adenomatous polyp at age ≥60 years, or two second-degree relatives affected with colorectal cancer	Same as average risk but starting at age 40 years
Two or more first-degree relatives[a] with colon cancer, or a single first-degree relative with colon cancer or adenomatous polyps diagnosed at an age <60 years	Colonoscopy every 5 years, beginning at age 40 years or 10 years younger than the earliest diagnosis in the family, whichever comes first
One second-degree or any third-degree relative[b,c] with colorectal cancer	Same as average risk
Gene carrier or at risk for familial adenomatous polyposis[d]	Sigmoidoscopy annually, beginning at age 10–12 years[e]
Gene carrier or at risk for HNPCC	Colonoscopy, every 1–2 years, beginning at age 20–25 years or 10 years younger than the earliest case in the family, whichever comes first

HNPCC, hereditary nonpolyposis colon cancer.
[a]First-degree relatives include patients, siblings, and children.
[b]Second-degree relatives include grandparents, aunts, and uncles.
[c]Third-degree relatives include great-grandparents and cousins.
[d]Includes the subcategories of familial adenomatous polyposis, Gardner syndrome, some Turcot syndrome families, and attenuated adenomatous polyposis coli (AAPC).
[e]In AAPC, colonoscopy should be used instead of sigmoidoscopy because of the preponderance of proximal colonic adenomas. Colonoscopy screening in AAPC should probably begin in the late teens or early 20s.
(From ref. 17 with permission.)

obscure gastrointestinal bleeding that remains after negative endoscopy. To date there have been no reported deaths and few side effects from CE. There have been a few efforts to look at CE for colorectal cancer screening, but further work is needed to determine if this method has potential for colorectal cancer screening.

COLORECTAL CANCER SCREENING FOR HIGH-RISK PATIENTS

Based on familial or hereditary risk factors, patients may be at higher-than-average risk of colorectal cancer. The screening recommendations specifically address high-risk individuals, but implementation is a challenge. In a recent study of randomly selected patients in a large multispecialty group practice, Fletcher et al.[61] found that less than half of the patients with a strong family history of colorectal cancer were appropriately screened. Known clinical conditions such as inflammatory bowel disease (Crohn disease or ulcerative colitis) or familial adenomatous polyposis put individuals at higher risk for disease. The term *screening* is not usually applied to such situations, and instead the term *surveillance* is applied. However, there are other high-risk conditions that nonetheless require screening, and these are genetic or phenotypic markers that elevate the chance of colorectal cancer to the extent that screening needs to occur earlier or with more certainty.[62] Another method proposed for identifying individuals at high risk for colorectal cancer to target screening programs is the use of a risk score based on risk factors such as age, alcohol use, smoking status, and body mass index.[63] In one such application using data from the Physicians Health Study, those in the highest risk group had an odds ratio of 15.3. For individuals who are suspected to have hereditary nonpolyposis colon cancer in their families, early and frequent screening with colonoscopy is recommended. Even if the patient does not meet these criteria, however, there are some situations in which the pattern of colorectal cancer in the family raises the risk to the point where earlier or more frequent screening may be necessary. Table 58.2[17] gives the guidelines for high-risk patients. It is important to carefully collect a full family cancer history when evaluating a screening regimen for an individual.

OTHER GASTROINTESTINAL CANCERS

Unfortunately, other gastrointestinal cancers are not associated with accepted methods of screening for asymptomatic disease. For stomach, small intestine, pancreas, and liver cancer, no viable options are on the horizon. For pancreatic cancer, the search for biomarkers has focused on the histology and molecular genetics of carcinogenesis. The need for large cohorts with stored biological samples and who are followed prospectively makes such research difficult.[64]

For liver cancer, work has focused on very high-risk individuals, such as those with cirrhosis.[65] Small study sizes and dependence on lead time biased case-survival rather than mortality comparisons make the results to date unreliable.

For esophageal cancer, most work has focused on endoscopic screening for those at high risk from chronic, severe gastroesophageal reflux disease.[66] If the condition known as Barrett's esophagus—which is characterized by the replacement of endothelial cells with squamous cells—is found, some physicians advocate implementing an endoscopic surveillance schedule, but there is neither any firm data to guide the clinician on how often such examinations should be done nor any evidence that such surveillance is effective in reducing cancer mortality. Thus, some promising research has been done, but the short-term horizon for new screening technologies is somewhat barren.

TABLE 58.3

AVERAGE RISK INDIVIDUAL COLORECTAL CANCER SCREENING RECOMMENDATIONS

Screening Test	Frequency
1. Fecal occult blood test	Annually
2. Flexible sigmoidoscopy	Every 5 years
3. Combined fecal occult blood test and flexible sigmoidoscopy	Fecal occult blood test annually; flexible sigmoidoscopy every 5 years
4. Colonoscopy	Every 10 years
5. Double-contrast barium enema x-ray examination	Every 5 to 10 years

(From refs. 20 and 21, with permission.)

SCREENING

In the United States and worldwide, cancer contributes significantly to morbidity and mortality. Recent declines in cancer incidence and mortality among U.S. residents have in part been due to declines in gastrointestinal cancer rates, especially those in colorectal cancer. Some of the decline is due to improvements in treatment, but screening for colorectal cancer has been shown by both well-designed observational studies as well as by rigorous randomized trials to save lives and prevent disease.

Screening methods for other gastrointestinal cancers are not in current use. Research into screening for esophageal, pancreas, and liver cancer is ongoing, but so far the evidence does not support routine use of endoscopic or molecular screening methods for these cancers. Limited availability of large cohorts with prospective tissue sample collection and the difficulties and expense of conducting large trials of endoscopic screening procedures will continue to challenge the eventual proof of such methods.

Colorectal cancer screening in the United States is well accepted, and rates of screening in the United States have increased to over 50% in the last decade. Five different methods of screening for average risk individuals are currently recommended by the U.S. Multisociety Task Force on Colorectal Cancer (Table 58.3).

Earlier or more intensive screening is necessary for individuals at higher risk due to familial or hereditary reasons. Careful evaluation of family history is essential to identify such individuals.

Newer screening methods are gaining acceptance. Immunochemical fecal occult blood tests provide greater specificity by reacting only to human blood, while maintaining the sensitivity of the older guaiac-based tests. Studies of DNA testing in stool samples have shown some promise from that technology. Newer imaging techniques improve on barium enema x-rays by employing spiral CT with three-dimensional reconstruction of the lumen of the bowel combined with stool-tagging as well as barium contrast media. This technology may provide even higher sensitivity than optical colonoscopy for some lesions. Continuing development of screening technology will improve the precision of the tests and drive wider acceptance among the targeted population.

Selected References

The full list of references for this chapter appears in the online version.

1. Jemal A, Siegel R, Xu J, Ward E. Cancer statistics, 2010. *CA Cancer J Clin* 2010;60(5):277.
2. Dukes CD. The classification of cancer of the rectum. *J Pathol Bacteriol* 1932;35:323.
3. Gilbertsen VA, Nelms JM. The prevention of invasive cancer of the rectum. *Cancer* 1978;41(3):1137.
4. Gilbertsen V. Colon cancer screening: the Minnesota experience. *Gastrointest Endosc* 1980;26(2 (Suppl):31S.
5. Selby JV, Friedman GD. Sigmoidoscopy in the periodic health examination of asymptomatic adults. *JAMA* 1989;261(4):595.
6. Selby JV, Friedman GD, Quesenberry CP Jr., Weiss NS. A case-control study of screening sigmoidoscopy and mortality from colorectal cancer. *N Engl J Med* 1992;326(10):653.
7. Flehinger BJ, Herbert E, Winawer SJ, Miller DG. Screening for colorectal cancer with fecal occult blood test and sigmoidoscopy: preliminary report of the Colon Project of Memorial Sloan-Kettering Cancer Center and PMI-Strang Clinic. In: Chamberlain J, Miller AB, eds. *Screening for Gastrointestinal Cancer*. Toronto: Huber, 1988:9.
9. Gohagan JK, Prorok PC, Kramer BS, Hayes RB, Cornett JE. The Prostate, Lung, Colorectal, and Ovarian Cancer Screening Trial of the National Cancer Institute. *Cancer* 1995;75(7 Suppl S):1869.
10. Lieberman D. Colonoscopy as a mass screening tool. *Eur J Gastroenterol Hepatol* 1998;10(3):225.
11. Zauber AG, Bushey MT, Khvatyuk O, et al. Familial risk in an asymptomatic general population cohort: preliminary results of the national colonoscopy study (NCS). *Gastroenterology* 2002;122(4 Suppl):1.
12. Greegor TH. Diagnosis of large bowel cancer in the asymptomatic patient. *JAMA* 1967;201:943.
13. Greegor D. Occult blood testing for detection of asymptomatic colon cancer. *Cancer* 1971;28:131.
15. Brandeau ML, Eddy DM. The workup of the asymptomatic patient with a positive fecal occult blood test. *Med Decis Making* 1987;7(1):32.
16. Eddy DM. Screening for colorectal cancer. *Ann Intern Med* 1990; 113(5):373.
17. Winawer S, Fletcher R, Rex D, et al. Colorectal cancer screening and surveillance: clinical guidelines and rationale-Update based on new evidence. *Gastroenterology* 2003;124(2):544.
18. Smith RA, von Eschenbach AC, Wender R, et al. American Cancer Society guidelines for the early detection of cancer: update of early detection guidelines for prostate, colorectal, and endometrial cancers. Also: update 2001—testing for early lung cancer detection [erratum appears in *CA Cancer J Clin* 2001;51(3):150]. *CA: Cancer J Clin* 2001;51(1):38.
20. Pickhardt PJ, Choi JR, Hwang I, et al. Computed tomographic virtual colonoscopy to screen for colorectal neoplasia in asymptomatic adults. *N Engl J Med* 2003;349(23):2191.
21. Burt RW. Colorectal cancer screening. *Curr Opin Gastroenterol* 2010; 26(5):466.
22. Shapiro S, Strax P, Venet L. Periodic breast cancer screening in reducing mortality from breast cancer. *JAMA* 1971;215(11):1777.
23. Mandel JS, Bond JH, Church TR, et al. Reducing mortality from colorectal cancer by screening for fecal occult blood [erratum appears in *N Engl J Med* 993;329(9):672]. *N Engl J Med* 1993;328(19):1365.
24. U.S. Preventive Services Task Force. *Guide to Clinical Preventive Services*. 2nd ed. Baltimore, MD: Williams & Wilkins, 1996.

25. Mandel JS, Church TR, Ederer F, Bond JH. Colorectal cancer mortality: effectiveness of biennial screening for fecal occult blood. *J Natl Cancer Inst* 1999;91:434.
26. Mandel JS, Church TR, Bond JH, et al. The effect of fecal occult-blood screening on the incidence of colorectal cancer. *N Engl J Med* 2000; 343(22):1603.
27. Hardcastle JD, Chamberlain JO, Robinson MH, et al. Randomised controlled trial of faecal-occult-blood screening for colorectal cancer. *Lancet* 1996;348(9040):1472.
28. Kronborg O, Fenger C, Olsen J, Jorgensen OD, Sondergaard O. Randomised study of screening for colorectal cancer with faecal-occult-blood test. *Lancet* 1996;348(9040):1467.
29. Hewitson P, Glasziou P, Irwig L, Towler B, Watson E. Screening for colorectal cancer using the faecal occult blood test, hemoccult. Cochrane Database Syst Rev2007(1):CD001216.
30. Atkin WS, Edwards R, Kralj-Hans I, et al. Once-only flexible sigmoidoscopy screening in prevention of colorectal cancer: a multicentre randomised controlled trial. *Lancet* 2010;375(9726):1624.
31. Winawer SJ, Zauber AG, Ho MN, et al. Prevention of colorectal cancer by colonoscopic polypectomy. *N Engl J Med* 1993;329(27):1977.
32. Robertson DJ, Greenberg ER, Beach M, et al. Colorectal cancer in patients under close colonoscopic surveillance. *Gastroenterology* 2005;129:34.
36. Allison JE, Tekawa IS, Ransom LJ, Adrain AL. A comparison of fecal occult-blood tests for colorectal-cancer screening. *N Engl J Med* 1996;334(3):155.
37. Levin B, Brooks D, Smith RA, Stone A. Emerging technologies in screening for colorectal cancer: CT colonography, immunochemical fecal occult blood tests, and stool screening using molecular markers. *CA: Cancer J Clin* 2003;53(1):44.
38. Rozen P, Knaani J, Samuel Z. Comparative screening with a sensitive guaiac and specific immunochemical occult blood test in an endoscopic study. *Cancer* 2000;89(1):46.
39. Saito H, Soma Y, Koeda J, et al. Reduction in risk of mortality from colorectal cancer by fecal occult blood screening with immunochemical hemagglutination test: a case-control study. *Int J Cancer* 1995;61(4):465.
42. Young GP, St John JB, Winawer SJ, Rozen P. Choice of fecal occult blood tests for colorectal cancer screening: recommendations based on performance characteristics in population studies. A WHO (World Health Organization) and OMED (World Organization for Digestive Endoscopy) report. *Am J Gastroenterol* 2002;97(10):2499.
43. Zappa M, Castiglione G, Paci E, et al. Measuring interval cancers in population-based screening using different assays of fecal occult blood testing: the district of Florence experience. *Int J Cancer* 2001;92(1):151.
45. Cole SR, Young GP, Esterman A, Cadd B, Morcom J. A randomised trial of the impact of new faecal haemoglobin test technologies on population participation in screening for colorectal cancer. *J Med Screen* 2003; 10(3):117.
46. Fraser CG, Matthew CM, Mowat NAG, Wilson JA, Carey FA, Steele RJ. Evaluation of a card collection based faecal immunochemical test in screening for colorectal cancer using a two-tier reflex approach. *Gut* 2007; 56(10):1415.
48. Hayes RB, Sigurdson A, Moore L, et al. Methods for etiologic and early marker investigations in the PLCO trial. *Mutati Res* 2005;592(1-2):147.
50. Levin TR. Flexible sigmoidoscopy for colorectal cancer screening: valid approach or short-sighted? *Gastroenterol Clin North Am* 2002; 31(4):1015.
51. Prorok PC, Andriole GL, Bresalier RS, et al. Design of the Prostate, Lung, Colorectal and Ovarian (PLCO) Cancer Screening Trial. Control Clin Trials 2000;21(6 Suppl):273S.
53. van Rijn JC, Reitsma JB, Stoker J, Bossuyt PM, van Deventer SJ, Dekker E. Polyp miss rate determined by tandem colonoscopy: a systematic review. *Am J Gastroenterol* 2006;101(2):343.
55. Trecca A, Gai F, DiLorenzo G, et al. Improved detection of colorectal neoplasms with selective use of chromoendoscopy in 2005 consecutive patients. *Tech Coloproctol* 2006;10:339.
56. Husband JE, Hodson NJ, Parsons CA. The use of computed tomography in recurrent rectal tumors. *Radiology* 1980;134(3):677.
57. Rosman AS, Korsten MA. Meta-analysis comparing CT colonography, air contrast barium enema, and colonoscopy. *Am J Med* 2007;120(3):203.
58. Florie J, Jensch S, Nievelstein RA, et al. MR colonography with limited bowel preparation compared with optical colonoscopy in patients at increased risk for colorectal cancer. *Radiology* 2007; 243(1):122.
60. Pennazio M. Capsule endoscopy: where are we after 6 years of clinical use? *Dig Liver Dis* 2006;38(12):867.
61. Fletcher R, Lobb R, Bauer M, et al. Screening patients with a family history of colorectal cancer. *J Gastroent Med* 2007;22:508.
62. Davidson N. Genetic testing in colorectal cancer: who, when, how and why. *Keio J Med* 2007;56:14-20.
63. Driver JA, Gaziano JM, Gelber RP, Lee I-M, Buring JE, Kurth T. Development of a risk score for colorectal cancer in men. *Am J Med* 2007; 120(3):257.
65. Kemp W, Pianko S, Nguyen S, Bailey MJ, Roberts SK. Survival in hepatocellular carcinoma: impact of screening and etiology of liver disease. *J Gastroenterol Hepatol* 2005;20(6):873.

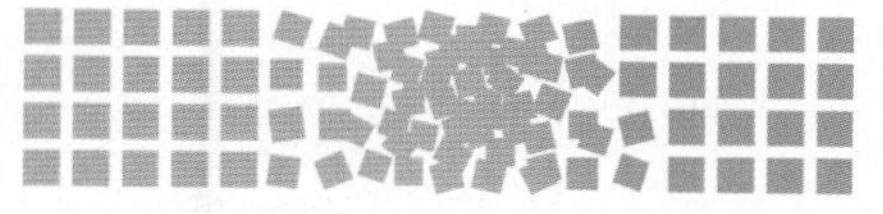

CHAPTER 59 SCREENING FOR GYNECOLOGIC CANCERS

MARY B. DALY AND JANET S. RADER

CERVICAL CANCER

Cervical cancer screening policies follow a triage system for detection, treatment, and follow-up. The principal screening test for cervical cancer in developed countries is the Pap smear, in which a cellular specimen from the cervix is fixed and stained on a slide for visual interpretation. Morphologic changes of precancerous cells, cervical intraepithelial neoplasia (CIN), are identified. Patients with abnormal findings on Pap smears are referred for colposcopy, in which 3% to 5% acetic acid is applied to the cervix and examined under magnification with a bright light to enhance lesions for biopsy. Women are then recalled for results and treatment. In some clinics a "see and treat" approach is taken, in which patients with an abnormal Pap smear are evaluated and treatment is determined by colposcopy in the same visit. The see and treat method is advantageous in low resource areas or when patient compliance is of concern. The overall cost of treatment should be less, but the possibility of overtreatment is disadvantageous.

It is well accepted that the Pap test has decreased the incidence of cervical cancer.[1] This is based on evidence that the decline in cervical cancer mortality closely parallels the implementation of the Pap smear during the past 50 years. However, controversy exists as to the frequency with which the test should be performed, how to implement human papillomavirus (HPV) DNA testing into screening procedures, and the lack of applicability for Third World countries.

Observational data suggest the effectiveness of screening increases when Pap tests are performed more frequently. Although a single Pap test may have a relatively low sensitivity, the cumulative sensitivity of several yearly tests should be high. Consensus guidelines on Pap smear frequency have been developed by the American Cancer Society (ACS),[2] the American College of Obstetricians and Gynecologists (ACOG),[3] and the National Comprehensive Cancer Network (www.nccn.org) (Table 59.1). Current recommendations favor initiation of screening by the age of 21 years or within 3 years of first sexual intercourse, whichever comes first. Up to the age of 30 years, screening is advised at 1- to 3-year intervals, depending on the specific recommendations being followed and the method of collection. After age 30 years, screening intervals may be extended to 2- to 3-year intervals if the patient meets specific low-risk criteria. Most recommendations stop screening by 65 or 70 years of age or after hysterectomy. Those women who test negative by cytology and HPV do not require retesting for 3 years. Women who have received HPV vaccination should continue cervical cancer screening according to the guidelines.

Cervical cytologic specimens can be collected with a variety of devices. The use of an ectocervical spatula and endocervical brush or swab together appears to be the best method for obtaining cervical cells for conventional specimens.[4] Both liquid-based and conventional exfoliate cytology Pap tests are acceptable for screening.[5] Liquid-based cytologic collection and analysis has the health care provider place the cervical cells in a small bottle containing fixative solution instead of making a direct slide preparation. The liquid-based/thin-layer preparation systems—ThinPrep Pap Test (Hologic, Inc., Marlborough, Massachusetts) and BD SurePath (BD, Franklin Lakes, New Jersey)—are designed to remove obscuring nonepithelial cells and distribute cells evenly on a slide. The sample is sent to the cytology laboratory where it is filtered or centrifuged to remove excess blood and debris. The cells are then transferred to the slide in a single layer. The slide is stained and examined manually. Two systems of computer-assisted screening are currently available: ThinPrep Imaging System (Hologic) and BD Focal-Point GS Imaging System (BD). Both are approved for use with liquid-based slide preparation. The ThinPrep Imaging System (www.thinprep.com/pap-test/thinprep-imaging.html) was developed for primary screening and presents computer images of 22 fields that contain cells of interest using a quantitative DNA stain. After the cytotechnologist has entered an opinion, the device reveals its determination based on a ranking as to whether manual review is warranted. When the human reviewer and the computer agree that no review is needed, a diagnosis of "within normal limits" is given. Manual review is required for any case if ranked by either the cytologist or the computer. With BD Focal-Point GS Imaging System (www.tripathimaging.com/physicians/focal_biblio.html), the device reviews the material on the slide and, based on an algorithm, scores the slide as to the likelihood of an abnormality being present. This algorithm includes a variety of visual characteristics, such as shape and optical density of the cells. The slides are prioritized for cytotechnologists review.

The Bethesda System used for reporting uniform cervical cytology results was initially developed in 1988. It was updated in 1991 and 2001 to incorporate laboratory and clinical experience.[6] These guidelines are endorsed by more than 40 international societies, and more than 90% of laboratories in the United States use the Bethesda System, as do laboratories in many other countries. The Bethesda System includes a descriptive diagnosis and an evaluation of specimen adequacy (Table 59.2). Bethesda 2001 adds a new category for atypical cells at higher risk of association with precancer, "atypical squamous cells—cannot exclude a high-grade lesion" or "ASC-H." This category highlights the 5% to 10% of atypical squamous cells of undetermined significance (ASCUS) that are more likely to contain high-grade squamous intraepithelial lesions. The classification of glandular abnormalities has been revised, eliminating the category "atypical glandular cells of undetermined significance" or "AGUS" to prevent confusion with ASCUS. The finding of atypical glandular cells is important clinically because 10% to 39% of cases are associated with underlying

TABLE 59.1

CONSENSUS GUIDELINES ON PAP SMEAR SCREENING

	ACS	NCCN	ACOG
Start screening	Within 3 years after initiating sexual activity, no later than ≥21 years		Age 21 years
≤30 years	Every year for conventional Pap; every 2 years for liquid Pap		Every 2 years
>30 years	Every 2–3 years after three consecutive normal Pap smears	Every 2–3 years after three consecutive normal Pap smears[a] or every 3 years when cytology is combined with HPV typing	Every 3 years after 3 consecutive normal Pap smears[a]
Stop screening[b]	Age 70 after three consecutive normal Paps and no abnormal results within 10 years	Age 70 after three consecutive normal Paps and no abnormal results within 10 years	Age 65–70 years after three consecutive normal Paps and no abnormal results within 10 years
After hysterectomy	None[c]	None[c]	None, except if a history of CIN 2–CIN 3
HPV DNA testing for screening	Option for women >30 years, performed every 3 years in conjunction with cytology		

ACS, American Cancer Society; NCCN, National Comprehensive Cancer Network; ACOG, American College of Obstetricians and Gynecologists; HPV, human papillomavirus; CIN, cervical intraepithelial neoplasia.

[a]More frequent screening may be required for higher-risk women: immunosuppressed, or human immunodeficiency virus-infected, exposed to diethylstilbestrol *in utero*, previously diagnosed with cervical cancer.

[b]Screening is recommended in older women who have not been screened or for whom information about previous screening is unavailable.

[c]Women with a history of CIN 2 or 3 should continue screening until three consecutive negative Pap tests.

high-grade disease. Glandular cell abnormalities are now classified as "atypical endocervical, endometrial or glandular cells—not otherwise specified (NOS) or favor neoplastic."

Overall, cervical cytology screening programs for the detection of CIN 3 or cancer have reported a range of sensitivities (50% to 75%) and specificities (69% to 94%).[7–9] The sensitivity of cytology is limited by sampling error, in which the abnormal cells do not get collected, and reading error, in which a few abnormal cells are not identified among the normal cells or obscured by blood or debris. Cytology also has problems with specificity. The screening program is overburdened by borderline smears of uncertain malignant potential, which are costly to follow and cause anxiety to the women involved. Moreover, the multicenter randomized National Cancer Institute ASCUS LSIL (low-grade squamous intraepithelial lesion) Triage Study (ALTS), which evaluated triaging methods for mildly abnormal Pap smears, confirmed the poor reproducibility of cytology readings by pathologists: 45% of referral Pap readings were disputed by the pathology quality control group. These studies point to the need for improvement in the screening system.[10]

The clinical utility of HPV-based screening for cervical disease results from its negative predictive value. A positive HPV result can indicate infection only rather than a high probability of cervical disease. Most HPV infections are transient, persisting for only 12 to 18 months.[11,12] However, women who develop a persistent infection with an oncogenic HPV have a much higher risk of developing neoplasia compared with uninfected patients.[13] Given the importance of HPV in the development of cervical cancer, clinical detection of HPV has become an important diagnostic tool for identifying patients at risk for cervical cancer. The ALTS clinical trial helped define the clinical utility of HPV testing in triaging annual cytology screening. This trial concluded that HPV testing of patients with ASCUS Pap smears before referral for colposcopy was more effective for detecting disease than repeat cytology or direct referral to colposcopy. The sensitivity of HPV DNA testing for the detection of biopsy-confirmed CIN 2 with ASCUS is 96% and is higher than the sensitivity of a single repeat cervical cytologic test.[14] Therefore, HPV testing can be used as an alternative approach for the follow-up of ASCUS in order to determine who is referred for further colposcopy. The test is performed on the original liquid-based cytology specimen to eliminate the need for the patient to return to the clinic. This "reflex HPV DNA testing" offers significant advantages because women do not need an additional clinical examination for specimen collection, and 40% to 60% of women will be spared a colposcopic examination.

Patients with ASCUS cytology and a positive HPV test result have a 15% prevalence of high-grade squamous intraepithelial lesions versus 1% or less for patients with ASCUS and a negative HPV test.[14] There are three tests approved by the U.S. Food and Drug Administration for HPV testing. Digene HC2 (Qiagen, Valencia, California) identifies any of 13 high-risk HPV types, Cervista HPV HR (Hologic) identifies any of 14-high risk types, and Cervista HPV 16/18 (Hologic) identifies HPV 16 and/or 18. The American Society for Colposcopy and Cervical Pathology has developed criteria in which testing for HPV DNA can be used for primary screening (http://www.asccp.org/pdfs/consensus/hpv_genotyping_20090320.pdf). High-risk HPV testing can be used in conjunction with a Pap smear for women over the age of 30. For those with negative results on both a Pap and an HPV test, repeat screening with both tests can be done after 3 years. If the tests are positive for any high-risk HPV, then the test for HPV types 16 and 18 is an option for further evaluation. Those women with positive results for HPV 16 and 18 should be examined with a colposcope. Those whose test for HPV 16 and 18 is negative should have a repeat Pap and HPV DNA test in 12 months.

An overview of studies on HPV testing in primary cervical cancer screening showed an average sensitivity for detection of CIN 2 or higher of 96%, which was unaffected by patient

TABLE 59.2

BETHESDA SYSTEM (2001)

Specimen Type
Indicate conventional smear (Pap smear) vs. liquid-based vs. other

Specimen Adequacy
Satisfactory for evaluation (*describe presence or absence of endocervical/transformation zone component and any other quality indicators [e.g., partially obscuring blood, inflammation]*)
Unsatisfactory for evaluation . . . (*specify reason*)
Specimen rejected/not processed (*specify reason*)
Specimen processed and examined, but unsatisfactory for evaluation of epithelial abnormality because of (*specify reason*)

General Categorization (*optional*)
Negative for intraepithelial lesion or malignancy
Epithelial cell abnormality: see "Interpretation/Result" (*specify "squamous" or "glandular" as appropriate*)
Other: see "Interpretation/Result" (*e.g., endometrial cells in a woman more than 40 years of age*)

Automated Review
If case examined by automated device, specify device and result.

Ancillary Testing
Provide a brief description of the test methods and report the result so that it is easily understood by the clinician.

Interpretation/Result
Negative for intraepithelial lesion or malignancy (*when there is no cellular evidence of neoplasia, state this in the "General Categorization" above and/or in the "Interpretation/Result" section of the report, whether or not there are organisms or other nonneoplastic findings*)
Organisms:
Trichomonas vaginalis
Fungal organisms morphologically consistent with *Candida* spp.
Shift in flora suggestive of bacterial vaginosis
Bacteria morphologically consistent with *Actinomyces* spp.
Cellular changes consistent with herpes simplex virus
Other nonneoplastic findings (*Optional to report; list not inclusive*):
Reactive cellular changes associated with
Inflammation (*includes typical repair*)
Radiation
Intrauterine contraceptive device
Glandular cells status posthysterectomy
Atrophy
Other
Endometrial cells (*in a woman more than 40 years of age*) (*Specify if "negative for squamous intraepithelial lesion"*)

Epithelial Cell Abnormalities
Squamous cell
Atypical squamous cells
Of undetermined significance (ASC-US)
Cannot exclude high-grade squamous intraepithelial lesion (HSIL; ASC-H)
Low-grade squamous intraepithelial lesion (LSIL)
Encompassing: HPV/mild dysplasia/CIN 1
HSIL Encompassing: moderate and severe dysplasia, CIS/CIN 2 and CIN 3
With features suspicious for invasion (if invasion is suspected)
Squamous cell carcinoma
Glandular cell
Atypical
Endocervical cells (NOS or specify in comments)
Endometrial cells (NOS or specify in comments)
Glandular cells (NOS or specify in comments)
Atypical
Endocervical cells, favor neoplastic
Glandular cells, favor neoplastic
Endocervical adenocarcinoma *in situ*
Adenocarcinoma
Endocervical
Endometrial
Extrauterine
NOS

Other Malignant Neoplasms (*specify*)

HPV, human papillomavirus; CIN, cervical intraepithelial neoplasia; NOS, not otherwise specified.

age.[15] Specificity (less than CIN 2) varied between 76% and 96% and was significantly on the lower end in young women. Adjusting for women 35 years and older, specificity was 93%. The majority of these studies were based on cross-sectional designs that assessed prevalent disease detected by either HPV testing or cytology. A randomized clinical trial for initial screening in rural India showed a significant reduction in advanced cervical cancers and deaths from cervical cancer after a single round of HPV testing followed by treatment.[16] The ultimate benefits, risks, and cost of HPV testing compared with cytology screening depend on the subsequent triage procedure, HPV typing assay, and primary testing frequency. It is also unclear whether HPV testing will become more or less important in a population of women vaccinated against HPV 16 and 18.

Cervicography and colposcopy have been evaluated as primary screening tests, but accuracy and technical requirements are suboptimal. Cervicography, in which a photograph of the cervix is examined at a central location for atypical lesions, has a sensitivity that is comparable to that of the Pap smear but a much lower specificity.[17] In addition, the performance of cervicography is poor in women more than 50 years of age, and about 10% to 15% of the cervigrams are unsatisfactory. Colposcopy, in which the cervix is magnified directly after the application of acetic acid, is widely performed on women with abnormal Pap smears, but this procedure has poor sensitivity (34% to 43%) and specificity (68%) when used as a screening test for cervical neoplasia in asymptomatic women.[18] Other disadvantages of colposcopy screening include its cost, the limited availability of the equipment, and the time and the skill required to perform the procedure. The ALTS trial also highlighted the lack of precision of colposcopy: 47% of the colposcopically directed cervical biopsies showed no pathologic lesion.[10]

Widespread cytology screening programs that function well in industrialized regions are simply not feasible in the developing world. They are far too expensive and do not attain adequate coverage. Moreover, poor countries often lack the manpower, technical support, and expertise to guarantee accurate results. In low-resource settings, direct visual inspection has been evaluated as a screening test alone or with cytology. The cervix is visualized with either the naked eye or a low-power magnification device after the application of 3% to 5% acetic acid. There is considerable variation in the mean sensitivity and specificity (80% and 80%) reported for direct visual inspection, probably because of the variation in the training and performance of the test and failure to adjust for verification bias.[17] The University of Zimbabwe and JHPIEGO evaluated visual inspection of the cervix with acetic acid (VIA) in a large-scale screening program.[19] In this study, 10,934 women were screened by six trained nurse-midwives using VIA. Colposcopy with biopsy, as indicated, was used as the reference test. VIA and Pap smears were done concurrently and their sensitivity and specificity compared. VIA was more sensitive but less specific than cytology. Sensitivity was 76.7% for VIA and 44.3% for cytology. Specificity was 64.1% for VIA and 90.6% for cytology. Belinson et al.[20] noted similar sensitivity (71%) and specificity (74%) in their study of approximately 2,000 women in rural China using trained gynecologists for the VIA. VIA has a role in areas of the world with limited resources. This procedure does not require laboratory infrastructure and provides immediate results and allows for screening, diagnosis, and treatment in a single visit.

Regular cervical cancer screening needs to be encouraged for all women, especially those likely to be exposed to HPV and human immunodeficiency virus infection. Special efforts are needed to reach those women less likely to be screened, like the elderly, poor, less educated, and recent immigrants. The National Breast and Cervical Cancer Early Detection Program, administered by the Centers for Disease Control and Prevention, is a nationwide comprehensive public health program that helps uninsured and underserved women gain access to screening services for the early detection of breast and cervical cancer (http://cdc.gov/gov/cancer/nbccedp/). The Centers for Disease Control and Prevention provides funds to qualifying health agencies (50 states, six U.S. territories, the District of Columbia, and 15 American Indian/Alaskan Native tribes and tribal organizations) to implement comprehensive screening programs. To maximize efficient use of limited resources, the program is focusing Pap screening on those who have not been tested for 5 years and is increasing the screening interval to every 3 years.

OVARIAN CANCER

Survival rates for epithelial ovarian cancer are directly related to stage at diagnosis and range from 80% to 90% for stage I to 25% for stage IV. Because more than 70% of women are diagnosed with advanced disease, the overall survival is approximately 30% at 5 years. The low rate of early detection has been attributed to a rapid aggressive growth pattern, the lack of an obvious precursor lesion, and/or to the lack of specific and reliable symptoms for early-stage disease. The high burden of cancer mortality associated with ovarian cancer, and the existence of curative strategies for early-stage disease, have led to extensive efforts during the past three decades to identify an effective population screening strategy. However, despite the strong rationale for population screening for ovarian cancer, there is currently no proven effective strategy for use in clinical practice. An effective screening test is defined as one that is safe and acceptable, cost-effective, and one that has high sensitivity, specificity, and positive predictive value (PPV). Because of the necessity to follow abnormal screening tests for ovarian cancer with an invasive procedure, usually laparoscopy or laparotomy, it has been estimated that an effective screening strategy for ovarian cancer requires a sensitivity of at least 75%, a specificity of more than 99.6%, and a PPV of at least 10%.[21] Efforts to find an effective screening test for ovarian cancer have focused to date on ultrasound imaging and tumor markers.

Early studies that used transabdominal ultrasonography to determine ovarian volume and morphologic characteristics had low PPVs, less than 2%. Transvaginal ultrasonography (TVUS), which achieves better resolution and visualization of the ovaries, has replaced the transabdominal approach. However, most studies report a high rate of false-positive results, with only the experience of van Nagell et al.[22] achieving a PPV above the recommended 10%.

Several attempts have been made to improve the evaluation of ovarian morphologic characteristics seen with ultrasonography, such as degree of cyst complexity and thickness of wall structure. However, these systems often lack validation. Nor has the addition of Doppler flow examination, which capitalizes on the presence of neovascularization in tumor masses, improved the ability to identify malignant masses. The latest addition to standard TVUS is three-dimensional Doppler, which has been shown by some investigators to be superior to two-dimensional Doppler.[23] However, its uptake among radiologists to date has been limited. Overall, lack of specificity of ultrasound alone for the detection of ovarian cancer in the general population argues against its adoption as a single screening approach.

Diagnosis of early-stage cancer by detection of a tumor biomarker in blood or other easily available body tissue would seem to be an ideal screening strategy. The most extensively studied biomarker of ovarian cancer is CA 125, a glycoprotein that is expressed by tissue derived from coelomic epithelium. Although not present in normal ovarian epithelium, CA 125 is overexpressed by serous papillary ovarian tumors, and less often in mucinous, clear cell, and borderline tumors. Retrospective analysis of serum bank data showed a prior CA 125 elevation in one-third to one-half of women who eventually developed ovarian cancer. Elevated levels were evident 18 months to 3 years prior to diagnosis.[24] Serum CA 125 levels are highly correlated with advanced-stage disease, with more than 90% of stage II–IV tumors presenting with elevated levels (usually defined as 35 U/mL or more). However, elevated CA 125 levels are found in only 50% of stage I tumors, when diagnosis would be optimal.[25] Conversely, CA 125 levels are also elevated in a variety of other benign and malignant conditions, significantly compromising its specificity.[21] As a result of these limitations, most screening programs rely on a multimodal approach.

Two early nonrandomized studies evaluated the role of CA 125 as a trigger for more intensive surveillance with ultrasonography and/or clinical evaluation. Einhorn et al.[26] screened more than 5,000 women aged 40 and older with two annual CA 125 screens. Six women eventually developed clinical ovarian cancer. Four of the six had elevated levels at the first screen, and all six had elevated levels at the second screen. The specificity of the test using a cutoff of 35 U/mL was 97.6%. A larger study screened 22,000 women with a single CA 125 level with TVUS as a follow-up for elevated levels, and reported a sensitivity of 78.6%, a specificity of 99.9%, and a PPV of 26.8%. Of 11 cancers found in women with elevated CA 125 levels, however, only 3 were stage I.[27] A subsequent study randomized postmenopausal women to three annual screens with CA 125 followed by ultrasonography if levels exceeded 30 U/mL. Women in the study arm with both elevated CA 125 levels and abnormal findings on ultrasounds were referred for surgical evaluation. Women in the control arm were followed with routine clinical care. Of 29 women in the screened group who underwent surgery, 6 had ovarian cancer, yielding a PPV of 20.7%. However, women in the control group had a similar incidence of ovarian cancer, and overall mortality between the two groups was not significantly different.[28] A large prospective trial in Japan randomized 80,000 women to annual TVUS and CA 125 versus usual care. At a mean follow-up of 9.2 years, the rates of ovarian cancer were similar in both arms, and although the proportion of early-stage cancers was higher in the screened group, the difference was not statistically significant.[29]

Two multimodal randomized trials that will provide more definite data in the efficacy of this approach are currently under way. The National Institutes of Health Prostate Lung Colorectal and Ovary (PLCO) Study has randomized 34,261women above age 55 years to annual concurrent CA 125, pelvic examination, and TVUS for 4 years, plus an additional 2 years of screening with CA 125 only, versus routine care. Any abnormal test prompts surgical referral. After four rounds of screening, the PPV of the two tests ranged from 1.0% to 1.3%. Seventy-two percent of the screen-detected cancers were stage III or IV.[30] The impact of screening on mortality is pending. The United Kingdom Collaborative Trial of Ovarian Cancer Screening (UKCTOCS) has recruited 200,000 postmenopausal women who are randomized to routine care, ultrasound screen only, or multimodal screening with ultrasound and CA 125. Preliminary results of the prevalent screen found a sensitivity, specificity, and PPV for primary invasive epithelial ovarian and tubal cancers of 89.5%, 99.8%, respectively, and 35.1% for the multimodal screen, and 75.0%. 98.2%, and 2.8%, respectively, for ultrasound alone. Also, 48.3% of the ovarian and tubal cancers found at the prevalent screen were stage I or II.[31] The primary outcome of the ongoing screening will be mortality from ovarian cancer.

An alternative strategy to improve the sensitivity of CA 125 is to take into account the rate of change over time. A computer algorithm has been developed that uses sequential values to estimate the risk of ovarian cancer on the basis of change point analysis. A prospective study randomized 13,000 women to screening with serial CA 125 levels with calculation of the "risk of ovarian cancer algorithm" or to a control group. Women with intermediate risk had a repeat level drawn at 3 months. Those with high risk underwent TVUS. Of 144 women in the elevated risk category, 16 underwent surgery and 3 primary ovarian cancers were found (2 stage I and 1 stage II). The specificity and PPV of this screening strategy were 99.8% and 19%, respectively.[32] The risk of ovarian cancer algorithm approach has been incorporated into the UKCTOCS trial.

Another approach to increase the sensitivity of CA 125 is to combine it with other complementary tumor markers. Several markers, including CA 19-9, carcinoembryonic antigen, human chorionic gonadotropin, CA 72-4, macrophage colony-stimulating factor, inhibin, alpha-fetoprotein, lysophosphatidic acid, osteopontin, mesothelin, and HE-4, among others, have been combined in a variety of studies. Increased sensitivity, however, is typically accompanied by a decrease in specificity. Proteomic analysis has been applied to the early detection of ovarian cancer with mixed results. This technology combines mass spectrometry profiling with artificial intelligence to identify unique protein fragments that form signatures of preclinical disease.[33] Several groups report high levels of sensitivity and specificity using banked sera, but lack of reproducibility and changes in technology have so far precluded the use of proteomic markers in the clinical setting. Both the PLCO and the UKCTOCS screening studies are creating biospecimen banks for use in further refinement of proteomic and other novel approaches.

There is a growing consensus that certain symptoms, including bloating, pelvic or abdominal pain, difficulty eating or early satiety, and urinary frequency may be associated with ovarian cancer. Sole reliance on symptom reporting as a screening tool, however, results in a very low PPV.[34]

Given the relatively low prevalence of ovarian cancer in the general population, resulting in the need for highly sensitive and specific tests for screening, another strategy is to focus on select populations characterized by an increased risk for ovarian cancer. One such group is women with a hereditary predisposition for ovarian cancer, including women with deleterious mutations in *BRCA1/2* or women from Lynch syndrome families with mutations in one of the DNA mismatch repair genes, in whom estimates of lifetime risk for ovarian cancer range from 16% to 60%. Hermsen et al.[35] summarized the results of a European multicenter observational study of 888 *BRCA1/2* mutation carriers who were screened annually with TVUS and CA 125 between 1993 and 2005. Of the ten incident ovarian cancers diagnosed, half were interval cancers and eight of the ten were advanced stage. Despite the lack of evidence that any of the screening modalities for ovarian cancer are effective for women with a hereditary predisposition, the National Comprehensive Cancer Network guidelines include recommendations for TVUS and CA 125 for these women until they undergo prophylactic oophorectomy. When offering ovarian cancer screening to this population, it is particularly important that the provider explore issues of false-positive and false-negative tests, and other preventive options.

Given the limitations of current screening modalities, the United States Preventive Services Task Force, American College of Obstetricians and Gynecologists, and the American College of Physicians all discourage routine screening for ovarian cancer for the general population.[36–38] And although guidelines have been proposed for women with a hereditary predisposition to ovarian cancer, they are not evidence-based.

ENDOMETRIAL CANCER

Most women (90%) who are diagnosed with endometrial cancer are postmenopausal and present with abnormal uterine bleeding, resulting in a high proportion (75%) of early-stage disease with an overall 5-year survival of 86%.[39] A number of risk factors have been identified that significantly increase a woman's risk for endometrial cancer, including menopausal status, obesity, diabetes, the use of unopposed estrogens, and the use of tamoxifen. Furthermore, women from Lynch syndrome families who are carriers of germ line mutations in the DNA mismatch repair genes have a lifetime risk of endometrial cancer that ranges from 20% to 60% with an average age at onset of 48 years, or 15 years earlier than the general population.[40] TVUS and endometrial sampling have been proposed as screening strategies, particularly in women with known risk factors.

Endometrial thickness, as determined by TVUS, has been used in several studies to evaluate women presenting with abnormal vaginal bleeding. These studies have established an upper limit of normal for endometrial thickness ranging from 4 to 6 mm. Fleischer et al.[41] screened 1,926 asymptomatic women with TVUS and aspiration endometrial biopsy for eligibility in a 2-year placebo-controlled trial using a selective estrogen receptor modulator to prevent osteoporosis. The use of a threshold of 6 mm for endometrial thickness had a low sensitivity (17%) and a low PPV of 2%. As part of the Postmenopausal Estrogen/Progestin Interventions trial, Langer et al.[42] performed annual concurrent TVUS and endometrial biopsies in 448 women. A threshold of 5 mm for abnormal endometrial thickness resulted in a sensitivity of 90%, a specificity of 48%, and a PPV of 9%. The authors found, however, that the highest values for endometrial thickness were not associated with the most serious diagnoses. This plus the high false-positive rate led them to conclude that ultrasonography is not a practical screening tool in asymptomatic women.

Endometrial biopsy is often used as a first-line diagnostic tool for women presenting with abnormal uterine bleeding. The detection rate using the Pipelle is 99.6% in postmenopausal women. However, issues of inadequate access to the endometrial cavity or sampling error have been reported with use of endometrial biopsy in asymptomatic women. A large study of 801 women in whom endometrial biopsy was performed prior to the initiation of hormone replacement therapy reported a rate of insufficient tissue in 24.5% of women. Furthermore, only one case of endometrial cancer was detected.[38]

The use of tamoxifen is associated with a two- to threefold increased risk of endometrial cancer. The National Surgical Adjuvant Breast and Bowel Project Breast Cancer Prevention Trial evaluated the role of concurrent ultrasound and endometrial biopsy in 257 women randomized to tamoxifen or placebo. Altogether these tests performed poorly, with a 27% sensitivity for ultrasound and the detection of only one invasive cancer by biopsy.[43] Gerber et al.[44] followed 247 tamoxifen-treated women and 98 controls with TVUS every 6 months for 2 to 5 years. A threshold of 10 mm triggered further evaluation with hysteroscopy and dilation and curettage; 1,265 ultrasounds were performed, and only 1 endometrial cancer was detected. Furthermore, four uterine perforations were reported. Markovitch et al.[45] found that increasing the cutoff value of endometrial thickness in tamoxifen-treated women to increase specificity led to unacceptable declines in the sensitivity of the test. Sonohysterography shows promise in improving the performance of TVUS in this patient population, but evidence at this time is insufficient to recommend its use in routine clinical care. Current studies are exploring the identification of serum biomarkers, which may be predictive of endometrial cancers.[46,47]

As in the general population, TVUS alone leads to a high false-positive and false-negative rate in women with Lynch syndrome mutations. The addition of endometrial biopsy to TVUS in mutation carriers has improved the detection rate.[48] Although data on the impact of this approach on survival are lacking, the ACS recommends annual screening with endometrial biopsy for Lynch syndrome women starting at age 35. For all other women, the ACS recommends that women be informed at menopause of the need to report any unexpected bleeding to their physician.[49]

References

1. Cardenas-Turanzas M, Follen M, Benedet JL, Cantor SB. See-and-treat strategy for diagnosis and management of cervical squamous intraepithelial lesions. *Lancet Oncol* 2005;6:43.
2. Saslow D, Runowicz CD, Solomon D, et al. American Cancer Society guideline for the early detection of cervical neoplasia and cancer. *CA Cancer J Clin* 2002;52:342.
3. ACOG Practice Bulletin no. 109: cervical cytology screening. *Obstet Gynecol* 2009;114:1409.
4. Sawaya GF, Washington AE. Cervical cancer screening: which techniques should be used and why? *Clin Obstet Gynecol* 1999;42:922.
5. Arbyn M, Bergeron C, Klinkhamer P, et al. Liquid compared with conventional cervical cytology: a systematic review and meta-analysis. *Obstet Gynecol* 2008;111:167.
6. Solomon D, Davey D, Kurman R, et al. The 2001 Bethesda System. Terminology for reporting results of cervical cytology. *JAMA* 2002;287:2114.
7. Kulasingam SL, Hughes JP, Kiviat NB, et al. Evaluation of human papillomavirus testing in primary screening for cervical abnormalities: comparison of sensitivity, specificity, and frequency of referral. *JAMA* 2002;288:1749.
8. Schiffman M, Herrero R, Hildesheim A, et al. HPV DNA testing in cervical cancer screening: results from women in a high-risk province of Costa Rica. *JAMA* 2000;283:87.
9. Fahey MT, Irwig L, Macaskill P. Meta-analysis of Pap test accuracy. *Am J Epidemiol* 1995;141:680.
10. Stoler MH, Schiffman M. Interobserver reproducibility of cervical cytology and histologic interpretations realistic estimates from the ASCUS-LSIL triage study. *JAMA* 2001;285:1500.
11. Richardson H, Kelsall G, Tellier P, et al. The natural history of type-specific human papillomavirus infections in female university students. *Cancer Epidemiol Biomarkers Prev* 2003;12:485.
12. Rodriguez AC, Burk R, Herrero R, et al. The natural history of human papillomavirus infection and cervical intraepithelial neoplasia among young women in the Guanacaste cohort shortly after initiation of sexual life. *Sex Transm Dis* 2007;34(7):494.
13. Koshiol J, Lindsay L, Pimenta JM, et al. Persistent human papillomavirus infection and cervical neoplasia: a systematic review and meta-analysis. *Am J Epidemiol* 2008;15:15.
14. Solomon D, Schiffman M, Tarone R. Comparison of three management strategies for patients with atypical squamous cells of undetermined significance: baseline results from a randomized trial. *J Natl Cancer Inst* 2001;93:293.
15. Cuzick J, Clavel C, Petry KU, et al. Overview of the European and North American studies on HPV testing in primary cervical cancer screening. *Int J Cancer* 2006;119:1095.
16. Sankaranarayanan R, Nene BM, Shastri SS, et al. HPV screening for cervical cancer in rural India. *N Engl J Med* 2009;360:1385.
17. Wright TC Jr. Cervical cancer screening using visualization techniques. *J Natl Cancer Inst Monogr* 2003;31:66.
18. Olatunbosun OA, Okonofua FE, Ayangade SO. Screening for cervical neoplasia in an African population: simultaneous use of cytology and colposcopy. *Int J Gynecol Obstet* 1991;36:39.
19. Visual inspection with acetic acid for cervical -cancer screening: test qualities in a primary-care setting. University of Zimbabwe/JHPIEGO Cervical Cancer Project. *Lancet* 1999;353:869.
20. Belinson JL, Pretorius RG, Zhang WH, et al. Cervical cancer screening by simple visual inspection after acetic acid. *Obstet Gynecol* 2001;98:441.
21. Rosenthal AN, Menon U, Jacobs IJ. Screening for ovarian cancer. *Clin Obstet Gynecol* 2006;49:433.
22. van Nagell JR, Depriest PD, Ueland FR, et al. Ovarian cancer screening with annual transvaginal sonography. *Cancer* 2007;109:1887.
23. Cohen LS, Escobar PF, Scharm C, Glimco B, Fishman DA. Three-dimensional power Doppler ultrasound improves the diagnostic accuracy for ovarian cancer prediction. *Gynecol Oncol* 2001;82:40.
24. Zurawski VR Jr, Orjaseter H, Andersen A, Jellum E. Elevated serum CA 125 levels prior to diagnosis of ovarian neoplasia: relevance for early detection of ovarian cancer. *Int J Cancer* 1988;42:677.
25. Bast RC Jr, Badgwell D, Lu Z, et al. New tumor markers: CA 125 and beyond. *Int J Gynecol Cancer* 2005;15(Suppl 3):274.
26. Einhorn N, Sjovall K, Knapp RC, et al. Prospective evaluation of serum CA 125 levels for early detection of ovarian cancer. *Obstet Gynecol* 1992;80:14.
27. Jacobs I, Davies AP, Bridges J, et al. Prevalence screening for ovarian cancer in postmenopausal women by CA 125 measurement and ultrasonography. *Br Med J* 1993;306:1030.
28. Jacobs IJ, Skates SJ, MacDonald N, et al. Screening for ovarian cancer: a pilot randomised controlled trial. *Lancet* 1999;353:1207.
29. Kobayashi H, Yamada Y, Sado T, et al. A randomized study of screening for ovarian cancer: a multicenter study in Japan. *Int J Gynecol Cancer* 2008;18:414.
30. Partridge E, Kreimer AR, Greenlee RT, et al. Results from four rounds of ovarian cancer screening in a randomized trial. *Obstet Gynecol* 2009;113:775.
31. Menon U, Gentry-Maharaj A, Hallett R, et al. Sensitivity and specificity of multimodal and ultrasound screening for ovarian cancer, and stage distribution of detected cancers: results of the prevalence screen of the UK Collaborative Trial of Ovarian Cancer Screening (UKCTOCS). *Lancet Oncol* 2009;10:327.
32. Menon U, Skates SJ, Lewis S, et al. Prospective study using the risk of ovarian cancer algorithm to screen for ovarian cancer. *J Clin Oncol* 2005;23:7919.
33. Kim G, Minig L, Kohn EC. Proteomic profiling in ovarian cancer. *Int J Gynecol Cancer* 2009;19:S2.
34. Rossing MA, Wicklund KG, Cushing-Haugen KL, et al. Predictive value of symptoms for early detection of ovarian cancer. *J Natl Cancer Inst* 2010;102:222.
35. Hermsen BBJ, Olivier RI, Verheijen RHM, et al. No efficacy of annual gynaecological screening in BRCA1/2 mutation carriers: an observational follow-up study. *Br J Cancer* 2007;96:1335.
36. Screening for ovarian cancer: recommendation statement. US Preventive Services Task Force. *Am Fam Phys* 2005;71:759.
37. ACOG committee opinion number 280, December 2002: the role of the generalist obstetrician-gynecologist in the early detection of ovarian cancer. *Obstet Gynecol* 2002;100:1413.
38. American College of Physicians. Screening for ovarian cancer: recommendations and rationale. *Ann Intern Med* 1994;121:141.
39. Sonoda Y, Barakat RR. Screening and the prevention of gynecologic cancer: endometrial cancer. *Best Pract Res Clin Obstet Gynaecol* 2006;20:363.
40. Lynch HT, Lynch PM, Lanspa SJ, et al. Review of the Lynch syndrome: history, molecular genetics, screening, differential diagnosis, and medicolegal ramifications. *Clin Genet* 2009;76(1):1.
41. Fleischer AC, Wheeler JE, Lindsay I, et al. An assessment of the value of ultrasonographic screening for endometrial disease in postmenopausal women without symptoms. *Am J Obstet Gynecol* 2001;184:70.
42. Langer RD, Pierce JJ, O'Hanlan KA, et al. Transvaginal ultrasonography compared with endometrial biopsy for the detection of endometrial disease: Postmenopausal Estrogen/Progestin Interventions Trial. *N Engl J Med* 1997;337:1792.

43. Runowicz C, Constantino J, Kavanah M, et al. National Surgical Adjuvant Breast and Bowel Project (NSABP) Breast Cancer Prevention Trial (BCPT) summary analysis of transvaginal sonography and endometrial biopsy in detecting endometrial pathology [abstract]. American Society of Clinical Oncology. 1999.
44. Gerber B, Krause A, Muller H, et al. Effects of adjuvant tamoxifen on the endometrium in postmenopausal women with breast cancer: a prospective long-term study using transvaginal ultrasound. *J Clin Oncol* 2000;18:3464.
45. Markovitch O, Tepper R, Fishman A, et al. The value of transvaginal ultrasonography in the prediction of endometrial pathologies in asymptomatic postmenopausal breast cancer tamoxifen-treated patients. *Gynecol Oncol* 2004;95:456.
46. Seko A, Kataoka F, Aoki D, et al. *N*-acetylglucosamine 6-*O*-sulfotransferase-2 as a tumor marker for uterine cervical and corpus cancer. *Glycoconj J* 2009; 26(8):1065.
47. Linkov F, Edwards R, Balk J, et al. Endometrial hyperplasia, endometrial cancer and prevention: gaps in existing research of modifiable risk factors. *Eur J Cancer* 2008;44:1632.
48. Gerritzen LH, Hoogerbrugge N, Oei ALM, et al. Improvement of endometrial biopsy over transvaginal ultrasound alone for endometrial surveillance in women with Lynch syndrome. *Fam Cancer* 2009;8:391.
49. Smith RA, Cokkinides V, Eyre HJ. American Cancer Society guidelines for the early detection of cancer, 2005. *CA Cancer J Clin* 2005;55:31.

CHAPTER 60 SCREENING FOR BREAST CANCER

LAURA J. ESSERMAN AND CHRIS I. FLOWERS

Finding a cancer before it has the potential to spread is the goal of screening for breast cancer. For most breast cancers, increasing tumor size is related to an increasing likelihood of regional and distant metastases and poor prognosis. Small tumors at diagnosis have an increased chance of survival. Women with cancers diagnosed at 5 mm or smaller have a 3% risk of nodal metastasis compared with 15% for tumors larger than 5 mm. Treating cancers at a smaller size also means less invasive surgery (lumpectomy vs. mastectomy) and less need for aggressive systemic treatment such as chemotherapy.

There is no question that breast screening by mammography picks up cancers at a smaller size and stage compared to a nonscreened population. The main questions are how much impact does screening have on reducing mortality, what are the limitations, and how can screening be improved by tailoring the recommendations based on the current understanding of breast cancer biology? This chapter will review the evidence of mortality benefit from randomized screening trials, a factor that is critical in terms of implementation of screening, the harms of screening, and potential limitations, as well as make suggestions for how to improve or tailor screening based on insights from breast cancer biology.

THE EVIDENCE OF MORTALITY BENEFIT FROM RANDOMIZED TRIALS OF MAMMOGRAPHY SCREENING

There is level 1 evidence to support population-based screening. However, there is considerable variability in how screening is implemented, and the ages at which to start and stop vary by country as does the frequency. Table 60.1 shows how screening is implemented across countries in the United States, Europe, and Canada.

Evidence of benefit comes from several randomized controlled trials (RCTs) of mammography, the most important of which is the Swedish two counties trial in the 1980s, which has many years of follow-up and for which much data are available.[1–5] Long-term follow-up of several of these controlled trials show a relative mortality reduction between 28% and 45%.[1] The larger percentage is claimed when women who actually had screening were considered compared with women invited for screening. The argument for including just the women undergoing screening is that RCTs underestimate the effect of women actually screened by approximately 25%, as not everyone in the screening cohort actually went for screening. However, these studies were designed to estimate the benefits of a national screening program, where half the women were invited to screen and half were not. The data are disputed by some authors and strongly supported by others. However, several meta-analyses, including the compilation of the Swedish screening studies as well as the U.S. Preventive Task Force analyses, have been performed confirming the mortality benefits.[5,6]

The analysis of these RCTs and their relevance to population screening is further complicated by the different intervals between screens used in the various trials. The interval between screens varied between 18 months and 33 months among the randomized screening trials. Of note, the two county trial from Sweden, where the benefits were among the highest, had a 24-month interval, but in service, the actual interval was 33 months.

The data that supports breast cancer screening are strong, with mature outcome data. The 2009 systematic review of updated evidence for the U.S. Preventive Services Task Force confirmed that mammography reduces breast cancer mortality in women aged 39 to 69 years.[6] The benefits are the most significant in women aged 50 to 74.

There are several aspects to screening that deserve further exploration with the goal of improving our understanding of the benefits and limitations of screening and the opportunities to improve and tailor population screening. These include how the advances in systemic therapy might impact screening, how the organization of screening can improve screening, and how the potential harms of screening might be mitigated, based on advances in our understanding of the biology of breast cancer. Screening is different from most interventions in medicine in that it targets a well population that does not have a disease. It attempts to balance risks and benefits to detect disease early enough to make a difference, while at the same time minimizing the harms, such as false-positive recall, biopsy, and unnecessary surgeries (e.g., in lung cancer screening with small pulmonary nodules). It is therefore essential to target screening to a population that will likely benefit and to have an open debate about the risks and benefits of screening tests.

CHANGES IN SYSTEMIC THERAPIES AND IMPACT ON SCREENING

Randomized trials were largely conducted in the 1980s and 1990s. At that time, the quality of mammography was beginning to improve and systemic therapies were just being tested for their impact on mortality. These include hormonally based therapies such as tamoxifen and chemotherapy. For the entire population of breast cancer patients, the relative chance of dying of breast cancer is reduced by 30% for chemotherapy and by 50% for hormonally based therapy.[7] Most of the randomized trials of screening were conducted prior to the widespread use of modern systemic therapy, so it is not clear whether screening mammography would continue to have as much impact on mortality in a contemporary treatment

TABLE 60.1

SCREENING POLICIES ACROSS NORTH AMERICA AND EUROPE

Country	Starting Age	Ending Age	Frequency
United States	40 (ACS, ACR) 50 (USPSTF)50 (shared decision making 40–50)	All >40 (ACS) 74 (USPSTF)	Q1 yr Q2 yr (USPSTF)
Canada	50	69	Q2 yr
United Kingdom	47 (from 2012)	74 (from 2012)	Q3 yr
Sweden	40	74	<50 18 months >50 Q2 yr
Netherlands	50	70	Q2 yr
France	50	74	Q2 yr
Spain	50	70	Q2 yr

ACS, American Cancer Society; ACR, American College of Radiology; USPSTF, United States Preventive Services Task Force.

setting. For specific types of cancers, such as triple negative cancers and human epidermal growth factor receptor 2 (HER2)–positive cancers, chemotherapy is more effective.[8] For HER2-positive cancers, targeted therapeutics are now available that dramatically improve outcome.[9] However, given that these cancers are the most aggressive, and that therapy is not 100% effective, early detection is likely to play a role. To better address all of these complexities, the CIS-NET (Cancer Intervention and Surveillance Modeling Network) modeling group has estimated the relative contributions of systemic therapy and screening on mortality reduction for breast cancer. A recent study suggests that two thirds of the benefit in mortality reduction, previously ascribed to screening, is now accomplished with modern adjuvant therapy.[10]

OPTIMIZING THE ORGANIZATION OF SCREENING

Screening is an expensive endeavor. In the United States, the annual cost of screening and diagnostic workup is in the range of $7 to 10 billion.[11] However, in the United States, screening is opportunistic, whereas in Europe screening is centrally organized in a more quality oriented and cost-effective manner. Programs are organized, targets for screening and implementation are set, women are invited to screen, and outcomes are tracked and reported by unit and for the program overall. The Institute of Medicine, in a recent review of mammography screening practices, highlighted the value of such an approach and recommended that the United States follow such practices.[12]

Setting Targets for Quality Management

Many European countries, like the United Kingdom, have centralized programs with designated screening centers that require a minimum volume of 5,000 (target of 7,000) screenings per year.[13] There are also variable ways of monitoring quality. In the United States, the Mammography Standards Quality Act (MSQA) mandates minimum requirements for equipment and reporting. Others require reporting on the major screening parameters, including invitations to screen, rate of acceptance, recall, biopsy rates, cancer to biopsy ratios, and the biology and stage of all cancers detected. The measurement and reporting of these outcome parameters enable the opportunity for analysis and improvement. In the United Kingdom a testing and training system is used to help mammographers continually assess and improve their performance, with a tool called the PERFORMS (PERsonal perFORmance in Mammographic Screening), a set of mammographic images used to assess sensitivity and specificity of the U.K. radiologists across the country. The test is taken twice per year and specialized training is given for problems identified.[13] This approach utilizes tools for quality improvement and skills maintenance not unlike the airline industry. Over time, quality has improved significantly in the United Kingdom, more so than in countries where such a systematic approach is not used.[14] Altough radiologists in the United States have led the development of standards and benchmarks for evaluation, there is no central commitment to applying and tracking the benchmarks in a uniform manner across the country.[15,16]

OPTIMIZING THE INTERPRETATION OF MAMMOGRAPHY

An ideal screening test would have a high sensitivity and high specificity, preferably 100%. However, sensitivity and specificity are trade-offs, as in order to maximize sensitivity ther must be a lower specificity, and vice versa. The trade-off can be measured in the form of a receiver operating characteristic (ROC) curve (Fig. 60.1).

A helpful analogy would be to consider a bug screen on a window and the fineness of the mesh used. The principle is to allow the desirable effects through (light and air) while keeping out what is bad (the bugs). The finer the screen, the less light and air get through, but no bugs get through. A coarser mesh will let an acceptable amount of light and air through, but some bugs will also get through. If the threshold for intervention is low, then many nonmalignant lesions will be caught, but many people will be harmed if there is a false-positive result. If the threshold is elevated to reduce these false positives, then small cancers will slip through and be missed. To be efficacious, screening has to balance the benefits and the risks.

Although there is a trade-off along the ROC curve for sensitivity and specificity, the most important factor is to be on the optimal ROC curve. A major determinant of the quality of screening is the person who interprets the mammogram. The most experienced mammographers find the most cancers and recall the fewest cancers. Less-experienced mammographers are on a different ROC curve and not only recall more women and recommend more biopsies (more false positives) but also miss the most cancers.[17] There is considerable variation among countries in terms of how they organize mammographic

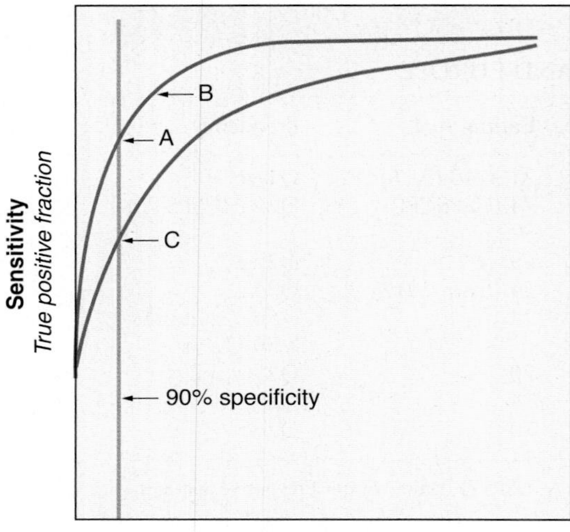

FIGURE 60.1 A receiver operating characteristic (ROC) curve schematic demonstrates that when specificity of a diagnostic test increases (false-positive fraction decreases), the ROC curve dictates an attendant decrease in sensitivity. As sensitivity increases, specificity will necessarily decrease if all operators area on the same ROC curve (movement from point A to point B). Another scenario, however, is that some operators (in this case, mammographers) will not be on the optimal curve, and both sensitivity and specificity will be lower (movement from point A to point C). For a screening test, such as mammography, which requires high specificity, it is most appropriate to assess sensitivity at a specificity of 90% (vertical line). (From Esserman L, et al. Improving the accuracy of mammography: volume and outcome relationships. *J Natl Cancer Inst* 2002;94(5), with permission.)

screening programs. When dedicated mammographers are used to interpret mammograms, and batch reading is used, and programs that support training and quality improvement, in both sensitivity and specificity, are higher.[14,16]

Setting the Optimal Screening Interval

The threshold for picking up a disease is partly based on the timing of the screening test, relative to the disease process. This is called the iceberg principle of continuous developing disease, where initially a tumor is too small to be seen until it reaches a detection threshold (which depends on the sensitivity of the test). The timing of the test matters, as the tumor needs to be big enough to be perceived, and depending on the sampling interval, will determine if it is detected at the screening visit or will wait until the next round when it will be more easily visible.

The longer the gap between screening examinations, the greater the likelihood that cancers can occur between screening rounds. These are known as interval cancers. The chance of interval cancers varies by age and by aggressiveness of the underlying disease. Interval cancers reported from the Norbotten Screening Program ranged from 43% in women aged 40 to 50 to 10% in women aged 70.[18] Aggressive cancers are more common in young women,[19] and a significant proportion of women who present with large aggressive cancers have cancers that appear between screens and are interval cancers even when the screening interval is 1 year.[20] Thus there are some cancers that may not be detectable early even in an annual screening program. When it becomes possible to predict which populations will be susceptible to more rapidly growing tumors, the screening interval can be altered. For example, in women with BRCA mutations, screening is recommended at 6 months intervals (magnetic resonance imaging [MRI] annually alternating with annual mammography, staggered by 6 months). Figure 60.2 shows how various tumor growth rates may be affected by screening over time.

In reality, the growth curves in Figure 60.1 represent the heterogeneity of breast cancer and tumors types vary in frequency across a population, so this is a stylized generalization, but it also illustrates that interval cancers are a fact of life. Even if a woman is screened every 6 months, some would present clinically with an interval cancer due to the rapid speed of growth in the interval screened. The CIS-NET modeling group, based on the data from clinical trials, estimates that the vast majority of the benefit is accrued by screening women aged 50 to 74 every 2 years, and this interval is associated with many fewer recalls and biopsies than annual screening.[21]

ADDRESSING THE POTENTIAL HARMS AND LIMITATIONS OF SCREENING

Overdiagnosis

Overdiagnosis is defined as the diagnosis of a cancer as a result of screening that would not have been diagnosed in the woman's lifetime had screening not taken place. This reflects

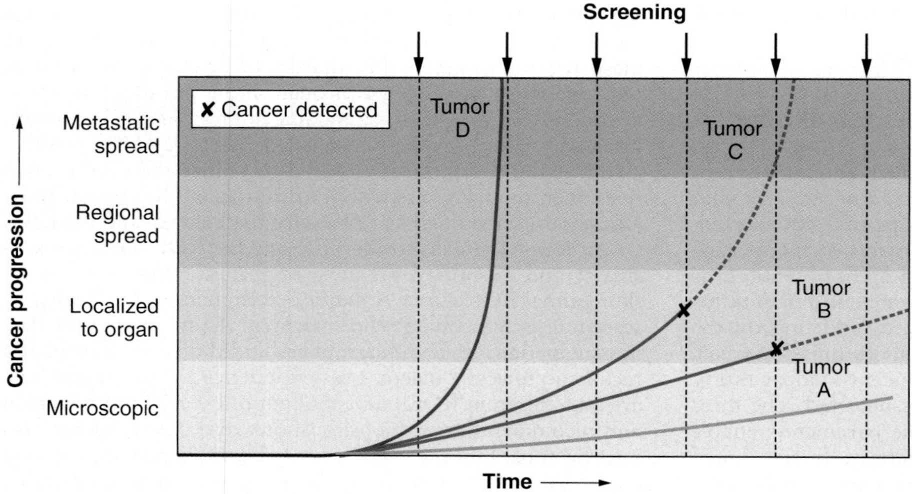

FIGURE 60.2 (From Esserman L, Shieh Y, Thompson I. Rethinking screening for breast cancer and prostate cancer. *JAMA* 2009;302(15):1685.)

diagnosing type A and possibly some type B disease as shown in Figure 60.1. This also may include the majority of *in situ* disease.

One regular criticism of screening in general is that it may lead to the surfacing of indolent disease that many have never come to clinical attention. Clearly, over the past 20 years, there has been an increase in the rate of detection of early stage disease, without the concomitant decrease in the detection of higher stage disease.[22] As women age, the types of cancers that develop are more likely to be of lower risk. Greater awareness has led to more early detection, both clinically and mammographically. It is possible that some of these cancers would not have come to clinical attention if not identified in screening.[23] It is not a problem if these lesions are identified. It is only a problem if they are not recognized as low-risk lesions at the time of diagnosis and inadvertently treated more aggressively than may be warranted. Fortunately, tools are now emerging that enable the classification of cancers as low risk, and these tools should enable testing of less aggressive treatments for women.[24–26]

Also combining the outcome data from both the U.K. National Health Service Breast Screening Programme (NHSBSP) and the Swedish two counties trials in women aged 50 to 69 years shows that high-grade cancers outnumber indolent cancers by a factor of 2 to 1, with an estimate of absolute benefit of screening of 8.8 and 5.7 breast cancer deaths prevented per 1,000 women screened for 20 years from age 50 from the Swedish and U.K. programs, respectively. Correspondingly, estimated overdiagnosed cases were 4.3 and 2.3 per 1,000 over 20 years.[27]

Detection of Ductal Carcinoma *In Situ*

Since the advent of mammographic screening the incidence of ductal carcinoma *in situ* (DCIS) has increased over 500%.[28,29] In spite of the detection and removal in over 60,000 cases per year, for almost a decade, there has not been a sustained drop in the incidence of invasive breast cancer. While there was a drop in cases from 2002 to 2005, this drop in incidence is most likely due to the precipitous drop in the use of hormone replacement therapy following the publication and reporting of the Women's Health Initiative study showing that hormone replacement therapy was associated with an increase in breast cancer and no improvement in cardiac mortality.[20] There is an ongoing debate about DCIS and its significance.[30] Although intervention clearly decreases the reoccurrence of DCIS and the incidence of invasive disease, there is no evidence of mortality benefit from early detection of DCIS, in spite of the fact that the standard of care includes lumpectomy, usually with radiation or mastectomy, as well as use of tamoxifen. Recent trends show that the rates of mastectomy have increased particularly for women with DCIS, and that the rates are as high as they are for women with stage I breast cancer.[31,32] As has been seen with invasive breast cancer, there is significant heterogeneity among DCIS lesions. High-grade lesions, if they are left to progress, are likely to do so in the first 5 years after diagnosis, whereas for low- and intermediate-grade lesions, the time period for spread may be 10 to 20 years. The risk of progression to invasive cancer for the low- to intermediate-grade lesions may be quite low after lumpectomy alone.[33] For DCIS, physicians must be more judicious with how they intervene and perhaps focus detection on the types of DCIS with shorter-term risk for invasion (e.g., high-grade DCIS). Certainly, a better understanding of the risks and the timing of progression of lower-grade *in situ* lesions may enable more judicious advising about biopsies for women with low-risk calcifications, which are likely to be low- to intermediate-grade DCIS at best.

In countries where the cancer to benign biopsy ratio is higher, the emphasis may already be on the detection of high grade DCIS. Data from the U.K. NHSBSP show that 87% of DCIS detected at screening is of high nuclear grade with necrosis and therefore more likely to be significant, compared with low-grade DCIS, which may take decades to progress to cancer and may be the precursor to more indolent disease. In the United States, where the cancer to benign biopsy ratios are lower, the rate of detection of lower-grade DCIS is much higher, in the range of 50% to 80% of DCIS detected.[34]

Biopsy Rates and Performance Measures

Biopsy rates are often cited as one of the potential harms of screening. Women who are screening annually for 10 years have a 50% chance of a recall and possible biopsy.[35] As has been noted under the section on the organization of screening, there are approaches to screening that can minimize the biopsy rates and improve the cancer to biopsy yield without losing sensitivity. So one of the critical opportunities to improve screening and avoid potential harms from screening is to adopt radiologist performance measures.[36] Unlike European countries, general radiologists interpret most mammography in the United States. There is significant variation in biopsy rates and cancer to biopsy yields across the United States and Europe. There is relatively poor performance from a proportion of the physicians, as identified in this recent study.[21] In population screening programs like that in the United Kingdom, biannual testing of radiologists is a mandatory requirement for screeners (PERFORMS). In a study conducted using the PERFORMS test in California,[20] only a third of the radiologists interpreting mammograms were considered high volume and dedicated mammographers. Their performance on the PERFORMS test (as shown in Fig. 60.3) was significantly higher for high volume, dedicated radiologists. Over time, the performance of radiologists in the United Kingdom has continued to improve.[14]

There is considerable variation in biopsy rates, as discussed above. Higher biopsy rates have consequences. There needs to be more concerted efforts to safely reduce the biopsy rates.[37]

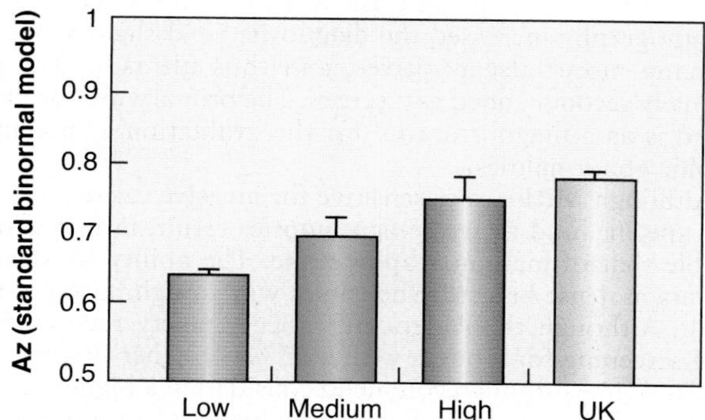

FIGURE 60.3 Sensitivity at specificity equals 0.90 with the use of the standard binormal model for different-volume mammography readers of the PERFORMS 2 test. Low-, medium-, and high-volume readers were from the United States. Low-volume radiologists read 100 or fewer mammograms per month. Medium-volume radiologists read 101 to 300 mammograms per month. High-volume radiologists read 301 or more mammograms per month. All U.K. radiologists were high-volume readers. Two Swedish radiologists, included as a high-volume control (data not shown), were high-volume readers who demonstrated a sensitivity of 88%. Bars represent the mean and standard error of the mean for the sensitivity at specificity equal to 0.90. (From Esserman L, Shieh Y, Thompson I. Rethinking Screening for Breast Cancer and Prostate Cancer. *JAMA* 2009;302(15):1685, with permission.)

Psychological Impact of Recall from Screening

It has long been known that there is substantial and measurable anxiety following recall from screening, which persists even after the workup has ruled out cancer. In the setting of a new diagnosis of cancer, one or more prior biopsies have been shown to be associated with a higher rate of mastectomy, presumably to avoid the anxiety of screening and biopsy. The use of MRI has also been associated with higher rates of mastectomy[38–40] and contralateral prophylactic mastectomy.[41,42] Therefore, clinicians need to be aware of the potential long-term consequences of biopsy and strive to improve specificity.[37]

HIGH-RISK SCREENING

Familial breast cancer represents a small, but important, group of breast cancers. Familial cancers are thought to affect 10% to 15% of women with breast cancer. Approximately half of those cancers are caused because of mutations in either of two genes that regulate DNA repair, *BRCA1* and *BRCA2* on chromosomes 17 and 13, respectively. Women with known mutations in BRCA have an estimated lifetime risk of developing breast cancer in the range of 45% to 85% as well as for ovarian cancer, in the range of 15% to 30%.[43]

MRI has been shown to have significantly higher sensitivity in mutation carriers compared to mammography and ultrasound.[44,45] The frequency of cancers detected in this population is indeed very high, 28.5 of 1,000. Women who have MRI compared to mammography screening had a smaller chance of lymph node involvement. The optimal combination of tests was found to be MRI, mammography, and clinical breast examination.[44] Given the aggressive nature of many of these tumors, especially *BRCA1* carriers who most commonly develop high-grade hormone receptor negative tumors, most high-risk programs recommend that annual mammogram and MRI examinations be staggered by 6 months to enable some type of imaging every 6 months. Women are also advised to be familiar with their breast self-examination and bring any new masses to clinical attention.

For high-risk women, an American College of Radiology Investigation Network (ACRIN) trial (6666)[46] showed that the use of ultrasound for high-risk women in combination with mammography increased the diagnostic yield slightly but led to many more false positives, and thus ultrasound is not routinely recommended as a screen. The primary use for ultrasound is as a diagnostic tool for the evaluation of mammographic abnormalities.

Although MRI is very sensitive for invasive cancer, it is not very specific, and many benign biopsies result, in fact almost double that of mammography alone. The ability to identify cancers in dense breast tissue comes with a high false-positive result. Although the American Cancer Society recommends MRI screening for women with a 25% or higher lifetime risk of cancer, the authors recommend considering a higher threshold or perhaps a risk model, like the Breast Cancer Screening Consortium model,[47] which integrates breast density into their models of assessing risk. One can also use the Gail model[48] and apply a multiplication factor based on underlying breast density, or use a threshold of 45% or greater lifetime risk for the basis for recommending MRI screening.[49]

WHAT HAS BIOLOGY TAUGHT US?

How does the improved understanding of biology help clinicians understand the impact of screening? Screening is complex because the biology of breast cancer is complex. There are likely some whose tumors are very slow growing, and early detection does not afford a benefit. There are some women who have aggressive disease that metastasizes very early and their systemic risk is not dependent as much on the size of the tumor detected but on the biology of the tumor that arises. As a result of the varying growth patterns, a proportion of women have their disease diagnosed years before it would have presented as a palpable finding. In Figure 60.1 only tumor B would likely show a good effect of screening. Depending on the age at which the woman with tumor A was screened, she may never die of the slow growing cancer detected in this screening, with subsequent possible overtreatment (length bias).

There is currently a lack of data about these slow growing, more indolent (idle) tumors that may never progress to disease that would kill a patient, yet there are risks of overtreatment.[23] There is emerging evidence that a higher fraction of screening detected cancers (may be as much as 67%) may have low-risk biology, half of which meet criteria for being ultralow risk. Fortunately, there are molecularly based tools that can help distinguish these cancers at the time of diagnosis. Effort and attention should be dedicated to documenting, in a large population of patients, the frequency of these tumors and whether molecular characterization can identify a subset of tumors that can be treated much less aggressively.[19]

Early detection will not be the answer to reducing mortality for all breast cancers. That does not mean that no one benefits from screening. Quite the contrary, some will benefit more than others, and it is important to focus on doing a better job of understanding who is at risk for what disease in order to tailor the screening.

Unfortunately, there are no tools to determine which populations are at risk for which types of cancers. However, some general comments can be made.

1. Certain populations may be more at risk for aggressive disease and at young age. It is known, for example, that African American women have double the risk of developing triple negative disease relative to the white population. Latina women also have a higher risk. Women with *BRCA1* mutations are principally at risk for triple negative tumors, which largely occur at young age.[50]
2. The fraction of biologically good risk tumors (as defined by low risk by the 70 gene prognostict structure) increases with age.[19] Young women are more likely to have aggressive biology if they develop cancer and can have high interval cancer rates. Although there are no good data to state that a more frequent interval is better in younger women, given that the disease is more likely to have a faster growth rate, it makes sense to use an annual screening interval if one chooses to screen.
3. Breast cancer risk generally increases with age. Look for women with high-risk features where rates indicate a three- to fivefold increase in the chance of getting breast cancer over other women of their age. The rate of cancer detection in the average woman in her 40s is 1 per 100. But in moderate- to high-risk women (nonmutating cancers) the risk is 5 to 8 per 1,000, which makes screening compelling even if a significant fraction (46%) would have interval cancers.[16]
4. Older women are more likely to have lower risk disease. As women age, and especially if they have competing comorbidities, the benefits of screening will be substantially reduced (disease may be just as treatable if detected clinically, and other health risks may be much more significant). Certainly, there is no need to look for DCIS in these patients, which confers risk over the next 5 to 20 years. So if older women are to be screened, the goal should be to

detect invasive cancers and not focus on or attempt to detect noninvasive disease.

The balance of screening interval is important and probably should also mirror the differences in biology and breast cancer incidence at different ages. Cancer is less common in premenopausal women, and mammography is less sensitive due to breast density, but grows more quickly usually due to hormonal influences, so an annual mammogram is likely the best option. This is likely to persist through menopause, after which time tumors tend to grow more slowly, and the interval can likely be extended without decreasing the benefit of screening significantly.

In the United States, guidelines published by the American Cancer Society recommend annual mammography at all ages from 40 years.[51] This is mirrored by the American College of Radiology and Society of Breast Imaging. The U.S. Preventive Services Task Force (PSTF) guidelines recommend starting routine mammography at 50 (and shared decision making for women aged 40 to 50 and over age 75 to weigh risks and benefits). The recommended screening interval of every 2 years is in line with the European model, where screening is population based and funded by the government and generally starts at age 49 to 50. European screening is based on both effectiveness and cost-effectiveness. In the United Kingdom screening is limited to 3 years based on cost limitations.

CONCLUSION AND CONSIDERATIONS FOR SCREENING

1. The degree of benefit for an individual woman will vary based on age and risk. For women less than age 50, breast cancer is less common (1 in 1,000), unless she has moderate or high risk (5 to 7 per 1,000),[45] the frequency of call backs as high or higher, and the chance of discovery of premalignant conditions is high, women and physicians should understand the risks and benefits of screening in their 40s and proceed with screening where it is an appropriate informed decision.
2. Screening should be performed once every 2 years for women aged 50 to 75. Screening over the age of 75 should again be individualized and based on health. For older women, the target of screening should be invasive cancers and not *in situ* disease.
3. For women in their 40s, if screening is to be pursued, annual screening is probably the proper interval, given that faster growing tumors are more common in younger women.
4. Finally, screening is ideally performed in a population-based manner with data on performance and outcomes captured as a routine by product of care and used to support learning and quality improvement.

References

1. Tabár L, Vitak B, Chen HH, et al. Beyond randomized controlled trials: organized mammographic screening substantially reduces breast carcinoma mortality. *Cancer* 2001;91(9):1724.
2. Tabár L, Vitak B, Chen HH, et al. The Swedish two-county trial twenty years later. Updated mortality results and new insights from long-term follow-up. *Radiol Clin North Am* 2000;38(4):625.
3. Smith RA, Duffy SW, Gabe R, et al. The randomized trials of breast cancer screening: what have we learned? *Radiol Clin North Am* 2004;42(5):793.
4. Tabár L, Fagerberg G, Duffy SW, et al. Update of the Swedish two-county program of mammographic screening for breast cancer. *Radiol Clin North Am* 1992;30(1):187.
5. Nyström L, Andersson I, Bjurstam N, et al. Long-term effects of mammography screening: updated overview of the Swedish randomised trials. *Lancet* 2002;359(9310):909.
6. Nelson HD, Tyne K, Naik A, et al., Screening for breast cancer: an update for the U.S. Preventive Services Task Force. *Ann Intern Med* 2009;151(10):727.
7. Early Breast Cancer Trialists' Collaborative Group. Effects of chemotherapy and hormonal therapy for early breast cancer on recurrence and 15-year survival: an overview of the randomised trials. *Lancet* 2005;365(9472):1687.
8. Hayes DF, Thor AD, Dressler LG, et al. HER2 and response to paclitaxel in node-positive breast cancer. *N Engl J Med* 2007;357(15):1496.
9. Romond EH, Perez EA, Bryant J, et al. Trastuzumab plus adjuvant chemotherapy for operable HER2-positive breast cancer. *N Engl J Med* 2005;353(16):1673.
10. Kalager M, Zelen M, Langmark F, et al. Effect of screening mammography on breast-cancer mortality in Norway. *N Engl J Med* 2010;363(13):1203.
11. Burnside E, Belkora J, Esserman L. The impact of alternative practices on the cost and quality of mammographic screening in the United States. *Clin Breast Cancer* 2001;2(2):145.
12. Joy JE, Penhoet EE, Petitti DB, eds. *Saving women's lives. Strategies for improving breast cancer detection and diagnosis*. Washington, DC: National Academies Press, 2005.
13. National Health Service Breast Screening Programme. Quality assurance guidelines for breast cancer screening radiology. Sheffield: NHSBSP, 2005.
14. Smith-Bindman R, Chu PW, Miglioretti DL, et al. Comparison of screening mammography in the United States and the United Kingdom. *JAMA* 2003;290(16):2129.
15. Sickles EA, Miglioretti DL, Ballard-Barbash R, et al. Performance benchmarks for diagnostic mammography. *Radiology* 2005;235(3):775.
16. Burnside ES, Park JM, Fine JP, Sisnay GA. The use of batch reading to improve the performance of screening mammography. *AJR Am J Roentgenol* 2005;185(3):790.
17. Esserman L, Cowley H, Eberle C, et al. Improving the accuracy of mammography: volume and outcome relationships. *J Natl Cancer Inst* 2002;94(5):369.
18. Bordás P, Jonsson H, Nystöm L, Lenner P. Interval cancer incidence and episode sensitivity in the Norrbotten Mammography Screening Programme, Sweden. *J Med Screen* 2009;16(1):39.
19. Shieh Y, Esserman L, Rutgers EJ, et al. *Effect of screening on the detection of good and poor prognosis breast cancers*. Chicago: American Society of Clinical Oncology, 2010.
20. Lin C, Moore D, DeMichele A, et al. Detection of locally advanced breast cancer in the I-SPY TRIAL (CALGB 150007/150012, ACRIN 6657) in the interval between routine screening. Orlando, FL: American Society Clinical Oncology, 2009.
21. Mandelblatt JS, Cronin KA, Bailey S, et al. Effects of mammography screening under different screening schedules: model estimates of potential benefits and harms. *Ann Intern Med* 2009;151(10):738.
22. Esserman L, Shieh Y, Thompson I. Rethinking screening for breast cancer and prostate cancer. *JAMA* 2009;302(15):1685.
23. Welch HG, Black WC. Overdiagnosis in cancer. *J Natl Cancer Inst* 2010;102:605.
24. Knauer M, Mook S, Rutgers EJ, et al. The predictive value of the 70-gene signature for adjuvant chemotherapy in early breast cancer. *Breast Cancer Res Treat* 2010;120(3):655.
25. Mook S, Knauer M, Bueno-de-Mesquita JM, et al. Metastatic potential of T1 breast cancer can be predicted by the 70-gene MammaPrint signature. *Ann Surg Oncol* 2010;17(5):1406.
26. Paik S, Shak S, Tang G, et al. A multigene assay to predict recurrence of tamoxifen-treated, node-negative breast cancer. *N Engl J Med* 2004;351(27):2817.
27. Duffy SW, Tabar L, Olsen AH, et al. Absolute numbers of lives saved and overdiagnosis in breast cancer screening, from a randomized trial and from the Breast Screening Programme in England. *J Med Screen* 2010;17(1):25.
28. Ernster VL, Ballard-Barbash R, Barlow WE, et al. Detection of ductal carcinoma in situ in women undergoing screening mammography. *J Natl Cancer Inst* 2002;94(20):1546.
29. Ernster VL, Barclay J, Kerlikowske K, Grady D, Henderson C. Incidence of and treatment for ductal carcinoma in situ of the breast. *JAMA* 1996;275(12):913.
30. Evans AJ, Pinder SE, Ellis IO, Wilson AR. Screen detected ductal carcinoma in situ (DCIS): overdiagnosis or an obligate precursor of invasive disease? *J Med Screen* 2001;8(3):149.
31. Gomez SL, Lichtensztajn D, Kurian AW, et al. Increasing mastectomy rates for early-stage breast cancer? Population-based trends from California. *J Clin Oncol* 2010;28(10):e155; author reply e158.
32. Tuttle TM, Jarosek S, Habermann EB, et al. Increasing rates of contralateral prophylactic mastectomy among patients with ductal carcinoma in situ. *J Clin Oncol* 2009;27(9):1362.
33. Hughes LL, Wang M, Page DL, et al. Local excision alone without irradiation for ductal carcinoma in situ of the breast: a trial of the Eastern Cooperative Oncology Group. *J Clin Oncol* 2009;27(32):5319.

34. Li CI, Daling JR, Malone KE. Age-specific incidence rates of in situ breast carcinomas by histologic type, 1980 to 2001. *Cancer Epidemiol Biomark Prev* 2005;14(4):1008.
35. Elmore JG, Barton MB, Moceri VM, et al. Ten-year risk of false positive screening mammograms and clinical breast examinations. *N Engl J Med* 1998;338(16):1089.
36. Carney PA, Sickles EA, Monsees BS, et al. Identifying minimally acceptable interpretive performance criteria for screening mammography. *Radiology* 2010;255(2):354.
37. Esserman L, Thompson I. Solving the overdiagnosis dilemma. *J Natl Cancer Inst* 2010;102(9):582.
38. McGuire KP, Santillan AA, Kaur P, et al. Are mastectomies on the rise? A 13-year trend analysis of the selection of mastectomy versus breast conservation therapy in 5865 patients. *Ann Surg Oncol* 2009;16(10):2682.
39. Turnbull L, Brown S, Harvey I, et al. Comparative effectiveness of MRI in breast cancer (COMICE) trial: a randomised controlled trial. *Lancet* 2010;375(9714):563.
40. Katipamula R, Degim AC, Hoskin T, et al. Trends in mastectomy rates at the Mayo Clinic Rochester: effect of surgical year and preoperative magnetic resonance imaging. *J Clin Oncol* 2009;27(25):4082.
41. Sorbero ME, Dick AW, Beckjord EB, Ahrendt G. Diagnostic breast magnetic resonance imaging and contralateral prophylactic mastectomy. *Ann Surg Oncol* 2009;16(6):1597.
42. Tuttle TM. Magnetic resonance imaging and contralateral prophylactic mastectomy: the "no mas" effect? *Ann Surg Oncol* 2009;16(6):1461.
43. Brose MS, Rebbeck TR, Catzone KA, et al. Cancer risk estimates for BRCA1 mutation carriers identified in a risk evaluation program. *J Natl Cancer Inst* 2002;94(18):1365.
44. Warner E, Plewes DB, Hill KA, et al. Surveillance of BRCA1 and BRCA2 mutation carriers with magnetic resonance imaging, ultrasound, mammography, and clinical breast examination. *JAMA* 2004;292(11):1317.
45. Kriege M, Brekelmans CT, Boetes C, et al. Efficacy of MRI and mammography for breast-cancer screening in women with a familial or genetic predisposition. *N Engl J Med* 2004;351(5):427.
46. Berg WA, Blume JD, Cormack JB, et al. Combined screening with ultrasound and mammography vs mammography alone in women at elevated risk of breast cancer. *JAMA* 2008;299(18):2151.
47. Barlow WE, White E, Ballard-Barbarash R, et al. Prospective breast cancer risk prediction model for women undergoing screening mammography. *J Natl Cancer Inst* 2006;98(17):1204.
48. Cummings S, Ziv E, Kerlikowske K. Mammographic breast density and the Gail model for breast cancer risk prediction in a screening population. *Breast Cancer Res Treat* 2005;94:115.
49. Zakhireh J, Gomez R, Esserman L. Converting evidence to practice: a guide for the clinical application of MRI for the screening and management of breast cancer. *Eur J Cancer* 2008;44(18):2742.
50. Chlebowski RT, Chen Z, Anderson GL, et al. Ethnicity and breast cancer: factors influencing differences in incidence and outcome. *J Natl Cancer Inst* 2005;97(6):439.
51. Smith RA, Cokkinides V, Eyre HJ. American Cancer Society guidelines for breast cancer screening: update 2003. *CA Cancer J Clin* 2003;53(3):141.

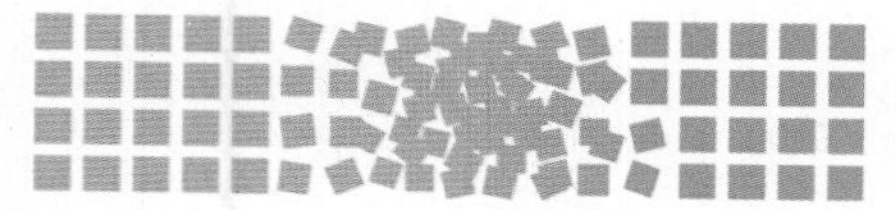

CHAPTER 61 SCREENING FOR PROSTATE CANCER

PETER C. ALBERTSEN

Few cancers generate as much controversy surrounding screening, diagnosis, and treatment as prostate cancer. This controversy has escalated ever since prostate-specific antigen (PSA) was introduced as a prostate cancer tumor marker in the United States in 1986 and was rapidly embraced by clinicians as a test to screen for this disease.[1] As of 2009 investigators believe that in the United States over 55% of men age 50 years and older are undergoing annual PSA testing and that over 75% have been tested at least once.[2,3] From 1977 to 2005 the lifetime risk of prostate cancer diagnosis in the United States increased from 7.3% to 17%.[4,5] During this same period the lifetime risk of dying from prostate cancer fell from 3.0% to 2.4%.

Prostate cancer is a major public health problem affecting 679,000 men and causing 221,000 deaths annually worldwide.[6] As a consequence of testing for PSA, the incidence of prostate cancer in the United States is now 50% higher than that seen in the early 1980s and is now the highest rate in the world.[7] Mortality from prostate cancer peaked in the United States in 1994 at almost 35,000 deaths and has since declined. In 2009, over 192,000 men were diagnosed with prostate cancer and over 27,000 men died from this disease (Figs. 61.1 and 61.2).[8]

This chapter reviews the evidence surrounding the benefits and harms of screening for prostate cancer using PSA testing.

IS PROSTATE CANCER A SUITABLE DISEASE FOR SCREENING?

The medical community has advocated early detection and treatment for prostate cancer for over a century. As early as 1905, Hugh Hampton Young suggested that a careful digital rectal examination could identify changes in prostate gland texture that could lead to the early diagnosis of cancer and appropriate intervention.[9] Unfortunately, several issues confound the belief that early diagnosis prevents death from this disease.

The natural history of prostate cancer is extraordinarily variable. Some men have aggressive disease that may benefit from early detection and intervention, but many others harbor cancers that grow slowly and never progress to clinical significance. Several key studies have helped shape our understanding of the natural history of prostate cancer progression. Between 1989 and 2004, Johansson et al. published a series of four articles that documented the outcomes of untreated prostate cancer in a population-based cohort of patients diagnosed with prostate cancer in Sweden.[10–13] No screening for prostate cancer took place during the period when this study population of 648 consecutive cases was assembled. Initially the authors found relatively low 5- and 10-year mortality rates among men with clinically localized disease and challenged the use of aggressive initial treatment for all patients with low-grade early stage prostate cancer. Long-term follow-up of the study cohort, however, suggested a rising mortality rate from prostate cancer for those men surviving 15 to 20 years following diagnosis.

In 1994 Chodak et al.[14] published a report describing the results of conservative management of clinically localized prostate cancer. Unlike the Johannson report, this study consisted of a pooled analysis of 828 case records from six nonrandomized studies published during the decade preceding the report. Patients with poorly differentiated cancers had a significantly lower cancer-specific survival rate (34%) when compared with men who had well or moderately differentiated cancers (87%). In addition, men with poorly differentiated tumors were much more likely to develop metastases when compared to men who were diagnosed with well-differentiated disease.

In 1998 and 2005, Albertsen et al.[15,16] reported long-term outcomes of a competing risk analysis of 767 men diagnosed between 1971 and 1984 who were managed expectantly for clinically localized prostate cancer. The results of this study are presented in Figure 61.3. Few men (4% to 7%) with Gleason 2 to 4 tumors identified by prostate biopsy had progression leading to death from prostate cancer within 20 years of diagnosis. Men with Gleason 5 and 6 tumors identified by prostate biopsy experienced a somewhat higher risk of death from prostate cancer when managed expectantly (6% to 11% and 18% to 30%, respectively). Men with Gleason scores 7 and 8 to 10 tumors identified by prostate biopsy experienced a very high rate of death from prostate cancer regardless of their age at diagnosis (42% to 70% and 60% to 87%, respectively). Very few of these men of any age survived more than 15 years.

These studies reveal that there is a pool of men with high grade disease (Gleason score ≥7) that face a substantial risk of death from prostate cancer in the absence of treatment. These are the men who could potentially benefit from prostate cancer screening. These studies also reveal that many men, especially older men with low-grade disease (Gleason score ≤6), have a relatively low risk of disease progression. These men are unlikely to benefit from PSA testing but would suffer harm associated with screening and treatment.

Prostate cancer is also unique in that many men harbor multiple foci of indolent disease. Autopsy studies have revealed a high prevalence of prostate cancer even among men under age 50.[17] Estimates suggest that anywhere from 14% to 70% of men in their 60s and 31% to 83% of men in their 70s have evidence of prostate cancer. Results from the Prostate Cancer Prevention Trial published in 2003 confirmed the high prevalence of disease.[18] Researchers designing the trial estimated the prevalence of prostate cancer to be 6% and powered the trial to detect a 25% reduction in incidence. After 7 years of follow-up, prostate cancer was detected in 24.4% of men in the control arm and 18.4% in the treatment arm. These substantially higher

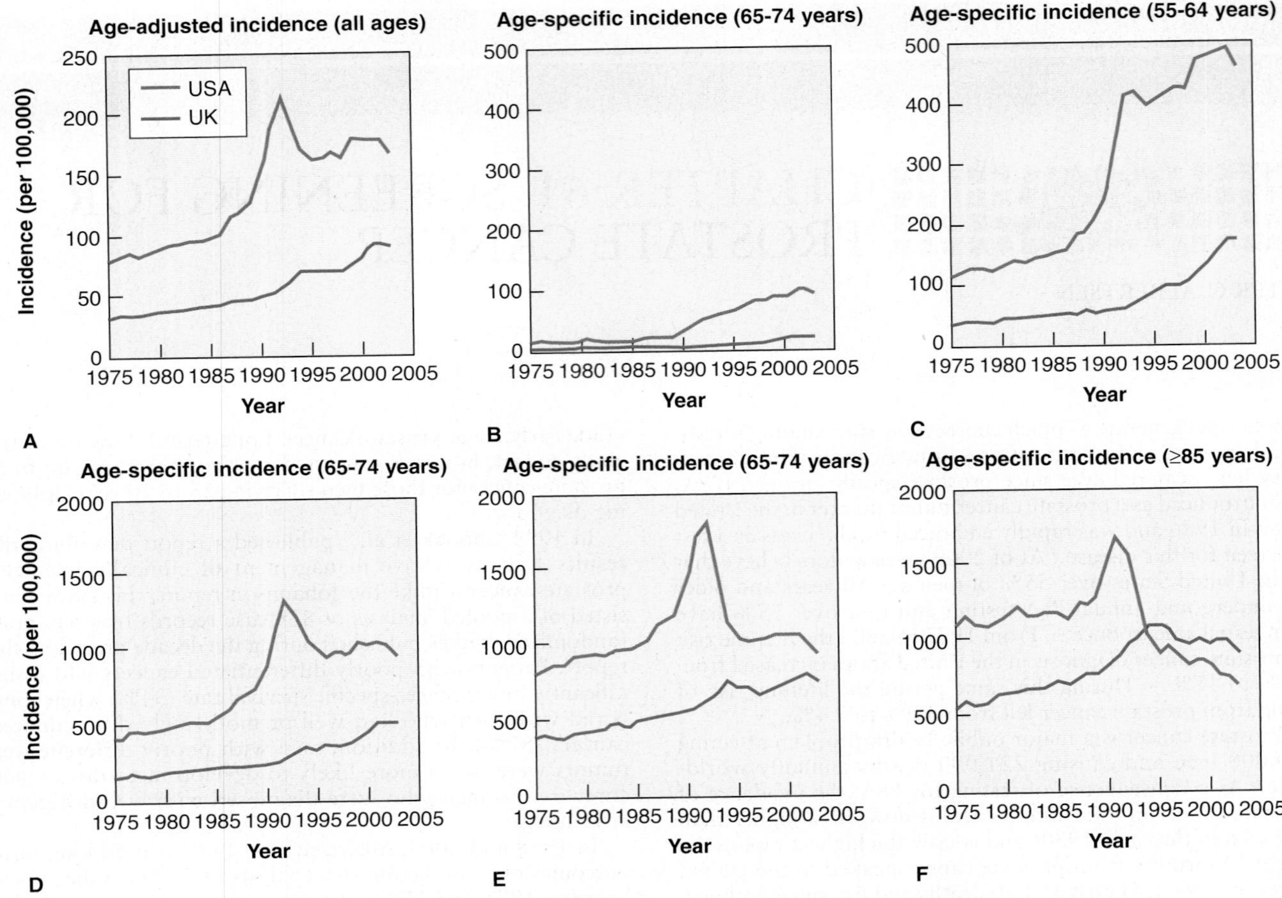

FIGURE 61.1 U.S. and U.K. prostate cancer incidence rates, by age group 1975 to 2003. (From ref 36.)

rates were the result of a decision to biopsy as many men as possible in each arm regardless of their clinical findings or PSA levels. The trial demonstrated that clinically significant prostate cancers were present even among men with serum PSA values less than 4.0 ng/mL. Equally important was the observation that most of the cancers detected were low grade Gleason score 3 + 3 = 6 tumors. Many of these incidental cancers would never have been discovered if men had not undergone a transrectal ultrasound and biopsy.

Understanding the threat posed by prostate cancer has also been confounded by pathologists' changing interpretation of the Gleason scoring system. When Gleason originally developed his scoring system, based on low power analysis of glandular architecture, men were commonly diagnosed with prostate cancer following a transurethral resection, an open prostatectomy performed to treat obstructive urinary symptoms, or a needle biopsy with an 18-gauge needle.[19] Before 2000 most pathologists used all five patterns described by Gleason. Since then they have become increasingly hesitant to grade prostate cancers any lower than Gleason score 3 + 3. This stems from a report by Epstein who commented that Gleason score assignments following radical prostatectomy were frequently higher for those men who had biopsies assigned Gleason scores less than 6.[20] Thus many low grade tumors previously recorded as Gleason score 2 to 5 are now classified as Gleason score 6 and many Gleason score 6 tumors are now classified as Gleason score 7. Reclassification during the past two decades has been so extensive that clinical outcomes are significantly improved if historical classifications are replaced by contemporary classifications.[21] Death from prostate cancer appears to be rare among men with contemporary low and moderate grade T1c prostate cancers during the first 10 years following diagnosis.[22]

IS TREATMENT FOR PROSTATE CANCER EFFECTIVE?

The goal of screening is to lengthen life or prevent morbidity through early detection. For screening to be effective, treatment must be available that alters disease outcomes. Mortality from prostate cancer has been falling in both the United States and the United Kingdom since the early 1990s.[23] These trends can be explained by several factors, including earlier detection and treatment, improved treatment, changes in exposure to risk factors, other environmental factors such as the growing use of statins, or changes in the attribution of cause of death.[23,24] Two studies from Sweden have recently provided important data concerning the efficacy of two common therapies used to treat localized prostate cancer: surgery and radiation.

In 2008, Bill-Axelson et al.[25] published findings from an 11-year follow-up of the Scandinavian Prostate Cancer Group-4 (SPC-4) randomized trial comparing surgery against watchful waiting for men presenting with clinically localized prostate cancer. They recruited 695 men between 1989 and 1999 to participate in the study: half were randomized to receive a radical prostatectomy, the other half were followed. Most of the men included in the trial presented with clinically localized disease, only 12% were identified on the basis of PSA testing. Approximately 60% of the patients randomized had tumors with Gleason scores 6 or less, 23% had Gleason 7, 5% had Gleason 8 or higher, and 12% had tumors with unknown scores. At 12 years, 12.5% of the

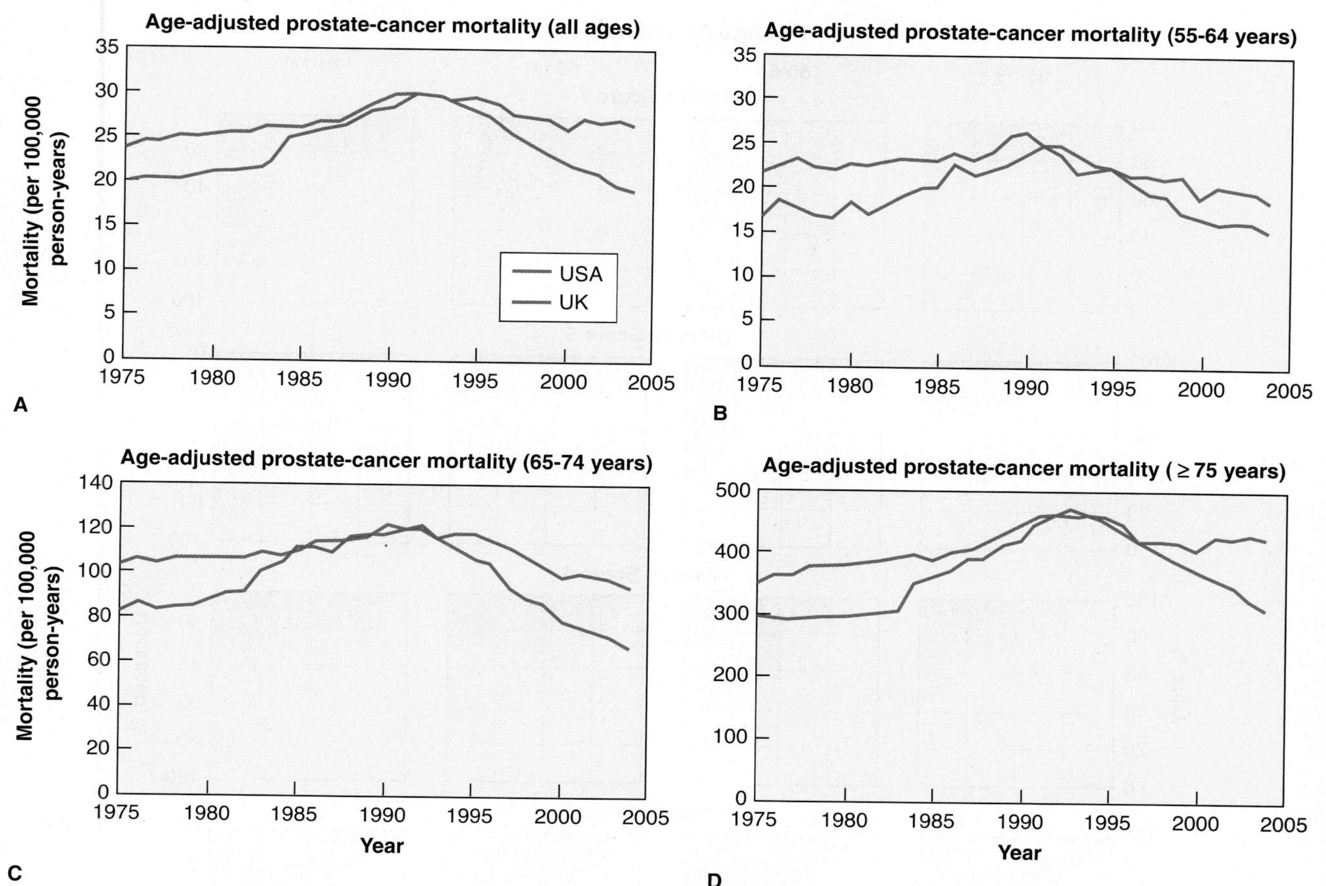

FIGURE 61.2 U.S. and U.K. prostate cancer mortality rates, by age group 1975 to 2004. (From ref 36.)

surgery group and 17.9% of the watchful waiting group had died of prostate cancer. Men undergoing surgery had a relative risk reduction of 0.65 from dying from prostate cancer. Interestingly, there was no significant difference in overall survival between the surgical group and the observation group. After a median follow-up of 10.8 years, approximately 42% of the patients had died in each arm (137 in the surgery group and 156 in the watchful waiting group, $p = .09$).

A careful subset analysis of the data revealed several interesting findings. Radical prostatectomy reduced the risk of prostate cancer mortality and the risk of metastases, but this benefit was limited to the first decade following treatment. The cumulative incidence of death from prostate cancer remained constant beyond 9 years of follow-up, and the cumulative incidence of metastases remained constant after 7 years. Furthermore, only patients younger than age 65 years appeared to benefit from the intervention. For men aged 65 years and older, there was no discernible difference between the groups in any outcome.

How would these results have differed if the majority of patients had been identified on the basis of PSA testing? Because of the lead time introduced by PSA testing, the relative reduction in risk of death following radical prostatectomy might be similar or larger than documented in the SPC-4 study, but the absolute reduction would likely be smaller. In the SPC-4 study the absolute risk reduction was 5.4%, implying that 19 men needed to be treated to avert one prostate cancer death after 12 years of follow-up. If the study had included a substantial population of men identified by PSA testing, the number needed to treat to prevent one cancer death would have been considerably higher.

In 2009, Widmark et al.[26] published findings from the Scandinavian Prostate Cancer Group-7 (SPC-7) study that compared endocrine treatment for men with locally advanced prostate cancer with or without radiotherapy. This studied accrued 875 patients between 1996 and 2002 and randomized them to a protocol of 3 months of total androgen blockade followed by continuous flutamide therapy either with or without radiation therapy. Of note, over three quarters of the patients had locally advanced T3 disease and only 16 patients (2%) had disease identified by PSA testing.

After 8 years of follow-up the 10-year prostate cancer mortality rate was 23.9% in the endocrine alone group and 11.9% in the endocrine plus radiation therapy group for a relative risk reduction of 0.44. The overall mortality rate also favored combined therapy. At 10 years the cumulative mortality was 39.4% in the endocrine alone group and 29.6% in the endocrine plus radiation therapy group ($p = .004$)

How would these results have differed if the majority of patients had been identified on the basis of PSA testing? Once again because of the effect of lead time introduced by PSA testing, very few patients would have advanced localized disease. As a result the absolute risk reduction of 12% at 10 years would likely be substantially less. In the SPC-7 study, eight men needed to be treated to avert one prostate cancer death after 10 years of follow-up. Changing the population to reflect contemporary patients identified by PSA testing would increase this number substantially. The SPC-4 study and the SPC-7 study clearly show that surgery and radiation can lower prostate cancer mortality. The impact appears to be greatest when applied to men with advanced localized disease. How large an impact these treatments would have on men identified with prostate cancer as a consequence of PSA testing is less clear.

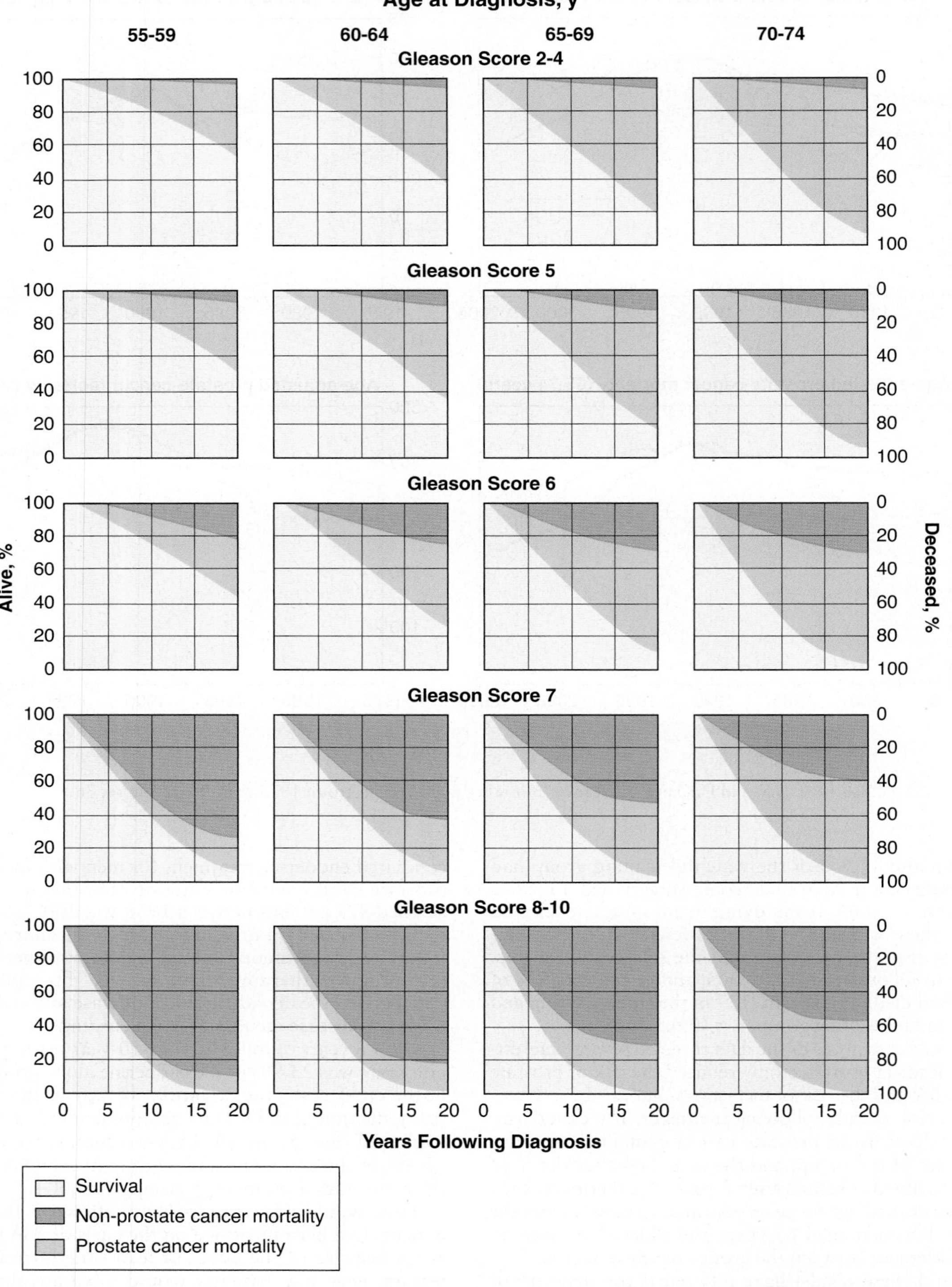

FIGURE 61.3 Survival and cumulative mortality from prostate cancer and other causes up to 20 years after diagnosis, stratified by age at diagnosis and Gleason score. (From ref. 16.)

IS PROSTATE-SPECIFIC ANTIGEN AN EFFECTIVE SCREENING TEST?

PSA is a glycoprotein produced almost exclusively by the epithelial component of the prostate gland. Men with prostate diseases may have high serum PSA levels because of enhanced production of PSA or from architectural distortions in the gland that allow PSA greater access to the bloodstream. Several conditions can produce a rise in serum PSA levels. These include benign prostatic enlargement, inflammation, urethral or prostatic trauma, and the presence of prostate cancer. Unfortunately, PSA screening cannot differentiate between benign conditions and indolent and lethal prostate cancer. Androgen deprivation will lower PSA levels dramatically, while 5-alpha reductase inhibitors will lower PSA levels by approximately 50% regardless of the dose.[27] A prostate biopsy will usually cause a substantial increase in PSA levels.

Several issues confound the ability of PSA testing to identify lethal prostate cancers. PSA values may fluctuate for physiologic reasons, including a recent ejaculation. In a retrospective analysis of an unscreened population of 972 men with a median age of 62 years, Eastham et al.[28] demonstrated substantial year-to-year variation in PSA levels. They encouraged patients to repeat minimally elevated PSA values before considering prostate ultrasound and biopsy. As many as 21% of PSA values over 4.0 ng/mL will return to normal during a 1-year follow-up.

Repeated PSA testing is imprecise. Laboratory variability can range from 20% to 25% depending on the type of standardization used. PSA assays are not interchangeable and, therefore, the same assay should be used for longitudinal monitoring.[29] An abnormal PSA value should be confirmed before recommending a prostate biopsy.

Gann et al.[30] assessed the relationship between PSA levels in baseline serum samples and the subsequent development of clinically significant prostate cancer in a case control analysis of men participating in the Physician's Health Study. They found that at a cutoff point of 4.0 ng/mL, testing for PSA had a sensitivity of 46% for identifying prostate cancer that was clinically important within the next 10 years and a sensitivity of 56% to detect prostate cancer diagnosed clinically within 2 years. The specificity in this population of 63-year-old men was 91%. In the European Randomized Study of Screening for prostate cancer, the sensitivity of PSA to detect prostate cancer was 71%, with an average positive predictive value of 24%.

Researchers have explored various forms of PSA that can be detected in the circulation.[31] PSA exists both free and in complexes with macromolecules. For reasons that are uncertain, men with prostate cancer have a lower percentage of circulating free PSA than men with benign prostate hypertrophy. Unfortunately, these tests are also relatively poor discriminators of men with clinically significant prostate cancer.

RECENT EVIDENCE FROM RANDOMIZED TRIALS

Results from two long awaited randomized trials on PSA screening were published in 2009: the Prostate, Lung, Colorectal and Ovarian (PLCO) Cancer Screening Trial conducted by the National Cancer Institute and the European Randomized Study of Screening for Prostate Cancer (ERSPC) supported by grants from Europe Against Cancer and multiple European agencies and health authorities.[32,33] Both trials have strengths and weaknesses. The PLCO trial followed a common protocol conducted at ten study centers located within the United States. The ERSPC study was a collection of seven PSA screening trials that employed different study designs, screening tests, screening intervals, and different ages of patient at entry and choices of controls. Both of these trials are ongoing. The results reported last spring represent interim analyses. Several more years of follow-up will be needed before the full impact of PSA testing can be determined.

The PLCO trial was initiated in 1993 and recruited 76,693 men at ten study centers within the United States before closing to accrual in 2001. Men were randomly assigned to receive annual PSA tests for 6 years and digital rectal examinations for 4 years (n = 38,343) or were assigned to usual care (n = 38,350). Study coordinators notified primary caregivers whenever a study participant was found to have a PSA greater than or equal to the threshold of 4.0 ng/mL.

Compliance with the screening protocol was 85% for PSA testing and 86% for digital rectal examination. Unfortunately, the rate of PSA testing in the control arm was 40% in the first year and increased to 52% by the sixth year. Compliance was monitored through random surveys. After 7 to 10 years of follow-up the rate of death from prostate cancer was very low in both groups and did not differ significantly between the two study groups.

The report of the ERSPC trial represents a combined analysis of seven separate PSA screening trials conducted from 1991 to 2003 in the Netherlands, Belgium, Sweden, Finland, Italy, Spain, and Switzerland. All study centers included a core age group of men aged 55 to 69 years old who became the subject of the report (n = 162,387). The recruitment and randomization procedures differed among countries. In Finland, Sweden, and Italy, trial subjects were identified from population registries and underwent randomization before written informed consent was provided. In the Netherlands, Belgium, Switzerland, and Spain, the target population was identified from population lists, but only those who agreed to participate were randomized. Finland contributed about 50% of the study subjects (n = 80,379) and the Netherlands about 20% (n = 34,833).

The screening protocol used in the trials varied both by site and by calendar year. In the early 1990s the Dutch and Belgium sites relied on a combination of digital rectal examination, transrectal ultrasonography, and PSA tests. Later, most centers relied on a PSA test alone except in Finland and Italy where rectal examinations were used to identify men for biopsy who had marginally normal values (i.e., PSA values between 2.5 and 3.9 ng/mL). Initially most sites used a cutoff point of 4.0 ng/mL, but this was lowered to 3.0 ng/mL as the study progressed. Most countries used a 4-year screening interval. Sweden screened men every 2 years, and Belgium screened men every 4 to 7 years because of funding problems. Unlike the PLCO trial, all of the screening protocols mandated a subsequent transrectal ultrasound and biopsy. Most centers used a sextant biopsy protocol, but this was later amended in several centers to include 10 to 12 cores.

After a median follow-up of 9 years, the cumulative incidence of prostate cancer was 8.2% in the screening group and 4.8% in the control group. The rate ratio for death from prostate cancer in the screening group as compared to the control group was 0.80 (p = .04). The absolute risk difference was 0.71 deaths per 1,000 men. This means that one prostate cancer death was averted for every 1,410 men screened and 48 prostate cancers diagnosed.

The PLCO trial was designed to test the public health impact of annual PSA testing as compared to standard of care in practice at the inception of the study. As a consequence it was a trial comparing more thoroughly screened men with less thoroughly screened men in an environment that allowed men to choose how they would deal with a positive study. The trial was biased in favor of healthy men because it relied on recruits to participate in the trial. The strength of the trial was the common study protocol. The primary weakness was its power. As the rate of contamination in the control arm increased during the study, the power to detect a difference in mortality decreased. Although significantly more cancers were found in the screening arm, after 7 years of follow-up, only 50 deaths had occurred in the screening arm and 44 deaths occurred in the control arm (rate ratio 1.13; 95% CI [confidence interval], 0.75 to 1.70). The wide confidence interval suggests that it will be many more years before the study might have the power to identify a difference.

The lack of a common design and protocol makes the ERSPC report more difficult to interpret. The trials in Finland, Sweden, and Italy were designed as population-based effectiveness trials, while the other centers were designed as efficacy trials. The populations recruited in the former centers are less biased in favor of healthy patients. As a consequence they test whether PSA testing is an effective public health initiative.

The other centers test whether PSA testing and subsequent biopsy lowers prostate cancer mortality in a group of healthier volunteer patients. The strength of the ERSPC analysis is its much greater power, the weakness stems from the variable protocols used. Unfortunately, this is the third interim analysis of the ERSPC data. Results from the 2009 analysis were marginally significant (95% CI, 0.65 to 0.98). This study will require several more years to have the power to detect a definitive difference in the final analysis. Many more deaths may be required if this study is to have sufficient statistical significance in subsequent analyses.

Unfortunately, both of these analyses have failed to resolve the controversy surrounding the benefit of PSA testing. Insufficient time has elapsed to determine whether men aged 55 to 74 years benefit from PSA screening. Neither of these studies provides support for PSA testing for those men who have a life expectancy of 10 years or less. Both trials have issues related to statistical power that may prevent making a conclusive statement 5 to 10 years from now. Both studies suggest that PSA testing leads to a substantial increase in prostate cancer incidence and treatment. In the ERSPC trials, men in the screened groups were 2.77 times more likely to undergo a radical prostatectomy and twice as likely to receive radiation when compared to men in the control groups.

ARE THERE SUBSTANTIAL RISKS ASSOCIATED WITH PROSTATE-SPECIFIC ANTIGEN SCREENING?

Widespread testing for PSA has changed the clinical characteristics of men presenting with localized disease. Since the introduction of PSA screening, more than 1 million additional men have been diagnosed with this disease in the United States. Prior to PSA testing it was rare to diagnose prostate cancer before age 55 years. While some men now present in their late 40s and early 50s, there has been a dramatic increase in the number of men diagnosed with prostate cancer in their late 50s and early 60s.[34] Compared to 1986, the relative incidence of prostate cancer is 1.91 times greater among men aged 60 to 69 years, 3.64 times greater among men aged 50 to 59 years, and 7.23 times greater among men younger than 50 years. Draisma et al.[35] estimate that PSA testing has advanced the date of diagnosis by approximately 12.3 years for men aged 55 years and by 6.0 years for men aged 75 years.

Testing for PSA is still relatively uncommon in the United Kingdom. Long-term age-adjusted and age-specific prostate cancer incidence rate trends were similar in the United States and the United Kingdom from 1975 to 2003, although the rates in the United States were consistently higher by a factor of 2.5.[36] Because of PSA testing prostate cancer was diagnosed 8.2 times more frequently in the United States when compared to the United Kingdom for men aged 45 to 54 years and 6.7 times more frequently for men aged 55 to 64 years (Figs. 61.1 and 61.2).

Most men identified through screening are not destined to die of their prostate cancer and therefore do not benefit from screening. Draisma et al.[35] estimate that overdiagnosis can be as high as 50%. In the ERSPC trial and in the finasteride chemoprevention trial most men in the screening group were diagnosed with Gleason 2 to 6 cancers. Many of these lesions are indolent and do not require treatment. Unfortunately, no molecular or pathologic markers exist that can discriminate clinically significant disease from indolent disease. Therefore, a man with newly diagnosed disease faces the uncomfortable dilemma of choosing between aggressive interventions or monitoring his disease on an active surveillance program. This is not an issue for men with Gleason 7 to 10 cancers (approximately 28% of the men in the ERSPC trial), but treatments are less effective in men with high-grade prostate cancer, and many of these men will experience a rising PSA value after treatment and require additional intervention including androgen deprivation therapy.

Aggressive treatment of localized disease comes at a price. The side effects of surgery and radiation therapy are well known and often include problems with urinary function, bowel function, and especially sexual function. Sanda et al.[37] recently reported results from surveys completed by 1,201 men and 625 spouses concerning quality of life and satisfaction with outcomes following either surgery or radiation to treat localized prostate cancer during the period 2003 to 2006. Long-term incontinence persists in 2% to 22% of patients depending upon the definition of incontinence used and the age of the patient. Erectile dysfunction affects 20% to 90% of men depending on factors such as patient baseline sexual function, age, and surgical technique. In a study of 964 eligible men Miller et al.[38] demonstrated that men undergoing radiation therapy, either in the form of external beam radiation or brachytherapy, continued to experience significant concerns related to sexual, urinary, and bowel dysfunction. Overall health-related quality of life was significantly worse in at least one of four domains (urinary irritative-obstructive, urinary incontinence, bowel and sexual) for men in the therapy groups compared with controls.

Widespread PSA testing has also led to an increase in the use of androgen deprivation therapy. The role of androgen deprivation therapy in men with advance prostate cancer is well recognized, but its role among men with localized disease is more controversial. Bolla et al.[39] have clearly demonstrated that androgen deprivation therapy can improve survival among men undergoing radiation therapy for advanced localized disease; however, many men with much earlier stage disease also receive this treatment. No clinical trials support the use of androgen deprivation therapy as a primary treatment for localized disease. Despite this fact, a 1999 to 2001 survey by Cooperberg et al.[40] demonstrated that primary androgen deprivation therapy has become the second most common treatment after surgery for localized prostate cancer. Androgen deprivation therapy is not benign. Several medical conditions are adversely impacted, including osteoporosis, cardiovascular disease, lipid profiles, diabetes mellitus, cognitive impairment, and functional losses. Prolonged use of androgen deprivation therapy among the elderly has led geriatricians to coin a new term: androgen deprivation syndrome.[41]

HOW SHOULD PHYSICIANS ADVISE THEIR PATIENTS?

Unfortunately, data are still insufficient to make a definitive recommendation concerning the value of screening for prostate cancer. Based on current data the European Association of Urology has stated that the costs and benefits remain insufficient to support population-based screening.[42] Early detection of prostate cancer by selective PSA testing, however, is encouraged by the American Urological Association because PSA measurement is still the single best test for early detection of prostate cancer.[43]

Because of the significant new data published since the last guideline update in 2001, the American Cancer Society (ACS) released new prostate cancer screening recommendations in 2010.[44] The ACS no longer supports routine annual PSA testing. The 2010 recommendations clearly state that any reduction in the likelihood of dying from prostate cancer from PSA testing must be "weighed against the serious risks incurred by early detection and subsequent treatment and particularly

TABLE 61.1

AGE-SPECIFIC REFERENCE RANGES FOR SERUM PROSTATE-SPECIFIC ANTIGEN

Age Range (years)	Asian Americans (ng/mL)	African Americans (ng/mL)	Caucasians (ng/mL)
40–49	0–2.0	0–2.0	0–2.5
50–59	0–3.0	0–4.0	0–3.5
60–69	0–4.0	0–4.5	0–4.5
70–75	0–5.0	0–5.5	0–6.5

(From ref. 43)

against the risk of treating many men for screen-detected prostate cancer who would not have experienced ill effects from their disease if it had been left undetected." As a consequence the ACS now recommends that men must be involved in the decision whether to initiate and continue testing. Clinicians should not simply order a PSA test as part of an annual check-up. The ACS suggests that health care providers can and should play a critical role in helping men to make an informed decision, but recognizes that the complexity of the issue may overwhelm the average patient–clinician encounter. The ACS therefore suggests that patients and providers turn to many of the prostate cancer decision aids outlined in their report.

In view of the delay between diagnosis through screening and the expected mortality benefit, the ACS recommends against screening men who have less than a 10-year life expectancy. They conclude that the risks of treatment outweigh any benefits in this group of men. While not actually recommending that younger patients be screened, the ACS suggests that "men at higher risk of developing prostate cancer at earlier ages—African American men and men with a family history of prostate cancer in non-elderly relatives—be provided the opportunity for informed decision making at an earlier age than average-risk men." Men at average risk should receive information about the "uncertainties, risks and potential benefits" associated with prostate cancer screening beginning at age 50 years.

PSA values are known to increase with age. Carter et al.[45] demonstrated that men with benign prostatic hyperplasia can have a rise of 0.75 ng/mL/year. In order to improve the sensitivity and specificity of PSA testing, some clinicians have suggested varying the threshold value used to recommend prostate biopsy by patient age and ethnicity.[46] A recent report by the American Urological Association suggests that the median PSA value for men in their 40s is 0.7 ng/mL; for men in their 50s, 0.9 ng/mL; for men in their 60s, 1.2 ng/mL; and for men in their 70s, 1.5 ng/mL. Age specific reference ranges are listed in Table 61.1.

Since the long-term impact of screening for prostate cancer with PSA testing remains unknown, the American Urological Association has suggested that men should have an initial PSA test at age 40 in order to establish a baseline value. Men at this age do not have significant prostatic enlargement and therefore benign enlargement should not confound results. Men with a value above 0.7 ng/mL are at greater risk for being diagnosed with prostate cancer.[47]

The appropriate frequency of repeated PSA testing also remains controversial. There is no evidence to support annual PSA testing. The ERSPC trial demonstrated that 90% of men with a PSA value less than 1.9 ng/mL will have a value less than 3.0 ng/mL 4 years later.[48] Few clinically important interval cancers are identified using a more frequent screening interval. Furthermore, because of the long natural history of most prostate cancers and the increasing frequency of competing diseases associated with aging, any benefits of PSA testing decline rapidly with age.[49] For this reason the U.S. Preventative Services Task Force recommends against screening men over the age of 75 years.[50]

Screening for prostate cancer using PSA testing has resulted in a dramatic increase in the incidence of this disease. Unfortunately, to date this has not led to dramatic declines in prostate cancer mortality. Screening is inappropriate for men over the age of 75 years, but potentially could benefit men much younger. Data from randomized trials have demonstrated that PSA testing can lower prostate cancer mortality, but this success comes at a significant price. The ERSPC study has demonstrated that 1,410 men need to be screened to indentify 48 men with prostate cancer. Treatment of these 48 men prevents one prostate cancer death. Until researchers develop better tools to distinguish men with clinically significant disease from those who have indolent disease, screening for prostate cancer will produce a modest public health benefit at a very large cost.

References

1. Stamey TA, Yang N, Hay AR, et al. Prostate-specific antigen as a serum marker for adenocarcinoma of the prostate. *N Eng J Med* 1987;317:909.
2. Smith RA, Cokkinides, Brawley OW. Cancer screening in the United States, 2008: a review of current American Cancer Society guidelines and cancer screening issues. *CA Cancer J Clin* 2008;58:161.
3. Ross LE, Berkowitz Z, Ekwueme DU. Use of the prostate specific antigen test among US men: findings from the 2005 National Health Interview Survey. *Cancer Epidemiol Biomarkers Prev* 2008;17:636.
4. Ries LAG, Melbert D, Krapcho M, et al., eds. *SEER cancer statistics review, 1975–2005. Surveillance, Epidemiology and End Results*. Bethesda, MD: National Cancer Institute, 2008.
5. Merrill RM, Weed DL. Measuring the health burden of cancer in the United States through lifetime and age-conditional risk estimates. *Ann Epidemiol* 2001;11:547.
6. Parkin DM, Bray F, Ferlay J, et al. Global cancer statistics 2002. *CA Cancer J Clin* 2005;55:74.
7. Brawley OW, Ankerst DP, Thompson IM. Screening for prostate cancer. *CA Cancer J Clin* 2009;59:264.
8. Jemal A, Siegel R, Ward E, et al. Cancer statistics, 2009. *CA Cancer J Clin* 2009;59:225.
9. Young HH. Early diagnosis and radical cure of carcinoma of the prostate. *Bull Johns Hopkins Hosp* 1905;16:314.
10. Johansson JE, Adami HO, Andersson SO, et al. Natural history of localized prostatic cancer. A population-based study in 223 untreated patients. *Lancet* 1989;1(8642):799.
11. Johansson JE, Adami HO, Andersson SO, et al. High 10 year survival rate in patients with early, untreated prostatic cancer. *JAMA* 1992;267:2191.
12. Johansson JE, Holmberg, Johansson S, Bergrstrom R, Adami HO. Fifteen year survival in prostate cancer. A prospective, population-based study in Sweden. *JAMA* 1997;277:467.
13. Johansson JE, Andren O, Andersson SO, et al. Natural history of early, localized prostate cancer. *JAMA* 2004;291:2713.

14. Chodak GW, Thisted RA, Gerber GS, et al. Results of conservative management of clinically localized prostate cancer. *N Engl J Med* 1994;330:242.
15. Albertsen PC, Hanley JA, Gleason DF, Barry MJ. Competing risk analysis of men aged 55 to 74 years at diagnosis managed conservatively for clinically localized prostate cancer. *JAMA* 1998;280:975.
16. Albertsen PC, Hanley JA, Fine J. 20 year outcomes following conservative management of clinically localized prostate cancer. *JAMA* 2005;293:2095.
17. Sakr WA, Haas GP, Cassin BF, Pontes JE, Crissman JD. The frequency of carcinoma and intraepithelial neoplasia of the prostate in young male patients. *J Urol* 1993;150:379.
18. Thompson IM, Goodman PJ, Tangen CM, et al. The influence of finasteride on the development of prostate cancer. *N Engl J Med* 2003;349:215.
19. Gleason DF, Mellinger GT for the Veterans Administration Cooperative Urological Research Group. Predication of prognosis for prostatic adenocarcinoma by combined histologic grading and clinical staging. *J Urol* 1974;111:58.
20. Epstein JI. Gleason score 2-4 adenocarcinoma of the prostate on needle biopsy. *Am J Surg Pathol* 2000;24:477.
21. Albertsen PC, Hanley JA, Barrows GH, et al. Prostate cancer and the Will Rogers phenomenon. *J Natl Cancer Inst* 2005;97:1248.
22. Lu-Yao GL, Albertsen PC, Moore DF, et al. Outcomes of localized prostate cancer following conservative management. *JAMA* 2009;302:1202.
23. Collin SM, Martin RM, Metcalfe C, et al. Prostate cancer mortality in the USA and UK in 1974–2004: an ecological study. *Lancet Oncol* 2008;9:445.
24. Murtola TJ, Tammela TL, Maattanen L, et al. Prostate cancer and PSA among statin users in the Finnish prostate cancer screening trial. *Int J Cancer* 2010;127(7):1650.
25. Bill-Axelson A, Holmber L, Filen F, et al. Radical prostatectomy versus watchful waiting in localized prostate cancer: the Scandinavian prostate cancer group-4 trial. *J Natl Cancer Inst* 2008;100:1144.
26. Widmark A, Klepp O, Solberg A, et al. Endocrine treatment, with or without radiotherapy, in locally advanced prostate cancer (SPCG-7/SFUO-3): an open randomized phase III trial. *Lancet* 2009;373:301.
27. Kramer BS, Hagerty KL, Justman S, et al. Use of 5-alpha reductase inhibitors for prostate cancer chemoprevention: American Society of Clinical Oncology/American Urological Association 2008 Clinical Practice Guideline. *J Clin Oncol* 2009;27:1502.
28. Eastham JA, Riedel E, Scardino PT, et al. Variation of serum prostate-specific antigen levels: an evaluation of year-to-year fluctuations. *JAMA* 2003;289:2695.
29. Slev PR, La'ulu SL, Roberts WL. Intermethod differences in results for total PSA, free PSA, and percentage of free PSA. *Am J Clin Pathol* 2008;129:952.
30. Gann PH, Hennekens CH, Stampfer MJ. A prospective evaluation of plasma prostate-specific antigen for detection of prostatic cancer. *JAMA* 1995;273:289.
31. Catalona WJ, Partin AW, Slawin KM, et al. Use of the percentage of free prostate-specific antigen to enhance differentiation of prostate cancer from benign prostatic diseases. *JAMA* 1998;279:1542.
32. Andriole GL, Grubb RL, Buys SS, et al. Mortality results from a randomized prostate-cancer screening trial. *N Engl J Med* 2009;360:1310.
33. Schroeder FH, Hugosson J, Roobol MJ, et al. Screening and prostate cancer mortality in a randomized European study. *N Engl J Med* 2009;360:1320.
34. Welch AG, Albertsen PC. Prostate cancer diagnosis and treatment after the introduction of prostate specific antigen screening: 1986–2005. *J Natl Cancer Inst* 2009;101:1325.
35. Draisma G, Boer R, Otto SJ, et al. Lead times and over detection due to prostate-specific antigen screening: estimates from the European Randomized Study of Screening for Prostate Cancer. *J Natl Cancer Inst* 2003;95:868.
36. Collin SM, Martin RM, Metcalfe C, et al. Prostate-cancer mortality in the USA and UK in 1975–2004: an ecological study. *Lancet Oncol* 2008; 9:445.
37. Sanda MG, Dunn RL, Michalski J, et al. Quality of life and satisfaction with outcome among prostate-cancer survivors. *N Engl J Med* 2008; 358:1250.
38. Miller DC, Sanda MG, Dunn RL, et al. Long-term outcomes among localized prostate cancer survivors: health-related quality of life changes after radical prostatectomy, external radiation, and brachytherapy. *J Clin Oncol* 2005;23:2772.
39. Bolla M, deReijke TM, Tienhoven GV, et al. Duration of androgen suppression in the treatment of prostate cancer. *N Engl J Med* 2009;360:2516.
40. Cooperberg MR, Grossfeld GD, Lubeck DP, Carroll PR. National practice patterns and time trends in androgen ablation for localized prostate cancer. *J Natl Cancer Inst* 2003;95:981.
41. Shahinian VB, Kuo YF, Freeman JL, Goodwin JS. Risk of the "androgen deprivation syndrome" in men receiving androgen deprivation for prostate cancer. *Arch Intern Med* 2006;166:465.
42. Abrahamsson PA, Artibani W, Chapple CR, Wirth M. European Association of Urology position statement on screening for prostate cancer. *Eur Urol* 2009;56:270.
43. Greene KL, Albertsen PC, Babaian RJ, et al. Prostate specific antigen best practice statement: 2009 update. *J Urol* 2009;182:2232.
44. Wolf AMD, Wender RC, Etzioni RB, et al. American Cancer Society Guideline for the early detection of prostate cancer: update 2010. *CA Cancer J Clin* 2010;60:70.
45. Carter HB, Pearson JD, Metter J, et al. Longitudinal evaluation of prostate specific antigen levels in men with and without prostate disease. *JAMA* 1992;267:2215.
46. Loeb S, Roehl KA, Catalona WJ, Nadler RB. Is the utility of prostate-specific antigen velocity for prostate cancer detection affected by age? *BJU Int* 2008;101:817.
47. Loeb S, Roehl KA, Antenor JA, et al. Baseline prostate-specific antigen compared with median prostate-specific antigen for age group as a predictor of prostate cancer risk in men younger than 60 years old. *Urology* 2006;67:316.
48. Schroeder FH, Raaijmakers R, Postma R, van der Kwast TH, Roobol MJ. 4-year prostate specific antigen progression and diagnosis of prostate cancer in the European Randomized Study of Screening for Prostate Cancer, Section Rotterdam. *J Urol* 2005;174:489.
49. Ross KS, Guess HA, Carter HB. Estimation of treatment benefits when PSA screening for prostate cancer is discontinued at different ages. *Urology* 2005;66:1038.
50. Screening for prostate cancer: U.S. Preventive Services Task Force recommendation statement. *Ann Intern Med* 2008;149:185.

CHAPTER 62 SCREENING FOR LUNG CANCER

DAVID E. MIDTHUN AND JAMES R. JETT

For most patients, detection of lung cancer occurs when they present with symptoms. By the time lung cancer causes symptoms, the disease is usually advanced and noncurable. Earlier detection is preferred, but no test had proven efficacy in screening for lung cancer. Chest radiography (CXR) and sputum cytology showed the ability to identify more cancers, more cancers in early stage, and improve survival, but failed to show a reduction in deaths from lung cancer. Advances in computed tomography (CT) allow for scanning of the entire chest in less than 15 seconds and in a single breath hold. Prospective single-arm studies of low-dose spiral CT (LDCT) screening created considerable excitement about the potential to effectively screen for lung cancer. Usual clinical practice identifies only about 20% of lung cancer in stage I, the earliest stage, when surgery results in cure in approximately 70%. CT screening series report 58% to 93% of prevalence cancers and 25% to 100% of incidence cancers identified were stage I.[1–12] Findings like these suggested that screening with CT may have the ability to shift stage of detection from late stage to early stage. Randomized controlled trials are underway, and the recently announced findings from the National Lung Screening Trial (NLST) indicate a 20% reduction in lung cancer deaths compared to chest x-ray.[13] The study is not yet published. This review will examine the issues presented by screening for lung cancer, and the results of past and recent studies of lung cancer screening.

THE OPPORTUNITY

The role of screening in lung cancer management has been a subject of controversy, but there is no controversy about the amount of devastation caused by this disease. More women and men die of lung cancer annually in the United States and the world than any other cancer.[14] More people die of lung cancer—over 400 people per day—than from breast, colon, and prostate cancer combined.[15] The high frequency and lethality of lung cancer presents an opportunity for intervention. Prevention is key, but improving outcomes from lung cancer will result from early detection and effective treatment. The 5-year survival of 16% for lung cancer pales in comparison to 88% for breast cancer, 65% for colon cancer, and 99% for prostate cancer.[15] Part of the reason lung cancer lags so far behind in survival is that there has not been an established screening test. As has been shown with mammography for breast cancer and with fecal occult blood testing for colon cancer, proving mortality reduction with CT for lung cancer screening is required before widespread application is pursued. The persistence of smoking prevalence rates, and the fact that more lung cancers are diagnosed annually in former smokers than in current smokers, implies that the problem of lung cancer will have a secure hold for a number of decades. An effective screening tool is desired.

The 2010 American Cancer Society (ACS) guidelines for the early detection of cancer states: "At present neither the ACS, nor any other medical/scientific organization, recommends testing for early lung cancer detection in asymptomatic individuals."[16] Why were we not screening when we knew that screening with CXR or CT leads to the detection of more cancers, more early-stage cancers, and marked improvement in survival? The answer lies within issues introduced by screening—each of those measures is a necessary outcome, but together are insufficient to show efficacy from screening.

Use of a screening test introduces biases that are inherent in screening. The most significant of these include lead time, length time, and overdiagnosis bias. These screening issues are not specific for lung cancer. Because of these biases inherent in screening, survival would be expected to be more favorable after screening even if earlier detection and intervention did not alter the course of the disease. For this reason, mortality reduction rather than improvement in survival is the ultimate measure of a screening tool's effectiveness and requires performance of randomized controlled trials (RCTs).

CHEST RADIOGRAPHY AND SPUTUM CYTOLOGY

The National Cancer Institute (NCI) supported three randomized trials screening for lung cancer in the 1970s and early 1980s involving Johns Hopkins University, Memorial Sloan-Kettering, and Mayo Clinic.[17–23] These studies involved over 30,000 men over age 45 who were current or former smokers. At Johns Hopkins and Memorial Sloan-Kettering, the screening algorithm investigated the addition of sputum cytology every 4 months to annual CXR. These two trials showed that adding sputum cytology every 4 months to annual CXR screening did not improve mortality rates of lung cancer when compared with the use of annual CXRs alone. The 5-year survival in these two studies was nearly 35%, which was considerably above the historical average at the time of 13%.[18–21]

The Mayo Lung Project (MLP) compared every-4-month CXR and sputum cytology to standard care. After baseline screening, those patients without cancer were randomized to the group that received CXR and sputum cytology every 4 months or to the group that was advised to have yearly CXR and sputum cytology. In the screened group, 206 cancers were detected, and 160 were detected in the control group.[22] Surgical resection was feasible in 46% of the cancers in the intervention group compared with 32% of cancers in the control group. The anticipated stage shift in diagnosis from advanced stage to earlier stage was not found in the more frequently screened group. There were 112 participants with unresectable lung cancer identified in the group screened every 4 months compared with 109 unresectable cancers identified in the control group. The MLP showed that the screened group had a 5-year survival of nearly 35%, whereas the 5-year survival in the nonscreen group was 15%. However, the mortality from lung cancer in the screen group was 3.2 per 1,000 person-years and not statistically different from the 3.0 per 1,000 person-years in the control group.[23] Considerable controversy has resulted from the interpretation of these trials, but the lack of improvement in mortality in all three of the NCI-sponsored studies failed to prove that screening for lung cancer was appropriate.[16] In the MLP, over half of the control group had a CXR in the last year of the study and 75% within the last 2 years. The lack of mortality reduction has been interpreted as showing that screening was of no benefit, but these studies evaluated screening at different frequencies rather than screening versus no screening. A meta-analysis showed that more frequent screening with CXR led to an increase in mortality when compared with less frequent screening. In other words, screening resulted in more harm than good.[24]

Further randomized controlled study information on CXR screening has been reported from the Prostate Lung Colon and Ovary (PLCO) screening trial. Beginning in 1993, 77,464 participants, more than half of whom were current or former smokers, were randomized to receive a CXR at baseline and for 3 years.[25] The control group received no screening radiology. In the screened arm, 564 (0.7%) participants were diagnosed with lung cancer, although only 306 (54%) were screen-detected; the remainder were interval cancers (diagnosed after a negative screen and before the next screen study) or in those who had not yet received a screen study. Of the screen-detected cancers, 59.6% were stage I or II.[25] Results from the control arm have not been reported; information regarding mortality in the two arms is anticipated in 2015.

Although the CXR is easy to perform, is of low risk, and is well accepted by patients, it is not very sensitive. From the results of the NCI trials, Flehinger and Melamed[26] estimated that the probability of detecting the presence of a stage I lung cancer by CXR was only 16%. Within the MLP, 90% of the peripheral lung cancers detected using every 4-month CXRs were evident in retrospect despite the fact that three radiologists had interpreted the previous radiograph findings as normal.[27] Several studies screening simultaneously with both CT and CXR showed that about three of four cancers seen on CT will be missed on CXR.

CT SCREENING

Single-Arm Studies

Conventional chest CT uses a radiation dosage and image-acquisition time that is impractical for screening purposes. The development of low-dose, fast spiral CT greatly reduced the radiation dose and the scan time, making screening feasible. Conventional CT images are obtained at 140 to 300 mA and are performed over many minutes using multiple breath holds. In contrast, LDCT images may be obtained at 20 to 50 mA and the entire scan completed in 15 seconds during a single breath hold. LDCT is comparable in sensitivity and specificity of lung nodule detection when compared with conventional CT mode.

Initial studies from Japan created excitement in support of LDCT as a tool for early lung cancer detection. The first report was from Kaneko et al.[1] comparing LDCT scanning with CXR in screening a high-risk population for lung cancer. CT scans and CXRs were obtained every 6 months in 1,369 participants who were over age 50 years and had a greater than 20-pack-year history of smoking. CT detected 15 cases of peripheral lung cancer, and 11 of these were missed on CXR. An amazing 93% of the non–small cell carcinomas identified were stage I. The second report in the literature was from Sone et al.,[2] who screened 3,958 participants with low-dose spiral CT. There were 19 lung cancers detected by CT, and only four of these were seen on CXR. Remarkably, 16 of the 19 (84%) were stage I at resection

CT screening efforts in the United States were lead by Henschke et al.[3] with the Early Lung Cancer Action Project (ELCAP). They enrolled 1,000 current or former smokers aged 60 years or more and screened with LDCT and CXR. Prevalence results were reported in 1999. CT detected a total of 27 prevalence lung cancers, and only 7 were also seen by CXR. CT detected 4 times more lung cancers and 6 times the number of stage I lesions than did CXR. At surgery, 23 of the 27 (85%) malignancies were stage IA.

Since these initial studies in Japan and the United States, multiple additional single-arm observational CT screening studies in current or former smokers have been reported worldwide (Table 62.1). Each of these studies has identified a high percentage of early-stage cancers. Rates of cancer detection at baseline (prevalence) ranged from 0.48% to 2.7%, and 58% to 93% prevalence cancers detected were surgical stage I.[1–12] Cancers detected with subsequent screening that were not present on the baseline scan are incidence cancers. Studies report incidence rates of cancer detection from 0.2% to 1.4%, and 53% to 100% of incidence cancers were surgical stage I.[1–12] The largest single-arm observational report of CT screening is a combination of results of ELCAP with that of the International Early Lung Cancer Action Program (IELCAP).[11] The 31,567 participants received a baseline scan, and 27,456 repeat scans were performed. A total of 484 cancers were found, 412 (85%) of these were clinical stage I non–small cell carcinomas and 375 (77%) were surgical stage I. The actuarial 10-year survival for those with clinical stage I was 88%; however, median follow-up in this study was only 40 months.[11] The high percentage of cancer found in stage I suggested that LDCT may have the potential to shift detection of lung cancer from a more advanced stage to stage I.

A subsequent report challenged this premise. Investigators applied a validated lung cancer prediction model to three prospective single-arm observational studies of CT screening combining 3,246 participants.[28] CT screening found 3 times the number of expected cancers, resulted in 10 times the expected number of resections (109 of 144 cancers were resectable), and identified more than the expected number of advanced-stage cancers. Despite having a 94% actual 4-year survival for participants with clinical stage I cancers, CT screening did not result in a reduction in the expected number of deaths from lung cancer. These results emphasize the need to evaluate the effectiveness of screening by mortality rather than survival.

Randomized Trials

Several RCTs are underway to address the question of whether or not screening with CT reduces mortality from lung cancer. The National Lung Screening Trial (NLST) is a study of 53,457 participants in the United States, aged 55 to 74 years with 30 or more pack-year smoking history, that were randomized between low-dose CT (LDCT) and CXR.[29] Enrollment began in 2002 and final screening was completed in January 2007; in November 2010, preliminary results of this trial were released and revealed a 20% reduction in lung cancer mortality with CT screening.[13] There were 354 lung cancer deaths among those in the CT arm versus 442 deaths among those in the chest x-ray arm indicating in a 20.3% reduction with CT screening. The trial was stopped by the independent Data and Safety Monitoring Board because the trial met the primary endpoint. Other findings from the NLST indicate that all-cause

TABLE 62.1

PROSPECTIVE, SINGLE-ARM OBSERVATIONAL LOW-DOSE SPIRAL COMPUTED TOMOGRAPHY (CT) SCREENING STUDIES

Study (Ref.)	No. of Participants	Participants with Noncalcified Nodules	No. of CT-Detected Prevalence NSCLC	Prevalence Surgical Stage I	No. of CT-Detected Incidence NSCLC	Incidence Surgical Stage I
Kaneko et al. (1)	1,369	588[a] (17%)	15	14 (93%)	—	—
Sone et al. (2)	3,967	217[b] (5%)	19	16 (84%)	—	—
ELCAP (3,4)	1,000	233 (23%)	27	23 (85%)	7	5 (71%)
Sobue et al. (5)	1,611	186 (12%)	14	10 (71%)	18	15 (83)
Mayo (6)	1,520	782 (51%)	31	22 (71%)	34	17 (61%)
Diederich et al. (7)	817	350 (43%)	12	7 (58%)	10	7 (70%)
Nawa et al. (8)	7,956	2,099 (26%)	36	31 (86%)	4	4 (100%)
McWilliams et al. (9)	561	431 (46%)	10	7 (70%)	—	—
Pastorino et al. (10)	1,035	199 (19%)	11	6 (55%)	11	11 (100%)
IELCAP (11)	31,567	4,186 (13%)[c]	405	85%[d]	74	85%[d]
PLuSS (12)	3,642	1,477 (40.6)	52	30 (60%)	17	9 (53%)

NSCLC, non–small cell lung cancer; ELCAP, early lung cancer action project; IELCAP, international early lung cancer action project; PLuSS, Pittsburgh Lung Screening Study.
[a]CT findings described as abnormal shadows.
[b]CT findings described a suspicious or indeterminate.
[c]Not reported for nodules <5 mm.
[d]Only pooled prevalence and incidence clinical stage information reported.
[e]Two cancers were clinical stage IA but not resected because of medical reasons, and therefore not surgically staged.

mortality was 7% lower in the CT group, and 25% of all deaths in the trial were due to lung cancer. About 25% of the participants had false positive CT scans. Publication of this study is anticipated in 2011.

The Dutch-Belgian randomized lung cancer screening trial known as the Nederlands-Leuvens Longkanker Screenings Onderzoek (NELSON) trial is underway. The baseline information was reported for the 7,557 participants randomized to receive CT screening.[30] Over 50% of the particpants had one or more nodules identified, and evaluation led to the diagnosis of 70 cancers giving a prevalence rate of 0.9%; 64% of the cancers were stage I. During the second round of screening an additional 57 cancers were identified in 54 participants; 74% were surgical stage I cancers. To date, no information has been provided for the control group, so mortality information is unknown.

The Danish Lung Cancer Screening Trial (DLCST) randomized 4,104 participants to CT versus no screening.[31] Among those who received CT screening, there were 17 cancers found at baseline (prevalence rate of 0.8%); 9 of these (53%) were stage I and 8 (47%) were stage III or IV. No information was provided on the control group.

In the ITALUNG study in Italy, 3,206 participants, current or former smokers aged 55 to 69 years, were randomized to LDCT versus no screening.[32] The baseline CT was positive (nodules ≥5 mm) in 426 (30.3%) of 1,406 subjects, and 21 lung cancers were diagnosed in 20 participants (prevalence, 1.5%) and 10 (47.6%) were stage I. Control group findings have not been reported and outcomes will likely be pooled for greater power with other RCTs in Europe.

Two small RCTs of CT screening have also reported data on the control group. The Lung Screening Study was the pilot study to determine feasibility of the NLST. A total of 1,660 subjects were randomized to the LDCT arm and 1,658 to the CXR arm.[33] Cancer yield for LDCT was 1.9% at baseline and 0.57% for year 1. Cancer yield for CXR was 0.45% at baseline and 0.68% for year 1. Forty lung cancers in the LDCT arm and 20 in the CXR arm were diagnosed over the study period. Stage I cancers comprised 48% of cases in the LDCT arm and 40% in the CXR arm. A total of 16 stage III-IV cancers were observed in the LDCT arm versus 9 in the CXR arm.[33] No mortality information was presented for the study; however, the finding of a nearly twofold higher number of advanced-stage cancers in the CT arm suggests there was to be no measured mortality benefit from CT screening. In the French Depiscan study, 621 participants were randomized and received either CT or CXR.[34] At least one nodule was seen on LDCT in 152 (45%) of 336, and 8 lung cancers were identified, with only one seen in the CXR arm.

The only other RCT that has published data on both the screen and control group is the DANTE trial. In this study a total of 2,472 participants were enrolled and randomized to a CT screen versus no CT following a baseline CXR, with the plan for annual scanning for 4 years in the screen group.[35] After a mean of 33 months of follow-up, 60 participants in the CT arm had lung cancer identified versus 34 in the control group. Stage I cancers were 60% of the CT screen group and 15% of the controls; however, there were 23 cancers in stage IIIA/B or IV in the screen group and 21 in the control group. No mortality or survival data are presented. The results are preliminary; however, they suggest that despite finding many more cancers and more early-stage cancers, CT screening did not show a shift in stage by finding fewer advanced-stage cancer, suggesting that mortality may not be reduced through CT screening in this study.

THE PROBLEMS WITH CT SCREENING

Although LDCT shows promise in reducing death from lung cancer, problems include false-positive findings resulting in unnecessary surgery, overdiagnosis, and the risk of radiation.

The prevalence data from these prospective, single-arm CT studies show a rate of nodule detection among participants between 23% and 60%.[1–12] Frequency of nodule detection appears to be a function of slice thickness rather than the

TABLE 62.2

RANDOMIZED, CONTROLLED LOW-DOSE SPIRAL COMPUTED TOMOGRAPHY (CT) SCREENING STUDIES

Study (Ref.)	Participant Randomization	Noncalcified Nodules (%)	No. of Cancers Detected	Surgical Stage I (%)	Prevalence Cancer Rate (%)
LSS (33)	CT: 1,660	25.8[a]	40	48	2.4
	CXR: 1,658	8.7[a]	20	40	1.2
Depiscan (34)	CT: 336	45.2	8	37.5	2.4
	CXR: 285	7.4	1	100	0.4
DANTE (35)	CT: 1,276	15.6[b]	28	57	2.2
	None: 1,196	3.1	8	50	0.7
DLSCT (31)	CT: 2,052	29	17	59	0.8
	None: 2,052	—	—	—	—
ITALUNG (32)	CT: 1,613	30[b]	21	48	1.5
	None: 1,593	—	—	—	—
NELSON (30)	CT: 7,557	51	70	64	0.9
	None: 8,265	—	—	—	—
NLST (29)[c]	CT: 26,724	—	—	—	—
	CXR: 26,733	—	—	—	—

LSS, Lung Screening Study; CXR, chest radiography; DLSCT, Danish Lung Cancer Screening Trial; NELSON, Nederlands-Leuvens Longkanker Screenings Onderzoek; NLST, National Lung Screening Trial.
[a]Reported as positive if a nodule ≥4 mm was detected.
[b]Reported as positive if a nodule ≥5 mm was detected.
[c]Now announced 20.3% reduction in lung cancer deaths with CT screening compared to chest x-ray screening.[13]

geographic location of screening. To reduce the number of false-positive findings, some researchers have decided to call the scan negative if the largest nodule detected is less than 5 mm.[11] The result will be to reduce the false-positive findings, but this will be at the expense of increasing the number of false-negative findings. In the study by McWilliams et al.,[36] 18% of the cancers identified were first detected when less than 4 mm and these would have been considered "negative" if the threshold of 5 mm for a positive had been applied.

Although there may be some psychological impact of having any abnormality seen on one's scan, the harm from false-positive findings evolves primarily around unnecessary invasive procedures or surgery. In the Mayo study, 10 of 55 participants (18%) underwent resection for benign disease.[37] Similarly in the German study, benign nodules represented 20% of resections.[7] Benign nodules comprised 34% of the resections by thoracotomy or video-assisted thoracoscopic surgery in the Pittsburgh Lung Screening Study.[12] Bach et al.[28] found that there were 10 times the number of surgeries expected and only 3 times the number of cancers expected as a result of CT screening. Careful evaluation of detected nodules with old images, serial examinations, positron emission tomography, or needle biopsy may allow avoiding removal of benign nodules in most but not all circumstances. Invasive procedures for baseline abnormalities identified benign disease 27.2% of the time in the participants randomized to CT in the NELSON trial.[30]

Contrary to the concern that spiral CT might not be able to identify lung cancers early enough in their course is the notion of overdiagnosis. Although the issue of overdiagnosis may initially raise eyebrows in the context of lung cancer, clinicians are quite familiar with it in prostate cancer and breast ductal carcinoma *in situ*. Support for presence of overdiagnosis in lung cancer was found within an extended follow-up of the Mayo Lung Project. Marcus et al.[38] reported on participant follow-up through 1996 (median follow-up time, 20.5 years). The median survival for patients with resected early-stage cancer was 16.0 years in the intervention arm versus 5.0 years in the control arm. However, lung cancer mortality was 4.4 deaths per 1,000 person-years in the intervention arm and 3.9 in the control arm ($P = .09$). The improvement in survival and the lack of reduction in mortality for participants in the screening arm suggested that some cancers with limited clinical significance were identified; in other words, there were overdiagnosed cancers. Using the results from the MLP, one author calculated the risk that a CXR and/or sputum cytology–detected cancer represented overdiagnosis was about 51%.[39]

CT data regarding tumor-doubling times lend further evidence that overdiagnosis is a factor in the apparent survival improvement with LDCT screening. Aoki et al.[40] reported on 34 patients with peripheral adenocarcinoma less than 3 cm in size who had undergone CT and CXR before surgery but also had CXR or CT more than 6 months before surgery. Tumor-doubling times were calculated based on the tumor growth pattern in comparing the films. Those with bronchoalveolar cell carcinomas had tumor-doubling times ranging from 662 to 1,486 days with a mean of 880 days. A mean doubling time of 880 days would take a 1 cm bronchoalveolar cell cancer 19 years to grow to a size of 2 cm. Adding to the concern of overdiagnosis was the report from Nawa et al.[8] that found 23 of 40 (58%) prevalence cancers in a CT-screened population were in never smokers. Further support for overdiagnosis with CT screening came from an analysis of the cancers identified in the Mayo CT screening study. Volume doubling times were retrospectively calculated for 48 screen-detected cancers and 13 (27%) were slow-growing cancers with doubling times over 400 days.[41]

Radiation from CT scans has the potential to increase risk for cancer. The absorbed dose of radiation is expressed in grays (Gy) or milligray (mGy) but is often expressed as an effective dose in Sievert (Sv) or milliseverts (mSv) for dose distributions that are not homogeneous for x-ray radiation (1 mSv =1 mGy). Effective dose is a generic estimate of overall harm to the patient from radiation exposure and is used for comparison of risks from different imaging techniques. The risks of ionizing radiation depend on age and sex, with women estimated to have an increase in cancer-related mortality for solid tumors than men with similar levels of exposure.[42] The average effective dose for CT of the chest is 7 mSv.[43] Authors estimated that the number of CT scans of the chest that it would require to cause one radiation-induced cancer would be 720 for a 40-year-old woman and 1,566 for a man. If scanned at age 60 years, the numbers would be 1 in 1,090 for women and 1 in 2,080 for men.[44]

Using the low-dose CT screening parameter from the NLST of 1.3 and 1.0 mSv for women and men, investigators estimated the mortality reduction required to outweigh the radiation-induced cancer risk from three annual CT scans at varying ages.[45] The mortality reduction needed was higher with younger age and for never smokers. For a current smoker screened at age 50 to 52 years, the radiation-induced lung cancer mortality was 5 per 10,000 for women and 2 per 10,000 for men. The reduction in lung cancer mortality to outweigh the radiation risk would be 4% and 2%, respectively, for women and men. As the NLST is now indicating a 20% reduction in deaths, then the benefit of screening with low-dose CT would greatly outweigh any cancer radiation risks. Even though the radiation risk of screening is very low, it is difficult to quantify exactly. The radiation from diagnostic CT scans is 7 to 10 times the amount of that used for CT screening with low dose. Early efforts are underway by the U.S. Food and Drug Administration to develop and disseminate patient medical imaging cards to help track patients' radiation exposure.

OTHER METHODS OF SCREENING

Although CT screening has generated the most clinical trial data, there have been efforts in a number of areas to define high-risk individuals and biomarkers for early detection. Genomewide association studies have attempted to identify single nucleotide polymorphisms (SNPs) for susceptibility to development of lung cancer. There is a strong association with the nicotine acetylcholine receptor subunit genes on *15q24-25*.[46–48] Two SNPs were reported to yield an odds ratio of 1.32 for both SNPs and account for 14% attributable risk of lung cancer cases. There is some question if these genes (*15q24–25*) may be associated with nicotine dependence only. Other investigators evaluated SNPs in 377 cases and control matched pairs of never smokers and identified that chromosome *13q31.3* had an odds ratio of 1.46 and an estimated attributable risk of at least 10% for lung cancer in never smokers.[49]

A tremendous amount of research has been performed evaluating biomarkers in airway epithelial cells, sputum, blood, breath, and urine for early diagnosis and prediction of persons at high- risk. An 80-gene biomarker performed in cytologically normal large airway epithelial cells was able to distinguish smokers with and without lung cancer with an accuracy of 83%.[50] Another group has evaluated expression of 14 antioxidant, DNA repair, and transcription factor genes in normal bronchial epithelioma and reported a receiver operating characteristic (ROC) of 0.82 for separating lung cancer from normals.[51] Both groups are evaluating these gene biomarker panels in prospective trials as potential screening tools. In a case-control study, fluorescence *in situ* hybridization (FISH) detection of chromosomal aneusomy (CA) in sputum cytology had an adjusted odds ratio of 29.9 for specimens collected within 18 months before diagnosis of lung cancer.[52] The CA-FISH assay was far superior to cytologic atypia or gene promoter methylation for predicting risk of lung cancer. The CA-FISH test was most useful for centrally located squamous cell cancers.

Blood biomarkers have included a panel of serum proteins that may correctly classify lung cancer from controls and may be useful in predicting individuals at high risk.[53] Connective tissue-activating peptide III/neutrophil activating protein-2 was elevated in blood of lung cancer patients and improved the accuracy of lung cancer risk prediction in a Canadian model.[54] Autoantibodies to tumor antigens have been reported to precede the diagnosis of cancer by as much as 3 to 5 years.[55–57] The cancer antigens reported have included annexin-1, *p53*, cancer-associated antigen (CAGE), SOX2, 14-3-3 theta, and others.[55,57,58] Efforts are directed at developing a panel of autoantibodies that would be able to detect lung cancer with adequate sensitivity (≥50%) and high specificity (≥90%). In a case-control study, using three autoantibodies, a sensitivity of 51% and specificity of 82% was reported with an ROC of 0.73 for predicting lung cancer up to 1 year before the clinical diagnoses.[57]

Volatile organic compounds such as alkanes, alkine derivatives, and benzene derivatives can be detected in exhaled breath via a variety of sensing techniques and are under investigation for their ability to detect early lung cancers.[59,60] A 2-minute breath test that used six volatile organic compounds was able to predict lung cancer from normals with a sensitivity of 85% and 80% specificity and ROC of 0.88. If used as a screening test in a population with 2% prevalence of lung cancers, it would have a negative predictive value of 0.98 and a positive predictive value of 0.16.[59]

Urinary levels of NNAC (methylnitrosamine butanol) in smokers were significantly associated with risk of lung cancer in a dose-dependent manner after adjusting for cigarette smoking and urinary cotinine. Urinary levels of NNAC were associated with as high as an eightfold risk of lung cancer in smokers relative to comparable smokers with the lowest NNAC levels.[61] Urinary NNAC is not useful in never or former smokers.

FUTURE DIRECTIONS

The findings from the NLST trial confirming the effectiveness of LDCT screening in reducing lung cancer mortality are likely to be practice changing. It would appear that CT screening will be the centerpiece for future research in combination with one or more biomarkers. Risk models are likely to be used to help decide who to screen.[62–64] Published risk models have been developed based on somewhat different population but have generally included age, smoking history, and asbestos exposure; others have included family history of lung cancer. The inclusion of pulmonary function data, the degree of chronic obstructive pulmonary disease, and use of a biomarkers in these models will further enhance their utility.[54,65–67] The risk-prediction models may help in decision making regarding screening tests; if estimated lung cancer risk was to be 5% to 10% over 5 years, then one might elect to undergo screening studies; however, if risk was 1%, then one may decide not to be screened. Now that mortality reduction has been demonstrated, studies will be needed to help define the optimal risk-benefit breakpoint in screening for the number-one lethal cancer.

Selected References

The full list of references for this chapter appears in the online version.

1. Kaneko M, Eguchi K, Ohmatsu H, et al. Peripheral lung cancer: screening and detection with low-dose spiral CT versus radiography. *Radiology* 1996;201:798.
2. Sone S, Takashima S, Li F, et al. Mass screening for lung cancer with mobile spiral computed tomography scanner. *Lancet* 1998;351:1242.
3. Henschke CI, McCauley DI, Yankelevitz DF, et al. Early lung cancer action project: overall design and findings from baseline screening. *Lancet* 1999;354:99.
4. Henschke CI,Naidich DP, Yankelevitz DF, et al. Early lung cancer action project: initial findings on repeat scanning. *Cancer* 2001;92:153.
5. Sobue T, Moriyama N, Kaneko M, et al. Screening for lung cancer with low-dose helical computed tomography: Anti-Lung Cancer Association project. *J Clin Oncol* 2002;20:911.
6. Swenson SJ, Jett JR, Hartman TE, et al. CT screening for lung cancer: five-year prospective experience. *Radiology* 2005;235:259.
7. Diederich S, Wormanns D, Semik M, et al. Screening for early lung cancer with low-dose spiral CT: prevalence in 817 asymptomatic smokers. *Radiology* 2002;222:773.
8. Nawa T, Nakagawa T, Suzushi S, et al. Lung cancer screening using low-dose spiral CT: results of baseline and 1-year follow-up studies. *Chest* 2002;122:15.
9. McWilliams A, Mayo J, MacDonald S, et al: Lung cancer screening: a differentparadigm. *Am J Respir Crit Care Med* 2003;168:1167.
10. Pastorino U, Bellomi M, Landoni C, et al. Early lung cancer detection with spiral CT and positron emission tomography in heavy smokers: 2-year results. *Lancet* 2003;362:593.
11. The International Early Lung Cancer Action Program Investigators. Survival of patients with stage I lung cancer detected on CT screening. *N Engl J Med* 2006;355:1763.
12. Wilson DO, Weissfeld JL, Fuhrman CR, et al. The Pittsburgh Lung Screening Study (PLuSS): outcomes within 3 years of a first CT scan. *Am J Respir Crit Care Med* 2008;178:956.
13. National Cancer Institute Lung Cancer trial results show mortality benefit with low-dose CT. Twenty percent fewer lung cancer deaths seen among those who were screened with low-dose spiral CT than with chest x-ray. Available at: http://www.cancer.gov/newscenter.pressreleases/NLSTresultsRelease. Accessed Nov 5, 2010.
28. Bach PB, Jett JR, Pastorino U, et al. Computed tomography screening and lung cancer outcomes. *JAMA* 2007;297:953.
29. Gierada DS, Garg K, Nath H, et al. CT quality assurance in the lung screening study component of the National Lung Screening Trial: implications for multicenter imaging trials. *AJR Am J Roentgenol* 2009;193:419.
30. van Klaveren RJ, Oudkerk M, Prokop M, et al. Management of lung nodules detected by volume CT scanning. *N Engl J Med* 2009;361:2221.
31. Pedersen JH, Ashraf H, Dirksen A, et al. The Danish randomized lung cancer CT screening trial–overall design and results of the prevalence round. *J Thorac Oncol* 2009;4:608.
32. Lopes Pegna A, Picozzi G, Mascalchi M, et al. ITALUNG Study Research Group. Design, recruitment and baseline results of the ITALUNG trial for lung cancer screening with low-dose CT. *Lung Cancer* 2009;64:34.
33. Gohagan JK, Marcus PM, Fagerstrom RM, et al., The Lung Screening Study Research Group. Final results of the Lung Screening Study, a randomized feasibility study of spiral CT versus chest X-ray screening for lung cancer. *Lung Cancer* 2005;47(1):9.
34. Blanchon T, Brechot JM, Grenier PA, et al., for the "Depiscan" Group. Baseline results of the Depiscan study: a French randomized pilot trial of lung cancer screening comparing low dose CT scan (LDCT) and chest X-ray (CXR). *Lung Cancer* 2007;58:50.
35. Infante M, Lutman FR, Cavuto S, et al. DANTE Study Group. Lung cancer screening with spiral CT: baseline results of the randomized DANTE trial. *Lung Cancer* 2008;59:355.
36. McWilliams AM, Mayo JR, Ahn MI, et al. Lung cancer screening using multi-slice thin-section computed tomography and autofluorescence bronchoscopy. *J Thorac Oncol* 2006;1:61.
37. Crestanello JA, Allen MS, Jett JR, et al. Thoracic surgical operations in patients enrolled in a computed tomographic screening trial. *J Thorac Cardiovasc Surg* 2004;128:254.
38. Marcus PM, Bergstralh EJ, Fagerstrom RM, et al. Lung cancer mortality in the Mayo Lung Project: the impact of extended follow-up. *J Natl Cancer Inst* 2000;92:1308.
40. Aoki T, Nakata H, Watanabe H, et al. Evolution of peripheral lung adenocarcinomas: CT findings correlated with histology tumor doubling time. *AJR Am J Roentgenol* 2000;174:763.
41. Lindell RM, Hartman TE, Swensen SJ, et al. Five-year lung cancer screening experience: CT appearance, growth rate, and histologic features of 61 lung cancers. *Radiology* 2007;242:555.
43. Mettler FA, Huda W, Yoshizumi TT, Mahesh M. Effective doses in radiology and diagnostic nuclear medicine: a catalog. *Radiology* 2008;248:254.
44. Berrington de Gonzalez A, Mahesh M, Kim K, et al. Projected cancer risks from computed tomographic scans performed in the United States in 2007. *Arch Intern Med* 2009;169:2071.
45. Berrington de Gonzalez A, Kim KP, Berg CD. Low-dose lung computed tomography screening before age 55: estimates of the mortality reduction required to outweigh the radiation-induced cancer risk. *J Med Screen* 2008;15:153.
46. Thorgeirsson TE, Geller F, Sulem P, et al. A variant associated with nicotine dependence, lung cancer, and peripheral arterial disease. *Nature* 2008; 452:638.
47. Hung RJ, McKay JD, Gaborieau V, et al. A susceptibility locus for lung cancer maps to nicotinic acetylcholine receptor subunit genes on 15q25. *Nature* 2008;452:633.
48. Amos CI, Wu X, Broderick P, et al. Genome-wide association scan of tag SNPs identifies a susceptibility locus for lung cancer at 15q25.1. *Nat Genet* 2008;40:616.
49. Li Y, Sheu CC, Ye Y, et al. Genetic variants and risk of lung cancer in never smokers: a genome-wide association study. www.thelancet.com/oncology. Published March 22, 2010.
50. Spira A, Beane JE, Shah V, et al. Airway epithelial gene expression in the diagnostic evaluation of smokers with suspect lung cancer. *Nat Med* 2007; 13:361.
51. Blomquist T, Crawford EL, Mullins DíAnna, et al. Pattern of antioxidant and DNA repair gene expression in normal airway epithelium associated with lung cancer diagnosis. *Cancer Res* 2009;69:8629.
52. Varella-Garcia M, Schulte AP, Wolf HJ, et al. The detection of chromosomal aneusomy by fluorescence in situ hybridization in sputum predicts lung cancer incidence. *Cancer Prev Res* 2010;3:447.
53. Patz EF, Campa MJ, Gottlin EB, et al. Panel of serum biomarkers for the diagnosis of lung cancer. *J Clin Oncol* 2007;25:5578.
54. Yee J, Sadar MD, Sin DD, et al. Connective tissue-activating peptide III: a novel blood biomarker for early lung cancer detection. *J Clin Oncol* 2009; 27:2787.
55. Chapman CJ, Murray A, McElveen JE, et al. Autoantibodies in lung cancer: possibilities for early detection and subsequent cure. *Thorax* 2008;53:228.
56. Zhong L, Coe SP, Stromberg AJ, et al. Profiling tumor-associated antibodies for early detection of non-small cell lung cancer. *J Thorac Oncol* 2006; 1:513.
57. Qiu J, Choi G, Lin L, et al. Occurrence of autoantibodies to annexin I, 14-3-3 Theta and LAMR1 in prediagnostic lung cancer sera. *J Clin Oncol* 2008;26:5060.
58. Murray A, Chapman CJ, Healey G, et al. Technical validation of an autoantibody test for lung cancer. *Ann Oncol* 2010; doi:10.1093/annonc/mdp606.
59. Phillips M, Altorki N, Austin JHM, et al. Prediction of lung cancer using volatile biomarkers in breath. *Cancer Biomarkers* 2007;3:95.
60. Mazzone PJ. Analysis of volatile organic compounds in the exhaled breath for the diagnosis of lung cancer. *J Thorac Oncol* 2008;3:774.
61. Yuan JM, Koh WP, Murphy SE, et al. Urinary levels of tobacco-specific nitrosamine metabolites in relation to lung cancer development in two prospective cohorts of cigarette smokers. *Cancer Res* 2009;69:2990.
62. Bach PB, Kattan MW, Thornquist MGK, et al. Variations in lung cancer risk among smokers. *J Natl Cancer Inst* 2003;95:470.
63. Spitz MR, Hong WK, Amos CI, et al. A risk model for prediction of lung cancer. *J Natl Cancer Inst* 2007;99:715.
64. Cassidy A, Myles JP, van Tongeren M, et al. The LLP risk model: an individual risk prediction model for lung cancer. *Br J Cancer* 2008;98:270.
65. Wasswa-Kintu S, Gan WQ, Man SFP, et al. Relationship between reduced forced expiratory volume in one second and the risk of lung cancer: a systematic review and meta-analysis. *Thorax* 2005;60:570.
66. Turner MC, Chen Y, Krewski D, et al. Chronic obstructive pulmonary disease is associated with lung cancer mortality in a prospective study of never smokers. *Am J Respir Crit Care Med* 2007;176:285.
67. Jiang F, Todd NW, Liu Z, et al. Combined genetic analysis of sputum and computed tomography for noninvasive diagnosis of non-small-cell lung cancer. *Lung Cancer* 2009;66:58.

CHAPTER 63 GENETIC COUNSELING

ELLEN T. MATLOFF AND DANIELLE CAMPFIELD BONADIES

In the past 15 years clinically based genetic testing has evolved from an uncommon analysis ordered for the rare hereditary cancer family to a widely available tool ordered on a routine basis to assist in surgical decision making, chemoprevention, and surveillance of the patient with cancer, as well as management of the entire family. The evolution of this field has created a need for accurate cancer genetic counseling and risk assessment. Extensive coverage of this topic by the media and widespread advertising by commercial testing laboratories have further fueled the demand for counseling and testing.

Cancer genetic counseling is a communication process between a health care professional and an individual concerning cancer occurrence and risk in his or her family.[1] The process, which may include the entire family through a blend of genetic, medical, and psychosocial assessment and intervention, has been described as a bridge between the fields of traditional oncology and genetic counseling.[1]

The goals of this process include providing the client with an assessment of individual cancer risk, while offering the emotional support needed to understand and cope with this information. It also involves deciphering whether the cancers in a family history are likely to be caused by a mutation in a cancer gene and, if so, *which one*. There are more than 30 hereditary cancer syndromes, many of which can be caused by mutations in different genes. Therefore, testing for these syndromes can be complicated. Advertisements by genetic testing companies bill genetic testing as a simple process that can be carried out by health care professionals who have no training in this area; however, there are many genes involved in cancer, the interpretation of the test results is often complicated, the risk of result misinterpretation is great and associated with potential liability, and the emotional and psychological ramifications for the patient and family can be powerful. A few hours of training by a company generating a profit from the sale of these tests does not adequately prepare providers to offer their own genetic counseling and testing services. Furthermore, the delegation of genetic testing responsibilities to office staff is alarming[2] and likely presents a huge liability for these ordering physicians, their practices, and their institutions. *Providers should proceed with caution before taking on the role of primary genetic counselor for their patients.*

Counseling about hereditary cancers differs from "traditional" genetic counseling in several ways. Clients seeking cancer genetic counseling are rarely concerned with reproductive decisions, which are often the primary focus in traditional genetic counseling, but are instead seeking information about their own and other relatives' chances of developing cancer.[1] Additionally, the risks given are not absolute but change over time as the family and personal history changes and the patient ages. The risk reduction options available are often radical (e.g., chemoprevention or prophylactic surgery) and are not appropriate for every patient at every age. The surveillance and management plan must be tailored to the patient's age, childbearing status, menopausal status, risk category, ease of screening, and personal preferences and will likely change over time with the patient. The ultimate goal of cancer genetic counseling is to help the patient reach the decision best suited to his or her personal situation, needs, and circumstances.

There are now a significant number of referral centers across the country specializing in cancer genetic counseling, and the numbers are growing. However, some experts insist that the only way to keep up with the overwhelming demand for counseling will be to educate more physicians and nurses in cancer genetics. The feasibility of adding another specialized and time-consuming task to the clinical burden of these professionals is questionable, particularly with average patient encounters of 19.5 and 21.6 minutes for general practitioners and gynecologists, respectively.[3,4] A more practical goal may be to better educate primary care providers in the area of generalized risk assessment so that they can screen their patient populations for individuals at high risk for hereditary cancer and refer them on to comprehensive counseling and testing programs. Access to genetic counseling is no longer an issue because there are now Internet, phone, and satellite-based telemedicine services available and several major health insurance companies now cover these services.[5–7]

WHO IS A CANDIDATE FOR CANCER GENETIC COUNSELING?

Only 5% to 10% of most cancers are due to single mutations within autosomal dominant inherited cancer susceptibility genes.[8] The key for clinicians is to determine which patients are at greatest risk to carry a hereditary mutation. There are seven critical risk factors in hereditary cancer (Table 63.1). The first is early age of cancer onset. This risk factor, *even in the absence of a family history,* has been shown to be associated with an increased frequency of germline mutations in many types of cancers.[9] The second risk factor is the presence of the same cancer in multiple affected relatives on the same side of the pedigree. These cancers do not need to be of similar histological type in order to be caused by a single mutation. The third risk factor is the clustering of cancers known to be caused by a single gene mutation in one family (e.g., breast/ovarian/pancreatic cancer or colon/ovarian/uterine cancers). The fourth risk factor is the occurrence of multiple primary cancers in one individual. This includes multiple primary breast or colon cancers as well as a single individual with separate cancers known to be caused by a single gene mutation (e.g., breast and ovarian cancer in a single individual). Ethnicity also plays a role in determining who is at greatest risk to carry a hereditary cancer mutation. Individuals of Jewish ancestry are at increased risk to carry three specific *BRCA1/2* mutations.[10] The presence of a cancer that presents unusually, in

TABLE 63.1

RISK FACTORS THAT WARRANT GENETIC COUNSELING FOR HEREDITARY CANCER SYNDROMES

1. Early age of onset (e.g., <45 years for breast cancer; <50 years for colon and uterine cancer)
2. Multiple family members on the same side of the pedigree with the same cancer
3. Clustering of cancers in the family known to be caused by a single gene mutation (e.g., breast/ovarian/pancreatic; colon/uterine/ovarian; colon cancer/polyps/desmoid tumors/osteomas)
4. Multiple primary cancers in one individual (e.g., breast/ovarian cancer; colon/uterine; synchronous/metachronous colon cancers; >15 gastrointestinal polyps; >5 hamartomatous or juvenile polyps).
5. Ethnicity (e.g., Jewish ancestry for breast/ovarian cancer syndrome)
6. Unusual presentation of cancer/tumor (e.g., breast cancer in a male; medullary thyroid cancer; retinoblastoma; even one sebaceous carcinoma or adenoma)
7. *Pathology** (e.g., medullary breast cancer and triple negative breast cancer are overrepresented in women with hereditary breast and ovarian cancer; a colon tumor with an abnormal microsatellite instability (MSI) or immunohistochemistry (IHC) result increases the risk for a hereditary colon cancer syndrome)

*An evolving area of risk assessment.

this case breast cancer in a male, represents a sixth risk factor and is important even when it is the only risk factor present. Finally, the last risk factor is pathology. This risk factor is listed in Table 63.1 in italics because it is a new and evolving entity. It appears that certain types of cancer are overrepresented in hereditary cancer families. For example, medullary breast cancer appears to be overrepresented in *BRCA1* families[11] and early data suggest that the triple negative breast cancer phenotype (ER-, PR-, her2-) may also be overrepresented in *BRCA1* families[12]; however, breast cancer patients without these pathological findings are *not* necessarily at lower risk to carry a mutation. In contrast, patients with a borderline or mucinous ovarian carcinoma appear to be at lower risk to carry a *BRCA1* or *BRCA2* mutation[13] and may instead carry a mutation in a different gene. It is already well established that medullary thyroid carcinoma, sebaceous adenoma or carcinoma, adrenocortical carcinoma before the age of 25, and multiple adenomatous, hamartomatous, or juvenile colon polyps are indicative of other rare hereditary cancer syndromes.[14,15] These risk factors should be viewed in the context of the entire family history and must be weighed in proportion to the number of individuals who have not developed cancer. Risk assessment is often limited in families that are small or have few female relatives; in such families, a single risk factor may carry more weight.

A less common, but extremely important, finding is the presence of unusual physical findings or birth defects that are known to be associated with rare hereditary cancer syndromes. Examples include benign skin findings, autism, large head circumference[16,17] and thyroid disorders in Cowden syndrome, ontogenic keratocysts in Gorlin syndrome,[18] and desmoid tumors or dental abnormalities in familial adenomatous polyposis (FAP).[19] These and other findings should prompt further investigation of the patient's family history and consideration of a referral to genetic counseling.

In this chapter, the breast or ovarian cancer counseling session with a female patient will serve as a paradigm by which all other sessions may follow broadly.

COMPONENTS OF THE CANCER GENETIC COUNSELING SESSION

Precounseling Information

Before coming in for genetic counseling, the counselee should be given some basic information about the process. This information, which can be imparted by telephone or in the form of written material, should outline what the counselee can expect at each session and what information he or she should collect before the first visit. The counselee can then begin to collect medical and family history information and pathology reports that will be essential for the genetic counseling session.

Family History

An accurate family history is undoubtedly one of the most essential components of the cancer genetic counseling session. Optimally, a family history should include at least three generations; however, patients do not always have this information. For each individual affected with cancer, it is important to document the exact diagnosis, age at diagnosis, treatment strategies, and environmental exposures (i.e., occupational exposures, cigarettes, other agents).[19] The current age of the individual and laterality and occurrence of any other cancers must also be documented. Cancer diagnoses should be confirmed with pathology reports whenever possible. A study by Love et al.[20] revealed that individuals accurately reported the primary site of cancer only 83% of the time in their first-degree relatives with cancer, and 67% and 60% of the time in second- and third-degree relatives, respectively. It is common for patients to report a uterine cancer as an ovarian cancer, or a colon polyp as an invasive colorectal cancer. These differences, although seemingly subtle to the patient, can make a tremendous difference in risk assessment. Individuals should be asked if there are any consanguineous (inbred) relationships in the family, if any relatives were born with birth defects or mental retardation, and whether other genetic diseases run in the family (e.g., Fanconi anemia or Cowden syndrome), as these pieces of information could prove important in reaching a diagnosis.

The most common misconception in family history taking is that somehow a maternal family history of breast, ovarian, or uterine cancer is more significant than a paternal history. Conversely, many still believe that a paternal history of prostate cancer is more significant than a maternal history. Few cancer genes discovered thus far are located on the sex chromosomes, therefore, both maternal and paternal history are significant and must be explored thoroughly. It has also become necessary to elicit the spouse's personal and family history of cancer. This has bearing on the cancer status of common children, but may also determine if children are at increased risk for a serious genetic disease such as Fanconi anemia.[21] Children who inherit two copies of a *BRCA2* mutation are now known to have this serious disorder characterized by defective DNA repair and high rates of birth defects, aplastic anemia, leukemia, and solid tumors.[21] Patients should be encouraged to report changes in their family history over time (e.g., new cancer diagnoses, genetic testing results in relatives), as this may change their risk assessment and counseling.

A detailed family history should also include genetic diseases, birth defects, mental retardation, multiple miscarriages, and infant deaths. A history of certain recessive genetic diseases (e.g., ataxia telangiectasia, Fanconi anemia) can indicate that healthy family members who carry just one copy of the genetic mutation may be at increased risk to develop cancer.[21,22] Other genetic disorders, such as hereditary hemorrhagic telangiectasia, can be associated with a hereditary cancer syndrome caused by a mutation in the same gene, in this case juvenile polyposis.[23]

Dysmorphology Screening

Congenital anomalies, benign tumors, and unusual dermatologic features occur in a large number of hereditary cancer predisposition syndromes. Examples include osteomas of the jaw in FAP, palmar pits in Gorlin syndrome, and papillomas of the lips and mucous membranes in Cowden syndrome. Obtaining an accurate past medical history of benign lesions and birth defects and screening for such dysmorphology can greatly impact diagnosis, counseling, and testing. For example, *BRCA1/2* testing is inappropriate in a patient with breast cancer who has a family history of thyroid cancer and the orocutaneus manifestations of Cowden syndrome.

Risk Assessment

Risk assessment is one of the most complicated components of the genetic counseling session. It is crucial to remember that risk assessment changes over time as the person ages and as the health statuses of their family members change. Risk assessment can be broken down into three separate components:

1. What is the chance that the counselee will develop the cancer observed in his or her family (or a genetically related cancer)?
2. What is the chance that the cancers in this family are caused by a single gene mutation?
3. What is the chance that we can identify the gene mutation in this family with our current knowledge and laboratory techniques?

Cancer clustering in a family may be due to genetic or environmental factors or may be coincidental because some cancers are very common in the general population.[24] Although inherited factors may be the primary cause of cancers in some families, in others, cancer may develop because an inherited factor increases the individual's susceptibility to environmental carcinogens. It is also possible that members of the same family may be exposed to similar environmental exposures, due to shared geography or patterns in behavior and diet, that may increase the risk of cancer.[25] Therefore, it is important to distinguish the difference between a familial pattern of cancer (due to environmental factors or chance) and a hereditary pattern of cancer (due to a shared genetic mutation). Emerging research is also evaluating the role and clinical utility of more common low-penetrance susceptibility genes and single nucleotide polymorphisms (SNPs) that may account for a proportion of familial cancers.[26]

Several models are available to calculate the chance that a woman will develop breast cancer. Each model has its strengths and weaknesses, and the counselor must decide which model is most appropriate for each individual family. The most commonly used models to assess breast cancer risk are the Gail and Claus models.[27,28] Computer-based models are also available to help determine the chance that a *BRCA* mutation will be found in a family.[29] However, these models have many limitations and cannot factor in other risks that may be essential in hereditary risk calculation (e.g., a sister who was diagnosed with breast cancer after radiation treatment for Hodgkin's lymphoma).

DNA Testing

DNA testing is now available for a variety of hereditary cancer syndromes. However, despite misrepresentation by the media, testing is feasible for only a small percentage of individuals with cancer. DNA testing offers the important advantage of presenting clients with *actual risks* instead of the empiric risks derived from risk calculation models. DNA testing can be very expensive (full sequencing of the *BRCA1/2* genes currently costs more than $3,300). Patients deemed high risk should also be offered *BRCA* rearrangement testing (BART), which looks for large structural rearrangements within these genes. It is the clinician's responsibility to discuss and order this test separately (an additional $700). Importantly, testing should begin in an affected family member, whenever possible. Most insurance companies now cover cancer genetic testing in families where the test is medically indicated.

The results of DNA testing are generally provided in person in a result disclosure session. It is recommended that patients bring a close friend or relative with them to this session who can provide them with emotional support and who can help them listen to and process the information provided.

One of the most crucial aspects of DNA testing is accurate result interpretation. One study found that test results for the hereditary colon cancer syndrome FAP were misinterpreted more than 30% of the time by those ordering the testing.[30] More recent data have shown that many medical providers have difficulty interpreting even basic pedigrees and genetic test results.[31–33] In a survey of over 2,000 physicians, only 13% of internists, 21% of obstetricians or gynecologists, and 40% of oncologists correctly answered four basic knowledge questions about genetic aspects of breast cancer and *BRCA* testing. This deficiency in knowledge did not necessarily deter them from discussing or ordering testing.[4] Misinterpretation of results is now the greatest risk of genetic testing, and it is very common.[34] Interpretation is becoming increasingly complicated as more tests become available. For example, one study demonstrated that approximately 12% of high-risk families who test negative by standard *BRCA1* and *BRCA2* testing are found to carry a deletion or duplication in one of these genes or a mutation in another gene.[35] This is particularly concerning in an era in which testing companies are canvassing physicians' offices and are encouraging them to perform their own counseling and testing. The potential impact of test results on the patient and his or her family is great, therefore, accurate interpretation of the results is paramount. The U.S. Preventive Services Task Force recommends that women whose family history is suggestive of a *BRCA* mutation be referred for genetic counseling before being offered genetic testing.[36]

Results of genetic testing fall into five categories:

1. *True positive:* an individual is found to carry a mutation that is known to be deleterious;
2. *True negative:* an individual does not carry the deleterious mutation found in her family, therefore, her cancer risks are reduced to the population risks;
3. *Negative:* a mutation was not detected and the cancers in the family are not likely to be hereditary based on the personal and family history assessment;
4. *Uninformative:* a mutation cannot be found in affected members of a family in which the cancer pattern appears to be hereditary; there is likely an undetectable mutation within the gene, or the family carries a mutation in a different gene. These results are not "true negative" and do *not* mean that the cancers are not hereditary;

5. *Variant of uncertain significance:* a genetic change is identified whose significance is unknown. It is helpful to test other *affected* family members to see if the mutation segregates with disease in the family. If it does not segregate, the variant is less likely to be significant. If it does, the variant is more likely to be significant. Other tools, including a splice site predictor, in conjunction with data on species conservation and amino acid difference scores, can also be helpful in determining the likelihood that a variant is significant. It is rarely helpful (and can be detrimental) to test *unaffected* family members for such variants.

In order to pinpoint the mutation in a family, an affected individual most likely to carry the mutation should be tested first, whenever possible. This is most often a person affected with the cancer in question at the earliest age. Test subjects should be selected with care, as it is possible for a person to develop sporadic cancer in a hereditary cancer family. For example, in an early onset breast cancer family, it would not be ideal to first test a woman diagnosed with breast cancer at age 65, as she may represent a sporadic case.

If a mutation is detected in an affected relative, other family members can be tested for the same mutation with a great degree of accuracy. Family members who do not carry the mutation found in their family are deemed "true negative." Those who are found to carry the mutation in their family will have more definitive information about their risks to develop cancer. This information can be crucial in assisting patients in decision making regarding surveillance and risk reduction.

If a mutation is not identified in the affected relative, this usually means that either the cancers in the family (1) are not hereditary or (2) are caused by an undetectable mutation or a mutation in a different gene. A careful review of the family history and the risk factors will help to decipher whether interpretation (1) or (2) is more likely. Additional genetic testing may need to be ordered at this point. In cases in which the cancers appear hereditary and no mutation is found, DNA banking should be offered to the proband for a time in the future when improved testing may become available. A letter indicating exactly who in the family has access to the DNA should accompany the banked sample.

The penetrance of mutations in cancer susceptibility genes is also difficult to interpret. Initial estimates derived from high-risk families provided very high cancer risks for *BRCA1* and *BRCA2* mutation carriers.[37] More recent studies done on populations that were not selected for family history have revealed lower penetrances.[38] Because exact penetrance rates cannot be determined for individual families at this time, and because precise genotype and phenotype correlations remain unclear, it is prudent to provide patients with a range of cancer risk and to explain that their risk probably falls somewhere within this spectrum.

Female carriers of *BRCA1* and *BRCA2* mutations have a 50% to 85% lifetime risk to develop breast cancer and between a 15% to 60% lifetime risk to develop ovarian cancer.[10,37,38] It is important to note that the classification "ovarian cancer" also includes cancer of the fallopian tubes and primary peritoneal carcinoma.[39,40] *BRCA2* carriers also have an increased lifetime risk of male breast cancer, pancreatic cancer, and possibly melanoma.[41,42] Carriers of Lynch syndrome mutations (also known as hereditary nonpolyposis colorectal cancer [HNPCC]) have a 65% to 85% lifetime risk to develop colon cancer, and female carriers have at least a 40% to 60% lifetime risk of uterine cancer and as great as a 10% to 12% risk of ovarian cancer.[43,44] Individuals with Lynch syndrome may also be at some increased risk for a variety of other types of cancers, including head and neck and other gastrointestinal, urinary tract, and hematological malignancies.

Options for Surveillance and Risk Reduction

The cancer risk counseling session is a forum to provide counselees with information, support, options, and hope. Mutation carriers can be offered earlier and more aggressive surveillance, chemoprevention, or prophylactic surgery. Surveillance recommendations are evolving with newer techniques and additional data.

At this time, it is recommended that individuals at increased risk for breast cancer, particularly those who carry a *BRCA* mutation, have annual mammograms beginning at age 25, with a clinical breast examination by a breast specialist, a yearly breast magnetic resonance imaging (MRI) with a clinical breast examination by a breast specialist, and a yearly clinical breast examination by a gynecologist.[45,46] It is suggested that the mammogram and MRI be spaced out around the calendar year so that some intervention is planned every 6 months. Recent data suggest that MRI may be safer and more effective in *BRCA* carriers younger than 40 years and may someday replace mammograms in this population.[47]

BRCA carriers may take tamoxifen or raloxifene (Evista) in hopes of reducing their risks of developing breast cancer. Both of these medications are selective estrogen receptor modulators (SERMs) that have been proven effective in women at risk due to a positive family history of breast cancer.[48,49] There are limited data on the effectiveness of prophylactic SERMs in *BRCA* carriers[50–52]; however, there are some data to suggest that *BRCA* carriers taking tamoxifen as treatment for a breast cancer reduce their risk of a contralateral breast cancer.[53] Additionally, the majority of *BRCA2* carriers who develop breast cancer develop an estrogen-positive form of the disease,[54] and it is hoped that this population will respond especially well to chemoprevention. Further studies in this area are necessary before drawing conclusions about the efficacy of SERMs in this population. Prophylactic bilateral mastectomy appears to reduce the risk of breast cancer by greater than 90% in women at high risk for the disease.[55] Before genetic testing was available, it was not uncommon for entire generations of cancer families to have at-risk tissues removed without knowing if they were *personally* at increased risk for their familial cancer. Fifty percent of unaffected individuals in hereditary cancer families will *not* carry the inherited predisposition gene and can be spared prophylactic surgery or invasive high-risk surveillance regimens. Therefore, it is clearly not appropriate to offer prophylactic surgery until a patient is referred for genetic counseling and, if possible, testing.[56]

Women who carry *BRCA1/2* mutations are also at increased risk to develop second contralateral and ipsilateral primaries of the breast.[57] These data bring into question the option of breast-conserving surgery in women at high risk to develop a second primary within the same breast. For this reason, *BRCA1/2* carrier status can have a profound impact on surgical decision making,[56] and many patients have genetic counseling and testing immediately after diagnosis and before surgery or radiation therapy. Those patients who test positive and opt for prophylactic mastectomy can often be spared radiation and the resulting side effects that can complicate reconstruction. Approximately 30% to 60% of previously irradiated patients who later opt for mastectomy with reconstruction report significant complications or unfavorable aesthetic results.[58,59]

Women who carry *BRCA1/2* mutations are also at increased risk to develop ovarian, fallopian tube, and primary peritoneal cancer, even if no one in their family has developed these cancers. Surveillance for ovarian cancer is complex, with the recommended interventions being annual transvaginal ultrasounds and cancer antigen 125 (CA 125) levels beginning between the ages of 25 to 35 years.[60] The effectiveness of such surveillance in detecting ovarian cancers at early, more treatable stages has not been proven in any population. Some data have indicated that oral contraceptives reduce the risk of ovarian cancer in women carrying *BRCA* mutations.[61] Recent data indicate that the impact of this intervention on increasing breast cancer risk, if any, is low.[52,62] Given the difficulties in screening and treatment of ovarian cancer, risk–benefit analysis likely favors the use of oral contraceptives in young carriers of *BRCA1/2* mutations[25] who are not yet ready to have their ovaries removed. Prophylactic bilateral salpingo-oophorectomy (BSO) is currently the most effective means to reduce the risk of ovarian cancer and is recommended to *BRCA1/2* carriers by the age of 40 or when child bearing is complete.[63] Specific operative and pathologic protocols have been developed for this prophylactic surgery.[64] In *BRCA1/2* carriers whose pathology comes back normal, this surgery is highly effective in reducing the subsequent risk of ovarian cancer.[65] A decision analysis comparing various surveillance and risk-reducing options available to *BRCA* carriers has shown an increase in life expectancy if BSO is pursued by age 40.[66] A relatively small percentage of women who undergo this procedure may develop primary peritoneal carcinoma.[39,67] There has been some debate about whether *BRCA1/2* carriers should opt for total abdominal hysterectomies (TAH) versus BSO due to the fact that small stumps of the fallopian tubes remain after BSO alone. The question of whether or not *BRCA* carriers are at increased risk for uterine serous papillary carcinoma (USPC) has also been raised.[68–70] If a relationship does exist between *BRCA* mutations and uterine cancer, the risk appears to be low and not elevated over that of the general population.[71] Removing the uterus may make it possible for a *BRCA* carrier to take unopposed estrogen or tamoxifen in the future without risk of uterine cancer, but this surgery is associated with a longer recovery time and has more side effects than does BSO. Each patient should be counseled about the pros and cons of each procedure.

A secondary, but important, reason for female *BRCA* carriers to consider prophylactic oophorectomy is that it also significantly reduces the risk of a subsequent breast cancer, if they have this surgery before menopause.[72,73] The reduction in breast cancer risk remains even if a healthy premenopausal carrier elects to take low-dose hormone replacement therapy (HRT) after this surgery.[74] Early data suggest that tamoxifen in addition to premenopausal oophorectomy in *BRCA* carriers may have little additional benefit in terms of breast cancer risk reduction.[75] Research is needed in balancing quality of life issues secondary to estrogen deprivation with cancer risk reduction in these young female *BRCA1/2* carriers.

The standard surveillance method in carriers of Lynch syndrome mutations is full colonoscopy to the cecum every 1 to 2 years beginning between the ages of 20 to 25 years.[76] While several studies are investigating chemopreventive options for colorectal cancer, no agents are currently approved for clinical use. Total colectomy with ileorectal anastomosis is an option for patients upon a diagnosis of colon cancer. *Prophylactic* colectomy is *usually* not recommended as regular screening and polypectomy is generally effective; however, a decision analysis revealed that this procedure may offer slightly greater gains in life expectancy for young Lynch syndrome carriers than surveillance alone.[77,78] Quality of life issues must be weighed against the rate of detecting cancer at an early, treatable stage with surveillance alone.

Options for endometrial and ovarian cancer surveillance include educating patients about the symptoms of endometrial cancer and consideration of endometrial biopsies, transvaginal ultrasound, and CA 125 tumor marker screening beginning at age 30.[79] The efficacy of such surveillance in Lynch syndrome carriers is unknown. Oral contraceptives are known to reduce the risk of both ovarian and endometrial cancer in the general population,[80] but the impact of this intervention in Lynch syndrome carriers, or on colon cancer risk, is currently unknown. Prophylactic total hysterectomy is also an option. Recent data suggest that this surgery is effective in significantly reducing the risk of both ovarian and uterine cancer in women with Lynch syndrome and should be considered after the age of 35 or once childbearing is completed.[44,79] Screening should also be considered for cancers of the upper gastrointestinal, urinary tract, central nervous system, and hepatobiliary tract as well as dermatologic findings.[79] Breast cancer is commonly misperceived as part of the spectrum of cancers seen in Lynch syndrome. Although it is a common cancer and can be seen with colon cancers in other rare syndromes (e.g., Peutz-Jeghers), the rate of breast cancer is not increased in Lynch syndrome mutation–positive families.[81]

Genetic counseling and testing are also available for many rare cancer syndromes, including von Hippel-Lindau, multiple endocrine neoplasias, and FAP. Surveillance and risk reduction for patients who are known mutation carriers for such conditions may decrease the associated morbidity and mortality of these syndromes.

Follow-Up

A follow-up letter to the patient is a concrete means of documenting the information conveyed in the sessions so that the patient and his or her family members can review it over time. This letter should be sent to the patient and health care professionals to whom the patient has granted access to this information. A follow-up phone call or counseling session may also be helpful, particularly in the case of a positive test result. Some programs provide patients with an annual or biannual newsletter updating them on new information in the field of cancer genetics or patient support groups. It is now recommended that patients return for follow-up counseling sessions months, or even years, after their initial consult to discuss advances in genetic testing and changes in surveillance and risk-reduction options. This can be beneficial for individuals who have been found to carry a hereditary predisposition, for those in whom a syndrome or mutation is suspected but yet unidentified, and for those who are ready to move forward with genetic testing. Follow-up counseling is also recommended for patients whose life circumstances have changed (e.g., preconception, after child bearing is complete), are preparing for prophylactic surgery, or are ready to discuss the family genetics with their children.

ISSUES IN CANCER GENETIC COUNSELING

Psychosocial Issues

The psychosocial impact of cancer genetic counseling cannot be underestimated. Just the process of scheduling a cancer risk counseling session may be quite difficult for some individuals with a family history who are not only frightened about their own cancer risk but are reliving painful experiences associated with the cancer of their loved ones.[8] Counselees may be faced with an onslaught of emotions, including anger, fear of developing cancer, fear of disfigurement and dying, grief, lack of control, negative body image, and a sense of isolation.[19] Some counselees are wrestling with the fear that insurance companies, employers, family members, and even future partners will react negatively to their cancer risks. For many it is a double-edged sword as they balance their fears and apprehensions about dredging up these issues with the possibility of obtaining reassuring news and much needed information.

A person's perceived cancer risk is often dependent on many "nonmedical" variables. They may estimate that their risk is higher if they look like an affected individual or share some of their personality traits.[19] Their perceived risks will vary depending on whether their relatives were cancer survivors or died painful deaths from the disease. Many people wonder not *if* they are going to get cancer but *when*.

The counseling session is an opportunity for individuals to express why they believe they have developed cancer or why their family members have cancer. Some explanations may revolve around family folklore, and it is important to listen to and address these explanations rather than dismiss them.[19] In doing this the counselor will allow the clients to alleviate their greatest fears and to give more credibility to the "medical" theory. Understanding a patient's perceived cancer risk is important in that fear may *decrease* surveillance and preventive health care behaviors.[82] For patients and families who are moving forward with DNA testing, a referral to a mental health care professional is often very helpful. Genetic testing has an impact not only on the patient but also on his or her children, siblings, parents, and extended relatives. This can be overwhelming for an individual and the family and should be discussed in detail prior to testing.

To date, studies conducted in the setting of pre- and postgenetic counseling have revealed that, at least in the short term, most patients do not experience adverse psychological outcomes after receiving their test results.[83,84] In fact, preliminary data have revealed that individuals in families with known mutations who seek testing seem to fare better psychologically at 6 months than those who avoid testing.[83] Among individuals who learn they are *BRCA* mutation carriers, anxiety and distress levels appear to increase slightly after receiving their test results but returned to pretest levels in several weeks.[85] Although these data are reassuring, it is important to recognize that genetic testing is an individual decision and will not be right for every patient or every family.

Presymptomatic Testing in Children

Presymptomatic testing in children has been widely discussed, and most concur that it is appropriate only when the onset of the condition regularly occurs in childhood or there are useful interventions that can be applied.[86] For example, genetic testing for mutations in the *BRCA* genes and other adult-onset diseases is generally limited to individuals who are older than 18 years of age. The American College of Medical Genetics states that if the "medical or psychosocial benefits of a genetic test will not accrue until adulthood . . . genetic testing generally should be deferred."[87] In contrast, DNA-based diagnosis of children and young adults at risk for hereditary medullary thyroid carcinoma (MTC) is appropriate and has improved the management of these patients.[88] DNA-based testing for MTC is virtually 100% accurate and allows at-risk family members to make informed decisions about prophylactic thyroidectomy. FAP is a disorder that occurs in childhood, and mortality can be reduced if detection is presymptomatic.[89] Testing is clearly indicated in these instances.

Questions have been raised about parents' right to demand testing for adult-onset diseases. Parents may have a constitutionally protected right to demand that unwilling physicians order this test, but there is little risk for liability for damages unless the child suffers physical harm as a direct result of this refusal.[86] The child's right *not* to be tested must be considered. Whenever childhood testing is not medically indicated, it is preferable that testing decisions are postponed until the children are adults and can decide for themselves whether or not to be tested.

Confidentiality

The level of confidentiality surrounding cancer genetic testing is paramount due to concerns of genetic discrimination. Some programs opt to keep shadow files, keep their databases offline, limit patient information in e-mails, and take precautions to protect confidentially when leaving voice mail messages for patients. Genetic counseling summary letters are often sent directly to patients and are copied to the referring physicians only with the explicit permission of the patient. These measures are taken because confidentiality and genetic discrimination are a grave concern for many of the patients seen in the cancer genetic counseling clinic.[90]

Confidentiality of test results *within* a family can also be of issue, as genetic counseling and testing often reveal the risk statuses of family members other than the patient. Under confidentiality codes, the patient needs to grant permission before at-risk family members can be contacted. It has been questioned whether or not a family member could sue a health care professional for negligence if they were identified at high risk yet not informed.[91] Most recommendations have stated that the burden of confidentiality lies between the provider and the patient. However, more recent recommendations state that confidentiality *should* be violated if the potential harm of not notifying other family members outweighs the harm of breaking a confidence to the patient.[92] There is no patent solution for this difficult dilemma, and situations must be considered on a case-by-case basis with the assistance of the in-house legal department and ethics committee.

Patients should be counseled about the benefits to other family members of knowing testing results, but, at the present time, the decision is ultimately the patient's. Extended family members who are notified, with the patient's consent, may not always be grateful to receive this information and may feel that their privacy has been invaded by being contacted.

Insurance and Discrimination Issues

When genetic testing for cancer predisposition first became widely available, the fear of health insurance discrimination—by both patients and providers—was one of the most common concerns.[90,93] It appears that the risks of health insurance discrimination were overstated and that almost no discrimination by health insurers has been reported.[94] In May 2008 Congress passed the Genetic Information Nondiscrimination Act (GINA) (HR 493) that provides broad protection of an individual's genetic information against health insurance and employment discrimination.[95] Health care providers can now more confidently reassure their patients that genetic counseling and testing will not put them at risk of losing group or individual health insurance. In addition, the 2010 Heath Care reform (HR 4872) will prohibit group health plans from denying insurance based on pre-existing conditions and from increasing premiums based on health status.[96] These protections have been enacted for children and are slated to take effect in 2010 for adults.

More and more patients are choosing to submit their genetic counseling or testing charges to their health insurance companies. In the past few years, more insurance companies have agreed to pay for counseling or testing,[97] perhaps in light of decision analyses that show these services and subsequent prophylactic surgeries to be cost-effective.[98] The risk of life or disability insurance discrimination, however, is more realistic.

Patients should be counseled about such risks before they pursue genetic testing.

FUTURE DIRECTIONS

The field of cancer genetic counseling and testing has grown tremendously over the past 15 years. Although cancer genetic counseling has traditionally been targeted at individuals with strong personal or family histories of cancer, this focus has broadened. Genetic counseling and testing is now offered to patients who have been diagnosed with early onset breast and colon cancer as a critical tool to guide surgical and radiation decision making, as the risk of new primaries is greater in individuals who carry germline mutations.[56,57]

Clinicians should be aware that research continues to identify new cancer susceptibility genes and SNPs that may be associated with cancer risks. Therefore, the clinician should elicit and update a family history from each patient, determine if they are at increased risk for a hereditary cancer syndrome, and, if so, refer them to genetic counseling. Low-penetrance, highly prevalent genes and SNPs continue to be identified and have been associated with breast, colon, prostate, and other cancers.[99–104] The clinical utility of germline genetic testing for these mutations is under investigation because they are modifying markers with relatively low risks, and it is unclear whether they will be useful in guiding decisions regarding prevention and early detection. For example, the risks associated with most of these markers confer a one- to twofold increased risk of cancer, compared with up to 50-fold risk seen with mutations in the *BRCA* genes. Therefore, surveillance recommendations in lower-risk families can often be made based on the family history alone, without the need for genetic testing. Individuals with *no* family history of cancer may actually derive the most benefit from such testing, as a positive test result would elucidate which patients in that population would benefit from increased surveillance. A shift in emphasis from rare, high-penetrance mutation screening in high-risk families to broad screening for lower-penetrance mutations in lower risk populations could change the face of the field of cancer genetic counseling.

Additionally, technology to perform whole exome and whole genome sequencing is becoming more wildly available. These tests can identify mutations associated with rare and common disorders that may be overlooked by targeted, single-gene testing. The cost of this technology continues to decrease and now costs, roughly, just a few hundred dollars more than full testing for *BRCA1* and *BRCA2*. However, the feasibility of translating millions of base pairs into clinically useful information and ways to deliver and utilize that information in a patient-care setting need to be further investigated.

A remarkable limitation of this technology in the field of cancer genetics are specific gene patents that prohibit testing and reporting of genetic variants found in these regions. In particular, the U.S. Patent and Trademark Office issued patents on the *BRCA1* and *BRCA2* genes. Although various researchers contributed to the identification of these genes, patent rights were granted to the privately owned biotech firm Myriad Genetics.[105] As the exclusive patent holder, Myriad has opted to strictly enforce its monopoly rights and is the only laboratory in the country where diagnostic testing can be performed. In 2009, the American Civil Liberties Union filed suit against Myriad and the U.S. Patent and Trademark Office, arguing that the patents are illegal because genes are "products of nature." According to the lawsuit, researchers and scientists are prevented from studying testing and developing alternative tests because of the strict control of these genes. Several of the patents were overturned in a March 29, 2010, ruling. Judge Robert Sweet stated that purification of DNA does not change the essential characteristic of DNA and is therefore not a patentable product.[106] If the ruling is upheld, precedent will be set about how gene patents are issued and genetic counselors, clinicians, and researchers will be able to engage freely in research, testing, and clinical practice involving these genes. Patients would also have access to genetic testing services from multiple, and perhaps more affordable, sources.

New developments are also emerging in the treatment and possibly prevention of *BRCA*-related cancers. Several small studies have evaluated the effect of poly adenosine diphosphate [ADP]-ribose polymerases (PARP) inhibitors in combination with chemotherapy for cancer treatment. It appears that PARP inhibitors are particularly effective in patients with *BRCA* mutations.[107–108] Future studies will focus on the use of PARP inhibitors in earlier stage cancers in *BRCA* carriers, cancers in women with triple negative breast cancers, and *BRCA* carriers in the prevention setting.

Reproductive technology in the form of preimplantation genetic diagnosis is also an option[109] for men and women with a hereditary cancer syndrome, but one that is requested by few patients for adult-onset conditions in which there are viable options for surveillance and risk reduction. The option of sperm selection to increase the likelihood of having a male fetus (or vice versa for a condition that affects mostly males) can be discussed if parents are looking for preconception options. If a *BRCA2* carrier is considering having a child, it is important to assess the spouse's risk of also carrying a *BRCA2* mutation. If the spouse is of Jewish ancestry or has a personal or family history of breast, ovarian, or pancreatic cancer, *BRCA* testing should be considered and a discussion of the risk of Fanconi anemia in a child with two *BRCA2* mutations should take place.[110]

The combination of technological advances in genetic testing, new pharmacological developments for cancer risk reduction, and increased utility for testing in high- and moderate-risk populations will result in a significant expansion in the field of cancer genetic counseling. Maintenance of high standards for thorough genetic counseling, informed consent, and accurate result interpretation will be paramount in reducing potential risks and maximizing the benefits of this technology in the next century.

CANCER SCREENING

Selected References

The full list of references for this chapter appears in the online version.

1. Peters J. Breast cancer genetics: relevance to oncology practice. *Cancer Control* 1995;2(3):195.
4. Doksum T, Bernhardt BA, Holtzman NA. Does knowledge about the genetics of breast cancer differ between nongeneticist physicians who do or do not discuss or order BRCA testing? *Genet Med* 2003;(2):99.
8. Claus E, Schildkraut J, Thompson W, et al. The genetic attributable risks of breast and ovarian cancer. *Cancer* 1996;77:2318.
10. Struewing J, Hartge P, Wacholder S. The risk of cancer associated with specific mutations of BRCA1 and BRCA2 among Ashkenazi Jews. *N Engl J Med* 1997;336:1401.
11. Eisinger F, Jacquemier J, Charpin C, et al. Mutations at BRCA1: the medullary breast carcinoma revisited. *Cancer Res* 1998;58:1588.
12. Kandel M, Stadler Z, Masciari S, et al. Prevalence of BRCA1 mutations in triple negative breast cancer. Presented at the 42nd Annual ASCO Meeting, Atlanta, Georgia, 2006.
15. Matloff E, Brierley K, Chimera C. A clinician's guide to hereditary colon cancer. *Cancer J* 2004;10(5):280.

16. Pilarski R. Cowden syndrome: a critical review of the clinical literature. *J Genet Couns* 2009;18(1):13.
19. Schneider K. *Counseling about cancer: strategies for genetic counseling*, 2nd ed. New York: Wiley-Liss, 2001.
26. Stratton MR, Rahman N. The emerging landscape of breast cancer susceptibility. *Nat Genet* 2008;40(1):17.
30. Giardiello F, Brensinger J, Petersen G. The use and interpretation of commercial APC gene testing for familial adenomatous polyposis. *N Engl J Med* 1997;336:823.
31. Brierley K, Kim K, Matloff E, et al. Obstetricians' and gynecologists' knowledge, interests, and current practices with regard to providing breast and ovarian cancer genetic counseling. *J Genet Couns* 2001; 10:438.
34. Friedman S. Thoughts from FORCE: comments submitted to the Secretary's Advisory Committee on Genetics Health and Society, 2008. World Wide Web URL: http://facingourrisk.wordpress.com/2008/12/03/comments-submitted-to-the-secretarys-advisory-committee-on-genetics-health-and-society/.
35. Walsh T, Casadei S, Coats K, et al. Spectrum of mutations in BRCA1, BRCA2, CHEK2, and TP53 in families at high risk of breast cancer. *JAMA* 2006;295(12):1379.
36. Genetic risk assessment and BRCA mutation testing for breast and ovarian cancer susceptibility. Topic page. September 2005. U.S. Preventive Services Task Force. Agency for Healthcare Research and Quality, Rockville, MD. World Wide Web URL: http://www.ahrq.gov/clinic/uspstf/uspsbrgen.htm.
37. Ford D, Easton D, Bishop D, et al. Risks of cancer in BRCA1 mutation carriers. *Lancet* 1994;343:692.
38. Antoniou A, Pharoah P, Narod S, et al. Average risks of breast and ovarian cancer associated with BRCA1 or BRCA2 mutations detected in case series unselected for family history: a combined analyses of 22 studies. *Am J Hum Genet* 2003;72:1117.
41. van Asperen C, Brohet R, Meijers-Heijboer, et al. Cancer risks in BRCA2 families: estimates for sites other than breast and ovary. *J Med Genet* 2005;42:711.
43. Aarnio M, Mecklin J-P, Aaltonen L. Lifetime risk of different cancers in hereditary non-polyposis colorectal cancer (HNPCC) syndrome. *Int J Cancer* 1995;64:430.
44. Schmeler K, Lynch H, Chen L, et al. Prophylactic surgery to reduce the risk of gynecologic cancers in the Lynch syndrome. *N Engl J Med* 2006;354(3):261.
45. Warner E, Plewes D, Hill K, et al. Surveillance of BRCA1 and BRCA2 mutation carriers with magnetic resonance imaging, ultrasound, mammography, and clinical breast examination. *JAMA* 2004;202(11):1317.
46. Kriege M, Brekelmans CT, Boetes C, et al. Efficacy of MRI and mammography for breast-cancer screening in women with a familial or genetic predisposition. *N Engl J Med* 2004;29:351(5):427.
51. King M, Wieand S, Hale K. Tamoxifen and breast cancer incidence among women with inherited mutations in BRCA1 and BRCA2. *JAMA* 2001;286:2251.
52. Narod S, Brunet J, Ghadirian P. Tamoxifen and risk of contralateral breast cancer in BRCA1 and BRCA2 mutation carriers: a case-control study. *Lancet* 2000;356:1876.
53. Metcalfe K, Lynch H, Ghadirian P, et al. Contralateral breast cancer in BRCA1 and BRCA2 mutation carriers. *J Clin Ocol* 2004;22:2328–35.
54. Lakhani S, van de Vijver M, Jacquemier J, et al. The pathology of familial breast cancer: predictive value of immunohistochemical markers estrogen receptor, progesterone receptor, HER-2, and p53 in patients with mutations in BRCA1 and BRCA2. *J Clin Oncol* 2002;20(9):2310.
55. Hartmann L, Schaid D, Woods J. Efficacy of bilateral prophylactic mastectomy in women with a family history of breast cancer. *N Engl J Med* 1999;340:77.
56. Matloff E. The breast surgeon's role in BRCA1 and BRCA2 testing. *Am J Surg* 2000;180(4):294.
57. Turner B, Harold E, Matloff E, et al. BRCA1/BRCA2 germline mutations in locally recurrent breast cancer patients after lumpectomy and radiation therapy: implications for breast-conserving management in patients with BRCA1/BRCA2 mutations. *J Clin Oncol* 1999;17(10):3017.
59. Forman DL, Chiu J, Restifo RJ, et al. Breast reconstruction in previously irradiated patients using tissue expanders and implants: a potentially unfavorable result. *Ann Plast Surg* 1998;40(4):360.
62. Milne R, Knight J, John E, et al. Oral contraceptive use and risk of early-onset breast cancer in carriers and noncarriers of BRCA1 and BRCA2 mutations. *Cancer Epidemiol Biomark Prev* 2005;14(2):350.
63. Domchek S, Friebel T, Neuhausen S, et al. Mortality reduction after risk-reducing bilateral salpingo-oophorectomy in a prospective cohort of BRCA1 and BRCA2 mutation carriers. *Lancet Oncol* 2006;7(3):223.
64. Powel CB, Kenley E, Chen LM, et al. Risk-reducing salpingo-oophorectomy in BRCA mutation carriers: role of serial sectioning in the detection of occult malignancy. *J Clin Oncol* 2005;23(1):127.
65. Finch A, Beiner M, Lubinski J, et al. Salpingo-oophorectomy and the risk of ovarian, fallopian tube, and peritoneal cancers in women with a BRCA1 or BRCA2 mutation. *JAMA* 2006;296(2):185.
66. Kurian AW, Sigal BM, Plevritis SK. Survival analysis of cancer risk reduction strategies for BRCA1/2 mutation carriers. *J Clin Oncol* 2010: 10;28(2):222.
72. Rebbeck T, Lynch H, Neuhausen S, et al. Prophylactic oophorectomy in carriers of BRCA1 or BRCA2 mutations. *N Engl J Med* 2002; 346(21):1616.
73. Kauff N, Satagopan J, Robson M, et al. Risk-reducing salpingo-oophorectomy in women with a BRCA1 or BRCA2 mutation. *N Engl J Med* 2002;346(21):1609.
74. Rebbeck T, Friebel T, Wagner T, et al. Effect of short-term hormone replacement therapy on breast cancer risk reduction after bilateral prophylactic oophorectomy in BRCA1 and BRCA2 mutation carriers: the PROSE study group. *J Clin Oncol* 2005;23(31):7804.
75. Gronwald J, Tung N, Foulkes W, et al. Tamoxifen and contralateral breast cancer in BRCA1 and BRCA2 carriers: an update. *Int J Cancer* 2006;118(9):2281.
76. Lindor NM, Petersen GM, Hadley DW, et al. Recommendations for the care of individuals with an inherited predisposition to Lynch syndrome: a systematic review. *JAMA* 2006;296:1507.
77. Syngal S, Weeks J, Schrag D. Benefits of colonoscopic surveillance and prophylactic colectomy in patients with hereditary nonpolyposis colorectal cancer mutations. *Ann Intern Med* 1998;129:787.
78. Kohlman W, Gruber SB. Hereditary non-polyposis colon cancer. World Wide Web URL: http://www.ncbi.nlm.nih.gov/bookshelf/br.fcgi?book=gene&part=hnpcc.
79. Burt RW, Barthel JS, Dunn KB, et al. NCCN clinical practice guidelines in oncology. Colorectal cancer screening. *J Natl Compr Cancer Netw* 2010;8(1):8.
87. ASHG/ACMG. 1995. Points to consider: ethical, legal, and psychosocial implications of genetic testing in children and adolescents. American Society of Human Genetics Board of Directors, American College of Medical Genetics Board of Directors. *Am J Hum Genet* 1995; 57:1233.
88. Ledger G, Khosia S, Lindor N, et al. Genetic testing in the diagnosis and management of multiple endocrine neoplasia type II. *Ann Intern Med* 1995;122(2):118.
89. Rhodes M, Bradburn D. Overview of screening and management of familial adenomatous polyposis. *Br J Surg* 1992;33(1):125.
95. Library of Congress. Genetic Information Nondiscrimination Act of 2008 (H.R. 493). World Wide Web URL: http://thomas.loc.gov/cgi-bin/bdquery/z?d110:h.r.00493:.
96. Library of Congress. Health Care and Education Affordability Reconciliation Act of 2010 (H.R. 4872). World Wide Web URL: http://thomas.loc.gov/cgi-bin/bdquery/z?d111:HR4872:.
100. Easton DF, Pooley KA, Dunning AM, et al. Genome-wide association study identifies novel breast cancer susceptibility loci. *Nature* 2007;447(7148):1087.
106. Kesselheim AS, Mello MM. Gene patenting—Is the pendulum swinging back? *N Engl J Med* 2010;362(20):1855.

PART SEVEN
SPECIALIZED TECHNIQUES IN CANCER MANAGEMENT

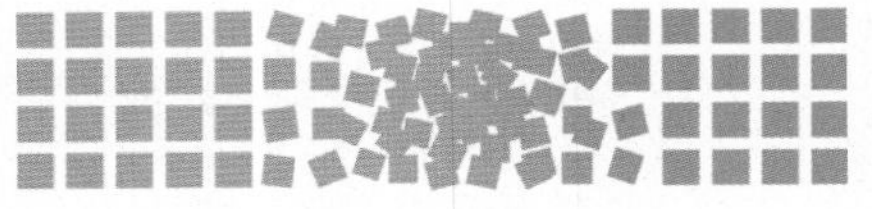

CHAPTER 64 VASCULAR ACCESS AND SPECIALIZED TECHNIQUES

JAMES F. PINGPANK, Jr.

The development of increasingly complex treatment regimens for patients with advanced malignancies has led to a greater reliance on a variety of intra-arterial and intravenous delivery systems. Long-term access may be required for chemotherapy, total parenteral nutrition, or analgesics. Since the introduction of indwelling catheters and infusion systems in 1973, changes and improvements in design have resulted in the development of a diverse group of products to meet specific treatment goals.[1,2] A basic understanding of the selection and maintenance of these devices is important for all clinicians who care for cancer patients. This chapter reviews the issues surrounding catheter selection, insertion techniques, maintenance, and management of frequent catheter-related complications.

CATHETER TYPES

A diverse group of catheters is available, each with their own strengths and weaknesses. Issues critical to the selection of a specific catheter include the number and type of agents to be infused, the length and frequency of the proposed treatment, the use of bolus versus continuous-infusion administration schedules, the potential need for frequent blood draws or the administration of blood products, along with patient and physician preference. Most catheters are venous, all designed for access to the central venous system. The most useful division of catheter systems is between those with an external component and completely implanted devices, which are accessed percutaneously (Table 64.1). Intra-arterial delivery systems are considered separately.

External Catheters

Catheters with external components are most frequently used in hospitalized patients and acute care. They are the simplest to insert, exchange, and remove and may be safely used for all aspects of patient care. The most basic of these is the single or multilumen 16-gauge catheter positioned via the internal jugular, subclavian, or femoral vein, and it may be used for intraoperative and acute care as well as longer-term administration of chemotherapy or supportive care. Although these catheters are not tunneled, when inserted under sterile conditions, they may be safely used for 7 to 14 days, but are not appropriate for long-term or outpatient use. In addition, these catheters are considered to have the highest risk for migration and infection because of the minimal subcutaneous catheter length and the absence of a subcutaneous cuff.

External catheters designed for more long-term use include Hickman, Groshong, and Broviac (Bard Access Systems, Salt Lake City, Utah) catheters, each of which possesses subtle differences in design. These catheters are available in single-, double-, and triple-lumen systems and in a variety of sizes for adult and pediatric patients and are designed to be inserted in an operating room or interventional radiology suite. The longer length of these devices allows for the creation of a subcutaneous tunnel between the skin insertion site and the central vein, which aids in catheter fixation and infection control. In addition, a Dacron cuff is affixed to the catheter, designed to be positioned in the subcutaneous tissue near the skin insertion site. The cuff is intended to promote tissue ingrowth and scarring and serve as an additional protection against catheter infection and migration. Several modifications to the basic design of these Silastic catheters have been marketed in an attempt to improve the function and durability of the catheter. Early data suggest that the use of antibiotic- or silver ion–impregnated cuffs could decrease the incidence of catheter-associated infections,[3] but larger, random-assignment trials failed to confirm a benefit.[4] Among different catheters, the most significant design modification is the slit valve design to the Groshong catheter tip (Fig. 64.1). This slit valve is designed to stay in a closed position, except in the presence of positive or negative pressure, to prohibit passive blood reflux and subsequent catheter infection or thrombosis, decrease catheter maintenance, and avoid frequent heparin-containing flushes. However, the frequent loss of valve competence does not obviate the need for regular heparin flushes to prevent device-associated clot.[5]

More recently, an increasing number of central access devices are being placed through more peripheral access sites. These peripherally inserted central catheters (PICC lines) are inserted through a peripheral vein using a Seldinger technique, with the catheter tip positioned in the subclavian, or more central, vein.[6,7] PICC lines offer the potential for long-term access, with a decrease in insertion-associated complications such as pneumothorax or arterial injury. Catheters may be inserted and maintained by a committed, skilled nursing team, bypassing the need for surgical or interventional radiology directed line placement and decreasing cost and resource use. Several studies demonstrate safety and durability of these systems for outpatient antibiotic and nutritional therapy when managed by experienced nursing teams.[6,8] Additional studies to examine the utility of peripherally placed lines in the acute setting have revealed a greater rate of thrombophlebitis and venous thrombosis over standard centrally placed lines in hospitalized patients as well as in those undergoing hemodialysis.[9]

Implanted Devices

The development of completely implantable infusion catheters has greatly simplified the management of patients who require long-term chemotherapy or nutritional support. The catheter itself is unchanged, but it is connected to a subcutaneously implanted reservoir, or port, constructed from

TABLE 64.1

CATHETER-SPECIFIC ADVANTAGES AND DISADVANTAGES

Catheter Type	Advantages	Disadvantages
Central indwelling catheter	Low device profile Durable Low routine maintenance	Operating room with sedation for insertion Increased insertion-associated risks (pneumothorax, arterial injury)
Central externalized catheter	Large catheter lumen for cellular therapy and transfusion Durable, low catheter thrombosis rate	Shorter catheter life vs. indwelling ? Increased rate of catheter infections Increased insertion-associated risks (pneumothorax, arterial injury) Ongoing, routine care required
Peripheral port	Local anesthesia for insertion Decreased insertion-associated risks (pneumothorax, arterial injury) Low device profile	? Decreased durability ? Increased rate of catheter infections Increased rates of catheter-associated thrombosis
PICC line	Local anesthesia for insertion Decreased insertion-associated risks (pneumothorax, arterial injury) Easily exchanged for new catheter Ease of use	? Decreased durability ? Increased rate of catheter infections Increased rates of catheter-associated thrombosis Ongoing, routine care required

PICC line, peripherally inserted central catheter.

titanium or plastic (Fig. 64.2). These ports contain 1 to 3 mL of heparinized saline and incorporate a compressed, self-sealing silicone diaphragm just below the patient's skin. The diaphragm allows repeated puncture with a noncoring Huber needle, designed with a hole along the side of the needle shaft. When not in use, the entire system is contained below the skin. Single- and double-lumen devices are available. The majority of these ports are placed under fluoroscopic guidance in the operating room or interventional radiology suite with local anesthesia or intravenous sedation. The hub of the port is placed along the chest wall, often directly inferior and medial to the deltopectoral groove, where it may be easily palpated and accessed while preserving patient modesty. It is important to fix the port to the underlying pectoralis fascia with interrupted sutures to avoid flipping or migration, which may kink the catheter. Devices placed in interventional radiology (Passport, Sims Deltec; St. Paul, Minnesota) often have the device hub placed in the subcutaneous tissue of the upper arm or forearm. Creation of the subcutaneous port pocket should be accomplished with a minimum of dissection to reduce the risk for seroma formation and subsequent port site infection. Unlike external devices, malfunction or infection of an implanted device requires operative revision or removal. Management of catheter infections is discussed later, in "Infections," but infections of the port pocket or overlying skin require device removal, with primary skin closure achieved once the pump pocket is excised. Modern ports are low-profile devices with an expected lifespan of far more than a year when properly cared for. They are compatible with both magnetic resonance imaging and computed tomography scan. Most recently, Power Port devices (CR Bard, Murray Hill, New Jersey) allow rapid infusion of contrast for patients who undergo interval imaging studies.

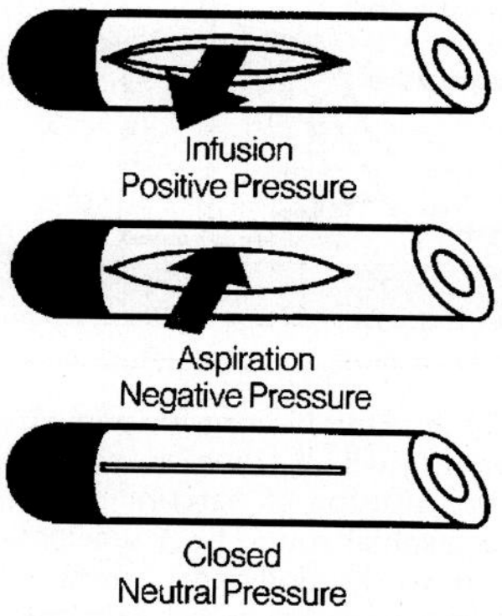

Infusion
Positive Pressure

Aspiration
Negative Pressure

Closed
Neutral Pressure

FIGURE 64.1 The slit valve along the side of the Groshong catheter tip is designed to prevent passive reflux of blood into the lumen.

Several studies have compared complication rates and overall performance of implantable ports and external catheters. Overall, there has consistently been little difference between the two systems with respect to infection rate, catheter-associated thrombosis, and catheter patency, although the implantable devices tend to be more durable.[10,11] Overwhelming studies point to the positive impact of a well-trained, diligent catheter-care staff in preserving long-term function.[12] As noted in "External Catheters," recent data suggest increased rates of thrombotic complications in peripherally placed central lines, most certainly related to the relative size of extremity veins. Careful patient selection, including lifestyle, body habitus, and planned therapeutic regimen, remains a central component of catheter durability. Proper matching of patients and catheter types, along with the standardization of catheter care, results in high rates of long-term catheter function (see "Catheter Selection"). A recent series of 368 patients reported a short-term complication rate (arterial puncture, pneumothorax, and catheter malposition) in 3% of patients, and long-term complication rate (infection, thrombosis) of 1.6%.[5,9]

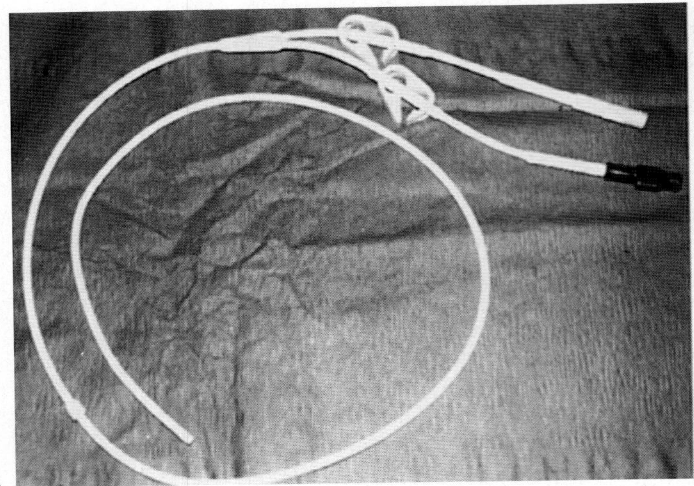

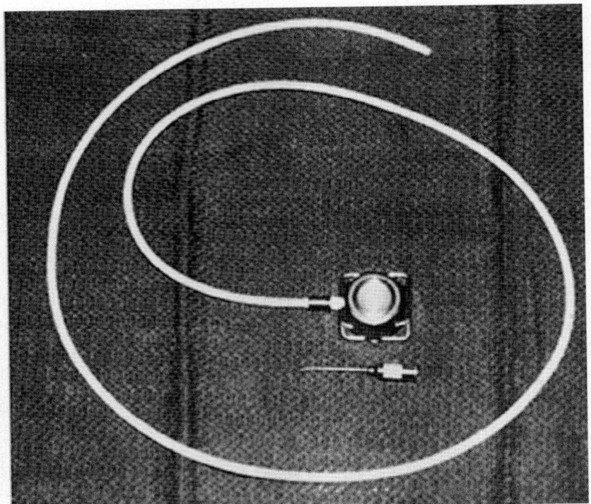

FIGURE 64.2 **A:** Dual-lumen 10 Fr. Hickman catheter showing the Dacron cuff. **B:** Implantable venous device. A noncoring Huber needle is also shown. The housing of the port can be made of titanium (pictured) or plastic.

Implantable Infusion Pumps

Implantable ports offer the advantage of a completely contained system between medication doses. For patients who undergo continuous-infusion therapy, an external pump was necessary. The development of completely implantable subcutaneous infusion pumps has helped patients break the reliance on external pumps. Initially developed for the long-term delivery of heparin to patients with venous thrombosis,[13] these pump or catheter systems are now used for a variety of conditions in which continuous drug administration is desired. Infusion pumps are manufactured by Codman/Johnson & Johnson (Raynham, Massachusetts) and Medtronic (Minneapolis, Minnesota) and are available for intravenous or intra-arterial drug delivery. Modern pumps are constructed from titanium and weigh between 98 and 173 g when empty. Reservoir volumes range from 16 to 60 mL, with available constant infusion rates of 0.3 to 4.0 mL/d.

Pumps are surgically implanted in the subcutaneous tissue, usually on the anterior abdominal wall, and accessed percutaneously using noncoring needles. Bolus or sustained administration of a given agent for therapeutic or diagnostic intervention is possible with both pumps, albeit through different mechanisms (Fig. 64.3). The main pump chamber contains a reservoir surrounded by a chamber of gas-phase fluorocarbon, which is compressed into a fluid phase on filling of the drug reservoir. With time, the fluid expands at a constant rate at body temperature, serving as a propellant. These systems may be used for intravenous administration of medications such as insulin, intrathecal administration of narcotics, or intra-arterial administration of regional chemotherapy.[14–17] In the care of cancer patients, the administration of systemic and intrathecal narcotics and intrahepatic chemotherapy via the gastroduodenal artery have been the most common uses of these devices.

Implantable systems capable of delivery of medication at variable rates are under investigation. Early studies regarding these programmable implantable medication systems report successful euglycemic control in dogs using a battery-powered solenoid pump capable of pulsatile administration of intraperitoneal administration of insulin. Bidirectional communication between the pump and an external transmitter allows for monitoring and regulation of drug delivery.[18] Studies in small numbers of human subjects report reductions in hemoglobin

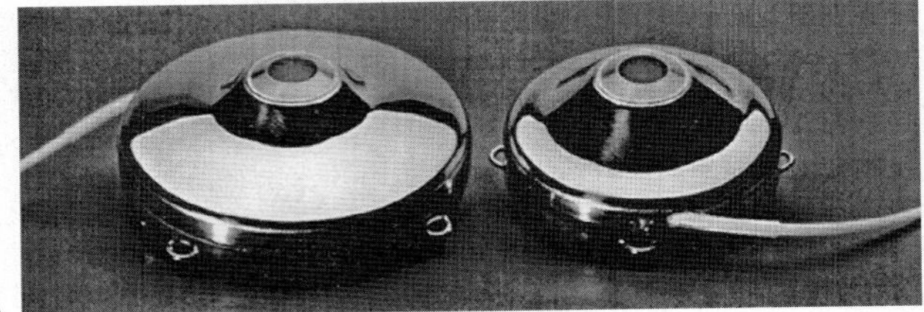

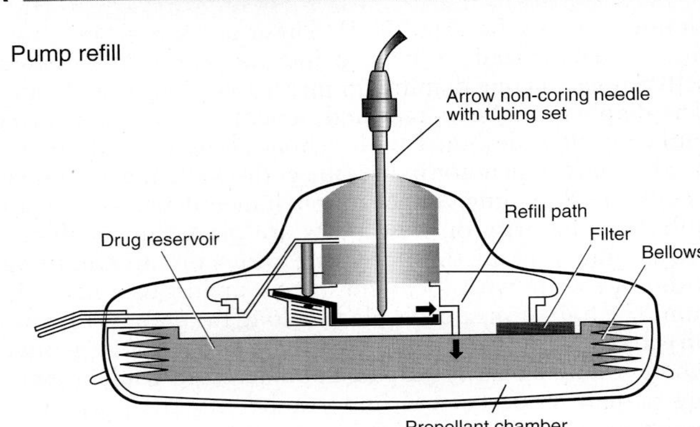

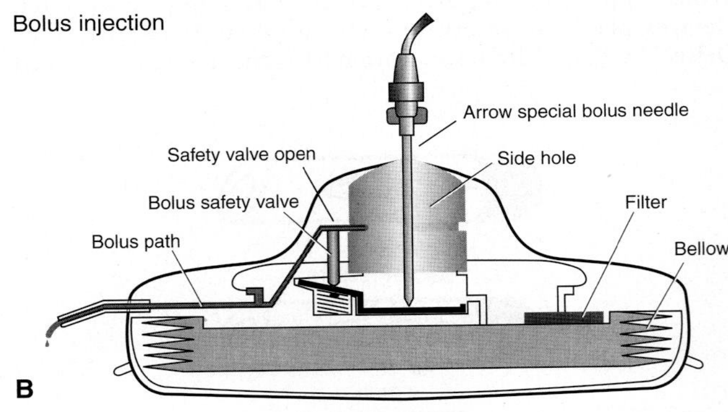

FIGURE 64.3 **A:** The implantable infusion pump (Arrow International, Reading, Pennsylvania), which comes in various sizes. The smaller pump is used for the infusion of narcotic analgesics either intravenously or via an intraspinal route. **B:** A schematic representation of how the pump system works. Body heat causes the propellant to shift from a liquid to a gaseous phase, which compresses the bellows and allows for the drug to be dispensed. When the drug reservoir is refilled, the propellant is compressed and shifts back into a liquid phase.

A_{1C}, no episodes of insulin overdelivery, and good patient quality of life.[19] At present, all subcutaneously placed pumps are hampered by the increased cost associated with operative placement and the absence of available data supporting a benefit over conventional therapy.

CATHETER SELECTION

Careful matching of patients with appropriate vascular access systems is essential to avoid patient exposure to unnecessary risks and financial expense. The selection of the proper catheter must take into account numerous factors, including the proposed length of treatment, the number of agents to be used, the need for frequent blood draws or transfusions, and the patient's vascular anatomy. For example, a patient scheduled for a short, 1- to 2-week course of total parenteral nutrition could be adequately treated with a percutaneously placed single- or double-lumen catheter, which may be inserted and removed more easily. Patients with the potential for more aggressive transfusion support or in need of cell transplants are best served by larger external catheters, which are easily accessed and enable infusion of blood products, chemotherapy, and nutritional support. Although these catheters need to be inserted in the operating room, removal is easier than with implanted ports, and more rapid infusion is possible. By contrast, patients who require prolonged administration of chemotherapy with serial blood draws are ideal candidates for implanted ports, which are low-profile and require little maintenance between treatments.

At present, the choice of catheter is often based on the specialization of the physician responsible for line insertion. PICC lines are placed by nurses with or without the assistance of interventional radiologists, whereas peripheral implanted ports are the responsibility of interventional radiologists. Central catheters, with the exception of single-lumen percutaneous lines, are inserted in the operating room by surgeons, often with fluoroscopic assistance. In the highest-volume centers, the establishment of a vascular access team responsible for catheter selection, insertion, and long-term care has resulted in prolongation of catheter life, a decreased infection rate, and improved efficiency.[20] Such a team approach aids in hospital-wide standardization as well as accurate assessment of catheter-related complications. Additional factors to consider before selecting a specific access device include a history of previous indwelling catheter, central vein patency, patient age and size, patient immune status, and the need for frequent blood draws. In those patients with a history of multiple previous catheters or catheter-related complications, or both, duplex Doppler examination may be needed to ensure vein patency. Other patient factors such as the potential for superior vena cava narrowing or obstruction from mediastinal tumors or the increased risk of thrombosis and cellulitis in postmastectomy and post-axillary dissection patients may limit access sites. Recent data would suggest that establishing central venous access ipsilateral to a breast cancer may be performed safely and effectively.[21] Ample data exist to support an evidence-based approach for catheter selection for a variety of clinical scenarios. Percutaneously placed, nontunneled central catheters are the primary choice for patients who undergo major surgical procedures or in whom a significant intensive care unit stay can be reasonably anticipated. These catheters allow rapid administration of drugs, blood products, and volume resuscitation and are routinely inserted, changed, and removed at the bedside. Triple lumen catheters allow concurrent administration of multiple medications, blood, or nutritional support and are associated with low rates of infectious, thrombotic, or mechanical complications when maintained by experienced clinical teams.[22] Discontinuation of central catheters in favor of PICC lines is recommended once the need for multiple medications and potential volume resuscitation has dissipated, as multilumen PICC lines are associated with increased thrombotic complications versus standard multilumen catheters.[23] For prolonged inpatient and limited outpatient use, however, single- or double-lumen PICC lines are associated with lower infection rates for the administration of medications and total parenteral nutrition (TPN).[24,25] A recent report details a high level of patient satisfaction and successful catheter maintenance for terminally ill cancer patients who need ongoing home hospice care.[26] Once the transition to long-term maintenance chemotherapy has been made, indwelling ports are the access of choice. As previous PICC line placement has been associated with higher complication rates in patients needing long-term central venous access,[5,27] all PICC lines should be removed as soon as clinically indicated and not maintained for prophylaxis or intermittent long-term use.

PEDIATRIC PATIENTS

Pediatric patients account for a small, but significant percentage of oncology patients in need of long-term totally implanted venous access devices. Several recent series have examined this group of patients. Five hundred consecutive pediatric patients (mean age; 44 months) who underwent central venous ultrasound-guided Hickman catheter placement at a single institution experienced a 99.8% successful cannulation rate with perioperative complication rate of 2.4% (all conservatively managed).[28] Dillon and Foglia reported 296 port placements and 175 port removals on 301 pediatric patients. The overall complication rate was 5.1%, and included 11 leaks, most frequently arising from a needle perforation from the port base. Six patients had complications associated with the port-catheter connection, including two leaks and four disrupted connections. The functional duration of the ports averaged 425 days, for those ports not electively removed at the completion of therapy.[22] Similar durable rates of catheter function were observed in a group of 200 consecutive treated at the Royal Children's Hospital, in Victoria, Australia.[23] Infectious and thrombotic events were the most common complications observed in this group of patients,[29,30] occurring at a rate of 0.56 and 0.33 episodes per 1,000 catheter days, resulting in catheter removal in less than 5% of patients. In patients with indwelling catheters who experience febrile episodes, one-third had catheter-associated infections. Risk factors for such infections include the duration of access and the need for blood transfusions or TPN.[31]

INSERTION TECHNIQUES

The preferred arena for the insertion of long-term venous access is either the operating room or the interventional radiology suite, where sterility can be ensured. Adequate lighting, analgesia, and staffing are essential to ensure proper catheter placement and maximize catheter life. Although local anesthesia is all that is required for catheter placement, the use of intravenous sedation provides better patient comfort, especially in difficult insertions. Sedation is mandatory in pediatric patients, and general anesthesia is often preferred. Real-time fluoroscopy is helpful in directing guidewires in difficult cases and should be used to confirm catheter tip placement at the junction of the superior vena cava and the right atrium before fixing the catheter to the skin or chest wall. Calibrated guidewires are available to facilitate accurate measurement for proper catheter positioning.

The most commonly used insertion technique is that initially described by Seldinger, in which a catheter is placed over a percutaneously placed wire.[32] This technique may be used to access any deep or central vein, but in patients with long-term access needs, the internal jugular and subclavian veins are preferred. In difficult cases, access to the central venous system can be obtained via a femoral vein approach, with the port or the catheter exit site placed on the abdominal wall at the level of the umbilicus.

Accessing the subclavian vein demonstrates general technical points. A rolled towel is placed longitudinally between the patient's shoulders to increase the distance between the clavicle and the chest wall. A wide sterile preparation and drape are mandatory to allow access to the ipsilateral internal jugular vein if cannulation of the subclavian vein is unsuccessful. It is the author's practice to consent the patient for both sides, in the event of unanticipated difficulty accessing either vein on a given side. Comfortable patient positioning and liberal infiltration with local anesthesia, including along the periosteum of the clavicle, ensure a minimum of patient movement and discomfort. Trendelenburg's position aids in vein access. A finder needle attached to a 5-mL syringe is advanced, bevel up, under the clavicle in the direction of the sternal notch. A constant gentle aspiration is applied until blood freely enters the syringe, indicating venous access. If bright red blood or pulsatile flow is noted, the syringe is withdrawn and pressure is held. Once the vein has been located, an introducer needle is placed in the same fashion as the finder needle. On access to the vein, the needle hub is rotated 90 degrees, and a flexible guidewire is advanced through the needle into the superior vena cava. If the wire is placed too far, cardiac irritation develops, usually a supraventricular tachycardia, and the wire should be pulled back. If resistance to threading the wire is encountered immediately, the needle is likely not in the vein and the syringe should be used to ensure proper position. Resistance after several centimeters of wire has been threaded may indicate entrance into a smaller vein or central vein stenosis. Fluoroscopy should be used with or without contrast to thread the wire and examine potential venous narrowing. A wire should never be advanced against resistance.

Once the wire has been successfully inserted, fluoroscopy should confirm its location in the vena cava and not in the contralateral subclavian vein or other feeding vessel. Subsequently, a catheter exit site or port placement site should be selected on the anterior chest wall. The skin and subcutaneous tissue surrounding the proposed catheter exit site or port site should be infiltrated with local anesthesia and a skin incision performed. If a single- or double-lumen external catheter is to be inserted, the incision should be made in a location cosmetically favorable that also allows for easy catheter care. In this circumstance, a second 5-mm incision is made at the site where the guidewire exits the skin. A subcutaneous tunnel is then fashioned between the two incisions, and the catheter is advanced from the exit site to the wire exit site. The catheter should be advanced until the cuff is 1 cm past the skin incision and then measured for proper placement. It is the author's practice to assess proper catheter length with a calibrated guidewire before trimming the catheter length. After establishing the proper catheter length, attention is turned toward accessing the subclavian vein. A peel-away sheath and dilator are advanced over the guidewire into the vein with care. Once the dilator/sheath combination is inside the vein, the sheath should be advanced over the dilator the remainder of its length. This is done to minimize the risk of significant venous injury by the rigid dilator. Once the sheath is completely inside the vein, the dilator is withdrawn and blood return confirmed, and only then is the wire completely removed. If blood return is not observed after removal of the dilator, fluoroscopy should confirm sheath placement and the catheter checked for kinking. For this reason, it is best to maintain the wire inside the vein until blood return is ensured.

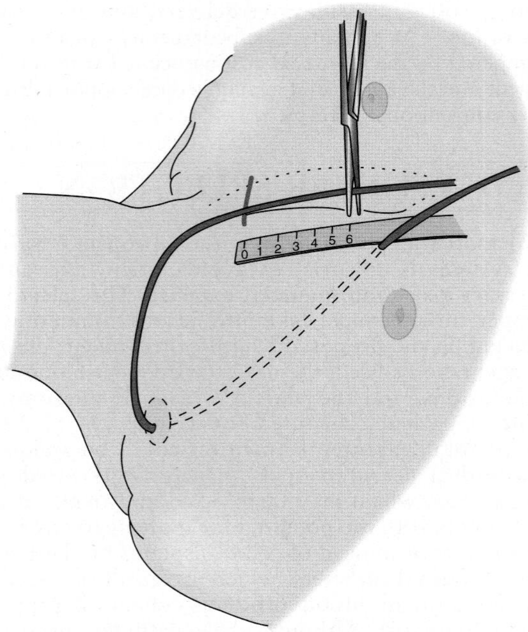

FIGURE 64.4 The length of the catheter can be estimated by simulating its course through the subclavian vein and superior vena cava along the clavicle and right border of the sternum. If the catheter is cut 6 cm inferior to the angle of Louis, it approximates a final position at the superior vena caval and atrial junction. Tip position should be confirmed using fluoroscopy.

Once the sheath is in place, the catheter is inserted into the vein through the lumen and the sheath is split and peeled away. To avoid losing access to the vein, the entire length of the catheter should be advanced into position, with placement confirmed via fluoroscopy before removal of the sheath, rather than pulling the sheath back as the catheter is advanced. During sheath removal, the catheter is steadied at the skin with a pair of forceps. Improper placement of the catheter tip increases the rate of associated complications, including cardiac arrhythmias from cardiac irritation and catheter failure associated with thrombosis.[33] The ideal catheter tip position is just inside the right atrium or at the junction of the superior vena cava and the right atrium, keeping in mind that the tip migrates up 1 to 3 cm when the patient is upright. Catheter placement in the subclavian vein is associated with a higher rate of venous thrombosis and catheter failure versus placement in the right atrium or vena cava. The author's technique for using external bony landmarks to estimate proper catheter length is described in Figure 64.4. The usual location of the junction of the right atrium and the superior vena cava is 4 to 6 cm below the angle of Louis, but fluoroscopic confirmation of location is essential. An upright chest x-ray should be obtained at the completion of the procedure to document catheter placement and confirm the absence of a pneumothorax, a complication of less than 1% of catheters placed by the subclavian or jugular approach.[34] If an implanted pump is being placed, similar technique is used, except the second incision is placed higher on the chest, just medial to the deltopectoral groove, in a vertical orientation. A subcutaneous pocket is fashioned to accommodate the port after it is attached to the catheter. Care should be taken to ensure the orientation of the port does not kink the catheter at the port hub before placing the anchoring sutures.

Increasingly, real-time ultrasound guidance has been used to aid in catheter insertion, predominantly via a cervical approach. Several recent randomized series have noted decreased rates of arterial puncture and cervical hematoma, shorter procedure times, and increased rates of successful catheter insertion when ultrasound guidance is used versus a more traditional technique based solely on anatomic landmarks.[35,36] In a large nonrandomized series of 493 patients, the overall success rate of ultrasound-guided internal jugular vein cannulation was 94.5%, with cervical hematoma and arterial puncture rates of 4.3% and 1.4%, respectively.[37] In experienced hands, the use of real-time ultrasonography is associated with an index central vein cannulation failure rate of 4.8% and ultimate procedure failure rate of 0.3% in 2,456 consecutive patients examined.[7] Such a benefit does not appear to extend to subclavian vein catheter insertion, where surface landmarks are more consistent and ultrasonic venous examination is more difficult.[38] Although routine use of real-time ultrasonography may not be necessary in experienced hands, its use in patients with poorly defined surface landmarks, thrombocytopenia or coagulation abnormalities, or a history of multiple indwelling central catheters should be encouraged. In the author's institution, the majority of surgically placed venous access devices are performed via the subclavian vein, utilizing a shorter subcutaneous tunnel, and removing the utility for ultrasound guidance. Transcervical approaches are more common when placing short- and intermediate-term lines, and ultrasound use is routine. A nonrandomized series of 1,222 patients who underwent central venous catheter placement at 5 teaching institutions demonstrated successful first-attempt access in 86% of procedures. Ultrasound guidance was utilized in 41% of initial attempts, and although not associated with ultimate success rates, did lead to a significant reduction in the number of total puncture attempts ($P < .02$).[39]

Alternatives to subclavian vein access are available when catheter insertion is not possible secondary to anatomic or safety concerns. If subclavian vein access is not successful, ultrasound can be helpful in assessing vein patency and location. Alternative sites include the ipsilateral internal jugular and cephalic veins. The internal jugular vein may be cannulated percutaneously or via a cutdown procedure. With either approach, the port or catheter exit site should remain on the anterior chest wall. Cephalic vein isolation is an especially appealing approach for patients who need subcutaneous ports, in whom a single incision in the deltopectoral groove may be used to isolate the vein and create the pump pocket while virtually eliminating the risk of pneumothorax and inadvertent arterial puncture.[40] In a series of 318 patients who underwent placement of an indwelling subcutaneous catheter, cephalic vein cutdown was successful in 79.5% and was associated with a lower rate of procedure-associated complications compared with those who underwent placement via the Seldinger technique.[24] A comparative study between two groups of surgeons within the same institution confirmed the decrease in complications (hemothorax, pneumothorax, catheter fragmentation) using the cutdown approach.[25] In situations of stenosis, obstruction, or thrombosis of the subclavian or internal jugular systems, alternatives include the femoral vein or accessed percutaneously or via the saphenous vein using a cutdown procedure.[41] Investigators from the Cathedia Study Group examined a group of 750 bedbound patients in need of central venous for dialysis access. Patients were randomized to cervical versus femoral approaches, and when controlled for patient body mass index (BMI), there was no observed difference in catheter-related infectious complications.[42] Similar conclusions were reported in short-term access for critically ill patients.[43] In rare circumstances, insertion sites may include the gonadal, intercostals, and azygous veins or direct placement into the inferior vena cava.[36,44–46]

CATHETER-RELATED COMPLICATIONS

Venous Thrombosis

Catheter-associated thrombosis is the most common complication associated with long-term indwelling catheters, reported in 30% of 70% of patients, the majority of whom are asymptomatic. Symptomatic thrombosis is reported in 5% to 10% of patients with central catheters.[47,48] When present, thrombi remain a source of catheter infection as well as pulmonary emboli and permanent venous obstruction.[49] The latter complication must always be considered when planning to attempt venous access at or distal to sites previously used. Chronic irritation of the venous endothelium, at the catheter tip, the area of venous entry, or another area of sustained contact, is thought to be the inciting event in the development of catheter-associated thrombi. Recent data suggest that thrombi develop early in the life of the catheter and do not become clinically apparent unless collateral veins do not compensate for the progressive decrease in venous flow.[44] Routine utilization of scheduled heparin flushes are recommended to preserve catheter patency, as demonstrated by a recent report detailing the increase in PICC line thrombotic complications observed during a national heparin shortage.[50]

Management of catheter-associated thrombosis is geared toward catheter preservation and prevention of secondary complications. Immediate catheter removal before attempted salvage is rare, and completion of therapy is often possible. Prompt relief of symptoms through elevation of the affected the extremity and decreased risk of pulmonary emboli and clot propagation with therapeutic anticoagulation are the most pressing interventions. Traditional strategies based on therapeutic heparinization followed by oral warfarin therapy proved effective in catheter preservation and prevention of clot extension.[46] The true risk of pulmonary emboli from catheter-associated thrombi is unknown, but reviews of upper extremity deep venous thrombosis report an incidence of pulmonary emboli in 10% to 15% of affected patients, some of which were fatal.[51,52] The significance of asymptomatic catheter-associated thrombi is not clear, as few complications of catheter removal were noted in patients with small, asymptomatic clots. Furthermore, modern silicone and polyurethane catheters appear to be less likely associated with severe pulmonary emboli. These risks, and those of chronic venous insufficiency secondary to thrombotic complications, must be weighed in light of the life-threatening malignancy necessitating therapy.

Treatment of clinically significant catheter-associated thrombus is similar to that for other deep venous thrombosis and is centered around long-term anticoagulation. Initial trials were performed using bolus and continuous-infusion intravenous heparin for 24 to 48 hours before initiation of warfarin therapy.[51,52] Presently, initial therapy with low molecular-weight heparin therapy followed by warfarin allows complete management in the outpatient setting and allows prolonged catheter preservation. Recommendations regarding the length of therapy are based on small, nonrandomized trials and include continuation of therapy for the length of the remaining catheter life and possibly for several weeks after catheter removal.[53] Thrombolytic therapy has been reported as a salvage strategy for maintaining a vital catheter or vein. Low-dose recombinant tissue plasminogen activator injected directly into the catheter and clot has been shown to be effective when used in combination with long-term anticoagulation after catheter removal.[54]

Prophylaxis against catheter-associated thrombosis has been examined using low molecular-weight heparin or low-dose warfarin. Both strategies appeared effective when compared in randomized, controlled trials of high-risk patients.[55,56] Both trials were conducted in small groups of high-risk patients, leaving questions as to the benefit of such therapy on the majority of cancer patients with indwelling catheters. At present, the author's practice is to individualize therapy based on the patient's risk for thrombosis, the length of therapy, and a history of catheter-related complications.

Infections

Although subclinical thrombosis is a frequent complication of long-term indwelling catheter, infection is the greatest cause of catheter loss.[57] Risk factors for infectious complications include the type of catheter used, the absence of a skilled team caring for catheters, the lack of antibiotic-coated catheters, and the length and frequency of catheter use.[58,59] Percutaneously placed short-term catheters are associated with the highest rate of infectious complications but are also accessed more often and for greater periods of time than other types of catheters. Site selection for short-term catheter placement was found to impact the risk of infectious complications, with the risk greatest in femoral lines, followed by internal jugular and then subclavian sites of access.[26] A nonrandomized series of patients treated within a single intensive care unit demonstrated an apparent decrease in infection rates between patients with central lines (6.0 per 1,000 cath days) versus those with PICC lines (2.2 per 1,000 cath days). Upon multivariate analysis, only duration of catheter placement was associated with increased infection rate.[60] The establishment of dedicated care teams and protocols and the use of antibiotic-coated catheters have proven beneficial. Among those catheters designed for long-term use, tunneled catheters with externalized hubs are more likely to develop infections (40%) than implanted subcutaneous devices (5% to 10%).[54,55] Infectious complications decrease in frequency with time. This is thought to be the result of the restoration of the skin integrity after insertion. Recently, the use of antiseptic barrier caps has been shown to decrease the incidence of central venous catheter associated infections.[61]

Skin flora, either the patient's own or transferred from a caregiver, are the most common contaminating organisms.[62] In the period immediately after catheter insertion, infections have the pattern of standard postoperative infections, most commonly presenting as cellulitis or deeper infections in the port pocket or along the catheter. These complications may be treated conservatively with antibiotics if discovered early in their course. The presence of a postoperative abscess mandates catheter removal. Inability to clear acute or chronic infections may indicate the presence of a bacterial biofilm surrounding the catheter, secreted by the infecting organism. Such a film makes delivery of antibiotics difficult, often necessitating catheter removal.[63]

Infectious complications of established venous access devices include those at the catheter exit or access site, infections of the catheter subcutaneous tunnel, and catheter-associated bacteremia. Tenderness or erythema at the catheter skin exit site or the port access site is frequently due to *Staphylococcus epidermidis* and may be associated with localized purulent discharge. Signs of systemic infection or sepsis are rare. Catheter preservation is the rule, and local treatment with antibiotic ointment usually is indicated. Cultures of any purulent discharge should be obtained before initiation of therapy. In cases of infection with *Pseudomonas* or atypical mycobacterium species or when blood cultures reveal the offending organism, catheter removal is indicated.[64,65] In the presence of systemic symptoms but negative blood cultures, oral or intravenous antibiotics are usually effective. More deep-seated infections manifest by erythema, tenderness, and fluctuance overlying the port pocket or subcutaneous catheter tunnel. These infections are more difficult to control, even with intravenous antibiotics. Catheter salvage is possible with several weeks of antibiotics, but in the absence of prompt clinical improvement, catheter removal is inevitable.[66]

The presence of a catheter-related source of bacteremia must be documented by blood cultures obtained through the line as well as from a peripheral site. The most common pathogen in catheter-related bacteremia is a coagulase-negative staphylococci, and it is usually readily treated with vancomycin administered via all lumens of the infected line.[56,62] After 2 to 3 days of antibiotic therapy, peripheral and catheter cultures should be repeated to ensure adequate treatment. After a total of 14 days of therapy, antibiotics should be discontinued and cultures repeated after 48 to 72 hours.[62] Additional effective eradication of catheter-based infection has been reported using antimicrobial lock or dwell solutions for 48 hours. Although this strategy was successful in 69% of patients treated, prophylaxis with a similar approach did not decrease catheter complication rates versus standard heparin flush protocols.[27,28] Indications for catheter removal include the inability to clear the infection after antimicrobial therapy, continued signs and symptoms of bacteremia, or recurrent infection after completion of a full course of therapy. Before catheter removal, patients with persistent or recurrent catheter infections may benefit from a short course of low-dose recombinant tissue plasminogen activator designed at treating infections associated with catheter tip fibrin sheath or thrombus. Adequate delivery of antibiotics to the septic focus is not possible without destruction of the associated sheath or thrombus.[67] At the National Institutes of Health, the presence of such a sheath or thrombus is confirmed with a catheter venogram before initiating therapy.

Selected References

The full list of references for this chapter appears in the online version.

1. Broviac JW, Cole JJ, Scribner BH. A silicone rubber atrial catheter for prolonged parenteral alimentation. *Surg Gynecol Obstet* 1973;136:602.
2. Hickman RO, Buckner CD, Clift RA. A modified right atrial catheter for access to the venous system in marrow transplant recipients. *Surg Gynecol Obstet* 1979;148:791.
3. Flowers RH, Schwenzer KJ, Koper RF, et al. Efficacy of an attachable subcutaneous cuff for the prevention of intravascular catheter-related infection. A randomized, controlled trial. *JAMA* 1989;261:878.
4. Groeger JS, Lucas AB, Coit D, et al. A prospective, randomized evaluation of the effect of silver impregnated subcutaneous cuffs for preventing tunneled chronic venous access infections in cancer patients. *Ann Surg* 1993; 218:206.
5. Mayo DJ, Horne MK, Summers BL, et al. The effects of heparin flush on patency of the Groshong catheter: a pilot study. *Oncol Nurs Forum* 1996; 23:1401.
6. Cardella JF, Cardella K, Bacci N, Fox PS, Post JH. Cumulative experience with 1,273 peripherally inserted central catheters at a single institution. *J Vasc Interv Radiol* 1996;7:5.
7. Banton J. Using midlines and PICC lines for chemotherapy regimens. *Oncol Nurs Forum* 1999;26:514.
8. Alhimyary A, Fernandez C, Picard M, et al. Safety and efficacy of total parenteral nutrition delivered via a peripherally inserted central venous catheter. *Nutr Clin Pract* 1996;11:199.
9. Allen AW, Megargell JL, Brown DB, et al. Venous thrombosis associated with the placement of peripherally inserted central catheters. *J Vasc Interv Radiol* 2000;11:1309.

10. May GS, Davis C. Percutaneous catheters and totally implantable access systems: a review of reported infection rates. *J Intraven Nurs* 1988;11:97.
11. Ross MN, Hasse GM, Poole MA, et al. Comparison of totally implanted reservoirs with external catheters as venous access devices in pediatric oncology patients. *Surg Gynecol Obstet* 1988;167:141.
12. Viale PH. Complications associated with implantable vascular access devices in the patient with cancer. *J Infus Nurs* 2003;26:97.
14. Kemeny N, Jarnagin W, Gonen M, et al. Phase I/II study of hepatic arterial therapy with floxuridine and dexamethasone in combination with intravenous irinotecan as adjuvant treatment after resection of hepatic metastases from colorectal cancer. *J Clin Oncol* 2003; 21:3303.
15. Rougier P, Laplanche A, Huguier M, et al. Hepatic arterial infusion of floxuridine in patients with liver metastases from colorectal carcinoma: long-term results of a prospective randomized trial. *J Clin Oncol* 1992;10:1112.
16. Hassenbusch SJ, Pillay PK, Majdinec M, et al. Constant infusion of morphine for intractable cancer pain using an implantable pump. *J Neurosurg* 1990;73:405.
18. Saudek CD, Fischell RE, Swindle MM. The programmable implantable medication system (PIMS): design features and pre-clinical trials. *Horm Metab Res* 1990;22:201.
20. Hunter MR. Development of a vascular access team in an acute care setting. *J Infus Nurs* 2003;26:86.
22. Al Raiy B, Fakih MG, Bryan-Nomides N, et al. Peripherally inserted central venous catheters in the acute care setting: a safe alternative to high-risk short-term central venous catheters. *Am J Infect Control* 2010;38(2):149.
23. Trerotola SO, Stavropoulos SW, Mondschein JI, et al. Triple-lumen peripherally inserted central catheter in patients in the critical care unit: prospective evaluation. *Radiology* 2010;256(1):312.
24. Haider G, Kumar S, Salam B, et al. Determination of complication rate of PICC lines in oncological patients. *J Pak Med Assoc* 2009;59(10):663.
25. Pittiruti M, Hamilton H, Biffi R, et al. ESPEN guidelines on parenteral nutrition: central venous catheters (access, care, diagnosis and therapy of complications). *Clin Nutr* 2009;28(4):365.
26. Yamada R, Morita T, Yashiro E, et al. Patient-reported usefulness of peripherally inserted central venous catheters in terminally ill cancer patients. *J Pain Symptom Manage* 2010;40(1):60.
27. Butler PJ, Sood S, Mojibian H, Tal MG. Previous PICC placement may be associated with catheter-related infections in hemodialysis patients. *Cardiovasc Intervent Radiol* 2010; (in press).
28. Arul GS, Lewis N, Bromley P, Bennett J. Ultrasound-guided percutaneous insertion of Hickman lines in children. Prospective study of 500 consecutive procedures. *J Pediatr Surg* 2009;44(7):1371.
29. Ruggiero A, Barone G, Margani G, et al. Groshong catheter-related complications in children with cancer. *Pediatr Blood Cancer* 2010;54(7):947.
30. Nam SH, Kim DY, Kim SC, Kim IK. Complications and risk factors of infection in pediatric hemato-oncology patients with totally implantable access ports (TIAPs). *Pediatr Blood Cancer* 2010;54(4):546.
31. Wylie MC, Graham DA, Potter-Bynoe G, et al. Risk factors for central line-associated bloodstream infection in pediatric intensive care units. *Infect Control Hosp Epidemiol* 2010;31(10):1049.
32. Jansen RF, Wiggers T, van Geel BN, et al. Assessment of insertion techniques and complication rates of dual-lumen central venous catheters in patients with hematological malignancies. *World J Surg* 1990;14:100.
34. Miller JA, Singireddy S, Maldjian P, Baker SR. A reevaluation of the radiographically detectable complications of percutaneous venous access lines inserted by four subcutaneous approaches. *Am Surg* 1999;65:125.
35. Slama M, Novara A, Safavian A, et al. Improvement of internal jugular vein cannulation using an ultrasound-guided technique. *Intensive Care Med* 1997;23:916.
36. Teichgraber UK, Benter T, Gebel M, Manns MP. A sonographically guided technique for central venous access. *AJR Am J Roentgenol* 1997;169:731.
37. Mey U, Glasmacher A, Hahn C, et al. Evaluation of an ultrasound-guided technique for central venous access via the internal jugular vein in 493 patients. *Support Care Cancer* 2003;11:148.
38. Bold RJ, Winchester DJ, Madary AR, et al. Prospective, randomized trial of Doppler-assisted subclavian vein catheterization. *Arch Surg* 1998; 133:1089.
39. Balls A, LoVecchio F, Kroeger A, et al. Ultrasound guidance for central venous catheter placement: results from the Central Line Emergency Access Registry Database. *Am J Emerg Med* 2010;28(5):561.
40. Povoski SP. A prospective analysis of the cephalic vein cutdown approach for chronic indwelling central venous access in 100 consecutive cancer patients. *Ann Surg Oncol* 2000;7:496.
42. Parienti JJ, Thirion M, Mégarbane B, et al. Femoral vs jugular venous catheterization and risk of nosocomial events in adults requiring acute renal replacement therapy: a randomized controlled trial. *JAMA* 2008; 299(20):2413.
43. Nakae H, Igarashi T, Tajimi K. Catheter-related infections via temporary vascular access catheters: a randomized prospective study. *Artif Organs* 2010;34(3):E72.
47. Horne MK, May DJ, Alexander HR, et al. Venographic surveillance of tunneled venous access devices in adult oncology patients. *Ann Surg Oncol* 1995;2:174.
48. De Cicco M, Matovic M, Balestreri L, et al. Central venous thrombosis: an early and frequent complication in cancer patients bearing long-term Silastic catheter. A prospective study. *Thromb Res* 1997;86:101.
49. Raad I, Luna M, Khalil SA, et al. The relationship between the thrombotic and infectious complications of central venous catheters. *JAMA* 1994; 271:1014.
50. Jonker MA, Osterby KR, Vermeulen LC, et al. Does low-dose heparin maintain central venous access device patency?: a comparison of heparin versus saline during a period of heparin shortage. *JPEN J Parenter Enteral Nutr* 2010;34(4):444.
52. Hicken GJ, Ameli FM. Management of subclavian-axillary vein thrombosis: a review. *Can J Surg* 1998;41:13.
54. Horne MK, Mayo DJ, Cannon RO, et al. Intra-clot recombinant tissue plasminogen activator in the treatment of deep venous thrombosis of the lower and upper extremities. *Am J Med* 2000;108:251.
56. Bern MM, Lokich JJ, Wallach SR, et al. Very low doses of warfarin can prevent thrombosis in central venous catheters. A randomized prospective trial. *Ann Intern Med* 1990;112:423.
58. Mirro J, Rao BN, Kumar M, et al. A comparison of placement techniques and complications of externalized catheters and implantable port use in children with cancer. *J Pediatr Surg* 1990;25:120.
59. Darouiche RO, Raad II, Heard SO, et al. A comparison of two antimicrobial-impregnated central venous catheters. Catheter Study Group. *N Engl J Med* 1999;340:1.
60. Gunst M, Matsushima K, Vanek S, et al. Peripherally inserted central catheters may lower the incidence of catheter-related blood stream infections in patients in surgical intensive care units. *Surg Infect (Larchmt)* 2010; (in press).
61. Menyhay SZ, Maki DG. Preventing central venous catheter-associated bloodstream infections: development of an antiseptic barrier cap for needleless connectors. *Am J Infect Control* 2008;36(10):S174.e1.
64. Benezra D, Kiehn TE, Gold JW, et al. Prospective study of infections in indwelling central venous catheters using quantitative blood cultures. *Am J Med* 1988;85:495.
66. Jones GR. A practical guide to evaluation and treatment of infections in patients with indwelling central venous catheters. *J Intraven Nurs* 1998;21:S134.

CHAPTER 65 INTERVENTIONAL RADIOLOGY

CHRISTOS S. GEORGIADES AND JEAN-FRANCOIS H. GESCHWIND

Interventional radiology (IR) is a specialty heavily dependent on technological advancements, one that avails itself to the creativity of its members and one that offers ever-expanding research horizons. These factors make IR a continuously evolving and increasingly indispensable member of the multidisciplinary cancer care team. Its contributions cover the entire spectrum of cancer care, including diagnosis, staging, prevention, treatment, resolving complications of treatment, and follow-up.

The objective of this chapter is to showcase the technical and clinical contributions of IR and answer the question, "what can interventional radiology do for your cancer patient?" keeping in mind that the "your" refers to nonradiologists. The discussion is organized according to a system-based approach and technical descriptions are limited to those required to understand the clinical contribution of each procedure.

Finally, although most services offered by IR are now standard treatments, one does well to understand that IR physicians are adept at finding solutions to unusual clinical problems. Presenting the IR physician with an atypical clinical dilemma is always a welcome challenge and may very well result in an equally atypical but effective solution.

PULMONARY

Lung cancer is the leading cause of cancer-related mortality in the Western world.[1,2] Despite a recent decrease in its incidence (which currently stands at approximately 54 per 100,000 in the United States), lung cancer remains a serious epidemiologic problem because of the high mortality rate (nearly identical to incidence).[1] In the United States alone, lung cancer will cause 160,000 deaths per year, which accounts for 28% of all cancer deaths.[2] At presentation, 27% of patients are stage I, 13% stage II, 41% stage III, and 19% stage IV.[3] Many of the early-stage cancer patients are unresectable because of comorbidities. Overall, only 15% of lung cancer patients are candidates for resection at presentation.[4]

Percutaneous Ablation

Computed tomographic (CT)-guided, percutaneous thermal ablation of lung cancer is a relatively new approach in treating early-stage disease. It is currently reserved for patients whose operative risks are too high. Although resection is still considered the treatment of choice, a multicentered, prospective, randomized trial comparing radiofrequency ablation (RFA) and surgery for stage IA is currently under way in the U.S. ACOSOG (American College of Surgeons Oncology Group) trial. The procedure takes less than an hour and is mostly performed under conscious sedation, which is a major advantage because the majority of patients are referred for RFA of lung cancer because their pulmonary status is too poor for general anesthesia. The ablation probe is guided to the lesion under CT visualization, and when in the proper position, the probe ablates a variable volume of tissue around its tip. The volume depends on the type of needle and, by extension, lesion size. Figure 65.1 shows the steps for CT-guided, percutaneous RFA of a lung lesion. The efficacy of CT-guided, percutaneous RFA for lung cancer depends on two variables: the size and location of the lesion. Percutaneously accessible lesions that are 3 cm or less in diameter are likely to show complete response.[5] The efficacy of RFA for larger lesions, however, drops precipitously, with those larger than 5 cm unlikely to show complete response.[5] Figure 65.2 summarizes the efficacy of RFA for lung cancer. Follow-up requires serial CT imaging at 1-, 3-, and 6-month intervals and, if negative findings, then the patient follows the standard follow-up for lung cancer.

Recent evidence[5] suggests that positron emission tomography (PET)/CT is superior to CT alone for follow-up. Follow-up interval is the same; however, the combined metabolic and anatomic information of PET/CT improves the negative and positive predictive values. Figure 65.3 shows a PET/CT follow-up for a lung cancer patient treated with RFA. Lung RFA-related complications include bleeding, infection, and pneumothorax. The first two are rare (<5%) with proper patient preparation, that is, correction of coagulation abnormalities and periprocedural antibiotics. The reported rate of RFA-related pneumothorax is 25% to 40%. Only a small minority of these patients (10%–20%) will require a chest tube, which can be easily placed during the procedure using CT guidance. For incompletely responsive lesions, the procedure can be repeated without any additional risks.

Because the major determinant of favorable response to RFA is size, treatment should be sought as soon as possible. The "wait and see" approach is no longer valid because nearly all patients can undergo this minimally invasive procedure irrespective of most comorbidities. The results of the RUPTURE trial—a prospective, multicenter trial on the safety and efficacy of RFA for primary and metastatic lung cancer—were recently published and support a high efficacy and low complication rate for lesions 3 cm or smaller.[6]

Cryoablation has been increasingly used to treat primary or secondary pulmonary neoplasms. Comparative data as to the relative efficacy of cryoablation versus RFA are lacking; however, there is no theoretical reason why one should be more efficacious than the other. There are some safety considerations that must be included in the risk-benefit analysis though. Specifically, cryoablation does not cause vessel coagulation as effectively as RFA does. This can be clinically significant, especially considering that many of the patients presenting for pulmonary ablation do so because their chronic obstructive pulmonary disease is the reason they are not surgical candidates (Fig. 65.4). A large pulmonary hemorrhage may be

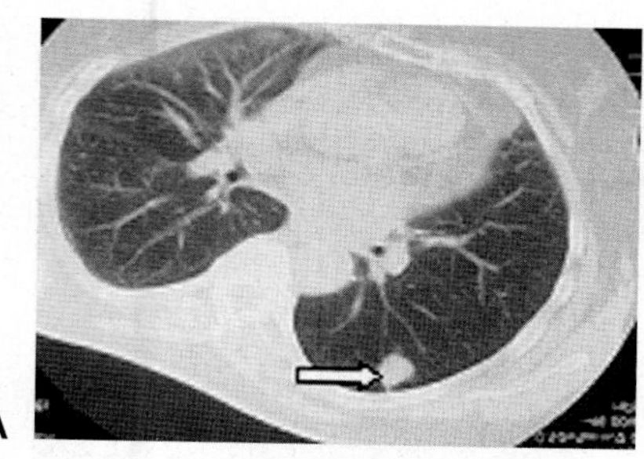

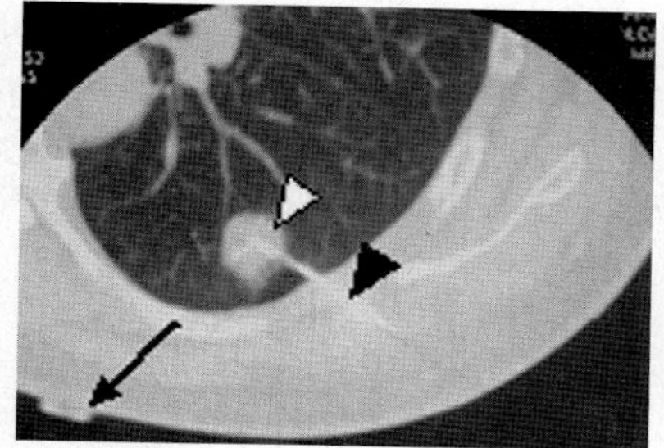

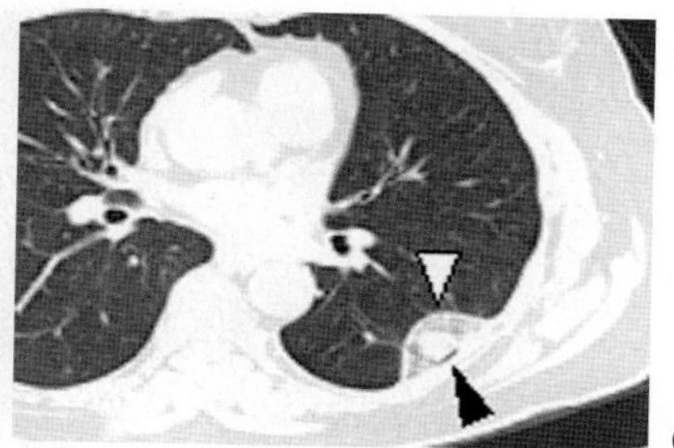

FIGURE 65.1 Pre–radiofrequency ablation (RFA) computed tomographic (CT) image (**A**) shows a 1.5-cm lesion (*arrow*) in the superior segment of left lower lobe. Intraprocedure CT image (**B**) shows the RFA probe (*black arrowhead*) directed percutaneously and its tines (*white arrowhead*) opening up in the lesion. The lesion margins are fuzzy because of the increased temperature and resultant tissue changes. The placement of radio-opaque skin markers (*black arrow*) helps select the proper access. One-month post-RFA CT image (**C**) shows sharp delineation of the ablated zone (*white arrowhead*). The lesion is still visible (*black arrowhead*) within the ablated zone, which indicated complete ablation. Because of cicatricial atelectasis and retraction, the ablated zone is now pleural-based.

life-threatening to patients with borderline pulmonary function. On the other hand, ablating lesions attached to the pleura is much better tolerated using cryoablation as RFA can result in significant pain/intercostal neuralgia.

Embolization

Transarterial embolization for pulmonary malignant disease should be reserved for specific situations and with a clear objective. It is not the standard of treatment. However, in selected cases it can offer significant benefits and indeed be life-saving. The most common indication for bronchial embolization of pulmonary malignant disease is hemoptysis, which is a very common complication of lung cancer, and sometimes the terminal event. Lung cancers, whether primary or metastatic, recruit blood vessels from the bronchial arteries rather than the pulmonary arteries via a process termed *tumor angiogenesis*. This allows catheter selection of the hypertrophied bronchial artery branch and embolization without risk for pulmonary embolism. Once selected, the artery supplying the lung tumor can be embolized to occlusion. The choice of embolization method is particles. Coils result in proximal occlusion, which allows for distal collateralization. When this occurs, further treatment is impossible because the coils do not allow access to the tumor. Gelfoam, another choice for embolization, is temporary and should be avoided. Therefore, particle embolization is the ideal choice as the particles travel distally, embolize in the rumor bed, and permanently stop blood flow. The main risk associated with bronchial embolization is inadvertent embolization of the spinal artery, which occasionally comes off one of the bronchial arteries. Therefore, bronchial embolization should be performed by experienced interventionalists only.

Another indication for bronchial tumor embolization is for a rapidly growing lung cancer refractory to systemic chemotherapy. This, although novel compared with other treatment methods, has been used both with particles alone as well as with chemotherapy (i.e., chemoembolization). Again, in selected patients and performed by experienced interventionalists, these procedures can offer substantial benefits to the patients that cannot be realized otherwise. Figure 65.5 shows a patient with metastatic chondrosarcoma to the lungs and life-threatening hemoptysis successfully treated with embolization.

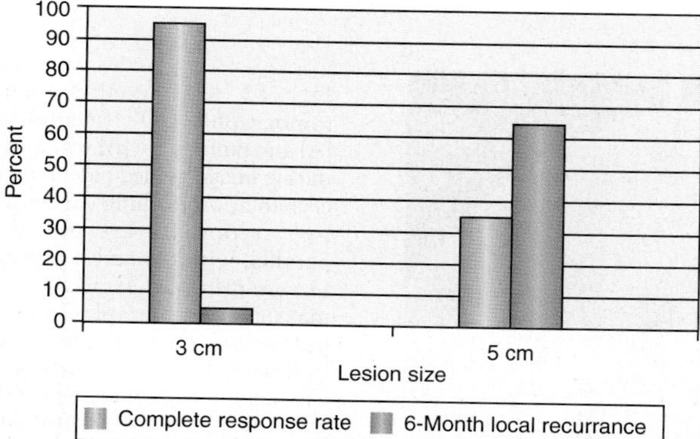

FIGURE 65.2 The efficacy of radiofrequency ablation (RFA) for lung cancer is mostly dependent on lesion size. Literature generally shows that lesions 3 cm or less respond favorably to RFA with a high primary complete response rate approaching 90% to 100%. On the other hand, lesions 5 cm or larger are unlikely to show complete response and generally require reintervention. Lesions 4 to 5 cm show variable response rates between these extremes that generally depend on operator experience and accessibility.

HEPATICOBILIARY

Hepatocellular Carcinoma

Liver cancer is the most common solid, nonskin cancer worldwide. Hepatocellular carcinoma (HCC) is on the rise both in the Western world as well as in areas that have been witnessing an endemic.[7,8] Its incidence has been steadily increasing over the past few years.[7] It is expected to continue increasing as its main underlying causes (hepatitis C in the West and hepatitis B in the east) continue to show an increase in incidence as well. Obesity-related liver disease is also increasing and likely to become a significant cause of liver cirrhosis and HCC in the next few decades. Irrespective of the cause, HCC is rarely a surgical disease as 75% to 85% of patients present with advanced, nonresectable lesions and/or cirrhosis.[9,10] In those patients whose cancer are deemed resectable, the disease will recur at a high rate (60%–80%) even when surgery is undertaken with curative intent.[9,10] Transplant has been shown to be the treatment offering the best chance for long-term survival, but very few patients with HCC are candidates because of unresectable lesions or comorbid conditions. Traditional systemic chemotherapy has been tried, but with disappointing results. Relevant studies show minimal or no survival benefit and significant chemotherapy-related toxicities. In this environment of limited and mostly ineffective choices for patients with HCC, interventional oncology has found its niche by developing techniques such as

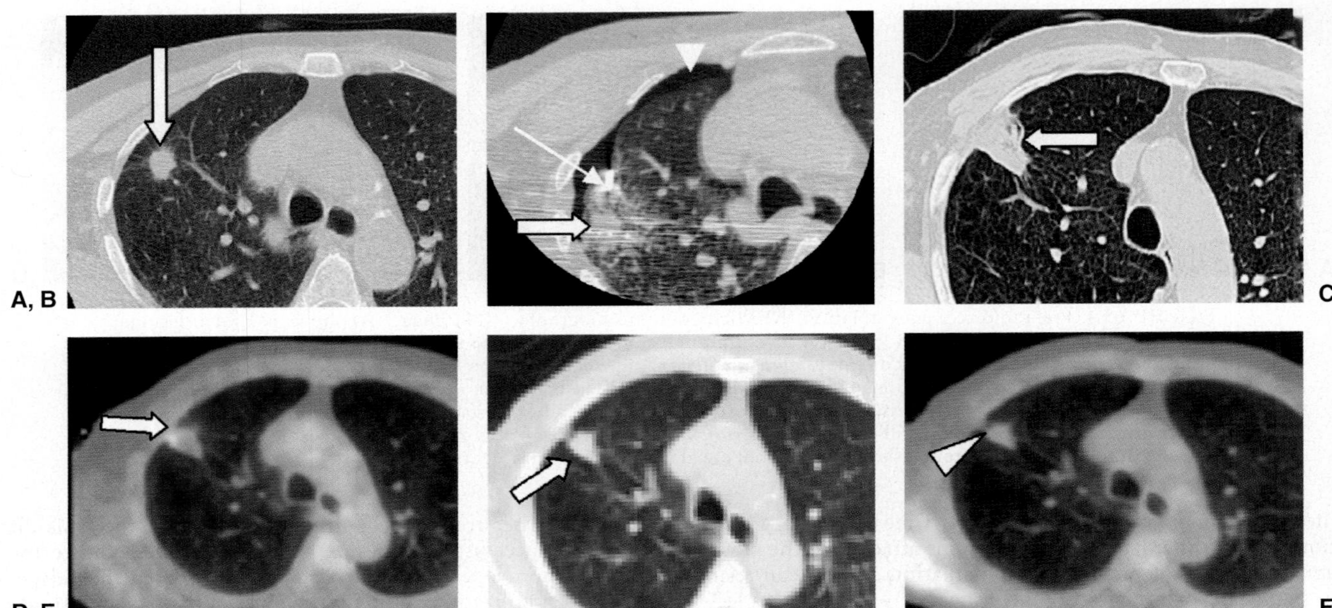

FIGURE 65.3 Pre–radiofrequency ablation (RFA) computed tomographic (CT) (**A**) shows a 1.5-cm speculated mass in the right upper lobe (*block arrow*). Intraprocedure CT image (**B**) shows the dense probe (*white arrow*) and the lesion (*block white arrow*) obscured by RFA-associated ground-glass opacities around it. A small pneumothorax (*white arrowhead*) is also noted. One-month post-RFA CT image (**C**) shows a wedge defect signifying cicatricial atelectasis (*block white arrow*), which includes the nonvisualized lesion. A 3-month post-RFA positron emission tomography (PET)/CT image (**D**) shows a focus of activity (*block white arrow*) peripherally in the treated lesion of unknown clinical significance at the time. Six-month CT (**E**) and PET/CT (**F**) follow-up show the treated area (*block white arrow*) diminished in size and no activity (*white arrowhead*) confirming complete response. The focus of activity in the previous PET/CT was thus inflammatory.

intra-arterial, tumor-targeted, and percutaneous thermal ablation treatments.

Transarterial Chemoembolization

Transarterial chemoembolization (TACE) has been shown to provide a significant survival benefit in selected patients with unresectable HCC.[11–13] The 1- and 2-year survival is typically 57% to 82% and 31% to 63% in the TACE-treated group, respectively, whereas it is 32% to 63% and 11% to 27% in patients receiving supportive care alone. A meta-analysis of five randomized controlled trials also concluded that TACE reduced the 2-year mortality of patients with unresectable HCC (odds ratio, 0.54; 95% confidence interval, 0.33–0.89; P = .015). Given these encouraging results, TACE has become the mainstay of treatment for unresectable HCC. TACE takes advantage of the fact that liver neoplasms receive their blood supply nearly exclusively from the hepatic artery, whereas normal liver parenchyma is mostly fed via the portal vein. Nevertheless, TACE does cause transient liver dysfunction. Therefore patient selection is crucial. Exclusion criteria are shown in Table 65.1. The treatment protocol has not been standardized yet; in general, it consists of selective intra-arterial delivery of a highly concentrated

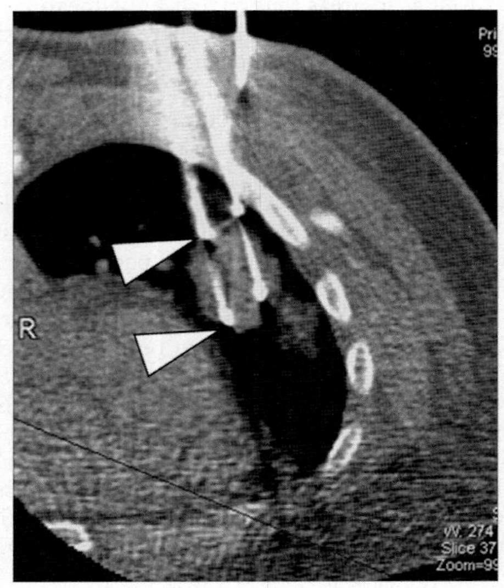

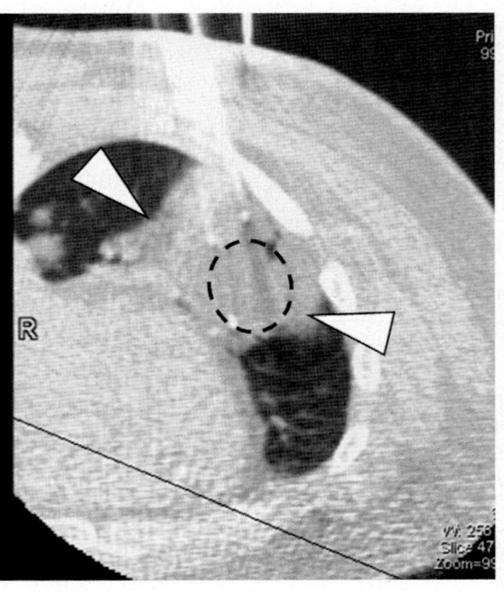

FIGURE 65.4 Axial computed tomographic (CT) (mediastinal [**A**] and pulmonary [**B**] windowed) during image-guided percutaneous cryoablation for lung cancer. The two cryoprobes are placed in parallel, with the active portions (*arrowheads*, **A**) straddling the mass. Soon after placement a pulmonary hemorrhage ensued indicated by *arrowheads* in **B**. The hemorrhage remained stable and the patient asymptomatic. This could have been a major clinical concern if the patient had significant pulmonary dysfunction (as many who are referred for lung ablation do) and the bleeding was not self-limiting. Many authors prefer radiofrequency ablation of lung lesions in order to minimize this risk.

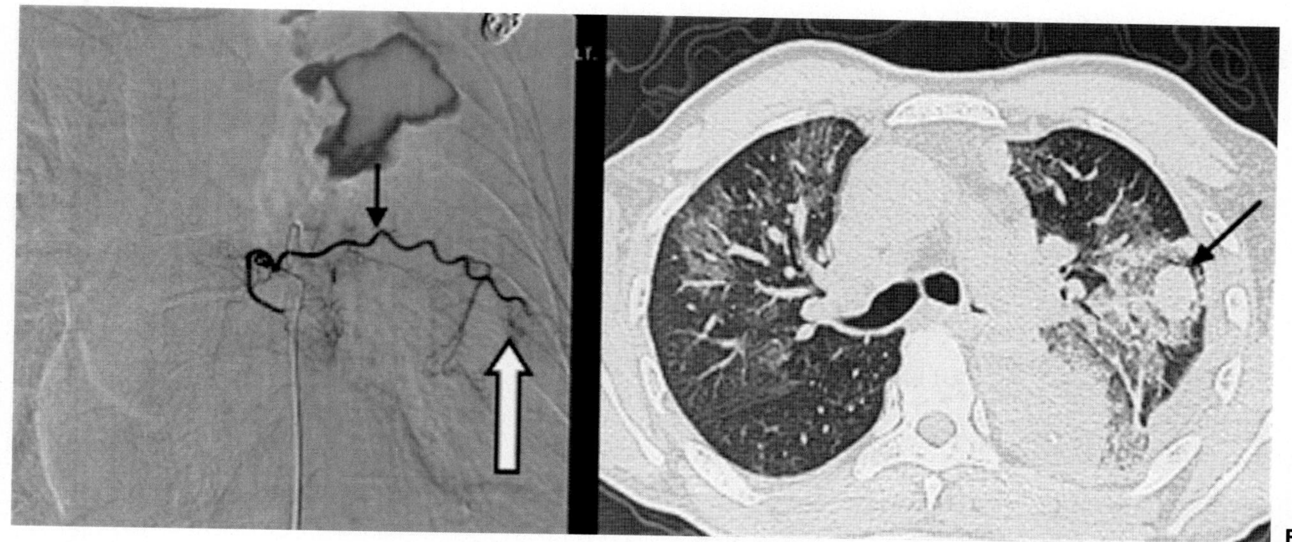

FIGURE 65.5 Digital subtraction angiogram (**A**) of left intercostal artery (*arrow*) in a patient with metastatic chondrosarcoma and life-threatening hemoptysis shows the blush at the bleeding site. Axial computed tomographic scan (**B**) shows the metastasis (*arrow*) surrounded by alveolar hemorrhage. Hemoptysis resolved after particle embolization of the bleeding intercostal.

chemotherapy mixture (single-, double-, or triple-agent mixture) into the hepatic artery supplying the tumor. Follow-up should include dual-phase magnetic resonance imaging (MRI) and repeat TACE every 4 to 6 weeks until tumor shows nearly 100% response or the patient develops a contraindication to TACE. Figure 65.6 shows pre- and intraprocedure images of a patient treated with TACE.

Drug-Eluding Beads

Drug-eluding beads (DEB) have been increasingly used in lieu of standard TACE. Studies attribute significant advantages to the use of DEB over TACE. The pharmacokinetic profile of DEB is superior to that of standard TACE, with studies showing a significantly lower plasma concentration and area under the curve.[14] Pathologic studies on liver explants have confirmed that the pharmacologic advantage of DEB does indeed translate to better tumor response. The rate of complete tumor necrosis after DEB embolization is about 77%, compared with 27% after standard TACE.[15] Survival has also been shown to improve with DEB over standard TACE.[16] Most institutions have already shifted to using DEB (loaded with doxorubicin) instead of standard TACE.

TABLE 65.1

EXCLUSION CRITERIA FOR TRANSARTERIAL CHEMOEMBOLIZATION (TACE)[a]

1. Child-Pugh C cirrhosis
2. Uncorrectable bleeding diathesis
3. Poor performance status (ECOG 3)
4. Resectable disease
5. Total bilirubin >4 mg/dL
6. Significant encephalopathy

ECOG, Eastern Cooperative Oncology Group.
[a]Patients with advanced liver disease may suffer acute liver failure because TACE transiently raises liver function tests, whereas early and intermediate cirrhosis patients recover from TACE-related injury. Additionally, Child-Pugh C patients will likely expire from their liver disease and not from their tumor; therefore, treatment is unlikely to offer a survival benefit. High bilirubin is an independent risk factor for liver failure after TACE and patients with levels above 4 mg/dL should avoid TACE unless it can be performed in a superselective manner to avoid inordinate liver injury. Also excluded are patients with poor performance status and clinical picture such as those with encephalopathy.

Radioembolization

Radioembolization, like TACE, takes advantage of the liver's dual blood supply to deliver the therapeutic agent to the liver tumor, which is predominantly supplied via the hepatic artery, while mostly sparing normal liver parenchyma. The therapeutic agent in this case, instead of chemotherapy, is a radioactive isotope coupled to a carrier particle. There are two types of radioembolization particles. Theraspheres (MDS Nordion, Ottawa, Ontario, Canada), which are glass microspheres with a diameter of 25 ±10 mcm, impregnated with yttrium-90 (^{90}Y), a radioactive element, and SIRspheres (Sirtex, Medical Limited, Wilmington, MA) are resin-based microspheres with a diameter of 29 to 35 mcm also attached to ^{90}Y. Following intra-arterial infusion, most Theraspheres embolize at the arteriolar level because of their relative size. ^{90}Y is a pure beta emitter (937 KeV) that decays to zirconium-90 with a half-life of 64.2 hours. The emitted electrons have an average tissue penetration of 2.5 mm (effective max, 10 mm).[17,18]

Histologic studies have shown that there is a disproportionate accumulation of ^{90}Y microspheres along the vascular periphery of the hepatic tumor, with a relative concentration of 2.4 to 50 times more than in the normal liver parenchyma.[19,20] Although the exact reason for this is not understood (perhaps the altered blood vessel flow and diameter that results from tumor angiogenesis allows preferential embospheres flow), this phenomenon can be used to deliver large doses of radiation to the tumor, while relatively sparing the normal liver. Radioactive microspheres are considered second-line intra-arterial treatment for HCC if TACE results are poor, and first or second line for colorectal metastases. Because of the use of radiation, this method has unique possible complications, which are nontarget radiation injury and radiation pneumonitis. Radiation duodenitis or gastritis is possible because of the proximity of the gastroduodenal artery and gastric arteries to the hepatic arteries, but avoidable with meticulous technique

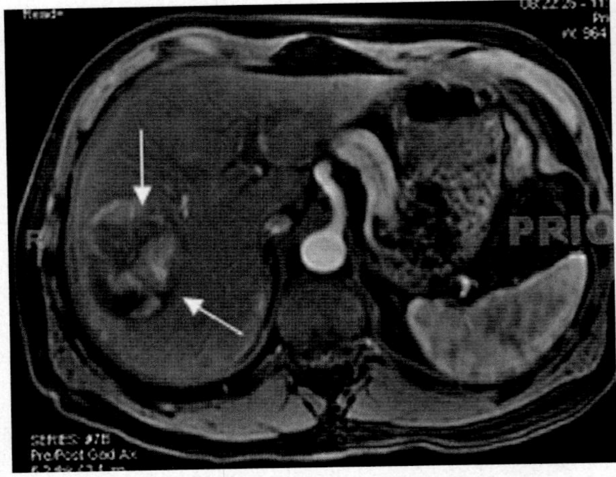

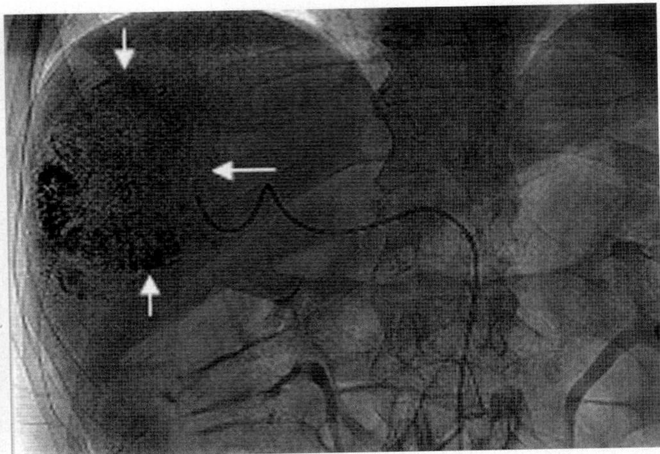

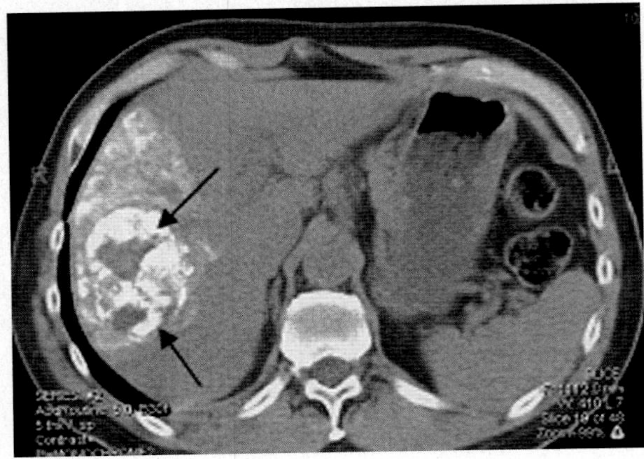

FIGURE 65.6 Sixty-two-year-old man with biopsy-proven hepatocellular carcinoma. Pretreatment, contrast-enhanced magnetic resonance imaging (MRI) of the liver (**A**) shows a right lobe mass with central necrosis and peripheral enhancement (*arrows*). Transarterial chemoembolization with doxorubicin, mitomycin C, and cisplatin was performed (**B**),which shows excellent deposition of chemoembolization mixture within the tumor (*arrows*). Follow-up computed tomographic scan of the liver (**C**) shows dense chemoembolization mixture distribution corresponding to the vascular regions of the tumor (*arrows*) and correlating well with the MRI findings on Figure 65.5A.

and good anatomic knowledge. Radiation pneumonitis results from shunting of blood from the hepatic artery to the hepatic vein through large tumor vessels. Quantification and elimination of the shunting, if necessary, is essential prior to radioembolization in order to prevent this complication. Thus, all patients undergo shunt calculation prior to radioembolization. Follow-up of patients treated with radioembolization is centered on establishing tumor viability and is thus identical to that of TACE-treated patients. A dual-phase liver MRI in 4 to 6 weeks posttreatment is obtained. Retreatment or merely continued follow-up is dependent on tumor residual.

Percutaneous Ablation

Several methods for percutaneous treatment for liver tumors exist, including RFA, microwave coagulation therapy, cryoablation (Cryo), and ethanol or acetic acid injection. The most widely used are RFA and Cryo, which use heat and cold, respectively, to cause tissue necrosis. The efficacy of both methods depends on lesion size, location, and operator experience and is independent of histology or organ. The efficacy of RFA in liver tumors has been established and for lesions 3 cm or less, is at or near 100% complete response.[21,22] As in the lung, efficacy decreases with lesion size, and lesions larger than 5 cm are unlikely to be eradicated. For relatively small lesions (3 cm or less), the median survival is the same between RFA and surgically treated patients.[23]

Percutaneous ablation, whether RFA or Cryo, is performed under conscious sedation, has minimal risks, and usually is an outpatient procedure and can be repeated, all of which are obvious advantages over surgery. Figure 65.7 shows pre- and post-RFA images for metastatic colon cancer to liver. Figure 65.8 shows the risk of HCC recurrence after RFA according to lesion size, and Figure 65.9 compares the efficacy of RFA and resection for HCC 3 cm or smaller.

CHOLANGIOCARCINOMA

Intrahepatic cholangiocarcinoma (ICC) is primary liver cancer with cholangiocytic molecular and histopathologic characteristics located peripheral to the biliary ductal confluence and is usually a mass-forming tumor. Cholangiocarcinomas in general represent only 15% of primary liver cancers,[24] with ICC comprising only about 15% of those. Thus, 85% of cholangiocarcinomas are not mass-forming, involve the central ducts, and present with biliary obstruction. The distinction between the two types of cholangiocarcinoma is crucial from a treatment point of view. The common intraductal type presents with obstructive jaundice and treatment by IR is placement of a biliary stent for decompression, whereas the rarer mass-forming peripheral type presents usually with pain and other constitutional symptoms and can be treated with locoregional techniques.

Common Type Cholangiocarcinoma

Catheter Drainage

In the case of a centrally obstructing cholangiocarcinoma, the objective is to decompress the obstructed biliary system.

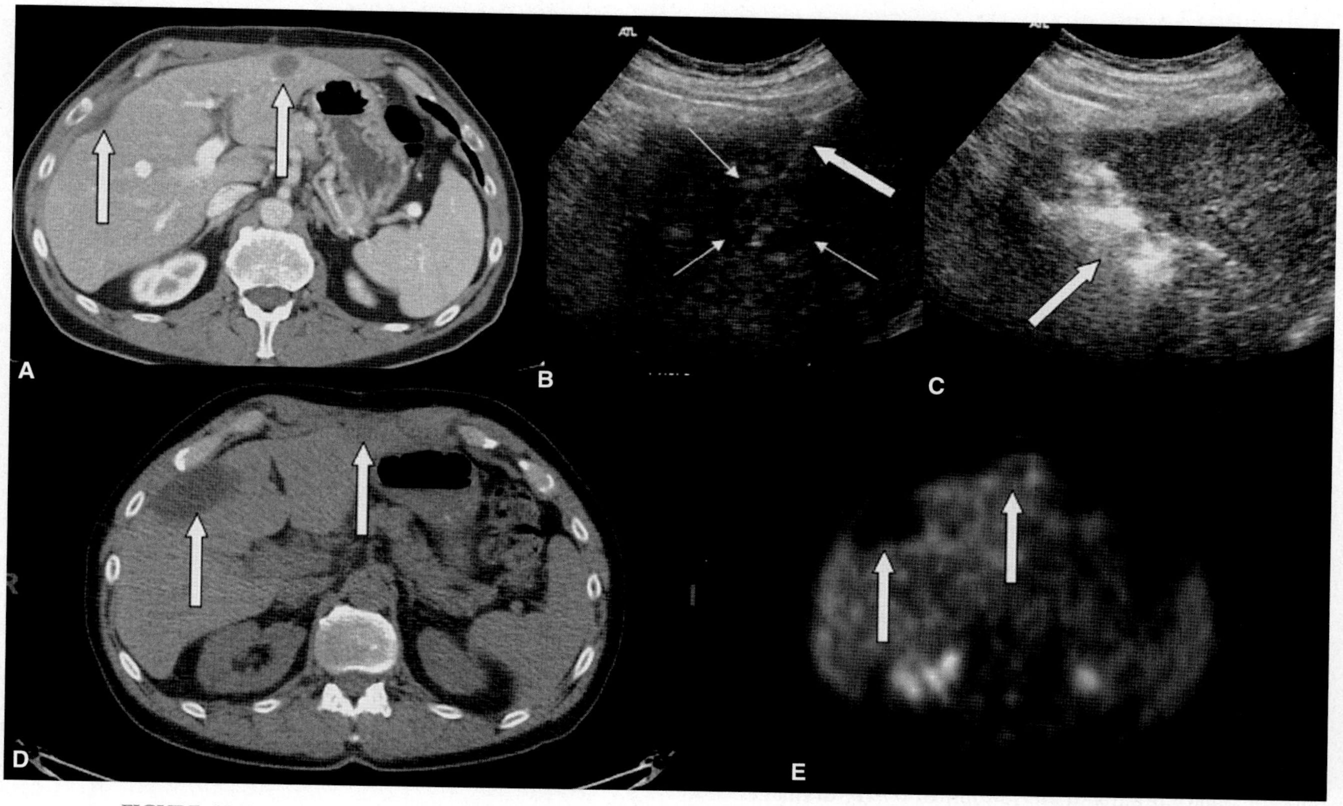

FIGURE 65.7 Sixty-one-year-old man presenting 2 years status post colectomy for colon cancer with two metastatic colon cancer lesions (*block arrows*) to the liver seen on surveillance computed tomography (CT) (**A**). Intraprocedure ultrasound images (**B**) during radiofrequency ablation (RFA) show the RFA probe (*block arrow*) placed within the lesion (*arrows*). At the end of the ablation (**C**), microbubbles (*block arrow*) resulting from tissue overheating cause artifact rendering the lesion no longer discernible. Repeated CT (**D**) and positron emission tomography/CT studies (**E**), the last 18 months postablation, show large inactive defects (*block arrows*) in the location of the tumors confirming complete response and no residual viable tumor.

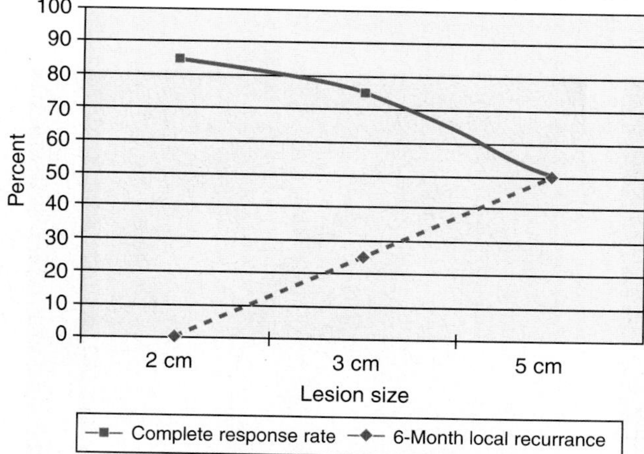

FIGURE 65.8 Graph showing the efficacy of percutaneous, image-guided radiofrequency ablation (RFA) of hepatocellular carcinoma according to lesion size. The solid line (*blue*) indicates the percentage of lesions showing complete response to RFA. Lesions smaller that 3 cm respond excellently to percutaneous RFA. Similarly, the risk of local recurrence indicated by the dashed line (*red*) increases with lesion size. As supported in the relevant literature, percutaneously accessible lesions measuring 3 cm or less in diameter can be effectively treated with percutaneous RFA with an efficacy similar to that of surgical resection (see Fig. 65.9).

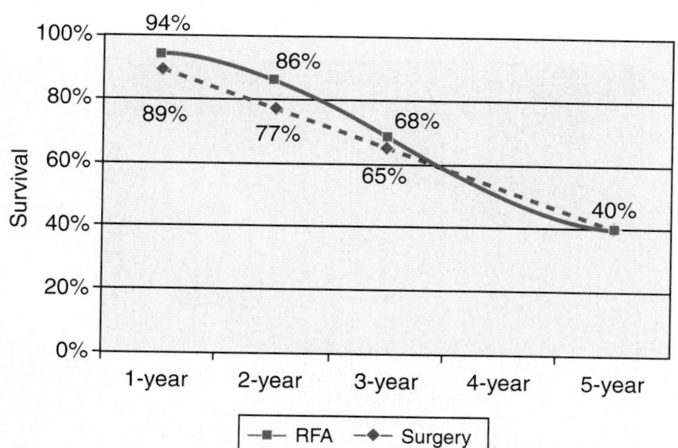

FIGURE 65.9 Graph shows the 1-, 2-, 3-, and 5-year survival rates for hepatocellular carcinoma lesions treated with radiofrequency ablation (RFA) (*solid blue line*) versus surgery (*dashed red line*) for lesions 3 cm in diameter or less and Child-Pugh class A or B patients. Irrespective of risk of local or distal recurrence, the survival of the two groups is the same (not statistically significant). Given that surgical resection invariably results in significant normal liver parenchymal loss and that most patients have limited liver reserve owing to their cirrhosis, RFA becomes a very attractive alternative even in resectable patients.

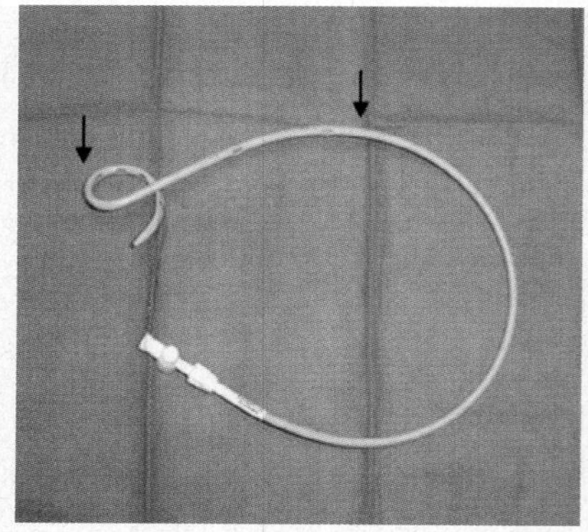
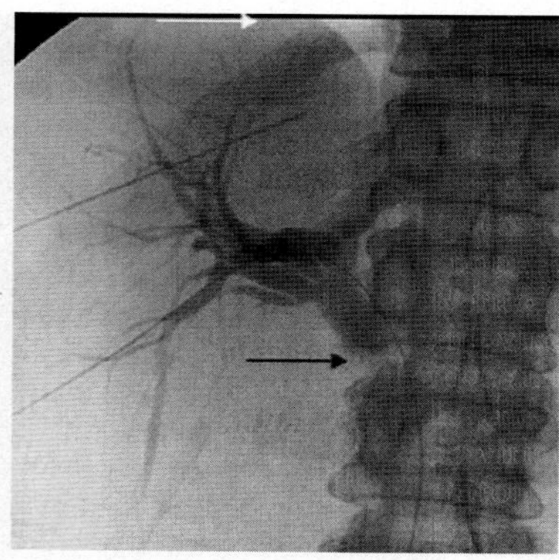
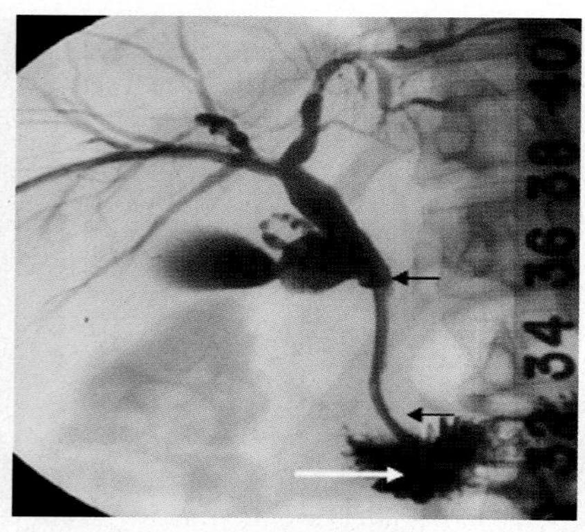

FIGURE 65.10 Placement of a percutaneous biliary drainage catheter. The catheter (**A**) has multiple side holes (between arrows) that collect the bile and drain it into the small bowel, thus bypassing the bile duct obstruction. A common bile duct obstruction (*arrow*, **B**) is bypassed by the biliary catheter (*black arrows*, **C**) draining the bile into the duodenum (*white arrow*).

Because of the infiltrating nature of this type of cholangiocarcinoma, no effective intra-arterial treatment method has been developed. Approximately 20,000 new cases are diagnosed annually in the United States, with a nearly identical mortality rate resulting in a median survival of less than 1 year.[25] Proper biliary catheter placement can result in dramatic improvement in quality of life and significant survival benefit. The biliary catheter's location should be such that the whole system is adequately decompressed. Figure 65.10 shows the internal external type biliary drain and an example of biliary drainage.

Internal Biliary Stent

The placement of an internal metallic stent has the advantage of not requiring maintenance, or exchanges, and causes no discomfort to the patient. Because of tumor overgrowth, however, all internal stents will eventually occlude. Because of this, stents are reserved for patients whose life expectancy is shorter than the patency rate of the stent.

Figure 65.11A shows such a stent that is covered with expanded polytetrafluoroethylene (ePTFE), a material resistant to bile penetration. The median patency rate of ePTFE-covered biliary stents is about 18 months (Fig. 65.12) and the 3-, 6-, and 12-month patency rate is 90%, 76%, and 76%, respectively.[26] Because of the limited patency rate, candidates for this procedure are generally patients with unresectable pancreatic cancer and advanced cholangiocarcinoma involving the common bile duct. Patients with benign biliary strictures should not be treated with internal stent placement. Figure 65.11B shows an example of biliary decompression after internal stent placement.

Transbiliary Biopsy, Cholangioplasty, Choledochoscopy

A percutaneous biliary drain catheter offers itself as a conduit for biliary biopsy and other procedures. Once a stricture (benign or malignant) is identified, the catheter is exchanged for a sheath (a hollow tube) through which many intrabiliary procedures can be performed, such as biopsies, balloon cholangioplasty, and choledochoscopy. The brush or clamshell biopsy set is advanced under fluoroscopic guidance and samples are obtained at the stricture site. The sensitivity and specificity of these biopsies depend on the type of biopsy (brush vs. clamshell) and the number of specimens obtained (Table 65.2). Figures 65.13

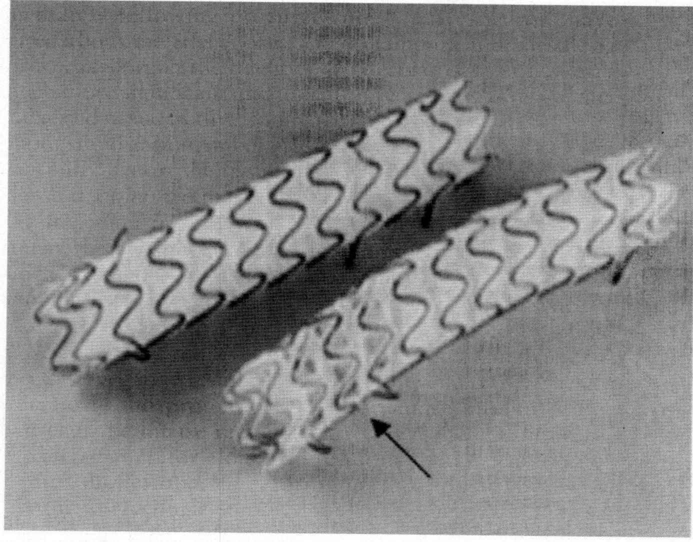
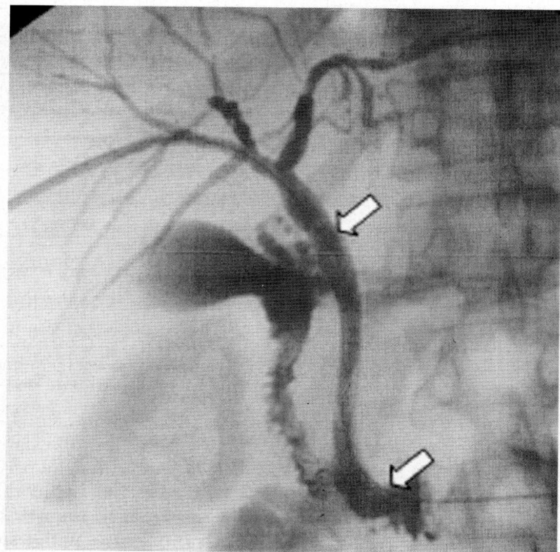

FIGURE 65.11 Covered biliary stents (**A**) with (*arrow*) and without proximal side holes. The stent with side holes is chosen when the gallbladder is still present to avoid cystic duct obstruction. Percutaneous cholangiogram (**B**) after placement of an internal, metallic-covered biliary stent (*white arrows*) shows decompression of contrast into the duodenum.

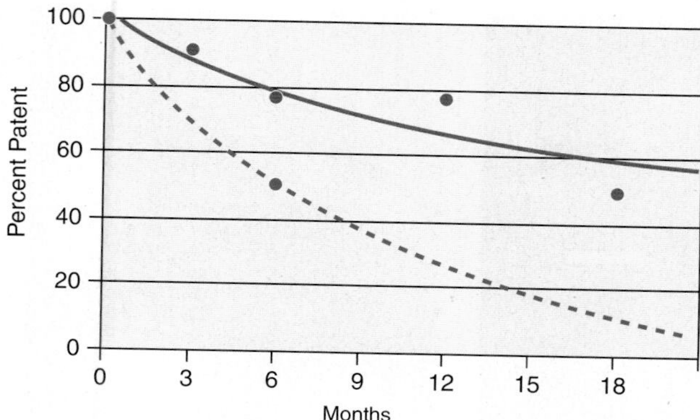

FIGURE 65.12 Patency rates for internal biliary stents. Stents covered with expanded polytetrafluoroethylene (*solid red line*) show a much better patency rate with more than 50% being open at 2 years. On the other hand, bare stents (*dashed blue line*) have a mean patency rate of 6 months. Because the life expectancy of unresectable pancreatic cancer is less than 1 year, covered stents offer a significant advantage over bare stents.

through 65.15 showcase the types of procedures that can be performed via a percutaneous transbiliary route.

Mass-Forming, Intrahepatic Cholangiocarcinoma

Even though mass-forming cholangiocarcinoma is a rare entity, its incidence has been increasing over the past few years. Currently there are 3,000 new cases per year of mass-forming ICC in the United States,[25] most of which are unresectable at presentation and with universally poor survival. Because of its peripheral nature, ICC is technically amenable to locoregional treatment modalities. In addition, because these patients do not usually suffer from underlying liver cirrhosis, they are better able to tolerate TACE and/or percutaneous ablation than their HCC counterparts.

TACE and RFA

Both of these treatment modalities have been used to treat mass-forming cholangiocarcinomas. Early data suggest similar safety and efficacy as in patients with unresectable HCC. One advantage of the cholangiocarcinoma patients is that they do not generally have associated liver cirrhosis and thus are better able to complete the treatment protocol with minimal complications. TACE has been shown to improve median survival from 16 to 23 months and convert 10% to 15% of patients into surgical candidates after tumor shrinkage.[27] RFA has also been shown to be effective in treating mass-forming cholangiocarcinomas, with tumors 3 cm or less showing complete response nearly 100% of the time.[28,29] Figure 65.16 shows the results of TACE for a mass-forming cholangiocarcinoma.

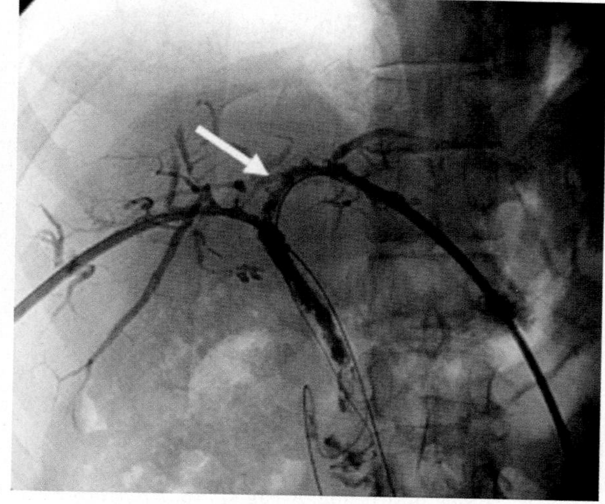

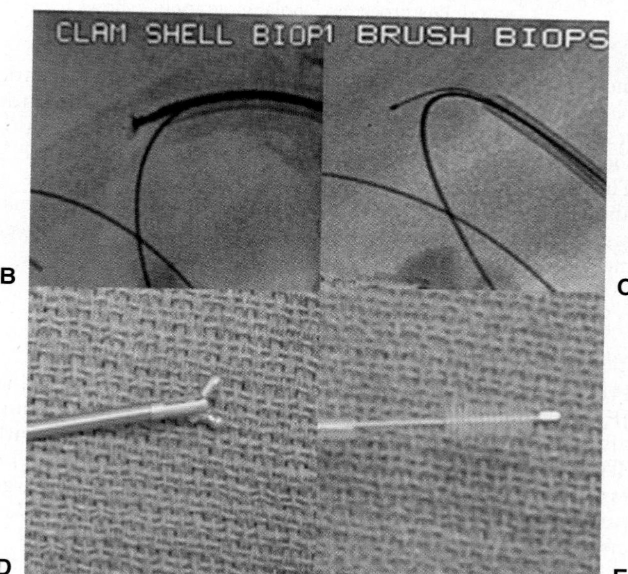

FIGURE 65.13 Percutaneous cholangiogram (**A**) shows abnormal biliary epithelium of the left main duct near the biliary confluence (*arrow*). Brush biopsy (**C** and **E**) and clamshell biopsy (**B** and **D**) of the suspicious lesion were performed under fluoroscopy to ensure proper sampling. Biopsy results were positive for cholangiocarcinoma.

TABLE 65.2

ACCURACY DATA FOR PERCUTANEOUS BILIARY BIOPSY[a]

Biopsy Type	Sensitivity (%)	Negative Predictive Value (%)	Specificity (%)
Brush (×3)	70	50	45
Clamshell (×3)	90	80	95

[a]Performing brush biopsies of a suspicious lesion alone is unreliable and most of the time nondiagnostic. When, however, it is combined with clamshell biopsies, the sensitivity and specificity of percutaneous biliary biopsy is dramatically increased. The endoscopic approach does not offer itself for clamshell biopsy and thus suffers from low accuracy.

LIVER METASTASES

Colon Cancer Liver Metastases

Of the nearly 20% of colon cancer patients who present with metastatic disease, the majority will have liver involvement. Eventually more than 50% of patients will develop liver

SPECIALIZED TECHNIQUES IN CANCER MANAGEMENT

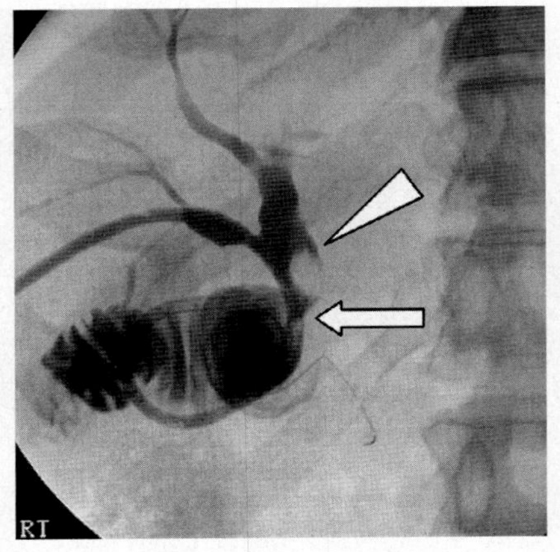

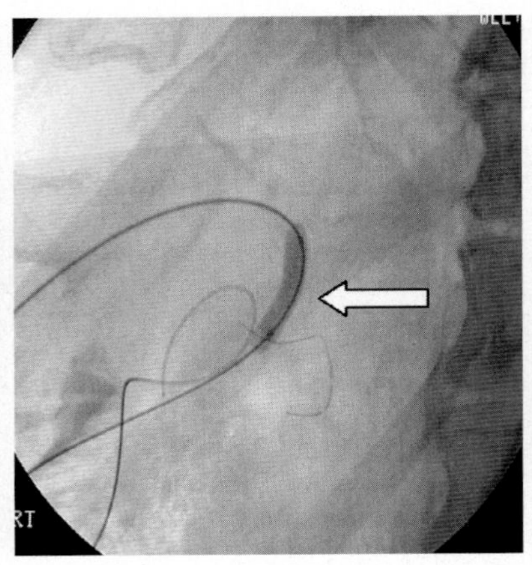

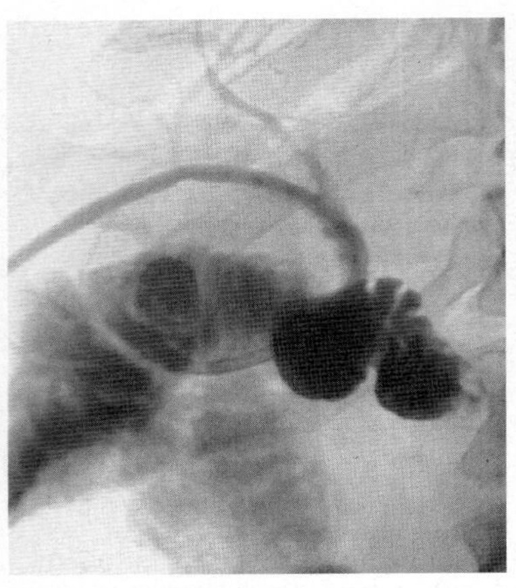

FIGURE 65.14 Percutaneous cholangiogram (**A**) of a patient with obstructive jaundice 1 year after hepatojejunostomy (HJ) for pancreatic cancer. A stone (*white arrowhead*) is impacted against the HJ anastomotic stricture (*white arrow*) causing obstruction. A balloon (**B**, *white arrow*) is used to dilate the stricture and to push the stone into the small bowel. Postprocedure cholangiogram (**C**) shows the stone has passed and the stricture has resolved.

metastases and only a minority, those with excellent hepatic reserve and minimal liver involvement, are candidates for resection. Despite the introduction of new effective chemotherapy agents, mortality is still close to 40% of incidence.[30] The annual incidence of colon cancer in the United States is about 150,000 with 20,000 of the patients having liver metastases at presentation and many of the rest developing liver metastases in the future.[31]

TACE, Radioembolization, RFA

Preliminary data from Johns Hopkins Hospital (Geschwind JF, et al, unpublished data, 2006) suggest a 10-month survival benefit for patients with liver metastases treated with TACE (Figure 65.17). The study was limited to patients who failed first-, second-, and third-line chemotherapy, with large tumors (mean 10 cm) and extrahepatic disease, which makes any survival benefit extraordinary.

RFA for colorectal metastases is no different, as far as efficacy and safety is concerned, from any other neoplasm in the liver. The most crucial variables are size, location, and number of lesions. Lesions 3 cm or less, visible using CT, ultrasound, or MR for guidance can be effectively treated, offering the patient significant survival benefit.

Neuroendocrine Liver Metastases

Neuroendocrine cancers are relatively rare tumors of the gastrointestinal tract with about 4,000 new cases annually in the United States. At presentation 10% to 20% of patients have metastatic disease mostly in the liver with a 5-year survival of 20%.[31] Resection of primary and liver metastases is the treatment of choice and has been shown to improve survival.[32] TACE is recommended if there is bulky liver disease prior to resection or if the disease is unresectable but liver-dominant. For lesions less than 3 cm, RFA has shown promising results with 100% response in most cases.[33] Even for patients with multifocal disease, RFA can result in disease control and an extended median survival of 53 months.[34]

Other Liver Metastases

The condition of a large number of patients with primary lung, breast cancer, or melanoma (as well as other epidemiologically less significant cancers) is complicated by liver metastases. Many of these patients, that is, those with liver-dominant disease, will likely die from liver failure. Although current research is lacking, TACE or RFA concurrent with systemic

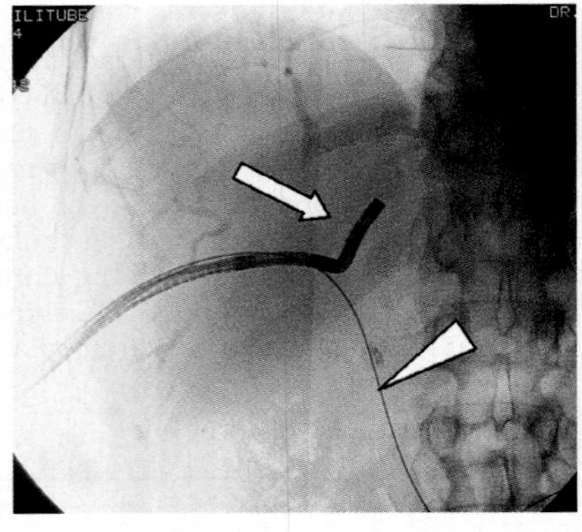

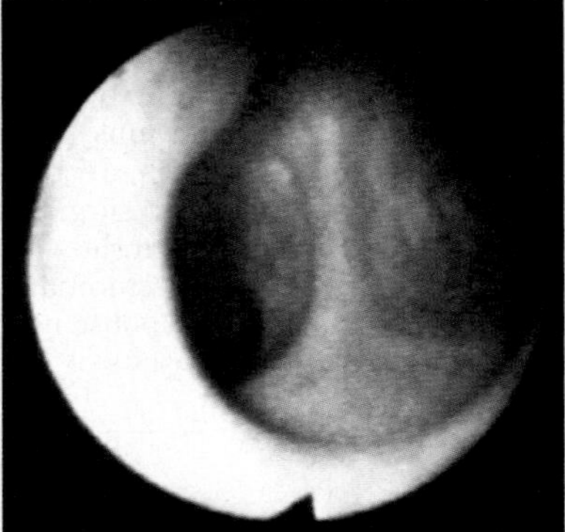
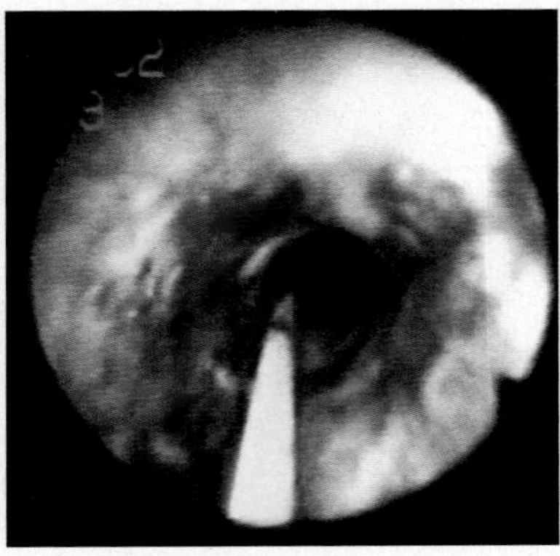

FIGURE 65.15 Although access into the biliary tree is maintained with a wire (**A**, *white arrowhead*) a choledochoscope is inserted percutaneously to establish biliary pathology. The scope has been inserted via a right-sided bile duct and its tip (*white arrow*) advanced into the left bile duct. A choledochoscopic view of a healthy biliary epithelium is shown in **B**. **C** shows a diffusely inflamed biliary epithelium in a patient with primary sclerosing cholangitic. Choledochoscopy can be useful in diagnosing bile duct cancers, stones, and evaluation for bleeding.

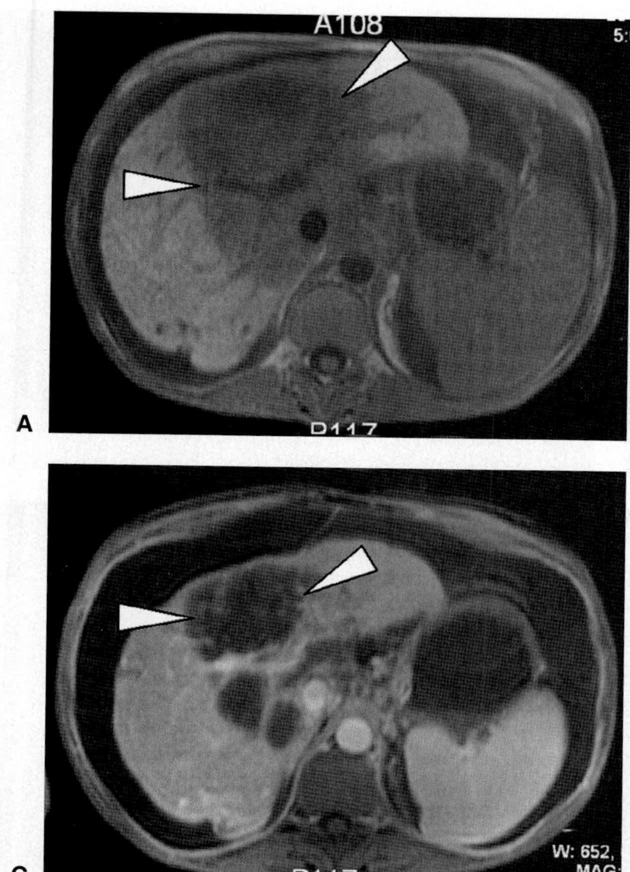

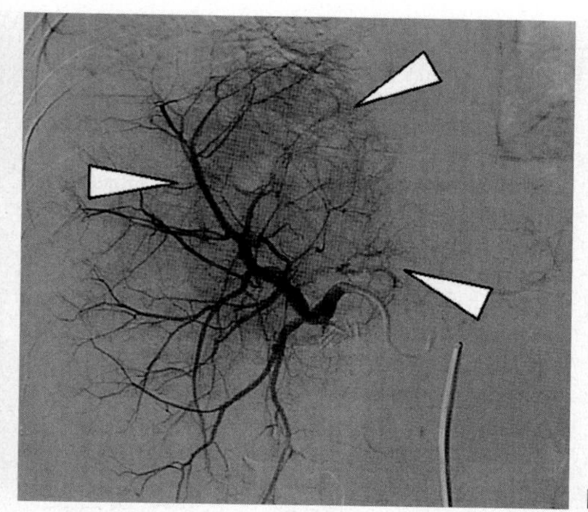

FIGURE 65.16 Axial magnetic resonance (MR) image of the liver (**A**) shows a central low signal lesion in the liver (*arrowheads*), which was a biopsy-proven cholangiocarcinoma. Angiogram during transarterial chemoembolization (**B**) shows the hypervascular blush (*arrowheads*) representing this lesion. One-month post-treatment follow-up MR image (**C**) shows the previously solid lesion is now mostly cystic (*arrowheads*); 80% to 90% of the tumor is necrotic.

chemotherapy or after chemotherapy failure can result in significant tumor cytoreduction. Irrespective of tumor histology, TACE and RFA can reasonably be expected to effect a tumor response rate of 50% to 75%, many times even close to 100%. Evidence is currently emerging that cytoreduction may extend survival in many patients. Because of the lack of prospective randomized studies, liver-directed therapies for metastatic liver disease should be reserved for those patients with liver-dominant disease and for whom standard of treatment has either failed or can be administered concurrently with TACE or ablation.

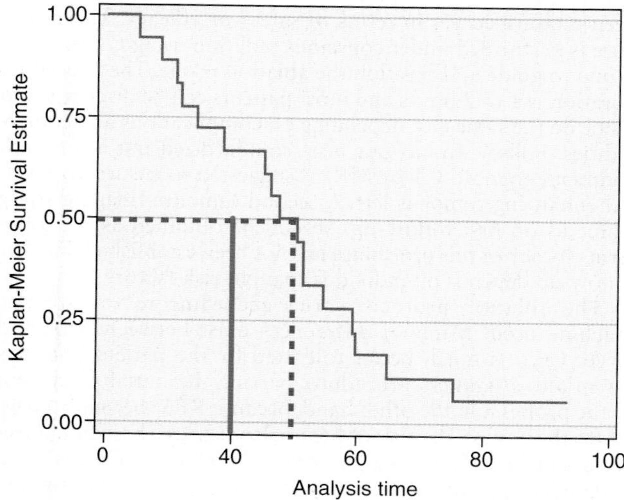

FIGURE 65.17 Survival of patients treated with transarterial chemoembolization (TACE) for colon cancer metastases to the liver. Even though the treatment group consisted of patients who failed all other treatments, they still enjoyed nearly 10-month survival benefit (*dashed red line*) compared with those who did not receive TACE (*solid green line*).

Special Topic: Portal Vein Embolization

Partial liver resection is a curative option for patients with HCC and unable or unwilling to be considered for transplantation. The role of liver resection has also expanded to include patients with certain types of oligometastatic disease in whom metastectomy has been shown to improve survival (colorectal, sarcoma). However, even in technically resectable patients, partial liver resection can only be performed if adequate liver function remains after surgery. In general the minimum liver volume required to sustain life is 20% to 25% and higher for patients with liver dysfunction. Portal vein embolization has been shown to induce contralateral liver parenchyma hypertrophy, thus improving the chances of resection (Fig. 65.18). Studies report a remnant liver hypertrophy of 10% to 69% from its original volume,[35,36] and improved probability of undergoing resection without subsequent complications.[37]

GENITOURINARY

Renal Cancer

Renal cell carcinoma (RCC) is the 7th and 12th most common malignancy in men and women, respectively, in the United

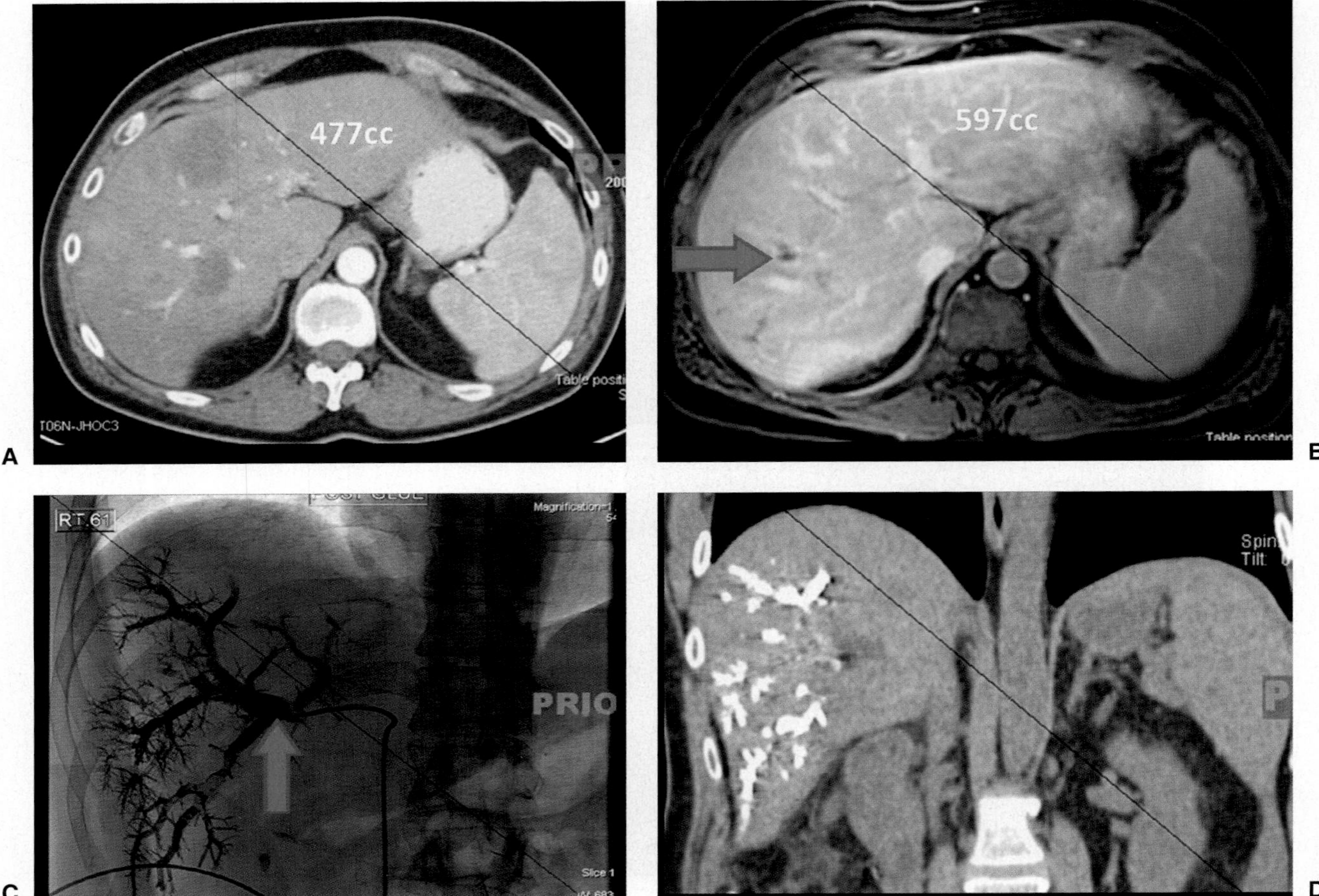

FIGURE 65.18 Patient with metastatic colorectal cancer to the right liver who could benefit from liver resection. Projected remnant liver calculated on baseline contrast enhanced computed tomography (CT) (**A**) was calculated at 477 cc and not adequate. Right portal vein embolization was performed, which resulted in left lobe hypertrophy to 597 cc 1 month later (**B**). The right portal vein branches are occluded (*arrow*). The intaprocedural angiogram (**C**) shows the cast of the glue used to embolize the right portal vein (*arrow*). Postprocedure, coronal-reconstructed CT (**D**) again shows the glue casting the embolized right portal vein branches.

States, with an annual incidence of about 36,000. Mortality is about one-third of incidence, translating to 12,000 per year.[35] The majority of cases are sporadic (97%) with only 2% to 3% being attributed to inherited conditions.[35,36] Risk factors include obesity and cigarette smoking and possibly hypertension, which account for one-fourth of all cases.[36] Despite the decrease in cigarette smoking, the incidence of RCC has been on the rise. This is, to a large degree, because of earlier or incidental detection with the widespread use CT and MRI.[35] Because of the smaller size at presentation and technological advancements, the past few years have witnessed a trend toward less invasive interventions. Open surgery is reserved for larger or technically challenging lesions, whereas the number of laparoscopic nephrectomies is increasing. Nephron-sparing interventions have been developed such as laparoscopic partial nephrectomy and laparoscopic ablations, which have the obvious advantage of sparing normal renal parenchyma. The contribution of IR has been the performance of image-guided percutaneous cryoablation or RFA of renal cancer as well as transarterial embolization.

Percutaneous Ablation for RCC

Percutaneous ablation using either RFA or Cryo is a minimally invasive procedure that can effectively treat RCC and other renal tumors. Similar to ablations elsewhere, the safety and efficacy of RCC ablation depend on tumor size, location, and operator experience. No difference between RFA and Cryo has been established yet in terms of safety or efficacy. The procedure is performed under conscious sedation using CT or ultrasound to guide and position the ablation probe. The procedure duration is 1 to 2 hours and most patients can be discharged to home on the same day, depending on complications and comorbidities. Follow-up has not been standardized but a 3-month contrast-enhanced CT or MRI is suggested to ensure no residual enhancing tumor is left. A second 6-month imaging study (same as on first follow-up) should be obtained as the long-term efficacy of this procedure has not been established. Further follow-up depends on individual patient risk factors.

The ablation protocol varies according to the specific machine used. Minimal differences exist between RFA and Cryo. Cryo is much better tolerated by the patient and it is essentially a painless procedure, barring the initial placement of the probes. On the other hand, because RFA thermally coagulates the tissues, the risk of hemorrhage is less, based on anecdotal evidence. Figure 65.19 shows the procedure steps for a CT-guided, percutaneous Cryo of an RCC and its follow-up. Early results are very promising, indicating near 100% response for lesions 3 cm or less,[37,38] with larger lesions showing a precipitous drop in efficacy with size.[35] Even if the lesion to be treated is too large to expect complete response, it has been shown that cytoreduction of RCC with metastases prolongs

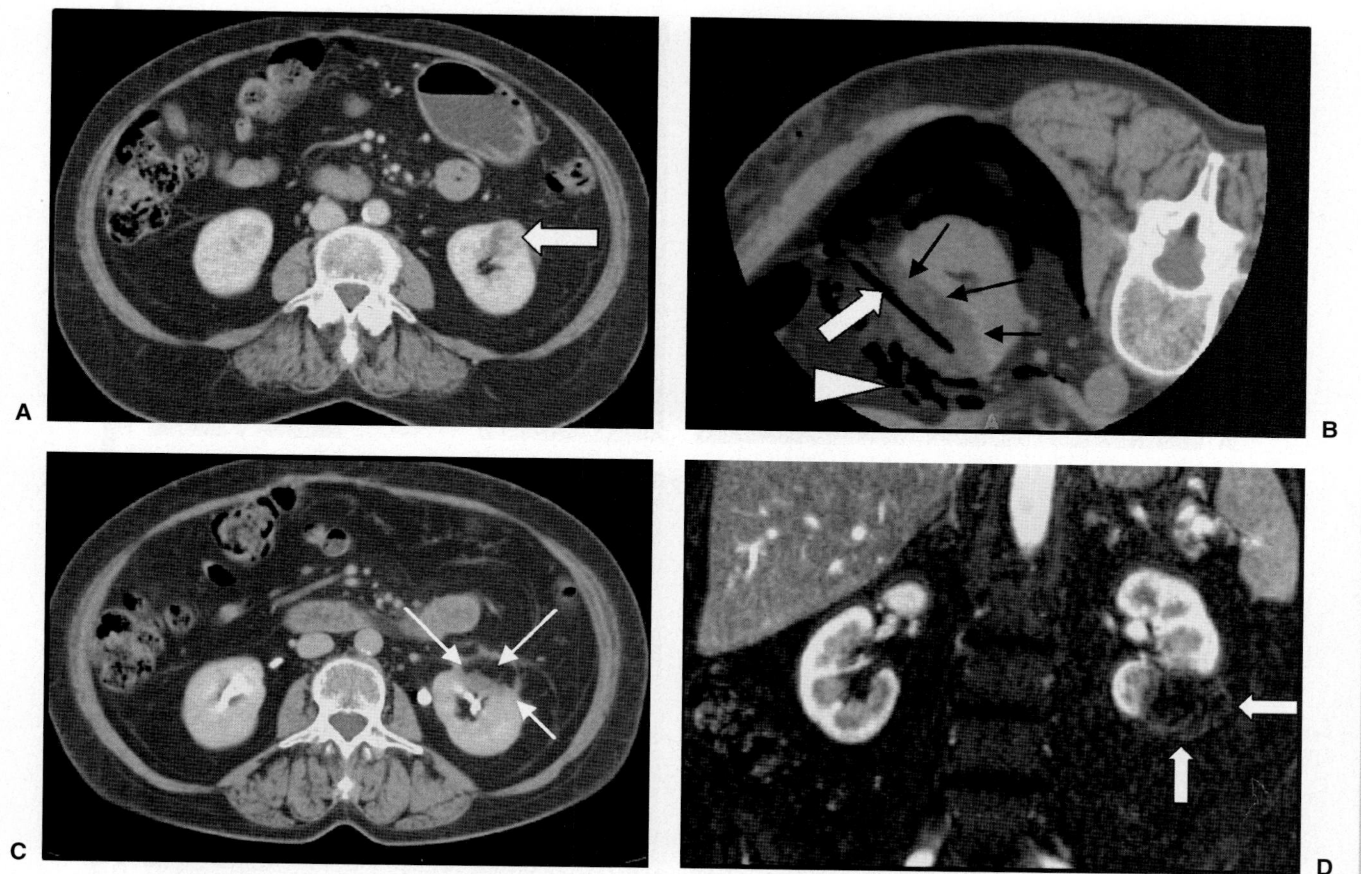

FIGURE 65.19 Axial, contrast enhanced computed tomography (CT) image (**A**) shows a 2-cm enhancing left renal mass (*arrow*), which was biopsy-proven renal cell carcinoma. Intraprocedural CT image during percutaneous cryoablation (**B**) shows the ablation probe tract (*white arrow*) and the surrounding ablation zone (*black arrows*), which is hypodense compared to rest of renal parenchyma. The ablation zone covers the mass seen on **A**. *White arrowhead* shows air injected through a separate needle to push the adjacent bowel away from the ablation zone and avoid collateral injury. Axial contrast-enhanced CT 1-month postablation (**C**) shows minimal inflammatory changes (*arrows*) and no residual enhancing lesion. Coronal T1-weighted gadolinium enhanced MR image 3-months postablation (**D**) shows a round defect in the left kidney (*arrows*) confirming complete resolution of the tumor.

survival. The development of MR interventional software and hardware will likely increase the use of this procedure.

Transarterial Embolization

Transarterial embolization (TAE) for renal tumors can be used alone or in conjunction with percutaneous ablation for larger tumors. Early reports (mean follow-up, 16 months) show that TAE and ablation for lesions 3.5 to 9 cm show complete response in nearly all cases, which is significantly better than ablation alone.[39] TAE on its own can reduce intraoperative hemorrhage during nephrectomy as well as tumor-related hematuria in unresectable patients,[40] but there are no data yet as to improving survival for unresectable patients. TAE is also useful in treating nonmalignant renal tumors such as angiomyolipomas. Arterial embolization has been shown to significantly improve symptoms related to tumor size and minimize the risk of bleeding.[41–43] Figure 65.20 shows arterial embolization for symptomatic angiomyolipoma and follow-up.

MUSCULOSKELETAL CANCER

There are many indications for percutaneous or intra-arterial treatment of musculoskeletal neoplasms; however, as most represent metastatic disease, treatment objectives are limited to local tumor control, pain alleviation, or preoperative embolization to minimize intraoperative blood loss. Nevertheless, in properly selected patients such minimally invasive procedure can result in significant improvement in quality of life. The selection of the specific intervention is equally crucial for a good outcome. TAE is quite effective in minimizing intraoperative blood loss, especially when dealing with hypervascular metastatic lesions such as renal cell and thyroid carcinoma. On the other hand, percutaneous ablation procedures are effective in alleviating pain related to the local effects of tumor that result in painful lytic lesions and/or associated pathologic fractures. A physical examination is necessary prior to any intervention because the ablation must target the actual cause of the pain. Therefore, generalized pain is unlikely to respond to locoregional treatments, whereas focal pain that is elucidated during a physical examination is very likely to respond favorably to percutaneous ablation. The choice of Cryo versus RFA is operator-dependent; however, in general Cryo is better tolerated and shows faster recovery. On the other hand, RFA has less bleeding complications, which may be important in large vascular lesions.

Finally, a specific lesion may require a combination treatment to respond. Figure 65.21 shows one such patient with debilitating pain, who responded very well after a combined percutaneous RFA and cementoplasty procedure for a pathologic bone

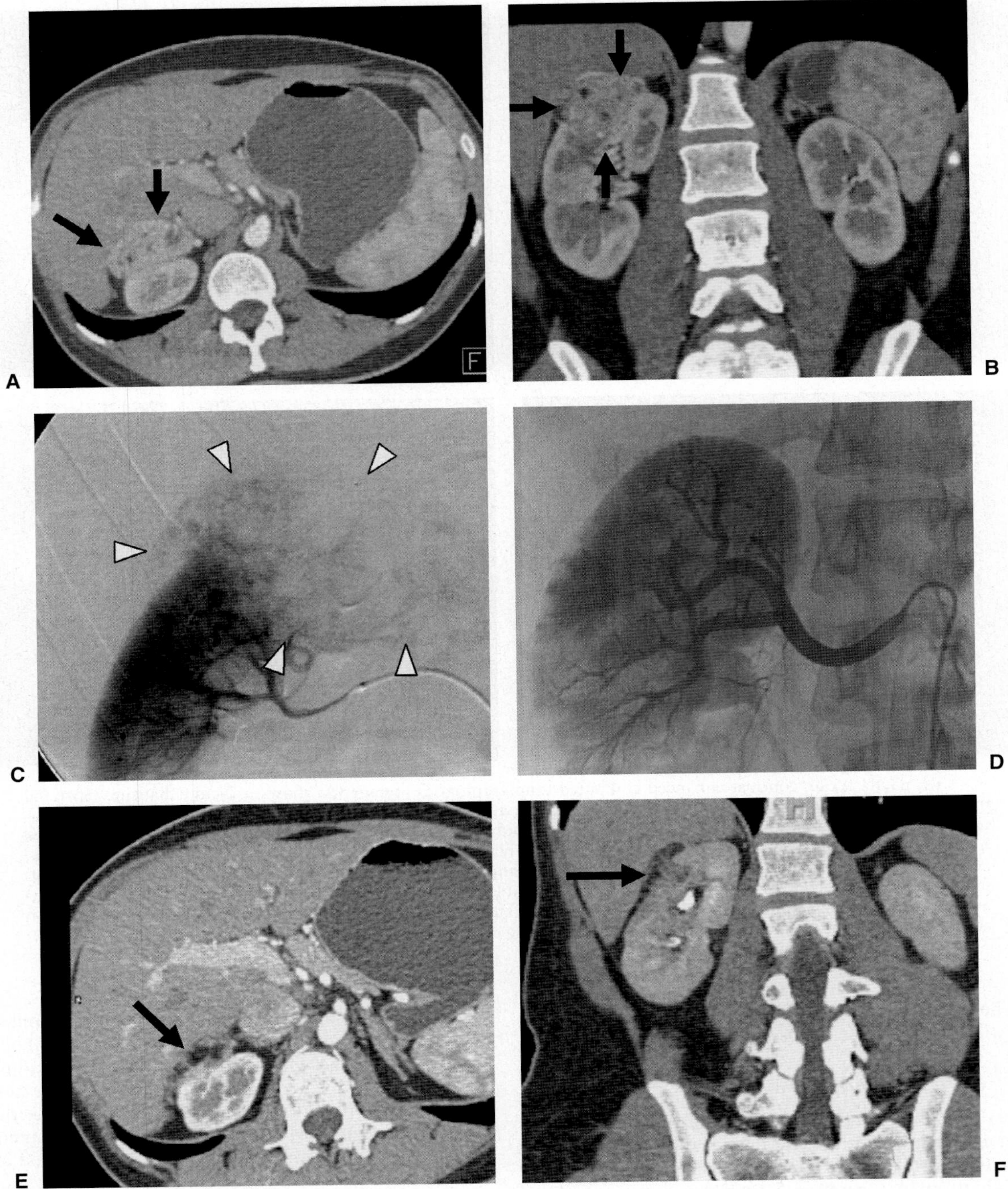

FIGURE 65.20 Thirty-six-year-old woman presenting with hematuria and right flank pain. Axial (**A**) and coronal reconstructed (**B**) contrast-enhanced computed tomography (CT) images show a hypervascular pedunculated mass (*black arrows*) from the upper pole of the right kidney. Selective right renal angiogram pre-embolization (**C**) shows the hypervascular mass (*white arrowheads*) to be supplied by branches of the renal artery. Renal arteriogram after embolization (**D**) shows no residual blood supply to the mass and an intact renal circulation. Axial (**E**) and coronal reconstructed (**F**) contrast-enhanced CT images 1 month after embolization show near complete resolution of the mass with mostly the fatty portion of the angiomyolipoma remaining. The patient's pain and hematuria resolved completely.

fracture. Figures 65.22 and 65.23 show patients with painful musculoskeletal metastases before and after treatment with cryoablation and intra-arterial embolization, respectively. In summary, RFA and/or cryoablation can significantly reduce pain associated with musculoskeletal lesions via multiple mechanisms (tumoricidal, debulking, denervation), while cementoplasty can stabilize a weight-bearing or mobile fracture thus further to pain control.

Vertebroplasty

Vertebroplasty, that is, the stabilization of a fractured vertebral body by injection of bone cement, can have dramatic and immediate benefits in patients with fracture-related pain. If indeed the culprit vertebral body is identified and treated promptly, then the majority of patients will walk away with

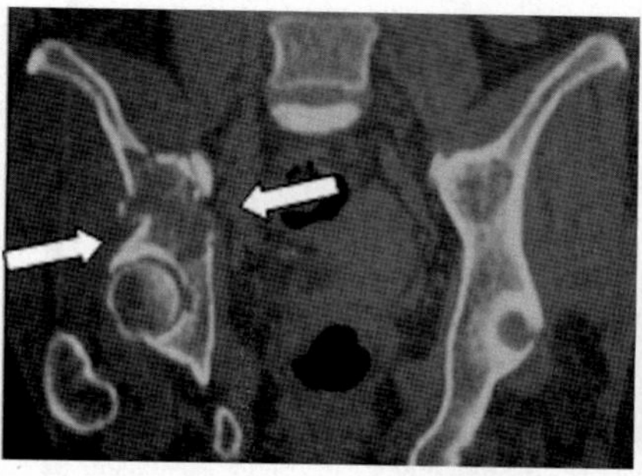

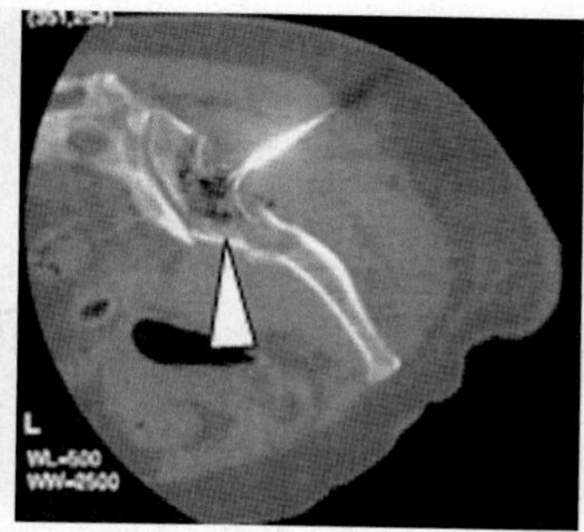

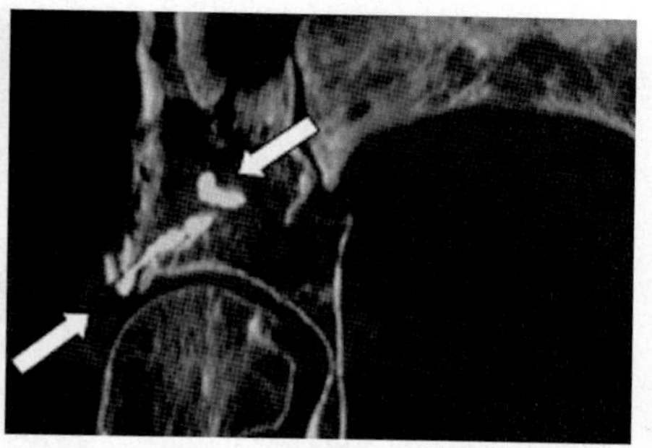

A, B C

FIGURE 65.21 Fifty-four-year-old woman with metastatic disease to the right iliac bone from unknown primary. Coronal computed tomography (CT) reconstruction (**A**) shows the metastasis localized at a weight-bearing region and resulted in a pathologic fracture (*white arrows*). The patient suffered from severe, continuous pain unresponsive to high-dose, combination analgesics and was confined to bed. Axial CT of the pelvis (**B**) shows the percutaneous radiofrequency ablation (RFA) probe causing desiccation of the bone tumor, indicated by gasses released during tissue superheating (*white arrowhead*). After RFA, the pathologic fracture was stabilized with injection of bone cement. Coronal-reconstructed CT image (**C**) shows the cement along the fracture line. Within 5 days the patient's pain decreased significantly and was easily managed with single oral analgesic agent. She was discharged to home and able to walk with minimal support.

significant-to-complete pain resolution after vertebroplasty. The pain results not from the fracture itself—many patients have vertebral body fractures without pain—but from the continuous movement of the fragments as a result of instability. The injection of bone cement stabilizes these fragments and results in pain relief. Although pain relief is achieved for most patients irrespective of causation, the majority of fractures treated with vertebroplasty are osteoporotic in nature (90%). Because of this, about 75% of patients are women suffering from osteoporosis. The associated pain of unstable vertebral body fracture results in significant lifestyle limitations and occasionally renders the patient bedridden. Figure 65.24 shows images during a vertebroplasty procedure, and Figure 65.25 shows the indications of vertebroplasty procedures and their relative distribution by level.

Many patients have bone pain as a result of metastatic disease to the vertebral column. Symptoms are related to unstable pathologic fractures or sometimes because of the local lytic tumor effects even in the absence of fracture. Vertebroplasty is equally efficacious whether the pain is from fracture or tumor mass/lytic effects. Additionally, there are reports of strong tumoricidal effect of vertebroplasty. This is thought to be because during the solidification of the injected cement the local temperature increases for a few minutes. Recovery from vertebroplasty is almost immediate and the procedure is usually performed as an outpatient procedure. The results also are almost immediate and in many patients dramatic with respect to pain relief and improvement in mobility.

FIGURE 65.22 Axial computed tomographic image of a patient with lytic metastatic lesion to right iliac bone near sacroiliac joint. The cryoablation zone (*arrows*) is covering the lytic lesion. The cryoablation probe tract is also seen (*block arrow*). The patient went from a continuous pain rated 10/10 to being pain-free with occasional 1/10 pain.

SPECIAL TOPIC: INFERIOR VENA CAVA/PORTAL VEIN OCCLUSION

Both the inferior vena cava (IVC) and portal vein are frequently compromised by direct tumor extension, extrinsic compression, or thrombosis as a result of cancer-related coagulopathy. IVC occlusion in cancer patients is most commonly seen with HCC extension through the hepatic veins or by direct compression of the tumor, especially if it involves the caudate lobe (Figure 65.26). The patient presents with gradual pelvic congestion and lower extremity edema. This may initially respond to diuretics; however, the disease is progressive and inevitably the symptoms will recur or worsen. IVC stenting is a very effective intervention that can provide almost immediate and sustain relief of the related symptoms. Compromise of the portal vein, most commonly seen with pancreatic cancer or thrombosis of the portal vein, results in presinusoidal portal hypertension and is complicated by ascites.

Portal vein interventions are technically more challenging than IVC intervention because of lack of direct access. The interventionalist must choose either the transjugular, intrahepatic route (similar to transjugular intrahepatic portosystemic shunt) or the direct percutaneous route. The choice depends on specific risks and the operator's experience. Nonetheless, the objective is to relieve the portal vein occlusion, restore portal flow, and by doing so eliminate ascites. If the cause of portal vein occlusion is thrombosis, then percutaneous intervention is difficult and risky as it may require catheter-directed thrombolysis. With few exceptions, portal vein recanalization should be reserved for patients with short segment occlusion, amenable to focal angioplasty/stent placement (Figure 65.27).

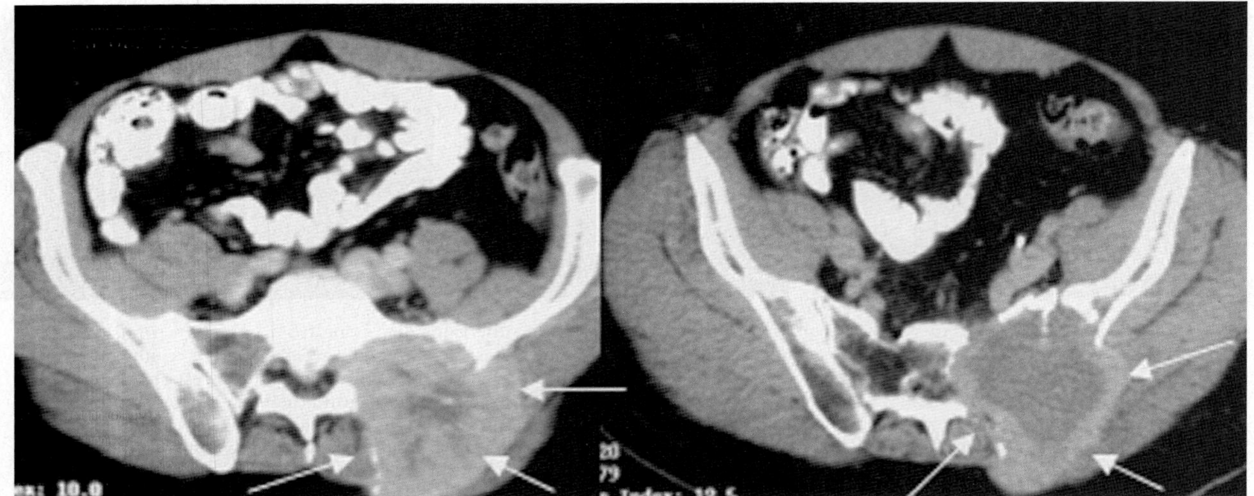

FIGURE 65.23 Fifty-two-year-old woman with large lytic metastasis to the left iliac bone from renal cell carcinoma. Axial contrast-enhanced computed tomographic (CT) image (**A**) shows a large hypervascular solid mass eroding the left iliac bone and invading the ischium (*arrows*). The lesion was the cause of severe, uncontrolled pain. Axial contrast-enhanced CT image 6 weeks postembolization (**B**) shows the tumor to be mostly necrotic with a thin rim of enhancing tissue (*arrows*). The patient's pain resolved completely.

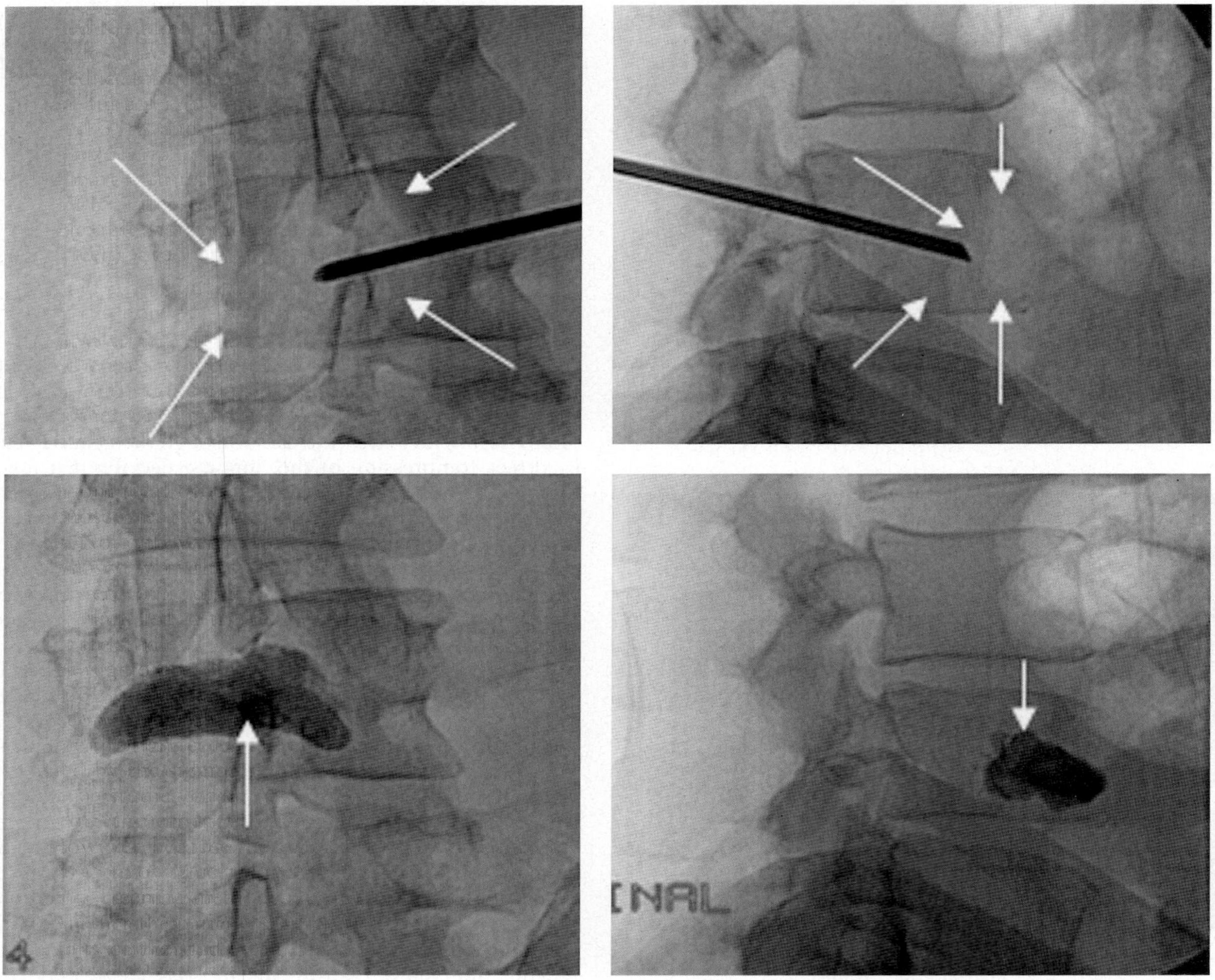

FIGURE 65.24 Seventy-three-year-old man with metastatic lung cancer to body of L4 causing severe intractable pain. Frontal (**A**) and lateral (**B**) fluoroscopic views during vertebroplasty show the cement needle placed into a lytic lesion (*arrows*) via a transpedicular approach. Postvertebroplasty frontal (**C**) and lateral (**D**) views show the radio-opaque cement (*arrows*) filling the area of the lytic lesion. The patient's pain resolved immediately after vertebroplasty and he resumed normal activities.

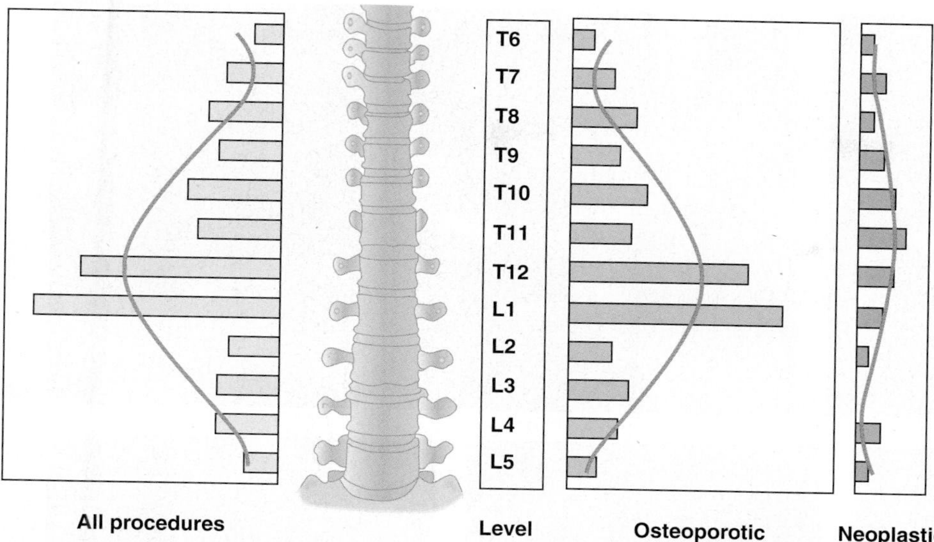

FIGURE 65.25 Bar graphs showing the distribution of the vertebroplasty procedures according to vertebral level. The first graph shows the distribution of all procedures (osteoporosis-related fractures and neoplastic involvement). The second and third graphs show the relative frequency of vertebroplasty for osteoporosis (90%) and neoplastic involvement (10%), respectively. Rarely, vertebroplasty can be performed for acute traumatic fractures.

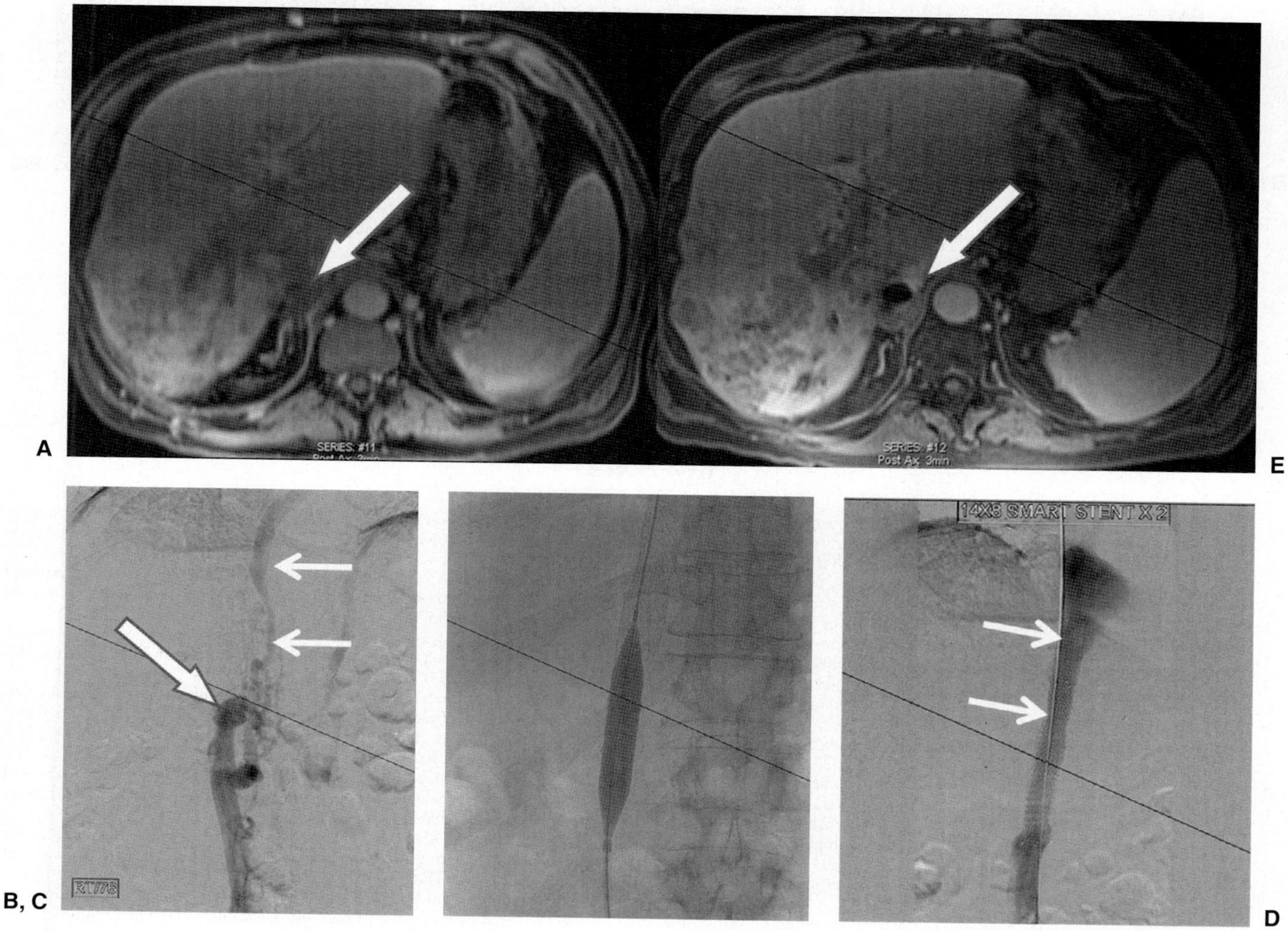

FIGURE 65.26 A 66-year-old patient with hepatocellular carcinoma. Axial magnetic resonance (MR) image (**A**) shows the tumor invading the portal vein and the inferior vena cava (IVC, *arrow*). The IVC occlusion resulted in severe pelvic and lower extremity edema with the patient being barely mobile. Digital subtraction angiogram (DSA) of the patient's IVC venogram (**B**) shows complete occlusion of the IVC (*block arrow*) with drainage via paravertebral collateral (*arrows*). Stent placement and balloon venoplasty (**C**) were performed across the occlusion, which completely restored the flow (**D**) through the IVC (*arrows*). The patient's edema completely resolved within 1 week, and 6 months postintervention the patient remained symptom-free. Last MR follow-up (**E**) shows a signal void in the region of the IVC stent (*arrow*). The metal artifact precludes evaluation of stent's patency on MRI, therefore follow-up should be based on clinical findings.

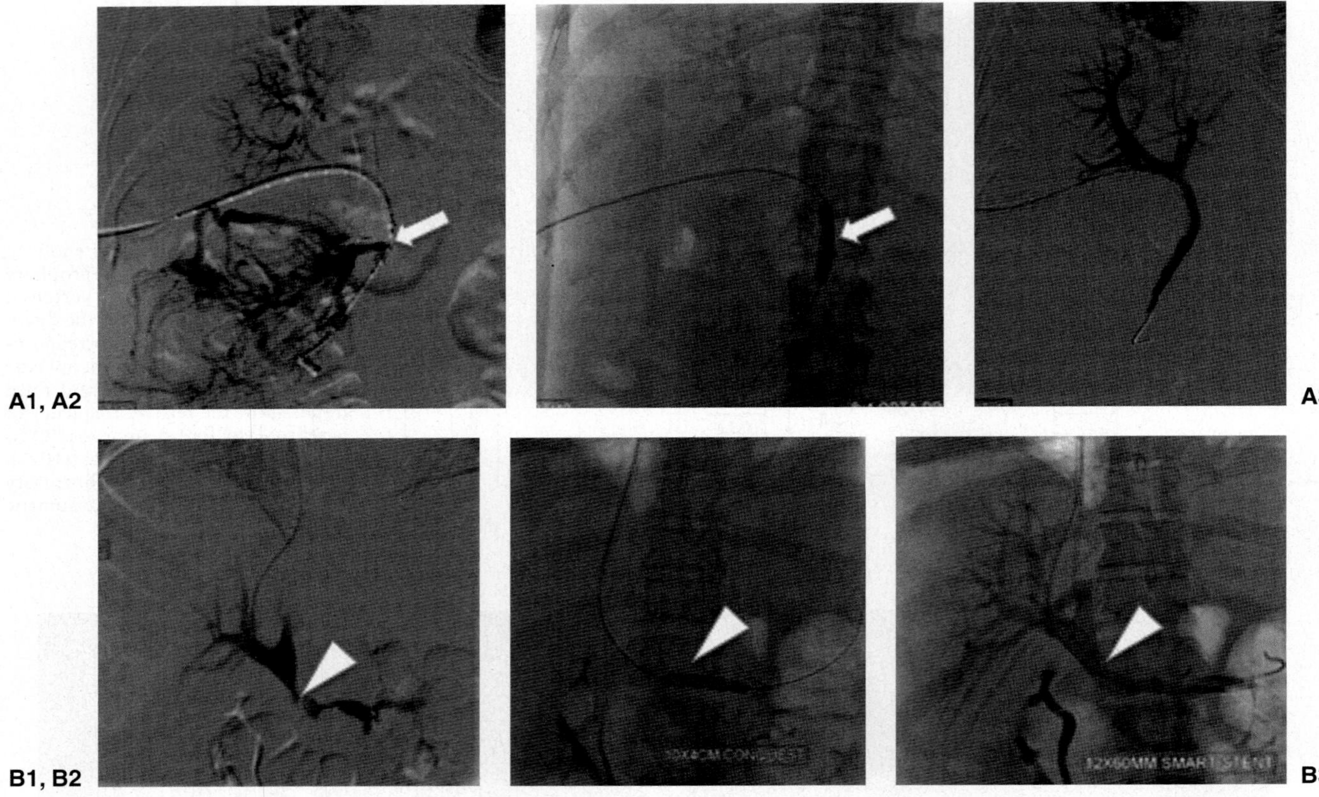

FIGURE 65.27 Percutaneous, transhepatic direct portal venogram (**A**) shows a complete occlusion of the portal vein (*arrow*) in a patient with pancreatic cancer and ascites. The contrast flow is hepatofugal, giving rise to colonic varices. After balloon angioplasty (*arrow*, A2) the occlusion has resolved and the flow is again hepatopedal. Ascites resolved within a few days and patient returned to work. Transjugular, intrahepatic, portal venogram in another patient with pancreatic cancer (**B**) and ascites, shows a high-grade stricture of the main portal vein (B1, *arrow*). After balloon angioplasty (B2, *arrow*) and stenting (B3, *arrow*), the flow is restored. Ascites again completely resolved in a timely fashion.

References

1. Alberg AJ, Samet JM. Epidemiology of lung cancer. *Chest* 2003;123 (1 Suppl):21S.
2. Lobrano MB. Partnerships in oncology and radiology: the role of radiology in the detection, staging and follow-up of lung cancer. *Oncologist* 2006;11 (7):774.
3. Radzikowska E, Glaz P, Roszkowski K. Lung cancer in women: age, smoking, histology, performance status, stage, initial treatment and survival: population-based study of 20 561 cases. *Ann Oncol* 2002;13:1087.
4. Suh R, Reckamp K, Zeidler M, Cameron R. Radiofrequency ablation in lung cancer: promising results in safety and efficacy. *Oncology (Williston Park)* 2005;19(11 Suppl 4):12.
5. Rose SC, Thistlethwaite PA, Sewell PE, Vance RB. Lung cancer and radiofrequency ablation. *J Vasc Interv Radiol* 2006;17(6):927.
6. Lencioni R, Crocetti L, Cioni R, et al. Response to radiofrequency ablation of pulmonary tumours: a prospective, intention-to-treat, multicentre clinical trial (the RAPTURE study). *Lancet Oncol* 2008;9(7):621.
7. Yu MC, Yuan JM, Govindarajan S, et al. Epidemiology of hepatocellular carcinoma. *Can J Gastroenterol* 2000;14:703.
8. El-Serag HB, Mason AC. Risk factors for the rising primary liver cancer in the United States. *Arch Intern Med* 2000;27:3227.
9. Vogl JT, Trapp M, Schroeder H, et al. Transarterial chemoambolization for hepatocellular carcinoma: volumetric and morphologic CT criteria for assessment of prognosis and therapeutic success-results from a liver transplantation center. *Radiology* 2000;214:349.
10. De Sanctis TJ, Goldberg NS, Mueller RP. Percutaneous treatment of hepatic neoplasms: a review of current techniques. *Cardiovasc Intervent Radiol* 1998;21:273.
11. Llovet JM, Real MI, Montana X, et al. Arterial embolization or chemoembolization versus symptomatic treatment in patients with unresectable hepatocellular carcinoma: a randomized controlled trial. *Lancet* 2002;359:1734.
12. Camma C, Schepis F, Orlando A, et al. Transarterial chemoembolization for unresectable hepatocellular carcinoma: meta-analysis of randomized controlled trials. *Radiology* 2002;224:47.
13. Lo CM, Ngan H, Tso WK, et al. Randomized control trial of transarterial lipiodol chemoembolization for unresectable hepatocellular carcinoma. *Hepatology* 2002;35:1164.
14. Varela M, Real MI, Burrel M, et al. Chemoembolization of hepatocellular carcinoma with drug eluting beads: efficacy and doxorubicin pharmacokinetics. *J Hepatol* 2007;46(3):474.
15. Nicolini A, Martinetti L, Crespi S, et al. Transarterial chemoembolization with epirubicin-eluting beads versus transarterial embolization before liver transplantation for hepatocellular carcinoma. *J Vasc Interv Radiol* 2010;21(3):327.
16. Dhanasekaran R, Kooby DA, Staley CA, Kauh JS, Khanna V, Kim HS. Comparison of conventional transarterial chemoembolization (TACE) and chemoembolization with doxorubicin drug eluting beads (DEB) for unresectable hepatocelluar carcinoma (HCC). *J Surg Oncol* 2010;101(6):476.
17. Carr IB. Hepatic Arterial ^{90}yttrium glass microspheres (therasphere) for unresectable hepatocellular carcinoma: interim safety and survival data on 65 patients. *Liver Transplant* 2004;10(2)(Suppl 1):S107.
18. Geschwind JF, Salem R, Carr BI, et al. Yttrium-90 microspheres for the treatment of hepatocellular carcinoma. *Gastroenterology* 2004;127(5 Suppl):S194.
19. Cao X, He N, Sun J, et al. Hepatic radioembolization with yttrium-90 glass microspheres for the treatment of primary liver cancer. *Chin Med J (Engl)* 1999;112(5):430.
20. Campbell AM, Bailey IH, Burton MA. Analysis of the distribution of intra-arterial microspheres in human liver following hepatic yttrium-90 microsphere therapy. *Phys Med Biol* 2000;45(4):1023.
21. Chow DH, Sinn LH, Ng KK, et al. Radiofrequency ablation for hepatocellular carcinoma and metastatic liver tumors: a comparative study *J Surg Oncol* 2006;94(7):565.

22. Machi J, Bueno RS, Wong LL. Long-term follow-up outcome of patients undergoing radiofrequency ablation for unresectable hepatocellular carcinoma. *World J Surg* 2005;29(11):1364.
23. Hong SN, Lee SY, Choi MS, et al. Comparing the outcomes of radiofrequency ablation and surgery in patients with a single small hepatocellular carcinoma and well-preserved hepatic function. *J Clin Gastroenterol* 2005; 39(3):247.
24. Parkin DM, Ohshima H, Srivatanakul P, Vatanasapt V. Cholangiocarcinoma: epidemiology, mechanisms of carcinogenesis and prevention. *Cancer Epidemiol Biomarkers Prev* 1993;2(6):537.
25. Shaib Y, El-Serag HB. The epidemiology of cholangiocarcinoma. *Semin Liver Dis* 2004;24(2):115.
26. Schoder M, Rossi P, Uflacker R, et al. Malignant biliary obstruction: treatment with ePTFE-FEP-covered endoprostheses initial technical and clinical experiences in a multicenter trial. *Radiology* 2002;225(1):35.
27. Burger I, Hong K, Schulick R, et al. Transcatheter arterial chemoembolization in unresectable cholangiocarcinoma: initial experience in a single institution. *J Vasc Interv Radiol* 2005;16:353.
28. Zgodzinski W, Espat NJ. Radiofrequency ablation for incidentally identified primary intrahepatic cholangiocarcinoma. *World J Gastroenterol* 2005;11(33): 5239.
29. Chiou YY, Hwang JI, Chou YH, Wang HK, Chiang JH, Chang CY. Percutaneous ultrasound-guided radiofrequency ablation of intrahepatic cholangiocarcinoma. *Kaohsiung J Med Sci* 2005;21(7):304.
30. Natarajan N, Shuster TD. New agents, combinations, and opportunities in the treatment of advanced and early-stage colon cancer. *Surg Clin North Am* 2006;86(4):1023.
31. Taal BG, Visser O. Epidemiology of neuroendocrine tumours. *Neuroendocrinology* 2004;80(Suppl 1):3.
32. Osborne DA, Zervos EE, Strosberg J, et al. Improved outcome with cytoreduction versus embolization for symptomatic hepatic metastases of carcinoid and neuroendocrine tumors. *Ann Surg Oncol* 2006;13(4):572.
33. Sutcliffe R, Maguire D, Ramage J, Rela M, Heaton N. Management of neuroendocrine liver metastases. *Am J Surg* 2004;187(1):39.
34. Gillams A, Cassoni A, Conway G, Lees W. Radiofrequency ablation of neuroendocrine liver metastases: the Middlesex experience. *Abdom Imaging* 2005;30(4):435.
35. Nanashima A, Sumida Y, Abo T, et al. Clinical significance of portal vein embolization before right hepatectomy. *Hepatogastroenterology* 2009;56 (91–92):773.
36. de Baere T, Teriitehau C, Deschamps F, et al. Predictive factors for hypertrophy of the future remnant liver after selective portal vein embolization. *Ann Surg Oncol* 2010;17(8):2081.
37. Haghighi KS, Glenn D, Gruenberger T, Morris DL. Extending the limits for curative liver resections by portal vein embolization. *Int Surg* 2009;94(1):43.
38. Cohen HT, McGovern FJ. Renal-cell carcinoma. *N Engl J Med* 2005; 353(23):2477.
39. Lipworth L, Tarone RE, McLaughlin JK. The epidemiology of renal cell carcinoma. *J Urol* 2006;176(6 Pt 1):2353.
40. Chiou YY, Hwang JI, Chou YH, Wang JH, Chiang JH, Chang CY. Percutaneous radiofrequency ablation of renal cell carcinoma. *J Chin Med Assoc* 2005;68(5):221.
41. Merkle EM, Nour SG, Lewin JS. Imaging follow-up after percutaneous radiofrequency ablation of renal cell carcinoma: findings in 18 patients during first 6 months. *Radiology* 2005;235(3):1065.
42. Yamakado K, Nakatsuka A, Kobayashi S, et al. Radiofrequency ablation combined with renal arterial embolization for the treatment of unresectable renal cell carcinoma larger than 3.5 cm: initial experience. *Cardiovasc Intervent Radiol* 2006;29(3):389.
43. Christensen SW, Berg J, Brynitz S, Rasmussen MS. Arterial embolization in patients with renal carcinoma. *Int Urol Nephrol* 1989;21(6):575.
44. Ewalt DH, Diamond N, Rees C, et al. Long-term outcome of transcatheter embolization of renal angiomyolipomas due to tuberous sclerosis complex. *J Urol* 2005;174(5):1764.

CHAPTER 66 FUNCTIONAL IMAGING

BRIAN D. ROSS, CRAIG J. GALBÁN, AND ALNAWAZ REHEMTULLA

The introduction of magnetic resonance imaging (MRI) into clinical practice has been among the most important advances in the radiologic diagnosis of oncology patients. Excellent soft tissue differentiation, rapid technologic advancements, and widespread availability of clinical MR scanners have resulted in crucial roles performed by routine anatomic MRI. Through specific MR acquisition sequences, images of fundamental biophysical, physiologic, metabolic, or functional properties of tissues can be obtained. MR images for characterization of tissue perfusion,[1] vascular permeability,[2,3] tissue oxygenation,[4] cellular status,[5] cellular density,[6] and microstructural organization,[7,8] all of which are used in clinical and research studies, can now be routinely acquired. Extension of MRI applications for prediction of outcome in the clinical management of individual cancer patients could improve the therapeutic index through the development and validation of MRI biomarkers for predicting the biology and behavior of tumors. This is especially warranted as standard risk factors currently used cannot account for the variable and unpredictable treatment responses of patients with a similar risk profile. This chapter will highlight several of these key, emerging functional and molecular imaging approaches as they are applied to clinical oncologic imaging.

DIFFUSION MAGNETIC RESONANCE IMAGING

Molecular imaging is commonly defined as the ability to localize and measure biologic processes on the cellular and molecular levels in the living organism. An imaging probe or readout that serves as a biomarker for a cellular event, such as the presence of an enzyme expressed from a targeted gene, qualifies as a molecular imaging modality. Although diffusion-sensitive MRI techniques do not reach this level of biologic specificity, diffusion is often discussed within the context of molecular imaging. The rationale for this is that diffusion MR is sensitive to molecular water interactions that occur at the cellular level. The central contrast mechanism in diffusion-based imaging is molecular mobility. With rare exception, water molecules are the signal source; therefore, water mobility is probed in diffusion-weighted imaging (DWI). In pure water, temperature is the only significant modulator of molecular mobility, and, in fact, diffusion MRI has been used to measure temperature noninvasively.[9] However, cancer tissue is not composed of pure water, and biologic factors on the cellular level have a strong impact on molecular mobility, which makes DWI a unique diagnostic tool.[10,11] Indeed, DWI is readily available and increasing in its use in clinical practice due to its exquisite sensitivity to cellular status, cytotoxic edema, cellular density, and cellular organization of tissues.[12–15] The objective of this section will be to provide a broad overview of basic methods and applications of diffusion MRI as applied to cancer imaging.

Principles Involved in Diffusion Imaging of Cancer

Diffusion-weighted MRI of *in vivo* systems was initially reported in the 1980s,[11,16,17] and reviews on the technical aspects and consensus biomarker recommendations using diffusion imaging are available.[15,18,19] Molecular diffusion is a thermally driven random translational motion of molecules in media and is also referred to as *Brownian motion*. Key factors that exert their influence on the mobility of a diffusing molecule include media viscosity, temperature, and its molecular mass. Diffusion is not a magnetization-related process such as, for example, T1 and T2 magnetization relaxation that drives conventional MRI contrast. Nevertheless, MRI can be used to noninvasively quantify (image) water diffusion values spatially *in vivo*. This is accomplished in part through the use of magnetic gradients that allow for the "encoding" of initial locations of constituent water molecules in the tissue. Following a brief interval, the same gradients are used to "decode" the molecular locations. For those water molecules in which displacement has occurred during the time interval, decoding will be incomplete, resulting in the loss of signal through spin dephasing. The dephasing amount increases in proportion to the distance translated between encode/decode diffusion gradient pulses. Highly mobile water molecules will have a larger loss of signal relative to immobile water in more restricted or cellular tissue environments, which will produce a relatively strong signal on diffusion-weighted sequences. Determination of the degree of signal loss at various diffusion gradient settings provides for the ability to calculate molecular mobility in complex systems, such as tumor tissue. However, because tumor tissue is composed of water located within a variety of intra- and extracellular compartments separated by semipermeable membranes, the concept of a single diffusion coefficient is not valid; thus the measured value is reported as an "apparent diffusion coefficient" (ADC) when performing diffusion-sensitive sequences on tissues.[11,15] ADC measurements can be used to assess myriad effects that impede molecular motions, including cell membrane integrity, cell density, interactions with macromolecules, as well as processes that enhance mobility via active transport, convective motion, and perfusion.

The diffusion coefficient of pure water at body temperature is approximately 3×10^{-3} mm^2/s; therefore, free water molecules normally migrate a displacement distance of 0.03 mm, or 30 microns, in 50 ms, which is on the order of the typical MR time interval used clinically. Because the diameter of a tumor cell is on the order of a few microns to tens of microns, and that of other structures such as membranes, organelles, myelin layers, and macromolecules span yet smaller dimensions, a given water molecule will likely encounter many interactions with cellular or subcellular entities over this measurement interval. Transient association of water with large, slow-moving macromolecules and cell membranes, as well as impediment by membranes and other structures, effectively reduce water mobility to an ADC lower than free water diffusion. The greater the bulk density of structures within a tumor tissue that impedes water mobility, the lower the ADC value for that tumor. For this reason, ADC is considered a noninvasive imaging biomarker of cellularity or cell density. However, if two tissues have different ADC values, the lower ADC tissue may not necessarily have the greater number of cells per unit volume. Other factors such as cell size, relative extra- versus intracellular volume, and membrane permeability also affect water mobility and ADC. Within a given tissue or cell type, ADC is useful as an indicator of the relative cellularity, such as in the evolution of tumor over time following therapy. Cellular alterations due to disease or intervention, as well as changes in cellular organization or integrity of cellular elements, are available for study by diffusion imaging.

Diffusion measurement on the order of cellular distances is measurable in spite of the presence of other much larger physiologic motions. A single-shot echo-planar imaging (EPI) approach[20] is typically used in these studies as its rapid acquisition speed allows the entire set of echoes for an image to be collected within one single scan period, thereby essentially eliminating bulk tissue motion that would otherwise overwhelm measurement of molecular motion. However, images generated by EPI are sensitive to other artifacts such as distortion and signal loss due to magnetic susceptibility. These limitations aside, EPI is the most commonly used clinical sequence combined with diffusion-sensitization gradient pulses to perform DWI.

Applications of Diffusion Imaging

Diffusion Imaging in Tissue Characterization

Tumor ADC maps generated from DWI data have proved helpful in defining solid enhancing tumor, noncontrast-enhancing lesions, peritumoral edema, and necrotic or cystic regions from normal surrounding tissue. Observations of progressively increasing ADC values from dense cellular tumors to necrotic cysts have been widely observed and are consistent with known histologic properties of tumors. The ADCs for exceptionally cellular dense tumors are 0.6 to 0.8×10^{-3} mm^2/s, whereas the ADCs for solid enhancing high-grade glioma span a range from 0.8 to 1.3×10^{-3} mm^2/s.[21] ADC values of edematous brain are in the range of 1.3 to 1.4×10^{-3} mm^2/s, and a necrotic tumor core typically has an ADC of 1.8 to 2.4×10^{-3} mm^2/s. Diffusion MRI has also been shown to reliably obtain ADC measurements of abdominal organs and tumors within these organ sites, such as renal, liver, and pancreas.[22] Studies have also evaluated ADC values in colorectal hepatic metastases.[23,24] The ability to reliably obtain ADC measurements of internal organs has allowed investigation as to whether the pretreatment ADCs of hepatic metastatic lesions from colorectal cancer are predictive of chemotherapeutic response.[24] A significant increase in mean pretreatment ADC values was found in metastatic lesions that responded to chemotherapy, which may have implications for future development of individualized therapy.

Applications of diffusion also include differentiation of benign and malignant lesions in liver, breast, and prostate, where increased cellularity of malignant lesions restricts water motion in a reduced extracellular space.[25] Whole-body diffusion MRI has recently been reported for screening malignancies in the body.[26] This approach has been shown to be able to obtain displays of whole-body diffusion images on freely breathing patients. Figure 66.1 shows whole-body MRI, including DWI of a 60-year-old man with stage III diffuse large B-cell lymphoma. Coronal T1-weighted, short-T1 inversion recovery (STIR), and slab maximum intensity projection DWI are shown, revealing lymph node involvement on both sides of the diaphragm (see arrows). Note that whole-body DWI provides the highest lymph node-to-background contrast. Applications of whole-body diffusion MRI for tumor detection and monitoring of treatment response will continue to be an active area of investigation.

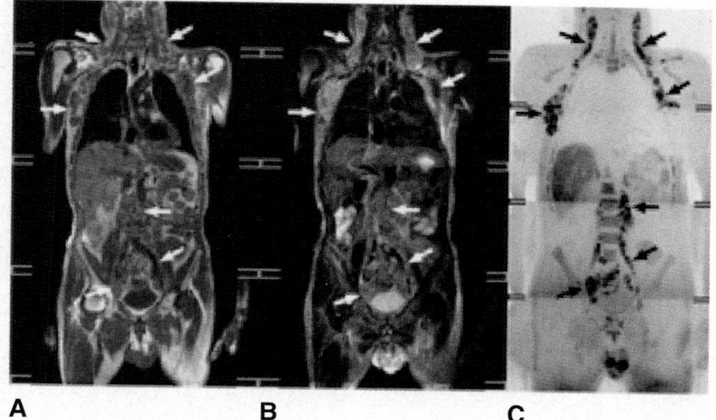

FIGURE 66.1 Whole-body magnetic resonance image (MRI), including diffusion-weighted imaging (DWI), in a 60-year-old male with stage III diffuse large B-cell lymphoma. Coronal T1-weighted (**A**), short-T1 inversion recovery (STIR) (**B**), and slab maximum intensity projection DWI (**C**) obtained with a b-value of 1,000 s/mm^2 show lymph node involvement on both sides of the diaphragm (*arrows*). Note that whole-body DWI provides the highest lymph node-to-background contrast. (Figure kindly provided by Dr. Thomas Kwee, Department of Radiology, University Medical Centre Utrecht, Utrecht.)

Diffusion Imaging in Tumor Grading

The possibility of differentiating the type and grade of a tumor has also been explored using DWI and diffusion tensor imaging (DTI) in adult as well as pediatric populations. Preliminary diffusion MRI results have also been reported on detection of pancreatic adenocarcinoma with high sensitivity and specificity[27] as well as for providing useful diagnostic information for discriminating poorly differentiated from undifferentiated carcinomas[28] and benign from malignant salivary gland tumors.[29] Several studies have also shown that low-grade astrocytoma has high ADC values, whereas high-grade malignant glioma has low ADC values, findings reflecting more restricted diffusion with increasing tumor cellularity.[6,30] It remains uncertain whether anisotropy indices will be able to differentiate tumor type and grade. Tumor cytoarchitecture is predominantly random; therefore, anisotropy tends to be low in tumor. In addition, the large variation in normal tissue anisotropy depends heavily on its location in the brain,[31] which implies that the contrast of tumor to normal background, as depicted by anisotropy, will depend on lesion location. There is justifiable optimism that anisotropy will be valuable in assessing the effect of tumor on normally omnidirectional white matter structures. Mass effects that displace and compress white matter tracks as well as destruction of track organization by tumor infiltration have been documented by anisotropy-based diffusion imaging, suggesting that this technology may have a role in presurgical planning.[32–34]

Diffusion Imaging to Assess Tumor Cellularity and Treatment Response

It is traditionally believed that as cellular density increases, the added tortuosity to extracellular mobility paths also reduces water mobility. The inverse relationship between ADC and cellular density has been noted by several groups.[6,33,35,36] A

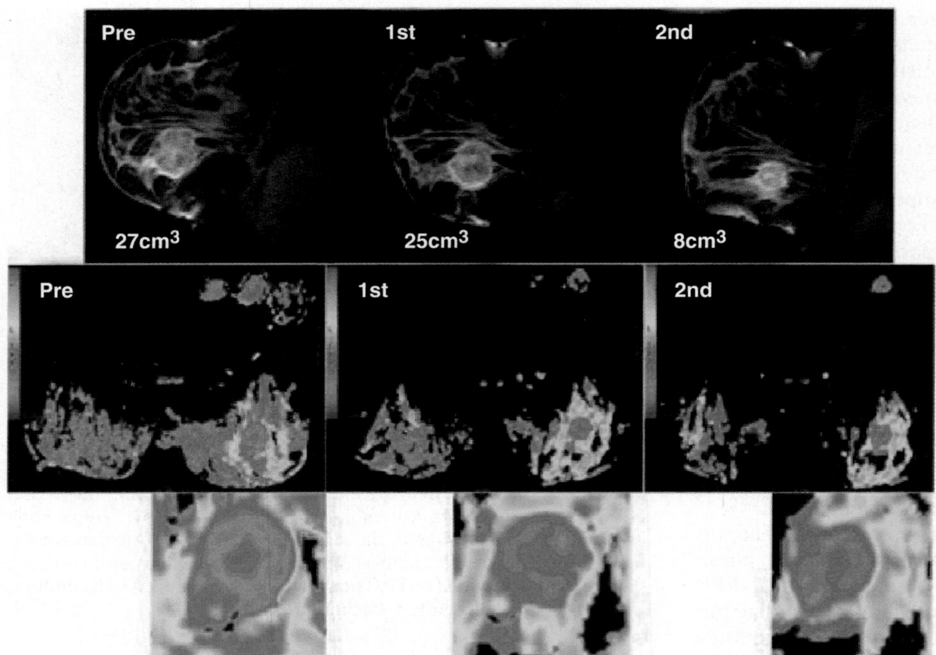

FIGURE 66.2 **Top panel:** T1-weighted, fat-saturated postcontrast images of a breast tumor patient before and following one and two cycles of chemotherapy. **Middle panel:** Color apparent diffusion coefficient (ADC) maps during the same time intervals. Note the increased diffusion signal in the tumor following the first cycle of therapy with no significant change in tumor volume. **Bottom panel:** Expanded region of the tumor region of the ADC maps. Blue areas on the ADC map represent low ADC values, whereas green-red areas represent higher ADC values. (Images kindly provided by Dr. Martin D. Pickles, ref. 56.)

recent proposed biphasic model relating ADC values to cellularity is based on the notion of two pools of water within tissue, a fast diffusion and a slow diffusion pool.[37] The slow diffusion pool is proposed to consist of a water layer trapped by electrostatic forces of the protein membranes and associated cytoskeleton. The fast diffusion pool is thought to belong to a combination of intra- and extracellular compartments that are, however, slower than free water. Both the traditional and biphasic diffusion models provide for the rationale that water diffusion will decrease during cell swelling or cell proliferation and increase during treatment-induced loss of cellular viability or density. Whatever the specific underlying mechanism is for these differing diffusion pools, the fact remains that tumor diffusion values increase as tumor tissue progresses from a solid, cellular lesion to an acellular, necrotic tumor during successful cytotoxic therapy. This characteristic of tumor water diffusion values provides a key opportunity to use this biophysical and quantifiable ADC parameter as a sensitive biomarker for detecting the underlying changes of tumor cytoarchitecture associated with treatment.[38]

Because treatment-induced molecular and cellular changes precede macroscopic changes in tumor size, diffusion MRI can be used to detect early changes in tumor structure, thus providing the possibility of using this imaging biomarker as an early response indicator in preclinical and clinical cancer studies. Fourteen years of research in preclinical studies have supported this notion, revealing that diffusion MR can be used to noninvasively detect cellular changes associated with treatment-induced cell killing in animal models.[6,33,35,39–45] Key findings were that changes in ADC values were observed to precede changes in tumor volume regression, changes were observed to be treatment independent and dose dependent, all supporting the claim that this imaging biomarker may indeed be used as an early surrogate for treatment outcome.

Comparisons of tumor burden are usually made between pretreatment scans and those obtained weeks to months after the conclusion of a therapeutic protocol.[46,47] Clinical studies have found a correlation between early changes in tumor ADC values and a delayed clinical response to therapy, as summarized in Table 66.1.[36,48–83] Results from clinical studies have shown a significant difference in the mean ADC between responders and nonresponders to therapy, as well as a linear correlation between the relative change in ADC and the normalized change in tumor volume.[61] Early increasing ADC values during therapy are attributed to therapy-induced necrosis. Shown in Figure 66.2 are MRIs of a breast cancer patient treated with two cycles of neoadjuvant therapy. ADC maps clearly reveal an increase in the tumor diffusion values occurred at the end of the first treatment cycle, indicating that the treatment is causing a reduction in the tumor cell density but, at this time, no significant reduction in tumor size. Following the second cycle of treatment, a significant decrease in tumor volume was noted. Although initial increases in tumor values during treatment are typically associated with cell death, a drop in ADC values can occur later within the tumor, even to pretreatment levels. If this occurs, it can be an indicator of tumor regrowth or fibrosis. This present understanding is supported by observations of lower ADC values in contrast-enhancing portions of recurrent high-grade gliomas when compared with those obtained in patients with radiation injury and necrosis and higher diffusion values in necrotic regions of osteosarcomas.[50,84]

Tumor heterogeneity is a major confounding factor in assigning a single indicator to patient or tumor response. A given lesion often contains wide gradations of viable cellularity and necrosis, and the response of tumor subregions to treatment is nonuniform and dependent on many factors. Histogram analysis of ADC values throughout the tumor is one approach to address heterogeneity. The magnitude of regional changes may be underestimated by whole-tumor averages. An alternative approach to deal with intrinsic heterogeneity of diffusion values within a tumor is referred to as *functional diffusion mapping* (fDM).[58] A key element of fDM is spatial registration of all three-dimensional image sets into a common geometrical framework. In this way, diffusion changes are measurable on a voxel-by-voxel basis from spatially aligned pretreatment, during treatment, and posttreatment image sets. Tumors are segmented into three categories representing (1) voxels for which ADC increased by a specified threshold (red voxels), (2) voxels for which ADC decreased (blue voxels), and (3) voxels that did not change outside this threshold range (green voxels). A series of fDM color overlays

TABLE 66.1

CLINICAL DIFFUSION MAGNETIC RESONANCE IMAGING STUDIES

Site	N[a]	Treatment[b]	Timing[c]	Conclusion	Ref.
Bladder	20 (20)	Chemoradiation	10 d	DWI predicted pathologic complete response	48
Bone	24 (24)	RT	1–6 mo	Increased ADC in with clinical response	82
Breast	10 (10)	Chemotherapy	3 wk	Increased ADC after first/second cycle	56
Breast	11 (11)	Chemotherapy	15–18 wk	Increased ADC following treatment ($P <.05$)	49
Cervical	20 (20)	Chemoradiation	2 wk	Increased ADC correlated with response	75
Cervical	17 (17)	Chemoradiation	4 & 8 wk	ADC may predict response	62
CNS	2 (2)	Chemo/RT	Serial	Increase in ADC preceded tumor response	36
CNS	20 (20)	Avastin	6 wk	DWI may be used for early response	72
CNS	3 (3)	CED	Serial	Changes in ADC preceded tumor response	60
CNS	10 (8)	RT	3–10 d	Increased ADC preceded tumor response	61
CNS	20 (20)	Stereotactic RT	2–4 wk	Differential ADC change between outcomes	51
CNS	6 (3)	Chemotherapy/RT	NA	Increased ADC in responding lesions	54
CNS	20 (20)	Chemotherapy/RT	3 wk	fDM discriminates later radiographic response	58
CNS	34 (34)	RT +/− chemo	3 wk	fDM predicts OS ($P <.01$) and PFS ($P <.04$)	76
CNS	60 (60)	RT +/− chemo	1, 3 & 10 wk	fDM predicts OS at 3 weeks	130
CNS	6 (6)	Radiosurgery	8 wk	fDM's of DTI allows early treatment detection	63
HNSCC	28 (28)	Neoadjuvant therapy	NA	ADCs had weak correlation with regression	69
HNSCC	40 (40)	Chemoradiation	1 wk	ADC can serve as early response biomarker	68
HNSCC	15 (15)	Radiotherapy	3 wk	DW-MR shows potential for early response	79
HNSCC	15 (15)	Radiochemotherapy	3 wk	PRM/fDM yields prognostic information	77
Liver	60 (13)	Chemotherapy	4 and 11 d	Correlation of ADC with radiographic response	52
Liver	23 (87)	Chemotherapy	3 and 7 d	ADC increased by week 1	81
Liver	12 (48)	Arterial infusion	9 d	Corelation of ADC with responders	59
Liver	38 (38)	TACE	4–6 wk	Increased ADC ($P <.03$) and fall in AFP	71
Liver	6 (6)	^{90}Y microspheres	6 wk	Increased ADC, no response by RECIST	80
Liver	19 (13)	^{90}Y microspheres	4 wk	Increased ADC in treated ($P <.001$) lesions	70
Liver	18 (18)	Radiotherapy	1,2 & 4 wk	ADC increased in proportion to response	83
Liver	20 (20)	^{90}Y microspheres	4 wk	ADC increase preceded tumor shrinkage	55
Lung	17 (20)	Radiofreq. ablation	3 d	ADC predicted responders	57
Rectum	14 (14)	Chemo/RT	NA	Decreased ADC correlated with response	78
Rectum	37 (37)	Chemo/RT	1 wk	Increased ADC indicated response	53
Rectum	8 (8)	Chemo/RT	1 wk	Increased ADC at week 1 predicts response	65
Rectum	40 (40)	Chemoradiation	2 wk	DWI adds to accuracy of response	67
Sarcoma	18 (18)	Chemotherapy	NA	Increased ADC greater in those with response	74
Sarcoma	8 (8)	Chemotherapy	NA	Higher ADC in necrotic vs. non-necrotic areas	50
Solid tumors	16 (16)	CA4P/Avastin	3 h	ADC promising for antivascular drugs	66
Uterus	32 (11)	Embolization	99–239 d	Decrease in ADC late after treatment	64
Uterus	14 (14)	Ultrasound	Early and 6 mo	Initial fall in ADC followed by late rise	73

ADC, apparent diffusion coefficient; RECIST, response evaluation criteria in solid tumors; NA, not available in text; fDM, functional diffusion mapping; OS, overall survival; PFS, progression free survival, CNS, central nervous system; HNSCC, head and neck squamous cell carcinoma.

[a]Number of lesions and number of patients in parentheses.

[b]RT, radiation therapy, CED, convection enhanced delivery of chemotherapy, TACE, trans-arterial chemo-embolization, CA4P, combretastatin A-4 phosphate.

[c]Timing of response evaluation relative from start of treatment.

and corresponding voxel-wise scatterplots of ADC pretreatment compare 1, 3, and 10 weeks of treatment, as illustrated in Figure 66.3 for a therapeutically responding and nonresponding patient. The fractional volume of tumor representing the relative volume of tumor that exhibited a significant increase in ADC is shown as red voxels in the color overlay and scatterplots and are used as a metric to predict treatment outcome.

A key finding of these early studies was that tumors that exhibit a significant change in fDM values measured at 3 weeks into treatment were predictive of the radiographic response measured at 10 weeks.[58,76] Moreover, tumor assessment by fDM at 3 weeks into treatment provided an early indicator of the eventual clinical responses of disease time to progression and overall survival in patients with malignant glioma.[58,76] The use of fDM for quantification of tumor response provides for the possibility of a standardized approach for treatment response assessment using diffusion MRI. This approach can be extended to other tumor types. While further validation of DW-MRI measurements as a biomarker for early treatment response is needed, recent studies have shown promising results.

Summary

MRI methods such as DWI and DTI based on tissue biophysical properties are rapidly being incorporated in routine imaging protocols to improve the diagnosis, characterization, and management of cancer patients. In the future, these methods combined with other physiology-based methods, such as MR perfusion and magnetic resonance spectroscopy (MRS) metabolite mapping, as well as excellent anatomic images are anticipated to improve tumor diagnosis, biopsy guidance, pretreatment and presurgical planning, and the assessment of early therapeutic efficacy in individuals. Research is ongoing to

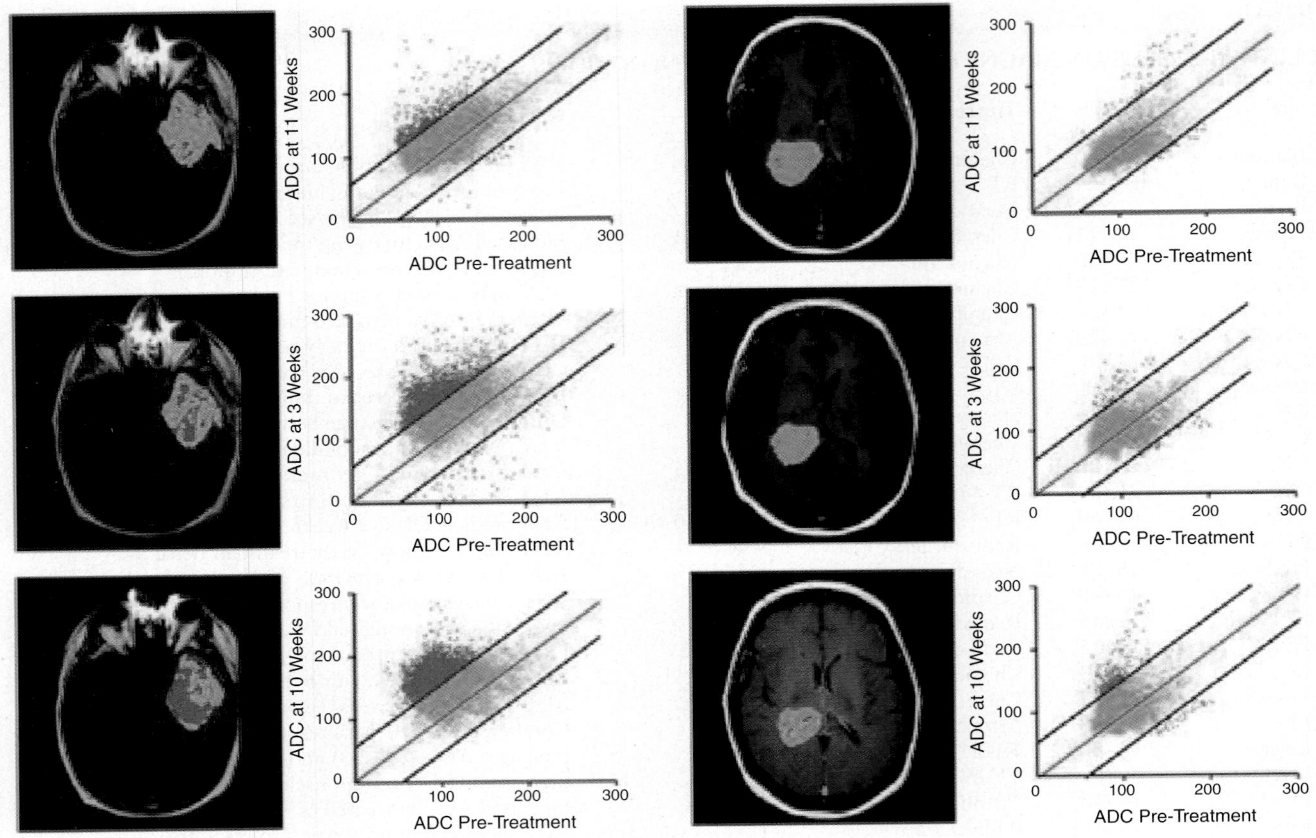

FIGURE 66.3 Representative functional diffusion map (fDM) analysis over time. Functional diffusion maps at 1, 3, and 10 weeks for two patients treated with fractionated radiation therapy. The patient on the left was scored as responsive by fDM at 3 weeks but progressive disease by radiologic response at week 10 and had overall survival (OS) of more than 33 months. The patient on the right was scored as nonresponsive by fDM at 3 weeks but stable disease by Macdonald criteria and OS of 7 months. Depicted images are single slices of the T1 postcontrast scans at each time point with a pseudocolor overlay of the fDM. Red voxels indicate regions with a significant rise in apparent diffusion coefficient (ADC) at each time point compared with pretreatment, green regions had unchanged ADC, and blue voxels indicate areas of significant decline in ADC. The scatter plots display data for the entire tumor volume and not just for the depicted slice at each time point, with the pretreatment ADC on the *x*-axis and post-treatment ADC on the *y*-axis. The central red line represents unity, and the flanking blue lines represent the 95% confidence intervals. (From ref. 130, with permission.)

determine how to best use diffusion information to impact patient management in a positive fashion.

PERFUSION MAGNETIC RESONANCE IMAGING

Treatment of tumors with targeted compounds against the vascular support network is an active area of drug development. Development and validation of imaging biomarkers for tumor angiogenesis are under investigation for detection and quantification of pharmacodynamic drug activity. The application of dynamic contrast–enhanced magnetic resonance imaging (DCE-MRI) for assessment of tumor pathophysiology and treatment response against radiotherapy as well as antiangiogenic and vascular disruption agents is rapidly progressing as a noninvasive imaging-based biomarker for drug efficacy studies in clinical trials.[85–101]

General Principles of Dynamic Contrast-Enhanced Magnetic Resonance Imaging

DCE-MRI provides a means to investigate microvascular structure and function by following the pharmacokinetics of injected low-molecular-weight contrast agents as they pass through the tumor vasculature. Following an intravenous bolus injection of a paramagnetic contrast agent, the contrast agent enters the tumor arterioles, passes through capillary beds, and finally drains via the veins within the tumor. A gadolinium contrast agent is commonly used, which shortens the T1 relaxation time of blood and results in a concentration-dependent spatially varying enhanced signal intensity (contrast) on T1-weighted images. Collection of rapid serial T1-weighted images during a few second intervals across time provides the initial area under the contrast-agent concentration time curve, which can be analyzed for kinetic information. The degree of signal enhancement depends on a variety of physiological and physical factors such as tissue perfusion, arterial input function, capillary surface area, capillary permeability, and the volume of the extracellular extravascular space (EES). Data are collected from a defined region of interest that encompasses all or part of the tumor. Compartmental modeling of tumor microvasculature generates parameters that describe the shape of the contrast agent time-dependent concentration curve, which represents a combination of flow, blood volume, vessel permeability, and EES. A set of standardized terms for the kinetic variables of DCE-MRI are commonly used in these studies.[102] The two-compartment model regards the EES and plasma as the two compartments that are well mixed with contrast agent and which have a constant permeability.

Transport between these compartments is determined by the parameter K^{trans} (volume transfer constant between the blood plasma and the EES) and κ_{ep} (rate constant between the EES and the blood plasma). The EES fractional volume (v_e) is related via the equation, $v_e = (K^{trans}/\kappa_{ep})$. K^{trans} is one of the key primary end points used in clinical trials, but changes in this parameter may represent different physiological processes in different individuals within a patient population (e.g., a reduction of K^{trans} could represent reduced permeability, reduced blood flow, or a combination of the two). There are various analytical approaches that are used for data analysis; however, a consensus has been reached that recommends that simple models that describe the volume transfer coefficient of contrast between the blood plasma and the EES (K^{trans}), and the size of the EES (v_e) should be used along with initial area under the contrast-agent concentration time curve in assessing antiangiogenic and vascular disrupting agents in clinical trials.[103]

Dynamic Contrast-Enhanced Magnetic Resonance Imaging for Detection of Residual Disease

The use of DCE-MRI following therapy has been proposed to assist with the detection of residual disease or early recurrence, which can be difficult to detect in tissue regions exposed to radiotherapy. DCE-MRI measurements following radiotherapy have been investigated in cervix, lung, head and neck, and bladder tumors wherein high enhancement has been associated with an increase in local recurrence and poor survival.[104–107] The persistence or early return of a contrast agent enhancement pattern is attributed to viable tumor cells following treatment completion. An early DCE-MRI enhancement in cervical cancer has been shown to be associated with early recurrence and poor survival.[107]

As shown in Figure 66.4, a large cervical tumor is detected using T2-weighted MRI (Fig. 66.4*A*), which had a robust signal enhancement (Fig. 66.4*B*). At 6 to 8 weeks following radiotherapy, the tumor had decreased in size (Fig. 66.4*C*) but there remained a significant region of postcontrast signal enhancement, indicating that a region of viable tumor remained. This patient was determined to be a nonresponder and died within 7 months following radiotherapy.

In another study, head and neck tumor patients were also found to have a positive correlation between the presence of lesion enhancement and viable tumor cells in postradiation surgical specimens.[104] Finally, in meningioma patients examined using DCE-MRI following radiotherapy, pharmacokinetic analysis revealed that patients who responded had a decrease in the exchange rate constant relative to nonresponders. Overall, although there is emerging evidence as to the potential utility of DCE-MRI for detection of posttreatment residual disease, further studies are required in order to adequately validate this approach for routine clinical use.

Dynamic Contrast-Enhanced Magnetic Resonance Imaging as Predictor of Treatment Response

DCE-MRI can provide anatomic and physiological information using commonly available clinical MRI systems. The required DCE imaging sequences are incorporated into standard imaging protocols for treatment assessment. There have been many studies that have evaluated the prognostic value of DCE-MRI in assessing treatment response to radiotherapy,

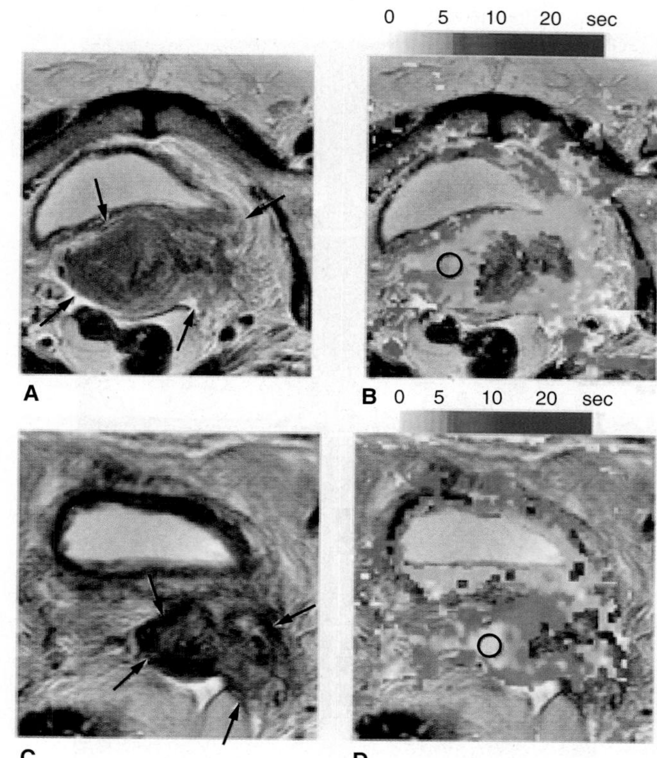

FIGURE 66.4 **A:** An axial T2-weighted turbo spin-echo (TSE) image of a large cervical tumor (*arrows*) with invasion into the parametrium is visible. **B:** A time image, with information about start of enhancement projected over (B) in color. The fastest-enhancing tumor region (within *circle*) starts to enhance 4 seconds after the artery. **C:** Axial postradiotherapy T2-weighted TSE image. The tumor has decreased in size; however, residual tumor is present (*arrows*). **D:** Time image in the fastest-enhancing part (within *circle*). Tumor enhancement occurs only 2 seconds after the artery. This patient proved to be a nonresponder and died 7 months after radiotherapy. (From ref. 107, with permission.)

antivascular, and antiangiogenic therapies.[85,86] Most studies consisted of small cohort single-center phase 1 trials, although a few phase 2 trials have also incorporated DCE-MRI.[108] Overall, evidence of drug efficacy has been demonstrated with DCE-MRI in clinical trials of antiangiogenic drugs. For example, a rapid tumor vascular shutdown induced by the vascular disrupting agent combretastatin in colorectal cancer was observed 4 hours after the first dose (Fig. 66.5).[109] Maps of area under gadolinium contrast medium curve at 60 seconds ($AUGC_{60}$; second row images in Fig. 66.5) revealed significant decreases in perfusion. In addition, the inflow transfer constant (K^{trans}; third row images in Fig. 66.5) and extracellular leakage space (v_e; bottom row images in Fig. 66.5) revealed that a significant vascular shutdown was induced by this drug by darker regions on the color overlay maps with the absence of morphologic change.

DCE-MRI biomarkers have been used to provide early indicators of efficacy, dose, and outcome and to assist in defining the biologically active and maximum tolerated doses. However, few trials have actually demonstrated a correlation between DCE-MRI measurements and clinical outcome measures; thus, observations of changes in DCE-MRI biomarkers should not be considered a guarantee of success in randomized phase 3 trials. Further advancement of the diagnostic and predictive value of DEC-MRI will require attention to the designing of a clinical protocol that has acquired the imaging data at a well-conceived scanning interval after administration of the agent.

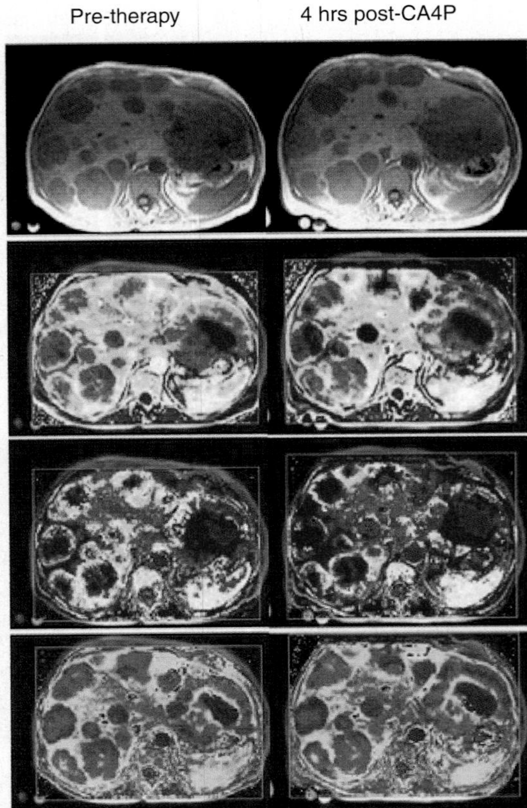

FIGURE 66.5 Rapid tumor vascular shutdown induced by the vascular disrupting agent, combretastatin, in colorectal cancer. Columns represent an examination acquired before treatment and 4 hours after the first dose, given intravenously. Rows show morphological T1-weighted images (**top row**) and maps of area under gadolinium contrast medium curve at 60 seconds ($AUGC_{60}$; **second row**), inflow transfer constant (K^{trans}; **third row**) and extracellular leakage space (v_e; **bottom row**) acquired at the three imaging time points. Vascular shutdown induced by drug is observed as darker colors on $AUGC_{60}$ and K^{trans} maps with the absence of morphologic change. Note marked inter- and intratumoral heterogeneity with great antivascular effects within the center of some lesions only. (Figure kindly provided by Dr. Anwar Padhani, Mount Vernon Cancer Centre, London, UK.)

For example, a vascular disrupting agent may require a baseline image, a 4- to 6-hour image, and a 24-hour image, in comparison to an antiangiogenic (or radiotherapy) trial in which images may be more sensitive to treatment-induced effects at longer interscan intervals of days to weeks or months in order to reach maximal change in the DCE-MRI biomarkers.

Another important area for potential improvement may be in the choice of the specific imaging biomarker(s) or parameters selected for a given therapeutic intervention. Moreover, the criteria used in the selection of regions of interest along with the specific method used in analysis of the imaging data that provides for the quantification of the DCE-MRI biomarkers can also impact the final results, and alternative methods may have a significant role, especially in tumors with significant regions of heterogeneity.

Summary

As with any biomarker, the routine application of DCE-MRI as a noninvasive biomarker of tumor angiogenesis and response to therapy requires validation through statistical correlation with traditional clinical outcome measures (i.e., radiologic response, overall survival). Overall, there is currently a lack of clinical data correlating changes in quantified DCE-MRI biomarkers with outcome measures to adopt this measurement as a surrogate end point in drug efficacy studies. Further developments of new contrast agents, higher magnetic fields (7 and 9.4 T), and image acquisition and analysis tools are in development, which may help to improve the prognostic value of DCE-MRI in cancer trials.

MAGNETIC RESONANCE SPECTROSCOPY

MRS is used to detect metabolites in tissues that contain protons (^{1}H), phosphorus (^{31}P), or enriched carbon (^{13}C) using the same equipment that is used for MRI. MRI produces images from ^{1}H nuclei in tissue water (or lipids) that are present in the molar concentration range, but MRS measures signals from nuclei of tissue metabolites about a 1,000-fold less in concentration (millimolar range). This brief overview will highlight applications of ^{1}H MRS and discuss the emerging possibilities offered by hyperpolarized ^{13}C.[110]

Unlike radiotracer techniques, different metabolites detected using ^{1}H MRS can be distinguished based on differences in their chemical shift, which is expressed in parts per million (ppm) of the main precession frequency (63 MHz at 1.5 T), allowing for spectral results from different magnetic fields to be compared. Moreover, compounds typically detected using ^{1}H MRS are naturally present in tissue; thus, administration of labeled compounds is unnecessary. Naturally present tissue metabolites detectable by ^{1}H MRS include choline-containing compounds (Cho: 3.2 ppm), creatine (Cr: 3.02 ppm), lactate (Lac: 1.33 ppm), lipids (Lip: 1.3, 0.9 ppm), myo-inositol (mI: 3.52 ppm), *N*-acetyl aspartate (NAA: 2.01 ppm), and citrate (Citrate: 2.6 ppm). The reported uses of MRS in cancer trials includes diagnostic functions such as identification of tumor presence and extent, distinguishing between tumor grades and tissue types as well as uses in monitoring response to therapy and identification of recurrence.[111,112]

^{1}H Spectroscopy in Preoperative Diagnosis

The use of ^{1}H MRS is promising for guidance of tumor biopsy, for example, in brain, prostate, and breast. Brain tumors are usually characterized by increasing Cho/Cr ratios with increasing tumor grade, whereas mI/Cr ratios decrease with increasing grade. A spectroscopic map of the Cho/Cr ratio registered with an anatomic image can be used to guide the surgeon to the most probable location of the central region of the tumor. In a study of 164 patients, ^{1}H MRS was reported to be a very sensitive technique for differentiating high-grade gliomas from low-grade lesions.[113] Similar studies have been accomplished in prostate cancer patients wherein the use of ^{1}H MRS has been found to be useful in predicting tumor presence with up to 91% specificity and 95% sensitivity.[114] Finally, in a combined study of 50 patients after positive mammography but prior to biopsy, MRI had 100% sensitivity and 62.5% specificity for detection of malignant breast tumors. Addition of ^{1}H MRS for quantification of choline levels improved the specificity to 87.5%.[115]

Treatment Guidance, Response, and Progression

A recent preliminary study of neoadjuvant therapy in locally advanced breast cancer patients revealed that a decrease in Cho levels within 24 hours of treatment following the first course of chemotherapy has the potential for predicting clinical response.[116]

The relatively low levels of ^{1}H metabolites (millimolar) present within tissue limits the overall voxel size that can be used to obtain adequate signal-to-noise levels, resulting in a lower resolution of MRS relative to anatomic MRI. Nevertheless, the use of ^{1}H MRS is actively being evaluated as a clinically prognostic factor in many different tumor types. Overall, it appears that generally increased choline levels can be used to identify lesion extent for malignant tumors that tend to decrease in lesions that respond to therapy with an increase in lipid/lactate resonances.[112,117,118] These changes can occur immediately following or up to 6 months after completion of treatment. It is hoped that this (and other) metabolic feature of cancer can be exploited as an imaging biomarker for the detection and response monitoring of cancer using ^{1}H MRS.

Hyperpolarized ^{13}C Magnetic Resonance Spectroscopy

Dynamic nuclear polarization was recently introduced as a method for increasing the sensitivity of detecting a ^{13}C metabolite using MRI by 10,000-fold or more.[119] This technology is undergoing investigation in animal models with U.S. Food and Drug Administration (FDA) approval received for trials in prostate cancer patients.[120] Studies have shown that this approach allows for detection of real-time metabolic images of the metabolic disposition of [1-^{13}C]-labeled pyruvate in animals with implanted tumors.[110,121–124] This approach has been expanded to additional molecules including bicarbonate ($H^{13}CO_3^-$), [1,4-$^{13}C_2$] fumarate, 3,5-difluorobenzoyl-L-glutamic acid, [5-$^{13}C_1$] glutamine, and ^{13}C-succinate in animals with exquisite sensitivity.[125–129] Following intravenous injection of hyperpolarized ^{13}C-labeled molecules in animal tumor models, metabolic images corresponding to metabolites are generated due to the availability of MR chemical shift information. Metabolic conversion of injected substrates into metabolites can be used to detect therapeutic-induced changes in tumor metabolic pathways that are involved with such pathways as oxidative phosphorylation and glycolysis. This technology has primarily been investigated in animal models and clinical trials have recently been initiated. Future applications may see the use of potentially many other hyperpolarized molecules for tumor imaging, expanding the opportunities in both animal studies and in the clinic.

References

1. Rosen BR, Belliveau JW, Vevea JM, et al. Perfusion imaging with NMR contrast agents. *Magn Reson Med* 1990;14(2):249.
2. Tofts PS, Kermode AG. Measurement of the blood–brain barrier permeability and leakage space using dynamic MR imaging. 1. Fundamental concepts. *Magn Reson Med* 1991;17(2):357.
3. Schwickert HC, Stiskal M, Roberts TP, et al. Contrast-enhanced MR imaging assessment of tumor capillary permeability: effect of irradiation on delivery of chemotherapy. *Radiology* 1996;198(3):893.
4. Su FC, Chu TC, Wai YY, et al. Temporal resolving power of perfusion- and BOLD-based event-related functional MRI. *Med Phys* 2004;31(1):154.
5. Warach S, Gaa J, Siewert B, et al. Acute human stroke studied by whole brain echo planar diffusion-weighted magnetic resonance imaging. *Ann Neurol* 1995;37(2):231.
6. Guo AC, Cummings TJ, Dash RC, et al. Lymphomas and high-grade astrocytomas: comparison of water diffusibility and histologic characteristics. *Radiology* 2002;224(1):177.
7. Pierpaoli C, Basser PJ. Toward a quantitative assessment of diffusion anisotropy. *Magn Reson Med* 1996;36(6):893.
8. Basser PJ, Pierpaoli C. Microstructural and physiological features of tissues elucidated by quantitative-diffusion-tensor MRI. *J Magn Reson B* 1996;111(3):209.
9. Gellermann J, Wlodarczyk W, Feussner A, et al. Methods and potentials of magnetic resonance imaging for monitoring radiofrequency hyperthermia in a hybrid system. *Int J Hyperthermia* 2005;21(6):497.
10. Sorensen AG, Buonanno FS, Gonzalez RG, et al. Hyperacute stroke: evaluation with combined multisection diffusion-weighted and hemodynamically weighted echo-planar MR imaging. *Radiology* 1996;199(2):391.
11. Le Bihan D, Breton E, Lallemand D, et al. Separation of diffusion and perfusion in intravoxel incoherent motion MR imaging. *Radiology* 1988; 168(2):497.
12. Moseley ME, et al. Diffusion-weighted MR imaging of acute stroke: correlation with T2-weighted and magnetic susceptibility-enhanced MR imaging in cats. *AJNR Am J Neuroradiol* 1990;11(3):423.
13. Moseley ME, Cohen Y, Kucharczyk J, et al. Diffusion-weighted MR imaging of anisotropic water diffusion in cat central nervous system. *Radiology* 1990;176(2):439.
14. Le Bihan D, Douek P, Argyropoulou M, et al. Diffusion and perfusion magnetic resonance imaging in brain tumors. *Top Magn Reson Imaging* 1993;5(1):25.
15. Le Bihan D. Molecular diffusion nuclear magnetic resonance imaging. *Magn Reson Q* 1991;7(1):1.
16. Thomsen C, Henriksen O, Ring P. In vivo measurement of water self diffusion in the human brain by magnetic resonance imaging. *Acta Radiol* 1987;28(3):353.
17. Merboldt KD, Bruhn H, Frahm J, et al. MRI of "diffusion" in the human brain: new results using a modified CE-FAST sequence. *Magn Reson Med* 1989;9(3):423.
18. Bammer R. Basic principles of diffusion-weighted imaging. *Eur J Radiol* 2003;45(3):169.
19. Padhani AR, Liu G, Koh DM, et al. Diffusion-weighted magnetic resonance imaging as a cancer biomarker: consensus and recommendations. *Neoplasia* 2009;11(2):102.
20. Edelman RR, Wielopolski P, Schmitt R. Echo-planar MR imaging. *Radiology* 1994;192(3):600.
21. Provenzale JM, McGraw P, Mhatre P, et al. Peritumoral brain regions in gliomas and meningiomas: investigation with isotropic diffusion-weighted MR imaging and diffusion-tensor MR imaging. *Radiology* 2004;232(2):451.
22. Yoshikawa T, Kawamitsu H, Mitchell DG, et al. ADC measurement of abdominal organs and lesions using parallel imaging technique. *AJR Am J Roentgenol* 2006;187(6):1521.
23. Koh DM, Scurr E, Collins DJ, et al. Colorectal hepatic metastases: quantitative measurements using single-shot echo-planar diffusion-weighted MR imaging. *Eur Radiol* 2006;16(9):1898.
24. Koh DM, Scurr E, Collins D, et al. Predicting response of colorectal hepatic metastasis: value of pretreatment apparent diffusion coefficients. *AJR Am J Roentgenol* 2007;188(4):1001.
25. Charles-Edwards EM, deSouza NM. Diffusion-weighted magnetic resonance imaging and its application to cancer. *Cancer Imaging* 2006;6:135.
26. Takahara T, Imai Y, Yamashita T, et al. Diffusion weighted whole body imaging with background body signal suppression (DWIBS): technical improvement using free breathing, STIR and high resolution 3D display. *Radiat Med* 2004;22(4):275.
27. Ichikawa T, Erturk SM, Motosugi U, et al. High-b value diffusion-weighted MRI for detecting pancreatic adenocarcinoma: preliminary results. *AJR Am J Roentgenol* 2007;188(2):409.
28. Sumi M, Ichikawa Y, Nakamura T. Diagnostic ability of apparent diffusion coefficients for lymphomas and carcinomas in the pharynx. *Eur Radiol* 2007;17(10):2631.
29. Eida S, Sumi M, Sakihama N, et al. Apparent diffusion coefficient mapping of salivary gland tumors: prediction of the benignancy and malignancy. *AJNR Am J Neuroradiol* 2007;28(1):116.
30. Bulakbasi N, Guvenc I, Onguru O, et al. The added value of the apparent diffusion coefficient calculation to magnetic resonance imaging in the differentiation and grading of malignant brain tumors. *J Comput Assist Tomogr* 2004;28(6):735.
31. Shimony JS, McKinstry RC, Akbudak E, et al. Quantitative diffusion-tensor anisotropy brain MR imaging: normative human data and anatomic analysis. *Radiology* 1999;212(3):770.
32. Mori S, Frederiksen K, van Zijl PC, et al. Brain white matter anatomy of tumor patients evaluated with diffusion tensor imaging. *Ann Neurol* 2002; 51(3):377.
33. Chenevert TL, McKeever PE, Ross BD. Monitoring early response of experimental brain tumors to therapy using diffusion magnetic resonance imaging. *Clin Cancer Res* 1997;3(9):1457.
34. Brunberg JA, Chenevert TL, McKeever PE, et al. In vivo MR determination of water diffusion coefficients and diffusion anisotropy: correlation with structural alteration in gliomas of the cerebral hemispheres. *AJNR Am J Neuroradiol* 1995;16(2):361.

35. Lyng H, Haraldseth O, Rofstad EK. Measurement of cell density and necrotic fraction in human melanoma xenografts by diffusion weighted magnetic resonance imaging. *Magn Reson Med* 2000;43(6):828.
36. Chenevert TL, Stegman LD, Taylor, JM, et al. Diffusion magnetic resonance imaging: an early surrogate marker of therapeutic efficacy in brain tumors. *J Natl Cancer Inst* 2000;92(24):2029.
37. Le Bihan D. The "wet mind": water and functional neuroimaging. *Phys Med Biol* 2007;52(7):R57.
38. Chenevert TL, Sundgren PC, Ross BD. Diffusion imaging: insight to cell status and cytoarchitecture. *Neuroimaging Clin North Am* 2006;16(4): 619, viii.
39. Ross BD, Moffat BA, Lawrence TS, et al. Evaluation of cancer therapy using diffusion magnetic resonance imaging. *Mol Cancer Ther* 2003;2 (6):581.
40. Lee KC, Sud S, Meyer CR, et al. An imaging biomarker of early treatment response in prostate cancer that has metastasized to the bone. *Cancer Res* 2007;67(8):3524.
41. Lee KC, Moffat BA, Schott AF, et al. Prospective early response imaging biomarker for neoadjuvant breast cancer chemotherapy. *Clin Cancer Res* 2007;13(2 Pt 1):443.
42. Lee KC, Hamstra DA, Bullarayasamudram S, et al. Fusion of the HSV-1 tegument protein vp22 to cytosine deaminase confers enhanced bystander effect and increased therapeutic benefit. *Gene Ther* 2006;13(2):127.
43. Lee KC, Hamstra DA, Bhojani MS, et al. Noninvasive molecular imaging sheds light on the synergy between 5-fluorouracil and TRAIL/Apo2L for cancer therapy. *Clin Cancer Res* 2007;13(6):1839.
44. Lee KC, Hall DE, Hoff BA, et al. Dynamic imaging of emerging resistance during cancer therapy. *Cancer Res* 2006;66(9):4687.
45. Hamstra DA, Lee KC, Tychewicz JM, et al. The use of 19F spectroscopy and diffusion-weighted MRI to evaluate differences in gene-dependent enzyme prodrug therapies. *Mol Ther* 2004;10(5):916.
46. Therasse P, Arbuck SG, Eisenhauer EA, et al. New guidelines to evaluate the response to treatment in solid tumors. European Organization for Research and Treatment of Cancer, National Cancer Institute of the United States, National Cancer Institute of Canada. *J Natl Cancer Inst* 2000;92 (3):205.
47. Sorensen AG, Patel S, Harmath C, et al. Comparison of diameter and perimeter methods for tumor volume calculation. *J Clin Oncol* 2001;19 (2):551.
48. Yoshida S, Koga F, Kawakami S, et al. Initial experience of diffusion-weighted magnetic resonance imaging to assess therapeutic response to induction chemoradiotherapy against muscle-invasive bladder cancer. *Urology* 2010;75(2):387.
49. Yankeelov TE, Lepage M, Chakravarthy A, et al. Integration of quantitative DCE-MRI and ADC mapping to monitor treatment response in human breast cancer: initial results. *Magn Reson Imaging* 2007;25(1):1.
50. Uhl M, Saueressig U, van Buiren M, et al. Osteosarcoma: preliminary results of in vivo assessment of tumor necrosis after chemotherapy with diffusion- and perfusion-weighted magnetic resonance imaging. *Invest Radiol* 2006;41(8):618.
51. Tomura N, Narita K, Izumi J, et al. Diffusion changes in a tumor and peritumoral tissue after stereotactic irradiation for brain tumors: possible prediction of treatment response. *J Comput Assist Tomogr* 2006;30(3):496.
52. Theilmann RJ, Borders R, Trouard TP, et al. Changes in water mobility measured by diffusion MRI predict response of metastatic breast cancer to chemotherapy. *Neoplasia* 2004;6(6):831.
53. Sun YS, Zhang XP, Tang L, et al. Locally advanced rectal carcinoma treated with preoperative chemotherapy and radiation therapy: preliminary analysis of diffusion-weighted MR imaging for early detection of tumor histopathologic downstaging. *Radiology* 2010;254(1):170.
54. Schubert MI, Wilke M, Müller-Weihrich S, et al. Diffusion-weighted magnetic resonance imaging of treatment-associated changes in recurrent and residual medulloblastoma: preliminary observations in three children. *Acta Radiol* 2006;47(10):1100.
55. Rhee TK, Naik NK, Deng J, et al. Tumor response after yttrium-90 radioembolization for hepatocellular carcinoma: comparison of diffusion-weighted functional MR imaging with anatomic MR imaging. *J Vasc Interv Radiol* 2008;19(8):1180.
56. Pickles MD, Gibbs P, Lowry M, et al. Diffusion changes precede size reduction in neoadjuvant treatment of breast cancer. *Magn Reson Imaging* 2006;24(7):843.
57. Okuma T, Matsuoka T, Yamamoto A, et al. Assessment of early treatment response after CT-guided radiofrequency ablation of unresectable lung tumours by diffusion-weighted MRI: a pilot study. *Br J Radiol* 2009;82 (984):989.
58. Moffat BA, Chenevert TL, Lawrence TS, et al. Functional diffusion map: a noninvasive MRI biomarker for early stratification of clinical brain tumor response. *Proc Natl Acad Sci U S A* 2005;102(15):5524.
59. Marugami N, Tanaka T, Kitano S, et al. Early detection of therapeutic response to hepatic arterial infusion chemotherapy of liver metastases from colorectal cancer using diffusion-weighted MR imaging. *Cardiovasc Intervent Radiol* 2009;32(4):638.
60. Mardor Y, Roth Y, Lidar Z, et al. Monitoring response to convection-enhanced taxol delivery in brain tumor patients using diffusion-weighted magnetic resonance imaging. *Cancer Res* 2001;61(13):4971.
61. Mardor Y, Pfeffer R, Spiegelmann R, et al. Early detection of response to radiation therapy in patients with brain malignancies using conventional and high b-value diffusion-weighted magnetic resonance imaging. *J Clin Oncol* 2003;21(6):1094.
62. Liu Y, Bai R, Sun H, et al. Diffusion-weighted imaging in predicting and monitoring the response of uterine cervical cancer to combined chemoradiation. *Clin Radiol* 2009;64(11):1067.
63. Lin YC, Wang CC, Wai YY, et al. Significant temporal evolution of diffusion anisotropy for evaluating early response to radiosurgery in patients with vestibular schwannoma: findings from functional diffusion maps. *AJNR Am J Neuroradiol* 2010;31(2):269.
64. Liapi E, Kamel IR, Bluemke DA, et al. Assessment of response of uterine fibroids and myometrium to embolization using diffusion-weighted echoplanar MR imaging. *J Comput Assist Tomogr* 2005;29(1):83.
65. Kremser C, Judmaier W, Hein P, et al. Preliminary results on the influence of chemoradiation on apparent diffusion coefficients of primary rectal carcinoma measured by magnetic resonance imaging. *Strahlenther Onkol* 2003;179(9):641.
66. Koh DM, et al. Reproducibility and changes in the apparent diffusion coefficients of solid tumours treated with combretastatin A4 phosphate and bevacizumab in a two-centre phase I clinical trial. *Eur Radiol* 2009;19 (11):2728.
67. Kim SH, Blackledge M, Collins DJ, et al. Locally advanced rectal cancer: added value of diffusion-weighted MR imaging in the evaluation of tumor response to neoadjuvant chemo- and radiation therapy. *Radiology* 2009; 253(1):116.
68. Kim S, Loevner L, Quon H, et al. Diffusion-weighted magnetic resonance imaging for predicting and detecting early response to chemoradiation therapy of squamous cell carcinomas of the head and neck. *Clin Cancer Res* 2009;15(3):986.
69. Kato H, Kanematsu M, Tanaka O, et al. Head and neck squamous cell carcinoma: usefulness of diffusion-weighted MR imaging in the prediction of a neoadjuvant therapeutic effect. *Eur Radiol* 2009;19(1):103.
70. Kamel IR, Reyes DK, Liapi E, et al. Functional MR imaging assessment of tumor response after 90Y microsphere treatment in patients with unresectable hepatocellular carcinoma. *J Vasc Interv Radiol* 2007;18(1 Pt 1):49.
71. Kamel IR, Bluemke DA, Eng J, et al. The role of functional MR imaging in the assessment of tumor response after chemoembolization in patients with hepatocellular carcinoma. *J Vasc Interv Radiol* 2006;17(3):505.
72. Jain R, Scarpace LM, Ellika S, et al. Imaging response criteria for recurrent gliomas treated with bevacizumab: role of diffusion weighted imaging as an imaging biomarker. *J Neurooncol* 2010;96(3):423.
73. Jacobs MA, Herskovits EH, Kim HS. Uterine fibroids: diffusion-weighted MR imaging for monitoring therapy with focused ultrasound surgery—preliminary study. *Radiology* 2005;236(1):196.
74. Hayashida Y, Yakushiji T, Awai K, et al. Monitoring therapeutic responses of primary bone tumors by diffusion-weighted image: initial results. *Eur Radiol* 2006;16(12):2637.
75. Harry VN, Semple SI, Gilbert FJ, et al. Diffusion-weighted magnetic resonance imaging in the early detection of response to chemoradiation in cervical cancer. *Gynecol Oncol* 2008;111(2):213.
76. Hamstra DA, Chenevert TL, Moffat BA, et al. Evaluation of the functional diffusion map as an early biomarker of time-to-progression and overall survival in high-grade glioma. *Proc Natl Acad Sci U S A* 2005;102(46): 16759.
77. Galban CJ, Mukherji SK, Chenevert TL, et al. A feasibility study of parametric response map analysis of diffusion-weighted magnetic resonance imaging scans of head and neck cancer patients for providing early detection of therapeutic efficacy. *Transl Oncol* 2009;2(3):184.
78. Dzik-Jurasz A, Domenig C, George M, et al. Diffusion MRI for prediction of response of rectal cancer to chemoradiation. *Lancet* 2002;360(9329): 307.
79. Dirix P, Vandecaveye V, De Keyzer F, et al. Dose painting in radiotherapy for head and neck squamous cell carcinoma: value of repeated functional imaging with (18)F-FDG PET, (18)F-fluoromisonidazole PET, diffusion-weighted MRI, and dynamic contrast-enhanced MRI. *J Nucl Med* 2009; 50(7):1020.
80. Deng J, Miller FH, Rhee TK, et al. Diffusion-weighted MR imaging for determination of hepatocellular carcinoma response to yttrium-90 radioembolization. *J Vasc Interv Radiol* 2006;17(7):1195.
81. Cui Y, Zhang XP, Sun YS, et al. Apparent diffusion coefficient: potential imaging biomarker for prediction and early detection of response to chemotherapy in hepatic metastases. *Radiology* 2008;248(3):894.
82. Byun WM, Shin SO, Chang Y, et al. Diffusion-weighted MR imaging of metastatic disease of the spine: assessment of response to therapy. *AJNR Am J Neuroradiol* 2002;23(6):906.
83. Eccles C, Haider MA, Dawson LA. Change in diffusion weighted MRI during liver cancer radiotherapy: preliminary observations. *Acta Oncol* 2009;48(7):1034.
84. Hein PA, Eskey CJ, Dunn JF, et al. Diffusion-weighted imaging in the follow-up of treated high-grade gliomas: tumor recurrence versus radiation injury. *AJNR Am J Neuroradiol* 2004;25(2):201.
85. Zahra MA, Hollingsworth KG, Sala E, et al. Dynamic contrast-enhanced MRI as a predictor of tumour response to radiotherapy. *Lancet Oncol* 2007;8(1):63.

86. O'Connor JP, Jackson A, Parker GJ, et al. DCE-MRI biomarkers in the clinical evaluation of antiangiogenic and vascular disrupting agents. *Br J Cancer* 2007; 96(2):189.
87. Ah-See ML, Makris A, Taylor NJ, et al. Early changes in functional dynamic magnetic resonance imaging predict for pathologic response to neoadjuvant chemotherapy in primary breast cancer. *Clin Cancer Res* 2008;14(20):6580.
88. Baar J, Silverman P, Lyons J, et al. A vasculature-targeting regimen of preoperative docetaxel with or without bevacizumab for locally advanced breast cancer: impact on angiogenic biomarkers. *Clin Cancer Res* 2009;15 (10):3583.
89. Batchelor TT, Sorensen AG, di Tomaso E, et al. AZD2171, a pan-VEGF receptor tyrosine kinase inhibitor, normalizes tumor vasculature and alleviates edema in glioblastoma patients. *Cancer Cell* 2007;11(1):83.
90. Bauerle T, Bartling S, Berger M, et al. Imaging anti-angiogenic treatment response with DCE-VCT, DCE-MRI and DWI in an animal model of breast cancer bone metastasis. *Eur J Radiol* 2010;73(2):280.
91. Jain RK, et al. Biomarkers of response and resistance to antiangiogenic therapy. *Nat Rev Clin Oncol* 2009;6(6):327.
92. Jarnagin WR, Schwartz LH, Gultekin DH, et al. Regional chemotherapy for unresectable primary liver cancer: results of a phase II clinical trial and assessment of DCE-MRI as a biomarker of survival. *Ann Oncol* 2009;20 (9):1589.
93. Kamoun WS, Ley CD, Farrar CT, et al. Edema control by cediranib, a vascular endothelial growth factor receptor-targeted kinase inhibitor, prolongs survival despite persistent brain tumor growth in mice. *J Clin Oncol* 2009;27(15):2542.
94. Kim S, Loevner LA, Quon H, et al. Prediction of response to chemoradiation therapy in squamous cell carcinomas of the head and neck using dynamic contrast-enhanced MR imaging. *AJNR Am J Neuroradiol* 2010; 31(2):262.
95. Lockhart AC, Rothenberg ML, Dupont J, et al. Phase I study of intravenous vascular endothelial growth factor trap, aflibercept, in patients with advanced solid tumors. *J Clin Oncol* 2010;28(2):207.
96. Meyer T, Gaya AM, Dancey G, et al. A phase I trial of radioimmunotherapy with 131I-A5B7 anti-CEA antibody in combination with combretastatin-A4-phosphate in advanced gastrointestinal carcinomas. *Clin Cancer Res* 2009;15(13):4484.
97. Sorensen AG, Batchelor TT, Zhang WT, et al. A "vascular normalization index" as potential mechanistic biomarker to predict survival after a single dose of cediranib in recurrent glioblastoma patients. *Cancer Res* 2009;69 (13):5296.
98. van Laarhoven HW, Fiedler W, Desar IM, et al. Phase I clinical and magnetic resonance imaging study of the vascular agent NGR-hTNF in patients with advanced cancers (European Organization for Research and Treatment of Cancer Study 16041). *Clin Cancer Res* 2010;16(4): 1315.
99. Vriens D, van Laarhoven HW, van Asten JJ, et al. Chemotherapy response monitoring of colorectal liver metastases by dynamic Gd-DTPA-enhanced MRI perfusion parameters and 18F-FDG PET metabolic rate. *J Nucl Med* 2009;50(11):1777.
100. Wong CI, Koh TS, Soo R, et al. Phase I and biomarker study of ABT-869, a multiple receptor tyrosine kinase inhibitor, in patients with refractory solid malignancies. *J Clin Oncol* 2009;27(28):4718.
101. Zahra MA, Tan LT, Priest AN, et al. Semiquantitative and quantitative dynamic contrast-enhanced magnetic resonance imaging measurements predict radiation response in cervix cancer. *Int J Radiat Oncol Biol Phys* 2009;74(3):766.
102. Tofts PS, Brix G, Buckley DL, et al. Estimating kinetic parameters from dynamic contrast-enhanced T(1)-weighted MRI of a diffusable tracer: standardized quantities and symbols. *J Magn Reson Imaging* 1999;10(3): 223.
103. Leach MO, Brindle KM, Evelhoch JL, et al. The assessment of antiangiogenic and antivascular therapies in early-stage clinical trials using magnetic resonance imaging: issues and recommendations. *Br J Cancer* 2005; 92(9):1599.
104. Semiz Oysu A, Ayanoglu E, Kodalli N, et al. Dynamic contrast-enhanced MRI in the differentiation of posttreatment fibrosis from recurrent carcinoma of the head and neck. *Clin Imaging* 2005;29(5):307.
105. Ohno Y, Nogami M, Higashino T, et al. Prognostic value of dynamic MR imaging for non-small-cell lung cancer patients after chemoradiotherapy. *J Magn Reson Imaging* 2005;21(6):775.
106. Dobson MJ, Carrington BM, Collins CD, et al. The assessment of irradiated bladder carcinoma using dynamic contrast-enhanced MR imaging. *Clin Radiol* 2001;56(2):94.
107. Boss EA, Massuger LF, Pop LA, et al. Post-radiotherapy contrast enhancement changes in fast dynamic MRI of cervical carcinoma. *J Magn Reson Imaging* 2001;13(4):600.
108. Wedam SB, Low JA, Yang SX, et al. Antiangiogenic and antitumor effects of bevacizumab in patients with inflammatory and locally advanced breast cancer. *J Clin Oncol* 2006;24(5):769.
109. Goh V, Padhani AR, Rasheed S. Functional imaging of colorectal cancer angiogenesis. *Lancet Oncol* 2007;8(3):245.
110. Golman K, Zandt RI, Lerche M, et al. Metabolic imaging by hyperpolarized 13C magnetic resonance imaging for in vivo tumor diagnosis. *Cancer Res* 2006;66(22):10855.
111. Payne GS, Leach MO. Applications of magnetic resonance spectroscopy in radiotherapy treatment planning. *Br J Radiol* 2006;79(Spec No 1):S16.
112. Kwock L, Smith JK, Castillo M, et al. Clinical role of proton magnetic resonance spectroscopy in oncology: brain, breast, and prostate cancer. *Lancet Oncol* 2006;7(10):859.
113. Moller-Hartmann W, Herminghaus S, Krings T, et al. Clinical application of proton magnetic resonance spectroscopy in the diagnosis of intracranial mass lesions. *Neuroradiology* 2002;44(5):371.
114. Scheidler J, Hricak H, Vigneron DB, et al. Prostate cancer: localization with three-dimensional proton MR spectroscopic imaging—clinicopathologic study. *Radiology* 1999;213(2):473.
115. Huang W, Fisher PR, Dulaimy K, et al. Detection of breast malignancy: diagnostic MR protocol for improved specificity. *Radiology* 2004;232(2):585.
116. Meisamy S, Bolan PJ, Baker EH, et al. Neoadjuvant chemotherapy of locally advanced breast cancer: predicting response with in vivo (1)H MR spectroscopy—a pilot study at 4 T. *Radiology* 2004;233(2):424.
117. Nelson SJ, Graves E, Pirzkall A, et al. In vivo molecular imaging for planning radiation therapy of gliomas: an application of 1H MRSI. *J Magn Reson Imaging* 2002;16(4):464.
118. Chan AA, Lau A, Pirzkall A, et al. Proton magnetic resonance spectroscopy imaging in the evaluation of patients undergoing gamma knife surgery for grade IV glioma. *J Neurosurg* 2004;101(3):467.
119. Goetz M, Fottner C, Kiesslich R. Molecular imaging with endogenous substances. *Proc Natl Acad Sci U S A* 2003;100(18):10435.
120. Kurhanewicz J, Bok R, Nelson SJ, et al. Current and potential applications of clinical 13C MR spectroscopy. *J Nucl Med* 2008;49(3):341.
121. Ward CS, Venkatesh HS, Chaumeil MM, et al. Noninvasive detection of target modulation following phosphatidylinositol 3-kinase inhibition using hyperpolarized 13C magnetic resonance spectroscopy. *Cancer Res* 2010;70(4):1296.
122. Park I, Larson PE, Zierhut ML, et al. Hyperpolarized 13C magnetic resonance metabolic imaging: application to brain tumors. *Neuro Oncol* 2010; 12(2):133.
123. Harris T, Eliyahu G, Frydman L, et al. Kinetics of hyperpolarized 13C1-pyruvate transport and metabolism in living human breast cancer cells. *Proc Natl Acad Sci U S A* 2009;106(43):18131.
124. Day SE, Kettunen MI, Gallagher FA, et al. Detecting tumor response to treatment using hyperpolarized 13C magnetic resonance imaging and spectroscopy. *Nat Med* 2007;13(11):1382.
125. Jamin Y, Gabellieri C, Smyth L, et al. Hyperpolarized (13)C magnetic resonance detection of carboxypeptidase G2 activity. *Magn Reson Med* 2009; 62(5):1300.
126. Gallagher FA, et al. Production of hyperpolarized [1,4-13C2] malate from [1,4-13C2] fumarate is a marker of cell necrosis and treatment response in tumors. *Proc Natl Acad Sci U S A* 2009;106(47):19801.
127. Gallagher FA, Kettunen MI, Hu DE, et al. 13C MR spectroscopy measurements of glutaminase activity in human hepatocellular carcinoma cells using hyperpolarized 13C-labeled glutamine. *Magn Reson Med* 2008;60 (2):253.
128. Gallagher FA, Kettunen MI, Day SE, et al. Magnetic resonance imaging of pH in vivo using hyperpolarized 13C-labelled bicarbonate. *Nature* 2008; 453(7197):940.
129. Bhattacharya P, Chekmenev EY, Perman WH, et al. Towards hyperpolarized (13)C-succinate imaging of brain cancer. *J Magn Reson* 2007;186(1):150.
130. Hamstra DA, Galbán CJ, Meyer CR, et al. Functional diffusion map as an early imaging biomarker for high-grade glioma: correlation with conventional radiologic response and overall survival. *J Clin Oncol* 2008;26(20): 3387.

CHAPTER 67 MOLECULAR IMAGING

STEVEN M. LARSON, HEIKO SCHÖDER, AND JAN GRIMM

Molecular imaging for oncology can be defined as imaging the key molecules and molecular events that are fundamental to the development and progression of cancer. Table 67.1 is one way to organize some of these molecules and biochemical pathways that are currently under investigation. Among the various molecular imaging techniques, nuclear-based methods have the advantage of great versatility because radiotracers can be developed for a myriad of functions. This chapter will emphasize nuclear techniques that will likely continue to dominate molecular imaging in the near term.[1–5] In particular, positron emission tomography (PET) is a nuclear medicine imaging technology that uses compounds labeled with positron-emitting radioisotopes to image and measure biochemical processes.[6] Commonly used positron emitters in medicine include the isotopes ^{11}C carbon, ^{15}O oxygen, ^{13}N nitrogen, and ^{18}F fluorine. Since many naturally occurring compounds contain the atoms of oxygen, carbon, or nitrogen (e.g., H_2O, CO_2, or ammonia), it is potentially possible to replace these nonradioactive atoms with their positron-emitting isotope. The resulting labeled compound will be biochemically identical to the original compound. In other cases, natural substances can be labeled with ^{18}F, for instance, by replacing the OH group with ^{18}F fluorine in producing FDG from deoxyglucose. The resulting compound may show somewhat different biochemical behavior but will still reflect distribution of the natural compound to such a degree that part of the normal metabolism is traced. Usually, PET and computed tomography (CT) are now operated within a hybrid machine, thus combining accurate structural and functional assessment in one imaging session.[7–11] In oncology, the vast majority of studies are performed using the radiotracer [^{18}F] 2-fluoro-2-deoxyglucose (FDG), which takes advantage of the Warburg effect (see below).

CHARACTERIZING THE CANCER CELL PHENOTYPE

Cancer cells have a characteristic phenotype that distinguishes them from their benign counterparts,[12] including an altered intermediary metabolism and increased proliferation. This requires nutrients and basic substrates as building blocks for proteins, DNA and RNA, lipids, and other macromolecules. A number of these processes can be studied with PET imaging for both clinical and research purposes.

Warburg Effect

Glycolysis is the dominant means of energy production in cancer cells, even in the presence of oxygen,[13,14] leading to increased lactate production. This phenomenon, first reported by the biochemist Otto Warburg (after whom is it named) and his group in the 1920s, occurs because of the need to control redox state in the cell and to obtain carbon backbone for macromolecular synthesis.[15,16] Several other metabolic processes are also altered in the cancer cell, including lipid synthesis and glutamine dependent anaplerosis.[17] Signal transduction molecules and gene expression are regulators of many cancer pathways. For instance, phosphatidylinositol 3-kinase (PI3K) and Akt[18–20] regulate glucose uptake and metabolism, and hypoxia-induced factor-1α (HIF-1α), *RAS*, and *MYC* oncogenes are other mediators of metabolism.[21] Further, the tumor suppressor protein p53 stimulates the gene encoding the enzyme synthesis of cytochrome-C oxidase; accordingly, low p53 causes inhibition of mitochondrial oxidative phosphorylation.[22] The altered metabolism contributes to increased biosynthesis of nucleotides, proteins, phospholipids, and fatty acids, and it inhibits apoptosis by neutralizing reactive oxygen species through the production of nicotinamide adenine dinucleotide phosphate (NADPH). However, toxic metabolites, such as lactate and some nucleotides, need to be removed. In the clinic, the Warburg effect can be imaged with FDG-PET. Of note, in many malignancies there is a relationship between intensity of FDG uptake and tumor aggressiveness.[23–33] FDG uptake depends on glucose transporters (GLUT); GLUT-1 and -3 are overexpressed in many cancers. In the cell, FDG is phosphorylated by hexokinase (HK) to FDG-6-phosphate. HK-II is the isoform found in most cancers. Overexpression of HK-II protein and increased enzyme activity are common events in rapidly growing, poorly differentiated tumors (sometimes as early event).[34–36] The underlying molecular mechanisms include overexpression of the HK gene, increased gene transcription, gene duplication and amplification, and promotor activation.[34] In contrast to many normal tissues, in the cancer cell, HK binds to channels in the outer mitochondrial membrane (voltage-dependent anion channels [VDAC]). By so doing, hexokinase (1) has rapid access to mitochondrially generated adenosine triphosphate (ATP); (2) is protected against feedback inhibition by glucose-6-phosphate as well as against proteolytic degradation; and (3) can inhibit Bax-induced cytochrome-C release and apoptosis.[36] Interestingly, binding of HK-II to VDAC in the outer mitochondrial membrane is enhanced by overexpression of Akt[18] by negatively regulating the activity of glycogen synthase kinase-3-β (GSK-3-β).[19] Conversely, inhibition of Akt leads to activation of GSK-3-β and phosphorylation of VDAC. HK-II is then unable to bind to these phosphorylated VDAC and therefore dissociates from the mitochondria. Of note, many cancers show a correlation between HK expression and FDG uptake on PET imaging.[37–40] The resulting decline in glycolysis, which can also be imaged by PET, is associated with an increase in chemotherapy-induced cell death.[19] Akt may also promote glycolysis indirectly through its repressive effect on fatty acid oxidation, thereby eliminating a potential

TABLE 67.1

POSITRON EMISSION TOMOGRAPHY RADIOTRACERS AND BIOCHEMICAL PRINCIPLES FOR MOLECULAR CANCER IMAGING

Tracers	Molecular Mechanism	Molecular Target or Principle	Cancer Example
^{18}F FDG	GluT, hexokinase	Increased aerobic glucose metabolism in cancer (Warburg effect)	NSCLC, HNSCC, colorectal, esophagus, lymphomas
^{18}F fluoromisonidazole	Electrochemical reduction	Hypoxia	HNSCC, cervix uteri
^{11}C methionine ^{18}F FACBC, ^{18}F FET ^{18}F DOPA	AA transporter	AA uptake into tumor	GBM, prostate, some neuroendocrine tumors
^{11}C acetate	Fatty acid synthetase	Fatty acid metabolism, membrane synthesis	GBM, prostate
^{11}C/^{18}F choline	Choline kinase activity	Membrane synthesis, cell turnover, increased cell density	Prostate, gliomas
^{18}F FLT	Thymidine kinase	Proliferation	Lung, esophagus, lymphoma, sarcoma
^{18}F FDHT	Receptor binding and internalization	Androgen receptor	Prostate
^{18}F estradiol	Receptor binding	Estrogen receptor	Breast
^{124}I NaI	NIS	Retained only in NIS+ thyroid tissue	Thyroid
^{124}I cG250	Chimeric antibody, antibody binding	Carbonic anhydrase-IX (overexpressed in renal cancer; also in hypoxia)	Renal clear cell
^{124}I A33	Antibody binding	A33 receptor	Colorectal
^{68}Ga trastuzumab	Antibody or antibody fragment binding	*HER2* receptor	Breast, prostate
^{68}Ga DOTATOC	Receptor binding	SSR-2, SSR-5	SSR expressing neuroendocrine tumors
^{18}F RGD peptide	$\alpha_v\beta_3$ integrins	Angiogenesis (integrins overexpressed on neovascular endothelium)	Investigational with clinical promise

GluT, glucose transporters; FDG, ^{18}-F-fluoro-2-deoxy-D-glucose; NSCLC, non–small cell lung cancer; HNSCC, head and neck squamous cell carcinoma; AA, amino acid; GBM, glioblastoma multiforme; FLT, ^{18}-F-fluoro-thymidine; FDHT, ^{18}F-fluoro-dihydrotestosterone; NIS, Na iodide symporter; DOTATOC, ^{90}Y-DOTA-D-Phe^1-Tyr^3-octreotide; RGD, arginine-glycine-aspartate; SSR, somatostatin receptor.

alternative pathway for energy production in the cancer cell.[20] In some malignancies, other oncogenic enzymes have been identified, such as fumarate hydratase (in leiomyosarcomas) and succinate dehydrogenase (in paragangliomas). Defects in these enzymes lead to accumulation of fumarate and succinate with subsequent overexpression of HIF-1α, which promotes tumor vascularization and increased glycolysis. Similarly, 70% of gliomas have mutations in the isocitrate dehydrogenase enzymes (IDH-1 and IDH-2), suggesting their possible role in cancer development and progression.[41]

In clinical practice, it is possible to take advantage of some of the aforementioned metabolic abnormalities and use them for imaging the cancer cell and its microenvironment. FDG is now the most commonly used positron-labeled tracer in clinical practice worldwide, accounting for more than 90% of all PET studies. Note that unlike glucose, the fraction of FDG not taken up by tissues will be excreted by the kidneys (the predominant route of excretion for many other radiotracers is the hepatobiliary system), and this results in improved imaging contrast between tumor and normal tissues. FDG is taken up into cells by the same GLUT family of transporter molecules as normal glucose and is then phosphorylated by hexokinase to FDG-6-phosphate. However, in contrast to unlabeled glucose, FDG-6-phosphate does not enter any further metabolic processes, such as glycolysis, the hexose monophosphate shunt, or glycogen synthesis. Thus, for practical purposes, FDG is metabolically trapped within the cell. HK-II expression and activity is generally considered the rate limiting step. Of note, the Warburg effect promotes survival and biologic aggressiveness of the cancer cell. Accordingly, there is a high correlation of FDG uptake and biologic aggressiveness in many human cancers.[23–33]

Cellular Proliferation and Apoptosis

Unrestrained growth of cancer cells requires DNA, for which thymidine is an essential building block. For PET imaging, the thymidine analogue ^{18}F-3′deoxy-3′-flurothymidine (FLT) is used.[42–48] FLT is phosphorylated intracellularly by thymidine kinase-1 (TK-1) and enters the salvage pathway but is not incorporated into DNA. However, since TK-1 activity and incorporation into DNA are linked in most situations, there is a good correlation between tissue markers of proliferation and the intensity of FLT uptake *in vitro* and *in vivo*.[49–54] FLT uptake correlates well with the expression of ki-67, a tissue marker of cellular proliferation,[49,55] and early changes in FLT uptake may be a marker of effective treatment in patients undergoing chemotherapy (Fig. 67.1).[56–59] FLT is taken up avidly within the bone marrow, and metabolites of FLT are

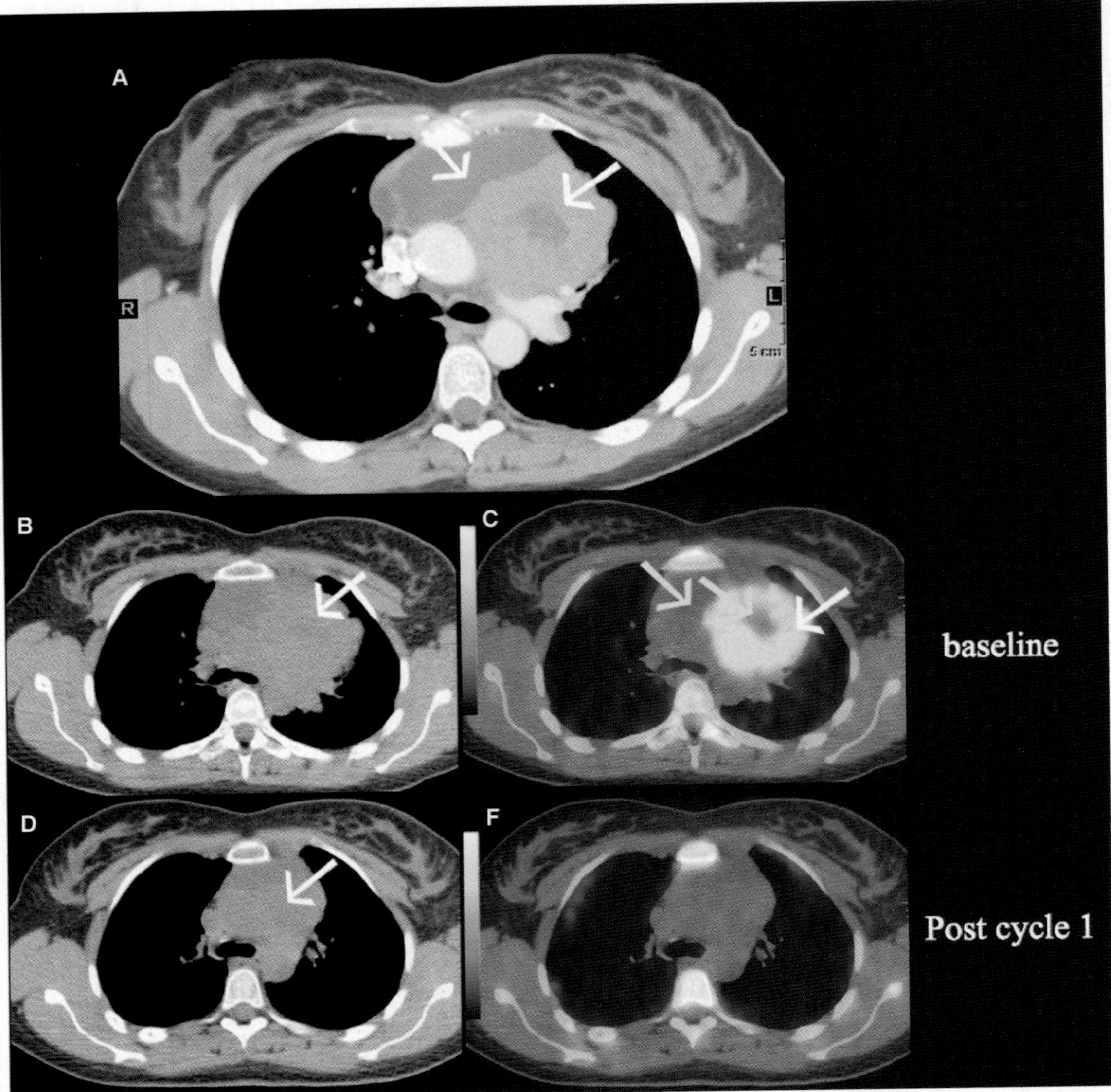

FIGURE 67.1 Treatment response assessment with [18]-F-fluoro-thymidine (FLT) positron emission tomography computed tomography (PET-CT) in patient with diffuse large cell lymphoma at baseline and after one cycle of chemotherapy. **A:** Contrast-enhanced CT shows large anterior mediastinal mass. **B, C:** Low dose CT and PET-CT fusion images at baseline. There is intense FLT uptake prior to treatment in this mass (*white arrow*); mass also shows areas of necrosis (*yellow arrow*). **D, E:** After one cycle of R-CHOP (rituximab, cyclophosphamide, doxorubicin, vincristine, prednisolone) chemotherapy, the size of the mass has declined only slightly, but FLT uptake has already resolved, indicating response to therapy. The patient continued standard chemotherapy and remains disease free 14 months later.

accumulated within the liver. Thus, the biodistribution of FLT in normal organs is very different from that of FDG. Because the intensity of uptake in cancer cells, and therefore the sensitivity for detection, is generally lower for FLT than for FDG, FLT is not an agent for cancer detection, but rather for measuring proliferation and treatment response.

Amino Acid Transport

L-type amino acid transport is strongly up-regulated in most human cancers, and thus labeled amino acids can serve as PET tracers for cancer imaging. Most data are reported for brain tumors and prostate cancer.[60,61] Agents under study include ^{18}F-fluorocyclobutane-1-carboxylic acid (FACBC)[62] and fluoroethyltyrosine (FET).[63–65]

Androgen and Estrogen Receptor Expression

Targeted therapy for endocrine responsive tumors (breast, prostate) requires knowledge if and to what degree the targeted receptor is present, whether it is functionally active, and whether its activity is critical for tumor progression. ^{18}F-estradiol[66] and ^{18}F-fluoro-dihydrotestosterone (FDHT)[67] have emerged as useful PET tracers in these settings (Fig. 67.2).

Sodium Iodide Symporter

Molecular targeting of key molecules in the cancer cell with radiolabeled compounds is an emerging concept. It is hoped that the likelihood for response may be predicted by calculating the radiation dose that can be delivered. For instance,

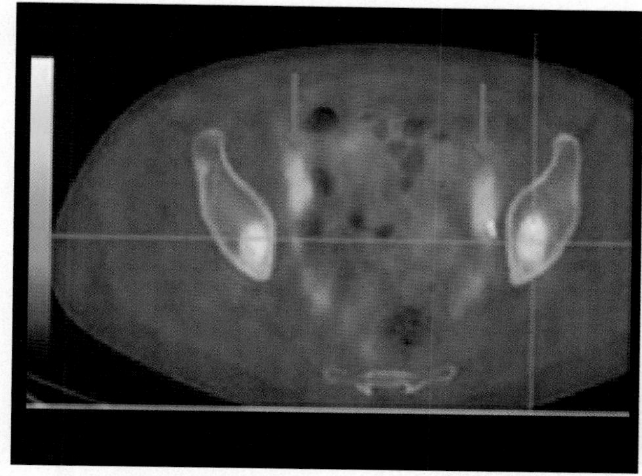

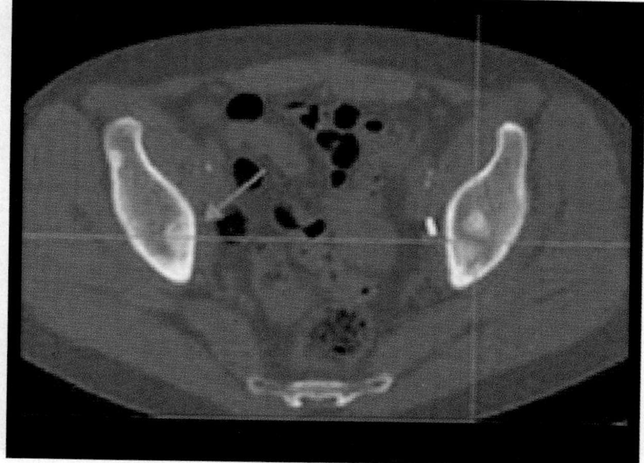

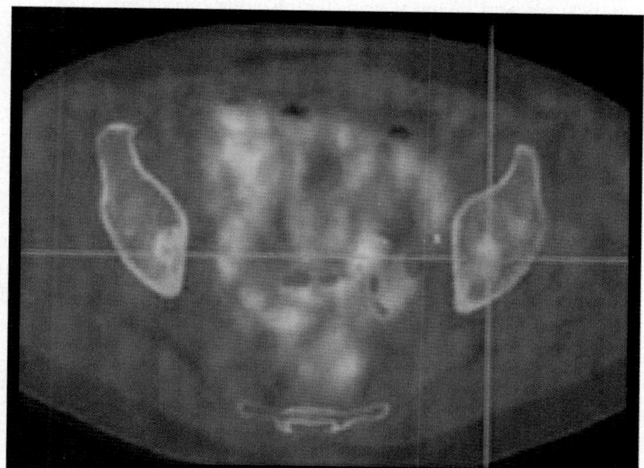

FIGURE 67.2 Androgen receptor imaging. ^{18}F-fluoro-dihydrotestosterone (FDHT) and ^{18}F-fluoro-2-deoxy-D-glucose (FDG) imaging in a patient with castrate-resistant metastatic prostate cancer to bone. **A:** Transaxial FDHT positron emission tomography computed tomography (PET-CT) fusion image shows abnormal radiotracer accumulation in bilateral supra-acetabular iliac bones (*crosshair*). Note relatively high blood pool activity in iliac vessels (*blue arrows*), which, however, does not interfere with imaging of the metastatic lesions. **B:** Corresponding CT image showing sclerotic osseous metastases bilaterally. **C:** FDG PET-CT also shows uptake in the bilateral iliac bone metastasis. However, the intensity of FDG uptake is much lower than that of the FDHT uptake. Normal intestinal activity is seen in the center of the pelvis.

quantitative PET with ^{124}I can be used to determine the dose and dose distribution for subsequent treatment with the beta-emitter ^{131}I in thyroid cancer.[68]

Imaging the Human Epidermal Growth Factor Receptor 2 Oncogene

In some breast cancers, human epidermal growth factor receptor 2 (HER-2) oncogene overexpression causes increased production of the ERBB-2 (Her-2) growth factor receptor, which can be imaged with a ^{68}G-labeled trastuzumab antibody fragment.[69] In animal models, this agent rapidly binds to the receptor, and the level of binding is proportional to the level of receptor expression. Of note, changes in receptor number can be quantified using this technique. It is hoped that this technique will enable us to determine the effectiveness of drug response more rapidly than with other imaging tests.[70]

Gene Expression Imaging

In gene expression imaging, a reporter gene, which has a selective action to concentrate or localize a substrate (reporter substrate) when the gene is active, is used. A classic example is the use of the herpes simplex thymidine kinase (*HSV-TK*) gene, which inserts into the DNA of the transfected cell and becomes activated under the control of a constitutively active promoter (always active). The radiotracer ^{124}I-FIAU (1-(2′-deoxy-2′-fluoro-β-D-arabinofuranosyl-5-iodouracil) and many others serve as reporter substrates to image gene expression. Since FIAU is not a substrate for mammalian TK, only transfected cells will phosphorylate and retain the agent.[71] PET imaging of gene expression has been used in pilot studies in humans after intratumoral vector injection in brain or liver lesions.[72,73] It is likely that gene expression imaging will be used increasingly in the clinic to monitor gene therapy or therapy with stem cells or immunocompetent cells.

Hypoxia

Solid tumors have a tendency to outgrow their blood supply and to become hypoxic, which renders them resistant to radiation and chemotherapy.[74,75] For this reason, radiation oncologists have long sought a noninvasive method for evaluating the extent of tumor hypoxia. Hypoxia can for instance be

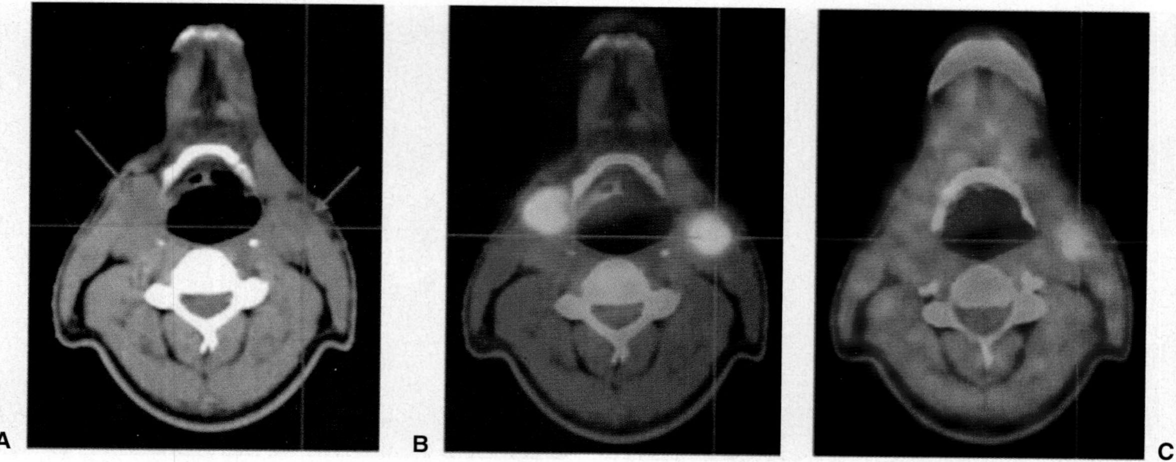

FIGURE 67.3 Hypoxia imaging. A patient with base of tongue cancer and bilateral neck lymph node metastases. **A:** Low-dose computed tomography (CT) of the combined positron emission tomography CT (PET-CT) shows enlarged lymph nodes (*arrows*). **B:** ^{18}F-fluoro-2-deoxy-D-glucose (FDG) PET-CT fusion image shows localization of FDG to the enlarged metastatic nodes. **C:** fluoromisonidazole (FMISO) PET/CT fusion image.

imaged with labeled nitroimidazoles, for example, ^{18}F-fluoromisonidazole (FMISO)[76–78] (Fig. 67.3) or ^{18}F-FAZA (^{18}F-fluroazomycinarabinoside)[79]. This may be helpful in guiding the use of radiation sensitizers in patients with hypoxic tumors or guiding radiation dose boost to hypoxic subvolumes.

CLINICAL APPLICATIONS

Accepted clinical indications for oncologic PET imaging, mostly with FDG, are listed in Table 67.2 and clinical examples are shown in Figures 67.4 and 67.5. When PET is added

TABLE 67.2

CLINICAL APPLICATIONS FOR POSITRON EMISSION TOMOGRAPHY IMAGING

Tumor	N Staging	M Staging	Recurrence	Treatment Monitoring	Monitoring Neoadjuvant Therapy
NSCLC	+ +	+ +	+ +	+	+
SCLC	+ +	+ +	+ +	+	N/A
HNSCC	+ +	+ + (for locally advanced disease)	+ +	+	+
Esophagus	(+)	+ +	+ +	+ +	+ +
Stomach	(+)	+	+	N/A	+
Colorectal	(+)	+ +	+ +	+	+
Breast	+ (for internal mammary nodes)	+	+ +	+	+
Cervix uteri	+ +	+	+	+	N/A
Ovarian	–	–	+	(+)[a]	(+)[a]
Sarcomas	–	+	+ +	+ +	+
RCC	–	–	+	–	N/A
Bladder	–	–	+	N/A	–
Prostate	–[b]	–	+ +[c]	+	–
Testicular	–	–	+ (rising marker, equivocal CT)	+ (assess residual mass >3 cm in seminoma)	N/A
Melanoma, stage III, IV	+	+	+ +	+	N/A

(+), limited value; +, valuable, may impact patient care; + +, strongly recommended. NSCLC, non–small cell lung cancer; SCLC, small cell lung cancer; HNSCC, head and neck squamous cell carcinoma; RCC, renal cell carcinoma; CT, computed tomography; N/A, not available. The radiotracer is ^{18}-F-fluoro-2-deoxy-D-glucose (FDG), unless otherwise noted.
[a]Probably helpful, but currently only limited data are available.
[b]FDG not helpful in nodal staging of prostate cancer; possible role of acetate and choline is under investigation.
[c]In patients with prostate-specific antigen relapse, choline and acetate show higher sensitivity than FDG and are therefore preferred where available.

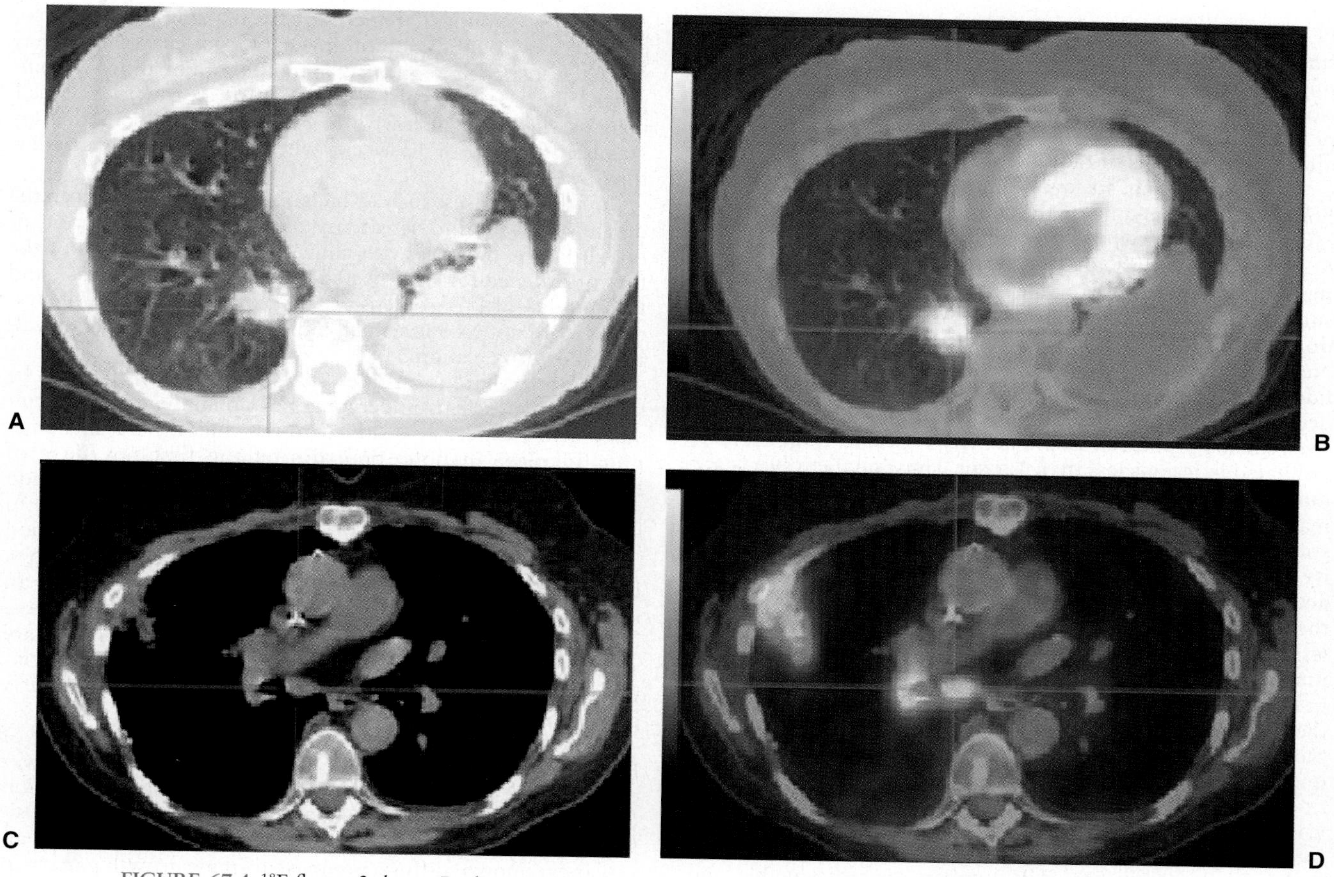

FIGURE 67.4 ^{18}F-fluoro-2-deoxy-D-glucose (FDG) positron emission tomography computed tomography (PET-CT) images in a patient with metastatic non–small cell lung cancer. **A, B:** CT, transaxial PET, and PET-CT fusion images of a tumor mass in the right lower lobe. Note FDG uptake in the left ventricular myocardium, which is seen to variable degrees in some patients. **C, D:** CT, PET, and PET-CT fusion images of mediastinal lymph node metastases and a separate lesion in the periphery of the right midlung.

to the standard clinical management and structural imaging with CT or MRI, unknown distant metastases are detected in 10% to 20% of cases with locally advanced disease.[80–84] In many instances, PET imaging may replace a battery of other tests. An area of growing interest is the use for PET imaging for radiotherapy planning. Although some technical details are still under investigation (e.g., Should the metabolic target volume be defined by visual analysis, based on absolute quantitation of glucose metabolism in the tumor, or based on thresholding algorithms?), preliminary data support a role for

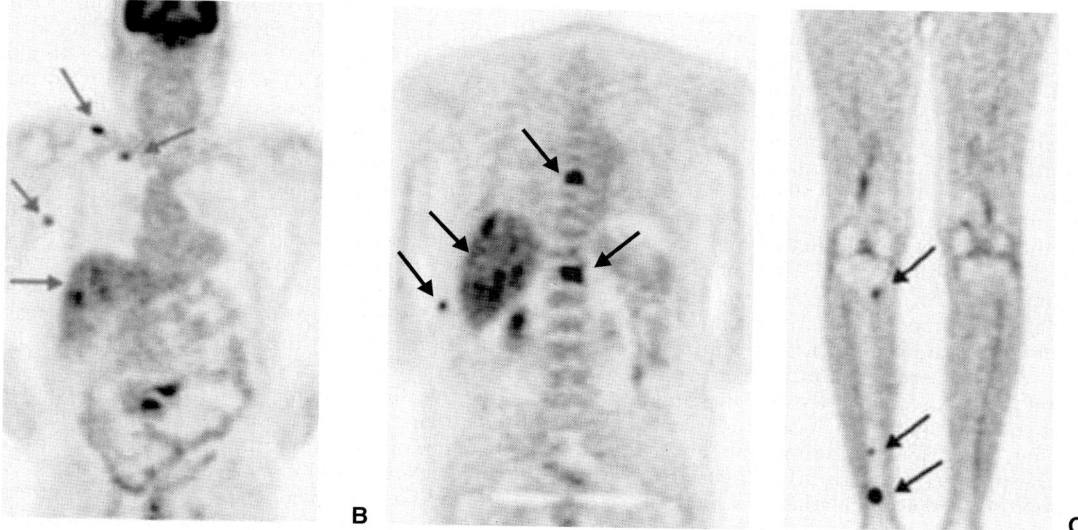

FIGURE 67.5 **A–C:** Coronal ^{18}F-fluoro-2-deoxy-D-glucose (FDG) positron emission tomography (PET) images in a patient with widespread metastatic melanoma involving lymph nodes, liver, and bone marrow. Arrows indicate the location of the FDG and metastases.

PET in radiation treatment planning because it improves the staging accuracy, improves interobserver agreement, may distinguish active disease from benign structural abnormalities (such as postobstructive atelectasis in lung cancer), and may provide an early readout of treatment response when applied after a few fractions of radiotherapy.

In cancer staging, structural imaging has many limitations. For instance, depending on the chosen size, lymph node metastases are detected with either high sensitivity/low specificity (e.g., 6–7 mm cutoff) or vice versa (e.g., only nodes greater than 1.5 cm are considered metastatic). PET, in contrast, measures the metabolism of tumor cells within a lymph node and does not suffer from this method-inherent limitation. Nevertheless, while metastasis can be excluded with high confidence in an enlarged lymph node without FDG uptake, the detection of small volume disease in lymph nodes of normal size remains problematic, and activity concentration is underestimated in lesions less than 1.5 cm. Thus, smaller objects are more difficult to distinguish from background activity in normal tissues. However, a very small object (e.g., 2 to 3 mm) may still be detectable by the PET camera as long as the radioactivity concentration in the object is very high and background activity concentration is low (e.g., a melanoma metastasis in the lung). For practical purposes, the detectability of a small lesion will therefore depend on the combination of (1) the volume of metabolically active disease, (2) the intensity of radiotracer uptake in this volume, (3) the resolution limits of the PET camera, (4) background activity in normal tissues and blood pool, and (5) the degree of lesion motion during the image acquisition.

In the clinic, PET imaging studies are interpreted either visually or by using a semiquantitative score, termed standardized uptake value (SUV). When PET studies are performed under similar conditions, SUV numbers are reproducible, and an SUV change greater than 20% is considered significant,[85] which is of increasing importance in modern chemotherapy trials.[86–88] In addition, both absolute SUV number as well as the magnitude of change under therapy may provide prognostic information.[30,38,89–92] There is now increasing emphasis on early PET for response assessment before structural changes have occurred. The "optimal" time point for early PET response is under study for hematologic malignancies[29] as well as some solid tumors. Solid tumors differ from hematologic malignancies by their lower response rates to standard chemotherapies. Here, PET has been used mainly for assessing the response to neoadjuvant regimens. For instance, in gastric and gastroesophageal-junction cancers a decrease in tumor SUV by more than 35% at 2 weeks[87] or more than 50% at 6 weeks[93] of chemotherapy can distinguish between metabolic responders and nonresponders, and these PET findings correlate with disease-free survival. Continuing chemotherapy in metabolic nonresponders does not improve survival, but it is currently unclear if the prognosis of these patients can be improved meaningfully with alternate drug regimens. Instead neoadjuvant therapy may be terminated and these patients should proceed directly to surgery.[94] After the end of therapy, the optimal time point for response assessment may depend on the tumor histology, modality of treatment (chemotherapy vs. chemoradiation), and chemotherapy regimen. In general, inflammatory changes are most intense after concurrent chemoradiation therapy, so that early PET imaging (less than 10 weeks after end of treatment) will cause a larger number of false-positive interpretations. In animal models, a transient increase in FDG uptake, secondary to cellular stress, energy-dependent apoptosis, and accumulation of white cells responsible for removal of cellular debris, has been observed during the early treatment phase. On the other end of the spectrum, a PET may rarely be false negative when performed too early after radiation or chemotherapy. It is believed that some tumor cells may be "stunned" temporarily as a result of therapy, for instance, due to inhibition of the hexokinase enzyme, but may not have lost their replicative potential.[95] For practical purposes, the time interval between end of treatment and PET imaging should be at least 6 to 8 weeks when chemotherapy was used and 10 to 12 weeks when combined chemoradiotherapy was used.

In other diseases, such as melanoma or cervical cancer, the diagnostic yield and sensitivity of PET for the detection of nodal disease increase with clinical stage.[96–98] Because of the low prevalence for unexpected nodal or distant disease and the inability of PET to detect microscopic cancer foci, the test is therefore not recommended in patients with clinically localized (N0M0) melanoma.[96,99]

Metabolic flare is an interesting phenomenon that can be seen in some patients undergoing hormonal therapy for metastatic breast cancer. It is similar to the clinical flare phenomenon (increase in bone pain during the first few days of hormonal therapy), or the well-documented flare phenomenon on bone scan (increase in intensity of radiotracer uptake in previously shown osseous metastasis or even the visualization of apparently new lesions early during the course of therapy). Likewise, on FDG-PET early during hormonal therapy, an increase in SUV or the appearance of new spots of FDG uptake in the skeleton can be seen in some patients. Both clinical flare and metabolic flare on PET herald a future response to continued therapy with the same drug and are thus indicators of a good prognosis.[100]

Some primary malignancies show relatively low uptake of FDG, which reflects their low glucose metabolism, lower expression of GLUT, a high rate of FDG dephosphorylation (e.g., hepatocellular carcinoma), and the histologic composition of the lesion (e.g., little solid tissue in a true bronchoalveolar carcinoma; diffuse, nonmass-forming growth pattern in invasive lobular breast cancer; predominantly cystic mucinous tumors, including some pancreatic and ovarian primaries). As a rule, most well-differentiated malignant tumors, including differentiated, iodine-avid thyroid cancer, and many primary prostate cancers, also show low FDG uptake. Similarly, indolent lymphomas, in general, also show relatively low FDG uptake.[101] As these aforementioned malignancies become more aggressive and clinical disease progresses, they will become detectable on FDG-PET, and this test can then help in monitoring the response to chemotherapy or experimental therapies (e.g., in castration-resistant metastatic prostate cancer) and also provide prognostic information.[102] Finally, since the brain almost exclusively metabolizes glucose as a fuel, FDG uptake will be high. Therefore, tumors with glucose metabolism lower than or even equal to that in normal cortex (e.g., low-grade astrocytomas) may not be detected on FDG-PET, but instead only with labeled amino acids. Similar to other diagnostic test, false-positive findings may also occur with FDG-PET. For instance, high FDG uptake in brown adipose tissue is a frequent normal variant[103]; granulomatous diseases or reactions (e.g., sarcoidosis; talc pleurodesis) and some benign tumors (e.g., paragangliomas, meningiomas, many benign bone lesions such as eosinophilic granuloma, nonossifying fibroma, fibrous dysplasia, Paget's disease), as well as sites of infection (which can be used clinically for diagnosis of patients with fever of unknown origin), may show false-positive FDG uptake. Finally, since FDG undergoes renal excretion, it is not a good agent for imaging primary kidney, bladder, or prostate cancer. Alternate PET tracers for cancer imaging are shown in Table 67.1. One of these is the proliferation marker FLT, which appears promising for early response assessment and tumor grading. In addition, positron-labeled antibodies and antibody fragments (Fig. 67.6) appear promising for very specific cancer imaging. One example is ^{124}I-labeled cG250 for renal clear cell carcinoma, which recognizes

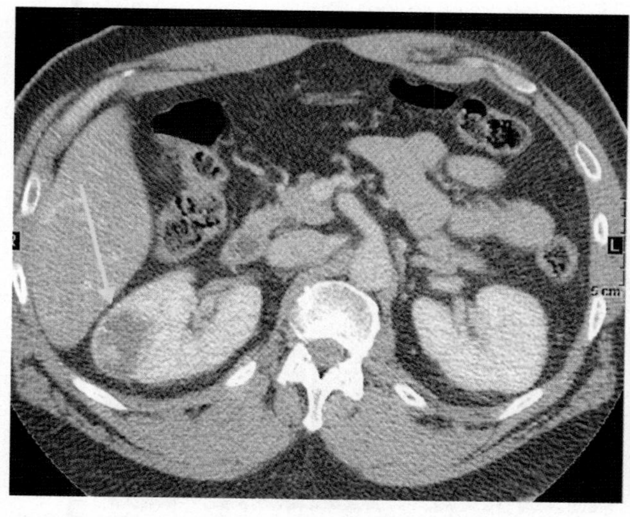

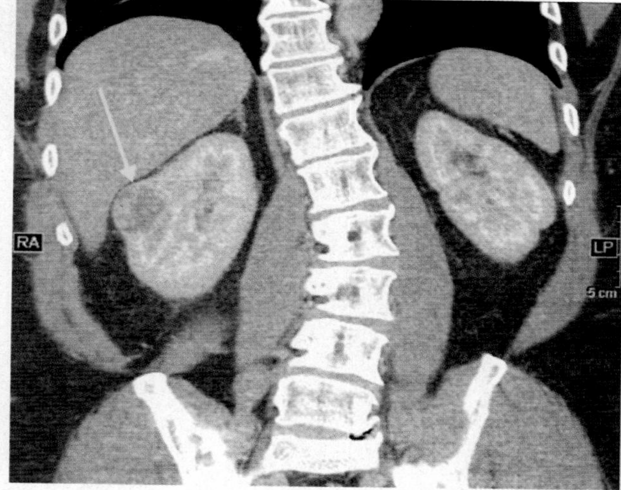

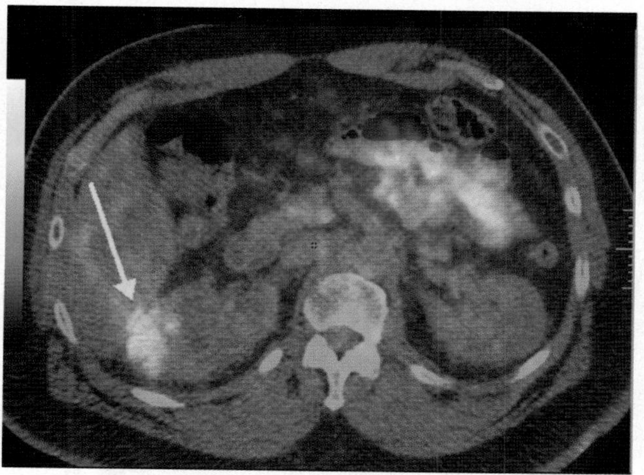

A B C

FIGURE 67.6 Transaxial (**A**) and coronal (**B**) contrast enhanced computed tomography (CT) images show a nodular lesion in the lateral parenchyma of the right kidney. PET image (**C**) shows specific accumulation of ^{124}I cG250 only in the renal lesion, consistent with binding to histologically proven carbonic anhydrase-IX expressing clear cell renal carcinoma (note nonspecific excreted activity in intestines).

carbonic anhydrase-IX (Ca-IX), a commonly expressed antigen on clear cell renal cell carcinoma. Since Ca-IX is not expressed by other renal lesions, this method proved highly useful in preliminary studies for the presurgical assessment of renal tumors.[104] Therefore, some patients may qualify for partial nephrectomy, whereas other patients with more benign tumors, such as oncocytoma which does not generally express Ca-IX, could be watched. Of note, because of the superior imaging characteristics of PET, high-contrast images can be obtained even if there is as little as 50% difference between tumor and background activity. Recently, a phase 3 study with ^{124}I cG250 was completed successfully, and the agent is now under review by the U.S. Food and Drug Administration for consideration as a diagnostic radiopharmaceutical for the presurgical evaluation of renal masses (Fig. 67.6).

OPTICAL IMAGING

Optical imaging is an inexpensive and rapid way to image molecular processes *in vitro* and *in vivo*.[105] Activatable optical probes, which minimize background fluorescence, appear particularly promising.[106] Due to light scattering, there is no linearity between the signal captured at the surface of the studied animal and the actual, true signal intensity emanating from within the depth of the animal. Fluorescence tomography is one way to account for this and to allow allowing for quantitative measurements throughout the target tissue. Two main approaches for optical imaging are fluorescence and bioluminescence. Both employ a signal of a specific frequency generated at the tissue site of interest and then detected by sensitive cameras using filters specific to the generated signal. *Fluorescence* takes advantage of fluorophores that are excited by a specific wavelength to emit light shifted to a longer wavelength. These fluorochromes can be organic dyes, fluorescent proteins, or quantum dots (QD). QDs are nanocrystals that can act as fluorophores; they have unique optical properties that make them particularly suitable for imaging. Newer (nontoxic) QDs are undergoing first preclinical and clinical testing. Fluorescence imaging has been used for receptor-targeted[107] or antibody-mediated imaging of tumors in mice.[108] A probe activated by cathepsins has been used in mouse models to detect lung tumors smaller than 1 mm in diameter.[109] Annexin-V labeled with cyanine 5.5 has been used to image apoptosis very early after initiation of chemotherapy treatment in an animal model.[110] Nanoparticles labeled with cyanine 5.5 have been used to image gene expression via maker genes. Since optical imaging suffers from limited depths of penetration, in the clinic it may be applied best for superficial lesions, on the body surface, or internally using near-infrared endoscopy.[111,112]

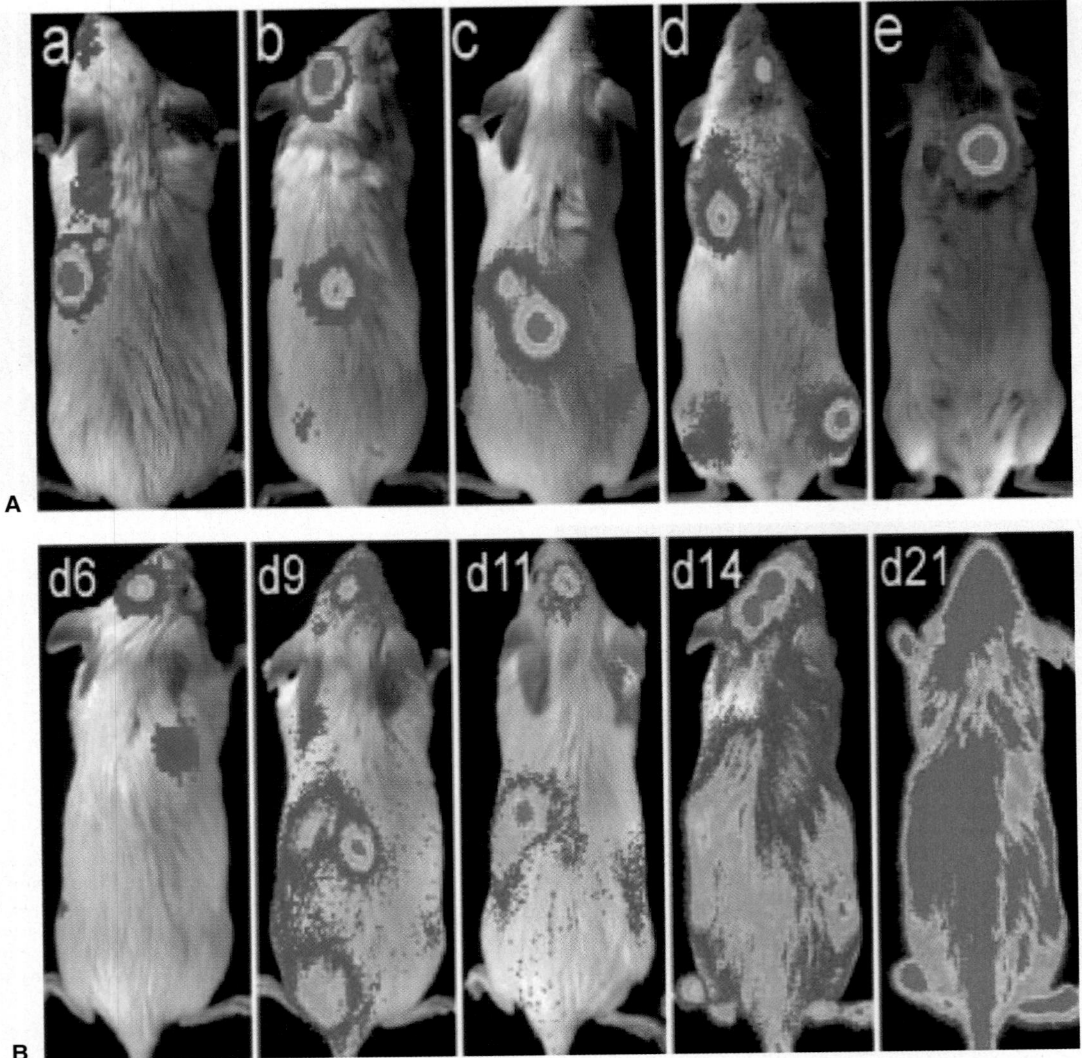

FIGURE 67.7 Bioluminescence imaging (BLI), using the luciferase gene as a marker gene for gene expression, shows the dynamics of hematopoietic stem cell (HSC) engraftment. Luciferase-positive HSCs were transplanted into lethally irradiated nontransgenic recipients. BLI was used to monitor the engraftment of HSC. All images are displayed at the same scale. **A:** Bioluminescent foci derived from 50 transplanted HSC were apparent in individual animals at anatomic sites corresponding to the location of the spleen, skull, vertebrae, femurs, and sternum (*a to e, respectively*) at 6 to 9 days after transfer. **B:** The pattern of engraftment is dynamic with formation and expansion or formation and loss of the bioluminescent foci. In this animal, some foci of engraftment disappear over time, others remain. By day 21, a significant degree of engraftment had been achieved. (From ref. 116, with permission.)

In contrast to fluorescence, *bioluminescence* is an energy-consuming biological process catalyzed by the enzyme luciferase (or its relatives) that oxidizes its substrate, thereby emitting light. In order to use this system, the luciferase gene has to be expressed in cells and its substrate, luciferin, has to be injected. Bioluminescence also has limited depth of penetration and resolution of only several millimeters. To overcome these limitations, luciferase with a QD has been used,[113] whereby bioluminescent emission excites the QD to emit light in the near infrared spectrum, allowing imaging of deeper tissues. Bioluminescence is commonly used in the laboratory for tumors imaging, response assessment,[114] imaging of gene expression,[115] and biodistribution of transfected cells (Fig. 67.7).[116,117]

Selected References

The full list of references for this chapter appears in the online version.

1. Gambhir SS, Herschman HR, Cherry SR, et al. Imaging transgene expression with radionuclide imaging technologies. *Neoplasia* 2000;2:118.
3. Serganova I, Blasberg R. Reporter gene imaging: potential impact on therapy. *Nucl Med Biol* 2005;32:763.
6. Phelps M. Positron emission tomography provides molecular imaging of biological processes. *Proc Natl Acad Sci U S A* 2000;97:9226.
7. Schöder H, Erdi YE, Larson SM, Yeung HW. PET/CT: a new imaging technology in nuclear medicine. *Eur J Nucl Med Mol Imaging* 2003;30:1419.
8. Antoch G, Saoudi N, Kuehl H, et al. Accuracy of whole-body dual-modality fluorine-18-2-fluoro-2-deoxy-D-glucose positron emission tomography and computed tomography (FDG-PET/CT) for tumor staging in solid tumors: comparison with CT and PET. *J Clin Oncol* 2004;22:4357.

10. Schöder H, Yeung HW, Gonen M, Kraus D, Larson SM. Head and neck cancer: clinical usefulness and accuracy of PET/CT image fusion. *Radiology* 2004;231:65.
12. Hanahan D, Weinberg RA. The hallmarks of cancer. *Cell* 2000;100:57.
13. Gatenby RA, Gillies RJ. Why do cancers have high aerobic glycolysis? *Nat Rev Cancer* 2004;4:891.
14. Warburg O. *The metabolism of tumors.* New York: Richard R. Smith, 1931.
16. Hsu PP, Sabatini DM. Cancer cell metabolism: Warburg and beyond. *Cell* 2008;134:703.
17. Wise DR, DeBerardinis RJ, Mancuso A, et al. Myc regulates a transcriptional program that stimulates mitochondrial glutaminolysis and leads to glutamine addiction. *Proc Natl Acad Sci U S A* 2008;105:18782.
20. Buzzai M, Bauer DE, Jones RG, et al. The glucose dependence of Akt-transformed cells can be reversed by pharmacologic activation of fatty acid beta-oxidation. *Oncogene* 2005;24:4165.
21. DeBerardinis RJ, Lum JJ, Hatzivassiliou G, Thompson CB. The biology of cancer: metabolic reprogramming fuels cell growth and proliferation. *Cell Metab* 2008;7:11.
24. Downey RJ, Akhurst T, Gonen M, et al. Preoperative F-18 fluorodeoxyglucose-positron emission tomography maximal standardized uptake value predicts survival after lung cancer resection. *J Clin Oncol* 2004;22(16):3255.
26. Robbins RJ, Wan Q, Grewel RK, et al. Real-time prognosis for metastatic thyroid carcinoma based on 2-[18F]fluoro-2-deoxy-D-glucose-positron emission tomography scanning. *J Clin Endocrinol Metab* 2006; 91(2):498.
29. Schöder H, Moskowitz C. PET imaging for response assessment in lymphoma: potential and limitations. *Radiol Clin North Am* 2008; 46(2):225.
30. Wong RJ, Lin DT, Schöder H, et al. Diagnostic and prognostic value of [(18)F]fluorodeoxyglucose positron emission tomography for recurrent head and neck squamous cell carcinoma. *J Clin Oncol* 2002;20:4199.
31. Lee YY, Choi CH, Kim CJ, et al. The prognostic significance of the SUVmax (maximum standardized uptake value for F-18 fluorodeoxyglucose) of the cervical tumor in PET imaging for early cervical cancer: preliminary results. *Gynecol Oncol* 2009;115:65.
32. Grigsby PW. The prognostic values of PET and PET/CT in cervical cancer. *Cancer Imaging* 2008;8:146.
34. Pedersen PL, Mathupala S, Rempel A, Geschwind JF, Ko YH. Mitochondrial bound type II hexokinase: a key player in the growth and survival of many cancers and an ideal prospect for therapeutic intervention. *Biochim Biophys Acta* 2002;1555:14.
35. Rempel A, Mathupala SP, Griffin CA, Hawkins AL, Pedersen PL. Glucose catabolism in cancer cells: amplification of the gene encoding type II hexokinase. *Cancer Res* 1996;56:2468.
36. Mathupala SP, Ko YH, Pedersen PL. Hexokinase II: cancer's double-edged sword acting as both facilitator and gatekeeper of malignancy when bound to mitochondria. *Oncogene* 2006;25:4777.
37. Bos R, van Der Hoeven JJ, van Der Wall E, et al. Biologic correlates of (18)fluorodeoxyglucose uptake in human breast cancer measured by positron emission tomography. *J Clin Oncol* 2002;20:379.
39. Mamede M, Higashi T, Kitaichi M, et al. [18F]FDG uptake and PCNA, GluT-1, and hexokinase-II expressions in cancers and inflammatory lesions of the lung. *Neoplasia* 2005;7:369.
42. Shields AF, Grierson JR, Dohmen BM, et al. Imaging proliferation *in vivo* with [F-18]FLT and positron emission tomography. *Nat Med* 1998;4:1334.
50. Rasey JS, Grierson JR, Wiens LW, Kolb PD, Schwartz JL. Validation of FLT uptake as a measure of thymidine kinase-1 activity in A549 carcinoma cells. *J Nucl Med* 2002;43:1210.
52. Barthel H, Cleij MC, Collingridge DR, et al. 3′-deoxy-3′-[18F]fluorothymidine as a new marker for monitoring tumor response to antiproliferative therapy *in vivo* with positron emission tomography. *Cancer Res* 2003;63:3791.
54. Chen W, Cloughesy T, Kamdar N, et al. Imaging proliferation in brain tumors with 18F-FLT PET: comparison with 18F-FDG. *J Nucl Med* 2005;46:945.
55. Vesselle H, Grierson J, Muzi M, et al. *In vivo* validation of 3′deoxy-3′-[(18)F]fluorothymidine ([(18)F]FLT) as a proliferation imaging tracer in humans: correlation of [(18)F]FLT uptake by positron emission tomography with Ki-67 immunohistochemistry and flow cytometry in human lung tumors. *Clin Cancer Res* 2002;8:3315.
57. Yue J, Chen L, Cabrera AR, et al. Measuring tumor cell proliferation with 18F-FLT PET during radiotherapy of esophageal squamous cell carcinoma: a pilot clinical study. *J Nucl Med* 2010;51:528.
58. Everitt S, Hicks RJ, Ball D, et al. Imaging cellular proliferation during chemo-radiotherapy: a pilot study of serial 18F-FLT positron emission tomography/computed tomography imaging for non-small-cell lung cancer. *Int J Radiat Oncol Biol Phys* 2009;75:1098.
65. Schuster DM, Votaw JR, Nieh PT, et al. Initial experience with the radiotracer anti-1-amino-3-18F-fluorocyclobutane-1-carboxylic acid with PET/CT in prostate carcinoma. *J Nucl Med* 2007;48:56.
66. Dehdashti F, Mortimer JE, Siegel BA, et al. Positron tomographic assessment of estrogen receptors in breast cancer: comparison with FDG-PET and *in vitro* receptor assays. *J Nucl Med* 1995;36:1766.
67. Larson SM, Morris M, Gunther I, et al. Tumor localization of 16beta-18-F-fluoro-5alpha-dihydrotestosterone versus 18F-FDG in patients with progressive, metastatic prostate cancer. *J Nucl Med* 2004;45:366.
69. Smith-Jones PM, Solit DB, Akhurst T, et al. Imaging the pharmacodynamics of *HER-2* degradation in response to Hsp90 inhibitors. *Nat Biotechnol* 2004;22:701.
73. Penuelas I, Mazzolini G, Boan JF, et al. Positron emission tomography imaging of adenoviral-mediated transgene expression in liver cancer patients. *Gastroenterology* 2005;128:1787.
75. Vaupel P, Mayer A. Hypoxia in cancer: significance and impact on clinical outcome. *Cancer Metastasis Rev* 2007;26:225.
76. Rajendran JG, Mankoff DA, O'Sullivan F, et al. Hypoxia and glucose metabolism in malignant tumors: evaluation by [18F]fluoromisonidazole and [18F]fluorodeoxyglucose positron emission tomography imaging. *Clin Cancer Res* 2004;10:2245.
87. Ott K, Weber WA, Lordick F, et al. Metabolic imaging predicts response, survival, and recurrence in adenocarcinomas of the esophagogastric junction. *J Clin Oncol* 2006;24:4692.
89. Vansteenkiste JF, Stroobants SG, Dupont PJ, et al. Prognostic importance of the standardized uptake value on (18)F-fluoro-2-deoxy-glucose-positron emission tomography scan in non–small cell lung cancer: an analysis of 125 cases. Leuven Lung Cancer Group. *J Clin Oncol* 1999; 17:3201.
91. Downey RJ, Akhurst T, Ilson D, et al. Whole body ^{18}FDG-PET and the response of esophageal cancer to induction therapy: results of a prospective trial. *J Clin Oncol* 2003;21:428.
94. Lordick F, Ott K, Krause BJ, et al. PET to assess early metabolic response and to guide treatment of adenocarcinoma of the oesophagogastric junction: the MUNICON phase II trial. *Lancet Oncol* 2007;8:797.
96. Wagner JD, Schauwecker D, Davidson D, et al. Prospective study of fluorodeoxyglucose-positron emission tomography imaging of lymph node basins in melanoma patients undergoing sentinel node biopsy. *J Clin Oncol* 1999;17:1508.
100. Mortimer JE, Dehdashti F, Siegel BA, et al. Metabolic flare: indicator of hormone responsiveness in advanced breast cancer. *J Clin Oncol* 2001;19:2797.
104. Divgi CR, Pandit-Taskar N, Jungbluth AA, et al. Preoperative characterisation of clear-cell renal carcinoma using iodine-124-labelled antibody chimeric G250 (124I-cG250) and PET in patients with renal masses: a phase I trial. *Lancet Oncol* 2007;8:304.
105. Ntziachristos V, Bremer C, Graves EE, Ripoll J, Weissleder R. *In vivo* tomographic imaging of near-infrared fluorescent probes. *Mol Imaging* 2002;1:82.
109. Grimm J, Kirsch DG, Windsor SD, et al. Use of gene expression profiling to direct *in vivo* molecular imaging of lung cancer. *Proc Natl Acad Sci U S A* 2005;102:14404.
113. So MK, Xu C, Loening AM, Gambhir SS, Rao J. Self-illuminating quantum dot conjugates for *in vivo* imaging. *Nat Biotechnol* 2006;24:339.
116. Cao YA, Wagers AJ, Beilhack A, et al. Shifting foci of hematopoiesis during reconstitution from single stem cells. *Proc Natl Acad Sci U S A* 2004;101:221.

CHAPTER 68 PHOTODYNAMIC THERAPY

KEITH A. CENGEL, SMITH APISARNTHANARAX, AND STEPHEN M. HAHN

Photodynamic therapy (PDT) has its origins in early observations that certain chemicals have the ability to cause light-dependent cytotoxicity in living tissues. The term photodynamic was first used in a report on the effects of topically applied eosin and white light on tumors of the skin in 1903. Despite the fact that these observations are over 100 years old, the use of PDT as a cancer treatment modality remained relatively underexplored until the mid- to late 1970s.[1] Since that time, PDT has become increasingly common in clinical use for the treatment of both benign and malignant conditions. Indeed, the fact that PDT now represents the standard of care for treatment of macular degeneration speaks well for its efficacy and relatively safe toxicity profile. As a cancer treatment, PDT has been approved for use in patients with esophageal, lung, and skin neoplasms in both the United States and the European Union. In the European Union, PDT is also approved for treatment of some head and neck cancers. There are also numerous ongoing preclinical and clinical studies that seek to optimize the efficacy and extend the spectrum of PDT as a cancer treatment. In this chapter, the preclinical rationale, the clinical experience to date, and the prospects for future improvements in PDT as a cancer treatment modality will be presented.

COMPONENTS OF PHOTODYNAMIC THERAPY: PHOTOSENSITIZERS, LIGHT, AND OXYGEN

In PDT, the photosensitizer must absorb light energy and transfer this energy to cellular substrates for cytotoxicity to occur (Fig. 68.1).[2] The nature of the cellular damage and the phenotype of the cellular cytotoxicity depends on the predominant subcellular localization of the photosensitizer, the presence and concentration of molecular oxygen, and the underlying molecular abnormalities of the target cell. For example, photosensitizers that localize primarily to the mitochondria rapidly and efficiently stimulate intrinsic apoptosis (see the section "Mechanisms of Photodynamic Therapy Cytotoxicity"). In addition, the time interval between photosensitizer administration and light delivery can alter the type of tissue damage. For relatively short time intervals, when the photosensitizer is primarily located within the vascular compartment, the initial PDT damage is preferentially vascular. For longer time intervals, the initial damage occurs at the level of cells and tissues where the photosensitizer is retained.

First-Generation Photosensitizers

The most extensively studied photosensitizers are porphyrin-type structures and are often referred to as first-generation photosensitizers (Table 68.1). Hematoporphyrin derivative (HPD) was initially developed in 1955 by Samuel Schwartz, but was not used to treat cancers until 1975, when the efficacy of HPD-mediated PDT was reported for mammary and bladder tumors in mice.[1] Later a partially purified formulation of hematoporphyrin monomers, dimmers and oligomers was produced called porfimer sodium (Photofrin). Porfimer sodium is the best-characterized agent for PDT of neoplasms. With a 630 nm light source, porfimer sodium is U.S. Food and Drug Administration (FDA) approved for the definitive treatment of Barrett's esophagus with high-grade dysplasia and microinvasive bronchial cancers, as well as the palliative treatment of cancers that obstruct the esophagus and bronchi. The major photosensitizer-specific toxicity of porfimer sodium is a potentially severe sensitivity of skin to sunlight that typically lasts 4 to 6 weeks, but may last as long as 3 months. Other toxicities are related to the specific location of light delivery.

Second-Generation Photosensitizers

The pro-drug photosensitizer 5-aminolevulinic acid (ALA) is also an intermediate in the biosynthesis of heme. Exogenously administered ALA is converted into protoporphyrin IX (PpIX), which accumulates intracellularly, preferentially in rapidly dividing cells. For clinical use, either 630 nm (red) or 400 to 450 nm (approximately 417 nm polychromatic blue from Blu-U DUSA Pharmaceuticals, Inc, Wilmington, Massachusetts) light is used to produce PDT cytotoxicity. ALA is extremely flexible in its route of administration and can be given orally, intravenously, intraperitoneally, or topically. In order to avoid body-wide cutaneous photosensitivity, ALA is often given topically for skin cancer treatments.[3] Topical ALA and blue light are FDA-approved treatments for actinic keratosis. Photobiologically, the subcellular distribution and tissue effects ALA induced PpIX are similar to porfimer sodium, but interestingly, somewhat different from exogenously administered PpIX. PDT using ALA or its esther derivatives such as mALA (5-ALA methylesther, Metvix (Photocure ASA, Oslo Norway), recently approved in the United States for treatment of skin cancers using red 634 nm light) has been performed in clinical trials with promising results in treating cancers of the skin (basal cell), head and neck, and bladder, as well as vulvar neoplasms such as Paget's disease and vulvar intraepithelial neoplasia. In addition, the ability of ALA-induced PpIX to concentrate in cancer cells has been used for photodiagnosis of head and neck cancers, peritoneal micrometastases from ovarian and gastrointestinal cancers, and malignant brain tumors.[4,5] Despite these results, concern has been raised over preclinical data that show the efficiency of a tumor converting ALA to PpIX may be inversely proportional to the degree of differentiation of the tumor cells.[6]

Other second-generation photosensitizers that are approved for use in the United States or the European Union include

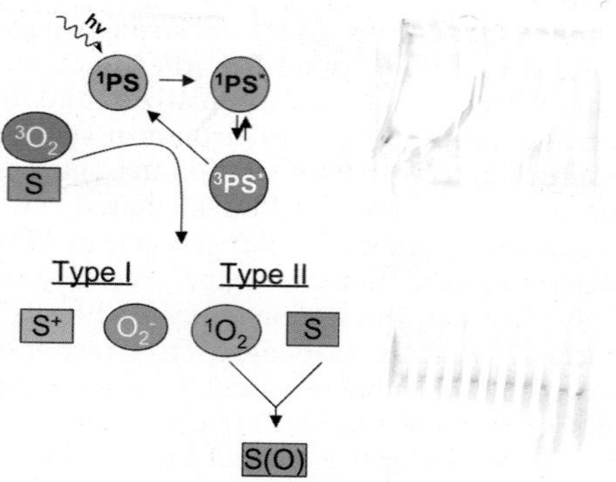

FIGURE 68.1 The ground state (unexcited) photosensitizer (^1PS) can absorb light energy to produce an excited singlet state photosensitizer ($^1PS^*$) molecule. This can decay back to ground state or reconfigure into the relatively long-lived excited triplet state photosensitizer ($^3PS^*$). Under aerobic conditions, $^3PS^*$ transfers energy to ground state oxygen $^3O_2$ to produce singlet oxygen ($^1O_2$). $^1O_2$ then reacts with bio-organic, cellular substrates (S) to make oxygenated adducts (S(O)). In relatively hypoxic environments, $^3PS^*$ can react directly with substrates to produce oxidized substrate (S^+) or with oxygen to produce superoxide anions (O^{2-}).

benzoporphyrin derivative monoacid (BPD, verteporfin, Visudyne) and meso-tetro-(hydroxyphenyl)-chlorin (mTHPC, Foscan). BPD is approved in the United States and the European Union for the treatment of age-related macular degeneration, likely representing the most common clinical use of PDT to date. The safety profile of the drug is excellent, and the cutaneous photosensitivity following administration is generally less than 5 days duration. PDT using mTHPC is approved in the European Union for the treatment of head and neck cancer. Clinical trials have been performed using mTHPC-mediated PDT in the treatment of mesothelioma, pancreatic cancer, and prostate cancer. The length of cutaneous photosensitivity for mTHPC is approximately 15 days. Second-generation photosensitizers that are currently under investigation in clinical trails include phthalocyanine-4,[7] HPPH (Photochlor),[8] SnET2 (Purlytin),[9] and LS11 (Talaporfin).[10]

Light Delivery and Dosimetry

PDT has the potential to combine partially selective destruction of cancerous tissue compared to normal tissues with the ability to treat and conform to relatively large surface areas. Specific wavelengths of visible light can be focused on areas of clinical concern for malignant involvement and the light dose accurately measured using a variety of available technologies. Moreover, the intrinsic physical limitation in the depth of effective visible light penetration through tissue (2 to 10 mm for red light) limits PDT damage to deeper structures and thereby provides additional potential for tumor cell selectivity.

In most clinical settings, monochromatic laser light is used. The wavelength is selected by matching the absorbance peaks of the photosensitizer being used with the desired tissue penetration for the light. For the visible and near infrared range, longer wavelengths penetrate more deeply into tissues. For example, when 630 nm (red) light is used with porfimer sodium, the light penetrates to a depth of 3 to 5 mm in tissues. In contrast, when 532 nm (green) light is used, the light penetrates to a depth of 1 to 2 mm. Light delivery systems are designed to provide uniform illumination of the desired target using a variety of optical fibers and applicators. However, the goal of uniform light delivery is complicated by the inherent inhomogeneities introduced by the variability in both intrapatient's and interpatient's tissues' optical properties. Moreover, these properties can change significantly over the course of light delivery.

Currently approved PDT methods use a combination of photosensitizer dose and the incident light fluence that are administered to the patient. Newer techniques are being developed to more accurately determine PDT effects, with the eventual goal of being able to modulate the light delivery in real time to achieve the desired level of PDT tissue cytotoxicity. One approach to explicitly estimate the tissue cytotoxic effects of PDT is to measure the tissue concentrations of oxygen and photosensitizer and combine these with measurements of the absorbed light dose. An estimate of tissue oxygen concentration can be determined using the difference in absorption spectra for oxy- versus deoxyhemoglobin. In addition, it is also possible to estimate local photosensitizer tissue concentration using fluorescence or absorbance spectroscopy. Finally, the light dose delivered to tissue can be measured using isotropic (spherical, incident plus scattered light) or nonisotropic (flat, incident light only) detector systems. Alternatively, the cytotoxic effect of PDT on tissues can be estimated implicitly by measuring the generation of singlet oxygen in tissues. However, both explicit and implicit dosimetric methods suffer from limitations in spatial resolution and complexity of clinical interpretation. Further preclinical and clinical studies are needed to more fully develop and implement these technologies in PDT.

TABLE 68.1

PHOTOSENSITIZER PROPERTIES

Photosensitizer	Excitation Wavelength	Clinical Uses
Porfimer sodium (Photofrin)	630 nm	Barrett's esophagus+*, endobroncheal cancer*+, esophageal+, serosal cancers (pleural peritoneal), bladder cancer, skin cancer Bowen's disease or AK), breast cancer metastases, head and neck cancer, brain
ALA (Levulan), mALA (Metvixv)	400–450 nm 635 nm	AK*+, BCC+, Bowen's disease, bladder cancer, vulvar cancer
BPD (Visudyne)	690 nm	Macular degeneration+*, BCC
mTHCP (Foscan)	652 nm	Head and neck+, pancreatic cancer, cancer, pleural cancers, brain
HPPH (Photochlor)	665 nm	BCC, pleural cancers
Silicon pthalocyanine-4 (Pc-4)	672 nm	Cutaneous and subcutaneous metastases malignancies
SnET2 (Purlytin)	664 nm	BCC, Kaposi's sarcoma, prostate cancer, cancer cutaneous

Note: All treatments are in clinical development, unless noted with an * (approved in United States) or + (approved in European Union).
ALA, 5-aminolevulinic acid; BPD, benzoporphyrin derivative monoacid; BCC, basal cell carcinomas; mTHCP, meso-tetro-(hydroxyphenyl)-chlorin.

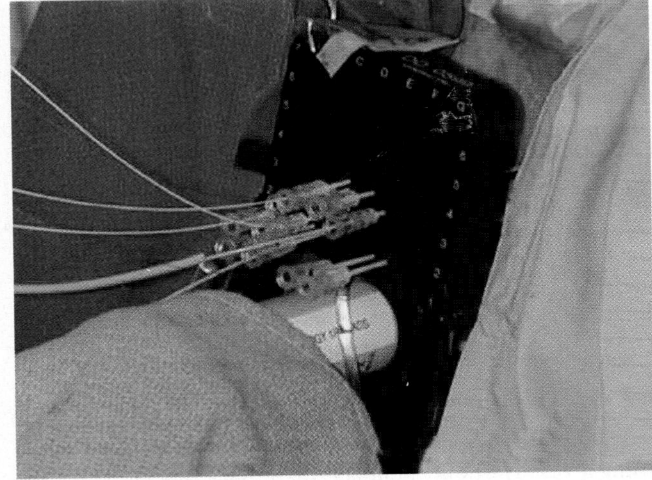

FIGURE 68.2 Prostate photodynamic therapy using interstitially implanted, cylindrically diffusing linear fibers to deliver light.

In addition to developing real-time PDT dosimetry systems, the ability to deliver light to deeply located (greater than 1 cm) tumors without the need for surgical exposure would significantly help to extend the spectrum of PDT clinical applicability. Clinical trials are currently under way to test the use of tissue-implanted (interstitial) light sources and detectors for PDT of solid malignancies such as prostate cancer (Fig. 68.2).[11] In addition, the development of light emitting or reflecting nanoparticles may allow for PDT without surgical exposure.

Oxygen Effects

Experiments on oxic and hypoxic cells and tissues show that pretreatment tumor hypoxia significantly decreases the efficacy of PDT. Limited studies of PDT and tumor hypoxia in clinical samples confirm this relationship between hypoxia and decreased PDT efficacy, but suggest that the heterogeneity in tumor hypoxia, both within the same patient and between patients with similar tumor types, precludes a universal or one-fit solution to this problem. In addition, since PDT itself consumes oxygen and can lead to vascular collapse, it is important to consider these effects in PDT. The rate at which PDT consumes molecular oxygen depends on the fluence rate of the light (amount of light energy delivered to an area as a function of time). One way to help with both of these hypoxia issues would be to monitor tumor blood flow and tissue oxygenation in real time and modify the light doses accordingly. Along with real-time light dosimetry and fluoresce-based methods to detect photosensitizer levels, such technology is currently under development and testing and would likely revolutionize the field of PDT.

MECHANISMS OF PHOTODYNAMIC THERAPY CYTOTOXICITY

Indirect Photodynamic Therapy Cytotoxicity

The antitumor efficacy of PDT stems from a combination of indirect and direct tumor cell killing. Indirect tumor effects can only be observed and measured *in vivo* and result from PDT-mediated changes in tumor microenvironment, including vessel leakage, vasoconstriction, and vascular thrombosis. The antivascular effects of PDT are strongly dependent on the photosensitizer used as well as the time interval between the administration of photosensitizer and light. In addition, changes in tumor microenvironment such as hypoxia prior to and during PDT administration may have a profound impact on the overall level of PDT-mediated cell killing due to the requirement for molecular oxygen in PDT. This effect also determines the minimum time necessary to deliver a specific light dose (see the section "Oxygen Effects"). Following PDT, there is an acute vasoconstrictive response that is later followed by thrombosis, vascular collapse, and tumor hypoxia. Although these vascular effects are very important contributors to the indirect effects of PDT on tumors, there are likely other, more subtle alterations in tumor microenvironment that similarly facilitate tumor regression.

In addition to altering the tumor microenvironment, PDT may act to stimulate an antitumor immune response. The mechanism for this effect has been postulated to involve the release of pro-inflammatory cytokines and fixation of complement in response to PDT. In addition, PDT may result in the release of immunogenic, tumor-associated antigens. These are thought to stimulate infiltration of lymphocytes, monocytes, and granulocytes into tumors and initiate an antitumor immune response. The potential immunological component of PDT is perhaps most dramatically demonstrated in experiments by Korbelik et al.[12] who compared the efficacy of PDT in Balb/C (immunocompetent) versus SCID (immunocompromised) mice. In these experiments, despite similar efficacy of PDT in initial ablation of EMT6 mammary sarcomas from both Balb/C and SCID mice, long-term tumor cure occurred in all of the Balb/C and none of the SCID mice. Importantly, the long-term efficacy of PDT in SCID mice was dramatically improved if bone marrow transplant from Balb/C donors was performed prior to PDT. Recently, increased antibasal cell cancer antigen reactivity has been found in lymphocytes isolated from patients treated with PDT as compared to surgery.[13] Nevertheless, the immunologic effects of PDT in humans remain incompletely understood.

Direct Photodynamic Therapy Cytotoxicity

In addition to indirect mechanisms of tumor cell kill, PDT also results in direct tumor cell killing due to PDT-mediated damage of cellular macromolecules. For these effects, the subcellular localization of photosensitizer is important because the lifetime or diffusion radius for the reactive oxygen species that mitigate PDT cytotoxicity is very short. Indeed, the lifetime of singlet oxygen is estimated at 0.03 to 0.18 mcs, which corresponds to a diffusion distance of less than 0.2 mcm, or about 1/50th of a cell diameter. Thus, the macromolecular damage inside the cell occurs very close to the location of photosensitizer activation or singlet oxygen production. Different photosensitizers are know to localize to the plasma membrane, lysosome, mitochondria, Golgi apparatus, endoplasmic reticulum, or nuclear membrane, and this localization appears to influence the cell death phenotype. For example, photosensitizers that localize to the mitochondria, such as porfimer sodium and BPD, rapidly and effectively stimulate intrinsic mitochondrially mediated apoptosis both *in vivo* and *in vitro* in many cell lines. However, the extent to which tissue microenvironment or other cellular inputs can influence the predominant photosensitizer subcellular localization remains unclear.

Although apoptotic cell death appears to play a highly important role in PDT cytotoxicity induced by a variety of photosensitizers, PDT cytotoxicity can also involve nonapoptotic mechanisms. In general, apoptotic cell death tends to predominate in the most PDT-sensitive cell lines at lower light or photosensitizer doses, and necrotic or nonapoptotic mechanisms tend to predominate at higher light or photosensitizer

doses. When PDT kills cells by apoptosis, the percentage of apoptosis achieved, as well as the mechanism of apoptosis (extrinsic vs. intrinsic), appears to be both tumor cell line and the photosensitizer dependent.[14] However, PDT can also stimulate necrotic cell death at relatively low light or photosensitizer doses under certain circumstances, and this may stimulate a strong bystander effect.[15,16] Recent studies indicate low-dose PDT effectively stimulates autophagy, leading to increased cytotoxicity in cells with deficient apoptotic pathways (e.g., cancer cells) as compared to cells with normal apoptotic pathways (e.g., normal cells).[17]

CLINICAL INDICATIONS FOR PHOTODYNAMIC THERAPY FOR EARLY STAGE CANCERS IN THE DEFINITIVE SETTING

In the definitive setting, PDT is currently approved in the United States and the European Union for the treatment of actinic keratosis, basal cell carcinoma (EU only), Barrett's esophagus, microinvasive endobronchial lung cancer, and head and neck cancer (EU only). These indications will be discussed in detail in this section, along with the results of clinical trials for investigational uses of PDT.

Nonmelanoma Skin Cancers and Actinic Keratosis

PDT using porfimer sodium and ALA and its derivatives has been extensively studied in the treatment of both premalignant and malignant skin tumors. For the treatment of nonhyperkeratotic actinic keratosis of the scalp and face, a 20% solution of ALA is applied directly to the lesion and polychromatic blue light (approximately 417 nm) is given to a dose of 10 J/cm^2. The complete response rate at 8 weeks from therapy is 70% to 90%, depending on the lesion thickness. The drug light interval for this application is 14 hours, although an interval of 3 to 6 hours has been tested in multiple trials with similar results. The results of ALA PDT in the treatment of Bowen's disease (squamous cell carcinoma *in situ*) have been similarly positive. Recently, the esther derivative mALA (5-ALA methylesther, Metvix, Photocure ASA, Oslo Norway) was approved in the United States for treatment of actinic keratosis, basal cell cancer, and Bowen's disease using a more deeply penetrating red (634 nm) light. Overall, PDT has shown to be similar or superior in efficacy for the treatment of actinic keratosis and Bowen's disease compared to either cryotherapy or topical 5-fluorouracil creams, but with a superior toxicity profile.

PDT using either topical ALA or intravenous porfimer sodium (1 mg/kg, 48 hours prior to light delivery) has been successfully used to treat basal cell carcinomas (BCC). For both nodular and superficial BCC, a single porfimer sodium-mediated PDT treatment with 200 J/cm^2 630 nm light has an 85% to 90% complete response rate, with a recurrence rate of less than 10% at 4 years.[5] Similar results can be obtained using ALA PDT with a red light source (approximately 630 nm), but the response rates for single ALA PDT treatments for nodular BCC are considerably lower. Long-term data from multiple randomized trials comparing surgery to multifractionated topical ALA PDT indicate that although surgical excision should remain the standard of care for nodular BCC, ALA PDT is also an effective treatment for select tumors. Surgery had superior efficacy with recurrence rates less than 5% compared to 14% to 30% with ALA PDT.[18,19] Cosmesis, however, is consistently shown to be more favorable with ALA PDT. PDT has been used in the past to treat squamous cell carcinomas (SCC) of the skin, but the two largest trials of PDT for SCC have demonstrated unacceptably high recurrence rates following therapy (greater than 50%). The reason for this difference in PDT efficacy for BCC versus SCC is unclear, but may relate to differences in lesion thickness or keratinization. In summary, either single fraction porfimer sodium–mediated PDT or multifraction ALA-mediated PDT are appropriate and effective treatment alternatives for BCC.

Early Stage, Endobronchial Lung Cancer

Porfimer sodium–mediated PDT has been used with efficacy in the treatment of medically or surgically (multiple lesions in separate locations) unresectable early stage endobronchial lung cancer. In a phase 2 trial, porfimer sodium (2 mg/kg) was administered to 51 patients with 61 total carcinoma lesions, and PDT was performed 48 hours later using 150 to 200 J/cm^2 630 nm light.[20] In this trial the complete response rate was 85% and no grade 3 or 4 toxicities were reported. With a median follow-up of 20.2 months, only five of the patients who achieved a complete response had relapsed at the initial site. The results of this trial have been upheld in subsequent clinical experience, and this treatment is now approved in both the United States and the European Union. Trials using second-generation photosensitizers that exhibit less prolonged cutaneous photosensitivity have been performed and show similar results.

Barrett's Esophagus

Barrett's esophagus is characterized by columnar metaplasia of the normally squamous epithelium of the esophagus and predisposes affected patients to the development of esophageal carcinoma, especially in cases where severe dysplasia is identified. The standard approach for medically resectable patients with Barrett's esophagus and high-grade dysplasia (BE-HGD) has been esophagectomy. However, the significant morbidity and mortality associated with surgery has stimulated interest in the nonoperative management of BE-HGD. Nonoperative therapies have been tested in single institution, nonrandomized trials, including proton pump inhibitors (PPI) plus frequent surveillance endoscopies, coagulation with thermal laser or multipolar electrode, and photodynamic therapy. All have been shown to result in regression or complete elimination of BE-HGD. The results of a phase 3 multicenter randomized trial of porfimer sodium–mediated PDT combined with PPI therapy versus PPI therapy alone were recently updated.[21] In this trial 208 patients were randomly assigned to receive either PDT with PPI or PPI alone on a two-to-one basis. PDT patients received porfimer sodium (2 mg/kg) 40 to 50 hours prior to the first light delivery. Areas of BE were exposed to 130 J/cm 630 nm light using a cylindrical fiberoptic diffuser encased in an inflated esophageal balloon so that the fiber would be centered and the esophageal folds flattened. Ninety-six to 120 hours later, a repeat endoscopy was performed to assess response and an additional 50 J/cm could be given to areas of insufficient mucosal damage. If BE was found to persist on follow-up endoscopy, additional PDT treatments could be performed as described above to a maximum of three total treatments given at least 3 months apart. All patients (in both arms) received omeprazole therapy at a dose of 20 mg given twice daily. The results of this trial showed that PDT plus PPI was superior to PPI alone, both in terms of ablation of BE-HGD and progression to adenocarcinoma. At 5 years of follow-up, 77% of patients treated with PDT-PPI showed ablation of HGD versus 39% of patients treated with PPI alone ($P <.0001$). In addition, this response was shown to be durable at 5 years. The probability of maintaining complete ablation of HGD was 48% with PDT-PPI versus 4% with PPI alone. Finally, 15% of the patients in the PDT-PPI arm showed progression to cancer versus 29% of patients on the PPI arm ($P < .006$). The most serious toxicity of the PDT-PPI treatment was esophageal stricture, but the majority of these were successfully managed with esophageal dilatation. These results suggest that PDT is a relatively safe and effective management option of patients with BE-HGD.

Early Stage Head and Neck Cancer

The rationale for using PDT in premalignant or early stage head and neck cancer (HNC) is similar to that of using PDT for BE-HGD. However, it is important to note that this therapy is approved in the European Union but is not approved by the FDA. Multiple institutions have published small series demonstrating the efficacy of PDT for T0 to T2 N0 HNC, the largest of which represents a 15-year clinical experience treating over 200 patients with definitive porfimer sodium–mediated PDT.[22] In this series patients with either recurrent or primary T0 to T2, N0 HNC were given porfimer sodium (2 mg/kg) 48 hours prior to delivery of 50 to 80 J/cm^2 630 nm light. Patients with invasive disease to a depth of less than 3 mm were treated with light from a fiber fitted with a microlens applicator. Patients with more deeply invasive disease were treated with implantable, cylindrically diffusing fibers to ensure homogenous light delivery to the tissues. For 110 patients with T0 to T2 laryngeal lesions, 100% of patients achieved a complete response following PDT, and the 5-year local recurrence rate was 10% with a mean follow-up of 84 months. For 112 patients with T0 or T1 oral cavity lesions with 80-month mean follow-up, there were six local failures and two additional regional failures (recurrent nodal disease), all of which were salvaged with either repeated PDT or surgical resection. Complications seen in this series were limited to cutaneous photosensitivity, and local pain following therapy was controlled by oral analgesics. Several series have also reported on the use of the second-generation photosensitizers ALA and mTHPC. A multi-institutional phase 2 trial of mTHPC-PDT in 114 patients with T0 to T2 oropharyngeal cancer showed a complete response rate of 85% with up to three PDT treatments.[23] Moreover, 77% of complete responders were free of disease at 2 years. Taken together, these results suggest that PDT shows significant promise in the treatment of early stage HNC, and that further research in this area, including randomized trials, is needed.

CLINICAL INDICATIONS FOR PHOTODYNAMIC THERAPY IN THE LOCALLY ADVANCED AND PALLIATIVE SETTINGS

Intraperitoneal Photodynamic Therapy for Carcinomatosis or Sarcomatosis

In a phase 1 clinical trial for treatment of patients with disseminated intraperitoneal malignancies, intraoperative PDT following maximal surgical debulking resulted in a 76% complete cytologic response rate with tolerable toxicity. In the follow-up phase 2 study, patients were enrolled, stratified according to cancer type (ovarian, gastrointestinal, or sarcoma), and given doses of porfimer sodium and light at the maximally tolerated dose that was defined in the phase 1 trial.[18] As in the phase 1 trial, intraperitoneal PDT was associated with a postoperative capillary leak syndrome that necessitated massive fluid resuscitation in the immediate postoperative period that was in excess of the typical fluid needs of patients who receive surgery alone.[24] Other than the capillary leak syndrome and the skin photosensitivity, the complication rates are similar to the complication rates that are observed after similarly extensive surgery in the absence of PDT. With a 51-month median follow-up, the median failure-free survival and overall survival rates for the patients who received PDT were: for ovarian cancer, 3 months and 22 months; for gastrointestinal cancers, 3.3 months and 13.2 months; for sarcoma, 4 months and 21.9 months, respectively. At 6 months after therapy, the pathologic complete response rate was 3 of 33 (9.1%), 2 of 37 (5.4%), and 4 of 30 (13.3%) for the patients with ovarian cancer, gastrointestinal cancer, and sarcoma, respectively. Although most patients had disease at early follow-up between 3 and 6 months, the median survival of almost 2 years in the ovarian patients and over 1 year in the gastrointestinal patients suggests some benefit from this treatment. In the patients with sarcoma the prolonged overall survival was primarily due to patients with sarcomatosis from gastrointestinal stromal tumors who were treated with imatinib when it became available. Analysis of the patterns of treatment failure in this study suggests that a significant percentage of patients experienced treatment failure at sites not initially involved by gross disease. Moreover, patients with gross residual disease (who received a PDT boost to these sites) showed similar recurrence kinetics as compared to patients without gross residual disease, suggesting a dose–response relationship in intraperitoneal PDT. However, given the presence of fairly significant toxicities at PDT doses that were not adequate to fully control local disease, the therapeutic window for intraperitoneal PDT appears to be quite narrow. Thus, undirected PDT dose escalation is unlikely to result in a significant improvement in treatment outcomes, and other means to improve the therapeutic index are worthy of future study.

Postoperative Photodynamic Therapy for Pleural-Based Spread of Non–Small Cell Lung Cancer and Mesothelioma

Non–small cell lung cancer (NSCLC) with pleural spread is incurable, with median survival rates ranging from 6 months to 9 months, and surgery alone fails to locally control this disease or extend survival beyond the accepted treatment of palliative chemotherapy. Based on promising phase 1 results, a pilot phase 2 trial of porfimer sodium–mediated PDT was performed to investigate the efficacy of combined surgery and PDT for either recurrent or primary NSCLC with pleural spread.[25] Twenty-two patients were enrolled in this study and 5 did not receive light delivery due to unresectability. The 17 remaining patients who received porfimer sodium (2 mg/kg) 24 hours prior to gross tumor resection and the hemithorax was illuminated with 630 nm light to a measured dose of 30 J/cm^2. In order to facilitate homogenous delivery of light to the entire pleural cavity, the pleural cavity was filled with a solution of diluted intralipid prior to light delivery (Fig. 68.3). The majority of this population had poor prognostic features, including N2 nodes and bulky pleural disease. Local control of pleural disease at 6 months was achieved in 11 of 15 (73%) of evaluable patients and median overall survival for all 22 patients was 21.7 months. Two patients died in the immediate postoperative period, one of which was from adult respiratory distress syndrome that could have been related to PDT, surgery, or both. The other patient died of pneumonia in the contralateral lung following a difficult 2-month postoperative course. These results are highly encouraging in this population of patients and suggest that additional investigation in this area is warranted.

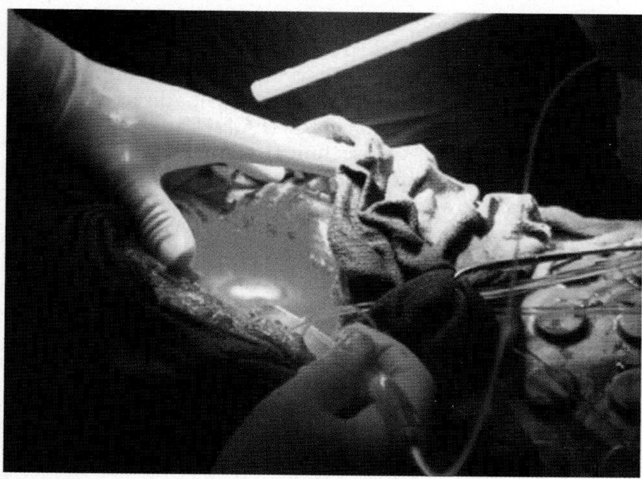

FIGURE 68.3 Pleural photodynamic therapy using intralipid to diffuse light.

Malignant pleural mesothelioma (MPM) is a cancer of the pleura that has no currently available curative options. In a phase 2 study of porfimer sodium–mediated PDT following extrapleural pneumonectomy for MPM, patients were given porfimer sodium 48 hours prior to surgery.[26] Patients with stage I and II disease experienced a median survival of 36 months with a 2-year survival rate of 61%. Patients with stage III and IV disease experienced a median survival rate of 10 months. Both of these are significantly improved compared to historical series of surgery alone. However, in a randomized phase 3 study of surgery versus surgery with PDT, patients received similar treatment as described above, but did not appear to benefit from the addition of PDT to surgery.[27] This trial was potentially underpowered and also involved surgical debulking that could leave disease of up to 5-mm thickness as opposed to a marcoscopically complete resection. Two trials of intraoperative PDT using the second-generation photosensitizer mTHPC have been performed.[28,29] These trials show that mTHPC PDT is feasible and has potentially acceptable toxicity. One important finding is that a lung-sparing, tumor-debulking surgery can be combined with PDT to achieve local control rates similar to those observed with extrapleural pneumonectomy. Indeed, a more recent study of macroscopically complete, lung-sparing surgical debulking followed by intraoperative porfimer sodium–mediated PDT for patients with locally advanced MPM found a median survival that had not been reached with a 2.1 year median follow-up in patients following radical pleurectomy with PDT. Thus, PDT for MPM needs to be further evaluated in clinical trials of lung-sparing surgery.

Palliation of Obstructing Lesions

PDT is approved in the United States and European Union for palliation of obstructive tumors of the esophagus and bronchi and has shown some success in maintaining bile duct patency in the face of partially obstructive lesions. For esophageal lesions, a multicenter trail that compared porfimer sodium–mediated PDT to neodymium:yttrium aluminum garnet (Nd:YAG) laser therapy for palliation of esophageal obstruction showed that the two treatments are equally effective for palliation of dysphagia; there was a trend toward improved objective tumor responses with PDT.[30] A similar randomized trial of PDT versus Nd:YAG laser therapy for obstructing NSCLC lesions showed equal initial efficacy for these two treatments, with a longer duration of response for PDT.[31]

Multiple clinical series have shown that intraluminal PDT for bile duct obstruction due to malignancy (usually unresectable pancreatic cancer or cholangiocarcinoma) can be performed safely and may improve bile duct patency rates compared to historical controls. Finally, two randomized trials of stent placement followed by porfimer sodium–mediated PDT versus stent placement alone showed a three- to fivefold increase in median survival for PDT-treated patients.[32] Taken together, these results suggest that PDT is a highly effective treatment for palliation of obstructing malignancies.

Hepatocellular Carcinoma

Multiple preclinical studies have been performed using hepatocellular carcinoma cells that suggest PDT may be able to stimulate decreased chemotherapy resistance and increased antitumor immune reactions in addition to promoting direct cellular cytotoxicity. Indeed, early clinical results using Talaporfin (LS11) and interstitially placed light-emitting diode (LED) light sources have shown promising results.[10] Currently, a phase 3 study is under way to evaluate the efficacy of Talaporfin-mediated PDT using interstitial LEDs as compared to institution-specific standard treatment that can include percutaneous ethanol injection, transcatheter arterial chemoembolization, or radio frequency ablation or cryotherapy with or without systemic chemotherapy.

Prostate and Bladder Cancers

For patients who receive definitive radiation therapy for prostate cancer and experience a local recurrence of disease, salvage options are limited. In phase 1 studies of second-generation photosensitizer-mediated PDT in patients with biopsy proven, locally recurrent prostate cancer following definitive radiotherapy, PDT was relatively well tolerated.[11,33] The major toxicities in these studies were mild to moderate urinary toxicities, including stress incontinence. One patient in each study experienced urethrorectal fistula, in one study this occurred following a nonprotocol, full thickness rectal biopsy performed 1 month after therapy and in the other study this occurred as a likely result of light inhomogeneity during treatment. Although not designed to measure efficacy, these studies provided some evidence of biochemical and pathologic disease response to PDT. Currently, this remains an active area of clinical investigation, with several institutions performing phase 1 and 2 studies of PDT for either locally recurrent or primary prostate cancer.

Bladder cancers are often superficial and multifocal that can be assessed and debulked endoscopically. In clinical trials, bladder cancer has been treated with porfimer sodium or ALA-mediated PDT with some success. Treatment of superficial bladder cancer with PDT is generally well tolerated, with dysuria, hematuria, and skin photosensitivity being the most common acute toxicities. Early response rates (2 months to 3 months) to PDT have been about 50% to 80% of patients with longer term (1year to 2 years) durable responses in 20% to 60% of patients. It should be noted that many of the patients treated in these studies had disease that had recurred after standard therapies such as BCG. Early studies combining intravesical immunotherapies such as BCG or chemotherapies such as mitomycin-C with PDT show that these therapies may significantly enhance the PDT responsiveness of bladder tumors.[34]

Brain Tumors

PDT has been used postoperatively to treat malignant gliomas, metastatic brain tumors from solid malignancies, and meningiomas. Intracavitary porfimer sodium or mTHPC-mediated PDT performed postoperatively is safe, and phase 2 studies suggest that PDT may prolong the survival of patients compared with maximal resection alone.[35] However, these data await confirmation from completed phase 3 trials. As with all PDT treatments, damage to normal tissue limits the dose of PDT that can be safely delivered in a single fraction. Interestingly, a recent preclinical study suggests that by using protracted, continuous delivery of photosensitizer (ALA given for 5 days in drinking water) followed by protracted delivery of light (50 J every 24 hours) with implanted laser-emitting diodes, high PDT doses can be given without increasing the toxicity of treatment.[36] Thus, PDT remains under active investigation and shows promise as a treatment for brain tumors.

MOLECULARLY TARGETED PHOTODYNAMIC THERAPY

Newly emerging data suggest that signaling through growth factor receptors and postreceptor signaling partners may be important in the survival of cancer cells following PDT and therefore may be methods that can be used clinically to improve therapeutic index. As the signaling mechanisms of PDT-mediated cytotoxicity are further elucidated, new molecular targets will continue to develop that may improve the therapeutic index of PDT. Currently, agents directed against epidermal growth factor receptor (EGFR) and angiogenesis have shown promise in preclinical testing.[37] Although the mechanism for these effects remains incompletely understood, these studies show that there is tremendous potential for increasing PDT efficacy by combining PDT with molecularly targeted therapy.

Another potential mechanism for enhancing the efficacy of PDT is through targeted photosensitizer delivery. Recent evidence suggests that the tumor-to-normal-tissue uptake ratios for relevant normal tissues may not be as high as was originally supposed.[24] There is also significant intra- and interpatient variability in photosensitizer uptake in both tumor and normal tissues. Initial studies of an anti-EGFR antibody (OC125) that is covalently lined to a photosensitizer showed superior PDT efficacy in a mouse model of ovarian carcinomatosis as compared to PDT using the unbound photosensitizer.[37] Another potential method to target photosensitizers would be to use nanoparticle technology. Early studies have demonstrated PDT-mediated cancer cell killing using various photosensitizer-nanoparticle designs and that these nanoparticles can allow for targeted delivery of photosensitizer to cancer cells.

References

1. Dougherty TJ, Grinday GB, Fiel R, Weishaupt KR, Boyle DG. Photoradiation therapy. II. Cure of animal tumors with hematoporphyrin and light. *J Natl Cancer Inst* 1975;55:115.
2. Weishaupt KR, Gomer CJ, Dougherty TJ. Identification of singlet oxygen as the cytotoxic agent in photoinactivation of a murine tumor. *Cancer Res* 1976;36:2326.
3. Blume JE, Oseroff AR. Aminolevulinic acid photodynamic therapy for skin cancers. *Dermatol Clin* 2007;25:5.
4. Löning MC, Diddens HC, Holl-Ulrich K, et al. Fluorescence staining of human ovarian cancer tissue following application of 5-aminolevulinic acid: fluorescence microscopy studies. *Lasers Surg Med* 2006;38:549.
5. Marcus SL, Sobel HC, Golub L, et al. Photodynamic therapy (PDT) and photodiagnosis (PD) using endogenous photosensitization induced by 5-aminolevulinic acid (ALA): current clinical and development status. *J Clin Laser Med Surg* 1996;14:59.
6. Ortel B, Chen N, Brissette J, et al. Differentiation-specific increase in ALA-induced protoporphyrin IX accumulation in primary mouse keratinocytes. *Br J Cancer* 1998;77:1744.
7. Miller JD, Baron ED, Scull H, et al. Photodynamic therapy with the phthalocyanine photosensitizer Pc 4: the case experience with preclinical mechanistic and early clinical-translational studies. *Toxicol Appl Pharmacol* 2007;224:290.
8. Bellnier DA, Greco WR, Loewen GM, et al. Clinical pharmacokinetics of the PDT photosensitizers porfimer sodium (Photofrin), 2-[1-hexyloxyethyl]-2-devinyl pyropheophorbide-a (Photochlor) and 5-ALA-induced protoporphyrin IX. *Lasers Surg Med* 2006;38:439.
9. Rostaporfin: PhotoPoint SnET2, Purlytin, Sn(IV) etiopurpurin, SnET2, tin ethyl etiopurpurin. *Drugs R D* 2004;5:58.
10. Wang S, Bromley E, Xu L, Chen JC, Keltner L. Talaporfin sodium. *Expert Opin Pharmacother* 2010;11:133.
11. Nathan TR, Whitelaw DE, Chang SC, et al. Photodynamic therapy for prostate cancer recurrence after radiotherapy: a phase I study. *J Urol* 2002;168:1427.
12. Korbelik M, Krosl G, Krosl J, Dougherty GJ. The role of host lymphoid populations in the response of mouse EMT6 tumor to photodynamic therapy. *Cancer Res* 1996;56:5647.
13. Kabingu E, Oseroff AR, Wilding GE, Gollnick SO. Enhanced systemic immune reactivity to a basal cell carcinoma associated antigen following photodynamic therapy. *Clin Cancer Res* 2009;15:4460.
14. Oleinick NL, Morris RL, Belichenko I. The role of apoptosis in response to photodynamic therapy: what, where, why, and how. *Photochem Photobiol Sci* 2002;1:1.
15. Chakraborty A, Held KD, Prise KM, Liber HL, Redmond RW. Bystander effects induced by diffusing mediators after photodynamic stress. *Radiat Res* 2009;172:74.
16. Dahle J, Bagdonas S, Kaalhus O, et al. The bystander effect in photodynamic inactivation of cells. *Biochim Biophys Acta* 2000;1475:273.
17. Reiners JJ Jr, Agostinis P, Berg K, Oleinick NL, Kessel D. Assessing autophagy in the context of photodynamic therapy. *Autophagy* 2010;6:7.
18. Mosterd K, Thissen MR, Nelemans P, et al. Fractionated 5-aminolaevulinic acid-photodynamic therapy vs. surgical excision in the treatment of nodular basal cell carcinoma: results of a randomized controlled trial. *Br J Dermatol* 2008;159:864.
19. Rhodes LE, de Rie MA, Leifsdottir R, et al. Five-year follow-up of a randomized, prospective trial of topical methyl aminolevulinate photodynamic therapy vs surgery for nodular basal cell carcinoma. *Arch Dermatol* 2007;143:1131.
20. Furuse K, Fukuoka M, Kato H, et al. A prospective phase II study on photodynamic therapy with photofrin II for centrally located early-stage lung cancer. The Japan Lung Cancer Photodynamic Therapy Study Group. *J Clin Oncol* 1993;11:1852.
21. Overholt BF, Wang KK, Burdick JS, et al. Five-year efficacy and safety of photodynamic therapy with photofrin in Barrett's high-grade dysplasia. *Gastrointest Endosc* 2007;66:460.
22. Biel MA. Photodynamic therapy of head and neck cancers. *Methods Mol Biol* 2010;635:281.
23. Hopper C, Kübler A, Lewis H, Tan IB, Putnam G. mTHPC-mediated photodynamic therapy for early oral squamous cell carcinoma. *Int J Cancer* 2004;111:138.
24. Hahn SM, Fraker DL, Mick R, et al. A phase II trial of intraperitoneal photodynamic therapy for patients with peritoneal carcinomatosis and sarcomatosis. *Clin Cancer Res* 2006;12:2517.
25. Friedberg JS, Mick R, Stevenson JP, et al. Phase II trial of pleural photodynamic therapy and surgery for patients with non–small cell lung cancer with pleural spread. *J Clin Oncol* 2004;22:2192.
26. Moskal TL, Dougherty TJ, Urschel JD, et al. Operation and photodynamic therapy for pleural mesothelioma: 6-year follow-up. *Ann Thorac Surg* 1998;66:1128.
27. Pass HI, Temeck BK, Kranda K, et al. Phase III randomized trial of surgery with or without intraoperative photodynamic therapy and postoperative immunochemotherapy for malignant pleural mesothelioma. *Ann Surg Oncol* 1997;4:628.
28. Friedberg JS, Mick R, Stevenson J, et al. A phase I study of Foscan-mediated photodynamic therapy and surgery in patients with mesothelioma. *Ann Thorac Surg* 2003;75:952.
29. Schouwink H, Ruevekamp M, Oppelaar H, et al. Photodynamic therapy for malignant mesothelioma: preclinical studies for optimization of treatment protocols. *Photochem Photobiol* 2001;73:410.

30. Lightdale CJ, Heier SK, Marcon NE, et al. Photodynamic therapy with porfimer sodium versus thermal ablation therapy with Nd:YAG laser for palliation of esophageal cancer: a multicenter randomized trial. *Gastrointest Endosc* 1995;42:507.
31. Diaz-Jimenéz JP, Martínez-Ballarín JE, Llunell A, et al. Efficacy and safety of photodynamic therapy versus Nd-YAG laser resection in NSCLC with airway obstruction. *Eur Respir J* 1999;14:800.
32. Ortner MA. Photodynamic therapy for cholangiocarcinoma: overview and new developments. *Curr Opin Gastroenterol* 2009;25:472.
33. Du KL, Mick R, Busch TM, et al. Preliminary results of interstitial motexafin lutetium-mediated PDT for prostate cancer. *Lasers Surg Med* 2006;38:427.
34. Pinthus JH, Bogaards A, Weersink R, Wilson BC, Trachtenberg J. Photodynamic therapy for urological malignancies: past to current approaches. *J Urol* 2006;175:1201.
35. Kostron H. Photodynamic diagnosis and therapy and the brain. *Methods Mol Biol* 2010;635:261.
36. Bisland SK, Lilge L, Lin A, Rusnov R, Wilson BC. Metronomic photodynamic therapy as a new paradigm for photodynamic therapy: rationale and preclinical evaluation of technical feasibility for treating malignant brain tumors. *Photochem Photobiol* 2004;80:22.
37. Solban N, Rizvi I, Hasan T. Targeted photodynamic therapy. *Lasers Surg Med* 2006;38:522.

CHAPTER 69 BIOMARKERS

DANIEL F. HAYES

A tumor marker is a molecular or tissue-based process that provides future behavior of a cancer but requires a special assay that is beyond routine clinical, radiographic, or pathologic examination.[1] Biomarkers can be the result of changes in malignant tissue compared to normal tissue, changes in one type of malignancy that distinguish it from another, or changes within a tumor type that distinguish one behavior from the other. Tumor markers can be measured at multiple levels: DNA, RNA, protein, cell, and tissue. For example, DNA-based marker assays might detect gene mutations, deletions, amplifications, or methylation. RNA-based marker assays, which include a recently described class of molecules designated micro-RNAs (miRNA) might detect over- or underexpression of the message, splice differences in the message, or inhibitory miRNAs that prevent translation of other transcripts. Protein-based markers can include overexpression, underexpression, or qualitative abnormalities. One might detect cancer cells in tissues or fluid in which they do not belong, such as regional lymph nodes, circulation, or distant organs (like bone marrow). Detection of abnormal tissue processes induced by an existing cancer, such as neovascularization, can also serve as a marker. An assay for a marker might be for a single molecule, such as amplification of a specific gene or overexpression of a single protein, or it might include a multiparameter analysis, resulting in an index (analogous to using TNM [tumor, necrosis, metastasis] to create a tumor stage) or a profile or "signature," most commonly developed within gene expression microarray technologies. Each of these might provide evidence of the presence of cancer or insight into whether the patient might benefit from a change in clinical course, such as application of subsequent therapy.

A biomarker might be identified and evaluated in the tissue of origin or, as noted, in regional lymph nodes or distant tissues. Markers can also be identified in circulation, either as soluble molecules, such as DNA, RNA, or protein, or as whole cells. Finally, the same "biomarker" may have very different implications, depending on what molecule is measured, how it is measured, and where it is measured. For example, the protooncogene *HER2* (also designated as *c-erbb-2* and c-*neu*) has been shown to be very important in breast cancer biology and is a critical target for at least two therapies: trastuzumab and lapatinib.[2–8] *HER2* gene amplification and its expression can be measured by many different assays, either in primary or metastatic breast cancer tissue or in blood, either as a soluble protein or expressed on circulating tumor cells.[9–11] Gene amplification can be assayed using fluorescent or chromogenic *in situ* hybridization, high resolution comparative genomic hybridization, or by dot blot technology. Breast cancer tissue HER2 message can be evaluated using reverse transcription-polymerase chain reaction (RT-PCR) or microarray based assays, and HER2 protein overexpression can be quantified by Western blot, immunohistochemistry (IHC), immunofluorescence, or enzyme-based immunosorbent assays (ELISA). The circulating extracellular domain of HER2 can be detected in serum, plasma, and saliva. HER2 protein expression in circulating cancer cells can be measured by immunohistochemistry or immunofluorescence, and amplification of *HER2* gene in these cells can be measured by fluorescent *in situ* hybridization. Each of these assays for the same fundamental marker may give very different indications of the biology of the tumor and may differ for one type of tumor (i.e., breast cancer) compared to another (i.e., gastric, lung, or ovary cancer). These considerations illustrate the enormous complexity of biomarker biology, research, and clinical use. Thus, it is critical that each end-user (i.e., the biologist, investigator, and clinician) has a thorough understanding of the important concepts and pitfalls of tumor marker results and applications.

WHAT IS A BIOMARKER USED FOR?

There are several possible clinical uses for a tumor marker (Table 69.1). A marker might be used to adjust risk categorization for an individual not affected by the disease. Such a marker could then be used to more efficiently apply screening or prevention methods, if these are known to be effective. Tumor markers might also be used for screening to detect an established cancer earlier than it would have been using standard clinical signs and symptoms.

Markers in tissue and serum have also been used to establish the tissue of origin of a newly diagnosed cancer (differential diagnosis). This utility requires that the marker be tissue specific. One of the better examples of this use is analysis of either tissue-expression or circulating α-fetoprotein (AFP) or β–human chorionic gonadotropin (β-hCG) in males with poorly differentiated malignancies of uncertain origin. Although other conditions can cause elevated serum levels of these markers, they are rare. Most oncologists would feel comfortable treating such a patient with chemotherapy directed toward germ cell malignancy.[12,13]

The most frequent use of a biomarker is to determine prognosis in a patient with an established cancer. However, it is important to distinguish the difference between a prognostic factor and a predictive factor. A pure prognostic factor is associated with risk of invasion and metastasis in the absence of a therapy one might apply if the patient's prognosis is sufficiently poor. For almost every tumor, the presence of involved local-regional lymph nodes, as determined by routine hematoxylin and eosinophilic staining, is highly associated with subsequent distant recurrence in death, especially in the absence of systemic therapy.[14] A prognostic factor may determine future risk of an event

TABLE 69.1

POTENTIAL USES FOR TUMOR MARKERS

Risk determination
Screening
Differential diagnosis
Prognosis
Prediction
Monitoring

in the absence of any therapy, or residual risk of an event assuming some therapy (e.g., such as surgery), but in anticipation of other therapy if appropriate (e.g., systemic therapy).

In contrast, a pure predictive factor is associated with the likelihood of sensitivity or resistance to a specific therapy, assuming the patient's prognosis is sufficiently poor to justify its toxicity and cost. A marker can be predictive because it is the direct target of the anticipated therapy (such as breast cancer tissue estrogen-receptor content for endocrine therapy), or it is indicative of a pathway or process that is involved in activity of the drug (such as KRAS mutations and antiepidermal growth factor receptor [EGFR] antibody therapies). Perhaps the best example of a predictive factor in all of oncology is the presence or absence of estrogen receptor in breast cancer and response to antiestrogen therapy, such as tamoxifen.[15]

In fact, few markers are pure prognostic or predictive factors, but, rather, they are mixed. Again, using breast cancer as an example, amplification or overexpression of HER2 is associated with a worse prognosis in the absence of therapy. HER2 is also a predictive factor, but its effects are enigmatic. HER2 may be a favorable predictive factor for some types of therapy, such as anthracycline or taxane-based chemotherapy, and anti-HER2 therapies (trastuzumab and lapatinib), while it is a negative predictive factor for others, such as all or certain types of endocrine treatments.[16–19] Therefore, it is important for both the investigator and the clinician to understand a study that claims that a given marker is "prognostic" cannot be considered valid unless all systemic therapies are considered. If these issues are not considered, it is likely that a marker will either never be found to be useful, or, worse, it will be misused clinically.[20]

The final potential utility of a marker is to monitor patients either during or after therapy to determine the status of the cancer. Of course, monitoring is classically performed using clinical and radiographic procedures, especially for solid tumors. Patients might be monitored during primary therapy or during therapy for established metastatic disease to determine if the current treatment should be continued or an alternative strategy might be indicated. Patients who are free of detectable disease after primary therapy might be monitored to detect "occult," or impending, recurrence prior to classic clinical signs and symptoms of metastases. Several markers have been evaluated for this use in a variety of malignancies. Since serial biopsies are inconvenient and logistically problematic, most of these are detected in the circulation. For example, circulating carcinoembryonic antigen (CEA), the first reported circulating tumor-associated antigen, tracks reliably with tumor status in patients with colorectal carcinoma.[21] Serial CEA levels are recommended for patients who have been rendered disease free after primary therapy, since resection of those with isolated hepatic metastases appears to improve survival and for monitoring patients with established metastases.[22] Likewise, AFP and β-hCG for germ cell malignancies in men, prostate-specific antigen (PSA) for prostate cancer, cancer antigen 125 (CA 125) for ovarian cancer, and MUC-1 assays (CA 15-3 and CA 27.29) for breast cancer have all gained widespread use to monitor patients with these respective malignancies. Serial assays for malignant cells in blood or bone marrow have also been used to monitor patients with a number of malignancies.[23] However, it is important to note that while monitoring patients who are free of disease for occult recurrence may be clinically indicated in some cancers, such as in colorectal[22] and male germ cell malignancies,[24] it is not recommended in others, such as breast cancer.[11,25]

WHAT ARE THE CRITERIA TO INCORPORATE A TUMOR MARKER INTO CLINICAL PRACTICE?

In 1996 the American Society of Clinical Oncology convened an expert panel to establish guidelines for the use of tumor markers in breast and colon cancers. In spite of the impressive explosion in molecular biological and technical knowledge about these cancers, the recommendations of the panel have been quite conservative because the members have attempted to base their recommendations on evidence as much as possible (Table 69.2).[11,22] To do so, they developed a tumor marker utility grading system in which was embedded a scale that defined levels of evidence required to accept a marker for routine clinical use.[1] Recently, this scale has been modified and updated to address the hierarchy of types of studies that might lead to sufficiently high levels of evidence that one can determine if a marker does or does not have clinical utility (Tables 69.3 and 69.4).[26]

The following three fundamental criteria must be met for a marker to be of use (Table 69.5): (1) the precise use must be well defined, as described above; (2) the magnitude in the differences in outcomes between those patients who are positive for a given marker must be sufficiently large compared to those who are negative that the clinician and patient would elect to follow a different clinical course than they would have otherwise; and (3) the estimate of that magnitude must be accurate. The latter criterion can be divided into three subcategories: Is the assay technically reliable? Is the clinical study designed to address the clinical question properly and has the observation been validated in a separate, equally well-designed clinical study? Is the statistical analysis of the clinical results appropriate and robust?

These three criteria can be summarized using the increasingly used terms *analytical validity*, *clinical validity*, and *clinical utility*.[27] Before a tumor marker assay can be used to care for patients, it must be technically and analytically stable and highly validated, including accuracy and reproducibility. Preanalytical concerns, such as type and time of fixation and storage, may fundamentally alter tumor marker results, giving spurious data, and these must be considered carefully. Clinical validity suggests that the marker does, indeed, separate a population of patients into two groups for whom some outcome, such as disease-free, progression-free, or overall survival, is different. However, these observations do not translate into clinical utility. Rather, the latter requires carefully designed, conducted, analyzed, and validated studies that demonstrate that clinical application of the assay results in improved outcomes, related to one of the uses described in Table 69.1, for the patient when compared to not knowing the assay data.

These concerns bring us back to the levels of evidence (LOE) scale described in Tables 69.3 and 69.4. Ideally, a tumor marker assay will have been investigated with the same rigor as one would study a new therapeutic agent, generating level I evidence. In this regard, the precise use of the marker should be determined from preliminary studies before the definitive

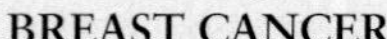

TABLE 69.2

AMERICAN SOCIETY OF CLINICAL ONCOLOGY TUMOR MARKER GUIDELINES RECOMMENDATIONS FOR BREAST AND COLON CANCER

Marker	Recommendation
BREAST CANCER	
Estrogen receptors and progesterone receptors	ER and PgR should be measured on every primary invasive breast cancer to identify patients most likely to benefit from endocrine forms of therapy.
Tissue HER2	HER2 expression or amplification should be evaluated in every primary invasive breast cancer either at the time of diagnosis or at the time of recurrence, principally to guide selection of trastuzumab in the adjuvant or metastatic setting and lapatinib in the metastatic setting.
uPA and PAI-1	uPA/PAI-1 measured by ELISAs on a minimum of 300 mg of fresh or frozen breast cancer tissue may be used for the determination of prognosis in patients with newly diagnosed, node negative breast cancer.
Multiparameter gene expression analysis for breast cancer	In newly diagnosed patients with node-negative, estrogen receptor–positive breast cancer, the Oncotype DX™ (Genomics Health, Inc., Redwood City, CA) assay can be used to predict the risk of recurrence in patients treated with tamoxifen. The precise clinical utility and appropriate application for other multiparameter assays, such as the MammaPrint™ (Agendia, Inc., Irvine, CA) assay, the Rotterdam Signature, and the Breast Cancer Gene Expression Ratio are under investigation.
DNA flow cytometry-based parameters	Present data are insufficient to recommend use of DNA content, S phase, or other flow cytometry–based markers of proliferation for management of patients with breast cancer.
Markers of proliferation	Present data are insufficient to recommend measurement of Ki67, cyclin D, cyclin E, p27, p21, thymidine kinase, topoisomerase II, or other markers of proliferation for management of patients with breast cancer.
p53	Present data are insufficient to recommend use of p53 measurements for management of patients with breast cancer.
Cathepsin D	Present data are insufficient to recommend use of cathepsin D for management of patients with breast cancer.
Cyclin E	Present data are insufficient to recommend use of cyclin E for management of patients with breast cancer.
Proteomic analysis	Present data are insufficient to recommend use of proteomic patterns for management of patients with breast cancer.
CA 15-3 and CA 27.29 and CEA	Present data are insufficient to recommend CA 15-3 or CA 27.29 or CEA for screening, diagnosis, and staging or for monitoring patients for recurrence after primary breast cancer therapy. For monitoring patients with metastatic disease during active therapy, these assays can be used in conjunction with diagnostic imaging, history, and physical examination. Caution should be used when interpreting a rising marker level during the first 4–6 weeks of a new therapy, since spurious early rises may occur.
Circulating extracellular domain of HER2	Measuring circulating extracellular domain of HER2 is not currently recommended for management of patients with breast cancer.
Bone marrow micrometastases as markers for breast cancer	Present data are insufficient to recommend assessment of bone marrow micrometastases for management of patients with breast cancer.
Circulating tumor cell assays as markers for breast cancer	The measurement of circulating tumor cells (CTC) should not be used to make the diagnosis of breast cancer or to influence any treatment decisions in patients with breast cancer.
COLORECTAL CANCER	
CEA	CEA is not recommended to be used as a screening test for colorectal cancer. CEA may be ordered preoperatively in patients with colorectal carcinoma if it would assist in staging and surgical treatment planning. Postoperative serum CEA testing should be performed every 3 months in patients with stage II or III disease for at least 3 years after diagnosis, if the patient is a candidate for surgery or systemic therapy. CEA is the marker of choice for monitoring metastatic colorectal cancer during systemic therapy.
CA 19-9	Present data are insufficient to recommend CA 19-9 for management of patients with colorectal cancer.
DNA ploidy or flow cytometric proliferation analysis	Present data are insufficient to recommend flow cytometrically derived DNA index or S phase for management of patients with early stage colorectal cancer.
p53	Present data are insufficient to recommend the use of p53 expression or mutation for screening, diagnosis, staging, surveillance, or monitoring treatment of patients with colorectal cancer.
Ras	Present data are insufficient to recommend the use of the r*Ras* oncogene for screening, diagnosis, staging, surveillance, or monitoring treatment of patients with colorectal cancer.
TS, DPD, TP	TS, DPD, and TP are not useful for screening, determining the prognosis, predicting, or monitoring response to therapy.
MSI	MSI ascertained by PCR is not recommended at this time to determine prognosis or to predict the effectiveness of adjuvant chemotherapy.
18q-LOH/DCC	Assaying for loss of heterozygosity (LOH) on the long arm of chromosome 18 (18q) or DCC protein determination by immunohistochemistry should not be used to determine the prognosis of operable colorectal cancer, nor to predict response to therapy.
KRAS mutations	All patients with metastatic colorectal carcinoma who are candidates for anti-EGFR antibody therapy should have their tumor tested for KRAS mutations in a CLIA-accredited laboratory. If KRAS mutation in codon 12 or 13 is detected, then patients with metastatic colorectal carcinoma should not receive anti-EGFR antibody therapy as part of their treatment.

TABLE 69.2

(CONTINUED)

PANCREATIC CANCER	
CA 19-9	CA 19-9 is not recommended for use as a screening test for pancreatic cancer, nor is it, alone, recommended for use in determining operability or the results of operability. CA 19-9 itself cannot provide definitive evidence of disease recurrence without seeking confirmation with imaging studies for clinical findings or biopsy. Present data are insufficient to recommend the routine use of serum CA 19-9 levels alone for monitoring response to treatment. However, CA 19-9 can be measured at the start of treatment for locally advanced metastatic disease and every 1 to 3 months during active treatment as an indication of progressive disease and confirmation with other studies should be sought.

ER, estrogen receptor; PgR, progesterone receptor; ELISA, enzyme-linked immunosorbent assay; CA, cancer antigen; CEA, carcinoembryonic antigen; TS, thymidine synthase; DPD, dihydropyrmidine dehydrogenase; TP, thymidine phosphorylase; MSI, microsatellite instability; CLIA, clinical laboratory improvement amendments; EGFR, epidermal growth factor receptor.
(Modified from refs. 11, 22, 28.)

TABLE 69.3

ELEMENTS OF TUMOR MARKER STUDIES THAT CONSTITUTE LEVELS OF EVIDENCE DETERMINATION

Category	A	B	C	D
Trial Design	**Prospective**	**Prospective Using Archived Samples**	**Prospective/ Observational**	**Retrospective/Observational**
Clinical trial	PRCT designed to address tumor marker	Prospective trial not designed to address tumor marker, but design accommodates tumor marker utility Accommodation of predictive marker requires PRCT	Prospective observational registry, treatment, and follow-up not dictated	No prospective aspect to study
Patients and patient data	Prospectively enrolled, treated, and followed in PRCT	Prospectively enrolled, treated, and followed in clinical trial and, especially if a predictive utility is considered, a PRCT addressing the treatment of interest	Prospectively enrolled in registry, but treatment and follow-up standard of care	No prospective stipulation of treatment or follow-up; patient data collected by retrospective chart review
Specimen collection, processing, and archival	Specimens collected, processed and assayed for specific marker in real time	Specimens collected, processed, and archived prospectively using generic SOPs. Assayed after trial completion.	Specimens collected, processed, and archived prospectively using generic SOPs. Assayed after trial completion.	Specimens collected, processed, and archived with no prospective SOPs
Statistical design and analysis	Study powered to address tumor marker question	Study powered to address therapeutic question; underpowered to address tumor marker question Focused analysis plan for marker question developed prior to doing assays	Study not prospectively powered at all. Retrospective study design confounded by selection of specimens for study. Focused analysis plan for marker question developed prior to doing assays	Study not prospectively powered at all. Retrospective study design confounded by selection of specimens for study. No focused analysis plan for marker question developed prior to doing assays
Validation	Result unlikely to be play of chance Although preferred, validation not required	Result more likely to be play of chance that A, but less likely than C. Requires one or more validation studies	Result very likely to be play of chance Requires subsequent validation studies	Result very likely to be play of chance Requires subsequent validation

PRCT, prospective, randomized, controlled trial; SOPs, standard operating procedures.
(From ref. 26.)

TABLE 69.4

REVISED DETERMINATION OF LEVELS OF EVIDENCE USING ELEMENTS OF TUMOR MARKER STUDIES

Level of Evidence	Category from Table 69.1	Validation Studies Available
I	A	None required
I	B	One or more with consistent results
II	B	None or Inconsistent results
II	C	2 or more with consistent results
III	C	None or 1 with consistent results or Inconsistent results
IV–V	D	NA[a]

[a]NA, not applicable, since levels of evidence IV and V studies will never be satisfactory for determination of medical utility.
(From ref. 26.)

study is performed, and that study should be a prospective, hypothesis-based clinical trial in which the marker use is the primary objective of the trial. Such a trial has rarely been performed, although there are currently a few ongoing within the cooperative groups in both North America and Europe in patients with breast and colorectal cancers.

However, trials such as these are cumbersome and expensive. A more common approach is to conduct a clinical trial addressing a therapeutic strategy in which biologic specimens are collected and the marker is a secondary objective of the study, either prospectively defined or, alternatively, retrospectively conducted after the study is complete using the archived specimens. Several of these studies, designated LOE II, have been conducted, and most cooperative groups have large specimen banks designed to collect, process, and store material for these types of investigations. Of note, arguably, several LOE II studies can be pooled (assuming they ask the same clinical use question using similar techniques) to generate an LOE I study. LOE III studies are, on the most part, investigations of convenience, in which archived samples are collected, stored, and available and are linked to patient outcomes, but eligibility, treatment, and follow-up are not prospectively directed. The level of evidence scale has recently been updated to reflect the use of archived specimens to determine clinical utility.[26] These studies can be used to develop valuable hypotheses, but they are rarely if ever sufficient to direct patient care.

TABLE 69.5

CRITERIA NEEDED FOR TUMOR MARKER TO BE ACCEPTED FOR CLINICAL USE

1. The intended use must be clearly delineated (Table 69.1)
2. The magnitude of differences in outcomes between "positive" and "negative" populations must be sufficient that a clinical decision would be changed based on the results
3. The estimate of that magnitude must be reliable and validated
   a. The assay must be technically stable, reproducible, and accurate
   b. The clinical study must be appropriately designed and powered to address the intended use
   c. The analysis of the study must be statistically rigorous

PROGNOSIS VERSUS PREDICTION

As described previously, one of the most frequent uses of a tumor marker is to predict outcome of the patient after diagnosis in order to guide future treatment. This situation provides ample examples of the issues of "use," "magnitude," and "accuracy" to define clinical utility and deserves further discussion. Figure 69.1 is a hypothetical schematic that illustrates the differences between a pure prognostic factor (Fig. 69.1*A*), a pure predictive factor (Fig. 69.1*B*), and a mixed factor that, in this example, is a favorable prognostic factor but a negative predictive factor for a specific systemic therapy. Within each category, an example of a strong factor is contrasted with a weak one. In each case, the study that generated the hypothetical data was sufficiently robust to determine that, indeed, the "positive" curves are clearly distinct from the "negative" curves; in other words, the curves are statistically significantly different by conventional criteria. However, in each case, it is unlikely the clinician would use the "weaker" factor (factor 2 in each figure) to treat patients differently. In contrast, if the therapy is toxic or very expensive, patients who are "negative" for the strong prognostic factor (i.e., they have a very favorable prognosis; Fig. 69.1*A*) or "negative" for the strong predictive factor (i.e., the therapy is unlikely to be active against their cancer; Fig. 69.1*B*) might forgo the small chances of benefit.

Figure 69.1C illustrates how confounded an LOE III study can be by treatment. Before a marker can be accepted into routine clinical use, it is essential to be certain that the clinical studies have been well designed to address a specific question with sufficiently robust technical and statistical considerations to be certain that the estimates of magnitude between those who are positive or negative are reliable. For example, recently, several investigators have demonstrated that monoclonal antibodies (cetuximab or panitumumab) directed against EGFR provide no benefit to patients with colorectal cancer if mutations in codon 12 or 13 of KRAS are discovered, while these agents appear quite effective in patients with wild type tumors.[28] Thus, these monoclonal antibodies (cetuximab, panitumumab) should not be administered to patients whose cancers harbor the KRAS mutations.

PHARMACOGENOMICS: A SPECIAL CIRCUMSTANCE

In addition to tumor-related somatic changes, inherited, germline differences in genes either responsible for metabolism of drugs or that act as the direct or indirect target of drugs may also play an important role in assessing benefits and risks for specific therapeutic strategies.

Several examples highlight the importance that pharmacogenomic alterations may exert on the treatment of adult solid tumors. The drug 5-fluorouracil (5-FU) and its related oral agent, capecitabine, are both cleared by the enzyme dihydropyrimidine dehydrogenase (DPD). Patients who are homozygous for selective inactive alleles of the *DPD* gene are unable to clear these agents, and very small doses are associated with severe and often life-threatening toxicities.[24] Unfortunately, a convenient and accurate assay for this inherited condition is not widely available. Likewise, recently reported data have demonstrated a similar deficiency in the UDP glucuronosyltransferase 1A1 (*UGT1A1*) gene, which

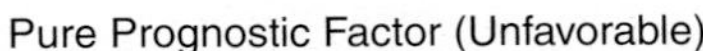

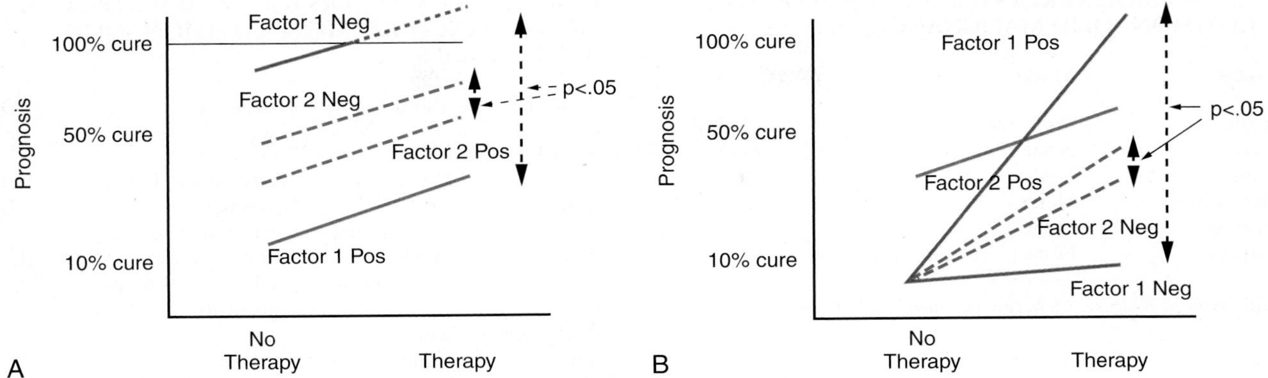

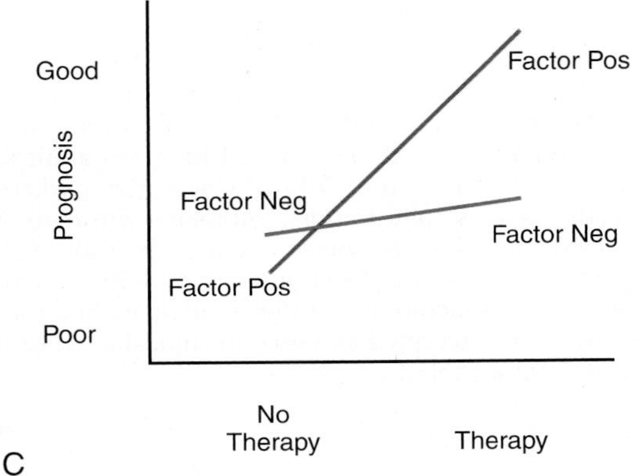

FIGURE 69.1 Schematic representation of prognostic and predictive factors. **A:** Illustration of a pure prognostic factor that is associated with unfavorable prognosis. **B:** Illustration of pure predictive factor that is associated with response to specific therapy. **C:** Illustration of mixed factor that is associated with unfavorable prognosis and favorable response to therapy. (Modified from ref. 20.)

renders carriers unable to metabolize irinotecan, also exposing them to unacceptable toxicities.[29] Although the clinical utility of these findings is controversial, the U.S. Food and Drug Administration has recently changed the package insert for irinotecan to recommend testing for this genetic abnormality in patients who appear to be candidates for this agent.

Antiestrogen therapies have been the mainstay for prevention and treatment of women with estrogen receptor–rich breast cancer. Of these, the selective estrogen receptor modulator (SERM) tamoxifen has been the most widely used. Tamoxifen is a prodrug, but it is metabolized to both active and inactive metabolites. Of these, 4-hydroxy-*N*-desmethyl tamoxifen

TABLE 69.6

ACCEPTED BIOMARKERS USEFUL FOR DIFFERENTIAL DIAGNOSIS OF COMMON SOLID MALIGNANCIES

Cancer	Marker	LOE
Breast	Tissue ER, PgR (some uterine and lung cancers are weakly positive)	III
	Gross cystic disease protein	
Colon/intestine	Tissue CDX2	III
Lung	Tissue TTF1 (also positive in thyroid cancer, but thyroid also positive for thyroglobulin)	III
Melanoma	Tissue S100, Melan-A, HMB45, MITF	III
Ovarian	WT1	III
Prostate	Circulating or tissue PSA, urinary PCA3	III
Male germ cell	Tissue or circulating α-fetoprotein, β–human chorionic gonadotropin (β-hCG)	II–III
	Tissue PLAP	
Female choriocarcinoma	Tissue or circulating β-hCG (also elevated in pregnancy)	III

ER, estrogen receptor; PgR, progesterone receptor; LOE, levels of evidence; PSA, prostate-specific antigen; PLAP, placental-like alkaline phosphatase.

TABLE 69.7

ACCEPTED BIOMARKERS USEFUL FOR PROGNOSIS OF COMMON SOLID MALIGNANCIES

Cancer	Marker	LOE
Breast	See Table 34.8.6	I, II
Colon	None (? circulating CEA)	
Lung	None	
Melanoma	None	
Ovarian	None	
Prostate	None	

LOE, levels of evidence; CEA, carcinoembryonic antigen.

(designated endoxifen) is the most abundant active compound. Tamoxifen is converted to endoxifen via activity of cytochrome P-450 2D6 enzymatic activity.[30] Preliminary data suggest that patients who are homozygous for inactivating single-nucleotide polymorphism (SNP) in CYP2D6 are less likely to benefit from tamoxifen than those who are wild type for this gene, although the results of several subsequent studies have been mixed, and it is not clear if patients considering tamoxifen therapy should or should not be genotyped for CYP2D6 SNPs.[31]

MARKERS THAT ARE ACCEPTED FOR ROUTINE CLINICAL UTILITY

Using the preceding concepts, one can now review several markers that are routinely incorporated into standard clinical care.

TABLE 69.8

ACCEPTED BIOMARKERS USEFUL AS PREDICTIVE FACTORS FOR TREATMENT COMMON SOLID MALIGNANCIES

Cancer	Marker	Treatment	LOE
Breast	ER	Endocrine	I
	HER2	Trastuzumab; lapatinib	I–II
Colon	KRAS mutations	Cetuximab; panitumumab	I–II
Lung	EGFR mutations	Tyrosine kinase inhibitors (erlotinib, gefitinib)	II
Melanoma	None		
Ovarian	None		
Prostate	None		

ER, estrogen receptor; LOE, levels of evidence.

Although the principles described above relate to any malignancy, the remainder of this chapter will focus on adult solid tumors. Tables 69.6 through 69.9 list the accepted markers by use within the various solid tumors, with some effort to state the level of evidence that supports these uses. Not all of these markers and their uses have been addressed by the American Society of Clinical Oncology or other guidelines bodies, but since they are widely accepted and used in clinical practice they are included in these tables.

TABLE 69.9

ACCEPTED BIOMARKERS USEFUL FOR MONITORING OF COMMON SOLID MALIGNANCIES

Cancer	Marker	Specific Situation	LOE
Breast	CA 15-3, CA 27.29 CEA Circulating Tumor Cells	Monitor selected patients with metastatic disease	II–III
Colon	CEA	Monitor patients after primary and systemic adjuvant chemotherapy to detect resectable relapse Monitor selected patients with metastatic disease	II–III
Lung	None		
Melanoma	None		
Ovarian	CA 125	Monitor patients after primary and adjuvant chemotherapy for relapse Monitor patients with metastatic disease	II–III
	HE-4	Monitor patients with metastatic disease who are CA 125 negative	
Prostate	PSA	Monitor patients after primary and adjuvant chemotherapy for relapse Monitor patients with metastatic disease	II–III
Male germ line malignancy	β-hCG; AFP	Monitor patients after primary and adjuvant chemotherapy for relapse Monitor patients with metastatic disease	II–III
Female choriocarcinoma	β-hCG	Monitor patients after primary and adjuvant chemotherapy for relapse Monitor patients with metastatic disease	II–III

CA, cancer antigen; CEA, carcinoembryonic antigen; LOE, levels of evidence; PSA, prostate-specific antigen; β-hCG, β–human chorionic gonadotropin; AFP, α-fetoprotein.

References

1. Hayes DF, Bast RC, Desch CE, et al. Tumor marker utility grading system: a framework to evaluate clinical utility of tumor markers. *J Natl Cancer Inst* 1996;88:1456.
2. Slamon DJ, Clark GM, Wong SG, et al. Human breast cancer: Correlation of relapse and survival with amplification of the HER-2/neu oncogene. *Science* 1987;235:177.
3. Slamon DJ, Leyland-Jones B, Shak S, et al. Use of chemotherapy plus a monoclonal antibody against HER2 for metastatic breast cancer that overexpresses HER2. *N Engl J Med* 2001;344:783.
4. Yamauchi H, Stearns V, Hayes DF. When is a tumor marker ready for prime time? A case study of c-erbB-2 as a predictive factor in breast cancer. *J Clin Oncol* 2001;19:2334.
5. Piccart-Gebhart MJ, Procter M, Leyland-Jones B, et al. Trastuzumab after adjuvant chemotherapy in HER2-positive breast cancer. *N Engl J Med* 2005;353:1659.
6. Romond EH, Perez EA, Bryant J, et al. Trastuzumab plus adjuvant chemotherapy for operable HER2-positive breast cancer. *N Engl J Med* 2005; 353:1673.
7. Geyer CE, Forster J, Lindquist D, et al. Lapatinib plus capecitabine for HER2-positive advanced breast cancer. *N Engl J Med* 2006;355:2733.
8. Di Leo A, Gomez HL, Aziz Z, et al. Phase III, double-blind, randomized study comparing lapatinib plus paclitaxel with placebo plus paclitaxel as first-line treatment for metastatic breast cancer. *J Clin Oncol* 2008;26:5544.
9. Slamon D, Godolphin W, Jones L, et al. Studies of the HER-2/neu proto-oncogene in human breast and ovarian cancer. *Science* 1989;244:707.
10. Wolf A, Hammond EH, Schwartz JN, et al. Human epidermal growth factor receptor 2 testing in breast cancer [reply]. *J Clin Oncol* 2007;25:4021.
11. Harris L, Fritsche H, Mennel R, et al. American Society of Clinical Oncology 2007 update of recommendations for the use of tumor markers in breast cancer. *J Clin Oncol* 2007;25:5287
12. Horwich A, Shipley J, Huddart R. Testicular germ-cell cancer. *Lancet* 2006; 367:754.
13. Greco FA, Hainsworth JD. Cancer of unknown primary site. In: DeVita VT Jr, Hellman S, Rosenberg SA, eds. *Cancer: principles and practice of oncology*, 4th ed. Philadelphia: JB Lippincott, 1993:2072.
14. American Joint Committee on Cancer. *AJCC cancer staging manual*, 6th ed. New York, Berlin, Heidelberg: Springer-Verlag, 2009.
15. Early Breast Cancer Trialists' Collaborative Group. Effects of chemotherapy and hormonal therapy for early breast cancer on recurrence and 15-year survival: an overview of the randomised trials. *Lancet* 2005;365:1687.
16. Pritchard KI, Messersmith H, Elavathil L, et al. HER-2 and topoisomerase II as predictors of response to chemotherapy. *J Clin Oncol* 2008;26:736.
17. Hayes DF, Thor AD, Dressler LG, et al. HER2 and response to paclitaxel in node-positive breast cancer. *N Engl J Med* 2007;357:1496.
18. Press MF, Finn RS, Cameron D, et al. HER-2 gene amplification, HER-2 and epidermal growth factor receptor mRNA and protein expression, and lapatinib efficacy in women with metastatic breast cancer. *Clin Cancer Res* 2008;14:7861.
19. Yamauchi H, Stearns V, Hayes DF. The role of c-erbB-2 as a predictive factor in breast cancer. *Breast Cancer* 2001;8:171.
20. Henry NL, Hayes DF. Uses and abuses of tumor markers in the diagnosis, monitoring, and treatment of primary and metastatic breast cancer. *Oncologist* 2006;11:541.
21. Gold P, Freedman SO. Specific carcinoembryonic antigens of the human digestive system. *J Exp Med* 1965;122:467.
22. Locker GY, Hamilton S, Harris J, et al. ASCO 2006 update of recommendations for the use of tumor markers in gastrointestinal cancer. *J Clin Oncol* 2006;24:5313.
23. Hayes DF, Smerage J. Is there a role for circulating tumor cells in the management of breast cancer? *Clin Cancer Res* 2008;14:3646.
24. Gilligan TD, Seidenfeld J, Basch EM, et al. American Society of Clinical Oncology 2009 clinical practice guideline on uses of serum tumor markers in adult males with germ cell tumors. *J Clin Oncol* 2010;28(20):3388.
25. Khatcheressian JL, Wolff AC, Smith TJ, et al. American Society of Clinical Oncology 2006 update of the breast cancer follow-up and management guidelines in the adjuvant setting. *J Clin Oncol* 2006;24:5091.
26. Simon RM, Paik S, Hayes DF: Use of archived specimens in evaluation of prognostic and predictive biomarkers. *J Natl Cancer Inst* 2009;101:1446.
27. Teutsch SM, Bradley LA, Palomaki GE, et al. The Evaluation of Genomic Applications in Practice and Prevention (EGAPP) Initiative: methods of the EGAPP Working Group. *Genet Med* 2009;11:3.
28. Allegra CJ, Jessup JM, Somerfield MR, et al. American Society of Clinical Oncology Provisional Clinical Opinion: testing for KRAS gene mutations in patients with metastatic colorectal carcinoma to predict response to anti-epidermal growth factor receptor monoclonal antibody therapy. *J Clin Oncol* 2009;27(12):2091.
29. Innocenti F, Ratain MJ. Pharmacogenetics of irinotecan: clinical perspectives on the utility of genotyping. *Pharmacogenomics* 2006;7:1211.
30. Stearns V, Johnson MD, Rae JM, et al. Active tamoxifen metabolite plasma concentrations after coadministration of tamoxifen and the selective serotonin reuptake inhibitor paroxetine. *J Natl Cancer Inst* 2003;95:1758.
31. Higgins MJ, Rae JM, Flockhart DA, et al. Pharmacogenetics of tamoxifen: who should undergo CYP2D6 genetic testing? *J Natl Compr Canc Netw* 2009;7:203.

PART EIGHT
PRACTICE OF ONCOLOGY

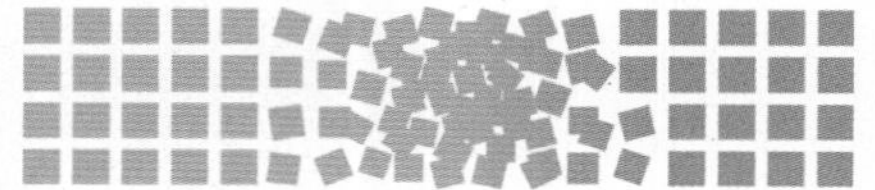

CHAPTER 70 DESIGN AND ANALYSIS OF CLINICAL TRIALS

RICHARD SIMON

Clinical trials are experiments. The purpose of a therapeutic clinical trial is to determine the value of a treatment. There are two key components to the experimental approach. First, results rather than plausible reasoning are required to support conclusions. Second, experiments should be prospectively planned and conducted under controlled conditions to provide definitive answers to well-defined questions. Using tumor registry data to compare the survival rates of prostate cancer patients treated with surgery with those of patients receiving radiotherapy is an example of an *observational study*, not a clinical trial. In an observational study, the investigators are passive observers. Treatment assignments, staging workup, and follow-up procedures are out of the control of the investigators and are conducted with no considerations about the validity of the subsequent attempt at comparison. The statistical associations resulting from such studies are, consequently, a weak basis for causal inferences about relationships between the treatments administered and the outcomes observed. Treatments are usually selected on the basis of subjective assessment of the prognosis of the patient, specialties of the physician, and diagnostic evaluations. Unknown patient selection factors generally are more important determinants of patient outcome than are differences between treatments. For example, Subramanian and Simon[1] found that, in observational studies that developed gene expression prognostic signatures for early stage non–small cell lung cancer patients, those who received chemotherapy had poorer survivals than those who did not, even after adjusting for all recorded prognostic factors.

Clinical trials require careful planning. The first result of the planning process is a written protocol. Typical subject headings for the protocol are shown in Table 70.1, and the protocol development process is discussed in more detail by Green et al.[2] The protocol should define treatment and evaluation policies for a well-defined set of patients. It also should define the specific questions to be answered by the study and should directly justify that the number of patients and the nature of the controls are adequate to answer these questions. Some clinical trials are really only guidelines for clinical management supplemented by lofty objectives with no scientific meaning and no realistic chance of providing a reliable answer to a well-defined medical question. Such studies are a disservice to the patients who are undergoing some inconvenience to contribute to the welfare of future patients.

PHASE 1 CLINICAL TRIALS

The main objectives of phase 1 trials have traditionally been to determine a dose that is appropriate for use in phase 2 and 3 trials and to determine information about the pharmacokinetics of distribution of the drug. Patients with advanced disease that is resistant to standard therapy but who have normal organ function are usually included in such trials.

Drugs in phase 1 trials are usually initiated at a low dose that is not expected to produce serious toxicity. A starting dose of one-tenth the lethal dose (expressed as milligrams per square meter of body surface area) in the most sensitive species is usually used.[3] The dose is increased for subsequent patients according to a series of preplanned steps. Dose escalation for subsequent patients occurs only after sufficient time has passed to observe acute toxic effects for patients treated at lower doses. Cohorts of three to six patients are treated at each dose level. Usually, if no dose-limiting toxicity (DLT) is seen at a given dose level, the dose is escalated for the next cohort. If the incidence of DLT is 33%, then three more patients are treated at the same level. If no further cases of DLT are seen in the additional patients, then the dose level is escalated for the next cohort. Otherwise, dose escalation stops. If the incidence of DLT is greater than 33% at a given level, then dose escalation also stops. The phase 2 recommended dose often is taken as the highest dose for which the incidence of DLT is less than 33%. Usually, six or more patients are treated at the recommended dose.

The dose levels themselves are commonly based on a modified Fibonacci series. The second level is twice the starting dose, the third level is 67% greater than the second, the fourth level is 50% greater than the third, the fifth is 40% greater than the fourth, and each subsequent step is 33% greater than that preceding it. Escalating doses for subsequent courses in the same patient are generally not done, except at low doses before any DLT has been encountered.

Accelerated Titration Designs

There is no compelling scientific basis for the approach just outlined, except that experience has shown it to be safe. Traditional phase 1 trials have three limitations:

1. They sometimes expose too many patients to subtherapeutic doses of the new drug.
2. The trials may take a long time to complete.
3. They provide very limited information about interpatient variability and cumulative toxicity.

New trial designs have been developed to address these problems.[4] The *accelerated titration designs*[5] permit within-patient dose escalation and use only one patient per dose level until grade 2 or greater toxicity is seen. Doses are titrated within patients to achieve grade 2toxicity. The analysis consists of fitting a statistical model to the full set of data that includes all grades of toxicity for all courses of a patient's treatment. The model includes parameters that represent the steepness of the dose-toxicity curve, the degree of interpatient variability in the location of the dose-toxicity curve, and the degree (if any) of cumulative toxicity. All these parameters are estimated from the data.

TABLE 70.1

SUBJECT HEADINGS FOR A PROTOCOL

Introduction and scientific background
Objectives
Selection of patients
Design of study (including schematic diagram)
Treatment plan
Drug information
Toxicities to be monitored and dosage modifications
Required clinical and laboratory data and study calendar
Criteria for evaluating the effect of treatment and end point definition
Statistical considerations
Informed consent and regulatory considerations
Data forms
References
Study chairperson, collaborating participants, addresses, and telephone numbers

In developing the accelerated titration designs, Simon et al.[5] fit a stochastic model to data from 20 phase 1 trials of 9 different drugs. New data were then simulated using the model with the parameters estimated from the actual trials, and the performance of alternative phase 1 designs on this simulated data was evaluated. Design 1 was a conventional design using cohorts of three to six patients with 40% dose-step increments and no intrapatient dose escalation. Design 2 uses conventional 40% dose steps during the initial accelerated phase, whereas designs 3 and 4 use 100% dose steps until one patient experiences DLT or two patients experience grade 2 toxicity. At that point, acceleration ceases and standard cohorts of three to six patients with 40% dose-step increments are used.

In the 20 phase 1 trials initially evaluated, only 3 showed any evidence of cumulative toxicity. The average number of patients required was reduced from 39.9 for the standard design to 24.4, 20.7, and 21.2 for designs 2, 3, and 4, respectively. The average number of patients who had grade 0 to 1 toxicity as their worst toxicity grade over three cycles of treatment was 23.3 for design 1 but only 7.9, 3.9, and 4.8 for designs 2, 3, and 4, respectively. The average number of patients with a worst toxicity grade of 3 increased from 5.5 for design 1 to 6.2, 6.8, and 6.2 for designs 2, 3, and 4, respectively. The average number of patients with a worst toxicity grade of 4 increased from 1.9 for design 1 to 3.0, 4.3, and 3.2 for designs 2, 3, and 4, respectively. Accelerated titration designs appear to be effective in reducing the number of patients necessary for finding the maximum-tolerated dose, for reducing the number who are undertreated, and for providing increased information. They do not necessarily reduce the length of time necessary for completion of the trial. They increase the information yield if investigators analyze the results of the trial using the model developed by Simon et al.[5] Software for fitting the model is available at http://brb.nci.nih.gov. Software for determining dose assignments and for recording the data in a spreadsheet format are also available at that Website. The model of Simon et al. uses actual worst grade toxicity for each course of treatment of each patient and it enables one to determine whether there is cumulative toxicity and to estimate the variability among patients in toxic effects. The use of the accelerated titration design has recently been reviewed.[6,7]

Other Methods

O'Quigley et al.[8] used a dose-toxicity model to guide the dose escalation, as well as to determine the maximum tolerated dose. A Bayesian prior distribution is established for the steepness of the dose-toxicity curve and the distribution is updated after each patient is treated. The model is based on using only first-course treatment data and whether the patient experiences DLT. This approach is called the *continual reassessment method*. For each new patient, the model is used to determine the dose predicted to cause DLT to a specified percentage of the patients. That dose is assigned to the next patient. Many modifications of the original continual reassessment method have been subsequently proposed.[9–11]

For some tumor vaccines and molecularly targeted drugs, toxicity may not be dose-limiting[12] and the dose selected may be based on preclinical findings or on practical considerations. For some molecularly targeted drugs, preclinical studies provide a target serum concentration of the active moiety necessary to maximally inhibit the target, and drug administration can be titrated for each patient to the targeted serum concentration. This approach can be complex because it involves developing a population pharmacokinetic model relating dose to concentration as the study progresses. A simpler approach is to have separate cohorts of patients who are treated at each of several dose levels without intrapatient dose titration. A population pharmacokinetic model relating dose to concentration is fit to the data.

Ideally, a trial design should provide the smallest dose that gives maximum biologic effect. For molecularly targeted therapeutics, the biologic effect might be a measure of the degree of inhibition of the target. Because it can be very difficult to obtain tumor samples before and after treatment, biologic effect is sometimes measured in an accessible surrogate tissue, such as peripheral blood lymphocytes or skin, or by using functional imaging.[13] For therapeutic vaccines, the biologic effect might be a measure of stimulation of tumor reactive T cells.

Finding the dose that provides maximum biological effect is often not practical in a phase 1 trial, as it may require a large number of patients. For example, to have 90% power for detecting a 1 standard error difference in mean response between two dose levels at a one-sided 10% significance level requires 14 patients per dose level. A more limited objective is to identify a dose that is biologically active. Korn et al.[14] developed a sequential procedure for finding such a dose when the measure of biologic response is binary. During an initial accelerated phase they treat one patient per dose level until a biologic response is seen. Then, they treat cohorts of three to six patients per dose level. With 0 to 1 biologic responses among three patients at a dose level, they escalate to the next level. With 2 to 3 responses among three patients, they expand the cohort to six patients. With 5 to 6 biologic responses from the six patients, they declare that dose to be the biologically active level and terminate the trial. With four or fewer biologic responses at a level, they continue to escalate.

Designs have recently been developed for phase 0 proof-of-concept trials.[15,16] Patients are treated with single doses of a new drug at very low concentrations not expected to cause toxicity. This enables the investigator obtain an early assessment of whether the molecular target of the drug is being inhibited by measuring a pharmacodynamic end point before and after drug administration. These trials require prior development of an assay for measuring the pharmacodynamic end point and an adequate database for estimating the variability of measurement for independent tissue samples of the same patient. This estimate should reflect variability of tissue sampling as well as technical variability of the assay. The approach developed depends on having a good estimate of assay variability and in having assay sufficiently reproducible to be able to reliably classify individual patients as responders or nonresponders based on the observed change in the level of the pharmacodynamic end point. The designs described by Rubinstein et al.[16] use a small number of patients for establishing whether the drug causes target inhibition in a substantial proportion of patients

PHASE 2 CLINICAL TRIALS

Patient Selection

Phase 2 trials have traditionally been performed separately by tumor type in patients with the least amount of prior therapy for whom no effective therapy is available. With cytotoxics, full-dose chemotherapy is often impossible in patients debilitated by prior treatment, and lack of chemotherapeutic activity in previously treated patients may not indicate lack of clinical usefulness in earlier disease. The development of molecularly targeted drugs has introduced new complexities with regard to selection and evaluation of patients for phase 2 trials. When the target of the drug is clearly known, it may be more appropriate to select patients based on target expression than based on primary site of disease. Even if target expression is not used as an eligibility criterion, the drug should be evaluated in an adequate number of patients whose tumors express the target. Consequently, it is important to have an adequate assay for the target available at the time that phase 2 development begins.

In many cases, the drug will have multiple targets; there may be several candidate assays available for each target. Expression of the target often will prove to be only part of the relevant genomic information. For example, the effectiveness of anti-*EGFR* antibodies cetuximab and panitumumab turned out to depend on whether the tumor had an activating *K-RAS* mutation.[17–19]

Whereas the major objective of phase 2 trials have traditionally been to identify the primary tumor sites in which a new drug was active, a new important objective is to develop promising predictive biomarkers that identify the patients whose tumors are most (or least) likely to respond to the drug. The phase 2 development stage is also the time to select the assay(s) that will be used in the phase 3 trials of the new drug and to define the criteria that will be used to either select patients for such trials or to structure the analysis, as will be described later in this chapter.

It is often undesirable to restrict entry to phase 2 trials based on what one thinks one knows about the drug target, at least in cases where this knowledge is uncertain. It is important, however, to ensure that the activity of the drug is not missed because the phase 2 trials did not accrue enough of the right kinds of patients. The decision of whether or not to restrict entry based on the presumed mechanism of action will depend in part on the adverse effects of the drug.

If tumor specimens are archived for the patients entered on broad eligibility phase 2 trials, then one avoids the need to develop assays in advance for all candidate targets, but it is not possible to ensure adequate accrual for subsets of patients whose tumors are positive for the candidate markers. Pusztai et al.[20] described a hybrid approach that begins with conducting a standard single-arm, two-stage design for evaluating whether the overall response rate for unrestricted patients is sufficiently large. If the overall response rate is sufficient in the first stage of the standard phase 2 trial, then the second stage is completed with accrual of additional unrestricted patients. If there are too few responses overall in the first stage, then one starts a two-stage phase 2 study restricting entry to patients who have positive markers. If there are multiple markers of interest, then one restricts entry to patients positive for one of the markers and ensures that each marker has sufficient number of positive patients for evaluation. LeBlanc et al.[21] have described how multiple primary sites can be incorporated in a single-phase 2 trial.

In some cases, the list of candidate targets can be narrowed using mRNA transcript expression profiling of the pretreatment specimens. By comparing pretreatment expression levels of responders to nonresponders, one can potentially prioritize targets for assay development. If one does not have a good list of candidate targets, genomewide expression profiling can be used to develop a classifier of the tumors likely to respond to the drug. Dobbin et al.[22] have provided sample size guidelines for genomewide expression profiling studies and generally recommend at least 20 responders for developing a classifier. Pusztai et al.[20] performed a computer simulation study to indicate that *HER2* transcript overexpression would have been missed as a predictive biomarker for treatment of advanced breast cancer with trastuzumab in whole-genome expression profiling with only five responders to analyze. They recommend analysis based on candidate genes if the number of responders is very limited.

Single-Arm Phase 2 Trials

Single Agents

For most single-agent phase 2 trials, the objective is simply to determine whether the drug has activity against the tumor type in question. For this objective, response rate based on the RECIST guidelines may provide a satisfactory approach.[23] A variety of statistical accrual plans and sample size methods have been developed for single-arm phase 2 trials. One of the most popular approaches is the optimal two-stage design.[24] n_1-evaluable patients are entered into study in the first stage of the trial. If no more than r_1 responses are obtained among these n_1 patients, then accrual terminates and the drug is rejected as being of little interest. Otherwise, accrual continues to a total of n-evaluable patients. At the end of the second stage, the drug is rejected if the observed response rate is less than or equal to r/n, where r and n are determined by the design used.

Tables 70.2 and 70.3 illustrate some of these optimized designs, and a Web-based interactive computer program is available at http://linus.nci.nih.gov/brb. To select a design, the investigator specifies the target activity level of interest, p_1, and also a lower activity level, p_0, representing inadequate activity. The first row of each triplet of optimal designs provides designs with probability 0.10 of accepting drugs worse than p_0 and probability 0.10 of rejecting drugs better than p_1. Subject to these two constraints, the optimal designs minimize the average sample size. The average sample size is calculated at the lower activity level p_0 to optimize protection of patients from exposure to inactive drugs. The tables show for each design the optimal values of r_1, n_1, r, and n; the average sample size; and the probability of stopping after the first stage for a drug with activity level p_0.

These tables also show the "minimax" designs, which provide the smallest maximum sample size n that satisfies the two constraints just described. Although minimax designs have somewhat larger average sample sizes than do optimal designs, in some instances they are preferable because the small increase in average sample size is more than compensated for by a large reduction in maximum sample size.

The designs shown in Tables 70.2 and 70.3 are two-stage designs with the potential for early stopping for lack of activity. Optimized three-stage designs have been described by Ensign et al.[25] Others have extended the design to incorporate toxicity or tumor progression information.[26–28]

Some authors have recommended use of progression-free survival instead of response[29] for evaluating molecularly targeted drugs that may be cytostatic. Single-arm phase 2 trials can be designed using Tables 70.2 and 70.3 for testing whether the proportion of patients with stable disease at a specified landmark time like 12 months after the start of

TABLE 70.2

SIMON TWO-STAGE PHASE 2 DESIGNS FOR $p_1 - p_0 = .20^a$

		Optimal Design				Minimax Design			
		Reject Drug if Response Rate				Reject Drug if Response Rate			
p_0	p_1	r_1/n_1	r/n	EN (p_0)	PET (p_0)	r_1/n_1	r/n	EN (p_0)	PET (p_0)
.05	.25	0/9	2/24	14.5	.63	0/13	2/20	16.4	.51
		0/9	2/17	12.0	.63	0/12	2/16	13.8	.54
		0/9	3/30	16.8	.63	0/15	3/25	20.4	.46
.10	.30	1/12	5/35	19.8	.65	1/16	4/25	20.4	.51
		1/10	5/29	15.0	.74	1/15	5/25	19.5	.55
		2/18	6/36	22.5	.71	2/22	6/23	26.2	.62
.20	.40	3/17	10/37	26.0	.55	3/19	10/36	28.2	.46
		3/13	12/43	20.6	.75	4/18	10/33	22.3	.50
		4/19	15/54	30.4	.67	5/24	13/45	31.2	.66
.30	.50	7/22	17/46	29.9	.67	7/28	15/39	35.0	.36
		5/15	18/46	23.6	.72	6/19	16/39	25.7	.48
		8/24	24/63	34.7	.73	7/24	21/53	36.6	.56
.40	.60	7/18	22/46	30.2	.56	11/28	20/41	33.8	.55
		7/16	23/46	24.5	.72	17/34	20/39	34.4	.91
		11/25	32/66	36.0	.73	12/29	27/54	38.1	.64
.50	.70	11/21	26/45	29.0	.67	11/23	23/39	31.0	.50
		8/15	26/43	23.5	.70	12/23	23/37	27.7	.66
		13/24	36/61	34.0	.73	14/27	32/53	36.1	.65
.60	.80	6/11	26/38	25.4	.47	18/27	24/35	28.5	.82
		7/11	30/43	20.5	.70	8/13	25/35	20.8	.65
		12/19	37/53	29.5	.69	15/26	32/45	35.9	.48
.70	.90	6/9	22/28	17.8	.54	11/16	20/25	20.1	.55
		4/6	22/27	14.8	.58	19/23	21/26	23.2	.95
		11/15	29/36	21.2	.70	13/18	26/32	22.7	.67

[a]For each value of (p_0, p_1), designs are given for three sets of error probabilities (α, β). The first, second, and third rows correspond to error probability limits (.10, .10), (.05, .20), and (.05, .10), respectively. α is the probability of accepting a drug with response probability p_0. β is the probability of rejecting a drug with response probability p_1. For each design, EN (p_0) and PET (p_0) denote the expected sample size and the probability of early termination when the true response probability is p_0.

treatment is greater than a specified value p_0, but that is only meaningful if the value p_0 is a stable, robust, and well-characterized stable disease rate that results from multiple large studies with control regimens. Single-arm studies using stable disease are rarely planned or analyzed with that care, and hence conclusions of single-arm phase 2 trials claiming that molecularly targeted agents cause disease stabilization are often dubious.[30] Vidaurre et al.[30] have questioned, however, whether molecularly targeted drugs are any more cytostatic than conventional chemotherapy drugs. El-Maraghi and Eisenhauer[31] have also recommended that objective response is a useful end point for screening molecularly targeted agents.

Combination Regimens

Determination of whether a new drug adds anticancer activity to an active regimen is inherently comparative. In using Tables 70.2 and 70.3 to design a single-arm trial, p_0 should represent the level of activity of existing standard regimens. If this response probability is not well determined, however, because it varies among studies and varies based on patient prognostic factors, then a single-arm trial based on an assumed known p_0 may not be appropriate.

Several approaches to single-arm study design have been developed that attempt to either account for or control the variability in p_0. One approach to controlling this variability is to base the analysis of the single-arm trial on comparison to a specific set of control patients, matched for prognostic factors, and treated at the same institution as those for the new study. This can be a better approach than just using an assumed known value of p_0 as previously described, but it still assumes that adjustment for known prognostic factors is sufficient to ensure comparability. Although such historical control comparisons are not considered reliable enough to eliminate the need for phase 3 trials, if done carefully, they may provide an adequate basis for decisions about which new regimens are worthy of phase 3 evaluation.

For comparative trials of response rates using specific historical controls, the sample size should be planned using the formulas appropriate for randomized clinical trials. By inserting the number of historical controls to be used, one can compute the number of patients needed to treat on the new regimen in the single-arm phase 2 trial.[32] For binary end point data, the results of these calculations are presented in Table 70.4 for 80% power with a one-sided 10% significance level. The tabulated entries indicate that a 25 percentage point difference can be detected with fewer than 40 new patients if there are at least 30 appropriate historical controls.

TABLE 70.3

SIMON TWO-STAGE PHASE 2 DESIGNS FOR $p_1 - p_0 = .15^a$

		Optimal Design				Minimax Design			
		Reject Drug if Response Rate				Reject Drug if Response Rate			
p_0	p_1	r_1/n_1	r/n	EN (p_0)	PET (p_0)	r_1/n_1	r/n	EN (p_0)	PET (p_0)
.05	.20	0/12	3/37	23.5	.54	0/18	3/32	26.4	.40
		0/10	3/29	17.6	.60	0/13	3/27	19.8	.51
		1/21	4/41	26.7	.72	1/29	4/38	32.9	.57
.10	.25	2/21	7/50	31.2	.65	2/27	6/40	33.7	.48
		2/18	7/43	24.7	.73	2/22	7/40	28.8	.62
		2/21	10/66	36.8	.65	3/31	9/55	40.0	.62
.20	.35	5/27	16/63	43.6	.54	6/33	15/58	45.5	.50
		5/22	19/72	35.4	.73	6/31	15/53	40.4	.57
		8/37	22/83	51.4	.69	8/42	21/77	58.4	.53
.30	.45	9/30	29/82	51.4	.59	16/50	25/69	56.0	.68
		9/27	30/81	41.7	.73	16/46	25/65	49.6	.81
		13/40	40/110	60.8	.70	27/77	33/88	78.5	.86
.40	.55	16/38	40/88	54.5	.67	18/45	34/73	57.2	.56
		11/26	40/84	44.9	.67	28/59	34/70	60.1	.90
		19/45	49/104	64.0	.68	24/62	45/94	78.9	.47
.50	.65	18/35	47/84	53.0	.63	19/40	41/72	58.0	.44
		15/28	48/83	43.7	.71	39/66	40/68	66.1	.95
		22/42	60/105	62.3	.68	28/57	54/93	75.0	.50
.60	.75	21/34	47/71	47.1	.65	25/43	43/64	54.4	.46
		17/27	46/67	39.4	.69	18/30	43/62	43.8	.57
		21/34	64/95	55.6	.65	48/72	57/84	73.2	.90
.70	.85	14/20	45/59	36.2	.58	15/22	40/52	36.8	.51
		14/19	46/59	30.3	.72	16/23	39/49	34.4	.56
		18/25	61/79	43.4	.66	33/44	53/68	48.5	.81
.80	.95	5/7	27/31	20.8	.42	5/7	27/31	20.8	.42
		7/9	26/29	17.7	.56	7/9	26/29	17.7	.56
		16/19	37/42	24.4	.76	31/35	35/40	35.3	.94

[a]For each value of (p_0, p_1), designs are given for three sets of error probabilities (α, β). The first, second, and third rows correspond to error probability limits (.10, .10), (.05, .20), and (.05, .10), respectively. α is the probability of accepting a drug with response probability p_0. β is the probability of rejecting a drug with response probability p_1. For each design, EN (p_0) and PET (p_0) denote the expected sample size and the probability of early termination when the true response probability is p_0.

The table entries indicate that detecting a 15 percentage point difference is almost never feasible with this single-arm approach and that detecting a 20 percentage point difference generally requires at least 50 appropriate historical controls and up to 60 or more new patients.

Thall et al.[33] and Estey and Thall[34] have developed and used Bayesian methods for planning and conducting single-institution trials comparing one or more new regimens to a specific set of historical controls who received a control treatment at the same institution. The Bayesian designs provide for continual analysis of results with either tumor response or time to event end points or for joint monitoring of efficacy and toxicity. Their methods require a substantial number of patients who have been treated on protocol with an appropriate control regimen and who have been staged comparably to the patients to be treated with the new regimen.

Korn et al.[35] developed an approach for using historical control data in phase 2 multicenter trials of metastatic melanoma. They reviewed 42 previous phase 2 trials in melanoma conducted by the U.S. cancer cooperative oncology groups. They found that after adjustment for performance status, sex, presence of visceral disease, and presence of brain metastases, there was little interstudy variability in survival among the arms of the phase 2 trials. Consequently, for any single-arm phase 2 trial of metastatic melanoma, one can use their results in conjunction with the prognostic makeup of the patients in the new study, to synthesize a benchmark overall survival curve or a benchmark 1-year overall survival rate for use in evaluating the new regimen. They provide an example of planning a phase 2 trial using this approach that required 72 patients to have 85% to 90% power for detecting a 15 percentage point improvement in the 1-year overall survival rate with a one-sided type 1 error of 10%. They found that this approach was less satisfactory for use with progression-free survival because interstudy variability remained substantial after adjustment for prognostic factors.

Mick et al.[36] proposed that the time to progression of a patient on a phase 2 trial be compared with the time to progression of the same patient on his or her previous trial. The ratio of these times was called a *growth modulation index*, and the agent was considered active if the index was greater than 1.3 on average. In practice, however, follow-up intervals on different protocols are different and there may be substantial variability and bias in computing the ratio of progression times. As tumors

TABLE 70.4

NUMBER OF PATIENTS TO TREAT IN SINGLE-ARM PHASE 2 TRIAL USING HISTORICAL CONTROLS AND BINARY END POINT[a]

Proportion of Success for Historical Controls	Number of Historical Controls				
	30	40	50	75	100
0.10	94[b]	69	59	50	46
	36	32	30	28	27
	21	20	19	18	18
0.20	c	226	126	80	67
	68	49	43	36	33
	29	25	24	21	21
0.30	c	c	307	113	86
	132	69	54	41	37
	36	29	26	23	21
0.40	c	c	c	137	95
	267	83	59	43	37
	39	29	25	22	20
0.50	c	c	c	136	91
	370	80	54	38	33
	34	25	22	18	17
0.60	c	c	910	104	72
	178	56	39	28	25
	22	17	14	12	12

[a]One-sided significance level of 10% and power of 80%.
[b]First entry is number of new patients required to detect 15 percentage point difference. Second and third entries are for detecting 20 and 25 percentage point differences, respectively.
[c]Number of required new patients exceeds 1,000..

grow larger, the doubling time may increase, and hence in some cases the chance of false-positive findings may be inflated.[37]

Randomized Phase 2 Trials

Time till tumor progression or disease-free survival has been recommended for evaluation of single-agent phase 2 trials of drugs that may be cytostatic and for trials adding a new drug to an active regimen. Even single-agent phase 2 trials of cytotoxics have been criticized on the basis that they do not provide much evidence that the drug will be able to prolong survival when incorporated into a regimen with other active drugs. Demonstrating that the regimen incorporating the new drug prolongs progression-free survival compared with the control regimen may provide a stronger basis for conducting a phase 3 trial of the new regimen.

Simon et al.[12] suggested two key design differences between such randomized phase 2 designs and phase 3 designs. A randomized phase 2 design may use an end point that is a sensitive indicator of antitumor effect although it may not be an acceptable phase 3 end point that directly reflects patient benefit. Such an end point does not need to be "validated." It is not claimed to be a valid surrogate for survival; no regulatory approval or practice standard decisions should be based on the phase 2 trials using such an intermediate end point. The purpose of the phase 2 trial is merely to determine whether to conduct a phase 3 trial that will evaluate the new regimen with an accepted phase 3 end point The phase 2 trial may also serve to optimize the regimen that might be carried forward to phase 3 and to provide information about the best target population. The second key difference noted by Simon et al. is that the type I error "alpha level" for planning and analyzing the phase 2 trial can be increased from the two-sided 5% level used for phase 3 trials. By letting this alpha level increase to a one-sided 10%, meaningful savings in number of patients required can be achieved.

How large should a randomized phase 2 design comparing a new treatment to a control regimen be? Consider for example a randomized phase 3 trial comparing a new regimen with a control in a patient population in which the median time to progression on the control is 6 months and the median survival is 2 years. A 25% reduction in the hazard of death amounts to a 4 month prolongation of median survival with exponential distributions. A phase 3 trial with 90% statistical power for detecting this effect at a two-sided 5% significance level would require about 510 deaths (see Table 70.7). With an average follow-up time of 2 years, 50% of the patients would have events, so the number of patients required for randomization would be just in excess of 1,000. A randomized phase 2 trial with 90% power for detecting a 33% reduction in hazard of progression corresponding to a 2-month increase in median progression-free survival at a one-sided 10% significance level would require observing 164 progression events (Table 70.5). With an average follow-up time of 2 years, over 90% would have progression events, so a sample size of 180 total randomized patients would

PRACTICE OF ONCOLOGY

TABLE 70.5

NUMBER OF TOTAL EVENTS TO OBSERVE IN TWO-ARM RANDOMIZED PHASE 2 TRIAL BASED ON PROGRESSION-FREE SURVIVAL

Reduction in Hazard (%)	Ratio of Medians	Equal Randomization				2:1 Randomization[a]			
		$\alpha = 0.05$[b]		$\alpha = 0.10$[b]		$\alpha = 0.05$[b]		$\alpha = 0.10$[b]	
		Power = .8	Power = .9	Power = .8	Power = .9	Power = .8	Power = .9	Power = .8	Power = .9
25	1.33	301	417	219	319	339	469	246	358
30	1.43	195	270	141	206	219	303	159	232
33	1.5	155	215	113	164	175	242	127	185
40	1.67	96	132	70	101	108	149	78	114
50	2.0	52	72	38	55	59	81	43	62

[a]Two-thirds of patients are randomized to the new treatment group.
[b]One-sided significance level.

TABLE 70.6

NUMBER OF PATIENTS IN EACH ARM OF RANDOMIZED PHASE 2 TRIAL PROPORTION WITHOUT PROGRESSION AT T IN CONTROL ARM TO NEW TREATMENT ARM[a]

T Month DFS for Control Group	5% One-Sided Significance Level Increase in T Month DFS				10% One-Sided Significance Level Increase in T Month DFS			
	0.10	0.15	0.20	0.25	0.10	0.15	0.20	0.25
0.05	129	72	48	35	99	56	38	28
0.10	176	91	58	41	133	70	45	32
0.15	216	108	66	46	163	82	51	36
0.20	250	121	73	50	188	92	56	39
0.25	278	132	79	53	208	100	60	41
0.30	300	141	83	55	224	106	63	42
0.35	315	146	85	56	235	110	65	43
0.40	324	149	86	56	243	112	65	43

DFS, disease-free survival.
[a]80% statistical power.

suffice. Accrual to the randomized phase 2 study could potentially be stopped early based on futility monitoring if results are not promising for the new regimen. The results in Table 70.5 show that if an imbalanced randomization is used in which two-thirds of the patients are randomized to the new treatment, then the number of progression events needed increases to 185 instead of 164. So although a larger total sample size would be required, somewhat fewer patients would receive the control regimen.

The randomized phase 2 design with control regimen has also been discussed by Korn et al.[38] and by Rubinstein et al.[39] Randomized phase 2 trials can require fewer patients than phase 3 trials, but they generally require more patients than single-arm phase 2 trials. Nevertheless, they are generally necessary for evaluating time to event end points or for evaluating combination regimens. Table 70.6 shows the number of patients required for randomized phase 2 trials where the primary end point is either response rate or the proportion of patients without progression by a specified landmark time.

Randomized Screening Designs

Phase 2 trials are generally viewed as a means of determining whether a particular regimen is worthy of phase 3 evaluation. They can, however, be viewed as ways to screen a wide range of new regimens in order to select those most promising for phase 3 evaluation. Traditional single-arm phase 2 designs are problematic for screening when there is substantial interstudy variation in patient selection and outcome evaluation. Simon et al.[40] proposed the randomized phase 2 design in which multiple new regimens are randomized against each other as one way of avoiding such interstudy variability in prioritizing the candidate regimens. This randomized design can provide more interpretable results if it also incorporates a control arm. This design is more efficient than separate randomized phase 2 trials because the control arm does not have to be replicated in all of the randomized phase 2 trials. Using the example previously described, if it takes 90 patients per arm to conduct a randomized phase 2 trial, instead of $180 \times 5 = 900$ patients to conduct randomized phase 2 trials of five new regimens, one would require only $90 \times 6 = 540$ patients, a savings of 40%. The savings in number of patients can be even more dramatic if one takes the position that the objective is not to evaluate all five new regimens, but rather the select the best one and determine whether it is worthy of phase 3 evaluation. For this selection objective, one does not require 90 patients per arm.[40] These designs have been discussed and extended by others.[41–44]

Simon et al.[12] showed that one can take advantage of the nontoxic nature of some molecularly targeted drugs to efficiently evaluate multiple regimens in the same study. They propose using a factorial design in which concurrent randomizations are made for each drugs. For example, if there are three drugs (A, B, C) being evaluated, then some patients will receive all three, some will receive pairs (AB, AC, or BC), some will receive single drugs (A, B, C), and one group will receive none of the drugs. In evaluating each drug, the time to progressions for all patients receiving that drug are compared with the times for all patients not receiving that drug. The trial can be sized as if it were a single two-arm trial. The design is effective as long as there are not negative interactions among drugs. Negative interactions would result from the toxicity of one drug interfering with the full dose administration of other drugs, which may not be a problem for many molecularly targeted drugs. The design is also useful for attempting to identify combinations that are therapeutically synergistic, a circumstance of particular importance with molecularly targeted drugs.

Rosner et al.[45] describe a "randomized discontinuation design" for phase 2 studies of therapeutically targeted drugs. All eligible patients are administered the drug and given two to four courses of treatment. Patients are then evaluated: Those with progression are removed from study, those with objective tumor response are continued on treatment, and the remaining patients are randomized to either continue or discontinue the drug. The continued and discontinued groups of randomized patients are compared with regard to time to progression. Freidlin and Simon[46] evaluated and further developed this design. It may require as large a number of patients started on treatment as a straightforward randomized phase 2 design. The advantage of the design is that because all patients begin the new regimen, accrual rate may be better with the randomized discontinuation design.

Seamless Phase 2/3 Designs

Hunsberger, Zhao and Simon developed a design for a seamless phase 2/3 design. Patients are randomized between a new regimen and control. An interim analysis is performed using a phase 2 end point such as response rate or time to progression to decide whether the results with the new treatment as sufficiently promising to continue to a phase 3 sample size. If accrual continues, then the final analysis is performed using an acceptable phase 3 end point. A similar approach was described by Goldman et al.[47] Phase 2/3 designs using Bayesian methods have been discussed by Inoue et al.[48] and by Thall.[49] Sher and Heller[50] proposed conducting phase 3 trials with multiple experimental regimens, a control arm, and early termination of all experimental arms that are not promising. They used the statistical design of Schaid et al.[51] for time to event data. Thall et al.[52] had studied such designs when the end point was binary. A similar approach was recently recommended by Parmar et al.[53] Freidlin et al.[54] have discussed statistical and practical aspects of conducting clinical trials with a control arm and multiple new treatment arms.

DESIGN OF PHASE 3 CLINICAL TRIALS

Good therapeutic research requires asking important questions and getting reliable answers. The most important clinical trials are often the most difficult to conduct.[55] They may involve withholding a treatment established by tradition, potentially transferring patient management responsibility across specialties, standardizing procedures among physicians who believe that their way is best, and sharing recognition with a large group of collaborators.

End Points

Phase 3 trials attempt to provide guidance to practicing physicians to help them make treatment decisions with their patients. Consequently, the trials should provide reliable information concerning end points of relevance to the patients. The major end points for evaluating the effectiveness of a treatment should be direct measures of patient welfare. Survival and symptom control are two such end points. The latter is not routinely used because of the difficulty of measuring it reliably and because it may be influenced by concomitant treatments.

Although durable complete regression of metastatic disease is usually a good surrogate for prolonged survival, partial tumor shrinkage usually is not an appropriate end point for phase 3 trials. Torri et al.[56] performed a meta-analysis of the relationship between difference in response rates and difference in median survivals for randomized clinical trials of advanced ovarian carcinoma. They found that large improvements in response rates corresponded to very small improvements in median survival. Hence, use of response rate as an end point results in giving patients increasingly intensive and toxic therapy with little or no net benefit to them. Proper validation of an end point as a surrogate for clinical benefit requires a series of randomized clinical trials in which treatment differences with regard to the candidate surrogate are related to treatment differences with regard to clinical benefit.[57–59] It is not sufficient to show that clinical outcome is related to the candidate surrogate measured on the same treatment arm as this may just reflect the known responder versus nonresponder bias.

Disease-free survival is often accepted as an important measure of clinical benefit to be used as an end point for adjuvant treatment trials. There is more controversy, however, about the use of time to progression in metastatic disease trials. The controversy relates to whether prolonged time to progression provides clinical benefit and whether it can be measured without bias. With unblinded evaluation of time to progression there could be a reduced threshold for declaring progression for control patients so that they can cross over to the new treatment.[60] Central party blinded review of progression is often used to avoid such potential bias. Because the review is not performed in real-time, however, it can introduce additional biases of "informative censoring." Freidlin et al.[61] proposed an approach to adjusting for increased surveillance of the control group. Dodd et al.[62] proposed that central review be performed only for a subset of patients to evaluate whether local assessments were biased, not to replace local assessments.

Patient Eligibility

To ensure that the results of phase 3 trials are applicable to patients seen in the community outside the clinical research settings, the trials themselves involve numerous centers and extensive community participation. In order to ensure broad generalization of conclusions, most multicenter phase 3 trials have employed broad eligibility criteria. In the United Kingdom, many trials are designed using the *uncertainty principle*, an approach that leaves much of the decision making about eligibility to the treating physician. There may be guidelines for eligibility, but the ultimate decision is made by the treating physician; if he or she is uncertain about which treatment is more appropriate for the patient, then the patient is eligible.

There is a growing recognition, however, that one of the key hallmarks of cancer is intertumor heterogeneity. Tumors that arise in the same primary site are often quite different with regard to their oncogenesis, pathophysiology, and drug sensitivity. Consequently, conducting broad eligibility clinical trials with drugs expected to be effective for most patients is in many cases no longer an appropriate research strategy.[63–65] Particularly with molecularly targeted drugs, effectiveness is likely to be limited to a sensitive subset of tumors. Even with cytotoxics, many patients are generally treated for each patient who benefits. The high cost of many molecularly targeted drugs makes this approach increasingly unsustainable.

Clinical trials can be conducted with fewer patients if patients are selected based on assays that identify the tumors likely to be sensitive to the drug in question. Simon and Maitournam[66,67] have evaluated the efficiency of such targeted designs. When fewer than half of the patients are "test positive" and when the new treatment has little benefit for test-negative patients, the required sample size can be dramatically reduced by restricting eligibility to test-positive patients. Simon and Zhao have made available a Web-based computer program to enable investigators to compare such designs with standard broad eligibility designs (http://linus.nci.nih.gov/brb).

This targeted approach was effectively used for the development of trastuzumab in patients with metastatic breast cancer. In that case, about 450 patients whose tumors overexpressed *HER2* participated in a randomized clinical trial that provided convincing evidence that trastuzumab prolonged survival. Had the study been conducted without evaluating *HER2* expression, more than 8,000 patients would have been needed for similar statistical power.[66] Even if a huge study of unselected patients had been conducted and given a statistically significant result, the size of the benefit would have been very small as the benefit in the 25% of patients with *HER2* overexpression would have been diluted by lack of benefit from the remaining 75%. It is questionable whether such a small benefit overall would have justified approval or use of a drug with clear and serious toxicities.

In many cases in which the biological credentials of a predictive biomarker are less compelling, one will want to use the marker as a key part of the primary analysis plan; that is, to evaluate the treatments in the marker-positive patients separately, and to size the study accordingly, even if one does not restrict eligibility based on the marker. Simon and his colleagues have described a variety of designs of this type and provided

PRACTICE OF ONCOLOGY

Web-based computer programs at http://linus.nci.nih.gov/brb to facilitate the design of clinical trials for the prospective co-development of new drugs and companion diagnostics.[68–72] Because of the complexity of cancer biology, it is not always possible to have the right predictive biomarker identified by the start of a phase 3 trial of a new drug, as was shown in the case of *K-RAS* and anti-*EGFR* antibodies. Simon et al.[73] described a prospective-retrospective approach to using archived tumor specimens for a focused reanalysis of a randomized phase 3 trial with regard to a predictive biomarker. The approach requires that archived specimens be available on most patients, and that an analysis plan focused on a single marker be developed prior to performing the blinded assays. Friedlin et al.[74] have also discussed design issues for the phase 3 evaluation of prognostic and predictive markers.

In many cases there is a role for both randomized and nonrandomized trials in drug development. The nonrandomized format can in some cases be used for determining which regimens are sufficiently promising for randomized phase 3 evaluation and in clinical settings in which outcome is uniformly poor. For major questions of public health importance, unless the treatment effects are huge, the need for reliable answers dictates the use of randomized phase 3 trials.

Randomization of a patient should be performed after the patient has been found eligible and has consented to participate in the trial and to accept either of the randomized options. A truly random and nondecipherable randomization procedure should be used and implemented by calling a central randomization office staffed by individuals who are independent of participating physicians.

Randomization

History is a satisfactory control in determining whether a new treatment cures any patients with a disease that is uniformly and rapidly fatal. Once we leave this setting of complete determinism, however, the definition of an adequate nonrandomized control group becomes problematic. In studies using nonrandomized controls, often diagnostic and staging procedures, supportive care, secondary treatments, and methods of evaluation and follow-up are different for the controls and for the new patients. Current patients sometimes are excluded from analysis for not meeting eligibility criteria, not receiving "adequate" treatment, refusing treatment, or committing a major protocol violation. The control group, on the other hand, generally contains all the patients. There may be differences in the distribution of known and unknown prognostic factors between the controls and the current treatment group. There is often inadequate information to determine whether such differences are present, and current known prognostic factors may not have been measured for the controls. It generally is difficult or impossible to determine whether the controls would have been eligible for the current study and in what way they represent a selection of all eligible patients.

Formation of the control group by random treatment assignment as an integral part of the planned study can avoid most of the systematic biases just mentioned.[75–78] Randomization does not ensure that the study will include a representative sample of all patients with the disease, but it does help to ensure an unbiased evaluation of the relative merits of the two treatments for the types of patients entered.

It is sometimes said that randomization is unnecessary because matched historical or concurrent controls can be selected. However, matching can be done only with regard to known prognostic factors, and those factors often do not account for enough of the variation in patient outcome to assure that an unbiased historical control group can be constructed. It also is sometimes said that randomization is not effective in ensuring that the treatment groups are similar with regard to unknown prognostic factors unless the number of patients is large. This is true but reflects a misunderstanding of the purpose of randomization. Randomization does not ensure that the groups are medically equivalent, but it distributes the unknown biasing factors according to a known random distribution so that their effects can be rigorously allowed for in significance tests and confidence intervals. This is true regardless of the study size. A significance level represents the probability that differences in outcome can be the result of random fluctuations. Without a randomized treatment allocation, a "statistically significant difference" may be the result of a nonrandom difference in the distribution of unknown prognostic factors.

Stratification

When important prognostic factors are known for patients in a randomized trial, it is often advisable to stratify the randomization to ensure equal distribution of these factors. This is usually accomplished by preparing a separate randomization list for each stratum of patients. Each list must be balanced so that after each block of four to ten patients within the stratum, the treatment groups contain equal numbers of patients. Within the blocks, the sequence of treatment assignments is random. The stratification factors must be known for each patient at the time of randomization.

It is generally best to limit stratification to those factors definitely known to have important independent effects on outcome. If two factors are closely correlated, only one needs to be included. Peto et al.[79,80] believe that stratification is an unnecessary complication because adjustment for imbalances of known factors can be made in the analysis. This is true for most phase 3 clinical trials but stratification helps to ensure balance for interim analyses when the sample sizes may be limited and provides the medical audience with confidence in the results, which often is not available when depending on complex adjustment methods to deal with prognostic imbalances. Stratification also is a convenient way of specifying *a priori* what are considered the important prognostic factors.

Many clinical trials use adaptive stratification methods. The most popular such method is that conceived by Pocock and Simon,[81] which permits effective balancing with regard to many prognostic factors. There has been some concern about the effect of adaptive stratification on analysis of treatment differences. Multiple studies, including those by Kalish and Begg[82] have demonstrated that if the stratification factors are included in the model used for final analysis, then the effect of adaptive stratification is to make the true type I error less than the nominal rate; hence, the analyses are slightly conservative. Simon[83] showed that model-based analyses are not necessary to use with adaptive stratification methods. One can define a linear test statistic that reflects the treatment effect difference on the outcome adjusted for the stratification variables and generate the null distribution of the test statistic by reapplying the adaptive stratification method. The Pocock-Simon[81] method of adaptively stratified treatment assignment is not deterministic. Consequently, one can replicate the stratified treatment assignments, holding fixed the order of patient registrations and the stratification variables of the patients, recompute the value of the test statistic for the rerandomized treatment assignment, repeat this process a thousand times, and thereby generate the null distribution of the test statistic. Consequently, although the use of adaptive stratification methods, like the use of all stratification methods, are not essential, the criticisms of their effect on final analyses are unjustified.

Sample Size

The protocol for a phase 3 trial should specify the number of patients to be accrued and the duration of follow-up after the close of accrual when the final analysis will be performed. Methods of sample size planning are usually based on the assumption that at the conclusion of the follow-up period, a statistical significance test will be performed comparing the experimental treatment with the control treatment with regard to a single primary end point. A statistical significance level of .05 means that if there is no true difference in treatment effectiveness, the probability of obtaining a difference in outcomes as extreme as that observed in the data is .05. The significance level does not represent the probability that the null hypothesis is true; it represents a probability of an observed difference, assuming that the null hypothesis is true. Conventional statistical theory ascribes no probabilities to hypotheses, only to data.

A one-sided significance level represents the probability, by chance alone, of obtaining a difference as large as and in the same direction as that actually observed. A two-sided significance level represents the probability of obtaining by chance a difference in either direction as large in absolute magnitude as that actually observed. The two-sided significance level is usually twice the one-sided significance level. Controversy exists over the appropriateness of one-sided or two-sided significance levels. Although this is a somewhat trivial issue, a two-sided significance level of .05 has become widely accepted as a standard level of evidence.

The probability of obtaining a statistically significant result when the treatments differ in effectiveness is called the *power* of the trial. As the sample size and extent of follow-up increases, the power increases. The power depends critically, however, on the size of the true difference in effectiveness of the two treatments. Generally, one sizes the trial so that the power is either .80 or .90 when the true difference in effectiveness is the smallest size that is considered medically important to detect.

Statisticians have developed useful methods for planning sample size to compare survival curves or disease-free survival curves in phase 3 trials. Table 70.7 shows the number of total events needed assuming that the *hazard ratio*—the ratio of forces of mortality for the two treatment groups—is constant over time.[84] The table shows the total number of events that must occur in a given cohort to provide 90% power for detecting a specified reduction in the hazard for the experimental treatment relative to the control treatment. For exponential distributions, the percentage reduction in hazard of death can be expressed as a ratio of median survivals, which is displayed in the second column of Table 70.7. When the primary end point is overall survival, the events are deaths; for disease-free survival curves, *events* are deaths or recurrences. The translation of the number of deaths or events required to the number of patients required depends on the actual shape of the survival distributions, the rate of accrual, and the duration of follow-up after close of accrual. Generally, however, it is best to specify the time of the final analysis as the time when the specified number of deaths or events is obtained—not in terms of absolute calendar time.

In some cases, it may be convenient to think in terms of the proportion of patients without progression or death beyond some landmark time, such as 5 years. Tables 70.8 and 70.9 provide required numbers of patients for clinical trials planned on this basis. This approach is less flexible for studies in which survival or disease-free survival is the end point, as it presumes that all patients will be followed for the landmark time as a minimum. These tables can, however, be used generally for detecting differences in a binary end point, denoted *success rate* in the tables. For comparing treatments in phase 3 trials, differences of more than 15 to 20 percentage points usually are considered unrealistic. Establishing a sample size that provides good statistical power for detecting realistically expected treatment improvements is important. Many published "negative" results are actually uninterpretable because the sample sizes are too small.[85]

TABLE 70.7

NUMBER OF EVENTS NEEDED FOR COMPARING SURVIVAL CURVES

Percentage Reduction in Hazard of Death	Ratio of Median Survival for Exponential Distributions	No. of Total Deaths to Observe[a]
25	1.33	508
30	1.43	330
33	1.50	257
40	1.67	162
50	2.0	88

[a]Total number of deaths in both groups to have power .90 for detecting ratio of median survival. Type I error $\alpha = .05$ (two-sided).

FACTORIAL DESIGNS

The 2^K factorial design was described earlier in the section "Randomized Screening Designs" for phase 2 trials but it can also be used for phase 3 trials. The two-by-two factorial design is the version most often used. There are four treatment groups; one receiving neither of the two drugs A or B, one receiving A, one receiving B, and one receiving both. Although there are four treatment groups, the average effect of each treatment factor can be evaluated using all of the patients. To evaluate the effect of A, one compares outcomes for patients receiving A with outcomes for those not receiving A, ignoring B. Usually, the sample size for a two-by-two factorial trial is computed assuming that there is no interaction between the effects of the two drugs. The sample size is approximately the same as for a simple two-arm trial. The factorial design offers the possibility of answering two questions for the cost of one, but there is a risk of ambiguity in the interpretation of results.[86] For situations in which negative interactions are unlikely or in which it is unlikely that both factors will have substantial effects, the factorial design can provide a substantial improvement in the efficiency of clinical trials.

Simon and Freedman[87] developed a Bayesian method for the design and analysis of factorial trials. Their approach avoids the need to dichotomize one's assumptions that interactions either do or do not exist and provides a flexible approach to the design and analysis of such clinical trials. The Bayesian approach also avoids a preliminary test of interaction; such tests have poor power and basing the analysis on such tests is problematic. The Bayesian model suggests that in planning a factorial trial in which interactions are unlikely but cannot be excluded, the sample size should be increased by approximately 30%, as compared with a simple two-arm clinical trial for detecting the same size of treatment effect. The 30% figure allows for a 5% prior probability of a medically important, qualitative interaction between the treatment effects.

Noninferiority Trials

Noninferiority trials often compare a standard treatment with a less invasive or more convenient therapy that is not expected

TABLE 70.8

NUMBER OF PATIENTS IN EACH OF TWO TREATMENT GROUPS TO COMPARE PROPORTIONS (ONE-SIDED TEST)

Smaller Success Rate	Larger Minus Smaller Success Rate									
	0.05	0.10	0.15	0.20	0.25	0.30	0.35	0.40	0.45	0.50
0.05	512[a] 381[b]	172 129	94 72	62 48	45 35	35 27	28 22	23 18	19 15	16 13
0.10	786 579	236 176	121 91	76 58	54 41	40 31	31 24	25 20	21 16	17 14
0.15	1026 752	292 216	144 108	88 66	60 46	44 34	34 26	27 21	22 17	18 14
0.20	1231 900	339 250	163 121	98 73	66 50	48 37	36 28	29 22	23 18	19 15
0.25	1402 1024	377 278	178 132	105 79	70 53	50 38	38 29	29 23	23 18	19 15
0.30	1539 1122	407 300	189 141	111 83	73 55	52 39	38 30	30 23	23 18	19 15
0.35	1642 1196	429 315	197 146	114 85	74 56	52 40	38 30	29 23	23 18	18 14
0.40	1711 1246	441 324	201 149	115 86	74 56	52 39	38 29	29 22	22 17	17 14
0.45	1745 1271	446 327	201 149	114 85	73 55	50 38	36 28	27 21	21 16	16 13
0.50	1745 1271	441 324	197 146	111 83	70 53	48 37	34 26	25 20	19 15	15 12

[a]Upper figure: significance level = .05, power = .90.
[b]Lower figure: significance level = .05, power = .80.

to be superior to the standard treatment with regard to the primary end point. For such trials, the secondary benefits of the new regimen, although important, is not worth reductions in effectiveness in the primary end point. Unfortunately, it is not possible to establish that the two treatments are completely equivalent with regard to the primary end point. The usual approach is to plan the trial to have high statistical power for detecting small reductions in effectiveness, and this requires a large sample size. Because failure to reject the standard null hypothesis of no treatment difference results in adoption of a new, and potentially inferior regimen, misinterpretation of the results of noninferiority trials can result in serious problems. For the analysis of such trials, confidence intervals rather than statistical significance tests should be emphasized.[88] The confidence interval for the true difference of effectiveness gives a much clearer picture of which differences are consistent with the data. Makuch and Simon[89] and Durrleman and Simon[90] discuss this approach for planning and monitoring therapeutic equivalence trials.

Noninferiority trials are generally planned to distinguish the null hypothesis that the treatments are equivalent from the alternative that the new treatment is inferior by an amount δ. One of the key problems in designing a noninferiority trial is specification of δ. A small value of δ leads to a large trial. A large value of δ can lead to a small but meaningless trial. The reduction in effectiveness that the trial will be able to detect should be some fraction of the effectiveness of the standard treatment. For example, suppose the standard treatment is 12 months of a chemotherapy regimen that increases 5-year survival by 10 percentage points relative to no chemotherapy, and the new regimen of interest is use of the same regimen for only 6 months. If we want to have high power for detecting a reduction in effectiveness by half, then δ should represent a difference of 5 percentage points in 5-year survival. If we want high power for detecting a reduction in effectiveness by one quarter, then δ should represent a difference of 2.5 percentage points in 5-year survival. An appropriate value of δ can be determined only on the basis of a careful review of the studies that established the effectiveness of the standard treatment.

Another problem in the design of noninferiority trials is the lack of internal validation of the assumption that the control treatment is actually effective for the patient population at hand. If the effectiveness of the standard treatment is highly variable among studies, then there is the risk that a new regimen will be found noninferior to the standard because the standard is not effective in the current study. Consequently, noninferiority trials are only appropriate when the standard regimen is highly and reproducibly effective.

None of the conventional frequentist approaches to the design and analysis of therapeutic equivalence trials satisfactorily account for the uncertainty in estimation of the effectiveness of the standard treatment. Simon[91] developed a Bayesian approach that addresses this problem. The effectiveness of the control treatment C relative to the previous standard (P) is represented by a prior distribution, which is normal with mean μ and standard deviation λ and these values are obtained from a random-effects meta-analysis of the previously conducted randomized trials comparing C to P. The result of the noninferiority trial is summarized by an estimate $\hat{\delta}$ with standard error σ of the effectiveness of E relative to C. With some simplifying

TABLE 70.9

NUMBER OF PATIENTS IN EACH OF TWO TREATMENT GROUPS TO COMPARE PROPORTIONS (TWO-SIDED TEST)

Smaller Success Rate	Larger Minus Smaller Success Rate									
	0.05	0.10	0.15	0.20	0.25	0.30	0.35	0.40	0.45	0.50
0.05	620[a]	206	113	74	54	42	33	27	23	19
	473[b]	159	88	58	43	33	27	22	18	16
0.10	956	285	146	92	64	48	38	30	25	21
	724	218	112	71	50	38	30	24	20	17
0.15	1250	354	174	106	73	53	41	33	26	22
	944	269	133	82	57	42	32	26	21	18
0.20	1502	411	197	118	79	57	44	34	27	22
	1132	313	151	91	62	45	34	27	22	18
0.25	1712	459	216	127	84	60	45	35	28	23
	1289	348	165	98	65	47	36	28	22	18
0.30	1880	495	230	134	88	62	46	36	28	22
	1414	375	175	103	68	48	36	28	22	18
0.35	2006	522	239	138	89	63	46	35	27	22
	1509	395	182	106	69	49	36	28	22	18
0.40	2090	537	244	139	89	62	45	34	26	21
	1571	407	186	107	69	48	36	27	21	17
0.45	2132	543	244	138	88	60	44	33	25	19
	1603	411	186	106	68	47	34	26	20	16
0.50	2132	537	239	134	84	57	41	30	23	17
	1603	407	182	103	65	45	32	24	18	14

[a]Upper figure: significance level = .05, power = .90.
[b]Lower figure: swignificance level = .05, power = .80.

assumptions, the posterior distribution of the effectiveness of E relative to P is a normal distribution with mean $\mu + \hat{\delta}$. and variance $\lambda^2 + S^2$. Simon[91] also shows how the sample size of the therapeutic equivalence trial may be planned and how the size depends critically on the strength and consistency of the evidence that the active control C is superior to P and on the size of that difference in effectiveness.

Bayesian Methods

Conventional statistical methods regard the data collected in an experiment as being random; they test hypotheses about parameters that represent fixed but unknown treatment effects. For example, *frequentist methods*, derive probability statements about differences in observed response rates under an assumed null hypothesis that the true response probabilities are equal. *Bayesian* statistical methods consider the parameters, as well as the data, as being random; consequently they require us to specify these *prior distributions*. What does the assumption that the true treatment effect is a random draw from a prior distribution mean? One interpretation is that we regard the prior distribution as expressing our subjective beliefs about the value of the treatment effect based on previous experience with this treatment and other similar treatments. Such subjective prior distributions would vary among individuals based on their experience, biases, circumstances, and perhaps economic interests. Bayesian methods use Bayes' theorem to update the prior distributions of the parameters based on data from the study to produce the posterior distributions of the parameters. Using the posterior distributions, hypotheses about whether the treatments are equivalent or not can be tested. Consequently, Bayesian methods can derive direct probability statements about the parameters, such as "the probability that the treatment effect is zero is .04." The probability statements about the parameters seem to tell us what we want to know, but the results may depend as much on our prior distributions as on the data.

Many Bayesian statisticians use "noninformative" prior distributions. For example, a noninformative prior distribution for the difference in response probabilities might be constant for all differences between −1 and +1. That noninformative prior represents the belief that huge differences are just as likely as small differences. Consequently, methods based on apparently innocuous noninformative prior distributions may not be appropriate for real-world studies. In some cases, the treatment being evaluated can be considered "exchangeable" with other treatments that have been previously evaluated and a prior distribution can be defined based on that previous experience. Spiegelhalter et al.[92] have suggested analysis of a clinical trial with regard to both an "enthusiastic" prior and a "skeptical" prior. The former might be held by a developer of the treatment and the later by a regulator. Robust conclusions are obtained when the data are so extensive and strong that the posterior distributions are little changed regardless of whether you use an enthusiastic or skeptical prior.

Unfortunately, such robustness generally requires a huge sample size, much larger than indicated by use of standard frequentist methods. For some parameters, there may be a consensus prior distribution. For example, for evaluating cytotoxics there was generally broad consensus that large treatment effect by patient-subset interactions were unlikely, and Simon.[93] used this in a Bayesian approach to subset analysis. Generally, however, there is no meaningful prior consensus about the effect of treatment. Randomized clinical trials are done because the opinions of experts are often wrong. The subjective nature of the prior distribution is problematic for the interpretation of phase 3 clinical trials.

There are several important misconceptions about the use of Bayesian methods for clinical trials. First, some people believe that Bayesian methods provide an adequate alternative to randomized treatment assignment. In fact, however, randomization is just as important for the validity of Bayesian methods as for frequentist methods.[94] Second, some people mistakenly believe that Bayesian clinical trials require fewer patients than frequentist trials. Bayesian sample size calculations depend on the prior distribution used. Using *skeptical priors,* the sample size needed with Bayesian methods may be much larger than the conventional sample size. Third, some statisticians believe that the main impediment to use of Bayesian methods in clinical trials has been the difficulty of computing posterior distributions. The main limitation has been the fact that subjectivity of analysis is problematic for phase 3 clinical trials.

Bayesian methods can be very useful for phase 1 and phase 2 trials. For such trials, the prior distribution need only be appropriate for the investigator or sponsor. For phase 3 trials, the situation is more complex. Bayesian methods are applicable to phase 3 problems in which a consensus prior is appropriate. Such priors are possible for parameters representing interaction effects,[93] for the effectiveness of active controls in noninferiority trials,[91] and for unexpected findings with multiple safety end points.[95] As previously indicated, however, subjective opinion of the investigator or sponsor should have no role in testing the primary hypothesis of whether the new treatment is better than the control for the prespecified target population. Once the basic effectiveness of the treatment is established, however, there are many other analyses that can help physicians decide how to use the new treatment. Those analyses generally cannot be answered as precisely or with as little chance of error as the testing of the primary null hypothesis. Different physicians may have different prior beliefs about the treatment and how its effectiveness might vary among patients, and Bayesian methods may be useful for physicians in determining how to implement the results in the context of the patients they see. One must recognize, however, that Bayesian models can be overfit to data like any other models and can produce poor predictions. Simon[69] has developed a cross-validation based approach to evaluating the prediction accuracy of models that predict treatment preference for individual patients based on results of a randomized clinical trial.

ANALYSIS OF PHASE 3 CLINICAL TRIALS

Intention-to-Treat Analysis

The *intention-to-treat* principle indicates that all randomized patients should be included in the primary analysis of the trial. For cancer trials, this has often been interpreted to mean all "eligible" randomized patients. Excluding patients from analysis because of treatment deviations, early death, or patient withdrawal can severely distort the results.[80,96,97] Often, excluded patients have poorer outcomes than do those who are not excluded. Investigators frequently rationalize that the poor outcome experienced by a patient was from lack of compliance to treatment, but the direction of causality may be the reverse. For example, in the Coronary Drug Project, the 5-year mortality for poor adherents to the placebo regimen was 28.3%, significantly greater than the 15.1% experienced by good adherents to the placebo regimen.[98] In randomized trials, there may be poorer compliance in one treatment group than the other, or the reasons for poor compliance may differ. Excluding patients, or analyzing them separately (which is equivalent to excluding them), for reasons other than eligibility is generally considered unacceptable. The intention-to-treat analysis with all eligible randomized patients should be the primary analysis. If the conclusions of a study depend on exclusions, then these conclusions are suspect. The treatment plan should be viewed as a policy to be evaluated. The treatment intended cannot be delivered uniformly to all patients, but all eligible patients should generally be evaluable in phase 3 trials.

Interim Analyses

If statistical significance tests are performed repeatedly, the probability that the difference in outcomes will be found to be statistically significant (at the .05 level) at some point may be considerably greater than 5%. This probability is called the *type I error* of the analysis plan. Fleming et al.[99] have shown that the type I error can be as great as 26% if a statistical significance test is performed every 3 months of a 3-year trial that compares two identical treatments. Some trials are published without stating the target sample size, without indicating whether a target sample size was stated in the protocol, and without describing whether the published analysis represented a planned final analysis or was one of multiple analyses performed during the course of the trial. In such cases, one must suspect that the investigators were not aware of good statistical practices and of the dangers of informal multiple analyses.

Interim analyses can be very misleading and interfere with a physician's attempt to state honestly to the patient that there is no reliable evidence indicating that one treatment option or the other is preferable. Consequently, it has become standard in phase 3 multicenter clinical trials to have a data-monitoring committee review interim results, rather than having the monitoring done by participating physicians. This approach helps to protect patients by having interim results carefully evaluated by an experienced group of individuals and helps to protect the study from damage that ensues from misinterpretation of interim results.[100,101] Generally, interim outcome information is available to only the data-monitoring committee. The study leaders are not part of the data-monitoring committee because they may have a perceived conflict of interest in continuing the trial. The data-monitoring committee determines when results are mature and should be released. These procedures are used mostly for phase 3 trials.

A number of useful statistical designs have been developed for monitoring interim results. The simplest is that of Haybittle.[102] Interim differences are discounted unless the difference is statistically significant at the two-sided $P < .0025$ level. If the interim differences are not significant at that level, the trial continues until its originally intended size. The final analysis is performed without regard to the interim analyses, and the type I error is almost unaffected by the monitoring. Many others have developed group-sequential methods for interim monitoring based on a prespecified number of planned interim analyses. One of the most commonly used methods is that of O'Brien and Fleming.[103] The critical P value for determining whether an interim difference should be judged statistically significant depends on the number of analyses that will be performed during the trial. For a five-stage trial—four interim analyses and one final analysis—the critical P values are shown in Table 70.10. The experience of the U.S. cancer

TABLE 70.10

NOMINAL TWO-SIDED SIGNIFICANCE LEVELS FOR EARLY STOPPING IN INTERIM MONITORING METHODS THAT MAINTAIN AN OVERALL TYPE I ERROR LEVEL OF .05

Analysis Number	Pocock[78]	Haybittle[102]	O'Brien and Fleming[103]	Fleming et al.[49]
1	.016	.0027	.00001	.0051
2	.016	.0027	.0013	.0061
3	.016	.0027	.008	.0073
4	.016	.0027	.023	.0089
Final	.016	.049	.041	.0402

cooperative groups with interim analysis of phase 3 clinical trials was reviewed by Korn et al.[104]

Extreme treatment differences at an interim analysis are less usual in cancer clinical trials than finding that interim results do not support the hypothesis that the experimental treatment is substantially better than the control. Futility analyses are important in order to avoid exposing patients to a more toxic and debilitating new treatment *E* once the essential outcome of the trial is well assured.[105] Data-monitoring committees are charged with helping to make these difficult judgments. A variety of statistical approaches to "futility monitoring" have been developed.[106] Goldman et al.[47] have shown that futility analyses based on intermediate end points like disease-free survival can be particularly effective even in trials in which the primary end point is survival.

The method of stochastic curtailment[107] is widely used for futility analyses. At any interim analysis, the probability of rejecting the null hypothesis at the end of the trial is computed. This probability is calculated as being conditional on the data already obtained and on the assumption that the alternative hypothesis of superiority of the experimental treatment used initially in planning the sample size for the trial is true. If this conditional power is less than approximately 0.20, then the trial may be terminated with acceptance of the null hypothesis. The 0.20 cutoff can be raised substantially to at least 0.40 if this type of interim analysis is performed only a few times during the course of the trial. With stochastic curtailment, interim analyses need not be equally spaced, and the number of interim analyses need not be specified in advance.

Significance Levels, Hypothesis Tests, and Confidence Intervals

Medical decision making is complicated, and clinicians frequently misinterpret statistical significance tests in search of clear-cut answers from ambiguous data. A statistical significance level for comparing outcomes represents the probability of obtaining a difference as large as that actually observed if the treatments were actually of equal efficacy and differences occur merely by chance. After significance tests had been used for many years, Neyman and Pearson formalized a mathematical theory of hypothesis testing. In this theory, a study must prespecify a null hypothesis, an alternative hypothesis, and a decision rule for accepting one hypothesis and rejecting the other based on the data obtained. The theory has appealed to clinicians because it simplifies complex medical decision making by providing yes or no answers; either the difference is statistically significant or it is not. The distinction between one- and two-sided decision rules becomes crucial because a one-sided $P = .05$ is simply nonsignificant if a type I error of .05 based on a two-sided decision rule is prespecified.

The concept of prespecification of hypotheses is important for medical experimentation. However, the accept–reject nomenclature of the Neyman-Pearson theory provides an oversimplified and sometimes misleading interpretation of the data. Significance levels can serve as useful aids to interpretation of results, but quibbling about whether a one-sided $P = .04$ is significant makes little sense. Significance levels are influenced by sample sizes, and failure to reject the null hypothesis does not mean that the treatments are equivalent. There is no simple index of truth for interpreting results. Some attempt to use the notion of statistical significance in this way, but thorough presentation, skeptical evaluation, and cautious interpretation of results always are required.

Confidence intervals are generally much more informative than are significance levels. A confidence interval for the size of the treatment difference provides a range of effects consistent with the data. The significance level tells nothing about the size of the treatment effect because it depends on the sample size. However, it is the size of the treatment effect, as communicated by a confidence interval, that should be used in weighing the costs and benefits of clinical decision making. Many so-called negative results are actually noninformative, and confidence intervals help to determine when this is the case. Simon[88] has presented a nontechnical discussion of how to calculate confidence intervals for treatment differences with the types of end points commonly used in cancer clinical trials.

Calculation of Survival Curves

Most cancer clinical trials display results by showing survival curves or disease-free survival curves. Survival curves display the probability of surviving beyond any specified time, with time shown on the horizontal axis. In disease-free survival curves, it is the time until recurrence or death that is shown. Other time-to-event distributions can be similarly represented using the same methods. The usual statistical methods are not appropriate for analyzing survival because they ignore the fact that surviving patients have a limited follow-up period after which their survivals are "censored."

The most satisfactory way of representing such data is to estimate the survival function $S(t)$. This function represents the probability of surviving more than t time units. Time t is measured from diagnosis, start of treatment, or some other meaningful time point. For randomized studies, it is best to measure time from the date of randomization. There are basically two satisfactory methods for estimating $S(t)$. The first is the life-table or actuarial method[108,109] and is appropriate when the number of patients is large. The other method is the product limit method of Kaplan and Meier.[110] This method is appropriate for any number of patients, but it involves more effort than the life-table method when the number of patients is large.

The first step in the application of either method is the calculation of survival time for all patients. Survival is the duration from the chosen baseline (e.g., date of randomization) until death or date last known to be alive for patients who are not known to have died. To use the life-table method, intervals for the grouping of survival times are determined. The life table, shown in Table 70.11, is then filled out. This sample life table is prepared with yearly intervals in the first column. The number of patients alive at the beginning of the interval is entered in column 2. The number who died in the interval is entered in column 4. Patients dying exactly at a time that represents a boundary between two intervals (e.g., 365 days) are considered to have died in the preceding interval (e.g., 0 to 1 year). Column 3 contains the number of patients who are lost to follow-up during the interval or who are alive with maximum follow-up duration included in the interval. These latter patients are referred to as *withdrawn alive* in the conventional

TABLE 70.11

LIFE-TABLE METHOD FOR ESTIMATING A SURVIVAL DISTRIBUTION

Years after Randomization	No. Alive at Beginning of Interval l_x	No. Lost to Follow-Up or Withdrawn Alive during Interval w_x	No. Died during Interval d_x	At Risk during Interval 2 (Col 2 – 1/2 Col 3)	Proportion Dying (Col 4/Col 5) q_x	Proportion Surviving (1 – Col 6) p_x	Cumulative Proportion Surviving (S_x) ($p_1 \times p_2 \times \ldots \times p_x$)
0–1	252	38	94	233	0.40	0.60	0.60
1–2	120	34	10	103	0.10	0.90	0.54
2–3	76	30	4	61	0.07	0.93	0.50
3–4	42	18	4	33	0.12	0.88	0.44
4–5	20	12	0	14	0.00	1.00	0.44
5–6	8	8	0	4	0.00	1.00	0.44

Col, column.

life-table terminology. The life-table method assumes that patients lost to follow-up or withdrawn alive during the interval are at risk of death for one-half of the interval. Hence, column 5—the number alive at the start of the interval minus half the number lost or withdrawn during the interval—represents an approximate number of patients at risk of death during the interval. Column 6 gives the ratio of the number of patients who died during the interval to the number at risk during the interval. Column 7 gives the estimated probability of surviving the interval for patients alive at the start of the interval.

Column 8 should be studied carefully, because it provides the life-table estimate of the survival distribution and indicates the logic behind the method. The probability of surviving more than 3 years after randomization, for example, equals the entry in the third row of column 8 (0.50). The logic is as follows: To survive 3 full years, the patients must survive through the first year; given that they have survived the first year, they must survive the second year; and given that they have survived the second year, they must survive the third year. Consequently, the probability of surviving for at least 3 years is estimated by the product $p_1 \times p_2 \times p_3$ of factors in column 7. By using this product, the life-table method takes maximal advantage of the mortality experience of patients with limited follow-up. The entry S_x in column 8, row x, represents the life-table estimate of the probability of surviving more than x years from randomization. Computational shortcuts to observe are those for column 8: $S_x = p_x \times S_{x-1}$ and for column 2: $l_{x+1} = l_x - w_x - d_x$.

The product limit method of Kaplan and Meier is similar in concept to the life-table method. With the Kaplan-Meier approach, however, the intervals are defined by the actual survival times of patients who have died. Suppose, for example, that the survivals are 3, 3, 3+, 5, 6, 8+, 8+, 10, 10, and 12+ months, where a plus sign follows survivals for patients still alive. Then the intervals are 0 to 3, 3 to 5, 5 to 6, and 6 to 10 months, as shown in Table 70.12. With the Kaplan-Meier method, deaths occur only at the ends of intervals. The entry in column 5 equals $l_x - w_x$ rather than $l_x - 2w_x$ for the life-table method. This is because deaths occur only at the ends of intervals here, and the number of patients at risk of death just before the interval end is $l_x - w_x$. In the entry w_x in column 3 for the Kaplan-Meier method, patients who are lost to follow-up or withdrawn alive at the end of an interval are considered not lost or withdrawn until the following interval. These differences between the Kaplan-Meier and life-table methods render the former more appropriate for studies with fewer patients.

Once the values S_x have been calculated for the Kaplan-Meier method, they may be graphed with time on the horizontal axis. The graph is a step function that starts at time zero and ordinate 1.0. It drops to value S_x at time x, where x is the time at the right end of an interval. The survival curve corresponding to Table 70.12 is shown in Figure 70.1. The tic marks are placed on the curve at 3, 8, and 12 months to represent the follow-up times of living patients. The step function can be extended horizontally out to 12 months to represent follow-up of the last patient, but the right-hand end of the curve usually is very imprecisely estimated, and concluding that a plateau exists at the level shown on the curve is often erroneous.

TABLE 70.12

KAPLAN-MEIER METHOD FOR ESTIMATING A SURVIVAL DISTRIBUTION

Months after Randomization	No. Alive at Beginning of Interval l_x	No. Lost to Follow-Up or Withdrawn Alive during Interval w_x	No. Died during Interval d_x	Effective No. Exposed to Risk of Dying Just Before End of Interval (Col 2 – Col 3)	Proportion Dying (Col 4/ Col 5) q_x	Proportion Surviving (1 – Col 6) p_x	Cumulative Proportion Surviving ($p_1 \times p_2 \times \ldots \times p_x$) S_x
0–3	10	0	2	10	0.2	0.8	0.8
3–5	8	1	1	7	0.14	0.86	0.68
5–6	6	0	1	6	0.17	0.83	0.57
6–10	5	2	2	3	0.67	0.33	0.19

Col, column.

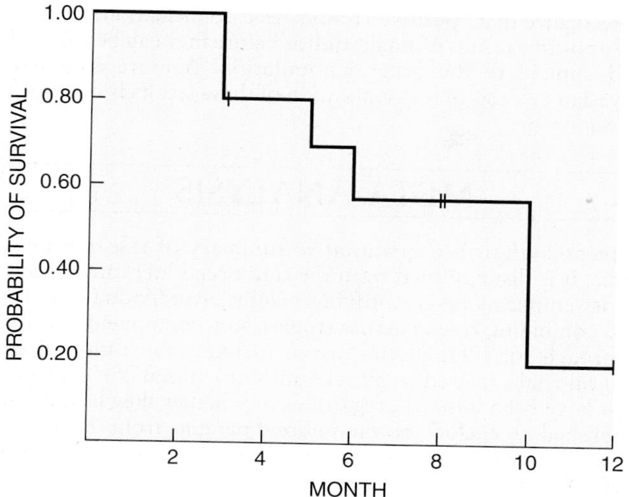

FIGURE 70.1 Example of estimated survival distribution.

For any time t, the Kaplan-Meier curve is an estimator of the true unknown value of $S(t)$. The Kaplan-Meier estimate of a survival distribution is based on the assumption that censoring is noninformative, which means that the censoring time is independent of the prognosis of the patient. Most censoring in a randomized clinical trial results from the fact that some patients are alive and still being followed at the time of analysis. This is noninformative censoring. However, if patients are lost to follow-up—if they fail to return to clinic when they are too sick to travel—then the censoring is informative and all the usual methods of survival analysis are invalidated. Consequently, it is essential to obtain follow-up information actively on *all* patients before analysis. If some patients have not been contacted for many months and their status is unknown, that information should be obtained before any analysis is performed. Examining the distribution of time since the last contact for patients not known to have died is a good way to examine the adequacy of follow-up.

The issue of informative censoring also arises in considering end points other than death. For example, one may be attempting to estimate the distribution of time until tumor recurrence in the CNS in a pediatric leukemia trial. How should one handle patients whose disease recurs in the marrow without evidence of CNS recurrence? One may be tempted to censor the time to CNS recurrence of such patients at their time of marrow recurrence, but that implicitly assumes that the censoring is noninformative. Because CNS and marrow recurrence may be biologically linked, the assumption of noninformative censoring may not be valid. Other issues of informative censoring can be similarly problematic. Clearly, one should never censor patients because of lack of compliance with therapy, as this can severely bias results. More extensive discussions of statistical methods for the analysis of clinical trial data are given by Marubini and Valsecchi.[111]

Multiple Comparisons

Table 70.13 shows the probability of obtaining one statistically significant ($P < .05$) difference by chance alone as a function of the number of independent comparisons of two equivalent treatments. With only five comparisons, the chance of at least one false-positive conclusion is 22.6%. When the number of end points, interim analyses, and patient subsets

TABLE 70.13

PROBABILITY OF OBTAINING AT LEAST ONE STATISTICALLY SIGNIFICANT ($P < .05$) DIFFERENCE BY CHANCE ALONE IN MULTIPLE COMPARISONS OF TWO EQUIVALENT TREATMENTS

Comparisons	Probability of at Least One "Significant" Difference (%)
1	5
2	9.7
3	14.3
4	18.5
5	22.6
10	40
20	64.1

are considered in the analysis of clinical trials, these results are disturbing.[112] The comparisons performed in clinical trials are not entirely independent, but this does not have much effect on ameliorating the problem. Fleming and Watelet[113] performed a computer simulation to determine the chance of obtaining a statistically significant treatment difference when two equivalent treatments in six subsets determined by three dichotomous variables are compared. The chance of a statistically significant difference between treatments in at least one subset was 20% at the final analysis and 39% in the final or one of the three interim analyses. Subset analysis, comparison of treatments with regard to multiple end points, and multiple interim analyses are common sources of erroneous conclusions. The primary end point should be defined in the protocol. Subset analyses and analyses with regard to secondary end points should be specified in advance, and statistical significance should be declared only for significance levels much more extreme than the conventional .05. The simplest approach to multiple comparisons is to declare statistical significance only if the P value is $< .05/n$, where n denotes the number of comparisons to be made. For example if $n = 10$, then .005 should be the threshold for declaring significance for a secondary analysis. The number of comparisons planned in the protocol is represented by n. Comparisons that are not preplanned should not be considered significant in any case and represent hypothesis generation to be tested in subsequent trials.

Interaction tests are statistical procedures that test for lack of homogeneity of treatment effect across subsets of patients. A statistically significant interaction should be documented before claiming that treatment effects vary among subsets unless the test of treatment effect in the subset were prespecified in the protocol and part of the overall 5% type I error level reserved for it. Qualitative interaction tests are described by Gail and Simon.[114]

Generally, it is not valid to adjust the analysis by characteristics measured after the start of treatment (e.g., compliance, dose delivered, toxicity). New approaches to subset analysis and multiple end point analysis using Bayesian methods have been described by Dixon and Simon.[93, 115]

REPORTING RESULTS OF CLINICAL TRIALS

Effective reporting of results is an integral part of good research. Unfortunately, numerous reviews have indicated that the quality of reporting of clinical trial results is poor.[97, 116,117] Pocock et al. concluded that "overall, the reporting of clinical trials appears to

TABLE 70.14

SUMMARY OF GUIDELINES FOR REPORTING CLINICAL TRIALS

- Quality control of data and response evaluations should be discussed.
- All patients registered on study should be accounted for.
- Inevaluability rate for major end points should not exceed 15%.
- No exclusions of eligible patients in comparing outcomes by treatment group.
- The sample size should be large enough to establish or conclusively rule out effects of clinically important magnitude. Confidence limits for size of treatment vs. control effectiveness should be given.
- Publication should provide protocol specified sample size and interim analysis plan as well as actual timing of analyses.
- Claims of therapeutic effectiveness should not be based on phase 2 trials
- Generalizability of conclusions should be carefully discussed. Subset-specific claims should be justified based on prospective planning and statistical control of studywise type I error.

be biased toward an exaggeration of treatment differences." Tannock and Murphy[97] and Tannock[112] have given clear illustration of how this is easily done. Simon[118] developed a set of methodologic guidelines for reports of clinical trials, and these guidelines have been adopted by several cancer journals. These nine guidelines are summarized in Table 70.14.

FALSE-POSITIVE REPORTS IN THE LITERATURE

Many of the positive results reported in the literature for small clinical trials are probably false-positive results.[119,120] In 100 trials, suppose that there are 10 in which the experimental treatment is sufficiently better than the control, such that there is a 90% chance of the difference being detected in a small or moderate-sized clinical trial. Of these ten trials, obtaining a statistically significant difference is expected in nine. Of the remaining 90 trials, we assume that the treatments are approximately equivalent to the control. A statistically significant difference could be expected in 5% (4.5) of these. Hence, of the 13.5 (9 + 4.5) trials that yield statistically significant results, the finding is false-positive in 4.5 or 33% of the cases. The 33% false discovery rate is striking but it depends on the assumption that only 10 percent of the trials study new treatments with large treatment effects. For large clinical trials, the size of treatment effect that can be detected with high statistical power is likely to be larger. The Eastern Cooperative Oncology Group reported that about one-third of their phase 3 clinical trials resulted in statistically significant results.[121] Assuming that most of these trials are conducted with 90% power and a 5% statistical significance level, then the false discovery rate is about 9%.

An additional factor to consider is that of publication bias,[122] which denotes the preference of journals to publish positive rather than negative results. A negative result may not be published at all, particularly from a small trial. If it is published, it is likely to appear in a less widely read journal than it would if the result were positive.

These observations emphasize that results in the medical literature often cannot be accepted at face value. It is important to recognize that "positive" results need confirmation, particularly positive results of small studies, before they can be believed and applied to the general population. A more complete Bayesian analysis of the implication of these results is described by Simon.[121]

META-ANALYSIS

A *meta-analysis* is a quantitative summary of research on a topic. It is distinguished from the traditional literature review by its emphasis on quantifying results of individual studies and combining results across studies. Key components of this approach for therapeutics are to include only randomized clinical trials, to include all relevant randomized clinical trials that have been initiated, regardless of whether they have been published, to exclude no randomized patients from the analysis, and to assess therapeutic effectiveness based on the average results pooled across trials.[123]

Attention is restricted to randomized trials, because the bias from nonrandomized comparisons may be larger than the small to moderate therapeutic effects likely to be present. Including all relevant randomized trials that have been initiated in a geographic area (e.g., the world, or the Americas and Europe) represents an attempt to avoid publication bias. Avoiding exclusion of any randomized patients also functions to avoid bias. Assessing therapeutic effectiveness based on average pooled results is an attempt to make the evaluation on the totality of evidence rather than on extreme isolated reports. In calculating average treatment effects, a measure of difference in outcome between treatments is calculated separately for each trial. For example, an estimate of the logarithm of the hazard ratio can be computed for each trial. A weighted average of these study-specific differences then is computed, and the statistical significance of this average is evaluated. This approach to meta-analysis requires access to individual patient data for all randomized patients in each trial. It also requires collaboration of the leaders of all the relevant trials and is very labor-intensive. Nevertheless, it represents the gold standard for meta-analysis methodology.

A major issue of concern in meta-analyses is whether the individual trials are sufficiently similar to make calculation of average effects medically meaningful. If the therapeutic interventions or control treatments differ too greatly or if the patient populations are too different, then the results may not be medically meaningful as a basis for making treatment decisions for individual patients. Often in cancer therapeutics, the studies will not be identical in their treatment regimens or their patient populations, but they will not be so different as to make the results meaningless. In this case, the meta-analysis may be useful for answering important questions about a class of treatments that the individual trials cannot address reliably. For example, trials evaluating adjuvant treatment of primary breast cancer often are designed to detect differences in disease-free survival, and a meta-analysis is often required to evaluate survival. Similarly, subset analysis can usually be meaningfully evaluated only in the context of a meta-analysis, because individual trials are not sized for this objective.

Meta-analysis is not an alternative to properly designed and sized randomized clinical trials. Some have suggested that one need not be concerned about computing sample size in the traditional ways because small, randomized trials can be pooled for meta-analysis. Because most investigators would prefer to "do their own thing," this would lead to a proliferation of diverse trials of inconsequential individual size that may be too heterogeneous to permit a meaningful meta-analysis. Given that sufficient large, randomized clinical trials of very similar treatment regimens have been conducted, meta-analysis can provide supplemental information about a given class of treatments that is not available from the individual trials.

Selected References

The full list of references for this chapter appears in the online version.

1. Subramanian J, Simon R. Gene expression-based prognostic signatures in lung cancer: Ready for clinical use? *J Natl Cancer Inst* 2010;102(7): 464.
2. Green S, Benedetti J, Crowley J. *Clinical Trials in Oncology,* 2nd ed. Boca Raton, FL: CRC, 2003.
3. Leventhal BG, Wittes RE. *Research Methods in Clinical Oncology*. New York: Raven Press, 1988.
4. Eisenhauer EA, O'Dwyer PJ, Christian M, Humphrey JS. Phase I clinical trial design in cancer drug development. *J Clin Oncol* 2000;18(3): 684.
5. Simon R, Freidlin B, Rubinstein L. Accelerated titration designs for phase I clinical trials in oncology. *J Natl Cancer Inst* 1997;89:1138.
9. Babb J, Rogatko A, Zacks S. Cancer phase I clinical trials: efficient dose escalation with overdose control. *Stat Med* 1998;17:1103.
10. Goodman SN, Zahurak ML, Piantadosi S. Some practical improvements in the continual reassessment method for phase I studies. *Stat Med* 1995;14:1149.
12. Simon RM, Steinberg SM, Hamilton M, et al. Clinical trial designs for the early clinical development of therapeutic cancer vaccines. *J Clin Oncol* 2001;19:1848.
15. Kummar S, Kinders R, Rubinstein L, et al. Compressing drug development timelines in oncology using phase '0' trials. *Nat Rev Cancer* 2007;131.
17. Karapetis CS, Khambata-Ford S, Jonker DJ, et al. K-ras mutations and benefit from cetuximab in advanced colorectal cancer. *N Engl J Med* 2008;359(17):1757.
20. Pusztai L, Anderson K, Hess KR. Pharmacogenomic predictor discovery in phase II clinical trials for breast cancer. *Clinical Cancer Research* 2007;13:6080-6.
21. LeBlanc M, Rankin C, Crowley J. Multiple histology phase II trials. *Clin Cancer Res.* 2009;15:4256.
22. Dobbin KK, Zhao Y, Simon RM. How large a training set is needed to develop a classifier for microarray data? *Clin Cancer Res* 2008;14:108.
23. Eisenhauer EA, Therasse P, Bogaerts J, et.al. New response evaluation criteria in solid tumors: revised RECIST guideline (version 1.1). *Eur J Cancer* 2009;45:228.
24. Simon R. Optimal two-stage design for phase II clinical trials. *Control Clin Trials* 1989;10:1.
29. Seymour L, Ivy SP, Sargent D, et.al. The design of phase II clinical trials testing cancer therapeutics: consensus recommendations from the clinical trial design task force of the National Cancer Institute investigational drug steering committee. *Clin Cancer Res* 2010;16(6):1764.
30. Vidauurre T, Wilkerson J, Simon R, Bates SE, Fojo T. Stable disease is not preferentially observed with targeted therapies and as currently defined has limited value in drug development. *Cancer J* 2009;15(5):366.
31. El-Maraghi RH, Eisenhauer EA. Review of phase II trial designs used in studies of molecular targeted agents: outcomes and predictors of success in phase III. *J Clin Oncol* 2008;26(8):1346.
34. Estey EH, Thall PF. New designs for phase 2 clinical trials. *Blood* 2003;102(2):442.
35. Korn EL, Liu PY, Lee SJ, et al. Meta-analysis of phase II cooperative group trials in metastatic stage IV melanoma to determine progression-free and overall survival benchmarks for future phase II trials. *J Clin Oncol* 2008;26 (4):527.
38. Korn EL, Arbuck SG, Pluda JM, Simon R, Kaplan RS, Christian MC. Clinical trial designs for cytostatic agents: are new approaches needed? *J Clin Oncol* 2001;19:265.
39. Rubinstein LV, Korn EL, Freidlin B, Hunsberger S, Ivy SP, Smith MA. Design issues of randomized phase 2 trials and a proposal for phase 2 screening trials. *J Clin Oncol* 2005;23:7199.
40. Simon R, Wittes RE, Ellenberg SS. Randomized phase II clinical trials. *Cancer Treat Rep* 1985;69:1375.
45. Rosner G, Stadler W, Ratain M. Randomized discontinuation design: application to cytostatic antineoplastic agents. *J Clin Oncol* 2002;20(22): 4478.
46. Freidlin B, Simon R. An evaluation of the randomized discontinuation design. *J Clin Oncol* 2005;23:1.
47. Goldman B, LeBlanc M, Crowley J. Interim futility analysis with intermediate endpoints. *Clin Trials* 2008;5:14.
50. Sher HI, Heller G. Picking the winners in a sea of plenty. Clinical Cancer *Research* 2002;8:400.
53. Parmar MKB, Barthel FMS, Sydes M, et.al. Speeding up the evaluation of new agents in cancer. *J Natl Cancer Inst* 2008;100(17):1204.
54. Freidlin B, Korn EL, Gray R, Martin A. Multi-arm clinical trials of new agents: some design considerations. *Clin Cancer Res* 2008;14:4368.
55. Simon R. Randomized clinical trials: Principles and obstacles. *Cancer* 1994;74:2614.
56. Torri V, Simon R, Russek-Cohen E, Midthune D, Freidman M. Relationship of response and survival in advanced ovarian cancer patients treated with chemotherapy. *J Natl Cancer Inst* 1992;84:407.
57. Buyse M, Molensberghs G, Burzykowski T, Renard D, Geys H. The validation of surrogate endpoints in meta-analyses of randomized experiments. *Biostatistics* 2000;1:49.
59. Korn EL, Albert PS, McShane LM. Assessing surrogates as trial endpoints using mixed models. *Stat Med* 2004;24:163.
60. Fleming TR, Rothmann MD, Lu HL. Issues in using progression-free survival when evaluating oncology products. In; 2009:2874.
61. Freidlin B, Korn EL, Hunsberger S, Gray R, Saxman S, Zujewski JA. Proposal for the use of progression-free survival in unblinded randomized trials. In; 2007:2122.
62. Dodd LE, Korn EL, Freidlin B, et al. Blinded independent central review of progression-free survival in phase iii clinical trials: important design element or unnecessary expense? In; 2008:3791.
63. Simon R. An agenda for clinical trials: clinical trials in the genomic era. *Clin Trials* 2004;1:468.
64. Simon R. A roadmap for developing and validating therapeutically relevant genomic classifiers. *J Clin Oncol* 2005;23:7332.
65. Simon R. New challenges for 21st century clinical trials. *Clin Trials* 2007;4:167.
66. Simon R, Maitournam A. Evaluating the efficiency of targeted designs for randomized clinical trials. *Clin Cancer Res* 2005;10:6759.
67. Simon R, Maitournam A. Correction and supplement: Evaluating the efficiency of targeted designs for randomized clinical trials. *Clin Cancer Res* 2006;12:3229.
68. Simon R. Using genomics in clinical trial design. *Clin Cancer Res* 2008;14: 5984.
69. Simon R. Clinical trials for predictive medicine: new challenges and paradigms [published online ahead of print March 25, 2010]. *Clin Trials* doi:10.1177/1740774510366454.
70. Freidlin B, Jiang W, Simon R. The cross-validated adaptive signature design for predictive analysis of clinical trials. *Clin Cancer Res* 2010;16(2):691.
71. Jiang W, Freidlin B, Simon R. Biomarker adaptive threshold design: A procedure for evaluating treatment with possible biomarker-defined subset effect. *J Natl Cancer Inst* 2007;99:1036.
72. Freidlin B, Simon R. Adaptive signature design: an adaptive clinical trial design for generating and prospectively testing a gene expression signature for sensitive patients. *Clin Cancer Res* 2005;11:7872.
73. Simon RM, Paik S, Hayes DF. Use of archived specimens in evaluation of prognostic and predictive biomarkers. *J Natl Cancer Inst.* 2009;101(21):1446.
74. Freidlin B, McShane LM, Korn EL. Randomized clinical trials with biomarkers: design issues. *J Natl Cancer Inst* 2010;102(3):152.
79. Peto R, Pike MC, Armitage P. Design and analysis of randomized clinical trials requiring prolonged observation of each patient: I. Introduction and design. *Br J Cancer* 1976;34:585.
80. Peto R, Pike MC, Armitage P. Design and analysis of randomized clinical trials requiring prolonged observation of each patient: II. Analysis and examples. *Br J Cancer* 1977;35:1.
81. Pocock S, Simon R. Sequential treatment assignment with balancing for prognostic factors in the controlled clinical trial. *Biometrics* 1975;31:103.
83. Simon R. Restricted randomization designs in clinical trials. *Biometrics* 1979;35:503.
84. Rubinstein L, Gail M, Santner T. Planning the duration of a comparative clinical trial with loss to follow-up and a period of continued observation. *J Chronic Dis* 1981;34:469.
88. Simon R. Confidence intervals for reporting results from clinical trials. *Ann Intern Med* 1986;105:429.
91. Simon R. Bayesian design and analysis of active control clinical trials. *Biometrics* 1999;55:484-7.
92. Spiegelhalter DJ, Freedman LS, Parmar MKB. Bayesian approaches to randomized trials. *J R Stat Soc Ser A* 1994;157:357.
93. Simon R. Bayesian subset analysis: application to studying treatment-by-gender interactions. *Stat Med* 2002;21:2909.
94. Rubin DB. Bayesian inference for casual effects: the role of randomization. *Ann Stat* 1978;6(1)34–58.
95. Simon R. Discovering the truth about tamoxifen: problems of multiplicity in the evaluation of biomedical data. *J Natl Cancer Inst* 1995;87:627.
96. Barr J, Tannock I. Analyzing the same data two ways: a demonstration model illustrate the reporting and misreporting of clinical trials. *J Clin Oncol* 1989;7:969.
97. Tannock I, Murphy K. Reflections on medical oncology: an appeal for better clinical trials and improved reporting of their results. *J Clin Oncol* 1983;1:66.
100. Ellenberg S, Fleming TR, DeMets D. *Data Monitoring Committees in Clinical Trials: A Practical Perspective*. New York: Wiley, 2002.
101. Smith M, Ungerleider R, Korn E, Rubinstein L, Simon R. The role of independent data monitoring committees in randomized clinical trials sponsored by the National Cancer Institute. *J Clin Oncol* 1997;15:2736.
102. Haybittle JL. Repeated assessment of results in clinical trials of cancer treatment. *J Radiol* 1971;44:793.
103. O'Brien PC, Fleming TR. A multiple testing procedure for clinical trials. *Biometrics* 1979;35:549.

105. Freidlin B, Korn EL. Monitoring for lack of benefit: a critical component of a randomized clinical trial. In; 2009:629.
107. Lan KKG, Simon R, Halperin M. Stochastically curtailed test in long-term clinical trials. *Commun Stat Seqen Anal* 1982;1:207.
110. Kaplan EI, Meier P. Nonparametric estimation from incomplete observations. *J Am Stat Assoc* 1958;53:457.
112. Tannock IF. False-positive results in clinical trials: multiple significance tests and the problem of unreported comparisons. *J Natl Cancer Inst* 1996;88:206.
113. Fleming TR, Watelet L. Approaches to monitoring clinical trials. *J Natl Cancer Inst* 1989;81:188.
114. Gail M, Simon R. Testing for qualitative interactions between treatment effects and patient subsets. *Biometrics* 1985;41:361.
115. Dixon DO, Simon R. Bayesian subset analysis. *Biometrics* 1991;47:871.
120. Ioannidis JPA. Why most published research findings are false. *PLOS Med* 2005;2(8):696.
122. Begg CB, Berlin JA. Publication bias and dissemination of clinical research. *J Natl Cancer Inst* 1989;81:107.
123. Collins R, Gray R, Godwin J, Peto R. Avoidance of large biases and large random errors in the assessment of moderate treatment effects: the need for systematic overviews. *Stat Med* 1987;6:245.

CHAPTER 71 MOLECULAR BIOLOGY OF HEAD AND NECK CANCERS

NISHANT AGRAWAL, JOSEPH CALIFANO, AND PATRICK HA

Research regarding head and neck squamous cell carcinoma (HNSCC) has shifted from the detection of individual gene mutations and deletions to detailing the complex interactions of networks of genes altered by genetic alterations, including sequence alterations, chromosomal aberrations, epigenetic modifications, microRNA changes, and even mitochondrial mutations. High throughput, whole-genome–based discovery approaches that have been successful in other tumor types are currently being employed in the study of HNSCC.

With improved understanding of HNSCC has come the solidification of several different mechanisms of carcinogenesis. Although the majority of these cancers still come from mutagenic environmental exposures, namely tobacco (smoking or chewing) and use of betel products, the rise in prevalence of oropharyngeal cancer in the United States is largely related to human papillomavirus (HPV) type 16. With the different etiologies of cancer development, we have seen distinctions in clinical behavior and thus can directly see how the underlying molecular mechanisms may have important clinical implications.

In this chapter, we highlight some of the newer developments in HNSCC research that have special relevance to clinical therapeutics. As we further understand the underlying genetic basis of this disease, we can transition this knowledge into developing targeted therapy and refine treatment paradigms. These data are by no means comprehensive, as the expansion in detailed knowledge regarding HNSCC biology has dramatically expanded.

GENETIC SUSCEPTIBILITY

Despite the well-established association between HNSCC and smoking, heavy ethanol use, and betel use, the overall incidence of HNSCC remains relatively low. Thus, there must be elements of genetic susceptibility that predispose certain patients to disease progression while in others there is relative resistance to cancer formation. Several case-control studies have demonstrated that first-degree relatives of patients with HNSCC were 3.5- to 3.8-fold more likely to also develop HNSCC even when controlling for factors such as age, gender, ethnicity, tobacco, and alcohol use.[1–3] Likewise, HNSCC patients were found to be 3.8 times more likely to develop a second primary tumor if one or more first-degree relatives suffered from upper aerodigestive tract cancer.[4]

These familial susceptibilities provide evidence that there are likely underlying genetic mechanisms that preclude one to cancer formation. However, direct evidence of heritable HNSCC syndromes is rare. The most common direct, genetic association with HNSCC exists with Fanconi anemia, a rare, autosomal recessive disease associated with aplastic anemia, congenital anomalies, and a predisposition for cancer development, especially head and neck and anogenital squamous cell carcinoma.[5] There has been suggestion that one of the mechanisms of cancer development in Fanconi anemia is HPV-related, but recent studies show that the precise mechanism of susceptibility remains unknown and that the presence of high-risk HPV viruses in Fanconi anemia–related HNSCC is variable.[6] There have also been associations with HNSCC and other syndromes such as Lynch-II, Bloom, xeroderma pigmentosum, ataxia telangiectasia, and Li-Fraumeni,[7] all of which have specific genetic aberrations that link them to cancer. The fact that a consistent genetic mechanism remains elusive in HNSCC highlights its heterogeneity.

Building on the link between these known syndromes and gene alterations, investigators have looked to other genetic polymorphisms, such as single nucleotide polymorphisms (SNPs), to evaluate whether patterns of HNSCC susceptibility can be detected. It is important to note that it is generally not known what the exact differential function is of these SNPs and whether they have a direct link toward carcinogenesis. Many of the single-institution studies also suffer from smaller sample sizes and lack the ability to control for the potential ethnic or geographic variability inherent in these polymorphisms.

The general families of gene alterations have focused on carcinogen-detoxifying mechanisms (cytochrome p450 members [CYP], glutathione-S-transferases [GSTs], alcohol and ethanol dehydrogenases [ADH and ALDH]), DNA damage repair, nucleotide excision repair enzymes (NER), excision repair cross-complementing rodent repair deficiency complementation genes (ERCC), x-ray repair complementing defective repair in Chinese hamster cells (XRCC), and RecA homolog, *Escherichia coli* (Rad51), inflammation/angiogenesis (cyclooxygenase-2 [COX-2], hypoxia-inducible factors [HIF], cytokines), apoptosis, cell cycle, and many other pathways salient to cancer formation.

Larger cooperative studies, across institutions, help to further refine the most important polymorphisms and provide the greatest evidence for their role in carcinogenesis. A cooperative European group (ARCAGE) surveyed 115 polymorphisms in 62 selected genes in a cohort of 1,511 cases and 1,457 controls.[8] Several genes showed promise (*CYP2*, murine double-minute 2 [*MDM2*], and tumor necrosis factor [*TNF*]), but there still remains work to be done in looking at the mechanisms and applicability of these markers. Another multinational study pooled patient samples from several institutions and used a cohort of over 3,000 HNSCC patients along with over 5,000 controls and discovered a protective effect from two of the studied ADH polymorphisms.[9]

Despite the numerous studies looking at these relationships, the effects of polymorphic variants seem to be quite modest, and there are often conflicting studies reported on the same polymorphisms, underscoring the complexity of HNSCC as well as the role of these DNA changes. Further study to validate the previously studied SNPs with a relationship to HNSCC as well as mechanistic confirmation of an altered function would help to further our understanding of carcinogenesis. With newer technology, there will be an opportunity to perform further genome-wide screens to discover new targets as well in an effort to make sense of the complicated pathway associations that these SNPs have in the context of specific patient variables.

MOLECULAR NETWORKS ALTERED IN HNSCC

Tumorigenesis in the head and neck is the result of multiple genetic and epigenetic alterations of molecular pathways in the squamous epithelium.[10,11] The progression of head and neck cancer is thought to result from multistep alterations in tumor suppressor genes and oncogenes.[10,12–18] A variety of genetic changes have been reported for squamous cell carcinomas (SCCs) including loss of heterozygosity or amplification of specific chromosomal regions, although tumor suppressor genes have not been characterized for most of the regions that are commonly lost in HNSCC. Nevertheless, several signaling pathways have been implicated and are described in the following sections (Table 71.1).

P16/p53/Cyclin D

Loss of 9p21, resulting in inactivation of the *p16* gene, is the most common genetic alteration in the progression of head and neck cancer.[19,20] P16 is an inhibitor of cyclin-dependent kinase (CDK), which is intimately involved in G1 cell-cycle regulation. Phosphorylation and inactivation of pRb by unbridled CDK4 and CDK6 enable cells to escape senescence. Loss of chromosome 9p21 occurs in the majority of invasive tumors and is also present at a high frequency in the earliest definable lesions, including dysplasia and carcinoma *in situ*.[19] Loss of p16 appears necessary for immortalization of keratinocytes.[21] Loss of p16 protein has been observed in most advanced premalignant lesions.[22] In addition to deletions and point mutations, p16 is also inactivated by methylation of the 5′CpG region.[23] This methylation is associated with complete block of *p16* transcription and appears to be a common mechanism for p16 inactivation. The notion that p16 inactivation is directly involved in the progression of primary tumors has been strengthened. Lack of p16 protein was detected by immunostaining in most primary invasive lesions, and tumors with absent p16 protein contained a homozygous deletion, methylation, or point mutation of p16.[24]

Loss of *p53* on chromosomal region 17p13 and subsequent point mutation within the remaining allele is another critical step in tumor progression. Inactivation of *p53* now represents the best-described and most common genetic change in all of human cancer.[25] Initially by analysis of exons 5-8, *p53* mutations were observed in approximately 50% of head and neck tumors.[26,27] The *p53* gene can be inactivated by a large variety of distinct mutations and more thorough sequence analyses of exons 2-11, a *p53* mutation rate of almost 80% has been observed in head and neck tumors.[28] *p53* normally halts cell-cycle progression in the setting of DNA damage and induces apoptosis with inadequate DNA repair. *p53* mutations result in a progression from preinvasive to invasive lesions, while increasing the probability of further progression. If 17p loss or *p53* mutation is present in early lesions, the chance of progression to cancer within 10 years approaches 80% (33-fold relative risk). In a large definitive collaborative group study, disruptive *p53* mutations were an independent prognostic marker and predicted a worse outcome in surgically resected primary tumors.[29]

Carcinogens in tobacco and alcohol have a causal role as the prevalence of *p53* mutations is greater in patients who smoke and drink alcohol.[30] HPV16- and HPV18-induced SCC of the oropharynx is more common in nonsmokers and is not associated with *p53* mutations. Instead, the viral oncoprotein E6 promotes the accelerated, ubiquitin-mediated, degradation of *p53*.

Amplification of chromosome region 11q13 containing cyclin D1 is seen in approximately one-third of head and neck

TABLE 71.1

COMMON GENETIC ALTERATIONS IN HEAD AND NECK SQUAMOUS CELL CARCINOMA

Alteration	Frequency	Comments
p16 inactivation	70%	Via homozygous deletion and less frequently promoter methylation
p53 mutation	50%	Predominantly mutation
High-risk HPV integration	25%	Found predominantly in oropharyngeal sites
EGFR axis alteration	80%–90%	Via amplification, overexpression, and downstream target activation
PI3-K/AKT/mTOR	>40%	
(DIME-6), ATM, p15, TIMP-3, MGMT, RARB-2, DAP-K, E-cadherin, cyclin A1, RASSF1A, CDKN2A, CDH1, and DCC	Variable, up to 60% (DCC)	Inactivated by promoter hypermethylation
HIF-1α	60%	Proliferation, angiogenesis
VEGF and other angiogenic pathways	Variable	
E-cadherin, matrix metalloproteinases	Variable	Invasion, anoikis, and metastasis
TKTL1, cancer testes antigens	50%	Protooncogenes activated by promoter hypomethylation

HPV, human papillomavirus; EGFR, epidermal growth factor receptor; *DCC*, deleted in colon cancer; HIF-1α, hypoxia-inducible factor-1-α; VEGF, vascular endothelial growth factor; *TKTL1*, transketolase-like-1.

tumors.[31] The role of cyclin *D1* in the progression of human cancer is now well established and constitutive activation of oncogene cyclin D1 has been shown to confer a growth advantage in SCCs.[32] Other tumor suppressor genes, including *Rb* and *p16*, are negative regulators of the *cyclin D1* pathway and often are inactivated in human neoplasms. Cyclin *D1* amplification is independent of *p16* inactivation in head and neck cancers.[33]

PI3-K/AKT/mTOR

Mutation in the PI3-K signaling pathway are found in up to 30% of all human cancers, and activation of the PI3-K/AKT/mTOR pathway has also been implicated in tumorigenesis of HNSCC.[34] Mutations of the PI3-K network have shown to confer a growth advantage, transforming capacity, and drug resistance.[35] The PI3-K family is divided into three different classes based on structure and substrate specificity. Class I P13-Ks are heterodimers of a p85 regulatory subunit and a p110 catalytic subunit, which is mutated in many cancers. The class I P13-Ks are activated by tyrosine kinase receptors, including epidermal growth factor receptor (EGFR) and oncogenic proteins, and lead to the production of the lipid second messenger, phosphatidylinositol 3-phosphatase (PIP3), which in turn facilitates phosphorylation and subsequent activation of AKT. The PI3-K pathway also leads to activation of the serine/threonine kinase, mammalian target of rapamycin (mTOR), which in turn phosphorylates p70S6K, a kinase that modulates protein synthesis.

Invasion/Metastasis

Metastasis is a complicated, multistep process in which selective pressures select for a clone of malignant cells selected to survive in a distant, permissive environment. The multistep process includes angiogenesis, altered cellular adhesion, cellular motility, disruption of the base membrane/extracellular matrix, and anchorage-independent proliferation.

Up-regulation of hypoxia-inducible factor 1-α (HIF-1α), induced by intratumor hypoxia, has been documented in invasive HNSCC and correlates with progression to a more invasive and aggressive phenotype.[36,37] HIF-1α is a master regulator of oxygen homeostasis and activates genes involved in angiogenesis, glucose metabolism, cell survival, invasion, cell renewal, and immortalization.[38–40]

The vascular endothelial growth factor (VEGF) pathway is critical in angiogenesis in HNSCC. Increased expression of VEGF and its receptors is regulated by HIF-1α–dependent and -independent pathways, both of which converge on the PI3-K/AKT pathway.

Diminished cell-to-cell adhesion, through down-regulation of cellular adhesions molecules such as E-cadherin, is integral to invasion.[41,42] In addition to cell-to-cell adhesion mediated by cadherins, integrins that mediate cell-to-extracellular matrix interaction also play a fundamental role in tumor cells gaining access to the angiolymphatic system.[43] Laminins, which are extracellular glycoproteins, are one of the ligands for integrins. Laminin 5 is overexpressed in invasive fronts, is associated with poorer prognosis, and downstream activates mitogen-activated protein kinase, which leads to cell survival and proliferation.[44–51] In addition to altered cell adhesion, migration mediated by the Rho family of GTPases is an important step in the multistep process of metastasis.[52] Cancer cells also actively disrupt the base membrane through the proteolytic activity of zinc-dependent endopeptidases, matrix metalloproteinases (MMPs), to disseminate. MMPs degrade most components of the base membrane, including collagen. Evasion from anchorage-dependent survival is a feature of metastatic HNSCC, and anoikis resistance is crucial in the process of metastasis as a defense against microenvironmental death stimuli. E-cadherin has been implicated in conferring anoikis resistance in HNSCC by physically associating with a number of signaling effectors such as PI3-K and EGFR.[53,54]

Epidermal Growth Factor Receptor

The *EGFR* is one of the best-studied oncogenes in HNSCC. This receptor tyrosine kinase belongs to the ErbB family of cell surface receptors and has many downstream signaling targets associated with carcinogenesis. Once phosphorylated, the receptor can signal via the MAPK, Akt, ERK, and Jak/STAT pathways (Fig. 71.1). These pathways are related to cellular proliferation, apoptosis, invasion, angiogenesis, and metastasis.[55–57] Expression of *EGFR* is a normal finding in many tissues including the dermis, gastrointestinal tract, and kidneys. However, dysfunction of this receptor and its associated pathways occurs in most epithelial cancers[55] and 80% to 90% of HNSCC specifically.[9,56] The story of *EGFR* is promising in that our understanding of its molecular biology has led directly to clinically beneficial targeted therapies and its use as a marker and prognosticator of disease.

Initially, EGFR was first found to be up-regulated in HNSCC cell lines and in a high percentage of primary HNSCC.[58–60] Further study showed that histopathologically normal mucosa adjacent to cancer had a high degree of overexpression[61] and that the up-regulation of EGFR occurs in the transition from dysplasia to HNSCC.[62] Now it is well known that elevated levels of expression predict a worse disease-free and cause-specific survival.[63] Studies looking at copy number amplification have also been shown to be associated with poorer prognosis in HNSCC. One study has demonstrated that the overexpression of *EGFR* is a biomarker for an improved response to therapy and could serve as a predictive marker to separate patients into different arms of therapeutic trials.[64]

In addition to serving as a marker for prognosis, EGFR axis alterations are currently under investigation as markers for response to treatment and as therapeutic targets. Several strategies exist for targeting the EGFR pathway including the use of specific tyrosine kinase inhibitors (TKIs), monoclonal antibodies blocking receptor dimerization, and antisense oligodeoxynucleotides or siRNA blocking mRNA expression.

Cetuximab is one of the most well studied monoclonal antibodies directed against EGFR. A recently published phase 3 clinical trial examined the effects of this drug in conjunction with radiotherapy in the treatment of locoregionally advanced HNSCC. This study demonstrated an overall survival benefit (49 vs. 29 months) and increased duration of locoregional control (24.4 vs. 14.9 months) in the cetuximab plus radiotherapy arm versus the arm receiving radiotherapy alone. This was the first randomized study showing a survival benefit with an EGFR targeting agent in locally advanced HNSCC.[65,66] Conversely, the TKI gefitinib has shown no survival benefit for recurrent or metastatic HNSCC.[66,67] There are, however, several phase 1 and 2 trials under way studying the concomitant use of chemoradiation with gefitinib and two other TKIs (erlotinib and lapatinib) in the treatment of HNSCC.[68] There are several other studies currently investigating the role of EGFR targeting agents, three of which are mentioned here. The first trial is evaluating gefitinib plus docetaxel versus placebo on recurrent or metastatic disease. The second trial is examining the role of cetuximab as an adjuvant to cisplatin and 5- fluorouracil therapy in recurrent/metastatic disease. The last notable trial is studying cetuximab as an adjuvant to radiotherapy and cisplatin treatment for locally advanced disease.[66] A shortcoming of all these clinical trials is that they fail to incorporate the presence of *EGFR*-activating mutations, *EGFR* gene copy number, or both,

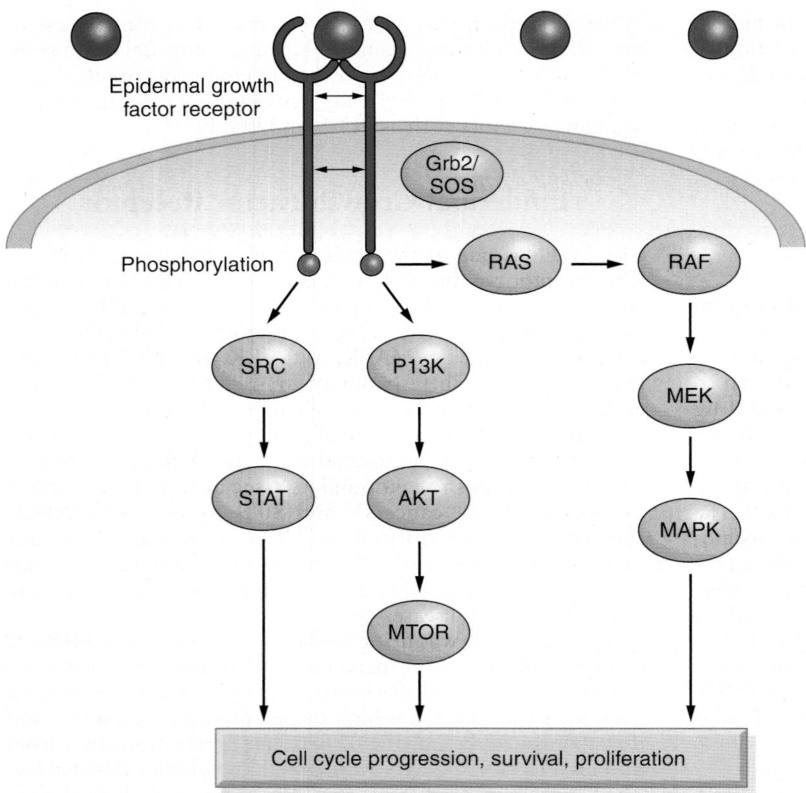

FIGURE 71.1 Cell-cycle progression, survival, and proliferation.

into their primary analyses, although both of these factors have recently emerged as predictors of efficacy.[66] However, retrospective analysis of these factors within the context of prospective therapeutic trials should provide some information.

As mentioned previously, increased *EGFR* expression correlates with a poor prognosis; conversely, the presence of activating somatic mutations in the EGFR-TK domain have been shown to be a positive predictor for a patient's response to treatment. These mutations, which are present in ~10% of NSCLC[69,70] and 1% to 7% in non–small cell lung cancer (HNSCC),[71,72] correlated with prolonged survival in patients with advanced NSCLCs treated with chemotherapy regardless of EGFR-TKI.[73] Several other studies in NSCLCs did show that *EGFR* mutations were predictive of survival in patients treated with EGFR-TKIs.[74–76] Multiple clinical trials are under way to evaluate the use of EGFR-TKIs in chemotherapy-naive patients with advanced NSCLC and *EGFR*-activating mutations.[66,77,78] Both gefitinib and erlotinib have demonstrated response rates of 75% to 82%.[66,77,78] It is yet to be determined whether the same correlation and response to therapy will be found in HNSCC with *EGFR*-activating mutations.

Human Papillomavirus in HNSCC

Although it is well known that tobacco and alcohol are the two primary environmental risk factors associated with the development of HNSCC, it is now recognized that HPV infection plays an important role in the pathogenesis of a unique subset of oropharyngeal HNSCCs.[79–85] These tumors primarily emerge from the lingual and palatine tonsils in the oropharynx.[80,83,86–91] HPV-related HNSCC has distinguished itself as a separate entity with an improved prognosis and response to therapy from non-HPV–related HNSCC. It has also been proposed that it is the reason for the increasing incidence of oropharyngeal HNSCC relative to all other anatomic sites in the head and neck. This section will first briefly review what is known about the molecular biology of HPV as this topic is covered in other chapters within this edition, and then move on to how HPV-related HNSCC affects everyday clinical practice.

HPV is an ~7.9-kb, nonenveloped, double-stranded, circular DNA virus that has a specific tropism for squamous epithelium.[92] Although the sequences for over 320 different types of HPV have been identified, HPV-16 and -18 are the two types most pertinent to the development of HNSCC. The E6 and E7 oncoproteins contained within the viral genome, if overexpressed, are able to disrupt the function of *Rb* and *p53*, well-known tumor suppressor genes, leading to development of a malignant phenotype (Fig. 71.2).[93] It is now established that histopathologically, HPV-positive tumors tend to have a poorly differentiated and frequently basaloid histology that often lacks keratin.[79,80,85,94] Researchers have also discovered that human keratinocytes expressing E6 and E7 genes from HPV-16 become immortal,[95] as do oral epithelial cells.[96–98]

In a recent meta-analysis, HPV genomic DNA was detected in approximately 26% of all HNSCC by sensitive polymerase chain reaction–based methods.[99] However, in the majority of studies, 50% or more of oropharyngeal tumors contained the HPV genome.[100] A multinational study conducted by the International Agency for Research on Cancer (IARC), only 18% of oropharyngeal tumors were HPV-positive, indicating that this proportion likely varies by geography.[101] Regardless of the study population, high-risk HPV-16 accounts for the overwhelming majority (90% to 95%) of HPV-positive tumors.[99]

Our knowledge of HPV and its causal relationship with oropharyngeal cancer has improved our ability to diagnose and locate disease in patients with occult primary tumors.[102] Tonsillectomy has been shown in retrospective analyses to identify the primary site of cervical metastases as the contralateral or ipsilateral tonsil in approximately 10% and 30% of cases, respectively.[103–106] Therefore, HPV-related cancer is a distinct established entity that can be reliably diagnosed.

On average, patients with HPV-positive HNSCC are approximately 5 years younger than HPV-negative HNSCC patients,

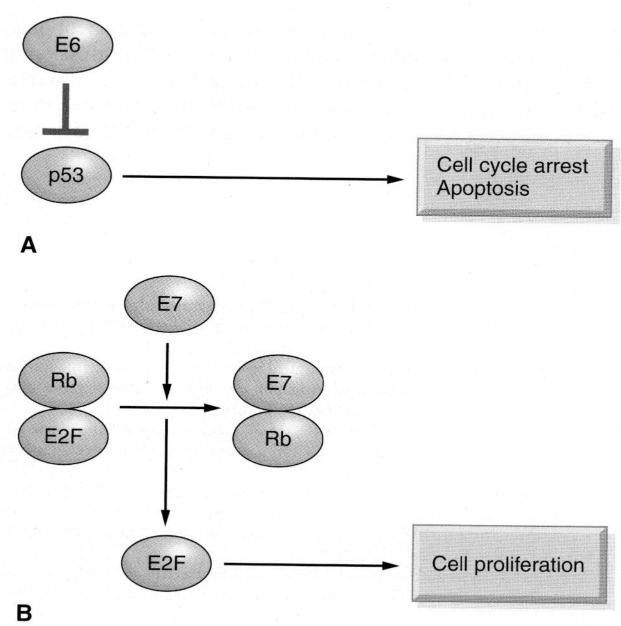

FIGURE 71.2 **A:** E6 binds p53, targets it for degradation, and promotes cell-cycle progression. **B:** E7 binds Rb and releases E2F, which promotes cellular proliferation.

with equal distribution among the sexes.[90,107–110] HPV-positive HNSCC is more likely than HPV-negative HNSCC to occur in the nonsmoker and nondrinker.[80,81,88,89] Risk factors for HPV-related HNSCC include a high lifetime number of vaginal-sex partners (26 or more), a high lifetime number of oral-sex partners (6 or more),[111] and seropositivity for HPV-16 viral capsid protein antibodies,[82] which carries a 15-fold increased risk for HNSCC. In a study restricted to patients with oropharyngeal cancers, nonsmokers were approximately 15-fold more likely to have a diagnosis of HPV-positive HNSCC than smokers.[112]

Our knowledge of the HPV status of our patients' tumors also improves our ability to provide an accurate prognosis. Patients with HPV-positive tumors have improved prognosis when compared with patients with HPV-negative tumors in the majority of studies, with as much as 60% to 80% reduction in risk of dying from their cancer when compared with the HPV-negative patient after controlling for other risk factors.[80,108,112–115] The reason for the improved survival is unclear; however, improved radiation responsiveness, immune surveillance to viral antigens, and the absence of field cancerization in these patients who tend to be nonsmokers have been postulated as possibilities. In addition, E6-related degradation of *p53* in HPV-positive cancers may not be functionally equivalent to HPV-negative *p53* mutations, and therefore HPV-positive tumors may have an intact apoptotic response to radiation and chemotherapy.

Therapeutic implications of an HPV-positive diagnosis are an active area of investigation. The Eastern Cooperative Oncology Group is studying the impact of HPV presence on oropharyngeal organ-preservation therapy. It is believed that HPV-HNSCC will perform better than HPV-negative HNSCC. A clinical trial of an HPV-16–specific therapeutic vaccine is also currently being evaluated. The vaccine is administered in the adjuvant setting and is intended to enhance the cytotoxic T-cell response to the HPV-16 oncoproteins.[116] With regard to prevention, a prophylactic vaccine composed of the HPV-16 viral capsid protein has recently been shown to prevent persistent HPV-16 infection and the development of cervical dysplasia.[117,118] However, the clinical trials have not included an evaluation of the impact of the vaccine on oral HPV infection. The vaccine does have the potential to have an impact on HNSCC incidence because the current vaccines are targeted to HPV-16 and there are animal models that demonstrate a protective effect and a reduction in the development of HPV-related oral lesions.

Possible future diagnostic tests that would likely have high specificity but low sensitivity for a diagnosis of HPV-associated HNSCC will include the detection of HPV-16 DNA in plasma,[119] which can be used for surveillance. Other screening tests like fluorescence *in situ* hybridization (FISH) on Papanicolaou smears obtained directly from tumors and HPV-16 E6 and E7 seroreactivity are other tests currently being tested.

EPIGENETICS

Regulation of gene expression by DNA methylation was first recognized in development, where the coordinated expression and silencing of genes needs to take place in an organized fashion.[120] As a novel mechanism of gene regulation, it was quickly proposed that epigenetic control of tumor suppressor genes could be an important mechanism of carcinogenesis.[121,122] To date, methylation has been primarily considered as a mechanism of tumor suppressor gene inactivation, and one of the earliest genes to be characterized as being epigenetically controlled was the retinoblastoma gene. Primary tissue analysis showed that 10% of the retinoblastomas analyzed were hypermethylated at the Rb promoter[123] in the absence of any other mutations. In recent years, new assays such as sodium bisulfite treatment of DNA, which converts nonmethylated cytosines to uracil and methylation-sensitive quantitative polymerase chain reaction, have further advanced our ability to evaluate the methylation status of tissue samples.[124–126] With these advances, many different tumor suppressor genes in various tumor types have been shown to be down-regulated by methylation. The utilization of comprehensive whole-genome profiling approaches to promoter hypermethylation has identified novel putative tumor suppressor genes silenced by promoter hypermethylation. These *in vitro* techniques employ treatment of cultured cells with pharmacologic demethylating agents and subsequent expression array analysis with validation of tumor suppressor gene targets.[127]

Promoter hypermethylation of p16 is a frequent event in HNSCC and this mechanism of gene silencing accounts for the low levels of expression.[23,24,123,128,129] Thus, Knudsen's two-hit hypothesis could include promoter hypermethylation as one of the "hits" along with the more traditional sequence mutation or chromosomal deletion.

Studies of promoter methylation have uncovered many other putative tumor suppressor genes in HNSCC including lhx-6 (*DIME-6*), *ATM*, *p15*, *TIMP-3*, *MGMT*, *RARB-2*, *DAP-K*, E-cadherin, cyclin A1, *RASSF1A*, *CDKN2A*, *CDH1*, and *DCC*. These genes are known to function in pathways that control cell-cycle progression, apoptosis, cell-cell adhesion, DNA repair, and tumor invasion.[130–141] With the advent of new molecular techniques and whole-genome screening strategies, the list of tumor suppressor genes that are silenced through promoter hypermethylation continues to grow at a rapid pace. For instance, in the relatively young field of microRNA research, it has been demonstrated that those microRNAs having tumor-suppressor function also undergo DNA methylation-associated silencing in cancer.[137,142,143]

LOSS OF HETEROZYGOSITY AND RISK OF MALIGNANT PROGRESSION

Premalignant lesions of the head and neck are often characterized by large patches of clonally related precursors, often demonstrating dysplastic changes. Increased risk of progression to

PRACTICE OF ONCOLOGY

malignancy is also associated with prior head and neck cancer, advanced histologic grade, and evidence of genetic instability including chromosomal loss and aneuploidy. Those patients with moderate or severe dysplasia are noted to have a risk of progression to malignancy of approximately 60%, in a study with median 7-year follow up. Likewise, a prior history of head and neck cancer resulted in a similar 60% risk of progression in the same study.[6] Approximately 40% of patients with mild dysplasia or hyperplasia combined with 3p or 9p loss of heterozygosity demonstrated progression to malignancy within 5 years.

Selected References

The full list of references for this chapter appears in the online version.

1. Foulkes WD, Brunet JS, Sieh W, Black MJ, Shenouda G, Narod SA. Familial risks of squamous cell carcinoma of the head and neck: retrospective case-control study. *BMJ* 1996;313:716.
6. van Zeeburg HJ, Snijders PJ, Wu T, et al. Clinical and molecular characteristics of squamous cell carcinomas from Fanconi anemia patients. *J Natl Cancer Inst* 2008;100:1649.
12. Califano J, van der Riet P, Westra W, et al. Genetic progression model for head and neck cancer: implications for field cancerization. *Cancer Res* 1996;56:2488.
16. Mao L, Lee JS, Fan YH, et al. Frequent microsatellite alterations at chromosomes 9p21 and 3p14 in oral premalignant lesions and their value in cancer risk assessment. *Nat Med* 1996;2:682.
23. Reed AL, Califano J, Cairns P, et al. High frequency of p16 (CDKN2/MTS-1/INK4A) inactivation in head and neck squamous cell carcinoma. *Cancer Res* 1996;56:3630.
28. Poeta ML, Manola J, Goldwasser MA, et al. TP53 mutations and survival in squamous-cell carcinoma of the head and neck. *N Engl J Med* 2007;357:2552.
36. Hoogsteen IJ, Marres HA, Bussink J, van der Kogel AJ, Kaanders JH. Tumor microenvironment in head and neck squamous cell carcinomas: predictive value and clinical relevance of hypoxic markers. A review. *Head Neck* 2007;29:591.
41. Mandal M, Myers JN, Lippman SM, et al. Epithelial to mesenchymal transition in head and neck squamous carcinoma: association of Src activation with E-cadherin down-regulation, vimentin expression, and aggressive tumor features. *Cancer* 2008;112:2088.
55. Kalyankrishna S, Grandis JR. Epidermal growth factor receptor biology in head and neck cancer. *J Clin Oncol* 2006;24:2666.
64. Bonner JA, Harari PM, Giralt J, et al. Radiotherapy plus cetuximab for squamous-cell carcinoma of the head and neck. *N Engl J Med* 2006;354:567.
78. Andl T, Kahn T, Pfuhl A, et al. Etiological involvement of oncogenic human papillomavirus in tonsillar squamous cell carcinomas lacking retinoblastoma cell cycle control. *Cancer Res* 1998;58:5.
79. Gillison ML, Koch WM, Capone RB, et al. Evidence for a causal association between human papillomavirus and a subset of head and neck cancers. *J Natl Cancer Inst* 2000;92:709.
80. Hafkamp HC, Speel EJ, Haesevoets A, et al. A subset of head and neck squamous cell carcinomas exhibits integration of HPV 16/18 DNA and overexpression of p16INK4A and p53 in the absence of mutations in p53 exons 5-8. *Int J Cancer* 2003;107:394.
81. Mork J, Lie AK, Glattre E, et al. Human papillomavirus infection as a risk factor for squamous-cell carcinoma of the head and neck. *N Engl J Med* 2001;344:1125.
82. Schwartz SM, Daling JR, Doody DR, et al. Oral cancer risk in relation to sexual history and evidence of human papillomavirus infection. *J Natl Cancer Inst* 1998;90:1626.
110. D'Souza G, Kreimer AR, Viscidi R, et al. Case-control study of human papillomavirus and oropharyngeal cancer. *N Engl J Med* 2007;356:1944.
120. Feinberg AP, Vogelstein B. Hypomethylation of ras oncogenes in primary human cancers. *Biochem Biophys Res Commun* 1983;111:47.
127. El-Naggar AK, Lai S, Clayman G, et al. Methylation, a major mechanism of p16/CDKN2 gene inactivation in head and neck squamous carcinoma. *Am J Pathol* 1997;151:1767.
140. Ha PK, Califano JA. Promoter methylation and inactivation of tumour-suppressor genes in oral squamous-cell carcinoma. *Lancet Oncol* 2006;7:77.

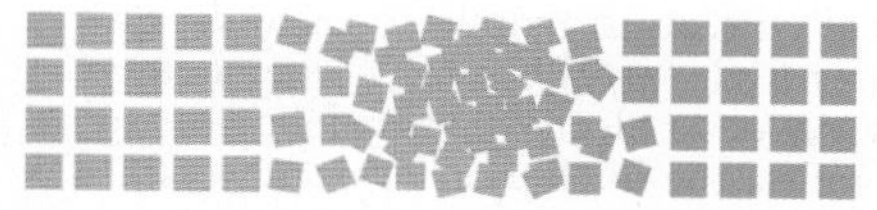

CHAPTER 72 TREATMENT OF HEAD AND NECK CANCER

WILLIAM M. MENDENHALL, JOHN W. WERNING, AND DAVID G. PFISTER

EPIDEMIOLOGY OF HEAD AND NECK CANCER

The estimated number of new head and neck cancer cases (excluding skin cancer) in the United States in 2009 was 48,010; this represents 3.2% of the total new cancer cases.[1] Approximately 27% of these patients are women.[1] African Americans have a higher age-adjusted incidence than other ethnic groups. The usual time of diagnosis is after the age of 40, except for salivary gland and nasopharyngeal cancers (NPCs), which may occur in younger age groups. For many primary sites, tobacco use is associated with an increased risk. Alcohol has also been implicated as a causative factor; the effects of alcohol and tobacco may be synergistic.[2] Head and neck cancer patients have an increased risk for developing a second primary tumor (SPT), both within the head and neck and elsewhere (e.g., esophageal and lung cancers),[3] attributed to the field defect associated with tobacco and alcohol use.[4] Human papillomavirus infection (HPV; most commonly HPV-16) plays a role in the development of certain head and neck cancers, particularly those in the oropharynx.[5,6] Patients with high-risk HPV (HR-HPV) positive head and neck cancers tend to be younger and less likely to have a strong history of tobacco and ethanol use, have a history of multiple sex partners (particularly oral-genital sex), and have a better prognosis.[6,7] There is a long-standing association between Epstein-Barr virus (EBV) and NPC.[8] Occupational exposures are associated with the development of sinonasal tract tumors.[9]

ANATOMY

The anatomy pertaining to a particular primary site is described in subsequent sections. To facilitate communication, lymph nodes are organized into levels. Level I includes the submental and submandibular areas; levels II–IV include the internal jugular vein lymph nodes; level V includes the posterior triangle (Fig. 72.1).[10] Furthermore, which lymph node levels are involved are predictive of the primary site. For example, lip, oral cavity, and facial skin tumors typically spread to level I initially; larynx and pharynx cancers have a predilection for spread to levels II and III.

There are no capillary lymphatics in the epithelium. Tumor must penetrate the lamina propria before lymphatic invasion can occur. One can predict the richness of the capillary network in a given head and neck site by the relative incidence of lymph node metastases at presentation. The nasopharynx and pyriform sinus have the most profuse capillary lymphatic networks. The paranasal sinuses, middle ear, and vocal cords have few or no capillary lymphatics. Muscle and fat contain few capillary lymphatics, as do bone and cartilage within the periosteum or perichondrium. There are no capillary lymphatics in the eye, and few in the orbit.

PATHOLOGY

Most head and neck malignant neoplasms arise from the surface epithelium and are squamous cell carcinoma (SCC) or one of its variants, including lymphoepithelioma, spindle cell carcinoma, verrucous carcinoma, and undifferentiated carcinoma. Lymphomas and a wide variety of other malignant and benign neoplasms make up the remaining cases.[11-13]

Lymphoepithelioma is an SCC with a lymphoid stroma and occurs in the nasopharynx, tonsillar fossa, and base of tongue; it may also occur in the salivary glands. In the spindle cell variant, found in 2% to 5% of upper aerodigestive tract malignancies, there is a spindle cell component that resembles sarcoma intermixed with SCC. It is generally managed like other high-grade SCCs. Verrucous carcinoma is a low-grade SCC found most often in the oral cavity, particularly on the gingiva and buccal mucosa. It usually has an indolent growth pattern and is often associated with the chronic use of snuff or chewing tobacco.

Small cell neuroendocrine carcinoma occurs rarely throughout the head and neck. Upper aerodigestive tract lymphomas almost always show a diffuse non-Hodgkin's histologic pattern.

NATURAL HISTORY OF SQUAMOUS CELL CARCINOMA

Patterns of Spread

Primary Lesion

SCCs usually begin as surface lesions, but occasionally originate below the surface of the mucosa. Superficial tumors arising in Waldeyer's ring may be difficult to distinguish from normal lymphoid tissue. Very early surface lesions may show only erythema and a slightly elevated mucosa.

Spread is dictated by local anatomy, and thus varies by each site. Muscle invasion is common, and tumor may spread along muscle or fascial planes for a surprising distance from the palpable or visible lesion. Tumor may attach early to the periosteum or perichondrium, but bone or cartilage invasion is usually a late event.

Bone and cartilage usually act as a barrier to spread; tumor that encounters these structures will often be diverted and spread along a path of less resistance. Slow-growing gingival neoplasms may produce a smooth pressure defect of the underlying bone without bone invasion.

Tumor extension into the parapharyngeal space allows superior or inferior spread from the skull base to the low neck.

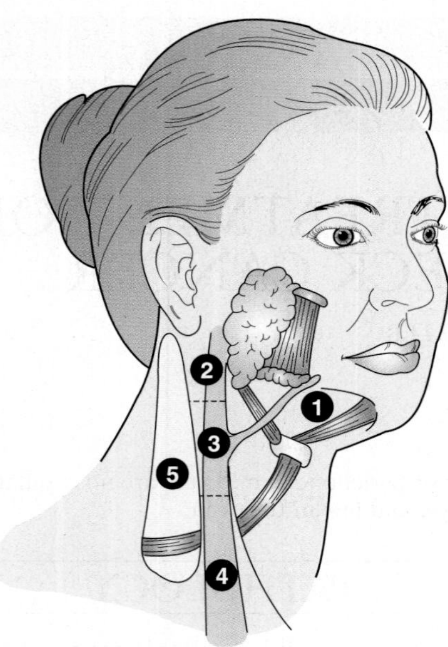

FIGURE 72.1 Head and neck lymph node levels.

Spread inside the lumen of the sublingual, submandibular, and parotid gland ducts is uncommon. The nasolacrimal duct, however, is often invaded in ethmoid sinus and nasal carcinomas.

Perineural invasion (PNI) is observed in SCCs as well as salivary gland tumors, especially adenoid cystic carcinomas. The presence of PNI predicts a poorer rate of local control when managed by surgery[14]; there are no specific data for definitive radiotherapy (RT). Tumors may track along a nerve to the skull base and central nervous system (CNS). Peripheral PNI is also observed. Patients with PNI may develop neurologic symptoms secondary to nerve invasion or, less frequently, entrapment of the nerve.

Vascular space invasion is associated with an increased risk for regional and distant metastases.

Lymphatic Spread

The differentiation of the tumor, size of the primary lesion, presence of vascular space invasion, and density of capillary lymphatics predict the risk of lymph node metastasis. Recurrent lesions have an increased risk.

Although access to the capillary lymphatics is a central event, histology further impacts on the likelihood of lymphatic spread. Low-grade minor salivary gland tumors and sarcomas have a lower risk of lymph node metastases than SCCs arising in similar mucosal sites.

A patient may present with SCC in a cervical lymph node, and despite an extensive workup, the site of origin may remain undetermined in approximately 50% of patients.[15] If the neck only is treated, a primary lesion may appear later, but sometimes the primary site is never found.[16]

The relative incidence of clinically positive lymph nodes on admission is determined by primary site and T stage.[17] Well-lateralized lesions spread to ipsilateral neck nodes.[18] Lesions on or near the midline, tongue base and nasopharyngeal lesions (even when lateralized), may spread to both sides of the neck, although the risk is higher to the side occupied by the bulk of the lesion. Patients with clinically positive ipsilateral neck nodes are at risk for contralateral disease, especially if the nodes are large or multiple. Obstruction of the lymphatic pathways by surgery or RT also shunts the lymphatic flow to the opposite neck. This shunting is mainly through anastomotic channels that cross through the submental space.[19]

When contralateral metastases occur from well-lateralized lesions, the level II nodes are the most commonly involved but may be bypassed, with level III or level IV next affected. When lymph node metastases appear at an unusual site, a careful search must be made for a second primary.

The likelihood of retropharyngeal adenopathy is related to the presence of clinically involved lymph nodes and primary site, and is particularly high for NPCs.[20] The percentage of patients with positive nodes reflects the incidence of radiographically positive nodes; the likelihood of occult disease is probably higher.

Distant Spread

The risk of distant metastasis is related more to N stage, and location of involved nodes in the low neck, than T stage.[21] The risk is less than 10% for N0 or N1 disease and rises to approximately 30% for N3 disease as well as N1 or N2 nodes with disease below the level of the thyroid notch. The lung is the most common site, accounting for half of the first recognized distant metastases. Almost 50% of the metastases are recognized by 9 months, 80% by 2 years, and 90% by 3 years.[22]

DIAGNOSTIC EVALUATION

A general medical evaluation is performed, including a thorough head and neck examination. The location and extent of the primary tumor and any clinically positive lymph nodes is documented. Almost all patients undergo contrast enhanced computed tomography (CT) and/or magnetic resonance imaging (MRI) to further define the extent of locoregional disease. The authors prefer to use CT and reserve MRI for situations in which further information is required. The scan(s) should be obtained prior to biopsy so that biopsy changes are not confused with tumor. A chest radiograph is obtained to determine the presence of distant metastases and/or a synchronous primary lung cancer. Patients with N3 neck disease, as well as those with N2 disease with nodes below the level of the thyroid notch, have a 20% to 30% risk of developing distant metastases and are considered for a chest CT or positron emission tomography (PET).

Tumors amenable to transoral biopsy may be biopsied using local anesthetics in the clinic. Otherwise direct laryngoscopy under anesthesia is performed to determine the extent of the tumor and to obtain a tissue diagnosis. Given the risk of synchronous cancers, some advocate routine triple endoscopy (i.e., laryngoscopy/pharyngoscopy, bronchoscopy, and esophagoscopy). The additional yield is low, unless diffuse mucosal abnormalities or a malignant lymph node without an identified primary site, particularly in the low neck, are present. Patients presenting with a metastatic node from an unknown primary site undergo fine-needle aspiration (FNA) of the node. Excisional biopsy is not routinely performed unless lymphoma is suspected or FNA results are equivocal. If SCC is a consideration, the excision should be done in a manner to facilitate subsequent management, including neck dissection. Occasionally the diagnosis may be made by clinical and radiographic evaluation, and biopsy is avoided in situations in which the treatment is definitive RT and obtaining tissue is risky (i.e., paragangliomas or juvenile nasopharyngeal angiofibromas).[11,23]

Before initial treatment, the patient should be evaluated by members of the team who may be involved in the initial management as well as possible salvage therapy. Head and neck surgeons, radiation oncologists, medical oncologists, diagnostic radiologists, plastic surgeons, pathologists, dentists, speech and swallowing therapists, and social workers may all play a role. The treatment options are discussed and recommendations are presented to the patient who makes the final decision.

TABLE 72.1

2010 AMERICAN JOINT COMMITTEE ON CANCER STAGES OF REGIONAL LYMPH NODE (N) INVOLVEMENT

NX	Regional lymph nodes cannot be assessed
N0	No regional lymph node metastasis
N1	Metastasis in a single ipsilateral lymph node, 3 cm or less in greatest dimension
N2	Metastasis in single ipsilateral lymph node, more than 3 cm but no more than 6 cm in greatest dimension; or in multiple ipsilateral lymph nodes, none more than 6 cm in greatest dimension; or in bilateral or contralateral lymph nodes, no more than 6 cm in greatest dimension
N2a	Metastasis in single ipsilateral lymph node, more than 3 cm but no more than 6 cm in greatest dimension
N2b	Metastasis in multiple ipsilateral lymph nodes, none more than 6 cm in greatest dimension
N2c	Metastasis in bilateral or contralateral lymph nodes, none more than 6 cm in greatest dimension
N3	Metastasis in a lymph node more than 6 cm in greatest dimension

From ref. 24, with permission.

STAGING

The staging for the primary lesions is given in the discussion of each primary site. The American Joint Committee on Cancer (AJCC) neck staging is common to all head and neck sites, except the nasopharynx (Table 72.1).[24] Lesions may be clinically or pathologically staged; the former is designated by cN and the latter is designated by pN. Clinical staging is more commonly used for treatment planning and the reporting of results. The format for combining T and N stages into an overall stage is depicted in Table 72.2 and is common to all sites except the nasopharynx.[24]

Stage IV represents a wide spectrum of disease. One patient may have a T1, T2, or T3 lesion with treatable N2 neck disease and represent a reasonable candidate for curative therapy, whereas another may have a T4b primary cancer and/or N3 neck disease and a relatively low chance of cure.[25]

PRINCIPLES OF TREATMENT FOR SQUAMOUS CELL CARCINOMA

General Priniciples for Selection of Treatment

Surgery and RT are the only curative treatments for head and neck carcinomas. Although chemotherapy alone is not curative, it enhances the effects of RT, and thus is routinely used as part of combined modality treatment, particularly in patients with stage III or IV disease. Indications for the use of chemotherapy are discussed in subsequent sections.

The advantages of surgery compared with RT, assuming similar cure rates, may include (1) a limited amount of tissue is exposed to treatment, (2) treatment time is shorter, (3) the risk of immediate and late RT sequelae is avoided, and (4) RT is reserved for a head and neck SPT, which may not be as suitable for surgery.

The advantages of RT may include (1) the risk of a major postoperative complication is avoided; (2) no tissues are removed, so the probability of a functional or cosmetic defect may be reduced; (3) elective neck RT can be included with little added morbidity, whereas the surgeon must either observe the neck or proceed with an elective neck dissection(s); and (4) the surgical salvage of RT failure is probably more likely than the salvage of a surgical failure.

Salvage of a surgical failure may be attempted by operation or RT, or both. Surgical recurrences usually develop at the resection margins, in or near the suture line. It is difficult to distinguish the normal surgical scarring from recurrent disease, and diagnosis of recurrence is often delayed. Tumor response to RT under these circumstances is poor. Surgery or RT, or both, however, may salvage small mucosal recurrences and some neck recurrences.

TABLE 72.2

2010 AMERICAN JOINT COMMITTEE ON CANCER OVERALL STAGE GROUPING

Stage 0	Tis	N0	M0
Stage I	T1	N0	M0
Stage II	T2	N0	M0
Stage III	T3	N0	M0
	T1-T3	N1	M0
Stage IVA	T4a	N0-N1	M0
	T1-T4a	N2	M0
Stage IVB	Any T	N3	M0
	T4b	Any N	M0
Stage IVC	Any T	Any N	M1

From ref. 24, with permission.

MANAGEMENT

Primary Site

The management of the primary cancer will be considered separately for each anatomic site. Patients who are in poor nutritional condition may require a nasogastric tube or a percutaneous gastrostomy (PEG) before initiating RT, particularly if concomitant chemotherapy is used. If external-beam radiotherapy (EBRT) is selected, it may be given with either conventional once-daily fractionation to 66 to 70 Gy at 2 Gy per fraction, 5 days a week in a continuous course, or with an altered fractionation schedule. Whether an altered fractionation schedule is better than conventional fractionation depends on the altered fractionation technique that is selected. Two altered fractionation schedules shown to result in improved locoregional control rates are the University of Florida hyperfractionation and the M. D. Anderson Cancer Center concomitant boost techniques.[26]

TABLE 72.3

ALTERED FRACTIONATION: 5-YEAR OUTCOMES FROM THE RADIATION THERAPY ONCOLOGY GROUP 90-03 TRIAL

	Fractionation Schedule			
Parameter	Conventional (70 Gy/35 Fx/7 wk)	Hyperfractionation (81.6 Gy/68 Fx/7 wk)	Accelerated Split Course (67.2 Gy/42 Fx/6 wk)	Accelerated Concomitant Boost (72 Gy/42 Fx/6 wk)
Number patients	268	263	274	268
Locoregional failure (%)	59.1	51.2 (*P* = .037)	57.8 (*P* = .042)	51.7
Disease-free survival (%)	21.2	30.7 (*P* = .013)	26.6 (*P* = .042)	28.9
Overall survival (%)	29.5	37.1 (*P* = .063)	30.8	33.5
Cause-specific survival (%)	42.9	45.5	40.9	43.4
Grade 3 late toxicity (%)	25.2	27.4	26.8	33.3 (*P* = .066)

Fx, fractions.
P values reflect comparison of the experimental arms with standard fractionation.
From ref. 26, with permission.

The results of a prospective randomized Radiation Therapy Oncology Group (RTOG) trial comparing these schedules with conventional fractionation and the Massachusetts General Hospital accelerated split-course schedule are shown in Table 72.3. Acute toxicity is increased with altered fractionation; late toxicity is comparable with conventional fractionation.[27]

Conventional EBRT techniques and/or brachytherapy will be discussed in the subsequent site-specific sections. EBRT may also be delivered with intensity-modulated radiation therapy (IMRT) to produce a more conformal dose distribution and reduce the dose to the normal tissues.[28–30] The disadvantages of IMRT are that it is much more time-consuming to plan and treat the patient, the dose distribution is often less homogenous so that "hot spots" may increase the risk of late complications, the risk of a marginal miss may be increased because the fields are more conformal, the total body RT dose is higher because of increased "beam on" time and scatter irradiation, and it is more costly. Therefore, it is essential that a clear reason for using IMRT versus conventional RT be identified. The usual indication for IMRT is to reduce the dose to the contralateral parotid gland and thus limit long-term xerostomia. Another indication is to reduce the CNS dose in patients with NPC. Finally, it may be used to avoid a difficult low neck match in patients with laryngeal or hypopharyngeal cancers and a low lying larynx.

NECK

In a classic *radical neck dissection*, the superficial and deep cervical fascia with its enclosed lymph nodes (levels I to V) is removed in continuity with the sternocleidomastoid muscle, the omohyoid muscle, the internal and external jugular veins, cranial nerve XI, and the submandibular gland. The incisions used by the surgeon will be governed largely by the primary lesion. The radical neck dissection can be *modified* to spare certain structures with the intent of decreasing morbidity and improving functional outcome without compromising disease control. There are three main types of modified radical neck dissections: type I—cranial nerve XI is spared; type II—cranial nerve XI and the internal jugular vein are spared; type III (functional)—cranial nerve XI, the internal jugular vein, and the sternocleidomastoid muscle are spared. Radical and modified radical neck dissections, which remove lymph node levels I through V, are comprehensive neck dissections. *Selective* neck dissections are more limited and include the resection of lymph node levels that are at greatest risk for nodal metastatic spread. Types include the lateral, posterolateral, and supraomohyoid, which include resections of lymph node levels II–IV, II–V, and I-III, respectively.

A modified or selective neck dissection is recommended for the cN0 neck, for selected clinically positive necks (mobile, 1–3 cm lymph nodes), and for removing residual disease after RT when there has been excellent regression of N2 or N3 disease.[31,32]

The more extensive the neck dissection, the higher the risk of complications. Complications after neck dissection include hematoma, seroma, lymphedema, wound infections and dehiscence, damage to the 7th, 10th, 11th, and 12th cranial nerves, carotid exposure, and carotid rupture. The last-mentioned complication can be minimized by covering the carotid artery with a dermal graft at the time of surgery.[31]

Clinically Negative Neck

The estimated incidence of subclinical disease in the regional lymphatics when the neck is cN0 is presented in Table 72.4.[33] Both RT and neck dissection are approximately 90% efficient in eradicating subclinical regional.[31] Alternatively, a policy of close observation may be adopted for the cN0 neck to avoid unnecessary treatment, and the neck is managed by surgery and/or RT if cervical metastases develop. The salvage rate for patients developing clinically positive lymph nodes with the primary lesion controlled is 50% to 60%.[33]

Elective neck irradiation (ENI) results in in-field control rates that exceed 90%.[33] The regional control rates versus extent of ENI at the University of Florida were no ENI, 22 of 28 patients (79%); partial ENI, 82 of 88 patients (93%); and total ENI, 72 of 74 patients (97%).[33] ENI and elective neck dissection are equally effective in the management of the N0 neck.[33,34] Partial neck treatment is suboptimal for primary lesions of the base of tongue, soft palate, supraglottis, and hypopharynx; treatment of the entire neck is advised for sites with a high rate of subclinical disease. Patients with lateralized T1–T2 tonsillar cancers do not require elective treatment for the contralateral N0 neck.[18] Those with significant extension into the tongue and/or soft palate, as well as those with T3 or T4 cancers, should receive bilateral neck treatment to the entire neck.

When the primary tumor is to be treated surgically, an elective neck dissection should be performed when the risk of regional lymph node metastasis is 10% to 15% or greater.

TABLE 72.4

DEFINITION OF RISK GROUPS FOR THE CLINICALLY N0 NECK

Group	Estimated Risk of Subclinical Neck Disease (%)	T Stage	Site
I, low risk	<20	1	Floor of mouth, oral tongue, retromolar trigone, gingiva, hard palate, buccal mucosa
II, intermediate risk	20–30	1	Soft palate, pharyngeal wall, supraglottic larynx, tonsil
		2	Floor of mouth, oral tongue, retromolar trigone, gingiva, hard palate, buccal mucosa
III, high risk	>30	1–4	Nasopharynx, pyriform sinus, base of tongue
		2–4	Soft palate, pharyngeal wall, supraglottic larynx, tonsil
		3–4	Floor of mouth, oral tongue, retromolar trigone, gingiva, hard palate, buccal mucosa

From ref. 33, with permission.

Modified neck dissection has a good rate of disease control; patients who are found to have multiple positive nodes or extracapsular extension (ECE) are then referred for postoperative RT,[35] and concurrent chemotherapy is recommended in the latter circumstance.[36–38] If the primary lesion is to be treated with EBRT, ENI adds relatively little cost and modest morbidity.

Clinically Positive Neck Lymph Nodes

The rates of neck failure by N stage and treatment group reported from the M. D. Anderson Cancer Center and the University of Florida are shown in Tables 72.5 and 72.6, respectively.[34,39] In general, RT precedes surgery if the primary site is to be treated by RT or if the node was immobile. The operation precedes RT if the primary site is to be treated surgically.

Modified neck dissection is sufficient treatment for the ipsilateral neck for patients with N1 or N2a disease without ECE. RT, often combined with concurrent chemotherapy, is added for N2b and N3 disease, control of contralateral subclinical disease, ECE, and/or multiple positive nodes.[35]

When the primary lesion is to be managed by RT or chemoradiotherapy (chemoRT), then RT-based therapy alone is sufficient for patients in whom the node(s) regresses completely as documented on CT obtained 4 weeks after RT.[32,40] RT is followed by a neck dissection for patients with residual nodes that are 1.5 cm or larger, as well as those that demonstrate focal defects, enhancement, and/or calcification.[40] A PET scan obtained 3 months after RT is completed is often helpful in assessing whether there is persistent disease.[41]

Many have condemned excisional or incisional biopsy of a neck mass for diagnosis. McGuirt and McCabe[42] compared results of definitive surgery with and without a prior open biopsy and concluded the risks of neck failure, distant metastases, and complications were all increased. Ellis et al.[43] studied the results of therapy following open biopsy of a lymph node before treatment. Patients received definitive RT to the primary site and neck; a subset of patients underwent a neck dissection after RT. Open biopsy had no adverse impact on these patients compared with those who did not undergo an open biopsy.[43] Therefore, after open biopsy of the neck, RT-based therapy is recommended as the initial treatment. If the primary tumor is to be managed by RT or chemoRT, no further neck treatment is needed if the neck node has been removed. If there is residual gross tumor in the neck after open biopsy, a planned neck dissection should be added, depending on the results of a restaging CT scan 3 to 4 weeks after RT.[40] If the primary tumor is to be managed by surgery, preoperative RT is followed by resection of the primary site with or without a neck dissection.

Once the normal lymphatic pathways have been surgically interrupted by the open biopsy procedure, shunting of lymph nodes to the contralateral side of the neck may occur, placing it at risk for lymph node spread when the opposite neck would not normally be at risk.[19]

TABLE 72.5

FAILURE OF INITIAL NECK TREATMENT[a]

	Stage							
	N0							
Treatment	No Treatment	Partial	Complete	N1	N2a	N2b	N3a	N3b
Radiation	55% (16/29)	15%	2%	15%	27%	27%	38%	34%
Surgery		35%	7%	11%	8%	23%	42%	41%
Combined		1/5	0/6	0	0	0	23%	25%

[a]Results of 596 patients with carcinoma of the tonsillar fossa, base of tongue, supraglottic larynx, or hypopharynx, M. D. Anderson Cancer Center, 1948–1967.
Adapted from ref. 34.

TABLE 72.6

FIVE-YEAR RATE OF NECK CONTROL ACCORDING TO THE 1983 AMERICAN JOINT COMMITTEE ON CANCER[350] STAGE AND TREATMENT

	RT Alone		RT + Neck Dissection		
Stage	No. of Heminecks	Control (%)	No. of Heminecks	Control (%)	Significance (P)
N1	215	86	38	93	.28
N2a	29	79	24	68	.6
N2b	138	70	80	91	<.01
N3a	29	33	40	69	<.01

Includes 459 patients, 593 heminecks; excludes 67 heminecks that received incisional or excisional biopsies before treatment.
Note: The University of Florida data, patients were treated October 1964 to October 1985; analysis December 1988 by Eric R. Ellis, MD.
From ref. 39, with permission.

CHEMOTHERAPY

Drug therapy may be administered to prevent the development of SPTs (chemoprevention); to palliate symptoms in patients with incurable disease; to improve the odds of cure or organ preservation when combined with definitive locoregional therapy; or to decrease treatment toxicity. The first two indications are discussed here; the last two are discussed in a subsequent section.

Chemoprevention

Chemoprevention is the administration of natural or synthetic agents to reduce the risk of developing SPTs. Patients who have a head and neck SCC have an increased risk of developing an upper aerodigestive tract SPT because of exposure to carcinogens and/or genetic predisposition.[3] The risk of developing a SPT is approximately 2.7% to 4% per year[44] and may impact survival. Of note, current data indicate that HR-HPV–related head and neck cancers are not associated with this increased risk.[6] Analogues of vitamin A, particularly of the retinoids, have been a particular focus of clinical investigations.

Retinoids and beta carotene both may cause regression of oral leukoplakia; the former appear more efficacious.[45] Lesions commonly recur after cessation of drug therapy. Chemoprevention agents do not reduce the risk of recurrence of the index cancer. Reversal of moderate to severe dysplasia is unlikely with single-agent chemoprevention.[46,47]

13-*cis*-Retinoic acid has been shown in a randomized, placebo-controlled trial to reduce the risk of SPTs in patients previously treated for stage I–IV, M0, head and neck cancer. This study used a high-dose schedule of the drug (100 mg/m^2) daily for 12 months.[48] However, a large, placebo-controlled, randomized trial of 1,190 survivors of stage I and II head and neck SCC found no difference in the rate of SPTs or survival after 3 years of a low-dose schedule of this agent (30 mg/day).[49] Similarly, etretinate was not shown to be efficacious in decreasing SPTs.[50]

With regard to other agents, vitamin A, *N*-acetylcysteine, both or neither were evaluated using a factorial design in the EUROSCAN study. No significant improvement in survival or SPTs was observed.[51] Bairati et al.[52] randomized head and neck cancer survivors to 3 years of therapy with alpha-tocopherol and beta carotene versus placebo; the rate of SPTs was actually higher during the period of treatment, a difference that did not persist with longer follow-up.

There is an interest in cyclooxygenase 2 inhibitors as chemopreventive agents because cyclooxygenase 2 is up-regulated in oral cancers and premalignant lesions; however, a randomized phase 2, placebo-controlled trial demonstrated no significant benefit of celecoxib at 100 mg or 200 mg, both twice daily, on the control of oral premalignant lesions.[53] Similarly, targeting the epidermal growth factor receptor pathway is receiving attention, as there is an association between progressive epidermal growth factor receptor dysregulation and the transition from normal mucosa to dysplasia to SCC.[54] Finally, the concept of bioadjuvant therapy, whereby drug combinations intended to reduce both the risk of SPTs and of relapse from the index cancer, is being investigated.[49]

Although of interest, there is no standard role for the use of HR-HPV vaccination in the prevention of head and neck cancer at this time.[55]

Chemotherapy for Recurrent or Metastatic Disease

Single Agents

Patients with recurrent or metastatic head and neck SCCs have a median survival of 6 to 9 months, and a 1-year survival rate of 20% to 40% when treated with chemotherapy alone.[46,56] The survival benefit associated with the use of chemotherapy compared to best supportive care only in these patients has not been well studied. Although selected patients may derive apparent significant prolongations in survival, average survival improvements appear small at best. Morton et al.[57] reported a 2-month improvement in median survival after treatment with cisplatin, with or without bleomycin, compared with no treatment. The duration of responses is typically measured in weeks to months, not years; survival beyond 2 years is infrequent; cures are anecdotal. Thus, the primary intent of chemotherapy in this setting is to achieve tumor regression with the hope that the potential palliative benefit and possible modest survival improvement will outweigh the side effects of treatment. Unfortunately, most clinical trials have historically used response rate and toxicity reporting as surrogate measures for outcomes of greater priority to the patients, such as palliation of specific symptoms (e.g., pain), improvement in function (e.g., swallowing), or overall quality of life.

A number of drugs have been demonstrated in clinical trials to have activity in head and neck SCCs, and the list is well summarized in prior reviews.[46,56] The most commonly used include methotrexate, cisplatin, carboplatin, 5-fluorouracil, paclitaxel, and docetaxel, with reported major response rates ranging from 15% to 42%. Among other drugs with reported major response rates of 15% or greater are bleomycin, cyclophosphamide, doxorubicin, hydroxyurea, ifosfamide, irinotecan, oral uracil, and ftorafur (with leucovorin), pemetrexed, vinblastine, and vinorelbine. Some of these agents (e.g., cyclophosphamide, doxorubicin, hydroxyurea) have their activity based on reported assessment in a limited number of patients from over 2 decades ago, an era when methods and criteria for response assessment may have differed from current standards. Anticipated response rates and toxicity profiles may vary based on patient selection and drug schedule. Poor performance status is associated with both lower response rates and greater potential for toxicity. The larger the amount of prior treatment also adversely affects response rates.[56]

Methotrexate is a historic standard drug used in the recurrent or metastatic disease setting. The typical standard dosing is 40 mg/m^2 intravenously weekly, with dose attenuation or increase (up to 60 mg/m^2) based on toxicity, with mucositis being a frequent reason for dose adjustment. The favorable side effect profile and convenience of administration of methotrexate make it well suited for use in this patient population in which medical comorbidity is common, as is more advanced age. Higher doses have been compared to standard dosing in randomized trials: response rates increase as does toxicity, without a significant improvement in overall survival.[58,59] Similarly, newer analogues of methotrexate (e.g., edatrexate) have not been shown in phase 3 trials to offer a therapeutic advantage.[60]

Cisplatin is a cornerstone drug in the modern management of head and neck cancer. Cisplatin is customarily dosed at 75 to 100 mg/m^2 intravenously every 3 to 4 weeks. The potential for renal (i.e., increase in creatinine, electrolyte abnormalities), otologic (i.e., high-frequency hearing loss, tinnitus), neurologic (i.e., peripheral neuropathy), and gastrointestinal (i.e., nausea and vomiting) toxicity are widely appreciated, but these risks are manageable if patients are appropriately screened for therapy, monitored closely during it, and state of the art antiemetics are applied. Further dose escalation of cisplatin has not been established to improve outcome. A randomized trial comparing 60 mg/m^2 versus 120 mg/m^2 of cisplatin failed to demonstrate a significant improvement in response or survival.[61] Carboplatin is the best studied and most commonly used platinum analogue in head and neck cancer. It has less renal, otologic, neurologic, and gastrointestinal toxicity than the parent drug, and is also easier to administer. The tradeoff is that it is more bone marrow-suppressive and may be somewhat less active. This last issue is more of a concern in the definitive treatment setting in which cure is a central end point, as opposed to the palliative setting, when patients often seek a less toxic alternative treatment.

Although taxanes as a class have significant activity in head and neck SCCs, hopes of clinically significant improvement in survival in the palliative setting with the introduction of these agents have yet to be realized. Neither paclitaxel or docetaxel has been demonstrated in random assignment trials to be clearly superior to methotrexate with regard to survival as an end point.[62] Initial studies with paclitaxel used a dose of 250 mg/m^2 intravenously over 24 hours with growth factor support. In an Eastern Cooperative Oncology Group (ECOG) trial, 12 of 30 patients (40%) had a partial (8 patients) or complete (4 patients) response. However, grade 3 or greater neutropenia occurred in 91% of patients, and there were two deaths.[63] Less cumbersome to administer and less toxic schedules are commonly used in practice (e.g., 135–225 mg/m^2 intravenously over 3 hours every 3 weeks; 80–100 mg/m^2 weekly), although their relative efficacies have not been well evaluated. A paclitaxel schedule that provides more prolonged exposure to the drug may be more efficacious,[64] although a phase 2 trial of 120 to 140 mg/m^2 every 96 hours yielded disappointing results even in treatment-naïve patients (major response rate, 13%).[65] Other toxicities, besides myelosuppression, include sensory neuropathy, alopecia, allergic reactions, and arrhythmia, although cardiac monitoring is not required.

Docetaxel appears less neuropathic than paclitaxel, but fluid retention and hematologic toxicity may be more problematic. A typical dose is 60 to 100 mg/m^2 intravenously over 1 hour. Initial studies evaluated the efficacy of the 100 mg/m^2 dose level, with major response rates ranging from 21% to 42%[66]; an excellent performance status is required for this higher dose. Lower doses may offer similar efficacy and better tolerance. A multicenter study evaluating a 60 mg/m^2 dose level reported a major response rate of 22%.[67] As with paclitaxel, weekly schedules are applied in practice, but the relative efficacy of a weekly versus every-3-weeks schedule is not well studied.

Although initial studies evaluated a bolus schedule for 5-fluorouracil, an infusional program of 1,000 mg/m^2/day over 96 to 120 hours appears more efficacious in head and neck cancer.[68] Infusional 5-fluorouracil is associated with more mucositis and diarrhea than a bolus schedule, so the shorter infusion (i.e., 96 hours) is typically applied in patients who are pretreated and have received prior head and neck RT.

EGFR is highly expressed in most head and neck SCCs, and the degree of expression is inversely associated with prognosis.[69–71] As such, there has been keen interest in drugs that target the receptor itself or steps downstream. Cetuximab, a chimeric immunoglobulin G antibody that binds the receptor, has been approved by the U.S. Food and Drug Administration for use in patients with disease refractory to platin-based therapy. As summarized in Table 72.7, the response rates in this refractory setting are similar, 10% to 13%, whether cetuximab is used alone or combined with platin-based therapy.[72–75] Disease stabilizations were more common, but median survivals remained disappointing, ranging from 5.2 to 6.1 months.[72–74]

The small molecule tyrosine kinase inhibitors gefitinib and erlotinib offer no efficacy advantage in similar refractory

PRACTICE OF ONCOLOGY

TABLE 72.7

CETUXIMAB FOR RECURRENT OR METASTATIC HEAD AND NECK CANCER

Study	No. of Patients	Cancer	Chemotherapy	RR (%)	Median PFS (mo)	Median OS (mo)
Herbst et al.[73a]	79	SCC—POD on CDDP-based	CDDP-based + cetuximab	6–20	2.0–3.0	4.3–6.1
Baselga et al.[72a]	96	SCC—POD on platin-based	CDDP-based + cetuximab	10–11	2.4–2.8	4.9–6.0
Trigo et al.[74]	103	SCC—POD on platin-based	Cetuximab	13	2.3	5.9
Burtness et al.[75b]	117	SCC—no chemo for R/M	CDDP	10	2.7	8.0
			CDDP + cetuximab	26	4.2	9.2

RR, response rate; PFS, progressive-free survival; OS, overall survival; SCC, squamous cell cancer; POD, progression of disease; CDDP, cisplatin; R/M, recurrent or metastatic disease.

[a]Range related to how POD was defined in different subgroups.

[b]Response rates were significantly different (P = .03): PFS (P = .09) and OS (P = .21) did not reach statistical significance.

patients. Major response rates and median survivals ranged from 0% to 15% and 5.9 to 8.1 months, respectively.[71,76–78] A large randomized trial (486 patients) compared gefitinib (250 or 500 mg daily) to methotrexate and demonstrated no survival improvement with either gefitinib dose. There were more tumor hemorrhage-type events on the gefitinib arms (8.9% and 11.4% vs. 1.9%).[79]

With both of these classes of agents, the development of rash was associated with clinical benefit, but this association is not fully explained by simple pharmacokinetics.[71] There is no established molecular predictor of response to these agents currently in head and neck SCC. Higher-quality data evaluating the activities of standard chemotherapy drugs versus these newer targeted therapies are limited at present.

The successful development and approval of cetuximab in head and neck SCC highlights the potential for therapies to exploit specific molecular pathways with therapeutic effect. There is a good rationale for agents that target angiogenesis in head and neck SCC.[80] However, the development of bevacizumab has been cautious, given reported toxicity concerns, specifically bleeding, in patients with squamous cell lung cancer.[81] A number of other new agents, often with multitarget capability, are entering clinical trials. Cancer gene therapy, whereby genetic sequences are introduced via viral or nonviral vectors, is well suited to head and neck tumors, given the locoregional character of head and neck tumors that facilitates direct injection and the monitoring of gene expression. The tumor suppressor gene *p53* has been one target, as somatic mutations of it are common in head and neck cancers, particularly among patients who have smoked cigarettes and used alcohol.[82] For example, in a phase 2 study of Onyx-015, a replication-competent adenovirus absent the *E1B* gene, major responses, including some complete regressions, occurred in 10% to 14% of treated patients.[83] In other studies, treatment with Onyx-015, or a similar virus H101, improved the efficacy of chemotherapy.[84,85] The latter trial led to the approval in China of the first oncolytic therapy for cancer treatment. The therapeutic potential for cancer gene therapy in head and neck cancer is further discussed in other reviews.[86]

Combination Therapy

Given the disappointing track record for single-agent therapy in the palliative setting, combinations of drugs have been extensively evaluated. Cisplatin lends itself for combination with other drugs and modalities (i.e., RT), as it typically does not cause significant mucositis or severe bone marrow suppression. In the early 1980s, investigators from Wayne State University, building on potential synergy between cisplatin and 5-fluororuacil, reported a major response rate of 70% with a complete response rate of 27% using a regimen of cisplatin 100 mg/m^2 intravenously and 5-fluorouracil 1,000 mg/m^2/day continuous infusion over 96 hours recycled every 3 weeks in patients with recurrent or disseminated disease.[87] Other investigators confirmed the significant activity of the regimen, albeit with a somewhat lower major and complete response rate on average (50% and 16%, respectively).[88] A meta-analysis of randomized studies from the pretaxane era concluded that the combination of cisplatin and infusional 5-fluorouracil was superior to other combinations, further establishing it as the standard regimen to which new therapies are compared.

Despite improvement in response rates associated with the use of combination therapies like cisplatin and 5-flurouracil, demonstrating a statistically or clinically significant improvement in survival compared to single-agent therapy has proven elusive. Table 72.8 summarizes the results of three randomized trials that compared treatment with cisplatin and infusion 5-fluorouracil to that with different single agents.[89–91] All three studies yielded similar results.[89–91] Treatment with combination chemotherapy led to a significant increase in response rate, albeit at the cost of greater toxicity. Overall survival did not significantly improve. The meta-analysis reported by Browman and Cronin[92] yielded similar conclusions: higher response rates but more toxicity with cisplatin and infusional 5-fluorouracil compared with

TABLE 72.8

CHEMOTHERAPY FOR RECURRENT OR METASTATIC HEAD AND NECK CANCER: SELECTED PHASE 3 TRIALS OF CISPLATIN/5-FLUOROURACIL VERSUS OTHER OPTIONS

Study	No. of Patients	Agents	Response Rates[a] (%)	Median Survival[b] (mo)
Jacobs et al.[90]	249	CDDP/FU	32	5.5
		CDDP	17	5.0
		FU	13	6.1
Forastiere et al.[89]	277	CDDP/FU	32	6.6
		CBDCA/FU	21	5.0
		MTX	10	5.6
Clavel et al.[91]	382	CDDP/MTX/BLEO/VCR	34	8.2
		CDDP/FU	31	6.2
		CDDP	15	5.3
Schrijvers et al.[102]	122	CDDP/FU/IFNa-2b	38	6.0
		CDDP/FU	47	6.3
Gibson et al.[100]	218	CDDP/FU	27	8.7
		CDDP/PAC	26	8.1

CDDP, cisplatin; FU, 5-fluorouracil; CBDCA, carboplatin; MTX, methotrexate; BLEO, bleomycin; VCR, vincristine; IFNa-2b, interferon alpha-2b; PAC, paclitaxel.

[a]The following response rate differences were statistically significant at $P < .05$: Jacobs et al. (1992), CDDP/FU versus both CDDP and FU; Forastiere et al. (1992), CDDP/FU versus MTX; Clavel et al. (1994), both combinations versus CDDP.

[b]All survival differences were not statistically significant.

single-agent therapy, and a difference in median survival of less than 1 month. These data do not support the routine use of cisplatin-based combinations for patients with recurrent or metastatic SCC. Combination therapy seems most appropriate for patients with a good performance, who will be able to tolerate the added toxicity, and have significant symptoms (e.g., pain) for which the higher anticipated response rate will translate into better palliation.

The activity of paclitaxel and docetaxel in head and neck cancer has fostered the development and evaluation of taxane and cisplatin combinations. Docetaxel with cisplatin is associated with a major response rate of 40% to 53%, with complete response rates approximating 6% to 18%[93-95]; a weekly schedule of paclitaxel (80 mg/m^2) and carboplatin (area under concentration-versus-time curve [AUC] 2) appeared more efficacious than every 3 weeks dosing (paclitaxel 175–200 mg/m^2 intravenously over 3 hours followed by carboplatin AUC 6) in two separate phase 2 studies.[96-98] ECOG compared high-dose (200 mg/m^2) and moderate-dose (135 mg/m^2) paclitaxel, both by 24-hour infusion and followed by the same dose of cisplatin (75 mg/m^2) in a randomized study (E1393). No significant difference in response rate or survival was found between the arms; grade 3–4 neutropenia occurred in 70% and 78% of patients, respectively.[99] Another randomized trial done under the auspices of ECOG compared standard cisplatin and 5-fluorouracil with paclitaxel 175 mg/m^2 intravenously over 3 hours and cisplatin 75 mg/m^2 (E1395).[100] Objective major response rates (27% vs. 26%) and median survivals (8.7 vs. 8.1 months) were no different between the arms. Overall, the magnitude of treatment toxicities was similar, although there was more gastrointestinal and hematologic toxicity with cisplatin and 5-fluorouracil, which was also more cumbersome to administer. Reported quality of life was also better on the paclitaxel arm over the first 16 weeks of treatment.[101]

Attempts have been made to improve the efficacy of combination chemotherapy through the development of a variety of triplets. The addition of interferon-alpha2b to cisplatin and 5-fluorouracil failed to significantly improve response or survival in a randomized trial.[102] Phase 2 studies of a taxane with cisplatin or carboplatin and a third drug (e.g., 5-fluorouracil, ifosfamide), have yielded major response rates of 55% to 86%[103-107]; two studies have reported 1-year survival rates exceeding 50%.[103,104] Whether these regimens translate into better survival outcomes compared with a cisplatin-based doublet that may be less toxic awaits further evaluations.

There is great interest in the combination of standard chemotherapy with newer targeted agents. Available randomized data evaluating the incremental impact of this approach are limited. One ECOG study compared cisplatin versus cisplatin and cetuximab as first-line treatment in 123 patients. The arm including the cetuximab had a significantly higher response rate (10% vs. 26%; P = .03), but no significant difference was found in the primary end point of progression-free survival (2.7 vs. 4.2 months; P = .09) nor in overall survival (8.0 vs. 9.2 months; P = .21), although the trends favored the combination arm.[75] In a larger trial (EXTREME),[108] 442 patients were randomized to cisplatin or carboplatin and 5-fluorouracil with or without cetuximab for six cycles. Patients with stable disease or no response stopped therapy at that point on the platin and 5-fluorouracil arm, while maintenance cetuximab alone was continued on the investigational arm. No crossover was allowed. Both median progression-free (5.6 vs. 3.3 months) and overall (10.1 vs. 7.4 months) survivals were significantly improved on the triplet arm, at the cost of more sepsis (9 vs. 1 patient; P = .02), grade 3 skin reactions (9%), and grade 3 or higher infusion reactions. There were, however, no cetuximab-related deaths. This trial is noteworthy because demonstrating an improvement in overall survival in this study population has proven elusive despite multiple randomized trials designed with that intent over the past 30 years. Of interest, data from Taamma et al.[109] and Vermorken et al.[110] suggest that the therapeutic effect of cetuximab, when combined with chemotherapy, is mainly additive rather than synergistic. Whether allowing patients to cross over to cetuximab on the doublet arm at progression would have decreased or eliminated the observed survival difference is of interest for future research.

Long-term survival with chemotherapy alone is anecdotal. With advances in RT techniques that facilitate reirradiation with acceptable morbidity, this approach has been increasingly explored in patients with unresectable local or regional recurrence, often with integrated chemotherapy. The observed median survivals in these series are similar to those obtained in phase 2 trials of chemotherapy alone, but more durable responses occur in selected patients and there is a clearer plateau on the survival curve. In two larger series involving 169 and 115 patients, respectively, among patients treated with a variety of RT fractionation schedules and concurrent chemotherapy regimens, 2-year survival rates exceeded 20%.[108,111] In two sequential RTOG studies, a regimen of daily paclitaxel (20 mg/m^2) and cisplatin (15 mg/m^2) added concurrently to split-course RT (total dose 60 Gy, 1.5 Gy twice-daily fractions; granulocyte colony-stimulating factor support during off weeks) (RTOG 96–11) yielded a better 2-year survival rate than concurrent 5-fluororuacil and hydroxyurea added to the same RT schedule (RTOG 96–10) (24.9% vs. 16.9%; P = .44).[112,113] The reported 2-year survival rates exceed the rate of 10.5% observed in a subgroup of 124 patients with local disease only who had previously received RT and participated in E1393 or E1395.[114] However, the results of randomized trials comparing chemotherapy alone with reirradiation and chemotherapy are not available.

Nasopharynx Cancer

Many of the same drugs and regimens used in the treatment of head and neck SCC are also active in NPC. There is an impression that NPC, particularly World Health Organization (WHO) types II and III, is more responsive to chemotherapy than other upper aerodigestive tract cancers. Consistent with this impression is that there are reports of a small proportion of patients with recurrent or metastatic disease being controlled long term with chemotherapy alone.[115] Available data support the use of cisplatin-based combination chemotherapy (e.g., cisplatin/5-fluorouracil; cisplatin/bleomycin/5-flurouracil ± epirubicin), although there is a lack of randomized studies to clarify the relative efficacies and toxicities of different options. Site-specific phase 2 studies report major response rates of 70% or higher with regimens containing cisplatin.[116-118] In a review of the Princess Margaret Hospital experience, single-agent or non-cisplatin–based combination chemotherapy was associated with major and complete response rates of 25% and 8%, respectively, in 40 patients, while cisplatin-based combination therapy produced major and complete response rates of 70% and 23%, respectively, in 30 patients.[116] Substitution of carboplatin may be associated with less activity.[117]

With regard to newer agents, paclitaxel as a 175 mg/m^2 3-hour infusion is active with a response rate of 22% in a series of 24 patients with undifferentiated NPCs.[118] The combination of it with carboplatin has yielded response rates consistently greater than 50%.[119-121] Surprisingly, the combination of docetaxel and cisplatin yielded a response of only 22%, albeit in a small series (n = 9) reported from the Princess Margaret Hospital.[122] Gemcitabine appears particularly active in NPCs,[123,124] and combinations including it appear promising with response rates exceeding 70%.[125,126] Capecitabine, prolonged 5-fluorouracil infusion, and cetuximab all have modest activity in the refractory setting, and no major responses were seen in one study with gefitinib.[127-130] There is keen interest in looking to exploit for therapeutic purpose the association NPC has with the EBV. Potential gene therapy approaches are discussed elsewhere.[131,132]

GENERAL PRINCIPLES OF COMBINING MODALITIES

Surgery Plus Radiation Therapy

Either preoperative or postoperative RT-based therapy may be used; there are advocates of each. Analysis of available data suggests there is no compelling difference in the locoregional control or survival rates comparing the two sequences.[35]

Combined modality therapy should be avoided for lesions with a high cure rate (70% or greater) by either surgery or RT alone. The increased morbidity from combined treatment is not associated with a significantly improved control rate, and many patients with local or regional failure can be salvaged by secondary procedures.

The advantages of postoperative compared with preoperative RT include less operative morbidity, more meaningful margin checks at the time of the surgery, a knowledge of tumor spread for RT planning, safe use of a higher RT dose, and no chance the patient will refuse surgery. The disadvantages of postoperative RT include the larger treatment volume necessary to cover surgical dissections, a delay in the start of RT with possible progression, and the higher dose required to accomplish the same rates of locoregional control.

Preoperative Radiation Therapy

Preoperative RT should be considered for the following situations: (1) fixed neck nodes, (2) initiation of postoperative RT will be delayed more than 8 weeks, (3) use of the gastric pull-up for reconstruction, and (4) open biopsy of a positive neck node.

Postoperative Radiation Therapy

Postoperative RT is considered when the risk of recurrence above the clavicles exceeds 20%. The operative procedure should be one stage and of such magnitude that RT is started no later than 6 to 8 weeks after surgery. The operation should be undertaken only if it is believed to be highly likely that all gross disease will be removed and margins will be negative.

Although no definitive randomized trials have addressed the efficacy of postoperative RT in the treatment of head and neck cancer, excellent data that have bearing on this issue are available from the Medical College of Virginia. Two groups of surgeons operated on patients with head and neck cancer: general surgical oncologists who used surgery alone and reserved RT for treatment of recurrent disease, and otolaryngologists who routinely sent patients with locally advanced disease for postoperative RT.[133] One hundred twenty-five of 441 patients treated surgically between 1982 and 1988 had ECE and/or positive margins; 71 were treated with surgery alone and 54 received postoperative RT. Patients were irradiated once daily at 1.8 to 2.0 Gy per fraction to doses of 50 to 50.99 Gy in 26 patients and to 60 Gy or more in the remainder. Local control rates at 3 years after surgery alone compared with surgery and RT were ECE, 31% and 66% ($P = .03$); positive margins, 41% and 49% ($P = .04$); and ECE and positive margins, 0% and 68% ($P = .001$). A multivariate analysis of local control was performed evaluating the impact of T stage, N stage, use of postoperative RT, the number of positive nodes, the number of nodes with ECE, primary site, microscopic and macroscopic ECE, and margin status. For the end point of local control, use of postoperative RT ($P = .0001$), macroscopic ECE ($P = .0001$), and margin status ($P = .09$) were of independent significance. Disease-free survival at 3 years was 25% after surgery alone and 45% after combined-modality treatment ($P = .0001$). Cause-specific survival rates at 3 years were 41% for surgery alone and 72% for surgery and postoperative RT ($P = .0003$). Multivariate analysis of cause-specific survival showed that postoperative RT ($P = .0001$) and the number of nodes with ECE ($P = .0001$) significantly influenced this end point.

In another series, Lundahl et al.[134] reported on 95 patients with node-positive SCC who were treated with a neck dissection and postoperative RT at the Mayo Clinic. A matched-pair analysis was performed using a series of patients treated with surgery alone; 56 matched pairs of patients were identified. The recurrence rates in the dissected neck (relative risk [RR] = 5.82; $P = .0002$), recurrence in either side of the neck (RR = 2.21; $P = .0052$), and death from any cause (RR = 1.67; $P = .0182$) were significantly higher for patients treated with surgery alone.

Thus, it appears that postoperative RT may significantly improve both locoregional disease control and survival for patients who are at high risk for failure after surgery.

Indications for postoperative RT include close (<5 mm) or positive margins, ECE, multiple positive nodes, invasion of the soft tissues of the neck, endothelial-lined space invasion, PNI, and more than 5 mm of subglottic invasion.[35] The authors currently recommend 60 Gy in 6 weeks to 66 Gy in 6.5 weeks for patients with negative margins and fewer than three indications for RT. For patients with close (<5 mm) or positive margins, the authors recommend 70 Gy in 7 weeks or 74.4 Gy at 1.2 Gy twice a day. Concomitant cisplatin chemotherapy should be considered for patients with positive margins and/or ECE.[36–38]

CHEMOTHERAPY AS PART OF CURATIVE TREATMENT

Systematically designed randomized studies have established a role for drug therapy as part of the standard combined modality management of head and neck SCC in several settings. These include the therapy of unresectable disease, for organ preservation, and for patients with poor-risk pathologic features after surgery. Chemotherapy has been shown to improve the likelihood of disease control compared to RT alone in patients with advanced disease, albeit with increased acute toxicity, particularly within the RT field, which may necessitate temporary PEG placement. In certain circumstances, chemotherapy response to it has been used to triage patients to different locoregional treatments.

Chemotherapy has been integrated with surgery or RT in a variety of ways including induction, concurrent with RT, and/or maintenance. Unlike outcome studies of surgery and/or RT in which site-specific results are reported, albeit typically using a retrospective methodology, many of the trials evaluating the role of chemotherapy enrolled patients with a variety of head and neck SCCs, even when site-specific, although prospective, subsites are combined. This is less of an issue for studies evaluating therapy for NPC.[135,136] Nonetheless, important lessons have been learned from these studies, further enhanced by use of a random assignment methodology. In this section, general principles for the integration chemotherapy with locoregional treatment will be discussed with a focus on the results of randomized trials.

The Meta-Analysis of Chemotherapy on Head and Neck Cancer (MACH-NC) included 63 randomized trials published from 1965 through 1993, all of which compared locoregional treatment with or without chemotherapy.[137] Individual patient data were available on 10,741 patients. The absolute improvement in 5-year survival overall was 4% ($P < .001$). However, the significant improvement appeared limited to those patients who received concomitant treatment (absolute difference of 8% at 5 years, $P < .001$). Neither the difference seen at 5 years with induction (2%, $P = .10$) or maintenance (1%, $P = .74$) chemotherapy was statistically significant.[137] An update of this analysis was recently reported, including trials through 2000, totaling 17,346 patients.[138] The superior efficacy of concurrent therapy was confirmed, and was greater than that seen with induction chemotherapy.

Recently, tumor HPV status has emerged as an important predictor of favorable treatment response and survival.[7] This observation is well illustrated in the analysis of ECOG 2399. Patients received induction paclitaxel and carboplatin, followed by weekly paclitaxel during RT. Most patients enrolled had oropharynx cancer. Response to chemotherapy, to all protocol treatment, progression free-survival, and overall survival were all improved in the HPV-positive group.[7]

Induction Chemotherapy

In untreated patients with local or regionally advanced, M0 head and neck SCC, treatment with cisplatin-based combination chemotherapy will yield major response rates approximating 90%, with clinical complete response rates in the 30% range.[139] Enthusiasm that response rates of this magnitude should translate into survival benefit when induction chemotherapy was combined with surgery or RT is understandable. Yet in the original report of the MACH-NC analysis, which included 31 induction studies, all but 2 suggested no survival benefit.[137]

However, a more careful look at these and other data do provide grounds for continued interest in this approach. Many of the included studies had significant methodologic limitations with regard to the prognostic heterogeneity of the patients entered, sample sizes that were inadequate to rule out false-negative results, and the use of drug therapy insufficiently active by current standards. A subset analysis, limited to the 15 trials that used cisplatin and infusional 5-fluorouracil, suggested survival benefit (hazard ratio, 0.88; 95% confidence interval [CI], 0.79 to 0.97).[137] In a randomized trial limited to patients with locoregionally advanced, oropharyngeal cancer reported by Domenge et al.,[140] induction chemotherapy with cisplatin and 5-fluorouracil significantly improved survival ($P = .03$) compared to locoregional treatment alone (i.e., surgery plus RT or RT alone). Even in the absence of survival improvement, there seemed to be a correlation between response to chemotherapy and subsequent response to RT, which provided a basis for subsequent organ preservation initiatives.[141,142] Finally, patterns of failure were affected with less distant metastases in certain studies when induction chemotherapy was incorporated. There is a growing appreciation that, as locoregional control improves, the rate of clinically apparent distant metastases is increasing,[143] and induction chemotherapy is on average better tolerated than maintenance therapy as a way to give additional systemic therapy.

The study reported originally by Paccagnella et al.[144] and Zorat et al.[145] is illustrative of these types of trials and provides further insights. Two hundred thirty-seven patients with stage III or IV head and neck cancer were randomized to four cycles of induction cisplatin and infusional 5-fluorouracil followed by standard locoregional treatment (i.e., surgery plus RT if resectable, RT alone if unresectable). Resectability was assessed pretreatment, not after chemotherapy, and was a stratification criteria. Overall, there was no significant difference between the arms with regard to overall survival or locoregional control, although the incidence of distant metastases was lower among patients treated with chemotherapy. On subset analysis, however, patients with unresectable disease benefited from the incorporation of induction chemotherapy for all outcomes, including locoregional control, distant control, and overall survival (3-year survival 24% vs. 10%; $P = .04$). Among resectable patients, improvement in distant control was offset by a decrement in locoregional control with the integration of induction chemotherapy, and reported survival rates in this subgroup were similar on both treatment arms.

Historically, then, despite the initial enthusiasm, there was no role for induction chemotherapy prior to planned surgery and postoperative RT, and a limited role only in selected settings prior to RT. However, with the incorporation of taxanes into induction regimens containing cisplatin and 5-fluororuacil, newer data suggest that the indications for induction chemotherapy may evolve in the near future.

Three randomized trials have compared the relative efficacies of induction chemotherapy with standard cisplatin and 5-fluorouracil versus a triplet including a taxane and these same two drugs with one or both being dose adjusted.[110,146,147] All three studies randomized patients with advanced M0 head and neck cancer to either cisplatin and 5-fluororuacil or a triplet, followed by the same RT-based treatment. In one study, this was RT alone, while in the other two studies, concurrent therapy with carboplatin and cisplatin, respectively, were employed. In general, the taxane-containing triplet was associated with a higher response rate to induction chemotherapy and improved both progression-free and overall survival. More neutropenia was observed with triplet therapy but, overall, it was as well tolerated as standard cisplatin and 5-fluorouracil.

These studies were designed to determine which induction chemotherapy was more efficacious and provide convincing evidence that the triplet of a taxane with cisplatin and 5-flurouracil is superior to standard cisplatin and 5-fluorouracil alone as induction therapy. However, an alternative design is necessary to define the role of induction with such triplets in standard practice. For this population, as discussed in the next section, concurrent chemotherapy and RT alone without induction chemotherapy is the more established standard therapy. Randomized studies will be necessary to determine whether a sequential approach using induction with a triplet followed by RT-based treatment (typically with concurrent chemotherapy) is superior to concurrent chemotherapy and RT alone. One recently presented randomized study failed to yield a clear answer as interpretation was confounded by the lack of an intention-to-treat analysis with unequal exclusions among treatment arms.[148]

The optimal role of induction chemotherapy is currently controversial. A review of the National Comprehensive Cancer Network (NCCN) guidelines highlights this reality, as concurrent chemoRT alone and induction followed by RT-based therapy are both listed as treatment options for certain disease scenarios. Although concurrent chemoRT alone remains the standard to which new treatments are compared for local or regionally advanced disease, induction is well suited for certain settings in patients who are medically fit. Examples include when immediate therapy is needed in the hope of avoiding a tracheostomy or PEG, in organ-preservation settings in which the degree of response affects the decision to proceed with surgery versus RT-based therapy, or in patients with advanced neck disease at high risk for distant metastases.

Concurrent Chemotherapy and Radiation for Gross Disease

Although there are a number of ways to integrate chemotherapy with RT, available data most strongly support concurrent chemotherapy. Given proven efficacy in patients with poor prognostic, unresectable disease, more recent investigations have applied the approach in better prognostic, organ preservation, and adjuvant settings.

Concurrent chemoRT programs vary in many ways, of which the type of chemotherapy (i.e., specific agents, single agent, or combination) and RT schedule (i.e., dose, fractionation) are the most apparent variables. In general, three main approaches can be discerned: single-agent or combination chemotherapy with continuous-course RT; combination chemotherapy with split-course RT, often with altered fractionation; and chemotherapy alternating with RT.[149] Although continuous-course RT may be desirable and more attractive from a radiobiologic perspective, local toxicities may preclude it, depending on the concurrent agents used. The first two approaches are the most common.

A variety of drugs and combinations have been used concurrently with RT. When only one drug is used, the MACH-NC indicates that the impact is largest with a platin, of which cisplatin is the predominant one studied, a conclusion shared in another meta-analysis reported by Browman et al.[150] Of interest, platin plus 5-fluorouracil (hazard ratio, 0.75) offered no advantage compared with platin alone (hazard ratio, 0.74).[138]

A three-arm study reported by Adelstein et al.,[151] E1392, is consistent with the previously mentioned analysis. In this trial, 295 patients with unresectable SCC were randomized to RT alone (70 Gy, 2-Gy fractions); cisplatin 100 mg/m^2 on days 1, 22, and 43 concurrent with the same RT schedule; or split-course RT (60–70 Gy, 2-Gy fractions) with three planned cycles of concurrent cisplatin and infusional 5-fluorouracil, although resection was considered after two cycles. Treatment with concurrent cisplatin RT yielded a significantly higher 3-year survival rate compared to RT alone (37% vs. 23%; P = .014). Despite the added chemotherapy agent and the option of possible surgery, the split-course arm offered no advantage (27% 3-year survival).

Although daily,[152] weekly,[153] and every-3-week schedules of cisplatin intravenously concurrent with RT have been applied, the last schedule is the one most studied and is a widely accepted standard. Attempts to improve the efficacy of concurrent cisplatin through intra-arterial administration[154,155] have not been proven more efficacious. The preliminary report of a randomized European study comparing intra-arterial versus intravenous cisplatin showed no significant difference in locoregional control (62% vs. 68%, respectively) or survival (61% vs. 63%, respectively) at 2 years, although toxicity profiles differed: more neurologic and leukopenia with intra-arterial administration, but less renal and skin toxicity.[156] In the absence of a proven efficacy advantage with intra-arterial delivery, intravenous cisplatin is preferred as it is logistically easier to administer and less expensive.

Most randomized trials to date have compared chemoRT with RT alone. As such, studies evaluating the efficacy of different chemoRT programs are limited. For example, for purposes of the MACH-NC analysis, "platin" included both cisplatin and carboplatin. Yet the relative efficacy of these agents, when given concurrently, is not well studied. In one three-arm, randomized study by Jeremic et al.[152] using a daily schedule for each drug with RT and a control arm of RT alone, both the cisplatin (6 mg/m^2/day) and carboplatin (25 mg/m^2/day) arms appeared comparable, and superior in efficacy to RT alone. However, in a randomized study reported by the Hellenic Cooperative Oncology Group using an every-3-week schedule for each drug (cisplatin 100 mg/m^2, carboplatin AUC 6), their equivalence seemed less clear.[157] The RTOG reported a randomized phase 2 study comparing three different chemotherapy regimens, all delivered concurrently with 70 Gy in 2-Gy fractions: arm 1, cisplatin 10 mg/m^2/day and 5-fluorouracil 400 mg/m^2/day continuous infusion for the final 10 days of treatment; arm 2, hydroxyurea 1 g every 12 hours and 5-fluorouracil 800 mg/m^2/day continuous infusion every other week; or arm 3, weekly paclitaxel 30 mg/m^2 and cisplatin 20 mg/m^2. Among 231 analyzable patients, 2-year disease-free and overall survival rates were arm 1, 38.2% and 57.4%; arm 2, 48.6% and 69.4%; and arm 3, 51.3% and 66.6%, respectively.[158]

Concurrent chemotherapy may increase hematologic toxicity, including anemia. Anemia may adversely affect the efficacy of RT; the integration of an appropriate hematopoietic growth factor is a consideration. In this regard, a multicenter, double-blind, randomized, placebo-controlled trial evaluating the addition of erythropoietin 300 IU/kg three times weekly during postoperative RT is of interest.[159] Three hundred fifty-one patients with head and neck SCC were randomized to erythropoietin or placebo starting 10 to 14 days before and then concurrently with 60 to 70 Gy of RT. Although target hemoglobin levels were reached in 82% of patients receiving erythropoietin compared with 15% receiving placebo, locoregional progression-free survival (adjusted relative risk, 1.62; 95% CI, 1.22 to 2.14; P = .0008), locoregional progression (relative risk, 1.69; 95% CI, 1.16 to 2.47; P = .007), and survival (relative risk, 1.39; 95% CI, 1.05 to 1.84; P = .02) were all inferior on the erythropoietin arm, raising concerns that disease control may be adversely affected with concurrent use of the growth factor. Consistent with the current U.S. Food and Drug Administration alert, an erythropoietin-stimulation agent is contraindicated during curative-intent RT-based therapy.[160]

An important question is whether the use of newer, more efficacious, altered fractionated RT programs[161] obviates the benefits accrued with the addition of chemotherapy. A single-institution study reported by Brizel et al.[162] compared a more aggressive RT schedule with or without concomitant 5-fluorouracil and cisplatin. Patients who underwent RT alone received 75 Gy in 60 twice-daily fractions; those who underwent concomitant chemotherapy received 70 Gy in 56 twice-daily fractions with a 7-day split. Chemotherapy consisted of two cycles of concomitant cisplatin 12 mg/m^2/day and 5-fluorouracil 600 mg/m^2/day each for 5 days, followed by two cycles of maintenance chemotherapy. Among the 116 patients included, chemoRT was associated with improved 3-year rates of locoregional control (70% vs. 40%; P = .01), relapse-free survival (61% vs. 41%; P = .08), and overall survival (55% vs. 34%; P = .07). In another randomized study reported by Jeremic et al.,[163] the addition of daily cisplatin to hyperfractionated RT also led to incremental benefits. The results of these studies are consistent with the MACH-NC analysis, which demonstrated significant hazard ratios consistent with benefit among patients receiving postoperative RT (hazard ratio, 0.79), conventional RT (hazard ratio, 0.83), or altered fractionated RT (hazard ratio, 0.73), suggesting a benefit for adding concomitant chemotherapy regardless of the type of RT schedule.[138]

For patients who are not cisplatin candidates, using a carboplatin-based (e.g., carboplatin/5-fluorouracil)[164] or other concurrent programs that have withstood the scrutiny of a randomized trial is recommended. A newly available option is cetuximab and concurrent RT, which was shown to be superior to RT alone.[165] Patients with locoregionally advanced head and neck cancer were randomized to RT alone (213 patients) or combined with cetuximab (211 patients); median follow-up was 54 months. The initial dose of cetuximab was 400 mg/m^2 followed by 250 mg/m^2 weekly for the duration of RT. The median duration of survival was 49 months after combined therapy compared with 29 months after RT alone (P = .03). Further, the addition of cetuximab was associated with significantly improved progression-free survival (P = .006). Other than an acneiform rash and infusion reactions, grade 3 or greater complications were similar in the two groups of patients. The results of this trial have been confirmed with longer follow-up.[166] Randomized data comparing cetuximab and RT with other chemoRT programs are not available. Investigators at Memorial-Sloan Kettering reported a phase 2 trial of cisplatin and cetuximab concurrent with RT in patients with locoregionally advanced head and neck SCC. Efficacy was impressive, although there were toxicity concerns.[167] The RTOG has completed accrual to a randomized trial to better assess the efficacy and safety of this regimen compared with concurrent cisplatin and RT. The paradigm of combining chemotherapy and newer targeted therapies with RT is currently an active area of investigation.

Choosing among the numerous concurrent programs can be difficult. In the NCCN guidelines,[168] concurrent cisplatin with RT is the preferred choice, although several other options are listed. It is important to emphasize that concurrent chemoRT may be associated with significant toxicity; treatment-related mortality, albeit infrequent (<5% in the cooperative group setting), may occur. Morbidity from chemotherapy (dependent on the agent chosen) and RT are possible and there are both acute (e.g., mucositis, blood count suppression) and chronic (e.g., dry mouth, swallowing dysfunction, fibrosis) toxicities. Selected studies have begun to report long-term, not just acute, toxicities.[169] Appropriate infrastructure, an experienced multidisciplinary team, and a cooperative patient are necessary to optimize both efficacy and safety.

Nasopharynx Cancer

Given that NPCs are responsive to both RT and chemotherapy, and have the high rate of distant metastases among the WHO types II and III, there has been keen interest in chemoRT approaches to the disease. Current practice has been particularly affected by the Intergroup Study 0099 (Table 72.9).[170] In it, 147 patients with stage III or IV NPC were randomized to definitive RT (70 Gy, 35 fractions over 7 weeks) versus cisplatin 100 mg/m^2 intravenously on days 1, 22, and 43 concurrent with the same dose of RT followed by three planned cycles of cisplatin and infusional 5-fluorouracil. Although only 63% and 53% of patients received all the planned concurrent and maintenance treatments, respectively, locoregional control, distant control, progression-free, and overall survivals were all significantly improved with chemoRT.

One of the potential limitations of the Intergroup Study was how generalizable its results would be to endemic NPCs, because 24% of patients entered in the trial had WHO type I histology. However, subsequent reports of randomized trials in which WHO types II and III predominated have similarly shown a survival advantage with concurrent cisplatin-based concurrent chemotherapy without[171–173] or with maintenance chemotherapy.[174,175]

Another limitation of the Intergroup Study was that is was not designed to delineate the proportional benefits of concurrent and maintenance chemotherapy. Although current NCCN guidelines recommend concurrent and maintenance chemotherapy in M0 patients with more advanced disease based on the Intergroup experience,[168] in reviewing available data, the benefits of maintenance chemotherapy appear more controversial. As noted, other randomized studies have demonstrated a survival improvement with concurrent therapy alone.[171,176] Earlier randomized trials, summarized elsewhere, failed to demonstrate a survival benefit when either maintenance or induction chemotherapy was added to definitive RT.[177,178] Furthermore, a meta-analysis of updated individual patient data on 1,753 patients enrolled in eight randomized trials, besides confirming an absolute survival benefit of 6% at 5 years with incorporation of chemotherapy with RT (hazard ratio, 0.82; 95% CI, 0.71 to 0.91; P = .006), also reported a significant association between the timing of chemotherapy and overall survival (P = 0.005), with the largest benefit being attributed to concomitant therapy.[179]

There is a resurgence of interest in induction chemotherapy for advanced NPC as part of a sequential strategy prior to concurrent treatment, given that distant failure is relatively common. Selected randomized studies have demonstrated evidence of a positive biologic effect with the use of induction chemotherapy, but no survival benefit has been documented.[178,180–182] Such promising results have engendered interest in the potential for enhanced efficacy with newer drugs and combinations. A randomized phase 2 trial evaluating induction with docetaxel and cisplatin prior to concurrent cisplatin and RT was

PRACTICE OF ONCOLOGY

TABLE 72.9

RANDOMIZED TRIALS EVALUATING CONCURRENT CHEMORADIOTHERAPY VERSUS RADIOTHERAPY FOR ADVANCED NASOPHARYNX CANCER

Study	No. of Patients	Maintenance Chemotherapy	Treatment Arms	PFS[a,b] (*P* Value)	OS[a,b] (*P* Value)
Al-Sarraff et al.[170]	147	Yes, on CDDP/RT arm	RT CDDP/RT	24% 69% (<.001)	47% 78% (.005)
Lin et al.[171]	284	No	RT CDDP/FU/RT	53% 72% (.0012)	54% 72% (.0022)
Chan et al.[176]	350	No	RT CDDP/RT	52% 60% (.06)	59% 70% (.049)
Wee et al.[174]	221	Yes, on CDDP/RT arm	RT CDDP/RT	53% 72% (.0093)	65% 80% (.0061)
Lee et al.[175]	348	Yes, on CDDP/RT arm	RT CDDP/RT	62% 72% (.027)	78% 78% (.97)

PFS, progression-free survival; OS, overall survival; CDDP, cisplatin; RT, radiation therapy; FU, 5-fluorouracil.
[a]Five-year rates for Lin et al. (2002) and Chan et al. (2005), otherwise 3-year rates.
[b]Disease-free rate provided for Wee et al. (2005) and failure-free rate for Lee et al. (2005).

consistent with benefit compared with concurrent cisplatin and RT alone.[178] Programs incorporating newer taxane- and cisplatin-based triplet induction regimens warrant further study.[183] There is also interest in the role of plasma EBV-DNA assays as a way to assess disease and monitor response.[177]

Organ Preservation

Organ-preservation therapy is intended to control disease without compromise in survival, while optimizing function or cosmesis.[184] The term implies that the tumor is potentially resectable for cure, and that the morbidity from surgery is significant. Although conservation-surgical procedures can achieve the same goals, more commonly, the label of *organ preservation* is applied to nonsurgical approaches. In that regard, the role of chemotherapy integrated with RT is best established for more advanced primary tumors. In this setting, conservation-surgical procedures become less feasible, and local control rates with RT alone are lower than those seen with earlier stage disease.

Total laryngectomy is one of the surgical procedures most feared by patients[185] and is associated with both functional (i.e., loss of spoken voice) and cosmetic (i.e., presence of a stoma) deficits. Thus, larynx preservation has been a central focus of many organ-preservation studies, including those that established integrated chemotherapy and RT as a standard organ-preservation treatment option. Studies commonly focused on patients with advanced tumors of the larynx, hypopharynx, and oropharynx (particularly base of tongue) in whom primary surgical management would jeopardize the glottis.[186]

Initial chemoRT approaches to larynx preservation used induction chemotherapy. The response to initial chemotherapy was used to triage patients to either definitive RT (a partial response or better at the primary site; surgery to the primary site was reserved for salvage) or primary surgical management (less than a partial response). The randomized and landmark Veterans Administration Larynx Preservation Study demonstrated that such an approach could be pursued in patients with advanced laryngeal cancer without compromise in survival when compared with primary treatment with surgery and RT.[141] Over 60% of patients on the chemoRT arm avoided total laryngectomy. Among long-term survivors, patients treated on the chemoRT arm had better emotional well-being and were less depressed, and also reported less pain.[187]

A similarly designed randomized trial in patients with pyriform sinus and aryepiglottic fold tumors reported by the European Organisation for Research and Treatment of Cancer (EORTC) confirmed these findings.[142] However, a small randomized study (n = 68) limited to patients with T3 disease with a fixed cord done by the Groupe d'Etude des Tumeurs de la Tete et du Cou (GETTEC) reported that survival was superior on the primary surgery arm (84% vs. 69% at 2 years; $P = .006$).[188]

When the MACH-NC performed a collective analysis of the Veterans Administration, EORTC, and GETTEC studies, the rate of larynx preservation among survivors was 58%. A nonsignificant, 6% decrement in survival at 5 years was seen in the chemoRT group (39% vs. 45%; pooled hazard ratio, 1.19; 95% CI, 0.97 to 1.46; $P = .10$).[137] These data indicate that the outlined approach with chemoRT allowed for larynx preservation in a significant proportion of patients without compromise in survival. Clearly, there was no evidence that survival was improved compared to primary surgical management. Whether the induction chemotherapy had an independent therapeutic effect or simply served a selection purpose was uncertain.

The data reviewed in the prior section highlighting the therapeutic benefits of a concurrent chemoRT relative to an induction or RT alone approach have obvious implications for the larynx preservation setting. RTOG 91–11 was designed to assess the impacts of adding chemotherapy to RT, and its timing (concurrent vs. induction), with regard to achieving larynx preservation. Four hundred ninety-seven patients with larynx cancer were randomized to one of three arms: primary RT, 70 Gy to the primary site, 50 to 70 Gy to nodes; induction chemotherapy with cisplatin and infusional 5-fluorouracil for three cycles followed by RT in responders, surgery in nonresponders; and cisplatin 100 mg/m^2 days 1, 22, and 43 concurrent with RT. Surgical salvage was an option on all three arms. The results are summarized in Table 72.10.[136,189] As anticipated, the rate of grade 3 or 4 mucosal toxicity was highest on the concurrent arm; however, this did not translate into more significant speech or swallowing impairment at 2 years compared to the other treatment arms. Noteworthy is that, while the larynx preservation rate and locoregional control were highest and statistically superior with concurrent treatment, there was no significant difference in overall survival rates among the arms.

In another randomized larynx-preservation study, induction chemotherapy followed by RT and alternating chemotherapy and RT approaches were compared in 450 patients with advanced larynx or hypopharynx cancer. Both treatment arms used cisplatin and 5-flourouracil and allowed surgical salvage. Overall and progression-free survival rates were similar on both arms. Survival with a functional larynx in place

TABLE 72.10

INTERGROUP 91-11: UPDATED RESULTS AT 5 YEARS

RX Arms	No. of Patients	LP Rate (%)	LRF (%)	DMF[a] (%)	DFS (%)	OS (%)
RT only	171	65.7 $P<.0002$	49.0 $P = .0005$	22.3	27.3[b]	53.5
Induction PF→RT	173	70.5 $P = .0029$	45.1 $P = .0018$	14.3	38.6 $P = .016$	59.2
Concurrent P/RT	171	83.6[a]	31.2[b]	13.2	39.0 $P = .0058$	54.6

RX, treatment; LP, larynx preservation; LRF, locoregional failure; DMF, distant metastatic failure; DFS, disease-free survival; OS, overall survival; RT, radiation therapy; PF, cisplatin/5-fluorouracil; P, cisplatin.
[a]Trend, but not statistically significant; P values of .069 and .064 for RT versus induction and concurrent arms, respectively.
[b]Comparison group.
Data from ref. 189.

was higher with alternating, chemoRT, although the difference was not statistically significant (median, 2.3 years vs. 1.6 years; hazard ratio, 0.85; 95% CI, 0.68 to 1.06).[190]

A non–site-specific trial from the Cleveland Clinic yielded similar results.[191] One hundred patients with stage III or IV resectable SCC of the oral cavity (4%), oropharynx (44%), larynx (36%), or hypopharynx 16%) were randomized to either RT (66–72 Gy) or the same RT program plus two cycles of concurrent cisplatin and 5-fluorouracil. The 3-year survival rate with organ preservation was superior with concomitant of chemotherapy (57% vs. 35%; $P = .02$). However, the contribution of salvage surgery negated any survival advantage. Given the large proportion of patients with oropharynx cancer in this trial, a concurrent chemotherapy-RT strategy administered with organ preservation intent is supported by these data for this site. A randomized study from the Groupe d'Oncologie Radiothérapie Tête et Cou (GORTEC) also demonstrated improved locoregional control (66% vs. 42% at 3 years; $P = .03$) in patients with advanced oropharynx cancer who received concurrent chemotherapy (carboplatin and 5-fluorouracil) and RT (70 Gy) compared with RT alone.[164]

Although concurrent chemotherapy is the current cornerstone of organ-preservation treatment of advanced disease, other paradigms deserve mention. Usually, a response to chemotherapy is used as a selection tool to target patients for RT-based treatment. However, in an Italian study, 195 patients with T2–T4 oral cavity cancer were randomized to either primary surgical management or induction chemotherapy with cisplatin and 5-fluorouracil followed by a surgical procedure which could be modified based on response. Overall survival was similar on both arms, but less postoperative RT was necessary (33% vs. 46%) and fewer mandible resections were performed (31% vs. 52%) on the chemotherapy arm.[192] As a further extension of this concept, Laccourreye et al.[193] have pioneered the selective observation without locoregional treatment of patients with laryngeal cancer who have a complete response to induction chemotherapy. Durable tumor control without the addition of surgery or RT has been reported in a small subset of patients with early-stage tumors. The University of Michigan has developed a larynx-preservation program whereby the triage to RT-based treatment or surgery occurs after only one cycle of chemotherapy.[194] The intent is to improve survival and minimize morbidity through timely selection of appropriate therapy, including referral to surgery, if indicated; the implication is that induction chemotherapy has little other therapeutic benefit, and some patients who are slow to respond may be triaged unnecessarily to total laryngectomy.[195] Conversely, newer sequential strategies of induction chemotherapy followed by planned concurrent chemotherapy are looking to optimize both locoregional and distant control. Induction with more efficacious triplet chemotherapy, including a taxane combined with cisplatin and 5-fluorouracil, is already being incorporated into larynx-preservation strategies with evidence of improved larynx-preservation rates.[196]

Adjuvant Therapy after Surgery

The use of maintenance chemotherapy after the completion of locoregional treatment has been evaluated in several randomized trials, but with disappointing results. Suboptimal compliance with maintenance treatment may partly explain the lack of benefit, as tolerance of chemotherapy can be poor after surgery and RT.[197] Also, the potential inclusion of patients unlikely to benefit from systemic therapy and thus diluting the potential impact of the maintenance intervention is a methodologic challenge. Despite these limitations and the lack of convincing survival benefit, patterns of failure were affected in selected studies, with a decrease in distant metastases, consistent with a biological effect of chemotherapy.[197,198]

The results of Intergroup 0034 highlight these points. In this trial, 442 analyzable patients were randomized after definitive surgical therapy to either postoperative RT alone (50–60 Gy) or three cycles of standard-dose cisplatin and 5-fluorouracil by infusion followed by the same RT-dosing scheme. The randomization was stratified by risk, with surgical margins less than 5 mm, cancer *in situ* (CIS) at the margins, and ECE being considered high-risk features. Even though the chemotherapy was administered prior to RT, which should improve tolerance, 37% of patients on the adjuvant chemotherapy arm either failed to receive chemotherapy or had a major protocol violation. Overall, there was no significant difference in overall survival, disease-free survival, or locoregional control between the treatment arms, although there was a significant decrease in incidence of distant metastases on the investigational arm ($P = .03$). Interestingly, on subset analysis, adjuvant chemotherapy had no significant impact in the low-risk group, but a more dramatic impact on survival and tumor control was seen among high-risk patients. This trial highlighted the importance of defining risk in trial design, and important work, summarized elsewhere, focused on better defining and standardizing poor risk features.

Given the success of concurrent chemoRT as definitive treatment, its application in the adjuvant setting was a logical extension. A pilot study done by the RTOG demonstrated that concurrent high-dose cisplatin every 3 weeks with RT was feasible in the adjuvant setting.[199] Early randomized studies demonstrated an improvement in locoregional control with the incorporation of concurrent mitomycin.[200,201] A study comparing weekly cisplatin concurrent with postoperative RT versus RT alone with ECE yielded a significant improvement in both locoregional control and survival with combined modality treatment.[153]

Two randomized studies, both published in 2004, have further clarified the indications for postoperative chemoRT in the poor-risk adjuvant setting. RTOG 9501 and EORTC 22931 had very similar designs.[36–38,186] Patients were randomized after surgery if they had poor-risk features to either standard postoperative RT alone (60–66 Gy, over 6–6.5 weeks, standard fractionation) or the same RT with three planned cycles of concurrent cisplatin at 100 mg/m^2 every 3 weeks. What constituted poor risk differed somewhat between the studies: the RTOG required the presence of two or more positive lymph nodes, ECE, or positive margins; the EORTC required ECE, positive margins, pT3 or pT4 with any N, N2, or N3 disease, level IV nodes or stage IV disease in patients with oral cavity or oropharynx primaries, PNI, or vascular embolism.[36–38] Both studies demonstrated a significant improvement in locoregional control and disease-free or progression-free survival with combined modality therapy. These improvements translated into a significant advantage in overall survival in the EORTC study ($P = .02$), but only a trend ($P = .19$) in the RTOG study. Interestingly, neither study showed a significant impact on distant control with the addition of chemotherapy. Acute toxicity was greater with the addition of the cisplatin, but there was no difference in late toxicity. A randomized study from Germany using concurrent cisplatin and 5-fluorouracil instead of cisplatin alone yielded similar results to the RTOG study: significant improvement in locoregional control and disease-free survival, with a nonsignificant survival trend favoring combined modality adjuvant therapy.[202]

A subsequent analysis of these two studies was performed to better understand which pathologic subgroups may benefit the most from the concurrent addition of cisplatin to RT.[203] Patients having evidence of ECE or a positive margin derived the largest benefit from combined modality adjuvant therapy. Conversely, patients in whom their only poor-risk factor was two or more positive lymph nodes without ECE seemed to do just as well with RT alone.

The EORTC and RTOG studies focused on patients who were previously untreated, with the exception of prior surgery. Recent data presented by Janot et al.[204] on behalf of the GETTEC and GORTEC groups addresses the potential role of concurrent chemotherapy and reirradiation after salvage surgery. In this randomized study enrolling 65 patients, the standard arm was salvage surgery alone. The combined modality treatment significantly improved disease-free survival (hazard ratio, 1.68; 95% CI, 1.13 to 2.5; $P = .01$), although overall survival was not significantly improved and both acute and chronic toxicities were worse.

Toxicity Reduction

Xerostomia is one of the most troubling side effects of RT-based treatment. Extraoral fluids, artificial saliva, other topical measures, and humidity are commonly used. Available data indicate that IMRT applied with salivary-sparing intent decreases this symptom.[205–207] Pharmacotherapy may also help. The cholinomimetic, muscarinic agent pilocarpine at a dose of 5 mg three times a day was shown in a randomized trial to improve production of saliva as well as symptoms of dry mouth compared with placebo in patients treated with at least 40 Gy to the head and neck.[208] Excessive sweating was the most common side effect. Cevimeline, a similar agent with a more selective mechanism of action, was associated with a significant increase in unstimulated salivary flow at dosing of 30 to 45 mg three times a day.[209] Amifostine is a thiol with chemo- and radioprotectant properties. Objective and subjective measures of salivary function were improved in an open-label, randomized study among patients who received 200 mg/m^2 of amifostine intravenous daily 15 to 30 minutes before RT.[210] Grade 3 toxicities were infrequent, but nausea, vomiting, hypotension, and allergic reactions were more common among patients treated with amifostine. Alternative, more convenient, and better tolerated ways to deliver this medication (i.e., subcutaneous dosing) are being evaluated. Finally, acupuncture may be of benefit in selected patients.[211,212]

Mucositis is a troubling symptom typically exacerbated by aggressive altered fractionated RT programs and the use of concurrent chemoRT. A variety of rinses (e.g., topical anesthetics, antifungals) and systemic pain medications are used for symptomatic relief. Concurrent amifostine with RT has not been clearly shown to decrease mucositis.[210] Iseganan hydrochloride, a synthetic peptide with broad-spectrum antibacterial activity, was evaluated in a multinational, double-blind, placebo-controlled trial among patients receiving definitive or postoperative RT-based therapy. No improvement in oral mucositis was found compared with placebo.[213] Recombinant human keratinocyte growth factor has been shown to decrease the incidence and duration of mucositis in the transplant setting.[214] However, its role is not established to decrease mucositis in patients being treated with RT-based therapy for head and neck cancer.[215]

FOLLOW-UP

How to optimally follow patients after treatment for head and neck cancer is less well studied than how to treat it. Approaches are informed by patterns of failure. Most relapses occur within the first 3 years and are front-loaded; relapses above the clavicles are potentially curable; the lung is the most common site of distant spread.

The schedule proposed in the NCCN practice guidelines is reasonable.[168] Patients are seen for follow-up head and neck examinations every 1 to 3 months during year 1, every 2 to 4 months during year 2, every 4 to 6 months during years 3 through 5, and every 6 to 12 months thereafter. Thyroid function tests are obtained every 6 to 12 months, if the neck was irradiated. Many practitioners obtain annual chest radiographs or other chest imaging to monitor for a second primary lung cancer and to document distant metastases. The impact of this imaging on outcome is not well established, consistent with a vague recommendation from the NCCN of chest imaging "as clinically indicated." Additional studies such as CT, MRI, and PET may be necessary to determine whether there is a recurrence or a complication, but are not routinely performed in surveillance. Speech and swallowing evaluations and rehabilitation are obtained as indicated. Counseling is indicated for patients in whom tobacco or alcohol contributed as a risk factor for tumor development.

ORAL CAVITY

The oral cavity consists of the lips, floor of mouth, anterior two-thirds of the tongue, buccal mucosa, upper and lower alveolar ridges, hard palate, and retromolar trigone.

The AJCC staging system for primary tumors of the oral cavity is depicted in Table 72.11.[216]

LIP

The ratio between men and women with lip cancer is approximately 15:1.[217] Persons with light-colored skin and/or prolonged exposure to sunlight are most prone to develop lip carcinoma.

Anatomy

The lips are composed of the orbicularis oris muscle with skin on the external surface and mucous membrane on the internal surface. The transition from skin to mucous membrane is the lip vermilion. The blood supply is from the labial artery, a branch of the facial artery. The motor nerves are branches of

TABLE 72.11

2010 AMERICAN JOINT COMMITTEE ON CANCER STAGING FOR ORAL CAVITY PRIMARY TUMORS (T)

TX	Primary tumor cannot be assessed
T0	No evidence of primary tumor
Tis	Carcinoma *in situ*
T1	Tumor 2 cm or less in greatest dimension
T2	Tumor more than 2 cm but no more than 4 cm in greatest dimension
T3	Tumor more than 4 cm in greatest dimension
T4a	(Lip-vermillion border) Tumor invades through cortical bone, inferior alveolar nerve, floor of mouth, or skin of face (i.e., chin or nose)
T4a	(Oral cavity) Tumor invades adjacent structures (e.g., through cortical bone, into deep [extrinsic] muscle of tongue [genioglossus, hyoglossus, palatoglossus, and styloglossus], maxillary sinus, skin of face)
T4b	Tumor invades masticator space, pterygoid plates, or skull base and/or encases internal carotid artery

Note: Superficial erosion alone of bone or tooth socket by gingiva primary is not sufficient to classify a tumor as T4.
From ref. 216, with permission.

the seventh cranial nerve. The sensory nerve to the upper lip is the infraorbital branch of the fifth cranial nerve (V 2), and the mental nerve (V 3) supplies the lower lip.

Pathology

The most common neoplasms are SCCs. Basal cell carcinomas start on the skin of the lip and may secondarily invade the vermilion. Keratoacanthoma occurs on the skin of the lips and may be mistaken grossly and histologically for SCC.

Leukoplakia and CIS are common problems on the lower lip and may precede the appearance of carcinoma by many years. Primary lesions arising from the moist mucosa of the lip are considered under the section "Buccal Mucosa."

Patterns of Spread

SCC can originate from the skin of the lip or the vermilion, which may invade the adjacent skin and orbicularis muscle. Advanced lesions invade the adjacent commissures of the lip, the buccal mucosa, the skin and wet mucosa of the lip, the adjacent mandible, and eventually the mental nerve. PNI occurred in 2% of the cases reported by Byers et al.[218] and was related to recurrent lesions, large tumor size, mandibular invasion, and poorly differentiated histology. Lymphatic spread is to the submental (IA) and submandibular (IB) lymph nodes and then to the jugular chain. The risk for lymph node metastases is approximately 5% at diagnosis and is increased by high-grade histology, large lesions, invasion of the mucosa of the lip and buccal, and for patients with recurrent disease.

Clinical Picture

The vermilion of the lower lip is the most common site of origin. SCC may present as an enlarging discrete lesion that is not tender until it ulcerates. Some lesions develop slowly on a background of leukoplakia or CIS and present as superficially ulcerated lesions with little or no bulk. Erythema of the adjacent skin suggests dermal lymphatic invasion. Palpation of the lip will reveal the extent of induration. Paresthesia of the skin of the lip indicates PNI.

Treatment

Selection of Treatment Modality

Early lesions may be cured equally well with surgery or RT. The length of the relaxed lower lip is approximately 7 cm but tends to be shorter in edentulous patients. Surgical excision is preferred for the majority of lower lip lesions up to 2 cm in diameter that do not involve the commissure; the treatment is simple and the cosmetic result is satisfactory. Removal of more of the lip with simple closure usually results in a poor cosmetic and functional result and therefore requires reconstructive procedures. RT is often preferred for lesions involving the commissure, for lesions over 2 cm in length, and for upper lip carcinomas. Advanced lesions with bone, nerve, or node involvement frequently require a combined modality approach.

The regional lymphatics are not treated electively for early cases. Advanced lesions, high-grade lesions, and recurrent lesions should be considered for elective neck treatment. Clinically positive nodes are managed as previously discussed in "Clinically Positive Neck Lymph Nodes."

Surgical Treatment

Surgical treatment for early lesions (0.5–1.5 cm) uses a V- or W-shaped excision, depending on the size of the defect, which facilitates cosmetic primary closure. If the vermilion is diffusely involved with little or no involvement of the muscle, a vermilionectomy may be performed and the mucosa from the labial vestibule of the oral cavity advanced to cover the defect.

Irradiation Technique

Lip cancer may be successfully treated by EBRT, interstitial brachytherapy, or a combination of both. Interstitial brachytherapy may be accomplished with removable sources such as iridium-192. EBRT techniques use orthovoltage (55.8 Gy at 1.8 Gy per fraction) or electrons (60–66 Gy at 2 Gy per fraction) with lead shields behind the lip to limit exit EBRT. IMRT is not indicated except for the occasional patient with advanced neck disease and/or clinical PNI, when it is necessary to extend the dose distribution to the skull base and reduce the dose to the contralated parotid. For more advanced lesions, combining chemotherapy with EBRT is appropriately considered.[148]

Results of Treatment

MacKay and Sellers[219] reviewed 2,864 patients with all stages of lip cancer, of whom 92% were managed initially by RT. The primary lesion was controlled by the initial treatment in 84% of cases; an additional 8% were salvaged by later treatment for an overall local control rate of 92%. Fifty-eight percent of those who presented with clinically involved nodes had control of disease, but only 35% had control of disease when neck nodes appeared later. The 5-year cause-specific survival rate was 89%; the 5-year absolute survival rate was 65%.

Mohs and Snow[220] reported the results for 1,448 patients treated with microscopically controlled surgery for SCCs of the lower lip between 1936 and 1976. Eighty-three percent had cancers less than 3 cm in diameter, with a 5-year cure rate of 96.6%. For 192 patients with cancers that measured 2 cm or more, the cure rate dropped to 60%. For patients with grade 1 or 2 SCC, the 5-year cure rate was 96%, as contrasted with 67% for 81 patients with grade 3 or 4 SCC.

Complications of Treatment

Oral competence, which permits patients to control oral secretions and effectively suck, speak, and swallow, requires the sphincteric function of an intact orbicularis oris muscle. Hence, disruption of the sphincteric function resulting from division of the orbicularis oris should be restored. Microstomia and drooling secondary to oral incompetence may occur after a large flap reconstruction. If the oral opening is too small, the patient may not be able to inset a denture.

There will be some atrophy of the irradiated tissues; this progresses with time. Soft tissue necrosis may occur; this problem is reduced by schemes that prolong the treatment.

FLOOR OF THE MOUTH

Anatomy

The floor of the mouth is a U-shaped area bounded by the lower gum and the oral tongue; it terminates posteriorly at the insertion of the anterior tonsillar pillar into the tongue. The paired sublingual glands lie immediately below the mucous membrane; the paired genioglossus and geniohyoid muscles separate them.

Bony protuberances, the genial tubercles, occur at the point of insertion of these two muscle groups at the symphysis and may interfere with the placement of interstitial sources. The mylohyoid muscle arises from the mylohyoid ridge of the mandible and is the muscular floor for the oral cavity; it ends posteriorly at about the level of the third molars. The submandibular gland rests on the external surface of the mylohyoid muscle between the mandible and the insertion of the mylohyoid. The submandibular duct (Wharton's duct) is about 5 cm long. It courses between the sublingual gland and the genioglossus muscle and exits in the anterior floor of the mouth near the midline.

Pathology

Most neoplasms are SCC, usually of moderate grade. Adenoid cystic and mucoepidermoid carcinomas account for about 5% of malignant tumors in this area.

Patterns of Spread

Primary

Approximately 90% of neoplasms originate within 2 cm of the anterior midline floor of the mouth, penetrating early beneath the mucosa into the sublingual gland and eventually into the genioglossus and geniohyoid muscles. The mylohyoid muscle acts as an effective barrier until the lesion becomes advanced. Extension toward the gingiva and periosteum of the mandible occurs early. When tumor reaches the periosteum, the tumor usually spreads along the periosteum rather than through it. Mandible invasion is a late manifestation. The skin of the lower lip may be involved in advanced cases. Posterior extension occurs into the muscles of the root of the tongue. One or both submandibular ducts are frequently obstructed by tumor or after biopsy; it may be difficult to distinguish between tumor extension and infection in an obstructed duct. Tumor rarely grows inside the duct but may grow along the path of the duct. The submandibular gland frequently enlarges, becoming firm and occasionally painful when the duct is obstructed. CT is useful to distinguish between tumor directly invading the gland and chronic infection related to obstruction.

Extensive lesions may escape the oral cavity by following the anatomic plane of the mylohyoid muscle to its posterior extremity, emerging in the submandibular space of the neck.

Lymphatics

Approximately 30% of patients will have clinically positive nodes on admission; 4% will have bilateral nodes. The reported incidence of conversion from N0 to N+ with no neck treatment varies from 20% to 35%.[33,221] For T1 or superficial T2 lesions, the risk for occult metastasis is probably 10% to 15%.[33,221]

The first nodes involved are the level I and the level II nodes; the midline submental nodes are bypassed. Because most lesions either approach or cross the midline, the risk for bilateral spread is fairly high.

Clinical Picture

On physical examination, the earliest lesions appear as a red area, slightly elevated, with ill-defined borders and very little induration. As the lesion enlarges, the edges of the tumor become distinct, elevated, and "rolled," with a central ulceration and induration. Some lesions start with a background of leukoplakia. Bimanual palpation will determine the extent of the induration and the degree of fixation to the periosteum. Large lesions bulge into the submental space and rarely grow through the mylohyoid muscle into the soft tissues of the neck. Gross invasion of the mandible may be detected, especially when the anterior teeth have been removed. A tumor may grow through the mandible to involve the gingivolabial sulcus and lip. The submandibular duct and gland are evaluated by bimanual palpation.

Treatment

Selection of Treatment Modality

Early Lesions. Surgery or RT is equally effective treatment for T1 or T2 lesions. Most patients are treated surgically because of the risk of soft tissue or bone necrosis after RT.

A few patients are seen after excisional biopsy of a tiny lesion, and the only finding is a surgical scar with varying degrees of induration or nodularity under the scar (TX). The margins are often equivocal. These patients are sometimes treated with an interstitial implant or, more commonly, re-excision.

Moderately Advanced Lesions. The usual recommendation for moderately advanced anterior midline lesions is rim resection or segmental mandibulectomy and osteomyocutaneous free flap reconstruction; postoperative RT is added, with the addition of concurrent chemotherapy in some cases, as dictated by the findings in the specimen. The clinically N0 neck is usually managed by a bilateral functional neck dissection for midline lesions.

Advanced Lesions. Massive lesions have a poor prognosis with combined surgery, RT, with or without chemotherapy. Only palliation can be offered in some cases.

Surgical Treatment

Wide Local Excision. Small lesions (≤5 mm in size) may be excised transorally with a 1-cm margin with primary closure or a skin graft. If the duct is involved, the submandibular gland and duct are removed in continuity.

Rim Resection. Rim resection of the mandible in continuity with excision of the primary lesion preserves the arch and may be combined with postoperative RT. Periosteal invasion is often an indication for this procedure. Patients who have been edentulous for a long time may have an atrophic mandible and are not suitable because the mandible is likely to fracture.

Segmental Mandibulectomy. Lateral floor of mouth: a modified neck dissection is performed and the specimen remains attached to the mandible. Partial segmental mandibulectomy with resection of the floor of the mouth is done through a lip-splitting incision or by using a visor flap. A cheek flap is elevated to the level of the mandibular condyle to provide exposure. The mandible is separated at the mental foramen anteriorly and the neck of the condyle posteriorly. The primary lesion and neck specimen are then removed in continuity. An osteomyocutaneous flap is usually used to repair the defect.

For lesions of the anterior floor of mouth, a full-thickness resection of the anterior mandible (arch) is required. Techniques for reconstruction include the use of trapezius myocutaneous flap with a portion of the scapular spine to bridge the bony gap, or the use of a free flap.

Irradiation Technique

Superficial T1 cancers are treated with either brachytherapy or intraoral cone RT to approximately 65 Gy and the neck is observed. Larger lesions are treated with EBRT to 45 to 50 Gy over 5 weeks followed by an interstitial implant for an additional 20 to 30 Gy. Lesions that are suitable for intraoral cone RT may be boosted with this technique prior to EBRT of the primary lesion and upper neck. Use of EBRT alone results in suboptimal cure rates and is discouraged.[222]

External-Beam Irradiation. Opposed lateral EBRT portals are used to treat anterior floor of mouth carcinomas. The entire width of the mandibular arch is included and the superior border is shaped to spare part of the parotid gland. The level I and level II nodes are included to the level of the thyroid notch if the neck is clinically negative; the lower neck may be electively irradiated. If the neck is clinically positive, the portals are enlarged to include all of the upper neck nodes, and en face low neck field is added. IMRT may be useful to reduce the dose to the contralateral parotid in patients with positive nodes.

Interstitial Irradiation. Implantation of T1–T2 lesions confined to the floor of the mouth with minimal extension to the mucosa of the tongue can be accomplished with iridium using the plastic tube technique.

Intraoral Cone Irradiation. Intraoral orthovoltage or electron cone RT requires daily positioning by the physician and is preferable to interstitial RT because there is little or no irradiation of the mandible.[223] An intraoral cone can be used for well-circumscribed anterior superficial lesions and is easiest to perform in the edentulous patient.

Combined Treatment Policies

Postoperative RT is preferred, because the risk of bone complications and fistulae is higher with preoperative RT. Concurrent chemotherapy may be necessary based on pathologic findings. Preoperative RT may be used if the patient has a large fixed node.

Management of Recurrence

RT failures are treated by an operation. The salvage rate is good for patients with T1–T2 lesions and poor for those with more advanced lesions.

Surgical treatment failures may be treated by a repeat operation and postoperative RT.

Results of Treatment

Rodgers et al.[224] reported on 194 patients treated with surgery and/or RT at the University of Florida between 1964 and 1987. The local control rates after RT versus surgery alone or combined with RT were T1, 32 of 37 (86%) versus 10 of 11 (91%); T2, 25 of 36 (69%) versus 16 of 19 (84%); T3, 11 of 20 (55%) versus 9 of 9 (100%); and T4, 2 of 5 (40%) versus 6 of 10 (60%).[224] The local control rates are similar for T1 and T2 tumors for the various treatment groups; those with T3 and T4 cancers have better local control after surgery and RT compared with RT alone. The 5-year cause-specific survival rates were comparable for the treatment groups.[224] Mild to moderate and severe complications were observed as follows: RT alone, 49 of 117 (42%) and 6 of 117 (5%); surgery alone, 3 of 36 (8%) and 6 of 36 (17%); and surgery and RT, 8 of 41 (20%) and 6 of 41 (15%), respectively.[224]

Two hundred seven patients treated with RT alone at the Centre Alexis Vautin between 1976 and 1992 were reviewed by Pernot et al.[225] Local control and cause-specific survival rates at 5 years were as follows: T1, 97% and 88%; T2, 72% and 47%; and T3, 51% and 36%, respectively. Six percent of patients developed complications necessitating surgical intervention and one patient experienced a fatal complication.

Follow-Up

There are two major difficulties in follow-up after RT: soft tissue ulcers and enlarged submandibular glands. An ulcer in the floor of the mouth within 2 years of treatment can be either recurrence or necrosis. If the lesion appears to be soft tissue necrosis, a trial of conservative therapy is adequate. Failure to stabilize or resolve is an indication for biopsy. A negative biopsy does not rule out recurrence, and repeat deep biopsies may be necessary. An enlarged submandibular gland(s) may be a sequel to obstruction of the submandibular duct; contrast-enhanced CT is useful to distinguish between an enlarged submandibular gland and tumor in a lymph node.

Follow-up of surgical cases may be difficult if skin grafts or flaps have been used because of the associated induration and thickness of the flaps. If the submandibular ducts have been reimplanted, stenosis may occur with subsequent enlargement of the submandibular glands.

Complications of Treatment

Radiation Therapy. A small soft-tissue necrosis may develop, usually in the site of the original lesion where the dose is highest. These are moderately painful and respond to local anesthetics, antibiotics, and the tincture of time. Treatment with pentoxifylline 400 mg three times daily may be beneficial.

If the ulceration develops on the adjacent gingiva, the underlying mandible is exposed. These areas are mildly painful. They are managed by discontinuing dentures, local anesthetics, antibiotics, and smoothing of the bone by filing if needed. These small bone exposures do not often progress to osteoradionecrosis (ORN) and either sequestrate a small piece of bone or are simply recovered by mucous membrane. Severe ORN may require daily hyperbaric oxygen treatments for 4 to 6 weeks, either alone or in conjunction with surgical intervention.

Surgical. These include bone exposure, orocutaneous fistula, and failure of osteomyocutaneous flaps. Salvage procedures after RT are associated with an increased risk of complications.

ORAL TONGUE

Anatomy

The circumvallate papillae locate the division between oral tongue and base of tongue. The arterial supply is mainly by way of paired lingual arteries that are branches of the external carotid. The sensory pathway is by the way of the lingual nerve to the gasserian ganglion.

Pathology

More than 95% of oral tongue lesions are SCCs. Coexisting leukoplakia is common. Verrucous carcinoma and minor salivary gland tumors are uncommon. Granular cell myoblastoma is a benign tumor of uncertain origin that occurs on the dorsum of the tongue and may be confused histologically with carcinoma.

Patterns of Spread

Primary

Nearly all SCCs occur on the lateral and ventral middle and posterior thirds of the oral tongue. They tend to remain in the tongue until large, unless they originate near the junction with the floor of the mouth. PNI and vascular space invasion may occur.

Anterior third (tip) lesions usually are diagnosed early. Advanced lesions invade the floor of the mouth and root of the tongue, producing ulceration and fixation. Middle-third lesions invade the musculature of the tongue and later invade the lateral floor of the mouth.

Posterior-third lesions grow into the musculature of the tongue, the floor of the mouth, anterior tonsillar pillar, base of tongue, and glossotonsillar sulcus.

Lymphatics

The first-echelon nodes are the level Ib and II nodes.[17] The submental and level V lymph nodes are seldom involved. Rouviére[10] describes lymphatic trunks that bypass the level I–II nodes and terminate in the level III lymph nodes. Byers et al.[226] evaluated nodal spread patterns in 277 patients treated surgically at the M. D. Anderson Cancer Center and observed skip metastases to the level III or IV nodes without involvement of levels I and II in 16% of patients. Thirty-five percent of patients with oral tongue cancer have clinically positive nodes on admission; 5% are bilateral. The incidence of occult disease is approximately 30%. The incidence of positive nodes increases with T stage. Patients with N1 or N2 ipsilateral nodes have a significant risk of developing node metastasis in the opposite neck.

Clinical Picture

Mild irritation of the tongue is the most frequent complaint. As ulceration develops, the pain worsens and is referred to the external ear canal. Extensive infiltration of the muscles of the tongue affects speech and deglutition and is associated with a foul odor.

Extent of disease is determined by visual examination and palpation. The tongue protrudes incompletely and toward the side of the lesion as fixation develops. Posterior oral tongue lesions may grow behind the mylohyoid, and present as a mass in the neck at the angle of the mandible. Invasion of the hypoglossal nerve is rare.

Differential Diagnosis

The differential diagnosis includes granular cell myoblastomas, which are usually slow growing, nontender masses, and 0.5 to 2.0 cm in size. The lesions are well circumscribed, firm, and slightly raised; they may be multiple. Aggressive behavior is rare, and wide local excision is preferred. Pyogenic granulomas mimic small exophytic carcinomas. Tuberculous ulcer and syphilitic chancre are rare.

Treatment

Selection of Treatment Modality

Both surgery and RT result in cure rates that are similar for similar stages. The disadvantages of surgery include removal of part of the tongue and the decision of whether or not to do a neck dissection for the N0 neck. The disadvantage of RT is the risk of necrosis.

Excisional Biopsy (TX). Excisional biopsy of a small lesion may show inadequate or equivocal margins. An interstitial implant or re-excision will produce a high rate of local control.

Early Lesions (T1 or T2). A partial glossectomy with primary closure or a skin graft may be done transorally and is usually the preferred therapy. Depending on the depth of invasion, an elective neck dissection may be indicated. Postoperative RT would only be added for indications previously discussed.

Moderately Advanced Lesions (T2 or T3). The preferred treatment for the majority of these patients is partial glossectomy, neck dissection, and postoperative RT-based treatment.

Advanced Lesions (T4). Bi- or trimodality treatment will cure the minority of these patients. Some patients are best treated with palliative intent.

Surgical Treatment

Early Lesions (T1 or T2). Partial glossectomy and primary closure is performed.

Moderately Advanced Lesions (T2 or T3). Deeply infiltrative lesions are managed by partial glossectomy followed by postoperative RT or chemoRT based on pathologic features. Frozen section control is an essential part of the procedure; positive margins are an indication for excision of additional tissue.

Advanced Lesions (T4). Advanced lesions would require a total glossectomy and sometimes a laryngectomy combined with postoperative RT or chemoRT.

Irradiation Technique

The ability to control the primary lesion is enhanced by giving all or part of the treatment by interstitial RT or by intraoral cone.[227–229] Superficial T1 tumors may be treated with iridium-192 brachytherapy alone using the plastic tube technique. Larger lesions that have an increased risk for subclinical neck disease may be treated with EBRT and a brachytherapy boost or with brachytherapy combined with an elective neck dissection. The time factor is critical for oral tongue cancer, and the EBRT part of the treatment is shortened (30 Gy in ten once-daily fractions or 38.4 Gy in 1.6 Gy twice-daily fractions) in order to increase the proportion of the RT given by either interstitial or intraoral cone therapy. The interstitial therapy is given after the EBRT; the intraoral cone therapy should be done prior to the EBRT. The authors favor elective neck RT for nearly all lesions.

Combined Treatment Policies

Postoperative RT is administered to the primary site and neck for indications previously outlined; chemoRT may be indicated based on pathologic findings. IMRT may be useful to reduce the dose to one or both parotids. Preoperative RT, often with chemotherapy, is advised when fixed nodes are present.

Management of Recurrence

Local recurrence after RT or surgery is heralded by ulceration, pain, or increased induration. Recurrences have a slightly elevated or rolled border, whereas necroses do not. Biopsy should be done as soon as ulceration appears, if it is within the original tumor site. Ulcers that appear on adjacent normal tissues are likely due to RT and not cancer.

RT failure is managed by surgery. Surgical failure occasionally is salvaged by re-resection and postoperative RT-based treatment. Recurrence in the soft tissues of the neck is rarely eradicated by any procedure.

Nodes appearing in a previously untreated neck are managed by neck dissection with or without postoperative RT; chemoRT is indicated if ECE is present.

Results of Treatment

The local control rates for 170 patients treated with RT alone versus surgery alone or with RT between 1964 and 1990 at the

University of Florida were T1, 79% versus 76% (P = .76); T2, 72% versus 76% (P = .86); T3, 45% versus 82% (P = .03); and T4, 0% versus 67% (P = .08).[230] Local control rates for T1 or T2 cancers are comparable after RT versus surgery; patients with T3 or T4 lesions have improved local control if surgery is part of the treatment. The differences in 5-year survival between the two treatment groups were not statistically significant.

The results of brachytherapy alone or combined with EBRT for 448 patients treated at the Centre Alexis Vautin were reported by Pernot et al.[231] and revealed the following 5-year local control and survival rates: T1, 93% and 69%; T2, 65% and 41%; and T3, 49% and 25%, respectively. Shorter time intervals between brachytherapy and EBRT were associated with significantly improved local control and survival for those who received both modalities.

Complications of Treatment

Surgical. Orocutaneous fistula, flap necrosis, and dysphagia are the most common complications after surgery of the tongue. Damage to the lingual nerve or the hypoglossal nerve, although rare, is associated with difficulty in swallowing and/or speaking. Fistula and flap necrosis must be handled judiciously because the danger of carotid artery hemorrhage increases with either of these complications. Enunciation difficulties occur whenever the tongue is bound down by scarring. The incidence of complications increases for surgical salvage attempts after RT failure. Thirteen of 65 patients (20%) treated with surgery alone or combined with RT at the University of Florida developed significant complications.[230]

Radiation Therapy. A minor soft tissue necrosis is fairly common; considerable patience is required for healing. Broad-spectrum antibiotics, local anesthetics such as viscous lidocaine, and analgesics are prescribed as needed. Pentoxifylline 400 mg three times daily may be beneficial. Hyperbaric oxygen treatment may be tried in difficult cases. If the necrosis is persistent and pain is uncontrollable, the lesion must be resected.

Radiation-Induced Bone Disease. The edentulous person is less likely to develop serious RT-induced mandibular damage than a person with teeth.[232] The most frequent problem involving the mandible is a bone exposure. The gingiva disappears, exposing the underlying bone. If the exposed area is small, the patient is often unaware of the problem. If the patient has dentures, those dentures should be discontinued or altered to relieve the pressure over the exposed bone. If sharp bony edges appear, they are filed and the bone edge lowered to speed healing. Healing may require months or even years.

If ORN develops, hyperbaric oxygen has been used with some success. Conservative measures should be given a fair trial, but if unsuccessful, segmental mandibulectomy and an osteomyocutaneous flap reconstruction is performed.

Severe complications were observed in 9 of 105 patients (9%) treated with RT at the University of Florida.[230] Pernot et al.[231] observed the following soft tissue and/or bone complications in a series of 448 patients: grade 1, 19%; grade 2, 6%; and grade 3, 3%.

BUCCAL MUCOSA

Epidemiology

SCC is relatively uncommon in the United States. In southern India it is common and is related to chewing a combination of tobacco mixed with betel leaves, areca nut, and lime shell.[233]

Anatomy

The buccal mucosa is the mucous membrane covering the inner surface of the cheeks and lips, ending above and below with a transition to the gingiva. It ends posteriorly at the retromolar trigone. The parotid duct opens into the buccal mucosa opposite the second upper molar. It is innervated by a branch of the mandibular nerve, which is sensory to the buccal mucosa, and the skin of the cheek that covers the buccinator muscle.

Pathology

Most malignant tumors are low-grade SCCs, frequently appearing on a background of leukoplakia or lichen planus. Verrucous carcinoma occurs. Minor salivary gland tumors and melanomas are rare.

Patterns of Spread

Almost all SCCs originate on the mucosa lining the cheeks; primary lesions seldom originate from the wet mucosa of the lips. Early lesions are usually discrete and exophytic. As they enlarge, they penetrate the underlying muscles and eventually extend to the skin. Peripheral growth occurs into the gingivobuccal sulci and eventually onto the gingiva and into bone.

The lymphatic spread is first to the level I and level II nodes. The incidence of positive nodes on admission is 9% to 31%, and the risk of occult disease is 16%.[17,221]

Clinical Picture

Small lesions produce the sensation of a lump that is felt with the tongue. Pain is minimal, unless there is posterior extension to involve the lingual and dental nerves. Pain may be referred to the ear. Obstruction of the Stensen's duct will produce parotid enlargement. Extension posteriorly, behind the pterygomandibular raphe or into the buccinator and masseter muscles, causes trismus.

Differential Diagnosis

The differential diagnosis includes lues and tuberculosis; both are rare. If the first biopsy reveals chronic inflammation or pseudoepitheliomatous hyperplasia, repeat biopsy may be necessary.

Treatment

Selection of Treatment Modality

Small lesions (≤1 cm) may be excised with primary closure; small lesions that involve the lip commissure are sometimes treated by RT. Lesions 2 to 3 cm in size can be treated with surgery or by RT, usually the former. Larger lesions are usually treated with surgery, and postoperative RT or chemoRT.

Surgical Treatment. Lesions that invade the mandible or maxilla require bone resection along with the soft tissues. Repair may require a maxillary prosthesis. A myocutaneous flap repairs full-thickness removal of the cheek.

Irradiation Technique. Buccal mucosa lesions are suited for treatment with electrons, intraoral cone, and interstitial techniques to spare the contralateral normal tissues. When tumors extend into one of the gingivobuccal gutters or onto bone, treatment must be entirely by EBRT.

Results of Treatment

Diaz et al.[234] recently reported the M. D. Anderson experience for 119 patients treated with surgery alone (84 patients) or combined with adjuvant RT (35 patients) between 1974 and 1993. Tumor recurrence developed in 54 patients (45%): local recurrence in 27 patients (23%); regional recurrence in 13 patients (11%); local and regional recurrence in 11 patients (9%); and distant metastases in 3 patients (3%). The 5-year survival rates versus stage were stage I, 78%; stage II, 66%; stage III, 62%; stage IV, 50%; and overall, 63%.

Nair et al.[233] reported the definitive RT results for 234 cases of buccal mucosa cancer treated in southern India during the 1982 calendar year. The 3-year disease-free survival rates were stage I, 85%; stage II, 63%; stage III, 41%; and stage IV, 15%. Thirty-two patients had verrucous carcinoma; the 3-year disease-free survival rate was 47%, similar to that for other grades of SCC.

Complications of Treatment

The buccal mucosa is tolerant of high-dose RT, and complications are uncommon. Bone exposure may appear on the mandible or maxilla. Trismus may develop if the muscles of mastication receive high doses.

Surgical injury of Stensen's duct may cause obstruction and parotitis. Injury to branches of the VII nerve may occur. Split-thickness skin grafts may shrink and produce partial trismus. Resection of the lip commissure may produce oral incompetence.

GINGIVA AND HARD PALATE (INCLUDING RETROMOLAR TRIGONE)

Anatomy

The lower gingiva includes the keratinized masticatory mucosa covering the mandible from the gingivobuccal gutter to the origin of the nonkeratinized lining mucosa covering the floor of the mouth. The retromolar trigone lies behind the third molar and is contiguous superiorly with the maxillary tuberosity. Beneath the keratinized mucosa of the retromolar trigone is the tendinous pterygomandibular raphe, which is attached to the pterygoid hamulus and the posterior mylohyoid ridge of the mandible and serves as the insertion of the buccinator, orbicular oris, and superior pharyngeal constrictor muscles. Behind the pterygomandibular raphe and between the medial pterygoid muscle and the ascending ramus is the pterygomandibular space, containing the lingual and dental nerves; it is related posteriorly to the deep lobe of the parotid and the parapharyngeal space. There are no minor salivary glands in the mucous membranes of the alveolar ridges.

Pathology

Most neoplasms of the lower alveolar ridge and retromolar trigone are SCCs; SCC is relatively uncommon on the upper alveolar ridge and hard palate, where minor salivary gland tumors, usually adenoid cystic carcinomas, are more frequent.[235] Verrucous carcinomas occur, usually on the lower gingiva. Melanoma has been reported.[236]

SCC may arise within the body of the mandible or maxilla either from odontogenic epithelium or from epithelium trapped during embryonic development. It is more frequent in the mandible than the maxilla, and is most common in the molar regions. It must be distinguished from metastatic SCC and ameloblastoma.

Ameloblastoma is a rare, benign, locally aggressive odontogenic tumor with an incidence of about 1% of all tumors of the maxilla and mandible; about 80% of cases occur in the mandible with the molar–ramus region most commonly involved.

Patterns of Spread

Lower Gum

SCC invades the periosteum and the adjacent buccal mucosa and floor of the mouth. Slow-growing, low-grade lesions tend to produce a smooth, saucerized defect before invading the mandible. Moderate to high-grade lesions invade the bone directly or through recently opened dental sockets and produce a lytic defect.

Lymphatic spread is to the level I and level II nodes. Eighteen percent to 52% have clinically positive nodes on admission; occult disease occurs in 17% to 19%.[17,221]

Ameloblastoma expands and destroys the bone and extends to adjacent areas by contiguous growth. Ameloblastic carcinoma, a rare malignant variant of ameloblastoma, may give rise to regional and distant metastasis.[237]

Upper Alveolar Ridge and Hard Palate

Most SCCs originate on the gingiva and spread secondarily to the hard palate, soft palate, buccal mucosa, and underlying bone. The maxillary antrum is invaded late unless there are recent extractions providing access. The risk for positive lymph nodes at diagnosis is 13% to 24%, and the incidence of occult disease is 22%.[17,221]

Retromolar Trigone

Carcinomas spread to the adjacent buccal mucosa, anterior tonsillar pillar, and maxilla early. Posterior spread occurs into the pterygomandibular space and the medial pterygoid muscle. Posterolateral spread occurs into the buccinator muscle and fat pad. The first echelon lymphatics are the level I and level II nodes. The incidence of clinically positive nodes on presentation is about 30%; the risk for occult disease is 15% to 25%.[238]

Clinical Picture

The patient with SCC may present to the dentist first with ill-fitting dentures, pain, loose teeth, or a sore that will not heal. A history of inappropriate dental extractions or root canal therapy is common. Invasion into the mandible may involve the inferior dental nerve and produce paresthesia of the lower lip. A background of leukoplakia is frequently present.

Retromolar trigone lesions have pain referred to the external auditory canal and preauricular area. Invasion of the pterygoid muscle produces trismus. Intra-alveolar SCC presents with a submucosal mass and dental symptoms. Roentgenograms show a lytic lesion in the mandible.

Ameloblastoma exhibits few symptoms in the early stages. Patients may notice a gradually increasing facial deformity or loosening of teeth. An intraoral submucosal mass may be present initially; ulceration occurs as the mass increases in size. On roentgenograms, a radiolucent area is seen with the following: expansion of the overlying cortical plate, scalloped margins, a multilocular appearance, and/or resorption of the roots of adjacent teeth.[237]

Minor salivary gland tumors present as a submucosal mass, enlarge slowly, and may develop a central ulceration.[239]

Differential Diagnosis

The differential diagnosis includes dental disease and underlying bony cysts or tumors.

Treatment

Selection of Treatment Modality

Lower Alveolar Ridge. The majority of lesions are managed by operation. Postoperative RT or chemoRT may be indicated depending on pathologic findings.

Ameloblastoma. The treatment for ameloblastoma is surgery; however, local recurrence is a problem. Sehdev et al.[240] reported curettage was followed by local recurrence in 90% of mandibular and in all maxillary ameloblastomas. Subsequent resection controlled 80% of the mandibular but only 40% of the maxillary tumors. The initial use of segmental mandibular resection controlled 78% (18 of 23 patients) with subsequent resection controlling those that recurred. The use of partial maxillectomy as the first treatment controlled 100% (7 of 7 patients) of maxillary ameloblastomas as opposed to only 40% when partial maxillectomy was performed for recurrence.

Limited experience with RT suggests that it may reduce the probability of progression and result in long-term local control in the occasional patient with incompletely resectable disease.[237]

Retromolar Trigone. Surgery is preferred for discrete early lesions. RT is recommended for superficial lesions involving a large surface area.[241] Advanced carcinomas are treated with surgery and postoperative RT with or without chemotherapy.

Upper Alveolar Ridge and Hard Palate. Resection is the usual treatment for most lesions; postoperative RT or chemoRT is added as needed. However, if the lesion is superficial and extensively involves the hard palate or involves a significant portion of the soft palate, then an RT-based approach should be considered for the initial therapy. If the lesion is small and discrete and there is no bone involvement, resection includes the periosteum or occasionally some underlying bone. Bone invasion requires a maxillectomy that is tailored to optimally resect the cancer. The resulting defect is usually rehabilitated with a removable prosthesis that restores midfacial contour and palatal function so that speech articulation, mastication, and deglutition are normalized.

Surgical Treatment

Rim Resection (Marginal Mandibulectomy). For discrete T1–T2 carcinomas with minimal cortical bone invasion, at least 1 cm of the inferior border of the mandible is preserved, maintaining its biomechanical integrity.

Segmental Mandibulectomy. For lesions with transcortical bone invasion into the medullary space, a segment of the mandible is removed in continuity with the tumor. Massive anterior lesions may necessitate removal of the mandible from angle to angle; tumors that invade the mandible posterior to the angle may require condylar resection. Reconstruction is ideally accomplished with a revascularized osteomyocutaneous flap.

Irradiation Technique

Small lesions of the lower alveolar ridge and retromolar trigone may be treated by intraoral cone for all or part of their therapy. Well-lateralized lesions of the retromolar trigone and posterior alveolar ridge may be treated by either an ipsilateral mixed beam or IMRT; the latter is preferred. Parallel-opposed portals treat anterior gum lesions.

Carcinomas that involve a large surface area with little or no bone invasion may be treated by EBRT. T1–T2 carcinomas are treated with altered fractionation; larger tumors are treated with combined EBRT and concomitant chemotherapy.

Management of Recurrence

RT failures are managed by operation. Surgical failures may be managed by surgery and postoperative RT.[242] Salvage procedures frequently are not attempted because of the advanced nature of the recurrence and the low chance of cure.

Results of Treatment

Mandibular Gingiva. Overholt et al.[243] reported 155 patients with SCCs of the lower alveolar ridge treated at M. D. Anderson between 1970 and 1990. Surgery alone was used for 131 patients and the remainder received surgery and RT. Five-year survival for patients with T1 and T2 cancers were 85% and 84%, respectively, compared with 66% and 64%, respectively, for those with T3 and T4 malignancies. Local control at 2 years was impacted by tumor size ($P = .021$) and margin status ($P = .027$), whereas 5-year cause-specific survival was influenced by tumor size ($P = .001$), margin status ($P = .011$), mandibular invasion ($P < .05$), and the presence of lymph node metastases ($P < .001$).

Retromolar Trigone. Byers et al.[238] reported the M. D. Anderson results for 110 previously untreated patients with SCC of the retromolar trigone treated between 1965 and 1977, with a minimum 5-year follow-up. Surgery was often selected for patients with leukoplakia, poor teeth, mandible invasion, large neck nodes, or trismus. RT was selected for poorly differentiated tumors, for mainly exophytic lesions, and lesions involving the faucial arch or soft palate, or lesions having ill-defined borders, and for patients who had poor surgical risk. The local control rates were as follows: T1, 12 of 13 (92%); T2, 50 of 57 (88%); T3, 18 of 20 (90%); and T4, 15 of 20 (75%). Local control was similar after surgery and/or RT. The absolute 5-year survival rate was 26%.

Mendenhall et al.[241] reported on 99 patients with retromolar trigone SCCs treated between 1966 and 2003 with RT alone (35 patients) or combined with surgery (64 patients). The 5-year locoregional control rates after RT versus surgery and RT were stages I–III, 51% and 87%; stage IV, 42% and 62%; and overall, 48% and 71%, respectively. The 5-year cause-specific survival rates after RT versus surgery and RT were stages I–III, 56% and 83%; stage IV, 50% and 61%; and overall, 52% and 69%, respectively. Multivariate analysis revealed that the likelihood of cure was better after surgery and RT compared with definitive RT.

Hard Palate. Shibuya et al.[244] reported the results for 38 cases of carcinoma of the hard palate and 82 cases of carcinoma of the upper alveolar ridge treated between 1953 and 1982 in Japan. Sixty-six patients were managed initially by RT alone to the primary lesion, and 54 patients were managed by RT and surgery. The 5-year actuarial survival rate by stage was the following: stage I, 56%; stage II, 41%; stage III, 32%; and stage IV, 12%. There was no difference in survival when comparing hard palate versus upper alveolar ridge, SCC versus minor salivary gland tumors, or RT alone versus RT plus surgery as the initial therapy. The overall risk for metastatic lymph nodes was 47% for hard palate and 49% for the upper alveolar ridge. Thirty patients were recorded as having "slight bone invasion" and no metastases and had a 5-year survival rate of 75% when treated by RT.

Complications of Treatment

Surgical complications include orocutaneous fistula, bone exposure, extrusion of a metal tray, and loss of graft or flap. Following hemimandibulectomy, the edentulous patient usually cannot wear dentures.

The complications of RT include soft tissue necrosis, bone exposure, and ORN. The risk is greatest for patients with advanced lesions of the lower gum and retromolar trigone. Huang et al.[245] reported the following rates of grade 3 bone and soft tissue complications in 65 patients treated for retromolar trigone carcinomas: preoperative RT, 0 of 10 patients (0%); surgery and postoperative RT, 5 of 39 patients (13%); and RT alone, 2 of 16 patients (13%).

OROPHARYNX

ANATOMY

The base of tongue is bounded anteriorly by the circumvallate papillae, laterally by the glossotonsillar sulci, and posteriorly by the epiglottis. The vallecula is a strip of mucosa that is the transition from the base of the tongue to the epiglottis; it is considered part of the base of tongue. The musculature of the base of tongue is contiguous with that of the oral tongue.

The tonsillar fossa is bounded anteriorly by the anterior tonsillar pillar (palatopharyngeal muscle), posteriorly by the posterior tonsillar pillar (palatopharyngeal muscle), and inferiorly by the glossotonsillar sulcus and pharyngoepiglottic fold. The pharyngeal constrictor muscle and its fascia, the mandible, and the lateral pharyngeal space bound the tonsillar region laterally. The tonsillar area is separated from the base of the tongue by the glossotonsillar sulcus, which extends from the anterior tonsillar pillar to the pharyngoepiglottic fold. Beneath the mucous membrane of the sulcus are the styloglossal muscle and the stylohyoid ligament.

The soft palate is a thin, mobile muscle complex separating the nasopharynx from the oropharynx. The epithelium of the oral side of the soft palate is squamous; the epithelium of the nasopharyngeal surface is respiratory. It is contiguous laterally with the tonsillar pillars.

Pathology

SCC accounts for 95% of cancers. Lymphoepitheliomas occur in the tonsillar fossa and base of tongue. Basaloid features suggest a HR-HPV–related tumor. Lymphomas account for 5% of tonsillar and 1% to 2% of base of tongue malignancies. Minor salivary gland malignancies, plasmacytomas, and other rare tumors make up the remainder.[246,247]

Patterns of Spread

Base of Tongue

Primary. Base of tongue SCC usually remains in the tongue unless it begins at the peripheral margin. Vallecular lesions spread along the mucosa to the lingual surface of the epiglottis, laterally along the pharyngoepiglottic fold, and then to the lateral pharyngeal wall and anterior wall of the pyriform sinus. Vallecular lesions frequently penetrate through the hyoepiglottic ligament to enter the pre-epiglottic space.

Lesions beginning on the lateral base of tongue may invade the glossotonsillar sulcus and eventually escape into the neck because there is no effective musculature barrier at this point. Advanced lesions tend to spread toward the larynx, oral tongue, and parapharyngeal space.

Lymphatics. The first-echelon nodes are in level II; spread is then along the jugular chain to the level III and level IV nodes. The level IB nodes may become involved if the tumor extends anteriorly into the oral tongue or if massive upper neck disease is present. The level V nodes are involved often enough to be included in treatment plans. Approximately 75% of patients will have clinically positive neck nodes at diagnosis; 30% will have bilateral nodes.[17] The risk of occult disease in the clinically negative neck is probably 40% to 50%.

Tonsillar Area

Anterior Tonsillar Pillar. Almost all malignancies are SCCs; they tend to be diagnosed early when they are relatively superficial. Their borders are usually indistinct; they may be red, white, or a mixture of both. As the lesions progress, they may develop a central ulcer with a rolled margin and infiltrate the palatoglossus. Superior medial spread occurs onto the soft palate, the posterior hard palate, and the maxillary gingiva. Anterolateral spread to the retromolar trigone is frequent, with later spread to the posterior gingivobuccal sulcus. Extension to the buccal mucosa facilitates occult anterior extension in the buccal pouch. Invasion of the adjacent tongue is frequent; palpation is necessary to detect the early submucosal nodule. As these lesions advance, they adhere to the mandible and eventually invade bone. Extension to the skull base and nasopharynx occurs late and is often associated with invasion of the medial pterygoid muscle and plate; such lesions produce trismus and temporal pain.

Tonsillar Fossa. There are differences in the early development and spread patterns for SCC of the tonsillar fossa compared with anterior tonsillar pillar lesions. Leukoplakia rarely occurs within the fossa, and asymptomatic red mucosa lesions are infrequent. The initial lesions tend to be exophytic with central ulceration plus an infiltrative component. However, some lesions develop submucosally and present with neck nodes and no obvious tonsillar lesion. Extension to the posterior tonsillar pillar and the oropharyngeal wall occurs early. Invasion into the glossotonsillar sulcus and base of tongue occurs in approximately 25% of cases. As the lesions advance, they penetrate to the parapharyngeal space and gain access to the skull base. Cranial nerve involvement is uncommon. Advanced lesions may invade the mandible, nasopharynx, and pyriform sinus.

Posterior Tonsillar Pillar. Early posterior tonsillar pillar lesions are uncommon. They may spread inferiorly along the palatopharyngeal muscle to its insertions into the middle pharyngeal constrictor, the pharyngoepiglottic fold, and the posterior border of the thyroid cartilage. Also, the lymphatic trunks of the posterior tonsillar pillar are theoretically more likely to spread to the junctional (parapharyngeal) and level V nodes.

Lymphatics. Retromolar trigone/anterior tonsillar pillar lesions have a lower risk of clinically positive lymph nodes (45%) compared with the tonsillar fossa (76%). The distribution for the retromolar trigone/anterior tonsillar pillar on the ipsilateral side is to the jugular and level IB lymph nodes with a very low risk for junctional and level V nodes. Contralateral spread is uncommon (5%) and is confined to the jugular chain. The risk of occult disease in the clinically negative neck (N0) is 10% to 15%. The incidence of positive nodes increases with T stage.

Tonsillar fossa lesions have a high risk of clinically positive lymph nodes on admission (76%). The lymph node distribution for tonsillar fossa lesions on the ipsilateral side includes the jugular, junctional, level V, and level IB lymph nodes. Contralateral spread occurs in only 11% of patients and is mainly to the jugular chain lymph nodes, but there is some risk for level V and level IB involvement. The risk of contralateral spread is related to invasion of the tongue, spread near or across the midline of the soft palate, and large lymph nodes in the ipsilateral neck that produce lymphatic obstruction. The incidence of occult disease is probably 50% to 60%.

There is no information about lymphatic spread for posterior tonsillar pillar lesions.

Soft Palate

Primary. Nearly all SCCs occur on the oral side of the palate; the nasopharyngeal side is rarely involved. The earliest tumors are red lesions with ill-defined borders. White lesions are common on the soft palate and may be leukoplakia, CIS, or early SCC. Multiple sites of involvement with normal-appearing intervening mucosa may occur. Most SCCs are diagnosed while still confined to the soft palate. Spread occurs first to the tonsillar pillars and hard palate. Lateral spread may eventually penetrate the superior constrictor muscle and skull base, and may rarely extend to cranial nerves in the parapharyngeal space. Involvement of the lateral wall(s) of the nasopharynx may occur in advanced lesions.

Lymphatics. The spread pattern is first to the level II nodes and then along the jugular chain. The level IB and level V nodes are less commonly involved.

Approximately 56% of patients will have clinically positive nodes on admission; 16% are bilateral.[17] Lindberg et al.[248] noted an approximate 20% incidence of occult disease following either no or partial neck RT with the primary lesion controlled. The incidence of clinically positive nodes increases with T stage.[17]

Clinical Picture

Base of Tongue

Often, the earliest symptom is a mild sore throat. Because many early lesions are relatively silent, a level II neck mass is often the first sign. Difficulty swallowing, a nasal voice quality, and ear pain occur as the lesion enlarges. Advanced lesions fix the tongue. Ulceration and necrosis result in foul breath.

Flexible fiberoptic endoscopy, digital palpation, and a high level of suspicion are necessary for diagnosis of early lesions of the base of tongue.

Lymphomas are usually large, mostly submucosal masses. Minor salivary gland tumors are also usually submucosal, but more discrete and firm than lymphomas.

Tonsillar Area

Anterior Tonsillar Pillar. Early symptoms include sore throat; pain is referred to the ear as soon as ulceration takes place. As the lesion progresses, it may cause ill-fitting dentures, trismus, and temporal pain.

Tonsillar Fossa. Ipsilateral sore throat is common. Detection by visual examination with a tongue depressor is sufficient for most lesions; however, a few cancers arise in the lower pole of the tonsil and are only visible by indirect examination. A few patients present with a node in the neck. Lymphomas tend to be large submucosal masses, but may ulcerate and appear similar to carcinomas.

TABLE 72.12

OROPHARYNX 2010 AMERICAN JOINT COMMITTEE ON CANCER STAGING SYSTEM FOR THE PRIMARY TUMOR

T1	Tumor 2 cm or less in greatest dimension
T2	Tumor more than 2 cm but not more than 4 cm in greatest dimension
T3	Tumor more than 4 cm in greatest dimension
T4a	Tumor invades the larynx, deep/extrinsic muscles of the tongue, medial pterygoid, hard palate, or mandible
T4b	Tumor invades lateral pterygoid muscle, pterygoid plates, lateral nasopharynx, or skull base or encases the carotid artery

From ref. 216, with permission.

Soft Palate

The earliest symptom is usually a mild sore throat that is not well localized. Advanced lesions interfere with swallowing and may cause voice change. Regurgitation of food and liquid into the nasopharynx occurs with destruction or fixation of the soft palate. Lateral and superior spread to the nasopharynx and parapharyngeal space is associated with trismus, otitis media, temporal headache, and, rarely, cranial nerve involvement.

Staging

The staging system for the primary tumor is depicted in Table 72.12. Bone involvement is uncommon and may be seen on radiographic studies. Invasion of soft tissues of the neck is best assessed by CT and/or MRI. Invasion of the deep musculature of the tongue is diagnosed if the tongue is partially fixed. Lesions that produce trismus or cranial nerve palsy are classified as T4. Pathologic staging usually results in "upstaging." Stage migration renders a meaningful comparison of outcomes between clinically and pathologically staged patients nearly impossible.

Treatment: Base of Tongue

Selection of Treatment Modality

Surgery and RT produce similar cure rates. Because excision of the base of tongue generally causes greater disability and because of the high risk for bilateral lymphatic involvement, RT or chemoRT is the treatment of choice for almost all lesions.[249]

Surgical Treatment

The occasional patient with a low-volume T1 or early T2 cancer may be suitable for transoral laser excision in combination with a neck dissection.[250] Otherwise, the surgical approach requires an incision that splits the lip and a mandibulotomy, which permits lateral rotation of the mandible. Suprahyoid, transhyoid, and infrahyoid approaches also can be used to resect small lesions. After the tumor has been removed, the mandibular edges are reapproximated and stabilized with a titanium reconstruction plate. Only one lingual artery may be sacrificed. A neck dissection is done in continuity with excision of the primary lesion. Removal of a large tumor requires simultaneous removal of part or the entire larynx.

Irradiation Technique

Parallel opposed EBRT portals encompass the primary site and bilateral cervical nodes. Interstitial brachytherapy with flexible sources, such as ^{192}Ir ribbons, may be used for part of the treatment if the lesion is relatively limited. In contrast to oral tongue cancer, there is no proven advantage in local control for interstitial boosts as opposed to EBRT alone. Concomitant chemotherapy is indicated for most patients with stage III–IV tumors.

One of the common errors in planning EBRT portals is failure to recognize anterior extension of cancers into the lateral floor of the mouth; this is usually appreciated on CT and/or MRI. The inferior border of the lateral portals is usually the thyroid notch unless tumor has extended into the upper pyriform sinus, lateral pharyngeal wall, or pre-epiglottic space.

The primary portals include the level II, posterior level I, and level V nodes when the neck is N0. The superior border is approximately 2 cm above the tip of the mastoid even with clinically negative nodes to ensure coverage of the nodes near the skull base.

The bilateral lower neck nodes are always treated with a separate anterior portal. If the upper neck is clinically negative, the lower neck portals include the level III and level IV nodes and are tailored to exclude as much normal tissue as possible. If the upper neck is clinically positive, the lower neck portals are more generous.

Patients treated with conventional fields receive 1.2 Gy per fraction twice daily to 74.4 to 76.8 Gy. Most patients with a N0 neck or ipsilateral positive nodes are treated with IMRT to reduce the dose to the contralateral parotid. The low neck is irradiated with a separate anterior field to reduce the dose to the larynx. The M. D. Anderson concomitant boost technique is selected if IMRT is employed for logistical reasons.

Management of Recurrence

RT treatment failures are treated surgically; salvage is infrequent except for T1 and early T2 lesions. Surgical treatment failures are rarely salvaged, except for the early lesion with a discrete local recurrence. Palliative management is often preferred.

Results of Treatment: Base of Tongue

The 5-year local control rates after definitive RT in a series of 333 patients treated at the University of Florida were T1, 98% (n = 46); T2, 92% (n = 125); T3, 82% (n = 92); and T4, 53% (n = 70).[249] The 5-year locoregional control, distant metastasis-free survival, and survival are depicted in Table 72.13. Severe, acute, late, and/or postoperative complications developed in 52 patients (16%).

Follow-Up: Base of Tongue

RT failures may present as an ulcer and must be distinguished from necrosis. Most necroses appear in the vallecula or glossotonsillar sulcus. Deep biopsies usually must be done under general anesthesia to obtain adequate tissue and control bleeding.

Complications of Treatment: Base of Tongue

Surgical Complications

Surgical complications include an operative mortality of about 5%; fistula, mandibular necrosis, dysphagia, aspiration pneumonia, hoarseness, trismus, and carotid rupture are nonfatal complications.

Complications of Irradiation

Bone exposure and ORN are uncommon. Mild to moderate soft tissue necroses occur in approximately 10% of patients, and mild to moderate bone exposures occur in 5% of patients treated solely by EBRT. Many necroses persist several months and may respond to pentoxifylline. Hypoglossal nerve palsy occurs rarely.

Occasionally, patients may have difficulty swallowing solid foods. The action of the base of tongue is to force the bolus of food into the hypopharynx, and loss of full motion impedes swallowing. This is probably a result of some fibrosis of the base of tongue compounded by xerostomia. Significant aspiration is unusual. It is uncommon for a patient to develop severe swallowing disability requiring a PEG.[251]

Treatment: Tonsillar Area

Selection of Treatment Modality

The cure rates are similar after definitive RT-based treatment compared with surgery alone or combined with adjuvant RT.[252] Because the morbidity is generally higher after surgery, definitive RT or chemoRT is usually preferred.

Surgical Treatment

Surgery for early cancers of the tonsillar pillars consists of a transoral wide local excision, including a tonsillectomy. Larger lesions may require removal of the adjacent mandible as well

TABLE 72.13

BASE OF TONGUE: 5-YEAR OUTCOMES AFTER RADIOTHERAPY AT THE UNIVERSITY OF FLORIDA (333 PATIENTS)

Stage	No. of Patients	Locoregional Control (%)	Ultimate Locoregional Control (%)	Distant Metastasis-Free Survival (%)	Cause-Specific Survival (%)	Survival (%)
I–II	26	100	100	92	91	67
III	58	82	87	90	77	66
IVA	124	87	90	92	84	67
IVB	125	58	62	69	45	33

From ref. 249, with permission.

as a portion of the tongue and soft palate. Depending on the size of the defect, a tongue, deltopectoral, or osteomyocutaneous flap may be required. Speech may be impaired if a significant portion of the tongue or palate has been removed. A prosthesis may be needed for the palatal defect.

Irradiation Technique

The portal arrangement depends on the extent of locoregional disease. The risk for contralateral lymph node metastases is low unless there is tongue invasion, soft palate invasion within 1 cm of midline, or extensive ipsilateral positive nodes.[18] If these risk features are absent, an ipsilateral IMRT technique is employed. The major advantage of this technique is a lower incidence of xerostomia.

More advanced lesions, as well as those with N3 neck disease, have a higher risk for nodes in the contralateral side of the neck and are treated with parallel opposed photon portals, usually weighted 2 to 1 or 3 to 2 to the involved side. If there are positive contralateral nodes or extension across the midline, the portals usually are equally weighted. The inferior border is placed 2 cm below the primary tumor. IMRT may be employed to irradiate both sides of the neck and reduce the dose to the contralateral parotid in patients with a N0 neck or ipsilateral-positive neck nodes. The low neck is treated with a separate anterior field with a thin midline block over the larynx. Small, discrete lesions of the anterior tonsillar pillar may have part of the RT by intraoral cone.

The dose for tonsillar lesions is 74.4 to 76.8 Gy (1.2 Gy twice daily) for T1 to T3 lesions, and 76.8 Gy for T4 lesions. Concomitant boost RT (72 Gy in 42 fractions for 30 treatment days) is used when IMRT is employed.

Management of Recurrence

Surgery will salvage a good portion of T1 or T2 RT failures, but only an occasional advanced lesion is salvaged.

Results of Treatment: Tonsillar Area

The 5-year local control rates after definitive RT in a series of 503 patients treated at the University of Florida between 1964 and 2003 for cancer of the anterior tonsillar pillar versus tonsillar fossa/posterior tonsillar pillar were T1, 70% versus 94%; T2, 74% versus 90%; T3, 72% versus 79%; and T4, 57% versus 62%.[252] The local control rates are better for tonsillar fossa/posterior tonsillar pillar cancers compared with those arising in the anterior tonsillar pillar. The 5-year locoregional control, distant metastases-free survival, and survival rates are depicted in Table 72.14.[252]

Complications of Treatment: Tonsillar Area

Radiation Therapy

The risk for a severe complication, usually a bone or soft tissue necrosis, requiring surgical intervention is low. The probability of a fatal complication is remote. An occasional patient, usually one treated for advanced disease, may have long-term swallowing problems. Other complications include trismus, hypoglossal nerve entrapment, and a remote risk of an RT-induced malignancy and/or myelitis. Severe late complications occurred in 46 of 503 patients (9%).[252]

Surgery

Complications of operation include impaired swallowing, fistula, flap failure, poor wound healing, and aspiration occasionally leading to laryngectomy. The risk of severe and/or fatal complications is higher after surgery compared with RT.[252]

Treatment: Soft Palate

Selection of Treatment Modality

Although small, well-defined lesions may be excised and the neck observed, the risk of subclinical regional disease is high. Therefore, definitive RT is indicated for nearly all soft palate carcinomas; neck dissection is added as needed. Concomitant chemotherapy is indicated for patients with T3–T4 and/or N2–N3 disease.

Surgical Treatment

Small, discrete lesions can be managed by transoral excision and repaired by a pharyngeal flap to prevent any velopharyngeal incompetence. Tonsillectomy may also be necessary in order to obtain an adequate margin. If full-thickness resection is required, prosthesis is often required.

Irradiation Technique

The RT technique involves equally weighted parallel opposed EBRT portals that include the primary lesion and the bilateral first-echelon upper neck nodes. A separate anterior portal is used to treat the low neck. If the primary lesion is discrete and the neck is clinically negative, a portion of the treatment may be given with an intraoral cone prior to EBRT.

Patients are treated with 4- to 6-MV photons to 74.4 to 76.8 Gy at 1.2 Gy per fraction, twice daily, in a continuous

TABLE 72.14

TONSILLAR REGION: 5-YEAR OUTCOMES AFTER DEFINITIVE RADIOTHERAPY AT THE UNIVERSITY OF FLORIDA (503 PATIENTS)

Stage	No. of Patients	Locoregional Control (%)	Ultimate Locoregional Control (%)	Distant Metastasis-Free Survival (%)	Cause-Specific Survival (%)	Survival (%)
I	22	66	92	100	100	54
II	83	75	88	95	86	61
III	95	85	88	97	84	62
IVA	184	76	84	85	73	57
IVB	119	58	66	68	46	33

From ref. 252, with permission.

course. IMRT using the concomitant boost technique may be used to reduce the dose to one or both parotids.

Management of Recurrence

A persistent ulcer after RT is indicative of recurrent disease. Patients with a limited local recurrence after RT for a T1 or T2 lesion may be suitable for surgical salvage.

Results of Treatment: Soft Palate

Chera et al.[253] reported on 145 patients treated with definitive RT at the University of Florida between 1963 and 2004. Local control rates at 5 years were T1, 90%; T2, 90%; T3, 67%; T4, 57%; and overall, 81%. The 5-year locoregional control and cause-specific survival rates were stage I, 84% and 89%; stage II, 85% and 87%; stage III, 66% and 88%; stage IVA, 59% and 57%; and stage IVB, 43% and 0%, respectively.[253]

Complications of Treatment: Soft Palate

Surgical Complications

Nasal speech and regurgitation of food into the nasopharynx are sequelae of full-thickness soft palate resection. A prosthesis is partially successful in correcting the functional deficit.

Complications of Irradiation

Soft-tissue necrosis is uncommon. The soft palate may become retracted following successful treatment of advanced lesions and may result in regurgitation into the nasopharynx and a slight alteration in speech. ORN requiring surgical management is rare. Severe late complications were observed in 8 of 145 patients (6%) treated with definitive RT.[253]

LARYNX

Cancer of the larynx is related primarily to cigarette smoking.[254] The importance of alcohol remains unclear, but it is probably less important than in the other head and neck sites.[254]

ANATOMY

The larynx is composed of several cartilages connected by ligaments and muscles, divided anatomically into the supraglottis, glottis, and subglottis. The supraglottis consists of the epiglottis, false vocal cords, ventricles, aryepiglottic folds, and arytenoids; the arytenoids are cartilages that articulate on the cricoid. The glottis includes the true vocal cords and the anterior commissure. The subglottis is 2 cm long and extends from 5 mm below the free edge of the true vocal cords to the lower margin of cricoid cartilage.

The pre-epiglottic space is bounded by the epiglottis posteriorly, the hyoepiglottic ligament and vallecula superiorly, and the thyroid cartilage and thyrohyoid membrane anteriorly and laterally. It can be seen as a low-density area on a CT scan.

The supraglottis has a moderately rich capillary lymphatic plexus. The lymphatic trunks pass through the pre-epiglottic space and the thyrohyoid membrane to the level II nodes. A few trunks drain directly to the level III or level IV nodes. There are essentially no capillary lymphatics of the true vocal cords; thus, lymphatic spread from glottic cancer rarely occurs unless tumor extends to supraglottis or subglottis. The subglottis area has relatively few capillary lymphatics. The lymphatic trunks pass through the thyrocricoid membrane to the pretracheal (Delphian) node(s) in the region of the thyroid isthmus, and/or to the level IV nodes. The pretracheal nodes are midline and, even when clinically positive, are 1 cm or less in diameter. The subglottis also drains posteriorly through the cricotracheal membrane with some trunks going to the paratracheal (level VI) nodes while others pass to the level IV nodes.

PATHOLOGY

Nearly all laryngeal cancers arise from the surface epithelium and are SCCs. Minor salivary gland tumors are rare; even rarer are soft tissue sarcomas, lymphomas, neuroendocrine carcinomas, and plasmacytomas. Hemangiomas, chondromas, and osteochondromas are reported, but their malignant counterparts are rare.

CIS is common on the vocal cords. Distinction between CIS and invasive SCC is often challenging because focal biopsies of the vocal cords can miss an area of microinvasion and mucosal stripping of a vocal cord lesion results in a disoriented specimen that precludes complete evaluation of the basement membrane region. However, the distinction between CIS and microinvasive SCC is academic as either diagnosis is treated with endoscopic transoral laser resection or RT.

Most vocal cord SCCs are either well or moderately well differentiated. In a few cases, SCCs with a spindle cell component may be observed. Verrucous carcinoma occurs on the vocal cords in about 1% to 2% of patients with carcinoma. Supraglottic SCCs are less differentiated; verrucous cancers are rare.

Patterns of Spread

Supraglottic Larynx

Suprahyoid Epiglottis. Lesions may exhibit an exophytic growth pattern with little tendency to destroy cartilage or spread to adjacent structures. Others may infiltrate and destroy cartilage and eventually amputate the tip. They tend to invade the vallecula, pre-epiglottic space, lateral pharyngeal walls, and the remainder of the supraglottis.

Infrahyoid Epiglottis. Lesions tend to produce irregular tumor nodules with invasion through the porous epiglottic cartilage into the pre-epiglottic space. They grow circumferentially to involve the false cords, aryepiglottic folds, and eventually the medial wall of the pyriform sinus and the pharyngoepiglottic fold. Invasion of the anterior commissure and cords is usually a late phenomenon, and subglottic extension occurs only in advanced lesions. Lesions that extend onto or below the vocal cords are at a high risk for cartilage invasion, even if the cords are mobile.[255]

False Vocal Cord. Early SCCs usually have the appearance of a submucosal mass and are difficult to delineate accurately. They extend toward the thyroid cartilage and medial wall of the pyriform sinus. Extension to the infrahyoid epiglottis is common. Initial invasion of the vocal cord may occur submucosally and may be difficult to detect. Vocal cord invasion is often associated with thyroid cartilage invasion. Subglottic extension is uncommon.

Aryepiglottic Fold and Arytenoid. Early lesions are usually exophytic. As the lesions advance, they extend to adjacent sites and eventually cause laryngeal fixation by invasion of the cricoarytenoid muscle and joint. Advanced lesions invade the base of tongue, pharyngeal wall, and postcricoid region of the hypopharynx.

Vocal Cord

The majority of lesions begin on the free margin and upper surface of the vocal cord and are easily visible. When diagnosed, about two-thirds are confined to one cord, usually the anterior two-thirds of the cord. Extension to the anterior commissure is frequent. As the lesion enlarges, it extends to the ventricle, false cord, vocal process of the arytenoids, and subglottis. Infiltrative lesions invade the vocal ligament and thyroarytenoid muscles, eventually reaching the thyroid cartilage. As cancers reach the cartilage, they tend to grow up or down the paraglottic space rather than invade cartilage. The conus elasticus initially acts as a barrier to subglottic extension. Advanced glottic lesions eventually invade through the thyroid cartilage or thyrocricoid membrane to enter the neck and/or thyroid gland.

Subglottic Larynx

Subglottic cancers are uncommon. It is difficult to determine whether a tumor started on the undersurface of the vocal cord or in the subglottis with extension to the cord. They involve the cricoid cartilage early, because there is no intervening muscle layer. Cord fixation is common.

Lymphatic Spread

Supraglottic. Lymphatic drainage is initially to the level II nodes, and then to levels III and IV.[17] The incidence of clinically positive nodes is 55% at diagnosis; 16% are bilateral.[17] Elective neck dissection will show pathologically positive nodes in 16% to 26% of cases; observation of the neck will be followed by the appearance of positive nodes in approximately 33% of cases. Delphian node involvement is rare.

Glottic. The incidence of clinically positive nodes at diagnosis varies with T stage: T1, 1% or less; T2, 5% or less; and T3 and T4, 20% to 30%.[256] Supraglottic spread is associated with metastasis to the level II nodes. Anterior commissure and subglottic invasion is associated with level III, level IV, and Delphian node involvement.[257]

Subglottic. Lederman[258] reported a 10% incidence of clinically positive lymph nodes on admission. Spread is primarily to the Delphian nodes and the level IV nodes.

Clinical Picture

Presenting Symptoms

Vocal Cords. Carcinoma produces hoarseness at a very early stage. Pain, dysphagia, and airway obstruction may be observed with advanced cancers.

Supraglottic Larynx. Hoarseness is not a prominent symptom until the lesion becomes extensive. Pain on swallowing, referred to the ear by the vagus nerve and the auricular nerve of Arnold, is a frequent initial symptom. A neck mass may be the first sign of a supraglottic cancer. Late symptoms include weight loss, foul breath, dysphagia, and aspiration.

Physical Examination

In addition to the laryngeal mirror, flexible fiberoptic endoscopes are routinely used to complement the examination. Determination of laryngeal mobility frequently requires multiple examinations because the subtle distinctions between mobile, partially fixed, and fixed cords are often difficult. Preepiglottic space invasion is best appreciated on CT.

Postcricoid extension may be suspected when the laryngeal "click" disappears on physical examination. Localized pain or tenderness to palpation over the thyroid cartilage is suggestive of invasion. Advanced tumors may penetrate through the thyroid ala and be felt as a bulge on the cartilage. CT scan may detect cartilage invasion, but irregular calcification of the cartilage, coupled with volume averaging of the CT slice, creates technical problems in appreciating early cartilage invasion.

Differential Diagnosis and Staging

The differential diagnosis includes papillomas, polyps, vocal nodules, fibromas, and granulomas. Papillomas generally occur in children and young adults, and may persist into adulthood. Vocal polyps and nodules occur at the junction of the middle and anterior third of the true vocal cords. There is usually a history of voice abuse followed by hoarseness. Vocal cord granulomas usually occur as a result of intubation and are located on or near the posterior commissure. Endoscopic removal may be necessary if medical therapy for gastroesophageal reflux provides no improvement, although this is rare.

The staging system for the primary tumor is depicted in Table 72.15.

Treatment: Vocal Cord Carcinoma

Selection of Treatment Modality

Carcinoma in situ. Vocal cord stripping may sometimes control CIS. Recurrence is frequent, and the vocal cord may become thickened and the voice hoarse with repeated stripping. The authors recommend RT for patients with multiple recurrences.[259]

Early Vocal Cord Lesion (T1, T2). In most centers, RT is the initial treatment, with operation reserved for salvage of RT failure.[260] Although open partial laryngectomy will produce comparable cure rates for selected T1 or T2 vocal cord lesions, RT is generally preferred because it is less expensive and voice quality is better. Endoscopic transoral laser resection is increasingly being used.[260] Using this technique, small midcord lesions may be treated; voice quality depends on the extent of tissue removal and whether surgical resection involves the anterior commissure. Open partial laryngectomy or total laryngectomy may be used as a salvage operation after RT failure. Although there have been reports that anterior commissure involvement predicts for RT failure, the data do not support this finding.[256]

Verrucous carcinomas are treated with transoral laser resection or open partial laryngectomy. Definitive RT is employed if the alternative is total laryngectomy.

Advanced Vocal Cord Lesions (T3, T4). Low-volume cancers (≤3.5 cc) with stage III–IV disease are treated with definitive RT and concomitant chemotherapy.[261,262] Higher-volume carcinomas are usually treated with total laryngectomy, neck dissection, and postoperative RT or chemoRT.

Surgical Treatment

Stripping of the cord implies transoral removal of the mucosa of the edge of the cord.

Cordectomy is an excision of the vocal cord and is usually performed via transoral laser. It is used for well-defined lesions of the midthird of the vocal cord. The major advantages of laser excision are that it requires a day, as opposed to the 5.5 weeks necessary for RT, and RT may be reserved if the patient develops a second head and neck cancer.

Hemilaryngectomy is a partial laryngectomy allowing removal of limited cord lesions with voice preservation. Restrictions

TABLE 72.15

2010 AMERICAN JOINT COMMITTEE ON CANCER STAGING FOR LARYNGEAL CANCER

PRIMARY TUMOR (T)	
TX	Primary tumor cannot be assessed
T0	No evidence of primary tumor
Tis	Carcinoma *in situ*
SUPRAGLOTTIS	
T1	Tumor limited to one subsite of supraglottis with normal vocal cord mobility
T2	Tumor invades mucosa of more than one adjacent subsite of supraglottis or region outside the supraglottis (e.g., mucosa of base of tongue, vallecula, medial wall of pyriform sinus) without fixation of the larynx
T3	Tumor limited to larynx with vocal cord fixation and/or invades any of the following: postcricoid area, preepiglottic tissues, paraglottic space, and/or minor thyroid cartilage erosion (e.g., inner cortex)
T4a	Tumor invades through the thyroid cartilage and/or invades tissues beyond the larynx (e.g., trachea, soft tissues of neck including deep extrinsic muscles of the tongue, strap muscles, thyroid, or esophagus)
T4b	Tumor invades prevertebral space, encases carotid artery, or invades mediastinal structures
GLOTTIS	
T1	Tumor limited to one (T1a) or both (T1b) vocal cord(s) (may involve anterior or posterior commissure) with normal mobility
T2	Tumor extends to supraglottis and/or subglottis, and/or with impaired vocal cord mobility
T3	Tumor limited to the larynx with vocal cord fixation, and/or invades paraglottic space, and/or minor thyroid cartilage erosion (e.g., inner cortex)
T4a	Tumor invades through the thyroid cartilage and/or invades tissues beyond the larynx (e.g., trachea, soft tissues of neck including deep extrinsic muscles of the tongue, strap muscles, thyroid, or esophagus)
T4b	Tumor invades prevertebral space, encases carotid artery, or invades mediastinal structures
SUBGLOTTIS	
T1	Tumor limited to the subglottis
T2	Tumor extends to vocal cord(s) with normal or impaired mobility
T3	Tumor limited to larynx with vocal cord fixation
T4a	Tumor invades cricoid or thyroid cartilage and/or tissues beyond the larynx (e.g., trachea, soft tissues of neck including deep extrinsic muscles of the tongue, strap muscles, thyroid, or esophagus)
T4b	Tumor invades prevertebral space, encases carotid artery, or invades mediastinal structures

From ref. 216, with permission.

include involvement of one cord and up to 5 mm of the opposite cord, partial fixation of one cord, and up to 9 mm of subglottic extension anteriorly and 5 mm posteriorly (to preserve the cricoid cartilage). Extension to the epiglottis, false cord, or interarytenoid area is a contraindication. One arytenoid may be sacrificed; the reconstructed vocal cord must be fixed in the midline to prevent aspiration. The patient must have adequate pulmonary function. More extensive open partial laryngectomies have been described, such as the supracricoid partial laryngectomy.[263]

The last surgical alternative is total laryngectomy with or without a neck dissection. The entire larynx is removed, the pharynx is reconstituted, and a permanent tracheostoma is created.

There are several options to accomplish voice rehabilitation after total laryngectomy. Prosthetic devices (e.g., the Blom-Singer Voice Prosthesis) have been developed for insertion into a tracheoesophageal fistula which permits the patient to speak without aspiration.[264] Voice rehabilitation was evaluated in 173 patients who underwent a total laryngectomy and postoperative RT at the University of Florida; 118 patients were evaluable 2 to 3 years after treatment and 69 patients were evaluated for 5 years or longer.[264] Methods of voice rehabilitation at 2 to 3 years and 5 years or more after surgery were: tracheoesophageal speech, 27% and 19%; artificial ("electric") larynx, 50% and 57%; esophageal, 1% and 3%; nonvocal, 17% and 14%; and no data, 5% and 7%, respectively.[264]

Irradiation Technique

RT for early vocal cord cancer is delivered by portals including only the primary lesion. Portals for T1 lesions extend from the thyroid notch superiorly to the inferior border of the cricoid; the posterior border depends on posterior extension of the tumor. Portals larger than this increase the risk of edema without increasing the cure rate. Portals for T2 lesions are slightly larger, depending on the anatomic extent of the lesion. Patients receive 2.25 Gy per fraction once daily to 63 Gy (T1 and T2a) or 65.25 Gy (T2b).[256,265]

RT for T3 and T4 lesions include the primary lesion and the level II–IV, and Delphian lymph nodes. The initial treatment is delivered at 1.2 Gy per fraction twice daily to 45.6 Gy. The portals are then reduced to include only the primary lesion; the final tumor dose is 74.4 Gy. The low neck is treated through a separate anterior portal. IMRT may be useful to avoid a difficult low neck match in patients with a low-lying larynx.

Management of Recurrence

Worsening laryngeal edema suggests recurrence. Cord fixation usually implies local recurrence; fixation may rarely develop in the absence of recurrent disease.

RT failures (T1–T2) are almost always salvaged by cordectomy, partial laryngectomy, or total laryngectomy. The salvage rate for T3 lesions recurring after RT is approximately 60%.[262]

Salvage by RT-based treatment for recurrences or new tumors appearing after partial laryngectomy is about 50%. Isolated tracheostomal recurrences may be managed by RT, chemoRT, or surgery and postoperative RT-based treatment; the chance of cure is relatively low. A multi-institutional surgical experience in the management of stomal recurrence was reported by Gluckman et al.[266] Forty-one patients came to operation. The 2-year cause-specific survival was 24%. Patients with localized recurrences had a 45% 5-year survival rate.

Treatment: Supraglottic Larynx Carcinoma

Selection of Treatment Modality

T1, T2, and low-volume (≤6 cc) T3 lesions are favorable and can be treated with definitive RT or supraglottic laryngectomy. It is seldom necessary to combine RT and surgery for the management of the primary lesion; however, combined treatment may be indicated to control neck disease.

Following are guidelines for selection of either supraglottic laryngectomy or RT. Patients who are candidates for supraglottic laryngectomy must have lesions that are anatomically suitable, resectable neck disease, and adequate pulmonary reserve to withstand aspiration. Because the likelihood of local control after RT is related to primary tumor volume calculated on pretreatment CT, lesions larger than 6 cc are treated with partial laryngectomy.[267,268] The anatomic constraints include no extension inferior to the apex of the ventricle, minimal or no involvement of the medial wall of the pyriform sinus, mobile cords, no cartilage invasion, and limited lateralized extension to the tongue base. Patients who are not candidates for the supraglottic laryngectomy are treated with RT; concomitant chemotherapy is added for those with stage III–IV disease.

When a patient presents with an early-stage primary lesion and N2b–N3 neck disease, combined treatment is necessary to produce a high rate of neck control. Thus, the primary lesion is preferably treated with chemoRT, with neck dissection(s) added to the involved side(s) of the neck if necessary. If the patient has N1 or N2a neck disease and surgery is elected for the primary site, postoperative RT or chemoRT is only added because of unexpected findings (e.g., positive margins, multiple positive nodes, or ECE). The probability of a good functional result is improved if the dose to the remaining larynx is limited to 55 Gy at 1.8 Gy per once-daily fraction. The involved neck may be boosted to a higher dose without irradiating the larynx.

Selected unfavorable T3 and T4 lesions that are mainly exophytic can be treated by chemoRT. Lesions unsuitable for RT are endophytic, high-volume cancers often associated with vocal cord fixation and are managed by total laryngectomy. If the neck disease is resectable, surgery is followed by postoperative RT or chemoRT. If the neck disease is unresectable, preoperative RT or chemoRT is used.

Surgical Treatment

Supraglottic Laryngectomy. The incision is usually an apron flap. The neck dissection is completed and left attached to the thyrohyoid membrane. The perichondrium of the larynx is elevated in continuity with the strap muscles and used to close the surgical defect. Saw cuts are made through the thyroid cartilage and the pharynx is entered above the hyoid bone through the vallecula so the pre-epiglottic space is included in the specimen. The arytenoids and true vocal cords are preserved. If one arytenoid is sacrificed, the vocal cord is fixed in the midline to prevent aspiration. Suturing the perichondrium and muscle to the base of tongue closes the defect. After the tracheostomy is removed the patient is retrained in the act of swallowing. The extended supraglottic laryngectomy may include resection of the base of tongue to the level of the circumvallate papillae as long as one lingual artery is spared.

Total Laryngectomy. The entire larynx and pre-epiglottic space are resected *en bloc* and a permanent tracheostoma is fashioned. A portion of the thyroid gland is also removed if there is extralaryngeal or subglottic extension. The pharyngeal defect is closed, re-establishing a conduit from the pharynx into the esophagus and resulting in complete separation of the digestive tract from the respiratory tract.

Irradiation Technique

The primary lesion and both sides of the neck are included with opposed lateral portals. The inferior border of the portals depends on the inferior extent of the primary tumor; it is usually at the inferior border of the cricoid. The dose is 74.4 Gy in 62 twice-daily fractions; the lower neck nodes are irradiated through a separate anterior portal. Patients with ipsilateral positive nodes may be treated with IMRT to reduce the dose to the contralateral parotid and/or to avoid a difficult low neck match. The concomitant boost technique is employed if IMRT is used.

Patients develop a sore throat, loss of taste, and moderate dryness during RT. Arytenoid edema may occur and produce the sensation of a lump in the throat. Tracheostomy is seldom necessary before the start of RT. Laryngeal edema may persist for up to a year. Neck dissection increases the degree of lymphedema; bilateral neck dissection should be avoided, if possible.[269]

Combined Treatment Policies

If total laryngectomy is required and the lesion is resectable, postoperative RT or chemoRT are preferred and are added for indications previously discussed. The high-risk areas are usually the base of tongue and neck. The stoma is at risk when subglottic extension is present or there is tumor in the low neck lymph nodes. Complications related to postoperative RT are relatively uncommon.

RT or chemoRT is used prior to total laryngectomy for patients with unresectable neck nodes, or when scheduling problems require a long delay to operation.

Management of Recurrence

Failures after supraglottic laryngectomy or RT frequently can be salvaged by further treatment. Salvage of recurrences that develop after total laryngectomy and adjuvant RT is uncommon.

Treatment: Subglottic Larynx Carcinoma

Early lesions are treated with RT; advanced lesions are usually managed by total laryngectomy and postoperative RT or chemoRT.

Results of Treatment

Vocal Cord Cancer

Surgical Results. Garcia-Serra et al.[259] reviewed ten series containing 269 patients with CIS of the vocal cord treated with stripping; the weighted average 5-year local control and ultimate local control rates were 71.9% and 92.4%, respectively. Similarly, ten series containing 177 patients treated with carbon dioxide laser revealed the following weighted average 5-year local control and ultimate local control rates: 82.5% and 98.1%, respectively.[259]

Thomas et al.[270] reported on 159 patients who underwent an open partial laryngectomy at the Mayo Clinic between 1976 and 1986. Seventeen of 159 patients had CIS; the remaining patients had T1 SCCs. Local recurrence developed in 11 patients (7%), and 9 eventually required laryngectomy. Ten patients developed recurrent cancer in the neck; distant metastases were observed in ten patients.

Hemilaryngectomy including the ipsilateral arytenoid was reported by Som[271] for 130 cases of vocal cord carcinoma extending to the vocal process and face of the arytenoid. The cure rate was 74% for 104 patients with T2 lesions and 58% for 26 patients with T3 cancers.

Foote et al.[272] reported on 81 patients who underwent a laryngectomy for T3 cancers at the Mayo Clinic between 1970 and 1981. Seventy-five patients underwent a total laryngectomy and 6 underwent a near-total laryngectomy; 53 received a neck dissection. No patient underwent adjuvant RT or chemotherapy. The 5-year rates of locoregional control, cause-specific survival, and absolute survival were 74%, 74%, and 54%, respectively.

Radiation Therapy Results. Garcia-Serra et al.[259] reviewed 22 series containing 705 patients with CIS of the vocal cord treated with RT and observed that the weighted average 5-year local control and ultimate local control rates were 87.4% and 98.4%, respectively.

TABLE 72.16

T1-T2N0 GLOTTIC LARYNX—5-YEAR OUTCOMES AFTER RADIOTHERAPY IN 585 PATIENTS

Stage	No. of Patients	Local Control (%)	Ultimate Local Control (%)	LC with Larynx Preservation (%)	CSS (%)	Survival (%)
T1a	253	94	98	95	97	82
T1b	72	93	97	94	99	83
T2a	165	80	96	81	94	76
T2b	95	70	93	74	90	78

LC, local control; CSS, cause-specific survival.
Data from ref. 256.

The results of RT for 585 patients with T1 and T2 N0 SCC of the glottis treated by RT are presented in Table 72.16. The 5-year rates of neck control for the overall groups and for the subsets of patients who remained continuously disease-free at the primary site were T1a, 98% and 100%; T1b, 99% and 100%; and T2a, 96% and 98%; and T2b, 88% and 94%, respectively.[256]

The 5-year outcomes after RT alone (53 patients) versus surgery alone or combined with RT (65 patients) in a series of 118 patients with T3 fixed cord glottic carcinomas treated at the University of Florida were locoregional control, 62% versus 75% (*P* = .10); ultimate locoregional control, 84% versus 82% (*P* = .95); cause-specific survival, 75% versus 71% (*P* = .26); overall survival, 55% versus 45% (*P* = .119); and severe complications, 16% versus 15% (*P* = .558), respectively.[261] Hinerman et al.[273] recently updated the University of Florida experience and reported a 5-year local control rate of 63% for 87 patients with fixed cord T3 glottic carcinomas. The likelihood of local control after RT is related to primary tumor volume and cartilage sclerosis.[274]

Treatment results for T4 glottic carcinomas are shown in Table 72.17.[275-280]

Treatment: Supraglottic Larynx Cancer

The 5-year local control rates after definitive RT in a series of 274 patients treated between 1964 and 1998 at the University of Florida were T1, 100% (n = 22); T2, 86% (n = 125); T3, 62% (n = 99); and T4, 62% (n = 28).[281] The likelihood of local control and local control with a functional larynx is related to tumor volume; those with tumors 6 cc or less have a more favorable outcome than those with larger primary tumors.[268] The 5-year rates of locoregional control and cause-specific survival were stage I, 100% and 100%; stage II, 86% and 93%; stage III, 64% and 81%; stage IVA, 61% and 50%; and stage IVB, 28% and 13%, respectively.[281] Twelve of 274 patients (4%) experienced a severe acute or late complication; 2 patients (1%) died as a consequence.

Lee et al.[282] reported on 60 patients who underwent a supraglottic laryngectomy and modified neck dissection at the M. D. Anderson Hospital between 1974 and 1987; 50 of 60 patients (83%) received postoperative RT. Local control was 100% and locoregional control was obtained in 56 of 60 patients (93%). The 5-year disease-free survival rate was 91%. Three of 60 patients (5%) required a completion laryngectomy for intractable aspiration.

Ambrosch et al.[283] reported on 48 patients treated with transoral laser resection for T1N0 (12 patients) and T2N0 (36 patients) supraglottic carcinoma. Twenty-six patients underwent a unilateral (11 patients) or bilateral (15 patients) neck dissection. Postoperative RT was administered to two patients (4%). The 5-year local control rates were 100% for pT1 cancers and 89% for pT2 malignancies. The 5-year recurrence-free survival and overall survival rates were 83% and 76%, respectively. No patient developed severe aspiration.

Complications of Treatment

Surgical

Repeated stripping of the cord may result in vocal cord fibrosis and hoarseness. Neel et al.[284] reported a 26% incidence of

TABLE 72.17

GLOTTIC CANCER: RESULTS OF TREATMENT

Study	Stage	No. of Patients	Method of Treatment	Results (NED)
Jesse[275]	T4 N0–N+	48	Laryngectomy	54% at 4 years
Ogura et al.[276]	T4 N0	11	Laryngectomy	45% at 3 years
Skolnick et al.[277]	T4 N0	7	Laryngectomy	30% at 5 years
Vermund[278]	T4 N0	31	Laryngectomy	35% at 5 years
Stewart and Jackson[279]	T4 N0	13	RT with surgery for salvage	38% at 5 years
Harwood et al.[280]	T4 N0	56	RT with surgery for salvage	49% at 5 years[a]
Hinerman et al.[351]	T4 N0–N+	22	RT with surgery for salvage	81% local control at 5 years

NED, no evidence of disease; RT, radiotherapy.
[a]Actuarial survival, uncorrected for deaths due to intercurrent disease.
Modified from ref. 280.

nonfatal complications for cordectomy. Immediate postoperative complications included atelectasis and pneumonia, severe subcutaneous emphysema in the neck, bleeding from the tracheotomy site or larynx, wound complications, and airway obstruction requiring tracheotomy. Late complications included removal of granulation tissue by direct laryngoscopy to exclude recurrence, extrusion of cartilage, laryngeal stenosis, and obstructing laryngeal web.

The postoperative complications of hemilaryngectomy include aspiration, chondritis, wound slough, inadequate glottic closure, and anterior commissure webs.

The complication rate following supraglottic laryngectomy is about 10%, including fistula formation, aspiration, chondritis, dysphagia, dyspnea, and carotid rupture.[281]

The postoperative complications of total laryngectomy may include perioperative death, hemorrhage, fistula, chondritis, wound breakdown, carotid rupture, dysphagia, and pharyngoesophageal stenosis.

Radiation Therapy

After RT, the quality and volume of the voice tend to diminish at the end of the day. Laryngeal edema is the most common sequela. Steroids may be used to reduce edema secondary to RT after recurrence has been ruled out. If ulceration and pain occur, antibiotics are used.

Soft tissue necrosis leading to chondritis occurs in about 1% of patients. Soft tissue and cartilage necroses mimic recurrence with hoarseness, pain, and edema; a laryngectomy may be recommended for fear of recurrent cancer, even though biopsies show only necrosis. Chera et al.[256] recorded severe complications after definitive RT in 10 (1.7%) of 585 patients treated for T1–T2N0 glottic SCCs.

Combined Treatment

Preoperative RT is associated with an increased risk of an operative complication and prolonged hospitalization. The major late effects of combined treatment are an increased fibrosis of soft tissues, stomal stenosis, and pharyngeal stricture.

HYPOPHARYNX: PHARYNGEAL WALLS, PYRIFORM SINUS, AND POSTCRICOID PHARYNX

Both the oropharyngeal and hypopharyngeal walls will be considered together because there is no distinct difference in the presentation or treatment. The majority of hypopharyngeal lesions originate in the pyriform sinus. Postcricoid carcinomas are uncommon.

Anatomy

The epithelium of the pharyngeal mucous membrane is squamous; it is continuous with the mucous membrane of the nasopharynx. The dividing point between the nasopharynx and posterior pharyngeal wall is Passavant's ridge, a muscular ring that contracts to close the nasopharynx during swallowing. The thin constrictor muscles surround the posterior and lateral walls. Between the constrictor muscles and the prevertebral fascia covering the longitudinal prevertebral muscles (longus colli and longus capitis) is a thin layer of loose areolar tissue, the retropharyngeal space. The entire thickness of the posterior pharyngeal wall from the mucous membrane to the anterior vertebral body is no more than 1 cm in the midline. Lateral to the pharyngeal wall are the vessels, nerves, and muscles of the parapharyngeal space. The constrictor muscles are relatively thin, especially the superior constrictor, and do not present much of an obstacle to tumor penetration. There is a variable weak spot in the lateral pharyngeal wall just below the hyoid where the middle and the inferior constrictor muscles fail to overlap. The lateral wall in this area is composed of the thin thyrohyoid membrane, which is penetrated by the vessels, nerves, and lymphatics of the laryngopharynx.

The pharyngeal walls are continuous with the cervical esophagus below; the transition to cervical esophagus is below the arytenoids (C4). The transition zone, 3 to 4 cm in length, is the postcricoid hypopharynx.

The lateral pharyngeal wall is a narrow strip of mucosa that lies behind the posterior tonsillar pillar in the oropharynx, is partially interrupted by the pharyngoepiglottic fold, and then continues into the hypopharynx, where it becomes the lateral wall of the pyriform sinus. The posterior cornu of the hyoid bone may protrude into the lateral pharyngeal wall on one or both sides, producing a submucosal bulge. The posterior pharyngeal wall is 4 to 5 cm wide and 6 to 7 cm in height.

The superior margin of the pyriform sinus is the pharyngoepiglottic fold and the free margin of the aryepiglottic fold. The superolateral margin of the pyriform sinus is an oblique line along the lateral pharyngeal wall opposite the aryepiglottic fold. Thus, the pyriform sinus has three walls: the anterior, lateral, and medial (there is no posterior wall). The pyriform sinus tapers inferiorly to the apex and terminates variably at a level between the superior and inferior borders of the cricoid cartilage. The superior limit of the pyriform sinus is opposite the hyoid. The thyrohyoid membrane is lateral to the upper portion of the pyriform sinus, and the thyroid cartilage, cricothyroid membrane, and cricoid cartilage are lateral to the lower portion. The internal branch of the superior laryngeal nerve, a branch of the vagus, lies under the mucous membrane on the anterolateral wall of the pyriform sinus. The auricular branch is sensory to the skin of the back of the pinna and the posterior wall of the external auditory canal.

The postcricoid pharynx is funnel-shaped, to direct food into the esophagus. The superior margin begins just below the arytenoids. The anterior wall lies behind the cricoid cartilage and is the posterior wall of the lower larynx. The posterior wall is a continuation of the hypopharyngeal walls. The recurrent laryngeal nerve ascends in the tracheoesophageal groove, entering the larynx posterior to the cricothyroid articulation at the junction of the hypopharynx and esophagus. Internal branches of the superior laryngeal nerve extend inferiorly anterior to the mucosa of the piriform sinuses.

Pathology

More than 95% of malignant tumors are SCCs. CIS is commonly seen in surgical specimens at the edge of pharyngeal wall SCCs; multifocal skip areas of CIS may make it difficult to obtain clear margins if excision is done. Minor salivary gland tumors are rare.

Patterns of Spread

Posterior Pharyngeal Wall

SCCs of the posterior wall have a tendency to remain on the posterior wall, grow up or down the wall, and infiltrate posteriorly; they seldom spread circumferentially to the lateral walls, even when advanced. Early lesions are red, sometimes with white areas sprinkled over the involved area. As the lesion progresses, the tumor bulges into the pharyngeal cavity and a linear midline ulceration appears. The tumor may spread up the pillars, eventually reaching the palate. Advanced lesions tend to terminate inferiorly at the level of the arytenoids without growing into the postcricoid region. Superiorly, they may extend into the nasopharynx. Direct invasion of the cervical vertebrae or skull base is uncommon.

Lateral Pharyngeal Wall

Early tumors may be well-defined exophytic lesions. As they advance, they tend to penetrate laterally through the constrictor muscle, thus entering the lateral pharyngeal space or the soft tissues of the neck.

The muscles of the pharynx originate from the skull base, eustachian tube, styloid process, pterygomandibular raphe, and hyoid bone; tumor may spread along muscle and fascial planes to all muscular points of origin.[285] Tumor also follows a course along cranial nerves IX and X and the sympathetic chain. Tumor secondarily invades the pharyngoepiglottic fold, the vallecula, and the anterior and lateral walls of the pyriform sinus.

Pyriform Sinus

Early lesions usually appear as nodular mucosal irregularities. Medial wall lesions may grow superficially along the aryepiglottic fold and arytenoids, or invade directly into the false cord and aryepiglottic fold. Medial wall lesions also extend posteriorly to the postcricoid region, cricoid cartilage, and to the opposite pyriform sinus. Extensive submucosal spread is characteristic. There is frequently an area of central ulceration. The vocal cord becomes fixed because of infiltration of the intrinsic muscles of the larynx, the cricoarytenoid joint or muscle, or less commonly, the recurrent laryngeal nerve. Spread into the cervical esophagus is a late event.

Lesions arising on the lateral wall tend toward early invasion of the posterior thyroid cartilage and the posterior superior cricoid cartilage. The ipsilateral superior lobe of the thyroid gland may be invaded after tumor penetrates the cartilage, or when tumor penetrates behind the thyroid cartilage or through the cricothyroid membrane. Kirchner[286] reported that thyroid cartilage invasion was associated with involvement of the apex of the pyriform sinus, and the extent of invasion was unrelated to extent of visible disease. Lesions of the lateral walls tend to spread submucosally to the posterior pharyngeal wall.

Advanced lesions of the pyriform sinus invade all three walls, fix the larynx, involve the ipsilateral posterior pharyngeal wall, invade the thyroid cartilage and thyroid gland, and often escape into the soft tissues of the neck. The pre-epiglottic space often is involved. PNI of the recurrent laryngeal nerve may be seen in whole organ sections.

Postcricoid Pharynx

Early postcricoid lesions are rare. Lesions arising from the posterior wall tend to remain on the posterior wall. Lesions arising from the anterior wall tend to invade the posterior cricoarytenoid muscle and the cricoid and arytenoid cartilages. Advanced tumors eventually encircle the lumen. Some lesions secondarily invade the apex of the pyriform sinus early.

Lymphatics

Pharyngeal Walls. The lymphatics of the pharyngeal walls terminate primarily in the jugular chain and secondarily in the level V nodes. The level II nodes are most often involved. Lindberg[17] reported 59% clinically positive nodes on admission; 17% were bilateral. Retropharyngeal lymph node involvement is frequent.

Pyriform Sinus. The drainage is mainly to the jugular chain with a relatively small proportion to the level V nodes. The level II nodes are most commonly involved, but level III involvement occurs without level II metastases. On admission, 75% of patients have clinically positive nodes and at least 10% have bilateral nodes. There is no difference in the risk of lymph node metastases by T stage. Ogura et al.[287] reported a 62% incidence of subclinical disease; some of the patients had 15 to 30 Gy of preoperative RT.

Clinical Picture

Tumors that are lateralized to the lateral pharyngeal wall or pyriform sinus produce a unilateral sore throat. Dysphagia, sensation of foreign body, ear pain, blood-streaked saliva, and voice change occur later. A neck mass may be the presenting complaint.

Lesions of the apex of the pyriform sinus or postcricoid area produce pooling of secretions, indicating obstruction of the gullet. Arytenoid edema and inability to see into the apex of the pyriform sinus may be observed. Invasion of the palatopharyngeal muscle at its insertion into the inferior constrictor can cause shortening of the muscle and asymmetry of the posterior tonsillar pillars. An extensive postcricoid tumor may push the larynx anteriorly and the thyroid click, produced by the superior thyroid cornu hitting against the spine while rocking the thyroid cartilage back and forth, is lost.

Staging

The staging system for the primary tumor is depicted in Table 72.18.

TABLE 72.18

HYPOPHARYNX: 2010 AMERICAN JOINT COMMITTEE ON CANCER STAGING SYSTEM FOR THE PRIMARY TUMOR

T1	Tumor limited to one subsite of hypopharynx and 2 cm or less in greatest dimension
T2	Tumor invades more than one subsite of hypopharynx or an adjacent site, or measures more than 2 cm but not more than 4 cm in greatest diameter without fixation of the hemilarynx
T3	Tumor more than 4 cm in greatest dimension or with fixation of the hemilarynx or extension to esophagus
T4a	Tumor invades thyroid/cricoid cartilage, hyoid bone, thyroid gland, or central compartment soft tissue[a]
T4b	Tumor invades the prevertebral fascia, encases the carotid artery, or involves mediastinal structures

[a]Central compartment soft tissue includes the prelaryngeal strap muscles and subcutaneous fat.
From ref. 216, with permission.

Treatment

Selection of Treatment Modality

Posterior Pharyngeal Wall. RT produces cure rates similar to those produced by surgery alone or combined with RT, and with less morbidity. Thus, almost all cancers are treated with RT.

Lateral Pharyngeal Wall. The preferred treatment is definitive RT.

Pyriform Sinus. T1 and low-volume (≤6 cc), exophytic T2 cancers with normal cord mobility can be treated either by RT or partial laryngopharyngectomy.[288] RT is preferred because it is associated with less morbidity.

Selected high-volume endophytic T2 and T3 lesions extending with normal or reduced mobility may be suitable for chemoRT. The swallowing outcomes after chemoRT may be less optimal than those seen in the oropharynx and larynx.[289]

The remaining lesions are best treated with total laryngopharyngectomy, neck dissection, and postoperative RT or chemoRT. Patients presenting with an extensive primary lesion and extensive neck metastases are frequently offered palliative therapy.

Surgical Treatment

Posterior Pharyngeal Wall. If the lesion is high on the posterior wall, a transoral approach can be used. Lower lesions were traditionally accessed via a transhyoid approach, a lateral pharyngotomy, or a midline mandibulolabial glossotomy. More recently, transoral laser microsurgical resection has been employed to reduce the morbidity associated with the aforementioned open approaches, which also frequently require tracheotomy. Dissection extends deep to the tumor down to the prevertebral fascia; smaller defects heal by secondary intention without a skin graft, whereas larger defects may require radial forearm free flap placement.

Pyriform Sinus

Partial laryngopharyngectomy. A partial laryngopharyngectomy removes the false cords, epiglottis, aryepiglottic fold, and pyriform sinus; one arytenoid may be removed when necessary. The vocal cords are preserved. The following findings contraindicate partial laryngopharyngectomy: extension to the apex of the pyriform sinus, fixed cord, extension to contralateral arytenoid, poor pulmonary function, and large, fixed lymph nodes. There is a greater tendency to aspirate after partial laryngopharyngectomy compared with supraglottic laryngectomy.

Total laryngopharyngectomy. Total laryngopharyngectomy removes the larynx and varying amounts of pharyngeal wall. Advanced lesions require excision of nearly the entire circumference. The pharynx is re-established by primary closure after a partial pharyngectomy; reconstruction with a pectoralis major myocutaneous flap or radial forearm free flap is typically required.

Postcricoid Pharynx. Total laryngopharyngectomy with immediate reconstruction, generally using a pectoralis major myocutaneous flap or free flap, is performed. If the lesion extends into the cervical esophagus, a gastric pullup or jejunal free flap may be necessary.

Irradiation Technique

Posterior Pharyngeal Wall. The RT technique for lesions of the posterior pharyngeal wall is opposed lateral fields to include the primary lesion and the regional nodes. Because these lesions tend to "skip" areas, the entire posterior pharyngeal wall is included initially. If the lesion extends near the arytenoids, the postcricoid pharynx, pyriform sinuses, and upper cervical esophagus are included. The retropharyngeal nodes are included even if the neck is N0. When the field is reduced at 45 Gy to avoid the spinal cord, the posterior border of the portal is placed just anterior to the spinal cord.[290] The dose is 74.4 to 76.8 Gy, 1.2 Gy per fraction twice daily in a continuous course. IMRT is useful to reduce the dose to one or both parotids; the concomitant boost technique is employed if IMRT is used. Concomitant chemotherapy should be included for stage III–IV cancers.

Pyriform Sinus. Parallel opposed lateral portals are used to encompass the primary lesion and regional nodes on both sides. The superior border is placed 2 cm above the tip of the mastoid to cover the most superior jugular chain and the retropharyngeal lymph nodes. The posterior border encompasses the level V nodes. Clinically positive nodes behind the plane of the spinal cord require an electron boost. The anterior border is usually placed about 0.5 to 1 cm behind the anterior skin edge, if it is possible to do so, and adequately encompass the tumor. The inferior border is 2 cm below the inferior border of the cricoid. The remaining lower neck lymph nodes are treated through an *en face* portal. The doses are the same as for the posterior pharyngeal wall. IMRT is an option if the tumor can be adequately encompassed while sparing the contralateral salivary gland(s) and/or to avoid a difficult low neck match.

Combined Treatment Policies

Posterior Pharyngeal Wall. An operation should usually precede RT when a combination is selected, unless a gastric pull-up is planned.

Pyriform Sinus. Following total laryngopharyngectomy with or without neck dissection, RT is usually recommended for indications previously outlined.

RT or chemoRT is used prior to operation for patients with a large fixed node. The dose to the primary tumor ranges from 45 to 50 Gy; the fixed node(s) is boosted to 60 to 75 Gy.

Management of Recurrence

Posterior Pharyngeal Wall. Recurrence after RT may be limited to the posterior pharyngeal wall and suitable for surgical excision, with occasional salvage. There is frequently a persistent ulcer after RT for advanced lesions; it should be considered evidence of persistent disease if it does not heal. Surgical excision is limited posteriorly by the prevertebral fascia. RT salvage of a surgical failure is unusual.

Pyriform Sinus. The hallmark of local recurrence after RT is persistent edema, pain, and fixation of laryngeal structures. Direct laryngoscopy is required, but biopsy may be negative. CT or PET is often helpful for distinguishing local recurrence from necrosis. It may be necessary to recommend total laryngopharyngectomy for salvage without a positive biopsy.

Recurrence after total laryngopharyngectomy is usually in the soft tissues of the neck, the untreated opposite neck, the base of tongue, or stoma. Surgical failures after partial laryngopharyngectomy for early lesions may be salvaged by total laryngopharyngectomy. Failures after total laryngopharyngectomy are rarely salvaged.

Results of Treatment

Pharyngeal Wall

The 5-year local control rates and ultimate local control rates after RT at the University of Florida for 148 patients were T1 (n = 15), 93% and 93%; T2 (n = 45), 82% and 87%; T3 (n = 6), 59% and 61%; and T4 (n = 12), 50% and 50%, respectively.[290] The 5-year locoregional control and cause-specific survival rates were stage I, 89% and 89%; stage II, 83% and 88%; stage III, 58% and 44%; and stage IV, 47% and 34%, respectively.[290]

Pyriform Sinus

The results of treatment for 80 patients with carcinoma of the pyriform sinus treated at Washington University by preoperative RT followed by partial laryngopharyngectomy are shown

PRACTICE OF ONCOLOGY

TABLE 72.19

CARCINOMA OF THE PYRIFORM SINUS: RESULTS OF TREATMENT BY LOW-DOSE RADIATION THERAPY PLUS PARTIAL LARYNGOPHARYNGECTOMY OR TOTAL LARYNGECTOMY AND PARTIAL PHARYNGECTOMY (WASHINGTON UNIVERSITY, ST. LOUIS, MISSOURI, 1964–1974)

Result	PLP (80 Patients)[a] (%)	TLP (57 Patients)[b] (%)
Local recurrence ± neck recurrence	14[c]	14
Neck recurrence ± distant metastases (primary controlled)	9	23
Distant metastases alone	11	21
5-year actuarial survival (no evidence of disease)	40	22

PLP, partial laryngopharyngectomy; TLP, total laryngopharyngectomy.
[a]T1, 70 patients; T2-T4, 10 patients (American Joint Committee on Cancer staging).
[b]T1, 35 patients; T2-T4, 22 patients (American Joint Committee on Cancer staging).
[c]Four patients salvaged.
Data from ref. 291.

in Table 72.19.[291] Seventy patients had the equivalent of AJCC T1 lesions (disease limited to the pyriform sinus) and ten patients had disease extending beyond the pyriform sinus; none had invasion of the apex of the pyriform sinus. The cause of death was cancer in 26%, complications of treatment in 14%, and intercurrent disease in 20%. The 5-year absolute survival was 25 of 66 patients (38%) (J. E. Marks, personal communication, 1979).

The results of treatment for 57 patients from the same institution who were treated by preoperative RT followed by total laryngectomy and partial pharyngectomy are depicted in Table 72.19.[291] Thirty-five patients had lesions confined to the pyriform sinus (AJCC T1) and the remainder had extension beyond the pyriform sinus (AJCC T2–T4). The cause of death was cancer in 56% of patients, complications of treatment in 11% of patients, and intercurrent disease in 18% of patients.

The 5-year local control rates for 123 patients treated with definitive RT for T1 (23 patients) and T2 (100 patients) pyriform sinus SCCs were T1, 85%, and T2, 85%, respectively.[289] The 5-year rates of locoregional control and cause-specific survival were stage I–II, 86% and 85%; stage III, 65% and 73%; stage IVA, 83% and 62%; and stage IVB, 24% and 22%, respectively.[289] The 5-year distant metastasis-free survival rates were N0, 96%; N1, 88%; N2, 68%; and N3, 55%.

Complications of Treatment

Posterior Pharyngeal Wall

Surgical Complications. Marks et al.[292] reported a 14% operative mortality plus major complications including pharyngocutaneous fistula (31%) and carotid rupture (14%) for patients treated with preoperative RT, 25 to 30 Gy.

Radiation Therapy Complications. Hull et al.[290] observed 8 fatal complications (5%) in 148 patients who were treated at the University of Florida. These included aspiration pneumonia (4 patients), soft tissue or cartilage necrosis (3 patients), and laryngeal edema (1 patient). Twenty-three patients (16%) experienced nonfatal severe complications including permanent PEG (15 patients), soft tissue and/or bone necrosis (7 patients), and carotid rupture, orocutaneous fistula, tracheostomy, and brachial plexopathy (1 patient).

Pyriform Sinus

Surgical Complications. The complications of partial laryngopharyngectomy included a 12% operative mortality, fistula, aspiration, and dysphagia.[291] The complications of total laryngopharyngectomy included a treatment-related mortality of 11%, fistula, and pharyngeal stenosis.[291] The complication rate is increased by the addition of RT.

Radiation Therapy Complications. The major RT complication is laryngeal necrosis. Rabbani et al.[289] reported the following rates of moderate to severe complications in 123 patients: acute (2%); late (9%); and postoperative (5%).

Complications of Salvage Treatment. Attempted surgical salvage of RT failures has a significant operative morbidity and mortality; few patients are cured.

NASOPHARYNX

NPCs are uncommon in the United States. The Chinese have a high frequency; American-born second-generation Chinese maintain the risk of NPC. NPC has been shown to have an association with elevated titers of EBV, which is independent of geography.[293] There is a 3:1 ratio of predominance in men. The age distribution for NPC is younger than for other head and neck sites; about 20% of patients are younger than 30 years of age.

ANATOMY

The nasopharynx is roughly cuboidal in shape. It is contiguous with the nasal cavity, inferiorly with the oropharynx, and laterally with the middle ears by way of the eustachian tubes.

The mucosa of the roof and posterior wall is often irregular because of the pharyngeal bursa, adenoids, and pharyngeal hypophysis; it tends to become smooth with age.

The lateral walls include the eustachian tube openings with the fossa of Rosenmuller located behind the torus tubarius. The superolateral muscular wall of the nasopharynx is incomplete. The floor of the nasopharynx is incomplete and consists of the upper surface of the soft palate.

Lymphatics

There is an extensive submucosal lymphatic capillary plexus. Tumor spreads along three different pathways: the jugular chain, the spinal accessory chain, and the retropharyngeal pathway.[294] The lateral retropharyngeal nodes lie in the retropharyngeal space medial to the carotid artery. Directly behind the nodes are the lateral masses of C1 and C2. Inconstant lymphatic vessels may drain directly to the level III and level V nodes.[10]

PATHOLOGY

Carcinomas compose about 85% and lymphomas about 10% of the malignant lesions. The WHO has classified NPCs as follows: WHO type I, SCC; WHO type II, nonkeratinizing carcinoma; and WHO type III, undifferentiated carcinoma. Lymphoepithelioma is included in the WHO III category. A miscellaneous group of malignant tumors includes melanoma, plasmacytoma,[247] juvenile angiofibroma,[11] carcinosarcoma, sarcomas, nonchromaffin paragangliomas, and minor salivary gland tumors.

PATTERNS OF SPREAD

Primary

Inferior extension along the lateral pharyngeal walls and tonsillar pillars occurs in almost one-third of patients. Extension into the posterior nasal cavity is frequent but usually limited to less than 1 cm. Invasion of the posterior ethmoids, maxillary antrum, and/or orbit occurs fairly often. Skull base invasion is recognized radiographically in at least 25% of patients. The sphenoid sinus frequently is invaded. Tumor may erode through the foramen an ovale, lacerum, and/or spinosum. Tumor eventually reaches the cavernous sinus and has access to cranial nerves II to VI.

The lateral muscular wall of the nasopharynx is incomplete superiorly. The defect, termed the *sinus of Morgagni*, is transversed by the cartilaginous eustachian tube and the levator palatine muscle, providing access for NPC to the lateral pharyngeal space and skull base.

Lymphatics

There is an 80% to 90% incidence of metastatic neck nodes on presentation; approximately 50% are bilateral. Low-grade SCCs produce fewer metastases (73%) than high-grade carcinomas (92%). Metastases to submental and occipital nodes may appear when there is blockage of the common lymphatic pathways either by massive neck disease or by an untimely neck dissection.

CLINICAL PICTURE

The most common presenting complaint is a painless upper neck mass. Nasal obstruction, epistaxis, and otitis media may be observed. Sore throat occurs in about 15% of patients and is related to spread into the oropharyngeal wall. Facial pain may be referred from any of the three divisions of the trigeminal nerve, usually V3. Occipital or temporal headache frequently is seen. Pain in the scalp over the left mastoid area is related to involvement of a high jugular lymph node that has become fixed to the skull and spine. Pain in lifting the head and neck extension is due to infiltration of the prevertebral muscles. Proptosis occurs with posterior orbital invasion. Trismus is due to the invasion of the pterygoid region.

Neurologic symptoms and signs occur in about 25% of patients. Involvement of cranial nerves II to VI indicates extension into the cavernous sinus. Cranial nerves IX to XII and the sympathetic chain are involved in the lateral pharyngeal space.

Examination of the nasopharynx will show a lesion on the lateral wall or roof; the nasopharyngeal surface of the soft palate is rarely involved. Early lesions may be submucosal and difficult to detect. Lymphomas tend to remain submucosal until quite large.

Fiberoptic examination may show tumor growing into the posterior nasal cavity. Tumor may be seen infiltrating submucosally along the posterior tonsillar pillars but infrequently grows very far down the posterior pharyngeal wall. The posterior tonsillar pillars may bulge into the oropharynx if an enlarged node develops in the lateral pharyngeal space. Cranial nerve VI is the one most commonly involved. The eyes should be evaluated for proptosis. Ear examination may show findings of otitis media or, rarely, gross tumor.

STAGING

The AJCC staging system is depicted in Table 72.20.

TABLE 72.20

2010 AMERICAN JOINT COMMITTEE ON CANCER STAGING FOR NASOPHARYNGEAL CANCER

PRIMARY TUMOR (T)

T1	Tumor confined to the nasopharynx, or tumor extends to oropharynx and/or nasal cavity without parapharyngeal extension[a]
T2	Tumor with parapharyngeal extension[a]
T3	Tumor involves bony structures of skull base and/or paranasal sinuses
T4	Tumor with intracranial extension and/or involvement of cranial nerves, hypopharynx, orbit, or with extension to the infratemporal fossa/masticator space

REGIONAL LYMPH NODES (N)

NX	Regional lymph nodes cannot be assessed
N0	No regional lymph node metastasis
N1	Unilateral metastasis in lymph node(s), 6 cm or less in greatest dimension, above the supraclavicular fossa and/or unilateral or bilateral, retropharyngeal lymph nodes, 6 cm or less, in greatest dimension[b]
N2	Bilateral metastasis in cervical lymph node(s), 6 cm or less in greatest dimension, above the supraclavicular fossa[b]
N3	Metastasis in a lymph node(s)[b] >6 cm and/or to supraclavicular fossa
N3a	Greater than 6 cm in dimension
N3b	Extension to the supraclavicular fossa[c]

STAGE GROUPING

0	Tis	N0	M0
I	T1	N0	M0
II	T1	N1	M0
	T2	N0	M0
	T2	N1	M0
III	T1	N2	M0
	T2	N2	M0
	T3	N0	M0
	T3	N1	M0
	T3	N2	M0
IVA	T4	N0	M0
	T4	N1	M0
	T4	N2	M0
IVB	Any T	N3	M0
IVC	Any T	Any N	M1

[a]Parapharyngeal extension denotes posterolateral infiltration of tumor.
[b]Midline nodes are considered ipsilateral nodes.
[c]Supraclavicular zone or fossa is relevant to the staging of nasopharyngeal carcinoma and is the triangular region originally described by Ho. It is defined by three points: (1) the superior margin of the sternal end of the clavicle, (2) the superior margin of the lateral end of the clavicle, and (3) the point where the neck meets the shoulder. Note that this would include caudal portions of levels IV and VB. All cases with lymph nodes (whole or part) in the fossa are considered N3b.
From ref. 216, with permission.

TREATMENT

Selection of Treatment Modality

The treatment of almost all NPCs is RT-based because complete surgical resection is usually not feasible. Neck dissection is used less often in the management of neck disease because of the relatively high success rate with RT or chemoRT alone, particularly for lymphoepithelioma. A small adenocarcinoma or sarcoma may be excised. Juvenile angiofibromas are preferably excised because of the young age of the patient, although the tumors are quite successfully cured by RT when complete resection is unlikely or dangerous.[11] Patients with advanced disease should receive concomitant chemotherapy.[170,172,179,295,296] Adjuvant chemotherapy may be considered according to the NCCN practice guidelines[168] based on available randomized studies.[167,171,172]

Irradiation Technique

If the tumor is thought to be limited to the nasopharynx or to have minimal soft-tissue extension, the following areas are included in the treatment volume: (1) nasopharynx, (2) posterior 2 cm of the nasal cavity, (3) posterior ethmoid sinuses, (4) entire sphenoid sinus and basioccipital bone, (5) cavernous sinus, (6) base of skull (7–8 cm width encompassing the foramen ovale, carotid canal, and foramen spinosum laterally), (7) pterygoid fossae, (8) posterior third of maxillary sinus, (9) oropharyngeal wall to the level of the midtonsillar fossa, (10) retropharyngeal nodes, and (11) neck nodes on both sides.

Extension to the skull base or involvement of cranial nerves II to VI requires the superior border to be raised to include the entire pituitary, the base of the brain in the suprasellar area, the adjacent middle cranial fossa, and the posterior portion of the anterior cranial fossa. Patients with anterior invasion into the orbit, ethmoids, or maxillary sinus require an individualized plan to produce a satisfactory dose distribution. Three-dimensional CT-based treatment planning allows for the use of more conformal fields. IMRT is useful to improve coverage of the poststyloid parapharyngeal space and reduce the dose to parotid glands and the temporal lobes to reduce long-term morbidity. The authors currently treat patients to 74.4 at 1.2 Gy per fraction twice daily.

Neck Nodes. The entire neck is irradiated to the level of the clavicles. The retropharyngeal nodes are included in the treatment of the primary lesion. The upper neck nodes are included in the primary fields to the level of the thyroid notch. In the case of a neck with N0 lesion, the posterior margin is placed about 1 to 2 cm behind the posterior border of the sternocleidomastoid to encompass the high level V nodes and level II nodes. The portals are extended to include the submental area only if there is disease in the level IB nodes or if the patient had a neck dissection prior to RT. The lower neck is treated through an anterior portal with a shield over the larynx.

Acute Sequelae. Sore throat begins at the end of the second week of therapy and persists for 2 to 3 months after the completion of RT. Xerostomia is always present. Loss of taste and appetite is often profound; both return 1 to 6 months after completion of RT. Obstruction of the eustachian tubes may occur with secondary otitis media and hearing loss. Polyethylene tubes inserted through the eardrums to drain the middle ears can correct this condition. The obstruction often improves after a few months. Severe nausea and vomiting are uncommon.

Management of Recurrence

The majority of recurrent SCCs are diagnosed within 2 years, but lymphoepithelioma may recur many years after treatment. Headache and cranial nerve palsies usually indicate recurrence. Retreatment for local recurrences with limited RT portals and/or intracavitary brachytherapy may be rewarding, particularly if the recurrence is due to a marginal miss or low dose.[297,298]

Results of Treatment

Lee et al.[299] reported the following 10-year outcomes in a series of 5,037 patients treated with RT at the Queen Elizabeth Hospital, Hong Kong, between 1976 and 1985: local control, 61%; regional control, 64%; distant metastasis-free survival, 59%; and survival, 42%. Leung et al.[300] reported the following 5-year local control rates in a series of 1,070 patients: T1, 88%; T2a, 87%; T2b, 82%; T3, 69%; and T4, 69%. Chua et al.[301] evaluated 290 patients and found that primary tumor volume of more than 60 cc was associated with a lower likelihood of local control after RT. Teo et al.[302] evaluated a series of 903 patients treated at the Prince of Wales Hospital, Hong Kong, and observed that local control was adversely affected by advanced patient age, skull base invasion, and cranial nerve involvement. Prognostic factors associated with an increased rate of distant metastases and poor survival were male sex, skull base and cranial nerve(s) involvement, advanced neck stage, nodal fixation, and bilateral neck nodes.[302] The 5-year outcomes for 82 patients treated at the University of Florida were local control, 78%; regional control, 90%; locoregional control, 76%; distant metastasis-free survival, 80%; cause-specific survival, 66%; and survival 57%.[303] Table 72.9 summarizes the results of selected randomized trials comparing chemoRT versus RT alone.

Follow-Up Policy

Follow-up includes careful observation and laboratory testing for possible thyroid and/or pituitary hypofunction. Dental care must be closely monitored because of xerostomia.

Complications of Treatment

Primary or secondary hypopituitarism (from a hypothalamic lesion) has been reported. Brain necrosis is rare. Hypothyroidism may result from either a direct effect on the thyroid gland or an indirect effect on the pituitary. Delayed bone age and growth failure may be seen in young patients. A transient CNS syndrome may appear 2 to 3 months after RT and may require several months to resolve. General weakness and extreme fatigue may be symptoms of low serum cortisol levels. Radiation myelitis of the cervical cord or brainstem is the most severe CNS complication. IMRT may be used to reduce the dose to the CNS, particularly the temporal lobes.

Trismus may occur because of fibrosis of the pterygoid muscles; this is more likely in those treated with two opposing portals for the entire course. Palsy of cranial nerves IX to XII may occur several years after RT and is related to nerve entrapment in the lateral pharyngeal space. Eye complications (e.g., retrobulbar optic neuritis) may develop because of RT of the optic nerve.[304] RT of the posterior eyeball to high doses may produce a retinopathy.[305]

NASAL VESTIBULE, NASAL CAVITY, AND PARANASAL SINUSES

Tumors of the nasal vestibule are considered separately from nasal cavity tumors because they are essentially skin cancers and have a different natural history. Primary tumors arising from the nasal cavity and paranasal sinuses are considered together because the lesions are frequently advanced when first seen and it is not always possible to determine the site of origin.

Cancer of the nasal cavity or paranasal sinuses is a relatively rare problem, with a yearly risk factor estimated at approximately one case for every 100,000 people. They occur more often in men and usually appear after the age of 40 except for minor salivary gland tumors and esthesioneuroblastomas, which may appear before the age of 20.[306] Nasal cavity and ethmoid sinus adenocarcinomas have been linked to occupations associated with wood dust: the furniture industry, sawmill work, and carpentry. Other occupations with dust-filled work environments such as shoe making, baking, and flour milling industry also have been implicated.[9]

Carcinomas of the sphenoid and frontal sinuses are rare.

Anatomy

The nasal vestibule is the entrance to the nasal cavity. It is lined by skin in which there are numerous hair follicles and sebaceous glands. The vestibule is a three-sided, pear-shaped cavity about 1.5 cm in diameter that ends posteriorly at the limen nasi. The alar cartilages form the anterolateral wall. The medial wall is the columella, formed by the medial wing of the alar cartilage and the anterior portion of the cartilaginous septum. The floor is the maxilla.

The nasal cavity begins at the limen nasi and ends at the posterior nares, where it communicates with the nasopharynx. The lateral walls are composed of thin bony folds that project into the nasal cavity: the inferior, medial, and superior turbinates. The nasolacrimal duct enters the nasal cavity beneath the inferior turbinate. The frontal sinus and ethmoid bullae connect to the nasal cavity with openings that lie under the middle turbinate. The sphenoid sinus communicates with the nasal cavity by an opening on the anterior wall of the sinus. Approximately 20 branches of the olfactory nerves enter the nasal cavity through the cribriform plate; nerve fibers are distributed over the upper third of the septum and superior nasal turbinate. The epithelium is nonciliated columnar. The lower half of the nasal cavity is the respiratory portion, and the epithelium is ciliated columnar. There are numerous collections of lymphoid tissue and mucous glands beneath the epithelium.

The maxillary sinuses are single pyramidal cavities. The medial wall is the lateral wall of the nasal cavity and has one or two openings communicating with the middle meatus under the medial turbinate. The inferior wall is the hard palate. The posterolateral wall is related to the zygomatic process and the pterygomaxillary space. The superior wall is the orbital floor.

The frontal sinuses are two irregular, asymmetrical air cavities separated by a thin bony septum. They connect to the middle meatus of the nasal cavity by the frontonasal duct. They are separated from the anterior ethmoid cells by thin bony walls. The posterior wall separating the frontal sinus from the anterior cranial fossa is relatively thick.

The ethmoid sinuses consist of a number of air cells lying between the medial walls of the orbits and the lateral wall of the nasal cavity. The lateral wall is the thin porous lamina papyracea. Medially, the ethmoid air cells bulge into the lateral wall of the nasal cavity. The ethmoid cells communicate with the nasal cavity in the middle meatus. These bony walls are thin and easily traversed by tumor. The ethmoid air cells extend far anteriorly; the lacrimal bone covers the anterior cells laterally. The midline perpendicular plate of the ethmoid separates the right and left ethmoid cells anatomically. There is no anatomic barrier between the anterior, middle, and posterior ethmoids.

The sphenoid sinus is a midline structure in the body of the sphenoid bone. The pituitary lies above, the cavernous sinuses laterally, the nasal cavity and ethmoid sinuses in front, and the nasopharynx beneath. The clivus and brainstem lie posteriorly. The pneumatization is variable and can extend into all portions of the sphenoid bone. The right and left sinuses are partially separated by an incomplete septum. The sphenoid sinus connects anteriorly with the nasal cavity in the sphenoethmoidal recess.

Lymphatics

Nasal Vestibule. The lymphatic trunks run to the level IB nodes. There is a small risk for involvement of the intercalated facial nodes just behind the commissure of the lip along the course of the facial neurovascular bundle.

Nasal Cavity and Paranasal Sinuses. The lymphatics of the nasal cavity are separated into the olfactory group and the respiratory group. According to Rouviére,[10] they do not communicate with each other. There is a connection between the lymphatic network of the olfactory region and the subarachnoid spaces, which allows some absorption of cerebrospinal fluid (CSF) into the lymphatic system. The lymphatics of the olfactory region of the nasal cavity run posteriorly to terminate in lymph nodes alongside the jugular vein at the skull base in the lateral pharyngeal space. The lymphatics of the respiratory nasal cavity terminate in the lateral retropharyngeal nodes or the level II nodes. The capillary lymphatic plexus of the nasal mucosa is probably not very profuse, judged by the relatively low incidence of metastatic nodes.

The mucosa of the paranasal sinuses has either no or very sparse capillary lymphatics.

Pathology

Benign Tumors

Inflammatory polyps, giant cell reparative granulomas, benign odontogenic tumors, and necrotizing sialometaplasia may appear in this area. Inverted papilloma is a benign, aggressive neoplasm that is associated with carcinoma in 5% to 15% of cases.[307]

Malignant Tumors

Nasal Vestibule. Almost all malignant tumors are SCCs; basal cell carcinoma and adnexal carcinomas are also reported.

Nasal Cavity and Paranasal Sinuses. SCC or one of its variants is the most common neoplasm. Minor salivary gland tumors account for about 10% to 15% of neoplasms in this region. Lymphoma and melanoma account for approximately 5% and 1% of cases, respectively. Esthesioneuroblastoma is a neuroendocrine carcinoma that originates from the olfactory mucosa. Sinonasal undifferentiated carcinoma, a more aggressive neuroendocrine malignancy, is sometimes encountered.[308] Soft tissue and bone sarcomas may occur in the nasal cavity and paranasal sinuses, including chondrosarcoma, osteosarcoma, and Ewing sarcoma.[309]

Midline lethal granuloma is a nonkiller nasal T-cell lymphoma. Unchecked, the disease is fatal. Death results from extension to the CNS, hemorrhage, sepsis, or inanition. Treatment is usually RT; often combined with chemotherapy.[310]

Patterns of Spread

Nasal Vestibule

Primary. Lesions of the nasal vestibule invade the alar and septal cartilages and may extend to the nasal skin. The upper lip is frequently invaded. Posterior growth into the nasal cavity is frequent. Early cancers originating on the columella and anterior septum are often superficial lesions that ulcerate and produce a crust or scab and often present with septal perforation.

Lymphatics. Lymph node spread is usually to a solitary ipsilateral level IB node, but may be bilateral. The facial, preauricular, and submental nodes are at small risk. Wallace et al.[311] reported only 4 of 79 patients (5%) with clinically positive lymph nodes at diagnosis, but 9 patients (11%) later developed positive lymph nodes.

Nasal Cavity and Paranasal Sinuses

Nasal Cavity. The routes of spread are essentially the same for various histologies, with the exception of esthesioneuroblastoma and minor salivary gland tumors. The latter have a greater propensity for PNI.

Lesions arising in the olfactory region invade the ethmoids and the orbit, spread through the cribriform plate to the anterior cranial fossa, and spread between bone and dura. Eventually they penetrate dura and invade the frontal lobes. These lesions also tend to destroy the septum and may invade through nasal bone to the skin. Lesions arising on the lateral wall of the nasal cavity invade the maxillary sinus, ethmoids, and orbit.

Esthesioneuroblastomas may show submucosal spread and may grow along olfactory nerves and penetrate through an intact dura to the frontal lobes.

The nasopharynx and sphenoid sinus are secondarily invaded in advanced lesions. Tumor may follow nerves posteriorly and superiorly toward the sphenopalatine ganglion near the skull base or along V2.

Maxillary Sinus. All walls of the sinus may be penetrated by tumor; the pattern of spread and bone destruction depends on site of origin within the sinus. Lesions arising in the anterolateral infrastructure tend to invade through the lateral inferior wall or grow through dental sockets, causing loosening of the teeth or improper seating of a denture. Ulceration follows, with the development of an oral-antral fistula. Lesions arising on the medial infrastructure readily extend into the nasal cavity.

Posterior infrastructure lesions erode through the posterolateral wall and into the infratemporal fossa and extend superiorly to the skull base. Orbital extension occurs either through the roof of the maxillary sinus, through the ethmoids and lamina papyracea, or by way of the infratemporal fossa and then through the infraorbital fissure.

Tumors arising in the suprastructure of the antrum have two general patterns of development. One group extends laterally, invades the malar bone, and produces a mass below the lateral floor of the orbit that may ulcerate through to the skin. The orbit is invaded laterally and displaces the eye superomedially. The temporal fossa is often involved, as is the zygomatic bone in advanced lesions. Suprastructure cancers that extend medially invade the nasal cavity, ethmoid and frontal sinuses, lacrimal apparatus, and medial inferior orbit.

Ethmoid Sinuses. The lamina papyracea is the lateral wall of the middle and posterior ethmoid air cells; invasion through it into the medial orbit is common. The anterior ethmoid cells are covered laterally by the thin lacrimal bone and the frontal process of the maxilla. Thus, the ethmoid air cells extend anteriorly within a centimeter of the inner canthus. The medial surfaces of the ethmoid labyrinth are the middle and superior nasal conchae, which are formed by thin, convoluted bone; spread into the nasal cavity is common. More advanced lesions invade the maxillary antrum, nasopharynx, sphenoid sinus, and anterior cranial fossa.

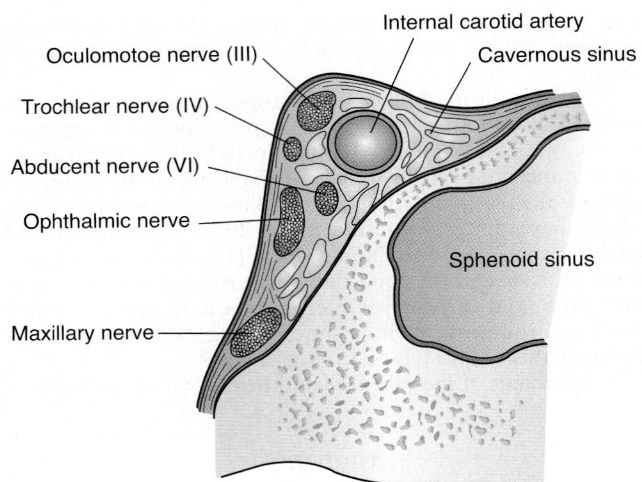

FIGURE 72.2 Coronal section of the cavernous sinus. (Adapted from Mendenhall WM, Million RR, Mancuso AA, Stringer SP. Nasopharynx. In: Million RR, Cassisi NJ (eds). *Management of Head and Neck Cancer: A Multidisciplinary Approach*, 2nd ed. Philadelphia: JB Lippincott Company, 1994: 606 [Figure 23-10]).

Sphenoid Sinus. The sphenoid sinus is closely related to the cranial nerves in the cavernous sinus: III, IV, V1, V2, and VI (Fig. 72.2). Cranial nerve palsies and headache are frequently the first clinical evidence of a sphenoid sinus tumor. Diagnosis is usually made, however, when tumor eventually breaks through into the nasopharynx or nasal cavity where it can be seen.

Inverted Papilloma. A report of 223 cases of inverted papillomas showed the lateral nasal wall was the most commonly involved site (68%), with ethmoid and maxillary sinus involvement also being common (57%), as was involvement of the septum (28%). However, ethmoid and maxillary sinus involvement without tumor of the lateral nasal wall occurred in 4%. Intracranial extension was usually associated with a carcinoma. Tumor occurred bilaterally when there was spread through the nasal septum; multicentric sites of origin were observed.[312]

Lymphatics. The incidence of lymphatic metastases at diagnosis is 10% to 15% for nasal cavity and ethmoid sinus tumors and probably lower for antral and sphenoid tumors. The risk of lymphatic metastases is related to extension of tumor outside the sinus to areas with capillary lymphatics. Maxillary sinus tumors that invade the oral cavity and involve the buccal mucosa, maxillary gingiva, or hard palate may spread to the level IB and level II nodes. Lesions that invade the nasal cavity or nasopharynx spread posteriorly to the parapharyngeal nodes and then to the level II nodes. Minor salivary gland tumors, melanoma, and sarcomas have an unknown rate of lymph node metastasis. The risk of cervical node involvement for esthesioneuroblastoma is approximately 20%.[306]

Clinical Picture

Nasal Vestibule

These lesions present with symptoms of a slow-growing mass with attendant crusting, and occasional minor bleeding. Pain, if it occurs, is usually modest, even with destruction of cartilage or involvement of the lip. Septal perforation may occur.

Nasal Cavity and Paranasal Sinuses

Nasal Cavity. The earliest symptoms of nasal cavity neoplasms are a low-grade chronic infection with discharge, obstruction, and minor, intermittent bleeding. Subsequent symptoms depend on pattern of growth. Lesions arising in the olfactory region may cause unilateral or bilateral nasal expansion of the bridge of the nose; a mass may appear near the inner canthus and eventually ulcerate. Obstruction of the nasolacrimal system may be a presenting complaint. Extension through the cribriform plate or into the ethmoid sinuses is accompanied by frontal headache. Aberration of smell is rare. Invasion of the medial orbit produces proptosis and diplopia; a mass may be palpated in the orbit. Indirect examination of the nasopharynx may show early submucosal invasion through the posterior nares.

Maxillary Sinus. These cancers develop silently when they are confined to the sinus and produce symptoms after extension through the walls. If the tumor invades toward the oral cavity, the presenting symptoms include pain and loosening or loss of teeth. Palpation and observation of the face may show a mass. Posterior invasion of the orbit will produce proptosis, diplopia, and conjunctival edema. Invasion of V2 in the floor of the orbit may cause paresthesia. Nasal obstruction and bleeding are common complaints, along with "sinus pain" or "fullness" over the antrum. Trismus and headache are associated with invasion posteriorly into the pterygopalatine fossa, pterygoid muscles, infratemporal fossa, and skull base.

Cancers developing in the medial suprastructure of the antrum present with nasal symptoms of discharge or bleeding, mild infraorbital pain, infected lacrimal sac, and displacement of the eye superolaterally with proptosis, diplopia, and conjunctival edema.

Cancer developing in the lateral suprastructure produces a mass below the lateral canthus with associated pain. The eye may be deviated medially and upward when orbital invasion occurs. There is conjunctival edema narrowing of the palpebral opening, diplopia, and proptosis. Tumor may extend to the temporal fossa, producing a diffuse fullness.

Ethmoid Sinuses. Mild to moderate sinus pain referred to the frontonasal area is an early symptom. A painless mass may present near the inner canthus. Diplopia and proptosis develop with invasion of the medial orbit. Nasal discharge, epistaxis, and obstruction are frequent presenting complaints. Paresthesia may occur over the distribution of sensory nerves.

Early invasion of the nasal cavity may produce submucosal bulging into the superior or medial meatus. Invasion into the nasopharynx is usually submucosal and appears on the roof and lateral wall. Advanced lesions may obstruct the eustachian tube.

Staging

The AJCC staging system for the nasal cavity and paranasal sinuses is depicted in Table 72.21. Nasal vestibule tumors are staged according to the AJCC staging system for skin cancers.

Treatment

Selection of Treatment Modality

Nasal Vestibule. RT is usually the preferred treatment because of the deformity produced by excision.[311] Surgery alone is preferred for the occasional very small lesion, the removal of which will not produce cosmetic deformity or require reconstruction.

TABLE 72.21

2010 AMERICAN JOINT COMMITTEE ON CANCER STAGING SYSTEM FOR NASAL CAVITY AND PARANASAL SINUS CANCERS

MAXILLARY SINUS	
TX	Primary tumor cannot be assessed
T0	No evidence of primary tumor
Tis	Carcinoma *in situ*
T1	Tumor limited to the maxillary sinus mucosa with no erosion or destruction of bone
T2	Tumor causing bone erosion or destruction including extension into the hard palate and/or middle nasal meatus, except extension to posterior wall of maxillary sinus and pterygoid plates
T3	Tumor invades any of the following: bone of the posterior wall of maxillary sinus, subcutaneous tissues, floor or medial wall of orbit, pterygoid fossa, ethmoid sinuses
T4a	Tumor invades anterior orbital contents, skin of cheek, pterygoid plates, infratemporal fossa, cribriform plate, sphenoid or frontal sinuses
T4b	Tumor invades any of the following: orbital apex, dura, brain, middle cranial fossa, cranial nerves other than maxillary division of trigeminal nerve (V2), nasopharynx, or clivus
NASAL CAVITY AND ETHMOID SINUS	
TX	Primary tumor cannot be assessed
T0	No evidence of primary tumor
Tis	Carcinoma *in situ*
T1	Tumor restricted to any one subsite, with or without bony invasion
T2	Tumor invading two subsites in a single region or extending to involve an adjacent region within the nasoethmoidal complex, with or without bony invasion
T3	Tumor extends to invade the medial wall or floor of the orbit, maxillary sinus, palate, or cribriform plate
T4a	Tumor invades any of the following: anterior orbital contents, skin of nose or cheek, minimal extension to anterior cranial fossa, pterygoid plates, sphenoid or frontal sinuses
T4b	Tumor invades any of the following: orbital apex, dura, brain, middle cranial fossa, cranial nerves other than V2, nasopharynx, or clivus

From ref. 216, with permission.

A subset of patients best treated by surgery and adjuvant RT or chemoRT is those with invasion of the premaxilla.

Surgical Treatment. Excision of lesions in the nasal vestibule usually involves removal of cartilage as well as skin. Depending on the site of the lesion, the columella, the septum, or the alar cartilages will have to be removed, with a resulting cosmetic deformity that is difficult to reconstruct. If the alar cartilage has been sacrificed, either a composite graft consisting of skin and cartilage from the ear or a nasolabial flap can be used to repair the defect. If the entire external nose is resected, a prosthesis is used.

Irradiation Technique. EBRT, brachytherapy, or a combination of both may be used. EBRT is usually administered with a single anterior portal technique that uses a combination of photons and electrons; a wax bolus ensures a homogenous dose.

The dose ranges from 66 to 70 Gy at 2 Gy per fraction, once daily in a continuous course.

Interstitial brachytherapy of the nasal vestibule and nasal cavity is highly individualized and employs afterloaded ^{192}Ir needles. The implant is usually composed of two, three, or four planes of sources inserted perpendicularly through the skin surface of the external nose with crossing needles placed in the dorsum of the nose, floor of the nasal cavity, and upper lip. The dose varies depending on the size of the lesion.[311]

Inverted Papilloma. Inverted papilloma is treated initially by surgery. Depending on the procedure, the local recurrence rate may be fairly high, and subsequent excisions may be required. When the lesion begins to act aggressively with rapid recurrences and invasion of the sinuses, orbit, and anterior cranial fossa, it should be considered a low-grade cancer and treated by a more radical removal. RT is recommended for lesions that are incompletely resected, for multiple recurrences, and for those in whom carcinoma is found.[307]

Nasal Cavity. SCC and adenocarcinoma of the nasal cavity can be treated with surgery, RT, or both. Surgery is indicated for early lesions, in which good margins can be expected without cosmetic or functional loss. Combined surgery and adjuvant RT is preferred for more advanced lesions because local control is probably better than after single modality treatment, and a lower dose can be used compared with definitive RT, thus reducing the risk of damage to the visual apparatus.[313] Definitive RT is used for incompletely resectable tumors.

Surgical Treatment. Lateral rhinotomy provides the best access for resection of lesions of the nasal cavity. Generally, reconstruction is not necessary unless the entire cartilaginous septum has been removed, in which case there will be a saddle deformity of the nose. The lateral wall of the nose may be removed by this approach for resection of inverted papilloma and other localized neoplasms. More advanced lesions require removal of involved sinuses and orbit. A craniofacial procedure may be required.

Irradiation Technique. The EBRT technique emphasizes an anterior portal with one or two lateral portals. Contiguous structures such as the maxillary sinus, ethmoid sinus, medial orbit, nasopharynx, skull base, and sphenoid sinus are generally included in the initial treatment volume as required. The treatment volume is reduced after 50 Gy to include the original gross disease with a margin. IMRT may be employed if feasible.

Advanced lesions may require inclusion of an entire orbit; loss of vision usually occurs, but an operation would require visual loss in any case. Treatment planning should protect the opposite eye and optic nerve.

Combined Treatment Policies

If combined treatment is planned, the authors prefer surgery first; RT or chemoRT is started 4 to 6 weeks afterward. The dose is usually 60 to 65 Gy for clear margins; patients with positive margins or for gross residual tumor after operation receive 74.4 at 1.2 Gy per twice daily fraction.

Management of Recurrence

Once the patient has had surgery or RT, it is difficult to determine the extent of recurrent disease because of changes from the previous therapy. The most common situation for salvage is a patient with RT or surgical failure who can be treated successfully by a craniofacial resection. Tumor extension to the sphenopalatine fossa with definite destruction of a pterygoid plate is a relative contraindication to craniofacial resection. Cranial nerve involvement, posterior invasion near the optic chiasm, and sphenoid sinus or cavernous sinus invasion are contraindications to resection. MRI can distinguish between exudate and gross tumor in a sinus. The anterior wall of the sphenoid sinus may be removed, but the sinus itself cannot be completely resected. Postoperative RT should be considered whether or not margins are positive.

Maxillary Sinus

Selection of Treatment Modality. Surgery gives the best results. Early infrastructure lesions may be cured by surgery alone, but, for most other cases, RT is given postoperatively even if margins are negative. ChemoRT should be considered for a positive margin. Extension of cancer to the skull base, nasopharynx, or sphenoid sinus contraindicates excision. The pterygoid process below the foramen rotundum may be removed along with the attached pterygoid muscles, but destruction of the sphenoid bone above this point is a contraindication to operation. Procedures to resect portions of the skull base are described for special situations.

Surgical Treatment. Surgery for maxillary sinus carcinoma depends on which walls are involved. If the floor of the orbit is free of disease, then the eye and orbital rim may be left undisturbed. If, however, there is involvement through the orbital floor, then a maxillectomy with resection of the floor with or without an orbital exenteration must be performed. If the posterior wall or the pterygoid plates are involved, they too must be included in the resection. A split-thickness skin graft is used to line the cavity, and a removable dental prosthesis is then used to fill the resulting deformity in the palate. An interim prosthesis is constructed prior to surgery so it can be placed at the time of operation and act as a stent. The permanent prosthesis is constructed about 6 months after the operation.

Irradiation Technique. RT treatment planning includes the entire maxilla, the adjacent nasal cavity, ethmoid sinus, nasopharynx, and pterygopalatine fossa. All or part of the orbit is included in patients with extension into or near the orbit. Target volume definition is aided by the use of treatment planning CT, combined with image-fusion MRI. The prescribed dose is 74.4 Gy at 1.2 Gy per fraction twice daily for RT alone. The dose for preoperative RT varies from 50 to 60 Gy, and the dose for postoperative RT varies from 60 to 74.4 Gy.

Ethmoid Sinus

Selection of Treatment Modality. Ethmoid sinus lesions are usually extensive when first diagnosed. If resection is feasible, surgery is followed by postoperative RT, even if the margins are clear, and chemoRT should be considered for a positive margin. Unresectable tumors are treated with chemoRT.

Surgical Treatment. Localized lesions require resection of the ethmoids with or without the ipsilateral maxilla and/or orbit. Extensive lesions require a craniofacial procedure. Endonasal endoscopic resection of selected malignant tumors involving the nasal cavity, ethmoid sinuses, and anterior skull base is being performed with increasing frequency. Limited published results regarding the treatment outcomes that have been achieved with this minimally invasive surgical approach, which circumvents the need for craniotomy, are promising.

Irradiation Technique. RT treatment is entirely by EBRT, emphasizing treatment through an anterior field combined with one or two lateral fields. This field arrangement, weighted 2:1 or 3:1 in favor of the anterior field, provides adequate treatment of the tumor volume while avoiding excessive RT to the contralateral eye and optic nerve. Wedges are added to achieve a satisfactory dose distribution. Electrons should not be used for the anterior portal. IMRT should be considered if a more conformal dose distribution can be achieved.

Management of Recurrence. Recurrent disease is heralded by recurrent pain and cranial nerve palsies. Localized recurrence after surgery only may be managed by chemoRT or craniofacial resection and postoperative RT or chemoRT. RT failures may be suitable for maxillectomy or craniofacial resection.

Sphenoid Sinus

The treatment is with RT, and the technique is similar to that used for advanced NPC.

Results of Treatment

Nasal Vestibule

Goepfert et al.[314] reviewed the M. D. Anderson Cancer Center experience of 26 patients with nasal vestibule SCCs. The absolute 5-year survival was 78%. Ten patients were treated initially by surgery; one developed a local recurrence that was salvaged by RT. Sixteen patients were treated by RT; three developed local recurrence and two were salvaged by an operation.

Wallace et al.[311] reviewed 71 patients treated by RT at the University of Florida for SCC of the nasal vestibule (Table 72.22). The 5-year local control and cause-specific survival rates were: T1–T2, 95% and 95% (N = 43); T4, 71% (N = 28); and overall, 86% and 91% (N = 71), respectively.[311] Eight additional patients with unfavorable T4 cancers were treated with resection and adjuvant RT. All eight patients treated with surgery and RT were locally controlled; three of eight patients experienced severe complications.

Nasal Cavity and Ethmoid Sinus

Inverted Papilloma. Weissler et al.[312] reported 233 cases of inverting papilloma seen over a 35-year period. One hundred thirty-four patients had at least 1 year of follow-up. The risk of recurrence was 71% in patients who had an intranasal procedure and 56% for those having a Caldwell-Luc approach. Patients having a lateral rhinotomy had the lowest incidence of recurrence (29%).

Weissler et al.[312] also reported six patients who received RT for benign inverting papilloma and nine for inverting papilloma associated with malignant disease. Twelve of the 15 patients had a complete response to RT and were free of disease for long periods of follow-up. Gomez et al.[307] reported ten patients with advanced and/or recurrent inverting papillomas who were treated with definitive RT. Local recurrence developed in four patients (40%) at 1.5, 6.5, 12, and 13 years after treatment. Six patients remained continuously disease-free at 7, 8.5, 8.5, 9, 9, and 20.5 years after RT.

TABLE 72.22

FIVE-YEAR OUTCOMES OF SQUAMOUS CELL CARCINOMA OF THE NASAL VESTIBULE AFTER DEFINITIVE RADIOTHERAPY AT THE UNIVERSITY OF FLORIDA (71 PATIENTS)

T Stage	No. of Patients	Local Control %	Cause-Specific Survival %
T1-T2	43	95	95
T4	28	71	No Data
Overall	71	86	91

Data from ref. 311.

Carcinoma. Mendenhall et al.[313] reviewed 109 patients treated at the University of Florida for carcinomas of the nasal cavity (69 patients), ethmoid sinus (33 patients), sphenoid sinus (6 patients), and frontal sinus (1 patient). Fifty-six patients were treated with definitive RT, 45 with surgery and postoperative RT, and 8 with preoperative RT and surgery. The 5-year local control rates were: T1–T3, 82%; T4, 50%; and overall 63%. Local control at 5 years was 43% after definitive RT and 84% after surgery and adjuvant RT ($P < .0001$). Multivariate analysis revealed that both overall stage and treatment group (definitive RT vs. surgery and adjuvant RT) impacted this end point. Cause-specific survival rates at 5 years were stages I–III, 81%; stage IV, 54%; and overall, 62%. Multivariate analysis of cause-specific survival revealed that T stage, N stage, and treatment group significantly impacted this end point. Thirty-one (20%) of 109 patients sustained severe complications: 17 (16%) of 56 patients had complications after definitive RT and 14 (25%) of 53 patients after surgery and adjuvant RT.

Esthesioneuroblastoma. Elkon et al.[315] reviewed the literature on esthesioneuroblastoma and compiled the results of 78 cases. They concluded that either RT or surgery was sufficient treatment for early-stage disease, but combined treatment might be advantageous for late-stage presentations. The 5-year absolute survival rate was 75% for lesions confined to the nasal cavity, 60% for those involving the nasal cavity and paranasal sinuses, and 41% for tumors extending beyond the nasal cavity and paranasal sinuses.

Monroe et al.[306] reported on 22 patients treated with curative intent at the University of Florida and observed the following 5-year outcomes: local control, 59%; cause-specific survival, 54%, and survival, 48%. The 5-year cause-specific survival rate was lower after definitive RT (17%) compared with craniofacial resection and postoperative RT (56%). Cervical metastases occurred in 6 of 22 patients (27%). Recurrence in the neck was observed in 4 of 9, initially N0 patients, who did not receive elective neck RT compared with none of 11 patients who were electively treated ($P = .02$).

In the University of Virginia experience (n = 50) using surgery and RT only for Kadish A and B tumors, and adding chemotherapy for Kadish C and D tumors, disease-free survival was 82.6% at 15 years. Most relapses were locoregional.[316]

Maxillary Sinus

Waldron et al.[317] reported on 110 patients treated with curative intent at the Princess Margaret Hospital with definitive RT (83 patients) or surgery and adjuvant RT (27 patients). The 5-year rates of local control and cause-specific survival were 42% and 43%, respectively. Sixty-three patients developed a local recurrence and 25 of 63 underwent salvage surgery with a subsequent 5-year cause-specific survival of 31%.

Complications of Treatment

Surgery

Complications of maxillectomy include failure of the split-thickness skin graft to heal, trismus, CSF leak, and hemorrhage. Complications of ethmoid sinus surgery include hemorrhage, meningitis, CSF leak, cellulitis and pansinusitis, brain abscess, and stroke. Complications of craniofacial resection include meningitis, subdural abscess, CSF leak, diplopia, and hemorrhage.

Radiation Therapy

The most frequent and significant complications of RT involve the eye.[313,318,319] When only a portion of the ipsilateral eye is irradiated (medial third), it is possible to preserve vision in the majority of patients. When there is extensive disease in the orbit, however, the entire eye is irradiated to a high dose with almost certain loss of vision; however, these same patients would require orbital exenteration if treated by surgery. The risk for bilateral blindness can be reduced by use of CT and MRI scans for improved treatment planning and knowledge of the tolerance of the optic nerve.

A few patients will experience a transient CNS syndrome that includes vertigo, headaches, decreased cerebration, and lethargy. This syndrome usually appears 2 to 3 months after completion of treatment, but may occur as late as 12 to 15 months. The early-appearing CNS syndromes usually last 1 to 2 months; the late-appearing syndromes last 6 to 12 months before slowly resolving. Aseptic meningitis, chronic sinusitis, or serous otitis media can occur. High-dose RT of the nasal cavity can cause narrowing and synechiae of the nasal cavity. Douching with salt water and daily self-dilations with petrolatum-coated cotton swabs will reduce the problem. Septal perforations occur when tumor has destroyed part of the septum; these do not usually require treatment. Destruction of the nasal bone and septum by tumor may result in cosmetic deformity. Maxillary necrosis may develop, particularly if teeth are extracted.

PARAGANGLIOMAS

Paragangliomas are an uncommon group of neoplasms that may originate anywhere glomus bodies are found. The lesions are rare before the age of 20, there is a female predominance in some series, and the lesions may occur in multiple sites in about 10% to 20% of cases, especially in patients with familial history. Carotid body tumors are associated with conditions producing chronic hypoxia, such as high-altitude habitation.

Anatomy

The normal glomus bodies in the head and neck vary from 0.1 to 0.5 mm in diameter. Tumors in glomus bodies (i.e., paragangliomas) arise most often from the carotid and temporal bone glomus bodies, with rare reports of tumors arising in the orbit, nasopharynx, larynx, nasal cavity, paranasal sinuses, tongue, and jaw. The temporal bone glomus bodies are not found consistently in any location. At least half of the glomus bodies are found in the general region of the jugular fossa and are located in the adventitia of the superior bulb of the internal jugular vein. The remaining glomus bodies are distributed along the course of the nerve of Jacobson (a branch of cranial nerve X). Approximately 20% of all temporal bone glomus bodies lie in the tympanic canaliculus and approximately 10% in relation to the cochlear promontory. A few glomus bodies are located in the descending part of the facial canal. The carotid bodies are located adjacent to the bifurcation of the common carotid. Orbital bodies are in relation to the ciliary nerve, and vagal bodies are adjacent to the ganglion nodosum of the vagus nerve.

Pathology

Paragangliomas are histologically benign tumors resembling the parent tissue and consist of nests of epithelioid cells within stroma-containing, thin-walled blood vessels and nonmyelinated nerve fibers. Although the tumor is well circumscribed, a true capsule is not seen. The criterion of malignancy is based on the development of metastases rather than the histologic appearance.

Patterns of Spread

These lesions usually grow slowly; it is usual to have a history of symptoms for a few years and occasionally for 20 years or longer.

Carotid Body Tumors

Carotid body tumors are usually located at the common carotid bifurcation and, as they expand, tend to displace and encircle the internal and external carotid vessels. The tumor begins in the adventitia of the artery and initially derives its blood supply from the vaso vasorum. An accessory blood supply may come from branches of the vertebral artery and ascending cervical artery. The tumor is usually closely adherent to the wall of the carotid adjacent to the vascular pedicle, and there may be thinning of the arterial wall from pressure by the mass. Large masses extend toward the cervical spine, skull base, angle of the mandible, and the lateral pharyngeal space.

Temporal Bone Tumors

Glomus tympanicum lesions tend to be small when diagnosed because they produce symptoms early in their course. Tumor may involve the ossicles, tympanic membrane, mastoid, external auditory canal, semicircular canal, and the seventh, Jacobson's, and Arnold's nerves.

Glomus jugulare tumors invade the skull base, petrous apex, jugular vein, middle ear, and middle and posterior cranial fossae. Cranial nerves V to XII may be involved.

Lymphatics

Lymphatic metastases occur in about 5% of carotid body tumors but are very rare for temporal bone tumors. An upper neck mass may be an inferior extension of a jugular fossa or vagal tumor rather than a lymph node metastasis.

Distant Metastases

Distant metastases have been rarely reported for temporal bone tumors; carotid body tumors have a low risk for distant metastases, probably in the range of 5% or less.

Clinical Picture

Carotid Body Tumors

The most common presenting symptom is an asymptomatic, slow-growing mass in the upper neck near the carotid bifurcation. Large masses may encroach on the parapharyngeal space and produce dysphagia, pain, and cranial nerve palsies. Carotid sinus syndrome may occur because of the pressure of the mass.

On examination, the mass usually lies deep to the sternocleidomastoid muscle and is tethered to surrounding structures. Fixation occurs only in large tumors extending to the spine and skull base. A submucosal bulge may be seen in the tonsillar area. A bruit may be heard.

Temporal Bone Tumors

Because glomus bodies are distributed throughout the temporal bone, the initial symptoms and signs depend on the site of origin. Tumor arising in or near the middle ear presents with an insidious conductive hearing loss, pulsatile tinnitus, vertigo, and headache. Patients with lesions developing in or around the jugular fossa develop headache, often pulsatile in nature, referred to the orbit or temple. Cranial nerves V to XII and the sympathetic nerves become affected. Lesions developing in the facial canal present with facial nerve symptoms. Otorrhea and hemorrhage may occur when tumor extends into the external auditory canal.

A characteristic blue-red mass may be seen bulging the tympanic membrane. A mass may be appreciated in the upper neck between the mandible and mastoid. Paralysis of cranial nerves V to XII and sympathetic nerves may occur.

Differential Diagnosis

Carotid Body Tumors

The differential diagnosis includes enlarged lymph nodes, carotid artery aneurysm, branchial cleft cyst, benign tumors (e.g., lipoma), and direct extension of a lateral pharyngeal wall or pyriform sinus cancer into the soft tissues of the neck.

CT and/or MRI scan with contrast provides the diagnosis. A biopsy usually produces serious hemorrhage and is not recommended. Angiography is usually unnecessary unless resection is anticipated.

Temporal Bone Tumors

The differential diagnosis includes an internal carotid artery in the middle ear either as an aberrant vessel or as an aneurysm. These patients also present with hearing loss, pulsatile tinnitus, and a pulsatile mass behind the eardrum. A high jugular bulb may present as a vascular mass in the middle ear and mimic a glomus tumor. Other possibilities include ear canal polyp, NPC with extension to the temporal bone, acoustic neuroma, middle ear carcinoma, metastatic carcinoma, cholesteatoma, histiocytosis, chronic serous otitis, and mastoiditis.

Staging

There is no accepted staging system for paragangliomas.

Treatment

Selection of Treatment Modality

Temporal Bone Tumors. Excision is satisfactory for small lesions that can be removed without risk of operative death or damage to normal structures. Stereotactic radiosurgery is an option for early lesions, although long-term results are limited.

Early lesions of the tympanic cavity are managed successfully by excision without loss of hearing or vestibular function. The remainder of the lesions are managed best by RT, with a very high success rate and minimal morbidity with current techniques. Partial removal of the tumor prior to RT does not improve the results and only increases the overall morbidity. Local control after RT is defined as stable disease or partial regression with no evidence of growth.

Carotid Body Tumors. Small lesions (1–5 cm) may be successfully removed with little risk to the patient. However, if resection of the carotid vessels is anticipated or if a large lesion is fixed or unresectable because of size, RT is the preferred initial treatment. These lesions are identical histologically to temporal bone paragangliomas, and the response to RT is similar.

Surgical Treatment

Temporal Bone Tumors. Small glomus tympanicum lesions are approached through the eardrum or mastoid area and are removed. Hearing loss may occur from the operation, but if there is conductive hearing loss from the tumor, it may be correctable.

For the glomus jugulare tumors, surgery is reserved for RT failure, in which case a radical mastoidectomy or a subtotal temporal bone resection would be required. Some surgeons advocate a skull base approach.

Carotid Body Tumors. A standard neck incision is made in a skin crease at the level of the carotid bulb, and the carotid sheath and its contents are identified. The tumor is usually lying at the bifurcation of the internal and external carotid arteries, often displacing these vessels. Marked drops in blood pressure and bradycardia can be avoided by injecting the bulb area with lidocaine. Bleeding may be avoided by using the bipolar electrode before excising the mass. The mass is then removed, preserving the carotid arteries. Preoperative embolization of feeder vessels is frequently employed to minimize intraoperative blood loss.

Irradiation Technique

RT consists of 45 Gy in 25 fractions over 5 weeks. The dose is below the tolerance of the normal tissues included in the treatment volume. Patients are treated with CT-based treatment planning and either stereotactic RT or IMRT.

Acute RT sequelae are almost nonexistent. The patient will have temporary hair loss in the entrance and exit areas beginning about the third week. Mild nausea may occur. There are few late sequelae. The patient may develop otitis media, especially if tumor involves the middle ear.

Management of Recurrence

Patients have follow-up with annual CT or MRI scans. Recurrence after surgery usually is treated by RT. Recurrence after RT should be treated by operation if feasible; if surgery is not possible, reirradiation may be considered.

Results of Treatment

Woods et al.[320] observed a local control rate of 89% in 71 patients with temporal bone paragangliomas who were treated surgically and followed from 1 to 22 years. Green et al.[321] reported a local control rate of 89% after surgery for 18 patients who had a mean follow-up of 8 years.

Hinerman et al.[23] reported on 104 patients with 121 paragangliomas who were treated with RT (115 tumors) or radiosurgery (6 tumors) and followed for a median of 8.5 years. The 10-year actuarial local control and cause-specific survival rates were 94% and 95%, respectively.

Complications of Treatment

Surgery

The major risks during operation are hemorrhage and injury to the cranial nerves. Other complications include hemiparesis, spinal fluid leak, and hearing loss.

Irradiation

Complications include cholesteatoma and sequestrum of the mastoid and otitis media. Detectable damage to the hearing mechanism and vestibular apparatus is unlikely after 45 Gy in 25 fractions.[322]

MAJOR SALIVARY GLANDS

Tumors of the major salivary glands account for 3% to 4% of all head and neck neoplasms. The average age of patients is 55 years for malignant neoplasms, and about 40 years for benign tumors. Approximately 25% of parotid tumors and 50% of submandibular tumors are malignant.

Anatomy

The parotid gland is formed by the muscles, bones, vessels, and nerves that come in contact with the gland. The bulk of the parotid gland is superficial, extending superiorly to the zygomatic arch and anterior aspect of the external auditory canal. The anterior border is variable, but does not extend beyond the opening of the parotid duct into the oral cavity opposite the second molar. Inferiorly, the gland extends between the mastoid and the angle of the mandible. The gland lies in front of and below the external auditory canal. A deep lobe extends into the parapharyngeal area, where it is in relationship to the lateral process of C1, the styloid process, and the parapharyngeal space.

The parotid gland is encompassed by fascia that is sufficient to contain most parotid infections in addition to benign tumors and low-grade malignancies. However, the fascia between the parotid gland and the conchal and tragal cartilages is thin; this is a weak spot that tumor quickly traverses. The fascia separating the deep lobe from the parapharyngeal space (stylomandibular fascial membrane) may be sufficiently thin to allow tumor or infection easy access to the parapharyngeal space and pharynx.

The sensory nerve supply to the parotid area and part of the pinna is from the greater auricular nerve (C2–3). This nerve is severed in removal of the parotid gland with permanent loss of sensation. The facial nerve (VII) penetrates the parotid gland almost immediately on leaving the stylomastoid canal and forms an extensive anatomic network within the gland and gives off branches to the muscles of expression.

The parotid gland is richly supplied from several arteries that freely anastomose and create arteriovenous bleeding during parotidectomy. The external carotid, the internal maxillary and superficial temporal arteries, and the posterior facial vein lie deep to cranial nerve VII.

The superficial preauricular nodes lie outside the fascia of the parotid gland and immediately in front of the tragus. They drain the skin of the anterior ear, temple, and upper face, including the eye and nose. They are involved most frequently by metastatic skin cancer and lymphoma, but not usually from parotid neoplasms. The preauricular nodes empty into the external jugular chain nodes, or they may communicate with the internal jugular chain nodes.

There are two nodal groups within the parotid fascia. Within the substance of the parotid gland are numerous lymph follicles and four to ten small lymph nodes scattered along the posterior facial and external jugular veins. Thus, they may lie deep to cranial nerve VII. Outside the gland but within the fascia are subparotid nodes that lie in front of the tragus and between the inferior aspect of the parotid tail and the anterior border of the sternocleidomastoid muscle.

Pathology

Benign Tumors

Benign Mixed Tumors. Also called *pleomorphic adenoma*, these slow-growing neoplasms are surrounded by an imperfect pseudocapsule traversed by fingers of tumor. The age of appearance begins in the early 20s with a mean age of 40.

Papillary Cystadenoma Lymphomatosum. Also called Warthin tumor, it is encased by a thin but complete capsule, occurs predominantly in older men, is bilateral in approximately 10% of cases, and may be multiple on one or both sides.

Benign Lymphoepithelial Lesions. Benign lymphoepithelial lesions account for about 5% of benign lesions. The tumor may be bilateral and is more common in women.

Oncocytoma. Oncocytoma is a benign, slow-growing tumor found mostly in the older age group. The encapsulated tumor has a dark appearance similar to melanoma.

Basal Cell Adenoma. The basal cell adenoma is an uncommon benign lesion, usually appearing in older people. It is cured by simple excision. Basal cell adenoma must be distinguished from basal cell carcinoma of the skin metastatic to parotid lymph nodes.

Malignant Tumors

Low-Grade Malignancy. Acinic cell carcinoma. Acinic cell carcinomas typically are indolent low-grade neoplasms appearing in all age groups and are most common in women. Metastases occur in a small percentage of cases and cannot be predicted by the histologic picture.

Mucoepidermoid carcinoma, low grade. Most mucoepidermoid carcinomas are indolent lesions readily cured by adequate excision. They may appear in any age group and grow slowly; there is little or no capsule. They are usually well circumscribed, but they may widely infiltrate the normal gland or become fixed to skin.

High-Grade Malignancy. Mucoepidermoid carcinoma, high grade. High-grade mucoepidermoid carcinomas behave aggressively, widely infiltrating the salivary gland and producing lymph node and distant metastases. They may be difficult to distinguish from SCC.

Adenocarcinoma; poorly differentiated carcinoma; anaplastic carcinoma; SCC. These histologies tend to appear late in life and have an aggressive behavior. True SCC arising from the salivary gland occurs rarely. Almost all of the so-called SCCs of the parotid are metastatic from skin cancer, especially from the temple area.[323]

Malignant mixed tumor. A small percentage of benign mixed tumors may develop into frank malignancy (carcinoma expleomorphic adenoma).

Adenoid cystic carcinoma. This is uncommon in the major salivary glands. Its growth rate is variable. Metastases to regional lymph nodes and distant sites occur; PNI is characteristic; and recurrences may appear many years after initial treatment.

Lymphoepithelioma (malignant lymphoepithelial lesion, "eskimoma"). Lymphoepithelioma occurs rarely in the parotid and submandibular gland. The histologic picture is that of lymphoepithelioma with varying degrees of nonmalignant lymphoid stroma.

Patterns of Spread

Benign Mixed Tumors

Benign mixed tumors of the parotid gland grow by expansion and local infiltration. Most tumors begin in the superficial lobe. Because of their slow growth, they rarely cause cranial nerve VII palsy, although the nerve may be stretched by large masses. When incompletely excised, multiple tumor nodules develop within the tumor bed. Skin invasion may occur in recurrent lesions; bone invasion does not occur, but a mass may cause pressure defects of adjacent bone.

Malignant Tumors

Malignant neoplasms infiltrate the parotid gland, invade cranial nerve VII and the auriculotemporal nerve, and spread along nerve sheaths. Tumor may invade the adjacent skin, muscles, and bone. Deep lobe lesions invade the parapharyngeal space, infratemporal fossa, and skull base and compromise additional cranial nerves.

Malignant tumors of the submandibular gland invade the gland, fix the tumor to the adjacent mandible, and invade the mylohyoid muscle and eventually the tongue, hypoglossal nerve, and oral cavity or oropharynx. Skin invasion occurs in advanced cases.

Sublingual gland neoplasms usually present as a submucosal mass in the floor of the mouth. The advanced lesions show an ulcerated mass in the floor of the mouth with extension to the tongue, mandible, and submental soft tissues.

Lymphatic Spread

Lymph node metastases may occur from all of the malignant neoplasms. Approximately 20% to 25% of patients with malignant tumors will have clinically positive or occult metastases in lymph nodes at the time of diagnosis. Low-grade mucoepidermoid carcinoma and acinic cell adenocarcinoma have a low rate of lymph node metastasis. There is little difference in the rate of lymph node metastasis among the various high-grade lesions. The risk for lymph node metastasis increases with recurrent disease and increased size of the primary lesion.

Clinical Picture

Parotid Gland

The majority of patients with either benign or malignant parotid tumors present with a mass. Mild, intermittent pain is occasionally present, but does not distinguish between benign and malignant tumors. Facial nerve palsy is an infrequent presenting complaint and indicates malignancy. Deep lobe tumors may produce dysphagia. The mobility of the mass depends on its size and location. Fixation or reduced mobility may occur in both benign and malignant neoplasms. Tumors presenting in the deep lobe may cause bulging of the palate and tonsil. Advanced malignant lesions may rarely affect cranial nerves IX to XII and the sympathetic chain if the parapharyngeal space is invaded. The mandibular branch of cranial nerve V may be involved when tumor tracks along the auriculotemporal nerve to the skull base; pain is an associated finding.

Submandibular Gland

Both benign and malignant neoplasms present as a mass usually associated with mild pain. Nerve palsy is rarely present. The skin may be infiltrated in advanced lesions. The tumor mass usually is partially fixed to the mandible unless it is quite small. Loss of mobility occurs with both benign and malignant lesions.

Sublingual Gland

Sublingual gland lesions are clinically similar to floor of the mouth SCCs. They produce a mass, submucosal at first, that may be felt by the tongue. There is mild discomfort, if any, in the early stages.

Differential Diagnosis

Parotid Gland

Gallia and Johnson[324] reviewed 140 patients who eventually underwent parotidectomy for diagnosis. Only 11% had malignant masses; the remainder had benign neoplasms (62%) or nonneoplastic conditions (27%). Conditions that may be confused with a parotid tumor include: (1) metastatic cancer, lymphoma, or leukemia involving parotid-area lymph nodes; (2) fatty replacement, tail of parotid; (3) chronic parotitis; (4) Boeck's sarcoid; (5) stone in duct; (6) cysts (branchial cleft, dermoid); (7) hypertrophy associated with diabetes; (8) hypertrophy of masseter muscle; (9) mandibular neoplasms; (10) prominent transverse process of C1; (11) penetrating foreign bodies; (12) hemangiomas/lymphangioma; and (13) lipoma.

Submandibular Gland

The differential diagnosis of a submandibular mass includes inflammatory disease, SCC metastatic to a lymph node, and a primary neoplasm of the submandibular gland.

Gallia and Johnson[324] reviewed 110 submandibular lesions in patients who underwent biopsy. Ninety-three lesions (85%) were nonneoplastic, usually inflamed glands, and nine lesions (8%) were benign tumors. Eight patients (7%) had malignant lesions, of which three lesions were lymphoma, three were metastatic carcinoma, and two were primary submandibular gland carcinoma.

Biopsy Technique

Parotid Gland. The biopsy and definitive surgical treatment are often the same for parotid masses. Lesions lying in the superficial lobe are biopsied best by performing a superficial parotidectomy. Lesions involving both the superficial and deep lobes or just the deep lobes are "biopsied" by total parotidectomy. Incisional and excisional biopsy may contaminate the tumor bed, increasing the risk of tumor recurrence and facial nerve damage as well as increasing the extent of the definitive surgical procedure by necessitating wide removal of the biopsy site.

FNA cytology can be performed for diagnosis. A negative finding on FNA does not necessarily mean that there is no tumor, so surgical decisions often rely heavily on clinical and radiographic findings. FNA can be used in the inoperable or recurrent lesions when RT is the initial treatment.

Submandibular Gland. FNA is helpful when positive for tumor, but may delay diagnosis when falsely negative. When needle biopsy is negative, but history, physical examination, and radiographic studies suggest neoplasm, and a careful search of the head and neck area fails to reveal a primary mucosal lesion, the submandibular triangle is dissected as the biopsy procedure.

Staging

The AJCC staging system is depicted in Table 72.23.

Treatment

Selection of Treatment Modality

Parotid Gland. The initial management of resectable superficial lobe parotid masses is *en bloc* superficial lobectomy. The tumor usually can be dissected free of the facial nerve. If the tumor involves the deep portion of the gland, the nerve is

TABLE 72.23

2010 AMERICAN JOINT COMMITTEE ON CANCER STAGING FOR MAJOR SALIVARY GLAND PRIMARY TUMORS (T)

TX	Primary tumor cannot be assessed
T0	No evidence of primary tumor
T1	Tumor 2 cm or less in greatest dimension without extraparenchymal extension[a]
T2	Tumor more than 2 cm but not more than 4 cm in greatest dimension without extraparenchymal extension[a]
T3	Tumor more than 4 cm and/or tumor having extra parenchymal extension[a]
T4a	Tumor invades skin, mandible, ear canal, and/or facial nerve
T4b	Tumor invades skull base and/or pterygoid plates and/or encases carotid artery

[a]Extraparenchymal extension is clinical or macroscopic evidence of invasion of soft tissues. Microscopic evidence alone does not constitute extraparenchymal extension for classification purposes.
From ref. 216, with permission.

retracted and the deep portion excised (i.e., total parotidectomy). Skin, bone, and muscle may also be resected as needed.

Low-grade malignant neoplasms are usually managed by operation only. RT is given postoperatively for nearly all high-grade lesions. RT is advised for low-grade malignant lesions that are recurrent and those with close or positive margins on the facial nerve. Postoperative RT is advised for selected benign mixed tumors when there is microscopic residual disease after operation and for nearly all patients after surgery or recurrent disease. RT alone is unlikely to control gross disease; if possible, resection of any gross residual benign mixed tumor should be performed prior to RT. Inoperable malignancies are treated by RT with occasional success. Data are limited with regard to the use of chemoRT.

Submandibular Gland. If frozen section diagnosis shows a malignant lesion and there is no involvement of nerves, mandible, or soft tissues, submandibular triangle dissection is performed and postoperative RT is given to the submandibular bed and ipsilateral neck. If there is PNI, bone invasion, a clinically positive node, or extension to contiguous soft tissues, resection is enlarged to encompass the necessary areas. Postoperative RT is added in nearly all cases.

Surgical Treatment

Superficial Parotidectomy. The incision is made in the preauricular crease and then curves under the earlobe posteriorly, and extends into the neck. The facial nerve is identified and the dissection is carried out between the mass and the facial nerve. Ideally, a 1-cm circumferential cuff of "normal" parotid tissue should be resected along with the tumor. However, close margins of less than 1 mm are frequently encountered as most parotid gland tumors lay close to branches of the facial nerve. In such cases, completely encapsulated tumors can frequently be resected with confidence. On the other hand, facial nerve sacrifice must be considered if the nerve branch courses directly through the tumor or when there is gross extracapsular extension into the parotid gland. The adequacy of resection is determined by frozen sections.

Total Parotidectomy. A superficial parotidectomy is performed, the nerve is dissected free from the underlying deep lobe, and the deep lobe and tumor are removed. Occasionally, the mandible must be divided to gain access to the retromandibular portion of the deep lobe. A partial mandibulectomy is required when the mandible is invaded by tumor.

The intraparotid nodes are removed with the primary lesion. If the nodes are positive, a neck dissection is added. Neck dissection is always included for clinically positive nodes. Elective neck dissection is not done for low-grade lesions.

A radical parotidectomy implies removal of the entire parotid, the facial nerve, and other involved tissues such as skin, bone, or muscle. Part or all of the seventh nerve must be sacrificed, and an immediate autologous nerve graft may be done. If frozen section examination of the facial nerve is positive at the stylomastoid foramen, mastoidectomy may be required to complete the resection. Postoperative RT is delayed for 6 weeks, and the chance of successful function is reported to be good.[325]

Radiation Therapy

The minimum treatment volume for parotid lesions includes the parotid bed and upper neck nodes. PNI indicates enlargement of the portals to cover the nerve pathways. The entire ipsilateral neck is included for high-grade lesions or for clinically positive nodes in the neck dissection specimen. The tumor dose to the primary area is 60 to 65 Gy over 6 to 7 weeks if there is no gross residual disease. Higher doses employing altered fractionation are used for patients with microscopically positive margins or gross disease.

Submandibular space EBRT portals are tailored to the extent of disease found in the surgical dissection. The entire ipsilateral neck is included. The postoperative dose is 65 to 70 Gy because the rate of recurrence, even with combined treatment, is substantial. Neutron therapy has been used in the management of unresectable salivary gland cancers.[326]

Chemotherapy for Salivary Gland Cancers

There is no established role for chemotherapy as part of the definitive treatment of salivary gland cancers. Historically, chemotherapy has been primarily used for patients with incurable disease or on prospective clinical trials. The safety and dosing of concurrent chemotherapy and RT has been established for this body region from the experience in patients with upper aerodigestive tract SCCs and, as such, this approach is sometimes applied to patients with unresectable disease or in the poor risk adjuvant setting. Available efficacy data for such an approach in this setting are limited.[327,328]

Results of Treatment

Parotid Gland

Benign Mixed Tumors. Enucleation or excision with a narrow rim of normal tissue will result eventually in a local recurrence rate of approximately 20% after 10 to 15 years of follow-up. Superficial parotidectomy will result in a recurrence rate of approximately 5%.[329]

The surgical success rate for recurrent lesions depends on the number of previous operations and the size and extent of recurrence. It may be necessary to sacrifice one or several branches of cranial nerve VII and to repair the defect with a nerve graft. Postoperative RT of 66 to 70 Gy is added in selected cases in which there are close margins or microscopic residual disease, or in cases in which a subsequent recurrence would be almost impossible to manage surgically or would result in loss of the facial nerve.[330] Death because of benign mixed tumors is unlikely.

Malignant Tumors. The likelihood of cure after surgery alone for low-grade tumors is high, and adjuvant RT is usually unnecessary. The local recurrence rate for operation alone is approximately 50% to 60% for high-grade tumors.[331,332]

Garden et al.[333] reported 166 patients treated with surgery and postoperative RT for parotid malignancies at the M. D. Anderson Hospital between 1965 and 1989. Forty patients (24%) developed a recurrent disease that was local in 9% and regional in 6%. Histologic type did not significantly influence the likelihood of local control (P = .36). Twenty-five patients (15%) developed distant metastases with disease control above the clavicles. The 10- and 15-year survival rates were 60% and 52%, respectively.

Submandibular Gland

Byers et al.[334] reported the results of treatment for 22 malignant tumors of the submandibular gland with no prior therapy. Treatment was resection followed selectively by postoperative RT. The local control rate was 64% and the survival rate was 50%.

Spiro[329] reported the results of surgery for 129 malignant submandibular gland carcinomas seen between 1939 and 1973. All patients had a minimum of 10 years of follow-up. Adenoid cystic carcinoma occurred in 35%, mucoepidermoid carcinoma in 29%, and malignant mixed tumor in 19%. Cervical lymph nodes were malignant in 28%. The locoregional control rate was 40% and the cause-specific cure rate was 31% at 5 years and 22% at 10 years.

Benign tumors of the submandibular gland were resected in 106 patients; only 2 patients developed a local recurrence.[329]

Chemotherapy Results

The heterogeneity and relative rarity of malignant salivary gland tumors have complicated the evaluation of systemic therapies. Prospective clinical trials are infrequent; different histologies are often combined, as are the results for major and minor salivary gland tumors. Over the past 2 decades, fewer than 500 patients with adenoid cystic cancer have been the subject of studies evaluating drug therapy.[335] Drugs like doxorubicin and 5-fluorouracil with reported activity have this claim largely based on retrospective case series, not prospective clinical trials.

Cisplatin, paclitaxel, vinorelbine, epirubicin, and mitoxantrone have major response rates in the 10% to 20% range in prospective studies in the recurrent or metastatic disease setting.[336–340] The potential importance of histology in trial design is well illustrated with the case of paclitaxel, in which 3 of 12 and 4 of 17 patients with mucoepidermoid and adenocarcinoma responded, respectively, yet none of 14 with adenoid cystic cancer responded.[341] Treatment with gemcitabine also did not yield any major response in patients with adenoid cystic carcinoma.[130] Cisplatin- or anthracycline-containing combinations (e.g., cyclophosphamide/doxorubicin/cisplatin; cisplatin/vinorelbine; cisplatin/5-fluorouracil) will increase this rate to 20% or 30% at the expense of greater toxicity.[335] The relative efficacies of single-agent versus combination chemotherapies have not been well studied. It should be emphasized that the natural history of some salivary gland cancers, of which the adenoid cystic subtype is perhaps the best example, can be quite indolent, making initial observation a prudent course.

Given the previous response rates, clinical trials are often an attractive option for patients, and there has been interest in the potential utility of newer targeted agents. Expression of potential molecular targets varies by pathologic subtype. For example, c-kit is commonly expressed in adenoid cystic cancer, but variably or not at all in other salivary cancer subtypes.[335] Although there have been reported responses to imatinib in case reports,[342,343] demonstrating objective responses in clinical trials with the agent has proved elusive, and so the drug remains investigation for this disease.[344,345] Data thus far for EGFr pathway and *Her-2* targeted agents are limited and not compelling.[346] Of note, the androgen receptor is commonly expressed in patients with salivary duct carcinoma, and there are reports under these circumstances of response to antiandrogen therapy.[347]

Complications of Treatment

Surgery

Facial paralysis is the most important complication associated with parotid surgery. Temporary facial nerve palsy may occur due to manipulation of the nerve during operation, and function will gradually return over a few months' time. Isolated persistent weakness of the lower lip may occur due to division of the platysma muscle. Incomplete eyelid closure requires protective measures such as artificial tears, Lacri-Lube (Allergan Inc., Irvine, CA), and eye patches to prevent corneal abrasion. A variety of surgical techniques can be employed to address facial nerve deficits if functional recovery is not expected, including nerve grafting, browlift, gold weight implantation into the upper eyelid, lower eyelid tightening, and facial suspensory procedures. Gustatory sweating (Frey syndrome) occurs in about 10% of patients after parotidectomy and rarely requires treatment. Persistent salivary fistula is rare.

Radiation Therapy

Xerostomia is avoided by techniques that spare the contralateral salivary tissues. There may be trismus due to fibrosis of the masseter and pterygoid muscles and the temporomandibular joint.

Otitis media may occur if the ear is irradiated. Localized hair loss may occur with some techniques. Osteoradionecrosis may rarely occur with high doses.

MINOR SALIVARY GLANDS

Tumors of minor salivary gland origin are uncommon, accounting for about 2% to 3% of all malignant neoplasms of the upper aerodigestive tract. They may appear at any age, but are uncommon before age 20 and rare under age 10. They tend to occur most often in the hard palate, nasal cavity, and paranasal sinuses, areas infrequently involved by SCCs. Thus, the site of origin is related more to the density of the minor salivary glands in a particular tissue than to an environmental factor.

Anatomy

Minor salivary glands are ubiquitous in mucosa of the upper aerodigestive tract with the exception of the gingivae and the anterior portion of the hard palate, which are free of minor salivary glands. They are distributed on the undersurface of the anterior and lateral oral tongue and the base of the tongue. Aberrant salivary tissue sometimes is seen in lymph nodes, in the body of the mandible just behind the third molar teeth, in the vestigial remnant of the nasopalatine canal in the anterior maxilla, middle ear, lower neck, sternoclavicular joint, thyroglossal duct, and other sites.

Pathology

Approximately half of minor salivary gland tumors are malignant. The histologic varieties of malignant tumors include adenoid cystic carcinoma, mucoepidermoid carcinoma, adenocarcinoma, malignant mixed, acinic cell, and oncocytic carcinomas.

About two-thirds of these tumors are adenoid cystic. Mucoepidermoid carcinomas and adenocarcinomas arise predominantly in the oral cavity.

The benign tumors are pleomorphic adenomas in the great majority of cases, with a few cases of intraductal papillomas, papillary cystadenomas, basal cell adenomas, and benign oncocytomas.

Patterns of Spread

There are no minor salivary glands in the anterior half of the hard palate, so tumors arise on the posterolateral hard palate and all of the soft palate. The site of origin for floor of mouth salivary gland tumors is either the sublingual gland or a minor salivary gland.

These tumors grow by local infiltration with eventual invasion of muscle, bone, and cartilage. PNI is a common feature, particularly for adenoid cystic carcinoma. Tumor may track both centrally and peripherally along nerves, but the central spread is the more common event. Extension along nerves eventually may traverse the skull base and surface intracranially, although this spread pattern may not become manifest for several years after the original treatment. Tumor growth along a nerve may be characterized by skip areas, so that a normal nerve segment is no assurance of free margins. Adenoid cystic carcinoma may grow along the Haversian systems of bone without showing bone destruction.

The risk of positive lymph nodes is related to the site of origin and the histology. Lymph node metastases are most likely from sites with a dense capillary lymphatic network, similar to the pattern for SCC. Adenoid cystic carcinoma, low-grade mucoepidermoid carcinoma, and acinic cell carcinoma are at low risk to spread to lymph nodes; about 20% of adenoid cystic carcinomas spread to lymph nodes, but this low incidence may be partly related to their frequent site of origin in the hard palate and paranasal sinuses, areas that infrequently produce lymph node metastases. The high-grade tumors carcinomas have a 30% incidence of lymph node involvement on admission, and eventually half will develop lymph node metastases.

Clinical Picture

The clinical picture depends on the site of origin. The signs and symptoms differ from those of SCC arising in the same area. Many of the lesions are indolent, and the history may go back many months or even years. Because lesions develop under the epithelium, the initial lesion is a submucosal mass that is often painless until ulceration develops. PNI is expressed as pain or paresthesias. Otherwise, the clinical picture resembles that for SCCs for a given size and site. Lymph node metastases occur at predictable sites. The clinically positive nodes are usually small and mobile, but neck dissection on such a patient may show numerous small, clinically undetectable positive nodes. The same staging systems applied to SCCs may be used.

Treatment

Selection of Treatment Modality

Benign mixed grade tumors are managed by operation; postoperative RT sometimes is advised in cases in which margins are close or positive.[348]

The low-grade carcinoma is treated initially by an operation when feasible, but RT is sometimes used as the primary treatment for inaccessible lesions or where the functional loss would be considerable. Postoperative RT is added for close margins or for those lesions that have recurred more than once. If the patient presents after excisional biopsy of a small lesion, RT is an alternative to re-excision, particularly if the procedure would produce significant cosmetic or functional loss.

The treatment of high-grade lesions varies immensely, depending on the site of origin, stage of disease, and willingness of the patient to accept a major cosmetic or functional change subsequent to an operation. Surgery and postoperative RT are preferred; RT alone is used for unresectable cancers. There are data that support the use of neutron therapy.[326]

Surgical Treatment

Benign tumors are removed by wide local excision that includes a cuff of normal tissue. Small low-grade lesions with a long history of slow growth may be treated with a wide local excision including a shell of normal tissue. Large low-grade lesions and high-grade lesions require a more radical resection. When PNI is present, it is not possible to remove all the nerves potentially involved, but the nerves that are involved should be sacrificed wherever it is reasonable to do so. As an alternative, postoperative RT may be used to cover the perineural routes of spread.

Irradiation Technique

The RT techniques and doses are similar to those for SCCs of the same anatomic site and similar tumor size, with the exception that nerve pathways must be covered for adenoid cystic carcinomas. Subclinical PNI for adenoid cystic carcinomas must be considered to be present even though not seen on the biopsy or surgical sections.

Results of Treatment

Spiro et al.[349] reported the Memorial Sloan-Kettering Cancer Center results for 434 malignant minor salivary gland tumors, of which 90% were treated surgically. The cause-specific 5-, 10-, and 15-year cure rates were 44%, 32%, and 21%, respectively; 51% of patients died of the original cancer. Patients with adenoid cystic carcinoma had the poorest prognosis, with about 20% surviving without recurrence. Those with adenocarcinoma had an intermediate outlook, about 35% surviving without recurrence, and mucoepidermoid carcinomas had the best control rate with about 70% long-term cures.

Cianchetti et al.[15] reported on 140 patients treated at the University of Florida for minor salivary gland carcinomas between 1966 and 2006. The 10-year local control rate was 66%; multivariate analysis revealed that treatment group and T stages significantly influenced this end point. Patients treated with RT alone had a lower local control rate compared with those treated with surgery and RT. The 10-year outcomes were distant metastasis-free survival, 67%; cause-specific survival, 56%; and overall survival, 45%.

Benign mixed tumors of minor salivary gland origin have a good prognosis. Spiro[329] reported on 81 benign tumors; 60 occurred on the palate and 13 on the lip or cheek. With a minimum follow-up of 10 years, the local recurrence rate was 6%.

Hodge et al.[330] reported on 17 patients treated with RT alone (2 patients) or combined with surgery (15 patients) for pleomorphic adenoma and followed for a median of 9.6 years. Local control was obtained in eight of ten patients with subclinical disease and three of seven patients irradiated for gross disease. The 10-year overall local control rate was 61%.

In a small randomized trial of inoperable primary or recurrent salivary gland cancers (both major and minor salivary gland cancers were allowed), neutron therapy ($n = 25$) improved locoregional control significantly ($P = .009$) but at the expense of more severe morbidity.[326]

Selected References

The full list of references for this chapter appears in the online version.

3. Erkal HS, Mendenhall WM, Amdur RJ, et al. Synchronous and metachronous squamous cell carcinomas of the head and neck mucosal sites. *J Clin Oncol* 2001;19:1358.
5. Gillison ML, Koch WM, Capone RB, et al. Evidence for a causal association between human papillomavirus and a subset of head and neck cancers. *J Natl Cancer Inst* 2000;92:709–720.
6. Mendenhall WM, Logan HL. Human papillomavirus and head and neck cancer. *Am J Clin Oncol* 2009;32:535–539.
10. Rouvière H. *Anatomy of the Human Lymphatic System*. Tobias MJ, trans-ed. Ann Arbor, MI: Edwards Brothers, 1938:44–56.
15. Cianchetti M, Mancuso AA, Amdur RJ, et al. Diagnostic evaluation of squamous cell carcinoma metastatic to cervical lymph nodes from an unknown head and neck primary site. *Laryngoscope* 2009;119:2348.
17. Lindberg RD. Distribution of cervical lymph node metastases from squamous cell carcinoma of the upper respiratory and digestive tracts. *Cancer* 1972;29:1446.
18. O'Sullivan B, Warde P, Grice B, et al. The benefits and pitfalls of ipsilateral radiotherapy in carcinoma of the tonsillar region. *Int J Radiat Oncol Biol Phys* 2001;51:332–343.
20. McLaughlin MP, Mendenhall WM, Mancuso AA, et al. Retropharyngeal adenopathy as a predictor of outcome in squamous cell carcinoma of the head and neck. *Head Neck* 1995;17:190–198.
21. Al-Othman MOF, Morris CG, Hinerman RW, et al. Distant metastases after definitive radiotherapy for squamous cell carcinoma of the head and neck. *Head Neck* 2003;25:629–633.
23. Hinerman RW, Amdur RJ, Morris CG, et al. Definitive radiotherapy in the management of paragangliomas arising in the head and neck: a 35-year experience. *Head Neck* 2008;30:1431–1438.
26. Trotti A, Fu KK, Pajak TF, et al. Long term outcomes of RTOG 90–03: a comparison of hyperfractionation and two variants of accelerated fractionation to standard fractionation radiotherapy for head and neck squamous cell carcinoma. [Abstr.] *Int J Radiat Oncol Biol Phys* 2005;63:S70–S71.
27. Mendenhall WM, Riggs CE, Vaysberg M, et al. Altered fractionation and adjuvant chemotherapy for head and neck squamous cell carcinoma. *Head Neck* 2010;32(7):939.
28. Mendenhall WM, Amdur RJ, Palta JR. Intensity-modulated radiotherapy in the standard management of head and neck cancer: promises and pitfalls. *J Clin Oncol* 2006;24:2618.
32. Yeung AR, Liauw SL, Amdur RJ, et al. Lymph node-positive head and neck cancer treated with definitive radiotherapy: can treatment response determine the extent of neck dissection? *Cancer* 2008;112:1076–1082.
33. Mendenhall WM, Million RR. Elective neck irradiation for squamous cell carcinoma of the head and neck: analysis of time-dose factors and causes of failure. *Int J Radiat Oncol Biol Phys* 1986;12:741–746.
34. Barkley HT Jr, Fletcher GH, Jesse RH, et al. Management of cervical lymph node metastases in squamous cell carcinoma of the tonsillar fossa, base of tongue, supraglottic larynx, and hypopharynx. *Am J Surg* 1972; 124:462–467.
36. Cooper JS, Pajak TF, Forastiere AA, et al. Postoperative concurrent radiotherapy and chemotherapy for high-risk squamous cell carcinoma of the head and neck. *N Engl J Med* 2004;350:1937–1944.
37. Bernier J, Domenge C, Ozsahin M, et al. Postoperative irradiation with or without concomitant chemotherapy for locally advanced head and neck cancer. *N Engl J Med* 2004;350:1945–1952.
38. Cooper JS, Pajak TF, Forastiere AA, et al. Long-term survival results of a phase III intergroup trial (RTOG 95–01) of surgery followed by radiotherapy vs. radiochemotherapy for resectable high risk squamous cell carcinoma of the head and neck. [Abstr.] *Int J Radiat Oncol Biol Phys* 2006; 66:S14–S15.
40. Liauw SL, Mancuso AA, Amdur RJ, et al. Postradiotherapy neck dissection for lymph node-positive head and neck cancer: the use of computed tomography to manage the neck. *J Clin Oncol* 2006;24:1421.
43. Ellis ER, Mendenhall WM, Rao PV, et al. Incision or excisional neck-node biopsy before definitive radiotherapy, alone or followed by neck dissection. *Head Neck* 1991;13:177–183.
48. Hong WK, Lippman SM, Itri LM, et al. Prevention of second primary tumors with isotretinoin in squamous-cell carcinoma of the head and neck. *N Engl J Med* 1990;323:795–801.
49. Khuri FR, Lee JJ, Lippman SM, et al. Randomized phase III trial of low-dose isotretinoin for prevention of second primary tumors in stage I and II head and neck cancer patients. *J Natl Cancer Inst* 2006;98:441–450.
50. Bolla M, Lefur R, Ton VJ, et al. Prevention of second primary tumours with etretinate in squamous cell carcinoma of the oral cavity and oropharynx. Results of a multicentric double-blind randomised study. *Eur J Cancer* 1994;30A:767–772.
135. Calais G, Alfonsi M, Bardet E, et al. Randomized trial of radiation therapy versus concomitant chemotherapy and radiation therapy for advanced-stage oropharynx carcinoma. *J Natl Cancer Inst* 1999;91: 2081–2086.
136. Forastiere AA, Goepfert H, Maor M, et al. Concurrent chemotherapy and radiotherapy for organ preservation in advanced laryngeal cancer. *N Engl J Med* 2003;349:2091–2098.
137. Pignon JP, Bourhis J, Domenge C, et al. Chemotherapy added to locoregional treatment for head and neck squamous-cell carcinoma: three meta-analyses of updated individual data. MACH-NC Collaborative Group. Meta-Analysis of Chemotherapy on Head and Neck Cancer. *Lancet* 2000; 355:949–955.
138. Bourhis J, Le Maitre A, Baujat B, et al. Individual patients' data meta-analyses in head and neck cancer. *Curr Opin Oncol* 2007;19:188–194.
140. Domenge C, Hill C, Lefebvre JL, et al. Randomized trial of neoadjuvant chemotherapy in oropharyngeal carcinoma. French Groupe d'Etude des Tumeurs de la Tete et du Cou (GETTEC). *Br J Cancer* 2000;83:1594–1598.
141. The Department of Veterans Affairs Laryngeal Cancer Study Group. Induction chemotherapy plus radiation compared with surgery plus radiation in patients with advanced laryngeal cancer. *N Engl J Med* 1991; 324:1685–1690.
142. Lefebvre J-L, Chevalier D, Luboinski B, et al. Larynx preservation in pyriform sinus cancer: preliminary results of a European Organization for Research and Treatment of Cancer phase III trial. EORTC Head and Neck Cancer Cooperative Group. *J Natl Cancer Inst* 1996;88:890–899.
147. Posner MR, Hershock DM, Blajman CR, et al. Cisplatin and fluorouracil alone or with docetaxel in head and neck cancer. *N Engl J Med* 2007;357: 1705–1715.
153. Bachaud JM, Cohen-Jonathan E, Alzieu C, et al. Combined postoperative radiotherapy and weekly cisplatin infusion for locally advanced head and neck carcinoma: final report of a randomized trial. *Int J Radiat Oncol Biol Phys* 1996;36:999–1004.
156. Rasch CRN, Salverda GJ, Schornagel JH, et al. Intra-arterial versus intravenous chemoradiation for advanced head and neck cancer, early results of a multi-institutional trial [abstract]. *Int J Radiat Oncol Biol Phys* 2006; 66:S1.
161. Bourhis J, Overgaard J, Audry H, et al. Hyperfractionated or accelerated radiotherapy in head and neck cancer: a meta-analysis. *Lancet* 2006;368: 843–854.
162. Brizel DM, Albers ME, Fisher SR, et al. Hyperfractionated irradiation with or without concurrent chemotherapy for locally advanced head and neck cancer. *N Engl J Med* 1998;338:1798–1804.
163. Jeremic B, Shibamoto Y, Milicic B, et al. Hyperfractionated radiation therapy with or without concurrent low-dose daily cisplatin in locally advanced squamous cell carcinoma of the head and neck: a prospective randomized trial. *J Clin Oncol* 2000;18:1458–1464.
164. Calais G, Alfonsi M, Bardet E, et al. Randomized trial of radiation therapy versus concomitant chemotherapy and radiation therapy for advanced-stage oropharynx carcinoma. *J Natl Cancer Inst* 1999;91:2081–2086.
165. Bonner JA, Harari PM, Giralt J, et al. Radiotherapy plus cetuximab for squamous-cell carcinoma of the head and neck. *N Engl J Med* 2006;354: 567–578.
170. Al-Sarraf M, LeBlanc M, Shanker Giri PG, et al. Chemoradiotherapy versus radiotherapy in patients with advanced nasopharyngeal cancer: phase III randomized Intergroup study 0099. *J Clin Oncol* 1998;16:1310–1317.
171. Lin JC, Jan JS, Hsu CY, et al. Phase III study of concurrent chemoradiotherapy versus radiotherapy alone for advanced nasopharyngeal carcinoma: positive effect on overall and progression-free survival. *J Clin Oncol* 2003;21:631–637.
172. Chan AT, Teo PM, Ngan RK, et al. Concurrent chemotherapy-radiotherapy compared with radiotherapy alone in locoregionally advanced nasopharyngeal carcinoma: progression-free survival analysis of a phase III randomized trial. *J Clin Oncol* 2002;20:2038–2044.
174. Wee J, Tan EH, Tai BC, et al. Randomized trial of radiotherapy versus concurrent chemoradiotherapy followed by adjuvant chemotherapy in patients with American Joint Committee on Cancer/International Union against cancer stage III and IV nasopharyngeal cancer of the endemic variety. *J Clin Oncol* 2005;23:6730–6738.
175. Lee AW, Lau WH, Tung SY, et al. Preliminary results of a randomized study on therapeutic gain by concurrent chemotherapy for regionally-advanced nasopharyngeal carcinoma: NPC-9901 Trial by the Hong Kong Nasopharyngeal Cancer Study Group. *J Clin Oncol* 2005;23:6966–6975.
178. Chua DT, Ma J, Sham JS, et al. Long-term survival after cisplatin-based induction chemotherapy and radiotherapy for nasopharyngeal carcinoma: a pooled data analysis of two phase III trials. *J Clin Oncol* 2005;23: 1118.
179. Baujat B, Audry H, Bourhis J, et al. Chemotherapy in locally advanced nasopharyngeal carcinoma: an individual patient data meta-analysis of eight randomized trials and 1753 patients. *Int J Radiat Oncol Biol Phys* 2006;64:47–56.
184. Pfister DG, Laurie SA, Weinstein GS, et al. American Society of Clinical Oncology Clinical Practice Guideline for the Use of Larynx-Preservation Strategies in the Treatment of Laryngeal Cancer. *J Clin Oncol* 2006;24: 3693–3704.

190. Lefebvre JL, Rolland F, Tesselaar M, et al. Phase 3 randomized trial on larynx preservation comparing sequential vs alternating chemotherapy and radiotherapy. *J Natl Cancer Inst* 2009;101:142–152.
191. Adelstein DJ, Lavertu P, Saxton JP, et al. Mature results of a phase III randomized trial comparing concurrent chemoradiotherapy with radiation therapy alone in patients with stage III and IV squamous cell carcinoma of the head and neck. *Cancer* 2000;88:876–883.
192. Licitra L, Grandi C, Guzzo M, et al. Primary chemotherapy in resectable oral cavity squamous cell cancer: a randomized controlled trial. *J Clin Oncol* 2003;21:327–333.
193. Laccourreye O, Veivers D, Hans S, et al. Chemotherapy alone with curative intent in patients with invasive squamous cell carcinoma of the pharyngolarynx classified as T1-T4N0M0 complete clinical responders. *Cancer* 2001;92:1504–1511.
203. Bernier J, Cooper JS, Pajak TF, et al. Defining risk levels in locally advanced head and neck cancers: a comparative analysis of concurrent postoperative radiation plus chemotherapy trials of the EORTC (#22931) and RTOG (# 9501). *Head Neck* 2005;27:843–850.
210. Brizel DM, Wasserman TH, Henke M, et al. Phase III randomized trial of amifostine as a radioprotector in head and neck cancer. *J Clin Oncol* 2000;18:3339–3345.
215. Brizel DM, Murphy BA, Rosenthal DI, et al. Phase II study of palifermin and concurrent chemoradiation in head and neck squamous cell carcinoma. *J Clin Oncol* 2008;26:2489–2496.
218. Byers RM, O'Brien J, Waxler J. The therapeutic and prognostic implications of nerve invasion in cancer of the lower lip. *Int J Radiat Oncol Biol Phys* 1978;4:215–217.
223. Wang CC, Biggs PJ. Technical and radiotherapeutic considerations of intra-oral cone electron beam radiation therapy for head and neck cancer. *Semin Radiat Oncol* 1992;2:171.
225. Pernot M, Hoffstetter S, Peiffert D, et al. Epidermoid carcinomas of the floor of mouth treated by exclusive irradiation: statistical study of a series of 207 cases. *Radiother Oncol* 1995;35:177–185.
226. Byers RM, Weber RS, Andrews T, et al. Frequency and therapeutic implications of "skip matastases" in the neck from squamous carcinoma of the oral tongue. *Head Neck* 1997;19:14–19.
227. Mendenhall WM, Van Cise WS, Bova FJ, et al. Analysis of time-dose factors in squamous cell carcinoma of the oral tongue and floor of mouth treated with radiation therapy alone. *Int J Radiat Oncol Biol Phys* 1981;7:1005–1011.
231. Pernot M, Malissard L, Hoffstetter S, et al. The study of tumoral, radiobiological, and general health factors that influence results and complications in a series of 448 oral tongue carcinomas treated exclusively by irradiation. *Int J Radiat Oncol Biol Phys* 1994;29:673–679.
232. Chang DT, Sandow PR, Morris CG, et al. Do pre-irradiation dental extractions reduce the risk of osteoradionecrosis of the mandible? *Head Neck* 2007;29:528–536.
234. Diaz EM Jr, Holsinger FC, Zuniga ER, et al. Squamous cell carcinoma of the buccal mucosa: one institution's experience with 119 previously untreated patients. *Head Neck* 2003;25:267.
235. Mendenhall WM, Morris CG, Amdur RJ, et al. Radiotherapy alone or combined with surgery for adenoid cystic carcinoma of the head and neck. *Head Neck* 2004;26:154.
238. Byers RM, Anderson B, Schwarz EA, et al. Treatment of squamous carcinoma of the retromolar trigone. *Am J Clin Oncol* 1984;7:647–652.
239. Cianchetti M, Sandow PS, Scarborough LD, et al. Radiation therapy for minor salivary gland carcinoma. *Laryngoscope* 2009;119:1334–1338.
241. Mendenhall WM, Morris CG, Amdur RJ, et al. Retromolar trigone squamous cell carcinoma treated with radiotherapy alone or combined with surgery. *Cancer* 2005;103:2320–2325.
243. Overholt SM, Eicher SA, Wolf P, et al. Prognostic factors affecting outcome in lower gingival carcinoma. *Laryngoscope* 1996;106:1335–1339.
249. Mendenhall WM, Morris CG, Amdur RJ, et al. Definitive radiotherapy for squamous cell carcinoma of the base of tongue. *Am J Clin Oncol* 2006;29:32.
251. Al-Othman MOF, Amdur RJ, Morris CG, et al. Does feeding tube placement predict for long-term swallowing disability after radiotherapy for head and neck cancer? *Head Neck* 2003;25:741.
252. Mendenhall WM, Morris CG, Amdur RJ, et al. Definitive radiotherapy for tonsillar squamous cell carcinoma. *Am J Clin Oncol* 2006;29:290–297.
253. Chera BS, Amdur R, Hinerman RW, et al. Definitive radiotherapy for squamous cell carcinoma of the soft palate. *Head Neck* 2008;30:1114–1119.
256. Chera BS, Amdur R, Morris CG, Kirwan JM, Mendenhall WM. T1N0 to T2N0 squamoud cell carcinoma of the glottic larynx treated with definitive radiotherapy. *Int J Radiat Oncol Biol Phys* 2010; 78(2):461.
259. Garcia-Serra A, Hinerman RW, Amdur RJ, et al. Radiotherapy for carcinoma in situ of the true vocal cords. *Head Neck* 2002;24:390–394.
260. Mendenhall WM, Werning JW, Hinerman RW, et al. Management of T1-T2 glottic carcinomas. *Cancer* 2004;100:1786–1792.
261. Mendenhall WM, Parsons JT, Stringer SP, Cassisi NJ, Million RR. Stage T3 squamous cell carcinoma of the glottic larynx: a comparison of laryngectomy and irradiation. *Int J Radiat Oncol Biol Phys* 1992;23:725–732.
264. Mendenhall WM, Morris CG, Stringer SP, et al. Voice rehabilitation after total laryngectomy and postoperative radiation therapy. *J Clin Oncol* 2002;20:2500.
265. Yamazaki H, Nishiyama K, Tanaka E, et al. Radiotherapy for early glottic carcinoma (T1N0M0): results of prospective randomized study of radiation fraction size and overall treatment time. *Int J Radiat Oncol Biol Phys* 2006;64:77.
267. Mendenhall WM, Morris CG, Amdur RJ, et al. Parameters that predict local control following definitive radiotherapy for squamous cell carcinoma of the head and neck. *Head Neck* 2003;25:535–542.
272. Foote RL, Olsen KD, Buskirk SJ, et al. Laryngectomy alone for T3 glottic cancer. *Head Neck* 1994;16:406–412.
273. Hinerman RW, Mendenhall WM, Morris CG, et al. T3 and T4 true vocal cord squamous carcinomas treated with external beam irradiation: a single institution's 35-year experience. *Am J Clin Oncol* 2007;30:181–185.
274. Pameijer FA, Mancuso AA, Mendenhall WM, et al. Can pretreatment computed tomography predict local control in T3 squamous cell carcinoma of the glottic larynx treated with definitive radiotherapy? *Int J Radiat Oncol Biol Phys* 1997;37:1011–1021.
283. Ambrosch P, Kron M, Steiner W. Carbon dioxide laser microsurgery for early supraglottic carcinoma. *Ann Otol Rhinol Laryngol* 1998;107:680–688.
288. Pameijer FA, Mancuso AA, Mendenhall WM, et al. Evaluation of pretreatment computed tomography as a predictor of local control in T1/T2 pyriform sinus carcinoma treated with definitive radiotherapy. *Head Neck* 1998;20:159–168.
289. Rabbani A, Amdur R, Mancuso A, et al. Definitive radiotherapy for T1–T2 squamous cell carcinomas of the pyriform sinus. *Int J Radiat Oncol Biol Phys* 2008;72:351–355.
290. Hull MC, Morris CG, Tannehill SP, et al. Definitive radiotherapy alone or combined with a planned neck dissection for squamous cell carcinoma of the pharyngeal wall. *Cancer* 2003;98:2224–2231.
293. Ho JH. An epidemiologic and clinical study of nasopharyngeal carcinoma. *Int J Radiat Oncol Biol Phys* 1978;4:182–198.
294. Fletcher GH, Million RR. Malignant tumors of the nasopharynx. *Am J Roentgenol Radium Ther Nucl Med* 1965;93:44–55.
297. Leung TW, Tung SY, Sze WK, et al. Salvage radiation therapy for locally recurrent nasopharyngeal carcinoma. *Int J Radiat Oncol Biol Phys* 2000;48:1331.
298. Mendenhall WM, Mendenhall CM, Malyapa RS, et al. Re-irradiation of head and neck carcinoma. *Am J Clin Oncol* 2008;31:393–398.
300. Leung TW, Tung SY, Sze WK, et al. Treatment results of 1070 patients with nasopharyngeal carcinoma: an analysis of survival and failure patterns. *Head Neck* 2005;27:555–565.
301. Chua DT, Sham JS, Kwong DL, et al. Volumetric analysis of tumor extent in nasopharyngeal carcinoma and correlation with treatment outcome. *Int J Radiat Oncol Biol Phys* 1997;39:711–719.
304. Bhandare N, Monroe AT, Morris CG, et al. Does altered fractionation influence risk of radiation-induced optic neuropathy? *Int J Radiat Oncol Biol Phys* 2005;62:1070–1077.
305. Monroe AT, Bhandare N, Morris CG, et al. Preventing radiation retinopathy with hyperfractionation. *Int J Radiat Oncol Biol Phys* 2005;61:856–864.
311. Wallace A, Morris CG, Kirwan J, et al. Radiotherapy for squamous cell carcinoma of the nasal vestibule. *Am J Clin Oncol* 2007;30:612.
322. Bhandare N, Antonelli PJ, Morris CG, et al. Ototoxicity after radiotherapy for head and neck tumors. *Int J Radiat Oncol Biol Phys* 2007;67:469–479.
323. Hinerman RW, Amdur RJ, Morris CG, et al. Cutaneous squamous cell carcinoma metastatic to parotid-area lymph nodes. *Laryngoscope* 2008;118:1989–1996.
333. Garden AS, El-Naggar AK, Morrison WH, et al. Postoperative radiotherapy for malignant tumors of the parotid gland. *Int J Radiat Oncol Biol Phys* 1997;37:79–85.
334. Byers RM, Jesse RH, Guillamondegui OM, et al. Malignant tumors of the submaxillary gland. *Am J Surg* 1973;126:458–463.
348. Mendenhall WM, Mendenhall CM, Werning JW, et al. Salivary gland pleomorphic adenoma. *Am J Clin Oncol* 2008;31:95–99.
349. Spiro RH, Koss LG, Hajdu SI, et al. Tumors of minor salivary origin: a clinicopathologic study of 492 cases. *Cancer* 1973;31:117–129.
351. Hinerman RW, Mendenhall WM, Morris CG, et al. T3 and T4 true vocal cord squamous cell carcinomas treated with external beam irradiation: a single institution's 35-year experience. *Am J Clin Oncol* (CCT) 2007;30(2):181.

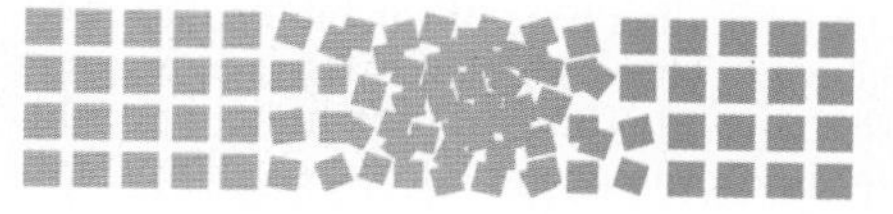

CHAPTER 73 REHABILITATION AFTER TREATMENT OF HEAD AND NECK CANCER

DOUGLAS B. CHEPEHA, MARK J. HAXER, AND TERESA H. LYDEN

Progress has been made in the past several years with survival for patients with head and neck cancer.[1] The current challenge is how to balance intensity of treatment and preserve function. Conservation surgery, radiation strategies, autogenous revascularized tissue transplantation, and treatment selection protocols continue to be used in an attempt to maintain or reestablish functional speech, voice, and swallowing in head and neck cancer patients. The ideal multidisciplinary team requires interaction among the surgical oncologists, radiation oncologists, medical oncologists, reconstructive surgeons, speech pathologists, physical therapists, maxillofacial prosthodontists, dental oncologists, nutritionists, nurse oncologists, psychologists, audiologists, and social workers during pretreatment assessment and posttreatment intervention. As radiation and chemotherapy protocols are being initiated in smaller centers, steps must be taken to ensure that the patient benefits from a multidisciplinary approach.

This chapter will focus on the rehabilitation of the whole patient. Pretreatment counseling is essential for all patients with aerodigestive tract cancer. Patients benefit from discussions regarding swallowing, voice, and speech difficulties that can result from radiation and chemotherapy regimens. Regrettably, patients who undergo radiation and chemotherapy protocols often are inadequately counseled, if at all. For rehabilitation to be effective, the patient's social, psychological, and addictive behaviors must be assessed and treated. Many of these patients have addictions to tobacco and alcohol at presentation and may lack social support. All these issues should be comprehensively addressed, and in so doing, the provider and the patient are often rewarded by the productive role the patient assumes for him- or herself, as well as within his or her family and in the workplace.

PRETREATMENT COUNSELING

The education process begins during the initial consultation with the physician. Each team member has a specific, yet overlapping, role in preparing the patient for his or her intervention. The physicians are essential for providing information to the patient with respect to diagnosis, prognosis, and treatment options. This includes providing education to the patient on his or her specific treatment plan. Patients who are previously untreated and receive single modality treatment are going to do much better than patients who are recurrent or are going to undergo multimodality therapy. In order to design the best intervention for the patient, the physicians must also remain flexible and integrate feedback from the team. Once the plan is established, the physician team has to clearly communicate the treatment plan to the remaining members of the team so they can provide appropriate counseling.

Nursing will provide education on feeding tube and tracheotomy management. The placement of a gastrostomy or a tracheotomy is associated with the poorest patient reported quality of life.[2] Because the patient will have little or no familiarity with these interventions, specific explanation of the anatomy and postoperative care is important.

Preoperative counseling with the speech pathologist is an essential part of patient education and shaping expectations. The speech pathologist is often regarded by the patient as the individual who will restore function posttreatment. The greatest counseling challenge in this patient group is overcoming poor coping skills.[3] Quality-of-life assessment has correlated low scores in emotional well-being domains with increased "overall bother" scores.[4] The speech pathologist must contend with the patient's coping mechanisms in order to facilitate rehabilitation. Psychosocial counseling, which speech pathologists often do on an *ad hoc* basis, has been shown to benefit head and neck cancer patients when compared to controls.[5] The speech pathologist must describe the expected long-term functional outcomes, the communicative and swallowing strategies that will be necessary, and indicate his or her interest in supporting the patient throughout treatment and rehabilitation.

The patient must also be counseled on smoking and alcohol cessation. This is a central piece of the rehabilitation efforts that ideally should be handled by a cessation specialist. Smoking cessation interventions, particularly those that take into consideration alcohol intake and depression, have been shown to be efficacious for this patient population.[6] This is encouraging as smoking is highly correlated with alcohol intake and depression. An addicted patient is unlikely to be effectively rehabilitated. Therefore, the patient must understand that continuation of addictive behaviors represents the greatest risk to patient survival and future functioning. It is important to emphasize to the patient that there are many different ways to quit smoking. The patient should understand that alcohol is a facilitator and nicotine is a lower level carcinogen than tobacco products.

The use of patient volunteers who have completed treatment is an invaluable resource. They provide education and experience with regard to what one may experience during treatment, posttreatment recuperation, and long-term quality of life to patients who are preparing for treatment.

SUPPORT DURING TREATMENT AND REHABILITATION OF THE CHEMORADIATION PATIENT

Radiation alone or concurrent with chemotherapy is the most common treatment approach for pharyngeal and laryngeal cancers. This approach will likely be refined to more customized approaches that involve treatment selection.[1] Even so, the majority of patients with disease involving these sites will have undergone radiation as part of their treatment. Swallowing and voice are affected by radiation, but the effect is variable and depends on the radiation field, the radiation dose, and the concomitant chemotherapy agents. After treatment there can be stiffness, edema, fibrosis, xerostomia, and stenosis. The severity of these effects is proportional to the aggressiveness of the treatment. To help reduce the effects of chemotherapy and radiation therapy, mobility of the aerodigestive tract should be maintained during treatment.[7]

This is facilitated by good supportive care, which includes appropriate treatment of mucositis, adequate analgesia, management of depression, maintenance of nutrition, and monitoring by the treatment team. The treatment of mucositis involves use of a mouthwash and oral care. There are many different "recipes" for mouthwashes but the common components are an antifungal such as nystatin (Mycostatin), an antihistamine such as diphenhydramine (Benadryl), and a barrier agent such as an antacid. The approach to analgesia is a sustained release agent that covers 80% to 90% of the analgesia needs and a shorter acting agent to cover breakthrough pain. To address issues relating to depression, the creation of an environment where depressive emotions or issues can be addressed is important. At present, serotonin reuptake inhibitors are the first-line antidepressants and modafinil is added if the patient has significant symptoms of fatigue. Clonazepam is added to the antidepressant regimen if there is a significant component of anxiety or to support the withdrawal of alcohol. Transdermal testosterone is also useful for symptoms of fatigue. A free testosterone serum level should be obtained to verify that testosterone levels are low. If unable to maintain adequate nutrition orally, particularly for the patient who is receiving radiation therapy, supplemental or primary nutrition can be met via a temporary gastrostomy tube. It is important to keep the patient swallowing even if the patient is only able to take sips of liquids. If a patient is unable to swallow anything, then a nasogastric feeding tube should be inserted as a stent for the pharynx. Removal of the stent is recommended only when the lumen is patent and the patient is able to swallow again. The consequence of "resting" the digestive tract during chemoradiation is possible complete pharyngeal stenosis or a nonfunctional upper aerodigestive tract. If pharyngeal stenosis occurs, management is achieved through dilation in the operating room or a program of self-dilation.

Rehabilitation after treatment usually focuses on relief from xerostomia or mucositis, maintenance of mobility of the oropharyngeal musculature, improved swallowing function, including reducing the risk of aspiration, and improvement with communication or voice. The posttreatment examination usually reveals edema, decreased sensation, and thick secretions. The thick secretions and xerostomia are managed with regular intake of liquids. In addition, medications designed to improve salivary flow such as pilocarpine and cevimeline can be taken daily. Pilocarpine is indicated in the radiated patient, but a minority of patients report subjective efficacy.[8] Cevimeline is indicated for Sjogren's disease but is often used off label for xerostomia. Artificial saliva can be taken as a gel, spray, or a lozenge and contains methylcellulose as a lubricating agent. However, in lieu of using salivary substitutes most patients choose to take frequent sips of water to thin secretions and keep their aerodigestive tract lubricated. The most recent advancement to reduce the incidence of xerostomia is intensity modulated radiation (IMRT), which is a radiation delivery technique that uses selective targeting. In cases where it is safe to spare the parotid from radiation it has been shown that there is improved salivary flow, relief from xerostomia, and improved quality of life.[9–11] Even with better salivary flow, patients frequently need to use liquid washes to improve swallowing function by moisturizing dry foods and lubricating the aerodigestive tract to allow for easier bolus passage. Reduction of aspiration is facilitated by aggressive swallowing exercises[7] and use of strategies, postures, or maneuvers. Incidence of aspiration can increase during and posttreatment. Exercises are introduced focusing on improving strength, range of motion, and coordination of movement. Areas that are commonly focused on include improving mandibular, labial, and lingual range of motion and improving strength and coordination of the lips, tongue (including base of tongue), palate, and posterior pharyngeal wall. There are several strategies that may be of benefit that include, but are not limited to, the effortful swallow, supra- and supersupraglottic swallows, and the Mendelsohn maneuver.[12–14]

There are several patient factors that also affect outcome. These include continued smoking, continued alcohol consumption, gastroesophageal reflux disease, and tissue reaction to the oxidative effects of radiation. As previously mentioned, in order to facilitate optimal rehabilitation, these factors need to be addressed as part of the patient's rehabilitation.

Posttreatment Speech and Swallowing Assessment

The team should understand which aspects of communication and swallowing functions have been compromised by treatment. Because of their training in the areas of communication and swallowing, the speech pathologist assumes a leading role in the evaluation and treatment of deficits in these areas. The site of lesion, extent of resection, type of reconstruction, and use of adjunct treatment modalities will influence the extent and severity of the communication and swallowing disorder. In addition, these factors will help guide the selection of assessment tools to be used as well as which strategies may be of benefit to the patient. In order to better understand the rehabilitation process with respect to swallowing, it may be useful to briefly review the four phases or stages of the normal swallow. The oral preparatory phase involves mastication and bolus formation. During this phase, the lips are closed anteriorly while the posterior tongue is closed against the soft palate, which keeps the bolus from prematurely spilling into the pharynx. The bolus is formed, shaped, and readied for swallowing.[15] During the oral phase, the bolus is propelled into the oropharynx as a result of the oral tongue rolling posteriorly in a pistonlike motion. Once this occurs, the swallow is voluntarily initiated, which facilitates the beginning of the pharyngeal stage of the swallow. This phase involves palatal closure, bolus transport through the pharynx as a result of base of tongue retraction along with sequential contraction of the pharyngeal constrictor musculature, laryngeal elevation, which results in glottic closure to prevent aspiration, and relaxation of the upper esophageal sphincter to allow for delivery of the bolus into the esophagus. The latter results in initiation of the esophageal phase of the swallow. Thus, the swallowing mechanism can be thought of as a series of valves that, when functioning normally, results in safe and efficient delivery of food or liquid into the stomach.[14] Any alteration of this valve system will result in compromised swallowing. Normal transmit times for the oral and pharyngeal phases of the swallow are 1.5 seconds or less. These increase slightly as bolus viscosity increases.[14] Transit times for the esophageal phase of the swallow vary between 8 and 20 seconds.[14]

Swallowing can be assessed subjectively or objectively. Subjective assessment is a clinical examination that involves evaluation of oral motor skills along with presentation of various consistencies of foods or liquids. Observations are made with regard to oral competency, timeliness of the swallow, laryngeal elevation, and clinical signs or symptoms of aspiration. Objective measures include fiberoptic endoscopic evaluation of swallowing (FEES) and videofluoroscopic swallow study (VFSS).[14,16] The VFSS is performed using c-rays (cineradiography or fluoroscopy) with barium as a contrast agent to visualize swallowing movements. The VFSS is an objective evaluation of swallowing function that includes all stages of the swallow during presentation of varying food consistencies. This procedure allows measured amounts of barium boluses to be followed from the lips to the stomach and, if needed, can incorporate the effects of compensatory strategies, such as postural assists or maneuvers. The VFSS is ideal for patients with oropharyngeal dysphagia as it allows for assessment of strategies and diagnosis of severity of aspiration. VFSS is expensive and time consuming. It requires at least 30 minutes to perform, involves radiation exposure, and requires a radiologist and a speech pathologist.[14] FEES utilizes a fiberoptic nasoendoscope to observe the pharyngeal and laryngeal structures directly during the pharyngeal phase of the swallow. A bolus of contrasting color is used to note premature spillage into the hypopharynx or laryngeal vestibule before swallow initiation along with the presence of residuum in the hypopharynx and laryngopharynx after a swallow. Vocal fold movement patterns can be assessed during FEES but need to be visualized independent of swallows. This examination yields minimal information relative to the oral preparatory and oral phases of the swallow. However, there are advantages to FEES completion, including a shorter assessment time, avoidance of radiation, and less expensive instrumentation. The Fiberoptic Endoscopic Evaluation of Swallowing with Sensory Testing (FEESST)[17] combines the FEES with a technique that determines laryngopharyngeal sensory discrimination thresholds by endoscopically delivering air pulse stimuli to the mucosa.

VFSS and FEES integrate diagnosis and intervention. During these diagnostic interventions the food bolus size, consistency, and maneuvers are all assessed to identify the safest and most efficient method for bolus transport and clearance and to reduce or eliminate aspiration events. At the most basic level, the assessment and interventions allows for the potential to continue with oral intake with or without use of a modified consistency and implementation of strategies, maneuvers, or posture. At the most sophisticated level, efficient eating in social situations can only be accomplished if the patient understands the consistencies, the bolus size, and the maneuvers that are appropriate to the speed of consumption in particular social situations. As a result, the VFSS and FEES are only as good as the knowledge and training of the speech pathologist providing the rehabilitation to this patient group. If the speech pathologist lacks this experience and training in the completion or the interpretation of either the VFSS or FEES of head and neck cancer patients, the physician must recognize and manage this situation by encouraging the patient to make the effort to go to an institution where the assessment and plan will be appropriate to the patient's needs.

The speech pathologist rehabilitates swallowing disorders with use of postural assists, maneuvers, control of bolus size or rate of intake, modification of bolus consistencies, and exercises.[14,18] Postures are body positions that the patient utilizes to improve bolus control and transport. Most of the postures involve the alteration of head or body position to direct the bolus to sensate native tissue, direct the bolus to more functional tissue, or to open the pharynx or close the larynx. Maneuvers are used to alter swallow physiology. These maneuvers are designed to improve laryngeal closure, increase base of tongue contact with the posterior pharyngeal wall, elevate the larynx, and open the hypopharynx. Postural assists and maneuvers may be prescribed to reduce penetration, which is entry of the bolus into the supraglottis, and aspiration, which is entry of the bolus into the trachea, with the goal of achieving safe and efficient oral intake. Many patients who have been treated for advanced head and neck cancer and are in need of evaluation and rehabilitation are actively aspirating. Successful rehabilitation is reduction but not necessarily elimination of aspiration. Optimization of the bolus type and consistency is an art. The bolus size and type of consistencies consumed evolve during rehabilitation. Management of swallowing requires understanding of the pre- versus posttreatment physiology and the probability of improvement during the first year following treatment. Swallowing exercises are important for strengthening, improving mobility, and coordination of movement. They involve both passive and active range of motion exercises. Exercises are designed to improve labial seal, mandibular movement or mouth opening, oral tongue mobility, base of tongue mobility, velopharyngeal closure, posterior pharyngeal wall strength or movement, and laryngeal elevation.

Speech generation involves assessment of respiration, phonation, resonance, and articulation. For optimum phonatory function there has to be adequate pulmonary reserve for breath support, an intact sound generator, and an intact vocal tract. Respiratory support is the driver of sound generation. Head and neck cancer patients frequently have impaired respiratory support secondary to chronic lung disease or pulmonary resection for second primary tumors. Reduced respiratory support decreases sound volume, increases vocal fatigue, and makes select consonants difficult to produce. Phonation can occur in the glottic or supraglottic larynx, the pharynx, or from an external source such as an artificial larynx. An important component of speech production is vocal resonance. If the soft palate and the lateral or posterior pharyngeal walls are not functioning properly, the voice may sound hyper- or hyponasal. Hypernasality is associated with too much sound (air leakage) into the nasopharynx during speech. Whereas hyponasality is associated with inadequate nasal resonance during speech. For the sound to be shaped into intelligible speech, there must be coordination between and adequate contact of the articulators. Much of the shaping of speech occurs in the oral cavity. For articulation to be optimized, the patient has to have an intact oral sphincter, tongue tip to premaxilla contact, maxillary alveolar contact with the lateral tongue and a mobile tongue tip, obliteration of dead space within the oral cavity, and soft palate contact with the base of the tongue.

Assessment of speech after treatment of head and neck cancer is varied depending on the site of the lesion, treatment completed, extent of surgical resection, and type of reconstruction, if any. Speech deficits commonly occur in postsurgical patients. However, it is important to be aware that even without surgical resection, patients can have imprecise articulation, altered nasality, or disruption in phonation as a result of tissue loss and nerve impairment pretreatment due to tumor size or location or posttreatment after chemoradiation therapy. Access to the surgeon's template of the surgical defect, including the involved muscles and nerves, is useful for the assessment of the postoperative patient.[19] For assessment of resonance and velopharyngeal competence, a thorough evaluation includes articulation assessment, oral motor assessment, and measurement of nasal airflow. A nasometer (Zoo Passage, Rainbow Passage and Nasal Sentences) is used to measure nasal airflow during recitation of standard passages. This is a relatively simple and noninvasive test. The results are compared to normative data. In addition, periodic retesting can be useful to monitor patient progress with interventions. VFSS and FEES can also be useful for the assessment of articulatory precision and velopharyngeal competency, but are better suited to the evaluation of swallowing. Articulation can be assessed by a number of survey instruments, including those that can be used for the assessment of intraoral prostheses.[21] These instruments are useful in the research setting and should be used in conjunction with the clinical examination. An interesting area of development is assessment using pressure-sensing electrode arrays. These electrodes are placed on the hard and soft palate to determine the exact location of tongue contact points during articulation. The contact points are then viewed as contrasting colored dots in a line drawing of the palate on a computer screen. This display can be used to assess and treat articulation problems particularly after tongue resection or reconstruction.

To determine candidacy for tracheoesophageal puncture insufflation testing[20] is an available objective measure to assist this process. This test provides information relative to the pressure generated within the pharyngoesophageal segment during production of structured speech tasks. It has never gained widespread use among speech pathologists due to the fact that more patients are undergoing TEP at the time of laryngectomy.

Just as with assessment, the treatment of communication disorders after the treatment of head and neck cancer is varied depending on site of lesion, treatment rendered, surgical management, and reconstruction. A laryngeal speech can be achieved with the use of a tracheoesophageal prosthesis, an artificial larynx or esophageal speech. Rehabilitation of the velum involves a multidisciplinary approach.[22] The speech pathologist can ensure that respiratory support is optimized, increase the precision of articulation, increase or decrease vocal intensity, slow the rate of articulation, and use biofeedback for frequently spoken words. If the patient is unable to optimize speech production with these interventions, then further evaluation for reconstruction or prosthetic management is warranted. The rehabilitation of oral articulation involves maximizing the coordination of the articulators to improve accuracy of contact particularly after ablation and reconstruction. Therapy may also focus on use of contrastive drills (words that sound similar but need to be contrasted for clarity of speech), use of drills of sound isolated or in combination with other sounds, and implementation of speech strategies such as decreasing the rate of speech or increasing volume.

Rehabilitation After Neck Dissection

Neck dissection is performed for the diagnosis or treatment of neck metastasis. The clinical sequela are secondary to postoperative weakness of the trapezius muscle, which include neck stiffness, shoulder girdle weakness, and chronic pain. The extent of the neck dissection (selective versus modified), radiation, age, and weight all affect the patient's ability to rehabilitate after neck dissection.[2] Patients who undergo selective neck dissection have significantly better shoulder function than patients who undergo modified radical neck dissection with the same regional control rates.[23,24] To reduce pain and discomfort and improve mobility, passive and active range of motions have been shown to significantly improve long-term function and quality of life.[25]

Rehabilitation of the Oral Cavity

Surgery and postoperative radiation therapy remain the most common treatment approach in the oral cavity. Reconstructive surgeons must be versed in optimization of oral function. The general approach for oral cavity reconstruction is to perform an anatomic reconstruction (Figs. 73.1 and 73.2). The goals of oral cavity reconstruction are:

1. Obliteration of the oral cavity. This is achieved when all oral cavity mucosal surfaces are in contact with one another when the mouth is closed. This goal is important as it should decrease the likelihood of food getting lost in a "dead space" in the oral cavity. Additionally, it should improve the handling of secretions by bringing the revascularized free tissue transfer in contact with the remaining native mucosa.

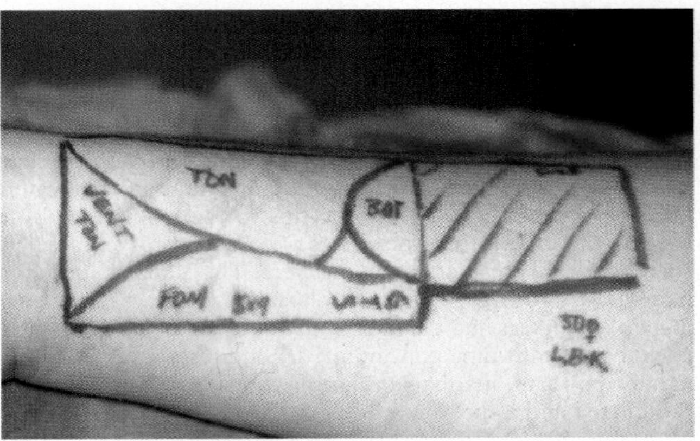

FIGURE 73.1 This is the preoperative "rectangle tongue" template for reconstruction of a hemiglossectomy defect. The template is marked out on the patient's forearm, will be excised, implanted, and revascularized to reconstruct the tongue.

2. Maintain premaxillary contact. This is an extension of the goal of obliteration of the oral cavity. In terms of speech generation, premaxillary and palatal contact is important for maintaining precision of articulation for a number of speech sounds. Generally, reduced precision of linguadental, alveolar, palatal, and velar sounds will occur if adequate contact is not achieved. The surgeon needs to ensure that some of the volume of the reconstructive flap is concentrated anteriorly to allow for obliteration of the oral cavity.
3. Maintain the "finger function" of the tongue. This is the ability of the tongue to sweep and clear the buccal, labial, and alveolar sulci and protrude past the coronal plane of the incisors.
4. Maintain movement of secretions from the anterior to the posterior aspect of the oral cavity.
5. Optimize sensation of the remaining native tissue and the revascularized free tissue transfer.

In general, these goals are best met with local tissue and revasularized autogenous tissue reconstruction. Traditional regional flaps, such as the pectoralis flap, are less commonly used as they are associated with higher gastrostomy tube rates.[26] There are published studies that suggest that autogenous revascularized free tissue transplantation is a disadvantage.[27] These data are not general to present day reconstruction because, in this historic cohort, free flaps were used for large defects and skin grafts were used for smaller defects. The differences related more to the size of the defect than the reconstructive approach.

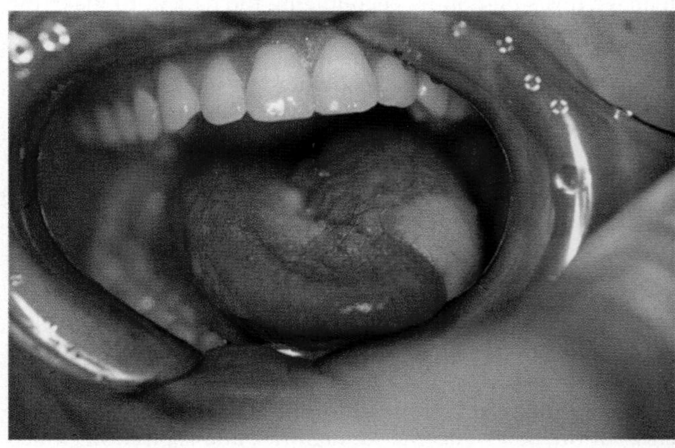

FIGURE 73.2 Postoperative reconstructed hemiglossectomy defect 22 months after implantation.

For oral cavity rehabilitation the speech pathologist will perform an oral motor assessment. Assessment includes evaluation of oral sphincter competence, the patient's ability to handle secretions, tongue to premaxillary/palatal contact, anterior-posterior movement of the tongue, location of sensate tissue, and identification of areas where food will collect (dead space). A clinical swallow examination is used to assess swallowing function with focus on the oral phase of the swallow. The patient's ability to remove the bolus from an eating utensil (i.e., spoon), create a labial seal, manipulate and control the bolus, and clear the bolus is assessed. The challenge for the speech pathologist is to modify the treatment plan and strategies used to compensate for the changing reconstruction during the first year of rehabilitation.

During the immediate postoperative period, the reconstruction will frequently be bulky and edematous; with radiation, the reconstruction will become smaller and the native tissue will undergo fibrosis. During the recovery period after treatment, the patient may develop xerostomia. However, there may also be recovery of some sensory and motor function that was lost during treatment. The objective throughout the first year is to maximize and maintain mobility of the tongue, focusing on the use of the remaining native tissue. In this patient group, after surgery and radiation, use of liquid washes to add moisture and aid in bolus passage with dry and solid consistencies should be considered the norm and not a failure of oral rehabilitation.

Maintenance of remaining native dentition is important for communication, swallowing, and for general health, so including a dentist as part of the treatment team is critical. Poor oral hygiene can result in dental caries, which could rapidly progress to tooth loss if left untreated. As a result of this tooth loss, osteoradionecrosis can result, and this is often a difficult condition to treat. The best approach is prevention, which involves reduction of radiation dose to the mandible when possible, removal or restoration of carious teeth prior to treatment, regular fluoride trays before and after treatment, and treatment of inflamed gingival tissue with antibiotics or antifungals. Should a patient develop osteoradionecrosis, surgical excision and reconstruction is the mainstay, as hyperbaric oxygen therapy has been shown to lack efficacy in controlled clinical trials.[28]

The maxillofacial prosthodontist makes important contributions to the rehabilitation of the patient with an oral cavity defect. Dental rehabilitation with dental prostheses is important for function and cosmesis. When introducing dental prosthetics it is important to consider the patient's ability to masticate and prevent bolus loss. Introduction of a dental prosthesis can impair bolus control by covering sensate tissue, preventing glossal-labial contact, and decreasing the functional oral opening. It is also important to ensure that the patient can perform a "tongue sweep" of the labial sulci to clear food residue, especially if a lower (mandibular) dental prostheses is introduced. If the patient is unable to perform this maneuver, then use of a digit may be required to clear food particles while eating. Even if the patient is a good candidate for a dental prosthesis, implants may be required to assist in retention of a lower dental prosthesis. Implants can be placed in the native mandible or in an osseous free flap for the purpose of supporting and retaining a dental prosthesis. An individual knowledgeable of the use of implants in radiated bone is important as the rate of implant failure is high and there is a risk of osteoradionecrosis.[29] Prostheses can also be useful for the rehabilitation of soft tissue deficits. For example, if the patient does not have good palatal-maxillary contact, a "palatal drop" prosthesis can be fashioned facilitating obliteration of dead space within the oral cavity, which allows the tongue to contact the prosthetically reconstructed palate. This may result in improved clarity of speech sounds, thus improving overall speech intelligibility. In addition, the palatal drop prosthesis may assist in improved bolus manipulation, control, and oral transfer.

Rehabilitation After Partial Laryngeal Procedures

Both communication and swallowing function can be adversely affected with partial surgical resection of the larynx. Supraglottic laryngectomy, hemilaryngectomy, and supracricoid laryngectomy all result in some degree of compromised phonatory function. Subsequent to these surgical procedures, swallowing function is generally adversely affected in the short term, but improvement can be anticipated with the process of healing and implementation of swallowing therapy. Postoperative dysphagia after partial laryngeal procedures is common due to a decrease in sensation and alteration of normal laryngeal anatomy. As a result, the patient is at risk for penetration and aspiration secondary to the compromise in airway protection that completion of these procedures brings about. Postoperatively, the patient will be trained on swallowing strategies to improve laryngeal closure in an attempt to prevent aspiration. In the early stages of recovery, liquids are usually the most difficult consistency to consume due to reduced sensation in and around the laryngeal complex and incomplete laryngeal closure, reducing airway protection. Therefore, consumption of a modified diet (thickened liquids and purees) with or without the use of alternative means of nutrition is not uncommon until adequate airway protection can be achieved. Implementation of swallowing maneuvers, such as the supra- and supersupraglottic swallow maneuvers are helpful in facilitating airway protection.[12–14]

Rehabilitation After Laryngectomy or Laryngopharyngectomy

After total laryngectomy, the patient has a tracheostoma in the lower neck and a separated digestive tract. The stoma and lungs require management to prevent stomal stenosis, prevent stomal trauma, enhance humidification, and reduce tracheal crusting. There are a variety of products that prevent tracheostomal stenosis, protect the stoma from digital trauma, and enhance humidification (Fig. 73.3). Many of these tracheal stomal prosthetics are designed to be used with or without tracheoesophageal prostheses.

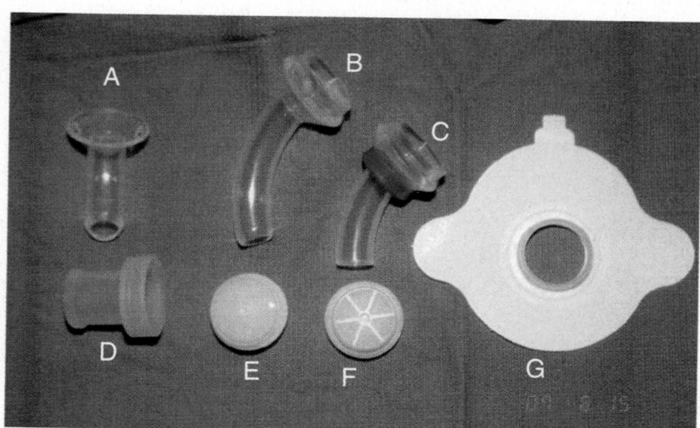

FIGURE 73.3 Laryngectomy tubes with filters. Inhealth laryngectomy tube for treatment of tracheal stenosis but will not retain a filter (**A**). Provox laryngectomy tubes (**B, C**) which retain Provox tracheostomy filters (**E, F**). Tracheostomy filters are used for pulmonary humidification. Barton Mayo button is a self-retaining laryngectomy tube that will retain a filter and does not need neck ties to aid in retention of the tube within the laryngostomy (**D**). Provox FLEXDERM oval adhesive retention collar for retention of tracheostomy filters (**G**).

PRACTICE OF ONCOLOGY

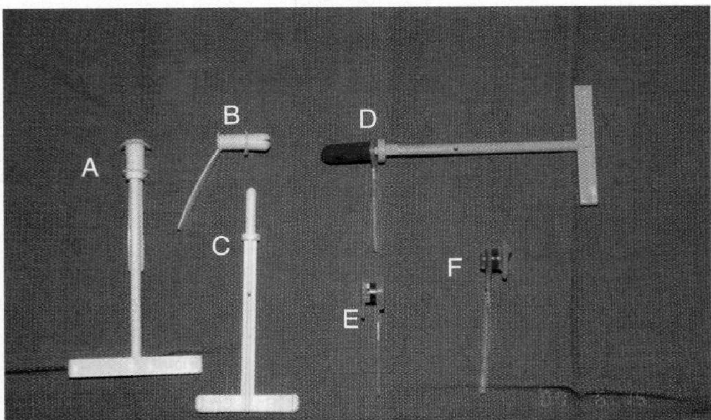

FIGURE 73.4 Patient changeable (**A, B, C**) and indwelling tracheal esophageal voice prosthesis (**D, E, F**). Inhealth low pressure voice prosthesis mounted on introducer (A). Inhealth duckbill prosthesis (**B**). Inhealth duckbill prosthesis introducer (**C**). Inhealth indwelling voice prosthesis mounted on introducer and inserted into gelcap. The prosthesis is inserted into the tracheal esophageal fistula and as the gelcap dissolves, the retention collar unfurls within the esophagus (**D**). Inhealth indwelling advantage prosthesis (**E**). Atos medical Provox 2 indwelling prosthesis (**F**).

Rehabilitation of speech after total laryngectomy has improved. Options for alaryngeal communication are tracheoesophageal voice, voice generated by an artificial larynx, and esophageal voice. Tracheoesophageal voice has become the gold standard for voice rehabilitation after total laryngectomy. The challenge with prosthetic rehabilitation is a customized solution as one size does not fit all. An experienced speech pathologist is essential for long-term patient compliance (Fig. 73.4). The artificial larynx is a device that produces mechanical sound. This sound is transferred into the oral cavity via placement of the device on the cheek or neck. Additionally there is an intraoral adapter, allowing for direct transmission of sound into the oral cavity. This device can be used short term until a patient achieves functional esophageal or tracheoesophageal speech. In some cases it is used long term, as the primary means of communication. This device can be difficult to use. Training of and practice by the patient are essential to become adept for daily communication requirements (Fig. 73.5). Another alaryngeal speech option is esophageal speech, which does not utilize devices or implants. It involves trapping air in the pharynx distal to the cricopharyngeus with subsequent controlled release of air through the pharyngoesophageal segment to produce sound. Learning esophageal speech is time intensive and can take up to a year

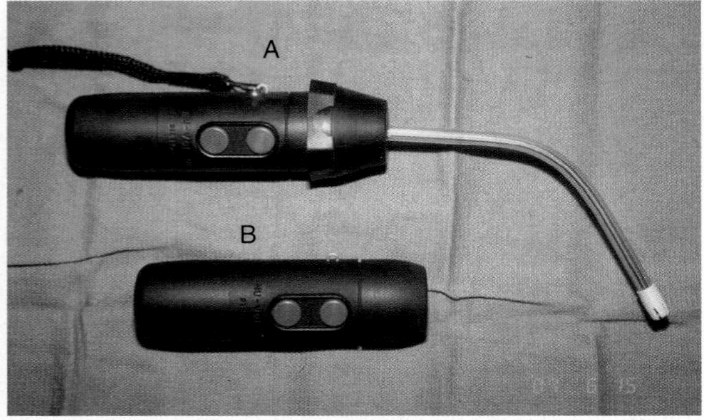

FIGURE 73.5 Artificial larynx with intraoral adaptor (**A**) and for neck and cheek placement (**B**).

or longer to achieve a functional result. In some cases, fluent sound is never realized. As a result, esophageal speech is not commonly used. Whereas, voice production with a tracheoesophageal voice prosthesis, in many instances, can be achieved on the day of insertion.

A wide variety of tracheoesophageal voice prostheses are available. Prosthesis selection is related to many factors. It is important to know that prostheses come in different diameters, lengths, amount of valve resistance, and size of tracheal and esophageal retention collars. Additionally, there are standard prostheses and yeast-resistant prostheses. The type of voice prosthesis that is chosen will depend upon the diameter, length, and integrity of the tissue that makes up the tracheoesophageal puncture. Yeast colonization also affects prosthesis selection. Yeast can cause a prosthesis to prematurely fail, as a result increased frequency of replacement may be required. Therefore, consideration for transition to a yeast-resistant prosthesis may be indicated. There are patient changeable and clinician placed (indwelling) prostheses. The voice prosthesis selected will be based on each individual's need. In addition, social and financial factors need to be considered. Some patients have to pay for their own prosthesis out of pocket or need to travel long distances to visit the speech pathologist for replacement. Therefore, cost in combination with replacement interval and travel time has to be considered along with the clinical indication for prosthesis selection. Patient-changeable prostheses can last from less than 1 month to 6 months on average, whereas, clinician-placed prosthetics can last 3 to 6 months on average. The goal is for the patient to be independent with care. This includes daily cleaning and maintenance. However, this may also include replacement of the prosthesis, if the patient is judged to be a candidate to do so. The advantages of the patient-changeable prosthesis is that it is less expensive than the clinician-placed prosthesis. In addition, in the event of prosthesis failure, the patient can replace the prosthesis independently. The clinician-placed (indwelling) prosthesis comes with added options (yeast resistant, large tracheal or esophageal flanges, dual valves). However, the indwelling prosthesis can cost two to three times more than a patient changeable. Additionally, if the prosthesis fails, the patient may have to wait 1 to 3 days to get an appointment to have the prosthesis replaced.

Voice production can be difficult for some patients even when there is a properly fitting tracheoesophageal prosthesis. There are several causes of aphonia following placement of a voice prosthesis. These include posttreatment edema, spasm of the cricopharyngeus, and pharyngeal stenosis. A VFSS is utilized for the evaluation of spasm versus stenosis. If a stenosis is present then dilation is appropriate. If there is hypertonicity of the pharyngoesophageal segment or cricopharyngeal spasm, this can be treated with botulinum toxin injection in a clinic setting or administered under fluoroscopy.

Sound production with a tracheoesophageal voice prosthesis requires adequate occlusion of the tracheostoma. The tracheostoma can be occluded directly with a digit, an object such as a table tennis ball, using a stoma filter with application of digital pressure (Fig. 73.6), or with a mechanical valve that fits over the stoma. A mechanical valve is considered to be "hands free" and fit into a tracheostomal housing that can be adhered to the skin adjacent to the stoma or inserted into a button or tube that is placed in the stoma (Fig. 73.7). The hands-free devices most closely duplicate an intact larynx because the patient does not have to use a digit to occlude the stoma. Use of forced exhalation closes off the valve, shunting air through the voice prosthesis. The challenges with these devices are retention while speaking, avoiding obstruction due to secretions, and maintaining optimal respiratory support for valve closure. For effective long-term use of a tracheostomal housing used with a hands-free device, the peristomal skin must be able to withstand wound breakdown. An alternative to the adhesive tracheostomal housing is a

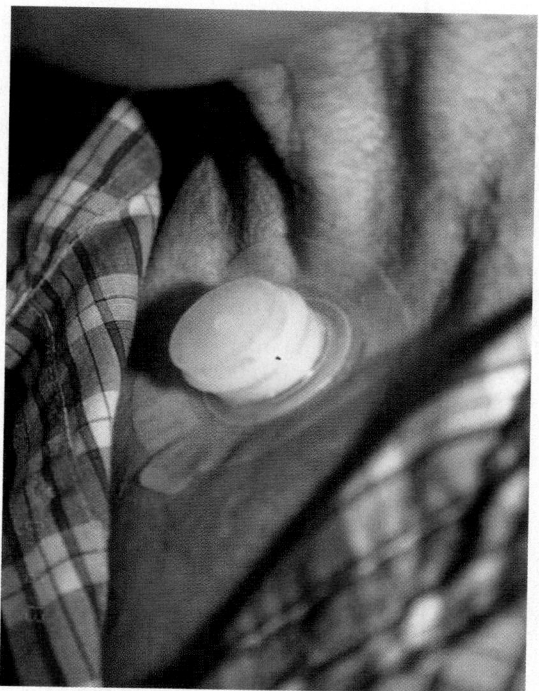

FIGURE 73.6 Patient with adhesive tracheostoma baseplate heat and moisture exchange system with cassette in position. The patient will push on the cassette for tracheoesophageal voice production.

stoma button. The button fits in the tracheostoma, and retention is facilitated by a slightly stenotic stoma and a small retention collar on the distal end of the button. There are stoma buttons that include attachments on the face that allow the button to be secured via a strap to the peristomal skin in an attempt to further improve retention. For those patients who are not able to use a stoma button but require use of a tube to maintain stoma patency, another option is a combination of the adhesive housing and the laryngectomy tube. If the retention and secretion issues can be overcome, the hands-free device is a major step forward in the rehabilitation of the head and neck cancer patient (Fig. 73.8).

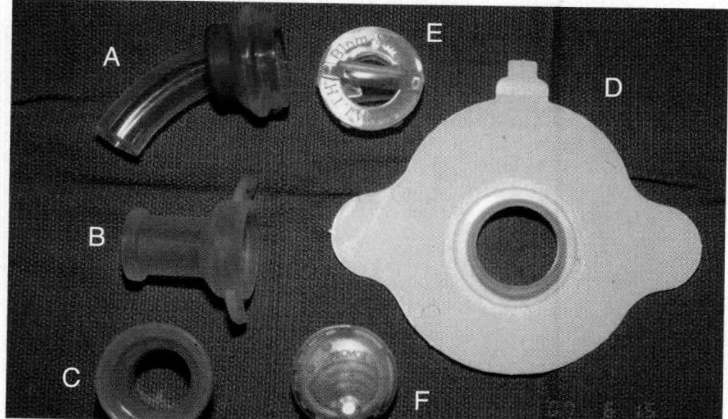

FIGURE 73.7 Self-retaining laryngectomy tubes and buttons, hands-free speaking valves, and baseplate. To use a hands-free speaking valve, a patient needs to use either a peristomal housing or an intrastomal button to retain the valve. The retention devices include the Provox laryngectomy tube with a retention ring (**A**) to be used with a Provox FLEXDERM oval (**D**), the Provox self-retaining laryngectomy button (**B**), and Medical Innovations Barton Mayo self-retaining laryngectomy button (**C**). The hands-free speaking valve include the Inhealth adjustable speaking valve (**E**) and the Provox hands-free speaking valve (**F**).

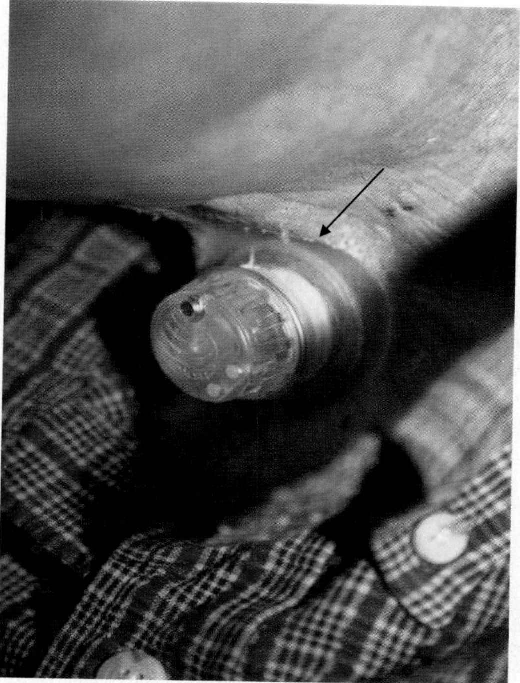

FIGURE 73.8 Patient with modified tracheostoma housing with hands-free speaking valve.

RESOURCES FOR REHABILITATION OF HEAD AND NECK CANCER PATIENTS

For the clinician, there are a number of useful references for the rehabilitation of head and neck cancer patients:

Doyle PC, Keith RL. *Contemporary considerations in the treatment and rehabilitation of head and neck cancer.* Austin, TX: PRO-ED, 2005.

Fried MP. *The larynx—a multidisciplinary approach.* Vol. 15. Boston: Little, Brown, 1988.

Logemann JA. *Evaluation and treatment of swallowing disorders.* 2nd ed. Vol. 13. Austin, TX: PRO-ED, 1998.

Perlman AL, Schulze-Delrieu KS. *Deglutition and its disorders—anatomy, physiology, clinical diagnosis, and management.* Vol. 13. San Diego: Singular, 1997.

Sullivan P, Guilford A. *Swallowing intervention in oncology.* Vol. 21. San Diego: Singular, 1999.

Many larger communities have support groups. However, there are few, if any, in small rural areas. Most large head and neck oncology programs are associated with support groups. It may be helpful for a newly diagnosed head and neck cancer patient to have the opportunity to speak with a member of the support group prior to treatment. For additional information about support groups:

Support for People with Oral and Head and Neck Cancer (SPOHNC) has a listing of support groups in the United States. In addition, it has a useful list of Web links for the head and neck cancer patient. SPOHNC can be located at www.spohnc.org, PO Box 53, Locust Valley, NY, 11560-0053, 1-800-377-0928

Web Whispers is a laryngectomy online support group that provides information, has a monthly online newsletter, conducts an annual meeting, and provides loaner artificial electric larynx for members. It is located at www.webwhispers.org.

The International Association of Laryngectomees (IAL) is an international association with educational materials, meetings and links to medical equipment companies. IAL can be located at www.larynxlink.com, 1203 Wolf Swamp Rd., Jacksonville, NC, 28546. The site is also available in Spanish.

Cancercare provides educational programs, counseling, information, and financial assistance. There are useful links and documents on recent cancer-related research. Patients can call and obtain a free counseling from a social worker. It is located at www.cancercare.org. To contact telephone counseling call 1-800-813-4673.

The Head and Neck Cancer Alliance has a link to a blog where patients can ask other patients about their experiences. The site is located at www.headandneckcancer.org.

For the patient there is an "official" Web site for information:

Medline Plus is a patient health information site supported by the National Library of Medicine and the National Institutes of Health. It is located at www.nlm.nih.gov/medlineplus/headandneckcancer.html#cat26. This site is also available in Spanish.

Cancer.net offers information on a variety of topics for the head and neck cancer patient. The site is located at www.cancer.net.

National Cancer Institute offers information on head and neck cancer treatment, prevention, causes, and screening. The site can be accessed at www.cancer.gov/cancertopics/types/head-and-neck.

References

1. Urba SG, Moon J, Giri PG, et al. Organ preservation for advanced resectable cancer of the base of tongue and hypopharynx: a Southwest Oncology Group Trial. *J Clin Oncol* 2005;23(1):88.
2. Taylor RJ, Chepeha JC, Teknos TN, et al. Development and validation of the neck dissection impairment index: a quality of life measure. *Arch Otolaryngol Head Neck Surg* 2002;128(1):44.
3. Henderson JM, Ord RA. Suicide in head and neck cancer patients. *J Oral Maxillofacial Surg* 1997;55(11):1217.
4. Terrell JE, Nanavati K, Esclamado RM, et al. Health impact of head and neck cancer. *Otolaryngol Head Neck Surg* 1999;120(6):852.
5. Hammerlid E, Persson LO, Sullivan M, et al. Quality-of-life effects of psychosocial intervention in patients with head and neck cancer. *Otolaryngol Head Neck Surg* 1999;120(4):507.
6. Duffy SA, Ronis DL, Valenstein M, et al. A tailored smoking, alcohol, and depression intervention for head and neck cancer patients. *Cancer Epidemiol Biomarkers Prev* 2006;15(11):2203.
7. Gaziano JE. Evaluation and management of oropharyngeal dysphagia in head and neck cancer. *Cancer Control* 2002;9(5):400.
8. Scarantino C, LeVeque F, Swann RS, et al. Effect of pilocarpine during radiation therapy: results of RTOG 97-09, a phase III randomized study in head and neck cancer patients. *J Support Oncol* 2006;4(5):252.
9. Eisbruch A, Ship JA, Dawson LA, et al. Salivary gland sparing and improved target irradiation by conformal and intensity modulated irradiation of head and neck cancer. *World J Surg* 2003;27(7):832.
10. Lin LC, Wang SC, Chen SH, et al. Efficacy of swallowing training for residents following stroke. *J Adv Nurs* 2003;44(5):469.
11. Malouf JG, Aragon C, Henson BS, et al. Influence of parotid-sparing radiotherapy on xerostomia in head and neck cancer patients. *Cancer Detect Prevent* 2003;27(4):305.
12. Lazarus C, Logemann JA, Gibbons P. Effects of maneuvers on swallowing function in a dysphagic oral cancer patient. *Head Neck* 1993;15(5):419.
13. Fujiu M, Logemann JA. Effect of a tongue-holding maneuver on posterior pharyngeal wall movement during deglutition. *Am J Speech Lang Pathol* 1996;5:23.
14. Logemann JA. *Evaluation and treatment of swallowing disorders*. 2nd ed. Vol. 13. Austin, TX: PRO-ED, 1998.
15. Dodds WJ, Stewart ET, Logemann JA. Physiology and radiology of the normal oral and pharyngeal phases of swallowing [comment]. *AJR Am J Roentgenol* 1990;154(5):953.
16. Murray J, Langmore SE, Ginsberg S, et al. The significance of accumulated oropharyngeal secretions and swallowing frequency in predicting aspiration. *Dysphagia* 1996;11(2):99.
17. Aviv JE, Murry T, Zschommler A, et al. Flexible endoscopic evaluation of swallowing with sensory testing: patient characteristics and analysis of safety in 1,340 consecutive examinations. *Ann Otol Rhinol Laryngol* 2005;114(3):173.
18. Logemann JA. Role of the modified barium swallow in management of patients with dysphagia. *Otolaryngol Head Neck Surg* 1997;116(3):335.
19. Jacobson MC, Franssen E, Fliss DM, et al. Free forearm flap in oral reconstruction. Functional outcome. *Arch Otolaryngol Head Neck Surg* 1995;121(9):959.
20. Lewin JS, Baugh RF, Baker SR. An objective method for prediction of tracheoesophageal speech production. *J Speech Hear Disord* 1987;52(3):212.
21. Mahanna GK, Beukelman DR, Marshall JA, et al. Obturator prostheses after cancer surgery: an approach to speech outcome assessment. *J Prosthetic Dentistry* 1998;79(3):310.
22. Doyle P, Keith R. *Contemporary considerations in the treatment and rehabilitation of head and neck cancer (voice, speech, and swallowing)*. Austin, TX: PRO-ED, 2005.
23. Chepeha DB, Taylor RJ, Chepeha JC, et al. Functional assessment using Constant's Shoulder Scale after modified radical and selective neck dissection. *Head Neck* 2002;24(5):432.
24. Chepeha DB, Hoff PT, Taylor RJ, et al. Selective neck dissection for the treatment of neck metastasis from squamous cell carcinoma of the head and neck. *Laryngoscope* 2002;112(3):434.
25. Salerno G, Cavaliere M, Foglia A, et al. The 11th nerve syndrome in functional neck dissection. *Laryngoscope* 2002;112(7 Pt 1):1299.
26. Chepeha DB, Annich G, Pynnonen MA, et al. Pectoralis major myocutaneous flap vs revascularized free tissue transfer: complications, gastrostomy tube dependence, and hospitalization. *Arch Otolaryngol Head Neck Surg* 2004;130(2):181.
27. Pauloski BR, Logemann JA, Colangelo LA, et al. Surgical variables affecting speech in treated oral/oropharyngeal cancer patients. *Laryngoscope* 1988;108:908.
28. Annane DD, Aubert P, Villart M, et al. Hyperbaric oxygen therapy for radionecrosis of the jaw: a randomized, placebo-controlled, double-blind trial from the ORN96 Study Group. *J Clin Oncol* 2004;22(24):4893.
29. Visch LL, van Waas MA, Schmitz PI, et al. A clinical evaluation of implants in irradiated oral cancer patients. *J Dental Res* 2002;81(12):856.

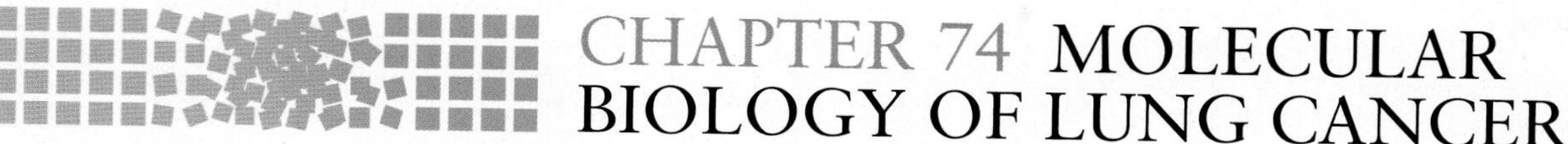

CHAPTER 74 MOLECULAR BIOLOGY OF LUNG CANCER

JACOB KAUFMAN, LEORA HORN, AND DAVID CARBONE

Lung cancer tumorigenesis is a multistep process of transformation from normal bronchial epithelium to overt lung cancer. Various molecular events that result in gain or loss of function cause dysregulation of key genetic pathways involved in cellular proliferation, differentiation, apoptosis, migration, invasion, and other processes characteristic of the malignant phenotype. Mutations, including single nucleotide substitution or deletion, and translocation, deletion, or amplification of larger portions of genetic material may result from environmental factors, inherited susceptibility, or random events. Many genes are involved in tumorigenesis of both small cell lung cancer (SCLC) and non–small cell lung cancer (NSCLC) (Table 74.1, Fig. 74.1), but there are also unique genetic aberrations associated with each tumor type. Following the development of overt cancer, continued accumulation of genetic abnormalities influences the processes of invasion, metastases, and resistance to cancer therapy. Identification of the nature and frequency of these molecular abnormalities is necessary to determine their clinical implications (e.g., associations with smoking, histological type, stage, survival, response to therapy) and define their clinical utility for prevention and early diagnosis of lung cancer, as well as for the development of therapeutic targets.

SUSCEPTIBILITY TO LUNG CANCER: GENETIC SUSCEPTIBILITY AND CARCINOGENS IN TOBACCO SMOKE

Tobacco use is the most important environmental factor associated with the development of lung cancer. Approximately 85% of lung cancer occurs in current or former smokers, which corresponds to a greater than tenfold increase in risk of lung cancer compared to never-smokers. Cigarette smoke contains more than 60 known carcinogens, 20 of which have been convincingly shown to cause lung tumors in laboratory animals or humans.[1] Of these, polycyclic aromatic hydrocarbons, such as benzo(a)pyrene, tobacco-specific nitrosamines, such as 4-(methylnitrosamino)-1-(3-pyridyl)-1-butanone (NNK), and aromatic amines, such as 4-aminobiphenyl, appear to have an important role in cancer causation. Nitrosamines such as NNK induce lung tumors, primarily adenomas and adenocarcinomas, in mice independent of the route of administration. Among the polycyclic aromatic hydrocarbons, benzo(a)pyrene is the most extensively tested and the first to be detected in tobacco smoke. Its role in cancer tumorigenesis is well described, and its diol epoxide metabolite has been implicated as the cause of mutation in the *TP53* gene.[2] One of the carcinogenic effects of tobacco smoke in the lung is the formation of DNA adducts, leading to errors in DNA replication and resulting mutations. DNA adducts have been identified in the bronchial tissue of patients with lung cancer. In current smokers, adduct levels correlate with the amount of tobacco smoke exposure.[3,4] Smoking cessation for at least 5 years results in adduct levels similar to nonsmokers.[4] In addition, in former smokers, age at smoking initiation has been inversely associated with levels of DNA adducts, suggesting that prevention of smoking in adolescence is of utmost importance in decreasing lung cancer risks.

Although tobacco use can account for the majority of lung cancers, most chronic smokers still do not develop lung cancer. Differences in inherent susceptibility may be related to variations in carcinogen metabolizing enzymes, DNA repair mechanisms, chromosome fragility, and other homeostatic mechanisms. Among genes for carcinogen-metabolizing enzymes, polymorphisms in the cytochrome P-450 genes *CYP1A1*, *CYP2D6*, and *CYP2E1* and in mu-class glutathione S-transferase (*GSTM1*) have received the most attention. Although studies have suggested that there may be a modest association of *GSTM1* null polymorphism with lung cancer, knowledge of the state of single candidate genes may not be adequate to predict lung cancer risk due to the complexity of carcinogen metabolism, gene–gene and gene–environment interactions, and the relatively small effect of an individual gene. In addition to inherent susceptibility to the carcinogenic effects of tobacco smoke, large genome-wide association studies have identified lung cancer susceptibility loci at 15q25, 5p15, and 6p21.[5,6] In particular, polymorphisms in and around nicotinic cholinergic receptors at chromosome 15q25 appear to correlate with messenger RNA (mRNA) and protein expression of these receptors as well as functional changes in the calcium ion channel of the A5 nicotine receptor; these differences confer susceptibility to smoking behaviors.[7]

Researchers are optimistic that molecular epidemiology will help identify individuals at the highest risk of developing lung cancer. Such information, in addition to the smoking history, will be of great value in new lung cancer screening trials and in chemoprevention trials to identify persons at highest risk of developing lung cancer.

MOLECULAR CHANGES IN PRENEOPLASIA

Before lung cancer is clinically recognizable, a series of morphologically distinct changes (hyperplasia, metaplasia, dysplasia, and carcinoma in situ) are thought to occur. Whether one

TABLE 74.1

MOST FREQUENTLY ACQUIRED MOLECULAR ABNORMALITIES IN LUNG CANCER

Abnormalities	Small Cell Lung Cancer	Non–Small Cell Lung Cancer
Microsatellite instabilities	~35%	~22%
Autocrine loops	GRP/GRP receptor; SCF/KIT	TGF-α/EGFR; heregulin/ERBB2; HGF/MET
RAS point mutation	<1%	15%–20%
EGFR mutation	<1%	<10% (West), ~40% (Asia)
EML4-ALK	0%	3%–7%
MYC family overexpression	15%–30%	5%–10%
p53 inactivation	~90%	~50%
RB inactivation	~90%	15%–30%
$p16^{INK4A}$ inactivation	0%–10%	30%–70%
LKB1 inactivation	~40%–60% (IHC)	20%–40%
Frequent allelic loss	3p, 4p, 4q, 5q, 8p, 10q, 13q, 17p, 22q	3p, 6q, 8p, 9p, 13p, 17p, 19q
Telomerase activity	~100%	80%–85%
BCL2 expression	75%–95%	10%–35%

EGFR, epidermal growth factor receptor; GRP, gastrin-releasing peptide; HGF, hepatocyte growth factor; RB, retinoblastoma protein; SCF, stem cell factor; TGF-α, transforming growth factor-α; IHC, immunohistochemistry.

cell of origin leads to all histological variants is unclear. It is believed that dysplasia and carcinoma *in situ* represent true preneoplastic changes. These sequential changes found within squamous cell cancers that arise from central bronchi have long been recognized. Although the exact cell of origin for lung cancer is unknown, it is thought that type II epithelial cells have the capacity to give rise to lung adenocarcinomas, while cells of neuroendocrine origin are likely precursors of SCLC.

It is evident that preneoplastic cells contain several genetic abnormalities identical to some of the abnormalities found in overt lung cancer cells. For squamous cell cancers, immunohistochemical analysis has confirmed abnormal expression of protooncogenes (cyclin D1) and tumor suppressor genes (TSGs) (p53).[8] Allelotyping of precisely microdissected, preneoplastic foci of cells shows that 3p allele loss is currently the earliest known change, suggesting that one or more 3p TSGs may act as gatekeepers for lung cancer pathogenesis.[9] This is followed by 9p, 8p, and 17p allele loss and p53 mutation. Even histologically normal bronchial epithelium has been shown to have genetic losses. Similarly, atypical alveolar hyperplasia, the potential precursor lesion of adenocarcinomas, can harbor Kristen rat sarcoma viral oncogene homolog (*KRAS*) mutations and allele losses of 3p, 9p, and 17p.[10] Other genetic alterations, such as inactivation of *LKB1*, whose germline mutations cause Peutz-Jeghers syndrome, have also been implicated in the development of adenocarcinoma. These observations are consistent with the multistep model of carcinogenesis and a field cancerization process, whereby the whole tissue region is repeatedly exposed to carcinogenic damage (tobacco smoke) and is at risk for development of multiple, separate foci of neoplasia.[11]

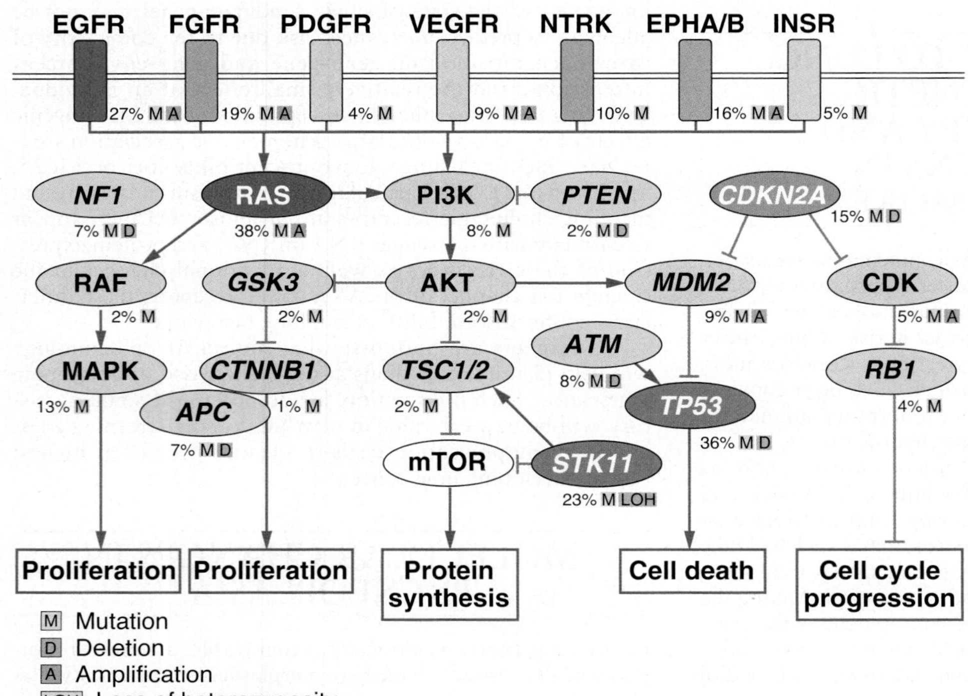

FIGURE 74.1 Significantly mutated pathways in lung adenocarcinomas. Genetic alterations in lung adenocarcinoma frequently occur in genes of the mitogen-activated protein kinase (MAPK) signaling, p53 signaling, Wnt signaling, cell cycle, and mammalian target of rapamycin (mTOR) pathways. Oncoproteins are indicated in pink to red and tumor suppressor proteins are shown in light to dark blue. The darkness of the colors is positively correlated to the percentage of tumors with genetic alterations. Frequency of genetic alterations for each of these pathway members in 188 tumors is indicated. (From Macmillan Publishers Ltd, ref. 113, copyright 2007, with permission.).

Although all types of lung cancers have associated molecular abnormalities in their normal and preneoplastic lung epithelium, SCLC patients in particular appear to have multiple genetic alterations occurring in their histologically normal-appearing respiratory epithelium. Molecular changes have been found not only in the lungs of patients with lung cancer but also in the lungs of current and former smokers without lung cancer. These molecular alterations are thus important targets for use in the early detection of lung cancer and for use as surrogate biomarkers in following the efficacy of lung cancer chemoprevention. In this regard, it appears that the smoking-damaged respiratory epithelium has thousands of clonal patches, each containing clones of cells with 3p and other allele loss abnormalities.[12] The challenge is to identify not only the prevalence and temporal sequence of molecular lesions in lung preneoplasia, but to determine which are rate limiting and indispensable and thus represent potential candidates for intermediate biomarker monitoring and therapeutic efforts.

GENETIC AND EPIGENETIC ALTERATIONS IN LUNG CANCERS

Genomic Instability and DNA Repair Genes

Similar to other epithelial tumors, lung cancer cells typically display chromosomal instability—both numeric abnormalities (aneuploidy) of chromosomes and structural cytogenetic abnormalities.[13] Allele loss on chromosome 3p is thought to be the among the earliest genetic change occurring in both NSCLC and SCLC.[14] In addition, nonreciprocal translocations and recurrent losses involving 1p, 4p, 4q, 5q, 6p 6q, 8p, 9p, 11p, 13q, 17p, 18q, and 22q may occur, representing changes in known and potential tumor suppressor genes.[15] Polysomies or regions of gene amplifications also occur and often involve protooncogenes such as epidermal growth factor receptor (*EGFR*) and myelocytomatosis viral oncogene homolog (*MYC*).[16,17] Simple reciprocal translocations are uncommonly observed in lung cancer, although translocations that give rise to BRD4-NUT,[18] CRCT1-MAML2,[19] SLC34A2–ROS,[20] and EML4-ALK[21] fusion proteins have been reported, and for the case of EML4-ALK this has been shown to drive the development and proliferation of tumors. Alterations in microsatellite polymorphic repeat sequences are found in 35% of SCLC and 22% of NSCLC.[22] The underlying mechanism for this chromosomal instability has not yet been discovered.

The most powerful tumor surveillance mechanism is involved in DNA damage response and repair of errors in DNA replication.[23] The DNA glycosylase 8-Oxo guanine (OGG1) specifically excises the oxidatively damaged mutagenic base 8-hydroxyguanine, which causes G:C→T:A transversions frequently found in lung cancer. Lung adenocarcinoma spontaneously develops in Ogg1 knockout mice and 8-hydroxyguanine accumulates in their genomes.[24,25] Individuals with low OGG activity have a greatly increased risk of developing lung cancer. Polymorphisms in other DNA repair genes *ERCC1*, *XRCC1*, *ERCC5/XPG*, and *MGMT/AGT* have been correlated with reduction of polyaromatic hydrocarbon DNA adduct formation as well as with lower lung cancer risks in case-control studies. High expression of excision repair cross-complementation gene-1 (ERCC1) is associated with decreased response to platinum-based chemotherapy, but in contrast, overexpression of ERCC1 correlates with better overall prognosis in NSCLC,[26] reflecting improved repair of lethal DNA damage by platinum, on the one hand, and greater DNA stability with less aggressive disease course, on the other. Similarly, ribonucleotide reductase M1 (RRM1) overexpression correlates with better *de novo* prognosis but resistance to gemcitabine. Assays of both ERCC1 and RRM1 are commercially available and are marketed as tools to guide cytotoxic therapy in NSCLC; treatment based on these assays has not yet been prospectively validated, but may prove important.

PROTOONCOGENES, GROWTH FACTOR SIGNALING, AND GROWTH FACTOR TARGETED THERAPIES

EGFR and *KRAS* are the two most commonly mutated protooncogenes in lung adenocarcinomas; these mutations appear to be mutually exclusive. EGFR is a transmembrane tyrosine kinase, which, when activated by binding with one of its ligands, members of the EGF family, stimulates cell proliferation. When mutated, EGFR tyrosine kinase is constitutively activated, resulting in uncontrolled proliferation, invasion, and metastasis. Coexpression of EGFRs and their ligands, especially transforming growth factor-α, by lung cancer cells indicates the presence of an autocrine (self-stimulatory) growth factor loop. Activating *EGFR* mutations are observed in approximately 10% of North American and European populations and 30% to 50% of Asian populations[27–32] and are significantly more common in never-smokers (100 or less cigarettes per lifetime) or light former smokers (quit 1 year or more ago and less than ten-pack per year smoking history). The leucine to arginine substitution at position 858 (L858R) in exon 21 and short in-frame deletions in exon 19 are the most common mutations seen in adenocarcinomas of the lung. These mutations result in prolonged activation of the receptor and downstream signaling through phosphorylated Akt, in the absence of ligand stimulation of the extracellular domain. *EGFR* mutations are both prognostic for response rate to chemotherapy and survival irrespective of therapy and are predictive of response to specific inhibitors of the EGFR tyrosine kinase—gefitinib and erlotinib.[31,33,34] *EGFR* mutations are found almost exclusively in adenocarcinomas and occur much more frequently in tumors from never-smokers, women, and in Asian populations, explaining the increased clinical response to gefitinib noted in these subpopulations before the association with *EGFR* mutation was discovered.[31,33,34] A recent review by Rosell et al.[32] suggested patients with adenocarcinoma who are never or light remote smokers, especially women and Asians, should be screened for the presence of an *EGFR* mutation. The IPASS (Iressa Pan-Asia Study) trial demonstrated an improved outcome with up-front treatment with gefitinib compared with chemotherapy for patients with *EGFR* mutation, but on the other hand, much worse outcome compared with chemotherapy in patients with wild type *EGFR*.[35,36] Previous suggestions that *EGFR* gene amplification by detected by fluorescence *in situ* hybridization (FISH) or immunohistochemistry may correlate with response to therapy with an EGFR tyrosine kinase inhibitor[28] have not been corroborated. Cetuximab, a human murine chimeric immunoglobulin G subclass-1 (IgG-1) antibody that binds to the extracellular domain of EGFR and affects ligand-induced phosphorylation and degradation has been evaluated in patients with NSCLC. Contrary to data from colon cancer studies, neither expression of nor mutations in EGFR or KRAS appear to predict response or survival to this agent.[37]

ERBB2 (formerly human epidermal growth factor receptor 2 [HER2]/neu) is also a member of the erbB receptor family, along with *EGFR*. The ERBB2 receptor is unusual in that it does not interact with the EGF ligand family; its activation depends on heterodimerization with other erbB receptors following ligand binding. *ERBB2* mutations have been detected with low frequency in lung adenocarcinomas.[30] Similar prevalence of gene amplification of *ERBB2* can be observed.[38] A meta-analysis suggested that overexpression of ERBB2 is a poor prognostic indicator for survival in NSCLC.[39] Several clinical trials examining trastuzumab (Herceptin), a recombinant humanized monoclonal antibody against ERBB2, as a single agent or in combination with chemotherapy, have failed to demonstrate a survival benefit.[40] A new generation of dual irreversible EGFR/ERBB2 inhibitors is under development. These agents form a covalent bond with CYS-733 in EGFR and may be effective in patients with resistance to reversible EGFR tyrosine kinase inhibitors.[41]

c-KIT belongs to the PDGF/c-Kit receptor tyrosine kinase family that results in activation of the Janus-associated tyrosine kinase/signal transducers and activators of transcription (JAK-STAT), phosphoinositide 3-kinase (PI3K), and mitogen-activated protein kinase (MAPK) pathways important in cell growth and differentiation. Along with its ligand, stem cell factor (SCF), it is preferentially expressed in many SCLCs and is thought to have prognostic implications.[42–45] Activation of this putative autocrine loop may also mediate chemoattraction and may provide a growth advantage in tumor cells. Although the c-KIT tyrosine kinase inhibitor imatinib reduces cell proliferation and induces cell death in several preclinical SCLC models,[46] it failed to demonstrate any objective response in clinical trials.[47–49] Another receptor tyrosine kinase, c-MET and its ligand, hepatocyte growth factor (HGF), play an important role in fetal lung development. Coexpression of this putative loop is observed in both NSCLC and SCLC. High HGF levels have also been associated with a poor outcome in resectable NSCLC patients; furthermore, elevated expression of MET is associated with resistance to EGFR targeted therapy,[50] and improvement in patient outcome has recently been reported when monoclonal antibodies inhibiting MET are combined with erlotinib.[51] The insulin-like growth factor receptor 1 (IGFR1) signaling pathway plays an important role in cancer growth and progression and has been associated with resistance to therapy. IGFR1 monoclonal antibodies and small molecule inhibitors are currently in clinical testing in patients with NSCLC. A phase 3 clinical trial of figitumumab (CP-751871) was closed early due to excess toxicities, including treatment-related deaths, in the experimental arm, so the possible role of these agents in the treatment of NSCLC remains to be determined.

In addition to protooncogene products, other growth stimulatory loops are found in lung cancer. The best known is that governed by gastrin-releasing peptide and other bombesin-like peptides, together with their receptors, which participate in lung development and repair and promote SCLC growth in cell culture via an autocrine loop. Immunohistochemical studies showed that gastrin-releasing peptide is expressed in 20% to 60% of SCLC but less frequently in NSCLCs. Although this loop is a possible therapeutic target, a phase 1 clinical trial of the anti–gastrin-releasing peptide monoclonal antibody 2A11 did not result in an objective antitumor response in patients with lung cancer.[52]

Other signaling pathways historically linked to embryonic development likely to be relevant for lung carcinogenesis include the Sonic hedgehog (Shh) and Notch signaling pathways. Extensive activation of the hedgehog pathway has been demonstrated within the airway epithelium during repair of acute airway injury and in a subset of SCLC.[53] Notch 3 has been found to be overexpressed in about 40% of lung cancers. Inhibition of this pathway *in vitro* has resulted in the loss of tumor phenotypes.[54] Clinical trials are under way to determine whether targeting these pathways has any clinical utility.

As downstream effectors are required for intracellular transduction of incoming growth factor or receptor signals, it is not surprising that proteins important in cytoplasmic signal transduction cascades are also implicated in carcinogenesis. Mutation of *KRAS* is the most frequently reported alteration in the downstream EGFR signaling pathways. The *RAS* gene family, in particular *KRAS*, can be activated by point mutations at codons 12 or 13 in exon 2 in approximately 20% to 30% of NSCLCs, with 90% of the RAS mutations observed in lung adenocarcinomas and with approximately 85% of the *KRAS* mutations affecting codon 12.[55] *KRAS* mutations are rarely observed in SCLCs. Transgenic mice with oncogenic Kras alleles that are activated by spontaneous recombination events in the whole animal are highly predisposed to early onset lung cancer, further supporting the hypothesis that *KRAS* mutation is an early oncogenic event in lung cancer.[56] Interestingly, the remaining wild type Ras allele appears to function as a potential tumor suppressor, because mice susceptible to the chemical induction of lung tumors frequently lose wild type Kras2 during lung tumor progression.[57] *KRAS* mutations more commonly occur in patients with a significant smoking history.[58] Approximately, 70% of *KRAS* mutations are G→T transversions, with the substitution of glycine by either cysteine or valine. Similar G→T transversions are observed in the mutated p53 gene, representing similar DNA damage as a result of bulky DNA adducts caused by the polycyclic hydrocarbons and nitrosamines in tobacco smoke. This observation provides further evidence for a causative role for tobacco smoke in *KRAS* mutations. In a meta-analysis of 3,779 lung cancer patients, 18.4% of whom had *KRAS* mutations detected by polymerase chain reaction (PCR), mutant *KRAS* was associated with worse prognosis in adenocarcinoma but not in squamous histology.[59] However, a prospective study failed to show a survival difference correlated with *KRAS* mutation in advanced NSCLC.[60] Although the oncogenicity of aberrant *KRAS* mutation appears to be well established, all attempts to inhibit mutant KRAS have failed to demonstrate objective responses in clinical trials, including attempts to prevent binding to the inner cell membrane by inhibiting farnesyltransferase or geranylgeranyltransferase.[61]

Direct downstream effectors of RAS are the RAF1 and BRAF protooncogenes. Unlike *RAS*, mutations in the RAF1 gene have not been detected in human lung cancers. Its role is complex, as growth arrest of SCLC by activated RAF1 suggests that it has a TSG-like function, and one copy of *RAF1* is frequently lost in lung cancer.[62] Although *BRAF*, another member of the RAF family, is commonly mutated in malignant melanomas and colon cancers, mutations in this gene are found in fewer than 5% of lung cancers.

Activation of nuclear protooncogene products, such as those encoded by the myc family genes (*MYC*, *MYCN*, and *MYCL*) is often the end point for many signaling cascades. MYC, when heterodimerized with MAX, functions as a transcription factor, and this functional complex is necessary for normal cell cycle progression and differentiation, as well as programmed cell death. *MYC* gene amplification or transcriptional dysregulation is often observed in SCLC and to a lesser degree in NSCLC. One member of the *MYC* family is amplified in 18% of SCLC tumors and 31% of cell lines, compared to 8% of NSCLC tumors and 20% of cell lines. Amplification appears more frequently in SCLC patients previously treated with chemotherapy, giving rise to the "variant" subtype of SCLC, and its presence correlates with adverse survival.[63] There are no MYC-specific drugs in development.

EML4-ALK fusion protein is a recently identified activating oncogenic driver of lung adenocarcinomas occurring in less than 5% of all NSCLC. It is formed by fusion of the N-terminal portion of the protein encoded by the echinoderm microtubule-associated protein-like 4 (*EML4*) gene with the intracellular signaling portion of the receptor tyrosine kinase encoded by the anaplastic lymphoma kinase (*ALK*) gene, resulting from a t(2:5) translocation.[21] Multiple *EML4-ALK* variants have been identified in lung cancer.[64–67] Similar to EGFR mutations, *EML4-ALK* fusions appear to occur almost exclusively in adenocarcinomas, specifically with acinar histology, in never or former light smokers.[65,68–70] *EML4-ALK* fusions do not occur in tumors with mutations in *EGFR* or *KRAS*, and patients appear to be of younger age compared to patients with *EGFR* mutations.[70] A variety of methods are currently being used to assess for the presence of the *EML4-ALK* fusion, including immunohistochemistry, FISH, and reverse transcription PCR (RT-PCR), however, each method has its own attributes and flaws and none has been adopted to date as a standard for testing. Several novel selective inhibitors of ALK kinase are in clinical development. A trial of crizotinib (PF-02341066), a dual MET/ALK inhibitor, in heavily pretreated patients with tumors that harbor the ALK fusion protein has resulted in a 57% response rate and 72% 6-month progression-free survival (PFS) with median PFS not reached at the time of report.[71] Phase 2 and 3 trials with this agent are currently under way.

TUMOR SUPPRESSOR GENES AND GROWTH SUPPRESSION

A number of TSGs have been identified that inhibit lung tumorigenesis or suppress key phenotypes in developed lung carcinomas. Germline mutations in some TSGs such as LKB1, *p53*, and *RB1* give rise to inherited tumor syndromes; however, somatic loss of TSGs within sporadic cancers is more commonly seen. Such genes can be lost through multiple mechanisms, such as inactivating mutations, chromosomal loss, methylation, or overexpression of other proteins that inhibit the suppressive gene's expression or activity. Many classical tumor suppressors, such as the three identified above, have been identified by decades of work examining genes involved in human-inherited cancer syndromes and elucidating their role in sporadic cancers. Many additional suppressor gene candidates have been identified as a result of profiling large numbers of tumors for loss of heterozygosity (LOH) using high-resolution comparative genomic hybridization systematically to look for recurrent regions of chromosomal loss. Results are expected in the next few years from whole genome sequencing of hundreds of tumors to identify novel mutations.

p53 PATHWAY

The *p53* gene, located at chromosome 17p13, is crucial for maintaining genomic integrity in the face of cellular stress from DNA damage through gamma and ultraviolet irradiation, carcinogens, and chemotherapy. It is the most frequently mutated TSG in human malignancies, and mutations affect approximately 90% of SCLCs and 50% of NSCLCs. In NSCLCs, p53 alterations occur more frequently in squamous cell (51%) and large cell (54%) carcinoma than adenocarcinomas (39%).[72] *p53* mutations have been linked to poorer prognosis retrospectively; however, they were not shown to correlate with survival in a prospective randomized clinical trial.[60,73] Most p53 mutations are G→T transversions, which correlate with cigarette smoking. A major cigarette smoke carcinogen, benzo(a)pyrene, selectively forms adducts at *p53* mutational hot spots.[2] The Li-Fraumeni syndrome of inherited germline *p53* mutation may also lead to increased susceptibility to lung cancer in adults; this risk is magnified by tobacco smoking, as carriers who smoked had a 3.16-fold higher risk for lung cancer than nonsmokers.[74] The majority of missense mutations occur in the DNA-binding domain of the protein, and five of the six most prevalently mutated sites are arginine residues that are involved with electrostatic interactions with DNA strands.[75] Missense mutations prolong the half-life of the p53 protein, leading to increased protein levels detectable with immunohistochemistry. Also, because p53 exerts its cellular actions as a tetramer, mutant forms of the protein appear to exert dominant negative effects on wild type p53 and have also been shown to inhibit the function of p63 and p73 family members.[76]

In addition to mutational or deletional loss of p53, other regulatory components of the p53 pathway are altered in lung cancer, including the ataxia-telangiectasia (*ATM*) gene, the p53 binding protein MDM2, and the p14[ARF] tumor suppressor. *ATM* and the related protein ATR are tumor suppressive serine/threonine kinases that activate cell cycle checkpoints in response to DNA damage and ultimately activate and stabilize p53.[77] Although ATR and the downstream checkpoint kinases (CHEK) are mutated in less than 1% of lung adenocarcinomas, ATM has been found to have deleterious mutations in 7% of lung adenocarcinomas; these mutations were largely mutually exclusive with p53 mutations, likely indicating that mutations in both genes would have redundant effects, especially since it has been shown that gain-of-function mutations in p53 can inactivate ATM.[78,79] Conversely, the MDM2 oncogene product negatively regulates p53 by binding its transcriptional activation domain, inducing its nuclear export, and by polyubiquitinating p53, marking it for proteasomal degradation.[80] Abnormal overexpression of MDM2 is found in NSCLC, where it is amplified in a significant number of tumors. MDM2 activity is inhibited by other tumor suppressor genes in the p53 pathway, including ATM and also the p14[ARF] tumor suppressor gene, which is often lost in lung cancer.[81]

When p53 is functional, it is activated by phosphorylation in response to cellular stress (e.g., DNA damage). Once activated, p53 strongly induces the expression of other tumor suppressor genes that control cell cycle checkpoints (e.g., *p21*[WAF1/CIP1]), apoptosis (*BAX*), DNA repair (*GADD45*), and angiogenesis (thrombospondin).[82] p53 activation has also been found to alter microRNA expression and maturation,[83] and some effects of p53 are mediated by the induced expression of the microRNA miR-34.[84] The high frequency of p53 loss across the entire spectrum of human tumors is a strong testament to its importance in inhibiting tumor development and growth. Restoring p53 activity in tumors is effective in halting their growth and could represent an effective therapy, although development of this strategy is challenging.[85] Several gene therapy clinical trials have been reported in which lung cancers are treated by intratumoral injection (endobronchially or by computed tomography–guided needle injection), introducing a wild type *p53* gene using retroviral or adenoviral vectors. Future therapeutic gains may come from combining gene and conventional therapies, but this approach may be limited to locoregional disease control.[86] Other strategies have been developed to restore p53 activity without attempting to reintroduce the entire gene into tumor cells. These include the use of small molecule inhibitors of the MDM2–p53 interface that prevent the degradation of wild type p53 and the use of peptides and small molecules that are intended to restore wild type conformation to mutated p53.[85,87] Immunologic targeting of cancer with vaccines is a different strategy that is potentially nontoxic and specific. Such a strategy takes advantage of novel protein sequences that result from p53 mutations, which can potentially be recognized as foreign epitopes by cytotoxic T cells mounting an immune response against a tumor. Vaccination of patients with advanced cancer with a custom vaccine corresponding to their tumor's mutation in *p53* or *RAS* has demonstrated the generation of mutant oncogene specific immune responses associated with prolonged survival.[88] A trial of p53 vaccination in SCLC produced measurable increases in tumor-specific immune response that was associated with improved outcome and response to therapy in some patients.[89,90]

CYCLINS AND CELL CYCLE REGULATORY PATHWAYS

p16^{INK4A} is a cyclin-dependent kinase (CDK) inhibitor important for the integrity of the G_1 checkpoint. Loss of p16^{INK4A} frees CDKs from inhibition, permitting constitutive phosphorylation of retinoblastoma (RB) protein and inactivation of its growth suppressive function. Approximately 40% of primary NSCLCs lose *p16^{INK4A}*, located on chromosome 9p21, making it the most common component of the p16^{INK4A}–cyclin D1–CDK4–RB pathway to be inactivated in NSCLC. Other CDK inhibitors are also lost at a lower prevalence in NSCLC, and the *RB* gene is mutated or lost in a significant minority of cases.[79] In contrast, a strikingly different pattern of pathway dysregulation is observed in SCLC, in which abnormalities in *p16* are rarely observed but *RB* itself is nearly always abnormal. Although *p16^{INK4A}* point mutations in NSCLCs were observed in only 14% of tumors, homozygous deletions or aberrant promoter methylation are common mechanisms for *p16^{INK4A}* inactivation.[22] Indeed, aberrant *p16^{INK4A}* methylation is a frequent, early preneoplastic event in the pathogenesis of squamous cell carcinomas.[91] Furthermore, *p16^{INK4A}* and *p14^{ARF}* are alternative splice forms of RNA transcripts from the same DNA locus. p14^{ARF} is also a tumor suppressor gene and functions to stabilize p53. Thus, alteration at the *p16^{INK4A}* locus may not only abrogate *p16^{INK4A}* function but also disrupt p53 pathway through *p14^{ARF}*.[92]

In the absence of inhibitory regulation by the CDK inhibitors, cyclins and their catalytic partners, the CDKs, phosphorylate the retinoblastoma protein, a growth-suppressive nuclear phosphoprotein located on chromosomal region 13q14. When in its active, unphosphorylated form, RB binds and inactivates proteins such as transcription factor E2F-1 preventing G_1/S transition. Mutations of one *RB* allele together with loss of the other wild type *RB* allele are frequently observed in SCLC. The RB protein is absent or structurally abnormal in more than 90% of SCLCs and 15% to 30% of NSCLCs. Lung-targeted, conditional deletion of *Rb* and *p53* in mice leads to development of SCLC that recapitulated that observed in humans.[93] Although the *p16* and *RB* tumor suppressive components of this pathway are frequently lost in lung cancer, the growth promoting cyclin and CDK components of the pathway are often overexpressed and cyclin D1, cyclin E1, and CDK4 have each been shown to be amplified in a subset of lung cancers[94] and are overexpressed by immunohistochemical evaluation.

LKB1, AMPK, mTOR Pathway

LKB1 is a serine/threonine kinase that serves as a "master regulator" of several key intracellular pathways through phosphorylation of downstream regulatory kinases. Its tumor suppressive role became apparent when it was discovered that inherited mutations in *LKB1* gave rise to a rare autosomal dominant polyposis/cancer susceptibility disease, Peutz-Jeghers syndrome. This disease is characterized by the development of many hamartomas polyps throughout the intestinal tract, abnormalities in mucocutaneous pigmentation, and a 20-fold increase in lifetime risk for cancer, including gastrointestinal, breast, and pancreatic neoplasia.[95,96] Subsequent to this discovery it was found that *LKB1* is somatically mutated and deleted in a range of other carcinomas, most prevalently in non–small cell lung carcinoma, where approximately 20% to 30% of adenocarcinomas exhibit *LKB1* loss.[97–99] Squamous cell and large cell lung carcinomas also exhibit *LKB1* loss, but at a lower frequency, and immunohistochemical analysis revealed absent LKB1 expression in two-thirds of SCLC.[100] In a mouse model, tumors rapidly develop when conditional *Lkb1* knockout was combined with conditional expression of oncogenic *Kras*, using inhaled adenovirus-expressing Cre recombinase. High penetrance and multiple tumors per animal were noted. More than half of the incident tumors are associated with metastases. Additionally, whereas most other mouse models of lung tumorigenesis (e.g., oncogenic *Kras* with conditional *p53* deletion) cause only lung adenocarcinomas, more than half of the tumors that result from *Kras* with conditional *Lkb1* deletion showed squamous or mixed histology, and large cell histology was also observed.[98]

LKB1 regulates a key metabolic checkpoint through its phosphorylation of the AMP activated protein kinase AMPK. AMPK is sensitive to conditions of hypoxia and nutrient deprivation; under these conditions, AMPK is phosphorylated by LKB1, resulting in suppression of tumor growth and metabolic activity by direct phosphorylation of metabolic enzymes and by activation of the tuberous sclerosis complex tumor suppressors, which block activation of the mammalian target of rapamycin (mTOR) pathway.[101] In tumors that have lost LKB1, this growth suppressive checkpoint is defunct. Resultant tumors show elevated activity of the mTOR pathway and may be selectively dependent on this pathway for growth, and pharmacologic activation of AMPK may also be a therapeutic target in these cancers.[102,103] Metformin, an oral hypoglycemic drug commonly used for diabetes, activates AMPK and has been found to inhibit proliferation and colony formation *in vitro*.[104] Retrospective analyses demonstrate reduced incidence of cancer among diabetics treated with metformin.[105–107] In addition, metformin treatment for diabetes is associated with higher rates of complete response among neoadjuvantly treated breast cancer patients.[108] Although metformin appears to require functional LKB1 in order to effect AMPK activation, other compounds have been identified that circumvent this requirement. Thus, direct pharmacologic reactivation of the downstream tumor suppressive functions of AMPK may be a viable therapeutic strategy for LKB1 deficient tumors.

In addition to its role in regulating the AMPK metabolic checkpoint, LKB1 has many other distinct roles dependent on other downstream effector kinases, such as salt-inducible kinase, NUAK, and microtubule-affinity regulating kinase. These actions play a role in regulating a variety of cellular phenotypes important to cancer, such as cellular motility and transcriptional regulation, and LKB1 has been shown to exert profound effects in maintaining cellular polarity.[109,110] However, the relative importance of these various phenotypes in the biology of LKB1-deficient lung cancers is poorly understood.

Other Putative Tumor Suppressors

Several other genes that are less well characterized than the tumor suppressor genes detailed above have been identified as targets of recurrent mutational inactivation, chromosomal loss, and epigenetic repression in lung cancer. These candidate suppressor genes are often identified as regions of copy number loss or LOH that occur in multiple tumors in large genome-wide studies of chromosomal architecture in lung cancer. Further experimentation is required to elucidate which molecular pathways and cellular phenotypes are affected and to define the functional importance of these candidates. Common regions of genomic loss surround the chromosomal regions of classical tumor suppressors *CDKN2A*, *CDKN2B*, *LKB1*, and *RB1* (in SCLC). Other areas of recurrent loss in NSCLC occur at 9p23, 3p14.2, 3p21.3 16q23.1, 2q21.2, 4q35, 5q12.1, and

13q12.11.[94] Many of these regions are also altered in SCLC, although there are fewer data available for this tumor type. Areas of deletion may encompass many genes in any individual tumors. Determining the functional roles of each individual gene can be challenging. However, peak regions can be identified that are most frequently included in the deleted region across multiple tumors, and key genes are thought to be most likely to be included in these regions. Furthermore, integrating multiple types of data can reveal genes that are somatically inactivated by methylation or mutation, in addition to chromosomal loss; these are also likely to be the key suppressive genes within a deleted region. Of genes included in the regions listed above, missense mutations have been identified in *PTPRD* (9p23), *LRP1B* (2q21.2), *BLU* (3p21.3), and WWOX (16q23.1).[111,112] Experimental reexpression of candidate genes has been shown to inhibit proliferation in tumor cell lines for many of these putative tumor suppressors, including *PTPRD*, *LRP1B*, *WWOX* (16q23.1), *FHIT* (3p14.2), *SMARCA4* (19p13.2), *PTEN* (10q23), and *RASSF1*, *FUS1*, *BLU*, and *SEMA3B* (3p21.3).[113,114] However, for most of these candidates the biological implications of gene loss in a tumor is uncertain. More research devoted to these targets is required to further elucidate the roles they may play in lung cancer biology with the goal of identifying driver pathways that may become activated in the absence of particular TSGs and may thus be effective targets for therapeutic intervention.

OTHER BIOLOGIC ABNORMALITIES IN LUNG CANCER

Cellular Immortality Resulting from Increased Telomerase Activity

Cellular senescence is mainly regulated by telomerase, a ribonucleoprotein enzyme responsible for maintaining telomere length by *de novo* synthesis of telomeres and elongation of existing telomeres. The human telomerase reverse transcriptase (hTERT) catalytic subunit is the major determinant of telomerase activity *in vitro* and *in vivo*. During normal cell division, telomere shortening leads to cell senescence and thus governs normal cell mortality. Telomerase reverse transcriptase maintains telomere ends via the synthesis of TTAGG nucleotide repeats. Telomerase activation is considered mandatory for tumor cells to escape senescence and contributes to immortalization and cancer pathogenesis. For example, immortalization of primary human airway epithelial cells can be achieved by the successive introduction of the simian virus SV40 early region and *hTERT*.[115] Malignant transformation is seen when these immortalized cells are transfected by an activated *RAS* oncogene. Approximately 100% of SCLCs and 80% to 85% of NSCLCs have been demonstrated to express high levels of telomerase activity. Furthermore, hTERT gene amplification occurs in 57% of NSCLCs, suggesting that this pathway is commonly targeted in lung cancer.[116] The prognostic significance of hTERT expression or activity remains controversial, although a recent study demonstrated that the copy number of serum *hTERT* mRNA was independently correlated with tumor size, tumor number, presence of metastasis, likelihood of recurrence, and smoking.[117] Furthermore, elevated telomerase activity and hTERT levels have been associated with worse disease-free and overall survival in patients with stage I NSCLC.[118] In preneoplastic lesions, telomerase activity or expression of its RNA component, or both, are observed *in situ* in lesions with the expression proportional to the severity of histology grade, supporting a temporal role for telomerase activation during lung preneoplasia.[119] Thus, telomerase activity or expression can be used as a potential biomarker to detect premalignant as well as tumor cells. For these reasons, there is much interest in developing antitelomerase drugs as new therapeutics. GV1001 and HR2882 are telomerase peptide vaccines that are being evaluated in clinical trials in patients with NSCLC.[120]

Deregulation of Apoptosis

Loss of normal apoptosis commonly occurs in many cancer types and is associated with expansion of viable cells and the development of resistance to chemotherapy and radiation therapy. Many members of both the mitochondrial (intrinsic) and the death receptor (extrinsic) apoptotic signaling pathways are found to be abnormal in lung cancer. A member of the intrinsic pathway, the antiapoptotic gene *BCL2* originally described in follicular lymphomas, is abnormally overexpressed in SCLC (75% to 95%) and some NSCLCs (25% of squamous cell carcinoma and approximately 10% of adenocarcinoma).[121–123] BCL2 expression was associated with good prognosis in NSCLC.[124] Cytotoxicity of many chemotherapeutic agents is induced through the BCL2 apoptotic pathway; overexpression of BCL2 is associated with increased resistance to these agents.[125,126] Given the role of BCL2 in suppressing apoptosis and in reducing the efficacy of chemotherapy and radiotherapy, considerable effort is being made to develop BCL2-targeted therapeutics in combination with chemotherapy. In early phase 1 studies in patients with SCLC, *BCL2* antisense was found to be well tolerated when combined with chemotherapy.[127] However, randomized phase 2 trials found no difference in outcome compared with that of chemotherapy alone.[128] Despite these discouraging results, a new class of oral BCL2 antagonists is current being developed.

In the extrinsic pathway, death receptors are members of the tumor necrosis factor (TNF) receptor gene superfamily that consists of more than 20 proteins with a broad range of biological functions, including regulation of cell death and survival, differentiation, or immune regulation. The best-characterized death receptor, Fas (CD95), and its ligand (FasL) have also been implicated in lung cancer. In general, lung cancers express FasL but not the receptor. However, as T cells express Fas, one model that may help explain the resistance of lung cancer cells to immune surveillance involves the clonal deletion of immune T cells that would otherwise be directed against lung cancer antigens by this Fas–FasL interaction. Both caspase-8 and caspase-10 expression appears to be decreased in lung cancer. Homozygous deletion or methylation of *CASP8* gene has been observed in SCLC cell lines, with 79% demonstrating loss of expression.[129] Polymorphisms in the promoter region of caspase-9 have been shown to contribute to risk of lung cancer development.[130] Inhibitors of apoptosis (IAPs) impede cell death through caspase function, especially caspase-3 and -7. IAPs also inhibit apoptosis via modulation of the transcription of nuclear factor κB. One of the best-known members of this class of protein is survivin. Its expression is high in tumor but nearly nonexistent in adult normal tissue. Suppression of survivin has been shown to sensitize lung cancer cells to radiation, suggesting that it can be a potential target for intervention.[131]

Invasion, Metastasis, and Angiogenesis

Investigation of the molecular mechanisms of invasion and metastasis has yielded a variety of candidate genes, including cell adhesion molecules such as the cadherins, integrins, and

CD44. The E-cadherin–catenin complex is critical for intercellular adhesiveness and maintenance of normal and malignant tissue architecture. Epigenetically reduced expression of this complex in malignant disease is associated with tumor invasion, metastasis, and unfavorable prognosis in lung cancer. Another family of adhesion molecules are the integrins. Integrin α_3 has been shown to be important for normal lung development and diminished expression correlated with a poor prognosis of patients with lung adenocarcinoma. Specific isoforms of CD44 may also be associated with lung cancer metastasis. Matrix metalloproteinases (MMPs) are zinc-dependent proteases that belong to a family of endopeptidases, which degrade the extracellular matrix and basement membrane, necessary first steps in angiogenesis. Increased expression of MMPs has been strongly implicated in tumor growth, invasion, and metastasis. MMP2 and MMP9 have been associated with poorer prognosis. However, despite its established role in invasion and metastasis, many randomized phase 3 trials of MMP inhibitors have failed to demonstrate a survival benefit in patients with advanced lung cancer.[132] This is perhaps related to the lack of specificity of these inhibitors and recent findings that some MMPs actually inhibit tumor growth.[133] Many of the genes that confer invasive and metastatic phenotypes are coordinately regulated by transcription factors such as ZEB and SNAIL, which can be activated by several stimuli, especially the actions of transforming growth factor-beta.[134] It has recently been shown that a key set of microRNAs of the miR-200 family plays a crucial role in regulating this phenotype.[135] The stimuli that regulate tumor cell invasiveness are often generated or influenced by surrounding stromal or inflammatory cells, and as such, the invasive phenotype seems to be quite plastic, complex, and highly dependent on the context of the tumor microenvironment.[136]

Angiogenesis, the formation of new blood capillaries, is necessary for a tumor mass to grow beyond a few millimeters in size. The angiogenic switch results from perturbation in the balance between inducers and inhibitors, both of which are produced by tumor and host cells. Vascular endothelial growth factor (VEGF), basic fibroblast growth factor (bFGF), and angiogenic cytokines, such as interleukin-8, have all been implicated in lung cancer.[137] Furthermore, high microvessel density (MVD) and VEGF overexpression are predictive of poor outcome. Thus, tumor angiogenesis has become a major new therapeutic target for lung cancer.[138] Clinical trials in lung cancer with agents targeting angiogenesis have shown great promise and have demonstrated that the addition of bevacizumab, the humanized monoclonal antibody to VEGF, to chemotherapy prolongs progression-free survival in phase 3 clinical trials, although improvements in overall survival were not always observed.[139–141]

CANCER STEM CELL HYPOTHESIS

The cancer stem cell hypothesis proposes that a self-renewing undifferentiated stem cell population that comprises a small fraction of the total tumor burden gives rise to more numerous and more differentiated progeny that populate the tumor.[142] Among the characteristics reported to distinguish stem-like cell from cells constituting the bulk of tumors include the potential for supporting the continued growth of the local tumor mass, for seeding metastases throughout the body, and resistance to cytotoxic therapies that allow the residual viable stem cells to repopulate the tumor after treatment. Because of their resistance to treatment and potential for seeding distant metastatic disease, the study of cancer stem cell and development of strategies effectively to eradicate all residual stem cells is of critical importance in cancer treatment.

Cancer stem-like cells can be isolated from a variety of tumor types using antibodies to unique cell surface proteins. They are capable of forming xenograft tumors at a high frequency after injection into immunocompromised mice. Empirically selected surface markers have been used to isolate putative stem cells from human breast cancer, glioblastoma multiforme, colon cancer, and other carcinomas, and these cells have demonstrably greater potential for xenograft formation than do unselected tumor cells. The resulting tumors recapitulate the histological appearance of the primary tumor as well as the heterogeneous expression of various surface and intracellular molecular markers.[142]

Putative lung progenitor cells have been described as cells that reside at the bronchoalveolar duct junction that express both Clara cell and pneumocyte markers or as lung resident cells of hematopoietic origin that express CD133.[143,144] These cells have not been conclusively shown to be lung adult stem cell populations but are intriguing and have been shown to be involved in repair of lung tissue after injury and may be involved in cancer development. In lung tumors, CD133[145–148] and other commonly used markers of stem-like tumor cells—Hoechst dye efflux and aldehyde dehydrogenase activity[149]—have been shown to identify subsets of tumor cells that display characteristics consistent with the cancer stem cell hypothesis. CD133 has been shown to segregate with template DNA in lung cells undergoing asymmetric cell division.[150] However, conflicting reports suggest that CD133 may not define a specific subset of cells, as interconversion between CD133+ and CD133− populations is observed, and CD133 expression may be associated with specific stages of cell cycle progression[151]; furthermore, some studies show no association between CD133 expression and propensity to initiate tumors.[152] The cancer stem cell hypothesis has other important gray areas as well; it is not yet certain whether a consistent developmental hierarchy would exist for every individual tumor or only in certain cases; whether or not lineage differentiation in a tumor can be a reversible; and which basic properties should be required to define a stem-like phenotype in a given population of cells. A highly increased propensity for xenograft formation is one of the most convincing features that can be demonstrated experimentally for proposed cancer stem-like cells. However, even the reliability of this evidence is called into question by the observation that a much higher rate of tumor formation is observed when mouse tumor lines are propagated in isogenic immunocompetent mice, which raises the possibility that the xenograft initiation phenotype may be related to the ability to adapt to the tissue environment of an immunocompromised mouse, rather than a general property of enhanced tumor formation.[153]

Nevertheless, the balance of evidence from diverse tumor types favors the hypothesis that stem-like cells are present within tumors and may play a key role in certain aspects of tumor biology. Furthermore, developmental pathways that are proposed to be important in governing cancer stem cell biology may be important oncogenic drivers of proliferation and invasion for unselected tumor cell populations in certain subsets of tumors, and are important avenues of research in their own right. For instance, the activity of particular genes—achaete-scute complex homologue 1[148] and OCT4 transcription factors[146]—have been implicated in regulating this subset of lung tumor cells. Given the far-reaching implications of the cancer stem cell hypothesis, and especially the concept that targeting developmental pathways cancer stem cells or in particular subsets of cancer could represent an important therapeutic strategy, these complex and exciting areas warrant further study in lung cancer.

GENOMIC ANALYSIS OF LUNG CANCER

In recent years technological advances in high-throughput sequencing approaches have enabled the comprehensive analyses of gene expression, copy number alterations, mutations, and other genetic perturbations across a large number of tumors. A number of studies have employed cDNA microarray chips to profile transcriptional expression in large sets of tumors. The largest such study of 443 lung adenocarcinomas from four institutions determined that clusters of coexpressed genes were consistently associated with patient outcome.[154] Prognostic profiles have been derived in several independent studies, although it is unclear how reproducible their associations are when applied to independent datasets. Associations with patient prognosis and response to treatment are potentially useful as an adjunct to classical staging approaches to help inform clinical decision making. For instance, when treating early stage tumors, adjuvant treatment may be more likely to benefit patients with a poor prognostic profile; whereas, a good prognostic profile could justify avoidance of adjuvant therapy. Although gene expression profiling of breast cancers has been validated and are widely used for making adjuvant treatment decisions, so far gene expression assays in lung cancer have not been validated prospectively as a useful guide for treatment planning.

Beyond prognostic associations, global approaches to the study of lung cancer have great potential as discovery tools that can increase the understanding of cancer biology and the molecular mechanisms underlying key cancer phenotypes. Arguably the most important outcome of such studies will be the identification of subsets of tumors whose biology can be affected by interventions targeted against key dysregulated genes or pathways. Hypotheses regarding such relationships can be derived from statistical associations between patterns of transcriptional regulation, copy number alterations, and mutations and tumor characteristics such as proliferative rate, tendencies for invasion and metastasis, response to therapy, and survival. Several large studies have already begun in search of clinically important genetic patterns. High-resolution analysis of copy number alterations has led to the identification of chromosomal regions that are frequently amplified or deleted in subsets of lung cancer encompassing regions containing key oncogenes and tumor suppressor genes such as *EGFR*, *KRAS*, *myc*, *p53*, and *LKB1*, as well as other candidate genes whose importance may become apparent after further study.[79,94] Microarray data from large cohorts of patients may reveal coordinately regulated sets of genes potentially associated with underlying dysregulation of particular pathways or cellular phenotypes. Such gene sets can be subjected to computational analyses to discover the biological and clinical significance (e.g., elucidation of specific oncogenic pathways, regulation of a transcription factors) *inter alia*. Furthermore, a greater depth of understanding may arise from coordinated analysis of multiple types of data from the same samples, greatly adding to the ability to interpret the significance of these data. For example, gene expression profiling has been carried out on tumors that have additionally been characterized by comparative genomic hybridization and extensive mutational sequencing[112,155] or by microRNA expression profiling.[156] It then becomes apparent that common mutations such *p53* and *EGFR*, as well as regions of amplification and deletion, are consistently associated with altered expression of particular sets of genes.

A special case regarding the value of confluence of multiple types of data is seen with the analysis of large panels of lung cancer cell lines. Complete microarray expression profiling of the available lung cancer cell lines is complemented by independent knowledge of chromosomal changes, sequencing of mutations in common and novel cancer-associated genes, and profiling of microRNA expression, characterization of promoter methylation patterns and protein expression, and other molecular data. These molecular data can then be integrated with phenotypic observations such as sensitivity to targeted or cytotoxic therapies,[157–159] pathway activation,[160] or response to various perturbations.[161] High throughput approaches have also been applied to genetic perturbations using short interfering RNA screens and to drug treatment of cell lines, and these data can give additional detail regarding functional significance of particular genes.[162,163] Discovery efforts in cell lines may then generate hypotheses that can be applied back to enhance the understanding of data from primary tumors. For instance, expression profiles altered by oncogenic HRAS have been shown to be similar to profiles observed in lung cancer patients with *KRAS* mutations.[160] Profiles thought to be associated with activation of PI3K seem to be up-regulated in normal bronchial epithelia from smokers with cancer compared with smokers without cancer.[164] However, caution must be taken in generating these signatures and interpreting published associations, since a particular set of genes may be nonspecifically associated with the phenotype of interest, or the association may only be observed in the context of the *in vitro* system used in the experiments.

Global analysis of cancer biology is now poised to make an important step forward as massively parallel sequencing technologies become less expensive and more widespread. These technologies enable the sequencing of entire cancer genomes, allowing comprehensive determination of somatic mutations, polymorphisms, alternative splicing events, and chromosomal fusions. When this has been applied to a sufficient number of lung cancer samples, recurrent genetic alterations should become evident that may represent pharmaceutical targets or may highlight deregulated pathways where therapeutic intervention could be effective. The Cancer Genome Atlas represents a large-scale implementation of this strategy, and when it is complete it will combine gene expression, copy number alterations, single nucleotide polymorphisms, methylation status, microRNA expression, and mutation sequencing into a single compendium of data from several hundred clinically annotated tumors from multiple sites, including squamous cell lung carcinoma.

MOLECULAR TOOLS IN THE LUNG CANCER CLINIC

The understanding of the molecular genetic changes in lung cancer pathogenesis is advancing rapidly. Many genetic abnormalities identified in lung cancer are common to other human cancers, while others appear more specific for lung cancer, perhaps because of characteristics of the cells of origin and the unique nature of carcinogen exposure. Where their biochemical function is known, the proteins rendered abnormal appear to fall into several growth regulatory pathways.[160] Thus, understanding of the fundamental workings and diverse molecular drivers of lung cancer is becoming clearer. A substantial effort has been made to translate the current scientific knowledge of these abnormalities from the bench to the bedside in order to improve patient outcomes. These approaches fall into three general categories:

1. Development of early detection tools to identify primary and recurrent disease to enable effective early treatment. Because lung cancer eventually develops in only one of ten cigarette smokers, the identification of persons with a

genetic susceptibility to lung cancer should allow targeting and intensification of smoking cessation, early detection, and chemoprevention efforts. To date screening trials applied to smokers at high risk for the development of lung cancer, including the use of spiral computed tomography scans, have not been documented to decrease mortality. The identification of genetic epidemiologic markers and acquired respiratory genetic alterations may help to identify the most at-risk individuals for screening and chemoprevention trials.

2. Development of new cancer-specific therapies based on knowledge of genetic abnormalities. These may include replacing or pharmacologically reactivating mutant tumor suppressor genes, development of new drugs targeting activated protooncogenes, interfering with autocrine or paracrine growth stimulatory loops, and inhibiting angiogenesis, metastasis, and antiapoptotic. Some new therapies may be highly effective as single agents in some patients. However, it is likely that for many patients combinations of two or more targeted or cytotoxic agents will be required to maximize clinical benefit; and determining the optimal combination of therapy for a given patient will be an additional challenge in the field.
3. Identification of prognostic and predictive biomarkers, such as the *EGFR* mutation and *ALK-EML4* fusion, previously described, that predict the response to specific therapies and prognosticate outcomes. Such tools will play an increasingly important role in selecting optimal treatment strategies as the number of molecularly targeted therapies expands.

Selected References

The full list of references for this chapter appears in the online version.

6. Truong T, Hung RJ, Amos CI, et al. Replication of lung cancer susceptibility loci at chromosomes 15q25, 5p15, and 6p21: a pooled analysis from the International Lung Cancer Consortium. *J Natl Cancer Inst* 2010;102:959.
11. Braakhuis BJ, Tabor MP, Kummer JA, Leemans CR, Brakenhoff RH. A genetic explanation of Slaughterís concept of field cancerization: evidence and clinical implications. *Cancer Res* 2003;63:1727.
12. Park IW, Wistuba, II, Maitra A, et al. Multiple clonal abnormalities in the bronchial epithelium of patients with lung cancer. *J Natl Cancer Inst* 1999;91:1863.
15. Virmani AK, Gazdar AF. Tumor suppressor genes in lung cancer. *Methods Mol Biol* 2003;222:97.
21. Soda M, Choi YL, Enomoto M, et al. Identification of the transforming EML4-ALK fusion gene in non–small cell lung cancer. *Nature* 2007;448:561.
32. Rosell R, Moran T, Queralt C, et al. Screening for epidermal growth factor receptor mutations in lung cancer. *N Engl J Med* 2009;361:958.
40. Swanton C, Futreal A, Eisen T. Her2-targeted therapies in non–small cell lung cancer. *Clin Cancer Res* 2006;12:4377s.
44. Potti A, Moazzam N, Ramar K, et al. CD117 (c-KIT) overexpression in patients with extensive-stage small-cell lung carcinoma. *Ann Oncol* 2003;14:894.
51. Schiller JH, Akerley WL, Brugger W, et al. Results from ARQ 197-209: a global randomized placebo-controlled phase II clinical trial of erlotinib plus ARQ 197 versus erlotinib plus placebo in previously treated EGFR inhibitor-naive patients with locally advanced or metastatic non–small cell lung cancer (NSCLC). *J Clin Oncol* 2010;28: (abst LBA7502).
59. Mascaux C, Iannino N, Martin B, et al. The role of RAS oncogene in survival of patients with lung cancer: a systematic review of the literature with meta-analysis. *Br J Cancer* 2005;92:131.
62. Ravi RK, Weber E, McMahon M, et al. Activated Raf-1 causes growth arrest in human small cell lung cancer cells. *J Clin Invest* 1998;101:153.
65. Koivunen JP, Mermel C, Zejnullahu K, et al. EML4-ALK fusion gene and efficacy of an ALK kinase inhibitor in lung cancer. *Clin Cancer Res* 2008;14:4275.
68. Inamura K, Takeuchi K, Togashi Y, et al. EML4-ALK lung cancers are characterized by rare other mutations, a TTF-1 cell lineage, an acinar histology, and young onset. *Mod Pathol* 2009;22:508.
80. Klein C, Vassilev LT. Targeting the p53-MDM2 interaction to treat cancer. *Br J Cancer* 2004;91:1415.
84. Raver-Shapira N, Marciano E, Meiri E, et al. Transcriptional activation of miR-34a contributes to p53-mediated apoptosis. *Molecular Cell* 2007;26:731.
88. Carbone DP, Ciernik IF, Kelley MJ, et al. Immunization with mutant p53- and K-ras-derived peptides in cancer patients: immune response and clinical outcome. *J Clin Oncol* 2005;23:5099.
89. Antonia SJ, Mirza N, Fricke I, et al. Combination of p53 cancer vaccine with chemotherapy in patients with extensive stage small cell lung cancer. *Clin Cancer Res* 2006;12:878.
91. Belinsky SA, Nikula KJ, Palmisano WA, et al. Aberrant methylation of p16(INK4a) is an early event in lung cancer and a potential biomarker for early diagnosis. *Proc Natl Acad Sci U S A* 1998;95:11891.
92. Zhang Y, Xiong Y, Yarbrough WG. ARF promotes MDM2 degradation and stabilizes p53: ARF-INK4a locus deletion impairs both the Rb and p53 tumor suppression pathways. *Cell* 1998;92:725.
97. Carretero J, Medina PP, Pio R, Montuenga LM, Sanchez-Cespedes M. Novel and natural knockout lung cancer cell lines for the LKB1/STK11 tumor suppressor gene. *Oncogene* 2004;23:4037.
100. Amin RMS, Hiroshima K, Iyoda A, et al. LKB1 protein expression in neuroendocrine tumors of the lung. *Pathol Int* 2008;58:84.
102. Mahoney CL, Choudhury B, Davies H, et al. LKB1/KRAS mutant lung cancers constitute a genetic subset of NSCLC with increased sensitivity to MAPK and mTOR signalling inhibition. *Br J Cancer* 2009;100:370.
106. Evans JMM, Donnelly LA, Emslie-Smith AM, Alessi DR, Morris AD. Metformin and reduced risk of cancer in diabetic patients. *BMJ* 2005;330:1304.
109. Baas AF, Kuipers J, van der Wel NN, et al. Complete polarization of single intestinal epithelial cells upon activation of LKB1 by STRAD. *Cell* 2004;116:457.
117. Miura N, Nakamura H, Sato R, et al. Clinical usefulness of serum telomerase reverse transcriptase (hTERT) mRNA and epidermal growth factor receptor (EGFR) mRNA as a novel tumor marker for lung cancer. *Cancer Sci* 2006;97:1366.
118. Marchetti A, Pellegrini C, Buttitta F, et al. Prediction of survival in stage I lung carcinoma patients by telomerase function evaluation. *Lab Invest* 2002;82:729.
120. Brunsvig PF, Aamdal S, Gjertsen MK, et al. Telomerase peptide vaccination: a phase I/II study in patients with non–small cell lung cancer. *Cancer Immunol Immunother* 2006;55:1553.
121. Adams JM, Cory S. The Bcl-2 apoptotic switch in cancer development and therapy. *Oncogene* 2007;26:1324.
122. Pezzella F, Turley H, Kuzu I, et al. Bcl-2 protein in non–small cell lung carcinoma. *N Engl J Med* 1993;329:690.
129. Shivapurkar N, Reddy J, Matta H, et al. Loss of expression of death-inducing signaling complex (DISC) components in lung cancer cell lines and the influence of MYC amplification. *Oncogene* 2002;21:8510.
130. Park JY, Park JM, Jang JS, et al. Caspase 9 promoter polymorphisms and risk of primary lung cancer. *Hum Mol Genet* 2006;15:1963.
142. Jordan CT, Guzman ML, Noble M. Cancer stem cells. *N Engl J Med* 2006;355:1253.
143. Germano D, Blyszczuk P, Valaperti A, et al. Prominin-1/CD133+ lung epithelial progenitors protect from bleomycin-induced pulmonary fibrosis. *Am J Respir Crit Care Med* 2009;179:939.
144. Kim CFB, Jackson EL, Woolfenden AE, et al. Identification of bronchioalveolar stem cells in normal lung and lung cancer. *Cell* 2005;121:823.
149. Jiang F, Qiu Q, Khanna A, et al. Aldehyde dehydrogenase 1 is a tumor stem cell-associated marker in lung cancer. *Mol Cancer Res* 2009;7:330.
150. Pine SR, Ryan BM, Varticovski L, Robles AI, Harris CC. Microenvironmental modulation of asymmetric cell division in human lung cancer cells. *Proc Natl Acad Sci U S A* 2010;107:2195.
158. Sos ML, Fischer S, Ullrich R, et al. Identifying genotype-dependent efficacy of single and combined PI3K- and MAPK-pathway inhibition in cancer. *Proc Natl Acad Sci U S A* 2009;106:18351.
162. Luo J, Emanuele MJ, Li D, et al. A genome-wide RNAi screen identifies multiple synthetic lethal interactions with the Ras oncogene. *Cell* 2009;137:835.
163. Whitehurst AW, Bodemann BO, Cardenas J, et al. Synthetic lethal screen identification of chemosensitizer loci in cancer cells. *Nature* 2007; 446:815.
164. Gustafson AM, Soldi R, Anderlind C, et al. Airway PI3K pathway activation is an early and reversible event in lung cancer development. *Sci Transl Med* 2010;2:26ra25.

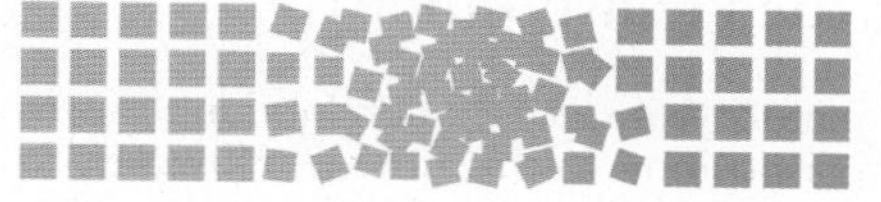

CHAPTER 75 NON–SMALL CELL LUNG CANCER

DAVID S. SCHRUMP, DARRYL CARTER, CHRISTOPHER R. KELSEY, LAWRENCE B. MARKS, AND GIUSEPPE GIACCONE

INCIDENCE

Lung cancer is one of the most common malignancies worldwide. During 2009, approximately 219,440 of an estimated 1,449,350 (15%) new cancer cases, and 159,390 of 562,340 (28%) total cancer deaths in the United States were attributable to lung cancer.[1] In the 40 countries comprising Europe, lung cancer accounts for 391,000 (12%) of approximately 3.2 million new cancer cases, and 19.9% (342,000) of cancer-related deaths.[2] Lung cancer is rapidly emerging as a major cause of mortality in the Middle East, Africa, and Asia as well.[3] Approximately 70,000 annual cancer-related deaths are currently attributed to lung cancer in Japan. More than 130,000 lung cancer deaths occur annually in China[4]; death rates attributable to this disease are expected to increase substantially over the next several decades.[5,6]

The incidence of lung cancer varies considerably among different ethnic populations throughout the world. Analysis of data from 22 cancer registries in 5 continents revealed that cumulative lung cancer risks were higher in males than females.[7] Among men, African Americans had the highest incidence of lung cancer risk (approximately 7.5%), whereas Swedes had the lowest cumulative risk (approximately 2%). Among women, cumulative lung cancer risk was highest in African Americans (approximately 3.5%), whereas French and Korean women had very low cumulative risks (approximately 1%). More recent data indicate that lung cancer rates for African Americans are converging with that of whites in the United States.[8] Lung cancer risks in East Asian female immigrants within the United States appear comparable to those observed in native populations.

ETIOLOGY

Smoking

Approximately 80% of cases of non–small cell lung cancer (NSCLC) in men and 50% of these neoplasms in women worldwide are directly attributable to cigarette smoking.[5] Age-adjusted lung cancer incidence rates range from 174 to 362, and 149 to 293 per 100,000 person-years for male and female active smokers, compared with 45 to 141 and 65 to 179 per 100,000 person-years for male and female former smokers, respectively. In contrast, age-adjusted lung cancer incidence rates range from 4.8 to 13.7 and 14.4 and 20.8 for male and female never-smokers, respectively.[9,10]

An estimated 1.3 billion people smoke worldwide.[11] In general, the incidence of lung cancer throughout the world reflects the prevalence of cigarette smoking, and evolving patterns of lung cancer appear attributable at least in part to filters, tar content, and other variations in tobacco blends.[12] Whereas tobacco consumption is decreasing in many industrialized nations, cigarette smoking has risen dramatically in developing countries, which lack resources for tobacco control and cancer care.[5,13]

The effects of cigarette smoke on respiratory epithelial cells are mediated by a complex mixture of organic as well as inorganic carcinogens present in the air/liquid interphase such as 4-(methylnitrosamino)-1-(3-pyridyl)-1-butanone (NNK) nicotine, benzo(a)pyrene, and cadmium, or vapor phase such as formaldehyde and ethylcarbamate.[14] Cigarette smoke condensate or purified activated tobacco carcinogens such as benzo(a) pyrene-diolepoxide-1 induce progressive genetic as well as epigenetic alterations coinciding with malignant transformation in cultured human respiratory epithelia.[15,16] Furthermore, purified tobacco carcinogens including NNK and ethylcarbamate induce pulmonary carcinomas in rodents exhibiting histologic and molecular genetic profiles virtually identical to human lung cancers.[17] NNK induces expression of type 1 insulin growth factor receptor and activates AKT signaling in respiratory epithelial cells[18,19]; in addition, NNK activates *k-ras*, and up-regulates DNA methyltransferase activity in pneumocytes *in vitro* and *in vivo*.[17,20] Polyaromatic hydrocarbonsin tobacco smoke forms DNA adducts, inducing mutations within tumor suppressor genes such as the *p53*, *RASSF1A*, and *FHIT*, thereby disrupting cell cycle regulation, DNA repair, and apoptosis. The carcinogenic effects of tobacco smoke are not simply related to NNK and polycyclic aromatic hydrocarbon (PAH), but are also directly attributable to nicotine as well as inorganic metals such as nickel, arsenic, and chromium.[14] For example, nickel and arsenic induce cancer-associated epigenetic alterations, whereas nicotine activates AKT, ERK, and PKC signaling,[21] and enhances beta arrestin-1–mediated activation of Src as well as c-fos. Furthermore, nicotine activates raf-1 kinase, promoting cell-cycle progression in respiratory epithelial cells.

During the past 3 decades, the prevalence of smoking in the United States has declined significantly. In 2008, the smoking rate for persons older than 18 years was approximately 20%, compared to 42% in 1965.[22] Prevalence of cigarette abuse varies among population groups, being highest in Native Americans and Alaskan natives (37%), intermediate for whites and African Americans (25%), and lowest among Hispanic Americans (18%) and Asian Americans (16%). In general, smoking is more prevalent in males, and is associated with low socioeconomic status and educational level.[22] In the European Union, prevalence of smoking varies among different populations and coincides with low socioeconomic status, particularly in women.[23] In Asia, smoking continues to be far more prevalent in males.[5]

Most cigarettes consumed worldwide contain filters, which reduce tar within inhaled smoke, resulting in deposition of carcinogens deeper in the lungs. In addition, modern tobacco blends contain higher amounts of nitrates, which on burning, form nitrosamines such as NNK. Smokers who convert to low-tar and nicotine (low-yield) cigarettes often compensate by smoking more cigarettes, puffing more vigorously, and inhaling deeper.[24] These data account, in part, for the emergence of adenocarcinomas as the dominant lung cancer histology during these past several decades. The cancer prevention study II trial, which involved more than 940,000 individuals 30 years of age or older who were either current, former, or never-smokers, revealed that lung cancer risk is highest in people smoking high-tar (22 mg or more) nonfilter brands, compared to medium tar (>15 mg) cigarettes.[25] Surprisingly, lung cancer risk for smokers of low-tar or very low-tar cigarettes appears comparable to risk in smokers of medium-tar blends. Menthol does not appear to increase lung cancer risk.

Lung cancer risk is related to duration as well as intensity of smoking. Persistent smokers exhibit a 16-fold increase in cumulative lung cancer risk; this risk is doubled for individuals who initiate smoking before age 15.[26] Data from the cancer prevention study II trial indicate that smoking one pack of cigarettes per day for 30 years increases the risk of lung cancer–specific mortality 20- to 60-fold in men, and 14- to 20-fold in women compared with never-smokers; the risk nearly doubles if consumption persists for 40 years.[27] Lung cancer risk depends more on duration rather than intensity of smoking in individuals with comparable pack-year tobacco exposures; whereas the relationship between the number of cigarettes smoked per day and lung cancer risk appears relatively linear, lung cancer risk varies exponentially with duration of tobacco exposure.[28]

Lung cancer risk in smokers can be significantly diminished in a time-dependent manner following smoking cessation. Analysis of a large cohort of U.S. veterans revealed that the relative risk of lung cancer in former smokers compared with never-smokers is approximately 16 for the first 5 years of abstinence, 8 for the next 5 years, and gradually declines to 2 during the next 30 years.[27,29] More recent studies confirm that cessation of smoking in middle life reduces risk of subsequent lung cancer.[30]

Whereas the link between tobacco and lung cancer risk is well established for people who actively smoke, the relationship between environmental tobacco smoke (ETS) exposure (passive smoking) and lung cancer risk in nonsmokers appears somewhat more controversial.[31,32] Individuals exposed to ETS inhale tobacco carcinogens at levels significantly lower than active smokers. Nonsmokers exposed to ETS excrete tobacco-specific carcinogens in the urine at levels 1% to 5% of those detected in active smokers.[33,34] Nevertheless, ETS is genotoxic[35]; numerous case-control as well as cohort studies indicate that ETS increases lung cancer risk, and currently contributes to 20% to 50% of lung cancers in never-smokers in the United States.[32,36]

Incontrovertible evidence linking cigarette smoking with lung cancer and the devastating social and economic impact of tobacco abuse[13,37] have prompted many countries to initiate programs to decrease tobacco addiction. These efforts have included legislation regulating tobacco components, increasing taxes on cigarettes, banning of tobacco advertisements and smoking in public places, and development of smoking-cessation clinics. In addition, educational programs have been implemented in schools to limit the number of adolescents who start smoking, because if individuals do not initiate smoking as adolescents, they are unlikely to smoke thereafter. Such tobacco control efforts appear to be impacting favorably on smoking prevalence in the United States as well as other developed countries.[22] Smoking prevalence and lung cancer death rates in the United States correlate inversely with state tobacco control efforts.[38] From 1988 to 2004, lung cancer death rates in California fell four times faster that the rest of the United States, and teenage smoking prevalence was the second lowest in the United States from a combination of cigarette taxation and evolving social norms.[39] Additional studies suggest that full implementation of simple population measures to curtail cigarette smoking could dramatically reduce lung cancer mortality in the United Kingdom.[40] Worldwide implementation of tobacco control will be a formidable and expensive undertaking.[13]

Genetic Predisposition

The fact that only a minority of smokers develop lung cancer suggests a genetic predisposition to this disease. However, to date, the genes conferring susceptibility to this disease have not been fully elucidated. A two- to threefold increased risk of lung cancer has been observed among first-degree relatives of probands with this disease[41]; risk appears most pronounced in individuals with nonsmoking family members who develop lung cancer at an early age, and in families with multiple afflicted members.[42] An ill-defined gene locus mapping to chromosome 6q confers susceptibility to lung cancer, particularly in never-smokers, and individuals with cumulative tobacco exposures to 20 or less pack-years; additional susceptibility loci map to 1q, 8q, and 9p.[43] Several recent genome-wide association studies have identified major susceptibility loci at 15q25, 5p15, and 6p21.[44,45] The 15q25 locus contains genes encoding the nicotinic acetylcholinergic receptor subunits CHRNA3 and CHRNA5; interestingly, the association of this locus with lung cancer risk persists after adjusting for smoking.[44]

Individuals with germ line mutations affecting expression of genes regulating cell-cycle progression or response to DNA damage appear to have increased lung cancer risk. For example, a threefold increase in lung cancer risk has been observed in patients with Li-Fraumeni syndrome who smoke relative to smokers without *p53* germ line mutations.[46] Survivors of hereditary retinoblastoma, particularly those treated with chemotherapy as well as radiation, have significantly elevated risks of lung cancer, which cannot be attributed solely to tobacco use.[47–49] A germ line *EGFR* T790M mutation has been observed in a family with multiple members, some of whom were smokers that developed bronchoalveolar carcinomas. Interestingly, lung tumors from these patients exhibited a second activating mutation in *cis* with the T790M mutation.[50]

A variety of single nucleotide polymorphisms (SNPs) affecting expression and/or function or enzymes regulating metabolism of tobacco carcinogens, DNA repair, or inflammation appear to influence lung cancer risk. In some studies, the effects of individual polymorphisms appear to be more evident in female nonsmokers, or patients with prolonged ETS exposure.[51–53] For example, the *CYP1B1* SNPre1056836 correlates with early-onset lung cancer in women.[54] In contrast, a polymorphism that results in complete loss of *CYP2A6* expression appears to be associated with reduced lung cancer risk.[55] Additional studies have demonstrated an eightfold higher lung cancer risk in patients with *CYPA1*23* or *CYP1A1*4* with double deletion of *GSTM1* and *GSTT1*. Among never-smokers, the combination of *CYP1A1*4* with double deletion of *GSTM1* and *GSTT1* was associated with a 16-fold increased risk of lung cancer relative to nonsmokers who did not exhibit these polymorphisms.[56] An SNP involving 13q31.3 that results in decrease expression of *GPC5* in normal lung tissues correlates with increased lung cancer risk in never-smokers.[57]

Additional studies indicate that polymorphisms involving genes that regulate DNA repair such as *XRCC1* (x-ray cross-complementing group 1) and *ERCC2* (excision repair cross complementing group 2) may also be associated with increased risk of lung cancer. For example, a polymorphism of *XRCC3* producing a variant T allele genotype appears to significantly increase lung cancer risk in African Americans and Mexican Americans (odds ratio = 5.2, 1.6–17); lung cancer risk in these individuals is markedly increased by heavy smoking (odds ratio = 37.3).[58] Analysis of more than 100 SNPs in 300 lung cancer patients in central and eastern Europe revealed modest but statistically significant associations regarding lung cancer risk and SNPs involving genes mediating DNA damage response (such as *ATM*) and mismatch repair (*LIG1, LIG3, MLH1,* and *MSH6*).[59] A more recent study of 37 SNPs in 23 genes regulating DNA damage repair identified three variants (XRCC1 194 Trp homozygotes, RAD 239 Arg heterozygotes, and POL delta 1 194 His homozygotes) that were associated with increased risk of lung cancer.[60]

Several polymorphisms affecting genes regulating chromatin structure also influence lung cancer risk. For example, skewed X chromosome inactivation in peripheral blood cells correlates with early development of lung cancer in women.[61] In addition, a polymorphism regulating expression of *DNA methyltransferase 3b (DNMT3b)* is associated with increased lung cancer risk.[62] Furthermore, several polymorphisms involving *methyl CpG binding domain 1* (*MBD1*) correlate with increased risk of lung cancer, particularly adenocarcinoma,[63] whereas a polymorphism within the 3′ UTR of *SUV39H2*, which encodes a histone lysine methyltransferase, correlates with increased risk of squamous cell carcinomas in Asian patients.[64]

Occupational/Environmental Exposure

A variety of occupational and environmental exposures have been implicated in the pathogenesis of lung cancer. These include asbestos and silica fibers, organic compounds such as chloral methyl ether and PAHs, diesel fumes and air pollution, metals such as chromium and nickel, arsenic, and ionizing radiation. Assessment of risk related to individual occupational/environmental factors is difficult because of imprecise methodologies for quantifying prolonged low-level exposure, the latency between exposure and cancer, and exposure to other factors such as smoking, which confound the analysis. In general, cigarette smoking potentiates the effects of many occupational/environmental carcinogens. These issues are comprehensively reviewed in several recent articles.[32,65,66]

Numerous studies have demonstrated a significant increase in lung cancer risk in individuals with occupational exposure to asbestos or silica.[67,68] All of the common types of commercial asbestos have been associated with lung cancer, with an apparent dose-response relationship and a long latency period. Smokers with lung cancer have higher pulmonary asbestos levels compared to nonsmokers with lung cancer,[69] a phenomenon that might explain the multiplicative effects of cigarette smoking and asbestos on lung cancer risk. Lung cancer risk increases with cumulative exposure to silica.[68] However, unlike asbestos, silica exposure does not appear to exhibit multiplicative effects with smoking.

A variety of metals including nickel, cobalt, cadmium, and chromium have been implicated as potential pulmonary carcinogens.[66,70] Exposure to these metals typically occurs among foundry workers and welders, with lung cancer risk appearing to be increased in individuals with high levels of exposure. The mechanisms by which these metals induce lung cancer appear complex, and the effects of these agents may be potentiated by cigarette smoke.[71] Nickel and cobalt induce oxidative stress in cultured cells, and up-regulate expression of hypoxia-inducible factor and downstream hypoxia-related genes through reactive oxygen species-independent mechanisms.[72] Furthermore, nickel enhances mutagenesis mediated by benzo-a-pyrene-diol epoxide, the active metabolite of benzo-a-pyrene via inhibition of nucleotide excision repair.[73] Nickel also mediates epigenetic silencing of tumor suppressor genes.[74,75] These recent observations explain, in part, the mechanisms by which nickel and tobacco smoke exhibit multiplicative effects regarding lung cancer risk.[76]

Inhalation or ingestion of arsenic increases lung cancer risk. Inhalation often occurs in foundry workers, whereas ingestion typically results from drinking well water; arsenic-induced lung cancers exhibit a long latency period.[77] A recent 50-year study of lung cancer mortality in Chile revealed a relative risk of approximately 3.5 for men and women living in regions containing high levels of arsenic in well water.[78] Additional studies pertaining to arseniasis-endemic areas in the United States and Asia have demonstrated similar dose-dependent relative risks.[79,80] Arsenic mediates a variety of epigenetic alterations including aberrant DNA as well as histone lysine methylation,[81] and appears to exhibit synergistic effects with cigarette smoking regarding risk of lung cancers, squamous cell and small cell lung cancers, but not adenocarcinomas.[82–84]

Ionizing radiation resulting from high-energy transfer agents such as neutrons, plutonium, or radon, as well as low-energy transfer sources such as x-rays and gamma rays increases lung cancer risk. An increased incidence of lung cancer has been observed among atomic bomb survivors.[85] Furthermore, uranium miners have markedly increased rates of lung cancer development, with radon (an inert gas resulting from radioactive decay of uranium) and cigarette smoking exhibiting synergistic effects.[86] Alpha particles emitted by radon progeny induce DNA mutations, epigenetic alterations, and chromosomal breaks. Of particular concern is radon exposure in household dwellings. Although residential radon levels are 50- to 100-fold less than the lowest levels in uranium mines, indoor radon exposure contributes to 10% to 14% of lung cancer cases per year in the United States.[32,87]

The effects of low-energy transfer radiation appear variable. Minimal increases in lung cancer risk have been observed in patients with ankylosing spondylitis who received radiation treatments over prolonged periods. In contrast, lymphoma and breast cancer patients receiving high doses of external-beam radiation to axillary, supraclavicular, or mediastinal lymph nodes exhibit increased susceptibility to lung cancer.[88] The latency period for radiation-induced lung cancers is approximately 5 to 10 years, and these tumors typically are highly aggressive. Lung cancer risk in Hodgkin's lymphoma or breast cancer correlates with doses and fields of radiation, and is significantly increased by exposure to alkylating agents and smoking history.[88] A recent case control study revealed a 4.3- to sevenfold increase in lung cancer risks in Hodgkin's lymphoma patients receiving alkylating agents and more than 0.05 Gy to the region of the lung that developed lung cancer, relative to those patients who had minimal lung exposure and were never or light smokers. Relative risk increased to 17- to 20-fold in patients who smoked more than one pack per day. Relative risk of lung cancer increased 50-fold in patients who smoked one pack per day, and received more than 0.05 Gy to the affected lung as well as alkylating agents.[89,90]

Breast cancer patients undergoing radiation therapy exhibit a 1.5- to threefold increased risk of lung cancer in the ipsilateral lung. Risk appears most associated with patients who received postmastectomy radiation therapy, and is compounded by cigarette smoking.[88,91] A recent population-based case-control study revealed an adjusted odds ratio of 5.9 (2.7–12.8) for average smokers who did not receive postmastectomy radiation therapy, compared to 18.9 (95% confidence interval: 7.9–45.4) for average smokers receiving postmastectomy radiation therapy. Adjusted odds ratios were 10.5 for the contralateral lung and 37.6 for the ipsilateral lung.[92] The impact of external-beam radiation on lung cancer risk is expected to diminish because of recent decreases in radiation therapy doses and improved delivery techniques.

Numerous studies have been performed to define the risk of lung cancer associated with exposure to specific pollutants in environmental air such as metals from smelting and refining industries, as well as PAH and particulate carcinogens resulting from combustion of fossil fuels. These studies have been difficult to control for all potential confounding variables. A well-designed, prospective, cohort study involving more than 8,000 men from six United States cities demonstrated a positive correlation between air pollution and lung cancer risk (adjusted mortality rate ratio = 1.26). Although several studies have suggested a correlation between increasing vehicle density and lung cancer risk, others studies have failed to demonstrate a consistent correlation between diesel exhaust and lung cancer risk.[93] Recent analysis of an ongoing Netherlands Cohort Study on Diet and Cancer involving more than 114,000 subjects revealed no apparent association between nitrogen dioxide or sulfur dioxide exposure and lung cancer risk, although a relative risk of 1.1 to 1.5 was observed for chronic exposure to black smoke or traffic.[94] An increased lung cancer risk has been reported for people living in U.S. counties with lead, copper, or zinc smelting and refining industries. Increased lung cancer risk has also been observed in individuals working in, or residing near, nonferrous smelters.[95,96]

Diet

Observations in the 1970s that lung cancer patients had low levels of vitamin A prompted intense interest in the potential role of diet in modulating lung cancer risk. Subsequent studies suggested that by inhibiting DNA damage, antioxidant micronutrients might reduce lung cancer risk. As with occupational/environmental risk factors previously addressed, the potential impact of dietary factors in terms of reducing lung cancer risk is difficult to assess because of the overwhelming carcinogenic effects of tobacco smoke.[32,97] Of particular interest in this regard are the effects of fruits and vegetables, as well as micronutrients such as retinols, carotenoids, vitamin C, and folate.

Data regarding fruit and vegetable consumption and lung cancer risk are somewhat contradictory. A protective effect of fruit consumption has been suggested in some, but not all, studies.[27,32] Recent analysis of more than 450,000 participants in the European Prospective Investigation into Cancer and Nutrition Study revealed an inverse correlation between variety of fruit and vegetable consumption and lung cancer risk among current smokers (hazard ratio [HR] = 0.77; 95% CI: 0.64–0.94).[98] Tang et al.[99] observed a significant inverse correlation between cruciferous vegetable intake and risk of lung cancer, particularly squamous cell carcinoma in smokers, implying that isothiocyanates modulate the effects of tobacco carcinogens. In a pooled analysis of seven cohort studies, Mannisto et al.[100] observed no association between α-carotene, β-carotene, lutein/zeaxanthin, lycopene, and lung cancer risk. Intake of β-cryptoxanthin, present in citrus fruits, was associated with moderate reduction in lung cancer risk.

Zinc, copper, and selenium intake appears to be associated with reduced lung cancer risk, although associations appear to be modest and differ in terms of minerals and patient subgroups.[101,102] The effects of folate intake and lung cancer risk are controversial. Pooled analysis of eight prospective studies revealed no association between folate intake and lung cancer risk.[103] A recent prospective cohort study of more than 55,000 Danish men revealed an unexpected, significant positive correlation between dietary folate intake and lung cancer risk.[104] On the other hand, Shen et al.[105] observed that dietary folate intake in lung cancer patients was significantly lower in lung cancer patients compared with matched normal controls ($P < .001$), and that dietary intake above the control median value was associated with a 40% reduction in lung cancer risk. The inverse correlation between dietary folate intake and lung cancer risk appeared most pronounced in patients who drank alcohol, smoked more, did not take supplemental folate, and had a family history of lung cancer. Consistent with these observations, a recent study involving more than 1,000 current and former smokers in the Lovelace Smokers Cohort revealed that folate levels and use of multivitamins protected against promoter methylation in respiratory epithelia.[106]

PATHOLOGY

The designation *non–small cell carcinoma of the lung* refers to a large group of disparate pulmonary neoplasms that are often associated with cigarette smoking and share the common property of being less responsive to small cell carcinoma treatment protocols (Table 75.1). Through the 1960s, the predominant type of NSCLC was squamous cell carcinoma, but adenocarcinoma has increased in both relative and absolute incidence, a phenomenon that has been temporally associated with changes in tobacco blends and the use of filters on cigarettes.[107]

Adenocarcinoma

The shift to adenocarcinoma has changed the clinical presentation and means of detection of early stage NSCLC. Nearly all adenocarcinomas arise in the smaller airways histologically, and can be detected radiographically, especially with computed tomography (CT) scan, in the periphery of the lung. They are less likely to present with cough and hemoptysis, and are less amenable to detection by sputum cytology or bronchoscopy, but more accessible to CT-guided fine-needle aspiration (FNA). The 2004 World Health Organization (WHO) Histologic Typing of Lung Cancers recognizes 14 subtypes of adenocarcinoma of the lung, but only a few types account for the great majority of cases (Fig. 75.1). Most adenocarcinomas of the

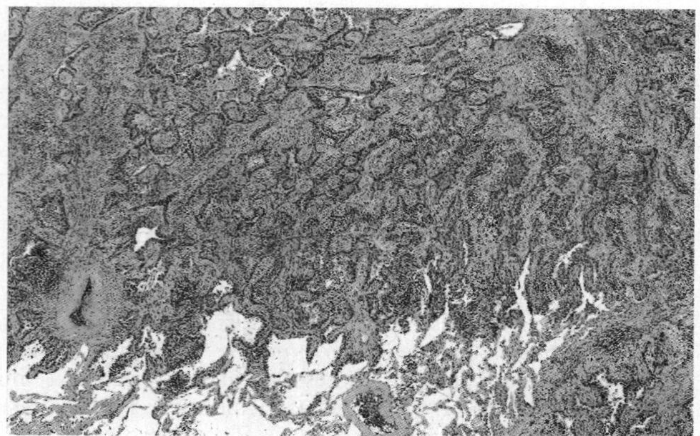

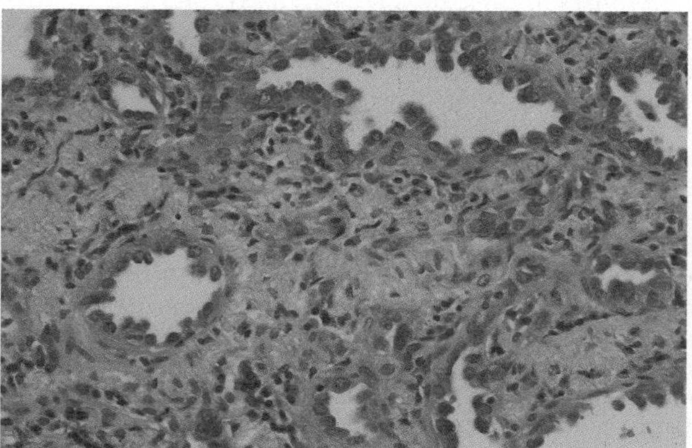

FIGURE 75.1 Adenocarcinoma. **A:** Mixed type including acinar pattern with evidence of stromal invasion and a peripheral bronchoalveolar carcinoma pattern. **B:** At higher magnification, the proliferating fibroblasts in the stroma of the acinar component of the carcinoma are evident.

TABLE 75.1

WORLD HEALTH ORGANIZATION HISTOLOGIC CLASSIFICATION OF EPITHELIAL TUMORS OF THE LUNG

PREINVASIVE LESIONS
Squamous dysplasia/carcinoma *in situ*
Atypical adenomatous hyperplasia
Diffuse idiopathic pulmonary neuroendocrine cell hyperplasia
INVASIVE MALIGNANT LESIONS
Squamous cell carcinoma
Variants
Papillary
Clear cell
Small cell
Basaloid
Small cell carcinoma
Variant
Combined small cell carcinoma
Adenocarcinoma
Acinar
Papillary
Bronchioloalveolar carcinoma
Nonmucinous (Clara cell/type II pneumocyte) type
Mucinous (goblet cell) type
Mixed mucinous and nonmucinous (Clara cell/type II pneumocyte and goblet cell) type, or indeterminate cell type
Solid adenocarcinoma with mucin formation
Adenocarcinoma with mixed subtypes
Variants
Well-differentiated fetal adenocarcinoma
Mucinous ("colloid") adenocarcinoma
Mucinous cystadenocarcinoma
Signet ring adenocarcinoma
Clear cell adenocarcinoma
Large cell carcinoma
Variants
Large cell neuroendocrine carcinoma
Combined large cell neuroendocrine carcinoma
Basaloid carcinoma
Lymphoepitheliomalike carcinoma
Clear cell carcinoma
Large cell carcinoma with rhabdoid phenotype
Adenosquamous carcinoma
Carcinomas with pleomorphic, sarcomatoid, or sarcomatous elements
Carcinomas with spindle or giant cells
Pleomorphic carcinoma
Spindle cell carcinoma
Giant cell carcinoma
Carcinosarcoma
Pulmonary blastoma
Carcinoid tumors
Typical carcinoid
Atypical carcinoid
Carcinomas of salivary gland type
Mucoepidermoid carcinoma
Adenoid cystic carcinoma
Others
Unclassified

From Travis WD, Colby TD, Corrin B. *Histologic Typing of Lung and Pleural Tumors—The World Health Organization (WHO) Classification of Lung Cancer 1999* (rev. 10 October 1998). Geneva: World Health Organization, 1999, with permission.

lung immunostain in the nucleus for thyroid transcription factor-1 and in the cytoplasm for carcinoembryonic antigen.

The histologic precursor to pulmonary adenocarcinoma is considered to be atypical adenomatous/alveolar hyperplasia (AAH).[108] Typically found incidentally in pulmonary specimens removed for other, more advanced, neoplasms, AAH measures less than 5 mm in diameter, and is composed of atypical type II pneumocytes proliferating on an alveolar wall that is either normal in thickness or altered by inactive fibrous scarring. There is a histologic spectrum between AAH and small nonmucinous bronchioloalveolar carcinoma (BAC), and these neoplasms are difficult to differentiate in small samples by cytologic, histologic, and genetic techniques. Lesions 5 mm in diameter or less are usually made up of relatively small cells with limited nuclear atypia in comparison to larger lesions, which exhibit correspondingly greater degrees of pleomorphism. The frequency and rate of progression of AAH to adenocarcinoma is uncertain, but considered to be low.

Bronchioloalveolar Carcinoma

BAC is a term that has been used loosely over the years, but the 1999 WHO Classification of Lung Tumors specified BAC as a noninvasive carcinoma spreading on the surface of alveolar walls without invasion. It is found in mucinous and nonmucinous variants. Mucinous BAC is an unusual variant characterized by the presence of malignant mucus-containing goblet cells on the surface of normal alveolar walls; it has a tendency to be multifocal or to spread through the airways and carries a high mortality rate. Nonmucinous BAC is much more commonly found, is composed of type II pneumocytes or Clara cells exhibiting nuclear anaplasia and pleomorphism greater than AAH, but less than invasive adenocarcinoma. The malignant cells spread over the alveolar walls in a monolayer, which presents a barrier to gas exchange in the affected alveolar sac, leading to right to left intrapulmonary shunt (Fig. 75.2). Although relatively uncommon, BACs have been the focus of intense research during recent years. These cancers, particularly those arising in nonsmoking females of Asian descent, exhibit unique epidermal growth factor (EGFR) mutations that confer exquisite sensitivity to EGFR-tyrosine kinase inhibitors (EGFR-TKI) such as erlotinib and gefitinib.[109]

Early-stage peripheral adenocarcinomas have also been studied and reported as having a good prognosis. Noguchi et al.[110] reported five different subtypes (A through E) of small, stage I adenocarcinomas. In type A, BAC proliferates on the alveolar surface of essentially normal alveolar walls, whereas

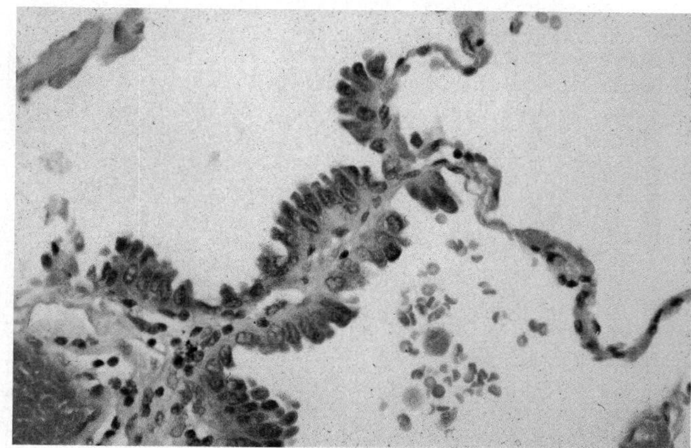

FIGURE 75.2 Bronchoalveolar carcinoma (BAC). Malignant columnar cells spread on the surface of a normal alveolar wall. The alveolar wall shows no evidence of reaction to or invasion by the carcinoma.

in type B, alveolar walls are scarred with well-established collagen or elastotic fibers, which are considered evidence of parenchymal collapse, but they are free of proliferating fibroblasts.[111] Types A and B were associated with a 100% survival rate and are considered noninvasive or carcinoma *in situ*, and therefore incapable of metastasizing because they have not invaded the stroma or angiolymphatic vessels of the lung. Their lepidic growth pattern, however, allows for spread within the airways. When invasive carcinoma is present, the term *BAC* should not be used. Thus defined, BAC is an uncommon type of adenocarcinoma of the lung.

However, a BAC pattern is much more often seen at the periphery of invasive types of adenocarcinoma in a *mixed subtype*, which includes acinar (gland-forming), papillary, and solid patterns. Vazquez et al.[111] named these mixed carcinomas as type C, with the discriminating feature of a desmoplastic stroma, considered evidence of invasion. Five-year mortality rates for patients with Noguchi type C adenocarcinomas approximate 20%, indicating a capacity of these neoplasms to invade angiolymphatic spaces, and to metastasize to lymph nodes and other sites. Types D and E adenocarcinomas have progressively higher nuclear and histologic grades in an invasive stroma and correspondingly higher mortality rates. Other authors have confirmed this work. Adenocarcinomas with a predominant BAC pattern, but limited areas of invasion also have a good prognosis, analogous to microinvasive carcinomas described in other organs.

Fetal adenocarcinomas are rare tumors that resemble the developing lung in the pseudoglandular period and are characterized by primitive bronchilike structures lined by columnar cells with subnuclear vacuoles rich in glycogen.[112]

Three other subtypes of primary pulmonary adenocarcinoma stress the ever-present differential diagnosis of primary from metastatic adenocarcinoma. Primary mucinous adenocarcinomas are composed of goblet cells and may mimic colon cancers both histologically and immunohistochemically; signet ring carcinomas with single cells and small groups with anaplastic nuclei and eccentric intracellular vacuoles of mucous resemble gastric carcinomas.[113] Clear cell carcinoma with centrally placed nucleus in a clear cytoplasm may be mistaken for renal cell carcinoma.[114] Distinctions are often made on clinical grounds with recognition of a prior or concurrent extrapulmonary carcinoma, and may be aided by the use of immunohistochemical staining.[115] Immunostains for carcinoembryonic antigen, BER EP4, MOC 31, and B72.3 are usually positive in adenocarcinomas of the lung, but fail to distinguish primary lung cancer from primaries in other organs. The antibody to thyroid transcription factor-1 and cytokeratin 7 (CK7) are useful as markers of origin for adenocarcinomas in the lung (or thyroid), whereas CK20 antigen is characteristic of adenocarcinomas of the gastrointestinal tract (especially colon), and GCDFP-15 is observed in breast cancers.[116]

Poorly differentiated adenocarcinomas are composed of a solid type of large cell carcinoma in which mucin production is limited and can only be demonstrated with the aid of histochemical stains. Differential diagnosis in these lesions is between adenocarcinoma and undifferentiated carcinoma of the lung or other organs.

Large Cell Carcinoma

Large cell carcinomas are composed of large cells that are similar in many ways to those of an adenocarcinoma or a squamous cell carcinoma, but the cytoplasm lacks the differentiating features of mucin production or dense keratinization and the cells form no glandular structures. They account for approximately 15% of all lung cancers. With extensive sampling and electron microscopy, many large cell carcinomas can be classified appropriately as poorly differentiated adenocarcinoma or, less often, squamous cell carcinoma.

Although the WHO classification recognizes basaloid, lymphoepithelioma-like, and clear cell types, they differ little in clinical presentation or course,[117,118] and in most clinical trials, large cell carcinoma and adenocarcinoma are grouped together.

Squamous Cell Carcinoma

Squamous cell carcinoma may present clinically in the periphery of the lung as a small subpleural nodule with the radiographic appearance and overall prognosis of a peripheral adenocarcinoma (Fig. 75.3), but squamous cell carcinoma classically arises in proximal (segmental or larger) bronchi via progression

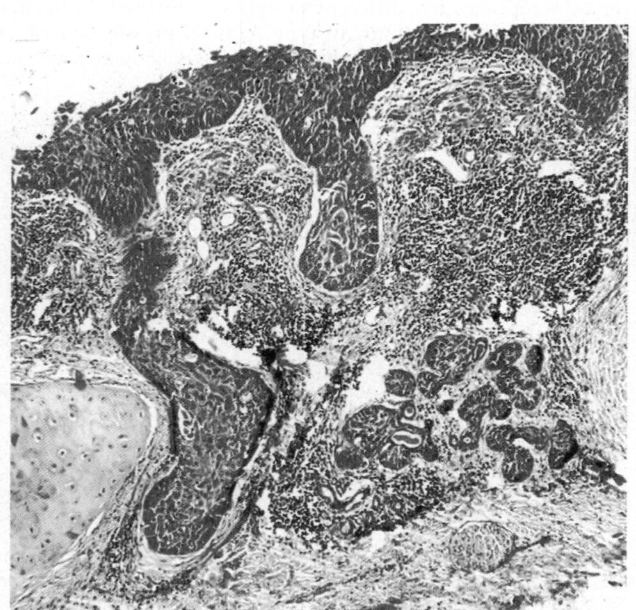

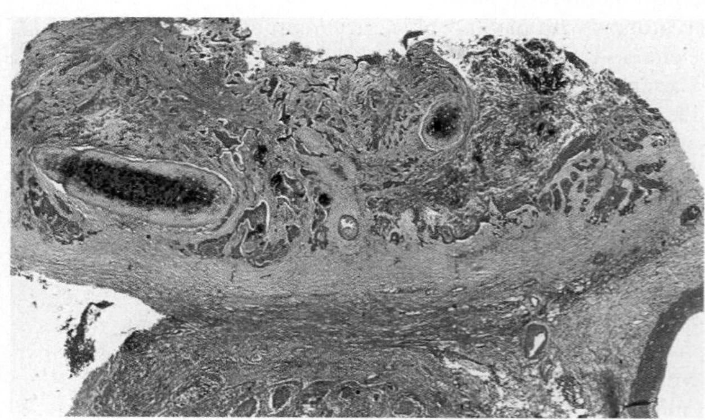

FIGURE 75.3 Squamous cell carcinoma. **A:** Carcinoma *in situ* in the surface epithelium with involvement of the submucosal glands. **B:** Invasive carcinoma confined to the bronchial wall.

through stages of dysplasia. In its earliest form (carcinoma *in situ*), malignant squamous cells spread over the bronchial surface, and may involve submucosal glands. Because there is exfoliation of the malignant cells from the bronchial surface, squamous cell carcinoma can rarely be detected by cytologic examination in an occult stage before it is evident on chest radiograph because of its origin in the large and dense proximal bronchi. With further growth, squamous cell carcinoma invades the basement membrane and extends into the parenchyma and bronchial lumen, producing obstruction with resultant atelectasis or pneumonia. Histologically, squamous cell carcinoma is composed of sheets of epithelial cells with individual cell keratinization, intercellular bridges, and/or pearl formation.[119] Squamous cell carcinoma tends to be slow-growing; it is estimated that the progression of *in situ* carcinoma to a clinically apparent tumor takes 3 to 4 years. Because of the proximal location and growth pattern, surgical resection may be compromised and local failure in the chest is more common. Most squamous cell carcinomas immunostain in the nucleus for p63 and in the cytoplasm for CK5/6.

Adenosquamous Carcinomas

Adenosquamous carcinomas have histologic areas differentiated as both squamous cell carcinoma and adenocarcinoma, are predominantly found in the periphery of the lung, and have clinical behavior much like that of adenocarcinoma. However, studies suggest that they are a cytogenetically distinct entity.[120]

Pleomorphic Carcinomas

This grouping of tumors includes carcinomas with giant and usually multinucleated cells, or with spindle cell, pseudosarcomatous configuration, and those with both carcinoma and sarcoma morphology, including the rare pulmonary blastoma.[121,122] All are aggressive malignancies, and typically are advanced when diagnosed; survival is stage-dependent.

Carcinomas of Salivary Gland Type

These tumors are predominantly found in large bronchi and thought to arise from submucosal gland epithelium. Mucoepidermoid carcinomas are recognized by their characteristic intermediate or transitional cells and are divided into low grade and high grade, based on nuclear morphology and degree of squamous cell differentiation. Mortality rates have been reported as distinctly worse for the high-grade mucoepidermoids in some series. Adenoid-cystic carcinomas share the aggressiveness of their salivary gland counterparts. Rare low-grade, acinic cell carcinomas have been reported.[123,124]

Carcinoids

These neoplasms manifest a prominent neuroendocrine phenotype in morphology, immunohistochemistry, and ultrastructure. Histology is characterized by insular, ribbon or festoon, pseudorosette, and sometimes spindle cell patterns of cuboidal cells with small and hyperchromatic nuclei. Immunohistochemically, they are usually positive for synaptophysin, chromogranin A, and/or CD56 and ultrastructurally, they contain dense core granules. Typical carcinoids are usually found in large bronchi and most often feature an organoid pattern. Peripheral carcinoids are often spindle-cell tumors, which may be mistaken for metastatic sarcomas, especially of the endometrial stroma.

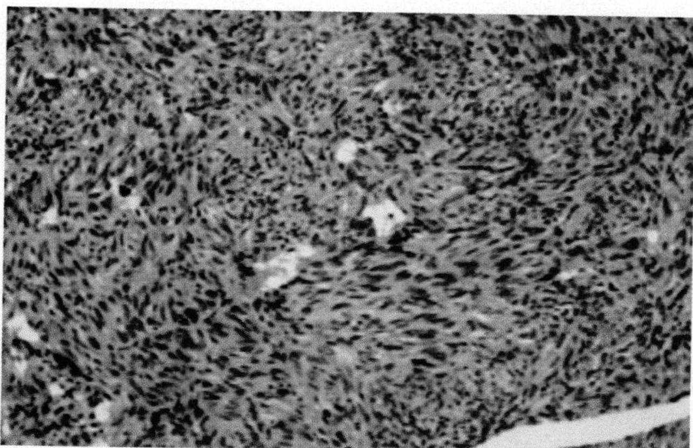

FIGURE 75.4 Benign peripheral carcinoid with a spindle cell pattern.

Typical and spindle cell carcinoids have a very low incidence of metastases (Fig. 75.4). Tumors with carcinoid histology altered by tumor necrosis, mitotic figures, and/or nuclear anaplasia are classified as atypical carcinoids and have a distinctly higher rate of metastases and mortality.[125] The very mitotically active, necrotic, and anaplastic carcinoids are classified with the large cell carcinomas as large cell neuroendocrine carcinomas, and have a very poor prognosis approaching that of small cell carcinoma, which they resemble histologically.[126]

MOLECULAR MARKERS OF PROGNOSIS

Lung cancers exhibit a variety of mutations involving genes that regulate cell-cycle progression and apoptosis, as well as invasion and metastasis, that could influence the malignant phenotype of these neoplasms. Numerous studies have been undertaken to ascertain the clinical relevance of mutations involving protooncogenes such as *k-ras*, *EGFR*, *erbB2*, *cyclin D*, and *Bc1-2*, or tumor suppressor genes such as *p53*, *p16*, *RASSF1A*, or *FHIT* in primary lung cancers. None of these "markers" of malignancy have proven to be sufficiently robust for establishing prognosis.

Additional recent studies have focused on global gene and protein expression profiles, which correlate with treatment response and overall prognosis in lung cancer patients. Miura et al.[127] identified 45 genes that distinguished smokers and nonsmokers, and 27 genes that were differentially expressed in long-term survivors relative to nonsurvivors following lung cancer resections. Interestingly, a number of these differentially expressed genes regulate the mitotic spindle checkpoint and maintain genomic stability. Additional investigators have identified gene expression signatures correlating with disease recurrence and survival in patients with early-stage adenocarcinomas[128,129]; significant interinstitution variability regarding gene expression profiling currently limits the routine use of gene expression signatures for ascribing prognosis or predicting response to therapy in lung cancer patients.[130] Roepman et al.[131] identified a 72-gene profile enriched with genes encoding immunoglobulins, interferon, and multiple cytokines that correlated with prognosis in 172 radically resected lung cancer patients. Additional studies indicate that DNA methylation profiles coincide with tumor histology and stage, as well as response to therapy, and overall survival in lung cancer patients.[132] Recently, Brock et al.[133] examined DNA methylation status of 7 genes in 51 patients with stage I NSCLC who had recurrence within 40 months and a comparative control of 166 patients with no recurrence during this period. Promoter methylation of *p16*, *CDH13*, *RASSF1A*, and *APC* were strongly associated with tumor recurrence.

Additional efforts have focused on the development of proteomic techniques development of diagnosing and staging primary lung cancers.[134] Using quantitative two-dimensional gel electrophoresis, Chen et al.[135] observed that aberrant intratumoral expression of 11 proteins associated with the glycolysis pathway correlated with poor survival. Using matrix-assisted laser desorption ionization time of flight (MALDI-TOF) mass spectroscopy techniques, Yanagisawa et al.[136] observed a pattern of 15 distinct protein peaks that distinguished patients with poor prognosis from those with much more favorable outcomes (median survival, 6 vs. 33 months; $P < .001$). In an additional study, Kikuchi and Carbone[137] observed that MALDI-TOF profiles could discriminate tumor versus normal cells with an accuracy approaching 95%, and could predict nodal metastases in 80% of disseminated lung cancers. Collectively, these data suggest that with further refinement and validation, proteomic profiling may prove useful for diagnosis and therapy of lung cancer.

MODES OF METASTASIS

After variable periods of growing within lung parenchyma or within the bronchial wall, primary tumors invade the vascular and lymphatic channels, metastasizing to regional lymph nodes and distant sites. In most instances, regional lymph node metastases precede systemic dissemination. The regional lymphatic drainage of the lung is outlined in Figure 75.5. Pulmonary lymphatic drainage parallels the bronchoarterial system, with lymph nodes situated adjacent to the segmental or lobar bronchi. In general, left and right lower lobe as well as right middle lobe lymphatics drain to the posterior mediastinum and subcarinal lymph nodes. Right upper lobe lymphatics drain toward the superior mediastinum, whereas the left upper lobe lymphatics typically course lateral to the aorta and subclavian artery in the anterior mediastinum, as well as along the left main bronchus to the superior mediastinum. Ultimately, all of these lymphatic channels drain into the right lymphatic or left thoracic ducts, which empty into the subclavian veins. Although skip metastases can occur in up to 25% of lung cancers, particularly upper lobe tumors and adenocarcinomas,[138,139] antegrade lymphatic metastases most commonly exhibit sequential involvement of bronchopulmonary (N1), mediastinal (N2 and N3), and supraclavicular (N3) lymph nodes. Retrograde lymphatic spread to the pleural surface can occur, particularly with peripheral tumors.

By direct extension, the primary tumor can invade contiguous structures, such as the mediastinal pleura, great vessels, heart, esophagus, diaphragm, or chest wall. Once vascular or lymphatic invasions occur, metastatic dissemination to distant sites is common. Whereas bone, liver, adrenals, and brain are the most frequent sites of distant disease, lung cancers metastasize to virtually every organ of the body. Metastases within the lung result from a variety of mechanisms including endobronchial embolization, retrograde lymphatic, as well as hematogenous dissemination.

CLINICAL MANIFESTATIONS

The signs and symptoms manifested by patients suffering from lung cancer depend on the histology of the tumor and the extent of locoregional invasion, as well as the location, size, and number of distant metastases. Many patients present with an asymptomatic lesion discovered incidentally on chest radiography or CT scan.

Tumors arising in the larger airways may cause persistent cough, wheezing, or hemoptysis (Table 75.2). Typically, patients with hemoptysis experience blood-streaked sputum; massive bleeding is rarely seen at presentation. Continued growth of endobronchial tumors frequently results in atelectasis with or without pneumonia and abscess. Pleural involvement by tumor or associated infection may cause pleuritic pain with or without effusion. Diminished lung function may result in dyspnea, the severity of which depends on the amount of lung involved and the patient's underlying pulmonary reserve.

Tumors invading the chest wall typically produce either stabbing or burning radicular pain with or without pleural effusion. Tumors arising within the superior sulcus may be associated with a classic Pancoast syndrome from invasion of the lower brachial plexus (T1 and C8 nerve roots), stellate ganglion, and chest wall or vertebral bodies. Invasion or encasement of structures within the mediastinum may cause superior vena cava (SVC) syndrome, recurrent or phrenic

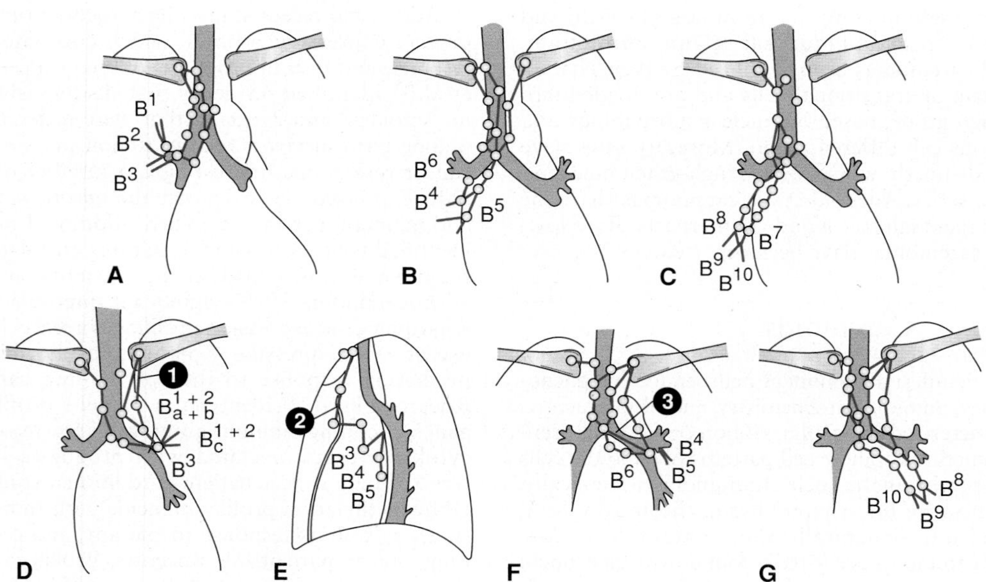

FIGURE 75.5 The regional lymphatic drainage of the lung. Most of the lymphatic drainage ultimately reaches the right superior mediastinum and right supraclavicular regions. (Reprinted with permission from Shields TW, LoCicero J III, Reed CE, et al., eds. *General Thoracic Surgery*, 7th ed. Lippincott Williams & Wilkins; 2009.)

TABLE 75.2

COMMON SIGNS AND SYMPTOMS OF LUNG CANCER

Symptoms secondary to central or endobronchial growth of the primary tumor
Cough
Hemoptysis
Wheeze and stridor
Dyspnea from obstruction
Pneumonitis from obstruction (fever, productive cough)
Symptoms secondary to peripheral growth of the primary tumor
Pain from pleural or chest wall involvement
Cough
Dyspnea on a restrictive basis
Lung abscess syndrome from tumor cavitation
Symptoms related to regional spread of the tumor in the thorax by contiguity or by metastasis to regional lymph nodes
Tracheal obstruction
Esophageal compression with dysphagia
Recurrent laryngeal nerve paralysis with hoarseness
Phrenic nerve paralysis with hemidiaphragm elevation and dyspnea
Sympathetic nerve paralysis with Horner's syndrome
Eighth cervical and first thoracic nerves with ulnar pain and Pancoast's syndrome
Superior vena cava syndrome from vascular obstruction
Pericardial and cardiac extension with resultant tamponade, arrhythmia, or cardiac failure
Lymphatic obstruction with pleural effusion
Lymphangitic spread through lungs with hypoxemia and dyspnea

From Cohen MH. Signs and symptoms of bronchogenic carcinoma. In: Straus MJ, ed. *Lung Cancer: Clinical Diagnosis and Treatment*. New York: Grune & Stratton, 1977:85, with permission.

TABLE 75.3

PARANEOPLASTIC SYNDROMES IN PATIENTS WITH LUNG CANCER

Endocrine
Hypercalcemia (ectopic parathyroid hormone)
Cushing syndrome
Syndrome of inappropriate antidiuretic hormone
Carcinoid syndrome
Gynecomastia
Hypercalcitoninemia
Elevated growth hormone
Elevated prolactin, follicle-stimulating hormone, luteinizing hormone
Hypoglycemia
Hyperthyroidism
Neurologic
Encephalopathy
Subacute cerebellar degeneration
Progressive multifocal leukoencephalopathy
Peripheral neuropathy
Polymyositis
Autonomic neuropathy
Eaton-Lambert syndrome
Optic neuritis
Skeletal
Clubbing
Pulmonary hypertrophic osteoarthropathy
Hematologic
Anemia
Leukemoid reactions
Thrombocytosis
Thrombocytopenia
Eosinophilia
Pure red cell aplasia
Leukoerythroblastosis
Disseminated intravascular coagulation
Cutaneous
Hyperkeratosis
Dermatomyositis
Acanthosis nigricans
Hyperpigmentation
Erythema gyratum repens
Hypertrichosis lanuginosa acquisita
Other
Nephrotic syndrome
Hypouricemia
Secretion of vasoactive intestinal peptide with diarrhea
Hyperamylasemia
Anorexia or cachexia

Adapted from Maddaus M, Ginsberg RJ. Diagnosis and staging. In: Pearson FG, Deslauriers J, Ginsberg R, eds. *Thoracic Surgery*. New York: Churchill Livingstone, 1995:671.

nerve palsy, esophageal dysphagia, tracheoesophageal fistula, or pericardial effusion. In addition to experiencing specific symptoms directly related to the tumor or associated lymphadenopathy, many patients complain of vague chest discomfort, which is usually of visceral origin.

Nearly all patients with advanced NCSLC exhibit symptoms referable to their disease on initial presentation. Fatigue and decreased activity are reported by more than 80% of individuals, and most patients also experience cough, dyspnea, anorexia, and weight loss. The presenting complaints of patients with metastatic disease are largely determined by the specific sites involved, such as bone, brain, liver, and adrenal glands. In addition, patients may exhibit a variety of paraneoplastic syndromes (Table 75.3), which may improve following treatment of the underlying malignancy.

STAGING AND DIAGNOSIS

The current system for lung cancer is based on recently revised tumor, node, and metastasis (TNM) criteria, emanating from review of an international database pertaining to 81,015 analyzable lung cancer patients. This updated staging system has been endorsed by the American Joint Committee on Cancer as well as the Union International Contre le Cancer (Table 75.4; Fig. 75.6). In this staging system, the primary tumor is defined using four major descriptors (T1 to T4), with various subdescriptors depending on size, location, extent of local extension, presence of atelectasis/pneumonia, or satellite nodules. Lymph node involvement has been subdivided into bronchopulmonary (N1), ipsilateral mediastinal (N2), and contralateral hilar or mediastinal or ipsilateral or contralateral supraclavicular disease (N3); metastases are absent (M0) or present (M1). The newly revised TNM system still identifies four major stages of lung cancer with subclassifications that correlate with significant differences in 5-year survival rates (Table 75.5).[140,141] The TNM system includes clinical as well as pathologic criteria; using clinical parameters alone, a significant percentage of patients are understaged relative to true pathologic stage. The

TABLE 75.4

DEFINITIONS FOR TNM DESCRIPTORS

TUMOR AND SUBGROUP[a]	DEFINITION
T (primary tumor)	
T0	No primary tumor
T	Tumor ≤3 cm,[b] surrounded by lung or visceral pleura, not more proximal than the lobar bronchus
T1a	Tumor ≤2 cm[b]
T1b	Tumor >2 but ≤3 cm[b]
T2	Tumor >3 but ≤7 cm[b] or tumor with any of the following:[c] invades visceral pleura, involves main bronchus ≥2 cm distal to the carina, atelectasis/obstructive pneumonia extending to hilum but not involving the entire lung
T2a	Tumor >3 but ≤5 cm[b]
T2b	Tumor >5 but ≤7 cm[b]
T3	
$T3_{>7}$	Tumor >7 cm[b]
$T3_{Inv}$	Directly invading chest wall, diaphragm, phrenic nerve, mediastinal pleura, parietal pericardium
$T3_{Centr}$	Tumor in the main bronchus <2 cm distal to the carina[d] or atelectasis/obstructive pneumonitis of entire lung
$T3_{Satell}$	Separate tumor nodule(s) in the same lobe
T4	
$T4_{Inv}$	Tumor of any size with invasion of: heart, great vessels, trachea, recurrent laryngeal nerve, esophagus, vertebral body, or carina;
$T4_{Ipsi\ Nod}$	Separate tumor nodule(s) in a different ipsilateral lobe
N (regional lymph nodes)	
N0	No regional node metastasis
N1	Metastasis in ipsilateral peribronchial or perihilar lymph nodes and intrapulmonary nodes, including involvement by direct extension
N2	Metastasis in ipsilateral mediastinal or subcarinal lymph node(s)
N3	Metastasis in contralateral mediastinal, contralateral hilar, ipsilateral or contralateral scalene, or supraclavicular lymph node(s)
M (distant metastasis)	
M0	No distant metastasis
M1a	
$M1a_{Contr\ Nod}$	Separate tumor nodule(s) in a contralateral lobe
$M1a_{Pl\ Dissem}$	Tumor with pleural nodules or malignant pleural dissemination[e]
M1b	Distant metastasis
Special situations	
TX, NX	T or N status not able to be assessed
T*is*	Focus of *in situ* cancer
T1[d]	
$T1_{SS}$	Superficial-spreading tumor of any size but confined to the wall of the trachea or mainstem bronchus

[a]These subgroup labels are not defined in the International Association for the Study of Lung Cancer publications[1–4] but are added for clarity.
[b]In greatest dimension.
[c]T2 tumors with these features are classified as T2a if ≤5 cm.
[d]The uncommon superficial-spreading tumor in central airways is classified as T1.
[e]Pleural effusions that are cytologically negative, nonbloody, transudative, and clinically judged not to be due to cancer are excluded.

TABLE 75.5

SURVIVAL BY CLINICAL AND PATHOLOGIC STAGES PROPOSED BY THE INTERNATIONAL ASSOCIATION FOR THE STUDY OF LUNG CANCER

	Clinical			Pathologic		
Stage	Median Survival (mo)	5-Year Survival Rate (%)	*P* Value Relative to Preceding Row	Median Survival (mo)	5-Year Survival Rate (%)	*P* Value Relative to Preceding Row
IA	60	50		119	73	
IB	43	43	.0035	81	58	<.0001
IIA	34	36	.0020	49	46	<.0001
IIB	18	26	<.0001	31	36	<.0001
IIIA	14	19	<.0001	22	24	<.0001
IIIB	10	7	<.0001	13	9	<.0001
IV	6	2	<.0001	17	13	.0974

Lung Cancer Stage According to TNM Descriptor and Subgroups

T/M	Subgroups	N0	N1	N2	N3
T1	T1a	IA	IIA	IIIA	IIIB
	T1b	IA	IIA	IIIA	IIIB
T2	T2a	IB	IIB	IIIA	IIIB
	T2b	IIA	IIB	IIIA	IIIB
T3	T3 >7	IIB	IIIA	IIIA	IIIB
	T3 *Inv*	IIB	IIIA	IIIA	IIIB
	T3 *Satell*	IIB	IIIA	IIIA	IIIB
T4	T4 *Inv*	IIIA	IIIA	IIIB	IIIB
	T4 *Ispi Nod*	IIIA	IIIA	IIIB	IIIB
M1	M1a *Contr Nod*	IV	IV	IV	IV
	M1a *Pl Dissem*	IV	IV	IV	IV
	M1b	IV	IV	IV	IV

FIGURE 75.6 New international lung cancer staging system. Categories of TNM criteria descriptors and stage of disease. (Reprinted with permission Detterbeck, et al. *Chest* 2010;137(5):1172–1180.)

newly revised system provides better prognostic information regarding survival of resected patients than the previous system, with approximately 15% of patients being staged differently in the new system relative to the previous system, with most shifts being from IB to IIA, and IIIB to IIIA.[142] For example, tumors with chest wall invasion without lymph node metastases (T3N0) are no longer stage IIIA, but are stage IIB cancers. Furthermore, cancers with malignant pleural effusions with or without nodal disease, but no distant metastases, which previously were categorized as T4 (wet IIIB), are now defined as M1 (stage IV) tumors. In addition, satellite nodules in the same lobe or a different ipsilateral lobe relative to the primary cancer, which previously were defined as M1, are now categorized as T3 or T4 lesions, respectively. Specific potential issues/nuances regarding the new staging system, such as the proposed T descriptor for lesions containing solid and lepidic ground glass opacity components, the minimum number of lymph nodes samples/resected necessary for valid staging, and a variety of optional descriptions have been articulated recently and are a focus of ongoing evaluations/validation.[143] In addition, a revised lymph node map (Fig. 75.7), which includes levels of mediastinal lymph node involvement, has been proposed to enhance uniformity and further prognostic validation of mediastinal staging.[144]

TABLE 75.6

BIOLOGICAL PREDICTORS OF RADIATION THERAPY (RT)-INDUCED LUNG INJURY

Study (Ref.)/Affiliation	No. of Patients	Cytokine	Predictive of Radiation Pneumonitis?
Chen et al. (574) Rochester	24	IL-1α, IL-6	Yes, for patients with high levels pre-, during, and post-RT
		TGF-β, bFGF, MCP-1, E/L selectin	No
DeJaeger et al. (575) Netherlands Cancer Institute	68	TGF-β1	No
Novakova-Jiresova et al. (576)	46	TGF-β1	Weakly, for patients who exhibit significant increase in levels at week 3 of RT as compared to pre-RT
Evans et al. (577) Duke University	121	TGF-β1	Yes, for patients with high V30
Hart et al. (578) Duke University	55	IL-8	Yes, for patients who exhibit lower levels of IL-8 pre-RT
		TGF-β, IL-6[a]	No
Wang et al. (579) Beijing	42	TGF-β	No
		IL-6	Weakly, for patients with higher post-RT levels as compared to pre-RT
		ACE	Yes, for patients with lower levels pre- or during-RT
Hauer-Jensen et al. (580) Arkansas	17	TM	Yes, for patients who did not exhibit a significant reduction in TM levels during RT

IL, interleukin; TGF-β, transforming growth factor-beta; bFGF, basic fibroblast growth factor; MCP, monocyte chemotactic protein; ACE, angiotensin-converting enzyme; TM, thrombomodulin.
[a]Many other interleukins were negative.

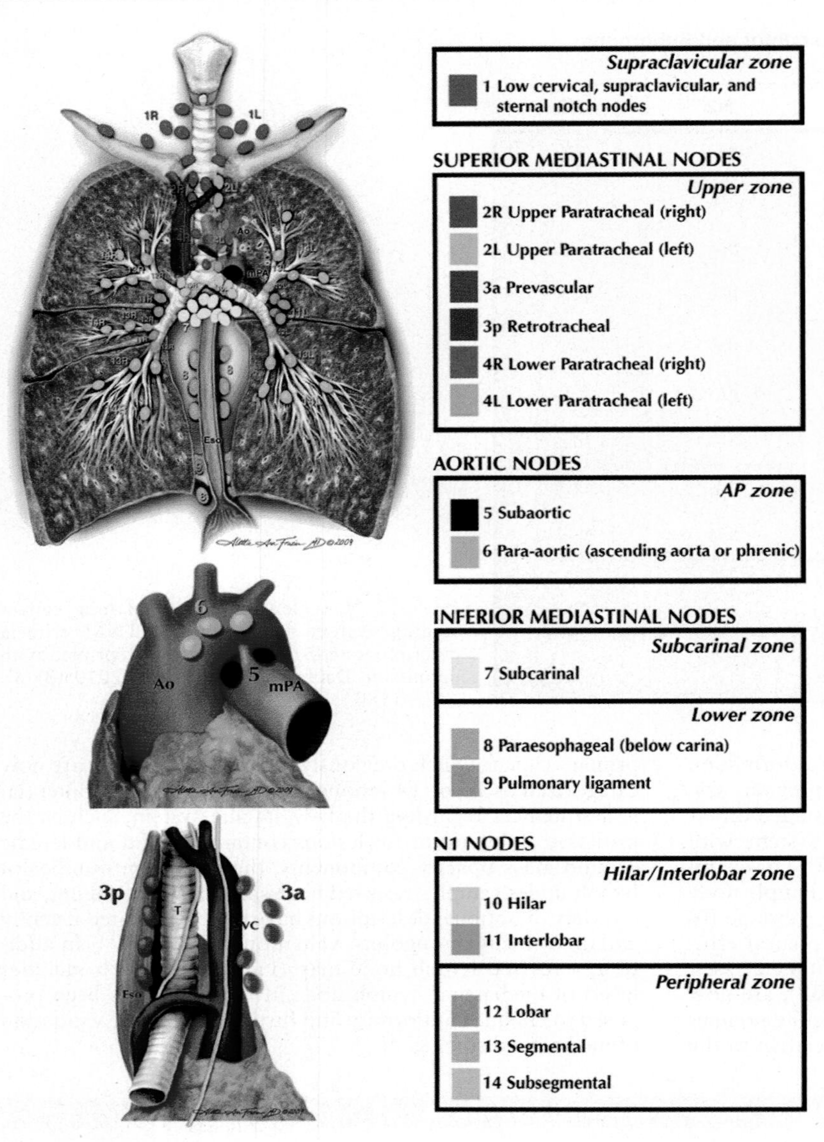

FIGURE 75.7 Proposed lymph node map for the new lung cancer staging system. Mediastinal nodes are designated by station as in previous maps, but are also classified in terms of levels/zones for possible further prognostic evaluation. (Reprinted with permission Rusch VW, Asamura H, Watanabe H, et al. The IASLC lung cancer staging project: a proposal for a new international lymph node map in the forthcoming seventh edition of the TNM classification for lung cancer. *J Thorac Oncol* 2009;4(5):568–570.)

Evaluation of any patient suspected of having lung cancer should proceed in an expeditious, cost-efficient manner (Fig. 75.8). A detailed history and physical examination remain the most important steps in initially assessing a patient with possible lung cancer. Smoking history, occupational/environmental exposures, and family history should be documented.

Once the physical examination has been completed, posteroanterior and lateral chest radiographs as well as CT scans of the chest and upper abdomen should be obtained. Routine chest radiographs will generally reveal large peripheral lung cancers, central obstructing lesions, and potentially malignant effusions; however, a normal chest radiograph does not exclude a primary lung cancer. In fact, conventional chest radiographs fail to detect nearly 80% of histologically proven CT-detected lung cancers 2.0 cm or more in diameter.[145] In general, conventional CT scans have a sensitivity of 60% and specificity of approximately 80% for the detection of lung cancer. The diagnostic accuracy of CT scans can be further improved by utilization of super high-resolution scanning techniques, which have a sensitivity and specificity of approximately 85% and 100%, respectively, for the detection of malignant endoluminal or obstructive lesions involving the airway.[146]

Although important for the preliminary assessment of patients with suspected lung cancers, CT scans are unreliable for detection of mediastinal lymph node metastases. Whereas the presence of lymph nodes more than 1 cm in transverse diameter suggests malignant lymphadenopathy, enlarged but histologically benign lymph nodes are frequently observed in the context of tumors associated with volume loss or postobstructive pneumonitis. Similarly, lymph nodes less than 1 cm may contain foci of malignant cells; the frequency of micrometastases depends on the size, histology, and location of the primary tumor. Therefore, any patient with a newly diagnosed lesion suspicious for lung cancer should undergo whole-body [^{18}F]fluorodeoxyglucose positron emission tomography (FDG-PET) imaging.

A variety of studies have compared FDG-PET with standard CT scans for staging of mediastinal lymph nodes in lung cancer patients. The overall accuracy, sensitivity, and specificity of PET scans approximates 70%, 70%, and 80%, respectively, compared with 70%, 50%, and 70%, respectively, for CT scans for the detection of histologically confirmed mediastinal lymph node (N2 and N3) metastases. Furthermore, FDG-PET scans are considerably superior to CT scans for the detection of N1 disease (42% vs. 13%; $P = .017$) in patients with potentially operable lung cancers. Whereas the positive predictive value of PET scans for detection of N1 or N2 nodal metastases is only 65%, the negative predictive value of PET imaging exceeds 90%.[147,148] Granulomatous inflammation, silicosis, and sinus histiocytosis contribute to false-positive PET results, whereas bronchoalveolar or mucoepidermoid carcinomas

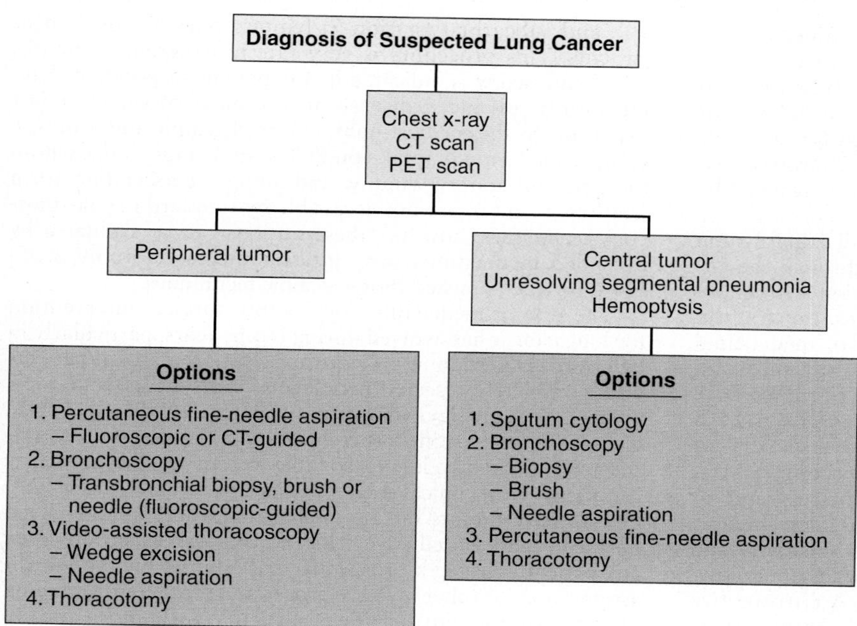

FIGURE 75.8 Schema to indicate the diagnostic procedures depending on the presenting lesion. CT, computed tomography; PET, positron emission tomography.

produce false-negative results. Integrated PET-CT scans are superior to either of these modalities for staging lung cancers. In a recent study, Ventura et al.[149] reported sensitivities, specificities, positive predictive values, and negative predictive values of 94%,73%, 66%, and 96% for PET/CT compared to 90%, 31%, 64%, and 71%, and 81%, 50%, 69%, and 66%, for PET and CT scans, respectively. Despite the superiority of integrated PET-CT scans for initial staging of lung cancers, this imaging modality has not consistently proven to be better than conventional CT scans for assessing response to chemotherapy and/or radiation therapy in patients with these neoplasms.[150,151]

Endoscopic ultrasound (EUS) is a relatively noninvasive method for evaluating mediastinal lymph nodes in lung cancer patients.[152] EUS can detect lesions 3 mm or more in the paratracheal (R2, R4, L2, L4), aortopulmonary window (L5), subcarinal (station 7), and paraesophageal (station 8) regions, but cannot assess prevascular (station 3) or ascending aorta (station 6) lymph node status. Size, shape, and echogenicity correlate with metastatic disease in mediastinal lymph nodes. Several recent studies have demonstrated sensitivities, specificities, and accuracies of 57%, 74%, and 67% for CT scans, 73%, 83%, and 79% for PET scans, and 94%, 71%, and 92% for EUS.[153,154] Additional studies have revealed sensitivities and specificities of 57% and 47% for CT scans, 84% and 89% for PET imaging, and 78% and 71% for EUS.[155] Despite advances regarding imaging technology, tissue confirmation is mandatory for determining the histology and stage of any lung cancer.

METHODS TO ESTABLISH TISSUE DIAGNOSIS

Sputum Cytology

Cytologic analysis of exfoliated cells in sputum is a rapid, relatively inexpensive means to establish a tissue diagnosis in an individual with an apparent pulmonary carcinoma. Sputum can be either spontaneously collected or induced with hypertonic saline; three daily pooled specimens increase the diagnostic yield. Sputum samples are considered representative if alveolar macrophages as well as bronchial epithelial cells are present. Previous reports have indicated that the sensitivity of sputum cytology is 65% (range, 22% to 98%) in the setting of established cancers. The diagnostic yield of sputum cytology is enhanced in the context of centrally located lesions, squamous cell carcinomas, and large tumors, particularly if multiple sputum samples are examined.[156]

A variety of molecular techniques have been evaluated as a means to increase the diagnostic yield of sputum cytology. These include nuclear image analysis, immunohistochemical evaluation of *p53,* and heterogeneous nuclear riboprotein A2/B1 expression, analysis of *k-ras* and *p53* mutations, as well as loss of heterozygosity, aberrant promoter methylation, and DNA adduct levels in genomic DNA. Additional studies have focused on the evaluation of automated sputum cytology techniques and analysis of gene or microRNA expression profiles in exfoliated tumor cells.[157–159] Overall, the feasibility and efficacy of these newer methodologies in the context of sputum cytology for detection of occult pulmonary malignancies, particularly peripheral adenocarcinomas and monitoring treatment responses in established carcinomas, have yet to be determined.

Percutaneous Fine-Needle Aspiration

FNA is an excellent method for establishing tissue diagnosis of pulmonary nodules. This can be performed using fluoroscopic or CT-guided techniques. The positive yield in experienced hands exceeds 95% even if lesions are less than 1 cm in diameter. Indeterminate biopsies must be interpreted with caution; FNA cannot rule out malignancy unless a true/positive benign diagnosis (i.e., hematoma or infectious process) is definitively established. Abnormalities involving bone, liver, and adrenal glands, suggestive of metastatic disease on staging studies, can be readily confirmed by FNA using ultrasonographic or CT-guided techniques. Frequently, biopsy of one of these sites simultaneously establishes tissue diagnosis and stage of disease.

Bronchoscopy

Fiberoptic bronchoscopy (FOB) can be performed with or without sedation, and with minimal morbidity and exceptional safety. FOB enables visualization of the tracheobronchial tree to the second or third segmental divisions; cytologic or histologic specimens can be obtained from identified lesions. In general, the diagnostic yield of FOB with cytologic brushings or biopsy of visible lesions exceeds 90%. Even when no visible lesion is identified, the bronchus draining the area of suspicion can be lavaged, and effluent obtained for cytologic analysis. With the use of FOB combined with fluoroscopy or CT imaging techniques, peripheral lesions can be reached by cytology brushes, needle, or biopsy forceps.

FOB also be used to evaluate hilar and mediastinal lymph nodes; transbronchoscopic needle aspiration through the airway wall, particularly when used in conjunction with endoscopic bronchial ultrasound (EBUS) techniques, can confirm the presence of malignancy in enlarged hilar or mediastinal lymph nodes without the need for mediastinoscopy, thoracoscopy, or EUS/FNA.[161] Two recent prospective studies have demonstrated sensitivities of 77% to 87% versus 68% to 85% and negative predictive values of 78% to 86% versus 59% to 90% for EBUS-FNA and cervical mediastinoscopy (CME), respectively.[160,161] Of note, the negative predictive value of EBUS-FNA needs to be confirmed in additional large studies.

Several recent studies have evaluated the sensitivity and accuracy of EBUS-FNA for restaging the mediastinum following induction therapy in lung cancer patients. A retrospective study involving 61 consecutive patients with confirmed stage IIIA/N2 disease who underwent induction chemotherapy followed by EBUS-FNA and extended CME, revealed sensitivity, specificity, accuracy, positive predictive value, and negative predictive value of restaging EBUS-FNA procedures of 67%, 86%, 80%, 91%, and 78%, respectively.[162] In contrast, evaluation of 124 consecutive patients with stage IIIA/N2 NSCLC treated with induction chemotherapy revealed that 28 of 35 patients with no apparent mediastinal nodal disease by EBUS-FNA had residual N2 lymph node metastases at thoracotomy; the vast majority of these false-negative results were due to sampling rather than detection errors. The overall sensitivity, specificity, positive predictive value, negative predictive value, and accuracy were 76%, 100%, 100%, 20%, and 77%, respectively.[163] These data suggest that given the potentially low negative predictive value, EBUS-FNA may not be a reliable means of confirming sterilization of mediastinal lymph node metastases following induction therapy in lung cancer patients.

Endoscopic Ultrasound–Fine-Needle Aspiration

EUS-FNA is a minimally invasive and safe means to assess subcarinal (station 7) lymph nodes typically biopsied by CME or transbronchial techniques, and lower mediastinal lymph nodes (stations 8 and 9) that are not accessible via standard CME. Meta-analysis of 18 studies revealed that EUS-FNA correctly identified 83% and 97% of patients with positive and negative mediastinal lymph nodes, respectively. Sensitivity and specificity were 90% and 97%, respectively, for patients with abnormal mediastinal lymph nodes on CT scans. Sensitivity was 58% for patients without mediastinal lymphadenopathy.[164] More recent analysis revealed that EUS-FNA has sensitivity, negative predictive value, and accuracy of 74%, 73%, and 85%, respectively, for N2/N3 disease; these values increase to 92%, 85%, and 85%, respectively, when EUS-FNA is combined with CME. EUS-FNA can reduce the number of patients requiring CME for documentation of mediastinal metastases, and decrease the number of patients undergoing potentially unwarranted thoracotomy.[165,166]

Mediastinoscopy/Mediastinotomy, and Thoracoscopy

CME remains the most accurate technique to assess paratracheal (stations 2, 3, and 4), proximal peribronchial (station 10), and subcarinal (station 7) lymph nodes in lung cancer patients. This procedure is very safe in experienced hands. Mediastinoscopy is indicated in any patient suspected of having locally advanced disease on the basis of direct tumor extension to the mediastinum, enlarged lymph nodes on CT scan, or mediastinal uptake on PET scan. Lymph nodes within the aortopulmonary window and along the ascending aorta (stations 5 and 6) are not accessible by standard mediastinoscopy techniques; however, these stations can be evaluated by extended mediastinoscopy, anterior mediastinotomy, EUS-FNA, or video-assisted thoracoscopic techniques.

The role of mediastinoscopy before surgical intervention for lung cancer has evolved during recent years, particularly in light of data pertaining to adjuvant chemotherapy in patients with completely resected neoplasms. With mediastinoscopy, inoperable supraclavicular or contralateral mediastinal (N3) disease can be identified, thereby avoiding unnecessary thoracotomies. Currently, it is reasonable to forgo mediastinoscopy in patients with clinical stage I disease, particularly those with PET-positive tumors but no mediastinal tracer uptake, given the high negative predictive value of FDG-PET scans. However, any patient entering a prospective trial should undergo mediastinoscopy (or other invasive procedure) for definitive staging of their tumor. Furthermore, patients with more locally advanced disease (clinical stage II or III), particularly those potentially requiring pneumonectomy, should undergo mediastinoscopy to rule out N3 disease, and to identify those individuals with N2 disease for whom induction therapy should be considered prior to surgery.

Several studies have examined the feasibility and safety of CME for mediastinal restaging following induction therapy in potentially resectable patients. Sensitivity of CME in this setting ranges from 30% to 70%; fibrosis resulting from prior CME or induction therapy may limit the number of nodal stations accessible on repeat CME. Two recent prospective studies have demonstrated sensitivity of 77% to 87% versus 68% to 85% per EBUS-FNA and CME, respectively, and a negative predictive value of 78% to 86% versus 59% to 90% for EBUS versus CME.[160] Presently, a reasonable approach for patients with high likelihood of requiring induction therapy prior to surgery is to use EBUS-FNA or EUS-FNA techniques to initially stage the mediastinum with the caveat that a negative EBUS-FNA will need confirmation by other more invasive techniques; CME should be performed prior to resection to accurately assess response to therapy.

Video-assisted thoracoscopic surgery (VATS) is frequently used for the diagnosis, staging, and resection of lung cancer. Peripheral nodules can be identified and excised using video-assisted, minimally invasive techniques, and mediastinal lymph nodes can be sampled for histologic examination. VATS is also extremely useful for evaluation and palliation of suspected pleural disease, particularly when thoracentesis has been nondiagnostic. Thoracoscopy is ideal for assessment of mediastinal nodes not accessible by standard mediastinoscopy or EUS-FNA techniques, and for evaluation of suspected T4 lesions.

Thoracentesis

Needle drainage of a pleural effusion associated with a presumed lung cancer can identify inoperable, pleural disease (M1a). Typically, a bloody pleural effusion is malignant; however, unless malignant cells are identified, a bloody pleural effusion should be considered traumatic. In general, a diagnosis of cancer can be established in 70% of malignant effusions by thoracentesis. If the initial thoracentesis is negative, additional percutaneous thoracenteses improve the diagnostic yield; otherwise, thoracoscopy can be used to simultaneously collect pleural fluid for cytologic examination, and obtain pleural as well as lymph node biopsies for tissue diagnosis.

Thoracotomy

Typically, more than 95% of tumors can be accurately diagnosed and staged prior to thoracotomy. Nevertheless, in a small minority of cases, the diagnosis of lung cancer is made only at thoracotomy. In general, these are cases in which there is a large, inflammatory component associated with a small focus of cancer that obscures diagnosis. During thoracotomy the diagnosis often can be obtained via multiple FNAs with immediate cytologic analysis, or incisional (or preferably excisional) biopsy with frozen section. Additional intraoperative biopsies of hilar and mediastinal lymph nodes should be obtained with resection of the primary lesion and complete mediastinal lymph node dissection performed, if indicated on the basis of intraoperative staging.

Lung Cancer Screening

Considerable efforts have focused on the evaluation of sputum cytology, chest radiographs, and more recently, screening CT scans for early detection of lung cancer. Whereas previous trials using sputum cytology and/or chest radiographs were negative, recent studies suggest that serial CT scans are useful for early detection of early-stage lung cancers, and have the potential of reducing lung cancer-specific mortality in high-risk individuals.[167–169] However, results of large randomized studies are still eagerly awaited. These issues are discussed in detail in Chapter 62.

Chemoprevention

Despite encouraging preclinical data, the results of large chemoprevention trials evaluating primary prevention (healthy high-risk smokers), secondary prevention (premalignant lesions), and tertiary prevention (second primary tumors in previously treated individuals) have been disappointing. Well-designed phase 2 or phase 3 trials have failed to demonstrate efficacy of retinoids including retinal, retinal palmitate, isotretinoin, or β-carotene, for primary, secondary, or tertiary prevention of lung cancer. Vitamin E (α-tocopherol) or selenium supplements do not appear to be affective chemopreventive agents.[170]

Recent data indicate that erbB1/erbB2, ras, cox-2, AKT, and PI3-kinase signaling modulate growth and metastasis of lung cancer cells[171]; as such, inhibitors of these pathways are attractive agents for evaluation in lung cancer prevention trials. A variety of drugs targeting these aforementioned signaling abnormalities, as well as DNA demethylating agents and histone deacetylase inhibitors, prevent lung cancers in mice exposed to tobacco carcinogens.[172] The efficacy of these compounds alone or in combination for chemoprevention of human lung cancers has not been established.

OVERVIEW OF INVASIVE LUNG CANCER MANAGEMENT: TREATMENT MODALITIES

Historically, surgery has provided the best chance of cure for patients with resectable NSCLC. Whenever surgery has not been an option for patients with resectable cancers, radiotherapy (RT) has been used for control of the primary tumor and regional lymphatics. In general, chemotherapy is rarely curative in lung cancer patients; however, complete responses and prolonged survivals occasionally have been seen in patients with advanced locoregional, as well as metastatic disease. Combined-modality therapies have been extensively evaluated as a means to enhance survival in patients with resectable as well as unresectable disease.

Surgery

Surgery remains the best treatment modality for patients whose lung cancers are limited to the hemithorax and can be totally encompassed by excision. In stage I and stage II disease, when the tumor has not extended beyond the bronchopulmonary lymph nodes, complete (R0) resections are almost always feasible. Currently, controversy arises regarding the management of N2 disease. Ipsilateral N2 mediastinal lymph node involvement, despite being potentially resectable, typically portends limited survival following surgery alone. Historically, patients in whom N2 disease is identified preoperatively have a much poorer prognosis than individuals with occult N2 disease discovered at the time of thoracotomy (<10% vs. 30% 5-year survival rates, respectively). Randomized trials indicate that combined-modality approaches using either induction (preoperative) or adjuvant chemotherapy with or without radiation improves survival in patients with resectable stage IIIA lung cancers.

In general, stage IIIB lung cancers, by virtue of contralateral (N3) lymph node metastases or invasion of vital structures such as carina, heart, or great vessels (T4), particularly in the presence of N2 disease are inoperable. Similarly, lung cancers that are associated with malignant pleural effusion or presence of contralateral nodules (M1a), or have metastasized to distant organs (M1b) are generally incurable by surgery; however, individuals with oligometastases involving brain or adrenal gland occasionally experience long-term survival following resection of the primary and metastatic lesions[173] (Fig. 75.9).

Patient Selection

The preoperative evaluation of patients considered for surgical management of lung cancer includes clinical staging of the disease to determine resectability, and assessment of cardiopulmonary reserve to ascertain if the intended pulmonary resection can be performed with acceptable perioperative risk. Studies best suited to assess cardiopulmonary reserve include spirometry with diffusion capacity, arterial blood gases, quantitative ventilation-perfusion scans, oxygen-consumption studies, echocardiography, cardiac radionuclide scans, and cardiac MRI.[174] Traditionally, patients have been deemed suitable candidates for pulmonary resection if the predicted postoperative forced expiratory volume in 1 second (FEV_1) and/or carbon monoxide diffusion capacity (DLCO) equal or exceed 40% predicted, and the patient does not suffer from hypercapnia or pulmonary hypertension. More recent data suggest that individuals in whom preoperative FEV_1 and DLCO values exceed 60% predicted are at low risk for pulmonary resection, including pneumonectomy, and need no additional pulmonary studies. In contrast, patients with preoperative FEV_1 and DLCO values less than 60% should undergo quantitative ventilation-perfusion scans to predict the impact of the intended resection on overall pulmonary reserve. Patients in whom postoperative predicted FEV_1 and/or DLCO values are less than 40%, or individuals with PCO_2 45% or more should undergo exercise testing (oxygen-consumption studies) using cycle ergometry with increasing workloads to further assess perioperative risk.

In general, patients with postoperative predicted FEV_1/DLCO values less than 40% predicted but with a VO_2 max more than 15 mL/kg can undergo pulmonary resection with acceptable risk. Patients with predicted postoperative FEV_1/DLCO values less than 40% predicted and a VO_2 max less than 15 mL/kg have increased risk of perioperative pulmonary complications and death, and should be considered for nonsurgical, palliative therapy. However, some individuals with small peripheral lesions and VO_2 max less than 15 mL/kg are

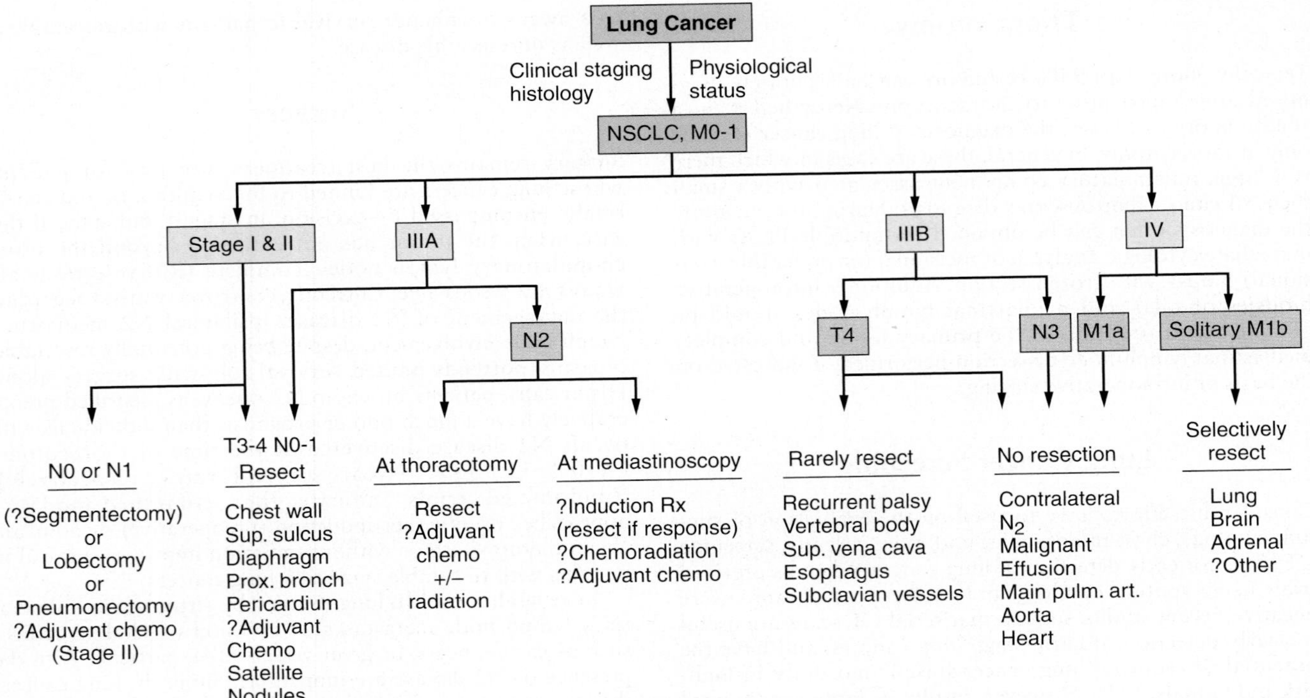

FIGURE 75.9 Algorithm of treatment for various stages of non–small cell lung cancer (NSCLC). See text for details. Chemo, chemotherapy; Sup., superior; Prox. bronch, proximal bronchus; Rx, therapy; pulm. art., pulmonary artery.

candidates for limited resection, although such interventions should be individualized, and patients informed regarding increased risk of these procedures.

Surgical Procedures

Lobectomy is currently the standard of care, providing this will result in complete resection of the tumor mass. If the tumor extends across a fissure, lobectomy with *en bloc* segmentectomy, bilobectomy, or pneumonectomy should be performed if the patient can tolerate a larger resection. Recently, there has been a resurgence of interest in smaller resection for early-stage node-negative carcinomas. For proximally situated (T3) tumors, parenchymal-preserving operations using bronchoplastic or angioplastic techniques should be performed whenever possible, as patients undergoing these resections have comparable survival rates and improved quality of life relative to patients with similarly staged tumors undergoing pneumonectomy.

The most common complications after lung cancer surgery are not related to technical failures of the operation, but rather are due to cardiopulmonary issues, particularly supraventricular arrhythmias and respiratory failure. Because of improved surgical and anesthetic techniques and perioperative care, postoperative mortality rates for surgical resection for lung cancer patients have decreased remarkably during the past 50 years. Presently, pneumonectomy can typically be performed with a mortality rate of less than 6%, lobectomy less than 3%, and smaller resections with 1% or less. Kozower et al.[175] used the Society of Thoracic Surgeons database containing 18,800 lung cancer resections performed at 100 centers between January 1, 2002, and June 30, 2008, to develop three multivariate risk models (major morbidity, mortality, and combined major morbidity/mortality). The overall perioperative mortality rate was 2.2%; the composite major morbidity/mortality rate was 8.6%. Significant predictors of mortality included pneumonectomy or bilobectomy, performance status, American Society of Anesthesiologists score, induction chemoradiation therapy, age, steroids, male gender, FEV_1, body mass index, and urgent procedures.

Radiation Therapy

Techniques

External-beam radiation therapy consists of high-energy photon beams generated by a linear accelerator or proton beams generated by a cyclotron. Therapeutic doses of radiation must be delivered to the target while minimizing incidental irradiation of surrounding normal tissues. A planning session is necessary before treatment can begin. This process typically requires a planning CT scan with the patient in the treatment position, often in an immobilization device to limit day-to-day setup errors. The radiation oncologist defines the target and surrounding normal tissues on the CT images using special treatment-planning software. New imaging modalities such as FDG-PET can be helpful in discriminating between tumor and atelectasis, and involved versus uninvolved lymph nodes. A three-dimensional (3D) map is constructed, which delineates the location of the target and normal surrounding organs (Fig. 75.10). A treatment plan is then developed. This involves choosing beam orientations, the number of beams, energy, and weighting. Multiple plans can be compared using dose-volume histograms, which display the dose received by the target and critical structures.

Photon energies between 4 and 10 MV are preferred for patients with peripheral tumors surrounded by low-density lung parenchyma, given dose build-up issues at the interface of the lung and tumor. Higher-energy photons (15–18 MV) may be necessary for optimal dose homogeneity in larger patients or when oblique fields are utilized.

Respiratory Motion

Lung tumors, especially peripheral tumors in the lower lobes, invariably move during the respiratory cycle. This motion must be taken into account during the planning process. Multiple methods, some simple and others more complex, are available to manage respiratory motion.[176–178] One approach is to determine the motion trajectory of the tumor during the respiratory

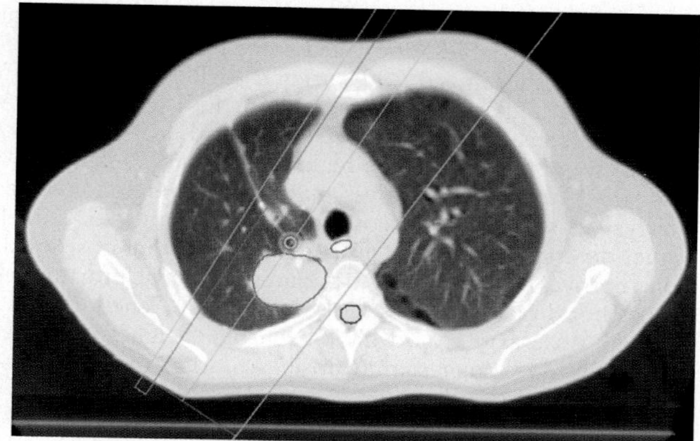

A

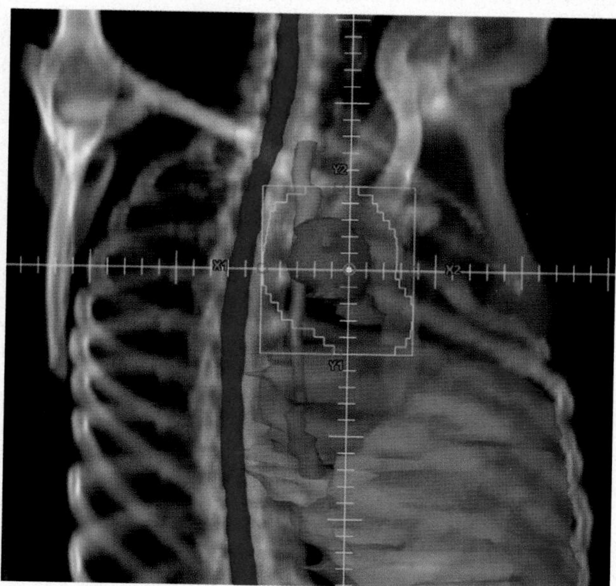

B

FIGURE 75.10 **A:** Three-dimensional axial image of a lung tumor and a right posterior oblique beam. **B:** A "beam's eye" view of this field. Red, tumor; blue, spinal cord; green, esophagus; aqua, liver; brown, heart.

cycle and design radiation fields that encompass this entire volume. This includes such methods as slow CT scanning during quiet respiration, obtaining a breath-hold CT in inspiration and expiration and combining these volumes, obtaining a four-dimensional CT (4D CT), and creating a maximum-intensity projection dataset. The magnitude of respiratory motion can be dampened using an abdominal compression device.

An alternative approach is to only treat the tumor when it is in a certain phase of the respiratory cycle. This is termed *respiratory gating* and requires technology that turns the beam on and off at the desired portions of the respiratory cycle.[178] A signal acting as a surrogate for respiratory motion is required. Although internal fiducial markers can be used, external markers of respiratory motion are more commonly employed (e.g., a beacon placed on the abdomen). It is essential to have CT images corresponding to the desired phase of the respiratory cycle for treatment planning. This is often accomplished with a 4D CT scan.

Another option is treating patients while they are holding their breath. In deep inspiratory breath hold, treatment planning and delivery are performed with the patient holding his or her breath in deep inspiration. This reduces tumor motion from respiration and can decrease the volume of normal lung in the field. Deep inspiratory breath hold requires a compliant patient who has sufficient pulmonary function to hold his or her breath for a moderate length of time. A potential downside is uncertainty whether the tumor is in the same position from day to day. Treating in breath-hold position can also be performed using an active breathing control device, in which the airflow of the patient is temporarily blocked by the device for a period of time that is comfortable for the individual patient.[179,180]

Finally, tumor tracking can also be performed whereby the radiation beam moves (i.e., tracks) the tumor as it moves during the respiratory cycle. This requires a fiducial marker in the tumor that can be used to match the motion. This technique is not widely used in clinical practice. Whatever method is used, the radiation oncologist must be comfortable that the position of the tumor during the planning phase is identical to the position of the tumor during the treatment phase.

Image-Guided Radiation Therapy

The most common method used today to confirm proper position of the isocenter and shape of individual radiation fields is megavoltage port films, typically obtained once a week during the course of therapy. Image-guided radiation therapy refers to newer methods and technologies that allow the patient, and in many cases the actual tumor, to be imaged prior to each fraction. Real-time shifts are then made making the delivery of radiation therapy even more accurate. With improved accuracy and less set-up error, treatment margins can also be safely reduced.

Several methods of imaging can be performed prior to treatment to increase accuracy of radiation therapy for lung cancer patients. Diagnostic-quality kilovolt images of the treatment isocenter, using on-board imaging equipment, can be performed prior to each fraction. This allows bony anatomy, or radio-opaque fiducial markers within the tumor, to be aligned before each treatment. A cone-beam CT scan can also be performed, which allows soft-tissue matching. This is particularly helpful when stereotactic body radiation therapy is performed for stage I NSCLC.

Intensity-Modulated Radiation Therapy

Intensity-modulated radiation therapy (IMRT) is a relatively new radiation delivery technique in which the fluence of individual beams is modulated to allow better conformality of the high-dose volume to the target (Fig. 75.11). Dose to adjacent normal structures is not eliminated with IMRT, rather it is redistributed. In fact, IMRT *increases* the volume of lung receiving a low dose of RT, and may actually *increase* the rate

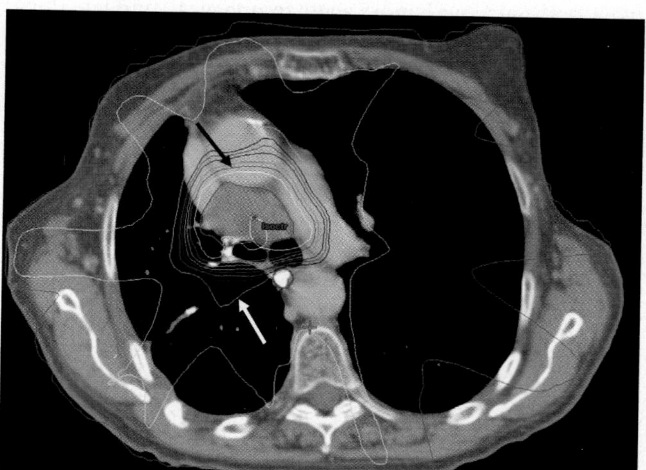

FIGURE 75.11 Axial image showing a treatment plan for a patient with IIIA non–small cell lung cancer treated with intensity-modulated radiation therapy. Note how the high-dose distribution avoids the esophagus (contoured in *green*). The 95% (*black arrow*) and 65% (*white arrow*) isodose lines are shown.

of injury.[181–183] Furthermore, because IMRT is typically delivered using moving multileaf collimators, where each region of the field is not treated simultaneously, one needs to be careful to consider the possible confounding impact of respiratory motion on IMRT dose delivery.[184,185]

Under clinical circumstances when IMRT is deemed necessary (e.g., when avoidance of critical structures such as the spinal cord cannot be accomplished using standard radiation fields) several factors must be explicitly addressed. Assessment of tumor motion, ideally with a 4D CT scan, is mandatory. The target volumes and surrounding organs at risk must be contoured and appropriate constraints placed to both adequately treat the tumor and minimize dose to critical surrounding structures. Procedures must be put in place to verify accurate patient-setup prior to treatment. This may include kilovolt onboard imaging, cone beam CT, or (at a minimum), verification of the isocenter weekly using megavoltage portal images. Finally, quality assurance measurements of the IMRT plan should be performed.

The M. D. Anderson Cancer Center has published the largest clinical experience using IMRT for lung cancer. Among 290 lung cancer patients (68 treated with IMRT and 222 treated with standard 3D techniques), the incidence of grade 3 or more radiation pneumonitis was significantly lower in those patients treated using IMRT versus 3D (8% vs. 32% at 12 months, P = .002). In the IMRT group, patients with V5 values (volume of lung receiving 5 Gy or more) greater than 70% appeared to be at higher risk of pneumonitis. Other dosimetric parameters (MLD, V20) were not assessed for their association with pneumonitis.[182] Similarly, a report from Memorial Sloan-Kettering Cancer Center noted resonable outcomes with IMRT.[183] Further investigation will be necessary to understand the utility and risks of IMRT relative to conventional conformal approaches.

Elective Nodal Irradiation

The conventional approach for locally advanced NSCLC is to treat sites of known intrathoracic disease (based on imaging and pathologic findings), as well as lymph node regions in the mediastinum and ipsilateral hilum at risk of harboring microscopic disease (elective nodal irradiation [ENI]). Although standard for several decades, this practice has been challenged in recent years.

Opponents of ENI have argued that until RT can effectively control known gross disease, treatment of *possible* microscopic disease seems unjustified.[186] Larger fields are likely associated with more acute (esophageal) and late (lung) toxicity, and may hinder the ability to escalate dose to gross disease. Furthermore, PET is being used increasingly in NSCLC staging and, as previously discussed, is more sensitive and has a higher negative predictive value than CT. The reported rates of isolated nodal failure in patients who did not receive (intentional) ENI are modest (5% to 10%).[187] Finally, most patients receive chemotherapy, which helps control microscopic disease.

Proponents of ENI assert that the technical limitations of PET limit its ability to identify *all* sites of microscopic tumor extension within the chest,[188–191] and cure is impossible without control of regional disease. Although the reported risk of an isolated mediastinal recurrence is low in absolute terms (5% to 10%), this rate is high relative to the overall cure rate. In other words, if the cure rate with RT can be increased by 5% to 10% with the addition of ENI, this would be a clinically meaningful benefit. Furthermore, while several studies have shown low rates of isolated nodal failures when ENI is omitted,[192] this relies principally on radiographic findings that may underestimate the true risk of uncontrolled regional disease, which can lead to subsequent distant dissemination.

A recent randomized study from China, although complicated by two variables, does shed some light on this issue.[193] This study randomized 200 patients to RT with ENI (60–64 Gy) or a higher dose of RT without ENI (68–74 Gy). All patients received concurrent cisplatin and etoposide. Local control was improved in the higher-dose arm (51% vs. 36%, P = .032) and there was less pulmonary toxicity. Five-year survival was 18% in the conventional arm and 25% in the higher-dose arm (P = .2). This study suggests that dose escalation improves local control and perhaps survival. Unfortunately, it does not directly address the value of ENI. Whether ENI in the high-dose arm would have been beneficial is unknown. This study does suggest that dose escalation may add more value than ENI.

It is reasonable to suppose that ENI does not need to be an all-or-nothing phenomenon. Surgical series have shown that NSCLC spreads in a fairly predictable pattern.[194,195] The judicious use of ENI, treating sites most at risk in the mediastinum based on the involved lobe and other features, seems reasonable.[196] Although dose escalation has potential to improve outcomes in locally advanced NSCLC, this does not necessarily preclude the prudent use of ENI.

Radiation Therapy Toxicity

Treating lung cancer with RT is challenging. Tumors are often large, irregularly shaped, move with respiration, and are in close proximity to several critical normal tissues. High-energy photons unavoidably deliver incidental dose to normal tissues throughout their trajectory, including tissues on the entrance and exit side of the beam. Proton beams are not immune from these complexities and have their own, and even unique, challenges. Sophisticated treatment planning (3D conformal, intensity modulation) and delivery (tomotherapy, radiosurgery) can reduce/redistribute, but not eliminate, normal tissue exposure.

Acute versus Late Injury

Reactions developing during or shortly after RT are termed *acute* and involve tissues with a relatively rapid cell turnover. For example, most patients will develop odynophagia from esophageal mucositis. Acute effects are typically transient, and resolve within weeks after completing RT. Conversely, *late* normal tissue injury occurs because of effects on more mature/slower-growing tissues, manifesting clinically months to years post-RT, and is typically chronic and irreversible (e.g., lung fibrosis, esophageal stricture). It appears that some late effects occur as a consequence of severe acute reactions.[197,198] In general, acute effects are relatively common. Late effects are more serious, but fortunately less common.

Clinical versus Subclinical Injury

It is important to recognize that there are often different methods to assess injury, and that the reported toxicity rate depends on the specific end points (Table 75.7). For example, abnormalities in radiographs or laboratory tests are more common than clinical symptoms.

Pulmonary Toxicity

Radiation-induced lung injury is relatively common, and traditionally is divided into early (acute) and late (chronic) toxicity. Early toxicity (radiation pneumonitis) is typically manifested as shortness of breath, dry cough, and occasionally fever, occurring 1 to 6 months after treatment.[199] Plain radiographs are often normal, but can demonstrate increased tissue density within the radiation field. Thus, pneumonitis is a *clinical*

TABLE 75.7

RADIATION-ASSOCIATED NORMAL TISSUE INJURY: DIFFERENT TYPES OF END POINTS (AND THEIR APPROXIMATE FREQUENCY)[a]

Organ	Subclinical	Clinical
Lung	Decline in PFTs (variable) Radiographic abnormalities (>50%–100%)	Dyspnea (5%–25%)
Esophagus	Dysmotility on barium swallow Thickened wall on CT	Acute/transient dysphagia (common) Late stricture (rare; more common with higher doses)
Heart	ECG abnormalities SPECT perfusion defects ECHO abnormalities	Symptomatic pericarditis (~3%[b])
Brachial plexus	None	Neuropathy (rare)
Spinal cord	None	Myelitis (<0.1%)

PFTs, pulmonary function tests; CT, computed tomography; ECG, electrocardiogram; SPECT, single photon emission computed tomography; ECHO, echocardiogram.
[a]Values in parentheses are the approximate incidence of the toxicity listed.
[b]Unpublished data from an ongoing prospective study at Duke University.

diagnosis. Radiographic abnormalities without symptoms do not warrant intervention. Pneumonitis typically responds well to oral prednisone,[200] typically 40 to 60 mg daily for 1 to 2 weeks, followed by a slow taper (reducing approximately 10 mg every 1 to 2 weeks). Symptoms recur with a rapid taper. The differential diagnosis of radiation pneumonitis is broad and includes tumor progression, infection, drug toxicity, cardiac disease, pulmonary embolus, and anemia. Because steroids can exacerbate an infection, an initial short course of antibiotics be considered. The majority of patients with pneumonitis recover; however, symptoms can be serious enough to require oxygen or hospitalization, and can be potentially fatal.

Late toxicity (fibrosis) is often detected on radiographic studies, but is usually asymptomatic.[201] If present, however, dyspnea can be progressive and difficult to manage, often requiring long-term steroids, oxygen, or rehabilitation. The severity of radiographic abnormalities is not well correlated with the presence or severity of pulmonary symptoms.[201] In patients treated with high doses of radiation (e.g., 70 Gy or more), unusual pulmonary complications, such as bronchial stenosis, bronchopleural fistula, and fatal hemoptysis, have been reported.[202,203]

After RT, pulmonary function can transiently improve as tumor regresses, especially for central tumors obstructing the major airways. However, eventual decline in pulmonary function is common after RT. Pulmonary function tests typically show a decline in FEV_1 by 3 to 6 months post-RT. DLCO typically is reduced to a greater degree than FEV_1.[204] In the few patients with long-term changes in pulmonary function tests who have been studied in a systematic manner, there appears to be long-term continued diminution in pulmonary function tests 2 to 8 years post-RT.[205]

Accurately predicting the risk of RT-associated pulmonary toxicity is challenging. Several clinical factors have been suggested to increase the risk of pneumonitis, including performance status,[206] lower lobe tumor,[207,208] as well as pre-RT pulmonary function,[206,209] among others. Many studies have also addressed the role of potential biologic predictors of RT-induced lung injury. These are markers found in the blood prior to or during RT and are thought to reflect a predisposition for, or the ongoing evolution of, RT-induced lung injury. A host of cytokines have been implicated, including transforming growth factor-beta (TGF-β). This is a multifunctional regulator of cell growth and differentiation that stimulates connective tissue formation and decreases collagen degradation, which can induce fibrosis.[210] In patient subsets, TGF-β has been shown to predict for RT-induced lung injury.[211,212] However, further investigation will be necessary before biological predictors of lung injury can be used clinically. The present data regarding such cytokines are conflicting (Table 75.6).

The risk of symptomatic lung injury has also been associated with a variety of dosimetric parameters including mean lung dose[207,213–219] and percentage of lung receiving a specified amount of radiation[207,213,215,220,221] (Fig. 75.12). These parameters are readily extractable from a dose-volume histogram. Determining the optimal parameter is difficult as there is extremely high correlation between the different dosimetric parameters. Strict dose-volume guidelines are difficult to define and implement clinically. Because tumors often cause lung dysfunction, such as a central tumor obstructing a major bronchus, function actually improves following RT. Further, traditional dose-volume histograms do not consider regional differences in

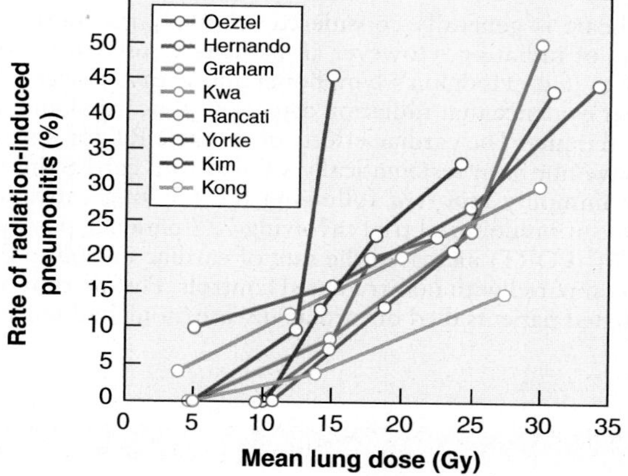

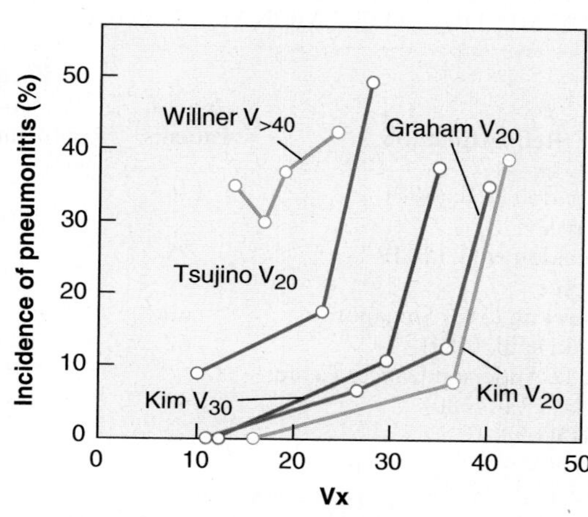

FIGURE 75.12 The rate of radiation-induced pneumonitis has been related to dosimetric parameters that can be extracted from a dose-volume histogram, such as the mean lung dose (**A**), or the volume of lung receiving at least a specified dose (**B**), such as 20, 30, or 40 Gy (denoted as V20, V30, and V40, respectively).

lung function, which might arise from diseases such as chronic obstructive pulmonary disease. With these caveats, limiting the volume of lung receiving over 20 Gy (V20) to 30% to 35%,[207] and limiting the mean lung dose to 20 to 22 Gy[213,214] are recommended. Recent data suggest that the volume of lung exposed to relatively low doses of RT (e.g., 5 to 15 Gy) be more predictive for pneumonitis than the V20 to 30.[222–224]

Esophageal Toxicity

Odynophagia secondary to esophagitis occurs in most patients receiving mediastinal RT. Utilization of conformal radiation therapy techniques, and movement away from elective nodal irradiation, have reduced the length of esophagus incidentally irradiated. Nevertheless, for most patients with stage III disease, the target volume is close to the esophagus and some degree of esophagitis is unavoidable. Esophagitis is typically managed with narcotic analgesics, topical agents such as viscous lidocaine, and occasionally antifungal agents if a candidal infection is suspected. Late esophageal injury, typically manifesting as a stricture or dysmotility, is relatively uncommon with conventional doses of RT (60–66 Gy). However, with more aggressive treatment (RT dose escalation, accelerated RT, concurrent chemotherapy), esophageal stricture has become somewhat more common.[202,225] The incidence of late esophageal injury appears to be related to the severity of the acute reaction.[197]

Cardiac Toxicity

The heart is generally considered relatively resistant to the effects of radiation. However, in patients irradiated for other diseases (e.g., Hodgkin's lymphoma and breast cancer), there is clear evidence that radiation can cause pericardial and myocardial injury. The cardiac effects of thoracic RT for lung cancer have not been systematically studied, and cardiac injury is not commonly *reported* following RT for lung cancer. In a European randomized trial involving 728 patients, postoperative RT (PORT) increased the rate of cardiac mortality threefold compared with nonirradiated controls. Five percent of the irradiated patients died of cardiac disease; nonlethal morbidity was not addressed.[226] In a prospective study of RT-induced lung injury at Duke University, the incidence of cardiac events was 1% (2 of 126) in patients with a mean heart dose less than 25 Gy versus 11% (5 of 47) in patients receiving a mean heart dose more than 25 Gy, respectively.[227] In patients with Hodgkin's lymphoma, Carmel and Kaplan[228] noted pericarditis requiring treatment in 1.5%, 10%, 7%, and 36% of patients receiving whole-heart doses of less than 6, 6 to 15, 15 to 30, and more than 30 Gy, respectively. Based on the available data, it seems prudent to limit the mean cardiac dose to less than 20 to 30 Gy. Depending on the location of the tumor, this may not be practical, and portions of the heart often receive the full prescription dose.

Radiation Protectors

A variety of agents have been used to mitigate the effects of radiation on normal tissue. The most widely tested agent is amifostine (Ethyol, WR-2721), which is believed to scavenge free radicals produced by the interaction of ionizing radiation and water molecules. Multiple randomized studies, and a meta-analysis,[229] have tested the utility of amifostine in patients receiving RT for lung cancer with conflicting results (Table 75.8). The largest study was performed by the Radiation Therapy Oncology Group (RTOG).[230] The incidence of grade 3 or more esophagitis (the primary end point of the study), was 30% with amifostine versus 34% without ($P = .9$). The incidence of grade 3 or more pulmonary toxicity was lower in patients receiving amifostine (9% vs. 16%), but this was not statistically significant. This study has been criticized because the drug was given *once* daily (4 days/week) and the RT was given *twice* daily (5 days/week); thus, 60% of the RT fractions were delivered without the protector. Presently, given the acute toxicity associated with amifostine (nausea/vomiting, hypotension, infection, rash), and the mixed clinical results, amifostine is not widely used for patients receiving thoracic RT.

In a small study of 40 patients irradiated for lung or breast cancer, the addition of pentoxifylline appeared to reduce the incidence of lung injury.[231] Additional evaluation of this approach may be warranted.

TABLE 75.8

RANDOMIZED TRIALS TESTING THE UTILITY OF AMIFOSTINE TO PREVENT RADIATION THERAPY-INDUCED PULMONARY TOXICITY[a]

Study (Ref.)/Affiliation	No. of Patients	Pneumonitis (≥Grade 2) (%) Amifostine vs. Placebo	Fibrosis (%) Amifostine vs. Placebo	Acute Toxicity of Amifostine (%) Hypotension	Nausea/Vomiting
Antonadou et al. (581) Greece	146	12 vs. 52[b] ($P < .001$)	28 vs. 53 ($P < .05$)	7	3
Antonadou et al. (582) Greece	73	30 vs. 67[b] ($P = .009$)	29 vs. 50 ($P = .15$)	22	8
Leong et al. (583) Singapore	60	—	—	70	30
Komaki et al. (584) M. D. Anderson Cancer Center	62	0 vs. 16[c] ($P = .02$)	—	65	—
Movsas et al. (230) RTOG 98-01	243	8 vs. 16.7[c] ($P > .05$)	—	—	23

RTOG, Radiation Therapy Oncology Group.
[a]Radiation therapy doses variable, 1.2 Gy twice daily to 69.6 Gy (Komaki et al. [584], Movas et al. [230]) or 2 Gy daily to 55–66 Gy (Antonadou et al. [581], Leong et al. [583]). Chemotherapy usage variable, no chemotherapy (Antonadou et al. [581]), concurrent therapy (Antonadou et al. [582]), Komaki et al. [584]), and induction + concurrent (Movsas et al. [230], Leong et al. [583]).
[b]Rates at 3-month follow-up.
[c]Grade ≥3.
(Some of the data are estimated from data, figures, and tables provided in the citations.)

Chemotherapy

Platinum-based combinations have become the standard of care for treating unselected advanced NSCLC, and chemotherapy has been advocated as an integral part of combined modality approaches to earlier stages of disease. In 1988, Rapp et al.[232] reported that cisplatin-based chemotherapy improved survival of patients with advanced NSCLC. Several additional trials comparing chemotherapy versus best supportive care (BSC) have confirmed these findings, prompting widespread use of chemotherapy for palliation in patients with advanced disease. Cisplatin- or carboplatin-based doublets (in combination with paclitaxel, gemcitabine, pemetrexed, docetaxel, or vinorelbine) are now standard for patients with stage IV disease (Table 75.9).

Recently, EGFR tyrosine kinase inhibitors have been introduced in second- and third-line treatment of advanced disease and in selected patients in first-line treatment. Recent evidence indicates that patients who have an activating mutation of EGFR benefit more from an EGFR inhibitor than from chemotherapy in first-line treatment of advanced disease.[233,234]

Chemotherapy also improves outcome for patients with locoregional disease. When used either in sequence or concurrently with radiation, platinum-based therapy prolongs survival and increases the fraction of patients with stage III disease who are long-term survivors. Whereas some of this benefit may be the result of improved local control, eradication of micrometastatic disease appears to be the principal mechanism by which chemotherapy improves survival of patients with locally advanced lung cancer.

Neoadjuvant (induction) chemotherapy, in which a specified number of cycles are administered before definitive local therapy with surgery or radiation, appears to be beneficial in patients with locally advanced NSCLC. The simultaneous use of chemotherapy and RT (concomitant chemoradiotherapy) has also been intensively investigated. In theory, adjuvant and induction chemotherapy are administered to improve control of occult metastatic disease. Decreasing the size (downstaging) of the locoregional tumor burden may also be observed after induction therapy. The delay of RT to allow administration of induction chemotherapy has been of theoretic concern because this could lead to the proliferation of clonogenic tumor cells in an unresponsive tumor. Concomitant chemoradiotherapy also results in systemic antitumor activity. However, this will be realized only if systemically active doses and schedules of the drugs are administered. In clinical practice, the latter has been challenging because radiation-related toxicities (i.e., esophagitis and radiation pneumonitis) are usually increased in the presence of chemotherapy. Therefore, the primary goal of concomitant chemoradiotherapy should be to enhance the antitumor activity of radiation and increase locoregional control (radiation sensitization or enhancement).

Induction chemotherapy followed by RT prolongs the overall survival in patients with unresectable stage III disease compared with patients receiving RT alone.[235] Trials by Furuse et al.[236] and the RTOG[237] support the use of concurrent chemotherapy and radiation compared with sequential chemotherapy when treating locally advanced disease. However, the toxicity of concurrent chemoradiotherapy is substantial, and for patients with an impaired performance status, sequential chemotherapy and radiation is preferable.

Chemotherapy has an emerging role in stage IIIA (N2) disease. The use of induction chemotherapy in the surgical setting (stage IIIA)[238,239] alone or in conjunction with RT,[240] results in a 5-year survival of 20% to 30% compared with 5% to 10% for surgery alone for clinical N2 disease. Intergroup data indicated a significant increase in progression-free survival in patients treated with chemoradiotherapy followed by surgery, but the anticipated improvement in survival of 10% was not evident.[240]

Before 2003 there was little evidence to support the routine use of adjuvant chemotherapy after potentially curative resections in lung cancer patients. Several large randomized studies now support the use of adjuvant cisplatin-based chemotherapy in radically resected stage II and IIIA NSCLC.

TABLE 75.9

SELECTED RESULTS OF RANDOMIZED TRIALS OF FIRST-LINE CHEMOTHERAPY FOR ADVANCED LUNG CANCER

Study (Ref.)	Regimen	No. of Patients	RR (%)	Survival	
				Median (mo)	1 Year (%)
Le Chevalier et al. (433)	Cisplatin and vinorelbine	206	30	9.3	35
	Cisplatin and vindesine	206	19	7.4	27
	Vinorelbine	206	14	7.2	30
Bonomi et al. (435)	Cisplatin and etoposide	150	12	7.7	32
	Cisplatin and paclitaxel, 135 mg/m²/24 hr	150	26.5	9.6	37
	Cisplatin and paclitaxel, 250 mg/m²/24 hr	150	32.1	10.0	39
Kelly et al. (452)	Carboplatin and paclitaxel	208	25	8	38
	Cisplatin and vinorelbine	202	25	8	36
Schiller et al. (585)	Cisplatin and paclitaxel, 135 mg/m²/24 hr	288	21.3	7.8	31
	Cisplatin and gemcitabine	288	22	8.1	36
	Cisplatin and docetaxel	289	17	7.4	31
	Carboplatin and paclitaxel	290	17	8.1	34
Smit et al. (444)	Cisplatin and gemcitabine	160	37	8.9	33
	Carboplatin and paclitaxel	159	32	8.1	36
	Cisplatin and vinorelbine	161	28	6.7	27

RR, response rate.

SPECIFICS OF LUNG CANCER MANAGEMENT

Localized "Resectable" (Stages I, II, and IIIA) Disease

When disease is localized to the lung or includes only regional lymphatics, the primary treatment modality is surgery. However, despite undergoing potentially curative resections, most patients with locally advanced lung cancer succumb to distant metastases. In light of these observations, combined-modality treatments presently are being evaluated in an attempt to improve survival of patients with potentially curable disease.

Primary Surgery

Surgical excision is the treatment of choice for all stage I and II, as well as selected T3N1 (stage IIIA) lung cancers. In most instances, lobectomy with node dissection is sufficient for local control. When the primary tumor or lymph node involvement extends to the proximal bronchus or proximal pulmonary artery (T3), or crosses the major fissure, lobectomy with *en bloc* segmentectomy, sleeve lobectomy, or pneumonectomy should be performed. When resectable adjacent structures (chest wall, diaphragm) are involved, an *en bloc* resection encompassing all sites of disease is necessary.

The role of mediastinal lymphadenectomy as part of the surgical procedure remains controversial. Increasing tumor size is associated with diminished survival after resection.[241,242] Watanabe et al.[243] observed mediastinal lymph node involvement in 11% of patients undergoing resection of clinical T1N0M0 lung cancers smaller than 2 cm in diameter; the majority of lymph node metastases were associated with adenocarcinomas. Nonaka et al.[244] detected lymph node metastases in 28% of patients with lung cancers less than 2 cm in diameter. Konaka et al.[245] observed lymph node metastases in 18% of 171 patients (6% N1, 12% N2) with peripheral clinical T1N0M0 carcinomas smaller than 2 cm in diameter; nodal metastases were more frequently associated with tumors 1.5 to 2.0 cm compared with those less than 1.5 cm in diameter. In another retrospective study, Miller et al.[246] observed lymph node metastases in 7 of 100 patients undergoing resection of lung carcinomas 1 cm or less in diameter.

Complete ipsilateral or bilateral mediastinal lymphadenectomy improves accuracy of staging.[247] Furthermore, some studies suggest that aggressive lymph node dissections improve survival. Keller et al.[248] randomly assigned 373 lung cancer patients to receive pulmonary resections with either systematic sampling or complete ipsilateral mediastinal lymph node dissection (MLND). Although the percentages of patients with N1 and N2 disease were comparable in the two arms, more patients were found to have multilevel N2 disease in the MLND group. Patients who underwent MLND had significantly longer survivals compared with those evaluated by systematic sampling (64 vs. 25 months, respectively). Interestingly, the survival advantage in the MLND group was restricted to individuals with right-sided cancers, possibly because of the lack of complete resection of L2 and L4 lymph node stations in the MLND group. A large study demonstrated significant improvement in survival of patients with stage I, II, and IIIA NSCLC undergoing pulmonary resection with MLND compared with those undergoing mediastinal lymph node sampling.[249]. In contrast, a large retrospective cohort study demonstrated no survival difference in patients undergoing complete MLND relative to those having selective lymph node dissections based on anticipated lobe-specific lymph node metastases.[250] A more recent prospective randomized trial involving over 1,000 patients with N0N1 nonhilar lung cancers revealed no significant differences regarding local or regional recurrence rates, or overall survival in patients undergoing complete mediastinal lymph node dissection versus lymph node sampling.[251] In light of the fact that in experienced hands, MLND does not significantly increase operative time or morbidity,[252] it is reasonable to consider complete ipsilateral MLND for resection of all lung cancers except small, peripheral PET-positive tumors with negative mediastinal uptake.

Although lobectomy remains standard of care, the role of lesser resections (anatomic segmentectomy, wedge excision, or precision cautery dissection) for early-stage lung cancer has yet to be fully defined.[253] A randomized trial conducted by the Lung Cancer Study Group demonstrated that after long-term follow-up, the locoregional recurrence rate was threefold higher with limited resection compared with lobectomy (15% vs. 5%), although morbidity and mortality rates were equal in both arms.[254] This trial was underpowered and included patients with tumors more than 3 cm, as well as patients undergoing wedge resections rather than anatomic segmentectomy. In a retrospective review, Warren and Faber[255] observed no survival difference in patients with T1N0 carcinomas resected via lobectomy compared with segmentectomy. More recently, Kodama et al.[256] compared segmentectomy with lobectomy for treatment of T1N0 carcinomas in patients with adequate pulmonary reserve for lobectomy. Overall 5-year survivals, recurrence rates, and lung cancer–related deaths were comparable in the two treatment arms; of note, however, the average tumor diameter was significantly larger in the lobectomy group than in the segmentectomy group (2.29 vs. 1.67 cm). Koike et al.[257] compared the results of limited resection in 74 patients with lobectomy in 159 patients with peripheral lung cancers less than 2 cm in diameter. All patients had adequate pulmonary reserve for lobectomy. No significant differences were noted in 5-year survival rates for these individuals. Similar results have been published by Okada et al.[258] in a large study examining outcomes of radical sublobar resections for lung cancers less than 2 cm in diameter. Results of these studies are consistent with data from the SEER registry pertaining to 1,165 patients with stage I lung cancers 2 cm or less in diameter, which revealed no significant differences in overall or lung cancer–specific survival for patients undergoing segmentectomy/wedge resection compared to lobectomy.[259]

Although current data do not clearly support the routine use of limited resection for all stage I lung cancers in patients who are candidates for lobectomy, anatomic segmentectomy is reasonable for individuals with peripheral tumors 2 cm or less in diameter that exhibit no endobronchial extension or intrapulmonary metastases, and do not involve N1 or N2 lymph node stations on the basis of intraoperative staging. A large randomized Intergroup trial (CALGB 140503) is currently under way to compare recurrence and survival rates in patients undergoing lobectomy versus anatomic segmentectomy for peripheral early stage lung cancers. A similar trial (JCOG 0802) is ongoing in Japan.

Whereas most lobectomies/segmentectomies are performed via thoracotomy, an increasing number of surgeons have advocated that video-assisted techniques be used for these resections.[260–262] In experienced hands, pulmonary resections and MLNDs performed by VATS techniques are comparable to those performed via thoracotomy. Typically, VATS lobectomies are performed via several port sites as well as a 5- to 8-cm "utility" incision, through which instruments are placed for hilar dissection.

Because VATS resections are less invasive, patients undergoing these procedures return to normal activity sooner than those undergoing thoracotomy. Recent studies indicate that hospital stay and postoperative pain are decreased, frequency of blood transfusion and arrhythmias is lower, and chest tubes

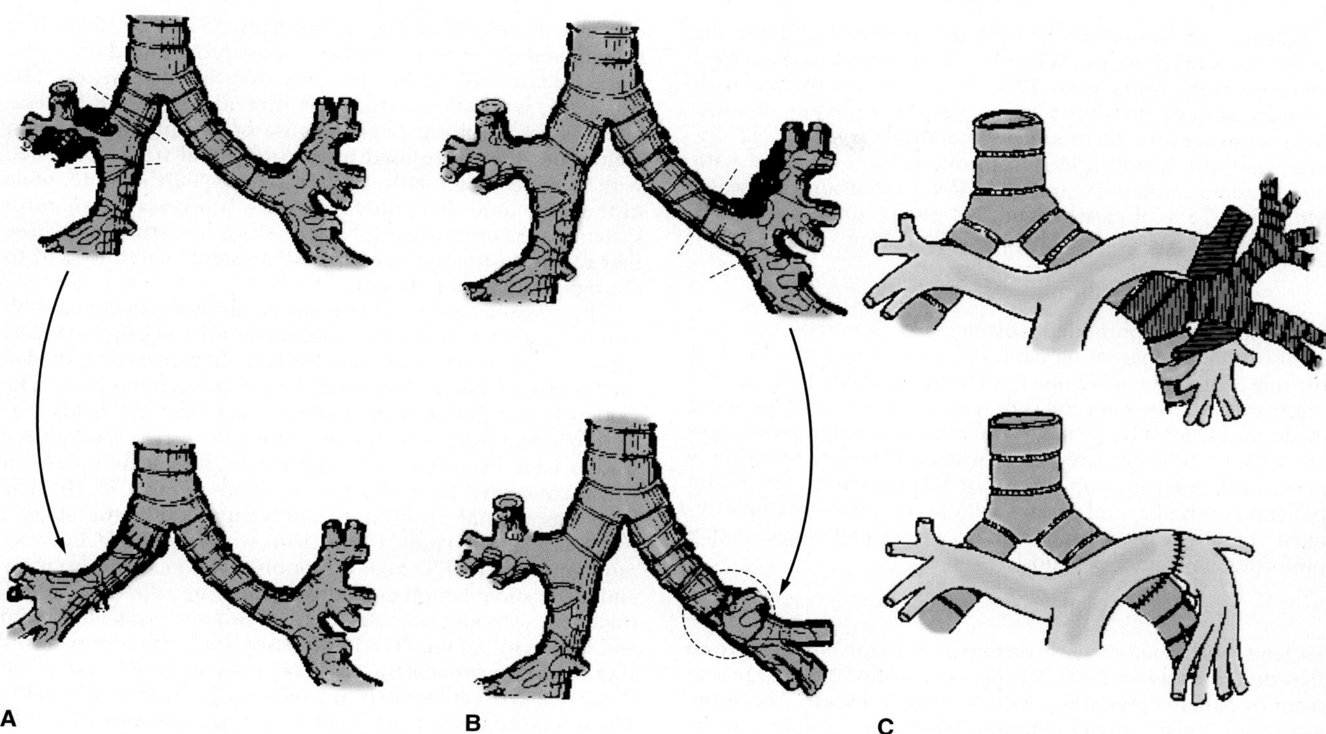

FIGURE 75.13 Bronchoplastic and bronchovascular sleeve resections to preserve pulmonary function. **A:** Right upper lobe sleeve resection. **B:** Left upper lobe sleeve resection. **C:** Left upper lobe bronchovascular sleeve resection.

are removed sooner in patients undergoing VATS procedures than those undergoing thoracotomy.[263,264] Furthermore, several recent studies suggest that survival rates following VATS resections are comparable if not better than those performed by thoracotomy.[260,263,265]

In the new staging system, lung cancers with satellite lesions in the same lobe are defined as T3 tumors, which if not associated with lymph node metastases are classified as stage IIB. Lobectomy with hilar and mediastinal lymph node dissection is the standard of care for these lesions. Similarly, lung cancers invading the chest wall, diaphragm, phrenic nerve, mediastinal pleura, or pericardium are designated T3 tumors. In all instances, it is recommended that these tumors be resected *en bloc* within all involved structures. Prognosis is related to completeness of resection, depth of invasion, and lymph node status. For example, 5-year survival rates approximate 40% for radically resected T3N0 tumors involving chest wall; survival rates of 25% and 15% have been reported for T3 tumors involving chest wall with N1 or N2 lymph node metastases, respectively.[266] Similar results have been observed in patients undergoing resection of T3N0 and T3N1 tumors invading the diaphragm without an associated malignant effusion.[267]

Invasion of the mediastinal pleura, pericardium, or mediastinal fat occasionally may be seen in lung cancer patients. The results of surgery for these lesions are not well known because most of these tumors involve major vascular structures (T4) as well as mediastinal (N2) lymph nodes. Survival is contingent on completeness of resection and nodal status. A 30% 5-year survival rate can be seen in patients with completely resected T3N0 disease involving the mediastinum.[268]

Tumors within 2 cm of the carina are also designated T3. Although these neoplasms can be resected by pneumonectomy, parenchyma-preserving operations using bronchoplastic or angioplastic techniques are preferable alternatives (Fig. 75.13). Numerous cohort studies have indicated that sleeve lobectomy yields similar if not better survival rates with improved quality of life compared with standard pneumonectomy[269]; nodal status is the major determinant of survival in patients undergoing complete resection. In some studies, patients requiring bronchovascular reconstruction fare worse than those having bronchoplasty alone.[270] A recent single-institution study comparing 157 sleeve lobectomies with 257 pneumonectomies revealed significantly lower operative mortality in the sleeve lobectomy group (1% vs. 8%), with similar morbidity, and significantly improved survival in the sleeve lobectomy group (58% vs. 32%). Interpretation of this as well as other retrospective cohort studies is difficult because some pneumonectomy patients may have had more extensive disease and may not have been appropriate candidates for sleeve resections. Despite these limitations, cohort studies as well as a recent meta-analysis[271] indicate that sleeve lobectomy is associated with a lower perioperative mortality and affords comparable if not superior overall survival rates and improved quality of life compared with pneumonectomy for centrally located tumors.

Stage IIIA Disease

T3-4N1 Disease

Stage IIIA disease includes T3N1/N2 and T4N0-1 tumors. As with any other T status, once lymph nodes are involved, the prognosis is much worse. Historically, fewer than 25% of patients with T3 lesions associated with N1 metastases survive 5 years, and few if any survive 5 years when mediastinal nodes are involved.

T1-3N2 Disease

The existence of N2 disease remains the most controversial area for primary surgical management of lung cancer. Although such tumors are potentially resectable, once ipsilateral mediastinal or subcarinal lymph nodes (or both) are involved by tumor, the prognosis is much worse. When N2 nodal disease is diagnosed preoperatively, fewer than 10% of all patients treated with primary surgery survive 5 years, despite adjuvant therapy. Adverse prognostic factors include multiple levels of N2 disease, multiple lymph nodes from one station involved with tumor, adenocarcinoma, and extranodal extension of disease. More than 75% of patients with N2 disease present with disease extending beyond one lymph node station.

"Minimal" N2 Disease

Single-station lymph node involvement with microscopic foci of disease not apparent on clinical staging constitutes most of the subset of minimal N2 disease. This stage of disease is usually discovered at the time of thoracotomy or at pretreatment mediastinoscopy. Five-year survival rates after surgical resection are 10% to 20% and are higher when a complete resection is performed. After incomplete (R1 or R2) resections, few if any patients survive beyond 3 years. Patients found to have involvement of multiple lymph node stations at final pathologic staging uniformly have poor prognosis.

"Bulky" N2 Disease

Patients with tumors with mediastinal involvement beyond that described as minimal N2 disease constitute the large segment of patients presenting with stage IIIA disease. This more advanced, bulky, or multistation N2 disease usually can be identified preoperatively and is termed *clinical N2 disease.* It is considered by many surgeons to be inoperable as few individuals are cured by resection alone.[272,273] As such, induction chemotherapy or induction chemoradiotherapy have been evaluated in select patients. For many patients, however, definitive chemoradiotherapy is the preferred treatment.[274]

Postoperative Radiation Therapy

Locoregional recurrence after resection of NSCLC is common, occurring in approximately 20% to 25% of patients with stage I–II disease,[275,276] and in up to 50% of patients with stage III disease.[277–279] These observations were the rationale behind multiple randomized studies, initiated in the 1960s through the 1980s, examining the role of PORT.[226,279–283] A meta-analysis was performed by the Medical Research Council pertaining to 2,128 patients enrolled on 9 trials.[586]. PORT was associated with an increase in local control but a 7% absolute decrease in survival at 2 years (48% vs. 55%; P = .001). The detrimental effect on survival was most pronounced for early-stage disease (N0-1). For patients with N2 disease, the HR was 0.96, with wide confidence intervals. The PORT meta-analysis has been criticized because of antiquated radiation techniques that were used in the individual trials combined with relatively high daily and total doses. Furthermore, none of the trials used chemotherapy, which is necessary to control systemic micrometastases. Nevertheless, this study did show that radiation therapy must be administered carefully and to the right patient population.

The stage-dependent detriment in survival associated with PORT suggests that improved local control and cancer-specific survival were offset (in the case of stage III disease) or exceeded (in the case of stage I–II disease) by RT-induced mortality. The studies in the PORT meta-analysis used large RT fields that were planned using fluoroscopic simulation. Two randomized studies have been reported since the PORT meta-analysis in which conformal RT techniques were used (Table 75.10). The first was a trial from Italy analyzing PORT for stage I NSCLC.[276] In this study, 104 patients with stage I NSCLC were randomized to PORT (50.4 Gy) or observation after lobectomy and mediastinal lymph node dissection. Three-dimensional RT treatment planning was used to treat only the bronchial stump and ipsilateral hilum. PORT was associated with a statistically significant improvement in local control (98% vs. 77%; P <.01), and overall survival at 5 years (67% vs. 58%; P = .048). The second trial was from Austria; 155 patients with stage I–III NSCLC were randomized to PORT (50–56 Gy) or observation.[285] Modern RT machines and 3D treatment planning appeared to improve 5-year recurrence-free survival (27% vs. 16%; P = .07), and perhaps overall survival (30% vs. 20% at 5 years; P = NS), without any severe late complications. The small size of this trial rendered it insufficiently powered to detect a statistically significant result. When these more recent studies are considered in the context of the PORT meta-analysis, they suggest that improvements in RT techniques (e.g., conformal techniques, reduced target volumes) improve the therapeutic ratio of PORT and allow the improvement in local control to be translated into a survival benefit.

Recent studies that have suggested that modern RT methods may improve outcomes include the Adjuvant Navelbine International Trialist Association (ANITA) study and a SEER study from a more modern period. The ANITA trial randomized 840 patients to adjuvant chemotherapy (cisplatin and vinorelbine) or observation. PORT was not randomized but given at the discretion of the participating center after completing

TABLE 75.10

POSTOPERATIVE RADIATION THERAPY (PORT) FOR NON–SMALL CELL LUNG CANCER

Study (Ref.)	No. of Patients	Stage	Planning	Gy/Day	Total Dose (Gy)	Treatment	Local Control (Crude) (%)	Overall Survival (5 Years[a]) (%)
PORT meta-analysis (586)	2128	I–III	Conventional	1.8–3	30–60	S	74	55
1966–1992						S → RT	82	48[b]
STUDIES NOT IN THE PORT META-ANALYSIS								
Mayer et al. (285)	155	I–III	Conformal	2	50–56	S	76	20
NS						S → RT	94	30
Trodella et al. (276)	104	I	Conformal	1.8	50.4	S	77	58
1989–1997						S → RT	98	67

S, surgery; RT, radiation therapy; NS, not stated.
[a]Unless otherwise noted.
[b]Two years.

chemotherapy. It was noted that in patients with stage III disease randomized to receive chemotherapy, 5-year survival for those who received PORT was 47% versus 34% for those who did not receive RT.[286] PORT was not a randomized variable and therefore no definitive conclusions concerning the effectiveness of RT can be drawn from these data. A SEER study examined 7,500 patients with stage II–III NSCLC (including approximately 2,000 with N2 disease) between 1988 and 2002.[326] The study found that PORT was beneficial for those with N2 disease (HR = 0.855; 95% CI: 0.762–0.959). These retrospective analyses provide a compelling rationale for prospective trials evaluating the role of PORT for patients with N2 disease in the modern era.

In light of criticisms of the PORT meta-analysis,[586] PORT is not currently considered standard therapy despite the high risk of local recurrence after complete resection of lung cancer. Phase 2 trials in which conformal RT was combined with systemic chemotherapy have shown promising results,[289,290] but attempts to re-evaluate PORT in the context of a randomized trial have been difficult. For patients with microscopic disease at the bronchial resection margin, vascular margin, or chest wall, general oncologic principles would suggest that further local therapy is warranted. In addition, patients with high-risk features such as mediastinal lymph node involvement,[286] inadequate mediastinal dissection, close margins, or extracapsular extension should also be considered for PORT. Additional evaluation of the utility of PORT in the context of modern RT techniques and systemic therapy is warranted.

Local Recurrence after Surgery

Depending on pathologic stage, locoregional recurrence of NSCLC after surgical resection occurs in 20% to 50% of patients.[276,277] Although distant failure is more common than local failure, approximately 25% of all failures are confined to the involved lung and mediastinum without radiographic evidence of distant metastatic disease.[275,292,293] Salvage RT, in this otherwise fatal circumstance, is reasonably successful with survival at 2 and 5 years being approximately 30% and 5%, respectively.[294,295] For many patients, concurrent chemotherapy would also be recommended.

Adjuvant Chemotherapy

In the 1980s, the Lung Cancer Study Group conducted two large randomized trials evaluating the cyclophosphamide plus doxorubicin and cisplatin (CAP) regimen. The first trial included patients with completely resected stage II or III adenocarcinoma or large cell carcinoma.[296] Patients were randomly assigned to receive either CAP chemotherapy or immunotherapy with intrapleural bacille Calmette-Guerin and levamisole administered for 18 months. In 141 randomly assigned patients, there was a significant 6-month delay in median time to recurrence and a 15% survival advantage at 1 year favoring chemotherapy. The survival of the control immunotherapy group was similar to that of earlier patients treated with surgery alone, and the authors attributed the improved survival in the experimental arm to the effects of chemotherapy.

Another Lung Cancer Study Group study involved 164 patients with incompletely resected disease who were randomly assigned to PORT, or RT and six cycles of CAP.[297] Incomplete resection was defined as postoperative residual microscopic or macroscopic disease, or disease in the highest resected paratracheal lymph node. The chemotherapy group had a longer time to progression (*P* = .066), but median survival was only marginally improved with chemotherapy, and there was no 5-year survival benefit.

Major limitations of these initial studies included the use of ineffective chemotherapy regimens and small numbers of patients, which precluded detection of a relatively small improvement in survival attributable to adjuvant chemotherapy. Additional studies indicated that concurrent chemoradiotherapy is superior to sequential therapy in nonsurgical treatment of stage III disease.[236,298,299] These data provided the rationale for examining the efficacy of adjuvant concurrent chemoradiotherapy after resection of lung cancer.

Keller et al.[300] randomly assigned 488 patients with stage II and IIIA disease to receive either radiation alone (50.4 Gy) or radiation (50.4 Gy) administered concurrently with four cycles of cisplatin and etoposide. There was no difference in overall survival between the two groups: the median survival was 39 months for the radiation-alone arm versus 38 months for the chemotherapy plus RT arm (*P* = .56).

In 1995 the Non–Small-Cell Lung Cancer Collaborative Group published a meta-analysis examining survival in 9,387 patients (7,151 deaths) in 52 randomized clinical trials.[301] Included in this analysis were data from 14 randomized trials pertaining to 4,357 patients receiving surgical resection alone or surgery plus adjuvant chemotherapy. Cisplatin-based chemotherapy regimens appeared to improve survival in patients undergoing resection by 5%. Whereas the benefit was not statistically significant, this observation prompted additional evaluation of adjuvant chemotherapy in patients with resected lung cancer in clinical trials sufficiently large to enable detection of the survival difference observed in the meta-analysis. Table 75.11 summarizes the results from the most important studies presented after the 1995 meta-analysis. An updated meta-analysis[302] included 17 additional studies and confirmed the benefit from adjuvant chemotherapy (HR = 0.86; *P* <.0001), which represents an absolute benefit of 4% at 5 years, from 60% to 64%. Results obtained with tegafur and uracil or tegafur alone appeared to impart the same benefit as those containing platinum-based therapies.

The Adjuvant Lung Project Italy trial enrolled more than 1,200 patients who were randomly assigned to receive surgery with or without three cycles of adjuvant mitomycin, vindesine, and cisplatin.[303] At 5 years, the group receiving adjuvant chemotherapy had a nonsignificant (2% to 3%) improvement in overall survival. However, this trial was limited by the fact that compliance was poor, with only 69% of patients receiving the full three cycles of chemotherapy. The use of mitomycin C may have contributed to poor compliance of chemotherapy patients.

In the International Adjuvant Lung Cancer (IALT) study, patients with completely resected stage I, II, or IIIA NSCLC were randomly assigned to observation, or three or four cycles of cisplatin-based chemotherapy.[304] A unique feature of the trial was that each participating facility chose one of the following chemotherapy regimens: cisplatin plus vindesine, cisplatin plus etoposide, cisplatin plus vinorelbine, or cisplatin with vinblastine. Radiation treatment was also left to the discretion of each institution, but a consistent standard had to be maintained. Patients were enrolled at 148 centers in 33 countries, with 36% of individuals having pathologic stage I disease, 25% having stage II disease, and 39% having stage III disease. Although the initial accrual target was 3,300 patients, the trial was closed after 1,867 patients had been enrolled because a planned interim analysis revealed a significant impact of therapy on survival (the primary end point). The HR for death in patients receiving adjuvant chemotherapy was 0.86 (95% CI: 0.76–0.98). The median overall survival improved from 44 months to 50 months. This translated into a 4% improvement in overall survival at 5 years (44.5% vs. 40.4%; *P* <.03). Approximately 1% of individuals receiving chemotherapy died as a result of this intervention. Subset analysis revealed no trend for benefit based on either stage of

TABLE 75.11

RECENT LARGE RANDOMIZED STUDIES OF ADJUVANT CHEMOTHERAPY

Study (Ref.)	Chemotherapy Arm	No. of Patients (Chemotherapy vs. Control)	Pathologic Stages	% Compliance	Median Disease-Free Survival (mo)	*P*	HR	Median Survival (mo)	% 5-Year Survival	*P*	HR
ALPI (303)	Mitomycin C 8 mg/m^2 day 1, vindesine 3 mg/m^2 days 1 and 8, cisplatin 100 mg/m^2 day 1, every 3 weeks for 3 cycles	606 vs. 603	I–III	69	36.5 vs. 28.9	.128	0.89	55.2 vs. 48	NR	.59	0.96
IALT (304)	Cisplatin 80–120 mg/m^2 day 1 and vindesine, or vinblastine, or vinorelbine or etoposide, for 3–4 cycles	932 vs. 935	I–III	74	39.4% vs. 34.3% (5-year)	<.003	0.83	NR	44.5 vs. 40.4	<.03	0.86
BR10 (306)	Cisplatin 50 mg/m^2 days 1 and 8 every 4 weeks, vinorelbine 25 mg/m^2 weekly, for 4 cycles	242 vs. 240	IB–II	50	61% vs. 49% (5-year)	<.001	0.60	94 vs. 73	69 vs. 54	.009	0.69
ANITA (291)	Cisplatin 100 mg/m^2 days 1 and 8 every 4 weeks, vinorelbine 30 mg/m^2 weekly, for 4 cycles	407 vs. 433	IB–IIIA	50	36.3 vs. 20.7	.002	0.76	65.7 vs. 43.7	NR	.017	0.80
CALGB 9633 (308)	Carboplatin AUC = 6, paclitaxel (253) for 4 cycles 200 mg/m^2, every 3 weeks	173 vs. 171	IB	NR	89 vs. 52	.030	0.74	95 vs. 78	59 vs. 57	.10	0.80
Kato et al. (310)	UFT 250 mg/m^2 daily for 2 years (255)	491 vs. 488	I	61	50 vs. 42 (2-year)	.14	NR	NR	88 vs. 85	.047	0.71

HR, hazard ratio; NR, not reported.

disease or chemotherapy regimen. Long-term results of this study have recently been reported.[305] With a median follow-up of 7.5 years, there was still a beneficial effect of adjuvant chemotherapy on overall survival, which however lost significance (P = .10); median survivals were 54 and 45 months in the adjuvant chemotherapy and control arms, respectively. There was a higher death rate not due to lung cancer after 5 years of follow-up in the adjuvant chemotherapy arm. Disease-free survival remained significantly in favor of adjuvant chemotherapy (P = .02). This study points to the necessity of having prolonged follow-up in NSCLC cancer adjuvant studies, like in other tumor types, and may suggest late toxicity of cisplatin-based adjuvant chemotherapy.

The North American Intergroup, led by the National Cancer Institute of Canada, performed the BR.10 study, in which completely resected stage IB or stage II NSCLC patients with good performance status were randomly assigned to observation, or vinorelbine 25 mg/m^2 weekly for 16 weeks, plus cisplatin 50 mg/m^2 on days 1 and 8, every 4 weeks for four cycles.[306] Four hundred eighty-two patients underwent randomization; 45% had pathologic stage IB disease, 55% had stage II disease, and 53% had adenocarcinomas. Toxicity of the chemotherapy regimen was as expected, with chemotherapy-related deaths observed in two patients (0.8%). Overall and relapse-free survivals were significantly prolonged in the chemotherapy group relative to the observation group. An update of this trial with a median follow-up of 9.3 years has been reported[307]; survival and disease-free survival were still significantly improved in the adjuvant treatment arms (HR = 0.78; P = .04, and HR = 0.73: P = .02, respectively), although the benefit seemed limited to N1 disease in this update. Within stage IB only tumors 4 cm or more derived benefit from adjuvant chemotherapy. Five-year survival rates were 67% and 56%, in the adjuvant and control arms, respectively. There was no increase in deaths from other causes in the chemotherapy arm in this study.

A large international study (ANITA) also investigated the cisplatin-vinorelbine regimen in patients with stage IB–IIIA NSCLC. Patients were randomized to receive adjuvant chemotherapy consisting of 30 mg/m^2 vinorelbine plus 100 mg/m^2 cisplatin (n = 407) or observation (n = 433). Postoperative RT was optional and was initiated according to the policy of individual centers. Three hundred one (36%) patients had stage IB disease, 203 (24%) had stage II disease, and 325 (39%) had stage IIIA disease. Toxicity of chemotherapy primarily included neutropenia (92%); seven (2%) toxic deaths were observed. Compliance was greater with cisplatin than with vinorelbine (median dose intensity, 89% [range, 17% to 108%] vs. 59% [17% to 100%]). After a median follow-up of 76 months, median survival was 65.7 months in the chemotherapy group and 43.7 months in the observation group (HR = 0.80; P = .017). Chemotherapy improved overall survival at 5 years by 8.6%; this survival benefit was maintained at 7 years.[291]

A randomized study (CALGB 9633) involving only patients with stage IB was conducted by Cancer and Leukemia Group B (CALGB), RTOG, and North Central Cancer Treatment Group (NCCTG). Stage IB patients were randomized following resection to receive paclitaxel 200 mg/m^2 and carboplatin (area under the curve [AUC] = 6 every 3 weeks for four cycles) or observation. Although the initial accrual target was 500 patients, the accrual rate was less than 50% expected. Because slow accrual allowed longer observation times, the accrual target was reduced to 384 patients. In 2004, the study was terminated early on recommendation by the Data Safety Monitoring Board as a result of a planned interim analysis that indicated statistically significant improvement in disease-free and overall survivals in patients receiving adjuvant paclitaxel and carboplatin. Overall, 344 patients were randomized to this trial. With a longer median follow-up of 74 months, however, there was no significant difference in overall survival between the arms (HR = 0.83; P = .12), or disease-free survival (HR = 0.80; P = .065). An exploratory analysis demonstrated a significant survival difference in favor of adjuvant chemotherapy for patients with tumors 4 cm or more in diameter (HR = 0.69; P = .043).[308] These results highlight the hazards of terminating a trial early based on short follow-up, and the need for sufficient sample sizes to detect small but potentially significant improvements in survival in patients receiving adjuvant chemotherapy. As such, data from this study do not support the use of chemotherapy in patients undergoing resection of stage IB NSCLC; no significant improvement was observed in stage IB patients treated on the BR.10 and the IALT studies. Another consideration is that the carboplatin/paclitaxel treatment regimen might be inferior to cisplatin-based chemotherapy in the adjuvant setting.

A meta-analysis based on individual patient data pooled from the five largest trials (ALPI, ANITA, BLT, IALT, and JBR10) of cisplatin-based chemotherapy in completely resected patients, which had been initiated after the 1995 NSCLC meta-analysis, was recently reported.[309] With a median follow-up of 5.2 years, the overall HR of death was 0.89 (95% CI: 0.82–0.96; P = .005) corresponding to a 5-year absolute benefit of 5.4% with chemotherapy. The benefit varied with stage, with the HR for stage IA = 1.40 (95% CI: 0.95–2.06), stage IB = 0.93 (95% CI: 0.78–1.10), stage II = 0.83 (95% CI: 0.73–0.95), and stage III = 0.83 (95% CI: 0.72–0.94). Because most positive studies used cisplatin and vinorelbine as adjuvant chemotherapy, this regimen appears preferable to other doublets in the absence of clear equivalence of other agents.

UFT is an oral antimetabolite composed of a fixed ratio of uracil and tegafur. This compound has been studied extensively in Japan as adjuvant treatment after complete surgical resection. Kato et al.[310] randomly assigned 979 patients with stage I disease to observation alone or 2 years of postoperative UFT (250 mg/m^2/day). At a median follow-up of 70 months, adjuvant UFT therapy was associated with a small (3%) but statistically significant improvement in 5-year survival. Subgroup analysis suggested that the magnitude of benefit was substantial for patients with T2N0 carcinomas (84.9% vs. 73.5%) but not for patients with T1N0 tumors. Several other smaller studies have been performed with UFT in Japan, and a meta-analysis of those studies revealed a reduction in mortality for adjuvant chemotherapy relative to surgery alone (HR = 0.77; P =.015), results which are very similar to those reported for cisplatin-based doublets.[311]

On the basis of the aforementioned studies, adjuvant chemotherapy has become standard for many patients with completely resected stage II and IIIA disease. However, questions remain regarding compliance because patients who have undergone thoracic surgery appear to be in worse shape than other individuals (e.g., breast cancer patients) who typically receive postoperative chemotherapy. Presently, it is reasonable to restrict treatment to patients with good performance status and adequate end-organ function. There is also no indication that patients with stage IA should be treated, as these individuals have relatively good survival rates without adjuvant therapy and have mainly been excluded from adjuvant chemotherapy trials. Furthermore, present data do not fully support the use of adjuvant chemotherapy in completely resected stage IB patients. Age alone should not be a criterion for treatment because there are no data indicating that older patients do not benefit from adjuvant chemotherapy. On the contrary, patients older than 65 benefit from cisplatin-based adjuvant chemotherapy, even if they may receive significantly lower doses and fewer cycles.[312,313]

Preoperative (Neoadjuvant) Chemotherapy

Induction (neoadjuvant) chemotherapy before resection has several theoretic advantages, including reducing tumor volume, enhancing local control, treating micrometastatic disease, and being better tolerated than postoperative chemotherapy. The only large randomized phase 3 study demonstrated a significant increase in time to progression, but not overall survival. In this study, the French Thoracic Cooperative Group randomly assigned a total of 355 patients to one of two arms: two courses of MIC (mitomycin C, ifosfamide, and cisplatin) followed by surgery and two postoperative chemotherapy cycles in responding patients, or surgery alone.[314] In both arms, patients with pT3 or pN2 disease received thoracic RT. Overall response to induction chemotherapy was 64%. The median survival was 37 months for the combined modality arm, and 26 months for the surgical arm (P = .15). Survival differences between arms increased from 3.8% at 1 year to 8.6% at 4 years. Interestingly, a survival benefit was observed in patients with stage I or II (P = .027), but not in patients stage IIIA disease. Despite an excess death rate during treatment, overall as well as disease-free survivals were statistically superior in the neoadjuvant chemotherapy arm (P = .044 and P = .033, respectively) in stage I and II. A major limitation of this study was the chemotherapy regimen, which resulted in poor compliance and excess toxicities in the initial phases of treatment. This group of investigators has recently completed another randomized trial in this patient population, comparing different chemotherapy regimens, that appear better tolerated.

The role of induction chemotherapy in early-stage (IB to IIIA) NSCLC has also been evaluated by the Bimodality Lung Oncology Team trial. In this phase 2 study, 94 patients with stage IB, II, and selected IIIA NSCLC received two courses of paclitaxel (225 mg/m^2 in a 3-hour infusion) and carboplatin (AUC = 6) administered every 21 days, followed by surgery. Patients with completely resected tumors received three additional courses of paclitaxel-carboplatin therapy. Ninety-two patients completed preoperative chemotherapy, with major responses observed in 59% of the enrolled individuals. Of the 92 patients potentially eligible for surgery, 80 (93%) underwent exploration and 70 (82%) underwent complete resection. The 1-year survival was estimated at 85%.[315] This trial demonstrated that induction chemotherapy with the North American standard of carboplatin-paclitaxel could be administered with acceptable toxicities in patients with early-stage lung cancers who were potentially curable with surgery alone. Based on this study, a randomized Intergroup trial (S9900) comparing three cycles of induction paclitaxel-carboplatin plus surgery to surgery alone in early-stage NSCLC was initiated, but closed early because of the positive data pertaining to adjuvant chemotherapy. A total of 354 patients with stage IB–IIIA lung cancers were accrued in this trial.[316] Major radiographic response to chemotherapy was 41%. Progression-free survival and overall survival were not significantly different between the arms; however, there was a trend in favor of neoadjuvant chemotherapy. Median survival was 41 months in the surgery-only arm and 62 months in the preoperative chemotherapy arm (P = .11). Median progression-free survival was 20 months and 33 months, respectively (P = .10).

Interpretation of numerous phase 2 studies of neoadjuvant chemotherapy for stage IIIA patients is very difficult because of differences in the chemotherapeutic regimens, mediastinal staging procedures, and radiation therapy used in these trials. Overall, the results of these phase 2 trials indicate an average response rate of 60%, with 55% of individuals undergoing thoracotomy and 49% of patients having complete resections. Median survival has been reported to be 16 months, with a 5-year survival rate of 30% in chemoresponsive patients and 50% in patients exhibiting pathologic complete response. In general, neoadjuvant chemotherapy-RT results in higher rates of down-staging of the primary tumor.

In a phase 3 trial, Rosell et al.[239] randomly assigned 60 patients with stage IIIA NSCLC to receive induction chemotherapy (three courses of cisplatin 50 mg/m^2 per cycle, mitomycin C, and ifosfamide) followed by resection and postoperative radiation therapy (50 Gy), or to resection plus PORT. A threefold survival advantage was seen in patients receiving induction chemotherapy (median survival, 26 vs. 8 months). Long-term results of this study confirmed a survival difference (median survival, 22 months for chemotherapy plus surgery vs. 10 months for surgery alone).[317] In an additional phase 3 trial, Roth et al.[238] randomly assigned 60 patients with stage IIIA lung cancer to surgery alone or to induction chemotherapy (three cycles of cyclophosphamide, etoposide, and cisplatin) plus surgery. Although not included in the formal protocol, radiation was administered to more than half the patients in both groups. Induction chemotherapy was associated with a sixfold increase in median survival (64 vs. 11 months) and significantly better 3-year survival (56% vs. 15%). In a subsequent report, 32% of patients who underwent neoadjuvant chemotherapy versus 16% of those who had surgery alone remained alive with a median follow-up of 82 months.[318] Although less than initially reported, the median survival in the perioperative chemotherapy arm (21 months) was consistent with that observed by Rosell et al.[317]

In the trial conducted by the French Thoracic Cooperative Group discussed previously, no improvement in survival was seen in patients with N2 disease who received chemotherapy.[314] A retrospective analysis suggested that preoperative chemotherapy was associated with a better prognosis for patients with bulky N2 disease; 5-year survival rates were 18% and 5% for patients treated with and without preoperative chemotherapy, respectively (P <.001). However, a similar advantage could not be demonstrated for those with minimal N2 disease.[319] Based on the contradictory results and limitations of phase 2 and 3 clinical trials, the benefit of induction chemotherapy in patients with resectable stage IIIA (N2) disease remains uncertain, and additional studies are warranted to further address this issue. A recent meta-analysis of 13 studies with 3,224 randomized patients revealed that individuals receiving neoadjuvant chemotherapy had improved survival compared with those who were treated by surgery alone (HR = 0.84; 95% CI: 0.77–0.92; P = .00001). These results were the same when considering only stage III disease.[320]

A few targeted agents have been assessed in the neoadjuvant setting before surgery. Gefitinib was tested in 36 patients with clinical stage I NSCLC. Gefitinib was given up to 28 days before performing mediastinoscopy and surgical resection.[321] Response was observed in 11% of cases and EGFR mutations were the best predictor of response. This setting provides a useful window of opportunity to study novel agents, and access to histologic material to perform biological studies.

Preoperative Radiation Therapy

Poor results with surgery or RT alone for patients with NSCLC led to several randomized trials in the 1970s to 1980s evaluating the role of a combined approach. Acceptance of this strategy was based on studies showing improved resectability and pathologic complete responses after preoperative RT.[322] Reports of long-term survival in patients with superior sulcus tumors after preoperative RT bolstered enthusiasm for this approach. The first major randomized trial was performed by the U.S. Veterans Administration.[323] Men with central lung tumors (all stages, all histologies) were randomized to preoperative RT (40–50 Gy) or immediate resection. There was no

TABLE 75.12

RANDOMIZED TRIALS OF INDUCTION CHEMOTHERAPY VERSUS CHEMORADIOTHERAPY FOR NON–SMALL CELL LUNG CANCER

Study (Ref.)[a]	No. of Patients	Patient Stage	Treatment	Resection Rate (%)	Survival/Tumor Control
Fleck et al. (329)	96	T4 or N2	CT → S	31	21%
			CT-RT → S	52	40%
					(Crude FFP)
Sauvaget et al. (330)	92	T4 or N2	CT → S	55	40%
			CT → CT-RT → S	66[b]	33%
					(4-year OS)
Thomas et al. (331)	558	IIIA/IIIB	CT → S → RT	32	21
			CT → CT-RT → S	37[c]	18
					(5-year OS)

CT, chemotherapy; S, surgery; RT, radiation therapy; FFP, freedom from progression; OS, overall survival.
[a]Fleck: Cisplatin (CDDP), mitomycin C (MMC), vinorelbine (VLB) in arm 1; CDDP, 5-FU with RT (30 Gy) in arm 2. Sauvaget: Induction MMC, vindesine (VDS), CDDP in both arms; CDDP, 5-FU concurrent with RT (40 Gy) in arm 2. Thomas: Induction CDDP, etoposide in both arms with postoperative RT (54 Gy) in arm 1; carboplatin, VDS concurrent with RT (45 Gy) in arm 2.
[b]IIIA only.
[c]Complete resection.
(Adapted from ref. 439.)

difference in the complete resection rate. Overall survival was 12.5% in the preoperative RT arm compared with 21% in the immediate resection arm. A similar trial conducted by the National Cancer Institute[324] also failed to demonstrate an improvement in local control or survival. Given these negative findings, most current trials are investigating the use of preoperative chemotherapy or chemotherapy combined with RT for patients with locally advanced, but potentially resectable, NSCLC.

Preoperative Chemotherapy and Radiation Therapy

Available data suggest that the risk of locoregional recurrence after cisplatin-based induction therapy followed by resection is 30% to 60%.[239,277,278] The addition of RT to chemotherapy in the preoperative setting may improve local control, facilitate a margin-negative resection, and help sterilize mediastinal disease. The principal drawback of preoperative chemoradiotherapy is increased surgical complications, principally bronchopleural fistula[331,376] and postpneumonectomy mortality.[240,331] In addition, when a patient fails to undergo resection, RT is typically resumed to a definitive dose after a lengthy break, which may hinder optimal disease control.

Several phase 2 studies have investigated the feasibility of preoperative chemoradiotherapy. Albain et al.[327] treated 126 patients with pN2-3 or T4 NSCLC with preoperative concurrent chemotherapy (cisplatin and etoposide) and RT (45 Gy). Overall, 76% of IIIA and 63% of IIIB patients underwent resection. Of resected patients, 21% were pT0N0 and 56% were pN0. The median and 3-year survivals for IIIA and IIIB patients were 13 and 17 months, and 27% and 24%, respectively. A pathologic complete response in mediastinal lymph nodes was associated with improved 3-year survival (18% for pN+ vs. 44% for pN0; $P = .0005$). Eberhardt et al.[328] treated 94 patients with IIIA/B NSCLC with preoperative chemotherapy (cisplatin and etoposide) followed by the same chemotherapy concurrent with RT (1.5 Gy twice daily to 45 Gy). Complete (R0) resections were achieved in 53% of patients, and of these, 39% were pT0N0. Of 60 patients with original involvement of mediastinal lymph nodes, 77% had a complete response in the mediastinum. The median and 4-year survival for IIIA and IIIB patients were 20 and 18 months, and 31% and 26%, respectively. An R0 resection and pathologic complete response in mediastinal lymph nodes were associated with improved survival.

Two small randomized trials[329,330] and one larger randomized trial[325] have compared preoperative chemotherapy versus preoperative chemotherapy and RT (Table 75.12). The largest study (N = 558) was conducted by the German Lung Cancer Cooperative Group.[331] All patients received three cycles of cisplatin and etoposide. The control group then underwent surgery followed by postoperative RT. The investigational arm received further chemotherapy with hyperfractionated RT (1.5 Gy twice daily to 45 Gy) followed by surgery. Although the addition of RT in the preoperative setting increased rates of mediastinal clearance (46% vs. 29%) and decreased the rate of positive surgical margins (8% vs. 14%), there was no difference in progression-free survival or overall survival. The risk of bronchopleural fistula (5% vs. 1%) and postpneumonectomy mortality (14% vs. 6%) was higher in patients receiving preoperative RT. Most patients in this study had T4 or N3 disease, a population that is not typically thought to be optimal for a surgical approach in the United States.

Preoperative Chemotherapy or Chemoradiation Therapy and Surgical Mortality

A major issue concerning the use of induction regimens in patients with potentially resectable NSCLC pertains to perioperative morbidity and mortality. Roberts et al.[332] reported that induction chemotherapy significantly increased life-threatening perioperative complications in patients undergoing potentially curative operations. Martin et al.[333] reported significantly increased risk of mortality in patients undergoing right pneumonectomy after preoperative chemotherapy with or without radiation therapy. On the other hand, Siegenthaler et al.[334] observed no increase in perioperative morbidity or mortality in patients undergoing resection for NSCLC after induction therapy compared with those treated with surgery alone. Ohta et al.[335] reported that induction chemoradiation therapy did not affect perioperative morbidity or mortality in lung cancer patients undergoing sleeve resection. Leo et al.[336]

PRACTICE OF ONCOLOGY

observed a threefold higher rate (19%) of pulmonary complications in patients undergoing pneumonectomy following induction chemotherapy compared with pneumonectomy patients who did not receive induction chemotherapy; however, no difference in overall survival rates was observed between the two groups. A similar experience has been reported by Thomas et al.[331] in a recent multi-institution study involving more than 500 patients. Daly et al.[337] observed a 13% postoperative mortality in patients undergoing pneumonectomy following high-dose radiation and concurrent chemotherapy. A recent review of the Society of Thoracic Surgeons database revealed that induction chemoradiation therapy as well as pneumonectomy or bilobectomy were significant predictors of mortality in patients undergoing lung cancer resections.[175] On the other hand, several recent studies suggest that in experienced centers, pneumonectomy after induction chemotherapy or chemoradiation can be performed with mortality rates of approximately 6% and long-term survival contingent on pathologic stage following induction therapy.[338,339] Collectively, these data indicate that induction therapy regimens (particularly those with radiation therapy) may increase perioperative morbidity and mortality, and that appropriate patient selection, as well as diligent intraoperative and postoperative management, can diminish this risk.

As experience with chemotherapy and RT increases, the role of surgery as an essential component of therapy in stage III disease has become more controversial.[340] Local failure remains a significant obstacle, even with concurrent chemoradiotherapy regimens. Theoretically, resection of residual disease will facilitate local control and improve survival. Indeed, surgery appears to improve long-term survival, particularly in patients exhibiting downstaging of nodal disease.[341,342] To date, four published randomized trials have compared a nonsurgical with a surgical regimen for patients with stage III NSCLC. Two small trials showed no advantage of surgery over radiation with or without chemotherapy.[343,344] EORTC 08941 randomized 333 patients to platinum-based chemotherapy with either surgery or definitive RT (60 Gy). Pathologic CR was observed in 5% of patients undergoing surgery. No difference in median overall survival (16.4 vs. 17.5 months) or progression-free survival (9.0 vs. 11.3 months) was observed. Although often cited as evidence for lack of benefit of surgery for stage IIIA (N2) NSCLC, this trial included patients with initially unresectable disease and had a high rate of pneumonectomies and bilobectomies.[345] The Intergroup 0139 trial[326] randomized 396 patients with T1-3pN2 disease to induction chemotherapy (cisplatin and etoposide) and RT (45 Gy) followed by resection versus definitive RT (61 Gy) with concurrent chemotherapy. All patients were required to have technically resectable disease. Pathologic CR was observed in 15% of patients undergoing surgery. The surgical arm had a higher progression-free survival (21% vs. 11%; $P = .008$) and a trend toward improved 5-year overall survival (27% vs. 20%; $P = .10$). Surgical mortality was high (>20%) in patients undergoing pneumonectomy. In an unplanned exploratory analysis, the addition of surgery improved survival in patients undergoing lobectomy.[240]

Surgery for Stage IIIB Disease

Stage IIIB NSCLC encompasses a heterogeneous group of neoplasms exhibiting invasion of the carina, great vessels, or vertebral bodies (T4), and tumors exhibiting ipsilateral supraclavicular or contralateral mediastinal lymph node metastases (N3). In general, tumors in patients with stage IIIB disease are inoperable. As such, combined-modality regimens using chemotherapy and radiation are most appropriate for patients with good performance status. Nevertheless, in highly selected patients, T4 tumors can be completely resected, with long-term survival achieved in some of these individuals who receive combined-modality treatment.[346,347]

Although generally unresectable, primary lung cancers invading the carina can occasionally be resected via pneumonectomy with tracheal sleeve resection and direct reanastomosis of the trachea to the contralateral main-stem bronchus. In some patients, "extended" sleeve lobectomy (resection of the carina) can be used to preserve pulmonary function. Survival is contingent on complete resection and nodal status. Mitchell et al.[348] reported 5-year survival rates of 51%, 32%, and 12% for patients undergoing resection of carinal tumors with N0, N1, and N2 disease, respectively. A more recent study revealed 5-year survival rate of 45% for patients with T4N0 NSCLC undergoing complete resection; no patients with N1 or N2 disease survived 5 years. Anastomotic dehiscence and postoperative pulmonary insufficiency are the most common postoperative problems in these individuals. Given the present survival rates, only highly selected patients without N2 disease should undergo carinal resection.

Tumors involving the SVC occasionally can be treated by *en bloc* resection and graft replacement. Patient survival is contingent on completeness of resection and nodal status. Preoperative differentiation of SVC invasion by direct tumor extension (T4) or via involved mediastinal lymph nodes (N2) can be difficult. Invasive staging of the mediastinum is mandatory in these individuals because patients with N2 disease typically do not benefit from SVC resection and reconstruction.[349,350]

En bloc resection of the lung with part of the involved aorta, esophagus, or vertebral body, not uncommon in the treatment of superior sulcus tumors, results in long-term survival for selected patients. PORT may be beneficial in these situations to augment local control. Long-term survival is limited to patients with minimal atrial or aortic adventitial involvement in tumors invading great vessels, and no mediastinal lymph node metastases.[351,352]

The role of surgery in preoperatively identified N3 disease previously considered totally inoperable has been examined in phase 2 trials. Hata et al.[353] investigated the use of two-field lymphadenectomy, including total mediastinal exenteration and supraclavicular node dissection. The exact role of postoperative therapies combined with this procedure was not discussed. The long-term results of such treatment are unknown. In addition, induction therapies (particularly chemoradiation) have been investigated by Southwest Oncology Group (SWOG) and other intergroups.[354] Overall, the data indicate that after intensive induction therapies, some patients survive long term; however, it does not appear that surgery improves survival in these individuals. In fact, in many phase 2 trials, no attempt was made to excise N3 lymph nodes. Instead, surgery was directed toward removal of the primary tumor and N2 nodes.

Adjuvant and Neoadjuvant Therapies

Because of the high incidence of locoregional failure, RT has been usually recommended as adjuvant treatment after complete resection in patients with T4 or N2-3 disease. However, the exact role of adjuvant RT in this context cannot be assessed because of the paucity of patients undergoing combined-modality treatment. It does appear that patients with T4 tumors (especially T4N0 disease) do reasonably well after neoadjuvant therapy and surgery.[355,356] In one such study,[356] patients with clinically evident T4 tumors, including SVC syndrome, tracheal involvement, and posterior mediastinal invasion, were treated with mitomycin, vinblastine, and cisplatin (MVP) chemotherapy followed by surgery. Sixty-three percent of patients underwent a complete resection, and overall survival at 4 years was 19.5%. Despite these encouraging results, most T4 and N3 tumors cannot be resected completely. In such instances, these tumors should be treated by combined-modality regimens, using RT to achieve local control.

SUPERIOR SULCUS TUMORS

Tumors arising in the apex of the lung that invade the first rib and involve the brachial plexus and stellate ganglion produce Pancoast syndrome. Failure to achieve local control of these neoplasms, which constitute less than 5% of all NSCLC, results in debilitating pain, loss of arm function, and high-level spinal cord compression. During the past 2 decades, treatment of superior sulcus carcinomas (SSCs) has evolved considerably, such that even tumors with vertebral body or subclavian vessel invasion are now considered for resection.[357]

Recent American College of Chest Physicians guidelines recommend that SSCs should be treated the same as similarly staged NSCLC located elsewhere in the chest. However the propensity of these tumors to invade local structures and cause significant symptoms mandates aggressive multimodality intervention, with surgery being an important component. Bruzzi et al.[358] proposed absolute and relative contraindications to surgery for SSCs. Absolute contraindications include distant metastases, invasion of trachea or esophagus, brachial plexus involvement above T1, more than 50% vertebral body involvement, and extensive N2 or contralateral N3 disease. Relative contraindications include invasion of subclavian, common carotid or vertebral artery, vertebral body invasion less than 50%, intraforamen extension, and N1 or ipsilateral supraclavicular (N3) disease. In contrast, Bilsky et al.[359] observed that completeness of resection, regardless of the extent of involvement of the spine, correlated with survival in patients with superior sulcus tumors with spinal or brachial plexus involvement. Bolton et al.[360] observed that nodal status and completeness of resection were determinants of survival in patients undergoing multimodality therapy including complete vertebrectomy for SSC.

Cisplatin-based therapy with concurrent radiation improves local control and possibly prolongs survival in patients undergoing surgery for SSC. Recent comprehensive literature reviews indicate 5-year survival rates of more than 45% versus 36% for SSC patients treated with tri-modality therapy relative to bi-modality therapy, respectively.[361,362] Although some institutions such as MDACC advocate up-front surgery with postoperative chemo-XRT, most academic centers utilize induction chemo-XRT regimens followed by surgery for operable SSCs.[361] The Intergroup trial 0160 evaluated induction chemotherapy plus radiation and surgical resection in 111 patients with mediastinoscopy-negative T3-4N0-1 NSCLC involving the superior sulcus.[363] Induction therapy consisted of two cycles of cisplatin-etoposide chemotherapy with concurrent RT (45 Gy). Eighty-three of 95 eligible patients underwent surgery, 76 of whom had complete resections. Pathologic complete response or minimal microscopic disease was observed in 61 (56%) resection specimens. Five-year survivals were 44% for all patients and 54% after complete resection, with no difference between patients with T3 versus T4 tumors. Most of the recurrences were systemic. Patients exhibiting pathologic complete responses had improved survivals compared with those with any residual disease ($P = .02$). In the Japan Clinical Oncology Trial 9806,[364] 76 patients with SSC (20 of whom had T4 disease) received two cycles of cisplatin, vindesine and mitomycin with concurrent RT (45 Gy). R0 resections were achieved in 51 of 57 patients undergoing surgery; 12 patients exhibited pathologic complete response. Three treatment-related deaths were observed. Five-year disease-free survival and overall survival rates were 45% and 56%, respectively. More recently, Kappers et al.[365] reported a remarkable pathologic complete response rate of 62% in 22 SSC patients undergoing cisplatin-based chemotherapy with hyperfractionated RT (66 Gy), with a 56% 5-year survival in patients with pathologic complete response compared to 17% for patients with residual disease following induction therapy. In this trial as in others, imaging studies have not reliably correlated with pathologic response to therapy. Collectively, these data indicate that aggressive multimodality therapy is feasible in patients with SSCs, and that complete resection affords significant palliation and prolongation of survival in properly selected patients.

UNRESECTABLE OR MEDICALLY INOPERABLE

Medically Inoperable (Stage I)

Conventional Radiation Therapy

In 1963, Morrison et al.[366] reported results of the only randomized trial comparing surgery with RT for early-stage lung cancer. Fifty-eight patients with squamous and small cell carcinomas were randomized. The primary tumor and hilar/mediastinal lymph nodes were treated to 45 Gy. Complete resection was performed in only 57% of patients randomized to surgery. Despite the obvious limitations of this small trial, survival was improved with surgery (32% vs. 7% at 4 years), which has since become the treatment of choice for patients with early-stage NSCLC.

However, the risks of general anesthesia and lung resection may be unacceptably high in many patients with significant cardiac and pulmonary comorbidities. Definitive RT has been used for many decades in these individuals. In early reports, Hilton[367] and Smart[368] described long-term outcomes in 38 patients with early-stage lung cancer treated with RT. Doses of 50 to 55 Gy were prescribed for squamous cell carcinomas delivered to the primary site only, and doses of 40 to 45 Gy were prescribed for small cell carcinomas, delivered to the primary site and mediastinum. Despite limited staging, inadequate doses, frequent treatment breaks to allow recovery of acute reactions, low-energy equipment, and a mix of tumor histologic types, the 5-year survival was 21%.

Table 75.13 summarizes large retrospective series in which patients with inoperable stage I NSCLC were treated with RT alone. Patients were generally treated with daily fractions of 1.8 to 2 Gy to a total dose of 60 to 66 Gy. Elective nodal irradiation was usually omitted. With this approach, 5-year survivals range between 10% and 20% and local failure is common. Higher RT doses,[369,370] smaller tumors,[371,372] and conformal treatment planning[373] have been shown to be associated with better outcomes. Compared with the surgical literature, series investigating RT for early-stage NSCLC often suffer from selection bias. Many of the medical contraindications that prohibit surgery, such as older age, poor performance status, severe intercurrent medical illness, and poor pulmonary function, are independent prognostic factors for survival. Furthermore, patients receiving RT are staged clinically. Surgical upstaging is known to occur in more than 20% to 25% of patients with clinical stage I disease.[374]

Stereotactic Body Radiation Therapy

RT techniques have evolved significantly in the past 10 years to treat medically inoperable NSCLC. Conventional radiation therapy has largely been supplanted with stereotactic body radiation therapy (SBRT) (Fig. 75.14). This unique approach

TABLE 75.13

SELECTED STUDIES OF RADIATION THERAPY ALONE FOR EARLY-STAGE NON–SMALL CELL LUNG CANCER

Study (Ref.)	No. of Patients	Median Dose (Gy)	5-Year Survival (%)	Local Failure[a] (%)
CONVENTIONAL RADIATION THERAPY				
Dosoretz et al. (587)	152	60–69	10	31
Graham et al. (557)	103	60	14	—
Krol et al. (372)	108	60	15	60
Sibley et al. (370)	141	64	13	19
Morita et al. (371)	149	65	22	44
STEREOTACTIC BODY RADIATION THERAPY (PROSPECTIVE STUDIES)				
Nagata et al. (588)	45	12 × 4	83 (T1)	5 (5-year actuarial)
			72 (T2)	0 (5-year actuarial)
Baumann et al. (406)	57	15 × 3	60 (3-year)	8 (3-year actuarial)
Fakiris et al. (407)	70	20–22 × 3	43 (3-year)	12 (3-year actuarial)
Ricardi et al. (408)	62	15 × 3	57 (3-year)	12 (3-year actuarial)
Timmerman et al. (589)	55	18 × 3	56 (3-year)	2 (3-year actuarial)

[a]Crude numbers; does not include regional failures.

involves a few very large fractions given within 7 to 10 days. Common prescriptions include 48 Gy in four fractions, 45 Gy in three fractions, and 54 to 60 Gy in three fractions. Biologically, 60 Gy delivered in 1 week is much more potent than 60 Gy delivered over 6 weeks. These large daily doses are feasible because only small volumes are treated with conformal techniques, which minimizes dose to surrounding critical structures. Appropriate patient immobilization, accurate daily setup, and some method to account for respiratory motion are critical. Table 75.13 contains several prospective trials in which SBRT was used for inoperable stage I disease. In general, reported rates of local control are 88% or higher. Whether SBRT can replace surgery for select patients, particularly those who cannot undergo lobectomy,[377] is currently being evaluated in prospective studies.

Although SBRT appears to be more efficacious than conventional RT techniques, the possibility of severe toxicity, given the high doses per fraction, is also increased. Although most patients tolerate treatment exceptionally well, and the overall risk of long-term toxicity is low, certain patient subgroups are at risk of complications. High rates of pulmonary toxicity, particularly with 60 Gy in three fractions, have been encountered when perihilar/central tumors are treated with SBRT.[375] A phase 1 dose-escalation study by the RTOG for this patient subgroup is ongoing. Patients with tumors in close proximity to the chest wall are at risk of developing severe pain and/or rib fractures.[377–379] Brachial plexopathy can occur when tumors in lung apex are treated.[378] Finally, thin patients with peripheral tumors in close proximity to the skin can develop significant skin toxicity.[379] For each of these circumstances, work is under way to define tolerance doses that will maintain excellent control rates while minimizing the risk of toxicity.

An alternative approach to SBRT for patients with inoperable stage I NSCLC, particularly for patients with central disease, is accelerated RT. A phase 1 study from the CALGB escalated the dose per fraction from 2.41 Gy to 4.11 Gy, to a total dose of 70 Gy.[396] Thus, in the final cohort, a 7-week course of conventional RT was delivered in 3.4 weeks. Treatment was well tolerated and survival rates were promising.

A

Tumor

30%

95%

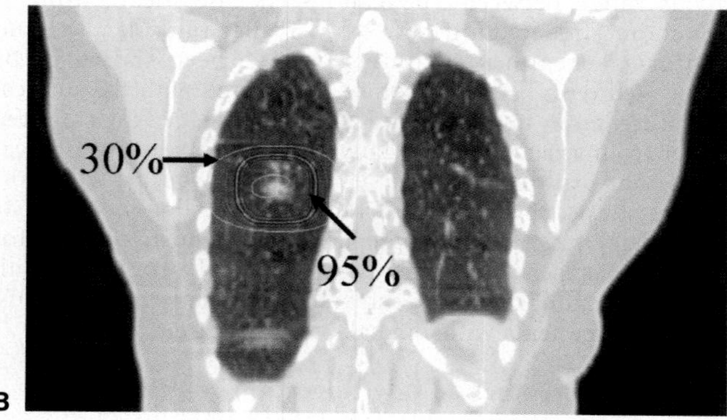

FIGURE 75.14 Axial (**A**) and coronal (**B**) images showing a treatment plan for medically inoperable stage I non–small cell lung cancer using stereotactic body radiation therapy. The 95% (*red*) and 30% (*light green*) isodose lines are shown.

LOCALLY ADVANCED

Combined-Modality Therapy

Prior to the 1990s, patients with locally advanced NSCLC were treated with RT alone. Based on a landmark dose escalation study by the RTOG,[381] a dose of 60 Gy in 1.8- to 2-Gy fractions became standard. Elective nodal stations in the ipsilateral hilum and mediastinum received 40 to 45 Gy. This approach yielded a median survival of approximately

TABLE 75.14

SELECT RANDOMIZED TRIALS OF RADIATION THERAPY (RT) ALONE VERSUS RT AND CHEMOTHERAPY (SEQUENTIAL)

Study (Ref.)[a]	No. of Patients	Patient Stage	Treatment	Overall Survival at 5 Years (%)
Dillman et al. (590)	155	IIIA/B	RT (60 Gy)	6
			CT → RT (60 Gy)	17
Sause et al. (386)	490	Unresectable II, IIIA/B	RT (60 Gy)	5
			CT → RT (60 Gy)	8
			RT (1.2 Gy bid to 69.6 Gy)	6
Le Chevalier et al. (591)	353	Unresectable	RT (65 Gy)	5
			CT → RT (65 Gy)	11[b]

CT, chemotherapy.
[a]Dillman et al.: cisplatin (CDDP), vinblastine (VBL). Sause et al.: CDDP, VBL. Le Chevalier et al.: vindesine, lomustine, CDDP, cyclophosphamide.
[b]Three-year data.
(Adapted from ref. 592.)

10 months, and a disappointing 5-year survival of approximately 5%. Local failure was a significant impediment to cure. Important prognostic factors included weight loss and poor performance status.

Sequential Chemotherapy and Radiation

Incorporation of chemotherapy into the treatment regimen was investigated in an attempt to improve outcomes in patients with medically inoperable or unresectable tumors. Initial randomized studies showed no clear benefit.[382,383] More recent studies, using modern staging techniques and cisplatin-based chemotherapy, have consistently demonstrated a modest improvement in survival with sequential chemotherapy and radiation[384–386] (Table 75.14). Patients with adverse prognostic factors, including weight loss, poor performance status, and malignant pleural effusions, were generally excluded from these studies. The median and 5-year survival with sequential chemotherapy and RT, while better than RT alone, are still only approximately 13 months and 10% to 15%, respectively.

Concurrent Chemotherapy and Radiation

Several studies were subsequently conducted in which sequential chemoradiotherapy was compared with concurrent chemoradiotherapy.[236,237,387,388] Concurrent cisplatin-based chemoradiotherapy was consistently shown to improve survival, at the cost of increased toxicity (Table 75.15). The primary limiting toxicity is grade 3–4 esophagitis, which occurs in 20% to 30% of patients.[387,388] Similar to the sequential chemotherapy studies, patients with poor prognostic factors were generally excluded from these trials. The median and 5-year survival with concurrent chemotherapy and RT are approximately 17 months and 15% to 20%, respectively. A meta-analysis of individual patient data identified seven trials where concomitant versus sequential RT were compared in locally advanced NSCLC.[389] Data from six trials were analyzed, with a total of 1,205 patients. There was a significant benefit of concomitant radiochemotherapy on overall survival (HR = 0.84; 95% CI: 0.74–0.95; P = .004), and an absolute benefit of 5.7% at 3 years (from 18.1% to 23.8%). The major effect was on reduction of local progression (HR = 0.77; 95% CI: 0.62–0.095; P = .01), at the cost of significantly more esophageal toxicity.

Induction and Consolidation Chemotherapy

Despite concurrent chemotherapy and RT for stage III disease, local and distant disease recurrence is common, and most patients die of progressive lung cancer. Early administration of full-dose systemic chemotherapy has the potential to improve

TABLE 75.15

SELECT RANDOMIZED TRIALS OF SEQUENTIAL VERSUS CONCURRENT CHEMORADIOTHERAPY

Study (Ref.)[a]	No. of Patients	Patient Stage	Treatment	Overall Survival (%)
Furuse et al. (236)	320	Unresectable IIIA/B	CT → RT (56 Gy, continuous)	9
			CT-RT (56 Gy, split course)	16 (5 years)
Fournel et al. (387)	212	Unresectable IIIA/B	CT → RT (66 Gy)	14
			CT-RT (66 Gy) → CT	21 (4 years)
Zatloukal et al. (388)	102	Unresectable IIIA/B	CT → RT (60 Gy)	10
			CT → CT-RT (60 Gy)	19 (3 years)
Curran et al. (237)	610	Unresectable IIIA/B	CT → RT (60 Gy)	12
			CT-RT (60 Gy)	21
			CT-RT (1.2 Gy bid to 69.6 Gy)	17 (4 years)

CT, chemotherapy.
[a]Furuse et al.: cisplatin (CDDP), vindesine, and mitomycin C. Fournel et al.: CDDP, vinorelbine (VNR) in sequential arm; CDDP, etoposide in concurrent arm followed by adjuvant CDDP, VNR. Zatloukal et al.: CDDP, VNR. Curran et al.: CDDP, vinblastine.
(Adapted from ref. 592.)

outcomes by early treatment of distant micrometastases and downstaging the primary tumor prior to chemoradiotherapy. A CALBG trial randomized 366 patients with stage III NSCLC to immediate chemoradiotherapy (carboplatin, paclitaxel, 66 Gy) or induction chemotherapy with two cycles carboplatin and paclitaxel prior to chemoradiotherapy.[390] Median and 1-year survivals were 11 months versus 14 months and 48% versus 54%, respectively, but these differences were not statistically significant. Grade 4 toxicity was more common with induction chemotherapy (24% vs. 41%; $P = .001$). Further follow-up and confirmatory trials will be necessary before induction chemotherapy replaces immediate concurrent chemoradiotherapy as standard therapy for unresectable stage III NSCLC.

Similarly, there are currently no phase 3 trial results demonstrating a benefit of consolidation chemotherapy after definitive chemoradiotherapy. The Hoosier Oncology Group randomized patients who had completed definitive cisplatin, etoposide and thoracic RT to consolidation docetaxel or observation.[391] Median survival was 21.2 months for the docetaxel arm compared to 23.2 months for the observation arm ($P = .88$). An RTOG phase 2 study randomized patients with unresectable stage III NSCLC to sequential chemotherapy and RT, induction chemotherapy followed by concurrent chemoradiotherapy, or chemoradiotherapy followed by consolidation chemotherapy.[392] Chemotherapy consisted of carboplatin and paclitaxel. Median survivals were 13, 12.7, and 16.3 months, respectively. Other phase 2 studies have demonstrated promising results with concurrent chemoradiotherapy followed by consolidation chemotherapy.[393] Whether consolidation chemotherapy is necessary in patients who have received lower doses of carboplatin and paclitaxel concurrent with thoracic RT, compared to full-dose cisplatin and etoposide, is unclear. Further randomized studies are necessary.

In conclusion, for favorable patients with medically inoperable, or unresectable, locally advanced NSCLC, the preferred treatment is platinum-based chemotherapy administered concurrent with RT. The American Society of Clinical Oncology (ASCO) 2003 guidelines[394] stipulate that good performance status patients with unresectable stage III NSCLC should receive two to four cycles of platinum-based chemotherapy combined with at least 60 Gy of RT. Current studies are evaluating the optimal dose of RT combined with chemotherapy as well as novel agents targeting EGFR and vascular endothelial growth factor.

Radiation Therapy and Targeted Agents

The most commonly used targeted agents in lung cancer include the oral tyrosine kinase inhibitors gefitinib (Iressa) and erlotinib (Tarceva), the EGFR monoclonal antibody cetuximab (Erbitux), and the vascular endothelial growth factor receptor monoclonal antibody bevacizumab (Avastin). Although these agents have been found to be efficacious in certain subsets of patients with metastatic NSCLC, their use has not been established in patients receiving radiation therapy and chemotherapy for locally advanced disease.

Maintenance gefitinib was evaluated in a phase 3 trial by the Southwest Oncology Group.[395] Patients with stage III NSCLC received concurrent radiation therapy (61 Gy) with cisplatin and etoposide followed by three cycles of docetaxel. Patients without evidence of progression were randomized to gefitinib 250 mg/day or placebo. Gefitinib was continued for 5 years or until disease progression. Median survival was 23 months for gefitinib and 35 months for placebo ($P = .013$). The inferior survival with maintenance gefitinib was due to tumor progression and not toxicity. In a phase 1, two-arm dose escalation trial, erlotinib was given concurrently with platinum-based chemotherapy and thoracic RT for patients with stage III NSCLC.[396] Median survival was 10.2 and 13.7 months, disappointing compared with historical outcomes. These studies do not support the use of either concurrent or adjuvant oral tyrosine kinase inhibitors in stage III NSCLC.

Bevacizumab has also been evaluated in patients with locally advanced lung cancer receiving radiation therapy. Unfortunately, this agent was associated with an increased risk of tracheoesophageal fistula formation.[391] Until further studies are completed, and the safety profile of bevacizumab better understood, it should not be combined with radiation therapy for lung cancer.

The concurrent use of cetuximab with chemotherapy and radiation therapy has been evaluated in two phase 2 studies. The CALGB evaluated cetuximab with thoracic RT (70 Gy) and carboplatin and pemetrexed.[397] The RTOG evaluated cetuximab with thoracic RT (63 Gy) and carboplatin and paclitaxel.[398] These combinations were thought to be feasible without excess toxicity. Outcomes data have not been published to date. An ongoing Intergroup study evaluating the optimal dose of thoracic RT (60 vs. 74 Gy) has a secondary randomization to concurrent cetuximab or placebo.

Radiation Dose and Fractionation

The standard treatment for inoperable NSCLC is concurrent chemotherapy and RT. Unfortunately, even with combined-modality therapy, local failure is common and most patients succumb to their disease. Various RT strategies have been investigated in an attempt to improve local control and survival. The U.S. Veterans Administration conducted a trial in the 1960s in which 554 men with locally advanced, inoperable lung cancer were randomized to RT (40–50 Gy) or observation. RT modestly improved survival at 1 year from 16% to 22% ($P = .05$).[399] Despite the limitations of staging and treatment techniques of the era, there was an apparent, albeit modest, gain with a relatively low dose of RT. A subsequent dose-escalation study conducted by the RTOG in the 1970s demonstrated an improvement in local control with 60 Gy relative to lower doses.[400] Three-year survivals were 15% for 60 Gy, 10% for 50 Gy, and 6% for 40 Gy. However, 5-year survivals were only 6% in all arms. Based on this study, the standard RT dose for locally advanced NSCLC remains 60 to 66 Gy in 1.8- to 2-Gy daily fractions. However, local control with 60 Gy is poor. Within the setting of a French randomized trial,[401] patients with locally advanced NSCLC in complete remission after RT (65 Gy) with or without chemotherapy underwent bronchoscopy every 6 months for histologic confirmation of local control. At 1 year, local control was only 17% for patients receiving RT and 15% with RT and chemotherapy. As such, there has been interest in further escalating the RT dose or intensity in order to diminish local recurrences.

Multiple phase 2 RT dose-escalation studies have been conducted. Interpretation of these single-arm studies is difficult because of heterogeneous eligibility criteria and treatment approach. For example, many studies included all stages of disease,[225,275,397] including inoperable stage I, which is currently approached most commonly with SBRT. Several studies used altered fractionation schemes that are rarely used today.[403,405] Few studies used concurrent chemotherapy, which is currently a standard of care for patients with inoperable stage III lung cancer. Dose escalation in this setting is most relevant. Several phase 1/2 studies have shown that 74 Gy in 2-Gy daily fractions is the maximally tolerated dose of RT when given with concurrent carboplatin and paclitaxel.[402–404] These single-arm studies are the basis for the current Intergroup randomized study comparing 60 Gy versus 74 Gy with concurrent and adjuvant carboplatin and paclitaxel. This study is also evaluating the benefit of concurrent cetuximab.

TABLE 75.16

SELECTED RANDOMIZED ALTERED FRACTIONATION TRIALS FOR INOPERABLE NON–SMALL CELL LUNG CANCER

Study (Ref.)	No. of Patients	Treatment	Survival (%)
RADIATION THERAPY (RT) ALONE			
Sause et al. (386)	310	RT (60 Gy, 2 Gy qd)	5
		RT (69.6 Gy, 1.2 Gy bid)	6 (5 years)
Ball et al. (593)	99	RT (60 Gy, 2 Gy qd)	10
		RT (60 Gy, 2 Gy bid)	13 (5 years)
Saunders et al. (594)	563	RT (60 Gy, 2 Gy qd)	13
		RT (54 Gy, 1.5 Gy tid)	20 (3 years, $P < .01$)
RADIATION THERAPY AND CHEMOTHERAPY (CT)[a]			
Belani et al. (595)	119	CT → RT (64 Gy, 2 Gy qd)	14
		CT → RT (57.6 Gy, 1.5 Gy tid[b])	34 (3 years, $P = .28$)
Schild et al. (596)	234	CT-RT (60 Gy, 2 Gy qd)	37
		CT-RT (60 Gy, 1.5 Gy bid[c])	40 (2 years)
Curran et al. (237)	397	CT-RT (60 Gy, 2 Gy qd)	21
		CT-RT (69.6 Gy, 1.2 Gy bid)	17 (4 years)

[a]Belani et al.: carboplatin and paclitaxel. Schild et al.: cisplatin and etoposide. Curran et al.: cisplatin and vinblastine.
[b]Second daily fraction 1.8 Gy.
[c]Split course.

Several randomized studies have evaluated altered fractionation regimens, with or without chemotherapy (Table 75.16). The CHART trial,[409] which treated patients 3 times a day for 12 consecutive days, is the only positive trial. However, for logistical reasons, and because chemotherapy was not used, this is rarely employed today. Currently, the standard dose of RT used in conjunction with concurrent chemotherapy is 60 to ~70 Gy in 2-Gy fractions.

Prophylactic Cranial Irradiation for Locally Advanced Disease

The hypothesis that prophylactic cranial irradiation (PCI) can improve survival is based on the assumption that isolated brain failures occur commonly after treatment of locally advanced NSCLC, and these can be effectively prevented by tolerable doses of RT. After definitive treatment of locally advanced NSCLC, the brain is frequently the site of first recurrence, and often is the sole site of treatment failure. Patients receiving RT alone on RTOG 73-01 had an initial CNS failure rate of 7% for squamous histology, 19% for adenocarcinoma, and 13% for large cell carcinoma.[381] The addition of chemotherapy does not appreciably decrease the risk of developing brain metastases.[236,385,410] A phase 2 German trial evaluated patients with stage III NSCLC treated with chemoradiotherapy followed by resection. PCI (30 Gy) was offered to patients in the latter period of the trial. At 2 years, the incidence of brain metastases as first site of failure was 35% for those who did not receive PCI versus 8% for those who did.[411] Although this nonrandomized study does not clarify the role of PCI in locally advanced NSCLC, it demonstrates the high actuarial risk of developing brain metastases in patients treated with multimodality regimens.

PCI has been extensively studied in patients with small cell lung cancer and has been shown to improve survival.[412] Three randomized trials have examined PCI after RT alone[413,414] or RT and chemotherapy[415] for locally advanced NSCLC. Collectively, these studies show a significant reduction in the risk of developing brain metastases, but no improvement in survival. It can be assumed that PCI will only improve survival if systemic and local therapy is sufficiently effective to render the brain the main site of clinical failure. Recent advances in lung cancer treatment have revived interest in PCI for NSCLC, and a randomized study by the RTOG has been completed. Final results remain pending. At present, PCI for NSCLC remains investigational and cannot be recommended off-study.

ADVANCED DISEASE

Chemotherapy

Over 50% of patients diagnosed with NSCLC present with stage IIIB or IV disease that is not amenable to curative treatment. More than half of the remaining individuals treated with curative intent will experience relapse, and eventually succumb to their disease. With the exception of the rare patient with oligometastases, patients with stage IV NSCLC typically die from their disease, with an overall median survival time of 10 to 12 months. The fraction of patients who are alive 1 year after diagnosis has increased slightly over the past decade; presently approximately one-third of patients with stage IIIB or IV disease are alive at 1 year, and 10% to 21% of these individuals are alive 2 years after diagnosis. Although these data reflect improvements in the care of patients with advanced NSCLC, treatment remains palliative, with the goal of compassionate and effective end-of-life care.

Prolongation of Survival by Chemotherapy

In the 1970s and 1980s, combination chemotherapy (usually cisplatin-based) was shown to reproducibly achieve objective responses in 20% to 30% of advanced NSCLC patients. Despite the fact that cytotoxic regimens appear to have activity in stage IV NSCLC, overall median survival of patients receiving chemotherapy was only 6 to 8 months, with few patients surviving longer than 1 year. Because of this, the value of chemotherapy in the routine management of patients with stage IV NSCLC was unclear.[416–421] At least 12 randomized

TABLE 75.17

SELECTED RANDOMIZED TRIALS OF CHEMOTHERAPY VERSUS BEST SUPPORTIVE CARE (BSC) IN ADVANCED NON–SMALL CELL LUNG CANCER

Study (Ref.)	Chemotherapy	No. of Patients BSC/Chemo	Median Survival (wk) BSC/Chemo	*P* Value
Rapp et al. (232)	CAP/VP	50/43/44[a]	17/25/33[a]	.05/.01[b]
Cartei et al. (597)	CCM	50/52	17/37	.0001
Woods et al. (598)	VP	91/97	17/27	.33
Cellerino et al. (599)	CEP/MEC	57/58	21/34	.135
Kaasa et al. (600)	VP	43/44	17/22	.28
ELVIS (424)	VNR	81/80	21/28	.03
Cullen et al. (427)	MIC	176/175	21/29	.03
Spiro et al. (423)	Platinum based	364/361	24.5/33.1	.0016

Chemo, chemotherapy; CAP/VP, cyclophosphamide (Cytoxan), doxorubicin (Adriamycin), cisplatin (platinum)/vinblastine, cisplatin; CCM, cisplatin, cyclophosphamide/mitomycin; VP, vindesine/platinum; CEP/MEC, cyclophosphamide, etoposide + platinum/mitomycin, etoposide + cisplatin; ELVIS, Elderly Lung Cancer Vinorelbine Italian Study Group; VNR, vinorelbine; MIC, mitomycin, ifosfamide, cisplatin.
[a]BSC/chemo/chemo.
[b]CAP vs. BSC/VP vs. BSC.

studies, involving more than 2,000 patients, were initiated to compare combination chemotherapy with BSC in patients with advanced NSCLC (Table 75.17). Seven of these trials showed a statistically significant survival benefit in favor of chemotherapy. In a pivotal Canadian study, 150 patients with advanced NSCLC were randomly assigned to receive cisplatin plus vindesine, the CAP regimen, or BSC.[232] The median survival times were significantly longer in the cisplatin plus vindesine and CAP groups than in the BSC arm (33 and 25 weeks, respectively); survival prolongation was achieved with acceptable costs.[422] In a subsequent Big Lung Trial, Spiro et al.[423] randomly assigned 725 patients to receive either short-term cisplatin-based chemotherapy (three cycles) or BSC and confirmed that chemotherapy improved median survival by 8 weeks. The Elderly Lung Cancer Vinorelbine Italian Study Group[424] randomly assigned 161 elderly patients (older than 70 years) to receive BSC with or without single-agent therapy with vinorelbine (30 mg/m^2 on days 1 and 8 of every 21-day cycle for up to six cycles), and observed a statistically significant prolongation of survival with a possible improvement in overall quality of life in the vinorelbine-treated group ($P = .03$). Anderson et al.[425] randomly assigned 300 patients to receive BSC with or without single-agent chemotherapy with gemcitabine (1,000 mg/m^2 on days 1, 8, and 15 of each 28-day cycle); the chemotherapy-arm patients scored better than control patients on the quality-of-life scale and reported fewer lung cancer–related symptoms.

An update of the 1995 meta-analysis included 2,714 patients enrolled in 16 randomized studies. Results confirmed a significant benefit of chemotherapy (HR = 0.77; 95% CI: 0.71–0.83; $P < .0001$),[426] equivalent to an increase in survival of 23%, and an absolute increase of 9% at 1 year, from 20% to 29%, and an increase in median survival of 1.5 months (from 4.5 to 6 months). As a result, the use of chemotherapy has become the standard for most patients with advanced NSCLC and good performance status.[394]

Quality of Life

With the limited survival benefit for patients with stage IV NSCLC, quality of life has been considered a relevant end point for chemotherapeutic trials involving these individuals. Validated questionnaires have been developed to accurately assess quality of life. Early randomized trials suggested that chemotherapy can improve quality of life. Typically, disease-related symptoms improved after chemotherapy, sometimes even in the absence of a measurable tumor response.[427–429] Quality-of-life scores improved with chemotherapy, whereas they declined over the first 6 weeks with BSC. Improved survival and quality of life were also demonstrated with single-agent chemotherapy in a population of patients older than age 70 years.[424]

Therapeutic Options for Patients with Advanced Disease

Although systemic chemotherapy is the standard treatment for advanced NSCLC, in some circumstances, the initial treatment may be a local modality. For example, brain metastases, spinal cord compression, and impending fractures of weight-bearing bones can and should be treated with radiation or surgery before systemic therapy commences. Patients who present with postobstructive pneumonia are often treated initially by RT with the addition of either an endobronchial stent or endobronchial brachytherapy. After resolution of the pneumonia, systemic therapy can be considered. The major consideration for having the local treatment precede systemic chemotherapy is related to the risk of chemotherapy-induced complications, such as infections.

Based on available data from randomized trials, optimal chemotherapy regimens for advanced NSCLC include a platinum drug (cisplatin or carboplatin) and a second drug, such as vinorelbine, gemcitabine, paclitaxel, docetaxel, or pemetrexed.[430] An extensive update of the ASCO guidelines for systemic treatment of advanced NSCLC has recently been published.[430] Performance status is the single best factor for identifying those individuals who can tolerate and are most likely to benefit from chemotherapy. Patients with an Eastern Cooperative Oncology Group (ECOG) performance status of 0 or 1 are the best candidates for chemotherapy and can achieve both prolongation of survival and improvement in quality of life. Patients with an ECOG performance status of 2 are at a substantial higher risk of chemotherapy complications and have a significantly poorer prognosis regardless of the use of palliative chemotherapy. Single-agent chemotherapy or regimens with a good tolerance, such as carboplatin and paclitaxel, are advised in performance status 2 patients with advanced NSCLC. Individuals with an ECOG performance status of 3 or 4 do not benefit from chemotherapy; because of this, BSC is the preferred means of palliation. Age does not predict adverse outcome; thus, patients who are elderly with a good performance status should be offered systemic treatment. However, one should bear in mind the presence of comorbidities, such as chronic obstructive pulmonary disease, and vascular and metabolic diseases, which are commonly present in elderly patients, and which are associated with a significantly higher complication rate.

First-Line Chemotherapy

In the 1990s, reproducible single-agent activity was demonstrated for paclitaxel, docetaxel, vinorelbine, gemcitabine, irinotecan, and more recently pemetrexed. Evaluation of these newer agents frequently has included a comparison of the drugs administered with cisplatin versus cisplatin alone. Currently, platinum-based combination chemotherapy regimens are preferred for the treatment of advanced NSCLC with good performance status. Etoposide, vindesine, and vinblastine have traditionally been considered as first-generation agents when combined with cisplatin. The second generation of regimens includes platinum combinations with vinorelbine, docetaxel, paclitaxel, gemcitabine, and pemetrexed and nonplatinum regimens. Current regimens (particularly those that are carboplatin-based) appear less toxic, especially in terms of nonhematologic toxicities; however, the overall outcome of patients treated with these newer drug combinations is only marginally better than that reported for patients treated with older regimens.

A number of large analyses have been performed to validate prognostic factors in patients with stage IV NSCLC disease receiving chemotherapy. The SWOG analyzed their database of 2,531 patients with advanced NSCLC using Cox modeling, recursive partitioning, and amalgamation techniques, and reported that good performance status, female gender, age of 70 years or older, low tumor burden, normal lactate dehydrogenase and serum calcium levels, and a hemoglobin level of more than 11 g/dL were associated with favorable response to chemotherapy.[431] The use of cisplatin was an additional, favorable predictor of survival. A European group conducted a similar analysis of 1,052 patients and observed that lower tumor burden, good performance status, older age, and female gender were associated with a more favorable response to therapy.[432]

Standard of Care: Platinum-Based Doublets

In 1993, Le Chevalier et al.[433] were the first to use a second-generation agent along with platinum, reporting that cisplatin plus vinorelbine was superior to cisplatin plus vindesine. The median survival time for patients receiving cisplatin and vinorelbine was significantly longer than that noted for patients treated with cisplatin and vindesine (40 vs. 30 weeks, respectively). This study also demonstrated that cisplatin was required in the doublet because cisplatin plus vinorelbine was superior to vinorelbine alone. In a more recent randomized trial, cisplatin plus vinorelbine (P-NVB) was compared with vinorelbine plus ifosfamide plus cisplatin (NIP). The overall response rate was 34.6% for P-NVB and 35.7% for NIP. Median survival time and 1-year survival rate were 10.0 months and 38.4% for P-NVB and 8.2 months and 33.7% for NIP, respectively. The SWOG randomly assigned 432 chemotherapy-naive patients to receive cisplatin and vinorelbine or single-agent cisplatin. The median progression-free and overall survival times were modestly yet significantly better in patients receiving combined therapy than in those treated with cisplatin alone (4 vs. 2 months and 8 vs. 6 months, respectively).[434]

The cisplatin-etoposide combination was initially developed as an effective regimen for patients with small cell lung cancer and remains the standard of care for this disease. The efficacy of cisplatin-etoposide for NSCLC has also been documented. In a phase 2 study of 94 patients with advanced NSCLC, the response rate was 38% and median survival was 7.5 months. In a phase 3 trial, the ECOG randomly assigned patients to one of three regimens: cisplatin plus etoposide; high-dose paclitaxel, cisplatin, and granulocyte colony-stimulating factor; or paclitaxel plus cisplatin. In the 559 patients enrolled, significantly improved survival was observed in the combined paclitaxel arms, compared to cisplatin-etoposide (median survivals 9.9 vs. 7.6 months), but there was no difference between the two paclitaxel doses. Toxicity in general was preferable with the lower-dose paclitaxel.[435] Gemcitabine has been evaluated in randomized phase 2 and 3 trials.[436–439] A European trial compared cisplatin and gemcitabine with cisplatin and etoposide, and suggested a favorable impact on survival.[437] Another randomized trial demonstrated that, compared with cisplatin alone, gemcitabine plus cisplatin improved median survival by 2 months but was associated with an increase in hematologic toxicities.[440] In a phase 3 trial comparing gemcitabine alone with gemcitabine plus carboplatin in 334 patients with advanced NSCLC, Sederholm et al.[441] observed overall response rates of 30% in the combination arm and 11% in the gemcitabine arm ($P < .0001$); the overall survival in the combination arm was superior to that in the arm receiving gemcitabine alone ($P = .02$) and the 2-year survival rates were 15% versus 5%, respectively ($P = .009$).

Two randomized phase 3 trials failed to demonstrate any difference in efficacy between gemcitabine plus cisplatin and the combination of mitomycin, ifosfamide, and cisplatin or between gemcitabine plus carboplatin and the combination of either mitomycin, ifosfamide, and cisplatin or mitomycin, vinblastine, and cisplatin in treatment of stage IIIB or stage IV disease.[442,443] In clinical trial 08975 of the EORTC, 480 chemotherapy-naive patients with advanced lung cancer were randomly assigned to receive one of three different chemotherapy regimens: paclitaxel and cisplatin, gemcitabine and cisplatin, or paclitaxel and gemcitabine. Median survival times were 8.1, 8.9, and 6.7 months, respectively, for these regimens, suggesting that non–platinum-based chemotherapy might be inferior to platinum-based chemotherapy.[444]

Numerous studies have indicated that paclitaxel has single-agent activity against NSCLC.[445–447] A European trial demonstrated that cisplatin plus paclitaxel resulted in a median survival of 10 months—a response similar to that for cisplatin and teniposide—and was better tolerated.[448] In the mid-1990s, several groups reported successful phase 2 trials using carboplatin combined with a 3-hour infusion of paclitaxel. Other randomized trials have confirmed the activity of regimens of cisplatin or carboplatin plus paclitaxel, and the favorable toxicity profile of the latter combination.[448–453] The first phase 3 cooperative group trial to compare two second-generation regimens was performed by SWOG. This trial compared vinorelbine plus cisplatin to paclitaxel plus carboplatin and found that these regimens resulted in comparable response rates and median survival times (approximately 8 months).[454] ECOG conducted a randomized study comparing two different doses of 24-hour infusion of paclitaxel (135 mg/m^2 or 250 mg/m^2 with granulocyte colony-stimulating factor support) plus cisplatin with cisplatin plus etoposide in chemotherapy-naive patients with stage IIIB or IV NSCLC. When data for the two paclitaxel-cisplatin arms were analyzed together, higher response rates as well as significantly longer median survival times were seen with the cisplatin-paclitaxel combination than with the etoposide-cisplatin regimen (9.9 vs. 7.6 months, respectively). The higher paclitaxel dose did not improve the response rate.[435,455] CALGB conducted a phase 3 randomized trial in which 584 patients with stage IV NSCLC were randomly assigned to receive carboplatin (AUC = 6) and paclitaxel (225 mg/m^2 during 3 hours) or paclitaxel alone every 3 weeks for up to six cycles. The response rate and

PRACTICE OF ONCOLOGY

median survival were significantly improved in the carboplatin-paclitaxel arm.[456] The ease of administration of carboplatin combined with 3-hour paclitaxel infusion established this as a treatment standard for many oncologists in the United States.

Docetaxel has been shown to have activity as second-line therapy in patients with cisplatin-refractory disease.[457,458] A docetaxel-platinum combination was evaluated in the TAX 326 trial in which 1,218 patients with advanced NSCLC were randomly assigned to receive docetaxel (75 mg/m^2) with either carboplatin (AUC = 6) or cisplatin (75 mg/m^2) every 3 weeks; or vinorelbine (25 mg/m^2/week) with cisplatin (100 mg/m^2) every 4 weeks. Although the response rates were higher in the docetaxel-cisplatin arm (31.6% vs. 24.5%; P = .029), the median survivals and 2-year survival rates in the docetaxel-cisplatin and vinorelbine-cisplatin arms were not significantly different (11.3 vs. 10.1 months and 21% vs. 14%, respectively); docetaxel plus carboplatin was not significantly better than either vinorelbine plus cisplatin or docetaxel plus cisplatin for any end point. Patients treated with either of the docetaxel-containing regimens reported improved quality of life, whereas the quality of life for those treated with cisplatin and vinorelbine generally decreased.[459,460] Kubota et al.[461] evaluated the combinations of cisplatin (80 mg/m^2) plus docetaxel (60 mg/m^2) or vindesine (3 mg/m^2 on days 1, 8, and 15). The docetaxel-cisplatin regimen was significantly better than the vindesine-cisplatin therapy (response rate, 37% vs. 21%, and median survival 11.3 vs. 9.6 months, respectively).

A few studies have investigated the schedule of administration of taxanes, three weekly versus weekly. A phase 3 study investigated carboplatin at AUC 6 and paclitaxel given 225 mg/m^2 every 3 weeks, or carboplatin at AUC 6 given on day 1, and paclitaxel given at 100 mg/m^2 3 of 4 weeks. After four cycles both arms were eligible to receive maintenance paclitaxel.[462] Outcomes were similar between the two arms, but nonhematologic toxicities were less severe in the weekly paclitaxel regimen.

Positive data also exist for irinotecan.[463–465] In phase 2 trials, irinotecan-cisplatin regimens produced response rates of 35%, with median survivals of 6 to 8 months and 1-year survivals from 40% to 60% in chemotherapy-naive patients with advanced NSCLC.[466–468] In a phase 3 trial of irinotecan with and without cisplatin versus cisplatin plus vindesine in previously untreated patients with advanced NSCLC, survival among patients with stage IV disease was significantly better in the group given irinotecan plus cisplatin than in the groups receiving irinotecan alone or vindesine plus cisplatin (median survival, 50 weeks vs. 46.0 and 45.6 weeks, respectively).[469] Multiple phase 1 and 2 studies have combined irinotecan with taxanes, either alone or in combination with carboplatin, and have found similar response and survival rates.

Pemetrexed is the last chemotherapeutic agent to be approved for the treatment of advanced NSCLC.[470] Pemetrexed has been demonstrated to have similar efficacy to docetaxel in a large noninferiority study in second-line treatment of advanced NSCLC,[471] which also demonstrated a better toxicity profile. Higher doses of pemetrexed have not yielded better results than the standard dose of 500 mg/m^2 every 3 weeks.[472,473] A large randomized study compared cisplatin-gemcitabine with cisplatin-pemetrexed.[474] A total of 1,725 patients were randomized to receive cisplatin 75 mg/m^2 either with gemcitabine 1,250 mg/m^2 on days 1 and 8 or pemetrexed 500 mg/m^2 on day 1, with cycles repeated every 3 weeks. The major end point of this study, noninferiority for survival, was achieved, with a median survival of 10.3 months in both arms. Progression-free survival was also not inferior. In a predefined analysis for survival by histology, patients with adenocarcinoma and large cell carcinoma had a significantly better survival with cisplatin-pemetrexed than with cisplatin-gemcitabine (nonsquamous n = 1,000; median survival, 11.8 vs. 10.4 months, respectively; HR = 0.81; 95% CI: 0.70–0.94; P = .005). Squamous cell histology, on the other hand, did significantly worse with cisplatin-pemetrexed than cisplatin-gemcitabine (n = 473; median survival, 9.4 vs. 10.8 months, respectively; HR = 1.23; 95% CI: 1.0–1.51; P = .05). In 2008 the FDA approved pemetrexed in combination with cisplatin for front-line treatment of advanced nonsquamous NSCLC patients. This study, together with retrospective analysis of other pemetrexed studies confirmed histology as an important selector for patients treated with this drug.

The standard of care for patients with advanced NSCLC has long been chemotherapy with a platinum-based doublet. At least four randomized clinical trials have compared cisplatin with carboplatin doublets in the treatment of advanced NSCLC. Only one of the four trials has shown a modest but significant improvement in median survival.[475] The EORTC 07861 protocol compared cisplatin plus etoposide with carboplatin plus etoposide. The response rates favored the cisplatin-etoposide arm, but the difference did not reach statistical significance, and median survival was similar in both arms.[476] Rosell et al.[475] randomly assigned 618 patients to paclitaxel plus cisplatin or paclitaxel plus carboplatin and observed that the response rates were similar in both arms. However, the median survival was better in the cisplatin-paclitaxel group (9.8 vs. 8.2 months). The ECOG 1594 trial demonstrated similar outcomes in patients treated with carboplatin plus paclitaxel, cisplatin plus docetaxel, cisplatin plus gemcitabine, or cisplatin plus paclitaxel,[477] and a European trial[444] observed similar activities for cisplatin plus gemcitabine, cisplatin plus paclitaxel, and paclitaxel plus gemcitabine, although progression-free survival with the nonplatinum combination was significantly inferior. Collectively, these randomized trials indicate that none of these regimens is superior to the others.

An individual patient data meta-analysis was performed of nine randomized trials (2,968 patients) in which cisplatin-based chemotherapy was compared with carboplatin-based chemotherapy.[478] Second-generation drugs were used in 80% of the total population. Cisplatin-based chemotherapy produced a higher response rate (30% vs. 24%; P <.001), but the survival advantage was not significant (HR = 1.07; 95% CI: 0.99–1.15; P = .100). Subgroup analysis revealed that combination chemotherapy based on carboplatin was associated with a significantly increase in mortality in patients with nonsquamous tumors and those treated with second-generation chemotherapy. Patients on cisplatin-based chemotherapy more frequently developed nausea and vomiting and nephrotoxicity, whereas severe thrombocytopenia was more frequent during carboplatin-based chemotherapy. No significant differences in treatment-related mortality were observed.

Non–platinum-based regimens using gemcitabine combinations such as paclitaxel plus gemcitabine, vinorelbine plus gemcitabine, and docetaxel plus gemcitabine have been evaluated in several phase 2 clinical trials. The EORTC 08975 study[444] randomly assigned 480 patients to three arms: two cisplatin-based and one non–cisplatin-based paclitaxel and gemcitabine regimens. Response rates ranged from 27.7% to 36.6%, and median survivals ranged from 6.7 to 8.9 months, with no statistically significant differences in any of the clinical end points among arms. Overall, phase 3 trial data indicate no statistically significant survival advantage for nonplatinum combinations over platinum-containing doublets, and the most recent ASCO guidelines recommend the use of a platinum doublet in patients who can tolerate platinum compounds.[430]

Chemotherapy and Targeted Agents in First Line

A large number of randomized studies have investigated the addition of a biological or targeted agent to standard chemotherapy. Several of these studies are summarized in Table 75.18.

TABLE 75.18

SELECTED PHASE 3 STUDIES OF FIRST-LINE CHEMOTHERAPY WITH OR WITHOUT A BIOLOGICAL AGENT

Study (Ref.)	Regimen	No. of Patients	RR (%)	PFS/TTP (mo)	Median Survival (mo)	1-Year Survival (%)
Herbst et al.	Carboplatin/paclitaxel/placebo	345	28.7	5	9.9	42
(601) [INTACT 2]	Carboplatin/paclitaxel/gefitinib 250 mg/day	345	30	5.3	9.8	41
	Carboplatin/paclitaxel/gefitinib 500 mg/day	347	30.4	4.6	8.7	37
Giaccone et al.	Cisplatin/gemcitabine/placebo	363	47.2	6	10.9	44
(602) [INTACT 1]	Cisplatin/gemcitabine/gefitinib 250 mg/day	365	51.2	5.8	9.9	41
	Cisplatin/gemcitabine/gefitinib 500 mg/day	365	50.3	5.5	9.9	43
Herbst et al. (603)	Carboplatin/paclitaxel/placebo	533	19.3	4.9	10.5	43.8
[TRIBUTE]	Carboplatin/paclitaxel/erlotinib	526	21.5	5.1	10.6	46.9
Gatzemeier et al.	Cisplatin/gemcitabine/placebo	579	31.5	23.7 wk	43 wk	41
(604) [TALENT]	Cisplatin/gemcitabine/erlotinib	580	29.9	24.6 wk	44.1 wk	42
Williamson et al.	Carboplatin/paclitaxel	186	35	5	9	NR
(605)	Carboplatin/paclitaxel/tirapazamine	181	26	5	9	NR
Bissett et al.	Cisplatin/gemcitabine/placebo	181	26	5.5	10.8	38
(606)	Cisplatin/gemcitabine/prinomastat	181	27	6.1	11.5	43
Bissett et al.	Carboplatin/paclitaxel/placebo	198	21	3.5	10.2	29
(606)	Carboplatin/paclitaxel/prinomastat 5 mg/day	84	27	3.6	9.3	30
	Carboplatin/paclitaxel/prinomastat 10 mg/day	197	19	3.3	8.6	35
	Carboplatin/paclitaxel/prinomastat 15 mg/day	198	18	4.3	9.1	40
Leighl et al.	Carboplatin/paclitaxel/placebo	387	33.7	5.3	9.2	NR
(607)	Carboplatin/paclitaxel/BMS-275291	387	25.8	4.9	8.6	NR
Paz-Ares et al.	Cisplatin/gemcitabine	328	35	5.2	10.4	44.8
(608)	Cisplatin/gemcitabine/aprinocarsen	342	28.9	5	10	41.8
Ramlau et al.	Cisplatin/vinorelbine	312	24.4	5	9.9	NR
(516) [SPIRIT1]	Cisplatin/vinorelbine/bexarotene	311	16.7	4.3	8.7	NR
			P = .0224			
Blumenschein et al.	Carboplatin/paclitaxel	306	23.5	4.9	9.2	NR
(609) [SPIRIT II]	Carboplatin/paclitaxel/bexarotene	306	19.3f	4.1	8.5	NR
Sandler et al. (482)	Carboplatin/paclitaxel	444	15	4.5	10.3	44
	Carboplatin/paclitaxel/bevacizumab	434	35	6.2	12.3	51
			P <.001	P <.001	P = .003	
Reck et al.	Cisplatin/gemcitabine	351	20.1	6.1	13.1	NR
(483, 610) (AVaiL)	Cisplatin/gemcitabine/bevacizumab 7.5 mg/kg	345	34.1*	6.7*	13.6	NR
	Cisplatin/gemcitabine/bevacizumab 15 mg/kg	347	30.4**	6.5**	13.4	NR
			*P <.001	*P = .003		
			**P = .0023	**P = .03		
Pirker et al.	Cisplatin/vinorelbine	568	29	4.8	10.1	42
(486) [FLEX]	Cisplatin/vinorelbine/cetuximab	557	36	4.8	11.3	47
			P = .010		P = .044	
Lynch et al.	Carboplatin/taxane	338	17.2	4.24	8.4	NR
(487) [BMS09]	Carboplatin/taxane/cetuximab	338	25.7	4.40	9.7	NR
			P = .0066			
Scagliotti et al.	Carboplatin/paclitaxel/placebo	462	24	5.4	10.6	NR
(474)	Carboplatin/paclitaxel/sorafenib	464	27.4	4.6	10.7	NR
Lee et al. (479)	Carboplatin/gemcitabine/placebo	350	42	5.7	8.9	38
	Carboplatin/gemcitabine/thalidomide	372	40	5	8.5	35

*,**Comparison between experimental arms and the control cisplatin/gemcitabine (without*).
PFS, progression-free survival; TTP, time to progression; NR, not reported.

The vast majority of these studies have used carboplatin and paclitaxel or cisplatin and gemcitabine as the standard chemotherapy backbones commonly used in the United States and Europe. Several studies of oral agents also included a placebo to the control the chemotherapy arm. Unfortunately most of these studies have been negative because they did not meet their primary end point, which most commonly was increase in overall survival. In a few of these studies histologic subgroups had significantly worse survival with the experimental treatment,[479,480] suggesting that biological characteristics underlying the different histologies may be important in treatment selection.

Of the few positive studies, those with bevacizumab merit special attention. A randomized phase 2 study demonstrated that bevacizumab, a monoclonal antibody against the vascular endothelial growth factor, can be combined with carboplatin and paclitaxel at full doses.[481] This initial study, investigating two doses of bevacizumab, suggested an advantage in progression-free survival with the addition of the antibody to chemotherapy. Patients with central squamous cell carcinomas had a higher tendency to form cavitation within their tumors after combined treatment, and four of these patients developed fatal hemoptysis. As a result of this study, a large phase 3 trial was initiated, with the higher dose of bevacizumab. A careful monitoring of the safety of the study was performed by interim analyses. Between July 2001 and April 2004, ECOG conducted a randomized study in which 878 patients with recurrent or advanced NSCLC were assigned to chemotherapy alone (paclitaxel 200 mg/m^2 and carboplatin at an AUC of 6) or paclitaxel and carboplatin plus bevacizumab (15 mg/kg).[482] Chemotherapy was administered every 3 weeks for six cycles, and bevacizumab was administered every 3 weeks until disease progression was evident or toxic effects were intolerable. Patients with squamous cell tumors, brain metastases, clinically significant hemoptysis, inadequate organ function, or ECOG performance status more than 1 were excluded. The primary end point was overall survival. A significant improvement in overall survival, time to progression, and response rate was observed by the addition of bevacizumab to standard chemotherapy. Rates of clinically significant bleeding were 4.4% and 0.7%, respectively ($P < .001$). There were 15 treatment-related deaths in the chemotherapy-plus-bevacizumab group, including 5 from pulmonary hemorrhage. There was also significantly more hematologic toxicity in the experimental arm (severe neutropenia 25.5% vs. 16.8%; $P = .002$; and thrombocytopenia 1.6% vs. 0.2%; $P = .04$). As a result of this study, bevacizumab has been approved by the FDA for the treatment of first-line advanced NSCLC in combination with carboplatin and paclitaxel, in patients with nonsquamous histology, without brain metastases, and without serious bleeding.

Another large randomized study including another chemotherapy regimen (cisplatin and gemcitabine) with or without bevacizumab has also been completed.[483] A total of 1,043 advanced-stage NCLC patients were randomized to receive standard chemotherapy consisting of cisplatin 80 mg/m^2 on day 1 and gemcitabine 1,250 mg/m^2 on days 1 and 8 every 3 weeks, or the same chemotherapy with the addition of bevacizumab at 7.5 or 15 mg/kg every 3 weeks. Progression-free survival, the major end point of this study, was significantly longer in the bevacizumab arms (although the differences are very small), and a higher response rate was also observed in the bevacizumab arms. However, no difference in overall survival was demonstrated in this study. Grade 3–4 pulmonary hemorrhage was 1.5% or more in all arms. Comparison of bevacizumab doses was not statistically allowed in this study, although there did not appear to be a major difference in efficacy between the low and the higher doses. This study may suggest that the synergizing effect of bevacizumab may be different on different chemotherapy regimens.

Following three small randomized phase 2 studies that suggested improvement of cetuximab (a monoclonal antibody against the EGFR) when added to standard chemotherapy, two large randomized phase 3 studies were performed with cetuximab.[484,485] A large randomized study (FLEX) compared chemotherapy with chemotherapy plus cetuximab in patients whose tumors expressed EGFR by immunohistochemistry (at least one positive tumor cell). Chemotherapy consisted of cisplatin given at 80 mg/m^2 on day 1 and vinorelbine given at 25 mg/m^2 on days 1 and 8, every 3 weeks for up to six cycles. Cetuximab was given at a loading dose of 400 mg/m^2 on day 1 and at 250 mg/m^2 weekly starting on day 8. Cetuximab was continued beyond chemotherapy, until progression or unacceptable toxicity.[486] This study included a total of 1,125 patients and reached its major end point of improving overall survival; median survival in the chemotherapy alone arm was 10.1 months and it was 11.3 months in the cetuximab arm (HR = 0.871; 95% CI: 0.762–0.996; $P = .044$). A survival advantage was seen in all histologic subgroups. An increase in response rate was also observed, but progression-free survival was the same in both arms. As expected, acnelike skin rash grade 3, diarrhea grade 3–4, and infusion-related reactions grade 3–4 were more common in patients on the cetuximab arm. Given the modest increase in survival and substantial toxicity and the lack of improvement in progression-free survival, FDA and European Medicines Agency (EMEA) have so far not approved cetuximab for NSCLC.

Another randomized phase 3 (BMS099), designed as a supportive study for the FLEX study, had progression-free survival as major end point. In this study patients were not selected based on expression of EGFR in their tumors.[487] A total of 676 patients were randomized to receive carboplatin at AUC of 6 with either paclitaxel at 225 mg/m^2 or docetaxel at 75 mg/m^2, every 3 weeks. Cetuximab was administered at the same dose until progression or excessive toxicity, like in the FLEX study. This trial failed to demonstrate an increase in progression-free survival or survival. In the BMS099 study 225 patients had available tumor material for molecular analysis. *EGFR* and *K-Ras* mutations, as well as immunohistochemistry and FISH for *EGFR* were performed. None of these markers were found to be related to progression-free survival, overall survival, or response rate.[488]

Several other agents in addition to those reported in Table 75.19 have been tested in single-arm or randomized phase 2 studies and are at present running or have completed accrual of randomized phase 3 trials after promising results of phase 2 randomized studies.[489–495] Results of many of these studies will become available in the next few years.

EGFR Tyrosine Kinase Inhibitors in First-Line Treatment

For patients who have a higher frequency of *EGFR* sensitizing mutations (light or never-smokers, women, East Asians, adenocarcinoma histology), a high response rate to EGFR tyrosine kinase inhibitors, erlotinib and gefitinib, has been shown in first-line phase 2 studies.[496,497] Patients who are selected for EGFR mutations have a very high response rate of approximately 70%. For these patients, treatment with an EGFR inhibitor instead of chemotherapy may be suggested. On the contrary for unselected patients, chemotherapy is a more appropriate first-line therapy, as demonstrated by a randomized phase 2 study in advanced NSCLC with performance status of 2.[498] This study randomized 103 patients to either standard carboplatin-paclitaxel (carboplatin at AUC of 6, paclitaxel at 200 mg/m^2, every 3 weeks) or erlotinib 150 mg/daily. Response rate (12% vs. 4%), progression-free survival (median, 3.52 vs. 1.91 months; HR = 1.45; 95% CI: 0.98–2.15; $P = .063$), and overall survival (median, 9.7 vs. 6.6 months; HR = 1.73; 95% CI: 1.09–2.73; $P = .018$) all favored chemotherapy. This study demonstrates that chemotherapy is a better treatment for unselected patients than erlotinib.

A randomized phase 2 study compared gefitinib 250 mg/day with placebo in previously untreated advanced NSCLC with performance status 2–3, unfit for chemotherapy.[499] There were no differences in response rate, progression-free survival, or overall survival between the two arms; median survival was 3.7 and 2.8 months in the gefitinib and placebo arms, respectively. Progression-free survival was better in gefitinib-treated arm in patients with FISH-positive tumors; however, mutation analysis was not performed.

A large randomized study performed in several countries in East Asia (IPASS study) compared gefitinib 250 mg/day with standard carboplatin-paclitaxel (carboplatin AUC of 5–6, paclitaxel 200 mg/m^2 every 3 weeks), in untreated patients with stage IIIB or IV adenocarcinoma of the lung, light (stopped smoking at least 15 years before and had a history of smoking of $\leq$10 pack-years), or never-smokers (<100 cigarettes in their lifetime). A total of 1,217 patients were randomized 1:1 to gefitinib or chemotherapy.[234] The primary objective of noninferiority for progression-free survival was met. Actually, progression-free survival was significantly longer

TABLE 75.19

SELECTED PHASE 3 STUDIES OF SECOND-LINE THERAPY

Study (Ref.)	Regimen	No. of Patients	RR (%)	PFS/TTP (mo)	Median Survival (mo)	1-year Survival (%)
Shepherd et al. (458)	Docetaxel	104	5.8	10.6 wk	7	29
	BSC	100	0	6.7 wk	4.6	19
				P = .001	P = .047	
Fossella et al. (457)	Docetaxel 100 mg/m²	125	10.8*	19 wk*	5.5	21
	Docetaxel 75 mg/m²	125	6.7**	17 wk**	5.7	32*
	Vinorelbineifosfamide	123	0.8	8 wk	5.6	19
			*P = .001	*P = .013		*P = .025
			**P = .036	**P = .031		
Hanna et al. (471)	Docetaxel	288	8.8	2.9	7.9	29.7
	Pemetrexed	283	9.1	2.9	8.3	29.7
Shepherd et al. (526) [BR.21]	Erlotinib	488	8.9	2.2	6.7	31
	BSC	243	1	1.8	4.7	22
			P <.001	P <.001	P <.001	
Thatcher et al. (528) [ISEL]	Gefitinib	1129	8	7.2	5.6	27
	BSC	563	1.3	3	5.1	21
			P <.0001	P = .0006		
Kim et al. (529) [INTEREST]	Gefitinib	723	9.1	2.2	7.6	32
	Docetaxel	710	7.6	2.7	8	34
Maruyama et al. (531) [V-15-32]	Gefitinib	245	22.5	2	11.5	47.8
	Docetaxel	244	12.8	2	14	53.7
			P = .009			
Lee et al. (532)	Gefitinib	82	28.1	3.3	NR	NR
	Docetaxel	79	7.6	3.4	NR	NR
			P = .0007	P = .0441		
Krzakowski et al. (517)	Vinflunine	274	4.4	2.3	6.7	NR
	Docetaxel	277	5.5	2.3	7.2	NR

*,**Comparison between the docetaxel arms and the control arm (without *).
PFS, progression-free survival; TTP, time to progression; NR, not reported.

with gefitinib (HR = 0.74; 95% CI: 0.65–0.85; *P* <.001). Interestingly, the curves crossed each other at about 6-month time point and then the gefitinib curve remained on top of the chemotherapy curve for the rest of the observation period. The median progression-survival times were very similar at 5.7 and 5.8 months in the gefitinib and chemotherapy arms, respectively; however, the 1-year progression-free survivals were 24.9% and 6.7%, respectively. Response rate was significantly higher with gefitinib (43.0% vs. 32.2%; *P* <.001). Survival was similar in the two groups, with 37% of the patients reported dead at the time of this analysis (median, 18.6 vs. 17.3, respectively). *EGFR* mutation data was assessed in 437 patients (35.9% of the whole population), and 261 (59.7%) were positive for mutation. There was a significant interaction between presence of *EGFR* mutations and treatment. Progression-free survival was strikingly longer for gefitinib versus chemotherapy in *EGFR* mutants (HR = 0.48; 95% CI: 0.36–0.64; *P* <.001), where curves were widely separated all along, and significantly shorter in wild type EGFR patients who received gefitinib (HR = 2.85; 95% CI: 2.05–3.98; *P* <.001). Results in the unknown *EGFR* status were similar to the overall population. Toxicities were those commonly reported with these agents. The conclusion of this important study is that gefitinib is a better treatment for patients with *EGFR* mutations than chemotherapy in first line. Based on this study gefitinib was registered in Europe for advanced NSCLC with *EGFR* mutations.

A phase 3 study from Japan randomized 177 chemotherapy-naïve patients with advanced NSCLC and EGFR mutations to receive either gefitinib 250 mg/day or chemotherapy consisting of cisplatin 80 mg/m² plus docetaxel 60 mg/m² every 3 weeks.[233] The primary end point of this study, progression-free survival, was significantly in favor of gefitinib (median, 9.2 vs. 6.3 months, respectively; HR = 0.489; 95% CI: 0.336–0.710; *P* <.001). Response rate was also better in the gefitinib arm (62.1% vs. 32.2%; *P* <.0001). Overall survival has not been reported as yet. This study confirms the IPASS study in that patients with EGFR mutations fare better on gefitinib than chemotherapy.

Elderly Patients and Chemotherapy Treatment

Randomized trials have demonstrated that elderly patients receiving chemotherapy do not have worse outcomes than younger patients.[434,435,440] Furthermore, randomized trials restricted to elderly patients have shown that single-agent vinorelbine is superior to BSC,[424] but there are conflicting data regarding whether doublet chemotherapy regimens are superior to single-agent therapy in those individuals. Frasci et al.[500] reported that, compared with vinorelbine alone, gemcitabine-vinorelbine therapy prolonged median survival time and 1-year survival rates (29 vs. 18 weeks and 30% vs. 13%, respectively). Contrasting results were observed in the Multicenter Italian Lung Cancer in the Elderly Study in which 698 patients older than 70 years of age were randomly assigned to receive gemcitabine alone (1,200 mg/m² days 1 and 8 every 3 weeks), vinorelbine alone (30 mg/m² on days 1 and 8, every 3 weeks), or gemcitabine (1,000 mg/m²) plus vinorelbine (25 mg/m²), both administered on days 1 and 8 every 3 weeks. The response rates, times to progression, and survival in the group receiving the combination were not significantly better than those observed for patients treated with single-agent chemotherapy.[501]

A Japanese study compared vinorelbine with docetaxel in 182 patients who were age 70 or older.[502] Although there was no significant increase in survival, docetaxel significantly prolonged progression-free survival and increased response rate.

A randomized phase 2 study performed in chemotherapy-naive white elderly (>69 years of age) patients with advanced NSCLC, compared gefitinib versus vinorelbine.[503] Increase in progression-free survival with gefitinib was the primary end point of the study. A total of 196 patients were enrolled. There was no difference in terms of progression-free survival, overall survival, or response rate between the two treatment arms.

In a large analysis of the SEER-Medicare database which included 21,285 patients over 65 years of age, only 25.8% received first-line chemotherapy.[504] Although more often patients received single-agent chemotherapy, receipt of chemotherapy was associated with reduction in the adjusted hazard of death (0.558; 95% CI: 0.547–0.569), indicating that age should not be considered a limiting factor for chemotherapy in this category of patients. A randomized phase 2 study suggested that lower doses of cisplatin doublets are feasible and active in elderly patients.[505]

Optimal Duration of Chemotherapy

The goal of chemotherapy is to maximize survival benefit and palliate symptoms. It is intuitive that the duration of chemotherapy should be short to minimize potential toxicity. Socinski et al.[506] attempted to address the issue of optimal duration of chemotherapy in a study of 230 patients with advanced NSCLC. Individuals were randomly assigned to four courses of paclitaxel plus carboplatin, followed by salvage therapy with single-agent paclitaxel at the time of progression, or to continuous treatment with both agents until radiographically determined progression. Overall response rates as well as median and 1-year survival rates were similar, but the incidence of treatment-related grade 2 or higher neurotoxicity increased from 20% to 43% between the fourth and eighth cycles of continuous treatment. Four cycles of carboplatin-paclitaxel chemotherapy were as effective as continuous treatment until progression.

A Korean study demonstrated noninferiority of giving two additional cycles instead of four, after the initial two cycles of platinum-based chemotherapy had shown nonprogressive disease, in a total of 452 patients registered and 314 randomized.[507] The 1-year survival rates were 59% and 62.4%, respectively, in patients who received four versus two additional cycles, which met the predefined criteria for noninferiority. However, the time to progression was significantly longer in the patients who received four additional cycles (median, 6.2 vs. 4.6 months; $P = .001$).

Currently there is no evidence that continuing the same chemotherapy prolongs survival of patients exhibiting response or stabilization of disease after four or six cycles of chemotherapy. For this reason, it is recommended that chemotherapy be given for two cycles, at which point response should be assessed with appropriate imaging. Patients who show a clear response and those who have stable disease should receive two additional cycles before response is again evaluated. A maximum of six cycles should be administered, after which the standard of care would be to follow patients carefully and allow a treatment break.

Maintenance Therapy

Bevacizumab and cetuximab have been investigated in combination with chemotherapy and their administration has been continued after the end of chemotherapy until progression or tolerability as maintenance, although their role in prolonging survival or progression-free survival in this setting has not been confirmed.

Several agents have been tested as maintenance therapy after induction chemotherapy treatment. A significant improvement in survival has recently been documented with pemetrexed, erlotinib, and marginally with docetaxel. Pemetrexed and erlotinib have recently been approved for this indication by the FDA for patients who did not progress after induction chemotherapy for advanced NSCLC.

A randomized phase 3 study allocated patients who responded to mitomycin C-ifosfamide-cisplatin to receive maintenance vinorelbine (25 mg/m^2 every week for 6 months) versus no further treatment. This study registered 573 patients and randomized 181.[508] There were no differences in overall and progression-free survival between the two arms. The two-year survival rates were 20.1% and 20.2% in the vinorelbine and observation arms, respectively ($P = .48$).

A relatively large randomized phase 2 study allocated patients with stage IIIB and IV disease who responded to chemotherapy or chemoradiotherapy to receive BLP25 liposome vaccine or BSC.[509] BLP25 is a liposome vaccine that targets MUC1, which is overexpressed and aberrantly glycosylated in NSCLC. Patients on the BLP25 arm received a single intravenous dose of cyclophosphamide at 300 mg/m^2 followed by eight weekly subcutaneous vaccinations with 1,000 mcg of L-BLP25. Subsequent immunizations were delivered at 6-week intervals. A total of 171 patients were randomized. Although overall there was only a trend in improvement in survival in the vaccination arm (median survival, 17.4 vs. 13 months; adjusted $P = .112$), in patients with stage IIIB locoregional disease (no pleural effusion) the 2-year survival was 60% for the L-BLP25 arm (median not reached) versus 36.7% in the observation arm (median survival, 13.3 months; adjusted $P = .069$). Vaccination was well tolerated and a phase 3 study was initiated in patients with locally advanced stage III NSCLC, whose results are awaited.

A large randomized double-blind study allocated patients with advanced NSCLC who had not progressed on four cycles of platinum-based chemotherapy to receive intravenous pemetrexed at 500 mg/m^2 every 3 weeks or placebo.[510] Both arms received BSC. A total of 663 patients were randomized in a 2:1 ratio (434 in the pemetrexed arm and 222 in the placebo arm), and progression-free survival was the primary end point of this study. The median progression-free survival was significantly longer in the pemetrexed arm (4.3 vs. 2.6 months; HR = 0.50; 95% CI: 0.42–0.61; $P < .0001$). Median overall survival was also improved with pemetrexed (13.4 vs. 10.6 months; HR = 0.79; 95% CI: 0.65–0.95; $P = .012$). The improvements in progression-free and overall survival were recorded mainly in patients with nonsquamous histology. Treatment was well tolerated. Postdiscontinuation systemic anticancer therapies were given in 51% and 67% of the pemetrexed and placebo arms, respectively. In the placebo arm only 18% of patients received pemetrexed. Pemetrexed was approved by the FDA in 2009 for maintenance for patients with nonsquamous histology.

A phase 3 study randomized advanced NSCLC patients not progressing after four cycles of front-line therapy with carboplatin and gemcitabine to immediate compared with delayed docetaxel 75 mg/m^2 given up to a maximum of six cycles.[511] Patients in the delayed docetaxel arm received docetaxel on progression if they were fit for chemotherapy. Major end point of the study was an improvement in survival by administering immediate docetaxel over delayed docetaxel. In total, 556 patients were enrolled on induction chemotherapy and 309 were randomized. Overall survival in the immediate docetaxel arm was greater by 2.6 months (median, 12.3 vs.

9.7 months; $P = .0853$), and progression-free survival was significantly greater in the immediate docetaxel arm (5.7 vs. 2.7 months; $P = .0001$). Interestingly, patients who actually received delayed docetaxel had identical survival of the immediate docetaxel arm. Only 98 of 156 patients allocated to delayed docetaxel actually received drug. This study suggests that the difficulty of administering chemotherapy on progression may be the major reason for efficacy of maintenance chemotherapy.

A very large randomized study compared erlotinib maintenance with placebo in advanced NSCLC patients who did not progress after four cycles of platinum-based chemotherapy doublet (SATURN study).[512] Of 1,949 patients who were registered before start of chemotherapy, 889 were randomized 1:1, 438 to erlotinib and 451 to placebo. Coprimary end points were progression-free survival and progression-free survival in patients with EGFR-positive tumors by immunohistochemistry. Progression-free survival was significantly in favor of maintenance erlotinib (median, 12.3 vs. 11.1 months, respectively; HR = 0.71; 95% CI: 0.62–0.82; $P < .0001$) irrespective of immunohistochemical results for EGFR expression. Response rates were 11.9% versus 5.4% ($P = .0006$). The largest difference in progression-free survival was observed in *EGFR* mutant cases (HR = 0.10; 95% CI: 0.04–0.25; $P < .0001$), although a significant difference was also observed in *EGFR* wild type cases (HR = 0.78; 95% CI: 0.63–0.96; $P = .0185$). Overall survival was also significantly prolonged with erlotinib (median, 12.0 vs. 11.0 months; HR = 0.81; 95% CI: 0.70–0.95; $P = .0088$) in the whole population. Survival results in EGFR mutants are not mature as yet. Interestingly, patients with stable disease after first-line chemotherapy had overall survival benefit with maintenance erlotinib (median, 11.9 vs. 9.6 months; HR = 0.72; 95% CI: 0.59–0.89; $P = .0019$) but not those with a response (median, 12.5 vs. 12.0 months; $P = .618$). Based on these results, the FDA approved erlotinib for maintenance in patients who did not progress on first-line chemotherapy. Interestingly, EMEA limited the approval to patients who had stable disease after chemotherapy.

A Japanese study randomized 604 patients to receive platinum-based chemotherapy up to six cycles versus three cycles followed by gefitinib 250 mg/day until progression.[513] The primary end point of this study was improvement of overall survival with maintenance gefitinib. The study failed to prove an advantage in overall survival (12.9 vs. 13.7 months median survival, respectively), but progression-free survival was significantly longer in the gefitinib arm (median, 4.3 vs. 4.6 months; HR = 0.68; 95% CI: 0.57–0.80; $P < .001$). The randomization before start of chemotherapy and the high frequency of EGFR tyrosine kinase inhibitors given in second line may have influenced the results.

Second-Line Chemotherapy

In a landmark study, Shepherd et al.[458] demonstrated that second-line chemotherapy with docetaxel can improve outcome in patients who have received cisplatin therapy. Table 75.19 summarizes some of the most important randomized studies in second-line treatment. Individuals receiving docetaxel had better overall survival, with median and 1-year survivals of 7.5 versus 4.6 months and 37% versus 11%, compared with those receiving BSC, respectively. These results were confirmed by another randomized study that demonstrated that patients receiving docetaxel had significantly increased response and survival rates relative to patients receiving either vinorelbine or ifosfamide.[457] Two randomized studies investigated whether weekly docetaxel might be more effective or less toxic, but conflicting results were reported.[514,515] In a large study involving 571 patients who had failed platinum chemotherapy, pemetrexed, a multitargeted antifolate, had a similar efficacy to docetaxel but with less myelosuppression.[471] Pemetrexed has therefore been approved for the second-line treatment of advanced NSCLC.

A noninferiority study randomized 829 patients who had received only one line of prior chemotherapy, to receive docetaxel 75 mg/m² every 3 weeks or oral topotecan 2.3 mg/m²/day on days 1 to 5 every 3 weeks.[516] The 1-year survival was 25.1% and 28.7% for topotecan and docetaxel, respectively, which met the predefined criteria for noninferiority. Oral topotecan was approved in 2007 by the FDA for relapsed small cell lung cancer.

Vinflunine, a novel microtubule inhibitor, was compared with docetaxel in advanced NSCLC after failure of first-line platinum-based chemotherapy. A total of 551 patients received either vinflunine at 320 mg/m² or docetaxel at 75 mg/m² every 3 weeks.[517] This was yet another noninferiority study for progression-free survival. A total of 551 patients were randomized, and the progression-free survival was 2.3 months in both arms, confirming the noninferiority. Overall survival and response rates were also similar between the two arms. Some side effects, such as abdominal pain, fatigue, anemia, and constipation, were more common with vinflunine, but overall the toxicities were manageable.

A randomized phase 2 study investigated chemotherapy alone (docetaxel or pemetrexed) to the same chemotherapy with bevacizumab 15 mg/kg every 3 weeks, to bevacizumab and erlotinib 150 mg/day, in patients with advanced NSCLC who were eligible for bevacizumab and who progressed after one prior platinum-based chemotherapy regimen.[518] A total of 120 patients were randomized. Although this study was underpowered, both bevacizumab arms had longer progression-free survivals than the chemotherapy alone arm, and 1-year survival rate was 57.4% for bevacizumab-erlotinib and 53.8% for bevacizumab-chemotherapy, versus 33.1% for chemotherapy alone. The incidence of grade 5 hemorrhage in patients receiving bevacizumab was 5.1%. Based on these results a number of large randomized studies were performed with the combination of bevacizumab and erlotinib and with bevacizumab and chemotherapy. Final results of these studies are awaited.

A meta-analysis of single-agent versus combination chemotherapy as second-line treatment in advanced NSCLC based on individual patient data identified six trials with data available.[519] This analysis included 847 patients and showed that although progression-free survival is significantly improved by combination chemotherapy (median, 14 vs. 11.7 weeks; HR = 0.79; $P = .0009$), and response rate is increased (15.1% vs. 7.3%; $P = .0004$), survival was not improved and toxicity was substantially increased.

Several studies with targeted agents have been performed in patients with advanced NSCLC in second-line setting or later line of treatment. Many randomized studies have been preceded by relatively successful phase 2 studies.[520,521]

EGFR Inhibitors in Advanced NSCLC

EGFR is expressed in 40% to 80% of lung cancers, which makes this an attractive target for molecular intervention in this disease. Gefitinib and erlotinib were the first two agents to target the tyrosine kinase of the EGFR. Both of these agents have activity in NSCLC. Phase 1 trials of gefitinib showed that this oral agent was well tolerated, with rash and diarrhea as the major side effects. In the phase 1 series, encouraging activity was seen in patients with NSCLC. This led to phase 2 trials in patients who had previously been treated with chemotherapy. In the Iressa Dose Evaluation in Advanced Lung 1 (IDEAL-1) trial conducted in Japan and Europe,[522] a response rate of 18% was observed among patients who were mostly receiving gefitinib as second-line therapy. In the IDEAL-2 study conducted in the United States, gefitinib was administered to patients who had received prior cisplatin and docetaxel therapy (hence, therapy was mostly third line). The response rate was 11% in this trial.[523] In both of these trials, gefitinib was well tolerated; once again, rash and diarrhea were the principal side effects. The speed of response was remarkable; the median time to response was 8 days. Both of these studies randomized two doses, 250 mg and 500 mg per day. No differences in response rate, symptom control, or survival end points were observed between the doses, and because of less severe toxicities, the 250 mg/day dose was chosen for further evaluation.

The ability of gefitinib to provide meaningful benefit to patients with lung cancer who had received prior first-line therapy with a platinum-based regimen and second-line therapy with docetaxel led to FDA approval for this setting based on phase 2 data only. Enthusiasm for gefitinib has been somewhat tempered by the development of interstitial pneumonitis in approximately 1.0% of patients receiving this drug. The frequency of this complication appears considerably higher in Japan. In a retrospective study of 1,976 patients treated with gefitinib, 3.5% developed interstitial pneumonitis, which was fatal in 1.6% of patients. A higher incidence of pneumonitis was associated with male gender, smoking history, and coincidental interstitial pneumonia.[524]

Erlotinib is an EGFR tyrosine kinase inhibitor that has activity in NSCLC. In a phase 2 study of patients with previously treated lung cancer, erlotinib produced a response rate of 13%.[525] The toxicity profile is very similar to that of gefitinib, with rash and diarrhea being the most common side effects. At the chosen dose of 150 mg/day, erlotinib is close to the maximum tolerated dose, and the frequency and severity of side effects are higher than those observed in patients receiving the 250 mg/day dose of gefitinib.

A large randomized study (BR.21), performed by the National Cancer Institute of Canada, randomized patients who had received prior chemotherapy to compare erlotinib with BSC.[526] Patients were randomly assigned to treatment or placebo in a 2:1 ratio. A total of 731 patients were randomized. The response rate to erlotinib was 8.9% compared with less than 1% in the placebo arm ($P < .001$). Progression-free and overall survival durations were significantly greater in the erlotinib arm (2.2 vs. 1.8 months, $P < .001$; and 6.7 vs. 4.7 months, $P < .001$). Erlotinib also improved tumor-related symptoms and important aspects of quality of life.[527] Treatment was relatively well tolerated, although 5% of patients discontinued treatment because of side effects. Main toxicities included rash and diarrhea, which were severe in less than 10% of patients. Cox regression analysis indicated erlotinib therapy was associated with a longer survival ($P = .002$), as was Asian origin ($P = .01$), adenocarcinoma histology ($P = .004$), and never-smoking status ($P = .048$). This study brought erlotinib to registration in the United States and Europe. Immunohistochemistry, FISH, and mutation analyses were performed to examine *EGFR* expression in a subset of patients from this study. Univariate analysis revealed that high-level *EGFR* expression (HR for death = 0.68; $P = .02$), and *EGFR* gene amplification (HR = 0.44; $P = .008$) correlated with prolonged survival in erlotinib-treated patients. However, multivariate analysis revealed that survival after treatment with erlotinib was not influenced by the level of *EGFR* expression, or *EGFR* amplification/mutation status.

Another very large placebo-controlled phase 3 study investigated the effect on survival of gefitinib as second-line or third-line treatment for patients with locally advanced or metastatic NSCLC.[528] Nearly 1,700 patients who were refractory to, or intolerant of, their latest chemotherapy regimen were randomly assigned in a 2:1 ratio to receive either gefitinib (250 mg/day) or placebo, plus BSC. The primary end point was survival in the overall population of patients, and those with adenocarcinoma. At median follow-up of 7.2 months, median survivals did not differ significantly between the groups in the overall population or among the 812 patients with adenocarcinoma (6.3 vs. 5.4 months). Preplanned subgroup analyses showed significantly longer survival in the gefitinib-treated group than the placebo group for never-smokers (n = 375; HR 0.67; $P = .012$; median survival, 8.9 vs. 6.1 months) and patients of Asian origin (n = 342; HR 0.66; $P = .01$; median survival 9.5 vs. 5.5 months). Gefitinib was well tolerated, as in previous studies. The results of this study were surprising because despite the very large sample size (double that of the BR.21), no significant improvement in survival was detected with gefitinib, whereas a significant survival benefit was observed with erlotinib in the BR.21 study. Discrepant results of these two studies have been attributed in part to the use of a relatively high dose of erlotinib, compared to a well-tolerated and biologically active dose of gefitinib. Following publication of these negative results, the use of gefitinib has been restricted in the United States. The drug remains widely available in Asia, where clinical activity and patient tolerance appear to be higher than in the Western world.

A very large noninferiority study (INTEREST) was performed comparing docetaxel with gefitinib in 1,466 patients with advanced NSCLC who had at least one prior line of chemotherapy including platinum.[529] Gefitinib was given at 250 mg/daily, and docetaxel was given at 75 mg/m^2 every 3 weeks. The major goal of the study was to prove noninferiority of gefitinib in terms of overall survival. The study met its primary objective, and median survivals of docetaxel and gefitinib were 8 and 7.6 months, respectively, not statistically different. Median progression-free survival was 2.7 and 2.2 months, also not statistically different. Response rates were 7.6% and 9.1%, also not statistically different. Quality of life was better with gefitinib as assessed by FACT-L total score ($P < .0001$) and FACT-T TOI ($P = .0026$). This partly reflects the better tolerability of gefitinib compared with docetaxel.

Molecular predictors of outcome were investigated retrospectively in 451 (31%) samples with one marker only and all four markers in 253.[530] The four biomarkers were EGFR expression by immunohistochemistry, copy number by FISH, and mutation analysis of *EGFR* and *K-Ras*. Overall 15% of assessable patients had EGFR mutations, and 18% had K-Ras mutations. *EGFR* mutation-positive patients had significantly longer progression-free survival (7 vs. 4.1 months; HR = 0.16; 95% CI: 0.05–0.49; $P = .001$) and a higher objective response rate (42.1% vs. 21.1%; $P = .04$) with gefitinib than with docetaxel. Also, high EGFR copy number was associated with higher response rate with gefitinib (13.0% vs. 7.4%; $P = .04$). All other markers were not predictive or prognostic. No marker was predictive of overall survival.

Two other smaller randomized studies compared gefitinib with docetaxel. Study V-15-32 performed in Japan as a noninferiority study for survival included 489 advanced NSCLC patients who had failed one or two prior lines of chemotherapy. The noninferiority was not achieved in this study, although overall survivals, progression-free survival, and response rates were similar between the arms.[531] Another smaller Asian phase 3 study with the primary end point of progression-free survival randomized a total of 161 patients who failed one prior platinum-based chemotherapy to receive gefitinib at 250 mg/day or docetaxel at 75 mg/m^2 every 3 weeks.[532] Progression-free survival was longer with gefitinib in this study ($P = .0441$), although the median was very similar. Response rate was also significantly better with gefitinib. Survival was not reported as too few deaths had occurred at the time of the analysis of this study. A randomized phase 2 study investigated the same comparison of gefitinib 250 mg daily versus docetaxel 75 mg/m^2 every 3 weeks, in a total of 141 randomized patients after failure of one line of prior chemotherapy.[533] This small study confirmed the results of the INTEREST trial[529] in that there were no major differences in terms of response rate, progression-free survival, and overall survival between the two arms, with a better toxicity profile for gefitinib.

The selection of patients for treatment with EGFR tyrosine kinase inhibitors (EGFR-TKI) has received much attention. Clinical characteristics including never-smoker status, female gender, adenocarcinoma, BAC carcinoma histologies, and East Asian ethnicity have been recognized as powerful positive selection criteria, but are far from perfect. Among the biological factors investigated, mutations within the tyrosine kinase domain of EGFR are the most powerful predictor for dramatic responses, and in some studies, overall survival in patients receiving EGFR-TKIs. Also, *EGFR* copy number has been shown in several retrospective studies to have some value. At present, immunohistochemistry analysis of EGFR expression does not appear to be a reliable method of selecting patients for treatment with EGFR-TKI.

Selection of patients who have *EGFR* mutations represents the best predictor for response to EGFR TKIs. In a prospective Japanese study 118 patients were screened; 32 were found to have sensitizing mutations and 28 were prospectively treated with gefitinib at 250 mg/day. Response rate was 75%, median progression-free survival was 11.5 months, and median survival was not reached at time of publication, but 1-year survival was 79%.[534] A combined analysis of prospective studies performed in Japan in patients with advanced NSCLC and *EGFR* mutations treated with gefitinib identified 148 patients, of whom 87 received gefitinib as first-line treatment. There was a response rate of 76.4% (95% CI: 69.5–83.2), a median progression-free survival of 9.7 months, and median survival of 24.3 months.[535] *EGFR* mutations identify a separate category of patients for whom long survival can be achieved with treatment with EGFR TKIs.

Although preclinical data suggested that inhibition of EGFR activity potentiates the effects of cytotoxic chemotherapy agents, combining gefitinib or erlotinib with standard chemotherapy regimens has not been successful. More than 4,000 patients have been entered onto four large randomized trials of chemotherapy combined with either erlotinib or gefitinib. Unfortunately, none of these studies has demonstrated that combining an EGFR–TKI with standard chemotherapy is beneficial in lung cancer patients.[536]

Cetuximab (IMC-C225, Erbitux) is a human-mouse chimeric monoclonal antibody that binds specifically to human EGFR. In a phase 2 study, cetuximab was given to patients with EGFR-positive or -negative tumors and who had not responded to at least one prior chemotherapy regimen.[537] The response rate was 4.5% of 66 patients enrolled, with a median survival of 8.9 months. Several randomized studies of cetuximab in combination with chemotherapy have been performed in first-line treatment and have been described previously.

Many other agents that target EGFR are under development. Some of these target EGFR only, whereas others (e.g., ZD6474) also target tyrosine kinases involved in angiogenesis.

INVESTIGATIONAL AGENTS IN DEVELOPMENT FOR NSCLC

A large number of targeted and nontargeted agents have been tested in advanced NSCLC in recent years. Among these are small molecules that inhibit multiple tyrosine kinases, such as sunitinib and sorafenib. Other approaches involve the use of vaccinations targeting MAGE-3, Tol-9 receptor, TGF-β, and MUC-1. Numerous large randomized studies are ongoing or have been completed in several settings, including early stages of disease. Results of these studies are anticipated to be available over the next several years.

Of interest is the development of second-generation EGFR inhibitors. Several irreversible inhibitors of EGFR have been developed, which are usually also potent inhibitors of other kinases of the Erb-B family, such as PF-00299804 and BIBW2992.[538,539] Both agents are more potent than erlotinib and gefitinib on wild type EGFR and sensitizing mutants of EGFR. They are preclinically also more active on the T790M-resistant mutation of EGFR, which represents approximately 50% of the mechanism of resistance to EGFR TKIs.[540] Both agents are being investigated in phase 3 clinical studies.

Another well-described mechanism of acquired resistance to EGFR TKIs is amplification of c-Met.[541] Several Met inhibitors are being presently tested either alone or in combination with chemotherapy and EGFR inhibitors.

PERSONALIZED MEDICINE IN NSCLC

The use of traditional chemotherapy in advanced disease is in general not tailored based on molecular characteristics of the tumor. However, there is some indication that a few markers are associated with sensitivity to specific chemotherapeutic agents. In particular, expression of *excision repair cross-complementing 1 (ERCC1)* has been associated with cisplatin resistance. This marker has been shown to be both prognostic and predictive of response to cisplatin-based chemotherapy in a large randomized study of adjuvant chemotherapy.[542] A large Spanish randomized study showed that response rate was significantly higher in patients who received chemotherapy based on *ERCC1* mRNA expression.[543] Response was also highly associated with levels of *RRM1* and *ERCC1* in a prospective study of gemcitabine versus gemcitabine plus carboplatin, although it did not predict survival.[544] This study confirms the feasibility of performing the assessment of these markers in the community setting. Nevertheless, these markers so far have not been introduced into standard decision-making strategies.[542,545–547]

EGFR mutations have been reported as the most predictive marker for response to EGFR TKIs.[548] They are present in only 10% to 15% of whites, but they are present in 30% to 35% of East Asians and are more common in women, in those with adenocarcinoma histology, and never-smokers. They are reciprocally exclusive of *K-Ras* mutations. In a large prospective study, 217 patients with *EGFR* mutations who received erlotinib experienced a progression-free survival of 14 months and a median survival of 27 months.[549] Deletions in exon 19 are more predictive of response and prolonged survival than the L858R mutations in exon 21. *EGFR* copy number appears less well correlated with response and survival than mutations. There is an overlap of increased copy number and presence of *EGFR* mutations. Presence of *K-Ras* mutations has been found to be usually correlated to lack of activity of EGFR TKIs.[550]

In 2007 Soda et al.[551] identified a potential driver mutation in NSCLC, the fusion of the N-terminal portion of the protein encoded by the *echinoderm microtubule-associated protein like 4* (*EML4*) gene and the intracellular signaling portion of the receptor tyrosine kinase encoded by the anaplastic lymphoma kinase (*ALK*) gene. To date, multiple variants of *EML4-ALK* have been found in NSCLC, and these fusions demonstrate gain of function. Their frequency is 3% to 7%, they are more common in adenocarcinoma, light smokers (<10 pack years) or never-smokers, and younger age. Interestingly *EML4-ALK* fusions have also been associated with lack of *EGFR* or *K-Ras* mutations. Preliminary results of a phase 1 study of PF-02341066, a MET/ALK inhibitor, showed impressive responses in patients with *EML4-ALK*–positive

NSCLC.[552] Patients with *EML4-ALK* fusion gene appear to be resistant to EGFR inhibitors and have similar sensitivity to chemotherapy.[553]

Abundant information is becoming available by high-throughput screening studies of mutations and other genetic alterations using several platforms.[554] The use of next-generation sequencing and other emerging technologies will allow in the near future real-time analysis of patient tumors for multiple genetic variations, which may prove useful for selecting patients for targeted therapies, predicting response to therapy, or establishing prognosis.

LOCAL THERAPIES AND PALLIATION

Metastatic Disease

Palliation of Intrathoracic Disease

Surgery. A variety of surgical interventions are required to palliate symptoms in patients with advanced NSCLC: bronchoscopic ablation of tumor with or without stent placement to relieve endobronchial obstruction or hemoptysis, and pleurodesis to relieve symptomatic malignant pleural effusions, or pericardial fenestration for malignant pericardial effusions. On rare occasions, resection of primary tumors and lung parenchyma are required to control septic complications or massive hemoptysis, or to palliate unstable vertebral body involvement.

Bronchoscopic removal of endobronchial tumor is an efficient way of relieving endobronchial obstruction. Simple mechanical debridement with the use of the bronchoscope is often sufficient. Coagulative techniques such as use of a carbon dioxide, argon, or neodymium:yttrium aluminum garnet laser, electrocautery, and cryotherapy have been used in conjunction with mechanical debridement.[555] There has been increased interest in the use of photodynamic therapy for relieving endobronchial obstructions.[556] Massive hemorrhage is infrequently seen because of the judicious use of coagulative techniques. Frequently, endobronchial stents are used for long-term palliation. Malignant pleural and pericardial effusions, which are frequently observed in patients with advanced NSCLC, can be effectively palliated with a variety of techniques as outlined in Chapter 151.

Radiation Therapy. RT plays an important role in the palliation of symptomatic intrathoracic disease. Such symptoms include dyspnea, cough, hemoptysis, and/or chest pain. The optimal fractionation scheme in this setting has been the subject of many randomized trials as well as a meta-analysis.[557] Common schemes include 10 Gy in a single fraction, 17 Gy in two fractions, and 30 Gy in ten fractions. More conventional 5- or 6-week courses have also been investigated. In general, for symptomatic patients with metastatic disease or locally advanced tumors not suitable for curative therapy, abbreviated RT courses have provided similar symptom control and survival to more protracted regimens.

A trial from Norway is representative.[558] Patients (n = 421) with advanced NSCLC were randomized to 17 Gy in two fractions on days 1 and 8 (arm A), 42 Gy in 2.8-Gy fractions (arm B), and 50 Gy in 2-Gy fractions (arm C). There was no difference in median survival (8.2, 7, and 6.8 months, respectively) or quality of life. Furthermore, symptom control, reported separately by physicians and patients, was similar between the three arms. As expected, esophagitis occurred earlier in arms A and B.

Numerous trials have demonstrated the palliative benefit of RT in patients with advanced NSCLC.[559–561] RT is especially effective in controlling hemoptysis with 75% to 85% of patients improving after treatment.[560,561] RT regimens used for curative intent typically consist of at least 6 weeks of daily therapy. This is generally not appropriate for patients with metastatic disease with limited expected survival. Short fractionation schemes are attractive for obvious reasons. However, concerns of late toxicity and reduced efficacy have dissuaded many from using extremely hypofractionated regimens (10 Gy in one fraction or 17 Gy in two fractions). Radiation myelitis has been reported when 17 Gy has been given in two fractions.[560–562] The crude incidence of this complication is small, but the effects can be devastating. Acute toxicity to large fractions, including fever, nausea, and/or chest pain, is common but seems to be mitigated with prophylactic corticosteroids. Finally, there are some data suggesting that survival is better in patients with good performance status and limited disease burden who undergo more protracted regimens. In the Norwegian trial,[558] for patients with good performance status and stage III disease, there was a trend ($P = .06$) toward improved survival when patients were treated with more conventional schemes as opposed to 17 Gy in two fractions. In a Medical Research Council study,[559] median survival was 9 months with 39 Gy in 3-Gy fractions versus 7 months with 17 Gy in two fractions.

Endobronchial brachytherapy is rarely used in a curative setting but is often used to palliate endobronchial tumors, especially in patients who have previously received external-beam radiation therapy.[563,564] During bronchoscopy, the endobronchial tumor is identified, its distance from the carina is measured, and an afterloading catheter is inserted through the brush channel of the bronchoscope and guided past the lesion. The bronchoscope is carefully removed, leaving the wire in place. A plan is generated to treat the tumor with a 1- to 2-cm margin proximally and distally. Patients generally receive one to four fractions, which is generally well tolerated and performed on an outpatient basis. Symptoms from endobronchial tumor such as hemoptysis and dyspnea improve in most patients. Late effects of treatment are unusual but can include bronchial stenosis, radiation bronchitis, and fatal hemoptysis.

Brain Metastases from NSCLC

The development of brain metastases in patients with NSCLC is high. Autopsy series have shown an incidence exceeding 25%.[565] Appropriate management depends on multiple factors including performance status, status and extent of extracranial disease including the primary tumor, and number of lesions.[566] With rare exceptions, hematogenous spread of lung cancer outside the thorax represents an incurable situation, and brain metastases are nearly always a fatal development. However, long-term survivals, on the order of 10% to 20%, have been reported with resection[567] as well as stereotactic radiosurgery (SRS)[568] of a synchronous or metachronous solitary brain metastases, usually followed by whole-brain radiation therapy (WBRT). A metachronous presentation typically has a better prognosis. For synchronous solitary brain metastases, especially with an early-stage primary tumor, resection of both sites is indicated in the context of multimodality therapy including systemic chemotherapy and radiation.

For patients with good performance status and a single brain metastasis, especially when extracranial disease is controlled, resection followed by WBRT is superior to WBRT alone (40 vs. 15 weeks).[569] SRS provides similar outcomes to surgery. Many patients present with multiple lesions in the setting of either an uncontrolled primary or extensive extracranial disease. In this setting, corticosteroids and WBRT are standard, with a median survival of approximately 4 months. In select patients, notably those with one to three metastases, an SRS boost can improve intracranial control.[570]

Bone Metastases from NSCLC

Painful bone metastases are common in patients with lung cancer and require immediate and appropriate pain management using narcotic analgesics, anti-inflammatory medications, and occasionally a referral to a pain management specialist. Pathologic fractures or impending fractures, especially in weight-bearing bones, require orthopedic fixation. Symptomatic compression fractures in the spine can be palliated with vertebroplasty or kyphoplasty. RT is especially effective in palliating pain from bone metastases. Single 8-Gy fractions are often sufficient, usually well tolerated, and convenient for patients and providers.[571] More protracted regimens (30 Gy in 3-Gy fractions) are used for large fields or when there is interest in minimizing long-term toxicity.

Metastasis (M1) to the Adrenal Gland

Adrenal metastases from bronchogenic carcinoma are found in approximately one-third of patients at autopsy. Routine preoperative upper abdominal CT scanning reveals an adrenal mass in approximately 10% of patients.[572] In selected patients, excision of the primary lung tumor and of an isolated adrenal metastasis improve survival.[573] The ultimate role of such an approach in the context of multimodality therapy has yet to be defined.

Selected References

The full list of references for this chapter appears in the online version.

7. Sano H, Marugame T. International comparisons of cumulative risk of lung cancer, from cancer incidence in five continents Vol. VIII. *Jpn J Clin Oncol* 2006;36(5):334.
9. Wakelee HA, Chang ET, Gomez SL, et al. Lung cancer incidence in never smokers. *J Clin Oncol* 2007;25(5):472.
25. Harris JE, Thun MJ, Mondul AM, Calle EE. Cigarette tar yields in relation to mortality from lung cancer in the cancer prevention study II prospective cohort, 1982–8. *BMJ* 2004;328(7431):72.
31. Clement-Duchene C, Vignaud JM, Stoufflet A, et al. Characteristics of never smoker lung cancer including environmental and occupational risk factors. *Lung Cancer* 2010;67(2):144.
32. Samet JM, vila-Tang E, Boffetta P, et al. Lung cancer in never smokers: clinical epidemiology and environmental risk factors. *Clin Cancer Res* 2009;15(18):5626.
43. Amos CI, Pinney SM, Li Y, et al. A susceptibility locus on chromosome 6q greatly increases lung cancer risk among light and never smokers. *Cancer Res* 2010;70(6):2359.
45. Landi MT, Chatterjee N, Yu K, et al. A genome-wide association study of lung cancer identifies a region of chromosome 5p15 associated with risk for adenocarcinoma. *Am J Hum Genet* 2009;85(5):679.
57. Li Y, Sheu CC, Ye Y, et al. Genetic variants and risk of lung cancer in never smokers: a genome-wide association study. *Lancet Oncol* 2010;11(4):321.
133. Brock MV, Hooker CM, Ota-Machida E, et al. DNA methylation markers and early recurrence in stage I lung cancer. *N Engl J Med* 2008;358(11):1118.
140. Chansky K, Sculier JP, Crowley JJ, Giroux D, van MJ, Goldstraw P. The International Association for the Study of Lung Cancer Staging Project: prognostic factors and pathologic TNM stage in surgically managed non-small cell lung cancer. *J Thorac Oncol* 2009;4(7):792.
141. Rami-Porta R, Chansky K, Goldstraw P. Updated lung cancer staging system. *Future Oncol* 2009;5(10):1545.
143. Detterbeck FC, Boffa DJ, Tanoue LT, Wilson LD. Details and difficulties regarding the new lung cancer staging system. *Chest* 2010;137(5):1172.
149. Ventura E, Islam T, Gee MS, Mahmood U, Braschi M, Harisinghani MG. Detection of nodal metastatic disease in patients with non-small cell lung cancer: comparison of positron emission tomography (PET), contrast-enhanced computed tomography (CT), and combined PET-CT. *Clin Imaging* 2010;34(1):20.
162. Szlubowski A, Herth FJ, Soja J, et al. Endobronchial ultrasound-guided needle aspiration in non-small-cell lung cancer restaging verified by the transcervical bilateral extended mediastinal lymphadenectomy—a prospective study. *Eur J Cardiothorac Surg* 2010;37(5):1180.
172. Hecht SS, Kassie F, Hatsukami DK. Chemoprevention of lung carcinogenesis in addicted smokers and ex-smokers. *Nat Rev Cancer* 2009;9(7):476.
175. Kozower BD, Sheng S, O'Brien SM, et al. STS database risk models: predictors of mortality and major morbidity for lung cancer resection. *Ann Thorac Surg* 2010;90(3):875.
193. Yuan S, Sun X, Li M, et al. A randomized study of involved-field irradiation versus elective nodal irradiation in combination with concurrent chemotherapy for inoperable stage III nonsmall cell lung cancer. *Am J Clin Oncol* 2007;30(3):239.
207. Graham MV, Purdy JA, Emami B, et al. Clinical dose-volume histogram analysis for pneumonitis after 3D treatment for non-small cell lung cancer (NSCLC). *Int J Radiat Oncol Biol Phys* 1999;45(2):323.
233. Mitsudomi T, Morita S, Yatabe Y, et al. Gefitinib versus cisplatin plus docetaxel in patients with non-small-cell lung cancer harbouring mutations of the epidermal growth factor receptor (WJTOG3405): an open label, randomised phase 3 trial. *Lancet Oncol* 2010;11(2):121.
234. Mok TS, Wu YL, Thongprasert S, et al. Gefitinib or carboplatin-paclitaxel in pulmonary adenocarcinoma. *N Engl J Med* 2009;361(10):947.
235. Sause WT, Scott C, Taylor S, et al. Radiation therapy oncology group (RTOG) 88-08 and eastern cooperative oncology group (ECOG) 4588: preliminary results of a phase III trial in regionally advanced, unresectable non-small-cell lung cancer. *J Natl Cancer Inst* 1995;87(3):198.
236. Furuse K, Fukuoka M, Kawahara M, et al. Phase III study of concurrent versus sequential thoracic radiotherapy in combination with mitomycin, vindesine, and cisplatin in unresectable stage III non-small-cell lung cancer. *J Clin Oncol* 1999;17(9):2692.
237. Curran W, Scott C, Langer C, et al. Long-term benefit is observed in a phase III comparison of sequential vs concurrent chemo-radiation for pateints with unresected stage III nonsmall cell lung cancer: RTOG 9410. *Proc Am Soc Clin Oncol* 2003;22.
240. Albain KS, Swann RS, Rusch VW, et al. Radiotherapy plus chemotherapy with or without surgical resection for stage III non-small-cell lung cancer: a phase III randomised controlled trial. *Lancet* 2009;374(9687):379.
250. Ishiguro F, Matsuo K, Fukui T, Mori S, Hatooka S, Mitsudomi T. Effect of selective lymph node dissection based on patterns of lobe-specific lymph node metastases on patient outcome in patients with resectable non-small cell lung cancer: a large-scale retrospective cohort study applying a propensity score. *J Thorac Cardiovasc Surg* 2010;139(4):1001.
251. Darling GE, Allen MS, Decker DA, et al. Randomized trial of mediastinal lymph node sampling versus complete lymphadenectomy during pulmonary resection in patients with N0 or N1 (less than hilar) non-small cell lung carcinoma: results of the ASCOSOG Z0030 trial. Abstract presented at the 90th annual meeting of the American Association for Thoracic Surgery. 2010.
253. Rami-Porta R, Tsuboi M. Sublobar resection for lung cancer. *Eur Respir J* 2009;33(2):426.
259. Kates M, Swanson S, Wisnivesky JP. Survival following lobectomy and limited resection for the treatment of stage I non-small-cell lung cancer <= 1cm in Size: A review of SEER data. *Chest* 2010.
264. Paul S, Altorki NK, Sheng S, et al. Thoracoscopic lobectomy is associated with lower morbidity than open lobectomy: a propensity-matched analysis from the STS database. *J Thorac Cardiovasc Surg* 2010;139(2):366.
269. Yang HC, Kim HK, Kim K, Shim YM, Choi YS, Kim J. Sleeve lobectomy as an alternative procedure to pneumonectomy for non-small cell lung cancer. *J Thorac Oncol* 2010;5(4):517.
285. Mayer R, Smolle-Juettner FM, Szolar D, et al. Postoperative radiotherapy in radically resected non-small cell lung cancer. *Chest* 1997;112(4):954.
286. Douillard JY, Rosell R, De Lena M, Riggi M, Hurteloup P, Mahe MA. Impact of postoperative radiation therapy on survival in patients with complete resection and stage I, II, or IIIA non-small-cell lung cancer treated with adjuvant chemotherapy: the adjuvant Navelbine International Trialist Association (ANITA) Randomized Trial. *Int J Radiat Oncol Biol Phys* 2008;72(3):695.
291. Douillard JY, Rosell R, De Lena M, et al. Adjuvant vinorelbine plus cisplatin versus observation in patients with completely resected stage IB-IIIA non-small-cell lung cancer (Adjuvant Navelbine International Trialist Association [ANITA]): a randomised controlled trial. *Lancet Oncol* 2006;7(9):719.
301. Chemotherapy in non-small cell lung cancer: a meta-analysis using updated data on individual patients from 52 randomised clinical trials. Non-small Cell Lung Cancer Collaborative Group. *BMJ* 1995;311(7010):899.
302. Arriagada R, Auperin A, Burdett S, et al. Adjuvant chemotherapy, with or without postoperative radiotherapy, in operable non-small-cell lung cancer: two meta-analyses of individual patient data. *Lancet* 2010;375(9722):1267.
304. Arriagada R, Bergman B, Dunant A, Le Chevalier T, Pignon JP, Vansteenkiste J. Cisplatin-based adjuvant chemotherapy in patients with completely resected non-small-cell lung cancer. *N Engl J Med* 2004;350(4):351.
306. Winton T, Livingston R, Johnson D, et al. Vinorelbine plus cisplatin vs. observation in resected non-small-cell lung cancer. *N Engl J Med* 2005; 352(25):2589.
308. Strauss GM, Herndon JE, Maddaus MA, et al. Adjuvant paclitaxel plus carboplatin compared with observation in stage IB non-small-cell lung

PRACTICE OF ONCOLOGY

cancer: CALGB 9633 with the Cancer and Leukemia Group B, Radiation Therapy Oncology Group, and North Central Cancer Treatment Group Study Groups. *J Clin Oncol* 2008;26(31):5043.
310. Kato H, Ichinose Y, Ohta M, et al. A randomized trial of adjuvant chemotherapy with uracil-tegafur for adenocarcinoma of the lung. *N Engl J Med* 2004;350(17):1713.
313. Fruh M, Rolland E, Pignon JP, et al. Pooled analysis of the effect of age on adjuvant cisplatin-based chemotherapy for completely resected non-small-cell lung cancer. *J Clin Oncol* 2008;26(21):3573.
314. Depierre A, Milleron B, Moro-Sibilot D, et al. Preoperative chemotherapy followed by surgery compared with primary surgery in resectable stage I (except T1N0), II, and IIIa non-small-cell lung cancer. *J Clin Oncol* 2002; 20(1):247.
316. Pisters K, Vallieres E, Bunn P, et al. S9900: a phase III trial of surgery alone or surgery plus preoperative (preop) paclitaxel/carboplatin (PC) chemotherapy in early stage non-small cell lung cancer (NSCLC): preliminary results. *J Clin Oncol* 2005;23(16S), abstract 7012.
317. Rosell R, Gomez-Codina J, Camps C, et al. Preresectional chemotherapy in stage IIIA non-small-cell lung cancer: a 7-year assessment of a randomized controlled trial. *Lung Cancer* 1999;26(1):7.
318. Roth JA, Atkinson EN, Fossella F, et al. Long-term follow-up of patients enrolled in a randomized trial comparing perioperative chemotherapy and surgery with surgery alone in resectable stage IIIA non-small-cell lung cancer. *Lung Cancer* 1998;21(1):1.
331. Thomas M, Rube C, Hoffknecht P, et al. Effect of preoperative chemoradiation in addition to preoperative chemotherapy: a randomised trial in stage III non-small-cell lung cancer. *Lancet Oncol* 2008;9(7):636.
336. Leo F, Solli P, Veronesi G, et al. Does chemotherapy increase the risk of respiratory complications after pneumonectomy? *J Thorac Cardiovasc Surg* 2006;132(3):519.
338. Krasna MJ, Gamliel Z, Burrows WM, et al. Pneumonectomy for lung cancer after preoperative concurrent chemotherapy and high-dose radiation. *Ann Thorac Surg* 2010;89(1):200.
340. Vandenbroucke E, De Ryck F, Surmont V, van Meerbeeck JP. What is the role for surgery in patients with stage III non-small cell lung cancer? *Curr Opin Pulm Med* 2009;15(4):295.
345. van Meerbeeck JP, Kramer GW, Van Schil PE, et al. Randomized controlled trial of resection versus radiotherapy after induction chemotherapy in stage IIIA-N2 non-small-cell lung cancer. *J Natl Cancer Inst* 2007;99(6): 442.
358. Bruzzi JM, Komaki R, Walsh GL, et al. Imaging of non-small cell lung cancer of the superior sulcus: part 2: initial staging and assessment resectability and therapeutic response. *Radiographics* 2008;28(2):561.
361. Peedell C, Dunning J, Bapusamy A. Is there a standard of care for the radical management of non-small cell lung cancer involving the apical chest wall (Pancoast tumours)? *Clin Oncol (R Coll Radiol)* 2010;22(5):334.
363. Rusch VW, Giroux DJ, Kraut MJ, et al. Induction chemoradiation and surgical resection for superior sulcus non-small-cell lung carcinomas: long-term results of Southwest Oncology Group Trial 9416 (Intergroup Trial 0160). *J Clin Oncol* 2007;25(3):313.
375. Timmerman R, McGarry R, Yiannoutsos C, et al. Excessive toxicity when treating central tumors in a phase II study of stereotactic body radiation therapy for medically inoperable early-stage lung cancer. *J Clin Oncol* 2006;24(30):4833.
381. Perez CA, Pajak TF, Rubin P, et al. Long-term observations of the patterns of failure in patients with unresectable non-oat cell carcinoma of the lung treated with definitive radiotherapy. *Cancer* 1987;45:1874.
384. Dillman RO, Herndon J, Seagren SL, Eaton WL Jr, Green MR. Improved survival in stage III non-small-cell lung cancer: seven-year follow-up of cancer and leukemia group B (CALGB) 8433 trial. *J Natl Cancer Inst* 1996;88(17):1210.
385. LeChavelier T, Arriagada R, Quoix E, et al. Radiotherapy alone versus combined chemotherapy and radiotherapy in nonresectable nonsmall cell lung cancer: first analysis of a randomized trial in 353 patients. *J Natl Cancer Inst* 1991;83:417.
386. Sause W, Kolesar P, Taylor S, et al. Five-year results: phase III trial of regionally advanced unresectable nonsmall cell lung cancer. *Proc Am Soc Clin Oncol* 1998;7.
387. Fournel P, Robinet G, Thomas P, et al. Randomized phase III trial of sequential chemoradiotherapy compared with concurrent chemoradiotherapy in locally advanced non-small-cell lung cancer: Groupe Lyon-Saint-Etienne d'Oncologie Thoracique-Groupe Francais de Pneumo-Cancerologie NPC 95-01 Study. *J Clin Oncol* 2005;23(25):5910.
388. Zatloukal P, Petruzelka L, Zemanova M, et al. Concurrent versus sequential chemoradiotherapy with cisplatin and vinorelbine in locally advanced non-small cell lung cancer: a randomized study. *Lung Cancer* 2004;46(1):87.
390. Vokes EE, Herndon JE 2nd, Kelley MJ, et al. Induction chemotherapy followed by chemoradiotherapy compared with chemoradiotherapy alone for regionally advanced unresectable stage III non-small-cell lung cancer: Cancer and Leukemia Group B. *j clin oncol* 2007;25(13):1698.
391. Hanna N, Neubauer M, Yiannoutsos C, et al. Phase III study of cisplatin, etoposide, and concurrent chest radiation with or without consolidation docetaxel in patients with inoperable stage III non-small-cell lung cancer: the Hoosier Oncology Group and U.S. Oncology. *J Clin Oncol* 2008;26(35): 5755.
395. Kelly K, Chansky K, Gaspar LE, et al. Phase III trial of maintenance gefitinib or placebo after concurrent chemoradiotherapy and docetaxel consolidation in inoperable stage III non-small-cell lung cancer: SWOG S0023. *J Clin Oncol* 2008;26(15):2450.
409. Saunders M, Dische S, Barrett A, Harvey A, Griffiths G, Palmar M. Continuous, hyperfractionated, accelerated radiotherapy (CHART) versus conventional radiotherapy in non-small cell lung cancer: mature data from the randomised multicentre trial. CHART Steering committee. *Radiother Oncol* 1999;52(2):137.
426. Chemotherapy in addition to supportive care improves survival in advanced non-small-cell lung cancer: a systematic review and meta-analysis of individual patient data from 16 randomized controlled trials. *J Clin Oncol* 2008;26(28):4617.
430. Azzoli CG, Baker S Jr, Temin S, et al. American Society of Clinical Oncology Clinical Practice Guideline update on chemotherapy for stage IV non-small-cell lung cancer. *J Clin Oncol* 2009;27(36):6251.
433. Le Chevalier T, Brisgand D, Douillard J-Y, et al. Randomized study of vinorelbine and cisplatin versus vindesine and cisplatin versus vinorelbine alone in advanced non-small-cell lung cancer: results of a European multi-center trial including 612 patients. *J Clin Oncol* 1994;12:360.
458. Shepherd FA, Ramlau R, Mattson K, et al. Prospective randomized trial of docetaxel versus best supportive care in patients with non-small-cell lung cancer previously treated with platinum-based chemotherapy. *J Clin Oncol* 2000;18(10):2095.
459. Fossella F, Pereira JR, von Pawel J, et al. Randomized, multinational, phase III study of docetaxel plus platinum combinations versus vinorelbine plus cisplatin for advanced non-small-cell lung cancer: the TAX 326 study group. *J Clin Oncol* 2003;21(16):3016.
471. Hanna N, Shepherd FA, Fossella FV, et al. Randomized phase III trial of pemetrexed versus docetaxel in patients with non-small-cell lung cancer previously treated with chemotherapy. *J Clin Oncol* 2004;22(9):1589.
477. Schiller JH, Harrington D, Belani CP, et al. Comparison of four chemotherapy regimens for advanced non-small-cell lung cancer. *N Engl J Med* 2002;346(2):92.
478. Ardizzoni A, Boni L, Tiseo M, et al. Cisplatin- versus carboplatin-based chemotherapy in first-line treatment of advanced non-small-cell lung cancer: an individual patient data meta-analysis. *J Natl Cancer Inst* 2007;99(11):847.
482. Sandler A, Gray R, Perry MC, et al. Paclitaxel-carboplatin alone or with bevacizumab for non-small-cell lung cancer. *N Engl J Med* 2006;355(24):2542.
486. Pirker R, Pereira JR, Szczesna A, et al. Cetuximab plus chemotherapy in patients with advanced non-small-cell lung cancer (FLEX): an open-label randomised phase III trial. *Lancet* 2009;373(9674):1525.
498. Lilenbaum R, Axelrod R, Thomas S, et al. Randomized phase II trial of erlotinib or standard chemotherapy in patients with advanced non-small-cell lung cancer and a performance status of 2. *J Clin Oncol* 2008;26(6):863.
501. Gridelli C, Perrone F, Gallo C, et al. Chemotherapy for elderly patients with advanced non-small-cell lung cancer: the Multicenter Italian Lung Cancer in the Elderly Study (MILES) phase III randomized trial. *J Natl Cancer Inst* 2003;95(5):362.
509. Butts C, Murray N, Maksymiuk A, et al. Randomized phase IIB trial of BLP25 liposome vaccine in stage IIIB and IV non-small-cell lung cancer. *J Clin Oncol* 2005;23(27):6674.
510. Ciuleanu T, Brodowicz T, Zielinski C, et al. Maintenance pemetrexed plus best supportive care versus placebo plus best supportive care for non-small-cell lung cancer: a randomised, double-blind, phase 3 study. *Lancet* 2009;374(9699):1432.
511. Fidias PM, Dakhil SR, Lyss AP, et al. Phase III study of immediate compared with delayed docetaxel after front-line therapy with gemcitabine plus carboplatin in advanced non-small-cell lung cancer. *J Clin Oncol* 2009;27(4):591.
512. Cappuzzo F, Ciuleanu T, Stelmakh L, et al. Erlotinib as maintenance treatment in advanced non-small-cell lung cancer: a multicentre, randomised, placebo-controlled phase 3 study. *Lancet Oncol* 2010;11(6):521.
518. Herbst RS, O'Neill VJ, Fehrenbacher L, et al. Phase II study of efficacy and safety of bevacizumab in combination with chemotherapy or erlotinib compared with chemotherapy alone for treatment of recurrent or refractory non small-cell lung cancer. *J Clin Oncol* 2007;25(30):4743.
522. Fukuoka M, Yano S, Giaccone G, et al. Multi-institutional randomized phase II trial of gefitinib for previously treated patients with advanced non-small-cell lung cancer. *J Clin Oncol* 2003;21(12):2237.
524. Ando M, Okamoto I, Yamamoto N, et al. Predictive factors for interstitial lung disease, antitumor response, and survival in non-small-cell lung cancer patients treated with gefitinib. *J Clin Oncol* 2006;24(16):2549.
526. Shepherd FA, Rodrigues PJ, Ciuleanu T, et al. Erlotinib in previously treated non-small-cell lung cancer. *N Engl J Med* 2005;353(2):123.
528. Thatcher N, Chang A, Parikh P, et al. Gefitinib plus best supportive care in previously treated patients with refractory advanced non-small-cell lung cancer: results from a randomised, placebo-controlled, multicentre study (Iressa Survival Evaluation in Lung Cancer). *Lancet* 2005;366(9496):1527.
529. Kim ES, Hirsh V, Mok T, et al. Gefitinib versus docetaxel in previously treated non-small-cell lung cancer (INTEREST): a randomised phase III trial. *Lancet* 2008;372(9652):1809.
541. Engelman JA, Zejnullahu K, Mitsudomi T, et al. MET amplification leads to gefitinib resistance in lung cancer by activating ERBB3 signaling. *Science* 2007;316(5827):1039.

548. Eberhard DA, Giaccone G, Johnson BE. Biomarkers of response to epidermal growth factor receptor inhibitors in Non-Small-Cell Lung Cancer Working Group: standardization for use in the clinical trial setting. *J Clin Oncol* 2008;26(6):983.
549. Rosell R, Moran T, Queralt C, et al. Screening for epidermal growth factor receptor mutations in lung cancer. *N Engl J Med* 2009;361(10):958.
551. Soda M, Choi YL, Enomoto M, et al. Identification of the transforming EML4-ALK fusion gene in non-small-cell lung cancer. *Nature* 2007; 448(7153):561.
553. Shaw AT, Yeap BY, Mino-Kenudson M, et al. Clinical features and outcome of patients with non-small-cell lung cancer who harbor EML4-ALK. *J Clin Oncol* 2009;27(26):4247.
554. Ding L, Getz G, Wheeler DA, et al. Somatic mutations affect key pathways in lung adenocarcinoma. *Nature* 2008;455(7216):1069.
570. Andrews DW, Scott CB, Sperduto PW, et al. Whole brain radiation therapy with or without stereotactic radiosurgery boost for patients with one to three brain metastases: phase III results of the RTOG 9508 randomised trial. *Lancet* 2004;363(9422):1665.
586. Postoperative radiotherapy in non-small-cell lung cancer: systematic review and meta-analysis of individual patient data from nine randomised controlled trials. PORT Meta-analysis Trialists Group. *Lancet* 1998; 352(9124):257.
589. Timmerman R, Paulus R, Galvin J, et al. Stereotactic body radiation therapy for inoperable early stage lung cancer. *JAMA* 2010;303(11):1070.
590. Dillmam RO, Herndon J, Seagren SL, Eaton WL, Green MR. Improved survival in stage III non-small-cell lung cancer: seven-year follow-up of cancer an leukemia group B (CALGB) 8433 trial. *J Natl Cancer Inst* 1996; 88(17):1210.
591. Le Chevalier T, Arriagada R, Quoix E, et al. Radiotherapy alone versus combined chemotherapy and radiotherapy in nonresectable non-small-cell lung cancer: first analysis of a randomized trial in 353 patients. *J Natl Cancer Inst* 1991;83(6):417.
593. Ball D, Bishop J, Smith J, et al. A randomised phase III study of accelerated or standard fraction radiotherapy with or without concurrent carboplatin in inoperable non-small cell lung cancer: final report of an Australian multi-centre trial. *Radiother Oncol* 1999;52(2):129.
594. Saunders M, Dische BA, Harvey A, Gibson D, Parmar M. Continuous hyperfractionated accelerated radiotherapy (CHART) versus conventional radiotherapy in non-small-cell lung cancer: a randomised multicentre trial. *Lancet* 1997;350:161.
595. Belani CP, Wang W, Johnson DH, et al. Phase III study of the Eastern Cooperative Oncology Group (ECOG 2597): induction chemotherapy followed by either standard thoracic radiotherapy or hyperfractionated accelerated radiotherapy for patients with unresectable stage IIIA and B non-small-cell lung cancer. *J Clin Oncol* 2005;23(16):3760.
596. Schild SE, Stella PJ, Geyer SM, et al. Phase III trial comparing chemotherapy plus once-daily or twice-daily radiotherapy in stage III non-small-cell lung cancer. *Int J Radiat Oncol Biol Phys* 2002;54(2):370.

CHAPTER 76 SMALL CELL AND NEUROENDOCRINE TUMORS OF THE LUNG

LEE M. KRUG, M. CATHERINE PIETANZA, MARK G. KRIS, KENNETH ROSENZWEIG, AND WILLIAM D. TRAVIS

SMALL CELL LUNG CANCER

Incidence and Etiology

Although the incidence of small cell lung cancer (SCLC) is declining, it remains a worldwide public health problem. The Surveillance, Epidemiologic, and End Results (SEER) database reports the proportion of SCLC cases among all lung cancers in the United States decreased from 17% to 13% in the past 30 years (Fig. 76.1).[1] Among the predicted 219,000 lung cancer cases in the United States in 2009,[2] an estimated 28,000 cases of SCLC were diagnosed.

Tobacco exposure causes SCLC in over 95% of cases, and as a result, the incidence rates mirror smoking patterns. Peak cigarette consumption occurred in the 1960s but began to decline following the Surgeon General's report linking smoking to cancer and the subsequent ban on tobacco advertising on television.[3] The percentage of men who smoke decreased from 50% in 1965 to 21% in 2005, a much greater proportional reduction than in women, who went from a rate of 32% to 18% during the same years.[3,4] Correspondingly, the incidence of SCLC in men peaked in 1984 and has since been trending steadily down. The incidence in women peaked later and has only declined slightly.[5] The gender gap has narrowed such that currently about half of the patients diagnosed with SCLC are women (Fig. 76.1).

Anatomy and Pathology

Neuroendocrine tumors of the lung encompass a spectrum of tumors, including low-grade typical carcinoid, intermediate-grade atypical carcinoid, high-grade large cell neuroendocrine carcinoma (LCNEC), and SCLC (Table 76.1).[6] Because of their shared neuroendocrine properties, these tumors have common morphologic, ultrastructural, immunohistochemical, and molecular features. Despite this, there are also important differences in clinical, epidemiologic, histologic, and molecular characteristics.

SCLC is readily diagnosed on small specimens such as bronchoscopic biopsies, fine-needle aspirates, core biopsies, and cytology. The diagnosis of SCLC is based primarily on light microscopy (Fig. 76.2). Immunohistochemistry may be helpful, but if the histologic features are classic, it may not be needed. Necrosis is common and frequently shows large areas. The tumor cells usually measure less than the diameter of three small resting lymphocytes. They are round to fusiform in shape and have scant cytoplasm. The nuclear chromatin is finely granular and nucleoli are inconspicuous or absent.[6,7] The mitotic rate is characteristically high, averaging 60 to 80 per 2 mm^2. Crush artifact is a frequent finding in small transbronchial or mediastinal biopsy specimens and can make pathologic interpretation difficult. The tumor cells of SCLC also have a tendency to show a streaming artifact. This can also occur with non–small cell lung cancer (NSCLC), lymphoma, and chronic inflammation. In surgically resected specimens where the tumor cells achieve better fixation, the cells of SCLC appear larger than in small biopsies.[7,8] When a component of NSCLC, including adenocarcinoma, squamous cell carcinoma, large cell carcinoma, spindle cell carcinoma, and giant cell carcinoma, is present, the term combined SCLC is used with mention of the specific histology of the non–small cell component.[6,7] In resected specimens, combined SCLC may occur in up to 28% of cases.[7] To diagnose combined SCLC and large cell carcinoma, the large cell carcinoma component must comprise at least 10% of the overall tumor.[6,7]

The following immunohistochemical stains are helpful in difficult cases. A pancytokeratin antibody such as AE1/AE3 is useful to confirm if the tumor is a carcinoma. If this is negative, stains for lymphoma, such as CD45 and CD20, or stains for primitive neuroectodermal tumors (PNET), such as CD99, may be helpful. Neuroendocrine differentiation can be demonstrated using a panel of markers such as CD56, chromogranin, and synaptophysin. A high proliferation rate of 80% to 100% should be seen with Ki-67. Thyroid transcription factor-1 (TTF-1) is positive in 70% to 80% of small cell carcinomas.[9–11]

SCLC must be separated from other primary lung cancers, carcinoid tumors, malignant lymphoma, and sarcomas such as PNET. This differential diagnosis can be very difficult in small, crushed biopsy specimens. Since cytology is often obtained at the time of bronchoscopic biopsy and SCLC shows characteristic cytologic features, comparison of biopsy material with the cytology specimen can be helpful. In particular, large cell neuroendocrine carcinoma and the basaloid variant of large cell carcinoma can be difficult to distinguish from SCLC. In the differential diagnosis with NSCLC, reproducibility studies among expert lung cancer pathologists have shown interobserver disagreement in approximately 5% of cases,[12] so these cases may require special scrutiny using a consensus approach among other pathology colleagues. If a consensus diagnosis cannot be reached, it may be appropriate to refer the case for extramural consultation. Immunohistochemical markers can be of assistance in crushed specimens, as SCLC may demonstrate positive staining for cytokeratin, chromogranin, CD56, synaptophysin, TTF-1, and a high proliferation index with Ki-67.[13] However, some preserved tumor cells with characteristic morphology should be seen on light microscopy to confirm the diagnosis.

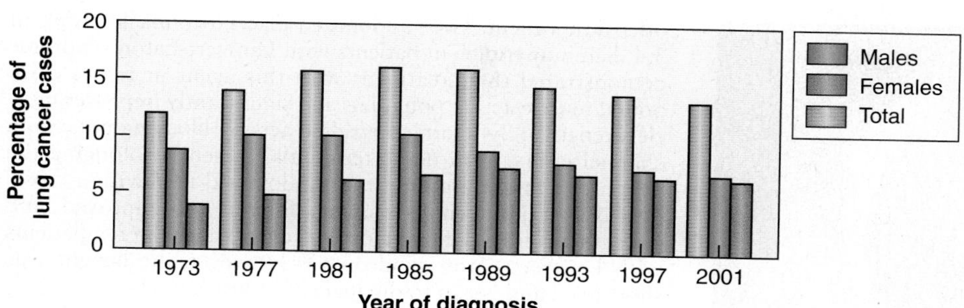

FIGURE 76.1 Patients diagnosed with small cell lung cancer as a percentage of all lung cancer cases and the breakdown by gender. (Adapted from ref. 1.)

Up to 10% of SCLC may be negative for all neuroendocrine markers if a panel of antibodies, including CD56, is utilized.[14] TTF-1 can be positive in extrapulmonary small cell carcinomas, so it is not useful in determining the primary site of small cell carcinomas.[15]

Screening

The natural history of SCLC is characterized by rapid tumor growth and early metastatic spread. For this reason, the diagnosis of SCLC in an asymptomatic patient is rare. In one study, SCLC was diagnosed in only 9 of 31,567 (0.02%) asymptomatic patients undergoing baseline lung cancer screening CT scans.[16] Screening for SCLC by any method is not recommended.

Diagnosis

Presenting symptoms in patients with SCLC can be constitutional, pulmonary, the result of extrathoracic spread, or due to paraneoplastic disorders.[17,18] In one series in which patient-reported symptoms were recorded using the Lung Cancer Symptom Scale, fatigue was the most common symptom with decreased physical activity, cough, dyspnea, decreased appetite, weight loss, and pain occurring sometime in the course of the illness in the majority of patients.[18] Hemoptysis was noted in 14% in the same series.[18] The primary tumor often presents as a large central mass invading or compressing the mediastinum. Superior vena cava obstruction is present at diagnosis in 10% of patients with SCLC[19] (Fig. 76.3), and in these cases, the symptoms are often worsened by associated thrombosis in the compromised blood vessel. Chest imaging typically shows hilar and mediastinal adenopathy. One-third of patients have some degree of atelectasis present.[17] A peripheral location or chest-wall involvement by the tumor is uncommon. Rarely SCLC presents as a solitary pulmonary nodule.[20,21] No more than 2% of SCLC present as a superior sulcus tumor.[22]

Most patients with SCLC have metastases at diagnosis. Bone involvement is usually characterized by osteolytic lesions, often in the absence of bone pain, or elevations in the serum alkaline phosphatase.[23] However, osteoblastic bone metastases can occur as well in some patients. Hepatic and adrenal lesions are typically asymptomatic. Brain metastases can be detected in at least 10% of patients at diagnosis; these may cause neurologic symptoms, such as motor weakness or seizures, but they are often asymptomatic.

The paraneoplastic syndromes associated with SCLC differ from those observed with NSCLC. Only 5% of patients with lung cancer diagnosed with hypertrophic pulmonary osteoarthropathy have SCLC. Hypercalcemia is very rare as well. On the other hand, the vast majority of lung cancer patients in whom the syndrome of inappropriate antidiuretic hormone (SIADH), Cushing syndrome, or neurologic paraneoplastic syndromes develop have SCLC.

SCLC accounts for approximately 75% of the tumors associated with SIADH. Although serum concentrations of antidiuretic hormone are elevated in the majority of those with

TABLE 76.1

THE SPECTRUM OF PULMONARY NEUROENDOCRINE (NE) PROLIFERATIONS AND NEOPLASMS[a]

I. NE cell hyperplasia and tumorlets
   A. NE cell hyperplasia
      1. NE cell hyperplasia associated with fibrosis or inflammation
      2. NE cell hyperplasia adjacent to carcinoid tumors
      3. Diffuse idiopathic NE cell hyperplasia with or without airway fibrosis/obstruction
   B. Tumorlets (less than 0.5 cm)

II. Tumors with NE morphology
   A. Typical carcinoid (0.5 cm or larger)
   B. Atypical carcinoid
   C. Large cell neuroendocrine carcinoma
      Combined large cell neuroendocrine carcinoma[b]
   D. Small cell carcinoma
      Combined small cell carcinoma[b]

III. Non–small cell carcinomas with NE differentiation (NED)

[a]Modified from ref. 6.
[b]The histologic type of the other component of non–small cell carcinoma should be specified.

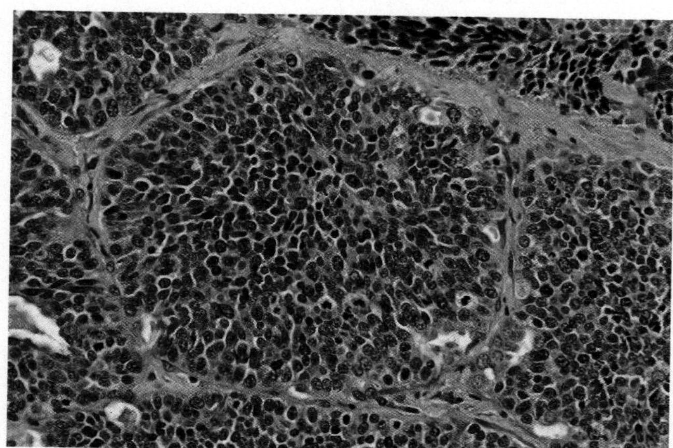

FIGURE 76.2 Small cell carcinoma. This tumor consists of dense sheets of small cells with scant cytoplasm, finely granular nuclear chromatin, frequent mitoses, and inconspicuous or absent nucleoli.

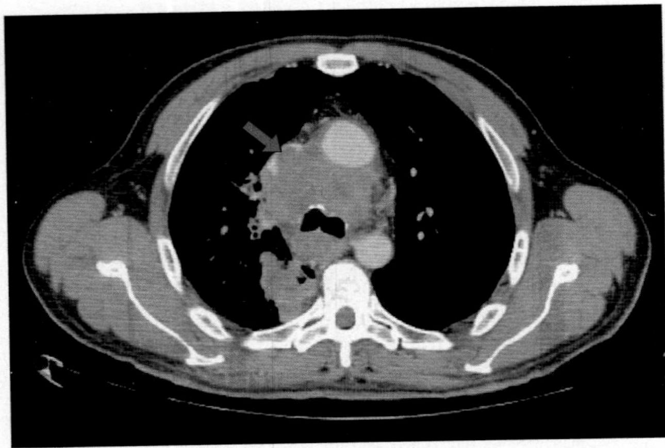

FIGURE 76.3 Computed tomography scan showing small cell lung cancer with an infiltrative mediastinal mass causing compression of the superior vena cava (*arrow*).

SCLC, only approximately 10% of patients fulfill the criteria of SIADH, and symptoms are present in no more than 5%. In some cases, ectopic production of atrial natriuretic factor contributes to the disorder in sodium homeostasis. The primary treatment for hyponatremia in SCLC patients is treatment of the disease with chemotherapy. Otherwise it is managed as with other etiologies with fluid restriction in mild cases or with intravenous hypertonic saline (in a monitored setting) in severe, symptomatic cases. Demeclocycline, a tetracycline derivative that induces a nephrogenic diabetes insipidus, can be used in refractory SIADH.

Increased serum levels of adrenocorticotropic hormone can be detected in up to 50% of patients with lung cancer, but Cushing syndrome develops in only 5% of patients with SCLC. In approximately one-half of these cases, it is present at diagnosis. Low serum sodium is an adverse prognostic factor,[24] and patients with Cushing syndrome have a very limited survival.[25]

Paraneoplastic neurologic disorders seen in patients with SCLC include sensory, sensorimotor, and autoimmune neuropathies and encephalomyelitis.[26] These syndromes are thought to occur through autoimmune mechanisms, and antinuclear antibodies that bind to SCLC and to neuronal tissues have been identified. Symptoms may precede the diagnosis by many months and are often the presenting complaint. They may also be the initial sign of relapse from remission. An aggressive search may be required to discover small tumor nodules causing profound neurologic syndromes. Subacute peripheral sensory neuropathy associated with the anti-Hu antibody may be the most frequent paraneoplastic neurologic disorder seen in those with SCLC. Less common is the Lambert-Eaton syndrome, characterized by proximal muscle weakness that improves with continued use, hyporeflexia, and dysautonomia. Classic electromyographic findings confirm the diagnosis. The cause is related to autoantibody impairment of voltage-gated calcium channels. Rarer neurologic disorders seen in patients with SCLC include cerebellar degeneration or retinopathy. Two studies conflicted when evaluating whether the presence of paraneoplastic antibodies have prognostic implications.[27,28]; the utilization of different techniques to measure antibody levels may account for the discrepant results.[29]

In contrast to the endocrine syndromes, for which successful treatment of the tumor effectively controls the symptoms, the occurrence and severity of the neurologic symptoms is unrelated to tumor bulk and usually does not resolve with antineoplastic therapy. Various therapies such as plasma exchange and immunosuppressive therapy with agents such as corticosteroids, cyclophosphamide, and tacrolimus have been tried, but generally offer little benefit. Two randomized placebo-controlled trials of 3,4 diaminopyridine in patients with Lambert-Eaton syndrome demonstrated that treatment with this agent increases compound muscle action potentials and significantly improves muscle strength[30]; 3,4 diaminopyridine acts by blocking potassium channel efflux from nerve terminals, thereby prolonging the action potential duration. In a randomized trial with a cross-over design, intravenous immunoglobulin also improved limb strength as measured by myometry over placebo in ten patients with Lambert-Eaton syndrome.[30] However, the benefit was short-lived and began to dissipate after just 8 weeks.

Staging

Staging determines prognosis and treatment. Surgery plays a small role in the management of this disease. Fewer than 10% of patients, only those with lung-confined disease, are candidates for thoracotomy. As a result, a simpler two-stage system, introduced by the Veterans' Administration Lung Study Group (VALSG), has historically been utilized instead of the TNM (tumor, node, metastasis) system employed for most other cancer types.[31] In the VALSG system, limited stage is defined as disease confined to one hemithorax that can be "encompassed" in a "tolerable" radiation field. These patients are currently treated with a combined modality approach. All other patients are considered to have extensive-stage disease. At presentation, approximately two-thirds of patients with SCLC have extensive disease and one-third limited-stage disease.[1]

In the VALSG staging system, the appropriate classification of ipsilateral pleural effusion, supraclavicular lymphadenopathy (ipsilateral or contralateral), or contralateral mediastinal lymphadenopathy as either limited or extensive stage remains controversial. Some large series have not found a survival difference between patients with an isolated ipsilateral pleural effusion and other patients with limited SCLC,[32] and some groups have included patients with ipsilateral pleural effusions within their definition of limited-stage disease.[33,34] However, analyses of two large cooperative group databases, which included *in toto* more than 4,000 patients, showed that the survival of individuals with an isolated effusion was similar to that of patients with extensive disease.[33,35] In clinical practice, it is assumed that an effusion is malignant unless three criteria are met: the fluid must be a transudate, nonhemorrhagic, and cytologically negative on repeated examinations. Patients with a malignant effusion are appropriate to exclude from combined modality treatment because hemithoracic radiotherapy to encompass the entirety of the pleura is impractical.

Although most trials to evaluate the role of combined modality therapy in limited-stage SCLC have excluded patients with an ipsilateral pleural effusion, they have usually included those with ipsilateral, and sometimes contralateral, supraclavicular lymph node metastases. The presence of supraclavicular lymphadenopathy is commonly associated with extensive disease but, when encountered in patients with otherwise limited disease (5% of cases), carries a trend toward poorer survival.[35] Contralateral mediastinal involvement is also usually classified as limited-stage disease. However, two studies that evaluated twice-a-day radiation regimens excluded patients with contralateral hilar disease to reduce the normal lung volume irradiated and the risk for toxicity.[36,37] Patients with limited-stage disease who present with superior vena cava syndrome have a similar prognosis to other patients with limited-stage disease[34] and have been included in randomized studies investigating the role of combined modality therapy.

For patients who appear to have limited-stage SCLC, some additional tests may be appropriate to confirm this assessment. Unilateral iliac crest bone marrow aspiration and biopsy are still a routine part of staging for many oncologists and should

TABLE 76.2

TUMOR, NODE, METASTASIS STAGING AND SURVIVAL

Stage	N	1-Year Survival Rate (%)	5-Year Survival Rate (%)	Median Survival (mo)
IA	55	91	56	78
IB	45	82	57	77
IIA	56	78	38	32
IIB	25	76	40	34
IIIA	68	49	12	11
IIIB	12	33	0	9

From ref. 41.

be performed in limited-stage patients with elevations of serum lactate dehydrogenase (LDH)[38,39] and evidence of myelophthisis (nucleated red blood cells, leukopenia, or thrombocytopenia) on the peripheral blood smear. If there is evidence of a pleural effusion, a thoracentesis or thoracoscopy may help confirm that the effusion is nonbloody, a transudate, and cytologically negative. Effusions too small to permit image-guided sampling should not be considered in staging.[40] Bony abnormalities seen on positron emission tomography (PET) or bone scan require confirmation with magnetic resonance imaging (MRI) or computed tomography (CT) scan if they represent the only disease site that makes a patient extensive stage.

For the American Joint Committee on Cancer (AJCC) seventh edition, the use of a TNM staging system for SCLC has been revisited. To establish the accuracy of outcomes based on stage, cases of completed resected SCLC were staged using the same definitions as used for NSCLC. Survival rates based on stage are shown in Table 76.2.[41] The use of pathologic stage was necessary to accurately stage the patients used for this analysis; however, most patients with limited SCLC are managed with chemotherapy and radiation. Nonetheless, more favorable outcomes of patients have been reported in patients previously classified as "very limited" disease (no evidence of mediastinal metastases by CT or mediastinoscopy) treated with chemotherapy and radiation, as compared with other patients with limited-stage disease.[42–44] The use of the TNM system is best applied for cases of early stage disease and may have less relevance for the majority of patients presenting with metastatic disease.

Clinical and Serologic Predictive and Prognostic Factors

Multivariable analyses suggest that performance status is a strong and reproducible predictive and prognostic factor.[35,45,46] Poorer performance status can additionally identify individuals at higher risk for treatment-related complications. Several other clinical parameters have been proposed. Female gender has been associated with improved response and survival in patients with SCLC.[35,45,46] In patients 70 years and older, response and survival rates with multimodality therapy were similar to younger individuals but toxicity was greater.[47] Older age (variably defined) has not been identified an adverse prognostic factor in patients with SCLC in most[47–50] but not all[24,33,35] series. Older age has been associated with decreased performance status and more comorbid illnesses and often results in compromised chemotherapy dose intensity,[51,52] which may partially explain its prognostic implications. Although the majority of patients with SCLC in the United States are over age 65, they comprise only 39% of individuals enrolled on lung cancer clinical trials. Clinicians need to be aware of this fact as they attempt to apply clinical trial data to the actual care of this growing population. Certain metastatic sites, such as liver,[53–55] brain,[54,56] bone marrow,[55] and bone,[56] as well as the total number of metastatic sites involved,[35] have been found to be of prognostic significance for patients with extensive-stage disease. Paraneoplastic Cushing syndrome has been correlated with a poor response to therapy and short survival.[25] Continued use of tobacco during combined modality therapy was identified as an adverse prognostic factor in a group of 186 patients with limited disease.[57]

Elevation of serum LDH is found in 33% to 57% of all patients with SCLC and up to 85% of patients with extensive-stage disease and is a strong prognostic and predictive factor.[33,34,45,53,54,56,58,59] Elevation of serum LDH is associated with the presence of bone marrow involvement.[38] In one study, 20 of 20 patients with bone marrow involvement had elevation of serum LDH.[38] In contrast, 0 of 33 patients with a normal LDH had bone marrow involvement. Although many other serum markers have been proposed to have prognostic significance, including neuron-specific enolase,[49,54] chromogranin, and precursors of gastrin-releasing peptide,[60,61] none have been strong and reliable enough to warrant general use. In one report, the use of neuron-specific enolase provided no additional benefit over the widely available serum LDH.[58] Carcinoembryonic antigen (CEA) has been found to predict outcome in SCLC in multiple series.[45,62,63]

Management by Stage

General Recommendations for Initial Management

Once the pathologic diagnosis of SCLC is confirmed, a complete history and physical examination is the next step. Special attention should be paid to the cigarette smoking history. If a patient is a current smoker, he or she should be advised to quit immediately in the strongest terms and offered the most aggressive smoking cessation intervention available.[57] If the patient is a never-smoker, the pathologic diagnosis of SCLC should be reviewed as only 1% of never-smokers develop SCLC. The National Comprehensive Cancer Network has compiled consensus guidelines for the initial evaluation of individuals with SCLC.[40] A complete blood cell count (CBC) with platelet count, electrolytes, calcium, creatinine, serum urea nitrogen (BUN), liver function tests, and LDH are recommended. All patients should undergo a contrast-enhanced CT scan of the chest, a gadolinium enhanced MRI of the head, and whole-body PET or a bone scan. If disease is suspected clinically at other sites, those should be imaged as well. A PET scan can identify sites of metastases undetected by other modalities[64–66] and can replace the bone scan.[67]

All fit patients (Karnofsky performance status greater than 60% or Eastern Cooperative Oncology Group [ECOG] performance status 0, 1, or 2) should initially receive combination chemotherapy with etoposide plus either cisplatin or carboplatin for four to six cycles (Fig. 76.4).[40] Supportive data, specifics of chemotherapy regimens, duration of therapy, and alternatives for patients with contraindications or special needs are discussed in the sections below. Patients with limited-stage disease should receive the chemotherapy concurrently with twice-daily thoracic irradiation beginning with the first or second cycle.[37] Patients who achieve a response to chemotherapy should receive prophylactic whole-brain radiotherapy at the conclusion of chemotherapy or chemoradiotherapy.[68] There is no routine recommendation for treatment of patients who have a Karnofsky performance status of 50% or less or ECOG performance status 3 or 4. Since the toxicity of all treatment

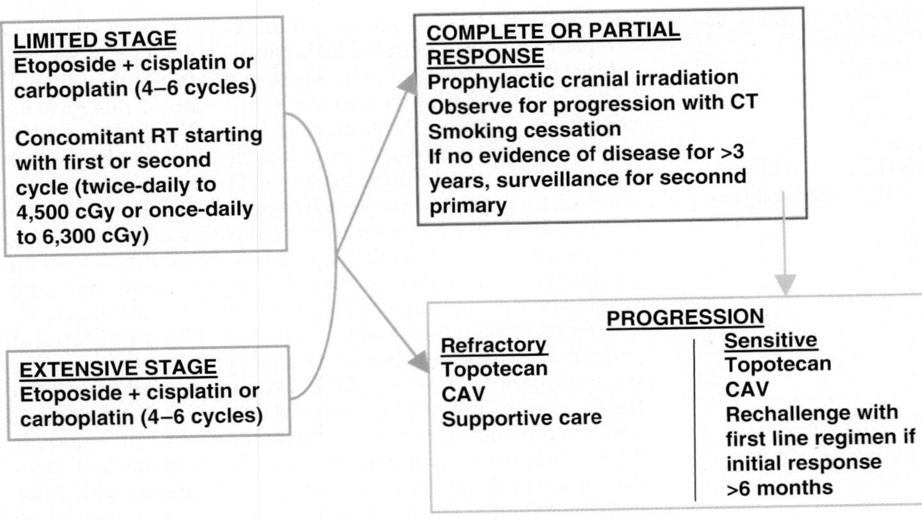

FIGURE 76.4 General treatment paradigm for small cell lung cancer.

worsens and effectiveness lessens in patients with a low performance status, clinicians must carefully evaluate the agent(s) used and the appropriateness and goals of therapy individually. For many patients in this low performance status group, supportive care only and referral to hospice are the best options.

Chemotherapy

Evolution of Chemotherapy Regimens. Due to the rapid growth rate of SCLC and its propensity for developing metastases early in the disease course, outcomes reported in studies from the 1960s for patients treated with surgery or radiation therapy alone were dismal. As the field of medical oncology evolved, the sensitivity of SCLC to chemotherapy agents was recognized, and the primary role of systemic treatment in SCLC was established. In a series of studies conducted four decades ago to test alkylating agents, cyclophosphamide was shown to double survival compared with supportive care in patients with extensive disease.[69] Thereafter, the Medical Research Council showed that a combination of cyclophosphamide with radiation improved survival compared to radiation alone in patients with limited-stage disease.[70] An extensive evaluation of the drugs then available demonstrated that anthracyclines and vinca alkaloids, along with certain alkylating drugs, produced single-agent response rates of up to 50%. The antimetabolites appeared to be less active with response rates of 20% to 30%. In the 1980s, the epipodophyllotoxin, etoposide, and the platinum analogues, cisplatin and carboplatin, were introduced, and their activity ranged from 40% to 60% in previously untreated patients.[71] Since then, numerous other chemotherapeutic agents have demonstrated activity in SCLC, but aside from the camptothecins, the drugs identified in the 1970s and 1980s remain the backbone of therapy.

After the activity of cyclophosphamide was established in SCLC, multidrug combinations were tested. Randomized trials of combinations demonstrated superior activity to single-agent cyclophosphamide. The combination of cyclophosphamide, doxorubicin, and dacarbazine produced a higher response rate and survival when compared with an equally toxic dose of single-agent cyclophosphamide.[72] Hansen et al.[73] demonstrated that the addition of vincristine to the combination of cyclophosphamide, methotrexate, and lomustine improved survival compared to the three-drug combination, highlighting the usefulness of this relatively nonmyelotoxic agent in combination therapy. Livingston et al.[74] developed the CAV (cyclophosphamide, doxorubicin, vincristine) combination, and reported on 358 patients who received this combination followed sequentially by thoracic and brain irradiation. For patients with extensive disease, the complete response rate was 14%, the overall response rate was 57%, and the median survival was 26 weeks. For patients with limited disease, the rates were 41%, 75%, and 52 weeks, respectively. With these data, CAV became the standard chemotherapy regimen.

With the identification of etoposide as perhaps the most active agent, several modifications of the CAV regimen that included etoposide were tested. A randomized trial showed greater response duration and survival with CAE compared with CAV.[75] Hong et al.[76] compared intensive CV (with the dose of cyclophosphamide increased from 1,000 to 2,000 mg/m^2) to CAV and to CEV (cyclophosphamide, etoposide, and vincristine) and reported that patients treated with CV had a shorter survival and experienced more myelosuppression than those treated on the other two arms.

Five randomized trials have evaluated the addition of etoposide (CAVE) to the CAV regimen.[77–81] In three studies, the doses of CAV were equivalent in each arm.[77–79] Although a better response rate was evident in the arm that contained etoposide, in at least some patient subsets in each of these studies, an improvement in response duration (of 3 months) and survival (of 6 weeks, $P = .08$) was seen in only one study.[77] In these studies, the addition of etoposide resulted in increased hematologic toxicity. Jett et al.[79] compared CAVE to CAV in 231 patients with limited disease. Despite a reduction of the dose of cyclophosphamide by 33%, there was still greater myelosuppression in the CAVE arm. A numerical improvement in median and 2-year survival was seen with CAVE, which was not statistically significant. Two studies intensified components of this regimen: in one the cyclophosphamide was increased from 1,000 to 1,200 mg/m^2, and the dose of doxorubicin increased from 40 to 75 mg/m^2 in the CAV arm compared to the CAVE arm.[80] The regimens produced equivalent myelotoxicity, response rates, and survival. These results were comparable to the outcomes with less-intensive CAV regimens in patients with extensive disease.

The etoposide/cisplatin (EP) regimen was tested in SCLC because this combination produced synergistic activity in preclinical systems. In addition, both agents could be given at full doses because of less myelosuppression with cisplatin. The first report by Sierocki et al.[82] at Memorial Sloan-Kettering Cancer Center in 1979 demonstrated the activity of this combination in

TABLE 76.3

RANDOMIZED CLINICAL TRIALS COMPARING ETOPOSIDE AND CISPLATIN TO OTHER CHEMOTHERAPY REGIMENS

Study (Ref.)	Stage	Treatment Arm	No. of Patients	Overall Response Rate (%)	Median Survival (mo)	1-Year Survival (%)	2-Year Survival (%)
Fukuoka et al. (86)	Limited and extensive	EP	97	78	9.9	NR	12
		CAV	97	55	9.9	NR	10
		CAV/EP alternating	94	76	11.8 (P = .056)	NR	21
Roth et al. (87)	Extensive	EP	159	61	8.6	NR	NR
		CAV	156	51	8.3	NR	NR
		CAV/EP alternating	162	59	8.1	NR	NR
Sundstrom et al. (88)	Limited and extensive	EP	218	NR	10.2 (P = .0004)	NR	14
		Cyclophosphate, epirubicin, vincristine	218	NR	7.8	NR	6
Skarlos et al. (93)	Limited and extensive	EP	71	69	12.5	NR	NR
		Etop/carboplatin	72	78	11.8	NR	NR
Noda et al. (97)	Extensive	EP	77	52	9.4	58	20
		Irinotecan/cis	77	65	12.8 (P = .002)	38	5
Hanna et al. (98)	Extensive	EP	110	44	10.2	35	8
		Irinotecan/cis	221	48	9.3	35	8
Lara et al. (99)	Extensive	EP	327	57	9.1	34	NR
		Irinotecan/cis	324	60	9.9	41	NR
Eckardt et al. (105)	Extensive	EP	395	69	9.4	31	NR
		Oral topotecan/cis	389	63	9.2	31	NR
Miyamoto et al. (120)	Limited and extensive	EP	45	78	12.8	53	15
		Ifosfamide/etop/cis	47	74	13.0	62	17
Loehrer et al. (121)	Extensive	EP	84	67	7.3	27	5
		Ifosfamide/EP	87	73	9.1 (P = .045)	36	13
Mavroudis et al. (125)	Limited and extensive	EP	71	48	10.5	37	NR
		Paclitaxel, etop, cis	62	50	9.5	38	NR
Niell et al. (126)	Extensive	EP	282	68	9.9	37	8
		Paclitaxel, etop, cis	283	75	10.6	38	11

EP, etoposide and cisplatin; CAV, cyclophosphamide, doxorubicin, vincristine; NR, not reported; etop, etoposide; cis, cisplatin.

SCLC. EP was given for two cycles followed by CAV. Subsequent studies by Evans et al.[83,84] reported response rates of 55% in patients previously treated with CAV and 86% in newly diagnosed patients. Einhorn et al.[85] reported that two cycles of consolidation with EP, when added to the treatment of patients with limited disease who were responding to six cycles of CAV, produced longer survival than with CAV only. Three randomized trials have compared EP to cyclophosphamide, vincristine, and an anthracycline.[86–88] Less myelosuppression occurred with EP, and, if given with radiation, patients experienced less esophagitis and interstitial pneumonitis. Furthermore, the largest trial showed that EP produced a better median (15 months vs. 10 months) and 5-year (10% vs. 3%) survival for patients with limited disease.[88] Retrospective analyses and meta-analyses also support the superiority of cisplatin- or carboplatin-containing chemotherapy for SCLC.[89–91] As a result, EP is now the standard first-line chemotherapy regimen for SCLC (Table 76.3).

Carboplatin has been substituted for cisplatin in SCLC chemotherapy regimens in an effort to lessen nonhematologic toxicities. In combination with etoposide, Bishop et al.[92] reported response rates of 77% and 58% and median survival times of 15.3 months and 8.1 months for limited and extensive disease, respectively. Randomized trials comparing cisplatin and carboplatin suggest that they may have similar efficacy, but the design of those studies limits interpretation. The Hellenic Cooperative Oncology Group randomized 147 patients with either limited or extensive disease to receive etoposide 100 mg/m^2 days 1 to 3, and cisplatin, 100 mg/m^2, or carboplatin, 300 mg/m^2.[93] Concurrent radiation was also administered to responding patients starting with the third cycle. Response and survival were similar in the two arms. Nausea, vomiting, nephrotoxicity, and neurotoxicity were significantly lower in the patients who received carboplatin. Grade 4 leukopenia was also less in the carboplatin arm. However, the sample size of this study is inadequate to confirm equivalent efficacy. In a larger three-arm randomized trial, induction with teniposide, vincristine, and either carboplatin or cisplatin produced equivalent activity and toxicity.[94] The survival was also similar for the two treatment arms, but relative differences between the two platinum drugs may not be apparent because six other drugs were included in the regimen. Based on these data, etoposide and carboplatin can be considered an appropriate first-line regimen, particularly in patients who cannot tolerate cisplatin.

More recently, platinum combinations with topotecan and irinotecan have emerged as potential regimens for initial therapy. Japanese studies first demonstrated the activity of irinotecan as a single agent,[95] and the subsequent phase 2 results of the irinotecan and cisplatin combination[96] prompted interest in a randomized trial. The Japan Clinical Oncology Group compared cisplatin and irinotecan to EP as initial treatment in extensive disease.[97] The study was terminated after 154 of the planned 230 patients were enrolled because median (12.8 months vs. 9.4 months) and 2-year (19.5% vs. 5.2%) survival were significantly better in the group treated with cisplatin and irinotecan. Myelosuppression was the most common severe toxicity in both groups and was more frequently observed with EP. Significant diarrhea occurred only in the irinotecan group and was observed in 16% of the patients. Two confirmatory studies were subsequently launched in the United States. In the first trial, the irinotecan/cisplatin schedule was modified in an effort to decrease toxicity; the day 15 irinotecan dose was eliminated, and the cisplatin was split between days 1 and 8. Hanna et al.[98] reported that the response rate (48% for irinotecan/cisplatin vs. 44% for EP), median time to progression (4 months vs. 5 months), and overall median survival (9 months vs. 10 months) were equivalent. The Southwest Oncology Group compared these two regimens with the same dose and schedule used in the Japanese trial and also showed, in a well-powered study, that outcomes are equivalent with the two regimens in Caucasian patients.[99] High response rates have been reported in several trials using irinotecan and carboplatin with varied dosing schedules.[100,101] A phase 3 trial comparing that regimen with etoposide/cisplatin showed improved survival, but the median survival of 7 months in the control arm, which used oral etoposide, is lower than expected.[102] Many hypothesize that population-based polymorphisms in uridine 5′-diphospho (UDP)-glucuronosyltransferase (UGT1A1), the enzyme responsible for detoxifying SN-38, the active metabolite of irinotecan, may account for differences in toxicity and efficacy between Japanese and Americans.[103] The regimen of topotecan plus cisplatin has also undergone phase 2 and 3 testing.[104,105] Eckardt et al.[105] reported the results of a randomized trial including 784 patients in which patients received oral topotecan (1.7 mg/m²/d for 5 days) plus cisplatin, or standard etoposide and cisplatin. The response rates, median survival, and 1-year survival were identical. Severe neutropenia occurred more often with EP, but oral topotecan and cisplatin caused more anemia and thrombocytopenia.

Strategies to Improve Outcomes with Chemotherapy Regimens

Alternating Cycles of Combination Chemotherapy Regimens. The recognition of clonal heterogeneity within a tumor and the intolerability of treatment regimens that included more than four drugs due to overlapping toxicity led to trials of alternating chemotherapy combinations. The somatic mutation model developed by Goldie et al.[106] predicted that the best probability of cure was achieved by the earliest possible introduction and most rapid alternation of all active agents. If two equally effective non–cross-resistant regimens were available, the model predicted that alternating between regimens every other cycle would be more effective than alternating after every three cycles or giving one regimen continuously for five cycles before switching to the second regimen.

Many randomized clinical trials have tested the concept of alternating multidrug combinations.[87,107–111] The fact that the EP regimen was effective in patients who had progressed after cyclophosphamide-based chemotherapy suggested that these drug combinations were non–cross-resistant.[112] With this in mind, the National Cancer Institute of Canada conducted a study in which 289 patients were randomized to CAV or CAV alternating with EP.[109] Chemotherapy was given for a total of six cycles. The response rate (65% vs. 47%), progression-free survival, and median survival time (10 months vs. 8 months) favored the patients who had received alternating therapy. The authors postulated that these findings could be the result of inclusion of a more active regimen (EP) within the alternating arm, an advantage due to greater drug diversity with five effective drugs rather than three, or support of the Goldie et al. concept. A Japanese study compared CAV to EP to alternating CAV/EP.[86] Patients with limited disease received four cycles of chemotherapy followed by thoracic irradiation. Patients with extensive disease who responded to chemotherapy continued treatment for 1 year. A total of 288 patients were enrolled. No differences in survival were noted in the patients with extensive disease. Patients with limited disease had improved survival, even after adjusting for other prognostic factors with the alternating regimen compared with CAV ($P = .058$) or EP ($P = .032$). Roth et al.[87] evaluated 437 patients with extensive disease in a randomized trial comparing EP for four cycles, CAV for six cycles, or CAV alternating with EP for a total of six cycles. Although a slight improvement occurred in progression-free survival ($P = .052$) with the alternating regimen, there was no difference in response rate or overall survival among the treatment arms. The patients whose tumors did not respond to CAV and were crossed over to EP were twice as likely to benefit as individuals who initially received EP and were crossed over to CAV, although these differences were not significant (28% vs. 14% for induction responders who relapsed and 15% vs. 8% for patients with primary resistance, respectively). The modest activity seen when refractory patients were crossed over from one of these regimens to the other suggests that the CAV and EP combinations are not entirely cross-resistant, which works against a primary assumption of the Goldie et al. hypothesis. Taking all of these studies together, alternating regimens appears to have slight or no benefit over initial treatment with EP alone.

Additional studies have evaluated alternating chemotherapy introduced after achieving a response to an induction regimen.[113–115] The National Cancer Institute of Canada designed a randomized trial in which 300 patients with limited disease received either CAV for three cycles followed by EP for three cycles or CAV alternating with EP for a total of six cycles.[116] Response rates, time to treatment failure, or survival did not differ. Wolf et al.[113] randomized 321 patients to treatment with ifosfamide plus etoposide given until a response plateau, followed by CAV or ifosfamide plus etoposide alternating with CAV. A total of six cycles of chemotherapy were delivered in each arm. No difference in outcome was noted.

Studies have also evaluated alternating more intensive regimens. For example, a German multicenter trial demonstrated that an alternating eight-drug regimen was superior to CAV.[117] Two other European trials testing three drugs regimens alternating with four drug regimens found no survival advantage to that approach.[110,118] Again, the median survival times observed in these studies were no different from those that used EP alone.[86,87]

Addition of a Third Chemotherapeutic Agent to Etoposide Plus Cisplatin. All efforts to add a third drug to the standard EP regimen have resulted in more toxicity with little or no improvement in survival. The three-drug regimen of etoposide, ifosfamide, and cisplatin (VIP), developed initially for refractory germ cell tumors, has also been evaluated in SCLC.[119] In randomized trials comparing VIP to EP, one study, which included patients with limited and extensive disease, found no difference in survival between the two treatment groups,[120] while another, which was larger and enrolled only patients with extensive disease, identified a significant difference in median survival (9 months vs. 7 months) and 2-year survival rates (13% vs. 5%).[121] In both studies, myelosuppression was more severe in the ifosfamide-containing arm. Carboplatin has been substituted for cisplatin in this regimen (ICE), and in single-arm studies impressive response rates and cumulative myelosuppression have been reported.[122,123] A large trial comparing ICE plus a midcycle dose of vincristine to other standard therapy demonstrated an improvement in the median and 1-year survival rates.[124] However, an increased rate of septicemia was noted with ICE-V (15% vs. 7% in the control arm).

Studies that added paclitaxel to EP reach the same conclusion: enhanced toxicity with similar efficacy. Two studies that compared EP to EP plus paclitaxel showed that the addition of the third drug increased toxicity without improving survival.[125,126] Notably, despite the addition of granulocyte colony-stimulating factor (G-CSF), these studies reported a treatment-related mortality in the three-drug arm of 7%[126] and 13%.[125] This led to early termination of one of the studies.[125] A German study that added paclitaxel to etoposide and carboplatin demonstrated a significantly better median survival (13 months vs. 12 months) and 3-year (17% vs. 9%) survival only in patients with limited disease as compared to treatment with etoposide, carboplatin, and vincristine.[127]

Maintenance Therapy. Throughout the 1970s, chemosensitive tumors were often treated for as long as 2 years. For SCLC, this meant that most patients continued chemotherapy until disease progression or death. In 1984 Feld et al.[128] demonstrated that six cycles of CAV and thoracic irradiation produced survival comparable to the results of a previous treatment program that included 12 months of maintenance therapy. Subsequently, a large number of randomized studies examined whether maintenance chemotherapy prolonged survival.[107,129–139]

Three studies that randomized patients in complete remission after induction therapy to maintenance treatment or observation identified improved survival with the prolonged treatment program in some patient groups.[107,132,135] The Cancer and Leukemia Group B (CALGB) randomized 258 patients to one of four chemotherapy regimens, and 57 patients in complete remission underwent a second randomization to maintenance therapy or observation. Among the 46 patients with limited disease who proceeded to the second randomization, the median survival was improved with maintenance chemotherapy (17 months vs. 7 months).[135] However, the initial regimens used in this study might be considered inferior to currently used treatments. In a second study, patients treated with six cycles of CAV and in complete remission were randomized to six additional cycles of the same chemotherapy or observation.[132] For the patients with extensive disease, the median survival was improved by approximately 4 months with maintenance treatment. An additional trial, organized by the ECOG, randomized patients to CAV alternating with another three-drug combination or CAV alone.[107] After six to eight cycles of induction, patients in complete remission underwent a second randomization to maintenance treatment or observation. Patients assigned to CAV and maintenance therapy had a longer progression-free survival and overall survival (P = .09) than patients who received only CAV with no maintenance. In contrast, for the patients who received the six-drug regimen, those who were given no maintenance survived longer than the patients who received maintenance treatment. These studies suggest that there may be patients, perhaps those with particularly chemotherapy-sensitive disease, who derive a benefit from maintenance if they are treated with a CAV induction regimen. In unselected patients, however, clinical trials that have evaluated treatment programs that extend beyond six cycles of chemotherapy have not demonstrated an advantage in survival.

The Medical Research Council randomized 265 patients who had responded to six cycles of induction chemotherapy to an additional six cycles of maintenance or observation.[129] Overall, there was no difference in survival between patients treated with 6 or 12 cycles of chemotherapy, although for patients in complete remission at the time of randomization a subset analysis suggested that maintenance provides a survival benefit. Three other large studies that randomized patients responding to 5 or 6 cycles of induction to a total of 12 cycles of chemotherapy or observation found no difference in outcome.[133,134,137] Another study that randomized patients with limited disease from the start of chemotherapy to a total of 6 or 12 cycles identified inferior survival in the arm treated with the longer course of therapy.[131]

Other studies have evaluated whether four cycles of chemotherapy are adequate.[130,136,140] Spiro et al.[140] designed a study that included a double randomization at diagnosis. Patients received four or eight cycles of CEV and on relapse were given additional chemotherapy or supportive care. Of the four treatment arms, patients who received four cycles of chemotherapy and only supportive care at relapse had a significantly inferior median survival of 30 weeks. Thus, in this study, four cycles of treatment were adequate, provided that chemotherapy was offered to patients appropriate for additional therapy at relapse. Two additional studies evaluated four cycles of induction with longer treatment programs. A European trial randomized patients who responded to four cycles of EP to CAV for up to ten additional cycles or to observation.[130] No survival differences were identified, but the study had limited power based on a small sample size that included limited and extensive disease. The ECOG enrolled 402 eligible patients with extensive-stage disease into a trial that delivered four cycles of EP followed by a randomization of patients with at least stable disease to four additional cycles of topotecan or to observation.[136] Although maintenance therapy increased the time before documentation of disease progression, there was no difference in overall survival. Despite a predicted favorable distribution into the cerebrospinal fluid, topotecan maintenance did not reduce the incidence of central nervous system (CNS) metastases.

In summary, four to six cycles of chemotherapy appear to be optimal in the management of limited and extensive SCLC. After completion of this initial treatment, patients should be monitored closely and then offered further chemotherapy at the time of progression.

Dose Intensification. In experimental models, numerous chemotherapy drugs display log-linear or near linear dose–response curves,[141] and high-dose chemotherapy has been proven effective in treating hematologic diseases. It seemed reasonable to test the hypothesis that more intensive chemotherapy could improve outcomes in SCLC given the known chemosensitivity of that disease. Methods used have included use of higher chemotherapy doses without or with hematopoietic growth factor support, shortened cycle length, or extreme dose intensification with marrow or peripheral blood stem cell support.

Several investigators evaluated whether increasing the dose of drugs beyond the usual dose improves survival.[142–147] Three randomized trials comparing standard versus high-dose CAV (two studies)[144,146] or EP[145] found no difference in response rates or median survival. Furthermore, no hematopoietic growth factors were used in these three trials, and, as such, myelosuppression and infections were significantly more severe in the high-dose arms. A randomized trial that did utilize granulocyte-macrophage colony-stimulating factor (GM-CSF) to dose escalate cyclophosphamide, 4′-epidoxorubicin, etoposide, and cisplatin found that excess toxicity actually resulted in lower drug delivery and poorer response and survival rates in the dose-intense arm.[147] The only study that has suggested that the administration of higher drug doses was beneficial was a French study with 105 limited-stage patients.[142] Despite improvements in progression-free survival at 2 years (28% vs. 8%) and overall survival (43% vs. 26%), few oncologists have embraced this regimen. Many question this result since the doses of cisplatin (100 vs. 80 mg/m^2) and cyclophosphamide (1,200 vs. 1,000 mg/m^2) were increased modestly only for the first of six cycles and in a regimen that also included doxorubicin and etoposide.

A number of studies have evaluated whether shortening the interval between chemotherapy cycles improves survival. A multicenter study randomized 300 patients mostly with limited-stage disease to six cycles of ICE-V delivered every 4 weeks or every 3 weeks.[148] In a second randomization, patients were given GM-CSF or placebo after each chemotherapy cycle. In the group receiving chemotherapy every 3 weeks, the delivered dose intensity was increased by 26% over the entire treatment program compared with the group treated every 4 weeks. The median survival (443 days vs. 351 days) and the 2-year survival rate (33% vs. 18%) were better in the intensified arm ($P = .0014$), even after adjustment in a multivariable analysis. The addition of GM-CSF did not reduce the incidence or the duration of febrile neutropenia, and there was no difference in survival between the patients who received GM-CSF or placebo. In a subsequent study, ICE given every 4 weeks was compared to ICE given every 2 weeks with support of G-CSF, and autologous blood collected before the cycle was reinfused 24 hours after the chemotherapy.[177] Although the median delivered dose intensity was increased by 82% without significant increased toxicity, no survival benefit was identified. Two studies compared treatment with cyclophosphamide, doxorubicin, and etoposide given either every 3 weeks, or every 2 weeks with G-CSF support.[149,150] The larger trial,[150] which also included a higher percentage of limited-stage patients, showed an improvement in complete response rate and overall survival, but the other trial did not. No fewer than four randomized trials have shown that intensive multidrug weekly regimens are no better yet significantly more toxic than standard regimens.[151–154]

Numerous reports cite the use of high-dose chemotherapy with autologous bone marrow or stem cell rescue for treating SCLC.[155–173] All of these studies have included small numbers of highly selected patients.[169,170,174–177] Only a fraction of patients can complete high-dose chemotherapy, and treatment-related toxicity is severe in this group of patients who are older and have other smoking-related comorbid illnesses. Even in a highly selected subset that is younger and healthier than the general population of patients with SCLC, it is not clear whether survival is better than would have been expected with conventional treatment. As in other chemosensitive solid tumors like breast cancer, high-dose chemotherapy with stem cell support does not appear to have a role in SCLC. Escalating chemotherapy doses in SCLC does not overcome the development of drug resistance.

Treatment After Relapse Following Initial Therapy. The strongest predictor of outcome for patients with relapsed SCLC is the duration of remission. As such, patients are distinguished as having "sensitive" or "refractory" disease. The term *sensitive* implies an appropriate response to initial therapy that is maintained for 3 months or more. These patients have a higher likelihood of response to any additional chemotherapy, although at best it is approximately half that expected in the first-line setting. Survival from the start of a second regimen averages around 6 months. Patients with *refractory* disease either had no response to initial therapy or progressed within 3 months after completing treatment. Their chance of response to additional therapy is less than 10%, and their median survival from the start of a second regimen is 4 months.

In contrast to the tremendous number of phase 3 trials conducted in the first-line setting, surprisingly few large trials have been conducted in relapsed patients. The most studied agent in this setting is topotecan. Ardizzoni et al.[178] reported a phase 2 trial in which topotecan, administered at a dose of 1.5 mg/m^2 daily for 5 days, yielded a response rate of 38% in sensitive patients and 6% in refractory patients. Median survival from the start of second-line therapy was 7 and 5 months, respectively. A randomized trial compared topotecan, administered at that same dose and schedule, to CAV in patients who relapsed at least 2 months after initial therapy.[179] The response rates for topotecan (24%) and for CAV (18%) were similar. The median survival was 6 months in both arms. Trilineage myelosuppression was severe, with grade 4 neutropenia occurring at a higher rate with CAV than topotecan (51% vs. 38% of courses), but the reverse for grade 3 or 4 anemia (1% vs. 7%) and thrombocytopenia (10% vs. 18%). Symptom improvement was better with topotecan for four of the eight symptoms queried. This study led to the U.S. Food and Drug Administration's approval of intravenous topotecan with an indication for sensitive relapsed SCLC. Oral topotecan has also undergone extensive testing in patients with relapsed SCLC. In a randomized phase 2 study, oral topotecan at a dose of 2.3 mg/m^2 daily for 5 days was comparable to intravenous topotecan 1.5 mg/m^2 daily for 5 days with regards to response rate (23% vs. 15%), median survival (32 weeks vs. 25 weeks), and symptom control.[180] Oral topotecan caused less severe neutropenia, but the rates of infection were similar in both arms. Subsequently, the Medical Research Council showed that oral topotecan improved survival in relapsed SCLC over best supportive care alone.[181] In this trial, which included patients with sensitive and refractory disease, the median survival was 26 weeks after treatment with oral topotecan and 14 weeks without, and there was a slower deterioration of quality of life and symptomatology. The response rate to oral topotecan was 7%. In a subgroup analysis, patients with disease progression within 2 months of their initial therapy derived a survival advantage similar to the patients with a longer time to progression. Oral topotecan has also received regulatory approval for second-line therapy of SCLC.

Apart from those studies, only small phase 2 trials have been conducted of other agents. A list of single agents and their activity in relapsed SCLC is found in Table 76.4. These drugs have also been tested in multiple combination trials. The agent with the highest response rates is amrubicin, an anthracycline that has primarily been studied in Japan. A randomized phase 2 trial conducted there showed higher response rates and progression free survival compared with topotecan.[191] A North American phase 2 trial of amrubicin showed lower response rates than observed in the Japanese studies, though still encouraging considering the refractory population.[190] A phase 3 trial comparing amrubicin to topotecan is being conducted.

In summary, the optimal drug or combination of drugs in relapsed SCLC has not been established. Single agent topotecan or CAV are appropriate for patients with sensitive relapse. These regimens could also be used for patients with refractory SCLC, although the response rates are lower. For patients with relapse 6 months or more after initial therapy, rechallenging with the same regimen as used in first-line treatment is also a consideration.[40]

Immunotherapy and Other Targeted Therapies

In light of the therapeutic plateau achieved with current chemotherapy, investigators have studied a wide range of novel therapies in the hopes of improving outcomes (Table 76.5). The association of SCLC with immunogenic effects, such as the prolonged survival of patients with autoantibodies (i.e., Hu) and neurologic paraneoplastic syndromes,[27] has generated interest in studying immunomodulators as treatment. Perhaps the most extensively studied agent in this regard is interferon. The expression of major histocompatibility complex antigens is reduced in SCLC and thus may play a role in this tumor's ability to escape immune surveillance.[192,193] Interferon has been shown to increase the expression of major histocompatibility antigens on SCLC cells *in vitro* and *in vivo*.[194] Small studies in newly diagnosed patients treated with either interferon-alfa or interferon-gamma, however, showed a total absence of activity. Because immune augmentation may be most effective in patients with low disease burden, larger studies have evaluated interferons as maintenance treatment in patients responding to chemotherapy. Mattson et al.[195] conducted a study in which

TABLE 76.4

ACTIVITY OF SINGLE AGENT CHEMOTHERAPY IN RELAPSED SMALL CELL LUNG CANCER

Drug (Ref.)	Dose/Schedule	N	Sensitive/Refractory	Response Rate (%)	Median Survival (mo)
Topotecan (178)	1.5 mg/m² daily × 5	45	Sensitive	38	6.9
		47	Refractory	6	4.7
Topotecan (IV) (179)	1.5 mg/m² daily × 5	107	Sensitive (60 days)	24	6.0
Topotecan (IV) (180)	1.5 mg/m² daily × 5	54	Sensitive	15	5.8
Topotecan (oral) (180)	2.3 mg/m² daily × 5	52	Sensitive	23	7.5
Topotecan (oral) (181)	2.3 mg/m² daily × 5	71	Sensitive + refractory	7	6.0
		30	Sensitive	3	
		41	Refractory	10	
Irinotecan (95)	100 mg/m² weekly	16	Sensitive*	47	6.2
Paclitaxel (182)	175 mg/m² every 3 wk	24	Refractory	29	3.0
Docetaxel (183)	100 mg/m² every 3 wk	34	Not specified**	25	Not reported
Gemcitabine (184)	1,000 mg/m² d1, 8, 15 every 4 wk	46	Both	12	7.1
Gemcitabine (185)	1,250 mg/m² d1, 8 every 3 wk	27	Both	0	6.4
Gemcitabine (186)	1,000 mg/m² d1, 8, 15 every 4 wk	38	Refractory	13	4.0
Vinorelbine (187)	25 mg/m² weekly	24	Both	13	5.0
Vinorelbine (188)	30 mg/m² weekly	26	Sensitive	16	Not reported
Amrubicin (189)	40 mg/m² daily × 3 every 3 wk	44	Sensitive	52	10.3
		16	Refractory	50	11.6
Amrubicin (190)	40 mg/m² daily × 3 every 3 wk	75	Refractory	21	6.0

*All but one patient had a chemotherapy-free interval of >90 days.
**Previously untreated patients also included.
IV, intravenous.

patients responding to induction chemotherapy were randomized to a maintenance chemotherapy, natural interferon-alfa, or observation. Although there were no differences overall, a subset analysis showed improved survival for patients with limited disease who received interferon. Another study that administered interferon-alfa along with induction chemotherapy and as maintenance reported a higher complete response rate and improved median survival.[196] Due to poor accrual, however, the study was stopped prematurely, and only 77 patients were evaluable. Two other randomized trials, one in which interferon-alfa was included as part of the induction and maintenance regimen and a second cooperative group trial in which interferon-alfa maintenance was evaluated in patients with limited disease who had responded to induction chemotherapy, showed no survival advantage.[197,198] Interferon-gamma maintenance therapy in patients with complete or near complete remissions has also been evaluated in two randomized trials.[199,200] Although the dose and schedule selected from one trial were confirmed to be biologically active as demonstrated by a significant increase in the expression of human leukocyte antigen (HLA)-DR and Fc receptors on monocytes,[201] neither study demonstrated an impact on survival. In addition to the typical constitutional side effects and myelosuppression, a few of the studies in lung cancer have suggested that the interferons may enhance radiation-induced lung injury, and at least one case of fatal pneumonitis occurred.[200] High-dose interleukin-2 has also been evaluated in a group of patients with extensive disease who experienced less than a complete remission to induction chemotherapy.[202] The overall response rate was 21%, but the toxicity was severe, and treatment was discontinued in 11 of 24 patients because of life-threatening side effects.

Vaccination therapy conceptually could stimulate the host immune response to eradicate microscopic residual cancer after maximal response has been achieved by standard therapy. One potential immunologic target is the ganglioside GD3 expressed on most SCLC tumors and cell lines. Using an anti-idiotype approach, the mouse monoclonal antibody BEC2 was developed against the binding region of the mouse monoclonal antibody R24, which binds to GD3. Injection of BEC2 into humans generates an antibody response that could cross-react with the GD3 on tumor cells. A small pilot study suggested that patients with SCLC who had a major response to induction chemotherapy immunized with BEC2 plus BCG adjuvant enjoyed superior survival rates compared to historical control.[203] This led to a randomized phase 3 trial conducted by the European Organisation for Research and Treatment of Cancer (EORTC) in which patients with limited SCLC who completed initial therapy were randomized to vaccination with BEC2 plus BCG or best supportive care.[204] Despite a humoral immune response in one-third of the patients, no improvement in overall or progression-free survival was observed after vaccination. Vaccination strategies against other gangliosides[205] and alternate targets such as p53[206] continue to be explored.

A potential role of the coagulation system in the propagation of SCLC has been recognized for many years. Thrombin is generated *in situ* and may function as a growth factor for the tumor.[207] Initial studies to evaluate whether the addition of warfarin to a chemotherapy regimen improved survival yielded mixed results. In a randomized trial involving 50 patients, the addition of warfarin significantly improved progression-free and overall survival.[208] In a larger cooperative group study, patients who received warfarin with chemotherapy had a higher response rate ($P = .012$) and a 6-week improvement in median progression-free and overall survival, although the difference for the latter two end points was not significant.[209] The addition of 1 g/d aspirin, a dose sufficient to inhibit platelet aggregation, failed to demonstrate a benefit.[210] A subsequent trial by the same group of investigators demonstrated that the subcutaneous administration of unfractionated heparin at therapeutic doses given during the first 5 weeks of chemotherapy resulted in a higher complete remission rate and improved survival.[207]

Small molecule kinase inhibitors are now established therapies for several diseases, but as yet, have not proven efficacious in SCLC. This includes imatinib, which, in addition to its inhibition of bcr/abl kinase that provides remarkable success

TABLE 76.5

IMMUNOTHERAPIES AND OTHER TARGETED AGENTS THAT HAVE UNDERGONE TESTING IN SMALL CELL LUNG CANCER

Agent (Ref.)	Mechanism of Action	Study Design	Result
Interferon-alfa (187–190)	Immunomodulator	Phase 3 (multiple)	Two studies with improved survival in limited-stage patients, two studies with no survival benefit
Interferon-gamma (191,192)	Immunomodulator	Phase 3 (multiple)	No improvement in survival
Interleukin-2 (194)	Immunomodulator	Phase 2	21% response rate but excessive toxicity
Marimastat (212)	Matrix metalloproteinase inhibitor	Phase 3	No improvement in progression-free or overall survival
Bay 12-9566 (213)	Matrix metalloproteinase inhibitor	Phase 3	No improvement in progression-free or overall survival
Imatinib (203,206,207)	c-kit tyrosine kinase inhibitor	Phase 2 (multiple)	No responses
Gefitinib (208)	Epidermal growth factor receptor (EGFR) tyrosine kinase inhibitor	Phase 2	No responses
Temsirolimus (CCI-779) (218)	Mammalian target of rapamycin (mTOR) inhibitor	Randomized phase 2	Improved survival at higher dose but no improvement in outcome compared with prior trials
Tipifarnib (R115777) (209)	Farnesyl transferase inhibitor	Phase 2	No responses
Oblimersen (G3139) (218)	Bcl-2 antisense	Randomized phase 2	No improvement in response rate
Bortezomib (PS-341) (219)	Proteosome inhibitor	Phase 2	One response in refractory patient (2% overall response rate)
BEC-2 + BCG adjuvant (196)	Ganglioside (GD3) anti-idiotype vaccine	Phase 3	No improvement in progression-free or overall survival
Thalidomide (220,221)	Multiple immunomodulatory effects, also inhibits vascular endothelial growth factor (VEGF)	Phase 3	Improved survival from 8.7 to 11.7 months but not significant (hazard ratio 0.74; $P = .16$)
		Phase 3	No improvement in any parameters
Vandetanib (222)	Tyrosine kinase inhibitor of VEGFR-2 and EGFR	Randomized phase 2	No improvement in progression-free survival
Bevacizumab (223–225)	Monoclonal antibody to VEGF	Phase 2 (multiple)	No increased risk of hemorrhage. Favorable survival compared with historical control

in chronic myelogenous leukemia, also blocks c-kit signaling. C-kit protein expression has been reported in 28% to 93% of SCLC tumors.[211] *In vitro* studies support the role of c-kit and its ligand, stem cell factor (SCF), on SCLC autocrine and paracrine growth stimulation,[212] and imatinib has demonstrated growth inhibition of multiple SCLC cell lines.[213] Nonetheless, three phase 2 studies in SCLC failed to demonstrate a single radiologic response to imatinib, even when enrollment was restricted to patients with tumors expressing c-kit protein by immunohistochemistry.[211,214,215] Likewise, the oral tyrosine kinase inhibitor of the epidermal growth factor receptor (EGFR), gefitinib, proved inactive in SCLC.[216] Since activating mutations in target genes (c-kit for gastrointestinal stromal tumors, and EGFR for NSCLC) confer sensitivity to these tyrosine kinases, the lack of those mutations in SCLC likely explains their inactivity. Similarly, *kras* mutations are lacking in SCLC, yet, based on preclinical data suggesting the farnesyl transferase inhibitor tipifarnib (R115777) induced SCLC growth inhibition, a phase 2 study was conducted in patients with sensitive relapse.[217] No responses were observed. Temsirolimus (CCI-779) is a novel small molecule inhibitor of the downstream mammalian target of rapamycin (mTOR). The ECOG randomized patients after initial chemotherapy to maintenance therapy with either high-dose or low-dose temsirolimus.[218] Although the progression-free survival (1.8 months vs. 2.5 months) and overall survival were better for the high dose arm (6.5 months vs. 9.0 months), these results were no better than those observed in the previous ECOG trial of topotecan maintenance therapy,[136] suggesting no added benefit from temsirolimus.

Matrix metalloproteinases (MMPs) are extracellular enzymes that degrade connective tissue and stroma, allowing tumor cells to penetrate basement membranes, invade blood vessels, and colonize distant sites. High MMP expression levels have been reported in SCLC and identified as a negative predictor of survival.[219] However, in two randomized placebo-controlled phase 3 trials, the use of the MMP inhibitors marimastat or BAY12-9566 in the maintenance setting failed to improve survival or time to progression.[220,221]

The antiapoptotic gene product, bcl-2 protein, is expressed in 80% to 90% of SCLC tumor samples and as such is a potential therapeutic target.[222,223] Oblimersen (G3139) is an antisense oligonucleotide that suppresses bcl-2 expression. The CALGB conducted a series of studies with oblimersen in combination with chemotherapy for SCLC.[224,225] In a randomized phase 2 study of etoposide/carboplatin with or without oblimersen, survival was inferior in the patients receiving oblimersen (hazard ratio [HR] for overall survival 2.13; $P = .02$).[226] Insufficient suppression of bcl-2 by this agent may explain its lack of efficacy. More potent small molecule inhibitors of bcl-2 that act as BH3 mimetics are now in development. Bortezomib has also been studied based on the rationale that proteasome inhibition regulates the apoptotic pathway through inhibition of nuclear factor-κB and bcl-2; however, only one response was seen among 28 refractory patients and no responses were observed among 28 sensitive patients.[227]

Angiogenesis inhibitors have entered into standard clinical practice for numerous malignancies, and they are being tested in SCLC as well. Two phase 3 trials that tested thalidomide as maintenance therapy after first-line chemotherapy showed no significant effect on overall survival.[228,229] Likewise, vandetanib, an oral tyrosine kinase inhibitor of vascular endothelial growth factor receptor 2 (VEGFR-2) and EGFR, failed to improve progression-free survival in a randomized phase 2 maintenance trial.[230] In all of these cases, toxicity was significantly greater in the treatment arms. Multiple phase 2 studies adding the VEGF monoclonal antibody, bevacizumab, to chemotherapy have not shown any increased risk of pulmonary hemorrhage in this cohort of patients who commonly have central tumors.[231–233] These studies have also yielded favorable survival rates when compared to historical controls, but this may have been due to selection bias since patients with brain metastases were excluded.

Radiation

Role of Radiotherapy in Limited Disease. Despite being exquisitely chemo- and radioresponsive, neither modality alone controls all aspects of disease. The CALGB trial of the late 1980s demonstrated that 90% of patients treated with chemotherapy alone failed locally.[234] The meta-analysis of Pignon and Arriagada[235] provided more data to mandate thoracic radiotherapy, but a number of treatment issues remained to be determined, including sequencing of radiation with chemotherapy, early versus late radiotherapy, altered fractionation, and prophylactic cranial irradiation.

Concurrent combined modality therapy is the standard treatment for SCLC patients with limited-stage disease.[40] It requires close coordination between medical and radiation oncologists. Selection for combined modality treatment requires patients with an excellent performance status. Because not all patients are sufficiently fit for combined modality treatment, single modality therapy may be appropriate for those who are debilitated or have serious comorbidities. Because single modality therapy is suboptimal, reassessment after initial chemotherapy or radiotherapy may allow for sequencing of the other modality if the patient's condition sufficiently improves to warrant this. A substantial clinical challenge continues to be inadequate control of local and systemic disease, in addition to failure in sanctuary sites. In the past 15 years, gains have been realized, with better integration of radiotherapy with CT-aided targeting and beam delivery and fewer cycles of chemotherapy, each of which contributes to lower morbidity.

Sequencing of Radiation with Chemotherapy. Concurrent therapy is defined as combined modality treatment in which chemotherapy and radiation therapy are administered throughout the same time period. Sequential therapy is defined as the administration of chemotherapy and radiotherapy separately in time, with one modality begun only after completion of the other, often associated with a delay for the second modality to allow the patient an adequate recovery from the initial treatment modality. A 1992 meta-analysis evaluated randomized trials in which more than 2,100 patients with limited-stage SCLC were randomized to receive either chemotherapy alone or in combination with chest irradiation.[236] Patients given combined modality therapy had a 14% reduction in death rate and an absolute 5.4% improvement in 3-year survival compared with those who received chemotherapy alone. Both differences were highly significant in this meta-analysis. This study reinforces the results of individual studies that demonstrated modest but statistically significant improvement in survival after combined modality treatment. A second and independent meta-analysis reached similar conclusions.[237]

The trials included in the meta-analysis used cyclophosphamide- and doxorubicin-based chemotherapy, combinations that are incompatible with concurrent thoracic radiotherapy due to excess toxicity. Therefore, multiple strategies were attempted to avoid giving chemotherapy and radiation simultaneously, such as sequential chemoradiation, interdigitated chemoradiation, and using different chemotherapy regimens during the concurrent phases. However, with the current standard chemotherapy regimen, consisting of cisplatin and etoposide, these issues are not as much of a concern since these drugs can be used safely with concurrent radiotherapy.

Thoracic Radiation Dose and Fractionation. Due to the observed radioresponsiveness of SCLC, traditionally modest total doses of radiation, ranging from 45 to 50 Gy, have been used. However, with modest-dose radiation therapy there is a high rate of local failure. For example, in the Intergroup trial, the control arm of 45 Gy given once daily had a 75% rate of intrathoracic relapse.[238] Therefore, higher doses of radiation or different methods of radiation delivery (i.e., acceleration) appear to be needed to improve local control. A retrospective review from Massachusetts General Hospital suggested that there may be continued dose response beyond 50 Gy.[239] The maximum tolerated dose of thoracic irradiation concurrent with chemotherapy seems to be 45 to 51 Gy with a twice-daily approach and 70 Gy when the radiation is given daily.[240]

CALGB-39808 determined that 70 Gy delivered with daily fractions of 2 Gy with concurrent chemotherapy is feasible in the cooperative group setting.[241] They reported a median survival of 22.4 months and acceptable rates of esophagitis and pneumonitis. Other CALGB trials have examined the use of 70 Gy of thoracic irradiation with concurrent chemotherapy. For example, in CALGB-30002, induction therapy consisted of paclitaxel, topotecan, and etoposide followed by concurrent chemoradiation utilizing carboplatin and etoposide.[242] This radiation dose has the advantage of being delivered in fractionation that most radiation oncologists are familiar with. Additionally, daily fractionation is more convenient for patients especially on days when concurrent chemotherapy is to be delivered. The prolonged course of radiation causes the radiation to overlap with three cycles of chemotherapy. In addition, the delay of radiation until the third cycle of chemotherapy might have an impact on outcome. However, a retrospective analysis of radiation therapy interruptions of greater than 3 days due to hemotologic toxicity did not adversely affect outcome.[243]

Delivering chest irradiation in multiple daily fractions was theorized on experimental grounds to reduce long-term pulmonary toxicity while still maintaining antitumor efficacy. In fact, using even smaller doses per fraction has a theoretic basis because small cells are exponentially killed with very low doses and very low-dose rates.[244] SCLC would appear to be an ideal neoplasm for twice-daily treatment in that it has a high growth fraction, short cell cycle time, and small to absent shoulder on the *in vitro* cell survival curve. Pilot studies in the late 1980s combining etoposide and platinum plus twice-daily chest irradiation were promising, with median survivals greater than 2 years and in most series low rates of associated pneumonitis.[238,245,246] An Intergroup study randomized 417 patients with limited-stage SCLC to a program that included EP for four cycles and radiation therapy beginning on day 1 of the first cycle.[37] The cumulative dose was 45 Gy in both arms, with one arm receiving the radiation in 1.8 Gy fractions daily and the other arm receiving 1.5 Gy fractions on a twice-daily basis. Although the fractionation might be the obvious variable, the duration of therapy (total time) varied between the arms as well (3 weeks vs. 5 weeks). Of importance, higher doses using conventional fractions lengthen time of treatment, and longer treatment times may exert selective pressure on the emergence of resistant clones. The target volume included the primary tumor plus bilateral mediastinal nodes and the ipsilateral hilum but included the supraclavicular nodes only when involved. Local failure was reduced from 52% with the daily schedule to 36% with the twice-daily schedule ($P = .06$). Of interest, patients who failed in local and in distant sites had a frequency of 23% with daily treatment, versus only 6% with the twice-daily approach ($P = .01$). More important, although statistically significant differences in survival were not seen at 24 months,[246] the curves deviated so that at 5 years the survival was only 16% with once-a-day treatment, as opposed to 26% with the twice-daily schedule ($P = .04$).[37] All patients who achieved less than complete response were scored as local failures, but some of those treated with the accelerated scheme who achieved only a partial response survived, as well as those with a complete response, implying that the local failure rate was overcalled by imaging on that arm. Overall long-term morbidities were not significantly different between the two arms, although there was a higher frequency of grade 3 esophagitis with twice-daily treatment.

A North Central Cancer Treatment Group trial attempted to reduce morbidity of twice-daily radiation by inserting a 2.5-week pause between two equally balanced 24 Gy split courses.[36,247] After three cycles of induction chemotherapy, fit and responding patients were randomized to receive either 48 Gy delivered in a twice daily regimen as split courses of 24 Gy or 54 Gy in a once daily regimen in 6 weeks. Chemotherapy was delivered every 28 days for two additional cycles. Thus, the 48 Gy dose was delivered in 5.5 weeks, longer than standard time, *not* an accelerated regimen.[247] The 20% 5-year survival percentage was notably less than the benchmark 26% from the Intergroup trial when 45 Gy was delivered in 3 weeks. However, a follow-up of this trial used a higher dose of radiation, 60 Gy also given via 1.5 Gy twice daily with a 2-week treatment break and reported a favorable 5-year survival of 24%.[248]

A phase 1 trial conducted by the Radiation Therapy and Oncology Group (RTOG) and CALGB evaluated the use of 70 Gy delivered in daily fractionation or 45 Gy given in twice a day fractionation.[249] Although it was a trial to establish the maximum-tolerated does (MTD) of irinotecan given with cisplatin and thoracic radiation therapy, it was the first trial to evaluate 70 Gy delivered at cycle one. Two of 15 patients treated to 70 Gy had dose-limiting toxicities (diarrhea, esophagitis, and cardiovascular complications).

RTOG-9712 was a phase 1 trial to establish the MTD of radiation therapy with delayed accelerated hyperfractionation.[250] With this technique a large field encompassing the gross tumor and mediastinum was treated to 45 Gy. A smaller field that encompassed only the gross tumor was treated as a second daily treatment in a fraction size of 1.8 Gy for the last 3, 5, 7, and 11 days. The MTD was found to be 61.2 Gy utilizing nine twice-daily fractions at the end of treatment. This regimen was subsequently evaluated in RTOG-0239, a phase 2 trial.[251] It reported a 2-year overall survival of 37%, short of the predicted survival of 60%. However, the regimen demonstrated an excellent local control of 80%.

Currently, a three-armed randomized phase 3 trial is being conducted by the RTOG and CALGB to evaluate three radiation therapy fractionation schemes: 45 Gy in 1.5 Gy twice-daily fractions (standard), 70 Gy in 2 Gy fractions, and 61.2 Gy with delayed accelerated hyperfractionation. In the first part of this trial, toxicity will be assessed and the less toxic of arms B and C will be compared head to head with the standard arm.

Early versus Late Radiotherapy. Randomized trials have yielded conflicting results on whether concurrent irradiation is best given early or late in the chemotherapy program. Although the CALGB study reported by Perry et al.[234] found better results with delayed irradiation, the immediate concurrent arm had markedly attenuated subsequent dose intensity of chemotherapy. Perhaps because the use of cyclophosphamide and etoposide caused marked myelosuppression, investigators were reluctant to push onward with full doses of chemotherapy. Moreover, these results really show that, using 1980s staging and treatment techniques, all treatment arms produced unacceptable survival by today's benchmarks, and therefore it is not at all clear that the intended focus of timing has any relevance to today's treatment. The National Cancer Institute of Canada trial came to the opposite conclusion.[252] This trial used full doses with EP, randomizing the radiotherapy to be concurrent with cycle two or cycle six. The radiotherapy delivered 40 Gy in 3 weeks and added an additional week for recovery in the early treatment. Indirect comparisons from the meta-analysis could not resolve this issue.[236] This study was replicated by the London Lung Cancer Group and no difference in survival was reported.[253] This was felt to be due to the decreased ability to deliver full-dose chemotherapy in the early radiotherapy group. The Japanese Clinical Oncology Group randomized patients to concurrent cycle one EP with sequential therapy after four cycles, with twice-daily radiotherapy delivering 45 Gy in 3 weeks.[254] Unfortunately, the trial was underpowered, but it points toward early concurrent therapy being superior to sequential therapy. This trial verifies that only four cycles of EP and 45 Gy delivered in an accelerated fraction scheme produce credible response, survival, and local control.

There have been multiple meta-analyses of the timing of thoracic irradiation.[253,255–258] One meta-analysis[255] reviewed seven randomized trials with a total of 1,524 patients that addressed timing of radiotherapy relative to chemotherapy. Early radiation therapy was defined as beginning before 9 weeks after the initiation of chemotherapy and before the third cycle of chemotherapy. Late radiation therapy began 9 weeks or more after the initiation of chemotherapy or after the beginning of the third cycle. They reported a small but statistically significant improvement in 2-year survival for patients receiving early radiation therapy. A greater benefit was observed in patients receiving hyperfractionated radiation.

Another meta-analysis[259] evaluated four randomized trials consisting of 1,056 patients to determine whether the time from the start of chemotherapy until the end of radiotherapy (SER) was a predictor of survival. They found that there was a significantly higher 5-year survival rate in the treatment arms with a shorter SER. In addition, a low SER was associated with a higher incidence of severe esophagitis. This suggests that an important factor in the treatment of SCLC involves counteracting accelerated repopulation that occurs after treatment with chemotherapy.

Radiation Therapy Treatment Volumes. An early randomized trial by Southwest Oncology Group showed no difference in recurrence rate whether pre- or postchemotherapy imaging was used to determine radiation therapy treatment fields.[260] Of course, if early radiation therapy is used, then there is no postchemotherapy treatment volume. The Intergroup trial[37] included gross disease, the bilateral mediastinum, and the ipsilateral hilum in the treatment field. The uninvolved supraclavicular area was excluded. RTOG-9712[250] allowed for treatment of the uninvolved supraclavicular area in the setting of apical tumors. A small phase 2 trial suggested that there may be increased elective nodal failure in the supraclavicular area if it is included from the treatment field.[261] Currently, there is no standard treatment technique regarding the use of elective nodal irradiation.[262]

Toxicity of Radiation Therapy. Although minimizing the toxicities of the combined modality approach without compromising therapeutic efficacy is worthy of further research, the addition of chest irradiation has increased myelosuppressive, pulmonary, and esophageal complications of treatment, particularly with concurrent cyclophosphamide-based regimens.[263–265] Esophagitis is a difficult toxicity to compare since trials often use a unique criteria system and even the Common Terminology Criteria for Adverse Events (CTCAE) version 3.0 grades the severity of the esophagitis on the treatment offered (e.g., the use of intravenous hydration). However, most trials with concurrent chemoradiation therapy that used a cisplatin-based regimen report a 10% to 25% rate of severe esophagitis.[266] A retrospective review revealed that various radiation dosimetric parameters, such as mean esophageal dose and volume of esophagus receiving 15 Gy, were associated with a higher incidence of grade 3 or worse esophagitis in patients receiving twice-daily radiation.[267]

Radiation pneumonitis (RP) has not been as well studied in SCLC as it has in NSCLC most likely due to the fact that most trials have used a moderate dose of radiation therapy, below which high rates of radiation pneumonitis are seen. Recent trials report a clinical radiation pneumonitis rate of approximately 10%.[241,268] This is lower than some of the trials reported in the 1980s and 1990s probably due to improved radiation therapy techniques and better determination of pneumonitis as opposed to other etiologies of respiratory distress such as infection or tumor recurrence. The volume of lung receiving 20 Gy (V20) is a standard parameter used to assess the predicted lung toxicity in patients with NSCLC. It has been shown to have value in patients receiving concurrent accelerated hyperfractionated treatment for SCLC as well, with a V20 less than 25% associated with a lower rate of radiation pneumonitis.[269]

Role of Chest Irradiation in Extensive Disease. Retrospective reviews of the literature demonstrate that the addition of chest irradiation plus chemotherapy for patients who have extensive-stage SCLC may reduce the frequency of progressive disease in the thorax, but the overall response rates, median survival, and 2-year disease-free survival figures remain unchanged.[270,271] Because patients with extensive disease generally achieve complete response rates of only 20% to 25% with current chemotherapy regimens and frequently relapse in distant metastatic sites, it is logical that an additional localized form of treatment would have minimal impact on survival. Successive large studies by the Southwest Oncology Group also confirm that, although thoracic radiotherapy can substantially reduce the frequency of initial relapse at the primary tumor site, it has no apparent effect on survival.[108,272]

Several clinical trials have randomized patients with extensive disease to chemotherapy alone or in combination with irradiation to the chest disease as well as to some or all sites of overt distant metastases.[272–275] With one exception,[273] no worthwhile advantages in survival have been seen with the addition of radiotherapy for patients with extensive disease. At present, except as part of a clinical trial, there is no indication for chest irradiation in extensive SCLC other than symptomatic palliation, such as in patients presenting with superior vena cava syndrome.

In the setting of improved survival with the use of prophylactic cranial irradiation (PCI) in the setting of extensive-stage SCLC, a new trial is evaluating the role of chest irradiation after systemic therapy and PCI. These patients will be randomized to either 40 Gy in ten fractions or observation.

Prophylactic Cranial Irradiation. Brain metastases are detected in fewer than 10% of SCLC patients at the time of presentation and are subsequently diagnosed during life in another 20% to 25%, with an increasing likelihood of development seen with lengthening survival.[276,277] In the absence of radiation therapy to the CNS, actuarial analysis reveals a probability of brain metastases ranging from 50% to 80% in terms of those patients who survive 2 years.[276,278] At postmortem examination, they are found in up to 65% of patients.[279] Because these metastases are sometimes the sole site of clinical relapse from complete remission and are frequently clinically disabling, PCI has been recommended by many,[280] but not all,[281] over the past 15 to 20 years to curtail their development. The rationale is essentially an extrapolation from original strategies used in acute lymphocytic leukemia of childhood.

A large number of early prospective randomized trials assessed the benefit of PCI given at or within a few months of diagnosis in patients who were initially free of CNS involvement.[135,282–285] When these trials were considered together, doses of PCI ranging from 20 to 40 Gy reduced the frequency of clinically detectable brain metastases from 24% to 6%. In most of these trials, a significant reduction of intracranial tumor spread was observed. However, no significant impact of PCI on survival was seen in any of those studies. Retrospective analyses suggested that virtually all benefit in preventing intracranial metastases with PCI was confined to patients who achieved a complete remission from their initial treatment.[278] In actuarial analysis, partial responders or nonresponders have similar risks of recurrence in the brain regardless of whether or not PCI was administered. This is not surprising because persistent systemic cancer could readily metastasize to the CNS after completion of PCI.

In a meta-analysis of almost 1,000 patients in seven trials between 1977 and 1995, patients were evaluated with and without PCI after initially obtaining a complete response.[286] The primary end point was overall survival, and the analysis was based on intent to treat. PCI doses ranged from 24 to 40 Gy in most patients, although the meta-analysis did include one series of 25 patients who received only 8 Gy in one fraction. The meta-analysis suggested that a significant gain in survival was seen with PCI in patients who achieved complete remission, with 3-year survival figures increasing from 15% to almost 21%. PCI significantly decreased the probability of brain metastases and increased the likelihood of disease-free survival. Going to higher doses appeared to have no obvious impact on survival, although it seemed to have an increasing effect of eliminating brain metastases. A trend was also seen toward a decreased risk of brain metastases when PCI was administered earlier. The meta-analysis was not able to assess the impact of PCI on cognitive function, because most of the studies did not include neurocognitive assessments, at baseline or beyond 2 years. Two studies that assessed baseline neuropsychological function before treatment demonstrated that many patients appear to have abnormalities of cognitive function as initial manifestations of their cancer, even when brain metastases were not detected and before any treatment.[287,288]

An Intergroup trial evaluated standard-dose versus higher-dose prophylactic cranial irradiation after complete response for limited-stage disease.[289] Seven hundred twenty patients were randomized to either 25 Gy in 10 fractions or 36 Gy delivered in either 18 daily fractions of 2 Gy or 24 twice-daily fractions of 1.5 Gy. There was no significant difference in incidence of brain metastases between the standard-dose group and the high-dose group. The overall survival was significantly worse in the higher-dose group, although this was due to disease progression and not toxicity. The conclusion of this study was that 25 Gy in ten fractions should be the standard dose of prophylactic cranial irradiation for limited-stage patients.

A recent EORTC randomized trial demonstrated a survival benefit with PCI in patients with extensive-stage SCLC who had had a response to chemotherapy.[68] The use of PCI significantly improved the rate of 1-year freedom from symptomatic brain metastases from 14.6% to 40.4% and the 1-year survival from 13.3% to 27.1% in the 286 randomized patients. Various fractionation schemes were used, but the most common ones were 20 Gy in five fractions and 30 Gy in ten fractions.

A major factor that produces considerable controversy about recommending PCI is the significant risk of toxicity associated with it. Because the 5-year survival appears to have improved, it is evident that some patients have neurologic and intellectual impairment as well as abnormalities on CT scan that may be related to PCI.[290,291] In one study, CT scan and CNS abnormalities were significantly more frequent in patients who had received PCI or therapeutic brain irradiation than in those who had not.[292] These findings were especially disturbing because complete responders are at greater risk for possible complications. Many deficits on neuropsychological testing have been unsuspected on casual examination, but a few patients have obvious major impairments. CT scan abnormalities continue to worsen for several years after treatment has ended, although the abnormalities may eventually stabilize.[293] Neurologic abnormalities were most prominent in one series of patients who were given PCI concurrently with high-dose chemotherapy or in individual radiation fractions of 4 Gy.[290] Some authorities suggest that PCI should be administered only in standard fractions of 2 Gy after completion of chemotherapy.[238]

After PCI, the neuropsychological and imaging abnormalities may or may not be due to PCI. Chemotherapy, possible paraneoplastic syndromes, micrometastases, and the effects of chronic cigarette and alcohol abuse are some of the factors that may be important contributors. In one study that evaluated cognitive function in patients before and after chemoradiation but before any PCI, deficits were discovered in verbal memory, frontal lobe function, and motor coordination within both groups of patients.[108] Administration of methotrexate, procarbazine, and lomustine has decreased over the past 15 years; these particular agents have been incriminated in neuropsychological dysfunction.

One of the studies included in the meta-analysis had almost 300 patients who were randomized to receive PCI after having achieved a complete remission to initial treatment.[282] Twenty percent of these patients had extensive-stage disease, virtually all of whom were ultimately expected to relapse and die. The mean time between the initiation of treatment and the randomization was 5 months. The actuarial likelihood of isolated brain metastasis as the first site of treatment failure was 19% in patients given PCI and 45% in those who did not receive PCI. Corresponding figures for total brain metastases were 40% and 67%, respectively; both differences were highly significant. However, in this one study overall survival was not significantly improved. The important observation was that there were no obvious differences in the neuropsychological function between the two groups, but only 33 patients underwent a complete reassessment at 18 months. Inasmuch as neuropsychological abnormalities possibly due to PCI progress over time, these data are insufficient to exclude radiation-associated cognitive damage, but they are nonetheless relevant.

A recent decision analysis suggests that for patients who have had a complete response to initial therapy, PCI offers a better quality-adjusted life expectancy, even if a mild to moderate neurotoxicity rate was assumed.[294]

If PCI is administered at a time when no chemotherapeutic agents are being administered, radiation-induced permeability alterations that allow more chemotherapeutic agent into brain parenchyma should be obviated. The authors' guidelines for PCI, after thorough discussion with the patient of potential risks and benefits, are: (1) PCI is typically recommended 2 weeks after completion of all chemotherapy to complete and partial responders after induction therapy, and (2) radiotherapy fractions of 2 to 3 Gy are given over 2 to 3 weeks to a total dose of 24 to 30 Gy.

Role of Chemotherapy and Radiation Therapy to the Neuraxis. For overt metastatic lesions within the CNS, doses of 3 Gy daily to doses of 30 to 36 Gy typically are used. Overt intracranial metastases appear to be more difficult to sterilize than intrathoracic disease.[295] If there are only one or two clinically documented intracranial lesions, a boost to 50 Gy can be considered if the patient has excellent performance status. Based on experience in other clinical settings, stereotactic treatment can also be used, although unlike some cases of NSCLC, whole-brain irradiation should not be omitted due to the high rate of micrometastatic disease.

Chemotherapy is also a therapeutic option for brain metastases, perhaps because the blood–brain barrier is disrupted in the setting of macroscopic metastatic disease. Small series of patients in whom brain metastases were present at diagnosis have been treated with standard chemotherapy regimens without radiation, and the majority have demonstrated clinical and radiographic improvement.[296] Chemotherapy has also been used at the time of relapse, and response rates of 33% to 43% have been reported.[296–298] In previously treated patients, the response to chemotherapy in the brain appears to be comparable to the response rates in other organs, and it is not dissimilar from the activity of irradiation, which in one series produced a partial response rate of 50%; the median survival was 4.7 months in a series of 22 patients.[299] Thus, although brain irradiation remains the standard for patients who have not been previously irradiated, chemotherapy is a reasonable option for those in whom recurrent disease develops after prior brain radiation, particularly if active systemic disease is also present.

Surgery

Even before the advent of combination chemotherapy for SCLC, the poor outcomes in various case series clearly indicated that surgery is not advisable as a sole treatment modality in this disease. In 1975, Martini et al.[300] reviewed the cases of SCLC treated surgically at Memorial Hospital; the resectability rate was 7% and he identified only two 5-year survivors over a 40-year period.[300] Around the same time, Mountain[301] highlighted the differences in outcomes between patients with resectable SCLC and NSCLC and reported that patients with SCLC who had surgical resection had the same median survival as those who did not have surgery. The British Medical Research Council published a 144-patient trial that demonstrated superiority of radiotherapy as primary treatment for operable SCLC.[302] Even woefully inferior chemotherapy regimens by today's standards can improve survival in patients with resected SCLC.[303]

Reports that address the role of surgery for limited-stage SCLC can be categorized based on the sequence of therapies. Since most patients at diagnosis present with bulky unresectable disease, studies using surgery first followed by chemotherapy primarily include stage I and II patients. In some cases, patients who undergo thoracotomy for an abnormal pulmonary nodule are unexpectedly diagnosed with SCLC.[43] About 4% of solitary pulmonary nodules are diagnosed as SCLC.[20,21] In these cases, a complete surgical resection should be performed and the patient should be referred for adjuvant therapy. Based on current recommendations, patients with N0 disease should then receive adjuvant chemotherapy, while patients with nodal involvement should receive chemotherapy and mediastinal radiation.[40] It is difficult to assess the outcomes for this group of patients since it is an uncommon situation, making prospective studies difficult. Previous reports used a variety of treatment regimens.[43] Furthermore, the long survival times reported in some series for patients with resected stage I SCLC may be due to more favorable tumor biology.

Nodal status and primary tumor (T) status have significant effects on the survival of patients who have undergone resection. Angeletti et al.[304] and Shepherd et al.[305] reported increased survival of node-negative compared to N1 and N2 patients after surgical resection and postoperative chemotherapy, whereas Macchiarini et al.[306] found a decrease in 5-year survival with increasing T category in surgically resected patients without nodal metastases. Retrospective reviews published by Rea et al.[307] and Lucchi et al.[308] have reinforced the importance of surgical staging in evaluating the outcomes for surgery and SCLC. Rea et al. reported that 51 stage I or II SCLC patients resected and given chemotherapy after resection had 5-year survival rates of 52% (stage I) and 30% (stage II). In the review by Lucchi et al., stage I or II resected SCLC patients who underwent postoperative chemotherapy had 5-year survival rates of 47% and 15%, respectively. Stage III patients from this series who underwent surgery followed by adjuvant therapy had a 5-year survival of 14%. The largest experience examining the role of surgery followed by adjuvant therapy in SCLC was a cooperative group trial conducted by the International Society of Chemotherapy Lung Cancer Study Group.[42] Four-year survival rates for completely resected, pathologically staged SCLC patients with N0 (n = 69), N1 (n = 58), and N2 (n = 36) who received postoperative therapy were 60%, 36%, and 33%, respectively. Based on these studies, most authorities believe that surgery may have a role as part of a multimodality approach, but only for patients with stage I disease.[40] Mediastinoscopy should be performed in all patients who are being considered for resection of known SCLC. In a large series from the University of Toronto, surgery followed by chemotherapy had the same outcome as treatment in the reverse order.[305]

Surgical resection has also been studied as a way of reducing the risk of local recurrence in patients with limited disease after completion of chemoradiation. Although most patients with SCLC succumb to metastatic disease, local recurrence occurs in 35% to 50%.[37] Furthermore, tumors may have a mixed histology such that residual NSCLC remains after treatment of the more chemosensitive SCLC component. Of 38 cases resected after chemoradiation in a University of Toronto study, 29 had pure SCLC but 4 were pure NSCLC, 2 had a mixed histology, and 3 had no residual tumor.[309] Several groups have reported the feasibility of this approach, though notably in these prospective studies, only about half of the cases were resectable and pneumonectomies were frequently required.[283–285] One randomized trial attempted to address the question of whether surgical resection of persistent local disease adds any benefit to the usual approach of chemoradiation for limited-stage patients.[310] The Lung Cancer Study Group enrolled 328 patients who were first treated with CAV for five cycles. Fit patients with at least a partial response were then randomized to surgical resection or not. All patients were then intended to receive thoracic and prophylactic cranial irradiation. As with the previously reported studies, only a fraction of the patients were eligible for surgery after induction therapy; only 146 patients were randomized, and this diminished the power of the statistical analysis. Nonetheless, no differences in overall survival or even in local control rates were noted between the two groups. NSCLC or mixed NSCLC/SCLC comprised 11% of the resected specimens. These data suggest that surgical resection of residual disease in limited-stage SCLC does not improve outcomes. The use of surgery for patients with SCLC should be restricted to patients with stage I tumors.

Palliative Care

Survivorship Issues

Although minor advances have transpired over the past three decades, there has been no dramatic change in outcomes for SCLC since the introduction of etoposide plus cisplatin chemotherapy in the late 1970s. Although this therapy significantly changes the natural history of SCLC, and the use of twice-daily concomitant radiotherapy and prophylactic cranial irradiation adds incremental benefit in patients with limited disease, the number of persons cured remains small. Few patients with extensive disease attain long-term survival. Patients are at greatest risk of dying from SCLC during the first 24 months after diagnosis. This risk declines between years 2 and 3 and is further reduced beyond the year 3. In the SEER program database, overall survival at 2, 3, and 5 years was 12%, 7%, and 5%, respectively.[311]

Excessive mortality in long-term survivors is due primarily to the development of second primary tumors, mainly NSCLC, and other illnesses associated with cigarette smoking.[55,312–315] Late relapse can occur in approximately 10% of patients at 5 years.[316] Overall, the relative risk of a second primary tumor in patients who survive beyond 2 years is increased 3.5-fold. The second lung cancer risk is increased 13-fold among those who received chest irradiation.[312] Since most of the second primary tumors are NSCLC or other malignancies of the upper aerodigestive tract, it is likely that field cancerization due to tobacco exposure has occurred.[312,313] The risk of a second primary tumor increases significantly over time and with continued smoking. Treatment with alkylating agents further magnifies this risk.[312] For example, the risk of a second lung cancer in patients who continue to smoke was approximately fourfold more than those who stopped before the diagnosis of SCLC and twofold greater in patients who received chest irradiation compared to nonirradiated patients. The cumulative risk of a second lung cancer was 32% at 12 years and continued to increase beyond that time point. Secondary leukemias have been seen as well.[314,315] Patients successfully treated for SCLC constitute an extraordinarily high-risk group for second malignancies and require close surveillance. The cigarette smoking status of every long survivor of SCLC should be assessed at every visit. Aggressive smoking cessation efforts should be marshaled for any patient who expresses an interest in quitting. In addition, this population should be considered for studies evaluating new surveillance technologies and chemoprevention.

Long-term survivors are also at increased risk for non–cancer-related problems, including complications of treatment (pulmonary fibrosis in patients receiving thoracic irradiation, neurologic impairment both as a consequence of treatment with cranial irradiation and paraneoplastic effects of SCLC, and the acceleration of coronary artery disease following thoracic irradiation) as well as tobacco-related illnesses like heart disease, stroke, and chronic obstructive pulmonary disease. In a French study of patients surviving beyond 30 months, treatment-related sequelae included neurologic impairment in 13% of the patients, pulmonary fibrosis in 18%, and cardiac disorders in 10%.[317] Return to work was possible in 40% of these patients and was not influenced by the presence of late treatment-related complications. In a Danish analysis of patients surviving 5 years or more, there was a sixfold increased risk of death from noncancer causes, particularly cardiovascular and pulmonary diseases.[318] Physicians who care for survivors of SCLC should aggressively implement all strategies to reduce cardiovascular disease. These patients should be considered high risk and managed like any other high-risk individual.

TYPICAL CARCINOID AND ATYPICAL CARCINOID TUMORS

Incidence and Etiology

Although over 60% of carcinoid tumors originate in the gastrointestinal system, about 25% of all carcinoids have a pulmonary origin, representing the second most common involved site.[319] Pulmonary carcinoids comprise about 2% of all primary lung tumors.[320] Over the past 30 years, the age-adjusted incidence rate in pulmonary carcinoids has significantly increased, which may represent the improvement in classification of these tumors, as well as the rise of imaging techniques.[319] There is a higher incidence of pulmonary carcinoids in women compared to men and whites compared to blacks.[321,322]

Atypical carcinoids, which have a higher likelihood of metastatic spread or relapse after surgery, are distinguished from the typical carcinoids, which have a more favorable prognosis. Ten percent to 30% of pulmonary carcinoids are atypical.[323–325] Patients with typical carcinoids are approximately 10 years younger than those with atypical carcinoids, which occur in the sixth decade of life.[322,326] Carcinoids are not clearly caused by smoking like SCLC and LCNEC, though some series suggest that a higher percentage of patients with atypical carcinoid smoke as compared to patients with typical carcinoid tumors.[322,323,327]

Pulmonary carcinoids occur rarely in association with multiple endocrine neoplasia type 1 (MEN-1) syndrome. Some sporadic pulmonary carcinoid tumors demonstrate inactivation of the *MEN-1* gene located on chromosome 11q13.[328]

Anatomy and Pathology

All carcinoids are malignant. Typical carcinoids are low grade and atypical carcinoids are intermediate grade. Although carcinoid tumors can be diagnosed by small biopsies or cytology, it is difficult to separate typical from atypical carcinoid. This distinction usually requires a surgical biopsy or resection specimen. The histologic appearance of typical and atypical carcinoids is similar with a uniform population of tumor cells arranged in organoid nests with a moderate amount of cytoplasm with an eosinophilic hue (Figs. 76.5 and 76.7). The finely granular nuclear chromatin frequently has a salt-and-pepper appearance. There are a wide variety of histologic patterns in these tumors, including spindle cell, oncocytic, glandular, follicular, clear cell, and melanocytic. Stromal ossification can occur as well. Atypical carcinoids show increased mitoses (Fig. 76.7) with 2 to 10 mitoses per 2 mm^2 or necrosis that is typically punctuate.[329] Mitotic activity is the most important way to distinguish typical from atypical carcinoid. The most useful immunohistochemical neuroendocrine markers are chromogranin, synaptophysin, and CD56.

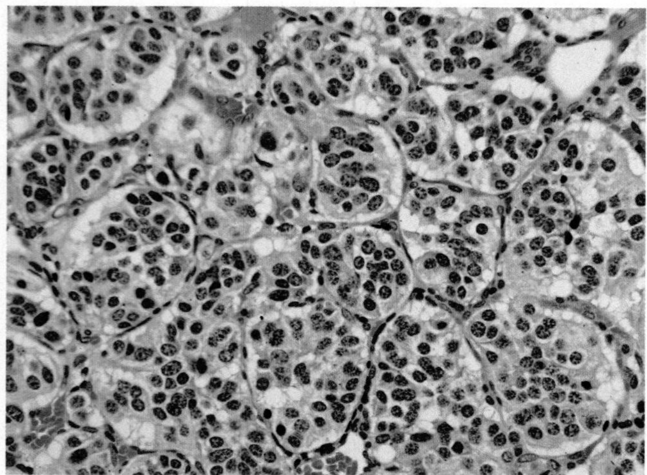

FIGURE 76.5 Typical carcinoid. The tumor shows an organoid nesting pattern of uniform cells with a moderate amount of eosinophilic cytoplasm and finely granular nuclear chromatin.

A mitotic count of 11 or more mitoses per 2 mm^2 (10 high power fields) is the main criterion for separating atypical carcinoids from LCNEC and SCLC.[329,330] LCNEC and SCLC usually have very high mitotic rates, with an average of 70 to 80 per 2 mm^2 (10 high power fields in some microscope models). LCNEC and SCLC also generally have more extensive necrosis than atypical carcinoids. In small specimens where mitotic figures are difficult to demonstrate, it may be helpful to use Ki-67 staining because most typical carcinoids show less than 5% staining, atypical carcinoids are usually 10% to 30%, and most LCNEC or SCLC have a proliferation index of 80% to 100%.[331]

Tumorlets are separated from carcinoid tumors by size. Nodular neuroendocrine proliferations 0.5 cm or larger are called *carcinoid tumors*. Smaller proliferations are called *tumorlets*. The morphology of the cells of tumorlets is identical to that seen in carcinoid tumors. Tumorlets are usually incidental histologic findings of no clinical significance, although they can be seen in interstitial or airway inflammatory and fibrosing conditions. A very rare condition called *diffuse idiopathic pulmonary neuroendocrine cell hyperplasia* is regarded as a preinvasive condition for pulmonary carcinoids. These patients have widespread neuroendocrine cell hyperplasia and tumorlets in their airways and can develop multiple carcinoid tumors.[332]

Screening

Screening for pulmonary carcinoids is not useful. They represent a very small percentage of all lung malignancies and have an indolent natural history. In one study, atypical carcinoid was diagnosed in only 2 of 31,567 (0.006%) asymptomatic patients undergoing baseline lung cancer screening CT scans.[16]

Diagnosis

Two-thirds of carcinoids develop in the major bronchi. As a result, the most common presenting symptoms include obstructive pneumonia, pleuritic pain, atelectasis, dyspnea, and cough.[323,333] Hemoptysis may occur in 10% to 20%. Up to 30% of patients with pulmonary carcinoid tumors are asymptomatic at presentation. In contrast to carcinoids of gastrointestinal origin, carcinoid syndrome (facial flushing, diarrhea, wheezing) is rare in pulmonary carcinoids, occurring in only about 2% of cases.[323,333] Cushing syndrome due to ectopic corticotropin production has been reported in approximately 2% of pulmonary carcinoids.[334] A rare manifestation of pulmonary carcinoids is acromegaly due to ectopic production of growth hormone–releasing hormone (GHRH); yet these tumors are the most common cause of extrapituitary secretion of GHRH.[335]

Initial workup proceeds in a similar fashion as with other lung tumors, but once a diagnosis of carcinoid is confirmed, more specific radiologic and serologic evaluations for these neuroendocrine tumors may be employed. Biopsy of central tumors can be easily obtained by bronchoscopy. Biopsy of peripheral lesions by fine needle can be performed, but a definitive diagnosis may be difficult to ascertain in small cytology samples. In addition to routine chest imaging with CT scans, nuclear medicine studies are helpful adjuncts for staging (Fig. 76.7). Due to the overexpression of somatostatin receptors, immunoscintigraphy by somatostatin analogues such as octreotide is widely used. In one series, the sensitivity and specificity was 90% and 83%, respectively.[336] In patients with somatostatin receptor–positive pulmonary carcinoids, octreotide scans have been found to be useful for follow-up and detection of recurrent disease, as well as for guiding treatment options.[337] Fluorine 18-fluorodeoxyglucose (FDG) PET scanning may be less accurate since these indolent tumors generally have a low standard

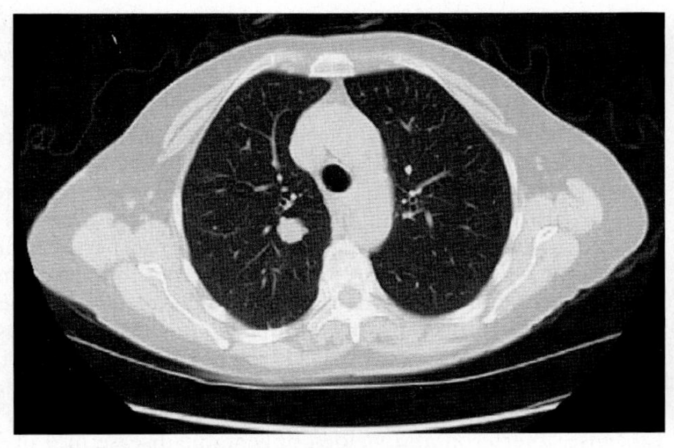

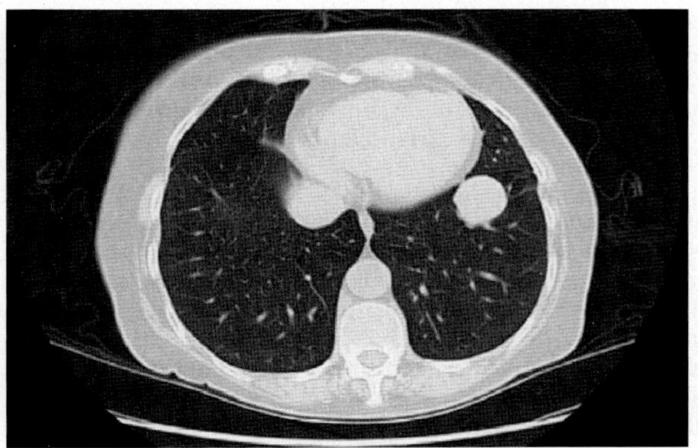

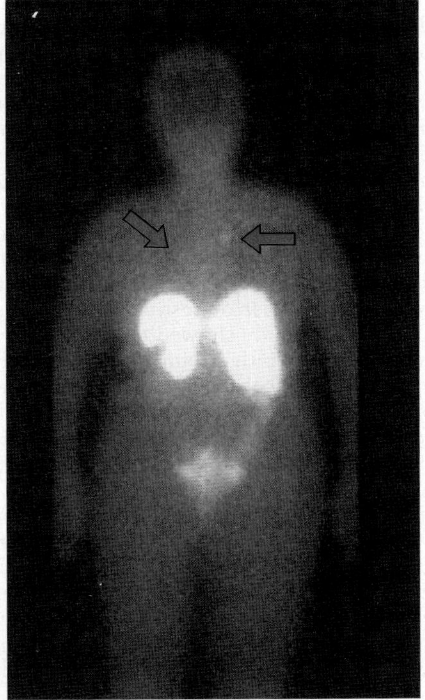

FIGURE 76.6 Computed tomography scan of a patient with bilateral typical carcinoid. These masses are well defined and spherical, as often seen with these tumors. They are also seen faintly on an ^{111}In Octreotide scan (*arrows*, posterior view).

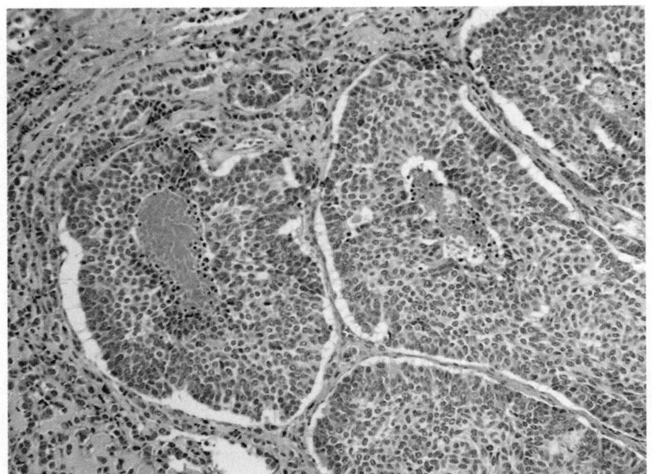

FIGURE 76.7 Atypical carcinoid. The tumor shows a punctate focus of necrosis within sheets and nests of carcinoid tumor cells. Mitoses are few.

uptake value (SUV),[338] but some still advocate its potential use.[339] Recent series have shown that FDG-PET is useful for the assessment of intermediate- and high-grade neuroendocrine tumors and may have prognostic value.[340,341] Elevated chromogranin A levels have been measured in serum or plasma, although they have been found to be lower in pulmonary carcinoids compared to gastroenteropancreatic endocrine tumors.[342,343] In the setting of advanced or metastatic disease, chromogranin A levels can be useful to follow disease activity.[343] Urinary 5-hydroxyindoleacetic acid (5-HIAA) may be elevated in patients with carcinoid syndrome.

Staging

Pulmonary carcinoid tumors are staged according to the TNM classification used for NSCLC in the AJCC seventh edition. The International Association for the Study of Lung Cancer (IASLC) proposed and approved this in 2009 when it was determined that the TNM staging system was helpful in predicting prognosis for pulmonary carcinoids.[344] Applying this staging system to cases in the National Cancer Institute SEER registry and cases submitted to the IASLC database, it was determined that 5-year overall survival for patients with stage I was 93%, stage II was 74% to 85%, stage III was 67% to 75%, and stage IV was 57%.[344] Survival is significantly better for typical carcinoid than for atypical carcinoid. Five-year and 10-year survival rates have been reported at 87% and 87%, respectively, for typical carcinoid, while they were 56% and 35%, respectively, for atypical carcinoid.[329] Predictors of survival include stage, tumor size, higher mitotic rates (i.e., atypical subtype), and age greater than 60.[327,344,322] Importantly, patients with multiple nodules have a very favorable prognosis, likely reflected by the fact that these individuals tend to have the underlying preinvasive lesion, diffuse idiopathic pulmonary neuroendocrine cell hyperplasia.[344]

Several series have shown that the majority of patients with typical carcinoid present with stage I disease (up to 90%), whereas those with atypical carcinoid present with more advanced disease.[323,325,345]

Management by Stage

Stages I, II, and III

Surgery is the primary treatment modality and the only curative option for patients with pulmonary carcinoids. Because carcinoids often present centrally, pneumonectomy or bilobectomy is frequent, but most patients undergo a lobectomy.[320,327] For patients with favorable prognostic features, such as typical histology and absence of lymph node involvement, a more limited resection has been proposed.[333] Patients with atypical carcinoids should be resected using the same principles guiding surgery for NSCLC.[346]

Mediastinal lymph node metastases occur in patients with pulmonary carcinoids. Therefore, a complete mediastinal lymph node dissection at the time of surgery is advocated, with surgical resection of nodal metastases when feasible.[326,345,347–351] Multiple series have found decreased incidence of local recurrence[347,349] and improved survival when complete mediastinal lymph node dissection is performed.[325,345]

Adjuvant chemotherapy after surgical resection for patients with typical carcinoid with or without regional lymph node metastases (stages I, II, and III) is not recommended,[352] as the risk of recurrence has been shown to be low.[326] Similarly, following surgical resection, patients with stage I atypical carcinoid are followed expectantly. However, as systemic recurrence occurs more frequently in patients with atypical carcinoid with N1 or N2 involvement (stages II and III), adjuvant chemotherapy after surgical resection has been advocated by some,[352] but it is unknown whether this is beneficial. There is no defined adjuvant regimen for atypical carcinoid, yet due to similarities with SCLC, etoposide and platinum (cisplatin or carboplatin) combinations are used generally.[352]

The use of radiation therapy for carcinoid tumors is most similar to its pattern of use in NSCLC. For tumors that are resectable, adjuvant radiation therapy is typically recommended in situations of residual disease (R1 resection) and mediastinal lymphadenopathy (N2 disease). The use of adjuvant radiation therapy for nodal disease is probably of greater utility in the more aggressive atypical carcinoid.[352] In patients with unresectable disease, radiation therapy can be used after induction chemotherapy or concurrently.[353] Doses of 60 Gy are typical. Carcinoid tumors are less responsive to radiation therapy than SCLC.[354]

Stage IV

Data regarding the efficacy of chemotherapy specifically in pulmonary carcinoid (as opposed to gastrointestinal carcinoids) are lacking, as this tumor type has not been studied independently of other neuroendocrine tumors and occasionally has been omitted from such trials. Further, many of the studies used older classification systems for carcinoids and different criteria for response. Various chemotherapeutic agents have been used, including doxorubicin, 5-fluorouracil, dacarbazine, cisplatin, carboplatin, etoposide, and streptozocin.

Patients with gastrointestinal carcinoids often are treated with streptozotocin combinations, although the data for this in pulmonary carcinoids are sparse. In an older prospective study that included all types of carcinoid tumors, 2 of the 17 patients (12%) with pulmonary carcinoid responded to streptozotocin plus either 5-fluororuracil or cyclophosphamide.[355] In a subsequent retrospective series, seven patients treated with streptozotocin plus 5-fluorouracil had progression and two treated with streptozotocin plus doxorubicin had stable disease.[342] Likewise, interferon-alfa yielded only stable disease in 4 of 27 patients.[342] Many of these patients were also given octreotide, and while it helped patients symptomatically and induced some biochemical responses, it did not shrink tumors. An Italian group reported on seven patients with atypical carcinoid metastatic to the liver with carcinoid syndrome that were treated with octreotide. The patients had improvement in their symptoms and prolonged survival; three patients were noted to have a reduction in tumor burden.[356] In a more recent retrospective series, somatostatin analogues were given to six patients as first-line therapy for either antitumor effect or symptom control, with a median time to progression of 10.5 months (range, 3 months to 24 months).[357] These results are similar to the experience with octreotide in gastrointestinal carcinoids.[358] Notably, the recent PROMID study showed that long acting–release octreotide acetate significantly prolonged time to tumor progression compared with placebo in patients with newly diagnosed functionally active or inactive well-differentiated midgut neuroendocrine tumors (14.3 months vs. 6 months, HR 0.34; 95% confidence interval [CI], 0.20 to 0.59; $P = .000072$). However, there was no improvement in overall survival.[359]

Regimens typically used for SCLC often are recommended.[352,360] However, typical carcinoid and atypical carcinoid are clearly less chemosensitive than SCLC. In two small series that included 26 patients in total treated with chemotherapy (mostly etoposide and cisplatin), the response rate was about 20%.[342,353] Cisplatin and etoposide were administered to 18 patients with foregut-origin carcinoids (lung and thymus) who had progressed after first- or second-line treatment in a prospective study. Radiographic response was noted in 2 of the 5 patients with atypical carcinoid (40%) and in 5 of the 13 with typical carcinoid (39%). The median response duration was 9 months (range, 6 months to 30 months).[361]

Newer agents are being studied actively in neuroendocrine carcinoma. Temozolomide, a nonclassical oral alkylating agent, has been evaluated either alone or in combination with other agents such as thalidomide and bevacizumab. Thirteen patients with pulmonary carcinoids (10 typical, 3 atypical) were included in a retrospective study using single-agent temozolomide. Four of these patients (31%) had a partial response to treatment (3 typical, 1 atypical), and 62% derived clinical benefit (response or stable disease) with temozolomide.[362] However, in two prospective trials that included patients with carcinoid tumors, a 7% response rate was noted using temozolomide with thalidomide and no response was observed using temozolomide and bevacizumab.[363,364] Four patients with pulmonary carcinoid were included in a phase 2 clinical trial evaluating everolimus, an mTOR inhibitor, and long acting–release octreotide acetate, in which the response rate was 20%.[365] In a phase 2 study in low- to intermediate-grade neuroendocrine tumors, patients were randomized to receive either bevacizumab or pegylated interferon-alfa-2b. Again, only four patients with pulmonary carcinoids were included in this trial, where an 18% partial response rate was observed in the bevacizumab group compared with no responses in the pegylated interferon-alfa-2b arm.[366] Fourteen patients with foregut carcinoids of the lung and stomach were included in a phase 2 study using sunitinib, a multitargeted oral tyrosine kinase inhibitor. The overall response rate for patients with carcinoid tumors was only 2.4% with a median time tumor progression of 10.2 months.[367]

In the approach to metastatic carcinoid tumors, many advocate using somatostatin analogues as first-line treatment in patients with well-differentiated tumors with little tumor bulk in the setting of a positive octreotide scan[337,356] and chemotherapy for those with more rapidly progressing tumors or those who have progressed on less toxic treatments.[368,369] Additional studies are needed for both traditional cytotoxic and molecularly targeted agents in this disease. Palliative radiation therapy can be used for symptomatic lesions.[354]

LARGE CELL NEUROENDOCRINE CARCINOMA

Incidence and Etiology

LCNEC of the lung was first described in 1991 as a form of high-grade non–small cell neuroendocrine carcinoma.[370] LCNEC accounts for about 3% of surgically resected lung cancers.[371] In previously reported series, LCNEC patients have a median age of 62 years (range, 33years to 87 years) and the vast majority of patients are male cigarette smokers.[322,371]

Anatomy and Pathology

In the 2004 World Health Organization (WHO) classification, LCNEC is classified as a variant of large cell carcinoma.[6,371,372] There are four ways neuroendocrine differentiation can be manifest within large cell carcinomas: (1) if both neuroendocrine morphology by light microscopy as well as neuroendocrine differentiation by immunohistochemistry or electron microscopy are seen, the tumor is classified as LCNEC, (2) if there is no neuroendocrine morphology by light microscopy and neuroendocrine differentiation is seen by immunohistochemistry or electron microscopy, the tumor is classified as large cell carcinomas with neuroendocrine differentiation (LCC-NED), (3) if the tumor lacks both neuroendocrine morphology by light microscopy and neuroendocrine differentiation by immunohistochemistry or electron microscopy, it is classified as a classic large cell carcinoma, and (4) large cell carcinoma with neuroendocrine morphology (LCNEM) that have neuroendocrine morphology but lack neuroendocrine differentiation by electron microscopy or immunohistochemistry.[6,371,372] Little is known about the latter category.

LCNEC are diagnosed based on the following criteria (Fig. 76.8): (1) neuroendocrine morphology with organoid nesting, palisading, or rosettelike structures, (2) high mitotic rate greater than 10 mitoses per 2 mm^2 (average 60 to 80 mitoses per 2 mm^2), (3) non–small cell cytologic features, including large cell size, low nuclear or cytoplasmic ratio, nucleoli, or vesicular chromatin, and (4) neuroendocrine differentiation by immunohistochemistry (chromogranin, CD56, or synaptophysin) or electron microscopy.[6,329]

When LCNEC has components of adenocarcinoma, squamous cell carcinoma, giant cell carcinoma, or spindle cell carcinoma, it is called combined LCNEC and the specific components present should be mentioned.[6,329] Adenocarcinoma is the histologic type found most often in combined large cell carcinomas. When SCLC is combined with LCNEC, the tumor becomes a combined SCLC and LCNEC and should be regarded as a SCLC.

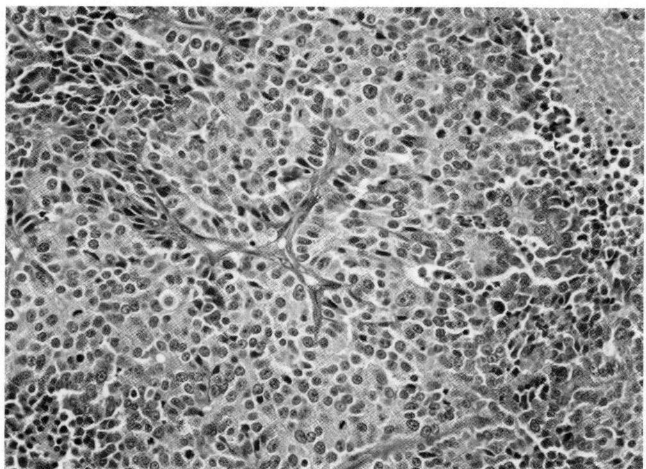

FIGURE 76.8 Large cell neuroendocrine carcinoma. The tumor grows in organoid nests with peripheral palisading and rosettelike structures. The tumor cells have abundant cytoplasm, prominent nucleoli, and frequent mitoses.

LCNEC will be positive for pancytokeratin and at least one neuroendocrine marker such as chromogranin, CD56, or synaptophysin. TTF-1 will be positive in 60% to 80% of cases. There is a very high proliferation index with 80% to 100% positive tumor cells.[13,371] When the differential diagnosis of basaloid carcinoma is a consideration, diffuse strong staining for p63 or 34βE12 would favor this diagnosis over LCNEC.[10]

It is difficult to make the diagnosis of LCNEC on small biopsies or cytology since the characteristic neuroendocrine morphologic pattern and neuroendocrine differentiation by immunohistochemistry are difficult to demonstrate in minute pieces of tissue.[13,371] Therefore, in the vast majority of cases a definite diagnosis of LCNEC will require a surgical biopsy. Separation of LCNEC from SCLC requires consideration of multiple histologic features such as cell size, nucleoli, chromatin pattern, and nuclear to cytoplasmic ratio, rather than a single criterion. Artifacts, such as those introduced by frozen sections, can distort cellular morphology, resulting in confusion with SCLC.[13,371]

Screening

Clinically, LCNEC is characterized by similar behavior to SCLC, with rapid tumor growth and early metastatic spread.[322] Further, LCNEC represents a small percentage of all lung malignancies. In one study, LCNEC was diagnosed in only 15 of 31,567 (0.05%) asymptomatic patients undergoing baseline lung cancer screening CT scans.[16] Therefore, screening for LCNEC is not useful.

Diagnosis

In patients with LCNEC, presenting symptoms mimic those of SCLC and other NSCLC. For example, in one series of 83 patients, the main symptoms were hemoptysis (30%), chest pain (22%), dyspnea (16%), cough (16%), and weight loss (13%); only 4% of patients were asymptomatic.[373] Ectopic hormone production and paraneoplastic syndromes are typically absent.[322]

LCNEC generally present as peripheral tumors. When centrally located, endobronchial growth and obstructive pneumonia can be found.[374] On CT scan these tumors are often well defined and lobulated, without air bronchograms or calcifications; spiculated margins are less commonly observed.[374,375] Inhomogenous enhancement is found in larger diameter (33 mm or larger) tumors secondary to necrosis.[374] LCNEC typically have homogenously high FDG uptake on PET scans, which is helpful in locating extrathoracic metastases.[375] These tumors also contain somatostatin receptors and can be Ocreoscan (Covidien, Mansfield, Massachusetts) positive, yet this imaging modality is not used frequently for the evaluation of this malignancy.

Although a biopsy specimen can be obtained via bronchoscopy or CT guidance, a definitive diagnosis may be difficult to determine in small specimens or by cytology, as indicated above.[13,371] Therefore, a surgical biopsy is often needed in LCNEC.

Staging

The TNM classification used for NSCLC in the AJCC seventh edition is used for the staging of LCNEC.

Survival for LCNEC is poor and appears to be significantly worse than that of nonneuroendocrine NSCLC.[376] In a series of 335 pathologic stage IA NSCLC comprising 259 adenocarcinomas, 65 squamous cell carcinomas, and 11 large cell neuroendocrine carcinomas, LCNEC histology was found to have a significant adverse prognostic impact and was predictive of poorer overall survival.[376] Asamura et al.[322] found that the survival curve of LCNEC can be superimposed on that for SCLC, with no difference in survival stage for stage between the two, confirming the findings of multiple other series. Reported overall 5-year survival after surgical resection of LCNEC ranges between 15% and 57%,[371] indicating that the recurrence rate after surgery is high. Data from different series reveal that the 5-year survival rate ranges between 33% to 62% in stage I patients, 18% to 75% in stage II patients, and 8% to 45% in stage III patients; and 0% in stage IV patients.[322,373,376,378,379] Factors significantly related to survival among clinicopathologic parameters are tumor stage and size (less than 3 cm vs. 3 cm or greater).[373]

Management by Stage

Patients with LCNEC are managed as if they have NSCLC with the same treatment algorithm stage for stage. The controversy in LCNEC centers on the choice of chemotherapy. Based on the neuroendocrine features, should LCNEC be treated with the same chemotherapy regimens used for SCLC? Certainly the aggressive natural history and propensity to metastasize are similar to SCLC, yet LCNEC clearly does not demonstrate the same chemosensitivity. Published reports about LCNEC are not instructive since essentially all are retrospective series with a focus on patients who underwent surgery. Details regarding chemotherapy treatment, such as the agents used or the response rates, are generally not provided. Only small series include these specifics.

Stages I, II, and III

For patients with early stage LCNEC, resection is recommended. The modalities of choice are either lobectomy or pneumonectomy, with systematic nodal dissection.[380] After careful mediastinal lymph node sampling, patient without lymph node metastases seem to experience improved survival.[380]

Given the aggressive nature of LCNEC, surgery alone is not sufficient for its treatment. Several studies have attempted to discern the role of adjuvant chemotherapy in LCNEC; yet the majority of these are retrospective and include small numbers of patients. A Japanese group compiled data on 16 patients who received postoperative chemotherapy and 57 who did not.[379] For most patients, the chemotherapy regimens administered included combinations typically used for SCLC, such as cisplatin or carboplatin with etoposide, or cyclophosphamide, doxorubicin, and vincristine. For all patients, the 5-year survival was 62% for stage I, 18% for stage II, and 17% for stage III. The authors note that the 5-year survival for the five patients with stage I disease who received adjuvant chemotherapy was 100%, while it was 51% for the 23 patients who did not. Postoperative chemotherapy did not affect survival for other stages.[379] In a retrospective analysis of 144 surgical cases, Veronesi et al.[378] showed a trend toward improved survival in stage I patients who received neoadjuvant or adjuvant chemotherapy. Preoperative and postoperative chemotherapy was given to 21 and 24 patients, respectively, with half receiving standard SCLC regimens and the other half receiving regimens recommended for NSCLC. A statistically significant survival benefit was found for patients with LCNEC who received perioperative chemotherapy compared to surgery alone across all stages ($P = .04$). In a retrospective review of 45 surgically resected patients with LCNEC, 23 received perioperative chemotherapy, 91% of which was cisplatin based. Further, surgery with or without chemotherapy demonstrated an independent prognostic influence on survival in multivariate analysis; patients who did not receive chemotherapy after surgery were more likely to die than patients who underwent surgery plus chemotherapy (HR 9.472; 95% CI, 1.050 to 85.478; $P = .0457$).[381]

Importantly, several studies support the use of SCLC-based regimens in the adjuvant treatment of LCNEC. Iyoda et al.[382] performed a prospective analysis on 15 LCNEC patients who received adjuvant chemotherapy with cisplatin and etoposide and compared outcomes to a historic cohort of LCNEC patients treated without platinum-based adjuvant therapy. Prolonged survival was noted for the patients that received at least two cycles of SCLC-based regimens; the 5-year overall survival rates were 88.9% and 47.4% in the adjuvant chemotherapy group and in the control group, respectively. Further, those receiving platinum-based adjuvant chemotherapy were noted to have a significantly lower rate of tumor recurrence when compared to patients receiving nonplatinum-based adjuvant chemotherapy or no adjuvant chemotherapy.[383] Finally, in an Italian retrospective series of 83 LCNEC cases, the 13 patients who received SCLC-based regimens had significantly better survival than the 15 patients who received drug combinations used in NSCLC (median survival, 42 months vs. 11 months, respectively; $P < .0001$). The best prognosis was noted in stage I LCNEC patients who received SCLC-based adjuvant chemotherapy. In univariate and multivariate analyses, the administration of adjuvant chemotherapy with cisplatin or carboplatin plus etoposide was the most important variable correlating with survival.[373]

Interpretation of these reports is limited by their retrospective nature and the small sample size. However, these data, along with the known poor natural history and the routine use of adjuvant chemotherapy for SCLC and NSCLC, suggest that postoperative treatment with etoposide and cisplatin is appropriate in patients with completely resected LCNEC, including patients with stage I disease.

Data regarding use of radiation therapy in this disease are sparse, but its role in the adjuvant setting is likely similar to that in NSCLC. As per the National Cooperative Cancer Network guidelines, definitive radiation therapy is recommended for patients who are unable to undergo surgical resection.[384]

Adjuvant treatment with octreotide for patients with LCNEC was evaluated by Filosso et al.[385] Retrospectively, 18 patients were identified who had surgery for LCNEC. Ten patients had positive octreotide scans preoperatively and were given octreotide as adjuvant therapy. No patient received adjuvant chemotherapy, but patients with greater than stage

IB disease received radiation. At the time of their report, 90% of patients were alive and free of disease.

Stage IV

The optimal chemotherapeutic regimen in relapsed or stage IV disease is not defined. For example, in the study by Mazieres et al.,[386] 13 patients with relapsed disease received chemotherapy with etoposide plus cisplatin or carboplatin. Partial responses were noted in only two of the ten evaluable patients. Kozuki et al.[387] described five patients with stage IV disease treated with chemotherapy. Three of these patients received platinum-based regimens, without any objective response. Subsequent regimens, including paclitaxel, docetaxel, irinotecan, gemcitabine, vinorelbine, or amrubicin, were equally ineffective. Five patients were treated with gefitinib, an epidermal growth factor tyrosine kinase inhibitor, and one (a male with a 114-pack per year smoking history) achieved a partial response.

In contrast, several studies have shown that the response rate of LCNEC to cisplatin-based chemotherapy is comparable to SCLC. A retrospective series of 20 patients with advanced LCNEC (stage IIIA, 3; stage IIIB, 6; stage IV, 6; postoperative recurrence, 5) treated with platinum-based therapy showed a response rate of 50% (complete response, 1; partial response, 9).[388] Interestingly, the response rate for chemotherapy-naive patients (64%) was better than those patients that were previously treated (17%).[388] Rossi et al.[373] showed that in metastatic disease, the 12 patients who received SCLC-based chemotherapy (3 also received radiation therapy) had a significantly better survival than the 15 patients who received common NSCLC regimens (gemcitabine and carboplatin, 10; carboplatin and paclitaxel, 3; gemcitabine, 2; 6 also received radiation therapy); median survival was 51 months versus 21 months, respectively ($P < .001$). Only the patients who received SCLC-based chemotherapy had a complete ($n = 2$) or partial ($n = 4$) response.

As can be seen from the above, information regarding the treatment of LCNEC has been derived from small retrospective studies for the most part. Larger, randomized prospective studies are needed to determine the optimal treatment regimen for this disease.

PRACTICE OF ONCOLOGY

Selected References

The full list of references for this chapter appears in the online version.

1. Govindan R, Page N, Morgensztern D, et al. Changing epidemiology of small-cell lung cancer in the United States over the last 30 years: analysis of the surveillance, epidemiologic, and end results database. *J Clin Oncol* 2006;24:4539.
6. Travis WD, Brambilla E, Muller-Hermelink HK, et al. *Pathology and genetics: tumours of the lung, pleura, thymus and heart.* Lyon: IARC, 2004.
7. Nicholson SA, Beasley MB, Brambilla E, et al. Small cell lung carcinoma (SCLC): a clinicopathologic study of 100 cases with surgical specimens. *Am J Surg Pathol* 2002;26:1184.
17. Chute CG, Greenberg ER, Baron J, et al. Presenting conditions of 1539 population-based lung cancer patients by cell type and stage in New Hampshire and Vermont. *Cancer* 1985;56:2107.
26. Darnell RB, Posner JB. Paraneoplastic syndromes involving the nervous system. *N Engl J Med* 2003;349:1543.
31. Zelen M. Keynote address on biostatistics and data retrieval. *Cancer Chemother Rep* [3] 1973;4:31.
33. Albain KS, Crowley JJ, LeBlanc M, et al. Determinants of improved outcome in small-cell lung cancer: an analysis of the 2,580-patient Southwest Oncology Group data base. *J Clin Oncol* 1990;8:1563.
37. Turrisi AT 3rd, Kim K, Blum R, et al. Twice-daily compared with once-daily thoracic radiotherapy in limited small-cell lung cancer treated concurrently with cisplatin and etoposide. *N Engl J Med* 1999;340:265.
38. Doll DC. Serum lactate dehydrogenase and bone marrow involvement in small-cell carcinoma of the lung. *N Engl J Med* 1985;312:1262.
39. Van den Brande P, Demedts M. Serum lactate dehydrogenase in small-cell lung cancer. *N Engl J Med* 1989;320:61.
40. Johnson BE, Crawford J, Downey RJ, et al. Small cell lung cancer clinical practice guidelines in oncology. *J Natl Compr Canc Netw* 2006;4:602.
41. Vallieres E, Shepherd FA, Crowley J, et al. The IASLC Lung Cancer Staging Project: proposals regarding the relevance of TNM in the pathologic staging of small cell lung cancer in the forthcoming (seventh) edition of the TNM classification for lung cancer. *J Thorac Oncol* 2009;4:1049.
42. Karrer K, Ulsperger E. Surgery for cure followed by chemotherapy in small cell carcinoma of the lung. For the ISC-Lung Cancer Study Group. *Acta Oncol* 1995;34:899.
47. Yuen AR, Zou G, Turrisi AT, et al. Similar outcome of elderly patients in intergroup trial 0096: cisplatin, etoposide, and thoracic radiotherapy administered once or twice daily in limited stage small cell lung carcinoma. *Cancer* 2000;89:1953.
55. Lassen U, Osterlind K, Hansen M, et al. Long-term survival in small-cell lung cancer: posttreatment characteristics in patients surviving 5 to 18+ years—an analysis of 1,714 consecutive patients. *J Clin Oncol* 1995;13:1215.
58. Quoix E, Purohit A, Faller-Beau M, et al. Comparative prognostic value of lactate dehydrogenase and neuron-specific enolase in small-cell lung cancer patients treated with platinum-based chemotherapy. *Lung Cancer* 2000;30:127.
63. Sculier JP, Feld R, Evans WK, et al. Carcinoembryonic antigen: a useful prognostic marker in small-cell lung cancer. *J Clin Oncol* 1985;3:1349.
64. Bradley JD, Dehdashti F, Mintun MA, et al. Positron emission tomography in limited-stage small-cell lung cancer: a prospective study. *J Clin Oncol* 2004;22:3248.
67. Cheran SK, Herndon JE 2nd, Patz EF Jr. Comparison of whole-body FDG-PET to bone scan for detection of bone metastases in patients with a new diagnosis of lung cancer. *Lung Cancer* 2004;44:317.
68. Slotman B, Faivre-Finn C, Kramer G, et al. Prophylactic cranial irradiation in extensive small-cell lung cancer. *N Engl J Med* 2007;357:664.
79. Jett JR, Everson L, Therneau TM, et al. Treatment of limited-stage small-cell lung cancer with cyclophosphamide, doxorubicin, and vincristine with or without etoposide: a randomized trial of the North Central Cancer Treatment Group. *J Clin Oncol* 1990;8:33.
86. Fukuoka M, Furuse K, Saijo N, et al. Randomized trial of cyclophosphamide, doxorubicin, and vincristine versus cisplatin and etoposide versus alternation of these regimens in small-cell lung cancer. *J Natl Cancer Inst* 1991;83:855.
87. Roth BJ, Johnson DH, Einhorn LH, et al. Randomized study of cyclophosphamide, doxorubicin, and vincristine versus etoposide and cisplatin versus alternation of these two regimens in extensive small-cell lung cancer: a phase III trial of the Southeastern Cancer Study Group. *J Clin Oncol* 1992;10:282.
88. Sundstrom S, Bremnes RM, Kaasa S, et al. Cisplatin and etoposide regimen is superior to cyclophosphamide, epirubicin, and vincristine regimen in small-cell lung cancer: results from a randomized phase III trial with 5 years' follow-up. *J Clin Oncol* 2002;20:4665.
89. Chute JP, Venzon DJ, Hankins L, et al. Outcome of patients with small-cell lung cancer during 20 years of clinical research at the US National Cancer Institute. *Mayo Clin Proc* 1997;72:901.
93. Skarlos DV, Samantas E, Kosmidis P, et al. Randomized comparison of etoposide-cisplatin vs. etoposide-carboplatin and irradiation in small-cell lung cancer. A Hellenic Co-operative Oncology Group study. *Ann Oncol* 1994;5:601.
97. Noda K, Nishiwaki Y, Kawahara M, et al. Irinotecan plus cisplatin compared with etoposide plus cisplatin for extensive small-cell lung cancer. *N Engl J Med* 2002;346:85.
98. Hanna N, Bunn PA Jr, Langer C, et al. Randomized phase III trial comparing irinotecan/cisplatin with etoposide/cisplatin in patients with previously untreated extensive-stage disease small-cell lung cancer. *J Clin Oncol* 2006;24:2038.
99. Lara PN Jr, Natale R, Crowley J, et al. Phase III trial of irinotecan/cisplatin compared with etoposide/cisplatin in extensive-stage small-cell lung cancer: clinical and pharmacogenomic results from SWOG S0124. *J Clin Oncol* 2009;27:2530.
105. Eckardt JR, von Pawel J, Papai Z, et al. Open-label, multicenter, randomized, phase III study comparing oral topotecan/cisplatin versus etoposide/cisplatin as treatment for chemotherapy-naive patients with extensive-disease small-cell lung cancer. *J Clin Oncol* 2006;24:2044.
107. Ettinger DS, Finkelstein DM, Abeloff MD, et al. A randomized comparison of standard chemotherapy versus alternating chemotherapy and maintenance versus no maintenance therapy for extensive-stage small-cell lung cancer: a

phase III study of the Eastern Cooperative Oncology Group. *J Clin Oncol* 1990;8:230.

121. Loehrer PJ Sr, Ansari R, Gonin R, et al. Cisplatin plus etoposide with and without ifosfamide in extensive small-cell lung cancer: a Hoosier Oncology Group study. *J Clin Oncol* 1995;13:2594.
126. Niell HB, Herndon JE 2nd, Miller AA, et al. Randomized phase III intergroup trial of etoposide and cisplatin with or without paclitaxel and granulocyte colony-stimulating factor in patients with extensive-stage small-cell lung cancer: Cancer and Leukemia Group B Trial 9732. *J Clin Oncol* 2005;23:3752.
133. Giaccone G, Dalesio O, McVie GJ, et al. Maintenance chemotherapy in small-cell lung cancer: long-term results of a randomized trial. European Organization for Research and Treatment of Cancer Lung Cancer Cooperative Group. *J Clin Oncol* 1993;11:1230.
134. Lebeau B, Chastang C, Allard P, et al. Six vs twelve cycles for complete responders to chemotherapy in small cell lung cancer: definitive results of a randomized clinical trial. The "Petites Cellules" Group. *Eur Respir J* 1992; 5:286.
136. Schiller JH, Adak S, Cella D, et al. Topotecan versus observation after cisplatin plus etoposide in extensive-stage small-cell lung cancer: E7593—a phase III trial of the Eastern Cooperative Oncology Group. *J Clin Oncol* 2001;19:2114.
142. Arriagada R, Le Chevalier T, Pignon JP, et al. Initial chemotherapeutic doses and survival in patients with limited small-cell lung cancer. *N Engl J Med* 1993;329:1848.
145. Ihde DC, Mulshine JL, Kramer BS, et al. Prospective randomized comparison of high-dose and standard-dose etoposide and cisplatin chemotherapy in patients with extensive-stage small-cell lung cancer. *J Clin Oncol* 1994; 12:2022.
146. Johnson DH, Einhorn LH, Birch R, et al. A randomized comparison of high-dose versus conventional-dose cyclophosphamide, doxorubicin, and vincristine for extensive-stage small-cell lung cancer: a phase III trial of the Southeastern Cancer Study Group. *J Clin Oncol* 1987;5:1731.
154. Murray N, Livingston RB, Shepherd FA, et al. Randomized study of CODE versus alternating CAV/EP for extensive-stage small-cell lung cancer: an Intergroup study of the National Cancer Institute of Canada Clinical Trials Group and the Southwest Oncology Group. *J Clin Oncol* 1999;17:2300.
170. Humblet Y, Symann M, Bosly A, et al. Late intensification chemotherapy with autologous bone marrow transplantation in selected small-cell carcinoma of the lung: a randomized study. *J Clin Oncol* 1987;5:1864.
179. von Pawel J, Schiller JH, Shepherd FA, et al. Topotecan versus cyclophosphamide, doxorubicin, and vincristine for the treatment of recurrent small-cell lung cancer. *J Clin Oncol* 1999;17:658.
181. O'Brien ME, Ciuleanu TE, Tsekov H, et al. Phase III trial comparing supportive care alone with supportive care with oral topotecan in patients with relapsed small-cell lung cancer. *J Clin Oncol* 2006;24:5441.
190. Ettinger DS, Jotte R, Lorigan P, et al. Phase II study of amrubicin as second-line therapy in patients with platinum-refractory small-cell lung cancer. *J Clin Oncol* 2010;28:2598.
191. Inoue A, Sugawara S, Yamazaki K, et al. Randomized phase II trial comparing amrubicin with topotecan in patients with previously treated small-cell lung cancer: North Japan Lung Cancer Study Group trial 0402. *J Clin Oncol* 2008;26:5401.
200. van Zandwijk N, Groen HJ, Postmus PE, et al. Role of recombinant interferon-gamma maintenance in responding patients with small cell lung cancer. A randomised phase III study of the EORTC Lung Cancer Cooperative Group. *Eur J Cancer* 1997;33:1759.
204. Giaccone G, Debruyne C, Felip E, et al. Phase III study of adjuvant vaccination with Bec2/bacille Calmette-Guérin in responding patients with limited-disease small-cell lung cancer (European Organisation for Research and Treatment of Cancer 08971-08971B; Silva Study). *J Clin Oncol* 2005; 23:6854.
209. Chahinian AP, Propert KJ, Ware JH, et al. A randomized trial of anticoagulation with warfarin and of alternating chemotherapy in extensive small-cell lung cancer by the Cancer and Leukemia Group B. *J Clin Oncol* 1989; 7:993.
211. Krug LM, Crapanzano JP, Azzoli CG, et al. Imatinib mesylate lacks activity in small cell lung carcinoma expressing c-kit protein: a phase II clinical trial. *Cancer* 2005;103:2128.
226. Rudin CM, Salgia R, Wang X, et al. Randomized phase II study of carboplatin and etoposide with or without the bcl-2 antisense oligonucleotide oblimersen for extensive-stage small-cell lung cancer: CALGB 30103. *J Clin Oncol* 2008;26:870.
231. Horn L, Dahlberg SE, Sandler AB, et al. Phase II study of cisplatin plus etoposide and bevacizumab for previously untreated, extensive-stage small-cell lung cancer: Eastern Cooperative Oncology Group Study E3501. *J Clin Oncol* 2009;27:6006.
234. Perry MC, Eaton WL, Propert KJ, et al. Chemotherapy with or without radiation therapy in limited small-cell carcinoma of the lung. *N Engl J Med* 1987;316:912.
236. Pignon JP, Arriagada R, Ihde DC, et al. A meta-analysis of thoracic radiotherapy for small-cell lung cancer. *N Engl J Med* 1992;327:1618.
241. Bogart JA, Herndon JE 2nd, Lyss AP, et al. 70 Gy thoracic radiotherapy is feasible concurrent with chemotherapy for limited-stage small-cell lung cancer: analysis of Cancer and Leukemia Group B study 39808. *Int J Radiat Oncol Biol Phys* 2004;59:460.
247. Schild SE, Bonner JA, Shanahan TG, et al. Long-term results of a phase III trial comparing once-daily radiotherapy with twice-daily radiotherapy in limited-stage small-cell lung cancer. *Int J Radiat Oncol Biol Phys* 2004; 59:943.
252. Murray N, Coy P, Pater JL, et al. Importance of timing for thoracic irradiation in the combined modality treatment of limited-stage small-cell lung cancer. The National Cancer Institute of Canada Clinical Trials Group. *J Clin Oncol* 1993;11:336.
253. Spiro SG, James LE, Rudd RM, et al. Early compared with late radiotherapy in combined modality treatment for limited disease small-cell lung cancer: a London Lung Cancer Group multicenter randomized clinical trial and meta-analysis. *J Clin Oncol* 2006;24:3823.
254. Takada M, Fukuoka M, Kawahara M, et al. Phase III study of concurrent versus sequential thoracic radiotherapy in combination with cisplatin and etoposide for limited-stage small-cell lung cancer: results of the Japan Clinical Oncology Group Study 9104. *J Clin Oncol* 2002;20:3054.
255. Fried DB, Morris DE, Poole C, et al. Systematic review evaluating the timing of thoracic radiation therapy in combined modality therapy for limited-stage small-cell lung cancer. *J Clin Oncol* 2004;22:4837.
286. Auperin A, Arriagada R, Pignon J, et al. Prophylactic cranial irradiation for patients with small-cell lung cancer in complete remission. *N Engl J Med* 1999;341:476.
296. Kristensen CA, Kristjansen PE, Hansen HH. Systemic chemotherapy of brain metastases from small-cell lung cancer: a review. *J Clin Oncol* 1992; 10:1498.
310. Lad T, Piantadosi S, Thomas P, et al. A prospective randomized trial to determine the benefit of surgical resection of residual disease following response of small cell lung cancer to combination chemotherapy. *Chest* 1994;106:320S.
322. Asamura H, Kameya T, Matsuno Y, et al. Neuroendocrine neoplasms of the lung: a prognostic spectrum. *J Clin Oncol* 2006;24:70.
323. Fink G, Krelbaum T, Yellin A, et al. Pulmonary carcinoid: presentation, diagnosis, and outcome in 142 cases in Israel and review of 640 cases from the literature. *Chest* 2001;119:1647.
326. Thomas CF Jr, Tazelaar HD, Jett JR. Typical and atypical pulmonary carcinoids: outcome in patients presenting with regional lymph node involvement. *Chest* 2001;119:1143.
327. McCaughan BC, Martini N, Bains MS. Bronchial carcinoids. Review of 124 cases. *J Thorac Cardiovasc Surg* 1985;89:8.
337. Granberg D, Sundin A, Janson ET, et al. Octreoscan in patients with bronchial carcinoid tumours. *Clin Endocrinol (Oxf)* 2003;59:793.
344. Travis WD, Giroux DJ, Chansky K, et al. The IASLC Lung Cancer Staging Project: proposals for the inclusion of broncho-pulmonary carcinoid tumors in the forthcoming (seventh) edition of the TNM Classification for Lung Cancer. *J Thorac Oncol* 2008;3:1213.
345. Garcia-Yuste M, Matilla JM, Cueto A, et al. Typical and atypical carcinoid tumours: analysis of the experience of the Spanish Multi-centric Study of Neuroendocrine Tumours of the Lung. *Eur J Cardiothorac Surg* 2007; 31:192.
356. Filosso PL, Ruffini E, Oliaro A, et al. Long-term survival of atypical bronchial carcinoids with liver metastases, treated with octreotide. *Eur J Cardiothorac Surg* 2002;21:913.
362. Ekeblad S, Sundin A, Janson ET, et al. Temozolomide as monotherapy is effective in treatment of advanced malignant neuroendocrine tumors. *Clin Cancer Res* 2007;13:2986.
371. Travis WD, Krug LM, Rusch V. Large cell neuroendocrine carcinoma. In: Raghavan D, Brecher ML, Johnson DH, et al. eds. *Textbook of uncommon cancer*. 3rd ed. New York: Wiley, 2006.
373. Rossi G, Cavazza A, Marchioni A, et al. Role of chemotherapy and the receptor tyrosine kinases KIT, PDGFRalpha, PDGFRbeta, and Met in large-cell neuroendocrine carcinoma of the lung. *J Clin Oncol* 2005;23: 8774.
378. Veronesi G, Morandi U, Alloisio M, et al. Large cell neuroendocrine carcinoma of the lung: a retrospective analysis of 144 surgical cases. *Lung Cancer* 2006;53:111.
379. Iyoda A, Hiroshima K, Toyozaki T, et al. Adjuvant chemotherapy for large cell carcinoma with neuroendocrine features. *Cancer* 2001;92:1108.
380. Zacharias J, Nicholson AG, Ladas GP, et al. Large cell neuroendocrine carcinoma and large cell carcinomas with neuroendocrine morphology of the lung: prognosis after complete resection and systematic nodal dissection. *Ann Thorac Surg* 2003;75:348.
382. Iyoda A, Hiroshima K, Moriya Y, et al. Prospective study of adjuvant chemotherapy for pulmonary large cell neuroendocrine carcinoma. *Ann Thorac Surg* 2006;82:1802.

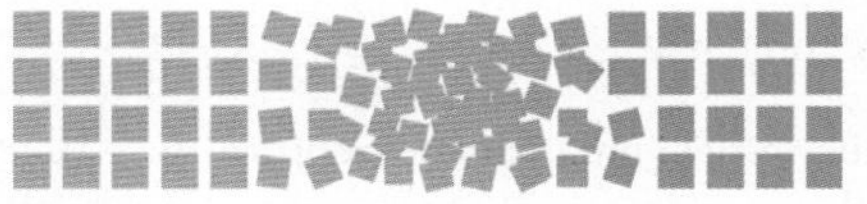

CHAPTER 77 NEOPLASMS OF THE MEDIASTINUM

ROBERT B. CAMERON, PATRICK J. LOEHRER, AND CHARLES R. THOMAS, Jr.

THYMIC NEOPLASMS

Incidence and Etiology

Thymic neoplasms, predominantly thymomas, constitute 30% and 15% of anterior mediastinal masses in adults and children, respectively. Surveillance, Epidemiology, and End Results (SEER) data suggest that thymomas occur in 15 of every 100,000 person-years, are more common in males and Pacific Islanders, and increase in frequency into the eighth decade of life.[1] Other studies document a lower incidence—as low as 0.15 to 0.32 per 100,000 population. Outside of an association with myasthenia gravis (MG), the etiology of these uncommon malignancies and any associated risk factors are completely unknown. Thymic carcinoma, on the other hand, is a rare, aggressive thymic neoplasm that is occasionally associated with paraneoplastic syndromes[2] and has a poor prognosis. Like thymoma, it is an epithelial tumor, but cytologically it exhibits malignant features. It is unclear if thymoma and thymic carcinoma share a common stem cell of origin. Thymic carcinoma is most often located in the anterior mediastinum, although like thymoma, other sites have been reported.[3] Extensive local invasion and distant metastases are common. Suster and Rosai[4] reported on 60 patients ranging in age from 10 to 76 years and with a slight male predominance. Nearly 70% of patients had symptoms of cough, chest pain, or superior vena cava syndrome. Myasthenia and other thymoma-associated syndromes are rare in this more aggressive thymic malignancy.

Anatomy and Pathology

The thymus is an incompletely understood lymphatic organ functioning in T-lymphocyte maturation. It is composed of thymocytes, lymphocytes, and an epithelial stroma. Although lymphomas, carcinoid tumors, and germ cell tumors all may arise within the thymus, only thymomas, thymic carcinomas, and thymolipomas arise from true thymic elements.[5,6] The thymus develops from a paired epithelial anlage in the ventral portion of the third pharyngeal pouch and is closely associated with the developing parathyroid glands.[7] The thymic epithelial stromal cells are likely derived from both ectodermal and endodermal components.[8] During weeks 7 and 8 of development, the thymus elongates and descends caudally and ventromedially into the anterior mediastinum. Lymphoid cells arrive during week 9 and are separated from the perivascular spaces by a flat epithelial cell layer that creates the blood–thymus barrier. Maturation and differentiation occurs in this antigen-free environment and during the fourth fetal month, lymphocytes begin to circulate to peripheral lymphoid tissue.[8]

Six subtypes of epithelial cells have been identified in mature thymus.[8] Four exist primarily in the cortical region and two in the medullary region. Type 6 cells form Hassall corpuscles that are characteristic of thymus. These cells have an ectodermal origin and are displaced into the thymic medulla, where they hypertrophy, form tonofilaments, and finally appear as concentric cells without nuclei.[7,8]

At maturity, the thymus gland is an irregular, lobulated organ. It attains its greatest relative weight at birth, but its absolute weight increases to 30 to 40 g by puberty. During adulthood, it slowly involutes and is replaced by adipose tissue. Ectopic thymic tissue has been found to be widely distributed throughout the mediastinum and neck, particularly the aortopulmonary window and retrocarinal area, and often is indistinguishable from mediastinal fat.[9] This ectopic tissue is the likely explanation for thymomas outside the anterior mediastinum and possibly for failure in some cases of simple thymectomy to improve MG.

THYMOMA

Ninety percent of thymomas occur in the anterior mediastinum and the remainder arise in the neck or other areas of the mediastinum, including, rarely, the heart.[10] The normal contour of the thymus is biconcave or flat. The diseased thymus gland displays a more convex margin. Thymomas grossly are lobulated, firm, tan-pink to gray tumors that may contain cystic spaces, calcification, or hemorrhage. They may be encapsulated, adherent to surrounding structures, or frankly invasive. Microscopically, thymomas arise from thymic epithelial cells, although thymocytes or lymphocytes may predominate histologically. True thymomas contain cytologically bland cells and should be distinguished from thymic carcinomas, which have malignant cytologic characteristics. Originally, in 1976, Rosai and Levine[11] proposed that thymomas be divided into three types: lymphocytic, epithelial, or mixed (lymphoepithelial). In 1985, Marino and Muller-Hermelink[12] proposed a histologic classification system determined by the thymic site of origin—that is, cortical thymomas, medullary thymomas, and mixed thymomas—which were later subdivided further.[13,14] To unify the pathology of thymic neoplasms[15–17] the World Health Organization (WHO) adopted a new classification system for thymic neoplasms (Table 77.1).[17] WHO type A-B2 tumors are more likely to present with locoregional disease, compared with WHO type B3-C tumors.[18,19]

Although Suster and Moran[20] have proposed a simpler classification schema that separates thymic tumors into three categories of thymic carcinoma: well-differentiated (WHO types A, AB, B1, and B2), moderately differentiated (WHO type B3), and poorly differentiated (WHO type C), the full WHO classification system remains more broadly accepted.

TABLE 77.1

WORLD HEALTH ORGANIZATION CLASSIFICATION SYSTEM FOR THYMIC EPITHELIAL TUMORS

Tumor Type	Cells	Clinicopathologic Classification	Histologic Terminology
A	Spindle or oval	Benign thymoma	Medullary
B	Epithelioid or dendritic	Category I malignant thymoma	Cortical; organoid
B1			Lymphocyte-rich; predominately cortical
B2			Cortical
B3			Well-differentiated thymic carcinoma
AB		Benign thymoma	Mixed
C		Category II malignant thymoma	Nonorganotypic; thymic carcinoma, epidermoid keratinizing and nonkeratinizing carcinoma, lymphoepithelioma-like carcinoma, sarcomatoid carcinoma, clear cell carcinoma, basaloid carcinoma, mucoepidermoid carcinoma, undifferentiated carcinoma

From ref. 21 with permission.

Currently, the terms *noninvasive* and *invasive* thymoma are preferred over *benign* and *malignant* designations. Noninvasive thymomas have an intact capsule, are movable, and are easily resected, although they can be adherent to adjacent organs. In contrast, invasive thymomas involve surrounding structures and can be difficult to remove without *en bloc* resection of adjacent structures, despite their benign cytologic appearance. Metastatic disease may occur in both noninvasive (less common) and invasive thymoma and is most commonly seen as pleural implants and pulmonary nodules. Metastases to extrathoracic sites, such as liver, brain, bone, and kidney, infrequently occur.[21]

In 1981, Masaoka et al.[22] developed a surgical staging system shown in Table 77.2. An update of this series of 273 patients confirmed that both WHO histology and clinical staging were independently predictive of 20-year survival.[23] The Groupe d'Etudes des Tumeurs Thymiques (GETT) has another surgically oriented staging system.[24] The Istituto Nazionale Tumori system combines the Masaoka classifications in three distinct stage groupings (locally restricted, locally advanced, and systemic disease) and may better encompass all WHO subtypes.[25] Although the Masaoka thymoma staging system[26] and a proposed tumor-node-metastasis (TNM) classification system[27] (Table 77.3) have been used in staging thymic carcinoma, their utility largely is unproven.

TABLE 77.2

THYMOMA STAGING SYSTEM OF MASAOKA

Stage	Description	Survival (%)
I	Macroscopically completely encapsulated and microscopically no capsular invasion	96
II	Macroscopic invasion into surrounding fatty tissue or mediastinal pleura	86
	Microscopic invasion into capsule	69
III	Macroscopic invasion into neighboring organs (pericardium, great vessels, lung)	50
IVa	Pleural or pericardial dissemination	
IVb	Lymphogenous or hematogenous metastasis	

Adapted from ref. 22.

THYMIC CARCINOMA

The histologic classification of thymic carcinoma was proposed by Levine and Rosai[28] and revised by Suster and Rosai.[4] The tumors are classified broadly as low or high grade. Low-grade tumors include squamous cell carcinoma, mucoepidermoid carcinoma, and basaloid carcinoma. High-grade neoplasms include lymphoepithelioma-like carcinoma and small cell, undifferentiated, sarcomatoid, and clear cell carcinomas.[4,26,29,30] Although the histologic classification of thymic carcinomas was designed to be descriptive, correlations with prognosis have been made. For instance, low-grade tumors may have a more favorable clinical course (median survival rates of 25.4 months to more than 6.6 years) because of lower local and systemic recurrence rates, when compared with higher grade malignancies (median survival of only 11.3 months to 15.0 months).[4,26]

Molecular profiling of rare solid tumors such as thymic neoplasms has taken place over the past decade.[31] Emerging analysis does suggest that mutations in genes of the epidermal growth factor receptor (EGFR) and KIT pathways have documented a progressive increase in observed genomic aberrations from WHO subtype A thymoma to WHO subtype C thymic carcinoma.[32]

Diagnosis

A meticulous history and physical examination, along with myriad imaging, serological, and invasive tests, usually confirm the suspected diagnosis. With improved imaging, core needle biopsy, and pathological techniques, the majority of patients no longer require open surgical biopsy.

Symptoms and Signs

Approximately 40% of mediastinal masses are asymptomatic and discovered incidentally on routine chest imaging.[1] The

TABLE 77.3

ISTITUTO NAZIONALE TUMORI TUMOR-NODE-METASTASIS (TNM)-BASED STAGING SYSTEM

TNM	Description
T1	No capsular invasion
T2	Microscopic invasion into the capsule, or extracapsular involvement limited to the surrounding fatty tissue or normal thymus
T3	Direct invasion into the mediastinal pleura and/or anterior pericardium
T4	Direct invasion into neighboring organs, such as sternum, great vessels, and lungs; implants to the mediastinal pleura or pericardium, only if anterior to phrenic nerves
N0	No lymph nodes metastasis
N1	Metastasis to anterior mediastinal lymph nodes
N2	Metastasis to intrathoracic lymph nodes other than anterior mediastinal
N3	Metastasis to prescalene or supraclavicular nodes
M0	No hematogenous metastasis
M1a	Implants to the pericardium or mediastinal pleura beyond the sites defined in the T4 category
M1b	Hematogenous metastasis to other sites, or involvement of lymph nodal stations other than those described in the N categories
Stage Grouping	**Description**
I	Locally restricted disease T1-2 N0 M0
II	Locally advanced disease T3-4 N0 M0 Any T N1-2 M0
III	Systemic Any T N3 M0 Any T any N M1
Classification	**Description of Residual Disease**
R0	No residual tumor
R1	Microscopic residual tumor
R2a	Local macroscopic residual tumor after reductive resection (more than 80% of the tumor)
R2b	Other features of residual tumor

TNM, tumor, node, metastasis.
Adapted from ref. 27.

remaining 60% have symptoms related to either compression or direct invasion of surrounding mediastinal structures or to paraneoplastic syndromes. Asymptomatic patients are more likely to have benign lesions, whereas symptomatic patients more often harbor malignancies. Davis et al.[33] found that 85% of patients with a malignancy were symptomatic, but only 46% of patients with benign neoplasms had identifiable complaints. The most common symptoms are chest pain, cough, and dyspnea. Superior vena cava syndrome, Horner syndrome, hoarseness, and neurologic deficits are less common and often signal a malignancy.[33] Systemic syndromes associated with mediastinal neoplasms are shown in Tables 77.4 and 77.5.

Associated Systemic Syndromes

A wide variety of associated systemic disorders may be identified in up to 71% of patients, including autoimmune diseases (MG, systemic lupus erythematosus, polymyositis, myocarditis, Sjögren syndrome, ulcerative colitis, Hashimoto thyroiditis, rheumatoid arthritis, sarcoidosis, and scleroderma), endocrine disorders (hyperthyroidism, hyperparathyroidism, stiff-person syndrome, Addison disease, and panhypopituitarism), blood disorders (red cell aplasia, hypogammaglobulinemia, T-cell deficiency syndrome, erythrocytosis, pancytopenia, megakaryocytopenia, T-cell lymphocytosis, and pernicious anemia), neuromuscular syndromes (myotonic dystrophy, myositis, and Eaton-Lambert syndrome), as well as other disorders (hypertrophic osteoarthropathy, nephrotic syndrome, minimal change nephropathy, pemphigus, and chronic mucocutaneous candidiasis).[34] Symptoms of one or more of these disorders may lead to the original discovery of the mediastinal tumor.

Myasthenia Gravis. MG is the most common autoimmune disorder associated with thymoma, occurring in 30% to 50% of patients.[35] Younger women and older men usually are affected, with a female-to-male ratio of 2:1. Myasthenia is a disorder of neuromuscular transmission. The temporal association is variable and a prolonged interval between the diagnosis of myasthenia and development of a visible thymic tumor can occur.[36] Symptoms (e.g., diplopia, ptosis, dysphagia, fatigue) begin insidiously and result from the production of antibodies to the postsynaptic nicotinic acetylcholine receptor at the myoneural junction. Ocular

TABLE 77.4

SYSTEMIC SYNDROMES ASSOCIATED WITH MEDIASTINAL NEOPLASMS

Tumor	Syndrome
Thymoma	Acute pericarditis, Addison disease, agranulocytosis, alopecia areata, Cushing syndrome, hemolytic anemia, hypogammaglobulinemia, limbic encephalopathy, myasthenia gravis, myocarditis, nephrotic syndrome, panhypopituitarism, pernicious anemia, polymyositis, pure red cell aplasia, rheumatoid arthritis, sarcoidosis, scleroderma, sensorimotor radiculopathy, stiff-person syndrome, thyroiditis, ulcerative colitis
Hodgkin's lymphoma	Alcohol-induced pain, Pel-Ebstein fever
Neurofibroma	von Recklinghausen disease, osteoarthritis
Thymic carcinoid	Multiple endocrine neoplasia
Neuroblastoma	Opsomyoclonus, erythrocyte abnormalities
Neurilemoma	Peptic ulcer

symptoms are the most frequent initial complaint, eventually progressing to generalized weakness in 80%. The role of the thymus in myasthenia remains unclear, but autosensitization of T lymphocytes to acetylcholine receptor proteins or an unknown action of thymic hormones remain likely possibilities.[37]

The altered microenvironment may adversely impact the output of T-regulatory (Treg) cells, altering the autoimmune homeostasis.[38] Pathologic changes in the thymus are noted in 70% of patients with MG. Lymphoid hyperplasia, characterized by the proliferation of germinal centers, is most commonly seen. Thymomas are identified in only about 15% of patients with MG.[37]

The treatment of MG involves the use of anticholinesterase mimetic agents (i.e., pyridostigmine bromide [Mestinon]). In severe cases, plasmapheresis may be required to remove high antibody titers. Thymectomy has become an increasingly accepted procedure in the treatment of MG, although the indications, timing, and surgical approach remain controversial.[39] Some improvement in myasthenic symptoms almost always occurs after thymectomy, but complete remission rates vary from 7% to 63%.[39] Patients with MG and thymomas do not respond as well to thymectomy as MG patients without thymomas. Age 55 years and older and a duration of symptoms of less than 1 year also are associated with poor outcome.[40] It does not appear that MG portends to a poorer outcome.[41]

Red Cell Aplasia. Pure red cell aplasia is considered an autoimmune disorder and is found in approximately 5% of patients with thymomas.[42] Thirty percent to 50% of patients with red cell aplasia have associated thymomas. Ninety-six percent of the patients affected are older than 40 years of age. Examination of the bone marrow reveals an absence of erythroid precursors and, in 30%, an associated decrease in platelet and leukocyte numbers. Thymectomy has produced remission in 38% of patients. For patients with recurrent disease, octreotide and prednisone were effective in case reports.[42,43] The pathologic basis of these responses is poorly understood.

Hypogammaglobulinemia. Hypogammaglobulinemia is seen in 5% to 10% of patients with thymoma (Good syndrome), and 10% of patients with hypogammaglobulinemia have been shown to have thymoma. Recurrent sinusitis is a common associated symptom in such patients. Defects in both cellular and humoral immunity have been described, and many patients also have red cell hypoplasia.[44] Thymectomy has not proven beneficial in this disorder.

Radiographic Imaging Studies

Imaging studies initially localize mediastinal neoplasms.[45] The posteroanterior and lateral chest radiographs define the location, size, density, and calcification of a mass, which helps

TABLE 77.5

SYSTEMIC MANIFESTATIONS OF HORMONE PRODUCTION BY MEDIASTINAL NEOPLASMS

Symptoms	Hormone	Tumor
Hypertension	Catecholamines	Pheochromocytoma, chemodectoma, neuroblastoma, ganglioneuroma
Hypercalcemia	Parathyroid hormone	Parathyroid adenoma
Thyrotoxicosis	Thyroxine	Thyroid
Cushing syndrome	ACTH	Carcinoid tumor
Gynecomastia	HCG	Germ cell tumor
Hypoglycemia	? Insulin	Mesenchymal tumors
Diarrhea	VIP	Ganglioneuroma, neuroblastoma, neurofibroma

ACTH, adrenocorticotropic hormone; HCG, human chorionic gonadotropin; VIP, vasoactive intestinal polypeptide.

focus the initial diagnostic testing; however, an intravenous contrast-enhanced spiral computed tomography (CT) scan remains the best imaging modality to accurately assess the nature of the lesion (cystic vs. solid), detect fat and calcium, determine the relationship to surrounding anatomic structures, and, in some instances, predict invasiveness of tumors.[46,47]

Recent advances in electrocardiogram-gating and real-time magnetic resonance imaging (MRI) and angiography have dramatically increased the usefulness of this modality in the evaluation of mediastinal masses. Not only is it superior to CT in defining vascular involvement, MRI can detect subtle differences in tumor contour, capsule clarity, and intratumoral signal (low), which correlate with the WHO classification of thymomas.[48]

Positron emission tomography (PET) is well established for the assessment of mediastinal lymphoma, and its utility in clarifying the nature of other mediastinal masses, including invasive thymoma, is gaining general acceptance, and standardized uptake value may partially correlate with histological subtype.[49–51] Although transesophageal ultrasonography can assess invasiveness of posterior mediastinal tumors,[52] other imaging modalities generally have limited utility.

Serology and Chemistry

Many germ cell neoplasms release chemical markers into the serum that may be measured to confirm a diagnosis, evaluate response to therapy, and monitor for tumor recurrence. Lactate dehydrogenase, α-fetoprotein (AFP), and human chorionic gonadotropin-β (β-hCG) are common tumor markers that should be obtained in male patients with anterior mediastinal masses. Also, adrenocorticotropic hormone, thyroid hormone, and parathormone may help differentiate certain mediastinal masses (Table 77.4).

Invasive Diagnostic Tests

An accurate histologic diagnosis is essential for appropriate treatment of nearly all mediastinal neoplasms. Although some patients may still require open surgical biopsies, CT- or ultrasound-guided percutaneous needle biopsy now is standard in the initial evaluation of mediastinal masses.[10] Although fine-needle specimens are often adequate to distinguish carcinomas, core biopsies are recommended for most mediastinal neoplasms, especially lymphoma and thymoma. Recent series report diagnostic yields for percutaneous needle biopsy in excess of 90%.[53] Complications include simple pneumothorax (25%), hemoptysis (7% to 15%), and pneumothorax, requiring chest tube placement (5%).[53] In some circumstances, fine-needle aspiration of posterior and middle mediastinal tumors can be performed endoscopically using transesophageal ultrasonography.[52,54]

Surgical procedures occasionally are still required in the diagnosis of mediastinal tumors. Mediastinoscopy is a relatively simple procedure with a diagnostic accuracy of more than 90% for biopsies of the upper middle and, in some surgeons' hands, the anterior and posterior mediastinum.[55] Anterior parasternal mediastinotomy (Chamberlain procedure) yields a diagnosis in 95% of anterior mediastinal masses and may be accomplished under local anesthesia.[55,56] Thoracoscopy is a minimally invasive procedure that provides a diagnostic accuracy of nearly 100% in most areas of the mediastinum.[55] Currently, thoracotomy rarely is necessary solely as a diagnostic procedure.

Management by Stage

Thymomas, albeit slow-growing, should be considered potentially malignant neoplasms. Surgery, radiation, and chemotherapy all may play a role in their management.[41,57] Few prospective, well-designed clinical trials in the management of thymoma have been conducted, particularly evaluating the role of surgery and radiotherapy; however, the newly formed International Thymic Malignancy Interest Group is planning cohort studies to help guide diagnostic and therapeutic interventions.[58]

Masaoka Stage I/II Thymoma

Complete surgical resection is the mainstay of therapy for stage I/II thymomas and is the most important predictor of long-term survival.[59–62] Although median sternotomy with a vertical or submammary skin incision is most commonly used, bilateral anterolateral thoracotomies with transverse sternotomy, or "clam-shell procedure," is useful with advanced or laterally displaced large tumors. Video-assisted thoracoscopy and, more recently, robotic-assisted surgery have been used with increasing frequency and acceptable outcomes, but long-term results with this highly specialized approach are still a number of years away.[63] During any surgery, a careful assessment of areas of possible invasion and adherence should be made. Extended total thymectomy, including all tissue anterior to the pericardium from the diaphragm to the neck and laterally from one phrenic nerve to the other, including *en bloc* pericardium, phrenic nerve, chest wall, lung, and diaphragmatic resection (with reconstruction) in up to two-thirds of cases in order to achieve an R0 resection is recommended in all good performance status patients.[41,59–61] Operative mortality is less than 3% in experienced centers.[41]

Thymomas harbor variable radio sensitivity to ionizing radiation.[64] Consequently, radiation has been used to treat various tumor stages as well as recurrent disease.[59,62,65] Furthermore, modern imaging, three-dimensional treatment planning, and delivery techniques have allowed thoracic radiotherapy to be prescribed in a safer fashion than noted in the past century. Radiation therapy is delivered in doses ranging from 30 to 60 Gy in 1.8 to 2.0 Gy fractions during 3 to 6 weeks.[59,64,66,67] There are suggestions of a dose–response relationship with local control in some patients, albeit from retrospective data, although it is not clear that doses exceeding 60 Gy offer any consistent advantage[68,69]; however, completely resected and microscopic residual disease can be well controlled with only 40 to 45 Gy.[62,70] Emerging data suggest that certain histological subtypes (WHO type B1 and B2) are more likely to respond to preoperative radiotherapy compared to others subtypes (WHO type B3),[71] although whether outcome is related to WHO subtype is inconclusive.[41,72,73] Treatment portals have included single anterior field, unequally weighted (2:1 or 3:2) opposed anterior-posterior fields, wedge-pair, and multifield arrangements.[68] The gross tumor volume is defined by visible tumor or surgical clips seen on a treatment-planning CT scan. Areas of possible microscopic disease and a small border to account for daily variability and respiratory motion are added to define the clinical and planning target volumes. Gating techniques to minimize respiratory variation and intensity-modulated radiation therapy are new techniques that can minimize the dose heterogeneity, increase total dose and fraction size, and minimize toxicity.[70,74] Prophylactic supraclavicular and hemithorax fields have been used but are not warranted because of increased risks of pulmonary fibrosis, pericarditis, and myelitis.[62,68,75,76] This is clearly a disease that warrants a prospective, multi-institutional clinical trial to further define the role of thoracic radiotherapy.

Masaoka Stage III/IV Thymoma

The role of subtotal surgical resection or "debulking" surgery in stage III and IV disease remains highly controversial.[77] Several studies have documented improved 5-year survival rates after subtotal resection compared to biopsy alone.[59,62] Another study suggested no survival advantage to debulking surgery followed by radiation when compared with radiation alone; and a more recent report reached the opposite conclusion.[77] The use of surgery in recurrent disease remains to be defined.

Radiation therapy has proven beneficial in the treatment of extensive disease.[62,64,66,68,78] Large variations in the amount of tumor treated, radiation delivered, and tumor biology, however, make interpretation of these results difficult.[62,68,79,80]

Cytotoxic chemotherapy has been used with increasing frequency in the treatment of invasive thymomas.[81] Both single-agent and combination therapy have demonstrated activity in the adjuvant and neoadjuvant settings. Doxorubicin, cisplatin, ifosfamide, corticosteroids, and cyclophosphamide all have been used as single-agent therapy.[82] The most active agents are cisplatin, doxorubicin, ifosfamide, and corticosteroids; however, only a few single agents, such as cisplatin, ifosfamide, pemetrexed, gefitinib, and imatinib have undergone formal phase 2 trials.

A number of molecular targets have been identified in thymic tissue.[83] Overexpression of the epidermal growth factor receptor has been found in more than two-thirds of patients, mostly WHO B2–3 subtypes.[84–86] The overexpression of *c-kit* is common in thymic carcinoma, although *c-kit* mutations are less frequent.[85,87,88]

Thymic Carcinoma

The optimal treatment of thymic carcinoma remains undefined, but currently a multimodality approach, including surgical resection, postoperative radiation, and chemotherapy, is recommended.[89] Initial surgical resection followed by radiation has been used in most studies.[4,26,27,29,90] Complete resection should be attempted, but often is not possible.[26,91] One analysis noted a 9.5-month median survival after resection and postoperative electron-beam radiation therapy,[90] with a trend toward improved survival in other studies.[4,26,29] Chemotherapy with cisplatin-based regimens similar to those used with thymomas have produced variable responses in small numbers of patients.[4,26,29] Combinations of doxorubicin, cyclophosphamide, and vincristine also have generated partial responses, as has the combination of 5-fluorouracil and leucovorin. Use of neoadjuvant chemotherapy has been reported in a small number of patients.[89,92]

Results of Treatment

Thymoma

In nearly 700 patients in the SEER database treated between 1973 and 1998, advanced disease was associated with decreasing survival.[42] According to various retrospective series, the 5- and 10-year survival rates for stage I, III, and IV tumors are reported to be 89% to 95% and 78% to 90%; 70% to 80% and 21% to 80%; and 50% to 60% and 30% to 40%, respectively.[59,93] Ten-year disease-free survival rates of 74%, 71%, 50%, and 29% also have been reported for stage I, II, III, and IV disease, respectively.[59] Long-term results from an experienced Indiana University group has yielded a 66% 1-year overall survival.[41] Although Maggi et al.[59] reported a 10% overall recurrence rate in 241 patients, less than 5% of noninvasive thymomas and 20% of invasive thymomas were noted to recur. A large Japanese multi-institutional experience with 1,320 patients reported 5-year survival rates of 100%, 98.4%, 88.7%, 70.6%, and 52.8% for Masaoka stages I, II, III, IVa, and IVb, respectively.[60] Although MG once was considered an adverse prognostic factor, this is no longer the case because of improved perioperative care, and in fact, MG actually may be associated with an improved survival owing to earlier tumor detection.[41,94] Complete surgical resection of thymomas is associated with an 82% overall 7-year survival rate, whereas survival with incomplete resection is 71% and with biopsy is only 26%.[59] Survival after complete tumor resection has been similar in patients with noninvasive and invasive thymomas in several studies.[60,61] Patients with MG and thymoma have a 56% to 78% 10-year survival rate and a 3% recurrence rate with 4.8% (1.7% since 1980) operative mortality after extended thymectomy.[62,95] Rarely, a syndrome of myasthenia crisis may occur following surgery and lead to increased perioperative morbidity.[95]

While the data on whether outcome is related to WHO subtype is inconclusive,[41,72,73] it may be that when coupled with other factors such as completeness of resection, WHO subtype may be prognostic in some patients.[96]

For example, in stage I thymomas, adjuvant radiotherapy has been administered but has not improved on the excellent results with surgery alone (more than 80% 10-year survival rate).[59,62] In stage II and III invasive disease, adjuvant radiation can decrease recurrence rates after complete surgical resection from 28% to 5%.[68] In addition, Pollack et al.[66] reported an increase in 5-year disease-free survival for stage II to IVa from 18% to 62% with the addition of adjuvant radiation. Stage II patients with cortical tumors[97,98] and invasion of pleura or pericardium are most likely to benefit from postoperative radiation.[78] Preoperative radiotherapy for extensive tumors has been reported in limited studies that suggest a decreased tumor burden and potential for tumor seeding at the time of surgery.[59,62] Data suggest that not all Masaoka stage II patients may necessarily require postoperative radiotherapy.[57,101] Indeed, a review of SEER registry data from 1975 to 2003 demonstrated a worse cancer-specific survival for patients with resected, localized thymoma who received postoperative radiotherapy (PORT) compared to those without (91% vs. 98%; $P = .03$). For patients with regional disease, PORT had a slight but nonstatistically significant difference (91% vs. 86%; $P = .12$).[102]

Masaoka Stage III/IV Thymoma

The role of subtotal surgical resection or "debulking" surgery in stage III and IV disease remains highly controversial.[77] Several studies have documented 5-year survival rates from 60% to 75% after subtotal resection and 24% to 40% after biopsy alone.[59,62] Although one study did suggest no survival advantage to debulking followed by radiation when compared with radiation alone, another more recent experience reached the opposite conclusion.[77] The use of surgery in recurrent disease remains to be defined. Maggi et al.[59] reported a 71% 5-year survival rate in 12 surgery patients and a 41% survival rate in 11 patients treated with radiation and chemotherapy alone. Prolonged tumor-free survival also was reported by Kirschner[75] in 23 patients. Urgesi et al.,[79] however, noted a 74% 5-year survival rate in 11 patients undergoing surgery and radiation, compared with 65% in ten patients treated with radiation alone (not statistically different). In 71 patients with thymoma (WHO types A-B3) with stage I to IVA disease, 54 (75.3%) patients are alive and free of disease with six additional patients alive with disease with a mean follow-up of 66 months.[41]

Radiation therapy has proven beneficial in the treatment of extensive disease.[62,64,66,69,78] Radiotherapy after incomplete surgical resection produces local control rates of 35% to 74% and 5-year survival rates ranging from 50% to 70% for stage III and 20% to 50% for stage IVa tumors.[62,67,68] In addition, Ciernik et al.[68] and others[79] have reported similar survival rates (87% 5-year and 70% 7-year) in patients treated with radiation alone compared with partial surgical resection and adjuvant radiation in small numbers of stage III and IV patients and patients with intrathoracic recurrences. Large variations in the amount of tumor treated, radiation delivered, and tumor biology, however, make interpretation of these results difficult at best.[62,68,79,80]

Cytotoxic chemotherapy has been used with increasing frequency in the treatment of invasive thymomas.[81] Both single-agent and combination therapy have demonstrated activity in the adjuvant and neoadjuvant settings. Doxorubicin, cisplatin, ifosfamide, corticosteroids, and cyclophosphamide all have been used as single-agent therapy.[82] The most active agents are cisplatin, doxorubicin, ifosfamide, and corticosteroids; however, only a few single agents, such as cisplatin, ifosfamide, pemetrexed, gefitinib, and imatinib, have undergone formal phase II trials. Cisplatin, at doses of 100 mg/m^2, has produced complete responses lasting up to 30 months, but lower doses (50 mg/m^2) have associated response rates of only 11%.[82] Ifosfamide (with mesna) at a single dose of 7.5 g/m^2 or as a continuous infusion of 1.5 g/m^2/d for 5 days every 3 weeks has resulted in 50% complete and 57% overall response rates. Duration of complete remission ranged from 6 to 66 months.[103] Varying regimens of corticosteroids have shown effectiveness in the treatment of all histologic subtypes of thymoma (with and without myasthenia), with a 77% overall response rate in limited numbers of patients.[82,104,105] Corticosteroids also have been effective for patients unsuccessful with chemotherapy[82]; however, the actual impact may only be on the lymphocytic and not the malignant epithelial component of the tumor.

Combination chemotherapy regimens have shown higher response rates and have been used in both neoadjuvant and metastatic settings in the treatment of advanced invasive, metastatic, and recurrent thymoma. Cisplatin-containing regimens appear to be the most active. Fornasiero et al.[93] reported a 43% complete and 91.8% overall response rate with a median survival of 15 months in 37 previously untreated patients with stage III or IV invasive thymoma treated with monthly (median, 5 months) cisplatin, 50 mg/m^2 on day 1; doxorubicin, 40 mg/m^2 on day 1; vincristine, 0.6 mg/m^2 on day 3; and cyclophosphamide, 700 mg/m^2 on day 4. Loehrer et al.[106] documented 10% complete and 50% overall response rates with a median survival of 37.7 months in 29 patients with metastatic or locally progressive recurrent thymoma treated with cisplatin, 50 mg/m^2; doxorubicin, 50 mg/m^2; and cyclophosphamide, 500 mg/m^2, given every 3 weeks for a maximum of eight cycles after radiotherapy. Park et al.[107] retrospectively described 35% complete and 64% overall response rates with a median survival of 67 months in responding and 17 months in nonresponding patients in 17 patients with invasive stage II and IV thymoma initially treated after relapse with cyclophosphamide, doxorubicin, and cisplatin, with or without prednisone. The European Organisation for Research and Treatment of Cancer noted 31% complete and 56% overall response rates with a median survival of 4.3 years in a small study of 16 patients with advanced thymoma treated with cisplatin and etoposide.[108] The addition of ifosfamide to cisplatin and etoposide had a lower than anticipated response rate (approximately 32%) in patients with thymoma and thymic carcinoma.[90]

The Eastern Cooperative Oncology Group conducted a prospective trial in patients with thymoma (n = 25) and thymic carcinoma (n = 21) who were treated with carboplatin plus paclitaxel with a 33% objective response rate for the former group and 24% for the latter.[109] In total, these data suggest higher objective response rates achieved with anthracycline-based regimens.

Combined Modality Approaches

The use of neoadjuvant (induction or preoperative) chemotherapy is part of a multimodality approach to stage III and IV thymoma.[82] Six combined reports document 31% complete and 89% overall response rates in 61 total patients treated with a variety of neoadjuvant chemotherapy regimens (80% cisplatin-based). Twenty-two patients (36%) underwent surgery, with 11 (18%) achieving a complete resection (all treated with cisplatin). Nineteen patients were treated with radiotherapy, but only five patients had disease-free survivals exceeding 5 years.[82] Rea et al.[110] reported 43% complete and 100% overall response rates with median and 3-year survival rates of 66 months and 70%, respectively, in 16 stage III and IVa patients treated initially with cisplatin, doxorubicin, vincristine, and cyclophosphamide, followed by surgery. At surgery, 69% were completely resected and the other 31% received postoperative radiation. A recent report from the Amsterdam team noted a 50% objective response rate, using the Response Evaluation Criteria in Solid Tumors (RECIST) criteria in 16 patients with locally advanced tumors.[108] Macchiarini et al.[111] reported similar findings. Recently, the Japan Clinical Oncology Group reported a phase 2 trial (JCOG 9606) that treated 23 patients with unresectable stage III thymoma with 9 weeks of CODE chemotherapy, including cisplatin 25 mg/m^2 on weeks 1 through 9; vincristine 1mg/m^2 on weeks 1, 2, 4, 6 and 8; and doxorubicin 40 mg/m^2 and etoposide 80 mg/m^2 on days 1–3 of weeks 1, 3, 5, 7 and 9.[112] Twelve patients (57%) completed the planned 9-week therapy without mortality. Of 21 eligible patients, 0, 13 (62%), and 7 achieved a complete response, partial response, and stable disease, respectively. Subsequently, 13 (62%) underwent thoracotomy with 9 (39%) undergoing complete R0 resection and postoperative radiotherapy (48 or 60 Gy in completely or incompletely resected disease, respectively). Progression-free survival at 2 and 5 years was 80% and 43% and overall survival at 5 and 8 years was 85% and 69%, respectively. Survival was not improved by surgical resection. Finally 25% complete (3 patients) and 92% overall response rates (11 patients) with a remarkable 83% 7-year disease-free survival rate (10 patients) were reported in only 12 patients at the M. D. Anderson Cancer Center who received cisplatin, doxorubicin, cyclophosphamide, and prednisone induction chemotherapy followed by surgical resection (80% complete) and adjuvant radiotherapy for locally advanced (unresectable) thymoma.[113] The degree of chemotherapy-induced tumor necrosis correlated with Ki-67 expression.

A multi-institutional prospective trial demonstrated a 22% complete and 70% overall response rate with a median survival of 93 months and a Kaplan-Meier 5-year failure-free survival rate of 54.3% in 23 patients with stage III (22/23) unresectable thymoma (GETT stage IIIA/IIIB) stage IV (1/23) thymoma, and thymic carcinoma (2/23) treated with two to four cycles of cisplatin, doxorubicin, and cyclophosphamide chemotherapy and sequential radiation therapy (54 Gy).[114] Just more than 25% had MG. Although these results compare favorably with those obtained with neoadjuvant therapy followed by surgical resection and radiation, further data are required. Postoperative (adjuvant) chemotherapy is not recommended.[41]

Molecularly Targeted Therapy

A case report demonstrated brief response to imatinib in a patient with thymic carcinoma, but two additional trials failed to find any activity in an additional 20 patients.[115] Further trials with gefitinib as a single agent and erlotinib plus bevacizumab in previously treated patients had minimal to no activity. Cetuximab has been demonstrated to have some durable stable disease.[116] Furthermore, antitumor activity has been reported with dasatinib, a small molecule oral, multitargeted kinase inhibitor of *Bcr-Abl* and *src* kinases, ephrin receptor kinases, platelet-derived growth factor receptor, and c-kit, in thymoma.[94] With more time, molecular therapy will likely be integrated into current systemic cytotoxic therapy. In addition, coamplification of the *HER-2/neu* topoisomerase 2-alpha gene may correlate with response to the cyclophosphamide, doxorubicin, and cisplatin chemotherapy regimen.[117]

Thymus-specific targeted therapy has shown promise in small clinical trials.[84] Somatostatin analogues have shown activity in thymic neoplasms. Although the mechanism of action is not clear, inhibition of the insulin-like growth factor– or epidermal growth factor receptor–related pathways are possible. Response rates were seen in more than one-third (37%) of patients with tumors that were resistant to cytotoxic chemotherapy and received octreotide plus prednisone.[118] The median and progression-free survival of 15 months and 14 months, respectively, is encouraging. In a North American Cooperative Group trial in thymoma patients with positive radionuclide octreotide scans, one-eighth (12.5%) of the patients demonstrated a partial response to octreotide alone, which increased to almost one-third (32%) with the addition of prednisone.[118]

Nearly 15% of patients with thymoma develop a second malignancy, such as Kaposi sarcoma, chemodectoma, multiple myeloma, acute leukemia, non-Hodgkin's lymphoma, sarcomas, and various carcinomas (e.g., lung, colon).[1]

Thymic Carcinoma

The prognosis of thymic carcinoma is poor because of early metastatic involvement of mediastinal, cervical, and axillary lymph nodes; pleura; lung; brain; bone; and liver.[4,92,119] The overall survival rate at 5 years is approximately 35%.[4,26] The recently reported Japanese experience noted a 88.2%, 51.7%, and 37.6% 5-year survival in patients with stages I/II, III, and IV, respectively.[60] Improved survival has been correlated with encapsulated tumors, lobular growth pattern, low mitotic activity, early-stage tumors, low histologic grade, lymphoepithelioma-like histology, and complete surgical resection.[4,87,91] In addition, patients with stage IVa disease appear to benefit more from treatment than those with more disseminated disease (stage IVb).[88]

THYMIC CARCINOID

Thymic carcinoid tumors are rare, male-predominant tumors that are associated with Cushing syndrome, multiple endocrine neoplasia, and, rarely, carcinoid syndrome.[120–126] Complete surgical resection with adjuvant radiotherapy for incompletely resected tumors is recommended.[121–124] Chemotherapy rarely has been used.[127,128] Although a 5-year survival rate of 60% has been reported with complete surgical resection,[122] the long-term prognosis is generally poor and is correlated with the extent of disease and the degree of differentiation of the tumor.[129]

THYMOLIPOMA

Thymolipomas are rare, benign neoplasms composed of mature adipose and thymic tissue, and they account for 1% to 5% of thymic neoplasms.[130] These tumors are also known as *lipothymomas, mediastinal lipomas with thymic remnants, and thymolipomatous hamartomas*.[130,131] In a review of 27 patients, Rosado-de-Christenson et al.[131] noted an equal gender distribution and a mean age of 27 years. Approximately 50% of patients presented with symptoms of vague chest pain, dyspnea, and tachypnea. Others have reported, in adults only, an association with MG, red cell aplasia, hypogammaglobulinemia, lichen planus, and Graves' disease, but less commonly than with thymoma.[130,132–134]

Thymolipomas are soft, lobulated, encapsulated tumors that originate in the anterior mediastinum. They often attain a large size before becoming symptomatic.[135] They frequently conform to the shape of the cardiac and mediastinal structures and are found in the anterior-inferior mediastinum "draped along the diaphragm" and connected to the thymus by a small pedicle.[131] Microscopically, the tumors comprise thymic tissue, often with calcified Hassall corpuscles, and more than 50% adipose tissue.[131] Histologically, thymolipomas do not appear malignant, and malignant transformation does not occur. Treatment involves complete resection.[135]

GERM CELL TUMORS

Incidence and Etiology

Although most germ cell tumors arise within gonadal tissue, the most common site for the development of extragonadal germ cell tumors is the mediastinum. Mediastinal germ cell neoplasms account for only 2% to 5% of all germinal tumors, but they constitute 50% to 70% of all extragonadal tumors.[136] They are most commonly seen in the anterior mediastinum and account for 10% to 15% of all primary mediastinal tumors. Mediastinal germ cell tumors are most commonly diagnosed in the third decade of life, but patients as old as 60 years of age have been reported. The incidence of these neoplasms is equal in all races.

Benign teratomas are the most common mediastinal germ cell tumor, accounting for 70% of the mediastinal germ cell tumors in children and 60% of those in adults. They can be seen in any age group but most commonly occur in adults from 20 to 40 years of age.

Primary pure mediastinal seminomas account for approximately 35% of malignant mediastinal germ cell tumors and are principally seen in men aged 20 to 40 years.[137]

Although in adults benign germ cell tumors have no sex predilection, 90% of malignant germ cell tumors occur in men with a mean age of 29. In the pediatric population, both benign and malignant extragonadal germ cell tumors occur with equal sex distribution.

Anatomy and Pathology

Extragonadal germ cell tumors are found along the body's midline from the cranium (pineal gland) to the presacral area. This line corresponds to the embryologic urogenital ridge. It is presumed that these tumors arise from malignant transformation of germ cells that have abnormally migrated during embryonic development.[136] Mediastinal germ cell tumors are broadly classified as benign or malignant. Benign tumors include mature teratomas and mixed teratomas with an immature component of less than 50%. Malignant germ cell tumors are divided into seminomas (dysgerminomas) and nonseminomatous tumors. In addition, mediastinal germ cell tumors have a propensity to develop a component of non–germ cell malignancy (e.g., rhabdomyosarcoma, adenocarcinoma, permeative neuroectodermal tumor), which can become the predominant histology.

Teratomas

Teratomas contain elements from all three germ cell layers, with a predominance of the ectodermal component in most tumors, including skin, hair, sweat glands, sebaceous glands, and teeth. Mesoderm is represented by fat, smooth muscle, bone, and cartilage. Respiratory and intestinal epithelium are often seen as the endodermal component. Teratomas may be solid or cystic in appearance and are often referred to as *dermoid cysts* if unilocular. The majority of mediastinal teratomas are composed of mature ectodermal, mesodermal, and endodermal elements and exhibit a benign course. Immature teratomas phenotypically may appear as a malignancy derived from these ectodermal, mesodermal, and endodermal elements. These latter tumors behave aggressively and generally are not responsive to systemic therapy.

Seminomas

Seminomas less commonly may exist in a pure form, but any elevation of serum AFP levels indicates the presence of at least a small element of nonseminomatous tumor.

Nonseminomatous Tumors. Mediastinal nonseminomatous germ cell tumors are most commonly found in the anterior mediastinum and appear grossly as often invasive, lobulated masses with a thin capsule. Nonseminomatous tumors include embryonal carcinomas, choriocarcinomas, yolk sac tumors, and immature teratomas.[138] They may occur in pure form, but in approximately one-third of cases, multiple cell types are present. Other malignant components, including adenocarcinoma, squamous cell carcinoma, small cell undifferentiated carcinoma, neuroblastoma, rhabdomyosarcoma as well as other sarcomas, may be present or even represent the predominant tissue type, as usually occurs in immature teratomas.[136] Other hematologic malignancies, such as acute myeloid leukemia, acute nonlymphocytic leukemia, erythroleukemia, myelodysplastic syndrome, malignant histiocytosis, thrombocytosis, and one of the most interesting, acute megakaryocytic leukemia, have also been reported. Hematologic malignancies may antedate the discovery of the germ cell tumor or occur synchronously.

Karyotypic abnormalities, particularly the 47XXY pattern of Klinefelter syndrome, have been found in up to 20% of patients.[139]

Eighty-five percent to 95% of patients have obvious distant metastases at the time of diagnosis. Common metastatic sites include lung, pleura, lymph nodes, liver, and, less commonly, bone.[137]

Diagnosis

Many patients with benign tumors, including 50% of teratomas, are asymptomatic; however, 90% to 100% of patients with malignant tumors have symptoms of chest pain, dyspnea, cough, fever, or other findings related to compression or invasion of surrounding mediastinal structures.[139,140]

Seminomas grow slowly and metastasize later than their nonseminomatous counterparts, and they may have reached a large size by the time of diagnosis. Twenty percent to 30% of mediastinal seminomas are asymptomatic when discovered,[137] symptoms are usually related to compression or even invasion of surrounding mediastinal structures. Pulmonary and other intrathoracic metastases are present in 60% to 70% of patients. Extrathoracic metastases usually involve bone.[137]

Determination of serum tumor markers is important in the diagnosis and follow-up of mediastinal germ cell tumors. Immunoassays for serum β-hCG and AFP should be obtained in all patients who have mediastinal masses suspicious for germ cell tumors. Elevation of β-hCG and AFP confirm a malignant component to the tumor. AFP or β-hCG, or both, are elevated in 80% to 85% of nonseminomatous germ cell tumors, with AFP being detected in 60% to 80% of these tumors and β-hCG in 30% to 50%.[140] Patients with benign teratomas have normal markers, and patients with pure seminoma may have low levels of β-hCG, but AFP is not detected.

Mediastinal germ cell tumors are most often detected on the basis of standard chest radiographs. More than 95% of the chest films are abnormal, with almost all masses noted in the anterior mediastinum. Three percent to 8% of tumors arise within the posterior mediastinum.[139] Chest CT scans demonstrate the extent of disease, relationship to surrounding structures, and presence of cystic areas and calcification within the tumor. They appear on CT scans as large inhomogeneous masses containing areas of hemorrhage and necrosis. Sonographic patterns may improve the diagnostic accuracy of CT alone in mediastinal teratomas.[141] Abdominal imaging should be performed to assess for possible liver metastases. Although careful examination of the testes, including a testicular ultrasound, should always be performed, it is not necessary to perform blind orchiectomy or testicular biopsy in patients with normal physical examinations and unremarkable ultrasound findings,[136] since an isolated tumor mass in the anterior mediastinum without retroperitoneal nodal involvement is not consistent with a primary testicular tumor.

The diagnosis of nonseminomatous germ cell tumors can often be made without tissue biopsy.[142] In many centers, the presence of an anterior mediastinal mass in a young male with elevated serum tumor markers (AFP and β-hCG) is adequate to initiate treatment. If a tissue diagnosis is deemed necessary, fine- or core-needle–guided aspiration with cytologic staining for tumor markers may be used for confirmation. An anterior mediastinotomy provides the best approach for open biopsy if necessary.[142]

Management by Histology

Mediastinal germ cell tumors are not formally staged according to the American Joint Committee on Cancer (AJCC) staging system but can be localized, locally advanced, and metastatic. Due to the lack of a widely accepted staging system, these tumors will be discussed by histologic subtype.

Teratoma

Treatment of "benign" mediastinal teratoma consists of complete surgical resection, which results in excellent long-term cure rates. Radiotherapy and chemotherapy play no role in the management of this tumor. The tumor may be adherent to surrounding structures, necessitating resection of pericardium, pleura, or lung. Resection of mature teratomas has been shown to result in prolonged survival with little chance of recurrence.[138] Currently, a trial of cisplatin-based combination chemotherapy (up to four cycles of cisplatin, etoposide, and bleomycin or vinblastine, ifosfamide, and cisplatin, if responding) is frequently administered before attempted surgical resection.[138]

Seminoma

The treatment of mediastinal seminoma has evolved since the early 1970s. Seminomas are extremely radio-sensitive tumors, and for many years, high-dose mediastinal radiation has been used as initial therapy, resulting in long-term survival rates of 60% to 80%.[142] A review of recommendations for radiation therapy treatment in extragonadal seminoma was reported by Hainsworth and Greco.[137] The most commonly used radiation dose is 35 to 45 Gy. Doses as low as 20 Gy have been reported to be curative, but most reports note a significant local recurrence rate with doses of less than 45 Gy.[137] Radiation portals should include a shaped mediastinal field and both supraclavicular areas.[137]

Mediastinal seminoma often presents as bulky, extensive, and locally invasive disease, requiring large radiotherapy portals. These portals can result in excessive irradiation of surrounding normal lung, heart, and other mediastinal structures. Additionally, 20% to 40% of patients who achieve local control fail at distant sites.[137] Because of these limitations, the use of cisplatin-based combination chemotherapy, which was previously used only in advanced gonadal seminoma, was explored in earlier-stage disease with encouraging results. Lemarie et al.[140] reported that 12 of 13 patients treated experienced complete remission, with two recurrences after treatment. Bokemeyer et al.[143] reported an international analysis of 51 patients with mediastinal seminoma. Chemotherapy was primarily cisplatin based (45, 88%) but also included carboplatin (3, 5.9%), which had a lower objective response rate (80% vs. 93%) and was thus not recommended for treatment. In this study, patients were treated with chemotherapy (38, 74.5%), chemotherapy and radiation (10, 19.6%), or radiation alone (3, 5.9%). The progression-free survival and overall survival were 77% and 88%, respectively. Patients with extrathoracic metastases (6, 11.8%) had a worse prognosis. A collective review of 52 patients was undertaken by Hainsworth and Greco.[137] Fourteen patients had received prior radiation therapy, but all underwent chemotherapy with cisplatin and various combinations of cyclophosphamide, vinblastine, bleomycin, or etoposide. Complete responses to treatment were noted in 85% of patients, and 83% were long-term disease-free survivors.

Pure mediastinal seminoma, even with visceral metastases, falls into the intermediate-risk category of the new International Staging System for Germ Cell Tumors, and all patients should be treated with curative intent. Currently, isolated mediastinal seminoma with minimal disease is most often managed with radiotherapy alone, with excellent long-term survival. Locally advanced and bulky disease should be treated initially with cisplatin-based combination chemotherapy, usually four cycles of cisplatin and etoposide with or without supradiaphragmatic radiotherapy. Patients with distant metastases should undergo chemotherapy alone as initial treatment. Salvage chemotherapy (vinblastine, ifosfamide, and cisplatin) may be required for persistent or recurrent disease.[144]

Despite a recent report of 76.9% long-term survival using primary surgical resection followed by adjuvant therapy,[145] most authors believe that surgery does not play a role in the definitive treatment of seminoma.[142] In addition, surgical debulking of large tumors has not been shown to be of benefit in improving local control or survival.[137]

The management of patients with residual radiographic abnormalities after chemotherapy is controversial. Studies have shown that the residual mass is a dense scirrhous reaction or fibrosis in 85% to 90% of patients, and the presence of viable seminoma is rare. Others have shown a 25% incidence of residual viable seminoma in these patients treated with chemotherapy followed by resection of residual masses larger than 3 cm.[145] Close observation without surgery is recommended for residual masses after chemotherapy unless the mass enlarges.[137,142] Evaluation with PET scans is superior to CT alone with a sensitivity and specificity of 80% and 100, respectively, versus 73% and 73% for CT alone. There were no false-positive scans in lesions larger than 3 cm, and all 11 lesions greater than 3 cm with residual tumor were PET avid, making this a useful modality to avoid unnecessary surgery and empiric radiation therapy.[137,142]

Nonseminomatous Germ Cell Tumors

The mainstay of treatment of nonseminomatous germ cell tumors is cisplatin-based chemotherapy, identical to that of gonadal nonseminomatous germ cell tumors and is discussed more completely in Chapter 99. Overall complete remission rates of 40% to 64% are obtained in most series.[137,138,140,143] In an international review of 287 patients, responses were noted in 178 (64%) and the progression-free and overall survival were 62% and 45%, respectively.[143] Patients with relapsing mediastinal nonseminomatous germ cell tumors do extraordinarily poorly even with salvage therapy, such as vinblastine, ifosfamide, and cisplatin,[144] with only 9 of 79 patients (11%) becoming disease free in one study.[143] Surgical resection of residual disease despite persistently elevated tumor markers has been reported by several authors to be beneficial.[145–147]

Prognosis

Immature teratomas are potentially malignant tumors; their prognosis is influenced by the anatomic site of the tumor, patient age, and the fraction of the tumor that is immature.[138] In patients younger than 15 years, immature teratomas behave similarly to their mature counterparts. In older patients, they may behave as highly malignant tumors. Nonseminomatous mediastinal germ cell tumors carry a poorer prognosis than either pure extragonadal seminoma or their gonadal nonseminomatous counterparts, and all patients with primary mediastinal nonseminomatous germ cell tumors fall into the poor-risk category of the new International Germ Cell Consensus Classification.[148]

Selected References

The full list of references for this chapter appears in the online version.

4. Suster S, Rosai J. Thymic carcinoma: a clinicopathologic study of 60 cases. *Cancer* 1991;67:1025.
5. Tomaszek S, Wigle DA, Keshavjee S, et al. Thymomas: review of current clinical practice. *Ann Thorac Surg* 2009;87:1973.
20. Suster S, Moran CA. Thymoma classification: current status and future trends. *Am J Clin Pathol* 2006;125: 542.
31. Marchevsky AM, Gupta R, McKenna RJ, et al. Evidence-based pathology and the pathologic evaluation of thymomas: the World Health Organization classification can be simplified into only 3 categories other than thymic carcinoma. *Cancer* 2008;112:2780.
41. Okereke IC, Kesler KA, Morad MH, et al. Prognostic indicators after surgery for thymoma. *Ann Thorac Surg* 2010;89:1071.
45. Nasseri F, Eftekhari F. Clinical and radiologic review of the normal and abnormal thymus: pearls and pitfalls. *Radiographics* 2010;30(2):413.
49. Sun YM Lee, KS, Kim T, et al. 18F-FDG PET/CT of Thymic epithelial tumors: usefullness for distinguishing and staging tumor subgroups. *J Nucl Med* 2006;47(10):1628.
57. Falkson CB, Bezjak A, Darling G, et al. The management of thymoma: a systematic review and practice guideline. *J Thorac Oncol* 2009;4(7):911.
58. Detterbeck F, Giaccone G, Loehrer P, et al. International Thymic Malignancy Interest Group. *J Thorac Oncol* 2010;5(1):1.
60. Kondo K, Monden Y. Therapy for thymic epithelial tumors: a clinical study of 1,320 patients from Japan. *Ann Thorac Surg* 2003;76:878.
63. Rea F, Marulli G, Bortolotti L, et al. Experience with the "Da Vinci" robotic system for thymectomy in patients with myasthenia gravis: report of 33 cases. *AnnThorac Surg* 2006;81(2):455.
64. Eng TY, Thomas CR Jr. Radiation therapy in the management of thymic tumors. *Semin Thorac Cardiovasc Surg* 2005;17(1):32.
72. Wright CD, Wain JC, Wong DR, et al. Predictors of recurrence in thymic tumors: importance of invasion, World Health Organization histology, and size. *J Thorac Cardiovasc Surg* 2005;130:1413.
73. D'Angelillo RM, Trodella L, Ramella S, et al. Novel prognostic groups in thymic epithelial tumors: assessment of risk and therapeutic strategy selection. *Int J Radiat Oncol Biol Phys* 2008;71(2):420.
81. Tiseo M, Ardizzoni A. Chemotherapy in the treatment of thymic tumors. *Oncol Rev* 2008;2:95.

83. Hammond-Thelin LA, Thomas CR Jr. Systemic therapeutic options in thymic malignancies: a glimmer of hope. *Rev Recent Clin Trials* 2007;2:191.
89. Magois E, Guigay J, Blancard PS, et al. Multimodal treatment of thymic carcinoma: report of nine cases. *Lung Cancer* 2008;59:126.
95. Fang W, Chen W, Chen G, et al. Surgical management of thymic epithelial tumors: a retrospective review of 204 cases. *Ann Thorac Surg* 2005;80:2002.
101. Korst RJ, Kansler AL, Christos PJ, et al. Adjuvant radiotherapy for thymic epithelial tumors: a systematic review and meta-analysis. *Ann Thorac Surg* 2009;87:1641.
106. Loehrer PJ, Kim KM, Aisner SC, et al. Cisplatin plus doxorubicin plus cyclophosphamide in metastatic or recurrent thymoma: final results of an intergroup trial. *J Clin Oncol* 1994;12:1164.
108. Giaccone G, Ardizzoni A, Kirkpatrick A, et al. Cisplatin and etoposide combination chemotherapy for locally advanced or metastatic thymoma: a phase II study of the European Organization for Research and Treatment of Lung Cancer Cooperative Group. *J Clin Oncol* 1996;14:814.
112. Kunitoh H, Tamura T, Shibata T, et al. A phase II trial of dose-dense chemotherapy followed by surgical resection and/or thoracic radiotherapy in locally advanced thymoma: report of a Japan Clinical Oncology Group trial (JCOG 9606). *Br J Cancer* 2010;103(1):6.
129. Moran CA, Suster S. Neuroendocrine carcinomas (carcinoid tumor) of the thymus. *Am J Clin Pathol* 2000;114:100.
143. Bokemeyer C, Nichols CR, Draz J, et al. Extragonadal germ cell tumors of the mediastinum and retroperitoneum: results from an international analysis. *J Clin Onocol* 2002;20:1864.
144. Becherer A, De Santis M, Karanikas G, Szabó M, et al. FDG PET is superior to CT in the prediction of viable tumour in post-chemotherapy seminoma residuals. *Eur J Radiol* 2005;54(2):284.
146. Nakamura Y, Matsumura A, et al. Cisplatin-based chemotherapy followed by surgery for malignant nonseminomatous germ cell tumor of mediastinum: one institution's experience. *Gen Thorac Cardiovasc Surg* 2009; 57(7):363.
147. Kesler KA, Einhorn LH. Multimodality treatment of germ cell tumors of the mediastinum. *Thorac Surg Clin* 2009;19(1):63.
148. International Germ Cell Collaborative Group. International germ cell consensus classification: a prognostic factor-based staging system for metastatic germ cell cancers. *J Clin Oncol* 1997;15:594.

SECTION 3: CANCERS OF THE GASTROINTESTINAL TRACT

CHAPTER 78 MOLECULAR BIOLOGY OF THE ESOPHAGUS AND STOMACH

ANIL K. RUSTGI

This chapter will deal with the molecular biology of esophageal and gastric cancers. The reader is referred to Chapters 79 and 80 for detailed information about the epidemiology, etiology, pathology, clinical manifestations, diagnosis, and therapy of esophageal and gastric cancers. There are several key aspects in the elucidation of the genetic basis of esophageal and gastric cancers through molecular biology approaches. These include, but are not limited to, new insights into underlying pathogenesis, possibilities for risk stratification and prognosis, correlations with traditional pathology classification schemes, development of new diagnostics, and potential applications in imaging and therapy. In considering the genetic underpinnings of esophageal and gastric cancers, or for any cancer, critical appraisal is required of oncogenes, tumor suppressor genes, and DNA mismatch repair genes as they modulate, either positively or negatively, growth factor receptor–mediating signaling cascades, transcription of target genes, and cell-cycle progression. These molecular networks conspire to influence cellular behaviors, such as proliferation, differentiation, apoptosis, senescence, and response to stress and injury. The exquisite equilibrium that is the signature of normal cellular homeostasis is perturbed in uncontrolled cell growth, resulting in eventual evolution of premalignant stages and malignant transformation. However, the time required for malignant transformation varies, depending on cellular- and tissue-specific context, and is affected by environmental factors.

The salient features of tumorigenesis and acquisition of the malignant phenotype that are required, as described by Hanahan and Weinberg,[1] include growth signal autonomy, ability to surmount antigrowth signals, evasion of apoptosis, unlimited replicative ability, angiogenesis, and invasion and metastatic potential. More recently, the role of inflammation in carcinogenesis has gained much attention.

MOLECULAR BIOLOGY OF ESOPHAGEAL CANCER

The vast majority of esophageal cancers are of two subtypes: esophageal squamous cell cancer (ESCC) and esophageal adenocarcinoma (EAD). ESCC is preceded by squamous dysplasia, whereas EAD is preceded by Barrett's esophagus or incomplete intestinal metaplasia of the normal squamous epithelium of the esophagus (Fig. 78.1). Barrett's esophagus undergoes transition from low-grade and high-grade dysplasia before converting into EAD. ESCC and EAD have common and divergent genetic features as manifest by alterations in canonical oncogenes and tumor suppressor genes in somatic cells of tumors (Table 78.1). However, inherited predisposition to ESCC is rare, as described in tylosis palmaris et plantaris. Although the gene mutation for tylosis has remained elusive, the region of allelic deletion is on chromosome 17p.[2] Similarly, there is no classic syndrome that distinguishes familial Barrett's esophagus or familial EAD. That being said, studies continue to analyze families with Barrett's esophagus in an effort to identify relevant genes or single-nucleotide polymorphisms. It is estimated that about 7% of patients with Barrett's esophagus may have a family history. As a separate consideration, ESCC or EAD does not appear to emerge from infectious etiologies, although a small subset of ESCC is associated with human papillomavirus in some endemic regions of the world.

The Epidermal Growth Factor Receptor

The epidermal growth factor receptor (EGFR) family of receptor tyrosine kinases stimulates a number of signal transduction cascades (e.g., *Ras/Raf/MEK/ERK, PI3K/AKT*) that regulate diverse cellular processes, such as proliferation, differentiation, survival, migration, and adhesion.[3] These signaling pathways are important in normal cellular homeostasis, but aberrant activation of the EGFR members is crucial in esophageal carcinogenesis. This family of receptors comprises EGFR (also referred to as *erbB1*), *erbB2*, *erbB3*, and *erbB4*. The receptors have the ability to homo- or heterodimerize on engagement with one of several ligands: TGF (transforming growth factor)-α, EGF (epidermal growth factor), amphiregulin, heparin-binding EGF-like growth factor, betacellulin, and epiregulin. Tyrosine phosphorylation of homo- or heterodimers of EGFRs creates docking sites for signaling proteins or adapter proteins. EGFR is commonly overexpressed in early-stage esophageal cancer, and overexpression correlates with a poor prognosis.[4–7] EGFR overexpression is typically due to increased engagement with ligands and decreased turnover. However, mutation of a tyrosine residue in the cytoplasmic domain is rare. Increased expression of TGF-α and EGF has been detected in Barrett's esophagus, EAD, and ESCC.[8–12] EGFR overexpression may predict a poor response to chemoradiotherapy[13,14] and is associated with decreased survival in patients with squamous cell carcinoma.[13] Furthermore, EGFR overexpression was associated with recurrent disease and diminished overall survival in patients undergoing esophagectomy for ESCC.[14,15] In contrast to EGFR, it is not clear if *erbB2* overexpression is consistently found either in ESCC or EAD.

Normal esophagus → Squamous dysplasia → Squamous cell cancer

Normal esophagus → Intestinal metaplasia → Low-grade dysplasia → High-grade dysplasia → Adenocarcinoma

FIGURE 78.1 Progression of stages in esophageal squamous cell cancer and esophageal adenocarcinoma.

Cyclin D1 and *p16INK4a*

The mammalian cell cycle is regulated exquisitely by cyclins, cyclin-dependent kinases (CDK), and cyclin-dependent kinase inhibitors (CDKi such as p15, p16, p21, and p27). During G1 phase, the cyclin D1 oncogene complexes with either CDK4 or CDK6 to phosphorylate the retinoblastoma (pRb) tumor suppressor protein and, in so doing, relieves the negative regulatory effect of pRb, allowing the E2F family of transcription factors to propel the cell cycle toward the G_1/S phase transition.[16] Toward the late G_1 phase, cyclin E complexes with CDKs to phosphorylate p107, which is related to pRb, and liberate more E2F members to navigate the cell cycle into S phase. As with EGFR, cyclin D1 overexpression is found in premalignant lesions, such as esophageal squamous dysplasia or Barrett's esophagus, and the majority of early-stage ESCC or EAD.[17,18] Additionally, cyclin D1 overexpression correlates with poor outcomes and survival as well as poor response to chemotherapy.[19,20]

Although cyclin D1 overexpression accounts for cyclin D1 dysregulation, other mechanisms include mutations in cyclin D1 and mutations in Fbx4, which is the E3 ligase for cyclin D1, thereby preventing degradation of cyclin D1 in the cytoplasm and reimportation into the nucleus, where it exerts its oncogenic effects.[21]

In a similar vein, *p16INK4a* is an early genetic alteration, via promoter hypermethylation, point mutation, or allelic deletion, in Barrett's esophagus and EAD, but interestingly, a late event in ESCC. Loss of heterozygosity of 9p21, the locus for both p16 and p15, has been demonstrated with high frequency in both dysplastic Barrett's epithelium and Barrett's adenocarcinoma (90% and more than 80% of cases, respectively).[22,23] Promoter hypermethylation, which prevents tumor suppressor function by blocking transcription, has been documented and correlates with the degree of dysplasia in Barrett's esophagus. It is present in up to 75% of specimens with high-grade dysplasia and is found in almost 50% of patients with adenocarcinoma of the esophagus.[24] Point mutations of p16 in ESCC have been found and promoter hypermethylation has been noted in up to 50% of these tumors.[25,26] *Rb* gene mutation is not found in either type of esophageal neoplasm, but allelic loss of 13q where the locus of the *Rb* gene resides is found in up to 50% of patients with Barrett's adenocarcinoma and squamous cell carcinoma.[18,27] This can correlate with diminished or loss of pRb protein in Barrett's esophagus with dysplasia, EAD, and ESCC.[28,29]

TABLE 78.1

COMMON MOLECULAR GENETIC ALTERATIONS OBSERVED IN ESOPHAGEAL AND GASTRIC CANCERS

Oncogenes
Epidermal growth factor receptor (*EGFR*)
Cyclin D1
Tumor suppressor genes
P16INK4a
p53
E-cadherin
DNA mismatch repair genes (*hMLH1, hMSH2*)
Mismatch repair instability

p53 Tumor Suppressor Gene

p53 is one of the most commonly mutated genes in human cancer.[22–24] *p53* (molecular weight approximately 53 kDa) is a tumor suppressor that interrupts the G_1 phase to evaluate and permit repair of damaged DNA, which may arise from environmental exposure (e.g., irradiation, ultraviolet light) or cellular stress.[30] In the face of irreparable damage, *p53* induces apoptosis. The *p53* transcription factor binds DNA to activate or suppress a large repertoire of target genes.[31] *p53* mutations induce loss of cell-cycle checkpoints and promote genomic instability. The majority of *p53* mutations occur in the DNA-binding region, and more than 80% of them are missense mutations resulting in loss of wild type *p53* function.[32] Wild type *p53* has a short half-life and is difficult to detect by immunohistochemistry; mutation in *p53* results in stabilization of the protein and allows for easier detection by immunohistochemistry.

Detection of mutated p53 protein by immunohistochemistry has been demonstrated with increasing frequency during histologic progression from Barrett's esophagus (5%) through dysplasia (65% to 75%) to frank adenocarcinoma (up to 90%).[33–36] Thus, *p53* mutation or loss of heterozygosity appears early in Barrett's esophagus and EAD. Both mutant p53 protein detected by immunohistochemistry and specific *p53* gene mutations detected by genomic sequencing have been identified in 40% to 75% of patients with ESCC.[37–40] The presence of a *p53* point mutation correlates with response to induction chemoradiotherapy and predicted survival after esophagectomy in patients with either ESCC or EAD.[41]

Telomerase Activation

Maintenance of telomere length allows DNA replication to be sustained indefinitely. Aberrant expression of telomerase has been observed in most esophageal cancers examined to date.[42] Morales et al.[43] observed increased telomerase expression in 100% of adenocarcinoma and Barrett's esophagus cases with high-grade dysplasia. Telomerase activation is important, but alternative mechanisms to maintain the length of telomeres may operate in these cancers as well.[44]

Tumor Invasion and Metastasis

Loss of cell-cell adhesion can lead to both invasion and metastases. Alterations in expression of E-cadherin, a cell-cell adhesion molecule, or its associated catenins disrupt cell-cell interactions, which results in the potential for tumor progression.[45] Reduced expression of E-cadherin has been correlated with progression from Barrett's esophagus to dysplasia and finally to adenocarcinoma, and also observed in ESCC.[46,47]

Models of ESCC and EAD

Advances in diagnosis and therapy of esophageal neoplasms will ultimately be fostered through cell lines, xenotransplantation mouse models, surgically based rodent models, and genetically engineered mouse models. There is a vast array of cell lines established from primary and metastatic human esophageal cancers that allow perturbation of gene expression to gauge effects on cellular behavior. Recently, organotypic (three-dimensional) cell culture models, which mimic human tissue, have revealed that the combination of EGFR and mutant *p53* results in transformation of human esophageal epithelial cells immortalized with hTERT.[48] A classic rodent model involves total gastrectomy followed by esophagojejunostomy.[49] This creates a milieu whereby the esophagus is exposed to high concentrations of bile ("nonacid reflux") with the development of Barrett's esophagus and EAD. In transgenic mice in which cyclin D1 is targeted to the esophagus, esophagi reveal evidence of dysplasia that evolves into squamous cell cancer on crossbreeding the mice with *p53* haploinsufficiency or loss.[50] Rodents have also been treated with nitrosamines to yield esophageal papillomas and ESCC.[51,52]

The underlying fate switch between ESCC and EAD may be influenced as well by the expression and function of "lineage"-specific transcriptional factors as demonstrated through functional genomics. To that end, *SOX2*, found to be part of an amplicon on chromosome 3q26.33 in human ESCC, fosters growth of these cancers. This may have implications in the therapy of human ESCC.[53]

MOLECULAR BIOLOGY OF GASTRIC CANCER

The most common type of gastric cancer is adenocarcinoma, of which there are two subtypes: intestinal and diffuse. They are distinguished by different anatomic locations within the stomach, variable clinical outcomes, and different pathogenesis. The intestinal type of sporadic gastric adenocarcinoma has a hallmark progression from normal gastric epithelium to chronic atrophic gastritis (typically due to *Helicobacter pylori* infection) to intestinal metaplasia (which has some overlapping but also different features than intestinal metaplasia of Barrett's esophagus) to dysplasia to cancer (Fig. 78.2). Diffuse-type gastric adenocarcinoma is even more invasive and aggressive in its behavior, has overlap with lobular-type breast cancer, and may be highlighted by loss of E-cadherin.

Inherited Susceptibility

Case-control studies have observed consistent, up to threefold, increases in risk for gastric cancer among relatives of patients with gastric cancer.[54,55] Studies of monozygotic twins have even shown a slight trend toward increased concordance of gastric cancers compared with dizygotic twins.[56,57] Large families with an autosomal dominant, highly penetrant inherited predisposition for the development of gastric cancer are rare. However, early-onset diffuse gastric cancers have been described and linked to the *E-cadherin/CDH1* locus on chromosome 16q and associated with mutations in this gene.[58] This seminal finding has been confirmed in other studies with gastric cancers at a relatively high (67% to 83%) penetrant rate.[59–62] Thus, E-cadherin mutation testing should be considered in the appropriate clinical setting. In fact, prophylactic gastrectomy should be considered strongly in families with germ line E-cadherin mutation even without gross mucosal abnormalities by endoscopic examination of the stomach.[63]

Lynch syndrome or hereditary nonpolyposis colon cancer involves germ line mutations of DNA mismatch repair genes.[64] Gastric adenocarcinoma may be observed in some families with Lynch syndrome. Gastric cancers have also been noted to occur in patients with familial adenomatous polyposis and Peutz-Jeghers syndrome.

The Role of *Helicobacter pylori* Infection and Other Host-Environmental Factors

As a commensal organism, *H. pylori* infection is widely prevalent throughout the world. Despite its classification by the World Health Organization as a class I carcinogen, infection with *H. pylori* does not typically lead to gastric cancer. This underscores the importance of other factors, such as virulence, environmental, and host factors, as well as genetic polymorphisms (e.g., in interleukin-1β, a potent inhibitor of acid secretion).[65] The blood group A phenotype has been reported to be associated with gastric cancers.[66,67] *H. pylori* may adhere to the Lewis blood group antigen, indicating a factor for increased risk for gastric cancer.[68] Small variant alleles of a mucin gene, *Muc1*, were found to be associated with gastric cancer patients when compared with a blood donor control population.[69] Epstein-Barr virus infection has been noted in a certain type of gastric carcinoma (lymphoepithelioid type), although the importance of this is unclear.[70]

Molecular Genetic Alterations

In contrast to ESCC, EAD, pancreatic cancer, and colon cancer in which certain oncogenes and tumor suppressor genes are altered with high frequency, such degree of alteration is not observed in sporadic gastric cancers. A reasonably prevalent alteration is microsatellite instability, the result of changes in DNA mismatch repair genes (Table 78.1). Microsatellite instability and associated alterations of the *TGF*-beta *II receptor*, *IGFRII*, *BAX*, *E2F-4*, *hMSH3*, and *hMSH6* genes are found in a subset of gastric carcinomas.[71–75] Microsatellite instability has been found in 13% to 44% of sporadic gastric carcinomas.[76] A high degree of microsatellite instability occurs in gastric cancers of the intestinal type, reduced involvement of lymph nodes, enhanced lymphoid infiltration, and better prognosis.[77] This is reminiscent of colon cancers associated with Lynch syndrome.

The *p53* tumor suppressor gene is consistently altered in most gastric cancers.[78] In a study of the promoter region of p16 in gastric cancers, a significant number (41%) exhibited CpG island methylation.[79] Many cases with hypermethylation of promoter regions displayed the phenotype with a high degree of microsatellite instability and multiple sites of methylation, including the *hMLH1* promoter region.[80]

Many sporadic diffuse gastric cancers display altered E-cadherin, a transmembrane, calcium-dependent adhesion molecule important in epithelial cell homophilic and heterophilic interactions. E-cadherin may be down-regulated in gastric carcinogenesis (especially diffuse gastric adenocarcinoma) by point mutation, allelic deletion, or promoter methylation.[81,82] In addition, during epithelial-mesenchymal transition, E-cadherin transcription can be silenced by transcriptional factors such as Snail and Slug. However, it is not clear if epithelial-mesenchymal transition is an important process in gastric carcinogenesis, as is believed to be the case, for example, in breast cancer.

Alterations in a number of other oncogenes and tumor suppressor genes have been described in a very small subset of gastric cancers by polymerase chain reaction–based or immunohistochemical analysis, but the variability in methods and lack of uniformity in quality control make these observations less compelling. As with esophageal cancer, high-throughput assays, such as single-nucleotide polymorphism arrays, chromosomal genomic hybridization (to assess chromosomal gains

Normal gastric mucosa → chronic atrophic gastritis → Intestinal metaplasia → Low-grade dysplasia → High-grade dysplasia → Adenocarcinoma

FIGURE 78.2 Progression of stages in intestinal-type gastric adenocarcinoma.

and losses) arrays, gene expression profiling through microarrays, and tissue- and plasma-based proteomics may unravel molecular signatures (and even specific genes and/or pathways) that define subtypes of gastric cancers, different stages of gastric cancers, and correlations with clinical outcomes.

Models of Gastric Cancer

Genetically engineered mouse models of gastric cancer have emerged in rapid fashion in recent years, indicating that activated Wnt signaling and induced downstream effectors, *p53* inactivation, *APC* gene inactivation, *Smad4* gene inactivation, and gastrin are critical factors.[83–87] Gastric cancers in these protean mouse models are facilitated by concomitant infection with *Helicobacter*.[88,89] Furthermore, recruitment of bone marrow stem cells may augment the effects of *Helicobacter* infection during gastric carcinogenesis.[90]

Recently, it has been demonstrated that overexpression of interleukin-1β in mice results in gastric inflammation and cancer, with concomitant recruitment of immature myeloid cells (also referred to as *myeloid-derived suppressor cells*).[91]

Selected References

The full list of references for this chapter appears in the online version.

1. Hanahan D, Weinberg RA. The hallmarks of cancer. *Cell* 2000;100:57.
3. Schlessinger J. Cell signaling by receptor tyrosine kinases. *Cell* 2000;103(2): 211.
5. Torzewski M, Sarbia M, Verreet P, et al. The prognostic significance of epidermal growth factor receptor expression in squamous cell carcinomas of the oesophagus. *Anticancer Res* 1997;17(5B):3915.
8. Jankowski J, McMenemin R, Hopwood D, et al. Abnormal expression of growth regulatory factors in Barrett's oesophagus. *Clin Sci (Lond)* 1991;81: 663.
10. Jankowski J, Hopwood D, Wormsley KG. Flow-cytometric analysis of growth-regulatory peptides and their receptors in Barrett's oesophagus and oesophageal adenocarcinoma. *Scand J Gastroenterol* 1992;27:147.
12. Yacoub L, Goldman H, Odze RD. Transforming growth factor-alpha, epidermal growth factor receptor, and MiB-1 expression in Barrett's-associated neoplasia: correlation with prognosis. *Mod Pathol* 1997;10:105.
13. Itakura Y, Sasano H, Shiga C, et al. Epidermal growth factor receptor overexpression in esophageal carcinoma: an immunohistochemical study correlated with clinicopathologic findings and DNA amplification. *Cancer* 1994; 74:795.
17. Arber N, Lightdale C, Rotterdam H, et al. Increased expression of the cyclin D1 gene in Barrett's esophagus. *Cancer Epidemiol Biomarkers Prev* 1996; 5:457.
19. Shamma A, Doki Y, Shiozaki H, et al. Cyclin D1 overexpression in esophageal dysplasia: a possible biomarker for carcinogenesis of esophageal squamous cell carcinoma. *Int J Oncol* 2000;16:261.
20. Sarbia M, Bektas N, Muller W, et al. Expression of cyclin E in dysplasia, carcinoma, and nonmalignant lesions of Barrett esophagus. *Cancer* 1999;86: 2597.
21. Barbash O, Zamfirova P, Lin DI, et al. Mutations in Fbx4 inhibit dimerization of the SCF(Fbx4) ligase and contribute to cyclin D1 overexpression in human cancer. *Cancer Cell* 2008;14(1):68.
22. Barrett MT, Sanchez CA, Galipeau PC, et al. Allelic loss of 9p21 and mutation of the CDKN2/p16 gene develop as early lesions during neoplastic progression in Barrett's esophagus. *Oncogene* 1996;13:1867.
24. Klump B, Hsieh CJ, Holzmann K, et al. Hypermethylation of the CDKN2/ p16 promoter during neoplastic progression in Barrett's esophagus. *Gastroenterology* 1998;115:1381.
25. Xing EP, Nie Y, Wang LD, et al. Aberrant methylation of p16INK4a and deletion of p15INK4b are frequent events in human esophageal cancer in Linxian, China. *Carcinogenesis* 1999;20:77.
26. Maesawa C, Tamura G, Nishizuka S, et al. Inactivation of the CDKN2 gene by homozygous deletion and de novo methylation is associated with advanced stage esophageal squamous cell carcinoma. *Cancer Res* 1996;56:3875.
28. Coppola D, Schreiber RH, Mora L, et al. Significance of Fas and retinoblastoma protein expression during the progression of Barrett's metaplasia to adenocarcinoma. *Ann Surg Oncol* 1999;6:298.
29. Ikeguchi M, Oka S, Gomyo Y, et al. Clinical significance of retinoblastoma protein (pRB) expression in esophageal squamous cell carcinoma. *J Surg Oncol* 2000;73:104.
33. Hamelin R, Flejou JF, Muzeau F, et al. TP53 gene mutations and p53 protein immunoreactivity in malignant and premalignant Barrett's esophagus. *Gastroenterology* 1994;107:1012.
35. Younes M, Lebovitz RM, Lechago LV, et al. p53 protein accumulation in Barrett's metaplasia, dysplasia, and carcinoma: a follow-up study. *Gastroenterology* 1993;105:1637.
37. Gaur D, Arora S, Mathur M, et al. High prevalence of p53 gene alterations and protein overexpression in human esophageal cancer: correlation with dietary risk factors in India. *Clin Cancer Res* 1997;3:2129.
38. Kato H, Yoshikawa M, Miyazaki T, et al. Expression of p53 protein related to smoking and alcoholic beverage drinking habits in patients with esophageal cancers. *Cancer Lett* 2001;167:65.
40. Taniere P, Martel-Planche G, Saurin JC, et al. TP53 mutations, amplification of P63 and expression of cell cycle proteins in squamous cell carcinoma of the oesophagus from a low incidence area in Western Europe. *Br J Cancer* 2001;85:721.
41. Ribeiro U Jr, Finkelstein SD, Safatle-Ribeiro AV, et al. p53 sequence analysis predicts treatment response and outcome of patients with esophageal carcinoma. *Cancer* 1998;83:7.
43. Morales CP, Lee EL, Shay JW. In situ hybridization for the detection of telomerase RNA in the progression from Barrett's esophagus to esophageal adenocarcinoma. *Cancer* 1998;83:652.
44. Opitz OG, Suliman Y, Hahn WC, et al. Cyclin D1 overexpression and p53 inactivation immortalize primary oral keratinocytes by a telomerase-independent mechanism. *J Clin Invest* 2001;108(5):725.
45. Christofori G, Semb H. The role of the cell-adhesion molecule E-cadherin as a tumour-suppressor gene. *Trends Biochem Sci* 1999;24:73.
47. Takeno S, Noguchi T, Fumoto S, et al. E-cadherin expression in patients with esophageal squamous cell carcinoma: promoter hypermethylation, Snail overexpression, and clinicopathologic implications. *Am J Clin Pathol* 2004;122(1):78.
48. Okawa T, Michaylira CZ, Kalabis J, et al. The functional interplay between EGFR overexpression, hTERT activation, and p53 mutation in esophageal epithelial cells with activation of stromal fibroblasts induces tumor development, invasion, and differentiation. *Genes Dev* 2007;21(21):2788.
50. Opitz OG, Harada H, Suliman Y, et al. A mouse model of human oral-esophageal cancer. *J Clin Invest* 2002;110:761.
51. Siglin JC, Khare L, Stoner GD. Evaluation of dose and treatment duration on the esophageal tumorigenicity of *N*-nitrosomethylbenzylamine in rats. *Carcinogenesis* 1995;16(2):259.
53. Bass AJ, Watanabe H, Mermel CH, et al. SOX2 is an amplified lineage-survival oncogene in lung and esophageal squamous cell carcinomas. *Nat Genet* 2009;41(11):1238.
58. Guilford P, Hopkins J, Harraway J, et al. E-cadherin germline mutations in familial gastric cancer. *Nature* 1998;392:402.
59. Gayther SA, Gorringe KL, Ramus SJ, et al. Identification of germ-line E-cadherin mutations in gastric cancer families of European origin. *Cancer Res* 1998;58:4086.
62. Pharoah PD, Caldas C. Incidence of gastric cancer and breast cancer in CDH1 (E-cadherin) mutation carriers from hereditary diffuse gastric cancer families. *Gastroenterology* 2001;121:1348.
63. Lewis FR, Mellinger JD, Hayashi A, et al. Prophylactic total gastrectomy for familial gastric cancer. *Surgery* 2001;130(4):612.
64. Chung DC, Rustgi AK. The hereditary nonpolyposis colorectal cancer syndrome: genetics and clinical implications. *Ann Intern Med* 2003;138(7):560.
65. El Omar EM, Rabkin CS, Gammon MD, et al. Increased risk of noncardiac gastric cancer associated with proinflammatory cytokine gene polymorphisms. *Gastroenterology* 2003;124:1193.
69. Silva F, Carvalho F, Peixoto A, et al. MUC1 polymorphism confers increased risk for intestinal metaplasia in a Colombian population with chronic gastritis. *Eur J Hum Genet* 2003;11(5):380.
70. Lee HS, Chang MS, Yang HK, Lee BL, Kim WH. Epstein-Barr virus-positive gastric carcinoma has a distinct protein expression profile in comparison with Epstein-Barr virus-negative carcinoma. *Clin Cancer Res* 2004;10(5): 1698.
71. Kim SJ, Bang YJ, Park JG, et al. Genetic changes in the transforming growth factor beta (TGF-beta) type II receptor gene in human gastric cancer cells: correlation with sensitivity to growth inhibition by TGF-beta. *Proc Natl Acad Sci U S A* 1994;91:8772.
72. Yamamoto H, Sawai H, Perucho M. Frameshift somatic mutations in gastrointestinal cancer of the microsatellite mutator phenotype. *Cancer Res* 1997;57:4420.
76. Seruca R, Santos NR, David L, et al. Sporadic gastric carcinomas with microsatellite instability display a particular clinicopathologic profile. *Int J Cancer* 1995;64:32.

77. dos Santos NR, Seruca R, Constancia M, et al. Microsatellite instability at multiple loci in gastric carcinoma: clinicopathologic implications and prognosis. *Gastroenterology* 1996;110:38.
80. Toyota M, Ahuja N, Suzuki H, et al. Aberrant methylation in gastric cancer associated with the CpG island methylator phenotype. *Cancer Res* 1999;59:5438.
82. Grady WM, Willis J, Guilford PJ, et al. Methylation of the CDH1 promoter as the second genetic hit in hereditary diffuse gastric cancer. *Nat Genet* 2000;26:16.
83. Taketo MM. Wnt signaling and gastrointestinal tumorigenesis in mouse models. *Oncogene* 2006;25(57):7522.
84. Fox JG, Dangler CA, Whary MT, et al. Mice carrying a truncated Apc gene have diminished gastric epithelial proliferation, gastric inflammation, and humoral immunity in response to *Helicobacter felis* infection. *Cancer Res* 1997;57(18):3972.
85. Teng Y, Sun AN, Pan XC, et al. Synergistic function of Smad4 and PTEN in suppressing forestomach squamous cell carcinoma in the mouse. *Cancer Res* 2006;66(14):6972.
86. Watson SA, Grabowska AM, El-Zaatari M, Takhar A. Gastrin—active participant or bystander in gastric carcinogenesis? *Nat Rev Cancer* 2006;6(12):936.
87. Wang TC, Dangler CA, Chen D, et al. Synergistic interaction between hypergastrinemia and *Helicobacter* infection in a mouse model of gastric cancer. *Gastroenterology* 2000;118(1):36.
88. Rogers AB, Taylor NS, Whary MT, et al. *Helicobacter pylori* but not high salt induces gastric intraepithelial neoplasia in B6129 mice. *Cancer Res* 2005;65(23):10709.
89. Cai X, Carlson J, Stoicov C, et al. *Helicobacter felis* eradication restores normal architecture and inhibits gastric cancer progression in C57BL/6 mice. *Gastroenterology* 2005;128(7):1937.
90. Houghton J, Stoicov C, Nomura S, et al. Gastric cancer originating from bone marrow-derived cells. *Science* 2004;306(5701):1568.
91. Tu S, Bhagat G, Cui G, et al. Overexpression of interleukin-1beta induces gastric inflammation and cancer and mobilizes myeloid-derived suppressor cells in mice. *Cancer Cell* 2008;14(5):408.

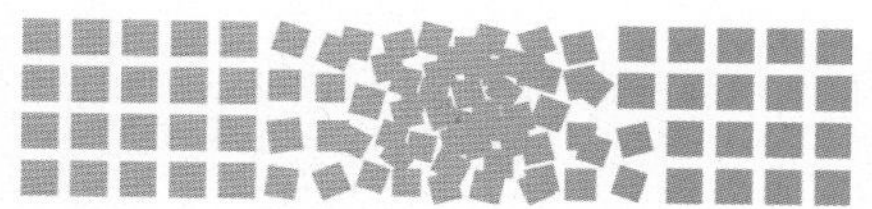

CHAPTER 79 CANCER OF THE ESOPHAGUS

MITCHELL C. POSNER, BRUCE D. MINSKY, AND DAVID H. ILSON

Esophageal cancer is unique among the gastrointestinal tract malignancies because it embodies two distinct histopathologic types: squamous cell carcinoma and adenocarcinoma. Which type of cancer occurs in a given patient or predominates in a given geographic area depends on many variables, including individual lifestyle, socioeconomic pressures, and environmental factors. The United States, along with many other Western countries, has witnessed in recent decades a profound increase in incidence rates of adenocarcinoma, whereas squamous cell carcinoma continues to predominate worldwide. Although it would seem appropriate to individualize treatment of these tumors, in the past they have often been managed as a single entity. While present-day therapeutic interventions have begun to have an impact, with statistically significant improvement in survival over the most recent three successive decades, cancer of the esophagus remains a highly lethal disease as evidenced by the case fatality rate of 90%. However, a more thorough understanding of the initiating events, the molecular biologic basis, and treatment successes and failures has begun to spawn a new era of therapy aimed at targeting both adenocarcinoma and squamous cell carcinoma of the esophagus.

EPIDEMIOLOGY

The epidemiology of esophageal cancer is defined by its substantial variability as a function of histologic type, geographic area, gender, race, and ethnic background.[1] Because of the recent increase in incidence rates of adenocarcinoma, especially in the Western hemisphere, epidemiologic studies are now distinguishing between histologic types when reporting results, whereas in the past, incidence rates of esophageal cancer reflected only squamous cell carcinoma. This remains true in high-incidence areas where published rates are not obtained from population-based tumor registries. These high-incidence areas include Turkey, northern Iran, southern republics of the former Soviet Union, and northern China, where incidence rates exceed 100 per 100,000 person-years. Incidence rates of squamous cell carcinoma may vary 200-fold between different populations in the same geographic area because of unique cultural practices. The highest incidence rates for males (more than 15 per 100,000 person-years) reported from population-based tumor registries were in Calvados, France; Hong Kong; and Miyagi, Japan; and the highest rates for females (more than 5 per 100,000 person-years) were in Mumbai, India; Shanghai, China; and Scotland.[2]

Esophageal cancer is relatively uncommon in the United States, and the lifetime risk of being diagnosed with the disease is less than 1%.[3] It was estimated that 16,470 new cases would be identified in 2009, with over 14,500 patients expected to die of the disease.[4] Age-adjusted incidence rates are highest among African American men, and the predominant histologic type is squamous cell carcinoma (Fig. 79.1). The incidence rates for African American men peaked in the early 1980s, and since then they have shown a marked decline to the current rate of approximately 9 per 100,000 person-years.[4] Incidence rates among white men continue to increase and now exceed 8 per 100,000 person-years, reflecting the marked increase in the incidence of adenocarcinoma of the esophagus of more than 400% in the past two decades.[1] Although the incidence of adenocarcinoma in white females (2 per 100,000) is lower than that in white men, rates of adenocarcinoma have increased in women by more than 300% during the past 20 years. Similar trends have been noted in Western European countries. This trend of increased incidence of adenocarcinoma of the esophagus has paralleled the upward trend in rates of both gastroesophageal reflux disease and obesity.

A steady decline in esophageal cancer mortality has been noted since the mid-1980s in the nonwhite U.S. population, whereas a marked increase in mortality was noted among white men and women during the same period[1] (Fig. 79.2). The mortality rates among African Americans exceed those for all other populations, and men fare more poorly than women. Although survival rates for all esophageal cancer patients are uniformly dismal, regardless of race or gender, 5-year relative survival rates have significantly improved since the 1970s (5% if diagnosed in 1975 to 1977 vs. 17% if diagnosed in 1996 to 2004) based on Surveillance, Epidemiology, and End Results population-based tumor registry reporting.[3] There is no survival difference related to cell type (squamous cell carcinoma vs. adenocarcinoma).

ETIOLOGIC FACTORS AND PREDISPOSING CONDITIONS

Squamous cell carcinoma and adenocarcinoma of the esophagus share some risk factors, whereas other risk factors are specific to one histologic type or the other.

Tobacco and Alcohol Use

Tobacco and alcohol use are considered the major contributing factors in the development of esophageal cancer worldwide. It is estimated that up to 90% of the risk of squamous cell carcinoma of the esophagus in Western Europe and North America can be attributed to tobacco and alcohol use.[5] Population-based studies demonstrate that tobacco and alcohol use are independent risk factors, and their effects are multiplicative, as evidenced by the association of the highest risk of developing esophageal cancer with heavy use of both agents.

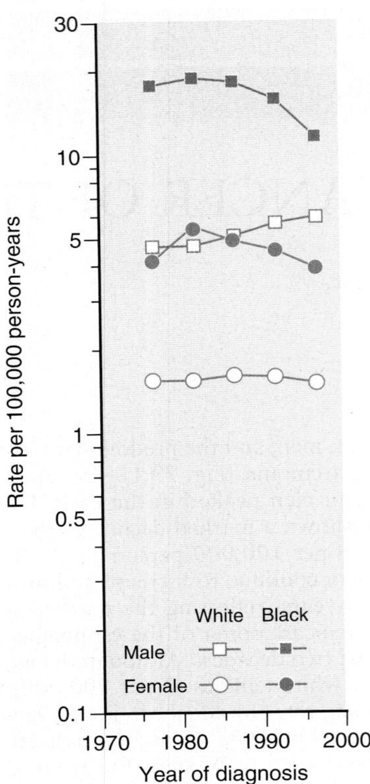

FIGURE 79.1 Trends in age-adjusted incidence rates for esophageal cancer in the United States by race.

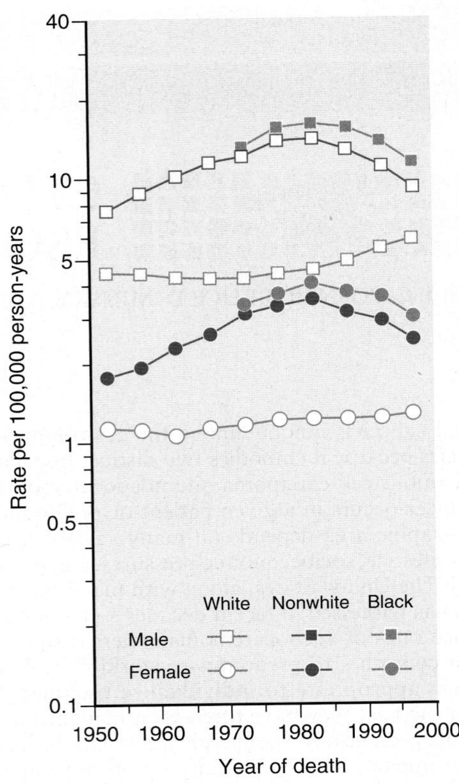

FIGURE 79.2 Trends in esophageal cancer mortality rates in the United States by race and gender.

Approximately 65% and 57% of squamous cell carcinomas of the esophagus have been attributed to smoking tobacco for longer than 6 months in white and African American men, respectively, in the United States.[6] There appears to be a dose–response effect related to the duration and intensity of smoking, and, importantly, there is an impressive (up to 50%) reduction in risk of developing squamous cell carcinoma of the esophagus for those who quit smoking and an inverse relationship between risk and the length of time since cessation of tobacco use.[7] Cigarette smoking in adenocarcinoma of the esophagus leads to a twofold increase in risk for heavy smokers (more than one pack per day).[7,8] Quitting smoking does not appear to decrease the risk of adenocarcinoma, which remains elevated for decades after smoking cessation.[7,8] This suggests that tobacco carcinogens may affect carcinogenesis early on in esophageal adenocarcinoma, and, therefore, the decline in prevalence of smoking in the United States has not had an impact on the risk for the disease.

Alcohol is a major contributing factor in the increased risk of esophageal squamous cell carcinoma in Western countries, likely accounting for 80% of squamous cell carcinoma of the esophagus in men in the United States.[6] A dose–response relationship exists between the amount of alcohol ingested and the risk of developing squamous cell carcinoma.[9,10] In most studies the most commonly consumed beverage in a specific geographic region is the one most frequently associated with increased risk.[1] Although specific carcinogens may be present in a variety of alcoholic beverages, in all likelihood it is alcohol itself, either as a mechanical irritant, promoter of dietary deficiency, or contributor to susceptibility to other carcinogens, that leads to carcinogenesis. Large population-based case-control studies in both the United States and Australia revealed no relationship between alcohol intake and risk of esophageal adenocarcinoma.[11]

Diet and Nutrition

For both squamous cell carcinoma and adenocarcinoma of the esophagus, case-control studies provide evidence of a protective effect of fruits and vegetables, especially those eaten raw.[7,12] These food groups contain a number of micronutrients and dietary components such as vitamins A, C, and E, selenium, carotenoids, and fiber that may prevent carcinogenesis. Deficiencies of the aforementioned nutrients and dietary components, in particular selenium, have been associated with increased risk of esophageal squamous cell carcinoma in some parts of the world.[13] Consumption of hot beverages has been suggested as a risk factor for esophageal cancer in South America.[14]

Socioeconomic Status

Low socioeconomic status as defined by income, education, or occupation is associated with increased risk for esophageal squamous cell carcinoma and, to a lesser degree, for adenocarcinoma.[8,15] In the United States it is estimated that 39% and 69% of squamous cell carcinomas of the esophagus in white men and African American men, respectively, are related to low annual income.[6] A number of occupational and industrial hazards, including exposure to perchloroethylene (dry cleaners, metal polishers), combustion products, and fossil fuels (chimney sweeps, printers, gas station attendants, asphalt and metal workers), silica and metal dust, and asbestos, as well as viral exposure via meat packing and slaughtering, have been suggested as possible risk factors for squamous cell carcinoma but not adenocarcinoma of the esophagus.[2]

Obesity

The prevalence of obesity in the United States markedly increased from 12.8% in the early 1960s to almost 23% between 1988 and 1994.[16] This upward trend parallels that seen for incidence rates of esophageal adenocarcinoma. Increased body mass index (BMI) is a risk factor for adenocarcinoma of the esophagus, and individuals with the highest BMI have up to a sevenfold greater risk of esophageal cancer than those with a low body mass index.[7,17–19] The mechanism by which obesity contributes to an increased risk of esophageal adenocarcinoma is uncertain, although the linkage between obesity and gastroesophageal reflux disease is presumed to be a chief, but not the sole, factor. Recent reports suggest that presence of abdominal or central obesity rather than BMI itself may increase the risk of Barrett's esophagus and subsequent esophageal adenocarcinoma.[20,21] Because of the influence of nutritional and socioeconomic factors, the risk of squamous cell carcinoma of the esophagus increases with decreasing BMI.

Gastroesophageal Reflux Disease

Gastroesophageal reflux disease has been implicated as one of the strongest risk factors for the development of adenocarcinoma of the esophagus.[22,23] Chronic reflux is associated with Barrett's esophagus, the premalignant precursor of esophageal adenocarcinoma. Population-based case-control studies that examined the relationship between symptomatic reflux and risk of adenocarcinoma of the esophagus have demonstrated that increased frequency, severity, and chronicity of reflux symptoms are associated with a 2- to 16-fold increased risk of adenocarcinoma of the esophagus, regardless of the presence of Barrett's esophagus.[22,23] Trends in incidence rates of gastroesophageal reflux disease during the past three decades parallel the time trends of increasing incidence of adenocarcinoma in the United States.

Helicobacter Pylori Infection

Infection with *Helicobacter pylori*, and particularly with cagA+ strains, is inversely associated with the risk of adenocarcinoma of the esophagus.[24,25] The mechanism of action is unclear, although *H. pylori* infection can result in chronic atrophic gastritis, leading to decreased acid production and potentially reducing the development of Barrett's esophagus. Although infection by *H. pylori* cagA+ strains by itself may not increase the risk of squamous cell carcinoma, the concurrent presence of gastric atrophy and *H. pylori* infection has been reported to significantly increase the risk of squamous cell carcinoma.[26] Atrophic gastritis may promote bacterial overgrowth, leading to intragastric nitrosation, with the production of nitrosamines increasing the risk of esophageal squamous cell carcinoma.

Barrett's Esophagus

Barrett's esophagus is defined by the presence of intestinal metaplasia (mucin-producing goblet cells) in columnar cell–lined epithelium that replaces the normal squamous epithelium of the distal esophagus.[27–29] The appearance at endoscopy of salmon-colored columnar epithelium extending about the gastroesophageal junction contrasts with the pale, pink-colored normal squamous epithelium of the esophagus. Although other types of mucosa (gastric fundic or junctional type) have been identified in Barrett's esophagus, specialized intestinal metaplasia confirmed by histologic examination of biopsy specimens is required for the diagnosis of Barrett's esophagus. A diagnosis of Barrett's esophagus confers a 40- to 125-fold higher risk of progressing to esophageal carcinoma compared with the risk in the general population and is the single most important risk factor for developing adenocarcinoma.[30,31] The absolute risk to develop adenocarcinoma in a year is approximately 1 in 200 (absolute risk, 0.5% per patient-year).[31–34] Patients with short- and long-segment Barrett's esophagus are at risk of developing dysplasia and subsequently adenocarcinoma.[35]

The prevalence of Barrett's esophagus in the general population undergoing endoscopy is approximately 1.5%[36]; for those with reflux symptoms, the presence of Barrett's esophagus is 2.3%, and in those without reflux symptoms it is 1.2%. The utility of screening patients with symptomatic reflux is unproven and unlikely to have a significant impact on reducing death from cancer because 40% of patients with adenocarcinoma of the esophagus have no history of reflux,[22] and fewer than 5% of patients undergoing resection for adenocarcinoma were documented to have Barrett's esophagus before seeking medical attention for their symptomatic cancer.[37] Appropriately, the American Gastroenterological Association Institute concluded that there was insufficient evidence supporting screening for Barrett's esophagus in patients with gastroesophageal reflux,[38] and the American College of Gastroenterology Guidelines no longer recommends endoscopic screening of patients with reflux.[39] Both medical and surgical antireflux therapies are effective at reducing or eliminating the symptoms of gastroesophageal reflux, but no clear-cut evidence exists that either therapy reduces the risk of esophageal adenocarcinoma. A randomized Veterans Affairs Cooperative Study of medical and surgical antireflux treatment in patients with severe gastroesophageal reflux disease demonstrated superior control of reflux symptoms in the surgical treatment group but no difference between medical and surgical therapy groups in the incidence of esophageal cancer.[33] Overall survival was significantly decreased in the surgical treatment group as a result of an unexpected excess of deaths from heart disease.

Practice guidelines published by the American College of Gastroenterology recommend surveillance endoscopy for patients with the diagnosis of Barrett's esophagus, and the grade of dysplasia determines the endoscopy interval.[29] Uncontrolled studies suggest that adenocarcinomas identified by surveillance methods are detected at an earlier stage and are associated with a more favorable outcome after esophagectomy.[40–42] However, the efficacy of surveillance endoscopy is unclear, and there are no convincing data demonstrating that surveillance prevents cancer or improves life expectancy.[32,43,44] Macdonald et al.[44] followed 143 patients with Barrett's esophagus for an average of 4.4 years with surveillance endoscopy and identified only one patient with asymptomatic esophageal adenocarcinoma. Similar findings were reported by O'Connor et al.[32] These studies suggest that routine surveillance of patients with Barrett's esophagus is unlikely to alter the natural history of this disease due to the low incidence of adenocarcinoma. Some authors suggest that surgical antireflux therapy causes regression of metaplastic epithelium or interrupts progression from Barrett's esophagus to low-grade and high-grade dysplasia,[45,46] but convincing evidence is lacking. A prospective, randomized trial of medical treatment versus open Nissen fundoplication in patients with Barrett's esophagus with or without low-grade dysplasia showed no statistically significant difference in progression to dysplasia or adenocarcinoma.[47] Progression from intestinal metaplasia to dysplasia in Barrett's esophagus signifies an unequivocal neoplastic change associated with the potential for malignant degeneration. Dysplasia is classified as low grade or high grade. The experience of the pathologist is crucial in correctly diagnosing high-grade dysplasia, which is the most important predictor for esophageal adenocarcinoma.[48] The differentiation of high-grade dysplasia from either low-grade dysplasia, indefinite dysplasia, or absence of dysplasia is straightforward (85% interobserver agreement). However, the diagnosis of low-grade dysplasia as differentiated from either indefinite dysplasia or findings negative for dysplasia is less reproducible (50% to 75% interobserver agreement).[49,50] Any degree of dysplasia warrants endoscopic surveillance. Annual endoscopy is recommended for those patients with low-grade dysplasia, and more frequent screening is recommended for those patients with high-grade dysplasia. The management of high-grade dysplasia is discussed in "Treatment of Premalignant and T1 Disease" later in this chapter.

The proposed stepwise carcinogenic sequence in which specialized intestinal metaplasia proceeds to low-grade dysplasia, high-grade dysplasia, and frank carcinoma suggests a potential opportunity for chemoprevention to disrupt the succession to cancer. Buttar et al.,[51] recognizing that carcinogenesis in Barrett's esophagus is associated with increased expression of cyclooxygenase-2 (COX-2), examined the effect of COX-2 inhibitors on the development of Barrett's esophagus and adenocarcinoma in a preclinical model. Both selective and nonselective COX-2 inhibitors were effective in inhibiting Barrett's esophagus–related adenocarcinoma. A meta-analysis of two cohort and seven case-control studies comprising 1,813 cancer cases demonstrated a protective association between aspirin or nonsteroidal anti-inflammatory drugs and esophageal cancer.[52] These findings suggest nonsteroidal anti-inflammatory drugs may act as potential chemopreventive agents. A small, phase 2b randomized placebo-controlled trial of celecoxib in 100 patients with Barrett's esophagus and low- or high-grade dysplasia failed to demonstrate a protective effect against progression of Barrett's dysplasia to adenocarcinoma.[53] The ongoing ASPECT trial in the United Kingdom, a phase 3 randomized study of aspirin and esomeprazole chemoprevention in Barrett's metaplasia, is evaluating the effect of high- and low-dose esomeprazole, with and without low-dose aspirin, on the progression of Barrett's esophagus to high-grade dysplasia or cancer. More than 2,500 patients have been enrolled in this chemoprevention trial with a planned follow-up of at least 8 years and an interim analysis due in 2011.

Tylosis

Tylosis (focal nonepidermolytic palmoplantar keratoderma) is a rare disease inherited in an autosomal dominant manner that is characterized by hyperkeratosis of the palms and soles and esophageal papillomas. Patients with this condition exhibit abnormal maturation of squamous cells and inflammation within the esophagus and are at extremely high risk of developing esophageal cancer.[54,55] The tylosis esophageal cancer (*TOC*) gene has been mapped to 17q25 by linkage analysis of pedigrees.[56] The *TOC* gene is also frequently deleted in sporadic human esophageal cancers.[57,58] Envoplakin, encoding a protein component of desmosomes that is expressed in esophageal keratinocytes, has been mapped to the *TOC* region[61]; however, no tylosis-specific mutations involving this gene have been observed.[59]

Plummer-Vinson/Paterson-Kelly Syndrome

Plummer-Vinson/Paterson-Kelly syndrome is characterized by iron-deficiency anemia, glossitis, cheilitis, brittle fingernails, splenomegaly, and esophageal webs. Approximately 10% of individuals with Plummer-Vinson/Paterson-Kelly syndrome develop hypopharyngeal or esophageal epidermoid carcinomas.[60] The mechanisms by which these tumors arise have not been fully defined, although nutritional deficiencies as well as chronic mucosal irritation from retained food particles at the level of the webs may contribute to the pathogenesis of these neoplasms.[61]

Caustic Injury

Squamous cell carcinomas may arise in lye strictures, often developing 40 to 50 years after caustic injury.[62] The majority of these cancers are located in the middle third of the esophagus. The pathogenesis of these neoplasms may be similar to that implicated in esophageal cancers arising in patients with Plummer-Vinson/Paterson-Kelly syndrome. These cancers are often diagnosed late because chronic dysphagia and pain caused by the lye strictures obscure symptoms of esophageal cancer.

Achalasia

Achalasia is an idiopathic esophageal motility disorder characterized by increased basal pressure in the lower esophageal sphincter, incomplete relaxation of this sphincter after deglutition, and aperistalsis of the body of the esophagus. A 16- to 30-fold increase in esophageal squamous cancer risk has been noted in achalasia patients.[63,64] In a retrospective analysis, Aggestrup et al.[65] observed the development of esophageal carcinomas in 10 of 147 patients undergoing esophagomyotomy for achalasia. These neoplasms are believed to result from prolonged irritation from retained food in the midesophagus and arise an average of 17 years after onset of achalasia. The chronic dysphagia and pain attributable to megaesophagus contributes to their late diagnosis in achalasia patients.[66]

Human Papillomavirus Infection

Human papillomavirus (HPV) infection may contribute to the pathogenesis of esophageal squamous cell cancer in high-incidence areas in Asia and South Africa.[67] This oncogenic virus encodes two proteins (E6 and E7) that sequester the *Rb* and *p53* tumor suppressor gene products. Using polymerase chain reaction techniques, de Villiers et al.[68] detected HPV DNA sequences in 17% of esophageal squamous cell cancers in patients from China. In an additional study using similar techniques, Lavergne and de Villiers[69] identified a broad spectrum of HPV in approximately one-third of esophageal cancer specimens obtained from patients living in high-incidence areas in China and South Africa. Shibagaki et al.[70] detected HPV sequences in 15 of 72 (21%) esophageal cancer specimens obtained from Japanese patients. In contrast, neither evidence of HPV infection nor HPV DNA sequences have been observed in cancers arising in low-incidence areas.[71–74]

Prior Aerodigestive Tract Malignancy

Patients with upper aerodigestive tract cancers develop second primary cancers at a rate of approximately 4% per year.[80] Nearly 10% of secondary neoplasms arising in patients with prior histories of oropharyngeal of lung carcinoma arise in the esophagus.[75–77] Interestingly, *p53* mutational analysis of multiple primary cancers of the aerodigestive tract in 17 patients demonstrated complete discordance of *p53* genotype between separate primary tumors from the same patient, which suggests that *p53* is not functioning as a tumor susceptibility gene in this setting.[78]

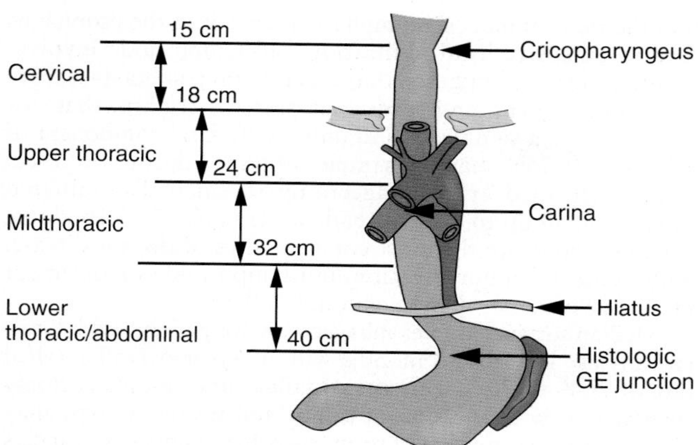

FIGURE 79.3 Anatomy of the esophagus with landmarks and recorded distance from the incisors used to divide the esophagus into topographic compartments. GE, gastroesophageal.

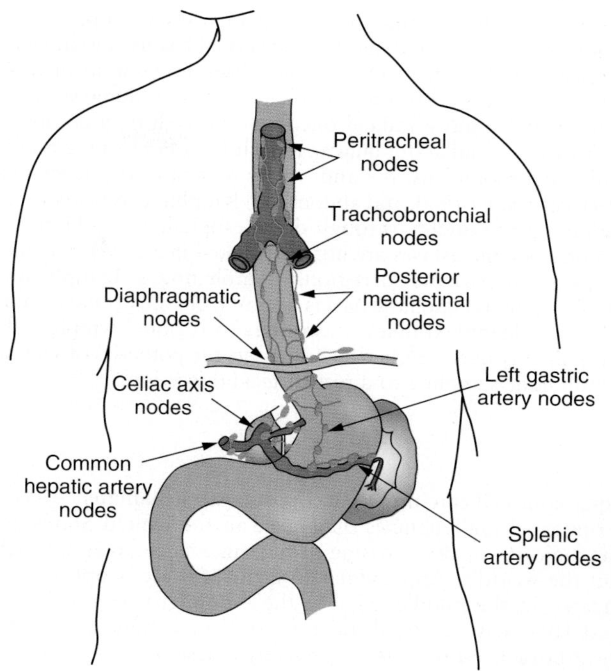

FIGURE 79.5 Lymphatic drainage of the esophagus with anatomically defined lymph node basins.

APPLIED ANATOMY AND HISTOLOGY

Anatomy

The esophagus bridges three anatomic compartments: the neck, thorax, and abdomen (Fig. 79.3). The esophagus extends from the cricopharyngeus muscle at the level of the cricoid cartilage to the gastroesophageal junction.[79] The borders of the cervical esophagus span from the cricopharyngeus to the thoracic inlet (approximately 18 cm from the incisors). The remainder of the esophagus is commonly divided into thirds, with the upper third extending from the thoracic inlet to the carina (approximately 24 cm from the incisors), the middle third extending from the carina to the inferior pulmonary veins (32 cm from the incisors), and the distal esophagus traversing the remaining distance into the abdomen to the gastroesophageal junction (40 cm from the incisors). Squamous cell carcinoma of the esophagus is the predominant histology in the cervical esophagus and upper and middle thirds (above the pulmonary vein) of the thoracic esophagus, whereas adenocarcinoma predominates in the distal esophagus.

Adenocarcinomas of the gastroesophageal junction present a unique challenge as appropriate management of these tumors as either esophageal or gastric cancers has been uncertain. Siewert et al.[80] have offered a classification system based on demographics, histopathologic variables, and patterns of lymphatic spread that provides clarity, is well established, and has been generally accepted worldwide (Fig. 79.4). In this classification scheme type I tumors are considered adenocarcinomas of the distal esophagus and type II and III lesions are classified as gastric cancers (cardia and subcardia). This classification system allows for a tailored and consistent surgical approach to these tumors as well as consistency in reporting outcome results associated with therapeutic interventions. However, it should be noted that in the most recent guidelines established by the American Joint Committee on Cancer, gastroesophageal junction tumors are included under the esophageal cancer staging classification.[81]

The pattern of lymphatic drainage of the esophagus influences the choice of surgical approach, based on tumor location in the esophagus (Fig. 79.5). Tumors of the cervical and upper third of the thoracic esophagus drain to cervical and superior mediastinal lymph nodes. Tumors of the middle third of the esophagus drain both cephalad and caudad with lymph nodes at risk in the paratracheal, hilar, subcarinal, periesophageal, and pericardial nodal basins. Lesions in the distal esophagus primarily drain to lymph nodes in the lower mediastinum and celiac axis region. Because of the extensive lymphatic network within

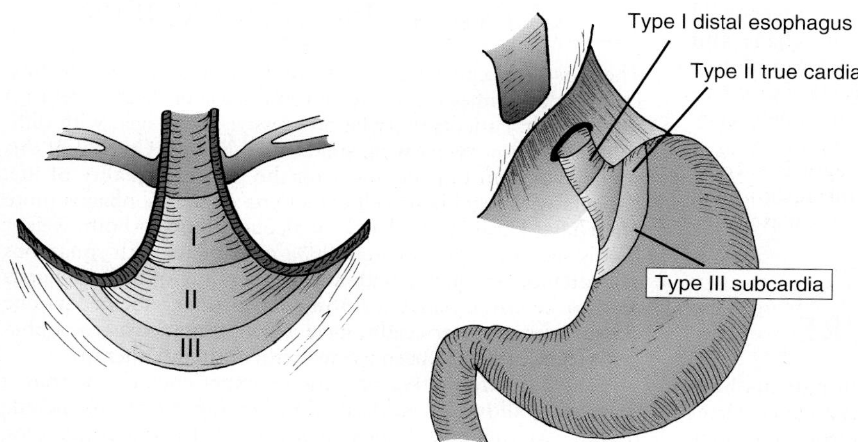

FIGURE 79.4 Anatomic classification of gastroesophageal junction tumors.

PRACTICE OF ONCOLOGY

the wall of the esophagus, skip metastases for upper third lesions have been noted in celiac axis nodal basins, and likewise, cervical lymph node metastases have been noted in as many as 30% of patients with distal esophageal lesions. Some surgeons recommend a more radical oncologic procedure, a combined transthoracic and abdominal approach for lesions of the middle and distal esophagus,[82,83] and others recommend a three-field (cervical, mediastinal, and abdominal) lymphadenectomy for all tumors of the middle through distal esophagus.[84,85] However, lymph node metastases are initially limited in an overwhelming majority of patients to regional lymph nodes. Lymph node involvement in lymphatic basins distant from the primary tumor are rarely identified unless metastases to regional lymph nodes have already occurred,[86] which suggests the potential of sentinel lymph node sampling to direct surgical dissection.[87]

Histology

Squamous cell carcinomas account for approximately 40% of esophageal malignancies diagnosed in the United States and the majority of cases arising in high-incidence areas throughout the world.[88] Approximately 60% of these neoplasms are located in the middle third of the esophagus, whereas 30% and 10% arise in the distal third and proximal third of the intrathoracic esophagus, respectively. These tumors are associated with contiguous or noncontiguous carcinoma *in situ* as well as widespread submucosal lymphatic dissemination.

Adenocarcinomas frequently arise in the context of Barrett's esophagus; because of this, these tumors occur in the distal third of the esophagus. No significant survival differences have been noted in adenocarcinoma patients compared with individuals with squamous cell cancers.

Rarer cancers of the esophagus include squamous cell carcinoma with sarcomatous features, adenoid cystic, and mucoepidermoid carcinomas. These neoplasms are indistinguishable clinically and prognostically from the more common types of esophageal carcinoma.

Small cell carcinomas account for approximately 1% of esophageal malignancies and arise from argyrophilic cells in the basal layer of the squamous epithelium. These neoplasms are usually located in the middle or lower third of the esophagus and may be associated with ectopic production of a variety of hormones, including parathormone, secretin, granulocyte colony-stimulation factor, and gastrin-releasing peptide; individuals with these cancers often present with systemic disease.[89–91] Recent series have reported patients with locally advanced disease treated with systemic chemotherapy in combination with either radiation therapy, surgery, or both, with some patients achieving long-term disease-free survival.[92]

Leiomyosarcoma is the most common mesenchymal tumor that affects the esophagus, still accounting for less than 1% of esophageal malignancies. These neoplasms are lower-third tumors presenting as bulky masses with hemorrhage and necrosis. Malignant lymphoma and Hodgkin's lymphoma rarely involve the esophagus and is usually secondary to extension from other sites. Patients with acquired immunodeficiency syndrome may exhibit Kaposi's sarcoma involving the esophagus. Malignant melanoma involving the esophagus is exceedingly rare and presents as a bulky polypoid intraesophageal tumor of varying color depending on melanin production.

NATURAL HISTORY AND PATTERNS OF FAILURE

At presentation, the overwhelming majority of patients have locally or regionally advanced or disseminated cancer, irrespective of histologic type.[4,93] The lack of a serosal envelope and the rich submucosal lymphatic network of the esophagus lead to extensive local infiltration and lymph node involvement. Evidence suggests that occult micrometastases are invariably present, and recurrence patterns confirm that distant failure is a significant and universally fatal component of relapse.[94–98] Bone marrow samples obtained during rib resections performed at esophagectomy revealed disseminated tumor cells in up to 90% of patients sampled.[99,100] The lung, liver, and bone are the most common sites of distant disease, with depth of tumor invasion and lymph node involvement predictive of tumor dissemination.[79,94,95]

Median survival after esophagectomy for patients with localized disease is 15 to 18 months with a 5-year overall survival rate of 20% to 25%. Patterns of failure after esophagectomy suggest that both location of tumor and histologic type may influence the distribution of recurrence. In patients with cancers of the upper and middle thirds of the esophagus, which are predominately squamous cell carcinomas, locoregional recurrence predominates over distant recurrence, whereas in patients with lesions of the lower third, where adenocarcinomas are more frequently located, distant recurrence is more common.[94,95] Only a very small percentage of patients (fewer than 5%) develop clinically evident recurrence at cervical sites.[86]

The addition of chemotherapy, radiotherapy, or chemoradiation to surgery alters patterns of failure, although reported results are not consistent. Preoperative radiotherapy and preoperative chemoradiation may reduce the rate of locoregional recurrence but have no obvious effect on the rate of distant metastases.[98–102] In two prospective randomized trials of preoperative chemotherapy plus surgery versus surgery alone, one study showed a slight but nonstatistically significant decrease in distant relapse with chemotherapy,[96] whereas the other demonstrated equivalent distant recurrence rates in both the preoperative chemotherapy and surgery-alone arms.[97] Treatment failure patterns after definitive chemoradiation without surgical resection reveal that concurrent administration of chemotherapy and radiotherapy provides better local control than radiotherapy alone, and that the administration of chemotherapy may reduce systemic recurrence; however, long-term follow-up of both randomized and nonrandomized patients treated with primary chemoradiation failed to indicate a clear reduction in distant disease recurrence compared with radiation therapy alone.[103] Although the addition of surgery further reduces local failure from 45% to 32%,[104] it does not diminish systemic recurrence and, in fact, may enhance it by allowing patients to manifest distant disease because they do not succumb to locoregional failure.[105,106] These patterns of relapse suggest that any further improvement in overall outcome for patients with esophageal cancer will be achieved through advances in systemic therapy.

CLINICAL PRESENTATION

The most noticeable symptoms are dysphagia and weight loss. Dysphagia signifies locally advanced disease or distant metastases, or both. Patients describe progressive dysphagia, with difficulty initially in swallowing solids, then liquids. Control of this single symptom impacts most on the patient's quality of life. Patients with squamous cell carcinoma of the esophagus more often have a history of tobacco or alcohol abuse, or both. Weight loss is seen in approximately 90% of patients with squamous cell carcinoma. Patients with adenocarcinoma of the esophagus tend to be white males from middle to upper socioeconomic classes who are overweight, have a symptomatic gastroesophageal reflux, and have been treated with antireflux therapy.

Approximately 20% of patients experience odynophagia (painful swallowing). Additional presenting symptoms include dull retrosternal pain, bone pain secondary to bone metastases, and cough or hoarseness secondary to paratracheal nodal or recurrent laryngeal nerve involvement. These types of symptoms suggest unresectable locally advanced disease or metastases. Unusual presentations are pneumonia secondary to tracheoesophageal fistula or exsanguinating hemorrhage due to aortic invasion.

DIAGNOSTIC STUDIES AND PRETREATMENT STAGING

Patients with symptoms of dysphagia should undergo upper endoscopy and biopsy to establish a tissue diagnosis. Biopsies or cytologic brushings have a diagnostic accuracy approaching 100%.[107,108] Targeted biopsy can be enhanced by the use of chromoendoscopy techniques using vital dyes, including indigo carmine, Lugol's iodine solution, methylene blue, and toluidine blue.[109,110] Autofluorescence imaging and narrow band imaging are emerging endoscopic techniques that allow for detailed inspection of mucosa.[111–114]

A focused history taking should elicit information on predisposing factors for esophageal cancer, including tobacco use, alcohol use, symptomatic reflux, diagnosis of Barrett's esophagus, and history of head and neck or thoracic malignancy. Prior surgery on the stomach or colon may influence the choice of reconstructive conduit to restore alimentary continuity at the time of esophagectomy. Findings on history and physical examination that would prompt further diagnostic testing include hoarseness, cervical or supraclavicular lymphadenopathy, pleural effusion, or new onset of bone pain.

Chest radiography and liquid oral contrast examination of the esophagus and stomach have been replaced by computed tomography (CT) and flexible endoscopy. Esophagogastroscopy allows precise evaluation of the extent of esophageal and gastric involvement and can precisely measure the distance of the tumor from the incisors to appropriately categorize the tumor's location. Upper endoscopy also allows identification of "skip" lesions or second primaries as well as indicates the presence and extent of Barrett's esophagus. Bronchoscopy should be reserved for those patients with tumors of the middle and upper esophagus to rule out invasion of the membranous trachea and possible tracheoesophageal fistula.

Pretreatment staging procedures establish the depth of esophageal wall penetration, regional lymph nodes, and the presence distant metastases so that patients can be guided to appropriate treatment. CT scan of the chest and abdomen is mandatory. A recent single institution review of 201 CT scans in 99 patients undergoing staging for esophageal cancer indicated that imaging of the pelvis did not contribute added staging information, and it may not need to be routinely performed.[115] CT scans are highly accurate (approaching 100%) in detecting liver or lung metastases and suggesting peritoneal carcinomatosis (e.g., ascites, omental infiltration, peritoneal tumor studding).[116–118] Accuracy for detecting aortic involvement or tracheobronchial invasion exceeds 90%.[117,119,120] CT is inaccurate in determining T stage and N stage.[116,117,119,121–123] The accuracy of endoscopic ultrasonography (EUS) in determining both T and N stage is a function of its ability to clearly delineate the multiple layers of the esophageal wall[124,125] and its use of multiple criteria, including shape, border pattern, echogenicity, and size, to determine lymph node involvement.[126,127] EUS is superior to CT in both T and N staging of esophageal cancer.[128,129] The overall accuracy for T staging is approximately 85% and for N staging it is approximately 75%.[130] The accuracy of determining lymph node involvement has been increased to 85% to 100% with the use of linear-array EUS with a channel that allows passage of a needle to perform tissue aspiration for cytology.[123,131,132] EUS is highly operator dependent and is limited in its ability to define relatively superficial lesions as either T1 or T2.[130,133,134] This distinction is critical to allow the use of minimal resection techniques for T1 lesions and to avoid preoperative chemoradiation for T1 and T2 tumors. Miniprobe high-frequency (20 MHz) sonographic catheters that can be passed through the working channel of the standard endoscope are now being used and provide improved accuracy.[135,136] A new generation of endoscopes that are thin caliber may traverse almost all obstructing lesions, allowing EUS assessment.[137] The accuracy of EUS in assessing response to induction chemoradiation is severely limited, and its use frequently leads to overstaging because the fibrotic changes induced by treatment mimic residual tumor,[138,139] although recent data may indicate some utility for posttherapy EUS.[140]

Fluorine-18 (^{18}F) fluorodeoxyglucose (FDG) positron emission tomography (PET) is being widely applied in the management of esophageal cancer. The accuracy of FDG-PET in assessing regional lymph nodes falls somewhere between the low and high accuracy of CT and EUS, respectively.[141,142] In the detection of distant metastases, FDG-PET is superior to CT, with a sensitivity, specificity, and accuracy all in the range of 80% to 90%.[142,143] PET in combination with CT (PET-CT fusion or hybrid FDG-PET/CT) further improves specificity and accuracy of noninvasive staging.[144] This leads to detection of unsuspected metastatic disease (up-staging) in 15% of patients, which leads to alteration of the intended treatment plan in at least 20% of patients. FDG-PET may also have value in evaluating response to chemotherapy and radiotherapy. Weber et al.[145] demonstrated that decreased FDG uptake significantly correlated with pathologically confirmed response in patients treated with induction chemotherapy before esophagectomy for esophageal adenocarcinoma.

A prospective validation study confirmed that a decrease in the standard uptake value of 35% or more during preoperative chemotherapy may predict histologic response and is associated with improved survival and decreased recurrence.[146] Brucher et al.,[147] from the same institution, Technische Universitat Munchen, showed a similar result of decreased FDG uptake in responders compared with nonresponders in patients with squamous cell carcinoma of the esophagus treated with preoperative chemoradiation. A recent trial from the Munich group led by Lordick et al.[148] examined PET scan response during induction chemotherapy in 110 patients with adenocarcinoma of the gastroesophageal junction. PET scan nonresponders (54 patients) assessed after 2 weeks of induction chemotherapy were referred for immediate surgery rather than continuing with the full 3-month course of preoperative chemotherapy. Survival in these patients (median 26 months) was comparable to nonresponding patients in a preceding trial (median 18 months) who continued the full 3 months of chemotherapy prior to surgery, indicating that discontinuation of an ineffective therapy and referral for earlier surgery did not compromise outcome. Survival, however, was inferior in the PET nonresponding patients compared with the PET responders. Although PET response may identify patients in whom ineffective preoperative therapy should be discontinued, whether or not referral of such patients for alternative chemotherapy, or chemoradiation, is warranted remains to be established. One series of patients treated with induction chemotherapy, followed with serial PET scans, identified some patients who progressed on induction chemotherapy. Several of these patients achieved durable disease control, including pathologic complete response, when changed to an alternative chemotherapy during radiation therapy, suggesting that salvage with alternative treatment may be possible.[92] Two recent systematic reviews of the current available literature that addressed the evaluation of tumor response by PET to neoadjuvant therapy concluded that while PET is the best imaging modality available to assess response, the current data do not support recommending the routine use of PET scans to guide therapeutic decisions.[149,150] Currently, the utility of PET to detect distant disease not identified by other imaging modalities confirms a role for PET that is complementary to other staging procedures, although it should not supplant them.

Minimally invasive surgical techniques (laparoscopy, thoracoscopy, or both) are being used for staging of both locoregional and distant disease. Performing laparoscopy as the initial procedure at the time of planned esophagectomy adds little in the way of time and cost to the procedure and allows detection of unsuspected distant metastases, which spares the morbidity of laparotomy in 10% to 15% of cases.[151,152] Although studies suggest improved pretreatment staging with minimally invasive surgical approaches,[153–155] such approaches have not been embraced because of the morbidity, length of hospital stay, and cost associated with what is considered an additional procedure.

A study comparing the health care costs and efficacy of staging procedures, including CT scan, EUS fine-needle aspiration (FNA), PET, and thoracoscopy or laparoscopy reported that CT plus EUS FNA was the least expensive and offered the most quality-adjusted life-years on average than all the other strategies. PET plus EUS FNA was somewhat more effective but also more expensive.[156]

PATHOLOGIC STAGING

The most recent guidelines established by the American Joint Committee on Cancer (AJCC) for staging of esophageal cancer are outlined in Tables 79.1 and 79.2.[81] Changes between the current (seventh edition) and immediate past staging guidelines are highlighted. Tumor location is now defined by the position of the proximal edge of the tumor and is designated as upper, middle, or lower esophagus. Esophagogastric junction tumors are now included in the esophageal cancer staging schema. The primary tumor (T) stage is based on depth of tumor invasion into and through the wall of the esophagus. T stage is now listed as high-grade dysplasia that includes all noninvasive neoplastic epithelium, which was formerly called carcinoma *in situ*. T1 tumors are now subclassified as T1a (tumor invades lamina propria or muscularis mucosae) and

TABLE 79.1

TUMOR (T), NODE (N), METASTASIS (M) STAGING SYSTEM FOR ESOPHAGEAL CANCER

PRIMARY TUMOR (T)	
TX	Primary tumor cannot be assessed
T0	No evidence of primary tumor
Tis	High grade dysplasia*
T1	Tumor invades lumina propria, muscularis mucosae, or submucosa
T1a	Tumor invades lamina propria or muscularis mucosae
T1b	Tumor invades submucosa
T2	Tumor invades muscularis propria
T3	Tumor invades adventitia
T4	Tumor invades adjacent structures
T4a	Resectable tumor invading pleura, pericardium, or diaphragm
T4b	Unresectable tumor invading other adjacent structures, such as aorta, vertebral body, trachea, etc.
	*High-grade dysplasia includes all noninvasive neoplastic epithelium that was formerly called carcinoma *in situ*, a diagnosis that is no longer used for columnar mucosae anywhere in the gastrointestinal tract
REGIONAL LYMPH NODES (N)	
NX	Regional lymph nodes cannot be assessed
N0	No regional lymph node metastasis
N1	Regional lymph node metastasis involving 1 to 2 nodes
N2	Regional lymph node metastases involving 3 to 6 nodes
N3	Regional lymph node metastases involving 7 or more nodes
DISTANT METASTASIS (M)	
M0	No distant metastasis (no pathologic M0; use clinic M to complete stage group)
M1	Distant metastasis

TABLE 79.2

CLASSIFICATION OF STAGE GROUPINGS FOR ESOPHAGEAL CANCER

Squamous Cell Carcinoma[a]

Group	T	N	M	Grade	Tumor Location[b]
0	Tis (HGD)	N0	M0	1	Any
IA	T1	N0	M0	1, X	Any
IB	T1	N0	M0	2–3	Any
	T2–3	N0	Mo	1, X	Lower, X
IIA	T2–3	N0	M0	1, X	Upper, middle
	T2–3	N0	M0	2–3	Lower, X
IIB	T2–3	N0	M0	2–3	Upper, middle
	T1–2	N1	M0	Any	Any
IIIA	T1–2	N2	M0	Any	Any
	T3	N1	M0	Any	Any
	T4a	N0	M0	Any	Any
IIIB	T3	N2	M0	Any	Any
IIIC	T4a	N1–2	M0	Any	Any
	T4b	Any	M0	Any	Any
	Any	N3	M0	Any	Any
IV	Any	Any	M1	Any	Any

[a]Or mixed histology including a squamous component or not otherwise specified.
[b]Location of the primary cancer site is defined by the position of the upper (proximal) edge of the tumor in the esophagus.

Adenocarcinoma

Group	T	N	M	Grade
0	Tis (HGD)	N0	M0	1, X
IA	T1	N0	M0	1–2, X
IB	T1	N0	M0	3
	T2	N0	M0	1–2, X
IIA	T2	N0	M0	3
IIB	T3	N0	M0	Any
	T1–2	N1	M0	Any
IIIA	T1–2	N2	M0	Any
	T3	N1	M0	Any
	T4a	N0	M0	Any
IIIB	T3	N2	M0	Any
IIIC	T4a	N1–2	M0	Any
	T4b	Any	M0	Any
	Any	N3	M0	Any
IV	Any	Any	M1	Any
Stage unknown				

T1b (tumor invades submucosa). T4 tumors that invade adjacent structures are now subclassified as T4a (resectable tumor invading pleura, pericardium or diaphragm) and T4b (unresectable tumor). The nodal (N) stage is determined by the presence of involved regional lymph nodes and is now subclassified according to the number of regional lymph nodes involved. The subclassification of metastasis (M) based on distant lymph node involvement (e.g., celiac node metastases for distal esophageal tumors) is no longer used. An analysis of 336 esophageal cancer patients who underwent resection alone recommended that the AJCC system be revised to take into account the number of involved lymph nodes, and that 18 lymph nodes should be the minimum harvested to provide accurate staging.[157] The current AJCC guidelines does not specify the number of lymph nodes to be removed, but instead suggests that the surgeon resect as many lymph nodes as possible while minimizing morbidity. Future refinements in the staging of esophageal cancer may result from incorporation of computational modalities such as nomograms and artificial neural networks that may predict outcome better than TNM-based staging systems.[158] Successive pathologically determined stage groups are predictive of length of survival.[79,93]

TREATMENT

The paucity of appropriately designed studies to scientifically determine the most effective therapeutic strategy in esophageal cancer fuels an ongoing debate and undermines the potential for achieving consensus. Although there is no disagreement that esophageal resection prevents progression from high-grade dysplasia to invasive carcinoma and is curative for T1 lesions limited to the mucosa, the morbidity and mortality associated with esophagectomy has created enthusiasm for alternative approaches such as mucosal ablation and endoscopic resection. Surgery has always been considered the most effective way of ensuring both locoregional control and long-term survival for patients with tumors invading into or beyond the submucosa with or without lymph node involvement. Some investigators suggest that extending the limits of resection will further improve outcome. However, surgery alone or any other single modality fails in most patients, which has led many oncologists to embrace chemoradiation and some to question the necessity for surgical intervention. Chemoradiation with or without resection is the most common therapeutic regimen offered to patients with esophageal carcinoma in the United States.[93]

Treatment of Premalignant and T1 Disease (Localized to the Mucosa Only)

High-grade dysplasia in Barrett's esophagus is the most powerful predictor of subsequent invasive adenocarcinoma and warrants therapy. The rationale for esophagectomy is that resection completely eradicates the mucosa at risk, which prevents progression to invasive carcinoma. This is supported by surgical series reporting previously unidentified invasive cancer, which is present in up to 40% of resected specimens.[159–162] The argument against esophagectomy is that most patients with high-grade dysplasia do not develop invasive carcinoma in their lifetimes. Those supporting endoscopic methods, ranging from surveillance to mucosal ablative and resection techniques, argue that this allows identification of patients with an early invasive lesion that is readily amenable to cure or elimination of the mucosa at risk, preventing progression. Indeed, patients with superficial invasive tumors confined to the mucosa, those with T1a disease in particular, have little or no risk of lymph node metastases[163] and are considered candidates for endoscopic therapies.

Surveillance

Endoscopic surveillance is based on the assumptions that the majority of patients will not progress to invasive carcinoma[164] and that actual cancers detected by surveillance are at an earlier stage and are therefore curable.[165] Studies demonstrating that patients with Barrett's esophagus–associated adenocarcinomas detected by surveillance have an earlier stage of disease and have better survival than those detected at initial endoscopy provide supportive evidence for surveillance.[40–42,159] Critics counter this argument with reports identifying invasive adenocarcinoma in up to 45% of esophagectomy specimens from patients with a diagnosis of high-grade dysplasia.[160–162] Proponents of surveillance management argue that these patients were not on an endoscopic surveillance program with strict biopsy criteria, and that strict pathologic criteria of invasive disease (submucosal invasion or beyond) were not utilized.[166]

Proposed guidelines for surveillance includes serial endoscopy at 3- to 6-month intervals with multiple four-quadrant biopsies at 1- to 2-cm intervals.[30] The downside of endoscopic vigilance is that in a certain percentage of patients invasive cancer goes undetected and the patients will not be candidates for potentially curative treatment.[167–169] This must be weighed against the morbidity and mortality of esophagectomy. It is important to note that the extent of high-grade dysplasia does not predict the presence of occult adenocarcinoma identified at esophagectomy and therefore cannot necessarily be applied to a subjective quantification of disease.[170]

Ablative Methods

The mechanism of action of all mucosal ablative techniques, including photodynamic therapy (PDT), laser ablation, multipolar electrocoagulation, argon plasma coagulation, and radiofrequency ablation, is destruction of the mucosal layer. The premise for managing high-grade dysplasia with endoscopic ablative therapy is that mucosal injury in an acid-controlled environment eliminates the premalignant mucosa and resurfaces the esophageal lining with regenerated squamous epithelium.[165]

PDT involves administration of an inactive photosensitizing agent that, when exposed to light of the proper wavelength, results in oxygen radical production and tissue destruction. The largest single institution experience with this technique has been reported by Overholt et al.[171] In their study, 80% of patients had eradication of high-grade dysplasia with PDT combined with acid-suppressive therapy during a mean follow-up period of 50 months. Eight percent of patients developed carcinomas, half of which were subsquamous adenocarcinomas detected during extended follow-up. PDT was also used in nine patients with "early-stage cancer," and treatment was declared to have failed in almost 60% of these patients. Results of a phase 3 multicenter study that randomized 208 patients on a two to one basis to either PDT plus omeprazole or omeprazole alone demonstrated improved eradication of high-grade dysplasia in the PDT arm (77% vs. 39%; $P < .0001$) at a 24-month follow-up.[172] A marked reduction in the occurrence of adenocarcinoma was noted in the PDT-treated group (13% vs. 28%); however, the results emphasize the risk of development of invasive cancer in a relatively short follow-up interval of 24 months. These results highlight the limitations of PDT, and because tissue is not obtained to properly stage the disease, at the present time this modality should only be offered to patients with comorbid disease who are not candidates for other more definitive therapy. Limited experience with thermal ablation for high-grade dysplasia has been reported. Small series of either laser ablation[173,174] or argon plasma coagulation[175,176] of high-grade dysplasia suggest that high-grade dysplasia can be eradicated; however, the follow-up period in these studies was short, and invasive carcinoma has subsequently been documented. A recent randomized trial in 127 patients with Barrett's esophagus and either low- or high-grade dysplasia assigned patients to either a sham endoscopic procedure or to treatment with radiofrequency ablation.[177] Patients assigned to receive radiofrequency ablation were treated with a circumferential ablation device employing an inflatable cylindrical balloon, bringing electrodes into contact with the esophageal lining, with four applications performed per session, and up to four sessions performed over 9 months. At 12 months, complete eradication of metaplasia occurred in 77.4% of the radiofrequency ablation patients compared to 2.3% in the control group. Although the development of cancer in either group was uncommon, progression to cancer in the ablation group was significantly less in the control group. More long-term follow-up beyond the 12 months in this trial as well as other confirmatory studies are required.

Endoscopic Mucosal Resection

Endoscopic mucosal resection (EMR) is a relatively recent addition to the endoscopic therapeutic options available for patients with either high-grade dysplasia or superficial esophageal cancers (T1a). EMR technique either involves submucosal injection of fluid to lift and separate the lesion from the underlying muscular layer or the use of suction to trap the lesion into a cylinder, which allows full resection and tissue retrieval for appropriate histologic examination. Ell et al.[178] prospectively examined the utility of endoscopic resection in 100 consecutive patients with low-risk adenocarcinoma (no ulceration, mucosal lesion, no vascular or lymphatic invasion, less than 20 mm, and not poorly differentiated). Complete local remission was achieved in 99 of 100 patients; at a median follow-up of 33 months, 11% of patients developed recurrent or metachronous carcinomas, all successfully treated with repeat endoscopic resection. The calculated 5-year survival rate was 98% and no patient died of esophageal cancer. In a previous study from the same group,[179] the complete remission rate in patients with less favorable lesions was 59%, which emphasizes the need to adhere to strict criteria to optimize disease eradication.

A report examining the value of EUS and EUS-guided FNA in patients with high-grade dysplasia or intramucosal cancer considered candidates for endoscopic therapy and demonstrated that 20% of patients had unsuspected lymph node metastases and were therefore deemed unsuitable for endoscopic intervention.[180] These results and similar findings in smaller series examining EMR[181,182] confirm that use of this technique is feasible for treatment of high-grade dysplasia and carcinoma limited to the mucosa (T1a) and provides an alternative to esophagectomy, especially in those patients considered at high risk for surgical intervention. Furthermore, one could justifiably conclude that patients carefully screened and confirmed to have mucosa-limited lesions should first be offered EMR prior to considering esophagectomy.[183]

Minimally Invasive Esophagectomy

In an attempt to reduce morbidity and mortality while achieving an equivalent oncologic outcome, minimally invasive techniques for esophageal resection have been designed and are being investigated. A variety of minimally invasive approaches have been used for esophagectomy, including laparoscopic, thoracoscopic, combined laparoscopic and thoracoscopic, and hand-assisted techniques.[184–187] These techniques have been described and are similar in conduct to open procedures of transthoracic and transhiatal esophagectomy (detailed in "Surgical Resection") except for the nuances of the minimally invasive approach (Figs. 79.6 and 79.7). These procedures have

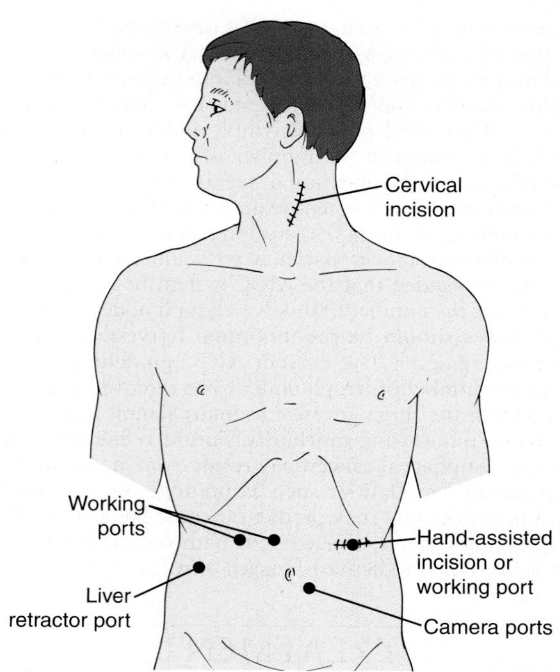

FIGURE 79.6 Abdominal port sites and incisions used for minimally invasive esophagectomy. If a thoracoscopic approach is not used to dissect and mobilize the thoracic esophagus, a 6-cm incision is used instead of the left-sided abdominal working port to perform a hand-assisted transhiatal esophagectomy.

been applied to the treatment of all stages of potentially resectable esophageal cancer but would seem to be most applicable in the management of premalignant and early-stage disease.

By far the largest single-institution experience with minimally invasive esophagectomy has been reported by Luketich et al.[188] in a study of 222 patients with high-grade dysplasia (n = 42) or cancer (n = 175), the majority of whom underwent a combined laparoscopic and thoracoscopic procedure. Median intensive care unit stay was 1 day, median length of hospital stay was 7 days, and 30-day perioperative mortality was 1.4%. Median follow-up was only 19 months, and stage-specific survival was similar to that reported in a series with open esophagectomy. The same group reported their experience with 100 consecutive patients with T1 esophageal cancer who underwent esophagectomy, 80% of which were performed via a minimally invasive approach. The 30-day mortality was 0% and a R0 resection was achieved in 99%. N1 disease was present in 21% of patients, the majority of whom (90%) had T1b lesions

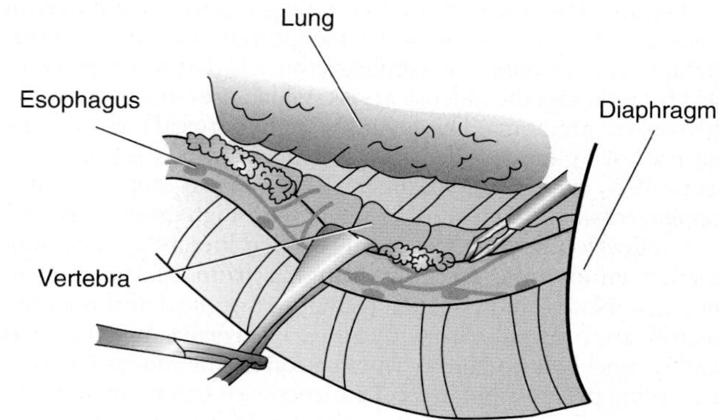

FIGURE 79.7 Thoracoscopic view and dissection of intrathoracic esophagus.

with submucosal invasion. At a median follow-up of 5.5 years, 5-year overall survival was 62% and 3-year disease-free survival was 80%. The authors concluded that esophagectomy remains the standard of care for patients with T1 esophageal cancer.[189] The results following minimally invasive esophagectomy reported by this group at the University of Pittsburgh are promising, but whether they are reproducible in other institutions and therefore more broadly applicable must be determined through further study.[190,191]

Initial experience with the hand-assisted laparoscopic esophagectomy technique has been reported. By providing tactile feedback to the surgeon, this approach closely mimics open esophagectomy and may be more widely applicable in the surgical community.[186]

There is limited experience with the use of radiation or chemoradiation in the curative setting for patients with cT1N0 disease. Sai et al.[192] from Kyoto University treated 34 patients who were either medically inoperable or refused surgery with either external beam alone (64 Gy) or external beam (52 Gy) plus 8 to 12 Gy with brachytherapy. With a median follow-up of 61 months, 5-year results were 59% survival, 68% local relapse-free survival, and 80% cause-specific survival. Treating a similar population of 63 patients with chemoradiation plus brachytherapy, Yamada et al.[193] reported 66% survival, 64% disease-free survival, and 76% cause-specific survival at 5 years.

Treatment of Localized Disease

Surgery has traditionally been the treatment of choice for patients with localized, resectable carcinoma of the esophagus and continues to be a component of a more comprehensive approach to esophageal cancer in a substantial number of patients. Failure of surgery alone to significantly alter the natural history of esophageal cancer has resulted in considerable enthusiasm for chemoradiation. The shift toward multimodal treatment, although theoretically sound, is supported by mixed results from phase 3 randomized trials, many of which are statistically underpowered and often come to both positive and negative conclusions about the worth of preoperative therapeutic regimens (radiation, chemotherapy, or chemoradiation) compared with surgery alone. Similarly, it is appropriate to question the role of surgery in a multimodal approach to treatment of esophageal cancer, with studies (almost exclusively in squamous cell cancer) suggesting the absence of a survival benefit for the addition of surgery after chemoradiation, despite potentially improved local disease control.

Surgical Resection

Decisions regarding surgical technique are routinely based on personal bias, comfort level of the surgeon, and a subjective view of tumor biology because solid evidence from scientifically designed trials is nonexistent. Studies that used health services–linked databases have demonstrated a statistically significant association between performance of surgery in hospitals designated as high-volume esophagectomy institutions with lower complication and mortality rates.[194–198] A recent study from the Netherlands noted a significant reduction in postoperative morbidity, decrease in length of stay, reduction in in-hospital mortality, and improved 2-year survival following centralization of esophageal resections in high volume units when compared to before the centralization project was introduced.[199]

Transhiatal Esophagectomy. The transhiatal route for esophageal resection has gained favor, especially among surgeons in the United States, concurrent with the rising incidence of adenocarcinoma of the distal esophagus, which is readily approachable and effectively dissected through the diaphragmatic hiatus

TABLE 79.3

CONVENTIONAL APPROACHES TO ESOPHAGEAL RESECTION FOR CANCER

TRANSHIATAL
Laparotomy and cervical approach
Peritumoral or two-field lymph node dissection
En bloc resection feasible for distal esophageal tumors
Cervical anastomosis
TRANSTHORACIC
Ivor Lewis
Right thoracotomy and laparotomy
Peritumoral or two-field lymph node dissection
En bloc resection feasible for middle/distal thoracic tumors
McKeown or "three hole"
Right thoracotomy, laparotomy, cervical approach
Peritumoral, two-field or three-field lymph node dissection
En bloc resection feasible for mid- or distal thoracic tumors
Cervical anastomosis
Left thoracotomy
Left thoracotomy with or without cervical approach
Peritumoral lymph nodes dissection
Intrathoracic or cervical anastomosis
Left thoracoabdominal
Left thoracoabdominal approach
Peritumoral or two-field lymph node dissection
Intrathoracic anastomosis

(Table 79.3). The technique is as follows.[200,201] It is prudent to initially perform laparoscopic exploration to rule out disseminated disease and, if it is confirmed, to abort the intended resection before exposing the patient to the risks of laparotomy. Through a midline incision, the stomach is mobilized by dividing all vascular attachments while preserving the right gastroepiploic and right gastric vessels on whose pedicle the reconstructive conduit will be based. The duodenum is fully mobilized via a Kocher maneuver and a pyloric drainage procedure is performed, which has been demonstrated in prospective randomized trials to reduce gastric stasis and minimize pulmonary complications such as aspiration.[202,203] Cautery division of the diaphragmatic crus allows wide access to the mediastinum and dissection under direct vision of the middle and lower third of the esophagus. A left cervical incision provides exposure to the cervical esophagus, and circumferential dissection of the cervical esophagus is carried down to below the thoracic inlet to the upper thoracic esophagus, with care to avoid injury to the recurrent laryngeal nerve. The remainder of the dissection at the level of and superior to the carina is completed by blunt dissection through the esophageal hiatus.

The cervical esophagus is then divided, the stomach and attached intrathoracic esophagus are delivered through the abdominal wound, and a gastric tube, which will serve as the reconstructive conduit, is fashioned using multiple applications of a linear stapling device. The gastric tube is then transposed through the posterior mediastinum to the cervical wound, where a cervical esophagogastric anastomosis is performed. The stomach is considered by most surgeons as the replacement conduit of choice for the resected esophagus. A segment of colon, usually based on the ascending branch of the inferior mesenteric artery, is an effective esophageal substitute if for any reason the stomach is deemed unsuitable for reconstruction or if it is the surgeon's preference. Although the original intent of this approach was not to perform a methodical lymph node dissection, a standard two-field lymphadenectomy (abdominal and lower mediastinal) can readily be achieved, and for that matter, if the surgeon is so inclined, a radical *en bloc* resection can be performed, as described by Bumm et al.[204]

The stated advantages attributed to the transhiatal approach to esophagectomy include avoidance of a thoracotomy incision, which thereby minimizes pain and subsequent postoperative pulmonary complications; elimination of the lethal complications of mediastinitis associated with an intrathoracic anastomotic leak; and a shorter duration of operation, which results in decreased morbidity and mortality.[201] Limitations and disadvantages of transhiatal esophagectomy include poor visualization of upper and middle thoracic esophageal tumors, increased anastomotic leak rate with subsequent stricture formation, possibility of chylothorax, and possibility of recurrent laryngeal nerve injury. The largest experience with transhiatal esophagectomy was reported by Orringer et al.[205] and included 1,525 patients with esophageal cancer, 79% of whom had adenocarcinoma and 21% of whom had squamous cell carcinoma. Tumors were located in the lower third of the esophagus in 82% and in the middle or upper third in 18%. In-hospital mortality was 3%. The most common complications were anastomotic leak (12%) and recurrent laryngeal nerve palsy (4.5%). Leak of a cervical esophageal gastric anastomosis was handled simply, in most patients with opening of the cervical wound, followed by local wound care. Hoarseness from recurrent laryngeal nerve injury resolved spontaneously in 99% of cases. Overall 5-year survival was 29%, and stage-specific 5-year survival was 65% for stage I, 28% for stage II, 29% for stage IIB, and 11% for stage III. These results reflect those reported from other surgical series of transhiatal esophagectomy (Table 79.4).[206–211]

Transthoracic Esophagectomy. Transthoracic esophagectomy has been the most common surgical approach used to resect carcinomas of the esophagus and is the standard procedure against which all other techniques are measured (Table 79.3). Although a left thoracotomy provides adequate exposure to tumors of the distal esophagus, a right thoracotomy affords access to upper, middle, and distal esophageal lesions and is the preferred route for transthoracic exposure. A right thoracotomy combined with an upper midline laparotomy (Ivor Lewis esophagectomy) is the technique most commonly used for esophageal resection and is briefly described here.[201] The abdominal portion of the procedure duplicates that of the transhiatal approach previously detailed and includes mobilization of the stomach and distal esophagus, upper abdominal lymphadenectomy, pyloromyotomy, and placement of a feeding jejunostomy before abdominal wound closure and repositioning for the thoracic component of the procedure. A muscle-sparing right lateral thoracotomy is performed through the fifth or sixth intercostal space. The azygos vein is divided, the mediastinal pleura incised, the intrathoracic esophagus mobilized, and a mediastinal lymph node dissection performed.

After division of the proximal esophagus in the chest to ensure an adequate margin, the gastroesophageal junction and stomach are pulled into the thoracic cavity. The stomach is then divided with a linear stapler, the specimen is removed, and an esophagogastric anastomosis is performed. An alternative approach has been described in which the right thoracotomy is the initial stage of the procedure followed by repositioning of the patient supine for an abdominal and left cervical incision to achieve a cervical esophagogastric anastomosis.[212,213] Initial experience with minimally invasive Ivor Lewis esophagectomy has also been reported.[214]

The transthoracic approach provides direct visualization and exposure of the intrathoracic esophagus, facilitating a wider dissection to achieve a more adequate radial margin around the primary tumor and more thorough lymph node dissection, which theoretically results in a more sound cancer operation. In patients with significant comorbid conditions, the combined effects of an abdominal and thoracic incision may compromise cardiorespiratory function. An intrathoracic anastomotic leak can lead to mediastinitis, sepsis, and death. In addition, esophagitis in the nonresected thoracic esophagus may occur secondary to bile reflux. The three-incision (cervical, thoracic, and abdominal) modification of the procedure effectively eliminates the potential for complications associated with an intrathoracic esophagogastric anastomosis.

Numerous authors have reported results of transthoracic esophagectomy; however, most, if not all, of these reports include patients who were resected via other surgical approaches and underwent a more extended lymphadenectomy (Table 79.5).[215–220] Both overall and stage-specific 5-year survival rates were similar to those seen with transhiatal esophagectomy. The most reliable data may be derived from prospective randomized trials in which there is a surgery-alone control arm. In only one of those trials[220] was a transthoracic approach the only surgical procedure allowed. In that trial, median survival time on the surgery alone arm was 18.6 months and 5-year survival rate was 26%.

Transhiatal versus Transthoracic Esophagectomy. The controversy regarding the optimal surgical approach for esophageal cancer remains unresolved. Two large meta-analyses have compared transhiatal esophagectomy with transthoracic esophagectomy based on collective reviews of numerous individual studies.[221,222] Both reports include studies that compared transhiatal with transthoracic esophagectomy, studies of transhiatal esophagectomy only, and studies of transthoracic esophagectomy only. Rindani et al.[221] reviewed 5,483 patients from 44 series published between 1986 and 1996. Perioperative mortality was significantly higher in the transthoracic

TABLE 79.4

RESULTS OF TRANSHIATAL ESOPHAGECTOMY FOR ESOPHAGEAL CANCER

Study (Ref.)	Year	No. of Patients (n)	Histologic Type	Perioperative Mortality (%)	5-Y Survival (%)
Gelfand et al. (207)	1992	160	A	0.9	21
Gertsch et al. (209)	1993	100	A/S	3	23
Vigneswaran et al. (208)	1993	131	A/S	2.3	21
Dudhat and Shinde (211)	1998	80	S	7.5	37
Orringer et al. (206)	1999	800	A/S	4.5	23
Bolton and Teng (210)	2002	124	A/S	1.6	27.3

A, adenocarcinoma; S, squamous cell carcinoma.

TABLE 79.5

RESULTS OF TRANSTHORACIC ESOPHAGECTOMY FOR ESOPHAGEAL CANCER

Study (Ref.)	Year	No. of Patients (n)	Histologic Type	Perioperative Mortality (%)	5-Y Survival (%)
Wang et al. (218)	1992	368	S	6.5	7.6
Lieberman et al. (219)	1995	258	A/S	5	27
Adam et al. (217)	1996	597	A/S	6.9	16.3
Sharpe and Moghissi (215)	1996	562	A/S	9	18
Bosset et al. (220)	1997	139	S	3.6	26
Ellis (216)	1999	455	A/S	3.3	24.7

A, adenocarcinoma; S, squamous cell carcinoma.

esophagectomy group than in the transhiatal group (9.5% vs. 6.3%), whereas overall perioperative complications were not significantly different. Transhiatal esophagectomy resulted in a higher incidence of anastomotic leak, anastomotic stricture, and recurrent laryngeal nerve injury. Overall 5-year survival was similar: 24% for transhiatal esophagectomy and 26% for transthoracic esophagectomy. Hulscher et al.[222] performed a collective review of 50 studies performed between 1990 and 1999 yielding 7,527 patients. Postoperative mortality was significantly greater in the transthoracic group than in transhiatal group (9.2% vs. 5.7%). Transthoracic esophagectomy was associated with a significantly higher risk of pulmonary complications (18.7% vs. 12.7%), whereas patients treated with transhiatal esophagectomy had a higher anastomotic leak rate (13.6% vs. 7.2%). Five-year survival was not significantly different, with 23% 5-year survival for transthoracic and 21.7% 5-year survival with transhiatal esophagectomy. A prospective database based on the Veterans Administration National Surgical Quality Improvement Program analyzed perioperative outcome in 945 patients, 562 who underwent transthoracic esophagectomy and 383 who underwent resection through a transhiatal approach.[223] There was no difference in overall mortality (10% for transthoracic approach vs. 9.9% for transhiatal approach) or morbidity (47% for transthoracic vs. 49% for transhiatal). A large population-based study evaluated transhiatal and transthoracic esophagectomy through the Surveillance, Epidemiology and End Results (SEER) Medicare-linked database from 1992 to 2002.[224] A lower operative mortality was found after transhiatal esophagectomy (6.7% vs. 13.1%). Although observed 5-year survival was higher after transhiatal esophagectomy, after adjusting for stage, patient, and provider factors, no significant 5-year survival difference was found.

Four phase 3 trials have prospectively examined the outcomes for patients randomly assigned to undergo either transhiatal or transthoracic esophagectomy.[225–228] No definitive conclusions can be drawn from three of these trials because of the extremely small sample size. The trial in the Netherlands, however, deserves special attention. Hulscher et al.[228] randomly assigned 220 patients with middle or distal esophageal carcinoma to undergo either transhiatal esophagectomy or transthoracic esophagectomy. The transthoracic group underwent a systematic mediastinal and upper abdominal lymph node dissection. Although the number of lymph nodes retrieved was significantly higher in the transthoracic group (31 vs. 16; $P < .001$), there was no difference in the radicality of the two procedures with equivalent R0, R1, and R2 resections. Postoperative pulmonary complications, ventilatory time, intensive care unit stay, and hospital stay were significantly higher in those patients assigned to the transthoracic group. Despite the higher perioperative morbidity, there was no statistically significant increase in in-hospital mortality (4% vs. 2% for transthoracic vs. transhiatal esophagectomy, respectively; $P = .45$). At a median follow-up of 4.7 years, there were no significant differences between the transhiatal and transthoracic esophagectomy groups with respect to median disease-free interval (1.4 years vs. 1.7 years) and median overall survival time (1.8 years vs. 2.0 years), respectively. Likewise, no significant differences were noted in locoregional recurrence, distant recurrence, and combined locoregional and distant recurrence for patients randomly allocated to the transthoracic or transhiatal esophagectomy arm. The investigators point out that a trend toward improved disease-free survival (39% vs. 27%) and overall survival (39% vs. 29%) at 5 years favored the transthoracic approach group. However, a recent update on this study that provided complete 5-year survival data demonstrated that survival was equivalent in patients randomized to either a transhiatal (34%) or transthoracic (36%) resection.[229]

Either the transhiatal or transthoracic procedure can be performed with acceptable morbidity and mortality in experienced hands and, with either technique, the outcome is remarkably similar.

Extended Esophagectomy. In an attempt to improve on the dismal results reflected in high local recurrence rates and poor overall survival with standard transhiatal and transthoracic esophagectomy techniques, some surgeons have examined extending the limits of resection to accomplish a more effective primary tumor excision and lymph node dissection. Two concepts guide the intent of these more extended resections: *en bloc* resection of the primary tumor with its adjacent surrounding tissue and systematic lymph node dissection, encompassing either two (mediastinal and abdominal) or three (cervical, mediastinal, and abdominal) lymph node basins (Fig. 79.8). Although some investigators have focused and reported separately on *en bloc* esophagectomy and extended lymphadenectomy, most of the techniques described encompass both components of this "radical" approach. *En bloc* esophagectomy involves resection of middle and lower esophageal tumors with an envelope of adjacent tissue that includes the mediastinal pleura laterally, the pericardium anteriorly, and the azygos vein and thoracic duct posterolaterally with the surrounding periesophageal tissue and lymph nodes. For tumors traversing the esophageal hiatus, a cuff of diaphragm is resected. In addition to a thorough mediastinal lymph node dissection extending from the tracheal bifurcation to the esophageal hiatus, an upper abdominal lymph node dissection incorporating lymph nodes along the portal vein, common hepatic artery, celiac trunk, left gastric artery, and splenic artery is included to achieve a two-field lymph node dissection.[230] A three-field lymph node dissection extends the lymphadenectomy to the superior mediastinum, including nodes

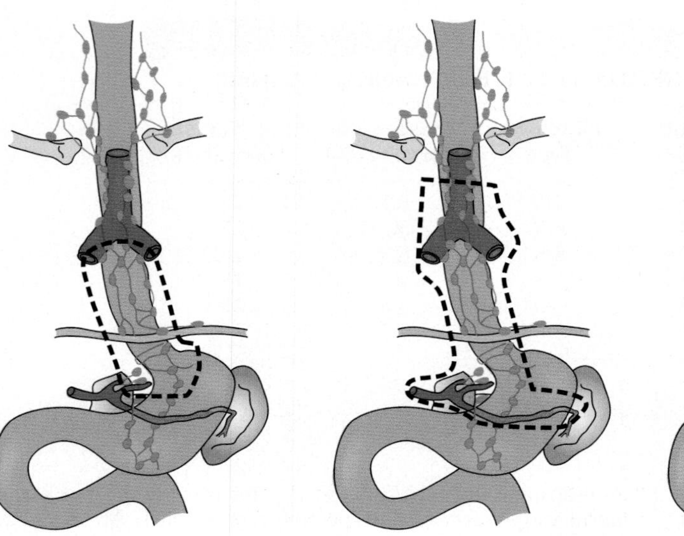

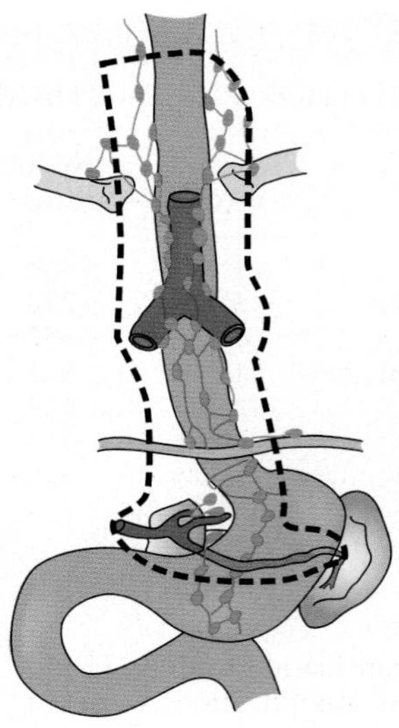

FIGURE 79.8 Left to right: Standard, two-field, and three-field lymphadenectomy.

along the course of the right and left recurrent laryngeal nerves, and, through a separate collar incision in the neck, completes the dissection with removal of the lower cervical nodes, including the deep external and lateral cervical lymph node basins.[84,85]

Most of the series that examine the utility of extended esophagectomy are retrospective and involve a single institution. Hagen et al.[82] reported on 100 consecutively treated patients who had undergone an *en bloc* esophagectomy with two-field lymphadenectomy; none of the patients received additional preoperative or postoperative chemotherapy or radiotherapy. The perioperative mortality was 6%, with the most common complications being pneumonia (19%), subphrenic abscess (13%), respiratory failure (9%), anastomotic leak (10%), and empyema (7%). Local recurrence was detected in only one patient and overall actuarial 5-year survival was 52%. Patients with stage III lesions had a 25% actuarial 5-year survival. Altorki et al.[83] reviewed the results for 128 patients who underwent esophagectomy at a single institution; 61% received an *en bloc* esophagectomy and the remainder underwent a standard esophageal resection. Approximately 40% of those undergoing the more extended resection had a three-field lymphadenectomy; the others had a systematic two-field lymphadenectomy. The in-hospital mortality for the *en bloc* resection group was 5.1%, similar to that for those undergoing a standard resection. The most common postoperative complications in the extended resection group were respiratory events (24%) and anastomotic leak (12.8%), but no significant differences were noted in comparison to the standard resection group. Four-year survival for the *en bloc* group was 41.5% overall and 34.5% for stage III patients, with both of these survival figures markedly better than those for the standard resection group. However, both of the studies described here are single-institution, retrospective analyses for which the results, at least in part if not completely, can be attributed to selection bias and enhanced staging, leading to stage migration. It is interesting to note that similar results have been achieved without thoracotomy using a transhiatal approach as described earlier in "Transhiatal Esophagectomy."[204]

A group at Cornell University also separately examined 80 patients who underwent esophagectomy with three-field lymphadenectomy.[85] Overall 30-day mortality was 5%, with 31% of patients developing major postoperative complications, including need for reintubation (16%), anastomotic leak (11%), and recurrent laryngeal nerve injury (9%). Overall 5-year survival was 51%. Cervical lymph node metastases were identified in 36% of patients, and the 5-year survival rate for those with positive cervical lymph nodes was 25%. Lerut et al.[231] reported on 174 patients, equally divided between squamous cell and adenocarcinoma histology, who underwent three-field lymphadenectomy. Hospital mortality was only 1.2%, with an overall mortality of 58%. Five-year survival for stage III patients was 36.8%. Twenty-three percent of patients with adenocarcinoma and 25% with squamous cell carcinoma had positive cervical nodes. Five-year survival for patients with positive cervical lymph nodes was 27% and 12%, respectively, for squamous cell and adenocarcinoma histology. The authors suggest that three-field lymphadenectomy may have a role in patients with squamous cell carcinoma but remains investigational for patients with adenocarcinoma. These results, although impressive, may also reflect both selection bias and stage migration. In addition, the expertise required to perform these technically demanding procedures effectively limits their application to specialized centers only and a fraction of the patients who might benefit from these procedures if an actual advantage were proven.

The Hulscher trial, discussed above, which also employed an *en bloc* resection of the esophagus compared to transhiatal esophagectomy, failed to improve outcome.[229] A small study by Nishihira et al.[232] of 62 patients showed an improved, but not statistically significant, survival advantage for extended lymphadenectomy (66.2% vs. 48%; $P = .19$). Patients in this study were also randomly assigned to receive either chemoradiation or chemotherapy alone after surgery, confounding the interpretation of the results.

The body of evidence confirms that extended resections improve staging and may enhance locoregional control; however, there are no reliable data confirming a survival benefit for these procedures.

Adjuvant Therapy

Preoperative Chemotherapy. Nearly three-fourths of patients newly diagnosed with esophageal cancer present with locally advanced (stage IIB or III) disease. The poor survival rate achieved with surgery alone, and given the patterns of both local and systemic disease recurrence, has provided the impetus for the evaluation of preoperative (induction) chemotherapy in patients with resectable esophageal cancer.

The benefits of induction chemotherapy include potential down-staging of the disease to facilitate surgical resection, improvement in local control, relief of dysphagia in patients responding to induction chemotherapy, and the potential eradication of micrometastatic disease. Esophagectomy after induction therapy enables comprehensive pathologic assessment of treatment response, which may be important in selecting patients for postoperative adjuvant therapy. The disadvantages of preoperative chemotherapy include the potential development of chemotherapy resistance and the delay in definitive treatment with the risk of further spread of disease. These are important concerns because approximately 50% of patients do not respond to current chemotherapeutic regimens. Further compromise of the patient's already marginal nutritional status due to a delay in local disease control is also of concern when surgery is not the initial treatment.

Trials evaluating the use of induction chemotherapy followed by surgery for treatment of esophageal cancer have been under way since the late 1970s. This strategy was evaluated in parallel with studies of concurrent chemoradiation followed by surgery or chemoradiation as definitive therapy. Early trials used cisplatin and bleomycin-based chemotherapy.[233–236] Use of cisplatin and 5-fluorouracil (5-FU)[237–241] led to the initiation of randomized trials in the 1980s. For lesions of squamous histology, the response rate to two or three cycles of cisplatin (100 mg/m^2 on day 1) and 5-FU (1,000 mg/m^2/d for 96 or 120 hours) every 3 weeks ranged between 42% and 66%, with a 0% to 10% pathologically confirmed complete-response rate; curative resection rates were between 40% and 80%, and median survival was from 18 to 28 months.[237–241] Lesions were staged with a barium esophagogram and CT scan initially and then again before surgery to assess response to induction therapy.

Seven randomized trials evaluating the use of preoperative chemotherapy in esophageal cancer patients are summarized in Table 79.6.[96,97,242–247] Four of the trials enrolled only patients with squamous cell carcinoma,[242–245] whereas half to two-thirds of patients enrolled in the two more recent and largest trials (U.S. Intergroup and Medical Research Council) had adenocarcinoma of the esophagus, gastroesophageal junction, or cardia.[96,97] Another large randomized trial treated mostly gastric cancer, although one-fourth of patients enrolled had adenocarcinoma of the distal esophagus or gastroesophageal junction.[246]

No improvement in survival was noted in three small trials enrolling fewer than 100 patients each, with the small sample size making study interpretation difficult.[242,244,245] Kok et al.[243] reported a survival advantage for preoperative chemotherapy in a preliminary communication. This study, enrolling 171 patients with squamous cell carcinoma, differed from other trials by requiring response assessment after two courses of preoperative chemotherapy. Patients showing no response underwent immediate surgery, whereas patients showing a response received two more courses of chemotherapy before surgery. The regimen consisted of cisplatin (80 mg/m^2 on day 1) and etoposide (100 mg/m^2 intravenously on days 1 to 2 and 200 mg/m^2 orally on days 3 to 5). In a preliminary communication, at a median follow-up for surviving patients of 15 months, the median survival of the preoperative chemotherapy group was significantly longer than for those randomly assigned to immediate surgery (18.5 months vs. 11.0 months; $P = .002$). However, a final report has never been published.

The U.S. Intergroup mounted a large, potentially definitive trial, INT-0113. A total of 467 patients with resectable esophageal cancer were randomly assigned to one of two treatment groups: (1) three cycles of cisplatin and 5-FU followed by surgery and then, for those patients whose resection was curative (R0), two additional cycles of cisplatin and 5-FU as adjuvant treatment; or (2) immediate surgery.[96] In contrast to other trials, barium esophagogram was the only test required to assess clinical response to preoperative chemotherapy. Thus, it is not surprising that only a 19% response rate was reported. Survival and pattern of failure were the major study end points. No differences were observed between the surgery control group and the preoperative cisplatin and 5-FU group in terms of curative resection rate (59% vs. 62%), treatment mortality (6% vs. 7%), overall median survival (16.1 months vs. 14.9 months),

PRACTICE OF ONCOLOGY

TABLE 79.6

RANDOMIZED TRIALS OF PREOPERATIVE CHEMOTHERAPY

Study (Ref.)	Treatment	No. of Patients (n)	Histologic Type	Survival		
				Median	2-Y (%)	3-Y (%) 5-Y (%)
Nygaard et al. (242)	Preop cisplat/bleo	50	S			3
	Surgery	41				9
Roth et al. (244)	Preoperative cisplat/VDS/bleo and adjuvant cisplat/VDS	19	S	9 mo		25
	Surgery	20		9 mo		5
Schlag (245)	Preop cisplat/5-FU	34	S	10 mo		
	Surgery	41		10 mo		
Kok et al. (243)	Preop cisplat/etoposide	86	S	18.5 mo		
	Surgery	85		11 mo		
Kelsen et al. (Intergroup 0013) (96)	Preop cisplat/5-FU and adjuvant cisplat/5-FU	213	S/A	15 mo	35	26
	Surgery	227		16 mo	37	23
Allum et al. (97, 247)	Preop cisplat/5-FU	400	S/A	16.8 mo	43	32 23
	Surgery	402	A	13.3 mo	34	25 17
Cunningham et al. (246)	Pre/postop ECF	250	A	24 mos	36	5
	Surgery	253		20 mos	23	

Preop, preoperative; cisplat, cisplatin; bleo, bleomycin; S, squamous cell carcinoma; VDS, vindesine; 5-FU, 5-fluorouracil; A, adenocarcinoma; ECF, epirubicin/cisplatin, 5-FU; postop, postoperative.

or 3-year survival (26% vs. 23%). Furthermore, the median survival of patients who had a curative resection was the same in both treatment groups (27.4 months vs. 25.0 months). The pattern of failure was also similar for the two treatment groups (local recurrence 31% vs. 32%, and distant recurrence of 50% vs. 41% in the surgery-alone group compared to those receiving induction chemotherapy followed by surgery, respectively). Tumor histologic type did not influence response to treatment.

Although no improvement in survival was demonstrated, the trial importantly provides a contemporary surgical experience in the treatment of esophageal squamous carcinoma and adenocarcinoma. Important outcomes in this trial include a postoperative death rate well below 10%, the lack of difference in survival for lesions of different histologic types, and the fact that an R0 curative resection (regardless of treatment) conferred a median survival time of more than 2 years. The trial results were reported at long-term follow-up, with a median follow-up of 55.4 months and a minimum follow-up of 29.5 months.

In contrast to the results of the 467-patient U.S. Intergroup trial, the Medical Research Council (MRC) Oesophageal Cancer Working Group demonstrated a statistically significant 9% improvement in 2-year survival rate (43% vs. 34%) with preoperative cisplatin and 5-FU.[97] A total of 802 patients, 31% with squamous lesions and 69% with adenocarcinoma or lesions of undifferentiated histologic type, were enrolled. Patients were randomly assigned either to receive two courses of cisplatin (80 mg/m^2) and 5-FU (1,000 mg/m^2/d, continuous infusion for 4 days) 3 weeks apart followed by surgery or to undergo immediate surgery. The curative resection (R0) rate (60% vs. 54%) and the percentage of randomly assigned patients undergoing surgery (92% vs. 97%) were similar for the two treatment groups, although the improvement in curative resection rate did reach statistical significance. Patients receiving preoperative chemotherapy had improved median survival (16.8 months vs. 13.3 months) and 2-year survival rate (43% vs. 34%). Overall survival was significantly improved with preoperative chemotherapy (P = .004; hazard ratio [HR] 0.79; 95% confidence interval [CI], 0.67 to 0.93). The estimated reduction in risk of death was 21%. The postoperative mortality rate was 10% in both treatment groups. Pathologic complete responses were rare and were reported in 4% of patients undergoing preoperative chemotherapy. These authors recently reported an update of this trial at a median follow-up of 6 years.[247] Although a survival benefit was maintained in the preoperative chemotherapy arm, it had diminished to only 6% at 5 years (23.0% for preoperative therapy vs. 17.1% for surgery; HR 0.84; P = .03). There was no difference in pattern of failure, in particular the development of distant metastatic disease, in the chemotherapy surgery versus surgery alone group, with the authors attributing the survival improvement with preoperative chemotherapy to the enhancement of rate of curative resection. The modest survival improvement with preoperative chemotherapy in this trial update is consistent with a 4.3% survival benefit observed in a recent meta-analysis of preoperative chemotherapy reported in abstract form, in which updated survival data from individual trials were obtained in over 2,000 patients in nine studies.[248]

There is no clear explanation for the discrepancy in survival outcome for the INT and MRC trials, whereas survival of the surgery control groups was essentially the same. The MRC study had the advantage of a larger sample size and greater power to observe a small difference. A greater proportion of patients who received chemotherapy underwent surgery in the MRC study, 92% compared with 80% in the INT trial. Although a microscopically complete resection (R0) was performed in similar proportions in the two trials, the MRC trial indicated a higher rate of R0 resection with preoperative chemotherapy compared to surgery alone. The duration of preoperative chemotherapy in the MRC trial was shorter and may have lessened the risk to patients of disease progression during induction therapy.

Positive results of another recent trial of perioperative chemotherapy in gastric and distal esophagus or gastroesophageal junction cancer have been reported. In a trial by Cunningham et al.,[246] 503 patients were assigned to three cycles of preoperative and three cycles of postoperative epirubicin/cisplatin/5-FU or surgery alone. Preoperative chemotherapy resulted in significant improvement in patient survival, with a 6-month improvement in progression-free survival, a 4-month improvement in median survival, and a 13% improvement in 5-year overall survival (23% to 36%), all statistically significant. Despite the survival improvement with pre- and postoperative chemotherapy, there was no improvement in rate of curative resection in patients treated with preoperative chemotherapy compared with surgery alone (66% to 69%), and there were no cases of pathologic complete response to preoperative chemotherapy. Down-staging was also observed with preoperative chemotherapy, with a shift to earlier T and N stage tumors with preoperative chemotherapy compared to surgery alone. As 26% of patients on this trial had tumors in the gastroesophageal junction and lower esophagus, the results may apply to locally advanced esophageal cancer. The median follow-up was 47 months in the surgery alone arm and 49 months in the chemotherapy arm.

As a consequence of these outcomes, preoperative cisplatin and 5-FU is now the standard of care for resectable esophageal cancer (squamous cell carcinoma and adenocarcinoma of the esophagus and gastroesophageal junction) in the United Kingdom, whereas this approach has not been generally accepted for esophageal cancer in the United States.

Preoperative Radiation Therapy. The high rate of local failure after esophagectomy engendered interest in the use of radiation therapy in conjunction with surgery. The incidence of local failure in the surgical control arms of randomized trials of preoperative radiation therapy reported by Mei et al.[249] and Gignoux et al.[250] was 12% and 67%, respectively. The local failure rate in the surgical control arm of the randomized trial of postoperative radiation therapy conducted by Teniere et al.[251] was 35% for patients with negative locoregional lymph nodes and 38% for patients with positive locoregional lymph nodes. The surgical control arm of INT-0113 provides a modern, more relevant baseline for the results of surgery alone. As discussed in "Preoperative Chemotherapy," there was a 31% local failure rate in patients undergoing an R0 resection and a total local failure rate (including the additional 30% of patients with persistent disease) of 61%. Six randomized trials of preoperative radiation therapy for patients with clinically resectable disease have been reported.[242,249,250,252–254] Overall, preoperative radiation therapy did not increase the resectability rate, and only two series reported local failure rates. Although Mei et al.[249] reported no difference in local failure, Gignoux et al.[250] observed a significantly lower local failure rate in patients who received preoperative radiation therapy than in those treated with surgery alone (46% vs. 67%, respectively).

Two trials have reported an improvement in survival. In the series of Nygaard et al.,[242] patients who received preoperative radiation therapy (with or without chemotherapy) had a significant improvement in overall 3-year survival (18% vs. 5%; P = .009). The 48 patients who received preoperative radiation therapy without chemotherapy had a 20% 3-year survival rate; however, this did not reach statistical significance. This was not a pure radiation study, and the benefit may have been partly because of the chemotherapy. A similar improvement in survival was reported by Huang et al.[254] (46% vs. 25%). A meta-analysis from the Oesphageal Cancer Collaborative Group also showed no clear evidence of a survival advantage with preoperative radiation therapy.[101]

Design flaws in these trials include the failure to use conventional doses of radiation therapy, the use of split-course radiation therapy, and failure to allow an adequate interval (4 to 8 weeks) between the completion of radiation therapy and surgery. The only study that allows analysis of the effect of radiation fractionation is a randomized trial performed in France involving patients with squamous cell carcinomas who received chemoradiation using continuous-course versus split-course radiation.[255] The 95 patients who received a continuous-course regimen had a significantly higher local control rate (57% vs. 29%) and 2-year event-free survival rate (33% vs. 23%), and a borderline significantly higher 2-year survival rate (37% vs. 23%). Because it is less effective than continuous-course therapy, split-course radiation therapy is not recommended.

In summary, because only two of the six series have reported local failure rates, it is difficult to draw firm conclusions regarding the influence of preoperative radiation therapy on local control. Nonrandomized trials[256,257] also reported no survival benefit. Based on the available data from randomized trials, preoperative radiation therapy does not appear to significantly decrease local failure rate or improve survival in esophageal cancer patients.

Preoperative Chemoradiation. The rationale for trimodal therapy, chemoradiation followed by surgery, is based on the pattern of both local and distant failure associated with surgery alone or chemoradiation without surgery, which are the two treatment options established as standards of care based on data from randomized controlled trials. The results for patients randomly assigned to the surgery control arm of the INT-0113 trial revealed a 61% rate of failure in controlling local disease.[96] Similarly, the two Intergroup trials (RTOG-85-01 and INT-0123) that evaluated nonsurgical treatment (concurrent cisplatin and 5-FU, and radiotherapy), discussed in greater detail later on in this chapter, showed unacceptably high rates of local failure (44% to 53%).[258,259] Most of the agents active against esophageal cancer (i.e., 5-FU, cisplatin, mitomycin C, paclitaxel, irinotecan, docetaxel, capecitabine, and oxaliplatin) are known to enhance radiosensitivity in cancer cells. Conceivably, chemotherapy in conjunction with radiotherapy may both sensitize radiation therapy to improve local control as well as impact a reduction on systemic disease recurrence. Treatment with chemoradiation followed by esophagectomy has the potential (1) to down-stage the disease, (2) to increase the rate of complete resection with negative circumferential margins, and (3) to eradicate occult micrometastatic disease.

Nonrandomized trials. Most trials have used 5-FU and cisplatin-based chemotherapy combined with radiation therapy (Table 79.7),[102,260–279] although more recent trials incorporate paclitaxel or irinotecan in two- or three-drug combination regimens (Table 79.8).[92,280–292]

The results of selected phase 2 series in which patients underwent preoperative chemoradiation followed by a planned operation are summarized in Table 79.7. Since the initial trials by Leichman et al.[293] and the Southwest Oncology Group (SWOG-8037),[260] results of many phase 2 single-institution or multicenter trials have been published.[294] Most trials used cisplatin (75 to 100 mg/m^2) and 5-FU (1,000 mg/m^2/d continuous infusion for 4 or 5 days) with concurrent radiotherapy followed by surgery in 4 to 8 weeks. In most series, the pathologic complete-response rate (based on total number treated) was approximately 25%. The highest pathologic complete-response rates have been reported in trials treating mainly squamous cancers, and as more modern series treat predominantly adenocarcinoma, pathologic complete-response rates are consistently lower. Intensive chemoradiation regimens using hyperfractionated radiotherapy were evaluated by Forastiere et al.,[262,263] Raoul et al.,[273] and Adelstein et al.[270] Some of these regimens achieved higher pathologically determined complete-response rates and survival rates, usually with corresponding increases in acute toxicity. However, no clear advantage to altered fractionation schedules has been shown. The total dose of radiotherapy with concurrent chemotherapy varied from 30 Gy in earlier series up to 60 Gy, followed by surgery. Pathologic complete-response rates are uniformly in the 15% to 20% range with lower doses of radiation,[260,264,275,276] whereas total doses exceeding 50 Gy are associated with increased toxicity and perioperative complications.[274] Doses of 44 to 50 Gy using standard fractionation and concurrent therapy with cisplatin plus 5-FU generally result in pathologic complete-response rates of 25% to 40%[102,262,264,265,268–270,273,277] and acceptable toxicity with postoperative mortality rates well below 10%.

Most trials use conventional fractionation and doses of radiotherapy (45.0 to 50.4 Gy) with concurrent chemotherapy. In addition to overall outcome, some investigators have sought to determine whether preoperative endoscopy with biopsy can accurately assess response to treatment and whether achievement of pathologically confirmed complete response after chemoradiation improves overall survival. Bates et al.[265] reported a 65% 3-year survival rate in patients who achieved a pathologic confirmed complete response, compared with a 25% survival rate in those who did not. In 106 of 262 (41%) patients who achieved a pathologic complete response with preoperative chemoradiation, the 5-year survival was 52% compared with 38% in partial responders (P <.001) and 19% in nonresponders (P <.001).[279]

In other trials with long-term follow-up, investigators observed 5-year survival rates of 60% to 67% and 27% to 32% for those with pathologic complete response and those with residual disease after induction therapy, respectively.[102,262] In addition, the fact that long-term survival was observed in approximately 30% of patients with residual tumor in the resected specimen suggests that surgery is an important component following chemoradiation.

At present, no methods short of surgical resection can accurately determine which patients will be found to have no residual tumor in the resected esophageal specimen after chemoradiation. Bates et al.[265] noted a 41% false-negative rate with preoperative endoscopy and biopsy. Sarkaria et al.[295] reported the correlation of post-chemoradiotherapy endoscopy findings and surgical pathologic findings in 156 patients with esophageal cancer. Although 76% had a biopsy-negative endoscopy after preoperative therapy, only 31% of these patients were found to be pathologic complete responders at subsequent surgery. Yang et al.[296] made similar observations about the accuracy of posttherapy biopsy. Jones et al.[297] reported that CT had a sensitivity of 65%, a specificity of 33%, a positive predictive value of 58%, and a negative predictive value of 41% in evaluating pathologic response after preoperative chemoradiation in esophageal cancer patients. Many studies show that EUS performed after chemoradiation is also a poor predictor of complete response because of the inability to distinguish postirradiation fibrosis and inflammation from residual tumor. Reported staging accuracy is below 50%.[298–300]

The value of FDG-PET for restaging after chemoradiation remains to be established. Several studies of esophageal cancer patients show that an early decrease in FDG uptake after chemotherapy can predict clinical response.[145,301,302] Flamen et al.[302] evaluated the predictive value of PET after chemoradiation in patients receiving preoperative treatment. The sensitivity and positive predictive value of PET for identifying a pathologically determined complete response were 67% and 50%, respectively. Both false-positive PET findings (residual FDG activity in an area of intense inflammatory activity on histopathologic analysis) and false-negative findings occurred at the primary tumor site. Vallbohmer et al.[303] treated 119 patients with preoperative chemoradiation (cisplatin, 5-FU,

TABLE 79.7

RESULTS OF PREOPERATIVE CHEMORADIATION FOR ESOPHAGEAL CANCER: SELECTED NONRANDOMIZED TRIALS

Study (Ref.)	No. of Patients (n)	Histology	Chemotherapy	RT (Gy)	Resection (%)	Pathologic CR (%)[a]	Survival	Operative Mortality (%)
Poplin et al., 1987 (260)	113	S	CF	30	49	16	12 mo (median), 28%(2-y)	11
Naunheim et al., 1992 (261)	47	S/A	CF	30–36	72	17	23 mo (median), 40% (3-y)	5
Forastiere et al., 1990 (263), 1993 (262)	43	S/A	CFV	38–45	91	23	29 mo (median), 46% (3-y), 34% (5-y)	2
Hoff et al., 1993 (264)	68	S/A	CFLE	30	75	18	24 mo (median), 51% (2-y)	2
Bates et al., 1996 (265)	39	S/A	CF	45	90	46	22 mo (median), 40% (3-y)	9
Malhaire et al., 1996 (266)	56	S	CF	37	79	38	37 mo (median), 55% (3-y), 30% (5-y)	11
Stahl et al., 1996 (267)	72	S/A	CFLE	40	67	22	17 mo (median), 33% (3-y)	15
Forastiere et al., 1997 (268)	50	S/A	CF	44	90	38	31 mo (median), 58% (2-y)	0
Jones et al., 1997 (269)	66	S/A	CF	45	82	33	19 mo (median), 32% (3-y)	7
Adelstein et al., 1997 (270)	72	S/A	CF	45	88	27	44% (4-y)	18
Posner et al., 1998 (271) , 2001 (272)	44	S/A	CFIfn	40–45	82	24	28 mo (median), 52% (2-y), 32% (5-y)	8
Raoul et al., 1998 (273)	32	S	CFL	45	81	56	52% (3-y)	10
Keller et al., 1998 (274)	46	A	FM	60	72	17	17 mo (median), 27% (2-y)	17
Bedenne et al., 1998 (275)	96	S	CF	30	82	20	17 mo (median), 40% (2-y), 25% (5-y)	9
Laterza et al., 1999 (276)	111	S	CF	30	78	15	14 mo (median), 32% (2-y)	10
Heath et al., 2000 (277)	42	S/A	CF	44	93	26	NR (median), 62% (2-y)	0
Kleinberg et al., 2003 (102)	92	S/A	CF	44	93	33	35 mo (median), 57% (2-y), 40% (5-y)	0
Roof et al. 2006 (278)	81	S/A	CF	58.5	73	37	(3-y) NS	
	83	S/A	PCF	58.5	65	31	(3-y) NS	
Meredith et al. (279)	262	S/A	CF	50.4	94	41	39% 5-y survival	

RT, radiation therapy; CR, complete response; S, squamous cell carcinoma; C, cisplatin; F, 5-fluorouracil; A, adenocarcinoma; V, vinblastine; L, leucovorin; E, etoposide; Ifn, interferon; M, mitomycin; NR, not reached; P, paclitaxel; NS, not stated.

[a]Percentage of patients enrolled.

TABLE 79.8

EARLY RESULTS OF SELECTED PHASE I AND II TRIALS OF PREOPERATIVE CHEMORADIATION

Study (Ref.)	No. of Patients (n)	Histologic Type	Preoperative Treatment	Outcome
Khushalani et al. (280)	38	S/A	Ph 1 Oxali F + RT 50.4 Gy	pCR, 38% (13 patients selected for resection)
Safran et al. (281)	41	S/A	Ph 2 C Pac + RT 39.6 Gy	pCR, 29%; 2-y survival, 42%
Adelstein et al. (282)	40	S/A	Ph 2 C Pac + RT 45 Gy (b.i.d.)[a]	pCR, 23%; 3-y survival, 30%
Wright et al. (283)	40	S/A	Ph 1–2 C F Pac + RT 58.5 Gy (b.i.d.)[a]	pCR, 35%; 2-y survival, 61%
Meluch et al. (284)	130	S/A	Ph 2 Carbo F Pac + RT 45 Gy	pCR, 36%; 3-y survival, 41%
Bains et al. (285)	41	S/A	Ph 2 C Pac × 2 then C Pac (96 h) + RT 50.4 Gy	pCR, 22%
Swisher et al. (286)	38	S/A	Ph 2 C F Pac × 2 then C F + RT 45 Gy	pCR, 21%; 3-y survival, 63%; 5-y survival, 39%
Ajani et al. (287)	43	S/A	Ph 2 C Irin then F Pac + RT	pCR, 28%
Van Meerten et al. (288)	54	S/A	Ph 2 Pac Carbo RT 41.4 Gy	pCR, 25%
Ku et al. (92)	55	S/A	Ph 2 C Irin then C Irin + RT 50.4 Gy	pCR, 17%
Spigel et al. (289)	59	S/A	Ph 1–2 Oxali, Doc, Cape + 45 Gy	pCR 49%, 2-y survival, 52%
Ajani et al.(290)	84	S/A	Randomized Ph 2: Pac, C +/– F then Pal, C +/– F + 50.4 Gy	F+: 2-y survival, 56% F-: 2-y survival, 37%
Ilson et al. (291)	18	A	Ph 1 C, Irin, Bev then C, Irin, Bev + 50.4Gy	pCR 10%
Rivera et al. (292)	23	S/A	Ph 2 C, Irin then C, Irin +45 Gy	pCR 9%, 2-y survival, 35%

S, squamous cell carcinoma; A, adenocarcinoma; Ph, phase; Oxali, oxaliplatin; F, 5-fluorouracil; RT, radiation therapy; pCR, pathologically confirmed complete response; C, cisplatin; Carbo, carboplatin; Pac, paclitaxel; Irin, irinotecan; Doc, docetaxel; Cape, capecitabine; Bev, bevacizumab.
[a]Regimen not recommended because of toxicity.

and 36 Gy) and reported a nonsignificant association between major responders and FDG-PET results ($P = .056$). However, there was no clear standardized uptake value threshold that predicted response. Possible reasons for discrepant findings include the inflammatory effect of chemoradiation as well as a lack of standardization of FDG-PET protocols and techniques and definitions of a pathologic response.

Few studies have reported long-term follow-up to determine actual survival rates at 5 years. Selected trials are seen in Table 79.7; rates range from 25% reported by Bedenne et al.[275] for a series of 96 patients with squamous cell esophageal cancer to as high as 39% reported by Meredith et al.[279]

Taken together, these nonrandomized data (Table 79.7) accumulated during nearly three decades suggest an approximate 5% to 10% improvement in survival compared with historical surgery controls. However, substantially greater improvement in survival is seen in patients who are down-staged to pathologically confirmed complete response or minimal residual disease.

Patterns of failure after chemoradiation and resection are influenced by histologic type, with a greater likelihood of local recurrence for patients with squamous cell carcinoma of the esophagus and predominantly distant recurrence for those with adenocarcinoma of the distal esophagus, gastroesophageal junction, and cardia. In a literature review of trials of preoperative chemoradiation published between 1980 and 2000, Geh et al.[294] found that the overall risk of relapse was 46%, but that the majority of relapses, 80%, were at distant sites; locoregional recurrence alone constituted only 9% of treatment failures. These cumulative data correspond with individual reports from other major centers[102,265,270,272] and suggest that preoperative chemoradiation followed by surgery leads to better locoregional control than does surgery alone or chemoradiation without surgery.

The preliminary results of selected phase 1 and 2 trials of preoperative chemoradiation that integrated newer cytotoxic and targeted agents such as oxaliplatin, paclitaxel, docetaxel irinotecan, capecitabine, cetuximab, and bevacizumab into combination chemotherapy regimens are listed in Table 79.8. In two phase 1 trials,[280] surgery was performed on selected patients only; otherwise, pathologically determined complete-response rates are based on the total number of patients initiating treatment and range from 9% to 49%.[281–292]

Overall the pathologic complete-response rates appear similar to those for previous cisplatin and 5-FU plus radiotherapy preoperative regimens, as do survival rates. Adelstein et al.[282] found less mucosal toxicity associated with a regimen of cisplatin and paclitaxel plus radiotherapy than with the cisplatin and 5-FU plus radiotherapy regimen they used earlier. However, the incidence of grade 3 or 4 neutropenia, fever, and unplanned hospitalizations was significantly higher with the paclitaxel regimen, without any improvement in either pathologic complete-response rate or survival estimates. This trial used a potentially more toxic schedule of twice daily, hyperfractionated radiation and a likely more myelosuppressive, once every 3 weeks, schedule of paclitaxel.

Meluch et al.[284] reported mature trial results for a combination of carboplatin, 5-FU, and paclitaxel plus concurrent radiotherapy. Among a total of 123 patients, the pathologic complete-response rate was 38%, and after a median follow-up of 45 months, the 3-year survival rate was 41%. Grade 3 or 4 leukopenia (73% of patients), esophagitis (43%), and hospitalization (57%) suggest that this regimen added toxicity without providing incremental improvement in survival. Toxicity on trials of paclitaxel and cisplatin on a once-weekly schedule, with conventional dose fractionation of radiation therapy, have reported lesser degrees of esophagitis.[281,286,304] McCurdy et al.[305] from the M. D. Anderson Cancer Center reported that the addition of taxanes to chemoradiation increased both the FDG-PET determined pulmonary metabolic response and the radiation pneumonitis response compared with nontaxane containing regimens. Weekly carboplatin combined with weekly paclitaxel and concurrent radiotherapy also appeared to have a favorable toxicity profile in a recent phase 2 trial treating 54 patients with adenocarcinoma and squamous cell carcinoma of the esophagus.[288] The rate of pathologic complete response was 25%. Rates of grade 3 and 4 neutropenia (15%) and esophagitis (8%) were relatively low, but were in agreement with other trials employing a weekly paclitaxel and platinum drug chemotherapy regimen.

Swisher et al.,[286] Ajani et al.,[287] Bains et al.,[285] Ku et al.,[92] and Rivera et al.[292] have published pilot experiences in administration of induction chemotherapy before chemoradiotherapy and then surgery as a strategy to increase pathologically determined complete-response rate and reduce distant failure. Some trials of induction chemotherapy have noted significant relief of patients' dysphagia and the rare need to place feeding tubes for nutritional support in patients.[92,285] The addition of bevacizumab to irinotecan, cisplatin, and radiation therapy resulted in no increase in hematologic or nonhematologic toxicity or surgical complications.[291] The RTOG-0113 performed a phase 2 randomized trial comparing paclitaxel and 5-FU to paclitaxel and cisplatin plus radiation therapy.[290] Both arms were associated with significant toxicity, and the study did not meet its 1-year survival end point.

In summary, some of these newer regimens appear to be more toxic than cisplatin and 5-FU plus radiotherapy, whereas others suggest a potentially more favorable toxicity profile; the pathologic complete-response rates and survival estimates show no consistent benefit, but longer follow-up is needed. Interpretation of survival rates from these studies must be done cautiously, given the likelihood of stage migration due to the incorporation of EUS and PET into routine staging evaluation. Roof et al.[278] reported a single-institution experience of 177 patients treated with either cisplatin, 5-FU, or paclitaxel in combination with cisplatin, 5-FU, and radiation therapy as preoperative treatment in esophageal cancer. The 3-year overall survival was similar for the 5-FU/cisplatin–treated patients (39%) compared with those receiving paclitaxel in combination with 5-FU/cisplatin (42%). Pathologic complete-response rates were also comparable for two-drug (42%) compared with three-drug therapy (37%). In two sequential trials from Urba et al.[306,307] that evaluated two-drug paclitaxel cisplatin therapy plus radiation in one trial, and three-drug 5-FU, cisplatin, and paclitaxel plus radiation in another trial, there was also no difference in pathologic complete-response rates (17% to 19%). These rates of pathologic complete response were significantly lower than other trials reporting pathologic complete-response rates of 37% to 38% for three-drug therapy.[278]

The Eastern Cooperative Oncology Group reported response[288] and survival[308] outcomes in a randomized phase 2 trial testing two of these combinations (E1201), limited to patients with resectable adenocarcinoma of the distal esophagus, gastroesophageal junction, and cardia (Fig. 79.9). The two preoperative treatments tested were (1) paclitaxel (50 mg/m^2, 1-hour infusion) followed by cisplatin (30 mg/m^2) on days 1, 8, 15, 22, 29, and concurrent radiotherapy (45 Gy); and (2) cisplatin (30 mg/m^2) followed by irinotecan (65 mg/m^2) on days 1, 8, 22, 29, and concurrent radiotherapy (45 Gy). Patients in each arm proceeded to esophagectomy followed by three cycles of adjuvant paclitaxel and cisplatin (arm 1) or cisplatin and irinotecan (arm 2). Staging with esophageal EUS was an eligibility requirement. A preliminary report indicated comparable rates of pathologic complete response for the two regimens of 15% to 16%, with the lower-than-expected pathologic complete-response rate likely partly due to the exclusive treatment of adenocarcinoma on this trial.[309] The median survival on the paclitaxel arm was 20.9 months, and 34.9 months on the irinotecan arm (difference nonsignificant). Although the results are comparable to other modern phase 2 trials in esophageal adenocarcinoma, neither regimen appeared superior to more conventional 5-FU and cisplatin-based therapy.

Randomized trials. Randomized trials comparing preoperative chemoradiation with surgery alone in patients with clinically resectable disease are listed in Table 79.9.[98,220,310–315] The series of Le Prise et al.[316] is not included because patients received sequential rather than concurrent chemotherapy and

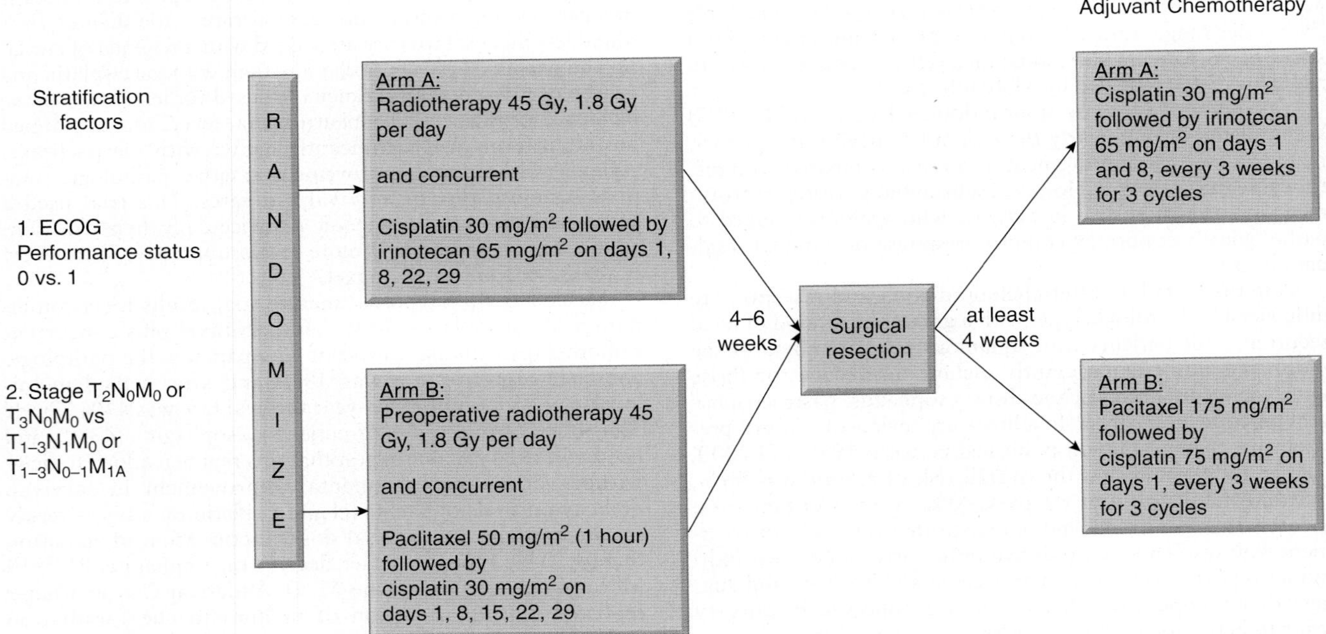

FIGURE 79.9 Schema of Eastern Cooperative Oncology Group (ECOG) trial E1201, a randomized phase 2 study of operable adenocarcinoma of the esophagus to measure response rate and toxicity of preoperative combined modality paclitaxel and cisplatin plus radiation therapy or irinotecan and cisplatin plus radiation therapy followed by postoperative chemotherapy.

TABLE 79.9

PREOPERATIVE CHEMORADIATION THERAPY FOR ESOPHAGEAL CANCER: RANDOMIZED TRIALS

Study (Ref.)	No. of Patients (n)	Histologic Type	Treatment	R0 Resection (%)	pCR (%)	Survival: Median	Survival: 3-Y (%)	Local Failure (%)
Urba et al. (98)	100	75% A, 25% S	Preop	90	28	1.46 y	30	19[a]
			CFV + RT					
			Surgery	90	0	1.48 y	16	39
Walsh et al. (310, 311)	113	A	Preop	NR	25	16 mo	32[a]	—
			CF + RT					
			Surgery	NR	0	11 mo	6	—
Bosset et al. (220)	282	S	Preop	81	26	19 mo	34	—
			C + RT					
			Surgery	69	0	19 mo	36	—
Burmeister et al. (312)	256	S/A	Preop	80	16	22 mo	35	—
			C + RT					
			Surgery	59	0	19 mo	30	—
Tepper et al. (313)	56	S/A	Preop	NR	33	4.5 y	39[b]	13
			CF + RT					
			Surgery	NR	0	1.8 y	16[b]	15
Stahl et al. (315)	119	A	Pre CF +	70	2	22 mo	28	41
Lee et al. (314)	101	S	Surgery	72	16	33 mo	47	23
			Pre CF +	100%	43	28 mo	57[c]	22
			EC + RT +	88%	0	27 mo	55[c]	12
			Surgery					
			Preop					
			C + Rt					
			Surgery					

pCR, pathologically confirmed complete response; A, adenocarcinoma; S, squamous cell carcinoma; Preop, preoperative; C, cisplatin; F, 5-fluorouracil; V, vinblastine; E, etoposide; RT, radiation therapy; NR, not reported.
[a]Difference statistically significant.
[b]5-year survival.
[c]*2-year survival.*

radiotherapy. Most trials combined cisplatin and 5-FU[310–312] or single-agent cisplatin[220] with concurrent radiotherapy.

The Bosset et al.[220] trial was limited to patients with stage I or II squamous cell carcinoma based on a previously defined CT staging system, whereas the trials of Urba et al.,[98] Burmeister et al.,[312] and Tepper et al.[313] treated adenocarcinoma and squamous cell carcinoma, and the trial of Walsh et al.[310,311] was designed for locally advanced, resectable adenocarcinoma. A significant difference in the median and 3-year survival rates was observed only in the Walsh et al. and Tepper et al. trials. It is noteworthy that the pathologically determined complete-response rate was consistent for all studies, 25% to 28%, with the exception of the Burmeister et al. trial, which indicated a statistically significant lower pathologic complete-response rate for adenocarcinoma (9%) compared to squamous cell carcinoma (27%). Comparable rates of 3-year survival for patients in each of the investigational treatment groups (30% to 40%) was also observed, with the exception of the Tepper et al. trial, which reported a 5-year overall survival of 39%.

Urba et al.[98] at the University of Michigan randomly assigned 100 patients (75 with adenocarcinoma, 25 with squamous cell carcinoma) to receive (1) preoperative cisplatin (20 mg/m^2 on days 1 to 5 and 17 to 21), vinblastine (1 mg/m^2 on days 1 to 4 and 17 to 20), 5-FU (300 mg/m^2/24 h on days 1 to 21), and concurrent radiotherapy (1.5 Gy twice a day to 45 Gy), followed on day 42 by a transhiatal esophagectomy or (2) immediate surgery. Survival analysis after a median follow-up of 8.2 years for surviving patients revealed a nonsignificant improvement favoring preoperative chemoradiation (3-year survival, 30% vs. 16%; $P = .15$). A significant decrease in locoregional recurrence as a component of first failure was observed (19% recurrence rate for the combined treatment group vs. 42% for the group undergoing immediate surgery; $P = .02$). However, there was no difference in the rates of distant metastases, 60% and 65%, respectively. Although overall survival rates were not significantly different, there was a 31% lower risk of death, after adjustment for other prognostic factors, for patients randomly assigned to receive trimodal therapy, which suggests a possible benefit and the need for a trial adequately powered to detect a smaller survival difference. Consistent with phase 2 trial data, patients who achieved a pathologically confirmed complete response had better survival outcome, with a median survival time of 50 months and 3-year survival rate of 64%, compared to those with residual disease in the resected specimen, who had a median survival time of 12 months and a 3-year survival rate of 19%. The low statistical power of this trial may have failed to detect a potential modest survival benefit for chemoradiation compared to surgery alone.

In their series, Walsh et al.[310] reported a significant survival advantage for patients receiving preoperative chemoradiation. A total of 113 patients with adenocarcinoma of the esophagus, gastroesophageal junction, and cardia were randomly assigned to receive (1) two cycles (weeks 1 and 6) of 5-FU (15 mg/kg/24 h on days 1 to 5), cisplatin (75 mg/m^2 on day 7), plus concurrent radiotherapy (2.67 Gy/d to 40 Gy) followed

PRACTICE OF ONCOLOGY

by esophagectomy; or (2) immediate surgery alone. Chemoradiation was well tolerated. The incidence of acute toxicity of grade 3 or higher was 15%. The operative mortality was 9% in the multimodality treatment arm compared with 4% in the surgery control arm. After a median follow-up of surviving patients of 18 months, a significant improvement in both median survival time (16 months vs. 11 months; *P* = .01) and 3-year survival rate (32% vs. 6%; *P* = .01) was observed in patients who received preoperative therapy compared with those treated with surgery alone. A major criticism of this trial was the low 3-year survival rate (6%) in the surgical control arm. This probably reflects a patient population with more advanced disease than in those enrolled in the other two trials. CT staging was not required. More than 80% of patients had lymph node metastases.[311]

A third randomized trial of preoperative chemoradiation was reported by Bosset et al.[220] of the European Organisation for Research and Treatment of Cancer (EORTC). A total of 282 patients with clinically resectable (early stage I and II) squamous cell carcinoma were randomly assigned to undergo either preoperative chemoradiation or surgery alone. The preoperative regimen consisted of five daily fractions of 3.7 Gy each followed by a 2-week rest and another 3.7 Gy for 5 days. Chemotherapy was limited to cisplatin, 80 mg/m^2, 0 to 2 days before starting each 5 days of radiotherapy. Rates of curative resection were significantly higher in patients undergoing preoperative chemoradiation (81%) compared with immediate surgery (69%). After a median follow-up of 55 months, patients who received preoperative chemoradiation had a significantly better 3-year disease-free survival rate (40% vs. 28%) and local disease-free survival (relative risk, 0.6), yet had no improvement in median survival time (19 months) or overall 3-year survival (36%) compared with patients treated with surgery alone. However, this chemoradiation regimen was unconventional in design; not only was the radiation split course and delivered with unusually high doses per fraction, but the doses of chemotherapy would not be considered adequate for systemic therapy. The threefold higher postoperative mortality in the combined modality arm (12%) compared with the surgery alone arm (4%) may have undercut any potential overall survival benefit for chemoradiation.

The trial reported by Burmeister et al.[312] treated 256 patients with adenocarcinoma and squamous cell carcinoma with either surgery alone, or preoperative cisplatin, 5-FU, and radiation followed by surgery. The combined modality arm received one cycle of 5-FU dosed at 800 mg/m^2/d during a 4-day continuous infusion in combination with cisplatin 80 mg/m^2 on day 1, plus concurrent radiotherapy (2.33 Gy/d to 35 Gy) followed by esophagectomy. Chemoradiation was well tolerated, with the most common toxicities grade 3 or 4 esophagitis (16%) or nausea and vomiting (5%). There was no difference in surgical complications in either treatment group, with an overall operative mortality of 5%. After a median follow-up of 65 months, no significant difference was seen in either median overall survival time (22 months vs. 19 months with surgery alone) or 3-year survival rate. The chemoradiation group had a higher rate or curative resection (80%) compared with the surgery alone arm (59%). Pathologic complete responses were significantly less common in adenocarcinoma (9%) compared with squamous cell carcinoma (27%). A univariate analysis indicated that patients with squamous cell cancer had significantly better progression-free and overall survival when treated with preoperative chemoradiation. The low rate of pathologic complete responses in patients with adenocarcinoma on this trial raises concern about the adequacy of chemotherapy delivered (one cycle) during radiotherapy.

A similar trial was reported by Lee et al.[314] from Korea. A total of 102 patients with squamous cell cancer were randomized to surgery alone versus preoperative therapy with 45.6 Gy (1.2 Gy twice a day) plus 5-FU/cisplatin. There was no difference in median survival (28 months vs. 27 months).

The sixth randomized trial by Tepper et al.[313] reported the results of an Intergroup trial led by the Cancer and Leukemia Group B (CALGB-9781), in which patients were randomly assigned to receive (1) immediate surgery or (2) two cycles of cisplatin, 5-FU, and concurrent radiotherapy (total dose, 50.4 Gy) followed by surgery. This trial, activated in July 1998 and projected to enroll 475 patients, was terminated early because of failure to meet accrual targets. However, follow-up was available in 56 patients ultimately randomized and treated on protocol. With a median follow-up of 6 years, 5-year survival was significantly improved with the addition of preoperative chemoradiation (39% vs. 16%; *P* = .005). Interpretation of this trial is confounded by the small number of patients treated.

Some additional insight may be obtained from a small trial reported by Stahl et al.,[315] a multicenter phase 3 trial directly comparing preoperative chemotherapy to combined chemoradiotherapy followed by surgery in patients with gastroesophageal junction adenocarcinoma. The trial did not meet accrual goals and randomized only 119 eligible patients with Siewert's I to III gastroesophageal junction adenocarcinoma. The strength of the trial was the rigorous pretherapy staging, including EUS and laparoscopy, and the balance in treatment arms by clinical stage. Patients were assigned to (1) two and a half cycles of a 6-week schedule of weekly 5-FU 2 g/m^2, 24-hour infusion and leucovorin 500 mg/m^2, 2-hour infusion plus biweekly cisplatin 50 mg/m^2, or (2) two cycles of the same regimen, followed by 3 weeks of radiotherapy given in 15 fractions at a dose of 2 Gy combined with cisplatin 50 mg/m^2 on day 1 and 8 and etoposide 80 mg/m^2 on days 3 to 5. The primary end point was 3-year overall survival. Comparable numbers of patients had R0 resection after chemotherapy (69.5%) compared to chemoradiotherapy (72%). More patients on the chemoradiotherapy arm achieved a pathologic complete response (15.6%) compared to the chemotherapy arm (2.0%), and more patients were node negative (64.4% compared to 36.7%, respectively). Three-year survival trended superior in the chemoradiotherapy group (47.4%) compared to the chemotherapy group (27.7%; *P* = .07), and freedom from local tumor progression also favored the chemoradiotherapy group (76.5% vs. 59%; *P* = .06). More in-hospital deaths occurred in the chemoradiotherapy arm (10.2% vs. 3.8%, not statistically significant). The authors concluded that preoperative chemoradiotherapy could be considered a standard of care based on the favorable comparison to preoperative chemotherapy alone.

Recently Dutch investigators led by van der Gaast et al.[317] published in abstract form the results of a multicenter, phase 3 randomized trial of surgery alone versus preoperative chemoradiotherapy in 363 patients with resectable, EUS staged, T2-3N0-1 squamous cell cancer or adenocarcinoma of the esophagus or gastroesophageal junction. The authors used a relatively simple and well-tolerated regimen of weekly carboplatin AUC = 2 and paclitaxel 50 mg/m^2 given for five doses during 41.4 Gy of radiotherapy administered in 23 fractions, based on their prior phase 2 experience. Grade 3 and 4 toxicities during chemoradiotherapy were uncommon. The median survival in the chemoradiotherapy group was 49 months compared to 26 months on the surgery alone arm (HR 0.67; *P* = .011). The rate of R0 resection was superior for chemoradiotherapy compared to surgery alone (90% vs. 65%), and a pathologic complete response of 33% was observed. Surgical mortality was similar in the surgery and chemoradiotherapy arms (3.7% to 3.8%). Once published, this trial will represent the largest positive trial reported for preoperative chemoradiotherapy in esophageal cancer. The majority of patients treated on the trial had adenocarcinoma (74%) and were node positive (67%).

The accumulated experience from phase 2 and 3 trials indicates the following concerning chemoradiation using cisplatin and infusional 5-FU-based therapy followed by esophagectomy:

1. In approximately two-thirds of patients, disease is downstaged.
2. A survival advantage exists for patients experiencing downstaging to pathologically confirmed complete response or minimal residual disease status.
3. Surgery appears to be an important component of treatment to eliminate persistent disease after chemoradiation, especially for adenocarcinoma. Twenty percent to 30% of this group will be long-term survivors.
4. Locoregional control is improved, whereas distant failure is frequent and is the major cause of death.
5. Rates of curative resection may be improved with preoperative chemoradiation.

In the absence of a much larger controlled trial than either the Urba et al.[98] or Walsh et al.[310,311] studies, preoperative chemoradiation, by strict criteria, has not been designated as "standard of care." However, the benefits outlined and the improved survival of patients in the studies by Urba et al. and Walsh et al. have led both academic centers and community practices to adopt this combined modality approach for locally advanced (stage IIB, III) disease, particularly distal esophageal and gastroesophageal junction adenocarcinoma. Meta-analyses lend support to inclusion of chemotherapy and radiation therapy as part of surgical management. Two studies evaluated in combined analysis randomized trials predominantly of preoperative chemotherapy[318] and preoperative chemotherapy and radiation therapy compared to surgery alone.[319] These studies pooled results of 11 to 18 randomized trials treating between 2,300 and nearly 3,000 patients. Preoperative chemotherapy improved 2-year survival by 6.3% to 7.0% for preoperative chemotherapy alone, and preoperative combined chemoradiation improved 2-year survival by 13%, with similar benefits seen for squamous cell and adenocarcinoma in patients treated with combined chemoradiation. Because of the toxicity and ongoing uncertainty about benefit associated with preoperative combined chemoradiation, it should be used cautiously and priority should be given to enrolling patients in clinical trials.

Although three of the seven randomized trials demonstrated a survival advantage for chemoradiation, the role of preoperative chemoradiation remains controversial. However, all studies have limited patient numbers, heterogeneous treatment regimens, and in some the dose of radiation may be insufficient based on a dose-response analysis by Geh et al.[294] Overall there may be a 5% to 10% survival benefit; however, a much larger randomized trial would be required to prove this with certainty.

Postoperative Chemotherapy. Administering chemotherapy after surgery to patients who have already received chemotherapy or chemoradiation preoperatively has not been easily achieved in phase 2[236,237,277] and phase 3 trials.[96,244] This is exemplified by the INT-0113 trial, in which only 38% of patients who were candidates for adjuvant cisplatin and 5-FU therapy received the two planned courses.[96]

In Japan, surgery includes removal of the primary lesion plus extended dissection of lymph nodes in the mediastinum, neck, and abdomen. The Japanese Oncology Group has evaluated postoperative chemotherapy in a series of randomized trials.[320–323] One study of 205 patients who had undergone resection compared observation with two courses of adjuvant cisplatin and vindesine.[322] Median follow-up was 59 months, and the 5-year survival rate was 45% in the control arm and 48% in the adjuvant treatment arm, which indicated no survival benefit from this chemotherapy regimen.

A second trial of adjuvant chemotherapy in 242 patients had the same study design, except that the chemotherapy was cisplatin and 5-FU administered for two courses after curative resection.[321,323] At a median follow-up of 40.4 months, no differences were observed in the 5-year survival estimates (51% vs. 61% for adjuvant chemotherapy; $P = .3$). The estimated 5-year disease-free survival rate was improved with chemotherapy (58% for the chemotherapy vs. 46% for observation; $P = .05$). Disease-free survival for node-negative patients was 77% in the surgery-alone group versus 82% in the adjuvant treatment group ($P = .3$), and for node-positive patients 35% in the surgery-alone group versus 53% in the adjuvant treatment group ($P = .06$). These data suggest that adjuvant chemotherapy may benefit node-positive patients, but this was an unplanned subset analysis on this trial. The Eastern Cooperative Oncology Group completed a phase 2 trial (E8296) to evaluate adjuvant therapy consisting of cisplatin (75 mg/m^2) and paclitaxel (175 mg/m^2 during 3 hours) every 3 weeks for four courses in 55 patients with completely resected, T3, or node-positive adenocarcinoma of the esophagus, gastroesophageal junction, or cardia.[324] The majority (89%) had lymph node involvement. The majority of these (84%) were able to complete all four cycles of chemotherapy. The 2-year survival rate was 60%, which compared favorably with results for contemporary historical controls.[96]

In summary, the available data for postoperative adjuvant chemotherapy suggest a possible prolongation of survival for patients who have had a potentially curative (R0) resection and have lymph node–positive (N1) disease. There are no data to indicate or suggest that administration of postoperative adjuvant chemotherapy will prolong survival for patients who have undergone a curative resection and have negative nodes (N0). Patients who have positive margins of resection should be considered for postoperative radiation. Those who have had R0 resections but have regional nodal metastases (stages IIB and III) should be enrolled in clinical trials to evaluate adjuvant therapies.

Postoperative Radiation Therapy. Several reports of nonrandomized trials have suggested that postoperative radiation therapy may be effective after esophagectomy. Yamamoto et al.[325] reported a 94% 2-year local control rate in node-positive patients. For patients who underwent a three-field dissection, Hosokawa et al.[326] added intraoperative radiation followed by 45 Gy postoperatively. The 5-year survival rate was 34%.

Two randomized trials were limited to patients treated in the adjuvant setting. Teniere et al.[251] reported the results for 221 patients with squamous cell carcinoma randomly assigned to receive either surgery alone or postoperative radiation therapy (45 to 55 Gy at 1.8 Gy per fraction). Postoperative radiation therapy was found to have no significant impact on survival. In the series of Fok et al.,[327] patients with both squamous cell carcinomas and adenocarcinomas receiving either curative or palliative resections were evaluated; although the total dose of radiation therapy was conventional, the dose per fraction (3.5 Gy) was unconventional. No significant decrease in local failure or distant failure or improvement in the median survival time was achieved with the addition of postoperative radiation therapy.

Postoperative Chemoradiation. The only randomized trial of postoperative chemoradiation is the Intergroup trial INT-0116.[328] Although the goal of this trial was to examine the role of postoperative adjuvant chemoradiation in gastric cancer, 20% of patients had adenocarcinoma of the gastroesophageal junction. Eligible patients included those with stage IB, II, IIIA, IIIB, or IV nonmetastatic adenocarcinoma of the stomach or gastroesophageal junction after curative resection. Patients were randomly assigned to receive either observation alone or postoperative chemoradiation consisting of four monthly cycles of bolus 5-FU and leucovorin plus 45 Gy concurrent radiation with cycle two. A total of 603 patients were registered. Pretreatment characteristics were similar in both arms, and most patients had locally advanced disease. Approximately two-thirds of the patients had pT3 or pT4 tumors and approximately 85% had positive locoregional nodes.

Patients randomly assigned to receive postoperative chemoradiation had a significant decrease in local failure as the first site of failure (19% vs. 29%) and an increase in median survival (36 months vs. 27 months), 3-year relapse-free survival (48% vs. 31%), and overall survival (50% vs. 41%; *P* = .005). Although 17% of patients could not complete all therapy as planned, there was only one treatment-related death. With a median follow-up of 10 years the improvement in survival with postoperative chemoradiation remains statistically significant.[328]

To minimize radiation-related toxicity, careful pretreatment review of the simulation films was performed. This frequently resulted in the recommendation to the treating radiation oncologist to modify the design or volume (or both) of the radiation fields. Because 20% had adenocarcinoma of the gastroesophageal junction, those patients should be considered to receive postoperative 5-FU-based chemoradiation if they have not received preoperative therapy.

The other role for postoperative radiation therapy is in cases of positive surgical margins. Based on the RTOG-85-01 trial, patients selected for treatment with postoperative radiation should receive chemoradiation.[258,329,330]

Definitive Chemoradiation

Although definitive chemoradiation is a treatment option for patients with localized resectable esophageal carcinoma, especially those with cervical esophageal squamous cell carcinoma or those not considered ideal resection candidates, this therapeutic approach is discussed in detail in "Chemoradiation" in the next section.

Treatment of Locally Advanced Disease

Radiation Therapy

The 1996 to 1999 patterns of care study examined 414 patients who received radiation therapy as part of definitive or adjuvant management at 59 institutions.[331] Overall, 51% had adenocarcinoma and 49% had squamous cell carcinoma. With a median follow-up of 8 months, multivariate analysis revealed that patients who received chemoradiation followed by surgery had a significant decrease in locoregional recurrence (HR 0.40; *P* <.0001) and survival (HR 0.32; *P* <.001) compared with those who did not undergo surgery. A similar significant decrease in locoregional recurrence (HR 1.36; *P* = .01) and survival (HR 1.32; *P* <.03) was seen in those patients who received their care at large radiation oncology centers (treating 500 or more new cancer patients per year) compared with small centers (treating fewer than 500 new cancer patients per year). In a similar patterns of care study of 767 patients treated in Japan from 1998 to 2001, 220 (29%) received preoperative or postoperative radiation, or both, with or without chemotherapy.[332] Various oncology groups have published treatment guidelines; however, there is still no consensus at the present time.[333,334]

The effect of histologic type (adenocarcinoma vs. squamous cell carcinoma) is unclear. Most series suggest that squamous cell cancers have a higher response rate compared with adenocarcinomas; however, no clear difference in outcome was found. The National Cancer Institute Intergroup has randomized trials that stratify patients by lesion histologic type. Until these data are available, the impact of histologic type cannot be adequately assessed, and it is reasonable to treat both types of lesions in a similar fashion.

Primary Nonsurgical Therapy. Primary therapy for esophageal cancer is either surgical or nonsurgical. The patient population selected for treatment with each modality is usually different. For several reasons, this results in a selection bias against nonsurgical therapy. Patients with unfavorable prognostic features are more commonly selected for treatment with nonsurgical therapy. These features include medical contraindications and primary unresectable or actual metastatic disease. Surgical series report results based on pathologic stage, whereas nonsurgical series report results based on clinical stage. Pathologic staging has the advantage of excluding some patients with metastatic disease not identified during clinical staging. Because some patients treated without surgery are approached in a palliative rather than a curative fashion, the intensity of chemotherapy and the doses and techniques of radiation therapy used may be suboptimal.

The difficulty of accurately staging esophageal cancer preoperatively is discussed in "Diagnostic Studies and Pretreatment Staging," earlier in this chapter. The efficacy of FDG-PET as a complement to CT and EUS must be emphasized. Undetected metastatic disease was identified by PET in 15% of patients in the series by Flamen et al.[302] and in 20% of patients in the series by Downey et al.[301]

Radiation therapy alone. Many series have reported results of external-beam radiation therapy alone. Most include patients with unfavorable features such as clinical T4 disease and multiple positive lymph nodes. For example, in the series of De-Ren,[335] 184 of the 678 patients had stage IV disease. Overall, the 5-year survival rate for patients treated with conventional doses of radiation therapy alone is 0% to 10%.[329,335,336] The use of radiation therapy as a potentially curative modality requires doses of at least 50 Gy at 1.8 to 2.0 Gy per fraction. Shi et al.[337] reported a 33% 5-year survival rate with the use of late-course accelerated fractionation to a total dose of 68.4 Gy. However, in the radiation-therapy–alone arm of the RTOG-85-01 trial in which patients received 64 Gy at 2 Gy/d with modern techniques, all patients were dead of their disease by 3 years.[258,330]

Collectively, these data indicate that radiation therapy alone should be reserved for palliation or for patients who are medically unable to receive chemotherapy. As is discussed in the following section, the results of chemoradiation are more favorable, and it remains the standard of care.

Definitive Chemoradiation

Conventional Approaches

Comparison of definitive chemoradiation and surgery. There are many single-arm, nonrandomized trials of chemoradiation alone, and they have included patients with disease at a variety of stages.[338–341] Few series examine patients with T1 or T2 disease.[340,342] In the series reported by Coia et al.,[340] patients received 5-FU and mitomycin C concurrently with 60 Gy of radiation therapy. When results for clinical stage I and II disease are combined, the local failure rate was 25%, the 5-year actuarial local relapse-free survival was 70%, and the 5-year actuarial survival was 30%.

Six randomized trials compared radiation therapy alone with chemoradiation.[103,242,258,343–347] Of these six trials, five used suboptimal doses of radiation and three used inadequate doses of systemic chemotherapy, and some studies used sequential chemotherapy and radiotherapy rather than concurrent therapy. For example, in the series of Araujo et al.,[347] patients received only one cycle of 5-FU, mitomycin C, and bleomycin. The EORTC trial used subcutaneous methotrexate.[343] In the Scandinavian trial reported by Nygaard et al.,[242] patients received low doses of chemotherapy (cisplatin, 20 mg/m^2, and bleomycin, 10 mg/m^2, for a maximum of two cycles). An analysis of pooled data from these trials reported a significant local control and survival benefit at 1 year for chemoradiation compared with radiation therapy alone.[333] Chemoradiation was associated with a significant increase in adverse effects, including life-threatening toxicities.

In the ECOG EST-1282 trial,[346] patients who received chemoradiation had a significantly increased median survival compared with those who received radiation alone (15 months vs. 9 months; $P = .04$) but experienced no improvement in 5-year survival (9% vs. 7%). However, this was not a pure nonsurgical trial because approximately 50% of patients in each arm underwent surgery after receiving 40 Gy of radiation. Furthermore, this decision depended on the individual investigator's preference. The operative mortality was 17%. Finally, the Pretoria trial reported by Slabber et al.,[345] which was limited to a total of 70 patients with T3 squamous cell cancers, used a low-dose (40 Gy) split-course radiation schedule.

The only trial that was designed to deliver adequate doses of systemic chemotherapy with concurrent radiation therapy was the RTOG-85-01 trial reported by Herskovic et al.,[258] and updated by Al-Sarraf et al.[344] (Fig. 79.10). This Intergroup trial primarily included patients with squamous cell carcinoma. Patients received four cycles of 5-FU (1,000 mg/m^2/24 h × 4 days) and cisplatin (75 mg/m^2 on day 1). Radiation therapy (50 Gy at 2 Gy/d) was given concurrently with day 1 of chemotherapy. Curiously, cycles three and four of chemotherapy were delivered every 3 weeks (weeks 8 and 11) rather than every 4 weeks (weeks 9 and 13). This intensification may explain, in part, why only 50% of the patients finished all four cycles of the chemotherapy. The control arm was given radiation therapy alone, albeit at a higher dose (64 Gy) than the chemoradiation arm.

Patients who received chemoradiation had a significant improvement in median survival (14 months vs. 9 months) and 5-year survival (27% vs. 0%; $P < .0001$).[344] There was a clear plateau in the survival curve. Minimum follow-up was 5 years, and the 8-year survival was 22%.[103,347] Histologic type did not significantly influence the results: 21% of patients with squamous cell carcinomas (n = 107) were alive at 5 years compared with 13% of patients with adenocarcinoma (n = 23) (*P* was not significant). Although African Americans had larger primary tumors, all of which were squamous cell cancers, there was no difference in their survival compared with that of whites.[348] The incidence of local failure as the first site of failure (defined as local persistence or recurrence) was also decreased in the chemoradiation arm (47% vs. 65%). The protocol was closed early because of the positive results; however, after this early closure, an additional 69 eligible patients were treated with the same chemoradiation regimen. In this nonrandomized combined modality group, the 5-year survival was 14% and local failure was 52%.

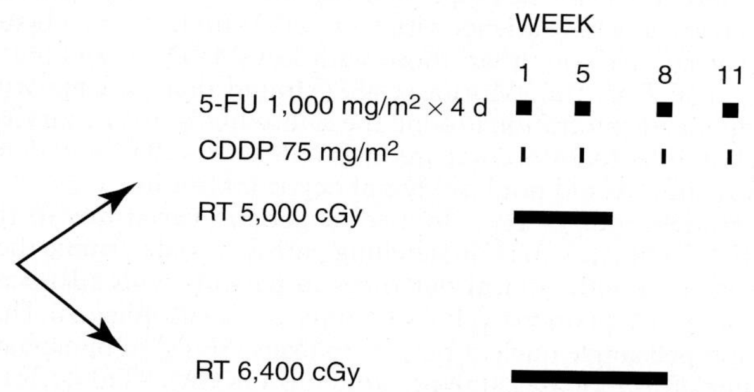

FIGURE 79.10 Phase 3 Intergroup trial Radiation Therapy Oncology Group 85-10 for patients with squamous cell and adenocarcinoma of the esophagus selected for a nonoperative approach. 5-FU, 5-fluorouracil; CDDP, cisplatin; RT, radiation therapy.

Chemoradiation not only improves the results compared with radiation alone but also is associated with a higher incidence of toxicity. In the 1997 report of the RTOG-85-01 trial, patients who received chemoradiation had a higher incidence of acute grade 3 toxicity (44% vs. 25%) and acute grade 4 toxicity (20% vs. 3%) compared with those who received radiation therapy alone. Including the one treatment-related death (2%), the incidence of total acute grade 3+ toxicity was 66%.[344] The 1999 report examined late toxicity. The incidence of late grade 3+ toxicity was similar in the chemoradiation arm and in the radiation-alone arm (29% vs. 23%).[103] However, grade 4+ toxicity remained higher in the combined modality arm (10% vs. 2%). Interestingly, the nonrandomized chemoradiation group experienced a similar incidence of late grade 3+ toxicity (28%) but a lower incidence of grade 4 toxicity (4%), and there were no treatment-related deaths.

Based on the positive results from the RTOG-85-01 trial, the conventional nonsurgical treatment for esophageal carcinoma is chemoradiation. Notwithstanding, the local failure rate in the RTOG-85-01 chemoradiation arm was 45%, and there is room for improvement. Therefore, new approaches such as intensification of chemoradiation and escalation of the radiation dose have been developed in an attempt to help improve these results.

Randomized trials. Although there are a number of trials comparing preoperative chemoradiation with surgery alone, there are only two trials that directly compare nonoperative treatment with surgery. One randomized trial compared surgery with radiation alone[349] and one compared surgery with chemoradiation.[350] Both series have small numbers of patients, limited follow-up, and neither report a difference in survival.

Nonrandomized trials. The positive results of RTOG-85-01, demonstrating a 27% 5-year survival rate for patients treated with definitive chemoradiation compared with no 5-year survival after treatment with radiotherapy alone, is a major advance. This treatment option has influenced the selection of patients for nonsurgical management because it provides an alternative for restoring swallowing function in patients with locally advanced disease for whom resection would likely be palliative.

For patients with earlier-stage disease that appears resectable, definitive chemoradiation may also be appropriate treatment; however, prospective trials comparing this approach with surgery, stratified by stage, have not been performed. Nonetheless, nonrandomized comparisons of contemporary series suggest that the nonsurgical approach offers a survival rate that is the same or better than that achievable with surgery alone. For example, the median survival time and 5-year survival rate were 14 months and 27%, respectively, in the chemoradiation arm of RTOG-85-01, and 20 months and 20%, respectively, in INT-0122.[351] In comparison, the median survival in the surgical control arm of the Dutch trial reported by Kok et al.[243] was 11 months, and the median survival time and 5-year survival rate in the surgical control arm of INT-0113 were 16 months and 20%, respectively. Likewise, the local failure rates were similar. The incidence of local failure (local recurrence plus local persistence of disease) as the first site of failure was 45% in RTOG-85-01 and 39% in INT-0122. If all patients, including patients failing to undergo surgery or patients having R2 resection are included, the local failure as the first site of failure was 61% on the surgical trial INT-0113, actually higher than the 45% reported on RTOG-85-01. The treatment-related mortality rates were also similar (2% in RTOG-85-01, 9% in INT-0122, and 6% in INT-0113).

In summary, the local failure, survival, and treatment-related mortality rates for nonsurgical and surgical therapies are similar. Although the results are comparable, it is clear that both the nonsurgical and surgical approaches have limited success.

Necessity for surgery after chemoradiation. Two randomized trials examine whether surgery is necessary after chemoradiation. In the Federation Francaise de Cancerologie Digestive (FFCD) 9102 trial, 444 patients with clinically resectable T3-4N0-1M0 squamous cell or adenocarcinoma of the esophagus received initial chemoradiation.[105] Patients initially received two cycles of 5-FU, cisplatin, and concurrent radiation (either 46 Gy at 2 Gy/d or split course 15 Gy weeks 1 and 3). The 259 patients who had at least a partial response were then randomized to surgery versus additional chemoradiation, which included three cycles of 5-FU, cisplatin, and concurrent radiation (either 20 Gy at 2 Gy/d or split course 15 Gy). Two-year local control was 66% in the surgery arm versus 57% in the chemoradiation-alone arm. There was no significant difference in 2-year survival (34% vs. 40%; $P = .44$) or median survival (17.7 months vs. 19.3 months) in patients who underwent surgery versus additional chemoradiation. These data suggest that patients who initially respond to chemoradiation should complete chemoradiation rather than stop and undergo surgery. Using the Spitzer index, there was no difference in global quality of life; however, a significantly greater decrease in quality of life was observed in the surgery arm during the postoperative period (7.52 vs. 8.45; $P < .01$, respectively).[352] A separate analysis revealed that compared with split course radiation, patients who received standard course radiation had improved 2-year local relapse-free survival rates (77% vs. 57%; $P = .002$) but no significant difference in overall survival (37% vs. 31%).[353]

The German Oesophageal Cancer Study Group compared preoperative chemoradiation followed by surgery versus chemoradiation alone.[106] In this trial, 172 eligible patients age 70 years or more with uT3-4N0-1M0 squamous cell cancers of the esophagus were randomized to preoperative therapy (three cycles of 5-FU, leucovorin, etoposide, and cisplatin, followed by concurrent etoposide, cisplatin, plus 40 Gy) followed by surgery versus chemoradiation alone (the same chemotherapy but the radiation dose was increased to 60 to 65 Gy with or without brachytherapy). The pathologic complete response (pCR) rate was 33%. Despite a decrease in 2-year local failure (36% vs. 58%; $P = .003$), there was no significant difference in 3-year survival (31% vs. 24%) for those who were randomized to preoperative chemoradiation followed by surgery versus chemoradiation alone.

In summary, although there is good rationale for its use, it is not clear that the combination of surgery and chemoradiation, regardless of the sequence, improves the survival results of either treatment alone. An alternative approach is to use "selective" surgery after preoperative chemoradiation. Swisher et al.[354] reported a retrospective analysis of patients who underwent a salvage compared with a planned esophagectomy at the M. D. Anderson Cancer Center from 1987 to 2000. The operative mortality was higher in those who underwent salvage versus planned surgery (15% vs. 6%) but there was no difference in survival (25%). Because only 13 patients were identified who had salvage, the results need to be interpreted with caution.

Tumor markers and predictors of response to chemoradiation. It would be helpful to predict which tumors have a higher likelihood of responding to radiation or chemoradiation. Geh et al.[294] performed a systematic review to identify factors associated with a higher rate of pCR in patients receiving preoperative chemoradiation. The analysis was limited to the 26 trials meeting four criteria: (1) at least 20 patients treated, (2) a single chemoradiation regimen was delivered, (3) 5-FU, cisplatin, or mitomycin C–based chemotherapy was used, and (4) there was information on patient numbers, age, resection, and pCR rates. Overall, the pCR rate was 24% and the probability of pCR increased with increasing radiation dose ($P = .006$) and the use of a 5-FU-based ($P = .003$) or cisplatin-based ($P = .018$) regimen. In contrast, increased radiation treatment time ($P = .035$) and median age ($P = .019$) both decreased the chance of a pCR.

Data from both Berger et al.[355] and Rohatgi et al.[356] suggest that patients who achieve a pCR had an improvement in survival compared with those who do not (5-year, 48% vs. 15%, and median, 133 months vs. 34 months, respectively). However, the ability to predict a pCR prior to surgery is variable, as discussed earlier. A multivariate analysis by Gaca et al.[357] reported that posttreatment nodal status ($P = .03$) but not the degree of primary tumor response predicted disease-free survival.

Posttreatment imaging does not consistently identify response. Ultrasound following chemoradiation does not accurately predict a pCR.[358] In contrast, Blackstock et al.[359] reported that the percentage of decrease in standard uptake value measured by 18F-FDG-PET predicted response, and Brucher et al.[360] found that it correlated with survival. McLoughlin et al.[361] treated 81 patients with preoperative chemoradiation and reported that FDG-PET was able to predict a pathologic complete response with 62% sensitivity, 44% specificity, and 56% accuracy.

The predictive ability of molecular markers has been examined. In 38 patients with squamous cell carcinoma who received chemoradiation with or without surgery, tumors without *p53* expression and tumors with weak *Bcl-*X_L expression showed a higher response to chemotherapy (56% and 53%, respectively) than tumors positive for *p53* or with strong *Bcl-*X_L expression (30% and 32%, respectively; *P* not significant).[362] After preoperative chemoradiation, patients with *p53*-negative tumors had a significantly better mean survival than those with *p53*-positive tumors (31 months vs. 11 months; $P = .0378$). By multivariate analysis, Pomp et al.[363] found that overexpression of p53 resulted in a decrease in survival in 69 patients with squamous cell carcinoma or adenocarcinoma treated with radiation alone. In one study, there was a correlation between decreasing levels of four phospholipids and increasing T stage and grade.[364]

Kishi et al.[365] reported that, of 77 patients treated with chemoradiation for squamous cell cancer, those with *p53*- and metallothionein-positive tumors had a poor response to treatment, whereas strong expression of CDC25B was associated with a good response. In 73 patients with T2 to T4 M0 esophageal cancer treated with 60 Gy of radiation plus 5-FU and cisplatin, Hironaka et al.[366] examined pretreatment biopsy specimens for a variety of markers, including *p53*, Ki-67, epidermal growth factor receptor, cyclin D1, vascular endothelial growth factor, microvessel density (MVD), thymidylate synthase, dihydropyrimidine dehydrogenase, and glutathione S-transferase. By multivariate analysis, MVD, T stage, and performance status were independent prognostic variables ($P = .002$, .02, and .02, respectively). Patients with high-MVD tumors had a better 3-year survival rate than those with low-MVD tumors (61% vs. 33%; $P = .02$). Morita et al.[367] found that patients with lymphocyte infiltration around the tumor had a 5-year survival rate of 46% to 76% compared with 28% ($P < .05$) in patients whose tumors did not have lymphocytic infiltration

Hildebrandt et al.[368] looked at genetic variations in the PI3K/PTEN/AKT/mTOR signaling pathway to determine their association with clinical outcomes in patients with adenocarcinoma or squamous cell carcinoma of the esophagus. They genotyped single nuclear polymorphisms (SNPs) in phosphatidylinositol-3-kinase catalytic subunit (PI3KCA), PTEN, AKT1, AKT2, and FRAP1 (encoding mammalian target of rapamycin [mTOR]) in esophageal cancer patients treated with chemoradiation and noted that AKT2 and FRAP1 were associated with a poor response to treatment, while heterozygosity for AKT1 was associated with good response to treatment. Understanding the mechanism of radioresistance through identification and targeting of molecular pathways by serum protein profiling[369] and identification of genes involved in apoptosis,[370] activated transcription factor nuclear factor κB,[371] and microvascular density[372] may offer new opportunities for therapeutic advances.

Intensification of chemoradiation. The phase 2 Intergroup trial 0122 (ECOG-PE289/RTOG-90-12) was designed to intensify treatment in the RTOG-85-01 combined modality arm.[352] Both the chemotherapy and radiation therapy in INT-0122 were intensified by 20%.[373] The median survival time was 20 months and the 5-year actuarial survival rate was 20%. Similar toxicities were reported by Ishikura et al.[374] for 139 patients with squamous cell cancers treated with 5-FU, cisplatin, and 60 Gy of radiation. However, the higher radiation dose (64.8 Gy) in INT-0122 was tolerated and compared with the 50.4 Gy of radiation in the Intergroup trial INT-0123 (Fig. 79.11), discussed below.

A limited number of phase 1 and 2 trials have tested the use of neoadjuvant chemotherapy before radiation therapy or chemoradiation with variable results, as discussed above. Dysphagia relief and a reduced need for feeding tube placement with induction therapy have been observed. A potential advantage of neoadjuvant chemotherapy is the early identification of those patients who may or may not respond to the chemotherapeutic regimen being delivered. The MUNICON trial, discussed earlier, indicated that PET nonresponding patients could be referred for earlier surgery rather than continue ineffective systemic therapy.[148] The potential to change to a salvage chemotherapy during radiotherapy has been reported with successful outcomes, but the use of PET scan to change chemotherapy remains investigational.[92,375]

Intensification of the radiation dose. Another approach to the dose intensification of chemoradiation is increasing the radiation dose above 50.4 Gy. There are two methods by which to increase the radiation dose to the esophagus: brachytherapy and external-beam radiation therapy.

Brachytherapy. Intraluminal brachytherapy allows the escalation of the dose to the primary tumor while protecting the surrounding dose-limiting structures such as the lung, heart, and spinal cord.[376] A radioactive source is placed intraluminally via bronchoscopy or a nasogastric tube. Brachytherapy has been used both as primary therapy (usually palliative)[377,378] and as a boost after external-beam radiation therapy or chemoradiation.[379–381] It can be delivered by high-dose rate or low-dose rate.[373] Although there are technical and radiobiologic differences between the two dose rates, there are no clear therapeutic advantages for either.

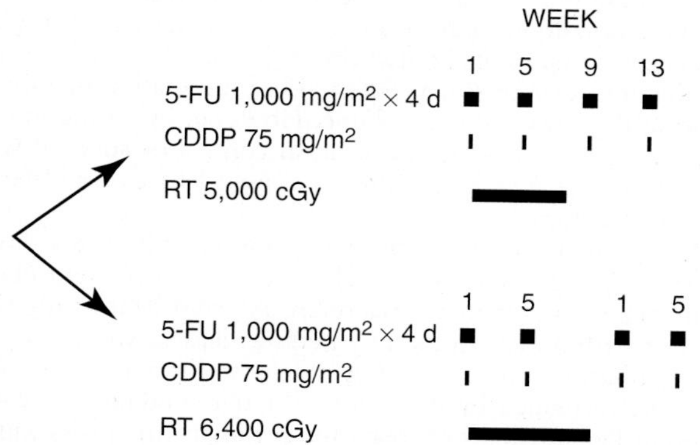

FIGURE 79.11 Phase 3 Intergroup trial 0123 (Radiation Therapy Oncology Group 94-05) for patients with squamous cell or adenocarcinoma of the esophagus. 5-FU, 5-fluorouracil; CDDP, cisplatin; RT, radiation therapy.

Series that combine brachytherapy with external-beam radiation therapy or chemoradiation report results similar to those for conventional chemoradiation. Yorozu et al.[381] reported a local failure rate of 57% and a 5-year actuarial survival of 28% in 46 patients with stage T2-3N0-1M0 disease. Even for a more favorable subset of patients with clinical T1 to T2 disease, Yorozu et al.[382] reported a local failure rate of 44% and a 5-year survival of 26%. In the series by Pasquier et al.[380] local failure was 23% and 5-year survival was 36%. In an updated series by Ishikawa et al.[383] 59 patients with submucosal esophageal cancer received external-beam therapy followed by brachytherapy in 36 patients with either low-dose rate ^{137}Cs (17 patients) or high-dose rate ^{192}Ir (19 patients). Patients selected to receive a brachytherapy boost had a significantly higher 5-year cause specific survival (86% vs. 62%; $P = .04$).

In the RTOG-92-07 trial, 75 patients with squamous cell cancers (92%) or adenocarcinomas (8%) of the thoracic esophagus received the RTOG-85-01 combined modality regimen (5-FU, cisplatin, and 50 Gy of radiation) followed by a boost during cycle three of chemotherapy with either low-dose– or high-dose–rate intraluminal brachytherapy.[384] Because of low accrual the low-dose–rate option was discontinued and the analysis was limited to patients who received the high-dose–rate treatment. High-dose–rate brachytherapy was delivered in weekly fractions of 5 Gy during weeks 8, 9, and 10. After the development of several fistulas, the fraction delivered at week 10 was discontinued. Although the complete-response rate was 73%, the rate of local failure was 27%. Rates of acute toxicity were 58% for grade 3, 26% for grade 4, and 8% for grade 5 (treatment-related death). The cumulative incidence of fistula was 18% per year and the crude incidence was 14%. Of the six treatment-related fistulas, three were fatal. Given the significant toxicity, this treatment approach should be used with caution.[385]

Based on these and other data the American Brachytherapy Society has developed guidelines for esophageal brachytherapy.[386–388]

External-Beam Therapy. Because almost all patients in both the INT-0122 trial who started radiation therapy were able to complete the full dose (64.8 Gy), this higher dose of radiation was used in the experimental arm of the Intergroup esophageal trial INT-0123 (RTOG-94-05).[259] In this trial, patients with either squamous cell carcinoma or adenocarcinoma who were selected for nonsurgical treatment were randomly assigned to receive a slightly modified RTOG-85-01 combined modality regimen with 50.4 Gy of radiation versus the same chemotherapy with 64.8 Gy of radiation (Fig. 79.10).

The modifications to the original RTOG-85-01 chemoradiation arm includes (1) using 1.8-Gy fractions to 50.4 Gy rather than 2-Gy fractions to 50 Gy; (2) treating with 5-cm proximal and distal margins for 50.4 Gy rather than treating the whole esophagus for the first 30 Gy followed by a cone down with 5-cm margins to 50 Gy; (3) cycle three of 5-FU and cisplatin did not begin until 4 weeks after the completion of radiation therapy rather than 3 weeks after; and (4) cycles three and four of chemotherapy were delivered every 4 weeks rather than every 3 weeks.

INT-0123 was closed to accrual in 1999 with 218 patients after an interim analysis revealed that it was unlikely that the high-dose arm would achieve superior survival compared with the standard-dose arm: there was no significant difference in median survival time (13.0 months vs. 18.1 months) or 2-year survival rate (31% vs. 40%) between the high-dose and standard-dose arms.[259] Although 11 treatment-related deaths occurred in the high-dose arm compared with 2 in the standard-dose arm, 7 of the 11 deaths occurred in patients who had received 50.4 Gy or less.

Although the crude incidence of local failure or persistence of local disease (or both) was lower in the high-dose arm than in the standard-dose arm (50% vs. 55%), as was the incidence of distant failure (9% vs. 16%), these were not significant. Although retrospective data from the M. D. Anderson Cancer Center suggest a positive correlation between radiation dose and locoregional control,[387] the results of the INT-0123 trial maintain, the standard dose of 50.4 Gy.

The modifications to the original RTOG-85-01 chemoradiation arm outlined earlier did not adversely affect the local control or survival rate in the control arm of INT-0123. Therefore, the radiation doses and field design used in the control arm of INT-0123 should be used.

Radiation can be intensified not only by increasing the total dose but also by using accelerated fractionation or hyperfractionation. Wang et al.[388] randomly assigned 101 patients with squamous cell cancer to receive either continuous accelerated hyperfractionated radiation (66 Gy) or late-course accelerated hyperfractionated radiation (68.4 Gy). Compared with patients who received late-course accelerated hyperfractionated radiation, those treated with continuous accelerated hyperfractionated radiation had a significantly higher incidence of grade 3+ esophagitis (61% vs. 10%; $P < .001$); however, no benefit was seen in local control or survival.[389,390] Most series report an increase in acute toxicity without any clear therapeutic benefit.

Proton therapy has been presented by Japanese investigators. Sugahara et al.[391] treated 46 patients with squamous cell cancers using protons with or without photons to a median total dose of 76 Gy. The 5-year local control rate was T1, 83%; T2 to T4, 29%, and survival was T1, 55% and T2 to T4, 13%. Koyama and Hirohiko[392] reported mean actuarial survival rates of 60% for patients with superficial lesions and 39% for those with advanced disease treated to mean total doses of 78 to 81 Gy. The incidence of esophageal ulcer was 67%.

New chemoradiation regimens. Because 75% to 80% of patients die of metastatic disease, advances in systemic therapies are necessary for further improvement of results. The most widely used chemotherapeutic regimen to be combined with radiation for the treatment of esophageal cancer is 5-FU and cisplatin. Most agents are being developed for use in preoperative regimens and are combined with radiation doses of 45 to 50.4 Gy. These include both cytotoxic and targeted small molecules. Phase 1 and 2 trials have been developed to examine the use of newer chemotherapeutic agents such as paclitaxel,[278,285,290,393,394] docetaxel,[289,395] irinotecan,[291–302,304,305,396,397] trastuzumab,[398] oxaliplatin,[280,291,399] bevacizumab,[291] and cetuximab[400,401] and are being used as the foundations for new regimens. As discussed above, to date there are no clear advantages to chemoradiotherapy protocols using some of the newer chemotherapy agents. However, as discussed above, a recent large phase 3 trial validated weekly carboplatin and paclitaxel as a well-tolerated and more modern alternative to 5-FU and cisplatin to use during radiation.[402] The ongoing RTOG-0436 trial is a randomized, phase 3 nonoperative trial to evaluate upfront use of cetuximab in combined chemoradiotherapy in esophageal cancer. Patients receive 50.4 Gy of radiotherapy combined with 6 weeks of weekly paclitaxel 50 mg/m^2 combined with weekly cisplatin 25 mg/m^2. Patients are randomized to receive, or not receive, cetuximab 400 mg/m^2 followed by weekly 250 mg/m^2. The primary end point is overall survival, and more than 400 patients will be accrued.

Palliation of esophageal cancer with radiation therapy

Palliation of Dysphagia and Bleeding. Many of the series examining dysphagia are retrospective, and most do not use objective criteria to define and assess dysphagia. Some do not report the number of patients presenting with dysphagia or the percentage who receive palliative treatment until the time of death. Furthermore, few series carefully examine other variables that may influence the results, such as histologic type, stage, and location of the primary tumor.

Options for palliation include stents, feeding tubes, chemotherapy, and external-beam radiation therapy or brachytherapy (or both). The selection of the technique is variable and commonly is based on physician preference. In a randomized trial from the Dutch SIREC Study Group of stent versus one 12-Gy fraction of brachytherapy, dysphagia, as measured by a variety of quality-of-life scales, improved more rapidly after stent placement; however, long-term relief was superior after brachytherapy.[378] Median survivals were similar (145 days vs. 155 days).

Patients for whom stents fail commonly are treated with palliative radiation. Li et al.[403] reported that the presence of a metal stent increases the radiation dose 5% to 10% at a 0.5-cm depth in the esophageal wall. Therefore, the radiation dose should be decreased by 5% to 10% when a metal stent is in the radiation field. Nishimura et al.[404] reported a high-grade 3+ complication rate in 47 patients who underwent stent placement before or during radiation treatment and recommend that stent placement be delayed until radiation therapy has failed.

As seen in Table 79.10, series have examined the palliative benefits of either radiation alone[343,405–408] or chemoradiation.[338,339,407,409–413] Overall, external-beam radiation therapy alone provides palliation of dysphagia in 70% to 80% of patients.

The most comprehensive and carefully performed analysis of swallowing function in patients receiving chemoradiation is by Coia et al.[413] Using a swallowing score modified from O'Rourke et al.,[414] they analyzed 102 patients treated with three 5-FU–based combined modality regimens. Before the start of therapy, 95% of patients had some degree of dysphagia. Within 2 weeks after the start of treatment, 45% had improvement in dysphagia, and by the completion of the 6-week therapy, 83% had improvement. Overall, 88% experienced an improvement in dysphagia. The median time to improvement was 4 weeks (range, 1 to 21 weeks), and all but two patients could swallow at least soft or solid foods. Harvey et al.[409] treated 106 patients and reported that 78% had improvement of at least one grade in their dysphagia score; 51% maintained swallowing improvement until the time of last follow-up.

Intraluminal brachytherapy is also an effective, albeit more limited, method, achieving palliation of dysphagia in 35% to 80% of patients and a median survival of 5 months. A major limitation of brachytherapy is the effective treatment distance. The primary isotope is ^{192}-Ir, which is usually prescribed to treat to a distance of 1 cm from the source. Any portion of the tumor that is more than 1 cm from the source will receive a suboptimal radiation dose, confirmed by pathologic analysis of surgical specimens.[415] Given its limited effective range, brachytherapy is usually not as successful as external-beam radiation therapy in treating the entire tumor volume. However, in a randomized trial there was no difference in local control or survival with high-dose–rate brachytherapy as opposed to external-beam radiation therapy.[415]

If a patient requires rapid palliation (within a few days), alternative approaches such as laser treatment or stent placement are recommended. Although external-beam radiation with or without chemotherapy takes at least 2 weeks to produce palliation, once palliation is achieved it is more durable than that provided by the other palliative modalities because external-beam radiation treats the problem (the gross tumor mass), not just the symptom. If external-beam radiation is not possible, then intraluminal brachytherapy should be considered because it is an effective modality for decreasing symptoms such as dysphagia and bleeding. Chemotherapy by itself

TABLE 79.10

PALLIATION OF DYSPHAGIA WITH RADIATION THERAPY WITH OR WITHOUT CHEMOTHERAPY

Study (Ref.)	No. of Patients	Palliation of Dysphagia[a]	
		At the End of Treatment (%)	Duration
RADIATION THERAPY ALONE			
Wara et al. (405)	103	89	6-mo average
Petrovich et al. (406)	133	87	34% ≥ 6 mo 18% ≥ 3 mo 35% ≤ 3 mo
Roussel et al. (343)	69	70	—
Caspers et al. (408)	127	71	54% until death
Whittington et al. (407)	25	—	5% at 9 mo
CHEMORADIATION			
Coia et al. (413)	102	88	67–100% until death
Seitz et al. (338)	35	100[b]	—
Whittington et al. (407)	26	—	87% 3-y actuarial
Algan et al. (410)	8	100	—
Gill et al. (411)	71	60	—
Urba et al. (412)	27	—	59% until death
Izquierdo et al. (339)	25	64	Median, 5 mo
Harvey et al. (409)	106	78	51% until lost follow-up

[a]See text for definition and number of patients presenting with dysphagia.
[b]Patients had dilation or neodymium yttrium-aluminum garnet laser treatment at the start of therapy.

may also substantially relieve dysphagia when used as an initial treatment of metastatic disease.

Treatment in the Setting of Tracheoesophageal Fistula

The presence of a malignant tracheoesophageal fistula usually results in poor survival, although occasionally patients may survive for a prolonged period. Historically, radiation therapy was believed to be contraindicated for these patients for fear of exacerbating the fistula as the tumor responded. More recently there have been reports to the contrary. In a Mayo Clinic series, ten patients with malignant tracheoesophageal fistulas received 30 to 66 Gy external-beam radiation, and the median survival time was 5 months.[416] A series from Japan that treated 24 patients with fistualization to the airway reported ultimate closure of the fistula after chemoradiotherapy in 17 patients, with time to closure ranging from 6 to 280 days.[417]

Although the experience is very limited, the data suggest that radiation treatment does not necessarily increase the severity of a malignant tracheoesophageal fistula and it can be administered safely. It is unclear if radiation treatment improves outcome.

Acute and Long-Term Toxicity of Radiation Therapy. The toxicity of radiation therapy is a function of what the total dose is, what technique is used, and whether the patient has received chemotherapy. Essentially all patients experience lethargy and esophagitis commencing 2 to 3 weeks after the start of radiation therapy; these symptoms usually resolve 1 to 2 weeks after completion of therapy.

The most carefully documented acute toxicity data for patients who receive radiation therapy alone (without chemotherapy) are from the control arm of RTOG-85-01 in which patients received radiation therapy alone to a dose of 64 Gy.[258,344] The incidence of acute grade 3 toxicity was 25% and the incidence of acute grade 4 toxicity was 3%. The incidence of long-term grade 3+ toxicity and long-term grade 4+ toxicity was 23% and 2%, respectively.[103]

Radiation therapy can produce esophageal strictures, as can surgery. The total incidence of stricture (benign plus malignant) in patients receiving radiation therapy alone or radiation combined with chemotherapy is 20% to 40% in a modern series and up to 60% in historical series,[418] with up to 50% malignant, associated with recurrence. The incidence of stricture is lower in series in which careful radiation techniques were used. Coia et al.[413] examined a subset of 25 patients who experienced local control and survived at least 1 year. The incidence of benign stricture was 12%. Radiation toxicity is related to dose–volume effects.[419]

One series examined the functional outcomes of benign and malignant strictures.[414] Patients received 45 to 56 Gy and 53% received some form of chemotherapy. Of the 24 patients (30%) who developed a benign stricture, 71% were able to tolerate a full or soft diet and required dilation, with a median interval between dilations of 5 months. Even in the subset of patients who develop a benign stricture, dilation is effective in the majority of patients. In contrast, in the 28% of patients who developed a malignant stricture, dilation was unsuccessful and esophageal intubation was required.

The high incidence of fistula reported in the RTOG-92-07 trial of chemoradiation plus intraluminal brachytherapy (18% actuarial, 14% crude) has not been seen in series using radiation therapy or chemoradiation. The incidence of other long-term grade 3+ toxicities such as pneumonitis or pericarditis is 5%.

The effect of radiation on pulmonary function was examined by Gergel et al.[420] Patients received 39.6 Gy with anterior-posterior fields followed by radiation with oblique fields to a total dose of 50.4 Gy, plus concurrent chemotherapy with oxaliplatin and 5-FU. Results of pulmonary function tests administered before and a median of 16 days after radiation revealed significant declines in diffusing capacity for carbon monoxide and total lung capacity. Investigators at the M. D. Anderson Cancer Center performed retrospective treatment-planning studies on ten patients and found that intensity-modulated radiotherapy (IMRT) reduced the dose volume of exposed normal lung but had no clinically meaningful differences on the irradiated volumes of spinal cord, heart, liver, or total body integral doses.[421] The impact of respiratory and organ movement on defining target volumes is being investigated.[422,423]

The issue of treatment-related deaths in patients who receive chemoradiation is complex. Although the incidence was only 2% in RTOG-85-01, subsequent trials have reported a higher treatment-related mortality rate (i.e., 9% in INT-0122 and 8% in RTOG-92-07). These mortality rates are lower than the 10% to 15% incidence reported in historical surgical series, although only slightly higher than the 6% reported in the surgical control arm of INT-0113.[96] It is interesting to note that, as the mortality rate with surgery has decreased, there has been a corresponding increase in the treatment-related mortality rate reported in the nonoperative trials. As discussed in "Primary Nonsurgical Therapy" above, this may be partly related to bias in selecting patients to be treated with the nonoperative approach.

Radiation Field Design and Treatment Techniques. Just as expert surgical skills are required for a successful esophagectomy, radiation field design for esophageal cancer requires careful planning.[424] Sensitive organs in the radiation field include, but are not limited to, skin, spinal cord, lung, heart, intestine, stomach, kidney, and liver. Minimizing the dose to these structures while delivering an adequate dose to the primary tumor and locoregional lymph nodes requires patient immobilization and CT-based treatment planning for organ identification, lung correction, and development of dose–volume histograms.

Although CT can identify adjacent organs and structures, it may be limited in defining the extent of the primary tumor. To assess the consistency of target volume delineation, Tai et al.[425] sent sample cases with CT scans to 48 radiation oncologists throughout Canada and asked them to complete questionnaires regarding treatment techniques as well as to outline the boost target volumes. There was substantial inconsistency in defining the planning target volume, both in the transverse and longitudinal dimensions. Therefore, in addition to a CT scan, it is helpful to obtain results of a barium swallow test at the time of radiation therapy simulation. The integration of other imaging modalities such as EUS, PET, and magnetic resonance imaging into radiation treatment planning is under active investigation. Hong et al.[426] provide a comprehensive review of technical considerations in treatment planning.

IMRT using nine equispaced fields provided no improvement over conformal radiation because the larger number of fields in the IMRT plan distributed a low dose over the entire lung.[427] IMRT using four fields equal to the conformal fields offered an improvement in lung sparing.

From a radiation treatment–planning viewpoint, tumors at or above the carina are treated as a cervical primary and the supraclavicular nodes are included in the radiation field. Tumors below the carina but not extending to the gastroesophageal junction are considered midesophageal, and the radiation field does not include the supraclavicular or celiac nodes. Tumors that involve the gastroesophageal junction are considered distal, and the celiac nodes are included. This simplistic but practical definition is helpful in designing radiation therapy fields.

The standard radiation dose for patients selected for curative nonoperative chemoradiation is 50.4 Gy at 1.8 Gy per fraction. The radiation field should include the primary tumor with 5-cm superior and inferior margins and 2-cm lateral margins. The primary locoregional lymph nodes should receive the same dose. An example of a CT-based plan for a midesophageal cancer is seen in Figure 79.12.

In the palliative setting there are a variety of radiation treatment regimens. The goal is rapid palliation of symptoms and the most common approach is to treat anteroposteriorly and posteroanteriorly, including the primary tumor with 2-cm margins, in ten 3-Gy fractions to a total dose of 30 Gy.

The most critical normal structures that lie in proximity to the esophagus are the spinal cord, heart, lungs, and kidneys. When radiation is combined with chemotherapy, the radiation fractionation should be 1.8 Gy/d. The spinal cord dose should be limited to 45.0 to 46.8 Gy. All fields should be treated each day. Doses to the heart, lungs, and kidneys depend to a large extent on the volume of these organs in the treatment field. Dose–volume histograms are the most effective way to modify

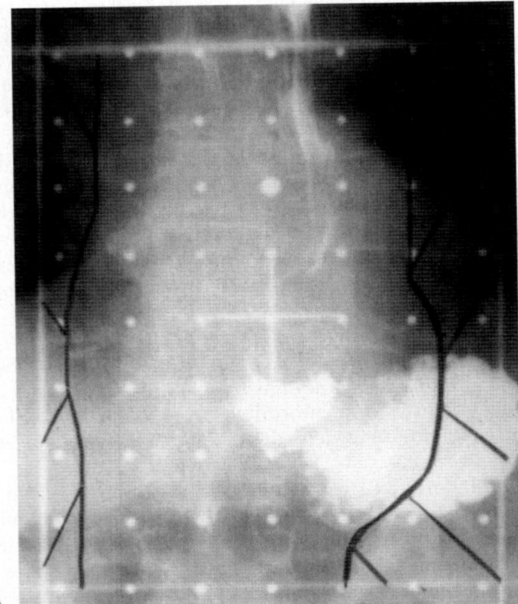

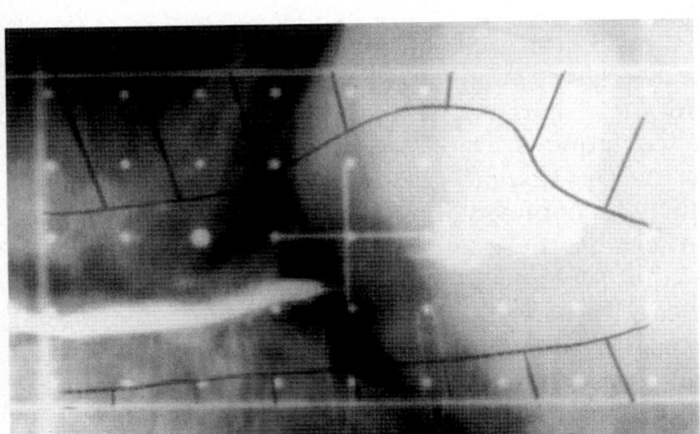

FIGURE 79.12 An example of a four-field technique for the treatment of a distal esophageal cancer

treatment techniques to decrease the acute and long-term radiation-related toxicity. The rate of symptomatic pneumonitis is related to dose and volume.[428] Fortunately, even with tumors as distal as the gastroesophageal junction, there is a limited amount of liver and kidney in the treatment fields.

Endoluminal Palliation Techniques

In the setting of either unresectable or disseminated disease, surgical approaches to palliation have been relegated to a historical footnote, citing the advances in endoscopic technology that achieve comparable or superior efficacy with less morbidity and mortality than the more invasive surgical techniques of resection and bypass.[429] These endoscopic techniques include dilation, stent placement, and ablation, mainly in the form of PDT or neodymium:yttrium-aluminum garnet (Nd:YAG) laser treatment.

Esophageal dilation can be effective in relieving dysphagia in up to 90% of patients.[430] However, the effect is transient (lasting 4 weeks or less) so that repeated dilations are required, and the procedure is associated with a 5% to 10% rate of complications, including perforation.[431] Because the duration of dysphagia relief is limited, dilation is most commonly performed to allow for proper placement of a self-expanding stent device.

Fixed-diameter plastic endoluminal prostheses, associated with significant morbidity and mortality and a low rate of dysphagia relief,[432] have largely been abandoned. Self-expandable metal stents are relatively easy to insert under fluoroscopic and endoscopic guidance, with a technical success rate of approximately 95% and an efficacy of 85% to 100% in relieving dysphagia.[429,433,434] The duration of response is 5 to 6 months, and complications occur in 10% to 15% of patients, the most common being stent migration and tumor ingrowth.[434] The use of stents coated with silicone or polyurethane may prevent or delay tumor ingrowth and subsequent esophageal obstruction.[435] Tumor ingrowth may be addressed by insertion of another stent or by tumor ablation. Placement of stents through proximally located tumors, especially those near the cricopharyngeus, is often not well tolerated by patients. Stents placed across the gastroesophageal junction have a greater tendency to migrate and may result in symptomatic acid reflux. Coated stents have been used with good success (more than 90%) for the treatment of tracheoesophageal fistula.[436] Finally, stents have been successfully deployed after chemoradiation to improve dysphagia, although exsanguinating hemorrhage has been reported with their use in patients with aortic invasion.[437]

Nd:YAG laser therapy delivers high-energy beams through an endoscopically introduced fiber to vaporize tumor tissue and create an esophageal lumen. Nd:YAG laser treatment is effective in relieving dysphagia in 70% to 90% of patients, with a duration of response of 1 to 3 months.[438–441] Tumors of the midesophagus are most amenable to laser therapy, although tumors in other locations can be treated. Complications occur in 2% to 4% of patients and include perforation and bleeding.[441]

PDT, as previously described, uses a photosensitizing agent that is introduced intravenously, is absorbed by tumor tissue, and, when activated with light of a certain wavelength, leads to tumor necrosis. Relief of dysphagia has been reported in 60% to 90% of patients, with a duration of response of 1 to 3 months.[442,443] Complications occur in 10% to 25% of patients and include chest pain, pleural effusion, tracheoesophageal fistula, and sun sensitivity. A multicenter randomized trial compared PDT with Nd:YAG laser therapy in 218 esophageal cancer patients with dysphagia.[444] Objective tumor response was significantly greater in those patients in the PDT arm; however, no differences were noted in dysphagia relief between the two treatment groups. Photosensitivity was noted in 19% of patients treated with PDT, and there was a significantly higher risk of perforation in the Nd:YAG group than in the PDT group (7% vs. 1%).

Other forms of ablative therapy, including argon plasma coagulation and electrocautery, produce tumor necrosis with efficacy rates similar to those of the ablative methods mentioned earlier.[429,445–447] Electrocautery is associated with higher perforation rates because it requires dilation, whereas argon plasma coagulation is most appropriate for smaller, vascular lesions.

Frequently more than one method is required to achieve effective palliation of symptoms during the patient's lifetime. Therefore, the endoluminal techniques described are considered complementary methods for palliation.

Treatment of Metastatic Disease

A variety of single agent and combination chemotherapy regimens have been evaluated in patients with recurrent or metastatic carcinoma of the esophagus. Phase 2 clinical trials in this population have identified drugs with activity that have been integrated into combined modality regimens for the treatment of earlier-stage disease. Standard criteria for evaluating treatment response require that serial measurement of disease be possible. For the esophageal cancer patient with metastatic disease to distant organ sites or lymph nodes, treatment response can be reliably assessed using spiral CT or magnetic resonance imaging. Serial tumor measurement for response assessment in patients with disease limited to the esophagus is less reliable. Endoscopy with brushings and biopsy may be performed to confirm a clinically determined complete response; however, biopsy is subject to sampling error, and biopsy findings are not a reliable indicator of complete histologic resolution of disease. Whole-body FDG-PET performed before and during or after chemotherapy may be a valuable noninvasive method of predicting tumor response and a favorable treatment outcome. Several studies have shown that a reduction in tumor FDG uptake (median decrease in standardized uptake value) correlates with response and longer survival.[144,147,301]

Until the mid-1990s, the accumulated experience with chemotherapy was almost entirely in patients with squamous cell tumors. With the rising incidence of adenocarcinoma of the distal esophagus, gastroesophageal junction, and cardia in the United States and Western industrialized countries, patients with this histologic type now make up well more than half of referrals for chemotherapy. Most trials of new agents and combined modality regimens now include patients with both tumor types.

Single-Agent Chemotherapy

Studies of single-agent chemotherapy for esophageal cancer are summarized here. Response data for many of the older drugs have come from broad phase 1 and 2 trials conducted in the early 1970s, which included small numbers of esophageal cancer patients.[448–457] Bleomycin, 5-FU, mitomycin, and cisplatin have been used most frequently because of their single-agent activity and additive or synergistic effects with radiation. Because of the potential for pulmonary toxicity, bleomycin is no longer included in combination regimens, having been replaced by 5-FU. Similarly, mitomycin is used less often because of its toxicity profile, which includes hemolytic-uremic syndrome and cumulative myelosuppression.

Seven trials examined the use of cisplatin for single-agent therapy in esophageal cancer patients,[455,458–463] six of which used dosages ranging from 50 to 120 mg/m^2 every 3 to 4 weeks. The cumulative response rate in patients with metastatic or recurrent disease was 21%. Vinorelbine is a semisynthetic vinca alkaloid that has less neurotoxicity than vincristine and vinblastine. Phase 2 trials in metastatic squamous cell cancer of the esophagus report response rates of 20% to 25% using weekly or biweekly dosing schedules.[464,465] In a subsequent trial, Conroy et al.[466] evaluated the doublet of vinorelbine and cisplatin. A total of 71 patients with metastatic squamous cell cancer were treated and a 34% response rate was observed. Vinorelbine was evaluated in a phase 2 trial in 29 patients with adenocarcinoma of the esophagus who had failed prior chemotherapy, with minor activity (7% response rate) observed.[467]

The taxane paclitaxel was the first entirely new compound to be tested in both adenocarcinoma and squamous cell carcinoma of the esophagus. Paclitaxel promotes the stabilization of microtubules and is a cycle-specific agent affecting cells in the G_2/M phase. Paclitaxel also enhances radiation effects and may be both concentration and schedule dependent.[468] Three trials of single-agent paclitaxel have been reported. One used the maximum tolerable dose of 250 mg/m², derived from initial phase 1 trials using a 24-hour infusion schedule.[469] The overall response rate was 32% (34% in 33 patients with adenocarcinoma, and 28% in 18 patients with squamous cell carcinoma). The second trial tested a regimen of 140 mg/m² infused during 96 hours in patients previously treated using a shorter infusion schedule of paclitaxel-containing combination chemotherapy.[470] No responses were observed. The third trial evaluated single-agent paclitaxel administered by a weekly 1-hour infusion at a dose of 80 mg/m² in a large multicenter phase 2 setting.[471] A modest response rate of 15% was observed in 65 patients without prior chemotherapy treatment (16% in the 50 patients treated with adenocarcinoma and 13% in the 15 patients treated with squamous cell carcinoma). Limited activity (5%) was seen in patients with prior chemotherapy. Despite the low response rate, the median survival was 274 days and toxicity, including hematologic toxicity, was minimal.

Docetaxel was evaluated at a dose of 100 mg/m², every 3 weeks in a combined esophageal and gastric cancer trial treating 33 patients with gastric cancer and 8 patients with esophageal adenocarcinoma.[472] Two of the eight patients (25%) with esophageal adenocarcinoma had a major response. Overall, grade 4 neutropenia occurred in 88% of patients and neutropenic fever in 46%. A larger trial of docetaxel 75 mg/m² in 22 patients with esophageal adenocarcinoma reported a response rate of 18% in chemotherapy-naive patients and no responses in previously treated patients.[472] Febrile neutropenia occurred in 32% of patients. A recent trial of 70 mg/m² every 3 weeks in 49 patients with squamous cell carcinoma reported a 20% response rate.[473] Eighty-eight percent of patients had grade 3 or 4 neutropenia and 18% febrile neutropenia.

Drugs that have been adequately tested in squamous cell cancer of the esophagus and have response rates of less than 5% are the methotrexate analogue dichloromethotrexate[474] and trimetrexate,[475,476] and etoposide,[477,478] ifosfamide,[402,479] and carboplatin.[480,481] A more contemporary study of etoposide in untreated patients with squamous cell carcinoma reported a response rate of 19% (5 of 26 patients).[482] Carboplatin has been studied in both adenocarcinoma and squamous cell carcinoma, and, in contrast to the activity of a single agent, responses to carboplatin were observed in only 3 of 59 chemotherapy-naive patients. Therefore, substitution of single-agent carboplatin for cisplatin is not recommended when treating patients with either adenocarcinomas or squamous cell carcinomas of the esophagus. Nonetheless, carboplatin combination regimens used as part of combination chemotherapy, in chemoradiation (as previously discussed) and in metastatic disease regimens (discussed later), appear to have comparable activity to cisplatin-based therapy.

Topotecan and gemcitabine have been separately evaluated in both histologic tumor types and have been shown to be inactive.[483–485] The topoisomerase II inhibitor irinotecan has been evaluated in two phase 2 trials in adenocarcinoma of the stomach and gastroesophageal junction, with a response rate of 15% observed.[486,487]

Combined-Agent Chemotherapy

Older trials (before the mid-1990s) and those in Europe were almost exclusively limited to patients with squamous cell carcinoma. Because esophageal cancer is a relatively uncommon malignancy, many studies include a heterogeneous population of treatment-naive patients with locally advanced intrathoracic disease as well as patients with recurrent or metastatic disease. Not only is there variation in the patient population, but more recent trials usually limit eligibility to patients with no prior chemotherapy and performance status of 0 or 1. Thus, in the absence of comparative trials, newer regimens may appear more effective.

The results for platinum-based combination chemotherapy regimens are detailed in Table 79.11. Most series consist of small numbers of patients; therefore, the 95% confidence intervals are large and nearly all responses are partial. On average, duration of response ranges from 3 to 6 months.

Trials conducted in the 1980s testing three-drug regimens such as cisplatin, bleomycin, and vindesine[234,488] and cisplatin and mitoguazone combined with vindesine[489] or vinblastine[490] yielded response rates of 30% to 40% in patients with squamous cell carcinoma. Toxicity was primarily moderate myelosuppression. Bleomycin and mitoguazone were subsequently replaced by 5-FU to reduce toxicity and to take advantage of its synergistic activity with cisplatin.

The two-drug combination of cisplatin (100 mg/m² on day 1) and 5-FU (1,000 mg/m²/d continuous infusion for 96 to 120 hours) has been the standard regimen for two decades to treat patients with either squamous cell carcinoma or adenocarcinoma. A 35% response rate was observed in patients with metastatic, recurrent, or locally advanced incurable squamous cell cancer of the esophagus.[459] Higher response rates (in the 40% to 60% range) were reported in trials administering two or three cycles of cisplatin and 5-FU as induction therapy before surgery. The difference in response rates may be related to better performance status, better nutrition, and smaller-volume disease in the surgical candidates. Despite the common use in the oncology community of the combination of 5-FU and cisplatin for the treatment of esophageal carcinoma, only one trial conducted by the EORTC has directly addressed the issue of the comparative efficacy of single-agent cisplatin and the combination of 5-FU and cisplatin.[459] Patients with locally advanced or metastatic squamous cell carcinoma were randomly assigned to receive either cisplatin (100 mg/m²) plus continuous-infusion 5-FU (1,000 mg/m²/d, days 1 to 5) or to cisplatin (100 mg/m²) alone, with both regimens repeated every 3 weeks. The cisplatin/5-FU arm had a higher response rate (35%) and better median survival (33 weeks) than the cisplatin arm (19% and 28 weeks, respectively), but these findings were not statistically significant. Cisplatin/5-FU was also more toxic, with 16% treatment-related deaths for the combination.

Cisplatin in combination with UFT, an oral 5-FU pro-drug combining tegafur with uracil, an inhibitor of the enzyme dihydropyrimidine dehydrogenase that degrades 5-FU, has also been evaluated in esophageal cancer. A response rate of 46% was reported.[491]

Recent phase 3 trials have compared the addition of a third agent to cisplatin/5-FU versus cisplatin/5-FU alone. The Royal Marsden group developed the ECF regimen, a combination of epirubicin (50 mg/m²) and cisplatin (60 mg/m²) every 3 weeks in combination with daily protracted continuous infusion 5-FU (200 mg/m²/d) in gastric cancer. The ECF regimen was compared, in a phase 3 trial in gastric and gastroesophageal junction adenocarcinoma, with a bolus regimen of 5-FU, doxorubicin, and methotrexate (FAMTX).[492] The ECF regimen

TABLE 79.11

SELECTED COMBINATION CHEMOTHERAPY REGIMENS FOR RECURRENT AND METASTATIC CARCINOMA OF THE ESOPHAGUS

Regimen	Evaluable Patients (n)	Histologic Type	% CR + PR	References
Cisplatin + bleomycin	17	S	17	233
Cisplatin + bleomycin + vindesine	51	S	31	234, 488
Cisplatin + mitoguazone + vindesine	20	S	40	489
Cisplatin + mitoguazone + vinblastine	36	S	11	490
Cisplatin + 5-FU	82	S	35	459
Oxaliplatin + 5-FU	34	A/S	40	494
Cisplatin + vinorelbine	71	S	34	466
5-FU + interferon-α_{2a}	57	S/A	26	501, 504
Cisplatin + 5-FU + interferon-α_{2a}	66	S/A	53 (62% S, 32% A)	502, 505
Cisplatin + etoposide	65	S	48	506
	27	A	48	508
Cisplatin + etoposide + 5-FU + leucovorin	69	S	34	507
Paclitaxel (24 h) + cisplatin every 3 wk	32	S/A	44 (25% S, 46% A)	511
Paclitaxel (3 h) + cisplatin every 2 wk	51	S/A	43	509
Paclitaxel (3 h) + cisplatin every wk × 6	24	A	50	510
Paclitaxel (3 h) + cisplatin + 5-FU every 4 wk	60	S/A	48 (56% S, 46% A)	513
Paclitaxel (1 h) + carboplatin every week	37	S/A	54%	512
Irinotecan + cisplatin every wk × 4, every 6 wk	35	S/A	57 (66% S, 52% A)	514
Irinotecan + cisplatin every wk × 4, every 6 wk	25	A	51	515
Docetaxel + irinotecan every wk × 3, every 4 wk	24	S/A	13	521
Docetaxel + irinotecan every 3 wk	46	A	26	518
Mitomycin + cisplatin + 5-FU vs.	285	A/G	46% A, 38% G	483
Epirubicin + cisplatin + 5-FU	289	A/G	44% A, 36% G	

CR, complete response; PR, partial response; S, squamous cell carcinoma; 5-FU, 5-fluorouracil; A, adenocarcinoma of esophagus, gastroesophageal junction, cardia; G, gastric cancer.

resulted in a superior response rate (45% vs. 21%), failure-free survival (7.4 months vs. 3.4 months), and median survival (8.9 months vs. 5.7 months) in comparison with FAMTX. The ECF regimen had a tolerable toxicity profile, with less than 10% rates of grade 3 or 4 diarrhea or stomatitis. A more recent trial treating nearly 600 patients with advanced esophageal squamous and adenocarcinoma and gastric adenocarcinoma compared the ECF regimen with a similar regimen substituting mitomycin (7 mg/m^2 every 6 weeks) for epirubicin.[493] This trial validated the previously reported response rate and median survival for the ECF regimen (42%, 9.4 months), but the response rate and median survival observed for the mitomycin combination regimen (44%, 8.7 months) were identical to those of ECF. Given that there was no difference in efficacy for the epirubicin- versus mitomycin-containing arms, this study raises the question of whether or not the addition of a third agent makes a difference in outcome when combined with cisplatin and protracted infusion 5-FU. Of the 533 patients enrolled in this trial, 40 had squamous cell carcinoma of the esophagus and the remainder had adenocarcinoma (125, esophagus; 125, gastroesophageal junction; 243, stomach). There was a significantly higher response rate among patients with gastroesophageal junction cancers than among those with distal gastric cancers (48% vs. 37%).

Oxaliplatin, as a potential substitute for cisplatin, and oral capecitabine, as a substitute for 5-FU, have been explored in phase 2[494] and more recently phase 3 randomized trials in esophageal and gastric adenocarcinoma. Cunningham et al.[495] reported results of a 1,000 patient phase 3 trial in esophageal squamous cell and adenocarcinoma and gastric cancer, evaluating the front-line use of oxaliplatin or capecitabine. This trial compared conventional ECF with the substitution of capecitabine for infusional 5-FU, and oxaliplatin for cisplatin. The trial employed a two-by-two design, with the control arm ECF, and the experimental arms including capecitabine (625 mg/m^2 twice daily) substituted for infusional 5-FU; oxaliplatin (130 mg/m^2) substituted for cisplatin; and a fourth arm with a substitution of both capecitabine and oxaliplatin. Capecitabine was found to be noninferior to 5-FU, and oxaliplatin noninferior to cisplatin, with comparable rates of antitumor response and progression-free survival across the four treatment arms. Toxicity analysis favored oxaliplatin over cisplatin for neutropenia, alopecia, renal toxicity and thromboembolism. In a planned comparison of ECF to EOX (epirubicin, oxaliplatin, capecitabine), median survival was superior for EOX (11.2 months vs. 9.9 months; HR 0.80; P = .02). A second phase 3 trial from the German AIO group compared infusional 5-FU (24-hour infusion) plus leucovorin combined with either oxaliplatin (85 mg/m^2) or cisplatin (50 mg/m^2) once every 2 weeks in 220 patients with metastatic gastroesophageal adenocarcinoma.[496] Like the Cunningham et al. trial, oxaliplatin was found to be noninferior to cisplatin. Oxaliplatin caused significantly less nausea and vomiting, fatigue, renal toxicity, and thromboembolism. Remarkable on both arms of this trial was the relatively low level of grade 3 or 4 toxicities in all categories, running less than 10% to 15%, likely due to the two weekly schedule of chemotherapy mimicking colorectal-like cancer scheduling of chemotherapy. Response rates (24.5% to 34.8%), progression-free (3.9 months vs. 5.8 months), and overall survival (8.8 months vs. 10.7 months) were comparable between the two treatment arms, although all end points trended higher on the oxaliplatin arm. Lastly, a third phase 3 trial reported by Kang et al.[497] compared capecitabine (1,000 mg/m^2) twice a day for 14 days to 5-FU (800 mg/m^2/d continuous infusion) for 5 days, cycled every 3 weeks with cisplatin (80 mg/m^2). Like the Cunningham et al. trial, capecitabine was found to be noninferior to 5-FU. Rates of toxicity on the treatment arms were similar, as were measures of progression-free (5.0 months vs. 5.6 months) and overall survival (9.3 months vs. 10.5 months). Based on the results of these three phase 3 trials, the substitution of oxaliplatin for cisplatin, or capecitabine for 5-FU, seems justified. The two-drug regimens in the Al-Batran et al.[496] and Kang et al.[497] trials had favorable toxicity profiles and efficacy compared to the three drug regimens of Cunningham et al., and whether or not epirubicin is required as part of therapy in metastatic disease is unclear.

An alternative oral 5-FU agent, S-1, combines the 5-FU pro-drug tegafur with a bowel protectant (oteracil) and an inhibitor of dihydropyrimidine dehydrogenase (gimeracil). A phase 3 trial conducted in Japan evaluated S-1 40 to 60 mg twice a day for 3 weeks as a single agent, versus S-1 plus cisplatin (60 mg/m^2), cycled once every 5 weeks, in advanced gastric cancer. S-1 plus cisplatin was superior to S-1 alone, with improved rates of response (54% vs. 31%), progression-free (6 months vs. 4 months), and overall survival (13 months vs. 11 months).[498] Based on encouraging data for S-1, a phase 3 superiority trial comparing S-1 50 mg/m^2 in two daily divided doses for 21 days was compared to infusional 5-FU 1,000 mg/m^2/d for 5 days, cycled every 28 days.[499] Both arms were combined with cisplatin, with a lower dose of cisplatin combined with S-1 (75 mg/m^2) compared to the 5-FU arm (100 mg/m^2). A lower dose of S-1 than that used in the Japanese trials was mandated due to greater toxicity for S-1 reported in Western patients in prior phase 1 and 2 trials. The trial failed to demonstrate superiority for the S-1 arm, with equivalent rates of overall survival (7.9 months vs. 8.6 months). The S-1 arm had less toxicity than 5-FU, but the lesser cisplatin dose likely accounted for much of the toxicity differences between the treatment arms. Whether or not S-1 will be adopted in practice in Western countries has yet to be established.

The addition of docetaxel as a third agent added to 5-FU and cisplatin has also recently been reported in a phase 3 trial of gastroesophageal junction and gastric cancer. 5-FU dosed at 1,000 mg/m^2 by continuous infusion during 5 days combined with cisplatin (100 mg/m^2) was compared with cisplatin (75 mg/m^2), 5-FU (750 mg/m^2) by continuous infusion during 5 days, and docetaxel (75 mg/m^2) in 445 patients with metastatic gastric or gastroesophageal junction adenocarcinoma.[500] Docetaxel resulted in a higher response rate and time to progression (36%, 5.6 months) compared with 5-FU and cisplatin (26%, 3.7 months), but only a marginal median survival improvement (0.6 months) was noted for three-drug therapy. Toxicity was substantial in both treatment arms, including hematologic and gastrointestinal toxicity, with 80% of patients receiving the three-drug combination experiencing grade 3 or 4 neutropenia. The recent trials of 5-FU infusion combination chemotherapy indicate improved therapy tolerance and potentially enhanced antitumor activity, employing either a once every two week or a more protracted infusion of 5-FU as in the ECF regimen. The addition of a third agent, including epirubicin or docetaxel, to 5-FU and cisplatin may modestly increase response rates and survival, but, in the case of docetaxel combination therapy, may result in substantial therapy-related toxicity. The use of relatively high and relatively toxic doses of cisplatin (75 to 100 mg/m^2) is also called into question, given data from the British phase 3 ECF trials that indicate potential better therapy tolerance for 60 mg/m^2 without evident compromising of treatment efficacy.

Five trials using interferon-α_{2a} as a biomodulator of 5-FU suggested possible benefit.[501–505] These phase 2 trials combined interferon-α_{2a} with 5-FU and with cisplatin combined with continuous-infusion 5-FU, with response rates reported ranging from 27% to 50%, with a suggestion of higher response rates seen in squamous cell carcinoma. Etoposide and cisplatin with or without 5-FU have also undergone phase 2 evaluation.[506–508] Combination regimens that include paclitaxel have been evaluated in esophageal cancer patients. In three phase 2 trials of paclitaxel and cisplatin, response rates ranged from 43% to 50%; activity was comparable in both histologic tumor types, often with severe hematologic toxicity.[509–511] A phase 1 trial of weekly carboplatin dosed from an area under the curve of 2 to 5 combined with a 1-hour infusion of paclitaxel, 100 mg/m^2, in 40 patients with advanced esophageal and gastroesophageal junction cancer had an overall response rate of 54%.[512]

The three-drug combination of paclitaxel (175 mg/m^2, 3-hour infusion), combined with cisplatin (20 mg/m^2/d^2 $\times$ 5) and 5-FU (1,000 mg/m^2/d continuous infusion $\times$ 120 hours) was evaluated in a multicenter 60 patient trial.[513] A 48% response rate was reported (56% in patients with squamous cell cancer and 46% in patients with adenocarcinoma). Toxicity resulted in unplanned hospitalizations for 48% of patients.

Although the dose and schedule of paclitaxel in combination with other active drugs varies among phase 2 trials, shorter infusion schedules of paclitaxel, in particular the weekly 1-hour schedule, result in less myelotoxicity.

Other regimens of interest include those containing irinotecan. First reported was the doublet of irinotecan and cisplatin administered in low dose on a weekly schedule.[514] *In vitro* studies demonstrated sequence-dependent synergy for cisplatin followed by irinotecan, which prevents removal of cisplatin-induced DNA interstrand cross-links. Two trials yielded encouraging results (51% to 57% response) with a regimen of cisplatin (30 mg/m^2) followed by irinotecan (65 mg/m^2) administered weekly for 4 weeks, repeated every 6 weeks in adenocarcinoma and squamous cancer.[514,515] Dysphagia and global quality of life were improved in the majority of patients in one of these trials.[514] In both studies, toxicity consisted of myelosuppression, diarrhea, and fatigue. Irinotecan 50 mg/m^2 combined with weekly cisplatin 25 mg/m^2 and docetaxel 30 mg/m^2, days 1 and 8 every 21 days, was studied in a phase 2 trial in 39 patients with esophagogastric cancer.[516] An encouraging response rate of 54% was observed, with tolerable rates of grade 3 and 4 neutropenia (21%) and diarrhea (26%).

Recent studies exploring non–cisplatin-containing combination regimens have employed the taxanes and irinotecan. Although these trials have indicated encouraging response rates in the phase 2 setting, substantial hematologic and diarrheal toxicities of these regimens may not offer an advantage over the older cisplatin-containing regimens.[517–521] Docetaxel has been evaluated in combination with irinotecan in four recent phase 2 trials. Two trials evaluated irinotecan doses of 100 to 160 mg/m^2 and docetaxel doses of 50 to 60 mg/m^2 administered once every 3 weeks. Two trials evaluated the day 1 and day 8 schedule of irinotecan (50 to 55 mg/m^2) and docetaxel (25 to 35 mg/m^2) cycled every 3 weeks. Response rates range from 13 to 30 hematologic toxicity, which exceeded 50% in patients treated on the schedule of once every 3 weeks, seemed to be less using the day 1 and day 8 schedule compared with the once every 3 week schedule.

Phase 3 comparison of cisplatin and infusional 5-FU to the combination of irinotecan and infusional 5-FU was recently reported in advanced esophagogastric cancer.[522] Response rates (25.8% to 31.8%), progression-free (4.2 months vs. 5.0 months), and overall survival (8.7 months vs. 9.0 months) were comparable for the two regimens. Toxicity favored the irinotecan 5-FU arm. Data from this trial, and the oxaliplatin-based studies conducted in Europe, have led to greater utilization of both irinotecan and oxaliplatin in combination with infusional 5-FU for the treatment of advanced esophagogastric cancer at European centers.

Docetaxel and either vinorelbine or capecitabine were evaluated in phase 2 trials in squamous cell carcinoma[523,524] with response rates of 46% to 60%. In summary, recent trials of combination regimens that include paclitaxel or irinotecan appear to have comparable response rates to previous regimens; however, duration of response remains brief. In addition, the toxicities recorded in some of these phase 2 single-institution experiences have been excessive.

Targeted Agents

Validation of the activity of a growth factor receptor targeted agent, trastuzumab, was recently achieved in esophagogastric cancer.[525] Over 3,800 patients with gastric or gastroesophageal junction adenocarcinoma were screened for overexpression of the HER2 receptor by fluorescence *in situ* hybridization (FISH) and immunohistochemistry; 22.1% tested positive. Five hundred eighty-four patients were ultimately randomized to chemotherapy alone with (1) capecitabine 1,000 mg/m^2 twice a day for 14 days or (2) infusional 5-FU 800 mg/m^2/d for 5 days, combined with cisplatin 80 mg/m^2 on day 1, cycled every 3 weeks, or to chemotherapy plus trastuzumab 6 mg/kg once every 3 weeks. All end points were improved with the addition of trastuzumab to chemotherapy, including antitumor response (47.3% vs. 34.5%), progression-free survival (6.7 months vs. 5.5 months), and overall survival (13.8 months vs. 11.1 months; HR 0.74; P = .0046). Toxicity was comparable for the two treatment arms, with no significant cardiotoxicity from trastuzumab other than an asymptomatic less than 10% drop in left ventricular ejection fraction, which was slightly higher on the trastuzumab arm compared to chemotherapy alone (4.6% vs. 1.1%). Based on these results, the inclusion of trastuzumab in the first-line treatment of HER2+ metastatic esophagogastric cancer should now be considered. Based on these data, and pilot data combining trastuzumab with chemoradiotherapy in esophageal cancer, RTOG has undertaken a phase 3 trial (RTOG-1010) comparing preoperative chemoradiotherapy with 5-FU and oxaliplatin with or without trastuzumab in locally advanced adenocarcinoma of the esophagus and gastroesophageal junction.

With evidence for effectiveness of agents targeting the epidermal growth factor receptor (EGFR) in non–small cell lung cancer (including receptor-associated tyrosine kinase inhibitors) and in colorectal cancer (including monoclonal antibodies blocking binding of the EGFR ligand), recent phase 2 trials have evaluated EGFR-targeted agents in esophageal squamous cell and adenocarcinoma. A recent phase 2 trial of the EGFR tyrosine kinase inhibitor gefitinib failed to indicate activity for esophageal adenocarcinoma, but limited activity was observed in squamous cell cancer.[526] A second trial indicated some limited activity for adenocarcinoma,[527] but in both trials most patients experienced early disease progression. A phase 2 trial of the EGFR tyrosine kinase inhibitor erlotinib reported a 9% response rate in 44 patients with adenocarcinoma of the gastroesophageal junction.[528] Monoclonal antibodies targeting the EGFR, including cetuximab, matuzumab, and panitumumab, are in phase 3 trial investigation combined with chemotherapy, based on promising data from phase 2 trials.[529–531] A randomized phase 2 trial conducted by the CALGB (80403) was recently completed, evaluating three modern chemotherapy regimens combined with cetuximab in the first-line treatment of esophageal and gastroesophageal junction cancer. The primary end point is antitumor response rate, and the regimens used were weekly irinotecan cisplatin, ECF, and FOLFOX (5-FU, leucovorin, and oxaliplatin). Data from this study that treated over 270 patients will be released in 2010. RTOG-0436, adding cetuximab to primary chemoradiotherapy in locally advanced esophageal cancer, was discussed earlier.

Another growth factor receptor pathway under active investigation is the vascular endothelial growth factor (VEGF) receptor pathway, based on trials that demonstrate improved effectiveness for chemotherapy in colorectal cancer when combined with the anti–VEGF-A ligand monoclonal antibody bevacizumab. A recent phase 2 trial combined bevacizumab at a dose of 15 mg/kg every 3 weeks in combination with a day 1 and day 8 schedule of irinotecan (65 mg/m^2) and cisplatin (30 mg/m^2).[532] The multicenter trial treated 47 patients treated with metastatic adenocarcinoma of the gastroesophageal junction and more distal gastric cancer. An encouraging response rate of 65% was observed, with a suggestion of improvement in time to tumor progression (8.9 months) compared with historical controls. A phase 3 trial combining bevacizumab with either 5-FU or capecitabine plus cisplatin in over 700 patients with esophagogastric adenocarcinoma has been completed and results from this trial will be reported in 2010. Incorporation of targeted agents into chemoradiation programs in locally advanced disease, including preoperative chemotherapy and chemoradiation, are the subject of ongoing and planned trials at the single institution and cooperative group level.

STAGE-DIRECTED TREATMENT RECOMMENDATIONS

Although level I evidence is lacking to support ironclad recommendations regarding the most effective treatment of patients grouped by stage in many clinical situations, reasonable trial-generated information exists to suggest appropriate therapeutic interventions for patients grouped under broad staging categories.

Resection remains the standard by which all other treatment options must be measured for patients with high-grade dysplasia in the setting of Barrett's esophagus or T1 disease limited to the mucosa, with the caveat that esophagectomy-associated mortality must be extremely low. Although more experience and longer follow-up are necessary to confirm efficacy, EMR may be considered an appropriate first step in addressing patients with mucosa-limited lesions. Intensive long-term endoscopic surveillance for patients with Barrett's esophagus–associated high-grade dysplasia is necessary to limit both cancer- and treatment-related mortality.

Esophagectomy is an appropriate method for treating patients with stage I, II, and III disease. Alternatively, definitive chemoradiation is a therapeutic option for patients with stage II and III disease, especially those who are not considered surgical candidates or who have squamous cell carcinoma at or above the carina. The high rate of persistent or recurrent locoregional disease after definitive chemoradiation suggests that additional local therapy in the form of surgery may be necessary and beneficial. This potential benefit may be realized only if perioperative mortality is minimized. Although preoperative chemoradiation has not been definitively proven to be more effective than surgery alone, it remains an attractive approach that has been embraced by oncologists for patients with resectable stage IIB and III esophageal cancers and should continue to be examined in well-designed clinical trials. Postoperative chemoradiation should be reserved for patients with resected adenocarcinoma of the gastroesophageal junction. Preoperative chemotherapy is an accepted standard of care in the United Kingdom but is still considered investigational in the United States. All patients with unresectable or stage IV disease are ideally suited for clinical trials exploring novel therapeutic agents and approaches.

Selected References

The full list of references for this chapter appears in the online version.

4. Jemal A, Siegel R, Ward E, et al. Cancer statistics 2009. *CA Cancer J Clin* 2009;59(4):225.
20. Edelstein ZR, Farrow DC, Bonner MP, et al. Central adiposity and risk of Barrett's esophagus. *Gastroenterology* 2007;133(2):403.
22. Lagergren, J, Bergstrom R, Lindgren A, et al. Symptomatic gastroesophageal reflux as a risk factor for esophageal adenocarcinoma. *N Engl J Med* 1999;340:825.
23. Chow WH, Finkle WD, McLaughlin JK, et al. The relation of gastroesophageal reflux disease and its treatment to adenocarcinomas of the esophagus and gastric cardia. *JAMA* 1995;274(6):474.
25. Kamangar F, Dawsey SM, Blaser MJ, et al. Opposing risks of gastric cardia and noncardiac gastric adenocarciomas associated with *Helicobacter pylori* seropositivity. *J Natl Can Inst* 2006;98(20):1445.
30. Cameron AJ, Ott BJ, Payne WS. The incidence of adenocarcinoma in columnar-lined (Barrett's) esophagus. *N Engl J Med* 1985;313(14):857.
33. Spechler SJ, Lee E, Ahnen D, et al. Long-term outcome of medical and surgical therapies for gastroesophageal reflux disease: follow-up of a randomized controlled trial. *JAMA* 2001;285(18):2331.
38. Kahrilas P, Shaheen NJ, Vaezi MF. American Gastroenterological Association Institute technical review on the management of gastroesophageal reflux disease. *Gastroenterology* 2008;135(4):1392.
39. Wang KK, Sampliner RE. Updated guidelines 2008 for the diagnosis, surveillance and therapy of Barrett's esophagus. *Am J Gastroenterol* 2008;103 (3):788.
42. Ferguson MK, Durkin A. Long-term survival after esophagectomy for Barrett's adenocarcinoma in endoscopically surveyed and nonsurveyed patients. *J Gastrointest Surg* 2002;6(1):29.
47. Faybush EM, Sampliner RE. Randomized trials in the treatment of Barrett's esophagus. *Dis Esophagus* 2005;18:291.
48. Haggitt RC. Barrett's esophagus, dysplasia, and adenocarcinoma. *Hum Pathol* 1994;25(10):982.
80. Siewert JR, Feith M, Werner M, et al. Adenocarcinoma of the esophagogastric junction. Results of surgical therapy based on anatomic-topographic classification in 1,002 consecutive patients. *Ann Surg* 2000;232:353.
81. Edge SB, Byrd DR, Compton CC, et al. American Joint Commission on Cancer. *AJCC cancer staging manual*. 7th ed. New York: Springer-Verlag, 2009.
96. Kelsen DP, Ginsberg R, Pajak RF, et al. Chemotherapy followed by surgery compared with surgery alone for localized esophageal cancer. *N Engl J Med* 1998;339(27):1979.
97. Medical Research Council Oesophageal Cancer Working Group. Surgical resection with or without preoperative chemotherapy in oesophageal cancer: a randomised controlled trial. *Lancet* 2002;359(9319):1727.
98. Urba SG, Orringer MB, Turrisi A, et al. Randomized trial of preoperative chemoradiation versus surgery alone in patients with locoregional esophageal carcinoma. *J Clin Oncol* 2001;19:305.
101. Arnott SJ, Duncan W, Gignoux M, et al. Preoperative radiotherapy in esophageal carcinoma: a meta-analysis using individual patient data (Oesophageal Cancer Collaborative Group). *Int J Radiat Oncol Biol Phys* 1998;41(3):579.
103. Cooper JS, Guo MD, Herskovic A, et al. Chemoradiotherapy of locally advanced esophageal cancer: long-term follow-up of a prospective randomized trial (RTOG 85-01). Radiation Therapy Oncology Group. *JAMA* 1999;281(17):1623.
105. Bedenne L, Michel P, Bouche O, et al. Chemoradiation followed by surgery compared to chemoradiation alone in squamous cancer of the esophagus: FFCD 9102. *J Clin Oncol* 2007;25(10):1160.
106. Stahl M, Stuschke M, Lehmann N, et al. Chemoradiation with and without surgery in patients with locally advanced squamous cell carcinoma of the esophagus. *J Clin Oncol* 2005;23:2310.
114. Wolfson HC, Crook JE, Krisha M, et al. Prospective, controlled tandem endoscopy study of narrow band imaging for dysplasia detection in Barrett's esophagus. *Gastroenterology* 2008;135(1):24.
140. Jost C, Binek J, Schuller JC, et al. Endosonographic radial tumor thickness after neoadjuvant chemoradiation therapy to predict response and survival in patients with locally advanced esophageal cancer: a prospective multicenter phase II study. Swiss Group for Clinical Cancer Research (SAKK 75/02). *Gastrointest Endosc* 2010;7:1114.
146. Ott K, Weber WA, Lordick F, et al. Metabolic imaging predicts response, survival, and recurrence in adenocarcinomas of the esophagogastric junction. *J Clin Oncol* 2006;24(29):4692.
148. Lordick F, Ott K, Krause BJ, et al. PET to assess early metabolic response and to guide treatment of adenocarcinoma of the oesophagogastric junction: the MUNICON phase II trial. *Lancet Oncol* 2007;8(9):797.
163. Stein HJ, Feiht M, Brucher BL, et al. Early esophageal cancer: pattern of lymphatic spread and prognostic factors for long-term survival after surgical resection. *Ann Surg* 2005;242(4):566.
166. Konda VJ, Ross AS, Ferguson MK. Is the risk of concomitant invasive esophageal cancer in high-grade dysplasia in Barrett's esophagus overestimated? *Clin Gastroenterol Hepatol* 2008;6(2):159.
170. Dar MS, Goldblum JR, Rice TW, et al. Can extent of high grade dysplasia in Barrett's oesophagus predict the presence of adenocarcinoma at oesophagectomy? *Gut* 2003;52(4):486.
172. Overholt BF, Lightdale CJ, Wang KK, et al. Photodynamic therapy with porfimer sodium for ablation of high-grade dysplasia in Barrett's esophagus: international, partially blinded, randomized phase III trial. *Gastrointest Endosc* 2005;62(4):488.
177. Shaheen NJ, Sharma P, Overhols BF, et al. Radiofrequency ablation in Barrett's esophagus and dysplasia. *N Engl J Med* 2009;360(22):2277.
178. Ell C, May A, Pech O, et al. Curative endoscopic resection of early esophageal adenocarciomas (Barrett's cancer). *Gastrointest Endosc* 2007;65 (1):3.
188. Luketich JD, Alvelo-Rivera M, Buenaventura PO, et al. Minimally invasive esophagectomy: outcomes in 222 patients. *Ann Surg* 2003;238(4):494.
189. Pennathur A, Farkas A, Krasinskas AM, et al. Esophagectomy for T1 esophageal cancer: outcomes in 100 patients and implications for endoscopic therapy. *Ann Thorac Surg* 2009;87(4):1048.
195. Begg CB, Cramer LD, Hoskins WJ, et al. Impact of hospital volume on operative mortality for major cancer surgery. *JAMA* 1998;280(20):1747.
196. Birkmeyer JD, Siewers AE, Finlayson EV, et al. Hospital volume and surgical mortality in the United States. *N Engl J Med* 2002;346(15):1128.
199. Wouters MW, Karin-Kos H, le Cessie S, et al. Centralization of esophageal cancer surgery: does it improve clinical outcomes? *Ann Surg Oncol* 2009; 16(7):1789.
200. Posner MC. Techniques of esophageal resection. In: Posner MC, Vokes EE, Weichselbaum, RR, eds. *Cancer of the upper gastrointestinal tract*. Hamilton, Ontario: BC Decker, 2002:1.
205. Orringer MB, Marshall B, Chang AC, et al. Two thousand transhiatal esophagectomies: changing trends, lessons learned. *Ann Surg* 2007;246(3): 363.
212. McKeown KC. Total three-stage oesophagectomy for cancer of the oesophagus. *Br J Surg* 1976;63(4):259.
220. Bosset JF, Gignoux M, Triboulet JP, et al. Chemoradiotherapy followed by surgery compared with surgery alone in squamous cell cancer of the esophagus. *N Engl J Med* 1997;337:161.
224. Chang AC, Ji J, Birkmeyer NJ, et al. Outcomes after transhiatal and transthoracic esophagectomy for cancer. *Ann Thorac Surg* 2008;85(2):424.
228. Hulscher JB, van Sandick JW, deBoer AG, et al. Extended transthoracic resection compared with limited transhiatal resection for adenocarcinoma of the esophagus. *N Engl J Med* 2002;347(21):1662.
229. Omloo JM, Lagarde SM, Hulscher JB, et al. Extended transthoracic resection compared with limited transhiatal resection for adenocarcinoma of the mid/distal esophagus: five-year survival of randomized clinical trial. *Ann Surg* 2007;246(6):992.
246. Cunningham D, Allum W, Stenning SP, et al. Perioperative chemotherapy versus surgery alone for resectable gastroesophageal cancer. *N Engl J Med* 2006;355:11.
247. Allum WH, STenning SP, Bancewicz J, et al. Long term results of a randomized trial of surgery with or without preoperative chemotherapy in esophageal cancer. *J Clin Oncol* 2009;27(30):5062.
251. Teniere P, Hay JM, Fingerhut A, et al. Postoperative radiation therapy does not increase survival after curative resection for squamous cell carcinoma of the middle and lower esophagus as shown by a multicenter controlled trial. French University Association for Surgical Research. *Surg Gynecol Obstet* 1991;173(2):123.
258. Herskovic A, Martz K, Al-Sarraf M, et al. Combined chemotherapy and radiotherapy compared with radiotherapy alone in patients with cancer of the esophagus. *N Engl J Med* 1992;326(24):1593.
259. Minsky B, Pajak T, Ginsberg RJ, et al. INT 0123 (Radiation Therapy Oncology Group 94-05) phase III trial of combined-modality therapy for esophageal cancer: high-dose versus standard-dose radiation therapy. *J Clin Oncol* 2002;20(5):1167.
301. Downey RJ, Akhurst T, Ilson D, et al. Whole body 18FDG-PET and the response of esophageal cancer to induction therapy: results of a prospective trial. *J Clin Oncol* 2003;21(3):428.
302. Flamen P, Van Cutsem E, Lerut A, et al. Positron emission tomography for assessment of the response to induction radiochemotherapy in locally advanced oesophageal cancer. *Ann Oncol* 2002;13(3):361.
308. Kleinberg L, Powell ME, Forastiere AA, et al. Survival outcome of E1201: an Eastern Cooperative Oncology Group randomized phase II trial of neoadjuvant preoperative paclitaxel/cisplatin/radiotherapy or irinotecan/cisplatin/radiotherapy in endoscopy with ultrasound stage esophageal adenocarcinoma. *J Clin Oncol* 2008;26(Suppl):4532.
310. Walsh TN, Noonan N, Hollywood D, et al. A comparison of multimodal therapy and surgery for esophageal adenocarcinoma. *N Engl J Med* 1996;335:462.
312. Burmeister BH, Smithers BM, Gebski V, et al. Surgery alone versus chemoradiotherapy followed by surgery for resectable cancer of the oesophagus: a randomised controlled phase III trial. *Lancet Oncol* 2005;6:659.
313. Tepper J, Krasna MJ, Niedzwiecki D, et al. Phase III trial of trimodality therapy with cisplatin, fluorouracil, radiotherapy, and surgery compared

with surgery alone for esophageal cancer: CALGB 9781. *J Clin Oncol* 2008;26(7):1086.
314. Lee J, Kim S, Jung H, et al. A single institutional phase III trial of preoperative chemotherapy with hyperfractionation radiotherapy plus surgery versus surgery alone for resectable esophageal squamous cell carcinoma. *Ann Oncol* 2004;15:947.
315. Stahl M, Walz MK, Stuschke M, et al. Phase III comparison of preoperative chemotherapy compared with chemoradiotherapy in patients with locally advanced adenocarcinoma of the esophagogastric junction. *J Clin Oncol* 2009;27(6):851.
316. Le Prise E, Etienne PL, Meunier B, et al. A randomized study of chemotherapy, radiation therapy, and surgery versus surgery for localized squamous cell carcinoma of the esophagus. *Cancer* 1994;73:1779.
317. Van Gaast A, van Hagen P, Hulshof M, et al. Effect of preoperative concurrent chemoradiotherapy on survival of patients with resectable esophageal or esophagogastric cancer; results from a multicenter randomized phase III study. *J Clin Oncol* 2010;28(18S): (abst 4004).
318. Kaklamanos IG, Walker GR, Ferry K, et al. Neoadjuvant treatment for resectable cancer of the esophagus and gastroesophageal junction: a meta-analysis of randomized clinical trials. *Ann Surg Oncol* 2003;10 (754):761.
319. Gebski V, Burmeister B, Smithers BM, et al. Survival benefits from neoadjuvant chemoradiotherapy or chemotherapy in oesophageal carcinoma: a meta-analysis. *Lancet Oncol* 2007;8:226.
327. Fok M, Sham JS, Choi D, et al. Postoperative radiotherapy for carcinoma of the esophagus: a prospective, randomized controlled study. *Surgery* 1993;113(2):138.
328. MacDonald J, Benedetti J, Smalley S, et al. Chemoradiation of resected gastric cancer: a 10-year follow-up of the phase III trial INT 0116 (SWOG 9008). *Proc Am Soc Clin Oncol* 2009;27:205s.
331. Suntharalingam M, Moughhan J, Cola LR, et al. Outcome results of the 1996–1999 patterns of care survey of the national practice for patients receiving radiation therapy for carcinoma of the esophagus. *J Clin Oncol* 2005;23:2325.
333. Wong RKS, Malthaner RA, Zuraw L, et al. Combined modality radiotherapy and chemotherapy in nonsurgical management of localized carcinoma of the esophagus: a practice guideline. *Int J Radiat Oncol Biol Phys* 2003;55:930.
344. Al-Sarraf M, Martz K, Herskovic A, et al. Progress report of combined chemoradiotherapy versus radiotherapy alone in patients with esophageal cancer: an Intergroup study. *J Clin Oncol* 1997;15:277.
349. Yu J, Ren R, Sun X, et al. A randomized clinical study of surgery versus radiotherapy in the treatment of resectable esophageal cancer. *Proc Am Soc Clin Oncol* 2006;24:181s.
350. Chiu PWY, Chan ACW, Leung SF, et al. Multicenter prospective randomized trial comparing standard esophagectomy with chemoradiotherapy for treatment of squamous esophageal cancer: early results from the Chinese University Research Group for Esophageal Cancer (CURE). *J Gastrointest Surg* 2005;9:794.
353. Crehange G, Maingon P, Peignaux K, et al. Phase III trial of protracted compared with split-course chemoradiation for esophageal cancer: Federation Francophone de Cancerologie Digestive 9102. *J Clin Oncol* 2007;25:4895.
354. Swisher SG, Hofsetter W, Wu TT, et al. Proposed revision of the esophageal cancer staging system to accommodate pathologic response (pP) following preoperative chemoradiation (CRT). *Ann Surg* 2005;241:810.
359. Blackstock AW, Farmer MR, Lovato J, et al. A prospective evaluation of the impact of 18-F-fluoro-deoxy-D-glucose positron emission tomography staging on survival for patients with locally advanced esophageal cancer. *Int J Radiat Oncol Biol Phys* 2006;64:455.
360. Brucher BLDM, Becker KR, Lordick F, et al. The clinical impact of histopathologic response assessment by residual tumor cell quantification in esophageal squamous cell carcinomas. *Cancer* 2006;106:2119.
361. McLoughlin J, Melis M, Siegel E, et al. Are patients with esophageal cancer who become PET negative after neoadjuvant chemoradiation free of cancer. *J Am Coll Surg* 2008;206:879.
368. Hildebrandt M, Yang H, Hung M, et al. Genetic variations in the PI3K/PTEN/mTOR pathway are associated with clinical outcomes in esophageal cancer patients treated with chemoradiotherapy. *J Clin Oncol* 2009; 27:857.
378. Homs MYV, Essink-Bot ML, Borsboom GJJM, et al. Quality of life after palliative treatment for oesophageal carcinoma—a prospective comparison between stent placement and single dose chemotherapy. *Eur J Cancer* 2004;40:1862.
384. Gaspar LE, Qian C, Kocha WI, et al. A phase I/II study of external beam radiation, brachytherapy and concurrent chemotherapy in localized cancer of the esophagus (RTOG 92-07): preliminary toxicity report. *Int J Radiat Oncol Biol Phys* 1997;37:593.
386. Gaspar LE, Nag S. Herskovic A, et al. American Brachytherapy Society (ABS) consensus guidelines for brachytherapy of esophageal cancer. *Int J Radiat Oncol Biol Phys* 1997;38:127.
404. Nishimura Y, Nagata K, Katano S, et al. Severe complications in advanced esophageal cancer treated with radiotherapy after intubation of esophageal stents: a questionnaire survey of the Japanese Society for Esophageal Diseases. *Int J Radiat Oncol Biol Phys* 2003;56:1327.
413. Coia LR, Soffen EM, Schultheiss TE, et al. Swallowing function in patients with esophageal cancer treated with concurrent radiation and chemotherapy. *Cancer* 1993;71:281.
415. Sur M, Sur R, Cooper K, et al. Morphologic alterations in esophageal squamous cell carcinoma after preoperative high dose rate intraluminal brachytherapy. *Cancer* 1996;77:2200.
418. Minsky BD. The adjuvant treatment of esophageal cancer. *Sem Radiat Oncol* 1994;4:165.
429. Nash CL, Gerdes H. Methods of palliation of esophageal and gastric cancer. *Surg Oncol Clin North Am* 2002;11(2):459.
436. Raijman I, Siddique I, Ajani J, et al. Palliation of malignant dysphagia and fistulae with coated expandable metal stents: experience with 101 patients. *Gastrointest Endosc* 1998;48(2):172.
459. Bleiberg H, Conroy T, Paillot B, et al. Randomised phase II study of cisplatin and 5-fluorouracil (5-FU) versus cisplatin alone in advanced squamous cell oesophageal cancer. *Eur J Cancer* 1997;33(8):1216.
492. Webb A, Cunningham D, Scarffe JH, et al. Randomized trial comparing epirubicin, cisplatin, and fluorouracil versus fluorouracil, doxorubicin, and methotrexate in advanced esophagogastric cancer. *J Clin Oncol* 1997; 15:261.
493. Ross P, Nicholson M, Cunningham D, et al. Prospective randomized trial comparing mitomycin, cisplatin, and protracted venous-infusion fluorouracil (PVI 5-FU) with epirubicin, cisplatin, and PVI 5-FU in advanced esophagogastric cancer. *J Clin Oncol* 2002;20(8):1996.
495. Cunningham D, Starling N, Rao S, et al. Capecitabine and oxaliplatin for advanced esophagogastric cancer. *N Engl J Med* 2008;358(1):36.
496. Al-Batran S, Hartmann J, Probst S, et al. Phase III trial in metastatic gastroesophageal adenocarcinoma with fluorouracil, leucovorin plus either oxaliplatin or cisplatin: a study of the Arbeitsgemeinschaft Internistische Onkologie. *J Clin Oncol* 2008;26(9):1435.
497. Kang YK, Kang KW, Shin DB, et al. Capecitabine/cisplatin versus 5-fluorouracil/cisplatin as first-line therapy in patients with advanced gastric cancer: a randomized phase III noninferiority trial. *Ann Oncol* 2009;20(4):666.
498. Koizumi W, Narahara H, Hara T, et al. S-1 plus cisplatin versus S-1 alone for first line treatment of advanced gastric cancer (SPIRITS Trial): a phase III trial. *Lancet Oncol* 2008;9(3):215.
499. Ajani JR, Correa A, Walsh G, et al. Multicenter phase II comparison of cisplatin/S-1 with cisplatin/infusional fluorouracil in advanced gastric or gastroesophageal adenocarcinoma study: the FLAGS Trial. *J Clin Oncol* 2010;28(9):1547.
500. Van Cutsem E, Moiseyenko VM, Tjulandin S, et al. Phase III study of docetaxel and cisplatin plus fluorouracil compared with cisplatin and fluorouracil as first-line therapy for advanced gastric cancer: a report of the V325 study group. *J Clin Oncol* 2006;24:4991.
514. Ilson DH, Saltz L, Enzinger P, et al. Phase II trial of weekly irinotecan plus cisplatin in advanced esophageal cancer. *J Clin Oncol* 1999;17(10):3270.
515. Ajani JA, Baker J, Pisters PW, et al. CPT-11 plus cisplatin in patients with advanced, untreated gastric or gastroesophageal junction carcinoma: results of a phase II study. *Cancer* 2002;94(3):641.
516. Enzinger PC, Ryan D, Clark J, et al. Weekly docetaxel, cisplatin, and irinotecan (TPC): results of a multicenter phase II trial in patients with metastatic esophagogastric cancer. *Ann Oncol* 2009;20(3):475.
522. Dank M, Zaluski J, Barone C, et al. Randomized phase III study comparing irinotecan combined with 5-fluorouracil and folinic acid to cisplatin combined with 5-fluorouracil in chemotherapy naive patients with advanced adenocarcinoma of the stomach or esophagogastric junction. *Ann Oncol* 2008;19(8):1450.
525. Van Cutsem E, Kang Y, Chung H, et al. Efficacy results from the TOGA trial: a phase III study of trastuzumab added to standard chemotherapy in first line human epidermal growth factor receptor 2 (HER2) positive advanced gastric cancer. *J Clin Oncol* 2009;27(18s):4509.
529. Pinto C, DiFabio F, Siena S, et al. Phase II study of cetuximab in combination with FOLFIRI in patients with untreated advanced gastric or gastroesophageal junction adenocarcinoma. *Ann Oncol* 2006;18(3):510.
530. Lorenzen S, Schuster T, Porschen R, et al. Cetuximab plus cisplatin 5-fluorouracil versus cisplatin 5-fluorouracil alone in first line metastatic squamous cell carcinoma of the esophagus: a randomized phase II trial. *Ann Oncol* 2009;20(10):1167.
532. Shah MA, Ramanathan RA, Ilson DH, et al. Multicenter phase II trial of irinotecan, cisplatin, and Bevacizumab in patients with metastatic gastric or gastroesophageal junction adenocarcinoma. *J Clin Oncol* 2006;24:5201.

CHAPTER 80 CANCER OF THE STOMACH

ITZHAK AVITAL, PETER W.T. PISTERS, DAVID P. KELSEN, AND CHRISTOPHER G. WILLETT

Adenocarcinoma of the stomach was the leading cause of cancer-related death worldwide through most of the 20th century. It now ranks second only to lung cancer, and an estimated 870,000 new cases are diagnosed annually, and 650,000 deaths (10% of all cancer deaths) worldwide.[1] In the West, the incidence of gastric cancer has decreased, potentially because of changes in diet, food preparation, and other environmental factors. The declining incidence has been dramatic in the United States, where this disease ranked sixth as a cause of cancer-related death (2000–2005).[2] It is estimated that in 2009, 21,130 new cases were diagnosed in the United States, with approximately 10,600 deaths.[2]

Prognosis remains poor except in a few countries. The explanations are multifactorial. The lack of defined risk factors, specific symptoms, and the low incidence has contributed to the late stage at diagnosis seen in most Western countries. In Japan, where gastric cancer is endemic, more patients are diagnosed at an early stage, which is reflected by higher overall survival rates.

The decline in incidence has been limited to noncardia gastric cancers.[3] The number of newly diagnosed cases of proximal gastric and esophagogastric junction adenocarcinomas has increased sixfold since the mid-1980s.[4] These tumors are thought to be biologically more aggressive and more complex to treat. The only chance at cure is surgical resection. However, even after what is believed to be a "curative" gastrectomy, disease recurs in the majority of patients. Efforts to improve these poor results have focused on developing effective pre- and postoperative systemic and regional adjuvant therapies. This chapter details the state of the art regarding the origins, diagnosis, and treatment of this worldwide health problem.

EPIDEMIOLOGY AND ETIOLOGY

The incidence and mortality rates for gastric cancer vary widely in different regions of the world. The highest incidences of stomach cancer can be found in Japan, Southeast Asia, South America, and Eastern Europe, with incidence rates as high as 30 to 85 cases per 100,000 population.[5] Almost two-thirds of the cases occur in developing countries with 42% in China alone.[5] In contrast, low-incidence areas such as the United States, Israel, Australia, New Zealand, and Kuwait have incidence rates of less than 10 cases per 100,000.[5] However, recent data suggest that the incidence of gastric cancer in the United States has increased by almost 60% over the past decade for ages 25 to 39 years.[3] Mortality figures approach incidence figures in many high-incidence countries. In Japan, there has been a continuous decline in mortality, perhaps as a result of mass screening and early detection.[6]

Immigrants gradually acquire the incidence rates of the country to which they move, suggesting that environmental factors are important in etiology.[7,8] Japanese persons migrating to lower risk areas had a risk of stomach cancer intermediate between that of the Western population and that of the Japanese population in Japan.[9] The risk of stomach cancer was high in second-generation offspring who continued to consume a Japanese-style diet but was low in those adopting a Western-style diet.[10] A study of Polish and Portuguese migrants living in the United States found that the incidence of gastric cancer decreased and became intermediate between the usual incidences in the countries of origin and adoption.[11] These studies suggest that environmental exposure in early life is essential in determining risk, but other environmental or cultural factors contribute to the predisposition to cancer.

In the United States, gastric cancer is now the sixth most common cause of cancer-related death, although a century ago it was the most common cause. Incidence rates increase and survival decreases with increasing age of the population.[2,12] There are substantial racial variations in incidence and death rates. The highest death rates are among African American men (11 cases per 100,000 population annually), followed by Asian American men (10 cases per 100,000), and American Indian and Alaskan men (9–10 cases per 100,000). The lowest incidence rates are recorded among white American women (2.5 cases per 100,000).

U.S. survival statistics have shown improvement in 5-year survival rates over the past two decades for all cancers from 50% in 1975 to 68% in 2006. The reason for this improvement is not clear. Surveillance, Epidemiology, and End Results (SEER) cancer statistics showed a 15.4% 5-year relative overall survival rate in 1973 compared with 26.7% by 2006. Survival rates are best in the groups with the lowest incidence of gastric cancer.

One of the most striking epidemiologic observations has been the increasing incidence of adenocarcinomas of the proximal stomach and distal esophagus.[4,13] These tumors are thought to have different etiologic factors than distal gastric cancers. Gastric body lesions are associated with low acid production and *Helicobacter pylori* infection, whereas cardia lesions are not associated with either. Potentially, the improvements in treatment for *H. pylori* resulted in decreased frequency of noncardia lesions while at the same time decreasing the protection for distal esophagus and cardia cancers due to decreased acid production and reflux in patients with *H. pylori* infection and atrophic gastritis.[14,15] Cardia lesions also have a higher male to female ratio and are more common in whites than in African Americans. In 2009, Wu et al.,[16] reviewing the SEER database, reported that between 1978 and 2005, total cases of gastric cancer decreased by 34%. Regardless of site, intestinal type rates decreased by 44%, whereas diffuse type increased by 62% up to 2000 and modestly declined in recent years. Cardia cancers increased by 23% mostly during the 1980s, and noncardia cancers declined consistently. When considered by type and site, diffuse type increased by 377% for cardia cancers. Intestinal-type rates decreased by 40% for all sites except cardia, which increased by 17%. Rates for all types were higher among males than females. Intestinal type and noncardia site were highest among blacks and lowest among white females. Diffuse type was highest among nonwhites. Cardia site were highest among white males and lowest among all females. Noncardia site among nonwhites were double to triple those among whites.[17-20] The majority of gastric cancers are adenocarcinomas. The "intestinal" type frequently arises in the body/antrum. Prior infection with *H. pylori*, especially cagA(+) A subtype, has been associated with an increased risk of the intestinal type.[21] Diffuse (signet cell) gastric cancer may develop in any part of the stomach, has no clear link to *H. pylori* infection, and is associated in a small percentage with *CDH1* mutation, which encodes for E-cadherin (hereditary diffuse gastric cancer). Silencing of CDH1 by methylation is also associated with the sporadic form of diffuse gastric cancer.

Although there are different epidemiologies and to a certain extent different histologic appearances, the clinical management of patients with gastric cancer does not currently take these differences into account. Strategies for prevention of gastric cancer are similar (with the exception of prophylactic gastrectomy for patients with inherited mutations of *CDH1*), nor do screening programs or therapeutic treatment plans differ among the three different subtypes. However, genomic analysis of the three histologic subtypes is being investigated and may show substantial differences between them.[22,23] One early finding supporting the hypothesis that there are at least three different subtypes of gastric cancer is the low incidence of *HER2* overexpression or amplification in the diffuse type.[24] For the endemic forms of gastric cancer, primarily the intestinal type, Correa,[25] as well as other authors, has postulated a progression from normal tissue to chronic atrophic gastritis, to intestinal metaplasia, and then to dysplasia. He has also suggested that this progression is associated with varying risk factors, with *H. pylori* and high salt intake associated with chronic atrophic gastritis and high nitrate intake leading to intestinal metaplasia.[26,27]

A list of risk factors associated with gastric cancer is outlined in Table 80.1. The following paragraphs address specific areas of interest in the literature addressing the etiology of gastric cancer.[28] The increasing prevalence of obesity in the United States may be one contributing factor for the increasing incidence of proximal gastric cancer. Elevated body mass index[29] and high caloric, high glycemic load diet[30] were associated with adenocarcinoma of the distal esophagus and gastric cardia. The risk of gastric cancer is increased directly with increasing body mass index.[29] Obesity is also associated with gastroesophageal reflux disease, another risk factor.[31] A population-based, case-control study performed in Sweden found that for persons with recurrent symptoms of reflux, as compared with those without such symptoms, the odds ratio (OR) was 7.7 (95% confidence interval [CI], 5.3 to 11.4) for esophageal adenocarcinoma and 2.0 (95% CI, 1.4 to 2.9) for developing adenocarcinoma of the gastric cardia.[32] Other studies have found tobacco use to be associated with tumors at these sites.[33] Steevens et al.[34] observed a relative risk (RR) of 1.6 (95% CI, 0.97 to 2.66) for gastric cancer in cigarette smokers that was enhanced with alcohol consumption to a RR of 8.5 (95% CI, 3.89 to 16.60). Conversely, the use of aspirin and nonsteroidal and anti-inflammatory drugs has been associated with a lower risk of esophageal and cardia cancers,[35] implicating inflammation in the etiology of gastric cancer

In 1965, Laurén[36] described two histologic types of gastric adenocarcinoma, intestinal and diffuse, which provided a model to understand better the etiology and epidemiology of the disease. The intestinal variant is corpus-dominant, arises from precancerous lesions (gastric atrophy or intestinal metaplasia), more common in men than in women, more frequent in older people, and represents the dominant histologic type in regions where stomach cancer is endemic, suggesting a predominantly environmental etiology. The diffuse form does not typically arise from recognizable precancerous lesions. It is more common in low-incidence regions, occurs more frequently in women and in younger patients, and has a higher association with familial occurrence (blood type A), suggesting a genetic etiology.[37] The intestinal type accounts for much of the geographical variation and the decline in the incidence of gastric cancer worldwide.[28,38]

Noncardia gastric cancer is thought to be a multistep progression related to chronic inflammation (e.g., *H. pylori* infection). This is a common infection in many parts of the world, associated with a doubled risk of such cancers.[39,40] The precise mechanism by which *H. pylori* infection increases gastric cancer incidence is unclear; it appears to increase the incidence of chronic atrophic gastritis, which produces a low-acidity environment, and the incidence of metaplasia and dysplasia.[41,42] However, because *H. pylori* infection is present in over 50% of the population in many parts of the world, it is clearly not a

TABLE 80.1

FACTORS ASSOCIATED WITH INCREASED RISK OF DEVELOPING STOMACH CANCER

ACQUIRED FACTORS

Nutritional
- High salt consumption
- High nitrate consumption
- Low dietary vitamin A and C
- Poor food preparation (smoked, salt cured)
- Lack of refrigeration
- Poor drinking water (well water)

Occupational
- Rubber workers
- Coal workers

Cigarette smoking

Helicobacter pylori infection

Epstein-Barr virus

Radiation exposure

Prior gastric surgery for benign gastric ulcer disease

Prior treatment for mucosa-associated lymphoid tissue (MALT) lymphoma

GENETIC FACTORS

- Type A blood
- Pernicious anemia
- Family history without known genetic factors (first-degree relative with gastric cancer)
- Hereditary diffuse gastric cancer (*CDH1* mutation)
- Familial gastric cancer
- Hereditary nonpolyposis colon cancer
- Familial adenomatous polyposis
- Li-Fraumeni syndrome
- *BRCA1* and *BRAC2*

Precursor lesions
- Adenomatous gastric polyps
- Chronic atrophic gastritis
- Dysplasia
- Intestinal metaplasia
- Menetrier disease

Ethnicity (in the United States, gastric cancer is more common among Asian/Pacific Islanders, Hispanics and African Americans)

Obesity (the strength of this link is not clear)

sufficient event for the development of gastric cancer.[43–45] Recent reports suggest that gastric cancer develops in 5% of *H. pylori*-positive persons over 10 years.[40] Multiple factors have been suggested that may interact with *H. pylori* in producing gastric cancer, including tobacco, age, gender, and diet (e.g., low intake of ascorbic acid, carotene, and vitamin E).[46] The risk and location of gastric cancer is associated with different serotypes of *H. pylori*. Recent studies evaluated the serostatus of patients for 15 different known *H. pylori* serotypes. These studies suggested that the cytotoxin-associated genes *cagA* and *VacA*, and the noncytotoxic proteins HyuA and GroEL in various *H. pylori* strains produce more gastric inflammation and have a strong association with gastric cancer. In addition, *cagA* and *GroEL* have stronger association with noncardia gastric cancer.[47,48] A number of other factors have been studied for their relationship with gastric cancer formation.

The only prospective study reporting on alcohol consumption, cigarette smoking, and gastric cancer did not find an association between alcohol and gastric cancer.[34] There was a moderate association between tobacco use and gastric cancer formation. The RR for current smokers is 1.86 (1.39 to 2.47) with a long time interval after smoking cessation necessary before a decrease in risk is seen.[34] There is fairly strong evidence that eating fruits and vegetables (especially raw) has a protective effect against gastric cancer, and there is a suggestion that foods high in antioxidants including vitamins C and E, carotenoids, and flavonoids may be beneficial. Green tea, which contains large amounts of phenols, could also be protective.[49] Nitrates (preserved foods) can be converted to nitrites and then to *N*-nitroso compounds, which produce gastric cancer in laboratory animals. Some studies showed a strong association between high intake of nitrates and gastric cancer, and other studies showed no association.[49,50] Radiation exposure, especially at a young age, has been shown to produce a high risk of gastric cancer.[51] Gastric ulcer disease, a condition sometimes related to *H. pylori* infection, is also associated with an increased risk of gastric cancer,[52] whereas duodenal ulcer disease is associated with a modest risk reduction.[53] Prevention of *H. pylori* infection did not decrease that risk.[54] Gastric surgery for benign disorders was also reported to increase the risk of gastric cancer.[55]

ANATOMIC CONSIDERATIONS

The stomach begins at the gastroesophageal junction and ends at the pylorus (Fig. 80.1). Cancers arising from the proximal greater curvature may directly involve the splenic hilum and tail of pancreas, whereas more distal tumors may invade the transverse colon. Proximal cancers may extend into the diaphragm, spleen, or the left lateral segment of the liver.

The blood supply to the stomach is extensive and is based on vessels arising from the celiac axis (Fig. 80.1). The right gastric artery is arising from the hepatic artery proper (50%–68%), left hepatic artery (29%–40%), and from the common hepatic artery (3.2%). The left gastric artery is arising from the celiac axis directly (90%), and may arise from the common hepatic (2%), splenic (4%), aorta (3%) arteries, or from the superior mesenteric artery. Both right and left gastric arteries course along the lesser curvature. Along the greater curvature are the right gastroepiploic artery, which originates from the gastroduodenal artery at the inferior border of the proximal duodenum (rarely from the superior mesenteric artery), and the left gastroepiploic artery (highly variable artery), branching from the distal (72%), inferior, middle splenic artery laterally. The short gastric arteries (*vasa brevia*, five to seven separate vessels) arise directly from the splenic artery or the left gastroepiploic. The posterior (dorsal) gastric artery (17%–68%) may arise from the splenic artery to supply the distal esophagus, cardia, and fundus. The preservation of any of these vessels in the course of a subtotal gastrectomy for carcinoma is not necessary, and the most proximal few centimeters of remaining stomach are well supplied by collateral flow from the lower segmental esophageal arcade. The rich submucosal blood supply of the stomach is an important factor in its ability to heal rapidly and produce a low incidence of anastomotic disruption. The venous supply of the stomach tends to parallel the arterial supply. The venous efflux ultimately passes the portal venous system and is reflected in the fact that the liver is a primary site for distant metastatic spread.

The lymphatic drainage of the stomach is extensive, and distinct anatomic groups of perigastric lymph nodes have

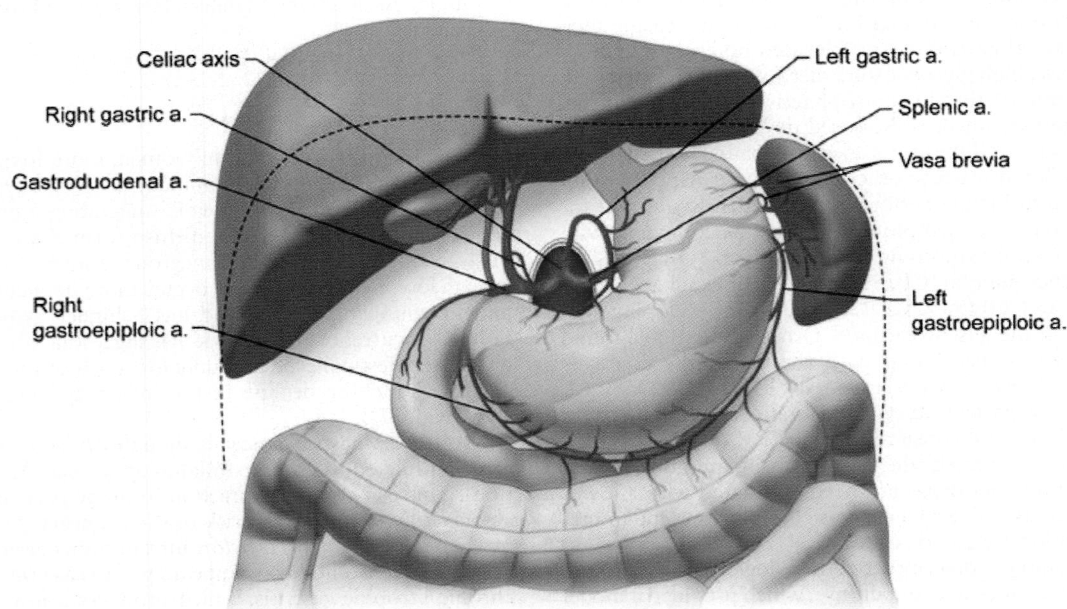

FIGURE 80.1 Blood supply to the stomach and anatomic relationships of the stomach with other adjacent organs likely to be involved by direct extension of a T4 gastric tumor.

been defined according to their relationship to the stomach and its blood supply. There are six perigastric lymph node groups. In the first echelon (stations 1 through 6) are the right and left pericardial nodes (stations 1 and 2). Along the lesser curvature are the lesser curvature nodes (station 3) and the suprapyloric nodes (station 5). Along the greater curvature, the gastroepiploic nodes or greater curvature nodes (station 4), and the subpyloric nodes (station 6). In the second echelon (stations 7 through 12) are the nodes along named arteries, which include the left gastric, common hepatic, celiac, splenic hilum, splenic artery, and hepatoduodenal lymphatics (stations 7 through 12, respectively), which drain into the celiac and periaortic lymphatics. The third echelon (stations 13 through 16) contains the posterior to pancreatic head, superior mesenteric artery, middle colic artery, and para-aortic lymphatics (stations 13 through 16, respectively). Proximally are the lower esophageal lymph nodes; extensive spread of gastric cancer along the intrathoracic lymph channels may be manifested clinically by a metastatic lymph node in the left supraclavicular fossa (Virchow's node) or left axilla (Irish's node). Tumor spread to the lymphatics in the hepatoduodenal ligament can extend along the falciform ligament and result in subcutaneous periumbilical tumor deposits (Sister Mary Joseph's nodes).

PATHOLOGY AND TUMOR BIOLOGY

Approximately 95% of all gastric cancers are adenocarcinomas. The term *gastric cancer* refers to adenocarcinoma of the stomach. Other malignant tumors are rare and include squamous cell carcinoma, adenoacanthoma, carcinoid tumors, small cell carcinoma, mucinous carcinoma, hepatoid adenocarcinoma, oncocytic (parietal gland) carcinoma, sarcomatoid carcinoma, lymphoepithelioma-like carcinoma, adenocarcinoma with rhabdoid features, gastric carcinoma with osteoclastlike giant cells, and leiomyosarcoma.[56] Although no normal lymphoid tissue is found in the gastric mucosa, the stomach is the most common site for lymphomas of the gastrointestinal tract. The increased awareness of association between mucosa-associated lymphoid tissue lymphomas and *H. pylori* may explain, in part, the rise in incidence,[57] although the incidence of mucosa-associated lymphoid tissue gastric lymphomas is decreasing likely because of effective treatment against *H. pylori*.[58]

In terms of pathogenesis, two new concepts are worth mentioning: bone marrow participation in gastric carcinogenesis and gastric cancer stem cells. It has been hypothesized that the gastric epithelial cells acquiring abnormal phenotype (resembling intestinal epithelium) originate from gastric stem cells localized to the only cell replication zone of the gastric glands (i.e., the isthmus). However, Houghton et al.,[59] Stoicov et al.,[60,61] and Li et al.[62] demonstrated in a rodent model of *Helicobacter*-induced gastric cancer that the entire cancer mass was derived from cells originating in the bone marrow. This interesting phenomenon was observed by other authors studying solid cancers in patients receiving bone marrow transplantation.[63] Recent evidence proposes the existence of cancer stem cells or stemlike cancer cells in various cancers. Although controversial, cancer stem cells are defined as cancer cells with the exclusive ability to initiate tumors, metastasize, and self-renew tumors. In gastric cancer, several investigators suggested the existence of gastric cancer stem cells (i.e., CD44+) and SP (side population) cells.[64,65] These cells showed relative resistance to chemotherapy and radiation, and exclusive ability to initiate tumors. These important observations might lead to novel approaches to the diagnosis and treatment of gastric cancer in the next decade.

HISTOPATHOLOGY

Several staging schemas have been proposed based on the morphologic features of gastric tumors. The Borrmann classification divides gastric cancer into five types depending on macroscopic appearance. Type I represents polypoid or fungating cancers, type II encompasses ulcerating lesions surrounded by elevated borders, type III represents ulcerated lesions infiltrating the gastric wall, type IV are diffusely infiltrating tumors, and type V gastric cancers are unclassifiable cancers.[66] The gross morphologic appearance of gastric cancer and the degree of histologic differentiation are not independent prognostic variables. Ming[67] has proposed a histomorphologic staging system that divides gastric cancer into either a prognostically favorable expansive type or a poor prognosis infiltrating type. Based on an analysis of 171 gastric cancers, the expansive-type tumors were uniformly polypoid or superficial on gross appearance, whereas the infiltrative tumors were almost always diffuse. Grossly ulcerated lesions were divided between the expansive or infiltrative forms. Broder's classification of gastric cancer grades tumors histologically from 1 (well-differentiated) to 4 (anaplastic). Bearzi and Ranaldi[68] have correlated the degree of histologic differentiation with the gross appearance of 41 primary gastric cancers seen on endoscopy. Ninety percent of protruding or superficial cancers were well differentiated (Broder's grade 1), whereas almost half of all ulcerated tumors were poorly differentiated or diffusely infiltrating (Broder's grades 3 and 4).

The most widely used classification of gastric cancer is by Laurén.[36] It divides gastric cancers into either intestinal or diffuse forms. This classification scheme, based on tumor histology, characterizes two varieties of gastric adenocarcinomas that manifest distinctively different pathology, epidemiology, genetics, and etiologies. The intestinal variety represents a differentiated cancer with a tendency to form glands similar to other sites in the gastrointestinal tract, but in particular the colon type; hence, intestinal type. In contrast, the diffuse form exhibits very little cell cohesion with a predilection for extensive submucosal spread and early metastases. Although the diffuse-type cancers are associated with a worse outcome than the intestinal type, this finding is not independent of tumor, node, and metastasis (TNM) stage. The molecular pathogenesis of these two distinct forms of gastric cancer is also different. Although the intestinal type represents *H. pylori*-initiated multistep progression with less defined progressive genetic alterations, the diffuse type main carcinogenic event is loss of expression of E-cadherin (*CDH1* gene). E-cadherin is a molecule involved in cell-to-cell adhesion; loss of its expression leads to noncohesive growth, hence the diffuse type. In tumors that display both intestinal and diffuse phenotypes the *CDH1* mutation and loss of E-cadherin function are observed only within the diffuse phenotype.[69]

PATTERNS OF SPREAD

Carcinomas of the stomach can spread by local extension to involve adjacent structures and can develop lymphatic metastases, peritoneal metastases, and distant metastases. These extensions can occur by the local invasive properties of the tumor, lymphatic spread, or hematogenous dissemination. The initial growth of the tumor occurs by penetration into the gastric wall, extension through the wall, within the wall longitudinally,[70] and subsequent involvement of an increasing percentage of the stomach. The two modes of local extension that can have a major therapeutic impact are tumor penetration through the gastric serosa, where the risk of tumor invasion of adjacent structures or peritoneal spread is increased, and lymphatic involvement. Zinninger[71] has evaluated the spread in the gastric wall and has found a wide variation in its extent. Tumor spread is often through the intramural lymphatics or in the subserosal layers.[70] Local extension can also occur into the esophagus or the duodenum.[72] Duodenal extension is rare (0.5%–1.8% of all resected cases),[73] portrays poor prognosis, and is principally through the muscular layer by direct infiltration and through the subserosal lymphatics, but is not generally of great extent.[74] Extension into the esophagus occurs primarily through the submucosal lymphatics.[75]

Local extension does not occur solely by radial intramural spread but also by deep invasion through the wall to adjacent structures[70] (omentum, spleen, adrenal gland, diaphragm, liver, pancreas, or colon). Many studies report that 60% to 90% of patients had primary tumors penetrating the serosa or invading adjacent organs and that at least 50% had lymphatic metastases. In the largest series reporting on 10,783 gastric cancer patients from Korea, 57% of the patients had lymph node metastasis, and the average number of involved lymph nodes was five.[76,77] Of the 1,577 primary gastric cancer cases admitted to Memorial Sloan-Kettering Cancer Center (MSKCC) between July 1, 1985, and June 30, 1998, 60% of the 1,221 resected cases had evidence of serosal penetration and 68% had positive nodes. Lymph node metastases were found in 18% of pT1 lesions, and 60% in pT2 lesions after R0 resection in 941 patients. The highest incidence of lymphatic metastasis was seen in tumors diffusely involving the entire stomach. Tumors located at the gastroesophageal junction also had a high incidence relative to other sites.[78]

The pattern of nodal metastases also varies depending on the location of the primary site. In a study, reporting on 1,137 patients with early gastric cancer, tumors located in the upper, middle, and lower third of the stomach had 12%, 10%, and 8% nodal involvement, respectively. The most common nodal station metastases for the upper, middle, and lower third of the stomach were stations 3 (lesser curvature), 3/4/7 (lesser/greater curvature and left gastric artery), and 3/4/6 (lesser/greater curvature and infrapyloric), respectively.[79] Earlier studies that included more advanced gastric cancers showed that the left gastric artery nodes were at increased risk for nodal metastases independent of tumor location.[79,80]

Gastric cancer recurs in multiple sites, locoregionally and systemically. Patterns of failure are variable. These differences are likely related to the patient cohorts evaluated, the time at which failure was determined, and the method of determination of failure patterns. Recent series from the MSKCC and Korea do shed light on modern patterns of failure.[78,81] In the report from MSKCC, recurrence patterns of 1,038 patients who underwent R0 gastrectomy with D2 lymphadenectomy (61%) were analyzed; complete data on recurrence were available in 367 (74%) of 496 patients who experienced recurrence. The locoregional area was involved in 199 (54%) patients. Distant sites were involved in 188 (51%) patients, and peritoneal recurrence was detected in 108 patients (29%). More than one site of recurrence was detected: distal, peritoneal, and locoregional recurrences in 9 (2.5%); locoregional and peritoneal in 34 (9.3%); locoregional and distant in 61 (16.6%); and distant and peritoneal in 15 (4.1%) patients. On multivariate analysis, peritoneal recurrence was associated with female gender, advanced T stage, and distal and diffuse type tumors; locoregional recurrence was associated with proximal location, early T stage, and intestinal type tumors. In the study from Korea, recurrence patterns were analyzed in 2,038 patients who were treated with potentially curative gastrectomy.[81] Of 508 patients who developed recurrence, 33% involved locoregional sites, 44% were peritoneal, and 38% were distant. At time of presentation, 35% of patients presented with distant metastasis, with 4% to 14% having liver metastases.[82,83]

CLINICAL PRESENTATION AND PRETREATMENT EVALUATION

Signs and Symptoms

Because of the vague, nonspecific symptoms that characterize gastric cancer, many patients are diagnosed with advanced-stage disease. Patients may have a combination of signs and symptoms such as weight loss (22%–61%)[84]; anorexia (5%–40%); fatigue, epigastric discomfort, or pain (62%–91%); postprandial fullness, heart burn, indigestion, nausea and vomiting (6%–40%); none of these unequivocally indicates gastric cancer. In addition, patients may be asymptomatic (4%–17%).[85] Weight loss and abdominal pain are the most common presenting symptoms at initial encounter.[86–88] Weight loss is a common symptom, and its clinical significance should not be underestimated. Dewys et al.[89] found that in 179 patients with advanced gastric cancer, more than 80% of patients had a greater than 10% decrease in body weight before diagnosis. Furthermore, patients with weight loss had a significantly shorter survival than did those without weight loss.[87]

In some patients, symptoms may suggest the presence of a lesion at a specific location. Up to 25% of the patients have history/symptoms of peptic ulcer disease.[86] A history of dysphagia or pseudoachalasia may indicate the presence of a tumor in the cardia with extension through the gastroesophageal junction.[90] Early satiety is an infrequent symptom of gastric cancer but is indicative of a diffusely infiltrative tumor that has resulted in loss of distensibility of the gastric wall. Later satiety and vomiting may indicate pyloric involvement. Significant gastrointestinal bleeding is uncommon with gastric cancer; however, hematemesis does occur in approximately 10% to 15% of patients, and anemia in 1% to 12% of patients. Signs and symptoms at presentation are often related to spread of disease. Ascites, jaundice, or a palpable mass indicates incurable disease.[87] The transverse colon is a potential site of malignant fistulization and obstruction from a gastric primary tumor. Diffuse peritoneal spread of disease frequently produces other sites of intestinal obstruction. A large ovarian mass (Krukenberg's tumor) or a large peritoneal implant in the pelvis (Blumer's shelf), which can produce symptoms of rectal obstruction, may be felt on pelvic or rectal examination.[84,91] Nodular metastases in the subcutaneous tissue around the umbilicus (Sister Mary Joseph's node) or in peripheral lymph nodes such as in the supraclavicular area (Virchow's node) represent areas in which a tissue diagnosis can be established with minimal morbidity.[92] There is no symptom complex that occurs early in the evolution of gastric cancer that can identify individuals for further diagnostic measures. However, alarm symptoms (dysphagia, weight loss, and palpable abdominal mass) are independently associated with survival; increased number and the specific symptom correlate with mortality.[87,88]

Screening

Mass screening programs for gastric cancer have been most successful in high-risk areas, especially in Japan.[6] A variety of screening tests have been studied in Japanese patients, with a sensitivity and specificity of approximately 90%.[93] Screening typically includes serology for *H. pylori*, the use of double-contrast barium radiographs, or upper endoscopy with risk stratification (OLGA staging system for gastric cancer risk; reviewed in refs. 6 and 94).

Ohata et al.[95] reported on 4,655 asymptomatic patients with an average age of 50 years old who were followed for 7.7 years. Atrophic gastritis was identified using pepsinogen and *H. pylori* testing; 2,341 (52%) were *H. pylori*-positive with nonatrophic gastritis, 967 (21%) were *H. pylori*-negative without atrophic gastritis, 1,316 (28%) were *H. pylori*-positive with atrophic gastritis, and 31 (0.7%) had severe atrophic gastritis. The rates of gastric cancer development per 100,000/population/year were 107, 0, 238, and 871, respectively. Thus the number of endoscopies needed to detect one cancer were 1/1,000, 0/1,000, 1/410, and 1/114. Similar data were reported on 6,985 patients by Watabe et al.[96] Surveillance in endemic populations is clinically important because early gastric cancer has a very high cure rate with surgical treatment. However, the fact that gastric cancer remains one of the top causes of death in Japan indicates the limitations of a mass-screening program when the entire population at risk is not effectively screened. However, more recent studies indicate that for surveillance programs to be effective and feasible from economical perspective they should be instituted only in high-risk populations (>20/100,000), and include the following components: detection and eradication of *H. pylori*, serum pepsinogen (pepsinogen I/II ratio), endoscopy with biopsy, and risk stratification before and after *H. pylori* eradication using a system like the OLGA. Such programs are expected to avoid long-term repeated screening of approximately 70% of the population who are at lower risk.[6,97–99] A U.S. study found that screening and eradication of *H. pylori* in Japanese Americans is cost-effective in preventing gastric cancer.[100] These findings were confirmed by two studies from the United Kingdom.[101,102]

PRETREATMENT STAGING

Tumor Markers

Most gastric cancers have at least one elevated tumor marker, but some benign gastric diseases show elevated tumor markers as well. Tumor markers in gastric cancer continue to have limited diagnostic usefulness, with their role more helpful in follow-up. The most commonly used markers are CEA, CA 19-9, CA 50, and CA 72-4. There is wide variation in the reported serum levels of these markers; positive CEA and CA 19-9 levels varied from 8% to 58% and 4% to 65%, respectively. Overall, the sensitivity of each tumor marker alone as a diagnostic marker of gastric cancer is low. However, when the levels are elevated, it does usually correlate with stage. Combining CEA with other markers, such as the CA 19-9, CA 72-4, or CA 50, can increase sensitivity compared with CEA alone.[103–109]

In a large study evaluating CEA, α-fetoprotein, human chronic gonadotropin-β (β-HCG), CA 19-9, CA 125, as well as tissue staining for *HER2* in gastric cancer patients, only β-HCG level greater than 4 IU/L, and a CA 125 level equal to or greater than 350 U/mL had prognostic significance. Elevated serum tumor marker levels in gastric cancer before chemotherapy may reflect not just tumor burden but also biology.

Endoscopy

Endoscopy is the best method to diagnose gastric cancer as it visualizes the gastric mucosa and allows biopsy for a histologic diagnosis. Chromoendoscopy helps identification of mucosal abnormalities through topical stains. Magnification endoscopy is used to magnify standard endoscopic fields by 1.5- to 150-fold. Narrow band imaging affords increased visualization of the microvasculature. Confocal laser endomicroscopy permits *in vivo*, three-dimensional microscopy including subsurface structures with diagnostic accuracy, sensitivity, and specificity of 97%, 90%, and 99.5%, respectively.[110–112]

Endoscopic ultrasound (EUS) is a tool for preoperative staging and selection for neoadjuvant therapy. It is used to assess the T and N stage. A study of 225 patients from MSKCC found that the concordance between EUS and pathology was lower than expected. The accuracy for individual T and N stage were 57% and 50%, respectively. However, the combined assessment of N stage and serosal invasion identified 77% of the patients at risk of death after curative resection.[113] Other investigators compared the accuracy of EUS with that of multidetector computed tomography (MDCT) and magnetic resonance imaging (MRI) and found that the overall accuracy was 65% to 92%, 77% to 89%, and 71% to 83% for T stage, and 55% to 66%, 32% to 77% for N stage, respectively. The corresponding sensitivity and specificity for serosal involvement were 78% to 100%, 83% to 100%, and 89% to 93% for T stage, and 68% to 100%, 80% to 97%, and 91% to 100% for N stage, respectively.[112,114]

Computed Tomography

Once gastric cancer is suspected, a triphasic CT with oral and intravenous contrast of the abdomen, chest, and pelvis is imperative. In a study of 790 patients who underwent MDCT prior to surgery, the overall accuracy in determining T stage was 74% (T1 46%, T2 53%, T3 86%, and T4 86%), and for N staging it was 75% (N0 76%, N1 69%, and N2 80%). The sensitivity, specificity, and accuracy for lymph node metastasis were 86%, 76%, and 82%, respectively.[115] MDCT with thin-sliced multiplanar reconstruction (MPR) and water filling is increasingly used. The accuracy rate for advanced gastric cancer was 96% and for early gastric cancer it was 41%. An improvement on axial CT and MPR-MDCT was the addition of staging with three-dimensional MPR-MDCT. The detection rate for MPR with virtual gastroscopy was 98%. MPR-MDCT with combined water and air distention is superior to conventional axial imaging.[116]

Magnetic Resonance Imaging

MRI is not used routinely in preoperative staging of gastric cancer. Several studies have demonstrated that CT and MRI are comparable in terms of accuracy and understaging.[117,118] However, MRI is a useful modality to further characterize liver lesions identified on preoperative CT staging workup.

Positron Emission Tomography

Whole-body 2-[^{18}F]-fluoro-2-deoxyglucose (FDG) positron emission tomography (PET) is being applied increasingly in the evaluation of gastrointestinal malignancies. In gastric cancer, approximately half of the primary tumors are FDG-negative; the diffuse (signet cell) subtype was most likely to be non-FDG avid, likely because of decreased expression of the glucose transporter-1 (Glut-1).[119] In patients with non-FDG avid primary tumor, FDG-PET/CT is not useful.[119–123] PET/CT was tested as a tool to predict response to neoadjuvant chemotherapy. Ott et al.[124] reported 90% 2-year survival in patients with PET-defined response (<35% decrease standardized uptake value [SUV]) versus 25% for patients not responding to PET. PET response could be detected as early as 14 days. At least 60% of the patients were PET-nonresponding patients and thus could have been spared further chemotherapy. Authors of the MUNICON trial reported on patients who were PET nonresponders by day 14 after cisplatin and fluorouracil (5-FU) neoadjuvant chemotherapy and subsequently were sent for surgery, and patients who were PET responders and continued 3 months of neoadjuvant therapy before surgery. The PET-responding patients had a survival benefit (hazard ratio [HR],

2.13; $P < 0.15$). In PET-nonresponding patients, stopping the chemotherapy did not affect long-term survival.[125] Recent studies, including one large meta-analysis, showed that in terms of diagnostic accuracy and lymph node staging EUS, MDCT, MRI, and PET/CT are comparable modalities. There were no significant differences between mean sensitivities and specificities.[126,127] Even in patients whose tumors were FDG-avid, FDG-PET/CT scans did not identify occult peritoneal disease (0 of 18) but did identify extraperitoneal M1 disease in nine patients with bone (n = 2), liver (n = 4), and retroperitoneal lymph node (n = 3) involvement. In patients with FDG-avid tumors, PET may be useful in detecting metastatic disease and follow-up for recurrence. Interestingly, the presence of glucose transporter-1 and FDG-avid gastric cancers may be associated with decreased overall survival.[119] The role of PET/CT in the primary staging of gastric cancer remains to be established; its role might be better defined in advanced disease.

Staging Laparoscopy and Peritoneal Cytology

Staging laparoscopy with peritoneal lavage should be an integral part of the pretreatment staging evaluation of patients believed to have localized gastric cancer. Current noninvasive modalities used in preoperative staging of gastric cancer have sensitivities significantly lower than 100%, particularly in cases of low-volume peritoneal carcinomatosis.[128–130] Current CT techniques cannot consistently identify low-volume macroscopic metastases that are 5 mm or less in size. Laparoscopy directly inspects the peritoneal and visceral surfaces for detection of CT-occult, small-volume metastases. Staging laparoscopy also allows for assessment of peritoneal cytology and laparoscopic ultrasound. Laparoscopic staging is done to spare nontherapeutic operations and for potential stratification in various trials.[131]

The rate of detection of CT-occult M1 disease by laparoscopy depends on the quality of CT scanning and interpretation.[132] Muntean et al.[132a] reported on 98 patients with primary gastric cancer, 45 underwent staging laparoscopy with subsequent surgery and 53 went directly to surgery. An unnecessary laparotomy was avoided in 38% of the patients. The overall sensitivity and specificity were 89% and 100%, respectively. Nonetheless, even high-quality MDCT is insufficiently sensitive for detection of low-volume extragastric disease and thus CT, EUS, and laparoscopy are complementary staging studies.[133,134]

The value of peritoneal cytology as a preoperative staging tool in patients with gastric cancer who are potential candidates for curative resection by EUS and CT has been examined by several investigators. Bentrem et al.[135] reported on 371 patients who underwent R0 resection, 6.5% of whom had positive cytology after staging laparoscopy. Median survival of patients with positive cytology was 14.8 versus 98.5 months for patients with negative cytology findings ($P < .001$). Positive cytology predicted death from gastric cancer (RR, 2.7; $P < .001$). Several groups confirmed these findings and concluded that staging laparoscopy with peritoneal cytology can change the management of gastric cancer in 6.5% to 52% of patients.[129,136–139]

Laparoscopy can be performed as a separate staging procedure prior to definitive treatment planning or immediately prior to planned laparotomy for gastrectomy. When performed as a separate procedure, laparoscopy has the disadvantage of the additional risks and expense of a second general anesthetic. However, separate procedure laparoscopy allows the additional staging information including cytology acquired at laparoscopy to be reviewed and discussed with the patient and multidisciplinary treatment group prior to definitive treatment planning. Laparoscopic ultrasound (LUS) and "extended laparoscopy" are techniques that may increase the diagnostic yield of laparoscopy. Preliminary results reveal conflicting data on the added benefit of LUS and extended laparoscopy.[140–142] Further prospective studies will be required to evaluate the cost-benefit relationship of LUS and extended laparoscopy in the routine or selective workup of patients with gastric cancer.

Although laparoscopic staging is thought to detect CT-occult metastatic disease in approximately 40% of patients and spares nontherapeutic operations in approximately one-third of gastric cancer patients, one needs to remember that tumor biology, not staging, will eventually guide outcomes. Clearly, not all patients benefit from preoperative laparoscopic staging; therefore, future studies should address the issue of selective laparoscopy based on noninvasive staging (i.e., patients with T1 tumors). Staging laparoscopy with or without cytology should be considered only if therapy will be altered consequent to information obtained by laparoscopy.[128]

STAGING, CLASSIFICATION, AND PROGNOSIS

For patients with surgically treated gastric adenocarcinoma, both pathologic staging (American Joint Committee on Cancer/International Union Against Cancer [AJCC/UICC] or Japanese system) and classification of the completeness of resection (R classification) should be done. Although not formal components of the stage grouping, the AJCC recommends collection of additional prognostic factors: tumor location, serum CEA and CA 19.9, histopathologic grade and type.[143]

AJCC/UICC Tumor, Node, Metastasis Staging

The AJCC/UICC TNM staging system for gastric cancer is outlined in Table 80.2.[143] The AJCC/UICC stage-stratified survival rates of 10,601 patients treated by surgical resection from SEER 1973–2005 public-use file diagnosed in years 1991–2000 are shown in Figure 80.2.

Several definitions in the most recent version of the AJCC (2010) differ from the previous version (2002). Tumors arising at the esophagogastric junction (EGJ) including Siewert type I or arising in the stomach 5 cm or less from the EGJ and crossing into the EJG including Siewert types II and III are staged using the TNM system for esophageal adenocarcinoma. Gastric tumors lying 5 cm or less from the EGJ but do not cross the EGJ into the esophagus are staged as gastric cancer.[143]

In the AJCC/UICC staging system, tumor (T) stage is determined by depth of tumor invasion into the gastric wall and extension into adjacent structures (Fig. 80.3). The relationship between T stage, the overall stage, and survival is well defined (Fig. 80.2). Nodal stage (N) is based on the number of involved lymph nodes, a criterion that may predict outcome more accurately than the location of involved lymph nodes.[144,145] Tumors with one to two involved nodes are classified as pN1, three to six involved nodes are classified as pN2, and those with more than seven involved nodes are classified as pN3 (N3a has 7–15 nodes and N3b has ≥16 nodes). The use of numerical thresholds for nodal classification has become increasingly more accepted, although the extent of lymphadenectomy and rigor of pathologic assessment may affect results.[146,147] The threshold approach is based on observations that survival decreases as the number of metastatic lymph nodes increases,[148,149] and that there are decreases in survival at three or more involved[148] lymph nodes and again at seven or more involved lymph nodes.[77,150]

Given the reliance on numerical thresholds for nodal staging, it is extremely important that adequate numbers of lymph

TABLE 80.2

AMERICAN JOINT COMMITTEE ON CANCER STAGING OF GASTRIC CANCER, 2010—DEFINITION OF TUMOR, NODES, METASTASIS

PRIMARY TUMOR (T)			
TX	Primary tumor cannot be assessed		
T0	No evidence of primary tumor		
Tis	Carcinoma *in situ*: intraepithelial tumor without invasion of the lamina propria		
T1	Tumor invades lamina propria, muscularis mucosae or submucosa		
T1a	Tumor invades lamina propria or muscularis mucosae		
T1b	Tumor invades submucosa		
T2	Tumor invades muscularis propria		
T3	Tumor penetrates subserosal connective tissue without invasion of visceral peritoneum or adjacent structures		
T4	Tumor invades serosa (visceral peritoneum) or adjacent structures		
T4a	Tumor invades serosa (visceral peritoneum)		
T4b	Tumor invades adjacent structures		
REGIONAL LYMPH NODES (N)			
NX	Regional lymph node(s) cannot be assessed		
N0	No regional lymph node metastasis		
N1	Metastasis in 1 to 2 regional lymph nodes		
N2	Metastasis in 3 to 6 regional lymph nodes		
N3	Metastases in more than 7 regional lymph nodes		
N3a	Metastasis in 7–15 regional nodes		
N3b	Metastasis in 16 or more regional nodes		
DISTANT METASTASIS (M)			
MX	Presence of distant metastasis cannot be assessed		
M0	No distant metastasis		
M1	Distant metastasis		
STAGE GROUPING			
O	Tis	N0	M0
IA	T1	N0	M0
IB	T2	N0	M0
	T1	N1	M0
IIA	T3	N0	M0
	T2	N1	M0
	T1	N2	M0
IIB	T4a	N0	M0
	T3	N1	M0
	T2	N2	M0
	T1	N3	M0
IIIA	T4a	N1	M0
	T3	N2	M0
	T2	N3	M0
IIIB	T4b	N0	M0
	T4b	N1	M0
	T4a	N2	M0
	T3	N3	M0
IIIC	T4b	N2	M0
	T4b	N3	M0
	T4a	N3	M0
IV	Any T	Any N	M1

From ref. 230, with permission.

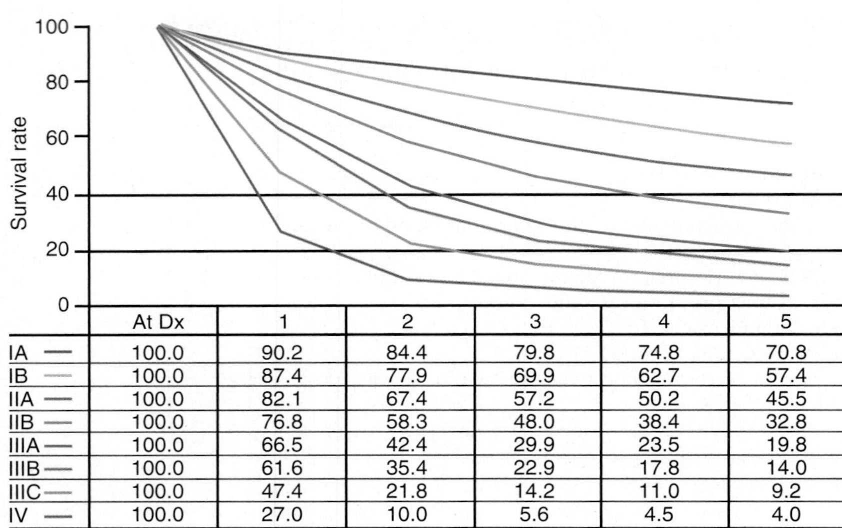

	At Dx	1	2	3	4	5
IA	100.0	90.2	84.4	79.8	74.8	70.8
IB	100.0	87.4	77.9	69.9	62.7	57.4
IIA	100.0	82.1	67.4	57.2	50.2	45.5
IIB	100.0	76.8	58.3	48.0	38.4	32.8
IIIA	100.0	66.5	42.4	29.9	23.5	19.8
IIIB	100.0	61.6	35.4	22.9	17.8	14.0
IIIC	100.0	47.4	21.8	14.2	11.0	9.2
IV	100.0	27.0	10.0	5.6	4.5	4.0

FIGURE 80.2 Disease-specific survival by American Joint Committee on Cancer stage grouping. Numbers beneath x-axis indicate patients at risk. (From ref. 230, with permission.)

nodes are retrieved and examined. However, recent reports document poor compliance with AJCC staging primarily because the number of lymph nodes removed and/or examined (15 or less) was insufficient.[149,151] Positive peritoneal cytology is classified as M1. Ratio-based lymph node classification is an alternative to the threshold-based system currently used for AJCC/UICC staging. It may minimize the confounding effects of regional variations in the extent of lymphadenectomy and pathologic evaluation on lymph node staging and thereby reduce stage migration.[152–154] Sun et al.[153] evaluated the ratio of metastatic to uninvolved lymph nodes (RML) in a group of 2,159 patients who underwent curative gastrectomy. The anatomic location, number of positive lymph nodes (AJCC/UICC), and RML were analyzed for staging accuracy and relationship to survival. RML was an independent prognostic factor for survival and reduced stage migration. These findings were confirmed by several investigators reporting on approximately 2,000 patients treated by R0 gastrectomy.[152,154–157]

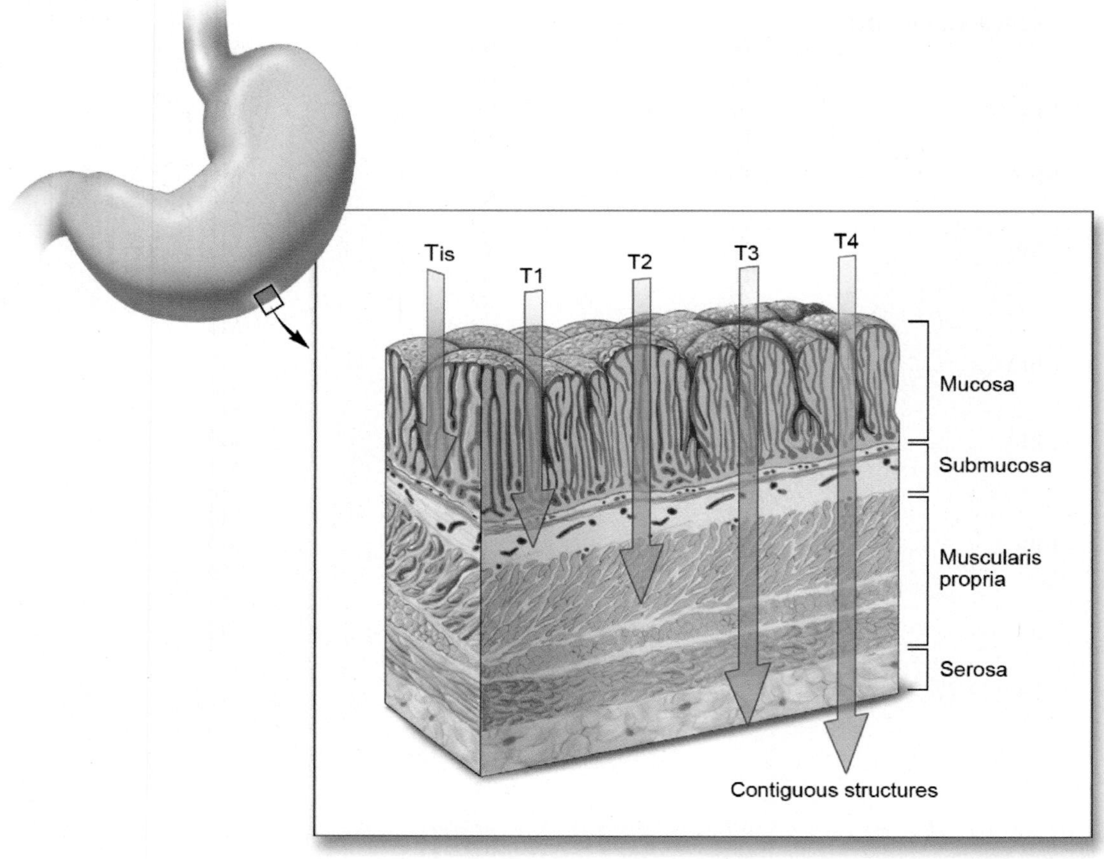

FIGURE 80.3 Definition of American Joint Committee on Cancer/International Union Against Cancer T stage based on depth of penetration of the gastric wall.

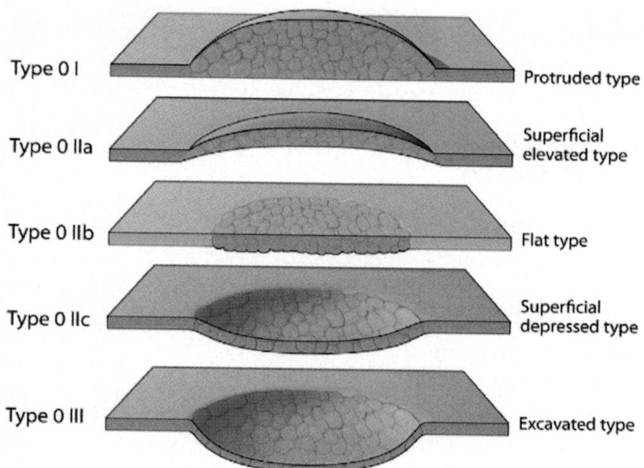

FIGURE 80.4 Japanese classification system for early gastric cancer. In the combined superficial types, the type occupying the largest area should be described first, followed by the next type (e.g., IIc + III). Type 0I and type 0IIa are distinguished as follows: type 0I, the lesion has a thickness of more than twice that of the normal mucosa; type 0IIa, the lesion has a thickness up to twice that of the normal mucosa.

Japanese Staging System

The most recent *Japanese Classification for Gastric Carcinoma* was published in 1998.[158–161] The Japanese classification and staging system is more detailed than the AJCC/UICC staging system and places more emphasis on the distinction between clinical, surgical, pathologic, and "final" staging (prefixes "c," "s," "p," and "f," respectively). For example, a surgically treated and staged patient with locally advanced, nonmetastatic gastric cancer might be staged as pT3, pN2, sH0, sM0, stage f-IIIB (where H0 denotes no hepatic metastases and the "f" prefix denotes final clinicopathologic stage). The Japanese classification system also includes a classification system for early gastric cancer (Fig. 80.4).

Similar to the AJCC/UICC staging system, primary tumor (T) stage in the Japanese system is based on the depth of invasion and extension to adjacent structures, as outlined in Table 80.3.[162] However, the assignment of lymph node (N) stage involves much more rigorous pathologic assessment than is required for AJCC/UICC staging. The Japanese system extensively classifies 18 lymph node regions into four N categories (N0 to N3) depending on their relationship to the primary tumor and anatomic location.[163] Most perigastric lymph nodes (nodal stations 1 through 6) are considered group N1. Lymph nodes situated along the proximal left gastric artery (station 7), common hepatic artery (8), celiac axis (9), splenic artery (11), and proper hepatic artery (12) are defined as group N2. Para-aortic lymph nodes (16) are defined as group N3. However, some lymph nodes, even perigastric nodes for specific tumor locations, can be regarded as M1 disease (i.e., involvement of station no. 2 in the case of antral tumors). This is because their involvement in antral tumors is rare and portrays a bad prognosis.[162]

The Japanese staging system also includes elements not included in the AJCC/UICC system (Table 80.3). These are macroscopic description of the tumor (early gastric cancer subtype or Borrmann type for more advanced tumors), extent of peritoneal metastases (classified as P0-1), extent of hepatic metastases (H0-1), and peritoneal cytology findings (CY0-1). Recent comparison of the Japanese and AJCC/UICC staging systems in 731 patients suggests that both are comparable.[164] However, older studies suggest that the AJCC/UICC system more accurately estimates prognosis.[146]

Classification of Esophagogastric Junction Cancers

EGJ cancers (i.e., tumors with a definitive component involving the EGJ) are no longer classified by the AJCC as gastric cancers per se. They are briefly reviewed here for historical reasons. Siewert and Stein[165] classified adenocarcinomas of the EGJ (Siewert classification) into three distinct clinical entities that arise within 5 cm of the EGJ: type 1 arises in the distal esophagus and may infiltrate the EGJ from above; type II arises in the cardia or the EGJ; and type III arises in the subcardial stomach and may infiltrate the EGJ from below. The assignment of tumors to one of these subtypes is based on morphology and the anatomic location of the epicenter of the tumor. The Siewert classification has important therapeutic implications.[166] The lymphatic drainage routes differ for type I versus types II and III lesions. The lymphatic pathways from the lower esophagus pass both cephalad and caudad. In contrast, the lymphatic drainage from the cardia and subcardial regions is caudad. Thus, the Siewert classification provides a practical means for choosing among surgical options. For type I tumors, esophagectomy is required, whereas types II and III tumors can be treated by transabdominal gastrectomy.[166,167]

Resection Classification

The R classification system indicates the amount of residual disease left after tumor resection.[168] R0 indicates no gross or microscopic residual disease; R1 indicates microscopic residual disease (positive margins); and R2 signifies gross residual disease. The R classification has implications for individual patient care and clinical research. Results of clinical trials that include surgery should include information on R status. Readers should be aware of the dual use of the "R" terminology in the gastric cancer literature. Prior to 1995, the Japanese staging and treatment vernacular included an "R level," which described the extent of lymphadenectomy. The latter is now classified by "D" (for dissection) level.

GASTRIC CANCER NOMOGRAMS: PREDICTING INDIVIDUAL PATIENT PROGNOSIS AFTER POTENTIALLY CURATIVE RESECTION

Kattan et al.[148] have developed a nomogram for predicting individual patient 5-year disease-specific survival using established prognostic factors derived from a population of 1,039 gastric cancer patients treated by R0 surgical resection without neoadjuvant therapy at a single institution (nomograms@mskcc.org). Clinicopathologic factors incorporated in the nomogram include age and gender, primary tumor site, Laurén classification, numbers of positive and negative lymph nodes resected, and depth of invasion. This nomogram was subsequently validated by several authors. Peeters et al.[169] found that the nomogram prognosticates better then the AJCC staging system. Novotny et al.[170] validated the nomogram in 862 patients from Germany and the Netherlands; Strong et al.[171] compared outcomes using the nomogram in 711 patients from the United

TABLE 80.3

JAPANESE GASTRIC CANCER ASSOCIATION STAGING SYSTEM FOR GASTRIC CANCER

TUMOR STAGE	
T1	Tumor invasion of mucosa and/or muscularis mucosa (M) or submucosa (SM)
T2	Tumor invasion of muscularis propria (MP) or subserosa (SS)
T3	Tumor penetration of serosal (SE)
T4	Tumor invasion of adjacent structures (SI)
TX	Unknown
NODAL STAGE	
N0	No evidence of lymph node metastasis
N1	Metastasis to group 1 lymph nodes, but no metastasis to groups 2 to 3 lymph nodes
N2	Metastasis to group 2 lymph nodes, but no metastasis to group 3 lymph nodes
N3	Metastasis to group 3 lymph nodes
NX	Unknown
HEPATIC METASTASIS STAGE (H)	
H0	No liver metastasis
H1	Liver metastasis
HX	Unknown
PERITONEAL METASTASIS STAGE (P)	
P0	No peritoneal metastasis
P1	Peritoneal metastasis
PX	Unknown
PERITONEAL CYTOLOGY STAGE (CY)	
CY0	Benign/indeterminate cells on peritoneal cytology[a]
CY1	Cancer cells on peritoneal cytology
CYX	Peritoneal cytology was not performed
OTHER DISTANT METASTASIS (M)	
M0	No other distant metastases (although peritoneal, liver, or cytological metastases may be present)
M1	Distant metastases other than the peritoneal, liver, or cytological metastases
MX	Unknown

STAGE GROUPING

	N0	N1	N2	N3	
T1	IA	IB	II		
T2	IB	II	IIIA		
T3	II	IIIA	IIIB		IV
T4	IIIA	IIIB			
H1, P1, CY1, M1					

[a]Cytology believed to be "suspicious for malignancy" should be classified as CY0.
(Adapted from ref. 460.)

States and 1,646 patients from Korea. This tool may be useful for individual patient counseling regarding the use of adjuvant therapy, follow-up scheduling, and clinical trial eligibility assessment and is available for personal hand-held computer devices at www.nomograms.org.

TREATMENT OF LOCALIZED DISEASE

Stage I Disease (Early Gastric Cancer)

Classification of Early Gastric Cancer and Risk for Nodal Metastases

The Japanese Research Society for Gastric Cancer has classified early gastric cancers (EGCs) based on endoscopic criteria first established for the description of T1 tumors. The current classification system is used for both *in situ* and invasive tumors and categorizes tumors based on endoscopic findings as follows: protruded, type 0I; superficial elevated, type 0IIa; flat, type 0IIb; superficial depressed, type 0IIc; and excavated, type 0III (Figure 80.4). The English-language version of the Japanese EGC classification contains excellent color photos of these subtypes.[172] This classification system is important in describing patients treated by newer gastric-sparing approaches for EGC, such as endoscopic mucosal resection (EMR).[159–161,173] The risk for lymph node metastasis is important when evaluating treatment options for patients with EGC. The frequency and anatomic distribution of nodal disease are related to the depth of tumor invasion. In a Japanese series of more than 5,000 patients who underwent gastrectomy with lymph node dissection for EGC, none of the 1,230 patients with well-differentiated intramucosal tumors less than 3 cm in diameter (regardless of ulceration) had lymph node metastases.[174] None of the 929 patients with EGC without ulceration had nodal metastases irrespective of tumor size. In contrast, in the subset of more than 2,000 patients with tumors that invaded the submucosa, the frequencies of lymph node involvement for tumors equal to or less than 1.0 cm, 1.1 to 2.0 cm, 2.1 to 3.0 cm, and greater than 3.0 cm were 7.9%, 13.3%, 15.55%, and 23.3%, respectively. Thus, once tumors penetrate into the submucosa, the risk for nodal metastasis increases with tumor size.[175–181] The estimates of the frequency of nodal disease in EGC are based on conventional light-microscopic histologic assessment. However, the use of more sensitive techniques such as serial sectioning of individual lymph nodes, immunohistochemistry, or reverse transcriptase-polymerase chain reaction may increase the frequency of detection of occult micrometastatic disease.[182] The clinical significance of micrometastases is unknown.

Endoscopic Mucosal Resection

A subset of patients with EGC can undergo an R0 resection without lymphadenectomy or gastrectomy. The Japanese have popularized EMR for EGC. This approach involves the submucosal injection of fluid to elevate the lesion and facilitate complete mucosal resection under endoscopic guidance. Most centers reporting significant experience with EMR are in Japan. There is less experience with EMR in Western countries. Only patients with tumors that have extremely low metastatic potential should be offered EMR. These are generally well-differentiated, superficial type IIa or IIc lesions smaller than 3 cm in diameter and located in an easily manipulated area. Tumors invading the submucosa are at increased risk for metastasizing to lymph nodes and are not usually considered candidates for EMR.

Recently, Bennett et al.[183] reviewed the available data reporting on EMR for EGC. No randomized controlled trial (RCT) reported on EMR. The indication for EMR are well-differentiated lesions, size 20 mm or less in elevated type, 10 mm or less in depressed type, no ulceration, and limited to the mucosa.[184] The incidence of lymph node metastases for such lesions is approximately 1.0%. Complete resection of selected EGCs can be accomplished in a majority of cases (73.4%–98%).[183,185,186]

Two retrospective reports indicated that EMR can reduce the risk of local residual tumor and repeat EMR is an effective option.[187,188] Recurrence after EMR varies with type. Ida et al.[189] reported on 412 patients; 8 of 199 (4.0%) had recurrence of lesions size 20 to 40 mm; five patients were retreated by EMR and three underwent open surgery; and none had lymph node metastases. Patients (0/305) with lesions 20 mm or less did not have recurrence. Complication rate associated with EMR is low. Bleeding and perforation are reported in 0% to 20.5% and 0% to 5.2 % of patients.[185,190–193] The reported complication and mortality rates in patients undergoing open surgery (n = 256) versus EMR (n = 56) were 0.8% and 7.8% versus 0% and 16%.[183,194]

Fukase et al.[195,196] reported on the long-term outcomes of patients undergoing open surgery (n = 116) versus EMR (n = 59). For patients age 65 year or under, the 5- and 10-year survival rates were 100% and 91.7% versus 92.8% and 92.8%, respectively. For patients older than 65 years of age, the 5- and 10-year survival rates were 100% and 75% versus 80.8% and 80.8%, respectively. The differences were not statistically significant. Similar results were reported by Park et al.[197] and Kim et al.[198]

There are emerging variations of EMR techniques, including the cap suction and cut versus a ligating device. As outcome studies accumulate demonstrating favorable survival, EMR is emerging as the definitive management of selected EGCs and is not just reserved for patients in whom gastrectomy cannot be considered. However, RCTs are needed to establish an outcome advantage over open surgery.[184,199–209]

Limited Surgical Resection

Given the low rate of nodal involvement for patients with EGC, limited resection may be a reasonable alternative to gastrectomy for some patients. There are no well-accepted pretreatment criteria for selection of patients for limited resection. Based on available pathology studies, patients with small (<3 cm) intramucosal tumors and those with nonulcerated intramucosal tumors of any size may be candidates for EMR or limited resection. Surgical options for these patients may include gastrotomy with local excision. This procedure should be performed with full-thickness mural excision (to allow accurate pathologic assessment of T status) and is often aided by intraoperative gastroscopy for tumor localization. Formal lymph node dissection is not required in these patients.

Gastrectomy

Gastrectomy with lymph node dissection should be considered for patients with EGC who cannot be treated with EMR or limited surgical resection and/or patients who have intramucosal tumors with poor histologic differentiation or size greater than 3 cm or who have tumor penetration into the submucosa or beyond. Gastrectomy with lymph node dissection allows for adequate pathologic staging and local therapy for these patients at higher risk. Dissection of level I lymph nodes is a reasonable minimum standard at this time. The roles for nodal "sampling" without formal node dissection (D0 dissection) and sentinel lymph node biopsy in the treatment of EGC remain undefined at this time.

Stage II and Stage III Disease

Surgery

Surgical resection is the cornerstone treatment for patients with localized gastric cancer. However, for stages II and III disease, surgery is necessary but often not sufficient for cure. The general therapeutic goal is to achieve a microscopically complete resection (R0). A complete discussion of all the technical details of gastric resection and reconstruction is beyond the scope of this chapter. However, specific surgical issues of oncologic significance are addressed here, including the extent of gastrectomy, extent of lymph node dissection, and role of partial pancreatectomy and splenectomy. Additional technical details can be found in surgical atlases and the section "Technical Treatment-Related Issues."

Extent of Resection for Mid- and Distal Gastric Cancers. The extent of gastrectomy required for satisfactory primary tumor treatment depends mostly on the gross and microscopic status of surgical margins. For most clinical situations, a 5-cm grossly negative margin around the tumor and microscopically negative surgical margins (R0) are the treatment goals. When gastrectomy is performed with curative intent, frozen-section assessment of proximal and distal resection margins should be used intraoperatively to improve the likelihood that an R0 resection has been performed. Three relatively small prospective RCTs have compared total gastrectomy with partial (subtotal) gastrectomy for distal gastric cancer.[210–212] Overall morbidity, mortality, and oncologic outcome were comparable in each of these RCTs. When the general oncologic goal of an R0 resection can be achieved by a gastric-preserving approach, partial gastrectomy is preferred over total gastrectomy. This is particularly relevant for distal gastric cancers, for which a gastric-preserving R0 approach may minimize the risks of specific sequelae of total gastrectomy such as early satiety, weight loss, and the need for vitamin B_{12} supplementation.

Extent of Resection for Proximal Gastric Cancer. There are many choices for surgical management of adenocarcinomas arising at the EGJ or in the proximal stomach (Siewert types II and III). Many abdominal surgeons have advocated transabdominal approaches with resection of the lower esophagus and proximal stomach or total gastrectomy. Surgeons trained in thoracic surgery have frequently advocated a combined abdominal and thoracic procedure (often termed *esophagogastrectomy*) with an intrathoracic or cervical anastomosis between the proximal esophagus and the distal stomach, or a procedure termed *transhiatal (or blunt) esophagectomy* (THE), which involves resection of the esophagus and EGJ with mediastinal dissection performed in a blunt fashion through the esophageal hiatus of the diaphragm. When THE is performed for adenocarcinoma of the EGJ, gastrointestinal continuity is restored by low cervical anastomosis of the stomach (usually advanced through the esophageal bed in the mediastinum) to the low cervical esophagus. Selection among the options has been dependent primarily on individual surgeon training and experience.

The optimal surgical procedure for patients with localized tumors of the EGJ and proximal stomach is a matter of considerable debate. A recently completed Dutch RCT compared transthoracic esophagogastrectomy (TTEG, with abdominal and thoracic incisions) with THE in 220 patients with adenocarcinoma of the esophagus and EGJ.[213] Although this trial was designed for patients with esophageal cancer, 40 (18%) of the patients had adenocarcinomas of the EGJ (Siewert type II), and the operations evaluated are among those considered for patients with Siewert type II or III cancers. Perioperative morbidity was higher after THE, but there was no significant difference in in-hospital mortality compared with TTEG. Although median overall, disease-free, and quality-adjusted survival did not differ significantly between the groups, there was a trend toward improved overall survival at 5 years with TTEG. These results are judged equivocal and there is currently no consensus on the optimal surgical approach for patients with Siewert type II tumors.[214] Until longer follow-up of the Dutch trial is available and/or additional RCTs are performed, the surgical approach to these patients will continue to be individualized and determined by a constellation of factors including surgeon factors (training and experience), patient factors (age, comorbidity, and performance status), and tumor factors (pretreatment T and N stage).

Extent of Lymphadenectomy. There has been intense debate surrounding the extent of lymphadenectomy. It involves at least two important issues: (1) adequate staging in terms of the number of lymph nodes resected and examined, and (2) adequate therapy (i.e., do some forms of lymphadenectomy result in better outcomes?).[215–226]

Single-institution reports suggest that the number of pathologically positive lymph nodes is of prognostic significance,[145,147,224,227–229] and that removal and pathologic analysis of at least 15 lymph nodes is required for adequate pathologic staging.[144,230] Indeed, the current AJCC staging system accounts for these issues and therefore requires analysis of 16 or more lymph nodes to assign a pathologic N stage.[231] The possible therapeutic benefit of extended lymph node dissection D2 versus D1 dissection has been the focus of six RCTs, which are summarized in Table 80.4.[211,232–236] These trials were performed because retrospective and prospective nonrandomized evidence suggested that extended lymph node dissection may be associated with improved long-term survival.[237] The RCTs tested the hypothesis that removal of additional pathologically positive lymph nodes (not generally removed as part of a standard lymph node dissection) improves survival. The larger RCTs attempted to follow what are referred to as the "Japanese rules" for lymph node classification and dissection that govern the extent of nodal dissection required based on anatomic location of the primary tumor.[238] Using these Japanese definitions, the RCTs compared limited lymphadenectomy of the perigastric lymph nodes (D1 dissection) to *en bloc* removal of second-echelon lymph nodes (D2 dissection). At least two of the completed trials are underpowered for their primary end point, overall survival.[211,232] The trials from the Medical Research Council (MRC) of the United Kingdom[233] and the Dutch Gastric Cancer Group-234 have received the most attention and discussion.

The MRC trial registered 737 patients with gastric adenocarcinoma; 337 (46%) patients were ineligible by staging laparotomy because of advanced disease, and 400 (54%) patients were randomized at the time of laparotomy to undergo D1 (200) or D2 (200) lymph node dissections. Postoperative morbidity was significantly greater in the D2 group (46% vs. 28%; $P < .001$), and in-hospital mortality rates were significantly higher in the D2 group than in the D1 group (13% vs. 6%, $P < .04$).[233] The most frequent postoperative complications were related to anastomotic leakage (D2 26% vs. D1 11%), cardiac complications (8% vs. 2%), and respiratory complications (8% vs. 5%). The excess morbidity and mortality seen in the D2 group were thought to be related to the routine use of distal (left) pancreatectomy and splenectomy. Partial pancreatectomy and splenectomy were performed to maximize clearance of lymph nodes at the splenic hilum, primarily for patients with proximal tumors; however, many surgeons now believe that adequate lymph node dissection can be performed with pancreas-and-spleen–preserving techniques. Long-term follow-up analysis of patients in the MRC trial demonstrated comparable 5-year overall survival rates of 35% and 33% in the D1 and D2 dissection groups, respectively. Survival based on death from gastric cancer as the event was also similar in the D1 and D2 groups (HR, 1.05; 95% CI, 0.79 to 1.39), as was recurrence-free survival (HR, 1.03; 95% CI, 0.82 to 1.29). The authors concluded that classic Japanese-style D2 lymphadenectomy (with partial pancreatectomy and splenectomy) offered no survival advantage over D1 lymphadenectomy.

The Dutch Gastric Cancer Group conducted a larger RCT with optimal surgical quality control comparing D1 to D2 lymph node dissection for patients with gastric adenocarcinoma that was updated in 2010 after 15-year follow-up.[239] Between 1989 and July 1993, 1,078 patients were entered, of whom 996 patients were eligible; 711 patients were randomized to D1 dissection (n = 380) or D2 dissection (n = 331). To maximize surgical quality control, all operations were monitored.[240] Initially, this oversight was done by a Japanese surgeon who trained a group of Dutch surgeons who in turn acted as supervisors during surgery at 80 participating centers. Notwithstanding the extraordinary efforts to ensure quality control of the two types of lymph node dissection, both noncompliance (not removing all lymph node stations) and contamination (removing more than was indicated) occurred, thus blurring the distinction between the two operations and confounding the interpretation of the oncologic end points.[239,241] The postoperative morbidity rate was higher in the D2 group (43% vs. 25%; $P < .001$), reoperation rate 18% (59/331) versus 8% (30/380), and the mortality rate was also significantly higher in the D2 group (10% vs. 4%; $P = .004$). Patients treated with D2 dissection also required a longer hospitalization.[242] As in the MRC trial, partial pancreatectomy and splenectomy were performed *en passant* in the D2 group. Five-year survival rates were similar in the two groups: 45% for the D1 group and 47% for the D2 group (95% CI for the difference, −9.6% to 5.6%). The subset of patients who had R0 resections, excluding those who died postoperatively, had cumulative risks of relapse at 5 years of 43% with D1 dissection and 37% with D2 dissection (95% CI for the difference, −2.4% to 14.4%).

The Dutch investigators concluded that there was no role for the routine use of D2 lymph node dissection in patients with gastric cancer. At 15-year follow-up, 174/711 (25%)

TABLE 80.4

PROSPECTIVE RANDOMIZED TRIALS COMPARING D1 VERSUS D2–3 RESECTION FOR POTENTIALLY CURABLE GASTRIC CARCINOMA

Study (Ref.)	Extent of Lymphadenectomy		
	D1	D2	*P* Value
Groote Schuur Hospital, Cape Town, 1988 (232)			
Number of patients	22	21	—
Length of operation (h)	1.7 ± 0.6	2.33 ± 0.7	<.005
Transfusions (units/group)	4	25	<.05
Postoperative stay (d)	9.3 ± 4.7	13.9 ± 9.7	<.05
5-y overall survival (log rank test)	0.69	0.67	NS
Prince of Wales Hospital, Hong Kong, 1994 (211)			
Number of patients	25	29	—
Length of operation (h)	140	260	<.05
Operative blood loss (mL)	300	600	<.05
Postoperative stay	8	16	<.05
Median survival (d)	1,511	922	<.05
Medical Research Council Trial, United Kingdom, 1999 (233, 461)			
Number of patients	200	200	—
Operative mortality (%)	6.5	13	<.04
Postoperative complications (%)	28	46	<.001
5-y overall survival (%)	35	33	NS
Dutch Gastric Cancer Trial, The Netherlands, 1999 (2009, 15-year follow-up update) (234, 239)			
Number of patients	380	331	—
Operative mortality rate (%)	4	10	.004
Postoperative complications (%)	25	43	<.001
Postoperative stay (d)	18	25	<.001
5-y overall survival (%)	45	47	NS
11-y F/U overall survival (%)	30	35	.53
11-y F/U survival (perioperative death excluded)	32	39	.10
15y F/U overall survival	21	29	.34
15y F/U gastric cancer specific death	48	37	.01
Italian Gastric Cancer Study Group (IGCSG), 2004 (235)			
Number of patients	76	86	—
Operative mortality rate (%)	1.3	0	NS
Postoperative complication (%)	10.5	16.3	.29
Postoperative stay (d)	12	12	NS
5-y overall survival	NS	NS	NS
Yang-Ming University, Taiwan, 2006 (236)			
Number of patients	110	111, D3	
Operative mortality rate (%)	0	0	
Postoperative complication (%)	10.1	17.1	.012
Postoperative stay (d)	15	19.6	.001
5-y overall survival	53.6	59.5	.041

NS, not stated; F/U, follow-up.

patients were alive, all but one without recurrence. The overall survival was 21% (82/711) and 29% (92 patients) for the D1 and D2 groups, respectively (P = .34). Interestingly, gastric cancer-specific death was higher in the D1 group 48% (182/380) versus 37% (123/331). Local recurrence was higher in the D1 group 22% (82/380) versus 12% (40/331), and regional recurrence 19% (73/380) versus 13% (43/331). The authors concluded that after 15 years of follow-up, D2 lymphadenectomy is associated with lower locoregional recurrence and gastric cancer-specific death rates than D1 lymphadenectomy. D2 resection is also associated with higher postoperative mortality, morbidity, and reoperation rates. Examining the results after 15-year follow-up and given the data regarding gastric cancer-specific mortality, local recurrence and regional recurrence, the authors revised their original conclusion: "Because spleen-preserving D2 resection is safer in high-volume centers, it is the recommended surgical approach for patients with potentially curable gastric cancer."[239]

Degiuli et al.[235] reported on the Italian Gastric Cancer Study Group (IGCSG) experience with a prospective randomized trial comparing pancreas-sparing D1 versus D2. There were 76 patients randomized to undergo D1 and 86 D2 resections. Complications rates were higher in the D2 group, 16.3% versus 10.5%. Postoperative mortality was higher in the D1 group, 1.3% versus 0%. Thus far, no survival data are available. The authors concluded that, in experienced hands, the morbidity and mortality can be as low as shown by Japanese surgeons.

Wu et al.[236] reported on a randomized trial comparing D1 versus D3 dissections.[242] There were no operative deaths and morbidity was only 12%. At median follow-up of 94.5 months, D3 showed better overall 5 = year survival 59.5% (95% CI, 50.3 to 68.7) versus 53.6% (95% CI, 44.2 to 63.0; *P* = .041), and a trend toward better disease-free survival at 5 years 40.3 % versus 50.6% (*P* = .197). Only 13% had pancreas or splenic resection as compared with 23% in the Dutch trial. The authors concluded that D3 as compared to D1 offers survival benefit. As far as the authors of this chapter understand, this is the first RCT to demonstrate survival advantage for more extensive lymphadenectomy (D3). As such, it requires a careful examination. Roggin and Posner[244] have critically reviewed the work by Wu et al. One controversial element of this trial was the use of overall survival versus gastric cancer-specific survival; 17/111 (15%) of the reported deaths were not related to tumor recurrence, resulting in very small survival benefit.

Interpretation of the existing level 1 evidence is encumbered by a number of issues that have been discussed in detail elsewhere.[215,216] The primary concerns relate to whether (1) the increased operative mortality associated with protocol-mandated partial pancreatectomy and splenectomy for patients with proximal tumors undergoing D2 dissection prevented identification of a potential therapeutic impact of extended lymph node dissection, and (2) the phenomena of noncompliance and contamination led to homogenization of the operative procedures to such an extent that the fundamental hypothesis was not tested. Owing to these interpretation issues, the question of a possible therapeutic benefit of D2 dissection remains unsettled.

Many Japanese gastric surgeons have considered the caveats associated with the MRC and Dutch trials and believe that, notwithstanding inherent patient selection and stage migration biases,[215,239,241,245,246] the existing retrospective data provide sufficient proof of a clinical benefit of D2 dissection. On this basis, D2 dissection has been adopted as the standard of care for patients with localized, higher-risk gastric cancer in many centers in Japan and some specialized centers in the West.[247] The Japanese Clinical Oncology Group (JCOG-9501) has investigated an even more aggressive surgical approach in an RCT evaluating standard D2 versus D2-plus (PAND, para-aortic node dissection) in the management of completely resected (R0) T2–4 gastric cancer.[248,249] Between July 1995 and April 2001, 523 patients from 25 institutions were registered. Patients were randomized intraoperatively to undergo D2 lymphadenectomy alone (263 patients) or D2 lymphadenectomy plus PAND (260 patients). The primary end point was overall survival. Postoperative morbidity was higher in the PAND group (28% vs. 21%; *P* = .07), and mortality was similar at 0.8% in each group. Five-year overall survival for patients undergoing PAND was 70.3% versus 69.2% (HR, 1.03; *P* = .85). There was no significant difference in recurrence-free survival. The authors concluded that, as compared to D2 lymphadenectomy, PAND does not improve survival rates.

Another Japanese study compared D2 with extended PAND (D4).[250] This trial randomized patients to undergo D2 (n = 135) or D4 (n = 134). The 5-year survival rates were 52.6% versus 55%, respectively (*P* = .8). The authors concluded that prophylactic D4 dissection is not recommended. In an RCT, a Western group from Poland investigated D2 dissection versus extended D2 dissection defined according to the Japanese gastric cancer association classification.[251] They randomized 275 patients, D2 (n = 141) versus D2+ (n = 134). The overall postoperative morbidity and mortality were similar and did not differ statistically. Survival data are not available at this time.[251] Thus, the limits of radical surgery have been reached in Japan and the pendulum has swung back toward D2 dissection in clinical settings in which this can be safely performed.[245]

In summary, lymph nodes should be considered as indicators that the gate was opened rather than as the gate keepers for cure.[252] None of the prospective RCT trials executed in the West demonstrated survival advantage for more extensive lymphadenectomy. However, none of these studies were powered enough to detect single-digit difference in 5-year survival. Several non *a priori* planned subgroup analyses were done and showed some survival advantage for certain subgroups. These analyses cannot be used to form evidence-based medicine but should be used to form hypotheses for further RCT studies. In high-volume specialty centers, spleen- and pancreas-preserving D2 dissection is performed safely, and can potentially result in decreased gastric cancer-specific–related death based on 15 years of follow-up from the Dutch study (D2 37% vs. 48%; *P* = .01).[239]

Partial Pancreatectomy and Splenectomy—Resect or Preserve? Partial (left, distal) pancreatectomy and splenectomy have been performed as part of D2 lymph node dissection to remove the lymph nodes along the splenic artery (station 11) and at the splenic hilum (station 12), primarily for patients with tumors located in the proximal and midstomach. Indeed, partial pancreatectomy and splenectomy were required for patients with proximal tumors in the D2 arm of the Dutch and MRC RCTs but were required only for direct tumor extension in the D1 arm. In the Dutch and MRC D1 versus D2 trials, splenectomy is associated with an increased risk for surgical complications and postoperative death. In addition, a multivariate analysis suggested that splenectomy is associated with inferior long-term survival. The frequent performance of splenectomy (e.g., 30% of patients in the D2 arm vs. 3% in the D1 arms of the Dutch trial), with its associated adverse effects on both short- and long-term mortality, confounds the interpretation of the Dutch and MRC RCTs. Thus, the hypothesis that spleen- and pancreas-preserving D2 lymph node dissection improves survival remains unproven. There is an evolving consensus that splenectomy should be performed only in cases with intraoperative evidence of direct tumor extension into the spleen or when the primary tumor is located in the proximal stomach along the greater curvature.[253] Partial pancreatectomy should be performed only in cases of direct tumor extension to the pancreas.

Recent reports have described pancreas- and spleen-preserving forms of D2 dissection.[254–260] This organ-preserving modification of classic D2 dissection allows for dissection of some station 11 and 12 lymph nodes without the potential adverse effects of pancreatectomy and/or splenectomy. In a small single-institution RCT recently reported from Chile, Csendes et al.[261] randomized 187 patients with localized proximal gastric adenocarcinoma to treatment by total gastrectomy with D2 lymph node dissection plus splenectomy or total gastrectomy with D2 lymphadenectomy alone. Operative mortality was similar in both groups (splenectomy group, 3%; control group, 4%). However, septic complication rates were higher in the splenectomy arm than in the control arm (*P* <.04). There was no difference in 5-year overall survival rates, although it is not clear that the trial was designed with survival as the primary end point. Other investigators confirmed these findings.[262–264]

The JCOG is conducting a multi-institutional RCT (JCOG 0110-MF) comparing D2 dissection with and without splenectomy for patients with proximal gastric cancer.[265] The hypothesis to be tested is that the 5-year overall survival of patients treated by D2 dissection without splenectomy is 5% less than that of patients treated by D2 dissection with splenectomy. With a planned accrual of 500 patients, this design will provide a 70% power to reject the null hypothesis when 5-year overall survival is 3% greater following splenic preservation compared with splenectomy.[265] The results of this trial will better define the short- and long-term effects of splenectomy for patients with proximal gastric cancers.

Individualized Assessments of Lymph Node Involvement. Recent attention has focused on methods of individual assessment of risk of lymphatic spread. These techniques offer the possibility of tailoring surgical therapy for an individual patient based on clinicopathologic risk assessment of the primary tumor and/or pre- or intraoperative identification of sentinel lymph nodes (SLNs) or primary draining lymph nodes. At present, at least three approaches to individual nodal risk assessment have been evaluated: computer modeling, preoperative endoscopic injection, and sentinel lymph node biopsy.

Preoperative Computer Modeling of Individual Patient Nodal Involvement. Kampschoer et al.[266] have developed a computer program to estimate the probability of spread to specific nodal regions for an individual patient using his or her pretreatment clinicopathologic data. The program incorporated data on tumor size, depth of infiltration, location, grade, type, and macroscopic appearance of primary tumors from 2,000 patients with surgically resected gastric cancers treated at the National Cancer Center of Tokyo. The data set used for matching individual patient data is continuously updated and now includes more than 8,000 patients. This computer model has been validated in non-Japanese patients in Germany[267] and Italy.[268] In the United States, Hundahl et al.[269] retrospectively applied this computer model to evaluate the surgical treatment of patients entered into the Intergroup trial of adjuvant fluorouracil-based chemoradiation. The Kampschoer et al. program was used to estimate the likelihood of disease in undissected regional node stations, defining the sum of these estimates as the Maruyama index of unresected disease. Fifty-four percent of participating patients underwent D0 lymphadenectomy. The median index was 70 (range, 0 to 429). In contrast to D level, the Maruyama index proved to be an independent prognostic factor of survival, even with adjustment for the potentially linked variables of T stage and number of positive nodes. More recent and smaller studies confirmed these findings.[270–272]

Preoperative Endoscopic Peritumoral Injection. The hypothesis that peritumoral injection of compounds designed to optimize lymph node dissection improves lymph node clearance was addressed in a small RCT evaluating preoperative endoscopic vital staining with CH40 prior to D2 dissection. The frequency of positive lymph nodes in patients injected with CH40 before D2 dissection was greater than that observed in patients treated by D2 dissection alone.[273] This approach optimized the yield of lymph node dissection presumably by directing surgeons to include specific lymph nodes in the dissection that would have otherwise been left *in situ* and/or by directing pathologists to examine specific areas of the lymphadenectomy specimens. Further prospective studies of this approach are required to confirm the feasibility of this technique and assess its impact on intraoperative decision making regarding the extent of lymphadenectomy.

Sentinel Lymph Node Biopsy. The goal of SLN biopsy is to identify the node or nodes believed to be the first peritumoral lymph nodes in the orderly spread of gastric adenocarcinoma from the primary site to the regional lymph nodes. Sampling of this lymph node may allow for prediction of the nodal status of the entire lymph node basin, possibly obviating node dissection and its attendant morbidity in patients found to have a negative SLN. Recent pilot studies have evaluated the feasibility, sensitivity, and specificity of SLN biopsy for patients with gastric cancer.[274–283] These pilot studies demonstrated that SLN identification is feasible in approximately 95% of patients. However, most patients with gastric cancer have multiple "sentinel" nodes, with mean numbers of SLNs per patient ranging from 2.6 to 6.3. The aggregate experience to date suggests that among patients with pathologically involved lymph nodes, SLN results in false-negative assessment of pathologic nodal status in 11% to 60% of patients. Thus, the preliminary data available suggest that SLN biopsy cannot reliably replace lymph node dissection as a means of accurately staging regional nodal basins.[284–288]

Volume Relationships for Gastrectomy. Recent studies have established a clear relationship between institutional gastrectomy volume and perioperative mortality rates. The recent analysis of a national database by Birkmeyer et al.[289–291] of 31,854 patients who underwent gastrectomy between 1994 and 1999 demonstrated an inverse relationship between institutional gastrectomy volume and operative mortality rates. The odds ratio for gastrectomy-related death was lowest among patients treated at the hospitals in the highest gastrectomy volume quintile (OR, 0.72; 95% CI, 0.63 to 0.83). A separate analysis evaluating surrogate end points for morbidity demonstrated that gastrectomy at high-volume centers was associated with the shortest duration of hospital stay and the lowest readmission rates.[292–295] Similar findings were noted by Hannan et al.[296] in an analysis of New York State's Department of Health's administrative database. Their analysis of 3,711 patients who underwent gastrectomy between 1994 and 1997 included adjustments for covariates such as age, demographic variables, organ metastasis, socioeconomic status, and comorbidities. Patients who had a gastrectomy at hospitals in the highest-volume quartile had an absolute risk-adjusted mortality rate that was 7.1% (P <.0001) lower than those treated at hospitals in the lowest-volume quartile, although the overall mortality rate for gastrectomy was only 6.2%.

These studies demonstrate that the risk-adjusted mortality rates for gastrectomy are significantly lower when gastrectomy is performed by high-volume providers.[297–300] It is likely that the variations in gastrectomy-related mortality rates relate in part to surgeon training and their age-volume[301–303] and experience with the procedure. Data on gastrectomy volume obtained from general surgeons undergoing recertification after a minimum of 7 years in practice demonstrate that the mean number of gastric resections performed by recertifying general surgeons in the United States is only 1.4 per year.[304,305] Thus, given the data supporting a relationship between hospital and provider volumes and the morbidity and mortality rate of gastric resection, there are reasons to consider regionalization of the surgical treatment of gastric cancers.

Outcome in Japan versus Western Countries. Stage-stratified survival rates for gastric adenocarcinoma are higher in Japan than in most Western countries. The reasons for this are complex, are incompletely understood, and cannot be fully addressed within the context of a chapter covering all aspects of gastric cancers.

Important differences in the epidemiology of gastric cancer may contribute to observed differences in outcome in Japan versus Western countries. First, the better-prognosis intestinal-type (Laurén classification)[306] tumors are seen more commonly in Japan, whereas the diffuse-type cancers (poorer prognosis) are more frequent in Western series. These regional differences in the frequencies of intestinal and diffuse cancers are believed to be related to the higher incidence of *H. pylori* infection and atrophic gastritis in Japan. Second, poorer-prognosis proximal gastric cancers are less frequent in Japan.[307–309] Indeed, the increase in proximal gastric cancers observed in the West has not been observed in Japanese populations.

Regional differences in the diagnostic criteria for EGC also may contribute to regional differences in observed outcome. In

Japan, gastric carcinoma is diagnosed based on its structural and cytologic features without consideration of invasion of the lamina propria. In contrast, Western pathologists consider invasion of the lamina propria to be an essential element of the diagnosis of carcinoma.[310–314] As a consequence, unequivocally neoplastic noninvasive lesions are classified as carcinoma in Japan but as dysplasia by Western pathologists.[310] To overcome these differences, the Padvova,[315] Vienna,[316] and Revised Vienna[316] classifications have recently been proposed. However, until there is worldwide consensus and implementation of uniform diagnostic criteria for EGC, comparative assessments of the outcome of patients with EGC treated in Japan and Western countries should acknowledge the selection bias associated with different diagnostic criteria.

Stage migration is a well-documented factor contributing to the stage-specific differences in outcome between Japanese and Western patients.[317] Stage migration arises because there is widespread use of extensive D2 or D3 lymphadenectomy combined with rigorous pathologic assessment of the lymphadenectomy specimen in Japan. More accurate stage assignment of Japanese patients leads to secondary stage migration—improvement in stage-specific survival without improvement in overall survival. The frequency and impact of stage migration were quantified by the Dutch Gastric Cancer Group in their RCT comparing D1 and D2 lymph node dissection.[234,318] Stage migration occurred in 30% of patients in the D2 group, and the stage-specific decreases in survival rates attributable to stage migration were 3% for AJCC/UICC stage I disease, 8% for stage II, 6% for stage III, and 12% for stage IIIB, with the more accurately staged D2 group having higher survival rates.[318]

In addition to regional differences in epidemiology, diagnostic criteria for EGC, and stage migration, other factors may contribute to the observed differences in stage-stratified survival. Such factors may include genetic, environmental, and biologic differences between Japanese and Western patients and tumors. These factors have been less well studied but were addressed in a comprehensive review by Davis and Sano.[319]

Minimally Invasive Surgery for Gastric Resection

The utilization of laparoscopy in gastric surgery has been increasing over the past decade. There are a plethora of non-RCTs reporting on laparoscopic distal gastrectomy, total gastrectomy, D2 dissection, and practically every open procedure has been tested using laparoscopy. We will review here the available data from RCT. There are no RCTs reporting on total gastrectomies.[320] None of the current RCTs reporting on laparoscopy in gastric cancer is of such quality and magnitude that it can be considered a "practice changing" trial. Huscher et al.[321,322] reported on the largest RCT testing laparoscopic (n = 29) versus open (n = 30) subtotal gastrectomy for distal gastric cancer. After 5 years of follow-up, overall morbidity and mortality were equivalent. Laparoscopic resection resulted in less blood loss, shorter hospital stay, longer operative time, and earlier resumption of oral intake; these were reported by other authors as well.[323,324] There was no difference in lymph nodes harvested. Overall 5-year and disease-free survival did not differ significantly. The authors concluded that laparoscopic subtotal gastrectomy is feasible and has similar short- and long-term outcomes as open surgery.

Kim et al.[325] reported on laparoscopy-assisted distal gastrectomy (LADG) versus open distal gastrectomy (ODG) for early gastric cancer. This trial was designed to test the 5-year survival in a noninferiority fashion. The interim analysis showed less blood loss (P <.001), amount of analgesic used (P <.019), hospital stay (P <.0001), lesser amount of lymph nodes harvested in the LADG arm (P <.05), and quality of life (QOL) parameters on global health (P <.0001). The authors concluded that comparison of LADG with ODG resulted in improved QOL outcomes in patients followed up to 3 months. Recently, Ohtani et al.[326] performed meta-analysis of RCT that compared LADG versus ODG for early gastric cancer. Their report confirmed the results from Kim et al.[325] and Lee and Han.[327]

Laparoscopy is another tool in the armamentarium of the surgical oncologist. The question is not whether it can be done laparoscopically, certainly it can; the question is whether it should be done. Whether the energy, time, and capital invested in developing laparoscopic surgery for gastric cancer is worth it is the question. Certainly, beyond the short term there seems to be no advantage of laparoscopic surgery in gastric cancer. In view of the reported morbidity and mortality in specialty centers, the advantage gained by laparoscopic gastric resection over the first few days underlines the question of whether we should invest more in innovative therapies to eradicate gastric cancer than the simple technical aspects of extirpative surgery.

Adjuvant Therapy

Patients with early-stage gastric cancers (e.g., AJCC stage I and some stage II patients) have a good chance of cure with surgery alone. However, the Japanese S-1 adjuvant study indicates that the prognosis for even stage II tumors can be improved with systemic chemotherapy.

Adjuvant therapy indicates a treatment after a potential curative resection. Therapy after resections that leave microscopic or gross disease are not adjuvant treatment, but rather therapy for known disease. Perioperative chemotherapy (or neoadjuvant chemotherapy) involves the use of systemic treatment before and/or after potentially curative surgery.

There are several theoretical reasons for beginning adjuvant therapy soon after operation. Studies have shown a rapid increase in cell growth of metastases after a primary tumor has been removed related to a decline in certain circulating factors, perhaps that block angiogenesis or other cell-cycle promotors, once the primary tumor is removed.

Perioperative or neoadjuvant chemotherapy has been studied because the ability to perform a R0 resection in gastric cancer is difficult. In addition, a substantial number of patients undergoing gastrectomy have a prolonged recovery. Neoadjuvant chemotherapy has a duel goal: allowing a higher rate of R0 resections and early treatment of micrometastatic disease.

Adjuvant Systemic Therapy. The results of selected recent RCT comparing adjuvant chemotherapy with surgery alone are summarized in Table 80.5. Japanese investigators studied S-1, an oral fluoropyrimidine, in a group of 1,059 patients (stages II to III B). S-1 was given for 12 months (4 weeks on/2 weeks off). Five hundred twenty-nine patients received S-1 plus operation and 530 patients underwent operation only. The 3-year overall survival was 80.1% and 70.1%, respectively (HR, 0.68).[328] In contradistinction to the positive results using S-1, and the MAGIC and ACCORD 07 trials described later, Di Costanzo et al.[329] did not find a benefit to the use of PELF (cisplatin, epirubicin, leucovorin, and fluorouracil) as adjuvant therapy.

Several meta-analyses of adjuvant chemotherapy in gastric cancer have been reported. Recently, Buyse et al.[330] reported on a meta-analysis that included individual patient data; 16 trials involving 3,710 patients were available for analysis. They found an overall survival benefit in favor of adjuvant chemotherapy (HR, 0.83; 95% CI, 0.76 to 0.91; P <.0001). The absolute benefit was 6.3% at 5 years. Shown in Table 80.5 are the results of recent trials in which adjuvant chemotherapy plus potentially curative resection was studied. The five most recent trials indicate that adjuvant therapy decreases the risk of recurrence by approximately 10%.[331] The use of systemic therapy plus

TABLE 80.5

ADJUVANT THERAPY FOR GASTRIC CANCER: PHASE 3 TRIALS

Study (Ref.)	No. of Patients	3-years DFS (%)	Overall 5-year Survival (%)	HR
S-1 (328)				
Surgery	530	60	70	
Adjuvant	529	72	80	0.38
INT-116 (366)				
Surgery	275	31	41	1.35
Adjuvant	281	48	50	
GOIRC (462)				
Surgery	128	42[a]	49	0.90
Adjuvant	130	43[a]	48	
MAGIC (356)				
Surgery	253	25	23	0.75
Neoadjuvant	250	38	36	
ACCORD-07 (350)				
Surgery	111	25	21	0.69
Neoadjuvant	113	40	34	

DFS, disease-free survival; HR, hazard ratio.
[a]Five-year DFS.

potentially curative resection is considered a standard of care for patients with locally advanced gastric cancers. The most effective regimen to use, whether or not it is best to give therapy perioperatively, and the role of postoperative radiation plus systemic therapy are the focus of ongoing clinical research trials.

Adjuvant Intraperitoneal Chemotherapy. Peritoneal recurrence is a common failure pattern for patients with gastric cancer even after curative resection.[78,332] The median survival time of patients with peritoneal recurrence is 3 to 6 months. The rationale is based on the observation that drug concentrations within the peritoneal cavity are much higher than those achievable intravenously or orally. The data are a mixture of retrospective reviews, pilot phase 2 trials, and several small phase 3 trials. No definitive conclusions can yet be drawn regarding the effectiveness of intraperitoneal postoperative chemotherapy in this setting.

There are several modes of administering intraperitoneal chemotherapy: hyperthermic intraoperative peritoneal chemotherapy (HIPEC), normothermic intraoperative chemotherapy (NIIC) given at the conclusion of the operation, early postoperative intraperitoneal chemotherapy (EPIC), or delayed postoperative intraperitoneal chemotherapy (DPIC). The theoretical advantage of intraoperative treatment is better drug distribution and the ability to use hyperthermia (HIPEC). Most trials in gastric cancer have used either fluorouracil or floxuridine, mitomycin C, or cisplatin.[333–342] Yan et al.[343] performed a meta-analysis of the randomized controlled trials reporting on adjuvant intraperitoneal chemotherapy for patients undergoing curative gastric resection; 10 trials involving 1,474 patients were included. A total of 775 patients had a resection alone and 873 patients had a resection plus intraperitoneal treatment. A significant improvement in survival was associated with HIPEC (HR, 0.6; 95% CI, 0.43 to 0.83; P = .002) or HIPEC plus EPIC (HR, 0.45; 95% CI, 0.29 to 0.68; P = .0002). There was only a trend toward survival benefit with NIIC (P = .06) but this was not significant with either EPIC alone or DPIC. The authors concluded that HIPEC with or without EPIC after curative resection is associated with modest improvement in survival and increased complication rate.

Recently, Kang et al.[344] reported on 640 serosal-positive gastric cancer patients who underwent resection and randomized to receive intraperitoneal cisplatin and early mitomycin-C plus long-term doxifluridine and cisplatin versus mitomycin-C plus short-term doxifluridine. Results indicated potential improvement in progression-free survival (PFS) and overall survival for the intraperitoneal therapy arm. Kuramoto et al.[345] reported in a retrospective fashion that extensive intraperitoneal lavage performed with 10 L of normal saline after curative resection and before NIIC is superior to surgery alone or to surgery plus NIIC.

Immunochemotherapy

The use of adjuvant immunostimulants given in association with cytotoxic chemotherapy has been studied primarily in Asia. The detailed results of these trials have been discussed in the previous edition of this textbook. Although the data available suggest that immunochemotherapy may be valuable, larger and well-powered studies are necessary to evaluate this approach.

Perioperative and Neoadjuvant Chemotherapy. Perioperative (pre- and postoperative) or neoadjuvant chemotherapy is an attractive concept in gastric cancer because many patients have locally advanced tumors at diagnosis. There are two goals of perioperative treatment: to increase the likelihood of an R0 resection, and treat micrometastatic disease early. After gastric resection many patients have a prolonged recovery, delaying initiation of adjuvant therapy. Phase 2 trials involving either purely preoperative or perioperative treatment demonstrated that there was no increase in anticipated surgical morbidity or mortality.[346,347] Brenner et al.[347] reported on locally advanced, high-risk gastric cancer patients who received preoperative cisplatin plus 5-FU followed by intraperitoneal chemotherapy after resection. At 43 months of follow-up, 39.5% of patients were still alive. Evaluating efficacy at the primary site is difficult in gastric cancer. Kelsen et al.[346] compared endoscopic ultrasonography with pathologic stage in assessing objective regression after neoadjuvant chemotherapy. They found that even though EUS was an accurate test in previously untreated patients following administration of chemotherapy, after chemotherapy and prior to surgery, EUS was inaccurate in measuring the depth of invasion (T stage) or lymph node involvement.

FDG-PET scans as a predictive marker of response to preoperative chemotherapy have been studied in patients with gastric cancer. Ott et al.[124] reported on 44 patients with locally advanced gastric cancer who underwent PET scans prior to and after receiving chemotherapy. A decreased SUV was able to differentiate between patients who responded to treatment and those who did not.[348] These data suggest that functional imaging may eventually prove to be a useful predictive marker for efficacy. Studies in which systemic therapy is changed on the basis of an early PET scan are now under way. As previously noted, for gastric cancer patients, approximately 20% to 25% of patients will not have an informative PET scan, so that this technique cannot be used as a predictive marker for these patients.

After phase 2 studies demonstrated safety and gave hints of efficacy, several perioperative phase 3 trials were performed (Table 80.5). English investigators led by Cunningham et al.[349] reported the final results of a well-designed, random assignment study comparing surgery alone with perioperative chemotherapy in patients with gastroesophageal junction and gastric cancers (the MAGIC trial). All patients had potentially resectable disease prior to entrance into the study. Patients assigned to perioperative chemotherapy were treated with the epirubicin-cisplatin-fluorouracil (ECF) regimen. Chemotherapy was given both before and after surgery. Five hundred three patients were entered into the study; three-quarters had gastric cancer and one-quarter had gastroesophageal junction or lower esophageal adenocarcinomas. The ECF chemotherapy was well tolerated, with no increase in surgical morbidity or mortality. There was a shift to an earlier stage overall in patients receiving perioperative chemotherapy, as well as an improved R0 resection rate. With a median follow-up of 4 years, there was a significant improvement both in disease-free and in overall survival for patients receiving perioperative chemotherapy: 5-year survival rate was 36% for those receiving chemotherapy and 23% for those receiving surgery alone (HR, 0.75; 95% CI, 0.6 to 0.9; P = .009). The authors concluded that ECF perioperative chemotherapy improves outcome for patients with resectable gastric cancer without increasing operative morbidity or mortality. This important trial was the well-designed, adequately powered study to demonstrate an advantage of systemic treatment plus operation when compared with operation alone.

More recently, French investigators reported the results of a similar trial (ACCORD 07-FFCD 9703) using cisplatin plus fluorouracil prior to surgery versus surgery alone.[350] Approximately half the patients receiving preoperative chemotherapy received postoperative treatment using the same regimen. The results were similar to those of the MAGIC trial, with 5-year overall survival being 24% for those undergoing operation alone versus 30% for those who received perioperative chemotherapy. There was a similar improvement in disease-free survival. The results of the ACCORD 07 trial support the results of the MAGIC study.

Summary for Neoadjuvant Chemotherapy. The results of the MAGIC and ACCORD 07 trials have shown that even regimens that are only modestly effective in palliating patients with advanced disease can have a small but real effect on survival when given in the perioperative setting. New effective cytotoxic agents and new biologic agents are now being introduced in the treatment of patients with gastric tumors. Studies involving perioperative chemotherapy using these agents are now in the advanced planning stage. As previously discussed, the results of the perioperative MAGIC and ACCORD 07 trials and of the postoperative S-1 and intergroup 116 chemoradiation studies support the use of systemic therapy as a portion of the treatment plan for patients with locally advanced gastric cancers. The best strategy to pursue—that is, whether to give systemic therapy first followed by operation or to proceed directly to operation followed by systemic treatment plus or minus radiation given after surgery—has not yet been determined.

Adjuvant Radiation and Chemoradiation Therapy. The recognition of the high rates of local and regional failure following surgery in patterns of failure analyses has served as the basis for clinical trials assessing the value of radiation therapy with and without chemotherapy as an adjuvant treatment. Although these studies have all addressed the important question of whether clinical outcome is enhanced by adjuvant radiation therapy, there has been marked variability in radiation dose and schedule, sequence with surgery (preoperatively, intraoperatively, or postoperatively), and the use of concurrent and maintenance chemotherapy. These differences in study design may explain in part the conflicting results observed in phase 3 studies.

Two randomized phase 3 trials have studied the use of external-beam radiation therapy (EBRT) alone with surgery.[351–353] Although both studies used similar radiation dose and schedule, sequence with surgery differed. In the British Stomach Cancer Group study, 436 patients were randomized to surgery alone; postoperative radiation therapy (45 to 50 Gy in 25 to 28 fractions); or cytotoxic chemotherapy with mitomycin, doxorubicin, and fluorouracil (FAM).[351,352] The 5-year survival for surgery alone was 20%, for surgery plus radiation therapy 12%, and for surgery plus chemotherapy 19%. In this study, no survival advantage was observed for patients who received postoperative EBRT, although there was an apparent improvement in local control, demonstrating that local disease could be affected by adjuvant radiation therapy. Locoregional failure was documented in only 15 of 153 (10%) in the irradiation arm versus 39 of 145 (27%) in the surgery-alone arm and 26 of 138 (19%) in the FAM group. Interpretation of these results is complicated by the inclusion of 171 patients undergoing resection with gross or microscopic residual carcinoma. These patients would not be candidates for current gastric surgical adjuvant trials in the United States. In addition, approximately one-third of patients randomized to receive adjuvant treatment did not receive the assigned therapy. Of 153 patients randomized to the irradiation arm, only 104 (68%) received a dose of 40.5 Gy or more, and 36 (24%) received none.

In contrast, the results of a phase 3 study from Beijing demonstrated a survival benefit for patients with gastric cardia carcinoma receiving preoperative irradiation and surgery versus surgery only.[353] In this study, 370 patients with gastric cardia carcinoma were randomized to 40 Gy in 20 fractions over 4 weeks of preoperative irradiation and surgery or surgery only. The 5-year survival rates of preoperative irradiation and surgery and the surgery-alone group were 30% and 20%, respectively (10-year, 20% and 13%, respectively; P = .009). Further, local and regional nodal control were improved in patients undergoing preoperative irradiation and surgery (61% and 61%, respectively) versus surgery (48% and 45%, respectively) only. Morbidity and mortality rates were not increased in patients receiving preoperative therapy.

An alternative approach to postoperative or preoperative irradiation is intraoperative radiation therapy (IORT).[354] The advantage of this technique is the ability to deliver a single large fraction (10 to 35 Gy) of radiation to the tumor or tumor bed while excluding or protecting surrounding normal tissue from the high-dose field. This approach permits high-dose irradiation with minimal normal tissue treatment. Two randomized trials have examined the efficacy of IORT in combination with surgery for patients with gastric carcinoma.[355,356] Abe et al.[355] from Kyoto University performed a randomized trial of 211 patients with gastric cancer comparing surgery alone with surgery and IORT (28 to 35 Gy). For patients with tumor confined to the gastric wall, 5-year survival rates were similar for IORT and for resection alone. However, patients with Japanese stages II to IV disease who received IORT in conjunction with resection showed improved survival over patients who underwent resection without irradiation. Among patients with stage IV disease (who usually had local residual disease after maximal resection), there were no 5-year survivors who received surgery alone, with 15% of the patients who received IORT alive at 5 years. The experience with IORT in gastric cancer at Kyoto University suggested that IORT may be beneficial in the treatment of locally advanced malignancies of the stomach.

To further evaluate this approach, Sindelar et al.[356] at the National Cancer Institute conducted a prospectively randomized controlled trial comparing surgical resection and IORT with conventional therapy in gastric carcinoma. Patients in the experimental group underwent gastrectomy, and IORT was administered to their gastric bed (20 Gy). Patients in the control group underwent resection and postoperative EBRT to the upper abdomen (50 Gy in 25 fractions) for advanced-stage lesions extending beyond the gastric wall. Of the 100 patients screened for the study, 60 were randomized and underwent exploratory surgery. Nineteen patients were excluded intraoperatively because of unresectability or metastases, leaving 41 patients in the study. The median survival for patients with tumors of all stages was 25 months for the IORT group and 21 months for the control group (P = NS). Locoregional disease relapse occurred in 7 of 16 IORT patients (44%), and in 23 of 25 patients (92%) control patients ($P < .001$). Complication rates were similar between IORT and control patients. Although IORT failed to afford a significant advantage over conventional therapy in overall survival, IORT did significantly improve control of locoregional disease. Based on these results, the use of IORT in gastric cancer remains investigational.

Because of the promising results in the early studies of combined-modality therapy for locally advanced (unresectable) or subtotally resected gastric cancer, investigators also have studied this combination in resectable gastric carcinoma. A small study from South Africa randomized 66 patients with resected gastric cancer (T1–3, N1–2, M0) to low-dose postoperative irradiation (20 Gy in eight fractions over 10 days) and 5-FU or no further therapy.[357] No difference in survival was observed between the patients undergoing surgery and adjuvant therapy and those undergoing surgery alone. Given the subtherapeutic doses of radiation used in this study, it is difficult to draw any conclusions as to the efficacy of adjuvant radiation therapy and 5-FU. In 1984, Moertel et al.[358] reported the results of a prospective randomized trial conducted at the Mayo Clinic with 62 patients with poor prognosis but completely resected gastric cancers who were randomized to either surgery alone or surgery followed by irradiation (37.5 Gy in 24 fractions over 4 to 5 weeks) with concurrent 5-FU. A nonstratified, prerandomization scheme was used with a 2:3 ratio favoring treatment. Ten of the 39 patients refused further therapy and were observed. When analyzed by intent to treat, the adjuvant arm had statistically significant improvement in both relapse-free and overall survival (overall 5-year survival 23% vs. 4%; $P < .05$). When patient outcome was compared with actual treatment received (29 adjuvant treatment, 33 surgery alone), 5-year survival continued to favor the adjuvant group (20% vs. 12%), but the differences were not statistically significant in view of the small patient numbers. The 10 patients who refused assignment to adjuvant treatment had more favorable prognostic findings than the other two groups of patients. When the two groups with equally poor prognostic factors were compared, the 5-year overall survival was 20% versus 4%, with an advantage to those receiving adjuvant treatment. When analyzed by treatment delivered, locoregional relapse was decreased with adjuvant treatments (54% with surgery alone vs. 39% with irradiation and 5-FU).

The Intergroup Trial (INT 0116) randomized patients to receive operation alone or operation plus postoperative 5-FU–based chemotherapy and irradiation.[359] Eligibility included patients with stages IB–IVA nonmetastatic adenocarcinoma of the stomach or GEJ. After an *en bloc* resection, 556 patients were randomized to either observation alone or postoperative combined-modality therapy consisting of one monthly 5-day cycle of 5-FU and leucovorin, followed by 45 Gy in 25 fractions plus concurrent 5-FU and leucovorin (4 days in week 1, 3 days in week 5) followed by two monthly 5-day cycles of 5-FU and leucovorin. Nodal metastases were present in 85% of the cases. With 5 years of median follow-up, 3-year relapse-free survival was 48% for adjuvant treatment and 31% for observation ($P = .001$); 3-year overall survival was 50% for treatment and 41% for observation ($P = .005$). The median overall survival in the surgery-only group was 27 months, compared with 36 months in the chemoradiotherapy group; the hazard ratio for death was 1.35 (95% CI, 1.09 to 1.66; $P = .005$). The hazard ratio for relapse in the surgery-only group as compared with the chemoradiotherapy group was 1.52 (95% CI, 1.23 to 1.86; $P < .001$). The median duration of relapse-free survival was 30 months in the chemoradiotherapy group and 19 months in the surgery-only group. Patterns of failure were based on the site of first relapse only and were categorized as local, regional, or distant. Local recurrence occurred in 29% of the patients who relapsed in the surgery-only group and 19% of those who relapsed in the chemoradiotherapy group. Regional relapse, typically abdominal carcinomatosis, was reported in 72% of those who relapsed in the surgery-only group and 65% of those who relapsed in the chemoradiotherapy group. Extra-abdominal distant metastases were diagnosed in 18% of those who relapsed in the surgery-only group and 33% of those who relapsed in the chemoradiotherapy group. Treatment was tolerable, with three (1%) toxic deaths. Grade 3 and 4 toxicity occurred in 41% and 32% of cases, respectively. The results of this large study demonstrate a clear survival advantage for the use of postoperative chemoradiation and strongly support the integration of postoperative chemoradiation into the routine care of patients with curatively resected high-risk carcinoma of the stomach and GEJ.

The U.S. Gastrointestinal Intergroup has recently completed a second randomized prospective trial (CALGB 80101) in patients with completely resected high-risk gastric cancer comparing two chemotherapy regimens given before and after 5-FU–based chemoradiation. This study examines the use of one cycle of postoperative ECF (epirubicin: 50 mg/m^2, cisplatin: 60 mg/m^2, and continuous infusion 5-FU: 200 mg/m^2 per day for 21 days) followed by radiation therapy with concurrent continuous infusion 5-FU (200 mg/m^2 per day) and two additional cycles of ECF. This will be compared with one cycle of postoperative 5-FU and leucovorin followed by concurrent continuous infusion 5-FU (200 mg/m^2 per day) and two additional cycles of 5-FU and leucovorin.

To address the role of adjuvant chemoradiation in light of the MAGIC trial, the Dutch Colorectal Cancer Group has initiated the CRITICS trial. This study is a phase 3 prospectively randomized trial that investigates whether chemoradiotherapy (45 Gy in 5 weeks with daily cisplatin and capecitabine) after preoperative chemotherapy (3 × ECC [epirubicin, cisplatin, and capecitabine]) and adequate (D1+) surgery lead to improved survival in comparison with postoperative chemotherapy alone (3 × ECC). Further evaluating the role of adjuvant radiation therapy, a Korean phase 3 trial (the ARTIST study) is randomizing patients undergoing D2 resection to adjuvant cisplatin and capecitabine, with or without radiation therapy.

Although no phase 3 trials have tested the value of preoperative radiation plus chemotherapy for patients with gastric cancer, two phase 2 trials for patients with esophagus cancer have included either lesions of the gastric cardia or the EGJ.[360,361] In both trials, the trimodality arm demonstrated an improvement in survival when compared with the control arm of surgery alone. The series by Walsh et al.[360] (adenocarcinoma of the esophagus or gastric cardia) demonstrated a median survival of 16 versus 11 months and 3-year survival of 32% versus 6% (P = .01), with the advantage to trimodality treatment. The U.S. GI Intergroup phase 3 trial (adenocarcinoma or squamous cell of esophagus or EGJ), which closed prematurely because of low accrual, resulted in a median survival of 54 versus 21.6 months and 5-year survival of 39% versus 16% (P = .008), with an advantage to the trimodality arm.[361] In addition, a recent phase 3 randomized German trial compared preoperative chemotherapy alone (5-FU, leucovorin, and cisplatin) versus the same regimen followed by low-dose radiation therapy (30 Gy) with concurrent cisplatin and etoposide in patients with adenocarcinoma of the lower esophagus or gastric cardia. Although the trial was closed early because of poor accrual (126 patients), patients receiving radiation therapy had significantly higher pathologic complete response rates (2% vs. 16%; P = .03) and trend toward improved survival (3-year survival 47% vs. 28%; P = .07).[362]

Preoperative chemoradiation data for patients with gastric cancer exclusively is limited to phase 2 studies from single institutions and cooperative groups. The M. D. Anderson Hospital has reported a study in which 33 patients completed a preoperative protocol that started with induction chemotherapy of 5-FU, leucovorin, and cisplatin, followed by 45 Gy of radiation therapy in 25 fractions over 5 weeks with concurrent infusional 5-FU. In 28 patients (85%), a gastrectomy was performed and D2 lymph node dissection was attempted. Pathologic complete and partial responses were found in 64% of all operated patients. These patients showed a significant longer median survival of 64 months in comparison with 13 months in patients with tumors not pathologically responders.[363] In a study from the same institution, 41 patients with operable gastric cancer received two cycles of continuous 5-FU, paclitaxel, and cisplatin followed by 45 Gy of radiation therapy with concurrent 5-FU and paclitaxel. An R0 resection was achieved in 78% of patients with pathologic complete response of 25% and pathologic partial response of 15%. Pathologic response, R0 resection, and postoperative T and N stage were correlated with overall and disease-free survival.[364]

The Radiation Therapy Oncology Group (RTOG 9904) reported the results of a phase 2 study of 49 patients undergoing induction 5-FU, leucovorin, and cisplatin followed by concurrent radiation therapy and infusional 5-FU and paclitaxel. Resection was attempted 5 to 6 weeks after radiation therapy and chemotherapy. The pathologic complete response and R0 resection rates were 26% and 77%, respectively. At 1 year, more patients with tumors exhibiting a pathologic complete response (89%) were living than patients with tumors having less favorable response (66%). Grade 4 toxicity occurred in 21% of patients. These data appear to support a study evaluating preoperative radiation therapy and chemotherapy versus postoperative radiation therapy and chemotherapy.[365]

TECHNICAL TREATMENT-RELATED ISSUES

Surgery

Surgery begins with careful laparoscopic staging and examination. Inspection for the presence of ascites, hepatic metastases, peritoneal seeding, disease in the pelvis (such as a "drop" metastasis), or ovarian involvement should be performed. Once distant metastases have been ruled out, depending on the location of the lesion, a bilateral subcostal incision or a midline abdominal incision can be used to gain adequate exposure to the upper abdomen. The stomach should be inspected to assess the location and extent of tumor. The size and location of the primary tumor dictate the extent of gastric resection. A D2 lymphadenectomy sparing the spleen and pancreas can be done safely and provides an excellent specimen for surgical and pathologic staging, but this procedure should only be performed by or with an experienced surgeon.

The D2 subtotal gastrectomy commences with mobilization of the greater omentum from the transverse colon. After the omentum is mobilized, the anterior peritoneal leaf of the transverse mesocolon is incised along the lower border of the colon, and a plane is developed down to the head of the pancreas. The infrapyloric lymph nodes are dissected and the origin of the right gastroepiploic artery and vein are ligated. With a combination of blunt and sharp dissection, the plane of dissection continues on to the anterior surface of the pancreas, extending to the level of the common hepatic and splenic arteries. This maneuver can be tedious, but theoretically it provides additional protection against serosal spread of tumor to the local peritoneal surface. The right gastric artery is ligated. At this point, the duodenum is divided distal to the pylorus. The stomach and omentum are then reflected cephalad. The gastrohepatic ligament is divided close to the liver up to the gastroesophageal junction. Dissection is then continued on the hepatic artery toward the celiac axis. Once near the celiac axis, the lymph node-bearing tissue is dissected until the left gastric artery is visualized and can be divided at its origin. The proximal peritoneal attachments of the stomach and distal esophagus can then be incised, and the proximal extent of resection is chosen. For tumors of the mid- and proximal stomach, dissection of the lymph nodes along the splenic artery and splenic hilum is important. This technique is not indicated for antral tumors, given the low rate of splenic hilar nodal metastases seen with these tumors. The stomach is then divided 5 cm proximal to the tumor, which dictates the extent of gastric resection. Despite the fact that the entire blood supply of the stomach has been interrupted, a cuff of proximal stomach invariably shows good vascularization from the feeding distal esophageal arcade. When feasible, most surgeons prefer to anastomose jejunum to stomach versus esophagus because of the technical ease and excellent healing. Reconstruction using a variety of techniques has been described and is a matter of personal choice.

Antibiotics Prophylaxis

One RCT (n = 501) tested single-dose cefazolin or ampicillin-sulbactam 30 minutes before surgery versus multiple dose regimen for 3 days postoperatively. There were no differences in surgical site infections or complication.[320,366]

Nasogastric Drainage After Gastrectomy

The Italian Total Gastrectomy Study Group reported on the largest RCT comparing total gastrectomy with Roux-en-Y with and without nasogastric tube (n = 237). There were no differences in overall morbidity, leak rate, hospital stay, and time to diet.[367] Other authors confirmed that nasogastric tube is not necessary after gastrectomy.[368–370]

Intraperitoneal Drains After Gastrectomy

As with other pathologies, two RCTs concluded that drains after gastrectomy are generally not indicated, and in certain situations can increase significantly morbidity.[371,372]

Reconstruction After Gastrectomy

Iivonen et al.[373] compared Roux-en-Y with and without pouch. They randomized 48 patients and found significantly less dumping syndrome and early satiety but no differences at 15 months of follow-up. Fein et al.[374] reported on 138 patients randomized in a similar fashion; they found similar QOL at 1 year but significantly improved QOL at 3-, 4-, and 5-year follow-up. It seems that reconstruction with pouch has long-term advantages and may be recommended as the standard reconstruction.[320]

Radiation Treatment

Technique of Radiation Therapy

Idealized portals generated from patterns of failure data should be modified on the basis of the individual patient's initial extent of disease.[375,376] Based on the likely sites of locoregional failure, the gastric/tumor bed, anastomosis and gastric remnant, and regional lymphatics should be included in most patients.[377–380] Major nodal chains at risk include the lesser and greater curvature; celiac axis; pancreaticoduodenal, splenic, suprapancreatic, and porta hepatis groups; and, in some, para-aortic to the level of mid-L3.

The relative risk of nodal metastases at a specific nodal location depends on both the site of origin of the primary tumor and other factors including width and depth of invasion of the gastric wall.[376] Tumors that originate in the proximal portion of the stomach and the GEJ have a higher propensity of spread to nodes in the mediastinum and pericardial region but a lower likelihood of involvement of nodes in the region of the gastric antrum, periduodenal area, and porta hepatis. Tumors that originate in the body of the stomach can spread to all nodal sites but have the highest likelihood of spreading to nodes along the greater and lesser curvature near the location of the primary tumor mass. Tumors that originate in the distal stomach, in the region of the gastric antrum, have a high likelihood of spread to the periduodenal, peripancreatic, and porta hepatis nodes, whereas they have a lower likelihood of spread to the nodes near the cardia of the stomach, the periesophageal and mediastinal nodes, or to the splenic hilar nodes. Any tumor originating in the stomach has a high propensity of spread to nodes along the greater and lesser curvature, although they are most likely to spread to those sites in close anatomic proximity to the primary tumor mass. Guidelines for defining the clinical target volume for postoperative irradiation fields have been developed based on location and extent of the primary tumor (T stage) and location and extent of known nodal involvement (N stage).[376] In general, for patients with node-positive disease, there should be wide coverage of tumor bed, remaining stomach, resection margins, and nodal drainage regions. For node-negative disease, if there is a good surgical resection with pathologic evaluation of at least 15 nodes, and there are wide surgical margins on the primary tumor (at least 5 cm), treatment of the nodal beds is optional. Treatment of the remaining stomach should depend on a balance of the likely normal tissue morbidity and the perceived risk of local relapse in the residual stomach.

Although parallel-opposed anteroposterior/posteroanterior (AP/PA) fields are a practical arrangement for tumor bed and nodal irradiation, three-dimensional multifield techniques should be used if they can improve long-term tolerance of normal tissues. Tightly contoured fields should be designed to spare as much normal tissue as possible. Over the past decade, a shift has occurred toward more sophisticated treatment techniques that use multiple and often noncoplanar beams including three-dimensional and intensity modulated radiation therapy. Attention has also been placed on accurate three-dimensional target delineated based on CT anatomy rather than only two-dimensional field design. In addition to refinements in radiation therapy target definition based on CT planning, technologic advances including study of and solutions for variability in target and normal organ location during a treatment course (day to day interfraction variability) and actual treatment delivered (intrafraction variability caused by respiration) have been undertaken. Interfraction variability in stomach location can be substantial, particularly among patients treated with neoadjuvant chemoradiation because of daily variations in gastric filling. Because of this, patients should generally be treated with an empty stomach. Intrafraction changes in target shape (deformation) and location are asymmetric and mainly from respiratory motion. Movement, particularly in the cranial-caudad dimension, frequently exceeds 1 to 1.5 cm. Image guidance, four-dimensional treatment planning, and respiratory gating have been developed to address these challenges.

More routine use of multiple field techniques should be considered when preoperative imaging exists to allow accurate reconstruction of target volumes. Single-institution data suggest that multiple field arrangements may produce less toxicity.[381] Although AP/PA fields can be weighted anteriorly to keep the spinal cord dose at acceptable levels using only parallel-opposed techniques, a four-field technique, if feasible, can spare spinal cord with improved dose homogeneity. Dependent on the posterior extent of the gastric fundus, either oblique or more routine lateral portals can be used to deliver a 10- to 20-Gy component of irradiation to spare spinal cord or kidney. When lateral fields are used, liver and kidney tolerance limits the use of lateral fields to 20 Gy or less. With the wide availability of three-dimensional treatment-planning systems, it may be possible to target more accurately the high-risk volume and to use unconventional field arrangements to produce superior dose distributions. To accomplish this without marginal misses, it will be necessary to both carefully define and encompass the various target volumes, given the use of oblique or noncoplanar beams could potentially exclude target volumes that would be included in AP/PA fields or nonoblique four-field techniques (AP/PA and laterals). In most patients, a portion of both kidneys is within the treatment field, but at least two-thirds to three-fourths of one kidney should be excluded beyond a dose of 20 Gy. For proximal gastric lesions, 50% or more of the left kidney is commonly within the irradiation portal, and the right kidney must be appropriately spared. For distal lesions with narrow or positive duodenal margins, a similar amount of right kidney often is included, and every effort must be taken to spare enough left kidney to maintain function. Late renal sequelae have not been encountered with these techniques, assuming normal renal function bilaterally.[382–384]

With proximal gastric lesions or lesions at the EGJ, a 3- to 5-cm margin of distal esophagus should be included; if the lesion extends through the entire gastric wall, a major portion of the left hemidiaphragm should be included. In these circumstances, blocking can decrease the volume of irradiated heart.

TREATMENT OF ADVANCED DISEASE (STAGE IV)

Treatment of Advanced Gastric Cancer: Palliative Systemic Chemotherapy

Chemotherapy versus Best Supportive Care

The modest activity and substantial toxicity of cytotoxic chemotherapy raised the question as to whether palliative use of

TABLE 80.6

CHEMOTHERAPY FOR ADVANCED GASTRIC CANCER: TREATMENT VERSUS BEST SUPPORTIVE CARE

Regimen	No. of Patients	Median Survival (mo)	Survival Rate (%) 1 Y	Survival Rate (%) 2 Y
FAMTX	30	10	40	6
BSC	10	3	10	0
FEMTX	17	12	—	—
BSC	19	3	—	—
ETOPLF	10	10	—	—
BSC	8	4	—	—
ELF	52	10.2	34.6	9.6
BSC	51	5	7.8	0
Irinotecan	21	123[a]	—	—
BSC	19	73[a]	—	—

A, doxorubicin (Adriamycin); BSC, best supportive care; E, epirubicin; ETOP, etoposide; F, fluorouracil; L, leucovorin; MTX, methotrexate.
[a]Median survival in days.
Modified from ref. 463.

the available agents was worth it; that is, there was controversy as to whether or not there was an advantage to early initiation of systemic therapy versus best supportive care. Although this is a difficult hypothesis to test because of patient's and physician's preferences and biases, several random assignment trials were performed in the 1990s in patients with advanced incurable gastric cancer addressing this issue.

Wagner et al.[385] performed a meta-analysis for the Cochrane collaboration. They included three random assignment trials involving a total of 184 patients in whom the study design was to initiate systemic chemotherapy plus best supportive care or to best supportive care alone. Median and overall survival were evaluated (Table 80.6). Patients receiving chemotherapy as part of their treatment had a better overall survival than those receiving best supportive care only, with an overall hazard ratio of 0.39 (95% CI, 0.28 to 0.52). The median survival was improved from 4.3 months for best supportive care to approximately 11 months for chemotherapy. Note that the median survival for patients receiving chemotherapy is consistent with several more recent trials. There was also a modest improvement in time to progression (7 months for patients receiving chemotherapy vs. 2.5 months for patients receiving best supportive care). Wagner et al. concluded that the evidence supporting initiating chemotherapy for patients with advanced incurable gastric cancer was convincing.

In a fourth trial, QOL was assessed. The average quality-adjusted survival for chemotherapy patients was superior to best supportive care patients (6 months vs. 12 months). Importantly, in those best supportive care trials that reported 2-year survival (24 months or greater) only chemotherapy patients survived. The 2-year survival rate was 5% to 14% for patients receiving combination chemotherapy versus 0% for patients receiving best supportive care. More recently, the preliminary results of a small study testing the use of single-agent chemotherapy versus best supportive care in patients who have already received chemotherapy were reported. Previously treated patients were randomly assigned to best supportive care or to single-agent irinotecan plus best supportive care. Although the study was initially powered to require 120 patients, accrual to this type of trial was difficult and a total of only 40 patients were eventually randomized. There was a modest improvement in overall survival, with median survival for those receiving irinotecan of 123 days, and median survival for those with best supportive care 73 days (HR, 2.85).[386] These results are in concert with the earlier studies in previously untreated patients, and indicate that systemic therapy has a modest but real effect on outcome. Many cytotoxic agents have been studied in patients with advanced gastric cancer; when used as single agents, modest activity has been identified for drugs from five different classes. More recently, targeted therapy has been tested. The following section summarizes the data for the use of systemic cytotoxic chemotherapy when given with palliative intent. An extensive discussion of older agents can be found in prior editions of this textbook.

Single-Agent Chemotherapy

For most drugs, a variety of doses and schedules have been studied. In the absence of comparative trials using the same agent with different doses and schedules, superiority of one regimen over the other cannot be assessed. Table 80.7 gives a listing of agents that have demonstrated at least modest activity in the treatment of gastric cancer and are routinely employed as part of standard care options. Drugs with little or no activity, especially if they were evaluated prior to 2000, are not included in this table.

Fluorouracil is the parent fluorinated pyrimidine, which has been the most extensively studied single agent in gastric cancer. An antimetabolite, the drug has been used in a variety of schedules and doses. One method involved the use of rapid intravenous injections on a weekly basis or daily for 5 consecutive days. In gastric cancer, continuous infusion fluorouracil has been used more recently. During the 1990s, in several studies, fluorouracil was the control arm of a random assignment trial or was studied as a single agent (with leucovorin) in a prospective phase 2 trial. This allowed an assessment using more modern criteria of activity. The studies from the 1990s suggest overall response rates of 10% to 20%, with a median duration of response, or time to progression, of approximately 4 months. As is the case in other diseases, the major toxicities reported in gastric cancer for fluorouracil are mucositis, diarrhea, or mild myelosuppression. Because continuous intravenous infusion schedules can be cumbersome, oral analogues of 5-FU have been studied in gastric cancer. Three oral drugs of this class have undergone study in gastric cancer. These are UFT (tegafur and uracil), S-1 (tegafur and two modulators,

TABLE 80.7

ACTIVITY OF SELECTED SINGLE AGENTS IN ADVANCED GASTRIC CANCER

Drug	Response Rate (%)
FLUORINATED PYRIMIDINES	
5-fluorouracil	21
UFT	28
S-1	49
Capecitabine	26
ANTIBIOTICS	
Doxorubicin hydrochloride	17
Epirubicin hydrochloride	19
HEAVY METALS	
Cisplatin	19
TAXANES	
Paclitaxel	17
Docetaxel	19
CAMPTOTHECANS	
Irinotecan hydrochloride	23

UFT, tegafur and uracil; S-1, tegafur and two modulators, 5-chloro-2, 4-dihydroxypyridine and potassium oxonate.
From van De Velde CJH, Kelsen D, Minsky B. Gastric cancer: clinical management. In: Kelsen D, Daly JM, Kern SE, et al., eds. *Principles and Practice of Gastrointestinal Oncology*, 2nd ed. Philadelphia: Lippincott Williams & Wilkins, 2008, with permission.

5-chloro-2,4-dihydroxypyridine and potassium oxonate), and capecitabine. The data for these agents are also shown in Table 80.7. S-1 has been most extensively studied in Japan. Although a response rate to single-agent S-1 of 44% to 54% was reported in Japanese patients, the response rate among European patients was substantially lower. Like capecitabine, S-1 is now undergoing study in combination with other agents, particularly cisplatin. UFT combines tegafur and uracil. In gastric cancer a response rate of 27.7% was seen in Japanese patients. In a small European study, Okines et al.[387] reported the results of a European Organisation for Research and Treatment of Cancer (EORTC) study combining UFT and leucovorin. A 16% response rate was seen in a group of 23 patients. Capecitabine has had fewer single-agent studies in gastric cancer. The data available suggest similar activity as seen with other oral fluorinated pyrimidines. Capecitabine has now been extensively studied in combination with cisplatin or oxaliplatin (see "The REAL-2 Trial").

Platinum compounds are an important part of treatment of gastric cancer. The parent analogue, cisplatin, was studied in the 1980s. In both previously treated and untreated patients, a response rate of approximately 15% was reported. The major toxicities for cisplatin are nausea and vomiting, peripheral neuropathy, ototoxicity, and nephropathy. The development of better antiemetics has significantly improved control of nausea and vomiting. An analogue, carboplatin, has been less well studied in gastric cancer; it appears to have less activity in this disease. Most recently, oxaliplatin, a diamino cyclohexane extensively used in the treatment of colorectal cancer, was included as part of combination chemotherapy for gastric cancer. The data for combination therapy, including oxaliplatin and data from the REAL-2 trial, are shown later.

A third class of cytotoxic agents with activity in gastric cancer is the taxanes. Both paclitaxel and docetaxel have been studied as single agents in gastroesophageal cancers. Docetaxel has been more extensively studied. De Cosimo et al.[388] reviewed trials in which docetaxel was used as single agent. Patients may have received prior treatment, and 262 patients were evaluable for response. The overall response rate was 19.1%. The major toxicities were neutropenia, alopecia, and edema. Allergic reactions were seen in about 25% of patients. The most common doses schedule was docetaxel 100 mg/m^2 every 3 weeks. When reported, the median time to progression was 6 months. A schedule using lower doses given once weekly has also been studied with similar activity. On the basis of a large randomized study comparing cisplatin plus fluorouracil to docetaxel-cisplatin-fluorouracil (DCF), docetaxel was approved by the U.S. Food and Drug Administration for treatment of advanced gastric cancer. Paclitaxel has also been studied in gastric cancer, although in smaller numbers of patients, and has a similar degree of activity.

A fourth class of active agent is represented by irinotecan. It has been studied both as a single agent and in combination. When used alone, response rates of 15% to 25% have been reported in both previously treated and untreated patients. Wagner et al.[385] reviewed the data for combinations, including irinotecan versus multidrug combination not including irinotecan. They concluded that irinotecan-containing multidrug chemotherapy combinations had a modest survival benefit, which was not statistically significant, when compared with regimens not including irinotecan. The major toxicities of irinotecan are myelosuppression and diarrhea.

Anthracyclines also have activity in gastric cancer. Single-agent data from the 1960s and 1970s show a response rate for doxorubicin of 17%, and for epirubicin a similar response rate of approximately 19%. The anthracyclines have undergone more extensive study in combination chemotherapy.

Single-Agent versus Combination Chemotherapy

The potential advantage of giving combination chemotherapy versus single agents has been evaluated by Wagner et al.[385] in an update of their original Cochrane review. They found that combination chemotherapy had a significant survival advantage when compared to single-agent chemotherapy (HR, 0.82; 95% CI, 0.74 to 0.90). The difference in average median survival, however, was modest, 8.3 months for combination chemotherapy versus 6.7 months for single agents. In the updated analysis, a test for heterogeneity was not statistically significant; they concluded that this indicated that the results of the different studies were consistent. A secondary analysis for response rate and for time to progression also favored combination chemotherapy. Not surprisingly, toxicity is higher when several agents are given together, although this was not statistically significant. Treatment-related mortality was only slightly higher (1.5%) for patients receiving combination chemotherapy versus 1.1% when single-agent therapy was used.

They also evaluated the role of several different combinations, including anthracyclines as part of combination chemotherapy. In this analysis, three studies with a total of 500 patients were included. Wagner et al.[385] found that including anthracyclines in a fluorouracil-cisplatin combination had a modest survival advantage over cisplatin-fluorouracil alone (HR, 0.77; 95% CI, 0.62 to 0.95). A similar advantage to anthracyclines in combination was found when fluorouracil-anthracyclines combinations without cisplatin were studied. In contrast to anthracyclines, there was a more modest, not statistically significant, benefit for irinotecan-containing combinations. Once again, there was a modest improvement in overall survival for docetaxel-containing regimens but this did not reach statistical significance. The response rate as a secondary objective was 36% for docetaxel-containing regimens versus 31% for non–docetaxel-containing regimens (not

TABLE 80.8

COMBINATION CHEMOTHERAPY IN ADVANCED GASTRIC CANCER: CISPLATIN-FLUOROURACIL–CONTAINING REGIMENS USED AS THE CONTROL ARM IN RANDOM ASSIGNMENT TRIALS

Study (Ref.)	Drug	Dose (mg/mL)	Schedule (d)	No. of Patients	RR (%)	Median TTP/ PFS (mo)	Med Survival (mo)	2-Y Survival (%)
EORTC (389)	C	100	1	127	20	4.1	7.2	~10
	F	1,000	1–5					
JCOG (390)	C	20	1–5	105	36	7.3	3.9	7
	F	800	1–5					
Dank et al. (392)	C	100	1	163	26	4.2	8.7	~10
	F	1,000	1–5					
TAX325 (391)	C	100	1	224	25	3.7	8.6	9
	F	1,000	1–5					
FLAGS (464)	C	100	1	508	32	5.5	7.9	~10
	F	1,000	1–5					
Kang et al. (402)	C	80	1	156	32	5.5	9.3	~10
	F	800	1–5					
REAL-2	E	50	1	289	41	6.2	9.9	~15
(387, 400, 465)	C	60	1					
	F	200	Daily					

RR, recovery rate; TTP, time to progression; PFS, progression-free survival; EORTC, European Organisation for Research and Treatment of Cancer; C, cisplatin; F, fluorouracil; JCOG, Japan Clinical Oncology Group; E, epirubicin.
Modified from van De Velde CJH, Kelsen D, Minsky B. Gastric cancer: clinical management. In: Kelsen D, Daly JM, Kern SE, et al., eds. *Principles and Practice of Gastrointestinal Oncology*, 2nd ed. Philadelphia: Lippincott Williams & Wilkins, 2008, with permission.

statistically significant). Oral fluoropyrimidines when compared to intravenous fluoropyrimidine therapy also showed no significant difference in median survival. The meta-analysis is in concert with the results of the REAL-2 trial, which indicated noninferiority for capecitabine when compared to intravenous fluorouracil. Similarly, oxaliplatin regimens were compared to cisplatin-containing regimens with modest superiority to oxaliplatin.

In summary, there are five classes of cytotoxic chemotherapy agents in which single agents have modest activity in gastric cancer. The response rates range from 10% to 25%, the median duration of response is relatively short. As a result of the single-agent trials, fluorouracil or capecitabine (or other oral fluoropyrimidines), cisplatin or oxaliplatin, docetaxel, and less commonly, paclitaxel, epirubicin, and irinotecan are the major components of conventional regimens contacting combination chemotherapy.

Like other malignancies, multidrug regimens using agents that have a single-agent activity have been extensively studied in gastric cancer. This section will focus on phase 3 random assignment trials. For some combinations, only phase 2 data are available. The recent Cochrane review summarizing a comparison of different regimens including three-drug versus two-drug combinations has already been discussed.[385]

Cisplatin-Fluorouracil. One of the most widely used combination chemotherapy regimens in upper gastrointestinal tract malignancies, including gastric cancer, is the two-drug combination of cisplatin and fluorouracil (CF). Although this regimen has been used for several decades, with a variety of doses and schedules employed, since 2000, several phase 3 random assignment trials have been performed in which CF was the control arm. This allowed an opportunity for an evaluation of the efficacy of this combination, in patients with advanced incurable gastric cancer both in terms of response rate and progression-free and overall survival, using currently accepted criteria for efficacy. Table 80.8 shows the data from six studies in which cisplatin-fluorouracil was the control arm. The doses of cisplatin used were 80 to 100 mg/m^2 per course. Fluorouracil was given as a continuous 24-hour infusion from days 1 through 5 at a dose of 800 to 1,000 mg/m^2 per day. Cycles were usually given on an every 28-day basis. Efficacy outcome was consistent across these trials. Response rates, PFS, and overall survival were quite similar. Major objective tumor regression was reported in 20% to 30% of patients; complete clinical remission was very uncommon. The median time to progression or PFS, depending on the study, ranged from 3.7 to 4.1 months, with median survival ranging from 7.2 to 8.6 months. Two-year survival was between 7% and 10%. Cisplatin-fluorouracil was compared to a variety of other agents in these trials.

Vanhoefer et al.[389] reporting for EORTC, compared cisplatin-fluorouracil to methotrexate, fluorouracil, and doxorubicin (FAMTX); a third group of patients received etoposide, leucovorin, and fluorouracil combination. There was no significant difference in outcome among the three arms. A Japanese study (JC 09205) also had three arms.[390] Fluorouracil was compared to cisplatin plus fluorouracil to a third arm of uracil/tegafur plus mitomycin. In this study, there was no advantage for the two-drug combination of cisplatin plus fluorouracil over fluorouracil alone. The final results of the TAX315 trial have recently been published.[391] The details of this study are described later. An advantage was seen for the DCF arm. The cisplatin-fluorouracil control arm gave results similar to that seen in the earlier trials previously described. The two-drug combination of fluorouracil plus irinotecan was compared to CF by Dank et al.[392] Cisplatin plus fluorouracil was equivalent to irinotecan plus fluorouracil. Kang et al.[393] reported the results of comparison between CF versus cisplatin-capecitabine. This study was design as a noninferiority trial with the hypothesis that capecitabine-cisplatin was not inferior to CF. The end point was PFS. The dose of cisplatin was slightly lower than in the studies described earlier (80 mg/m^2).

However, therapy was given on every-3-week basis; 316 patients were treated. The median PFS was 5.0 months for CF; median survival was 9.3 months. Ajani et al.[394] reported the results of the FLAGS trial described in more detail later. In this study involving 1,029 eligible patients, the control arm of cisplatin plus intravenous fluorouracil had a median overall survival of 7.9 months.

In summary, the random assignment trials discussed previously indicate consistent data for efficacy (and toxicity) for the two-drug combination of CF. The Japanese study raises the question as to whether there is a substantial clinical advantage to CF over fluorouracil alone, but the meta-analysis performed by Wagner et al.[385] supports the use of combination chemotherapy over single agents. Although, still commonly used as a conventional standard of care palliative treatment, the recent demonstration of modest superiority when docetaxel is added to CF (assuming that a more well-tolerated regimen using the three agents can be developed) as well as the noncomparative data using epirubicin-cisplatin-fluorouracil, which is discussed later, suggest that CF may not be the most effective option for therapy in patients with advanced gastric cancer. The slight advantage in longer-term survival (2-year survival) in the TAX325 and in the irinotecan-fluorouracil-leucovorin studies of 15% to 20% and 15% to 20% for ECF suggests that at least some patients may have longer-term survival with newer regimens.

Although toxicity is consistent across most CF trials and is generally tolerable, it can be severe on occasion. For example, in the EORTC trial, grade 3 or 4 neutropenia was seen in approximately one-third of patients; one-quarter of patients had grade 3 or 4 nausea or vomiting. Similarly, in the more recent TAX325 trial, overall grade 3 or 4 toxicity was seen in 75% of patients receiving CF; in the FLAGS trial, treatment-related mortality occurred in 4.9% of patients receiving CF. Some toxicity may be ameliorated by improved supportive care. For example, newer antiemetics such as aprepitant should improve control of severe nausea and vomiting. More widespread use of supportive cytokine agents may decrease the incidence of neutropenic fever. Nonetheless, it should be recognized that CF, using the doses and schedules described previously, is associated with substantial toxicity in some patients.

The use of oral fluoropyrimidines in place of intravenous fluorouracil has been studied in several phase 3 trials, including that of Kang et al.[393] described earlier, the REAL-2 trial described in more detail later, and the FLAGS trial comparing CF to cisplatin-S-1. In this trial, 1,029 patients received either cisplatin 100 mg/m^2 and fluorouracil 1,000 mg/m^2 as a continuous 5-day infusion or a slightly lower dose of cisplatin plus oral S-1.[394] Median overall survival was 8.6 months for patients receiving cisplatin plus S-1 versus 7.9 months in the CF arm, with less toxicity for the CS combination. These three trials indicate that oral fluoropyrimidine when given with a platinum compound is not inferior to intravenous fluorouracil plus cisplatin.

Docetaxel, Cisplatin, and Fluorouracil (DCF). Van Cutsem et al.[391] have reported the final results of a large-scale random assignment trial comparing the DCF combination with a control arm of cisplatin fluorouracil alone (the TAX325 trial). Previously untreated patients with advanced gastric cancer received either DCF (221 analyzable patients) or CF using the doses and schedules previously described (224 patients). The primary end point of the study was time to progression (TTP) and was powered to detect an increase in median TTP from 4 to 6 months. The two arms of the study were well balanced for prognostic factors, including weight loss, performance status, and extent of disease. The median TTP was 3.7 months for patients receiving CF, and 5.6 months for those receiving DCF (HR, 1.47; P = .0004). As a secondary end point, survival was also modestly increased from 8.6 months for CF to 9.2 months for DCF. The 2-year survival rate was, however, more than doubled for DCF (8.8% for CF and 18.4% for DCF). Another measure of efficacy favoring DCF was response (37% for DCF, 25% for CF). Although this study indicated an advantage to the three-drug combination of DCF, toxicity was also increased and was very substantial. Eighty-one percent of all patients receiving DCF had at least one grade 3 or 4 nonhematologic toxicity, as well as substantially more hematologic toxicity. Of the patients receiving CF, 13.5% had neutropenic fever, as did 30% of patients receiving DCF. However, there was no difference in the treatment-related mortality rate for the two arms. This study led to the recent approval of docetaxel by the U.S. Food and Drug Administration for the treatment of gastric cancer when given in association with CF.

Like epirubicin, docetaxel, when added to CF, has a modest improvement in efficacy. The very substantial toxicity seen with the DCF regimen, however, has led to concerns regarding its general use. A number of studies have been performed using modifications of DCF to develop a more tolerable regimen. Several strategies have been pursued, most of which involve using somewhat lower doses of docetaxel and fluorouracil, or modifications in the schedule as to length of fluorouracil infusion or timing of the cisplatin dose. The preliminary results of a phase 2 trial comparing one of these modified DCF regimes to the original DCF schedule indicate that modifications of the treatment schedule may decrease toxicity while efficacy was similar.[395]

Irinotecan Plus Fluorouracil-Leucovorin. A three-drug combination of irinotecan-fluorouracil-leucovorin (FOLFIRI) has been studied extensively in metastatic colorectal cancer. A random-assignment phase 2 study comparing irinotecan-fluorouracil-leucovorin with cisplatin-irinotecan indicated a potential advantage to the FOLFIRI-type regimen.[396] Therefore, a definitive phase 3 trial was performed with CF as the control arm.[392] One hundred seventy patients received IF (irinotecan-fluorouracil) and 163 received CF. The primary end point was TTP. The analysis allowed for a noninferiority comparison between the two arms. The study was reasonably well balanced for the usual prognostic indicators; approximately 20% of patients had EGJ tumors. There was no significant difference in the major objective response rate (31.8% for IF and 25.8% for CF) nor in median TTP (5 months for IF and 4.2 months for CF). Overall median survival was also not different (9 months for IF and 8.7 months for CF). Time to treatment failure was 4.0 versus 3.4 months for IF and CF, respectively (P = .018). IF was better in terms of toxic deaths (0.6% vs. 3%), discontinuation for toxicity (10% vs. 21.5%), neutropenia, thrombocytopenia, and stomatitis but not diarrhea. The investigator's final conclusion was that IF was not inferior to CF and was somewhat less toxic.

Epirubicin, Cisplatin, and Fluorouracil (ECF). English investigators have extensively studied the three-drug combination ECF. Two random-assignment phase 3 trials have compared the ECF with a noncisplatin-containing combination (FAMTX) or with a mitomycin-cisplatin-fluorouracil (MCF) combination.[397] In the first study, ECF was more effective than FAMTX both in terms of response rate and for median survival (8.7 vs. 6.1 months). Two-year survival was also superior for the ECF combination (14% vs. 5%). In the second study, Ross et al.[397] compared ECF with mitomycin-cisplatin-fluorouracil (MCF). In this larger study, 574 patients were treated. The primary end point was 1-year survival. The overall objective response rates were similar between the two arms (ECF 49.6%, MCF 55.4%). Toxicity was tolerable, although myelosuppression was greater for the experimental MCF arm. There was a slightly better median duration of survival for ECF (9.4 vs. 8.7 months) and for 1-year survival (40% for ECF, 32% for MCF). There was no difference in 2-year survival, approximately 15% for both arms. Several studies have demonstrated that a small percentage of patients may have 2-year survival, even with advanced unresectable gastric cancer. Data for the ECF regimen as the control arm of the REAL-2 trial are discussed later.

Cisplatin Plus Irinotecan. Cisplatin is a commonly used agent in gastric cancer, and irinotecan has been combined with this drug as well as with other agents. In single-arm phase 2 studies, response rates were encouraging and toxicity was tolerable. This observation led to a somewhat larger random-assignment phase 2 trial comparing irinotecan-cisplatin (IC) with the IF regimen previously described.[396] Sixty-two patients received IF and 61 received IC. The dose schedule used for the IC arm was higher than that from earlier IC regimens. In this study, the response rate was higher for IF than for IC, as was the TTP. Although IC in the dose and schedule used in the random-assignment phase 2 trial previously described was less effective than IF, other investigators have pursued this regimen using different schedules. These studies have been performed in patients with esophageal, gastroesophageal, and gastric cancers. One IC regimen was used with bevacizumab.[398]

Fluorouracil-Leucovorin-Oxaliplatin. As is the case for irinotecan-containing regimens, oxaliplatin plus fluorouracil is a standard care option for patients with both metastatic and locally advanced colon cancer. In part because of this data, fluorouracil-leucovorin-oxaliplatin (FOLFOX) regimens have also been studied in gastric cancer. The toxicity spectrum is similar to that seen in patients with colorectal cancer, with the dose-limiting toxicity of peripheral neuropathy (oxaliplatin). Myelosuppression, mucositis, and diarrhea typical for fluorouracil regimens were noted as well. Several FOLFOX phase 2 studies have now been reported in gastric cancer. Overall response rates of approximately 50% were reported, with median TTP of 5 to 6 months and median overall survival of 10 to 12 months.[399]

The REAL-2 Trial

Partly on the basis of these studies, a phase 3 trial comparing an oxaliplatin-based regimen with cisplatin-containing combinations was performed. Cunningham et al.[400] in the REAL-2 trial studied 1,002 patients who were randomized to one of four treatment groups: a control arm of ECF and three investigational arms. The central questions in this study were whether capecitabine could be substituted for fluorouracil and/or oxaliplatin substituted for cisplatin. The four arms were ECF (epirubicin-cisplatin-fluorouracil), EOF (epirubicin-oxaliplatin-fluorouracil), ECX (epirubicin-cisplatin-capecitabine), and EOX (epirubicin-oxaliplatin-capecitabine). The four regimens are shown in Table 80.9. Patients were stratified for performance status and extent of disease. The primary end point was in survival. The study was powered to show noninferiority for capecitabine compared with fluorouracil and oxaliplatin compared with cisplatin. There were approximately 250 patients per arm. The study design was a two-by-two comparison. Forty percent of patients had primary gastric cancer, and the remainder had either EGJ or esophageal cancers, with 10% of patients having squamous cell cancer of the esophagus. There was no difference in median overall survival between the arms (ECF 9.9 months, EOF 9.3 months, ECX 9.9 months, and EOX 11.2 months). The 1-year overall survival was also similar and ranged from 37.7% to 46.8%, the best outcome being seen with EOX and the lowest with the control arm of ECF. The authors concluded the oxaliplatin could be substituted for cisplatin, and capecitabine could be substituted for fluorouracil in the palliative setting.

Al-Batran et al.[401] reported the results of a trial comparing a FOLFOX regimen with fluorouracil-leucovorin-cisplatin (FLP). A modified FOLFOX-6 schedule was used for the experimental arm. The FLP regimen used slightly lower doses

TABLE 80.9

REAL-2 REGIMENS

Drug	Dose (mg/m²)	Day(s)	Week(s)[a]
ECF			
Epirubicin	50 mg/m² IV	1	Every 3 weeks
Cisplatin	60 mg/m² IV	1	
PVI 5-FU	200 mg/m²/d[b]	1	
EOF			
Epirubicin	50 mg/m² IV	1	Every 3 weeks
Oxaliplatin	130 mg/m² IV	1	
PVI 5-FU	200 mg/m²/d[b]	1	
ECX			
Epirubicin	50 mg/m² IV	1	Every 3 weeks
Cisplatin	60 mg/m² IV	1	
Capecitabine	625 mg/m²/BID	1	
EOX			
Epirubicin	50 mg/m² IV	1	Every 3 weeks
Oxaliplatin	130 mg/m² IV	1	
Capecitabine	625 mg/m² BID	1	

IV, intravenously.
[a]Planned treatment duration 24 weeks (8 cycles).
[b]PVI 5-FU delivered by central venous access catheter.
(Modified from ref. 400.)

of fluorouracil and cisplatin (50 mg/m^2) every 2 weeks. The study was powered for superiority of FOLFOX over cisplatin-fluorouracil-leucovorin. Two hundred twenty patients were randomized between the two arms. There was no significant difference in TTP (*P* = .08) and overall survival, 10.7 (FLO) months versus 8.8 (FLP) months. Although this study did not demonstrate superiority for oxaliplatin-containing regimen, it does support the results of the REAL-2 study for noninferiority comparing oxaliplatin and cisplatin. The FOLFOX regimen was slightly less toxic.

Finally, Kang et al.[402] compared capecitabine plus cisplatin with CF. One hundred sixty patients received capecitabine plus cisplatin (XP) and 156 patients received CF. The XP arm was not inferior, with a median PFS of 5.6 months versus 5 months for CF. Overall survival was 10.5 versus 9.3 months for XP versus CF (HR, 0.85; 95% CI, 0.64 to 1.13; *P* = .008 vs. noninferiority margin of 1.25). The authors concluded that XP can be considered an effective alternative to CF.

It is of note that FOLFOX, FOLFIRI, and capecitabine-containing regimens are widely used in colon cancer. In metastatic colorectal cancer, the median TTP using these regimens is approximately 7 to 8 months and the median survival (even without the use of bevacizumab) is 20 to 21 months. The 1-year survival for patients with stage IV unresectable colon cancer is approximately 70%, and, using these regimens, 2-year survival approaches 40%. As shown earlier, the same regimens used in patients with gastric or EGJ tumors result in substantially shorter times to progression and substantially shorter median survivals. There are more classes of active cytotoxic agents with demonstrated activity in EGJ than there are for colon tumors. In upper gastrointestinal tract malignancies, oxaliplatin, cisplatin, fluorouracil, irinotecan, capecitabine, taxane, and anthracyclines have at least modest single-agent activity, whereas the taxanes and anthracyclines are inactive in colon cancer. These differences in efficacy outcomes suggest biological differences between these malignancies, despite the histologic similarities (e.g., "intestinal-type" gastric cancers).

As is the case for other solid tumors, an important area of investigation is the development of better preclinical models, such as murine models, and the identification of predictive and prognostic biomarkers which may well be different between gastrointestinal tumors arising in the upper and lower gastrointestinal tract. On the other hand, using targeted therapies, predictive markers may be the same in different cancers; for example, overexpression or amplification of *HER2* is a predictive marker for the use of trastuzumab in both breast and now gastric cancers. It is also possible that the use of continued cytotoxic treatment after progression of disease on the first treatment regimen in gastroesophageal cancers would lead to a similar outcome as seen in colon cancers. For example, in the REAL-2 trial, only 15% of patients received additional therapy at the time of progression of disease. The irinotecan versus best supportive care study described previously suggests that at least some patients will have a modest survival benefit to second-line treatment.

Targeted Therapy

The Epidermal Growth Factor Receptor Superfamily: Monoclonal Antibodies

Trastuzumab. Overexpression or amplification of *HER2 (EGFR2)* occurs in approximately 20% of patients with gastric cancer; it varies with the subtype. A phase 3 study of trastuzumab plus chemotherapy versus chemotherapy alone was performed in patients with overexpression of *HER2*. The preliminary results of the ToGA trial have been recently reported.[403] Among 3,807 patients, 594 patients had *HER2*-positive gastric cancer. They were randomized to receive either CF or CX given every 3 weeks for six cycles, or the same chemotherapy plus trastuzumab. The median overall survival was 13.5 months for patients receiving trastuzumab plus chemotherapy versus 11.1 months for those receiving chemotherapy alone (HR, 0.74; *P* = .0048). The response rate was 47% versus 35%, respectively. There was no significant difference in toxicity. Trastuzumab has been approved in Europe for *HER2*-positive gastric cancer. The ToGA trial used a *HER2* scoring system similar to that used in breast cancer. *HER2* was more likely to be positive in patients with EGJ tumors than in more distal tumors (33% vs. 20%); patients with diffuse gastric cancer were much less likely to have a positive *HER2* (6%).[404]

Cetuximab. Cetuximab is an antibody against the EGFR. In a trial combining cetuximab plus FUFOX (weekly infusions of oxaliplatin and fluorouracil, and DL-folinic acid), 46 patients with advanced gastric cancer were treated. Toxicity was tolerable; the response rate was 56%; however, overall survival was 9.5 months. K-Ras mutations were rare.[405]

The Epidermal Growth Factor Receptor Superfamily: Tyrosine Kinase Inhibitors

Lapatinib. Lapatinib is the first dual inhibitor of *HER1 (EGFR1)* and *HER2 (EGFR2)*. Two phase 2 trials have evaluated lapatinib monotherapy in patients with advanced gastric cancer. In one study, 3 of 46 patients had partial responses. In the second study, 21 patients with EGJ carcinomas were treated without objective responses.

Gefitinib and Erlotinib. Both are epidermal growth factor receptor tyrosine kinase inhibitors. In a large study, a 9% response rate was seen for EGJ tumors versus no responses among patients with gastric cancer; other studies have failed to demonstrate activity even in EGJ tumors.

The Vascular Endothelial Growth Factor Superfamily: Monoclonal Antibodies

Bevacizumab. Bevacizumab is a humanized monoclonal antibody that binds the vascular endothelial growth factor ligand (VEGF-A). In gastric cancer, Shah et al.[398] reported on combining cisplatin plus irinotecan with bevacizumab (phase 2). Among 47 patients, the median TTP was 9.9 months. This trial demonstrated a potential efficacy with acceptable toxicity; follow-up phase 2 trials also demonstrated acceptable toxicity.[407] The AVAGAST multinational phase 3 trial comparing bevacizumab plus cisplatin-capecitabine versus cisplatin-capecitabine alone has now completed accrual.[406,407a]

The Vascular Endothelial Growth Factor Superfamily: Tyrosine Kinase Inhibitors

Sunitinib. Sunitinib is an oral inhibitor of VEGFR-1, -2, -3, and PDGFR-α, -β, and c-kit. Bang et al.[408] reported on a phase 2 trial of sunitinib as second-line treatment for advanced gastric cancer. Response rate, PFS, and overall survival were 2 of 72, 11.1, and 47.7 weeks, respectively. Sorafenib is another multi–tyrosine kinase inhibitor (VEGFR-2, -3, PDGFR-β, Flt-3, Raf-1, and c-kit). The ECOG5203, a phase 2 trial investigating docetaxel plus cisplatin plus sorafenib in gastric cancer, suggested clinical efficacy (RR, 38.6%; PFS, 5.8 months; and overall survival, 15.9 months).[409]

Inhibition of Mammalian Target of Rapamycin (mTOR Protein Kinase)

Everolimus. An oral inhibitor of the mTOR has shown activity against gastric cancer in preclinical phase 1 studies.[410,411] Doi et al.[412] reported on a phase 2 trial testing everolimus in

PRACTICE OF ONCOLOGY

metastatic gastric cancer. In 53 patients, the disease control rate (complete response rate plus partial response plus stable disease [CR+PR+SD]) was 56%, and the median PFS and overall survival were 2.7 and 10.1 months, respectively.

In summary, new agents targeting dysregulated pathways are now undergoing study in gastric cancer. At the present time, trastuzumab remains the only drug of this type that has demonstrated efficacy, in combination with cytotoxic chemotherapy, in gastric cancer.

Predictive Markers and Early Assessment of Response in Gastric and Gastroesophageal Tumors

The recognition that several different classes of cytotoxic anticancer agents and targeted agents have activity in subgroups of patients suggests the possibility that predictive markers or a gene signature might allow "customized" treatment that will spare patients from unnecessary toxicity from ineffective therapy, such as testing for *HER2* identified patients who would benefit from trastuzumab. Molecular markers that might indicate resistance or sensitivity to fluorouracil and cisplatin are reviewed elsewhere in this book.[413] Ooi et al.[414] and other investigators[415–417] have used gene expression arrays to identify pathways and gene signatures to predicting clinical prognosis. Ott et al.[124] reported that a drop in SUV of 35% after neoadjuvant chemotherapy was associated with significant pathologic response. Similar findings were reported by Shah et al.[418] and Weber.[419] Overall, PET may allow early identification of patients responding to chemotherapy.

SURGERY IN TREATMENT OF METASTATIC GASTRIC CANCER

Given the recent improvements in systemic therapy for gastric cancer, the question whether resection of limited metastases from gastric cancer can result in survival benefit remains open. To ask this question in a scientific manner, the surgery branch in the National Institutes of Health/National Cancer Institute is currently accruing patients to a prospective RCT comparing gastrectomy, metastasectomy plus systemic therapy versus systemic therapy alone (the GYMSSA Trial, Clinical Trials.gov ID. NCT00941655).[420]

Kerkar et al.[420,421] reviewed the published data reporting on liver resection for gastric cancer; 19 studies reported on 436 patients. The majority of the patients had synchronous isolated liver gastric metastases. Overall, the 1-, 3-, and 5-year survival rates were 62%, 30%, and 26.5%, respectively; 13.4% (48/358) were alive at 5 years, and in studies with more than 10 years of follow-up, 4% (48/358) survived for more than 10 years.[420]

Standard of care for patients with pulmonary gastric metastases is chemotherapy with a median survival of 6 months.[423] Kemp et al.[424] reviewed the published data reporting on lung resections for gastric cancer; 21 studies reported on 43 patients. Eighty-two percent of patients (34/43) had a solitary lesion. At a median follow-up of 23 months, 15 of 43 (35%) patients had no evidence of disease. The overall 5-year survival was 33%.

Gastric carcinomatosis occurs in 5% to 50% of patients undergoing surgery with curative intent.[425–432] The median survival for such patients is 1.5 to 3.1 months.[425,433–435] Overall data are limited; however, several investigators reported on cytoreductive surgery (CRC) plus HIPEC for gastric carcinomatosis; the median survival ranged from 6 to 21 months, 5-year survival ranged from 6% to 16% with 2% to 7.1% mortality. In patients with CCR-0/1 (no macroscopic or disease <5 mm), the 5-year survival was 16% to 30%. Complete cytoreduction was possible in only 44% to 51% of the patients.[342,443–447] In 2008 the Fifth International Workshop on Peritoneal Surface Malignancy indicated that peritonectomy, intraoperative and early postoperative hyperthermic intraperitoneal chemotherapy, potentially can be a powerful therapy against gastric cancer peritoneal carcinomatosis.[448–453]

Surgery for Palliation

Because the survival for patients with advanced gastric cancer is poor, any proposed operation should have a good chance of providing sustained symptomatic relief while minimizing the attendant morbidity and need for prolonged hospitalization. Ekbom and Gleysteen[454] have reviewed the results of palliative resection versus intestinal bypass (gastrojejunostomy) in 75 patients with advanced gastric cancer. The most frequent symptoms for which patients underwent operation included pain, hemorrhage, nausea, dysphasia, or obstruction. Operative mortality was 25% for gastrojejunostomy, 20% for palliative partial or subtotal gastrectomy, and 27% for total or proximal palliative gastrectomy. The most common and often fatal complication was anastomotic leak. After gastrojejunostomy, 80% of patients had relief of symptoms for a mean of 5.9 months compared with palliative resection, which provided relief of symptoms in 88% of patients for a mean of 14.6 months. Although the duration of palliation was significantly longer after resection (P <.01), the selection criteria for resection versus bypass were not controlled, and some bias against performing a palliative resection in high-risk patients with more advanced disease may have occurred. Meijer et al.[455] also reported on a retrospective analysis of 51 patients undergoing either palliative intestinal bypass or resection. In 20 of 26 patients (77%) undergoing resection, palliation was considered moderate to good with a mean survival of 9.5 months. After gastroenterostomy, some palliation was noted in 8 of 25 patients (30%), and survival was 4.2 months. Butler et al.[456] have presented the results of total gastrectomy for palliation in 27 patients with advanced gastric cancer. Operative mortality was only 4%, whereas morbidity occurred in 48% of patients. Median survival was 15 months, with a survival rate of 38% at 2 years. This substantial survival rate at 2 years reflects that, although all patients were symptomatic before surgery, only half had stage IV disease. Patients with linitis plastica present a very difficult therapeutic challenge. Resection may provide palliation of symptoms; however, survival after total gastrectomy is exceedingly poor, ranging from 3 months to 1 year.

Bozzetti et al.[457,458] have reviewed the outcomes of 246 patients with advanced gastric cancer who underwent simple exploratory laparotomy alone, gastrointestinal bypass, or palliative resection at the National Cancer Institute of Milan. When survival was compared in patients with similar type and extent of disease, a consistent trend was seen for improved median survival with palliative resection in patients with local spread (4.4 vs. 8 months) and distant spread of disease (3 vs. 8 months). Boddie et al.[459] have reported similar results in 45 patients undergoing palliative resection at the M. D. Anderson Cancer Center for advanced gastric cancer. Operative mortality for resection was 22%. In 21 patients who had undergone a palliative bypass procedure, survival was significantly shorter than for those undergoing resection (P <.01).

In select patients with symptomatic advanced gastric cancer, resection of the primary disease appears to provide symptomatic relief with acceptable morbidity and mortality, even in the presence of macroscopic residual disease.

RADIATION FOR PALLIATION

To date, no studies have evaluated the use of radiation therapy in patients with locally recurrent or metastatic carcinoma of the stomach. Its use is likely to be limited to palliation of symptoms such as bleeding or controlling pain secondary to local tumor infiltration. Although minimal data are available, radiation therapy seems to be anecdoticly effective in controlling bleeding, as is true in other sites. Pain from local tumor invasion can also be palliated. On rare occasions, a case may arise of a patient with a focal local recurrence without metastases who would be amenable to relatively high-dose radiation therapy to try to prolong survival or in whom radiation therapy would be given as an adjuvant to surgical resection. At present, however, no data support such an approach.

Selected References

The full list of references for this chapter appears in the online version.

3. Anderson WFC, Fraumeni FJ, Rosenberg PS, Rabkin CS. Age-specific trends in incidence of noncardia gastric cancer in US adults. *JAMA* 2010;303(17):1723.
36. Laurén P. The Two histological main types of gastric carcinoma: diffuse and so-called intestinal-type carcinoma: an attempt at a histo-clinical classification. *Acta Pathol Microbiol Scand* 1965;64:31.
94. Rugge M, Kim JG, Mahachai V, et al. OLGA gastritis staging in young adults and country-specific gastric cancer risk. *Int J Surg Pathol* 2008;16(2):150.
113. Bentrem D, Gerdes H, Tang L, et al. Clinical correlation of endoscopic ultrasonography with pathologic stage and outcome in patients undergoing curative resection for gastric cancer. *Ann Surg Oncol* 2007;14(6):1853.
124. Ott K, Fink U, Becker K, et al. Prediction of response to preoperative chemotherapy in gastric carcinoma by metabolic imaging: results of a prospective trial. *J Clin Oncol* 2003;21(24):4604.
125. Lordick F, Ott K, Krause BJ, et al. PET to assess early metabolic response and to guide treatment of adenocarcinoma of the oesophagogastric junction: the MUNICON phase II trial. *Lancet Oncol* 2007;8(9):797.
129. Conlon KC. Staging laparoscopy for gastric cancer. *Ann Ital Chir* 2001;72(1):33.
143. Edge SB, Compton CC. The American Joint Committee on Cancer: the 7th edition of the AJCC Cancer Staging Manual and the future of TNM. *Ann Surg Oncol* 2010;17(6):1471.
144. Karpeh MS, Leon L, Klimstra D, et al. Lymph node staging in gastric cancer: is location more important than Number? An analysis of 1,038 patients. *Ann Surg* 2000;232(3):362.
145. Smith DD, Schwarz RR, Schwarz RE. Impact of total lymph node count on staging and survival after gastrectomy for gastric cancer: data from a large US-population database. *J Clin Oncol* 2005;23(28):7114.
148. Kattan MW, Karpeh MS, Mazumdar M, et al. Postoperative nomogram for disease-specific survival after an R0 resection for gastric carcinoma. *J Clin Oncol* 2003;21(19):3647.
159. Kurihara M, Aiko T. The new Japanese classification of gastric carcinoma: revised explanation of "response assessment of chemotherapy and radiotherapy for gastric carcinoma." *Gastric Cancer* 2001;4(1):9.
165. Siewert JR, Stein HJ. Classification of adenocarcinoma of the oesophagogastric junction. *Br J Surg* 1998;85(11):1457.
183. Bennett C, Wang Y, Pan T. Endoscopic mucosal resection for early gastric cancer. *Cochrane Database Syst Rev* 2009(4):CD004276.
211. Robertson CS, Chung SC, Woods SD, et al. A prospective randomized trial comparing R1 subtotal gastrectomy with R3 total gastrectomy for antral cancer. *Ann Surg* 1994;220(2):176.
212. Bozzetti F, Marubini E, Bonfanti G, et al. Subtotal versus total gastrectomy for gastric cancer: five-year survival rates in a multicenter randomized Italian trial. Italian Gastrointestinal Tumor Study Group. *Ann Surg* 1999;230(2):170.
213. Hulscher JB, van Sandick JW, de Boer AG, et al. Extended transthoracic resection compared with limited transhiatal resection for adenocarcinoma of the esophagus. *N Engl J Med* 2002;347(21):1662.
216. Kodera Y, Schwarz RE, Nakao A. Extended lymph node dissection in gastric carcinoma: where do we stand after the Dutch and British randomized trials? *J Am Coll Surg* 2002;195(6):855.
232. Dent DM, Madden MV, Price SK. Randomized comparison of R1 and R2 gastrectomy for gastric carcinoma. *Br J Surg* 1988;75(2):110.
233. Cuschieri A, Weeden S, Fielding J, et al. Patient survival after D1 and D2 resections for gastric cancer: long-term results of the MRC randomized surgical trial. Surgical Co-operative Group. *Br J Cancer* 1999;79(9-10):1522.
234. Bonenkamp JJ, Hermans J, Sasako M, et al. Extended lymph-node dissection for gastric cancer. *N Engl J Med* 1999;340(12):908.
235. Degiuli M, Sasako M, Calgaro M, et al. Morbidity and mortality after D1 and D2 gastrectomy for cancer: interim analysis of the Italian Gastric Cancer Study Group (IGCSG) randomised surgical trial. *Eur J Surg Oncol* 2004;30(3):303.
236. Wu CW, Hsiung CA, Lo SS, et al. Nodal dissection for patients with gastric cancer: a randomised controlled trial. *Lancet Oncol* 2006;7(4):309.
239. Songun I, Putter H, Kranenbarg EM, et al. Surgical treatment of gastric cancer: 15-year follow-up results of the randomised nationwide Dutch D1D2 trial. *Lancet Oncol* 2010;11(5):439.
240. Bonenkamp JJ, Hermans J, Sasako M, et al. Quality control of lymph node dissection in the Dutch randomized trial of D1 and D2 lymph node dissection for gastric cancer. *Gastric Cancer* 1998;1(2):152.
242. Bonenkamp JJ, Songun I, Hermans J, et al. Randomised comparison of morbidity after D1 and D2 dissection for gastric cancer in 996 Dutch patients. *Lancet* 1995;345(8952):745.
245. Chen XZ, Hu JK, Zhou ZG, et al. Meta-analysis of effectiveness and safety of D2 plus para-aortic lymphadenectomy for resectable gastric cancer. *J Am Coll Surg* 2010(1):100.
247. Brennan MF. Lymph-node dissection for gastric cancer. *N Engl J Med* 1999;340(12):956.
250. Yonemura Y, Wu CC, Fukushima N, et al. Randomized clinical trial of D2 and extended paraaortic lymphadenectomy in patients with gastric cancer. *Int J Clin Oncol* 2008;13(2):132.
255. Doglietto GB, Pacelli F, Caprino P, et al. Pancreas-preserving total gastrectomy for gastric cancer. *Arch Surg* 2000;135(1):89.
259. Yao XX, Yan C, Yan M, et al. [A comparative study on the efficacy of spleen-preserving modified D2 radical gastrectomy and D2 radical gastrectomy with splenectomy]. *Zhonghua Wei Chang Wai Ke Za Zhi* 2010;13(2):111.
269. Hundahl SA, Macdonald JS, Benedetti J, et al. Surgical treatment variation in a prospective, randomized trial of chemoradiotherapy in gastric cancer: the effect of undertreatment. *Ann Surg Oncol* 2002;9(3):278.
328. Sakuramoto S, Sasako M, Yamaguchi T, et al. Adjuvant chemotherapy for gastric cancer with S-1, an oral fluoropyrimidine. *N Engl J Med* 2007;357(18):1810.
329. Di Costanzo F, Gasperoni S, Manzione L, et al. Adjuvant chemotherapy in completely resected gastric cancer: a randomized phase III trial conducted by GOIRC. *J Natl Cancer Inst* 2008;100(6):388.
330. Buyse ME, Pignon J. Meta-analyses of randomized trials assessing the interest of postoperative adjuvant chemotherapy and prognsotic factors in gastric cancer. *J Clin Oncol* 2009;27(15s):4539.
331. Paoletti X, Oba K, Burzykowski T, et al. Benefit of adjuvant chemotherapy for resectable gastric cancer: a meta-analysis. *JAMA* 303(17):1729.
346. Kelsen D, Karpeh M, Schwartz G, et al. Neoadjuvant therapy of high-risk gastric cancer: a phase II trial of preoperative FAMTX and postoperative intraperitoneal fluorouracil-cisplatin plus intravenous fluorouracil. *J Clin Oncol* 1996;14(6):1818.
347. Brenner B, Shah MA, Karpeh MS, et al. A phase II trial of neoadjuvant cisplatin-fluorouracil followed by postoperative intraperitoneal floxuridine-leucovorin in patients with locally advanced gastric cancer. *Ann Oncol* 2006;17(9):1404.
348. Downey RJ, Akhurst T, Ilson D, et al. Whole body 18FDG-PET and the response of esophageal cancer to induction therapy: results of a prospective trial. *J Clin Oncol* 2003;21(3):428.
351. Allum WH, Hallissey MT, Ward LC, et al. A controlled, prospective, randomised trial of adjuvant chemotherapy or radiotherapy in resectable gastric cancer: interim report. British Stomach Cancer Group. *Br J Cancer* 1989;60(5):739.
352. Hallissey MT, Dunn JA, Ward LC, et al. The second British Stomach Cancer Group trial of adjuvant radiotherapy or chemotherapy in resectable gastric cancer: five-year follow-up. *Lancet* 1994;343(8909):1309.
353. Zhang ZX, Gu XZ, Yin WB, et al. Randomized clinical trial on the combination of preoperative irradiation and surgery in the treatment of adenocarcinoma of gastric cardia (AGC)—report on 370 patients. *Int J Radiat Oncol Biol Phys* 1998;42(5):929.
354. Gunderson L, Willet G, Harrisson B, eds., et al. *Intraoperative Irradiation: Techniques and Results*. Totowa, NJ: Humana Press, 1999.
355. Abe M, Takahashi M, Ono K, et al. Japan gastric trials in intraoperative radiation therapy. *Int J Radiat Oncol Biol Phys* 1988;15(6):1431.
356. Sindelar WF, Kinsella TJ, Tepper JE, et al. Randomized trial of intraoperative radiotherapy in carcinoma of the stomach. *Am J Surg* 1993;165(1):178; discussion 186.
359. Macdonald JS, Smalley SR, Benedetti J, et al. Chemoradiotherapy after surgery compared with surgery alone for adenocarcinoma of the stomach or gastroesophageal junction. *N Engl J Med* 2001;345(10):725.
360. Walsh, TN, Noonan N, Hollywood D, et al. A comparison of multimodal therapy and surgery for esophageal adenocarcinoma. *N Engl J Med* 1996;335(7):462.
361. Tepper J, Krasna MJ, Niedzwiecki D, et al. Phase III trial of trimodality therapy with cisplatin, fluorouracil, radiotherapy, and surgery compared

with surgery alone for esophageal cancer: CALGB 9781. *J Clin Oncol* 2008;26(7):1086.
385. Wagner, AD, Unverzagt S, Grothe W, et al. Chemo therapy for advanced cancer. *Cochrane Database Syst Rev* 2010(3):CD004064.
386. Thuss-Patience PC, Kretzschmar A, Deist T, et al. Irinotecan versus best supportive care (BSC) as second-line therapy in gastric cancer: a randomized phase III study of the Arbeitsgemeinschaft Internistische Onkologie (AIO). *J Clin Oncol* 2009;27(15s):abstract 4540.
387. Okines AF, Norman AR, McCloud P, et al. Meta-analysis of the REAL-2 and ML17032 trials: evaluating capecitabine-based combination chemotherapy and infused 5-fluorouracil-based combination chemotherapy for the treatment of advanced oesophago-gastric cancer. *Ann Oncol* 2009;20(9):1529.
388. Di Cosimo S, Ferretti G, Fazio N, et al. Docetaxel in advanced gastric cancer—review of the main clinical trials. *Acta Oncol* 2003;42(7):693.
389. Vanhoefer U, Rougier P, Wilke H, et al. Final results of a randomized phase III trial of sequential high-dose methotrexate, fluorouracil, and doxorubicin versus etoposide, leucovorin, and fluorouracil versus infusional fluorouracil and cisplatin in advanced gastric cancer: a trial of the European Organization for Research and Treatment of Cancer Gastrointestinal Tract Cancer Cooperative Group. *J Clin Oncol* 2000;18(14):2648.
390. Ohtsu A, Shimada Y, Shirao K, et al. Randomized phase III trial of fluorouracil alone versus fluorouracil plus cisplatin versus uracil and tegafur plus mitomycin in patients with unresectable, advanced gastric cancer: the Japan Clinical Oncology Group Study (JCOG9205). *J Clin Oncol* 2003;21(1):54.
391. Van Cutsem E, Moiseyenko VM, Tjulandin S, et al. Phase III study of docetaxel and cisplatin plus fluorouracil compared with cisplatin and fluorouracil as first-line therapy for advanced gastric cancer: a report of the V325 Study Group. *J Clin Oncol* 2006;24(31):4991.
392. Dank M, Zaluski J, Barone C, et al. Randomized phase III study comparing irinotecan combined with 5-fluorouracil and folinic acid to cisplatin combined with 5-fluorouracil in chemotherapy naive patients with advanced adenocarcinoma of the stomach or esophagogastric junction. *Ann Oncol* 2008;19(8):1450.
393. Kang Y-K, Kang WK, Shin DB, et al. Capecitabine/cisplatin versus 5-fluorouracil/cisplatin as first-line therapy in patients with advanced gastric cancer: a randomised phase III noninferiority trial. *Ann Oncol* 2009;20(4):666.
395. Shah MA, Stoller R, Shibata S, et al. Random assignment multicenter phase II study of modified docetaxel, sisplatin, flourouracil (mDCF) versus DCF with growth factor support (GCSF) in metastatic gastroesophageal adenocarcinoma (GE). Poster session A Cancers of Esophagu and stomach abstract:46 *J Clin Oncol* 2010;28.
396. Pozzo C, Barone C, Szanto J, et al. Irinotecan in combination with 5-fluorouracil and folinic acid or with cisplatin in patients with advanced gastric or esophageal-gastric junction adenocarcinoma: results of a randomized phase II study. *Ann Oncol* 2004;15(12):1773.
397. Ross P, Nicolson M, Cunningham D, et al. Prospective randomized trial comparing mitomycin, cisplatin, and protracted venous-infusion fluorouracil (PVI 5-FU) with epirubicin, cisplatin, and PVI 5-FU in advanced esophagogastric cancer. *J Clin Oncol* 2002;20(8):1996.
398. Shah MA, Ramanathan RK, Ilson DH, et al. Multicenter phase II study of irinotecan, cisplatin, and bevacizumab in patients with metastatic gastric or gastroesophageal junction adenocarcinoma. *J Clin Oncol* 2006;24(33):5201.
399. Nardi M, Azzarello D, Maisano R, et al. FOLFOX-4 regimen as first-line chemotherapy in elderly patients with advanced gastric cancer: a safety study. *J Chemother* 2007;19(1):85.
400. Cunningham D, Okines AF, Ashley S, et al. Capecitabine and oxaliplatin for advanced esophagogastric cancer. *N Engl J Med* 2008;358(1):36.
401. Al-Batran SE, et al. Phase III trial in metastatic gastroesophageal adenocarcinoma with fluorouracil, leucovorin plus either oxaliplatin or cisplatin: a study of the Arbeitsgemeinschaft Internistische Onkologie. *J Clin Oncol* 2008;26(9):1435.
402. Kang YK, Hartmann JT, Probst S, et al. Capecitabine/cisplatin versus 5-fluorouracil/cisplatin as first-line therapy in patients with advanced gastric cancer: a randomised phase III noninferiority trial. *Ann Oncol* 2009; 20(4):666.
403. Van Cutsam E, Kang Y, Chung H, et al. Efficacy results from the ToGA trial: a phase III study of trastuzumab added to standard chemotherapy (CT) in first-line human epidermal growth factor receptor 2 (HER2)-positive advanced cancer (GC). *J Clin Oncol* 2009;27(18 Suppl): abstract LBA450.
404. Bang Y, Chung H, Sawaki A, et al. HER2-positivity rates in advanced gastric cancer (GC): results from a large international phase III trial. *J Clin Oncol* 2008;26(15S): abstract 4526.
405. Lordick F, Luber B, Lorenzen S, et al. Cetuximab plus oxaliplatin/leucovorin/5-fluorouracil in first-line metastatic gastric cancer: a phase II study of the Arbeitsgemeinschaft Internistische Onkologie (AIO). *Br J Cancer* 2010;102(3):500.

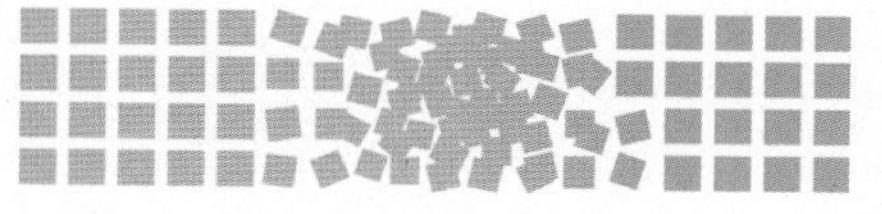

CHAPTER 81 MOLECULAR BIOLOGY OF PANCREAS CANCER

SCOTT E. KERN AND RALPH H. HRUBAN

Pancreatic ductal adenocarcinoma is a genetic disease. This perspective is supported by reproducible patterns of genetic mutations that accumulate during tumorigenesis. These patterns indicate the operation of a selective process favoring the emergence of specific constellations of genetic changes. Individuals who inherit a mutant form of certain genes have an increased risk of developing pancreatic cancer. According to this genetic theory, most pancreatic cancers share a common foundation of genetic mutations disrupting specific cellular regulatory controls. These shared abnormalities are responsible for the processes of growth, invasion, and metastasis in individual patients.

Four categories of mutated genes play a role in the pancreatic tumorigenesis: oncogenes, tumor-suppressor genes, genome-maintenance genes, and tissue-maintenance genes (summarized in Table 81.1). Some of these mutations are germ line, for example, they are transmitted within a family. Genetic mutations acquired during life, termed *somatic mutations*, contribute to tumorigenesis within a tissue but are not passed to offspring.

Very recently, techniques were developed to sequence all of the genes of individual cancers. Whole-exomic sequencing of pancreatic ductal cancers revealed an average of 63 somatic mutations per tumor.[1] Most of these mutations undoubtedly were nonfunctional "passenger" mutations, each mutated at a low frequency and not contributing to tumorigenesis. Indeed, most passenger mutations might arise as a normal aspect of tissue aging before tumorigenesis begins.[2] Smoking is associated with a doubling of the risk for pancreatic cancer, and remarkably is also associated with a 40% increase of the prevalence of low-frequency mutations in the cancers.[3] A subset of the mutations, however, is responsible for "driving" the neoplastic process in the ducts and is the focus here.

Telomere abnormalities and signs of chromosome instability are the most common alterations in pancreatic neoplasia. Four genes are mutated in most pancreatic cancers: the *KRAS*, *p16/CDKN2A*, *TP53*, and *SMAD4* genes. Other genetic abnormalities are seen at a much lower frequency, including mutations in the genes *BRCA2*, *PALB2*, *FANCC*, *FANCG*, *FBXW7*, *BAX*, *RB1*, the TGFβ (transforming growth factor-beta) receptors *TGFBR1* and *TGFBR2*, the activin receptors *ACVR1B* and *ACVR2*, *MKK4*, *STK11*, *GUCY2F*, *NTRK3*, *EGFR*, and cationic trypsinogen, alterations in the mitochondrial genome, amplifications, various chromosomal deletions, inactivation of DNA mismatch-repair genes, and rarely the presence of the Epstein-Barr virus genome as an episome.

Knowing the genes mutated in a cancer can have direct clinical impact. For example, many cancers occur from an inherited mutation, and these patients and their families could benefit from genetic counseling.[4–7] A distinct morphologic subtype of pancreatic cancer, the medullary cancer, can suggest such an inherited mutation.[8,9] Another example includes the analysis of the genetic alterations in precursors to invasive pancreatic neoplasia, which has indicated that most carcinomas arise by a process of progressive intraductal tumorigenesis.[10] Epigenetic changes in DNA methylation and in gene expression are also highly specific for the cancerous cells and can serve as diagnostic markers.

COMMON MOLECULAR CHANGES

Telomere shortening is the earliest and most prevalent genetic change identified in the precursor lesions.[11] Telomere shortening is thought to predispose to chromosome fusion (translocations) and the mis-segregation of genetic material during mitosis.[12] Later during tumorigenesis, telomerase is reactivated,[13,14] moderating the telomere erosive process while permitting continued chromosomal instability.[15]

The *KRAS* gene mediates signals from growth factor receptors and other signaling inputs (Fig. 81.1). The mutations convert the normal Kras protein (a protooncogene) to an oncogene, causing the protein to become overactive in transmitting the growth factor-initiated signals.[16] *KRAS* is mutated in over 90% of conventional pancreatic ductal carcinomas.[17] The first genetic change in the ducts is probably not (or not always) a *KRAS* gene mutation, for the prevalence of this mutation is highest in the more advanced lesions (Table 81.1).[18,19] *KRAS* is one of a family of *RAS* genes that can harbor mutations in human cancers. The other *RAS* genes include *NRAS* and *HRAS*, although it is possible that only *KRAS* is mutated in pancreatic carcinomas.

As one of the most commonly mutated genes in pancreatic cancer, Ras is an attractive target for the development of gene-specific therapies, and an understanding of the normal biology of the Ras protein should help in the development of these Ras targeted therapies. The Ras proteins require an attachment to the plasma membrane for activity. For many proteins, including Ras, a hydrophobic prenyl group is essential for the attachment. Either farnesyl (15-carbon) or geranylgeranyl (20-carbon) makes a covalent thioether linkage at a cysteine residue located near the C-terminal end of Ras proteins, termed the *CAAX motif*. Working mostly in artificial legacy models of the *HRAS* oncogene (rather than the more widely available but experimentally less tractable natural *KRAS*-mutant cancer cell lines), the farnesylation reaction was readily inhibited by various means; in these models, the Ras protein was rendered inactive and often accompanied by cytotoxicity limited to the mutant cells.

Although many types of compounds capable of blocking the farnesyltransferase enzyme were developed as drugs, they have not been successful anticancer agents. There are many reasons for this. Although Hras protein is linked predominantly through farnesyl groups, the Kras protein can be alternately prenylated by geranylgeranyl linkages. Unfortunately,

TABLE 81.1

GENETIC PROFILE OF PANCREATIC CARCINOMA

Gene	Gene Locations	Frequency in Cancers (%)	Timing During Tumorigenesis[a]	Mutation Origin
Oncogenes				
KRAS	12p	95	Early-mid	Som.
BRAF	7q	4		Som.
AKT2	19q	10–20		Som.
GUCY2F		3		Som.
NTRK3		1		Som.
EGFR		1		Som.
EBV genome		<1		
Tumor Suppressors/ Genome-Maintenance Genes				
p16	9p	>90	Mid-late	Som. > Germ.
TP53	17p	75	Late	Som.
SMAD4	18q	55	Late	Som.
BRCA2/PALB2	13q/16p	8	Late	Germ. > Som.
FANCC/FANCG	9q/9p	3		Germ. or Som.
MAP2K4	17p	4		Som.
LKB1/STK11	19p	4		Som. > Germ.
ACVR1B	12q	2		Som.
TGFBR1	9q	1		Som.[b]
MSI⁻/TGFBR2	3p	1		Som.[b]
MSI⁺/TGFBR2	3p	4		Som. > Germ.[c]
ACVR2	2q	4		Som. > Germ.[c]
BAX	19q	4		Som. > Germ.[c]
MLH1	3p	4		Som. > Germ.[c]
FBXW7/Cyclin E dereg.	4q	6		Som.[d]
Tissue-Maintenance Genes				
PRSS1	7q	<1	Prior	Germ.

Som., (prevalence of) somatic mutation or methylation; Germ., (prevalence of) germ line mutation.
[a]Stage of appearance of the genetic changes during the intraductal precursor phase of the neoplasm, where known. For *BRCA2*, most mutations are inherited, but the loss of the second allele is reported only in a single advanced pancreatic intraepithelial neoplasm.
[b]Single examples of homozygous deletion of the *TGFBR1* gene and *TGFBR2* gene have been identified in MSI-negative pancreatic cancer.
[c]In MSI-positive tumors, the mismatch repair defect is usually somatic in origin; the *TGFBR2*, *ACVR2*, and *BAX* alterations are somatic.
[d]A single example of homozygous mutation of the *FBXW7* gene is reported in a series having a 6% prevalence of cyclin E overexpression. Cyclin E amplification is reported to date only in cell lines.

the latter type of linkage is thought to be critical for a wider number of cellular proteins, and for fear of excessive toxicity, geranylgeranyl linkages have not usually been considered as an attractive drug target. Kras protein also appears to bind more tightly than Hras to the farnesyltransferase enzyme, requiring higher drug concentrations.[16] Additionally, the artificial models usually employed the engineered overexpression of the Ras protein, a situation in which the unattached Ras proteins would serve as a dominant-negative inhibitor, binding the necessary interacting proteins and sequestering them in

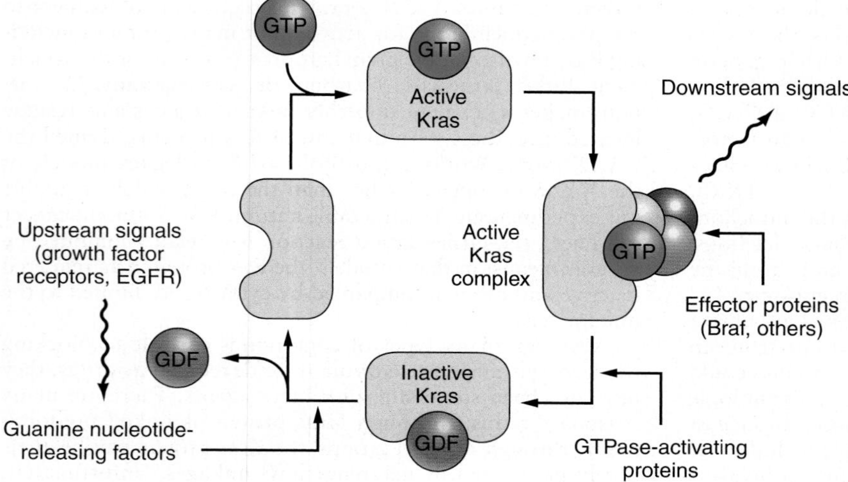

FIGURE 81.1 The *KRAS* pathway. *KRAS* normally integrates and regulates signals arising in the growth factor receptors that are passed to *KRAS* using the Grb2 and the Sos1 nucleotide exchange factor. The active GTP-bound form of *KRAS* recruits effector proteins such as Raf1 and Braf, in turn stimulating the downstream mitogen-activated protein kinases such as MEK and ERK and activating certain transcription factors. The EGF receptor can be overexpressed and occasionally mutated to provide inappropriately strong upstream signals, and the BRAF protein can be activated by point mutation, but more often in pancreatic cancer the Kras protein is mutated. These latter mutations impair the GAP (GTPase-activating protein)-stimulated reaction that normally returns Kras to the inactive state.

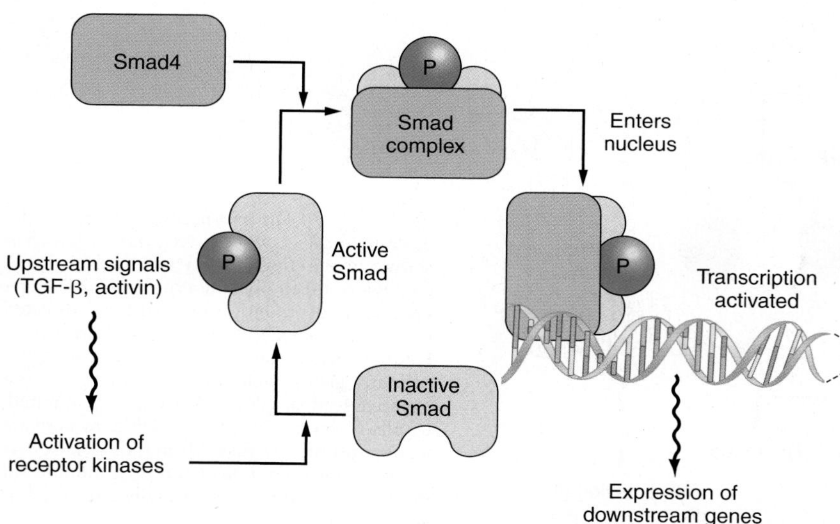

FIGURE 81.2 The transforming growth factor-beta (TGFβ)/Activin/Smad pathway. Dimeric kinase receptors of the TGFβ superfamily respond to extracellular ligands, causing phosphorylation of one or more of the receptor-associated Smad proteins and leading them to complex with the unphosphorylated common Smad, Smad4. This complex binds to specific DNA sequences and works with other transcription factors to stimulate gene expression. Mutations in pancreatic cancer can inactivate either partner of the dimeric receptors that respond to extracellular TGFβ or activin. More commonly, however, mutations and large deletions in the *SMAD4* gene destabilize its protein product or ablate gene expression.

the cytoplasm to ensure the inactivation of all three Ras pathways. Such a concentration-driven mechanism would presumably not occur under the normal levels of Ras proteins present in human cancers.[20] Indeed, it is proposed that the limited efficacy of farnesyltransferase inhibitors observed in some experimental models and in clinical trials may be attributable to a cellular target not yet identified.[21] Attention has turned to compounds that target the downstream mediators, such as Raf and Mek protein kinase inhibitors.

The Smad pathway mediates signals initiated on the binding of the extracellular proteins TGFβ and activin to their receptors (Fig. 81.2). These signals are transmitted to the nucleus by the Smad family of related genes, including *SMAD4 (DPC4)*.[22] Smad protein complexes bind specific recognition sites on DNA and cause the transcription of certain genes.[23] Mutations in the *SMAD4* gene are found in nearly half of pancreatic carcinomas, including both homozygous deletions and intragenic mutations combined with loss of heterozygosity (LOH).[24] Other Smad genes are also mutated occasionally.[1]

Homozygous deletions and mutation/LOH affecting the *TGFβ* receptor genes are seen in a few pancreatic cancers.[25] A more common abnormality, in pancreatic as well as in other tumor types, is the underexpression of TGFβ receptors, which results in cellular resistance to the usual suppressive effects of the TGFβ ligand.[26]

The *p16/RB1* pathway is a key control of the cell division cycle (Fig. 81.3). The retinoblastoma protein (Rb1) is a transcriptional regulator and regulates the entry of cells into S phase. A complex of cyclin D and a cyclin-dependent kinase (Cdk4 and Cdk6) phosphorylates and thereby regulates Rb1. The p16 protein is a Cdk-inhibitor that binds Cdk4 and Cdk6.[27–29] Virtually all pancreatic carcinomas suffer a loss of *p16* function, through homozygous deletions, mutation/LOH, or promoter methylation of the *p16/CDKN2A* gene associated

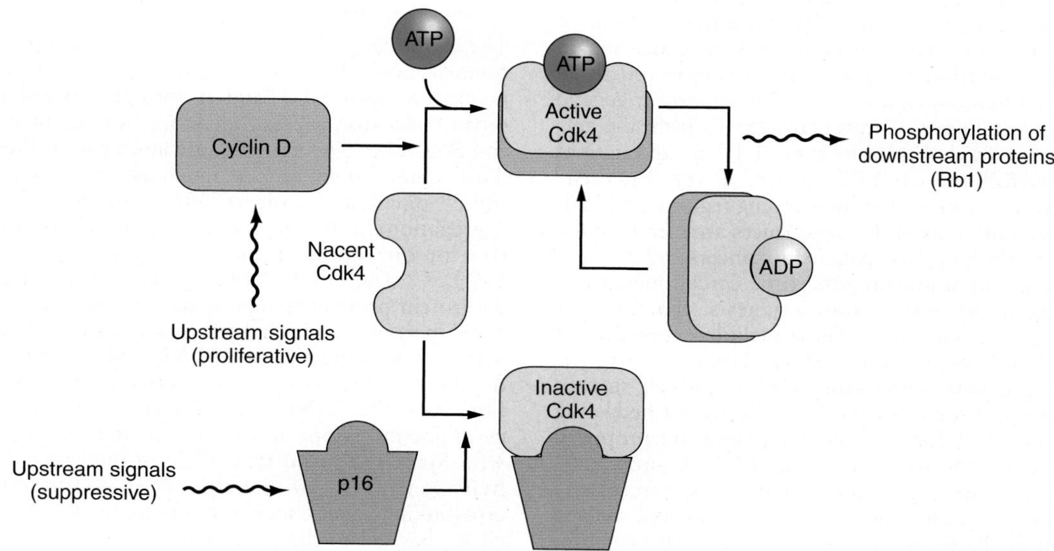

FIGURE 81.3 The *p16/RB1* pathway. *p16* binds to, inhibits, and thereby controls the availability of the cyclin-dependent kinases Cdk4 and Cdk6 (not shown). When activated by binding to cyclin D, these kinases phosphorylate and thereby inactivate the Rb1 tumor suppressor protein. The activity of *p16* is controlled in a complex manner, through changes in gene expression and by displacement reactions involving other similar kinase inhibitor proteins. *p16* mutations and deletions are nearly ubiquitous in pancreatic cancer, resulting in dysregulation of these cyclin-dependent kinases that regulate the cell division cycle.

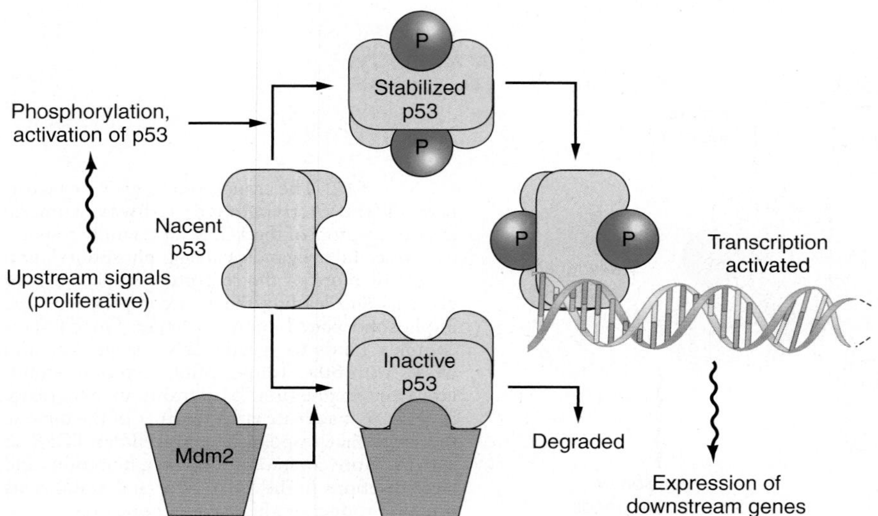

FIGURE 81.4 The *p53* pathway. Many modes of control affect *p53* activity, one of which is shown in the diagram. Stresses such as DNA damage result in phosphorylation of *p53*, preventing its degradation by an Mdm2-directed pathway. When stabilized, *p53* binds to specific DNA sequences and activates the transcription of many genes, including Mdm2 as part of a negative feedback loop. When *p53* is mutated, it fails to bind effectively to DNA to activate transcription. Because Mdm2 then lacks its transcriptional stimulus from *p53*, mutant but inactive p53 proteins are usually expressed at very high levels.

with a lack of gene expression.[30,31] In addition, inherited mutations of the *p16/CDKN2A* gene cause a familial melanoma/pancreatic cancer syndrome known as familial atypical multiple mole melanoma.[32–36] Occasional pancreatic cancers have inactivating mutations of the *RB1* gene.[37]

The protein product of the *TP53* gene binds to specific sites of DNA and activates the transcription of certain genes that control the cell division cycle and apoptosis.[38,39] Tp53 protein, normally a short-lived protein, becomes phosphorylated and stabilized after DNA damage and other cellular stresses (Fig. 81.4). In about 75% of pancreatic cancers the *TP53* gene has point mutations that inhibit the ability of p53 to bind DNA, or occasionally other types of inactivating mutation.[40–42]

Most human carcinomas have chromosomal instability (CIN), which produces changes in chromosomal copy numbers or aneuploidy.[43] Most pancreatic cancers have complex karyotypes including deletions of whole chromosomes and subchromosomal regions.[44–46] CIN is the process that causes most of the tumor deletions (LOH).[47] A few percent of pancreatic carcinomas, however, do not have significant gross or numerical chromosomal changes and instead have a different form of genetic instability; they have defects in DNA mismatch repair, producing high mutation rates at sites of simple repetitive sequences termed *microsatellites*.[8,9,48–51] The pattern of genetic damage in these carcinomas differs considerably from the pattern in carcinomas with CIN. The type II TGFβ and activin receptors (*TGFBR2*) and (*ACVR2*), as well as the *BAX* gene have a repetitive sequence within their coding regions, and biallelic inactivating mutations of these sequences are seen in many microsatellite instability (MIN) pancreatic cancers.[25,51–54]

There are also alterations in pancreatic carcinomas, some probably being important to tumorigenesis, that are not attributed to genetic mutations. These include expression of telomerase,[13,14] underexpression of TGFβ receptors,[26] overexpression of the growth-stimulating HER2/neu cell surface receptor,[55–58] a constitutive elevation of RelA and hedgehog pathway activities.[55,56] Some of these activities are proposed to be attractive as therapeutic targets, although supportive clinical evidence is not yet available. Pancreatic carcinomas also have reproducible alterations in gene expression, such as overexpression of the proteins mesothelin and prostate stem cell antigen that currently can serve as diagnostic aids in the histopathologic interpretation of biopsies and surgical resections.[57–59] The epigenetic patterns of gene hypermethylation in pancreatic cancers are considered promising for developing additional diagnostic markers for analysis of pancreatic secretions and for noninvasive diagnostic screening.[59]

The dominating genetic patterns previously described are altered among other diagnostic categories of pancreatic neoplasia. The precursor lesions, termed *PanIN* (pancreatic intraepithelial neoplasia), in their most advanced stage, closely resemble the genetic patterns of the conventional invasive ductal carcinomas. The intraductal papillary mucinous neoplasms, the mucinous cystic neoplasms, acinar cell carcinomas, neuroendocrine carcinomas, pancreatoblastomas, and solid pseudopapillary neoplasms, however, diverge significantly from the patterns of PanINs and typical invasive ductal carcinomas. Notable differences are the *PIK3CA* mutations present in some intraductal papillary mucinous neoplasms and the colloid carcinomas that can derive from them,[60] the *CTNNB1* (beta-catenin) mutations present in virtually all solid pseudopapillary neoplasms[61] and pancreatoblastomas,[62] and the *MEN1* mutations in many neuroendocrine neoplasms.[63]

LOW-FREQUENCY GENETIC CHANGES

The causative genes of *Fanconi anemia* play a role in human tumorigenesis. The *BRCA2* gene represents Fanconi complementation group D1 and is thought to aid DNA strand repair.[64] Because of this function, it is perhaps best to categorize *BRCA2* as a genome-maintenance gene rather than a standard tumor suppressor. As much as 7% of apparently "sporadic" pancreatic cancers (more, in instances of familial aggregation) harbor an inactivating intragenic inherited mutation of one copy of the *BRCA2* gene, accompanied by LOH.[1,2,66] The *PALB2* gene represents Fanconi group N, and its protein product functions by binding the Brca2 protein.[65] Three percent of familial pancreatic cancers had a germ line inactivating mutation of *PALB2*, and in a tumor studied in depth, the other copy was inactivated by a somatic mutation,[1,66,67] The *FANCC* and *FANCG* genes have somatic or germ line mutations in some pancreatic cancer patients, again with loss of the wild type allele in the cancer.[68] The known hypersensitivity of Fanconi cells to interstrand DNA-crosslinking agents, such as cisplatin, melphalan, and mitomycin C, has led to the hypothesis that pancreatic cancers with Fanconi pathway genetic defects should be especially susceptible to treatment with such agents.[69–72] Occasional complete remissions of pancreatic cancer have been reported with therapies that included DNA cross-linkers,[73–77] and there are recent reports of prolonged responses using such agents in patients having *BRCA2* mutations.[78,79] Cells made experimentally deficient for Fanconi genes are also hypersensitive to certain nongenotoxic compounds,[80] and patients having *BRCA2*-mutant cancers other than pancreatic cancer are reported to respond to therapeutic drug inhibition of the poly (ADP-ribose) polymerase enzyme, which normally becomes activated to facilitate DNA strand repair.[81] These opportunities are beginning to be explored clinically in pancreatic cancer.

BRCA1 gene mutations are not found in unselected pancreatic cancers or pancreatic cancer families.[82] Nonetheless, pancreatic cancers do occur in carriers of *BRCA1* inactivating mutations.[83,84] In these persons, the relatively high rate of LOH affecting the other *BRCA1* copy indicates that a loss of *BRCA1* function likely plays a role in tumorigenesis within these patients.[83]

The *mitochondrial genome* is mutated in a majority of pancreatic cancers.[85–87] These mutations most likely represent genetic drift, and perhaps do not directly contribute to the process of tumorigenesis.[87] Such mutations, however, could potentially serve as a diagnostic target because of the large number of copies of the mitochondrial genome in human carcinoma cells.[86,87]

The *MAP2K4* (*MKK4*) gene participates in a stress-activated protein kinase pathway.[81,82] It is stimulated by various influences, including chemotherapy, and its downstream effects include apoptosis and cellular differentiation. The *MKK4* gene is inactivated by homozygous deletions or mutation/LOH in about 4% of pancreatic cancers.[88,89] Experimental loss of one or both copies of the *MKK4* gene in cancer cells reduces Jun kinase activation and JUN expression; this is a rare example of a tumor-suppressor pathway affected by gene dosage. Such gene dose-dependent effects could rationalize the high rate of loss of chromosomal arm 17p affecting 90% of pancreatic cancers and more than half of the *TP53*-wild type cancers.[90]

Germ line mutations of the *STK11* (*LKB1*) gene, a serine-threonine kinase, are responsible for the Peutz-Jeghers syndrome (PJS).[91,92] PJS was anecdotally associated with pancreatic cancer.[93] A follow-up study examined lifetime risk, finding nearly a third of PJS patients to develop pancreatic cancer.[94] Sporadic pancreatic cancers, independent of PJS, also lose the gene by homozygous deletion or by somatic mutation/LOH in about 4% of cases.[95]

Kinase oncogenes are mutated at low frequency, including the *GUCY2F*, *EGFR*, and *NTRK3* genes.[91,92] This class of mutations is important in that these mutations can be targeted with antikinase drugs.[93]

Gene amplification also occurs in pancreatic cancer. Amplified regions include the *AKT2* gene within an amplicon on chromosome 19q, involving about 10% to 20% of cases studied.[94–96] About 6% of pancreatic cancers overexpress the oncogene, *CCNE1* (cyclin E). Two mechanisms have been demonstrated, cyclin E gene amplification and the genetic inactivation of the *FBXW7* (*AGO*) gene, which normally serves to degrade cyclin E during the normal phases of the cell division cycle.[1,96]

The patterns of *chromosomal deletion* in pancreatic cancer are complex. In one study, from 1.5% to 32% of all tested loci, in different cancers, had a deletion.[97] For most lost regions, we know of no particular tumor-suppressor genes targeted by the deletions. Conversely, in some regions known to harbor tumor-suppressor genes, the known mutated genes do not justify the high observed prevalence rates of LOH unless gene dose-dependent effects are postulated (90). Individual homozygous deletions are found at some additional genetic locations, again without a definitive target gene yet identified for most of these events.[98]

Defects in DNA mismatch repair (MIN) are seen in some pancreatic cancers. These cancers typically have a medullary histologic phenotype[8] and mutations of the type II TGFβ (*TGFBR2*) and activin (*ACVR2*) receptor genes.[25,52,53] They can also have mutations of the proapoptotic *BAX* gene[51] and of the growth factor pathway mediator *BRAF* gene (affecting the same pathway, presumably, as mutations of the *KRAS* gene).[8,9,51,96] The MIN tumors do not have the propensity for large chromosomal alterations and gross aneuploidy.[15,99] In a study of four cases of pancreatic cancers having MIN, all lacked expression of the Mlh1 protein.[9] Not all cancers with a medullary phenotype have MIN. Yet, medullary pancreatic carcinomas as a whole have a number of clinical and genetic differences as compared to those with conventional histologic appearance; the carcinomas have pushing rather than infiltrative borders, the *KRAS* gene often is wild type, and there is often a family history of malignancy.[5,6,47] A reported case of *Epstein-Barr virus (EBV)*–associated pancreatic cancer[9] had a medullary phenotype with heavy lymphocytic infiltration. Because of its distinctive features, it is advisable to separately designate the medullary category in the reporting of all clinical, genetic, and pathologic studies of pancreatic cancer.

Inherited mutations of the *cationic trypsinogen* (*PRSS1*) gene prevent the inactivation of prematurely activated trypsin within the ducts, causing a familial form of severe early-onset acute pancreatitis.[100] Some affected kindred have a cumulative risk of pancreatic cancer that approaches 40% by the time the affected individuals reach 60 years of age.[101] This cancer diathesis falls in a unique category of cancer susceptibility, in that the predisposition emanates from genetic alterations of a tissue-maintenance gene, one that is neither an oncogene, a tumor-suppressor gene, nor a genome-maintenance gene.

In summary, pancreatic cancer is fundamentally a genetic disease. An understanding of the genes altered in pancreatic cancer has led to a better understanding of the familial aggregation of pancreatic cancer, and, it is hoped, will lead to novel gene-specific targeted therapies for this deadly form of cancer.

Selected References

The full list of references for this chapter appears in the online version.

1. Jones S, Zhang X, Parsons DW, et al. Core signaling pathways in human pancreatic cancers revealed by global genomic analyses. *Science* 2008;321:1801.
4. Goggins M, Schutte M, Lu J, et al. Germline *BRCA2* gene mutations in patients with apparently sporadic pancreatic carcinomas. *Cancer Res* 1996;56:5360.
6. Murphy KM, Brune KA, Griffin C, et al. Evaluation of candidate genes MAP2K4, MADH4, ACVR1B, and BRCA2 in familial pancreatic cancer: deleterious BRCA2 mutations in 17%. *Cancer Res* 2002;62:3789.
8. Goggins M, Offerhaus GJA, Hilgers W, et al. Adenocarcinomas of the pancreas with DNA replication errors (RER+) are associated with wild-type K-ras and characteristic histopathology: poor differentiation, a syncytial growth pattern, and pushing borders suggest RER+. *Am J Pathol* 1998;152:1501.
10. Hruban RH, Wilentz R, Kern SE. Genetic progression in the pancreatic ducts. *Am J Pathol* 2000;156:1821.
13. Hiyama E, Kodama T, Shinbara K, et al. Telomerase activity is detected in pancreatic cancer but not in benign tumors. *Cancer Res* 1997;57:326.
17. Almoguera C, Shibata D, Forrester K, et al. Most human carcinomas of the exocrine pancreas contain mutant c-K-ras genes. *Cell* 1988;53:549.
18. Caldas C, Hahn SA, Hruban RH, et al. Detection of K-ras mutations in the stool of patients with pancreatic adenocarcinoma and pancreatic ductal hyperplasia. *Cancer Res* 1994;54:3568.
24. Hahn SA, Schutte M, Hoque ATMS, et al. DPC4, a candidate tumor-suppressor gene at 18q21.1. *Science* 1996;271:350.

26. Baldwin RL, Friess H, Yokoyama M, et al. Attenuated ALK5 receptor expression in human pancreatic cancer: correlation with resistance to growth inhibition. *Int J Cancer* 1996;67:283.
30. Caldas C, Hahn SA, da Costa LT, et al. Frequent somatic mutations and homozygous deletions of the p16 (MTS1) gene in pancreatic adenocarcinoma. *Nature Genetics* 1994;8:27.
34. Whelan AJ, Bartsch D, Goodfellow PJ. Brief report: a familial syndrome of pancreatic cancer and melanoma with a mutation in the CDKN2 tumor-suppressor gene. *N Engl J Med* 1995;333:975.
41. Redston MS, Caldas C, Seymour AB, et al. p53 mutations in pancreatic carcinoma and evidence of common involvement of homocopolymer tracts in DNA microdeletions. *Cancer Res* 1994;54:3025.
47. Hahn SA, Seymour AB, Hoque ATMS, et al. Allelotype of pancreatic adenocarcinoma using a xenograft model. *Cancer Res* 1995;55:4670.
48. Ionov Y, Peinado MA, Malkhosyan S, et al. Ubiquitous somatic mutations in simple repeated sequences reveal a new mechanism for colonic carcinogenesis. *Nature* 1993;363:558.
66. Jones S, Hruban RH, Kamiyama M, et al. Exomic sequencing identifies PALB2 as a pancreatic cancer susceptibility gene. *Science* 2009;324:217.
81. Fong PC, Boss DS, Yap TA, et al. Inhibition of poly(ADP-ribose) polymerase in tumors from BRCA mutation carriers. *N Engl J Med* 2009;361:123.
83. Al-Sukhni W, Rothenmund H, Borgida AE, et al. Germline BRCA1 mutations predispose to pancreatic adenocarcinoma. *Hum Genet* 2008;124:271.
88. Su GH, Hilgers W, Shekher M, et al. Alterations in pancreatic, biliary, and breast carcinomas support MKK4 as a genetically targeted tumor-suppressor gene. *Cancer Res* 1998;58:2339.
94. Giardiello FM, Brensinger JD, Tersmette AC, et al. Very high risk of cancer in familial Peutz-Jeghers syndrome. *Gastroenterology* 2000;119:1447.
95. Su GH, Hruban RH, Bova GS, et al. Germline and somatic mutations of the STK11/LKB1 Peutz-Jeghers gene in pancreatic and biliary cancers. *Am J Pathol* 1999;154:1835.
101. Lowenfels AB, Maisonneuve P, DiMagno EP, et al. Hereditary pancreatitis and the risk of pancreatic cancer. International Hereditary Pancreatitis Study Group. *J Natl Cancer Inst* 1997;89:442.

CHAPTER 82 CANCER OF THE PANCREAS

RICHARD E. ROYAL, ROBERT A. WOLFF, AND CHRISTOPHER H. CRANE

Adenocarcinoma of the pancreas remains a highly lethal disease despite advances in the surgical care of the resected patient, the proven benefit of adjuvant therapy, and the expansion of multidisciplinary care for patients in any stage. Moreover, recent advances in cytotoxic and molecular therapy for other solid tumors of the gastrointestinal tract have not been realized in pancreatic cancer. Patients often present with advanced disease complaining of vague, nonspecific symptoms. The combination of aggressive tumor biology and minimally effective therapies often results in rapid clinical decline, culminating in death within months of diagnosis. Overall survival remains poor, with approximately 23% of patients alive 12 months following diagnosis and only 5% alive at 5 years.[1]

Pancreatic neoplasms and malignancies arise from both the endocrine and exocrine portions of the organ. Pancreatic endocrine tumors are discussed elsewhere in this text (see Chapter 111). The most frequent type of exocrine pancreatic cancer is ductal adenocarcinoma of the pancreas, and except where clearly indicated, the discussion in this chapter focuses on this specific disease.

The genetic and molecular perturbations underlying pancreatic carcinogenesis, invasion, metastatic spread, and resistance to chemotherapy and radiation are covered in the previous chapter. Unfortunately, despite a greater understanding of these molecular mechanisms, no meaningful improvements in clinical outcomes have been achieved thus far. However, if investigators design clinical trials with more rigorous selection criteria, progress in the prevention, detection, and treatment of pancreatic cancer can be expected soon.

INCIDENCE AND ETIOLOGY

Epidemiology

An estimated 232,000 people were diagnosed worldwide with pancreatic cancer in 2002, with 227,000 people dying from the disease in that same year. Although pancreatic cancer ranks as the 13th most common type of cancer worldwide, it is the eighth most common cause of cancer-related death.[2]

The greatest impact on cancer-related deaths is in developed countries where pancreatic cancer is the fifth leading cause of cancer-related death after lung, stomach, colorectal, and breast cancers.[1] In developed countries the incidence and mortality rates range from 7 to 9 per 100,000 for men and 4.5 to 6 per 100,000 for women.[2] In Europe 64,000 people died from pancreatic cancer in 2006, representing 5.5% of cancer-related deaths, the fifth leading cause of cancer mortality.[3] In the United States, there were an estimated 42,470 new cases of pancreatic cancer in 2009 with approximately 35,240 deaths, the fourth most common cause of cancer-related death.[4] The lifetime risk of an American developing pancreatic cancer is 1.32% (95% confidence interval [CI], 1.29 to 1.34), with a current annual incidence for the entire population of 11.4 per 100,000; this has not changed over the past 10 years studied (1995 to 2004).[1] Of patients with available data in the United States diagnosed with pancreatic cancer in the years 1996 to 2004, less than 10% presented with local disease, 26% with regional disease, and over half had distant metastases.[4] The incidence of pancreatic cancer is lower in developing countries, which may be a reflection of lifespan and diagnostic limitations. Among the developing countries, the incidence is highest in Central and South America.

Pancreatic cancer tends to occur later in life. Only 10% of patients in Europe present before the age of 50, while those aged 50 to 54 experience an incidence of 9.8 per 100,000, and those 70 to 74, an incidence of 57 per 100,000. The median age of diagnosis with pancreatic cancer in the United States is 72, with less than 13% of cancers diagnosed prior to the age of 55 and greater than 69% of cancers diagnosed after the age of 65. Although the peak incidence is later in life, pancreatic cancer is the third leading cause of cancer-related death in the United States for those aged 40 to 59.

In the United States, blacks experience a higher rate of pancreatic cancer than whites, with an annual incidence of 16.7 per 100,000 versus 10.9 per 100,000, respectively. Death from pancreatic cancer is similarly elevated, with an annual rate of 14.6 per 100,000 versus 10.6 per 100,000.[5] Diagnosis is slightly but significantly earlier in African Americans, with a median age of diagnosis of 68 compared to median age of diagnosis of 73 for whites. In contrast, persons of nonwhite Hispanic/Latino descent and persons of Native American ancestry do not have disparate incidence of pancreatic cancer compared to persons of European descent, although these groups do differ in other cancer types.

Five-year survival from all stages of disease is 5%, which is a statistically significant increase from the 2% survival rate in 1975 to 1977.[1] However, the long-term survival rate often dissipates when examined carefully. Carpelon-Holstrom et al.[6] examined the records of 4,922 pancreatic cancer patients registered in the Finnish Cancer Registry from 1990 to 1996 and found 89 subjects who were 5-year survivors. Pathology was reviewed on all 89 subjects. In 59 cases, the diagnosis was found to be a histology other than pancreatic ductal adenocarcinoma, and 20 cases carried a clinical or cytological diagnosis or did not have pathology available for analysis. Only ten cases of long-term survival from pancreatic ductal carcinoma could be confirmed.

Etiologic Factors

Tobacco

Tobacco smoke exposure plays a significant role in the development of pancreatic adenocarcinoma. It has been estimated that tobacco smoking contributes to the development of 20% to 30% of pancreatic cancers.[7] The strongest associations between cigarette smoking and pancreatic cancer have been observed when the pack years smoked were within the previous 10 years.[8] Importantly, smoking cessation can reduce this risk, which in one study approached that of a never-smoker after 5 years of smoking cessation.[9]

Environmental tobacco smoke (ETS) contains the same toxins, irritants, and carcinogens, such as carbon monoxide, nicotine, cyanide, ammonia, benzene, nitrosamines, vinyl chloride, arsenic, and hydrocarbons, as primary cigarette smoke. Pancreatic cancer risk is increased particularly among never-smokers exposed to ETS in childhood and to a lesser extent, at work or home during adulthood.[9] Similar findings come from a prospective cohort in the Nurses' Health Study showing an increased risk of pancreatic cancer among women having ETS exposure from maternal smoking, but not paternal smoking.[10] This implies ETS exposure *in utero* or early life may result in pancreatic cancer in adulthood.

More recently, the role of smokeless tobacco in pancreatic cancer development has been suggested.[11] Other studies, including one supported by a tobacco company, claim that more rigorous methodology refutes these findings.[12] Nevertheless, investigators have demonstrated the presence of known carcinogens in three of the five most popular brands of moist snuff sold in the United States.[13]

Infectious Diseases

Previous reports have suggested an association between *Helicobacter pylori* and pancreatic cancer.[14,15] More recently, investigators performed a population-based, case-control study and found an association between risk of pancreatic cancer, *H. pylori* colonization, and ABO blood groups.[16]

Likewise, hepatitis B may also be a risk factor for pancreatic cancer. In a recent study involving 476 patients with pathologically confirmed adenocarcinoma of the pancreas and 879 age-, sex-, and race-matched healthy controls, a possible association between past exposure to hepatitis B virus (HBV) and pancreatic cancer was discovered.[17] The proximity of the liver to the pancreas and the fact that the liver and pancreas share common blood vessels and ducts may make the pancreas a potential target organ for hepatitis viruses. This is supported by the discovery of hepatitis B surface antigen (HBsAg) in pure pancreatic juice and pure bile juice.[18]

Occupational Factors

A meta-analysis of 20 population studies of occupational exposures and pancreatic cancer from journal publications during the period 1969 to 1998 showed exposure to chlorinated hydrocarbon solvents, nickel and nickel compounds, chromium compounds, polycyclic aromatic hydrocarbons, organochlorine insecticides, silica dust, and aliphatic solvents conveyed elevated risk ratios. Overall, the occupational etiologic fraction for pancreatic cancer was estimated at 12%, but it increased to 29% when the chlorinated hydrocarbon solvents were considered in a subpopulation.[19]

Elevated serum levels of organochloride compounds (dichlorodiphenyltrichlorethane, dichlorodiphenyldichloroethylene, and polychlorinated biphenyls) are also associated with the development of pancreatic cancer. Approximately 90% of pancreatic cancer patients have an acquired K-*ras* oncogene mutation. In a case-control study, pancreatic cancers with K-*ras* mutations had significantly higher levels of organochloride compounds compared to cancers without the K-*ras* mutation and to those in the control group.[20] These compounds are postulated to enhance the actions of K-*ras* rather than cause the mutation, suggesting a gene–environment interaction or effect modification.

Demographic and Host Risk Factors

A number of demographic risk factors have been associated with the development of this disease worldwide. These include older age (most cancers occur between the ages of 60 and 80), African American race, low socioeconomic status, and Ashkenazic Jewish heritage (related to germline mutations).[7] Host etiologic factors associated with an increased risk of pancreatic cancer include a history of diabetes mellitus, chronic cirrhosis, pancreatitis, a high-fat or cholesterol diet, and prior cholecystectomy.[7,8]

Diabetes Mellitus

Diabetes mellitus (DM) has been implicated as both predisposing to pancreatic cancer and a manifestation of the malignancy. Two meta-analyses have shown that pancreatic cancer occurs with increased frequency in patients with longstanding diabetes (diagnosed at least 5 years prior to the diagnosis of pancreatic cancer or death due to pancreatic cancer).[21,22] In contrast, a cohort study from Sweden found an increased risk of the diagnosis of pancreatic cancer after an initial hospitalization for diabetes that persisted for more than a decade but decreased with the duration of diabetes.[23] Although not uniformly accepted, it is estimated that DM doubles the risk of pancreatic cancer. Although longstanding diabetes mellitus appears to be a risk factor for pancreatic cancer, some studies also suggest new-onset diabetes as a potential manifestation.[24,25] Ductal adenocarcinoma can induce peripheral insulin resistance.[26] Furthermore, a putative cancer-associated diabetogenic factor has been isolated from conditioned medium of pancreatic cancer cell lines and patient serum.[27] The existence of such a factor is further supported by clinical observations showing diabetes can resolve after surgical resection of the primary tumor.[28]

Obesity, Physical Activity, and the Metabolic Syndrome

High body mass index (a measure of obesity), increased height, and a low level of physical activity all increased the risk of pancreatic cancer, as demonstrated in a cohort study of 160,000 health professionals.[29] Moderate physical activity resulted in decreased pancreatic cancer rates, and merely walking or hiking 1.5 hours or more per week was associated with a 50% reduction in pancreatic cancer, independent of smoking cessation.

Further evidence for a link between obesity, insulin resistance, and pancreatic cancer comes from emerging recognition of the metabolic syndrome. While definitions vary, this syndrome is characterized by type II DM, truncal obesity, hypertension, and dyslipidemia, which together increase the risk of cardiovascular disease.[30] More recent epidemiologic data have suggested the metabolic syndrome as a risk factor for pancreatic cancer.[31] Of note, fatty infiltration of the pancreas may lead to steatopancreatitis, suggesting a potential link between obesity, nonalcoholic fatty pancreatic disease, nonalcoholic steatopancreatitis, and pancreatic cancer.[32]

Pancreatitis

Although an association between pancreatitis and an increased risk of pancreatic cancer has long been suspected, the magnitude of the risk remains uncertain. Older clinical studies suggested that chronic forms of pancreatitis were most closely associated with the development of pancreatic cancer.[33] In contrast were the findings of Karlson et al.,[34] who found that the standardized incidence ratio (observed/expected) for the development of pancreatic cancer was increased in patients with pancreatitis (2.8; 95% CI, 2.5 to 3.2), after 10 years or more, the excess risk declined and was of borderline significance.

The incidence of pancreatic adenocarcinoma is also increased in patients with hereditary pancreatitis or tropical pancreatitis. Hereditary pancreatitis has an autosomal dominant pattern of transmission with 80% penetrance.[35] Symptoms usually arise by age 40 years, but can occur before age 5 years, and the cumulative risk of developing pancreatic cancer by age 70 in patients with hereditary pancreatitis has been estimated to be 40%.[36]

Inflammation and Pancreatic Cancer

No matter what the underlying cause, results from several sources detailed above implicate inflammation as a potential driver of pancreatic carcinogenesis. Whether the insult is precipitated by an infectious agent, results from steatopancreatitis related to obesity or the metabolic syndrome, or pancreatitis secondary to alcohol or genetic predisposition,[37] preclinical and epidemiologic studies suggest inflammation as a central mediator of the neoplastic process.[38]

Genetic Predispositions

Genetic predisposition plays a small but significant role in pancreatic cancer risk. Mutation and constitutive activation of the oncogene K-*ras* is present in approximately 95% of all pancreatic cancer with frequent inactivation of several tumor suppressor genes (p53, *DPC4*, p16, and *BRCA2*). Nearly 90% of all cases have p16 mutations, 55% to 75% have p53 mutations, and 50% have *DPC4* mutations.[39] The frequency of DNA repair gene inactivations, which include *BRCA2, MLH1, FANC-C,* and *FANC-G*, is relatively low.

It is estimated that 10% to 20% of pancreatic cancers are hereditary or have a familial link. Multiple lines of evidence support this. Cohort studies have shown an increased risk of developing the disease among individuals who report a family history of pancreatic cancer. Tersmette et al.[37] have shown that this risk increases with the number of affected members in the family. An 18-fold increased risk was found in familial pancreatic cancer kindreds compared to sporadic groups. When three or more family members were affected, there was a 57-fold increased risk.

Data from Familial Pancreas Tumor Registries: PALB2 Germline Mutations

The vast majority of cases in which there is a familial aggregation of pancreatic cancer are not explained by known genetic syndromes. The National Familial Pancreas Tumor Registry has therefore been established at the Johns Hopkins Medical Institutes (JHMI) with the hope of identifying the causes for the aggregation of pancreatic cancer in families. Early analyses of the kindreds enrolled in the registry showed that the risk of cancer is 18-fold greater in first-degree relatives of familial pancreatic cancer cases and also extends to second-degree relatives. Rates of pancreatic cancer are higher among second-degree relatives of familial cases compared with sporadic pancreatic cases (3.7% vs. 0.6%; $P < .0001$).[37]

More recently, the Hopkins group has identified mutations in the *PALB2* gene in 3 of 96 patients with familial pancreatic cancer (3.1%), defined as having at least one first-degree relative with pancreatic cancer.[40] These mutations each produced a different stop codon in the protein-coding regions of the gene. Shortly thereafter, other investigators interrogated European familial pancreatic cancer registries for *PALB2* mutations among index cases.[41] Three index patients from 81 families (3.7%) harbored truncating mutations within the exons of the *PALB2* gene. Of note, these three families also had a family history of breast cancer. Thus, traditional family registries, coupled with increasingly sophisticated genetic analyses, can be expected to identify novel germline mutations that drive pancreatic carcinogenesis.

TABLE 82.1

GENETIC SYNDROMES AND GENE ALTERATIONS ASSOCIATED WITH FAMILIAL PANCREATIC CANCER

Syndrome	Gene Alteration (Chromosomal Locus)
Hereditary pancreatitis	*PRSSI* (7q35)
Hereditary nonpolyposis colorectal cancer (Lynch II variant)	*hMSH2, hMLH1*, others
Hereditary breast and ovarian cancer	*BRCA2* (13q12q13)
Familial atypical multiple mole melanoma (FAMMM) syndrome	p16 (9p21)
Peutz-Jeghers syndrome	*STK11/LKB1* (19p13)
Ataxia-telangiectasia	*ATM* (11q22–23)

Inherited Syndromes

Although accounting for less than 20% of the familial aggregation of pancreatic cancer, several genetic syndromes (caused by germline mutations) associated with an increased risk of pancreatic cancer have been identified.[8,42] These are summarized in Table 82.1 and include:

1. Familial breast cancer with germline mutations in the *BRCA2* gene. Carriers of germline *BRCA2* mutations have a 3.5- to 10-fold increased risk of developing pancreatic cancer, and 17% (one in six) of patients with pancreatic cancer and a strong family history (at least three family members with pancreatic cancer) have been shown to have germline *BRCA2* mutations. *BRCA2* mutation is the most common germline mutation in patients with hereditary pancreatic cancer.
2. Familial atypical multiple mole melanoma syndrome with germline mutations in the p16 gene. Carriers of p16 germline mutations have a 12- to 20-fold increased risk of developing pancreatic cancer, as well as an increased risk of melanoma.
3. The Peutz-Jeghers syndrome, characterized by mucocutaneous melanocytic macules and hamartomatous polyps of the gastrointestinal tract. Patients with the Peutz-Jeghers syndrome have a greater than 100-fold increased risk of developing pancreatic cancer.
4. The hereditary nonpolyposis colorectal cancer syndrome, characterized by germline mutations in one of the DNA mismatch repair genes (*hMSH1, hMSH2*, etc.).
5. Hereditary pancreatitis with germline mutations in the *PRSS1* (cationic trypsinogen) gene. Patients develop severe pancreatitis at a young age (often affects children and adolescents) and have a 50-fold excess risk of developing pancreatic cancer.
6. Ataxia-telangiectasia, a rare autosomal recessive inherited disorder, characterized by cerebellar ataxia, oculocutaneous telangiectasias, and cellular and humoral immune deficiencies. The gene, *ATM*, is also associated with an increased risk of leukemia, lymphoma, and cancers of the breast, ovaries, biliary tract, stomach, and, occasionally, the pancreas.
7. Pancreatic cancer, pancreatic insufficiency, and DM have been described in a family (called *Family X*), and the phenotype has been linked to chromosome 4q32–34.[9]

Unfortunately, for most of the known genetic mutations listed above, therapeutic recommendations are not influenced by the verification of a germline mutation in any given patient. However, for patients with a documented *BRCA1* or *BRCA2* mutation, hypersensitivity to DNA damaging agents such as platinum analogues or mitomycin C may have clinically meaningful impact on the natural history of disease.[43]

ANATOMY AND PATHOLOGY

The pancreas is a soft yellowish gland fixed within the retroperitoneum. The majority of the gland is surrounded by the duodenal C-loop with a portion of the gland extending obliquely and superiorly to the left to the splenic hilum. The gland is divided into nonanatomic sections: the head with a posterior uncinate process, which is to the right of the superior mesenteric vein/portal vein (SMV-PV); the neck, which is that portion of the gland immediately anterior to the SMV-PV; the body, including the gland to the left of the SMV-PV to the left edge of the aorta; and the tail, which is the portion of the gland lateral to the left edge of aorta. The pancreas lies at the center of the retroperitoneum, and the anatomy of minor structures in the area is both complex and constant. A grasp of this anatomy is essential for operations of the pancreas.

Embryologically, two groups of cells migrate to fuse and form the mature pancreas. A dorsal anlagen arises from the portion of the foregut destined to be the duodenum, and the ventral anlagen buds off the developing common bile duct as part of the hepatic evagination. With organogenesis these migrate and fuse to form the mature pancreas.[44] The genetic and microenvironmental forces that lead to these embryological events are not fully elucidated, but some key insights have been established.

The most striking recent finding in pancreatic embryology is that all pancreatic cells types—ductal, acinar, and islet cells—develop from the same pancreatic precursors in the pancreatic anlagen.[45–47] This is in direct opposition to the longstanding assertion that pancreatic endocrine cells develop from neural crest cells that migrate into the developing pancreas. Expression of the transcription factor pancreatic duodenal homeobox-1 (PDX-1) is a key event in the differentiation of gut endoderm into pancreatic primordial cells.

Neoplasia that give rise to pancreas cancer progress from initial intraductal proliferative lesions to invasive carcinomas. This is similar to other carcinomas that arise from ductal epithelium, such as breast ductal carcinoma or prostate cancer. Pancreatic intraepithelial neoplasm (PanIN) is the term established for intraductal proliferative epithelial lesions.[48] PanINs are graded as 1A, 1B, 2, and 3 as they advance along a histologic continuum of progressive dysplasia, described in Table 82.2.[42]

TABLE 82.2

HISTOLOGIC CHARACTERISTICS OF THE PANCREATIC INTRAEPITHELIAL NEOPLASM

PanIN 1A	Columnar transition Retention of apical nuclei Intracellular mucin near the luminal aspect
PanIN 1B	Micropapillary or papillary transition
PanIN 2	Nuclear atypia/crowding/enlargement Loss of nuclear polarity
PanIN 3	Apical mitosis Prominent nucleoli Dystrophic goblet cells Cribriform architecture Luminal necrosis

PanIN, pancreatic intraepithelial neoplasm.

PanINs follow a stepwise progression of genetic mutational events that correlates with the stepwise progression of worsening neoplasia culminating in adenocarcinoma. PanIN-1 lesions show a predominance of K-*ras* mutations and overexpression of *HER2/neu*. In PanIN-2 lesions, p16 mutations are the typical mutational event and in PanIN-3 lesions, p53, *DPC4*, and *BRCA2* mutations predominate. The mutational pattern of PanIN-3 lesions is equivalent to mutations found in pancreatic adenocarcinoma. These events are the basis of a current progression model for pancreatic cancer in which point mutation of K-*ras* and overexpression of *HER2/neu* are initiating early events, p16 inactivation is an intermediate event, and p53, *DPCA*, and *BRCA2* inactivation follow just prior to invasion outside of the duct.[49]

SCREENING

Currently, no proven screening strategies exist for pancreatic cancer. But there is intense study into developing methods of early detection because cancer of the pancreas has curative potential in the setting of PanIN and small invasive ductal adenocarcinomas, which are amenable to surgical resection. For example, Japanese investigators compiled data for patients with early cancers, finding patients (n = 36) with resected tumors less than 1.0 cm in size experienced a 57% 5-year survival.[50] Unfortunately, early diagnosis is quite uncommon.

Prevalence of the disease is too low in the general population for screening with currently available techniques. Recent efforts in screening have focused on individuals considered to be at high risk for pancreatic cancer, such as those belonging to a familial pancreatic cancer kindred or having a known genetic syndrome.[51] Others have suggested that obese patients diagnosed with diabetes over the age of 60 may also be appropriate candidates for pancreatic cancer screening.[52] In general, pancreatic cancer screening has relied on endoscopic ultrasonography (EUS), which allows for excellent visualization of the gland and detection of subtle changes in pancreatic architecture. Although multidetector dynamic-phase computed tomography (CT) imaging has been improving in resolution, EUS maintains its advantage in detecting small abnormalities (less than 1 cm) within the pancreas. In addition, EUS-guided fine-needle aspiration (FNA) may provide a cytologic diagnosis for lesions measuring 2 to 5 mm.

To date screening programs for pancreatic cancer have been limited to single-institution studies. In a prospective trial conducted at the JHMI, 78 patients with a strong family history of pancreatic cancer or known Peutz-Jeghers syndrome were enrolled in addition to 149 control patients considered at average risk for pancreatic cancer. Baseline abdominal CT and EUS were performed and repeated 12 months later. If the EUS study was abnormal, an EUS-guided FNA and endoscopic retrograde cholangiopancreatography (ERCP) with aspiration of pancreatic juice for molecular analysis were obtained. Of the 78 high-risk patients, 8 patients (10%) were found to have pancreatic neoplasia confirmed by fine-needle aspirate or surgery. Six of these patients had benign intraductal pancreatic mucinous neoplasms (IPMNs), one patient had IPMN with progression to invasive ductal adenocarcinoma, and one patient had PanIN. This particular study implicated IPMN as a common early phenotype of familial pancreatic cancer.[53] In a separate trial conducted at the University of Washington, three high-risk families with unique phenotypic features (including DM and chronic pancreatitis) underwent screening. Of the 14 patients screened primarily with EUS, 7 were found to have EUS and ERCP abnormalities that suggested pancreatic ductal lesions. These seven patients underwent total pancreatectomy, and pathological analysis revealed diffuse, often high-grade PanIN.[54] Taken together, these two screening studies suggest that using EUS to screen high-risk patients will have relatively higher yield compared with broad screening of average-risk patients using serum tumor markers or transabdominal ultrasound. The cost-effectiveness of these strategies may remain prohibitive beyond small research-driven initiatives.

The currently accruing Cancer of the Pancreas Screening Study is a comprehensive multicentered trial that attempts to define the role of screening in high-risk individuals. Subjects are evaluated with CT, magnetic resonance imaging (MRI), and EUS along with a panel of biomarkers in serum or pancreatic juice. Among the aims of the trial is defining the rate of detectable lesions in high-risk individuals, comparing the utility of available imaging techniques, and evaluating a panel of DNA and protein markers for lesion detection.[55]

DIAGNOSIS AND STAGING

Presenting Symptoms

The clinical presentation of pancreatic cancer is often dependent on the location of the tumor within the gland, with most symptoms initially appearing vague and nonspecific.

The majority of pancreatic tumors develop in the head or uncinate process, putting the intrapancreatic portion of the bile duct at risk for obstruction. Jaundice is, therefore, a common presenting symptom and may be preceded by episodes of biliary colic, anorexia, or vague gastrointestinal distress.

Some tumors of the pancreatic head or body will not involve the bile duct but may invade the duodenum or neural structures, including the celiac or mesenteric plexi. Such invasion results in pain that may be characterized by aching, pressure, or burning. The presence of pain may have implications for operative treatment. In a prospective study conducted at Memorial Sloan-Kettering Cancer Center (MSKCC), pain, pain intensity, and location were evaluated among 77 patients appearing to have resectable pancreatic cancer.[56] The presence of pain prior to exploratory laparotomy was a predictor of unresectable tumor and the presence of metastatic disease. Moreover, for those patients undergoing surgery with curative intent, the presence of pain prior to surgery was associated with a worse survival (9.2 months vs. 21.9 months; $P = .045$). This implicates pain as a sign of more advanced disease, even when imaging suggests the primary tumor is potentially resectable.

Pancreatic exocrine insufficiency manifested by steatorrhea occurs relatively infrequently as a presenting symptom, and while it is often initially mild and easily manageable, it may worsen after surgical resection or radiation therapy. Pancreatic ductal obstruction may lead to acute pancreatitis, which is occasionally a presenting sign of pancreatic cancer.[57] When a patient without risk factors for pancreatitis experiences an acute attack, an underlying pancreatic cancer should be considered and thoroughly investigated. Importantly, it is increasingly recognized that glucose intolerance or overt DM is present in up to 70% of patients diagnosed with pancreatic cancer, and when diabetes develops in an older adult or when it is found in conjunction with other symptoms such as pain, anorexia, or weight loss, the possibility of an underlying pancreatic neoplasm should be raised.[52,58]

Other symptoms of pancreatic cancer include superficial or deep venous thromboses, anorexia, or weight loss. In some studies, weight loss is the most common symptom of pancreatic cancer. Unfortunately, initial symptomatology, to include weight loss, may be indicative of metastatic disease, such as night sweats, significant fatigue, or liver pain. Gastric outlet obstruction, increasing abdominal girth from ascites, and skin manifestations all occur in pancreatic cancer, but are fairly uncommon as presenting signs and symptoms.

Evaluation

The initial goals in the approach to the symptomatic patient are to confirm the diagnosis of a pancreatic mass, reestablish biliary tract patency, determine the extent of disease, determine the resectability of the primary tumor, and establish a histologic diagnosis. History, physical examination, and noninvasive and minimally invasive imaging often can accomplish all of these goals.

Physical Examination and Laboratory Findings

Patients with pancreatic cancer usually have an unremarkable physical examination, but the most common abnormal physical finding is jaundice, which may be accompanied by cutaneous excoriations related to pruritus. In patients with advanced disease, temporal muscle wasting, hepatomegaly or a nodular liver, left supraclavicular adenopathy (Virchow's node), periumbilical adenopathy (Sister Mary Joseph's nodes), or the unusual finding of a drop metastasis at Blumer's shelf may be discovered on digital rectal examination.[59]

Laboratory studies often reveal mild to moderate hyperglycemia[58] and abnormal liver enzymes but not necessarily hyperbilirubinemia. Hyperamylasemia and hyperlipasemia are uncommon in patients with ductal adenocarcinoma but may be seen in patients with IPMN. A normochromic anemia or mild hypoalbuminemia may reflect the chronic nature of the neoplastic process and its nutritional sequelae. Coagulation tests, particularly a prolonged prothrombin time, may be seen in deeply jaundiced patients due to malabsorption of fat-soluble vitamins.[59,60]

Diagnostic Imaging

In recent history, pancreatic lesions were evaluated with a combined treatment and diagnostic phase. Patients evaluated with this approach were surgically explored, and through palpation their tumors were deemed resectable or unresectable. In patients with resectable disease, tumor extirpation was then completed during the same procedure, while patients found to have unresectable tumors were treated with operative biliary and gastric bypass. This approach should be abandoned.

A separate diagnostic evaluation should precede operative resection of the tumor. The advantages to this approach are: (1) exploration can be limited to those patients with a high likelihood of resection, (2) objective criteria can be utilized to assess resectability rather than subjective imprecise tactile perception, (3) patients who will require venous reconstruction at time of resection can be identified, optimizing preoperative planning, (4) patients may move on to neoadjuvant therapy appropriate for their stage of tumor without an initial exploration, and (5) patients exhibiting an advanced tumor can be palliated with less morbid nonoperative procedures.

Multiphase Multidetector Helical Computerized Axial Tomography. Among diagnostic imaging techniques, abdominal CT scanning is the most common for confirming suspected pancreatic malignancy. Standard CT techniques are relatively insensitive for the assessment of resectability. However, vascular involvement and liver metastases can be most optimally assessed with newer CT imaging techniques. The cornerstone of diagnostic evaluation of a pancreatic tumor is the multiphase CT scan, coordinating intravenous contrast administration with subsequent rapid thin cut CT through the pancreas during arterial, portal venous, and parenchymal phases of enhancement. This must be obtained on a multidetector row helical CT scanner, allowing acquisition during a single breath-hold for each phase. With this type of CT, extension of the

TABLE 82.3

MULTIPHASE COMPUTED TOMOGRAPHY ACCURACY IN PREDICTING RESECTABILITY OF PANCREATIC CANCER

Group (Ref.)	Patients with Resectable Tumors by CT	Actually Resectable at Operation	Accuracy (%)
M. D. Anderson (246)	118	94	80.0
Beth Israel Deaconess (247)	68	52	76.0
Barcelona, Spain (248)	39	25	64.1
Liverpool, UK (64)	35	28	80.0
	N	Sensitivity (%)	Specificity (%)
UCLA (249)	25	84.0	98.0[a]
Montreal, Canada (63)	36	63.0	93.0[b]
Vienna, Austria (62)	20	85.5	85.2

CT, computed tomography.
[a]Based on vessel invasion only, including superior mesenteric vein/portal vein.
[b]Based on arterial invasion only.

tumor to the superior mesenteric artery (SMA), celiac axis, SMV-PV complex, and contiguous structures can be clearly determined, as well as an assessment of distant metastasis. Optimally, CT imaging should precede stent placement and biopsy due to the possibility of postprocedure inflammation from the biopsy and artifact from the stent, which can confound interpretation of the images.[61]

Resectability is defined on multiphase CT by (1) the absence of metastases outside the pancreas and the pancreatic nodal basin, (2) patency of the SMV-PV, and (3) presence of a definable fat plane between the SMA, celiac artery, and pancreatic mass. Some centers also include SMV-PV invasion as a criteria for unresectability, while others approach vein invasion with segmental resection of the SMV-PV and reconstruction (discussed below). Absence of a fat plane between the pancreatic mass and the right lateral margin of the SMV-PV identifies tumor invasion of the vein or fibrosis and defines the patient who may require a vein reconstruction at the time of resection.

Reports confirm the predictive power of preoperative multiphase CT scan in establishing resectability of pancreatic adenocarcinoma (Table 82.3). Some investigators recommend the use of curved planar reformations[62] and CT angiography[63] in addition to multiphase CT scanning to enhance detection of vessel invasion. Helical CT is poor at predicting nodal involvement,[64] and its accuracy is decreased following neoadjuvant therapy.[65]

Magnetic Resonance Imaging. To date, MRI has not been widely used to assess pancreatic cancer. This method was initially limited by long scanning times and the resultant artifact caused by organ motion. Dynamic MRI, with rapid scanning sequences and bolus intravenous contrast enhancement, however, is reported to have sensitivity and specificity comparable to those for helical CT.[66] Some investigators have found MRI more accurate at predicting malignancy of the pancreatic duct due to findings of concurrent magnetic resonance cholangiopancreatography,[67] but use of this imaging method for pancreatic cancer is currently not widespread.

Ultrasonography. Other investigators have found preoperative ultrasonography useful in assessing tumor characteristics and resectability of pancreatic adenocarcinoma. Calculli et al.[68] report that in 95 patients sonography had high sensitivity and specificity (92.3% and 72.7%, respectively) in defining SMV-PV invasion, although lower than helical CT (98% and 79%, respectively). Minniti et al.[69] found sonography to be superior to CT in identifying the primary tumor (95.3% vs. 89.1%, respectively) but less accurate in predicting resectability (81.4% vs. 86%, respectively) in blinded studies of 64 patients. In contrast, Morrin et al.[70] studied 23 patients with periampullary cancer using both multiphase helical CT and ultrasonography with Doppler and found close congruence both in the ability of the two studies to predict vascular involvement and in the poor ability to image metastases. Ultrasonography and CT were in agreement in all cases of unresectable disease. Ultrasonography in pancreatic cancer, as in other diseases, is particularly operator dependent, and in experienced hands may safely replace assessment with helical CT.

Endoscopic Ultrasonography

EUS can image the primary cancer and be a means of obtaining a FNA of pancreatic adenocarcinoma, but in general the procedure is noncontributory when CT scan characterizes the tumor. When a mass cannot be visualized on CT scan, sonography through the wall of the stomach or duodenum can image tumors in the body or tail and head of the pancreas, respectively.

Tissue diagnosis is not necessary prior to routine resection. A suspicious lesion by imaging should be treated with resection. But in specific patients a tissue diagnosis may be needed, such as in patients entering a clinical trial, prior to neoadjuvant therapy, and prior to chemotherapy in advanced tumors. In these patients, an EUS can be highly accurate. Raut et al.[71] found this evaluation has a sensitivity for histologic diagnosis of 91% with a specificity of 100% in testing 216 patients with a pancreatic mass. Like standard ultrasonography, this method is highly operator dependent, and only experienced groups can expect this level of accuracy.

Endoscopic Retrograde Cholangiopancreatography

ERCP delineates pancreatic duct and common bile duct anatomy from brushings and ductal lavage and is a means of obtaining cytologic diagnosis. But, similar to EUS, in the face of a defining CT scan, its findings are often redundant. Pancreatitis, bleeding, and perforation are severe complications associated with ERCP and preclude the routine use of this modality in all pancreatic cancer patients. ERCP should be reserved for patients in need of endoscopic stenting, equivocal findings on standard evaluation, or for patients in whom tissue diagnosis is needed, such as those in a clinical study, with advanced disease, or anticipating neoadjuvant therapy. Unfortunately, brushings during ERCP have a relatively low yield.[72] Farnell et al.[73] note that surgery may be delayed and rendered more difficult due to the complications that can accompany preoperative ERCP.

If neoadjuvant therapy is being considered, endoscopy of the upper gastrointestinal tract is the most valuable initial step in the management of patients who present with obstructive jaundice from presumed carcinoma of the pancreas. During this procedure, biliary outflow can be reestablished with the placement of an endobiliary stent, and EUS-FNA can be performed. Some centers prefer percutaneous CT-FNA; however, CT-FNA is operator dependent and is not possible if the lesion is not visible on CT. Although CT-FNA is generally safe, serious complications such as hemorrhage, pancreatitis, fistula, abscess, and death have been reported. Additionally, there have been reports of tumor seeding along the subcutaneous tract of the needle and concerns regarding tumor dissemination by the act of capsular disruption of the neoplasm.

Staging Laparoscopy

Laparoscopy and multiphase CT have evolved concurrently as methods to evaluate a pancreatic mass. Both have emerged as highly effective in evaluating the tumors, but CT as a noninvasive modality supplants the use of routine laparoscopy.

Laparoscopy that precedes planned resection can accurately identify metastases that avoid detection by CT, and when combined with laparoscopic ultrasound, can delineate vascular invasion as well as metastases within the hepatic parenchyma. Minnard et al.[74] found that 90 patients studied who had laparoscopy with sonography had accurate determination of resectability, and Pietrabissa et al.[75] found in 50 patients that laparoscopy with sonography identified hepatic metastases not seen by CT in 8% of patients.

Currently, routine use of laparoscopy is not warranted. Few patients will have findings on laparoscopy that add to information found at CT scanning. The group at JHMI retrospectively reviewed 188 cases of patients studied preoperatively using CT and treated through a laparotomy. Preoperative laparoscopy would have benefited a maximum of 2.3% of patients with a pancreatic head tumor. Lesions in the body and tail were more likely to have misleading CT scans (35.3%).[76] A consensus panel convened by the American Hepato-Pancreato-biliary Association[77] recommends laparoscopy be limited to select patients with primary tumors greater than 3 cm in diameter, body or tail tumors, equivocal findings of metastasis on CT, and CA 19-9 level greater than 100 U/mL. Using these criteria, the subset of patients with advanced tumors not identified on CT scan can be accurately assessed by laparoscopy, and patients likely to not have additional findings can be spared the expensive, time-consuming procedure.

STAGING

From a practical perspective, pancreatic cancer is often defined as resectable, locally advanced, or metastatic disease. Treatment and survival are defined for these three groups, although the boundaries defining the groups may vary slightly from one pancreatic specialist to another. Determining resectability is the most important aspect of clinical staging because surgical resection offers the only chance of cure.

The sixth edition of the American Joint Committee on Cancer's (AJCC) staging system (Table 82.4)[78] reflects a clinical definition of resectability based on CT assessment. The T-stage designation classifies T1 through T3 tumors as potentially resectable and T4 tumors as locally advanced (unresectable). Tumors with any involvement of the superior mesenteric or celiac arteries are classified as T4; however, tumors that involve the superior mesenteric, splenic, or portal veins are classified as T3 since these veins can be resected and reconstructed, provided that they are patent. Stage IV disease includes any disease at a distant site, or nodal metastases beyond N1 disease.[79] In this iteration of the AJCC staging system the stage of disease correlates with survival while previous versions did not.

TABLE 82.4

AMERICAN JOINT COMMITTEE ON CANCER: CANCER STAGING FOR EXOCRINE PANCREAS

PRIMARY TUMOR (T)	
TX	Primary tumor cannot be assessed
T0	No evidence of primary tumor
Tis	Carcinoma *in situ* (also PanIN 3)
T1	Tumor limited to pancreas, 2 cm or less in greatest dimension
T2	Tumor limited to pancreas, more than 2 cm in greatest dimension
T3	Tumor extends beyond the pancreas but without involvement of the celiac axis or the superior mesenteric artery
T4	Tumor involves the celiac axis or the superior mesenteric artery (unresectable primary tumor)
REGIONAL LYMPH NODES (N)	
NX	Regional lymph nodes cannot be assessed
N0	No regional lymph node metastasis
N1	Regional lymph node metastasis
DISTANT METASTASIS (M)	
MX	Distant metastasis cannot be assessed
M0	No distant metastasis
M1	Distant metastasis

STAGE GROUPING			
Stage 0	Tis	N0	M0
Stage IA	T1	N0	M0
Stage IB	T2	N0	M0
Stage IIA	T3	N0	M0
Stage IIB	T1	N1	M0
	T2	N1	M0
	T3	N1	M0
Stage III	T4	Any N	M0
Stage IV	Any T	Any N	M1

PanIN, pancreatic intraepithelial neoplasia.
(From ref. 78, with permission.)

TREATMENT OF POTENTIALLY RESECTABLE DISEASE: AMERICAN JOINT COMMITTEE ON CANCER STAGE I AND II

Operative Treatment

Rationale for Resection

Resectable pancreatic cancers are confined to the pancreas and draining lymph nodes with a patent SMV-PV and noninvolvement of the visceral arteries. Operative excision remains the

PRACTICE OF ONCOLOGY

standard of care in the United States, although justification for resection is based on few objective data. There has not been a randomized trial studying subjects with resectable tumors who are randomized to operative versus nonoperative treatment (just as there are no randomized trials for resection of any other type of primary gastrointestinal tumor). Without these trials, the impact of surgical removal is based on comparisons of disparate patient groups and small, single-institution experiences. It is therefore difficult to evaluate the oncologic aims for operative treatment, including cure of pancreatic cancer and prolongation of survival.

Although resection offers the only prospect of long-term survival or cure in this disease, it rarely accomplishes either of these. Conlon et al.[80] analyzed 357 patients with pancreatic cancer who were resected with curative intent from 1981 to 2001 at the Mayo Clinic. An 18% 5-year survival was observed with survival of 62 patients. Ten of these patients subsequently died of metastatic pancreatic cancer beyond the 5-year time point. Yeo et al.[81] at JHMI reviewed pancreatic head resections for pancreatic cancer showing 22 of 149 patients undergoing resection were alive at 5 years, noting most deaths later than 5 years were due to metastatic disease. Additionally, Cleary et al.[82] found 18 of 123 patients who were resected during the time period 1988 to 1996 were 5-year survivors. Four of these 18 patients died of metastatic disease after the 5-year time point. All of these studies reveal the 5-year survival of patients treated with pancreatic cancer resection is low. Many of the patients who surpass the 5-year survival target eventually die of the disease, and cure is realized in a very small number of patients who undergo resection.

If operative treatment rarely cures pancreatic cancer, resection can also be justified as a means to prolong survival; but there is a paucity of studies addressing whether removal of a primary pancreatic cancer prolongs life. Review of the National Cancer Data Base identified 9,559 patients with stage I pancreatic cancer. Of these 6,380 were likely eligible for resection based on age, comorbidities, or acceptance of surgery. Of these candidates for surgery, 2,736 were actually treated with pancreatectomy. Median survival in those patients with stage I disease treated with surgery was 10.9 months longer than those seemingly eligible patients who did not undergo surgery (19.3 months vs. 8.4 months). Similarly, 5-year survival rates were higher in the operative patients (24.6 vs. 2.9%).[83]

Operative Resection

Operative removal of a pancreatic cancer requires anatomic resections such as pancreaticoduodenectomy, distal pancreatectomy, or total pancreatectomy that includes contiguous structures (such as the duodenum, spleen, and common bile duct) and at least 15 draining lymph nodes.

The first description of pancreatic head resection with a portion of duodenum was by Codvilla in 1898.[84] This Italian surgeon, who is most known for advances in orthopedic surgery, operated on a jaundiced patient allegedly diagnosed with pancreatic cancer. In this case survival was limited to 24 days following the procedure. Kausch[85] described the first successful resection of the pancreatic head with a portion of the duodenum performed in 1909. Whipple[86] embarked on perfecting pancreas head resection in 1934, and in the subsequent 30 years he and contemporary surgeons of the period revised the resection to a technique resembling that used by most surgeons today. Early historical procedures utilized a two-stage approach with an initial biliary bypass. Patients demonstrated hepatic dysfunction due to biliary obstruction, and the initial drainage procedure allowed for normalization of coagulopathy prior to a second procedure during which varying amounts of the pancreatic head and duodenum were resected. An evolving understanding of the coagulopathy and the addition of vitamin K to the preoperative regimen of these patients allowed for single-stage procedures to be routinely completed in the 1940s.

The first description of a distal pancreatectomy was by Trendelenburg in 1882, allegedly for sarcoma involving the spleen and tail of pancreas.[87,88] The patient did not survive the procedure. In 1889, Ruggi[89] and Briggs[90] separately completed successful distal pancreatectomies for alleged malignant lesions, with patient survival at short-term follow-up.

Evans et al.[91] has described a stepwise methodology that can be applied to pancreaticoduodenectomy and is widely applicable to most resections. This can be summarized as six steps of resection followed by four steps of reconstruction (Figs. 82.1 and 82.2). An essential component to this resection is the approach to the SMA margin. This margin extends along the interface of the uncinate process and the length of the SMA, incorporating autonomic nerves at this interface. An R0 resection is defined by the absence of microscopic disease at this margin and is correlated with prolonged survival.[92,93] Although the extent of disease in some tumors precludes an R0 resection, a complete resection should be sought when at all feasible.

Intraperitoneal Drains

Intraperitoneal drains are usually placed intraoperatively in the vicinity of the pancreatic and biliary anastomosis following pancreas resection. A single study prospectively evaluated the contribution of this drainage to the postoperative course. One hundred seventy-nine patients who underwent pancreatic resection (pancreaticoduodenectomy: 139, distal pancreatectomy: 40)

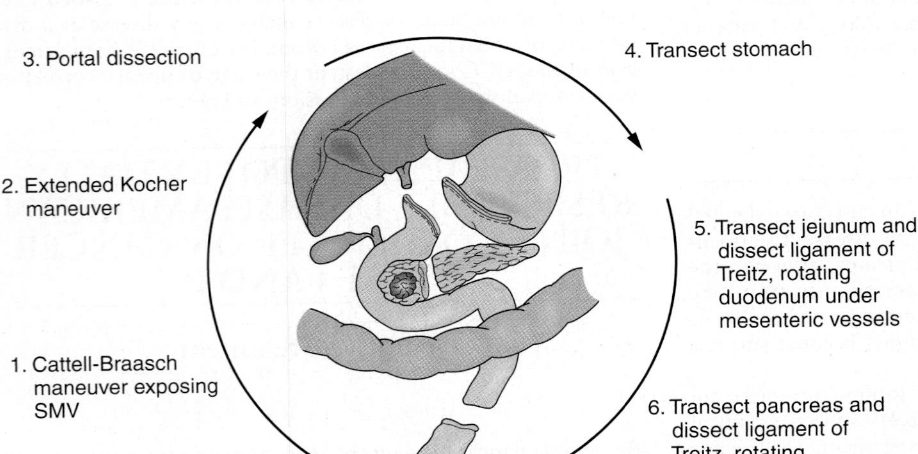

FIGURE 82.1 Six surgical steps of pancreaticoduodenectomy (clockwise resection). SMV, superior mesenteric vein. (Adapted from Evans DB, Abbruzzese J, Rich TA. In: DeVita VT, Hellman S, Rosenberg SA, eds. *Cancer: principles and practice of oncology*. 5th ed. Philadelphia: Lippincott-Raven, 1997:1071.)

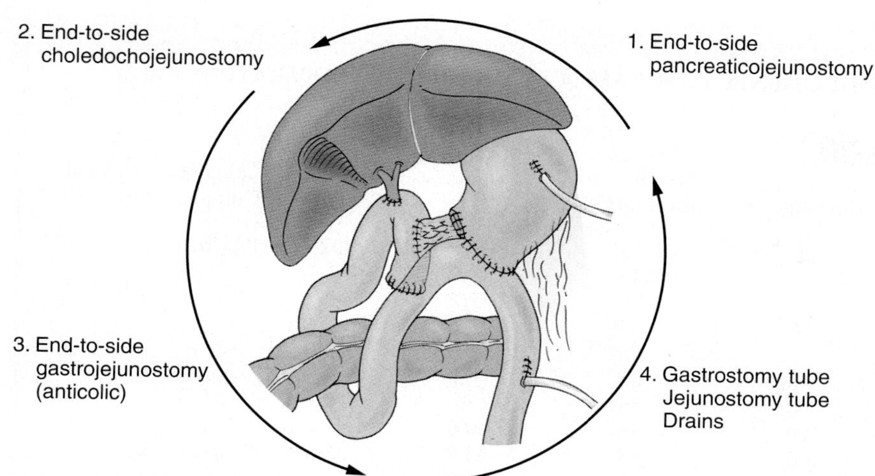

FIGURE 82.2 Four surgical steps of counterclockwise reconstruction following standard pancreaticoduodenectomy. (Adapted from Evans DB, Abbruzzese J, Rich TA. In: DeVita VT, Hellman S, Rosenberg SA, eds. *Cancer: principles and practice of oncology*. 5th ed. Philadelphia: Lippincott-Raven, 1997:1073.)

were randomized to have drains (88 patients) or no drains (91 patients) placed at the conclusion of the case. Placement of drains did not decrease the need for subsequent percutaneous drainage of an intra-abdominal collection (drain: eight patients, no drain: seven patients) and the incidence of intraperitoneal sepsis, fluid collection, or fistula was increased in the patients who were randomized to intraperitoneal drain (drain: 19 patients, no drain: eight patients).[94] Accordingly, the use of intraperitoneal drains is decreasing among pancreatic surgeons.

Biliary Stents

Seventy percent of resectable pancreatic cancers obstruct the distal common bile duct (CBD) at presentation. The intrapancreatic portion of the CBD passes behind or through the pancreatic head, rendering it susceptible to mass effect and obstruction from the tumor or associated desmoplasia. In many patients, hyperbilirubinemia precipitates the diagnosis of a mass in the pancreatic head.

Biliary stents relieve obstruction and are inserted using percutaneous transhepatic or endoscopic techniques, and their use in patients with resectable lesions can maintain a patent CBD during neoadjuvant therapy or referral to a regional center with a focus on pancreatic cancer. Soft silastic stents can be changed periodically and are most commonly used, but they can fail during a prolonged period of neoadjuvant therapy. Expandable metal stents do not have the interchangeability of silastic stents but are more durable. When placed in patients with resectable tumors, the most superior extent of the stent should be at the confluence of the cystic duct and the common bile duct, allowing division of the common bile duct above the cystic duct entrance in any subsequent procedure. A metal stent cannot be divided intraoperatively. Therefore, a metal stent cannot traverse a planned line of common bile duct division.

The morbidity associated with biliary stents has recently come into focus, raising questions regarding their safety in patients with resectable pancreatic head lesions. Povoski et al.[95] at MSKCC analyzed the clinical course of 240 patients treated by pancreaticoduodenectomy, 131 for pancreas adenocarcinoma. Overall, 175 patients were evaluated with biliary instrumentation, primarily ERCP, and 126 patients were treated with one or more drainage procedures using a stent (70.5% endoscopic and 19.9% percutaneous) or operative procedure (9.6%). Forty-eight percent of patients developed a postoperative complication, and biliary drainage by stent or operation was associated with an increased complication risk compared to those patients not treated with drainage (55% vs. 39% respectively; $P = .025$). Specifically, risk of infectious complication (41% vs. 25%; $P = .014$), intra-abdominal abscess (24% vs. 9%; $P = .020$), and death (8% vs. 3%; $P = .037$) were all increased with biliary drainage.

Several retrospective studies have recently challenged these findings, associating fewer complications with the use of preoperative stents (Table 82.5). These groups found no stent-related morbidity or an association between stents and wound infection or wound infection and pancreatic fistula during the postoperative period for pancreaticoduodenectomy. One of these investigators, Pisters et al.[96] at M. D. Anderson Cancer Center (MDACC) comprehensively scrutinized 300 consecutive patients treated with pancreaticoduodenectomy, finding 172 had been decompressed with a prosthetic stent, 35 with operative bypass, and 93 not drained. Only wound infection was found to be associated with preoperative biliary stenting (stent 13% vs. no stent 4%; $P = .029$). The bacterial species identified by intraoperative bile culture and at any subsequent wound infection are frequently the same, so the results of an intraoperative bile culture can direct antimicrobial choice when a wound infection is initially suspected.

Preoperative endobiliary stenting is a safe intervention that results in increased rates of postoperative wound infection, but should not be avoided when used to palliate patients for transfer to a high-volume center. Birkmeyer et al.[97,98] clearly establish that transfer of patients with pancreatic cancer to high-volume centers significantly decreases patient morbidity and mortality. Inasmuch as endobiliary stenting can facilitate this transfer, the maneuver should not be abandoned. Stenting additionally can temporize biliary obstruction for the completion of neoadjuvant therapy.

Extended Lymph Node Dissection

In general, pancreaticoduodenectomy includes *en bloc* resection of the duodenum, head of the pancreas, immediate peripancreatic nodal tissue, and possibly the pylorus and antrum of the stomach. Some have recommended a more extensive resection as a means of minimizing recurrence. Outcomes from these more radical operations have been the focus of recent randomized surgical trials. Three randomized prospective trials have evaluated the utility of an extended lymphadenectomy during pancreatic resection for pancreatic cancer.

A multi-institutional randomized surgical trial directed by Pedrazzoli et al.[99] at the University of Padova in Italy established no benefit from extended lymphadenectomy in the patients studied, although the group suggests a benefit may be conferred on patients with nodal disease. The study included 81 patients treated at six institutions randomized preoperatively to standard lymphadenectomy or extended dissection entailing piecemeal excision of additional hepatic hilar and periaortic nodes from

TABLE 82.5

MORBIDITY FOLLOWING PANCREATICODUODENECTOMY: ASSOCIATION WITH PREOPERATIVE BILIARY STENTS

Group (Ref.)	Stent	N	Mortality (%)	Overall Morbidity (%)	Wound Infection (%)	Wound Infection P	Other Stent-Related Complications
JHMI (250)	Y	408	1.7	35	10.0	.02	Pancreatic fistula
2000	N	158	2.5	30	4.0		
Univ. Amsterdam (251)	Y	232	1.2	50	7.3	NS	
2001	N	58	0.0	55	8.6		
M. D. Anderson (96)	Y	172	0.6	88	13.0	.029	
2001	N	93	1.0	86	4.0		
University of Bern[a] (252)	Y	50	4.0	56	13.0	NS	
2001	N	15	0.0	53	10.0		
SGP Institute[a] (253)	Y	54	15.0	48	43.0	.03	Pancreatic fistula
2001	N	41	10.0	55	24.0		Overall infection
Hines VA[a] (254)	Y	154	2.0	67	8.0	.039	
2003	N	58	2.0	57	0.0		

JHMI, Johns Hopkins Medical Institutes; SGP, Sanjay Ghandi Postgraduate; VA, Veterans Administration; NS, not significant.
[a]Jaundiced patients only in control and stented groups. No significant differences in mortality or overall morbidity for all groups.

the diaphragm to the inferior mesenteric arteries, encompassing the nodes of the renal hila, celiac, and SMA regions. Although overall survival was not affected, *post hoc*, unplanned, subset analysis showed the patients with node-positive disease had improved survival if treated with extended lymphadenectomy.

A larger prospective randomized trial from the group at JHMI suggests there is not a benefit to extended lymphadenectomy. The group studied 294 patients with periampullary adenocarcinoma who were randomized following a confirmed R0 resection intraoperatively. In 148 patients, a distal gastrectomy with sampling of the celiac nodes, resection of greater omental, lesser omental, portal, SMA, and periaortic nodes was completed for extended lymph node resection. Patients treated with an extended lymph node dissection experienced a prolonged operating time and greater frequency of postoperative complications. Survival in the group overall or in subset analysis of nodal involvement or primary histology was not improved by extended lymphadenectomy.[59,100]

Farnell et al.[101] at the Mayo Clinic conducted a randomized prospective trial involving 132 patients explored for suspected pancreatic cancer. When found at operation to have resectable disease, the patients were treated with pancreaticoduodenectomy (40 patients) or pancreaticoduodenectomy with extended lymph node dissection (39 patients). Patients treated with the extended resection did not experience prolonged similar median survival (19 months) to those undergoing standard resection (26 months; $P = .32$).

The Italian study, the JHMI, and the Mayo trials are commendable for the completion of a prospective randomized trial involving a rigorous operative treatment. Both the Italian and JHMI studies can be criticized for a lymphadenectomy that was not completed in continuity with the pancreas resection and the JHMI trial for an extended lymphadenectomy less extensive than most proponents of extended surgery would find appropriate. These limitations notwithstanding, extended lymphadenectomy currently has no role in pancreas resections, although the resection needs to be extensive enough to obtain at least 15 draining lymph nodes in the specimen.

Patterns of Failure in Resected Pancreatic Cancer

The pattern of failure in surgically resected pancreatic cancer has been well established. Prior to the routine delivery of adjuvant therapy, Tepper et al.[102] reviewed the records of 145 patients seen at Massachusetts General Hospital from 1963 to 1973. Thirty-one patients underwent surgery with curative intent, with an operative mortality rate of 16% and an overall median survival of 10.5 months. Of the patients who survived the operation 50% had evidence of local failure as a component of failure. More recently, autopsy data collected from 2003 to 2007 at JHMI demonstrate that the patterns of failure have not changed despite better preoperative imaging and more routine use of adjuvant therapy.[103] In a program established by Iacobuzio-Dohahue et al.[103] 76 patients with pancreatic cancer underwent rapid autopsy. Of these, 22 had undergone previous surgical resection of the primary tumor and 20 had gross evidence of disease at autopsy (91%). Local recurrence as the only site was found in 15% and an additional 65% had local disease as a component of failure. Metastatic disease was noted in 85% of patients with relapse after surgery. Of further note, among the six patients who underwent surgery with a positive surgical margin, 83% had local recurrence as a component of failure. Thus, patients with resected pancreatic cancer are at very high risk for both local recurrence and metastatic disease, with roughly 15% succumbing to local recurrence only.[103,104]

Adjuvant and Neoadjuvant Therapy

Adjuvant therapy, as properly defined, involves the delivery of anticancer therapy after surgical removal of all gross tumor to prevent tumor recurrence. Despite documented reductions in mortality related to surgery, improvements in radiation, and more active chemotherapy, little survival benefit has been demonstrated for adjuvant therapy in pancreatic cancer. Table 82.6 reviews the efficacy of adjuvant therapy.

Adjuvant Studies Using 5-Fluorouracil–Based Chemoradiation

Since resected pancreatic cancer has a propensity to recur locally, early studies of adjuvant therapy focused on radiation to prevent local relapse with delivery of systemic therapy to inhibit distant failure. There have been several randomized and nonrandomized trials of adjuvant 5-fluoroucil (5-FU)–based chemoradiotherapy. The three randomized trials that have received the most

TABLE 82.6

OVERALL SURVIVAL DATA FROM SEVERAL COMPLETED RANDOMIZED TRIALS OF ADJUVANT THERAPY IN PATIENTS WITH RESECTED PANCREATIC CANCER

Study (Ref.)	No. of Patients	Enrolled Patients with R1 Resection (%)	Treatment Assignment Median Survival Months	Treatment Assignment Median Survival Months	*P* Value
GITSG 1985 (258)	49	0	5-FU chemoradiation 21.0	Observation 10.9	.035
EORTC 40891 1999 (259)	114[a]	21	5-FU chemoradiation 17.1	Observation 12.6	.09
ESPAC-1 2004 (107)	289	18	5-FU/leucovorin chemotherapy 20.1	No chemotherapy 15.5	.009
			5-FU-based chemoradiation 15.9	No chemoradiation 17.9	.05
RTOG 9704 2006 (110)	380 (head lesions)	>35	Gemcitabine then 5-FU/EBRT then Gemcitabine 20.6	5-FU then 5-FU/EBRT then 5-FU 16.9	.033
CONKO-001[b] 2007 (116)	368	19	Gemcitabine 22.1	Observation 20.1	.06
			DFS = 13.9	DFS = 6.9	<.001

GITSG, Gastrointestinal Study Group; EORTC, European Organisation for Research and Treatment of Cancer; ESPAC, European Study Group for Pancreatic Cancer; RTOG, Radiation Therapy Oncology Group; CONKO, Charité Onkologie; EBRT, external beam radiotherapy; 5-FU, fluorouracil, DFS, disease-free survival.

[a]EORTC 40891 enrolled 214 patients, but only 114 had adenocarcinoma of the pancreas. Tabulated survival data are for patients with pancreatic primary tumors.

[b]In CONKO-001 there was a difference in disease-free survival between the gemcitabine arm and the control arm.

attention were conducted by the Gastrointestinal Study Group (GITSG), the European Organisation for Research and Treatment of Cancer (EORTC), and the European Study Group for Pancreatic Cancer (ESPAC).[105–107]

The first was the GITSG trial, which enrolled patients with completely resected pancreatic cancer and, importantly, microscopically negative margins (R0).[105] Forty-six patients were randomized to undergo observation or bolus 5-FU (500 mg/m^2 daily) during the first 3 days of each period of split course radiation (20 Gy in 10 fractions, 2 weeks break, and resumption of radiation to a total dose of 40 Gy), followed by up to 2 years of weekly bolus 5-FU. Survival was reported after only 43 patients had completed treatment and showed a striking survival advantage for patients receiving combined modality therapy compared with surgery alone (median 21.0 months vs. 10.9 months, respectively; one-tailed $P = .03$).

The GITSG findings could not be reproduced by a subsequent EORTC trial.[106] EORTC-40891 randomized 218 patients preoperatively for resection of tumors of the periampullary region (including pancreatic head, common bile duct, papilla of Vater, and duodenal cancers), to either undergo observation or receive 5-FU (25 mg/kg/d to a maximum dose of 1,500 mg/d) given concurrently during the first week of two split courses of radiation (total dose 40 Gy). Subgroup analysis for the 114 patients with cancer of the pancreatic head showed a trend toward improved overall survival for those receiving adjuvant therapy versus the observation group (median 17.1 months vs. 12.6 months, respectively), but the difference was not statistically significant ($P = .099$). Updated data from this trial were published in 2008 and again showed no survival advantage for the patients randomized to chemoradiation.[106a]

At about the same time, ESPAC launched an ambitious trial to determine the efficacy of chemotherapy versus chemoradiation on overall survival after surgery. ESPAC-1 enrolled 289 patients from 53 European hospitals.[107] After resection, patients were randomized to one of four arms: observation, chemotherapy with bolus 5-FU (425 mg/m^2) and leucovorin (20 mg/m^2) daily for 5 days every 28 days for 6 months, chemoradiation with bolus 5-FU 500 mg/m^2 during the first 3 days of split-course of radiation (as in the GITSG trial), or chemoradiation followed by 6 months of chemotherapy with bolus 5-FU and leucovorin. When overall survival of the four arms were directly compared, there was no statistically significant difference in survival. However, the study was designed to analyze survival outcomes using a two-by-two factorial design according to treatment assignment to chemotherapy (yes or no) or to chemoradiation (yes or no). Patients who received chemoradiation did worse (median survival of 15.9 months; hazard ratio [HR] for death 1.28; 95% CI, 0.99 to 1.66) than those who did not receive chemoradiation (median survival of 17.9 months; $P = .05$). Conversely, patients who received chemotherapy had a median survival of 20.6 months (HR for death 0.71; 95% CI, 0.55 to 0.92) versus 15.5 months for those patients who did not receive chemotherapy, a statistically significant improvement ($P = .009$). The investigators concluded that chemoradiation not only failed to benefit patients but also reduced survival when given before chemotherapy.

The merits of chemoradiation have been increasingly challenged over time, and the role of radiation as a component of adjuvant therapy should be considered an open question, with two current adjuvant trials trying to determine if there is a benefit. The EORTC is conducting a randomized trial comparing systemic gemcitabine therapy alone versus systemic gemcitabine followed by gemcitabine-based chemoradiation. The Radiation Therapy Oncology Group (RTOG) is delivering five cycles of gemcitabine with or without erlotinib as part of the first randomization. Thereafter, all patients will be restaged and for those without interval development of metastatic disease, a sixth cycle of gemcitabine will be delivered (with or without erlotinib) and a second randomization will occur to assign patients to no further therapy or to a standard course of 5-FU–based chemoradiation.

Radiation Technique: Postoperative Adjuvant Radiation Therapy

Postoperative radiation therapy has evolved from the early trials, and patients with resected disease are typically treated with 50.4 Gy, given in 1.8-Gy fractions. Field reductions are characteristic after 45 Gy. The boost volume should include the superior mesenteric vessels, the tumor bed, and the celiac axis.

A four-field technique using anterior, posterior, and opposed lateral fields allows sparing of critical tissues. Fields are weighted so that the dose contribution from the lateral fields is restricted to 20 Gy by weighting the anteroposterior–posteroanterior fields at twice that of the lateral fields. This approach prevents the liver and kidney tissue that are restricted to the lateral fields from receiving doses beyond their tolerance. In cases where the right kidney is receiving a toxic dose, the posterior field may be omitted or customized oblique fields used. Intensity modulated radiation therapy (IMRT) is not likely to result in a reduction of toxicity, but should be considered in cases where there are grossly enlarged lymph nodes or a positive margin. In these cases, a nested gross tumor volume can be used to deliver a higher dose. A simultaneous dose of 63 Gy in 28 fractions can be delivered to high-risk areas and 50.4 Gy to the microscopic areas at risk, avoiding the jejunal reconstruction. Although this practice is standard, there are no studies that demonstrate that higher doses of radiation compensate for a positive margin.

The celiac axis, which is most commonly located at T12, should be covered with a 2-cm margin superiorly. That superior border usually covers the porta hepatis as well. Inferiorly the tumor and duodenal bed should be covered with a 2-cm margin. The left border is usually placed 2 cm to the left of the vertebral body edge, as long as coverage of the preoperative tumor volume is adequate. The preoperative tumor volume and preoperative location of the duodenum define the right field border and the anterior extent of the lateral fields. The porta hepatis identified on the planning CT scans should be covered, and useful landmarks for the porta hepatis are the bifurcation of the portal vein and the hepatic artery. For lesions of the pancreatic body and tail, similar fields are used except that the splenic hilum is covered and the porta hepatis and duodenal bed are not covered. The right field border is typically located 2 cm from the right vertebral body edge.

Studies of Systemic Adjuvant Therapy without Radiation

Despite the ongoing debate about the role of radiation in resected pancreatic cancer, systemic chemotherapy without radiation has recently become firmly established as the standard of care after surgery. On a historical note, however, the first effort to show a benefit to adjuvant chemotherapy failed to provide a long-term survival advantage compared to treatment with surgery alone. In a European trial published in 1993, 61 patients with radically resected pancreatic cancer (47) or ampullary cancer (14), were randomized to receive no further therapy, or a combination of doxorubicin, mitomycin C, and 5-FU (AMF).[108] AMF postponed relapse of disease during the first 2 years after surgery compared with no treatment, however, long-term prognosis was the same, with an identical survival after 2 years.

Subsequent to this trial, three large randomized studies have shown the benefit of systemic chemotherapy for patients with pancreatic cancer resected with curative intent. First, as described above, the ESPAC-1 trial demonstrated a survival advantage for patients receiving chemotherapy compared with patients not receiving chemotherapy after surgery (20.6 months vs. 15.5 months).[107] Second, Neuhaus et al.[109] presented the long-term results of the CONKO-001 (Charité Onkologie) study. This study conclusively demonstrated the benefit of adjuvant gemcitabine compared with surgery alone in 368 patients with resected pancreatic adenocarcinoma. Gemcitabine was dosed at 1,000 mg/m^2 weekly for 3 of 4 weeks for six cycles in the adjuvant treatment group. Disease-free survival (DFS) and median overall survival were superior in the gemcitabine arm (13 months and 22.8 months, respectively) compared with the observation arm (6.9 months and 20.2 months, respectively). Furthermore, survival at 3 years and 5 years unequivocally favored the delivery of adjuvant gemcitabine over observation. Third, adjuvant chemotherapy was further supported by pooled data obtained by the investigators of ESPAC-1 and ESPAC-3. ESPAC-1 had an observation only arm and, initially, ESPAC-3 also had an observation arm. The observation arm of ESPAC-3 was subsequently closed after the results of CONKO-001 were released. A pooled analysis comparing observation after surgery with 6 months of postoperative 5-FU and leucovorin similarly demonstrated a statistically significant survival advantage for patients receiving adjuvant therapy (23.2 months vs. 16.8 months; HR for death = 0.70; P = .003).

Gemcitabine or 5-FU as Adjuvant Therapy

Given the modest superiority of gemcitabine over 5-FU for the treatment of patients with advanced disease, these two drugs have been compared head to head in the adjuvant setting. The RTOG performed a prospective randomized trial (RTOG 9704) comparing systemic gemcitabine with infusional 5-FU; patients in both arms also received 5-FU–based chemoradiation.[110] A total of 518 patients were enrolled in the study, with the majority of patients having tumors of the pancreatic head. There was no survival difference between patients randomized to gemcitabine and those who received infusional 5-FU. However, among the 380 patients with resected head lesions, survival was seemingly superior for patients randomized to gemcitabine compared with those who received infusional 5-FU (20.5 months vs. 16.9 months; HR for death 0.82; 95% CI, 0.65 to 1.03; P = .09).

The most recent results comparing systemic gemcitabine to systemic 5-FU come from the largest adjuvant phase 3 trial ever conducted, ESPAC-3. The results have not as yet been published, but they were presented at the 2009 ASCO Annual Meeting.[111] The original trial design randomized patients to one of three arms: observation, bolus 5-FU and leucovorin, or gemcitabine. A total of 1,088 patients were randomized to receive either five daily doses of 5-FU (425 mg/m^2 IV bolus) with leucovorin (20 mg/m^2 IV bolus) every 28 days for six cycles or gemcitabine (1,000 mg/m^2 weekly for 3 of 4 weeks). With a median follow-up of 34 months, there was no difference between the treatment arms. Median survival was 23.0 months in the 5-FU arm and 23.6 months in the gemcitabine arm (P = .39). As in ESPAC-1, these results lent credence to 5-FU and leucovorin as effective adjuvant chemotherapy. However, toxicity associated with gemcitabine was less than that observed using 5-FU and leucovorin. Taken together, the results from the RTOG trial and ESPAC-3 (v2) suggest that gemcitabine is either slightly better than 5-FU in terms of efficacy or slightly better tolerated, and at present, gemcitabine monotherapy has emerged as the standard of care for adjuvant therapy.

A New Standard Adjuvant Regimen, but No Real Progress

Table 82.6 summarizes the results of selected randomized adjuvant trials completed thus far. Based on these trials, six cycles of gemcitabine monotherapy should be considered the standard of care for patients with resected pancreatic cancer. No matter what treatment strategy is employed, overall survival ranges from 20 months to 23.6 months. This holds true from the first trial published in 1985 to the last one reported in 2009. Sadly, improved survival with adjuvant therapy rarely translates into cure. Currently, the realistic goal of adjuvant treatment is to delay relapse rather than to prevent it.

There are several reasons why adjuvant therapy research has failed to make any significant progress in comparison to the initial results in 1985. First, upfront surgery is not always linked to the subsequent delivery of adjuvant therapy. Reports from JHMI, the Mayo Clinic, and SEER/Medicare data sets all suggests that only about 60% of patients who undergo surgery with curative intent go on to receive adjuvant therapy. This suggests surgery is often being applied to a subset of patients with low potential to receive further therapy. Without more rigorous preoperative assessments, the number of patients eligible to enroll in adjuvant studies will be far lower than the number of patients who undergo resection.

Second, positive surgical margins portent poor survival, and most patients left with a positive surgical margin have a median survival of less than 12 months, with or without adjuvant therapy.[112–115] Recent studies have found positive surgical margins rates at university-based hospitals as high as 50%.[113] These rates may be underestimates, since strict assessment of the SMA margin (also known as the retroperitoneal margin or uncinate margin) has not been widely adopted. For example, in the RTOG trial,[110] no data were available regarding the surgical margin for roughly 25% of enrolled patients. In addition, in ESPAC-1[107] and CONKO-001,[116] although the proportion of patients who had a positive surgical margin was quite low, local failure rates as a component of failure were high, at 35% to 60%, implying a substantial proportion of patients had incomplete surgical resections. As previously discussed in this chapter, high-quality cross-sectional imaging can accurately predict tumor resectability. Unfortunately, none of the completed adjuvant trials has required high-quality imaging to define a resectable pancreatic cancer (one with high probability of being removed with negative surgical margins).

Third, early relapse can occur following pancreatic resection. Studies from the MDACC, the ECOG, and Duke University Medical Center have shown that about 15% to 20% of patients who enroll in preoperative trials with no evidence of distant disease will develop radiographic evidence of metastatic disease within several weeks.[117–121] Thus far, most adjuvant trials have not required postoperative imaging prior to the initiation of adjuvant therapy.

Given the local failure rates observed in completed adjuvant trials and the frequent development of metastatic disease noted in preoperative trials, it is reasonable to assume that a substantial subset of patients enrolled in past and current trials of adjuvant therapy do not receive adjuvant therapy as appropriately defined: some patients receive therapy for locally advanced disease (which was incompletely resected) or early metastatic relapse (which would be apparent on postoperative imaging before adjuvant therapy). Under these circumstances, progress in adjuvant therapy can be expected to remain slow.

An Alterative Approach to Resectable Disease: Preoperative Therapy

Some groups have investigated preoperative therapy, typically with chemoradiation (Table 82.7). Preoperative therapy has sound rationale: (1) initiation of local and systemic therapy shortly after diagnosis rather than weeks following surgery, (2) treatment of a relatively well-perfused tumor bed, and (3) provision of a time interval to assess for aggressive tumor biology with rapid onset of metastatic disease. Of further note, observation of the patient through a course of preoperative therapy provides a longitudinal assessment of the patient's potential to undergo the rigors of surgical intervention. The primary limitation of neoadjuvant therapy is the requirement for durable biliary drainage in those patients with biliary obstruction and a fully committed multidisciplinary care team.

Preoperative strategies for pancreatic cancer have not been widely adopted. A common reason for rejecting preoperative therapy centers on the potential for local tumor progression, which may preclude surgical intervention and a chance for

TABLE 82.7

SELECTED TRIALS OF NEOADJUVANT CHEMORADIATION FOR PATIENTS WITH POTENTIALLY RESECTABLE PANCREATIC CANCER

Author (Ref.)	Evaluable Patients	Resected	EBRT Dose (Gy)	Chemotherapy Regimen	Median Survival All Patients (Mo)	Median Survival Resected Patients (Mo)
Evans et al. (122)	28	17 (61%)	50.4 + IORT	CI 5-FU	NA	18
Hoffman et al. (118)	53	24 (45%)	50.4	Bolus 5-FU + MMC	9.7	15.7
Pisters et al. (119)	35	20 (57%)	30 + IORT	PVI 5-FU	7	25
White et al. (260)	53 resectable	28 (53%)	45	PVI 5-FU + MMC/CDDP	NR	NR
Moutardier et al. (261)	19	15 (79%)	30 or 45	Bolus 5-FU + CDDP	20	30
Arnoletti et al. (262)	26	14 (54%)	50.4	5-FU and/or MMC or Gem	NA	34
Pisters et al. (123)	35	20 (57%)	30 and 10 IORT	Paclitaxel	12	19
Wolff et al. (263)	86	64 (75%)	30	Gem	22	36
Magnin et al. (264)	32	19 (59%)	30 or 45	PVI 5-FU + CDDP	16	30
Talamonti et al. (127)	20	17 (85%)	36 Gy	Gem	NA	NA

EBRT, external beam radiotherapy; IORT, intraoperative radiotherapy; CI, continuous infusion; 5-FU, 5-fluorouracil; MMC, mitomycin C; PVI, protracted venous infusion; CDDP, cisplatin; Gem, gemcitabine; NA, not assessed; NR, not reached.

cure. However, none of the preoperative studies published to date suggests that this risk is substantial.[118,119,121–123] Moreover, in contrast to local recurrence rates when using adjuvant therapy, local failure after preoperative therapy has been relatively low, ranging from 10% to 25%.[119,123,124,125] In addition, R0 resection rates are higher using preoperative chemoradiation compared with upfront surgical resection.[126] Although 5-FU or paclitaxel-based preoperative regimens have not demonstrated superior survival results compared with adjuvant therapy, recent phase 2 trials of gemcitabine-based preoperative therapy have been encouraging.[124,125,127]

Borderline Resectable Tumors

There is growing recognition of a distinct group of tumors that are borderline resectable. Although a small localized pancreatic cancer should be resected, clinicians generally disagree whether or not a patient may derive benefit from resection of advanced tumors that involve vascular structures, but are technically resectable. As high-quality cross-sectional imaging is increasingly utilized and the implications of positive surgical margins appreciated, three distinct types of localized pancreatic tumors are now emerging: resectable, borderline resectable, and locally advanced (Fig. 82.3). Borderline resectable tumors are defined as those with (1) tumors confined to the pancreatic bed and draining nodes without distant metastases, (2) tumor involvement of the SMV or portal vein, including abutment, constriction of the lumen, and encasement; short segment occlusion from either thrombosis or constriction is included if vessels suitable for reconstruction exist proximal and distal to the occlusion, or (3) arterial involvement, including encasement of the gastroduodenal artery, short segment encasement or abutment of the hepatic artery (without celiac axis involvement), and abutment of the SMA with circumferential involvement of 180 degrees or less.[77]

Although tumor down-staging is often stated to be the goal of an initial course of cytotoxic therapy, pancreatic cancers uncommonly regress away from vascular structures, even if they respond to therapy. However, margin-negative resectability can be enhanced even if the tumor remains in close proximity to a vascular structure on imaging.[128] The treatment recommendations of patients with borderline resectable tumors are similar to the treatment of patients with locally advanced, unresectable disease. Often, the surgical procedure is more complex or the risk of systemic progression is greater in these patients, so longer courses of chemotherapy have been recommended in order to optimally select patients who are most likely to benefit from surgical resection.

The experience from MDACC using gemcitabine-based chemotherapy followed by chemoradiation (50.4 Gy in 28 fractions) with concurrent gemcitabine (400 mg/m^2 weekly) demonstrates the advantages of this hyperselection and the effect of therapy on the vascular margin. Approximately 40% of patients with borderline resectable disease were ultimately able to undergo surgical resection, with a median overall survival for the subset undergoing surgical resection of 40 months. Moreover, an R0 resection was achieved in 94% of resected patients, and 98% of patients with initial arterial involvement were able to undergo R0 resection. Compared to pretreatment studies, CT restaging evaluation may be less accurate following cytotoxic therapy and may underestimate the number of patients who can undergo resection since inflammation can obscure the fat plane between the vessel and the tumor, and scarring at the vessel margin may appear identical to tumor. The group at Duke reported that 11 of 49 patients deemed to have unresectable locally advanced tumors on restaging CT were successfully resected, 6 with R0 resection. Restaging CT scan suggested arterial involvement in these patients, when indeed no viable tumor was found histologically.[65] Therefore, for patients with borderline resectable or locally advanced disease, CT evaluation of the tumor–vessel interface following preoperative treatment requires prudent skepticism, and other surrogates of response to neoadjuvant therapy need to be considered including an overall decrease in the size of the mass, a substantial drop in CA 19-9 levels, or resolution of tumor-associated pain.

Patients who are treated with pancreas resection, including SMV-PV resection or reconstruction, exhibit survival similar to patients treated with standard pancreas resection (Table 82.8). Bold et al.[129] found that 71% of resected vein segments had histologic evidence of microscopic invasion. Noninvaded specimens exhibited perivascular fibrosis.

Practical Approaches to Neoadjuvant and Adjuvant Therapy

Early-stage tumors should be considered for resection and systemic therapy; and the nihilism that many clinicians feel

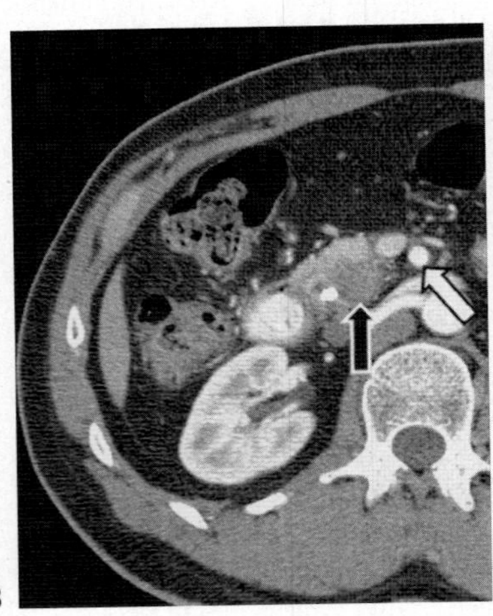
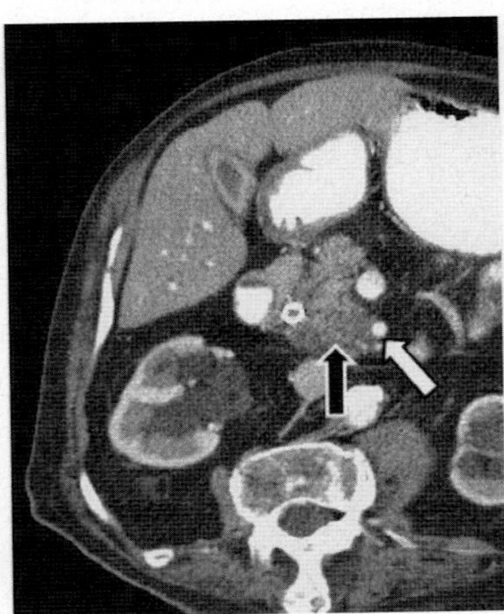
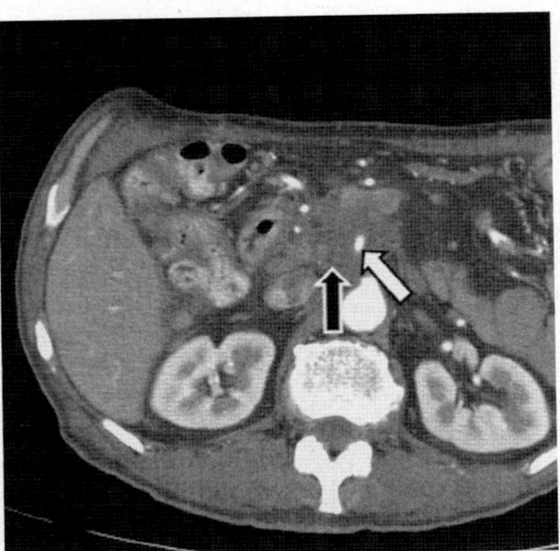
A,B C

FIGURE 82.3 Computed tomography images depicting spectrum of localized pancreatic cancer. Black arrows point to low-density tumors; white arrows point to superior mesenteric vein (SMA) and show the relationship of tumor to vessel. **A:** Resectable tumor with clear fat plane around the SMA. **B:** Borderline resectable pancreatic cancer with tumor abutting about half of the SMA circumference. **C:** Locally advanced, unresectable disease with completed encasement of the SMA.

TABLE 82.8

PANCREATICODUODENECTOMY WITH SUPERIOR MESENTERIC-PORTAL VENOUS RESECTION: EQUIVALENT SURVIVAL TO STANDARD RESECTION

Group[a] (Ref.)	Vein Resection	*N*	Survival		Median Survival (Mo)
			1 Y (%)	2 Y (%)	
MSKCC (255)	Y	58	NA	NA	13
1996	N	274	NA	NA	17
MDACC (256)	Y	31	84[b]	NA	22
1998	N	44	75[b]	NA	20
University of Hautepierre (257)	Y	21	NA	22	12
2001	N	66	NA	24	12

MSKCC, Memorial Sloan-Kettering Cancer Center; MDACC, M. D. Anderson Cancer Center; NA, not assessable.
[a]No statistically significant differences in survival for all studies.
[b]Approximate based on survival curves.

toward the treatment of early stage pancreas cancer is often a disservice to their patients. To identify tumors that are truly resectable, high-quality cross-sectional imaging is mandatory. Patients with resectable tumors should be considered for adjuvant chemotherapy following recovery from their surgery.

When adjuvant therapy is considered, some general principles must be considered. First, adjuvant therapy only applies to patients with adequate recovery from surgery, and whenever a patient continues to have compromised performance or nutritional status, the potential toxicity of chemoradiation, systemic therapy, or both may outweigh the modest anticipated benefits. Importantly, recent data from MDACC suggest that preoperative performance status is predictive of the potential to receive postoperative therapy, and obtaining an accurate assessment of preoperative functioning is critical to determining a patient's candidacy.[130] Second, whenever possible, enrollment in a well-designed clinical trial should be encouraged. Third, when no trial is available, the National Comprehensive Cancer Network clinical practice guidelines for pancreatic adenocarcinoma recommend acquisition of postoperative or prechemotherapy imaging studies and a serum CA 19-9 level to ensure no biochemical or radiographic evidence of persistent or early metastatic disease. Emerging evidence suggests that an elevated postoperative CA 19-9 level is associated with poor prognosis.[36] Once a decision to proceed with adjuvant therapy has been made, the National Comprehensive Cancer Network guidelines recommend that either 6 months of 5-FU or gemcitabine as systemic therapy are reasonable options. Although either agent is reasonable, gemcitabine monotherapy is both better tolerated and has slightly better efficacy, and this regimen should be considered the standard of care for patients with resected pancreatic cancer.

Those clinicians inclined to deliver adjuvant radiation should administer 5-FU–based chemoradiation. To date, the combination of gemcitabine with radiation as a component of adjuvant therapy should be considered nonstandard and at present cannot be endorsed.

Presently, preoperative therapy for resectable pancreatic cancer remains investigational and should be delivered only in the context of a clinical trial. Delivery of off-protocol preoperative therapy should be discouraged. However, for a patient who has been evaluated for surgery and considered to have a borderline resectable tumor, preoperative chemoradiation, systemic chemotherapy, or some sequence of these two modalities should be utilized.[131]

TREATMENT OF LOCALLY ADVANCED DISEASE: AMERICAN JOINT COMMITTEE ON CANCER STAGE III

Locally advanced disease is defined by more than 180-degree superior mesenteric arterial invasion or celiac axis invasion without gross disease outside the pancreatic primary. Traditionally, these nonresectable local tumors have been approached with a treatment strategy using radiotherapy plus a radiation sensitizer, resulting in a modest improvement in median survival.

Radiation-Based Therapies

Chemoradiation versus Radiation Alone

Several prospective randomized trials have shown a benefit from chemoradiation compared to either radiation or chemotherapy alone in the management of locally advanced disease (Table 82.9). The first trial was published in 1969 and included patients with various types of gastrointestinal cancers, 64 of whom had locally unresectable pancreatic cancer randomized to either 5-FU or placebo, combined with 35 to 40 Gy radiation.[132] Median survival in the combined modality arm was significantly higher than in the radiation therapy–only arm (10.4 months vs. 6.3 months). The GITSG subsequently randomized 194 patients with locally advanced pancreatic cancer to receive split-course external beam radiotherapy (EBRT), either alone (60 Gy) or combined (either 40 or 60 Gy) with 5-FU, 500 mg/m^2 on the first 3 days of each 20 Gy radiation.[133] The EBRT-alone arm was discontinued after an interim analysis showed improved median time to progression and overall survival in the combined modality arms. No significant differences were seen between the high- and low-dose EBRT chemoradiation arms, although there were trends favoring the higher-dose arm in time to progression and survival. Thus, these two randomized studies demonstrated a modest survival benefit for combined modality therapy over EBRT alone.

Chemotherapy Alone versus Chemoradiation Trials

Four randomized trials have been completed that have compared chemotherapy alone to chemoradiation. The first trial

TABLE 82.9

SELECTED RANDOMIZED TRIALS IN LOCALLY ADVANCED PANCREATIC CANCER

Study (Ref.)	Radiation (Gy)	Chemotherapy	No. of Patients	Median Survival (Mo)	1-Y Survival (%)
CHEMORADIATION VS. RADIATION ALONE					
Moertel et al. (132)	35–40	5-FU	32	10.4[a]	25[a,b]
	35–40	Placebo	32	6.3	6[b]
GITSG (133)	60	5-FU	111	11.4	44[a]
	40	5-FU	117	8.4	39[a]
	60	—	25	5.3	14
CHEMORADIATION VS. CHEMOTHERAPY ALONE					
ECOG (136)	40	5-FU	47	8.3	28[b]
	—	5-FU	44	8.2	31[b]
GITSG (134)	54	5-FU and SMF	22	9.7[a]	41[a]
	—	SMF	21	7.4	19
FFCD-SSRO (265)	60	5-FU and cisplatin[c]	59	9.1	24
	—	Gemcitabine	60	14.3	51

GITSG, Gastrointestinal Study Group; 5-FU, 5-fluorouracil; ECOG, Eastern Cooperative Oncology Group; FFCD-SSRO, Fondation Francophone de Cancérologie Digestive and Société Française de Radiothérapie Oncologique; SMF, streptozotocin, mitomycin, 5-FU.
[a]$P < .05$.
[b]Calculated from survival curve.
[c]Chemoradiation was followed by maintenance gemcitabine alone.
(Adapted from Earle CC, Agboola O, Maroun J, et al. The treatment of locally advanced pancreatic cancer: a practice guideline. *Can J Gastroenterol* 2003;17(3):161.)

was conducted by the Eastern Cooperative Oncology Group (ECOG) and randomly allocated patients to therapy with 5-FU alone (600 mg/m² in a weekly intravenous bolus) or to radiation therapy (40 Gy) with concurrent 5-FU (600 mg/m², days 1 to 3) followed by maintenance 5-FU (600 mg/m²). No difference was found between the arms in median survival, which could be explained either by inadequacies in the chemoradiation dose or schedule or because 22% of the patients did not follow the protocol or could not be evaluated.[133] A second study conducted by the GITSG compared SMF (streptozotocin, mitomycin, and 5-FU) chemotherapy alone versus SMF combined with EBRT (54 Gy) and showed a significant improvement in median survival (9.7 months vs. 7.4 months) for the chemoradiation arm.[134] It is not clear how relevant these studies are with advances in radiation techniques and imaging (leading to improved definition of disease extent and patient selection).

Two more recent phase 3 trials that compared initial chemotherapy to initial chemoradiation have reported conflicting results. The Fédération Francophone de Cancérologie Digestive and Société Française de Radiothérapie Oncologique (FFCD-SSRO) compared gemcitabine alone to an experimental chemoradiation regimen followed by gemcitabine.[135] Patients were treated with gemcitabine alone in one arm or radiation (total dose 60 Gy) with concurrent 5-FU and cisplatin, followed by gemcitabine, in the second arm. There were some notable aberrations in the results. The median survival in the gemcitabine alone arm was unusually high at 13 months compared to 9.1 months to 9.9 months in subsets of locally advanced patients in contemporaneous randomized trials to evaluate gemcitabine-based chemotherapy alone (ECOG 6201[136] and CALGB 80303[137]). A median survival greater than 10 months has rarely been reported in a multi-institutional phase 2 or 3 trial to evaluate chemotherapy alone for locally advanced disease. Conversely, a poor survival duration was observed among the patients treated with chemoradiation followed by gemcitabine (8.3 months compared to a more typical 10 to 12 months in most studies). One explanation is that the high rate of acute toxicity observed in the chemoradiation arm led to poor compliance with the regimen and declining performance status and probably contributed to the poor outcome. The chemoradiation regimen in this trial was experimental, consisting of cisplatin (which is not considered standard in this setting) combined with an unusually high dose of infusional 5-FU (300 mg/m²/d); moreover, the dose of radiation (60 Gy) to large volumes exceeded the tolerance of the duodenum. The hypothesis was that intensification of chemoradiation would improve outcomes, which it clearly did not. The important lessons from the FFCD-SFRO study are that chemoradiation regimens must be well tolerated, and phase 2 studies must be conducted to establish tolerance of experimental strategies prior to embarking on multi-institutional phase 3 trials.

In the United States, the only recent trial to compare chemotherapy to chemoradiation was ECOG 4201. It was designed to compare gemcitabine (600 mg/m² weekly) and concurrent radiation to regional nodal volumes (50.4 Gy in 28 fractions) followed by weekly gemcitabine (1,000 mg/m² weekly, 3 of 4 weeks) versus similar doses of gemcitabine alone. Although it closed prematurely after accruing only 74 of a planned 316 patients, a statistically significant median survival benefit was seen in the arm who received chemoradiation compared to the arm who received chemotherapy alone (11.0 months vs. 9.2 months; $P = .034$ two-sided, stratified log rank). This benefit came at the cost of increased gastrointestinal toxicity (grade 3 or 4, 38% vs. 14%; $P = .03$) and fatigue (32% vs. 6%).[138] Thus, the addition of chemoradiation prior to standard chemotherapy resulted in a modest prolongation of median survival at the cost of a modest increase in toxicity that remained manageable. The results in both arms of this trial are consistent with the results from other contemporaneous cooperative group studies.

Chemotherapy Alone versus Chemoradiation: An Important Controversy?

The reality is patients probably benefit modestly in different ways from both systemic therapy and chemoradiation. Selection of patients for chemoradiation is best accomplished with an initial strategy of gemcitabine-based chemotherapy for 2 to 4 months. Patients who tolerate chemotherapy and do not have rapidly progressive distant disease can then go on to consolidation with chemoradiation. Recent analyses indicate improved median survival among patients treated with chemotherapy followed by chemoradiation compared to those treated initially with chemoradiation. This is likely a reflection of the selection of patients who do not have rapidly progressive distant disease to receive chemoradiation.[139,140]

Investigation of Novel Radiosensitizers

Like many solid tumors, pancreatic cancer probably could be controlled locally with higher doses of radiation. However, the dose of radiation that can be safely given in patients (50.4 Gy in 28 fractions) is limited by the tolerance of the duodenum and stomach. Because of this, there has been an interest in the investigation of chemotherapeutic agents that can selectively enhance the effect of radiation beyond 5-fluorouracil.

Historical trials that examined the use of novel chemotherapeutic radiation sensitizers in the locally advanced setting led to little improvement over results achieved with fluorouracil-based chemoradiation. The first was a Southwest Oncology Group study published in 1980 randomizing 69 patients to mCCNU (methyl lomustine) and 5-FU with or without testolactone, combined with 60 Gy radiation.[141] No significant difference was found in overall survival, and myelosuppression (87%) and gastrointestinal toxicity (23%) were common. A subsequent GITSG study randomized 143 patients to EBRT with either weekly 5-FU or doxorubicin.[142] Median survival was similar in both arms (approximately 8 months), but the doxorubicin arm had more frequent severe toxicity. Finally, a randomized phase 2 study of 87 patients compared the radiation sensitizer hycanthone to 5-FU, both given with 60 Gy of split-course radiation, and found no difference in survival.[143] These three historical trials failed to demonstrate a therapeutic advantage of the addition of novel chemotherapeutic agents given with radiation therapy compared to 5-FU.

Gemcitabine-Based Chemoradiation

The approval of gemcitabine, which has radiosensitizing properties, for metastatic disease led to an interest in chemoradiation trials combining EBRT with gemcitabine.[144–147] Three multi-institutional studies have been completed to evaluate gemcitabine-based chemoradiation. In a small randomized study performed in Taiwan, 34 patients with locally advanced pancreatic cancer were randomized to receive 5-FU–based chemoradiation (500 mg/m^2 daily for 3 days, every 14 days, total radiation dose 50.4 to 61.2 Gy) or gemcitabine and radiation (600 mg/m^2 weekly with equivalent doses of radiation).[148] The objective response rate to gemcitabine and radiation was 50% and only 13% for 5-FU chemoradiation. In addition, median survival was substantially better using gemcitabine compared with 5-FU (14.5 months vs. 6.7 months; $P = .027$). These results must be interpreted with caution because of the limited accrual (34 patients) and the poor results in the control group. Although the authors concluded that there was no increase in toxicity in the gemcitabine arm, therapy was actually poorly tolerated in both arms. Only 75% of patients were able to complete the full dose of radiotherapy, and roughly one-third of the patients in both arms were hospitalized for 2 to 6 weeks due to the acute toxicity of treatment. A phase 2 study conducted in patients with locally advanced pancreatic cancer by the Cancer and Leukemia Group B evaluated gemcitabine given at 40 mg/m^2 twice weekly. There were 35% and 50% grade 3 or 4 gastrointestinal and hematologic toxicities, respectively, and the median survival was only 8.5 months.[131] Both of these studies used regional nodal fields that likely contributed to gastrointestinal toxicity. In contrast, an approach developed at the University of Michigan incorporates the manufacturer's recommended dose of gemcitabine (1 g/m^2) for metastatic disease and a slightly lower radiotherapy dose (36 Gy in 15 fractions at 2.4 Gy per fraction over 3 weeks) with conformal radiation fields encompassing the gross tumor volume alone. The irradiation of a smaller volume of normal tissue was reported to be well tolerated.[146] Investigators have since reported the results from a multi-institutional phase 2 study evaluating a similar chemoradiation regimen in patients with potentially resectable pancreatic cancer. Results from 20 patients treated indicated that only one patient experienced grade 3 acute gastrointestinal toxicity, only 35% of the patients had node-positive disease, and 23% had only microscopic or no residual disease in the specimen.[127] The same regimen was reported not to be tolerated as well (approximately 25% grade 3 gastrointestinal toxicity) by the same consortium when locally advanced patients were included in the analysis, reflecting the potential impact of inferior performance status among locally advanced patients.[149]

Other trials have illustrated the difficulty of combining chemotherapy agents with gemcitabine and radiation therapy. ECOG published a phase 1 study evaluating seven patients with locally advanced disease using 5-FU/gemcitabine combined with radiation therapy to a maximum dose of 59.4 Gy in 1.8-Gy fractions. In these patients 5-FU (200 mg/m^2/d as continuous infusion throughout radiation therapy) was administered with dose escalation weekly with gemcitabine beginning at 100 mg/m^2. Because of dose-limiting toxicities seen in two of the first three patients, the study was amended to lower the initial dose of gemcitabine to 50 mg/m^2.[150] However, dose-limiting toxicities were subsequently seen in three of four patients at the 50-mg/m^2 dose. Three of the five dose-limiting toxicities occurred at radiation doses less than 36 Gy. The study was subsequently closed.

Gemcitabine has also been combined with cisplatin and radiation in published phase 1 trials. A study based at the Mayo Clinic gave twice-weekly gemcitabine and cisplatin for 3 weeks during radiation (50.4 Gy in 28 fractions).[151] Dose-limiting toxicities consisted of grade 4 nausea and vomiting. The recommended phase 2 dose resulting from this study was gemcitabine, 300 mg/m^2, and cisplatin, 10 mg/m^2. Another trial delivered a novel schedule of gemcitabine (days 2, 5, 26, and 33) and cisplatin (days 1 to 5 and 29 to 33) combined with radiation, with a recommended phase 2 dose of 20 mg/m^2 for cisplatin and 300 mg/m^2 for gemcitabine.[152] The response to chemoradiation was reported to allow 10 of 30 initially unresectable patients to undergo surgery, with an R0 resection in nine cases and a complete response in two cases. The University of Michigan group also established a recommended dose of 40 mg/m^2 of cisplatin when combining full-dose gemcitabine with radiation therapy to the gross disease only in a phase 1 trial.[153]

Several points about gemcitabine-based chemoradiation are worth emphasizing. Similar to its value as a systemic agent,[154] gemcitabine is probably only modestly better than 5-FU when it is used with radiotherapy, but it is not tolerated as well.[155] The gastrointestinal toxicity reported in the initial phase 1 studies and the three multi-institutional studies using gemcitabine alone with radiation therapy demonstrate a narrow therapeutic index regardless of strategy. Typically either the radiation dose or the gemcitabine dose must be attenuated if the combination is to be given safely. Additionally, combining a second cytotoxic agent with gemcitabine-based chemoradiation leads to significant toxicity. Finally, compared with radiotherapy fields that target the gross tumor only, elective regional nodal irradiation results in increased gastrointestinal toxicity. Certainly, if gemcitabine is used in combination with irradiation on esophageal, gastric, or duodenal mucosa, the volume of mucosa being treated should be minimized or there will be a significant risk of severe acute toxicity. If investigators and clinicians with experience choose to use gemcitabine-based regimens, a dose and schedule that is well tolerated should be used. Table 82.10 presents the recommended combinations of radiation treatment volumes and

TABLE 82.10

RECOMMENDED RADIATION TREATMENT VOLUMES IN COMMONLY USED CHEMORADIATION REGIMENS FOR LOCALIZED PANCREATIC CANCER

Chemotherapy Choice	Chemotherapy Dose and Schedule (Ref.)	Radiation Dose and Schedule	No Arterial Involvement or Abutment with Likely Resectability (T3 or T4)	Extensive Arterial Involvement with Uncertain Resectability or Arterial Encasement/ Unresectable (T4)
Gemcitabine	400–500 mg/m² weekly (157)	50.4 Gy/5.5 wk (good PS) or 30 Gy/2 wk (poor PS)	GTV only	GTV only
	1 gm/m² weekly (147)	36 Gy/3 wk	GTV only	GTV only
	40 mg/m² twice weekly (266)	50.4 Gy/5.5 wk	GTV + ENI	GTV only
Capecitabine	800–825 mg m² b.i.d. on days of radiation (162)	50.4 Gy/5.5 wk (good PS) or 30 Gy/2 wk (poor PS)	GTV + ENI	GTV only
PVI 5-FU	225 mg/m² daily or 300 mg/m² on days of radiation (157,267)	50.4 Gy/5.5 wk (good PS) or 30 Gy/2 wk (poor PS)	GTV + ENI	GTV only

PS, performance status; GTV, gross tumor volume; ENI, elective nodal irradiation; PVI, protracted venous infusion; 5-FU, 5-fluorouracil.

doses, as well as chemotherapeutic agents, schedules, and doses.

Capecitabine-Based Chemoradiation

Capecitabine appears to have similar efficacy to intravenously administered 5-FU, and it is an appropriate substitute for infusional or bolus 5-FU when used with radiotherapy. It is an orally administered agent that has a clinical benefit response similar to that of gemcitabine in patients with locally advanced or metastatic pancreatic cancer[156] and unlike gemcitabine can be given at systemic doses with regional nodal irradiation with a favorable toxicity profile. In a recently published phase 1 trial, 800 mg/m² twice daily was the recommended dose when capecitabine was given on days of radiation only.[157] As demonstrated in a recently completed phase 1 trial conducted at MDACC, bevacizumab, capecitabine (825 mg/m² twice daily), and radiotherapy is a well-tolerated combination (discussed below), indicating that capecitabine may make an attractive chemoradiation platform upon which to integrate biologic agents. Only 2 of 47 (4%) patients developed grade 3 gastrointestinal toxicity, and there was no significant hematologic toxicity.[158]

Other Approaches

Novel Molecular-Targeted Approaches to Chemoradiation

Molecular-targeted therapies may be able to selectively enhance the effect of radiation on tumors compared to normal tissues. Agents that have a potential role in the metastatic setting are the most appealing candidates for investigation in locally advanced pancreatic cancer.

Capecitabine and bevacizumab were administered in combination with radiation (50.4 Gy) to 47 patients with locally advanced pancreatic cancer in a phase 1 dose escalation study conducted at MDACC. The study demonstrated that bevacizumab is generally safe when combined with chemoradiation. The acute toxicity was minimal and managed with dose adjustments of capecitabine alone. In addition, limiting radiotherapy fields to the gross tumor volume alone probably helped to minimize the incidence of grade 3 acute toxicity to 4.3%. Bevacizumab did not appear to enhance acute toxicity; however, tumors with invasion of the duodenum appeared to be at higher risk for bleeding or perforation. Importantly, there were no bleeding events in the final 18 patients who were accrued after a protocol modification excluded patients with duodenal invasion. Overall, the tumors in 9 of 46 (20%) evaluable patients had an objective partial response to initial therapy. This included 6 of 12 tumors treated at a dose of 5 mg/kg of bevacizumab. Additionally, 4 to 20 weeks after the last dose of bevacizumab, four patients underwent pancreaticoduodenectomy without perioperative complication.[159] The recommended dose of bevacizumab for further study is 5 mg/kg every 2 weeks with radiotherapy (50.4 Gy in 28 fractions) and concurrent capecitabine (825 mg/m² twice daily Monday through Friday).

The RTOG completed accrual on a phase 2 trial evaluating capecitabine-based chemoradiation with bevacizumab (RTOG PA04-11) followed by systemic therapy with concurrent gemcitabine and bevacizumab. Patients with tumor invasion of the duodenum were specifically excluded due to the risk of duodenal hemorrhage. The median survival was 11.9 months, which was not considered significantly different from previous RTOG trials and the regimen will not be further studied.[160]

Cetuximab has been shown to improve local tumor control and overall survival in combination with EBRT alone in locally advanced head and neck cancer.[161] But none of the currently available epidermal growth factor receptor (EGFR)inhibitors (gefitinib, erlotinib, or cetuximab) has been widely evaluated in combination with radiation for locally advanced pancreatic cancer. A phase 1 dose-escalation study from Brown University combined weekly gemcitabine (75 mg/m²), paclitaxel (40 mg/m²), and daily erlotinib with 50.4 Gy to the tumor and regional lymphatics. The maximum tolerated dose of erlotinib was 50 mg/m². The median survival was 14 months, and 6 of 13 (46%) locally advanced patients had a partial response.[162] The toxicity of the regimen was more severe than expected.

Another phase 1 study is ongoing at MSKCC to evaluate gemcitabine-based chemotherapy in combination with erlotinib.

Another novel biologic agent in development is TNFerade (GenVec Inc., Gaithersburg, Maryland), a replication-deficient adenovector carrying a transgene encoding human tumor necrosis factor-α regulated by a radiation-inducible promoter. Weekly intratumoral injections have been given in combination with chemoradiation (50.4 Gy with continuous infusion 5-FU, 200 mg/m^2 daily). A phase 3 trial designed to accrue 350 patients is comparing 50.4 Gy with 5-FU (225 mg/m^2/d continuous infusion) with or without TNFerade, followed by gemcitabine alone. Preliminary analysis of the first 51 patients indicates an encouraging 1-year survival rate in the experimental arm that has not reached statistical significance.[163] Interim analysis revealed no improvement in the TNFerade arm, and the trial was discontinued.

Radiation Technique for Locally Advanced Disease

Because patients with locally advanced tumors that are clearly unresectable probably do not clearly benefit from regional lymph node irradiation, and adequate coverage of the locoregional nodes usually leads to an increase in gastrointestinal toxicity, radiotherapy fields should be confined to the gross tumor. This strategy reduces the gastrointestinal toxicity of chemoradiation. Therefore, it is essential to identify the extent of the primary pancreatic tumor correctly on contrast-enhanced CT.

The pancreas and duodenum move a median of 1 cm with respiratory excursion.[164] If the gross tumor alone is to be treated, respiratory motion must be either controlled or accounted for in radiotherapy planning. Commonly, an additional margin to the planned radiation fields in the cranial and caudal directions is added to accomplish this. However, because axial tumor motion is negligible, an additional margin for motion in the axial directions is not necessary.

A three- or four-field technique is recommended with equally weighted anterior, posterior, and opposed lateral fields. A 2-cm block margin is used in the radial directions, and a 3-cm block margin is used in the cranial and caudal directions to account for respiratory motion. Delivery of greater than 50.4 Gy to the primary tumor while sparing the duodenum, stomach, and jejunum typically requires advanced radiation planning such as IMRT and delivery using active breathing control.[165]

Resection of Locally Advanced Tumors

There is a widespread perception that the delivery of preoperative or neoadjuvant therapy (generally using chemoradiation) may down-stage locally advanced, unresectable pancreatic tumors and allow for subsequent resection. Unfortunately, the data regarding the frequency of successful down-staging are confounded by inconsistent definitions of resectability and by inadequate preoperative imaging. Additionally, most tumors converted to resectable disease are actually borderline tumors (discussed above) when initially evaluated. Even with these caveats, the incidence of converting an advanced local tumor to a resectable tumor is extremely low (Table 82.11). Two large series from the MSKCC and MDACC reported that patients who had locally advanced tumors were rendered operable after chemoradiation in 1 of 87 and 6 of 114 patients, respectively.[155,166]

Survival in the rare patient who is treated with preoperative chemoradiation for locally advanced disease and ultimately undergoes an R0 resection is similar to survival for patients treated with neoadjuvant or adjuvant therapy for resectable disease.[167] But the goal of chemotherapy and chemoradiation for locally advanced disease is the small increase in survival rather than the conversion of a tumor to a resectable state.

Palliation in Locally Advanced Tumors

Surgery for advanced, nonresectable pancreatic adenocarcinoma can palliate obstruction of the common bile duct or duodenum as well as control visceral pain. Hepaticojejunostomy, choledochojejunostomy, or choledochoduodenostomy offers durable drainage of an obstructed bile duct. Cholecystojejunostomy is less reliable but can be employed when tumor bulk precludes a common duct procedure. Gastrojejunostomy palliates gastric outlet obstruction. Many surgeons utilize an antecolic anastomosis to avoid complications from an expanding lesser sac tumor, but a retrocollic anastomosis has been reliable when used by the group at JHMI.

Lillemoe et al.[168] at JHMI evaluated operative palliation at the time of diagnostic exploration, randomizing patients to gastric bypass (44 patients) versus observation (43 patients), and 19% of observed patients subsequently developed gastric outlet obstruction. The authors cite this finding as evidence that all patients with advanced pancreatic cancer should be palliated operatively with bypass; but groups using staging multiphase CT with selective laparoscopy suggest that with only a 19% rate of obstruction, bypass should be reserved for those who eventually obstruct. Espat et al.[169] at MSKCC investigated 155 patients staged with laparoscopy, finding that 152 patients did not require an open operation for palliation.

Less morbid, nonoperative techniques for palliation should be utilized when feasible. Endoscopic and percutaneous approaches result in satisfactory palliation. Common bile duct obstruction controlled with an endoscopically placed metal stent

PRACTICE OF ONCOLOGY

TABLE 82.11

LOCALLY ADVANCED PANCREAS ADENOCARCINOMA: LOW RATE OF RESECTION FOLLOWING CHEMORADIATION

		Preoperative Regimen[a]			
Group (Ref.)	*N*	Chemotherapy	Radiation	CR	R0 Resection
Duke University 1999 (268)	25	5-FU, CP, MMC	45 Gy	1	1
University of Erlangen, Germany 2000 (269)	27	5-FU, MMC	55.8 Gy	—	10
Vienna, Austria 2000 (270)	38	5-FU, LV, cisplatin	55 Gy	—	3
M. D. Anderson 2002 (155)	114	5-FU, Gem	30 Gy, hyperfractionated	—	6
Memorial Sloan-Kettering 2002 (169)	87	Various agents[b]	None or various doses	—	1

CR, complete response; 5-FU, 5-fluorouracil; MMC, mitomycin C; LV, leucovorin; Gem, gemcitabine.
[a]Few patients proceed to margin negative resection following preparative regimens for locally advanced pancreas adenocarcinoma.
[b]Majority of patients received 5-FU or Gem-based regimens. Other agents used in combination or as experimental treatments included carboplatin, MMC, taxol, topotecan, adriamycin, TNP-470, BB2516, or DX-8951F.

allows for endoluminal drainage of an obstructed biliary system. A percutaneous endoscopic gastrostomy tube can often decompress the stomach adequately for palliation of duodenal obstruction developing late in the clinical course. Although an operative approach can successfully palliate patients with pancreatic adenocarcinoma, this approach should be used sparingly when nonoperative approaches fail or cannot technically be completed.

Practical Approach to Patients with Locally Advanced Disease

The first consideration in the treatment of locally advanced disease is to differentiate between borderline resectable disease and true locally advanced tumors. Treatment goals and therefore treatment regimens will differ between the two groups of tumors, so evaluation of the extent of arterial involvement is essential to designing an individual treatment strategy.

Optimal treatment for true locally advanced pancreatic cancer remains controversial. Locally advanced disease is generally incurable, and all therapies have significant limitations. Systemic and local progression are common following treatment. Since the impact of standard therapies is limited, all patients should be considered for protocol-based therapy.

If enrollment on protocol is not possible, gemcitabine-based chemotherapy for 2 to 4 months followed by 5-FU or capecitabine-based chemoradiation is the most appropriate choice for the majority of patients with locally advanced, unresectable disease. If patients are responding to chemotherapy (objective radiographic response or CA 19-9 level decline) after 2 months and tolerating therapy well, it is reasonable to continue for 2 more months. When there is radiographic local progression, a CA 19-9 level plateau or increase, local symptomatic progression, or chemotherapy is poorly tolerated, chemoradiation should be initiated. In cases where distant progression has become evident during chemotherapy, a 2-week course of 30 Gy of 5-FU or capecitabine-based chemoradiation should be considered only in patients with symptomatic primary tumors. The patients who have not progressed after systemic therapy are most likely to benefit from chemoradiation, and typically a 5.5-week course is appropriate (50.4 Gy) with concurrent chemotherapy.

Although many novel concurrent chemotherapeutic radiation regimens have been investigated in clinical trials, none is clearly more efficacious than 5-FU or capecitabine-based chemoradiation, and they are typically more toxic. The use of concurrent gemcitabine with radiotherapy in this disease is also a reasonable choice for the experienced clinician since it is a proven systemic agent in pancreatic cancer and it has radiosensitizing properties. However, a decade of clinical experience has shown that treatment must be tailored to the patient to avoid toxicity. Table 82.10 summarizes the established chemoradiation regimens in localized pancreatic cancer with the doses of radiation, chemotherapy, and importantly, the radiation treatment volume recommendations. Although the AJCC staging system outlines objective radiographic criteria for resectability, it is not always clear to the treating clinician if the surgeon deems the tumor resectable. For this reason, various clinical scenarios are outlined that will help the clinician with individualization of therapy.

TREATMENT OF METASTATIC DISEASE: AMERICAN JOINT COMMITTEE ON CANCER STAGE IV

Most patients diagnosed with pancreatic cancer either present with metastatic disease or develop it during the course of their illness. When this occurs, anticancer therapy consists almost exclusively of systemic therapy. However, patients with metastatic pancreatic cancer are clinically dynamic and face significant morbidity, obligating clinicians to be mindful of palliation beyond the delivery of systemic therapy. This is particularly important since currently available cytotoxic therapy provides modest survival benefits. Recent efforts to improve survival have focused on the optimization of cytotoxic therapy and the integration of newer molecular agents into treatment. Unfortunately, several large randomized trials conducted over the past few years have yielded disappointing results, and no significant improvements in systemic therapy have been realized since the introduction of gemcitabine in the 1990s.

A History of Cytotoxic Chemotherapy for Pancreatic Cancer

Early trials of chemotherapy for advanced pancreatic cancer were based on 5-FU and later, on 5-FU combinations. In a review of trials dating back to the 1960s and 1970s, the overall response rate to 5-FU as a single agent was estimated to be 28%, but response assessments were based on fairly crude measurements: physical examination, liver–spleen scintillography, or ultrasonography.[170] With the advent of CT and MRI, more recent trials of 5-FU have shown virtually no activity when given as a bolus intravenous injection. For example, 31 patients with advanced pancreatic cancer were treated with a combination of bolus 5-FU and leucovorin given daily for 5 days; no objective responses were observed.[171] Furthermore, in the trial that led to approval of gemcitabine as front-line therapy for advanced pancreatic cancer in the United States, 57 patients with bidimensional, measurable disease were randomly assigned to receive weekly bolus 5-FU (600 mg/m^2); among these patients the response rate to bolus 5-FU was zero.[154]

Nevertheless, 5-FU does appear to have modest activity in pancreatic cancer when given as a prolonged infusion or in the form of capecitabine. In a randomized trial that compared infusional 5-FU with infusional 5-FU plus mitomycin C, a response rate of 8.6% was seen among the 105 patients who received infusional 5-FU alone, comparable to response rates reported for gemcitabine.[172] Similarly, capecitabine has some activity in pancreatic cancer based on a phase 2 trial that involved 42 patients. Of 41 patients with measurable disease 3 (7.3%) had an objective response rate.[156]

Older 5-Fluorouracil–Based Combinations Are No Better than Single-Agent 5-Fluorouracil

Predictably, since 5-FU was considered active in advanced pancreatic cancer based on early studies, 5-FU–based combination therapy was subsequently investigated. Commonly tested regimens included 5-FU, doxorubicin, and mitomycin C (FAM), 5-FU, streptozotocin, mitomycin C (SMF), and the Mallinson regimen, which consisted of induction therapy with 5-FU, cyclophosphamide, methotrexate, and vincristine followed by maintenance treatment with 5-FU and mitomycin C.[173–176] Initial results using these three regimens in phase 2 trials were encouraging, but none of them demonstrated any significant survival advantage over single agent 5-FU in larger randomized trials.[177,178] As mentioned above, a more recent trial tested infusional 5-FU and mitomycin C versus infusional 5-FU alone. Although the response rate was higher with combination therapy, 17.6% versus only 8.4% with infusional 5-FU alone, no survival advantage was observed for patients receiving the combination (median survival 6.5 months vs. 5.1 month, respectively; $P = .34$).[172] These investigations of 5-FU–based combinations reflect a common problem in chemotherapy trials in pancreatic cancer: encouraging results seen in phase 2 trials of new drug combinations have rarely been confirmed in larger, randomized phase 3 trials.

The Gemcitabine Era

For over a decade, gemcitabine has shown modest reproducible activity against advanced pancreatic cancer. Two of the initial phase 2 trials of gemcitabine, with a combined total of 72 evaluable patients, reported response rates ranging from 6% to 11%.[179,180] Importantly, symptomatic improvement was observed for some of these patients and led to a randomized trial of gemcitabine versus bolus weekly 5-FU as first-line therapy for patients with advanced pancreatic cancer. Patients assigned to receive gemcitabine had a higher response rate (5.4% vs. 0%), improved median survival (5.65 vs. 4.41 months; $P = .0025$), and 1-year survival rate (18% vs. 2%) compared with patients treated with bolus 5-FU. In addition, clinical benefit was also documented among patients subsequently treated with gemcitabine after disease progression with 5-FU.[154]

The clinical benefit and modest survival advantage produced by gemcitabine compared with bolus 5-FU led to its approval by the U.S. Food and Drug Administration in 1997 and its acceptance as standard treatment for advanced pancreatic adenocarcinoma. Since that time, few drugs given as single agents have been directly compared with gemcitabine, and to date, none of these has shown superiority. These agents include the matrix metalloproteinase inhibitors marimastat and BAY 12-9566 and the camptothecin, exatecan mesylate.[181–183] Thus, all recent large prospective randomized trials of front-line chemotherapy for pancreatic cancer have tested standard-dose gemcitabine against fixed-dose–rate gemcitabine, gemcitabine-based cytotoxic combinations, or molecular agents combined with gemcitabine.

Strategies to Optimize Gemcitabine Therapy

Fixed-Dose–Rate Gemcitabine. Gemcitabine is a pro-drug that requires intracellular phosphorylation for cytotoxic activity, either as an inhibitor of ribonucleotide reductase or for incorporation into an elongating chain of DNA. During early clinical trials of gemcitabine, the rate of gemcitabine phosphorylation was found to be subject to saturation kinetics.[184,185] Further studies demonstrated that the rate of intracellular gemcitabine triphosphate accumulation and peak intracellular concentrations was highest when it was delivered at a dose rate of 350 mg/m^2 per 30 minutes (approximately 10 mg/m^2/min). These pharmacokinetic findings suggested that by delivering gemcitabine at a fixed dose rate of 10 mg/m^2/min, increased intracellular levels of phosphorylated species of gemcitabine would be attained and provide dose intensification.

To test this hypothesis, a randomized phase 2 trial was conducted in 92 patients with advanced disease.[186] Patients received either fixed-dose–rate (FDR) gemcitabine or gemcitabine using the standard 30-minute bolus technique. Of note, in both arms gemcitabine was delivered at or near the maximum tolerated dose (FDR gemcitabine at 1,500 mg/m^2 over 150 minutes or standard-infusion gemcitabine at 2,200 mg/m^2 over 30 minutes).[187,188] Time to treatment failure was equivalent in both arms, but median overall survival was better for the patients randomized to FDR gemcitabine compared with those receiving dose-intense standard-infusion gemcitabine (8.0 months vs. 5.0 months; $P = .013$).[186] Among the patients with metastatic disease (91% of the enrolled patients) median survival was likewise better using FDR gemcitabine, but these differences were not statistically significant. This provocative result led to further investigation of FDR gemcitabine. In a subsequent phase 2 trial conducted by Louvet et al.,[189] FDR gemcitabine (1,000 mg/m^2 intravenous over 100 minutes) was given on day 1 followed by oxaliplatin (100 mg/m^2 over 100 minutes) on day 2 every 14 days (GemOx). The response rate to this combination was 30.6%, much higher than those previously reported for gemcitabine alone, and median survival for the group was 9.2 months, also better than historical data for gemcitabine alone. This trial allowed for enrollment of patients with locally advanced or metastatic disease.

GemOx was then tested in a larger, prospective, randomized trial and likewise found that it improved the response rate (26.8 vs. 17.3%; $P = .04$) and progression-free survival compared with standard-infusion gemcitabine (5.8 months vs. 3.7 months, respectively; $P = .04$), but the combination did not lead to a statistically significant improvement in overall survival (9.0 months vs. 7.1 months; $P = .13$).[190] Whether the higher response rate seen with GemOx was attributable to the addition of oxaliplatin or to the delivery of FDR gemcitabine was the subject of a subsequent ECOG trial. The ECOG trial enrolled 832 patients with advanced pancreatic cancer and randomized them to receive standard-infusion gemcitabine, FDR gemcitabine, or GemOx.[191] Published results showed a slight improvement in response rates for both GemOx and FDR gemcitabine (9% to 10%) compared with gemcitabine alone (6%), but there was no significant difference between gemcitabine, FDR gemcitabine, and GemOx in terms of overall survival. Table 82.12 summarizes phase 2 and 3 trials of FDR gemcitabine, delivered alone or in combination with a platinum analogue. Taken together, these results consistently show a trend toward improved survival when FDR gemcitabine is compared with standard-infusion gemcitabine, but to date, the delivery of FDR gemcitabine has not had a significant impact on overall survival. Importantly, FDR gemcitabine delivered at doses ranging from 1,000 mg/m^2 to 1,500 mg/m^2 has consistently led to higher rates of hematologic toxicity, and for reasons discussed later, further investigation of lower-dose FDR gemcitabine should be considered.

Cytotoxic Combinations. In addition to GemOx, other gemcitabine-based combinations have been evaluated over the past several years. In most phase 2 trials, gemcitabine has been combined with one other cytotoxic agent, including docetaxel, capecitabine, 5-FU, cisplatin, uracil-tegafur, irinotecan, pemetrexed, or epirubicin.[192–200] Generally, response rates to these combinations have been higher than those typically reported for gemcitabine alone, and overall survival durations have been longer than those historically reported for gemcitabine.

Unfortunately, just as 5-FU–based combinations have been disappointing when compared with 5-FU alone in large phase 3 trials, so too have gemcitabine-based regimens compared with gemcitabine alone (Table 82.13). Note that empiric combinations of gemcitabine with another cytotoxic agent have continued to the present, with recent trials reporting on combinations of gemcitabine with or without cisplatin and gemcitabine with or without capecitabine. For example, in a trial reported by Cunningham et al.,[201] the addition of capecitabine to gemcitabine was found to be superior to single-agent gemcitabine in regard to response rate and PFS. Although a trend toward improved overall survival was also observed with the combination compared with gemcitabine alone, this did not reach statistical significance (HR for death 0.88; $P = .077$). Further disappointment comes from the findings of the Gruppo Italiano Pancreas-1 (GIP-1) trial, which randomized 400 patients to received weekly gemcitabine plus cisplatin or gemcitabine alone.[202] Patients who received the doublet actually experienced inferior survival compared with patients randomized to gemcitabine (7.2 months vs. 8.3 months, respectively).

Careful review of Table 82.13 provides some important lessons. First, for most, but not all, combination regimens, overall survival has been somewhat improved compared with

TABLE 82.12

SUMMARY OF PHASE 2 AND PHASE 3 TRIALS INVESTIGATING FIXED-DOSE–RATE GEMCITABINE, WITH OR WITHOUT A PLATINUM ANALOGUE

Author (Ref.)	Study Design Disease Status of Patients Regimen Tested	STD Inf-Gem Median Survival (Mo)	FDR-Gem Median Survival (Mo)	FDR Gem + Platinum Median Survival (Mo)	*P* Value
Louvet et al. (189)	Phase 2 Locally advanced + Met dz GemOx	—	—	9.2	NA
Ko et al. (271)	Phase 2 Locally advanced dz only FDR Gem + CDDP	—	—	13.5	NA
Ko et al. (272)	Phase 2 Met dz only FDR Gem + CDDP	—	—	7.1	NA
Tempero et al. (186)	Randomized phase 2I Met dz only Gem vs. FDR Gem	5.0	8.0	—	.16
Louvet et al. (190)	Randomized phase 3 Locally advanced + Met dz Gem vs. GemOx	7.0	—	9.0	.09
Poplin et al. (273)	Randomized phase 3 Locally advanced + Met dz Gem vs. FDR Gem vs. GemOx	4.9	6.0	5.9	NS

Met dz, metastatic disease; Gem, gemcitabine; FDR, fixed dose rate; GemOx, fixed-dose–rate gemcitabine with oxaliplatin; CDDP, cisplatin; NA, not available; NS, not stated.

gemcitabine monotherapy, but no statistically significant improvements in survival have been observed. The reasons for this are not entirely clear, but may be explained in part by inadequate objective response rates (no matter what the therapy) and patient crossover from gemcitabine monotherapy to the experimental arm with a gemcitabine doublet. Second, although not shown in the table, the two Italian studies of gemcitabine/cisplatin combination conducted by Colucci et al.[202,203] used the same doses of gemcitabine and cisplatin. However, in the report from 2002, only 107 patients were enrolled patients and

TABLE 82.13

SELECTED RANDOMIZED TRIALS OF SINGLE-AGENT GEMCITABINE VERSUS GEMCITABINE-BASED CYTOTOXIC DOUBLETS IN THE TREATMENT OF ADVANCED PANCREATIC CANCER

Author (Ref.)	No. of Patients	Patients with Metastatic Disease (%)	Control Arm Median Survival (Mo)	Combination Therapy Median Survival (Mo)	*P* Value
Berlin et al. (274)	322	90	Gem 5.4	Gem/5-FU 6.7	.09
Colucci et al. (275)	107	58	Gem 5.4	Gem/cisplatin 7.0	.43
Heinemann et al. (276)	195	80	Gem 6.0	Gem/cisplatin 7.5	.12
Rocha Lima et al. (277)	342	80	Gem 6.6	Gem/irinotecan 6.3	NS
Louvet et al. (190)	313	70	Gem 7.0	GemOx 9.0	.13
Poplin et al.[a] (273)	555	88	Gem 4.9	GemOx 5.9	.16
Abou-Alfa et al. (278)	349	78	Gem 6.2	Gem/exatecan 6.7	.52
Hermann et al. (279)	319	80	Gem 7.2	Gem/capecitabine 8.4	.23

Gem, gemcitabine; 5-FU, 5-fluorouracil; GemOx, fixed-dose–rate gemcitabine with oxaliplatin; NS, not stated.
[a]The study by Poplin had three arms: standard-infusion Gem over 30 minutes, fixed-dose–rate gem, and GemOx. This table shows only the comparison between standard-infusion Gem and GemOx.

demonstrated a survival advantage for patients randomized to gemcitabine and cisplatin. Closer inspection of the table suggests this may be related to overall tumor burden and possibly overall performance status, since roughly 60% of patients enrolled in the smaller study had metastatic disease at time of entry, whereas in the more recent trial published in 2010, over 80% of patients had metastatic disease. This implies that the addition of cisplatin to gemcitabine may provide incremental benefit for patients with lesser tumor burden, or possibly better performance status.

This is supported by a recent meta-analysis of results from 15 evaluable randomized trials that has suggested a statistically significant survival advantage for patients randomized to receive a cytotoxic gemcitabine combination that contained either a platinum or a fluoropyrimidine analogue compared with patients who received gemcitabine alone.[204] (Patients who received gemcitabine/pemetrexed or gemcitabine/camptothecin did not benefit from combination therapy.) Importantly, the survival benefit conferred by combination therapy with a platinum analogue or a fluoropyrimidine was limited to patients with good performance status, having a Karnofsky score of 90% to 100% (HR 0.76; P <.0001). Patients with poor performance status (Karnofsky 80% or less) did not benefit from combination therapy (HR for death, 1.08; P = .4).[204] A similar meta-analysis has been performed using data from 935 patients enrolled in three separate trials of gemcitabine monotherapy versus a gemcitabine/capecitabine doublet. In this analysis the doublet conferred a statistically significant survival advantage over gemcitabine monotherapy (HR 0.86; P = .002).[201]

In summary, the addition of another cytotoxic agent to gemcitabine results in conflicting survival results. Many, but not all, studies show a trend toward improved survival when using a gemcitabine doublet. Of note, these improvements in survival remain quite modest and are usually measured in weeks. Furthermore, some data suggest that any survival advantage of a gemcitabine doublet will be limited to those patients with lower tumor burden or better performance status, and, currently, more aggressive doublet therapy should not be routinely advised to unselected patients.

Gemcitabine-Based Combinations Using Molecular Therapeutics The molecular defects responsible for pancreatic carcinogenesis, chemoresistance, invasion, metastatic potential, and angiogenesis are gradually being elucidated. Additionally, there is an expanding number of drugs specifically designed to inhibit the function of several important proteins. Recent efforts to improve on gemcitabine-based systemic therapy have focused on inhibition of several targets to include matrix metalloproteinases, RAS, EGFR, and vascular endothelial growth factor (VEGF).[183,205–207]

Table 82.14 summarizes the results of six large randomized clinical trials conducted to date. These studies have investigated marimastat, which inhibits matrix metalloproteinases 2 and 9; tipifarnib, which inhibits RAS farnesylation and abrogates RAS function; erlotinib, a tyrosine kinase inhibitor of the EGFR; cetuximab, a monoclonal antibody to EGFR; and bevacizumab, a monoclonal antibody to VEGF.[139,181,208–211]

Thus far only inhibition of EGFR with erlotinib combined with gemcitabine has led to a positive result; a small, but statistically significant improvement in survival compared with delivery of gemcitabine alone.[208] In this study, performed by the National Cancer Institute of Canada Clinical Trials Group, patients with advanced pancreatic cancer were randomized to receive gemcitabine alone at 1,000 mg/m^2 weekly for 7 weeks, then 1 week off, followed by gemcitabine days 1, 8, 15, every 28 days, or the combination of gemcitabine with erlotinib at a dose of 100 to 150 mg orally daily. Overall survival was improved for patients randomized to receive gemcitabine and erlotinib compared with patients receiving gemcitabine alone (median: 191 vs. 177 days, respectively; HR for death 0.82; P <.02).

This trial was important for two reasons: it was the first to demonstrate a very small, but statistically significant, survival advantage for a gemcitabine-doublet over gemcitabine monotherapy and also the first to show improved survival with the integration of a targeted agent into standard therapy for advanced pancreatic cancer. Although the improvement in survival provided by erlotinib was quite modest and considered by many to be clinically insignificant, the result was proof of principle regarding the potential of molecular agents to improve treatment for pancreatic cancer. Whether the small benefit

TABLE 82.14

RANDOMIZED PHASE 3 TRIALS OF GEMCITABINE PLUS A MOLECULAR AGENT VERSUS GEMCITABINE PLUS PLACEBO OR GEMCITABINE ALONE FOR THE TREATMENT OF ADVANCED PANCREATIC CANCER

Author (Ref.)	Delivered Therapy	No. of Patients	Patients with Metastatic Disease (%)	Response Rate (%)	Overall Survival (Median Days)	P Value	1-Y Survival Rate (%)
Van Cutsem et al. 2004 (209)	Gem + placebo	347		8	182		24
	vs.		76			.75	
	Gem + tipifarnib	314		6	193		27
Bramhall et al. 2002 (280)	Gem + placebo	119		11	164		18
	vs.		58			.95	
	Gem + marimastat	120		11	165.5		17
Moore et al. 2005 (208)	Gem	284		8.0	177		17
	vs.		75			.025	
	Gem + erlotinib	285		8.6	191		24
Kindler et al. 2007 (139)	Gem + placebo	300		10	180		20
	vs.		85			.40	
	Gem/bevacizumab	302		11	171		18
Philip et al. 2007 (210)	Gem	369		13	177		NR
	vs.		79			.14	
	Gem/cetuximab	366		12	192		NR

Gem, gemcitabine; NR, not reported.

observed with EGFR inhibitors can be predicted by the K-RAS mutational status of a patient's tumor is unknown in pancreatic cancer. EGFR inhibition has recently been shown to modulate tumor microenvironment, which is should be comprised of K-RAS wild type cells, and this might explain the meek improvements in survival observed in the clinic.[212]

Unfortunately, modulation of the tumor microenvironment through VEGF inhibition has not proven beneficial. Two large randomized phase 3 trials to investigate the addition of bevacizumab to gemcitabine or to gemcitabine and erlotinib have failed to show any survival benefit.[139,211]

Future Directions in Systemic Therapy

Efforts to Improve Cytotoxic Therapy

Revisiting Gemcitabine. Although molecular therapeutics are certain to be part of the future of systemic therapy for pancreatic cancer, the current foundation of systemic therapy, gemcitabine, must be refined and possibly begin with reevaluation of its dose and schedule. Currently, a standard regimen of gemcitabine consists of 1,000 mg/m^2 given over 30 minutes, on days 1, 8, and 15 of a 28-day cycle. However, results from a variety of sources suggest that gemcitabine can be effective, and likely better tolerated, at far lower than standard doses.

When gemcitabine was initially studied in phase 1, objective responses were observed in a patient with colorectal cancer at a dose of 180 mg/m^2 and another patient with non–small cell lung cancer who was given gemcitabine at 525 mg/m^2.[213] In this study, gemcitabine was infused over 30 minutes in all patients, and at doses higher than 350 mg/m^2, no further increases in intracellular concentrations of gemcitabine triphosphate were observed in mononuclear cells obtained from participating patients. The authors reported that intracellular accumulation of the gemcitabine nucleotide was saturated at higher doses of gemcitabine infused over 30 minutes. They further concluded that the maximum-tolerated dose of gemcitabine should be 790 mg/m^2.[213]

Other support for administration of lower doses of gemcitabine comes from a study in Japan that attempted to determine the individualized maximal repeatable dose (iMRD) of gemcitabine in a group of 18 patients with metastatic pancreatic cancer.[214] The iMRD ranged from 300 to 700 mg/m^2. These iMRDs (30% to 70% of the standard dose) led to objective responses in 16% of patients, with an overall median survival of 9.5 months; both end points are impressive in a cohort comprised of patients with metastatic disease.

Last are the data from the MDACC trial of preoperative GemXRT in patients with potentially resectable pancreatic cancer.[124] In this study, gemcitabine was given at a dose of 400 mg/m^2 over 30 minutes weekly for 7 weeks. The overall survival for all 86 patients was 23 months, although 25% of patients did not undergo surgery with curative intent. Among the 64 patients who did undergo resection, median survival was 34 months; superior to reports from other large trials of neoadjuvant or adjuvant therapy. Of interest, gemcitabine at 400 mg/m^2 was infused over 30 minutes (13 mg/m^2/min), approximating FDR gemcitabine. Of further note, the total cumulative dose of gemcitabine given to the patients in our preoperative trial (2,800 mg/m^2) is less than 20% of the total cumulative dose of gemcitabine delivered to patients in the CONKO-001 trial (18,000 mg/m^2), which proved the benefit of adjuvant gemcitabine.[116]

Taken together, these studies suggest gemcitabine at 1,000 mg/m^2 infused over 30 minutes lacks pharmacologic rationale and is not an optimal dose for efficacy or to minimize toxicity. In addition, gemcitabine doublets that rely on either standard gemcitabine dose and infusion or FDR gemcitabine given at 1,000 to 1,500 mg/m^2 have not shown any meaningful improvements in survival and imply that added toxicity may overwhelm any small clinical benefit. Thus, delivery of lower doses of FDR gemcitabine is an important research question. Further investigation of lower FDR gemcitabine may allow for the development of more tolerable and effective gemcitabine combinations (cytotoxic or molecular).

Other Cytotoxic Combinations. A number of other multidrug gemcitabine-based combinations have been tested in pancreatic cancer: gemcitabine, docetaxel, and capecitabine (known as GTX), G-FLIP (gemcitabine, 5-FU, leucovorin, irinotecan, and cisplatin), and GOFL (gemcitabine, oxaliplatin, 5-FU, leucovorin).[215–217] These combinations have all been reported to yield higher response rates than those typically observed with gemcitabine monotherapy with encouraging survival durations.

The best investment toward future systemic therapy is probably in the continued elucidation of targets linked to tumor cell proliferation, inhibition of apoptosis (to include chemo- and radioresistance), metastatic potential, and interactions with the surrounding microenvironment. Putative targets and new inhibitors have been extensively covered elsewhere in this book. However, a few targets worth mentioning are poly adenosine diphosphate-ribose polymerases (PARPs), nuclear factor kappa B (NF-κB), Src kinase, the Akt/phosphoinositol-3-kinase (PI3K), and secreted protein acidic and rich in cystein (SPARC).

Poly Adenosine Diphosphate-Ribose Polymerases

Some patients with pancreatic cancer are known to harbor *BRCA1* or *BRCA2* mutations, and a broader group likely has other germline or somatic mutations in DNA repair pathways. *BRCA1* and *BRCA2* mutations result in deficient homologous-recombination DNA repair. PARPs are DNA repair enzymes that provide an important alternative pathway that leads to repair of single-strand breaks in DNA. In tumors that have a deficiency in the homologous-recombination repair pathway, inhibition of PARPs can cause synthetic lethality. PARP inhibitors are now entering the clinic and already showing meaningful antitumor activity when given as single agents, or when combined with cytotoxic chemotherapy.[218,219]

Nuclear Factor Kappa B

NF-κB plays a major role in the proliferation, survival, angiogenesis, and chemoresistance of pancreatic cancer and is constitutively active in pancreatic cancer cells.[220] Agents that block NF-κB activation reduce chemoresistance to conventional cytotoxic agents. One agent of interest is curcumin (diferuloylmethane), a plant derivative of the spice turmeric (*Curcuma longa*). Curcumin has shown to suppress NF-κB and in one recent *in vitro* study, curcumin inhibited the proliferation of various pancreatic cancer cell lines, potentiated the apoptosis induced by gemcitabine, and inhibited constitutive NF-κB activation in the cells.[221] Furthermore, tumor xenografts injected with pancreatic cancer cells and treated with curcumin and gemcitabine showed significant reductions in tumor volume, Ki-67 proliferation index, NF-κB activation, and angiogenesis.[222]

A recent phase 2 clinical trial has evaluated the safety and efficacy of curcumin and its impact on biologic correlates when taken orally daily by patients with advanced pancreatic cancer.[223] In the 21 evaluable patients, low-circulating curcumin was detected in serum, suggesting poor oral bioavailability. However, two patients showed prolonged stable disease at 8 and 12 months or more.

Targeting Src Kinase

The tyrosine kinase Src is a nonreceptor protein that is overexpressed in 70% of pancreatic adenocarcinomas and implicated in pancreatic tumor progression and metastatic potential.[224] Inhibition of Src kinase *in vitro* leads to a decrease in the phosphorylation of Akt and p44/42 Erk mitogen-activated protein kinase and also decreases the synthesis of VEGF and interleukin-8. Dasatinib is an orally bioavailable Src/Abl selective inhibitor[225] that has been shown to decrease the size of tumors and the incidence of metastases in mice inoculated with human pancreatic cancer cells and in a genetically engineered mouse model of human ductal pancreatic carcinoma.[224,226] Dasatinib is now in phase 1 clinical investigation and is being combined with gemcitabine for the treatment of patients with advanced pancreatic cancer.

Targeting the Akt/Phosphoinositol-3-Kinase Pathway

Activation of the PI3K signal transduction pathway leads to downstream activation of Akt and NF-κB and has an important role in cell activation and inhibition of apoptosis. Constitutive activation of this pathway has been found in pancreatic cancer cell lines and tumor samples.[220] In addition, *in vitro* studies have shown that treating cells with gemcitabine or cisplatin activates Akt and NF-κB and leads to chemoresistance to cytotoxic agents. This chemotherapy-induced resistance is enhanced under hypoxic conditions.[227] PI3K inhibition has thus been studied as a way to block cellular activation and resensitize cells to chemotherapeutic agents.

Genistein is a soy isoflavone that inhibits PI3K activity. When combined *in vitro* with erlotinib, gemcitabine, or cisplatin, genistein leads to 60% to 80% growth inhibition of pancreatic cancer cells, while gemcitabine alone results in only 30% inhibition.[228] Furthermore, in studies of orthotopic mice, treatment with genistein decreased the size of pancreatic masses irrespective of the metastatic potential of the tumor.[229] These preclinical observations have led to a multicenter phase 2 trial conducted in previously untreated patients with metastatic pancreatic cancer.[230] Although genistein did not ultimately lead to a significant clinical improvement, interest in the development of more potent and specific inhibitors of the Akt/PI3K pathway remains.

Secreted Protein Acidic and Rich in Cystein

SPARC is an extracellular matrix protein that has gained notoriety as an important factor in the tumor microenvironment and is thought to foster the intense desmoplasia often observed in pancreatic cancer. SPARC overexpression in peritumoral fibroblasts has been associated with worse survival in a group of patients undergoing resection with curative intent.[231] Recently, Von Hoff et al.[232] reported on the combination of nanoparticle albumin-bound paclitaxel with gemcitabine for the treatment of advanced pancreatic cancer. Interestingly, the overexpression of SPARC was associated with very high response rates and longer progression-free survival, whereas SPARC-negative tumors were not as responsive and were associated with shorter progression-free survival.

Lessons from Four Decades of Chemotherapy for Pancreatic Cancer

Advances in therapy for pancreatic cancer have been extremely slow. This in large part may be explained by the impressive chemo- and radioresistance of this disease. Adding even more complexity, patients with pancreatic cancer can have a rapid decline in their clinical status due to venous thromboembolism, pulmonary embolus, cholangitis with biliary sepsis, worsening pain, declining performance status, gastrointestinal bleeding, and gastric outlet obstruction. Data from the Royal Marsden Hospital showed that 60-day all-cause mortality among pancreatic cancer patients enrolled in clinical trials was 13%, significantly higher than rates seen among patients with advanced colon cancer or even gastric cancer.[233] Despite these grim realities, learning from previous clinical trials may enable investigators to accelerate progress for patients:

1. Modern cross-sectional CT and MRI have been important advances, allowing for a clearer distinction between patients with locally advanced disease and patients with metastatic disease, and also providing better estimates of tumor burden. Moreover, although the primary tumor may not visibly respond to therapy, radiographic evidence of response in metastatic lesions is quite reliable.
2. Emerging evidence also suggests that CA 19-9 may have prognostic value at baseline,[234] and when CA 19-9 levels are driven substantially lower with therapy, survival is improved.
3. In general, patients who have locally advanced disease have a significantly better prognosis compared with patients who have metastatic disease.
4. Performance status at diagnosis is an independent predictor of survival.

These facts can be used to guide future trial designs, particularly in regard to eligibility criteria. In virtually all randomized trials of systemic therapy completed to date, eligibility criteria have led to enrollment of heterogeneous groups of patients. For example, most of the studies summarized in Tables 82.13 and 82.14 allowed for enrollment of patients with either locally advanced or metastatic disease. This makes results of individual trials difficult to generalize and comparisons between trials challenging. This has been further complicated by enrolling patients with varying levels of functional status (usually ECOG score 0 to 2), leading to inclusion of some marginal candidates for cytotoxic chemotherapy.

No matter what the direction of future clinical research, consideration should be given to the design of clinical trials with rigorous eligibility criteria, for example, trials where enrollment is limited to patients with metastatic disease with exceptionally good performance status (Karnofsky score greater than 80%).[235] In addition, it may be reasonable to use some defined parameters of tumor burden, such as response evaluation criteria in solid tumors (total measurable lesions 10 cm or less vs. greater than 10 cm), or to exclude patients with CA 19-9 levels above a predetermined cutoff. Such trials may allow for more robust distinctions between treatment arms and spur further investigation of the most promising drug regimens.

Whether resources should be focused on smaller, randomized phase 2 trials with novel drug combinations or on larger, randomized phase 3 trials with a bland control arm is currently a subject of some debate. Given the minimal progress observed since the advent of gemcitabine, a shift to smaller, well-designed randomized phase 2 trials may be a better strategy for the next several years.[235]

Practical Approach to Patients with Metastatic Disease

Although systemic therapy is often indicated for a patient with metastatic pancreatic cancer, a careful assessment of symptoms, biliary tract patency, and functional status is critical prior to making recommendations about anticancer therapy. Aggressive efforts to address pain control should be paramount. Patients requiring short-acting analgesics on a frequent basis should be prescribed long-acting oral or transdermal narcotics. For those patients with poor tolerance to their pain regimen, including nausea, sedation, delirium, or constipation, referral to a pain specialist is encouraged. These patients may benefit from neurolytic block of the celiac of splanchnic ganglion or parenteral medications.

Although not rigorously studied, patients with poor performance status (Karnofsky score less than 80%, ECOG score greater than 3), treated only with palliative interventions (without delivery of chemotherapy), probably survive as long as those patients offered best supportive care combined with chemotherapy. In general current data do not support the use of combination chemotherapy for patients with poor performance status.

For patients with good performance status (Karnofsky score greater than 80%), enrollment in a clinical trial should be encouraged, but off protocol, a gemcitabine doublet that contains erlotinib, a platinum analogue, or a fluoropyrimidine is a reasonable alternative to gemcitabine alone. When patients are offered systemic therapy, the goals of this therapy should be clearly explained, and careful follow-up during treatment is necessary. Patients with metastatic disease are extremely dynamic, and they may rapidly develop complications. Delivering treatment to overtly jaundiced patients may lead to excess toxicity, and efforts to optimize biliary drainage may be an important component of care. Additionally, frequent clinical assessments should include a careful history with emphasis on pain levels, nausea or vomiting, and functional status. Physical examinations should be performed to assess for superficial or deep venous thrombosis or evidence of tumor progression (ascites, new lymphadenopathy, or ongoing weight loss). Regular laboratory testing with complete blood tests, electrolytes, blood urea nitrogen and creatinine, and liver function tests are important to rule out worsening anemia, dehydration, and impending biliary obstruction with or without cholangitis. Gastric outlet obstruction can develop during the course of illness and is occasionally confused with chemotherapy-induced nausea and vomiting. For patients with a decline in clinical status in the face of cytotoxic therapy, clinicians must consider the possibility of disease progression versus excess toxicity from chemotherapy and discuss with the patient the pros and cons of continued treatment.

OTHER EXOCRINE NEOPLASMS

Ductal adenocarcinoma of the pancreas is the most common type of pancreatic exocrine neoplasm, but other exocrine neoplasms develop each year in small numbers of patients.

Solid Neoplasms or Malignancies

Acinar Cell Carcinoma

Acinar cell carcinoma presents with an estimated U.S. incidence of 300 cases per year, clinically presenting with pain or weight loss.[236] On imaging these appear to be a well-circumscribed heterogeneous solid mass. Pathologically these tumors exhibit clusters of acinar cells with luminal obliteration and at times endocrine differentiation. These tumors may secrete α-fetoprotein (AFP), endocrine products, or pancreatic enzymes, including lipase, into the circulation. A characteristic paraneoplastic syndrome has been described for 15% of patients, with these tumors due to elevated levels of circulating lipase. Patients experience parathyropathies, diffuse subcutaneous nodules, and sclerotic lesions in cancellous bone; the latter two findings are due to areas of fat necrosis in the subcutaneous tissue and bone.[237]

A resection is recommended when feasible; but metastases are frequent, with 50% of patients presenting with distant disease and those who have been resected experiencing a high rate of recurrence. Median survival for patients with localized disease and metastatic disease is 38 and 14 months, respectively.[238]

Pancreatoblastoma

Less than 60 cases of pancreatoblastoma have been reported in the literature. These tumors usually present in children with vague symptoms due to mass effect. On imaging the tumors are often large, multilobulated with heterogeneous attenuation. Pathologically they are similar to acinar cell carcinoma and can be considered a pediatric variant of acinar cell cancer. On histologic examination, these tumors have pathognomonic squamoid corpuscles. These tumors may secrete AFP and beta-human chorionic gonadotropin, either of which can be a marker for disease. Excision is the recommended treatment. In an isolated primary lesion an R0 resection is often feasible, but resection of metastatic disease and adjacent involved organs should be considered in advanced lesions.[239]

Lymphoplasmacytic Sclerosing Pancreatitis

Neither a neoplasm nor a malignancy, lymphoplasmacytic sclerosing pancreatitis is a solid pancreatic mass that is often mistaken as a pancreatic exocrine tumor. In several high-volume centers, 2% to 3% of pancreaticoduodenectomies are completed for this disease with diagnosis established at pathologic evaluation. These present as a localized mass or with diffuse involvement of the entire pancreas. Clinically, patients do not have risk factors for pancreatitis and may have other underlying autoimmune conditions such as Sjögren's syndrome or ulcerative colitis. Systemic extrapancreatic lesions may be present and have been described in the biliary system, salivary gland, lung, and kidney. Pathologically the disease may be centered on the pancreatic exocrine lobules or ducts, and plasmacytes expressing immunoglobulin subclass-4 (IgG-4) on immunohistochemistry are characteristic.[240]

Typically, these patients have elevated levels of IgG-4,[241] and this test should be considered in patients presenting with a new pancreatic mass. Clearly, this should be part of the workup for a mass that is a diagnostic dilemma after initial studies.

Lymphoplasmacytic sclerosing pancreatitis responds to treatment with corticosteroids, which is the preferred method of treatment when these are diagnosed preoperatively. If excised, the lesions tend to respond to the procedure alone, although a small proportion of patients may experience recurrence of inflammatory lesions following the operation.

Cystic Neoplasms or Malignancies

A wide range of benign conditions, including pancreatic pseudocysts and ductal carcinoma or neuroendocrine tumors, can all result in pancreatic cystic lesions. Four distinct pancreatic exocrine neoplasms also present as cystic lesions: (1) serous cystic neoplasm, (2) mucinous cystic neoplasm, (3) IPMN, alternatively known as intraductal pancreatic mucinous tumor, and (4) solid pseudopapillary cystic neoplasm. These tumors increasingly are identified incidentally, but may present with symptoms from mass effect, including nausea, early satiety, jaundice, bloating, and pain. For each disease entity, descriptions of unique demographics, appearance on radiologic imaging, and cyst characteristics have been described to differentiate the tumors.[242] In practice there is a wide variation of tumor characteristics, and the etiology of any cystic lesion may be elusive.

Serous cystic neoplasms tend to be comprised of microcystic disease with a honeycomb pattern on imaging. They have essentially no malignant potential. If a lesion is clearly a serous cystic neoplasm, it should be resected only to palliate symptoms from mass effect.

Mucinous cystic neoplasms have a clear malignant potential, with increasing incidence of malignancy as the patient ages. The lesions progress along a continuum: malignant transformation from mucinous cystadenoma to mucinous cystadenoma with dysplasia to mucinous cystadenocarcinoma. The median age for each condition is 48 years, 53 years, and 64 years, respectively, illustrating the advancing malignant nature of these cysts as age progresses. On imaging these cysts may communicate with the duct; histologically, they may exhibit discontinuous epithelium with ovarian-like stroma.

IPMN is often a multifocal disease involving the ductal epithelium of a major pancreatic duct and may be isolated to an interlobular duct (a side branch variant) or the main pancreatic duct. Patients with aberrantly separate ducts of Santorini and Wirsung may have IPMN involving only one ductal system. Grossly, the involved duct appears to have "roe" lining its luminal surface. These have multifocal malignant potential along the duct.

Solid pseudopapillary cystic neoplasms tend to affect young women and have a small malignant potential. Cysts are often unilocular, and scattered calcifications may be seen on imaging.

The approach to these lesions is in evolution, and several algorithms with disparate strategies have been recommended for these cystic lesions. The group at Massachusetts General Hospital, in a series of articles, recommends early evaluation of cystic fluid with cyst fluid aspiration and early excision of premalignant or malignant lesions in patients with a reasonable operative risk.[243] Conversely, considering similar data, the group at MSKCC recommends a more observational course, recommending serial imaging for small cystic lesions, intervening with cyst aspiration or resection only for a growing lesion in a patient with reasonable operative risk.[244]

While the authors favor the strategy proposed by MDACC,[245] the optimal approach to these tumors is not defined. Several points can be agreed on while designing an evaluation and treatment algorithm for these cystic tumors:

1. Mucinous tumors (mucinous cystic neoplasms and IPMN) and solid pseudopapillary cystic neoplasms are premalignant or malignant lesions. Serous cystic neoplasms are rarely malignant and should only be excised for symptoms from mass effect or equivocal diagnosis exists.
2. The risk of malignancy in a premalignant lesion increases with increasing age, lesion size, and cystic fluid carcinoembryonic antigen (CEA) level.
3. The end point of cystic mass evaluation is surgical resection of the tumor. Therefore, the risk–benefit ratio of surgical excision should be weighed prior to embarking on an invasive evaluation of a lesion.
4. One method of evaluating cystic lesions is serial cross-sectional imaging to observe the development of solid elements within the cyst or change in the cyst size. A lesion increasing in size should be excised if feasible.
5. Another method of evaluating cystic tumors is aspiration of the cyst fluid using percutaneous techniques, or preferably by endoscopic ultrasound. Analysis of cystic fluid obtained from aspiration yields the most useful diagnostic information of any diagnostic test. Mucin indicates a cyst with malignant potential, and cyst fluid CEA level is the most accurate measure to determine malignancy within the mass.

When the course of operative excision is chosen, anatomic excision should be used for large or symptomatic cystic tumors or for tumors where malignancy is suspected. Enucleation is acceptable for small tumors when the suspicion of malignancy is low. IPMN presents a unique problem for resection. Resections should always be anatomic and include the involved portion of pancreatic duct. Liberal use of frozen section evaluation of the duct margin and ductoscopy should be used to assess the remaining duct for tandem areas of involvement. If the entire duct is involved, a total pancreatectomy is indicated.

Selected References

The full list of references for this chapter appears in the online version.

1. Ries LAG, Melbert D, Krapcho M, et al. SEER cancer statistics review 1975–2004; based on November 2006 SEER data submission. World Wide Web URL: http://seer.cancer.gov/csr/1975_2004/. Bethesda, MD: National Cancer Institute, 2007.
4. Jemal A, Siegel R, Ward E, et al. Cancer statistics, 2009. *CA Cancer J Clin* 2009;59:225.
7. Lowenfels AB, Maisonneuve P. Epidemiology and risk factors for pancreatic cancer. *Best Prac Res Clin Gastroenterol* 2006;20(2):197.
8. Yeo TP, Hruban RH, Leach SD, et al. Pancreatic cancer. *Curr Probl Cancer* 2002;26(4):176.
10. Bao Y, Giovannucci E, Fuchs CS, Michaud DS. Passive smoking and pancreatic cancer in women: a prospective cohort study. *Cancer Epidemiol Biomarkers Prev* 2009;18(8):2292.
17. Hassan MM, Li D, El-Deeb AS, et al. Association between hepatitis B virus and pancreatic cancer. *J Clin Oncol* 2008;26(28):4557.
18. Hoefs JC, Renner IG, Askhcavai M, Redeker AG. Hepatitis B surface antigen in pancreatic and biliary secretions. *Gastroenterology* 1980;79(2):191.
25. Wang F, Gupta S, Holly EA. Diabetes mellitus and pancreatic cancer in a population-based case-control study in the San Francisco Bay Area, California. *Cancer Epidemiol Biomarkers Prev* 2006;15(8):1458.
29. Michaud DS, Giovannucci E, Willett WC, et al. Physical activity, obesity, height, and the risk of pancreatic cancer. *JAMA* 2001;286:921.
30. Eckel RH, Grundy SM, Zimmet PZ. The metabolic syndrome. *Lancet* 2005;365(9468):1415.
37. Tersmette AC, Petersen GM, Offerhaus GJA, et al. Increased risk of incident pancreatic cancer among first-degree relatives of patients with familial pancreatic cancer. *Clin Cancer Res* 2001;7:738.
39. Hruban RH, Maitra A, Schulick R, et al. Emerging molecular biology of pancreatic cancer. *Gastrointest Cancer Res* 2008;2(4 Suppl):S10.
44. Trede M. Embryology and surgical anatomy of the pancreas. In: *Surgery of the pancreas*. 2nd ed. Livingston, NY: Churchill, 1997.
47. Jensen J. Gene regulatory factors in pancreatic development. *Dev Dyn* 2004;229(1):176.
49. Hruban RH, Goggins M, Parsons J, Kern SE. Progression model for pancreatic cancer. *Clin Cancer Res* 2000;6:2969.
53. Canto MI, Goggins M, Yeo CJ, et al. Screening for pancreatic neoplasia in high-risk individuals: an EUS-based approach. *Clin Gastroenterol Hepatol* 2004;2(7):606.
54. Brentnall TA, Bronner MP, Byrd DR, Haggitt RC, Kimmey MB. Early diagnosis and treatment of pancreatic dysplasia in patients with a family history of pancreatic cancer. *Ann Intern Med* 1999;131:247.
56. Kelsen DP, Portenoy R, Thaler H, Tao Y, Brennan M. Pain as a predictor of outcome in patients with operable pancreatic carcinoma. *Surgery* 1997;122:53.
59. Yeo CJ, Cameron JL, Lillemoe KD, et al. Pancreaticoduodenectomy with or without distal gastrectomy and extended retroperitoneal lymphadenectomy for periampullary adenocarcinoma, part 2: randomized controlled trial evaluating survival, morbidity, and mortality. *Ann Surg* 2002;236:355.
61. Tamm EP, Silverman PM, Charnsangavej C, Evans DB. Diagnosis, staging, and surveillance of pancreatic cancer. *AJR Am J Roentgenol* 2003;180(5):1311.
65. White RR, Paulson EK, Freed KS, et al. Staging of pancreatic cancer before and after neoadjuvant chemoradiation. *J Gastrointest Surg* 2001;5(6):626–633.
71. Raut C, Grau A, Starkel G, et al. Diagnostic accuracy of endoscopic ultrasound-guided fine-needle aspiration in patients with presumed pancreatic cancer. *J Gastrointest Surg* 2002;7(1):118.
73. Farnell MB, Nagorney DM, Sarr MG. The Mayo Clinic approach to the surgical treatment of adenocarcinoma of the pancreas. *Surg Clin North Am* 2001;81(3):611.
74. Minnard EA, Conlon KC, Hoos A, et al. Laparoscopic ultrasound enhances standard laparoscopy in the staging of pancreatic cancer. *Ann Surg* 1998;228(2):182.
79. Tseng JF, Raut CP, Lee JE, et al. Pancreaticoduodenectomy with vascular resection: Margin status and survival duration. *J Gastrointest Surg* 2004;8:935.
80. Conlon KC, Klimstra DS, Brennan MF. Long-term survival after curative resection for pancreatic ductal adenocarcinoma; clinicopathologic analysis of 5-year survivors. *Ann Surg* 1996;223:273.

82. Cleary SP, Gryfe R, Guindi M, et al. Prognostic factors in resected pancreatic adenocarcinoma: analysis of actual 5-year survivors. *J Am Coll Surg* 2004;198(5):722.
86. Whipple AO. A reminiscence: pancreaticduodenectomy. *Rev Surg* 1963; 20:221.
91. Evans DB, Lee JE, Pisters PWT. Pancreaticoduodenectomy (Whipple operation) and total pancreatectomy for cancer. In: Baker RJ, Fischer FJ, eds. *Mastery of surgery.* 4th ed. Philadelphia: Lippincott Williams & Wilkins, 2001:1299.
94. Conlon KC, Labow D, Leung D, et al. Prospective randomized clinical trial of the value of intraperitoneal drainage after pancreatic resection. *Ann Surg* 2001;234(4):487.
96. Pisters PWT, Hudec WA, Hess KR, et al. Effect of preoperative biliary decompression on pancreaticoduodenectomy-associated morbidity in 300 consecutive patients. *Ann Surg* 2001;234:47.
98. Birkmeyer JD, Warshaw AL, Finlayson SR, Grove MR, Tosteson AN. Relationship between hospital volume and late survival after pancreaticoduodenectomy. *Surgery* 1999;126:178.
99. Pedrazzoli S, DiCarlo V, Dionigi R, et al. Standard versus extended lymphadenectomy associated with pancreatoduodenectomy in the surgical treatment of adenocarcinoma of the head of the pancreas: a multicenter, prospective, randomized study. Lymphadenectomy Study Group. *Ann Surg* 1998;228(4):508.
100. Yeo CJ, Cameron JL, Sohn TA, et al. Pancreaticoduodenectomy with or without extended retroperitoneal lymphadenectomy for periampullary adenocarcinoma: comparison of morbidity and mortality and short-term outcome. *Ann Surg* 1999;229(5):613.
101. Farnell MB, Pearson RK, Sarr MG, et al. A prospective randomized trial comparing standard pancreatoduodenectomy with pancreatoduodenectomy with extended lymphadenectomy in resectable pancreatic head adenocarcinoma. *Surgery* 2005;138(4):618.
105. Kalser MH, Ellenberg SS. Pancreatic cancer. Adjuvant combined radiation and chemotherapy following curative resection. *Arch Surg* 1985; 120(8):899.
106. Klinkenbijl JH, Jeekel J, Sahmoud T, et al. Adjuvant radiotherapy and 5-fluorouracil after curative resection of cancer of the pancreas and periampullary region: phase III trial of the EORTC gastrointestinal tract cancer cooperative group. *Ann Surg* 1999;230(6):776.
107. Neoptolemos JP, Stocken DD, Friess H, et al. A randomized trial of chemoradiotherapy and chemotherapy after resection of pancreatic cancer. *N Engl J Med* 2004;350:1200.
108. Bakkevold KE, Arnesjo B, Dahl O, Kambestad B. Adjuvant combination chemotherapy (AMF) following radical resection of carcinoma of the pancreas and papilla of Vater—results of a controlled, prospective, randomised multicentre study. *Eur J Cancer* 1993;29A(5):698.
109. Neuhaus P, Riess H, Post S, et al. Final results of the randomized, prospective, multicenter phase III trial of adjuvant chemotherapy with gemcitabine versus observation in patients with resected pancreatic cancer *J Clin Oncol* 2008;26(Suppl): (abst LBA4504).
110. Regine WF, Winter KW, Abrams R, et al. RTOG 9704: a phase III study of adjuvant pre and post chemoradiation 5-FU vs. gemcitabine for resected pancreatic adenocarcinoma. *J Clin Oncol* 2007;24(18 Suppl): (abst 4007).
111. Neoptolemos JP, Buchler MW, Stocken DD, et al. ESPAC-3(v2): a multicenter, international, open-label randomized, controlled phase III trial of adjuvant 5-fluoruracil/folinic acid versus gemcitabine in patients with resected pancreatic ductal adenocarcinoma. *J Clin Oncol* 2009;27(18 Suppl): (abst LBA4505).
114. Winter JM, Cameron JL, Campbell KA, et al. 1423 pancreaticoduodenectomies for pancreatic cancer: a single-institution experience. *J Gastrointest Surg* 2006;10(9):1199.
116. Oettle H, Post S, Neuhaus P, et al. Adjuvant chemotherapy with gemcitabine vs observation in patients undergoing curative-intent resection of pancreatic cancer: a randomized controlled trial. *JAMA* 2007;297(3):267.
117. Evans DB, Rich TA, Byrd DR, et al. Preoperative chemoradiation and pancreaticoduodenectomy for adenocarcinoma of the pancreas. *Arch Surg* 1992;127(11):1335.
119. Pisters PW, Abbruzzese JL, Janjan NA, et al. Rapid-fractionation preoperative chemoradiation, pancreaticoduodenectomy, and intraoperative radiation therapy for resectable pancreatic adenocarcinoma. *J Clin Oncol* 1998;16(12):3843.
120. Pisters PW, Wolff RA, Janjan NA, et al. Preoperative paclitaxel and concurrent rapid-fractionation radiation for resectable pancreatic adenocarcinoma: toxicities, histologic response rates, and event-free outcome. *J Clin Oncol* 2002;20(10):2537.
121. White RR, Tyler DS. Neoadjuvant therapy for pancreatic cancer: the Duke experience. *Surg Oncol Clin North Am* 2004;13(4):675.
122. Evans DB, Rich TA, Byrd DR, et al. Preoperative chemoradiation and pancreaticoduodenectomy for adenocarcinoma of the pancreas. *Arch Surg* 1992;127(11):1335.
126. Evans DB, Varadhachary GR, Crane CH, et al. Preoperative gemcitabine-based chemoradiation for patients with resectable adenocarcinoma of the pancreatic head. *J Clin Oncol* 2008;26(21):3496.
127. Varadhachary GR, Wolff RA, Crane CH, et al. Preoperative gemcitabine and cisplatin followed by gemcitabine-based chemoradiation for resectable adenocarcinoma of the pancreatic head. *J Clin Oncol* 2008;26(21): 3487.
128. Pingpank JF, Hoffman JP, Ross EA, et al. Effect of preoperative chemoradiotherapy on surgical margin status of resected adenocarcinoma of the head of the pancreas. *J Gastrointest Surg* 2001;5(2):121.
130. Katz MHG, Pisters PWT, Evans DB, et al. Borderline resectable pancreatic cancer: the importance of this emerging stage of disease. *J Am Coll Surg* 2008;206(5):833.
131. Bold RJ, Charnsangavej C, Cleary KR, et al. Major vascular resection as part of pancreaticoduodenectomy for cancer: radiologic, intraoperative, and pathologic analysis. *J Gastrointest Surg* 1999;3:233.
134. Moertel CG, Childs DS Jr, Reitemeier RJ, Colby MY Jr, Holbrook MA. Combined 5-fluorouracil and supervoltage radiation therapy of locally unresectable gastrointestinal cancer. *Lancet* 1969;2(7626):865.
135. Moertel CG, Frytak S, Hahn RG, et al. Therapy of locally unresectable pancreatic carcinoma: a randomized comparison of high dose (6000 rads) radiation alone, moderate dose radiation (4000 rads + 5-fluorouracil), and high dose radiation + 5-fluorouracil: the Gastrointestinal Tumor Study Group. *Cancer* 1981;48(8):1705.
138. Klaassen DJ, MacIntyre JM, Catton GE, Engstrom PF, Moertel CG. Treatment of locally unresectable cancer of the stomach and pancreas: a randomized comparison of 5-fluorouracil alone with radiation plus concurrent and maintenance 5-fluorouracil—an Eastern Cooperative Oncology Group study. *J Clin Oncol* 1985;3(3):373.
139. Kindler HL, Niedzwiecki D, Hollis D, et al. A double-blind, placebo-controlled randomized phase III trial of gemcitabine plus bevacizumab versus gemcitabine plus placebo in patients with advanced pancreatic cancer: a preliminary analysis of Cancer and Leukemia Group B. *J Clin Oncol* 2007;25(18 Suppl): (abst 4508).
142. Huguet F, Andre T, Hammel P, et al. Impact of chemoradiotherapy after disease control with chemotherapy in locally advanced pancreatic adenocarcinoma in GERCOR phase II and III studies. *J Clin Oncol* 2007;25(3): 326.
156. Burris HA 3rd, Moore MJ, Andersen J, et al. Improvements in survival and clinical benefit with gemcitabine as first-line therapy for patients with advanced pancreas cancer: a randomized trial. *J Clin Oncol* 1997;15:2403.
157. Crane CH, Abbruzzese JL, Evans DB, et al. Is the therapeutic index better with gemcitabine-based chemoradiation than with 5-fluorouracil-based chemoradiation in locally advanced pancreatic cancer? *Int J Radiat Oncol Biol Phys* 2002;52(5):1293.
158. Cartwright TH, Cohn A, Varkey JA, et al. Phase II study of oral capecitabine in patients with advanced or metastatic pancreatic cancer. *J Clin Oncol* 2002;20(1):160.
160. Crane CH, Ellis LM, Abbruzzese JL, et al. Phase I trial evaluating the safety of bevacizumab with concurrent radiotherapy and capecitabine in locally advanced pancreatic cancer. *J Clin Oncol* 2006;24(7):1145.
162. Crane CH, Winter K, Regine WF, et al. Phase II study of bevacizumab with concurrent capecitabine and radiation followed by maintenance gemcitabine and bevacizumab for locally advanced pancreatic cancer: Radiation Therapy Oncology Group RTOG 0411. *J Clin Oncol* 2009;27 (25):4096.
169. Chao C, Hoffman JP, Ross EA, Torosian MH, Eisenberg BL. Pancreatic carcinoma deemed unresectable at exploration may be resected for cure: an institutional experience. *Am Surg* 2000;66(4):378.
170. Lillemoe KD, Kaushal S, Cameron JL, et al. Distal pancreatectomy: indications and outcomes in 235 patients. *Ann Surg* 1999;229(5):693.
171. Espat NJ, Brennan MF, Conlon KC. Patients with laparoscopically staged unresectable pancreatic adenocarcinoma do not require subsequent surgical biliary or gastric bypass. *J Am Coll Surg* 1999;188(6):649.
177. Smith FP, Hoth DF, Levin B, et al. 5-Fluorouracil, adriamycin, and mitomycin C (FAM) chemotherapy for advanced adenocarcinoma of the pancreas. *Cancer* 1980;46:2014.
178. Bukowski RM, Balcerzak SP, O'Bryan RM, Bonnet JD, Chen TT. Randomized trial of 5-fluorouracil and mitomycin C with or without streptozotocin for advanced pancreatic cancer: a Southwest Oncology Group Study. *Cancer* 1983;52:1577.
179. Oster MW, Gray R, Panasci L, et al. Chemotherapy for advanced pancreatic cancer. A comparison of 5-fluorouracil, adriamycin, and mitomycin (FAM) with 5-fluorouracil, streptozotocin, and mitomycin (FSM). *Cancer* 1986;57:2.
180. Cullinan S, Moertel CG, Wieand HS, et al. A phase III trial on the therapy of advanced pancreatic carcinoma. Evaluations of the Mallinson regimen and combined 5-fluorouracil, doxorubicin and cisplatin. *Cancer* 1990;65: 2207.
185. Moore MJ, Hamm J, Dancey J, et al. Comparison of gemcitabine versus the matrix metalloproteinase inhibitor BAY 12-9566 in patients with advanced or metastatic adenocarcinoma of the pancreas: a phase III trial of the National Cancer Institute of Canada Clinical Trials Group. *J Clin Oncol* 2003;21(17):3296.
188. Tempero M, Plunkett W, Ruiz Van Haperen V, et al. Randomized phase II comparison of dose-intense gemcitabine: thirty-minute infusion and fixed dose rate infusion in patients with pancreatic adenocarcinoma. *J Clin Oncol* 2003;21(18):3402.
192. Louvet C, Labianca R, Hammel P, et al. Gemcitabine in combination with oxaliplatin compared with gemcitabine alone in locally advanced or

metastatic pancreatic cancer: results of a GERCOR and GISCAD phase III trial. *J Clin Oncol* 2005;23(15):3509.
193. Poplin E, Feng Y, Berlin J, et al. Phase III, randomized study of gemcitabine and oxaliplatin versus gemcitabine (fixed-dose rate infusion) compared with gemcitabine (30-minute infusion) in patients with pancreatic carcinoma E6201: a trial of the Eastern Cooperative Oncology Group. *J Clin Oncol* 2009;27(23):3778.
199. Kindler HL. The pemetrexed/gemcitabine combination in pancreatic cancer. *Cancer* 2002;95(4 Suppl):928.
203. Cunningham D, Chau I, Stocken DD, et al. Phase III randomized comparison of gemcitabine versus gemcitabine plus capecitabine in patients with advanced pancreatic cancer. *J Clin Oncol* 2009;27(33):5513.
204. Colucci G, Labianca R, Di Costanzo F, et al. Randomized phase III trial of gemcitabine plus cisplatin compared with single-agent gemcitabine as first-line treatment of patients with advanced pancreatic cancer: the GIP-1 study. *J Clin Oncol* 2010;28(10):1645.
205. Colucci G, Giuliani F, Gebbia V, et al. Gemcitabine alone or with cisplatin for the treatment of patients with locally advanced and/or metastatic pancreatic carcinoma: a prospective, randomized phase III study of the Gruppo Oncologia dell'Italia Meridionale. *Cancer* 2002;94(4):902.
206. Heinemann V, Boeck S, Hinke A, Labianca R, Louvet C. Meta-analysis of randomized trials: evaluation of benefit from gemcitabine-based combination chemotherapy applied in advanced pancreatic cancer. *BMC Cancer* 2008;8:82.
209. Kindler H, Friberg G, Stadler W, et al. Bevacizumab (B) plus gemcitabine (G) in patient (pts) with advanced pancreatic cancer (PC): updated results of a multi-center phase II trial. ASCO Annual Meeting Proceedings (Post-Meeting Edition). *J Clin Oncol* 2004;22(14 Suppl): (abst 4009).
210. Moore MJ, Goldstein D, Hamm J, et al. Erlotinib plus gemcitabine compared with gemcitabine alone in patients with advanced pancreatic cancer: a phase III trial of the National Cancer Institute of Canada Clinical Trials Group. *J Clin Oncol* 2007;25(15):1960.
211. Van Cutsem E, van de Velde H, Karasek P, et al. Phase III trial of gemcitabine plus tipifarnib compared with gemcitabine plus placebo in advanced pancreatic cancer. *J Clin Oncol* 2004;22(8):1430.
213. Philip PA, Benedetti J, Fenoglio-Preiser C, et al. Phase III study of gemcitabine plus cetuximab versus gemcitabine in patients with locally advanced or metastatic pancreatic adenocarcinoma: SWOG S0205 study. *J Clin Oncol* 2007;25(18 Suppl): (abst LBA 4509).
214. Van Cutsem E, Vervenne WL, Bennouna J, et al. Phase III trial of bevacizumab in combination with gemcitabine and erlotinib in patients with metastatic pancreatic cancer. *J Clin Oncol* 2009;27(13):2231.
218. Fine RL, Fogelman DR, Schreibman SM, et al. The gemcitabine, docetaxel, and capecitabine (GTX) regimen for metastatic pancreatic cancer: a retrospective analysis. *Cancer Chemother Pharmacol* 2008;61(1):167.
223. Wang W, Abbruzzese JL, Evans DB, et al. The nuclear factor-kappa B RelA transcription factor is constitutively activated in human pancreatic adenocarcinoma cells. *Clin Cancer Res* 1999;5(1):119.
236. Katopodis O, Ross P, Norman AR, Oates J, Cunningham D. Sixty-day all-cause mortality rates in patients treated for gastrointestinal cancers, in randomised trials, at the Royal Marsden Hospital. *Eur J Cancer* 2004;40(15):2230.
238. Philip PA, Mooney M, Jaffe D, et al. Consensus report of the national cancer institute clinical trials planning meeting on pancreas cancer treatment. *J Clin Oncol* 2009;27(33):5660.
242. Mortenson MM, Katz MH, Tamm EP, et al. Current diagnosis and management of unusual pancreatic tumors. *Am J Surg* 2008;196(1):100.
246. Brugge WR, Lauwers GY, Sahani D, Fernandez-del Castillo C, Warshaw AL. Cystic neoplasms of the pancreas. *N Engl J Med* 2004;351(12):1218.
247. Allen PJ, Jaques DP, D'Angelica M, et al. Cystic lesions of the pancreas: selection criteria for operative and nonoperative management in 209 patients. *J Gastrointest Surg* 2003;7(8):970.
248. Katz MH, Mortenson MM, Wang H, et al. Diagnosis and management of cystic neoplasms of the pancreas: an evidence-based approach. *J Am Coll Surg* 2008;207(1):106.
253. Sohn TA, Yeo CJ, Cameron JL, Pitt HA, Lillemoe KD. Do preoperative biliary stents increase postpancreaticoduodenectomy complications? *J Gastrointest Surg* 2000;4(3):258.
254. Sewnath ME, Birjmohun RS, Rauws EA, et al. The effect of preoperative biliary drainage on postoperative complications after pancreaticoduodenectomy. *J Am Coll Surg* 2001;192(6):726.
259. Leach SD, Lee JE, Charnsangavej C, et al. Survival following pancreaticoduodenectomy with resection of the superior mesenteric-portal vein confluence for adenocarcinoma of the pancreatic head. *Br J Surg* 1998;85(5):611.
261. Kalser MH, Barkin J, MacIntyre JM. Pancreatic cancer. Assessment of prognosis by clinical presentation. *Cancer* 1985;56(2):397.
262. Klinkenbijl JH, Jeekel J, Sahmoud T. Adjuvant radiotherapy and 5-fluorouracil after curative resection for the cancer of the pancreas and peri-ampullary region. Phase III trial of the EORTC Gastrointestinal Tract Cancer Cooperative Group. *Ann Surg* 1999;230:776.
276. Poplin E, Levy D, Berlin J, et al. Phase III trial of gemcitabine (30-minute infusion) versus gemcitabine (fixed-dose-rate infusion[FDR]) versus gemcitabine + oxaliplatin(GEMOX) in patients with advanced pancreatic cancer (E6201). 2006 ASCO Annual Meeting Proceedings Part I. *J Clin Oncol* 2006;24(18 Suppl): (abst LBA4004).
277. Berlin JD, Catalono P, Thomas JP, et al. Phase III study of gemcitabine in combination with fluorouracil versus gemcitabine alone in patients with advanced pancreatic carcinoma: Eastern Cooperative Group Trial E2297. *J Clin Oncol* 2002;20:3270.

CHAPTER 83 MOLECULAR BIOLOGY OF LIVER CANCER

SNORRI S. THORGEIRSSON AND JOE W. GRISHAM

Hepatocellular carcinoma (HCC) is one of the most common cancers worldwide, accounting for at least 600,000 deaths annually.[1] Although most frequent in southeast Asia and sub-Sahara Africa, the incidence and mortality rates of HCC have doubled in the United States and Europe in the past four decades and are expected to double again during the next 10 to 20 years.[2] As the incidence of HCC has increased, the age distribution of HCC has shifted toward relatively younger ages.[2] These observations make it clear that liver cancer is a major heath problem in the United States and Europe.

The etiologic agents responsible for the majority of HCC are known (e.g., infections with hepatitis B and C viruses [HBV and HCV], ethanol abuse), and additional causes are being identified (e.g., obesity, type 2 diabetes, nonalcoholic fatty liver disease).[3] Furthermore, the liver diseases that are associated with increased risk of HCC and the cellular alterations that precede HCC have been identified.[4–6] Research into the molecular pathogenesis of HCC currently focuses on the interrelationship of abnormal genomics and consequent alterations in molecular signaling pathways. Implicit in this research is the goal to integrate new data with clinicopathologic aspects of HCC in order to uncover new diagnostic, treatment, and prevention strategies.

Recent introduction of DNA microarray-based technologies makes it possible to measure simultaneously the expression of tens of thousands of genes in a tissue under a variety of conditions (reviewed in ref. 7). High-throughput microarray-based technologies and the recent advent of the next generation of whole genome DNA sequencers offer a unique opportunity to define the descriptive characteristics (i.e., "phenotype") of a biological system in terms of the genomic readout (e.g., gene expression, coding mutations, insertions and deletions in DNA, copy number variations and chromosomal translocations). Integrated views of biological systems have caused a paradigm shift in biological research methods, that is, from classic reductionism to systems biology.[8] Fundamental to the systems approach to the study of diseased biological systems is the hypothesis that disease processes are driven by aberrant regulatory networks of genes and proteins that differ from the normal counterparts. Application of multiparametric measurements promises to transform current approaches to diagnosis and therapy, providing the foundation for predictive and preventive personalized medicine.[8]

In this chapter we discuss the application of high-throughput genomic technologies to characterize HCC.

ALLELIC IMBALANCE IN LIVER CANCER

Chromosomal aberrations in tumors are regarded traditionally as evidence of gene deregulation and genome instability, and their detection may facilitate the identification of crucial genes and regulatory pathways that are perturbed in diseases. Several powerful analytical tools are currently available for analyzing chromosomal aberrations (reviewed in ref. 9). Comparative genomic hybridization (CGH), in particular array CGH, enables high-throughput analysis of DNA copy number and yields comprehensive information applicable to determining the molecular pathogenesis of human HCC. Meta-analysis of CGH studies of chromosome aberrations in human HCC shows that specific chromosomal gains and losses correlate with etiology and histologic grade (Table 83.1).[10] In HCC the most frequent amplifications of genomic material involve 1q (57.1%), 8q (46.6%), 6p (22.3%), and 17q (22.2%), whereas losses are most common in 8p (38%), 16q (35.9%), 4q (34.3%), 17p (32.1%), and 13q (26.2%). Deletions of 4q, 16q, 13q, and 8p correlate with HBV infection and lack of HCV infection. Chromosomes 13q and 4q are significantly underrepresented in poorly differentiated HCC, and gains of 1q correlate with other high-frequency alterations.[11] Amplifications and deletions often occur on chromosome arms at sites of oncogenes (e.g., *MYC* on 8q24) and tumor suppressor genes (e.g., *RB1* on 13q14), as well as at several loci that contain genes with known and/or suspected oncogenic functions (e.g., *FZD3*, *WISP1*, *SIAH-1*, and *AXIN2*, all of which modulate the WNT signaling pathway). In this meta-analysis, etiology and poor differentiation of HCC correlated with specific genomic alterations. In preneoplastic dysplastic nodules (DNs), amplifications are most frequent in 1q and 8q, whereas deletions occur in 8p, 17p, 5p, 13q, 14q, and 16q.[11] Gain of 1q appears to be an early event developing in DN, possibly predisposing affected cells to acquire additional chromosomal aberrations.

Bioinformatic analysis of CGH data was recently used to develop a progression model for human HCC.[11] Based on an evolutionary tree constructed from statistically significant CGH events, three subgroups of patients with different patterns of HCC progression were identified. The subgroups reflect the extent of tumor progression as indicated by the number of chromosomal aberrations, tumor stage, tumor size, and disease outcome. Gains of 1q21-23 and 8q22-24 appear to be early genomic events in development of HCC and gain of 3q22-24 a late genomic event, the latter associated with tumor recurrence and poor survival. The HCC progression model uncovered chromosomal imbalances associated with clinical pathologic characteristics of the disease and explained a significant part of the variations in clinical outcome among the HCC patients.[11]

These two studies illustrate the power of CGH analysis to identify the functional significance of genomic alterations in human HCC. Nevertheless, because CGH only analyzes

TABLE 83.1

FREQUENCIES IN CHROMOSOMAL ABERRATION IN HUMAN HEPATOCELLULAR CARCINOMA[a]

Chromosome	p-Arm Loss (%)	p-Arm Gain (%)	p-Arm High Frequency	p-Arm Genes	q-Arm Loss (%)	q-Arm Gain (%)	q-Arm High Frequency	q-Arm Genes
1	15.4	5.2	—	—	0.6	**57.1**	**q21.1–q44**	*WNT14, FASL*
2	1.4	7.1	—	—	2.9	8	—	—
3	3.9	5	—	—	1.9	8.8	—	—
4	10.6	6	—	—	**34.3**	1.7	**q21.1–q35**	*LEF1, CCNA*
5	1.7	13.6	—	—	7.8	11.1	—	—
6	1	22.3	—	*PIM1, CDKN1A*	15	7.9	—	—
7	0.9	15	—	—	3.1	16.8	—	—
8	**38**	4.6	**p21.1–p22**	*FZD3, PLK3*	1.9	**46.6**	**q22.1–q24.3**	*MYC, WISP1*
9	14	3.3	—	—	11.1	2.9	—	—
10	2.7	8.3	—	—	11.1	4.1	—	—
11	5.4	4.3	—	—	10.2	9.4	—	—
12	6.5	2.4	—	—	2.9	6.9	—	—
13	0	0	—	—	**26.2**	7.4	**q14.1–q22**	*RB1, BRCA3*
14	0	0	—	—	11.3	4.1	—	—
15	0	0	—	—	5.4	4.6	—	—
16	16.8	3.4	—	—	**35.9**	1.8	q12.1–q24	*SIAH1, CDH1*
17	**32.1**	2.9	**p13**	*p53, HIC1*	3.7	**22.2**	**q23–q25**	*AXIN2, TIMP2*
18	4.1	5.5	—	—	10.8	5	—	—
19	6.9	5	—	—	3.8	10.4	—	—
20	2	14.9	—	—	0.9	18.6	—	—
21	0	0	—	—	8.8	2.2	—	—
22	0	0	—	—	6.4	2.8	—	—
X	5	11.2	—	—	4.5	15	—	—
Y	5.1	2.3	—	—	5.6	2.3	—	—

[a]Summary of 785 different comparative genomic hybridization analyses of human hepatocellular carcinoma. Frequencies more than 20% are highlighted in bold. Region of highest frequency of imbalance on respective chromosomal arms are highlighted in bold. Examples of known tumor-relevant genes located on respective chromosomal high-frequency region are shown.
(Modified from ref. 10, with permission.)

genomic DNA, additional studies are required to measure and integrate data on global gene expression to confirm the roles of candidate genes. This can be accomplished by adapting the expression imbalance map method and array CGH analysis (reviewed in ref. 12). This approach was recently applied to human HCC.[13] Using regional pattern recognition approaches, the authors discovered the most probable copy number-dependent regions and 50 potential driver genes (Table 83.2). At each step of the gene selection process, the functional relevance of the selected genes was evaluated by estimating the prognostic significance of the selected genes. Further validation using small interference RNA-mediated knockdown experiments showed proof-of-principle evidence for the potential driver roles of the genes in HCC progression (i.e., *NCSTN* and *SCRIB*). In addition, systemic prediction of drug responses implicated the association of the 50 genes with specific signaling molecules (*mTOR*, *AMPK*, and *EGFR*). It was concluded that the application of an unbiased and integrative analysis of multidimensional genomic data sets can effectively screen for potential driver genes and provides novel mechanistic and clinical insights into the pathobiology of HCC.

It seems inevitable that new and improved array designs for both CGH and gene expression and the advent of whole genome sequencing combined with better software for statistical analysis of the data will continue to emerge.

CLASSIFICATION AND PROGNOSTIC PREDICTION OF HEPATOCELLULAR CARCINOMA

The application of microarray technologies to characterize tumors on the basis of global gene expression has had a significant impact on both basic and clinical oncology.[7] The goal of tumor microarray studies generally includes discovery of subsets of tumors (class discovery), which enables diagnostic classification (class comparison), prediction of clinical outcome (class prediction), and mechanistic analysis. Verification and validation of the primary results are essential for discovery of oncogenic pathways and identification of therapeutic targets (for technical details on microarray analysis see Chapter 2 and ref. 7). Analysis of global gene expression in selected tumors has successfully classified them into homogeneous groups and predicted the clinical outcome and survival (reviewed in ref. 7).

The goal of all staging systems is to separate patients into homogeneous prognostic groups to permit the selection of the most appropriate therapy for each group. Although much work has been devoted to establishment of prognostic models for HCC by using clinical information and pathologic classification,[6] many issues still remain unresolved. For example, a staging system that reliably separates patients into

TABLE 83.2

LIST OF 50 POTENTIAL DRIVER GENES[a]

Chr.	Cytoband	Gene Symbol	Correlation Coefficient	Correlation *P*-value	Copy Numbers	mRNA (Mean)	Chr.	Cytoband	Gene Symbol	Correlation Coefficient	Correlation *P*-value	Copy Numbers	mRNA (Mean)
chr1	q21.3	*C1orf43*	0.693	4.17E-03	0.366	0.324	chr8	q22.2	*POLR2K*	0.706	3.25E-03	0.291	0.805
chr1	q21.3	*HAX1*	0.668	6.47E-03	0.314	0.083	chr8	q22.3	*NCALD*	0.712	9.42E-03	0.086	0.204
chr1	q21.3	*ADAR*	0.803	3.14E-04	0.187	0.546	chr8	q22.3	*RRM2B*	0.788	8.23E-04	0.182	0.198
chr1	q22	*CCT3*	0.724	2.28E-03	0.313	1.084	chr8	q22.3	*AZIN1*	0.805	2.94E-04	0.205	0.271
chr1	q23.1	*CD1C*	0.716	2.70E-03	0.164	−0.432	chr8	q24.12	*TAF2*	0.659	7.56E-03	0.159	0.556
chr1	q23.2	*NCSTN*	0.668	6.48E-03	0.147	0.486	chr8	q24.13	*DERL1*	0.754	1.15E-03	0.209	0.224
chr1	q31.3	*CFHR2*	0.733	1.88E-03	0.106	−1.513	chr8	q24.13	*ZHX1*	0.672	8.49E-03	0.193	−0.08
chr1	q42.12	*PYCR2*	0.795	1.17E-03	0.201	0.751	chr8	q24.13	*TATDN1*	0.814	3.92E-04	0.229	0.654
chr6	p21.31	*C6orf107*	0.655	8.04E-03	0.198	0.075	chr8	q24.13	*NDUFB9*	0.754	1.15E-03	0.152	0.466
chr6	q16.3	*CCNC*	0.737	2.61E-03	−0.046	−0.315	chr8	q24.13	*KIAA0196*	0.678	5.46E-03	0.136	0.414
chr6	q22.31	*MAN1A1*	0.668	6.49E-03	−0.146	−1.293	chr8	q24.3	*TSTA3*	0.68	5.25E-03	0.153	0.401
chr6	q22.31	*SERINC1*	0.678	5.48E-03	−0.156	−0.825	chr8	q24.3	*SCRIB*	0.717	2.64E-03	0.163	1.102
chr7	q22.1	*EPHB4*	0.743	5.65E-03	0.286	0.189	chr8	q24.3	*HSF1*	0.654	8.12E-03	0.129	0.736
chr7	q22.1	*CUTL1*	0.73	1.99E-03	0.275	0.081	chr8	q24.3	*KIFC2*	0.677	7.76E-03	0.218	0.141
chr8	p22	*PCM1*	0.649	8.82E-03	−0.23	−0.225	chr16	q23.1	*KARS*	0.899	5.16E-06	0.012	0.072
chr8	p21.1	*ELP3*	0.745	2.23E-03	−0.204	−0.122	chr19	p13.12	*ILVBL*	0.914	1.86E-06	0.167	−0.253
chr8	p21.1	*HMBOX1*	0.771	7.57E-04	−0.204	−0.055	chr19	p13.12	*BRD4*	0.769	2.13E-03	0.163	0.209
chr8	q21.13	*MRPS28*	0.771	7.75E-04	0.087	−0.072	chr19	p13.12	*WIZ*	0.739	1.64E-03	0.163	0.463
chr8	q22.1	*KIAA1429*	0.699	3.76E-03	0.206	0.332	chr19	p13.12	*CYP4F11*	0.68	5.24E-03	0.109	−0.891
chr8	q22.1	*UQCRB*	0.676	5.67E-03	0.096	0.628	chr19	p13.12	*RAB8A*	0.722	2.38E-03	0.289	−0.081
chr8	q22.1	*PTDSS1*	0.818	1.96E-04	0.154	0.365	chr19	p13.11	*FAM32A*	0.769	8.09E-04	0.346	0.15
chr8	q22.1	*PGCP*	0.666	6.74E-03	0.041	0.388	chr19	p13.11	*C19orf42*	0.735	6.49E-03	0.3	0.366
chr8	q22.1	*MTDH*	0.669	6.37E-03	0.245	0.282	chr19	p13.11	*MYO9B*	0.825	1.75E-03	0.291	0.096
chr8	q22.2	*STK3*	0.686	4.78E-03	0.096	0.184	chr19	q12	*CCNE1*	0.76	1.62E-03	0.363	0.174
chr8	q22.2	*COX6C*	0.799	3.54E-04	0.172	0.508	chr19	q12	*C19orf2*	0.791	4.45E-04	0.069	0.437

[a]See ref. 13 for details.

homogeneous early and intermediate-to-advanced HCC groups with respect to prognosis does not exist. This is of particular importance because the natural course of early HCC is unknown, and the natural progression of intermediate and advanced HCC is known to be quite variable.[6] Because the accuracy of imaging techniques is rapidly evolving and affording detection of early HCC,[14] the inability to predict the prognosis of these early lesions poses a therapeutic dilemma. Although the accurate pathologic diagnosis of high-grade DNs and early HCC is currently difficult, it is likely that many HCC evolve from DN.[15]

A new insight on the transition of DN into early HCC was recently obtained.[16] A gene expression profiling on cirrhotic (regenerative) and DNs as well as early HCC was performed, and 460 differentially expressed genes were detected between DN and early HCC. Functional analysis of the significant gene set identified the *MYC* oncogene as a plausible driver gene for malignant conversion of the dysplastic nodules. In addition, gene set enrichment analysis revealed global activation of the *MYC* up-regulated gene set in early HCC versus dysplasia. Presence of the *MYC* signature significantly correlated with increased expression of *CSN5* gene as well as with higher overall transcription rate of genes located in the 8q chromosome region. Furthermore, a classifier constructed from *MYC* target genes could robustly discriminate early HCC from high- and low-grade DNs. Importantly, this study identified unique expression patterns associated with the transition of high-grade DNs into early HCC and demonstrated that activation of the *MYC* transcription signature is strongly associated with the malignant conversion of pre-neoplastic liver lesions.

Many studies on HCC gene expression profiling, as well as several reviews, have appeared during the last 5 years.[17] Interpretation of molecular profiling studies of HCC poses more challenges than other human tumors, mainly because of the complex pathogenesis of this cancer.[5] HCC arises in diverse settings ranging from infection with HBV or HCV, to chronic metabolic diseases as varied as diabetes, nonalcoholic fatty liver disease, and hemochromatosis. These different diseases represent complex assortments of genetic and epigenetic aberrations as well as altered molecular pathways.[5,6] Nevertheless, because of its extraordinary power of resolution, global gene expression profiling currently offers the most appropriate technology to resolve the complex molecular pathogenesis of HCC. Indeed, gene expression profiling of HCC has already generated impressive data sets that represent a remarkable progress toward the elucidation of the molecular pathogenesis of HCC, and may ultimately improve diagnosis and outcome prognosis for HCC patients.[17]

A class discovery approach applying hierarchical clustering of gene expression data from human HCC[18] revealed two subclasses of HCC that are strongly associated with survival of the patient. In this study, several independent prediction algorithms determined whether gene expression patterns could be used to predict survival. HCC patients were randomly divided into two equal groups, that is, a training set that was used to develop the HCC classifiers and a validation set that was used to evaluate the test. All the classifiers successfully separated patients with shorter survival from patients who survived longer. Gene expression patterns strongly associated with patient survival, and the reproducibility of these gene expression-based predictors, were robust. Moreover, application of a Cox regression model identified genes whose expression was highly correlated with the length of survival. Survival-associated genes could also be used for highly accurate subclass prediction without the application of sophisticated prediction models. The knowledge-based annotation of the survival genes provided insight into the underlying biological differences between the two subclasses of HCC.[18] Among several biological groups of the survival genes, the cell-proliferation group was the best predictor of an unfavorable outcome of the disease. Expression of proliferating cell nuclear antigen, a typical cell-proliferation marker, and cell cycle regulators such as *CDK4*, *CCNB1*, *CCNA2*, and *CKS2* was greater in the poor survival subclass (cluster A). Not surprisingly, many genes that were more highly expressed in the poor survival subclass had antiapoptotic functions. Higher expression of genes involved in ubiquitination and sumoylation also characterized the poor survival subclass. Enhanced activation of ubiquitin-dependent protein degradation may account for deregulation of cell cycle control and faster cell proliferation in the poor survival subclass. This study demonstrates that gene expression profiling can identify previously unrecognized, clinically relevant subclasses of HCC in a robust and reproducible manner.

Using a similar approach, Boyault et al.[19] further refined the transcriptome classification of HCC. Unsupervised transcriptome analysis identified six robust subgroups of HCC (G1-G6) associated with clinical and genetic characteristics of the tumors. G1 tumors had low HBV copy number and overexpressed genes controlled by parental imprinting in fetal liver. G2 tumors included HCC infected with a high copy number of HBV and mutations in *PIK3CA* and *TP53*. Specific activation of the AKT pathway was detected in both groups. G3 tumors were characterized by *TP53* mutations and overexpression of genes controlling the cell cycle. G4 was a heterogeneous subgroup of tumors that included both HCC and hepatocellular adenomas with *TCF1* mutations. G5 and G6 tumors contained β-catenin mutations that activate the WNT pathway. These results emphasize the genetic diversity of human HCC and provide specific identifiers for classifying the tumors. Also, this new classification shows that WNT and AKT pathways are activated in about 50% of the tumors, suggesting attractive potential therapeutic targets. Most recently Hoshida et al.[20] performed a meta-analysis of gene expression profiles in data sets from eight independent patient cohorts across the world. A total of 603 patients were analyzed, representing the major etiologies of HCC (hepatitis B and C) collected from Western and Eastern countries. Three robust HCC subclasses (termed S1, S2, and S3) were observed, each correlated with clinical parameters such as tumor size, extent of cellular differentiation, and serum alpha-fetoprotein levels. An analysis of the components of the signatures indicated that S1 reflected aberrant activation of the WNT signaling pathway, S2 was characterized by proliferation as well as MYC and AKT activation, and S3 was associated with hepatocyte differentiation. Functional studies indicated that the WNT pathway activation signature characteristic of S1 tumors was not simply the result of β-catenin mutation but rather was the result of transforming growth factor-β activation, thus representing a new mechanism of WNT pathway activation in HCC. These experiments establish the first attempt to develop consensus classification framework for HCC based on gene expression profiles and highlight the power of integrating multiple data sets to define a robust molecular taxonomy of the disease.

The transcriptomic analyses have also been used to address lineage heterogeneity of HCC. The two major adult liver cancers are HCC and cholangiocarcinoma (CC). The existence of combined hepatocellular-cholangiocarcinoma (CHC), a histopathologic intermediate form between HCC and CC, suggests phenotypic overlap between these tumors. Woo et al.[21] applied an integrative oncogenomic approach to address the clinical and functional implications of the overlapping phenotype between these tumors. By performing gene expression profiling of human HCC, CHC, and CC, the authors identified a novel HCC subtype, that is, cholangiocarcinoma-like HCC (CLHCC),

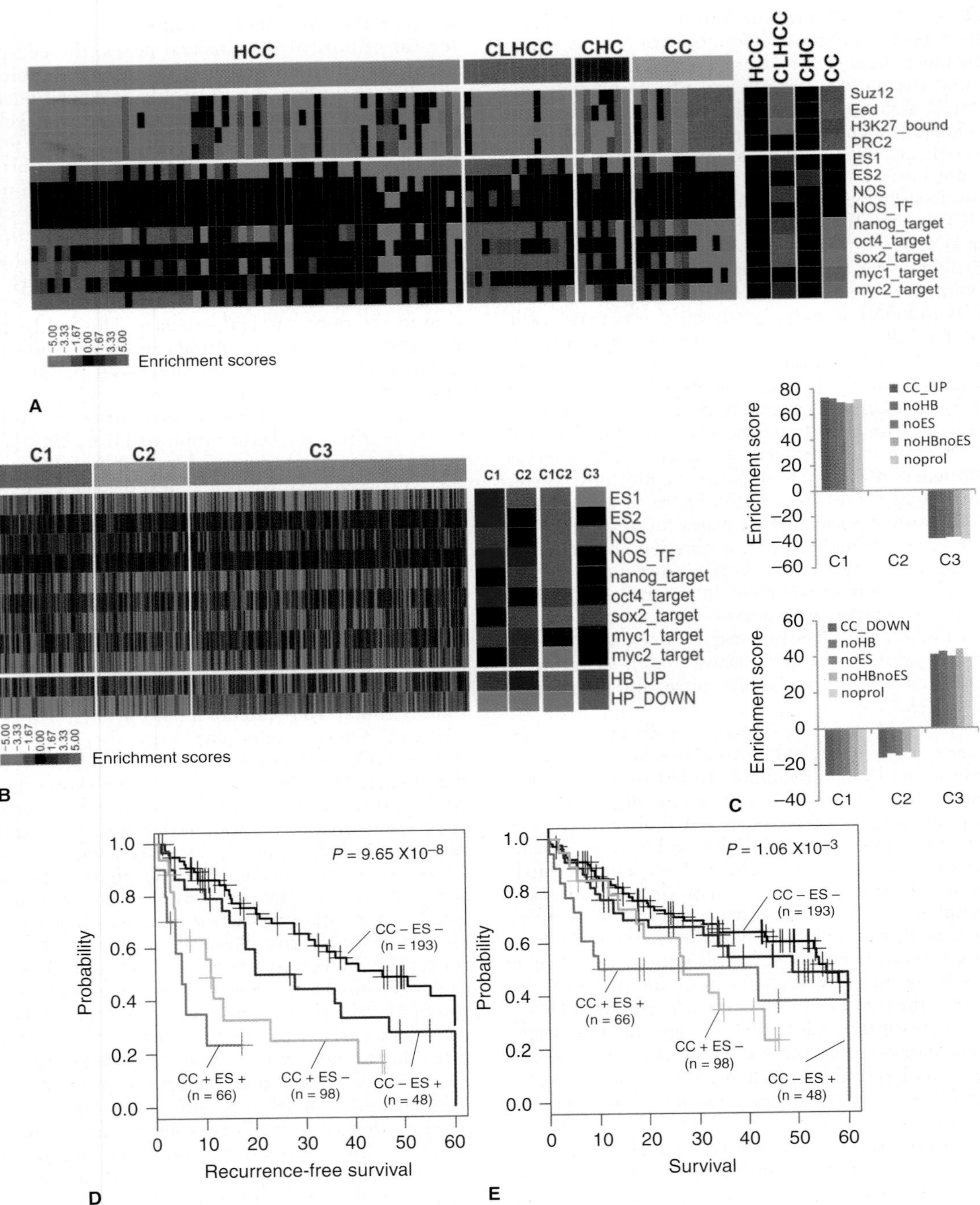

FIGURE 83.1 Comparison of the CC signature (cholangiocarcinoma-like traits) with ES signatures (embryonic stem cell-like expression traits). **A:** The enrichment of ES signatures and polycomb target gene sets in C1 and C2 classes in HCCcomp. The enrichment scores of ES signatures without proliferation signature (noprol; right bar). **B:** Bar plots for the enrichment scores of the CC_UP (**top**) and CC_DOWN (**bottom**) signatures and the CC_UP and CC_DOWN signatures subtracted by ES (noES), HB (noHB), or ES and HB (noESnoHB) signatures. **C:** The enrichment ES signatures in six independent data sets are shown. For each data set, the group enrichment in C1 and C2 tumors is indicated in the right bars ($P < .05$). **D:** Kaplan-Meier plots analyses for RFS (**left**) and OS (**right**) based on the expression status of CC and ES signatures in the integrated Laboratory of Experimental Carcinogenesis and Seoul National University data sets (n = 209). The CC+represents C1 tumors, and ES+ represents the tumors that express ES1 signature. RFS, recurrence-free survival; OS, overall survival. For details, see ref. 21. (From ref. 21, with permission.)

which expressed cholangiocarcinoma-like traits (CC signature). Similar to CC and CHC, CLHCC showed an aggressive phenotype with shorter recurrence-free and overall survival. In addition, CLHCC coexpressed embryonic stem cell-like expression traits (ES signature) suggesting its derivation from bipotent hepatic progenitor cells. By comparing the expression of CC signature with previous ES-like, hepatoblast-like, or proliferation-related traits, the authors demonstrated that the prognostic value of the CC signatures was independent of the expression of those signatures (Fig. 83.1). These data suggest that the acquisition of cholangiocarcinoma-like expression traits plays a critical role in the heterogeneous progression of HCC.

COMPARATIVE FUNCTIONAL GENOMICS

Despite the fact that transgenic and knockout mouse models have greatly enhanced the understanding of human cancers, in most cases we still rely on casual correlation between human and mouse models owing to lack of methods for direct comparisons.[22] Based on the neutral theory of molecular evolution, it is possible to identify both protein coding sequences and functional noncoding sequences in a genome.[22] Because regulatory elements of evolutionarily related species are conserved, it is likely that gene expression signatures reflecting similar phenotypes in different species could be also conserved. Based on this hypothesis, cross-comparison of global gene expression data from human HCC and mouse models of HCC has been undertaken to identify aberrant phenotypes that reflect evolutionarily conserved molecular pathways. Lee et al.[23] integrated gene expression data from human and transgenic mouse models of liver cancer. Hierarchical clustering analysis of integrated and standardized datasets revealed that HCC induced in mice by *Myc, E2f1,* and the combination of *Myc/E2f1* transgenes had the highest similarity with those of the better survival group of human HCC. However, the expression patterns in HCC induced by *Myc/Tgfa* transgenes or by the chemical carcinogen diethylnitrosamine were most similar to those of the poor survival group of human HCC. The results suggest that these mouse models might recapitulate the molecular patterns of the two subclasses of human HCC. In contrast, gene expression patterns of HCC from Acox1-/- and ciprofibrate-treated mice, in which development of HCC was driven by peroxisome proliferation in the liver, were least similar to those observed in either subclass of human HCC. These results suggest that the molecular pathways underlying hepatocarcinogenesis induced by peroxisome proliferation in mice are not frequent in humans.[23]

The similarity of gene expression profiles between human and mouse models is in good agreement with the phenotypic characteristics of the tumors,[23] that is, the human tumors with increased proliferation, decreased apoptosis, and worse prognosis pair with mouse models with the same features. The fact that these findings were first uncovered by unsupervised methods and later validated by supervised methods suggests that the underlying principles in gene expression changes are conserved between mouse and human HCC. These results strongly support the hypothesis that well-defined gene expression signatures from experimental conditions or animal models can be used to stratify human cancer patients into more homogeneous groups based on molecular similarity. The unique molecular identities of each subclass of HCC uncovered by comparative analysis of a genomewide survey of gene expression from human and animal models will facilitate the development of new therapeutic strategies.

Recent studies in different human tumors have provided further insights into how comparison of gene expression patterns from human and mouse tumors may permit the direct identification of common aberrant molecular pathways.[24,25] Comparison of gene expression profiles from a *Myc*-driven mouse prostate cancer model and human prostate cancer enabled Ellwood-Yen et al.[24] to identify a conserved expression module of human genes that corresponded to *Myc* signature genes defined in the mouse model. The *Myc* signature genes permitted the definition of a subset of *MYC*-like human cancers that are probably driven by *MYC* amplification or other mechanisms of *MYC* pathway activation. In a similar study, Sweet-Cordero et al.[25] detected a *KRAS2* gene expression signature by comparing a *KRAS2*-mediated mouse model of lung cancer with human lung cancer. It should be noted that when the investigators examined gene expression data from human lung adenocarcinomas alone, no statistically significant gene expression pattern correlated with *KRAS2* mutation status between wild type and mutated *KRAS2* tumors. The authors were able to identify a gene expression signature that reflected the *KRAS2* mutation in human adenocarcinomas only by comparing gene expression in tumors from humans and mice.

Functional genomics has the potential power to identify the cell of origin of cancer and the cellular pathway by which cancer subsequently evolves. This notion was recently tested in HCC.[26] Because HCC can originate from both adult hepatocytes and hepatic progenitor cells, our experimental strategy involved the integration of gene expression data generated from rat fetal hepatoblasts and adult hepatocytes with expression data from human HCC and mouse HCC models.[26] Patients with HCC that shared a gene expression pattern with fetal hepatoblasts had a poor prognosis. The gene expression program that distinguished this subtype from other types of HCC included markers of hepatic oval cells, suggesting that this HCC subtype may arise from hepatic progenitor cells. Furthermore, analyses of gene networks in these tumors showed that activation of AP-1 transcription factors in this newly identified HCC subtype might have a key role in tumor development.

CONCLUSION AND PERSPECTIVE

DNA microarray technology has provided an extraordinary opportunity for integrative analysis of the cancer transcriptome. Array-based gene expression profiling not only has advanced our understanding of cancer biology, but has begun to influence decisions in clinical oncology and ultimately may allow for the development of more effective therapies. The power of gene expression profiling of HCC can be further enhanced by cross-comparison analysis of multiple gene expression data sets from human HCC and the rich database of HCC in animal models.[22] The success of these new analytical approaches, comparative and/or integrative functional genomics, suggests that integration of independent data sets will enhance our ability to identify robust predictive markers. For example, a model to predict progression of mammary cancer has been recently developed based on a wound-healing gene expression signature.[27] Patients displaying the wound-healing signature had a significantly increased risk of metastasis compared with those without the signature, indicating that genomic data from normal physiological conditions may help to predict the prognosis of cancer patients. It is important to obtain additional tumor-independent signatures from multiple species that are unique for different physiological conditions, such as liver development, regeneration, hepatic stem cell activation, that can be integrated with gene expression patterns from human HCC. Although the clinical application of gene expression profiling to identify prognostic markers and therapeutic targets for HCC is still immature, the progress over the last few years suggest that prospective clinical studies are well justified and indeed needed.

It seems reasonable to predict that the genomic technologies will play an increasingly important role in clinical oncology. The immediate focus undoubtedly will be on using the current genomic technologies to improve the diagnosis and treatment of cancer. However, with the beginning of affordable whole genome sequencing and the current expansion of the cancer genome atlas,[28] one can certainly expect significant progress in the treatment of liver cancer.

References

1. Parkin DM, Bray F, Ferlay J, Pisani P. Global cancer statistics, 2002. *CA Cancer J Clin* 2005;55:74.
2. El Serag HB. Hepatocellular carcinoma: recent trends in the United States. *Gastroenterology* 2004,127: S27.
3. El-Serag HB, Hampel H, Javadi F. The association between diabetes and hepatocellular carcinoma: a systematic review of epidemiologic evidence. *Clin Gastroenterol Hepatol* 2006;4(3):369.
4. Libbrecht L, Desmet V, Roskams T. Preneoplastic lesions in human hepatocarcinogenesis. *Liver Int* 2005;25(1):16.
5. Thorgeirsson SS, Grisham JW. Molecular pathogenesis of human hepatocellular carcinoma. *Nat Genet* 2002;31:339.
6. Bruix J, Boix L, Sala M, Llovet JM. Focus on hepatocellular carcinoma. *Cancer Cell* 2004;5:215.
7. Quackenbush J. Microarray analysis and tumor classification. *N Engl J Med* 2006;354(23):2463.
8. Hood L, Heath JR, Phelps ME, Lin B. Systems biology and new technologies enable predictive and preventative medicine. *Science* 2004;306:640.
9. Pinkel D, Albertson DG. Array comparative genomic hybridization and its applications in cancer. *Nat Genet* 2005;37(Suppl):S11.
10. Moinzadeh P, Breuhahn K, Stutzer H, Schrmacher P. Chromosome alterations in human hepatocellular carcinomas correlate with aetiology and histological grade—results of an explorative CGH meta-analysis. *Br J Cancer* 2005;14:92:935.
11. Poon TCW, Wong N, Lai PBS, et al. A tumor progression model for hepatocellular carcinoma: bioinformatics analysis of genomic data. *Gastroenterology* 2006;131:1262.
12. Davies JJ, Wilson IM, Lam WL. Array CGH technologies and their applications to cancer genomes. *Chromosome Res* 2005;13: 237.
13. Woo HG, Park ES, Lee JS, et al. Identification of potential driver genes in human liver carcinoma by genomewide screening. *Cancer Res* 2009; 69(9): 4059
14. Kim CK, Lim JH, Lee WJ. Detection of hepatocellular carcinomas and dysplastic nodules in cirrhotic liver: accuracy of ultrasonography in transplant patients. *J Ultrasound Med* 2001;20:99.
15. Kojiro M, Roskams T. Early hepatocellular carcinoma and dysplastic nodules. *Semin Liver Dis* 2005;25:133.
16. Kaposi-Novak P, Libbrecht L, Woo HG, et al. Central role of c-Myc during malignant conversion in human hepatocarcinogenesis. *Cancer Res* 2009;69 (7):2775.
17. Thorgeirsson SS, Lee JS, Grisham JW. Molecular prognostication of liver cancer: end of the beginning. *J Hepatol* 2006;44(4):798.
18. Lee JS, Chu IS, Heo J, et al. Classification and prediction of survival in hepatocellular carcinoma by gene expression profiling. *Hepatology* 2004;40: 667.
19. Boyault S, Rickman DS, de Reynies A, et al. Transcriptome classification of HCC is related to gene alterations and to new therapeutic targets. *Hepatology* 2007;45(1):42.
20. Hoshida Y, Nijman SM, Kobayashi M, et al. Integrative transcriptome analysis reveals common molecular subclasses of human hepatocellular carcinoma. *Cancer Res* 2009;69(18):7385.
21. Woo HG, Lee JH, Yoon JH, et al. Identification of a cholangiocarcinoma-like gene expression trait in hepatocellular carcinoma. *Cancer Res* 2010; 70(8):3034.
22. Lee JS, Thorgeirsson SS. Comparative and integrative functional genomics of HCC. *Oncogene* 2006;25(27):3801.
23. Lee JS, Chu IS, Mikaelyan A, et al. Application of comparative functional genomics to identify best-fit mouse models to study human cancer. *Nat Genet* 2004;36(12):1306.
24. Ellwood-Yen K, Graeber TG, Wongvipat J, et al. Myc-driven murine prostate cancer shares molecular features with human prostate tumors. *Cancer Cell* 2003;4:223.
25. Sweet-Cordero A, Mukherjee S, Subramanian A, et al. An oncogenic KRAS2 expression signature identified by cross-species gene-expression analysis. *Nat Genet* 2005;37:48.
26. Lee JS, Heo J, Libbrecht L, et al. A novel prognostic subtype of human hepatocellular carcinoma derived from hepatic progenitor cells. *Nat Med* 2006;12(4):410.
27. Chang HY, Nuyten DS, Sneddon JB, et al. Robustness, scalability, and integration of a wound-response gene expression signature in predicting breast cancer survival. *Proc Natl Acad Sci U S A* 2005;102:3738.
28. International Cancer Genome Consortium. International network of cancer genome projects. *Nature* 2010;464(7291):993.

CHAPTER 84 CANCER OF THE LIVER

DAVID L. BARTLETT, ADRIAN M. DI BISCEGLIE, AND LAURA A. DAWSON

Primary tumors of the liver represent the sixth most common malignancy worldwide, and the third most common cause of death from cancer. The global incidence of the disease accounts for approximately 626,000 cases annually, with a male-to-female ratio of about 2.4:1. In the United States, approximately 19,160 new tumors of the liver and intrahepatic bile ducts are diagnosed each year, with 16,780 deaths estimated annually.[1] Primary liver cancers rank sixth among the most common cause of cancer deaths in males in the United States. In general these tumors have a poor prognosis, compounded by background liver disease in the majority of patients. Continued improvement in the management of liver cancers is expected. Better imaging studies have become available to screen for hepatic malignancies; liver transplantation has been increasingly applied with its role better defined; and newer therapies such as regional ^{90}Y-microspheres and systemic sorafenib have become available. It is likely that future advances in the control of these malignancies will be focused on prevention, immunization strategies for hepatitis B virus (HBV) and hepatitis C virus (HCV), as well as means to decrease cirrhosis of any origin. Earlier diagnosis by surveillance of patients at risk for hepatocellular carcinoma (HCC) development, improved regional therapy, and systemic targeted therapy will all lead to meaningful progress against this disease.

EPIDEMIOLOGY

The annual number of worldwide liver cancer cases (626,000) closely resembles the number of deaths (598,000). Long-term survival rates are 3% to 5% in most cancer registries. The variable geographic incidence of liver cancer (Fig. 84.1)[2] reflects the variable geographic incidence in HCV and HBV infections, which account for 75% of the world's cases. In Asia and Africa, high incidence rates have been associated both with high endemic HBV carrier rates as well as mycotoxin contamination of food, stored grains, drinking water, and soil. Ethnic factors also appear to be important because incidence rates can vary in the same population, according to ethnic origins. Ethnic Japanese in Japan have a higher incidence than those living in Hawaii, who in turn have a higher incidence than those living in California. Jews of European descent, when compared with Jews of African or Asian descent living in Israel, have a lower incidence. Differences have been found according to ethnic origin when examining an individual population. Los Angelinos of Japanese, Korean, and Chinese descent have a higher incidence of hepatoma than those of European or Hispanic descent.

HCC is 2.4 times more common in men than in women, and this difference is consistent globally. Higher levels of testosterone, lower levels of estrogens, and higher rates of liver disease are proposed explanations. In the United States, at all ages in both men and women, rates of HCC are two times higher in Asians than African Americans, which are two times higher than those in whites. There is a significant overall increase in the incidence of HCC in the United States during the past 25 years (Fig. 84.2).[3] This parallels the increase in HCV infection, the increase in immigrants from HBV endemic countries, and an increase in nonalcoholic fatty liver disease. The rate of increased incidence varies among different races in the United States (Table 84.1).[4] The widespread utilization of HBV vaccination is leading to a decrease in liver cancer in some areas. A dramatic demonstration of this is available from Taiwan, where HBV vaccine was introduced in 1984, and a reduction in the incidence of liver cancer was observed in children from 0.54 per 100,000 to 0.2 per 100,000 during a 16-year period.[5]

ETIOLOGIC FACTORS

Viral Hepatitis and Hepatocellular Carcinoma

Both case control studies and cohort studies have shown a strong association between chronic hepatitis B carriage rates and increased incidence of HCC. Beasley et al.[6] followed Taiwanese male postal carriers who were hepatitis B surface antigen (HBsAg)-positive and found an annual incidence of HCC of 495 per 100,000. This represented a 98-fold greater risk than observed in HBsAg-negative individuals. By evaluating apparently asymptomatic HBsAg-positive blood donors at American Red Cross centers, a minimum relative risk of 12.7 was noted for liver cancer compared with HBsAg-negative individuals. In men aged 30 to 35 years, three deaths due to HCC were noted, which relates to a 248-fold greater risk for such individuals compared with the general population. HBsAg-positive individuals who are at greatest risk are those who are male, who have a family history of the disease, whose age is more than 45 years, and who have cirrhosis. Multivariate analysis has been used to determine "risk scores" for the development of HCC.[7–9] Factors predictive of HCC include male gender, advanced age, specific promoter mutations, presence of cirrhosis, and higher viremia levels. If validated this may improve patient selection for surveillance.

The exact mechanism by which HBV infection causes HCC is not known.[10,11] Direct viral mechanisms may lead to HCC or, indirectly, the process of inflammation, regeneration, and fibrosis associated with chronic hepatitis and cirrhosis due to HBV infection may lead to HCC. HBV DNA may become integrated within the chromosomes of infected hepatocytes, and in some HCCs, this integration of viral genetic material may occur in a critical location within the cellular genome. For example, integration of HBV DNA has been observed within the retinoic acid receptor alpha gene and within the human cyclin A gene, both playing crucial roles in cellular growth. However, in most cases, the HBV DNA integration appears to be random. Furthermore, the HBV DNA integrant

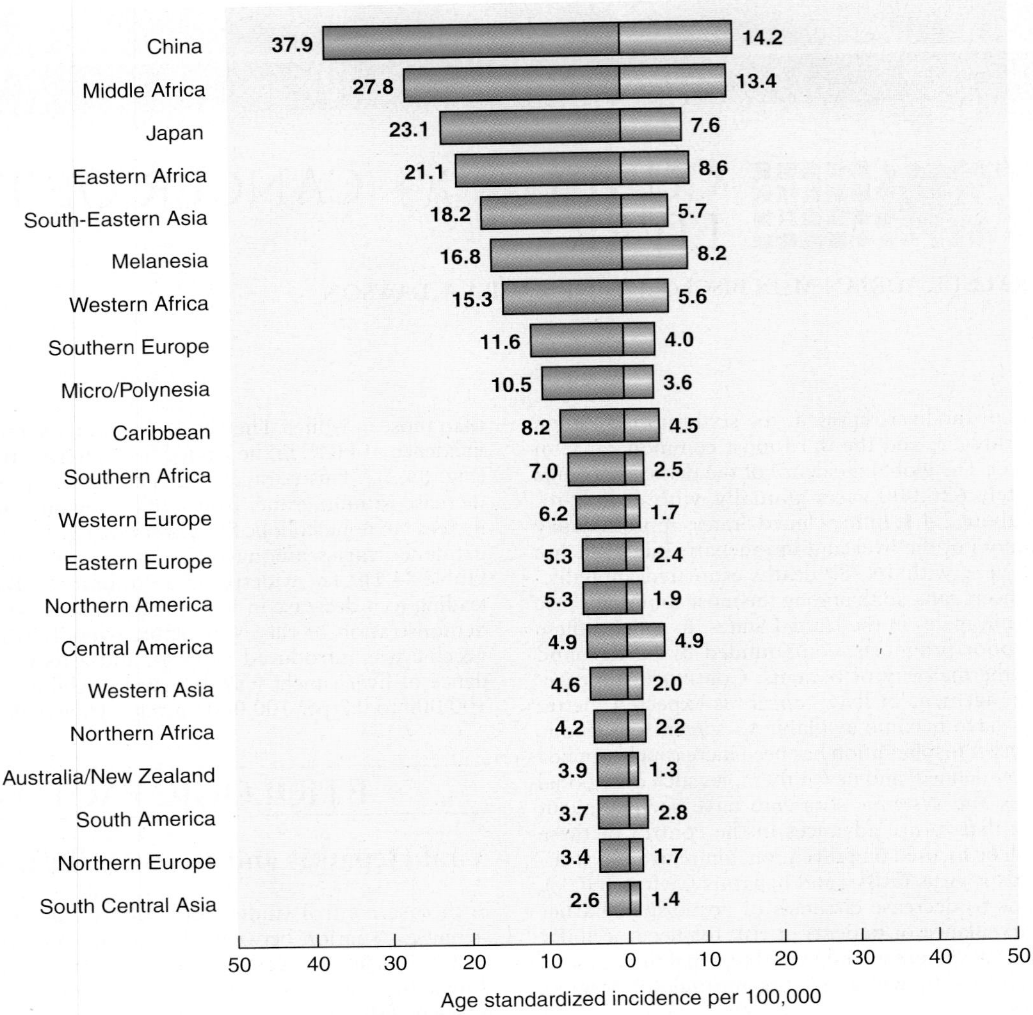

FIGURE 84.1 Age-standardized incidence rates for liver cancer. Data shown per 100,000. (From ref. 2, with permission.)

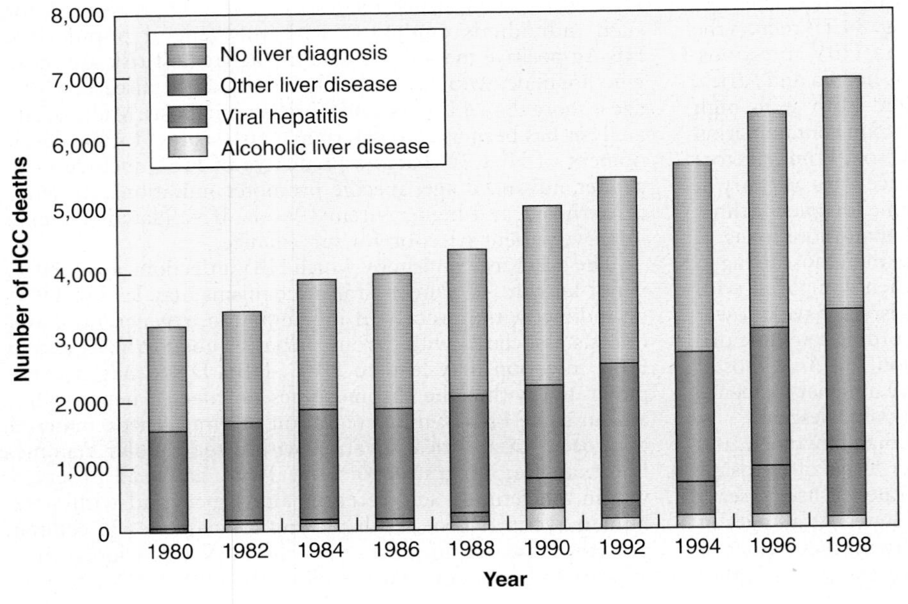

FIGURE 84.2 Number of hepatocellular carcinoma (HCC) deaths in the United States by identifiable coexistent liver disease by year, 1980 to 1998. (From ref. 3, with permission.)

TABLE 84.1

RANKING, INCIDENCE RATES, AND ANNUAL PERCENT CHANGES (A) AND RANKING, MORTALITY RATES, AND ANNUAL PERCENT CHANGES (B) OF HEPATOCELLULAR AND INTRAHEPATIC BILE DUCT CARCINOMAS IN THE UNITED STATES, 1992–2002

Group	Rank	Rate/100,000	Annual Percent Change
A			
All races			
Males	12	8.6	3.0
Females	18	3.3	3.0
Whites			
Males	15	6.8	2.9
Females	18	2.7	3.7
Blacks			
Males	14	10.8	4.5
Females	17	3.6	1.4
Asian/Pacific Islanders			
Males	5	20.9	1.0
Females	11	7.9	0.2
American Indian/Alaskan natives			
Males	8	9.0	—
Females	12	5.6	—
Hispanic/Latinos			
Males	8	13.4	2.2
Females	13	5.4	5.0
B			
Whites			
Males	12	5.9	2.1
Females	14	2.7	1.1
Blacks			
Males	8	9.2	1.3
Females	12	3.7	0.6
Asian/Pacific Islanders			
Males	3	15.9	−0.6
Females	6	6.5	−0.7
American Indian/Alaskan natives			
Males	4	7.6	1.6
Females	7	4.1	1.7
Hispanic/Latinos			
Males	4	10.3	1.6
Females	8	4.8	2.1

(From ref. 4, with permission.)

itself varies considerably and the integrated viral DNA may be rearranged, deleted, or present in repeats. This suggests that it is not the process of integration itself that leads to HCC.

The hepatitis B x gene (*HBx*) product has been implicated in causing HCC because it is a transcriptional activator of various cellular genes associated with growth control. S gene expression is also associated with activation of the Ras-Raf-MAP kinase pathway, an important cellular pathway that has been implicated in hepatocarcinogenesis. In addition, *HBx* has been found to interact with *p53*, interfering with its function as a tumor suppressor. Another viral gene product that has been implicated in causing HCC is the truncated surface gene product, although the mechanism by which this might result in HCC is not clear.

In keeping with the suggestion that HCC may be directly related to HBV infection is the observation from several studies that elevated serum levels of HBV DNA (a marker of higher levels of HBV replication) are associated with a higher risk of HCC.[12–15] Some genotypes of HBV appear to be associated with even higher rates of HCC than others. Thus, HBV genotype C is generally thought to increase the risk of HCC because these individuals are likely to remain seropositive for hepatitis B e antigen (HBeAg) and thus have higher serum levels of HBV DNA for a longer time. However, studies in some populations have found genotype B or even F to be more associated with HCC.[16,17]

Consistent with the hypothesis that HBV-related HCC may occur indirectly, via cirrhosis, is the observation that overall, approximately 70% of cases of HBV-related HCC occur in association with cirrhosis, although the rate of cirrhosis appears to be lower in younger patients with HCC. It is well known that cirrhosis of all causes, including hepatitis C and alcohol, may result in HCC.

In contrast to HBV, HCV is more likely to lead to chronic infection (10% vs. 60% to 80%), and cirrhosis (20-fold increase).[18] Also, in contrast to HBV, HCV is an RNA virus without a DNA intermediate form, and therefore cannot integrate into hepatocyte DNA. The mechanism for HCC induction is therefore more complicated. The precise timing of HCV infection from blood transfusions has allowed a comparison of latent periods for HCC development after HCV (transfusions) and after HBV (often at birth). The average age for HBV-associated HCC is around 52 years, compared with 62 years for HCV association. The typical interval between HCV-associated transfusion and subsequent HCC is only about 30 years (compared with 40 to 50 years for HBV). The state of the liver also differs in that HCV-associated HCC patients tend to have more frequent and more advanced cirrhosis. However, in HBV-associated HCC, only half the patients have cirrhosis; the remainder have chronic hepatitis with varying degrees of hepatic fibrosis. HCV is known to interact with the endoplasmic reticulum, causing stress and subsequent procarcinogenic effects. HCV core proteins have been shown to interact with the MAPK signaling pathway, directly modulating cell proliferation. The NS5A protein has been demonstrated to inactivate *p53* by sequestration, and the E1/E2 HCV proteins inhibit apoptosis through unknown mechanisms.[11] Chronic activation of the immune system in HCV infection may also play a significant role in tumor progression. Constant tissue destruction and regeneration lead to an accumulation of mutations leading to hepatocarcinogenesis.

A recent study of patients in the United States with advanced liver disease (cirrhosis or noncirrhotic fibrosis) due to hepatitis C found a 5-year incidence rate of HCC of about 5%. Although the rate of HCC was slightly higher among those with cirrhosis, patients with noncirrhotic livers had a significant rate of HCC. A multivariate model of risk factors was developed, indicating that older age, black race, lower platelet count, higher serum alkaline phosphatase, the presence of esophageal varices, and smoking were independent factors predictive of HCC.[19] There have been extensive efforts to establish the molecular pathways involved in the pathogenesis of HCC.[20,21] Some of the abnormalities that are commonly found in HCC include (1) cell-cycle dysregulation associated with somatic mutations or loss of heterozygosity in *TP53*, silencing of *CDKN2A* or *RB1*, or *CCND1* overexpression, (2) increased angiogenesis accompanied by overexpression or amplification of *VEGF, PDGF*, and *ANGPT2*, (3) evasion of apoptosis as a result of activation of survival signals such as NFκB, and (4) reactivation of *TERT*. In addition to these frequently occurring processes, there appears to be enormous molecular heterogeneity across HCC tumors. Some of this heterogeneity appears to be associated with race or etiology. Thus, cancer pathways seem to be different in white patients with HCV-related HCC compared with Asian patients with HBV-related HCC. Furthermore there is now good evidence that molecular signatures of HCC may identify tumors with good or poor prognoses. Finally, there is emerging evidence of the importance of microRNAs and epigenetic alterations such as hypermethylation in the pathogenesis of HCC.

Alcohol-Induced Hepatocarcinogenesis

There is a strong association between alcoholic cirrhosis and the development of HCC. Chronic alcohol consumption, by itself, has carcinogenic effects. Thus, chronic alcohol intake is known to lead to oxidative stress in the liver, inflammation, and cirrhosis. Ethanol is metabolized by alcohol dehydrogenases and cytochrome P-450, producing acetaldehyde and reactive oxygen species. Acetaldehyde binds directly to proteins and DNA. It damages mitochondria, initiating apoptosis. P-450 metabolism leads to reactive oxygen species, which lead to lipid consumption peroxidation, protein oxidation, and DNA adducts.[22] Alcohol leads to monocyte activation and inflammatory cytokine production. This leads to activation of Kupffer cells, which release chemokines and cytokines, leading to hepatocyte necrosis. Oxidative stress has been demonstrated in alcoholic cirrhosis through increased isoprostane, a marker of lipid peroxidation.[23] Oxidative stress promotes the development of fibrosis and cirrhosis, creating a permissive HCC microenvironment. Oxidative stress may also lead to decreased STAT1-directed activation of IFNγ signaling with consequent hepatocyte damage.[24] However, it may simply be the effects of cirrhosis itself that lead to the development of HCC.

Other Etiologic Considerations

The 60% to 80% association of HCC with underlying cirrhosis has long been recognized, more typically with macronodular cirrhosis in Southeast Asia, but also with micronodular cirrhosis in Europe and the United States. Approximately 20% of U. S. patients with HCC do not have underlying cirrhosis, and probably not more than 70% have associated viral hepatitis. In addition to alcoholic cirrhosis and viral hepatitis, several underlying conditions have been found to be associated with an increased risk for the development of HCC (Table 84.2). These include autoimmune chronic active hepatitis, cryptogenic cirrhosis, metabolic diseases, and nonalcoholic fatty liver disease (NAFLD). NAFLD is the hepatic manifestation of

TABLE 84.2

CONDITIONS ASSOCIATED WITH HUMAN HEPATOCELLULAR CARCINOMA

Condition	Risk
Cirrhosis	
Hepatitis B virus	High
Hepatitis C virus	High
Alcohol	High
Autoimmune chronic active hepatitis	High
Cryptogenic cirrhosis	High
Cirrhosis due to nonalcoholic fatty liver disease	High
Primary biliary cirrhosis	Low
Hereditary hemochromatosis	High
α_1-Antitrypsin deficiency	High
Wilson disease	Low
Metabolic diseases (without cirrhosis)	
Hereditary tyrosinemia	High
α_1-Antitrypsin deficiency	Moderate
Ataxia telangiectasia	Moderate
Types 1 and 3 glycogen storage disease	Moderate
Galactosemia	Moderate
Citrullinemia	Moderate
Hereditary hemorrhagic telangiectasia	Moderate
Porphyria cutanea tarda	Moderate
Orotic aciduria	Moderate
Alagille syndrome (congenital cholestatic syndrome)	Moderate
Environmental	
Thorotrast	Moderate
Androgenic steroids	Moderate
Cigarette smoking	Low to moderate
Aflatoxin	Moderate

the metabolic syndrome: obesity, insulin resistance, hypertriglyceridemia, and low high-density lipoprotein. It is the most common liver disorder in the Western world.[25] Increased free fatty acids in the liver leads to NFκB activation and inflammation. NAFLD can progress to cirrhosis and HCC. Diabetes itself is associated with an increased risk of HCC. It is not clear whether this is related to insulin resistance, or perhaps the effects of diabetes-associated NAFLD, as previously described, or some other, as yet unknown, mechanism.

Several other metabolic diseases are also associated with an increased risk for the development of HCC. These include hemochromatosis (iron accumulation), Wilson disease (copper accumulation), α_1-antitrypsin deficiency, tyrosinemia, porphyria cutanea tarda, glycogenesis types 1 and 3, citrullinemia, and orotic acid urea. In children, congenital cholestatic syndrome (Alagille syndrome) is associated with a familial type of HCC.

Chemical Carcinogens

Probably the best-studied and most potent ubiquitous natural chemical carcinogen is a product of the *Aspergillus* fungus, called aflatoxin B_1. *Aspergillus flavus* mold and aflatoxin product can be found in a variety of stored grains, particularly in hot, humid parts of the world, where grains such as rice are stored in unrefrigerated conditions. In the months following the monsoon in Southeast Asia, most village-based grains can be seen to be covered by a white layer that can easily be scraped off with the nails. This is highly enriched in aflatoxin and is consumed with the grain by most of the villagers over the following months. Data on aflatoxin contamination of foodstuffs correlate well with incidence rates of HCC in Africa and to some extent in China. In hyperendemic areas of China, even farm animals such as ducks have HCC.

Although some human medical compounds are hepatocarcinogens for rodents, there is little evidence that they play an important role in human hepatocarcinogenesis apart from sex hormones. There is considerable literature on the hepatocarcinogenicity of anabolic steroids as well as the induction of benign adenomas by estrogens.[26] Although estrogens are capable of causing HCC in rodents, an epidemiologic association in humans has never been clearly shown. In an industrial society, a large number of environmental pollutants, particularly pesticides and insecticides, are known rodent hepatic carcinogens.

PATHOLOGY

Primary tumors of the liver can be classified as either benign or malignant (Table 84.3) and by the tissue of origin, whether that represents mesenchymal tumors or the more common epithelial neoplasms. Malignant epithelial neoplasms constitute 85% to 95% of all tumors of the liver. Six percent to 12% are benign, and are largely of epithelial origin. Approximately 1% to 3% of liver tumors are malignant mesenchymal tumors.[27] Rare inflammatory pseudomasses and pseudotumors associated with either infarction or inflammation can be recognized and need to be distinguished from true tumors arising in the liver. Hepatic cysts and focal nodular hyperplasia are nonneoplastic processes that can mimic tumors.

The lymphatics of the liver course between lobules and drain primarily through vessels surrounding the portal veins directly into the liver hilum. About 20% of the liver is drained by vessels ascending along the vena cava and into the pericardial fat pad. HCC spreads most commonly to lymph nodes around the liver, then to the peritoneal cavity and lung. A characteristic feature of HCC is invasion of the portal vein, and to a lesser extent, the hepatic vein. After positive margins and lymph nodes, it is the most important negative prognostic factor for resection and for liver transplantation.

Many tumors have a propensity to metastasize to the liver or to the adjacent biliary tree. Metastases appear to obtain access to the liver by hematogenous spread through the portal vein.[28] Grossly, tumors metastatic to the liver are often peripheral and multiple and cause umbilication of the surface of the liver, whereas primary liver tumors are more often central and can be solitary and exophytic. By absolute number, the most frequent tumors of nonhepatic origin in the liver include lung cancer, colon cancer, pancreatic cancer, breast cancer, and gastric carcinoma, in decreasing order of frequency.[27] Melanoma and gallbladder cancer can also metastasize to the liver. Although rare, ocular melanoma has a unique propensity to metastasize hematogenously to the liver as an isolated site of metastases.

Pathologic classification involves a spectrum including dysplastic nodules, "very early HCC" and "small/progressed HCC," each with varying malignant potential and prognosis.[29] Specialized immunohistochemical staining can be used to distinguish primary tumors of the liver from metastatic deposits. Specifically, positive staining for α-fetoprotein (AFP), polyclonal

TABLE 84.3

HEPATIC NEOPLASMS

Benign tumors
Hepatocellular hyperplasia: macroregenerative nodule, nodular hyperplasia, mixed hamartoma
Hepatocellular adenoma: typical; associated with anabolic steroids
Hepatic cysts: simple, polycystic
Bile duct adenoma
Benign mesenchymal tumors and tumorlike conditions: mesenchymal hamartoma, hemangioma, infantile hemangioendothelioma, lymphangiomatosis, lipoma, leiomyoma, fibroma, inflammatory pseudotumor, myxoma
Tumor of heterotopic tissue and uncertain origin: adrenal rest tumors, pheochromocytoma, pancreatic rests, carcinoid, neuroendocrine infantile sinusoidal tumor, teratoma, yolk sac tumor, malignant trophoblastic tumor, hepatic malignant mixed tumor
Primary malignant epithelial tumors
Hepatocellular carcinoma variants: childhood, fibrolamellar, combined, spindle cell, clear cell, giant cell, carcinosarcoma, sclerosing hepatocellular carcinoma
Hepatoblastoma
Cholangiocarcinoma and cholangiocellular carcinoma
Biliary cystadenocarcinoma, squamous cell carcinoma
Primary malignant mesenchymal tumors

but not monoclonal carcinoembryonic antigen, and loss of reticulin staining are very useful. More specialized pathologic staining techniques, including flow-cytometric DNA analysis, are also useful in the evaluation of HCC.[30–33] Seventy-eight percent of HCCs are aneuploid and 22% are diploid. Elevated AFP has been shown to be significantly associated with aneuploid tumors, but appeared to provide no information regarding survival. This is different from what is observed with other gastrointestinal tumors, including gastric and esophageal cancers, for which clinical outcome is more clearly related to this DNA pattern. The rapidity of proliferation of cells within the HCC can be detected by the cell-cycle stains PCNA and Ki-67, which can be used to obtain additional prognostic information. Those individuals with low DNA synthetic capacity had greater 2-year survival after surgery and lesser incidence of intrahepatic metastases than those with high DNA synthetic capacity. This is similar to findings that have been observed in patients with breast cancer.

STAGING

Multiple clinical staging systems for hepatic tumors have been described. The most widely used is the American Joint Committee on Cancer/tumor-node-metastasis (AJCC/TNM) (Table 84.4).[34] However, the new Cancer of the Liver Italian Program (CLIP) system[35] and other systems[36,37] have been developed that take into account both tumor morphology and underlying hepatic disease and dysfunction. Comparison between these systems with external validation suggests that the Barcelona Clinic Liver Cancer staging system (BCLC) has the best prognostic value, and it has become widely used and serves both as a staging and treatment algorithm (Fig. 84.3).[38–40]

The best prognosis is clearly stage I, solitary tumors of less than 2 cm diameter without vascular invasion. Adverse prognostic features include multiple tumors, vascular invasion, and lymph node spread. Vascular invasion in particular has profound effects on prognosis. Vascular invasion may be macroscopic or microscopic. In general, large tumors often have microscopic invasion, which cannot be appreciated until after resection. As a consequence, full staging can usually be made only after surgical extirpation of the tumor. Stage III disease contains a mixture of lymph node-positive and -negative tumors. Stage III patients with positive lymph node disease have a poor prognosis, and few patients survive 1 year. The prognosis of stage IV is poor after either resection or transplantation, and there are few 1-year survivors. The prognosis in patients with HCC is very much influenced by the presence and severity of underlying liver disease. Thus in the presence of decompensated cirrhosis (Child Pugh class B or C), death may be more likely due to liver failure than it is due to cancer. The current TNM/AJCC/UICC (International Union Against Cancer) staging system still has some limitations and has been recently revised. This system should be used in research articles in order to compare treatment results between institutions.

Although staging is a valuable tool, the combination of molecular and clinical features of a tumor may prove more valuable. Marsh et al.[41] described 103 cases in which microdissection genotyping techniques were used to establish the "degree" of malignancy for each nodule by assessing the accumulated mutational load through loss of heterozygosity at ten different loci and by the calculation of the fractional allelic loss rate. By comparing the genotyping of multiple lesions in the liver, one can define whether these are multiple primary tumors or intrahepatic metastases, which have a much worse prognosis.[42]

A similar approach used microarray analysis for gene expression profiling of HCC. Certain expression signatures clearly distinguished tumors with poor prognosis from those with better outcomes.[43] These approaches need to be further validated in prospective studies, but provide the potential for better measurements of outcome using molecular characteristics.

TABLE 84.4

AMERICAN JOINT COMMISSION ON CANCER STAGING

PRIMARY TUMOR (T)	
TX	Primary tumor cannot be assessed
T0	No evidence of primary tumor
T1	Solitary tumor without vascular invasion
T2	Solitary tumor with vascular invasion, or Multiple tumors no more than 5 cm
T3a	Multiple tumors more than 5 cm
T3b	Tumor involving a major branch of the portal or hepatic vein(s)
T4	Tumor(s) with direct invasion of adjacent organs other than the gallbladder or with perforation of visceral peritoneum
REGIONAL LYMPH NODE (N)	
NX	Regional lymph nodes cannot be assessed
N0	No regional lymph node metastasis
N1	Regional lymph node metastasis
DISTANT METASTASIS (M)	
MX	Distant metastasis cannot be assessed
M0	No distant metastasis
M1	Distant metastasis

STAGE GROUPING			
I	T1	N0	M0
II	T2	N0	M0
IIIA	T3a	N0	M0
IIIB	T3b	N0	M0
IIIC	T4	N0	M0
IVA	Any T	N1	M0
IVB	Any T	Any N	M1

(From ref. 34, with permission.)

CLINICAL FEATURES

Common symptoms in patients affected with HCC include abdominal pain, weight loss, weakness, fullness and anorexia, abdominal swelling, jaundice, and vomiting. Common physical signs include hepatomegaly, hepatic bruit, ascites, splenomegaly, jaundice, wasting, and fever. There are some differences observed in presenting signs and symptoms between high- and low-incidence areas. The most common symptom is abdominal pain, particularly in high-risk areas. An abdominal mass or swelling may also be noticed by patients. Abdominal swelling may occur as a consequence of ascites because of the underlying chronic liver disease or may be due to a rapidly expanding tumor. Occasionally, central necrosis or acute hemorrhage into the peritoneal cavity leads to death. Hemoperitoneum from bleeding HCC is also a potential complication of needle biopsy of highly vascular hepatomas. Weakness, malaise, anorexia, and weight loss are common reported symptoms that should trigger the consideration of a diagnosis of HCC in a known cirrhotic patient. Jaundice is infrequent, and when present is usually the result of underlying liver disease. However, that can be attributed to the HCC in only 10% of patients presenting with jaundice. This may be because of obstruction of the main intrahepatic ducts, obstruction of the common hepatic duct at the porta hepatis, infiltration into the biliary radicals, or extremely rarely, blood in the biliary tree. Hematemesis may occur from esophageal varices from the underlying chronic

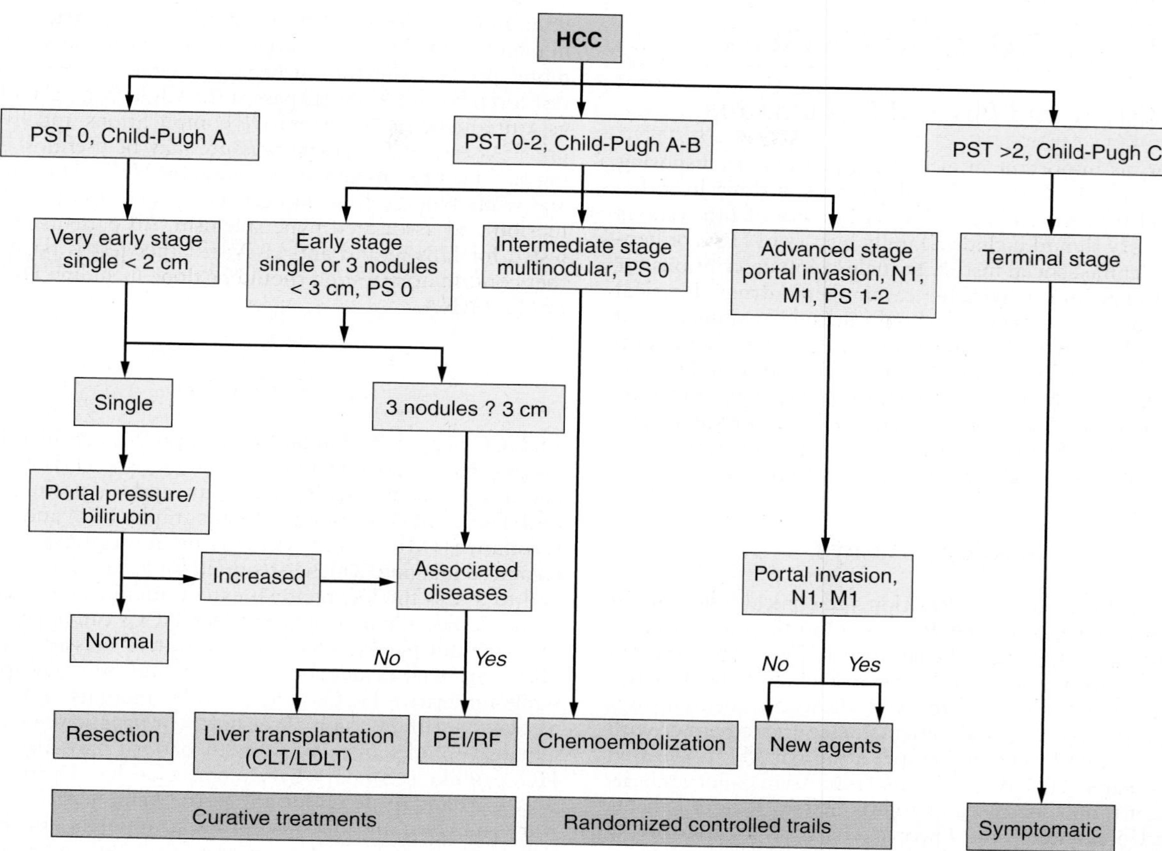

FIGURE 84.3 Strategy for staging and treatment assignment for patients with hepatocellular carcinoma (HCC) according to the Barcelona Clinic Liver Cancer (BCLC) staging system. PST, performance status; CLT, cadaveric liver transplantation; LDLT, living donor liver transplantation; PEI, percutaneous ethanol injection; RF, radiofrequency ablation.

liver disease with portal hypertension. Bone pain is seen in 3% to 12% of patients, but necropsies show pathologic bone metastases in approximately 20% of patients. Respiratory symptoms may occur on presentation, but are rare. They are usually due to elevated hemidiaphragm consequent to hepatomegaly or pain from rib metastases. Pleural effusions may occur, but symptomatic lung metastases are rare. In countries where there is an active surveillance program, such as Japan, HCC tends to be identified at an earlier stage, when symptoms may be few or attributable only to the underlying disease.

Physical Signs

Hepatomegaly is the most frequent physical sign, occurring in 50% to 90% of the patients. The size of the liver may be massive, particularly in endemic areas. Abdominal bruits arising from the HCC, presumably from the associated vascularity, have a variable incidence, ranging from 6% to 25%. Ascites occurs in 30% to 60% of patients. It is usually due to the underlying liver disease, although occasionally it may be caused by hemoperitoneum. Splenomegaly occurs commonly, mainly due to the associated portal hypertension from the underlying liver disease. Acute splenomegaly may be due to portal vein occlusion by the tumor. Weight loss and muscle wasting are common, particularly with rapidly growing or large tumors. Fever is found in 10% to 50% of patients with HCC. The cause is not clear, although tumor necrosis has been invoked as an explanation. The signs of chronic liver disease may often be present, including jaundice, dilated abdominal veins, palmar erythema, gynecomastia, testicular atrophy, and peripheral edema. The Budd-Chiari syndrome has been reported in several series because of HCC invasion of the hepatic veins. This causes tense ascites and a large tender liver. Virchow-Troisier nodes may occur in the supraclavicular region. Cutaneous metastases have also been reported as red-blue nodules.

Paraneoplastic Syndromes

A variety of paraneoplastic syndromes have been described. Most of these are biochemical abnormalities without associated clinical consequences. The most important ones include hypoglycemia (also caused by end-stage liver failure), erythrocytosis, hypercalcemia, hypercholesterolemia, dysfibrinogenemia, carcinoid syndrome, increased thyroxin-binding globulin, sexual changes (gynecomastia, testicular atrophy, and precocious puberty), and porphyria cutanea tarda. Hypoglycemia occurs in two settings. Relatively mild hypoglycemia occurs in rapidly growing HCC among the Chinese as part of a terminal illness. In the other setting, the HCC is more slowly growing, but the hypoglycemia may be profound. Its pathogenesis is unclear but may be related to production by the tumor of insulinlike growth factor-1. Erythrocytosis occurs in 3% to 12% of patients. Hypercholesterolemia may occur in 10% to 40% of patients. This has been shown to be due to an absence of normal feedback control in malignant hepatocytes and results from a deletion in β-hydroxy-methylglutaryl coenzyme A reductase.

CLINICAL EVALUATION

History and Physical Examination

The history is important in evaluating putative predisposing factors, including a history of viral hepatitis or other liver disease, blood transfusion, alcohol abuse, or use of intravenous drugs. History should include a family history of HCC or hepatitis and detailed social history to include job descriptions for industrial exposure to possible carcinogenic drugs. Physical examination is important and should include examination of underlying liver disease such as jaundice, ascites, peripheral edema, spider nevi, palmar erythema, and weight loss. Evaluation of the abdomen for hepatic size, presence of masses, hepatic nodularity, and tenderness, as well as presence of splenomegaly should be performed. Assessment of overall performance status is essential for management decisions.

Serologic Assays

The first serologic assay for detection and clinical follow-up of patients with HCC was AFP. It is found in the serum of animals bearing transplantable hepatomas and was later detected in humans. Improvements in this assay, including the development of radioimmunoassays for AFP, allowed sequential studies in high-risk patients and patients being treated either with surgical resection or chemotherapy. Although AFP is elevated in approximately 70% of individuals from Asian countries bearing HCC, it is only increased in approximately 50% of patients from the United States and Europe. AFP-L3 is an abnormally glycosylated fraction of AFP that is lectin-bound and appears to be more specific for HCC.[44] The other most widely used assay is that for des-γ-carboxy prothrombin protein induced by vitamin K abnormality (PIVKA-2). This protein is increased in as many as 80% of patients with HCC, but may also be elevated in patients with vitamin K deficiency.[45] It may even have prognostic value.[46] The elevations of both AFP and PIVKA-2 observed in chronic hepatitis and cirrhosis in the absence of HCC sometimes make it difficult to interpret these assays. Although many other assays have been developed, none have greater aggregate sensitivity and specificity.[47–51]

Assessment of liver function is an important component of evaluation of the patient with HCC or suspected HCC, for treatment decision making and for assessment of prognosis. The Child-Pugh classification of liver function, based on measurements of serum albumin, bilirubin, and prothrombin time, as well as presence or absence of ascites and encephalopathy, remains the most useful strategy for assessing liver function (Table 84.5). Other tests such as isocyanine green retention and 99m-Tc GSA (diethylenetriamine-penta-acetic acid-galactosyl human serum albumin) scintigraphy have been investigated as more specific indicators of hepatic reserve in preparation for resection, but have not surpassed the Child-Pugh classification as a predictor of postoperative complications and liver failure.[52] Assessment of portal pressure may be useful in evaluating patients prior to hepatic resection for HCC.[53] Platelet count and white blood cell count decreases may reflect portal hypertension and associated hypersplenism. All patients should be tested for HBsAg and anti-HCV; if either test is positive, further confirmatory testing should be done including HBV DNA or HCV RNA.

TABLE 84.5

CHILD-PUGH CLASSIFICATION OF CIRRHOSIS[a]

Measurement	1 Point	2 Points	3 Points
Bilirubin (mg/dL)	1–1.9	2–2.9	>2.9
Prolongation of PT	1–3	4–6	>6
Albumin (g/dL)	>3.5	2.8–3.4	<2.8
Ascites	None	Mild	Moderate/ severe
Encephalopathy	None	Grade 1 or 2	Grade 3 or 4

PT, prothrombin time.
[a]Grade A = 5–6 points; grade B = 7–9 points; grade C = 10–15 points.

Radiology

All HCC imaging techniques have improved considerably over the past few decades. High-resolution ultrasound (US) scans can detect liver lesions smaller than 1 cm, and is a useful screening tool. Fast multislice computed tomography (CT) and magnetic resonance (MR) scanners provide multiphasic contrast-enhanced imaging, which is required for lesion characterization and to assess the locoregional extent, number, and size of the lesions, especially in a cirrhotic liver. HCCs can appear as solitary or multiple expansive or infiltrative masses. Expansive HCCs are well demarcated, nodular, and often encapsulated, while infiltrative HCCs have irregular margins and are often associated with invasion of the portal or hepatic veins. A mixed expansive and infiltrative growth pattern may also be seen. HCC, unlike secondary liver metastases, has a propensity to invade to and grow within the portal vein, hepatic vein, inferior vena cava, and bile duct. To appropriately document the existence of HCC, a four-phase CT or MR imaging (MRI) study is required: unenhanced, arterial, venous, and delayed phases. A characteristic feature of HCC is rapid enhancement during the arterial phase of contrast administration and "washout" during the later portal venous and delayed phases. The presence of arterial hypervascularity alone is insufficient for diagnosis of HCC, while the presence of venous washout is essential.[54] Together, these findings are highly specific for HCC.[55] Hepatic tumors are usually hypervascular, show tortuosity of the vessels, vascular pooling, and often demonstrate rapid entry of contrast into the associated hepatic veins. Arterial portal shunting in the presence of portal hypertension can also be observed. These shunts can be mistaken for HCC in a cirrhotic liver. Typical imaging findings of the nontumorous shunts include small, peripherally located, wedge-shaped enhancing lesions seen on arterial phase CT[56] or MR scans[57]; however, the shunts do not show negative enhancement compared with the adjacent liver parenchyma during the portal and delayed phases.

The primary questions that need to be addressed with HCC imaging studies are the location and number of lesions in the liver, whether they have typical features of HCC, whether there is evidence of extrahepatic tumor spread, and whether the vessels are patent or not. Because performance of imaging studies is critical to the diagnosis of HCC, it is recommended that all imaging studies be performed in expert centers.

Ultrasound

Ultrasonography screening in prospective studies has been shown to be more sensitive than repetitive AFP testing, especially for small tumors in high-risk patients. Using transducers of 3.5 or 5.0 MHz, both diagnosis and biopsy of suspicious lesions can be performed. US is widely used in the diagnosis of HCC, particularly in surveillance programs for patients with chronic liver disease who are at risk for the development of HCC. The instrumentation is inexpensive and widely available.

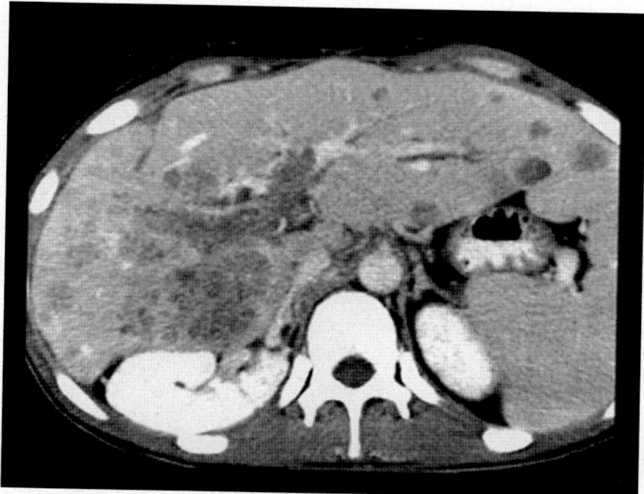

FIGURE 84.4 Portal venous phase of triphasic computed tomography scan demonstrating advance hepatocellular cancer involving the main portal vein.

HCCs have variable echogenicity on gray-scale US. Expansive HCCs are usually seen as discrete nodules with a heterogeneous echo, and a hypoechoic rim may be present, corresponding to a fibrous capsule. Infiltrative HCCs also demonstrate heterogeneous echogenicity and can be missed on US scans. Arterial hypervascularity of HCCs can be better evaluated using power Doppler US with a microbubble contrast agent. Microbubble-based contrast agents are available for clinical use in Europe, Asia, and Canada, but not in the United States. HCCs typically show strong, heterogeneous enhancement with irregular intratumoral vessels on arterial phase scans. Portal and delayed scans demonstrate negative enhancement, corresponding to "washout," and can diagnose portal venous thrombosis.

Computed Tomography Scans

The multislice, multiphasic (unenhanced, arterial, portal, and delayed phase) CT scan (Fig. 84.4) is the most commonly used standard imaging technique for determining the extent of HCC.[58,59] Like US, it can miss lesions smaller than 1 cm, especially in the presence of cirrhosis. The arterial phase scan demonstrates enhancement of hypervascular HCCs, and can also show hemodynamic changes associated with HCC or liver cirrhosis, such as arterioportal shunting. The portal phase scan is important for evaluation of venous invasion and distant metastases. The attenuation of HCCs on portal phase scans varies. A delayed-phase scan (at least 3 minutes after injection of contrast material) demonstrates negative enhancement of HCC (washout), compared with the adjacent liver parenchyma.

CT during arterial portography, in which contrast material is directly infused into the mesenteric vessels, and CT during hepatic arteriography have been shown to be superior to conventional dynamic CT in detecting very small lesions.[60] However, direct comparisons of individual imaging modalities are limited by the lack of a gold standard to define the number and size of lesions identified and the rapidly evolving standard imaging techniques. Drawbacks of CT portography include the detection of small abnormalities that represent flow voids or benign lesions (pseudolesions) and false-negative findings, especially in instances in which there is fatty infiltration of the liver. These invasive CT procedures are infrequently performed because of their invasiveness.

Magnetic Resonance Scan

MRI is particularly good at detecting intrahepatic lesions, especially T2-weighted spin-echo sequences that are the most efficient for tumor detection.[61,62] A nodule in a cirrhotic liver on T2-weighted images is highly suggestive of HCC; however, many well-differentiated HCCs may be seen as an isointensity or hypointensity. Some difficulty in distinguishing hemangiomas that have a very high T2 signal can be obviated because a less intense signal is observed with HCC.[63] The signal intensity of HCC on T1-weighted MR scan varies with tumor grade. Larger HCCs tend to show more hypointensity than hyperintensity on T1-weighted imaging. Most borderline malignant lesions and the majority of well-differentiated HCCs show hyperintensity, partly due to fatty metamorphosis in HCCs. The fibrous capsule is seen as a hypointense rim on both T1- and T2-weighted images. Improvements of fast MRI techniques allow imaging of the entire liver in multiple phases of contrast enhancement. Multiphasic (unenhanced, arterial, portal, and delayed phases) gadolinium-enhanced T1-weighted imaging shows findings similar to those of multiphasic contrast-enhanced CT and is important for detection and characterization of HCC, especially in a cirrhotic liver. Delayed-phase MRI can help distinguish between intrahepatic cholangiocarcinoma and HCC, as intrahepatic cholangiocarcinoma does not show washout in the venous delayed phases.[64] MRI with superparamagnetic iron oxide has been used to detect additional liver masses and can show higher diagnostic accuracy than multiphasic CT scan.[65–67] The use of MRI angiography has also been reported in HCC (Fig. 84.5).

Positron Emission Tomography

The role of [^{18}F]fluorodeoxyglucose (FDG) positron emission tomography (PET) scans in the evaluation of HCC has been studied. In one retrospective study, FDG-PET imaging was successful in detecting only 64% of lesions. Nevertheless, it had a clinically significant impact in 28% of patients above and beyond standard imaging, including the detection of unsuspected metastatic disease.[68] A prospective comparison of triphasic CT, gadolinium-enhanced MRI, US, and FDG-PET was reported and verified by explanted liver specimens after transplant. This study revealed similar results for CT, MRI, and US, while none of the lesions were detected by PET imaging.[69] At present, PET scans are not routinely used for staging or treatment decision making in HCC.

Obtaining a Diagnosis

The tests used to diagnose HCC include radiologic studies, as outlined earlier, and pathologic diagnosis with biopsy. Obtaining a pathologic diagnosis has substantial hazards in patients with HCC. Not only are bleeding studies often abnormal because of thrombocytopenia and a decrease in liver-dependent clotting factors, but these tumors tend to be hypervascular. Spillage of tumor has also been suggested as a problem following percutaneous biopsy, but is relatively rare. Fine-needle aspirates can provide sufficient material for diagnosis of cancer, but the hallmark feature of HCC, stromal invasion, may not be detected.[70] Core biopsies are most preferred because of the tissue architecture given by this technique. Laparoscopic approaches can also be used. For patients suspected of having portal vein involvement, a core biopsy of the portal vein may be performed.[70] In addition to morphologic features such as stromal invasion that help distinguish high-grade dysplastic nodules from HCC, several histologic staining characteristics may be helpful, including glypican 3[71] heat shock protein (HSP) 70[72] and glutamine synthetase.[72] Staining for vascular endothelium with CD34 is usually strongly positive in HCC, and cytokeratin stains for biliary epithelium (CK7 and CK19) should be negative.[73] It is recommended that the full panel of stains mentioned here be used to help distinguish high-grade dysplastic nodules from HCC.[74]

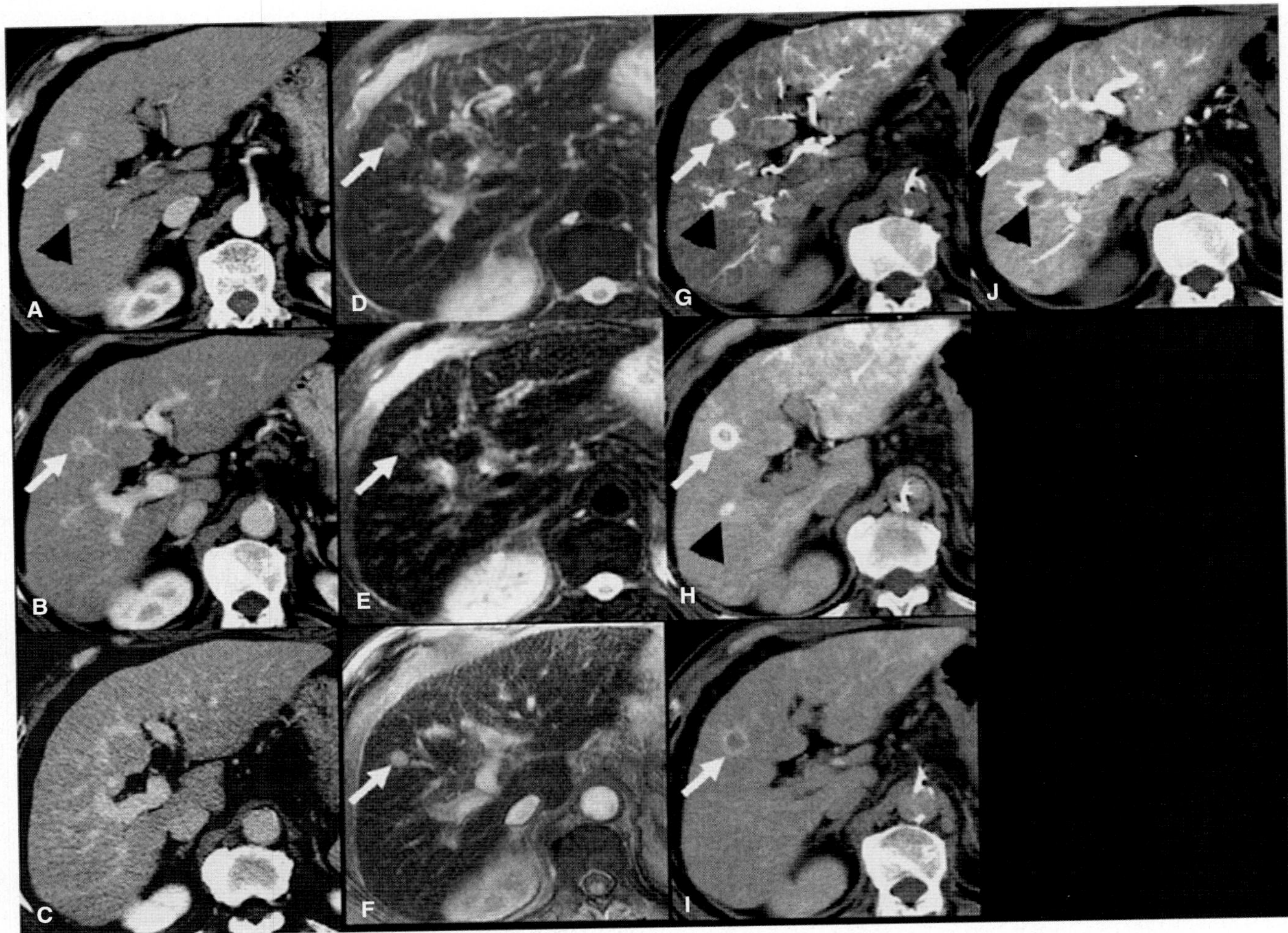

FIGURE 84.5 A comparison of imaging modalities to pick up multiple hepatocellular carcinoma (HCC) in a 69-year-old man. **A–C:** Transverse contrast-enhanced computed tomography (CT) scans (**A:** early phase; **B:** portal phase; **C:** delayed phase) show two lesions of high attenuation in segment 5 (*arrows* and *arrowhead* in **A** and **B**). **D–F:** Transverse magnetic resonance (MR) images: **D:** T2-weighted fast spin-echo MR image; **E:** superparamagnetic iron oxide (SPIO)-enhanced T2-weighted fast spin-echo MR image; **F:** SPIO-enhanced T2*-weighted MR image show one subtle high-intensity lesion in segment 5 (*arrows* in **D–F**). The other lesion was undetectable because of interference by signal intensity of overlying vascular structures. Transverse CT arterial portography (**G**) and CT during hepatic arteriography (**H:** first phase; **I:** second phase; **J:** third phase) show two HCCs in segment 5 (*arrows* and *arrowheads* in **G–J**), and these findings were pointed out by all observers. (From ref. 67, with permission.)

The American Association for the Study of Liver Diseases (AASLD) Practice Guideline on Management of Hepatocellular Carcinoma outlines criteria for diagnosis of HCC (2010 AASLD Guidelines).[74] Using this guideline, a biopsy can be avoided in most HCC patients, as there is substantial evidence that noninvasive diagnostic imaging can be used to make the diagnosis of HCC with high predictive value for many HCCs (Fig. 84.6).[74] AFP serology was used as a component of the HCC diagnostic criteria for many years. However, the most recent AASLD guideline recommends that it no longer be used for diagnosis as it is insufficiently sensitive or specific. AFP can be elevated in intrahepatic cholangiocarcinoma and in some metastases from colon cancer.[75,76] Detection of a hepatic mass on imaging within a cirrhotic liver is highly suspicious of HCC. Lesions larger than 1 cm on US should be investigated with a four-phase CT scan or MRI. If the lesion has the typical HCC features of arterial hypervascular and washout in the portal venous or delayed phase, the lesion should be treated as HCC. If the findings are not characteristic, a second contrast-enhanced study with another imaging modality should be performed, or the lesion should be biopsied. If the biopsy has negative findings, the lesion should be followed with imaging every 3 to 6 months until it disappears, enlarges, or demonstrates typical diagnostic characteristics of HCC. If the lesion enlarges but remains atypical, a repeat biopsy is recommended. Lesions less than 1 cm have a low likelihood of being HCC; therefore, it is recommended that these nodules be followed with US every 3 to 6 months for 2 years to detect changes suggestive of malignant transformation.

Screening Populations at High Risk of Hepatocellular Carcinoma

During the 1980s, it became apparent that early diagnosis of HCC was possible. Early approaches included identification of patients at risk for HCC and screening using measurement of serum AFP and imaging of the liver by US examination. During the 1990s, surveillance for HCC was adopted in several countries and regions, including Japan and parts of Europe. In the United States, surveillance was performed less frequently and in a nonstandardized way until recently, when the AASLD Practice

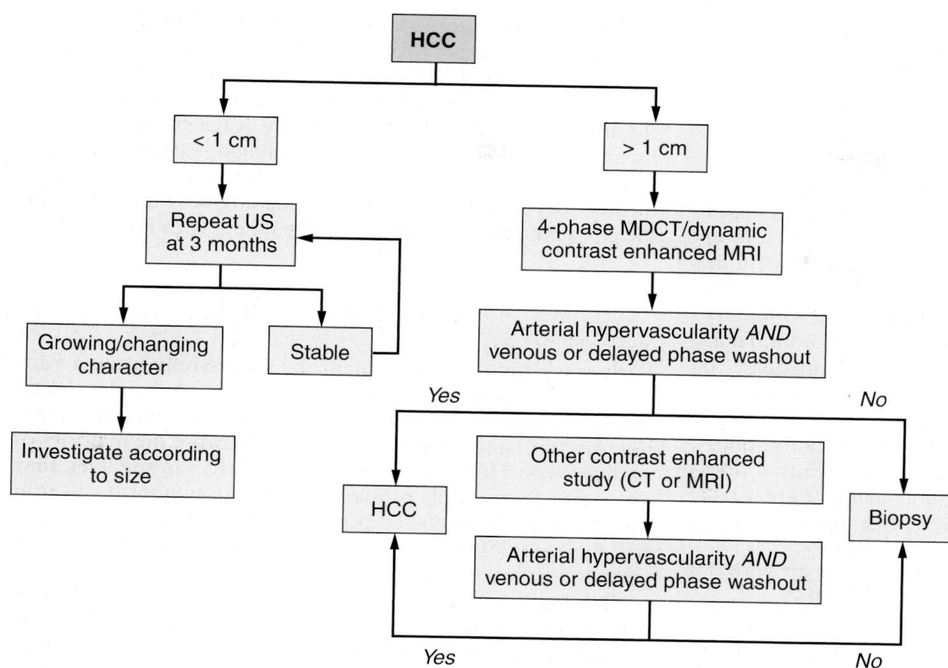

FIGURE 84.6 Algorithm for investigation of small nodules found on screening in patients at risk for hepatocellular carcinoma (HCC), from American Association for the Study of Liver Disease (AASLD) *Practice Guidelines* (2010 AASLD Guidelines). MDCT, multidetector computed tomography scan; US, ultrasound; MRI, magnetic resonance imaging; CT, computed tomography. (From ref. 74, with permission.)

Guideline was published, which provided evidence-based recommendations for identification of patients at risk, and recommended screening with periodic US examination with standardized recall policies and an algorithm for diagnosis of HCC.[74] Its authors acknowledge the paucity of data about the impact of screening but cite one large, randomized controlled trial of screening in China as being pivotal evidence of its benefit.[78]

When HCC presents with classic clinical features of abdominal pain and weight loss, the tumor is often very far advanced and few therapeutic options are available to the patient. Patient survival after diagnosis in this setting is dismal, on the order of 6 to 8 weeks on average. On the other hand, we have come to learn that HCC is potentially curable when treated at an early stage. Thus, results of liver transplantation for well-selected patients with stage I or II HCC show patient survival of 70% to 75% at 5 years.[77] Similarly, hepatic resection and local ablative therapies have been associated with good survival rates.[77] Early diagnosis is therefore the key to successful management of HCC. Because HCC is often associated with underlying liver disease, it is the physician who is providing care for these patients and who shoulders the burden of screening for HCC.

Although the term *screening* is used loosely, it actually refers to the application of diagnostic tests to someone at risk but with no evidence of HCC. *Surveillance,* on the other hand, refers to the repeated application of screening tests, as might be done as part of a systematic program in combination with standardized recall procedures and quality-control measures. The subject of screening for HCC has been somewhat controversial. On the one hand, there was wide recognition that patients with chronic liver disease were at risk of HCC and that screening with US and serum AFP allowed the detection of early tumors. On the other hand, there was not high-level evidence that such screening improved patient outcomes or survival of those with HCC.

Broadly speaking, populations at risk of HCC are divided into those with chronic HBV infection and those with cirrhosis of any other cause (Table 84.6).[74] Surveillance of patients waiting for liver transplantation is recognized as being in a special category because, at least in the United States, the development of HCC gives increased priority for orthotopic liver transplantation and because failure to screen means that patients may develop HCC that progresses beyond listing criteria while the patient is waiting.

Tests that have been used for surveillance for HCC include serologic tests (measurement of serum AFP) and radiologic tests (such as ultrasonography). However, the AASLD practice guideline recommends that surveillance for HCC should be performed using ultrasonography and that AFP alone should not be used for screening, unless US is suboptimal or not available. Thus, there appears to be little use for AFP in routine

TABLE 84.6

GROUPS RECOMMENDED TO BE UNDER SURVEILLANCE FOR HEPATOCELLULAR CARCINOMA (HCC)

Hepatitis B carriers
Asian men >40 y
Asian women >50 y
All cirrhotic hepatitis B carriers
Family history of HCC
Africans >20 y
Patients with high HBV DNA and ongoing hepatic injury remain at risk of HCC
Non–hepatitis B cirrhosis
Hepatitis C
Alcoholic cirrhosis
Genetic hemochromatosis
Primary biliary cirrhosis
Insufficient data to make recommendations
Cirrhosis due to α_1-anitrypsin deficiency
Cirrhosis due to nonalcoholic steatohepatitis
Cirrhosis due to autoimmune hepatitis

HBV, hepatitis B virus.
(Data derived from ref. 74.)

surveillance because of poor performance characteristics, depending on where the cutoff is set.[79,80] Ultrasonography has been widely used in surveillance for HCC, particularly in Japan and Europe.[81,82] The reported sensitivity of US is about 65% to 80% with a specificity approaching 90%, and it is very operator-dependent.[83]

Although the ideal surveillance interval is not known, a surveillance interval of 6 to 12 months has been proposed based on estimates of tumor doubling time.[84] There have been several estimates made of the growth rate of HCC. Tumor volume doubling times have ranged between 29 and 398 days (median, 117 days).[85,86] Thus, although there is considerable variability in growth rates, in general HCC is a slow-growing tumor. Thus, a screening interval of 6 to 12 months should be adequate to detect all but the fastest growing tumors before they exceed 5 cm in diameter. It is important to emphasize that the surveillance interval is determined by the growth rate of the tumor in question, not by the degree of risk of the individual.[74] Thus, it does not make sense to identify an individual as being at great risk of HCC and shorten the interval between screenings.

CLINICAL MANAGEMENT

The clinical management choices for HCC can be complex because of the numerous options that exist for treatment and the underlying liver disease that affects the majority of HCC patients (Table 84.7).[87] The natural history of HCC is variable, and prolonged survival without treatment has been reported.[88] Patients presenting with advanced tumors (vascular invasion, symptoms, extrahepatic spread) have a median survival of about 5 months with no treatment. Treatment results from the literature are difficult to interpret because survival as an end point may reflect the underlying liver disease more than progression of HCC. Treatment strategies may depend more on the underlying liver disease than the stage of the tumor. A focused multidisciplinary team, including a hepatologist, interventional radiologist, surgical oncologist, transplant surgeon, medical oncologist, and radiation oncologist, is important for the comprehensive management of patients with HCC.

TABLE 84.7

TREATMENT OPTIONS FOR HEPATOCELLULAR CARCINOMA

- Surgery
  - Partial hepatectomy
  - Liver transplantation
- Local ablative therapies
  - Cryosurgery
  - Microwave ablation
  - Ethanol injection
  - Acetic acid injection
  - Radiofrequency ablation
- Regional therapies: hepatic artery transcatheter treatments
  - Transarterial chemotherapy
  - Transarterial embolization
  - Transarterial chemoembolization
  - Transarterial ^{90}Y microspheres
  - Transarterial ^{131}I lipiodol
  - Proton or carbon ion therapy
  - Conformal radiation therapy
  - Stereotactic radiation therapy
  - Palliative low dose radiation therapy
- Systemic therapies
  - Chemotherapy
  - Targeted therapy (sorafenib)[a]
  - Immunotherapy
  - Hormonal therapy
- Supportive care

[a]Sorafenib is the only systemic therapy with level 1 evidence proving a survival benefit.

Stage I and II HCC

Early-stage tumors can be managed successfully using a variety of techniques, including surgical resection, local ablation (radiofrequency ablation), and local injection therapies (ethanol injection) and transplantation.[77,89] Because the majority of patients with HCC suffer from a field defect in the liver, they are at risk for multiple primary tumors throughout the liver in their lifetime. As discussed previously, the majority of patients will have significant underlying liver disease and may not tolerate major loss of hepatic parenchyma. Also, because of the underlying liver disease the patients may be eligible for liver transplantation in the future. Therefore, the most important principle to follow in early-stage HCC is to use treatment that allows for maximal sparing of the hepatic parenchyma. Avoiding major open surgery may also improve the results of subsequent transplant surgery, if required.

Surgical Excision

Open surgical excision is a reliable method for treating stage I HCC with 5-year survival exceeding 50%[90] (Table 84.8). The goal is to obtain a 1-cm margin of normal tissue around the tumor. Beyond that requirement, the type of excision may not have an impact on cancer treatment outcome, although this is controversial.[93,113] The excision of surface tumors may be best accomplished as a "nonanatomic wedge" excision, in which the tumor is simply excised with a 1-cm margin and no more. The hepatic parenchyma can be divided using a variety of techniques, with the goal to minimize blood loss and maintain adequate exposure to ensure accurate margins are obtained. This can be performed safely for tumors up to 5 cm in diameter with minimal blood loss. Deep tumors within the hepatic parenchyma and tumors greater than 5 cm must be managed by an anatomic resection, where the most distal portal triad to the region involved by the tumor is controlled and the segment or segments are resected. Centrally located tumors may require a lobectomy and large tumors may require an extended hepatectomy. The risk of major hepatectomy is high (5% to 10% mortality) because of the underlying liver disease and the potential for liver failure, but it is acceptable in selected cases.[114] Preoperative portal vein occlusion can be performed to cause atrophy of the HCC-involved lobe and compensatory hypertrophy of the noninvolved liver.[115–117] This allows for a safer resection. Intraoperative US is essential for planning the surgical approach for HCC.[118] The US can image the proximity of major vascular structures that may be encountered during the dissection. For deep tumors, the US may identify the portal pedicle supplying the segment involved with HCC, and early control of this triad can be obtained. Intraoperative US is also essential for screening the rest of the liver for small tumors.

The utility of inflow occlusion (Pringle maneuver) in liver resection in patients with cirrhosis has been studied. Concern exists regarding whether ischemic injury to the liver will lead to liver failure or result in worsening cirrhosis. Numerous reports, including a randomized trial, have demonstrated no ill effects to inflow occlusion. In fact, the most significant predictor of postoperative mortality is blood loss, and the Pringle

TABLE 84.8

LARGE SERIES OF SURVIVAL RESULTS AFTER LIVER RESECTION FOR HEPATOCELLULAR CARCINOMA

Study	No. of Patients	1-Year	3-Year Survival (%)	5-Year
Llovet et al., 1999[91]	77	85		51
Arii et al., 2000[a,92]				
T1 <2 cm	1,318	96	—	72
T1 2–5 cm	2,722	95	—	58
T2 <2 cm	502	92	—	55
T2 2–5 cm	1,548	95	—	58
Poon et al., 2000[93]				
Resection margin >1cm	150	54	34	22
Resection margin ≥1 cm	138	55	35	25
Grazi et al., 2001[94]	264	—	63	41
Wayne et al., 2002[95]	249	83	—	41
Yeh et al., 2002[96]	218	63	42	32
Ziparo et al., 2002[97]	81	75	62	51
Belghiti et al., 2002[98]	328	81	57	37
Kanematsu et al., 2002[99]	303	84	67	51
Grazi et al., 2003[100]				
Cirrhotic	308	86	64	42
Noncirrhotic	135	84	68	51
Lang et al., 2003[101]				
Major resection (cirrhotic)	84	90[b]	78[b]	73
Minor resection (cirrhotic)	134	85[b]	76[b]	60
Cha et al., 2003[102]	164	79	51	40
DeCarlis et al., 2003[103]	154	90[b]	65[b]	47
Chen et al., 2003[104]				
<3 cm	145	82	59	42
>3 cm	340	56	39	31
Vivarelli et al., 2004[105]	79	83	65	—
Liu et al., 2004[106]	229	73	—	33
El-Serag et al., 2006[107]	243	62	31	—
Bartlett et al., 2007[108]	53	74	54	43
Zhou et al., 2007[109]	81	78	47	39
Shimada et al., 2007[110]				
<4 cm	156	80	47	36
>4 cm	163	65	33	27
Shah et al., 2007[111]	193	85	68	53
Lo et al., 2007[112]				
<5 cm	39	95	84	76
>5 cm	41	88	66	66

[a]Nationwide survey in Japan.
[b]Estimated from article based on survival curves.

maneuver decreases blood loss, leading to an improvement in perioperative morbidity.[115,119,120] The morbidity and mortality of a simple wedge excision should be minimal, but even slight manipulation of a cirrhotic liver may lead to liver failure and other complications, such as respiratory failure (acute respiratory distress syndrome, pneumonia), cardiovascular compromise, ascites, and infection. Cirrhotic patients are fragile with respect to the tolerance of any major surgery. Any significant postoperative complications may lead to liver failure (Table 84.9). The Child-Pugh classification of liver failure is still the most reliable prognosticator for tolerance of hepatic surgery (Table 84.5). Only patients classified as Child-Pugh A should be considered for surgical resection and even then, those with significant portal hypertension may not tolerate surgery.[53] Child-Pugh B and C patients with stage I HCC tumors should be referred for transplant, if appropriate. Patients with ascites or a recent history of variceal bleeding should be treated with transplantation.

As discussed previously, a variety of hepatic functional tests have been described for a quantitative assessment of hepatic reserve, but these techniques have not been adopted in routine practices. The most validated is the indocyanine green clearance test. Indocyanine green is delivered systemically and the hepatic retention is measured at 15 minutes. When the retention rate is less than 10%, all resections are possible. If 10% to 20%, a bisegmentectomy is well tolerated; if 20% to 29%, a single segment can be excised safely; if 30% or more, the risk of liver failure with any form of resection is high. In one study, the operative mortality was reduced to 1% using these criteria.[127] The risk of recurrence after adequate resection of HCC remains high (>70% at 5 years). Predictors of recurrence include synchronous tumor sites and microvascular invasion.[128] Surgical re-resection or salvage transplantation for HCC recurrence is seldom an option because of the aggressive, multifocal nature of this recurrence.[129,130]

Even Child-Pugh A cirrhotic patients or noncirrhotic patients may be better served with a less-invasive option than

TABLE 84.9

HEPATIC RESECTION OPERATIVE MORTALITY IN CIRRHOTIC PATIENTS

Study	No. of Patients	Mortality (%)
Yeh et al., 2002[96]	218	8.8
Wei et al., 2003[114]	155	8.4[a]
Ziparo et al., 2002[97]	88	8.7
Belghiti et al., 2002[98]	328	6.4
Kanematsu et al., 2002[99]	303	1.6
Grazi et al., 2003[100]	308	5.0
Ferrero et al., 2005[121]		
>70 years old	64	3.1
>70 years old	177	9.6
Capussotti et al., 2005[122]		
Child A	169	5.0
Child B	47	21.0
Zhou et al., 2007[109]	81	1.2
Chik et al., 2007[123]	172	8.1[a]
Taketomi et al., 2007[124]	213	2.0
Dahiya et al., 2010[125]		
Minor hepatectomy	259	5.4
Major hepatectomy	114	8.8
Abdel-Wahab et al., 2010[126]	175	9.1

[a]Extended hepatectomy only.

open excision. Although open surgical excision is the most reliable, the patient may be better served with a laparoscopic approach to resection, laparoscopic radiofrequency ablation, percutaneous radiofrequency ablation, or percutaneous ethanol injection. Minimizing the damage to normal parenchyma may improve the outcome and allow for all options in the future. No adequate comparisons of these different techniques have been undertaken to determine their relative success. In general, the choice of treatment is based on physician and patient preference.

Laparoscopic Resection

Laparoscopic surgical resection is a minimally invasive technique for resecting liver tumors.[131–133] The abdomen can be insufflated with CO_2 or lifted with specialized retractors.[134] Visualization is accomplished with a camera, and instruments are placed through the abdominal wall for hepatic parenchymal dissection. A laparoscopic approach to small, surface liver tumors is safe and feasible with widely available laparoscopic instruments. Larger lobectomies and segmentectomies are more commonly performed as a minimally invasive approach in major liver centers. Many centers have reported major laparoscopic hepatectomies with the proposed advantage of less morbidity and quicker recovery.[135] Laparoscopic surgical resection has the advantage over local ablative techniques of being able to assess margins pathologically, but has the same risk of bleeding, hepatic failure, and ascites as open excision. Laparoscopic surgery for cancer has the theoretical downside of spreading tumor cells at the time of laparoscopy. In general, surgeons have been reluctant to adopt laparoscopic approaches for cancer resection until randomized studies fail to demonstrate a negative impact on tumor recurrence compared with open surgery. Trials of more common procedures for cancer such as colectomies have not demonstrated a negative impact of the laparoscopic technique to date.[136] This experience may translate to other procedures such as liver resection as long as the same oncologic principles of resection are used with the laparoscopic approach as they are with the open approach.

Local Ablation Strategies

Radiofrequency ablation is a technique that uses heat to thermally ablate tumors.[137–139] A thin probe (18 gauge) is inserted into the middle of a tumor, then needle electrodes are deployed to adjustable distances. An alternating electrical current (400 to 500 kHz) is delivered through the electrodes. The current causes agitation of the particles of the surrounding tissues, generating frictional heat. The heat leads to a reliable sphere of necrosis. The size of the sphere depends on the length of deployment of the electrodes. Currently, the maximum size of the probe arrays allows for a 7-cm zone of necrosis. This would be adequate for a 5-cm tumor. The heat reliably kills cells within the zone of necrosis. The lack of uniform success is because of the difficulty of positioning the probe accurately in three dimensions using US or CT guidance. Also, large blood vessels may act as heat sinks, preventing adequate cytodestruction of cells adjacent to these structures.[140] Finally, treatment of tumors close to the main portal pedicles can lead to bile duct injury and obstruction. This limits the location of tumors that are optimally suited for this technique.

In case series examining the results of treatment of HCC with radiofrequency ablation, the data suggest a uniformly excellent response, with a local recurrence rate (at the site of ablation) of between 5% and 20%.[138,141–145] The treatment can be performed percutaneously with CT or US guidance, or at the time of laparoscopy with US guidance. The downside of the laparoscopic approach is the requirement for general anesthesia, but some have suggested better results with this approach.[146] The percutaneous approach may also be limited by structures at risk for injury around the tumor, such as the diaphragm, colon, or gallbladder. These structures can be retracted free with a laparoscopic approach. In general, radiofrequency ablation is reliable as a single treatment. A single ablation can take up to 20 minutes for a 7-cm ablation. It is well tolerated and can be performed as an outpatient procedure. It can be repeated numerous times, especially if performed percutaneously. This technique is best suited overall to small tumors (<3 cm) deep within the hepatic parenchyma and away from the hepatic hilum. Complete preservation of hepatic parenchyma is possible with reliable tumor killing. A theoretical risk of needle tract tumor seeding exists.[147] The track can be thermally ablated while retracting the needle, which decreases this risk.

Local Injection Therapy

Numerous agents have been used for local injection into tumors, but the most widely used agent has been absolute ethanol. Ethanol injection into HCC is the most widely used therapy worldwide. The relatively soft HCC within the hard background cirrhotic liver allows for injection of large volumes of ethanol into the tumor without diffusion into the hepatic parenchyma or leakage out of the liver. Ethanol causes a direct destruction of cancer cells, but it is in no way selective for cancer, and will destroy normal cells in the vicinity. The key to success is the accuracy of the injection. This technique is associated with a 15% risk of recurrence at the site of treatment. It has the advantage of being minimally invasive—a very small needle can be used for injection—and it is quite inexpensive. The disadvantage is that a response usually requires multiple injections (average, three). The maximum size of tumor reliably treated is 3 cm, even with multiple injections. For this reason, radiofrequency ablation is preferable to most clinicians. Also, randomized trials have suggested an improved survival for radiofrequency ablation compared with percutaneous ethanol injection.[148–151] Nevertheless, the cost of radiofrequency ablation may be prohibitive in many places. Acetic acid is another agent with established success as a local injection for HCC. A randomized trial suggested that local recurrence is improved with acetic acid compared to ethanol.

TABLE 84.10

OVERALL SURVIVAL AFTER LIVER TRANSPLANTATION FOR NONSELECTED HEPATOCELLULAR CARCINOMA

Study	No. of Patients	3 Years	5 Years
O'Grady et al., 1988[152]	50	38	30
Olthoff et al., 1990[153]	16	NA	31
Iwatsuki et al., 1991[154]	105	39	36
Penn (Registry), 1991[155]	365	30	18
Ringe et al., 1991[156]	61	NA	15
Bismuth et al., 1993[157]	60	47	NA
Tan et al., 1995[158]	15 (<8 cm)	63	NA
Klintmalm (Registry), 1998[159]	422	50	44
Otto et al., 1998[160]	50	48	NA
Pichlmayr et al., 1998[161]	135	32	27
Hemming et al., 2001[162]	112	63	57

NA, not available.

Transplantation

A viable option for stage I and II tumors in the setting of cirrhosis is liver transplantation. The expected morbidity and mortality for transplantation for non–cancer-related liver disease has improved with appropriate patient selection and established expertise of liver transplant programs. With this acceptable morbidity and mortality, the major considerations for liver transplantation become the long-term outcome in terms of cancer recurrence. The National Institutes of Health Consensus Conference on liver transplantation in 1983 concluded that primary hepatic malignancy confined to the liver but not amenable to resection may be an indication for transplantation, although it was noted that the results had indicated a strong likelihood of recurrence of the malignancy. As predicted, recurrence proved to be the rule rather than the exception, and results were dismal (Table 84.10). As survival data gradually accumulated, advanced HCC cases were abandoned. However, no consensus existed among transplant surgeons and physicians as to the acceptable limits of HCC for which transplant could be beneficial, leaving each program's personnel free to transplant any patient it deemed deserving.

Staff at transplant centers realized over time that earlier tumors in the setting of severe cirrhosis could be treated successfully with transplantation. Originally proposed by Bismuth et al.[157] and then later studied prospectively by Mazzaferro et al.,[163] liver transplantation for patients with a single lesion of 5 cm or more, or multifocal disease limited to more than three nodules, each 3 cm or more, resulted in excellent tumor-free survival (70% or more at 5 years) (Table 84.11). These guidelines have become widely accepted, both in the United States and Europe, and were incorporated into United Network for Organ Sharing (UNOS) policy even though the Mazzaferro et al. study was based on a limited number of patients, and there were no data concerning the fate of those outside these criteria who did not receive a transplant. Subsequent studies from Pittsburgh,[175] the University of California at San Francisco, and Milan[176] have shown that acceptable tumor-free survival can be obtained for many patients outside these strict criteria who currently do not receive liver transplantation under current UNOS guidelines.

As of 2001, the indications for transplantation for HCC included the following: (1) the patient was not a liver resection candidate, (2) the tumor(s) was 5 cm or less in diameter, (3) there was no macrovascular involvement, and (4) there was no

TABLE 84.11

RESULTS OF LIVER TRANSPLANTATION FOR EARLY HEPATOCELLULAR CARCINOMA

Study	No. of Patients	Tumor (Size and No.)	Neoadjuvant Therapy	Survival (%)
Mazzaferro et al., 2009[164]	444	1 ≤5 cm; 3 ≤3 cm	None	73 (5-y)
	1,112	Beyond Milan criteria	None	54 (5-y)
Pelletier et al., 2009[165]	2,790	1≤5 cm; 3 ≤3 cm	None	61 (5-y)
	346	Beyond Milan criteria	None	32 (5-y)
Herrero et al., 2008[166]	47	1 ≤5 cm; 3 ≤3 cm	None	70 (5-y)
	26	Beyond Milan criteria	None	73 (5-y)
Onaca et al., 2007[167]	631	1 ≤5 cm; 3 ≤3 cm	None	62 (5-y RFS)
	575	Beyond Milan criteria	None	43 (5-y RFS)
Decaens et al., 2006[168]	279	1 ≤5 cm; 3 ≤3 cm	None	60 (5-y)
	44	UCSF criteria	None	46 (5-y)
	145	Beyond UCSF criteria	None	35 (5-y)
Bigourdan et al., 2003[169]	17	1 ≤5 cm; 3 ≤3 cm	TACE	71 (5-y)
Yao et al., 2001[170]	46	1 ≤5 cm; 3 ≤3 cm	TACE/ETOH	72 (5-y)
Tamura et al., 2001[171]	56	<5 cm	± TACE	71 (5-y)
Regalia et al., 2001[172]	122	1 ≤5 cm; 3 ≤3 cm	TACE	80 (5-y)
Jonas et al., 2001[173]	120	1 ≤5 cm; 3 ≤3 cm	None	71 (5-y)
Llovet et al., 1998[174]	58	<5 cm	None	74 (5-y)
Mazzaferro et al., 1996[163]	48	1 ≤5 cm; 3 ≤3 cm	TACE	75 (4-y)

RFS, recurrance-free survival; UCSF, University of California, San Francisco; TACE, trials involving transhepatic arterial chemoembolization; ETOH, alcohol.

TABLE 84.12

RESULTS OF LIVING DONOR LIVER TRANSPLANTATION FOR HEPATOCELLULAR CARCINOMA BASED ON THE MILAN CRITERIA

Study	Patients Meeting Milan Criteria		Patients Exceeding Milan Criteria	
	N	3-Year Survival (%)	N	3-Year Survival (%)
Todo et al., 2004[193]	137	80	172	60
Hwang et al., 2005[194]	151	91	62	62
Takada et al., 2006[195]	49	68	44	59
Sugawara et al., 2007[196]	68	79	10	60
Lee et al., 2008[197]	164	76	57	45

(From ref. 324, with permission.)

identifiable extrahepatic spread of tumor to surrounding lymph nodes, lungs, abdominal organs, or bone. Reports on the results of transplantation with these restrictions demonstrated 5-year survival rates in the range of 70% to 75%.[177] Even accepting the fact that preoperative imaging is far from perfect, 5-year tumor-free survival rates more than 70% can be expected by adhering to the current guidelines. In an evaluation of their living-donor transplants for HCC in which the only exclusion criteria were extrahepatic metastasis or vascular invasion detected during the preoperative evaluation, Kaihara et al.[178] reported 1- and 3-year survival rates of 73% and 55%, respectively. These results would have to be considered quite remarkable given that 54% of their patients were in pTNM stage IVA and 45% were outside the Milan/UNOS criteria at the time of transplantation. However, there are insufficient data in the literature to liberalize the current transplantation criteria.[164,166–168,179,180]

These strict criteria led to better results for those transplanted, but priority scoring for transplantation led to cancer patients waiting too long for their transplants. Tumors would often become too advanced during the patient's time on the waiting list for a donated liver. Survival statistics may be skewed because of selection of candidates who did not progress during their wait on the transplant list. A variety of nonresection therapies were used as a "bridge" to transplantation, including radiofrequency ablation, ethanol injection, and transarterial embolization procedures. At a minimum, it seems clear that these pretransplant treatment regimens allow patients to remain on the transplant waiting list longer, thereby giving them greater opportunities to be transplanted.[181] What remains unclear, however, is whether this translates into prolonged survival after transplant.[182–187] Further, it is not known whether patients who have had their tumor(s) treated preoperatively follow the recurrence pattern predicted by their tumor status at the time of transplant (i.e., after local ablative therapy), or if they follow the course set by their tumor parameters present before such treatment.

The UNOS system for prioritization scoring of liver transplant recipients now includes additional MELD (Model for End-Stage Liver Disease) points for patients with HCC.[188] This allows patients with early-stage disease to receive a priority score, which leads to rapid transplantation. Now, even patients who are resection candidates can be treated with transplantation. The controversy over appropriate management for these patients will exist until more data on the long-term results for transplantation of these early-stage patients are reported. To date, survival for early-stage disease treated with surgery is 50% to 75% versus transplantation, which is reportedly more than 70%. Longer-term intention-to-treat studies will be necessary to define the better treatment.[189,190]

The success of living related-donor liver transplantation programs has also led to patients receiving transplantation earlier for HCC. In the case of living related donations, the UNOS guidelines are often exceeded, accepting a lower potential of long-term survival in this setting where there is no competition for the organ. Gondolesi et al.[191] and Trotter[192] reported 2-year survival of 60% after living donor liver transplantation in 36 HCC patients, of which 53% exceeded UNOS priority criteria. Others have reported excellent results even in patients who exceed the Milan criteria (Table 84.12).

ADJUVANT THERAPY

The role of adjuvant chemotherapy for patients after resection or transplant with HCC remains undefined. Both adjuvant and neoadjuvant approaches have been studied. Two randomized controlled trials and seven nonrandomized trials have evaluated preoperative transarterial chemotherapy. No clear advantage in disease-free or overall survival was found in these studies.[198–200] Postoperative transarterial chemotherapy has been examined in four randomized controlled trials and three nonrandomized controlled trials. A meta-analysis of these trials revealed a significant improvement in disease-free and overall survival.[199,201] The regimens consisted of lipiodol and chemotherapy agents, including doxorubicin, mitomycin, and cisplatin. An analysis of postoperative adjuvant systemic chemotherapy trials demonstrates no consistent advantage in terms of disease-free or overall survival.[202–206] A recent report of a randomized trial of adjuvant interferon-α2b described an improved 5-year survival in patients with stage III/IVA tumor from 24% to 68% (P = .038).[112] Neoadjuvant approaches such as chemoembolization have been successful as a bridge to transplantation, and have decreased tumor burden in resection candidates to improve resectability. Numerous studies of postoperative adjuvants after resection and liver transplantation have been performed, but the results are not definitive.

Stage III and IV Tumors

Fewer surgical options exist for stage III tumors involving major vascular structures. In patients without cirrhosis, a major hepatectomy is feasible and provides the best chance of long-term survival, although prognosis is poor. Patients with Child-Pugh A cirrhosis may be resected, but a lobectomy is associated with significant morbidity and mortality, and long-term prognosis is poor. Nevertheless, a small percentage of patients will achieve long-term survival, justifying an attempt at resection when feasible. Preoperative portal vein occlusion in order to induce compensatory hypertrophy preoperatively may improve the results or help define which patients will tolerate a major hepatectomy. Because of the advanced nature of these tumors, even successful resection will be met with rapid recurrence. These patients are not considered candidates for transplantation because of the high tumor recurrence rates, unless their tumors can be downstaged with adjuvant therapy. Although unproven, these patients are ideal for neoadjuvant treatment approaches, such as embolization. Decreasing the size of the primary tumor allows for less surgery, and the delay in surgery allows for extrahepatic disease to manifest on imaging studies and avoid unnecessary surgery on the primary tumor. Successful regional therapy strategies may make the patient eligible for transplantation.[207] The prognosis is poor for stage IV tumors, and no surgical treatment is recommended. Care must be taken to differentiate multifocal disease from intrahepatic metastases, as the latter has a much worse prognosis. Molecular genotyping may be the best way to make this differentiation.

Radiation Therapy

Retrospective phase 1 and phase 2 studies have shown that tumoricidal doses of radiation therapy can be delivered safely to a wide spectrum of HCCs (early stage and locally advanced with portal vein thrombosis) using a variety of strategies. Although the potential for long-term tumor control has been demonstrated in selected patients, randomized trials are required to help define the role of radiation therapy in the management of HCC.

The low tolerance of the whole liver to irradiation limited the early application of radiation as a treatment for liver cancer. The first hepatic toxicity observed following liver irradiation was referred to as *radiation-induced liver disease* (RILD), a syndrome of anicteric ascites, hepatosplenomegaly, and elevated alkaline phosphatase, seen within 3 months following irradiation.[208] Pathologically, RILD is characterized by congestion of the central veins and central lobular sinusoids, followed by epithelial cell proliferation in the central lobulars zone, hepatocyte atrophy, and fibrosis. Proinflammatory cytokines such as transforming growth factor-β1 and interleukin-6 have been implicated in its development.[209] Elevation of transaminases, thrombocytopenia, variceal bleeding, and general decline of liver function have also been observed, most often in patients with cirrhosis. Reactivation of hepatitis B may occur because of interleukin-6 released by irradiated endothelial cells.[210] Changes in CT and MRI contrast enhancement[211] and perfusion[212] are seen within regions of the liver irradiated to high doses.

External-Beam Radiation Therapy

Whole-liver irradiation to doses above 32 Gy in 1.5 Gy per fraction twice daily, 25 Gy in ten fractions, or 21 Gy in seven fractions are associated with a risk of RILD greater than 5%.[213] However, far higher doses can be delivered safely to focal HCCs, as long as enough uninvolved liver can be spared.[135,136,214–216] In an analysis of 204 liver cancer radiation plans and complication data from patients treated on trials at University of Michigan (1.5 Gy twice daily to 90 Gy, with the hepatic arterial radiation sensitizers fluorodeoxyuridine or bromodeoxyuridine), the mean liver dose was found to be a reasonable estimate of RILD toxicity risk for patients with HCC, with 5% and 50% risks of toxicity for mean liver doses of 32 Gy and 40 Gy, in 1.5 Gy twice daily, respectively.[213]

The risk of toxicity and type of toxicity following liver irradiation varies in different patient populations.[215,216] In one series of 105 Korean patients with HCC, the incidence of grade 3 and 4 liver toxicity was 4.8% and 1%, respectively.[216] The tolerance of the liver to irradiation has also been found to be reduced with reduced liver reserve[217] and in the presence of hepatitis B.[218] Baseline indocyanine green retention rate at 15 minutes was found to correlate with hepatic insufficiency following carbon ion therapy.[219] No hepatic insufficiency was observed if the retention rate was less than 20%, whereas three of four patients with retention rates greater than 50% developed hepatic insufficiency.

Low-dose liver irradiation is an effective, safe, palliative therapy to reduce local symptoms of HCC such as pain, as well as symptoms due to HCC metastases to bone,[220,221] brain,[222] lymph nodes,[223,224] and other sites.[225]

Advances in liver cancer imaging, radiation planning, methods to account for breathing motion, and advances in image guidance at the time of radiation delivery make it possible for high doses of radiation to be safely delivered to focal HCCs, with a falloff in dose in the surrounding uninvolved liver, bringing with it the possibility of tumor eradication. At the University of Michigan, dose-escalated conformal hyperfractionated radiotherapy, with concurrent hepatic arterial fluorodeoxyuridine, has been used to treat unresectable small and bulky focal HCCs. An individualized prescription dose based on the volume of liver irradiated, up to 90 Gy (in 1.5 Gy per fraction, twice daily), was delivered safely in patients with Child-Pugh A liver function. In 1997, the median survival and 4-year survival rate of 20 patients with primary liver cancer was 16 months and 20%, respectively.[226] In subsequent phase 2 studies, the median survival was 15.2 months.[227] Hyperfractionated radiation therapy (45 to 75 Gy, 1.5 Gy twice daily) has also been used safely in combination with thalidomide in 121 Japanese HCC patients with 1- and 2-year survival rates of 60% and 45%, respectively. Portal vein thrombosis and AFP level were prognostic factors for survival.[228]

A French prospective phase 2 trial investigated conformal radiation therapy (66 Gy in 2 Gy per fraction) for small HCCs (one nodule 5 cm or less, or two nodules 3 cm or less), with a response rate of 92% in 27 patients with cirrhosis.[229] Two grade 4 toxicities occurred in 11 Child-Pugh B patients with pre-existing grade 3 liver abnormalities. Three hundred five Korean patients with HCC (80% Child-Pugh A, 88% >5 cm, and >50% with portal vein thrombosis) were treated with conventional fractionated conformal radiation therapy with systemic or hepatic chemotherapy in 41%.[230] The median survival was 11 months, and the 2-year survival rate was 24.5%. The TNM staging system was found best to predict prognosis in this series of predominantly Child-Pugh A patients. Increased local control and survival was observed with higher doses in this series and others.[223,231–233]

Shorter radiotherapy schedules (hypofractionation), with higher doses delivered at each radiation fraction (referred to as *stereotactic body radiation therapy* or *SBRT*) have also been used to treat HCCs (usually <8 cm in size), with local control at 1 to 2 years ranging from 73% to 93%.[233–240] In 98 patients with HCC, 48 to 63 Gy in six to nine fractions was associated with tumor remission in 86% of patients 6 months after therapy. The 1- and 2-year survival rates were 68% and 41%, respectively.[241] A phase 1 study of SBRT in 31 patients with advanced HCC (45% with portal vein thrombosis) ineligible for other local therapies (transhepatic arterial chemoembolization [TACE], radiofrequency ablation, surgery) was conducted in Canada.[236] Following 24 to 54 Gy in six fractions, toxicity was acceptable; 16% of cases had a decline in Child-Pugh score at 3 months, the majority of whom also had tumor progression. The median survival was 11.7 months. Another phase 1 study reported 100% local control after 36 to 48 Gy in three to five fractions. Patients with Child-Pugh B liver function were more likely to have liver toxicity following 42 Gy in three fractions, triggering a dose reduction in these patients to 40 Gy in five fractions.[242]

Radiation therapy has been combined with TACE. Following radiation therapy delivered either immediately prior to or following TACE,[243–246] 2- and 5-year survival rates ranged from 10% to 54% and 9% to 25%, respectively. In Korea, 38 of 73 patients with HCC who had an incomplete response to TACE were treated with radiotherapy while the remaining 35 patients received repeat TACE. A statistically significant improvement in survival was seen in patients treated with radiation therapy compared with TACE (2-year survival rate 37% vs. 14% for radiation therapy vs. TACE; P = .001). The difference in survival was greatest for large tumors, with 2-year survival rates of 63% versus 42% in 5- to 7-cm tumors, 50% versus 0% in 8- to 10-cm tumors, and 17% versus 0% in tumors larger than 10 cm, for radiation therapy and repeat TACE, respectively.[247]

Although phase 1 studies of radiation therapy with systemic therapies have not been conducted, a retrospective report in 23 patients with HCC treated with SBRT (median dose, 52.5 Gy in 15 fractions) with pretreatment, concurrent, and posttreatment sunitinib, found a median survival of 16 months. The time to progression was 10 months in patients who received continuous sunitinib following SBRT and 4 months in those who did not receive maintenance therapy.[248]

Charged particles (protons and heavy ions) are a specialized type of radiation that deposit little energy as they enter the patient and deposit the majority of energy at depth with a sharp falloff beyond the target, making them particularly well suited for HCC, and especially for patients with large HCC and/or Child-Pugh B or C cirrhosis who are at higher risk of toxicity.[249] In a retrospective review from Japan of 162 patients with 192 unresectable HCCs, the 5-year local control and survival rates following proton therapy (72 Gy in 16 fractions), with or without TACE or percutaneous ethanol injection, were 87% and 24%, respectively, with no grade 3 or higher toxicity.[250] These results were confirmed in a phase 2 proton study of 66 Gy in 10 fractions in 51 patients with one to three HCCs (≤10 cm), 20% Child Pugh class B. Five-year local control and survival were 88% and 39% respectively. In Child-Pugh class A patients with solitary tumors, 5-year survival was 46%. Liver function remained stable or improved in 84% of patients, and no radiation-induced liver disease was observed.[251] In a phase 1/2 study of carbon-ion radiation therapy in which the dose per fraction was escalated, 50 to 80 Gy in 15 fractions was used to treat 24 HCC patients. The 5-year local control and survival rates were 81% and 25%, respectively.[252] Another series of charged particles reported a 2-year local control rate of 96%.[219]

Proton and photon radiation therapy can be used to treat portal venous thrombosis, with recanalization observed in 39% to 83% of patients, and 3-year survival rates ranging from 15% to 21%.[253,254] Both proton and photon therapy have also been used as a bridge to liver transplantation, with pathologic complete responses observed.[242,249,255]

Brachytherapy

Although interstitial and intraluminal brachytherapy have been used to treat liver metastases and cholangiocarcinoma,[256] there is less experience in HCC perhaps because of the increased risk of intrahepatic hemorrhage in patients with underlying cirrhosis. Intraluminal iridium-192 has been used for intraductal HCC and following incomplete resection.[257,258]

Hepatic Arterial Radioisotopes

Another method of delivering radiation therapy to liver cancers is by hepatic arterial delivery of radioisotopes, or selective internal radiation therapy (SIRT). The most common radioisotope used in liver cancer is yttrium-90 (^{90}Y), incorporated into stable glass (TheraSphere, MDS Nordion Inc., Ottawa, Canada) or resin (SIRTex Medical, Inc., Lane Cove, New South Wales, Australia) microspheres. ^{90}Y is a pure beta emitter with a half-life of 64.5 hours and an effective path length of 5.3-mm; that is, 90% of the energy is deposited within a 5.3-mm radius of the microsphere. ^{90}Y microspheres may be delivered through the hepatic artery segmentally, subsegmentally, regionally, or to the whole liver, depending on the distribution of liver cancer. A typical prescribed dose is 150 Gy, in which the microspheres are primarily deposited at the periphery of the metastases.

In one of the first phase 1 studies of ^{90}Y, dose was escalated from 50 to 100 Gy in ten patients with HCC. All patients had stability of disease, with three patients living more than 1 year.[259] Since then, ^{90}Y microspheres have been assessed in several phase 2 studies, and more than 1,000 patients have received ^{90}Y microspheres therapy to date.[260] Reported median survival rates in patients with HCC treated with ^{90}Y microspheres range from to 9.4 to 21.6 months.[261,262] Goin et al.[263] reported outcomes of 121 patients treated with hepatic arterial ^{90}Y. Specific toxicities included liver toxicity (14 patients), pneumonitis (2 patients), and gastrointestinal bleeding (2 patients). Risk factors associated with early mortality included infiltrative tumor, tumor volume greater than 70% of liver, tumor volume greater than 50% of liver, and albumin 3 g/dL or less, bilirubin 2 mg/dL or more, aspartate aminotransferase/alanine aminotransferase five or more times normal, non-HCC diagnosis, and lung dose more than 30 Gy. Ninety-day mortality was 49% in 33 "high-risk" patients with at least one adverse variable and 7% in 88 "low-risk" patients with no adverse variables (P <.001). The median survival for high- and low-risk groups was 3.6 months and 15.5 months, respectively (P <.001). The most frequent toxicities in the low-risk patients were ascites, elevated bilirubin, and elevated transaminases, which were mostly transient. Although not common, fatal liver toxicity is possible.[264]

Another radioisotope that has been used to treat HCC is iodine-131 (^{131}I) tagged to ferritin antibodies[265,266] or lipiodol.[267–269] I antiferritin was studied in a randomized trial that compared ^{131}I antiferritin with chemotherapy in patients with HCC previously treated with whole-liver radiation therapy, doxorubicin, and 5-fluorouricil. In 98 of 180 potential patients randomized to ^{131}I antiferritin or further chemotherapy, there was no difference in response rate or survival.[266]

In a phase 2 study of ^{131}I lipiodol, the response rate of 40 patients with HCC was 48%, with all remaining patients having stability of disease. The median duration of response was 18 months, and 1- and 2-year survival rates were 90% and 60%, respectively.[269] There was no liver toxicity, but two patients developed fatal pneumonitis. In a randomized trial of ^{131}I lipiodol versus hepatic arterial cisplatin-based embolization in 142 patients with unresectable HCC, response rates and survival were similar (2-year survival, 22%).[267] The overall survival was also improved following adjuvant ^{131}I lipiodol studied in a randomized trial of 43 patients (3-year survival, 86% vs. 46%; hazard ratio, 3.1; 95% confidence interval, 1.0 to 9.9; P = .04),[201] although this trial has been criticized for ending too early.[270]

Holmium-166-chitosan complex is another therapy administered either by directly injecting the tumor (for HCC <3 cm) or using superselective arterial delivery for larger tumors. Long-term survivors were reported, with 3-year survival of 65% and 5-year survival of 51%.[271]

Challenges associated with hepatic arterial delivery of radioisotopes include the difficulty describing partial liver dosimetry, the possibility of a radiation hazard associated with lost radioisotopes, and the potential for not all the tumor being eradicated because of an inhomogeneous radiation dose distribution and/or vasculature heterogeneity. Safety of this treatment has been established, and outcomes following various hepatic arterial radioisotope therapies are excellent, providing rationale for randomized studies.

Regional Chemotherapy

A large number of encouraging reports have appeared concerning a variety of regional chemotherapies for HCC confined to the liver.[272] Much of the experience has come from Europe and Asia, where a large number of cases have allowed systematic studies to be performed. Despite the fact that increased hepatic extraction of chemotherapy has been shown for very few drugs, some drugs such as cisplatin, doxorubicin, mitomycin C, and others have been found to produce substantial objective responses when administered regionally. In contrast to the Western experience of metastatic colon cancer to the liver, few data are available on continuous hepatic arterial infusion for HCC, although recent pilot studies are suggestive.[273,274] Almost all studies have been done using bolus administration. Because almost none of the reports have stratified responses or survival based on TNM staging, it is difficult to know long-term prognosis in relation to tumor extent. Many, but not all, of the studies on regional intrahepatic arterial chemotherapy also use an embolizing agent such as lipiodol, gelatin (Gelfoam), starch (Spherex), microspheres, or polyvinyl alcohol (Ivalon).[275,276] The last is rarely used now because of increased hepatotoxicity.

Most centers in the United States now use commercially available degradable starch microspheres of defined size ranges. Consistently higher objective response rates appear to be reported for arterial administration of drugs together with some form of hepatic artery occlusion, compared with any form of systemic chemotherapy to date. The widespread use of some form of embolization (e.g., TACE) in addition to chemotherapy has added to its toxicities. These include the almost universal presence of high fever (>95%), abdominal pain (>60%), and anorexia (>60%). In addition, more than 20% of patients have increased ascites or transient elevation of transaminases. Cystic artery spasm and cholecystitis are also not uncommon.

Several studies have examined responses and survival, using mixtures of both chemotherapy and transhepatic arterial embolization or occlusion. Several studies have compared intrahepatic arterial chemotherapy, usually with addition of lipiodol and Gelfoam embolization, to either untreated controls or to embolization (with or without chemotherapy) or to other chemotherapy (Table 84.13). All of these studies used either doxorubicin or cisplatin at rather low doses when compared with what is employed systemically. None of the studies yielded response rates greater than 50%. As a consequence, few of these studies showed any survival advantage. Nonrandomized studies reported higher responses to platinum or showed greater survival, but only when compared with historical controls.[286] One study showing promising survival figures suggested decreased postresection recurrences.[198] The hepatic toxicities associated with embolization have been ameliorated by the use of degradable starch microspheres, with 50% to 60% response rates.[275,276] Similar results were achieved in a randomized study of doxorubicin and cisplatin with or without lipiodol or with doxorubicin and Gelfoam.[287,288]

Because there is no standard chemotherapy drug for HCC, combinations are used differently by different groups and often at suboptimal doses. The best strategy now is to take one step backward and find the optimum intra-arterial doses for each of our probable two current best drugs, cisplatin and doxorubicin, and then to combine a single drug at optimal dosing with an arterial-occluding agent. Once regimens that reliably and consistently induce more than 50% partial responses are available, effects on survival should be detectable. In addition, different studies report noncomparable patients. Tumor stage has been rarely given, so that different studies report responses of patients with differing tumor burdens and degrees of cirrhosis. Other reports have questioned the value of any chemotherapy added to embolization because of the lack of apparent survival advantages.[281,282] A high percentage of HCC patients die of their cirrhosis and not of their tumor. A reasonable target now should be to improve patient survival and quality of life,[289] with or without higher tumor response rates. In addition, it is not clear that the formal CT response criteria of oncologic partial responses are adequate for HCC. It appears that a loss of vascularity seen on CT without size change is also a reasonable index of loss of viability and thus tumor response to TACE.[290]

PRACTICE OF ONCOLOGY

TABLE 84.13

RANDOMIZED CLINICAL TRIALS INVOLVING TRANSHEPATIC ARTERIAL EMBOLIZATION/CHEMOEMBOLIZATION (TAE/TACE) CHEMOTHERAPY VERSUS NO TREATMENT OR OTHER LOCAL THERAPIES

Study	Agents	Effects on Survival
Pelletier et al., 1990[277]	TACE (doxorubicin + Gelfoam) vs. control (no treatment)	None
French Study[278]	TACE (cisplatin + Gelfoam) vs. control (no treatment)	None
Bruix et al., 1998[279]	TAE (coils and Gelfoam) vs. control (no treatment)	None
Pelletier et al., 1998[280]	TACE (cisplatin + lipiodol + Gelfoam) vs. control (no treatment)	None
Lo et al., 2002[281]	TACE (cisplatin + lipiodol + Gelfoam) vs. control (no treatment)	Yes (2-year survival TACE 31% vs. control 11%)
Llovet et al., 2002[282]	TACE (doxorubicin + lipiodol + Gelfoam) vs. control (no treatment) vs. TAE (Gelfoam alone)	Yes (2-year survival TACE 63% vs. control 27% vs. TAE 50%)
Ikeda et al., 2004[283]	TACE (cisplatin + lipiodol + embolization) vs. TACE (cisplatin + lipiodol)	None
Akamatsu et al., 2004[284]	TAE (lipiodol + Gelfoam) + PEI/RFA vs. PEI/RFA	None
Becker et al., 2005[285]	TACE (MMC + lipiodol + Gelfoam) + PEI vs. TACE (MMC + lipiodol + Gelfoam)	Yes (2-year survival TACE + PEI 39% vs. TACE 18%)

PEI, percutaneous ethanol injection; RFA, radiofrequency ablation; MMC, mitomycin C.

Two randomized controlled trials have shown a survival advantage for TACE, mainly in a selected subset of patients (Table 84.13).[281,282] However, these trials provide the first evidence of survival benefit for TACE, for surgically unresectable HCC. A recent systematic review and meta-analysis was performed on the trials of transarterial therapies for HCC, concluding that (1) no chemotherapeutic agent appears better than any other, (2) there is no benefit with lipiodol, and (3) transarterial embolization appears as effective as TACE.[207]

Systemic Therapy

A large number of controlled and uncontrolled clinical studies have been performed with most of the major classes of cancer chemotherapy, given intravenously as single agent or in combination (Table 84.14). Single-agent doxorubicin was one of the first agents studied, and with modest response rates (<25%). Combination gemcitabine and oxaliplatin (GEMOX) had a partial response rate of 18% and overall survival of 11.5 months in a phase 2 study of 32 patients.[291] However, these systemic therapies, and other chemotherapy combinations studied, have had no proven benefits on survival in HCC.[292,293] Furthermore, many chemotherapy agents are associated with a risk of liver toxicity, which could hasten liver failure, especially in the setting of cirrhosis. Thus, there appears to be little justification in treating patients with single or combination chemotherapy, unless in novel combinations in clinical trials.

Various other systemic therapies have been evaluated. The effects of systemic interferon therapy have been poor.[294–297] Postresection treatment with interferon has been suggested to reduce the risk of HCC recurrence. However, this outcome may have been partly due to the effect of viral suppression or viral eradication, and thus interferon is not recommended as an adjuvant therapy following HCC resection.[203,206] Similarly, tamoxifen was studied in HCC because of its low toxicity and the high male-to-female gender bias in HCC epidemiology. However, it and antiandrogens have been associated with poor response rates, and there is no support for their use from the evidence of randomized control trials.[298–302] Similarly, octreotide has been studied in HCC, with no proven benefits.

More recently, antiangiogenic agents have been studied, given the vascular nature of HCC, and that vascular endothelial growth factor (VEGF) promotes HCC development and metastasis. Increased levels of VEGF has been observed and have been associated with inferior survival.[303] Thalidomide was initially tried because of its proposed antiangiogenic properties, but results were disappointing.[304,305] A phase 2 study of GEMOX combined with bevacizumab, a monoclonal antibody inhibitor of VEGF ligand, in 33 patients resulted in a 20% partial response rate and a median survival of 9.6 months. Bevacizumab has also been investigated in other phase 2 studies.[306,307] One multi-institutional phase 2 study found 1- and 2-year survival rates of 53% and 28%, respectively, with serious bleeding occurring in 11% of patients.[308] TSU-68, an oral antiangiogenesis compound that blocks VEGFR-2, platelet-derived growth factor receptor, and fibroblast growth factor receptor, has been studied in a phase 1/2 study in Japan.[309] A phase 2 study of erlotinib, a receptor tyrosine kinase inhibitor with specificity for epidermal growth factor receptor, demonstrated a 9% response rate and median survival of 13 months.[310] Bevacizumab and erlotinib have been studied in another phase 2 study, with a median survival of 68 weeks and median progression-free survival of 39 weeks.[311]

A phase 2 study of sorafenib,[312] an oral multikinase inhibitor that has activity against Raf-1, B-Raf, VEGFR2, DGFR, c-Kit receptors, and other receptor tyrosine kinases, was performed in 137 patients with advanced HCC. The partial response rate was poor, 2.2%, yet the time to progression was 5.5 months, and median overall survival was 9.2 months, providing the basis for the SHARP (Sorafenib Hepatocellular Carcinoma Assessment Randomized Protocol) randomized trial. The SHARP trial was performed in 602 patients with advanced, predominantly hepatitis C–related, Child-Pugh A, HCC and demonstrated a survival advantage for sorafenib (n = 299) versus placebo (n = 303).[313] There was a 31% decrease in the risk of death, with a median survival of sorafenib and placebo arms of 10.7 months and 7.9 months, respectively (P = .00058). Sorafenib was also associated with a significant improvement in time to progression from 2.8 months for placebo to 5.5 months for sorafenib. Serious (grade 3 and 4) adverse events of diarrhea and hand-foot syndrome were more frequent with sorafenib (11% vs. 2% and 8% vs. 1%, respectively). Discontinuation of sorafenib because of adverse events occurred in 15% of patients. A second randomized trial conducted in Asia of predominantly hepatitis B patients confirmed a comparable hazard ratio for a survival benefit, but with substantial lower absolute benefit.[314]

In summary, sorafenib is established as the first-line treatment in patients with advanced HCC unsuitable for other established local and regional therapies. Other targeted therapies appear to have activity, and randomized trials of combinations of sorafenib with other therapies and of other targeted therapies are ongoing.

TABLE 84.14

VARIOUS NONCHEMOTHERAPY TREATMENTS FOR HEPATOCELLULAR CARCINOMA

Treatment	References
Tamoxifen	299–302, 325, 326
LHRH agonists	298
Interferon	294–297
Sandostatin	327, 328
Megestrol	329, 330
Vitamin K	331
Thalidomide	332
Interleukin-2	333
^{131}Iodine lipiodol	201, 334
^{131}Iodine ferritin	266
^{90}Yttrium microspheres	260, 335–337

LHRH, luteinizing hormone-releasing hormone.

TREATMENT OF OTHER PRIMARY LIVER TUMORS

In addition to HCC, which is the most frequent primary tumor of the liver, several other malignancies may arise in the liver (Table 84.3).

Fibrolamellar Hepatocellular Carcinoma

Fibrolamellar HCC is a rare histologic variant of HCC and differs in several respects from the usual HCC. Fibrolamellar HCC occurs in a much younger age group (peak incidence, third decade), is uncommonly associated with cirrhosis or viral hepatitis, and affects males and females equally. Additionally, a much higher percentage of patients with fibrolamellar HCC presents with positive lymph nodes than normal variant HCC.

Whether or not the diagnosis of fibrolamellar HCC portends a more favorable outcome after surgical treatment remains controversial.[315–318] As is true for essentially all malignant liver lesions, resection remains the first line of therapy. For those patients in whom the tumor is thought to be unresectable, liver transplantation provides a valuable alternative. Pinna et al.[319] described 13 patients with fibrolamellar HCC who received transplantation between 1968 and 1995 and reported 1-, 3-, and 5-year patient survival rates of approximately 90%, 75%, and 38%, respectively. Given that most patients transplanted presented with advanced disease, this is not an unacceptable survival rate, particularly given the young age of the patients. El-Gazzaz et al.[320] reported similar survival rates to those of Pinna et al.

Hepatoblastoma

Hepatoblastoma is the most common primary cancer of the liver occurring in childhood. The annual incidence of hepatoblastoma ranges from 0.5 to 1.5 cases per million children, with a peak incidence occurring within the first 2 years of life.[321] Hepatoblastoma is highly sensitive to chemotherapy and often renders unresectable tumors resectable. Surgical resection is considered the first line of therapy; however, for those tumors that cannot be converted to resectable lesions but without distant metastasis, most can be rescued with liver transplantation. Survival rates for these children after liver transplantation is excellent, with 1-, 3-, and 5-year survivals reported at 92%, 92%, and 83%, respectively.[322]

Epitheliod Hemangioendothelioma

Epithelioid hemangioendothelioma is a very rare tumor of vascular origin that can originate in the liver; it occurs predominantly in females. The tumor is often confused with other more aggressive cancers, particularly cholangiocarcinoma, angiosarcoma, and HCC. The clinical course of epithelioid hemangioendothelioma is quite variable. In the review by Makhlouf et al.,[323] 137 cases were described, and survival ranged from 4 months to 28 years. Of interest, one patient who received no treatment survived for 27 years without evidence of metastasis. Surgical resection is considered to be the treatment of choice; however, this particular cancer is often multifocal, making liver transplantation the only surgical option. The presence of metastatic disease does not seem to influence survival and should not be considered an absolute contraindication to either surgical resection or transplantation.

PRACTICE OF ONCOLOGY

Selected References

The full list of references for this chapter appears in the online version.

1. Jemal A, Siegel R, Ward E, et al. Cancer statistics, 2007. *CA Cancer J Clin* 2007;57:43.
4. Seeff LB, Hoofnagle JH. Epidemiology of hepatocellular carcinoma in areas of low hepatitis B and hepatitis C endemicity. *Oncogene* 2006;25:3771–3777.
6. Beasley RP, Hwang LY, Lin CC, Chien CS. Hepatocellular carcinoma and hepatitis B virus. A prospective study of 22 707 men in Taiwan. *Lancet* 1981;2:1129–1133.
8. Yang HI, Sherman M, Su J, et al. Nomograms for risk of hepatocellular carcinoma in patients with chronic hepatitis B virus infection. *J Clin Oncol* 2010;28:2437–2444.
10. Blum HE, Moradpour D. Viral pathogenesis of hepatocellular carcinoma. *J Gastroenterol Hepatol* 2002;17(Suppl 3):S413.
11. Farazi PA, DePinho RA. Hepatocellular carcinoma pathogenesis: from genes to environment. *Nat Rev Cancer* 2006;6:674.
12. Chen CJ, Yang HI, Su J, et al. Risk of hepatocellular carcinoma across a biological gradient of serum hepatitis B virus DNA level. *JAMA* 2006;295:65–73.
15. Yang HI, Lu SN, Liaw YF, et al. Hepatitis B e antigen and the risk of hepatocellular carcinoma. *N Engl J Med* 2002;347:168–174.
19. Lok AS, Seeff LB, Morgan TR, et al. Incidence of hepatocellular carcinoma and associated risk factors in hepatitis C-related advanced liver disease. *Gastroenterology* 2009;136:138–148.
20. Hoshida Y, Toffanin S, Lachenmayer A, et al. Molecular classification and novel targets in hepatocellular carcinoma: recent advancements. *Semin Liver Dis* 2010;30:35.
21. Villanueva A, Newell P, Chiang DY, Friedman SL, Llovet JM. Genomics and signaling pathways in hepatocellular carcinoma. *Semin Liver Dis* 2007;27:55.
29. ICGHN. Pathologic diagnosis of early hepatocellular carcinoma: a report of the international consensus group for hepatocellular neoplasia. *Hepatology* 2009;49:658–664.
34. Edge SB, Compton CC. The American Joint Committee on Cancer: the 7th edition of the AJCC cancer staging manual and the future of TNM. *Ann Surg Oncol* 2010;17:1471–1474.
36. Vauthey JN, Lauwers GY, Esnaola NF, et al. Simplified staging for hepatocellular carcinoma. *J Clin Oncol* 2002;20:1527–1536.
38. Forner A, Reig ME, de Lope CR, Bruix J. Current strategy for staging and treatment: the BCLC update and future prospects. *Semin Liver Dis* 2010;30:61–74.
41. Marsh JW, Finkelstein SD, Demetris AJ, et al. Genotyping of hepatocellular carcinoma in liver transplant recipients adds predictive power for determining recurrence-free survival. *Liver Transpl* 2003;9:664.
44. Marrero JA, Feng Z, Wang Y, et al. Alpha-fetoprotein, des-gamma carboxyprothrombin, and lectin-bound alpha-fetoprotein in early hepatocellular carcinoma. *Gastroenterology* 2009;137:110–118.
55. Forner A, Vilana R, Ayuso C, et al. Diagnosis of hepatic nodules 20 mm or smaller in cirrhosis: prospective validation of the noninvasive diagnostic criteria for hepatocellular carcinoma. *Hepatology* 2008;47:97–104.
61. Burrel M, Llovet JM, Ayuso C, et al. MRI angiography is superior to helical CT for detection of HCC prior to liver transplantation: an explant correlation. *Hepatology* 2003;38:1034.
65. Kang BK, Lim JH, Kim SH, et al. Preoperative depiction of hepatocellular carcinoma: ferumoxides-enhanced MR imaging versus triple-phase helical CT. *Radiology* 2003;226:79–85.
67. Yukisawa S, Okugawa H, Masuya Y, et al. Multidetector helical CT plus superparamagnetic iron oxide-enhanced MR imaging for focal hepatic lesions in cirrhotic liver: a comparison with multi-phase CT during hepatic arteriography. *Eur J Radiol* 2007;61:279.
69. Teefey SA, Hildeboldt CC, Dehdashti F, et al. Detection of primary hepatic malignancy in liver transplant candidates: prospective comparison of CT, MR imaging, US, and PET. *Radiology* 2003;226:533.
78. Zhang BH, Yang BH, Tang ZY. Randomized controlled trial of screening for hepatocellular carcinoma. *J Cancer Res Clin Oncol* 2004;130:417–422.
79. Lok AS, Sterling RK, Everhart JE, et al. Des-gamma-carboxy prothrombin and alpha-fetoprotein as biomarkers for the early detection of hepatocellular carcinoma. *Gastroenterology* 2010;138:493–502.
80. Forner A, Reig M, Bruix J. Alpha-fetoprotein for hepatocellular carcinoma diagnosis: the demise of a brilliant star. *Gastroenterology* 2009;137:26–29.
82. Sangiovanni A, Del Ninno E, Fasani P, et al. Increased survival of cirrhotic patients with a hepatocellular carcinoma detected during surveillance. *Gastroenterology* 2004;126:1005–1014.
84. Santagostino E, Colombo M, Rivi M, et al. A 6-month versus a 12-month surveillance for hepatocellular carcinoma in 559 hemophiliacs infected with the hepatitis C virus. *Blood* 2003;102:78–82.
88. Llovet JM, Bustamante J, Castells A, et al. Natural history of untreated nonsurgical hepatocellular carcinoma: rationale for the design and evaluation of therapeutic trials. *Hepatology* 1999;29:62–67.
91. Llovet JM, Fuster J, Bruix J. Intention-to-treat analysis of surgical treatment for early hepatocellular carcinoma: resection versus transplantation. *Hepatology* 1999;30:1434–1440.
102. Cha CH, Ruo L, Fong Y, et al. Resection of hepatocellular carcinoma in patients otherwise eligible for transplantation. *Ann Surg* 2003;238:315.
105. Vivarelli M, Guglielmi A, Ruzzenente A, et al. Surgical resection versus percutaneous radiofrequency ablation in the treatment of hepatocellular carcinoma on cirrhotic liver. *Ann Surg* 2004;240:102–107.
108. Bartlett AS, McCall JL, Koea JB, et al. Liver resection for hepatocellular carcinoma in a hepatitis B endemic area. *World J Surg* 2007;31:1775–1781.
110. Shimada K, Sakamoto Y, Esaki M, et al. Analysis of prognostic factors affecting survival after initial recurrence and treatment efficacy for recurrence in patients undergoing potentially curative hepatectomy for hepatocellular carcinoma. *Ann Surg Oncol* 2007;14:2337–2347.

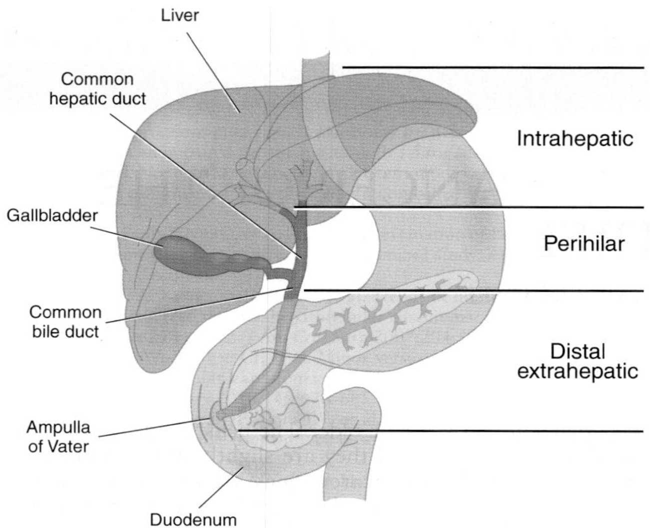

FIGURE 85.1 Terminology for biliary tract cancers based on anatomic site of involvement. (Adapted from ref. 3.)

infestation, early detection of bile duct malignancy is difficult. The prognosis if cancer develops appears similar to that reported in patients without liver fluke infestation.

Chronic calculi of the bile duct (outside the gallbladder) occurs very rarely and may predispose to cancer formation. In Southeast Asia, chronic portal bacteremia and portal phlebitis can lead to the development of intrahepatic pigmented stones. This is associated with about a 10% risk of cholangiocarcinoma. Anomalous pancreatic–biliary duct junction may lead to a chronic inflammatory state in the bile duct via reflux of pancreatic juice into the biliary tree. This has been associated with an increased risk of cholangiocarcinoma.[18]

Specific carcinogens that lead to cholangiocarcinoma have been reported. Exposure to thorotrast (thorium dioxide), a radio contrast agent used from 1930 to 1960, leads to cholangiocarcinoma after a latent period of 16 to 45 years.[19] The evidence is less clear for other environmental exposures. Cigarette smoking may increase the risk of cholangiocarcinoma.[20] Other potential carcinogens include radionuclides, radon, nitrosamines, dioxin, and asbestos. Patients with the acquired immune deficiency syndrome may have an increased risk of cholangiocarcinoma.[21] A case-control study for intrahepatic cholangiocarcinoma identified that prior bile duct disease, alcoholic liver disease, and diabetes may increase the risk of cholangiocarcinoma.[8] Obesity has also been defined as a risk factor for cholangiocarcinoma, as is true with many other cancers.[22] Recently, viral infections such as hepatitis C virus, hepatitis B virus, and even human immunodeficiency virus (HIV) have been reported as risk factors for cholangiocarcinoma.[23,24]

TABLE 85.1

RISK FACTORS FOR CHOLANGIOCARCINOMA

Primary sclerosing cholangitis (PSC)
Choledocholithiasis
Liver fluke infection
Choledochal cysts
Caroli's disease
Hepatitis C
Hepatitis B
Human immunodeficiency virus (HIV)
Cirrhosis
Biliary-enteric anastomosis
Thorotrast
Dioxin
Nitrosamines
Asbestos
Oral contraceptives
Isoniazid
Diabetes
Smoking
Obesity

Anatomy

The liver is divided into eight segments based on the blood supply and venous drainage of the liver. Bile ducts are included along with the hepatic artery and portal vein in the portal triad, which is directed to each segment of the liver. The main left hepatic duct exits the liver at the base of the umbilical fissure, and the main right hepatic duct exits the liver between segments 5 and 6. The caudate lobe drains directly into the left main hepatic duct via numerous small branches. The confluens of the right and left hepatic ducts occurs in the hilum of the liver. The cystic duct may enter the common duct near the confluens of the right and left ducts, or distally near the duodenum. It may also enter the right hepatic duct. This aspect of biliary anatomy is quite variable. The distal bile duct travels posterior within the head of the pancreas and then joins the pancreatic duct in a common channel leading to the ampulla of Vater. The type of surgery required for cholangiocarcinoma varies greatly depending on the location and extent of the tumor.

The porta hepatis consists of (from right to left) the bile duct, the portal vein, and the hepatic artery. At the hilum of the liver, the portal vein is posterior; the right hepatic artery generally passes between the common bile duct and the portal vein; and the cystic artery generally passes anterior to the bile duct. The proximity of the portal vein and hepatic artery to the bile duct leads to early vessel involvement or occlusion from cholangiocarcinoma, which affects the surgical resection options. Care must also be taken to map out the blood supply to the liver because arterial anomalies are common, and this can lead to inadvertent injury of the arterial system during dissection within the porta hepatis.

The lymph node drainage of the bile ducts involves the superior pancreaticoduodenal, retroportal, or proper hepatic nodes first, then the peripancreatic, celiac, and interaortocaval lymph nodes.[25] Lymph nodes in the porta hepatis may be difficult to remove because of attached venous branches from the portal vein or fixation of tumor-involved lymph nodes to the bile duct, portal vein, hepatic artery, or the head of the pancreas.

Pathology

More than 90% of cholangiocarcinomas are adenocarcinomas.[26] Other types, which account for less than 5% each, are squamous cell carcinomas, sarcomas, small cell cancer, and lymphomas. Local invasion within the porta hepatis is common, as well as metastatic or direct involvement of the liver and peritoneal carcinomatosis.[27] Cholangiocarcinomas may be divided into the following types: sclerosing, nodular (mass forming), or papillary, with the sclerosing type most frequently seen. The sclerosing type causes an intense desmoplastic reaction and is seen as diffuse thickening of the ducts without a defined mass. This form is the most difficult to treat. The nodular type tends to result in a mass lesion and usually arises within the liver. The papillary type is rare. It represents a low-grade adenocarcinoma

TABLE 85.2

FREQUENCY OF MUTATIONS DESCRIBED IN CHOLANGIOCARCINOMA AND GALLBLADDER CANCER

Mutated Genes	Cholangiocarcinoma	Gallbladder Cancer
ONCOGENES		
CTTNB1/β-catenin		5%–9%
K-ras	10%–54%	3%–38%
BRAF	22%	33%
EGFR	5%–20%	9%–12%
PIK3CA	9%	4%
ERBB2/Her-2	5%`	16%
SUPPRESSOR GENES		
P16Ink4A	55%–88%	31%–62%
TP53	33%–37%	36%
SMAD4	13%–55%	
STK11/LKB1	6%	

Data summarized from ref. 31.

that is represented by a polypoid mass filling the lumen of the bile duct, with minimal invasion and no desmoplastic reaction. It is associated with a favorable outcome.[28]

The reporting of cholangiocarcinoma should include the type and location of the tumor. The type often corresponds with the location. Intrahepatic forms are more likely to be nodular and mass forming, while hilar and extrahepatic cholangiocarcinomas are more likely to be sclerosing. Nevertheless, examples exist of sclerosing intrahepatic tumors and vice versa.

Histologically, cholangiocarcinomas are mucin-producing adenocarcinomas that consist of acinar and solid structures. The sclerosing type, which is the most common, is characterized by extensive fibrosis. Single tumor cells may be found within extensive fibrous stroma. The papillary form appears histologically as papillary fronds that extend into the lumen of the ducts. These may produce extracellular mucin. The nodular type demonstrates histologic heterogeneity at advanced stages. At early stages it appears similar to the sclerosing type, with abundant fibrous stroma and a tubular pattern. Satellites are common, representing spread distally down bile duct branches or invasion of small portal vein branches and metastases. Intrahepatic mass-forming nodular type cholangiocarcinomas are easily misinterpreted as metastatic cancers from other gastrointestinal primary tumors. Search for another primary tumor will be unproductive. Cytokeratin 20 staining may differentiate these tumors, as this staining is common and diffuse in colorectal cancers but focal and rare in cholangiocarcinoma.[29] The $\alpha v\beta 6$ integrin is highly expressed from cholangiocarcinoma but not hepatocellular cancer and can differentiate the two.[30]

An understanding of the molecular biology of cholangiocarcinomas is beginning to form. It is likely that the sequence of progression from normal mucosa to adenomatous hyperplasia, dysplasia, carcinoma *in situ*, and then invasive cancer takes place similar to the pathogenesis of other cancers, and that this progression is characterized by a number of genomic mutations.[31] Two precursor lesions are identified, biliary intraepithelial carcinoma neoplasia, which is more common, and intraductal papillary neoplasm of the bile duct.[31] Inflammation in PSC leads to activation of the nuclear factor κB (NF-κB) family which leads to increased tumor necrosis factor alpha (TNF-α) and interleukin-6 (IL-6). Similar to other cancers, the tumor suppressor genes *p53* and *K-ras* are mutated in the majority of biliary tract cancers.[32–35] Mutations of *Her-2/neu* and *c-met* have also been reported.[36] Autocrine growth loops have been identified, involving hepatocellular growth factor (HGF)/met and IL-6/glycoprotein 130 (gp130).[37] Alterations in the glycosylation of mucins (MUC proteins) and sialosyl-Tn antigen may be important in the pathogenesis of cholangiocarcinomas as well.[38] Table 85.2 summarizes the molecular alterations that have been described for cholangiocarcinomas. Different locations within the biliary tree may be associated with different mutations. For example, *K-ras* mutations are more common in extrahepatic cholangiocarcinomas.[39] Recently spontaneous animal models as well as engineered mouse models of cholangiocarcinoma have proved valuable and are increasingly used to understand relevant genetic events in pathogenesis and to test targeted agents for this disease.[31] In addition to genetic changes, epigenetic alterations have been described, such as hypermethylation of tumor suppressor genes and aberrant expression of microRNA.[40]

Staging

The tumor-node-metastasis (TNM) system devised by the American Joint Committee on Cancer should be used for staging cholangiocarcinoma.[41] The most recent version (seventh edition, 2010) has a number of revisions. Intrahepatic bile duct tumors are now separated from staging of primary hepatocellular cancer (Table 85.3). The TNM system for the extrahepatic potion of the bile duct has separate staging systems for perihilar bile duct (Table 85.4), and distal bile ducts (Table 85.5). It has been suggested that the TNM system is not helpful in defining surgical resectability and, therefore, may not adequately predict outcome.[27] Bismuth developed a classification system used by surgeons to define resectability and the extent of resection required for tumor eradication (Fig. 85.2). Staging that incorporates both the extent of vascular (unilateral versus bilateral) invasion and liver involvement may be most appropriate for hilar cholangiocarcinoma.[42]

Clinical Presentation

Early-stage tumors remain asymptomatic. In most patients, a diagnostic workup is initiated when there are signs and symptoms of obstruction of the biliary system. Painless jaundice is

TABLE 85.3

AMERICAN JOINT COMMITTEE ON CANCER STAGING OF INTRAHEPATIC CHOLANGIOCARCINOMA

T1 = Solitary tumor without vascular invasion
T2A = Solitary tumor with vascular invasion
T2B = multiple tumors with or without vascular invasion
T3 = Tumor perforating the visceral peritoneum or involving the local extra hepatic structures by direct invasion
T4 = Tumor with periductal invasion
N1 = Regional lymph node metastasis present
M1 = Any distant metastases

Stage I	T1	N0	M0
Stage II	T2	N0	M0
Stage III	T3	N0	M0
Stage IVA	T4	N0	M0
	Any T	N1	M0
Stage IVB	Any T	Any N	M1

Modified from ref. 41.

TABLE 85.5

AMERICAN JOINT COMMITTEE ON CANCER STAGING FOR DISTAL BILE DUCT CANCERS

T1 = Tumor confined to the bile duct histologically
T2 = Tumor invades beyond the wall of the bile duct
T3 = Tumor invades the gallbladder, pancreas, duodenum, or other adjacent organs without involvement of the celiac axis or the superior mesenteric artery
T4 = Tumor involves the celiac axis or the superior mesenteric artery
N1 = Regional lymph node metastasis
M1 = Distant metastasis

Stage IA	T1	N0	M0
Stage IB	T2	N0	M0
Stage IIA	T3	N0	M0
Stage IIB	T1-3	N1	M0
Stage III	T4	Any N	M0
Stage IV	Any T	Any N	M1

Modified from ref. 41.

most commonly a result of malignant obstruction. Pancreatic cancer is the most likely, followed by cholangiocarcinoma, then other parenchymal liver tumors. Painless jaundice is the most common complaint of patients with cholangiocarcinoma, seen in about 70% to 90% of patients, followed by pruritus (66%), abdominal pain, weight loss (30% to 50%), and fever in about 20%.[43] These symptoms, especially jaundice, tend to occur early with distal and hilar cholangiocarcinomas, but late with intrahepatic cholangiocarcinomas.[44] It is important to realize that obstruction of the right or left bile duct alone will usually not lead to jaundice or an elevated bilirubin. Other hepatic enzymes, such as alkaline phosphatase and γ-glutamyltransferase, will be markedly elevated because of cellular damage related to the obstruction, but the other lobe of the liver will compensate for the loss of bile drainage by producing enough bile to maintain a normal serum bilirubin. Over time the obstructed lobe may become atrophic, especially when the portal vein has also been blocked by the tumor. It is only when the unilateral tumor becomes large enough to cause pain or anorexia and weight loss that a diagnostic workup is initiated. The unilateral tumor may also extend down the bile ducts to involve the confluens of the right and left ducts, at which time the patient may become jaundiced.

On physical examination, a palpable liver may be noted in patients with intrahepatic cholangiocarcinoma. A palpable gallbladder, also called *Courvoisier's sign,* due to obstruction of the cystic duct (or common bile duct distal to the cystic duct), may be found. Obstruction of the bile duct and biliary stasis may lead to bacterial colonization and cholangitis. Patients with cholangitis present in a dramatic fashion, with high fever, pain, nausea, vomiting, and rigors. They will be bacteremic with typical biliary tract flora (*Escherichia coli,*

TABLE 85.4

AMERICAN JOINT COMMITTEE ON CANCER STAGING FOR PERIHILAR BILE DUCT CANCERS

T1 = Tumor confined to the bile duct, with extension up to the muscle layer or fibrous tissue

From ref. 41.

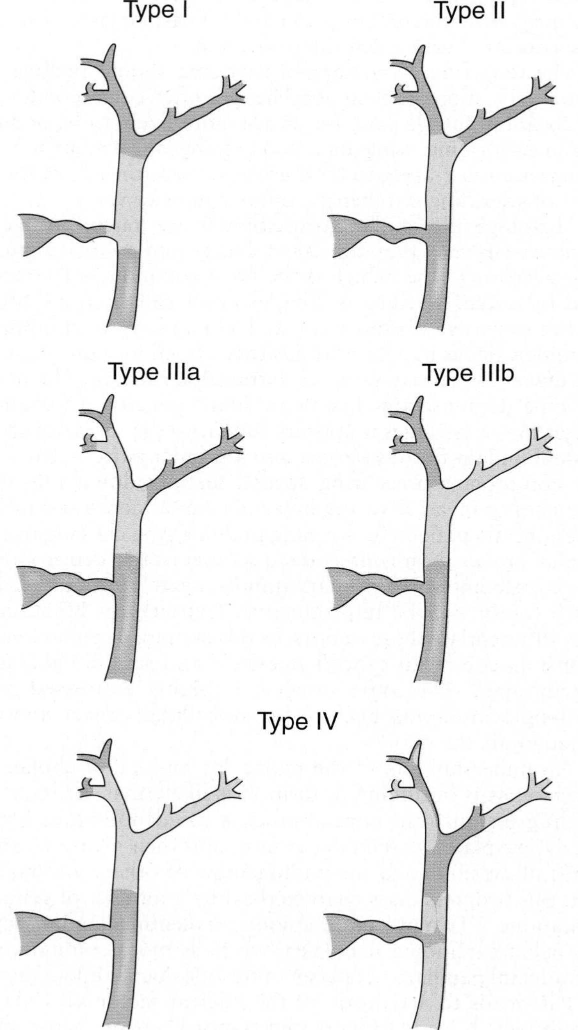

FIGURE 85.2 Bismuth classification of perihilar cholangiocarcinomas, designed to define resectability. Yellow areas represent tumor and green areas normal bile duct. (From ref. 3, with permission.)

Klebsiella, *Proteus*, *Pseudomonas aeruginosa*, *Serratia*, *Streptococcus*, and *Enterobacter*). In general, although bile is a rich medium for bacterial growth, it is sterile, and, therefore, obstruction should not lead directly to cholangitis. Once free communication is made between the gastrointestinal tract and the biliary system (as with a stent), the bile becomes contaminated and cholangitis is a more frequent problem. Patients with biliary stones are more likely to have contaminated bile and may present earlier with cholangitis in the face of biliary obstruction.

Diagnostic Evaluation

Laboratory Tests

Liver function tests generally reveal elevated markers of cholestasis—elevated bilirubin, alkaline phosphatase, and γ-glutamyltransferase. Serum aminotransferase levels may be normal or mildly elevated in the early stages. Serum tumor markers may aid in diagnosis. Serum carcinoembryonic antigen (CEA) and cancer antigen (CA) 19-9 levels are most commonly elevated in cholangiocarcinoma. CEA levels may be elevated but have a low predictive value for cholangiocarcinoma. The CEA level is therefore not helpful for diagnosis.[45] Most patients with cholangiocarcinomas have elevated CA 19-9 levels. CA 19-9 levels above 100 U/mL were found to be 89% sensitive and 86% specific for the diagnosis of bile duct carcinoma in patients with primary sclerosing cholangitis.[45] Other studies have demonstrated a lower predictive value of CA 19-9 for cholangiocarcinoma in patients with PSC.[46,47] Benign biliary tract disease may result in elevated CA 19-9 levels, and the optimal cutoff value for suspicion of cancer is not clear. High values (more than 180 U/mL) tend to be more specific at the expense of sensitivity.[45] CA 19-9 and CEA levels have also been measured in bile specimens and may be elevated in the presence of cancer.[48] A combined index of CA 19-9 and CEA has been proposed with studies showing mixed results in predicting cancer.[46] The presence of cholangitis or hepatolithiasis can cause elevations of tumor markers, and these tests should be repeated after symptoms have resolved. Also, CA 19-9 is a carbohydrate cell–surface antigen related to the Lewis blood group antigens. Patients with negative Lewis blood group antigen (representing 10% of the population) cannot synthesize CA 19-9 and cannot manifest an elevation in this marker.[49] Additional potential markers for cholangiocarcinoma include CA 242, CA 72-4, CA 50, CA 125, RCAS1, and serum MUC5AC. These have all been evaluated with mixed results.[47,50–54] CA 19-9 has also been defined as a poor prognostic factor in cholangiocarcinoma.[55]

Radiologic Evaluation

When a patient presents with jaundice or when the laboratory examination is consistent with biliary obstruction (elevated alkaline phosphatase and γ-glutamyltransferase), workup should begin with an ultrasound to rule out biliary stones as the cause. Ultrasound can be useful for the diagnosis of cholangiocarcinoma and with the addition of Doppler can aid in defining vascular invasion and thus respectability. Because it is operator dependent and difficult for the surgeon to interpret, further imaging is required. Magnetic resonance imaging (MRI)/magnetic resonance cholangiography for cholangiocarcinoma (MRCP) is an ideal imaging modality for cholangiocarcinoma (Fig. 85.3). Heavily T2-weighted MRI images of the liver and pancreas with projection images of the bile duct and pancreatic duct can provide three-dimensional images of the entire biliary tract. This is obviously less invasive for the patient and may provide better information than endoscopic retrograde cholangiography (ERCP) or percutaneous transhepatic cholangiography (PTC). In addition, associated masses and malignant thickening can be defined with the biliary obstruction. Hyperintense regions on T2-weighted MRI may be consistent with cholangiocarcinoma. If available and cost-effective, this test could replace computed tomography (CT) scans and other forms of cholangiography. The appearance and location of the bile duct stricture must be defined. Smooth, tapering strictures of the distal bile duct are more consistent with benign scarring, compared with irregular strictures at the confluens, which is more consistent with hilar cholangiocarcinoma. MRI has been demonstrated to have 66% accuracy for detection of lymph node metastases, 78% sensitivity and 91%

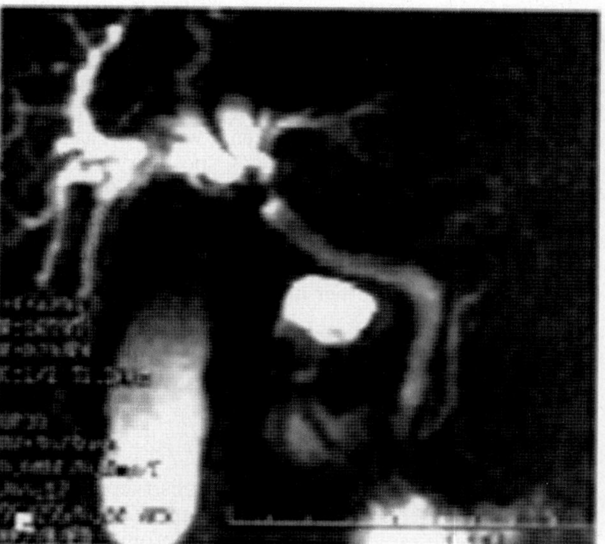

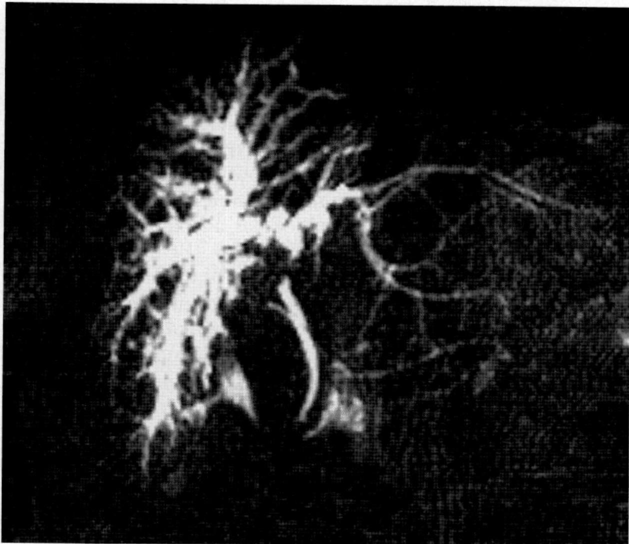

FIGURE 85.3 **A:** Magnetic resonance cholangiography for cholangiocarcinoma (MRCP) of a patient with resectable hilar cholangiocarcinoma. The *arrow* marks the clear definition of the proximal right and left main hepatic ducts. (Adapted from ref. 56.). **B:** MRCP of a patient with hilar cholangiocarcinoma. The *arrow* marks the hilum. There is no clear delineation of the main right or left hepatic ducts. This patient was explored and found to have disease which was unresectable for cure.

specificity for portal vein invasion, and 58% to 73% sensitivity and 93% specificity for arterial invasion.[9,57]

CT scan of the abdomen may be obtained as an alternative. A triple-phase helical CT scan with dynamic contrast and 5-mm cuts through the liver and head of the pancreas has 79% to 90% accuracy for the diagnosis of extrahepatic cholangiocarcinoma and 100% sensitivity and 90% specificity for portal vein invasion.[58–60] The CT scan will characteristically demonstrate thickening of the bile duct and dilated ducts proximal to the abnormality.[61] Attention should be given to associated portal vein patency and any evidence of liver atrophy. Three-dimensional reconstructions of the vascular anatomy can be performed to precisely detail the extent of vascular involvement. Three-dimensional helical CT cholangiography can also be performed to help in preoperative staging.[62] Also, attention should be given to lymphadenopathy in the periportal, celiac, and interaortocaval regions and any mass in the head of the pancreas or liver. On CT scans, intrahepatic cholangiocarcinoma usually presents as a hypodense mass with irregular margins, satellite tumors, and capsular retraction.

Once the location and characteristics of the obstruction is defined by MRCP or CT, decisions regarding the need for surgery, stenting, or biopsy should be made. In good operative candidates with resectable, atypical strictures in the absence of stones, it may be reasonable to proceed to surgery without stenting or further workup. Concern for liver failure after resection exists in patients with long-standing strictures manifested by extremely high bilirubin levels. In general, patients with bilirubin levels above 15 mg/dL will undergo biliary drainage preoperatively to allow the liver to recover before resection. For distal strictures in which a diagnosis is needed or where palliation is indicated, an ERCP is performed in which not only can the duct can be completely imaged but the obstruction can also be stented, with brushes of the duct obtained for pathologic evaluation. Hilar strictures may be managed with a PTC approach. This allows better visualization of the proximal bile ducts and a higher success rate for stenting and drainage of the biliary system. Failed stenting by ERCP can lead to severe cholangitis due to bacterial contamination of undrained bile. Some investigators have demonstrated an advantage to endoscopic nasobiliary decompression. This tube avoids the risk of sticking the liver directly and circumvents the risk of infection from duodenal contamination as seen with a standard internal drainage tube. Finally, it can be irrigated to keep it open and functioning.[63]

Although the anatomic definition of biliary obstruction can be identified with ultrasound, CT, ERCP, PTC, or MRCP, the differentiation of benign from malignant causes of obstruction can be difficult. The CA 19-9 and CEA levels can be helpful, as previously discussed. Endoscopic ultrasound may be useful for distal common bile duct cancers for defining a mass or abnormal thickening, which can direct biopsies and assess vascular invasion.[64] Positron emission tomography (PET) scans and PET/CT scans have been described as helpful in differentiating malignant from benign strictures of the bile duct; however, as with pancreatic cancer, the density of metabolically active cells in the setting of intense fibrosis is not always amenable to successful PET imaging.[65] The presence of inflammation from benign causes of biliary obstruction can provide falsely intense PET images. In a recent study, PET/CT was shown to have an overall sensitivity of 80% for identifying the primary tumor, and the results changed management in 25% of patients.[66]

Choledochoscopy and Intraductal Ultrasound

Direct visualization of the duct with directed biopsies is the ideal technique for workup of cholangiocarcinoma.[67] Techniques both at the time of ERCP or PTC have been described and developed. The technology has improved to allow biopsies to be obtained through a 1-mm port. As the technology becomes more widely available, more reports will define the utility of this technique. A visual assessment of proximal ducts at the time of PTC may be helpful to define resectability. Often, however, the tumor infiltrates within the wall of the bile duct and cannot be seen, involving the epithelium. Visual inspection may underestimate the true margin. A recent study demonstrated the utility of choledochoscopy for biliary strictures where the diagnosis was modified in 20 of 29 patients, and malignancy was demonstrated in 11 of 20 patients.[68] Intraductal ultrasound is performed by placing a probe into the bile duct using an ERCP scope. In a study of 62 patients, intraductal ultrasound had a sensitivity of 90% and specificity of 93%.[69] Another study demonstrated an increase in the diagnostic accuracy of ERCP from 58% to 90% in patients with biliary strictures.[70]

Biopsy and Cytology

Cells can be obtained for cytology using a variety of means. Bile can be collected for cytology, brushings of the bile duct can be obtained at the time of ERCP or PTC, and CT or endoscopic ultrasound-guided needle aspiration biopsy can be performed. The tumors are often hypocellular and difficult to diagnose by biopsy. A review of eight reports in the literature from 1980 to 1997 summarizes 223 cytologic examinations in patients with bile duct tumors.[71] The sensitivity for diagnosing cancer was 62%. This is unsatisfactory and leads to a resection to treat or rule out cancer regardless of the biopsy results. The consideration for neoadjuvant therapy may bring more importance to the preoperative pathologic assessment of cholangiocarcinoma. Endoscopic ultrasound-directed fine-needle aspiration has been reported to have an accuracy of 91%, sensitivity of 89%, and specificity of 100% in the diagnosis of patients with strictures at the hilum.[64] Newer techniques, such as mutational analysis of shed cells, may improve the sensitivity and usefulness of cytology. Studies have implicated *K-ras* mutations, $p16^{INK4a}/p14^{ARF}$ promoter methylation, and DNA aneuploidy as the most promising candidates for detecting early cholangiocarcinoma.[54] Using *K-ras* and fluorescence *in situ* hybridization (FISH) (for polysomy and trisomy 7) together the sensitivity for detecting cholangiocarcinoma from cytology specimens was still only 54%.[72]

Patients with primary sclerosing cholangitis have between a 10% and 36% chance of developing cholangiocarcinoma, as previously discussed. This high prevalence deserves special consideration for screening for cholangiocarcinoma, and much has been written about this. A recent study defined the optimal cutoff for serum CA 19-9 in patients with PSC as 20 U/mL, which provides a sensitivity of 78%, specificity of 67%, positive predictive value of 23%, and negative predictive value of 96%.[73] In addition to following serum CA 19-9, special consideration should be made for choledochoscopic biopsies and bile cytologic assessment of aneuploidy, *K-ras* mutations, promoter methylation, or other molecular assessments.[13,74]

Surgery for Cholangiocarcinoma

Preoperative Stenting of the Bile Duct

The utility of preoperative stenting for obstructive jaundice in the setting of resectable tumors is controversial. The major advantage is the rapid palliation of symptoms, the potential utility of transhepatic stents as postoperative stents,[75] and the potential decrease in the risk of postoperative liver failure. The disadvantage is the subsequent bacterial colonization of bile that leads to cholangitis, which may delay surgery or increase the risk of infectious complications postoperatively.[76] The stent itself may lead to a dense fibrous reaction that can be difficult to differentiate from the tumor. The common utilization of MRCP as a diagnostic modality and the ability to move rapidly to surgical resection could alleviate the need for more invasive cholangiography and stenting.

Five randomized trials have been performed to determine whether preoperative stenting is beneficial, and no benefit was demonstrated in these trials. Retrospective studies suggest a disadvantage to preoperative stenting, and a recent review and meta-analysis defined no advantage to preoperative stenting.[77] As flaws exist in all studies and all cases are not represented, questions remain for patients with high bilirubin levels (more than 10 mcg/dL) who undergo major hepatic resection as to whether preoperative stenting would decrease the risk of postoperative liver failure. As discussed earlier, there remains controversy over the best drainage method: percutaneous, endoscopic, or nasobiliary.

Intrahepatic Cholangiocarcinoma

The long-term results and natural history of surgery for intrahepatic cholangiocarcinomas are difficult to define because of its rarity; therefore, the indications for resectability are not well described. Subsequently, resectability is determined based on anatomic considerations. Intrahepatic metastases tend to occur as multiple satellites, and although their presence impacts prognosis, it should not define resectability (Fig. 85.4).

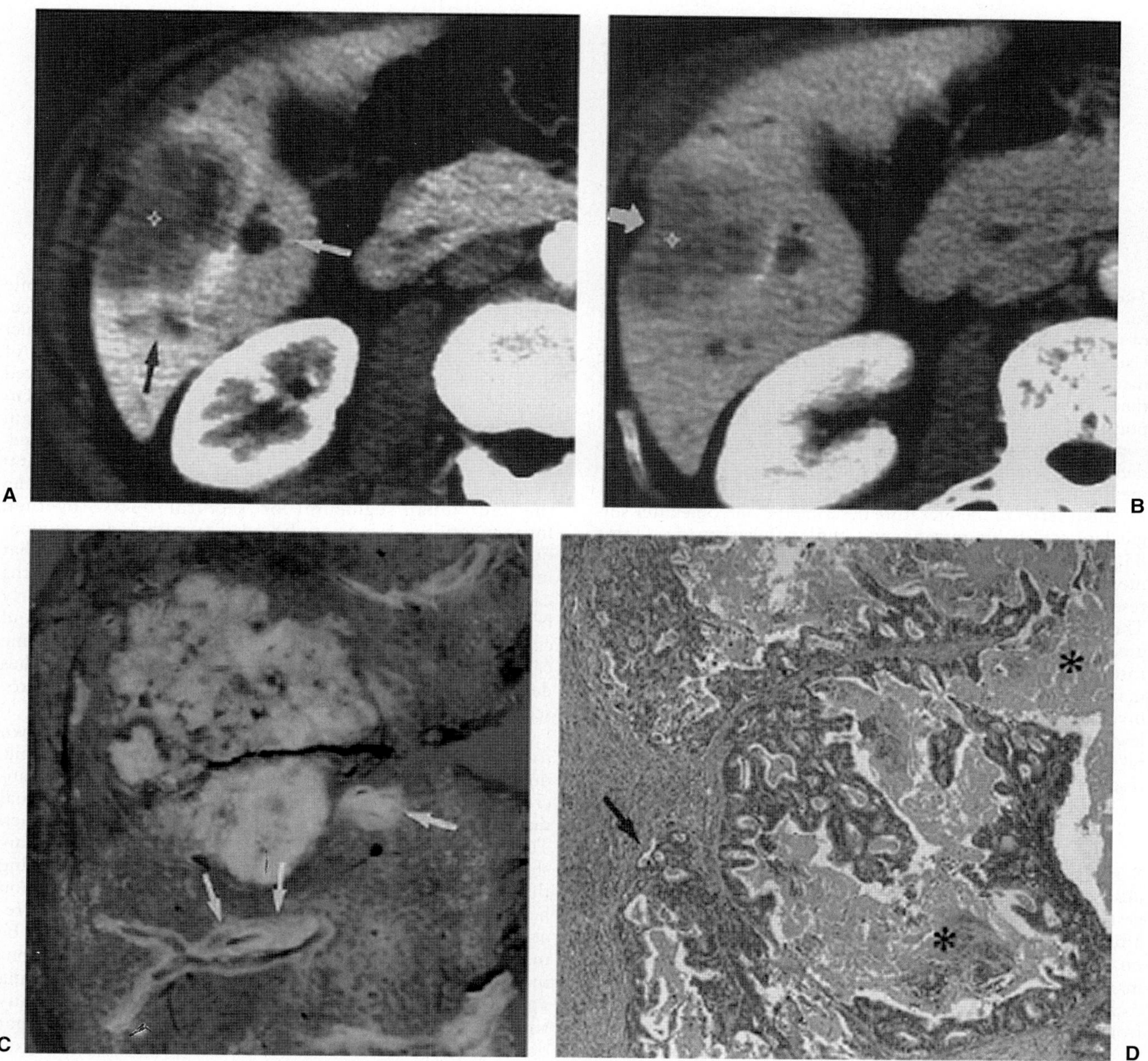

FIGURE 85.4 Intrahepatic cholangiocarcinoma. **A:** Arterial phase computed tomography (CT) scan demonstrating classic ring enhancement, central necrosis (*star*), satellitosis (*white arrow*), and dilated, thickened peripheral biliary ducts (*black arrow*). **B:** Portal venous phase CT scan demonstrates loss of enhancement, central necrosis (*star*), and dimpling of the surface of the liver (*arrow*). **C:** Gross pathologic photo of specimen demonstrating satellitosis and diffuse fibrous thickening of the peripheral bile ducts (*arrows*). **D:** Low-power microscopy with hematoxylin-eosin staining of same specimen demonstrating extensive necrosis (*star*) and invasion into the hepatic parenchyma (*arrow*). (From ref. 60, with permission.)

TABLE 85.6

PATIENT OUTCOME AFTER SURGICAL RESECTION FOR INTRAHEPATIC CHOLANGIOCARCINOMA

Study (Ref.)	Published Year	No. of Patients	Median Survival (months)	5-Year Survival (%)
Shimada et al. (79)	2001	49	26	28
Weber et al. (80)	2001	33	37	—
Ebata et al. (81)	2003	160	—	28
Ohtsuka et al. (82)	2003	50	26	23
Uenishi et al. (83)	2003	54	—	17
DeOliveira et al. (2)	2007	34	25	40
Hasegawa et al. (84)	2007	49	—	40
Paik et al. (85)	2008	97	—	31
Konstadoulakis et al. (86)	2008	54	—	25
Nakagohri et al. (87)	2008	56	—	32
Tamandl et al. (88)	2008	74	—	28
Endo et al. (89)	2008	82	36	—
Nathan et al. (90)	2009	598	—	18
Lang et al. (91)	2009	83	—	21
Choi et al. (92)	2009	64	—	39
Shimada et al. (93)	2009	104	—	34

The goal of resection is to remove all liver parenchyma at risk for intrahepatic metastases based on the most proximal extent of the tumor, while preserving adequate hepatic parenchyma. Usually this requires a lobectomy. For widespread hepatic metastases, curative resection is unlikely, and other forms of therapy should be considered. Extrahepatic spread portends a poor prognosis, and carcinomatosis should be considered a contraindication to resection. Staging laparoscopy can help define respectability prior to a full laparotomy and is recommended.[78]

Small series in the literature describe the outcome after surgical resection for intrahepatic cholangiocarcinoma (Table 85.6). The resectability rate ranges from 32% to 90%. The mortality of resection is slightly higher than series of hepatic resection for other indications, but is generally less than 10%. The median survival after resection for intrahepatic cholangiocarcinoma ranges from 15 to 59 months. Five-year survival rates range from 17% to 40%. Prognostic factors include margin status, satellite metastases, nodal metastases, vascular invasion (hepatic vein or portal vein), tumor size, and CA 19-9 level greater than 1,000. Although rare, intrahepatic intraductal papillary tumors have an excellent prognosis if completely resected.[94,95]

Hilar Cholangiocarcinoma

Surgery is indicated for hilar cholangiocarcinoma in the absence of distant metastases where preoperative workup suggests that an R0 resection is feasible. Periportal lymphadenopathy is not a contraindication, and resection with microscopic positive margins (R1) can provide significant palliation. The margin status will not be defined until the specimen is out and frozen-section pathology is examined. In a recent large series from 2001 to 2008, of 118 patients referred for surgery, 51% were resectable and 41% underwent R0 resection.[96] The surgical management of hilar cholangiocarcinoma is complex, usually requiring an *en bloc* resection of at least one lobe of the liver, the extrahepatic bile duct, and a complete periportal lymphadenectomy. The intraoperative assessment of extent of disease can be difficult because of the chronic inflammation that is associated with chronic biliary obstruction and the presence of a stent.

Based on preoperative assessment of the proximal bile ducts, a plan should be in place regarding the extent of resection. This usually involves hepatic lobectomy where the duct is abnormal past the first sectoral or segmental branches of the main right or left hepatic duct. The contralateral preserved bile duct should be transected at the level of the first segmental branch. This maximizes the chance of a negative margin while maintaining adequate drainage of the lobe. It is sometimes possible to extend the resection into the segmental branches, then re-create a main drainage channel by suturing the individual segmental or sectoral ducts together. Intraoperative decisions can be aided by pathologic examination of the transected duct margins. In the case of tumor that involves the left main hepatic duct, careful assessment of the caudate lobe branches needs to be made. Several early branches of the left hepatic duct drain the caudate lobe and can be involved early with tumor. Consideration for routine caudate lobectomy should be made in these cases.[97] Studies demonstrate that 46% of hilar cholangiocarcinomas microscopically involve the caudate lobe.[98]

The entire extrahepatic bile duct should be resected down to the level of the duodenum. A frozen section of the distal bile duct should be obtained for determination of margins. A pancreaticoduodenectomy may be required if the only residual disease is the distal intrapancreatic portion of the bile duct. This is rare for hilar cholangiocarcinoma. Lymphadenectomy should include all soft tissue in the porta hepatis, excluding the portal vein and hepatic artery. Assessment of the common hepatic artery nodes, the celiac artery nodes, the peripancreatic nodes, and the interaortocaval lymph nodes should be made. Under some circumstances, dissection of these regions may be indicated. The optimal node number for staging appears to be seven for hilar cholangiocarcinoma.[99] Many single-institution studies (mostly retrospective) exist that describe the results of surgical resection for hilar cholangiocarcinoma (Table 85.7). Approximately one-third of patients who present with the suspected diagnosis of cholangiocarcinoma will have resectable disease.[12] Operative mortality averaged about 8%, indicating the high-risk population that this tumor affects and the complexity of the procedure.[112] Ten percent to 35% of patients survived 5 years after surgical resection. Recurrences occurred most commonly at the bed of

TABLE 85.7

PATIENT OUTCOME AFTER SURGICAL RESECTION FOR HILAR CHOLANGIOCARCINOMA

Study (Ref.)	Published Year	No. of Patients	Median Survival (months)	5-Year Survival (%)
Gazzaniga et al. (100)	2000	74	17	11
Launois et al. (101)	2000	82[a]	22	10
Lee et al. (102)	2000	111[b]	37	22
Nimura et al. (97)	2000	142	25	21
Jarnagin et al. (42)	2001	80	—	—
Kawarada et al. (103)	2002	87	15	26
Kondo et al. (104)	2004	40	—	—
Rea et al. (105)	2004	46	—	26
Nishio et al. (106)	2005	301	—	22
Dinant et al. (107)	2006	99	—	27
Abdel et al. (108)	2006	73	—	13
DeOliveira et al. (2)	2007	173	14	10
Rocha et al. (96)	2009	48	74[c]	—
Miyazaki et al. (108)	2009	107	—	33
Shimizu et al. (110)	2010	224	—	29
Unno et al. (111)	2010	125	27	35

[a]Perioperative deaths excluded.
[b]Only examines those treated with liver resection, and median follow-up only 16 months.
[c]Only includes R0 resections.

PRACTICE OF ONCOLOGY

resection, followed by retroperitoneal lymph nodes. Distant metastases occur in one-third of cases. The most common sites are the lung or mediastinum, liver, and peritoneum. Comparisons of outcome over time suggest improved outcome in more recent series as a result of routine inclusion of liver resection. Prognostic factors for survival include negative microscopic margin status, lymph node metastases, tumor size, tumor grade, preoperative serum albumin, hepatic resection, and postoperative sepsis.[75,113] Even with positive microscopic margins, 5-year survival can be seen in up to 21% of cases.[114]

Distal Cholangiocarcinoma

The indication for resection of distal cholangiocarcinoma is the presence of any locally confined tumors without major vascular involvement or distant metastases. Extrahepatic cholangiocarcinoma not involving the confluens of the right and left main hepatic ducts involves the common hepatic duct and commonly involves the intrapancreatic portion of the duct. Complete surgical clearance of disease usually requires a pancreaticoduodenectomy with resection of the extrahepatic bile duct to the level of the confluens. Rarely the tumor may be confined to a small region of the duct, and an extrahepatic bile duct resection can then be performed without a pancreaticoduodenectomy. Intraoperative assessment with the help of the pathologist must dictate the extent of resection. In any case, the resection should again include a complete clearance of the peripancreatic and periportal lymph nodes with examination and consideration for resection of interaortocaval lymph nodes. For extensive involvement of the bile duct without distant spread, consideration can be made for *en bloc* combined hepatic and pancreatic resections. The morbidity of such extensive surgery is high, and the overall prognosis is poor with extensive disease, so careful consideration needs to be made before embarking on such extensive surgery.[97]

The incidence of distal common bile duct tumors compared with hilar cholangiocarcinomas is low, but the resectability rate is higher (89%).[109] A pancreaticoduodenectomy has a reasonable chance of providing a margin-negative resection for tumors of the distal bile duct. They less frequently involve the portal vein and are not limited by the liver involvement, as is seen with hilar cholangiocarcinomas. The risk of pancreaticoduodenectomy and distal bile duct resection is high, with morbidity rates between 40% and 60% and mortality rates between 2% and 10%. Probably because of the higher rate of resectability with negative margins, the outcome is improved although still poor. Median survival is expected to be between 18 and 36 months, and expected 5-year survival is between 23% and 50% (Table 85.8). Prognostic factors for poor survival include high p53 expression, nodal mets, positive margins, pancreatic invasion, and perineural invasion.[117,118]

Follow-Up after Resection

No clear guidelines exist for surveillance and follow-up after surgery. A physical examination with routine laboratory tests every 3 to 4 months for the first 3 years after surgery and then at longer interval of 6 months until year 5 is reasonable. The role of CA 19-9 as a surveillance indicator is not clear, but persistently rising levels often precede radiologic evidence of recurrence by a number of months. The role of CT scans for surveillance has not been evaluated in clinical trials, but because of the high risk of recurrence, radiological evaluation with CT scans of the abdomen every 6 months for 2 to 3 years after surgery may detect recurrent disease. In a recent study, PET/CT demonstrated a higher positive predictive value compared to CT alone (94% vs. 78%) for nodal metastases and a higher sensitivity (95% vs. 63%) for distant metastases.[120]

The pattern of failure after curative resection includes peritoneal spread, hepatic metastases, local extrahepatic recurrence, and distant metastases (most commonly lung). As with pancreatic, gallbladder, and hepatocellular cancer, cholangiocarcinomas have a propensity to seed and can recur in needle biopsy tracts, abdominal wall incision wounds, and the peritoneal cavity. Surgery is generally not indicated for recurrent cholangiocarcinoma. Close surveillance and early diagnosis of

TABLE 85.8

PATIENT OUTCOME AFTER SURGICAL RESECTION FOR DISTAL CHOLANGIOCARCINOMA

Study (Ref.)	Published Year	No. of Patients	Median Survival (months)	5-Year Survival (%)
Sasaki et al. (115)	2001	59	—	34
Yoshida et al. (116)	2002	26	20	37
DeOliveira et al. (2)	2007	229	18	23
Cheng et al. (117)	2007	112	36	25
Murakami et al. (118)	2007	36	—	50
Shimizu et al. (119)	2008	34	—	45

[a]Represents mean survival.
[b]Three-year survival.

recurrences may allow for eligibility for clinical trials, which may someday improve the outcome for this disease.

Adjuvant Therapy

The role of preoperative chemotherapy and radiation in cholangiocarcinomas remains investigational. This may be an option for patients with marginally resectable cancers; however, down-staging of a categorically unresectable cancer to an operable state, rarely, if ever occurs.[121,122] Newer regimens and biologic agents that are demonstrated to be effective in therapeutic trials for unresectable disease may find a role as a neoadjuvant treatment.

In general, postoperative adjuvant radiotherapy is administered after resection with curative intent to reduce the risk of local recurrence and potentially improve survival. Extrahepatic cholangiocarcinomas are characterized by a high rate of distant metastases as well as a very high rate of locoregional recurrence.[123] Postoperative adjuvant radiotherapy for biliary tract cancer can be administered either by external-beam radiotherapy (EBRT), brachytherapy, intraoperative radiotherapy (IORT), or a combination of radiotherapy modalities. EBRT is the most commonly used radiotherapy modality for biliary tract cancer. Advantages of EBRT include the widespread availability of this modality, its noninvasive nature, and the ability to deliver a homogeneous high dose to a large volume. Most commonly, radiotherapy is administered in a continuous course during 5 to 6 weeks. In most series, EBRT has been used to deliver a dose of 40 to 50 Gy (at 1.80 Gy/d) to the tumor bed and draining lymph node basin. In some series, a smaller volume (boost) was treated with additional EBRT, intraluminal brachytherapy, or IORT to a total dose of 60 Gy or more.

The targets for postoperative radiotherapy include the tumor bed and regional draining lymph node basin. Lymph from the gallbladder flows mainly through the cholecystoretropancreatic pathway, along the common bile duct to the superior retropancreaticoduodenal node or the retroportal node.[25] In approximately 50% of patients, the cholecystoceliac pathway drains lymph through the hepatoduodenal ligament to the celiac nodes. The posterior common hepatic node is the most prominent node on this pathway. The cholecystomesenteric pathway is another route by which some of the lymphatics run to the left in front of the portal vein and connect with the nodes at the superior mesenteric root. These three pathways converge with the aortocaval lymph nodes near the left renal vein. In addition, in approximately 20% of patients lymph ascends toward the hepatic hilum.

The upper abdomen contains a number of organs with relative low tolerance to radiation, such as the spinal cord, kidneys, liver, stomach, duodenum, and small bowel. The tolerance of these at-risk organs poses significant limitations to the dose used in postoperative radiotherapy of biliary cancers. Modern techniques, such as intensity-modulated radiation therapy, which can simultaneously reduce dose to normal structures and increase dose in the target volume, might prove beneficial.

The relative ease of placing a catheter through which radioactive sources can be placed into the involved portion of the biliary tract makes brachytherapy an attractive modality for treating a localized portion of the biliary tract. Brachytherapy has been used to administer a boost after EBRT or as the only form of radiotherapy for biliary tract tumors. A typical boost dose is 15 to 20 Gy at 0.5 to 1.0 cm from the sources over several days or, when the high-dose after-loading method is used, 5 Gy daily for 3 days. Higher doses have been used but caution should be exercised as the benefit of brachytherapy is questionable.[124] Brachytherapy has the advantage of providing a high dose to a localized, relatively small volume over several days. However, the disadvantage is that the falloff in dose is rather rapid. Thus, although a high dose is administered to the tissue immediately adjacent to the radioactive sources, the periphery of a larger tumor may be underdosed. Also, the insertion of a catheter into the biliary tract increases the risk of cholangitis and hemorrhage.

IORT, in which a single dose of radiation is administered using an electron beam at the time of surgery, usually immediately after resection and before closure of the abdominal cavity, offers the theoretical advantage of being able to deliver a high dose of radiation, usually more than 20 Gy, to the operative bed while at the same time sensitive structures such as the stomach and small intestine are displaced away from the beam. However, IORT presents a logistical problem unless a linear accelerator with high-energy electron-beam capabilities is situated within, or very close to, the operating room. This, as well as the lack of randomized clinical trials demonstrating benefit, has precluded the widespread use of IORT.

Extrahepatic cholangiocarcinoma is a rare disease, usually presenting at an advanced stage, precluding curative resection. Consequently, the efficacy of adjuvant radiotherapy has never been evaluated in prospective randomized trials. Data on the use of adjuvant radiotherapy for biliary tract cancer are derived from small retrospective reviews that include heterogeneous patient populations treated with a wide variety of modalities and techniques. Table 85.9 provides a summary of these reports with an emphasis on series that attempted to address the role of adjuvant radiotherapy.

TABLE 85.9

ADJUVANT RADIOTHERAPY OR CHEMORADIOTHERAPY FOR EXTRAHEPATIC CHOLANGIOCARCINOMA

Study (Ref.)	No. of Patients	R0 (%)	Radiotherapy	Chemotherapy	Locoregional Failure (%)	Median Survival (months)	P-Value
Kim et al. (125)	72	65	EBRT 40 Gy (split course, in 6 weeks)	Bolus 5-FU	47	25	—
Todoroki et al. (126)	29	4	IORT 21 Gy, EBRT 43 Gy, or the combination	None	20	32	.01
	20		No radiation	None	69	10	
Schoenthaler et al. (127)	6	0	EBRT 54 Gy, 1.8 Gy/fraction	None	—	21.5	.01
	15	60	No radiation	None		16	
Sagawa et al. (128)	39	49	EBRT 37 Gy + ILBT 37 Gy or EBRT 38 Gy	None	—	23	NS
	30		No radiation	None		20	
Gerhards et al. (124)	71	14	EBRT 46 Gy or EBRT 42 Gy + ILBT 10 Gy	None	—	24	<.01
	20		No radiation	None		8	
Pitt et al. (129)	14	68	EBRT ± Ir-192 13 Gy	None	—	20	NS
	17		No radiation	None		20	
Nakeeb et al. (130)	42	75	EBRT (no details)	Bolus and CI 5-FU; gemcitabine	—	16.4	—
Ben-David et al. (123)[b]	28	43	EBRT 54 Gy (median)	54% of patients; 5-FU, gemcitabine, floxuridine, bromodeoxyuridine	39	24.1 (R0) 15 (R1)	—

R0, resection with negative margins; EBRT, external-beam radiation therapy; CI, continuous infusion; 5-FU, 5-fluorouracil; IORT, intraoperative radiotherapy; ILBT, intraluminal brachytherapy; NS, not significant; R1, resection with microscopically positive margins.
[a]Includes patients with gallbladder cancer and intrahepatic cholangiocarcinoma.
[b]Includes patients with gallbladder cancer.

Most retrospective reviews of chemoradiotherapy have suggested superior outcomes for patients who receive adjuvant therapy.[130–134] In one randomized study, Klinkenbijl et al.[135] evaluated the effectiveness of adjuvant chemoradiotherapy for periampullary tumors. In this study, periampullary tumors were stratified separately from pancreatic cancers, and, following surgery, patients were randomized to observation or chemoradiation with 5-fluorouracil (5-FU). There were a total of 93 patients with periampullary tumors in this study; however, no differences in outcome were seen with adjuvant therapy.

Kim et al.[125] reported on a series of patients with hilar and distal cholangiocarcinoma treated between 1982 and 1994 with surgery and postoperative radiotherapy. Seventy-two patients had a gross total resection and margins of resection were negative in 47 (65%). Seventy-one patients were treated with a split-course regimen consisting of 20 Gy in ten fractions followed by a 2-week rest and then an additional 20 Gy in ten fractions using 10 × 10 cm anterior-posterior fields with blocks. Bolus 5-FU was given for the first 3 days of each course. The 5-year survival rates were 36%, 35%, and 0% for patients with complete surgical resection (R0), resection with microscopic residual tumor (R1), and resection with gross residual disease (R2), and the median survival times for these same groups were 25, 24, and 13 months, respectively. The observation that the 5-year survival rates and median survival times were equivalent for R1 and R0 patients suggests that postoperative adjuvant radiotherapy may have improved the outcome for the patients with microscopic residual tumor.

Todoroki et al.[126] reported on 63 patients with cholangiocarcinoma involving the main hepatic duct. Forty-nine patients had a potentially curative resection (2 R0 and 47 R1 resections) and of these, 29 were treated with adjuvant radiotherapy. Seventeen of the 29 were treated by both IORT and postoperative EBRT, 6 patients underwent resection and IORT, and 6 underwent resection and postoperative EBRT. IORT was administered using high-energy electron beams to a dose of 27.5 or 35 Gy. After observing a high complication rate, the investigators reduced the dose of IORT to 20 Gy and the electron energy beam to 8 MeV (from 16 or 18 MeV). The field diameter was also reduced to less than 6 cm. Subsequently, there were no severe complications related to the IORT. The median EBRT dose was 43.6 Gy in 1.8 to 3 Gy fractions. No description of the EBRT fields was provided. The 5-year survival rate after treatment with IORT and postoperative EBRT after resection was 39.2% compared with 16.7% for IORT alone and 0% for EBRT alone. The 5-year survival rate for patients treated with IORT and EBRT after resection was statistically significantly improved compared with that for patients undergoing resection alone (39.2% vs. 13.5%).

Gerhards et al.[124] reported on 91 patients with resectable hilar cholangiocarcinoma who were treated with either EBRT (30 patients, 46 Gy ± 11 Gy), a combination of EBRT (41 patients, 42 Gy ± 5 Gy) with intraluminal brachytherapy (20 patients, 10 Gy ± 2 Gy), or were observed with no further treatment. Only 14% of these patients had R0 resections. The median survival was superior in the adjuvant radiation arm (24 months vs. 8 months, respectively; $P < .01$).

Nakeeb et al.[130] reported on 44 patients who underwent resection of biliary malignancies (intrahepatic, perihilar, distal choledochal, and gallbladder). Of these, 42 received adjuvant chemotherapy (bolus and continuous 5-FU; gemcitabine) and EBRT. No details regarding radiotherapy were provided. The authors reported a median survival of 16.4 months in these patients.

PRACTICE OF ONCOLOGY

Ben-David et al.[123] reported on 28 patients who underwent resection of biliary malignancies and received adjuvant radiotherapy or chemoradiotherapy. Chemotherapy was given to 54% of patients and consisted mostly of 5-FU–based regimes. Some patients were treated with gemcitabine, floxuridine, or bromodeoxyuridine on institutional protocols. The median EBRT dose was 54 Gy. The median survival after R0 and R1 resections was 24.1 months and 15 months, respectively. Interestingly, there was no significant difference in survival between patients with microscopically positive margins and unresectable patients or those with grossly positive margins. It was suggested that surgery should be contemplated only when an R0 resection is likely and that borderline resectable patients might be better served by neoadjuvant therapy.

Nelson et al.[136] reported on 45 patients (13 with proximal duct and 32 with distal disease) who underwent resection plus radiotherapy (median dose 50.4 Gy). All but one patient received concurrent fluoropyrimidine-based chemotherapy. Of these, 33 underwent adjuvant radiotherapy, and 12 were treated neoadjuvantly. The 5-year actuarial overall survival, metastasis-free survival, and locoregional control rates were 33%, 42%, and 78%, respectively. The median survival was 34 months. Patients undergoing R0 resection had a significantly improved rate of local control but no survival advantage. Patients treated neoadjuvantly had a longer survival (5-year survival 53% vs. 23%; $P = .16$) and similar surgical morbidity. The authors suggested a possible local control benefit from adjuvant chemoradiotherapy and advocated a neoadjuvant approach.

Two analyses of the Surveillance, Epidemiology, and End Results (SEER) database were published recently. In one, 4,758 patients with extrahepatic cholangiocarcinoma were identified who underwent surgery (28.8%), surgery and radiotherapy (14.7%), radiotherapy alone (10%), and no therapy (46.4%).[137] The median overall survival time was significantly better in the surgery and radiotherapy group compared to surgery alone (16 months and 9 months, respectively; $P < .0001$). However, in a multivariate analysis, after adjusting for age, race, stage, and year of diagnosis, no significant improvement was found. There was also a significant survival benefit for palliative radiotherapy compared to no therapy (9 months vs. 4 months, respectively; $P < .0001$). In the other publication only 1,569 patients treated during the same time period were identified.[138] Median overall survival was 25 months for total or radical resection alone, 25 months for subtotal or debulking resection plus radiotherapy, 21 months for subtotal or debulking resection, 12 months for radiotherapy alone, and 9 months for those not receiving surgery or radiotherapy. The authors noted an early advantage but a late detriment to adjuvant radiotherapy.

Others have also not been able to demonstrate a survival advantage for adjuvant radiotherapy. Sagawa et al.[128] demonstrated similar outcomes with or without adjuvant radiation therapy in patients who underwent potentially curative resection (median survival of 23 months compared with 20 months, respectively).

In summary, despite the lack of conclusive evidence in support of adjuvant therapy, the authors recommend chemoradiotherapy for patients who have had a resection with curative intent, especially when the tumor has invaded into or through the muscularis layer, the margins of resection are involved, or regional lymph nodes are involved. Because of the small numbers of patients in reported series, possible selection bias, and lack of randomized data that show a benefit, routine adjuvant therapy cannot be considered standard. The authors recommend enrolling these patients in active clinical trials to examine the role of adjuvant therapy in this patient population. Newer regimens need to be explored. A common regimen used at the University of Michigan consists of four cycles of chemotherapy (gemcitabine 1,000 mg/m^2 intravenously for 30 minutes, days 1 and 8, and capecitabine 1,500 mg/m^2 daily in two divided doses, days 1 to 14, every 21 days) followed by chemoradiotherapy. A total of 54 to 60 Gy in 1.8- to 2-Gy daily fractions (five times per week) is delivered concurrently with capecitabine (1,330 mg/m^2 daily). Initially 45 Gy is delivered to the tumor bed and regional lymph node basin. This is followed by a boost dose of 9 to 15 Gy to the tumor bed. Three-dimensional CT-based treatment planning or intensity-modulated radiotherapy (IMRT) is used in all patients.

The role of adjuvant chemotherapy without radiation is even less clear. Because of the lack of randomized studies, there are few data on which to base treatment recommendations for adjuvant therapy, and clearly more studies are warranted. Only one randomized study has been published, evaluating the effect of chemotherapy alone after surgery. Takeda et al.[139] conducted a randomized study of chemotherapy consisting of mitomycin C and 5-FU compared with observation alone in patients with resected pancreaticobiliary cancers. A total of 508 patients were entered after surgery, with sites of disease being pancreas (n = 173), bile duct (n = 139), gallbladder (n = 140), and ampulla of Vater (n = 56). There were no apparent differences in 5-year disease-free survival or overall survival for patients with pancreatic, bile duct, or ampulla of Vater carcinomas. However, patients with gallbladder cancer had a significantly better 5-year survival with chemotherapy. Although when an intent-to-treat analysis was applied, the survival differences were no longer apparent.

Advanced Disease

Palliative Procedures

The prognosis for advanced cholangiocarcinoma is dismal. A recent review of 1,377 cases of cholangiocarcinoma undergoing palliative treatment alone revealed a median survival of 3.9 months, ranging from 3.0 months for intrahepatic cholangiocarcinoma to 5.9 months for hilar cholangiocarcinoma.[140] The goal of palliation for bile duct tumors is drainage of the biliary system to avoid jaundice. In many cases, patients will die of liver failure as a direct result of inadequate biliary drainage. The hepatocytes would otherwise function normally. In most cases it is unnecessary to drain both sides of the liver. However, this depends on the level of baseline hepatic dysfunction and any atrophy caused by long-term biliary obstruction or concomitant portal vein obstruction. Drainage of the bile ducts can be performed using ERCP-placed stents, PTC-placed stents, or with surgical bypass techniques.[141]

Hilar cholangiocarcinomas are best palliated using PTC-placed stents. An attempt should be made to drain the most functional lobe of the liver with a stent that traverses the malignant obstruction and allows for internal drainage. The catheter will exit the skin but can remain capped. This allows for irrigation and easy access for cholangiography and stent changes as needed. The downside is the exposed catheter that can be a factor in diminishing quality of life. Occasionally, a second stent draining the opposite lobe may be required to achieve normalization of bilirubin levels. Bilateral stents should not be performed routinely but considered if a unilateral stent is unsuccessful. A small, multicentered, randomized controlled trial was performed comparing PTC stents alone with PTC stents plus photodynamic therapy (39 patients total). Patients who received photodynamic therapy survived 493 days compared with 98 days for those treated with stenting alone.[142] This suggests a role for photodynamic therapy in these patients.

Operative drainage procedures for hilar cholangiocarcinomas can be technically challenging but quite effective. The best long-term palliation is performed using a bypass to intraparenchymal bile ducts, using a defunctionalized limb of jejunum. The segment 3 bile duct can be accessed through the liver parenchyma anteriorly, staying well away from the hilar region, which will be at risk from cancer progression.[143] The right lobe can be drained by a bypass to the anterior sectoral bile duct. Either bypass should be sufficient to avoid jaundice and maintain liver function. The obvious downside of operative drainage is the morbidity and recovery from surgery when overall life expectancy is limited. The best time for operative drainage would be at the time of exploration for presumed resectable tumors. The "cost" of surgery has already been paid, and the additional morbidity of the bypass is acceptable. The advantage of surgical bypass is the avoidance of long-term catheter presence within the bile duct, which leads to sludge and intermittent cholangitis. Cholangitis is a significant cause of morbidity and mortality in patients with cholangiocarcinoma.

Distal bile duct tumors can be successfully palliated with an ERCP-placed stent, which allows for completely internal drainage. Silastic stents need to be replaced every 3 months for best results and to minimize cholangitis.[144] This requires repeated endoscopy procedures. Surgical bypass to the common bile duct is easier than with hilar cholangiocarcinoma and as successful, but it still requires the morbidity and recovery of a laparotomy and bowel anastomosis. Again, this is best considered at the time of exploration for presumed resectable disease. Laparoscopic bypass of distal bile duct obstruction can be performed,[145] usually with a cholecystojejunostomy. This will be unsuccessful if the common bile duct at the level of the cystic duct is involved with tumor. This is often the case with unresectable cholangiocarcinoma.

Metal expandable stents can be placed both via PTC or ERCP to open malignant strictures of the bile duct. Physician preference often dictates whether these or silastic stents are used. The advantage of the metal stents is that they maintain biliary drainage longer than the silastic stents and, therefore, are associated with less cholangitis.[144] They do not require changing every 3 months. The disadvantage is that they cannot be removed, and they will eventually become obstructed from advancement of the tumor. It can be difficult or impossible to pass a new stent through an obstructed metal stent. A randomized controlled trial compared metallic stents with plastic stents, and the metallic stents were advantageous in patients who were expected to survive more than 6 months, whereas a plastic stent was advantageous in patients who were expected to survive 6 months or less.[144] In general, it is recommended that replaceable silastic stents be used for those with a life expectancy of less than 6 months, and metal stents be used for those with a longer life expectancy.[144]

Radiation Therapy

There are few data regarding the efficacy of radiotherapy or chemoradiotherapy in advanced-stage cholangiocarcinoma, either unresectable or resected with gross residual tumor. Table 85.10 provides a summary of the retrospective reviews reported. The median survival of approximately 1 year appears to be superior to the commonly reported 3 to 6 months with chemotherapy or supportive care alone, but formal comparative trials have never been conducted. Some authors reported a dose-dependent delay in local disease progression, but this has not been a uniform finding. Long-term survivors have been rarely described.

Morganti et al.[148] reported on a small series of 20 patients with unresectable tumor or gross residual tumor after resection, all treated with EBRT, 39.6 to 50.4 Gy, with 12 patients also receiving brachytherapy, 30 to 50 Gy administered at 1 cm from the sources. Two patients who had EBRT and brachytherapy for unresected tumors were 5-year survivors.

Shin et al.[149] reported on 31 patients with inoperable carcinoma of the extrahepatic bile ducts treated with EBRT alone (17 patients) or EBRT and high dose–rate brachytherapy (14 patients). The administered EBRT dose was 36 to 55 Gy (median, 50.4 Gy). Brachytherapy was administered in single doses of 5 Gy/d for 3 days using an after-loading technique. There was no statistically significant difference in local recurrence, but prolongation of the median time to tumor recurrence increased with the use of EBRT and brachytherapy

TABLE 85.10

DEFINITIVE RADIOTHERAPY OR CHEMORADIOTHERAPY FOR UNRESECTABLE CHOLANGIOCARCINOMA

Study (Ref.)	No. of Patients	Radiotherapy	Chemotherapy	Median Survival (months)
Hayes et al. (146)	14	63.5–108.2 Gy; EBRT + ILBT	None	12.8
Alden and Mohiuddin (147)	24	46 Gy EBRT + 25 ILBT	5-FU ± Adria; 5-FU ± Mito	12
Morganti et al. (148)	20	39.6–50.4 Gy EBRT ± 30–50 Gy ILBT (12 patients)	5-FU CI days 1–4 in 19 patients	21.2
Shin et al. (149)	31	50.4 Gy EBRT ± 15 Gy ILBT (14 patients)	None	7
Crane et al. (150)	52	30–85 Gy; EBRT ± ILBT	5-FU CI in 38 patients	10
Buskirk et al. (151)	34	45–55 Gy EBRT ± ILBT (20–25 Gy; 10 patients) or IORT (15–20 Gy; 7 patients)	5-FU in 7 patients	12
Urego et al. (131)	34	49.5 Gy (median) EBRT ± ILBT (4 patients)	5-FU + INF-alfa (27 patients)	14
Ben-David et al. (123)	52	23–86.3 Gy (median 60.2 Gy) EBRT	5-FU (21 patients); intrahepatic (21 patients); Gem (2 patients)	13.1
Nelson et al. (136)	45	50.4 Gy (median) EBRT; ILBT (4 patients)	5-FU-based (concurrent in 44 patients) and adjuvant (20 patients)	

EBRT, external-beam radiation therapy; ILBT, intraluminal brachytherapy; 5-FU, 5-fluorouracil; Adria, adriamycin; Mito, mitomycin C; Gem, gemcitabine; CI, continuous infusion; INF, interferon.

(9 months vs. 5 months; $P = .06$). The 2-year survival for patients treated with a combination of EBRT and brachytherapy was 21% versus 0% for those treated with EBRT alone ($P = .015$).

Alden and Mohiuddin[147] reported on 24 patients with advanced bile duct tumor treated with EBRT, brachytherapy, or both. The EBRT doses ranged from 27 to 60 Gy and the brachytherapy dose was 25 Gy at 1 cm. Nineteen patients also received chemotherapy. The 2-year survival rates and median survival intervals improved as the total dose of administered radiotherapy increased.

Crane et al.[150] reported on 52 patients with localized but unresectable biliary tract cancer treated with EBRT. Three patients also had brachytherapy and one patient had treatment with IORT. Total administered doses ranged from 30 to 85 Gy. The median time to local progression was not influenced by the total radiation dose administered.

Buskirk et al.[151] reported on 34 patients with subtotal resected or unresectable carcinoma of the extrahepatic bile ducts. All received EBRT to a minimum of 45 Gy with or without 5-FU. Seventeen patients received additional EBRT, 5 to 15 Gy; ten other patients received brachytherapy and seven other patients received additional IORT. Local control and length of survival seemed to be better in those patients who had EBRT plus brachytherapy or IORT.

Urego et al.[131] reported the experience of the University of Pittsburgh with radiotherapy for extrahepatic cholangiocarcinoma. The median survival of 34 patients with unresectable disease was 14 months. There was no impact of radiation dose on survival. Ben-David et al.[123] reported on 52 patients treated at the University of Michigan with EBRT. The dose ranged from 23 to 86.3 Gy (median, 60.2 Gy). Approximately half of these patients received concurrent chemotherapy (5-FU–based in 21, intrahepatic floxuridine in 21, gemcitabine in 2). The median survival was 13.1 months.

Although the data to support radiotherapy or chemoradiotherapy for unresectable extrahepatic cholangiocarcinoma are weak, patients with good performance should be considered for such therapy. One commonly used regimen consists of capecitabine (1,350 mg/m²/d) with concurrent EBRT. Forty-five Gy in 1.8-Gy fractions is delivered to the primary tumor and lymph node basin. Subsequently, a boost of 9 to 15 Gy in 1.8 to 2 Gy fractions is delivered to the primary tumor, to bring the total dose to 54 to 60 Gy.

Data are starting to emerge regarding the use of stereotactic body radiotherapy (SBRT) for unresectable cholangiocarcinoma. Kopek et al.[152] reported on 27 patients (of whom 18 were treated on a prospective phase 2 trial; 26 with hilar and 1 with intrahepatic cholangiocarcinoma) who received 45 Gy in three fractions over 5 to 8 days. The clinical target volume (CTV) was defined as the gross tumor volume plus any area of diagnostic uncertainty, and the CTV was expended 5 mm radially and 10 mm in the craniocaudal direction to form the treatment planning volume (PTV). This was encompassed by the 67% isodose line. With a median follow-up time of 5.4 years, the median overall survival was 10.6 months and the local control at 1 year was 84%. Six patients had severe duodenal or pyloric ulceration and three patients developed duodenal stenosis. Although no clear relationship could be established between duodenal dose–volume parameters and severe toxicity, the authors recommended limiting the volume of duodenum receiving 21 Gy to 1 cc or less. Interestingly, no such toxicity was observed in another group of 13 patients with Klatskin tumors treated at the University of Freiburg. Eight of these received 48 Gy in four fractions, the others a range of doses (32 to 56 Gy in 3 to 4 Gy per fraction).[153] The median survival was 33.5 months and treatment was tolerated very well, with nausea being the most common side effect. Taken together, SBRT for extrahepatic cholangiocarcinoma appears worthy of further investigation, but the authors advise caution against its use in routine practice, given the potential for severe toxicity.

Chemotherapy

Because of the rarity of these tumors, almost all clinical trials have broadened eligibility to include all tumors arising from the biliary tract. The small number of patients with biliary tract cancers in clinical trials makes it impossible to know whether there are differences in response to chemotherapy between anatomic sites of the biliary tract, such as gallbladder or cholangiocarcinomas.

Until recently, based on review of published studies (Table 85.11) of chemotherapy, there was no consensus on the "best agent or regimen" for unresectable or metastatic cholangiocarcinoma. Because of the rarity of the disease, few randomized studies have been conducted. In addition, a significant number of patients present with biliary obstruction and elevated liver function tests, which severely curtails the ability to administer chemotherapy. A major advance is that a new standard has now been established in 2010, based on a large randomized study that shows superior efficacy of gemcitabine in combination with cisplatin to gemcitabine alone for biliary tract cancer.[191]

As with most gastrointestinal malignancies, in the past 5-FU as a single agent or in combination is the most evaluated drug for gallbladder and bile duct malignancies and appears to have some activity. In addition, studies with agents such as cisplatin, mitomycin, and amsacrine (m-ANSA) have been disappointing.[192–194] Despite the wide range of activity reported with 5-FU, in most studies the time to tumor progression is a few months, and median survival of patients is in the range of 6 months. For locally advanced biliary tract cancers, concurrent chemotherapy and radiation are commonly used, although data for this approach are supported by a study only involving nine patients. In this study, continuous infusion of 5-FU with radiation therapy was found to be well tolerated.[155] Investigators have also evaluated older combination regimens used in gastric cancer (i.e., FAM: 5-FU, adriamycin, and doxorubicin) for biliary tract cancers,[195–197] which are not typically used in practice. A common regimen used in advanced gastric cancer is ECF (epirubicin, cisplatin, and infusional 5-FU).[156] The ECF regimen was compared to the FELV regimen (5-FU/leucovorin [LV] and etoposide) in a randomized trial. In this study, Rao et al.[157] randomized 27 patients to each arm. Response rates and overall survival (9 to 12 months) were comparable in each arm, with overall less acute toxicity for ECF.

The addition of LV to 5-FU generally results in a higher response rate in other tumors, and this combination has been evaluated in cholangiocarcinoma.[158,159,161,162] One study reported a response rate of 32% in 28 patients with cholangiocarcinoma; however, the median survival was only 6 months.[159] A weekly regimen of high-dose 5-FU with LV was reported to have a 33% response rate with a median survival of 7 months.[162] However, the same high-dose 5-FU/LV regimen with the addition of mitomycin proved intolerable, with severe toxicity.[163]

Combination chemotherapy with 5-FU has been reported to increase response rates, but at the expense of increased toxicity. Median survival rates in some of these studies appear to be promising, but the apparent benefit may be because of patient selection. In one study, Patt et al.[161] added cisplatin and doxorubicin to a modified 5-FU and interferon-alfa schedule (PIAF regimen). Forty-one patients were treated for an overall response rate of 21%. The median survival was 14 months, but most patients experienced significant toxicity. Other investigators have evaluated 5-FU with or without LV with carboplatin, cisplatin, doxorubicin, or epirubicin with similar results.[162,163]

TABLE 85.11

CHEMOTHERAPY TRIALS FOR ADVANCED BILIARY TREE CARCINOMAS

Study (Ref.)	No. of Patients: Gallbladder	Bile Duct	Total	Therapy	Response Rate (%)	Median Survival (months)
Falkson et al., 1984 (154)	18	12	30	Oral 5-FU	10	5.2–6.5
	16	10	36	Oral 5-FU + STZ	8	3.0–3.5
	19	12	31	Oral 5-FU + MeCCNU	10	2.0–2.5
Whittington et al., 1995 (155)	—	9	9	CI-5-FU + RT	—	11.9
Lee et al., 2004 (156)	—	24	24	Epirubicin + cisplatin + 5-FU	10	—
Rao et al., 2005 (157)	14	13	27	Epirubicin + CDDP + 5-FU	19	9.0
	12	15	27	5-FU + LV + etoposide	15	12.0
Sanz-Altamira et al., 1998 (158)	4	10	14	5-FU + LV + carboplatin	21	5.0
Choi et al., 2000 (159)	9	19	28	5-FU + LV	32	6.0
Patt et al., 1996 (160)	10	25	35	CI-5-FU + IFN	34	12.0
Patt et al., 2001 (161)	19	22	41	CI-5-FU + IFN + DOX + CDDP	21	14.0
Chen et al., 1998 (162)	6	13	19	CI-5-FU + LV	33	7.0
Chen et al., 2001 (163)	3	22	25	CI-5-FU + LV + MMC	26	6.0
Mani et al., 1999 (164)	0	13	13	UFT + LV	0	7.0
Kim et al., 2003 (165)	19	23	42	CDDP + capecitabine	21	9.1
Hong et al., 2007 (166)	15	17	32	CDDP + capecitabine	41	12.4
Kornek et al., 2004 (167)	7	19	26	MMC + capecitabine	31	9.3
	7	18	25	MMC + gemcitabine	20	6.7
Park et al., 2006 (168)	6	37	43	Epirubicin + CDDP + capecitabine	40	8.0
Jones et al., 1996 (169)	4	11	15	Paclitaxel	0	—
Pazdur et al., 1999 (170)	0	17	17	Docetaxel	0	—
Papakostas et al., 2001 (171)	16	10	26	Docetaxel	20	8.0
Sanz-Altamira et al., 2001 (172)	10	15	25	Irinotecan	8	10.0
Kubicka et al., 2001 (173)	—	23	23	Gemcitabine	30	9.3
Penz et al., 2001 (174)	10	22	32	Gemcitabine	22	11.5
Eng et al., 2003 (175)	9	6	15	Gemcitabine	0	5.0
Kuhn et al., 2002 (176)	26	17	43	Gemcitabine + Docetaxel	9	11.0
Lee et al., 2006 (177)	—	24	24	Gemcitabine + CDDP	21	9.3
Thongprasert et al., 2005 (178)	1	39	40	Gemcitabine + CDDP	28	9.0
Kim et al., 2006 (179)	10	19	29	Gemcitabine + CDDP	35	11.0
Valle et al., 2010 (122)	76	130	206	Gemcitabine	16	8.1
Knox et al., 2005 (180)	73	131	204	Gemcitabine + CDDP	36	11.7 (P <.001)
	22	23	45	Gemcitabine + capecitabine	31	14.0
Cho et al., 2005 (181)	7	37	44	Gemcitabine + capecitabine	32	14.0
Androulakis et al., 2006 (182)	15	14	29	Oxaliplatin	21	7.0
Andre et al., 2004 (183)	19	37	56	Oxaliplatin + gemcitabine	22–36	7.6–15.4
Harder et al., 2006 (184)	10	21	31	Oxaliplatin + gemcitabine	26	11.0
Dowlati et al., 2009 (185)	9	32	45	Rebeccamycin	5	6.3
Fiebiger et al., 2002 (186)	14	6	20	Lanreotide	5	4.5
Philip et al., 2006 (187)	16	26	42	Erlotinib	8	7.5
Ramanathan et al., 2009 (188)	5	12	17	Lapatinib	0	5.2
Bengala et al., 2010 (189)	14	32	46	Sorafenib	2	4.4
Zhu et al., 2010 (190)	10	25	35	Oxaliplatin + gemcitabine + bevacizumab	40	12.7

5-FU, 5-fluorouracil; STZ, streptozocin; MECCNU, methyl CCNU; RT, radiation therapy; CDDP, cisplatin; LV, leucovorin; MTX, methotrexate; IFN, interferon; CI–5-FU, continuous infusion of 5-FU; DOX, doxorubicin; MMC, mitomycin; UFT, uracil/tegafur. FAM–5-FU, adriamycin (doxorubicin), mitomycin.

Continuous infusion 5-FU, compared with bolus 5-FU schedules, is more active and better tolerated, especially in colorectal cancer. Oral formulations of 5-FU mimic a continuous infusion schedule and have the advantage of easy administration. A number of oral pro–5-FU drugs such as capecitabine, uracil/tegafur, S1, and eniluracil have been evaluated. In one study, uracil/tegafur in combination with LV was evaluated in 13 patients with cholangiocarcinoma, but no responses were reported. The median survival was 7 months.[164] In the United States, only capecitabine is commercially available. Capecitabine combinations have been evaluated in biliary tract cancer. Kornek et al.[167] randomized a total of 51 patients with biliary tract cancer to either mitomycin/capecitabine or mitomycin/gemcitabine arms. Both combinations were feasible and tolerable, with the mitomycin/capecitabine arm having a trend toward better efficacy. Capecitabine has also been evaluated in combination with cisplatin and substituted for 5-FU in the ECF regimen.[165,166,168]

During the past decade, newer chemotherapeutic agents have been evaluated without much success. The taxanes, both docetaxel and paclitaxel, have been evaluated in biliary tract cancers and overall single-agent activity appears to be low.[170,171] Irinotecan also had minimal activity in a phase 2 study of 25 patients.[172] Gemcitabine has proven activity in pancreatic cancer, which has led to a number of studies in biliary tract cancers, with mixed results.[173,198,176,175] Kubicka et al.[173] treated 23 patients with cholangiocarcinomas with gemcitabine; the response rate was 30%, with median survival of 9.5 months. In a study of gemcitabine given every 2 weeks, Penz et al.[174] found this regimen to be active with a response rate of 22% and median survival of 11.5 months. In contrast, Eng et al.[175] evaluated a fixed dose rate of gemcitabine (1,500 mg/m^2 during 150 minutes) in 14 patients with biliary tract cancers. No objective responses were documented, and the median survival was only 5 months.

Similar to advanced pancreatic cancer, gemcitabine combinations have been evaluated for biliary tract cancers. The combination of docetaxel and gemcitabine resulted in a response rate of 9.3% and a median survival of 11.0 months.[176] Phase 2 studies of gemcitabine in combination with cisplatin have shown activity with response rates of 21% to 35% and median survival of 9 to 11 months.[177–179] The combination of gemcitabine and cisplatin is now the reference regimen. In this study, 410 patients with locally advanced or metastatic biliary tract cancer (cholangiocarcinoma 36.3%, gallbladder cancer 56.3%, ampullary cancer 4.8%) were randomized to receive either cisplatin (25 mg/m^2) with gemcitabine (1,000 mg/m^2), administered on days 1 and 8, every 3 weeks for eight cycles, or gemcitabine alone (1,000 mg/m^2) on days 1, 8, and 15, every 4 weeks for six cycles for up to 24 weeks. The primary end point was overall survival. The combination of gemcitabine and cisplatin was superior to gemcitabine alone and resulted in a median overall survival of 11.7 months versus 8.1 months (hazard ratio, 0.64; 95% confidence interval [CI], 0.52 to 0.80; $P < .001$) and median progression-free survival of 8 months versus 5 months ($P < .001$), respectively. The cisplatin/gemcitabine regimen was tolerable with adverse events being similar in the two groups, with the exception of more neutropenia; however, the number of neutropenia-associated infections was similar in the two groups.[191]

Gemcitabine in combination with capecitabine also appears to have some degree of activity.[180,181] Knox et al.[180] treated 45 patients with advanced biliary tract cancer with the combination of gemcitabine and capecitabine. The response rate was 31% with a median survival 14 months. The regimen was well tolerated.

Oxaliplatin, a third-generation platinum drug, has been evaluated in biliary tract cancers. Single-agent oxaliplatin showed evidence of activity in a study with 29 patients.[182] In two phase 2 studies, oxaliplatin was combined with gemcitabine. The response rates in these studies ranged from 21% to 36% with median survival of 11.0 to 15.4 months.[183,184] In the study by Andre et al.,[183] patients were stratified to two groups. The median survival (15.4 months vs. 7.6 months) was much higher for patients with a good performance status, bilirubin less than 2.5 mg/dL, and no prior therapy.

A number of new combinations and novel drugs are undergoing evaluation in biliary tract cancers. One such agent is the somatostatin analogue lanreotide, which was found to be inactive.[186] The rebeccamycin analogue (NSC 655649), which is a novel antitumor antibiotic with both topoisomerase I and II activity as well as DNA intercalating properties, appeared to have promising activity, with median survival of 10 months in a phase 2 study, and results of a completed phase 3 study with the control arm being 5-FU/LV are awaited.[185]

The molecular pathogenesis of biliary tract cancers is now beginning to be understood (as previously discussed). The epidermal growth factor receptor (EGFR/HER-1) and its ligands are overexpressed in the majority of gallbladder and bile duct cancers.[199,200] Erlotinib is an orally active small-molecule inhibitor of EGFR. A phase 2 study was conducted by Philip et al.[187] in which 42 patients were treated with erlotinib. EGFR expression by immunohistochemistry was seen in 81%. The response rate was 8% and median survival was 7.5 months. Another phase 2 study evaluated lapatinib, a dual inhibitor of EGFR and *Her-2/neu*. However lapatinib did not show activity in 17 patients with biliary tract cancer.[188] Angiogenesis also appears to be important for tumor growth and metastasis in biliary tree cancers.[201,202] Sorafenib, an oral multitargeted small molecule against BRAF/vascular endothelial growth factor (VEGF) and AZD6244, a potent inhibitor of the RAS-RAF pathway have been evaluated in biliary cancer.[189,203,204] In these phase 2 studies minimal single agent activity was noted. Targeted agents in combination with cytotoxic therapy are being evaluated. Two phase 2 studies have evaluated cetuximab[205] (targeting EGFR) and bevacizumab[190] (targeting VEGF) in combination with the gemcitabine/oxaliplatin regimen. In particular the combination study with bevacizumab ($n = 35$) resulted in a response rate of 40% and a median survival of 10.7 months[190]; however, randomized trials are needed prior to incorporate targeted agents into the armamentarium for bile duct cancers.

Although hepatic arterial infusion therapy is widely used for primary hepatocellular cancers, its role in cholangiocarcinomas remains investigational, with few reported studies.[206] The blood supply to the biliary tract is primarily from the hepatic artery and hepatic arterial infusion is a logical approach. Tanaka et al.[207] reported a series of 11 patients with intrahepatic cholangiocarcinomas who received chemotherapy with 5-FU through an implanted hepatic arterial pump. Responses were noted, with a median survival of 26 months. Mezawa et al.[208] evaluated a carboplatin-coated percutaneous transhepatic biliary catheter in five patients with cholangiocarcinomas and noted activity. Photodynamic therapy is a new approach used to treat endoluminal lesions of the lung and esophagus. Tumors of the biliary tract frequently encroach the lumen of the bile ducts, and photodynamic therapy is being evaluated in cholangiocarcinoma, with preliminary evidence of activity in some patients.[209–211]

Transplantation for Cholangiocarcinoma

Transplantation as a primary treatment modality for hilar and intrahepatic cholangiocarcinoma is a viable option.[212] Organ availability has been the most limiting factor for this modality, but the success of living-related transplantation may rejuvenate the use of transplant for hilar and intrahepatic cholangiocarcinoma. Complete hepatectomy provides the best chance of a complete resection for these tumors and may be an alternative for patients who are unresectable by conventional means. The real possibility of achieving a cure for unresectable tumors exists only with liver transplantation. Meyer et al.[213] reported the results of liver transplantation for cholangiocarcinoma in 207 patients collected by the Cincinnati Transplant Tumor Registry. Fifty-one percent of the transplanted patients suffered recurrence; the median time from transplantation to recurrence was 9.7 months, and the median time between recurrence and death was 2 months. Several studies have focused on hilar cholangiocarcinoma, with 5-year survival rates from 12% to 36%.[214]

In 1993 a multimodality protocol was developed using EBRT and bolus 5-FU, followed by brachytherapy, protracted intravenous infusion of 5-FU, and liver transplantation for highly selected patients with early-stage cholangiocarcinoma.[215] Twenty-eight patients underwent exploratory surgery, at which time 11 were excluded because of metastatic disease. Seventeen patients proceeded to liver transplantation; seven patients had no identifiable tumor in the explanted specimen. Of the ten patients with identifiable tumor, two died of non–cancer-related causes. Of the remaining patients, two developed recurrent disease, one at 40 months and another at 54 months, after liver transplantation. The median duration of follow-up was 41.8 months (range, 2.8 to 105.5 months); the 5-year actuarial survival rate for those transplanted was 87%. A follow-up protocol from the same group was similarly designed, adding a transluminal boost of radiation with iridium seeds after EBRT and maintenance therapy with capecitabine until transplantation.[216] Of 56 patients enrolled, 28 received a transplant. The actuarial 1- and 5-year survivals were reported at 88% and 82%, respectively, after transplantation. A similar protocol that combined neoadjuvant brachytherapy and infusional 5-FU followed by transplantation was reported, with 5 of 17 patients (29%) achieving long-term disease-free survival.[93] Other small series have demonstrated 3-year survival rates from 0% to 53%.[217] A series of seven patients who underwent living-related transplant for cholangiocarcinoma demonstrated six of seven patients alive, with a median of 20-month follow-up. All of the intrahepatic cholangiocarcinoma patients had already recurred, however.[218] Extrahepatic nodal disease or metastases are a contraindication to transplant.

Treatment Recommendations

An algorithm for treatment is shown in Figure 85.5. The authors' practice is to enroll patients with biliary tract cancers into clinical trials, incorporating molecularly targeted agents and biomarkers whenever possible. Chemotherapy should be offered only to patients with a good performance status, as those who have significant cancer-related symptoms have a short life expectancy and are unlikely to benefit from therapy. In patients with evidence of locally advanced or metastatic disease, gemcitabine and cisplatin should be administered to those who meet eligibility criteria as described by Valle et al.[191] in their pivotal phase 3 study. Further support for this regimen comes from Eckel and Schmid,[219] who performed an analysis of 104 trials in biliary tract cancer with 2,810 patients. In this analysis, gemcitabine and platinum regimens had the highest activity. There is no proven benefit for second-line therapy, and in this setting, phase 1 studies or best supportive care would be appropriate.

TUMORS OF THE GALLBLADDER

Histologically, gallbladder cancers resemble other biliary neoplasms, and, therefore, it is appropriate that they be considered together. However, the epidemiology, clinical presentation, staging, and surgical treatment are distinct from cholangiocarcinoma, and, therefore, gallbladder cancers are considered separately within this chapter. Chemotherapy and radiation therapy trials often combine gallbladder cancers and cholangiocarcinoma, so there may be some overlap in the description of these treatments. Gallbladder cancer tends to be an aggressive tumor that spreads early and leads to rapid death. DeStoll[220] described the gross appearance and invasive nature of gallbladder cancer in 1788 based on his study of two autopsy cases. The clinical pessimism surrounding gallbladder cancer results from its late presentation and lack of effective therapy. Gallbladder cancer spreads early by lymphatic metastasis, hematogenous metastasis, direct invasion into the liver, and, as with cholangiocarcinoma, has a uniquely high propensity to seed the peritoneal surfaces after tumor spillage and cause tumor implants in biopsy tracts, abdominal wounds,

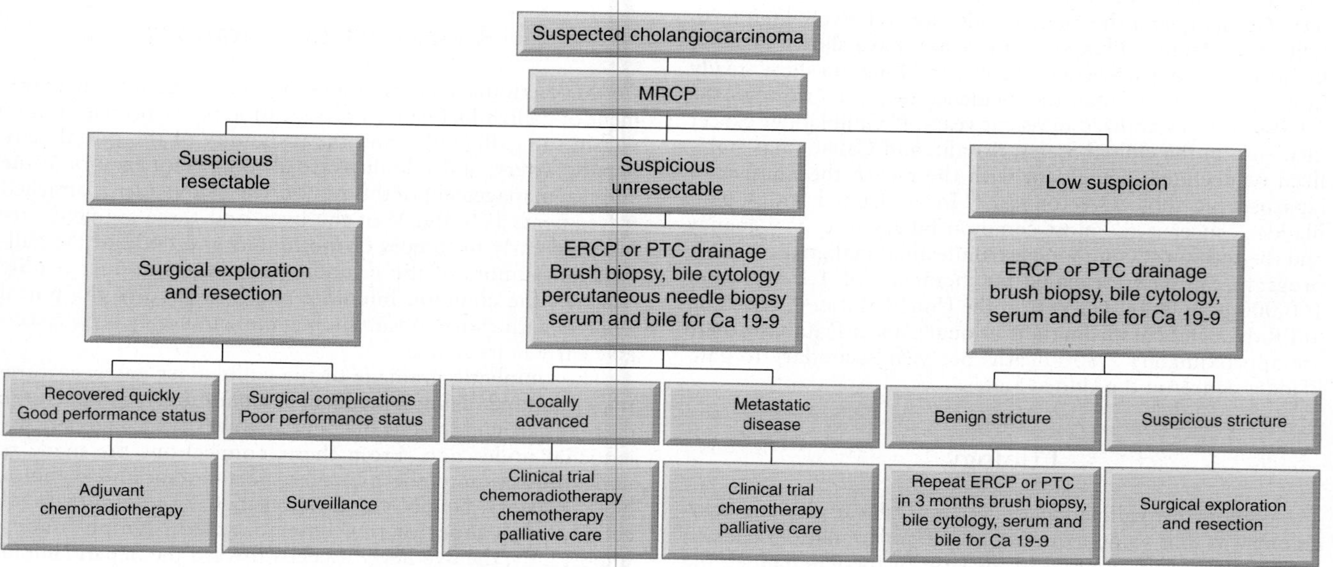

FIGURE 85.5 Algorithm for management of suspected cholangiocarcinoma. MRCP, cholangiography for cholangiocarcinoma; ERCP, endoscopic retrograde cholangiography; PTC, percutaneous transhepatic cholangiography.

and the peritoneal cavity. Classically, the 5-year survival in most large series is less than 5%, and the median survival is less than 6 months.[221] A recent summary of SEER data demonstrated a 15% 5-year survival rate with no improvement in overall survival since 1991.[222,223] It is important for the oncology clinician to understand the natural history, biology, staging, and surgical treatment of this tumor, so that appropriate decisions are made at the time of initial diagnosis. Given the high chance of these lesions being found incidentally at the time of cholecystectomy, the general surgeon must be familiar with the appropriate management in that setting. Inappropriate procedures may allow spread of this tumor throughout the abdominal cavity, to laparoscopic port sites, or biopsy needle tracts, rendering the disease untreatable. On the other hand, it is important to understand the limitations of surgical resection so that operations with unreasonably high morbidity but minimal chance of success are avoided.

Epidemiology

The incidence of gallbladder cancer varies by geographic region and racial-ethnic groups. Gallbladder cancer is up to 25 times more common in some geographic regions compared with others.[224] The highest incidences are reported in Indians, Pakistanis, Chileans, Bolivians, Central Europeans, Israelis, Native Americans, and Americans of Mexican origin.[225] Gallbladder cancer is the main cause of death from cancer among women in Chile. Japanese men have been reported to have the highest mortality rate from gallbladder carcinoma. The lowest rates are seen in the people of Spain and India, black Rhodesians, and black Americans. Within the United States and the United Kingdom, urban areas show higher incidences than rural regions.[181] It has been suggested that lower socioeconomic status may lead to delayed access to cholecystectomy, which may increase gallbladder cancer rates.[226]

In the United States, gallbladder cancer continues to be a rare cancer. It is the sixth most common gastrointestinal malignancy.[6] Women are two to six times more likely to develop gallbladder cancer than men. As with cholangiocarcinoma, the incidence steadily increases with age, reaching its maximum in the seventh decade of life. Nevertheless, reports exist of a 21-year-old Chilean woman[227] and an 11-year-old Native American girl[228] with the diagnosis of gallbladder cancer. Trends in gallbladder cancer mortality show a variable pattern. Germany and the Netherlands have relatively high mortality rates from gallbladder cancer and have shown declines in most age groups. Sweden, France, and Bulgaria show steady upward trends. In Japan the incidence increased through the 1980s but has stabilized in recent years.[224] Gallbladder cancer incidence in the United States, Britain, and Canada has stabilized or declined, coincident with the rise in the number of laparoscopic cholecystectomies.[229] In the United States, gallbladder cancer is the most common biliary tract malignancy and the fifth most common gastrointestinal malignancy. SEER program estimates revealed an incidence of 1.2 cases per 100,000 population per year in the United States.[230] Based on SEER data and data from the National Cancer Database, there are approximately 2,800 deaths per year secondary to gallbladder cancer in the United States.

Etiology

The etiology for gallbladder cancer is similar to cholangiocarcinoma, in that some form of chronic inflammation leads to malignant transformation. In the case of the gallbladder, the overwhelming inciting factor for chronic inflammation is gallstones. Seventy-five percent to 98% of all patients with carcinoma of the gallbladder have cholelithiasis. The epidemiology of gallbladder cancer is closely linked to the epidemiology of gallbladder stones. Calcification of the gallbladder (porcelain gallbladder) is associated with gallbladder cancer in 10% to 25% of cases. Calcification is the end stage of a long-standing inflammatory process and is therefore associated with an increased risk of gallbladder cancer.

Case control studies have identified a history of biliary problems, older age, and female gender as risk factors for the development of gallbladder cancer. The presence of anomalous pancreaticobiliary duct junction is a risk factor for gallbladder cancer independent of the presence of gallstones. This may establish a chronic inflammatory state of the gallbladder. Typhoid carriers may also suffer chronic inflammation of the gallbladder and have a sixfold higher risk of gallbladder cancer.[231] Multiple cohort studies have identified obesity as a risk factor for gallbladder cancer, but this parallels the risk for gallstone disease. *Helicobacter bilis* and *Helicobacter pylori* have been identified in bile specimens and have been demonstrated to increase the risk of biliary tract carcinoma (about sixfold higher risk).[232,233] Other rare associations with gallbladder cancer include inflammatory bowel disease and polyposis coli. Reports of family clusters of gallbladder cancer exist in the literature, but any inherited predisposition has not been found in large series of gallbladder cancer.[234] A recent cohort study from Sweden found an association among first-degree relatives, specifically among parents (relative risk, 5.1; 95% CI, 2.4 to 9.3) or offspring (relative risk, 4.1; 95% CI, 2.0 to 7.6).[235] Genetic variants in DNA repair pathways may be involved in gallbladder carcinogenesis.[236]

Although gallstones and chronic inflammation of the gallbladder are involved in the pathogenesis of this tumor, the incidence of gallbladder cancer in a population of patients with gallstones is only 0.3% to 3%. Chronic inflammation seems to act as a promoter for some other carcinogenic exposure. Experimentally, Kowalewski and Todd[237] show that carcinoma of the gallbladder was induced in 68% of hamsters who had cholesterol pellets inserted into the gallbladder and were given the carcinogen dimethylnitrosamine versus only 6% of controls fed the carcinogen alone. Chemicals implicated in carcinogenesis of gallbladder cancer include methyldopa,[238] oral contraceptives,[239] isoniazid,[240] and occupational exposure in the rubber industry,[241] but none of these associations have been proven.

Anatomic Considerations

Certain anatomic considerations are important in the management of gallbladder cancer. The location of the primary tumor within the gallbladder and the proximity of the portal vein, hepatic artery, and bile duct are all important factors in the surgical management of this tumor. The gallbladder is attached to segments IVb and V of the liver, and these segments are involved early in tumors of the fundus and body of the gallbladder. Tumors of the infundibulum or cystic duct readily obstruct the common bile duct and may involve the portal vein. As with cholangiocarcinoma, the tumor may be unresectable early in its course.

The lymphatic drainage of the gallbladder has been carefully mapped using a blue dye technique.[242] The lymph descends around the bile duct and involves cystic and pericholedochal nodes first. From there, connections are made to nodes posterior to the pancreas, portal vein, and common hepatic artery. Finally, the flow reaches the interaortocaval, celiac, and superior mesenteric artery lymph nodes. Importantly, the dye never ascends toward the hepatic hilum, whereas it stains node-bearing adipose tissue posterior to the head of the pancreas and portal vein as an early event. Some connections are made directly from the pericholedochal nodes to interaortocaval nodes, which explains the difficulty in controlling this disease with a regional lymph node dissection.

Pathology

Adenomas

Gallbladder cancers demonstrate progression from dysplasia to carcinoma *in situ* to invasive carcinoma. Severe dysplasia and carcinoma *in situ* are identified in surrounding gallbladder epithelium in more than 90% of gallbladder cancer cases. The rate of progression of precursor lesions to invasive carcinoma is 5 to 15 years.[243] Adenomas are present in up to 1.1% of cholecystectomy specimens.[244] The precancerous nature of adenomas of the gallbladder is controversial. Benign adenomas do not have the same association with cholecystitis as do invasive carcinomas; therefore, it is unlikely that the majority of carcinomas arise in adenomas. Nevertheless, 19% of invasive carcinomas are found to have adenomatous components. Papillary cancers may represent malignant degeneration of papillary adenomas.

Gross Pathology

Sixty percent of tumors originate in the fundus of the gallbladder, 30% in the body, and 10% in the neck. Tumors that arise in the neck and Hartman's pouch may infiltrate the cystic and common bile duct, making them clinically and radiographically indistinguishable from hilar cholangiocarcinomas. Gallbladder cancer can be categorized into infiltrative, nodular, and papillary forms. This directly parallels the forms of cholangiocarcinoma, as previously discussed. As with cholangiocarcinoma, the most common form is the infiltrative form, and the papillary forms have the best prognosis.

The infiltrative tumors cause thickening and induration of the gallbladder wall, sometimes extending to involve the entire gallbladder. These tumors spread in a subserosal plane, which is the same plane used by the surgeon for routine cholecystectomy. If the tumor is unrecognized at the time of cholecystectomy, this plane will be violated and tumor cells will seed the peritoneal cavity. As the infiltrative tumor becomes more advanced, it invades the liver and can result in a thick wall of tumor encasing the gallbladder. Nodular or mass-forming gallbladder cancers can show early invasion through the gallbladder wall into the liver or neighboring structures. Despite this invasiveness, it may be easier to control surgically than the infiltrative form, where the margins are less defined. Papillary carcinomas exhibit a polypoid or cauliflowerlike appearance and fill the lumen of the gallbladder with only minimal invasion of the gallbladder wall. Papillary carcinomas have a much improved prognosis compared with the other types.

Histology

The most common histologic type of gallbladder carcinoma is adenocarcinoma. However, unlike cholangiocarcinomas, the gallbladder can be involved with a number of different histologic types. The histologic types and incidences of gallbladder cancer as recorded in the SEER program of the National Cancer Institute are listed in Table 85.12. Primary malignant mesenchymal tumors of the gallbladder have been described, including embryonal rhabdomyosarcoma, leiomyosarcoma, malignant fibrous histiocytoma, angiosarcoma, and Kaposi's sarcoma. Other primary rare tumors of the gallbladder that have been described in the literature include carcinosarcoma, carcinoid, lymphoma, and melanoma. In addition, the gallbladder can be involved with metastatic cancers from numerous sites. Many tumors exhibit more than one histologic pattern. The only histologic type with clear prognostic significance is the papillary adenocarcinoma, which has a markedly improved survival compared with all other histologic types. There is also evidence to suggest that oat cell carcinomas, adenosquamous tumors, and carcinosarcomas have a poorer survival rate.[245]

TABLE 85.12

RELATIVE INCIDENCE OF GALLBLADDER CANCER BY HISTOLOGIC TYPE

Histologic Type	Relative Incidence (%)
Adenocarcinoma	80
Papillary adenocarcinoma	6
Mucinous and mucin-producing adenocarcinoma	5
Squamous cell carcinoma	2
Sarcoma	0.2
Other and unspecified	7

Data derived from ref. 193.

Metastases

Gallbladder cancer has a remarkable propensity to seed and grow in the peritoneal cavity, as well as along needle biopsy sites and in laparoscopic port sites. It can also spread early by direct extension into the liver and other adjacent organs. The gallbladder has a thin wall, a narrow lamina propria, and only a single muscle layer. Tumor invades into the liver at a thickness, whereas in other organs it would encounter a second muscle layer. Once it penetrates the thin muscle layer, it has access to major lymphatic and vascular channels. Gallbladder cancer therefore tends to have early lymphatic and hematogenous spread. At autopsy, gallbladder cancer patients have a 91% to 94% incidence of lymphatic metastasis, 65% to 82% incidence of hematogenous metastasis, and 60% incidence of peritoneal spread.[221,246] Hematogenous metastasis tends to be from invasion into small veins that extend directly from the gallbladder into the portal venous system, leading to hepatic metastases in segments IV and V of the liver. The incidence of regional invasion and metastasis at the time of diagnosis and treatment is summarized in Table 85.13. There is a high

TABLE 85.13

INCIDENCE OF REGIONAL INVASION AND METASTASIS AT THE TIME OF DIAGNOSIS AND TREATMENT

Pathologic Finding	Relative Incidence (%)
Confined to gallbladder wall	10
Liver invasion	59
Common bile duct infiltration	35
Lymphatic invasion and regional lymphatic metastases	45
Gallbladder vein infiltration	39
Portal vein or hepatic artery invasion	15
Adjacent organ invasion (excluding liver)	40
Perineural invasion	42
Liver metastasis	34
Distant metastasis (excluding liver)	20

Based on a literature review in ref. 247.

PRACTICE OF ONCOLOGY

propensity for intra-abdominal recurrence after resection, with distant metastasis occurring late in the course. The only common extra-abdominal site of metastasis is the lung. It is rare, however, to have metastasis to the lung in the absence of advanced locoregional disease.

Staging

Multiple staging systems have been described for gallbladder cancer, taking into account pathologic and clinical characteristics with prognostic significance. The different staging systems create confusion when attempting to compare the treatment results of different series in the literature. It is essential to standardize the staging system for the purpose of reporting and comparing treatment results. The main staging systems referred to in the literature include the modified Nevin system,[248,249] the Japanese Biliary Surgical Society system,[250] and the newly revised American Joint Committee on Cancer TNM staging system (Table 85.14).[41] It is the latter that should be reported uniformly for standardization.

The TNM system includes tumors that invade the lamina propria or muscle layer in stage I. It is important to realize that tumors can arise in Rokitansky-Aschoff sinuses and be considered stage I in a subserosal position. Tumors with invasion into the perimuscular connective tissue are considered stage II, and liver invasion is stage III. Extensive nodal metastasis to periaortic, pericaval, superior mesenteric artery, or celiac artery is now considered stage IVA. Stage IVB is patients with distant metastasis. It should be noted that although grade does not factor into staging, it does have prognostic significance. Gallbladder cancers undergo histopathologic grading from G1-well differentiated to G4-undifferentiated. High-grade tumors have a worse prognosis. The majority of patients present with grade 3, poorly differentiated tumors.

Molecular Genetics

Table 85.2 summarizes the known mutations in gallbladder cancer. *K-ras* and *p53* mutations are common in gallbladder cancer.[225,251] Mutant *p53* is found in 92% of invasive carcinomas, 86% of carcinoma *in situ*, and 28% of dysplastic epithelium.[252] *K-ras* mutations are identified in 39% of gallbladder carcinomas.[253] In one study, *b-RAF* mutations were evident in 33% of gallbladder cancers.[254] Overexpression of the *c-erbB-2* gene[255] and decreased expression of the nm23 gene product[256] have been reported to play an important role in the development of gallbladder cancer. A few studies have demonstrated that *CDKN2* (also known as *MTS1* or *p19*[ink4]) is an important gene in gallbladder carcinogenesis.[257] Another candidate suppressor gene implicated in the development of gallbladder cancer is fragile histidine triad (*FHIT*) gene.[258] A recent study defined epigenetic inactivation of tumor suppressor genes *SEMA3B* and *FHIT* in gallbladder cancers, suggesting a role in gallbladder cancer pathogenesis.[259] *EGFR* and *c-MET* may also be activated in some gallbladder cancers, warranting trials of small-molecule antagonists.[260,261] Cetuximab or panitumumab may be effective in the 50% of patients with wild type *K-ras*, as is seen in colon cancer.

TABLE 85.14

AMERICAN JOINT COMMITTEE ON CANCER STAGING SYSTEM FOR GALLBLADDER CANCER

Tis: Carcinoma *in situ*
T1: Tumor invades into the lamina propria or the muscle layer
  T1a: Tumor invades lamina propria
  T1b: Tumor invades the muscle layer
T2: Tumor invades perimuscular connective tissue
T3: Tumor perforates the serosa and/or directly invades the liver and/or one other adjacent organ.
T4: Tumor invades the main blood vessels leading into the liver or two or more organs outside the liver.
N1 = Metastasis to nodes along the cystic duct, common bile duct, hepatic artery, and/or portal vein
N2 = Metastasis to periaortic, pericaval, superior mesenteric artery, and/or celiac artery lymph nodes

Stage I	T1	N0	M0
Stage II	T2	N0	M0
Stage IIIA	T3	N0	M0
Stage IIIB	T1–3	N1	M0
Stage IVA	T4	N0-1	M0
Stage IVB		N2	M0
	Any T	Any N	M1

Modified from ref. 41.

Clinical Presentation

The clinical presentation of gallbladder cancer is identical to the symptoms of biliary colic or chronic cholecystitis. This leads to a low index of suspicion for cancer in most cases and leads to the incidental finding of gallbladder cancer at the time of surgery for cholecystitis or on pathologic review of the resected gallbladder. Patients older than 70 years with a history of recent weight loss and persistent right upper quadrant pain should be suspected of having gallbladder cancer. Careful history taking may reveal patients with gallbladder cancer to have a more continuous, diffuse abdominal pain compared with the crampy right upper-quadrant pain associated with biliary colic. Jaundice and anorexia are signs of advanced disease.

Diagnostic Evaluation

Laboratory Tests

As with cholangiocarcinoma, CA 19-9 is the best serum marker to detect gallbladder cancer. A level above 20 U/mL has 79% sensitivity and 79% specificity for the diagnosis of gallbladder cancer. This can be used to aid in the diagnosis in suspicious clinical situations but is not cost-effective as a general screen for all patients undergoing cholecystectomy. A CEA greater than 4 ng/mL is 93% specific for the diagnosis of gallbladder cancer compared with controls who undergo cholecystectomy or upper abdominal surgery for benign conditions, but it is only 50% sensitive for detecting cancer. CA 125 has also been reported to be a reasonable marker for gallbladder cancer in some small studies.[195] Increased alkaline phosphatase and bilirubin levels are found in cases of advanced gallbladder cancer. A trend toward anemia and leukocytosis has also been identified as an indicator of advanced disease.

Radiologic Evaluation

The most common initial radiologic evaluation for symptoms of right upper-quadrant pain is an ultrasound examination. An ultrasound typically demonstrates gallstones and gallbladder wall thickening, which is nonspecific for gallbladder cancer. A comparison of ultrasonographic features of early malignancy and benign gallbladder disease revealed some findings that were important in the differentiation. Discontinuous gallbladder mucosa, echogenic mucosa, and submucosal echolucency were significantly more common in gallbladder cancer than in benign gallbladder disease. A polypoid mass was present in

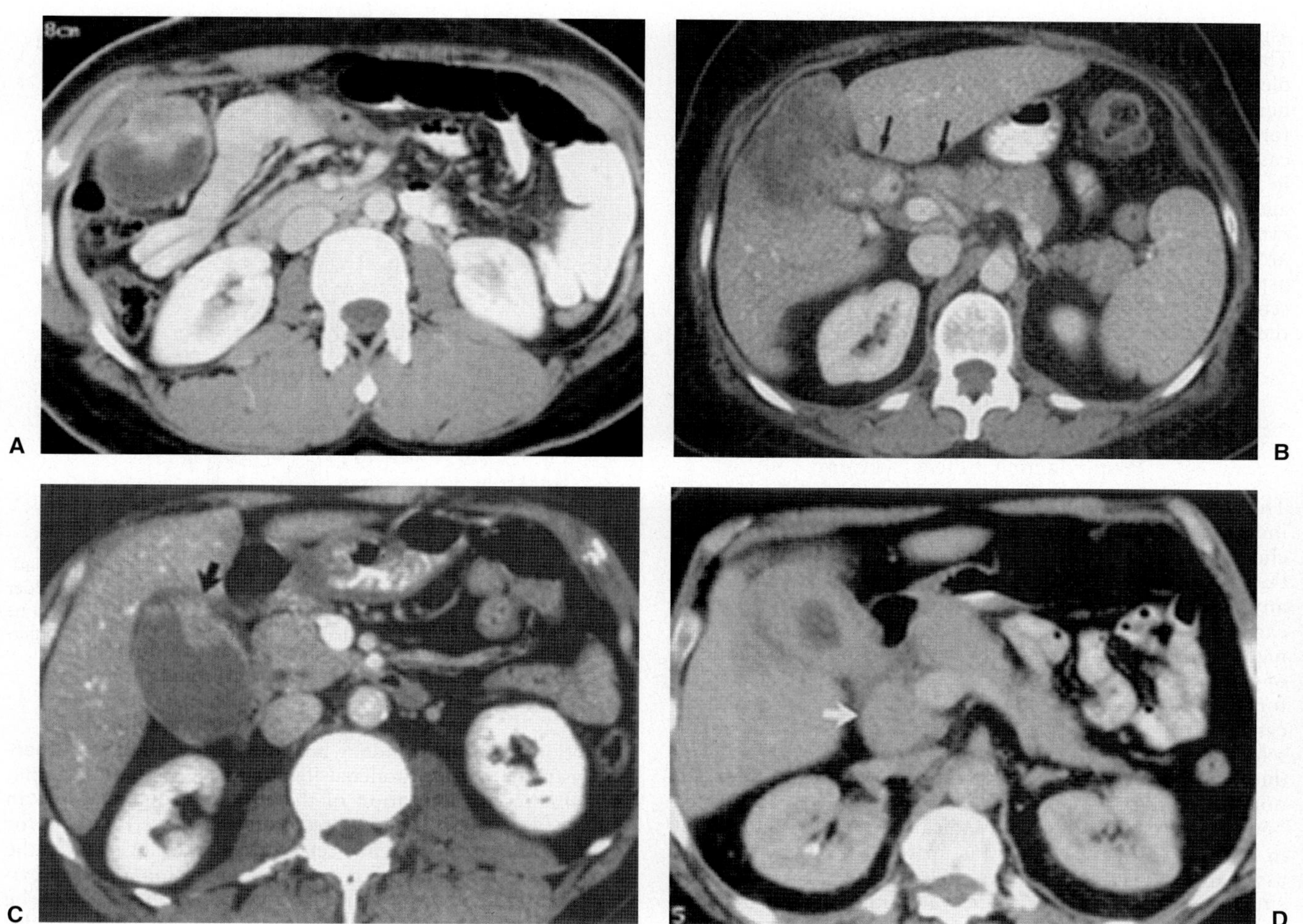

FIGURE 85.6 Classic contrast-enhanced computed tomography findings of gallbladder cancer. **A:** Focal mass in the gallbladder fundus, representing adenocarcinoma in a 35-year-old woman. **B:** Advanced diffusely infiltrative gallbladder cancer with hepatic invasion and periportal lymphadenopathy (*arrows*). **C:** Sessile, soft tissue mass in gallbladder, representing a moderately well-differentiated adenocarcinoma in a 55-year-old man. **D:** Diffusely thickened gallbladder with a mass extending into the adjacent liver parenchyma and a peripancreatic lymph node (*arrow*), representing poorly differentiated adenocarcinoma in a 67-year-old man. (From ref. 262, with permission.)

27% and a gallbladder-replacing or invasive mass was present in 50% of cases of gallbladder cancer examined.[196]

CT scanning will reveal a mass partially obliterating the gallbladder lumen in 42% of cases, a polypoidal mass in 26%, and diffuse wall thickening in 6% of cases (Fig. 85.6). However, only one-third of pathologically positive nodes are identified preoperatively by CT scan. Endoscopic ultrasound may be helpful as an adjunct to other imaging modalities for the evaluation of periportal and peripancreatic adenopathy. Unfortunately, large inflammatory lymph nodes are difficult to differentiate from metastatic tumor without pathologic confirmation. Endoscopic ultrasound-directed needle biopsy may be useful if the information would prevent a laparotomy. The use of MRI scanning for the diagnostic workup of gallbladder cancer can be helpful. MRCP may provide more detailed information than can be provided by ultrasound or CT scan.[197] Fluorodeoxyglucose (FDG)-PET scans have been examined in small studies with a sensitivity of 0.80 and a specificity of 0.82, positive predictive value of 0.67, and negative predictive value of 0.90 for suspicious lesions on ultrasound. For patients undergoing re-resection after an incidental finding of gallbladder cancer on routine cholecystectomy, FDG-PET was reported to change the management of 25% of patients.[65] As the availability of FDG-PET and PET/CT scans improves, more information will be reported on the accuracy of these studies to aid in the preoperative diagnosis of gallbladder cancer and to determine those to follow for residual or recurrent disease.[263]

Biopsy and Cytology

Once a mass suspicious for gallbladder cancer has been identified, it is controversial as to whether a biopsy should be performed prior to definitive exploration and resection. It is clear that cholecystectomy as a diagnostic biopsy prior to definitive resection is unacceptable, and all emphasis should be placed on being prepared for definitive resection at the time of initial exploration. Diagnosis by examination of bile cytology is one way to avoid violating the tumor and seeding cells into the peritoneal cavity or abdominal wound. The diagnostic accuracy of combined ERCP and bile cytology is 50% for gallbladder cancers. The sensitivity of bile cytology alone for the diagnosis of gallbladder cancer has been reported between 50% and 73%.[264] Any patient suspected of having gallbladder cancer who undergoes ERCP or PTC should have bile collected for cytologic examination.

Percutaneous fine-needle aspiration or core needle biopsy should be performed for masses that are not considered for surgical resection. The accuracy of percutaneous fine-needle aspiration has been reported at 88% for gallbladder cancers. The false-positive rate is negligible.[264] Percutaneous core needle biopsy has a higher chance of resulting in needle tract seeding than fine-needle aspiration and should be kept in reserve for cases in which fine-needle aspiration is unsuccessful. In cases in which a diagnosis of gallbladder cancer would result in referral to another institution for definitive surgical management, bile cytology or percutaneous fine-needle aspiration cytology would be preferable to any form of operative or laparoscopic biopsy. Endoscopic ultrasound-directed fine-needle aspiration for gallbladder lesions is associated with a 80% sensitivity and 100% specificity, and if available, is probably the best option for obtaining tissue for diagnosis.[265]

Surgery for Gallbladder Cancer

Prophylactic Cholecystectomy

The incidence of gallbladder cancer is low compared with the incidence of gallstones in the population, so prophylactic cholecystectomy for asymptomatic cholelithiasis to prevent the development of carcinoma is not indicated. Nevertheless, any abnormality in the gallbladder wall consistent with an early cancer needs to be taken seriously and consideration made for further workup. Only early diagnosis and treatment of gallbladder cancer are currently able to alter its natural history. High-risk situations may benefit from prophylactic cholecystectomy. For example, it has been suggested that patients with pancreaticobiliary maljunction and a normal-size bile duct may benefit from prophylactic cholecystectomy,[266] and northern Indian women may also benefit.[267] A calcified or "porcelain" gallbladder is an indication for cholecystectomy in the asymptomatic patient, as up to 25% of cases will be associated with gallbladder cancer. It may be in these high-risk situations that serum CA 19-9 evaluation and bile cytology will be helpful in making a preoperative diagnosis of cancer. Laparoscopic cholecystectomy could be reserved for those with normal markers and negative cytology. For those highly suspicious of cancer, the laparoscopic approach is not reasonable because of the risk for inadvertent seeding of the peritoneal cavity.

Benign Polyps

Benign tumors of the gallbladder are common and can be detected on ultrasound. They can be classified into epithelial tumors (adenoma), mesenchymal tumors (fibroma, lipoma, hemangioma), or pseudotumors (cholesterol polyps, inflammatory polyps, and adenomyoma). The majority of polyps are cholesterol polyps.[268] Four percent to 7% of patients with polypoid lesions of the gallbladder are found to have gallbladder cancer.[268] Malignant lesions were significantly more likely to be found in patients older than 50 years and more likely to be present as a solitary lesion more than 1 cm in diameter. A review of polypoid lesions recently demonstrated that 7.4% of polyps less than 10 mm in diameter were neoplastic with one adenocarcinoma (less than 2%).[269] Based on these findings, the indication for cholecystectomy for asymptomatic benign polyps includes any solitary polyp greater than 1 cm in diameter in a patient older than 50 years. For lesions that do not fit these characteristics, it is reasonable to obtain follow-up scans every 6 to 12 months, and any suspicious findings (focal thickening of the gallbladder wall) should be an indication for further workup, as previously described.

Extended (Radical) Cholecystectomy

A rational approach to surgery for gallbladder carcinoma was described by Glenn and Hays[270] in 1954 and included wedge resection of the gallbladder bed and regional lymphadenectomy of the hepatoduodenal ligament. Figure 85.7 is a diagrammatic representation of the extent of dissection in an extended or radical cholecystectomy. Definitive resection for gallbladder cancer depends on the stage and location of the tumor as well as whether it is a repeat resection after a previous simple cholecystectomy. T1 (stage IA) tumors can be treated with simple cholecystectomy. Any suspicious nodes should be removed for a frozen pathologic diagnosis. Stage IB, II, and selected stage III (T4N0) tumors should be treated with *en bloc* resection of the gallbladder, segments IVb and V of the liver, and regional lymph node dissection. Stage IV tumors should be treated with appropriate palliation as indicated. Patients who are being re-resected after simple cholecystectomy should undergo laparoscopic exploration for the diagnosis of small volume peritoneal and liver metastases. Twenty percent of patients will have findings that change the planned resection.[272] Because of the high incidence of locoregional recurrence, strict operative principles should be maintained for liver resection and lymph node dissection. Recommendations for liver resection for gallbladder cancer have ranged from a limited wedge excision of 2 cm of liver around the gallbladder bed to routine extended right hepatic lobectomy. The goal is to achieve a negative margin on the tumor, encompassing cells that have directly infiltrated the liver. The trend has moved away from aggressively resecting the liver toward using some technique to remove that part of the liver at the gallbladder bed that is contaminated with cancer cells.[273] Sometimes after prior cholecystectomy or biliary procedures, it can be difficult to differentiate scar and tumor in the porta hepatis. The best management in these cases may be an extended right hepatectomy and extrahepatic bile duct resection. The complication rate for extended resection can be as high as 50% with a mortality rate of 5%. The potential gain of the procedure must justify the risk. Good patient and tumor selection are essential in these cases.

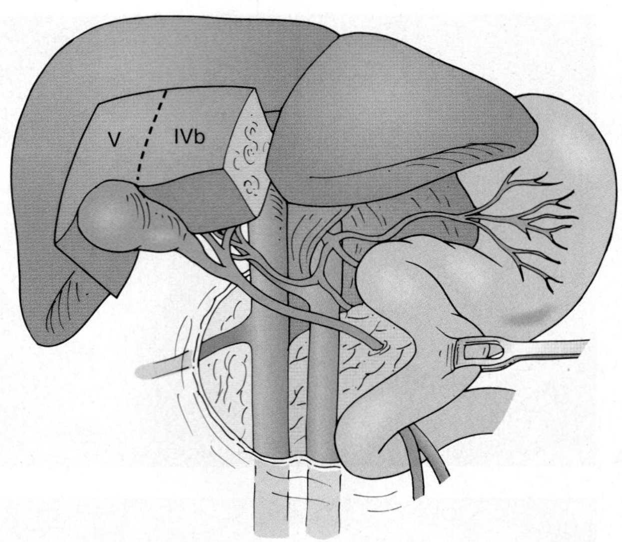

FIGURE 85.7 Schematic representing surgical treatment for gallbladder carcinoma. An extended cholecystectomy includes the gallbladder *en bloc* with segments IVb and V of the liver. Lymph nodes should be dissected completely from the shaded region. (From ref. 271, with permission.)

Recommendations for lymph node dissection for gallbladder cancer have ranged from excision of the cystic duct node alone to *en bloc* pancreaticoduodenectomy to clear the pancreaticoduodenal lymph nodes. In general, a full Kocher maneuver should be performed and lymphatic tissue should be dissected behind the duodenum and pancreas and swept superiorly. Any interaortocaval nodes or superior mesenteric nodes should be included in the specimen if possible. Also, the soft tissue anterior to the duodenum and pancreas should be swept superiorly. The portal vein and hepatic artery should be skeletonized and all tissue swept superiorly. Skeletonization should be continued as far into the liver hilum as possible. Resection of the common bile duct was thought to allow for a more reliable complete lymphatic clearance of the hepatoduodenal ligament, but it adds to the operative morbidity and does not increase the lymph node yield.[274,275] If the tumor is in the gallbladder neck and there is suspicion of mucosal spread into the common bile duct, or if inflammation and scarring compromise adequate skeletonization of the porta hepatis, then resection of the common bile duct with Roux-en-Y hepaticojejunostomy should be performed.

Surgical Results

Numerous studies have demonstrated that simple cholecystectomy is curative for stage I disease (T1N0) (Table 85.15). More recently, studies have suggested that the prognosis is different for pT1a and pT1b tumors after simple cholecystectomy.[286] Invasion of the muscular layer allows access to lymphatics and vessels, providing the rationale for extended cholecystectomy in this population. For accurate pathologic T1a staging, no extended cholecystectomy is indicated, and simple cholecystectomy should result in a 100% 5-year survival. These tumors are recognized incidentally at the time of pathologic review, and as long as the cystic duct margin is negative, no further surgery is indicated. The incidence of lymph node metastases is nonexistent in the setting of T1a disease.[287] If there is any doubt as to whether the pathologic staging is accurate, a more extensive re-resection is justified. For T1b staged tumors, an extended cholecystectomy is indicated, as these tumors have been reported to recur after simple cholecystectomy. In addition, there is a 10% incidence of residual disease in the gallbladder fossa and a 10% to 20% incidence of disease in lymph nodes discovered on re-resection for T1b cancers.[288]

Patients with stage II disease (T2N0) are best treated with an extended cholecystectomy. As previously discussed, ideally the cancer is recognized and diagnosed prior to disrupting the subserosal plane during simple cholecystectomy. Unfortunately, because most of these cases will be initially addressed laparoscopically, intraoperative diagnosis is uncommon for T2 disease. It is in these patients that radical repeat resection leads to the best chance of long-term cure. When an extended cholecystectomy is performed for T2 disease, the 5-year survival has been reported to be as high as 100%, but probably falls in the range of 70% to 90% (Table 85.16). Simple cholecystectomy alone is associated with a 5-year survival rate of 20% to 40.5%.[277,280] Lymph node metastases are seen in 46% of patients with T2 primary tumors, providing another reason in favor of radical repeat resection after simple cholecystectomy.[287]

For patients with stage IIb disease (T3N1), an extended cholecystectomy is the recommended treatment approach. This may include *en bloc* resection of the common bile duct for grossly positive periportal lymph nodes in order to improve periportal lymph node clearance. Patients with metastases to cystic duct or periportal lymph nodes can be cured, thus further justifying repeat resection for all tumors with transmural invasion. The 5-year survival ranges from 45% to 63% for patients having metastatic disease to N1 nodes. The 3-year survival has ranged from 38% to 80% in various trials (Table 85.17). Simple cholecystectomy or a lesser operation would not be expected to result in long-term survival.

TABLE 85.15

ACTUARIAL SURVIVAL RESULTS REPORTED IN RETROSPECTIVE REVIEWS AFTER RESECTION OF T1 GALLBLADDER CANCERS

Study (Ref.)	No. of Patients	Procedure	Survival (%) 3 Years	5 Years
Donohue et al., 1990 (248)	6	83% simple cholecystectomy	100	100
Ogura et al., 1991[a] (276)	366	Not specified	87	78
Shirai et al., 1992 (277)	39	Simple cholecystectomy	100	100
Yamaguchi and Tsuneyoshi, 1992 (278)	6	Simple cholecystectomy	100	100
Shirai et al., 1992 (279)	56	Simple cholecystectomy	100	100
	38	Extended cholecystectomy	100	100
de Aretxabala et al., 1997 (280)	32	69% simple cholecystectomy	94	94
Todoroki et al., 1999 (281)	13	Simple cholecystectomy	100	100
Wakai et al., 2002 (282)	12	Simple cholecystectomy	—	90
Toyonaga et al., 2003 (283)	23	Simple cholecystectomy	100	100
Yildirim et al., 2005 (284)				
(stage T1a)	5	40% simple cholecystectomy	100	100
(stage T1b)	8	62% simple cholecystectomy	100	80
Cangemi et al., 2006 (285)				
(stage T1a)	4	Simple cholecystectomy	100	100
(stage T1b)	11	73% simple cholecystectomy	—	55
Rodriguez Otero et al., 2006 (240)				
(stage T1a)	25	Simple cholecystectomy	100	100
(stage T1b)	26	Simple cholecystectomy	—	65

[a]Multi-institutional survey.

TABLE 85.16

ACTUARIAL SURVIVAL RESULTS REPORTED IN RETROSPECTIVE REVIEWS AFTER RESECTION OF T2 GALLBLADDER CANCERS

Study (Ref.)	No. of Patients	Procedure	Survival (%) 3 Years	5 Years
Donohue et al., 1990 (248)	12	67% extended cholecystectomy	58	22
Ogura et al., 1991[a] (276)	499	Not specified	53	37
Shirai et al., 1992 (279)	35	Simple cholecystectomy	57	40.5
	10	Extended cholecystectomy	90	90
Yamaguchi and Tsuneyoshi, 1992 (278)	25	Simple cholecystectomy	36	36
Cubertafond et al., 1994[a] (289)	52	88% simple cholecystectomy	20	—
Bartlett et al., 1996 (274)	8	Extended cholecystectomy	100	88
Todoroki et al., 1999 (281)	19	Extended cholecystectomy	—	78
Wakai et al., 2002 (282)	7	Extended cholecystectomy	100	100
Toyonaga et al., 2003 (283)	43	Extended cholecystectomy	68	54
Muratore et al., 2003 (290)	11	Extended cholecystectomy	—	64
Frena et al., 2004 (291)	5	Extended cholecystectomy	60	60
Yildirim et al., 2005 (284)	34	66% simple cholecystectomy	75	22
Foster et al., 2006 (292)	9	Extended cholecystectomy	78	78

[a]Multi-institutional survey.

Stage III gallbladder cancer represents an advanced malignancy that is generally beyond surgical treatment. However, patients with T4N0 disease, representing a mass-forming gallbladder cancer, may achieve long-term survival after an extended resection.[274] Patients with nodal metastases beyond the hepatoduodenal ligament have a poor prognosis, and in general for these cases the authors would advocate palliative care. Some investigators have reported anecdotal cases of long-term cures in patients with distant nodal disease (formerly N2 disease),[279] but most have reported a poor outcome, which does not justify the morbidity of the extended resection.

In series of extended cholecystectomies, the operative morbidity ranges from 5% to 46% and the mortality from 0% to 21%.[248,296,295] The morbidity and mortality rates of major liver resections have decreased in recent reports, even in the aged population, so with careful patient selection the extended cholecystectomy should be safe.[296] In a multiple-institution review of 1,686 gallbladder cancer resections from Japan, the authors reported a 12.8% morbidity for a simple cholecystectomy, 21.9% for extended cholecystectomy, and 48.3% for hepatic lobectomy.[276] The mortality rates were 2.9%, 2.3%, and 18%, respectively. The authors reported 150 hepatopancreaticoduodenectomies for gallbladder cancer, with 54% morbidity and 15.3% mortality rates. The risk of resection for each patient and for each type of resection needs to be weighed against the chance of benefiting from the procedure based on the tumor stage.

TABLE 85.17

ACTUARIAL SURVIVAL RESULTS REPORTED IN RETROSPECTIVE REVIEWS AFTER EXTENDED RESECTION OF T3 AND T4 GALLBLADDER CANCERS

Study (Ref.)	No. of Patients	T Stage	Survival (%) 3 Years	5 Years
Onoyama et al., 1995 (250)	12	T3	44	44
Bartlett et al., 1996 (274)	8	T3	63	63
Yildirim et al., 2005 (284)	10	T3	47	16
Foster et al., 2006 (292)	4	T3	25	25
Donohue et al., 1990 (248)	17	T3/T4	50	29
Shirai et al., 1992 (279)	20	T3/T4	—	45
Schauer et al., 2001 (293)	25	T3/T4	20	0
Kondo et al., 2002 (294)	68	T3/T4	44	33
Behari et al., 2003 (295)	29	T3/T4	35	28
Toyonaga et al., 2003 (283)	7	T3/T4	14	0
Frena et al., 2004 (291)	5	T3/T4	0	0
Ogura et al., 1991 (276)	453	T4	18	8
Onoyama et al., 1995 (250)	14	T4	8	8
Bartlett et al., 1996 (274)	7	T4	25	25
Todoroki et al., 1999 (281)	27	T4	7	—

Adjuvant Therapy

As with cholangiocarcinoma, reports on adjuvant radiotherapy after resection for gallbladder cancer are difficult to interpret. They consist of retrospective reviews and involve various combinations of resection (complete and incomplete), EBRT, brachytherapy, and IORT. Table 85.18 provides a summary of the larger reports. As shown, patients treated in the adjuvant setting have a median survival of approximately 2 years.

Kresl et al.[297] reported the Mayo Clinic experience with 21 gallbladder carcinoma patients who underwent surgery followed by EBRT to a median dose of 54 Gy in fractions of 1.8 to 2.0 Gy/d. One patient was also treated with 15 Gy of IORT after EBRT. All patients also received 5-FU with or without LV. For patients with gross residual tumor, microscopic residual tumor, and no residual disease, the median survival rates were 0.6, 1.4, and 15.1 years, respectively ($P = .02$). Two-year local control rates were 0%, 80%, and 88% for patients with gross residual tumor, microscopic residual tumor, and no residual tumor, respectively ($P < .01$). For six patients who received more than 54 Gy, the 3-year local control rate was 100% versus 65% for 15 patients who received less than 54 Gy. These results appear to be superior to surgery-alone historical results from the same institution.

Another report from the Mayo Clinic concentrated on 73 patients with stage I (T1-2N0M0) or stage II (T3N0M0 or T1-3N1M0) who underwent R0 resection.[301] Of these, 25 patients received adjuvant radiotherapy (median dose, 50.4 Gy in 28 fractions) with concurrent bolus 5-FU. The median overall survival for patients who received adjuvant chemoradiotherapy versus surgery alone was 4.8 years and 4.2 years, respectively (log-rank test, $P = .56$). However, patients who received adjuvant chemoradiotherapy had more advanced disease, and, on multivariate analysis, after adjusting for T and N category and histopathologic diagnosis other than adenocarcinoma, adjuvant chemoradiotherapy was found to be a significant predictor of improved overall survival (hazard ratio, 0.3; 95% CI, 0.13 to 0.69; $P = .0004$).

Balachandran et al.[299] reported on 117 patients with gallbladder cancer, of whom 80 underwent simple cholecystectomy and 37 underwent extended resections. Seventy-three patients received adjuvant chemoradiotherapy and 44 did not. No details were provided regarding this therapy or the selection criteria for adjuvant therapy. The median survival of all 117 patients was 16 months. On multivariate analysis, T stage and the use of adjuvant therapy were the only statistically significant independent predictors of survival. Median survival was 24 months, 11 months in patients with or without adjuvant chemoradiotherapy (P –.001), and this difference was most pronounced for patients with T3, node-positive disease or after a simple cholecystectomy.

Ben-David et al.[123] reported on 14 patients with gallbladder cancer treated at the University of Michigan with resection followed by radiotherapy or chemoradiotherapy. The median radiation dose was 54 Gy, and approximately half the patients received concurrent chemotherapy. The median survival was 23 months. Interestingly, there was no difference in survival between R0 and R1 resection patients. No differences were observed in survival or pattern of failure between patients with gallbladder cancer and patients with bile duct cancer (distal or hilar).

Czito et al.[298] reported on 22 patients with nonmetastatic gallbladder cancer treated at Duke University. R0, R1, and R2 resections were accomplished in 12, 6, and 4 patients, respectively. All patients received EBRT to a median dose of 45 Gy. This was followed by an external-beam boost of 5.4 to 10.8 Gy in four patients and intraluminal brachytherapy (50 Gy) in one patient. Concurrent 5-FU (bolus or continuous infusion) was administered to 18 patients. Median survival was 22.8 months and locoregional failure occurred in seven patients (35%).

To further clarify the potential role of adjuvant radiotherapy for gallbladder cancer, Wang et al.[302] analyzed the SEER data and identified 4,180 patients who underwent resection between 1988 and 2003. The authors constructed a multivariate Cox proportional hazards model for overall survival. Age, gender, papillary histology, stage, and adjuvant radiotherapy were significant predictors of survival. The model predicts that adjuvant radiotherapy provides a survival benefit in node-positive or T2 or higher disease. The unadjusted median overall survival in patients who received radiotherapy was 15 months compared to 8 months in those who did not ($P < .0001$).

The high risk of systemic spread and locoregional failure associated with gallbladder cancer that extends beyond the mucosa has led most cancer centers in the United States to recommend consideration of adjuvant chemotherapy and radiotherapy. For EBRT, the target volume should include the gallbladder fossa and adjacent liver, as well as the regional nodal areas (see earlier discussion on cholangiocarcinoma).

TABLE 85.18

ADJUVANT RADIOTHERAPY OR CHEMORADIOTHERAPY FOR GALLBLADDER CANCER

Study (Ref.)	No. of Patients	Radiotherapy	Chemotherapy	Median Survival (months)	*P*-Value
Kresl et al. (297)	21	54 Gy EBRT	5-FU bolus	31.2	—
Czito et al. (298)	22	45 Gy EBRT ± 5.4 to 50 Gy boost (5 patients)	5-FU bolus or CI (82% of patients)	22.8	—
Balachandran et al. (299)	44	None	None	11	.001
	73	Yes; no details	Yes; no details	24	
Ben-David et al. (123)	14	54 Gy EBRT	Mostly 5-FU-based (54% of patients)	23	—
Duffy et al. (300)	16	No details	Mostly 5-FU-based during radiotherapy; 8 received additional systemic therapy	23.4	.4
	99	None	None	30.3	
Gold et al. (301)	25	50.4 Gy EBRT	5-FU bolus	4.8 years	.56
	48	None	None	4.2 years	

EBRT, external-beam radiation therapy; 5-FU, 5-fluorouracil; CI, continuous infusion.

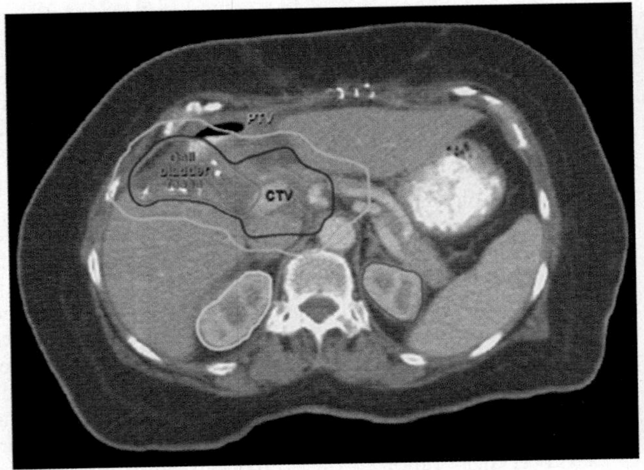

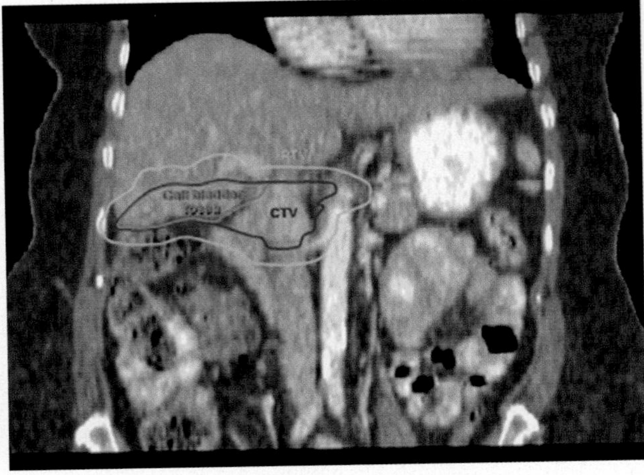

FIGURE 85.8 Target delineation for adjuvant radiotherapy for gallbladder cancer. The patient was a 70-year-old woman with *pT3N1* adenocarcinoma of the gallbladder, status after radical cholecystectomy with negative resection margins. The clinical target volume (CTV) includes the gallbladder fossa and the regional lymphatics. The planning target volume (PTV) includes a 5-mm expansion for setup error and appropriate expansions for breathing motion. The latter were determined in this case by diaphragmatic excursion as visualized on fluoroscopy. **A:** Target delineation in an axial plane. **B:** Target delineation in a coronal plane.

Using conformal three-dimensional treatment planning, doses of 45 to 50 Gy are delivered to the nodal basin, and doses of 54 to 60 Gy are delivered to the gallbladder fossa. The mean liver dose (the most common limiting factor) should not exceed 30 Gy. Small bowel dose should generally not exceed 45 Gy, although very small volumes can be taken to doses of 50 to 54 Gy if needed. Figure 85.8 depicts target delineation in the adjuvant setting, and Figure 85.9 shows a typical beam arrangement and the resulting dose distribution.

Advanced Gallbladder Cancer

The median survival for patients presenting with unresectable disease is 2 to 4 months, with a 1-year survival rate of less than 5%. This aggressive course needs to be considered when deciding on palliative management. The goal of palliation should be relief of pain, jaundice, and bowel obstruction and prolongation of life. These should be done as simply as possible, given

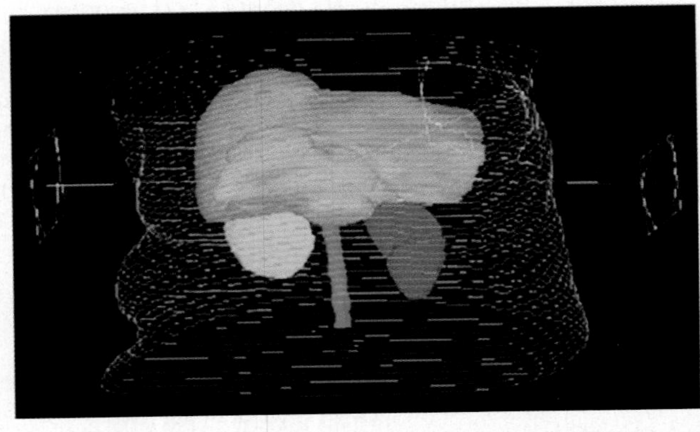

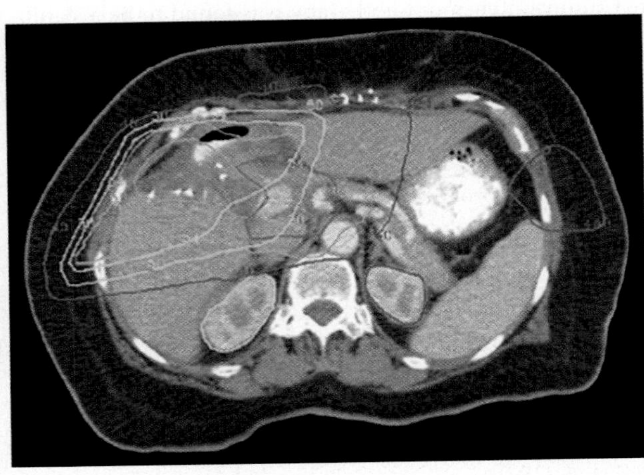

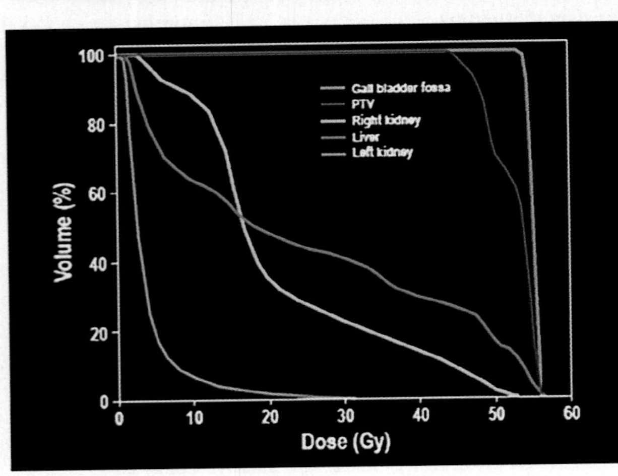

FIGURE 85.9 Treatment planning of adjuvant radiotherapy for gallbladder cancer. **A:** The beam arrangement used to treat the patient discussed in Figure 85.8. The liver is depicted in beige; the clinical target volume (CTV) is depicted in lavender, left kidney in red, right kidney in yellow, and spinal cord in green. **B:** The composite dose distribution in an axial plane. The planning target volume (PTV) was prescribed 45 Gy in 1.8 Gy fractions. This was followed by 9-Gy (in 5 fractions) boost to the gallbladder fossa. Radiotherapy was administered with concurrent capecitabine. **C:** The resulting cumulative dose-volume histogram.

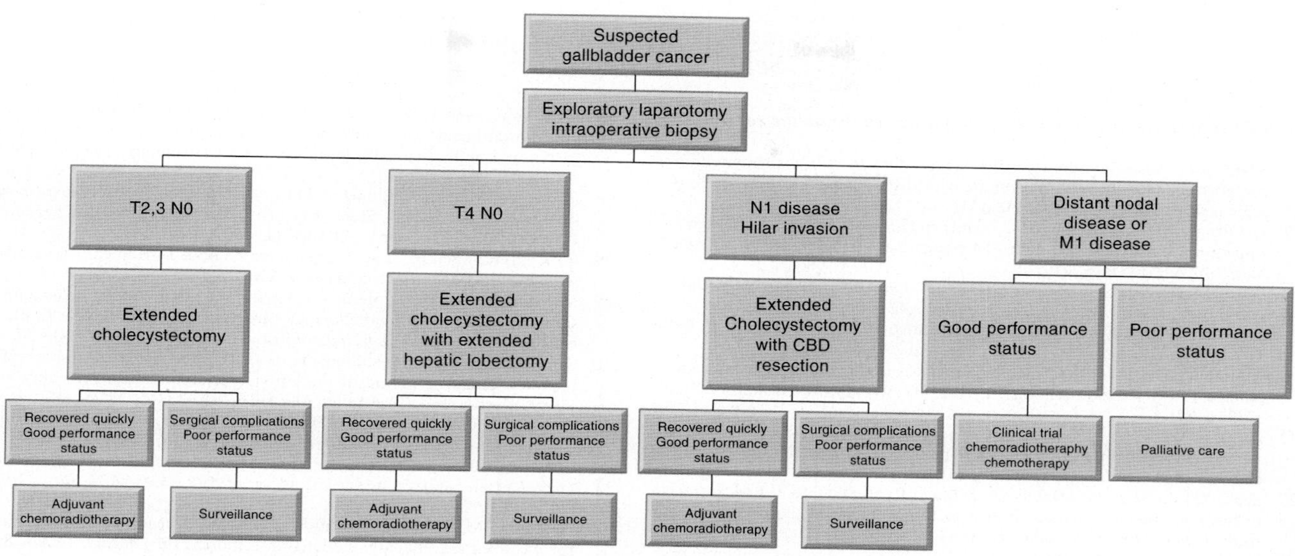

FIGURE 85.10 Algorithm for management of gallbladder carcinoma identified on preoperative imaging. T1 tumors should not be recognized preoperatively except for papillary tumors, which can be managed with simple cholecystectomy.

the aggressive nature of this disease. Resection of gross disease probably provides the best palliation and a chance for cure in some instances, but is usually not possible. Palliation of biliary obstruction is performed identical to that of cholangiocarcinoma, as previously discussed. Percutaneous stents are effective and should be used, as the expected survival does not usually warrant a surgical bypass.

Chemotherapy has been used for palliation of unresectable disease. Clinical trials have grouped gallbladder and bile duct cancers together. An analysis of 103 trials in biliary tree cancer suggests that gallbladder cancer may have a higher response to chemotherapy, but with lower median survival compared with bile duct cancers.[219] For practical purposes, chemotherapy recommendations are similar for both gallbladder and bile duct cancer, and the new reference regimen is gemcitabine and cisplatin, as described previously.[191] Regional therapy is possible for gallbladder cancer. In one study, intra-arterial mitomycin C was evaluated. A 48% overall response rate and a prolongation of median survival from 5 to 14 months compared with historical controls was reported.[192] Radiation therapy has also been examined in palliation for gallbladder cancer. The benefit is minimal, with a median survival of only 6 to 8 months. It does appear to be well tolerated, and although of unproven benefit, may improve symptoms and prolong survival in selected patients.

Gallbladder cancer is an aggressive disease with a dismal prognosis. Resection of hematogenous metastasis is not justified nor is resection of distant nodal disease. Patients with advanced disease should be considered for clinical trials. An algorithm for management is shown in Figures 85.10 and 85.11. It is unlikely that additional significant improvements in the survival of patients with biliary tract cancers will be seen with current available chemotherapeutic agents, and new approaches are needed. Understanding the molecular biology of the biliary tract cancers will be crucial, and future studies should be rationally designed based on the molecular profile of biliary tree cancers.[39]

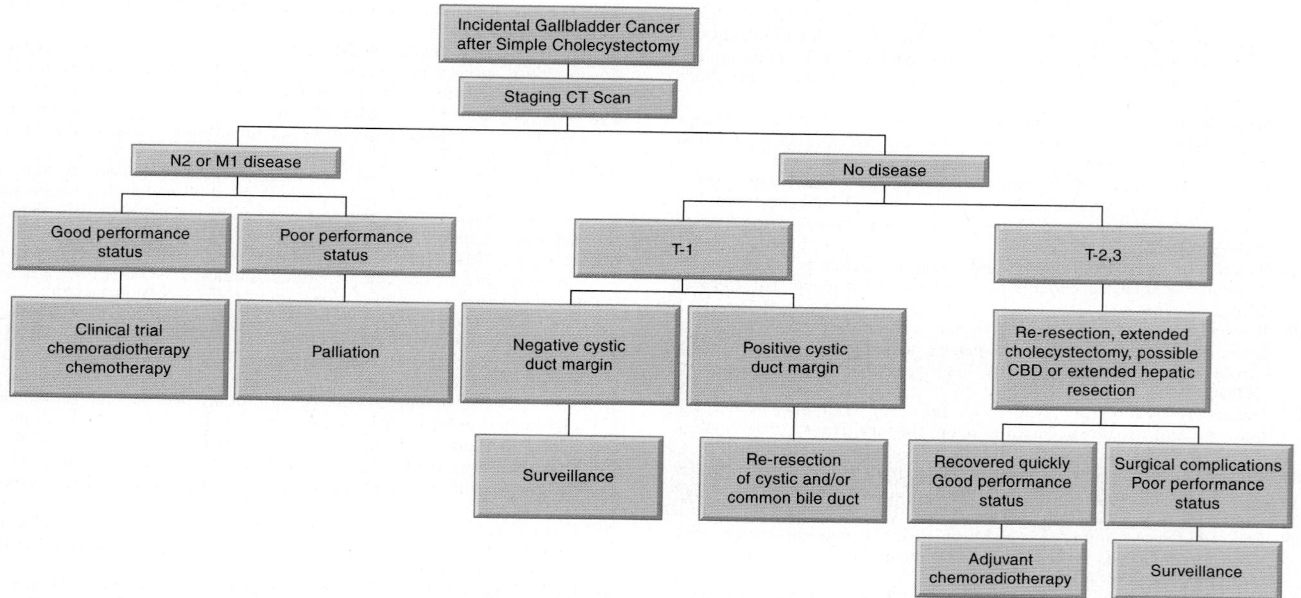

FIGURE 85.11 Algorithm for management of gallbladder cancer found as an incidental finding on pathologic examination of a cholecystectomy specimen. CT, computed tomography.

Selected References

The full list of references for this chapter appears in the online version.

1. Klatskin G. Adenocarcinoma of the hepatic duct at its bifurcation within the porta hepatis. An unusual tumor with distinctive clinical and pathologic features. *Am J Med* 1965;38:241.
2. DeOliveira ML, Cunningham SC, Cameron JL, et al. Cholangiocarcinoma: thirty-one-year experience with 564 patients at a single institution. *Ann Surg* 2007;245:755.
3. Gatto M, Bragazzi MC, Semeraro R, et al. Cholangiocarcinoma: update and future perspectives. *Dig Liver Dis* 2010;42:253.
6. Jemal A, Siegel R, Xu J, Ward E. Cancer statistics, 2010. *CA Cancer J Clin* 2010;60(5):277.
9. Aljiffry M, Walsh MJ, Molinari M. Advances in diagnosis, treatment and palliation of cholangiocarcinoma: 1990–2009. *World J Gastroenterol* 2009; 15(34):4240.
22. Grainge MJ, West J, Solaymani-Dodaran M, Aithal GP, Card TR. The antecedents of biliary cancer: a primary care case-control study in the United Kingdom. *Br J Cancer* 2009;100(1):178.
23. Shaib YH, El-Serag HB, Davila JA, Morgan R, McGlynn KA. Risk factors of intrahepatic cholangiocarcinoma in the United States: a case-control study. *Gastroenterology* 2005;128(3):620.
25. Uesaka K, Yasui K, Morimoto T, et al. Visualization of routes of lymphatic drainage of the gallbladder with a carbon particle suspension. *J Am Coll Surg* 1996;183:345.
31. Hezel AF, Deshpande V, Zhu AX. Genetics of biliary tract cancers and emerging targeted therapies. *J Clin Oncol* 2010;28:3531.
32. Hassid VJ, Orlando FA, Awad ZT, et al. Genetic and molecular abnormalities in cholangiocarcinogenesis. *Anticancer Res* 2009;29:1151.
40. Fevery J, Verslype C. An update on cholangiocarcinoma associated with primary sclerosing cholangitis. *Curr Opin Gastroenterol* 2010;26(3):236.
41. Edge SB, Byrd DR, Compton CC, et al. *AJCC cancer staging manual*. New York: Springer, 2010.
42. Jarnagin WR, Fong Y, DeMatteo RP, et al. Staging, resectability, and outcome in 225 patients with hilar cholangiocarcinoma. *Ann Surg* 2001; 234:507.
56. Manfredi R, Masselli G, Maresca G, et al. MR imaging and MRCP of hilar cholangiocarcinoma. *Abdom Imaging* 2003;28:319.
59. Seo H, Lee JM, Kim IH, et al. Evaluation of the gross type and longitudinal extent of extrahepatic cholangiocarcinomas on contrast-enhanced multidetector row computed tomography. *J Comput Assist Tomogr* 2009; 33(3):376.
63. Kawakami H, Kuwatani M, Onodera M, et al. Endoscopic nasobiliary drainage is the most suitable preoperative biliary drainage method in the management of patients with hilar cholangiocarcinoma. *J Gastroenterol* 2010; (in press).
66. Corvera CU, Blumgart LH, Akhurst T, et al. 18F-fluorodeoxyglucose positron emission tomography influences management decisions in patients with biliary cancer. *J Am Coll Surg* 2008;206(1):57.[dup ref 227]
70. Stavropoulos S, Larghi A, Verna E, Battezzati P, Stevens P. Intraductal ultrasound for the evaluation of patients with biliary strictures and no abdominal mass on computed tomography. *Endoscopy* 2005;37(8):715.
73. Charatcharoenwitthaya P, Enders FB, Halling KC, Lindor KD. Utility of serum tumor markers, imaging, and biliary cytology for detecting cholangiocarcinoma in primary sclerosing cholangitis. *Hepatology* 2008; 48(4):1106.
77. Sewnath ME, Karsten TM, Prins MH, et al. A meta-analysis on the efficacy of preoperative biliary drainage for tumors causing obstructive jaundice. *Ann Surg* 2002;236:17.
78. Goere D, Wagholikar GD, Pessaux P, et al. Utility of staging laparoscopy in subsets of biliary cancers: laparoscopy is a powerful diagnostic tool in patients with intrahepatic and gallbladder carcinoma. *Surg Endosc* 2006;20(5):721.
85. Paik KY, Jung JC, Heo JS, et al. What prognostic factors are important for resected intrahepatic cholangiocarcinoma? *J Gastroenterol Hepatol* 2008;23(5):766.
86. Konstadoulakis MM, Roayaie S, Gomatos IP, et al. Fifteen-year, single-center experience with the surgical management of intrahepatic cholangiocarcinoma: operative results and long-term outcome. *Surgery* 2008; 143(3):366.
87. Nakagohri T, Kinoshita T, Konishi M, Takahashi S, Gotohda N. Surgical outcome and prognostic factors in intrahepatic cholangiocarcinoma. *World J Surg* 2008;32(12):2675.
88. Tamandl D, Herberger B, Gruenberger B, et al. Influence of hepatic resection margin on recurrence and survival in intrahepatic cholangiocarcinoma. *Ann Surg Oncol* 2008;15(10):2787.
89. Endo I, Gonen M, Yopp AC, et al. Intrahepatic cholangiocarcinoma: rising frequency, improved survival, and determinants of outcome after resection. *Ann Surg* 2008;248(1):84.
91. Lang H, Sotiropoulos GC, Sgourakis G, et al. Operations for intrahepatic cholangiocarcinoma: single-institution experience of 158 patients. *J Am Coll Surg* 2009;208(2):218.
93. Shimada K, Sano T, Nara S, et al. Therapeutic value of lymph node dissection during hepatectomy in patients with intrahepatic cholangiocellular carcinoma with negative lymph node involvement. *Surgery* 2009; 145(4):411.
96. Rocha FG, Matsuo K, Blumgart LH, Jarnagin WR. Hilar cholangiocarcinoma: the Memorial Sloan-Kettering Cancer Center experience. *J Hepatobiliary Pancreat Sci* 2010;17(4):490.
99. Ito K, Ito H, Allen PJ, et al. Adequate lymph node assessment for extrahepatic bile duct adenocarcinoma. *Ann Surg* 2010;251(4):675.
109. Miyazaki M, Kimura F, Shimizu H, et al. One hundred seven consecutive surgical resections for hilar cholangiocarcinoma of Bismuth types II, III, IV between 2001 and 2008. *J Hepatobiliary Pancreat Sci* 2010;17(4):470.
110. Shimizu H, Kimura F, Yoshidome H, et al. Aggressive surgical resection for hilar cholangiocarcinoma of the left-side predominance: radicality and safety of left-sided hepatectomy. *Ann Surg* 2010;251(2):281.
114. Otani K, Chijiiwa K, Kai M, et al. Outcome of surgical treatment of hilar cholangiocarcinoma. *J Gastrointest Surg* 2008;12(6):1033.
117. Cheng Q, Luo X, Zhang B, et al. Distal bile duct carcinoma: prognostic factors after curative surgery. A series of 112 cases. *Ann Surg Oncol* 2007;14(3):1212.
123. Ben-David MA, Griffith KA, bu-Isa E, et al. External-beam radiotherapy for localized extrahepatic cholangiocarcinoma. *Int J Radiat Oncol Biol Phys* 2006;66:772.
124. Gerhards MF, van Gulik TM, Gonzalez GD, et al. Results of postoperative radiotherapy for resectable hilar cholangiocarcinoma. *World J Surg* 2003;27:173.
125. Kim S, Kim SW, Bang YJ, et al. Role of postoperative radiotherapy in the management of extrahepatic bile duct cancer. *Int J Radiat Oncol Biol Phys* 2002;54:414.
126. Todoroki T, Ohara K, Kawamoto T, et al. Benefits of adjuvant radiotherapy after radical resection of locally advanced main hepatic duct carcinoma. *Int J Radiat Oncol Biol Phys* 2000;46:581.
127. Schoenthaler R, Phillips TL, Castro J, et al. Carcinoma of the extrahepatic bile ducts. The University of California at San Francisco experience. *Ann Surg* 1994;219:267.
128. Sagawa N, Kondo S, Morikawa T, et al. Effectiveness of radiation therapy after surgery for hilar cholangiocarcinoma. *Surg Today* 2005;35:548.
129. Pitt HA, Nakeeb A, Abrams RA, et al. Perihilar cholangiocarcinoma. Postoperative radiotherapy does not improve survival. *Ann Surg* 1995; 221:788.
130. Nakeeb A, Tran KQ, Black MJ, et al. Improved survival in resected biliary malignancies. *Surgery* 2002;132:555.
131. Urego M, Flickinger JC, Carr BI. Radiotherapy and multimodality management of cholangiocarcinoma. *Int J Radiat Oncol Biol Phys* 1999; 44:121.
135. Klinkenbijl JH, Jeekel J, Sahmoud T, et al. Adjuvant radiotherapy and 5-fluorouracil after curative resection of cancer of the pancreas and periampullary region: phase III trial of the EORTC gastrointestinal tract cancer cooperative group. *Ann Surg* 1999;230:776.
136. Nelson JW, Ghafoori AP, Willett CG, et al. Concurrent chemoradiotherapy in resected extrahepatic cholangiocarcinoma. *Int J Radiat Oncol Biol Phys* 2009;73(1):148.
137. Shinohara ET, Mitra N, Guo M, Metz JM. Radiotherapy is associated with improved survival in adjuvant and palliative treatment of extrahepatic cholangiocarcinomas. *Int J Radiat Oncol Biol Phys* 2009;74(4):1191.
138. Fuller CD, Wang SJ, Choi M, et al. Multimodality therapy for locoregional extrahepatic cholangiocarcinoma: a population-based analysis. *Cancer* 2009;115(22):5175.
139. Takada T, Amano H, Yasuda H, et al. Is postoperative adjuvant chemotherapy useful for gallbladder carcinoma? A phase III multicenter prospective randomized controlled trial in patients with resected pancreaticobiliary carcinoma. *Cancer* 2002;95:1685.
140. Park J, Kim MH, Kim KP, et al. Natural history and prognostic factors of advanced cholangiocarcinoma without surgery, chemotherapy, or radiotherapy: a large-scale observational study. *Gut Liver* 2009;3(4):298.
157. Rao S, Cunningham D, Hawkins RE, et al. Phase III study of 5-FU, etoposide and leucovorin (FELV) compared to epirubicin, cisplatin and 5FU (ECF) in previously untreated patients with advanced biliary cancer. *Br J Cancer* 2005;92:1650.
167. Kornek GV, Schuell B, Laengle F, et al. Mitomycin C in combination with capecitabine or biweekly high-dose gemcitabine in patients with advanced biliary tract cancer: a randomised phase II trial. *Ann Oncol* 2004;15:478.
180. Knox JJ, Hedley D, Oza A, et al. Combining gemcitabine and capecitabine in patients with advanced biliary cancer: a phase II trial. *J Clin Oncol* 2005;23:2332.
185. Dowlati A, Posey J, Ramanathan RK, et al. Phase II and pharmacokinetic trial of rebeccamycin analog in advanced biliary cancers. *Cancer Chemother Pharmacol* 2009;65:73.
188. Ramanathan RK, Belani CP, Singh DA, et al. A phase II study of lapatinib in patients with advanced biliary tree and hepatocellular cancer. *Cancer Chemother Pharmacol* 2009;64:777.

190. Zhu AX, Meyerhardt JA, Blaszkowsky LS, et al. Efficacy and safety of gemcitabine, oxaliplatin, and bevacizumab in advanced biliary-tract cancers and correlation of changes in 18-fluorodeoxyglucose PET with clinical outcome: a phase 2 study. *Lancet Oncol* 2010;11:48.
191. Valle J, Wasan H, Palmer DH, et al. Cisplatin plus gemcitabine versus gemcitabine for biliary tract cancer. *N Engl J Med* 2010;362:1273.
203. El-Khoueiry AB, Rankin C, Lenz HJ, et al. SWOG 0514: a phase II study of sorafenib (BAY 43-9006) as single agent in patients (pts) with unresectable or metastatic gallbladder cancer or cholangiocarcinomas. *J Clin Oncol* 2007:25(Suppl 18s): (abst 4639).
205. Malka D, Trarbach T, Fartoux L, et al. A multicenter, randomized phase II trial of gemcitabine and oxaliplatin (GEMOX) alone or in combination with biweekly cetuximab in the first-line treatment of advanced biliary cancer: interim analysis of the BINGO trial. *J Clin Oncol* 2009;27(Suppl 15s): (abst 4520).
218. Jonas S, Mittler J, Pascher A, et al. Extended indications in living-donor liver transplantation: bile duct cancer. *Transplantation* 2005;80(1 Suppl):S101.
219. Eckel F, Schmid RM. Chemotherapy in advanced biliary tract carcinoma: a pooled analysis of clinical trials. *Br J Cancer* 2007;96:896.
221. Perpetuo MD, Valdivieso M, Heilbrun LK, et al. Natural history study of gallbladder cancer: a review of 36 years experience at M. D. Anderson Hospital and Tumor Institute. *Cancer* 1978;42:330.
223. Mayo SC, Shore AD, Nathan H, et al. National trends in the management and survival of surgically managed gallbladder adenocarcinoma over 15 years: a population-based analysis. *J Gastrointest Surg* 2010;14(10): 1578.
229. Saika K, Matsuda T. Comparison of time trends in gallbladder cancer mortality (1990–2006) between countries based using the WHO mortality database. *Jpn J Clin Oncol* 2010;40(4):374.
269. Zielinski MD, Atwell TD, Davis PW, Kendrick ML, Que FG. Comparison of surgically resected polypoid lesions of the gallbladder to their preoperative ultrasound characteristics. *J Gastrointest Surg* 2009;13(1):19.
270. Glenn F, Hays DM. The scope of radical surgery in the treatment of malignant tumors of the extrahepatic biliary tract. *Surg Gynecol Obstet* 1954;99:529.
275. D'Angelica M, Dalal KM, DeMatteo RP, et al. Analysis of the extent of resection for adenocarcinoma of the gallbladder. *Ann Surg Oncol* 2009; 16(4):806.
286. Rodriguez Otero JC, Proske A, Vallilengua C, et al. Gallbladder cancer: surgical results after cholecystectomy in 25 patients with lamina propria invasion and 26 patients with muscular layer invasion. *J Hepatobiliary Pancreat Surg* 2006;13:562.[dup ref 297]
288. Pawlik TM, Gleisner AL, Vigano L, et al. Incidence of finding residual disease for incidental gallbladder carcinoma: implications for re-resection. *J Gastrointest Surg* 2007;11(11):1478.
292. Foster JM, Hoshi H, Gibbs JF, et al. Gallbladder cancer: defining the indications for primary radical resection and radical re-resection. *Ann Surg Oncol* 2007;14:833.
297. Kresl JJ, Schild SE, Henning GT, et al. Adjuvant external beam radiation therapy with concurrent chemotherapy in the management of gallbladder carcinoma. *Int J Radiat Oncol Biol Phys* 2002;52:167.
298. Czito BG, Hurwitz HI, Clough RW, et al. Adjuvant external-beam radiotherapy with concurrent chemotherapy after resection of primary gallbladder carcinoma: a 23-year experience. *Int J Radiat Oncol Biol Phys* 2005;62:1030.
299. Balachandran P, Agarwal S, Krishnani N, et al. Predictors of long-term survival in patients with gallbladder cancer. *J Gastrointest Surg* 2006;10:848.
300. Duffy A, Capanu M, Abou-Alfa GK, et al. Gallbladder cancer (GBC): 10-year experience at Memorial Sloan-Kettering Cancer Centre (MSKCC). *J Surg Oncol* 2008;98(7):485.
301. Gold DG, Miller RC, Haddock MG, et al. Adjuvant therapy for gallbladder carcinoma: the Mayo Clinic experience. *Int J Radiat Oncol Biol Phys* 2009;75(1):150.
302. Wang SJ, Fuller CD, Kim JS, et al. Prediction model for estimating the survival benefit of adjuvant radiotherapy for gallbladder cancer. *J Clin Oncol* 2008;26(13):2112.

CHAPTER 86 CANCER OF THE SMALL INTESTINE

AMER H. ZUREIKAT, MATTHEW T. HELLER, AND HERBERT J ZEH, III

SMALL BOWEL CANCER

Small bowel cancer (SBC) is a rare entity that has increased in incidence in the past few decades. The diagnosis of SBC is often challenging due to its rarity, diversity, and the large variation in its clinical presentation. Consequently, a majority of these tumors are discovered at a late stage when available therapeutic interventions become limited. The following sections present a detailed account of the epidemiology, pathogenesis, diagnosis, and management of small bowel tumors, focusing on the four most common subtypes: adenocarcinomas, carcinoid, lymphoma, and sarcomas or gastrointestinal stromal tumors (GIST).

Epidemiology

SBCs are among the more rare types of cancer, accounting for only 2% of all gastrointestinal cancers. Incidence is approximately 6,100 new cases per year, causing approximately 1,100 deaths per year in the United States. The Surveillance, epidemiology, and End Results (SEER) database registries have documented an increased incidence in the past three decades.[1,2] More than 40 different histologically distinct tumors have been described in the small intestine; however, in more than 95% of them, pathology is consistent with adenocarcinoma carcinoid, lymphoma, or stromal tumors (GIST).

SBC occurs most commonly in the seventh decade, with a slight preponderance in men and whites. Until recently, adenocarcinoma of the small intestine comprised the most common histologic type of malignant tumors (45%), followed by carcinoid (29%), lymphoma (16%), and sarcoma (10%). The past decade witnessed an increased incidence of carcinoid tumors from 29% to 44%, surpassing adenocarcinoma as the most common tumors of the small intestine, with a decrease in incidence of adenocarcinoma from 45% to 33%.[3–16] The incidence of lymphoma and sarcoma remains unchanged.

Pathogenesis

Despite constituting 75% of the length of the gastrointestinal (GI) tract and 90% of its absorptive surface, SBC occurs with much less frequency than other GI tract malignancies (40- to 60-fold less than colon cancer). Arguments put forth to explain this include:

- *High levels of benzopyrene hydroxylase and folate receptors*: Benzopyrene is a well-known and potent mutagen that intercalates with DNA and interferes with transcription. It is present in cigarette smoke and may be found in high levels in barbecued food, canned food, and charbroiled (grilled) foods. Benzopyrene hydroxylase, an enzyme that converts this compound to a less toxic metabolite, is found in much higher levels in the small intestine compared to the colon. In addition, folate receptors, which are believed to play an antagonistic role in carcinogenesis, are found in high levels in the small intestine.
- *Low bacterial load*: Anaerobic bacteria, present in large quantities in the colon, are rare in the small bowel. Presence of bacteria may interact with bile salts and bile acids, and this milieu may act as a tumor promoter.
- *Fast transit time*: Almost 50% of the stomach's contents empty in 2.5 to 3 hours, which is the same amount of time it takes for the much longer small intestine to empty 50% of its contents. In contrast, the colon takes almost 30 to 40 hours for an entire transit. The much faster transit time provides less exposure to any carcinogenic stimulus in the lumen or its contents.
- *High cellular turnover*: The small intestine replaces its cellular mass at the rate of 90 g per day. This provides less chance for a certain "critical mass" to be reached within senescent cells, to provide any breeding ground for cancer.
- *Liquid and alkaline milieu*: Alkalinity of the small intestinal chyme renders most carcinogens less active.
- *Safe stem cells*: The small intestine has far fewer stem cells that could be exposed to carcinogens. Moreover, the stem cells in the small intestine are located deep in the intestinal glandular crypts, where they are least exposed to intraluminal carcinogenic stimuli.
- *Immune protection*: The small intestine has an abundance of lymphoid cells in Peyer's patches. It is also abundant in surface immunity due to the high levels of mucosal immunoglobulin A (IgA). This theory is also supported by other findings, such as the increased incidence of SBC in IgA deficient individuals and the remarkably low incidence of malignancy in the spleen, which is also an immune cell–rich organ.

Given the rare occurrence and diverse histologic makeup of cancers that arise in the small intestine, none of these theories has received sufficient study to be accepted as medical fact; however, they provide substrate for future research into these cancers.

Risk Factors

Although their etiology is still largely unknown, several genetic, autoimmune, and lifestyle factors (Table 86.1) have been recognized to predispose to an increased risk of small bowel cancers.[17–34]

- *Familial adenomatous polyposis (FAP)*: FAP is a condition caused by a germline mutation in the adenomatous polyposis coli (*APC*) gene, a tumor suppressor gene. Patients with FAP develop early onset of hundreds to thousands of adenomatous polyps primarily throughout the colon, as well as in the small intestine and duodenum. In effect, periampullary

TABLE 86.1

RISK FACTORS AND PREDISPOSING CONDITIONS IN THE DEVELOPMENT OF SMALL BOWEL CANCER

Risk Factor	Lifetime Risk	Small Bowel Cancer Type
GENETIC		
Familial adenomatous polyposis 2%–5%	2%–5%	Periampullary adenocarcinoma
Hereditary nonpolyposis colorectal cancer	1%–4%	Duodenal/jejunal adenocarcinoma
Peutz Jeghers syndrome	15-fold	Adenocarcinoma Gardner syndrome desmoid
AUTOIMMUNE/INFLAMMATORY		
Crohn's disease	(>10 yrs) 2%	Ileal adenocarcinoma Celiac disease (tropical sprue) Jejunal lymphoma/adenocarcinoma Cystic fibrosis Ileal adenocarcinoma Immunosuppression lymphoma *posttransplant lymphoproliferative disorder*/sarcoma Neurofibromatosis paraganglioma
MALIGNANCIES		
Colorectal cancer, pancreas, prostate, uterine, skin/soft tissues		
BENIGN CONDITIONS		
Cholecystectomy, peptic ulcer disease		
OTHER		
Male gender, African American, old age, high fat diet		

adenocarcinoma develops in 2% to 5% of patients with FAP following colectomy and is the leading cause of death in this patient group, with a lifetime risk of 330-fold over that of the general population.[18–22] Periodic screening with esophagogastroduodenoscopy is hence crucial in this patient population. In addition, patients with FAP have higher incidence of desmoid tumors in the small intestine as well as the mesentery.

- *Hereditary nonpolyposis colorectal cancer (HNPCC)*: HNPCC, also called Lynch syndrome, is an inherited condition characterized by mutations in the DNA mismatch repair genes. Affected individuals have about 80% lifetime risk for colon cancer. In addition, patients with HNPCC are at increased risk for development of other malignancies, such as SBC, occurring most commonly in the duodenum and jejunum, with a lifetime risk of 1% to 4% (or 100-fold increase).[23–27] Several recent reviews have suggested that small bowel tumors may often be the presenting tumor in these patients, which occur at a very young age.
- *Peutz-Jeghers syndrome (PJS)*: PJS is an autosomal dominant inherited disorder caused by a mutation in the *STK11* (*LKB1*) tumor suppressor gene. It is characterized by intestinal hamartomatous polyps in association with mucocutaneous melanocytic macules on the lips and oral mucosa. Although the intestinal polyps are benign hamartomas, patients with PJS have a 15-fold increased risk of development of small as well as large intestinal adenocarcinomas compared with that of the general population.[28]
- *Other genetic conditions*: Gardner syndrome, an autosomal dominant genetic disorder, is characterized by multiple colonic polyps, multiple osteomas, and skin and soft tissue tumors. Patients with this condition have a higher incidence of desmoid tumors compared to the general population. The neurofibromas in von Recklinghausen's disease have the potential of malignant transformation into paragangliomas. Patients with cystic fibrosis have also been noted to have increased incidence of ileal adenocarcinomas.
- *Crohn's disease (CD)*: Patients with CD have a recognized 10 to 66.7 increased risk of developing small intestinal adenocarcinomas compared to the general population. In effect, CD-associated adenocarcinomas occur in approximately 2% of patients with longstanding (more than 10 years) CD and are usually localized to the ileum.[29–31] Both medical and surgical management appears to decrease the risk of CD-associated adenocarcinomas.
- *Celiac disease*: Celiac disease is an autoimmune disorder characterized by villous atrophy of the small intestine caused by a reaction to gliadin, a gluten protein found in wheat. Refractory conditions are associated with lymphoma, referred to as *enteropathy-associated T-cell lymphoma* (EATL) in 39% of the cases.[32,33] These lymphomas are primarily localized to the jejunum and are T cell in origin. To a lesser extent, celiac disease can also be associated with adenocarcinoma of the jejunum.[34,35] The adherence to a gluten-free diet reduces the risk of all malignancies associated with celiac disease.
- *Immunosuppression*: Both iatrogenic, following transplantation, and acquired inflammatory states have been associated with increased rates of lymphomas and sarcomas. Lymphomas in the setting of immunosuppression are termed *posttransplant lymphoproliferative disorder* (PTLD) and are usually characterized by uncontrolled proliferation of B-cell lymphocytes following infection with Epstein-Barr virus.
- *Other malignancies*: Patients with other primary cancers, such as colon, rectum, pancreas, periampullary, uterine, ovarian, prostate, thyroid, skin, and soft tissue tumors are at a higher risk of developing SBC. The reverse is true with 30% to 40% of SBC patients harbouring another synchronous malignancy; the surgeon should, therefore, thoroughly explore the abdominal cavity before proceeding with a definitive resection for a small bowel malignancy.[36–38]

Clinical Presentation

The presentation of SBC is nonspecific. Despite this, some generalizations can be inferred from large case series: (1) although overall presentation is delayed, SBC is more likely to be symptomatic earlier in the course of illness as opposed to benign lesions[39]; (2) the most frequent presenting signs and symptoms include abdominal pain, nausea, vomiting, and weight loss, which are present in more than 45% of patients[9,11–13]; and (3) approximately 50% of all SBCs present acutely, which manifests as an obstruction or perforation in 77% of acute presentations.[24] With respect to various histologic subtypes, adenocarcinomas tend to be associated with pain and obstructions, while sarcomas and lymphomas are frequently associated with acute GI hemorrhage and perforation, respectively. In addition, different subtypes have predilection to different regions of the small intestine. Adenocarcinomas tend to involve mainly the duodenum, while carcinoids more commonly develop in the ileum. Sarcomas and lymphomas can affect the entire small bowel.

TABLE 86.2

DIAGNOSTIC MODALITY: DIAGNOSTIC ACCURACY

Plain abdominal radiographs: 50%–60% for small bowel obstruction
Small bowel follow through (SBFT): 33%–60% for small bowel lesions
Small bowel enteroclysis: sensitivity 90%–95%
Computed tomography scan with contrast: 70%–80% adenoca, 58% lymphoma, 33% carcinoid
Computed tomography enteroclysis: sensitivity 95%–100%, specificity 95%, accuracy 97%
Magnetic resonance imaging enteroclysis: sensitivity 86%, specificity 98%, accuracy 97%
Video capsule endoscopy: sensitivity 87%
Double balloon enteroscopy: sensitivity for obstruction or gastrointestinal bleed 74%–81%
Nuclear medicine (octreotide) scans: sensitivity for carcinoid 90%

Diagnosis

The lack of early and specific clinical symptoms and signs contributes to a delay in the diagnosis of SBC. Average delay in diagnosis is 8 to 12 months,[39–41] which is due to delays in patient reporting of symptoms, failure to obtain proper diagnostic workup, or the misinterpretation of test results. Accurate preoperative diagnosis is rarely established. A high index of suspicion is crucial for the adequate evaluation of patients with suspected small bowel malignancies, and no single diagnostic modality has been established as the gold standard. Table 86.2 lists the investigations and reported accuracy available in the diagnosis of small bowel pathology.[42–71]

Workup may begin with a plain abdominal radiograph, but its role is limited to diagnosis of small bowel obstruction (50% to 60% accuracy) only. Small bowel follow through (SBFT) is a time-honored test that is well suited for examination of luminal abnormalities and mucosal morphology but requires a considerable length of time. Reported accuracy of 33% to 60% can be improved to greater than 90% with the addition of enteroclysis.[42–46] This involves the delivery of contrast directly into the proximal small bowel via a nasoduodenal tube. The contrast is subsequently followed by fluoroscopy. Contrast consists of barium and methylcellulose, which distends the small bowel without altering peristalsis.

In most centers, computed tomography (CT) has become one of the initial modalities used for the evaluation of both vague or nonspecific abdominal complaints and acute abdominal pain. In addition to detecting the primary tumor and offering preoperative staging, CT scans allow for specific SBC diagnosis in 70% to 80% of adenocarcinoma, 58% of lymphomas, and 33% of carcinoids based on pathognomonic features.[47–53] Adenocarcinoma most commonly causes a discrete annular thickening with abrupt concentric or irregular overhanging edges. Eccentric thickening of the small bowel wall is usually present as well as potential narrowing of the lumen and dilation of the proximal small bowel. Duodenal adenocarcinoma frequently may present as intraluminal polyps, while more distal polypoid lesions can present with intussusception, which typically displays a "target sign"—low attenuation at the center with high attenuation in the periphery (Figs. 86.1 and 86.2).

Although differentiation from adenocarcinoma may be difficult, certain features of lymphoma (Fig. 86.3*A*,*B*) are commonly observed on CT: multiple filling luminal filling defects signifying lesions in the small bowel wall and a discrete mass that forms the lead point for an intussusception that can be identified as a target lesion on the CT scan; longer segments of small bowel involvement compared to adenocarcinoma; aneurysmal dilatation of the small bowel with intermittent obstruction; cavitary masses arising from the mesentery, which may be seen with aggressive large cell lymphoma; and absence of lymphadenopathy in other areas of the body.

Certain CT features also pertain to carcinoids. They appear as an intramural mass with increased enhancement due to

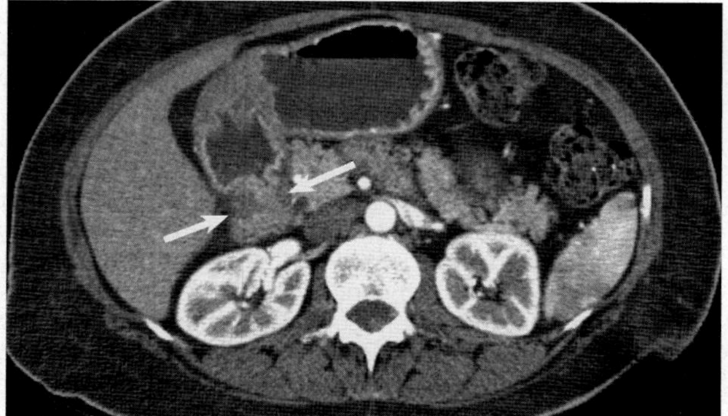

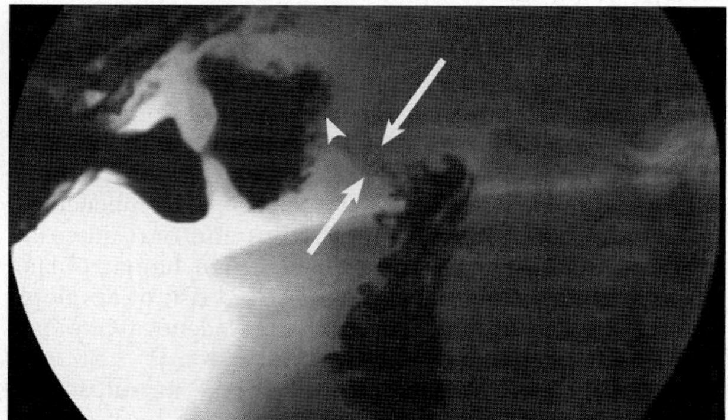

FIGURE 86.1 Moderately differentiated primary small bowel adenocarcinoma. A 59-year-old man presented with epigastric discomfort and weight loss. **A:** Contrast-enhanced axial computed tomography image shows an annular soft tissue lesion (*arrows*) in the duodenum, resulting in circumferential luminal narrowing and wall thickening. **B:** Lateral image from subsequent upper gastrointestinal series shows the annular "apple-core" lesion, resulting in advanced narrowing of the duodenal lumen (*arrows*). Note the compressed, overhanging edges (*arrowhead*) of the small bowel at the margin of the mass.

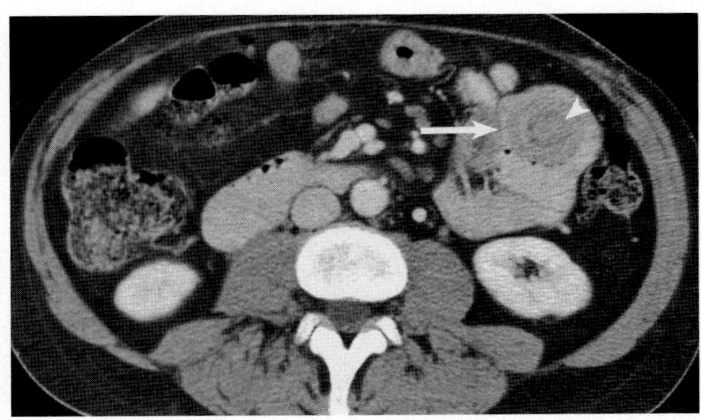

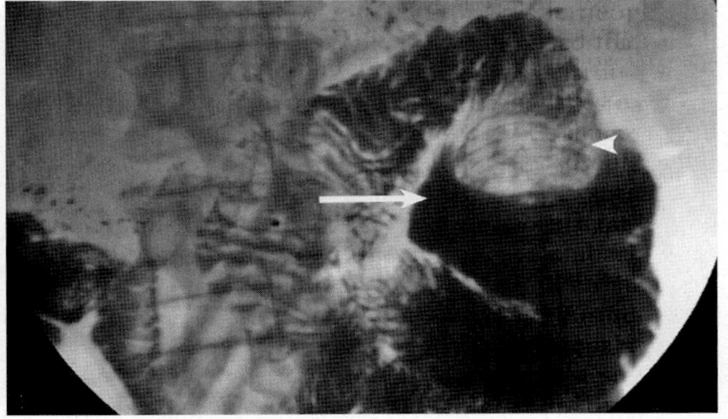

FIGURE 86.2 Small bowel intussusception due to primary small bowel adenocarcinoma. A 60-year-old woman presented with crampy left-sided abdominal pain. **A:** Contrast-enhanced axial computed tomography image shows a small bowel target sign consistent with intussusception; the intussusceptum (*arrowhead*) telescopes into the intussuscipiens (*arrow*). The lead point for the intussusceptions was a primary small bowel carcinoma. **B:** Image from small bowel follow through shows the "coiled spring" appearance of the intussusceptum (*arrowhead*) as it telescopes into the intussuscipiens (*arrow*).

vascularity. As these tumors progress they extend into the mesentery, producing a classic CT appearance of a stellate pattern of soft tissue stranding with a desmoplastic reaction. In 70% of cases some calcifications can be found in the mesentery, and this feature may be diagnostic in the correct setting (Fig. 86.4*A*,*B*).

GIST tumors appear as submucosal masses that are usually well circumscribed, hypervascular, and homogeneous on CT. They may be extrinsic or exocentric, and often, depending on the size, displace adjacent bowel loops. Larger lesions may have a necrotic center (Fig. 86.5*A*,*B*).

Due the success of CT, magnetic resonance imaging (MRI) and enteroclysis, their combined use has yielded high sensitivity and specificity (greater than 90%) and allowed the predication of various subtypes of small bowel lesions and their staging.[54–56] In a series of 219 patients suspected of having the diagnosis of small bowel neoplasm,[55] the overall sensitivity and specificity of CT enteroclysis was 84.7% and 96.9%, respectively. The negative and positive predictive values were 94.5% and 90.9%, respectively. Although multiple small institutional studies have reported similar results using this combined diagnostic modality, further larger comparative studies still need to confirm the advantage of CT/MRI enteroclysis over conventional enteroclysis as the imaging of choice in the evaluation of small intestinal pathologies.

More recently, double-balloon enteroscopy, also known as push enteroscopy, was developed in 2001. Although technically challenging, it allows visualization of the entire small bowel with the ability to biopsy any suspicious lesions. Diagnostic yield for occult GI bleeds and small bowel lesions ranges from 74% to 81%.[57–64] This diagnostic yield has been replicated with other endoscopic modalities such as video capsule endoscopy (VCE). Although VCE does not allow tissue sampling or precise localizations of lesions, it has demonstrated higher sensitivity and specificity than older techniques such as upper GI small bowel follow through.[65–69] In a large meta-analysis of 24 different studies (involving 590 patients) comparing capsule endoscopy to traditional radiographic or endoscopic evaluation of the small bowel, an average patient had undergone 6.77 diagnostic procedures prior to capsule endoscopy.[70] The comparison procedure was push enteroscopy in 300 patients, small bowel series in 140 patients, and colonoscopy with ileoscopy in 90 patients. Capsule endoscopy was found to be superior in identifying a new lesion in 50% of patient and was able to detect 87% of all lesions, versus 13% in any of the comparison methods alone. In addition, capsule endoscopy missed 146 disease instances, for a miss rate of 10%; while 989 were missed by the comparison methods, for a miss rate of 73%. In a large series of small bowel tumors identified by VCE, Schwartz and Barkin[67] reported the characteristics of 86 patients with small bowel tumors (52 malignant and 34 benign). Eighty-nine percent of these tumors were in the jejunum or beyond. These 86 patients had undergone an average of 4.6 negative diagnostic procedures per patient prior to VCE. One of the main risks associated with capsule endoscopy is retention of the capsule itself, which is clinically significant in about 1% of the cases, requiring surgical laparotomy for its removal.

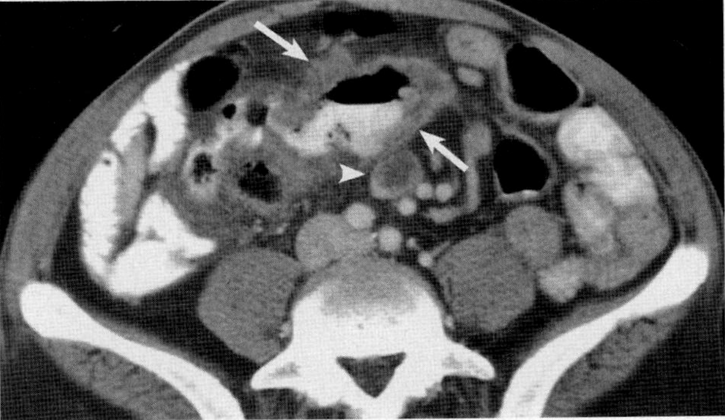

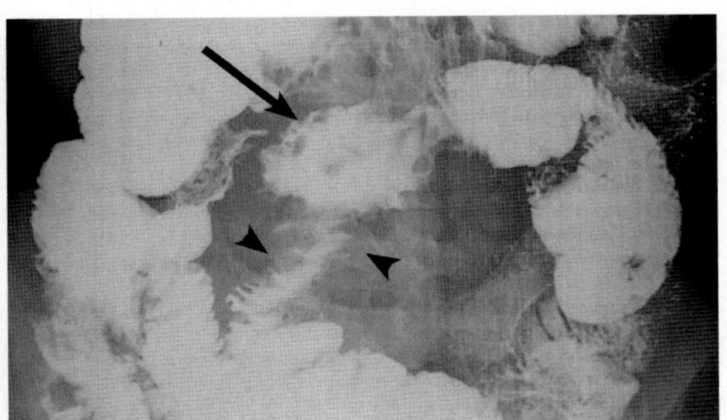

FIGURE 86.3 Primary small bowel lymphoma. A 58-year-old man presented with abdominal pain. **A:**) Contrast-enhanced computed tomography (CT) shows aneurysmal luminal dilatation and extensive wall thickening of a segment of small bowel (*arrows*). Note enlarged adjacent mesenteric node (*arrowhead*). **B:** Radiograph from small bowel follow through shows a small bowel segment with luminal dilatation (*arrow*) and extensive mural thickening and irregularity (*arrowheads*) corresponding to the diseased segment on CT.

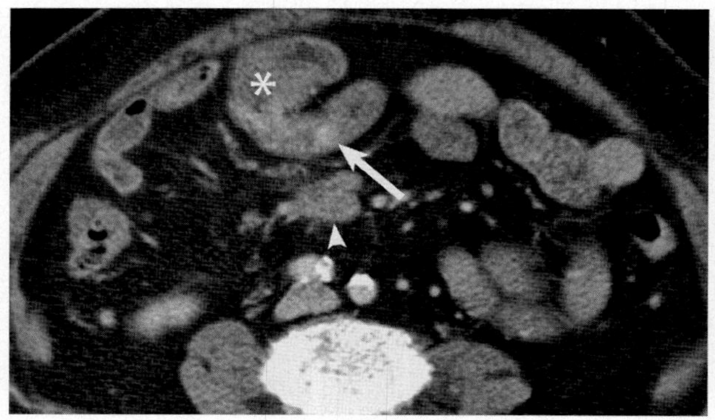
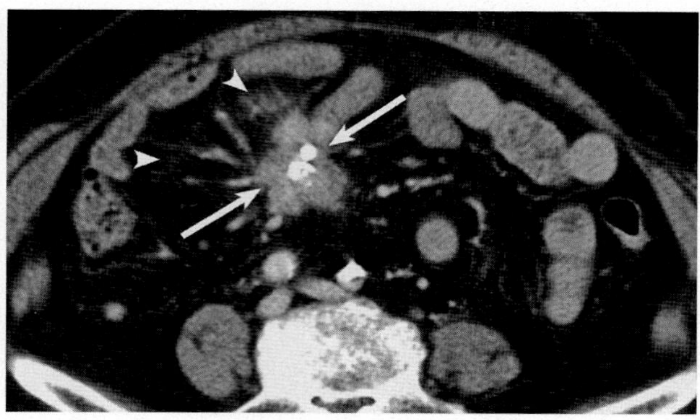

FIGURE 86.4 Primary ileal carcinoid. A 62-year-old woman presented with diarrhea and tachycardia. **A:** Contrast-enhanced computed tomography (CT) shows a tethered and thickened segment of ileum (*asterisk*) containing a small submucosal enhancing lesion (*arrow*), consistent with primary carcinoid. Note partially imaged metastasis (*arrowhead*) in the adjacent mesentery. **B:** More inferior CT image shows a stellate mesenteric carcinoid metastasis (*arrows*) with central calcification and desmoplastic reaction (*arrowheads*) in the adjacent fat.

Nuclear medicine also represents another modality available in the diagnosis of small bowel neoplasms. An Octreotide scan utilizes indium-11 octreotide,—a radioactive somatostatin analogue—in the detection of carcinoids. Sensitivity is reported to be greater than 90% for localization of primary or metastatic carcinoid tumors that express high levels of the somatostatin receptor. Moreover, technetium (99mTc) radionuclide scan in conjunction with angiography can be used in patients with active bleeding from hypervascular small bowel neoplasms such as carcinoids and leiomyosarcomas.

ADENOCARCINOMA

Historically, adenocarcinoma was the most common histological small bowel cancer subtype, representing 30% to 50% of small bowel tumors.[4–16] More recently, the National Cancer Data Base indicates that carcinoids have surpassed adenocarcinoma in incidence (44% vs. 33%, respectively).[71] Presentation is usually between the sixth and eighth decades, with earlier presentations observed in patients with predisposing genetic, inflammatory, or autoimmune conditions (Table 86.1). There is a slight predominance in men, with increased incidence in both black and white men. Distribution favors the duodenum with 50% to 65% of cases, followed by jejunum (16%) and ileum (13%). Duodenal adenocarcinoma tends to present in the elderly compared to more distal lesions. Most patients present as American Joint Committee on Cancer (AJCC) stage III or greater, leading to an overall 5-year disease-free survival of approximately 30% with mean survival of 20 months.[72] Outcomes are worse for duodenal tumors (28% 5-year survival) compared to jejunal and ileal lesions (38% 5-year survival).

Etiology

Despite being 40- to 50-fold less common than colorectal cancer (CRC), small bowel adenocarcinoma shares some genetic etiological pathways with its large bowel counterpart. This is substantiated by the occurrence of both SBC and CRC in patients with FAP, HNPCC, and inflammatory bowel disease. The first is the classic adenoma to carcinoma pathway were early lesions show mutations in the cyclooxygenase and APC genes followed later by K-ras, SMAD4, and p53. In the second pathway tumors arise in the setting of germline mutations in the DNA mismatch repair genes, the so-called replication error or RER phenotype. In one series by Blaker et al.[73] 17 cases of sporadic adenocarcinoma that arose in the jejunum were examined; 3 of 17 patients had mutations in the APC gene, which was similar to that of spontaneously arising colorectal cancer; 2 of 17 were found to have evidence of microsatellite instability; and 80% of them were found to have loss of the 18q21 through q22, an upstream gene from the *SMAD4* gene, which is also frequently lost in CRC. Planck et al.[74] examined 89 adenocarcinomas arising in the small intestine and found 15 of 89 were positive for microsatellite instability.

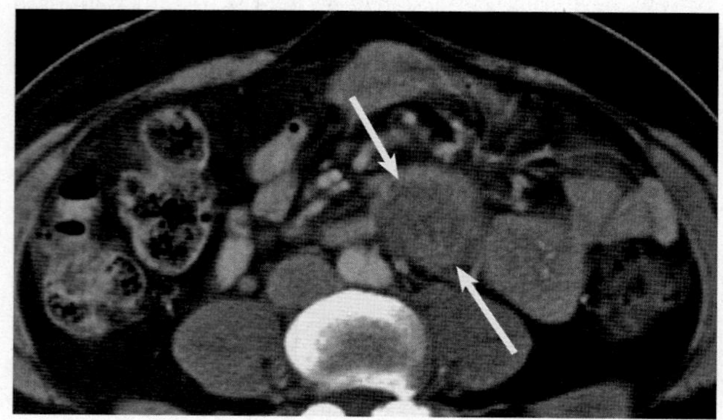
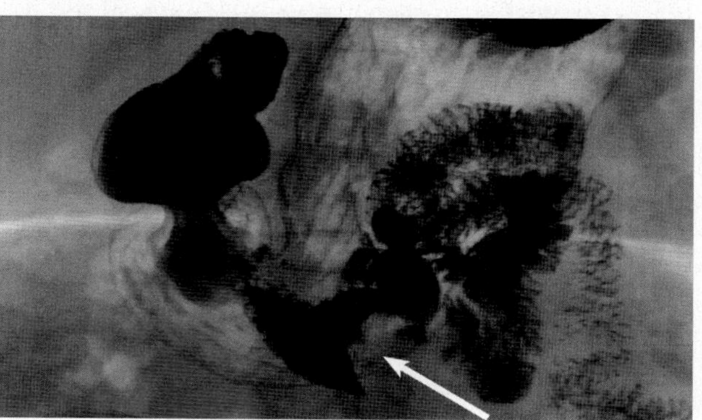

FIGURE 86.5 Gastrointestinal stromal tumor of the small bowel. A 57-year-old woman presented with vague abdominal pain. **A:** Contrast-enhanced computed tomography shows a solid, heterogeneously enhancing mass (*arrows*) arising from the submucosa of the third portion of the duodenum. **B:** Image from upper gastrointestinal series shows a filling defect (*arrow*) in the third portion of the duodenum due to the submucosal gastrointestinal stromal tumor.

Abnormalities in genes common in CRC (including the *APC, p53, K-ras, B-catenin,* and *E-cadherin* genes) are seen with small bowel adenocarcinoma, albeit with reduced frequency, suggesting that in addition to the genetic mechanisms observed in CRC pathogenesis, there is a distinct genetic pathway that does not follow the well-defined polyp-to-adenocarcinoma sequence found in colon cancer.[73–76] Whether small bowel enterocytes are inherently resistant to the development of APC mutations (as suggested by the above data and others) may explain the reason behind the rarity of small bowel adenocarcinoma compared to its large bowel counterpart.

Staging and Prognosis

The AJCC staging system is commonly used for small bowel adenocarcinoma (Table 86.3). SBA is diagnosed at a late stage (III, IV) in 58% of patients. Subsequently, only 50% of patients undergo surgery for curative intent. Survival by stage is 65% for stage I, 48% for stage II, 35% for stage III, and 4% for stage IV.[71] On multivariate regression analyses, poor prognostic factors include age greater than 55, men, African American ethnicity, T4 tumor, lymph node involvement (and ratio), duodenal or ileal primary, poor differentiation, metastatic disease, and positive margins.[71,77,78]

TABLE 86.3

AMERICAN JOINT COMMITTEE STAGING FOR SMALL BOWEL ADENOCARCINOMA

Primary Tumor (T) Staging	
Tx	Tumor cannot be assessed
T0	No evidence of primary tumor
Tis	Carcinoma *in situ*
T1	Invasion of lamina propria or submucosa
T2	Invasion of muscularis propria
T3	Invasion through muscularis propria into subserosa or into nonperitonealized perimuscular tissue (mesentery or retroperitoneum) with extension 2 cm or less
T4	Perforation of visceral peritoneum or direct invasion of other organs or structures (includes other loops of small intestine, mesentery or retroperitoneum more than 2 cm and the abdominal wall by way of serosa; for the duodenum only, includes invasion of pancreas)
Regional Lymph Nodes (N)	
Nx	Regional lymph nodes cannot be assessed
N0	No regional lymph node metastases
N1	Regional lymph node metastasis
Distant Metastasis (M)	
Mx	Distant metastasis cannot be assessed
M0	No distant metastasis
M1	Distant metastasis
Stage	**TNM**
0	Tis N0 M0
IA	T1 N0 M0
IB	T2 N0 M0
IIA	T3 N0 M0
IIB	T4 N0 M0
III	Any T N1 M0
IV	Any T Any N M1

(From Edge SB, Byrd DR, Compton CC (eds). *AJCC Cancer Staging Manual*, 7th ed. New York: Springer Publishers; 2010.)

Management

Surgical Resection

Surgery remains the mainstay of treatment of small bowel adenocarcinoma. Segmental resection with 5-cm margins and complete nodal extirpation of the segment have been advocated. Management of duodenal primaries is more controversial, with therapeutic options ranging from segmental duodenal resection to pancreaticoduodenectomy. Although several authors have reported improved overall survival with pancreaticoduodenectomy,.[79,80] segmental duodenal resection is curative if performed with negative margins and adequate lymphadenectomy. In the setting of FAP, isolated resection of individual polypoid lesions has high recurrence rates. More formal surgical procedures such as pancreas-preserving duodenectomy or segmental resection have been advocated. In advanced unresectable disease, options include palliative resection, diversion, and bypass. For peritoneal-based carcinomatosis, cytoreductive surgery with heated intraperitoneal chemotherapy in the form of mitomycin-C and fluorouracil (5-FU) has been performed with modest success.[81,82]

Adjuvant and Neoadjuvant Therapy

The recurrence pattern for small bowel adenocarcinoma is mainly systemic.[72,83–85] Duodenal adenocarcinoma, although having a higher local failure rate compared to jejunal or ileal adenocarcinoma, also recurs in a predominately systemic fashion.[86–89] Despite this compelling argument for systemic adjuvant therapy, evidence for its use is still lacking. Several series have reported adjuvant chemotherapy for jejunal or ileal adenocarcinoma,[72] while others have reported on adjuvant chemotherapy or radiation for duodenal cancer.[79,87–91] None have shown meaningful improvement in survival. The data, however, are limited by small numbers, single institutional selection bias, and its reliance on 5-FU as mainstay chemotherapy. Results with oxaliplatin in the systemic or palliative setting have been more encouraging, with response rates of 61%.[92] Its use in the adjuvant setting may reveal more promising results. The role of neoadjuvant therapy for SBC (mainly duodenal tumors) consists primarily of case reports or small case series. Its benefit remains largely unknown.

Systemic or Palliative Chemotherapy

Chemotherapy in the locally advanced or metastatic setting has shown some promising results. Although phase 3 trials of palliative chemotherapy versus best supportive care are lacking, a recent phase 2 trial from the M. D. Anderson Cancer Center, using capecitabine and oxaliplatin, has shown an overall response rate of 61% with median overall survival of 20.4 months.[92] This, in addition to other prospective and retrospective reports, indicates that combination regimens utilizing 5-FU and a platinum for advanced small bowel adenocarcinoma may yield improved response rates and survival.[92–94]

CARCINOID TUMORS

Carcinoid tumors are thought to arise from the neuroendocrine cells of Kulchitsky in the intestinal tract. These rare, slow growing tumors occur with the greatest frequency in the gastrointestinal tract (75% of all cases), followed by the lung and bronchus. They may occur with much less frequency in the liver, pancreas, or gonads. According to the SEER database, the majority of GI carcinoids occur in the small intestine (41.8%), followed by the rectum (27%), and the stomach and appendix (8.7%).[95,96] Within the small intestine, the majority are identified in the ileum, followed by the duodenum and then the jejunum. Carcinoid syndrome represents a constellation of symptoms, including flushing, diarrhea, and bronchospasm related to the secretion of a variety of hormonal peptides by the tumor (most notably serotonin, histamine, dopamine, and prostaglandins, to name a few). This syndrome occurs in 5% to 7% of patients with small bowel carcinoid.

Epidemiology

Carcinoid tumors have a slight preponderance to men (52.4%) and an average age of presentation of 66 years, which is within 2 years of the average age of diagnosis for noncarcinoid small intestinal tumors. White patients (80.4%) are significantly more affected compared to other ethnic groups. A fourfold increase in the incidence of carcinoids in the past two decades has made it the most common small bowel malignancy (37.4%), surpassing adenocarcinoma (36.9%). Although carcinoids follow an indolent course, a delay in their diagnosis leads to advanced presentation in more than two-thirds of cases. Interestingly, 29% of small bowel carcinoids are associated with other noncarcinoid neoplasms.

Prognosis

Despite their advanced presentation with localized and metastatic disease, overall 5-year survival is between 52% and 77%. Predictors of local-regional and metastatic spread are primarily the size of the lesion and its depth of invasion.[97–102] In a large series of 1,100 small bowel carcinoids, the risk of metastasis was highest for tumors larger than 10 mm (73.6%), compared to tumors 6 to 10 mm (31.5%) and small tumors less than 6 mm (15.8%). In addition, those lesions with transmural invasion were found to have metastasis 68.4% of the time, as opposed to those with just submucosal invasion (30.8%). Overall 5-year survival for all patients in this series was approximately 73.3%; patients without metastatic disease had a 5-year survival of 90.9% as opposed to 68.2% for patients with metastasis. Other small series have confirmed that size and depth of invasion are associated with locoregional spread, with findings of regional lymph node metastasis in 69%, 94% and 100%, for tumors less than 0.5 cm, 0.5 to 1.0 cm, and 1 to 2 cm or larger, respectively.

Diagnosis

Radiologic aids to the diagnosis of carcinoids have been discussed earlier; classic CT findings include an intramural mass with increased enhancement, propensity to extend into the mesentery, producing a classic stellate pattern of soft tissue stranding with "desmoplastic reaction," and calcifications in 70% of cases (Fig. 86.3). Octreotide scans can be diagnostic in 90% of cases. Biochemically, urinary 5-hydroxyindoleacetic acid (5-HIAA) levels and chromogranin A levels have been used as tumor markers for midgut carcinoids. They may be used to correlate with therapy.

Management of Localized Disease

Due to the propensity of locoregional spread in even the smallest of lesions, segmental resection of the tumor with accompanying draining lymph nodes is the treatment of choice for primary carcinoids arising in the small bowel. Five-year survival after resection of localized disease ranges between 50% and 85%. Thorough inspection of the bowel should be performed due to the increased risk of synchronous lesions. For appendiceal carcinoids management is dictated by size, as 30% of tumors larger than 2 cm in size are metastatic at the time of diagnosis, while smaller tumors almost never metastasize. Accordingly, appendiceal carcinoids smaller than 2 cm can be treated with simple appendectomy, while larger tumors require a right hemicolectomy. Surgical manipulation of carcinoids may precipitate a carcinoid crisis, and pretreatment with Octreotide is recommended prior to anesthesia induction.

Management of Advanced Disease

Due to the indolent course of most carcinoids, surgical resection of the primary and its associated lymph node basin—irrespective of the presence of widespread disease—has been shown to improve survival and control symptoms.[103–107] In the metastatic setting, resection of the primary and cytoreductive therapy in the appropriate circumstances can achieve (1) symptom control and reduction in octreotide dosing; (2) improved survival; and (3) prevention of fibrosing mesenteritis. The decision to perform palliative resection for disseminated carcinoid tumors should carefully balance the risks and benefits of the procedure. Different modes of cytoreductive treatments for metastatic carcinoid are available, including surgery or local ablative therapy, hepatic arterial chemoembolization, and systemic chemotherapy

Surgery or Local Ablative Therapy

The liver is the most common site of carcinoid metastasis. In resectable metastatic disease, formal liver resection in addition to the associated primary tumor should be attempted with curative intent. In patients with extensive bilobar liver disease, liver failure, or extensive metastatic disease, surgical debulking or cytoreductive surgery provides prolonged disease-free survival. A large series from the Mayo Clinic examined patients undergoing hepatic metastasectomy for neuroendocrine tumors, with major hepatectomy performed in 54% of patients.[108–110] Symptom control from carcinoid syndrome was effective in 96% of patients, 84% of patients eventually had tumor recurrence, and 59% of patients had recurrence of their symptoms in 5 years. Compared to historic controls, liver resection markedly improved the 5-year survival rate from 36% to 61%. Retrospective series comparing surgery (cytoreductive or debulking) to systemic therapy (octreotide or chemotherapy) or hepatic arterial embolization have found surgery to be superior to other modalities in providing symptom control and improved survival.[111] The role of orthotopic liver transplantation in unresectable liver disease still remains to be established with large studies. Local ablative techniques such as radiofrequency ablation (RFA) and cryoablation are some of the other cytoreductive options available for treatment of metastatic carcinoid tumors. They can be performed percutaneously or laparoscopically and allow reduction in octreotide dosing, although their long-term efficacy remains to be investigated.

Hepatic Arterial Therapy

Hepatic arterial embolization (HAE) with or without chemotherapy (HACE) can improve symptom control and survival in unresectable carcinoid liver metastasis. It is based on the assumption that most tumor cells derive their blood supply from the hepatic artery, while healthy hepatocytes derive it from the portal vein. Hepatic arterial embolization has been performed with gel foam, polyvinyl alcohol, and microspheres. The addition of hepatic arterial chemotherapy allows for much higher intratumoral concentrations than systemic levels.

At the M. D. Anderson Cancer Center 81 patients with carcinoid tumor underwent HAE with a response rate of 67%, with greater than a 50% reduction in their tumors, and median response duration of 17 months.[112] The addition of chemotherapy to hepatic artery embolization was not beneficial. Progression-free survival rates were 75%, 35%, and 11% at 1, 2, and 3 years, respectively. The probability of survival at 1 year was 93%, 60% at 2 years, and 24% at 5 years. The procedure may lead to transient or fulminant liver failure, liver abscess, or postembolization syndrome (fever, abdominal pain, leukocytosis, transient elevations in liver function tests).

Chemotherapy

The role of systemic chemotherapy in the treatment of metastatic carcinoid remains unclear. A variety of chemotherapeutic agents have been investigated, including 5-FU, streptozocin, and doxorubicin, yielding modest response rates of 20%. A combination of these agents has no impact on response rates or survival. Interferon-α (INF-α) has been reported to result in 40% to 50% biochemical responses and tumor stabilization in 20% to 40% of the cases.[113,114] Octreotide has also been reported to prevent progression of metastatic carcinoid tumors in multiple small case series.[115–117] The combination of IFN-α with octreotide or other chemotherapeutic agents has also been examined, but the superiority of these combinations compared to single agent therapy is not clear.

Poor responses have instigated the search for targeted agents in the treatment of metastatic carcinoid.[118] Imatinib or sunitinib, tyrosine kinase inhibitors, were observed to delay tumor cell growth in preclinical studies. They demonstrated disease stability in 83% of patients over a 1-year period. Similarly, bevacizumab, a humanized monoclonal antibody targeting vascular endothelial growth factor (VEGF), was shown to maintain disease stability in 95% of patients when combined with octreotide, compared to 68% with the combination of IFN-α and octreotide, in a recent phase 2 clinical trial. Carcinoids are highly vascular tumors, and the majority of these tumors overexpress VEGF and its receptors (VEGFR type 1 and 2). Everolimus, a molecule inhibiting the mammalian target of rapamycin (mTOR) pathway has also shown some promising results. The long-term benefit and safety of these and other novel agents needs to be established.

Carcinoid Syndrome

Carcinoid syndrome consists of a collection of symptoms, including cutaneous flushing, diarrhea, and wheezing mediated by the release into the circulation of tumor-derived humoral factors. Although more than 30 different polypeptides, biogenic amines, and prostaglandins have been identified serotonin, histamine, dopamine, tachykinins ,and prostaglandins are the most important. Since the liver usually metabolizes these substances, it follows that carcinoid syndrome develops in the presence of liver metastasis. Although a majority of patients with carcinoid syndrome (80%) have small bowel carcinoids, only 10% to 17% of patients with small bowel carcinoids present with carcinoid syndrome; however, symptoms develop in 60% to 70% of these patients at some point in their disease. Symptoms can be precipitated by alcohol ingestion, stress, and certain physical activities, including pressure to the right upper quadrant. Somatostatin, a 14 amino acid long peptide that binds to the somatostatin receptor found on the surface of carcinoid tumors prevents the secretion of hormones and is the most effective treatment for relieving symptoms of carcinoid syndrome.[119,120] At a dose of 150 mcg three times daily, around 80% of patients report improvement of flushing and diarrhea. Use of the long acting depot octreotide or lanreotide has been shown to be equally effective. Octreotide—as discussed earlier—has also been found to have a role in tumor growth control. For refractory symptoms, cyproheptadine, a nonselective potent antihistamine, improved severe diarrhea in a certain percentage of patients. IFN-α in addition to octreotide has also been found to alleviate symptoms in patients who did not respond to octreotide alone.

INTESTINAL LYMPHOMA

Lymphoma is the third most common malignant small bowel neoplasm (10% to 20%). Extranodal lymphoma (arising within a solid organ) constitutes 20% to 40% of all cases of lymphoma, and GI lymphomas are the most common extranodal form, accounting for up to half of all extranodal disease. In the Western world, the stomach harbors most GI lymphomas (75%), followed by the small intestine, the colon, and other organs such as the pancreas and the liver. Primary intestinal lymphoma has a peak incidence in the seventh decade, with a slight predominance in men (60%). They may present with perforation. The incidence of intestinal lymphoma has been reported to be increasing in the United States, doubling over the past two decades. This has been attributed to an upsurge in lymphoma among immunocompromised patients, as well as immigration from the Middle East and Near East, areas where primary intestinal lymphoma compromise the most common primary extranodal disease. Other predisposing factors for the development of intestinal lymphoma include Crohn's disease and prior radiation exposure.

Specific criteria used to differentiate primary intestinal lymphoma from secondary lymphomas are: (1) no superficial lymphadenopathy palpated on physical examination and the absence of mediastinal lymphadenopathy on chest radiograph; (2) both peripheral blood smears and bone marrow biopsies should have no evidence of disease involvement; (3) disease should be confined to the affected small bowel segment and the regional draining mesenteric lymph nodes only; and (4) no evidence of hepatic or splenic involvement except via direct extension from the primary tumor.

Staging

Because most GI lymphomas are of non-Hodgkin's type, staging is based on the Ann Arbor staging system adapted for non-Hodgkin's lymphomas. This staging system has undergone some modification and is currently as follows: stage I is a lymphoma limited to a single site; stage II is tumors confined to below the diaphragm and separated into two subgroups: those with regional (stage II 1E) and distant (stage II 2E) lymph node involvement; stage III is involvement of organs on both sides of the diaphragm; and stage IV is widespread dissemination, including the liver and the spleen. Tumor spread is thus the most significant prognostic indicator for intestinal lymphoma.

Subtypes

Most primary intestinal lymphoma is of B-cell origin and generally falls into one of four categories: (1) mucosal-associated lymphoid tissue (MALT) lymphomas, (2) diffuse large cell lymphoma, (3) Burkitt's lymphomas, and (4) mantle-cell lymphoma. Far less common are the T-cell intestinal lymphomas, with the enteropathy-associated T-cell lymphoma (EATL) being the most common type.

Mucosal-Associated Lymphoid Tissue Lymphoma

MALT lymphoma are the most common primary gastrointestinal lymphomas and occur more commonly in the stomach, followed by the small intestine (ileocecal region most commonly), the colon, and the esophagus. In the Revised European-American Lymphoma/World Health Organization (REAL/WHO) classification, MALT is now designated as *marginal zone B-cell lymphoma*. They have a predominance to men and peak in the sixth decade. Macroscopically, these tumors present as unifocal, ulcerated overhanging lesions. Microscopically, they are characterized by cellular heterogeneity, bearing close resemblance to normal gut associated lymphoid tissue (Peyer's patch and mesenteric nodal tissue). Nonneoplastic reactive lymphoid follicles surrounded by centrocytes are characteristic, with the neoplastic focus occupying the marginal zone or intrafollicular region. These tumor cells express elevated levels of IgM and B-cell–associated antigens (including CD19, CD20, CD22, and CD79a). They are usually CD5, CD10 and CD23 negative, while being CD43 variable. Unlike large diffuse B-cell lymphoma, they are not associated with Bcl-2 or Bcl-1 rearrangements. Clinically, these tumors are associated with chronic inflammatory conditions, including autoimmune disorders such as Sjögren syndrome and Hashimoto's thyroiditis. The majority of the patients present with localized stage I or II disease involving the small intestine. Therapy consists of multimodality treatment, including surgical resection and or chemoradiation therapy, with small intestinal lymphomas having better prognosis that tumors arising in the stomach. In addition, studies suggest that MALT tumors may be antigen driven, especially by *Campylobacter jejuni* and *Helicobacter pylori*.[121] Regression has been reported with eradication of *H. pylori* infection using antibiotics.

Immunoproliferative small intestinal disease (IPSID), also know as alpha heavy chain disease or Mediterranean lymphoma, is a subtype of MALT lymphomas that occurs exclusively in the Mediterranean area. It is characterized by defective secretion of alpha heavy chain. IPSID tends to present in younger men with more diffuse involvement, predominantly of the proximal small intestine. Similar to MALT lymphomas, IPSIDs are also thought to be antigen driven with an association to *C. jejuni*.

Diffuse Large B-Cell Lymphoma

Diffuse large B-cell lymphoma is the second most common non-Hodgkin's lymphoma occurring in the GI tract. It is also known as large cell immunoblastic, large-cleaved follicular center cell, centroblastic D immunoblastic cell, or diffuse mixed lymphocytic and histiocytic cell. It affects the ileocecal area predominately occurring more frequently in men, at a median age of 54 to 61 years. Macroscopically, it presents as a unifocal ulcerated lesion, while histologically, these tumors are composed of diffuse large B cells with large nuclei that are twice the size of a normal lymphocyte. These tumor cells are CD19, CD20, CD22, and CD79a positive. Bcl-2 gene mutation is present in approximately 30% of the cases. Similar to other lymphomas, immunosuppression is a major risk factor. For localized disease, surgery is the mainstay of treatment,[122] followed by adjuvant radiation or chemotherapy. Overall 5-year survival has been reported to be between 50% and 70% with multimodality therapy.[123]

Burkitt's Lymphoma

Burkitt's lymphoma of the small intestine accounts for less than 5% of all small intestinal lymphomas. It can occur endemically or sporadically and is highly aggressive. The endemic subtype is seen predominantly in Central Africa; it affects children with peak incidence at 8 years of age, is associated with Epstein-Barr virus (EBV) infection, and involves the gastrointestinal tract in only 20% to 30% of cases. Conversely, sporadic Burkitt's lymphoma occurs more commonly in Westernized countries; affects a broader age population; is not associated with EBV infections; and commonly affects the GI tract (ileocecal region). Clinically, they can mimic appendicitis by presenting as large masses. Microscopically, cells are monomorphic medium-sized cells with round nuclei and an abundant basophilic cytoplasm. It is a rapidly growing tumor with short doubling time; the high rate of proliferation gives it a "starry sky" pattern due to the numerous macrophages that have ingested apoptotic tumor cells. Treatment consists primarily of chemotherapy, usually vincristine, cyclophosphamide, doxorubicin, and methotrexate.[124]

Mantle Cell Lymphoma

This is a rare primary GI lymphoma that can either take an indolent or a very aggressive course. It commonly affects men (four to one) in their sixth and seventh decades and has a predilection to the small intestine and the colon. Macroscopically, there are multiple whitish polypoid lesions that share morphological features with nodal lymphomas. CD5+ B cells are located within the mantle zone that surrounds germinal centers. Four histologic subtypes have been described: nodular, diffuse, mantle zone, and blastic. Blastic type has the worst prognosis, while nodular and diffuse have the best prognosis. Mantle cell lymphoma has been associated with t(11:14) (q13; q32) chromosomal translocation, causing overexpression of cyclin D1. Most mantle cell lymphomas present as a stage IV disease.

T-Cell Lymphoma

T-cell lymphomas of the small intestine are less common than their B-cell counterparts, accounting for approximately 15% of all lymphomas arising in the small intestine. They affect men and women equally and most commonly arise in the jejunum or the proximal ileum. They tend to remain localized; however, dissemination is common. They typically present as large circumferential ulcers—in the absence of large masses—with associated mesenteric lymphadenopathy. As with other types of lymphomas, obstruction and perforation are common presentations. Microscopically, transmural replacement of the intestinal wall by highly pleomorphic lymphoid cells may be seen. A large number of surrounding intraepithelial lymphocytes may also show cellular atypia. Tumor cells stain positive for CD3, CD7, CD8, and CD103 and negative for CD4. T-cell lymphomas of the small intestine are known as enteropathy-associated T-cell lymphoma due to their association with long-standing enteropathy, primarily celiac disease. EATL is described in approximately 5% to 10% of all patients with celiac disease, and the relative risk of developing a lymphoma in the setting of celiac disease is 25- to 100-fold higher than in normal patients.[33] Prognosis is poor compared to B-cell lymphoma, with a 5-year survival rate of 10%.[125]

GASTROINTESTINAL STROMAL TUMORS

GIST arise from the intestinal cells of Cajal and are characterized by the presence of gain-of-function *c-kit* (CD117) mutation. The *c-kit* protein codes for a tyrosine kinase receptor involved in cellular proliferation, apoptosis, and differentiation. They most commonly involve the stomach and proximal small intestine and are the most common mesenchymal tumors of the small intestine. Approximately 80% to 90% of all GIST tumors arise because of the *c-kit* mutation, while the remainders have a mutation in another tyrosine kinase receptor gene; platelet derived growth factor (PDGF) receptor alpha. It is now recognized that a vast majority of the tumors that had been previously identified as leiomyomas and leiomyosarcomas are actually CD117+ GIST. The molecular discoveries have allowed the development of the specific c-*kit* tyrosine kinase inhibitor imatinib (Glivec/Gleevec), a drug initially designed to treat chronic myelogenous leukemia. Trials have proven imatinib to be effective in treating GIST tumors without many of the side effects associated with traditional chemotherapy

Epidemiology

Although GIST constitutes only 0.5% to 1% of all gastrointestinal tumors, it is the most common mesenchymal tumor of the small intestine. Due to the recent discovery in its molecular genetics and subsequent characterization, epidemiological data on GIST are limited to the past decade. Incidence is between 4,500 to 6,000 cases per year in the United States, or 10 to 20 cases per million population.[126–131] Incidence is equal in both genders and peaks between 50 and 60 years of age. In the small bowel, they are most commonly found in the jejunum, followed by the ileum, and lastly the duodenum. Presentation is with pain, intussusception, or bleeding.

Clinicopathologic Correlates of Malignant Potential

Although only approximately 30% to 50% of tumors are clinically malignant, all GIST tumors have malignant potential and approximately half of resected patients will recur within 5 years. The spectrum of clinical behavior exhibited by these tumors has been aided by the identification of the c-*kit* gain-of-function mutation characteristic of most GISTs and their subsequent classification. Several criteria have been found to predict the behavior of GIST tumors and to stratify them according to the risk of recurrence and metastasis.[132–135]

- *Tumor size*: In the National Institutes of Health 2002 consensus for risk stratification of GIST, tumor size represents one of the major criteria for recurrence and metastasis. This risk is noticeable for tumors larger than 2 cm and increases significantly for tumors larger than 5 cm in the largest dimension.
- *Mitotic rate*: Mitotic rate is the second major criteria for risk stratification of GIST tumors. Five or more mitoses per 50 high-powered field (HPF) indicates worse outcome, while mitotic rates higher than 10 per 50 HPF predicts high recurrence and metastases, irrespective of tumor size or location, with 5-year survival rates approximately 25%.
- *Tumor site*: Jejunal/ileal GISTs have more malignant behavior—irrespective of size—when compared to duodenal tumors, which in turn have more malignant potential compared to rectal and gastric lesions.
- Other histopathological criteria of malignant behavior have been examined, including cellularity and nuclear atypical, mucosal invasion, multiple genetic mutations, and ulceration, but none of these have been shown to correlate well with prognosis of mesenchymal tumors.

Management

Complete surgical resection with negative margins is the mainstay of GIST therapy. Wider resection of surrounding uninvolved tissue does not improve outcome. Similarly, and due to the fact that GIST rarely metastasizes to regional lymph nodes, routine lymphadenectomy is not recommended. Intraoperatively, great care should be taken to prevent tumor rupture and spillage, which has been associated with carcinomatosis. Metastatic and recurrent disease is mainly confined to the peritoneum and to the liver, and both should be carefully inspected at the time of surgical exploration. Laparoscopic GIST is safe, but should be limited to localized disease, and low risk tumors.[136–139]

In the localized setting adjuvant therapy with imatinib improves recurrence-free survival after complete surgical resection. In the phase 3 trial ACOSOGZ9001 adjuvant imatinib (400 mg daily for 1 year) improved progression-free survival at 1 year from 83% to 98%, leading to U.S. Food and Drug Administration approval in this setting (dose and duration not specified).[140] A phase 2 trial (Z9000) using a similar regimen and duration of imatinib in high-risk GIST yielded an overall survival of 97% at 3 years (compared to median overall survival of 2 years in historic controls), and progression-free survival of 61% at 3years.[141] In a significant number of patients with advanced (surgically unresectable) or metastatic disease, negative surgical margins may not be possible, greatly impacting disease-free survival and life expectancy, with median survival ranging from 9 months to 23 months. In this setting imatinib confers benefit in more than 80% of patients, extending median overall survival to 5 years (compared to 9 months) in the metastatic setting.[142] Furthermore, in the neoadjuvant setting, imatinib can successfully reduce tumor burden and facilitate margin-negative, organ-sparing resections.[143,144] Sunitinib, a relatively newer multitargeted receptor tyrosine kinase inhibitor initially approved for the treatment of renal cell carcinoma, is also now approved for the treatment of imatinib-resistant GIST.

OTHER MESENCHYMAL TUMORS

The majority of mesenchymal tumors arising in the small intestine are GISTs. Other less common mesenchymal neoplasms include leiomyomas and leiomyosarcomas, inflammatory fibroid polyps, desmoid tumors, inflammatory and myofibroblastic tumors, solitary fibrous tumors, schwannomas, and peripheral nerve sheath tumors.

Leiomyomas and Leiomyosarcomas

Leiomyomas and leiomyosarcomas of the small intestine arise from the muscularis propria and muscularis mucosa layers of the bowel wall. Leiomyosarcoma stains positive for desmin and actin and is negative for CD117 (*c-kit* and CD34). Obstruction is a late feature in presentation, as initial tumor growth is local and extraluminal. As tumor size increases, tumor ulceration and bleeding are observed. Metastasis is hematological, mainly to the liver and peritoneum. About a third of patients have metastasis at time of diagnosis and prognosis is very poor.

Inflammatory Fibroid Polyps

Inflammatory fibroid polyps are benign lesions infrequently encountered in the small intestine. They are typically submucosal and consist of a mixture of small granulation tissuelike vessels, spindle cells, and inflammatory cells. These lesions can stain positively for CD34; however, they do not stain for CD117 with the exception of very small areas of stroma within these tumors.

Desmoid Tumors

Desmoid tumors are histologically benign fibrous tumors originating from musculoaponeurotic structures throughout the body. They occur in higher incidence in patients with FAP and Gardner syndrome. These spindle cell tumors are frequently confused with GIST tumors. Histologically, they are characterized by fibroblastic proliferation and formation of bundles of spindle cells around blood vessels in a dense hypocellular fibrous stroma. Few mitotic figures are seen and necrosis is usually absent. They stain for vimentin, smooth muscle actin, and nuclear beta catenin. Although these tumors are histologically benign with no potential for metastasis, they tend to be locally aggressive and recur even after complete resection. Treatment is surgical resection with wide margin to ensure negative microscopic margins; however, this may be difficult due to anatomic location and involvement of vital structures. Other treatment modalities include chemotherapy (methotrexate and vinblastine, doxorubicin), radiation therapy, nonsteroidal anti-inflammatories, and antiestrogens (tamoxifen).

Inflammatory and Myofibroblastic Tumors

These inflammatory pseudotumors or inflammatory fibrosarcomas are uncommon inflammatory mesenchymal tumors that appear as solid white masses with infiltrative margins. They have been described in the small intestinal mesentery of young individuals and can also arise in the stomach where they can also be associated with peptic ulcer disease or chronic gastritis. Microscopically, they are characterized by spindle cells admixed with lymphocytes and plasma cells. These lesions are believed to be benign reactions to infectious processes, although local recurrence has been reported. They rarely behave in a malignant fashion. Unlike GIST, they stain negatively for CD117 and CD 34, but are positive for desmin, muscle-specific actin, and cytokeratin. Sixty percent of these lesions stain for anaplastic lymphoma kinase, a growth factor receptor.

Schwannomas

Schwannomas of the GI tract are more common in the stomach, colon, and esophagus, but rarely originate from the small intestine. These benign lesions are rubbery yellowish trabeculated tumors macroscopically. Microscopically, they are characterized by lymph node aggregates around their periphery, with nuclear palisading Verocay bodies and hyalinized vessels similar to schwannomas found elsewhere in the body. They stain strongly for S100 and glial fibrillary acidic protein but are CD117, CD 34, and smooth muscle actin negative.

Selected References

The full list of references for this chapter appears in the online version.

1. Jemal A, Siegel R, Ward E, et al. Cancer statistics, 2008. *CA Cancer J Clin* 2008;58:7196.
2. Haselkorn T, Whittemore AS, Lilienfeld DE. Incidence of small bowel cancer in the United States and worldwide: geographic, temporal, and racial differences. *Cancer Causes Control* 2005;16(7):781.
4. DiSario JA, Burt RW, Vargas H, McWhorter WP. Small bowel cancer: epidemiological and clinical characteristics from a population-based registry. *Am J Gastroenterol* 1994;89(5):699.
8. Severson RK, Schenk M, Gurney JG, Weiss LK, Demers RY. Increasing incidence of adenocarcinomas and carcinoid tumors of the small intestine in adults. *Cancer Epidemiol Biomarkers Prev* 1996;5(2):81.
10. Chow JS, Chen CC, Ahsan H, Neugut AI. A population-based study of the incidence of malignant small bowel tumours: SEER, 1973–1990. *Int J Epidemiol* 1996;25(4):722.
11. Cunningham JD, Aleali R, Aleali M, Brower ST, Aufses AH. Malignant small bowel neoplasms: histopathologic determinants of recurrence and survival. *Ann Surg* 1997;225(3):300.
15. Talamonti MS, Goetz LH, Rao S, Joehl RJ. Primary cancers of the small bowel: analysis of prognostic factors and results of surgical management. *Arch Surg* 2002;137(5):564.
18. Bjork J, Akerbrant H, Iselius L, et al. Periampullary adenomas and adenocarcinomas in familial adenomatous polyposis: cumulative risks and APC gene mutations. *Gastroenterology* 2001;121(5):1127.
41. Maglinte DD, O'Connor K, Bessette J, Chernish SM, Kelvin FM. The role of the physician in the late diagnosis of primary malignant tumors of the small intestine. *Am J Gastroenterol* 1991;86(3):304.
44. Buckley JA, Fishman EK. CT evaluation of small bowel neoplasms: spectrum of disease. *Radiographics* 1998;18(2):379.
45. Buckley JA, Siegelman SS, Jones B, Fishman EK. The accuracy of CT staging of small bowel adenocarcinoma: CT/pathologic correlation. *J Comput Assist Tomogr* 1997;21(6):986.
49. Horton KM, Juluru K, Montogomery E, Fishman EK. Computed tomography imaging of gastrointestinal stromal tumors with pathology correlation. *J Comput Assist Tomogr* 2004;28(6):811.
62. Zhong J, Ma T, Zhang C, et al. A retrospective study of the application on double-balloon enteroscopy in 378 patients with suspected small-bowel diseases. *Endoscopy* 2007;39(3):208.
65. Triester SL, Leighton JA, Leontiadis GI, et al. A meta-analysis of the yield of capsule endoscopy compared to other diagnostic modalities in patients with obscure gastrointestinal bleeding. *Am J Gastroenterol* 2005;100(11):2407.
68. Mazzarolo S, Brady P. Small bowel capsule endoscopy: a systematic review. *South Med J* 2007;100(3):274.
70. Lewis BS, Eisen GM, Friedman S. A pooled analysis to evaluate results of capsule endoscopy trials. *Endoscopy* 2005;37(10):960.
71. Bilimoria KY, Bentrem DJ, Wayne JD, et al: Small bowel cancer in the United States: changes in epidemiology, treatment, and survival over the last 20 years. *Ann Surg* 2009;249:63.
72. Dabaja BS, Suki D, Pro B, Bonnen M, Ajani J. Adenocarcinoma of the small bowel: presentation, prognostic factors, and outcome of 217 patients. *Cancer* 2004;101(3):518.
73. Blaker H, von HA, Penzel R, Gross S, Otto HF. Genetics of adenocarcinomas of the small intestine: frequent deletions at chromosome 18q and mutations of the SMAD4 gene. *Oncogene* 2002;21(1):158.
76. Arai M, Shimizu S, Imai Y, et al. Mutations of the Ki-ras, p53 and APC genes in adenocarcinomas of the human small intestine. *Int J Cancer* 1997;70(4):390.
77. Howe JR, Karnell LH, Menck HR, et al. The American College of Surgeons Commission on Cancer and the American Cancer Society. Adenocarcinoma of the small bowel: review of the National Cancer Data Base, 1985–1995. *Cancer* 1999;86:2693.
79. Sohn TA, Lillemoe KD, Cameron JL, et al. Adenocarcinoma of the duodenum: factors influencing long-term survival. *J Gastrointest Surg* 1998;2(1):79.
83. Agrawal S, McCarron EC, Gibbs JF, et al. Surgical management and outcome in primary adenocarcinoma of the small bowel. *Ann Surg Oncol* 2007;14:2263.
84. Wu TJ, Yeh CN, Chao TC, et al. Prognostic factors of primary small bowel adenocarcinoma: univariate and multivariate analysis. *World J Surg* 2006;30:391.
85. Bauer RL, Palmer ML, Bauer AM, et al. Adenocarcinoma of the small intestine: 21-year review of diagnosis, treatment, and prognosis. *Ann Surg Oncol* 1994;1:183.
88. Swartz MJ, Hughes MA, Frassica DA, et al. Adjuvant concurrent chemoradiation for node positive adenocarcinoma of the duodenum. *Arch Surg* 2007;142:285.
89. Barnes G Jr, Romero L, Hess KR, et al. Primary adenocarcinoma of the duodenum: management and survival in 67 patients. *Ann Surg Oncol* 1994;1:73.
90. Fishman PN, Pond GR, Moore MJ, et al. Natural history and chemotherapy effectiveness for advanced adenocarcinoma of the small bowel: a retrospective review of 113 cases. *Am J Clin Oncol* 2006;29:225.
91. Klinkenbijl JH, Jeekel J, Sahmoud T, et al. Adjuvant radiotherapy and 5-fluorouracil after curative resection of cancer of the pancreas and periampullary region: phase III trial of the EORTC gastrointestinal tract cancer cooperative group. *Ann Surg* 1999;230:776.
92. Overman MJ, Varadhachary GR, Kopetz S, et al. Phase II study of capecitabine and oxaliplatin for advanced adenocarcinoma of the small bowel and ampulla of Vater. *J Clin Oncol* 2009;27(16):2598.
93. Overman MJ, Kopetz S, Wen S, et al. Chemotherapy with 5-fluorouracil and a platinum compound improves outcomes in metastatic small bowel adenocarcinoma. *Cancer* 2008;113:2038.
95. Modlin IM, Lye KD, Kidd M. A 5-decade analysis of 13,715 carcinoid tumors. *Cancer* 2003;97(4):934.
96. Maggard MA, O'Connell JB, Ko CY. Updated population-based review of carcinoid tumors. *Ann Surg* 2004;240(1):117.
100. Shebani KO, Souba WW, Finkelstein DM, et al. Prognosis and survival in patients with gastrointestinal tract carcinoid tumors. *Ann Surg* 1999;229(6):815.
101. Soga J. Early-stage carcinoids of the gastrointestinal tract: an analysis of 1914 reported cases. *Cancer* 2005;103(8):1587.
104. Hellman P, Lundstrom T, Ohrvall U, et al. Effect of surgery on the outcome of midgut carcinoid disease with lymph node and liver metastases. *World J Surg* 2002;26(8):991.

105. Givi B, Pommier SJ, Thompson AK, Diggs BS, Pommier RF. Operative resection of primary carcinoid neoplasms in patients with liver metastases yields significantly better survival. *Surgery* 2006;140(6):891.
108. McEntee GP, Nagorney DM, Kvols LK. Cytoreductive hepatic surgery for neuroendocrine tumors. *Surgery* 1990;108:1091.
109. Sarmiento JM, Heywood G, Rubin J, et al. Surgical treatment of neuroendocrine metastases to the liver: a plea for resection to increase survival. *J Am Coll Surg* 2003;197(1):29.
111. Osborne DA, Zervos EE, Strosberg J, et al. Improved outcome with cytoreduction versus embolization for symptomatic hepatic metastases of carcinoid and neuroendocrine tumors. *Ann Surg Oncol* 2006;13(4):572.
112. Gupta S, Yao JC, Ahrar K, et al. Hepatic artery embolization and chemoembolization for treatment of patients with metastatic carcinoid tumors: the M. D. Anderson experience. *Cancer J* 2003;9(4):261.
114. Kulke MH, Kim H, Stuart K, et al. A phase II study of docetaxel in patients with metastatic carcinoid tumors. *Cancer Invest* 2004;22(3):353.
119. Kvols LK, Moertel CG, O'Connell MJ, et al. Treatment of the malignant carcinoid syndrome: evaluation of a long-acting somatostatin analogue. *N Engl J Med* 1986;315:663.
122. Fischbach W, Dragosics B, Kolve-Goebeler ME, et al. Primary gastric B-cell lymphoma: results of a prospective multicenter study. The German-Austrian Gastrointestinal Lymphoma Study Group. *Gastroenterology* 2000;119(5):1191.
123. Koniaris LG, Drugas G, Katzman PJ, Salloum R. Management of gastrointestinal lymphoma. *J Am Coll Surg* 2003;197(1):127.
126. Miettinen M, Lasota J. Gastrointestinal stromal tumors: review on morphology, molecular pathology, prognosis, and differential diagnosis. *Arch Pathol Lab Med* 2006;130(10):1466.
128. Perez EA, Livingstone AS, Franceschi D, et al. Current incidence and outcomes of gastrointestinal mesenchymal tumors including gastrointestinal stromal tumors. *J Am Coll Surg* 2006;202(4):623.
140. Dematteo RP, Ballman KV, Antonescu CR, et al. Adjuvant imatinib mesylate after resection of localised, primary gastrointestinal stromal tumour: a randomised, double-blind, placebo-controlled trial. *Lancet* 2009;373:1097.
141. DeMatteo RP, Antonescu CR, Chadaram V, et al. American College of Surgeons Oncology Group (ACOSOG). Adjuvant imatinib mesylate in patients with primary high risk gastrointestinal stromal tumor (GIST) following complete resection: safety results from the U.S. Intergroup phase II trial ACOSOG Z9000. *J Clin Oncol* 2005;23(16 Suppl):9009.
142. Blanke CD, Demetri GD, von Mehren M, et al. Long-term results from a randomized phase II trial of standard- versus higher-dose imatinib mesylate for patients with unresectable or metastatic gastrointestinal stromal tumors expressing KIT. *J Clin Oncol* 2008;26:620.

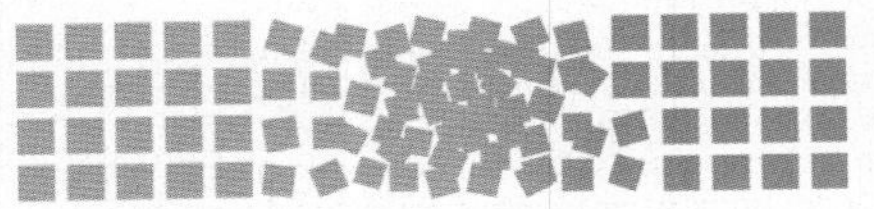

CHAPTER 87 GASTROINTESTINAL STROMAL TUMOR

GEORGE D. DEMETRI

Over the past decade, the approach to diagnosis and treatment of the sarcomas known as gastrointestinal stromal tumors (GISTs) has truly been revolutionized. GIST research and clinical care now represent a paradigm of translating discoveries in the molecular pathogenesis of cancer into highly effective new therapies that selectively inhibit these etiologic "driver" pathways in specific patients, leading to dramatically improved clinical outcomes. Rarely in the history of medicine does the opportunity arise to watch an entire field of investigation evolve so quickly and have such a major effect on the lives of patients with such a life-threatening malignancy. Differentiating GIST from all other abdominal and retroperitoneal sarcomas, poorly differentiated carcinomas, or lymphomas is a critically important scientific breakthrough, based on the molecular mechanisms of aberrant intracellular signaling pathways most often related to two receptor tyrosine kinases (KIT and platelet-derived growth factor receptor-alpha [PDGFRA]). From this fundamental mechanistic understanding of the disease, a series of highly collaborative worldwide investigations has developed novel and effective ways to approach patients with this disease, with attendant improvements in the recognition, diagnosis, imaging, staging, and treatment of GIST. In this chapter, the highlights of these advances are summarized, and the relevance to current clinical practice as well as future directions in basic and applied cancer research is discussed.

GIST AS A UNIQUE CLINICOPATHOLOGIC SUBSET OF SARCOMA

The diagnostic term *gastrointestinal stromal tumor* comprises several different molecularly distinct subtypes that collectively represent the most common form of sarcomas (i.e., mesenchymal malignancies) of the gastrointestinal (GI) tract. The incidence of GIST was vastly underrecognized (and therefore underreported in cancer registry databases) before the year 2000, but with improved diagnostic techniques and increased awareness among physicians, GIST is now estimated to account for approximately 1% to 3% of all malignant GI tumors, with a remarkably consistent annual incidence rate across the world of 10 to 15 cases per million people.[1] Before the late 1990s, the diagnostic categories of abdominal and retroperitoneal sarcomas were somewhat confusing and it was difficult to distinguish biologically distinct subtypes.[2,3] GIST was initially a purely descriptive term developed in 1983 by Mazur and Clark[4] to define intra-abdominal tumors that were definitely not carcinomas and that also failed to exhibit features of either smooth muscle or nerve cells. However, expert pathologists recognized that the expression of muscle or nerve antigenic markers, even in the most careful immunohistochemical analyses, could not reliably differentiate or subcategorize a certain class of mesenchymal tumors of the gut. Early diagnostic attempts to categorize GIST was plagued by the inherent variability of expression across many gut sarcomas of differentiation antigens used as markers for muscle cells (e.g., smooth muscle actin) and nerve cells (such as S100). Several names were applied to these tumors based on the variable patterns of cell lineage markers described by a variety of pathologists across the world (Table 87.1).

Before the current molecular understanding of GIST, these tumors were often previously diagnosed as leiomyomas or leiomyosarcomas because of their histologic resemblance to those forms of smooth muscle neoplasms. Despite this, it had long been recognized that a subset of these tumors that arose in the bowel wall had a number of uniquely characteristic histologic features and likely represented a different entity altogether.[2,3] The class of "leiomyosarcomas of the GI tract" was also noted to be exceptionally resistant to any standard chemotherapy regimens that had efficacy in the management of leiomyosarcomas arising in other anatomic sites (e.g., chemotherapy yielded far greater benefits for patients whose leiomyosarcomas originated in the uterus or extremities). Additional differences between GISTs and leiomyosarcomas became apparent with the application of modern immunohistochemical techniques in the 1980s. By these assays, a significant number of these tumors were noted to lack the characteristic muscle antigens that defined leiomyosarcomas located elsewhere in the body.

Based on these findings, Mazur and Clark[4] introduced the term *GIST* in 1983 in a descriptive effort to provide diagnostic guidance to subclassify these tumors. However, the term GIST remained controversial because it was not fully specific in its definition. Other terms were generated based on the fact that neural crest antigens such as neuron-specific enolase and S100 could be demonstrated in GIST cells; this led to the terms *plexosarcomas*[5] and *gastrointestinal autonomic nerve tumors*.[6] Additional research in immunohistochemical analysis of GISTs in the early 1990s revealed that a significant proportion of these tumors expressed the CD34 antigen (an antigen that is shared between hematopoietic stem cells as well as vascular and myofibroblastic cells). It was initially hoped that CD34 might prove to be a key differentiating feature between GISTs and other spindle cell tumors of the GI tract, such as schwannomas or leiomyomas. However, this was not the case. CD34 expression characterized only approximately half of all GIST cases, and a proportion of smooth muscle and Schwann cell tumors could also express CD34. Therefore, CD34 was neither a sensitive nor a specific marker to distinguish GIST from other mesenchymal neoplasms.[7,8]

Pathologists also proposed that some GIST cells differentiated along smooth muscle lineages, whereas others were neurogenic in origin; still, over a third of them lacked any detectable immunostaining for lineage-specific markers and were said to have a "null phenotype."[9–11]

TABLE 87.1

PATHOLOGY TERMS THAT ENCOMPASS THE SPECTRUM OF GASTROINTESTINAL STROMAL TUMORS

Gastrointestinal stromal tumor
Leiomyoblastoma
Gastrointestinal leiomyosarcoma
Gastrointestinal autonomic nerve tumor
Gastrointestinal pacemaker cell tumor
Plexosarcoma
Gastrointestinal neurofibrosarcoma

Before 2000, therefore, there were no reproducible, clearly defined, objective criteria to classify GIST, and it is likely that several types of epithelioid and spindle cell tumors were included in the early clinical and pathologic diagnoses of patients with GIST. Similarly, many true GIST cases were classified by other names, such as leiomyoblastomas, GI autonomic nerve tumors, leiomyosarcomas of the GI tract, or even as poorly differentiated carcinomas (especially for the epithelioid variants). This makes the interpretation of published clinical results before 2000 difficult, given the likely heterogeneity in the patients labeled with the diagnostic term GIST before the molecular definitions of these kinase-driven malignancies were developed.

GIST CELLS ARE RELATED TO THE MESENCHYMAL PRECURSOR CELLS THAT GIVE RISE TO NORMAL INTERSTITIAL CELLS OF CAJAL: ABERRANT DEVELOPMENTAL BIOLOGY

A conceptual advance in the thinking about GIST occurred in the late 1990s with the notion that these tumors bore certain histopathologic similarities to a specific cell type inherent in the GI tract, known as the *interstitial cells of Cajal* (ICC).[12] ICCs are the unique "pacemaker cells" that are normally present in the myenteric plexus and act to coordinate gut peristalsis by linking the smooth muscle cells of the bowel wall with the autonomic nervous system. GIST cells and ICCs were noted to have similar ultrastructural features combining neural and myogenic differentiation, and both cell types were documented to express the KIT receptor tyrosine kinase (KIT RTK); therefore, it has been widely accepted that the cells of both GISTs and normal ICCs share a common precursor cell.[13,14] The KIT RTK and its ligand, stem cell factor, are documented to play an essential role in the development and maintenance of normal ICCs as well as of other cells, including melanocytes, erythrocytes, germ cells, and mast cells. KIT expression is noted in the vast majority (more than 95%) of GISTs, but KIT is not expressed by other smooth muscle tumors of the GI tract nor by other stromal tumors outside the GI tract (e.g., there is no KIT expression in endometrial stromal tumors of the uterus).

The origin of the neoplastic cells of GIST remains a matter of active investigation. Certain data suggest that GISTs originate from CD34+ stem cells residing within the wall of the gut, which can then differentiate toward the ICC phenotype.[14–16] The recently identified association of different molecular subtypes of GIST with anatomically distinct regions of the GI tract (e.g., *KIT* exon 9-mutant GIST) is almost always noted as small bowel primary, while *PDGFRA*-mutant GIST most often occurs as gastric primary) is perhaps tied to the underlying differential migration and distribution of these ICC precursor cells along the length of the GI tract during embryonic and fetal development. Although the signaling pathways that are characteristically dysregulated in GIST have been identified to a great extent, the factors that are responsible for aggressive malignant behavior of certain forms of GIST are still poorly understood. This is particularly striking when one considers important studies that show that so-called micro-GISTs less than 1 cm are remarkably common and found in up to 35% of carefully studied gastric wall specimens of people who do not have any cancer.[17–19] These micro-GISTs appear to have no malignant potential at all, despite the fact that the tiny lesions generally harbor KIT mutations similar to aggressive malignant GIST, and it is very likely that an unknown "second hit" is altered in larger GISTs.

THE DEVELOPMENT OF A MOLECULAR UNDERSTANDING OF GIST

The molecular understanding of GIST pathogenesis was advanced greatly by a key observation made by Hirota et al.[20] in Japan in 1998. This group was interested in the role played by KIT in ICC and other cell growth and development signaling, and they went on to define the relationship between GIST and certain mutations in the *KIT* protooncogene that conferred uncontrolled activation to the KIT signaling enzyme. Normally, the KIT protein serves as a transmembrane RTK; the CD117 antigen can be detected by immunohistochemical staining as a marker for the presence of the KIT protein. In normal cell signaling, KIT binds its ligand, known also as stem cell factor or *Steel* factor, and this ligand binding brings together two molecules of KIT (the signaling cascade is summarized in Fig. 87.1). These two KIT receptors form a homodimer with cross-phosphorylation of critical tyrosine residues in the intracellular domains of KIT. These phosphorylation events then activate the signal transduction pathways downstream of KIT. The net physiologic effect of KIT activation is the stimulation of cell proliferation and enhanced cell survival; therefore, uncontrolled activation could theoretically lead to neoplastic growth of cells. The Japanese team provided the critical confirmation of this theory at both the cellular and molecular levels. This elegant work was derived from recognition of the key biologic similarities between GIST and ICC cells.[21–24] *KIT* gene mutations were identified in five of six cases of human GIST studied by this team, and they went on to document that the mutations led to uncontrolled, ligand-independent phosphorylation by the KIT kinase.[16] Genetically engineered cells harboring the mutant, overactive KIT proteins also grew into tumors when injected into nude mice, a proof of concept for the malignant phenotype induced by the aberrant signaling pathways associated with KIT overactivity.[20]

The oncogenic potential of mutant, uncontrollably active KIT in the pathogenesis of GIST in humans was further supported by the identification of a family that exhibited an autosomal dominant inheritance pattern of GIST. Genetic analysis of this kindred revealed that they harbored a germ line activating *KIT* mutation, similar to the mutations that were seen in sporadic cases of GIST.[25] Several other families have since been identified with germ line *KIT* mutations and an abnormally high incidence of GIST, usually occurring as multiple foci within any affected individual.[26,27] Often, these tumors may not present clinically until the second or third decade of life, and some even present in far advanced age. *KIT* mutations have also been documented in very small (<1 cm) GISTs that were detected incidentally and that appear morphologically benign.[17–19] These

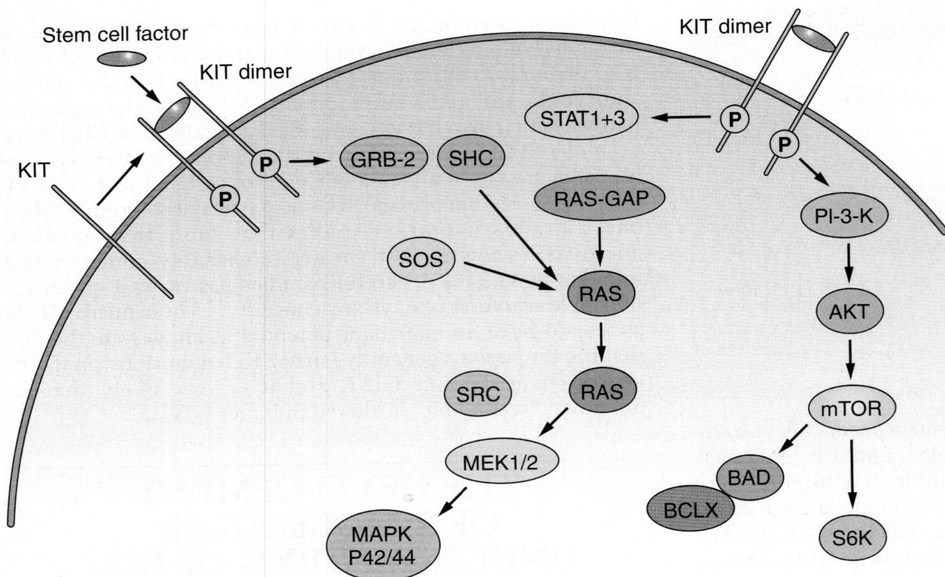

FIGURE 87.1 Simplified schema of the molecular cascade involved in KIT-mediated cell signaling. Other steps may be operative as well, and the relative contribution of each of these downstream signaling events to different aspects of aberrant KIT signaling in gastrointestinal stromal tumor remains the subject of active investigation. Each step may be a potential future target for therapeutic development. MAPK, mitogen-activated protein kinase; mTOR, mammalian target of rapamycin; P, phosphorus; PI-3-K, phosphatidylinositol 3 kinase; S6K, S6 kinase. (Modified from A. Fletcher, unpublished data, 2004, and ref. 29.)

findings support the hypothesis that activating mutations in the *KIT* protooncogene represent an early transforming mechanism in GIST oncogenesis. However, since many tumors harboring this mutation can remain small for years (or in the case of micro-GISTs, such cells may never have a risk of recurrence or metastasis), there must be other key signaling steps that confer an aggressive and malignant phenotype to GIST cells. These other molecular pathways remain poorly understood. Unique elements of the downstream signaling cascades in GIST are being actively elucidated, with prominent involvement of the PI-3-kinase, AKT, and mammalian target of rapamycin (mTOR) pathways. Importantly, these appear to differ from KIT signaling in hematologic neoplasia in that the STAT5 pathway prominent in leukemic cells is not typically activated in GIST, whereas STAT1 and STAT3 are activated at high levels.[28] New evidence also indicates that high level expression of the ETV1 transcription factor drives a unique pattern of genes whose expression is critical to formation of GIST through cooperativity with the mutant KIT oncoprotein.[29]

The literature before 2000 was somewhat confusing about whether mutations were relevant to the differentiation between "benign GIST" and "malignant GIST." With the recognition that *KIT* mutations can be found in even the smallest GISTs,[19] there is now consensus that *KIT* genotype alone cannot account for differences between GISTs that may behave in an indolent manner (and that may be functionally benign) and those that are clearly aggressive and malignant by any functional definition. Additionally, it is also clear that well-differentiated cell morphology (which might otherwise lead a pathologist to call the cells benign) cannot be used to ensure that any individual GIST will pursue a benign clinical course.

KIT mutations can be detected in approximately 85% of GIST lesions.[30–32] Constitutive activation of the KIT enzymatic function has been reported to characterize every GIST sample analyzed by immunoblotting technique, even in cases in which there are no detectable mutations in the *KIT* gene.[30] Defining the mechanisms by which wild type (nonmutant) KIT adopts an uncontrollably active and phosphorylated state is an important goal of current research. This is a poorly understood element of GIST biology and is the subject of active investigation, especially as wild type KIT characterizes most cases of pediatric GIST.

Importantly, virtually all GIST lesions with mutant *KIT* documented by conventional genomic technology at initial presentation in adults demonstrate only a single site of mutation in the *KIT* gene; complex genetic changes are truly rare until resistance to kinase inhibitors evolves. It remains to be seen whether next-generation "deep sequencing" will be able to detect low-copy number "TKI-resistance" mutations that likely already exist at the time of initial presentation but are below the limits of detection of current "standard" genomic detection methods. Gain-of-function mutations have been identified most commonly (up to 70% of cases) in exon 11 of *KIT*, which corresponds to the intracellular juxtamembrane domain of the KIT protein. Mutations in the *KIT* gene locus have also been described (in decreasing order of prevalence) in exon 9 (representing the KIT extracellular domain), exon 13 (first portion of split kinase domain), and exon 17 (separate portion of split kinase domain).[30–32] These genomic mutations lead to structural alterations in the KIT protein that alter enzymatic kinetics and favor a state of uncontrolled, ligand-independent activity.[33,34]

Another key advance in the understanding of GIST has been the recognition that signaling through other mutated kinases besides KIT could give rise to the neoplastic transformation of certain patients with GIST. Specifically, it is now recognized that approximately 15% of GIST patients do not demonstrate activation and aberrant signaling of the KIT receptor, with 10% instead harboring mutational activation of the structurally related kinase, PDGFRA[35,36] while very rare cases may have mutational activation of the *BRAF* kinase.[37] Overall, approximately 5% of GISTs will have no detectable kinase mutations (and are thus often referred to as wild type GIST). Although these may indeed be wild type for kinase, up to one-third of such GISTs may have mutations in non–tyrosine kinase metabolic pathway enzymes such as the Krebs-cycle enzyme subunits of succinate dehydrogenase.[38]

CLINICAL CONSIDERATIONS

Before 2000, the number of new GIST cases in the United States had been grossly underestimated and underreported; experts had proposed that there were perhaps only 300 to 500 new cases per year. However, it is now recognized that many GISTs were not captured in traditional cancer databases such as that of the Surveillance, Epidemiology, and End Results (SEER) program because of the problems of diagnostic techniques and terminology noted earlier. Given the significant progress made only recently in the diagnosis and reporting of these tumors and the extremely rapid rate of accrual to clinical trials in GIST, the estimated incidence of GIST has been revised upward to approximately 5,000 new cases per year in the United States alone.[39,40] It is important to note that not all of these cases will prove to be life-threatening, because many GISTs in cases of limited disease may be small and curable with appropriate surgery as the first-line therapy. A population-based study to define the incidence of GIST using current criteria has reported an incidence of approximately 15 cases per million population.[41]

GIST occurs predominantly in adults at a median age of 58 years but can occur across the age spectrum from infancy to old age. The incidence is slightly higher in men than in women. The majority of GISTs (60% to 70%) have been reported to arise in the stomach, whereas 20% to 30% originate in the small intestine, and fewer than 10% in the esophagus, colon, and rectum. GISTs can also occur in extraintestinal abdominopelvic sites such as the omentum, mesentery, or retroperitoneum.[42–44]

The clinical presentation of patients with GIST can vary tremendously based on the anatomic location of the tumor as well as the tumor size and aggressiveness. For many patients, the detection of GIST may occur from the evaluation of nonspecific symptoms or may even be an incidental finding. Symptoms tend to arise only when tumors reach a large size or are in critical anatomic localizations (e.g., constricting gastric outflow). Most symptomatic patients present with tumors that are larger than 5 cm in maximal dimension. Symptoms at presentation may include abdominal pain, an abdominal mass, nausea, vomiting, anorexia, and weight loss. Certain series have reported that up to 40% of patients present with acute hemorrhage into the intestinal tract or peritoneal cavity from tumor rupture, although this certainly depends on the size of the tumor. The vast majority of GIST metastases at presentation are intra-abdominal, either to the liver, omentum, or peritoneal cavity.[42] Metastatic spread to lymph nodes or to extra-abdominal sites via lymphatics is very rare; most lesions thought to be nodal metastases simply represent metastatic deposits of tumor nodules in the omentum or peritoneum rather than true lymphatic spread of the disease.

Diagnostic Evaluation and Approach to the Patient

The diagnostic evaluation of suspected or proven GIST is similar to that of other GI malignancies. The most important element is to keep GIST in the suspected differential diagnosis of an intra-abdominal nonepithelial malignancy. Computed tomography (CT) is essential for evaluating the primary tumor and for accurate staging of disease. Magnetic resonance imaging (MRI) can also be used to detect hepatic metastases, although CT is usually an adequate technology as long as appropriate techniques of both noncontrast and early and late visualization after intravenous contrast administration are used. On upper GI endoscopy, there may be a smooth, mucosa-lined protrusion of the bowel wall, which may or may not show signs of bleeding and ulceration.[45] Most GISTs arise below the layer of mucosa and grow in an endophytic fashion. This can make accurate detection of the tumor and assessment of the lesion size by visual endoscopy very challenging and can also make procurement of diagnostic tissue by endoscopy more difficult. Endoscopic ultrasound may be the ideal tool for localized GIST, with diagnosis through carefully considered endoscopic ultrasound-guided fine-needle aspiration for primary lesions.

Differential Diagnosis of Gastrointestinal Stromal Tumor: Dilemmas of Diagnostic Histopathology and Cytology

GIST was originally described as a monomorphic spindle cell neoplasm. However, it is very clear that this disease can exhibit a wide variety of appearances with characteristics of either an epithelioid (larger, rounder cells) or spindle cell histology. Because the accurate diagnosis of GIST is now critical for appropriate patient management, it is of crucial importance that pathologists consider GIST in the differential diagnosis of tumors arising anywhere along the GI tract or in the abdomen and pelvis. The spindle cell pattern of GIST is far more common, occurring in approximately 70% of cases. This subset corresponds to tumors often diagnosed before 2000 as GI leiomyosarcomas. The epithelioid, or round cell, pattern represents a majority of the remaining 30% and may have an admixture of spindle cell features. Tumors in the epithelioid subset generally were previously diagnosed as leiomyoblastomas, although some may have been mistaken for poorly differentiated carcinomas. GISTs account for approximately 80% of mesenchymal tumors of the GI tract. There are definitely true smooth muscle neoplasms of the GI tract, including true leiomyomas and leiomyosarcomas, which account for approximately 15% of GI nonepithelial neoplasms; schwannomas account for the remaining 5%. Rarely, other malignancies, such as melanomas of the GI tract, can occur. Therefore, the differential diagnosis is complex and requires expert pathologic review, as well as adequate and appropriately processed and fixed diagnostic tissues.

As noted earlier, GISTs characteristically exhibit expression of the CD117 antigen (KIT) by immunohistochemical assays, and the levels of expression can vary from generally diffuse and strong (most common in the spindle cell subtype) to focal and weakly positive in a dotlike pattern (characteristic of the epithelioid subtype).[39] CD34 expression is not specific for GIST because it can also be noted in desmoid tumors, and approximately 60% to 70% of GIST lesions are positive for CD34.[13,20,39] True leiomyosarcomas express the smooth muscle markers, smooth muscle actin, and desmin but fail to express CD117. Schwannomas are usually positive for the neural antigen S100 but are also negative for CD117.[39] Normal mast cells and ICCs in the surrounding stromal tissues serve as ideal positive internal controls because these normal cells strongly express CD117.

There remains a diagnostic challenge in the identification of CD117-negative GIST. Certainly, expert pathologists can define a rare subset (fewer than 5%) of GISTs that do not express CD117, and these are most likely to be driven by an alternative kinase such as PDGFRA.[35] The antigen known as DOG-1 (an acronym for "discovered on GIST-1") can help to identify certain KIT-negative GIST lesions as DOG-1 expression is quite selective for GIST.[46,47] DOG-1 is encoded by the gene *TMEM16A*, which encodes a calcium-dependent chloride ion channel whose roles in GIST pathophysiology remains obscure. Expert mutational analysis of the *KIT* and *PDGFRA* genotype may be useful to define with certainty the group of rare patients with CD117-negative GISTs in the future. There are no definitive diagnostic criteria of CD117-negative GIST unless the tumor genotype analysis indicates a *KIT* or *PDGFRA* mutation characteristic of GIST.

It is important to recognize that expression of KIT is not limited to GIST cells. Normal ICCs and mast cells express CD117 and are dependent on KIT for normal growth and development. A relatively limited number of other tumors may also express immunohistochemically detectable CD117. These include certain subsets of soft tissue sarcomas, including Ewing sarcoma and angiosarcoma, as well as other neoplasms such as occasional small cell lung cancers, melanomas, desmoid tumors, seminomas, ovarian carcinomas, mastocytomas, neuroblastomas, adenoid cystic carcinomas, and rare subsets of lymphoma and acute myeloid leukemia.[21,22,48,49] It is most important to recognize that expression alone of the CD117 antigen does not imply the activation of the KIT target, nor does it necessarily correlate with any *KIT* gene mutation. The same CD117 antigen is expressed by cells harboring normal (wild type) *KIT* as those that have activating *KIT* mutations. Additionally, expression of KIT protein does not necessarily mean that the protein is involved in the pathogenesis of that specific cancer. In all these regards, GIST was a very special example of a disease in which expression did correlate universally with kinase activation, and this activation was truly pathogenetically crucial to the malignancy. In general, with certain rare exceptions, there is little reason to expect that these other tumors would exhibit clinically important activity from an agent designed to block signaling through the KIT kinase.

PROGNOSTIC FEATURES OF GASTROINTESTINAL STROMAL TUMOR

What is the risk that a patient with primary GIST will develop metastases? The answer to this remains somewhat vague. However, it is clear that even reasonably small tumors (e.g., in the range of 3 cm) with benign-appearing cellular morphology can occasionally metastasize. Reports of patient outcomes in studies before 1999 are difficult to interpret, given the problems of diagnostic imprecision in that era. The current consensus among pathologists is to regard all GISTs, including those that seem to have a benign appearance by conventional histopathologic criteria, as having the potential to behave in a malignant fashion (i.e., to metastasize or to infiltrate sufficiently into surrounding tissues that resection for cure is impossible, or both), while recognizing that size and other features such as mitotic count strongly affect these risks.[39,50]

An early consensus reached among expert pathologists with experience in GIST identified the most reliable prognostic factors as the size of the primary tumor and the mitotic index, which measures the proliferative activity of the cells (Fig. 87.2). Recognizing that the recurrence and survival rates correlate with location of the primary GIST lesion (e.g., with small bowel and rectal primary GIST demonstrating worse prognosis than gastric lesions), subsequent risk stratification system revisions have incorporated primary site into the assessment of clinical risk for localized resected disease.[51] A nomogram predicting risk has been developed based on these factors, although the mitotic rate is a disproportionately "binary" variable for risk in the iteration of this risk assessment tool.[52]

Certain reports before the year 2000 suggested that GISTs showing *KIT* mutations were associated with a less favorable prognosis than cases of GIST with no detectable mutation.[53,54] However, these studies were technically limited, analyzing mutations solely in exon 11 of *KIT* and finding mutations in only 60% of samples (much lower than the 90% rate of *KIT* mutations seen in more recent series screening across more *KIT* exons so that 11, 9, 13, and 17 are included).[30] An early study showed that not all mutations in exon 11 of *KIT* are equivalent: deletions in this locus conferred a worse prognosis for GIST,[55] and this has now been confirmed with other studies and prospective data.[56,57] Larger prospective trials are pending to assess the degree to which *KIT* genotype may be an independent prognostic risk factor or whether this marker tracks with other clinical features to risk-stratify patients with primary resected GIST. Importantly, it is already quite clear that PDGFRA mutations in GIST (almost always in gastric primaries) appear to confer a very favorable prognosis with low risk of recurrence.[57]

DIAGNOSTIC IMAGING OF PATIENTS WITH GASTROINTESTINAL STROMAL TUMORS

Research studies have taken advantage of the remarkable visualization of GIST through functional imaging using ^{18}F-fluorodeoxyglucose (^{18}FDG) positron emission tomography (PET) to visualize the impact of molecularly targeted therapies in this disease. However, it must be emphasized that routine clinical practice rarely requires PET imaging of GIST for clinical care.[50] CT or MRI scanning can assess the size of GIST lesions quite accurately, and the decrease in lesion density on CT imaging can be an early marker of beneficial response in GIST patients treated with TKI drugs.[58] However, it is important to note that these eponymous "Choi criteria" representing density changes as well as smaller percentage changes in objective lesion size by CT imaging represent technically challenging metrics to apply across multiple centers with variable practice patterns of contrast administration and CT imaging; fundamentally, the Choi criteria are able to categorize "stable disease" as a "response to therapy." Once it is recognized that stable disease in GIST is a meaningful and beneficial outcome of therapy with TKI drugs, the prime value of this system is to recognize this biological imaging change as a "response."

In occasional cases, the functional imaging of GISTs with ^{18}FDG-PET can give information complementary to CT/MRI that can assist clinicians in the management of GIST patients. The actual mechanisms responsible for the high-level avidity of GISTs for the ^{18}FDG-PET tracer are not yet known; however, it is likely that there is a direct connection between signaling through the overactive KIT RTK and glucose transport proteins. In this way, one could explain the very rapid changes in PET imaging associated with inhibition of KIT signaling by pharmacologic means.[59–62] Large GISTs can demonstrate centers with predominately "cystic" or low attenuation characteristics noted on CT or MRI scans. It is clear by ^{18}FDG-PET scans that the

	Very low risk	Low risk	Intermediate risk	High risk	Metastatic or unresectable
Size of primary	< 2 cm	2–5 cm	< 3 cm	> 10 cm *or* > 5 cm + medium *or* ANY size + high	**ANY SIZE, ANY MITOTIC RATE**
Mitotic rate of primary	Low	Low	Medium		

FIGURE 87.2 Assessment of risk of recurrence or metastasis for localized, resectable primary gastrointestinal stromal tumors. (Adapted from ref. 39.)

internal mass of large GIST lesions can often be viewed as metabolically quiescent. This is likely because of the endogenous necrosis of very large lesions in their central portions; although GIST lesions can be very vascular, the internal portion can nonetheless represent a confluent mass of necrotic material, with the more viable aspects of the GIST pushing out toward the edges of the lesion. In addition, occasionally metastatic GIST lesions in the omentum can be subtle and easy to overlook on CT scans because small lesions can blend into the folds of the bowel walls and be difficult for even the most experienced radiologist to detect. ^{18}FDG-PET imaging can detect lesions at least 1 cm in size without difficulty because neither the normal bowel nor omentum takes up the ^{18}FDG tracer with excess avidity.

TREATMENT OPTIONS AND MANAGEMENT DECISIONS IN THE ERA OF MOLECULARLY TARGETED THERAPIES FOR GIST

Management of Metastatic, Unresectable, or Recurrent GIST: The Paradigm Changes for Advanced Disease

Failure of Traditional Systemic and Locoregional Cytotoxic Chemotherapy

New approaches to disease management in cancer medicine are often first tried in patients with advanced disease. This has certainly been true in the clinical development of therapies that target specific mutationally activated pathways for patients with GIST. In the case of GIST, the remarkably rapid translation of the molecular biologic and pathobiologic findings discussed earlier in the section "Histopathologic Features and Histogenesis" has led to dramatic changes in the management of patients with advanced GIST. Therefore, this chapter first discusses the management of patients with advanced disease and then moves to the management of patients with early-stage, full GIST.

In GIST, there was universal opinion that advanced disease represented a pressing unmet medical need before the advent of TKIs such as imatinib and sunitinib, which became known as "molecularly targeted therapy" for this disease. Efforts of medical oncologists to treat GISTs with conventional cytotoxic chemotherapy were recognized universally to be futile. The rates of objective antitumor response to a variety of chemotherapy agents for patients with GIST or abdominal leiomyosarcomas were routinely reported in the range of 0% to, at best, less than 5%.[61,63] Other investigators attempted to boost the benefits of chemotherapy by administering the drugs via an intraperitoneal route.[64] However, because few GISTs remain confined to the peritoneal surfaces, and because the majority of the life-threatening complications of GIST arise from hepatic involvement or other bulky sites of omental disease, this has been viewed as less than optimal.

Based on these disappointing results, conventional cytotoxic chemotherapy had generally been regarded as a dismal failure in the treatment of GIST prior to kinase inhibitors. There are limited data regarding the potential to control metastatic GIST by locoregional techniques such as hepatic artery embolization or chemoembolization. Although a subset of patients with metastatic GIST involving the liver can show antitumor responses and limited progression-free survival after chemoembolization, the benefits are generally measured in months rather than years, and this has not been viewed as a particularly promising strategy for management of most GIST patients.[65,66]

It is likely that the antiapoptotic impact of the aberrant KIT signaling interferes with the cytotoxic activity of even the most damaging chemotherapy to effect cell kill of GIST. Other mechanisms responsible for the extreme resistance to chemotherapy exhibited by GIST may also be invoked, for example, by the demonstration of the increased levels of P-glycoprotein (the product of the multidrug resistance-1 [*MDR-1*] gene) and the multidrug resistance protein-1 MRP1 that have been reported in GISTs and other intra-abdominal sarcomas. In one study evaluating the differences in outcome between GIST and leiomyosarcomas, significantly higher levels of expression of P-glycoprotein (38.4% vs. 13.4%) and MRP1 (35.4% vs. 13.3%) were demonstrated in the GIST cells.[67] It has been postulated that these cellular efflux pumps may prevent chemotherapy from reaching intracellular therapeutic concentrations in the target GIST cells.

Radiotherapy rarely plays any role in the management of patients with metastatic GIST. There are remarkably few instances in which radiotherapy has been carefully studied in this disease, most likely because the delivery of therapeutic doses of radiotherapy to the liver or the GI tract usually causes more morbidity than benefit. However, it is possible that targeting radiotherapy with newer techniques such as intensity-modulated radiotherapy or proton beam irradiation might be used for palliation in patients suffering from focal bleeding from a specific site of GIST recurrence. Radiotherapy may also be useful occasionally as a palliative maneuver for pain control in patients with bony involvement or those with a single large metastatic lesion fixed to the wall of the abdomen or pelvis. However, the diffuse pattern of disease recurrence in GIST does not allow radiotherapy to function as an effective therapeutic modality for the majority of patients with advanced disease. Similarly, surgery has traditionally not played a significant role in the management of patients with metastatic GIST because in most patients liver and peritoneal metastases from GIST are judged unresectable because of multifocal hepatic metastases or multiple sites of intra-abdominal metastatic disease.

Clearly, for patients with metastatic or unresectable GIST, the prognosis was dismal before the advent of mechanism-based molecularly targeted therapy. For patients with metastatic or recurrent GIST or GI sarcomas (the majority of which were likely to have been true GISTs), most studies have documented very poor survival rates, with fatal outcomes from disease progression generally occurring within 2 years from the date of first recurrence or metastasis.[42,63,68]

Development of the First Molecularly TKI Therapy for Gastrointestinal Stromal Tumor: Imatinib Mesylate

GIST represented a malignancy in which the stage was perfectly set for translational therapeutics. There was agreement among practitioners that no other systemic therapy was useful, and there was a pressing unmet medical need for thousands of patients across the world. There had been rapid and significant advances in understanding the critical molecular abnormalities that truly drove the neoplastic behavior of GIST and also served as a diagnostic biomarker for the majority of cases. There was also a tremendous stroke of serendipity in that a medication being developed for an entirely different purpose showed dramatic activity in inhibiting the uncontrollably activated KIT enzyme target, which was critical to the pathobiology of GIST. The rapid evolution of this therapeutic advance came from the collaborative efforts of many investigative teams sharing results across the world, with many patients being the beneficiaries of this rapid diffusion of technology and therapeutic knowledge.

The initial concept for this molecularly targeted approach came from studies of Druker et al.,[69] who were screening small molecules with the goal of inhibiting the constitutively active tyrosine kinase enzymatic function of the BCR-ABL oncopro-

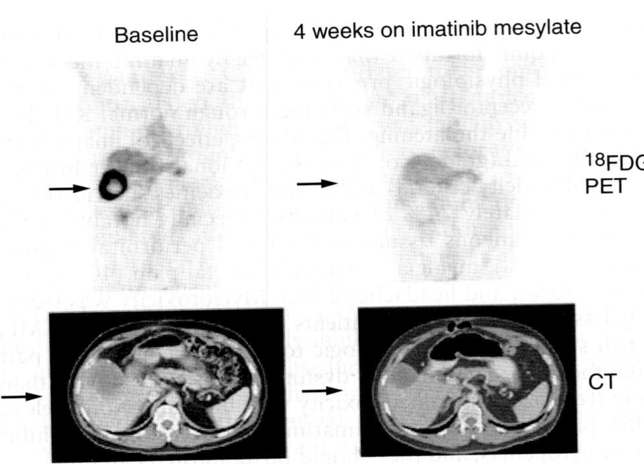

FIGURE 87.3 Rapid response to imatinib as imaged by ^{18}F-fluorodeoxyglucose–positron emission tomography (^{18}FDG-PET; *top*) and computed tomography (CT) scans (*bottom*). Baseline images (*left*) show large, ^{18}FDG-avid gastrointestinal stromal tumor metastasis in the right lobe of liver. After 4 weeks of daily imatinib therapy, there is no evidence of ^{18}FDG avidity remaining in the tumor, although the tumor is still prominent and hypodense on CT imaging. (Images from A. van den Abbeele and G. Demetri, Dana-Farber Cancer Institute, with permission.)

also be a very useful tool for future drug development efforts because the signal of drug activity can be detected clearly in patients within a very short period of time after drug dosing begins if effective target inhibition occurs.

Besides PET imaging, conventional CT imaging can also detect the clinical and biological activity of imatinib in GIST even in the absence of changes in tumor size. It is clear that imatinib therapy usually changes the density of tumor masses in GIST, inducing a hypodense appearance that is characteristic of the myxoid degeneration that is seen in the histopathologic sampling in clinical trials.[58,61,74,84]

The optimal dose of imatinib for treatment of most patients with advanced GIST has been accepted as 400 mg daily as the worldwide standard through large-scale collaborative trials, with documented benefit in terms of progression-free survival for the higher dose of 800 mg daily in the subset of GIST patients with *KIT* exon 9 mutation. Although there were no documented benefits to the higher dose of 600 mg/day in the United States–Finland trial, there were a few patients who regained disease control when crossed over from the lower dose (400 mg daily) to the higher dose level. Therefore, some marginal benefit might be obtained from modest dose escalation of imatinib in a subset of patients whose disease progresses on lower doses of imatinib. The pharmacologic levels of exposure to imatinib have also been proposed as a possible variable to explain why certain patients may be at risk for less durable disease control. In a retrospective analysis of systemic levels of imatinib in patients treated on the first United States–Finland trial of imatinib, those patients whose plasma levels were in the lowest 25% (below 1,100 ng/mL of parent drug) had the greatest risk of rapid disease progression, suggesting that inadequate kinase inhibitor levels may not be sufficient to silence the overactive kinase driving the malignancy.[85] This hypothesis is currently being tested in a properly powered prospective trial to assess whether individualized dose adjustments of the kinase inhibitor might improve the outcomes of patients with the lowest exposure levels of the TKI.

To explore more definitively whether there is a clinically significant dose response above the lowest recommended daily dose of 400 mg, two very large phase 3 randomized studies have been designed and conducted.[86–92] One of these studies has been performed by the North American Sarcoma Intergroup with the support of the U.S. National Cancer Institute and the National Cancer Institute of Canada, while the other has been conducted by the EORTC in conjunction with the Australasian GI Trials Group and the Italian Sarcoma Group. In both studies, patients with advanced metastatic and/or unresectable GIST were randomly assigned to receive imatinib at a dose of either 400 mg or 800 mg daily. Patients were allowed to cross over from the lower dose to the higher dose if there was progression of disease at the lower dose. These studies, which registered nearly 1,700 GIST patients across the two trials, were designed with adequate statistical power to determine whether this doubling of imatinib dose would translate into any clinically meaningful benefits in response rates, duration of disease control, or survival for patients with advanced unresectable or metastatic GIST. The results of these trials, designed in parallel and planned from the outset to be merged into a single meta-analysis database, are remarkably consistent, showing the same level of disease control demonstrated in earlier nonrandomized trials.[86–92] Although no survival difference was observed in either trial between patients receiving these two dose levels, there were somewhat discordant results in terms of the time to disease progression. The North American Sarcoma Intergroup trial demonstrated that the two doses were equivalent in terms of response rates and duration of disease control, as well as overall survival. The EORTC-led study noted a small but statistically significant benefit in favor of the higher-dose arm in progression-free survival, although this did not translate into any advantages in overall survival after patients were offered the option to cross over to the higher dose with progression. In both trials, the higher dose of imatinib was associated with greater incidence of adverse effects and led to higher dose reductions for toxicity. When primary data from these two large trials were pooled in a recent meta-analysis, the benefits in progression-free survival were identified solely in the subset of patients with KIT exon 9 mutations, confirming a prior observation made in the European study,[89] while all other GIST genotypes experienced identical outcomes with either imatinib dose level.[90] This work confirmed earlier observations[80] that patients with metastatic GIST harboring exon 11 *KIT* mutations exhibit improved outcomes compared with other molecular subtypes of GIST.[92] A small subset analysis of the study conducted outside North America suggested that there might be a particularly large impact of higher-dose imatinib to improve outcomes for GIST with exon 9 *KIT* mutations.[89] This requires larger numbers of patients to evaluate more fully, and a meta-analysis linking the data obtained globally from these two trials is being conducted to investigate this more completely.

The optimal duration of imatinib therapy for patients with metastatic GIST is an important question, as single-agent kinase inhibitor therapy does not appear to cure patients with metastatic GIST. Most experts consider kinase inhibition as lifelong therapy for advanced disease, based on studies of patients randomized either to stop or to continue imatinib dosing following disease control, which clearly demonstrate rapid disease progression within months after the imatinib is stopped.[93,94] These clinical data support the hypothesis that continuous and chronic exposure to imatinib is necessary to maintain control over a population of GIST cells that may remain quiescent in the long term as long as aberrant KIT signaling is inhibited. However, if the drug is withdrawn and the uncontrolled KIT activity is allowed to resume, the disease reactivates and progresses. Therefore, for GIST patients who achieve any measure of disease control, continued dosing with imatinib as long as the disease is not progressive appears to be the optimal course of management. However, future studies will be required to assess whether periodic pulse therapy might suppress emergence of multidrug-resistant GIST clones.

It is critical to emphasize the importance of multidisciplinary management in the care of GIST patients. For optimal management of metastatic disease, medical oncologists, surgeons, radiologists, and nuclear medicine imaging experts must all collaborate closely to determine the best course of action for any given patient. This important message has been emphasized in the Task Force Report on GIST Clinical Practice Guidelines of the National Comprehensive Cancer Network.[50] For example, disease that is initially judged as unresectable (or resectable only with unacceptable surgical morbidity) may become amenable to surgical excision after a major response induced by imatinib therapy; this "neoadjuvant" or preoperative use of imatinib for unresectable GIST has been supported for rectal GIST as well as other primary lesions in which function-sparing surgery could not be achieved because of disease size or location.[95] Most centers recommend surgical resection for such patients because it is feared that residual GIST may develop secondary mutations that could result in clinical resistance to imatinib and progression of disease. However, the role of surgery as an adjunct to imatinib therapy for patients for metastatic GIST remains unclear. Nonrandomized surgical series have noted that outcomes for patients who cannot achieve complete resection of all disease following kinase inhibitor therapy are less favorable than others for whom complete surgical excision of all disease is possible.[96] A prospective randomized trial is currently in progress under the auspices of the EORTC to assess rigorously whether aggressive surgical resection of advanced GIST adds any significant benefit to patients beyond the benefits induced by kinase inhibitor systemic therapy.

Resistance to Imatinib

Resistance to imatinib may be primary and manifest as rapid progression of disease despite imatinib dosing, although this appears in fewer than 15% of patients (Table 87.2). Alternatively, clonal evolution of resistant GIST may be detected after a year or more of durable objective response and disease control. Several mechanisms of resistance to imatinib in GIST have been described,[97,98] and these are somewhat similar to the resistance mechanisms that have been demonstrated in CML.[99] It is unclear what role should ideally be played by other modalities, such as surgery, radiofrequency ablation, embolization, or other locoregional approaches, in managing metastatic GIST once imatinib has achieved the optimal effect or after the appearance of limited resistance to imatinib with oligoclonal progression.[100] Certainly, it has been described that many GIST lesions may remain controlled, while limited clonal progression appears as the first sign of resistance to imatinib.[96,98,101] It may be feasible in such patients to resect the resistant clonal growth while maintaining control over the majority of the disease by continuation of imatinib dosing. These strategies will be tested in future trials, as new kinase inhibitors of varying target specificities are used to combat GIST that has become refractory to imatinib.

The mechanism of resistance to imatinib most often seen in GIST is the emergence of new secondary mutations in *cis* within a separate portion of the *KIT* kinase coding sequence.[97,98] It is likely that pre-existing double-mutant tumor cells slowly grow out under the influence of chronic imatinib selection pressure, much like the emergence of antibiotic-resistant strains of bacterial pathogens. In order to address the new challenge of a double-mutant KIT molecular target, new structurally dissimilar kinase inhibitors have been screened for differential activity against these new structural variants of the mutant kinase. In this way, sunitinib malate (previously known as SU11248) was identified as a particularly promising agent in preclinical screening against resistant human GIST cells *in vitro* (G. D. Demetri and J. A. Fletcher, unpublished observations, 2001). Sunitinib is also a very powerful antiangiogenesis agent by virtue of targeting multiple tyrosine kinases for inhibition, including the vascular endothelial growth factor receptors in addition to PDGFR. Phase 1 and 2 clinical trials of sunitinib in GIST patients following failure of imatinib showed that the majority of patients experienced diminution of GIST activity on ^{18}FDG-PET imaging, and a large fraction achieved stability of disease, although only a small minority actually experienced objective "response" by tumor size criteria.[102] Thus, a prospective, randomized, placebo-controlled trial was conducted worldwide to assess rigorously whether this agent could truly provide benefit to patients following therapeutic failure of imatinib. This large trial demonstrated that sunitinib definitely improved the progression-free survival of patients following imatinib failure due to resistance or intolerance.[103] The trial design allowed crossover to active drug from the placebo arm on progression, with the expectation that this would undoubtably confound any overall survival benefit; however, prior to the study being unblinded by successfully demonstrating the benefits of sunitinib, there was also a survival benefit noted at the first planned interim analysis. Based on these data, this agent was approved for treatment of GIST following failure of imatinib by the FDA in January 2006 and soon thereafter by worldwide regulatory authorities; sunitinib was the first kinase inhibitor to prove beneficial to patients after failure of a prior kinase-targeting agent (Table 87.3). This theme was extended to CML later that same year when another kinase inhibitor (dasatinib) was

PRACTICE OF ONCOLOGY

TABLE 87.3

DOSES AND SCHEDULES OF CURRENTLY APPROVED AGENTS IN THE MANAGEMENT OF GASTROINTESTINAL STROMAL TUMORS (GISTs)

Agent	Dose (mg)	Schedule	Duration
METASTATIC AND/OR UNRESECTABLE ADVANCED GIST			
Imatinib (Gleevec)	400 orally	Daily	Lifelong in absence of disease progression
Imatinib	800 orally[a]	Daily	Lifelong in absence of disease progression
Sunitinib	50 orally	Daily × 4 wk, off × 2 wk, then repeat cycle	Lifelong in absence of disease progression
Sunitinib[b]	37.5 orally	Daily continuously	Lifelong in absence of disease progression
ADJUVANT THERAPY FOR RESECTED PRIMARY GIST (NOT YET FDA-APPROVED)			
Imatinib (Gleevec)	400 orally	Daily	1 year, based on current evidence

FDA, U.S. Food and Drug Administration.
[a]Only if lower dose imatinib has failed to control disease; certain data support use of higher-dose imatinib in GISTs with KIT exon 9 mutation as well.
[b]Alternative dosing regimen.

approved in June 2006 as an effective therapeutic option for imatinib-resistant CML patients.

On the basis of improved understanding of the mechanisms of resistance to highly selective kinase inhibitors such as imatinib or more multitargeted kinase inhibitors such as sunitinib, many other new agents are currently in clinical trials for GIST patients. The structure of imatinib was modified as a scaffold to optimize its binding the ATP-binding domain of the BCR-ABL target, yielding a new molecule, nilotinib, with improved pharmacodynamic and clinical inhibitory properties for the CML target. Although nilotinib shows definite evidence of activity against GIST,[104] there has as yet not been sufficiently rigorous data to prove that this agent is superior to imatinib. A randomized phase 3 clinical trial of nilotinib versus a heterogenous control arm failed to show significant benefit for nilotinib, although the study was no doubt flawed by the lack of a single well-defined control arm. An ongoing trial is testing whether nilotinib might be superior in the first-line management of advanced GIST.

Some of the most promising new approaches to overcome resistance to TKIs in GIST include targeting multiple levels of the signal transduction cascade intracellularly by combining agents. This has been done, for example, by combining a kinase inhibitor such as imatinib with an inhibitor of the mTOR downstream signaling partner using the mTOR inhibitor everolimus.[105] Other strategies that are being explored include the inhibition of other pathways critical to the molecular processing of the mutant KIT or PDGFRA oncoproteins, such as the chaperone function of the heat shock protein-90 system. By inhibiting heat shock protein-90, preclinical and early clinical studies have already documented antineoplastic effects on kinase-inhibitor-resistant GIST both *in vitro* and in patients with progressive disease.[106,107]

EXTRAPOLATION OF EMERGING MANAGEMENT PARADIGMS TO EARLY-STAGE GIST

Definitive expert surgery remains the mainstay of treatment for patients with localized, primary GIST. It is important to recognize that surgical resection of advanced GIST should probably be performed first only if there is an acceptably low risk of functional deficit. If a very large GIST were diagnosed in an area that would present a challenge to complete resection (e.g., invading the pancreatic bed), it might be judicious to consider such a lesion unresectable for cure; in such a case, preoperative administration of imatinib could then serve as the initial therapeutic intervention, with follow-up at close intervals to ensure appropriate response to therapy. In this situation, early assessment of therapeutic response by ^{18}FDG-PET scanning could be very valuable to confirm that the patient's disease is indeed exhibiting the desired response to imatinib. This should minimize the risk of disease progression, which might put the patient at risk for further growth and invasion into other vital structures. After maximal response (usually occurring within 4 to 6 months), definitive surgery could be performed. A clinical trial has shown that preoperative imatinib is feasible in patients with resectable or potentially resectable GISTs.[95]

The surgical approach to resection of primary disease must take into account the specific growth and behavior characteristics of GIST. GIST rarely involves the locoregional lymph nodes, and so extensive lymph node exploration or resection is rarely indicated. GIST lesions may exhibit a fragile pseudocapsule, and intraoperative procedures must be optimized to minimize the risk of tumor rupture, which could increase the risk of peritoneal dissemination.[108] The margins of resection from the tumor specimen should be carefully oriented and examined, and biopsy samples from several different areas of the tumor should be evaluated by the surgical pathologist.

The natural history of early-stage, primary GIST has been examined in studies from single-institution referral centers. These are certainly prone to selection bias, and it is clear in this evolving field that many early-stage GIST patients have likely been managed by physicians in multiple specialties (including gastroenterology, general surgery, and others). However, one of the larger series that studied GISTs evaluated 200 patients followed prospectively at the Memorial Sloan-Kettering Cancer Center.[42] Eighty of these patients who had primary disease were managed with complete surgical resection. This group of patients with primary resected GIST demonstrated a 5-year disease-specific survival rate of 54%, which indicates the fact that GIST can recur and ultimately prove to be a life-threatening disease after recurrence. On multivariate analysis, large tumor size (>10 cm) was the only predictive factor that impacted negatively on disease-specific survival.[42]

In an earlier study of "GI leiomyosarcomas" (of which a sizable proportion were very likely to have been true GISTs), investigators at the M. D. Anderson Cancer Center reported that smaller tumor size (<5 cm), complete surgical resection without tumor rupture, and low grade of tumor were significant favorable prognostic factors in their series of 191 patients. The propensity of GIST to recur was confirmed by these data as well, because only 10% of these patients were disease-free with long-term follow-up.[108]

ADJUVANT THERAPY TO IMPROVE OUTCOMES FOR PATIENTS WITH RESECTED EARLY-STAGE GIST

To date, there have only been a limited number of case reports and small series that have investigated the role of adjuvant treatment using conventional cytotoxic modalities such as radiotherapy after surgical resection. As noted earlier in the section "Management of Metastatic, Unresectable, or Recurrent GIST," radiotherapy does not appear to have an important role in the treatment of GIST, with only minimal activity seen at doses that are safe to administer, given the toxicity to small bowel and other intra-abdominal structures. Because cytotoxic chemotherapy is not associated with disease control or objective responses in metastatic GIST, there have only been small series of patients who have received either adjuvant systemic or intraperitoneal chemotherapy, and these data have not clearly suggested any benefits. The standard of care after complete surgical resection of GIST has therefore been observation alone. Because there are now effective treatments for recurrent GIST, it is important that all GIST patients undergo regular surveillance after resection. In this way, any recurrent disease can be detected and treated at the earliest point, with, it is hoped, avoidance of complications that might stem from treatment of large, bulky disease such as intratumoral hemorrhage.

There are now prospective data to support the hypothesis that imatinib therapy offers clinical benefit to patients with larger, fully resected, primary localized GIST lesions at significant risk of relapse. Certainly, because imatinib exhibits such impressive activity in the treatment of advanced disease, it has been reasonable to imagine that this kinase inhibitor therapy might translate into benefit for the treatment of microscopic residual disease after complete surgical resection. However, this required prospective testing and confirmation. Additionally, because adjuvant therapy is generally time-limited, it is possible that the duration of drug exposure may determine the therapeutic impact. Specifically, too short a period of imatinib dosing in the adjuvant postresection setting may not confer optimal benefit to patients.

The activity of imatinib given for a 1-year period to patients with primary localized GIST following resection has been investigated in a large multicenter phase 3 trial sponsored by the National Cancer Institute and conducted under the auspices of the American College of Surgeons Oncology Group (ACOSOG study Z9001); this trial randomized patients with resected GIST (whose lesions were >3 cm) to receive either imatinib or placebo for 1 year.[109] The trial was stopped at an early, preplanned, event-based interim analysis because of the positive outcome: with a median of 15 months follow-up, only approximately 3% of patients in the study who received 1 year of imatinib after surgery exhibited a recurrence of GIST, compared with a 17% recurrence rate in patients who received the placebo. Despite this highly significant impact on prolonging recurrence-free survival, no benefit in overall survival was noted with short follow-up, perhaps because imatinib has such powerful effects at prolonging survival in the setting of advanced recurrent disease as well. More work is certainly needed to assist physicians and patients in using these data to optimize clinical practice. The FDA approved the use of imatinib as adjuvant therapy without any qualification or restriction following resection of primary GIST, but the European Medicines Agency approved adjuvant imatinib only for the subset of GIST patients with primary disease that is judged to be "at significant risk of recurrence" following resection.

Adjuvant imatinib for 1 year's duration certainly has a major impact on disease control rates, but these differences appear to fade with increased rates of recurrence noted on discontinuation of the imatinib dosing. It is certainly possible that a longer duration of adjuvant therapy might further improve clinical outcomes, and this is being tested in other trials that are ongoing in Europe and Scandinavia. A small study of adjuvant therapy for 2 years in Seoul, Korea, has shown much higher rates of disease control than in the 1-year experience, consistent with biological expectations.[110]

Additionally, it will be important to assess whether certain GIST genotypic subsets benefit more—or fail to benefit at all—from adjuvant therapy with imatinib or other drugs. A large analysis of the ACSOG Z9001 randomized trial has confirmed certain differences between the behavior of genetically different forms of GIST: specifically, the KIT exon 11 deletion mutations confer a much higher risk of relapse compared with other mutational subtypes in the placebo arm, but these exon 11 KIT mutants benefit greatly from adjuvant imatinib therapy to ablate this risk.[111] Additionally, although the PDGFRA-driven GIST is often very aggressive in the metastatic setting, the PDGFRA-mutant form of GIST is remarkably indolent with quite low risk for relapse following resection of limited-stage primary disease, as is wild type GIST. Given the potential toxicities and costs of imatinib, as well as the activity of imatinib as therapy for recurrent disease, it is very important that these well-designed adjuvant studies of imatinib be completed and analyzed in the context of molecular subtyping so that patients and physicians can manage GIST with the best knowledge of options, including potential risks and potential benefits for this therapeutic strategy.

SPECIAL CONSIDERATIONS IN GIST

Familial Syndromes of GIST

GIST can be associated with rare familial inheritance patterns in which several members of a kindred have the disease.[112–114] In several of these reported families, mutations in *KIT* loci have been reported. Additional characteristics of affected family members include cutaneous lesions such as hyperpigmentation or skin lesions that appear clinically like urticaria pigmentosa. These skin pigmentation abnormalities are no doubt due to the effect of the overactive mutated KIT RTK on melanocyte growth and development. The mechanisms by which such pigmentation disorders remain focal, rather than disseminated, may provide clues as to why GIST lesions may take decades to appear in these rare familial cases.

Relation of GIST to other Genetic Syndromes Predisposing to Neoplasms

Several syndromes that predispose to the development of neoplasms have been described in association with the occurrence of GIST. One of the more widely known of these is the Carney triad, which encompasses GIST (often multifocal) in addition to pulmonary chondromas and extra-adrenal paragangliomas.[115] A variant of this syndrome has been described with only GIST and familial paragangliomas.[116] Additionally, a linkage between neurofibromatosis type 1 and an increased incidence of GIST has been widely noted.[117,118] Molecular analysis of GIST lesions arising in patients with neurofibromatosis type 1 has documented that these GISTs are characterized by the wild type *KIT* gene.[118] It is unclear whether GISTs that arise in the setting of a genetic predisposition syndrome have the same response to imatinib as sporadically occurring GISTs.

NEW CHALLENGES AND ALTERNATIVE APPROACHES

The remarkable developments that have occurred in GIST research and clinical care in the past several years have only further intensified the research in this field. GIST remains a very informative disease for cancer biologists seeking the root causes of neoplastic transformation and maintenance of the malignant phenotype. Similarly, GIST has served as a paradigm for rationally designed translational therapeutics in a solid tumor. In many ways, GIST research is likely to inform many avenues of fundamental discovery research that can be applied to other more common malignancies.

Although imatinib has proven to be a highly effective treatment for patients with metastatic GIST, it is clear that this single agent is not curing the vast majority of patients with advanced disease. Although imatinib-associated control of GIST can be highly durable and last for years, a subset of patients may be either resistant to or intolerant of treatment with this drug. Very few patients with metastatic disease achieve a complete response, and it is important to seek out the mechanisms by which GIST cells go into a state of "hibernation" while still living under the selection pressure of chronic imatinib dosing. Most importantly, it has become clear that acquired resistance to imatinib will occur with increasing frequency over time, even in patients who benefit initially from outstanding clinical responses to this agent. Unusual patterns of recurrence have been seen in some patients, including development of isolated nodules within preexistent tumors[101] and the progression of individual disease sites, while the overall tumor burden remains stable and under good control. These findings are consistent with clonal evolution of GIST, with the outgrowth of resistant clones of tumor cells. Multidisciplinary approaches to control of these localized sites of imatinib-resistant disease, such as surgical resection, or other local therapies, such as tumor ablation, may have the best chance of offering some additional benefit to patients while continuing to allow control of the imatinib-sensitive tumor clones elsewhere by continuation of imatinib dosing despite limited progression. Molecular analyses of these resistant clones will provide an important opportunity to determine resistance mechanisms, perhaps even on an individual basis. This is an opportunity to meld structural biology and drug development to clinical medicine with unparalleled precision. Several clinical trials are already in progress using next-generation agents that target the KIT receptor via different mechanisms or that target alternate pathways thought to be important to the pathobiology of GIST. Many of these trials take advantage of the power of functional imaging with PET scanning to provide early signals of activity, along with correlative molecular analysis of tumor samples to explain clinical phenomena in a scientifically robust manner.

It is also clear that imatinib, as a therapy that targets the fundamental molecular pathophysiology of GIST and CML, does not have an obvious major impact in several other common diseases, such as carcinomas. This is quite different from the more broad-acting "multitargeted" agent sunitinib, which has activity against both GIST and renal cell carcinoma, presumably via the vascular endothelial growth factor-receptor inhibition of that agent. Studies are ongoing to define whether the PDGFR inhibitory activity of imatinib might prove therapeutically useful in some other ways. For the moment, imatinib has also proven highly effective in the PDGF-driven malignancies known as dermatofibrosarcoma protuberans and in certain myeloproliferative diseases in which aberrant PDGFR signaling drives the neoplastic cells.

In summary, it is clear that the acquisition of a deeper scientific understanding of GIST has led to the development of powerful new therapeutic tools such as imatinib and sunitinib to disable the malignant behavior of GIST cells. It is also clear, however, that new therapies will continue to be needed to improve outcomes for patients with this disease. With improved technology and rational molecular targeting, this translation of science into applied therapeutics should continue to move forward at a very rapid pace, aided by the efforts of collaborating investigators and physicians of multiple specialties around the world.

Selected References

The full list of references for this chapter appears in the online version.

1. Cassier PA, Ducimetière F, Lurkin A, et al. A prospective epidemiological study of new incident GISTs during two consecutive years in Rhône Alpes region: incidence and molecular distribution of GIST in a European region. *Br J Cancer* 2010;103(2):165–170.
13. Kindblom LG, Remotti HE, Aldenborg F, et al. Gastrointestinal pacemaker cell tumor (GIPACT): gastrointestinal stromal tumors show phenotypic characteristics of the interstitial cells of Cajal. *Am J Pathol* 1998;152:1259.
19. Corless CL, McGreevey L, Haley A, et al. KIT mutations are common in incidental gastrointestinal stromal tumors one centimeter or less in size. *Am J Pathol* 2002;160:1567.
20. Hirota S, Isozaki K, Moriyama Y, et al. Gain-of-function mutations of c-kit in human gastrointestinal stromal tumors. *Science* 1998;279:577.
25. Nishida T, Hirota S, Taniguchi M, et al. Familial gastrointestinal stromal tumours with germline mutation of the *KIT* gene. *Nat Genet* 1998;19:323.
29. Chi P, Chen Y, Zhang L, et al. ETV1 is a lineage survival factor that cooperates with KIT in gastrointestinal stromal tumours. *Nature* 2010;467:849.
30. Rubin BP, Singer S, Tsao C, et al. KIT activation is a ubiquitous feature of gastrointestinal stromal tumors. *Cancer Res* 2001;61:8118.
31. Lux ML, Rubin BP, Biase TL, et al. KIT extracellular and kinase domain mutations in gastrointestinal stromal tumors. *Am J Pathol* 2000;156:791.
34. Gajiwala KS, Wu JC, Christensen J, Deshmukh GD, et al. KIT kinase mutants show unique mechanisms of drug resistance to imatinib and sunitinib in gastrointestinal stromal tumor patients. *Proc Natl Acad Sci U S A* 2009;106(5):1542.
35. Heinrich MC, Corless CL, Duensing A, et al. PDGFRA activating mutations in gastrointestinal stromal tumors. *Science* 2003;299:708.
38. Janeway KA, Kim S, Lodish M, et al. Succinate dehydrogenase in KIT/PDGFRA wild-type gastrointestinal stromal tumors. *J Clin Oncol* 2010;28:15s (suppl; abstr 10008).
39. Fletcher CD, Berman JJ, Corless C, et al. Diagnosis of gastrointestinal stromal tumors: a consensus approach. *Hum Pathol* 2002;33:459.
41. Nilsson B, Bümming P, Meis-Kindblom JM, et al. Gastrointestinal stromal tumors: the incidence, prevalence, clinical course, and prognostication in the preimatinib mesylate era—a population-based study in western Sweden. 2005;103(4):821–829.
42. DeMatteo RP, Lewis JJ, Leung D, et al. Two hundred gastrointestinal stromal tumors: recurrence patterns and prognostic factors for survival. *Ann Surg* 2002;231:51.
47. Dei Tos AP, Rossi S, Flanagan A, et al. The diagnostic utility of DOG-1 in KIT-negative GIST. *J Clin Oncol* 2008;26 (May 20 suppl; abstr 10551).
50. Demetri GD, von Mehren M, Antonescu C, et al. NCCN task force report: Update on the management of patients with Gastrointestinal Stromal Tumors. *J Natl Compr Canc Netw* 2010;8:S-1.
51. Miettinen M, Lasota J. Gastrointestinal stromal tumors: pathology and prognosis at different sites. Sem Diagn Pathol 2006;23:70.
52. Gold JS, Gonen M, Gutierrez A, et al. Development and validation of a prognostic nomogram for recurrence-free survival after complete surgical resection of localised primary gastrointestinal stromal tumour: a retrospective analysis. *Lancet Oncol* 2009;10:1045.
56. Martin J, Poveda A, Llombart-Bosch A, et al. Deletions affecting codons 557-558 of the c-KIT gene indicate a poor prognosis in patients with completely resected gastrointestinal stromal tumors: a study by the Spanish Group for Sarcoma Research (GEIS). *J Clin Oncol* 2005;23(25):6190.
57. Corless CL, Ballman KV, Antonescu C, et al. Relation of tumor pathologic and molecular features to outcome after surgical resection of localized primary gastrointestinal stromal tumor (GIST): Results of the intergroup phase III trial ACOSOG Z9001. *J Clin Oncol* 28;15s:10006.
58. Choi H, Charnsangavej C, Faria SC, et al. Correlation of Computed Tomography and Positron Emission Tomography in Patients With Metastatic Gastrointestinal Stromal Tumor Treated at a Single Institution With Imatinib Mesylate: Proposal of New Computed Tomography Response Criteria. *J Clin Oncol* 2007;25(13):1753.
61. Demetri GD, von Mehren M, Blanke CD, et al. Efficacy and safety of imatinib mesylate in advanced gastrointestinal stromal tumors. *N Engl J Med* 2002;347:472.
69. Druker BJ, Tamura S, Buchdunger E, et al. Effects of a selective inhibitor of the Abl tyrosine kinase on the growth of Bcr-Abl positive cells. *Nat Med* 1996;2:561.
72. Heinrich MC, Griffith DJ, Druker BJ, et al. Inhibition of c-KIT receptor tyrosine kinase activity by STI 571, a selective tyrosine kinase inhibitor. *Blood* 2000;96:925.
73. Tuveson DA, Willis NA, Jacks T, et al. STI571 inactivation of the gastrointestinal stromal tumor c-KIT oncoprotein: biological and clinical implications. *Oncogene* 2001;20:5054.
74. Joensuu H, Roberts PJ, Sarlomo-Rikala M, et al. Effect of the tyrosine kinase inhibitor STI571 in a patient with a metastatic gastrointestinal stromal tumor. *N Engl J Med* 2001;344:1052.
75. van Oosterom AT, Judson I, Verweij J, et al. European Organization for Research and Treatment of Cancer soft tissue and bone sarcoma group. Safety and efficacy of imatinib (STI571) in metastatic gastrointestinal stromal tumours: a phase I study. *Lancet* 2001;358:1421.
76. Verweij J, van Oosterom A, Blay JY, et al. Imatinib mesylate is an active agent for gastrointestinal stromal tumors but does not yield responses in other soft-tissue sarcomas that are unselected for a molecular target. *Eur J Cancer* 2003;39:2006.
79. McArthur GA, Demetri GD, van Oosterom A, et al. Molecular and clinical analysis of locally advanced dermatofibrosarcoma protuberans treated with imatinib: Imatinib Target Exploration Consortium Study B2225. *J Clin Oncol* 2005;23(4):866.
80. Heinrich MC, Corless CL, Demetri GD, et al. Kinase mutations and imatinib response in patients with metastatic gastrointestinal stromal tumor. *J Clin Oncol* 2003;21:4342.
82. Force T, Krause DS, Van Etten RA. Molecular mechanisms of cardiotoxicity of tyrosine kinase inhibition. *Nat Rev Cancer* 2007;7(5):332.
85. Demetri GD, Wang Y, Wehrle E, et al. Imatinib Plasma Levels Are Correlated With Clinical Benefit in Patients With Unresectable/Metastatic Gastrointestinal Stromal Tumors (GIST). *J Clin Oncol* 2009:27(19):3141.
86. Blanke CD, Rankin C, Demetri GD, et al. Phase III randomized, intergroup trial assessing imatinib mesylate at two dose levels in patients with unresectable or metastatic gastrointestinal stromal tumors expressing the kit receptor tyrosine kinase: S0033. *J Clin Oncol* 2008;26(4):626.
87. Verweij J, Casali PG, Zalcberg J, et al. Progression-free survival in gastrointestinal stromal tumours with high-dose imatinib: randomised trial. *Lancet* 2004;364(9440):1127.
88. Zalcberg JR, Verweij J, Casali PG, et al. Outcome of patients with advanced gastro-intestinal stromal tumours crossing over to a daily imatinib dose of 800 mg after progression on 400 mg. *Eur J Cancer* 2005;41(12):1751.
90. Gastrointestinal Stromal Tumor Meta-Analysis Group. Comparison of two doses of imatinib for the treatment of unresectable or metastatic

gastrointestinal stromal tumors: a meta-analysis of 1640 patients. *J Clin Oncol* 2010;28:1247.

92. Heinrich MC, Owzar K, Corless CL, et al. Correlation of kinase genotype and clinical outcome in the North American Intergroup Phase III Trial of imatinib mesylate for treatment of advanced gastrointestinal stromal tumor: CALGB 150105 Study by Cancer and Leukemia Group B and Southwest Oncology Group. *J Clin Oncol* 2008;26(33):5360.
94. Le Cesne A, Ray-Coquard I, Bui BN, et al. Discontinuation of imatinib in patients with advanced gastrointestinal stromal tumours after 3 years of treatment: an open-label multicentre randomised phase 3 trial. *Lancet Oncology* 2010;11(10):942.
95. Eisenberg BL, Harris J, Blanke CD, et al. Phase II trial of neoadjuvant/adjuvant imatinib mesylate (IM) for advanced primary and metastatic/recurrent operable gastrointestinal stromal tumor (GIST): Early results of RTOG 0132/ACRIN 6665. *J Surg Oncol* 2009:99(1):42.
96. Raut CP, Posner M, Desai J, et al. Surgical management of advanced gastrointestinal stromal tumors after treatment with targeted systemic therapy using kinase inhibitors. *J Clin Oncol* 2006;24(15):2325.
97. Heinrich MC, Corless CL, Blanke CD. et al. Molecular correlates of imatinib resistance in gastrointestinal stromal tumors. *J Clin Oncol* 2006;24(29):4764.
98. Desai J, Shankar S, Heinrich MC, et al. Clonal evolution of resistance to imatinib in patients with metastatic gastrointestinal stromal tumors. *Clin Cancer Res* 2007;13(18):5398.
103. Demetri GD, van Oosterom AT, Garrett CR, et al. Efficacy and safety of sunitinib in patients with advanced gastrointestinal stromal tumour after failure of imatinib: a randomised controlled trial. *Lancet* 2006;368(9544):1329.
104. Demetri GD, Casali PG, Blay J-Y, et al. A Phase I Study of Single-agent Nilotinib (AMN107) or in Combination with Imatinib in Patients with Imatinib-Resistant Gastrointestinal Stromal Tumors. *Clin Cancer Res* 2009:15(18):5910.
105. Schöffski P, Reichardt P, Blay J, et al. A phase I–II study of everolimus (RAD001) in combination with imatinib in patients with imatinib-resistant gastrointestinal stromal tumors. *Ann Oncol* 2010;21(10):1990.
106. Bauer S, Yu LK, Demetri GD, Fletcher JA. Heat shock protein 90 inhibition in imatinib-resistant gastrointestinal stromal tumor. *Cancer Res* 2006;66(18):9153.
109. DeMatteo RP, Ballman KV, Antonescu CR, et al. Placebo-controlled randomized trial of adjuvant imatinib mesylate following the resection of localized, primary gastrointestinal stromal tumor (GIST). *Lancet* 2009:373(9669):1097–1104.
112. Nishida T, Hirota S, Taniguchi M, et al. Familial gastrointestinal stromal tumours with germline mutation of the *KIT* gene. *Nat Genet* 1998; 19:323.
115. Carney JA. Gastric stromal sarcoma, pulmonary chondroma, and extra-adrenal paraganglioma (Carney triad): natural history, adrenocortical component, and possible familial occurrence. *Mayo Clin Proc* 1999;74:543.

CHAPTER 88 MOLECULAR BIOLOGY OF COLORECTAL CANCER

RAMESH A. SHIVDASANI

The cumulative lifetime risk of developing colorectal cancer (CRC) in the United States is about 6%, and this increases about fourfold in persons with a history of CRC in first- or second-degree relatives. Although fewer than 5% of cases occur in patients with uncommon inherited predisposition syndromes and most CRCs are accordingly considered to be sporadic, 20% to 30% of cases might have a familial basis despite absence of a known germline defect. Characteristic somatic mutations, epigenetic alterations, and defects in DNA repair or chromosomal stability promote disease progression and malignant behaviors. Well-characterized predisposing conditions and somatic mutations profoundly inform the molecular understanding of CRC and serve as a paradigm for the genetic basis of cancer.

THE ADENOMA–CARCINOMA SEQUENCE AND MULTISTEP MODELS OF COLORECTAL TUMORIGENESIS

The genetic basis of CRC is best appreciated in light of the adenoma–carcinoma sequence and the premise that CRCs arise from benign precursor polyps. Most hyperplastic polyps harbor little potential for invasive cancer, although those of the sessile serrated variety may represent precursors of cancers with microsatellite instability.[1,2] By contrast, adenomatous polyps are known to be the important precursor lesions, with those larger than 1 cm carrying an estimated 15% risk of progression to adenocarcinoma over 10 years; endoscopic removal of such adenomas reduces CRC incidence and mortality.[3] Adenomas are marked by epithelial overgrowth, dysplasia, and abnormal differentiation, sometimes with small foci of invasive cells; residual areas of benign adenomatous tissue are frequently identified in surgical CRC specimens.

The prevalence of adenomas in the United States, estimated at 25% by age 50 and up to 50% by age 70,[4] dwarfs the 6% cumulative lifetime risk of CRC. This is because few adenomas progresses to invasive cancer, in a process that unfolds over one to three decades.[5] Alterations in three classes of genes drive tumors: oncogenes, tumor suppressor genes, and genes that prevent DNA damage. Although oncogenic events may have a genetic (mutational) or epigenetic basis, at present more is known about the somatic mutations that fuel step-wise increases in malignant potential.[6] The order of mutations can vary and most tumors do not carry every known genetic alteration. Nevertheless, certain mutations appear at appreciable frequency in different tumor stages, allowing assignment of a typical sequence (Fig. 88.1). Considered in light of the adenoma–carcinoma sequence, these mutations support the idea of cancer as a multifaceted disease that breaches natural checks on cell survival, growth, and invasion.[7] Individual mutations rarely correlate precisely with a particular feature, such as survival or angiogenesis, and common mutations often impinge on multiple cell functions. Nevertheless, the combination of somatic mutations defines cancer subtypes, their unique properties, and sensitivity to certain therapies. Specific mutations illuminate the normal controls on colonic epithelium, reveal key cellular pathways as rational targets for therapy, and may guide future prevention strategies. Furthermore, knowledge of the mutations classifies CRC into subgroups with distinctive features. For example, *KRAS* or *BRAF* gene mutations (together accounting for nearly half of all U.S. cases) predict for lack of response to epidermal growth factor receptor (EGFR) antibodies.[8,9] *KRAS* mutation status is now used to dictate EGFR antibody therapy in CRC, a practice likely to expand as the prognostic and predictive value of additional molecular features becomes apparent.

Global Events in Colorectal Cancer

In light of the central importance of somatic mutations, cellular conditions that elevate mutation rates might enable or accelerate tumor progression. Over 80% of CRCs display widespread chromosomal gains and losses, phenomena that favor amplification of oncogenes and loss of tumor suppressors.[10] Chromosomal segregation defects may account for this background of chromosomal instability (CIN), as illustrated by the segregation factor Bub1 in mice,[11] but few specific gene defects are implicated with confidence. The remaining fraction of CRCs appears euploid at the level of whole chromosomes but may carry thousands of point mutations, small deletions, and insertions near nucleotide repeat tracts, a defect known as microsatellite instability (MSI).[12] Molecular determinants of progression in MSI+ adenomas differ from those associated with CIN; for example, *BRAF V600E* mutations occur more commonly in MSI+ serrated adenomas than in other subtypes.[13] Hypermutability with CIN or MSI results in many inconsequential or detrimental "passenger" mutations, an important consideration that focuses attention on "driver" changes. Such changes are distinguished by their appearance in a significant proportion of tumor specimens and, ideally, by laboratory demonstration of their contribution toward malignancy.

Epigenetic mechanisms are probably as significant as mutations in cancer but also less well understood. Various covalent histone modifications and methylation of cytosine residues in DNA represent the principal means for gene regulation, the latter far better characterized in CRC than the former. The 5′-CpG-3′ dinucleotide pairs are particular targets for

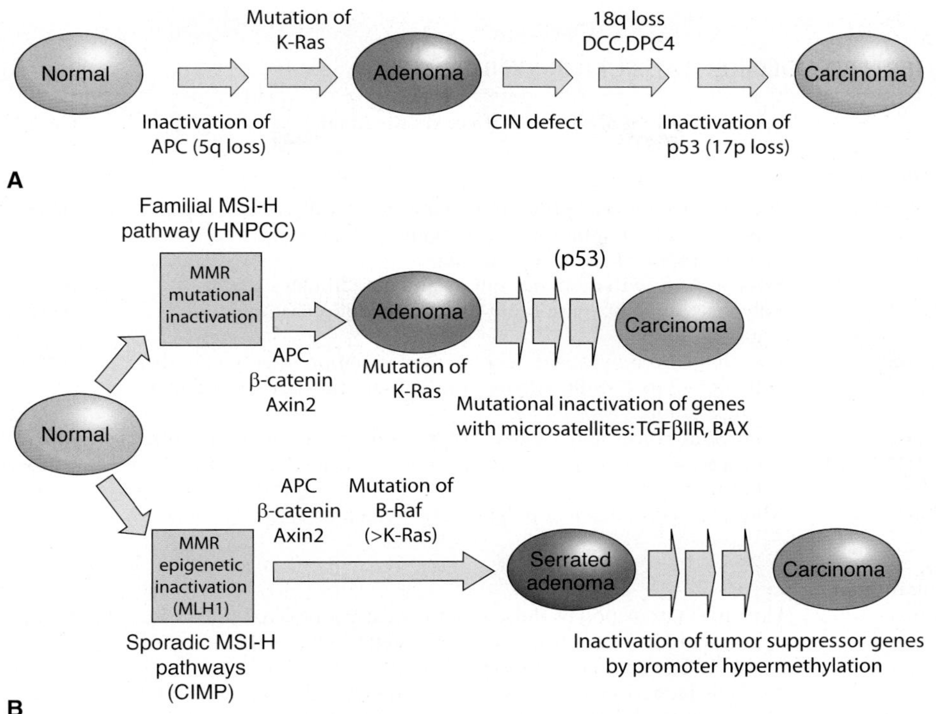

FIGURE 88.1 Genetic pathways to colorectal carcinoma. All colorectal cancers (CRCs) arise within benign adenomatous precursors, fueled by mutations that serially enhance malignant behavior. Mutations that activate the Wnt signaling pathway seem to be necessary initiating events, following which two possible courses contribute to accumulation of additional mutations. **A**: Chromosomal instability is a feature of up to 80% of CRCs and is commonly associated with activating *KRAS* point mutations and loss of regions that encompass *P53* and other tumor suppressors on 18q and 17p, often but not necessarily in that order. **B**: About 20% of CRCs are euploid but defective in DNA mismatch repair (MMR), resulting in high microsatellite instability (MSI-Hi). MMR defects may develop sporadically, associated with CpG island methylation (CIMP), or as a result of familial predisposition in hereditary nonpolyposis colorectal cancer (HNPCC). Mutations accumulate in the *KRAS* or *BRAF* oncogenes, *p53* tumor suppressor, and in microsatellite-containing genes vulnerable to MMR defects, such as *TGFβIIR*. Epigenetic inactivation of the MMR gene *MLH1* and activating *BRAF* point mutations are especially common in serrated adenomas, which progress in part through silencing of tumor suppressor genes by promoter hypermethylation. Progression from adenoma to CRC takes years to decades, a process that accelerates in the presence of MMR defects.

methylation in localized areas of high CpG content in promoters, where abundant methylation silences adjacent genes. Compared to normal tissue, CRCs show 8% to 15% lower total DNA methylation,[14] even in colorectal adenomas.[15] Reduced pericentromeric methylation might decrease the fidelity of chromosomal segregation, and altered methylation and loss of imprinting at the *IGF2* locus are associated with increased CRC risk,[16] suggesting broad effects of global hypomethylation on cell growth. However, because some animal models show increased tumor susceptibility with global hypomethylation,[17] whereas Apc^{Min} mice that lack or overexpress the *de novo* DNA methyltransferase DNMT3B show reduced or increased progression of small adenomas, respectively,[18,19] its precise significance is unclear. Against the background of genomewide hypomethylation, a subset of CRCs show coordinate hypermethylation of characteristic CpG-rich promoter islands, conferring the CpG island methylator phenotype (CIMP), with transcriptional attenuation of associated genes, including tumor suppressors such as *HIC1* and the secreted Wnt-inhibiting secreted Frizzled-related proteins (sFRPs).[20,21] Adenomatous precursors of CIMP cancers show the distinctive histology of sessile serrated adenomas, with dysplasia within an architectural pattern typical of hyperplastic polyps.

There are few variations to the adenoma–carcinoma sequence. A tenfold elevated risk of CRC in patients with longstanding inflammatory bowel disease, especially ulcerative colitis (UC),[22] probably reflects heightened mutation and tumorigenesis with repeated cycles of mucosal injury and repair. Such cancers arise not only from typical polyps but also within flat adenomatous plaques and nonadenomatous areas of dysplasia. A *p53* gene mutation tends to occur earlier in the cancer sequence,[23] and *APC* gene inactivation is less common than in sporadic CRC. Conversely, even in the absence of CIMP, methylation of the $p16^{INK4a}$ tumor suppressor gene, which is rare in sporadic CRC, is common in UC-associated cancers.[24]

EARLY EVENTS AND CRITICAL PATHWAYS IN COLORECTAL TUMORIGENESIS HIGHLIGHTED BY INHERITED SYNDROMES OF INCREASED CANCER RISK

Two uncommon but highly penetrant inherited syndromes, familial adenomatous polyposis (FAP) and hereditary nonpolyposis colorectal cancer (HNPCC), together account for about 5% of all CRC cases. Other rare syndromes, familial juvenile polyposis (FJP), Peutz-Jeghers syndrome (PJS), and Cowden disease, each occurring in fewer than 1 in 200,000

TABLE 88.1

GENETICS OF INHERITED COLORECTAL TUMOR SYNDROMES

Syndrome	Features Commonly Seen in Affected Individuals	Gene Defect
Syndromes with adenomatous polyps		
Familial adenomatous polyposis (FAP)	Multiple adenomas (>100) and colorectal carcinomas; duodenal polyps and carcinomas; gastric fundus polyps; congenital hypertrophy of retinal epithelium	*APC* (>90%)
Gardner syndrome	Same as FAP, with desmoid tumors and mandibular osteomas	*APC*
Turcot syndrome	Polyposis and CRC with brain tumors (medulloblastoma, glioblastoma)	*APC, MLH1*
Attenuated adenomatous polyposis (AAPC)	Less than 100 polyps, although marked variation in polyp number (from ~5 to >1,000 polyps) seen in mutation carriers within a single family	*APC* (5′ mutations)
Hereditary nonpolyposis colorectal cancer (HNPCC)	Colorectal cancer with modest polyposis; high risk of endometrial cancer; some risk of ovarian, gastric, urothelial, hepatobiliary, and brain cancers	*MSH2, MLH1, MSH6* (together >90%), may be *PMS2*
MYH-associated polyposis (MAP)	Multiple gastrointestinal polyps, autosomal recessive	*MYH*
Syndromes with hamartomatous polyps		
Peutz-Jeghers syndrome	Hamartomatous polyps throughout the gastrointestinal (GI) tract; mucocutaneous pigmentation; estimated 9- to 13-fold increased risk of GI and non-GI cancers	*STK11* (30%–70%)
Cowden disease	Multiple hamartomas involving breast, thyroid, skin, brain, and GI tract; increased risk of breast, uterus, thyroid, and some GI cancers.	*PTEN* (85%)
Juvenile polyposis syndrome	Multiple hamartomas in youth, predominantly in colon and stomach; variable increase in colorectal and stomach cancer risk; facial changes	*BMPR1A* (25%), *SMAD4* (15%), *ENG*

births, also elevate the risk of CRC, and some genes responsible for these autosomal dominant disorders have been identified (Table 88.1). Elucidation of the corresponding molecular defects serves not only in accurate molecular diagnosis, risk assessment, and disease prevention in affected families but also informs understanding of the considerably larger proportion of sporadic cases.

Familial Adenomatous Polyposis and the Central Importance of Wnt Signaling

In FAP, an autosomal dominant monogenic disorder that underlies about 0.5% of all CRCs, individuals develop hundreds to thousands of colonic polyps by their teens or early 20s, and the lifetime risk of progression to invasive cancer approaches 100%, with cancer diagnosed at a median age of 39. Extraintestinal manifestations include duodenal and gastric adenomas; congenital hypertrophy of the retinal pigmented epithelium; osteomas and mesenteric desmoid tumors in the Gardner syndrome variant[25]; and less commonly, brain tumors in the Turcot syndrome variant,[26] cutaneous cysts, thyroid tumors, and adrenal adenomas. Although most features are benign, rare patients develop hepatoblastoma or thyroid cancer. Reflecting the similar regulation of small bowel and colonic epithelia, patients have a 5% to 10% risk of developing duodenal or ampullary adenocarcinoma, mandating close endoscopic monitoring of the upper intestine after prophylactic colectomy.[27]

The gene affected by mutations in this disorder, adenomatous polyposis coli (*APC*) on chromosome 5q21, encodes a 2842-residue protein. Germline mutations occur throughout the locus but cluster in the 5′ half and exon 15,[28] mostly introducing stop codons or frame shifts that truncate the protein. Although a few mutations correlate with phenotypic severity or specific extraintestinal manifestations, identical mutations can produce different clinical features. In the attenuated APC (AAPC) variant, disease onset is delayed, individuals develop fewer colonic polyps or cancers, and mutations cluster in the extreme 5′ or 3′ ends of *APC* exons.[29] The *I1307K* allele, present in the Ashkenazi Jewish population, barely doubles the lifetime risk of CRC and does not affect APC protein function but replaces an $(A)_3T(A)_4$ coding sequence with an extended $(A)_8$ tract that is occasionally targeted for nearby truncating mutations.[30] Identification of an *APC* mutation in a proband allows reliable testing of family members. Carriers should have screening colonoscopy annually after age 10, gastroduodenoscopy after age 25, and treatment with nonsteroidal anti-inflammatory drugs to reduce the risk of progression to cancer.[31] Prophylactic colectomy is highly recommended, with subsequent monitoring of the rectal stump and other at-risk tissues.

The larger significance of the *APC* gene derives from its somatic inactivation in about 80% of sporadic CRCs and early colorectal adenomas.[32] Indeed, somatic *APC* mutations are found in tiny adenomas, containing few dysplastic glands. Attesting to the tumor suppressor function, tumors arising sporadically or in FAP patients show biallelic *APC* gene inactivation and loss of heterozygosity, with one copy usually lost by deletion. Except for the small bowel, *APC* mutations are rare in other cancers, including those in other digestive organs. *APC* gene inactivation is a rate-limiting step for development of adenomas, and its designation as a gatekeeper gene in CRC is now well supported by knowledge of its cellular functions. *APC* encodes several functional domains and proteins truncated by mutation that could in principle interfere with a wide range of cellular activities. Disruption of its known role in chromosome segregation might, for example, contribute to CIN.[33] However, attention on *APC* centers rightfully on its control of the Wnt signaling pathway. About half the sporadic

CRCs with intact *APC* function carry activating point mutations in the *CTNNB1* gene,[34,35] which encodes β-catenin, a transcriptional effector of Wnt signaling. Moreover, acute loss of APC function in mice produces intestinal defects identical to those observed upon Wnt pathway activation.[36]

The Wnt glycoproteins are secreted morphogens with diverse functions in development and homeostasis. In the absence of Wnt signaling, cells use a complex containing APC, Axin2, and other cytoplasmic proteins to promote phosphorylation, by casein kinase I and glycogen synthase kinase (GSK)-3β, of several conserved serine and threonine residues in the β-catenin N-terminus, thereby targeting β-catenin for ubiquitin-mediated proteasomal degradation.[37] When Wnt ligands bind a surface protein complex that contains a member of the Frizzled protein family and the obligate coreceptor LRP5/6, they antagonize APC/Axin2 activity and thereby stabilize β-catenin. *CTNNB1* mutations in CRC alter consensus residues for N-terminal phosphorylation and render the mutant protein resistant to degradation. Thus, inactivating *APC* or activating *CTNNB1* mutations, two alternative lesions in CRC, have the same effect: constitutive, Wnt-independent stabilization of β-catenin (Fig. 88.2). Accumulated β-catenin translocates to the cell nucleus, where it acts as a transcriptional coactivator for the T-cell factor/lymphoid enhancer factor (TCF/LEF) family of transcription factors. Nuclear β-catenin provides TCF/LEF proteins with an activating partner, resulting in transcription of target genes.[38] Of the four known TCF/LEF proteins, TCF4 is the most important in normal bowel epithelium and CRC.[34,39] Among the many components of the Wnt signaling cascade, rare *AXIN2* mutations of uncertain significance are reported in MSI+ cases,[40] but mutations in CRC are otherwise found only in *APC* and *CTNNB1*.

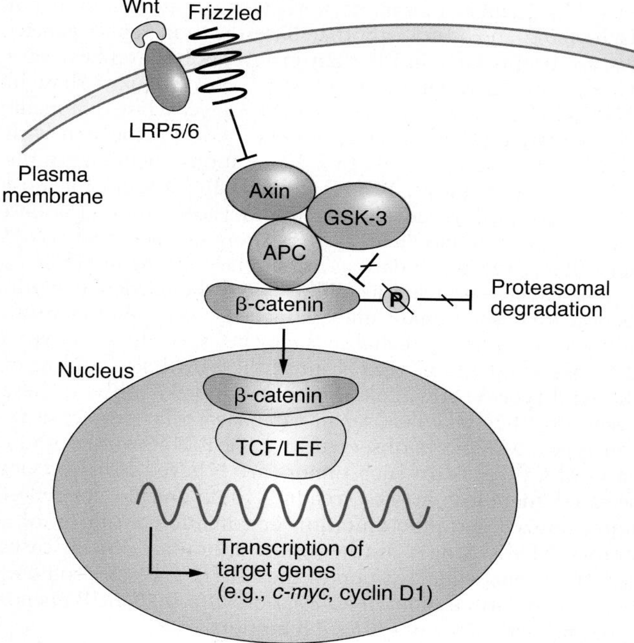

FIGURE 88.2 Outline of Wnt signaling, the key driver pathway in colorectal cancer. Members of the Wnt family of glycoprotein morphogens bind the cell surface co-receptors Frizzled and LRP5/6. In the absence of Wnt binding, normal cells use a complex containing adenomatous polyposis coli (APC), Axin, and other cytoplasmic proteins to promote glycogen synthase kinase (GSK)-3β-mediated phosphorylation of the β-catenin N-terminus, which targets β-catenin for proteasomal degradation (from ref. 37.). Binding of a Wnt ligand to Frizzled and its obligate coreceptor LRP5/6 antagonizes the APC/Axin destruction complex, stabilizing β-catenin (CTNNB1), which moves into the nucleus and coactivates genes through T-cell factor/lymphoid enhancer factor (TCF/LEF) transcription factors. Either of the two principal gatekeeper events in colorectal cancer, inactivating *APC* or activating *CTNNB1* mutations, results in constitutive, Wnt-independent stabilization of β-catenin and unregulated activation of the cognate transcriptional program. Wnt signaling in the intestine is normally confined to crypt progenitors, and its aberrant activation by *APC* or *CTNNB1* mutations confers a permanent cryptlike state that favors cell replication.

Although Wnt ligands signal in many tissues, intestinal homeostasis is particularly dependent on this pathway. Wnt signaling in the intestine is confined to proliferative crypt stem and progenitor cells. In mice, cycling crypt cells that express the surface marker LGR5 are far more susceptible to Wnt-induced transformation than their differentiated progeny, implying that CRC arises in a primitive stem or progenitor cell and not in mature descendants.[41] Moreover, the Wnt-dependent transcriptional program in CRC cell lines overlaps materially with that in intestinal crypts.[42] Wnt signaling is hence necessary for intestinal epithelial self-renewal, and constitutive, ligand-independent activation imposed by *APC* or *CTNNB1* mutations induces and sustains adenomas. Among the diverse transcriptional targets of the TCF-β-catenin complex identified to date, *CMYC* seems especially important because its absence in mice abrogates the effects of acute APC loss in the intestine.[43,44] Mice that lack CD44, another prominent Wnt-pathway target, develop fewer adenomas in an APC-deficient background.[45] Gene expression profiling offers an expanded list of over 100 candidate transcriptional targets,[42,46] but the individual significance of each will take many years to investigate.

Hereditary Nonpolyposis Colorectal Cancer and the Role of DNA Mismatch Repair

HNPCC, an autosomal dominant disorder that confers a nearly 80% lifetime risk of developing CRC, usually before age 50, is estimated to account for 2% to 4% of all CRC cases in the United States.[47] Affected individuals do not lack intestinal polyps (nearly all CRCs, syndromic or sporadic, arise within adenomatous precursors) but develop many fewer colonic polyps than patients with FAP, a condition that must be excluded to satisfy criteria for diagnosis of HNPCC (Table 88.2).[48] Cancers tend to develop in the ascending colon, and patients are further predisposed to develop tumors of the endometrium, small intestine, stomach, upper urothelium, ovary, biliary tract, and brain, a spectrum reflected in the revised Amsterdam II criteria (Table 88.2). The lifetime risk of endometrial cancer, in particular, is 35% to 50% and that of urologic and ovarian cancers is 7% to 8%.[49] Cancers in HNPCC show pronounced variation in the lengths of microsatellite DNA sequences in tumors compared with unaffected tissues. Cancers showing such MSI at two or more among a panel of five mono- and dinucleotide tracts (BAT26, BAT25, D5S346, D2S123, and D17S250) carry the MSI-Hi designation. Most other CRCs harbor CIN and show microsatellite stability (MSS) or, in a small fraction, instability at only one of the five test tracts (MSI-Lo), a finding of uncertain significance.

HNPCC results from germline mutations in any of several genes that enable DNA mismatch repair (MMR), a proofreading process that corrects base-pair mismatches and short insertions and deletions in the normal course of DNA replication. MMR in mammalian cells is mediated by homologs of bacterial and yeast repair proteins: MutS homologs (MSH) 1-6, MutL homologs (MLH) 1-3, and PMS1 and PMS2. MLH1 and PMS2 are recruited to sites of DNA mismatch as a MutLα complex and in turn recruit MSH2-MSH6 (MutSα) or MSH2-MSH3 (MutSβ) heterodimers to sites of 1-bp or 2- to 4-bp errors, respectively. These proteins excise the strand that

TABLE 88.2

CRITERIA FOR CLINICAL DIAGNOSIS OF HEREDITARY NONPOLYPOSIS COLORECTAL CANCER

A. *Revised Amsterdam criteria (clinical diagnosis)*
   1. Three or more family members with histologically verified hereditary nonpolyposis colorectal cancer (HNPCC)-related cancers, one of whom is a first degree relative of the other two.
   2. Two successive affected generations.
   3. One or more of the HNPCC-related cancers diagnosed before age 50.
   4. Exclusion of Familial adenomatous polyposis (FAP).

B. *Revised Bethesda guidelines (criteria to prompt MSI testing of tumors)*
   1. Diagnosis of colorectal cancer before age 50.
   2. Synchronous or metachronous presence of CRC or other HNPCC-associated cancer.
   3. CRC diagnosed before age 60 with histopathologic features associated with MSI-Hi.
   4. CRC in at least one first-degree relative with an HNPCC-related tumor, with one of the cancers diagnosed before age 50.
   5. CRC in 2 or more first-degree relatives with HNPCC-related tumors, regardless of age.

C. *Spectrum of sites for HNPCC-related cancers*

Colon and rectum, endometrium, stomach, ovary, pancreas, ureter and renal pelvis, biliary tract, small intestine, brain, sebaceous gland adenomas, and keratoacanthomas.

carries the mismatch, and they resynthesize and ligate the repaired DNA. Germline mutations in *MSH2*, *MLH1*, and *MSH6* together explain more than 90% of kindreds[50,51]; the significance of mutations in other canonical MMR pathway genes, *PMS1* and *PMS2*, is less certain.[52]

MSI-Hi colorectal cancers commonly show lymphocytic infiltrates, mucinous signet-ring differentiation, and a medullary growth pattern; Bethesda guidelines (Table 88.2) combine clinical and phenotypic features to facilitate diagnosis of HNPCC.[53] When these criteria are met, tumor DNA should either be tested for MSI in a simple, PCR-based assay or by immunohistochemistry for absence of the commonly implicated MLH1, MSH2, and MSH6 proteins.[54] A positive result should prompt genetic testing for *MLH1*, *MSH2*, or *MSH6* mutations; the personal and family history can predict the probability of identifying mutations.[55] Genetic testing identifies the mutant allele and carriers, allowing targeting of a recommendation for biannual colonoscopic screening between the ages of 20 and 40, with annual screening thereafter. Women should undergo annual endometrial evaluation soon after age 25, and carriers should consider prophylactic subtotal colectomy, hysterectomy, and oophorectomy.

In incipient cancers, random events first disrupt function of the wild type allele of a mutant MMR gene, and the resulting "mutator phenotype" induces brisk accumulation of DNA replication errors.[50] Consequently, adenomas progress into carcinomas over 3 to 5 years instead of two or more decades.[56] Paradoxically, the prognosis for patients with MSI-Hi colorectal cancers is better than for those with MSS disease, perhaps because many resulting somatic mutations are disadvantageous. Cancer develops, of course, because some mutations activate oncogenes or inactivate tumor suppressor genes. One frequently inactivated tumor suppressor gene in MSI-Hi colorectal cancers, *TGFβRII*, encodes the type II transforming growth factor-beta (TGF-β) receptor and contains a vulnerable mononucleotide tract in the coding sequence.[57] TGF-β inhibits proliferation of many normal epithelial cells, including intestinal cells, and biallelic *TGFβRII* inactivation is detected in over 90% of MSI-Hi and 15% of MSS, sporadic CRCs.[58] Other genes mutated in MSI-Hi colorectal cancers encode proapoptotic molecules, such as CASP5 and BAX,[59] transcription factors, including TCF4,[60] and the epidermal growth factor receptor.[61] Notably, all CRCs, regardless of MMR status, seem to require mutational deregulation of the gatekeeper APC-β-catenin pathway.[62]

Another recessively inherited syndrome of multiple adenomas and CRC, MUTYH-associated polyposis (MAP), is caused by germline mutations in *MYH*, the human homolog of *Escherichia coli MutY*, another base excision-repair gene.[63] Disease begins later in life than in FAP, polyp numbers vary widely, and extracolonic tumors are less frequent than in HNPCC. Because *MYH* encodes a DNA glycosylase that mediates oxidative DNA damage, tumors are not associated with MSI but with somatic G:C to T:A mutations, including in the *APC* gene. Two alleles, *Y165C* and *G382D*, account for most cases, and cancers develop in homozygotes or compound heterozygotes; monoallelic carriers show no increased risk.[64] Surveillance recommendations are similar to those in HNPCC.

The cancer spectrum in HNPCC and the particular predilection for CRC remain unexplained. Colonic, endometrial, and selected other epithelial cells may be especially sensitive to the class of mutations that occur in the MMR setting; loss of the wild type MMR allele may occur more readily in these tissues; or they may lack repair safeguards that protect other cell types. MSI-Hi is observed in 12% to 15% of sporadic cases of CRC.[65] Most such tumors are believed to arise from serrated adenomas in the ascending colon and do not reflect unrecognized germline mutation or somatic disruption of a known MMR gene.[66] Rather, most sporadic MSI-Hi cases reflect epigenetic inactivation of the *MLH1* gene by promoter hypermethylation, often in association with the CIMP phenotype and with activating *BRAF* mutations.[67–69]

Familial Juvenile Polyposis (FJP)

Patients with FJP develop three to ten or more premalignant hamartomatous polyps in the stomach or small or large intestine in childhood or adolescence.[70,71] Although affected individuals often have the appropriate family history, a significant minority represents the first case in their families. Germline mutations in genes that encode the bone morphogenetic protein (BMP) receptor *BMPR1A*, the accessory TGF-β receptor endoglin, *ENG*, or the *SMAD4* signal transducer point to the TGF-β signaling pathway in disease pathogenesis.[72,73] Indeed, sporadic CRCs are frequently insensitive to the growth inhibitory effects of TGF-β, and loss of BMP function in mice expands stem and progenitor cells, leading to polyposis or ectopic crypts.[74–76] Not all patients carry these mutations, indicating that additional genes remain undiscovered. Notably, conditional loss of *Smad4* in mouse intestinal cells does not affect growth, whereas selective loss in T lymphocytes causes intestinal mucosal thickening and polyposis.[77] These results complicate interpretation of TGF-β functions and implicate stromal inflammation in intestinal tumorigenesis.

Peutz-Jeghers Syndrome

Patients with PJS develop hamartomatous polyps, benign tumors containing differentiated but disorganized cells, mainly in the small intestine but also in the colon or stomach; these grow to variable size, often leading to hemorrhage or intussusception. PJS shows autosomal dominant inheritance and is associated with macular lesions on the skin and buccal mucosa; bladder and bronchial polyps; and a propensity to develop a range of cancers, including those of the lung, breast, and female reproductive organs. The lifetime risk for all cancers exceeds 90% and the incidence of digestive tract cancers, especially in the small intestine, stomach, and pancreas, is elevated 50- to 500-fold over the general population; CRC risk is nearly 100 times greater.[78]

Serine–threonine kinase 11 (*STK11*) or *LKB1* is a recessive oncogene that shows loss of heterozygosity in PJS tumors and somatic mutations in sporadic pulmonary, pancreatic and biliary carcinomas, and melanoma.[79] Its product is a complex protein that functions at the intersection of several cellular pathways and points to the central importance of cell polarity and metabolism in cancer. Although LKB1 is implicated in diverse functions, its principal activity, exerted through the adenosine monophosphate (AMP)-activated protein kinase AMPK, seems to be in linking nutrient and energy utilization to controls over cellular structure and, in particular, polarity.[80] LKB1 also modulates the Rheb-GDP:Rheb-GTP cycle and downstream activity of the tuberous sclerosis gene *TSC2* and the mammalian target of rapamycin (mTOR),[81] key regulators of protein synthesis and cell growth. Determining how LKB1's roles in cell polarity and metabolism contribute to tumor suppression is an intense and exciting area of cancer biology, likely to hold many surprises and useful clues for rational therapy.

Cowden Syndrome

In Cowden syndrome, the lifetime risk of developing colon or thyroid cancer approaches 10%, whereas the risk of breast cancer is nearly 50%. A diverse array of oral and gastrointestinal mucosal lesions, including lipomas, fibromas, ganglioneuromas, and hamartomas, occur together with specific cutaneous lesions (facial trichilemmomas and acral verrucous papules) and benign breast fibroadenomas, neurofibromas, lipomas, uterine leiomyomas, and meningiomas.[82] Cowden syndrome results from germline mutations in *PTEN*, the tumor suppressor gene encoding the phosphatase and tensin homolog deleted on chromosome 10.[83] PTEN is a lipid phosphatase that dephosphorylates key phosphoinositide signaling molecules[84] and is accordingly a negative regulator of intracellular growth signaling through PI-3 kinase and its downstream effectors AKT and mTOR. *PTEN* is the second most frequently mutated gene in cancers, after *TP53*. Although mutations are rarely seen in sporadic CRC, PTEN immunostaining is lost in about 40% of cases, often as a result of promoter hypermethylation in the MSI-Hi setting,[85] emphasizing its tumor suppressor function in this disease.

Significance of Inherited Syndromes of Elevated Colorectal Cancer Risk

Following a clinical diagnosis of the above syndromes, known germline mutations should be tested and patients provided with genetic counseling and advice on cancer prevention and screening. Elucidation of the corresponding molecular defects profoundly informs understanding of sporadic CRC, revealing in particular that *APC* gene inactivation or *CTNNB1* activation are early, rate-limiting events and the seminal role of the Wnt signaling pathway. Likewise, *LKB1* and *PTEN* loss in inherited and sporadic CRCs shed light on vital molecular pathways, and HNPCC helps in classifying the disease and appreciating the significance of MSI, a feature seen in 12% to 15% of sporadic cases. Even in the absence of a well-recognized predisposition syndrome, individuals with a history of CRC in a first-degree relative are up to four times more likely to develop CRC than those without a family history.

Specific environmental factors that compound the risk of developing CRC are complex and insufficiently characterized but might include obesity, excessive consumption of red meat, lack of exercise, and vitamin D deficiency.[86] As many of these factors converge on insulin signaling, some experts propose that insulin and insulinlike growth factors play a seminal role in CRC.[87] However, three of every four CRCs arise in individuals lacking a well-defined risk factor, and it is unknown to what extent particular genotypes confer sensitivity to environmental variables.

Insights from Genomewide Association Studies

The quarter or more of sporadic CRC cases with a familial component[88,89] probably have diverse molecular etiologies, with low risk conferred by some common genetic variants and interaction of individual risk alleles with other genes and with environmental factors. One early study linked colon cancer to chromosomal segment 9q22-31,[90] which reinforced the idea that single risk loci might contribute to susceptibility in nonsyndromic forms of familial disease; the authors recently narrowed the interval to a 7.7-cM distance covering five genes.[91] Genomewide association studies (GWAS) have interrogated thousands of genomes to uncover statistical association of CRC risk with at least seven distinct loci, including those linked to single nucleotide polymorphisms (SNPs) rs6983267 at 8q24.21, rs4939827 on 18q21, and rs3802842 at 11q23 (Table 88.3). Risk alleles typically elevate the rate of CRC 10% to 25% above the background in persons with the nonrisk allele.[92,93] Homozygosity for some risk alleles and combinations of risk alleles at different loci compound the risk, to 50% to 250% over the background.

The causal significance of most of these DNA sequence variants is unclear, and many localize in gene deserts or poorly characterized regions of the genome. Addressing the role of TGF-β in CRC, one group of risk polymorphisms on chromosome 18q21 is linked to the *SMAD7* locus.[94] Particularly strong association occurs with the SNP rs6983267 at 8q24.21, which lies in a gene desert near low-risk susceptibility alleles for breast and prostate cancers. Molecular studies indicate that each of the culpable regions acts as a tissue-specific enhancer, controlling expression of the nearest neighboring structural gene, *CMYC*,[95] a highly plausible factor in disease susceptibility. In summary, common predisposition alleles confer some risk of CRC with low penetrance. Their pathophysiologic functions should be studied in greater detail to inform prevention and screening strategies and to determine how risk alleles interact with particular habits or environmental factors.

ONCOGENE AND TUMOR SUPPRESSOR GENE MUTATIONS IN COLORECTAL CANCER PROGRESSION

Building on the foundation established upon loss of the *APC* gatekeeper function, somatic mutations in cellular protooncogenes and tumor suppressor genes contribute cumulatively to

TABLE 88.3

SINGLE NUCLEOTIDE POLYMORPHISMS (SNPs) CONFERRING INCREASED RISK OF COLORECTAL CANCER

Chromosomal Location	SNP-Risk Allele	Nearest Gene	Risk Allele Frequency in Controls	Odds Ratio [95% CI]	*P* Value
8q24.21	rs10505477-A	*MYC*	0.50	1.17 [1.12–1.23]	3×10^{-11}
	rs6983267-G		0.49	1.27 [1.16–1.39]	1×10^{-14}
	rs10795668-A		0.48	1.12 [1.10–1.16]	3×10^{-13}
	rs7014346-A	*POU5FIP1, DQ515897*	0.18	1.19 [1.15–1.23]	9×10^{-26}
18q21.1	rs4939827-T	*SMAD7*	0.53	1.2 [1.16–1.24]	8×10^{-28}
15q13.3	rs4779584		0.19	1.23 [1.14–1.34]	5×10^{-7}
10p14	rs10795668-A		0.48	1.12 [1.10–1.16]	3×10^{-13}
8q23.3	rs16892766-A	*EIF3H*	0.07	1.27 [1.20–1.34]	3×10^{-18}
11q23.1	rs3802842-C		0.43	1.11 [1.08–1.15]	6×10^{-10}
16q22.1	rs9929218-A	*CDH1*	0.29	1.1 [1.06–1.12]	1×10^{-8}
19q13.11	rs10411210-C	*RHPN2*	0.90	1.15 [1.10–1.20]	5×10^{-9}
14q22.2	rs4444235-C	*BMP4*	0.46	1.11 [1.08–1.15]	8×10^{-10}
20p12.3	rs961253-A		0.36	1.12 [1.08–1.16]	2×10^{-10}

the acquisition of malignant properties. The limited spectrum of recurring mutations in CRC provides a context for refined appreciation of the adenoma–carcinoma sequence and points to rational targets for therapy. The most frequent genetic events (Table 88.4) are discussed below, with reference to clinical associations and their impact on cell growth and differentiation.

KRAS, *BRAF*, and *PIK3CA* Oncogene Mutations

The Ras family of small G-proteins transduces growth factor signals and is aberrantly activated in a wide variety of cancers. *KRAS* gene mutations are detected in about 40% of colorectal carcinomas,[96] mostly clustered in codons 12 and 13, with fewer than 10% occurring at codon 61. These mutations can be present in small polyps, and their frequency increases with lesion size.[97] The significance of the same mutations in lesions of low malignant potential, such as hyperplastic polyps or aberrant crypt foci lacking dysplasia, is uncertain.[98] *KRAS* mutation is not required to initiate adenomas but almost certainly contributes to their progression, and disruption of mutant *KRAS* alleles in colon cancer cells impedes growth.[99,100]

Oncogenic *KRAS* mutations have the potential to deregulate several effector pathways for cell proliferation, survival, and metastasis (Fig. 88.3). Constitutive phosphorylation of

TABLE 88.4

SOMATIC MUTATIONS IN ONCOGENES AND TUMOR SUPPRESSOR GENES

Gene	Type of Mutation	Frequency of Alterations (%)
Oncogenes		
KRAS	Point mutation (codons 12, 13, 61)	40% (majority at codon 12)
PIK3CA	Point mutations activating kinase activity	14%–35%
BRAF	Point mutation (V600E)	5%–8%
CTNNB1	Point mutation and in-frame deletions (amino-terminus)	~5%
HER-2/ERBB2	Amplification	<5%
Tumor suppressor genes		
p53	Point mutation, LOH	>60% (most are missense mutations)
APC	Small insertion or deletion, point mutation, LOH	>80% (most result in a truncated protein)
SMAD4	LOH, point mutation	60% LOH; 10%–15% missense, nonsense mutations
SMAD2	LOH, point mutation, small deletion,	60% LOH; <5% missense mutations, small deletions
TGF-βRII	Small insertion or deletion	10%–15%; higher (>90%) in MSI-Hi disease
DCC	LOH, insertion, deletion	~60% LOH; 10%–15% microsatellite insertions in intron

LOH, loss of heterozygosity; MSI-Hi, high microsatellite instability.

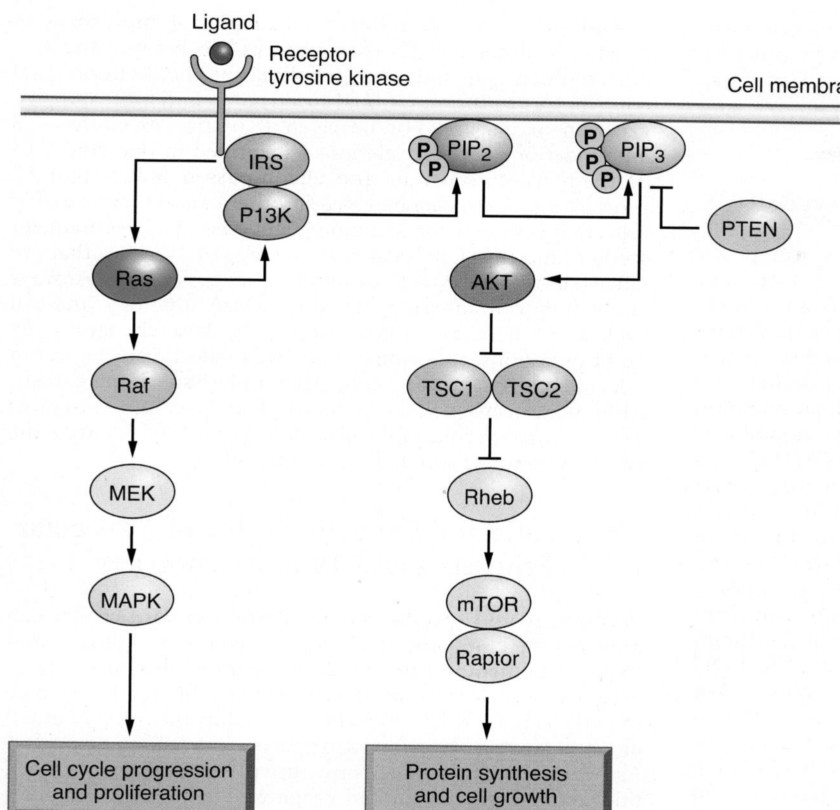

FIGURE 88.3 Signaling pathways, oncogenic mutations, and therapeutic opportunities in colorectal cancer (CRC). It is instructive to consider common genetic alterations in CRC in light of a common canonical outline of signaling through receptor tyrosine kinases, among which the epidermal growth factor receptor is a prime example. *KRAS*, the oncogene mutated in up to 40% of CRCs, signals receptor activation through RAF proteins (including BRAF, which is mutated in 5% to 8% of CRCs) and phosphatidylinositol 3-kinase (PI3K), whose catalytic PIK3CA subunit is mutated in 15% to 20% of CRCs. These transducers in turn activate the intracellular mitogen-activated protein kinase and AKT or mammalian target of rapamycin (mTOR) pathways, respectively. Common mutations hence confer growth factor independence on cells, resulting in dysregulated proliferation, protein synthesis, and metabolism. They also represent promising targets for therapeutic interference with aberrantly activated signaling cascades.

extracellular signal-regulated kinases, ERK-1 and ERK2, frequently accompanies *KRAS* mutation, reflecting activation of the mitogen-activated protein kinase (MAPK) pathway. This KRAS-mediated growth factor signaling cascade recruits RAF kinases to the plasma membrane and triggers ERK kinases MEK1 and MEK2 to activate ERK1 and ERK2, which phosphorylate factors that control the G_1-S cell cycle transition, among other substrates.[101] Although other, non-KRAS-mediated growth factor pathways also activate the MAPK cascade, signaling in cancer is most often deregulated through activating mutations in *KRAS* or *BRAF*. *BRAF* is mutated in 5% to 8% of CRCs, especially those associated with MSI-Hi or CIMP.[102,103] The most common *BRAF* mutation in colorectal and other cancers such as melanoma, *V599E*, affects a residue within the activation loop of the kinase domain and constitutively activates the kinase function, perhaps as a phosphomimetic.[104] Like mutant KRAS, activated BRAF also phosphorylates MEKs and ERKs, leading to dysregulated growth. Notably, KRAS and BRAF mutations are mutually exclusive in CRC,[102] reinforcing the role of the two oncogenes in a common cellular pathway and possibly reflecting alternative routes to the same end. However, patients with BRAF-mutant CRCs have a worse prognosis than those with KRAS-mutant tumors,[9] indicating the presence of distinctive features.

Besides the MAPK cascade, KRAS signals through the phosphatidylinositol 3-kinase (PI3K) pathway,[105] which phosphorylates the intracellular signaling lipid phosphatidylinositol-4,5-bisphosphate at the 3 position, triggering a cascade that promotes cell growth and survival.[106] Between 15% and 35% of CRCs carry activating mutations in *PIK3CA*, the gene encoding the catalytic p110 subunit of PI3K; most mutations cluster in exons 9 and 20 and seem to arise late in the adenoma–carcinoma sequence, perhaps coincident with invasion.[107] Curiously, although both PI3K and BRAF act downstream of KRAS, only the *BRAF-KRAS* mutant pair is mutually exclusive; *PIK3CA* mutations appear in nearly 10% of KRAS-mutant CRCs, implying that activation of both oncogenes may not be redundant. One reason could be that mutant KRAS activates PI3K signaling inefficiently[108]; more likely, oncogenic signaling pathways are less strictly linear than is convenient to depict. Indeed, the overtly parallel streams of KRAS signaling through RAF-MEK and PI3K (Fig. 88.3) interact extensively with one another and, in particular, both streams modulate mTOR, which coordinates cell growth with nutrient responses.[109] Such considerations notwithstanding, the recurrence of *KRAS*, *BRAF*, and *PIK3CA* mutations in CRC, at a collective frequency that rivals growth factor pathway aberrations in any carcinoma, appropriately places these oncogenes and their effectors at the center of research and drug development efforts.

The *p53* Tumor Suppressor

Allelic loss of chromosome 17p is observed in three of four colorectal carcinomas but fewer than 10% of adenomatous polyps.[97] The remaining *p53* allele is inactivated in most tumors with 17p loss of heterozygosity (LOH), most often at codons 175, 245, 248, 273, or 282.[110] LOH of 17p and mutations in *p53* thus appear to arise during the transition from adenoma to carcinoma, perhaps facilitating progression. When faced with stress from DNA damage, hypoxia, reduced nutrient access, and aneuploidy, cells with intact *p53* function undergo cell cycle arrest and apoptosis. The loss of *p53* may allow cells to overcome such barriers to tumor survival and progression.

Chromosome 18q Loss of Heterozygosity

LOH of chromosome 18q is rare in adenomas, except for large villous adenomas, observed in over 60% of primary CRCs, and present in nearly all liver metastases from colorectal primary tumors lacking MSI.[111] This sequence implicates loss of one or more genes on chromosome 18q in disease progression. Recent studies[112] challenge early ideas that 18q LOH conferred a poor prognosis.[113] The minimal common region of LOH on 18q21 contains two candidate tumor suppressor genes.[114] One of these genes, *SMAD4* (*DPC4*), is deleted in about one-third of cases and the remainder show loss of the other candidate gene, *DCC* (deleted in colorectal cancer), which encodes a cell surface receptor for the netrin family of axonal guidance proteins. *SMAD4/DPC4* and *SMAD2* are implicated as positive and negative regulators of TGF-β signaling, respectively, and lie close together on chromosome 18q. Somatic *SMAD4* deletions or localized mutations are present in 10% to 15% of CRCs, with 18q LOH and germline mutations noted in some FJP kindreds[115]; but *SMAD2* is somatically inactivated in fewer than 5% of CRCs.[116] Although *DCC* messenger RNA and protein are lost in more than 50% of CRCs,[117] few specific *DCC* coding mutations are known. Together with the low frequency of *SMAD4* or *SMAD2* mutations in 18q-deficient tumors, these findings suggest a complex, multifactorial basis for selection of 18q LOH in CRC.

INFREQUENT CHANGES AND CURRENT VIEWS OF THE MUTATIONAL LANDSCAPE OF COLORECTAL CANCER

Few cellular oncogenes besides *KRAS*, *BRAF*, and *PIK3CA* are common targets of point mutations in CRC (Table 88.4). Sequencing of the kinase domains in 133 tyrosine kinase (TK) and TK-like genes and 340 serine-threonine kinase (STK) genes revealed few recurrent nonsynonymous somatic mutations, including a handful in the *NTRK2*, *NTRK3*, and *FES* receptor TK genes[118] and the STK genes *MAPK24* and *MYLK2*.[119] Analysis of tyrosine phosphatases similarly identified scattered mutations of uncertain pathogenic significance in up to a quarter of CRCs.[120] In principle, increased expression by epigenetic mechanisms or gene amplification can have the same effect as activating point mutations, but oncogenes such as *HER-2* (*ErbB2*), *MYC*, *MYB*, and *CCND1* are amplified in fewer than 5% of cases in aggregate.

Most studies summarized in this chapter suffer from biased or opportunistic testing of genes, gene families, and pathways. To avoid such bias, groups have assessed copy number alterations (CNAs) by array hybridization and begun to sequence all exons and full genomes. Analysis of more than 13,000 genes in 11 CRCs revealed a substantially larger number of mutations than expected, with a conservative average estimate of 81 per tumor, but few of these mutations recur frequently and most may make small, if any, contribution to the neoplastic process.[121] The results are nevertheless informative because they reveal, for example, substantive differences in the nature of mutations in different tumor types, with CRCs showing a genomewide bias toward C:G to T:A transitions at 5′-CpG-3′ sites and a lower frequency of mutations in 5′-TpC-3′ dinucleotides than observed in breast cancer.[121] Such findings may find value in linking specific environmental contributors to the mutational spectrum in initiation and progression of disease. For nearly half of the 50 CNAs—28 amplifications and 22 deletions—identified in one study, 15 of them were recurrent and encompassed fewer than 12 genes[122] and were also detected in other cancers, presumably reflecting selection for common genetic events. A subsequent study found that CRCs carry an average of 17 genes that are deleted or amplified to 12 or more copies per cell.[123] Pathways controlling cell adhesion, signaling, DNA topology, and cell cycle were most commonly affected by these changes or by point mutations, confirming that CRCs reflect disturbances in selected pathways for replicative and tissue homeostasis. Although affected cellular processes may be common to most cancers, the specific molecular defects in CRC identify the best targets for rational, directed therapy.

Prognostic and Predictive Value of Molecular Properties and Tumor Genotypes

Phenotypes and specific genetic alterations in a cancer can hold useful clues about clinical behavior, prognosis, and response to therapy. Aneuploidy and tetraploidy confer a poor prognosis and MSI-Hi imparts a relatively favorable outcome in early stage CRC.[124] Benefit from adjuvant 5-fluorouracil monotherapy may be confined to patients with MSS tumors.[125,126] As nearly all CRCs have constitutive Wnt pathway activity, this factor alone has limited prognostic value, and outcomes seem unaffected by whether Wnt activity was stimulated by *APC* or *CTNNB1* mutations. The presence of *KRAS* or *BRAF* mutations and possibly also *PIK3CA* mutation or loss of PTEN expression predicts a lack of response to EGFR monoclonal antibodies.[8,127] These observations are important because they direct treatment decisions and because, unlike acute leukemia or breast cancer, CRC had previously resisted subgrouping on the basis of specific genetic alterations. For example, mutations in the two most frequently affected oncogenes, *KRAS* or *PIK3CA*, seem not to impact survival in stage III or IV disease treated with current drug regimens.[9,128] Patients with metastatic *BRAF*-mutant disease have especially low survival and respond poorly to current chemotherapy regimens.[9]

Mouse Models of Colorectal Cancer

The laboratory mouse has immense value in genetic analysis of CRC. The most informative mouse line, *multiple intestinal neoplasia* (*Min*), carries a mutagen-induced nonsense mutation in the murine homolog of *APC* and phenocopies human FAP with respect to intestinal adenomatosis,[129] although species' differences place the burden mainly in the small intestine instead of the colon. APC^{Min} mice serve as a cornerstone for genetic analysis of intestinal tumors and deregulated Wnt signaling. Modifications of the murine *APC* locus influence disease phenotypes, as detailed in other reviews[130]; the *D716* allele increases the number of adenomas, all showing LOH of the wild type copy,[131] whereas the APC^{1638N} mutation results in fewer adenomas, more of which appear in the colon.[132] Apc^{Pirc} rats carry a stop codon at position 1137 and develop more than half the tumors in the colon, similar to humans.[133] Deletion of the N-terminal degradation domain of β-catenin also stabilizes the protein and produces widespread intestinal polyposis in mice.[134] Expression of $Kras^{G12D}$ or $Kras^{G12V}$ in the intestinal epithelium of otherwise intact mice has subtle consequences on cell signaling and proliferation, whereas expression in mutant *Apc* backgrounds expands progenitor cell numbers and hastens adenoma progression,[135] modeling the sequence of mutations in human colon cancer. Finally, the *in vivo* requirements of each MMR gene have been analyzed by introducing inactivating mutations in all murine *mutS* and *mutL* homologs.[136] These mice generally develop lymphomas more often than intestinal tumors, and some mutants show neither MSI nor intestinal tumors, highlighting species differences. Nevertheless, the defects point to an essential role for some MMR genes in meiosis and underscore the importance of MMR in protecting cells from mutation and malignancy.

Selected References

The full list of references for this chapter appears in the online version.

1. Noffsinger AE. Serrated polyps and colorectal cancer: new pathway to malignancy. *Annu Rev Pathol* 2009;4:343.
3. Levin B, Lieberman DA, McFarland B, et al. Screening and surveillance for the early detection of colorectal cancer and adenomatous polyps, 2008: a joint guideline from the American Cancer Society, the US Multi-Society Task Force on Colorectal Cancer, and the American College of Radiology. *Gastroenterology* 2008;134:1570.
5. Jones S, Chen WD, Parmigiani G, et al. Comparative lesion sequencing provides insights into tumor evolution. *Proc Natl Acad Sci U S A* 2008;105:4283.
6. Vogelstein B, Kinzler KW. Cancer genes and the pathways they control. *Nat Med* 2004;10:789.
8. Van Cutsem E, Kohne CH, Hitre E, et al. Cetuximab and chemotherapy as initial treatment for metastatic colorectal cancer. *N Engl J Med* 2009;360:1408.
9. Souglakos J, Philips J, Wang R, et al. Prognostic and predictive value of common mutations for treatment response and survival in patients with metastatic colorectal cancer. *Br J Cancer* 2009;101:465.
12. Ionov Y, Peinado MA, Malkhosyan S, Shibata D, Perucho M. Ubiquitous somatic mutations in simple repeated sequences reveal a new mechanism for colonic carcinogenesis. *Nature* 1993;363:558.
14. Goelz SE, Vogelstein B, Hamilton SR, Feinberg AP. Hypomethylation of DNA from benign and malignant human colon neoplasms. *Science* 1985;228:187.
17. Eden A, Gaudet F, Waghmare A, Jaenisch R. Chromosomal instability and tumors promoted by DNA hypomethylation. *Science* 2003;300:455.
20. Toyota M, Ahuja N, Ohe-Toyota M, et al. CpG island methylator phenotype in colorectal cancer. *Proc Natl Acad Sci U S A* 1999;96:8681.
22. Jess T, Loftus EV Jr, Velayos FS, et al. Risk of intestinal cancer in inflammatory bowel disease: a population-based study from Olmsted county, Minnesota. *Gastroenterology* 2006;130:1039.
34. Morin PJ, Sparks AB, Korinek V, et al. Activation of beta-catenin-Tcf signaling in colon cancer by mutations in beta-catenin or APC. *Science* 1997;275:1787.
36. Sansom OJ, Reed KR, Hayes AJ, et al. Loss of Apc in vivo immediately perturbs Wnt signaling, differentiation, and migration. *Genes Dev* 2004;18:1385.
37. Clevers H. Wnt/beta-catenin signaling in development and disease. *Cell* 2006;127:469.
41. Barker N, Ridgway RA, van Es JH, et al. Crypt stem cells as the cells-of-origin of intestinal cancer. *Nature* 2009;457:608.
42. van de Wetering M, Sancho E, Verweij C, et al. The beta-catenin/TCF-4 complex imposes a crypt progenitor phenotype on colorectal cancer cells. *Cell* 2002;111:241.
43. He TC, Sparks AB, Rago C, et al. Identification of c-MYC as a target of the APC pathway. *Science* 1998;281:1509.
44. Sansom OJ, Meniel VS, Muncan V, et al. Myc deletion rescues Apc deficiency in the small intestine. *Nature* 2007;446:676.
48. Vasen HF, Watson P, Mecklin JP, Lynch HT. New clinical criteria for hereditary nonpolyposis colorectal cancer (HNPCC, Lynch syndrome) proposed by the International Collaborative group on HNPCC. *Gastroenterology* 1999;116:1453.
50. Fishel R, Kolodner RD. Identification of mismatch repair genes and their role in the development of cancer. *Curr Opin Genet Dev* 1995;5:382.
53. Umar A, Boland CR, Terdiman JP, et al. Revised Bethesda guidelines for hereditary nonpolyposis colorectal cancer (Lynch syndrome) and microsatellite instability. *J Natl Cancer Inst* 2004;96:261.
57. Markowitz S, Wang J, Myeroff L, et al. Inactivation of the type II TGF-beta receptor in colon cancer cells with microsatellite instability. *Science* 1995;268:1336.
62. Huang J, Papadopoulos N, McKinley AJ, et al. APC mutations in colorectal tumors with mismatch repair deficiency. *Proc Natl Acad Sci U S A* 1996;93:9049.
63. Sieber OM, Lipton L, Crabtree M, et al. Multiple colorectal adenomas, classic adenomatous polyposis, and germ-line mutations in MYH. *N Engl J Med* 2003;348:791.
65. Thibodeau SN, French AJ, Cunningham JM, et al. Microsatellite instability in colorectal cancer: different mutator phenotypes and the principal involvement of hMLH1. *Cancer Res* 1998;58:1713.
66. Liu B, Nicolaides NC, Markowitz S, et al. Mismatch repair gene defects in sporadic colorectal cancers with microsatellite instability. *Nat Genet* 1995;9:48.
69. Weisenberger DJ, Siegmund KD, Campan M, et al. CpG island methylator phenotype underlies sporadic microsatellite instability and is tightly associated with BRAF mutation in colorectal cancer. *Nat Genet* 2006;38:787.
73. Sweet K, Willis J, Zhou XP, et al. Molecular classification of patients with unexplained hamartomatous and hyperplastic polyposis. *J Am Med Assoc* 2005;294:2465.
79. Hemminki A, Markie D, Tomlinson I, et al. A serine/threonine kinase gene defective in Peutz-Jeghers syndrome. *Nature* 1998;391:184.
81. Shaw RJ, Bardeesy N, Manning BD, et al. The LKB1 tumor suppressor negatively regulates mTOR signaling. *Cancer Cell* 2004;6:91.
82. Rustgi AK. The genetics of hereditary colon cancer. *Genes Dev* 2007;21:2525.
83. Liaw D, Marsh DJ, Li J, et al. Germline mutations of the PTEN gene in Cowden disease, an inherited breast and thyroid cancer syndrome. *Nat Genet* 1997;16:64.
85. Goel A, Arnold CN, Niedzwiecki D, et al. Frequent inactivation of PTEN by promoter hypermethylation in microsatellite instability–high sporadic colorectal cancers. *Cancer Res* 2004;64:3014.
87. Slattery ML, Fitzpatrick FA. Convergence of hormones, inflammation, and energy-related factors: a novel pathway of cancer etiology. *Cancer Prev Res* 2009;2:922.
90. Wiesner GL, Daley D, Lewis S, et al. A subset of familial colorectal neoplasia kindreds linked to chromosome 9q22.2-31.2. *Proc Natl Acad Sci U S A* 2003;100:12961.
92. Tomlinson I, Webb E, Carvajal-Carmona L, et al. A genome-wide association scan of tag SNPs identifies a susceptibility variant for colorectal cancer at 8q24.21. *Nat Genet* 2007;39:984.
95. Ahmadiyeh N, Pomerantz MM, Grisanzio C, et al. 8q24 prostate, breast, and colon cancer risk loci show tissue-specific long-range interaction with MYC. *Proc Natl Acad Sci U S A* 2010;107:9742.
96. Bos JL, Fearon ER, Hamilton SR, et al. Prevalence of ras gene mutations in human colorectal cancers. *Nature* 1987;327:293.
97. Vogelstein B, Fearon ER, Hamilton SR, et al. Genetic alterations during colorectal-tumor development. *N Engl J Med* 1988;319:525.
101. Downward J. Targeting RAS signalling pathways in cancer therapy. *Nat Rev Cancer* 2003;3:11.
102. Rajagopalan H, Bardelli A, Lengauer C, et al. Tumorigenesis: RAF/RAS oncogenes and mismatch-repair status. *Nature* 2002;418:934.
104. Davies H, Bignell GR, Cox C, et al. Mutations of the BRAF gene in human cancer. *Nature* 2002;417:949.
107. Samuels Y, Wang Z, Bardelli A, et al. High frequency of mutations of the PIK3CA gene in human cancers. *Science* 2004;304:554.
110. Baker SJ, Fearon ER, Nigro JM, et al. Chromosome 17 deletions and p53 gene mutations in colorectal carcinomas. *Science* 1989;244:217.
115. Howe JR, Roth S, Ringold JC, et al. Mutations in the SMAD4/DPC4 gene in juvenile polyposis. *Science* 1998;280:1086.
121. Sjoblom T, Jones S, Wood LD, et al. The consensus coding sequences of human breast and colorectal cancers. *Science* 2006;314:268.
123. Leary RJ, Lin JC, Cummins J, et al. Integrated analysis of homozygous deletions, focal amplifications, and sequence alterations in breast and colorectal cancers. *Proc Natl Acad Sci U S A* 2008;105:16224.
127. Sartore-Bianchi A, Di Nicolantonio F, Nichelatti M, et al. Multideterminants analysis of molecular alterations for predicting clinical benefit to EGFR-targeted monoclonal antibodies in colorectal cancer. *PLoS One* 2009;4:e7287.
129. Moser AR, Pitot HC, Dove WF. A dominant mutation that predisposes to multiple intestinal neoplasia in the mouse. *Science* 1990;247:322.
134. Harada N, Tamai Y, Ishikawa T, et al. Intestinal polyposis in mice with a dominant stable mutation of the beta-catenin gene. *EMBO J* 1999;18:5931.

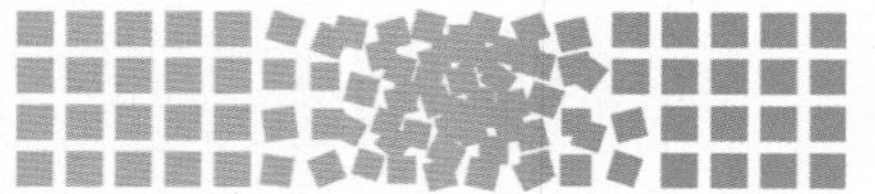

CHAPTER 89 CANCER OF THE COLON

STEVEN K. LIBUTTI, LEONARD B. SALTZ, AND CHRISTOPHER G. WILLETT

A more thorough understanding of the molecular basis for this disease, coupled with the development of new therapeutic approaches, has dramatically altered the way in which colorectal cancer patients are managed. This chapter and the one that follows will provide an up-to-date description of the current state of the science and outline a multidisciplinary approach to the patient with colon or rectal cancer.

EPIDEMIOLOGY

Incidence and Mortality

Globally, nearly 1,200,000 new colorectal cancer cases are believed to occur, which accounts for approximately 10% of all incident cancers, and mortality from colorectal cancer is estimated at nearly 609,000.[1] In 2010 there were an estimated 141,570 new cases of colorectal cancer and 51,370 deaths in the United States.[2] As such, colorectal cancer accounts for nearly 10% of cancer mortality in the United States. Prevalence estimates reveal that in unscreened individuals age 50 years or older, there is a 0.5% to 2.0% chance of harboring an invasive colorectal cancer, a 1.0% to 1.6% chance of an *in situ* carcinoma, a 7% to 10% chance of a large (1 cm or larger) adenoma, and a 25% to 40% chance of an adenoma of any size.[3]

Age impacts colorectal cancer incidence greater than any other demographic factor. To that end, sporadic colorectal cancer increases dramatically above the age of 45 to 50 years for all groups. In almost all countries, age-standardized incidence rates are less for women than for men. Although colorectal cancer incidence has been steadily decreasing in the United States and Canada, the incidence is rapidly increasing in Japan, Korea, and China.[1] In the United States from 2002 to 2006, the age-standardized incidence rates per 100,000 population was 59.0 for men and 43.6 for women when combined for all races.[2] Recognizing that decreases in age-standardized colorectal cancer incidence and mortality rates are apparent in the United States over the past 10 to 15 years, such trends may be counterbalanced by prolonged longevity.

Geographic Variation

The incidence rate for Alaskan Natives exceeds 70 per 100,000,[4] while that for Gambia and Algeria is less than 2 per 100,000.[5] Generally speaking, colorectal cancer incidence and mortality rates are the greatest in developed Western nations.[1,5] The reader is referred to the most recent detailed incidence and mortality rates in different countries over time according to gender, ethnicity, and anatomic site as established by the National Cancer Institute on their website.

As mentioned, there appears to be a recent decrease in age-standardized colorectal cancer incidence and mortality rates within the United States. From 1999 to 2006, colorectal cancer incidence and mortality both decreased.[2] Furthermore, 5-year survival improved. These trends are apparent regardless of gender, race, or ethnic group, except for Native Americans. Although at an initial glance one might invoke alterations in dietary and lifestyle factors, or the utilization of chemopreventive agents, it is clear that enhanced use of colonoscopy with polypectomy represents a significant reason for the improvements in trends in some areas.[6]

Emigration Patterns in Population Groups

Seminal studies have revealed that migrants from low-incident areas to high-incident areas assume the incidence of the host country within one generation.[7–10] For example, for Chinese who immigrate to the United States, higher colorectal cancer rates have been ascribed to greater meat consumption and diminished physical activity in contrast to controls within their original country.[8] These and other studies underscore the importance of environmental exposure in colorectal cancer incidence and provide a platform for attention to dietary and lifestyle modification as preventive measures.

Race and Ethnicity

Although dietary and lifestyle factors are of paramount importance in low incident regions of the world, especially Asia and Africa, nonetheless there are certain trends along racial or ethnic lines. For example, an inherited adenomatosis polyposis coli (APC) gene mutation, I1307K, confers a higher risk of colorectal cancer within certain Ashkenazi Jewish families that is not apparent in other ethnic groups.[11,12] Inherited mutations in the DNA mismatch repair genes may be more common among African Americans[13] in part accounting for anatomic variation in colon cancers among races in the United States,[14,15] an area that is receiving much attention in epidemiology- and biology-based research.

Socioeconomic Factors

Generally, cancer incidence and mortality rates have been higher in economically advantaged countries.[16,17] This may be related to consumption of a high fat and high red meat diet, lack of physical activity with resulting obesity, and variations in mortality causes over a longitudinal period of time.

Anatomic Shift

Classically, colon cancer was believed to be a disease of the left or distal colon. However, the incidence of right-sided or proximal colon cancer has been increasing in North America[15,18] and Europe.[19] Similar trends have been observed in Asian countries.[20] This anatomic shift is likely multifactorial: (1) due to increased longevity; (2) as a response to luminal procarcinogens and carcinogens, which can vary between different sites of the colon and rectum; and, (3) genetic factors, which can preferentially involve defects in mismatch repair genes with resulting microsatellite instability in proximal colon cancers and chromosomal instability pathway predominant in left-sided colon and rectal cancers. These developments in anatomic variation will necessarily impact considerably on screening procedures, response to chemoprevention, response to chemotherapy, and, ultimately, disease-specific survival.[21–23]

ETIOLOGY: GENETIC AND ENVIRONMENTAL RISK FACTORS

Inherited Predisposition

Family history confers an increased lifetime risk of colorectal cancer, but that enhanced risk varies depending on the nature of the family history (Table 89.1). Familial factors contribute importantly to the risk of sporadic colorectal cancer, depending upon the involvement of first- or second-degree relatives and the age of onset of colorectal cancer. Involvement of at least one first-degree relative with colorectal cancer serves to double the risk of colorectal cancer.[24] There is further enhancement of the risk if a case is affected prior to the age of 60. Similarly, the likelihood of harboring premalignant adenomas or colorectal cancer is increased in first-degree relatives of persons with colorectal cancer.[25,26] The National Polyp Study reveals compelling data; the relative risk for parents and siblings of patients with adenomas compared to spousal controls was 1.8, which increased to 2.6 if the proband was younger than age 60 at adenoma detection.[27]

Provocative assessments of population groups suggest a dominantly inherited susceptibility to colorectal adenomas and cancer, which may account for the majority of sporadic colorectal cancer, but this may have variable inheritance based on the degree of exposure to environmental factors.[28] What are these susceptibility factors? The answer has yet to emerge. Nonetheless, genetic polymorphisms may be of paramount importance, such as in glutathione-s-transferase,[29] ethylene tetrahydrofolate reductase,[30,31] and *N*-acetyltransferases, especially NAT1 and NAT2.[32] In fact, genetic polymorphisms can vary among different racial and ethnic groups, which may provide clues to the geographic variation of colorectal cancer as well.

TABLE 89.1

ETIOLOGY OF COLON CANCER: ENVIRONMENTAL FACTORS

Increased Incidence	Decreased Incidence
High-caloric diet	High-fiber diet
High red meat consumption	Antioxidant vitamins
Overcooked red meat	Fresh fruit/vegetables
High saturated fats	Nonsteroidal anti-inflammatories
Excess alcohol consumption	High calcium
Cigarette-smoking	
Sedentary lifestyle	
Obesity	
No effect on incidence with coffee or tea	

Environmental Factors

Seminal studies have underscored the importance of environmental factors as contributing to the pathogenesis of colorectal cancer. One has to take population-based studies into the context of methodologies employed, lead-time bias, time-lag issues, definition of surrogate and true end points, and the role of susceptibility factors.

Diet

Total Calories

Obesity and total caloric intake are independent risk factors for colorectal cancer as revealed by cohort and case-control studies.[33,34] Increased body mass may result in a twofold increase in colorectal cancer risk, with a strong association in men with colon but not rectal cancer.

Meat, Fat, and Protein

Ingestion of red meat but not white meat is associated with an increased colorectal cancer risk,[35,36] and as such, per capita consumption of red meat is a potent independent risk factor. Whether the total abstinence from red meat leads to a decreased colorectal cancer incidence has not been clarified, as there are studies with opposing results.[37] Fried, barbecued, and processed meats are also associated with colorectal cancer risk, especially for rectal cancer, with odds ratio of 6.[38]

Although high protein intake may augment carcinogenesis, definitive proof of this is lacking. Mechanistically, a high protein diet is associated with accelerated epithelial proliferation.[39] Fatty components of red meat may be tumor promoters, as fats may be metabolized by luminal bacteria to carcinogens,[35] which would cause abnormal colonic epithelial proliferation. There is controversy as to whether the type of fat is important. Some studies suggest that saturated animal fats may confer especially high risk,[17,35] and yet other investigations suggest that there is no evidence for increased risk for any specific dietary fat after adjustment for total energy intake.[35,40]

Fiber

Classically, a high fiber diet was associated with a low incidence of colorectal cancer in Africa,[41] with numerous studies substantiating this premise.[42] Protection was believed to be afforded from wheat bran, fruit, and vegetables.[36] A high-fiber diet was believed to dilute fecal carcinogens, decrease colon transit time, and generate a favorable luminal environment. However, these canonical concepts have been challenged by more recent, large, well-controlled studies that showed no inverse relationship between colorectal cancer and fiber intake.[43] In a study of nearly 90,000 women from ages 34 to 59 who were followed for 16 years, no protective effect was noted between fiber and incidence of either adenomatous polyp or colorectal cancer.[43] This was further corroborated by two large randomized controlled trials that evaluated high-fiber diets for moderate duration and discovered a lack of effect on the number, size, and histology of polyps found on colonoscopy.[44,45] At this point, therefore, the majority of evidence suggests that dietary fiber does not play a role in the risk of developing colorectal cancer.

Vegetables and Fruit

A protective effect of vegetables and fruits against colorectal cancer is generally believed to be true.[35] This has been observed with raw, green, and cruciferous vegetables. Whether certain agents such as antioxidant vitamins (E, C, and A), folate, thioethers, terpenes, and plant phenols may translate into effective chemopreventive strategies requires further investigation, although the data for folate intake are sound.[46]

Calcium also has been historically implicated as having a protective effect. Mechanistically, calcium can be viewed as being able to bind injurious bile acids with reduction of colonic epithelial proliferation.[47] This is supported through cell culture models. However, population-based studies are not definitive.

Lifestyle

Physical inactivity has been associated with colorectal cancer risk, for colon more than rectal cancer. A sedentary lifestyle may account for an increased colorectal cancer risk, although the mechanism is unclear. More recent data suggest that physical activity after the diagnosis of stages I to III colon cancer may reduce the risk of cancer-related and overall mortality, and that the amount of aerobic exercise correlates with a reduced risk of recurrence following resection of stage III colon cancer.[48]

Most studies of alcohol have demonstrated at most a minimally positive effect. Associations are strongest between alcohol consumption in men and risk of rectal cancer. Perhaps interference with folate metabolism through acetaldehyde is responsible.[49]

Prolonged cigarette smoking is associated with the risk of colorectal cancer.[35] Cigarette smoking for greater than 20 pack-years was associated with large adenoma risk and greater than 35 pack-years with cancer risk.

There has been no reproducible association in the chronic use of either coffee or tea with colorectal cancer risk.[50]

Drugs

Nonsteroidal Anti-Inflammatory Drugs

Population-based studies strongly support inverse associations between use of aspirin and other nonsteroidal anti-inflammatories (NSAIDs) and the incidences of both colorectal cancer and adenomas.[51–53] In a cohort study the relative risk of colorectal cancer was 0.49 (95% confidence interval [CI], 0.24 to 1.00) when comparing regular NSAID users with nonusers.[54] Duration of NSAID use is important, and right-sided colon cancers may benefit more than left-sided colorectal cancers. Interestingly, the type of NSAID was not important. As a result of this and other studies, NSAIDs and selective cyclooxygenase 2 (COX-2) inhibitors have been investigated intensively in familial adenomatous polyposis (FAP) and sporadic colorectal cancer.

FAMILIAL COLORECTAL CANCER

Familial Adenomatous Polyposis

FAP constitutes 1% of all colorectal cancers incidence (Table 89.2). Hallmark features include hundreds to thousands of colonic polyps that develop in patients in their teens to 30s, and if the colon is not surgically removed, 100% of patients progress to colorectal cancer. Extracolonic manifestations include benign conditions—congenital hypertrophy of the retinal pigment epithelium, mandibular osteomas, supernumerary teeth, epidermal cysts, adrenal cortical adenomas, desmoid tumors (although these tumors may lead to obstruction)—and malignant conditions—thyroid tumors, gastric small intestinal polyps with a 5% to 10% risk of duodenal or ampullary adenocarcinoma, and brain tumors.[55] The brain tumors may be of two types—glioblastoma multiforme or medulloblastoma—and the particular association of brain tumors and colonic

TABLE 89.2

FAMILIAL AND NONFAMILIAL CAUSES OF COLORECTAL CANCER

Syndromes with Adenomatous Polyps
***APC* Gene Mutations (1%):**
Familial adenomatous polyposis (FAP)
Attenuated APC
Turcot syndrome (two-thirds of families)
MMR Gene Mutations (3%):
Hereditary nonpolyposis colorectal cancer types I and II
Muir-Torre syndrome
Turcot syndrome (one-third of families)
Syndromes with Hamartomatous Polyps (<1%)
Peutz-Jeghers (*LKB1*)
Juvenile polyposis (*SMAD4, PTEN*)
Cowden (*PTEN*)
Bannayan-Ruvalcaba-Riley
Mixed polyposis
Other Familial Causes (up to 20%–25%)
Family history of adenomatous polyps (*MYH*)
Family history of colon cancer
Risk more than three times greater if two first-degree relatives or one first-degree relative <50 with colon cancer
Risk two times greater if second-degree relative affected
Familial colon-breast cancer
Nonfamilial Causes
Personal history of adenomatous polyps
Personal history of colorectal cancer
Inflammatory bowel disease (ulcerative colitis, Crohn's colitis)
Radiation colitis
Ureterosigmoidostomy
Acromegaly
Cronkhite-Canada syndrome

polyposis is called Turcot syndrome.[56] The colonic polyps in Turcot syndrome are fewer and larger than in classic FAP. An attenuated form of FAP harbors up to 100 colonic polyps and has a predisposition to colorectal cancer in patients when they are in their 50s or 60s.[57]

FAP is an autosomally dominant disorder with nearly 100% penetrance. However, about 30% of patients have *de novo* mutations and without an ostensible family history. Based on karyotypic analysis that reveals an interstitial deletion on human chromosome 5q and subsequent genetic linkage analysis to 5q21, the gene responsible for FAP was identified as *APC* (adenomatosis polyposis coli). FAP patients inherit a mutated copy of the *APC* gene, thereby predisposing them to early onset polyposis. During life, FAP patients acquire inactivation of the remaining *APC* gene copy, which accelerates the progression to colorectal cancer. Interesting genotypic-phenotypic associations exist between the location of the *APC* gene mutation and certain clinical manifestations, such as congenital hypertrophy of the retinal pigment epithelium (CHRPE), desmoid tumors, and classic FAP versus attenuated FAP.

The *APC* gene comprises 15 exons and encodes a protein of nearly 2,850 amino acids (310 kDa). Nearly all germline mutations in the *APC* gene lead to a truncated protein, which can be detected through molecular diagnostic assays that can be integrated into genetic counseling and genetic testing of affected patients and at-risk family members.[58,59] The functions of the APC protein and the interrelated pathways and regulatory molecules will be discussed later.

Hereditary Nonpolyposis Colorectal Cancer

Hereditary nonpolyposis colorectal cancer (HNPCC) accounts for about 3% of all colorectal cancers. Salient features include up to 100 colonic polyps (hence the term nonpolyposis), preferentially, albeit not exclusively, in the right or proximal colon.[60] There is an accelerated rate of progression to colorectal cancer in these diminutive, at times flat, polyps with mean age of onset of colorectal cancer being 43. This is designated HNPCC type I. HNPCC type II is distinguished by extra colonic tumors, originating in the stomach, small bowel, bile duct, renal pelvis, ureter, bladder, uterus and ovary, skin, and perhaps the pancreas. The lifetime risk of colorectal cancer in HNPCC is 80%, about 40% for endometrial cancer, and less than 10% for all other cancers.[61] Of note, a variant of HNPCC involves skin tumors and is designated as Muir-Torre syndrome. HNPCC is defined classically by the modified Amsterdam criteria (Table 89.3).

HNPCC is an autosomally dominant disorder with about 80% penetrance. Genetic and biochemical approaches led to the discovery of the involvement of human DNA mismatch repair genes in HNPCC. Recognized as the human orthologues of mismatch repair genes described in bacteria and yeast, human mismatch repair genes encode enzymes that repair errors during DNA replication that may occur spontaneously or upon exposure to an exogenous agent (e.g., ultraviolet light, chemical carcinogen). Mutations in one of these mismatch repair genes results in microsatellite instability, which creates a milieu of somatic mutations of target genes—*TGF-β2* receptor, *bax*, *IGF* type I receptor, among others—in HNPCC associated tumors.[60] About 60% of germline mutations in HNPCC are found in either the *hMLH1* gene or the *hMSH2* gene, but mutations in other members of this family—*hMSH6*, *hPMS1*, *hPMS2*—are rare, thereby indicating that other genes are involved but have yet to be discovered. Genetic testing is not facile for HNPCC as it is for FAP, but it involves sequencing both the *hMLH1* and *hMSH2* genes (Table 89.4). If a germline mutation is found, then the remaining at-risk family members can be genetically screened. Microsatellite instability (MSI) testing and hMLH1/hMSH2 immunohistochemistry can be performed on tumor specimens as a possible prelude to genetic testing.

TABLE 89.3

Amsterdam I Criteria
At least three relatives with colorectal cancer
One relative should be a first-degree relative of the other two
At least two successive generations should be affected
At least one colorectal cancer case before age 50
FAP should be excluded
Tumors should be verified histopathologically
Amsterdam II Criteria
At least three relatives with HNPCC-associated cancer (colorectal, endometrial, small bowel, ureter, or renal pelvis)
At least two successive generations should be affected
At least one case before age 50
FAP should be excluded
Tumors should be verified histopathologically
Bethesda Criteria (for Identification of Patients with Colorectal Tumor Who Should Undergo Testing for MSI)
Cancer in families that meet Amsterdam criteria
Two HNPCC-related cancers, including colorectal or extracolonic
Colorectal cancer and a first degree relative with colorectal cancer and/or HNPCC-related extracolonic cancer and/or colorectal adenoma: one cancer before age 45 and adenoma before age 40
Colorectal cancer or endometrial cancer before age 45
Right-sided colorectal cancer with an undifferentiated pattern on histopathology before age 45
Signet-ring cell type colorectal cancer before age 45
Adenoma before age 40

FAP, familial adenomatous polyposis; HNPCC, hereditary nonpolyposis colorectal cancer; MSI, microsatellite instability.

TABLE 89.4

GENETIC TESTING IN INHERITED COLORECTAL CANCER

FAP:	APC protein truncating testing (preferred) If APC mutation found, screen for mutation in family Less desirable alternatives: gene sequencing, linkage testing
HNPCC:	MSI testing in tumor[a] If MSI present, proceed to sequencing of both *hMLH1* and *hMSH2* genes If mutation found, screen for mutation in family

FAP, familial adenomatous polyposis; APC, adenomatosis polyposis coli; HNPCC, hereditary nonpolyposis colorectal cancer; MSI, microsatellite instability.
[a]Immunohistochemistry may be an option.
Peutz-Jeghers syndrome, juvenile polyposis, Cowden syndrome: Gene mutation analysis

Hamartomatous Polyposis Syndromes

Hamartomatous polyposis syndromes are rare syndromes, mostly affecting the pediatric and adolescent population, and represent less than 1% of colorectal cancers annually. Peutz-Jeghers syndrome involves large but few colonic and small bowel polyps that can manifest by gastrointestinal (GI) bleeding or obstruction and an increased risk of colorectal cancer. The polyps are distinguished by a smooth muscle band in the submucosa. Hallmark clinical features on physical examination include freckles on the hands, around the lips, in the buccal mucosa, and periorbitally. Associated characteristics include sinus, bronchial, and bladder polyps, and about 5% to 10% of patients have sex cord tumors. Patients can also develop lung and pancreatic adenocarcinomas. The gene responsible for this syndrome is *LKB1*, a serine threonine kinase.

Juvenile polyposis have overlapping clinical manifestations with Peutz-Jeghers, but the polyps tend to be confined to the colon, although cases of gastric and small bowel polyps have been described and there is an increased risk of colorectal cancer. Extracolonic manifestations are not prevalent. This is a polygenic disease, involving germline mutations in *PTEN*, *SMAD4*, *BMPR1*, or other genes yet to be identified.

Cowden syndrome harbors hamartomatous polyps anywhere in the GI tract, and surprisingly, there is no increased risk of colorectal cancer. However, about 10% of patients will have thyroid tumors and nearly 50% of patients have breast tumors. Germline *PTEN* mutations have been reported.

It is estimated that about 20% to 30% of colorectal cancers are compatible with an inherited predisposition, independent of known syndromes.[62] The identification of other responsible genes will have great clinical impact. Intensive approaches are being pursued through sibling-pair studies and other familial studies. As previously mentioned, patients may be predisposed to an increased risk of adenomatous polyps as well in the context of a family history of sporadic adenomatous polyps.

ANATOMY OF THE COLON

The colon and rectum make up the segment of the digestive system commonly referred to as the large bowel. Defined as the portion of intestine from the ileocecal valve to the anus, the large bowel is approximately 150 cm in length. It is divided into five segments defined by its vascular supply and by its extraperitoneal or retroperitoneal location: the cecum (with appendix) and ascending colon, the transverse colon, the descending colon, the sigmoid colon, and the rectum. The anatomy of the rectum will be discussed in detail in the chapter on rectal cancer. The large bowel has a muscular wall and can be distinguished from the small intestine by its increased diameter, the presence of haustra, appendices epiploicae, and tenia coli. The tenia consist of condensations of longitudinal muscle fibers starting near the base of the appendix and continuing throughout the abdominal colon to form a continuous longitudinal muscle coat in the upper rectum. Haustra are outpouchings of bowel wall separated by folds that give a classic appearance on radiography or barium enema.

The right colon is made up of the cecum (with appendix) and ascending colon. It is anterior to the right kidney and the duodenum. Its vascular supply is from branches of the superior mesenteric artery (SMA). The SMA divides into the middle colic artery and the trunk of the SMA. The middle colic artery immediately forms two to three large arcades in the transverse mesocolon. The SMA ileocolic arterial branches then extend from the SMA. The right colic artery arises as a separate branch from the SMA in 10.7% of cases.[63] The ileocolic artery gives off a right colic artery to the upper ascending colon and forms an anastomosis with branches from the middle colic artery. The ileal branch of the ileocolic artery gives off branches to the distal small bowel and cecum, whereas the colic branch supplies the ascending colon. An anastomosis occurs between the distal SMA and the ileal branch of the ileocolic artery at the junction of the terminal ileum and cecum. The right colon is a retroperitoneal structure.

The transverse colon is supplied by braches of the middle colic artery. It is the first portion of the colon considered to be intraperitoneal, and its length can vary. Its boundaries are defined by the hepatic flexure on the right and the splenic flexure on the left. Both of these points are fixed. The hepatic flexure abuts the gallbladder fossa, while the splenic flexure lies anterior to the splenic hilum and the tail of the pancreas. The descending colon is where the colon once again becomes a retroperitoneal structure, and it is defined as the segment of colon from the splenic flexure to the sigmoid colon. The descending colon is the first segment of the left side of the colon and receives its blood supply from the inferior mesenteric artery (IMA). The IMA arises from the aorta and gives off the left colic artery. It also gives off three to four sigmoidal arteries, which supply the intraperitoneal sigmoid colon. The anastomosis between the vessels of the middle colic artery and those of the left colic artery and right colic artery is known as the marginal artery of Drummond. The arcade, which effectively connects the left and right circulations, is known as the arc of Riolan. The arterial supply to the colon is depicted in Figure 89.1.

The venous and lymphatic drainage of the colon parallels the arterial supply, and all three vessels course and divide within the colonic mesocolon (Fig. 89.2). The mesocolon therefore contains the regional lymph nodes for the segment of colon it supplies and drains. The efferent lymphatic channels pass from the submucosa to the intramuscular and subserosal plexus of the bowel to the first tier of lymph nodes lying adjacent to the large intestine and known as *epicolic nodes*.[64] *Paracolic nodes* lie on the marginal vessels along the mesenteric side of the colon and are frequently involved in metastases. *Intermediate nodes* are found along the major arterial branches of the SMA and IMA in the mesocolon. The *principal nodes* are found around the origin of these vessels from the aorta, and

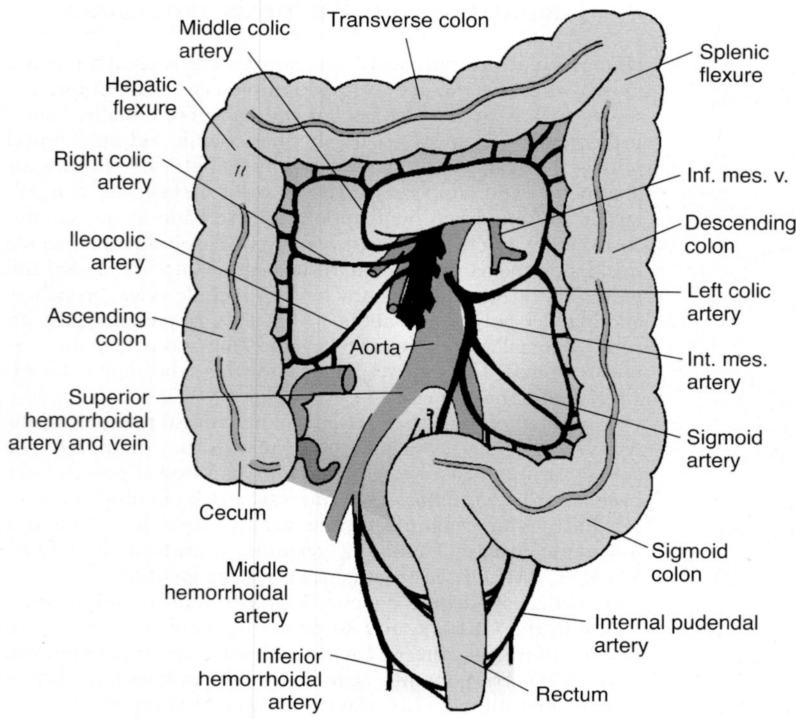

FIGURE 89.1 The anatomy of the colon with particular emphasis on the vascular supply.

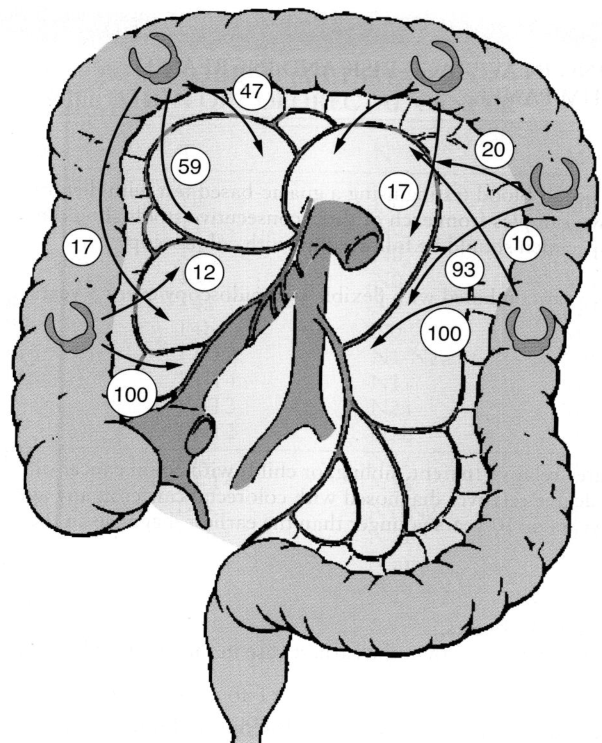

FIGURE 89.2 The lymphatic drainage of lesions in various anatomic locations throughout the colon.

they drain into retroperitoneal nodes. The drainage of the superior and inferior mesenteric veins, which drain the ascending, transverse, descending, and sigmoid colon, is to the portal vein. The rectum is drained by rectal tributaries to the vena cava.

The extent of resection of the colon is defined by the vascular supply and by the need to take the regional draining lymph nodes.[65,66] A careful understanding of the colonic anatomy, structure, location, and vascular supply is therefore critical in order to perform a safe and effective cancer operation. The segmental resections important for removal of lesions in various locations within the colon will be described in greater detail in later sections.

DIAGNOSIS OF COLORECTAL CANCER

Symptoms associated with colorectal cancer include lower gastrointestinal bleeding, change in bowel habits, abdominal pain, weight loss, change in appetite, and weakness, and in particular, obstructive symptoms are alarming.[67] However, apart from obstructive symptoms, other symptoms do not necessarily correlate with stage of disease or portend a particular diagnosis.[68]

Physical examination may reveal a palpable mass, bright blood per rectum (usually left-sided colon cancers or rectal cancer) or melena (right-sided colon cancers), or lesser degrees of bleeding (Hemoccult positive stool). Adenopathy, hepatomegaly, jaundice, or even pulmonary signs may be present with metastatic disease. Obstruction by colon cancer is usually in the sigmoid or left colon, with resulting abdominal distention and constipation; whereas right-sided colon cancers may be more insidious in nature. Complications of colorectal cancer include acute GI bleeding, acute obstruction, perforation, and metastasis with impairment of distant organ function.

Laboratory values may reflect iron-deficiency anemia, electrolyte derangements, and liver function abnormalities. The carcinoembryonic antigen (CEA) may be elevated and is most helpful to monitor postoperatively, if reduced to normal as a result of surgery.[69]

Evaluation should include complete history, family history, physical examination, and laboratory tests, colonoscopy, and pan-body computed tomography (CT) scan.[70] Upon completion of the diagnosis and staging (endoscopic ultrasound should be integrated for staging of rectal cancer), incorporation of expertise from medical, radiation, and surgical oncologists is required to formulate and implement a treatment plan.

With the advent of molecular biological techniques, attention has been drawn to stool-based tools and new blood-based tests. Technology now exists to extract genomic DNA or protein from stool and assay for evidence of genetic alterations.[71,72] Large-scale validation studies are in progress. One particularly attractive pathway for stool-based diagnostics would be able to stratify patients as high, moderate, or low risk for colorectal cancer and thus influence screening modalities and frequency of screening. In a complementary fashion, functional genomics are being applied to pair-wise comparisons of normal colon and colorectal cancers to sample the entire human genome of nearly 30,000 genes to discover those genes, known and novel, that may be up-regulated or down-regulated and possibly linked to detection, prognosis, and therapy.

SCREENING FOR COLORECTAL CANCER

Debate is vigorous as to the best approaches for screening, and multiple factors influence that decision: simplicity and rapidity so as to enhance patient compliance; benefit to risk ratio; sensitivity; specificity; and cost-effectiveness and other economic factors. To that end, currently, optical colonoscopy likely offers the most effective approach when one considers all of these factors.

The average-risk patient is defined as a man or woman above the age of 50 without personal or family history of adenomatous polyps or colorectal cancer and absence of any occult or acute GI bleeding. Screening recommendations or guidelines for average-risk and high-risk individuals are presented in Table 89.5.

Optical colonoscopy is currently the most sensitive method for screening. Advantages include direct visualization, with the ability to remove polyps (with rate-limiting factors of size and anatomic location) and to obtain biopsies. Disadvantages involve the preparation, invasive nature of the procedure, and potential side effects that include perforation (although this is less than 1%).

The digital rectal examination should be part of the general physical examination. Anorectal masses may be palpated. Flexible sigmoidoscopy does not require conscious sedation and hemodynamic monitoring and will typically allow visualization of the rectum, sigmoid colon, and descending colon to the splenic flexure. Flexible sigmoidoscopy should not be considered as a single screening measure but requires coupling with barium enema. Barium enema allows visualization of the entire colon, and experience is necessary to ensure proper visualization of the rectum. Barium enema affords advantages of ease of preparation, lack of conscious sedation and hemodynamic monitoring, and ability to visualize polyps and masses. However, small polyps may be missed. Furthermore, if a luminal polyp or mass is identified, then colonoscopy will be necessary for polypectomy or biopsies.

New noninvasive technologies are investigational but receiving attention in clinical studies, and these may provide some initial data demonstrating efficacy. These relate to CT-colonography (referred to as a *virtual colonoscopy*)[73–75]

and the resection is staged R1 (microscopic) or R2 (macroscopic). A positive CRM is highly predictive of local recurrence and should prompt consideration of adjuvant treatment.

Prognosis

Histologic Grade

Although histologic grade has been shown to have prognostic significance, there is significant subjectivity involved in scoring of this variable, and no one set of criteria for determination of grade are universally accepted.[77] The majority of staging systems divide tumors into grade 1 (well differentiated), grade 2 (moderately differentiated), grade 3 (poorly differentiated), and grade 4 (undifferentiated). Many studies collapse this into low grade (well to moderately differentiated) and high grade (poorly differentiated or undifferentiated). Greene et al.[79] demonstrated that this two-tiered split has important prognostic significance.

College of American Pathologists Consensus Statement. The College of American Pathologists (CAP) has published an expert panel consensus statement outlining their interpretation of the validity and usefulness of a large number of putatively prognostic and predictive factors in colorectal carcinoma.[80] Variables were categorized as belonging to categories I through IV. Category I was defined as those factors proven to be of prognostic import based on evidence from multiple, statistically robust, published trials and generally used in patient management. Category IIA included factors intensively studied biologically or clinically and repeatedly shown to have prognostic value for outcome or predictive value for therapy that is of sufficient import to be included in the pathology report, but that remains to be validated in statistically robust studies. Category IIB included factors shown to be promising in multiple studies but lacking sufficient data for inclusion in category I or IIA. Category III included factors felt to be not yet sufficiently studied to determine their prognostic value, and category IV includes those factors that are adequately studied to have convincingly shown no prognostic significance. A number of these factors are discussed in further detail below.

The T, N, and M categories of the current AJCC/UICC staging system were all classified as category I. Other category I inclusions were blood or lymphatic vessel invasion and residual tumor following surgery with curative intent (the R category). Although not assessed pathologically, an elevation of the preoperative CEA level was also felt to merit category I inclusion. Factors in category IIA included tumor grade, radial margin status (for resection of specimens with non peritonealized surfaces), and residual tumor in the resection specimen following neoadjuvant therapy. Factors in category IIB (many of which are discussed in further detail below) included histologic type, histologic features associated with MSI (i.e., host lymphoid response to tumor and medullary or mucinous histologic type), high degree of MSI (MSI-H), loss of heterozygosity of 18q (*DCC* [deleted in colon cancer] gene loss), and tumor border configuration (infiltrating versus pushing border). Factors grouped in category III included DNA content, all other molecular markers except for loss of heterozygosity of 18q/DCC and MSI-H, perineural invasion, microvessel density, tumor cell–associated proteins or carbohydrates, peritumoral fibrosis, peritumoral inflammatory response, focal neuroendocrine differentiation, nuclear organizing regions, and proliferation. Those factors in category IV (proven to be of no significance) included tumor size and gross tumor configuration.

Total Number of Lymph Nodes

It has been well established that an adequate number of lymph nodes must be sampled before a patient can be considered node negative. Metastases in lymph nodes may frequently be less than 5 mm in diameter, making them easy to overlook. Careful pathological technique has been demonstrated to be crucial to adequate nodal interpretation. Failure to adequately dissect and display the mesentery will lead to underreporting and understaging.[81,82] It should be noted that an insufficient number of lymph nodes reported could be due to a suboptimal nodal dissection at operation, a less than thorough search for nodes by the pathologist, or some combination of the two.

Wong et al.[82] analyzed the pathology of 196 colorectal cases and concluded that at least 14 nodes should be evaluated in each specimen in order to provide adequately reliable staging. Recently a much larger analysis was reported on outcome versus nodal sampling in the patients who participated in an Intergroup trial (INT-0089), a large four-arm trial of different fluorouracil-based adjuvant chemotherapies in colon cancer patients. Multivariate analyses were performed on the node-positive (2,768 patients) and node-negative (648 patients) groups separately. The median number of lymph nodes reported in the assessable patients on this trial was 11 (range, 1 to 87). Survival (overall, cancer-specific, and disease-free) was found to decrease with an increasing number of involved lymph nodes ($P = .0001$ for all three survival end points). However, after controlling for the number of involved nodes, survival increased with the total number of nodes (positive plus negative) reported ($P = .0001$ for overall survival, cancer-specific survival, and disease-free survival). Even in patients who were node negative, overall survival ($P = .0005$) and cancer-specific survival ($P = .007$) were significantly increased as the number of reported lymph nodes increased.

In a different secondary analysis of the Intergroup (INT-0089), a mathematical model was created to estimate the probability of a true node-negative result on the basis of the number of lymph nodes examined in a subset of patients who had at least ten lymph nodes reported in their resection specimen.[83] A total of 1,585 patients with stage III or high-risk stage II colon cancer were evaluated. This model concluded that when 18 nodes are examined, there is a less than 25% probability of true node negativity in T1 and T2 tumors. However, examination of fewer than 10 lymph nodes was needed in T3 and T4 tumors to achieve the same probability. The overall conclusions of this analysis were that a very significant proportion of patients are understaged, and that such understaging could have important implications for decisions regarding adjuvant therapy and for overall prognosis.

Tepper et al.[84] analyzed data from 1,664 patients with T3, T4, or node-positive rectal cancer treated in the national Intergroup trial INT-0114. The number of nodes reported was significantly associated with time to relapse and survival among patients who were node negative. For the first through fourth quartiles, the 5-year relapse rates were 0.37, 0.34, 0.26, and 0.19 ($P = .003$), and the 5-year survival rates were 0.68, 0.73, 0.72, and 0.82 ($P = .02$). No significant differences were found in this analysis by quartiles among patients who were node positive. The authors suggested that the differences noted were likely to be primarily related to erroneously declaring a patient node negative on the basis of insufficient analysis. These authors concluded that approximately 14 nodes need to be studied to define nodal status accurately.

The CAP consensus statement suggests that a minimum of 12 to 15 lymph nodes should be examined in order to determine node negativity.[80] Availability of fewer nodes should therefore be regarded as a relative high-risk factor in terms of prognosis and should be factored into decisions regarding adjuvant therapy.

Microscopic Nodal Metastases

The advent of improved pathologic techniques and sensitive methods such as immunohistochemistry or PCR may have an impact on the number of positive lymph nodes detected and may have important prognostic significance.[85,86] However, the prognostic value of these positive lymph nodes, which otherwise would not be detected, remains controversial. Jeffers et al.[87] evaluated lymph nodes from 77 patients who were found to have negative lymph nodes by routine examination with immunocytochemical staining for cytokeratin AE1:AE3. Nineteen patients (25%) were found to have immunohistochemical evidence of micrometastases; however, there was no difference in survival between the microscopically positive and negative patients. Of course the limited size of this analysis precludes detection of subtle differences in outcome. Although intuitively the presence of micrometastases detected by either immunohistochemical or reverse transcription-polymerase chain reaction (RT-PCR) techniques would seem to carry the prognostic risk associated with nodal positivity, to date such findings are not universally accepted as having prognostic significance, and for staging purposes nodes that harbor individual tumor cells or micrometastases are classified as being negative for tumor. It is currently recommended that tumor foci from 0.2 to 2.0 mm be classified as node positive, with an accompanying addendum stating that the biological and prognostic significance of this finding is unknown. If micrometastases are reported, the methodology by which they are detected should be specified, as it is likely that differences in reliability and reproducibility of different techniques will emerge. Although the actual TNM staging is not altered by the presence of micrometastases, many clinicians choose to regard the presence of such a finding as a poor prognostic variable in their consideration of adjuvant treatment.

Sentinel Node Analysis

Sentinel node analysis is an approach that has received attention in the management of cutaneous melanoma and breast cancer.[88,89] This technique has recently been proposed as a means of increasing the yield and the diagnostic information for colon cancer.[90,91]

The technique for sentinel node mapping and biopsy for colon cancer has been described by Saha et al.[92] Unlike sentinel node approaches for melanoma and breast, where the goal is to potentially limit the extent of an unnecessary formal dissection of a node basin, the goal of the sentinel node in colon cancer is to focus the pathologic analysis on fewer nodes so a more extensive study can be performed. The same extent of node dissection is performed regardless of the sentinel node procedure.

The initial studies of sentinel node biopsy demonstrated it was technically feasible, and in some cases, resulted in the upstaging of patients.[93,94] However, not all subsequent studies have shown equivalent results. False-negative rates as high as 60% have been reported and some studies have failed to demonstrate any change in the stage determination of the lesion.[95]

Based on the available data two conclusions can be reached. First, from a technical standpoint, sentinel node dissection at the time of a colon resection can be performed and the sentinel node accurately identified. Second, the utility of this technique has not yet been established and further large-scale trials are required to establish its role in the staging of colorectal cancer patients.

Blood or Lymphatic Vessel Invasion

Although there have been conflicting reports in the literature, the CAP consensus statement gave blood and lymphatic vessel invasion category I status, indicating that the preponderance of evidence strongly supports the reliability of these findings as indicators of poorer prognosis.[80] Unfortunately, considerable heterogeneity exists in the methodology for examining and reporting of vessel involvement. The finding of vessel involvement increases with the number of sections examined and differentiation of postcapillary venules from lymphatics is often not possible. These aspects can make interpretation of some older data on this topic potentially problematic. Current recommendations are that at least three blocks of tumor (optimally five or more) each have a single section examined using hematoxylin and eosin stain to look for tumor invasion of vessels. Vessels not definitively interpreted as venules or lymphatics should be reported as angiolymphatic vessels.

Histologic Type

Several histologic types of colorectal cancer carry specific independent prognostic significance. Signet ring carcinomas are characterized by greater than 50% of cells demonstrating the "signet ring" morphology in which intracellular mucin accumulation displaces the nuclei and cytoplasm toward the cellular periphery. This histology carries an adverse prognosis.[96,97]

The prognostic significance of the finding of mucinous (greater than 50% mucinous) carcinoma remains controversial. Although some reports list mucinous type as an adverse histology, this has not been consistently demonstrated. Most findings of adverse prognosis with mucinous histology are based on univariate analyses. The one finding in a multivariate analysis of a poor prognostic outcome with mucinous tumors was based on a study of tumors presenting with obstruction, a presentation that is in itself high-risk. Some reports have lumped mucinous and signet cell tumors together and found this to be a negative prognostic factor; however, this may simply reflect the negative impact of the signet cell tumors, and its meaning regarding the risk of a mucinous histology is unclear.

Small cell (extrapulmonary oat cell) tumors are high-grade neuroendocrine tumors with clearly adverse prognostic features. The prognostic significance of focal neuroendocrine differentiation is, however, unclear (CAP category III). Most data indicate that extensive neuroendocrine differentiation is associated with a poorer prognosis.[98]

Medullary carcinoma is a subtype characterized by an absence of glands and distinctive growth pattern that previously would have been classified as undifferentiated. It is typically infiltrated with lymphocytes. This histologic subtype is tightly associated with MSI-H and carries a more favorable prognosis.[99] Histologic types other than signet ring, small cell, and medullary carcinomas are routinely designated in the pathology report; however, the majority of these other histologic types carry no established independent prognostic significance.

Microsatellite Instability

As discussed earlier in this chapter, there are two distinct mutational pathways that can give rise to colorectal cancer: the microsatellite instability pathway or the chromosomal instability pathway. Microsatellites are sections of DNA in which a short sequence of nucleotides (most commonly a dinucleotide) is repeated multiple times.[100] MSI is a situation in which a microsatellite has gained or lost repeat units and so has undergone a change in length, resulting in frame shift mutations or base-pair substitutions. Approximately 15% of colorectal cancers display these mutations. This form of genetic destabilization is typically associated with defective DNA mismatch-repair function. Studies of HNPCC tumor specimens demonstrated mutations in mismatch repair genes such as MLH1 and MSH2. These genes encode proteins that repair nucleotide mismatches. The phenotype of tumors with this defect is termed the MSI-H-instability phenotype.

The majority (approximately 85%) of colorectal patients have cancers characteristic of the chromosomal instability pathway, typically having genetic alterations involving loss of heterozygosity (LOH), chromosomal amplifications, and chromosomal translocations. These are known as the microsatellite-stable (MSS) tumors. MSI-H tumors have a number of different features relative to low MSI (MSI-L) or MSS colorectal tumors.[101,102] MSI-L and MSS tumors tend to behave and present similarly. MSI-H tumors are more frequently right sided, high grade, and mucinous type.[21,103] They are characteristically associated with increased peritumoral lymphocytic infiltration and are characteristically diploid, while MSS tumors are more likely to be aneuploid.[104,105] MSI-H colorectal cancers are more likely to have a larger primary at the time of diagnosis but are more likely to be node negative. Patients with MSI-H colorectal cancers have a better long-term prognosis than stage-matched patients with cancers exhibiting MSS.[106]

Watanabe et al.[107] evaluated MSI status as well as allelic loss from chromosomes 18q, 17b and 8p, as well as cellular levels of p53 and p21$^{waf1/cip1}$ proteins as potential prognostic markers. Tumors were analyzed from 460 stage III and high-risk stage II patients who had been treated with fluorouracil-based adjuvant therapy. Sixty-two of 298 tumors evaluated for MSI status (21%) were found to be MSI-H. Of the MSI-H tumors, 38 (61%) had a mutation of the gene for type II receptor of transforming growth factor beta-1 (TGF-β1). In this analysis, MSI-H was a favorable prognostic indicator for 5-year disease-free survival (P = .02) and trended toward being a favorable independent prognostic indicator, but did not reach statistical significance for overall survival (P = .20). However, the 5-year survival among MSI-H patients was 74% in the presence of a mutated gene for the type II receptor of TGF-β1 and 46% in patients whose tumors lacked this mutation (relative risk 2.90; 95% CI, 1.14 to 7.34; P = .04). MSI-H cells are relatively resistant to 5-fluorourcil (5-FU) *in vitro*.[108] All of the patients in Watanabe's analysis received 5-FU-based chemotherapy. The TGF-β1 pathway inhibits tumor proliferation by causing a late G_1 cell cycle arrest. Therefore, a mutated and presumably nonfunctional *TGF-β1* gene could favor increased proliferation, which would be anticipated to confer increased susceptibility to cytotoxic chemotherapy.

Allelic Loss of 18q (*DCC* Gene Loss)

Allelic LOH that involves chromosome 18q occurs in half or more of all colorectal cancers. Allelic loss of 18q typically involves the *DCC* gene; however, other genes in this region, such as Smad2 and Smad4, may also be relevant to colorectal cancer development. DCC expression is greatly reduced or absent in many colorectal carcinomas, and loss of DCC is associated with metastasis and an adverse prognosis.[109] The specific product of the DCC gene has been shown to be the netrin-1 receptor. In the nonpathological state this receptor guides the migration of neuronal axons. DCC induces apoptosis in the absence of netrin-1 binding. DCC is cleaved by caspase, and mutation of the site at which caspase 3 cleaves DCC suppresses the proapoptotic effect of DCC completely. Binding of netrin-1 to DCC blocks apoptosis.[110] Loss of DCC as a result of allelic loss in 18q could therefore be anticipated to impair apoptosis, thereby resulting in greater resistance to chemotherapy. This hypothesized mechanism of action of 18q LOH is attractive, however, it should be emphasized that it is not at all clear to what extent DCC is the active moiety in the setting of 18q allelic loss.

Watanabe et al.[107] evaluated allelic loss from chromosome 18q as a potential prognostic indicator in archived specimens of tumors from patients who were treated in one of two national Intergroup adjuvant trials (INT 0035 or INT 0089). MSI status was also evaluated, as were 17p, 8p, and cellular levels of p53 and p21$^{waf1/cip1}$ proteins. Tumors were analyzed from 460 stage III and high-risk stage II patients who had been treated with fluorouracil-based adjuvant therapy. Allelic loss of 18q was present in 155 of 319 cancers (49%). Allelic loss in 18q was highly prognostically significant in this analysis (Table 89.7). In the stage III patients with allelic loss of 18q, 5-year overall survival was 50%, while in those with retained 18q alleles, 5-year survival was 69% (P = .005). Other markers evaluated in this analysis were not shown to be prognostically significant.

TABLE 89.7

LOSS OF HETEROZYGOSITY (ALLELIC LOSS) AT 18q AND PROGNOSIS IN PATIENTS WITH STAGE III COLON CANCER

Allelic Status of 18q	No. of Patients	5-Year Survival (%)	*P* Value
No loss	112	69	0.005
Loss	109	50	

From ref. 107.

In another series of 118 stage II and III colon cancer patients, 18q allelic loss was again shown to be an adverse indicator of prognosis. This was particularly true of the stage II patients, in whom the 5-year disease-free survival rate with chromosome 18q allelic loss was only 54%. Patients with stage II disease whose tumor had no chromosome 18q allelic loss demonstrated an excellent clinical outcome, with a 5-year disease-free survival rate of 96%. In a multivariate analysis, 18q allelic loss was a significant independent poor prognostic factor for both disease-free and overall survival.[111]

Host Lymphoid Response

Lymphocytic infiltration has been identified as a favorable prognostic indicator. Whether this is a truly independent predictor of outcome is not clear, however, since this finding is tightly associated with MSI-H, a favorable prognostic factor.

Tumor Border Configuration

The configuration of the tumor border (infiltrating versus pushing border) has been shown to have independent prognostic significance. An infiltrating border, characterized by an irregular, infiltrating pattern at the tumor edge (also known as focal dedifferentiation or tumor budding) has been shown in multivariate analyses to portend a poorer prognosis than tumors with smooth, pushing borders.

Carcinoembryonic Antigen

An elevated preoperative CEA is a poor prognostic factor for cancer recurrence. Although there is variability in the available data regarding the level that denotes a prognostic cutoff, a preoperative CEA level above 5 ng/mL is considered a category I poor prognostic indicator by the CAP consensus panel.[80] Patients in whom the elevated CEA fails to normalize after a potentially curative operation are at particularly high risk. Several authors have presented evidence that indicates that CEA is an independent prognostic factor. In a report of 572 patients who underwent curative resection for node-negative colon cancer the preoperative CEA level and the stage of disease predicted survival by both univariate and multivariate analyses.[112] Given the prognostic significance of the preoperative CEA, it is reasonable to recommend that all patients who undergo operation for colorectal cancer have a serum CEA drawn prior to operation.

No other serum markers have been demonstrated to be reliably prognostic or predictive in colorectal cancer. CA 19-9, a factor that has become widely used for pancreas cancer, has no role at this time in the routine management of colorectal cancer.

Obstruction and Perforation

Carcinoma of the colon that is complicated by obstruction or perforation has been recognized as having a poorer prognosis. Data obtained from 1,021 patients with Dukes stage B and C colorectal cancer, who were entered into randomized clinical trials of the National Surgical Adjuvant Breast and Bowel Project (NSABP) showed that the presence of bowel obstruction strongly influenced the outcome. The effect of bowel obstruction was more pronounced when the obstruction was located in the right colon. The larger-sized tumor needed to block the ascending colon completely might allow a longer time for these tumors to grow and spread when compared with tumors located in the descending colon.

A review of the Massachusetts General Hospital records compared patients who presented with obstruction or perforation with a control group who underwent curative resection. The actuarial 5-year survival rate seen in patients who present with obstruction was 31%, in contrast to 59% in historical controls. For patients with localized perforation, the 5-year actuarial survival rate was 44%. The Gastrointestinal Tumor Study Group (GITSG) multivariate analysis concluded that obstruction was an important indicator of prognosis, independent of Dukes stage. Bowel perforation was a poor prognostic factor only for disease-free survival.

Category III Factors

Multiple factors, while of investigational interest, are at this time not appropriate for routine clinical use and have so been designated as category III (defined as not sufficiently studied to prove their prognostic value) by the CAP consensus panel. These include DNA content, or ploidy, and proliferation indices. Also included in category III are all molecular markers other than MSI and 18q deletions, such as thymidylate synthase (TS), dihydropyrimidine dehydrogenase (DPD), and p53 mutational status. Perineural invasion, microvessel density, tumor cell–associated proteins or carbohydrates, peritumoral fibrosis, peritumoral inflammatory response, and focal neuroendocrine differentiation are also category III. The area of molecular prognostic markers is one of particular activity, however, and it is anticipated that clinical trials that are now ongoing will shed light on these important areas.

Perineural Invasion

The ability of colorectal cancers to invade perineural spaces as far as 10 cm from the primary tumor has long been described. Early reports suggest an increased disease recurrence rate and worse 5-year survival. Multivariate analyses have failed to show the prognostic significance of this finding. The CAP consensus panel classified perineural invasion as category III (insufficient evidence of determine prognostic significance).

Tumor Size and Configuration

Studies have consistently shown that both the size and configuration of the primary tumor in colorectal cancer do not carry prognostic significance (CAP category IV). In a review of 391 patients, the mean diameter of Dukes stage B2 tumors was actually greater than the mean diameter of stage C2 tumors ($P < .001$) and D tumors ($P < .05$). The size of the primary tumor showed no relationship to 5-year adjusted survival. These results were confirmed by the NSABP experience.[113] Tumor configuration is described as exophytic (fungating), endophytic (ulcerative), diffusely infiltrative (linitis plastica), or annular. The vast majority of studies have failed to show any of these configurations to have consistent independent prognostic significance. Linitis plastica has been related to a poor prognosis; however, this may be due to the signet cell and other high-grade features of the tumors that are typically associated with this morphology.

Hemorrhage or Rectal Bleeding

It has been speculated that tumors that present with bleeding might be found earlier and therefore might be associated with a better prognosis. This has not been confirmed by data. In the GITSG multivariate analysis, the presence of melena or rectal bleeding showed a trend as a prognostic factor for prolonged survival but failed to reach statistical significance ($P = .08$). One large study found bleeding to be a favorable prognostic indicator on univariate analysis; however, this finding disappeared on multivariate analysis. Bleeding at presentation does not appear to carry any significance.

Primary Tumor Location

Large retrospective reviews of data from the NSABP suggest that right-sided colon cancers carry a worse prognosis than left-sided ones. However, poorer prognosis for patients with disease in the left colon has also been reported. Several investigators report no difference based on the location of the primary tumor. The large GITSG colon cancer experience showed that tumor location (left, right, and rectosigmoid or sigmoid) was of low prognostic value.

Body Mass Index

Obesity is known to be a risk factor for the development of colon cancer. Influence of body mass index (BMI) on long-term outcomes and treatment-related toxicity was investigated in a group of colon cancer patients. A cohort study was conducted within a large randomized trial of 3,759 men and women with high-risk stage II or III colon cancer (INT-0089). Obese women with colon carcinoma had significantly worse overall mortality (hazard ratio [HR] 1.34; 95% CI, 1.07 to 1.67); BMI was not, however, related to long-term outcomes in men in this cohort. In both men and women, obese patients had significantly lower rates of grade 3 and 4 leucopenia and lower rates of any grade 3 or greater toxicity in comparison with those patients in normal weight categories.

Diabetes Mellitus

The same population of patients was studied to determine the influence of diabetes mellitus on outcome.[114] At 5 years, patients with diabetes mellitus compared with patients without diabetes mellitus experienced a significantly worse disease-free survival (48% vs. 59%; $P < .0001$). Overall survival was also worse for diabetic patients (57% vs. 66%; $P < .0001$) and recurrence-free survival was also worse (56% vs. 64%; $P = .012$). Median survival for diabetics was 6.0 years, while for nondiabetics it was 11.3 years.

Blood Transfusions

Considerable controversy has surrounded the question of an association between perioperative blood transfusions and the recurrence rate of colorectal cancer. Some investigators have reported worse disease-free survival in patients who require transfusions. By multivariate analysis in a large prospective study, however, no negative influence of transfusion on survival could be detected, and it does not appear that perioperative blood transfusions carry negative prognostic value. A retrospective analysis evaluating 1,051 patients treated with curative surgery for stage II or III colorectal adenocarcinoma at the Mayo Clinic demonstrated that the use of blood components probably had no impact on disease recurrence, and the documented adverse impact of transfusions is more likely due to other variables or to the underlying illness necessitating the transfusion.[115]

Oncogenes and Molecular Markers

Oncogenes and molecular markers are discussed extensively in another chapter. At present none of the markers under investigation has achieved adequate validity to permit routine clinical use. However, the study of molecular markers continues to progress and continues to advanced the understanding of the development and treatment of colorectal cancer.

TS continues to be a major area of investigation. Data are conflicting on its prognostic significance, however, preliminary studies suggest that high TS levels may be predictive for resistance to 5-FU-based therapies.[116] At present there is no role for TS determinations in routine clinical practice.

The *p53* gene located on chromosome 17p is a well-known tumor suppressor gene. The abnormal *p53* appears to be a late phenomenon in colorectal carcinogenesis. This mutation may allow the growing tumor with multiple genetic alterations to evade cell cycle arrest and apoptosis. In a retrospective review of 141 patients with resected stage II and III colon carcinoma, a *p53* mutation increased the risk of death by 2.82 times in patients with stage II disease and by 2.39 times in patients with stage III colon carcinoma. The Southwest Oncology Group (SWOG) assessed the prognostic value of p53 in 66 stage II and 163 stage III colon cancer patients. *p53* expression was found in 63% of cancers and was associated with favorable survival in stage III but not stage II disease. Seven-year survival with stage III disease was 56% with *p53* expression versus 43% with no *p53* expression ($P = .012$).[117] Overall, the data are conflicting on the utility of P53 as a prognostic variable, and it does not have a use at this time in standard practice.

Genetic Polymorphisms

Extensive preliminary work is indicating that genetic polymorphisms can potentially have important predictive implications in terms of both efficacy and toxicity with chemotherapy. For example, the UGT1A1 polymorphism has been correlated with CPT-11 toxicity, and TS and XRCC1 polymorphisms may predict efficacy for oxaliplatin or fluorouracil combinations.[118] Although a commercial assay is currently available for measurement of UGT1A1 polymorphisms, it is not, at this time, clear how, or if, this assay should be used in routine practice. Currently there are no specific guidelines for dose modifications on the basis of UGT1A1polymorphism, and the 7/7 mutation, associated with higher toxicity, has also been associated with greater antitumor activity. These approaches will require considerable more validation and exploration before they can be considered for standard management.[119]

APPROACHES TO SURGICAL RESECTION OF COLON CANCER

The management of colon cancer is best understood as a multimodality approach tailored to the stage of disease. However, there are certain basic tenets of surgical management for the resection of the primary lesion that can be applied across various pathologic stages. Therefore, in order to provide a clear description of these techniques they will first be described based on the type of surgical resection. These procedures will then be referred to throughout the discussion of stage specific treatment.

Colonoscopic Resection of Polyps

Many lesions of the colon are first detected during endoscopic procedures. These lesions can range from small hyperplastic polyps to large fungating invasive carcinomas. The appearance of these lesions often indicates their relative potential for malignancy. However, the only definitive way to make a diagnosis is through a pathologic examination of the tissue. Therefore, the goal of a colonoscopic biopsy or resection is to, whenever feasible, remove the lesion in its entirety and preserve a tissue architecture in order to achieve both a therapeutic resection and an accurate pathologic diagnosis. Various techniques can be employed for the removal of lesions in the colon depending on their size and location. Biopsy forceps and snares are the two most commonly employed instruments used during a colonoscopy. These devises are fashioned from flexible coated wires that can conform to the shape of the colonoscope and can also conduct bipolar electrical current in order to achieve coagulation and hemostasis.

Small polypoid lesions that are found during the course of a colonoscopic examination can often be removed in their entirety along with a small amount of normal mucosa using a biopsy forceps. Small amounts of bleeding can be controlled with bipolar electric cording. This is important, as bipolar cautery will avoid deep tissue injury that may put the patient at risk for colonic perforation or bleeding. Bleeding and perforation, while uncommon, are seen at an increased frequency during a therapeutic as opposed to a diagnostic colonoscopy.[120,121] Small polyps up to 5 to 8 mm in size can be removed very easily with these techniques. Larger well-pedunculated polyps can often be removed using a technique employing a snare and electrocautery. The snare is placed over the polypoid lesion and cinched down at the base of the polyp. Once tightened, an electrical current is applied and the polyp is resected. These polypoid lesions are often too large to be retrieved through the working port of the colonoscope and therefore are held in place with a snare just beyond the tip of the colonoscope where they can be kept in view and are then withdrawn with the scope from the patient. It is important, when sending these specimens to pathology, to properly orient the polyp so as to indicate the base where the resection took place as well as the other positions of the lesion. This will allow the pathologist to provide important information as to the margin status for the resection. Carcinoma *in situ* as well as stage I invasive carcinomas found in a well-pedunculated polyp can be treated with colonoscopic resection, as described above, and no further surgical management is needed as long as the margin of the invasive carcinoma can clearly be seen to be away from the electrocautery artifact at the base of the polyp. If this distinction cannot be clearly made, further therapy is required. It is for this reason that it is often helpful to mark the site of the polyp resection with an agent that will leave a "tattoo" at the point of resection.

Larger lesions with a broad base or sessile lesions are best biopsied to make a diagnosis rather than resected using the colonoscope. The risk of perforation or inadequate resection margins is greatly increased with broad-based and sessile lesions. Multiple biopsies should be taken in order to determine whether the lesion harbors an invasive cancer, and further resection decisions are made based on the pathologic findings. If such a lesion is left behind it is of critical importance to note the position of the lesion in order that it might be more easily found if the subsequent procedure is required. In addition to a determination of the depth of insertion of the scope, other landmarks should be utilized in order to more precisely pinpoint the lesion's location. Landmarks such as haustra, the appendiceal orifice or ileocecal valve in the cecum, or positions within the sigmoid loop can be especially helpful given the inaccuracies of a length measurement using a flexible instrument. In rare cases fluoroscopy can be used to precisely pinpoint the tip of the scope in relationship to its position within the colon.[122]

For lesions that cannot be resected through the scope or are found to be invasive carcinomas that are sessile or broad based, a variety of surgical resections can be employed depending on the position of the lesion and its T stage. It is important to keep in mind, however, that the formal staging of the lesion does not occur until after the resection is completed; therefore, if there is suspicion of an invasive carcinoma being present, a definitive oncologic resection should be performed.

For large polyps that are benign on biopsy but too large to resect through the scope a simple segmental resection can be performed at the time of an abdominal exploration. Typically, the polyp is located based on the preoperative colonoscopy reports and by careful palpation of the entire colon from the cecum to the peritoneal reflection. Once the lesion is palpated a small colotomy can be performed opposite the base of the lesion to confirm that the lesion is indeed the polyp that had been noted preoperatively. A resection encompassing 5 cm on either side of the polyp can then be easily accomplished without the need to isolate major vessels, removing just the portion of mesentery that supplies that segment of colon. A primary anastomosis can be performed using the surgeon's technique of choice. Discussion of hand-sewn versus stapled anastomoses have been extensively described elsewhere.[123]

Bowel Preparation

An important part of the preoperative regimen for a colon resection is the proper cleansing of the bowel in order to reduce the risk of postoperative complications as well as to allow for easier visualization during the procedure. A variety of regimens have been described and there are many that have demonstrated efficacy.[124,125] Although there are several choices described in the literature, the basic components of a bowel preparation are a mechanical cleansing of the bowel using a cathartic or volume-displacing agent and appropriate antibiotics both intraluminal as well as intravenously administered.[126,127] Recently, some studies have suggested that mechanical bowel preparation may be unnecessary; however, this remains controversial.[128,129]

Anatomic Resection

For invasive carcinomas of the colon, stages I through III, the surgical approach will be dictated by the lesions' size and location in the colon.[130,131] The location will determine what region of bowel is removed and the extent of its resection dictated by its vascular and lymphatic supply.

Resection of the Right Colon

Lesions in the cecum and ascending colon are managed with a right hemicolectomy (Fig. 89.3*A*,*B*). The right colon is mobilized from the retroperitoneum by incising its retroperitoneal attachments, taking care to avoid injury to the ureter, inferior vena cava, duodenum, and gonadal vessels. The colon is mobilized from the ileum to the transverse colon, taking care at the hepatic flexure not to injure the gallbladder or duodenum. The ileocolic, right colic, and right branch of middle colic vessels are then ligated and divided. A proximal ligation in order to allow for the removal of colonic mesentery along with lymph nodes is performed for staging purposes. Once the vascular supply is divided and the intervening mesenteric tissue ligated and divided, attention can be addressed to the resection of the colonic tissue.

There are a variety of techniques for dividing the colon. This can be done between clamps using scalpel or using a variety of stapling devices. One method would be to use a linear gastrointestinal anastigmatic (GIA) stapler. After making a small hole just below the colonic wall though the mesentery at the point chosen for resection, the stapler can be positioned across the colon and fired, thus dividing the tissue. This is then repeated across the ileum just proximal to the ileocecal valve. Once divided, all remaining mesenteric tissue is carefully ligated and divided and the colonic specimen can be removed. Although a no-touch "technique" has been advocated in the past, studies have demonstrated that this has no influence on recurrence or seeding of distant disease.[132] Once the right colon has been removed, intestinal continuity can be re-established by creating an anastomosis between the terminal ileum and the remaining transverse colon using either a hand-sewn or stapled technique.

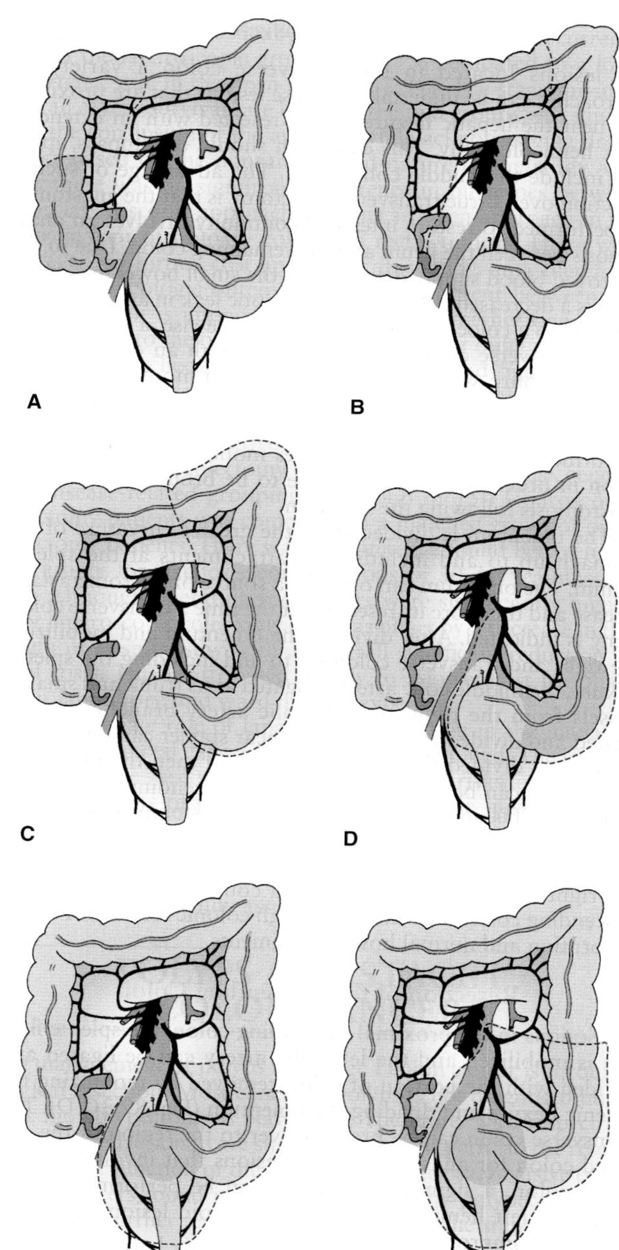

FIGURE 89.3 **A:** Surgical resection for a cecal or ascending colon cancer. **B:** Surgical resection for a cancer at the hepatic flexure. **C:** Surgical resection for a descending colon cancer. **D:** Preferred surgical procedure for cancer of the middle and proximal sigmoid colon. In poor-risk patients, the inferior mesenteric artery and the left colic artery may be preserved. **E:** Surgical resection for cancer of the rectosigmoid. **F:** A more radical surgical resection for cancer of the rectosigmoid. (Modified from Enker WE. Surgical treatment of large bowel cancer. In: Enker WE, ed. *Cancer of the colon and rectum*. Chicago: Year Book, 1978:73.)

PRACTICE OF ONCOLOGY

of anticancer agents that were available at that time. Many of these agents are now known to have no meaningful activity in metastatic colorectal cancer, and thus would not be studied in the adjuvant setting today.

The adjuvant trials of the 1950s through the mid-1980s tended to be small by current standards. Based perhaps on an unrealistically optimistic expectation of what magnitude of benefit might be achieved from the use of available chemotherapies, the size of the trials did not allow evaluation of more modest clinical benefits. A large meta-analysis of controlled randomized trials of adjuvant therapy published through 1986 indicated a nonsignificant trend toward an overall survival benefit, with a mortality odds ratio of 0.83 in favor of therapy (95% CI, 0.70 to 0.98).[151] This sobering analysis suggested that substantially larger trials would be needed to detect the modest advantages that available chemotherapies might afford.

Large-Scale Randomized Trials

The large-scale fluorouracil trials have been well summarized previously, and the reader who is interested in the details is referred to subject-relevant chapters in the previous edition of this book.[152] The outcome of numerous trials performed largely in the 1990s can be briefly summarized as follows. Trials comparing 5-FU-based therapy to surgery only demonstrated a clear benefit in terms of 5-year disease-free survival (essentially, an increased cure rate) for stage III patients who received chemotherapy.[153,154] Six months of chemotherapy was sufficient, and no further benefit was provided by extending treatment to either 9 or 12 months. Levamisole, an agent initially thought to be active, was, in fact inactive, and high-dose leucovorin did not confer superior efficacy over low-dose leucovorin, so comparisons of various 5-FU/leucovorin schedules did not demonstrate clear superiority of one schedule over the other in terms of efficacy. However, the Mayo Clinic daily times five schedule was substantially more toxic than either weekly bolus of biweekly infusion schedules. Alfa interferon conferred substantial toxicity and provided no benefit.[155–159]

Oral Fluoropyrimidine Therapies

Oral administration of fluorouracil proved to be problematic secondary to erratic bioavailability. This was likely due in large part to variable effects of DPD, the rate-limiting enzyme in catabolism of fluorouracil, on the first pass clearance of oral fluorouracil by the liver. Two oral 5-FU prodrugs, capecitabine and uracil/tegafur (UFT), have demonstrated efficacy in metastatic disease that is comparable to the Mayo Clinic schedule of parenteral 5-FU/leucovorin. Both of these agents have now been studied in the adjuvant setting in comparison to the now defunct Mayo Clinic 5-FU schedule. In a study designed to assess for noninferiority in 3-year disease-free survival, Twelves et al.[160] randomly assigned 1,987 resected stage III colon cancer patients to receive either oral capecitabine (1,004 patients) or Mayo Clinic bolus 5-FU plus leucovorin (983 patients). Each treatment was planned for 24 weeks. Disease-free survival in the capecitabine group was at least equivalent to that in the fluorouracil-plus-leucovorin group (in the intention-to-treat analysis [$P<.001$] for the comparison of the upper limit of the hazard ratio with the noninferiority margin of 1.20), and capecitabine resulted in significantly fewer adverse events than Mayo Clinic bolus 5-FU/leucovorin ($P<.001$). Overall, this trial demonstrates that capecitabine is a reasonable alternative to intravenous fluorouracil plus leucovorin in the adjuvant treatment of colon cancer in reliable, motivated patients who are able to comply with a complex schedule of oral medication. However, as discussed below, 5-FU/leucovorin alone is no longer the standard postsurgical adjuvant treatment for colon cancer. As such, the role of single-agent capecitabine in the adjuvant management of resected colon cancer remains limited at this time. Data supporting its use with concurrent intravenous oxaliplatin are discussed below.

The NSABP C-06 trial assessed the use of oral UFT plus oral leucovorin in the treatment of stage II and III colon cancer.[161] A total of 1,608 patients with stage II (47%) and stage III (53%) colon cancer were randomly assigned to receive either oral UFT with leucovorin or intravenous 5-FU with leucovorin. With a median follow-up of 62.3 months, there were no significant differences in disease-free or overall survival between the treatment groups. Toxicity and primary quality of life end points were similar in the two groups. As such, similar to the situation with capecitabine, the combination of oral UFT with leucovorin is an acceptable alternative to parenteral 5-FU/leucovorin, however, use of fluoropyrimidine plus leucovorin alone is no longer routine standard practice (see below) in the adjuvant treatment of at least stage III disease. Furthermore, UFT is not commercially available in the United States.

Combination Adjuvant Therapies

Clinical trials in the metastatic setting have established the antitumor activity of combinations of agents, including irinotecan, oxaliplatin, bevacizumab, cetuximab, and panitumumab (see discussion of treatment of metastatic disease below for more details). Although it had been assumed that activity in the metastatic setting would translate into an increased cure rate in the adjuvant setting, this assumption has turned out to be overly simplistic and often untrue. Of the agents listed above, only the addition of oxaliplatin to fluoropyrimidines has resulted in benefit in the adjuvant setting.

Oxaliplatin

Oxaliplatin plus biweekly infusional 5-FU/leucovorin was first evaluated in the adjuvant setting in the Multicenter International Study of Oxaliplatin/5-Fluorouracil/Leucovorin in the Adjuvant Treatment of Colon Cancer (MOSAIC) trial.[162] The results of this trial are summarized in Table 89.8. A total of 2,246 stage II and III patients were randomized to the LV/5-FU2 regimen, a biweekly infusional and bolus 5-FU/leucovorin regimen that has been demonstrated to have comparable efficacy to the Mayo Clinic daily times five bolus schedule in the adjuvant setting, or to the FOLFOX-4 regimen, which is LV/5-FU2 plus oxaliplatin on day 1.[155] The arms were well balanced for prognostic variables. For the combined stage II and III study population, the 5-year disease-free survival rates were 73.3% and 67.4% in the FOLFOX-4 and LV/5-FU2 groups, respectively (HR 0.80; 95% CI, 0.68 to 0.93; $P = .003$).[163] Six-year overall survival rates were statistically significantly improved by 2.5% (78.5% vs. 76.0% in the FOLFOX-4 and LV/5-FU2 groups, respectively; HR 0.84; 95% CI, 0.71 to 1.00; $P = .046$). For the stage III population, the 6-year overall survival rates were improved by 4.2% (72.9% vs. 68.7%, respectively; HR 0.80; 95% CI, 0.65 to 0.97; $P = .023$), while for the stage II population, the addition of oxaliplatin conferred no survival benefit (6-year survival 85.0% and 83.3%, respectively; $P = .65$). The toxicity of the FOLFOX-4 regimen was manageable but greater than that seen in the control arm, with 41% grade 3 or 4 neutropenia versus 5%, and 11% grade 3 or 4 diarrhea versus 7%. All-cause mortality in the first 60 days was 0.5% in each arm. Peripheral sensory neuropathy, a toxicity not present in the 5-FU/LV2 control arm, was a frequent occurrence on the FOLFOX-4 arm. Grade 2 neuropathy was reported in 32% of the patients, and grade 3 occurred in 12%. In some cases the duration of the neuropathy was substantial. One year after

TABLE 89.8

RESULTS OF THE MOSAIC TRIAL: BIWEEKLY INFUSIONAL 5 FU/LEUCOVORIN (LV5FU2) VERSUS LV5FU2 PLUS OXALIPLATIN (FOLFOX-4) IN PATIENTS WITH STAGE II AND III COLON CANCER

	FOLFOX (%)	5FULV2 (%)	*P* Value
5-year disease-free survival (stage II+III)	73.3	67.4	.003
6-year overall survival (stage II+III)	78.5	76.0	.046
6-year overall survival (stage III only)	72.9	68.7	.023
6-year overall survival (stage II only)	85	83.3	.65
Grade 3–4 neutropenia	41	5	
Grade 3–4 diarrhea	11	7	
Grade 3 neuropathy	12	0	
Grade 2 neuropathy	32	0	

completion of therapy, 27% of patients still experienced some grade of neuropathy (4% grade 2 and 1.3% grade 3). Four years after completion of therapy, 11% still had some degree of neuropathy, and 0.7% still had grade 3 neuropathy. It is reasonable to assume that the toxicity still present at 4 years out from the last treatment is essentially permanent.

Oxaliplatin has also been combined with a weekly bolus fluorouracil regimen in an adjuvant trial. The NSABP C-07 trial studied the FLOX regimen of oxaliplatin given on weeks 1, 3, and 5 plus weekly bolus 5-FU/leucovorin on weeks 1 through 6, repeated at 8-week cycles, versus the standard weekly Roswell Park regimen of 5-FU/leucovorin.[164] In this trial, 1,207 patients were randomized to FLOX and 1,200 to 5-FU/leucovorin. Twenty-nine percent of patients had stage II disease and 71% had stage III colon cancer. The median follow-up was 34 months. The hazard ratio of FLOX versus 5-FU/leucovorin was 0.79 (95% CI, (0.67 to 0.93), with a 21% risk reduction in favor of FLOX. Grade 3 neurotoxicity was reported in 8% of patients on FLOX and 1% on 5-FU/leucovorin. There were 15 deaths on treatment with FLOX and 14 deaths on 5-FU/leucovorin.

More recently, an evaluation of capecitabine plus oxaliplatin (Cape/Ox) versus bolus 5-FU/leucovorin in the adjuvant setting has been reported. A safety analysis comparing the 938 patients who received Cape/Ox to the 926 who received 5-FU/leucovorin showed similar overall rates of treatment-related adverse events in the two treatment arms, but with different toxicity patterns; patients who received Cape/Ox experienced less diarrhea and alopecia, but more sensory neuropathy, vomiting, and hand-foot syndrome than those who received 5-FU/leucovorin.[165] In the efficacy analysis, reported in abstract form only at the time of this writing, the Cape/Ox arm shows a 4% improvement in 3-year disease-free survival (71% vs. 67%; HR 0.80; *P* = .0045).[166] Overall survival data are not yet mature.

The efficacy results of the FOLFOX, FLOX, and Cape/Ox studies appear more similar than different at this point in time and appear to justify interchangeability of these regimens in the adjuvant setting, although data for FLOX and Cape/Ox are somewhat less mature. The higher degree of severe and life-threatening diarrhea seen with FLOX would appear to be a potential reason for favoring FOLFOX over FLOX, although in the absence of a head-to-head comparison, the relative safety and efficacy when comparing one or these regimens to the other is impossible to know with certainty. The Cape/Ox regimen is a reasonable consideration in highly reliable, motivated patients who can be expected to comply with taking multiple pills of capecitabine orally (typically three to five pills, twice daily) for 2 weeks on, 1 week off, in the setting of concurrent emetogenic intravenous chemotherapy.

Irinotecan

Based on improved overall survival in the first- and second-line metastatic settings, it was widely assumed that irinotecan would be beneficial to patients in the adjuvant setting.[167–169] This assumption has turned out to be incorrect, however, and the results of the adjuvant trials with this agent underscore the importance of both performing trials in the adjuvant setting and waiting for the results of those trials before adopting changes in practice.

The Cancer and Leukemia Group B (CALGB) studied the weekly schedule of irinotecan plus bolus fluorouracil and leucovorin (IFL). Early safety analysis of this trial identified an alarming elevation in early mortality for the experimental arm on this trial, with 18 deaths within the first 4 months of treatment on the IFL arm versus 6 deaths within the same time period on the control arm (*P* = .008).[170] At a median follow-up of 2.1 years in each arm, futility boundaries for both disease-free and overall survival had been crossed; thus the final result of this trial is that the addition of irinotecan provided no benefit, while increasing toxicity, including lethal toxicity.[171]

Results of adding irinotecan to biweekly infusional 5-FU/leucovorin (5-FU/LV2 vs. FOLFIRI) were also negative. In the ACCORD 02 trial, 400 patients with high-risk stage III disease (defined as four or more positive nodes or perforated or obstructed primary tumors) were randomly assigned to 5-FU/LV2 versus FOLFIRI. In this high-risk population, there was no benefit seen in the FOLFIRI group, and in fact the study trended insignificantly in favor of the non-irinotecan-containing arm (3-year disease-free survival 60% for 5-FU/LV2 vs. 51% for FOLFIRI).[172]

A second, larger trial of 5-FULV2 versus FOLFIRI was conducted by the PETACC-3 investigators.[173] The prespecified primary efficacy analysis of this trial was based on the 2,094 patients with stage III disease. At a median follow-up of 6.5 years, there was no statistically significant difference in the 5-year disease-free survival (56.7% vs. 54.3% for FOLFIRI vs. 5-FU/LV2, respectively; *P* = .1) or in 5-year overall survival (73.6% vs. 71.3%, respectively; *P* = .94). FOLFIRI was associated with an increased incidence of grade 3 or 4 gastrointestinal events and neutropenia.

Taken together, the results of these three trials to evaluate irinotecan in the adjuvant setting clearly establish that despite having substantial activity in the metastatic setting, irinotecan has no meaningful activity, and no role, in the adjuvant treatment of colon cancer. Of interest, an analysis from the CALGB trial suggested that patients with MSI-H showed a benefit from inclusion of irinotecan in their adjuvant treatment, however, a similar, substantially larger analysis from the PETACC-3 trial contradicted this and showed no benefit from adding irinotecan in MSI-H patients.[174,175]

Bevacizumab

As detailed below, bevacizumab has demonstrated the ability to favorably augment standard chemotherapy for metastatic disease and has become a part of standard management in that arena. This led to evaluation of this agent in the adjuvant setting. In the NSABP C-08 trial, 2,672 patients, 25% with stage II and 755 with stage III colon cancer, were randomized to receive modified FOLFOX-6, either alone or with bevacizumab.[176] In a design imbalance that could have been problematic had this been a positive trial, the FOLFOX was given for 6 months in each arm, while the bevacizumab was given both with the FOLFOX and then for an additional 6 months, for a total of 1 year of bevacizumab. The prespecified primary end point of the trial was 3-year disease-free survival, and this end point was not met, with a hazard ratio for FOLFOX plus bevacizumab versus FOLFOX alone of 0.89 (95% CI, 0.76 to 1.04; $P = .15$). There was a separation between the curves at the 1-year mark, however, this began to diminish a few months later and was all but absent by year 3. This finding suggests that bevacizumab did delay progression of micrometastases in some patients, but only for as long as it was continued. Bevacizumab did not contribute to the eradication of micrometastases and thus did not improve the cure rate in the adjuvant setting. Although some might choose to interpret these data to suggest that if bevacizumab were continued indefinitely, an improved survival *might* be seen, the long-term consequences of lifelong suppression of vascular endothelial growth factor, as well as the psychological, social, and economic considerations involved, render such an approach inappropriate, especially considering that only a very small percentage of patients so treated would actually have the potential to benefit, if there is a benefit. Thus, the available evidence suggests that bevacizumab is not beneficial in the treatment of colon cancer in the adjuvant setting, and until and unless data to the contrary emerge, bevacizumab should not be used in the nonresearch adjuvant treatment of stage II and III colon cancer.

Cetuximab

As outlined in detail below, cetuximab has demonstrated clinical activity in metastatic colorectal cancer, prompting investigation of its usefulness in the adjuvant setting. Intergroup trial N0147 randomized patients with stage III colon cancer to modified FOLFOX-6 with or without cetuximab. Once investigators became aware that the study included only patients whose tumors lacked mutations in the *KRAS* gene (see below), the study was modified to obtain KRAS genotyping on all patients and to only enroll those with wild type KRAS. At the time of this writing, the data from this trial have not been publically presented. However, the data safety monitoring committee for the trial has halted the trial and informed investigators that the trial shows no benefit for any subgroup of patients analyzed, with increased toxicity in the cetuximab-containing arm. Thus cetuximab too has failed to show activity in stage III colon cancer, even in patients with KRAS wild type tumors, and therefore cetuximab should not be used in adjuvant treatment outside of a research setting.

Panitumumab

Panitumumab, like cetuximab, is a monoclonal antibody that blocks ligand binding to the epidermal growth factor receptor (EGFR). Although no investigations have been reported to evaluate panitumumab in the adjuvant setting, results in the metastatic setting suggest that panitumumab and cetuximab are extremely similar in terms of target, mechanism of action, mechanisms of resistance, and clinical activity. It is therefore extremely unlikely that these agents would differ in the adjuvant setting, and statements regarding cetuximab in this setting may be reasonably applied to panitumumab.

TREATMENT OF STAGE II PATIENTS

The optimal management of stage II colon cancer patients remains undefined. Although the role of adjuvant therapy in stage II colon cancer patients has not been firmly established, it is interesting to see what practice patterns have been emerging. Using the Surveillance, Epidemiology, and End Results (SEER)-Medicare linked database, Schrag et al. identified 3,151 patients age 65 to 75 with resected stage II colon cancer and no adverse prognostic features. Using Medicare billing records, they identified those patients who did or did not receive chemotherapy within 3 months of operation. Their review identified that 27% of patients received chemotherapy during the 3-month postoperative period. Younger age, white race, unfavorable tumor grade, and low comorbidity were associated with a greater likelihood of receiving treatment. The 5-year survival was 75% for untreated patients and 78% for those patients who received therapy in this nonrandomized comparison. After adjusting for known between-group differences, the hazard ratio for survival associated with adjuvant treatment was 0.91 (95% CI, 0.77 to 1.09). Thus, despite the lack of proven benefit, a substantial percentage of Medicare beneficiaries have received adjuvant chemotherapy for stage II disease.

Because stage II patients as a group have a relatively favorable prognosis, benefits from treatment could only be expected if either a highly efficacious therapy were used or if extremely large trials were done to detect very subtle differences. The International Multicentre Pooled Analysis of B2 Colon Cancer Trials (IMPACT) meta-analysis provides one of the largest samples of stage II patients.[177] A total of 1,016 stage II patients were randomized between 5-FU/leucovorin and surgery alone. The surgery-only arm had a long-term overall survival rate of 81% versus 83% for those stage II patients who received adjuvant 5-FU/leucovorin. This absolute difference of 2% closely approached, but did not reach, statistical significance.

The NSABP reported a pooled analysis of the CO-1, CO-2, CO-3, and CO-4 trials. These trials do not lend themselves well for combination in a meta-analysis. Different regimens were used in the arms of the studies that were combined, and not all of the trials contained a surgery-alone arm. The analysis concluded that a statistically significant benefit for treatment was obtained for stage II patients who received therapy; however, the methodological flaws in the analysis limit its interpretability.

More recently the QUASAR group reported their results in 3,239 patients, 91% of whom had stage II disease and 71% of whom had colon, as opposed to rectal, cancer. Patients were randomly assigned to receive 5-FU and leucovorin ($n = 1,622$) or observation.[178] The relative risk of death from any cause with 5-FU/leucovorin versus observation was 0.82 (95% CI, 0.70 to 0.95; $P = .008$), and the relative risk of recurrence was 0.78 (95% CI, 0.67 to 0.91; $P = .001$). This relative risk of death translates into an absolute improvement in survival of 3.6% (95% CI, 1.0 to 6.0). It should be noted that high- versus low-risk individuals were not separated in this report, so, as with many other large trials, the impact of chemotherapy on patients with favorable risk stage II disease is difficult to ascertain.

Several prognostic indicators have been identified that correlate with a higher risk for subsequent failure in stage II patients. These include obstruction or perforation of the bowel wall as well as other less-established risk factors, such as elevated preoperative or postoperative CEA, poorly differentiated histology, and tumors not demonstrating high levels of MSI, or an 18q deletion in colorectal tumors, which may correlate with a poor prognosis.[107,179–181] It appears that stage II patients with one or more of these risk factors have a poorer prognosis, one closer to patients with stage III disease. Whether adjuvant chemotherapy can provide similar benefits in these patients as it does in stage III patients remains a matter of conjecture, and in the absence of definitive data, definitive recommendations on this topic cannot be made at this time. In fully informed high-risk stage II patients it is reasonable to consider adjuvant treatment, utilizing stage III treatment regimens. In the MOSAIC trial, a strong trend toward more favorable outcome in stage II patients with these poor risk factors was seen, while outcomes were identical with or without oxaliplatin for the overall stage II patients. Thus, oxaliplatin-containing regimens should not be used in stage II colon cancer patients who lack one or more of these high-risk factors.

Impact of Microsatellite Instability on Treatment

Ribic et al.[182] investigated the usefulness of MSI status as a predictor of benefit from fluorouracil-based adjuvant chemotherapy in 570 stage II and III patients from five randomized trials in which a no treatment control arm was used. MSI-H was exhibited in 95 patients (16.7%), MSI-L in 60 patients (10.5%), and MSS in 415 patients (72.8%). In the 287 patients who did not received adjuvant chemotherapy, those with tumors exhibiting MSI-H had superior 5-year survival compared to patients with MSI-L or MSS tumors (HR 0.31; *P* = .004). In the population of patients who received adjuvant chemotherapy there was no difference in survival between the MSI-H and non-MSI-H patients (*P* = .8). In the patients with MSI-L or MSS tumors, chemotherapy resulted in improved survival versus no chemotherapy (HR 0.72; *P* = .04). However, chemotherapy did not improve survival in the patients with MSI-H tumors (Table 89.9).

TABLE 89.9

MICROSATELLITE INSTABILITY STATUS VERSUS OUTCOME WITH FLUOROURACIL-BASED ADJUVANT CHEMOTHERAPY

	No. of Patients	5-Year Disease-Free Survival (%)	*P* Value
ALL PATIENTS			
Adjuvant chemotherapy	285	70	.06
No adjuvant chemotherapy	287	62	
PATIENTS WITH MSI-L/MSS			
Adjuvant chemotherapy	230	70	.01
No adjuvant chemotherapy	245	59	
PATIENTS WITH MSI-H			
Adjuvant chemotherapy	53	69	.11
No adjuvant chemotherapy	42	83	

MSI, microsatellite instability; MSS, microsatellite stable; MSI-H, high level of microsatellite instability; MSI-L, Low level of microsatellite instability.
(From ref. 182.)

Chemotherapy was associated with improved outcome in both stage II and III patients with MSS or MSI-L, with a hazard ratio of 0.67 (95% CI, 0.39 to 1.15) in stage II patients and 0.69 (95% CI, 0.47 to 1.01) in patients with stage III cancer. In contrast, in patients with MSI-H tumors, treatment did not improve survival, and in fact was associated with a trend toward worse outcome for both stage II (HR for death 3.28; 95% CI, 0.86 to 12.48) and stage III cancers (HR 1.42; 95% CI, 0.36 to 5.56). Of note, an analysis of MSI status from the NSABP failed to corroborate the results of the Ribic et al. study, and the authors concluded that in their trial there was no interaction between MSI status and treatment effect, and that their data do not support the use of MSI-H as a predictive marker for chemotherapy benefit.[183] However, an updated expansion on the data from the Ribic et al. report appears to corroborate the original findings, leading the authors of that study to suggest that MSI determinations should be performed on all stage II patients, and that stage II patients with high MSI should not be treated with fluoropyrimidines alone.[184] Currently the Eastern Cooperative Oncology Group I is leading a trial (ECOG 5202) in which patients with MSI-H and absence of LOH in chromosome 18q are being selected for observation, on the hypothesis that these patients will have a highly favorable prognosis with observation alone, while others are being assigned to FOLFOX chemotherapy and randomized to with or without bevacizumab. This trial is still accruing patients at the time of this writing.

The incidence of MSI has more recently been shown to vary with stage of disease presentation, with 22% of stage II patients, 12% of stage III, and only 3.5% of stage IV patients found to exhibit MSI, consistent with the data that MSI-H is a favorable *prognostic* factor. Data from the PETACC-3 trial suggest that it is a strong prognostic factor in stage II disease, however, it is less so in stage III.[185–187]

Other Molecular Markers

Since the majority of stage II, and even stage III, patients do not benefit from adjuvant therapy, it would highly desirable to be able to identify those patients who are both at risk for recurrent disease (i.e., harbor micrometastases) and those whose micrometastases are sensitive to, and will be eradicated by, a particular chemotherapy. At present there are no such validated markers, with the possible exception of MSI, as discussed above. KRAS mutations have no prognostic value in the adjuvant setting, and since there is no role for use of anti-EGFR agents in the adjuvant setting, the expense of genotyping patients with less than stage IV disease is difficult to justify.[187,188] BRAF mutations appear to be prognostic of poorer overall survival in stage II disease that is not MSI-H, however, this appears to be regardless of therapy, and so again it provides no information to inform treatment decision making.[187] At present, no molecular test has been validated as useful for making adjuvant treatment decisions, and none should be utilized outside of a clinical trial. Recently a genetic profiling assay utilizing 21-gene signature analysis has become available.[185] This assay has been shown to provide a risk stratification with stage II patients who are classified as having from 8% to 22% chance of recurrence. However, there was no interaction with treatment, meaning that the test is prognostic, identifying relatively lower or higher risk individuals, but it provided no guidance on whom or whom not to treat. Thus, it would appear to be of little value in decision making at this time.

The lack of clear direction on the matter of treatment of good risk stage II patients is reflected in a current consensus statement, which, while not recommending therapy for all stage II patients, does recommend a medical oncology consultation for the purpose of discussing the pros and cons of chemotherapy for all stage II patients.[189]

TREATMENT OPTIONS FOR STAGE III PATIENTS

It is clear that in the absence of medical or psychiatric contraindications, patients with node-positive colon cancer should receive postoperative chemotherapy. At the very least, a fluorouracil-based regimen would appear to be appropriate, and approximately 6 months of therapy would be supported by the majority of trials. The daily time five Mayo Clinic schedule or a variant has been shown to be more toxic than other 5-FU/leucovorin schedules and therefore daily time five schedules should not be used. Oral capecitabine or oral UFT/leucovorin are acceptable alternatives if a fluoropyrimidine-only approach is selected. At this time the data for incorporation of oxaliplatin into the routine adjuvant treatment of colon cancer appears compelling, and the FOLFOX schedule is now the most widely used adjuvant therapy. FLOX is an acceptable alternative, however, nonrandomized comparisons suggest that FLOX may carry a higher risk of serious diarrhea than FOLFOX. Cape/Ox is also an acceptable alternative in appropriately motivated and reliable patients. Although the pivotal adjuvant study was done with FOLFOX-4, in practice this regimen is rarely used, and the modified FOLFOX-6 regimen, which is the basis for the current National Cancer Institute Intergroup adjuvant and metastatic trials, is routinely used due to its greater convenience. The risk of peripheral neuropathy and the possibility of long-term neuropathy (27% persistent neuropathy 1 year after the last treatment and 1% persistent grade 3 neuropathy at 1 year) must be considered in the selection of therapy.

Irinotecan-based regimens should not be used in the adjuvant setting, as randomized data have shown increased toxicity and no long-term benefit. Bevacizumab, cetuximab, and panitumumab should also not be used in the adjuvant setting, as they add toxicity and expense, and do not add benefit.

Investigational Adjuvant Approaches

Portal Vein Infusion

The NSABP C-02 trial randomized 1,158 patients with Dukes A, B, or C colon cancers to either a 7-day portal vein infusion of 5-FU (600 mg/m²/d) or to surgery alone.[190] A modest, albeit statistically significant, advantage in disease-free survival (74% vs. 64% at 4 years) was demonstrated for the group who received intraportal chemotherapy, however, no difference was seen in the incidence of hepatic recurrences.

Similar findings were reported from a 533 patient trial performed by the Swiss Group for Clinical Cancer Research (SAKK).[191,192] In this trial intraportal chemotherapy included 10 mg/m² mitomycin C by 2-hour infusion followed by a 7-day infusion of 5-FU at a dose of 500 mg/m²/d. The 5-year disease-free and overall survivals were modestly improved in the intraportal treatment versus surgery-only groups (57% vs. 48% and 66% vs. 55%, respectively).

Subsequently a large meta-analysis of intraportal chemotherapy trials involving over 4,000 patients in ten randomized studies revealed only a 4% improvement in 5-year overall survival for the patients who received portal infusion. At present intraportal adjuvant chemotherapy has not been accepted as routine practice and remains limited to clinical investigations.

Intraperitoneal Chemotherapy

A small, single-arm study explored the feasibility of immediate postoperative intraperitoneal floxuridine and leucovorin plus systemic 5-FU and levamisole.[193] A randomized trial of 241 stage II and III patients compared intraperitoneal plus systemic 5-FU/leucovorin to systemic 5-FU/levamisole.[194] With 4 years' median follow-up, no benefit was seen for the stage II patients. Among the 196 eligible patients with stage III disease, however, a 43% reduction in mortality was seen. This small trial is encouraging but would require further corroboration before being accepted into standard practice.

Vaccines

Vaccination strategies endeavor to stimulate the patient's immune system to recognize and eradicate the patient's tumor cells. An ideal immunologic target molecule would be a highly antigenic epitope that is always expressed on the tumor and never expressed on normal tissue. Such an ideal target has yet to be identified, however, a number of approaches have been explored.

CEA is a commonly expressed antigen in colorectal carcinomas. Unfortunately, CEA does not appear to be particularly immunogenic. Several approaches have been pursued in an attempt to increase immune recognition of CEA. Thus, a number of avenues of investigation are being pursued, however, at this time the use of vaccine therapy for treatment of resected colon cancer remains highly investigational.

Active Specific Immunotherapy

Irradiated cancer cells maintain their immunogenicity, however, they are unable to proliferate. Active specific immunotherapy (ASI) is a maneuver in which patients are immunized with a preparation of their own irradiated tumor cells plus an immunostimulant such as BCG. This technique has been explored for some time now as a potential adjuvant immunotherapy for colorectal cancer. Overall, trials have failed to show a benefit for the use of ASI in the management of colon cancer, and its use should remain limited to investigational settings.

RADIATION THERAPY OF COLON CANCER

Patterns of Failure of and the Rationale for Radiation

The potential indications for adjuvant radiation therapy in colon cancer are based on analyses of patterns of failure following resection.[195–197] Advanced stage predicts for local failure in both colon and rectal cancers; however, local failure in colon cancer also depends on anatomic origin. The ascending and descending colon are considered anatomically immobile, and their close proximity to the retroperitoneal tissues often limits wide surgical resection. In contrast, the midsigmoid colon and midtransverse colon are relatively "mobile" with a wide mesentery, allowing the surgeon to obtain wide margins regardless of extent of disease invasion into the mesentery. Unless there is adjacent organ adherence or invasion by tumor, local failure at these sites is uncommon. Local failure rates for cecal, hepatic or splenic flexure, and proximal or distal sigmoid tumors are variable depending on the amount of mesentery present, tumor extension, and the adequacy of radial margins. When colon cancers adhere to or invade adjacent structures, local failure rates exceed 30% following surgery alone (Tables 89.10 and 89.11).

In summary, local failure occurs in patients with colonic tumors where there are anatomic constraints on radial resection margins, including tumors adherent to or invading adjacent structures.

TABLE 89.10

PATTERNS OF FAILURE AFTER POTENTIALLY CURATIVE SURGERY FOR COLON CANCER (ALL STAGES)

Series (Ref.)	Detection and Definition of Failure	Stage	No. of Patients	No. Experiencing Local Failure (%)		No. Experiencing Abdominal Failure (%)		No. Experiencing Distant Failure (%)	
				Only	Component	Only	Component	Only	Component
Gunderson et al. (196)	Reoperation, cumulative failure	All stages	91	22(030)	48 (0–64)	4 (0–9)	21 (0–36)	7 (0–16)	30 (0–38)
		T3–4 and/or N1–2	72	17	49	6	26	7	35
Willett et al. 197)	Clinical, cumulative failure	All stages	533	6 (0–12)	19 (0–49)	11(2–24)	21 (3–43)	4 (0–10)	13 (0–25)
		T3–4 and/or N1–2	395	8	26	14	25	5	16
Minksy et al. (362)	Clinical, first failure	All stages	284	6 (0–8)	9 (0–25)	8 (0–29)	13 (0–57)	3 (0–11)	6 (0–25)
		T3–4 and/or N1–2	229	4	10	10	15	5	6

Therapy Regimes

Until recently, data evaluating the use of adjuvant radiation therapy in high-risk colon cancer patients was limited to single-institution retrospective analyses.[195,198–202] To summarize, these studies have suggested that operative bed failures in high-risk patients who undergo resection alone is reduced by the administration of adjuvant radiation therapy.

A report from the Massachusetts General Hospital evaluated outcomes in high-risk patients who undergo resection followed by adjuvant radiation therapy and compared these to a similar cohort of patients treated over the same period who underwent surgery only (Table 89.11).[195] Irradiated patients included those with T4N0/N+, T3N+ disease (excluding mid-sigmoid and midtransverse colon) and T3N0 patients with margins of less than 1 cm. A total of 171 patients received postoperative radiation therapy, with 63 patients receiving concurrent chemotherapy, usually with bolus 5-FU (500 mg/m^2/d) for 3 consecutive days during the first and last weeks of radiation therapy. Radiation treatment was administered through parallel opposed or other multifield techniques to treat the tumor bed with an approximate 3- to 5-cm margin to a total dose of 45 Gy, followed by reduced fields to a total dose of 50.4 to 54 Gy. Draining nodes were included if they were thought to be at high risk for involvement. This cohort was compared to 395 patients with T3-4N0/N+ tumors who underwent surgery alone during the same time period. Table 89.11 shows 5-year actuarial local control and relapse-free survival in the adjuvant group compared to patients who underwent surgery alone. Local control rates in T4N0 and T4N+ patients treated with radiation therapy were 93% and 72%, respectively, versus 69% and 47%, respectively, in patients who underwent surgery alone. Similarly, relapse-free survivals were 79% and 53%, respectively, in T4N0/T4N+ patients who underwent adjuvant radiation, versus 63% and 38%, respectively, who underwent surgery alone. No significant outcome differences were observed in patients with T3N0 and T3N+ lesions; however, there may be an element of selection bias in the radiation group given most patients were referred because of concerns of adequacy of local control following surgery alone. There was a trend toward improved local control in patients who received 5-FU. The rate of acute enteritis in patients who received irradiation and 5-FU was 16% versus 4% in patients who underwent irradiation only. This rate of enteritis is similar to data from studies of concurrent 5-FU and radiation therapy in rectal cancer. Late bowel complication rates were not increased by concomitant 5-FU administration. The conclusion was that patients with T4 tumors or tumors with abscess or fistula formation or margin-positive resection may benefit from postoperative radiation.[195]

PRACTICE OF ONCOLOGY

TABLE 89.11

LOCAL ADJUVANT RADIATION THERAPY IN COLON CANCER

Group	Stage	Locoregional Failure[a]				5-Year Disease-Free Survival	
		No. of Patients	Surgery (%)	No. of Patients	Surgery + Radiation (%)	Surgery (%)	Surgery + Radiation (%)
Adjuvant therapy	T3N0	163	10	23	9[a]	70	72
	T4N0	83	31	54	7	63	79
	T3N1-2	100	35	55	30	44	47
	T4N1-2	49	53	39	28	37	53
Residual disease	All stages	—	—	30	47	—	37
Perforation or fistula	T4N0	21	48	23	6	43	91

[a]Actuarial component of total failure.
(From ref. 195.)

In an updated analysis from Massachusetts General Hospital, 152 patients with T4 tumors received adjuvant irradiation. On pathological examination, 42 patients had tumors with positive margins. For patients with negative margins the 10-year actuarial local control in T4N0 and T4N+ patients was 78% and 48%, respectively. In patients with node-negative tumors, the 10-year actuarial local control and relapse-free survival rates were 87% and 58%, respectively, compared to 65% and 33%, respectively, in patients with node-positive tumors. For patients with one involved lymph node, local control and relapse-free survival rates were similar to those without nodal involvement; however, with increasing numbers of nodes involved, survival steadily decreased.[200] Adjuvant tumor bed irradiation should be considered in patients with tumors (1) invading adjoining structures, (2) complicated by perforation or fistula, and (3) where incomplete excision is performed. Patients are generally given continuous 5-FU (225 mg/m²/24 h) 5 days per week or capecitabine throughout the course of radiation therapy.

Investigators from the Mayo Clinic described a series of 103 patients who received radiation therapy following surgery for locally advanced colon cancer.[201] Microscopic and gross residual disease was present in 18 and 35 patients, respectively. Over 90% of patients had T4N0/N+ disease. A median dose of 50.4 Gy was delivered through multifield techniques, and most patients received concurrent 5-FU-based chemotherapy. Eleven patients received an intraoperative boost of 10 to 20 Gy. Five-year actuarial overall local control was 40%. Patients with margin negative tumors had a 5-year local control rate of 90%, compared to 46% for patients with microscopic residual tumor, and 21% with gross residual tumor. In patients with residual disease, local control rates in patients who underwent intraoperative boost were 89% compared to 18% who underwent external irradiation alone. Similarly, 5-year survival rates were improved in patients who underwent margin negative resection (66%) compared to those with microscopic residual (47%) or gross residual (23%) tumors.

A report from the University of Florida of patients with locally advanced but completely resected colon cancers who received adjuvant radiation therapy reported a local control rate of 88%, similar to the 90% reported at the Mayo Clinic in patients who had completely resected tumors.[202] In addition, there appeared to be a dose–response relationship to local control. The 5-year rate of local control was 96% for patients who received 50 to 55 Gy versus 76% for patients who received less than 50 Gy (P = .0095).

To assess whether the addition of radiation therapy to adjuvant chemotherapy would result in superior survival and local regional failure rates in resected, high-risk colon cancer patients, the U.S. Intergroup[199] initiated a randomized prospective trial in 1992. In this trial, patients with resected colon cancer were randomized to postoperative irradiation with 5-FU and levamisole or 5-FU and levamisole alone. Eligibility criteria included margin negative tumors with adherence to or invasion of surrounding structures (i.e., T4N0 or N+ disease, excluding peritoneal invasion) or tumors arising in the ascending or descending colon with metastatic regional nodes (T3N+). Patients were randomized to receive (1) weekly 5-FU combined with levamisole for 12 months duration or (2) 5-FU and levamisole for 12 months with combined radiation therapy and chemotherapy beginning 1 month after the first 5-FU administration. The recommended total radiation dose was 45 Gy in 25 fractions over 5 weeks with an optional 5.4 Gy boost.

The initial trial accrual goal was 700 patients; however, the study was closed in 1996 due to poor accrual (222 patients; 189 evaluable). Therefore, total accrual was less than one-third of initial goals and there was decreased statistical power to detect any differences between the groups. Nonetheless, no difference in overall or disease-free survival was seen between the two groups. Five-year overall survival of patients who received chemotherapy only was 62% versus 58% for patients randomized to chemoirradiation (P >.50). Local recurrence rates were identical in both arms (18 patients each). Grade 3 or 4 hematologic toxicity was higher in patients who received radiation therapy.[199] Interpretation of study results was handicapped by decreased statistical power, high ineligibility rates, and lack of surgical clips or preoperative imaging to assist the definition of appropriate EBRT fields in a high percentage of patients. No definitive conclusions can be made regarding the efficacy of routine postoperative irradiation with 5-FU and levamisole based on this study; however, this study provides no data supporting its routine use.

Investigators have also examined the efficacy of hepatic irradiation following resection in high-risk patients. The combination of 5-FU and hepatic irradiation did not improve overall or disease-free survival over 5-FU alone.[198]

Relapse within the peritoneal cavity is also commonly observed in patients who undergo resection of locally advanced colon cancer. Investigators have reported outcomes and toxicities following adjuvant whole abdominal irradiation in high-risk patients. The SWOG reported the results of a pilot study to evaluate 41 patients with resected T3N1-2M0 colon cancer patients treated with continuous infusion 5-FU (200 mg/m²/24 h) with concomitant whole-abdominal irradiation. Patients received 30 Gy given at 1 Gy per fraction followed by a 16 Gy boost to the tumor bed at 1.6 Gy per fraction. Further 5-FU therapy was administered following completion of radiation. Five-year disease-free and overall survival estimates were 58% and 67%, respectively. Patients with tumors having more than four lymph nodes involved experienced 5-year disease-free and overall survival rates of 55% and 74%, respectively. Grade 3 and 4 toxicity was observed in 17% and 7% of patients, respectively. When compared to similarly staged patients from previous Intergroup trials treated with 5-FU/levamisole only, these survival results appeared favorable. The authors recommended that continuous infusion 5-FU and whole abdominal irradiation with tumor bed boost should be studied in a randomized trial.[203]

Estes et al.[204] reported a pattern of failure analysis in patients with T3N+ colon cancer treated with 5-FU/levamisole chemotherapy only (Intergroup), combined chemotherapy/whole abdominal irradiation (SWOG), and patients who underwent surgery only, from the previously described Massachusetts General Hospital study. Their analysis showed 5-FU/levamisole reduced the rate of lung metastases but was less effective at preventing local and peritoneal recurrence. In contrast, patients who received whole abdominal irradiation with continuous 5-FU experienced a 12% tumor bed relapse rate, 22% hepatic relapse rate, and 15% peritoneal relapse rate, all of which were superior to the nonirradiated arms. The use of whole abdominal irradiation should be considered investigational.

In summary, the use of adjuvant postoperative irradiation combined with systemic therapy for patients at high risk for local relapse is unlikely to ever be addressed in a definitive randomized trial. Treatment recommendations should be made on a case-by-case basis with existing data in the setting of an informed consent. Adjuvant tumor bed irradiation with concurrent 5-FU–based chemotherapy should be considered for patients with tumors (a) invading adjoining structures, (b) those complicated by perforation or fistula, and (c) where incomplete resection is performed.

FOLLOW-UP AFTER MANAGEMENT OF COLON CANCER WITH CURATIVE INTENT

Follow-up after definitive management has two primary goals. First, patients with a history of colorectal cancer are at higher risk than the general population for a second colon cancer primary.[205,206] A colonoscopic screening may benefit in the early detection of a second primary malignancy or detection of a benign polyp, which can then be resected, potentially preventing the development of an invasive cancer.

Second, surveillance may increase the chance of identifying local regional or distant recurrence that is potentially curable by surgery. It should be noted that it is this detection of potentially curable recurrent or second primary disease that justifies routine postoperative surveillance. To date there are no compelling data that indicate that early detection of unresectable asymptomatic metastatic disease is of benefit to the patient. In other words, if recurrent disease is unresectable and therefore incurable, there is no urgency to identify it; there is no compelling evidence that the early initiation of palliative chemotherapy is of benefit in the asymptomatic, incurable patient. The choice of follow-up routine and which studies to include in that follow-up have been the subject of much debate in the colon cancer literature.[207–210] Several studies and imaging modalities had been recommended as important components of a follow-up regimen. These include: (1) measurements of CEA, (2) a careful history and physical examination, (3) liver function tests including transaminase and lactate dehydrogenase (LDH), (4) complete blood cell count (CBC), (5) fecal occult blood tests, (6) chest x-ray, (7) CT, (8) pelvic imaging, (9) flexible proctosigmoidoscopy (rectal cancer), and (10) colonoscopy.

Various retrospective reviews and meta-analyses have argued the relative costs and benefits of each of these individual approaches.[211,212] In 2004 the American Society of Clinical Oncology undertook a review of these various strategies in order to update their 2000 recommendations. The panel examined outcomes, including overall and disease-free survival, quality of life, toxicity reduction, and cost-effectiveness.[213] The study reviewed all literature published on this subject using a Medline search for the 20 years preceding the initiation of the study. Levels of evidence were graded, possible consequences of false-positive and false-negative tests were examined, and an expert panel reviewed the data and made recommendations. Additional outside reviewers examined the final document and made additional recommendations. The panel's review included each of the aforementioned ten follow-up assessments, evaluating the costs and benefits, which resulted in a selection of those studies that were thought at the time to have the greatest potential yield in detecting new primaries and recurrent disease. The recommendations of the panel are based on the best surveillance guidelines for patients with stage II and III disease.

The role of CEA measurement in patients following definitive management of colorectal cancer has been controversial.[69,211,214] The American Society of Clinical Oncology (ASCO) carefully reviewed its utility in an additional panel guided in 1996.[215] Their recommendation for CEA monitoring then, which was confirmed in the surveillance guideline panel review, was postoperative serum CEA testing to be performed every 3 months in patients with stage II or III disease for up to 3 years after diagnosis. An elevated CEA level, if confirmed by retesting, warranted further evaluation for metastatic disease.

This further workup of an elevated CEA typically consists of a colonoscopy and a CT scan of the chest, abdomen, and pelvis. If these studies are negative the clinician is faced with a dilemma. The question of what to do in the face of a rising serum CEA level in the absence of imageable disease by conventional imaging modalities is one that has been addressed in clinical trials.[216–221] Strategies to image CEA expression might improve upon the detection capability of standard imaging studies. Several studies were performed using immunoscintigraphy with an antibody directed against CEA or Tag72, a CEA-like glycoprotein (CEA scan and OncoScint (Cytogen Corp, Lonza Biologics, Princeton, New Jersey) scan, respectively).[222–224] The results of these studies using antibody directed immunoscintigraphy were variable. In order to more directly address this clinical dilemma a prospective study was performed comparing CEA immunoscintigraphy to positron emission tomography (PET) using 18 fluorodeoxyglucose (^{18}FDG) and blind "second look" laparotomy.[219]

In this study patients with a rising CEA level without imageable disease by CT scan of the chest, abdomen, and pelvis as well as colonoscopy and abdominal ultrasound were enrolled along with patients with a single site of otherwise resectable disease. All patients had a CEA scan performed as well as a PET scan with FDG. All patients who failed to demonstrate evidence of disease outside of the abdominal cavity went on to have an exploratory laparotomy by a surgeon who had no knowledge of the CEA or the FDG scan results. A second surgeon participated in the remainder of the exploration after thoroughly reviewing all studies including the nuclear medicine scans. Twenty-eight patients were studied in this fashion and the trial demonstrated that PET scan with FDG was far superior to CEA scans in detecting recurrence and roughly 30% of the patients on the study potentially benefited by having recurrent disease treated at the time of surgery (Fig. 89.4).

Based on these findings it appears that serum CEA surveillance following definitive management of a primary colorectal cancer is a reasonable surveillance technique. If the CEA level is elevated on repeat testing, imaging studies should be performed consisting of CT scans and a through evaluation of the colon with colonoscopy performed as well. If no recurrence or second primary is detected a PET scan with FDG can be considered. If disease is discovered it should be managed as indicated. If no disease is detected, then continued surveillance is warranted with repeat CEA levels and CT or MR imaging at intervals.[219,225]

The role of physical examination has also been evaluated.[213] The ASCO panel noted that no formal examination of the contribution of physician's history and physical examination to help outcomes of colorectal cancer has been performed. However, data from the larger studies of surveillance showed that 80% of recurrences were found by CEA testing while only 20% were found by routine history and physical examination

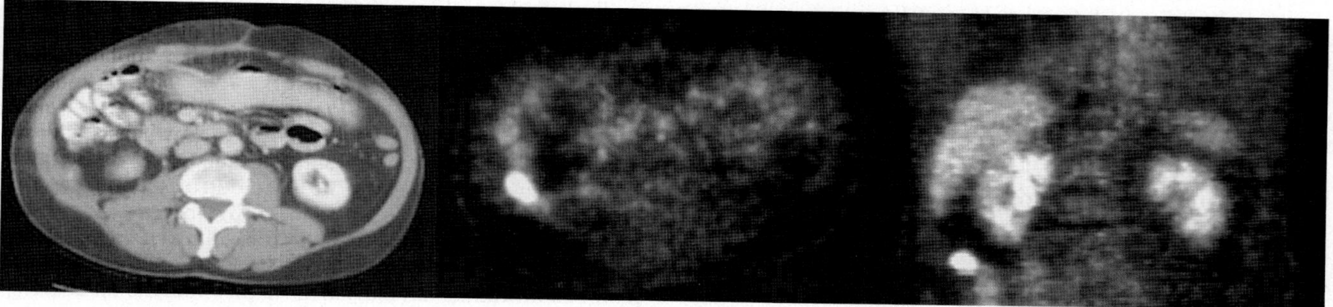

FIGURE 89.4 From left to right the first panel depicts a contrast enhanced computed tomography scan image of a patient with a rising carcinoembryonic antigen following a definitive resection of a right colon cancer. The middle and far panels show the same region imaged with fluorodeoxyglucose position emission tomography. (From ref. 219, with permission.)

done at the same time.[226] This has been confirmed by other studies.[227,228] Although no direct effects were shown on history or physical examination about the impact and detection or outcome in the surveillance period, a physician–patient encounter provides a vital link for other studies that may influence outcome. Therefore, while not in itself substantiated by the data in the literature, it is felt that routine postresection visits be performed every 3 to 6 months for the first 3 years following resection and every 6 months during years 4 and 5.

The role of liver function tests as a means for detecting colorectal recurrence has also been carefully evaluated. No studies that were reviewed by the ASCO panel demonstrated any benefit for the routine use of liver function test measurements in the postsurveillance period.[213,229] In fact studies suggest that other routine blood tests such as CEA detected recurrence far earlier than liver function test abnormalities.[69] Therefore, the 2005 ASCO consensus panel did not recommend the routine use of liver function test measurements in the postresection surveillance period.

Routine fecal occult blood testing, routine CBCs, and routine chest x-rays were all not thought to be of benefit in postoperative surveillance. Although the panel was not in uniform agreement with respect to chest x-ray, it was thought that all three of these modalities should be reserved for the evaluation of the patient with evidence of recurrence such as a rising CEA level or a positive endoscopy. Each of these modalities in and of itself was not found to be useful.

The panel recommended that annual CT of the chest and abdomen (with pelvis for rectal cancer) be performed for 3 years in those patients at higher risk for recurrence who could be candidates for curative-intent surgery of a recurrence. With respect to colonoscopy and flexible proctosigmoidoscopy, the panel, after reviewing the literature, recommended that all patients have a colonoscopy for the pre- or perioperative documentation of the cancer and to ascertain that the remainder of the colon is free from polyps. Further, the panel agreed that the data were sufficient to recommend colonoscopy at 3 years to detect new cancers and polyps and then every 5 years if normal. However, they did not recommend routine annual colonoscopy as follow-up following definitive management of patients with colorectal cancer. Further the panel concluded that colonoscopy was superior to flexible proctosigmoidoscopy and therefore should be performed as above for patients following both colon and rectal cancer surgery. Other studies have also supported the routine use of colonoscopic examination following definitive management of colorectal cancer.[230,231]

A meta-analysis and systematic review of randomized trials to address the impact of close postoperative surveillance on overall survival following definitive management of colorectal cancer was also performed by Renehan et al.[232] A total of five randomized trials that met their inclusion criteria were reviewed, representing 1,342 patients. For four of the studies, intensive follow-up consisted of blood work including serum CEA, colonoscopy, physical examination, abdominal ultrasound, and CT scans. In one study, no CEA measurements or CT scans were performed. Follow-up in the intensive arm was performed every 3 months for 2 years and then every 6 months thereafter up to 5 years, with yearly CT scans and endoscopy. All five studies had a control arm subjected to a less aggressive follow-up regimen, which varied from study to study ranging from no specific follow-up to interval laboratory tests and plain x-rays or ultrasound. They found that there was an absolute reduction in mortality of 9% to 13% by employing an aggressive follow-up regimen, consisting of serum CEA measurements and CT scans. Two studies in particular showed the greatest impact on survival.

In summary, a rational postoperative surveillance program would include CEA measurements every 3 to 6 months and a yearly CT scan of the chest, abdomen, and pelvis (for rectal cancer) for the first 3 years. Colonoscopy can be performed every 3 to 5 years following the resection. At the time of CEA measurements a physician encounter should be scheduled where a discussion of patient symptoms and a physical examination can be performed. If a rising serum CEA is detected on two consecutive measurements in the absence of imageable disease by CT scan, a PET scan with ^{18}FDG can be considered. Lesions found on colonoscopy should be managed appropriately either with colonoscopic resection or surgical management. These surveillance guidelines should allow for the early detection of either resectable recurrence or second primary lesions and therefore the potential to impact patient outcome.

SURGICAL MANAGEMENT OF STAGE IV DISEASE

For a select group of patients with metastatic colorectal cancer, complete surgical resection of stage IV disease may be an option and may provide a long-term survival advantage. This is especially true with respect to metastatic sites in the liver and lung. Resection of locoregional recurrence can also benefit the patient with respect to local control and overall outcome. Numerous regional approaches have also been explored for the treatment of stage IV colon cancer depending on the organ or body cavity involved. Organ-specific infusional therapy, isolated or continuous perfusion therapy, radio frequency ablation or cryotherapy, surgical debulking, and radiation are all technical approaches that have been performed. Many of these regional strategies as well as surgical metastasectomy will be discussed in separate chapters and therefore will not be specifically addressed here.

MANAGEMENT OF UNRESECTABLE METASTATIC DISEASE

Unresectable metastatic colorectal cancer is generally not curable with current technology. Management centers around palliation and control of symptoms, control of tumor growth, and attempts to lengthen progression-free and overall survival. Given the palliative nature of such treatments, extreme care must be taken to adequately assess each individual's potential for both benefit and harm from chemotherapy. Quality-of-life issues must be frankly and objectively discussed with patients and their caregivers so that informed decisions can be made and expectations can be contained within a realistic framework.

The chemotherapy options available and the developmental work that supports their utility are outlined below. It is of paramount importance to keep in mind that virtually all of the clinical trials done in patients with metastatic disease were performed by design on patients who were in good overall general medical condition. Entry criteria for most trials require a favorable performance status and acceptable bone marrow, renal, and hepatic function, and they often specify evidence of reasonable nutritional intake.

It is not reasonable to extrapolate the results of these trials to patients who do not conform to these entry criteria. The likelihood of benefit in a poor performance status patient is substantially diminished, and the likelihood of a serious adverse event is greatly increased. Patients with hepatic or renal dysfunction may be particularly prone to additional toxicity if the drug is cleared or metabolized by these organs. Patients with marginal nutritional intake may have their nutritional deficiencies further exacerbated by drugs that produce nausea or anorexia, and patients with partial or complete bowel obstruction or other causes of prolonged gastrointestinal transit time

TABLE 89.12

COMMONLY USED FLUOROURACIL REGIMENS

Name of Regimen	Author (Ref.)	Schedule (All Agents Administered Intravenously)
Roswell Park	Haller et al., 1998 (156)	LV 500 mg/m^2 over 2 hours; 5-FU 500 mg/m^2 by bolus 1 hour into LV infusion. Treatments given weekly for 6 consecutive weeks, repeated every 8 weeks
Low-dose weekly LV	Jager et al., 1996 (363)	LV 20 mg/m^2 over 5–15 minutes, followed by bolus 5-FU 500 mg/m^2; treatments given weekly for 6 consecutive weeks, repeated every 8 weeks
Protracted venous infusion (PVI)	Lokich et al., 1989 (364)	5-FU 300 mg/m^2/d by continuous infusion
AIO (weekly 24-hour infusion)	Kohne et al., 1998 (365)	LV 500 mg/m^2 over 2 hours, followed by 5-FU 2,600 mg/m^2 over 24 hours, repeated weekly
LV5FU2	de Gramont et al., 1997 (269)	LV 200 mg/m^2 over 2 hours days 1 and 2, followed by bolus 5-FU 400 mg/m^2 day 1 and 2, followed by 5-FU 600 mg/m^2 over 22 hours, day 1 and 2: cycle repeated every 14 days
Simplified LV5FU2	Adapted from Andre et al., 1999 (258)	LV 400 mg/m^2 over 2 hours, followed by bolus 5-FU 400 mg/m^2, followed by 5-FU 1,200 mg/m^2/d times 2 days (2,400 mg/m^2 over 46–48 hours); cycles repeated every 14 days

LV, leucovorin; 5-FU, 5-fluorouracil.
Note: Doses listed are recommended starting doses for good performance status patients with normal renal, hepatic, and bone marrow function. Individual dose adjustments may be required.

may have increased toxicity from those drugs that undergo an enterohepatic recirculation.

Thus, chemotherapy for patients with incurable metastatic disease should be approached with appropriate caution. Good performance status in well-motivated patients with good bone marrow reserve and good organ function portend a significant potential for substantial benefits from chemotherapy and should be strongly considered for aggressive therapy. Patients with poor performance status and significant comorbidities should be considered for either less aggressive therapies or for supportive care only.

Fluorouracil

Virtually the entire history of chemotherapy for colorectal cancer has revolved around the use of 5-FU. Developed by Heidleberger et al.[233] and patented in 1957, it is a source of frustration and humility for investigators working to move beyond it that over 50 years later this agent remains at the very core of most chemotherapeutic approaches to colorectal cancer.

Fluorouracil must be metabolized before it can exert cytotoxic activity. The details of 5-FU metabolism are covered in a separate chapter. The history of investigations of 5-FU in colorectal cancer treatment has been well summarized in previous editions of this book.[152] Fluorouracil remained the only drug available to treat colorectal cancer for almost four decades, during which time numerous agents were studied for their ability to "biomodulate" 5-FU. Of these, only leucovorin remains in use today, and it is debatable whether this reduced folate truly contributes to the efficacy of 5-FU. Most studies that evaluate the same dose of 5-FU with or without leucovorin find that both activity and toxicity are increased in the leucovorin arm, whereas studies that evaluate single-agent 5-FU versus an equitoxic schedule of a lower dose of 5-FU plus leucovorin find equivalent activity. Nevertheless, use of leucovorin persists in most standard regimens today. Data comparing bolus versus infusional schedules of 5-FU show a slight benefit for infusions. These infusional schedules achieved widespread acceptance in Europe sooner than in the United States. It was not until the advent of combination schedules of 5-FU plus other active agents that the benefits of infusional schedules, especially in terms of improved toxicity, asserted themselves in North American practice. A selection of commonly used 5-FU regimens is outlined in Table 89.12.

Capecitabine

Capecitabine is a 5-FU precursor that is administered orally. It is absorbed intact through the gut and then activated by a series of enzymatic alterations. Some data suggest that thymidine phosphorylase levels are higher in tumor than in normal tissue. This could, in theory, provide a degree of preferential intratumoral activation; however, clinical trials do not appear to support a substantially better therapeutic index than 5-FU.[234] Phase 2 studies demonstrate that this agent has substantial activity in colorectal cancer, with an acceptable toxicity profile.[235] Since the addition of leucovorin did not appear to show any benefit, clinical development went forward without additional biomodulation. Phase 3 randomized clinical trials, performed both in the United States and Europe, have now shown that this orally administered agent is at least as effective as intravenous 5-FU/leucovorin, and the side effect profile of capecitabine is superior to the daily times five Mayo Clinic schedule of 5-FU/leucovorin.[236,237] The dose used in these pivotal trials was 1,250 mg/m^2 given twice daily for 14 days followed by a 7-day rest. The major side effects of capecitabine appear to be palmar-plantar erythrodysesthesia, commonly called hand-foot syndrome, and to a lesser extent diarrhea. The hand-foot toxicity is frequently a dose-limiting side effect, and although the approved starting dose is 1,250 mg/m^2 twice daily, many clinicians choose to initiate therapy at a lower dose and escalate if little or no toxicity is seen.

Uracil/Tegafur with Leucovorin

UFT is a combination of uracil and the fluorouracil prodrug tegafur (Ftorafur) in a four to one molar ratio. Uracil reversibly and competitively inhibits DPD. Tegafur is a 5-FU prodrug that was previously shown to have antitumor activity in colorectal cancer; however, it produced a neurotoxic metabolite, which limited its clinical usefulness. By inhibiting DPD, uracil allows for reliable oral absorption of tegafur and allows small quantities to be used, greatly reducing the accumulation of metabolites and eliminating the neurotoxicity. Phase 2 schedules using low-dose leucovorin (5 mg three times daily) with 350 mg/m²/d of UFT divided over three doses daily and high-dose leucovorin (50 mg three times daily) with 300 mg/m² of UFT divided over three doses daily both showed acceptable tolerability and activity comparable to what can be achieved with intravenous 5-FU schedules.[238,239] Two large-scale randomized studies comparing UFT plus oral leucovorin to the parenteral Mayo Clinic schedule of 5-FU/leucovorin were conducted using 300 mg/m²/d of UFT and an intermediate leucovorin dose of 25 to 30 mg three times daily. Both of these trials show no significant differences in response rates, time to tumor progression, or overall survival between the oral and parenteral regimens.[240,241] The trials did not, however, fulfill the U.S. regulatory requirements for noninferiority of UFT/leucovorin and, therefore, this compound has not been registered in the United States. It is widely used in much of Asia and Europe.

Raltitrexed

Raltitrexed is a nonfluoropyrimidine TS inhibitor that is transported into the tumor-reduced folate carriers and then polyglutamated, resulting in retained intracellular levels and prolonged inhibition of TS. Large-scale trials have demonstrated similar response rates between raltitrexed at 3 mg/m² given once every 3 weeks, and standard 5-FU/leucovorin bolus schedules.[242–244] One trial, however, showed a statistically significantly worse survival for the raltitrexed arm versus the 5-FU/leucovorin arm (9.7 months vs. 12.7 months; $P = .01$). The drug is not approved for use in the United States, but is available and utilized in many other parts of the world.

Irinotecan

A published review of trials of new agents in colorectal cancer between 1960 and 1990 found that none of the 72 compounds tested was able to reproducibly exceed the response rate of 5-FU.[245] The first such agent to show substantial clinical activity in colorectal cancer was irinotecan.

Irinotecan (CPT-11) is a semisynthetic derivative of camptothecin, a plant alkaloid extracted from the wood of the Asian tree *Camptotheca acuminate*.[246] CPT-11 possesses a bulky dipiperidino side chain linked to the camptothecin molecule via a carboxyl-ester bond. This side chain provides solubility but greatly decreases anticancer activity. Carboxylesterase, a ubiquitous enzyme with primary activity in the liver and gut, cleaves the carboxyl-ester bond to form the more active metabolite 7-ethyl-10-hydroxycamptothecin (SN-38).[247] SN-38 is as much as 1,000-fold more potent in inhibiting topoisomerase I than irinotecan and is thus the predominant active form of the drug. CPT-11 is often considered to be a prodrug for SN-38, however, this concept may be a bit too simplistic, since achieved CPT-11 concentrations may be several logs higher than those of SN-38.

Camptothecin, CPT-11, and SN-38 function as inhibitors of topoisomerase I (topo I). Topo I is a nuclear enzyme that aids in DNA uncoiling for replication and transcription. When topo I binds to DNA, it causes a reversible single-stranded break in the DNA, allowing the intact strand to pass through the break to relieve torsional stress on the coiled helix, and then reseals the break. CPT-11 and SN-38 stabilize these single-stranded breaks. Although the stabilized breaks do not cause irreversible damage, the collision of replication forks with open single-stranded breaks results in double-stranded breaks, leading to lethal DNA fragmentation.

A phase 2 trial reported by Shimada et al.[248] found a 22% response rate in a population of previously treated colorectal cancer patients. A subsequent trial reported a 23% response rate and 31% stable disease rate in 43 patients with 5-FU-refractory colorectal cancer.[249] A combined analysis of 304 5-FU-refractory colorectal cancer patients from three trials using a 90-minute infusion of CPT-11 weekly for 4 weeks followed by a 2-week rest showed a major objective response rate of 13%, with 49% of patients having a minor response or stable disease.[250] Starting doses ranged from 100 to 150 mg/m²; however, 125 mg/m² was felt to have the best balance of efficacy and toxicity. Diarrhea and neutropenia were the primary dose-limiting toxicities encountered.

In a phase 2 trial conducted in France, investigators gave a 350 mg/m² starting dose of CPT-11 once every 3 weeks to colorectal cancer patients who were either previously treated with 5-FU or who were chemotherapy naive. An 18% response rate was seen, both in the 48 chemotherapy-naive patients and in the 165 patients who had previously progressed through a 5-FU-based regimen.[251] A U.S. phase 2 trial of CPT-11 in previously untreated colorectal cancer patients reported a 32% response rate, using a weekly 125 mg/m² starting dose of CPT-11 for 4 weeks followed by a 2-week break.[252] Another trial done in the United States with this same weekly schedule of CPT-11 found a response rate of 26% in 31 previously untreated colorectal cancer patients.[253]

The promising results seen in 5-FU-refractory colorectal cancer in phase 2 trials were confirmed in randomized phase 3 trials. Cunningham et al.[243] compared a 350 mg/m² starting dose of CPT-11 (300 mg/m² for patients age 70 and older) given every 3 weeks to best supportive care (BSC) in patients with 5-FU-refractory colorectal cancer. This trial showed a 36% 1-year survival for the CPT-11-treated group versus a 14% 1-year survival for the BSC group.

In a parallel trial 5-FU-refractory colorectal cancer patients were randomized to the same schedule of CPT-11 as the previously described trial or to an infusional 5-FU regimen.[254] In this trial as well, the survival of the patients who received CPT-11 was statistically superior, with the 1-year survival for the CPT-11-treated patients being 1.4 times that of the infusion 5-FU group.

Neutropenia and diarrhea were the major toxicities encountered in all of the initial trials of CPT-11, and diarrhea in particular threatened to greatly limit the clinical utility of this agent. Two different diarrheal syndromes were identified: early onset and late onset. The early-onset diarrhea, which occurs during or immediately after CPT-11 administration, is a cholinergic effect and is readily controlled by use of atropine.[255] In those patients who experience this symptom (and who do not have a contraindication to atropine administration), 0.5 to 1 mg of atropine gives rapid resolution, and subsequent CPT-11 doses can then be given with atropine as a premedication. The late-onset diarrhea is more problematic. Intensive loperamide is effective in the management of CPT-11-induced late-onset diarrhea.[256]

CPT-11 in First-Line Combination Regimens

Numerous phase 1 combinations of 5-FU, usually with leucovorin, plus CPT-11, were tried. Saltz et al.[257] reported a phase 1 trial built on the weekly CPT-11 schedule that had been selected for phase 1 development in North America. A low dose of weekly leucovorin was utilized in order to reduce the potential for 5-FU/leucovorin-induced diarrhea. The phase 1 trial showed that the full single-agent dose of 125 mg/m² of CPT-11 could be given with 500 mg/m² of 5-FU and 20 mg/m² leucovorin, with all drugs given weekly for 4 consecutive weeks followed by a 2-week break. This and other CPT-11/5-FU/leucovorin regimens are summarized in Table 89.13.

TABLE 89.13

COMMONLY USED IRINOTECAN/FLUOROURACIL COMBINATION REGIMENS

Name of Regimen	Author (Ref.)	Schedule (All Agents Administered Intravenously)
FOLFIRI	Douillard et al., 2000 (168)	Irinotecan 180 mg/m^2 over 2 hours; LV 200 mg/m^2 concurrently with irinotecan (can be given in same line through "Y" connector); followed by 5-FU bolus 400 mg/m^2, followed by 5-FU 600 mg/m^2 infusion over 22 hours. Irinotecan given day 1 only. All other meds given days 1 and 2. Cycle repeated every 14 days.
FOLFIRI (simplified)	Andre et al., 1999 (258)	Irinotecan 180 mg/m^2 over 90 minutes; LV 400 mg/m^2 concurrently with irinotecan (can be given in same line through "Y" connector); followed by 5-FU bolus 400 mg/m^2, followed by 5-FU 1,200 mg/m^2/d times 2 days (2,400 mg/m^2 infusion over 46–48 hours). Cycle repeated every 14 days.
FUFIRI	Douillard et al., 2000 (168)	Irinotecan 80 mg/m^2, then LV 500 mg/m^2, followed by 5-FU 2,300 mg/m^2; all drugs given weekly for 6 weeks, repeated every 7 weeks

LV, leucovorin; 5-FU, 5-fluorouracil.
Note: Doses listed are recommended starting doses for good performance status patients with normal renal, hepatic, and bone marrow function. Individual dose adjustments may be required.

This combination of irinotecan, 5-FU, and leucovorin (IFL) was compared to the Mayo Clinic schedule of 5-FU/leucovorin in a multicenter, multinational phase 3 trial.[169] For regulatory reasons, a single-agent CPT-11 arm was included as well. The IFL arm was found to be superior to Mayo Clinic 5-FU/leucovorin in terms of response rate, time to tumor progression, and overall survival. The CPT-11 alone arm appeared to be comparable in efficacy to the 5-FU/leucovorin arm. The overall incidence of severe toxicity was similar in all arms of this trial. More serious diarrhea and vomiting were seen with IFL, while more neutropenia, neutropenic fever, and stomatitis were seen with 5-FU/leucovorin. Treatment-related deaths occurred in 1% of patients in each arm of this trial. Although this IFL schedule represented a step forward over the Mayo Clinic 5-FU/leucovorin schedule, neither of these are recommended for current use. As outlined below, the infusional 5-FU schedules have a superior safety and efficacy profile and are preferred for use, especially in combination regimens.

In Europe a parallel study to investigate the benefit of adding irinotecan to a 5-FU-based schedule was undertaken.[168] Two high-dose intermittent infusional schedules were developed. In France, a biweekly treatment for 2 consecutive days was explored, while German investigators, building on their experience with weekly 24-hour high-dose infusions of 5-FU, combined CPT-11 with this schedule. A randomized phase 3 trial was performed in which a participating center chose which of these two schedules would be used, and then the patients were randomized to that 5-FU/leucovorin schedule plus or minus CPT-11. Again, response rate, progression-free survival, overall survival were superior in the CPT-11-containing arm of the trial. Of note, only the cohort treated with the biweekly schedule demonstrated a statistically superior survival over the 5-FU/leucovorin control arm, and the biweekly combination schedule is the only one registered for use in the United States.

More recently the biweekly schedule of leucovorin/5-FU2 plus irinotecan has been studied with a simplified leucovorin/5-FU2 infusion schedule.[258] This schedule known as FOLFIRI (FOL for folinic acid, F for 5-FU, and IRI for irinotecan), was initially studied as a salvage regimen; however, this has now gained widespread acceptance as a first-line treatment option, based on the data discussed below.

The BICC-C (Bolus, Infusional, or Capecitabine with Camptosar-Celecoxib) trial is the only trial to directly compare weekly bolus IFL to FOLFIRI.[259] This trial utilized a modified bolus IFL schedule, giving treatment on days 1 and 8, repeated on a 3-week cycle. This modified IFL was compared to FOLFIRI as well as to capecitabine/irinotecan (CapeIri). The first phase of this trial (430 patients) confirmed the superior safety and efficacy of FOLFIRI over IFL (median progression-free survival 7.6 months for FOLFIRI vs. 5.8 months; $P = .007$) and over CapeIri (progression-free survival 5.7 months; $P = .003$). The trial was halted when bevacizumab (see below) became commercially available, and a second phase randomized 117 patients to modified IFL plus bevacizumab versus FOLFIRI plus bevacizumab (CapeIri was dropped from the second phase of this trial). This second phase showed a significant overall survival advantage for FOLFIRI/bevacizumab over modified IFL/bevacizumab ($P = .002$). The BICC-C trial also had a second randomization of all patients to celecoxib versus placebo. Celecoxib was found to provide no benefit in terms of either safety or efficacy and does not appear to have a role as part of standard chemotherapy of this disease.

Oxaliplatin

Oxaliplatin (1,2-diaminocyclohexane (trans-l) oxalatoplatinum, OXAL) is a third-generation platinum compound of the diaminocyclohexane (DACH) family. Initial single-agent phase 1 studies established that oxaliplatin could be safely administered, with evidence of clinical activity.[260,261] No significant nephrotoxicity was seen. Nausea and vomiting, minimal leucopenia, and rare thrombocytopenia were observed. Extra et al.[260] were the first to describe in detail the most notable toxicity encountered with oxaliplatin: neurotoxicity. This neurotoxicity manifested as paresthesias and dysesthesias of the hands, feet, perioral region, and throat. Pharyngolaryngeal dysesthesia, a sensation of choking without overt airway blockage, was described as well. These neurologic toxicities were induced or worsened by exposure to cold. Using a 130 mg/m^2 starting dose over 2 hours every 3 weeks, Diaz-Rubio et al.[262] conducted a phase 2 trial of single-agent OXAL in chemotherapy-naive colorectal cancer patients. The investigator-reported response rate was 20%, however, an independent radiologic review identified a 12% major objective response rate. Neurotoxicity was common, with 92% of patients experiencing neuropathy and 75% experiencing laryngopharyngeal dysesthesias, but no grade 3 or 4 neurologic events were noted. No nephrotoxicity or ototoxicity was encountered. A second single-agent first-line study reported similar results, with a response rate of 24%.[263] Grade 3 neurotoxicity was encountered in 13% of the patients treated.

Machover et al.[264] reported two consecutive phase 2 trials of single-agent oxaliplatin given at 130 mg/m² every 3 weeks in previously treated colorectal cancer patients. The response rate for the total 106 patients was 10%. Neurotoxicity, which was cumulative both in severity and in incidence, was seen to some degree in over 95% of patients on both trials.

Other investigators explored the use of single-agent oxaliplatin using chronomodulation to exploit the potential influence of circadian rhythms on oxaliplatin activity and toxicity. A randomized phase 1 study indicated that a higher dose of oxaliplatin could be administered with manageable toxicity utilizing a chronomodulated schedule.[265] Patients received either a flat 5-day continuous infusion of oxaliplatin or a chronomodulated infusion. The chronomodulated group was able to achieve a 15% higher maximum tolerated dose, with substantially less neurotoxicity and less vomiting. A phase 2 trial was conducted in 29 chemotherapy-refractory colorectal cancer patients using this biomodulated regimen, using a starting dose of 30 mg/m²/d for 5 days repeated every 3 weeks, with peak administration at 4:00 P.M., and 5 mg/m² dose escalations over the first three cycles as tolerated. Despite the encouraging results from the previous phase 1 study, this phase 2 trial found a response rate of 10%, with 79% of patients experiencing some degree of neurotoxicity, 12% of which were grade 3.

Oxaliplatin/Fluorouracil/Leucovorin Combination Trials

Based on a series of phase 2 trials by Levi et al., Giachetti et al. from the same group reported a phase 3 trial of chronomodulated 5-FU/leucovorin alone or with oxaliplatin.[266–268] Two hundred patients were randomly assigned to receive a 5-day course every 3 weeks of chronomodulated 5-FU and leucovorin (700 and 300 mg/m²/d, respectively; peak delivery rate at 4 A.M.) with or without oxaliplatin on the first day of each course (125 mg/m², as a 6-hour infusion). The group who received oxaliplatin had a superior response rate (53% vs. 16%; $P < .001$). Progression-free survival was also superior, just reaching statistical significance (8.7 months vs. 7.4 months; $P = .048$). There were no differences in median overall survival (19.4 months and 19.9 months, respectively). Survival outcomes in this trial are somewhat difficult to interpret since extensive use of resection of metastatic disease was applied in both arms.

Most of the combination 5-FU/leucovorin/OXAL trials have used flat (nonchronomodulated) administration of agents, and have centered on variants of the FOLFOX regimen. The acronym FOLFOX (FOL for folinic acid (leucovorin), F for fluorouracil, OX for oxaliplatin) refers to a series of combinations of these agents. These are biweekly (every other week) regimens using 2 days of infusional 5-FU on a 14-day cycle (leucovorin/5-FU2).[269] The FOLFOX-1, -2, and -3 regimens employed various alterations in dosing of each oxaliplatin, 5-FU, and leucovorin.[270,271] They are of historical interest, but were never evaluated in randomized trials. FOLFOX-3 and FOLFOX-4 were reported in a combined series to have a response rate of 21% in a population of patients who had progressed on the same 5-FU/leucovorin schedule without OXAL.[270] The FOLFOX-4 regimen had a modestly higher response rate and lower toxicity than FOLFOX-3 (which used higher doses of 5-FU and leucovorin), and FOLFOX-4 appeared to be better tolerated. The more commonly used oxaliplatin/5-FU/leucovorin combinations are outlined in Table 89.14.

A randomized phase 3 trial was undertaken to evaluate FOLFOX-4 versus the leucovorin/5-FU2 schedule in previously untreated metastatic colorectal cancer patients (essentially a trial of leucovorin/5-FU2 with or without oxaliplatin).[272] Patients treated with FOLFOX-4 had a statistically significantly superior outcome in terms of response rate (51% vs. 22%; $P = .001$) and progression-free survival (9.0 months vs. 6.2 months; $P = .0003$). The FOLFOX arm had a 1.5-month improvement in median overall survival, however, this did not reach statistical significance (16.2 months vs. 14.7 months; $P = .12$). The number of patients experiencing grade 3 or 4 neutropenia was

TABLE 89.14

SELECTED COMMONLY USED OXALIPLATIN/FLUOROURACIL COMBINATION REGIMENS

Name of Regimen	Author (Ref.)	Schedule (All Agents Administered Intravenously)
FOLFOX-4	de Gramont et al., 2000 (272)	Oxaliplatin 85 mg/m² over 2 hours; LV 200 mg/m² concurrently with oxaliplatin (can be given in same line through "Y" connector); followed by 5-FU bolus 400 mg/m², followed by 5-FU 600 mg/m² infusion over 22 hours. Oxaliplatin given day 1 only. All other meds given days 1 and 2. Cycle repeated every 14 days.
FOLFOX-6	Tournigand et al., 2004 (275)	Oxaliplatin 100 mg/m² over 2 hours; LV 400 mg/m² concurrently with oxaliplatin (can be given in same line through "Y" connector); followed by 5-FU bolus 400 mg/m², followed by 5-FU 1,200 mg/m²/d times 2 days (2,400 mg/m² infusion over 46–48 hours). Cycle repeated every 14 days.
Modified FOLFOX-6 (mFOLFOX-6)	Widely used in current phase III trials, Wolmark et al. 2009 (176)	Oxaliplatin 85 mg/m² over 2 hours; LV 400 mg/m² concurrently with oxaliplatin (can be given in same line through "Y" connector); followed by 5-FU bolus 400 mg/m², followed by 5-FU 1,200 mg/m²/d times 2 days (2,400 mg/m² infusion over 46–48 hours). Cycle repeated every 14 days.
FUFOX	Grothey et al., 2002(366)	Oxaliplatin 50 mg/m² over 2 hours, followed by LV 500 mg/m², followed by 5-FU 2,000 mg/m² over 24 hours, weekly for 5 weeks, repeated every 6 weeks.

LV, leucovorin; 5-FU, 5-fluorouracil.
Note: Doses listed are recommended starting doses for good performance status patients with normal renal, hepatic, and bone marrow function. Individual dose adjustments may be required.

increased with FOLFOX-4 over leucovorin/5-FU2 (42% vs. 5% of patients). Grade 3 or 4 diarrhea (12% vs. 5%) was also increased in the FOLFOX arm. Neurotoxicity, virtually absent in the leucovorin/5-FU2 arm, was frequent in the FOLFOX arm, with 18% of patients experiencing grade 3 neurosensory toxicity.

The FOLFOX-4 regimen has also been evaluated in a multicenter randomized trial in second-line therapy following failure of first-line IFL chemotherapy.[273] Patients were randomly assigned to one of three arms: FOLFOX-4, leucovorin/5-FU2, or single-agent oxaliplatin. Response rates were 10% for FOLFOX, 0% for leucovorin/5-FU2, and 1% for oxaliplatin alone (P <.0001 for FOLFOX versus leucovorin/5-FU2). Time to tumor progression was also superior for FOLFOX-4 (4.6 months) versus leucovorin/5-FU2 (2.7 months) and oxaliplatin alone (1.6 months). These data confirm initial clinical impressions that oxaliplatin/5-FU combinations have superior activity to single-agent oxaliplatin, even in 5-FU-refractory disease. FOLFOX-4 has activity in IFL-refractory disease; however, single-agent oxaliplatin essentially does not.

Further modifications have been made to the FOLFOX schedule. FOLFOX-5 was designed with an increased dose of oxaliplatin to 100 mg/m^2 every 14 days, however, this regimen was never tested in clinical trials. FOLFOX-6 utilized this 100 mg/m^2 oxaliplatin dose with a simplified 5-FU/leucovorin schedule.[274] Oxaliplatin 100 mg/m^2 is given over 2 hours, with leucovorin 400 mg/m^2 given concurrently via a "T" connector. These are then followed by a 400 mg/m^2 bolus of 5-FU, and then a 46-hour infusion of 5-FU at 2,400 to 3,000 mg/m^2. More recently the FOLFOX-7 regimen has been reported, utilizing a 130 mg/m^2 dose of oxaliplatin every 14 days. The simplified leucovorin/5-FU administration of FOLFOX-6 is maintained, with deletion of the bolus 5-FU. Oxaliplatin is discontinued after 3 months, with planned reintroduction after 12 weeks or sooner if clinical progression occurred.[275] This rationale appears promising, both for treatment of metastatic disease and for potential use in the adjuvant setting. Given the similar response rates after 12 weeks, it would appear that the increased dose of oxaliplatin in FOLFOX-7 is unnecessary. A reasonable approach to standard use of FOLFOX in the metastatic setting is to use a modified FOLFOX-6, with 85 mg/m^2 of oxaliplatin and simplified 5-FU/LV2 at a dose of 2,400 mg/m^2 over 46 to 48 hours (1,200 mg/m^2/d for 2 consecutive days). As discussed below, the OPTIMOX trial data support cessation of oxaliplatin after 12 weeks and reintroduction of the oxaliplatin at a later date upon disease progression.

Comparisons of Oxaliplatin and Irinotecan-Based Combinations

With both oxaliplatin and irinotecan-based regimens showing encouraging activity, the question of which agent to use first was addressed by a number of investigators. Tournigand et al.[275] reported a phase 3 trial of FOLFOX-6 versus FOLFIRI. This trial utilized identical simplified leucovorin/5-FU2 schedules, with the only variable being oxaliplatin or irinotecan. All patients were planned to cross over to the other regimen at time of progression, and the primary end point was time to tumor progression after *both* chemotherapy regimens. Results are shown in Table 89.15. Although the study is somewhat underpowered at a total of 226 patients, the results show a striking consistency between regimens, suggesting that use of either FOLFOX-6 or FOLFIRI in first-line treatment is acceptable. A somewhat larger trial of 360 patients randomized to FOLFOX-4 versus the equivalent FOLFIRI schedule, utilizing the same leucovorin/5-FU2 dose and schedule in each arm, again shows comparable efficacy data, with differing and predictable toxicity profiles.[276]

The North Central Cancer Treatment Group–led U.S. Intergroup study N9741, a complex and important trial that underwent many iterations before its completion, initially opened as a four-arm trial comparing the Mayo Clinic 5-FU/leucovorin control arm to three different CPT-11/5-FU/leucovorin regimens: weekly bolus IFL as reported by Saltz et al.,[169] a "Mayo II" schedule of CPT-11 on day 1 and bolus 5-FU/low-dose leucovorin on days 2 to 5, or the biweekly infusional schedule of leucovorin/5-FU2 plus CPT-11 as reported by Douillard et al.[168] and Goldberg.[277] After accruing a small number of patients the trial was closed to incorporate three oxaliplatin-containing arms: FOLFOX-4, IROX (a once every 3 weeks combination of irinotecan and oxaliplatin, without 5-FU) and a modified Mayo Clinic schedule of bolus 5-FU plus low-dose leucovorin days 1 through 5, with oxaliplatin given on day 1. The infusional leucovorin/5-FU2 plus CPT-11 arm was dropped. This created a six-arm trial. In March 2000, the trial was again halted, based on presentation of evidence that the combination of CPT-11/5-FU/leucovorin, using either bolus or infusional schedules, was superior to 5-FU/leucovorin. The Mayo Clinic control arm of N9741 was now dropped, and weekly bolus IFL

TABLE 89.15

COMPARISON OF FIRST-LINE USE OF IRINOTECAN (FOLFIRI) VERSUS OXALIPLATIN (FOLFOX) IN CONJUNCTION WITH THE SAME SIMPLIFIED BIWEEKLY INFUSIONAL 5-FU/LEUCOVORIN SCHEDULE

	FOLFIRI (n = 109 Patients Treated)	FOLFOX-6 (n = 111 Patients Treated)	*P* Value
Major objective response rate (partial plus complete responses)	56%	54%	.68
Time to tumor progression (on first-line regimen)	8.5 months	8.1 months	.65
Time to tumor progression (after first- and second-line regimen)	14.4 months	11.5 months	.65
Overall survival (from initial randomization)	20.4 months	21.5 months	.9
2-year overall survival	41%	45%	
Grade 3–4 neutropenia	25%	44%	
Neutropenic fever	6%	1%	
Grade 3–4 diarrhea	14%	11%	
Neuropathy (grade 3)	0%	34%	
Alopecia (grade 2)	24%	9%	

From ref. 275.

became the control arm. At the same time, ongoing real-time monitoring of fatal toxicities identified unacceptably high rates of treatment-related mortality in the OXAL plus Mayo Clinic 5-FU/leucovorin and in the CPT-11 plus 5-FU/leucovorin arms. These schedules were also dropped from the trial and from further development, leaving a three-arm trial of CPT-11 plus bolus 5-FU/leucovorin (IFL), oxaliplatin plus infusional leucovorin/5-FU2 (FOLFOX-4), and oxaliplatin plus CPT-11 (IROX).

The trial was stopped a third time in April 2001, when monitoring of the trial indicated what appeared to be a higher than expected early mortality in the IFL control arm.[170] This observation, however, was based on utilization of a new metric, the 60-day all-cause mortality (ACM). This metric records death from *any* cause within 60 days of initial therapy. The 60-day ACM of the IFL arm was initially noted to be 4.5%. Because this was a new metric, however, there were no readily available historical controls; no one had ready access to data to say what the 60-day ACM had been in previous trials, either with IFL or with 5-FU/leucovorin regimens. The 4.5% ACM was therefore compared to the previously reported death rate for the IFL regimen, which was 0.9%. However the previously reported death rate was the treatment-related death rate, the percentage of deaths judged by the investigators to have been caused by treatment, not all deaths within 60 days of starting therapy. Of further concern to the safety monitoring committee, however, the experimental arms (FOLFOX-4 and IROX) each showed 60-day ACM's of 1.8% (compared to 4.5% for the IFL control arm). This information was difficult to put into context, however, because the efficacy of the two experimental arms had not yet been established.

In fact, the 60-day ACM on the original phase 3 trial of IFL (subsequently calculated after N9741 was halted) was 6.7%, and the 60-day ACM for the Mayo Clinic control arm of that trial was found to be 7.3%. Although the 7.3% 60-day ACM appeared subjectively to be unusually high, no historical baseline data on 60-day ACM in 5-FU-based regimens were readily available. To help interpret these data, an analysis was undertaken to determine the 60-day ACM in multiple large-scale randomized trials that had used 5-FU/leucovorin schedules over the prior decade. This analysis confirmed that 60-day ACM regularly was encountered at a rate of 5% to 8% in the treatment of metastatic colorectal cancer.[278] Thus the 60-day ACM for the IFL regimen was actually *lower* on N9741 than in previous trials and was *lower* than what had been seen consistently with 5-FU/leucovorin regimens alone. In the final analysis of N9741 the 60-day ACM seen in the IFL, FOLFOX-4, and IROX arms were 4.5%, 2.6%, and 2.7%, respectively, and these differences were not statistically significant.

The efficacy results of N9741, however, were statistically significant and showed superior outcome for the patients randomized to FOLFOX-4, as compared to those randomized to either IFL or IROX, in terms of response rate, time to tumor progression, and overall survival (Table 89.16).[279] Toxicity for FOLFOX-4 was also superior for virtually all parameters, except of course neurotoxicity. The results of the IROX arm did not statistically significantly differ from those of the IFL arm in terms of toxicity, response, or time to tumor progression, however, survival was borderline statistically significantly better in the IROX arm than the IFL arm ($P = .04$).

Taken together, where do these trials leave us in terms of first-line use of oxaliplatin and irinotecan-based regimens? Data from trial N9741 indicate that FOLFOX-4 is superior to IFL in both response rate and time to tumor progression. Overall survival was superior in the FOLFOX-4 arm versus IFL as well; however, interpretation of the survival results of N9741 is somewhat complicated due to imbalances between arms in availability of effective second-line therapy. Second-line CPT-11 was available to all patients who had received FOLFOX-4. Oxaliplatin, however, was not commercially available in the United States during the course of N9741. To what degree this imbalance in second-line therapy may have influenced the survival result is unknown. Also, since IFL contains bolus 5-FU, while FOLFOX-4 contains infusional leucovorin/5-FU2, it is difficult to isolate the irinotecan versus oxaliplatin component from the 5-FU bolus versus 5-FU infusion component.

Two other trials indicate that the FOLFOX and FOLFIRI regimens have similar safety and efficacy, with differing toxicity profiles.[275,276] Thus, FOLFOX has comparable efficacy to FOLFIRI, while FOLFOX has a superior response rate, time to tumor progression, and possibly some degree of survival benefit over IFL. Toxicity with irinotecan-based regimens shows a higher degree of alopecia. Diarrhea and neutropenia are increased on the bolus 5-FU schedule but are similar between FOLFOX and FOLFIRI. Oxaliplatin-based regimens, however, have neurotoxicity, absent from the irinotecan-based regimens, which can be problematic in some patients. It would therefore

TABLE 89.16

RESULTS OF INTERGROUP TRIAL N9741: IRINOTECAN PLUS BOLUS 5-FU/LEUCOVORIN (IFL), OXALIPLATIN PLUS INFUSIONAL 5-FU/LEUCOVORIN (FOLFOX-4), AND IRINOTECAN PLUS OXALIPLATIN (IROX) IN FIRST-LINE TREATMENT OF PATIENTS WITH METASTATIC COLORECTAL CANCER

	IFL ($N = 264$)	FOLFOX-4 ($N = 267$)	IROX ($N = 264$)	*P* Value (IFL vs. FOLFOX)
Major objective response rate (partial plus complete responses)	31%	45%	35%	.03
Time to tumor progression	6.9 months	8.7 months	6.5 months	.001
Overall survival	15.0 months	19.5 months	17.4 months	.0001
Received second-line therapy with active drug not included in first-line regimen	24% (oxaliplatin)	60% (irinotecan)	50% (fluorouracil)	Not given
Grade 3–4 neutropenia	40%	50%	36%	.35
Neutropenic fever	15%	4%	11%	.001
Grade 3–4 diarrhea	28%	12%	24%	.001
Grade 3–4 nausea	16%	6%	19%	.001
Grade 3 neuropathy	3%	18%	7%	.001
60-day all cause mortality	4.5%	2.6%	2.7%	Not significant

From ref. 279.

seem reasonable at this time to favor the use of a high-dose intermittent infusional 5-FU/leucovorin schedule plus either oxaliplatin (i.e., FOLFOX) or CPT-11 (i.e., FOLFIRI). Data do not support continued routine use of the bolus IFL schedule, nor are there randomized data to support the routine use of a bolus 5-FU/leucovorin schedule with oxaliplatin in the metastatic setting. Routine use of IROX is also not supported by the currently available body of data.

Whether to use an irinotecan-based or oxaliplatin-based combination in first-line treatment of good performance status patients can be considered a matter of patient preference, and discussion of the differing toxicity profiles is appropriate to help individuals decide. It is hoped that in the near-term future molecular prognostic indicators and pharmacogenomics will provide useful guidance for the individualization of therapies, but such approaches remain investigational at this time.

The only oxaliplatin schedule registered for use in the United States is FOLFOX-4, however, the modified FOLFOX-6 would appear at this time to be a very reasonable schedule for routine clinical use when the decision is made to use an oxaliplatin/fluorouracil combination.

The recognition of neurotoxicity as a major limitation of the FOLFOX regimens led to the investigation of optimization of oxaliplatin (the OPTIMOX study).[280] In this trial patients were randomly assigned to receive either standard FOLFOX-4 until progression or 12 weeks of FOLFOX-7, followed by planned cessation of oxaliplatin and continuation of the 5-FU/LV2. As designed, the study called for a reintroduction of oxaliplatin after 6 months of 5-FU/LV2, although this actually occurred in the minority of patients and outcomes were superior in those patients in whom reintroduction of oxaliplatin occurred.[281] The primary end point was duration of disease control, the time from initiation of treatment until either progression through all agents (including failure after reintroduction of oxaliplatin if this was done) or death. Duration of disease control as well as progression-free survival and overall survival were not statistically significantly different between the two arms. As anticipated, toxicity, including neurotoxicity, was substantially reduced in the OPTIMOX arm. This OPTIMOX strategy of planned interruption of oxaliplatin can be considered a standard care option in metastatic disease. It is important to discuss plans for such planned interruptions with patients at the beginning of therapy so that they will not be surprised or alarmed at the removal of one of the drugs.

Although a regimen of oxaliplatin, weekly bolus 5-FU, and low-dose weekly leucovorin (bFOL) appeared promising in an initial phase 2 trial, two sequential randomized phase 2 trials, known as TREE-1 and TREE-2, suggest modestly inferior activity for the bFOLF schedule compared with FOLFOX or CapeOx.[282,283] Thus, in the metastatic setting, oxaliplatin with bolus 5-FU schedules is therefore not recommended for routine use.

Use of planned sequential administration of FOLFOX and FOLFIRI has also been proposed, both in terms of pretreatment for potentially resectable patients with liver metastases and in terms of adjuvant treatment of earlier stage disease. Several groups are also exploring the use of "triple therapy" with OXAL, CPT-11, and 5-FU/leucovorin. Phase 1 and 2 trials have demonstrated high activity but also substantial toxicity.[284–286] Two modest-sized randomized studies have now been reported, with conflicting results; one study showed a survival advantage for the triple drug combination, while the other study showed no significant benefit in terms of response, progression-free survival, or overall survival.[287,288] At present this approach has not gained widespread acceptance and is little used in standard practice.

As discussed above, a trial comparing FOLFIRI to capecitabine/irinotecan suggested inferior outcome for the capecitabine-containing regimen.[259] However, a large randomized trial has now compared capecitabine plus oxaliplatin (CapeOx) versus FOLFOX. The study also had a two-by-two randomization to with or without bevacizumab (discussed below). This trial demonstrated the CapeOx regimen to be noninferior to FOLFOX, and each had acceptable toxicity, indicating that CapeOx is an acceptable alternative to FOLFOX.[289] It should be noted that the CapeOx regimen requires a motivated, reliable patients who will be able to take multiple pills of oral medication on a complex schedule, even in the setting of potentially emetogenic oxaliplatin.

Duration of Therapy

Controversy continues to exist regarding the optimal duration of chemotherapy for palliation of metastatic disease. Traditional practice for many years had been to continue chemotherapy until either unacceptable toxicity, clinical deterioration, or disease progression. When efficacy of treatment was more limited, with the duration of therapy typically limited to a small number of months, the issue of treatment breaks did not seem relevant. Now, with patients typically living multiple years with metastatic colorectal cancer and with some treatments maintaining control for more extended periods of time, the need for patients to have breaks (often referred to as "treatment holidays" or "chemotherapy-free intervals") is greater, and there is considerable interest in using these approaches. Both physically and psychologically, many patients appear to both need and derive benefit from these treatment interruptions.

The concept of noncontinuous chemotherapy has been investigated for some time now. Maughan et al.[290] conducted a randomized trial of continuous versus interrupted treatment in 354 patients who were responding or who had stable disease after receiving 12 weeks of either fluorouracil or raltitrexed-based chemotherapy. Patients were randomized to either continue chemotherapy until progression or to stop chemotherapy after the first 12 weeks, followed by a planned restarting on the same chemotherapy at the time of progression. At randomization, 41% of patients had achieved a major objective response and 59% had stable disease. There was no evidence of a difference in overall survival, the primary end point, between the two groups, with a hazard ratio of 0.87 ($P = .23$, favoring the intermittent arm).

More recently, the idea of planned early cessation of all chemotherapy was investigated in the OPTIMOX-2 trial.[291] Two hundred two previously untreated metastatic colorectal cancer patients were treated. All patients received six cycles of modified FOLFOX-7 followed by either continued leucovorin/5-FU2 until progression, or a complete cessation of all chemotherapy (a chemotherapy-free interval [CFI]). Patients on both arms were planned to receive retreatment with FOLFOX following tumor progression. The results of this study did not support the use of this planned, early interruption in therapy, as the median duration of disease control, progression-free survival, and overall survival were all inferior in the arm with the early planned CFI. This should not be misconstrued as evidence that CFIs are contraindicated, but rather that early planned CFIs for all patients is not an appropriate strategy. The authors suggest that this study indicates there are no pretreatment parameters that can identify *a priori* those patients who can successfully benefit from a CFI. Thus, specific decisions regarding use and timing of CFIs cannot be made in advance of starting treatment; rather clinical judgment must be exercised in deciding on treatment interruptions for CFIs in responding patients after a favorable response. In a retrospective review of 822 patients in the two OPTIMOX studies, after excluding those patients who had early progression within the first 3 months of treatment as well as those who underwent complete gross resection of metastatic disease within 3 months of stopping chemotherapy, Perez-Staub et al.[292] noted that there was no indication of a detriment in survival when comparing those patients who took a CFI versus those who did not. In fact, in this retrospective, nonrandomized analysis, the median survival was 37.5 months in patients who had a CFI versus 21.2 months in matched patients who did not have a CFI. Of note, median overall survival of patients who stopped chemotherapy earlier than 3 months was 24 months, whereas it was 42 months when a CFI was taken between 3 and 9 months into therapy, and 44 months when a CFI was taken later than 9 months into chemotherapy. The above studies were accomplished prior to the use of bevacizumab. Some clinicians have advocated the continuation of bevacizumab during CFIs. Such an approach is not supported by data, and given the absence of activity of single-agent bevacizumab in colorectal cancer, use of single-agent bevacizumab during otherwise CFIs is not recommended at this time.

Other investigators specifically addressed the question of whether rechallenge with fluorouracil after a planned treatment interruption could produce a response. A pooled analysis was conducted on 613 patients involved in three randomized trials of first-line 5-FU-based therapy.[293] All patients had a planned maximum treatment period of 6 months. Patients with responding or stable disease at the end of that period were observed off treatment with a plan for retreatment at the time of disease progression. Median time to rechallenge was 11.7 months. Seventeen percent of patients had an objective response to rechallenging. Median survival for the group was 14.8 months. These nonrandomized data indicate that patients have a meaningful response rate at time of reinstitution of chemotherapy.

A similar approach was explored in patients who received second-line irinotecan therapy.[294] A total of 333 patients entered into a trial to receive 24 weeks of irinotecan. Patients who remained in the study at the end of that time were to be randomized to either continue treatment or to stop therapy. Of the 333 patients, most came off the study due to progression or toxicity before reaching the 24-week mark. Fifty-five patients with responding or stable disease agreed to randomization. Although the numbers available for comparison were small, there were no differences between the arms in progression-free survival or overall survival, nor were there differences in quality-of-life scores.

Overall there appears to be no compelling evidence that continuation of chemotherapy indefinitely is necessary for optimal control of metastatic disease. The option of discontinuation of therapy after a reasonable period of time appears to be an appropriate consideration in standard practice.

Combination versus Single-Agent Chemotherapy

Given that combination regimens are invariably associated with more toxicity than single agents, the question of the need for universal upfront use of these combinations was investigated. The CAIRO (CApecitabine, IRinotecan, Oxaliplatin) trial randomized 820 patients to sequential versus concurrent therapies (Table 89.17).[295] In the sequential arm, first-line therapy was single-agent capecitabine. Upon failure, single-agent irinotecan was used, and then third-line therapy was oxaliplatin with capecitabine (since single-agent oxaliplatin is essentially inactive in fluorouracil-refractory colorectal cancer). The combination arm used CapeOx as first-line therapy and CapeIri as second-line therapy. The primary end point, median overall survival, was not statistically significantly different between the two arms (17.4 months for combination vs. 16.3 months for the sequential arm; $P = .33$). Dose-limiting toxicity (grade 3 or 4) was not significantly different between the two groups, in fact grade 3 hand-foot syndrome was somewhat more common in the sequential arm (13% vs. 7%; $P = .004$).

Similar findings were reported in the FOCUS study.[296] In this trial, a total of 2,135 patients were randomized to one of three arms. Arm A was sequential therapy, with initial treatment given with 5-FU on the leucovorin/5-FU2 (biweekly infusional) schedule until progression, at which point second-line therapy was given with single-agent irinotecan. Arm B also gave biweekly leucovorin/5-FU2 until failure, and then leucovorin/5-FU2 was continued with the addition of either oxaliplatin or irinotecan (this was a second randomization within this arm). Thus, second-line therapy was a change from biweekly leucovorin/5-FU2 to either FOLFOX or FOLFIRI in this arm. In arm C, patients began with combination chemotherapy, and within this arm were randomized to be treated with either FOLFOX or FOLFIRI. The primary end point, median overall survival, for arm A was 13.9 months. For arm B, survival was 15.0 months for irinotecan and 15.2 months for oxaliplatin. Arm C had a median overall survival of 16.7 months for the FOLFIRI patients and 15.4 months for those treated with FOLFOX. Only the difference between arm A and the irinotecan arm of arm C reached statistical significance ($P = .01$). Arm B (initial leucovorin/5-FU2 followed by FOLFOX or FOLIRI) was noninferior to arm C (initial FOLFOX or FOLIRI) (HR 1.06; 90% CI, 0.97 to 1.17).

Taken together, the CAIRO and FOCUS trials provide a strong argument that not all patients with unresectable metastatic disease require exposure to the toxicity of combination therapy, and that initial use of fluorinated pyrimidine alone in previously untreated metastatic colorectal patients is a treatment alternative that needs to be carefully considered.

Bevacizumab

Bevacizumab is a humanized monoclonal antibody that binds to vascular endothelial growth factor (VEGF), thereby substantially reducing the amount of circulating ligand and thus preventing receptor activation.[297,298] The first trial of bevacizumab in colorectal cancer was a modest-sized, three-arm, randomized phase 2 trial in which a total of 104 patients were

TABLE 89.17

SEQUENTIAL VERSUS COMBINATION CHEMOTHERAPY WITH CAPECITABINE (Cape), IRINOTECAN (Iri), AND OXALIPLATIN (Ox) IN ADVANCED COLORECTAL CANCER (CAIRO): EFFICACY END POINTS

	Overall Survival	1-Year Survival	Progression-Free Survival (First Line)	Response Rate
Sequential Cape, then Iri, then Cape/Ox (n = 401)	16.3 m	64%	5.8 m	20%
Combination Cape/Iri, then Cape/Ox (n = 402)	17.4 m	67%	7.8 m	41%
P value	.33	.38	.0002	.0001

From ref. 295.

TABLE 89.18A

EFFICACY OUTCOMES, FIRST-LINE TREATMENT OF METASTATIC COLORECTAL CANCER: IRINOTECAN PLUS BOLUS 5-FU/LEUCOVORIN (IFL) PLUS PLACEBO VERSUS IFL PLUS BEVACIZUMAB VERSUS FL PLUS BEVACIZUMAB

Regimen	No. of Patients	Response Rate	Progression-Free Survival	Overall Survival
IFL + placebo	411	34.8%	6.2 m	15.6 m
IFL + bevacizumab	402	44.8%	10.6 m	20.3 m
		P = .004	*P* <.001	*P* <.001

randomly assigned to either one of two different doses levels of bevacizumab (5 mg/kg or 10 mg/kg) plus weekly 5-FU/leucovorin or to 5-FU/leucovorin alone.[299] The response rate, time to tumor progression and overall survival were superior in the 5-FU/leucovorin with 5 mg/kg bevacizumab arm. Despite the small size and limited statistical power of this study, this result would served as the basis for design of the pivotal phase 3 trial of bevacizumab in colorectal cancer.

The initial design of the phase 3 pivotal trial was a comparison between 5-FU/leucovorin plus placebo to 5-FU/leucovorin plus 5 mg/kg of bevacizumab. However, as the randomized phase 2 trial, discussed above, was nearing completion, the randomized phase 3 trial was reported, which demonstrated a modest but statistically significant survival advantage for the IFL regimen (irinotecan plus weekly bolus 5-FU/leucovorin) compared with 5-FU/leucovorin alone.[169] As a result of this trial, the IFL regimen was then felt to be the appropriate control arm for subsequent phase 3 trials. There were no safety data at the time, however, on the combination of bevacizumab plus IFL. As a result of this, a three-arm trial was designed that contained (1) 5-FU/leucovorin/bevacizumab, (2) IFL/bevacizumab, and (3) IFL/placebo (the control arm).[300] The design included a preplanned analysis of safety on all arms when enrollment reached 100 patients per arm, with a further plan to close the 5-FU/leucovorin/bevacizumab arm at that time if the safety data indicated acceptable tolerability and safety of the IFL/bevacizumab arm.

In the final efficacy analysis, the IFL/bevacizumab cohort experienced superior outcome compared to the IFL/placebo group in response rate (45% vs. 35%; *P* <.003), progression-free survival (10.6 months vs. 6.2 months; *P* <.00001), and overall survival (20.3 months vs. 15.6 months; *P* = .00003) (Table 89.18*A*). It should be noted that no crossover to second-line bevacizumab in the IFL/placebo control arm was allowed in this trial.

In order to better understand the effects of bevacizumab in conjunction with 5-FU/leucovorin, Kavinibbar et al.[301] combined the data from three separate modest-sized trials to create a more robust data set. In this combined analysis of 5-FU/leucovorin with or without bevacizumab, there was a statistically significant survival advantage for the patients who received bevacizumab. Given the favorable aspects of the biweekly infusional leucovorin/5-FU2 schedule used in the FOCUS trial, the leucovorin/5-FU2 schedule would seem most appropriate for combination with bevacizumab.[302]

At the same time as the pivotal front-line study was accruing, ECOG also performed a trial (ECOG-3200) to evaluate the use of bevacizumab in the second-line setting.[303] This trial randomized patients who had failed irinotecan and fluorouracil but were naive to bevacizumab, to one of three arms: bevacizumab/FOLFOX, FOLFOX alone, or bevacizumab. The investigators chose to investigate a 10 mg/kg bevacizumab dose. Overall, a modest but statistically significant improvement in median overall survival was demonstrated for FOLFOX-4 with bevacizumab versus FOLFOX-4 alone (12.5 months vs. 10.7 months; *P* = .0024), and grade 3 or 4 toxicities were not increased. The bevacizumab-alone arm had substantially inferior progression-free survival and an investigator-adjudicated response rate of 3%, suggesting that single-agent bevacizumab does not have meaningful activity in colorectal cancer and should not be used. It is important to note that this trial was performed *exclusively* in patients who had *not* received bevacizumab in the first-line setting. This trial provides no data on whether use of bevacizumab with a second-line regimen after progression on a first-line bevacizumab-containing regimen is efficacious.

Although it was performed in second-line patients, the ECOG-3200 trial was the first trial to provide safety data for the combination of bevacizumab plus FOLFOX. As a result of this, even before front-line data were available, bevacizumab plus FOLFOX had become widely accepted as a front-line option in the United States for metastatic colorectal cancer. More recently, the NO16966 trial directly addressed the question of front-line bevacizumab plus oxaliplatin-based therapy (Table 89.18*B*).[304] In this trial, 1,400 previously untreated colorectal cancer patients were randomly assigned to either

TABLE 89.18B

EFFICACY OUTCOMES, FIRST-LINE TREATMENT OF METASTATIC COLORECTAL CANCER: CAPEOX/FOLFOX PLUS PLACEBO VERSUS CAPEOX/FOLFOX PLUS BEVACIZUMAB

Regimen	No. of Patients	Response Rate	Progression-Free Survival	Overall Survival
CapeOx/FOLFOX + Placebo	701	49%	8.0 m	19.9 m
CapeOx/FOLFOX + bevacizumab	699	47%	9.4 m	21.3 m
		P = .31	*P* = .0023	*P* = .078

CapeOx, capecitabine, oxaliplatin; FOLFOX, fluorouracil, leucovorin, oxaliplatin.
(From Saltz et al. Bevacizumab in combination with oxaliplatin-based chemotherapy as first-line therapy in metastatic colorectal cancer: a randomized phase III study. *J Clin Oncol* 2008:26(12):2013–2019.)

FOLFOX-4 or CapeOx and then to either placebo or bevacizumab, in a two-by-two randomization. Although the study did show a statistically significant progression-free survival advantage for the addition of bevacizumab (9.4 months vs. 8.0 months for chemo with bevacizumab vs. chemo with placebo, respectively; HR 0.83; $P = .003$), this difference was more modest than the 4.4-month progression-free survival difference seen in the initial bevacizumab with IFL front-line trial. Overall survival improvement with bevacizumab approached, but did not reach, statistical significance (21.3 months vs. 19.9 months; HR 0.89; $P = .077$) Also, in the NO16966 trial, the addition of bevacizumab to front-line oxaliplatin-based chemotherapy did not confer any response benefit. It is noteworthy that the majority of patients on this trial discontinued treatment, presumably due to nonbevacizumab-related toxicity issues, before progression. This may have diminished the impact of bevacizumab on survival and progression-free survival but would not have impacted the response rate.

Toxicity

In terms of toxicity, grade 3 hypertension was higher in the bevacizumab/IFL arm than in the placebo/IFL arm (11% vs. 2%) in the IFL/bevacizumab study.[300] Hypertension is now widely recognized as a common side effect of bevacizumab, and monitoring for and treatment of hypertension with antihypertensive medications is a routine part of bevacizumab management. Incidences of overall thromboembolic events and proteinuria were not statistically different between the two arms. However, two rare but extremely serious toxicities were encountered with increased frequency in the bevacizumab-containing arm: GI perforations and arterial thrombotic events.

The GI perforations were a group of events that included a perforated gastric ulcer, small bowel perforations, and free air under the diaphragm without identified source. Although these were somewhat heterogeneous in nature, it was noted that six such events occurred on the bevacizumab-containing arm (one fatal) compared with none on the chemotherapy alone arm. No clear risk factors for these perforations could be identified from this trial. Interestingly, GI perforations were not frequent occurrences in large cooperative group trials in lung cancer or breast cancer patients, however, an unusually high GI perforation rate has recently halted accrual on a trial of bevacizumab in ovarian cancer patients. These ovarian observations illustrate an important aspect about GI perforations in association with bevacizumab: there is not an association between the presence of an intact primary tumor in the colon and a GI perforation. Concerns have been expressed by some clinicians about the possibility of needing to remove an asymptomatic primary colorectal tumor in a patient with synchronous stage IV disease before using bevacizumab, out of an unsubstantiated fear that the primary will put the patient at risk for perforation. At present there are no data to support this assumption, and surgery for an asymptomatic primary tumor in a stage IV patient is not routinely indicated, regardless of whether there are plans to use a bevacizumab-containing chemotherapy regimen.[305]

The other rare but very serious identified increased risk with bevacizumab-containing treatment was that of arterial thrombotic events. Initially, no clear indication of this risk was detected in the pivotal phase 3 trial. However, in a combined analysis of several trials, an important observation was made. Here again, multiple events were combined into one metric. Thus, cerebral vascular accidents, myocardial infarctions, transient ischemic attacks, and angina were combined to create the metric of arterial thrombotic events. The observed incidence of these events was 2.5% in the nonbevacizumab-containing control arms versus 5.0% in the bevacizumab-containing experimental arms. It was noted that patients who had histories of cardiovascular or atherosclerotic disease appeared to be at greater risk for increased bevacizumab-related arterial thrombotic complications. In addition, a further analysis of these events suggested that the risk was essentially linear over time, indicating that the risk of a new arterial thrombotic event was the same in earlier versus later months of exposure.[306]

Cetuximab and Panitumumab

The EGFR, also called HER-1, is a transmembrane glycoprotein receptor. When the external binding domain of the EGFR binds specific ligands, such as epidermal growth factor (EGF) or transforming growth factor alpha (TGF-α), receptor dimerization occurs (either homodimerization with another EGFR or heterodimerization with another member of the EGFR family). This in turn stimulates phosphorylation of the tyrosine kinases on the intracellular domain of the receptor, which initiates a signaling cascade, which ultimately regulates cell proliferation, migration, adhesion, differentiation, and survival.[307–309] Cetuximab (c-mab), is a chimeric immunoglobulin G_1 (IgG_1) monoclonal antibody that recognizes and binds to the extracellular domain of the EGFR. Panitumumab (p-mab) is a fully human IgG_2 monoclonal antibody that also targets the EGFR. Binding of either c-mab or p-mab to this receptor does not cause receptor activation, but rather results in a steric interference with the ligand binding site.[310]

Preclinical models of cetuximab, or its murine precursor, demonstrated more substantial activity when given in combination with cytotoxic chemotherapy. Based on these observations, and on a single anecdotal report of a major response to cetuximab plus irinotecan in a young woman with irinotecan-refractory colorectal cancer, a multicenter phase 2 trial was initiated. This trial, reported in abstract form only, was conducted in patients who were determined by their treating investigator to have progressed on irinotecan.[311] Patients were treated with cetuximab at a dose of 400 mg/m^2 loading dose week 1 over 2 hours, followed by weekly 250 mg/m^2 over 1 hour. Irinotecan was given on the same dose and schedule as had previously failed. Irinotecan dose reductions made previously, prior to study entry, were maintained upon initiation of the study treatment.

One hundred twenty patients with irinotecan-refractory colorectal cancer were identified and enrolled. In addition, in a parallel portion of the trial, 28 patients with clinically and radiographically stable disease after receiving a minimum of 3 months of irinotecan therapy were also enrolled and treated by the addition of cetuximab to their ongoing irinotecan therapy. The response outcome of this "stable disease cohort" was not reported; only those patients who were felt to be irinotecan refractory were included in the initial report. As reported by an independent response assessment committee, 22.5% of irinotecan-refractory patients achieved a major objective response. The irinotecan-related toxicity was relatively mild in this population, at least in part because many patients had already had irinotecan dose modifications made prior to starting on this trial. Of the side effects specifically attributable to cetuximab, 3% of patients developed an allergic, anaphylactoid reaction requiring discontinuation of cetuximab therapy, and 75% of patients experienced a skin rash (12% grade 3), a rash now recognized to be characteristic of all EGFR inhibitors. This rash superficially resembles acne, leading to its initial description as an acneiform rash. However, microscopically this is not acne, and topical acne medications are ineffective in its management. An interesting observation from this trial, which has since been corroborated in multiple trials, is that the presence and severity of the rash appeared to be associated with response in this study.

The results seen in the phase 2 cetuximab plus irinotecan combination trial raised the question, both from a scientific and

TABLE 89.19

EFFICACY OUTCOMES: CETUXIMAB PLUS IRINOTECAN VERSUS CETUXIMAB ALONE IN IRINOTECAN-REFRACTORY COLORECTAL CANCER

	No. of Patients	Response Rate (95% CI)	Disease Control (95% CI)	Median TTP (months)	Median OS (months) (95% CI)
Cetuximab	111	11% (6%–18%)	32% (24%–42%)	1.5	6.9 (5.6–9.1)
Cetuximab + irinotecan	218	23% (18%–29)[a]	56% (49%–62%)[b]	4.1[c]	8.6 (7.6–9.6)

CI, confidence interval; TTP, time to progression; OS, overall survival.
[a]$P = .0074$.
[b]$P = .0001$.
[c]$P < .0001$.
(From ref. 167.)

from a regulatory perspective, of the activity of single-agent cetuximab in irinotecan-refractory colorectal cancer. A small phase 2 trial was therefore quickly designed and accrued. In this trial, 5 of 57 patients (9%) achieved a partial response confirmed by an independent radiologic review.[312]

Based on the preliminary results of the initial phase 2 cetuximab plus irinotecan study, described above, a subsequent larger trial, ultimately reported by Cunningham et al.,[167] was designed to provide confirmatory evidence of the activity of cetuximab in colorectal cancer (Table 89.19). This large, randomized phase 2 trial in irinotecan-refractory colorectal cancer patients, which has become known as the BOND trial, compared cetuximab plus irinotecan to cetuximab monotherapy. Three hundred twenty-nine patients were randomized in a two-to-one schema. The response rates of 22.9% for cetuximab plus irinotecan and 10.8% for cetuximab alone were virtually identical to the response rates that had been reported previously in the two U.S. phase 2 trials, confirming the activity of this agent in colorectal cancer. Time to tumor progression in the Cunningham et al. study was 4.1 months for the combination versus 1.5 months for single-agent cetuximab. Survival in the two arms was not significantly different, however, the study was neither designed nor powered to address the issue of a survival advantage for cetuximab, and cetuximab was given to all patients on both arms of the study.

A National Cancer Institute Canada (NCIC) phase 3 trial compared cetuximab plus best supportive care to best supportive care alone in 572 patients who had exhausted standard treatment options.[313] The median overall survival was improved by 1.5 months (from 4.6 months to 6.1 months) in the cetuximab group compared to supportive care alone. Partial responses occurred in 23 patients (8.0%) in the cetuximab group versus none in the supportive care group ($P < .001$).

Similar results were reported with panitumumab. As seen with single-agent cetuximab, phase 2 evaluations of panitumumab in colorectal cancer patients indicate approximately a 10% response rate, with over 90% of patients experiencing some degree of acneiform-like rash.[314,315] The fully human nature of this antibody appears to reduce the likelihood of anaphylactoid infusion reactions, with only 1 of the 148 patients treated after experiencing a dose-limiting allergic reaction. A randomized trial of panitumumab versus best supportive care in the salvage setting demonstrated a modest (8 weeks vs. 7.3 weeks) but highly statistically significant improvement in median progression-free survival for single-agent panitumumab over best supportive care (HR 0.54; $P < .000000001$). Response rate to p-mab was 10%. There was no difference in overall survival, however, there was extensive postprogression crossover, which obscures this end point.[316]

KRAS

Perhaps the most important development in the use of anti-EGFR agents over the past several years has been the recognition that these agents only have the potential to be beneficial to patients whose tumors have nonmutated, or wild type, *KRAS* gene. KRAS is a signal transduction protein that is a critical intermediate in transmission of growth and survival signals from the EGFR to the nucleus. Mutations in exon 2 of the gene that encodes for the KRAS protein lead to constitutive activation of this signaling pathway, which renders blocking of the EGFR-binding site on the surface useless. Several small retrospective series identified KRAS mutations as being incompatible with responses to cetuximab.[317,318] Subsequently, Amado et al.[319] demonstrated that the activity of panitumumab in the registration study referenced above was limited to those patients with wild type KRAS. In this trial, 92% of patients had tissue available for KRAS genotyping, and 43% of tumors were found to harbor a KRAS mutation. The objective response rate to single-agent panitumumab was 17% in KRAS wild type tumors and 0% in those tumors that had a KRAS mutation. The progression-free survival in the KRAS wild type tumor patients who received panitumumab was 12.3 weeks versus 7.3 weeks for best supportive care. In patients with KRAS-mutated tumors there was no difference in progression-free survival with panitumumab versus best supportive care. Again, overall survival in this trial could not be interpreted due to extensive postprogression crossover.

Similarly, analysis of the NCIC study, discussed above, demonstrated that activity of cetuximab as a single agent in chemotherapy-refractory disease was limited to the KRAS wild type patients only (Table 89.20).[320] Approximately 70% of patients on this trial had tissue available for KRAS genotyping and 42% were found to have mutated KRAS. Those with mutated KRAS showed no evidence of clinical benefit from cetuximab, while patients whose tumors had wild type K-ras showed a 4.7-month improvement in median overall survival with cetuximab versus best supportive care (9.5 months vs. 4.8 months; HR for death 0.55; 95% CI, 0.41 to 0.74; $P < .001$). In the control group who received best supportive care, KRAS mutation status had no impact on median overall survival ($P = .97$).

Genotyping for KRAS mutation status should now be regarded as standard practice in all patients with stage IV disease, and cetuximab and panitumumab should only be considered in patients with nonmutated KRAS.[321] It is prudent to obtain KRAS genotyping at the time that stage IV disease is diagnosed, not necessarily because the information is needed for first-line therapy, as only a minority of patients will be appropriate for first-line anti-EGFR therapy, but because whether or not a patient can consider the use of cetuximab or

TABLE 89.20

CETUXIMAB VERSUS BEST SUPPORTIVE CARE IN METASTATIC CHEMOTHERAPY-REFRACTORY COLORECTAL CANCER

	Overall Survival		Progression-Free Survival		Response Rate	
	KRAS Wt	KRAS Mut	KRAS Wt	KRAS Mut	KRAS Wt	KRAS Mut
Cetux	9.5 m	4.5 m	3.7 m	1.8 m	12.8%	1.2%
BSC	4.8 m	4.6 m	1.9 m	1.8 m	0%	0%
P value	.001	.89	.001	.96	NR	NR

Wt, wild type; Mut, mutant; Cetux, cetuximab; BSC, best supportive care; m, months
(From ref. 320.)

panitumumab in the course of multiple lines of therapy is easier to both determine and to deal with early on when there are multiple options, rather than waiting until all other options are exhausted. At present there is no role for determining KRAS status in stage I, II, or III disease, since there is no basis for use of EGFR agents in other than stage IV.

Cetuximab or Panitumumab in First-Line Therapy

An early trial of FOLFOX versus FOLFIRI with or without cetuximab in a two-by-two design was initiated by the CALGB (trial 80203) in 2003; however, this trial was halted early after the emergence of the front-line bevacizumab data precluded accrual to the chemotherapy-alone control arm of this trial. Almost 300 patients were accrued to this trial before accrual was suspended. A preliminary report by Venook et al.[322] demonstrated a significantly improved response rate but no improvement in progression-free survival with the addition of cetuximab to front-line chemotherapy. This modest-sized trial is too small to meaningfully assess impact on overall survival.

More recently, a 1,200-patient study of FOLFIRI with or without cetuximab, known at the CRYSTAL trial, has now been reported.[323] The primary end point of the trial, progression-free survival, was statistically significantly improved with the addition of cetuximab, albeit by only 0.9 month, or 27 days. When the study was analyzed in terms of KRAS genotype, those patients with mutated KRAS showed no benefit, while those with wild type KRAS showed a progression-free survival improvement of 1.2 months, or 37 days. Response rates were statistically significantly higher in the cetuximab arm for the KRAS wild type tumors. Skin rash and diarrhea were increased in the cetuximab arm. As has been noted in virtually all trials of anti-EGFR agents, there was a strong correlation between severity of skin rash and clinical benefit, with progression-free survival advantage being limited to those patients with grade 2 or 3 skin rash.

FOLFOX with or without cetuximab was investigated in a randomized phase 2 trial in which the primary end point was response rate.[324] A total of 337 patients were treated. The overall response rate was improved by the addition of cetuximab from 36% to 46%, a result that just missed statistical significance (P = .64). For the KRAS wild type patients, however, the result was more robust, with an improvement from 37% to 61% (P = .011). Progression-free survival was very modestly, albeit statistically significantly improved in the KRAS wild type patients by a median of 15 days, however, progression-free survival was statistically significantly *worse* in the cetuximab arm in those patients whose tumors had mutated KRAS.

In a phase 3 trial of FOLFOX with or without panitumumab (6 mg/kg every 14 days), 1,183 patients were randomized, of whom 60% had wild type KRAS.[325] Progression-free survival was modestly but statistically significantly improved with panitumumab in the KRAS wild type patients (9.6 months vs. 8.0 months; P = .02), and response rate was increased from 48% to 55%. However, as was seen with cetuximab, in the patients with KRAS-mutated tumors, the addition of panitumumab resulted in a statistically significant *worsening* of median progression-free survival from 8.8 months in the control arm to 7.3 months in the panitumumab-containing arm. The addition of panitumumab resulted in increased skin rash, diarrhea, and hypomagnesemia.

Also reported in abstract form is a phase 3 trial of second-line FOLFIRI with or without panitumumab.[326] Despite this being a second-line study, patients had an excellent performance status (ECOG 0 or 1 in 94% of patients). KRAS mutations were present in 45% of patients. For the patients with KRAS wild type tumors, the progression-free survival was statistically significantly improved in the panitumumab-containing arm (5.9 months vs. 3.9 months; P = .004), and response rate was improved as well (35% vs. 10%). Overall survival differences in favor of the panitumumab arm (14.5 months vs. 12.5 months) did not reach statistical significance (P = .1). There were no differences in efficacy outcomes with the addition of panitumumab in the patients with KRAS-mutated tumors. Again, skin rash, diarrhea, and hypomagnesemia were increased in the panitumumab arm.

The U.S. NCI cooperative groups have begun an ambitious 2,200-patient three-arm trial (80405), which began patient accrual in the fall of 2005. Physicians select either FOLFOX or FOLFIRI, and then patients are randomized to receive their chemotherapy with either bevacizumab, cetuximab, or both. Accrual to this trial continues at the time of this writing.

Toxicities of Anti–Epidermal Growth Factor Receptor Monoclonal Antibodies

The primary toxicity of cetuximab and panitumumab is an acne-like rash, which is seen to some degree in from 75% to 100% of patients treated. This rash is not acne, and it is accompanied by skin dryness and paronychial cracking. Other than moisturizers, which are recommended, no topical agents have been shown to be of benefit in the treatment of this rash. Drying agents and retinoids, such as are used in the treatment of acne, are contraindicated. Anecdotal reports of benefit for topical steroids or antibiotics do not have supportive randomized data, and since the natural history of the rash is to wax and wane, interpretation of these anecdotal reports is problematic. There are data suggesting that prophylactic use of oral antibiotics may somewhat mitigate the severity of the rash.[327] Importantly, it has been well established that there is a clear correlation between severity of skin rash and favorable outcome with EGFR agents.[328] The mechanism of this correlation has not yet been determined, however, it is clear that benefit from these agents is virtually confined to those patients who experience a grade 2 or 3 skin rash. A severe rash does not guarantee a response or clinical benefit, however, absence of a rash after the first month of therapy is virtually incompatible with clinical benefit from these agents. This is an important point to consider, especially in consideration of front-line use; only those patients with a very substantial rash stand a chance of benefit.

Hypersensitivity reactions, which are anaphylactoid in nature and are completely separate and distinct from the skin rash toxicity discussed above, occur in approximately 3% of patients with cetuximab and less than 1% of patients with panitumumab. Almost all of these reactions are first-dose events. Dramatic regional differences in the frequency of these reactions have been noted, with serious hypersensitivity reactions to cetuximab noted in up to 20% of patients in North Carolina and Tennessee, while the serious hypersensitivity reaction rate in the northeastern United States is less than 1%.[329] Subsequently it has been demonstrated that there is a high prevalence of cetuximab-specific IgE in Tennessee, suggesting cross-reactivity with an environmental allergen.[330] Panitumumab does not appear to exhibit this marked regional variation in incidence of hypersensitivity reaction, and would be the clearly preferred agent over cetuximab in these areas of high incidence of cetuximab hypersensitivity.

It should be noted that the incidence of skin rash appears to be quite similar between cetuximab and panitumumab, as does the degree of clinical activity. Thus, outside of the areas that see high frequency of cetuximab hypersensitivity reactions, there appears to be little reason to favor one agent over the other. Case reports and anecdotal evidence suggest that patients who experience hypersensitivity to cetuximab do typically tolerate panitumumab. There is no basis, however, for using one of these agents after clinical failure on the other.

Another more recently recognized toxicity of anti-EGFR therapy is hypomagnesemia.[331] This result is due to hypermagnesemia, presumably promoted by EGFR antagonism in the loop of Henle. Regular monitoring of serum magnesium levels, and intravenous magnesium supplementation, when indicated, should be practiced routinely with anti-EGFR therapies. Oral magnesium is unlikely to provide adequate supplementation, as diarrhea from this is often dose-limiting.

Cetuximab and Panitumumab in Epidermal Growth Factor Receptive–Negative Patients

From the outset of clinical development, the assumption was made that quantitative EGFR expression would be predictive of the activity, or lack thereof, of an anti-EGFR antibody, and that an absence of demonstrable EGFR expression would therefore preclude clinical activity of cetuximab or panitumumab. For this reason, all early trials with these agents required that the patient's tumor shows EGFR positivity by immunohistochemistry (IHC) as a criterion for study eligibility. This assumption, that EGFR expression would be predictive, has never been supported by clinical or preclinical data and has been refuted by all clinical data that have addressed the issue. All of the reported cetuximab trials to date, the earlier ones of which excluded EGFR-negative patients altogether, have demonstrated absolutely no correlation between the intensity of the EGFR expression and clinical response.[167,311] Additionally, in abstract form, the results of a small cohort of nine patients who were EGFR-negative and treated with cetuximab were reported.[332] Two major objective responses were reported by the investigators, one of which was confirmed as a major response by third-party review and one of which was not.

On the basis of the lack of correlation between EGFR staining intensity and response, as well as the small data set outlined above, a decision was made at Memorial Sloan-Kettering Cancer Center (MSKCC) in New York that EGFR-negative colorectal cancer patients would not be excluded from standard off-protocol treatment with cetuximab simply on the basis of EGFR status. Subsequently, a retrospective review was conducted using the computerized pharmacy records to identify all patients who had received nonresearch cetuximab-based therapy at MSKCC in the first 3 months of cetuximab's commercial availability. This review identified 16 irinotecan-refractory, EGFR-negative colorectal cancer patients who had been treated. Fourteen of these patients had received cetuximab in combination with irinotecan and two had received cetuximab alone. Of the 16, four patients experienced major objective (response rate 25%; 95% CI, 4% to 46%), demonstrating that the hypothesis that a negative EGFR stain would preclude the possibility of response to cetuximab is false.[333] A similar lack of correlation of EGFR staining and activity with panitumumab has also more recently been reported.[334]

Since current EGFR IHC techniques have no predictive value, these techniques have no role in current management of colorectal cancer. The exclusion of a patient from cetuximab-based or panitumumab-based therapy solely on the basis of EGFR IHC is not appropriate. Likewise, no patient, colorectal or otherwise, should be given an anti-EGFR treatment solely on the basis of a high EGFR IHC expression.

Bevacizumab Plus Anti–Epidermal Growth Factor Receptor Agents

Given the reported activity of both bevacizumab and cetuximab, investigators logically became interested in the idea of concurrent use of these agents. Both some limited preclinical data, as well as mechanistic understandings of potential interaction between anti-EGFR and anti-VEGF pathways, supported the concept. As will be discussed below, this concept serves as yet another example of perfectly logical, well-thought out assumptions, supported by preliminary clinical evidence, that turned out to be incorrect when subjected to the appropriately rigorous test of an adequately powered clinical trial.

The first study to attempt to administer bevacizumab and cetuximab concurrently was a small randomized phase 2 study of bevacizumab added to cetuximab alone or to cetuximab plus irinotecan, in patients with irinotecan refractory colorectal cancer.[335] This was a feasibility trial to assess the safety of concurrent administration of these agents and to look for preliminary evidence of efficacy. The study concluded that coadministration of these two monoclonal antibodies together was feasible, and that the preliminary data were encouraging. It should be noted, however, that this was a small feasibility trial with 41 and 40 patients, respectively, reported in each arm. Furthermore, this study was conducted in patients who were naive to both cetuximab and bevacizumab. Since now most patients receive bevacizumab with their first-line regimen, the results in the bevacizumab-naive population might not necessarily have a bearing on current practice today. A small follow-up trial in patients with prior progression on a front-line bevacizumab-containing regimen showed far less activity, with 3 of 33 patients (9%) achieving a partial response and a median time to tumor progression of 3.9 months.[336] These small trials were designed to served as the safety pilots for large-scale front-line studies that combined bevacizumab plus cetuximab with front-line chemotherapy. Two such studies have now been reported, with alarming results, which highlights the dangers of jumping to conclusions prior to the availability of mature, definitive data.

The CAIRO-2 study randomized 755 previously untreated metastatic colorectal cancer patients to CapeOx-bevacizumab with or without concurrent cetuximab (Table 89.21*A*).[337] Not only was there not a benefit to the addition of cetuximab, but the group receiving cetuximab actually had a worse median progression-free survival of 9.4 months, compared to 10.7 months in the CapeOx-bevacizumab alone arm (P = .01).

TABLE 89.21A

CAPECITABINE, OXALIPLATIN, AND BEVACIZUMAB WITH OR WITHOUT CETUXIMAB IN METASTATIC COLORECTAL CANCER

Overall	Median Progression-Free Survival	Median Response	Objective Survival Rates
COB (n = 332)	20.3 m	10.7 m	50%
COB plus cetux (n = 317)	19.4 m	9.4 m	52.7%
p value	.16	.01	.49

COB, capecitabine, oxaliplatin, bevacizumab; cetux, cetuximab; m, months.
(From ref. 337.)

Response rates were identical (44%) in the two arms. Furthermore, quality-of-life scores were lower in the cetuximab-containing arm. Overall survival was not statistically significantly different between the two groups. Even for the wild type KRAS patients, there was no benefit in progression-free survival with the addition of cetuximab. As might now be anticipated (Table 89.21*B*), within the cetuximab-containing arm, patients whose tumors had mutated KRAS had statistically significantly decreased progression-free survival compared to those with wild type KRAS tumors (8.1 months vs. 10.5 months; $P = .04$). However, for the patients with KRAS mutations, those who received cetuximab also had a worse outcome than those on the non-cetuximab-containing control arm (progression-free survival 8.1 months vs. 12.5 months; $P = .003$, and overall survival 17.2 months vs. 24.9 months; $P = .03$).

Another study that investigated the use of combined bevacizumab plus anti-EGFR monoclonal antibody was the Panitumumab in Advanced Colon Cancer Evaluation (PACCE) trial.[338] This trial used FOLFOX-bevacizumab (823 patients) or FOLFIRI-bevacizumab (230 patients) and randomized them with or without concurrent panitumumab. Again, the result of adding the anti-EGFR to chemotherapy plus bevacizumab was not only not beneficial, but was actually detrimental. The median progression-free survival for the overall study was 10.0 months versus 11.4 months for the panitumumab-containing versus chemo-bevacizumab alone arm. The median overall survival was decreased by 5.1 months, from 24.5 months in the control arm to 19.4 months in the panitumumab arm. Toxicity, including not only skin rash but also diarrhea, infections, and pulmonary embolisms, was more frequent in the panitumumab-containing arm, and worse outcomes were seen in the panitumumab-containing arm regardless of KRAS mutation status.

Clearly, the concurrent use of anti-EGFR monoclonal antibodies, bevacizumab, and cytotoxic chemotherapy, despite supportive encouraging preliminary data, is not an acceptable treatment strategy. The reasons for this unanticipated negative interaction remain unknown at this time.

Oral Epidermal Growth Factor Receptor, Vascular Endothelial Growth Factor, and Cyclooxygenase-2 Inhibitors

Thus far, no oral tyrosine kinase inhibitor has shown meaningful clinical activity in colorectal cancer, and none can be recommended for use at this time. The limited experiences with the oral EGFR tyrosine kinase inhibitors gefitinib (ZD1839) and erlotinib (OSI-774) in colorectal cancer have been essentially negative, and at present there is no role for these agents in this disease.[339,340] This is consistent with the findings that the activating mutation seen in lung cancer required for anti-EGFR tyrosine kinase activity does not appear to occur in colorectal cancer.

Oral VEGF tyrosine kinase inhibitors have been similarly disappointing. Sunitinib showed essentially no activity as a single agent in chemotherapy-refractory disease, and front-line trials of chemotherapy with or without sunitinib, as well as chemotherapy with or without sorafenib, have now been closed early by their respective data monitoring committees for futility.[341] Two large, randomized trials of FOLFOX with or without the investigational VEGF tyrosine kinase inhibitor PTK-787 have also been reported as negative trials.

Cyclooxygenase-2 Inhibitors. COX-2 catalyzes the synthesis of prostaglandins in the inflammatory response process. COX-2 has been frequently shown to be up-regulated in malignant and premalignant tissues. COX-2 expression has been correlated with increased invasiveness, resistance to apoptosis, and increased angiogenesis.[342] The science behind COX-2 inhibition appeared so compelling that many clinicians had chosen to add drugs such as celecoxib or rofecoxib (now withdrawn from the market for safety reasons) in the absence of efficacy data with the assumption that "it couldn't hurt." Evidence that use of either NSAIDs or selective COX-2 inhibitors has a beneficial role in the treatment of colorectal cancer is lacking. The large randomized BICC-C trial showed

TABLE 89.21B

IMPACT OF KRAS MUTATION STATUS ON ADDITION OF CETUXIMAB TO CAPECITABINE, OXALIPLATIN, AND BEVACIZUMAB

	Overall Survival COB+COB cetux	Progression-Free Survival COB+ COB cetux
KRAS-wild type	22.4 m 21.8 m ($P = .64$)	10.6 m 10.5 m ($P = .30$)
KRAS-mutated	24.9 m 17.2 m ($P = .03$)	12.5 m 8.1 m ($P = .003$)

COB, capecitabine, oxaliplatin-bevacizumab; cetux, cetuximab; m, months.
(From ref. 337.)

no benefit whatsoever for the use of celecoxib in terms of either safety or efficacy.[259] In the absence of any emerging data to the contrary, routine use of COX-2 inhibitors with chemotherapy is not recommended.

Other Novel Agents

The number of agents that are undergoing early evaluation in colorectal cancer is too large to allow a complete discussion of these in this chapter. Many are variations on the currently available agents and are unlikely to substantially move the field if successful in gaining approval. At present no new agent with a unique mechanism of action has been identified as having meaningful activity in colorectal cancer. Furthermore, all of these at this point are of research interest only and do not have a role in standard treatment of colorectal cancer at this time.

GENE THERAPY

Several aspects of colorectal cancer make the disease a reasonable potential target for gene therapy approaches.[343] Because colorectal cancer may progress within a confined space, such as the peritoneal cavity, or within a solitary organ, such as the liver, regional administration of a gene vector may be practical. Multiple trials of different gene therapy approaches, including virus directed enzyme prodrug therapy, immunogenic manipulation, gene correction, and viral therapy, have all been initiated. Major therapeutic benefits from gene therapy in colorectal cancer have yet to be realized, however, and these approaches remain highly investigational at this time.

MOLECULAR PREDICTIVE MARKERS

With the availability now of a number of active agents, the ability to prospectively select a particular drug or drug combination that would have an increased likelihood of efficacy or a decreased likelihood of toxicity would be clinically useful. Such means of rational selection do not yet exist.

One avenue of investigation has been the elucidation of markers of resistance to fluorouracil based on knowledge of its metabolic pathways. Studies have indicated that high levels of either TS, DPD,[344] or thymidine phosphorylase (TP), as measured in a tumor specimen by RT-PCR, predict for failure to respond to an infusional 5-FU regimen.[116,345,346] These observations are intriguing but are insufficient to exclude the use of 5-FU in a particular patient, and they need to be validated in large-scale prospective trials before being applied to routine practice. There is, at this time, no role for the use of these markers in standard practice. Others have investigated genomic analysis as an indicator of response or toxicity.[119,347] Although these approaches appear promising, they are not yet validated and should not be considered as part of standard care.

MANAGEMENT OF SYNCHRONOUS PRIMARY AND METASTATIC DISEASE

Patients who present with potentially resectable metastatic disease, such as those with metastases confined to the liver in a resectable distribution, should undergo resection of both the metastatic and primary tumors. PET scanning can be considered before undertaking such an aggressive surgical approach to ensure that other sites of metastatic disease are adequately ruled out.[348,349] Judgment must be exercised in terms of whether to perform both resections at once or to perform staged procedures.

Historical practice had previously favored routine palliative resection for patients who present with synchronous unresectable metastatic disease; however, more recent data indicate that the majority of such patients do not require surgical resection of their colorectal primary.

In an analysis of SEER-Medicare linked data, Temple et al.[350] assessed whether or not surgery was performed within 90 days of diagnosis in patients who presented with synchronous metastatic disease. The records of 5,235 patients over age 65 who presented with stage IV colorectal cancer from 1992 to 1996 were reviewed. Seventy-three percent of these stage IV patients were found to have undergone cancer-directed surgery with 90 days of diagnosis. Among patients over the age of 80, this rate was 68%. Twenty-four percent of all patients who underwent surgery received a colostomy or ileostomy. Of significant concern, 10% of patients who underwent these palliative resections died within 30 days of the operation. This perioperative mortality rose to 15% in patients over 80 years of age. The vast majority of surgeries were performed on the primary tumor. Surgical resection of metastases was rare, occurring in only 4.3% of patients. Overall, the prognosis for the entire cohort was poor, with 28% mortality at 90 days from diagnosis.

The risk of intestinal complications after chemotherapy for patients with unresected primary colorectal cancer and synchronous metastasis would appear to be low. Tebbutt et al.[351] have summarized the 10-year experience of patients at the Royal Marsden Hospital in London who have been treated with chemotherapy with or without palliative resection of the primary. Eighty-two patients received initial chemotherapy without surgery and 280 patients underwent surgery followed by chemotherapy. The incidences of peritonitis, fistula formation, and intestinal hemorrhage were not significantly different in the resected versus unresected patients. Intestinal obstruction occurred in 13% of both groups. Patients undergoing resection did have a lower incidence of requiring three or more blood transfusions (7.5% vs. 14.6%; $P = .048$), as well as lower rate of palliative abdominal radiotherapy (9.6% vs. 18.3%; $P = .03$).

More recently, Poultsides et al.[305] used a prospective institutional database to identify 233 consecutive patients with synchronous metastatic colorectal cancer and an unresected primary tumor who received chemotherapy containing oxaliplatin or irinotecan as initial therapy. Of these, 217 (93%) never required surgical palliation of their primary tumor. Sixteen patients (7%) required emergent surgery for primary tumor obstruction or perforation, 10 patients (4%) required nonoperative intervention (i.e., stent or radiotherapy), and 213 (89%) never required any direct symptomatic management for their intact primary tumor.

Current evidence would argue against the continued practice of routine noncurative resection for a majority of patients with synchronous metastatic disease. Response rates with initial chemotherapy using currently available combination regimens, as discussed above, are substantially higher than where achievable a decade ago. In following the patient's clinical course, the metastatic disease can serve as a clinical indicator of response to systemic chemotherapy. Response in the metastasis is extremely likely to correlate with disease control in the area of the primary as well. Patients felt to be at risk for obstruction within the time period necessary to evaluate the efficacy of first-line chemotherapy should be considered for mechanical stenting, utilizing expandable endoscopically placed metal stents.[352]

UNUSUAL COLORECTAL TUMORS

Carcinoid Tumors

Carcinoid tumors are neuroendocrine tumors characterized by the presence of neurosecretory granules. Histologically, these are typically characterized by bland, monotonous histology with small nuclei, few nucleoli, and ample cytoplasm. Tumors typically manifest a low-grade histology and an indolent clinical course. Approximately half of carcinoid tumors are hormonally nonfunctional in that they produce no clinical evidence of a hormonal syndrome. The hormone typically produced by functional carcinoid tumors is serotonin, and this is best detected by a 24-hour urine collection to measure the breakdown product, 5-hydroxy-indole acetic acid (5HIAA). Presentation and management of carcinoid tumors of the large bowel is discussed in detail in Chapter 90.

High-Grade Neuroendocrine Carcinoma

Neuroendocrine carcinomas comprise a spectrum, from well-differentiated carcinoid tumors on one end to high-grade, small cell or oat cell carcinomas on the other. Extrapulmonary small-cell or high-grade neuroendocrine tumors are very uncommon, accounting for fewer than 1,000 cases annually. Histologically, small cell cancers arising from different organs are indistinguishable from one another.[353,354] Since small cell lung cancer is far more common than an extrapulmonary neuroendocrine primary, chest imaging should be performed. The rectum is the most common presentation site within the large bowel, and the cecum is the next most common site.

The presentation of high-grade large bowel neuroendocrine tumors is nonspecific and similar to that of adenocarcinomas. Stage IV presentation is most common, with the liver being the most common site of distant spread. Recommendations for management of high-grade small cell colorectal tumors are based on extrapolation from small cell lung cancer paradigms. Systemic chemotherapy, utilizing small cell lung regimens, is the treatment of choice for patients with metastatic disease. Treatment of localized high-grade neuroendocrine carcinoma is controversial. Traditionally a combined modality approach similar to that used in rectal adenocarcinoma has been advocated; however, distant failure is a common occurrence. One reasonable approach would be to treat initially with small cell–directed chemotherapy, and then consider consolidation of patients with favorable responses with radiation or surgery.

Lymphoma

Although extranodal presentations of non-Hodgkin's lymphomas are rare, the GI tract is the most common site of extranodal involvement. The majority of colorectal lymphomas are non-Hodgkin's type and may present with low, intermediate, or high-grade histologies. B-cell diffuse large cell histology is most common, however, virtually all B-cell and T-cell types may occur. Approximately 13% to 18% of GI tract lymphomas arise in the large bowel, the majority being situated in the cecum or the rectum.[355–357]

Colorectal lymphomas usually present with nonspecific abdominal pain, weight loss, rectal bleeding, mass, or obstruction.[358] The clinical presentation is similar to that of common colorectal carcinoma, and the diagnosis is made on histologic examination of a biopsy specimen. Extensive workup for other sites of disease, including bone marrow biopsy and full body scanning, is necessary for both staging and for acceptance of the diagnosis of the GI site as primary.

Owing to the rarity of the disease, data regarding the optimal management of large bowel lymphomas are scarce. Patients with lymphoma of the colon are often treated initially with surgery, although the appropriateness of this has not been validated in randomized studies. A combined-modality approach, including surgery and chemotherapy, has been advocated by some investigators.[359] The role of radiation therapy also remains unclear, with some investigators favoring its use, especially in unresectable disease or bulky tumors. Chemotherapy use is based on the appropriate regimens for the particular histologic subtype that is present.

Selected References

The full list of references for this chapter appears in the online version.

1. Jemal A, Center MM, DeSantis C, Ward EM. Global patterns of cancer incidence and mortality rates and trends. *Cancer Epidemiol Biomarkers Prev* 2010;19:1893.
15. Nelson RL, Dollear T, Freels S, Persky V. The relation of age, race, and gender to the subsite location of colorectal carcinoma. *Cancer* 1997;80:193.
17. Wilmink AB. Overview of the epidemiology of colorectal cancer. *Dis Colon Rectum* 1997;40:483.
21. Thibodeau SN, French AJ, Cunningham JM, et al. Microsatellite instability in colorectal cancer: different mutator phenotypes and the principal involvement of hMLH1. *Cancer Res* 1998;58:1713.
27. Winawer SJ, Zauber AG, Gerdes H, et al. Risk of colorectal cancer in the families of patients with adenomatous polyps. National Polyp Study Workgroup. *N Engl J Med* 1996;334:82.
35. Potter JD. Colorectal cancer: molecules and populations. *J Natl Cancer Inst* 1999;91:916-32.
36. Willett WC, Stampfer MJ, Colditz GA, Rosner BA, Speizer FE. Relation of meat, fat, and fiber intake to the risk of colon cancer in a prospective study among women. *N Engl J Med* 1990;323:1664.
45. Alberts DS, Martinez ME, Roe DJ, et al. Lack of effect of a high-fiber cereal supplement on the recurrence of colorectal adenomas. Phoenix Colon Cancer Prevention Physicians' Network. *N Engl J Med* 2000;342:1156.
52. Thun MJ, Namboodiri MM, Heath CW Jr. Aspirin use and reduced risk of fatal colon cancer. *N Engl J Med* 1991;325:1593.
53. Rosenberg L, Louik C, Shapiro S. Nonsteroidal anti-inflammatory drug use and reduced risk of large bowel carcinoma. *Cancer* 1998;82:2326.
58. Powell SM, Petersen GM, Krush AJ, et al. Molecular diagnosis of familial adenomatous polyposis. *N Engl J Med* 1993;329:1982.
61. Marra G, Boland CR. Hereditary nonpolyposis colorectal cancer: the syndrome, the genes, and historical perspectives. *J Natl Cancer Inst* 1995;87:1114.
69. Rocklin MS, Senagore AJ, Talbott TM. Role of carcinoembryonic antigen and liver function tests in the detection of recurrent colorectal carcinoma. *Dis Colon Rectum* 1991;34:794.
72. Eguchi S, Kohara N, Komuta K, Kanematsu T. Mutations of the p53 gene in the stool of patients with resectable colorectal cancer. *Cancer* 1996;77:1707.
73. Fenlon HM, Nunes DP, Schroy PC 3rd, et al. A comparison of virtual and conventional colonoscopy for the detection of colorectal polyps. *N Engl J Med* 1999;341:1496.
76. Pickhardt PJ, Choi JR, Hwang I, et al. Computed tomographic virtual colonoscopy to screen for colorectal neoplasia in asymptomatic adults. *N Engl J Med* 2003;349:2191.
77. Compton CC. *Surgical pathology of colorectal cancer.* Totowa, NJ: Humana Press, 2002.
78. Edge SB, Byrd DB, Compton CC, et al., eds. *AJCC cancer staging manual.* 7th ed. New York: Springer, 2010.
84. Tepper JE, O'Connell M, Niedzwiecki D, et al. Adjuvant therapy in rectal cancer: analysis of stage, sex, and local control—final report of intergroup 0114. *J Clin Oncol* 2002;20:1744.
94. Turner RR, Nora DT, Trocha SD, Bilchik AJ. Colorectal carcinoma nodal staging. Frequency and nature of cytokeratin-positive cells in sentinel and nonsentinel lymph nodes. *Arch Pathol Lab Med* 2003;127:673.
100. de la Chapelle A. Microsatellite instability. *N Engl J Med* 2003;349:209.

103. Thibodeau SN, Bren G, Schaid D. Microsatellite instability in cancer of the proximal colon. *Science* 1993;260:816.
106. Gryfe R, Kim H, Hsieh ET, et al. Tumor microsatellite instability and clinical outcome in young patients with colorectal cancer. *N Engl J Med* 2000; 342:69.
107. Watanabe T, Wu TT, Catalano PJ, et al. Molecular predictors of survival after adjuvant chemotherapy for colon cancer. *N Engl J Med* 2001;344: 1196.
112. Harrison LE, Guillem JG, Paty P, Cohen AM. Preoperative carcinoembryonic antigen predicts outcomes in node- negative colon cancer patients: a multivariate analysis of 572 patients. *J Am Coll Surg* 1997;185:55.
119. McLeod HL. Individualized cancer therapy: molecular approaches to the prediction of tumor response. *Expert Rev Anticancer Ther* 2002;2:113.
124. Guenaga KF, Matos D, Castro AA, Atallah AN, Wille-Jorgensen P. Mechanical bowel preparation for elective colorectal surgery. *Cochrane Database Syst Rev* 2003; CD001544.
128. Ram E, Sherman Y, Weil R, et al. Is mechanical bowel preparation mandatory for elective colon surgery? A prospective randomized study. *Arch Surg* 2005;140:285.
138. Hartley JE, Monson JR. The role of laparoscopy in the multimodality treatment of colorectal cancer. *Surg Clin North Am* 2002;82:1019.
143. Delaney CP, Kiran RP, Senagore AJ, Brady K, Fazio VW. Case-matched comparison of clinical and financial outcome after laparoscopic or open colorectal surgery. *Ann Surg* 2003;238:67.
149. A comparison of laparoscopically assisted and open colectomy for colon cancer. *N Engl J Med* 2004;350:2050.
152. Libutti S, Saltz L, Tepper J. Cancer of the colon. In: DeVita VT, Hellman S, Rosenberg SA, eds. *Principles and practice of oncology*. 8th ed. Philadelphia: Lippincott Williams & Wilkins, 2008;.
156. Haller DG, Catalano PJ, Macdonald JS, et al. Phase III study of fluorouracil, leucovorin, and levamisole in high-risk stage II and III colon cancer: final report of Intergroup 0089. *J Clin Oncol* 2005;23:8671.
160. Twelves C, Wong A, Nowacki MP, et al. Capecitabine as adjuvant treatment for stage III colon cancer. *N Engl J Med* 2005;352:2696.
162. Andre T, Boni C, Mounedji-Boudiaf L, et al. Oxaliplatin, fluorouracil, and leucovorin as adjuvant treatment for colon cancer. *N Engl J Med* 2004;350: 2343.
163. Andre T, Boni C, Navarro M, et al. Improved overall survival with oxaliplatin, fluorouracil, and leucovorin as adjuvant treatment in stage II or III colon cancer in the MOSAIC trial. *J Clin Oncol* 2009;27:3109.
166. Haller D, Tabernero J, Maroun J, et al. First efficacy findings from a randomized phase III trial of capecitabine + oxaliplatin vs. bolus 5-FU/LV for stage III colon cancer (NO16968/XELOXA study). *Eur J Cancer Suppl* 2009;7:5 (abst 4LBA).
169. Saltz LB, Cox JV, Blanke C, et al. Irinotecan plus fluorouracil and leucovorin for metastatic colorectal cancer. Irinotecan Study Group. *N Engl J Med* 2000;343:905.
171. Saltz LB, Niedzwiecki D, Hollis D, et al. Irinotecan fluorouracil plus leucovorin is not superior to fluorouracil plus leucovorin alone as adjuvant treatment for stage III colon cancer: results of CALGB 89803. *J Clin Oncol* 2007;25:3456.
173. Van Cutsem E, Labianca R, Bodoky G, et al. Randomized phase III trial comparing biweekly infusional fluorouracil/leucovorin alone or with irinotecan in the adjuvant treatment of stage III colon cancer: PETACC-3. *J Clin Oncol* 2009;27:3117.
175. Bertagnolli MM, Niedzwiecki D, Compton CC, et al. Microsatellite instability predicts improved response to adjuvant therapy with irinotecan, fluorouracil, and leucovorin in stage III colon cancer: Cancer and Leukemia Group B Protocol 89803. *J Clin Oncol* 2009;27:1814.
178. QUASAR Collaborative Group et al. Adjuvant chemotherapy versus observation in patients with colorectal cancer: a randomised study. *Lancet* 2007;370:2020.
181. Willet CG, Tepper JE, Cohen AM. Obstructive and perforative colonic carcinoma: patterns of failure. *J Clin Oncol* 1985;3:379.
182. Ribic CM, Sargent DJ, Moore MJ, et al. Tumor microsatellite-instability status as a predictor of benefit from fluorouracil-based adjuvant chemotherapy for colon cancer. *N Engl J Med* 2003;349:247.
183. Kim GP, Colangelo LH, Wieand HS, et al. Prognostic and predictive roles of high-degree microsatellite instability in colon cancer: a National Cancer Institute-National Surgical Adjuvant Breast and Bowel Project Collaborative Study. *J Clin Oncol* 2007;25:767.
189. Benson AB 3rd, Schrag D, Somerfield MR, et al. American Society of Clinical Oncology recommendations on adjuvant chemotherapy for stage II colon cancer. *J Clin Oncol* 2004;22:3408.
190. Wolmark N, Rockette H, Wickerman DL, et al. Adjuvant therapy of Dukes' A, B, and C adenocarcinoma of the colon with portal vein fluorouracil hepatic infusion: preliminary results of National Surgical Adjuvant Breast and Bowel Project Protocol C-02. *J Clin Oncol* 1990;8:1466.
200. Willett CG, Goldberg S, Shellito PC, et al. Does postoperative irradiation play a role in adjuvant therapy of stage T4 colon cancer? *Cancer J Sci Am* 1999;5:242.
204. Estes NC, Giri S, Fabian C. Patterns of recurrence for advanced colon cancer modified by whole abdominal radiation and chemotherapy. *Am Surg* 1996;62:546
205. Muller AD, Sonnenberg A. Prevention of colorectal cancer by flexible endoscopy and polypectomy. A case-control study of 32,702 veterans. *Ann Intern Med* 1995;123:904.
206. Burt RW. Colon cancer screening. *Gastroenterology* 2000;119:837.
207. Mandel JS, Bond JH, Church TR, et al. Reducing mortality from colorectal cancer by screening for fecal occult blood. Minnesota Colon Cancer Control Study. *N Engl J Med* 1993;328:1365.
210. Atkin WS, Morson BC, Cuzick J. Long-term risk of colorectal cancer after excision of rectosigmoid adenomas. *N Engl J Med* 1992;326:658.
213. Desch CE, Benson AB 3rd, Somerfield MR, et al. Colorectal cancer surveillance: 2005 update of an American Society of Clinical Oncology practice guideline. *J Clin Oncol* 2005;23:8512.
219. Libutti SK, Alexander HR Jr, Choyke P, et al. A prospective study of 2-[18F] fluoro-2-deoxy-D-glucose/positron emission tomography scan, 99mTc-labeled arcitumomab (CEA-scan), and blind second-look laparotomy for detecting colon cancer recurrence in patients with increasing carcinoembryonic antigen levels. *Ann Surg Oncol* 2001;8:779.
225. Swanson RS. Is an FDG-PET scan the new imaging standard for colon cancer? *Ann Surg Oncol* 2001;8:752.
227. Makela J, Laitinen S, Kairaluoma MI. Early results of follow-up after radical resection for colorectal cancer. Preliminary results of a prospective randomized trial. *Surg Oncol* 1992;1:157.
230. Inadomi JM, Sonnenberg A. The impact of colorectal cancer screening on life expectancy. *Gastrointest Endosc* 2000;51:517.
233. Heidelberger C, Chanakari NK, Danenberg PV, et al. Fluorinated pyrimidines: a new class of tumor inhibitory compounds. *Nature* 1957;179:663.
237. Van Cutsem E, Twelves C, Cassidy J, et al. Oral capecitabine compared with intravenous fluorouracil plus leucovorin in patients with metastatic colorectal cancer: results of a large phase III study. *J Clin Oncol* 2001;19:4097.
240. Carmichael J, Popiela T, Radstone D, et al. Randomized comparative study of tegafur/uracil and oral leucovorin versus parenteral fluorouracil and leucovorin in patients with previously untreated metastatic colorectal cancer. *J Clin Oncol* 2002;20:3617.
246. Pizzolato JF, Saltz LB. The camptothecins. *Lancet* 2003;361:2235.
247. Kawato Y, Aonuma M, Hirota Y, Kuga H, Sato K. Intracellular roles of SN-38, a metabolite of the camptothecin derivative CPT-11, in the antitumor effect of CPT-11. *Cancer Res* 1991;51:4187.
252. Conti JA, Kemeny NE, Saltz LB, et al. Irinotecan is an active agent in untreated patients with metastatic colorectal cancer. *J Clin Oncol* 1996; 14:709.
254. Rougier P, Van Cutsem E, Bajetta E, et al. Randomized trial of irinotecan versus fluorouracil by continuous infusion after fluorouracil failure in patients with metastatic colorectal cancer. *Lancet* 1998;352:1407.
257. Saltz L, Kanowitz J, Kemeny N, et al. A phase I clinical and pharmacologic trial of irinotecan, 5-fluorouracil, and leucovorin in patients with advanced solid tumors. *J Clin Oncol* 1996;14:2959.
261. Raymond E, Chaney SG, Taamma A, Cvitkovic E. Oxaliplatin: a review of preclinical and clinical studies. *Ann Oncol* 1998;9:1053.
262. Diaz-Rubio E, Sastre J, Zaniboni A, et al. Oxaliplatin as single agent in previously untreated colorectal carcinoma patients: a phase II multicentric study. *Ann Oncol* 1998;9:105.
268. Levi F, Zidani R, Misset JL. Randomised multicentre trial of chronotherapy with oxaliplatin, fluorouracil, and folinic acid in metastatic colorectal cancer. International Organization for Cancer Chronotherapy. *Lancet* 1997;350:681.
269. de Gramont A, Bosset JF, Milan C, et al. Randomized trial comparing monthly low-dose leucovorin and fluorouracil bolus with bimonthly high-dose leucovorin and fluorouracil bolus plus continuous infusion for advanced colorectal cancer: a French Intergroup study. *J Clin Oncol* 1997;15:808.
272. de Gramont A, Figer A, Seymour M, et al. Leucovorin and fluorouracil with or without oxaliplatin as first-line treatment in advanced colorectal cancer. *J Clin Oncol* 2000;18:2938.
273. Rothenberg ML, Oza AM, Bigelow RH, et al. Superiority of oxaliplatin and fluorouracil-leucovorin compared with either therapy alone in patients with progressive colorectal cancer after irinotecan and fluorouracil-leucovorin: interim results of a phase III trial. *J Clin Oncol* 2003;21:2059.
276. Colucci G, Gebbia V, Paoletti G, et al. Phase III randomized trial of FOLFIRI vs FOLFOX4 in the treatment of advanced colorectal cancer: a multicenter study of the Grupo Oncologico Italia Meridionale. *J Clin Oncol* 2005;23:4866.
277. Goldberg RM. N9741: a phase III study comparing irinotecan to oxaliplatin-containing regimens in advanced colorectal cancer. *Clin Colorectal Cancer* 2002;2:81.
287. Falcone A, Ricci S, Brunetti I, et al. Phase III trial of infusional fluorouracil, leucovorin, oxaliplatin, and irinotecan (FOLFOXIRI) compared with infusional fluorouracil, leucovorin, and irinotecan (FOLFIRI) as first-line treatment for metastatic colorectal cancer: the Gruppo Oncologico Nord Ovest. *J Clin Oncol* 2007;25:1670.
290. Maughan TS, James RD, Kerr DJ, et al. Comparison of intermittent and continuous palliative chemotherapy for advanced colorectal cancer: a multicentre randomised trial. *Lancet* 2003;361:457.
291. Chibaudel B, Maindrault-Goebel F, Lledo G, et al. Can chemotherapy be discontinued in unresectable metastatic colorectal cancer? The GERCOR OPTIMOX2 Study. *J Clin Oncol* 2009;27:5727.

296. Seymour MT, Maughan TS, Ledermann JA, et al. Different strategies of sequential and combination chemotherapy for patients with poor prognosis advanced colorectal cancer (MRC FOCUS): a randomised controlled trial. *Lancet* 2007;370:143.
297. Ferrara N, Hillan KJ, Gerber HP, Novotny W. Discovery and development of bevacizumab, an anti-VEGF antibody for treating cancer. *Nat Rev Drug Discov* 2004;3:391.
303. Giantonio BJ, Catalano PJ, Meropol NJ, et al. Bevacizumab in combination with oxaliplatin, fluorouracil, and leucovorin (FOLFOX4) for previously treated metastatic colorectal cancer: results from the Eastern Cooperative Oncology Group Study E3200. *J Clin Oncol* 2007;25:1539.
304. Saltz LB, Clarke S, Diaz-Rubio E, et al. Bevacizumab in combination with oxaliplatin-based chemotherapy as first-line therapy in metastatic colorectal cancer: a randomized phase III study. *J Clin Oncol* 2008;26:2013.
310. Thomas SM, Grandis JR. Pharmacokinetic and pharmacodynamic properties of EGFR inhibitors under clinical investigation. *Cancer Treat Rev* 2004;30:255.
312. Saltz LB, Meropol NJ, Loehrer PJ Sr, et al. Phase II trial of cetuximab in patients with refractory colorectal cancer that expresses the epidermal growth factor receptor. *J Clin Oncol* 2004;22:1201.
313. Jonker DJ, O'Callaghan CJ, Karapetis CS, et al. Cetuximab for the treatment of colorectal cancer. *N Engl J Med* 2007;357:2040.
315. Hecht JR, Patnaik A, Berlin J, et al. Panitumumab monotherapy in patients with previously treated metastatic colorectal cancer. *Cancer* 2007;110:980.
316. Van Cutsem E, Peeters M, Siena S, et al. Open-label phase III trial of panitumumab plus best supportive care compared with best supportive care alone in patients with chemotherapy-refractory metastatic colorectal cancer. *J Clin Oncol* 2007;25:1658.
320. Karapetis CS, Khambata-Ford S, Jonker DJ, et al. K-ras mutations and benefit from cetuximab in advanced colorectal cancer. *N Engl J Med* 2008; 359:1757.
323. Van Cutsem E, Kohne C-H, Hitre E, et al. Cetuximab and chemotherapy as initial treatment for metastatic colorectal cancer. *N Engl J Med* 2009; 360:1408.
325. Douillard J, Siena S, Cassidy J, et al. Randomized phase 3 study of panitumumab with FOLFOX4 compared to FOLFOX4 alone as 1st-line treatment (tx) for metastatic colorectal cancer (mCRC): the PRIME trial. *Eur J Cancer Suppl* 2009;7:6 (abst 10LBA).
328. Perez-Soler R, Saltz L. Cutaneous adverse effects with HER1/EGFR-targeted agents: is there a silver lining? *J Clin Oncol* 2005;23:5235.
331. Schrag D, Chung KY, Flombaum C, Saltz L. Cetuximab therapy and symptomatic hypomagnesemia. *J Natl Cancer Inst* 2005;97:1221.
335. Saltz LB, Lenz H-J, Kindler HL, et al. Randomized phase II trial of cetuximab, bevacizumab, and irinotecan compared with cetuximab and bevacizumab alone in irinotecan-refractory colorectal cancer: the BOND-2 study. *J Clin Oncol* 2007;25:4557.
338. Hecht JR, Mitchell E, Chidiac T, et al. A randomized phase IIIB trial of chemotherapy, bevacizumab, and panitumumab compared with chemotherapy and bevacizumab alone for metastatic colorectal cancer. *J Clin Oncol* 2009;27:672.
345. Metzger R, Danenberg K, Leichman CG, et al. High basal level gene expression of thymidine phosphorylase (platelet-derived endothelial cell growth factor) in colorectal tumors is associated with nonresponse to 5-fluorouracil. *Clin Cancer Res* 1998;4:2371.
348. Desai DC, Zervos EE, Arnold MW, et al. Positron emission tomography affects surgical management in recurrent colorectal cancer patients. *Ann Surg Oncol* 2003;10:59.
355. Cheng P, L LS. Unusual tumors of the colon, rectum and anus. In: Raghavan D, Brecher M, Johnson D, et al., eds. *Textbook of uncommon cancer*. Chichester, UK: Wiley, 1999:439.
361. Winawer S, Fletcher R, Rex D, et al. Colorectal cancer screening and surveillance: clinical guidelines and rationale—update based on new evidence. *Gastroenterology* 2003;124:544.

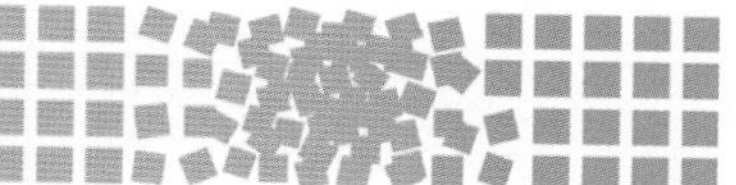

CHAPTER 90 CANCER OF THE RECTUM

STEVEN K. LIBUTTI, CHRISTOPHER G. WILLETT, AND LEONARD B. SALTZ

Information concerning epidemiology and systemic approaches to the management of both colon and rectal cancer was given in another chapter in this book. This chapter will focus on issues unique to rectal cancer with an emphasis on radiation, combined modality therapy, and sphincter-preserving surgery.

ANATOMY

The anatomy of the rectum can be very confusing as there are differing definitions of the relevant landmarks. In the upper portion of the rectum there are changes both in the musculature of the large bowel and in the relationship to the peritoneal covering that roughly coincide. In the lower portion of the rectum the mucosal changes occur at roughly the same location as the anal sphincter.

The anatomy of the rectum is usually divided into three portions (Fig. 90.1). The lower rectum is the area approximately from 3 to 6 cm from the anal verge. The midrectum goes from 5 to 6, to 8 to 10 cm, and the upper rectum extends approximately from 8 to 10, to 12 to 15 cm from the anal verge, although the retroperitoneal portion of the large bowel often reaches its upper limit approximately 12 cm from the anal verge. In some patients, especially elderly women, the peritonealized portion of the large bowel can be located much lower than these definitions. The determination of the location of the boundary between rectum and sigmoid colon is important in defining adjuvant therapy, with the rectum usually being operationally defined as that area of the large bowel that is at least partially retroperitoneal.

Externally, the upper extent of the rectum can be identified where the tenia spread to form a longitudinal coat of muscle. The upper third of the rectum is surrounded by peritoneum on its anterior and lateral surfaces but is retroperitoneal posteriorly without any serosal covering. At the rectovesical or rectouterine pouch, the rectum becomes completely extra/retroperitoneal. The rectum follows the curve of the sacrum in its lower two-thirds. It enters the anal canal at the level of the levator ani. The anorectal ring is at the level of the puborectalis sling portion of the levator muscles.

The location of a rectal tumor is most commonly indicated by the distance between the anal verge, dentate (pectinate or mucocutaneous) line, or anorectal ring and the lower edge of the tumor. These points of reference are all different for different individuals. Also, these measurements differ depending on the method of measurement. This can be important clinically, as the measurement from a flexible endoscopy can substantially overestimate the distance to the tumor from the anal verge or other landmark. The distance from the anal sphincter musculature is clinically of more importance than the distance from the anal verge, as it has implications for the ability to perform sphincter-sparing surgery. The lack of a peritoneal covering most of the rectum is a major reason for the higher risk for local failure after primary surgical management than for colon cancer. The mesorectum is usually used as the structure to define the extent of a total mesorectal excision, with most of the perirectal fatty tissue and perirectal lymph nodes contained within its boundaries.

Lymphatic Drainage

The lymphatic drainage of the upper rectum follows the course of the superior hemorrhoidal artery toward the inferior mesenteric artery. Lymph nodes that are above the midrectum and therefore drain along the superior hemorrhoidal artery are often part of the mesentery that is removed during resections of the intraperitoneal portion of the colon. Lesions that arise in the rectum below approximately 6 cm are in a region of the rectum that is drained by lymphatics that follow the middle hemorrhoidal artery. Nodes involved from a cancer in this region can include the internal iliac nodes and the nodes of the obturator fossa. These regions deserve particular attention during the resection and irradiation of lesions in this location. When lesions occur below the dentate line, the lymphatic drainage is via the inguinal nodes and external iliac chain, which has major therapeutic implications, especially for the radiation fields. The corollary of this high risk of inguinal node involvement for the very low-lying tumors is that tumors located above the dentate line are at low risk of inguinal node involvement, and these nodes as well as the external iliacs do not need to be treated.

Bowel Function

Fecal continence is maintained through the function of both sphincter control and the preservation of the normal muscular anatomy, which creates a neorectal angle or rectal sling. The pelvic floor is composed of the levator ani muscles, which separate the pelvis from the perineum and ischiorectal fossa. The urethra, vagina, and anus pass through the levator muscles.

Preservation of fecal continence during surgery for rectal cancer is therefore dependent on a thorough understanding of the anatomic relationships of the musculature and the sphincter mechanism. Maintenance of the sphincter apparatus without preservation of the muscular angles will not have the desired result. These anatomic constraints, especially with respect to lateral margins, make the use of adjuvant chemotherapy and radiation therapy critical to a successful surgical outcome. This is true from both an oncologic as well as a bowel function perspective.

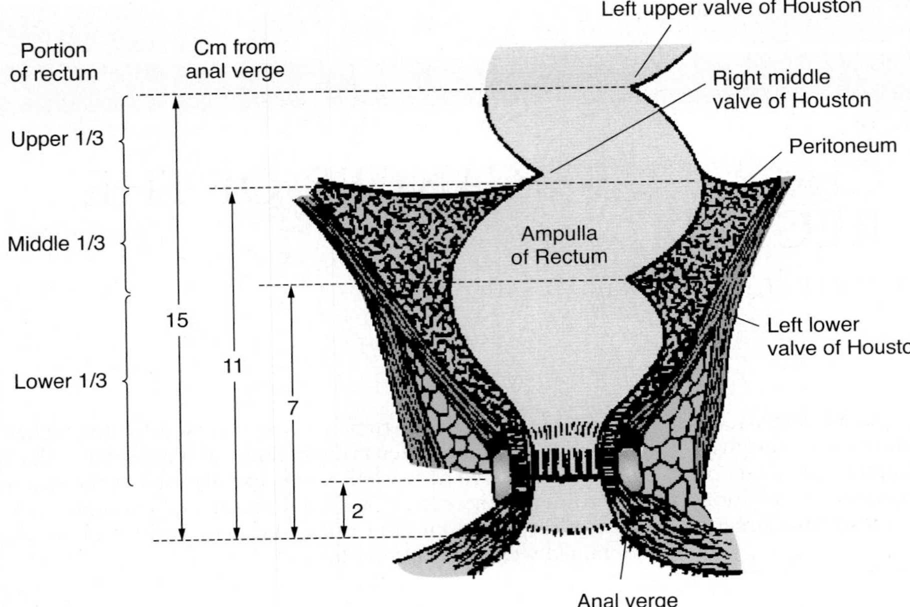

FIGURE 90.1 Division of the rectum into upper, middle, and lower thirds.

Autonomic Nerves

The preservation of both bladder and sexual function depends on the surgeon's understanding of the autonomic nerve supply to the pelvic organs.[1,2] The hypogastric plexus is formed from the sympathetic trunks as they converge over the sacral promontory. These sympathetic nerves are found beneath the pelvic peritoneum along the lateral pelvic sidewalls lateral to the mesorectum. The second, third, and fourth sacral nerve roots give rise to parasympathetic fibers to the pelvic viscera. The parasympathetic fibers proceed laterally as the nervi erigentes to join the sympathetic fibers at the site of the pelvic plexus that is just lateral and somewhat anterior to the tips of the seminal vesicle in men.[1,2] In order to preserve these structures and, therefore, sexual and bladder function, a sharp rather than a blunt technique should be used to dissect the mesorectum.[3–6]

STAGING

Standard clinicopathologic staging is the best indicator of prognosis for patients with rectal cancer. For rectal cancer, it is increasingly common to use clinical staging as the basis for the decision for neoadjuvant chemoradiation therapy. Therefore, the accuracy of that initial staging is critically important, both for management and for prognosis. There have been a large number of studies that have evaluated other prognostic markers, including pathologic, socioeconomic, and molecular, as described more fully in Chapter 89. However, even though many of these appear to have prognostic value, there are none that are commonly used to define management. This is related to the large number of tests that could be used, the lack of standardization of these tests, as well as the lack of knowledge as to how to incorporate them into the patient management scheme. The molecular marker that has engendered the most interest is the deletion of 18q.[7] These markers have been fully reviewed elsewhere.[8,9]

The staging system that should be used in the evaluation of patients with rectal cancer is the American Joint Committee on Cancer/International Union Against Cancer TNM (tumor, node, metastases) staging system (fully described in Chapter 14), which has been recently revised to subcategorize patients with stage III (node-positive) tumors. The Dukes staging system or its multiple modifications has been used for many years, but provides less information than the TNM system and should not be used. There have been gradual changes in the TNM system that primarily reflect the stage grouping rather than the system itself. The other systems should be acknowledged for their historical interest and for initially defining many of the high-risk factors for this disease.

Patients now often have both a clinical (preoperative) staging, which may define the use of neoadjuvant therapy, and a postoperative surgical stage. However, it is important to remember that initial therapy with radiation and chemotherapy can produce substantial downstaging (approximately 15% of patients will have a pathologic complete response), and that subsequent therapy should be based on the initial T and N staging determination. Specifically, a good tumor response locally to radiation and chemotherapy does not mean that a patient has any lower risk of having micrometastatic disease, and thus does not have a lesser need for adjuvant postoperative chemotherapy. Put another way, in a patient who receives preoperative radiation and chemotherapy, there is no decision point regarding whether or not postoperative chemotherapy should be given on the basis of the surgical pathology result. Until the data demonstrate otherwise, the plan for postoperative chemotherapy should be carried out even in the setting of a pathologic complete response.

The major change that has occurred in the newest version of the staging system is the acknowledgment that both the T stage and the N stage have independent prognostic importance for local control, disease-free survival, and overall survival.[10,11] Thus, for patients with N0 and N1 tumors viewed separately, the extent of the primary tumor in the rectum is of additional prognostic importance. Patients with T1-2N1 tumors have a relatively favorable prognosis and an outcome superior to that of other stage III patients. In fact, patients with T3N0M0 disease (stage II) have outcomes slightly inferior to those with T1-2N1M0, demonstrating the independent prognostic importance of T stage. These distinctions may allow future decisions to be more individualized as to the adjuvant therapy required.

Although at one level staging is very straightforward, the actuality of proper staging is much more difficult as it relies on multiple quality control issues that can mislead the clinician regarding proper therapy. For instance, it has been well demonstrated that for patients who are pathologically staged as N0, the prognosis is markedly improved for those in whom more than 12 to 14 nodes were identified by the pathologist compared with those in whom fewer nodes were identified.[12] This could be a surgical issue (fewer nodes were removed) or a pathologist issue (fewer nodes were identified), but it suggests that many patients were inappropriately staged lower, which could result in inappropriate therapy. Others have shown that staging accuracy continues to improve as the pathologist recovers more nodes, with accuracy leveling off at approximately 12 to 20 nodes recovered.[13,14] Likewise, as is true for colon cancer, the percentage of positive nodes is of substantial prognostic importance (M. Meyers, 2007, personal communication). The same issue relates to T-stage determination. If the pathologist does not look carefully for evidence of extension of tumor through the muscularis propria, the patient can be understaged, resulting in inappropriate treatment. Close or positive circumferential margins are a poor prognostic factor, which can only be found if the pathologist assiduously evaluates the radial margins.[15,16]

The standard staging procedure for rectal cancer entails a history, physical examination, complete blood cell count, liver and renal function studies, as well as carcinoembryonic antigen (CEA) evaluation. The routine laboratory studies are quite insensitive to the presence of metastatic disease, but they are usually ordered as a screen of organ function prior to surgery or chemoradiation therapy. High CEA levels are associated with poorer survival (see Chapter 14) and give an indication as to whether follow-up CEA determinations are likely to be useful. A careful rectal examination by an experienced examiner is an essential part of the pretherapy evaluation in determining distance of the tumor from the anal verge or from the dentate line, involvement of the anal sphincter, amount of circumferential involvement, clinical fixation, sphincter tone, and so forth, and has not been replaced by imaging studies or endoscopy. Colonoscopy or barium enema to evaluate the remainder of the large bowel is essential (if the patient is not obstructed) to rule out synchronous tumors or the presence of polyp syndromes.

Imaging studies including computed tomography (CT) or magnetic resonance imaging (MRI) to evaluate the pelvis, abdomen, and liver as well as a chest radiograph to screen for pulmonary metastases are routine. There has been much debate about the relative value of CT versus MRI without a clear resolution. This decision depends heavily on the institutional expertise and the equipment available. As the technology continues to change with fine-cut 64 detector row CT scans, improved MRI contrast agents, and so forth, one technique may become slightly better than another.

Conventional CT lacks sufficient accuracy to be used for preoperative staging of the primary tumor site. For example, in one series using air insufflation of the rectal ampulla and intravenous contrast, the overall T-stage accuracy was approximately 80%, with 18% overstaging in T2 disease and 21% understaging in T3 tumors.[17] As radiologists have usually defined node positivity on CT based on size (typically 1 cm or more), the overall accuracy of N staging by CT scan has been less than 80%, as nodes involved with rectal cancer are usually not markedly enlarged. The same study demonstrated the expected tradeoff between sensitivity and specificity, but with overall accuracy in a similar range. CT colonography is of increasing interest for screening, but at the present time has a minimal role in staging patients with known disease.

MRI suffers from some of the same limitations as CT for evaluating the primary tumor, although endorectal coil MRI allows discernment of the layers of the bowel wall and is similar in accuracy to endorectal ultrasound (see later discussion). Thin-section pelvic MRI with a surface coil allows for better visualization of the rectal wall layers and allows one to visualize the mesorectal fascia and thus to predict the likely distance of the surgical resection margin when using a total mesorectal excision (TME). Although there has been great interest in this technique, the studies to date still show a disappointing overall accuracy. In one study of 96 patients who had MRI followed by TME, of 22 patients classified as having T2 disease on MRI, 3 had T1, and 6 had T3 tumors. Of 61 patients classified as having T3 disease on MRI, 8 had T2 tumors and 2 had T4. Thus, 6 of 22 (27%) patients who might have benefited from preoperative therapy for T3 disease would not have received that therapy. Eight of 61 patients (13%) would have received preoperative treatment inappropriately based on the MRI T stage.[18] For nodal status, 8 of 33 MRI positive nodes were clinically negative, and 7 of 57 MRI negative nodes were pathologically positive.[19] The presence of nodal disease identified by MRI is also primarily determined by size, so the accuracy is similar to that of CT, although defining node positivity based on irregular border or mixed signal intensity could help improve sensitivity and specificity.[18]

CT, MRI, and positron emission tomography (PET) are all potentially useful for detecting metastatic disease, primarily in the liver. CT has an overall sensitivity of 70% to 85%,[20] which might be improved with multidetector-improved CT technology, although the data do not yet prove that contention. MRI is superior in characterizing liver lesions and distinguishing cysts and hemangiomas from tumor,[21] especially with the use of enhancement with gadolinium or other agents. PET with [^{18}F]fluorodeoxyglucose has engendered a great deal of interest as a method of possibly better defining patients with metastatic disease, especially in abdominal lymph nodes for which CT and MRI are relatively insensitive. However, PET is not standard in the preoperative staging and the incremental gain from routine PET scan appears to be small.[22] PET clearly can be of value in restaging patients with recurrence or suspected recurrence to detect additional metastatic sites prior to attempted resection of metastatic disease.

PET shows promise as the most sensitive study for the detection of metastatic disease in the liver and elsewhere. A meta-analysis of whole-body PET showed a sensitivity of 97% and a specificity of 76% in evaluating for recurrent colorectal cancer.[23] In the United States at the present time, contrast CT of the pelvis and the abdomen is the most commonly used imaging study, with MRI or PET being used to clarify abnormalities noted in the liver or abdomen. However, primary use of MRI is acceptable and could become standard with changing technology and availability.

There is much interest in the use of endorectal ultrasound (EUS) for staging of the primary tumor, and this, at present, is the most effective preoperative staging technique for T and N stage. Endorectal MRI provides similar information, but is not generally available and will not be discussed further here. EUS defines five interface layers of the rectal wall: mucosa, muscularis mucosa, submucosa, muscularis propria, and perirectal fat, as shown in Figure 90.2. Rectal tumors are generally hypoechoic and disrupt the interfaces depending on the level of tumor extension. The accuracy of EUS depends heavily on the experience and skill of the operator. The results mentioned later will not be obtained by an inexperienced examiner. However, in experienced hands EUS has an overall accuracy rate for T stage of 75% to 95% with an overstaging of approximately 10% to 20% in T2 disease because of an inability to distinguish a desmoplastic response and postbiopsy changes from local tumor invasion, and approximately a 10% rate of understaging because of an inability to detect microscopic tumor extension.[24–26]

EUS is less accurate in determining N stage than for T stage, with an overall accuracy rate of 62% to 83%.[24,25] Understaging occurs because many nodal metastases from rectal cancer are small, even micrometastatic, and not easily detected by EUS. In addition, some nodes are located beyond the range of the

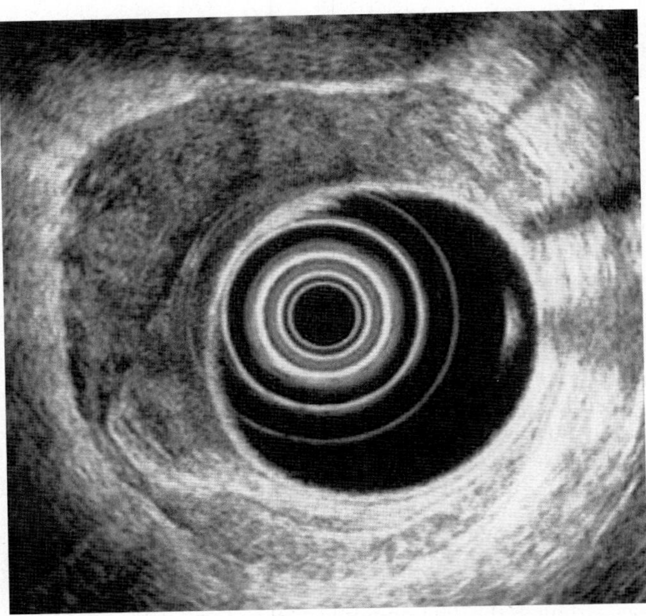

FIGURE 90.2 Endorectal ultrasound of a T3 tumor of the rectum, extension through the muscularis propria, and into perirectal fat. (From Ginsberg GG, Ahmad N. Endoscopic ultrasound for rectal cancer. *Vis Hum J Endosc* 2003;2(2):897, with permission.)

ultrasound transducer and thus cannot be seen during the procedure. Overstaging is often related to an inflammatory response, perhaps secondary to previous biopsy or manipulation. EUS is not accurate for determining tumor regression after preoperative radiation therapy and chemotherapy, as inflammatory changes and scarring can persist in the rectal wall or in perirectal soft tissue and may not reflect persisting tumor. Newer ultrasound techniques, such as three-dimensional ultrasound, are being explored but have not yet made it into standard practice.

SURGERY

The surgical management of primary rectal cancer presents unique problems for the surgeon based in large part on the anatomic constraints of the pelvis. Small early-stage lesions of the rectum that are diagnosed on physical examination or by colonoscopy/proctoscopy can often be managed with local resection. Local resection can be performed colonoscopically (as was described in the Chapter 89), or lesions can be removed via a transanal excision with the patient positioned in a prone or lithotomy position. Appropriate retractors can provide visualization, and resection should encompass a surrounding margin of normal mucosa[27] and should extend into the perirectal fat.

Stage I

The treatment of early-stage rectal cancer can be confusing as there are many approaches that can be used, and patient selection is critical to outcome. In addition, the risk of removal or damage to the anal sphincter is substantial for low-lying tumors and must be taken into consideration, along with the desire not to have a permanent colostomy for early-stage disease. Thus, the options for these patients are primarily those of local therapies without abdominal surgery, abdominal resection of the rectum with anastomosis and retention of the anal sphincter, and abdominal-perineal resection. The last two options are discussed in detail in "Stages II and III Rectal Cancer."

For selected T1 and T2 lesions without evidence of nodal disease, transanal excision often provides an adequate resection of the primary tumor mass and can spare the patient the morbidity of a more extensive rectal resection. However, it does not stage the nodal drainage areas and therefore cannot provide as complete staging and management of the tumor as a definitive resection. Tumors considered for local excision must meet a number of criteria to minimize the risk of local regional failure. Generally, local excision is limited to tumors within 8 to 10 cm of the anal verge, encompasses less than 40% of circumference of the bowel wall, is of well or moderately well-differentiated histology, and has no pathologic evidence of venous or lymphatic vessel invasion on biopsy. Although it has not been formally proven that these criteria need to be followed, small series have suggested a substantially higher risk of failure after local excision when these criteria have not been met, and most surgeons are reluctant to use local excision for the more extensive T1 or T2 lesions. Even when these criteria have been met, the local recurrence rate can be high after local excision (even when followed by postoperative radiation therapy and chemotherapy), so this approach must be used with caution. In the prospective phase 2 Cancer and Leukemia Group B study, local excision alone for T1 rectal cancer was associated with low recurrence and good survival rates that remain durable with long-term follow-up. T2 lesions treated via local excision and adjuvant therapy were associated with higher recurrence rates.[28] The American College of Surgeons Oncology Group has recently completed a phase 2 trial of neoadjuvuant capecitabine, oxaliplatin and radiation therapy followed by local excision for ultrasound T2 tumors (ACOSOG Protocol Z6041). This study should provide valuable data as to the role of neoadjuvant therapy versus adjuvant therapy in the setting of local excision approaches for rectal cancer.[29]

Performing a good transanal excision requires substantial surgical expertise as the surgeon must retain control over the primary tumor and obtain adequate mucosal margins as well as adequate deep resection into perirectal fat. Once removed, the tumor must be well laid out for the pathologist so that all relevant margins can be properly evaluated. There is some experience using preoperative radiation therapy and chemotherapy for small lesions, but care must be taken to have the site of the primary tumor well marked with a tattoo if this approach is taken, as excellent regression could make identification of the primary site difficult. The staging of such lesions should be performed using EUS to minimize the likelihood of doing a local excision for T3 tumors,[30] although there are inaccuracies with this approach.

A newer technique for transanal excision has gained popularity based on improved visualization of the lesion. Transanal endoscopic microsurgery (TEMS) makes use of a standard laparoscopic light source and monitoring system combined with specialized instruments and scopes. The technique allows for videoscopic magnification and the placement of instruments through an operating sigmoidoscope. TEMS is applied, in general, to the same patients who are candidates for standard transrectal resections. For lesions too large for colonoscopic removal, TEMS may be a viable alternative. Recurrence rates following TEMS resection as high as 30% have been reported[31] and therefore close endoscopic surveillance following TEMS is recommended.

A posterior proctotomy is useful for large posterior lesions and provides better access to more proximal lesions. This approach is known as a Kraske procedure and is performed by making a posterior longitudinal incision just above the anus to the inferior border of the gluteus maximus. The coccyx is removed and the underlying levator muscles are divided in a longitudinal fashion in the midline. This approach allows for the mobilization of the rectum and a full-thickness local excision. A transsphincteric excision (Bevan's or York-Mason) involves a similar approach as the posterior proctotomy, except the entire anal sphincter is divided posteriorly in the midline. Most investigators now believe that it is appropriate to use adjuvant pelvic radiation therapy with concurrent 5-fluorouracil (5-FU)-based chemotherapy for patients who have had a local excision for T2 tumors and also for selected patients with T1 tumors who have adverse prognostic factors (lymphovascular invasion, close margins, poorly differentiated histology), in order to decrease the risk of local recurrence.

Another approach that has been used sporadically for patients with early-stage disease is endocavitary radiation therapy. This technique is used for a similar category of patients who are treated with local excision; T1 or T2 tumors less than 3 cm, not poorly differentiated, with no evidence of nodal involvement. Patients are treated with a special low-energy x-ray machine (50 kVp) that is attached to a rigid endoscopic-type device that can be placed in the rectum directly over the tumor. Local control results with this approach have been very good in properly selected patients, but specialized equipment is required (which is not generally available) and less pathologic information is obtained than after a local excision. This approach is rarely used at the present time.

Stages II and III Rectal Cancer

The primary treatment of patients with stages II and III rectal cancer (T3-4 and/or node-positive) is surgical. However, in contrast to the treatment of patients with stage I disease, there is a strong body of information to suggest that combined modality therapy with radiation therapy and chemotherapy should be used in conjunction with surgical resection. This conclusion is based on both patterns of failure data, which demonstrate a substantial incidence of local, regional as well as distant disease failure, and the fact that this incidence of tumor recurrence at all sites is decreased with the use of trimodality therapy.

The desire when performing a resection for rectal cancer is to preserve intestinal continuity and the sphincter mechanism whenever possible while still maximizing tumor control. Therefore, careful preoperative screening is crucial in the determination of the location of the lesion and its depth of invasion. As previously described, it is convenient to think of the rectum as divided into thirds for the purposes of the evaluation and preoperative determination of the surgical approach for resection. The upper third of the rectum is often considered the region of large intestine from the sacral prominence to the peritoneal reflection. These lesions are in almost all cases managed with a low anterior resection in much the same way as a sigmoid colon cancer (see Chapter 89). An adequate 1- to 2-cm distal mucosal margin can be achieved for these lesions well above the sphincter mechanism, and intestinal continuity can be restored using either a hand-sewn technique or a circular stapling device inserted through the rectum.[30,32]

Tumors in the middle and lower thirds of the rectum can be considered as lying entirely below the peritoneal reflection. The resection of these tumors can be challenging because of the confines of the pelvic skeletal structure, and the ability to perform a resection with an adequate distal margin is significantly influenced by the size of the lesion. Nevertheless, tumors of the middle third of the rectum in most cases can be safely resected with a low anterior resection, with restoration of intestinal continuity and preservation of a continent sphincter apparatus.

Lesions in the distal third of the rectum, defined as those within 5 cm of the anal verge, can present the greatest challenge to the surgeon with respect to sphincter preservation. This is often influenced by the extent of lateral invasion of the lesion into the muscles of the sphincter apparatus and how close distally the tumor is to the musculature of the anal canal. The abdominal perineal resection (APR) has historically been considered the standard treatment for patients with rectal cancers located within 6 cm of the anal verge. This procedure requires a transperitoneal as well as a transperineal approach with removal of the entire rectum and sphincter complex. A permanent end colostomy is created and the perineal wound either closed primarily or left to granulate in after closure of the musculature.

Although an APR is associated with a relatively low rate of local recurrence, it is not without the obvious problems of the need for a permanent colostomy and loss of intestinal continuity and sphincter function. Therefore, intense interest has been focused on developing approaches to the resection of tumors in the distal third of the rectum that would both avoid local regional recurrence and preserve intestinal continuity and sphincter continence.

Tumors within 1 to 2 cm of the dentate line—that is, those that can be removed with at least a 1-cm distal margin—can be resected and intestinal continuity restored with a coloanal anastomosis.[33,34] When performing a very low coloanal anastomosis, it is often prudent to protect the healing suture line with a diverting loop ileostomy, which can be reversed in 4 to 6 weeks after the anastomosis has healed.

In order to increase the number of sphincter-preserving operations performed, several authors cite the use of preoperative chemoradiation as a means to decrease the local recurrence rate.[33,35] They cite statistics that rectal carcinoma responds to preoperative chemoradiation therapy with a 10% to 15% pathologic complete response rate and a substantial rate of tumor downstaging. The goal of such an approach would be to reduce the need for APR to an incidence of 10% or less.

When performing a sphincter-preserving operation, in order to preserve the lateral musculature and therefore a functional sphincter complex, the resection by necessity does not have as wide a margin as one performed during an APR. In order to improve on margin status, intersphincteric resections have been performed.[36] This approach includes a partial sphincteric resection designed to improve margin status without sacrificing sphincter function. In small series, functional results have been comparable to less aggressive sphincter-preserving operations. The impact on oncologic outcome is difficult to interpret and will require larger series.

The choice of a straight coloanal versus a pouch anastomosis is a decision that is based to a large degree on surgeon's preference and experience. Some advocate a pouch operation, citing improved anal function as measured by decreased stool frequency and urgency and improved continence.[4] Others have demonstrated that results are equivalent with a straight coloanal anastomosis.[37]

Chemoradiation should be used preoperatively when performing sphincter-preserving resections for T3 or T4 rectal lesions or for any node-positive disease stages II or III. There is some evidence that preoperative radiation results in less morbidity than postoperative radiation therapy when a coloanal anastomosis is planned. In a study of 109 patients treated with a low anterior resection and a straight coloanal anastomosis, those receiving preoperative radiation therapy had a lower incidence of adverse effects on anal function than those receiving postoperative radiation.[37] The authors attributed this to sparing of the neorectum from these effects. Relative benefits and outcomes for preoperative chemoradiation versus postoperative chemoradiation will be discussed in detail in following sections.

Total Mesorectal Resection

The goal of the resection of rectal tumors is the removal of the tumor with an adequate margin as well as removal of draining

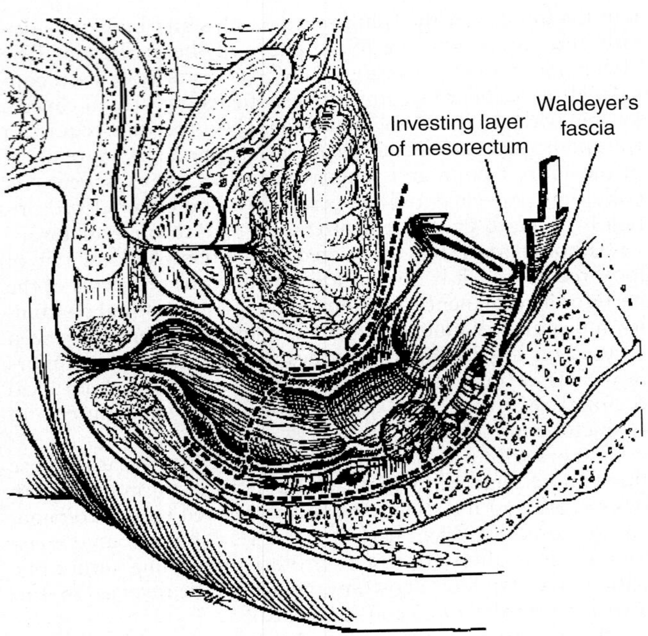

FIGURE 90.3 Total mesorectal excision.

lymph nodes and lymphatics to properly stage the tumor and to reduce the risk of recurrence and spread. For lesions in the intraperitoneal colon, the lymphatics and vascular supply are found in the mesentery associated with that region of bowel.

In the rectum the mesorectum is the structure that contains the blood supply and lymphatics for the upper, middle, and lower rectum. Most involved lymph nodes for rectal cancers are found within the mesorectum, with T1 lesions associated with positive lymph nodes in 5.7% of cases; T2 lesions having positive lymph nodes in 20% of cases; and T3 and T4 lesions having positive lymph nodes in 65% and 78% of cases, respectively.[38]

The anatomy and approach to mesorectal excision is depicted in Figure 90.3. This operation involves a sharp dissection occurring in an avascular plane beyond the perirectal fat that is beyond the region where most of the nodes are located. After a TME the specimen is typically shiny and bilobed in contrast to the irregular and rough surface after a blunt dissection where much of the mesorectal fat is left behind. TME attempts not only to clear involved lymph nodes but also to adequately manage the radial margins of the rectal tumor. These radial margins have been shown to be more important with respect to the risk of local regional recurrence than the distal mucosal margin.[35,39] Distal mucosal margins of 1 cm or greater are adequate for local control; however, the margin on the mesorectum should extend beyond the distal mucosal margin in order to ensure a successful surgical outcome.[34,35] A number of studies have demonstrated the benefit of TME, and it is thought by many that this is the procedure of choice for the management of middle- and lower-third rectal cancers.[5,40–42] Although some studies have suggested that an adequate TME might in and of itself be sufficient management for T2 and T3 rectal cancers, the majority of the literature still supports the use of adjuvant chemoradiation for stages II and III disease even when combined with TME.

Large studies of proctectomy with TME have demonstrated a reduction in the overall incidence of local recurrence to less than 10%.[4] The consequences of TME can be impairment in erectile and bladder function because of disruption of parasympathetic nerves that are located in proximity to the mesorectum. Several authors have stressed the importance of the experience of the surgeon performing the procedure, and some have suggested specific techniques for monitoring modalities that can be used during this procedure to minimize morbidity.[5,6] A careful understanding of the anatomy and adequate visualization during sharp dissection will help in minimizing injury to the parasympathetic nerves and the consequent morbidity.[3,4]

Adequate visualization in the deep pelvis can often be a challenge. This may be a situation where the visual magnification and ability to enter tight spaces that are unique to the laparoscopic approach may be an advantage. Several groups have demonstrated the feasibility of laparoscopic TME for low rectal cancer as part of a sphincter-preserving operation.[43–45] Some of the larger series, while demonstrating that TME using laparoscopic techniques can be performed safely, do not have adequate follow-up to demonstrate whether there were any oncologic disadvantages to such an approach. Unfortunately, the prospective random assignment trial conducted in the United States to evaluate the role of laparoscopic surgery for colon cancer excluded patients with low rectal lesions. Therefore, the ultimate role of the laparoscopic approach to TME will have to await prospective randomized trials using this technique and comparing it to the standard open approach.

Resection of Contiguous Organs and Total Pelvic Exenteration

Although aggressive surgical approaches to rectal cancer have resulted in improvement in locoregional recurrence rates, these rates can still be as high as 33%. Not infrequently, large rectal lesions will invade through the wall of the rectum into contiguous structures such as the bladder, prostate, vagina, and uterus. Carefully selected patients with recurrent or locally advanced rectal cancers may benefit from an aggressive approach such as a total pelvic exenteration. Local recurrences remain localized to the pelvis in a significant number of patients, with autopsy studies demonstrating the incidence of pelvic recurrence to be as high as 50%.[46]

Recurrences in the pelvis can result in significant morbidity such as tenesmus, pain, bowel obstruction, and fistula. Although some of these can be ameliorated with radiation, these problems are best managed by preventing their occurrence. Although the impact of total pelvic exenteration on survival has been debated, the potential benefits on controlling locoregional disease and preventing morbidity keeps this technique as one of the tools in the surgeon's armamentarium when approaching large rectal lesions.

Combined Modality Therapy (Stage II and III)

The use of adjuvant radiation therapy is based on the substantial incidence of locoregional failure with surgical therapy alone. Older studies demonstrate local failure rates of up to 50% in patients with T3-4 or node-positive disease[47–53] (Table 90.1). The locoregional recurrence rates in these studies are in the range of 25% to 50% for patients with T3-4 and/or node-positive disease and is a dominant pattern of failure, although distant recurrence is also of great importance. Local failure is related not just to the stage of the disease, but also the location of the tumor in the rectum (tumors located low in the rectum have a higher incidence of local failure) and the experience and ability of the surgeon. However, the relevance of these older local recurrence data has been brought into question with the advent of the use of TME, as previously described. It is important to realize that the data on local recurrence after primary surgical resection come from selected series with operations performed by experienced surgeons who have been

TABLE 90.1

LOCAL FAILURE OF RECTAL CANCER SURGERY ALONE (LOCAL FAILURE RATE PERCENTAGE/NO. OF PATIENTS IN COHORT)

	Gunderson and Sosin[50]	Rich et al.[52]	Minsky et al.[91]	Martling et al.[53]	Mendenhall et al.[47]	Pilipshen et al.[49]	Bonadeo et al.[107]
Analysis	Reoperation (Crude)	Clin Exam + Surgery (Crude)	First Failure—Clinical Exam + Surgery (5-y Actuarial)	Total Local Recurrence	Total Local Recurrence—5-y Follow-up Clinical	First Failure—Clinical	Total Local Recurrence—Clinical[a]
T1N0		8%/39	11%/11	9%/78	0/6	0%/5	3%/103
T2N0			3%/36		38%/16	14%/128	
T3N0	67%/6	24%/42	23%/60	34%/80	40%/30	30%/111	4%/181
T4N0		53%/15	11%/9				
T1-2N+	24%/17	50%/4	14%/11	37%/93	71%/17	22%/49	24%/133
T3N+	83%/40	47%/34	25%/31		65%/17	49%/89	
T4N+		67%/6	22%/10				
Total	64%/75	30%/142	15%/168	27%/251	46%/90		

[a]Local recurrence highly dependent on site in rectum—18% overall for tumors ≤7 cm from anal verge.

specially trained in TME and may not be relevant to the operations performed by general surgeons who perform the operation only occasionally and who are not specially trained.

Although initial studies reported locoregional failure rates of less than 5% after TME without the use of any adjuvant therapy,[40,42,54–56] there was concern that these excellent results could not be replicated in larger population-based studies. A number of European countries or regions have shown that the overall locoregional recurrence risks could be decreased by limiting the surgeons who were authorized to perform rectal surgery to those who were trained and certified in the procedure, and by having educational sessions for those who were performing the surgery.[5] This raised the question of what is the true rate of local failure after TME to help define which patients really require adjuvant therapy.

The most important analysis on local recurrence rates with TME are the data from the Dutch TME study in which patients were randomized to receive either TME alone or a short course of preoperative radiation therapy followed by TME.[42] All patients with rectal cancer were eligible, including those with early-stage disease. Special attempts were made to have good surgical and pathology quality control. The early results (2 years) relating to local tumor recurrence have been reported and are summarized in Table 90.2. The study demonstrates that there are subsets of patients in whom TME alone is likely sufficient for obtaining good pelvic control, including patients with high rectal tumors (some of these may have been sigmoid cancers, rather than rectal), and low-stage tumors (T1-2, N0). On the other hand, low-lying rectal tumors that are moderately advanced (T3-4 and/or node-positive) had a higher incidence of locoregional failure. Local failure after TME alone was 15% in node-positive patients at 2 years, not corrected for site of the primary, and longer-term follow-up will undoubtedly demonstrate higher local failure rates. In addition, as these results were obtained in a controlled setting, one would likely not obtain similarly good results when surgery is done with less careful quality control. There was a consistent decrease in local failure rate by the addition of preoperative radiation therapy, but the absolute magnitude of the effect varied by the tumor characteristics previously discussed.

A trial similar to the Dutch TME study was recently reported. This phase 3 trial randomized 1,350 patients with operable adenocarcinoma of the rectum to short-course preoperative radiotherapy (25 Gy in five fractions; n = 674) or to

TABLE 90.2

RESULTS OF DUTCH TOTAL MESORECTAL EXCISION TRIAL

Technique	Preop Radiotherapy (5 Gy × 5) + Total Mesorectal Excision	Total Mesorectal Excision Alone
PERCENTAGE OF PATIENTS		
Stage 0 or I		30
Local failure (2 y)	2.4	8.2
Local failure (4 y)	3	10
LOCAL FAILURE (DISTANCE FROM ANAL VERGE)		
0–5 cm	5.8	10
5–10 cm	1	10.1
10–15 cm	1.3	3.8
Stage III (4-y estimate)		20

(From ref. 41, with permission.)

TABLE 90.3

LOCAL CONTROL AND SURVIVAL WITH AND WITHOUT RADIOTHERAPY—PREOPERATIVELY, POSTOPERATIVELY, AND WITH OR WITHOUT CHEMOTHERAPY

Study/Institution[a] (Ref.)	No. of Patients	Local Failure (%)	Disease-Free Survival (%)	Survival (5 y)(%)
NSABP- RO-1 (61) Surg/ Surg + RT (Postop RT)	184/187	25/16	No difference	No difference
NSABP RO-2 (62) Surg + chemo/ Surg + chemo + RT (Postop RT)	348/346	13/8		
GITSG (59) Surg/Surg + RT/ Surg + chemo + RT (Postop RT)	58/50/46	25/20/10	44/50/65	26/33/45
Swedish (58) Surg/Surg + RT (Preop RT)		27/11		48/58
Stockholm II (53) Surg/Surg + RT (Preop RT)		34/16 Stage II 37/21 Stage II		
MRC (64) Surg/Surg + RT (Postop RT)	235/234	34/21		38/41

NSABP, National Surgical Adjuvant Breast and Bowel Project; RT, radiotherapy; GITSG, Gastrointestinal Study Group; MRC, Medical Research Council.
[a]Randomized studies in either all patients or patients with stage II and III disease.

initial surgery with selective postoperative chemoradiotherapy (45 Gy in 25 fractions with concurrent 5-FU) restricted to patients circumferential resection margin involvement (n = 676). The primary outcome measure was local recurrence. At the time of analysis, 330 patients had died (157 preoperative radiotherapy group vs. 173 selective postoperative chemoradiotherapy), and median follow-up of surviving patients was 4 years. Ninety-nine patients developed local recurrence (27 preoperative radiotherapy vs. 72 selective postoperative chemoradiotherapy). A reduction was noted of 61% in the relative risk of local recurrence for patients receiving preoperative radiotherapy (hazard ratio [HR], 0.39; 95% confidence interval [CI]: 0.27–0.58; P <.0001), and an absolute difference at 3 years of 6.2% (95% CI: 5.3–7.1) (4.4% preoperative radiotherapy vs. 10.6% selective postoperative chemoradiotherapy). A relative improvement in disease-free survival of 24% for patients receiving preoperative radiotherapy (HR, 0.76; 95% CI: 0.62–0.94;P = .013), and an absolute difference at 3 years of 6.0% (95% CI: 5.3–6.8) (77.5% vs. 71.5%) was observed. Overall survival did not differ between the groups (HR, 0.91; 95% CI: 0.73–1.13; P = .40). These findings provide further evidence that short-course preoperative radiotherapy is an effective treatment for patients with operable rectal cancer.[57]

The data are excellent that radiation therapy, especially when combined with chemotherapy, can decrease the local failure rate. This is shown by a Swedish study of preoperative radiation therapy compared with surgery,[58] the Dutch TME trial in the preoperative setting,[41] and by multiple studies in the postoperative setting.[59–64] There are also excellent data to show that locoregional failure is decreased by the use of radiation therapy and is further decreased by the use of concurrent 5-FU-based chemotherapy (Table 90.3).[59,60,65] Most studies have demonstrated that local failure decreases by about 50% with the use of adjuvant radiation therapy, with a greater effect when concurrent 5-FU is used with irradiation. This appears to provide a strong justification for the use of adjuvant radiation therapy. What is less clear is whether trimodality therapy with radiation therapy improves survival, if radiochemotherapy should be given preoperatively or postoperatively, and precisely which patients should be irradiated.

DOES ADJUVANT RADIATION THERAPY IMPACT SURVIVAL?

Although there have been multiple randomized trials addressing the use of adjuvant radiation therapy or chemoradiation therapy, and although they consistently show an improvement in local control with adjuvant radiation therapy, the survival outcome data have been mixed. In the past there have been two meta-analyses performed.[66,67] Table 90.4 shows the results of a meta-analysis by Camma et al.[67] showing a decreased

TABLE 90.4

RESULTS OF META-ANALYSIS, PREOPERATIVE RADIOTHERAPY VERSUS SURGERY ALONE

Result	Preop Radiotherapy versus Surgery
Overall 5-y mortality	OR 0.84 (P = .03)
5-y cancer mortality	OR 0.71 (P <.001)
5-y local recurrence	OR 0.49 (P <.001)
5-y distant metastases	OR 0.93 (P = .54)

OR, overall recovery.
(From ref. 67, with permission.)

TABLE 90.5

COLORECTAL CANCER COLLABORATIVE GROUP 2001 ADJUVANT RADIATION THERAPY IN RECTAL CANCER

	Preoperative RT versus Surgery	Postoperative RT versus Surgery
Yearly risk of local recurrence	46% decrease with RT	37% decrease with RT
Death rate	5% less than with surgery	No difference from surgery

RT, radiotherapy.
(From ref. 66, with permission.)

local recurrence rate, cancer mortality rate, and overall mortality rate with the use of preoperative radiation therapy, although without a decrease in distant metastasis rate. The Colorectal Cancer Collaborative Group study (Table 90.5) demonstrates no improvement in the likelihood of curative surgery with preoperative therapy or of overall survival with all types of radiation therapy combined.[66] Preoperative radiation therapy, however, was shown to improve local control, disease-free survival, and overall survival compared with surgery alone, although deaths within the first year after surgery were higher after radiation therapy. Local recurrence with preoperative radiation therapy was 46% lower than surgery alone, and cancer deaths were decreased from 50% to 45%. Postoperative radiation therapy was shown to improve local control (although less than preoperative therapy), but did not impact long-term survival. Lending substantial strength to the conclusion that there was a true advantage to radiation therapy is the fact that there was a dose response demonstrated for the radiation effect on local control (i.e., better control was obtained with higher radiation dose). This observation strengthens the conclusion, as it demonstrates a direct correlation between the amount of therapy and outcome. The data from this analysis are heavily influenced by the results of a single Swedish study that showed a long-term survival advantage to the use of preoperative radiation therapy compared with surgery alone.[58] Thus, these data show that improving local control with the use of radiation therapy (and presumably with concurrent chemoradiation therapy) is beneficial, and that trimodality therapy, especially when chemoradiation therapy is used preoperatively, can improve survival.

PREOPERATIVE RADIATION THERAPY

The second issue of importance is whether adjuvant therapy should be given preoperatively or postoperatively and the exact timing of the chemotherapy. Current data clearly favor the preoperative approach.

Perhaps the most important study addressing the issue of pre- versus postoperative adjuvant therapy is a German trial of preoperative versus postoperative chemoradiation with radiation therapy given at 1.8 Gy per fraction and using continuous-infusion 5-FU chemotherapy as a 120-hour infusion, for which results have been reported by Sauer et al.[68] This study demonstrates an advantage in sphincter preservation with the use of preoperative therapy. Of the patients thought to need an APR at initial assessment, only 19% had a sphincter-preserving surgery when operation was done immediately versus 39% after preoperative radiation therapy, although there was no difference in the overall sphincter preservation rate. There was a statistically significant decrease in local failure with preoperative radiation therapy compared to postoperative treatment (6% vs. 13%; $P = .006$). The relative risk of local failure in the pre- versus postoperative treatment group was 0.46. The 5-year disease-free survival showed a small advantage to preoperative therapy (68% vs. 65%; $P = .32$), which was not statistically significant. There was a decrease in late anastomotic strictures with preoperative therapy, and acute toxicity was also decreased by the use of preoperative radiation and chemotherapy, both statistically significant. This provides strong evidence of the superiority of preoperative adjuvant treatment in patients in whom it is determined that adjuvant therapy is needed.

Similar to the goals of the German trial, the NSABP R-03 (National Surgical Adjuvant Breast and Bowel Project R-03) trial compared neoadjuvant versus adjuvant chemoradiotherapy in the treatment of locally advanced rectal carcinoma. Patients with clinical T3 or T4 or node-positive rectal cancer were randomly assigned to preoperative or postoperative chemoradiotherapy. Chemotherapy consisted of fluorouracil and leucovorin with 45 Gy in 25 fractions with a 5.40-Gy boost within the original margins of treatment. In the preoperative group, surgery was performed within 8 weeks after completion of radiotherapy. In the postoperative group, chemotherapy began after recovery from surgery but no later than 4 weeks after surgery. The primary end points were disease-free survival and overall survival. Two hundred sixty-seven patients were randomly assigned to NSABP R-03. The intended sample size was 900 patients. Excluding 11 ineligible and 2 eligible patients without follow-up data, the analysis used data on 123 patients randomly assigned to preoperative and 131 to postoperative chemoradiotherapy. Surviving patients were observed for a median of 8.4 years. The 5-year disease-free survival for preoperative patients was 64.7% versus 53.4% for postoperative patients ($P = .011$). The 5-year overall survival for preoperative patients was 74.5% versus 65.6% for postoperative patients ($P = .065$). A complete pathologic response was achieved in 15% of preoperative patients. No preoperative patient with a complete pathologic response has had a recurrence. The investigators concluded that preoperative chemoradiotherapy, compared with postoperative chemoradiotherapy, significantly improved disease-free survival and showed a trend toward improved overall survival.[69]

In addition to improving survival, another reason for using preoperative chemoradiation therapy is to increase the chance for sphincter preservation for patients with low-lying tumors of the rectum, where an abdominoperineal resection would be conventionally used. The NSABP trial R-03 was able to obtain worthwhile information regarding this issue. When a patient was first seen, the surgeon was asked (for both preoperative and postoperative patients) what operation was needed. In the patients randomized to postoperative radiation therapy (i.e., immediate surgery), the determination in the office corresponded extremely well to the operation actually performed. However, in the patients who received preoperative radiation therapy, sphincter-preserving surgery was done in 50% of patients compared with 33% of those who had initial surgery.[70] However, the data have been inconsistent overall in demonstrating an advantage to preoperative therapy in terms of sphincter preservation. The analyses are complicated because the decision as to whether sphincter-preserving surgery should be done is heavily dependent on the biases of the surgeon. If the surgeon believes that the same operation should be done regardless of tumor regression, then clearly the same surgery will be done. There are some surgeons who will do sphincter-preserving operations after preoperative irradiation, when they would not have done so if the surgery had been done first.

If one is using preoperative radiotherapy to try to improve the likelihood of sphincter preservation, the radiation must be given in such a way as to maximize the likelihood of this occurring. Specifically, a "standard" long course of irradiation to a dose of approximately 50 Gy at 18 to 20 Gy per fraction over 5 to 5.5 weeks (as given in the German trial mentioned previously) has been thought by most U.S. investigators to be optimal. The short-course therapy with immediate surgery (typically 50 Gy for five fractions given over 1 week), as often used in Europe, followed by immediate surgery is not likely to produce enough tumor shrinkage to allow for sphincter preservation in patients with very low-lying tumors. Bujko et al.[71] have published data that suggest that the short course is as effective in producing local control as the longer course of therapy. Three hundred twelve patients were randomized to either 25 Gy in five fractions followed by surgery within 1 week, or 50.4 Gy in 28 fractions with concurrent bolus 5-FU and leucovorin and surgery 4 to 6 weeks later. Disease-free survival was respectively (short- vs. long-course therapy) 58.4% versus 55.6%; local recurrence, 9% versus 14.2%; severe late toxicity, 10.1% versus 7.1%; and acute toxicity, 3.2% versus 18.2%. There was no improvement in sphincter preservation with long-course treatment. Although this was a relatively small study, it provides important evidence to support the value of short-course preoperative therapy.

There are theoretical reasons to believe that radiation therapy delivered preoperatively would decrease the toxicity of therapy. With postoperative radiation therapy the soft tissues of the perineum are at risk for involvement after an APR because of surgical manipulation and, therefore, need to be irradiated with its attendant acute skin toxicity. This is not needed with preoperative therapy. With postoperative radiation therapy, normal bowel is moved into the pelvis for the anastomosis after a low anterior resection and therefore is irradiated and at risk for late toxicity. In the preoperative setting much of the irradiated bowel is removed with the surgical specimen and therefore is not at risk for producing late bowel injury. There is also likely to be a higher risk of having small bowel fixed in the pelvis after surgery secondary to adhesions, which could also lead to late toxicity. On the other hand, many studies have demonstrated that acute surgical morbidity and mortality are not substantially increased with the use of preoperative irradiation, although many surgeons routinely perform a temporary diverting colostomy in order to avoid the problems associated with an anastomotic leak. Except for the German trial previously mentioned, which shows decreased acute and late toxicity, data on late toxicity are not available to directly compare the two techniques when used with concurrent chemotherapy and the commonly used dose/fractionation schedules.

As the retrospective meta-analyses have generally shown better tumor control locally and better evidence of a survival advantage secondary to preoperative irradiation, many gastrointestinal oncologists prefer preoperative radiochemotherapy for the patient who clearly requires adjuvant radiation therapy. A reasonable strategy at present is to use preoperative radiochemotherapy for patients in whom there is little doubt about the advisability of adjuvant therapy (T3 node-positive or T4 disease) or patients with low-lying tumors in whom an APR may still be avoided, but to use initial surgery for other patient cohorts, with postoperative radiochemotherapy used based on the operative and pathologic findings.

Another issue of importance is the timing of chemotherapy. It has been assumed by many investigators that concurrent preoperative chemotherapy and postoperative adjuvant chemotherapy is the proper way of delivering treatment. A study by the European Organisation for Research and Treatment of Cancer, however, questions these assumptions.[72] Patients were randomized to receive either preoperative radiation therapy alone, preoperative chemoradiotherapy, preoperative radiation therapy and postoperative chemotherapy, or preoperative chemoradiotherapy and postoperative chemotherapy. Chemotherapy was bolus 5-FU (350 mg/m^2/d for 5 days) and leucovorin (20 mg/m^2 for 5 days) with two cycles given with radiation therapy and four cycles postoperatively for the appropriate groups. Local recurrence rates were roughly similar for all patients receiving chemotherapy regardless of timing (7% to 9%) and significantly improved compared with those patients not receiving any chemotherapy (17%). There was no difference in survival outcomes based on the timing of chemotherapy. The 5-year disease-free survival rates were 52.2% and 58.2% in the no adjuvant treatment groups and the adjuvant treatment groups, respectively (P = .13).

WHICH PATIENTS SHOULD RECEIVE ADJUVANT THERAPY?

For either pre- or postoperative therapy, the physician needs to address the issue of precisely which patients need to receive adjuvant radiation therapy and chemotherapy. At the present time these two modalities have been completely linked in U.S. clinical trials, so it is not possible to determine if there are subsets of patients who might benefit from one modality and not the other. In addition, recent U.S. trials have all used chemotherapy concurrent with the radiation therapy in addition to postradiation chemotherapy, so it is not possible to determine the relative importance of each modality.

Based on the historical patterns of failure data, which demonstrated high local failure rates with surgery alone for patients with T3 and/or node-positive disease, virtually all U.S. studies have evaluated this entire patient population. However, more detailed analyses have allowed us to define characteristics that help define relatively low-risk and relatively high-risk patient subsets. As mentioned earlier, among the patients conventionally treated with adjuvant chemoradiation therapy, a number of relatively lower risk categories have been identified. Those include patients with T3N0 or T1-2N1 disease,[10,11,73,74] those with primary tumors located high in the rectum, those with wide circumferential margins on the final pathology specimen,[15,16] those with node-negative disease after multiple (12 to 14 or more) nodes have been evaluated,[12–14,75] and those in whom TME surgery had been performed by an experienced colorectal oncologic surgeon.[76,77] In the preoperative setting only some of this information will be available at the time a therapeutic decision must be made, but some information will be available (including knowledge of the surgeon). In addition, one must consider the known inaccuracy of transrectal ultrasound in staging and the experience of the ultrasonographer.[26,31] However, if most of these conditions are met, it is possible that routine adjuvant radiation therapy, and perhaps chemotherapy, is not required for the lower-stage tumors. At the present time most patients treated outside clinical trials that have T3-4 and/or node-positive disease should probably receive adjuvant chemoradiation therapy if there are no extenuating circumstances. However, for patients who meet the previously mentioned favorable criteria, not using adjuvant radiation therapy and perhaps chemotherapy can be considered. Clinical trials will need to be performed to help resolve which subsets of patients do not require routine adjuvant radiation therapy.

CONCURRENT CHEMOTHERAPY

The use of adjuvant chemotherapy has centered on the use of 5-FU chemotherapy, although this drug has been in use for over 50 years and is not very effective for colon or rectal cancer. The initial trials of trimodality therapy in rectal cancer used bolus 5-FU at a dose of 500 mg/m²/d for 3 days during weeks 1 and 5 of the radiation therapy. This was the approach routinely used until the results of the North Central Cancer Treatment Group study testing the use of long-term continuous infusion 5-FU with postoperative radiation therapy (bolus 5-FU was used both before and after the radiation therapy) were reported.[65] This study demonstrated an advantage to continuous infusion 5-FU (only during radiation therapy) compared with bolus 5-FU in terms of local control, disease-free survival, and overall survival. Because of this result and the encouraging results found with more aggressive therapy in colon cancer, it was logical to think that further intensification of chemotherapy would be of value both for local and systemic control.

Unfortunately, this expectation has not been borne out. Two large U.S. Gastrointestinal Intergroup trials have been run testing intensification with either more aggressive 5-FU and leucovorin, additional continuous infusion 5-FU, and other combinations, with data demonstrating no advantage.[78,79] Thus, we are left with evidence that continuous infusion 5-FU during radiation therapy is of value in improving local control, distant metastases, and survival, but no evidence that anything other than simple 5-FU or 5-FU plus leucovorin should be used during the chemotherapy portion of the therapy. Whether newer agents including cytotoxins with clear efficacy against colon and rectal cancers in the metastatic disease setting, such as irinotecan or oxaliplatin, or biologics, such as bevacizumab or cetuximab, will be superior to standard 5-FU is at the present time unknown.

In practice, most gastrointestinal oncologists now use continuous-infusion 5-FU or capecitabine during radiation therapy. Preliminary data from a German randomized phase 3 trial of 401 patients with locally advanced rectal cancer comparing capecitabine versus 5-FU neoadjuvant chemoradiotherapy demonstrated a similar safety profile and a trend in improved downstaging in the capecitabine treated patients.[80]

The investigators concluded that capecitabine exhibits the potential to replace 5-FU as perioperative treatment of rectal cancer. The NSABP is nearing completion of a trial (R04) comparing continuous-infusion 5-FU with capecitabine, both with concurrent radiation therapy. Postresection use of adjuvant chemotherapy based on the results in colon cancer has become a widespread practice, with oncologists using primarily FOLFOX (biweekly oxaliplatin, 5-FU, and leucovorin; see Chapter 89) as the postradiation chemotherapy. This is based on the reasonable, albeit unproven, extrapolation from data showing that the addition of oxaliplatin to 5-FU/leucovorin improves disease-free and overall survival in the postoperative management of colon cancer patients (see Chapter 89).

In addition to studies that have substituted fluoropyrimidines, there is also substantial interest in the use of other agents added to fluoropyrimidines with concurrent radiation therapy. There have been studies with the addition of irinotecan,[81] but because of the overlapping toxicity of diarrhea with radiation therapy and 5-FU, plus the demonstrated lack of efficacy of irinotecan in the adjuvant treatment of colon cancer, use of irinotecan in the combined mode has not been, and most likely ought not be, heavily pursued. A small randomized phase 3 study showed no benefit to the addition of irinotecan to 5-FU/leucovorin in the nonradiation portion of the treatment.[82] The Radiation Therapy Oncology Group (RTOG) completed a small randomized phase 2 trial of concurrent capecitabine, irinotecan, and radiation therapy versus concurrent oxaliplatin, capecitabine, and radiation therapy.[83] Both on the basis of a lack of data supporting adjuvant irinotecan, and a superior pathologic complete response rate in the oxaliplatin-containing arm, no further development of the irinotecan-containing schedule is planned.

There has been greater interest in the use of oxaliplatin added to 5-FU and radiation therapy, although thus far the results have been disappointing. A phase 1/2 study performed by the Cancer and Leukemia Group B demonstrated the feasibility of concurrent oxaliplatin 5-FU and radiation therapy,[84] as did a German multicenter phase 2 trial,[85] and the previously mentioned RTOG randomized phase 2 trial.[83] The NSABP, as part of their R04 trial, is doing a second randomization to the use of weekly oxaliplatin (50 mg/m²/d) with an evaluation of pathologic complete response and local control as end points. However, phase 3 results have begun to emerge, and they are not as encouraging as had been hoped for. The French ACCORD cooperative group reported a trial in which 598 patients with locally advanced rectal cancer were randomly assigned to preoperative treatment with 5 weeks of radiation therapy (45 Gy in 25 fractions) with concurrent capecitabine 800 mg/m² twice daily 5 days per week or the same regimen plus oxaliplatin 50 mg/m² once weekly.[86]

There was not a statistically significant difference in the primary end point of the trial, the pathologic complete response rate, which was 13.9% without and 19.2% with oxaliplatin (P = .09). More preoperative grade 3–4 toxicity occurred in the oxaliplatin group (25% vs. 1%; $P < .001$). There were no statistically significant differences between groups in the rate of sphincter-preserving operations (75%), and no differences in terms of rates of serious medical or surgical complications or postoperative deaths at 60 days (0.3%). The authors concluded that the trial did not support the addition of oxaliplatin to this regimen, and that oxaliplatin should not be used with concurrent irradiation in standard practice. They did not detect an improvement in the frequency of clear circumferential radial margins, and speculated that further investigations are warranted in selected populations.

A large Italian cooperative group phase 3 trial reached a similar result.[87] A total of 747 patients were randomly assigned to either 5-FU infusion (225 mg/m²/d) concomitant with external-beam pelvic radiation (50.4 Gy in 28 daily fractions) or the same regimen plus weekly oxaliplatin (60 mg/m² × 6). The primary end point was overall survival. Data are not yet mature for this end point; however, a secondary end point of primary tumor response to preoperative treatment, as well as toxicity data, have been reported. Overall grade 3–4 toxicity rates on treated patients (mainly diarrhea) were 8% without oxaliplatin and 24% in the oxaliplatin-containing arm ($P < .001$). Eighty-two percent of patients receiving oxaliplatin got five or more doses of this drug. Pathologic complete response rates were 15% and 16% in the 5-FU only and 5-FU-oxaliplatin arms, respectively. The authors concluded that the addition of weekly oxaliplatin to standard 5-FU–based preoperative chemoradiation therapy significantly increases toxicity without affecting local tumor response. Survival data requires further maturation.

As biologic agents have a substantial appeal when used in combination with conventional cytotoxics, they also have a large appeal in combination with radiation therapy. There is evidence for a beneficial effect of both cetuximab and bevacizumab when combined with cytotoxics in patients with metastatic colon and rectal cancer (see Chapter 89). There are good laboratory data demonstrating radiation sensitization when these (and similar) agents are used *in vitro*, and a substantial improvement has been shown in survival in patients

PRACTICE OF ONCOLOGY

with head and neck cancer when cetuximab is added to radiation therapy.[88] Only preliminary studies have been done[89] but given the lack of encouraging complete responses and the negative results with cetuximab in adjuvant colon cancer (see Chapter 89), it is unlikely that there will be substantial further investigations in this area, and neither cetuximab nor panitumumab should be used in standard practice with radiation therapy for rectal cancer. Similarly, bevacizumab has failed to demonstrate a benefit in adjuvant colon cancer, and should not be used in the routine management of locally advanced rectal cancer.

SYNCHRONOUS RECTAL PRIMARY AND METASTASES

The use of pelvic radiotherapy in patients with synchronous presentation of primary and metastatic disease is controversial. Primary combination chemotherapy can provide substantial palliation and can be considered as initial therapy in many rectal patients with metastatic disease.[90] Endoscopically placed expandable metal stents can be considered for palliation or protection from impending obstruction. Control of disease in the pelvis can have important implications for patient quality of life; therefore, combined modality therapy, including radiation, chemotherapy, and in some cases palliative surgery, can be appropriate, especially when extrapelvic metastatic disease is small volume and the patient's prognosis is favorable enough that pelvic complications could be anticipated as a long-term problem. No firm guidelines can be made in the management of these complex patients, and treatment decisions must be made on an individual basis.

MANAGEMENT OF UNRESECTABLE PRIMARY AND LOCALLY ADVANCED DISEASE (T4)

Although the majority of patients who present with stage II and III disease have primary tumors that are technically easily resectable, there are a group of patients who have T4 tumors, with deep local invasion into adjacent structures, which makes primary resection for cure difficult, if not impossible. Some T4 tumors invade into the vagina, which is easily resectable, but others invade into pelvic sidewall or sacrum, where a complete surgical resection may be impossible (the coccyx and distal sacrum can be resected, if appropriate), and others invade into bladder or prostate, where a more extensive surgical resection can be done, but often at the expense of major morbidity or functional loss. Although there are few randomized trials to define optimal therapy in this group of patients, there are data suggesting that it is appropriate to treat these patients with preoperative radiation therapy combined with chemotherapy, in a manner similar to that described for T3 disease, generally with concurrent 5-FU–based chemotherapy. This will often result in a good clinical response that will allow for a potentially curative resection to be performed. It is preferable to treat a patient preoperatively to try to avoid leaving residual disease rather than attempting to salvage a patient after a clearly inadequate operation.

The use of adjuvant radiation therapy in this clinical situation also allows for treatment of the lymphatics draining the locally invaded organ, such as the internal or external iliacs, that are not typically resected in a low anterior resection or APR, but which may be at substantial risk of secondary involvement from an invaded organ, such as the bladder. Although the definition of "unresectable" is very subjective, a number of studies have shown that preoperative radiation therapy can convert a substantial number of these patients to having resectable disease with substantial cure rates.[91–94]

Although the use of preoperative radiation therapy with concurrent 5-FU–based chemotherapy, as described earlier in the adjuvant setting, appears of value in patients with locally advanced disease, there is still a substantial incidence of local failure. Therefore, a number of investigators have explored ways to increase the radiation dose to the highest risk region to try to improve local tumor control. Three main techniques have been used: supplemental postoperative external-beam radiation boost, intraoperative electron-beam radiation therapy boost, and intraoperative brachytherapy boost.

There are relatively few data on the use of postoperative external beam as a boost, largely because of concerns of normal tissue tolerance after the use of the relatively large fields delivered preoperatively, extensive surgical resection, and the prolonged delay between initial external-beam therapy and the final boost after recovery from surgery. The two intraoperative techniques are philosophically the same, although the technique of radiation delivery is different. After a high dose (50 Gy) of preoperative chemoradiotherapy and then a 4- to 6-week break, surgical resection is performed, the extent of which depends on the location and extent of tumor. Areas considered at high risk for residual tumor are determined both by the surgical findings and frozen section pathologic evaluation. For electron-beam intraoperative radiotherapy a treatment cylinder is placed over the high-risk region, often on a pelvic sidewall or the sacrum, and the cylinder is then aligned to the radiation machine, which is either in the operating room or in the radiation therapy department. The cylinder acts both to hold normal tissues outside the radiation beam and to confine the electron beam. The use of electrons allows the radiation oncologist to adjust the depth of penetration of the beam to conform to the local tumor extent. When using brachytherapy, carriers for the radioactive sources are placed over the high-risk region, and the radiation is then given either during the surgery (high-dose rate) or the radioactive sources are inserted approximately 5 days after surgery and left in place for 1 or 2 days (low-dose rate). In all situations the radiation dose is in the range of 10 to 20 (most commonly 15) Gy when used as a boost to conventional therapy. In both approaches care must be taken to ensure that normal tissues such as small bowel are out of the irradiated volume.

Techniques similar to this have been used for a number of years and have shown encouraging results, although formal randomized trials have not been performed. Data suggest fairly good levels of local control and long-term survival if a gross total resection can be accomplished, with poorer results if there is gross residual (Table 90.6).[95–98] Use of intraoperative radiotherapy boosts often requires specialized radiation facilities and expertise as well as an experienced team of radiation oncologists, surgical oncologists, urologists, and plastic surgeons. Similar types of surgical and radiation therapy approaches can produce surprisingly good results (35% 5-year survival) in patients with locally advanced nodal metastases, for instance in the para-aortic region,[99] from colon or rectal cancer.

For patients who still cannot have a surgical resection performed, either because of the tumor extent or because of coexisting medical problems, attempts should be made to maximize palliation and perhaps local control. Boost doses of radiation are appropriately delivered to the residual tumor to doses of greater than 60 Gy if sensitive normal tissues (primarily small bowel) can be removed from the radiation fields. Only a small percentage (5%) of patients with these advanced tumors will be locally controlled and cured by such an approach, but a substantial percentage will obtain good palliation.[100–102]

TABLE 90.6

INTRAOPERATIVE RADIATION THERAPY FOR LOCALLY ADVANCED RECTAL CANCER[a]

	Mayo Clinic			Massachusetts General Hospital		
Resection	No. of Patients	Local Failure (%)	Overall Survival (5 y) (%)	No. of Patients	Local Failure (%)	Disease-Specific Survival (%)
Complete resection	18[b]	7	69	40	9	63
Partial resection	35	~20	~40	24	37	35
No resection	1	—	0	—	—	—
Total	56	16	46	64	—	—
Recurrent locally advanced tumor	42	40	19	—	—	—

[a]External beam radiotherapy + resection + intraoperative radiotherapy, no prior radiation therapy.
[b]Two additional patients with no tumor in specimen—both without any tumor recurrence. These are included in the totals.

RADIATION THERAPY TECHNIQUE

There have been primarily two dosing schemes for radiation therapy that have been used in the treatment of rectal cancer. In the preoperative setting many European centers have favored a rapid short-course treatment of doses of approximately 25 Gy in five fractions followed by immediate surgery, while U.S. centers have generally favored doses of 50.4 Gy given at 1.8 Gy per fraction with a delay of 4 to 8 weeks until surgery. As previously mentioned, an advantage of the long-course therapy is that it provides time to have tumor regression, which appears to facilitate sphincter preservation, although it is more expensive and time-consuming for the patient. In addition, there was substantial late toxicity from the short-course treatment in earlier series, although this was most evident when the radiation therapy techniques were less sophisticated and simple anteroposterior/posteroanterior fields alone were used, which were at times quite large[103]; those techniques are not used at present.

Although major late toxicity is relatively uncommon, functional gastrointestinal disturbances are relatively common. These relate to both surgical effects on bowel with lack of a good reservoir function and possible nerve dysfunction, as well as long-term radiation effects on bowel compliance and neural functioning.[104,105] Many patients continue to have some rectal urgency and food intolerance (especially to roughage), but symptoms tend to improve over time and most patients can live a relatively normal life regarding their gastrointestinal tract. Detailed discussions with the patient on the type of foods likely to cause worsening bowel symptoms, attention to the superimposed problems that can occur from other difficulties such as lactose intolerance, and use of agents such as loperamide all can help the patient deal with bowel problems.

Small bowel–related complications are directly proportional to the volume of small bowel in the radiation field and the radiation dose. In patients receiving combined modality therapy, the volume of irradiated small bowel limits the ability to escalate the dose of 5-FU. A number of simple radiotherapeutic techniques are available to decrease radiation-related small bowel toxicity. First, small bowel contrast or CT scanning during treatment planning allows identification of the location of the small bowel so that fields can be designed to minimize its treatment. Multiple-field techniques (preferably a three- or four-field technique) are now standard to minimize normal tissue irradiation. The use of lateral fields for the boost as well as positioning the patient in the prone position can further decrease the volume of small bowel in the lateral radiation fields.

The treatment should be designed with the use of computerized radiation dosimetry and be delivered by high-energy linear accelerators that deliver a higher dose to the target volume while relatively sparing surrounding normal structures. The advantage of combining a multiple-field technique, high-energy photons, and computerized dosimetry produces a homogenous dose distribution throughout the target volume and minimizes the dose to the small bowel. Although not well studied to date, newer developments in intensity-modulated radiation therapy may allow more conformal radiation dose distributions and a decrease in the irradiation of small bowel. To date, intensity-modulated radiation therapy has not been shown to be of additional value in the adjuvant treatment of rectal cancer.

After pelvic surgery, the small bowel commonly fills the pelvis. Adhesions can form, resulting in fixed loops of small bowel in the radiation fields. In this situation, despite treatment of the patient in the prone position, the use of multiple-field techniques may be of limited value. In contrast, when radiation therapy is delivered preoperatively to a patient who has not undergone prior pelvic surgery, the small bowel is usually mobile. When no small bowel fixation is present, treatment in the prone position can exclude much of the small bowel from the posteroanterior field and completely from the lateral fields.

Various physical maneuvers to exclude small bowel from the pelvis have been examined. Gallagher et al.[106] determined the volume, distribution, and mobility of small bowel in the pelvis after a variety of maneuvers. Regardless of the prior surgical history, a significant decrease was seen in the average small bowel volume when the patients were treated in the prone position with abdominal wall compression and bladder distention compared with the supine position. Treatment in the prone position without abdominal wall compression was not consistently effective in displacing small bowel and, in some patients (most commonly, obese), the volume of small bowel increased.

Radiation Fields

The precise radiation fields that are used should depend on the individual clinical situation, although the principles of the radiation treatment remain the same. The locoregional failures in rectal cancer occur both because of residual disease in the soft tissues of the pelvis as well as from residual pelvic nodal disease. The nodal disease can be in the internal iliac chain for very low-lying lesions, but only involves the external iliac nodes if the anal canal or sphincter is involved or if an organ is involved that drains into the external iliac system. The internal iliac nodes are not usually dissected by the surgeon, so it is important to treat these for low rectal cancers, but the external iliacs should not be routinely irradiated. The proximal extent of nodal radiation is arbitrary, but the primary drainage of all rectal cancers is along the mesenteric system, and those nodes should primarily be treated surgically. Extending radiation fields to cover para-aortic nodes is not indicated unless there is evidence of disease in those chains.

Because many of the local recurrences occur in the soft tissues of the pelvis, the radiation oncologist must be sure to treat the regions that are least well treated by the surgeon. These include extension to the pelvic sidewall and presacral space, and to the prostate in men and vagina in women. The proximal extent of the radiation field should generally extend to the sacral promontory, as that is the level at which there is an attachment of the posterior peritoneum and where the retroperitoneal rectum becomes the intraperitoneal colon. Above this level there is little risk of pelvic soft tissue invasion for the standard rectal cancer.

The lower extent of the radiation field is more complex. Often the surgeon will rely on the radiation oncologist to sterilize the most distal extent of the primary tumor in order to perform a sphincter-preserving operation, so the distal margins should be at least a couple of centimeters below the primary tumor mass. Although rectal tumors tend to have only a minimal amount of longitudinal spread along the mucosal margin, they can spread further distally in the perirectal fat and in the lymph nodes in the mesorectum. In fact, this is part of the rationale for a total mesorectal excision. Attempts should thus be made for treatment to at least the level of the dentate line for most low-lying rectal cancers, although this is likely not necessary for rectal cancers in the proximal third. However, it is also likely true that a substantial part of the late toxicity from pelvic radiation therapy is related to dysfunction of the anal sphincter. Thus, it is important to try to minimize the amount of sphincter that is irradiated. Although many textbooks define the lower edge of the radiation field relative to the bones of the pelvis, this is not the proper way to think about irradiating such tumors. The locations of bony anatomic landmarks such as the ischial tuberosity have no consistent relationship to the anal sphincter, anal verge, dentate line, or the rectal cancer. The radiation oncologist must identify the location of these structures as best as possible using radio opaque markers and rectal contrast, and then determine the balance between adequate distal coverage of the tumor as well as minimizing irradiation of the anal sphincter and the perineum (acute toxicity). For anteroposterior or posteroanterior fields the lateral borders should extend to treat the pelvic sidewall, a possible region for soft tissue extension. The lateral fields should have a similar superior and inferior margin. The posterior border should include all of the presacral soft tissue so the posterior extent of the field should cover the anterior border of the sacrum with at least a 1.5-cm margin for patient motion and dosimetric variation. The anterior border of the lateral fields should cover at least the posterior border of the vagina or the prostate, the anterior extent of the primary rectal tumor, and the anterior edge of the sacral promontory. Examples of typical radiation fields as depicted by a CT simulation are shown in Figure 90.4.

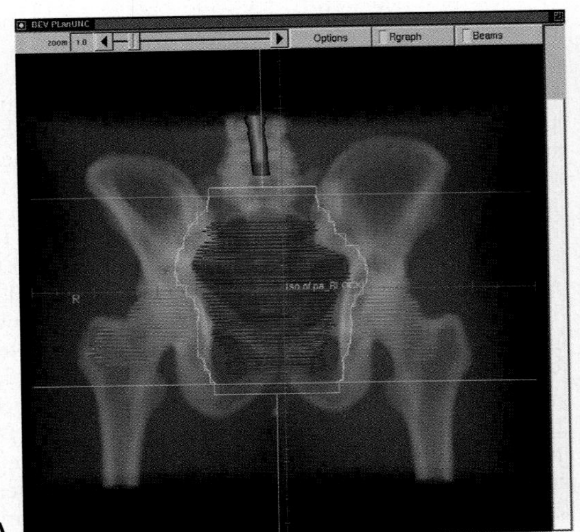

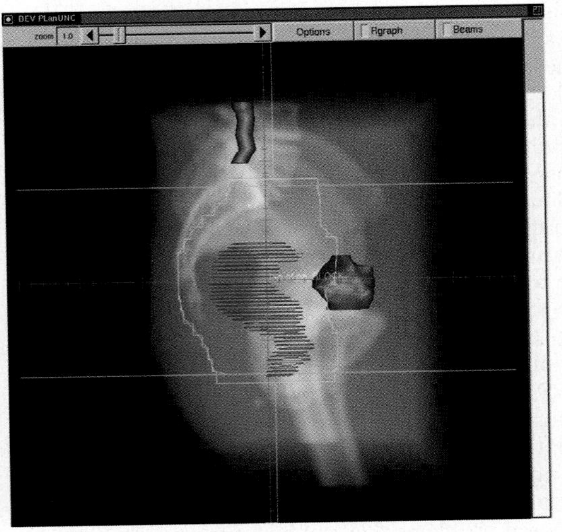

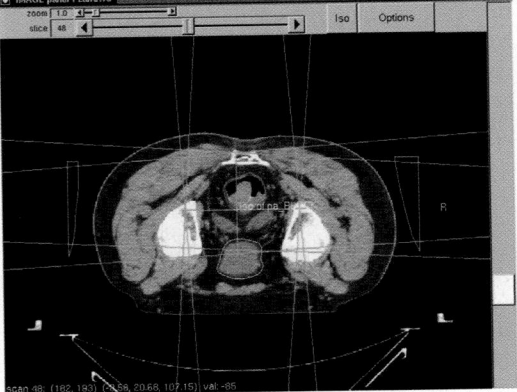

FIGURE 90.4 Posteroanterior (**A**) and lateral digitally (**B**) reconstructed radiograph of the radiation fields for preoperative radiation therapy of a T3N1 rectal adenocarcinoma. The clinical target volume and rectum are outlined. There is a marker at the anal verge to help avoid irradiating the entire anal canal. The field treats the mesorectum and the lymph nodes to the level of the sacral promontory. **C:** Transverse cut at the middle of the radiation field.

Selected References

The full list of references for this chapter appears in the online version.

4. McNamara DA, Parc R. Methods and results of sphincter-preserving surgery for rectal cancer. *Cancer Control* 2003;10:212.
5. Wibe A, Eriksen MT, Syse A, Myrvold HE, Soreide O. Total mesorectal excision for rectal cancer–what can be achieved by a national audit? *Colorectal Dis* 2003;5:471.
6. Hanna NN, Guillem J, Dosoretz A, Steckelman E, Minsky BD, Cohen AM. Intraoperative parasympathetic nerve stimulation with tumescence monitoring during total mesorectal excision for rectal cancer. *J Am Coll Surg* 2002;195:506.
7. Watanabe T, Wu TT, Catalano PJ, et al. Molecular predictors of survival after adjuvant chemotherapy for colon cancer. *N Engl J Med* 2001;344:1196.
10. Gunderson LL, Sargent D, Tepper J, et al. Impact of TN stage and treatment on survival and relapse in adjuvant rectal cancer pooled analysis. *Int J Radiat Oncol Biol Phys* 2002;54(2):386–396.
11. Greene FL, Stewart AK, Norton HJ. A new TNM staging strategy for node-positive (stage III) rectal cancer: An analysis of 5,988 patients. In: Steven M. Grunberg M, editor. Thirty-Ninth Annual Meeting of the ASCO; 2003; Chicago, IL: American Society of Clinical Oncology; 2003. p. 251.
12. Tepper JE, O'Connell MJ, Niedzwiecki D, et al. Impact of number of nodes retrieved on outcome in patients with rectal cancer. *J Clin Oncol* 2001; 19:157.
14. Wong JH, Severino R, Honnebier MB, Tom P, Namiki TS. Number of nodes examined and staging accuracy in colorectal carcinoma. *J Clin Oncol* 1999; 17:2896.
15. Quirke P, Durdey P, Dixon M, Williams N. Local recurrence of rectal adenocarcinoma due to inadequate surgical resection: histopathological study of lateral tumour spread and surgical excision. *Lancet* 1986;2:996.
18. Brown G, Richards CJ, Bourne MW, et al. Morphologic predictors of lymph node status in rectal cancer with use of high-spatial-resolution MR imaging with histopathologic comparison. *Radiology* 2003;227:371.
20. Haider MA, Amitai MM, Rappaport DC, et al. Multi-detector row helical CT in preoperative assessment of small (< or = 1.5 cm) liver metastases: is thinner collimation better? *Radiology* 2002;225:137.
23. Huebner RH, Park KC, Shepherd JE, et al. A meta-analysis of the literature for whole-body FDG PET detection of recurrent colorectal cancer. *J Nucl Med* 2000;41:1177.
24. Kim NK, Kim MJ, Yun SH, Sohn SK, Min JS. Comparative study of transrectal ultrasonography, pelvic computerized tomography, and magnetic resonance imaging in preoperative staging of rectal cancer. *Dis Colon Rectum* 1999;42:770.
26. Garcia-Aguilar J, Pollack J, Lee SH, et al. Accuracy of endorectal ultrasonography in preoperative staging of rectal tumors. *Dis Colon Rectum* 2002; 45:10.
27. Canter RJ, Williams NN. Surgical treatment of colon and rectal cancer. *Hematol Oncol Clin North Am* 2002;16:907.
28. Greenberg JA, Shibata D, Herndon JE 2nd, Steele GD, Jr, Mayer R, Bleday R. Local excision of distal rectal cancer: an update of cancer and leukemia group B 8984. *Dis Colon Rectum* 2008;51:1185.
29. Ota DM, Nelson H. Local excision of rectal cancer revisited: ACOSOG protocol Z6041. *Ann Surg Oncol* 2007;14:271.
31. Ganai S, Kanumuri P, Rao RS, Alexander AI. Local recurrence after transanal endoscopic microsurgery for rectal polyps and early cancers. *Ann Surg Oncol* 2006;13:547.
34. Moore HG, Riedel E, Minsky BD, et al. Adequacy of 1-cm distal margin after restorative rectal cancer resection with sharp mesorectal excision and preoperative combined-modality therapy. *Ann Surg Oncol* 2003; 10:80.
35. Kuvshinoff B, Maghfoor I, Miedema B, et al. Distal margin requirements after preoperative chemoradiotherapy for distal rectal carcinomas: are < or = 1 cm distal margins sufficient? *Ann Surg Oncol* 2001;8:163.
36. Tiret E, Poupardin B, McNamara D, Dehni N, Parc R. Ultralow anterior resection with intersphincteric dissection—what is the limit of safe sphincter preservation? *Colorectal Dis* 2003;5:454.
39. Willett CG. Sphincter preservation in rectal cancer. *Curr Treat Options Oncol* 2000;1:399.
41. Kapiteijn E, Marijne CAM, Nagtegaal ID, et al. Preoperative radiotherapy combined with total mesorectal excision for resectable rectal cancer. *N Engl J Med* 2001;345:638.
42. Tocchi A, Mazzoni G, Lepre L, et al. Total mesorectal excision and low rectal anastomosis for the treatment of rectal cancer and prevention of pelvic recurrences. *Arch Surg* 2001;136:216.
43. Zhou ZG, Wang Z, Yu YY, et al. Laparoscopic total mesorectal excision of low rectal cancer with preservation of anal sphincter: a report of 82 cases. *World J Gastroenterol* 2003;9:1477.
44. Tsang WW, Chung CC, Li MK. Prospective evaluation of laparoscopic total mesorectal excision with colonic J-pouch reconstruction for mid and low rectal cancers. *Br J Surg* 2003;90:867.
45. Morino M, Parini U, Giraudo G, Salval M, Brachet Contul R, Garrone C. Laparoscopic total mesorectal excision: a consecutive series of 100 patients. *Ann Surg* 2003;237:335.
46. Mukherjee A. Total pelvic exenteration for advanced rectal cancer. *S D J Med* 1999;52:153.
53. Martling A, Holm T, Johansson H, Rutqvist LE, Cedermark B. The Stockholm II trial on preoperative radiotherapy in rectal carcinoma: long-term follow-up of a population-based study. *Cancer* 2001;92:896.
57. Sebag-Montefiore D, Stephens RJ, Steele R, et al. Preoperative radiotherapy versus selective postoperative chemoradiotherapy in patients with rectal cancer (MRC CR07 and NCIC-CTG C016): a multicentre, randomised trial. *Lancet* 2009;373:811.
61. Fisher B, Wolmark N, Rockette H, et al. Postoperative adjuvant chemotherapy or radiation therapy for rectal cancer: results from NSABP protocol R-01. *J Natl Cancer Inst* 1988;80:21.
62. Wolmark N, Wieand HS, Hayams DM, et al. Randomized trial of postoperative adjuvant chemotherapy with or without radiotherapy for carcinoma of the rectum: national surgical adjuvant breast and bowel project protocol R-02. *J Natl Cancer Inst* 2000;92:388.
66. Colorectal Cancer Collaborative Group. Adjuvant radiotherapy for rectal cancer: a systematic overview of 8507 patients from 22 randomised trials. *Lancet* 2001;358:1291.
68. Sauer R, Becker H, Hohenberger W, et al. Preoperative versus postoperative chemoradiotherapy for rectal cancer. *N Engl J Med* 2004;351:1731.
71. Bujko K, Nowacki MP, Nasierowska-Guttmejer A, Michalski W, Bebenek M, Kryj M. Long-term results of a randomized trial comparing preoperative short-course radiotherapy with preoperative conventionally fractionated chemoradiation for rectal cancer. *Br J Surg* 2006;93:1215.
72. Bosset JF, Collette L, Calais G, et al. Chemotherapy with preoperative radiotherapy in rectal cancer. *N Engl J Med* 2006;355:1114.
73. Willett CG, Badizadegan K, Ancukiewicz M, Shellito PC. Prognostic factors in stage T3N0 rectal cancer: do all patients require postoperative pelvic irradiation and chemotherapy? *Dis Colon Rectum* 1999;42:167.
74. Gunderson LL, Sargent DJ, Tepper JE, et al. Impact of T and N substage on survival and disease relapse in adjuvant rectal cancer: a pooled analysis. *Int J Radiat Oncol Biol Phys* 2002;54:386.
80. Hofheinz H, Wenz F, Post S, et al. Capecitabine (Cape) versus 5-fluorouracil (5-FU)-based (neo-)adjuvant chemoradiotherapy (CRT) for locally advanced rectal cancer (LARC): Safety results of a randomized, phase III trial [abstract]. *J Clin Oncol* 2009;27:15 (Suppl; abstr 4014).
81. Mitchell EP. Irinotecan in preoperative combined-modality therapy for locally advanced rectal cancer. *Oncology (Williston Park)* 2000;14:56.
82. Kalofonos HP, Bamias A, Koutras A, et al. A randomised phase III trial of adjuvant radio-chemotherapy comparing Irinotecan, 5FU and Leucovorin to 5FU and Leucovorin in patients with rectal cancer: a Hellenic Cooperative Oncology Group Study. *Eur J Cancer* 2008;44:1693.
83. Wong SJ, Winter K, Meropol NJ, et al. RTOG 0247: A randomized phase II study of neoadjuvant capecitabine and irinotecan versus capecitabine and oxaliplatin with concurrent radiation therapy for locally advanced rectal cancer [abstract]. *J Clin Oncol* 2008;26: 2008 (May 20 suppl: abstr 4021.
84. Ryan DP, Niedzwiecki D, Hollis D, et al. Phase I/II study of preoperative oxaliplatin, fluorouracil, and external-beam radiation therapy in patients with locally advanced rectal cancer: Cancer and Leukemia Group B 89901. *J Clin Oncol* 2006;24:2557.
85. Rodel C, Liersch T, Hermann RM, et al. Multicenter phase II trial of chemoradiation with oxaliplatin for rectal cancer. *J Clin Oncol* 2007;25:110.
86. Gerard JP, Azria D, Gourgou-Bourgade S, et al. Comparison of two neoadjuvant chemoradiotherapy regimens for locally advanced rectal cancer: results of the phase III trial ACCORD 12/0405-Prodige 2. *J Clin Oncol* 2010;28:1638.
87. Aschele C, Pinto C, Cordio S. Preoperative fluorouracil (FU)-based chemoradiation with and without weekly oxaliplatin in locally advanced rectal cancer: pathologic response analysis of the Studio Terapia Adiuvante Retto (STAR)-01 randomized phase III trial [abstract]. *J Clin Oncol* 2009;27:18s (suppl; abstr CRA4008).
88. Bonner JA, Harari PM, Giralt J, et al. Radiotherapy plus cetuximab for squamous-cell carcinoma of the head and neck. *N Engl J Med* 2006;354:567.
89. Willett CG, Boucher Y, di Tomaso E, et al. Direct evidence that the VEGF-specific antibody bevacizumab has antivascular effects in human rectal cancer. *Nat Med* 2004;10:145.
90. Saltz L, Raben D, Minsky BD, et al. Rectal cancer: presentation with metastatic and locally advanced disease. American College of Radiology. ACR Appropriateness Criteria. *Radiology* 2000;215(Suppl):1491.
99. Haddock MG, Nelson H, Donohue JH, et al. Intraoperative electron radiotherapy as a component of salvage therapy for patients with colorectal cancer and advanced nodal metastases. *Int J Radiat Oncol Biol Phys* 2003;56:966.

CLINICAL PRESENTATION AND STAGING

The most common presentation of anal cancer is bleeding, which is reported in about 45% of patients.[2,4,22,23] Bleeding may be associated with pain, and is often mistakenly attributed to hemorrhoids. Approximately 30% of patients report an anal mass or as experiencing severe pruritus. Less frequently, a change in bowel habits or enlarged inguinal lymph nodes is reported and 20% of patients are initially asymptomatic.

Anal cancers are staged by physical examination and imaging studies. The current staging is adopted by the American Joint Committee on Cancer, seventh edition[24] (Table 91.1). Sigmoidoscopy provides information about the mucosal spread. Physical examination can determine the size, location, degree of fixation to adjacent structures, nodal enlargement, and sphincter function. It is often necessary to examine patients under anesthesia because of pain and sphincter muscle spasms. In contrast, tumors of the anal margin are easily identified, and local anesthesia to biopsy or excise it in its entirety is sufficient. Female patients should be subjected to a gynecologic examination to exclude other HPV-associated cancers.

Imaging studies should be performed to further assess the local extent of the disease and to detect regional adenopathy and/or distant metastases. Locoregional staging investigations include anal ultrasound, computed tomography (CT), or magnetic resonance imaging (MRI) of the pelvis, and these modalities can measure tumor dimensions and show invasion into the external sphincter and perirectal tissues. The advantage of MRI over CT is its ability to delineate the soft tissue planes better and demonstrate involvement of structures such as the male urethra or the vagina.

Of all patients presenting with palpable inguinal lymph nodes, only 50% are likely to have malignant nodes; therefore, fine-needle aspiration is recommended in all suspected cases. Patients who later develop inguinal nodal metastases typically do so in the ipsilateral groin.[25] Some oncologists have suggested a routine sentinel lymph node (SLN) evaluation as a staging technique. A systematic review of five published series evaluating the outcome of SLN biopsy of nonenlarged inguinal nodes has included 83 patients[26] and the success in identifying the SLN was 90%; however, only 21% of SLN were malignant. Usefulness of positron emission tomographic (PET)-CT to improve detection of nonenlarged involved nodes is under investigation. A study of 27 patients undergoing initial PET-CT then followed by SLN biopsy in patients with clinically normal inguinal nodes has been reported.[27] PET-CT detected inguinal metastasis in seven patients; however, histologic evaluation confirmed metastasis in only three of the seven patients, giving the positive predictive value of only 43%. Arguing against the routine evaluation of clinically normal nodes, it is unclear if elective lymphadenectomy of nodes containing micrometastases confers advantage over delayed lymphadenectomy performed when inguinal nodes become enlarged. The authors recommend an evaluation of enlarged nodes by palpation or by imaging techniques and histologic confirmation as indicated.

TABLE 91.1

TNM ANUS STAGING ACCORDING TO THE AMERICAN JOINT COMMITTEE ON CANCER

PRIMARY TUMOR (T)			
TX	Primary tumor cannot be assessed		
T0	No evidence of primary tumor		
Tis	Carcinoma *in situ* (Bowen disease, high-grade squamous intraepithelial lesion [HISL], AIN II–III)		
T1	Tumor 2 cm or less in greatest dimension		
T2	Tumor more than 2 cm but not more than 5 cm in greatest dimension		
T3	Tumor more than 5 cm in greatest dimension		
T4	Tumor of any size invades adjacent organ(s), e.g., vagina, urethra, bladder (direct invasion of rectal wall, perirectal skin, subcutaneous tissue or sphincter muscle is not classified as T4)		
REGIONAL LYMPH NODES (N)			
NX	Regional lymph nodes cannot be assessed		
N0	No regional lymph node metastasis		
N1	Metastasis in perirectal lymph nodes(s)		
N2	Metastasis in unilateral internal iliac and/or unilateral inguinal lymph node(s)		
N3	Metastasis in perirectal and inguinal lymph nodes and/or bilateral internal iliac and/or inguinal lymph nodes		
DISTANT METASTASES (M)			
M0	No distant metastasis		
M1	Distant metastasis		
ANATOMIC STAGE/PROGNOSTIC GROUP			
Stage 0	Tis	N0	M0
Stage I	T1	N0	M0
Stage II	T2	N0	M0
	T3	N0	M0
Stage IIIA	T1, T2, T3	N1	M0
	T4	N0	M0
Stage IIIB	T4	N1	M0
	Any T	N2, N3	M0
Stage IV	Any T	Any N	M1

AIN, anal intraepithelial neoplasia.
(From ref. 21, with permission.)

PROGNOSTIC FACTORS

Clinical

Baseline clinical stage is an established prognostic factor. In early surgical and radiation alone series, both tumor (T) stage and nodal (N) status were predictive of clinical outcomes. In a retrospective study from M. D. Anderson Cancer Center of 132 patients who underwent abdominoperineal resection (APR) for both squamous cell carcinoma and cloacogenic carcinoma of the anus,[28] there was no survival difference between the two histologic subtypes; however, the 10-year overall survival (OS) rate decreased with increasing baseline stage. Boman et al.[29] reviewed 114 patients treated with APR and demonstrated that tumor size inversely related to survival and was strongly associated with stage. This observation was further validated by a series of 270 patients treated with radiation reviewed by Touboul et al.[30]; larger tumors yielded inferior 10-year OS (T1, 86%; T2, 82.5%; T3, 56.8%; and T4, 45%). In addition, survival was significantly better in patients with tumors 4 cm or less in diameter as compared to tumors greater than 4 cm. However, in the multivariate analysis, nodal status, histology, age, total dose, overall treatment time, and irradiation technique were not predictive for outcome.

The prognostic value of T and N status in patients treated with primary chemoradiation is also demonstrated in randomized trials. Bilimoria et al.[31] performed a univariate analysis on 19,191 anal cancer cases from 1985 to 2000 in the National Cancer Data Base. Prognosticators of 5-year OS included T stage (T1, 68.5%; T2, 58.9%; T3, 43.1%; and T4, 34.3%; $P < .0001$), nodal involvement (node positive, 37.4%; node negative, 62.9%; $P < .0001$), and presence of distant metastases (metastases, 18.7%; no metastases, 59.4%; $P < .0001$). In the Cox multivariate analysis, patients did poorly if they were men, greater than 65 years of age, African American, lived in lower income areas, or had more advanced T stage, nodal involvement, or distant metastases. In the multivariate secondary analysis of the Radiation Therapy Oncology Group (RTOG) 98-11 trial, tumor-related prognosticators for poorer OS included node-positive cancer, large (>5 cm) tumor diameter, and male gender.[34] Tumors greater than 5 cm in diameter, regardless of nodal status, had a higher colostomy rate and inferior disease-free survival (DFS).

In addition to baseline clinical stage, other clinical prognostic factors include radiation total dose and treatment interruptions. Krieg et al.[35] have demonstrated significant improvement in local control (LC) for anal cancer patients who received more than 54 Gy within 60 days of starting treatment. These findings have also been corroborated from investigators at Boston Medical Center and M. D. Anderson Cancer Center.[36,37] The M. D. Anderson group showed LC rates of approximately 50% for patients receiving a total radiation dose of 45 to 49 Gy versus 90% for those receiving more than 55 Gy. The role of dose escalation is currently being addressed in the randomized French Féderation Nationale des Centres de Lutte Contre le Cancer ACCORD 03 trial. The study RTOG 92-08 investigated split-course therapy, or a planned treatment break, in attempts to decrease radiation-related toxicity associated with dose escalation.[38] In this phase 2 trial, 46 patients with tumors more than 2 cm in diameter received 5-FU for 4 days during weeks 1 and 7 of radiation and MMC on day 1 of each course of 5-FU. The radiation dose was 59.4 Gy in 9 weeks with a 2-week mandatory rest. The results were compared with the RTOG 87-04 trial in which patients were treated with 45 Gy in a continuous schedule plus the same chemotherapy regimen.[39,40] Although these toxicity profiles were similar to that of RTOG 87-04, the 2-year colostomy rate with 59.4 Gy and a 2-week break was increased (30% for RTOG 92-08 vs. 9% in RTOG 87-04). Thus, treatment break is generally associated with inferior outcomes.

Molecular

It would be an oversimplification to state that clinical prognostic factors reflect the biological behavior of the disease in its entirety. Attempts have been made to assess molecular prognostic factors for anal cancer. The majority of these studies are on small numbers of patients, and the biomarkers are not validated.

The largest molecular profiling study in anal cancer was reported by Mawdsley et al.,[41] but only as an abstract. Two-hundred forty of 577 anal cancer tissue samples were assessed from the United Kingdom Coordinating Committee on Cancer Research (UKCCCR) ACT I study for the expression level of p53, Bcl-2, thymidylate synthase, thymidine phosphorylase, and Ki-67. High expressions of p53 were associated with decreased DFS in the multivariate analysis. However, Bcl-2, thymidylate synthase, Ki-67, and thymidine phosphorylase expressions had no prognostic value. These results are being validated in the follow-up ACT II study (described later in "Definitive Chemoradiation"). RTOG 87-04 study confirmed that a trend of inferior LC at 5 years was found in tumors expressing a higher level of p53 (52% in tumors with >5% expression vs. 72% in tumors with <5%; $P = .27$).[42] A similar trend was observed for OS at 5 years (58% for tumors with >5% p53 vs. 78% <5%; $P = .14$). However, another study by Nilsson et al.[46] showed that p53 has no impact on prognosis. Ajani et al.[45] evaluated a panel of biomarkers including epidermal growth factor receptor (EGFR), p53, p16, Bcl-2, VEGF, nuclear factor kappa-B (NF-κB), Sonic hedgehog (SHH), and transcriptional factor Gli-1 in 30 anal cancer specimens. In the multivariate analysis, tumor diameter ($P = .003$), Ki-67 ($P = .005$), NF-κB ($P = .002$), SHH ($P = .02$), and Gli-1 ($P = .02$) were all significantly associated with DFS. Patients with a large tumor size and tumor with a high percentage of cells expressing NF-κB, SHH, or Gli-1 tended to have a shorter DFS, while patients with a high level of Ki-67 experienced a longer DFS.

It is clear that further investigation into the molecular prognostic factors of anal carcinoma is needed. Ongoing work with large prospective datasets such as ACT II and RTOG 98-11 will hopefully yield important hypothesis generating findings.

TREATMENT OF LOCALIZED SQUAMOUS CELL CARCINOMA OF THE ANAL CANAL

Surgery

In the 1970s, surgery was the gold standard to treat anal canal cancer. Local excision was reserved for well-differentiated, less than 2 cm in diameter cancers that were not invading the sphincter and had no enlarged lymph nodes. These patients had OS rates at 5 years of over 80%.[28,29,48,49] The standard of care for all other anal cancers was APR with removal of the rectum, ischiorectal fat, levator sling, perirectal and superior hemorrhoidal nodes, as well as a wide area of perianal skin. Beahrs et al.[50] analyzed 204 patients with anal neoplasms treated at the Mayo Clinic from 1950 to 1970. Of these 204 patients, 113 had squamous histology. Only 84 of these patients were analyzed for survival. The majority of the patients were treated with an APR, and 10 patients were treated with a local resection. The 5-year OS for superficial tumors was 90.9%, whereas it was 57.5% for muscle invasive, node-negative tumors, and further decreased to 31.8% in patients with muscle invasive, node-positive cancers. The work of Beahrs et al.[50] demonstrated that surgical resection is moderately effective in treating local-regionally confined anal cancer. Other reports have confirmed such results.[29,51]

Definitive Chemoradiation

In 1974, Nigro[52] reported the results of a preoperative chemoradiation therapy approach for anal canal squamous cell cancer. Radiation therapy (30 Gy in 15 fractions) with concurrent 5-FU and MMC was administered to three patients. Two patients underwent subsequent APR, and one patient refused surgery. Both patients who had surgery had no residual cancer in the surgical specimen and the patient who refused surgery remained without evidence of cancer for 14 months.[52] An additional 19 patients were treated with chemoradiation followed by APR or local resection, of these, 7 of the 12 APR specimens and all 7 patients treated with local excision after chemoradiation had no residual cancer in the surgical specimen.[53,54] Nigro[55] then continued with a definitive chemoradiation approach, and 38 of 45 patients were cured with 5-year OS of 67% and colostomy-free survival of 59%. These observations initiated the paradigm shift from radical surgery to sphincter and organ preservation, but the optimal treatment regimen remained controversial. Several large studies were subsequently conducted to compare the efficacy of radiation with chemoradiation in anal cancer; Table 91.2 summarizes the key findings.

TABLE 91.2

SELECTED PHASE 3 STUDIES IN ANAL CANCER

Study	Sample Size	Regimen	DFS	LF	OS
UKCCCR[56]	585	Radiation alone vs. MMC, 5-FU, radiation	Not provided	61% with radiation alone vs. 39% with chemoradiation at 3 years; *P* <.001	58% with radiation alone vs. 65% with chemoradiation at 3 years; *P* = .25
Bartelink et al.[33] EORTC	110	Radiation alone vs. MMC, 5-FU, radiation	Not provided	50% with radiation vs. 32% with 5-FU/MMC at 5 years; *P* = .02[a]	54% radiation vs. 58% with 5-FU/ MMC; *P* = .17
Flam et al.[40] RTOG 87-04	291	5-FU radiation vs. MMC, 5-FU, radiation	51% 5-FU vs. 73% with 5-FU/ MMC at 4 years; *P* = .0003	Colostomy-free survival: 59% with 5-FU vs. 71% with 5-FU/MMC at 4 years; *P* = .014 Colostomy rate: 22% with 5-FU vs. 9% with 5-FU, MMC; *P* = .002	71% with 5-FU vs. 78.1% with 5-FU/ MMC; *P* = .31
Ajani et al.[34] RTOG 98-11	644	5-FU/MMC radiation vs. induction 5-FU/ CDDP and 5-FU/ CDDP radiation	60% with 5-FU, MMC vs. 54% 5-FU/CDDP at 5 years; *P* = .17	25% with 5-FU/ MMC vs. 33% with 5-FU, cisplatin; *P* value not provided. Colostomy rate: 10% with 5-FU/MMC vs. 19% with 5-FU/CDDP; *P* = .02	75% with 5-FU, MMC vs. 70% with 5-FU, cisplatin; *P* = .10
James et al.[69] UKCCCR ACT II	940	MMC-based or CDDP-based chemoradiation +/− CDDP/5-FU maintenance	75% on both arms at 3 years	Similar on both arms (5% with maintenance vs. 4% without)	85% with maintenance at 3 years vs. 84% without; Not significant
Conroy et al.[67] ACCORD 03	307	A: Induction FUP/ RT + 15 Gy boost B: Induction FUP/ RT + 20–25 Gy boost C: FUP/RT + 15 Gy boost D: FUP/RT + 20–25 Gy boost	Not provided	A: 28% B: 21% C: 30% D: 30% *P* value NS	A: 79% B: 88.5% C: 89% D: 79% *P* value NS

DFS, disease-free survival; LF, local failure; OS, overall survival; MMC, mitomycin; 5-FU, 5-fluorouracil; CDDP, cisplatin; FUP, cisplatin and 5-FU; RT, radiation; NS, not stated.
[a]Estimated from figures in the original study.

The Benefit of Chemoradiotherapy Over Radiation Alone

The UKCCCR Anal Cancer Working Group compared radiotherapy alone with chemoradiation with 5-FU/MMC.[56] A total of 585 patients with anal canal or anal margin cancers were randomized to radiation alone with 45 Gy in 20 to 25 fractions versus the same radiation concurrent with 5-FU infusion over 5 days during weeks 1 and 5 of radiation, and MMC on day 1. Fifty-one percent had cT3 disease, 20% had positive nodes, and 23% had anal margin cancer. All patients were restaged 6 weeks after chemoradiation. Those with less than 50% response had salvage surgery, and those with more than 50% response received a boost of radiation: 15- to 20-Gy external-beam radiation or brachytherapy. The complete clinical response rates were similar between the two groups (39% for chemoradiation and 30% for radiotherapy alone; *P* = .08). However, the 3-year local failure rate was significantly lower in the chemoradiation group (39% for chemoradiation; 61% for radiotherapy alone; *P* <.0001), and the cancer-specific survival was superior with chemoradiation (relative risk, 0.71; *P* = .02). Although there was no statistically significant survival advantage (58% vs. 65%) for the addition of chemotherapy, chemoradiation reduced the risk of death from anal cancer. Acute toxicity, particularly hematologic, skin, gastrointestinal, and genitourinary, was higher in the combined-modality arm, but late morbidity was comparable in both groups. There were six treatment-related deaths (2%) in the chemoradiation arm and two (0.7%) in the radiation alone arm.

Bartelink et al.[33] confirmed that the addition of chemotherapy to radiotherapy is superior to radiotherapy alone in a phase 3 investigation conducted by the European Organisation for Research and Treatment of Cancer (EORTC 22861). A total of 110 patients were randomized to either radiotherapy alone or 5-FU/MMC concurrent with radiotherapy. Patients were administered 45 Gy of radiation with 5-FU and MMC. Notably, 83% of the patients had T3 disease, while 48% had involved lymph nodes at the time of diagnosis. Response was assessed 6 weeks after chemoradiation. Patients having a complete response or partial response received a 15- or 20-Gy radiation boost, respectively, and salvage surgery was reserved for patients with less than a partial response. A significant increase in complete clinical response was noted in the chemoradiation group (80% vs. 54% for radiation alone) and produced improved LC (68% vs. 50%) as well as lower 5-year colostomy rate (72% vs. 40% for radiation alone). Similar to the UK study, no difference in OS was seen.

Is Mitomycin a Necessary Component of Chemoradiation?

Although the benefit of the addition of chemotherapy is well demonstrated, the acute toxicity associated with MMC was significant. Therefore, the benefit of adding MMC to 5-FU or substituting with cisplatin concurrently with radiotherapy was investigated.

The U.S. Intergroup (RTOG 87-04/Eastern Cooperative Oncology Group [ECOG] 1289) was a prospective phase 3 study of 310 patients with stage I to IIIA (T1-4, N0-1) anal carcinoma randomized to radiation with 5-FU or 5-FU and MMC.[40] Primary tumors were assessed with a biopsy 4 to 6 weeks after chemoradiation. Patients who did not have a complete response received an additional cycle of cisplatin and 5-FU with radiotherapy. Twenty-eight patients had positive biopsies, of which 25 patients received salvage cisplatin, 5-FU, and radiation. Of the 22 evaluable patients, 12 had a negative biopsy. Ten patients had persistent disease and were offered APR. At 4 years, the MMC arm resulted in a significantly lower colostomy rate (9% vs. 22%; P = .002), reduced local failure (16% vs. 34%; P = .0008), higher colostomy-free survival (71% vs. 59%; $P < .05$), and higher DFS (73% vs. 51%; P = .0003). OS was similar in both arms. Both hematologic and nonhematologic toxicities, however, were significantly increased with MMC.

In the RTOG 98-11 trial, in which conventional radiation therapy techniques were employed (doses of 45 to 59.4 Gy), 87% of patients suffered National Cancer Institute Common Toxicity Criteria (CTC) version 2.0 grade 3 or 4 acute toxicity.[34] These toxicities included hematologic, moist desquamation, and gastrointestinal toxicity at rates of 61%, 48%, and 35%, respectively. Treatment breaks induced by or used to mitigate these morbidities are not uncommon and may compromise efficacy. Most large studies of combined modality have also reported a 2% mortality rate.[33,56] Although chemotherapy contributes to acute toxic effects, radiation contributes to late toxicities. However, overall data on late morbidities remain sparse and there are fewer reports from the patient's perspective.[59–62] In general, the rate of grade 1 to 2 late toxicities is estimated at 20% and includes anorectal dysfunction (urgency and frequency of defecation), anal and vaginal fibrosis, dyspareunia, and impotence.[34] A 5% to 15% rate of grade 3 to 4 late morbidities has been reported.[34,62] These toxicities include femoral head fracture and small bowel obstruction. Considerable progress has been made by refining radiation techniques to reduce acute and late complications.[63] Prospective studies of quality of life, patient reported symptoms, and physiological assessment of anorectal function after chemoradiation are warranted.

RTOG 98-11, a phase 3 trial compared standard concurrent chemoradiation with two cycles of 5-FU (1,000 mg/m²/day) CI on days 1 to 4 and 29 to 32 of radiation and MMC (10 mg/m²) IV bolus on days 1 and 29 of radiation versus two cycles of induction 5-FU (1,000 mg/m²/day) CI on days 1 to 4 and 29 to 32 and cisplatin (75 mg/m²) IV over 60 minutes on days 1 and 29 followed by concurrent chemoradiation with two cycles of 5-FU (1,000 mg/m²/day) CI on days 57 to 60 and 85 to 88 with radiation and cisplatin (75 mg/m²) IV over 60 minutes on days 57 and 85 with radiation.[34] The primary end point was an improvement in 5-year DFS for the cisplatin arm. A total of 644 patients were randomized. Radiation in this trial included a minimum dose of 45 Gy in 25 fractions to the primary tumor using nonconformal radiation delivery techniques with anteroposterior-posteroanterior or multifield arrangements. For T3, T4, node-positive disease or T2 tumors with residual disease after 45 Gy, a boost of 10 to 14 Gy could be delivered at the discretion of the treating physician in 2 Gy fractions for a total dose of 55 to 59 Gy. The results demonstrated that the two regimens were similar with regard to 5-year DFS (60% in the MMC arm; 54% in the cisplatin arm; P = .17), and 5-year OS (75% in the MMC arm; 70% in the cisplatin arm; P = .1). However, the colostomy rate was significantly higher in the cisplatin arm (19% vs. 10%; P = .02), as was the rate of locoregional recurrences (33% vs. 25%; P = .07). The rate of distant metastases was not reduced with the two induction cycles of cisplatin and 5-FU (19% in the cisplatin arm vs. 15% in the MMC arm). Even though the MMC arm was associated with an increased grade 3 or higher acute hematologic toxicity compared to cisplatin (61% vs. 42%; P <.001), the rate of acute nonhematologic toxicity was 74% in both arms. Induction chemotherapy did not appear to have any impact on advanced disease, as suggested in the CALGB study.

Role of Systemic Chemotherapy in Localized Disease

RTOG 98-11 results were confirmed by the ACCORD 03 study,[67] which randomized 307 patients in a 2 × 2 factorial fashion to address the role of induction chemotherapy (two cycles of cisplatin and 5-FU) followed by standard dose pelvic chemoradiation (with 5-FU and cisplatin), with or without a radiation dose escalation (radiation boost of 15 Gy). The primary end point was improved colostomy-free survival at 3 years with induction cisplatin or radiation dose escalation. At a median follow-up of 43 months, the overall local failure was 28%, without significant differences across the treatment arms. The 3-year colostomy-free survival (overall 83%) and OS (78%) were also similar across all four arms.

The role of postradiation "adjuvant" or "maintenance" chemotherapy has also been assessed. James et al.[69] reported on the United Kingdom Anal Cancer Trial (ACT) II. A total of 940 patients were randomized with a 2 × 2 factorial design to examine the role of MMC versus cisplatin with 5-FU chemoradiation, as well as the utility of maintenance 5-FU and cisplatin chemotherapy following chemoradiation. The primary end point was a 5% increase in complete response rate at 6 months from 90% to 95% for the cisplatin arm. A total dose of 50.4 Gy radiation was administered without a planned break. For the maintenance chemotherapy randomization, the primary end point was a decrease of recurrence from 25% without maintenance chemotherapy to 17.5% in the maintenance arm. One month after chemoradiation, patients were then randomized to either observation or maintenance therapy with cisplatin on days 1 and 29 and 5-FU on days 1 to 4 and 29 to 32. The clinical complete response rate was almost identical in the two arms (94% MMC vs. 95% cisplatin). Furthermore, there was no difference in DFS (hazard ratio, 0.89; 95% confidence interval: 0.68, 1.18; P = .42) and OS between the observation and maintenance chemotherapy groups (hazard ratio, 0.79; 95% confidence interval: 0.56, 1.12; P = .19). The 3-year colostomy rate was also similar in the two groups (13.7% MMC and 11.3% cisplatin). Grade 3 or 4 acute nonhematologic toxicity was 60% in the MMC group and 65% in the cisplatin group (P = .17). These preliminary study results suggest that there is no survival benefit to the use of maintenance chemotherapy following chemoradiation, and this trial also failed to confirm a benefit to chemoradiation with 5-FU and cisplatin over the standard regimen of 5-FU and MMC.

Novel Biological Radiosensitizing Agents

Cetuximab, a monoclonal chimeric antibody against EGFR, is effective in combination with radiotherapy in treating squamous cell carcinoma of the head and neck.[70] A small phase 1 study of anal cancer patients showed that the addition of cetuximab to cisplatin and 5-FU chemoradiation is safe and feasible.[71] This phase 1 study had patients with T2N2-3, T3N0-3, and T4N0. A 78% pathologic complete response rate was reported. KRAS and BRAF mutation appear to be infrequent, reinforcing the potential benefit of EGFR inhibitors.[72] Two phase 2 studies of cetuximab combined with 5-FU and cisplatin chemoradiation are being conducted by ECOG and AIDS Malignancy Clinical Trials Consortium.

Traditional Radiation and Intensity-Modulated Radiation Therapy

Radiotherapy has been the backbone of therapy of anal canal carcinoma since the original report by Nigro et al.[52] However, refinements in its planning and delivery continue to evolve, with the overall goal of improving outcomes, while reducing treatment-related complications.

The external beam radiation delivered in the aforementioned studies used conventional two-dimensional (2D) or three-dimensional (3D) techniques. In either approach, orthogonal beams of radiation covering gross primary and nodal tumor, as well as elective pelvic (mesorectal, presacral, internal, and external iliac, obturator) and inguinal nodal basins often use an anterior/posterior beam arrangement that also includes large volumes of bowel, bone, bladder, genitalia, and skin leading to considerable treatment-associated morbidity. With 2D planning, the design of the radiation field is based on known correlations between bony anatomy and soft tissue. Normal tissues adjacent to target structures cannot be spared. The 3D techniques are based on a CT simulation (planning session) of the patient immobilized in the treatment position. Some radiation oncologists use this technique to ensure that the radiation field adequately covers the tumor volume. The gross tumor volume (GTV) is delineated on each CT slice, but the radiation fields and blocks are based on bony landmarks, similar to the 2D technique. However, with a more optimal 3D approach, the radiation field delineates the clinical target volume (the GTV plus the draining nodal basins described previously; clinical target volume [CTV]) and the normal structures on each CT slice, and a planning tumor volume (PTV) is added around the CTV to account for beam penumbra and patient movement. A radiation dose is then prescribed to the target volume, and normal tissues receive dose limits. Treatment accuracy with highly conformal 3D is superior to 2D, but even with an optimal 3D plan, normal tissues cannot be adequately spared.

Intensity-modulated radiation therapy (IMRT) is a form of advanced external-beam radiation delivery that uses inverse planning with a computer-optimized algorithm to create radiation beam angles and fluctuating radiation beam intensities to meet strict requirements for target volume coverage and normal tissue protection. The radiation dose is highly conformal to the target volume with a steep dose gradient, thereby minimizing the radiation dose to the normal structures. There are several theoretical and practical advantages to the use of IMRT. First, IMRT holds the potential to reduce the significant acute and late toxicities. Second, IMRT may enable radiation dose escalation to high-risk tumors. Figure 91.2 shows the normal tissue sparing with IMRT over a 2D approach, even when considering a clinically node negative anal cancer.

Salama et al.[75] reported on the first multicenter experience of the use of IMRT for patients with anal canal cancer. Fifty-three patients were treated with IMRT to 45 Gy followed by a gross tumor boost to a median dose of 52 Gy and concurrent chemotherapy (48 receiving 5-FU and MMC). Acute grade 3+ gastrointestinal and dermatologic toxicity was 15% and 37.7%, respectively (as compared to 36% and 47% on the 5-FU/MMC arm of the RTOG 98-11 trial using conventional RT).[34] The only grade 4 toxicity was hematologic (34% grade 4 neutropenia). Encouragingly, 92.5% patients had a complete clinical response; one patient had a partial response and three had stable disease. Eighteen-month colostomy-free survival, OS, freedom from local failure, and freedom from distant failure were 83.7%, 93.4%, 83.9%, and 92.9%, respectively.

The only prospective trial of IMRT, RTOG 0529, has recently been completed, and its preliminary results have been

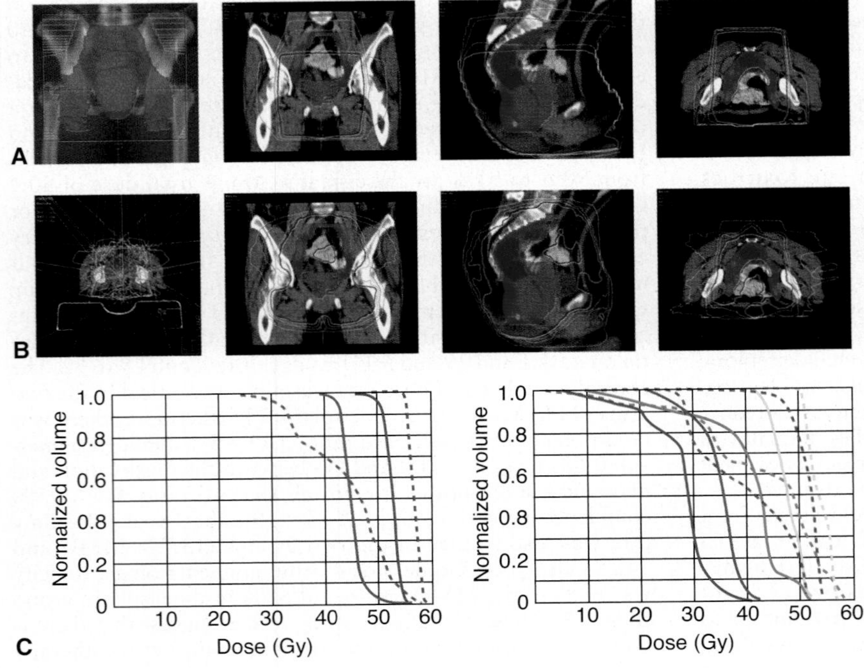

FIGURE 91.2 Comparison of two-dimensional (2D) and intensity-modulated radiation therapy (IMRT) for a T2N0 anal canal cancer. Planning target volume (PTV) for anal primary (*red*). PTV for elective nodes (*magenta*). **A:** 2D plan according to RTOG 98-11. **B:** IMRT plan according to RTOG 0529. From left to right: treatment fields and coronal, sagittal, and axial views. Isodose lines demonstrate the volumes receiving 42 Gy (*red*), 36 Gy (*yellow*), 30.6 Gy (*green*), and 20 Gy (*light blue*). **C:** Dose volume histograms (DVH) for anal primary PTV (*red*), elective nodal PTV (*magenta*), bladder (*yellow*), femoral heads (*purple*), genitals (*blue*), and small bowel (*green*). *Dotted lines* represent 2D plan according to RTOG 98-11. *Solid lines* represent IMRT plan according to RTOG 0529. Compared with 2D, IMRT shows better high-dose sparing of the critical normal structures and improved dose coverage of the superior portion of the elective nodal CTV. (Courtesy of David Kozono and John Willins.)

reported.[76] This phase 2 study combined concurrent 5-FU/MMC and IMRT to evaluate acute toxicity. The primary end point was to determine if the combined rate of acute grade 2 or higher gastrointestinal and genitourinary toxicity can be decreased by 15% with the use of IMRT, compared to the data reported in RTOG 98-11 as the benchmark.[34] All patients received 5-FU and MMC days 1 and 29 of IMRT. IMRT dose was prescribed based on the stage. For T2N0 cancers, the plan was for 42 Gy in 1.5 Gy per fraction to the elective nodal PTV and 50.4 Gy in 1.8 Gy per fraction to the anal tumor PTV. For T3-4N0-3 cancer, the dose was increased to 45 Gy in 1.5 Gy per fraction to the elective nodal PTV, and 54 Gy, 1.8 Gy per fraction to the anal tumor. Patients with nodal involvement included PTVs that received 50.4 Gy in 1.68 Gy per fraction for nodes 3 cm or less, and 54 Gy in 1.8 Gy per fraction for 3 cm or greater in size. Of 63 accrued patients, 52 were analyzable. Stage of cancer was 53% stage II, 25% IIIA, and 22% IIIB. Seventy-seven percent of patients experienced grade 2 or higher gastrointestinal/genitourinary (GI/GU) acute adverse events (AEs) that were equal to that noted in the MMC arm of RTOG 98-11 (76%). However, there was a statistically significant reduction in grade 3 or higher GI/GU AEs with IMRT, 21% versus 36% RTOG 98-11 ($P < .008$), and grade 3 or higher dermatologic AEs, 21% versus 47% RTOG 98-11 ($P < .0001$). Median radiation duration was 42.5 days (range, 32–59), as compared to 49 days (range, 0–102) on the MMC arm of 98-11 ($P < .0001$). Although in this study, the primary end point was not met, the use of IMRT with 5-FU and MMC resulted in significant reduction in grade 3+ dermatologic and GI/GU acute toxicity.

IMRT treatment planning for anal cancer relies on accurate delineation of the gross tumor and nodal regions at risk, as well as the normal surrounding organs. For each patient, a custom-made immobilization device is created to maintain the body in a reproducible position. The anal area and any gross tumor extension are marked. With patients in the treatment position, a CT scan is performed for high-resolution delineation of the tumor and surrounding structures; 2.5- to 5-mm slices are recommended. The use of small bowel contrast can be helpful to optimally delineate this normal structure. In addition, an [^{18}F]fluorodeoxyglucose (FDG)-PET scan may be obtained for planning purposes. The superiority of PET in demonstrating involved lymph nodes otherwise missed on CT scans has been shown.[77] The GTV is contoured on each axial CT slice based on the clinical examination, endoscopy, and correlation with pretreatment radiographic studies including CT and/or FDG-PET. Separate GTVs are specified for the primary tumor and for any grossly involved inguinal or pelvic lymph nodes. In general, a 2.0- to 2.5-cm expansion is added to the primary and anal canal and a 1.5-cm expansion is added to involved nodes, to create a preliminary CTV. Each preliminary CTV is then manually edited to avoid overlap into nontarget muscles or bone, which are considered natural barriers to tumor infiltration. A PTV (5–10 mm) is then generated around the CTV before planning is initiated.

Critical to the use of IMRT is an understanding of the elective CTV. Target volumes for anal cancer differ from those appropriate for gynecologic (GYN) or GU cancers. The rectum and its associated mesentery are to be avoided for IMRT planning of GYN or GU malignancies, but they represent the first echelon of nodal drainage for anal cancer, and therefore must be carefully contoured for treatment. To this end, an anorectal atlas (partly shown in Fig. 91.3) to assist radiation

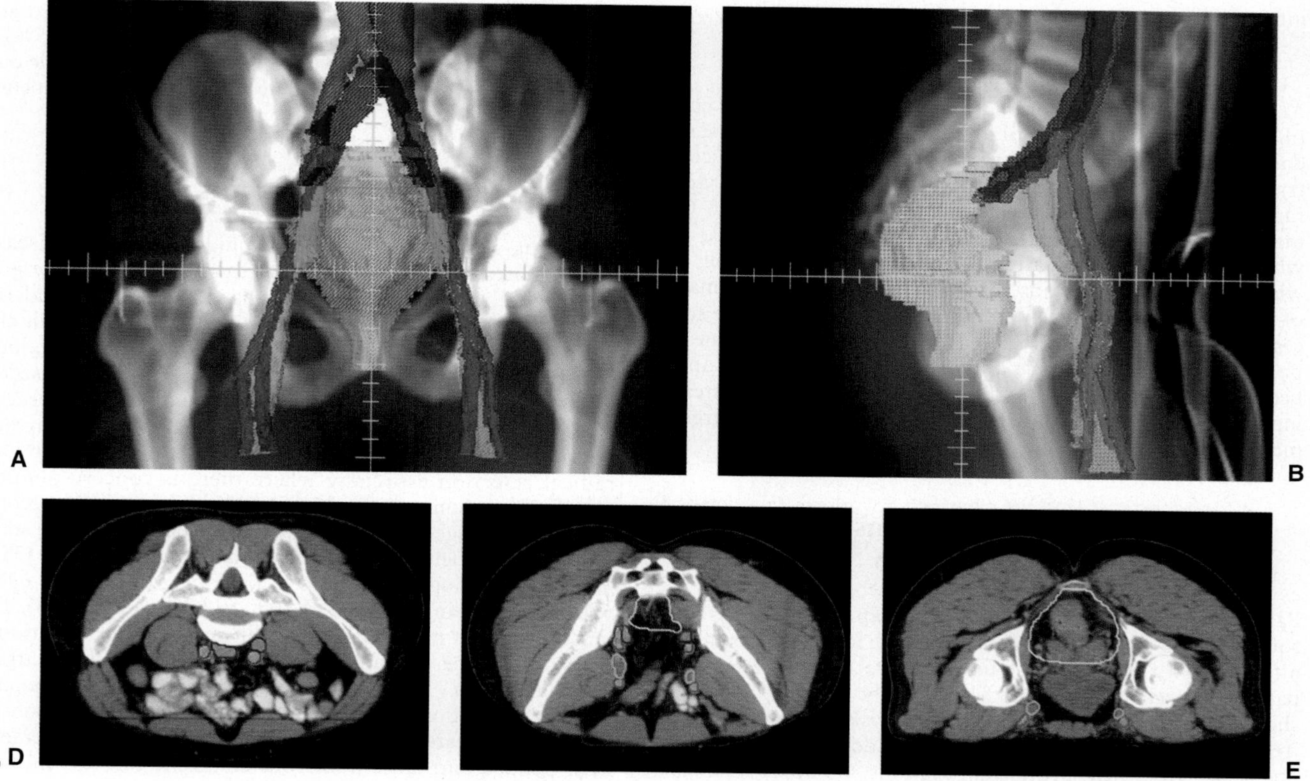

FIGURE 91.3 Anatomical considerations for elective nodal contouring. Aorta, common, and internal iliac arteries (*red*). External iliac and inguinal arteries (*magenta*). Inferior vena cava, common, and internal iliac veins (*blue*). External iliac and inguinal veins (*cyan*). Mesorectum (*yellow*). **A:** AP digitally reconstructed radiograph (DRR). **B:** Right lateral DRR. **C:** Axial computed tomographic (CT) slice at level of common iliac vessels. **D:** Axial CT slice at level of internal and external iliac vessels. **E:** Axial CT slice at level of external iliac-inguinal vessels. (Courtesy of David Kozono and John Willins.)

oncologists in delineating elective target volumes for anal cancer is available.[78]

Although IMRT was associated with improved acute toxicity in reports by Salama et al.[75] and RTOG 0529, an important educational need has been identified. Of the 52 cases of RTOG 0529, pretreatment central review revealed that 75% required planning revisions before commencing therapy. The majority of these revisions were due to incorrect contouring of the elective nodal volumes (mesorectal in approximately 50%). Incorrect contouring of areas that may harbor subclinical disease could result in marginal misses and poorer locoregional control rates. Until radiation oncologists become more educated on conformal target delineation, IMRT for anal cancer should not be considered as standard practice.

Currently, it is difficult to narrowly define a standard radiation technique and dose schedule based on the diversity of techniques used in the major phase 3 trials. However, general recommendations for non-IMRT delivery include the use of multiple radiation fields with 3D conformal techniques to deliver 30.6 to 45 Gy for elective nodal coverage and 45 to 59.4 Gy to gross anal and nodal disease. Total radiation doses should be based on response at 45 Gy and stage of disease. For more advanced disease, higher total doses are suggested. Radiation dose should also not exceed 45 Gy to the small bowel and femoral heads, and care should be taken to avoid excess dose to the genitalia.

Follow-Up Management

Squamous cell cancer of the anal canal can regress slowly, between 3 and 12 months, after completion of treatment.[79] As long as the cancer is not increasing, biopsies are not necessary and may lead to a nonhealing ulcer and chronic wound infection.[80]

Chemoradiation Summary

At the present time, chemoradiation with 5-FU/MMC and continuous radiation to a dose of 45 to 59.4 Gy remains the standard practice in the United States. For patients who have contraindications to chemotherapy or refuse drug therapy, radiation alone as initial treatment to doses of 60 to 66 Gy may be employed. Radical resection is reserved for patients who cannot tolerate radiation therapy or chemoradiation, or who are incontinent because of severe and prolonged damage of the sphincters or have an anovaginal fistula. Despite the success of chemoradiation, the 5-year locoregional failure rate in patients with node-positive and T3 or T4 disease can range between 58% and 64%.[81] IMRT may prove useful in decreasing morbidity of chemoradiation, and in turn, allow for treatment intensification.

Treatment Considerations for the HIV Population

Patients who are HIV-positive are at an increased risk of squamous cell cancer of the anus. Although it is not necessary to alter standard management recommendations, HIV-infected patients, especially those with a CD4 count less than 200/mcL, should be monitored for an increased risk of toxicity when treated with chemoradiation. Treatment modifications are based on the severity of the acute complications. OS appears similar to those achieved in HIV negative patients, while disease-free or colostomy-free survival rates are comparable or minimally inferior.

Retrospective reports suggest a high-grade 3+ acute toxicity profile in HIV-infected patients treated with chemoradiation. A multicenter analysis of patients treated at the George Washington University Medical Center and the affiliated Veterans Administration hospital revealed an 80% grade 3 or 4 major acute toxicity rate for patients with HIV treated with 5-FU, MMC, and radiation compared to 30% in patients without HIV.[82] Late complications were higher patients with HIV compared to patients without HIV (40% vs. 16%; NS). Other retrospective analyses show similar findings, most notably in patients with low pretreatment CD4 counts.[83–85]

In contrast, the reported DFS outcomes for patients infected with HIV are more variable. One multicenter retrospective study evaluating treatment outcomes in HIV-positive patients treated consecutively between 1997 and 2006, demonstrated a trend toward decreased cancer-specific survival at 5 years (HIV-positive, 68%; HIV-negative, 79%; $P = .09$).[85] Long-term LC was also worse in the HIV-positive group, with a 5-year LC rate of 38% in patients with HIV versus 87% in those who were HIV-negative.

However, in the era of improved antiviral therapy, the prognosis for HIV-positive patients may be improving. Wexler et al.[86] reported their experience of HIV-infected individuals treated in the era of highly active antiretroviral therapy at St. Vincent's Hospital in New York. Outcomes were comparable to patients without HIV, with 5-year locoregional relapse, anal cancer–specific survival, and OS rates of 16%, 75%, and 65%, respectively. Investigators at Northwestern Memorial Hospital also reported similar responses for HIV-positive and HIV-negative individuals,[83] with OS at 71% and 73%, respectively. Furthermore, no difference was found between CD4 count more than 200/mcL and CD4 count less than 200/mcL or between AIDS and non-AIDS patients with regard to colostomy, response to therapy, recurrence, or survival. Similarly, a large retrospective cohort study using the Veterans Administration administrative databases of 1,184 veterans reported 2-year observed survival rates to be similar among HIV-infected and noninfected patients (HIV-positive, 77%; HIV-negative, 75%).[87] Contemporary series using IMRT also suggest comparable outcomes between immunocompromised and immunocompetent patients.

Salvage Therapy for Local Recurrence

Following a careful workup to exclude extrapelvic disease, patients are then counseled about salvage surgery. The goal must be to achieve negative margins. Most patients undergo an APR and a permanent colostomy is established with creation of a large pelvic floor defect. Tumors that invade local structures such as the vagina or prostate should be resected with negative margins and this often involves multivisceral resection. The use of intraoperative radiotherapy or brachytherapy may decrease the chance of local recurrence following radical resection especially where there is concern about a positive resection margin. Most published series of outcome following salvage surgery for squamous cell cancer have small numbers of patients because of its relative rarity and the OS at 5 years following resection is in the range of 30% to 64%, with DFS rates in the range of 30% to 40% (Table 91.3). The most important prognostic factor of survival after resection is the status of the margin, and patients with negative margins (R0) have up to 75% 5-year OS.[88] Further predictors of a poor OS outcome following surgery are inguinal lymph node status, tumor size greater than 5 cm, adjacent organ involvement, male gender, and more numerous comorbidities.[89,90] In most series, the indication for salvage surgery is persistence of tumor following chemoradiotherapy in up to half of patients. Interestingly, these patients have a worse outcome following salvage surgery, even when resection is R0. The 5-year OS following salvage surgery for persistent disease is 31% to 33% compared to the outcome of surgery for true recurrence that is

TABLE 91.3

RESULTS OF SALVAGE SURGERY FOR RESIDUAL OR RECURRENT ANAL CANCER

Study	Patient No.	Negative Margin After Surgery (R0)	5-Year Survival Based on Margin Status	Overall 5-year Survival
Akbari et al. 2004[89]	62	53/62 85%	R0 = 38% R1/2 = 0%	33%
Nilsson et al. 2002[91]	35	32/35 91%	NS	52%
Ghouti et al. 2005[92]	36	NS	NS	69.4% (DFS 31.1%)
Renehan et al. 2005[93]	73	55/73 75%	R0 = 61.4% R1/2 = 0%	40%
Schiller et al. 2007[90]	40	33/40 83%	NS	39% (DFS 30%)
Ferenschild et al. 2005[95]	18	14/18 78%	NS	30%
Sunesen et al. 2009[88]	45	35/45 78%	R0 = 75% R1 = 40% R2 = 0%	61%

R0, clear margin; R1, microscopic positive margin; R2, grossly positive margin; NS, not stated; DFS, disease-free survival.

reported in 51% to 82% of patients.[89,91] It is thought that persistent tumors have a more aggressive tumor biology that is resistant to chemoradiotherapy leading to a worse outcome following salvage surgery. Overall, the length of time to recurrence after surgery varies from 1 to 50 months.[88,90,92,93]

Salvage surgery is associated with substantial morbidity in up to 72% of patients, particularly with delayed perineal wound healing, but also pelvic abscess, perineal wound hernia, urinary retention, and impotence.[90] The poor perineal wound healing is a result of both the large defect created to fully excise these low tumors as well as the prior radiotherapy received. Primary closure alone produces poor results when not combined with some type of a flap procedure. In a series of 22 patients undergoing salvage APR treated with primary closure, 59% experienced perineal wound breakdown, one requiring a reconstructive operation.[93] Commonly used tissue flaps include the pedicled omental flap and the vertical rectus abdominis myocutaneous flap (VRAM). In 95 patients undergoing salvage APR, a comparison of pedicled omental flap to VRAM reported fewer perineal wound complications and faster healing when the VRAM was employed.[94] In another series of 18 patients, the perineal wound breakdown rate was 36% in patients undergoing omental flap reconstruction versus 0% in patients having their perineal floor reconstructed with VRAM flap following salvage APR.[95] A final series of 48 patients undergoing salvage APR reported no delayed wound healing or infectious complications when VRAM flap was used.[88] Therefore, in patients who undergo salvage surgery for persistent or recurrent squamous cell cancer of the anal canal, a surgical strategy using a VRAM flap provides the optimal defect closure with the lowest complication rate.

In summary, salvage APR is the surgery of choice for persistent residual or recurrent cancer in which primary chemoradiotherapy has failed. A substantial portion of patients will be cured of their disease and outcomes may be optimized by careful selection of patients who will have negative margins following radical surgery. A concern following salvage surgery is the delay in perineal healing, and this morbidity may be greatly reduced by the use of tissue flaps.

Management of Metastatic Disease

Systemic chemotherapy for metastatic squamous cell carcinoma of the anus is generally similar to other metastatic squamous histology, such as lung or head and neck cancers. Agents including doxorubicin, vinblastine, bleomycin, and methotrexate have been used in some of the earlier studies.[96–98] Recently, platinum-based regimens have been adopted. For example, cisplatin and 5-FU have been reported to achieve an 11% complete response and 61% partial response rate[99] and the results are comparable with other reported studies.[100] Single-agent paclitaxel has also been assessed in small series and demonstrates a 60% response rate.[101] Hainsworth et al.[102] recently treated 60 patients with the combination of carboplatin, paclitaxel, and 5-FU in a phase 2 study with an overall response rate of 90%.

Most recently, cetuximab was employed in small series or anecdotal experiences. Cetuximab produces a 13% response rate in recurrent squamous cell carcinoma of the head and neck as a single agent in the second-line setting.[103] When used in combination with cisplatin as first-line therapy, an improvement in response rate (26%), progression-free survival, and OS was observed in head and neck cancers.[104] Data of cetuximab in anal cancer are limited. In a recent published small series, seven patients were treated with either cetuximab alone or cetuximab with irinotecan.[105] Five of seven patients achieved tumor control (three partial responses).

TREATMENT OF OTHER SITES AND PATHOLOGIES

Squamous Cell Cancer of the Anal Margin

Anal margin is usually defined as the area extending from the anal verge to 5 cm outward on the perineum.[106–108] The incidence of anal margin carcinoma is fairly low and the prognosis is more favorable than that of anal canal cancer.[109,110] The onset of the disease is usually in the seventh and eighth decade with a slight female predominance.[111–113] In most cases, these tumors are well differentiated and slow growing and distant metastases are rare. [112,116,117] Inguinal lymph nodes are the primarily nodal drainage for anal margin cancers,[117] and regional nodal metastasis is directly related to the size of the tumor. Tumors less than 2 cm rarely have lymph node metastasis, while tumors between 2 to 5 cm in size are associated with approximately a 23% positive nodal rate, and tumors larger than 5 cm have as high as approximately a 67% rate of lymph node metastasis.[109]

The treatment of anal margin cancer needs to be individualized based on the size and location. Wide local excision with a 1-cm margin is often sufficient for small and superficial tumors. When the tumor is advanced, or located close to the anal canal and sufficient surgical margin cannot be achieved, combined modality treatment or APR may have to be considered.[50,112,118,119]

Radiation or chemoradiation for anal margin cancer not amenable for local excision has been investigated, albeit in small case series. Papillon and Chassard[109] reported on eight patients with T1 or T2 lesions that were treated with either radium implant brachytherapy alone (six patients) or in combination with external-beam radiation (two patients).The local control rate was 100%. In this study, an additional 36 patients were treated with external radiation with 5-FU and MMC. The cure rate for T1, T2, and T3 lesions were 100%, 84%, and 50%, respectively. Cummings[120] compared radiation alone versus chemoradiation retrospectively in 29 patients; 11 patients were treated with radiotherapy alone and 18 patients received 5-FU, MMC, and radiotherapy. After a median of 7 years of follow-up, the local control rate was 64% for the radiation group and 88% for the chemoradiation group. The local control rate was inversely associated with larger cancers (T1-T2, 100%; T3 5–10 cm, 70%; T3 ≥10 cm, 40%).

Adenocarcinoma of the Anal Canal

Adenocarcinoma arises from the columnar epithelium of the anal canal and its incidence is low accounting for less than 5% of all anal malignancies.[122] Extension of rectal cancer into the anal canal is the more common presentation. Occasionally, adenocarcinoma may occur in patients with ulcerative colitis or Crohn disease who have ileal pouch-anal anastomosis.[123–125] Because of its rarity, the literature regarding treatment for anal canal adenocarcinoma is sparse. In general, these tumors should be treated similar to adenocarcinoma of the rectum. APR should be offered for early-stage disease. For locally advanced disease (T3 or any T with N+), a multimodality approach should be considered. Chang et al.[126] reviewed 34 cases treated at M. D. Anderson Cancer Center from 1984 to 2004. Among those patients, 46% of the patients were treated with local excision followed by either radiation alone or chemoradiation. Fifty-four percent of the patients were treated with radical surgery with either preoperative or postoperative chemoradiation. The median DFS was 13 months for local excision and 32 months for radical surgery ($P = .055$). There was also a nonsignificant trend toward a 5-year OS benefit for the radical surgery group (63% for radical surgery; 43% for local excision; $P = .30$). Kounalakis et al.[127] assessed 165 patients with adenocarcinoma from the Surveillance, Epidemiology, and End Results (SEER) registry and 30 patients were treated with APR, 42 patients were treated with APR, and radiation, and 93 patients were treated with radiation alone. Patients treated with APR had significantly improved 5-year OS than those treated with radiation alone.

Melanoma of the Anorectal Region

Anorectal melanoma is rare and accounts for less than 3% of all malignant melanomas and less than 1% of all anal canal tumors.[128–130] The 5-year OS rate is generally less than 20%.[130–132] The initial stage at presentation largely determines OS.[129,133–135] In addition, gender, tumor thickness, and perineural invasion are prognosticators.[136–139]

The optimal surgical approach for treating anorectal melanoma is controversial. Aggressive radical surgery such as APR with bilateral inguinal lymphadenectomy is no longer routinely recommended because of the lack of a survival advantage and its significant associated morbidity. As such, local resection with sphincter preservation is currently the preferred approach. Ross et al.[140] from the M. D. Anderson Cancer Center reviewed a series of 32 patients with melanoma treated with either APR or local resection. Local recurrence was lower in the APR group (29% for APR; 58% for local excision). However, there was no difference in OS between the two groups (19.5 months for APR; 18.9 months for local resection). Recently, Kiran et al.[141] reviewed 109 patients with anorectal melanoma from the SEER database between 1982 and 2002. Fifty-five percent of patients had local resection and 45% were treated with APR. The median OS was not statistically different in the two groups. However, patients treated with local excision were significantly older. Nillson and Ragnarsson-olding.[142] also retrospectively reviewed 251 patients with anorectal melanoma identified between 1960 and 1999 from the Swedish National Cancer Registry. Again, no OS difference was observed with these two surgical approaches. However, there was a trend toward improved LC in the group treated with APR. Patients with positive surgical margins experienced a significantly inferior OS.

In a review of the small case series, most authors recommend local excision of anorectal melanoma if adequate margins could be achieved. Although the technique of SLN mapping has been widely employed in the staging and management of cutaneous melanoma, there are not enough data to implicate its routine use in anorectal melanoma.[143]

Selected References

The full list of references for this chapter appears in the online version.

2. Bilimoria KY, Bentrem DJ, Rock CE, Stewart AK, Ko CY, Halverson A. Outcomes and prognostic factors for squamous-cell carcinoma of the anal canal: analysis of patients from the National Cancer Data Base. *Dis Colon Rectum* 2009;52(4):624.
9. Klencke B, Matijevic M, Urban RG, et al. Encapsulated plasmid DNA treatment for human papillomavirus 16-associated anal dysplasia: a phase I study of ZYC101. *Clin Cancer Res* 2002;8(5):1028.
11. Werness BA, Levine AJ, Howley PM. Association of human papillomavirus types 16 and 18 E6 proteins with p53. *Science* 1990;248(4951):76.
14. Mullerat J, Deroide F, Winslet MC, Perrett CW. Proliferation and p53 expression in anal cancer precursor lesions. *Anticancer Res* 2003;23 (3C):2995.
17. Smola S, Justice AC, Wagner J, Rabeneck L, Weissman S, Rodriguez-Barradas M. Veterans aging cohort three-site study (VACS 3): overview and description. *J Clin Epidemiol* 2001;54(Suppl 1):S61.
19. Frisch M. On the etiology of anal squamous carcinoma. *Dan Med Bull* 2002;49(3):194.
20. Fenger F, Marti M. Tumors of the anal canal. In: Hamilton SR AL, ed. *Pathology and Genetics of Tumors of Digestive System*. Lyon, France: IARC Press, 2000;145.

22. Horner MJ, Ries LAG, Krapcho M, et al. SEER Cancer Statistics Review, 1975–2006. http://seercancergov/csr/1975_2006/. Accessed
23. Surveillance, Epidemiology, and End Results. http://seer.cancer.gov/csr/1975-_2007/boNSds. Accessed
24. Edge SB, Compton CC. The American Joint Committee on Cancer: the 7th edition of the AJCC cancer staging manual and the future of TNM. *Ann Surg Oncol* 2010;17(6):1471.
26. Damin DC, Rosito MA, Schwartsmann G. Sentinel lymph node in carcinoma of the anal canal: a review. *Eur J Surg Oncol* 2006;32(3):247.
27. Mistrangelo M, Pelosi E, Bello M, et al. Comparison of positron emission tomography scanning and sentinel node biopsy in the detection of inguinal node metastases in patients with anal cancer. *Int J Radiat Oncol Biol Phys* 2010;77(1):73.
32. Das P, Bhatia S, Eng C, et al. Predictors and patterns of recurrence after definitive chemoradiation for anal cancer. *Int J Radiat Oncol Biol Phys* 2007;68(3):794–800.
33. Bartelink H, Roelofsen F, Eschwege F, et al. Concomitant radiotherapy and chemotherapy is superior to radiotherapy alone in the treatment of locally advanced anal cancer: results of a phase III randomized trial of the European Organization for Research and Treatment of Cancer Radiotherapy and Gastrointestinal Cooperative Groups. *J Clin Oncol* 1997;15(5):2040.
36. Constantinou EC, Daly W, Fung CY, Willett CG, Kaufman DS, DeLaney TF. Time-dose considerations in the treatment of anal cancer. *Int J Radiat Oncol Biol Phys* 1997;39(3):651.
37. Hughes LL, Rich TA, Delclos L, Ajani JA, Martin RG. Radiotherapy for anal cancer: experience from 1979–1987. *Int J Radiat Oncol Biol Phys* 1989;17(6):1153.
38. John M, Pajak T, Flam M, et al. Dose escalation in chemoradiation for anal cancer: preliminary results of RTOG 92-08. *Cancer J Sci Am* 1996;2 (4):205.
40. Flam M, John M, Pajak TF, et al. Role of mitomycin in combination with fluorouracil and radiotherapy, and of salvage chemoradiation in the definitive nonsurgical treatment of epidermoid carcinoma of the anal canal: results of a phase III randomized intergroup study. *J Clin Oncol* 1996;14(9): 2527.
48. Pyper PC, Parks TG. The results of surgery for epidermoid carcinoma of the anus. *Br J Surg* 1985;72(9):712.
49. Greenall MJ, Quan SH, Urmacher C, DeCosse JJ. Treatment of epidermoid carcinoma of the anal canal. *Surg Gynecol Obstet* 1985;161(6):509.
50. Beahrs OH, Wilson SM. Carcinoma of the anus. *Ann Surg* 1976;184(4): 422.
51. Hardcastle JD, Bussey HJ. Results of surgical treatment of squamous cell carcinoma of the anal canal and anal margin seen at St. Mark's Hospital 1928–66. *Proc R Soc Med* 1968;61(6):629.
52. Nigro ND, Vaitkevicius VK, Considine B Jr. Combined therapy for cancer of the anal canal: a preliminary report. *Dis Colon Rectum* 1974;17(3):354.
53. Nigro ND, Vaitkevicius VK, Buroker T, Bradley GT, Considine B. Combined therapy for cancer of the anal canal. *Dis Colon Rectum* 1981;24(2):73.
54. Nigro ND, Seydel HG, Considine B, Vaitkevicius VK, Leichman L, Kinzie JJ. Combined preoperative radiation and chemotherapy for squamous cell carcinoma of the anal canal. *Cancer* 1983;51(10):1826.
55. Leichman L, Nigro N, Vaitkevicius VK, et al. Cancer of the anal canal. Model for preoperative adjuvant combined modality therapy. *Am J Med* 1985;78(2):211.
56. Epidermoid anal cancer: results from the UKCCCR randomised trial of radiotherapy alone versus radiotherapy, 5-fluorouracil, and mitomycin. UKCCCR Anal Cancer Trial Working Party. UK Co-ordinating Committee on Cancer Research. *Lancet* 1996;348(9034):1049.
57. Bosset JF, Roelofsen F, Morgan DA, et al. Shortened irradiation scheme, continuous infusion of 5-fluorouracil and fractionation of mitomycin C in locally advanced anal carcinomas. Results of a phase II study of the European Organization for Research and Treatment of Cancer. Radiotherapy and Gastrointestinal Cooperative Groups. *Eur J Cancer* 2003;39(1):45.
58. Cummings BJ. Preservation of structure and function in epidermoid cancer of the anal canal. In: Rosenthal CJ, Rotman M, eds. *Infusion Chemotherapy Radiotherapy Interactions: Its Biology and Significance for Organ Salvage and Prevention of Second Primary Neoplasms*. Amsterdam: Elsevier Science Publishing Co, 1998:167.
59. Allal AS, Waelchli L, Brundler MA. Prognostic value of apoptosis-regulating protein expression in anal squamous cell carcinoma. *Clin Cancer Res* 2003;9(17):6489.
60. Vordermark D, Sailer M, Flentje M, Thiede A, Kolbl O. Curative-intent radiation therapy in anal carcinoma: quality of life and sphincter function. *Radiother Oncol* 1999;52(3):239.
61. Broens P, Van Limbergen E, Penninckx F, Kerremans R. Clinical and manometric effects of combined external beam irradiation and brachytherapy for anal cancer. *Int J Colorectal Dis* 1998;13(2):68.
62. Baxter NN, Habermann EB, Tepper JE, Durham SB, Virnig BA. Risk of pelvic fractures in older women following pelvic irradiation. *JAMA* 2005;294(20):2587.
63. Chen YJ, Liu A, Tsai PT, et al. Organ sparing by conformal avoidance intensity-modulated radiation therapy for anal cancer: dosimetric evaluation of coverage of pelvis and inguinal/femoral nodes. *Int J Radiat Oncol Biol Phys* 2005;63(1):274.
64. Hung A, Crane C, Delclos M, et al. Cisplatin-based combined modality therapy for anal carcinoma: a wider therapeutic index. *Cancer* 2003;97:1195.
65. Doci R, Zucali R, La Monica G, et al. Primary chemoradiation therapy with fluorouracil and cisplatin for cancer of the anus: results in 35 consecutive patients. *J Clin Oncol* 1996;14(12):3121.
67. Conroy T, Ducreux M, Lemanski C, et al. E. Treatment intensification by induction chemotherapy (ICT) and radiation dose escalation in locally advanced squamous cell anal canal carcinoma (LAAC): definitive analysis of the intergroup ACCORD 03 trial [abstract]. *J Clin Oncol* 2009;27:15s.
69. James R, Wan S, Glynne-Jones R, et al. A randomized trial of chemoradiation using mitomycin or cisplatin, with or without maintenance cisplatin/5FU in squamous cell carcinoma of the anus (ACT II) [abstract]. *J Clin Oncol* 2209;27:18s.
70. Bonner JA, Harari PM, Giralt J, et al. Radiotherapy plus cetuximab for squamous-cell carcinoma of the head and neck. *N Engl J Med* 2006;354 (6):567.
71. Olivatto LO, Meton F, Bezerra M, et al. Phase I study of cetuximab (CET) in combination with 5-fluorouracil (5-FU), cisplatin (CP), and radiotherapy (RT) in patients with locally advanced squamous cell anal carcinoma (LAAC) [abstract]. *J Clin Oncol* 2008;26:.
72. Evesque L, Etienne-Grimaldi M, Peyrottes I Sr, et al. KRAS and BRAF mutation status in squamous cell carcinoma (SCC) of the anal canal. In: Proceedings of the Gastrointestinal Cancers Symposium, American Society of Clinical Oncology; August 22-26, 2010; Orlando, FL. Abstract 326.
73. Eng C, Chang GJ, Das P, et al. E. Phase II study of capecitabine and oxaliplatin with concurrent radiation therapy (XELOX-XRT) for squamous cell carcinoma of the anal canal. *J Clin Oncol* 2009;27:15S.
74. Matzinger O, Roelofsen F, Mineur L, et al. Mitomycin C with continuous fluorouracil or with cisplatin in combination with radiotherapy for locally advanced anal cancer (European Organisation for Research and Treatment of Cancer phase II study 22011–40014). *Eur J Cancer*. 2009;45(16):2782.
76. Kachnic L, Winter K, Myerson R, et al. RTOG 0529: A phase II evaluation of acute morbidity in carcinoma of the anal canal. *Int J Radiat Oncol Biol Phys* 2009;74(Suppl 5):.
78. Myerson RJ, Garofalo MC, El Naqa I, et al. Elective clinical target volumes for conformal therapy in anorectal cancer: a Radiation Therapy Oncology Group consensus panel contouring atlas. *Int J Radiat Oncol Biol Phys* 2009;74(3):824.
79. Tanum G, Tveit KM, Karlsen KO. Chemoradiotherapy of anal carcinoma: tumour response and acute toxicity. *Oncology* 1993;50(1):14.
80. Cummings BJ, Keane TJ, O'Sullivan B, Wong CS, Catton CN. Epidermoid anal cancer: treatment by radiation alone or by radiation and 5-fluorouracil with and without mitomycin C. *Int J Radiat Oncol Biol Phys* 1991;21 (5):1115.
81. Gunderson L, Moughan J, Ajani J, et al. Impact of TN category of disease on survival, disease relapse, and colostomy failure in U.S. GI Intergroup RTOG 98-11 phase III trials. In: Proceedings of the Gastrointestinal Cancers Symposium, American Society of Clinical Oncology; August 22-26, 2010; Orlando, FL. Abstract 285.
82. Kim JH, Sarani B, Orkin BA, et al. HIV-positive patients with anal carcinoma have poorer treatment tolerance and outcome than HIV-negative patients. *Dis Colon Rectum* 2001;44(10):1496.
83. Hoffman R, Welton ML, Klencke B, Weinberg V, Krieg R. The significance of pretreatment CD4 count on the outcome and treatment tolerance of HIV-positive patients with anal cancer. *Int J Radiat Oncol Biol Phys* 1999; 44(1):127.
84. Hogg ME, Popowich DA, Wang EC, Kiel KD, Stryker SJ, Halverson AL. HIV and anal cancer outcomes: a single institution's experience. *Dis Colon Rectum* 2009;52(5):891.
94. Lefevre JH, Parc Y, Kerneis S, et al. Abdomino-perineal resection for anal cancer: impact of a vertical rectus abdominis myocutaneus flap on survival, recurrence, morbidity, and wound healing. *Ann Surg* 2009;250(5):707.
122. Deans GT, McAleer JJ, Spence RA. Malignant anal tumours. *Br J Surg* 1994;81(4):500.
124. Ota H, Yamazaki K, Endoh W, et al. Adenocarcinoma arising below an ileoanal anastomosis after restorative proctocolectomy for ulcerative colitis: report of a case. *Surg Today* 2007;37(7):596.
126. Chang GJ, Gonzalez RJ, Skibber JM, Eng C, Das P, Rodriguez-Bigas MA. A twenty-year experience with adenocarcinoma of the anal canal. *Dis Colon Rectum* 2009;52(8):1375.
128. Goldman S, Glimelius B, Pahlman L. Anorectal malignant melanoma in Sweden: report of 49 patients. *Dis Colon Rectum* 1990;33(10):874.

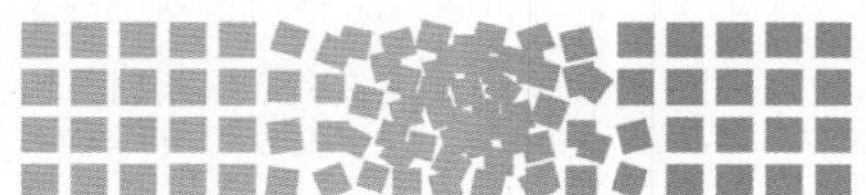

CHAPTER 92 MOLECULAR BIOLOGY OF KIDNEY CANCER

W. MARSTON LINEHAN AND LAURA S. SCHMIDT

Kidney cancer or renal cell carcinoma (RCC) affects more than 209,000 people annually worldwide, resulting in 102,000 deaths each year.[1] A variety of risk factors, including obesity, hypertension, tobacco smoking, and certain occupational exposures, have been shown to increase one's risk for developing RCC. Our current understanding of the molecular genetics of kidney cancer has come from studies of families with an inherited predisposition to develop renal tumors. Individuals with a family history of RCC have a 2.5-fold greater chance for developing renal cancer during their lifetimes[2] and comprise about 4% of all RCC.

Kidney cancer is not a single disease but is classified into tumor subtypes based on histology.[3] Over the past two decades, studies of families with inherited renal carcinoma enabled the identification of five inherited renal cancer syndromes, and their predisposing genes (Table 92.1), which implicate diverse biological pathways in renal cancer tumorigenesis.[4] The von Hippel-Lindau (*VHL*) tumor suppressor gene was discovered in 1993.[5] Subsequently, activating mutations were identified in the *MET* protooncogene in patients with hereditary papillary renal carcinoma (HPRC).[6] More recently, the gene for Krebs cycle enzyme fumarate hydratase (FH), responsible for hereditary leiomyomatosis and renal cell carcinoma (HLRCC),[7] and *FLCN*, the gene for Birt-Hogg-Dubé (BHD) syndrome, were identified.[8] Germline mutations in the gene encoding another Krebs cycle enzyme, succinate dehydrogenase subunit B (SDHB), have been found in patients with familial renal cancer.[9] Discovery of the genes for the inherited forms of renal cancer has enabled the development of diagnostic genetic tests for presymptomatic diagnosis and improved prognosis for at-risk individuals.

VON HIPPEL-LINDAU

VHL is an autosomal dominantly inherited multisystem neoplastic disorder that is characterized by clear cell renal tumors, retinal angiomas, central nervous system hemangioblastomas, tumors of the adrenal gland (pheochromocytoma), endolymphatic sac and pancreatic islet cell, and cysts in the pancreas and kidney. VHL occurs in about 1 in 36,000 and develops during the second to fourth decades of life with nearly 70% penetrance by age 60. Bilateral, multifocal renal tumors with clear cell histology develop in 25% to 45% of VHL patients[10] that can have metastatic potential when they reach 3.0 cm.

Genetics of Von Hippel-Lindau

Loss of heterozygosity (LOH) on chromosome 3p in clear cell renal tumors suggested the location of a predisposing gene for RCC.[11] Positional cloning in VHL kindreds defined the disease locus to chromosome 3p25-26, leading to the cloning of the *VHL* gene in 1993.[5] *VHL* is a tumor suppressor gene in which both copies of *VHL* must be inactivated for tumor initiation. Germline *VHL* mutations that predispose to VHL encompass the entire mutation spectrum, including large deletions, protein-truncating mutations, and missense mutations that exchange the amino acid in the VHL protein. Over 1,000 different *VHL* mutations have been identified in more than 945 VHL families worldwide. Mutations are located throughout the entire gene with the exception of the first 35 residues in the acidic domain.[10] With the development of new methods for detection of deletions, *VHL* mutation detection rates are approaching 100%.[12,13] VHL subclasses based on the predisposition to develop pheochromocytomas, and high or low risk of RCC are established with interesting genotype-phenotype associations.[14]

Gene Mutated in Renal Cancer Families with Chromosome 3p Translocations

In 1979 Cohen et al.[15] described a family with a constitutional t(3;8)(p14;q24) balanced translocation that cosegregated with bilateral multifocal clear cell renal tumors. Loss of the derivative chromosome carrying the 3p segment and different somatic mutations in the remaining copy of *VHL* were identified in the tumors from this translocation family. Based on these data Schmidt et al.[16] proposed a three-step tumorigenesis model in 3p translocation families: (1) inheritance of the constitutional translocation, (2) loss of the derivative chromosome bearing 3p25, and (3) mutation of the remaining copy of *VHL*, resulting in inactivation of both copies of *VHL* and predisposing to clear cell RCC. A number of chromosome 3 translocation families have been described.[17,18] Loss of the derivative chromosome concomitant with somatic mutation of the remaining copy of *VHL* in these families provides strong evidence for the three-step tumorigenesis model and implicates *VHL* loss in clear cell RCC that develops in chromosome 3 translocation kindreds.

Gene for Clear Cell Kidney Cancer

Mutation of the *VHL* gene is found in a high percentage of tumors from patients with clear cell kidney cancer.[19] Nickerson et al.[20] recently identified mutation or methylation of the *VHL* gene in 92% of clear cell kidney cancers. *VHL* gene mutation is not found in papillary, chromophobe, collecting duct, medullary, or other types of kidney cancer.

TABLE 92.1

HEREDITARY RENAL CANCER SYNDROMES

Syndrome	Chromosome Location	Predisposing Gene	Histology	Frequency of Gene Mutations: Germline (Ref.)	Frequency of Gene Mutations: Sporadic RCC (Ref.)
Von Hippel-Lindau (VHL)	3p25	*VHL*	Clear cell	100% (12)	92% (20)
Hereditary papillary renal carcinoma type 1 (HPRC)	7q31	*MET*	Type 1 papillary	100% (6,25,26)	13% (29)
Birt-Hogg-Dubé syndrome (BHD)	17p11.2	*FLCN*	Chromophobe, hybrid	90% (47)	11% (56)
Hereditary leiomyomatosis and renal cell carcinoma (HLRCC)	1q42–43	*FH*	Type 2 papillary	93% (71)	TBD
Succinate dehydrogenase (SDH)-associated familial renal cancer	1p35–36 11q23	*SDHB* *SDHD*	Clear cell, chromophobe	TBD	TBD

Function of the VHL Protein

The most well-understood function of the VHL protein pVHL is the substrate recognition site for the hypoxia-inducible factor (HIF)-α family of transcription factors targeting them for ubiquitin-mediated proteasomal degradation (Fig. 92.1).[14] pVHL binds through its α domain to elongin C and forms an E3 ubiquitin ligase complex with elongin B, cullin-2, and Rbx-1. Under normal oxygen conditions, HIF-α becomes hydroxylated on critical prolines by a family of HIF prolyl hydroxylases (PHD) that require 2-oxoglutarate, molecular oxygen, ascorbic acid, and iron as cofactors. pVHL then binds to hydroxylated HIF-α through its β domain, targeting HIF-α for ubiquitylation by the E3 ligase complex. Under hypoxic conditions when PHDs are unable to function or when pVHL is mutated, altering its binding to HIF-α or elongin C binding, HIF-α cannot be recognized by pVHL. HIF-α accumulates and transcriptionally up-regulates a number of genes important in blood vessel development (*EPO*, *VEGF*), cell proliferation (*PDGFβ*, *TGFα*), and glucose metabolism (*GLUT-1*).[14] HIF-α dependent up-regulation of target genes involved in neovascularization provides an explanation for the increased vascularity of central nervous system (CNS) hemangioblastomas and clear cell renal tumors in VHL. Germline *VHL* mutations frequently occur in the pVHL binding domains for HIF-α and elongin C.[21] HIF-2α, rather than HIF-1α, stabilization appears to be critical for renal tumor development.[22,23] Additional HIF-dependent and HIF-independent functions for pVHL have been reported.[10,14]

HEREDITARY PAPILLARY RENAL CARCINOMA TYPE 1

HPRC is an autosomal dominant hereditary cancer syndrome in which affected individuals are at risk for the development of multifocal, bilateral papillary type 1 kidney cancer.[24] HPRC

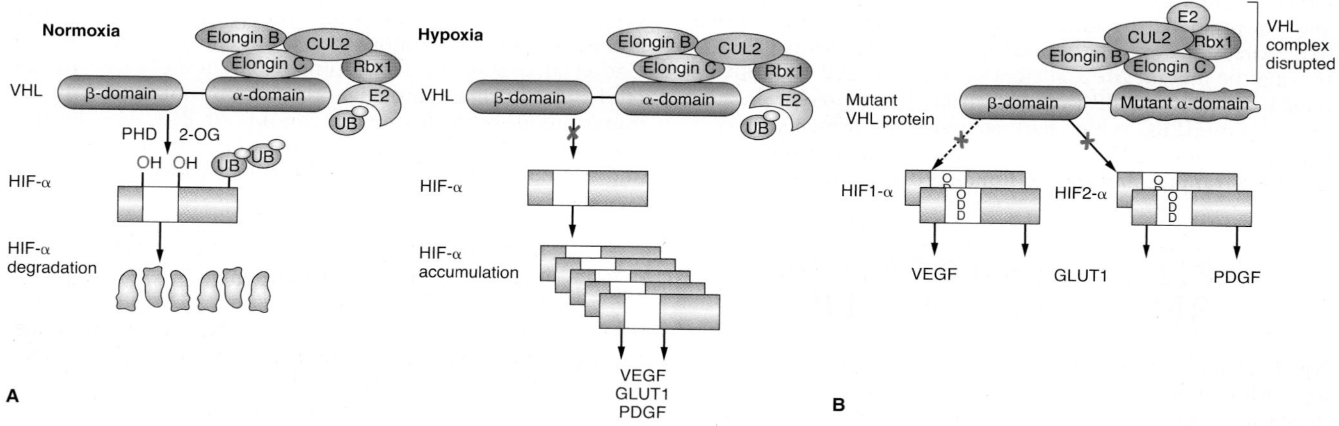

FIGURE 92.1 The von Hippel-Lindau (VHL) E3 ubiquitin ligase complex targets hypoxia-inducible factor (HIF)-α for ubiquitin-mediated degradation. **A:** Under normal oxygen conditions, HIF-α is hydroxylated on critical prolines by HIF prolyl hydroxylase (PHD), requiring molecular oxygen, 2-oxoglutarate, and iron as cosubstrates. The VHL protein (pVHL) can then recognize and bind hydroxylated HIF-α, enabling its ubiquitylation by the VHL E3 ligase complex and degradation by the proteasome. Under hypoxic conditions, PHD is unable to function properly, pVHL cannot recognize HIF-α, and HIF-α accumulates, leading to up-regulation of HIF-target genes (*VEGF, GLUT1, PDGF*) that support tumor growth and neovascularization. **B:** When *VHL* is mutated and pVHL is unable to bind HIF-α, HIF-α stabilization leads to transcriptional up-regulation of HIF target genes. (From ref. 4, with permission.)

develops in the fifth and sixth decades with age-dependent penetrance estimated at 67% by 60 years of age[25]; however, early onset HPRC has been described.[26] This rare disorder has been reported in less than 40 kindreds worldwide.[24]

Genetics of Hereditary Papillary Renal Carcinoma: *MET* Protooncogene

In 1995 Zbar et al.[27] described ten families in which multifocal, bilateral papillary renal tumors were inherited in an autosomal dominant fashion and suggested that these families might represent a hereditary counterpart to sporadic papillary tumors. Schmidt et al.[6] localized the HPRC disease locus to chromosome 7q31.1-34 by linkage analysis. Since trisomy of chromosome 7 was described as a hallmark feature of papillary renal tumors,[28] a gain-of-function oncogene seemed a likely candidate disease gene; in fact, germline missense mutations were identified in the tyrosine kinase domain of the *MET* protooncogene located at 7q31 in affected HPRC family members.[6] Mutations of the *MET* gene have been detected in 13% of sporadic papillary renal tumors.[6,29] Further studies to determine the role of *MET* and related genes in papillary type 1 kidney cancer are currently under way.

Hereditary Papillary Renal Carcinoma: Functional Consequences of *MET* Mutations

The *MET* protooncogene encodes the hepatocyte growth factor/scatter factor (HGF/SF) receptor tyrosine kinase. Binding of ligand HGF to MET triggers autophosphorylation of critical tyrosines in the intracellular tyrosine kinase domain, subsequent phosphorylation of tyrosines in the multifunctional docking site, and recruitment of a variety of transducers of downstream signaling cascades that regulate cellular programs, leading to cell growth, branching morphogenesis, differentiation, and "invasive growth."[30] Although MET overexpression has been demonstrated in a number of epithelial cancers,[31] HPRC was the first cancer syndrome for which germline *MET* mutations were identified. The missense *MET* mutations in HPRC are constitutively activating without ligand stimulation, display oncogenic potential *in vitro*,[32,33] and are predicted by molecular modeling to stabilize active MET kinase.[34] Nonrandom duplication of the chromosome 7 bearing the mutant *MET* allele was demonstrated in papillary renal tumors from HPRC patients[35] and may represent the second step in HPRC tumor pathogenesis. The presence of two copies of mutant *MET* may give kidney cells a proliferative growth advantage and lead to tumor progression.

XP11.2 TRANSLOCATION RENAL CELL CANCER

Xp11.2 translocation renal cell carcinomas, typically presenting with papillary architecture and clear or eosinophilic cytoplasm, are uncommon tumors often detected in young children and adolescents. Translocations involving Xp11.2 and 1q 21.2 associated with sporadic papillary renal carcinoma, and first described in a 2-year-old child,[36] generate a fusion between a novel gene, *PRCC*, and the basic helix-loop-helix family transcription factor gene, *TFE3*.[37] The encoded fusion protein, PRCC-TFE3, acts as a stronger transcriptional activator than native TFE3, and loss of the majority of native TFE3 transcripts is observed in these tumors. This deregulation of normal TFE3 transcriptional control caused by the chromosomal translocation may be important to the development of sporadic papillary renal cell carcinoma.[38,39] Xp11.2 translocation renal cell carcinomas involving at least five different TFE3 gene fusions and resulting in deregulation of TFE3 transcription activity have been described, including the identical ASPL-TFE3 fusion associated with alveolar soft part sarcoma.[40] Tsuda et al.[41] have shown that these TFE3 fusion proteins are strong transcriptional activators of the *MET* gene, resulting in inappropriate MET-directed cell proliferation and invasive growth. Given the physiologic consequences of TFE3 fusion protein expression, therapeutic targeting of MET may be an effective treatment for Xp11.2 translocation renal tumors.

BIRT-HOGG-DUBÉ SYNDROME

BHD syndrome is a rare autosomal-dominant inherited cancer syndrome characterized by benign tumors of the hair follicle (fibrofolliculoma), pulmonary cysts and spontaneous pneumothorax, and a sevenfold increased risk for renal cancers.[42–45] Fibrofolliculomas and lung cysts are the most common manifestations (>85% of BHD patients).[46–48] Renal tumors with variable histologies develop in about 30% of BHD-affected individuals (median age 48 to 50 years), most frequently chromophobe renal carcinoma and hybrid oncocytic tumors.[46,49] Metastases may develop from BHD renal tumors, but they are uncommon.

Genetics of Birt-Hogg-Dubé: Folliculin Gene

Linkage analysis performed in BHD kindreds led to localization of the disease locus to the short arm of chromosome 17[50,51] and the identification of the BHD gene, *FLCN*.[8] Almost all BHD-associated *FLCN* mutations are predicted to truncate the BHD protein, folliculin, including insertion or deletion, nonsense, and splice-site mutations,[8,46,47,52] but recently several missense mutations located in conserved amino acid residues have been described.[47,53] The mutation detection rate in several large BHD cohorts approached 90%, and germline mutations were distributed throughout the entire length of the *FLCN* gene with no clear genotype-phenotype correlations.[46,47,54] Vocke et al.[55] identified second "hit" somatic mutations or LOH in 70% of renal tumors from BHD patients, supporting a role for *FLCN* as a tumor suppressor gene that predisposes to renal tumors when both copies are inactivated. Gad et al.[56] detected *FLCN* mutations in 11% of chromophobe renal cell carcinomas; others found infrequent *FLCN* mutations in other histologic variants of RCC.[57–59] Further studies are currently in progress to evaluate the role of FLCN and related genes in chromophobe kidney cancer.

Function of the Birt-Hogg-Dubé Protein, Folliculin

The function of the BHD protein, FLCN, is currently under investigation. Baba et al.[60] identified a novel folliculin interacting protein, FNIP1, and showed that FNIP1 interacts with the γ subunit of 5′ adenosine monophosphate (AMP)-activated protein kinase (AMPK), an energy sensor in cells that negatively regulates mammalian target of rapamycin (mTOR), the master switch for protein translation and cell proliferation, through TSC1/2.[61,62] A second folliculin interacting protein, FNIP2, was subsequently identified that displayed similar biochemical properties to FNIP1.[63,64] FLCN, through FNIP1/2, may play a role in regulation of the AMPK-TSC1/2-mTOR signaling pathway (Fig. 92.2). Published data supporting mTOR

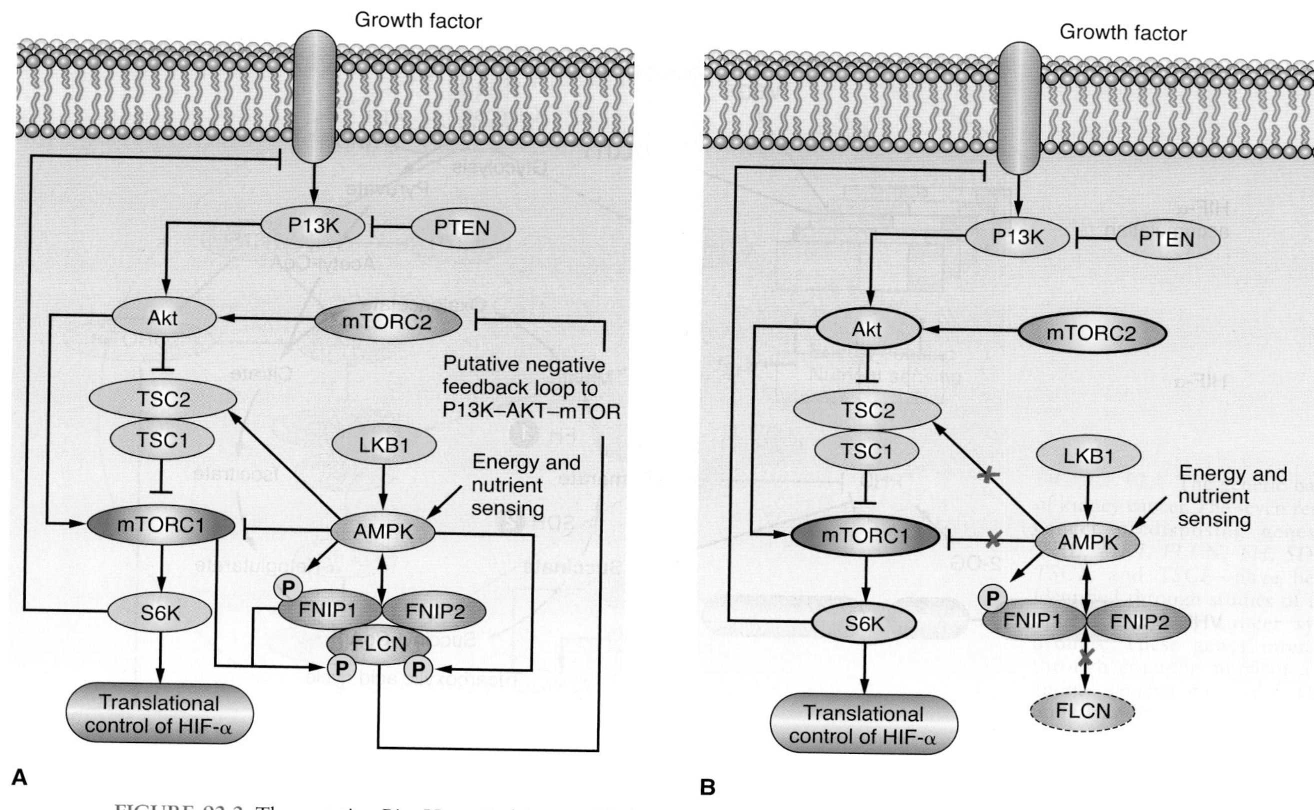

FIGURE 92.2 The putative Birt-Hogg-Dubé gene (*FLCN*) pathway. **A:** *FLCN* binds through FNIP1/2 to adenosine monophosphate (AMP)-activated protein kinase (AMPK) and may become phosphorylated by AMPK or by a rapamycin-sensitive kinase (i.e., mammalian target of rapamycin [mTOR]). **B:** When *FLCN* is inactivated and, presumably, FLCN protein is absent, mTOR is dysregulated, potentially driving kidney tumor formation in BHD patients. (From ref. 4, with permission.)

activation[65,66] as well as mTOR inhibition[67–69] as a consequence of *FLCN* inactivation in *in vivo* models and BHD renal tumors has led to the hypothesis that the mechanism by which FLCN interacts with and modulates mTOR is context dependent.[68]

HEREDITARY LEIOMYOMATOSIS AND RENAL CELL CARCINOMA

HLRCC is an autosomal dominantly inherited disorder that predisposes to the development of skin and uterine leiomyomas and an aggressive type 2 papillary renal carcinoma. Fewer than 150 HLRCC families have been reported worldwide.[70,71] Renal tumors, which are often unilateral and solitary,[70,72] may develop with early age of onset in 15% to 62% of affected individuals[70,71] and can be aggressive, metastasize, and cause death within 5 years of diagnosis.

Genetics of Hereditary Leiomyomatosis and Renal Cell Carcinoma: Fumarate Hydratase Gene

Linkage localized the HLRCC disease locus to chromosome 1q42-43,[73] but an association with renal cancer was not appreciated until Launonen et al.[74] demonstrated linkage to chromosome 1q in two Finnish MCUL kindreds with solitary, highly aggressive papillary type 2 renal tumors. The disorder was renamed *hereditary leiomyomatosis and renal cell carcinoma* and the locus was subsequently mapped to a 1.6Mb region of 1q42. Germline mutations were identified in the fumarate hydratase (*FH*) gene, a Krebs cycle enzyme that converts fumarate to malate in HLRCC-affected family members.[7] *FH* mutations in HLRCC include missense, frameshift, nonsense, and splice-site mutations as well as partial and complete gene deletions.[70,72,75,76] Missense mutations are most common (57%) and occur mainly at evolutionarily conserved residues.[72,75,76] Mutations are found throughout the entire length of the *FH* gene excluding exon 1, which encodes a mitochondrial signal peptide, and no clear genotype–phenotype associations have been reported.[70] *FH* acts as a classic tumor suppressor gene with loss or somatic mutation of the wild type *FH* allele at high frequency in renal tumors and skin and uterine leiomyomata.[7] *FH* mutations are rarely detected in sporadic uterine and skin leiomyomata or sporadic RCC.[77]

Functional Consequences of Fumarate Hydratase Mutations

FH mutations reduce FH activity by 20% to 80%[7,75,78] in lymphoblastoid cell lines from HLRCC patients. HLRCC-associated missense mutations significantly lowered FH activity compared with truncating mutations,[75] suggesting that mutant FH monomers might act in a dominant negative manner to alter proper conformation of FH tetramers. Loss of FH activity in HLRCC leads to accumulation of fumarate and, to a lesser extent, succinate, due to a block in the Krebs cycle.[79,80] Pollard et al.[79] have confirmed that the accumulation of fumarate and succinate resulted in elevation of

10. Nordstrom-O'Brien M, van der Luijt RB, van Rooijen E, et al. Genetic analysis of von Hippel-Lindau disease. *Hum Mutat* 2010;31(5):521.
14. Kaelin WG Jr. The von Hippel-Lindau tumor suppressor protein: O2 sensing and cancer. *Nat Rev Cancer* 2008;8:865.
15. Cohen AJ, Li FP, Berg S, et al. Hereditary renal-cell carcinoma associated with a chromosomal translocation. *N Engl J Med* 1979;301:592.
21. Stebbins CE, Kaelin WG Jr, Pavletich NP. Structure of the VHL-ElonginC-ElonginB complex: implications for VHL tumor suppressor function. *Science* 1999;284:455.
22. Kondo K, Kico J, Nakamura E, Lechpammer M, Kaelin W. Inhibition of HIF is necessary for tumor suppression by the von Hippel-Lindau protein. *Cancer Cell* 2002;1:237.
23. Maranchie JK, Vasselli JR, Riss J, et al. The contribution of VHL substrate binding and HIF1-alpha to the phenotype of VHL loss in renal cell carcinoma. *Cancer Cell* 2002;1:247.
24. Dharmawardana PG, Giubellino A, Bottaro DP. Hereditary papillary renal carcinoma type I. *Curr Mol Med* 2004;4:855.
27. Zbar B, Glenn G, Lubensky I, et al. Hereditary papillary renal cell carcinoma: clinical studies in 10 families. *J Urol* 1995;153:907.
29. Schmidt L, Junker K, Nakaigawa N, et al. Novel mutations of the MET proto-oncogene in papillary renal carcinomas. *Oncogene* 1999;18:2343.
30. Gentile A, Trusolino L, Comoglio PM. The Met tyrosine kinase receptor in development and cancer. *Cancer Metastasis Rev* 2008;27:85.
31. Birchmeier C, Birchmeier W, Gherardi E, Vande Woude GF. Met, metastasis, motility and more. *Nat Rev Mol Cell Biol* 2003;4:915.
34. Miller M, Ginalski K, Lesyng B, et al. Structural basis of oncogenic activation caused by point mutations in the kinase domain of the MET proto-oncogene: modeling studies. *Proteins* 2001;44:32.
35. Zhuang Z, Park WS, Pack S, et al. Trisomy 7: harboring non-random duplication of the mutant MET allele in hereditary papillary renal carcinomas. *Nat Genet* 1998;20:66.
37. Sidhar SK, Clark J, Gill S, et al. The t(X;1)(p11.2;q21.2) translocation in papillary renal cell carcinoma fuses a novel gene PRCC to the TFE3 transcription factor gene. *Hum Mol Genet* 1996;5:1333.
39. Weterman MA, van Groningen JJ, den Hartog A, Geurts van Kessel A. Transformation capacities of the papillary renal cell carcinoma-associated PRCCTFE3 and TFE3PRCC fusion genes. *Oncogene*. 2001;20:1414.
41. Tsuda M, Davis IJ, Argani P, et al. TFE3 fusions activate MET signaling by transcriptional up-regulation, defining another class of tumors as candidates for therapeutic MET inhibition. *Cancer Res* 2007;67:919.
42. Birt AR, Hogg GR, Dubé WJ. Hereditary multiple fibrofolliculomas with trichodiscomas and acrochordons. *Arch Dermatol* 1977;113:1674.
43. Toro JR, Glenn GM, Duray PH, et al. Birt-Hogg-Dubé syndrome: a novel marker of kidney neoplasia. *Arch Dermatol* 1999;135:1195.
44. Zbar B, Alvord WG, Glenn GM, et al. Risk of renal and colonic neoplasms and spontaneous pneumothorax in the Birt-Hogg-Dubé syndrome. *Cancer Epidemiol Biomarkers Prev* 2002;11:393.
46. Schmidt LS, Nickerson ML, Warren MB, et al. Germline BHD-mutation spectrum and phenotype analysis of a large cohort of families with Birt-Hogg-Dubé syndrome. *Am J Hum Genet* 2005;76:1023.
47. Toro JR, Wei MH, Glenn GM, et al. BHD mutations, clinical and molecular genetic investigations of Birt-Hogg-Dubé syndrome: a new series of 50 families and a review of published reports. *J Med Genet* 2008;45:321.
49. Pavlovich CP, Walther MM, Eyler RA, et al. Renal tumors in the Birt-Hogg-Dubé syndrome. *Am J Surg Pathol* 2002;26:1542.
50. Schmidt LS, Warren MB, Nickerson ML, et al. Birt-Hogg-Dubé syndrome, a genodermatosis associated with spontaneous pneumothorax and kidney neoplasia, maps to chromosome 17p11.2. *Am J Hum Genet* 2001;69:876.
55. Vocke CD, Yang Y, Pavlovich CP, et al. High frequency of somatic frameshift BHD gene mutations in Birt-Hogg-Dubé-associated renal tumors. *J Natl Cancer Inst* 2005;97:931.
60. Baba M, Hong SB, Sharma N, et al. Folliculin encoded by the BHD gene interacts with a binding protein, FNIP1, and AMPK, and is involved in AMPK and mTOR signaling. *Proc Natl Acad Sci U S A* 2006;103:15552.
61. Inoki K, Corradetti MN, Guan KL. Dysregulation of the TSC-mTOR pathway in human disease. *Nat Genet* 2005;37:19.
63. Hasumi H, Baba M, Hong SB, et al. Identification and characterization of a novel folliculin-interacting protein FNIP2. *Gene* 2008;415:60.
65. Baba M, Furihata M, Hong SB, et al. Kidney-targeted Birt-Hogg-Dubé gene inactivation in a mouse model: Erk1/2 and Akt-mTOR activation, cell hyperproliferation, and polycystic kidneys. *J Natl Cancer Inst* 2008;100:140.
66. Hasumi Y, Baba M, Ajima R, et al. Homozygous loss of BHD causes early embryonic lethality and kidney tumor development with activation of mTORC1 and mTORC2. *Proc Natl Acad Sci U S A* 2009;106:18722.
67. van Slegtenhorst M, Khabibullin D, Hartman TR, et al. The Birt-Hogg-Dubé and tuberous sclerosis complex homologs have opposing roles in amino acid homeostasis in Schizosaccharomyces pombe. *J Biol Chem* 2007;282:24583.
68. Hudon V, Sabourin S, Dydensborg AB, et al. Renal tumor suppressor function of the Birt-Hogg-Dubé syndrome gene product folliculin. *J Med Genet* 2010;47(3):182.
69. Hartman TR, Nicolas E, Klein-Szanto A, et al. The role of the Birt-Hogg-Dubé protein in mTOR activation and renal tumorigenesis. *Oncogene* 2009;28:1594.
70. Kiuru M, Launonen V. Hereditary leiomyomatosis and renal cell cancer (HLRCC). *Curr Mol Med* 2004;4:869.
71. Wei MH, Toure O, Glenn GM, et al. Novel mutations in FH and expansion of the spectrum of phenotypes expressed in families with hereditary leiomyomatosis and renal cell cancer. *J Med Genet* 2006;43:18.
73. Alam NA, Bevan S, Churchman M, et al. Localization of a gene (MCUL1) for multiple cutaneous leiomyomata and uterine fibroids to chromosome 1q42.3-q43. *Am J Hum Genet* 2001;68:1264.
74. Launonen V, Vierimaa O, Kiuru M, et al. Inherited susceptibility to uterine leiomyomas and renal cell cancer. *Proc Natl Acad Sci U S A* 2001;98:3387.
75. Alam NA, Rowan AJ, Wortham NC, et al. Genetic and functional analyses of FH mutations in multiple cutaneous and uterine leiomyomatosis, hereditary leiomyomatosis and renal cancer, and fumarate hydratase deficiency. *Hum Mol Genet* 2003;12:1241.
79. Pollard PJ, Briere JJ, Alam NA, et al Accumulation of Krebs cycle intermediates and over-expression of HIF1alpha in tumours which result from germline FH and SDH mutations. *Hum Mol Genet* 2005;14:2231.
80. Isaacs JS, Jung YJ, Mole DR, et al. HIF overexpression correlates with biallelic loss of fumarate hydratase in renal cancer: novel role of fumarate in regulation of HIF stability. *Cancer Cell* 2005;8:143–53.
82. Sudarshan S, Sourbier C, Kong HS, et al. Fumarate hydratase deficiency in renal cancer induces glycolytic addiction and hypoxia-inducible transcription factor 1alpha stabilization by glucose-dependent generation of reactive oxygen species. *Mol Cell Biol* 2009;29:4080.
85. Ricketts C, Woodward ER, Killick P, et al. Germline SDHB mutations and familial renal cell carcinoma. *J Natl Cancer Inst* 2008;100:1260.
90. Crino PB, Nathanson KL, Henske EP. The tuberous sclerosis complex. *N Engl J Med* 2006;355:1345.
91. van Slegtenhorst M, de Hoogt R, Hermans C, et al. Identification of the tuberous sclerosis gene TSC1 on chromosome 9q34. *Science* 1997;277:805.
92. The European Chromosome 16 Tuberous Sclerosis Consortium. Identification and characterization of the tuberous sclerosis gene on chromosome 16. *Cell* 1993;75:1305.
93. Shaw RJ, Bardeesy N, Manning BD, et al. The LKB1 tumor suppressor negatively regulates mTOR signaling. *Cancer Cell* 2004;6:91.

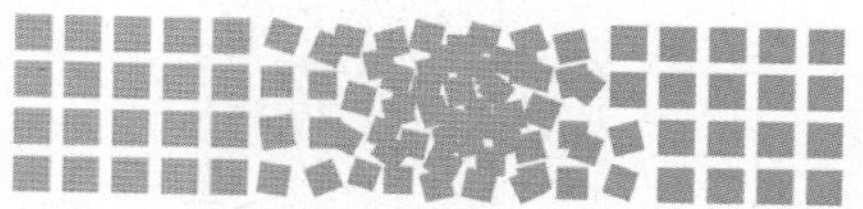

CHAPTER 93 CANCER OF THE KIDNEY

W. MARSTON LINEHAN, BRIAN I. RINI, AND JAMES C. YANG

Each year in the United States there are approximately 57,000 cases of kidney and upper urinary tract cancer, resulting in more than 12,900 deaths.[1] These tumors account for approximately 3% of adult malignancies and occur in a male-female ratio of 1.6:1. They are more common among urban than rural residents. Although most cases of renal carcinoma occur in persons aged 50 to 70 years, it has been observed in children as young as 6 months of age. Between 1975 and 1995 there was a steady and significant increase in the incidence of renal carcinoma, from 2% to 4% per year, an increase of 43% since 1973.[2,3]

Renal carcinoma was first described by Konig in 1826. As early as 1855 Robin concluded that the renal tubular epithelium was the most probable tissue of origin of the cancer, an observation that was confirmed by Waldeyer in 1867. In 1883 Grawitz, noting that the fatty content of the cancer cells was similar to that of adrenal cells, concluded that the tumors arose from adrenal rests within the kidney and introduced the term *stroma lipomatodes aberrata renis* for these clear cell tumors. The term *hypernephroid tumors* was introduced in 1984 by Birch-Hirschfeld. Since then the conceptually incorrect term *hypernephroma* has frequently been applied to renal tumors.[4,5]

HISTOLOGIC TYPES OF RENAL CARCINOMA

Kidney cancer is not a single disease; it is made up of a number of different types of cancer that occur in the kidney, including clear cell (75%), type 1 and type 2 papillary (15%), chromophobe (5%), and oncocytoma (5%). These cancers have different histologic types and different clinical courses, and they are caused by different genetic abnormalities (Fig. 93.1).[3]

Etiology

A number of environmental, hormonal, cellular, and genetic factors have been studied as possible causal factors in the development of renal carcinoma. In studies of risk of renal adenocarcinoma, cigarette smoking has been found to be a risk factor.[6] A statistically significant dose response has been observed in both genders for pack-years of cigarette use.[7] It has been estimated that 30% of renal carcinomas in men and 24% in women may be directly related to smoking.[8] Obesity is associated with an increased risk of development of renal carcinoma, particularly in women and particularly in patients with clear cell kidney cancer.[9,10] Analgesic abuse, which is known to be associated with renal pelvis cancer, is also associated with an increased incidence of kidney cancer. The increased risk for the development of renal carcinoma is observed primarily in patients who develop analgesic nephropathy associated with use of phenacetin-containing analgesics.[11–13]

Environmental and occupational factors have also been associated with the development of kidney cancer. Brauch et al.[14] demonstrated an association between the development of renal carcinoma and long-term exposure to high levels of the industrial solvent, trichloroethylene (TRI). There is an increased incidence of renal carcinoma among leather tanners, shoe workers, and workers exposed to asbestos.[15] Exposure to cadmium is associated with an increased incidence of kidney cancer, particularly in men who smoke.[16] An association between gasoline fume exposure and kidney cancer has been observed in animal studies. Although there is an increased incidence of renal carcinoma reported with exposure to petroleum, tar, and pitch products, studies of oil refinery workers and petroleum products distribution workers do not identify a definite relationship between gasoline exposure and renal cancer. There may be an increase risk of kidney cancer in older workers or in workers exposed to gasoline for prolonged periods of time.[17,18]

There is an increased incidence (100-fold) of renal carcinoma in patients with end-stage renal disease who develop acquired cystic disease of the kidneys.[19] Acquired cystic disease is a recently described phenomenon in which patients on long-term dialysis for renal failure develop renal cysts. Renal carcinoma has been found in association with the papillary hyperplasia observed in the cyst epithelium of these kidneys. The risk of developing kidney cancer has been estimated to be greater than 30 times higher in dialysis patients with cystic changes in their kidney than in the general population.[20] It is estimated that 35% to 47% of patients on long-term dialysis will develop acquired cystic disease, and that about 5.8% of the patients with acquired cystic disease will develop renal cancer. Kidney cancer can develop at any time in patients with end-stage renal disease, and it can occur in kidney transplant recipients. Kidney cancer can occur in patients with end-stage renal disease who are undergoing either hemodialysis or chronic ambulatory dialysis, and it has been reported to occur in patients with end-stage renal disease who are not being dialyzed.[19] Although many of these cancers are clinically insignificant and are found incidentally at autopsy or after bilateral nephrectomy, some will have an aggressive course.[21] Careful surveillance of patients with end-stage renal disease with ultrasonography and computed tomography is recommended. Family history is also associated with an increased risk of kidney cancer in both men and women.

HEREDITARY FORMS OF KIDNEY CANCER

Like breast cancer, colon cancer, and retinoblastoma, kidney cancer occurs in both sporadic (nonhereditary) as well as hereditary forms. There are six main forms of hereditary renal cell carcinoma (RCC): von Hippel-Lindau (VHL), hereditary papillary renal carcinoma (HPRC), Birt-Hogg-Dubé, hereditary

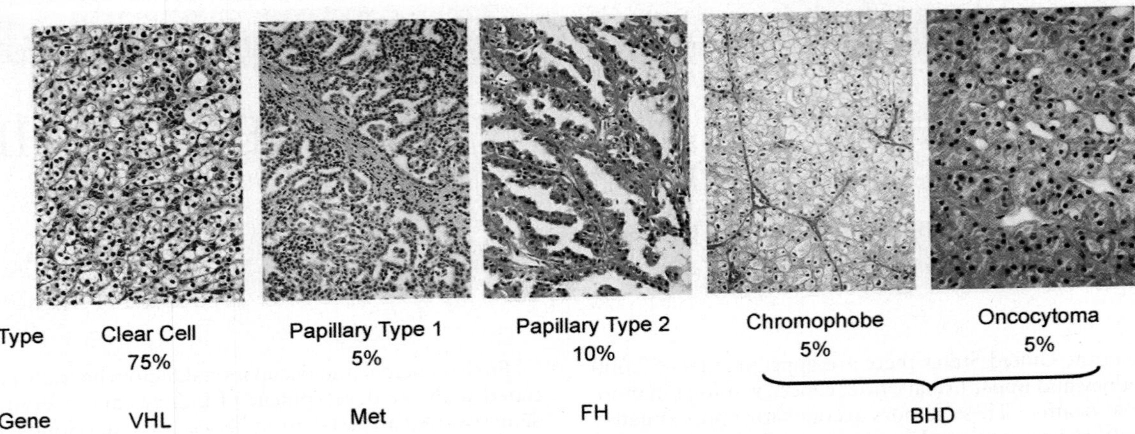

FIGURE 93.1 Kidney cancer is not a single disease; it is made up of a number of different types of cancers that occur in the kidney, each with a different histology, a different clinical course, and caused by a different gene. (From ref. 3.)

leiomyomatosis renal carcinoma (HLRCC), succinate dehydrogenase (SDH) familial renal carcinoma, and tuberous sclerosis complex (TSC) (Table 93.1).

Von Hippel-Lindau: Clear Cell Renal Carcinoma

VHL is a familial cancer syndrome in which affected individuals have a predisposition to develop tumors in a number of organs, including the kidneys, brain, spine, eyes, adrenal glands, pancreas, inner ear, and epididymis. Forty percent of VHL patients develop multiple, bilateral tumors or cysts in the kidneys. VHL patients acquire clear cell renal carcinoma; these patients can develop hundreds of small clear cell tumors and cysts in their kidneys. These tumors, which tend to occur early in life, are malignant and can metastasize. VHL patients can also develop pheochromocytoma, pancreatic cysts and islet cell tumors, retinal angiomas, central nervous system hemangioblastomas, inner ear tumors (endolymphatic sac tumors), and epididymal cystadenomas (Fig. 93.2).[22]

Genetic linkage analysis was used to identify the *VHL* gene in 1993.[23] Critical to management of VHL patients is the knowledge of who is affected and who is not. Early identification of at-risk individuals is essential for initiation of early intervention for potential prevention of life-threatening complications of the disease, such as metastatic kidney cancer. Identification of the *VHL* gene has allowed the detection of germline mutation in nearly 100% of VHL families.[24] VHL clinical features can be heterogeneous and manifestations, such as kidney cancer, occult. In some VHL families, particularly those with early onset pheochromocytoma, VHL can be confused with other hereditary cancer syndromes, such as multiple endocrine neoplasia-2 (MEN-2). The availability of germline mutation screening can aid in making the correct diagnosis as well as to perform presymptomatic screening in at-risk individuals.

TABLE 93.1

GENETIC BASIS OF INHERITED FORMS OF RENAL CARCINOMA

1. Von Hippel Lindau (VHL)
   Histology: Clear Cell RCC
   Gene: *VHL* Gene
2. Hereditary Papillary Renal Carcinoma (HPRC)
   Histology: Papillary Type 1 RCC
   Gene: *MET* Gene
3. Birt Hogg Dubé (BHD)
   Histology: Chromophobe RCC/Oncocytoma
   Gene: *FLCN* Gene
4. Hereditary Leiomyomatosis RCC (HLRCC)
   Histology: Papillary Type 2 RCC
   Gene: *FH* Gene
5. Succinate Dehydrogenase Familial Renal Cancer
   Histology: Clear Cell and Chromophobe RCC
   Gene: *Succinate Dehydrogenase D* Gene
6. Tuberous Sclerosis Complex (TSC)
   Histology: Angiomyolipoma, Clear Cell and Chromophobe RCC
   Gene: *TSC1/TSC2* Genes

Hereditary Clear Cell: Chromosome 3 Translocation

Families with multiple individuals who have clear cell kidney cancer have been reported to have germline-balanced reciprocal translocations involving chromosome 3. These patients are at risk to develop bilateral, multifocal clear cell kidney cancer. In these families, the derivative 3 chromosomal translocate is deleted and the somatic *VHL* allele is mutated, resulting in a VHL-deficient clear cell kidney cancer. The diagnosis is made by germline karyotypic analysis.[25]

The *VHL* Gene and Clear Cell Kidney Cancer

The *VHL* gene has been found to be mutated or methylated in over 90% of tumors from patients with sporadic (nonhereditary) clear cell renal carcinoma.[26,27] *VHL* gene mutations are not found in tumors from patients with non–clear cell kidney cancer or from the germline of patients with other hereditary cancers syndromes, such as HPRC (discussed below). Understanding the VHL gene pathway and how damage to this gene leads to clear cell kidney cancer has provided the basis for the development of disease-specific molecular therapeutic approaches, such as sunitinib, for clear cell kidney cancer (discussed below) (Fig. 93.3).

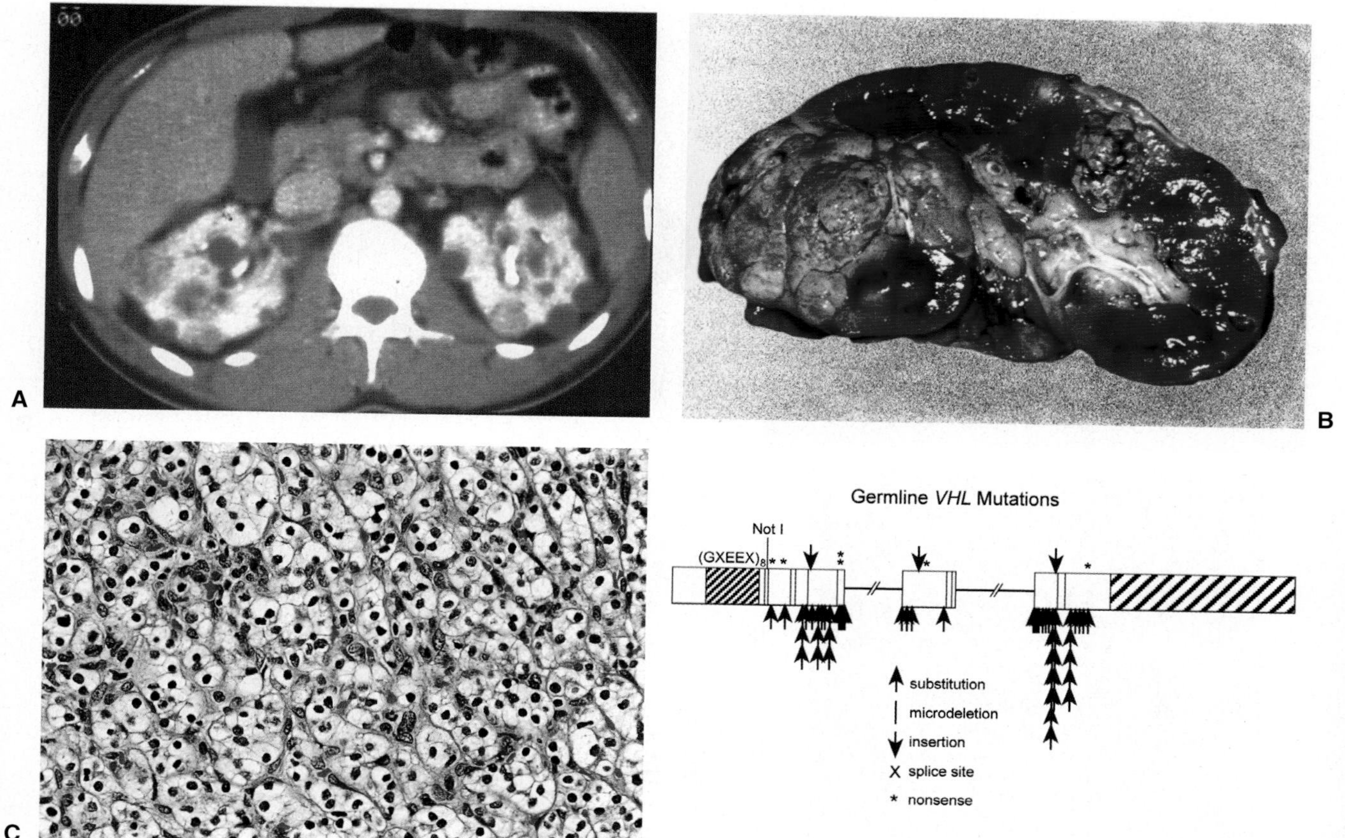

FIGURE 93.2 The von Hippel-Lindau (*VHL*) gene is responsible for the inherited form of clear cell kidney cancer associated with von Hippel-Lindau syndrome. Affected individuals in VHL families are at risk for the development of bilateral, multifocal (**A**), clear cell renal carcinoma (**B,C**). The *VHL* gene is mutated in the germline of affected individuals from VHL kindreds (**D**) and in tumor tissues from patients with sporadic, noninherited clear cell renal carcinoma (data not shown). (From ref. 3.)

Hereditary Papillary Renal Carcinoma: Type 1 Papillary Kidney Cancer

HPRC is a form of renal carcinoma in which affected individuals are at risk to develop bilateral, multifocal *papillary* renal carcinoma.[28,29] These tumors, which are often detected incidentally, can spread in a fashion similar to sporadic papillary renal carcinoma. Abdominal computerized tomography (CT) is recommended for evaluation of at-risk individuals as even large papillary renal tumors are frequently undetectable by renal ultrasound evaluation.[30]

The *MET* protooncogene is the gene responsible for HPRC.[31] Germline mutations in the tyrosine kinase domain of the *MET* gene are found in affected individuals in HPRC kindreds.[32] Germline *MET* mutation testing is recommended for patients at risk for HPRC. Individuals with HPRC kindreds, those with bilateral, multifocal papillary renal carcinoma, or those with a family history of papillary kidney cancer are considered candidates for germline testing (Fig. 93.4).[32]

Birt-Hogg-Dubé Syndrome: Chromophobe/Hybrid/Oncocytoma

Birt-Hogg-Dubé syndrome (BHD) is a hereditary cancer syndrome in which affected individuals are at risk for the development of benign hair follicle tumors (fibrofolliculoma), pulmonary cysts, and bilateral, multifocal renal tumors.[33] The renal tumors that occur in BHD can be chromophobe renal carcinoma (33%), oncocytic neoplasms (50%), clear cell renal carcinoma (10%), or oncocytoma (7%).[34] These tumors are malignant and can metastasize if not detected and treated.[35]

The *BHD* gene, *FLCN*, was recently identified and germline testing is recommended for individuals at-risk for BHDS.[36] The BHD-associated fibrofolliculomas tend to occur on the face and neck and can be very subtle. A biopsy positive for fibrofolliculoma or germline *BHD* gene mutation is considered diagnostic of the disease. The pulmonary cysts in BHD patients are best detected by high-resolution lung CT and have been found in 82% of gene carriers. Twenty-two percent of BHD patients have a history of pneumothorax.[33] Not all BHD patients or families have cutaneous fibrofolliculoma. In patients with bilateral, multifocal chromophobe or hybrid oncocytic renal carcinoma, germline *BHD* gene mutation testing is recommended.

Hereditary Leiomyomatosis Renal Carcinoma: Type 2 Papillary Renal Carcinoma

HLRCC is a hereditary cancer syndrome in which affected individuals are at risk for the development of cutaneous and uterine leiomyoma (uterine fibroids) and type 2 papillary renal carcinoma.[37] The type 2 papillary kidney cancer can be very aggressive and metastasize early. Affected females often develop significant

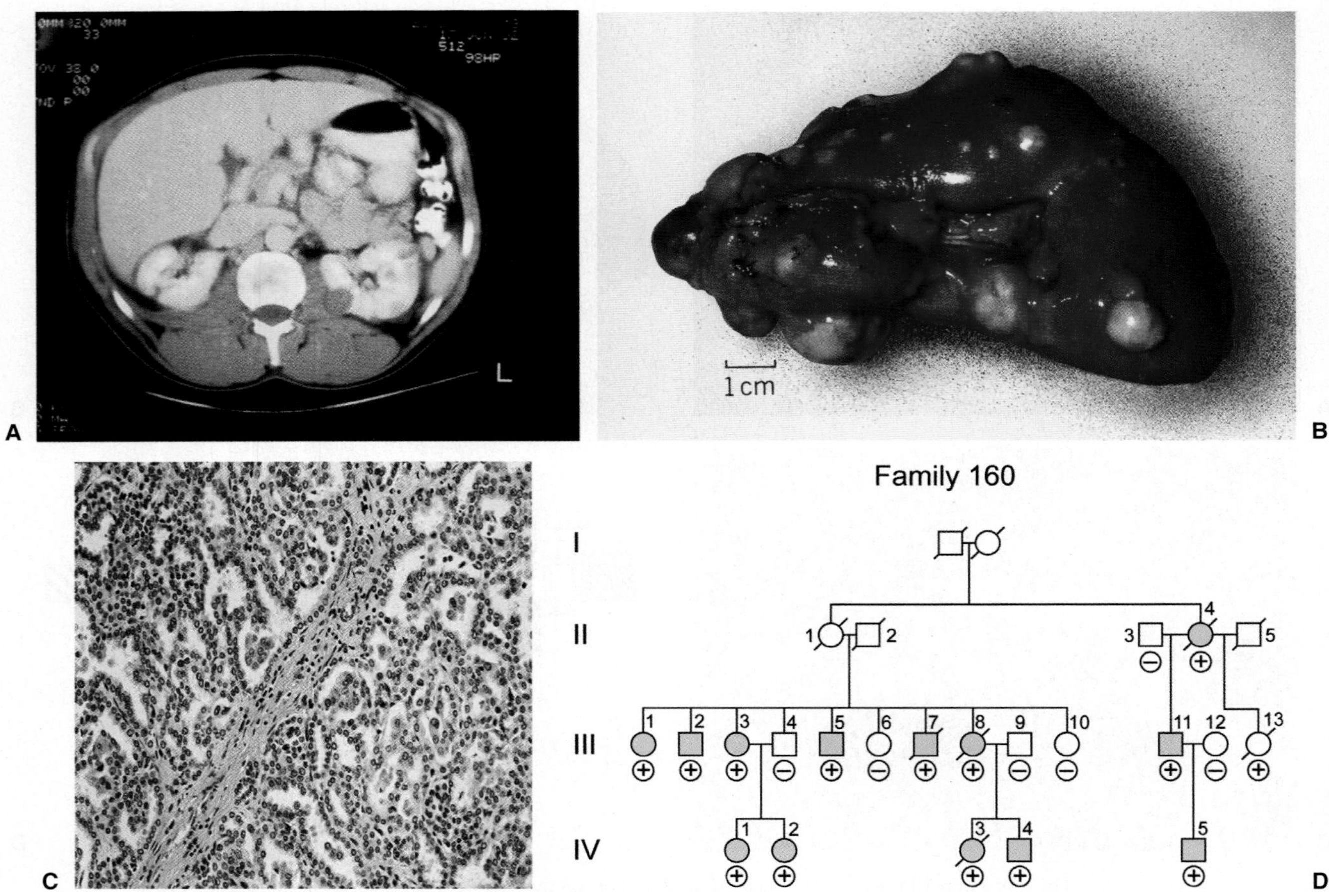

FIGURE 93.3 Hereditary papillary renal carcinoma (HPRC) is a hereditary cancer syndrome in which affected individuals are at risk for the development of bilateral (**A**), multifocal (**B**) type 1 papillary renal carcinoma (**C**). HPRC is a hereditary cancer syndrome (**D**) characterized by germline mutation of the c-Met protooncogene. (From ref. 3.)

uterine fibroids in their 20s. The gene for HLRCC is fumarate hydratase; mutations of this gene are found in the germline of affected individuals in HLRCC kindreds (Fig. 93.5).[38,39] In patients with a family history of papillary kidney cancer, cutaneous leiomyomas, or early onset uterine fibroids, germline fumarate hydratase mutation testing is recommended.[40]

Succinate Dehydrogenase Familial Renal Carcinoma

Germline mutations of the *SDH* gene have been found in the germline of patients affected with hereditary paraganglioma (PGL) or pheochromocytoma. Kidney cancer has been identified as a component of the hereditary PGL complex,[41] and germline SDH mutations have been found in patients with familial kidney cancer with no family history of pheochromocytoma, particularly those with early onset kidney cancer. Patients with bilateral, multifocal clear cell or chromophobe kidney cancer or those with early onset disease should be advised to have *succinate dehydrogenase* germline mutation testing.[42]

Tuberous Sclerosis Complex

TSC in an inherited condition in which affected individuals are at risk for the development of a number of manifestations, including renal tumors.[43] Although most TSC-associated renal tumors are angiomyolipomas, RCC has been detected in 1% to 3% of patients.[44] As the penetrance of TSC manifestations can be variable, TSC should be considered in those who have a history of familial renal cell with unknown genetic basis.

TRANSCRIPTION FACTORS AND KIDNEY CANCER

TFE3 and TFEB are transcription factors that are associated with the development of an aggressive, early onset form of kidney cancer.[45,46] TFE3 and TFEB are part of MiT family of transcription factors that have been found to be translocated in these forms of kidney cancer. The diagnosis of TFE3 or TFEB kidney cancer can often be made by histologic appearance of the tumor, immunohistochemical staining, or detection of the fusion protein in the tumor sample.

Pathology

Immunohistologic and ultrastructural analysis have suggested that the proximal renal tubular epithelium is the tissue of origin of most renal tumors. Renal tumors tend to be spherical, but may vary widely in size. The average diameter is approximately 7 cm; however, renal tumors can often grow to fill the entire retroperitoneum. Previously, renal lesions 2 cm or less in diameter were considered to be renal adenomas, while lesions 2 cm or more in diameter were considered to be carcinomas. The distinction between benign and malignant tumors is no

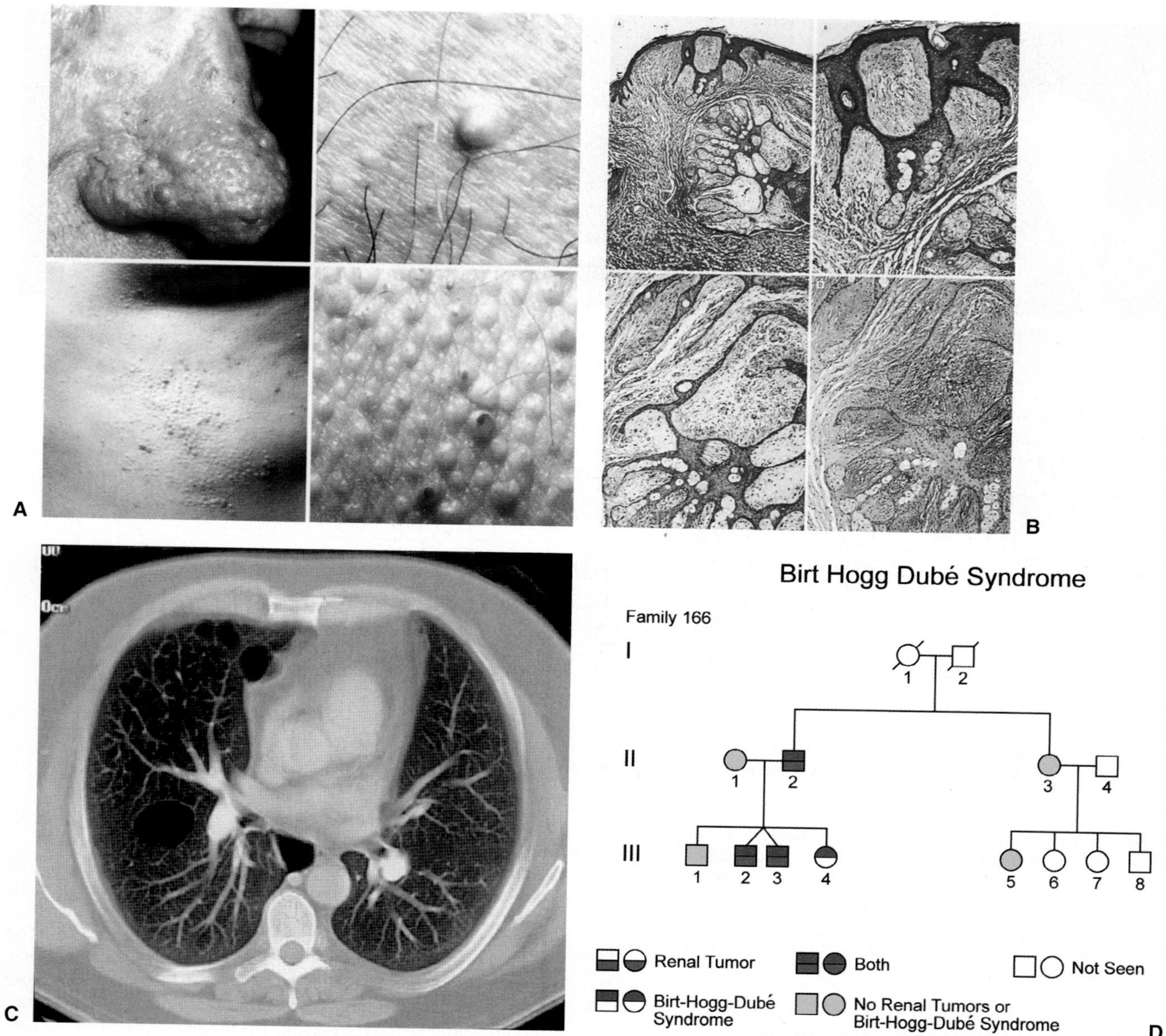

FIGURE 93.4 Birt-Hogg-Dubé syndrome is a hereditary kidney cancer syndrome in which affected individuals are at risk for the development of cutaneous (**A**) fibrofolliculoma (**B**), pulmonary cysts (**C**), and pneumothorax and bilateral, multifocal kidney tumors. The kidney tumors in this hereditary cancer syndrome (**D**) are predominantly chromophobe renal carcinoma, hybrid "oncocytic" renal carcinomas, and oncocytoma. (From ref. 3.)

longer made on the basis of size but rather on the basis of classic histologic criteria. Although renal carcinoma tends to arise in the cortex of the kidney, it can originate in the interior of the kidney. There is often a pseudocapsule formed around the tumor by compression of surrounding tissue. Hemorrhage and necrosis may be present, and frequently large areas of sclerosis and fibrosis are found within the tumor. Calcification and single or multiple fluid-filled cysts may be seen within the tumor. Sporadic renal carcinoma appears in either kidney with equal frequency; it is most often solitary and unilateral.

Renal tumors occur in six main cellular types: clear cell, papillary type 1, papillary type 2, chromophobe, oncocytoma, and collecting duct. Clear cell carcinomas, which make up 75% of kidney cancers, contain lightly staining cells with vacuolated cytoplasm containing cholesterollike substances, neutral lipids, phospholipids, and glycogen. Papillary renal carcinomas make up approximately 15%, with the remainder being chromophobe, collecting duct, and miscellaneous histologic types. Papillary renal carcinoma has been divided into two morphologic subtypes: type 1 and type 2.[47] Collecting duct carcinoma is an unusual variant of RCC that is characterized by a very aggressive clinical course. It is not uncommon for patients with collecting duct carcinoma to present with locally advanced or advanced disease. Chromophobe carcinoma, described by Thoenes et al.[48] in 1985, is characterized by large polygonal cells with pale reticular cytoplasm. Renal oncocytoma, which consists predominantly of eosinophilic cells in a characteristic nested or organoid pattern, is considered to be predominantly a benign lesion. Whether oncocytoma can occur in a malignant form or whether malignant oncocytoma is actually a variant of chromophobe renal carcinoma is not completely understood.

The sarcomatoid variant, which can occur with any histologic subtype, represents a localized dedifferentiation of the cancer and is associated with a significantly poorer prognosis

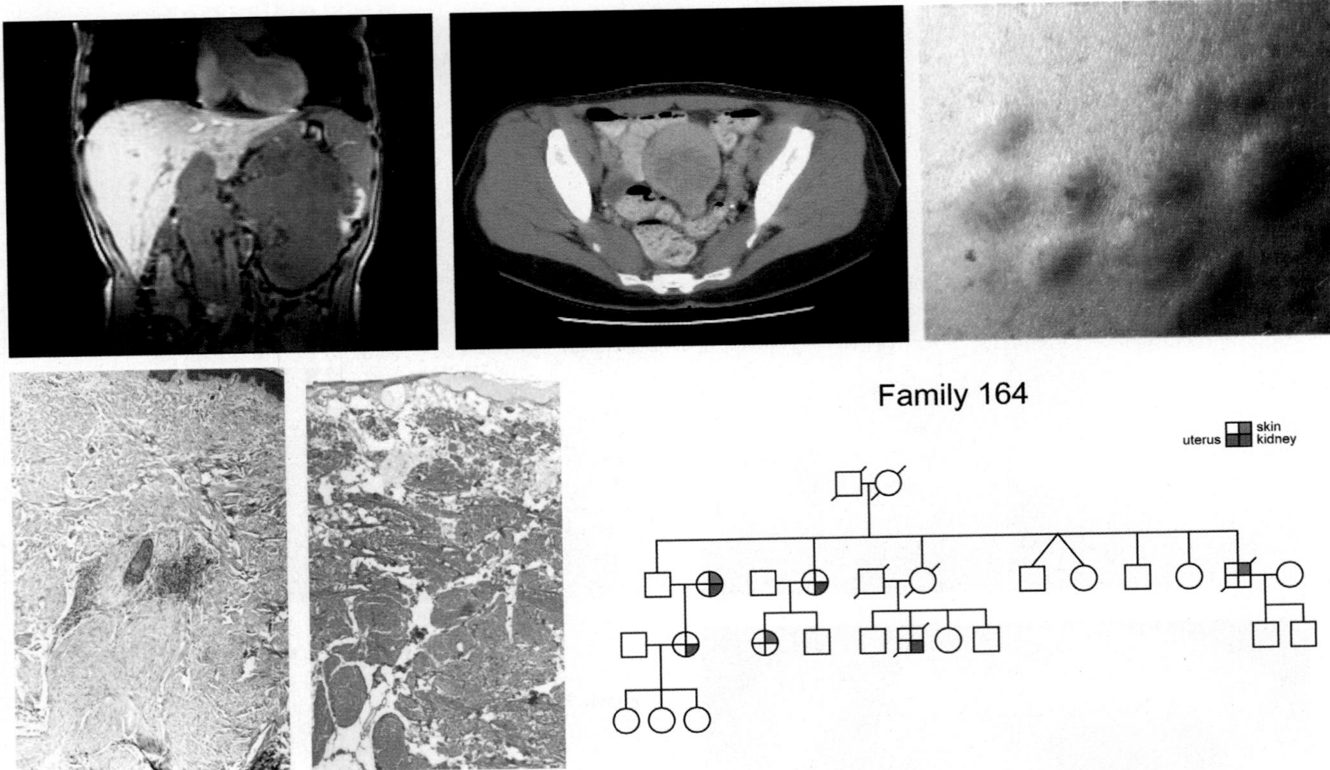

FIGURE 93.5 Hereditary leiomyomatosis renal cell carcinoma (HLRCC) is a hereditary cancer syndrome in which affected individuals are at risk for the development of cutaneous and uterine leiomyoma and type 2 papillary renal carcinoma. HLRCC is characterized by germline mutation of the Krebs cycle enzyme, fumarate hydratase (*FH*). Germline *FH* mutation testing is recommended for patients at risk for HLRCC. (From ref. 3.)

than are nonsarcomatous renal carcinomas.[49] A median survival of only 6.6 months in patients with sarcomatoid-type renal carcinoma is in contrast to a 19-month median survival in patients with nonsarcomatous renal carcinoma. Although infrequently used in renal carcinoma, tumor grading may correlate with survival, particularly in patients with nonmetastatic cancer.

Clinical Presentation

Renal carcinoma may remain clinically occult for most of its course. The classic presentation of pain, hematuria, and flank mass occurs in a minority of patients and often is indicative of advanced disease. A tumor in the kidney can progress unnoticed to a large size in the retroperitoneum until a metastasis appears. Approximately 30% of patients with renal carcinoma present with metastatic disease, 25% with locally advanced renal carcinoma, and 45% with localized disease.[50] Some 75% of patients with metastatic renal carcinoma have metastases to the lung, 36% to soft tissues, 20% to bone, 18% to liver, 8% to cutaneous sites, and 8% to the central nervous system.[51]

A considerable number of patients with renal carcinoma develop systemic symptoms of this disease. Hypochromic anemia, due to either hematuria or hemolysis, has been observed in 29% to 88% of patients with renal carcinoma. Pyrexia is observed in 20% and cachexia, fatigue, and weight loss in 33%. Secondary amyloidosis is observed in 3% to 5%. Nonmetastatic hepatic dysfunction, initially described by Stauffer in 1961, is a reversible syndrome associated with renal carcinoma that tends to occur in association with fever, fatigue, and weight loss and resolves when the primary tumor is removed. Nonmetastatic hepatic dysfunction, which is usually associated with poor long-term prognosis, occurs in up to 7% of patients with renal carcinoma.

One percent to 5% of patients with kidney cancer have polycythemia. Renin levels are often elevated in patients with renal carcinoma, but tend to return to normal after the kidney is removed. Whether the tumor itself produces renin or whether it induces renin production by compression of adjacent tissue is unclear. Immunocytochemical studies suggest that renal carcinoma may produce renin, which, however, may be biologically inactive. Plasma fibrinogen levels may be elevated in patients with renal carcinoma and may correlate with tumor stage, disease activity, and response to therapy.

Systemically Active Tumor Produced Factors

In many patients with RCC there is evidence of tumor-produced factors that have systemic effects. Pyrexia, cachexia, abnormal liver function, increased alkaline phosphatase levels, hypercalcemia, polycythemia, neuromyopathy, and amyloidosis have all been reported in association with RCC.[52,53]

Humoral hypercalcemia of malignancy, frequently observed in patients with advanced RCC, is thought to be caused by a tumor-produced, systemically active bone-resorbing factor. Kidney cancer produces a factor with parathyroid hormone–like bioactivity. A parathyroid hormone–related protein that has been implicated in malignant hypercalcemia has been cloned from a human lung cancer cell line and is expressed in mammalian cells. Thiede et al.[54] demonstrated that human renal carcinoma expresses a parathyroid hormone–like peptide with considerable similarity to parathyroid hormone. Humoral hypercalcemia of malignancy in patients with advanced RCC is associated with a poor prognosis.[55]

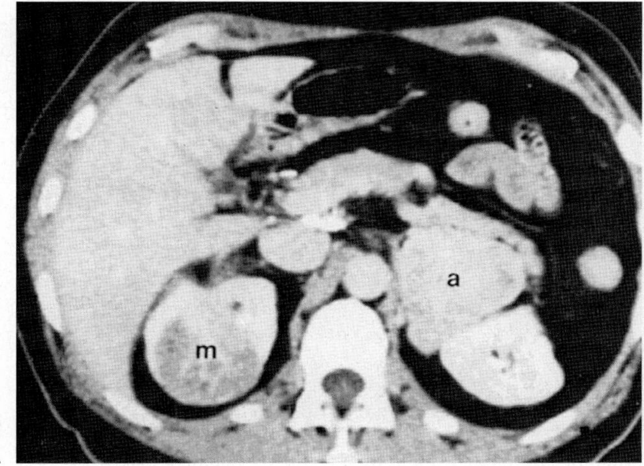

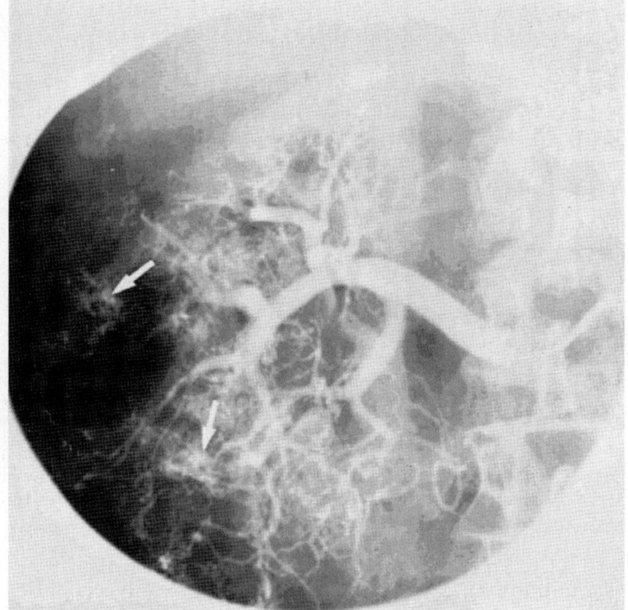

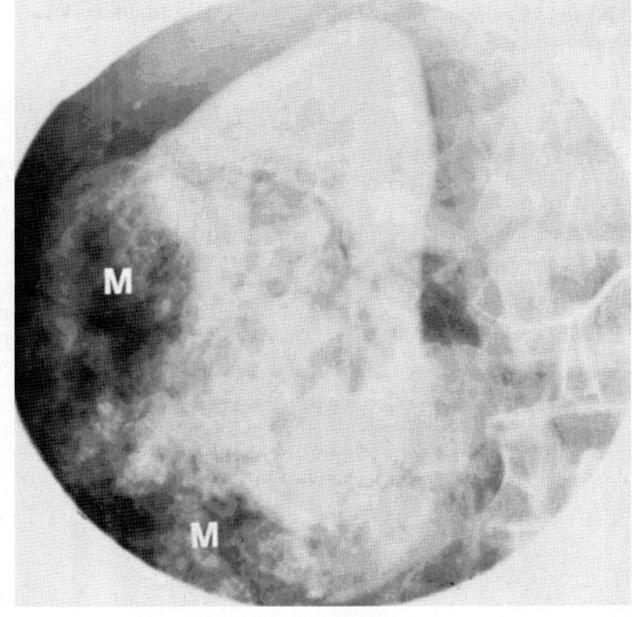

FIGURE 93.6 Angiographic appearance of a renal carcinoma. **A:** Computed tomography demonstrates a right renal carcinoma (*m*) with a large contralateral adrenal metastasis (*a*). **B:** Early phase of arteriogram demonstrates vascular changes indicative of a malignancy, with puddling and tortuosity (*arrows*). **C:** Late phase of the arteriogram demonstrates that the tumor (*M*) is relatively avascular despite its early appearance.

Radiographic Evaluation

Advances in imaging techniques have made much more accurate the determination of whether a space-occupying renal mass lesion is benign or malignant.[56] Diagnostic modalities used to evaluate and stage renal mass lesions have evolved from excretory urography to CT, ultrasound, and magnetic resonance imaging (MRI). CT and MRI are the mainstay of the initial evaluation of renal mass lesions. Although renal ultrasound is not a reliable modality for detection of renal tumors, it proves excellent staging and diagnostic information and can provide accurate anatomic detail of extrarenal extension of tumor, adrenal involvement, involvement of lymph nodes, and infiltration of adjacent viscera (Fig. 93.6).

Computed tomography is the modality of choice for imaging a renal mass (Fig. 93.7*A*). With newer techniques utilizing multidetector CT equipment and enhancement technology, it is now possible to obtain thinner cuts (approximately 1 mm) and to compare pre- and postcontrast enhancement of the suspected mass lesion.[56] The use of contrast agent enhancement has greatly increased the sensitivity of CT for abnormal renal mass lesions. Contrast-enhanced CT allows the clinician to detect very small changes in the density of a renal lesion that might indicate the presence of an early neoplastic lesion. Dynamic CT is superior to standard CT arteriography, ultrasonography, and radionuclide scanning and may correctly demonstrate tumor involvement of the kidney, involvement of the renal fascia, or extension into adjacent organs (Fig. 93.8).

There is no single imaging technique that is best for all patients with renal carcinoma. Depending on the size of the primary tumor and the extent of extrarenal disease, CT, ultrasound, MRI each can provide unique information in an individual case. Multiple imaging modalities are often used to provide the most complete information, particularly when surgical removal of a large tumor is being considered.

Staging and Prognosis

The American Joint Committee on Cancer's (AJCC) TNM (tumor, node, metastasis) classification proves an accurate method for classifying extent of tumor involvement.[57] In the TNM classification, T1 denotes a tumor that is 7 cm or less in greatest diameter and confined to the kidney. T1 is divided into two categories: T1a refers to a kidney tumor that is 4 cm or less, T1b is a tumor greater than 4 cm but not more than 7 cm in greatest dimension. T2 denotes a tumor more than 7 cm in greatest dimension but which is still confined to the kidney.

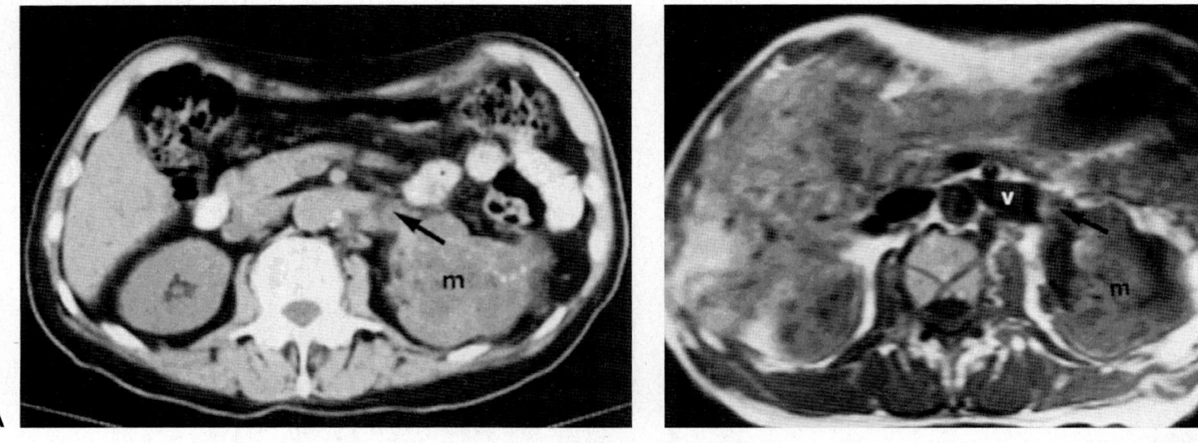

FIGURE 93.7 Renal vein invasion by a renal carcinoma as shown by computed tomography (CT) and magnetic resonance imaging (MRI). **A:** Nonenhanced CT scan shows large left renal mass with calcification (*m*) invading the left renal vein (*arrow*). **B:** T1-weighted MRI demonstrates tumor (*m*) and vascular invasion (*arrow*). Flowing blood (*v*) in the left renal vein is black on this scan.

T3 is a tumor that extends into the major veins or perinephric tissues but not beyond Gerota's fascia. T3 is divided into T3a, tumor that grossly extends into the renal vein or its segmental branches or perirenal or sinus fat but not beyond Gerota's fascia; T3b is tumor that extends into the vena cava below the diaphragm, and T3c is a tumor that grossly extends into the vena cava above the diaphragm or that invades the wall of the vena cava. T4 denotes tumor that has extended beyond Gerota's fascia (including contiguous extension into the ipsilateral adrenal gland (Table 93.2).

With the expanded use of CT scans and ultrasonography, the rate of incidentally found carcinomas of the kidney has increased. The prognosis for patients whose tumor was diagnosed incidentally is more favorable than that of those who present with symptoms, as the former group consists of patients with smaller tumors that usually tend to be confined to the kidney. The 5-year survival rates for 37,166 patients with kidney cancer, from the National Cancer Data Base for the years 2001 to 2002, classified by the current AJCC staging classification as stage I, II, III, and IV is 81%, 74%, 53%, and

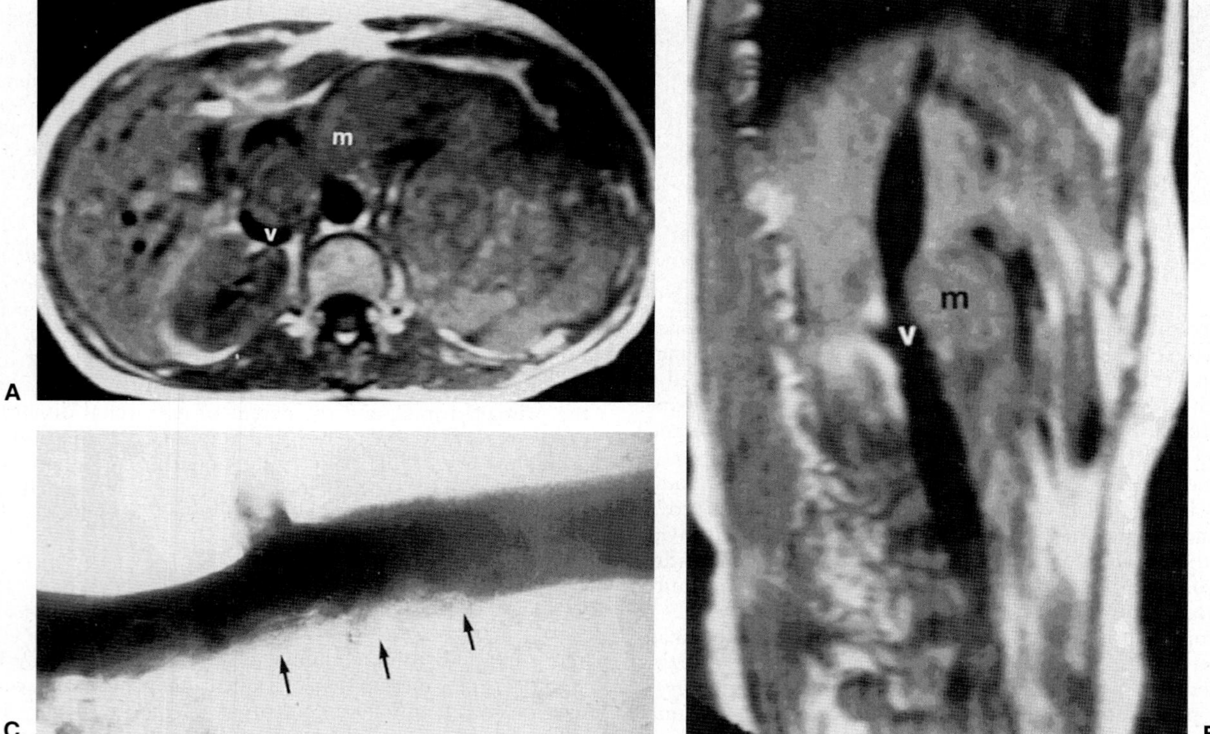

FIGURE 93.8 Invasion of inferior vena cava (IVC) by renal carcinoma demonstrated by magnetic resonance imaging and venography. **A:** Axial T1-weighted image demonstrates a large left renal carcinoma with extension into the left renal vein (*m*) with protrusion into the IVC (*v*). **B:** Sagittal T1-weighted image shows the relation of the tumor thrombus (*m*) to the IVC (*v*) in the lateral projection. **C:** An anteroposterior image of the interior cavagram demonstrates tumor in the medial aspect of the IVC.

TABLE 93.2

TUMOR, NODE, METASTASIS STAGE CLASSIFICATION DEFINITIONS FOR KIDNEY CANCER

PRIMARY TUMOR (T)

TX	Primary tumor cannot be assessed
T0	No evidence of primary tumor
T1	Tumor confined to kidney, less than 7 cm in greatest diameter
T1a	Tumor 4 cm or less in greatest dimension, limited to the kidney
T1b	Tumor more than 4 cm but not more than 7 cm in greatest dimension, limited to kidney
T2	Tumor more than 7 cm in greatest dimension, limited to the kidney
T2a	Tumor more than 7 cm but less than or equal to 10 cm in greatest dimension, limited to the kidney
T2b	Tumor greater than 10 cm, limited to the kidney
T3	Tumor extends into major veins or perinephric tissues but not into the ipsilateral adrenal gland and not beyond Gerota's fascia
T3a	Tumor grossly extends into the renal vein or its segmental (muscle containing) branches, or tumor invades perirenal and/or renal sinus fat but not beyond Gerota's fascia
T3b	Tumor grossly extends into the vena cava below the diaphragm
T3c	Tumor grossly extends into vena cava above the diaphragm or invades the wall of the vena cava
T4	Tumor invades beyond Gerota's fascia (including contiguous extension into the ipsilateral adrenal gland)

REGIONAL LYMPH NODES (N)

The regional lymph nodes are renal hilar, caval (paracaval, precaval, and retrocaval), interaortocaval and aortic (para-aortic, preaortic, and retroaortic). The juxtaregional lymph nodes are the pelvic nodes and the mediastinal nodes.

NX	Regional lymph nodes cannot be assessed
N0	No regional lymph node metastases
N1	Regional lymph node metastasis

DISTANT METASTASIS (M)

M0	No distant metastasis
M1	Distant metastasis

Anatomic Stage and Prognostic Groups

Group	T	N	M
I	T1	N0	M0
II	T2	N0	M0
III	T1 or T2	N1	M0
	T3	N0 or N1	M0
IV	T4	Any N	M0
	Any T	Any N	M1

From ref. 57, with permission.

8%, respectively. The 2-year survival rate for 7,859 patients with stage IV kidney cancer was 19%.[57]

Survival: Histology

Kidney cancer is not a single disease, it is made up of a number of cancers that occur in the kidney, each with a different histology, a different clinical course, and a different gene cause. Cheville et al.[58] evaluated outcome in 2,385 patients with sporadic kidney cancer who had a nephrectomy. Cancer-specific survival rates at 5 years were 68.9% for clear cell, 87.4% for papillary, and 86.7% for papillary renal carcinoma. When papillary renal carcinoma was stratified by type 1 and type 2 papillary renal carcinoma, Mejean et al.[59] found a significantly lower 10-year survival in patients with type 2 papillary renal carcinoma (59%) versus those with type 1 papillary renal carcinoma (80%). Other less frequent types of kidney cancer include collecting duct and medullary renal carcinoma. Collecting duct or Bellini duct carcinoma of the kidney is an uncommon, particularly aggressive form of papillary renal carcinoma. Medullary renal carcinoma is a rare and very aggressive tumor that has been reported in young patients with sickle cell trait. In most of the reported cases the disease has spread early and been fatal.[60]

LOCALIZED RENAL CARCINOMA

Surgical Treatment

Surgery is the only known effective therapy for localized renal carcinoma. The first nephrectomy was performed by Eratus B. Walcott in Milwaukee, Wisconsin, on June 4, 1861, on a 58-year-old man with a kidney tumor who died 15 days after surgery. Professor Gustave Simon, after completing a number of experimental nephrectomies on dogs, undertook the first deliberate, planned, and successful nephrectomy in Heidelberg on August 2, 1889, in a patient with a persistent ureteral fistula. The first successful nephrectomy in a patient with kidney cancer was performed in 1883 by Grawitz.[61] Since that first nephrectomy, there have been significant advances in surgical techniques involving the introduction of the thoracoabdominal approach to laparoscopic radical nephrectomy and changes in the surgical approach, including the use of laparoscopic and robotic partial nephrectomy for small renal tumors.

The most common procedure today for treatment of localized renal carcinoma greater than 4 cm is radical nephrectomy. Radical nephrectomy includes complete removal of Gerota's fascia and its contents, including the kidney and the adrenal gland, and provides a better surgical margin than simple removal of the kidney. However, in the 1990s a series of articles reported that partial nephrectomy resulted in better functional and equal oncologic outcome. As surgical techniques have improved, many are advocating partial nephrectomy even in patients with 4- to 7-cm tumors. Radical nephrectomy is associated with significant adverse effects compared with partial nephrectomy, and partial nephrectomy should be considered for most patients with small renal tumors.[62]

Laparoscopic nephrectomy has become the preferred method for removal of kidney tumors. As advances with this technique are growing, this approach has become the standard of care for management of most renal tumors not amenable to nephron-sparing surgery. The technique is associated with cancer control equivalent to open radical nephrectomy and is associated with decreased hospital stay, more rapid convalescence, decreased postoperative pain, and improved cosmesis.[63] Laparoscopic nephrectomy is most often used as a means of performing minimally invasive cytoreductive nephrectomy in patients with advanced RCC as preparation for immunologic therapy.[64]

In patients with locally advanced RCC (N+), there is currently no evidence to date that neoadjuvant or adjuvant surgical treatment of patients with agents such as sunitinib increases survival. In patients in whom all visible disease has been resected surgically, most physicians recommend treatment when residual or recurrent disease becomes detectable. It is not known whether agents such as sunitinib (in either the neoadjuvant or adjuvant setting) will decrease recurrence rates or increase survival.

Bilateral Renal Carcinoma, Tumors in Solitary Kidneys, and Renal Tumors

The treatment of patients with either bilateral renal carcinoma or renal carcinoma in a solitary kidney is evolving toward a more minimally invasive approach. Patients with tumor in a solitary kidney may be treated by either partial nephrectomy or nephrectomy followed by dialysis or transplantation if the tumor is too large for a partial nephrectomy. Nephron-sparing surgery may be recommended for patients with sporadic renal cell cancer, particularly those with a small tumor (7 cm or less) or a tumor in a solitary kidney. Nephron-sparing surgery for localized renal tumors has been found to be a safe procedure, providing long-term tumor control and preservation of renal function.[65] Laparoscopic and robotic partial nephrectomy provides a minimally invasive alternative for carefully selected patients with renal carcinoma. This technique has been shown to be a viable alternative for selected patients with renal tumors and is associated with excellent tumor control and preservation of renal function.[65,66]

Other approaches for minimally invasive nephron-sparing therapy of renal carcinoma, such as cryotherapy and radiofrequency ablation, are currently being evaluated. These techniques provide promise for the further development of effective forms of therapy with significant decrease in morbidity.[67] Currently these approaches are most appropriate for elderly patients or those who have significant comorbidities who would not be candidates for surgical intervention.

Surgical Management of Patients with Hereditary Forms of Renal Carcinoma

Patients with hereditary forms of renal carcinoma are often challenging to manage. Individuals with VHL, HPRC, or BHD can have widespread renal involvement. Surgical management in these patients involves careful parenchymal sparing surgery, which is recommended when the renal tumors reach a certain size threshold, generally 3 cm. The use of parenchymal sparing surgery in these patients is based on a strategy designed to maintain the patient's renal function as long as possible while decreasing the risk for metastasis.[35,68–72] Patients who are affected with HLRCC are at risk for the development of an aggressive form of type 2 papillary renal carcinoma that can metastasize early. In these patients early surgical intervention is recommended.[73]

Management of Small, Incidentally Detected Renal Masses

The experience with expectant management of small renal tumors in VHL, HPRC, and BHD patients has raised the question whether it might be appropriate to manage conservatively small incidentally detected renal masses in the nonhereditary patient population. A number of studies suggest that active surveillance of patients with renal tumors less than 4 cm may be appropriate for selected patients who are elderly or unsuited for surgery.[74,75] However, for patients who are surgical candidates, most experienced clinicians recommend surgical therapy. It is currently not possible to determine by preoperative imaging studies which small renal tumors will grow slowly and which will metastasize early. Tumors such as type 2 papillary renal carcinoma, collecting duct carcinoma, and medullary renal carcinoma are particularly aggressive and may spread from even a small-size renal tumor.

METASTATIC RENAL CARCINOMA

Cytoreductive Nephrectomy for Palliation

Adjuvant or palliative nephrectomy is not infrequently performed in patients with metastatic renal carcinoma, particularly those with pain, hemorrhage, malaise, hypercalcemia, erythrocytosis, or hypertension. Removal of the primary tumor may alleviate some or all of these abnormalities.[64] Although there are isolated reports of regression of metastatic renal carcinoma following removal of the primary tumor, only 4 of 474 (0.8%) patients in nine series who underwent nephrectomy experienced "regression" of metastatic foci.[76]

Cytoreductive Nephrectomy in the Management of Metastatic Renal Carcinoma

DeKernion et al.[77] reported results in 26 patients with metastatic renal carcinoma who underwent palliative nephrectomy and found no increase in survival, compared with survival in the entire group of 79 patients with metastatic renal carcinoma. In the context of metastatic disease, nephrectomy alone has not been associated with a survival benefit. Nephrectomy is not recommended for the purpose of inducing spontaneous regression; rather, it is performed to control symptoms or to decrease tumor burden in association with subsequent therapy.

Two large randomized trials have been performed to address the role of nephrectomy followed by interferon alfa–based immunotherapy compared with interferon alfa alone in metastatic RCC. Flanigan et al.[78] found the median survival of 120 patients assigned to surgery followed by interferon alfa to be 11.1 months compared to 8.1 months in 121 patients assigned to interferon alfa alone ($P = .05$). Mickisch et al.[79] found time to progression (5 months vs. 3 months) and median duration of survival to be better in patients randomized to surgery plus interferon alfa patients compared to those randomized to interferon alfa alone. Although there are no data to indicate that nephrectomy alone improves survival, these studies indicate that in well-selected patients with good performance status, nephrectomy plus interferon results in improved outcome among patients with metastatic renal carcinoma as opposed to interferon alone. Nephrectomy in patients with advanced RCC should be considered in the context of a treatment plan that includes systemic therapy. The use of laparoscopic nephrectomy in patients with advanced disease provides a potentially less-invasive method for cytoreduction as preparation for administration of systemic therapies.[80] Studies are currently in progress to evaluate the role of targeted therapy and nephrectomy in patients with advanced kidney cancer.

Resection of Metastases

Of the approximately 30% of patients with renal carcinoma who present with metastases, only 1.5% to 3.5% have a solitary metastasis.[81] Patients with a solitary metastasis synchronous with a primary lesion have decreased survival when compared with patients who develop metastasis after the primary tumor is removed.[82] Surgical resection is appropriate in selected patients with metastatic renal carcinoma. In one study, 59 patients with renal carcinoma who underwent surgical resection for a solitary metastasis had a 45% 3-year survival and a

34% 5-year survival.[81] O'Dea et al.[83] reported on patients who presented with primary tumor in place and a solitary metastasis. Of the patients who underwent nephrectomy and who later developed metastasis, 23% lived more than 5 years after removal of the metastatic lesions. Three of the 26 patients were alive 58, 94, and 245 months after resection of the metastatic lesions. In a report by van der Poel et al.,[82] better survival was found for lung metastases when compared with other sites of metastasis. In this study, 14% were free of disease at 45 months, while long-term (greater than 5 years) disease-free survival was observed in 7%. Resection of metastases will render few cures but will frequently produce some long-term survivors.

Debulking Nephrectomy

Debulking nephrectomy has become a standard of care in selected metastatic RCC patients on the basis of two prospective trials that randomized metastatic RCC patients to radical nephrectomy or no surgery, followed by interferon alfa for all patients.[78,79] A combined analysis of these trials demonstrated an overall survival advantage for the nephrectomy group (13.6 months survival with debulking nephrectomy versus 7.8 months for the interferon alone arm) despite no difference in objective response rate.[84] The mechanism of survival benefit related to debulking nephrectomy, however, remains obscure. Appropriate candidates for debulking nephrectomy include patients with (1) good performance status; (2) a resectable primary tumor that represents the majority of total tumor burden; (3) no evidence of rapidly progressing extrarenal disease; and (4) no prohibitive medical comorbidities. It is noteworthy that the selection criteria noted above are largely subjective, based on patients treated in the cytokine era, and very few prospective data with objective parameters exist. Delayed nephrectomy after systemic therapy is also a reasonable strategy, allowing assessment of response to systemic therapy and overall disease pace, thus allowing more appropriate patient selection for surgery and potential down-staging of the primary tumor. This latter strategy may be more relevant in the modern era with agents that have more overall antitumor effect and can have that effect in the primary tumor. The lack of insight into the biologic alterations of nephrectomy precludes definitive statements about the relative timing of debulking nephrectomy. Prospective clinical trials are planned to investigate this issue and will randomize metastatic RCC patients to upfront nephrectomy or not followed by sunitinib.

Surgical Resection of Metastatic Disease

The biology of RCC is unique and variable, including a small subset of patients who present with low-volume, radiographically solitary or limited metastases. These metastases may be present at the time of initial presentation or have been present many months to years after initial nephrectomy. Such patients with limited metastatic disease may be considered for surgery to remove all visible disease. This approach can yield a 30% 5-year disease-free survival. Characteristics that predict a more favorable outcome include a long interval between initial diagnosis and development of metastases, which reflects an indolent course and reinforces the likelihood that the metastasis is truly solitary, and the ability for complete resection (e.g., solitary lung metastasis).[85,86] Therefore, surgical resection of metastases can be considered in highly select RCC patients. However, whether metastasectomy is truly altering the natural history or extending survival of such patients, who by definition have low-volume, slow-growing disease, can be debated.

Angioinfarction

Angioinfarction refers to embolization of the renal artery in an attempt to reduce renal blood flow to the tumor. This procedure has historically been performed for symptomatic control of a primary tumor (e.g., bleeding control) if surgical intervention was not possible or was delayed. Refinements in surgical technique have made nephrectomy possible for the vast majority of patients. This, coupled with a decrease in symptomatic primary tumors due to earlier detection from widespread imaging (and thus reduced tumor size), has lessened the use of angioinfarction. It is an accepted current practice for palliation or if renal vessels are encased by tumor to facilitate subsequent surgery. In patients with metastatic disease, angioinfarction was attempted early as a replacement for debulking nephrectomy or in an attempt to induce antigen release to make subsequent immunotherapy more effective. Although no prospective, randomized data exist, no definitive benefit of this approach was realized.[87,88] Angioinfarction thus does not impact subsequent systemic therapy and should be undertaken only for palliative or surgical indications.

Chemotherapy

Based on the success in other solid tumors, chemotherapy for advanced RCC has been extensively studied. A summary of clinical trials from 1983 to 1993 noted a 6% overall response rate in 4,093 patients with advanced RCC.[89] Another report of 51 published phase 2 clinical trials (n = 1,347) involving 33 chemotherapeutic agents noted an overall response rate of 5.5%.[90] No single chemotherapeutic agent has reproducibly demonstrated response rates more than 10% (Table 93.3). Combinations of 5-fluorouracil and analogues with gemcitabine have produced modestly higher response rates on the order of 10% to 15% (Table 93.3).[103,104] Similarly, the addition

TABLE 93.3

CHEMOTHERAPY IN METASTATIC RENAL CELL CARCINOMA

Chemotherapeutic Agent (Ref.)	Objective Response Rate (%)
SINGLE AGENTS	
Bleomycin (91,92)	0
Cisplatin (93)	0
5-Fluorouracil (5-FU) and analogues (94–96)	0–20
Gemcitabine (97,98)	6–8
Vinblastine (99,100)	0–16
COMBINATION CHEMOTHERAPY	
Gemcitabine/5-FU (101)	17
Gemcitabine/5-FU/IL-2/IFNA (102)	15
Gemcitabine/capecitabine (103,104)	15
Gemcitabine/oxaliplatin (105)	14
PHASE 3 TRIALS OF CHEMOTHERAPY-CONTAINING REGIMENS	
IFNA/Vinblastine vs. IFNA (106)	8 vs. 12[a]
IFNA/Vinblastine vs. IFNA (99)	24 vs. 11[a]

IL, interleukin; IFNA, interferon alfa.
[a]No overall survival benefit demonstrated.

PRACTICE OF ONCOLOGY

of chemotherapy to cytokine regimens has not resulted in significant benefit over cytokine alones when investigated in phase 3 trials (Table 93.3).[99,106] A report of 18 metastatic RCC patients with sarcomatoid histologic features or rapidly progressing disease treated with doxorubicin and gemcitabine noted a 28% objective response rate, potentially identifying a subset of RCC patients where chemotherapy may have some utility.[107] Overall, chemotherapy currently has little to no role in the treatment of metastatic RCC pending further study of novel chemotherapeutic agents or combinations, or perhaps through additional patient selection efforts.

The mechanisms of chemotherapy resistance postulated in RCC include reduced drug accumulation due to the expression of transport proteins such as P-glycoprotein, increased detoxification, altered targets, and impaired apoptosis pathways. The best described is P-glycoprotein, a 170-kD membrane glycoprotein expressed on RCC cells that can act as an efflux pump, reducing intracellular concentrations of agents such as vinblastine.[108]

In view of this, compounds inhibiting P-glycoprotein such as toremifene, verapamil, nifedipine, and cyclosporin in combination with vinblastine have been investigated. To date, these combinations have not improved response rates, and it is likely that additional mechanisms are responsible for the resistance to chemotherapeutic agents in renal cancer patients.

Hormonal Therapy

The limited available data that would suggest the presence of steroid receptors in renal carcinoma tumors are rare.[109,110] A single animal model demonstrated that a progestational agent inhibited the growth of diethylstilbestrol-induced renal tumors in Syrian hamsters.[111] Despite this, the historic lack of other effective agents in RCC lead to the use of hormonal agents, mostly progestational agents such as medroxyprogesterone acetate (MPA), in metastatic RCC in the 1970s and 1980s.[112,113] These early reports documented some tumor regression and symptom reduction, largely applied to a very advanced, symptomatic population of RCC patients. These studies failed to correlate antitumor effect with the level of steroid receptor present within tumor tissue, and thus the mechanism of any effect is largely unproven. More recent multicenter randomized trials utilized oral MPA as an initial therapy for patients with metastatic renal cancer in comparison to cytokines.[114] Response rates to MPA were uniformly low (2.0% and 2.5%, respectively). In the current era of active drugs in RCC, progestational agents may be useful for symptom palliation, but they do not appear to have any significant antitumor effects.

Vascular Endothelial Growth Factor–Targeted Therapy

RCC presents a unique clinical setting for the application of antiangiogenic approaches. Through mutations in the *VHL* gene or other genetic events that result in the dysregulated expression of the hypoxia-inducible transcription factors (HIF-1α and HIF-2β), a large cohort of hypoxia-responsive genes is induced, including vascular endothelial growth factor (VEGF) as one of the classic transcriptional targets.[115] Cell culture model systems of RCC have demonstrated a direct link between *VHL* mutation and up-regulation of angiogenesis-promoting proteins including VEGF and platelet-derived growth factor (PDGF). Thus, increased expression of these proteins, and the consequences of that increased expression, is central in the development of most RCC tumors. VEGF is the major factor responsible for tumor angiogenesis, and PDGF is a critical signaling protein for pericytes, which serve as structural supporting cells for blood vessels. Several treatment strategies have thus been investigated in metastatic RCC to block components of the angiogenic signaling pathway components such as VEGF and PDGF.

Sunitinib

Sunitinib (Sutent) is an oral drug with potent *in vitro* and cellular inhibitory activity against several related protein tyrosine kinase receptors, including platelet-derived growth factor receptor (PDGFR) beta, stem cell factor receptor (KIT), and FMS-like tyrosine kinase-3 (FLT-3), as well as VEGF receptors 1, 2, and 3.[116,117] Sunitinib was initially studied in metastatic RCC in two sequential phase 2 trials in cytokine-refractory patients and demonstrated an objective response rate (ORR) of approximately 40% with a combined median progression-free survival (PFS) of 8.2 months (Table 93.4).[118,119] Additional patients in these studies had lesser degrees of overall tumor burden shrinkage (1% to 29%), thus not meeting the 30% Response Evaluation Criteria in Solid Tumors (RECIST) criteria[120] for an objective response, but nonetheless demonstrating an antitumor effect of the drug. The most common adverse events with sunitinib were fatigue, diarrhea, mucositis, hand-foot syndrome, and hypertension. A phase 3 randomized trial of first-line sunitinib versus interferon alfa in 750 patients with metastatic clear-cell RCC showed statistically significant improvements in ORR and PFS with sunitinib compared with interferon alone. Median PFS as assessed by an independent review was 11 months in the sunitinib arm versus 5 months in the interferon arm, and ORR was 31% versus 6%, respectively ($P < .000001$; Table 93.4).[121] Median overall survival was 26.4 months for sunitinib versus 21.8 months for interferon (P = .051).[122] The overall survival data are a reflection of not only sunitinib activity but also several other active drugs that patients received upon progression, thus the notably prolonged median survival times compared to historical controls. A *post hoc* analysis of overall survival for patients who did not have additional treatment after was 28.1 months versus 14.1 months in sunitinib versus interferon alfa, respectively. Sunitinib was approved by the U.S. Food and Drug Administration (FDA) as monotherapy for advanced RCC in January 2006 and is an initial standard of care in metastatic RCC.

Pazopanib

Pazopanib is an oral multitargeted tyrosine kinase inhibitor that targets VEGFR-1 through 3, PDGFR, and c-kit. A phase 2 study initially designed as a randomized discontinuation study was revised to an open-label study based on the response rate of a planned interim analysis. This study evaluated 255 patients with metastatic RCC who received pazopanib 800 mg once daily; 69% had no prior treatment and 31% had received one prior treatment. The ORR was 35%, the median PFS was 52 weeks, and the median duration of response was 68 weeks. The main adverse effects were diarrhea and fatigue, and the most common grade 3 or 4 side effect was hypertension. Aspartate aminotransferase/alanine aminotransferase (AST/ALT) elevation occurred in 54% of patients. In October 2009 the FDA approved pazopanib for the treatment of metastatic RCC, based on the results of a phase 3 trial. This study evaluated 435 patients with advanced clear cell RCC with either no previous treatment or with one prior cytokine treatment. Patients were randomized (2:1) to receive pazopanib 800 mg daily or placebo. The response rate for patients treated with pazopanib was 30% and the median duration of response was 58.7 weeks. Median PFS was 9.2 months in the pazopanib group and 4.2 months in the placebo group (hazard ratio [HR] 0.46; $P < .0001$; Table 93.4). PFS was prolonged in both treatment-naive patients (11.1 months vs. 2.8 months; $P < .0001$) and in cytokine-pretreated patients (7.4 months vs. 4.2 months; $P < .001$).

TABLE 93.4

SUMMARY OF TARGETED AGENTS IN METASTATIC RENAL CELL CARCINOMA

Treatment	Response Rate (%)	Progression-Free Survival	Overall Survival
VEGF RECEPTOR INHIBITORS			
Sunitinib	30–47	11 months in treatment-naive patients 8.4 months in cytokine refractory patients	26.4 months in treatment-naive patients (vs. 21.8 months for IFNA-treated patients; P = .051)
Pazopanib	30	9.2 months (11.1 months in treatment-naive patients)	21.1 months (vs. 18.7 months for placebo-treated patients)
Sorafenib	2–10	5.7 months in treatment-naive patients 5.5 months in treatment-refractory patients	17.8 months in treatment-refractory patients (vs. 15.2 months for placebo patients; P = .15) (vs. 14.3 months for placebo patients censored for crossover; P = .03)
VEGF LIGAND-BINDING AGENTS			
Bevacizumab	10–13 as monotherapy 26–31 in combination with IFNA	8.5 months in treatment-naive patients as monotherapy 8.5 to 10.2 months in treatment-naive patients in combination with IFNA 4.8 months in cytokine-refractory patients	18.3 months (vs. 17.4 months for interferon-treated patients; P = .097) and 23.3 months (vs. 21.3 months for interferon-treated patients; P = 0.13) for interferon-treated patients
mTOR-INHIBITING AGENTS			
Temsirolimus	7–9	3.7 months (vs. 1.9 months for IFNA monotherapy; P = .0001) in treatment-naive patients 5.8 months in treatment-refractory patients	10.9 months (vs. 7.3 months for IFNA; P = .008)
Everolimus	1	4.9 months (vs. 1.9 months for placebo-treated patients) in sunitinib/sorafenib-refractory patients	14.8 months (vs. 14.4 months for placebo-treated patients; p = 0.177)

VEGF, vascular endothelial growth factor; IFNA, interferon alfa; mTOR, mammalian target of rapamycin.

Sorafenib

Sorafenib (Nexavar) is an oral multikinase inhibitor that inhibits VEGF receptors 1 through 3, PDGFR-β, and the serine threonine kinase Raf-1, which acts through the canonical RAF/MEK/ERK signaling pathway and plays a role in cellular proliferation and tumorigenesis.[123,124] In an initial sorafenib trial, metastatic RCC patients (n = 202) were treated with 12 weeks of continuous oral sorafenib 400 mg twice daily, and patients with tumor burden increase or decrease within 25% of baseline were randomized to placebo or to continuation of sorafenib. A PFS advantage of 24 weeks versus 6 weeks (P = .0087) was demonstrated in the randomized cohort of 65 patients at 12 weeks postrandomization.[125] A subsequent 905 patient, placebo-controlled, randomized trial of sorafenib 400 mg twice daily in treatment-refractory, metastatic RCC was conducted. The trial investigators reported a PFS advantage in the sorafenib arm of 5.5 months versus 2.8 months (P <.000001; Table 93.4). A 2% RECIST-defined ORR was seen in the sorafenib arm, but 74% of patients overall had some degree of tumor burden shrinkage, thus accounting for the PFS benefit. The median overall survival was 19.3 months for patients in the sorafenib group and 15.9 months for patients in the placebo group (HR 0.77; 95% confidence interval [CI], 0.63 to 0.95; P = .02), which did not reach prespecified statistical boundaries for significance. However, there was a suggestion of improved survival with sorafenib after the censoring of placebo patients who crossed over to the sorafenib arm (17.8 months vs. 14.3 months; P = .03).[126] Common toxicity in the sorafenib trials has included dermatologic symptoms (hand-foot syndrome), fatigue, diarrhea, and hypertension. Sorafenib was approved by the FDA as monotherapy for advanced RCC in December 2005. A randomized phase 2 trial of sorafenib versus interferon alfa in untreated metastatic RCC has also been conducted to define the activity of sorafenib in this setting.[127] This trial failed to demonstrate a difference in median PFS between the two treatment arms. Thus, despite similarities in mechanism, sunitinib and sorafenib have different clinical effects. Sunitinib gives a higher ORR and a PFS advantage over interferon in the front-line setting, while sorafenib gives a lower ORR and no advantage over interferon. Sorafenib is likely to assume a second-line or later role in metastatic RCC based on these results.

Bevacizumab

Bevacizumab (Avastin) is a monoclonal antibody that binds and neutralizes circulating VEGF protein.[128] The activity of this agent in RCC was initially identified by small randomized trials.[126,129] More recently, two phase 3 trials have been reported and led to FDA approval of bevacizumab plus interferon for advanced RCC. One phase 3 trial randomized 649 untreated patients with metastatic RCC to treatment with interferon alfa (Roferon) plus placebo infusion or to interferon alfa plus bevacizumab infusion 10 mg/kg every 2 weeks.[130] A significant advantage for bevacizumab plus interferon alfa was observed for ORR (31% vs. 13%; P <.0001) and PFS (10.2 months versus 5.4 months; P <0.0001; Table 93.4). A second multicenter phase 3 trial, conducted in the United States and Canada through the Cancer and Leukemia Group B (CALGB), was

PRACTICE OF ONCOLOGY

nearly identical in design with the exception of lacking a placebo infusion and not requiring prior nephrectomy.[131] In this trial, the median PFS was 8.5 months in patients receiving bevacizumab plus interferon alfa (95% CI, 7.5 to 9.7) versus 5.2 months (95% CI, 3.1 to 5.6) for interferon alfa monotherapy (*P* <.0001; Table 93.4). Also, among patients with measurable disease, the objective response rate was higher in patients treated with bevacizumab plus interferon (25.5%) than for interferon alfa monotherapy (13.1%; *P* <.0001). Recent overall survival data are similar to the other agents with a numerical advantage in median survival not meeting statistical significance, reflecting the large proportion of patients who receive subsequent active therapy. The contribution of interferon alfa to the antitumor effect of this regimen is unclear at present, although preliminary results indicate a longer PFS and higher response rate than expected with bevacizumab monotherapy.[126] Combination interferon alfa and bevacizumab therapy is more toxic than either as monotherapy, notable for fatigue, anorexia, hypertension, and proteinuria. Thus, the use of interferon with bevacizumab with requires evaluation of the risk/benefit ratio for each patient.

Mammalian Target of Rapamycin–Targeted Therapy

Temsirolimus

Temsirolimus is an inhibitor of mammalian target of rapamycin (mTOR), a molecule implicated in multiple tumor-promoting intracellular signaling pathways, including regulation of HIF involved in VEGF expression. A phase 2 trial in patients with treatment-refractory, metastatic RCC randomized 111 patients to one of multiple dose levels (25 mg, 75 mg, or 250 mg intravenous [IV] weekly).[132] The overall response rate was 7%, with additional patients demonstrating minor responses (Table 93.4). Retrospective assignment of risk criteria to patients in this study identified a poor-prognosis group with a median overall survival of 8.2 months compare to 4.9 months for historical interferon alfa–treated patients.[133] Loss of PTEN or activation of Akt (upstream regulators of the mTOR expression) may be more common in poor risk patients and thereby potentially increase the relevance of mTOR-targeted therapy in this subgroup.

A subsequent randomized phase 3 trial was conducted in patients with metastatic RCC (n = 626) and three or more adverse risk features as defined by existing prognostic schema (Table 93.4).[133,134] Patients were randomized equally to receive interferon alfa 18 mU subcutaneous three times a week, temsirolimus 25 mg IV weekly, or temsirolimus 15 mg IV weekly plus interferon alfa 6 mU subcutaneous three times a week. The primary study end point was overall survival, and the study was powered to compare each of the temsirolimus arms to the interferon alfa arm. Both temsirolimus-containing arms demonstrated a PFS advantage versus interferon alfa (3.7 months for each arm vs. 1.9 months; *P* = .0001 for temsirolimus monotherapy and *P* = .0019 for temsirolimus plus interferon alfa). Patients treated with temsirolimus monotherapy had a statistically longer survival than those treated with interferon alfa alone (10.9 months vs. 7.3 months; *P* = .0069). Overall survival of patients treated with interferon alfa and temsirolimus plus interferon alfa were not statistically different (7.3 months vs. 8.4 months; *P* = .6912).

Everolimus

Everolimus is an oral rapamycin analogue that inhibits mTOR. A phase 3 study evaluated 410 patients who had previously been treated with sorafenib, sunitinib, or both and randomized them (2:1) to receive everolimus 10 mg once daily or placebo.[135] PFS was significantly longer in the everolimus group (HR 0.30; 95% CI, 0.22 to 0.40; *P* <.0001). Median PFS in the everolimus group was 4.9 months versus 1.9 months in the placebo group. Partial response in the everolimus group occurred in 1% of the patients, and 63% (vs. 32% in the placebo group) had disease stabilization for at least 56 days. The most common adverse effects of everolimus were stomatitis, rash, fatigue, asthenia, and diarrhea. Stomatitis, fatigue, infection, and pneumonitis were the most common grade 3 or 4 toxicities. On the basis of these results, everolimus was approved by the FDA for treatment of metastatic RCC that is refractory to sunitinib or sorafenib.

Prognostic Factors

A unique feature of the natural history of RCC is biologic variability in the natural history and in response to therapy. In this context, features that are associated with clinical outcome, loosely termed prognostic factors, have been described. It is acknowledged that, strictly speaking, prognostic factors relate to the natural history of a disease (in the absence of treatment or not affected by treatment) and that predictive factors describe features associated with outcome to a given therapy. The term *prognostic factors* will be used here in a general sense to describe factors associated with the clinical outcome in RCC.

Clinical Factors

Patient and disease characteristics are clinical characteristics that have been extensively studied as potential prognostic factors in metastatic RCC. Most studies have found that factors such as age and race were not associated with survival in metastatic RCC. Performance status is a measure of overall well-being and is the most consistently reported factor associated with survival in advanced RCC.[134,136–138] Some studies have found the presence of visceral (lung, liver, and adrenals), bone, and brain metastases to be associated with poor survival,[134,136,139] while others have found no relationship between these sites and prognosis.[138,140] A more reliable finding is the number of metastatic sites present, which provides a rough estimate of tumor burden. Most studies have found that patients with a higher number of metastatic sites (1 or 2 vs. more than 2) are independently associated with at least twofold greater probability of death. Similarly, patients with a short interval from initial RCC diagnosis to metastases have been found to have a worse outcome, possibly as a reflection of faster-growing disease.[133,134,137,141]

Laboratory Parameters

Investigators have evaluated the effects of several blood parameters in patients with advanced RCC. Erythrocyte sedimentation rate (ESR), C-reactive protein (CRP), hemoglobin, and white blood cell or platelet parameters were evaluated. Elevated ESR and CRP were found consistently to be independent poor prognostic factors.[141–144] Patients with thrombocytosis (defined as platelet counts greater than 400,000/mcL), another potential marker of inflammation, have been reported to have a negative survival outcome, mostly in patients with localized RCC. Studies overall have been inconsistent in the metastatic setting, especially when other markers of inflammation were considered. Anemia has also consistently been found to be an independent prognostic factor for an adverse outcome. Patients with pretreatment hemoglobin below the lower limit of laboratory normal (LLN) values were found to have twice the risk of death than patients with normal hemoglobin in several large studies.[134,138] The mechanism of effect of such blood parameters is unknown; whether these markers reflect an underlying inflammatory disease or somehow contribute to the disease process itself is unclear.

Biochemical factors most often studied include pretreatment serum lactate dehydrogenase (LDH) and calcium (corrected for albumin). Corrected serum calcium greater than 10 mg/dL and LDH greater than 1.5 times the upper limit of normal have been associated with a two- to threefold higher risk of death, respectively.[141,138,141] Other biochemical factors have been studied and found to not be of prognostic value, including serum alkaline phosphatase, creatinine, gamma glutamyltransferase (GGT), and triglycerides.

Prognostic Schema

Using the above-identified variables, investigators have combined these to stratify patients into risk groups to predict outcome. Such schema serve to aid in individual patient counseling, stratify patients for randomized clinical trial entry, and aid in interpretation of nonrandomized clinical trials. The most commonly employed schema from Memorial Sloan-Kettering Cancer Center (MSKCC) was developed from patients treated with interferon-based regimens.[133] This schema uses Eastern Cooperative Oncology Group (ECOG) performance status, anemia, LDH, corrected serum calcium, and time from diagnosis to metastatic disease to segregate patients into three risk groups. This schema is still widely used today, despite the current limited interferon use, and has been shown to also segregate patients treated with newer agents. More recent efforts have developed prognostic variables and risk groups based on patients treated with targeted agents. This schema uses hemoglobin, corrected calcium, performance status, and time from diagnosis to treatment, but additionally neutrophil and platelet count.[145]

Immunotherapy

Immunologic agents retain a critical and unique role in the armamentarium of agents used to treat widespread metastatic RCC. Their use in treating renal carcinoma was instrumental in demonstrating that biotherapies were capable of inducing complete and curative regressions of human cancer. In the treatment of common metastatic solid tumors, the potential for cure of disseminated cancer with systemic therapy in renal cancer is only exceeded by testicular cancer and matched by melanoma. It is true that this result is only attained by a small proportion of patients with advanced disease, and the factors that predict or produce dramatic, durable responses in such patients have not been clearly established. Nevertheless, the modest frequency of compete regression and the imperfect understanding of the biology of such results should not obscure the fact that biotherapy, and specifically interleukin-2, is the only systemic treatment that can consistently cures some patients with metastatic renal cancer. A more detailed understanding of the molecular interactions between renal cancer and the host immune system should lead to new approaches to enhance immune responses, overcome tolerance and immunosuppression, and facilitate the immunological rejection of this malignancy.

Spontaneous Tumor Regression

Much has been said of the rare but striking phenomenon of spontaneous tumor regression in patients with advanced renal cancer, and the mechanism is presumed to be immunological. Yet justifying nephrectomy in patients with metastatic disease based solely on the hope of inducing a spontaneous regression has been abandoned due to the disappointingly low incidence of this occurring.[146] In reviews of spontaneous tumor regression, another consistent feature is that the majority of regressions are short-lived. In one randomized study of interferon versus placebo in patients with RCC, the patients who received placebo demonstrated a singularly high response rate of 6%, but the duration of these regressions were 2 months to 13 months, with only one ongoing response of 9 months at the time of publication.[147] Other larger reviews show that the true incidence of this phenomenon is probably less than 1% and that the vast majority of documented spontaneous regressions will relapse with progressive metastatic disease and require other therapy.[148,149] A few well-documented cases of durable regressions have occurred in patients who had life-threatening infectious or inflammatory events as possible instigators of their regression.[150] These data indicate that spontaneous regression of RCC is rare, often transient, and not a phenomenon that should be relied upon as therapy.

Interferons

Early studies of leukocyte interferon in the treatment of cancer reported sporadic responses in patients with renal cell carcinoma.[151] Subsequently, increased dosages and larger studies were possible using recombinant interferon-α, and this experience was repeated and confirmed. The response rates in the largest studies ranged from 0% to 29% (Table 93.5), with few complete responses and few long-term survival data.[153] In

TABLE 93.5

TREATMENT OF METASTATIC RENAL CELL CANCER WITH INTERFERON

Author (Ref.)	IFN	Route and Schedule	N	RR (%)	CR(%)
deKernion (152)	IFN-α	6 MU im qd	48	15	2
Quesada et al. (151)	IFN-α	3 MU im qd	50	26	6[a]
Quesada et al. (153)	IFN-α	2 MU im qd	15	0	0
		20 MU im qd	41	29	2
Umeda and Niijima (154)	IFN-α	3–36 MU im qd	153	15	2
	Lymphoblastoid	5 MU im 2–7/wk	73	23	1
Muss (155)	IFN-α-2b	2–10 MU sc 3/wk	58	9	2
		30–50 MU iv qd	54	6	2
Motzer et al. (121)	IFN-α	3–9 MU sc 3/wk	327	6	0

IFN-α, interferon alfa; im, intramuscular; sc, subcutaneous; iv, intravenous;
[a]Duration of complete responses all less than 10 months.

a review of the literature, Moss[156] and Quesada[157] reported an ORR of 16% for 654 patients. Factors that seemed to increase the likelihood of responding included good performance status, prior nephrectomy, and metastases confined to the lungs. Nevertheless, these factors could not reliably exclude patients unable to benefit from interferon, and serve only as general guidelines. Few data exist on the long-term results from interferon therapy, but from the very small number of completely responding patients, it is safe to conclude there are only anecdotal cases of cures of metastatic disease from interferon. Recently, randomized prospective studies have been performed to measure the benefit of interferon alfa in patients with advanced renal cancer. A randomized comparison of interferon alfa versus medroxyprogesterone acetate in 335 patients demonstrated a significant prolongation of median survival (6 months for MPA and 8.5 months for interferon alfa).[158] This modest prolongation of survival was offset by greater symptoms and lesser quality of life in patients on interferon alfa. In addition, benefit did not appear durable, with estimated progression-free survival at 2 years 5% or less for both groups.

Many different types and preparations of interferons have been used in clinical trials. Early trials with "natural" interferon produced from donor leukocytes and subsequent trials with several different subtypes of recombinant interferon have not suggested a difference in efficacy between these preparations. Subsequent trials using interferon-α and interferon-α have indicated that these agents have either similar or less activity than interferon-α.[159]

One consideration in evaluating interferon therapy is that the optimal dose, schedule, and route of administration are not yet known, but in view of the limited benefit demonstrated to this point, it is unlikely that randomized studies will ever be done to effectively optimize these parameters. In summary, disseminated renal cell cancer shows a small but consistent response rate to interferon (primarily interferon-α), but these benefits must be weighed against the toxicity of chronic therapy and the poor evidence for long-term benefit.

Interleukin-2

After the discovery of interleukin-2 (IL-2) in 1976 and the demonstration of its activities as a T-cell growth factor and activator of T-cells and natural killer cells, it was utilized in clinical trials against a variety of malignancies. From the first trials in 1984, renal cell cancer was identified as a tumor that could respond to IL-2.[160,161] These early trials rapidly escalated the dose of IL-2 to the maximum tolerated dosage and then added lymphokine activated killer (LAK) cells to the therapy based on preclinical results. These trials initially reported response rates of 33% in RCC, and in a subsequent multicenter experience the response rate was 16%.[162] The remarkable feature of many of these responses is that they appear complete and durable (Fig. 93.9). Median follow-up of greater than 10 years is available from those early studies, and a review of these patients indicate that 7% to 9% of all

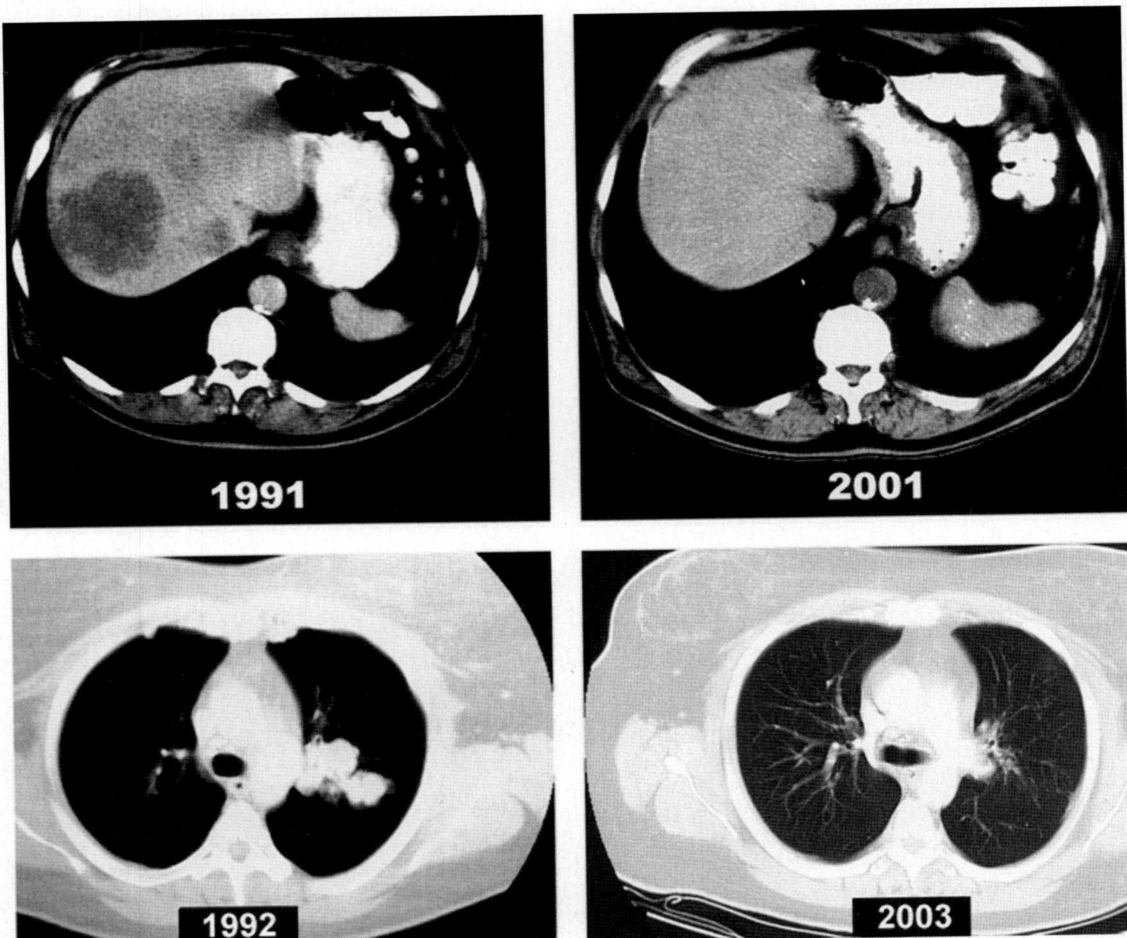

FIGURE 93.9 Two patients with visceral metastases from metastatic renal cancer who received high-dose interleukin-2 (IL-2) only and achieved complete responses. Patients showing initial resolution of all detectable disease rarely relapse as documented by follow-up that now exceeds 20 years for some patients.

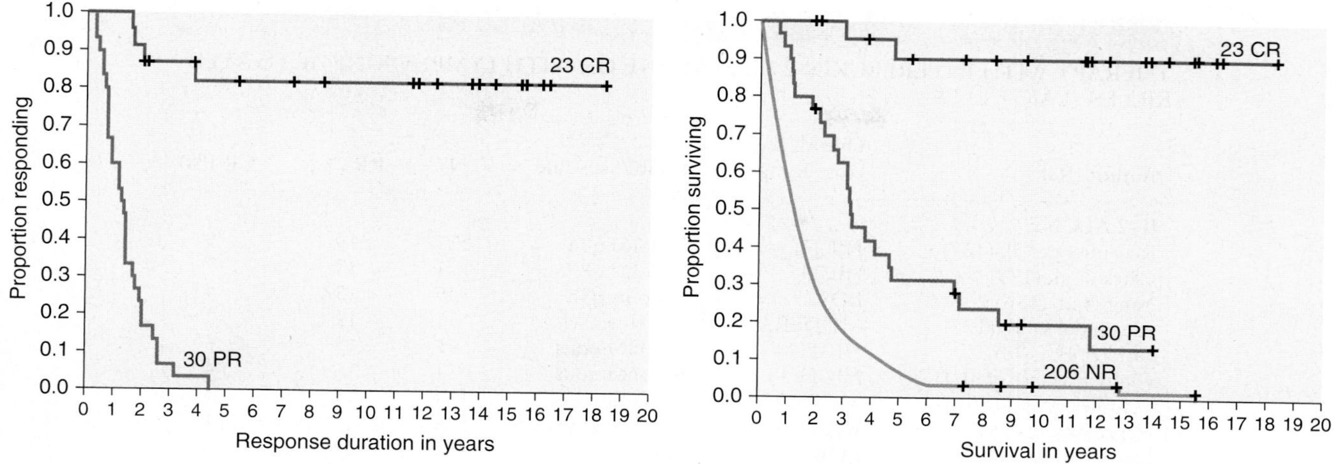

FIGURE 93.10 Experience with high-dose interleukin-2 (IL-2) in 259 patients with metastatic clear cell renal cancer. Response durations for complete and partial responders (**A**) and overall survival for responders and nonresponders are shown (**B**). Completely responding patients rarely experience relapse and nearly all long-term survivors had achieved an objective response to IL-2. The majority of patients who survived despite relapsing after a response were salvaged by surgical resection of a limited site(s) of recurrence, while maintaining their responses at other sites.

patients (nearly half of all responding patients) had a complete response, and the majority of those completely responding patients have never relapsed[163–166] (Fig. 93.10). These data (along with a similar experience with metastatic melanoma) constitute the first convincing evidence that immunotherapy can cure some patients with metastatic cancer. This was also the basis for the approval of IL-2 by the FDA for this disease. It should be emphasized that it is the curative potential of these responses, not their frequency, that is of note. These studies largely treated clear cell renal cancer and its variants and do not address whether other biologically distinct forms of renal cancer can respond. There is no consistent information documenting responses to IL-2 in patients with pure papillary, chromophobe, medullary, or collecting duct renal cancer. Although some controversy exists as to the response rates of sarcomatoid tumor variants of clear cell tumors, molecular analyses and published reports suggest that sarcomatoid, granular, and clear cell tumors with papillary features can all respond to IL-2 treatment.[49]

Following the initial studies with IL-2, several developments have occurred. The use of LAK cells with IL-2 has been critically examined in randomized studies. Although murine micrometastatic models predicted that the addition of LAK cells to IL-2 would substantially increase therapeutic efficacy, this has not proven to be true in clinical studies. A randomized comparison of high-dose intravenous bolus IL-2, with or without LAK cells, showed an insignificant difference in response rate (21% for IL-2 and 31% for IL-2 and LAK cells) with no difference in survival.[167] Other studies have confirmed this,[168] and currently there is no evidence to support the use of LAK cells in patients with RCC.

The initial rapid escalation of IL-2 to its maximum tolerated dose identified 600,000 to 720,000 IU/kg by intravenous bolus given every 8 hours as the maximum tolerated dose. On that schedule, patients tolerated approximately seven to nine consecutive doses before treatment had to be stopped for vascular leak syndrome, hypotension, multiorgan dysfunction, and a variety of other toxicities.[169] These effects rapidly reversed after therapy is stopped, but with hypotension requiring vasopressor support, pulmonary edema, and potential infectious complications, a 2% to 4% treatment-related mortality was initially encountered. Since then, increased experience with IL-2, prophylactic antibiotics when indicated, and patient screening for occult coronary disease have dramatically decreased this mortality rate. A recent report cites 809 consecutive patients who received high-dose bolus IL-2 without a treatment-related morality,[170] attesting to the safety of this treatment in experienced hands. Nevertheless, the expense of ICU care and the unpredictability of toxicities on high-dose IL-2 led many investigators to try lower-dose regimens. In particular, daily subcutaneous self-administration was adopted as a convenient and inexpensive route. In a scenario replayed many times during the development of IL-2, a multitude of small phase 2 studies were performed that reported short-term response rates similar to those seen with high-dose IL-2. An outpatient, daily, self-administered regimen using an initial week (Monday thru Friday) of 18 million IU (fixed dose) followed by 5 weeks at half that dose was well tolerated and produced a response rate of 23% in 26 evaluable patients.[171] Later, continued experience with a modification of this regimen showed a 20% ORR with one ongoing complete response in 47 patients[172] and an 18% response rate by others using a similar regimen.[173] Yet other investigators reported that high-dose continuous infusion IL-2 could achieve a similar response rate with less toxicity (and less overall IL-2 given for the same time period).[174] A review of the literature shows response rates to IL-2 delivered on many different schedules and at different doses, range from 8% to 35% (Table 93.6). Although it is clear that small nonrandomized studies cannot discern whether one schedule is more effective than another, low-dose schedules were widely adopted before being critically evaluated. A randomized study addressing this issue assigned patients to receive IL-2 at either 720,000 IU/kg or 72,000 IU/kg every 8 hours by intravenous bolus to maximum tolerance (or up to 15 consecutive doses).[190] The lower dose was selected as the maximal dose tolerated without intensive care unit care and vasopressor support. This two-arm comparison specifically addressed whether the dose of IL-2 was important. Subsequently, a third arm was added to the trial to evaluate the widely used daily, subcutaneous route of administration. This arm delivered 250,000 IU/kg daily for five days in the first week and then half that dose 5 days a week for the subsequent 5 weeks. Only concurrently randomized patients are compared in this two-stage trial. Although it is clear that the two lower dose regimens had lesser toxicity, especially in the areas of hypotension requiring pressors (36% of courses of high-dose IV IL-2 versus 3% of courses of low-dose IV IL-2 versus none with subcutaneous IL-2), thrombocytopenia, pulmonary distress, and disorientation, it is important to note that there were no deaths or major

TABLE 93.6

THERAPY WITH INTERLEUKIN-2 (IL-2) ALONE OR WITH LYMPHOKINE ACTIVATED KILLER (LAK) CELLS

Author (Ref.)	Overall IL-2 Dose Range[a]	Route/Schedule	N	RR (%)	CR (%)
IL-2 ALONE					
Rosenberg et al. (167)	HIGH	iv bolus q8h	227	19	9
Clark et al. (175)	HIGH	iv bolus q8h	71	17	7
Yang et al. (176)	LOW	iv bolus q8h	149	13	4
Alexander et al. (177)	MODERATE	iv 3 times/wk	41	12	2
Gold et al. (178)	HIGH	iv continuous	47	13	6
von der Maase et al. (179)	HIGH	iv continuous	51	16	4
Escudier et al. (180)	MODERATE	iv continuous	104	19	4
Negrier et al. (181)	HIGH	iv continuous	138	7	1
Lissoni et al. (182)	LOW	sc daily	91	23	2
Buter et al. (172)	LOW	sc daily	47	19	4
Kantor et al. (183)	LOW	sc 1-2/d	39	18	3
Yang et al. (176)	LOW	sc daily	93	10	2
			1098	15.4	4.5
IL-2 AND LAK CELLS					
Rosenberg et al. (184)	HIGH	iv bolus q8h	72	35	11
Fisher et al. (162)	HIGH	iv bolus q8h	35	14	6
Weiss et al. (185)	HIGH	iv bolus q8h	46	20	7
Parkinson et al. (186)	HIGH	iv continuous	47	9	4
Negrier et al. (187)	HIGH	iv continuous	51	27	10
Dillman et al. (187)	HIGH	iv continuous	46	15	N/A
Thompson et al. (188)	HIGH	iv continuous	76	22	8
Weiss et al. (185)	HIGH	iv continuous	48	15	4
			421	20.9	8.0

iv, intravenous; sc, subcutaneous.
[a]High dose indicates significant multiorgan toxicity and vasopressors with intensive care unit (ICU) support needed in over a quarter of treatments. Moderate dose indicates occasional multiorgan toxicity or significant single organ toxicity with occasional ICU support. Low dose indicates rare or mild multiorgan toxicity and rare ICU support, typically given in the outpatient setting.
(Adapted from ref. 189)

irreversible toxicities in any of the treatment arms. With a total of 400 patients randomized and a median follow-up of over 5 years, response rates are as shown in Table 93.7. In the two-arm comparison of high- and low-dose intravenous bolus IL-2, the respective response rates are 21% and 13% (P = .05). The duration of the responses are notable, as 8 of 11 patients completely responding to high-dose IL-2 remain in complete response beyond 4 years, while only 3 of 6 patients completely responding to low-dose IL-2 were maintaining their responses at 2 years (with a significant difference in the survival of completely responding patients in these two arms). The subset of patients randomized between three treatment arms showed response rates of 21%, 11%, and 10% for high-dose IV, low-dose IV, and subcutaneous IL-2, respectively, with the decrement in response rates of both low-dose regimens of borderline significance compared to high-dose therapy. As is common for IL-2 studies (where major benefit is manifested by a small minority of the patients treated), there were no significant differences when overall survival between any arms was assessed. Because the clinical benefit of IL-2 resides in the long-term complete responses attained by some patients, this study is most notable for the higher proportion of patients who attained complete responses when given high-dose therapy and the greater durability of those same complete responses. Very similar results were seen in another randomized study comparing high-dose bolus IV IL-2 (600,000 IU/kg/dose every 8 hours) to low-dose daily subcutaneous IL-2 with subcutaneous interferon alfa added.[191] This study compared the effect of IL-2 dose while also addressing whether the addition of interferon-α to low-dose outpatient IL-2 could compensate for any decrement in efficacy. After 95 evaluable patients were randomized to high-dose bolus therapy and 91 to low-dose IL-2 plus interferon, the response rates for these two groups were 23% and 10%, respectively (P = .02), with all seven durable complete responses found from high-dose bolus treatment.

Other studies have addressed the issue of continuous infusion IL-2 versus bolus IL-2. The initial nonrandomized studies that used continuous infusion IL-2 reported response rates similar to bolus IL-2 but lesser toxicities. In a subsequent randomized study (where all patients received LAK cells), patients received their IL-2 by either continuous infusion at 18 to 22.5 million IU/m^2/d or by intravenous bolus at 600,000 IU/kg/dose every 8 hours (the cumulative daily dose by bolus was over three times the dose by continuous infusion).[185] Both of these doses represented the maximally tolerated amounts for their respective routes of administration, and the few significant differences in toxicities did not favor either regimen. In this study, patients who received LAK cells and bolus IL-2 had a 20% major response rate compared to a 15% response rate for patients who were given LAK cells and continuous infusion IL-2 (P = N.S.). Other studies demonstrate the complete responses to high-dose continuous infusion IL-2 can also be of

TABLE 93.7

RANDOMIZED COMPARISONS OF HIGH- AND LOW-DOSE INTERLEUKIN-2

		National Cancer Institute (NCI) (ref. 50)			Cytokine Working Group (CWG) (ref. 189)	
		High-dose IV	Low-dose IV	Low-dose SC	High-dose IV	Low-dose SC + IFN
Patients (N)		156	150	94	96	96
Grade III/IV toxicity (%)[a]	Hypotension	36	3	0	57	1
	Neurological	10	4	2	15	3
	Cardiac	6	3	0	8	0
	Renal	1	3	1	14	3
IL-2 related deaths		0	0	0	1	1
Partial responses (N)		22	13	7	14	6
Complete responses (N)		11	6	2	8	3
Overall response rate (%)		21	13	10	23	10

IV, intravenous; SC, subcutaneous; IFN, interferon; IL, interleukin.
[a]Percentage of treatment courses for NCI, percent of patients for CWG (From ref. 189.)

long duration. A single institution study of 123 patients (some also receiving LAK cells) with follow-up of 1 to 109 months reported an ORR of 19%, with 7% complete responses, and 78% of those complete responses sustained at 42 to 109 or more months.[178]

A more complex issue is whether any combination of cytokine or chemotherapy added to interleukin-2 is superior to IL-2 alone. Here again, small, nonrandomized phase 2 studies have clouded this issue. Small studies combining IL-2 with interferon or chemotherapy (or both) reported improved short-term response rates but generated large, overlapping confidence intervals. The combination of interferon-α and IL-2 is especially appealing because both agents have single-agent activity against RCC, and preclinical animal models predict synergistic benefit from combining these agents. Early reports suggest that the response rate for patients with metastatic RCC might rise from 18% to 20% with high-dose IL-2 alone, to as much as 31% with high-dose IL-2 plus interferon.[184] However, further accrual and long-term follow-up of the patients in this study did not show sufficient improvement in either response rate or survival (when compared to historical controls from the same institution) to warrant the additional toxicity seen.[192] Other investigators have been utilizing this combination of cytokines in order to reduce the dose of IL-2 needed for a response and thus limit toxicity. Most have employed outpatient, subcutaneous schedules.[193] The initial nonrandomized reports on this regimen emphasized lesser toxicities, but similar response rates to high-dose IL-2 monotherapy. Yet when others have tried the same or similar regimens, their response rates as well as their toxicity profiles have not been as favorable. One randomized evaluation of IL-2 and interferon by Negrier et al.[194] randomized 425 patients to receive either continuous infusion, high-dose IL-2 alone, subcutaneous interferon-α three times a week or both agents simultaneously. There was a significantly higher response rate with the combination (18.6%) than with only IL-2 (6.5%) or interferon (7.5%), but this increased response rate did not translate into improved survival. This study demonstrated an unusually low response rate to IL-2 alone, and patients with tumor progression crossed over between therapy arms. Other small, randomized studies of IL-2 and interferon have also failed to demonstrate an advantage to combination therapy, but these studies are largely underpowered.[195,196]

In a further effort to enhance efficacy with other agents, investigators have added 5-fluorouracil (5-FU), which has a low, single-agent response rate against RCC, to IL-2 and interferon. Again early phase 2 studies report major increases in response rates,[197] but later studies do not always substantiate this.[198] In fact, an attempt to exactly reproduce the initial studies with 5-FU, interferon, and IL-2 (which had a reported response rate of 49%) resulted in a partial and complete response rate of 16%—exactly the same as with IL-2 alone.[199] Although some have reported favorable response durations, Dutcher et al.,[199] reviewing their sequential use of IL-2, IL-2 plus interferon, and IL-2 plus interferon plus 5-FU, saw no augmentation of response rate and a decrease in the percentage of patients attaining durable complete responses with the three-drug combination. Most recently, a large multicenter randomized comparison with over 1,000 patients with advanced RCC was performed, comparing IFN-α alone with IFN-α, subcutaneous IL-2, and 5-FU.[200] Although there was a modestly higher response rate with the combination regimen (23% vs. 16%; $P = .005$), overall and progression-free survival did not differ ($P = .55$ and $P = .81$, respectively), with only 2% of patients in each arm achieving complete responses. These data conclusively establish that such combination regimens do not offer clinical benefit over cytokine monotherapy and may have less curative potential than some alternatives.

Short-term gains could be achieved by simply defining patients who are more likely to respond to IL-2 prior to treatment. A retrospective study by one group has found that high expression of carbonic anhydrase IX (a protein controlled by the VHL/HIF pathway) is associated with a higher probability of response to IL-2.[201] A prospective evaluation of this parameter is under way. It remains unclear if this is simply a surrogate means of selecting true clear cell renal cancers or an independent predictor of response, but it may prove useful in either regard.

Vaccines, Immunomodulating Antibodies, and Cellular Therapy

There has been an ongoing effort to identify immune cells with reactivity to renal cancer. As described above, the use of nonspecific activated killer cells (NK or LAK cells) has largely been ineffective, but current efforts have concentrated on T cells and the induction of a T-cell response via vaccination. Following the lead of melanoma research, tumor infiltrating lymphocytes (TIL), isolated from renal cancer specimens and cells from mixed lymphocyte-tumor reactions, were examined for antitumor reactivity. With some notable exceptions,[202–204] little specific tumor reactivity was seen.[205] Attempts to use TIL clinically have showed some promising early results (usually combined with IL-2 and interferon-α),[206] but a randomized trial of IL-2 with and without CD8-enriched TIL was fraught with technical difficulties and showed no augmentation in response rate or survival with cell transfer.[207] Because of the relative scarcity of tumor-reactive specific T-cells against renal cancer, another approach has been the use of vaccines. Typically whole tumor preparations have been used because of the failure to identify broadly applicable common tumor antigens expressed by RCC. In one study, the gene for granulocyte-macrophage colony-stimulating factor (GM-CSF) was introduced into autologous cultured renal cell cancer lines by retroviral transduction in a concept based on preclinical studies.[208] Patients were then immunized with irradiated tumor cells that secreted large amounts of GM-CSF (or control nontransduced cells) and evaluated for immune responses and clinical tumor regression. One partial response was seen in 16 evaluable patients, but this approach is hampered by the requirement for an autologous cultured tumor line. Subsequently, two large randomized studies of this vaccine approach in patients with metastatic prostate cancer showed no clinical activity, dampening enthusiasm for further investigations in renal cancer.

A new area of investigation is the targeting of immunoinhibitory receptors with blocking antibodies and immunoenhancing receptors with agonist antibodies. Families of receptors expressed by lymphocytes that modulate their activity have been described and include agonist coreceptors such as CD28, 4-1BB, and OX40 and inhibitory receptors such as CTLA4, PD-1, and SOCS. Renal cancer cells themselves have even been described as expressing the ligands for some of these inhibitory lymphocyte receptors, and the expression of those ligands can be associated with an unfavorable prognosis. Therefore, agents that target these immunomodulating receptors are progressing to clinical testing, and monoclonal antibodies are being used as one approach. A monoclonal blocking antibody, ipilimumab, which targets the inhibitory receptor CTLA4, has been used in phase 1 through 3 trials in patients with melanoma and can causes responses in 10% to 15% of patients, with some complete responses of long duration. One phase 2 study in patients with metastatic renal cancer showed a response rate of 13% when given at 3 mg/kg every 3 weeks.[176] Treatment-related toxicities appeared immune mediated, and colitis and hypophysitis were the most common, with some patients experiencing perforation or hypopituitarism. As in patients with melanoma, there was a striking association between this apparent autoimmune toxicity and tumor regression. Two such antibodies against CTLA4 are currently in clinical testing and others targeting PD-1 are moving forward. The demonstration that this type of immunomodulation can induce tumor rejection in some patients with renal cancer will likely lead to further studies.

Another immunotherapeutic approach used against renal cancer is a nonmyeloablative allogeneic peripheral-blood stem cell transplant, with the hypothesis that a graft-versus-tumor response (as seen in leukemia) may lead to tumor regression. With this strategy, investigators saw tumor regression that did not occur until the onset of complete donor chimerism, tapering of immunosuppression, and, in most cases, the appearance of mild graft-versus-host disease (GVHD), supporting an immunological mechanism of action related to the allograft.[209] Response rates from different groups vary from 33% to 47%,[210,211] but they include patients who did not respond when given IL-2. It is still not clear if there is specific recognition of tumor-associated antigens by the matched allograft or if generalized GVHD leads to *in situ* production of cytokines, which then can treat an intrinsically cytokine-sensitive tumor. Clinical GVHD was highly associated with an improved probability of response but was not mandatory. The high frequency of GVHD also predictably led to substantial treatment-related mortality, ranging from 11% to 33%. As with IL-2 therapy, there are no data to document that this approach produces consistent responses in non–clear cell variants of renal cancer, nor indeed in any other tumor types, but this is still being investigated. This is an active modality that can produce major responses when other treatments have failed, but controlling toxicity and delineating the mechanism of action are important future goals.

Adjuvant Therapy

Despite the dramatic tumor regressions sometimes attained in patients with metastatic renal cancer given immunotherapy, frustration remains with the relatively low frequency of these successes. This has led to efforts to apply biotherapies earlier in the course of renal cancer and to the design of adjuvant strategies in the hope that smaller disease volumes might be more responsive. It is important to note that no retrospective analysis has identified lesser tumor burden as a predictor of the probability of responding in the metastatic setting, raising doubt as to the rationale for the adjuvant approach. Interferon is one agent that has been tested in a randomized adjuvant study following nephrectomy. Two hundred and eighty-three patients with completely resected T3 to T4a or N1, N2, or N3 disease were randomized to observation versus 9 months of subcutaneous lymphoblastoid interferon.[212] With a median follow-up of 10.4 years, patients who received interferon had similar recurrence rates, and they showed a trend toward poorer survival than patients randomized to observation only ($P = .09$). In view of these results and the limited response rate to interferon therapy of metastatic disease, there is currently no rationale for recommending adjuvant interferon outside of a protocol setting.

Another recent randomized study tested the administration of one course (two cycles) of high-dose bolus IL-2 versus no therapy in patients who had recently undergone resection of locally advanced or metastatic renal cancer.[175] After enrolling 69 patients, the study was stopped after interim analysis indicated that no significant differences could be demonstrated even if full accrual was attained. This result is not surprising in a study of this size in view of the finding that only a minority of patients with metastatic disease show any tumor regression with IL-2. A 200-patient randomized trial of adjuvant subcutaneous IL-2, interferon, and 5-FU versus observation after nephrectomy also failed to show a benefit in disease-free survival, and overall survival was significantly worse in the treated group.[213]

A large, randomized phase 3 adjuvant trial was undertaken to determine if vaccinating patients with autologous tumor-derived heat-shock proteins (chaperones for tumor antigens and activators of dendritic cells) can reduce the incidence of tumor recurrence when compared to observation in patients with high-risk primary tumors. Despite extensive supportive preclinical data for this approach, it has shown little evidence of efficacy in patients with measurable metastatic disease, and this phase 3 adjuvant trial that enrolled over 800 patients failed to show a significant progression-free or survival benefit.[214] In summary, for renal cancer, there are no data to support the application of immunotherapies in the adjuvant setting, and in view of the toxicity of some treatments, the lack of a relationship between tumor burden and response rate (in the metastatic setting), and uncertainties about the necessary duration of treatment, it seems currently preferable to reserve immunotherapy for patients with evaluable disease.

Selected References

The full list of references for this chapter appears in the online version.

1. Jemal A, Siegel R, Ward E, et al. Cancer statistics, 2009. *CA Cancer J Clin* 2009;59:225.
2. Chow WH, Devesa SS, Warren JL, Fraumeni JF Jr. Rising incidence of renal cell cancer in the United States. *JAMA* 1999;281(17):1628.
3. Linehan WM, Walther MM, Zbar B. The genetic basis of cancer of the kidney. *J Urol* 2003;170(6 Pt 1):2163.
9. Lowrance WT, Thompson RH, Yee DS, Kaag M, Donat SM, Russo P. Obesity is associated with a higher risk of clear-cell renal cell carcinoma than with other histologies. *BJU Int* 2010;105(1):16–20.
22. Linehan WM, Vasselli J, Srinivasan R, et al. Genetic basis of cancer of the kidney: disease-specific approaches to therapy. *Clin Cancer Res* 2004;10(18):6282S.
23. Latif F, Tory K, Gnarra JR, et al. Identification of the von Hippel-Lindau disease tumor suppressor gene. *Science* 1993;260(5112):1317.
25. Schmidt LS, Li F, Brown RS, et al. Mechanism of tumorigenesis of renal carcinomas associated with the constitutional chromosome 3;8 translocation. *Cancer J Sci Am* 1995;1(3):191.
26. Gnarra JR, Tory K, Weng Y, et al. Mutations of the VHL tumour suppressor gene in renal carcinoma. *Nat Genet* 1994;7(1):85.
27. Nickerson ML, Jaeger E, Shi Y, et al. Improved identification of von Hippel-Lindau gene alterations in clear cell renal tumors. *Clin Cancer Res* 2008;14(15):4726.
28. Zbar B, Tory K, Merino MJ, et al. Hereditary papillary renal cell carcinoma. *J Urol* 1994;151(3):561.
31. Schmidt LS, Duh FM, Chen F, et al. Germline and somatic mutations in the tyrosine kinase domain of the MET proto-oncogene in papillary renal carcinomas. *Nat Genet* 1997;16(1):68.
33. Zbar B, Alvord WG, Glenn GM, et al. Risk of renal and colonic neoplasms and spontaneous pneumothorax in the Birt-Hogg-Dube syndrome. *Cancer Epidemiol Biomarkers Prev* 2002;11(4):393.
34. Pavlovich CP, Walther MM, Eyler RA, et al. Renal tumors in the Birt-Hogg-Dubé syndrome. *Am J Surg Pathol* 2002;26(12):1542.
36. Schmidt LS, Nickerson ML, Warren MB, et al. Germline BHD-mutation spectrum and phenotype analysis of a large cohort of families with Birt-Hogg-Dubé syndrome. *Am J Hum Genet* 2005;76(6):1023.
38. Tomlinson IP, Alam NA, Rowan AJ, et al. Germline mutations in FH predispose to dominantly inherited uterine fibroids, skin leiomyomata and papillary renal cell cancer. *Nat Genet* 2002;30(4):406.
39. Toro JR, Nickerson ML, Wei MH, et al. Mutations in the fumarate hydratase gene cause hereditary leiomyomatosis and renal cell cancer in families in North America. *Am J Hum Genet* 2003;73(1):95.
41. Vanharanta S, Buchta M, McWhinney SR, et al. Early-onset renal cell carcinoma as a novel extraparaganglial component of SDHB-associated heritable paraganglioma. *Am J Hum Genet* 2004;74(1):153.
42. Linehan WM, Pinto PA, Bratslavsky G, et al. Hereditary kidney cancer: unique opportunity for disease-based therapy. *Cancer* 2009;115(10 Suppl):2252.
43. Crino PB, Nathanson KL, Henske EP. The tuberous sclerosis complex. *N Engl J Med* 2006;355(13):1345.
44. Lane BR, Aydin H, Danforth TL, et al. Clinical correlates of renal angiomyolipoma subtypes in 209 patients: classic, fat poor, tuberous sclerosis associated and epithelioid. *J Urol* 2008;180(3):836.
46. Davis IJ, Hsi BL, Arroyo JD, et al. Cloning of an Alpha-TFEB fusion in renal tumors harboring the t(6;11)(p21;q13) chromosome translocation. *Proc Natl Acad Sci U S A* 2003;100(10):6051.
62. Huang WC, Elkin EB, Levey AS, Jang TL, Russo P. Partial nephrectomy versus radical nephrectomy in patients with small renal tumors—is there a difference in mortality and cardiovascular outcomes? *J Urol* 2009;181(1):55.
66. Rogers CG, Metwalli A, Blatt AM, et al. Robotic partial nephrectomy for renal hilar tumors: a multi-institutional analysis. *J Urol* 2008;180(6):2353.
67. Gill IS. Minimally invasive nephron-sparing surgery. *Urol Clin North Am* 2003;30(3):551.
73. Grubb RL III, Franks ME, Toro J, et al. Hereditary leiomyomatosis and renal cell cancer: a syndrome associated with an aggressive form of inherited renal cancer. *J Urol* 2007;177(6):2074.
74. Volpe A, Panzarella T, Rendon RA, et al. The natural history of incidentally detected small renal masses. *Cancer* 2004;100(4):738.
75. Crispen PL, Viterbo R, Boorjian SA, et al. Natural history, growth kinetics, and outcomes of untreated clinically localized renal tumors under active surveillance. *Cancer* 2009;115(13):2844.
78. Flanigan RC, Salmon SE, Blumenstein BA, et al. Nephrectomy followed by interferon alfa-2b compared with interferon alfa-2b alone for metastatic renal-cell cancer. *N Engl J Med* 2001;345(23):1655.
148. Snow RM, Schellhammer PF. Spontaneous regression of metastatic renal cell carcinoma. *Urology* 1982;20:177.
153. Quesada JR, Rios A, Swanson D, et al. Antitumor activity of recombinant-derived interferon alpha in metastatic renal cell carcinoma. *J Clin Oncol* 1985;3:1522.
156. Moss HB. Interferon therapy for renal cell carcinoma. *Sem Oncol* 1987;14(2 Suppl 2):36.
158. Medical Research Council Renal Cancer Collaborators. Interferon-a and survival in metastatic renal carcinoma: early results of a randomized controlled trial. *Lancet* 1999;353:14.
160. Rosenberg SA, Lotze MT, Muul LM, et al. A progress report on the treatment of 157 patients with advanced cancer using lymphokine-activated killer cells and interleukin-2 or high-dose interleukin-2 alone. *N Engl J Med* 1987;316(15):889.
161. Lotze MT, Chang AE, Seipp CA, et al. High-dose recombinant interleukin 2 in the treatment of patients with disseminated cancer: responses, treatment-related morbidity and histologic findings. *JAMA* 1986;256:3117.
162. Fisher RI, Coltman CA, Doroshow JH, et al. Metastatic renal cancer treated with interleukin-2 and lymphokine-activated killer cells. *Ann Intern Med* 1988;108:518.
163. Fisher RI, Rosenberg SA, Sznol M, Parkinson DR, Fyfe G. High-dose aldesleukin in renal cell carcinoma: long-term survival update. *Cancer J Sci Am* 1997;3:S70.
164. Rosenberg SA, Yang JC, Topalian SL, et al. Treatment of 283 consecutive patients with metastatic melanoma or renal cell cancer using high-dose bolus interleukin-2. *JAMA* 1994;271:907.
165. Rosenberg SA, Yang JC, White DE, Steinberg SM. Durability of complete responses in patients with metastatic cancer treated with high-dose interleukin-2: identification of the antigens mediating response. *Ann Surg* 1998;228(3):307.
166. Gore ME, Griffin CL, Hancock B, et al. Interferon alfa-2a versus combination therapy with interferon alfa-2a, interleukin-2, and fluorouracil in patients with untreated metastatic renal cell carcinoma (MRC RE04/EORTC GU 30012): an open-label randomised trial. *Lancet* 2010;375(9715):641.
168. Law TM, Motzer R, Mazumdar M, et al. Phase III randomized trial of interleukin-2 with or without lymphokine activated killer cells in the treatment of patients with advanced renal cell carcinoma. *Cancer* 1995;76:824.
169. Margolin KA, Rayner AA, Hawkins MJ, et al. Interleukin-2 and lymphokine-activated killer cell therapy of solid tumors: analysis of toxicity and management guidelines. *J Clin Oncol* 1989;7(4):486.
170. Kammula US, White DE, Rosenberg SA. Trends in the safety of high dose bolus interleukin-2 administration in patients with metastatic cancer. *Cancer* 1998;83:797.
171. Sleijfer DT, Janssen RA, Buter J, et al. Phase II study of subcutaneous interleukin-2 in unselected patients with advanced renal cell cancer on an outpatient basis. *J Clin Oncol* 1992;10:1119.
172. Buter J, Sleijfer DT, Winette TA, et al. A progress report on the outpatient treatment of patients with advanced renal cell carcinoma using subcutaneous recombinant interleukin-2. *Sem Oncol* 1993;20:16.
174. West WH, Tayer KW, Yannelli JR, et al. Constant-infusion recombinant interleukin-2 plus lymphokine-activated killer cells in metastatic renal cancer. *N Engl J Med* 1987;316:898.
175. Clark JI, Atkins MB, Urba WJ, et al. Adjuvant high-dose bolus interleukin-2 for patients with high-risk renal cell carcinoma: a cytokine working group randomized trial. *J Clin Oncol* 2003;21(16):3133.
176. Yang JC, Hughes M, Kammula U, et al. Ipilimumab (anti-CTLA4 antibody) causes regression of metastatic renal cell cancer associated with enteritis and hypophysitis. *J Immunother* 2007;30(8):825.
178. Gold PJ, Thompson JA, Markowitz DR, Neumann S, Fefer A. Metastatic renal cell carcinoma: long-term survival after therapy with high-dose continuous-infusion interleukin-2 [comments]. *Cancer J Sci Am* 1997;3(Suppl 1):S85.
184. Rosenberg SA, Lotze MT, Yang JC, et al. Combination therapy with interleukin-2 and alpha-interferon for the treatment of patients with advanced cancer. *J Clin Oncol* 1989;7:1863.
185. Weiss GR, Margolin KA, Aronson FR, et al. A randomized phase II trial of continuous infusion interleukin-2 or bolus injection interleukin-2 plus lymphokine-activated killer cells for advanced renal cell carcinoma. *J Clin Oncol* 1992;10(2):275.
190. Yang JC, Sherry RM, Steinberg SM, et al. Randomized study of high-dose and low-dose interleukin-2 in patients with metastatic renal cancer. *J Clin Oncol* 2003;21(16):3127.
191. McDermott DF, Regan MM, Clark JI, et al. Randomized phase III trial of high-dose interleukin-2 versus subcutaneous interleukin-2 and interferon in patients with metastatic renal cell carcinoma. *J Clin Oncol* 2005;23(1):133.
192. Marincola FM, White DE, Wise AP, Rosenberg SA. Combination therapy with interferon alfa-2a and interleukin-2 for the treatment of metastatic cancer. *J Clin Oncol* 1995;13:1110.
193. Atzpodien J, Hanninen EL, Kirchner H, et al. Multi-institutional home-therapy trial of recombinant human interleukin-2 and interferon alfa-2 in progressive metastatic renal cell carcinoma. *J Clin Oncol* 1995;13:497.
194. Negrier S, Escudier B, Lasset C, et al. Recombinant human interleukin-2, recombinant human interferon alfa-2a, or both in metastatic renal-cell carcinoma. Groupe Francais d'Immunotherapie [comments]. *N Engl J Med* 1998;338(18):1272.

195. Atkins MB, Sparano J, Fisher RI, et al. Randomized phase II trial of high-dose interleukin-2 either alone or in combination with interferon alfa-2b in advanced renal cell carcinoma. *J Clin Oncol* 1993;11:661.
196. Jayson GC, Middleton M, Lee SM, Ashcroft L, Thatcher N. A randomized phase II trial of interleukin 2 and interleukin 2-interferon alpha in advanced renal cancer. *Br J Cancer* 1998;78:366.
197. Atzpodien J, Kirchner H, Hanninen EL, et al. Interleukin-2 in combination with interferon-alpha and 5-fluorouracil for metastatic renal cell cancer. *Eur J Cancer* 1993;29A(Suppl 5):S6.
198. Ravaud A, Audhuy B, Gomez F, et al. Subcutaneous interleukin-2, interferon alfa-2a, and continuous infusion of fluorouracil in metastatic renal cell carcinoma: a multicenter phase II trial. Groupe Francais d'Immunotherapie. *J Clin Oncol* 1998;16(8):2728.
199. Dutcher JP, Atkins M, Fisher R, et al. Interleukin-2-based therapy for metastatic renal cell cancer: the Cytokine Working Group experience, 1989–1997. *Cancer J Sci Am* 1997;3(Suppl 1):S73.
200. Klapper JA, Downey SG, Smith FO, et al. High-dose interleukin-2 for the treatment of metastatic renal cell carcinoma: a retrospective analysis of response and survival in patients treated in the surgery branch at the National Cancer Institute between 1986 and 2006. *Cancer* 2008;113(2):293.
202. Gaugler B, Brouwenstijn N, Vantomme V, et al. A new gene coding for an antigen recognized by autologous cytolytic T lymphocytes on a human renal carcinoma. *Immunogenetics* 1996;44(5):323.
205. Belldegrun A, Muul LM, Rosenberg SA. Interleukin 2 expanded tumor-infiltrating lymphocytes in human renal cell cancer: isolation, characterization, and antitumor activity. *Cancer Res* 1988;48(1):206.
207. Figlin RA, Thompson JA, Bukowski RM, et al. Multicenter, randomized, phase III trial of CD8(+) tumor-infiltrating lymphocytes in combination with recombinant interleukin-2 in metastatic renal cell carcinoma. *J Clin Oncol* 1999;17(8):2521.
209. Childs R, Chernoff A, Contentin N, et al. Regression of metastatic renal-cell carcinoma after nonmyeloablative allogeneic peripheral-blood stem-cell transplantation. *N Engl J Med* 2000;343(11):750.
211. Rini BI, Zimmerman T, Stadler WM, Gajewski TF, Vogelzang NJ. Allogeneic stem-cell transplantation of renal cell cancer after nonmyeloablative chemotherapy: feasibility, engraftment, and clinical results. *J Clin Oncol* 2002;20(8):2017.
212. Messing EM, Manola J, Wilding G, et al. Phase III study of interferon alfa-NL as adjuvant treatment for resectable renal cell carcinoma: an Eastern Cooperative Oncology Group/Intergroup trial. *J Clin Oncol* 2003; 21(7):1214.
214. Wood CG, Escudier B, Lacombe L, et al. A multicenter, randomized, phase 3 trial of a novel autologous therapeutic vaccine (vitespen) vs. observation as adjuvant therapy in patients at high risk of recurrence after nephrectomy for renal cell carcinoma. Paper presented at: Annual Meeting of the American Urological Association; May 21, 2007; Anaheim, California (abst 633).

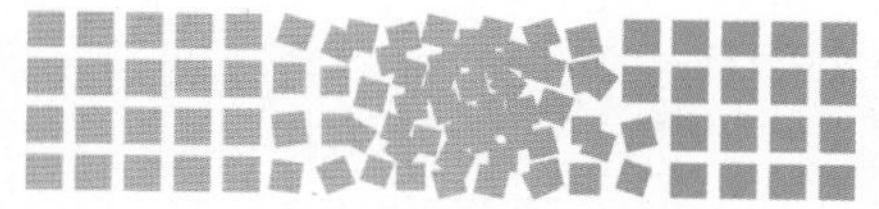

CHAPTER 94 MOLECULAR BIOLOGY OF BLADDER CANCER

MARGARET A. KNOWLES

Understanding of the molecular changes that underlie bladder cancer development has progressed rapidly.[1–4] Most studies have focused on urothelial carcinomas (UCs), which comprise the majority (>90%) of tumors diagnosed in the Western world. Where the parasite *Schistosoma haematobium* is endemic, squamous tumors predominate, and there is evidence that these differ at the molecular level.[5,6] This chapter will focus on somatic alterations identified in UC by genomic and RNA profiling. There is also much information about germline polymorphisms that confer increased risk of UC development and the reader is referred to recent reviews on this topic.[7–9]

At diagnosis more than 70% of UCs are noninvasive (Ta) or superficially invasive (T1) papillary lesions. These commonly recur, but progression to muscle invasion is infrequent (10% to 20%) and prognosis is good. In contrast, tumors that are muscle invasive at diagnosis (≥T2) have poor prognosis (<50% survival at 5 years). Carcinoma *in situ* (CIS) is a high-grade lesion, that is "superficial" in the strict sense, but has poor prognosis. It is not yet clear whether, or how often, papillary low-grade tumors become invasive. This has led to an ongoing debate, which is as yet unresolved.[1] The divergent behavior of these tumor groups is reflected in striking differences in their molecular profiles.[1–4]

MOLECULAR ALTERATIONS IN SUPERFICIAL UROTHELIAL CARCINOMA

Low-grade Ta papillary UCs are genetically stable and commonly contain point mutations or loss of entire chromosomes of chromosome arms rather than complex chromosomal rearrangements. Recent findings also indicate significant alteration or microRNA (miRNA) expression. Common alterations are deletions of chromosome 9 (>50%), mutations of FGF receptor 3 (*FGFR3*), and mutations of the p110α catalytic subunit of phosphatidylinositol-3-kinase (PI3K) (*PIK3CA*) (Table 94.1). These tumors are often near diploid. Loss of heterozygosity (LOH) of 11p is found in approximately 40% of UCs, including some Ta tumors, but is more common in tumors of higher grade and stage. Gains of 1q, 17, and 20q, amplifications of 11q, and loss of 10q have been identified but are not common (Table 94.1). Amplifications of 11q include the cyclin D1 gene (*CCND1*), which is involved in cell-cycle progression from G1 to S phase (Fig. 94.1).

Promoter hypermethylation of *APC*, *CDKN2A* (p14ARF), and *RASSF1A* has been found in DNA from urine of bladder cancer patients including those with low-grade/stage tumors.[10] However, this is more common in tumors of high tumor grade and stage.[11] Some hypermethylation in Ta/T1 tumors is associated with increased risk of progression.[12] A study that related regional gene expression to DNA copy number, identified genomic regions with altered expression that were copy number-independent, most showing down-regulation. Genes known to show promoter methylation in UC were not located in these regions, indicating other mechanisms of gene silencing.[13]

Low-grade Ta tumors are genetically stable. Thus, synchronous or metachronous tumors from the same patient show great genetic similarity, although some clonal evolution can be detected over time. LOH of chromosome 9 and mutation of *FGFR3* are the least divergent events, and widely believed to represent early genetic changes.[14,15] Flat urothelial hyperplasia, a predicted tumor precursor, shows more frequent chromosome 9 loss than *FGFR3* mutation, suggesting that this occurs earlier.[16]

Chromosome 9

More than 50% of UCs of all of grades and stages show chromosome 9 LOH, many with loss of an entire homologue.[17–19] A critical region on 9p21 and at least three regions on 9q (9q22, 9q32–q33, and 9q34) have been identified. Candidate genes within these regions are *CDKN2A* (p16/p14ARF) and *CDKN2B* (p15) at 9p21,[20–24] *PTCH* (Gorlin syndrome gene) at 9q22,[25,26] *DBC1* at 9q32–q33,[27–29] and *TSC1* (tuberous sclerosis syndrome gene 1) at 9q34[30–33] (Table 94.1).

CDKN2A (9p21) encodes the two cell-cycle regulators, p16 and p14ARF, which share coding region in exons 2 and 3 but have distinct exons 1. The protein products are translated in different reading frames to generate two entirely different proteins. p16 is a negative regulator of the Rb pathway and p14ARF, a negative regulator of the p53 pathway (Fig. 94.1). Inactivation of this locus in UC is commonly by homozygous deletion (HD). There are conflicting reports on association of 9p21 deletion with clinical parameters but HD appears to be associated with high tumor grade and stage.[34] Reduced copy number of 9p21 is present in approximately 45% of UC, indicating that, as suggested by knockout mice and *in vitro* experiments.[35,36] p16 and/or p14ARF may be haploinsufficient.[34]

On 9q, three genes are implicated. *PTCH*, the Gorlin syndrome gene (9q22) shows infrequent mutation,[26] but many tumors have reduced mRNA expression.[25] *DBC1* (9q33) shows HD in a few tumors[29,37] and no mutations, but is commonly silenced by hypermethylation.[27,38] LOH of 9q34 and mutation of the retained copy of *TSC1* is found in approximately 13% of UC.[39] The protein acts in complex with the TSC2 protein to negatively regulate mTOR, a central molecule in the control of protein synthesis and cell growth (Fig. 94.2).

FGFR3

Since the initial identification of *FGFR3* mutations in UC,[40] 11 different mutations have been identified.[41–54] These are in hotspot codons in exons 7, 10, and 15 (Fig. 94.3A) and are all

TABLE 94.1

GENETIC CHANGES IDENTIFIED IN Ta BLADDER TUMORS

Gene (Cytogenetic Location)	Alteration	Frequency (%) (Ref.)
ONCOGENES		
HRAS (11p15)/*NRAS* (1p13)/*KRAS2* (12p12)	Activating mutations	15 (60, 199–201)
FGFR3 (4p16)	Activating mutations	60–80 (40, 42, 43)
CCND1 (11q13)	Amplification/overexpression	10–20 (72, 202)
PIK3CA (3q26)	Activating mutations	27 PUNLMP; 16–30 Ta (39, 69)
MDM2 (12q13)	Overexpression	~30 overexpression (103, 203)
TUMOUR SUPPRESSOR GENES		
CDKN2A (9p21)	Homozygous deletion/ methylation/mutation	HD 20–30 (21, 23, 24) LOH ~60 (17)
PTCH (9q22)	Deletion/mutation	LOH ~60; mutation frequency low (25, 26)
DBC1 (9q32–33)	Deletion/methylation	LOH ~60 (38, 204)
TSC1 (9q34)	Deletion/mutation	LOH ~60; mutation ~12 (31, 33, 39)
DNA COPY NUMBER CHANGES[a]		
2q, 8p, 10p, 10q, 11p, 13q, 17p, 18q, Y	Deletion	~10 (186, 205, 206)
9p, 9q	Deletion	36–47 (186, 205, 206)
1q, 17q, 20q	Gain	11–17 (186, 205, 206)
8p12, 11q13 (including *CCND1*)	Amplification	Occasional (205, 206)

HD, homozygous deletion; LOH, loss of heterozygosity.
[a]Comparative genomic hybridization analyses.

predicted to constitutively activate the receptor.[55] Mutation is associated with low tumor grade and stage, with up to 80% of low-grade Ta tumors showing mutation.[42] Mutations are also found in urothelial papilloma, a likely precursor of superficial UC.[50] Mutation is not associated with tumor recurrence or progression in Ta tumors overall,[43,54,56] but there is evidence that mutant Ta grade 1 tumors show a higher risk of recurrence.[43] Tumors with *FGFR3* mutation show increased FGFR3 protein expression, as do a significant number of tumors without mutation.[57]

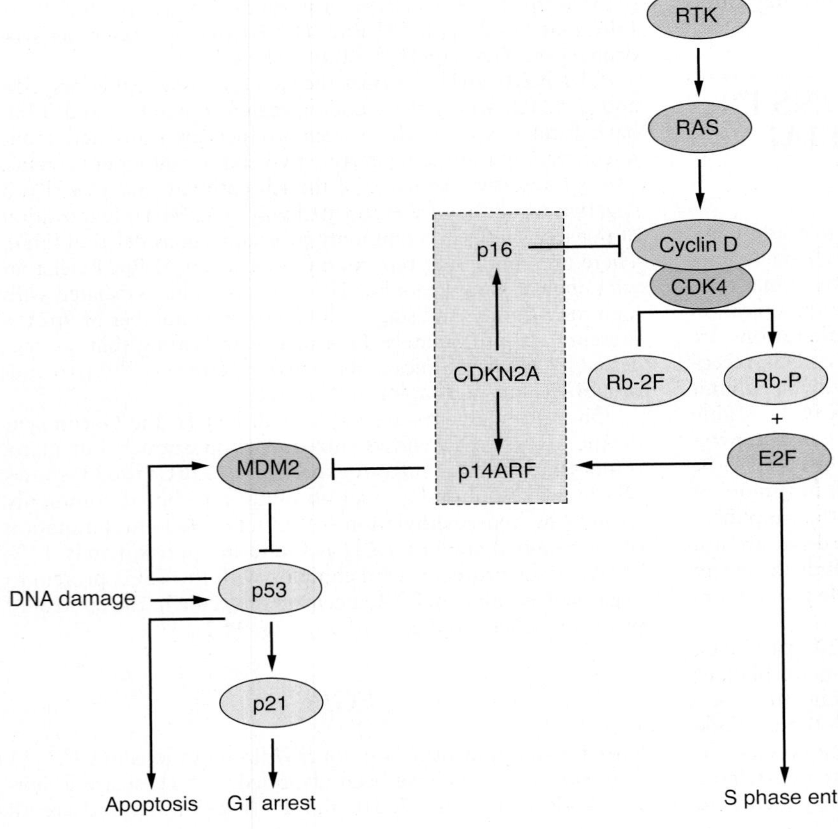

FIGURE 94.1 Key interactions in the Rb and p53 pathways. The *CDKN2A* locus encodes p16 and p14ARF that act as negative regulators of the Rb and p53 pathways, respectively. This interrelated signaling network is central to tumor suppression via the mechanisms of cell-cycle arrest and apoptosis. Stimulation by mitogens induces cyclin D1 expression. Phosphorylation of Rb by CDK4-cyclin D1 complexes releases E2F family members to induce expression of genes required for progression into S phase. The cyclin D-CDK4 complexes also sequester p27 and p21 (not shown). This allows formation of cyclin E-CDK2, which reinforces the inactivation of Rb. p16 negatively regulates this process by interacting with CDK4. The p53 pathway responds to stress signals (e.g., DNA damage). p21 expression is induced and this leads to cell-cycle arrest. MDM2 is a ubiquitin ligase responsible for inactivation of p53. In turn p53 regulates MDM2 expression providing a negative feedback loop. The p53 and Rb pathways are connected by p14ARF, which sequesters (inactivates) MDM2 in the nucleus and is up-regulated by E2Fs and in response to mitogenic signaling. Overexpression of E2Fs and oncogenes such as *MYC* can both result in p53-triggered cell-cycle arrest via p14ARF.

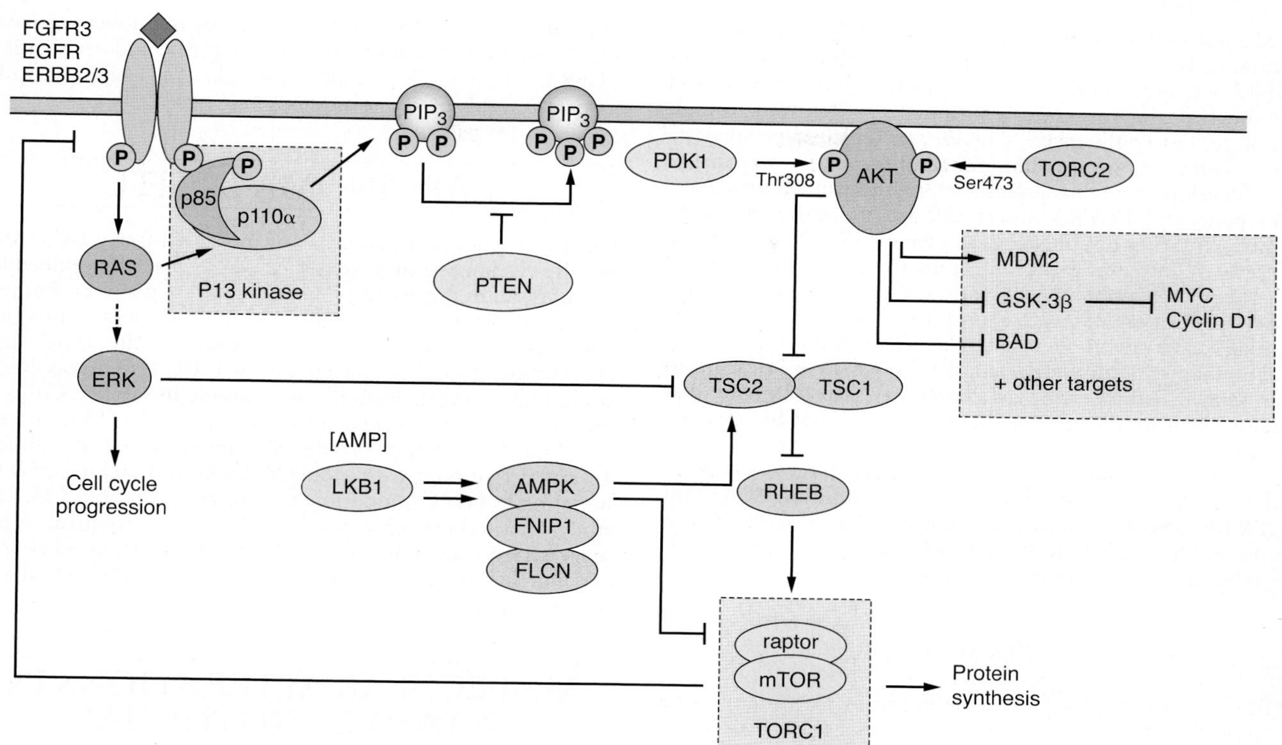

FIGURE 94.2 Oncogenic signaling via the RAS-MAPK and PI3K pathways. Growth factor-mediated signaling or mutational activation of Ras oncogenes can activate both of these pathways. Signaling via the RAS/RAF/MEK/ERK cascade leads to phosphorylation of many substrates that can have multiple cellular effects depending on the intensity and duration of signaling. In many situations proliferation is induced. Activated receptor tyrosine kinases bind p85, the regulatory subunit of PI3K, and recruit the enzyme to the membrane where it phosphorylates phosphatidyinositol-4, 5-bisphosphate (PIP2) to generate PIP3, which in turn recruits PDK1 and AKT to the membrane where AKT is activated by phosphorylation to regulate a wide range of target proteins (not all shown). Among these are cyclin D1 and MDM2, which are up-regulated either directly or indirectly, resulting in a positive stimulus via the Rb or p53 pathways, respectively. AKT also phosphorylates and inactivates tuberin the *TSC2* gene product, leading to activation of mTOR complex 1 (TORC1), which controls protein synthesis. The *TSC1* product hamartin forms an active complex with tuberin, and loss of function of either protein leads to dysregulated mTOR signaling. MYC expression is induced as a consequence of both by ERK and AKT signaling.

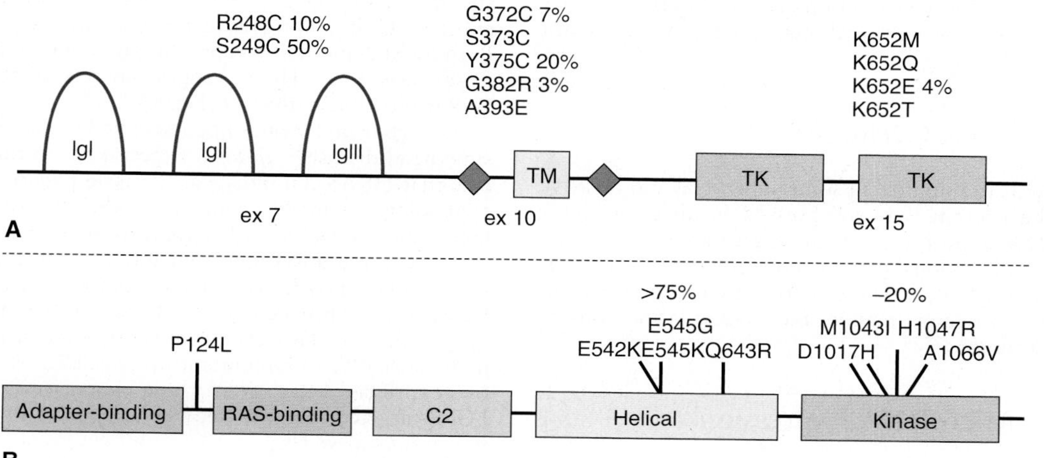

FIGURE 94.3 **A:** *FGFR3* mutations identified in bladder cancer. Positions of hot-spot mutations in exons 7, 10, and 15 that are found in bladder cancer are shown in relation to protein structure. The relative frequency of the more common mutations is given as a percentage. IgI, IgII, IgIII, immunoglobulinlike domains; TM, transmembrane domain; TK, tyrosine kinase domain. **B:** *PIK3CA* mutations identified in bladder cancer in relation to protein structure.

Mutant FGFR3 proteins are oncogenic in rodent mesenchymal cells.[58,59] In cultured normal urothelial cells, mutant FGFR3 activates the RAS-MAPK pathway, induces increased cell survival and stimulates continued proliferation to high cell density at confluence.[59] This *in vitro* phenotype suggests that *FGFR3* mutation could contribute to clonal expansion or the development of hyperplasia within the urothelium *in vivo*. RAS gene and *FGFR3* mutations are mutually exclusive events. Mutation of either a RAS gene or *FGFR3* was found in 82% of low-grade tumors, indicating that virtually all superficial UCs may share activation of the RAS-MAPK pathway.[60] Mutations of *FGFR3* and *TP53* are also somewhat mutually exclusive.[41,61] However, as *TP53* mutation is found predominantly in high-grade/stage UCs, which are thought to represent a distinct pathogenic pathway (see following discussion), it is predicted that these events are not biologically equivalent.

FGFR3 is considered a good therapeutic target in superficial UC.[62] Several studies indicate that inhibition of mutant *FGFR3* by knockdown or inhibition using small molecules or antibodies has a profound effect of UC cell phenotype including inhibition of xenograft growth *in vivo*.[58,63–68]

PIK3CA

PI3K plays a pivotal role in signaling from receptor tyrosine kinases (Fig. 94.2). Activating mutations of the p110α catalytic subunit (*PIK3CA*) are found in UC. One study identified mutations in 13%, with a significant association with low tumor grade and stage[69] and a second reported a frequency of 27%.[39] The development of a low-cost, high-throughput assay to detect the common variants should facilitate studies to clarify the exact frequency and clinical associations of these mutations.[70] The *PIK3CA* mutation spectrum (Fig. 94.3B) differs significantly from that in other cancers. Mutations E542K and E545K in the helical domain are most common (24% and 52%, respectively) and the kinase domain mutation H1047R, which is the most common mutation in other cancers, is less frequent (13% compared with 46% reported for other cancers in COSMIC, Catalogue of Somatic Mutations in Cancer [www.sanger.ac.uk/genetics/CGP/cosmic/]). The selective pressure for helical domain mutation in UC is not yet understood, although recent studies of the structure of p110α and the effect of the common activating mutations reveal different mechanisms of activation by helical domain and kinase domain mutations.[71]

Cyclin D1

CCND1 (11q13) is amplified in some superficial and invasive UCs[72] and the protein is overexpressed in an even larger number.[73–76] Overexpression in many cases may be the consequence of other alterations, such as activation of the MAPK or PI3K pathways (Fig. 94.2). There is no consensus on the clinical significance of overexpression, but up-regulation is more common in Ta tumors.[75,76]

MicroRNA Expression

There are several reports of altered miRNA expression in UC. Changes in apparently "normal" urothelium from UC patients indicate that such alterations may occur early in disease development.[77] Comparison of superficial and advanced UC indicates significant differences in profile.[77] Predominantly down-regulation of miRNAs was found in Ta tumors compared with normal urothelium. Interestingly, two of the down-regulated miRNAs, miR-99a and miR-100, were found to regulate FGFR3.[77] Low levels of miR-7 have also been reported to be associated with *FGFR3* mutation.[78]

CARCINOMA IN SITU

CIS is the predicted precursor of muscle-invasive UC.[79] It is usually recognized only retrospectively in paraffin-embedded samples, and few studies have assessed genetic changes. Alterations include *TP53* mutation, chromosome 9 loss, up-regulated ERBB2 expression, and a range of alterations similar to those found in muscle-invasive UC.[80–83] Array-based studies have revealed significant genomic instability. Gains of 5p, 6p22.3, 10p15.1, and losses of 5q and 13q13-q14 were common. The genomic profile was similar to that of high-risk Ta and T1 tumors with associated CIS and lacking *FGFR3* mutation.[84] *FGFR3* mutation has not been found in CIS. One study reported that chromosome 9 loss was infrequent in primary CIS but common in CIS associated with synchronous carcinoma,[84] indicating two forms of CIS with different developmental pathways.

MOLECULAR ALTERATIONS IN INVASIVE UROTHELIAL CARCINOMA

Many genetic alterations are found in muscle-invasive UC, including alterations to known genes and genomic alterations for which the target genes are currently unknown (Table 94.2).

Oncogenes

ERBB2 (17q23), a receptor tyrosine kinase of the *EGFR* gene family, is amplified in 10% to 20% and overexpressed in 10% to 50% of invasive UC.[85–89] The prognostic significance of these alterations is controversial.[90–94] As this receptor cannot bind ligand and relies on heterodimerization with ERBB3, it is likely that ERBB3 status and/or ligand expression may have significant influence.[95,96] Up to 70% of invasive tumors overexpress EGFR, and this is associated with poor prognosis.[97,98] Both ERBB2 and EGFR represent potential therapeutic targets in advanced UC.[99] These changes may activate the RAS-MAPK and/or the PI3K pathways (Fig. 94.2).

RAS gene mutation is not associated with either invasive or superficial disease.[60] *In vitro* experiments in tumor cells indicate that HRAS can induce an invasive phenotype.[100] In mice expressing mutant H-ras in the urothelium, superficial papillary tumors develop rather than muscle-invasive tumors.[101] Thus, RAS mutation may contribute to development of both forms of UC. *FGFR3* is mutated less frequently than in superficial UC. Approximately 15% of T2 tumors show mutation.[42,57,61] However, protein expression is up-regulated in 40% to 50% of nonmutant-invasive UC.[57,67] FGFR1 is also overexpressed in many of these cancers,[102] indicating that FGFR-targeted therapies may be applicable to both noninvasive and invasive UC.

Some UCs (4% to 6%) show amplification of *MDM2* (12q14).[103,104] MDM2 regulates p53 levels, and overexpression provides an alternative mechanism to inactivate p53 function (Fig. 94.1). There is no consensus on the relationship of up-regulated MDM2 to tumor grade, stage, or prognosis. MYC is up-regulated in many bladder tumors, although the

TABLE 94.2

GENETIC CHANGES FOUND IN INVASIVE (≥T2) BLADDER TUMORS

Gene (Cytogenetic Location)	Alteration	Frequency (%) (Ref.)
ONCOGENES		
HRAS (11p15)/*NRAS* (1p13)/*KRAS2* (12p12)	Activating mutations	10–15 (60, 199–201)
FGFR3 (4p16)	Activating mutations	0–34 (40, 42, 49, 54)
ERBB2 (17q)	Amplification/overexpression	10–14 amplification (87, 89, 207)
CCND1 (11q13)	Amplification/overexpression	10–20 amplification (72, 202, 208)
MDM2 (12q13)	Amplification/overexpression	4 amplification (103, 203)
E2F3 (6p22)	Amplification/overexpression	9–11 amplification in ≥T1 (108, 111)
TUMOR SUPPRESSOR GENES		
CDKN2A (9p21)	Homozygous deletion/ methylation/mutation	HD 20–30 (21, 23, 24) LOH ~60 (17)
PTCH (9q22)	Deletion/mutation	LOH ~60 (25, 26) Mutation frequency low
DBC1 (9q32–33)	Deletion/methylation	LOH ~60 (38, 204)
TSC1 (9q34)	Deletion/mutation	LOH ~60 (31, 33, 39) Mutation ~12
PTEN (10q23)	Homozygous deletion/mutation	LOH 30–35 (129–131, 133, 134); mutation 17 (132)
RB1 (13q14)	Deletion	37% (117–119)
TP53 (17p13)	Deletion/mutation	70% (209–211)
DNA COPY NUMBER CHANGES[a]		
2q, 5q, 6q, 8p, 9p, 9q, 10q, 11p, 11q, 13q, 15q, 16q, 17p, 18q, Y	Deletion in >12%	(186, 212)
1q, 3q, 5p, 7p, 8q, 10p, 17q, 20p, 20q	Gain in >12%	(186, 212)
1q22, 3p24, 6p22, 8p12, 8q21–22 and q24, 10p13–14, 12q15, 17q21, 20q13	Amplification <5% (5%–10% for 6p22)	(111, 186, 212)

HD, homozygous deletion; LOH, loss of heterozygosity.
[a]Comparative genomic hybridization analyses.

mechanism for this is unclear.[105] Although amplifications of 8q are found in some invasive UC, MYC is not the major target. However, additional copies of the whole of 8q are common and may lead to overexpression.[106,107] MYC may also be up-regulated in response to other molecular events (e.g., MAPK pathway stimulation). An amplicon on 6p in 14% of muscle-invasive UC and cell lines[108–110] contains *E2F3*, and functional studies indicate that *E3F3* can drive urothelial cell proliferation (Fig. 94.1).[111,112] E2F transcription factors interact with and are regulated by Rb and tumors with *E2F3* amplification have Rb inactivated.

Tumor Suppressor Genes

As in other aggressive cancers, the tumor suppressor genes *TP53*, *RB1*, *CDKN2A*, and *PTEN* are implicated in invasive UC. The pathways controlled by p53 and Rb regulate cell-cycle progression and responses to stress (Fig. 94.1). *TP53* mutation is common in invasive UC (mutations are listed in the International Agency for Research on Cancer *TP53* database).[113] Although immunohistochemical detection of p53 protein with increased half-life identifies many mutant p53 proteins and is commonly used as a surrogate marker for mutation, many *TP53* mutations (~20%) yield unstable or truncated proteins that cannot be detected in this way. Thus, p53 protein accumulation is not a useful prognostic marker. Two meta-analyses indicate only a small association between p53 positivity and poor prognosis.[114,115] A recent study that examined both protein expression and mutation of *TP53* confirmed limited concordance of these measurements but found that the combined measurements provided useful prognostic information.[116]

The Rb pathway regulates cell-cycle progression from G1 to S phase (Fig. 94.1). *RB1* has not been screened for mutations in UC but homozygous deletions, LOH of 13q14, and loss of Rb protein expression are detected in tumors of high grade and stage.[117–120] Altered Rb protein expression including both loss of expression, and the up-regulation which is associated with loss of p16 expression,[121] has been found in about 54% of cystectomy tumor samples.[122] *CDKN2A* (encoding p16 and p14ARF) is hemizygously deleted in more than 50% of UCs of all grades and stages, and homozygous deletion is associated with invasion.[34] These proteins link the Rb and p53 pathways (Fig. 94.1), and due to multiple regulatory feedback mechanisms, inactivation of both pathways together is predicted to have greater impact than inactivation of either pathway alone.[123] Assessment of Rb, p53, and p21 bear this out.[124] More recent studies indicate that broad analysis of changes that deregulate the G1 checkpoint achieves greater predictive power.[122,125–127] It is also reported that alterations of p53 and loss of p16 expression predict progression in Ta tumors.[128]

PTEN (phosphatase and tensin homologue deleted on chromosome 10) (10q23), a negative regulator of the PI3K pathway by virtue of its lipid phosphatase activity toward PtIns(3,4,5)P3 (Fig. 94.2), is deleted in 24% to 58% of invasive UCs.[129–131] Mutations of the retained copy are infrequent but HD has been detected in tumor cell lines.[39,132–134] Reduced expression is common[39,135] and is associated with p53 alteration. Many tumors (41%) with altered p53 show down-regulation of *PTEN*, and this combined alteration is associated with poor outcome.[136] As *PTEN* is haploinsufficient in mouse models,[137] loss of function of one allele in UC may lead to altered phenotype. In mice, conditional deletion of *Pten* in the urothelium led to early urothelial hyperplasia[135,138] and late development of tumors resembling human papillary superficial tumors. A study that induced stochastic deletion of *p53* and/or *Pten* in mice showed that deletion of either gene alone did not lead to tumor formation but dual deletion led to early development of aggressive UC, with frequent metastases.[136] PTEN loss may affect proliferation, apoptosis, and migration. Re-expression in PTEN-null UC cells has revealed effects on cell chemotaxis, anchorage independent growth, and tumor growth *in vivo*.[139–141] UC cell invasion can be inhibited by the protein phosphatase activity of PTEN alone.[141] Thus, loss of both lipid and protein phosphatase activities of PTEN may contribute in different ways to urothelial tumorigenesis. The *TSC1* product hamartin acts in the PI3K pathway downstream of PTEN (Fig. 94.2), providing an alternative mechanism of pathway activation in 13% of invasive UC.[31,39]

The Rho family GDP dissociation inhibitor RhoGDI2 has been implicated as a tumor suppressor in UC. Expression is reduced in an isogenic cell line model of metastasis[142] and low expression is associated with reduced survival in UC patients.[143] Phosphorylation by SRC appears to enhance the suppressive action of RhoGDI2 and down-regulation of SRC and RHOGDI2 are mutually exclusive in UC,[144] suggesting that SRC may play an important role in some cases.[145]

Other Genomic Changes in Invasive Urothelial Carcinoma

Large numbers of genomic changes have been detected in invasive UC. These include numerous losses and gains in DNA copy number and several regions of high-level amplification that may contain novel oncogenes (Table 94.2). To date the target genes within most of these regions have not been identified.

Invasive UC displays genetic instability with rapid genetic divergence of related tumors from the same patient. This is commonly chromosomal instability rather than microsatellite instability. No significant differences have yet been found between minimally invasive (T1) and deeply invasive tumors (T2 or greater), suggesting that T1 tumors with the ability to break through the basement membrane are aggressive lesions. Although T1 tumors often have good outcome, this may reflect complete resection rather than lack of tumor aggression. Some alterations, including gains of 3p22–25 and 5p and losses of 4p11–15, 5q15–23, 6q22–23, and 10q24–26, are associated with T1 tumor progression.[146] In one comparative genomic hybridization (CGH) study, muscle-invasive tumor samples and paired metastatic samples were compared, but no significant metastasis-associated markers were identified.[147]

MicroRNA Expression

Many miRNAs show altered expression in invasive UC.[78] In comparison with normal urothelium, invasive tumors are reported to show predominantly up-regulation of miRNAs rather than down-regulation.[77] Two studies have directly compared invasive and noninvasive samples[77] and several have shown association of specific changes with either poor outcome or the invasive phenotype.[78,148,149] Functional studies indicate potential roles for miR-145 and miR-221 in regulating urothelial cell survival,[150,151] miR-200 in regulating epithelial-mesenchymal transition,[152] miR-145 and miR-133a in regulating the cytoskeletal gene *FSCN1*,[153] and miR-101 in modulation of expression of the Polycomb Repressive Complex 2 gene *EZH1*.[154]

INFORMATION FROM EXPRESSION AND GENOMIC MICROARRAY PROFILING

Microarray analysis provides extensive information that is contributing to improved tumor classification and understanding of UC pathogenesis.[155] Molecular signatures for the known histopathologic subtypes (grade and stage), for CIS, the presence of metastases, and treatment response have been reported and some have been validated or are being validated in multicenter studies with the aim of introduction into clinical practice. Several reports have generated expression signatures for diagnostic classification.[156–161] Profiles of superficial tumors showed that the presence of *FGFR3* mutation has a major impact on expression profile.[162] One study[163] examined differences between normal urothelium, PUNLMP or low-grade Ta and high-grade Ta tumors.[164] Cytoskeletal genes differed most between normal urothelium and low-grade tumors, and changes in high-grade tumors were related to the cell cycle.

Signatures for prediction of recurrence in Ta grade 2 tumors and the presence of CIS in patients with Ta tumors have been generated.[165–168] Interestingly "normal" mucosa from cystectomy specimens with adjacent CIS contained the CIS signature, indicating that in such bladders there may be widespread urothelial alteration.[167] This CIS signature has been validated in a large multicenter study.[165] In another study a "no CIS" classification was correlated with *FGFR3* mutation.[54] Progression of superficial tumors has been predicted with relatively high sensitivity and specificity[159,169] and one of the signatures[169] validated in a multicenter study.[165] A recent study using large training and validation sets identified signatures for recurrence and progression in superficial and muscle-invasive tumors.[170] Real-time polymerase chain reaction confirmed an eight-gene predictor of progression in noninvasive disease. The other signatures were not confirmed, emphasizing the need for validation using an independent technique in a large sample set. The application of two forms of artificial intelligence to expression data from the study of Wild et al.[159] has also resulted in the identification of 11 genes associated with progression of noninvasive UC.[171] A panel of antibodies to six of these genes was predictive of outcome.

Muscle-invasive UC with known outcome have not been studied in large numbers, but in one study, tumors with good (survival ≥18 months) or bad (survival <18 months) prognosis were classified with 78% success.[158] Two other studies showed less ability to identify poor survival,[161,172] but one protein identified (synuclein) showed significant association with outcome.[172] Signatures for the presence of lymph node metastases have been presented[161,172] but robust predictors have not emerged.

Profiles of muscle-invasive UC reveal enrichment for markers of an epithelial-mesenchymal transition,[173] indicating that this may be an important feature of CIS->invasive UC progression. Immunohistochemistry results support this.[174,175] UC cell lines with epithelial-mesenchymal transition show resistance to EGFR inhibitors.[176,177] Tumor molecular profile may have profound effects not only on response to targeted therapies but to radiotherapy and conventional chemotherapy. Two studies

have examined response to neoadjuvant M-VAC (methotrexate, vinblastine, doxorubicin, and cisplatin) chemotherapy. Profiles from responders and nonresponders were used to generate a gene signature that correctly predicted response in eight of nine test cases.[178] In a second study, expression profiles from 30 patients yielded 55 genes that correlated with postchemotherapy survival, 2 of which (emmprin and survivin) were validated by immunohistochemistry and had significant correlation with therapeutic response and overall outcome in patients with no metastases.[179] Prediction models for response to both chemotherapy and targeted agents have also been developed using profiles of UC cell lines.[180,181] The same group developed a bioinformatics approach to predict drug sensitivity (COXEN), using expression profiles and known response of the NCI-60 panel of cell lines to predict response of cell lines based on expression profile. This predicted sensitivity of UC cell lines to several agents that was confirmed by *in vitro* testing[182] and has been shown to predict patients' response to chemotherapy.[183]

Genomic profiling has used array-based CGH (aCGH) and single nucleotide polymorphism (SNP) array analysis. aCGH provides high-resolution copy number profiles and has precisely defined regions of high-level amplification.[109,184–187] Used in concert with expression analysis, candidate "drivers" of these amplicons have been identified.[187] SNP array analysis has allowed novel chromosomal regions of allelic imbalance to be identified.[83,188] More regions of both copy number alteration and allelic imbalance have been found with increasing tumor stage. Despite a large body of data, no robust genetic markers to predict Ta tumor recurrence or progression of high-risk Ta tumors have been identified to date.

SIGNALING PATHWAYS IN UROTHELIAL CARCINOMA

There is overwhelming evidence for activation of the RAS-MAPK and PI3K pathways. In superficial UC, *FGFR3* and RAS mutation in almost all cases suggests dependence on RAS-MAPK pathway activation. As *FGFR3* activation does not activate the PI3K pathway in cultured normal urothelial cells,[59] the presence of *PIK3CA* mutations in superficial UC, including those with *FGFR3* mutation, implies that additional activation of the PI3K pathway is required. RAS mutation may activate both pathways. Inactivation of *TSC1* and activating mutations of *AKT1* in superficial and invasive UC, and *PTEN* inactivation in invasive UC, may also activate the PI3K pathway. Upstream activators of the pathway, including ERBB receptors, may also contribute. It is noteworthy that alterations in three of the key genes in the pathway (*PIK3CA, TSC1,* and *PTEN*) are not mutually exclusive,[39] implying that combined mutations have additive or synergistic effects and that noncanonical effects may be critical. This may be particularly important for *TSC1*. The widely studied functions of *TSC1* and *TSC2* are attributed to the *TSC1/TSC2* complex that regulates mTOR activity. Although independent functions have been ascribed to *TSC2*, independent function of *TSC1* is not clear. The finding of *TSC1* mutations in bladder but not other cancers and the lack of mutual exclusivity with *PIK3CA* and *PTEN* alterations may indicate an independent *TSC1* function in the urothelium. The known cross-talk between the MAPK and PI3K pathways via RAS and ERK (Fig. 94.2) could place the PI3K pathway at center stage and indicate utility of inhibitors of this pathway in treatment of both groups of UC. As targeted agents for inhibition of these pathways are now available or in development, it will be important to confirm these predictions by direct measurement of pathway activation in tumor samples.

UROTHELIAL TU… CELL… INITIATING

There is evidence for the existence wit… urothelial tumor cell populations of a highly… population with stem cell–like characteristics. …
other tumor types show resistance to che…
are predicted to be the cause of posttreatn…
there is great interest in characterizing these s…
tifying markers that may allow specific targe…
studies provide clear evidence for such a pop…
urothelial cancers.[189,190] He et al.[190] identified a …
tumor cells with urothelial basal cell-like charac…
reside at the tumor-stromal interface in tumors and…
and possess most of the tumor-forming ability of the…
tumor. A second study identified a CD44+ population o…
primary tumors that expressed the basal cell marker CK…
was enriched for tumor-initiating cells.[189] Expression profil…
both studies provides the basis for future attempts to iden…
tumor-initiating cells and examine relationships to therapeut…
response and outcome.[191]

MOLECULAR PATHOGENESIS AND TUMOR CLONALITY

UC are commonly multifocal and show frequent recurrence. In many cases, the macroscopically "normal" urothelium shows areas of microscopic dysplasia or CIS, and it is easy to envisage how new lesions may develop following resection of a primary tumor. The issue of clonality of UC has received much attention, and most studies have found only monoclonal tumors with shared genetic changes in multiple tumors resected from the same patient. However, there are some examples of more than one unrelated monoclonal tumor in the same bladder (oligoclonality) (reviewed in ref 192).

Macroscopically normal urothelium from tumor-bearing bladders has shown LOH in several genomic regions. Detailed mapping identified candidate genes whose involvement is predicted to be at a very early stage in tumor development. These have been termed "forerunner" genes and functional studies suggest that some regulate key cellular functions.[193,194]

Based on molecular and histopathological observations, a model for the molecular pathogenesis of UC has been developed (Fig. 94.4). *FGFR3* and *TP53* mutation are predominantly confined to one of the two major subgroups of UC and currently are the best molecular markers for these groups. It is not yet clear how often T1 tumors develop directly from flat dysplasia or from papillary Ta tumors. Similarly, the pathogenesis of high-grade papillary tumors and their relationship to flat dysplastic lesions is not well understood and is therefore represented as a potential third pathway in Figure 94.4. Further work is required to examine T1 tumors in more detail, to determine whether these are invasive tumors caught in their journey toward muscle, whether any develop from papillary Ta tumors or whether they represent a third distinct group. More detailed examination of differences between primary and UC-associated dysplasia/CIS may confirm the existence of a third pathway to urothelial neoplasia. To date, no molecular alterations can differentiate muscle invasive UC from their metastases. This may reflect early migration of cells to distant sites without requirement for additional changes, or that determinants of progression and metastasis are yet to be identified. Additional alterations may also remain to be identified in Ta tumors that show only one or two molecular events.

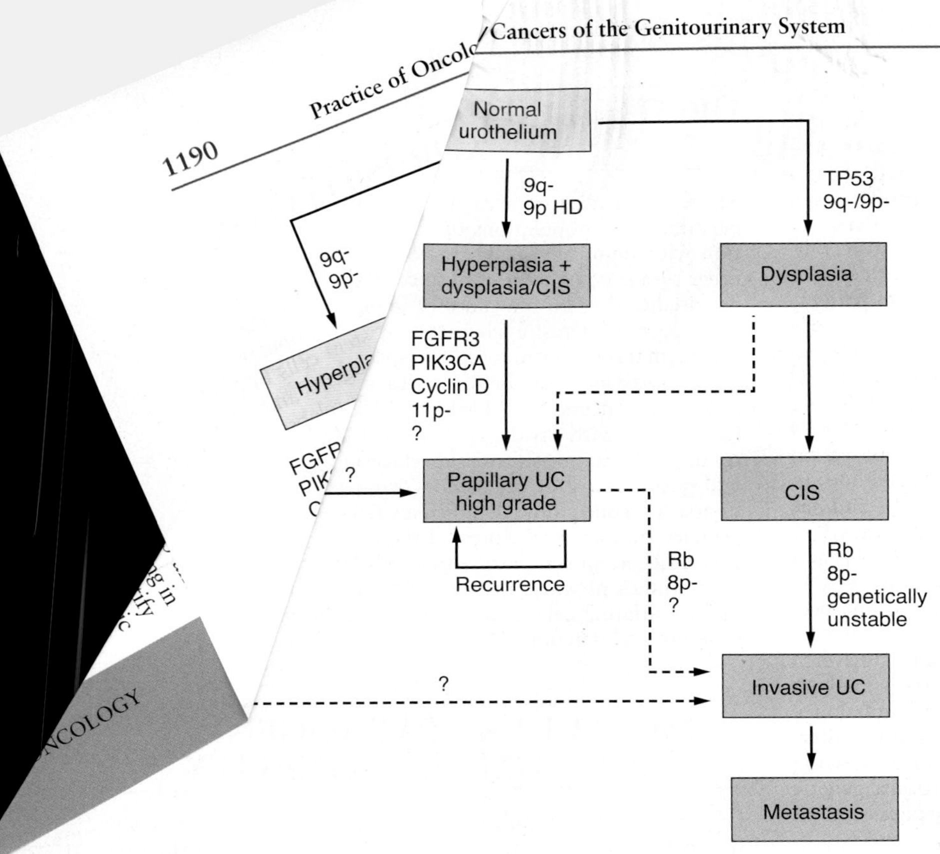

FIGURE 94.4 Potential pathways of urothelial tumorigenesis. Low-grade papillary tumors (*left*) may arise via simple hyperplasia and minimal dysplasia and are characterized at the molecular level by deletions of chromosome 9 and activating mutations of *FGFR3* and *PIK3CA*. Invasive carcinoma (*right*) is believed to arise via the flat high-grade lesion carcinoma *in situ* (CIS), and in this case *TP53* mutation occurs early, chromosome 9 deletions (9q) are less common, and *FGFR3* mutations are infrequent. These genetically unstable tumors accumulate genomic alterations, including *RB1* inactivation, 8p deletions, and many other genetic events. The finding of dysplasia in association with high-grade papillary tumors that lack *TP53* mutation but have frequent chromosome 9 losses suggests that an independent route to high-grade papillary tumors may exist (*center*).

Attempts have been made to apply bioinformatic modeling to define possible genetic pathways of UC development. Two potential cytogenetic pathways, one initiated by −9, followed by −11p and 1q+ and a second initiated by +7 followed by 8p− and +8q were identified, the latter group containing more aggressive tumors (T1–T3) and the former, Ta–T2 tumors.[195] A Bayesian network model using LOH data for 17 chromosomes in papillary UC (all grades) showed 9p and 9q loss as the most probable primary event with 8p− and 17− as major subsequent events[196] and a subsequent analysis based on cytogenetic data confirmed several of these associations and predicted two distinct pathways that ultimately converge, one initiated by +7 and the other by −9.[197]

Undoubtedly, application of array-based genomic and expression approaches in combination with high throughput mutation scanning will answer some of the outstanding questions relating to pathogenesis. Key to this will be appropriate selection of tissues for study, and there will be great advantages if archival samples from clinical trials can be used. It will be essential to test the effects of key molecular alterations on human urothelial cell phenotype. The recent development of immortal normal human urothelial cell lines will facilitate this.[198]

Selected References

The full list of references for this chapter appears in the online version.

1. Knowles MA. Molecular subtypes of bladder cancer: Jekyll and Hyde or chalk and cheese? *Carcinogenesis* 2006;27(3):361–373.
4. Cordon-Cardo C. Molecular alterations associated with bladder cancer initiation and progression. *Scand J Urol Nephrol Suppl* 2008:154–165.
7. Kiemeney LA, Grotenhuis AJ, Vermeulen SH, et al. Genome-wide association studies in bladder cancer: first results and potential relevance. *Curr Opin Urol* 2009;19:540–546.
9. Wu X, Hildebrandt MAT, Chang DW. Genome-wide association studies of bladder cancer risk: a field synopsis of progress and potential applications. *Cancer Metastasis Rev* 2009;28:269–280.
10. Cairns P. Gene methylation and early detection of genitourinary cancer: the road ahead. *Nat Rev Cancer* 2007;7:531–543.
14. Takahashi T, Habuchi T, Kakehi Y, et al. Clonal and chronological genetic analysis of multifocal cancers of the bladder and upper urinary tract. *Cancer Res* 1998;58:5835–5841.
30. Pymar LS, Platt FM, Askham JM, et al. Bladder tumour-derived somatic TSC1 missense mutations cause loss of function via distinct mechanisms. *Hum Mol Genet* 2008;17:2006–2017.
34. Chapman EJ, Harnden P, Chambers P, et al. Comprehensive analysis of CDKN2A status in microdissected urothelial cell carcinoma reveals potential haploinsufficiency, a high frequency of homozygous co-deletion and associations with clinical phenotype. *Clin Cancer Res* 2005;11:5740–5747.
39. Platt FM, Hurst CD, Taylor CF, et al. Spectrum of phosphatidylinositol 3-kinase pathway gene alterations in bladder cancer. *Clin Cancer Res* 2009;15:6008–6017.
40. Cappellen D, De Oliveira C, Ricol D, et al. Frequent activating mutations of FGFR3 in human bladder and cervix carcinomas. *Nat Genet* 1999;23:18.
42. Billerey C, Chopin D, Aubriot-Lorton MH, et al. Frequent FGFR3 mutations in papillary non-invasive bladder (pTa) tumors. *Am J Pathol* 2001;158:1955–1959.
54. Zieger K, Dyrskjot L, Wiuf C, et al. Role of activating fibroblast growth factor receptor 3 mutations in the development of bladder tumors. *Clin Cancer Res* 2005;11:7709–7719.
57. Tomlinson DC, Baldo O, Harnden P, et al. FGFR3 protein expression and its relationship to mutation status and prognostic variables in bladder cancer. *J Pathol* 2007;213:91–98.
58. Bernard-Pierrot I, Brams A, Dunois-Larde C, et al. Oncogenic properties of the mutated forms of fibroblast growth factor receptor 3b. *Carcinogenesis* 2006;27:740–747.
59. di Martino E, L'Hôte CG, Kennedy W, et al. Mutant fibroblast growth factor receptor 3 induces intracellular signaling and cellular transformation in a cell type- and mutation-specific manner. *Oncogene* 2009;28:4306–4316.
60. Jebar AH, Hurst CD, Tomlinson DC, et al. FGFR3 and Ras gene mutations are mutually exclusive genetic events in urothelial cell carcinoma. *Oncogene* 2005;24:5218–5225.

61. van Rhijn BW, van der Kwast TH, Vis AN, et al. FGFR3 and P53 characterize alternative genetic pathways in the pathogenesis of urothelial cell carcinoma. *Cancer Res* 2004;64:1911–1914.
63. Tomlinson DC, Hurst CD, Knowles MA. Knockdown by shRNA identifies S249C mutant FGFR3 as a potential therapeutic target in bladder cancer. *Oncogene* 2007;26:5889–5899.
65. Qing J, Du X, Chen Y, et al. Antibody-based targeting of FGFR3 in bladder carcinoma and t(4;14)-positive multiple myeloma in mice. *J Clin Invest* 2009;119:1216–1229.
68. Martinez-Torrecuadrada JL, Cheung LH, Lopez-Serra P, et al. Antitumor activity of fibroblast growth factor receptor 3-specific immunotoxins in a xenograft mouse model of bladder carcinoma is mediated by apoptosis. *Mol Cancer Ther* 2008;7:862–873.
69. Lopez-Knowles E, Hernandez S, Malats N, et al. PIK3CA mutations are an early genetic alteration associated with FGFR3 mutations in superficial papillary bladder tumors. *Cancer Res* 2006;66:7401–7404.
77. Catto JWF, Miah S, Owen HC, et al. Distinct microRNA alterations characterize high- and low-grade bladder cancer. *Cancer Res* 2009;69:8472–8481.
78. Veerla S, Lindgren D, Kvist A, et al. MiRNA expression in urothelial carcinomas: important roles of miR-10a, miR-222, miR-125b, miR-7 and miR-452 for tumor stage and metastasis, and frequent homozygous losses of miR-31. *Int J Cancer* 2009;124:2236–2242.
95. Memon AA, Sorensen BS, Meldgaard P, et al. The relation between survival and expression of HER1 and HER2 depends on the expression of HER3 and HER4: a study in bladder cancer patients. *Br J Cancer* 2006; 94:1703–1709.
96. Amsellem-Ouazana D, Bieche I, Tozlu S, et al. Gene expression profiling of ERBB receptors and ligands in human transitional cell carcinoma of the bladder. *J Urol* 2006;175:1127–1132.
99. Dovedi SJ, Davies BR. Emerging targeted therapies for bladder cancer: a disease waiting for a drug. *Cancer Metastasis Rev* 2009;28:355–367.
102. Tomlinson DC, Lamont FR, Shnyder SD, et al. Fibroblast growth factor receptor 1 promotes proliferation and survival via activation of the mitogen-activated protein kinase pathway in bladder cancer. *Cancer Res* 2009;69:4613–4620.
108. Oeggerli M, Tomovska S, Schraml P, et al. E2F3 amplification and overexpression is associated with invasive tumor growth and rapid tumor cell proliferation in urinary bladder cancer. *Oncogene* 2004;23:5616–5623.
109. Hurst CD, Fiegler H, Carr P, et al. High-resolution analysis of genomic copy number alterations in bladder cancer by microarray-based comparative genomic hybridization. *Oncogene* 2004;23:2250–2263.
111. Hurst CD, Tomlinson DC, Williams SV, et al. Inactivation of the Rb pathway and overexpression of both isoforms of E2F3 are obligate events in bladder tumours with 6p22 amplification. *Oncogene* 2008;27:2716–2727.
112. Olsson AY, Feber A, Edwards S, et al. Role of E2F3 expression in modulating cellular proliferation rate in human bladder and prostate cancer cells. *Oncogene* 2007;26:1028–1037.
116. George B, Datar RH, Wu L, et al. p53 gene and protein status: the role of p53 alterations in predicting outcome in patients with bladder cancer. *J Clin Oncol* 2007;25:5352–5358.
123. Mitra AP, Birkhahn M, Cote RJ. p53 and retinoblastoma pathways in bladder cancer. *World J Urol* 2007;25:563–571.
136. Puzio-Kuter AM, Castillo-Martin M, Kinkade CW, et al. Inactivation of p53 and Pten promotes invasive bladder cancer. *Genes Dev* 2009;23:675–689.
145. Said N, Theodorescu D. Pathways of metastasis suppression in bladder cancer. *Cancer Metastasis Rev* 2009;28:327–333.
148. Dyrskjot L, Ostenfeld MS, Bramsen JB, et al. Genomic profiling of microRNAs in bladder cancer: miR-129 is associated with poor outcome and promotes cell death in vitro. *Cancer Res* 2009;69:4851–4860.
152. Adam L, Zhong M, Choi W, et al. miR-200 expression regulates epithelial-to-mesenchymal transition in bladder cancer cells and reverses resistance to epidermal growth factor receptor therapy. *Clin Cancer Res* 2009; 15:5060–5072.
155. Orntoft TF, Dyrskjot L. Gene signatures for risk-adapted treatment of bladder cancer. *Scand J Urol Nephrol Suppl* 2008;(218):166–174.
162. Lindgren D, Liedberg F, Andersson A, et al. Molecular characterization of early-stage bladder carcinomas by expression profiles, FGFR3 mutation status, and loss of 9q. *Oncogene* 2006;25:2685–2696.
167. Dyrskjot L, Kruhoffer M, Thykjaer T, et al. Gene expression in the urinary bladder: a common carcinoma in situ gene expression signature exists disregarding histopathological classification. *Cancer Res* 2004;64:4040–4048.
169. Dyrskjot L, Zieger K, Kruhoffer M, et al. A molecular signature in superficial bladder carcinoma predicts clinical outcome. *Clin Cancer Res* 2005;11:4029–4036.
172. Sanchez-Carbayo M, Socci ND, Lozano J, et al. Defining molecular profiles of poor outcome in patients with invasive bladder cancer using oligonucleotide microarrays. *J Clin Oncol* 2006;24:778–789.
173. McConkey DJ, Choi W, Marquis L, et al. Role of epithelial-to-mesenchymal transition (EMT) in drug sensitivity and metastasis in bladder cancer. *Cancer Metastasis Rev* 2009;28:335–344.
179. Als AB, Dyrskjøt L, von der Maase H, et al. Emmprin and survivin predict response and survival following cisplatin-containing chemotherapy in patients with advanced bladder cancer. *Clin Cancer Res* 2007;13:4407–4414.
186. Blaveri E, Brewer JL, Roydasgupta R, et al. Bladder cancer stage and outcome by array-based comparative genomic hybridization. *Clin Cancer Res* 2005;11:7012–7022.
192. Hafner C, Knuechel R, Stoehr R, et al. Clonality of multifocal urothelial carcinomas: 10 years of molecular genetic studies. *Int J Cancer* 2002; 101:1–6.

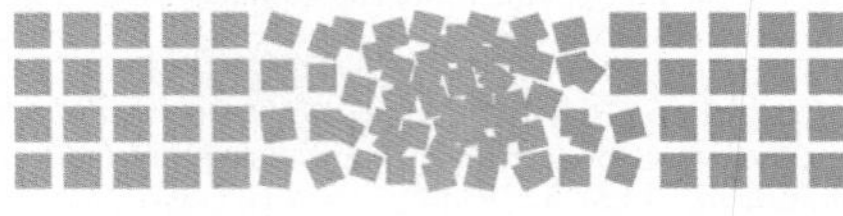

CHAPTER 95 CANCER OF THE BLADDER, URETER, AND RENAL PELVIS

W. SCOTT McDOUGAL, WILLIAM U. SHIPLEY, DONALD S. KAUFMAN, DOUGLAS M. DAHL, M. DROR MICHAELSON, AND ANTHONY L. ZIETMAN

This chapter details the incidence, epidemiology, pathology, and treatment of cancers of the bladder, ureter, and renal pelvis. Transitional cell carcinomas (TCCs) constitute 90% to 95% of all the urothelial tumors diagnosed in North America and Europe. TCCs occur throughout the lining of the urinary tract from the renal calyceal system to the proximal two-thirds of the urethra, at which point squamous epithelium predominates. In this ninth edition, cancers of the renal pelvis and ureter are grouped with bladder cancer rather than with cancers of the kidney. This is a natural fit as approximately 90% of the urothelial cancers of the renal pelvis, ureter, and bladder are transitional cell cancers, all of which share similarities in epidemiology, pathology, biology, patterns of spread, molecular tumor markers, and treatment. The chapter presents the common characteristics of urothelial cancers in an initial section and then deals in subsequent sections with the separate characteristics of these organs. The multidisciplinary treatment of this chapter reflects the current approach to patients with these diseases.

UROTHELIAL CANCERS

Epidemiology

Bladder cancer is almost three times more common in males than in females and more common in whites than in blacks. In 2007 there were approximately 69,000 new cases, a 20% increase from 20 years ago. The incidence increases with age and peaks in the sixth, seventh, and eighth decades of life.

Simultaneous or subsequent development of transitional cell cancer of the urethra in patients with transitional cell cancer of the bladder occurs with an incidence of 6% to 16% more common in women than men and in those with recurrent multifocal bladder cancers, and bladder neck or trigonal involvement with either invasive cancer or carcinoma *in situ* (CIS).[1,2]

The incidence of ureteral TCC is 0.7 per 100,000, whereas renal pelvic TCCs have an incidence of 1 per 100,000.[3] Renal pelvic tumors constitute 5% of all renal tumors, and 90% of them are TCCs. Squamous cell carcinoma and adenocarcinoma constitute the majority of the remainder. Renal pelvic transitional cell cancers constitute 5% of all TCCs of the urinary tract. Patients who have primary TCCs of the renal pelvis or ureter have a 20% to 40% incidence of either synchronous or metachronous bladder cancer. Conversely, patients with bladder cancer have a 1% to 4% incidence of synchronous or metachronous upper tract urothelial tumors.[4,5] However, if the bladder cancer is grade 3, there is associated CIS, or the patient has failed intravesical chemotherapy, some reports suggest a doubling of the incidence of upper tract tumors.[6] Patients with Balkan nephropathy have an increased incidence of upper tract tumors; these tumors are usually low grade and multiple.[7] There are specific areas of Taiwan where TCC of the renal pelvis accounts for 40% of all renal tumors, while in other nonendemic areas, the upper tract tumors account for only 1% or 2% of renal tumors.[8] The etiologic factor in the Taiwanese endemic region is still unknown.

Risk factors for urothelial cancer may be classified into one of three categories: (1) gene abnormalities that result in perturbations in cell cycle regulatory processes, (2) chemical exposure, and (3) chronic irritation. Those risk factors that involve genetic abnormalities include chromosome deletions or duplications, protooncogene expression, tumor suppressor gene mutation, and abnormalities of specific cell cycle regulatory proteins. In nonmuscularis propria invasive transitional cell cancers deletions of part or all of chromosome 9 and alterations in the gene encoding for fibroblast growth factor receptor 3 (FGFR-3) are often encountered. Other protooncogenes that have been implicated in bladder cancer include the RAS and p21 proteins.[9] Genetic abnormalities associated with CIS include alterations in the retinoblastoma gene (Rb), p53, and PTEN. In muscularis propria invasive disease the tumor suppressor genes that have been associated with an altered biology and more aggressive behavior include *p53* and the *Rb* gene.[10] Abnormalities in specific cell cycle regulatory proteins such as epidermal growth factor (EGF), Ki-67, cyclin D1, metalloproteinase(MMP), and inhibition of metalloproteinase (TIMP) have also been implicated.[10–15] At this time there is no single molecular marker that is capable of predicting the tumor with a high degree of accuracy, which may result in muscularis propria invasion or distant metastases.

Chemical exposure has perhaps the most epidemiologic evidence to support it as an inciting agent. Aromatic amines, aniline dyes, and nitrites and nitrates have all been implicated. There are genetic polymorphisms that appear to increase the susceptibility of affected patients exposed to carcinogens. *N*-acetyltransferase, which detoxifies nitrosamines and glutathione-S transferase, which conjugates reactive chemicals, have been implicated in increasing the risk for the development of bladder cancer in patients so afflicted. Tobacco use carries with it, for those who continue to smoke, a threefold increased risk of developing bladder cancer, and even ex-smokers have a twofold increased risk.[16] Numerous reports have shown strong associations between the development of both bladder and upper tract TCCs with industrial contact to chemicals, plastics, coal, tar, and asphalt. Cyclophosphamide administration over the long term, particularly in patients who have upper tract or bladder outlet obstructions, results in an increased risk of bladder cancer. These cancers when discovered tend to be particularly aggressive. Coffee, tea, analgesics, alcohol, and artificial sweeteners have not been shown to act as independent risk factors.

Chronic irritants include catheters, recurrent urinary track infections, *Schistosoma haematobium*, and irradiation. Chronic irritation due to indwelling catheters associated with chronic infection increases the risk for the development of squamous cell carcinoma; *S. haematobium* infestation results in an increased risk of squamous cell and TCCs; pelvic irradiation also carries with it an increased risk of developing a urothelial cancer.

There are many studies that suggest high water consumption, vitamin intake, and various diets as beneficial in preventing bladder cancer. However, none of these have shown any clear benefit with respect to prevention.

Screening and Early Detection

Screening has not been particularly useful in the detection of bladder cancer. The only test of proven usefulness is a urinalysis to detect microhematuria. If significant microhematuria is detected, then specific diagnostic studies are performed. When individuals are screened, 4% to 20% are found to have microhematuria. Of those with microhematuria, 0.1% to 6.6% have bladder tumors. This translates into a discovery rate of bladder cancer in the population at large varying from 0.005% to 0.2%. None of the patients who had bladder tumors incidentally discovered in these particular studies had invasive disease. In follow-up, no patient who had grade 1, stage Ta tumors discovered by disease screening progressed at 7 years of follow-up. Only those with CIS, T1, or high-grade tumors developed progressive disease, and that occurred only after 4 years of follow-up. However, some studies have suggested that routine screening results in a reduced mortality from bladder cancer. The data are, however, unconvincing as the studies are not randomized and the control arm consists of patients not comparable with those of the study population.[17] Others have suggested that screening in high-risk populations increases the early detection rate of high-grade cancers. Early treatment of these would be expected to be associated with an increased survival, although this hypothesis in this group of patients has not been substantiated. Screening does not generally improve the detection rate of low-grade tumors because the methods used for screening have a large number of false-negative findings for low-grade tumors. When urothelial cancer is suspected, noninvasive screening may be performed using cytology, nuclear matrix protein, telomerase, or fluorescence *in situ* hybridization analysis, but the definitive diagnosis is made only by cystoscopy and biopsy.

Cytology has been regarded as the gold standard for noninvasive screening of urine for bladder cancer. It has a sensitivity of 40% to 60% with a specificity in excess of 90%. Nuclear matrix protein[18] fibrin or fibrinogen degradation products,[19] urinary bladder cancer antigen,[20] and basic fetoprotein[21] have all been compared with cytology in bladder cancer screening studies. Other methods used include fluorescence *in situ* hybridization,[22] microsatellite analysis of free DNA,[23] and telomerase reverse transcriptase determination.[24] Unfortunately, all of these tests have a sensitivity that ranges from only 40% to 75% with a specificity of 50% to 90%, thus making it impossible to eliminate the need for cystoscopy by the use of these tests.[25] These urinary biomarkers have not been studied yet for sensitivity and specificity in detecting upper tract TCC.

Cytology remains the preferred bladder tumor marker for specificity[26]; however, many of the other bladder tumor markers have a better sensitivity.[27]

Pathology

More than 90% of the TCCs throughout the lining of the urinary tract occur in the urinary bladder and of the remaining 10%, most are in the renal pelvis and fewer than 2% are in the ureter and urethra. Squamous cell carcinomas, defined by the presence of keratinization, account for 5% of bladder tumors. Other even less-common bladder tumors include adenocarcinoma and undifferentiated carcinoma variants such as small-cell carcinoma, giant-cell carcinoma, and lymphoepitheliomas.[28–30] Tumors of mixed origin are quite common and consist of TCC, within which squamous and adenocarcinomatous elements are also identified. These are considered variants of TCC and they do not portend a worse prognosis. Adenocarcinoma may arise in the embryonal remnant of the urachus on or above the bladder dome. Other adenocarcinomas may closely resemble intestinal adenocarcinoma and must be distinguished from direct spread to the bladder from an intestinal primary by careful clinical evaluation. Rarely these demonstrate a signet ring cell or clear cell histology.

Primary Tumors of the Bladder

The differential diagnosis of TCC usually does not pose a diagnostic difficulty for experienced pathologists, but tumors that are grade 1 and invasive are occasionally difficult to distinguish from von Brunn's nests.[31] Also rarely, an invasive TCC may be overdiagnosed when the glandular component of a nephrogenic adenoma is mistaken for TCC with glandular differentiation or for a pure adenocarcinoma. When invasion of the lamina propria has occurred, the pathologist must report whether muscularis propria is present in the submitted tissue and whether there is invasion of the muscularis propria. If muscularis propria is not present in the submitted tissue, this should be noted by the pathologist. Identification of invasion of the muscularis propria by tumor may occasionally be difficult, as it may be confused with involvement of the muscularis mucosa, which is in the lamina propria.[32] More than two-thirds of newly diagnosed cases of bladder tumors are exophytic papillary TCCs that are confined to the epithelium (stage Ta) or invade only into the lamina propria (stage T1). These tumors are generally managed endoscopically and, in some cases, by intravesical therapy (discussed below). Approximately one-half to two-thirds of patients with such tumors have a recurrence or a new TCC in the bladder within 5 years.

Bladder tumors are also classified by their cytologic characteristics as low grade (G1) or high grade (G2, G3).[30] G1 tumors are also called papillary tumors at low malignant potential. Tumor grade is clinically more significant for noninvasive tumors because nearly all of the invasive neoplasms are high grade at diagnosis. Papillary carcinomas of low grade are considered to be relatively benign tumors that histologically resemble the normal urothelium. They show only very slight pleomorphism or loss of polarity and rarely progress to a higher stage. Primary CIS (stage Tis) that presents without a concurrent exophytic tumor constitutes only 1% to 2% of newly detected cases of bladder cancer, but CIS is found accompanying more than half of bladders presenting with multiple papillary tumors. CIS in this instance is either adjacent to or involving mucosal sites remote from papillary lesions.[33] CIS is believed to be an important precursor of invasive cancer and, if untreated, will develop into muscularis propria–invasive disease within 5 years from the initial diagnosis in more than 50% of patients.

Upper Tract Tumors

Like bladder tumors, 90% of upper tract tumors are TCCs with similar morphology.[34] Squamous cell carcinomas account for most of the remaining carcinomas, with adenocarcinoma representing at most 1% of upper tract malignancies. The cytologic characteristics for classification of TCC by grade are the same for upper tract TCC as they are for those in the bladder.

Molecular Tumor Markers

As the natural history of superficial urothelial tumors is that of recurrence, an area of controversy is whether tumors that occur at separate sites or at separate times in the urothelial tract are derived from the same clone or are polyclonal in origin. A report by Sidransky et al.[35] demonstrated the clonality of multiple bladder tumors from different sites. Miyao et al.[36] showed concordant genetic alterations in asynchronous tumors from individual patients. These studies suggest that urothelial TCCs appearing at different times and sites can be derived from the same neoplastic clone. Moreover, many studies have reported an increasing frequency of specific genetic abnormalities in bladder tumors of more advanced stages.[37–40] Many tumor suppressor gene modifications, including those of *p53*, *pRB*, *p16*, *p21*, thrombospondin-1, glutathione, and factors controlling the expression and function of the epidermal growth factor receptor (EGFR), have been shown in retrospective analyses to be adverse prognostic factors in patients with TCC after various treatments.[41–45] However, even in the most intensively studied tumor suppressor gene in advanced TCC, the *p53* gene, retrospective analyses give conflicting data on whether a mutation of *p53* confers an increased responsiveness or an increased resistance to chemotherapy or radiation.[42,43] Fortunately, this conflict in the predictability of the responsiveness to adjunctive chemotherapy of TCCs with a *p53* mutation is now being tested by a prospective phase 3 trial of postcystectomy methotrexate, vinblastine, doxorubicin, and cisplatin (MVAC) chemotherapy, funded by the National Cancer Institute.[46]

The enthusiasm engendered by the development of novel biologic agents targeted against tumor-specific growth factor pathways or against angiogenesis has been fortified by positive studies in a variety of solid tumors. Two classes of agents that have received great attention are inhibitors of EGFR, including EGFR1 and EGFR2 (or HER2/neu), and inhibitors of vascular endothelial growth factor (VEGF) or its receptors. Ample preclinical evidence has shown that (1) many, if not most, bladder tumors express products of the EGFR family, (2) overexpression correlates with an unfavorable outcome, and (3) inhibition of these pathways may have an antitumor effect.[47–52]

Evidence suggests that *p53*, *p16*, and *pRB* altered expression are of no prognostic significance in patients treated with chemoradiation, but that overexpression of *HER2* correlated with a significantly inferior complete response rate. EGFR overexpression, which occurred in only 19% of the patients, was associated with improved disease-specific survival.[53]

Another potential therapeutic avenue is the inhibition of angiogenic inducers, which are frequently present in bladder tumors. Several studies have correlated elevated VEGF levels or cyclooxygenase-2 expression with disease recurrence or progression, often as an independent prognostic factor by multivariate analysis.[52]

The major challenge for clinical and translational investigators is to design appropriate trials that will identify which molecular tumor markers will be prognostic of outcome *and* also be predictive of whether a patient will do better treated by surgery, radiation, chemotherapy, molecular targeted therapy, or a combination of these. Only then can molecular tumor markers be incorporated into clinical decision making and allow physicians to make better treatment choices on behalf of their patients.

CANCER OF THE BLADDER

Cancers of the bladder can be grouped into three general categories by their stages at presentation: those that do not invade the muscularis propria, muscularis propria–invasive cancers, and metastatic cancers. Each differs in clinical behavior, primary management, and outcome. When treating nonmuscularis invasive tumors, the aim is to prevent recurrences and progression to a stage that is life threatening. With muscularis propria–invasive disease, the main issue is to determine which tumors require cystectomy; which can be successfully managed by bladder preservation, using combined modality therapy; and which tumors, by virtue of a high metastatic potential, require an integrated systemic chemotherapeutic approach from the outset. Combination chemotherapy is the standard for treating metastatic disease. Despite reports of complete responses (CRs) in more than 40% of cases, the duration of response and overall cure rates remain low.

Clinical Presentations and Staging

Bladder cancer is rarely incidentally discovered at autopsy. Indeed, almost all cases show symptoms in the premortem period. The most common presentation is gross painless hematuria. Unexplained frequency and irritative voiding symptoms should alert one to the possibility of CIS of the bladder or, less commonly, muscularis propria–invasive cancer.

Workup

The workup of suspected bladder cancer should include cytology, a cystoscopy, and an upper tract study. The preference for the upper tract study is a renal computed tomography (CT) scan as both ureters and renal pelves as well as the relevant lymph nodes and the kidney parenchyma can be particularly well visualized.

Careful staging is important, as treatment depends on the initial stage of the disease. The clinical stage of the primary tumor is determined by transurethral resection of the bladder tumor (TURBT). This resection should include a sample of the muscularis propria for appropriate diagnosis, particularly if the tumor appears sessile or high grade. Once the specimen has been resected, the base of the resected area should be separately biopsied. Any suspicious areas in the remainder of the bladder should be biopsied, and many advocate additional selected biopsies of the bladder mucosa and a prostatic urethral biopsy as well. Urethral biopsies are clearly indicated in patients with risk factors for urethral involvement, as previously discussed, and in those who have persistent positive cytologies in the absence of a demonstrated bladder lesion. Alpha amino levulinic acid installation into the bladder, resulting in porphyrin-induced fluorescence of vascular lesions when viewed with blue light, and narrow band imaging, which increases the contrast between vascular lesions and normal mucosa, have been recommended by some to increase the yield of positive biopsies. Most studies show a slight advantage to these techniques, but it remains difficult to differentiate inflammatory lesions from urothelial carcinomas with either technique. Patients who have T1, G3 tumors on biopsy without muscularis propria in the specimen require a second biopsy in order to obtain muscularis propria to reduce the risk of understaging. Indeed, the authors rebiopsy all patients with T1, G3 disease, as it has been shown that even if muscularis propria is in the initial specimen, a finite number of patients will be upstaged (T2) on the second biopsy.

Staging

The primary bladder cancer is staged according to the depth of invasion into the bladder wall or beyond (Table 95.1).[53]

TABLE 95.1

AMERICAN JOINT COMMITTEE ON CANCER 2009 TNM BLADDER CANCER STAGING

PRIMARY TUMOR (T)	
Tis	Carcinoma *in situ*
Ta	Noninvasive papillary tumor
T1	Tumor invades the lamina propria, but not beyond
T2	Tumor invades the muscularis propria
pT2a	Tumor invades superficial muscle (inner half)
pT2b	Tumor invades deep muscle (outer half)
T3	Tumor invades perivesical tissue
pT3a	Microscopically
pT3b	Macroscopically (extravesical mass)
T4	Tumor invades any of the following: prostatic stroma, uterus, vagina, pelvis, or abdominal wall
T4a	Tumor invades prostate, uterus, vagina
T4b	Tumor invades pelvic or abdominal wall
REGIONAL LYMPH NODES (N)	
NX	Regional lymph nodes cannot be assessed
N0	No regional lymph node metastasis
N1	Metastasis in a single lymph node in primary drainage region
N2	Metastasis in multiple lymph nodes in primary drainage region
N3	Common iliac lymph node involvement
DISTANT METASTASIS (M)	
MX	Distant metastasis cannot be assessed
M0	No distant metastasis
M1	Distant metastasis

From ref. 54, with permission.

The urothelial basement membrane separates nonmuscularis propria bladder cancers into Ta (noninvasive) and T1 (invasive) tumors. Stage T2 and higher T-stage tumors invade the muscularis propria, the true muscle of the bladder wall. If the tumor extends through the muscle to involve the full thickness of the bladder and into the serosa, it is classified as T3. If the tumor involves contiguous structures such as the prostate, the vagina, the uterus, or the pelvic sidewall, the tumor is classified as stage T4 (nonstromal invasive urothelial tumors of the prostate are not classified as T4, as the prognosis in this group is quite good). In a fragmented TURBT specimen, in contrast to a cystectomy specimen, it is relatively infrequent for the pathologist to be able to make an accurate assessment as to the depth of invasion of the tumor into the muscularis propria. Thus the primary pathologic substages of the TNM (tumor, nodes, metastasis) staging system shown in Table 95.1, such as pT2a and pT2b, cannot be determined from TURBT specimens. CT scans or magnetic resonance images (MRIs), even those done prior to the TURBT, are not reliable for staging of the primary tumor. Neither scan can differentiate a Ta/T1 tumor from a T2/T3 tumor because neither can visualize the depth of invasion of the primary tumor into the bladder wall. These scans are helpful, however, when they show unequivocal tumor extension outside the bladder (stage T3, Fig. 95.1). CT scans or MRIs following a TURBT also are not reliable for staging of the primary tumor because either surgically induced edema in the resected portion of the bladder wall or postsurgical extravesical inflammatory stranding may be confused with extravesical tumor extension.

Patients who have documented muscularis propria–invasive bladder cancer require an additional set of studies: chest x-ray or CT scan, liver function studies, creatinine, and electrolytes, and a CT evaluation of the pelvic and retroperitoneal lymph nodes. Bimanual examination is also performed at the time the tumor is transurethrally resected to evaluate for possible extravesical extension of tumor and to determine mobility of the pelvic contents. MRI lymphangiography, using a lymphotropic iron nanoparticle administered intravenously, shows potential.[55] Nodes that appear to be enlarged on CT may be differentiated by this technique as to whether they are inflammatory or malignant. The sensitivity and specificity of the test are quite high.

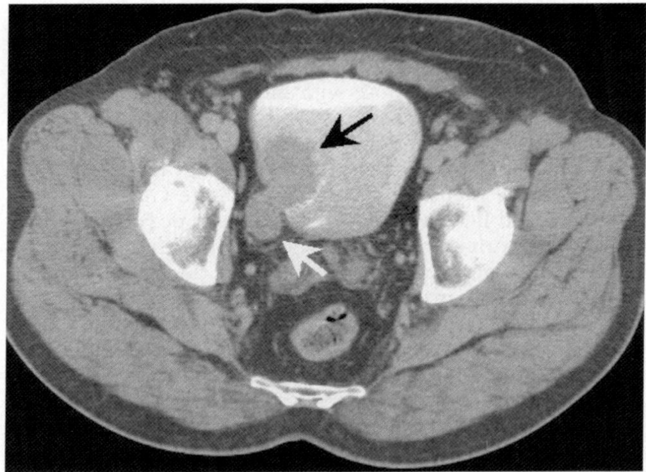

FIGURE 95.1 Computed tomography scan of a patient with a muscularis propria–invasive bladder cancer performed before a transurethral tumor resection, showing unequivocally an extravesical extension of tumor (stage T3). Tumor projecting into the bladder lumen (*black arrow*); portion of the tumor extending into the ureter outside the bladder (*white arrow*).

If there is a history of functional bowel abnormality, a barium study of the segment of bowel to be used for the diversion should be performed. It is the authors' practice when using colon in the reconstruction of the urinary tract to obtain a barium enema or colonoscopy so that there are no surprises at the time of surgery. Finally, patients with muscularis propria–invasive bladder cancer must have a prostatic urethra and bulbous urethra biopsy to determine whether an orthotopic bladder may be placed or whether the procedure should encompass the urethra: that is, a cystoprostatourethrectomy in males or a cystourethrectomy and anterior exenteration in females.

Treatment of Nonmuscularis Propria Invasive Bladder Cancer (Ta, Tis, T1)

Seventy percent of patients with bladder cancer have disease that does not involve the muscularis propria at presentation. Approximately 15% to 20% of these patients will progress to stage T2 disease or greater over time. Fifty percent to 70% of those presenting with Ta or T1 disease will have a recurrence following initial therapy. Low-grade tumors (G1 or G2) and low-stage (Ta) disease tend to have a lower recurrence rate at about 50% and a 5% progression rate, whereas high-risk disease (G3, T1 associated with CIS, and multifocal disease) has a 70% recurrence rate and a 30% to 50% progression rate to stage T2 disease or greater disease. Less than 5% of patients with nonmuscularis propria invasive bladder cancer will develop metastatic disease without developing evidence of muscularis propria invasion (stage T2 disease or greater) of the primary lesion.

Patients who are at significant risk for development of progressive disease or recurrent disease following TURBT are generally considered candidates for adjuvant intravesical drug therapy. This includes those with multifocal CIS, CIS associated with Ta or T1 tumors, any G3 tumor, multifocal tumors, and those whose tumors rapidly recur following TURBT of the initial bladder tumor. A number of drugs have been used intravesically, including bacillus Calmette-Guérin (BCG), interferon and BCG, thiotepa, mitomycin C, doxorubicin, and gemcitabine. Complications generally include frequency, dysuria, and irritative voiding symptoms. Over the long term, bladder contracture may occur with these agents. Other complications, which are specific for each drug, are as follows: BCG administration may result in fever, joint pain, granulomatous prostatitis, sinus formation, disseminated tuberculosis, and death; thiotepa may cause myelosuppression; mitomycin C may cause skin desquamation and rash; and doxorubicin may cause gastrointestinal upset and allergic reactions. The proposed benefit of intravesical chemotherapy is to lessen the rate of recurrences and reduce the incidence of progression. Unfortunately, it cannot be clearly stated that any of these drugs accomplish these goals over the long term.

A number of studies have compared one intravesical chemotherapeutic agent with another. For the most part, BCG in these comparisons has a slight advantage in reducing recurrences.[56] However, when the follow-up is more than 5 years, it appears that there is minimal overall effect in reducing the recurrence rate when compared with no treatment. Approximately 70% of patients with high-grade disease will experience recurrence whether or not they are treated with intravesical therapy. Moreover, there is no well-documented evidence that the use of these agents prevents disease progression, that is, from stage Ta/T1 disease to stage T2 or greater disease. One-third of patients who are at high risk for disease progression (those with G3, T1 disease) will progress to stage T2 or greater disease whether or not they are treated with BCG.[57] One-third of patients at 5 years who have disease progression and undergo a cystectomy die of metastatic disease. Thus, approximately 15% of patients with superficial disease at high risk for disease progression (CIS with associated Ta or T1 disease, rapidly recurrent disease, or G3 disease), irrespective of treatment modality, will die of their disease.[58] If definitive therapy (cystectomy) is performed when the disease is found to progress into the muscularis propria (T2 or greater), there is no difference in cure rate when these patients are compared with those who present with T2 or greater disease primarily. These statistics have encouraged some to perform a preemptive cystectomy in those patients at high risk for progression before muscularis propria invasion is documented. Ten-year cancer-specific survivals of 80% are given as justification for this approach, as compared with 50% in patients in whom the cystectomy is performed when the disease progresses to involve the muscularis propria.[59] Unfortunately, this approach subjects approximately two-thirds of these patients who are included in the 80% cancer-specific survival figure to a needless cystectomy, making it questionable as to whether there is in fact any survival advantage whatsoever.

Treatment of Muscularis Propria–Invasive Disease

Surgical Approaches

The standard of care for squamous cell carcinoma, adenocarcinoma, TCC, and spindle cell carcinoma that invade the muscularis propria of the bladder is a bilateral pelvic lymph node dissection and a cystoprostatectomy, with or without a urethrectomy in the male. In the female an anterior exenteration is performed, which includes the bladder and urethra (the urethra may be spared if uninvolved and an orthotopic bladder reconstruction is performed), the ventral vaginal wall, and the uterus. A radical cystectomy may be indicated in nonmuscularis propria–invasive bladder cancers when G3 disease is multifocal or associated with CIS or when bladder tumors rapidly recur, particularly in multifocal areas following intravesical drug therapy. When the prostate stroma is involved with TCC or when there is concomitant CIS of the urethra, a cystoprostatourethrectomy is the treatment of choice.[60] If the urethra needs to be removed, the type of urinary reconstruction is limited to an abdominal urinary diversion. In selected circumstances in the male, the neurovascular bundles coursing along the lateral side of the prostate caudally and adjacent to the rectum more cephalad may be preserved, sometimes preserving potency. Partial cystectomies may rarely be performed in selected patients, thus preserving bladder function and affording in the properly selected patient the same cure rate as a radical cystectomy. Patients who are candidates for such procedures must have focal disease located far enough away from the ureteral orifices and bladder neck to achieve at least a 2-cm margin around the tumor and a margin sufficient around the ureteral orifices and bladder neck to reconstruct the bladder. Practically, this limits partial cystectomies to those patients who have small tumors located in the dome of the bladder and in whom random bladder biopsies show no evidence of CIS or other bladder tumors.

Survival

The probability of survival from bladder cancer following cystectomy is determined by the pathologic stage of the disease. Survival is markedly influenced by the presence or absence of positive lymph nodes. Some have argued that the number of positive nodes impacts survival in that when resected, there is a potential for cure provided there are less than four to eight positive nodes.[61,62] Positive perivesical nodes have a less ominous prognosis when compared with involvement of iliac or para-aortic nodes. Pathologic type may also impact outcome, but in most series survival is more dependent on pathologic stage than on the cell type of the cancer. Most large series of survival statistics following treatment include all patients regardless of cell type. These series are generally constituted as to histologic type as follows: TCC, 85% to 90%; combination of TCC and either squamous cell or adenocarcinoma, 6%; pure squamous cell carcinoma, 3%; pure adenocarcinoma, 3%; small-cell and spindle cell carcinoma, 2% (Table 95.2).

TABLE 95.2

SURVIVAL AFTER RADICAL CYSTECTOMY ACCORDING TO PATHOLOGIC STAGE AT 10 YEARS

Pathologic Stage	Disease-Specific Survival (%)	Overall Survival (%)
pTa, Tis, T1 with high risk of progression	82	—
Organ confined, negative nodes (pT2, pN0)	73	49
Nonorgan confined (pT3–4a or pN1–2)	33	23
Lymph node-positive (any T, pN1–2)	28, 34	21

From refs. 61, 62, 63–65.

Types of Urinary Diversion

Urinary diversions may be divided into continent and incontinent. Incontinent urinary diversions or conduits involve the use of a segment of ileum or colon and, less commonly, a segment of jejunum. The distal end is brought to the skin and the ureters are implanted into the proximal end. The patient wears a urinary collection appliance. The advantages of a conduit (ileal or colonic) are its simplicity and the reduced number of immediate and long-term postoperative complications. In most series13% of patients who undergo a cystectomy and urinary diversion of this type will have a significant complication that impacts on hospital stay or recovery. Generally, the distal ileum is used for the urinary conduit or reservoir; however, if it has been irradiated or is otherwise involved, one may select the right colon or a short segment of jejunum. The latter is the least desirable choice as electrolyte problems may be significant. On occasion during exenterative surgery when an end colostomy is created, a segment of distal bowel is used, thus obviating the need for an intestinal anastomosis.

Continent diversions may be divided into two types: abdominal and orthotopic. Abdominal diversions require a continence valve, whereas an orthotopic neobladder depends on the urethral sphincter for continence. The reservoir is made of bowel that is fashioned into a globular configuration. In the abdominal type of continent diversion, the stoma is brought through the abdominal wall to the skin. The patient catheterizes the pouch every 4 hours. Orthotopic urinary diversions entail the use of bowel brought to the urethra, thus allowing the patient to void by Valsalva (Fig. 95.2). Patients must have the facility to catheterize themselves, as it is mandatory in the abdominal continent diversion and occasionally necessary in the orthotopic reconstruction. The advantage of continent diversions is the avoidance of a collection device. The advantage of an orthotopic bladder over all other types of continent diversions is that it rehabilitates the patient to normal voiding through the urethra, often without the need for intermittent catheterization or the need to wear a collection device.

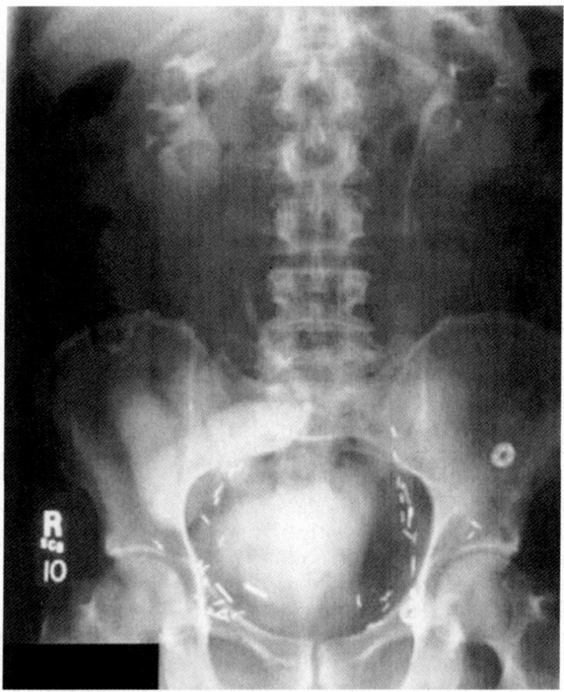

FIGURE 95.2 Intravenous urogram of a patient with an orthotopic bladder after radical cystoprostatectomy. The orthotopic bladder was constructed of the right colon and distal ileum.

Postoperative and long-term complications of continent diversion are increased over the conduit types of diversions. Indeed, in some series postoperative complications range from 13% to 30%. Long-term metabolic complications are also increased.

Complications of Cystectomy and Urinary Diversion

The complications of all types of urinary diversion may be divided into three groups: metabolic, neuromechanical, and surgical.

Metabolic Complications of Urinary Intestinal Diversion. When intestine is interposed in the urinary tract there is the potential for a number of metabolic complications.[66] These may involve electrolyte abnormalities and altered drug metabolism, which may result in altered sensorium, infection, osteomalacia, growth retardation, calculi both within the reservoir as well as in the kidney, short bowel syndrome, cancer, and altered bile metabolism.

Depending on the segment used, different specific electrolyte abnormalities may occur. When ileum and colon are used, hyperchloremic metabolic acidosis may result, when jejunum is used hypochloremic, hyperkalemic metabolic acidosis may follow.

Hypokalemia is more common when colon is used, hypocalcemia is more common when ileum and colon are used, and hypomagnesemia is more common when ileum and colon are used.

The most pervasive detrimental effect created by all urinary intestinal diversions is due to the acidosis. Acidosis may result in electrolyte abnormalities, osteomalacia, growth retardation, altered sensorium, altered hepatic metabolism, renal calculi, and abnormal drug metabolism. In general, patients with normal renal function as well as normal hepatic function are less prone to acidosis and its complications.

Treatment for the metabolic acidosis is straightforward and can be accomplished with bicarbonate or with Bicitra solution, which is sodium citrate and citric acid. Polycitra, which is a combination of potassium citrate, sodium citrate, and citric acid, may also be employed. It has the advantage of supplying potassium, which on occasion is deficient. Chlorpromazine and nicotinic acid have been used to block the chloride bicarbonate exchanger and thus lessen the potential for the acidosis.

Patients with conduits may have 3% to 4% incidence of renal calculi over the long term. Those with reservoirs have up to a 20% incidence of calculi within the reservoir. The pathogenesis may be a metabolic alteration or infection, whereas reservoir stones are most commonly due to a surgical foreign body or mucus serving as a nidus.

There is a high incidence of bacteriuria in patients with either conduits or pouches and the incidence of sepsis is 13%. There appears to be diminished antibacterial activity of the intestinal mucosa, with the immunoglobulins, which are normally secreted by the mucosa, being altered. In addition to this, when the bowel is distended there can be a translocation of bacteria from the lumen into the bloodstream.

Because the intestine is interposed in the urinary tract, drugs that are eliminated unchanged from the body through the kidney and have the potential to be reabsorbed by the gut can in fact result in significant alterations in metabolism of that drug. Patients with a urinary diversion, when given systemic chemotherapy, have a higher incidence of complications and are more likely to have their chemotherapy limited when compared with patients without diversion who receive the same drugs and dose.[67]

The loss of the distal ileum may result in vitamin B_{12} malabsorption and then manifest itself as anemia and neurologic abnormalities. Bile salt malabsorption may occur and result in diarrhea. Loss of the ileocecal valve may result in diarrhea with bacterial overgrowth of the ileum and malabsorption of vitamin B_{12} and fat-soluble vitamins A, D, E, and K. Loss of the colon may result in diarrhea and bicarbonate loss.

Neuromechanical Complications. Neuromechanical complications may be of two types: atonic, resulting in an atonic segment with urinary retention, and hyperperistaltic contractions. The latter is relevant in continent diversions, as this may result in incontinence and a low-capacity reservoir.

Surgical Complications. There are a number of complications that occur following any major surgical procedure, which include thrombophlebitis, pulmonary embolus, wound dehiscence, pneumonia, atelectasis, myocardial infarction, and death. Complications specific to cystectomy and urinary diversion are divided into short term and late. The short-term complications include acute acidosis (16%), urine leak (3% to 16%), bowel obstruction or fecal leak (10%), and pyelonephritis (5% to 15%). The longer-term complications include ureteral or intestinal obstruction (15%), renal deterioration (15%), renal failure (5%), stoma problems (15%), and intestinal stricture (10% to 15%).[68,69]

Selective Bladder-Preserving Approaches

The treatment options for muscularis propria–invasive bladder tumors can broadly be divided into those that remove the bladder and those that spare it. In the United States, radical cystectomy with pelvic lymph node dissection remains the standard method used to treat patients with this tumor. Several reports from North America and Europe have described long-term results using multimodality treatment of muscularis propria–invading bladder cancer, with appropriate safeguards for early cystectomy should this treatment fail. For bladder-conserving therapy to be more widely accepted, this treatment approach must have a high likelihood of eradicating the primary tumor, must preserve good organ function, and must not result in compromised patient survival.

Successful bladder-preserving approaches have evolved during the past two decades. They began with the use of radiation therapy but expanded when the National Bladder Cancer Group first demonstrated the safety and efficacy of cisplatin as a radiation sensitizer in patients with muscle-invasive bladder cancer that was unsuitable for cystectomy.[70] The long-term survival with stage T2 tumors (64%) and stage T3 to T4 tumors (22%) was encouraging. This was validated by the National Cancer Institute–Canada randomized trial of radiation (either definitive or precystectomy) with or without concurrent cisplatin for patients with T3 bladder cancer, which showed a significant improvement in long-term survival with pelvic tumor control (67% vs. 47%) in the patients who were assigned cisplatin.[71] Additional single-institution studies showed that the combination of a visibly complete TURBT followed by radiation therapy or radiation therapy concurrent with chemotherapy safely improved local control.[72,73] These findings led the Radiation Therapy Oncology Group (RTOG) to develop protocols for bladder preservation beginning with a TURBT of as much of the tumor as is safely possible, followed by the combination of radiation with concurrent radiosensitizing chemotherapy. One key to the success of such a program is the selection of patients for bladder preservation on the basis of the initial response of each individual patient's tumor to therapy. Thus, bladder conservation is reserved for those patients who have a clinical CR to concurrent chemotherapy and radiation. Prompt cystectomy is recommended for those patients whose tumors respond only incompletely or who subsequently develop an invasive tumor (Fig. 95.3). Up to one-third of the patients entering a potential bladder-preserving protocol with trimodality therapy (initial TURBT followed by concurrent chemotherapy and radiation) will ultimately require radical cystectomy.

For over two decades, the Massachusetts General Hospital (MGH), the RTOG, and several centers in Europe have evaluated in phase 2 and 3 protocols concurrent radiochemotherapy plus

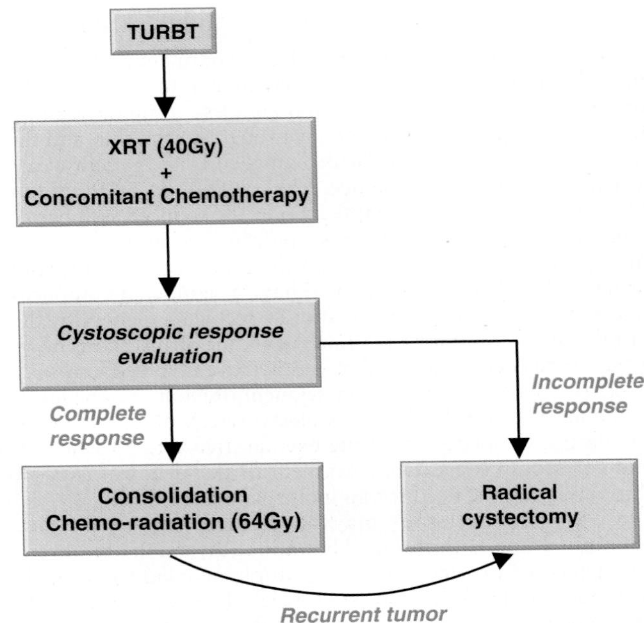

FIGURE 95.3 Schema for trimodality treatment of muscularis propria–invasive bladder cancer with selective bladder preservation. TURBT, transurethral resection of the bladder tumor; XRT, radiation therapy.

neoadjuvant or adjuvant chemotherapy (Table 95.3). Radiosensitizing drugs studied in these series, either singly or in various combinations, include cisplatin, carboplatin, paclitaxel, 5-fluorouracil (5-FU), and gemcitabine.[72] The first RTOG study of patients treated with once-daily radiation treatment and concurrent cisplatin yielded a 5-year survival of 52% (42% with intact bladder).[74] RTOG studies 8802 and 8903 used MCV (methotrexate, cisplatin, and vinblastine) chemotherapy as neoadjuvant treatment.[75] In the latter study the neoadjuvant therapy was tested in a randomized fashion.[76] No improvement was seen in survival or in local tumor eradication as a result of neoadjuvant therapy, although the trial was underpowered to give a definitive answer. The toxicity of the MCV arm was considerable, with only 67% of patients able to complete the planned treatment.

Other studies from Paris and Erlangen have reported their large experience with bladder sparing.[77,78] The CR rate at Erlangen was 72%, and local control of the bladder tumor after the CR without a muscle-invasive relapse was maintained in 64% of the patients at 10 years. The 10-year disease-specific survival was 42%, and more than 80% of these survivors preserved their bladder. This series reported the sequential use of radiation with no chemotherapy (126 patients), followed by concurrent cisplatin (145 patients), then concurrent carboplatin (95 patients), and finally concurrent cisplatin with 5-FU (49 patients). The CR rates in these four protocols were 51%, 81%, 64%, and 87%, respectively.[81,82] The 5-year actuarial survival with an intact bladder in these studies was 38%, 47%, 41%, and 54%, respectively. These results suggest strongly that radiochemotherapy, when given concurrently, is superior to radiation therapy alone, that carboplatin is less radiosensitizing than cisplatin, and that cisplatin plus 5-FU may be superior to cisplatin alone.

The RTOG protocols have subsequently explored both twice-daily radiation therapy and novel radiosensitization using cisplatin with or without 5-FU or paclitaxel.[45,83,79] Complete response and bladder preservation rates are consistently high, with no one regimen clearly superior.[45]

Gemcitabine has been also tested in bladder-treatment protocols. In a phase 1 trial from the University of Michigan, 23, mostly

TABLE 95.3

RESULTS OF MULTIMODALITY TREATMENT FOR MUSCLE-INVADING BLADDER CANCER

Series (Ref.)	Multimodality Therapy Used	No. of Patients	5-Year Overall Survival (%)	5-Year Survival with Intact Bladder (%)
RTOG 8512, 1993 (74)	External-beam radiation with cisplatin	42	52	42
RTOG 8802, 1996 (75)	TURBT, MCV, external-beam radiation with cisplatin	91	51	44 (4 y)
RTOG 8903, 1998 (76)	TURBT with or without MCV, external-beam radiation with cisplatin	123	49	38
U. Paris, 1997 (77)	TURBT, 5-FU, external-beam radiation with cisplatin	120	63	NA
Erlangen, 2002 (78)	TURBT, external-beam radiation, cisplatin, carboplatin, or cisplatin and 5-FU	415 (cisplatin, 82; carboplatin, 61; 5-FU/cisplatin, 87)	50	42
RTOG 9906 (79)	TURBT, TAX plus CP plus XRT; adj. CP plus GEM	80	56	47
MGH, 2009 (80)	TURBT, external beam radiation and cisplatin with or without 5-FU or TAX; neoadj. or adj. chemotherapy	348	52	42

RTOG, Radiation Therapy Oncology Group; TURBT, transurethral resection of bladder tumor; MCV, methotrexate, cisplatin, vinblastine; 5-FU, 5-fluorouracil; adj., adjuvant; TAX, paclitaxel; GEM, gemcitabine; CP, cisplatin; NA, not available; MGH, Massachusetts General Hospital.

T2, patients were treated with gemcitabine and concurrent daily radiation. At a median follow-up of 5.6 years, an impressive 91% CR rate was observed, and the 5-year actuarial estimates of survival include a bladder-intact survival of 62%, an overall survival of 76%, and a disease-specific survival of 82%.[84]

Cisplatin is not an ideal drug for bladder cancer patients, as many have impaired renal function. A British group therefore examined the combination of 5-FU and mitomycin C with pelvic radiotherapy. Having achieved high response rates, they are now testing, through a phase 3 trial, this chemoradiotherapy regimen compared with radiation therapy alone.[85]

Predictors of Outcome

A common feature of all the RTOG protocols was early bladder tumor response evaluation and the selection of patients for bladder conservation on the basis of their initial response to TURBT combined with chemotherapy and radiation.[86] Bladder conservation was reserved for those who had a complete clinical response at the midpoint in therapy (after a radiation dosage of 40 Gy). Approximately two-thirds of the total then received consolidation with additional chemotherapy and radiation to a total tumor dose of 64 to 65 Gy. Incomplete responders were advised to undergo radical cystectomy, as were patients whose invasive tumors persisted or recurred after treatment. The current schema for trimodality treatment of muscle-invading bladder cancer is provided in Figure 95.3. In the MGH series the median follow-up for all surviving patients is 7.7 years. The 10-year actuarial overall survival was 35% (T2, 43%; T3–T4a 27%) and the 10-year disease-specific survival was 59% (T2 67%; stage T3–T4a, 49%) (Figs. 95.4 and 95.5). Clinical stage was thus significantly associated with both overall survival and disease-specific survival, the use of neoadjuvant chemotherapy with MCV, however, was not. The 10-year disease-specific survival rate for the 102 patients undergoing cystectomy was 44%, illustrating the very important contribution of prompt salvage cystectomy. The 10-year disease-specific survival with an intact bladder

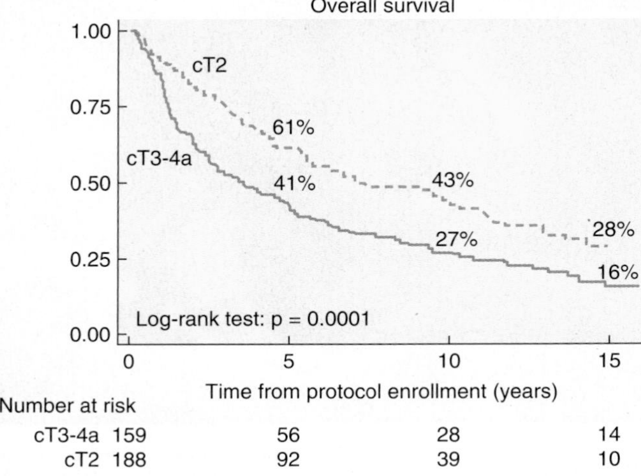

FIGURE 95.4 Massachusetts General Hospital Selective Bladder Preservation Series 1986 to 2002 reported by intention to treat. Overall survival.

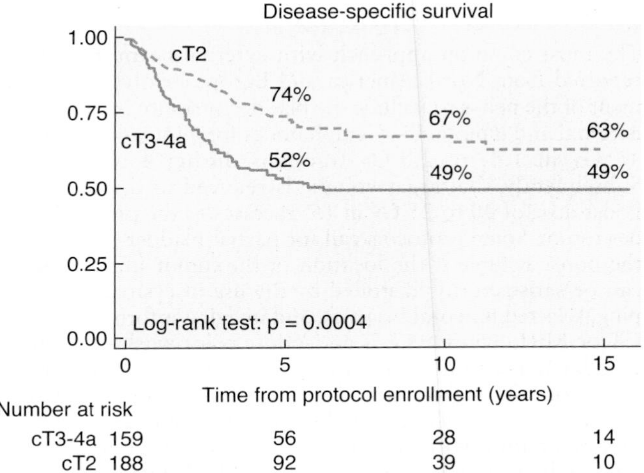

FIGURE 95.5 Massachusetts General Hospital Selective Bladder Preservation Series 1986 to 2002 reported by intention to treat. Disease specific survival.

TABLE 95.4

SURVIVAL OUTCOMES BY PATIENT AND TUMOR CHARACTERISTICS: MASSACHUSETTS GENERAL HOSPITAL[8]

		Overall Survival (%)				Disease-Specific Survival (%)			
Patient Group	*n*	5 Year	10 Year	15 Year	*P* value	5 Year	10 Year	15 Year	*P* value
All patients	348	52 ± 5.3[a]	35 ± 5.6[a]	22 ± 5.6[a]		64 ± 5.8[a]	59 ± 6.2[a]	57 ± 6.6[a]	
Age at entry (y)									
<75	262	54	39	27	0.004	65	59	58	0.59
>75	86	45	23	2.9		63	60	52	
Sex									
Female	91	55	37	17	0.72	64	55	55	0.59
Male	257	51	35	24		64	60	58	
Clinical stage									
T2	188	61	43	28	0.0001	74	67	63	0.0004
T3–T4a	159	41	27	16		52	49	49	
Hydronephrosis									
No	289	55	39	24	0.0004	68	63	61	0.0005
Yes	58	34	17	10		44	38	38	

NS, not stated.
[a]95% confidence interval.

was 45% (T2, 52%; T3–T4a, 36%). No patient required cystectomy due to bladder morbidity. The overall survival and disease-specific survival for all 348 patients and for some clinically important subgroups are shown in Table 95.4. The value of complete TURBT in bladder-sparing therapy is demonstrated in this report. Of the 348 patients followed, 227 underwent a complete TURBT and 116 had an incomplete TURBT. Patients who underwent a complete TURBT had improved CR, overall survival, disease-specific survival, and lower rates of cystectomy (22% vs. 42%) compared to those with an incomplete TURBT. In a review of the patients who were complete responders after induction therapy, 60% developed no further bladder tumors, 30% subsequently developed a superficial occurrence, and 10% developed an invasive tumor.[87] Most with superficial recurrence were treated conservatively by TURBT and intravesical chemotherapy. For these individuals the overall survival was comparable to those who had no failure. However, one-third of these patients required a salvage cystectomy.

Radiation Treatment

The most common approach with external-beam irradiation reported from North America and Europe involves the treatment of the pelvis to include the bladder, prostate (in men), and external and internal iliac lymph nodes for a total dose of 40 to 45 Gy in 1.8- to 2.0-Gy fractions during 4 to 5 weeks. Subsequently, the target volume is reduced to deliver a final boost dose of 20 to 25 Gy in 15 fractions to the primary bladder tumor. Some protocols call for partial bladder radiation as the boost volume if the location of the tumor in the bladder can be satisfactorily identified by the use of cystoscopic mapping, selected mucosal biopsies, and imaging information from CT or MRI. Figure 95.6 is an isodose color wash of a partial bladder boost in a three-dimensional–conformal plan. Plans using conventional fractionation that result in a whole bladder dose of 50 to 55 Gy and a bladder tumor volume dose of 65 Gy in combination with concurrent cisplatin-containing chemotherapy have been widely used. The available information suggests that higher doses per fraction may lead to a higher rate of serious late complications. Data from urodynamic and quality-of-life studies indicate that lower dose per fraction irradiation given once or twice a day concurrent with chemotherapy results in excellent long-term bladder function.[88]

Because the bladder is not a fixed organ, its location and volume can vary considerably from day to day. This results in a number of logistic problems to ensure adequate coverage of the bladder. Studies have identified substantial movement of the bladder during the course of external-beam radiation therapy, and as a result of these findings, the bladder must be empty when simulated and always emptied just prior to each treatment. A clinical target volume expansion of 2 cm is advised superiorly and 1 cm at the other borders.[89]

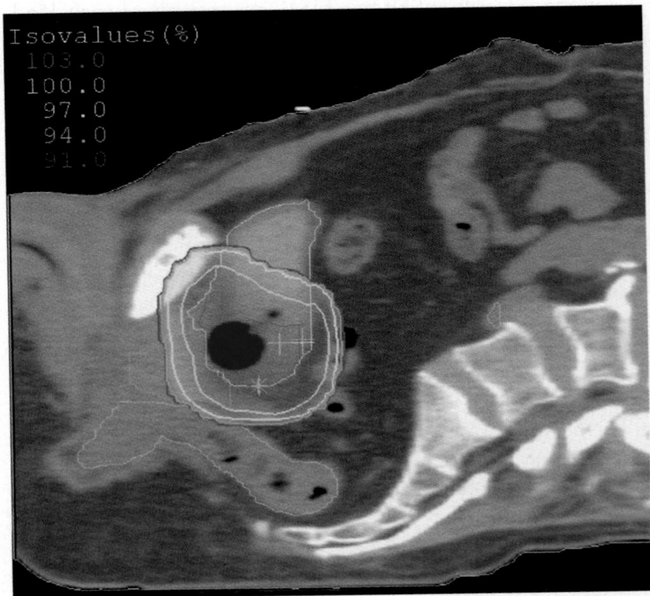

FIGURE 95.6 Display of a sagittal section through the three-dimensional data set, with dose displayed in color wash, for a patient with bladder cancer treated with a partial bladder tumor boost with three-dimensional conformal radiotherapy. Note sparing of the anterior, nontumor bearing portion of bladder.

Brachytherapy is another technique to deliver a higher dose of radiation to a limited area of the bladder within a short period. This approach has been reported from institutions in the Netherlands, Belgium, and France. It is reserved for patients with solitary bladder tumors and as part of combined modality therapy with transurethral resection and external-beam radiation therapy as well as interstitial radiation therapy. External-beam doses of 30 Gy are used in combination with an implant tumor dose of 40 Gy. These groups report that for patients with solitary clinical stage T2 to T3a tumors less than 5 cm in diameter, local control rates at 5 years range from 72% to 84% with disease-specific survivals of approximately 80%.[90]

Comparison of Treatment Outcomes of Contemporary Cystectomy Series with Contemporary Selective Bladder-Preserving Series

Comparing the results of selective bladder-preserving approaches with those of radical cystectomy series is confounded by the discordance between clinical (TURBT) staging and pathologic (cystectomy) staging. Clinical staging is more likely to understage the extent of disease with regard to penetration into the muscularis propria or beyond than is pathologic staging.[91] The University of Southern California and Memorial Sloan-Kettering Cancer Center have reported their large cystectomy experience.[90,64] A national phase 3 protocol by Southwest Oncology Group (SWOG), Eastern Cooperative Oncology Group, and Cancer and Leukemia Group B (CALGB) also reports valuable prospective data.[65] The overall survival rates from these contemporary cystectomy series are comparable to those reported from single-institution and cooperative group results using contemporary selective bladder-preserving approaches with trimodality therapy (Table 95.5).

Bladder-Preservation Treatments with Less than Trimodality Therapy

It has been argued that trimodality therapy might represent excessive treatment for many patients with invasive bladder cancer and that comparable results could be obtained by TURBT, either alone or with chemotherapy. Herr[92] reported the outcome of 432 patients initially evaluated by repeat TURBT for muscle-invasive bladder tumors. In that series, 99 patients (23% of the original 432 patients) initially treated conservatively without immediate cystectomy had a 34% rate of progression to a recurrent muscle-invading tumor at 20 years. In series combining TURBT and MVAC chemotherapy, only 50% of those found to have a clinical CR proved to be tumor-free at cystectomy.[93] By comparison one of the clearest examples of the improved success of trimodality treatment was reported in the study from the University of Paris.[92] TURBT followed by concurrent cisplatin, 5-FU, and accelerated radiation was used by this group initially as a precystectomy regimen. In the first 18 patients, all of whom demonstrated no residual tumor on cystoscopic evaluation and rebiopsy (a CR) but who all underwent a cystectomy, none had any tumor in the cystectomy specimen (100% had a pathologic CR). Comparing approaches by TURBT plus MVAC chemotherapy alone with trimodality therapy, the 5-year survival rates are comparable (50%), but the preserved bladder rate for all patients studied ranged from 20% to 33% when radiation therapy was not used and from 41% to 45% when radiation therapy was used.[94] Thus, trimodality therapy increases the probability of surviving with an intact bladder by 30% to 40% compared with the results reported with TURBT and chemotherapy alone.

Herr[95] reported on 63 patients who had achieved a complete clinical response to neoadjuvant chemotherapy with a cisplatin-based regimen, who then refused to undergo a planned cystectomy. He reported that the most significant predictor of improved survival was complete resection of the tumor before starting chemotherapy. Over 90% of surviving patients had small low-stage invasive tumors that were completely resected. Thus, he concluded, selected patients with T2 bladder cancers may do well after transurethral resection and chemotherapy.

Systemic Chemotherapy with Radical Therapy

Neoadjuvant Chemotherapy

The advantage of neoadjuvant chemotherapy is its potential to downsize and downstage tumors and to attack occult metastatic disease early. The disadvantages include the inherent

TABLE 95.5

MUSCLE-INVASIVE BLADDER CANCER: SURVIVAL OUTCOMES IN CONTEMPORARY SERIES

Series (Ref.)	Stages	No. of Patients	Overall Survival (%) 5 Year	10 Year
Cystectomy				
U. Southern California, 2001 (63)	pT2–pT4a	633	48	32
Memorial Sloan-Kettering, 2001 (64)	pT2–pT4a	181	36	27
SWOG/ECOG/CALGB,[a,b] 2003 (65)	cT2–cT4a	307	50	34
Selective bladder preservation				
U. Erlangen[a] (2002) (78)	cT2–cT4a	326	45	29
MGH[a] (2009) (86)	cT2–cT4a	348	52	35
RTOG[a] (1998) (76)	cT2–cT4a	123	49	—

SWOG, Southwest Oncology Group; ECOG, Eastern Cooperative Oncology Group; CALGB, Cancer and Leukemia Group B; MGH, Massachusetts General Hospital; RTOG, Radiation Therapy Oncology Group.

[a]These series include all patients by their intention to treat.

[b]Fifty percent of patients were randomly assigned to receive three cycles of neoadjuvant MVAC (methotrexate, vinblastine, doxorubicin, cisplatin).

difficulties in assessing response, the fact that clinical rather than pathologic criteria must be relied on, the debilitating effects of chemotherapy in some patients, increasing the risks of surgery and possibly complicating or delaying full recovery from surgery, and the possibility of the deleterious effects of the delay in cystectomy or radiation associated with neoadjuvant chemotherapy.[96]

Although downstaging of the primary tumor has been demonstrated, randomized studies using single-agent neoadjuvant chemotherapy have failed to demonstrate a survival benefit. Studies in patients with measurable metastatic disease clearly showed the superiority of MVAC over single-agent cisplatin on survival, inspiring further studies of multiagent neoadjuvant therapy.[97]

The study by Grossman et al.[92] randomly assigned patients with muscularis propria–invasive bladder cancer (stage T2 to T4a) to radical cystectomy alone or three cycles of MVAC followed by radical cystectomy. During an 11-year period, 317 patients were enrolled. The authors reported that MVAC can be given before radical cystectomy, but the side effects are appreciable. One-third of patients had severe hematologic or gastrointestinal reactions, but, on the positive side, there were no drug-related deaths nor did the chemotherapy adversely affect the performance of surgery. The authors concluded:

1. The survival benefit associated with MVAC appeared to be strongly related to downstaging of the tumor to pT0. Thirty-eight percent of the chemotherapy-treated patients had no evidence of cancer at cystectomy, as compared with 15% of patients in the cystectomy-only group. In both groups, improved survival was associated with the absence of residual cancer in the cystectomy specimen.
2. The median survival was 77 months for the chemotherapy-treated patients compared with 46 months for the cystectomy-only group.
3. The 5-year actuarial survival was 43% in the cystectomy group, which was not significantly different from 57% in the chemotherapy-treated group.

The authors point out that their study is different from seven previous negative studies that used either single-agent cisplatin (demonstrated to be inferior to MVAC in measurable metastatic disease) or a two-drug combination. They also acknowledged problems of interpretation created by slow accrual and a lack of pathologic review.

The Medical Research Council and the European Organisation for the Research and Treatment of Cancer (EORTC) performed a prospective randomized trial of neoadjuvant cisplatin, methotrexate, and vinblastine in patients undergoing cystectomy or full-dose external-beam radiotherapy for muscularis propria bladder cancer.[98,99] They reported with a median follow-up of 7.4 years.[99] The difference in 5-year survival between those who received chemotherapy (50%) and those who did not (44%) just reached clinical significance with a probability value of 0.048. The 7-year survival rates were 43% versus 37%. There was also an improved disease-free survival (P = .012). Based on their interpretation of the data as presented, Sharma and Bajorin[100] now recommend neoadjuvant chemotherapy, though others are concerned that the "number needed to treat" is very high.

A third randomized trial was the Nordic Cystectomy Trial 1.[101] Patients were treated with two cycles of neoadjuvant doxorubicin and cisplatin. All patients received 5 days of radiation followed by cystectomy. A subgroup analysis was performed and showed a 20% difference in disease-specific survival at 5 years in patients with T3 and T4 disease, but there was no difference in stages T1 and T2, nor a difference when all entered patients were compared.

The Nordic Cystectomy Trial 2 included only stage T3 or T4a patients in an attempt to confirm the positive results in Nordic I in this subgroup of patients.[102] This trial eliminated radiation therapy and substituted methotrexate for doxorubicin in order to lower toxicity. In 317 patients studied, no survival benefit was noted in the chemotherapy arm. The authors concluded that despite substantial downstaging, no survival benefit was seen with neoadjuvant chemotherapy after 5 years of follow-up.

Raghavan et al.[103] published a meta-analysis of all completed randomized trials of neoadjuvant chemotherapy for invasive bladder cancer (2,688 patients). They concluded that single-agent neoadjuvant chemotherapy is ineffective and should not be used; current combination chemotherapy regimens improve the 5-year survival by 5%, which reduces the risk of death by 13% compared with the use of definitive local treatment alone (i.e., from 43% to 38%).

Additional meta-analyses have been published[96,104–106] that showed a 4% to 6% absolute increase in 5-year survival. Many phase 2 studies are now investigating alternative neoadjuvant combinations, and time will tell whether any have superiority.[107–113]

In the 2008 National Comprehensive Cancer Network *Clinical Practice Guidelines in Oncology: Bladder Cancer*, neoadjuvant chemotherapy is only "considered," and that according to the National Cancer Data Base in the United States, only 11.6% of patients underwent any perioperative chemotherapy with most in the adjuvant setting.[113] Gene profiling may in the future identify those most likely to respond to chemotherapy.[114]

Adjuvant Chemotherapy

The advantage of adjuvant, as opposed to neoadjuvant, chemotherapy is that pathologic staging allows for a more accurate selection of patients. This approach facilitates the separation of patients in stage pT2 from those in stages pT3 or pT4 or node-positive disease, all at a high risk for metastatic progression.

Adjuvant chemotherapy has been studied in two major clinical settings: (1) following bladder-sparing chemoirradiation and (2) following radical cystectomy. In the former case, there is no guidance from pathologic staging, but experience has shown that up to 50% of those with invasive cancers have, in truth, a systemic disease.[115] Respecting this the RTOG studies have added adjuvant chemotherapy at first with MCV, later using cisplatin plus gemcitabine, and more recently adding paclitaxel.[116] The results thus far do not indicate whether adjuvant chemotherapy is affecting survival.

The place of adjuvant chemotherapy after cystectomy has been studied more thoroughly, but the results are again not clear. Investigators generally agree that in the face of positive nodes, and even with negative nodes and high pathologic stage of the primary tumor, adjuvant chemotherapy is likely to be important in improving survival. In reviewing existing reports of adjuvant trials in bladder cancer, there are five randomized trials using adjuvant chemotherapy.[117–121] Three studies found no difference between adjuvant chemotherapy and cystectomy alone, but all three were seriously flawed in design or accrual.[100] Two of the five studies[120,121] showed a survival benefit for cystectomy and adjuvant chemotherapy over cystectomy alone, but both are subject to criticism for both method considerations and small accrual.

Nonetheless, in a follow-up report by Stockle et al.[122] an analysis of 166 patients, including the 49 initially randomized patients, a difference was noted in the 80 patients who received adjuvant chemotherapy as compared with 86 patients who underwent cystectomy alone. The extent of nodal involvement proved important, and when patients were stratified by the number of nodes involved, adjuvant chemotherapy was most effective in patients with N1 disease.

In an important review of the current status of adjuvant chemotherapy in muscle-invasive bladder cancer, the Advanced Bladder Cancer Meta-Analysis Collaboration examined 491 patients from six trials, representing 90% of all patients randomized in cisplatin-based combination chemotherapy trials. They concluded that there is insufficient evidence on which to base reliable treatment decisions, and they recommended further research.[123]

Gallagher et al.[124] studied adjuvant, sequential chemotherapy in a nonrandomized design, using as a basis the improvement in survival in breast cancer when sequential adjuvant chemotherapy was used. In this study and others similarly designed,[125,126] adjuvant, sequential chemotherapy for patients with high-risk urothelial cancer did not appear to improve disease-specific survival over that observed with surgery alone.

Dreicer,[112] in reviewing the published literature, made the case for adjuvant chemotherapy as the standard of care given the lethality of radical cystectomy alone in muscle invasive bladder cancer, but he acknowledges that "suboptimal trial design, insufficient numbers of patients, and lack of standardization of the chemotherapy regimens used have plagued adjuvant studies."

Combined Modality Treatment of Locoregionally Advanced Disease

The place of combined modality therapy for advanced disease has not been settled. Several series have suggested an improvement in long-term survival in selected patients undergoing resection of persistent cancer deposits after MVAC or CMV (cisplatin, methotrexate, and vinblastine).[115,127]

In our experience, carefully selected patients with locally advanced unresectable bladder cancer, including some patients with pelvic nodal masses, may experience long-term survival with the combination of chemotherapy and radiation. To be selected for this combined modality treatment patients have to have (1) an excellent performance status, (2) locally advanced measurable disease, (3) normal kidney function tests, and (4) no evidence of distant metastases beyond the common iliac lymph nodes. The initial treatment consists of four to six cycles of combination chemotherapy. If significant regression of tumor is achieved, radiation treatment is administered in combination with radiosensitizing chemotherapy. These patients were carefully selected, but in the majority of patients so treated, excellent tumor shrinkage and long-term survival were achieved in patients who would otherwise have been expected to succumb rapidly if treatment had consisted of chemotherapy alone.

Quality of Life after Cystectomy or Bladder Preservation

Evaluating the quality of life in long-term survivors of bladder cancer has been difficult and only recently have attempts been made to assess this in an objective and quantitative fashion.[128–140] A number of problems arise in the interpretation of the published studies. Tools to assess quality-of-life variables were developed early for common prostate and gynecologic cancers, but until very recently no such instruments existed for bladder cancer. The instruments in use for bladder cancer have thus been adaptations of uncertain validity. The published studies are all cross-sectional and patients have follow-ups of varying lengths. This matters in a surgical series in which functional outcome improves with time and in a radiation series in which it may deteriorate. Despite these limitations, some conclusions can now be drawn.

Radical cystectomy causes changes in many areas of quality of life, including urinary, sexual, and social function, daily living activities, and satisfaction with body image.[117–122,141] Researchers have, during the past decade, concentrated on the relative merits of continent and incontinent diversions. Available data have been mixed with some groups, surprisingly, reporting few differences between the quality of life of those with an ileal conduit and those with continent diversions. Hart et al.[132] have compared outcome in cystectomy patients who have either ileal conduits, cutaneous Koch pouches, or urethral Koch pouches. Regardless of the type of urinary diversion, the majority of patients reported good overall quality of life, little emotional distress, and few problems with social, physical, or functional activities. Problems with their diversions and with sexual function were most commonly reported. After controlling for age, no significant differences were seen among urinary diversion subgroups in any quality-of-life area. It might be anticipated that those receiving the urethral Koch diversions would be the most satisfied, and the explanation why this is not so is unclear. It may be that the subgroups were too small to detect differences, but perhaps it is more likely that each group adapts in time to the specific difficulties presented by that type of diversion. Somani et al.[134] have recently reviewed 40 published studies that evaluated overall quality of life, reporting on 3,645 patients. Only two studies reported a better quality of life for those who had neobladder and only two reported a better body image.[134] Another prospective study reported by Mansson et al.[135] suggested that there may be a large cultural component to the response with big differences seen between Egyptian and Swedish men followed prospectively through trials of chemotherapy and cystectomy.

Porter and Penson[133] attempted a systematic review of the literature testing the premise that continent diversions result in improved health-related quality-of-life outcomes. They concluded that, whatever our assumptions, there is no literature to support the use of one urinary diversion over another. Reviews by Gerharz et al.[136] and Somani et al.[134] came to the same conclusion.

Zietman et al.[137] have performed a study on patients treated with chemoradiation for muscle–invasive bladder cancer. Patients underwent a urodynamic study and completed a quality-of-life questionnaire with a median time from therapy of 6.3 years. This long follow-up is sufficient to capture the majority of late radiation effects. Seventy-five percent of patients had normally functioning bladders by urodynamic studies. Reduced bladder compliance, a recognized complication of radiation, was seen in 22% but in only one-third of these was it reflected in distressing symptoms. The questionnaire showed that bladder symptoms were uncommon, especially among men, with the exception of control problems. These were reported by 19%, with 11% using incontinence products (all women). Distress from urinary symptoms was half as common as their prevalence. Bowel symptoms occurred in 22% with only 14% recording any level of distress. The majority of men retained sexual function. Global health-related quality of life was high. A study reported by Herman et al.[138] showed that when low doses of gemcitabine are used as an alternative radiation-sensitizer to cisplatin, then treatment is also very tolerable. Thus the great majority of patients treated by trimodality therapy retain good bladder function.

Two cross-sectional questionnaire studies, one from Sweden and one from Italy, have compared the outcome following radiation with the outcome following cystectomy.[139,140] The questionnaire results for urinary function following radiation were very similar to those recorded in the MGH study. More than 74% of patients reported good urinary function. Both studies compared bowel function in irradiated patients with that seen in patients undergoing cystectomy. In both, the bowel

PRACTICE OF ONCOLOGY

symptoms were greater for those receiving radiation than for those receiving cystectomy (10% vs. 3% and 32% vs. 24%, respectively), but in neither was this statistically significant.

Data on the assessment of sexual function are limited to men. The majority in the MGH series report adequate erectile function (full or sufficient for intercourse). These findings are in line with those obtained in the Swedish and Italian series in which three times as many men retained useful erections as compared with cystectomized controls.

A Bladder Cancer Index has recently been developed and validated.[142] It has been shown to have high internal and retest consistency and can be used regardless of local treatment type and across the genders. This is the first such tool developed and it holds great promise for comparative treatment studies in the future.

Metastatic Bladder Cancer

An estimated 12,500 deaths per year in the United States are due to metastatic bladder cancer.[143] Through lymphatic and hematogenous means, bladder cancer metastasizes to distant organs, most commonly the lungs, bone, liver, and brain. The prognosis of metastatic bladder cancer, as with other metastatic solid tumors, is poor, with a median survival on the order of only 12 months. Nevertheless, since the discovery that platinum-containing agents have significant antitumor effect in bladder cancer, there has been great interest in the use of chemotherapy for advanced disease.

Compared with other solid-tumor malignancies, transitional cell cancer is chemosensitive. In phase 2 clinical trials, radiographic response rates may be as high as 70% to 80%, and in phase 3 clinical trials, response rates are often on the order of 50%. Moreover, a small but substantial minority of responding patients manifest a CR, and among these patients some long-term, durable responses are observed. Overall, however, the duration of response in TCC is short, with a median of 4 to 6 months, and therefore the impact of chemotherapy on survival has been disappointing. As newer targeted agents come into clinical practice, the hope is that their incorporation into treatment regimens will lengthen duration of response and ultimately translate into a real change in survival.

Cisplatin

In 1976, a series of 24 patients with bladder cancer treated with single-agent cisplatin was reported.[144] The investigators observed eight partial responses in addition to four minor responses. Subsequent studies confirmed the activity of cisplatin in TCC, although the response rate to single-agent cisplatin has been lower than that of cisplatin-containing combination therapy.[145,146] Thus, most subsequent studies have explored combination regimens.

Cisplatin-Based Combination Chemotherapy

The standard chemotherapy regimen for advanced bladder cancer for more than a decade was MVAC.[147,148] MVAC is administered in 28-day cycles, with starting doses of methotrexate 30 mg/m^2 (days 1, 15, and 22), vinblastine 3 mg/m^2 (days 2, 15, and 22), doxorubicin 30 mg/m^2 (day 2), and cisplatin 70 mg/m^2 (day 2). Another commonly used regimen has been CMV, which omits the doxorubicin and has somewhat less toxicity.[149] The MVAC regimen has superior activity to cisplatin alone[145,146] and to other cisplatin-containing regimens.[150] The response rate to MVAC is 40% to 65%,[146,147,151] and there is improved progression-free and overall survival compared with either single-agent cisplatin or cisplatin, cyclophosphamide, and doxorubicin. Complete response is seen in 15% to 25% of patients, with an expected median survival of 12 months[145–150] (Table 95.6).

On the negative side, MVAC is associated with substantial toxicity, and most patients require dose adjustment at some point in their treatment. Toxic effects of MVAC in notable numbers of patients include neutropenia, anemia, thrombocytopenia, stomatitis, nausea, and fatigue.[99,100,151] The rate of chemotherapy-induced fatality among patients with metastatic disease may be as high as 3%, most often due to neutropenic sepsis.[151]

The doublet of gemcitabine and cisplatin showed encouraging results in phase 2 studies, with response rates of 42% to 66% and CR rates of 18% to 28%.[152,153] Primary toxicity was hematologic and was generally easily managed, with rare hospitalizations for febrile neutropenia and no toxic deaths. Based on these encouraging results, gemcitabine and cisplatin (GC) was compared with MVAC in a multicenter phase 3 study.[151,154] MVAC was administered as previously described, and GC was

TABLE 95.6

STANDARD CISPLATIN-CONTAINING REGIMENS FOR TRANSITIONAL CELL CARCINOMA

Regimen			Response			
Agents (Ref.)		Schedule	Composite No. of Assessable Patients	CR (%)	RR (%)	Median Survival (Mo)
MVAC (146,147,149)	Methotrexate Vinblastine Doxorubicin Cisplatin	30 mg/m^2 d 1, 15, 22 3 mg/m^2 d 2, 15, 22 30 mg/m^2 d 2 70 mg/m^2 d 2	374	12–35	39–65	12.5–14.8
CMV (160)	Cisplatin Methotrexate Vinblastine	70 mg/m^2 d 2 30 mg/m^2 d 1, 8 4 mg/m^2 d 1, 8	104	10	36	7
GC (161)	Gemcitabine Cisplatin	1000 mg/m^2 d 1, 8, 15 70 mg/m^2 d 2	203	12	49	13.8

CR, complete response; RR, response rate; MVAC, methotrexate, vinblastine, doxorubicin, cisplatin; CMV, cisplatin, methotrexate, vinblastine; GC, gemcitabine, cisplatin.

TABLE 95.7

PHASE 2 TRIALS OF TAXANE-CONTAINING CHEMOTHERAPY REGIMENS

Regimen	Composite No. of Patients	Response Rate (%)	Median Survival (Mo)	Reference
Carboplatin/paclitaxel	104	21–65	8.5–9.5	155,156,157
Cisplatin/paclitaxel	52	50	10.6	158
Cisplatin/docetaxel	129	52–60	8.0–13.6	159,160,161
Cisplatin/gemcitabine/paclitaxel	61	78	15.8	119, 162
Carboplatin/gemcitabine/paclitaxel	49	68	14.7	163
Cisplatin/gemcitabine/docetaxel	35	66	15.5	164
Gemcitabine/paclitaxel	94	54–60	14.4	165–167

administered in 28-day cycles with gemcitabine 1,000 mg/m^2 (days 1, 8, and15) and cisplatin 70 mg/m^2 (day 2). Four hundred five patients were randomized to one of the two treatment arms, and the two groups exhibited similar characteristics. Median survival was 14 months with GC and 15.2 months with MVAC, which were statistically comparable.[154] Patients treated with GC, however, had significantly less toxicity and improved tolerability. Patients receiving GC gained more weight, reported less fatigue, and had better performance status than patients who received MVAC. As a result of this study, GC is generally considered the current standard of care for metastatic bladder cancer.

Taxane- and Platinum-Containing Regimens

The addition of taxanes to cisplatin-based regimens has been the subject of numerous phase 2 trials in bladder cancer (Table 95.7). The doublets of cisplatin and paclitaxel and cisplatin and docetaxel appear to have response rates comparable to that of GC.[158–161] Trials with carboplatin suggest that this agent has good activity, although likely not the same level of activity as cisplatin.[156,168]

A phase 3 trial compared MVAC with carboplatin and paclitaxel.[157] The study failed to reach its accrual goal, with only 85 patients randomized, although no significant differences in efficacy were seen. It is of note that the MVAC group exhibited a trend toward higher response rate (36% vs. 28%), progression-free survival (8.7 vs. 5.2 months), and overall survival (15.4 vs. 13.8 months).

Omission of platinum completely has been studied as well. The doublet of gemcitabine and paclitaxel appears to have good activity, with phase 2 studies suggesting that this regimen has response rates and survival comparable to GC, with minimal toxicity.[165–167,169] Gemcitabine with paclitaxel may be a reasonable regimen to consider in patients unfit for platinum therapy. Gemcitabine and docetaxel demonstrated a response rate of 33% and median survival of 12 months in a trial of 27 patients with advanced TCC.[170]

Triplet Chemotherapy

Because of the activity of each of these agents in TCC, investigators then asked whether triplet combinations of platinum, taxanes, and gemcitabine might have increased activity over the doublets. In phase 2 trials, three such combinations, including cisplatin/gemcitabine/paclitaxel,[119] carboplatin/gemcitabine/paclitaxel,[171] and cisplatin/gemcitabine/docetaxel,[164] demonstrated high CR rates of 28% to 32%, and overall response rates of 66% to 78%, although the numbers of patients with visceral metastases was relatively low. A second study of carboplatin/gemcitabine/paclitaxel showed a more modest response rate of 43% and overall survival of 11 months in a more typical population of metastatic TCC.[163] A triplet of paclitaxel, cisplatin, and infusional high-dose 5-FU with leucovorin has also been studied. The response rate was 75%, with 28% CRs, and the median overall survival was 17 months. Significant toxicity included frequent myelosuppression, gastrointestinal disturbances, infections, and two treatment-related deaths.[172]

A randomized phase 3 trial compared the standard GC regimen with GC plus paclitaxel (PCG).[162] Preliminary results suggest that while the response rate was improved by the addition of paclitaxel, there will be no difference in progression-free survival or overall survival. Thus, GC remains the standard of care at this time for initial treatment of metastatic TCC.

Biologic Agents

The enthusiasm engendered by development of novel biologic agents targeted against tumor-specific growth factor pathways or angiogenesis has been fortified in recent years by positive studies in a variety of solid tumors. Two classes of agents that may be of interest in TCC are inhibitors of EGFR, including EGFR1 and EGFR2 (HER2/neu), and inhibitors of VEGF or its receptors. There is ample preclinical evidence that many bladder tumors express members of the EGFR family, that overexpression may correlate inversely with prognosis, and that inhibition of these pathways may have an antitumor effect.[46–52] A number of groups are conducting studies with inhibitors of EGFR1 and HER2/neu in the treatment of advanced bladder cancer. Similarly, the utility of angiogenesis inhibitors in TCC will be explored in upcoming years, as evidenced by a recently opened cooperative group trial in metastatic TCC studying GC with or without the addition of bevacizumab.

CANCERS OF THE RENAL PELVIS AND URETER

The majority of tumors of the upper urinary collecting system are TCCs. However, these are uncommon, with fewer than 3,000 cases diagnosed annually in the United States. The incidence has remained constant, but there has recently been a slight stage migration toward a higher proportion of earlier stage tumors.[173] Because of the challenge in gaining access to them, initial diagnosis and staging are less accurate than for cancer of the bladder. Histologically, 90% of upper tract tumors are TCC. Squamous cell carcinoma accounts for nearly all of the remainder. There is a predilection for these tumors to arise in the renal pelvis; primary tumors of the ureter occur only half as frequently as do tumors of the renal pelvis.[174] Men develop upper tract TCC two to three times more often than women, with the peak age of development of these tumors in the seventh and eighth decades of life.[158] Women, however, are more likely than men to have more advanced and higher grade tumor at nephroureterectomy.[175] As discussed in the first section of this chapter, the majority of these tumors arise as a result of, or at least in association with, environmental exposures and stresses.[6–8,15]

Clinical Presentation, Diagnosis, and Staging

Gross hematuria is the presenting symptom in 75% to 95% of all patients who present with tumors of the renal pelvis and ureter. Hematuria may be accompanied by colicky flank pain if the tumor or blood clots cause obstruction of the upper urinary tract. Patients often describe the passage of vermiform clots, which are unusual in bleeding from a lower tract source. Hydronephrosis may also be a presenting sign. Urinary cytology is an important part of the workup for an upper tract tumor. Voided urine cytology, though, has only 10% to 40% sensitivity in the detection of low-grade TCC lesions. Cytology is far more useful for high-grade tumors, for which the sensitivity may be as high as 70%.[176,177]

Improvements in endoscopic technology allow the urologist to view directly and to obtain tissue in many of the TCCs of the upper tract. Pathologic confirmation may be obtained prior to treatment. Also, grade may be a useful predictor of advanced stage disease.[178]

Intravenous urography was the mainstay of radiographic evaluation of upper tract tumors, but now in most major centers CT scan is preferred[179] (Fig. 95.7). MRI urography may also be useful in patients when sensitivity to iodinated contrast prevents the use of that agent.[180,181] When a patient is found or judged to have a TCC more aggressive than a G1 stage I tumor, additional staging of the patient is indicated, including CT scans of the chest, abdomen, and pelvis. Because standard therapy is radical excision of the kidney and the ipsilateral ureter, evaluation of the total remaining renal function prior to a proposed nephrectomy is indicated. Isotope renal scanning can accurately estimate the function of the uninvolved kidney.

The current American Joint Committee on Cancer TNM staging for tumors of the upper urinary tract is shown in Figure 95.8 and in Table 95.8. The staging is determined by

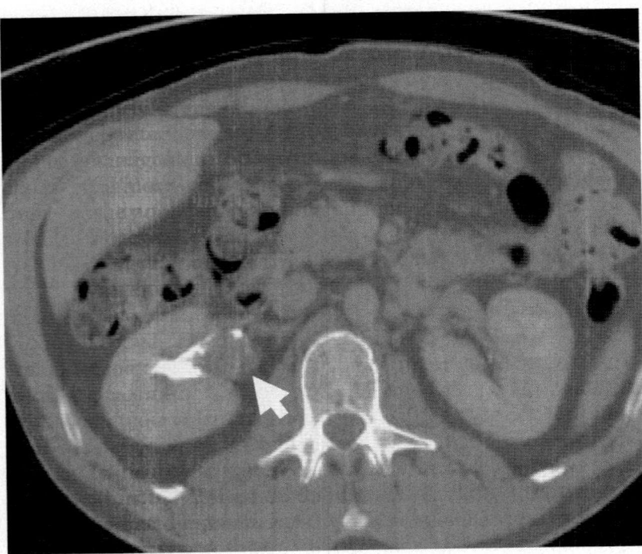

FIGURE 95.7 Abdominal computed tomographic scan of a stage T3 transitional cell carcinoma of the right renal pelvis, with intravenous contrast showing a large filling defect in the right renal pelvis (*arrow*).

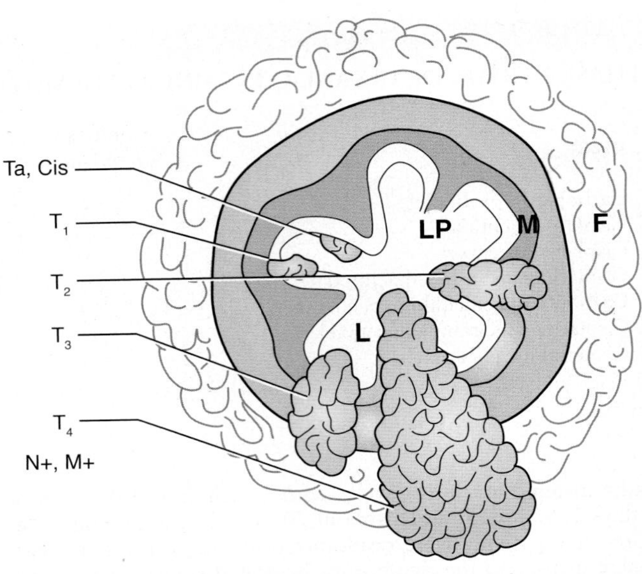

FIGURE 95.8 Schematic diagram of the American Joint Committee on Cancer TNM (tumor, necrosis, metastasis) staging of cancers of the renal pelvis. C, renal capsule; LP, lamina propria; M, muscularis propria; F, peripelvic fat; L, lumen.

TABLE 95.8

AMERICAN JOINT COMMITTEE ON CANCER 2009 TNM STAGING OF RENAL PELVIS AND URETER CANCERS: DEFINITION OF TNM

PRIMARY TUMOR (T)	
TX	Primary tumor cannot be assessed
T0	No evidence of primary tumor
Ta	Papillary noninvasive carcinoma
Tis	Carcinoma *in situ*
T1	Tumor invades subepithelial connective tissue
T2	Tumor invades the muscularis
T3	(For renal pelvis only) Tumor invades beyond muscularis into peripelvic fat or the renal parenchyma
T3	(For ureter only) Tumor invades beyond muscularis into periureteric fat
T4	Tumor invades adjacent organs or through the kidney into the perinephric fat.
REGIONAL LYMPH NODES (N)[a]	
NX	Regional lymph nodes cannot be assessed
N0	No regional lymph node metastasis
N1	Metastasis in a single lymph node 2 cm or less in greatest dimension
N2	Metastasis in a single lymph node more than 2 cm but not more than 5 cm in greatest dimension or multiple lymph nodes; none more than 5 cm in greatest dimension
N3	Metastasis in a lymph node, more than 5 cm in greatest dimension
DISTANT METASTASIS (M)	
MX	Distant metastasis cannot be assessed
M0	No distant metastasis
M1	Distant metastasis

[a]Laterality does not affect the N classification.
(From ref. 54, with permission.)

the extent of invasion by the primary tumor and by microscopic evaluation of the regional lymph nodes.

Surgical Treatment

The standard surgical treatment for patients with transitional cell cancer of the upper urinary tract of all grades and stages is radical nephroureterectomy. This involves a complete removal of the kidney with its surrounding perirenal fat contained within Gerota's fascia and *en bloc* removal of the ureter down to, and including, the portion of ureter within the urinary bladder (the ureteral orifice and the intramural ureter).[182] A retroperitoneal lymph node dissection along the ipsilateral great vessel (the vena cava for right-sided tumors; the aorta for left-sided tumors) is performed for more complete surgical staging, especially for higher grade and invasive cancers (Fig. 95.9). Lymphadenectomy and complete bladder cuff excision may not be necessary in cases of upper tract TCC, particularly at low stage and grade.[183] When TCC of the renal pelvis invades the renal vein or the vena cava, an extensive surgical procedure, including thrombus extraction or partial vena cava dissection, may be required. Nephroureterectomy traditionally is performed through open surgical techniques. Common approaches employ either a single extended midline abdominal incision or nephrectomy via a thoracoabdominal incision and a separate incision in the lower abdomen to accomplish the distal ureterectomy with a cuff of the contiguous urinary bladder.

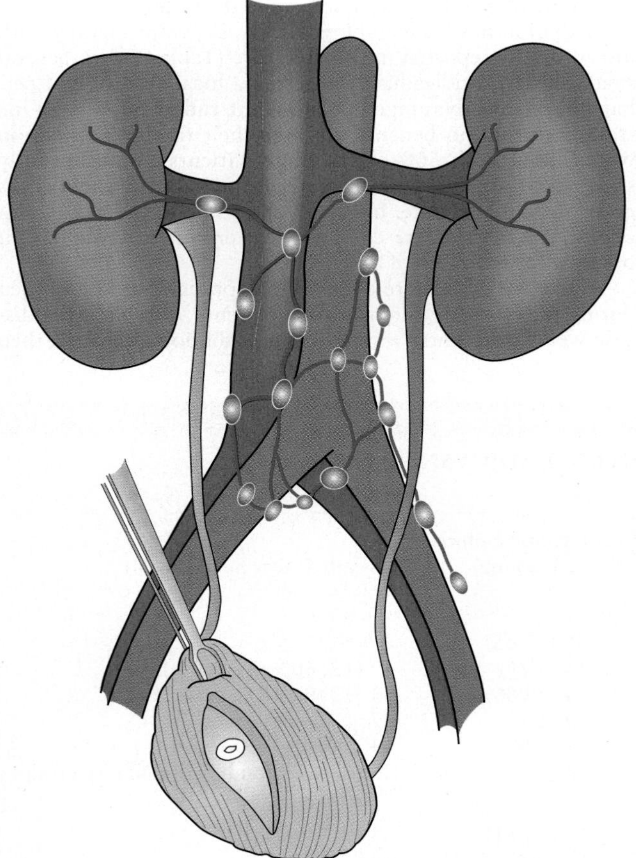

FIGURE 95.9 Diagram of the kidneys, ureters, bladder, and retroperitoneal lymph nodes to demonstrate that a nephroureterectomy for upper tract transitional cell carcinoma requires complete excision of the distal ureter, including the portion within the wall of the bladder. The bladder here is open to reveal the distal ureter, which tunnels within the wall of the bladder.

Open surgical approach has been the standard of treatment for the majority of patients with tumors of the renal pelvis and ureter, although morbidity may be reduced by using a laparoscopic technique.[184,185] The operative time and blood loss with the laparoscopic technique may be substantially less and the hospital stay shorter than those of an open surgical technique. With proper technique in resecting the distal ureter, laparoscopic nephroureterectomy is equally oncologically effective.[186] Invasive TCC may seed the abdomen if spilled, allowing tumor implantation, and this has led to concern among surgical oncologists about the laparoscopic approach. One group has reported three cases of laparoscopic port-site recurrence; however, in all three of these cases, the tumor was spilled from the operative specimen, allowing growth of the tumor tissue at the trocar sites.[187]

In patients in whom radical excision of the tumor would result in severe renal insufficiency that required dialysis (such as patients with a solitary kidney or in a patient with substantially diminished renal function), other surgical therapies may be considered. Endoscopic resection techniques have been developed and shown to be effective, when done selectively and in experienced hands.[188] It is now possible to endoscopically ablate small tumors of the ureter, particularly low-grade tumors, by fulguration or resection. TCCs of the renal pelvis and the calyceal system are more difficult to resect endoscopically. The success of focal resection is thwarted by the multicentricity of these tumors and the common concurrent existence of CIS.[189] Improvements in electrosurgical instruments and the development of neodymium:yttrium aluminum garnet (Nd:YAG) laser technology have added to the urologists armamentarium for focal treatment of upper tract TCC.

Percutaneous endoscopic surgery of renal pelvic and calyceal TCC with access via the flank has been developed as a treatment option in highly select patients who have poor renal function or who medically could not withstand an open surgical procedure.[190] Using standard endoscopic tools, it is possible to resect tumors in the fashion similar to that which is used for bladder tumors. All limited resection endoscopic procedures require vigilant follow-up with endoscopic reevaluation on a regular schedule. Recurrence is very common. In one study, 33% of patients ultimately required nephroureterectomy and 11% of patients died of TCC.[191]

A kidney-sparing approach may be advisable in selected cases of low-stage and low-grade distal ureteral tumors. Because recurrences and urothelial atypia are usually distal in the ureter to the index lesion, it is reasonable to spare the kidney without undue risk of recurrent disease. Surgically it is possible to remove approximately half of the distal ureter and reimplant it in the bladder. For upper ureteral tumors, replacement of the ureter with a segment of the ileum may be considered.

Results of Surgical Therapy

The success rate of surgical procedures is primarily influenced by the pathologic stage of the disease at the resection (Table 95.9). Tumors lower in the urinary tract have a better prognosis when matched by stage with tumors higher in the ureter and pelvis.[193] Within the upper tract, location of the tumor in the ureter versus the renal pelvis does not seem to affect the prognosis.[194,195] In a report with long follow-up from the University of Texas Southwestern Medical Center, of 252 patients treated surgically for upper tract TCC, disease-specific and overall survival were strongly influenced by the pathologic

TABLE 95.9

FIVE-YEAR DISEASE-SPECIFIC SURVIVAL BY PRIMARY TUMOR PATHOLOGIC STAGE AFTER SURGICAL RESECTION OF TRANSITIONAL CELL CARCINOMA OF THE UPPER URINARY TRACT

Tumor Stage	No. of Patients	Percentage
pTa/pTis	38	100
pT1	99	92
pT2	34	73
pT3	53	41
pT4	19	0

From ref. 192, with permission.

stage of the primary tumor.[192] The 5-year actuarial disease-specific survival rates by primary tumor pathologic stage were 100% for noninvasive tumors (Ta and Tis), 92% for pathologic stage T1, 73% for pathologic stage T2, and 41% for pathologic stage T3. There were no long-term survivors for those with stage T4 tumors (Table 95.9). The type of open surgical procedure used (nephroureterectomy in 77% of the patients compared with a kidney-sparing approach used in 17%) was evaluated by univariate and multivariate analysis. Patients undergoing nephroureterectomy were found to have a significantly improved recurrence-free and disease-specific survival on multivariate analysis but not on univariate analysis. However, in other series patients with ureteral cancers who were selected for kidney-sparing resections did not have a poorer outcome.

Adjuvant Topical Therapy Following Local Excision Only

In cases in which endoscopic resection is performed, topical immunotherapy or topical chemotherapy may be important in preventing or delaying local tumor recurrence. BCG appears to be useful in treating carcinomas of the upper tract that are stage Tis.[189] Adriamycin given prophylactically following conservative resection of upper tract TCCs, using an antegrade infusion, also has been judged to be of some benefit in reducing recurrence.[196] The risk of systemic absorption of BCG or the chemotherapeutic agents is substantially higher than in treatment of the bladder.

Adjuvant Combined-Modality Therapy: Advanced Primary Tumors

The most appropriate treatment for invasive transitional cell cancers of the upper urinary tract is nephroureterectomy. Despite aggressive surgery, cure rates are low when the disease has spread beyond the muscularis, with 5-year survival rates varying between 0% and 34%.[196–201] Whether these low survival rates can be improved by adjuvant therapy depends on the pattern of failure and the efficacy of the available treatment. Metastatic relapse appears to predominate over local relapse when systemic cisplatin-based chemotherapy has been used, extrapolating from the experience with locally advanced bladder cancer. The true rate of locoregional failure is, however, unknown because many of the published series are old and employed pre-CT methods of intra-abdominal evaluation. The available data suggest an overall locoregional failure of 2% to 27%, although these figures may be an underestimate.[202–204] Cozad et al.[205] report local failure rates of 50% in stage T3 disease, rising to 60% if the tumors were high grade. Brookland and Richter[206] have reported locoregional recurrence in 45% and 62%, respectively. Most series report a close association between local failure and distant metastasis, although whether the association is causal or simply synchronous cannot be determined from the small numbers in the series.

Radiation has been employed as an adjuvant therapy with mixed results reported in the literature (Table 95.10). Several small phase 2 studies have suggested a local control and perhaps survival advantage for adjuvant radiation.[206–211] One study reported no benefit, although their treated population was diluted with 30% early stage patients. Another study showed no advantage to radiation, but the radiation doses given were inadequate. In others chemotherapy was given in addition. It is therefore difficult to determine the true benefit of adjuvant radiation, if any.

At the MGH a more aggressive approach has been taken during the past 20 years in which patients with high-risk disease were treated first with adjuvant radiation alone and then

TABLE 95.10

LARGER PUBLISHED SERIES USING SURGERY WITH OR WITHOUT ADJUVANT RADIATION FOR CARCINOMA OF THE UPPER URINARY TRACT

Method/Study (Ref.)	No. of Patients	Median Dose (Gy)	Locoregional Failure % (Absolute)	Overall 5-Year Survival (%)
SURGERY WITH RADIOTHERAPY				
Ozsahin et al. (207)	45	50	38 (17/45)	21
Maulard-Durdux et al. (208)	26[a]	45	19 (5/26)	49 (T2, 60%; T3, 19%)
Catton et al. (209)	86[b]	35	34 (29/86)	43 (T3N0, 45%; N+, 15%)
Brookland and Richter (206)	11	50	9 (1/11)	27
Cozad et al. (205)	9	50	11 (1/9)	44
Czito et al. (210)	31	47	23 (7/31)	39 (67% in combined-modality group)
SURGERY ONLY				
Ozsahin et al. (207)	81		65 (53/81)	33
Cozad et al. (205)	17[c]		53 (9/17)	24
Brookland and Richter (206)	11		45 (5/11)	17

[a]Thirty percent stage T2.
[b]Twenty-seven percent stage T1 to T2.
[c]All stages ≥T3.

more recently with concomitant radiation-sensitizing chemotherapy and, if tolerable, further combination chemotherapy.[210] Although the authors' series of 31 patients is nonrandomized and small, local failure was lower if chemotherapy was combined with radiation and the survival rate at 5 years higher (Table 95.10). Kwak et al.[211] also suggested that cisplatin-based adjuvant chemotherapy may reduce the rate of relapse and death from disease at 5 years. The small size of these two series and the biases inherent in this kind of retrospective review make it difficult to draw conclusions.

Very little published data exist to guide physicians managing patients with a local relapse following nephroureterectomy. If the relapse is bulky and metastases are present elsewhere, then palliation with chemotherapy would be the most appropriate course. When the relapse appears isolated and the patient relatively vigorous, consideration can be given to an aggressive approach that holds out the chance for cure. The first step would be to downsize and perhaps improve the respectability of the recurrence using external radiation to a modest preoperative dose of 30 to 45 Gy along with sensitizing chemotherapy. An attempt could then be made at resection or debulking and, if the facility were available, intraoperative radiation could then be given directly onto the tumor bed or onto an unresectable mass, with the bowel and other critical organs displaced out of the field. Such an approach allows the delivery of high doses of radiation to the target without the risk of bowel injury that is present when managing such disease using external radiation treatment alone (Fig. 95.10).

Advanced Transitional Cell Carcinoma of the Upper Tract

Most patients with upper tract TCC have superficial disease, with a favorable prognosis.[212,213] However, patients with disease that invades beyond the muscularis propria have a significantly worse prognosis. The most consistent prognostic variables for the outcome of patients with upper tract TCC, including renal pelvic and ureteral carcinomas, are tumor stage and grade.[214–217] Molecular markers are being studied, and poor outcome may be predicted by overexpression of *p53* and higher Ki-67 labeling index.[218–220]

In a series of 252 patients with mostly localized disease, relapse occurred in 67 patients (27%) after a median of 12 months.[204] Survival was highly stage specific, with 5-year disease-specific survival of 92% for T1, 73% for T2, 41% for T3, and 0% for T4. In a series of 126 patients with nonmetastatic but more advanced renal pelvic or ureteral tumors, relapsed disease was noted in 81 patients (64%) after a median of 9 months.[207] Overall, 5- and 10-year survival rates were 29% and 19%, respectively. The most common sites of distant metastases were liver, bone, or lung. Utilization of postoperative radiation therapy did not impact on local or distant relapse. Factors that influenced survival outcome in multivariate analysis were initial tumor stage, residual postsurgery tumor, and location of initial tumor, with renal pelvic cancer being more favorable than ureteral cancer. The role of adjuvant chemotherapy in reducing relapse has not been explored in randomized fashion in this uncommon disease.

The biology of upper tract TCC is considered to be identical to that of bladder TCC. Consequently, the chemotherapy regimens recommended for advanced or metastatic upper tract TCC are the same as that for bladder cancer, as previously described. Standard treatment is cisplatin-based combination therapy, such as gemcitabine and cisplatin or methotrexate, vinblastine, doxorubicin, and cisplatin. As with bladder cancer, upper tract TCC is highly responsive to chemotherapy but has a short median duration of response.

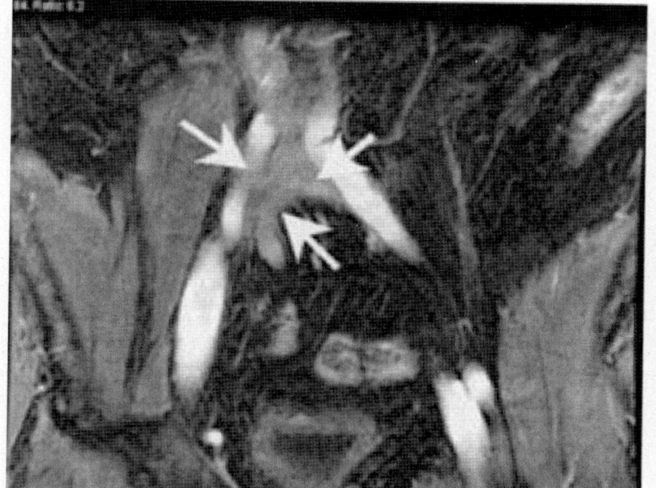

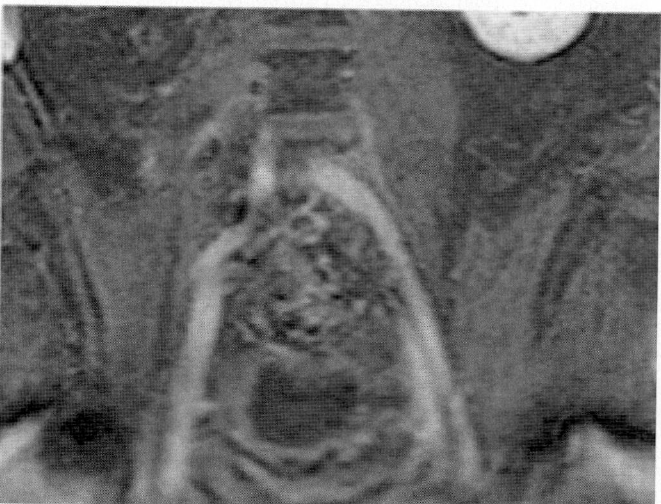

FIGURE 95.10 Sequential coronal magnetic resonance imaging (MRI) of a patient with an unresectable ureteral tumor mass. The mass shown on the MRI on the left (*arrows*) was at the bifurcation of the aorta; it was initially judged unresectable because of involvement of the vessels. Partial resection, however, became possible as part of a combined-modality treatment approach that included preoperative conformal external-beam radiation. Intraoperative electron-beam radiation was given to the entire tumor bed after resection. On the right is the repeat MRI 1 year after treatment without any visible tumor.

Selected References

The full list of references for this chapter appears in the online version.

2. Erckert M, Stenzl A, Falk M, et al. Incidence of urethral tumor involvement in 910 men with bladder cancer. *World J Urol* 1996;14(1):3.
5. Rabbani F, Perrotti M, Russo P, et al. Upper-tract tumors after an initial diagnosis of bladder cancer: argument for long-term surveillance. *J Clin Oncol* 2001;19(1):94.
6. Hurle R, Losa A, Manzetti A, et al. Upper urinary tract tumors developing after treatment of superficial bladder cancer: 7-year follow-up of 591 consecutive patients. *Urology* 1999; 53(6):1144.
10. Primdahl H, von der Masse H, Sorenson FB, et al. Immunohistochemical study of the expression of cell cycle regulating proteins at different stages of bladder cancer. *J Cancer Res Clin Oncol* 2002;128(6):295.
14. Santos LL, Amaro T, Pereira SA, et al. Expression of cell-cycle regulatory proteins and their prognostic value in superficial low-grade urothelial cell carcinoma of the bladder. *Eur J Surg Oncol* 2003;29(1):74.
16. Zeegers MP, Goldbohm RA, van den Brandt PA. A prospective study on active and environmental tobacco smoking and bladder cancer risk (The Netherlands). *Cancer Causes Control* 2002;13(1):83.
17. Messing, EM, Madeb, R, Young, T, et al. Long-term outcome of hematuria home screening for bladder cancer in men. *Cancer* 2006;107(9):2173.
26. Lokeshwar, VB, Habuchi, T, Grossman HB, et al. Bladder tumor markers beyond cytology: international consensus panel on bladder tumor markers. *Urology* 2005;66(6 Suppl 1):35.
27. Lotan Y, Roehrborn CG. Sensitivity and specificity of commonly available bladder tumor markers versus cytology: results of a comprehensive literature review and meta-analysis. *Urology* 2003;61(1):109.
30. Epstein JI, Amin MB, Reuter VE, et al. The World Health Organization/International Society of Urological Pathology consensus classification of urothelial (transitional cell) neoplasms of the urinary bladder. *Am J Surg Pathol* 1998;22:1435.
32. Younes M, Sussman J, True LD. The usefulness of the level of the muscularis mucosae in the staging of invasive transitional cell carcinoma of the urinary bladder. *Cancer* 1990;66:543.
35. Sidransky D, Frost P, Von Eschenbach A, et al. The clonal origin of bladder cancer. *N Engl J Med* 1992;326:737.
37. Williams SG, Buscarini M, Stein JP. Molecular markers for diagnosis, staging and prognosis of bladder cancer. *Oncology* 2001;15:1461.
40. Cordon-Cardo C. Molecular alterations associated with bladder cancer initiation and progression. *Scand J Urol Nephrol Suppl* 2008;218:154.
42. Cote RJ, Esrig D, Groshen S, et al. p53 and the treatment of bladder cancer. *Nature* 1997;385:123.
44. Roedel C, Grabenbauer GG, Rodel F, et al. Apoptosis, p53, bcl-2, Ki-67 in invasive bladder carcinoma: possible predictors for response to radiochemotherapy and successful bladder preservation. *Int J Radiat Oncol Biol Phys* 2000;46:1213.
52. Jimenez RE, Hussain M, Bianco FJ Jr, et al. Her-2/neu over-expression in muscle-invasive urothelial carcinoma of the bladder: prognostic significance and comparative analysis in primary and metastatic tumors. *Clin Cancer Res* 2001;7:2440.
53. Chakravarti A, Winter K, Wu CL, et al. Expression of the epidermal growth factor receptor and Her-2 are predictors of favorable outcome and reduced complete response rates, respectively, in patients with muscle-invading bladder cancers treated by concurrent radiation and cisplatin-based chemotherapy: a report from the Radiation Therapy Oncology Group. *Int J Radiat Oncol Biol Phys* 2005;62:309.
56. Bohle A, Jocham D, Bock PR. Intravesical bacillus Calmette-Guerin versus mitomycin C for superficial bladder cancer: a formal meta-analysis of comparative studies on recurrence and toxicity. *J Urol* 2003;169(1):900.
59. Yiou R, Patard JJ, Benhard H, et al. Outcome of radical cystectomy for bladder cancer according to the disease type at presentation. *BJU Int* 2002;89(4):374.
62. Stein JP, Cai J, Groshen S, et al. Risk factors for patients with pelvic lymph node metastases following radical cystectomy with en bloc pelvic lymphadenectomy: concept of lymph node density. *J Urol* 2003;170(1):35.
63. Stein JP, Lieskovsky G, Cote R, et al. Radical cystectomy in the treatment of invasive bladder cancer: long-term results in 1,054 patients. *J Clin Oncol* 2001;19:666.
64. Dalbagni G, Genega E, Hashibe M, et al. Cystectomy for bladder cancer: a contemporary series. *J Urol* 2001;165:1111.
65. Grossman HB, Natale RB, Tangen CM, et al. Neoadjuvant chemotherapy plus cystectomy compared with cystectomy alone for locally advanced bladder cancer. *N Engl J Med* 2003;349:859.
66. McDougal WS. Metabolic complications of urinary intestinal diversion. *J Urol* 1992;147:1199.
70. Shipley WU, Prout GR Jr, Einstein AB, et al. Treatment of invasive bladder cancer by cisplatin and radiation in patients unsuited for surgery. *JAMA* 1987;258:931.
71. Coppin CM, Gospodarowicz MK, James K, et al. Improved local control of invasive bladder cancer by concurrent cisplatin and preoperative or definitive radiation. The National Cancer Institute of Canada Clinical Trials Group. *J Clin Oncol* 1996;14:2901.
75. Tester W, Caplan R, Heaney J, et al. Neoadjuvant combined modality program with selective organ preservation for invasive bladder cancer: results of Radiation Therapy Oncology Group phase II trial 8802. *J Clin Oncol* 1996;14:119.
76. Shipley WU, Winter KA, Kaufman DS, et al. Phase III trial of neoadjuvant chemotherapy in patients with invasive bladder cancer treated with selective bladder preservation by combined radiation therapy and chemotherapy: initial results of Radiation Therapy Oncology Group 89-03. *J Clin Oncol* 1998;16:3576.
78. Rodel C, Grabenbauer GG, Kuhn R, et al. Combined-modality treatment and selective organ preservation in invasive bladder cancer: long-term results. *J Clin Oncol* 2002;20:3061.
79. Kaufman DS, Winter KA, Shipley WU, et al. Phase I-II RTOG study (99-06) of patients with muscle-invasive bladder cancer undergoing transurethral surgery, paclitaxel, cisplatin, and twice-daily radiotherapy followed by selective bladder preservation or radical cystectomy and adjuvant chemotherapy. *Urology* 2009;73(4):833.
87. Zietman AL, Grocela J, Zehr E, et al. Selective bladder conservation using transurethral resection, chemotherapy, and radiation: management and consequences of Ta, T1, and Tis recurrence within the retained bladder. *Urology* 2001;58:380.
90. Moonen LM, Horenblas S, van der Voet JC, et al. Bladder conservation in selected T1G3 and muscle-invasive T2-T3a bladder carcinoma using combination therapy of surgery and iridium-192 implantation. *Br J Urol* 1994;74:322.
92. Herr HW. Transurethral resection of muscle-invasive bladder cancer: 10-year outcome. *J Clin Oncol* 2001;19:89.
99. Hall RR. Updated results of a randomized controlled trial of neoadjuvant cisplatin, methotrexate and vinblastine chemotherapy for muscle invasive bladder cancer. *Proc Am Soc Clin Oncol* 2002;21:178.
101. Malmstrom PU, Rintala E, Wahlqvist R, et al. Five-year follow-up of a prospective trial of radical cystectomy and neoadjuvant chemotherapy: Nordic Cystectomy Trial I. The Nordic Cooperative Bladder Cancer Study Group. *J Urol* 1996;155:1903.
103. Raghavan D, Quinn D, Skinner DG, et al. Surgery and adjunctive chemotherapy for invasive bladder cancer. *Surg Oncol* 2002;11:55.
106. Winquist E, Waldron T, Segal R, et al. Neoadjuvant chemotherapy in transitional cell carcinoma of the bladder: a systematic review and meta-analysis. *J Urol* 2004;171:561.
116. Bellmunt J, Guillem V, Paz-Ares L, et al. Phase I–II study of paclitaxel, cisplatin and gemcitabine in advanced transitional-cell carcinoma of the urothelium. *J Clin Oncol* 2000;18(8):3247.
117. Studer UE, Bacchi M, Biedermann C, et al. Adjuvant cisplatin chemotherapy following cystectomy for bladder cancer: results of a prospective randomized trial. *J Urol* 1994;152:81.
118. Bono AV, Benvenuti C, Reali L, et al. Adjuvant chemotherapy in advanced bladder cancer. Italian Uro-Oncologic Cooperative Group. *Prog Clin Biol Res* 1989;303:533.
119. Freiha F, Reese J, Torti FM. A randomized trial of radical cystectomy versus radical cystectomy plus cisplatin, vinblastine and methotrexate chemotherapy for muscle invasive bladder cancer. *J Urol* 1996;155:495.
120. Skinner DG, Daniels JR, Russell CA, et al. The role of adjuvant chemotherapy following cystectomy for invasive bladder cancer: a prospective comparative trial. *J Urol* 1991;145:459.
121. Stockle M, Meyenburg W, Wellek S, et al. Advanced bladder cancer (stages pT3b, PT4a, pN1 and pN2): Improved survival after radical cystectomy and 3 adjuvant cycles of chemotherapy results of a controlled prospective study. *J Urol* 1992;148:302.
122. Stockle M, Meyenburg W, Wellek S, et al. Adjuvant polychemotherapy of nonorgan-confined bladder cancer after radical cystectomy revisited: long-term results of a controlled prospective study and further clinical experience. *J Urol* 1995;153:47.
123. Adjuvant chemotherapy in invasive bladder cancer: a systematic review and meta-analysis of individual patient data. Advanced bladder cancer (ABC) meta-analysis collaboration. *Eur Urol* 2005;48:189.
129. Mansson A, Johnson G, Mansson W. Quality of life after cystectomy: comparison between patients with conduit and those with caecal reservoir urinary diversion. *Br J Urol* 1988;62:240.
132. Hart S, Skinner EC, Meyerowitz BE, et al. Quality of life after radical cystectomy for bladder cancer in patients with an ileal conduit, or cutaneous or urethral Kock pouch. *J Urol* 1999;162:77.
134. Somani BK, Gimlin D, Fayers P, N'Dow J. Quality of life and body image for bladder cancer patients undergoing radical cystectomy and urinary diversion—a prospective cohort study with systematic review of the literature. *Urology* 2009;74:1138.
135. Mansson A, Al Amin M, Malmstrom PU et al. Patient-assessed outcomes in Swedish and Egyptian men undergoing radical cystectomy and orthotopic

bladder substitution—a prospective comparative study. *Urology* 2007;70:1086.

139. Caffo O, Fellin G, Graffer U, et al. Assessment of quality of life after cystectomy or conservative therapy for patients with infiltrating bladder carcinoma. *Cancer* 1996;78:1089.
140. Henningsohn L, Wijkstrom H, Dickman PW, et al. Distressful symptoms after radical radiotherapy for urinary bladder cancer. *Radiother Oncol* 2002;60:215.
144. Yagoda A, Watson RC, Gonzalez-Vitale JC, et al. Cis-dichlorodiammineplatinum(II) in advanced bladder cancer. *Cancer Treat Rep* 1976;60:917.
145. Saxman SB, Propert KJ, Einhorn LH, et al. Long-term follow-up of a phase III intergroup study of cisplatin alone or in combination with methotrexate, vinblastine, and doxorubicin in patients with metastatic urothelial carcinoma: a cooperative group study. *J Clin Oncol* 1997;15:2564.
154. Roberts JT, von der Maase H, Sengelov L, et al. Long-term survival results of a randomized trial comparing gemcitabine/cisplatin and methotrexate/vinblastine/doxorubicin/cisplatin in patients with locally advanced and metastatic bladder cancer. *Ann Oncol* 2006;17(Suppl 5):v118.
157. Dreicer R, Manola J, Roth BJ, et al. Phase III trial of methotrexate, vinblastine, doxorubicin, and cisplatin versus carboplatin and paclitaxel in patients with advanced carcinoma of the urothelium. *Cancer* 2004;100:1639.
162. Bellmunt J, von der Maase H, Mead GM, et al: Randomized phase III study comparing paclitaxel/cisplatin/gemcitabine and gemcitabine/cisplatin in patients with locally advanced or metastatic urothelial cancer without prior systemic therapy: EORTC 30987/intergroup study. *Proc Am Soc Clin Oncol* 2007;25: (abst LBA5030).
168. Dogliotti L, Carteni G, Siena S, et al. Gemcitabine plus cisplatin versus gemcitabine plus carboplatin as first-line chemotherapy in advanced transitional cell carcinoma of the urothelium: results of a randomized phase 2 trial. *Eur Urol* 2007;52(1):134.
171. Hussain M, Vaishampayan U, Du W, et al. Combination paclitaxel, carboplatin, and gemcitabine is an active treatment for advanced urothelial cancer. *J Clin Oncol* 2001;19:2527.
179. O'Malley ME, Hahn PF, Yoder IC, et al. Comparison of excretory phase, helical computed tomography with intravenous urography in patients with painless haematuria. *Clin Radiol* 2003;58(4):294.
180. Jung P, Brauers A, Nolte-Ersting CA, Jakse G, Günther RW. Magnetic resonance urography enhanced by gadolinium and diuretics: a comparison with conventional urography in diagnosing the cause of ureteric obstruction. *BJU Int* 2000;86(9):960.
186. Matin SF, Gill IS. Recurrence and survival following laparoscopic radical nephroureterectomy with various forms of bladder cuff control. *J Urol* 2005;173(2):395.
187. Ong AM, Bhayani SB, Pavlovich CP. Trocar site recurrence after laparoscopic nephroureterectomy. *J Urol* 2003;170(4):301.
190. Goel MC, Mahendra V, Roberts JG. Percutaneous management of renal pelvic urothelial tumors: long-term followup. *J Urol* 2003;169(3):925; discussion 929.
192. Hall MC, Womack S, Sagalowsky AI, et al. Prognostic factors, recurrence, and survival in transitional cell carcinoma of the upper urinary tract: a 30-year experience in 252 patients. *Urology* 1998;52:594.
205. Cozad SC, Smalley SR, Austenfeld M, et al. Transitional cell carcinoma of the renal pelvis or ureter: patterns of failure. *Urology* 1995;46:796.
210. Czito B, Zietman AL, Kaufman DS, et al. Adjuvant combined modality therapy in locally advanced upper urinary tract malignancies. *J Urol* 2004;172:1271.
215. Charbit L, Gendreau MC, Mee S, et al. Tumors of the upper urinary tract: 10 years of experience. *J Urol* 1991;146:1243.
217. Guinan P, Vogelzang NJ, Randazzo R, et al. Renal pelvic cancer: a review of 611 patients treated in Illinois 1975–1985. Cancer Incidence and End Results Committee. *Urology* 1992;40:393.
225. Mead GM, Russell M, Clark P, et al. A randomized trial comparing methotrexate and vinblastine (MV) with cisplatin, methotrexate and vinblastine (CMV) in advanced transitional cell carcinoma: results and a report on prognostic factors in a Medical Research Council study. MRC Advanced Bladder Cancer Working Party. *Br J Cancer* 1998;78:1067.

CHAPTER 96 MOLECULAR BIOLOGY OF PROSTATE CANCER

YU CHEN, VIVEK K. ARORA, AND CHARLES L. SAWYERS

Prostate cancer is the most common malignancy and the second leading cause of cancer death in Western men. It is highly heterogeneous with a disease specific mortality of one in seven. Many men survive decades without treatment, while others succumb quickly despite aggressive management. Among men who require systemic treatment, response rates to therapies are also highly variable—most notably some patients respond to androgen deprivation therapy for decades while a minority do not respond at all. Currently, the combination of clinical stage (tumor size on palpation), serum level of the prostate specific antigen (PSA), and histological grade (reported as Gleason score) is used to guide treatment decisions. Although useful for some clinical decisions, the modest predictive value of these parameters results both in overtreatment of many man and ineffective treatment for others. To achieve a "personalized medicine" approach to prostate cancer, it is important to define the repertoire of molecular lesions in prostate cancer, to identify the effect of these lesions on disease aggressiveness, and to identify therapies that have specific effectiveness against individual molecular lesions. Precedent for the ultimate success of this approach comes from other malignancies, such as the target specific kinase inhibitors erlotinib and PF-02341066 in lung cancers harboring epidermal growth factor receptor (EGFR) mutations and *EML4-ALK* fusions, respectively, the anti-HER2 antibody trastuzumab in breast cancers harboring HER2 amplification, and the kinase inhibitor PLX4032 in melanomas harboring BRAF mutations.[1–5] In prostate cancer, recent work is beginning to define disease subtypes driven by different oncogenic genetic lesions. Ongoing research is expected to result in a more personalized treatment approach in prostate cancer, including who to screen, who to treat, and what form of treatment to use.

GENETIC PREDISPOSITION

Prostate cancer has a significant genetic component. A large Nordic study of 44,788 pairs of twins concluded that 42% of prostate cancers are attributable to genetic risk.[6] Men with one, two, and three first degree relatives afflicted with prostate cancer have a 2-, 5-, and 11-fold risk of developing the disease, respectively.[7] Given that large-scale screening of the general population is associated with small overall survival benefit and excess morbidity from curative surgery or radiation therapy for low risk disease,[8,9] identification of genetic predispositions—especially of aggressive disease—could guide screening decisions.

Early work identified rare mutations of several genes—*ELAC2*, *MSR1*, *RNAseL*—that confer increased risk of prostate cancer development but affect a small group of patients. Polymorphisms of genes in the androgen signaling pathway have been extensively studied with conflicting results.[10] With the technology to detect single nucleotide polymorphisms (SNP), genome-wide association studies (GWAS) of large cohorts have discovered novel genomic regions associated with prostate cancer risk. A number of independent reports showed that polymorphisms of multiple loci on chromosome 8q24 account for 10% and 30% of prostate cancer cases among European and African ancestry, respectively.[11–15] One challenge is to identify mechanisms by which these SNPs confer prostate cancer susceptibility since the 8q24 loci are located at a "gene desert." Recent work suggests that at least one loci may serve as an enhancer for *MYC*, which is approximately 300 kb away.[16] In addition, other loci have been recently discovered,[17,18] but none have shown a significant enough increase in the odds ratio of developing cancer to warrant screening of the general population. There is some evidence that simultaneous presence of multiple risk-associated SNPs in the same individual is associated with a significantly higher risk of prostate cancer.[19]

GENETIC LANDSCAPE OF PROSTATE CANCER

Like other epithelial tumors, many prostate cancers have a large number of genetic and epigenetic lesions associated with hallmark properties of malignancies.[20] Types of lesions include overexpression of oncogenes and underexpression of tumor suppressor genes, genomic amplifications and deletions, translocations, and, more rarely, point mutations. One recent large-scale study that combines gene expression profiling, comparative genomic hybridization (array CGH) to characterize amplifications and deletions, and targeted resequencing for somatic mutations has shed light onto the genetic landscape of prostate cancer.[21] On average, prostate cancer is characterized by a relatively low mutation rate of genes commonly mutated in other malignancies, such as *KRAS*, *BRAF*, or *p53*, but a relatively large number of genomic alterations (Fig. 96.1). Recurrent amplifications and deletions, some focal, covering single to a handful of genes, and others spanning entire arms covering thousands of genes, are present in many tumors at diagnosis. On average, higher grade and stage tumors contain a greater number of genomic alterations. The most common genomic alteration is loss in the chromosomal arm 8p followed by a gain of chromosomal 8q. Some focal genomic alterations, such as deletion of *PTEN* or deletion of the interstitial region between *TMPRSS2* and *ERG* that creates the TMPRSS2-ERG fusion gene, results in a clearly established oncogenic driver lesion. But for most genomic alterations, the specific genes responsible for oncogenesis are a subject of speculation.

Although many individual genes are rarely affected in prostate cancer, several key oncogenic and tumor suppressor pathways are commonly involved when the individual genes in each pathway are considered collectively. Four pathways—the phosphatidylinositol 3-phosphate kinase (PI3K)/AKT pathway, the RAS/MAP kinase pathway, the retinoblastoma pathway, and

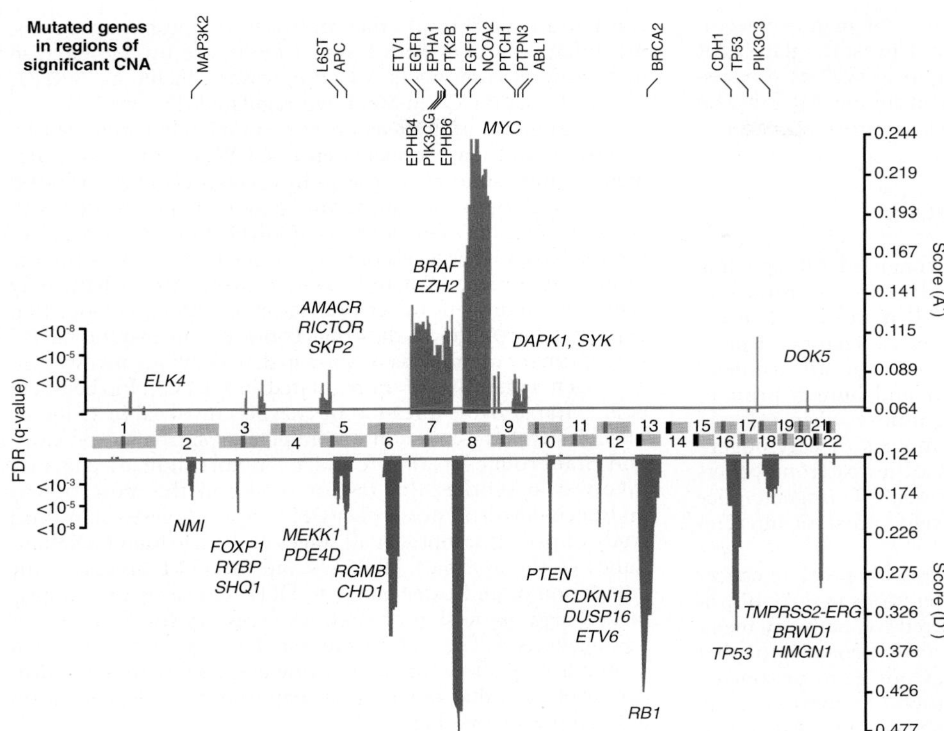

FIGURE 96.1 Genomic aberrations in prostate cancer. Regions of amplification (*red*) or deletion (*blue*) with false discovery rate (FDR) 10% or less are plotted, with chromosomes indicated at the center and centromeres in red. Genes with somatic nonsynonymous mutations are listed on top (*black*). Additional genes of interest targeted by copy-number alterations alone are also indicated (*gray*). (From ref. 21 with permission.)

the androgen receptor (AR) pathway—are altered in one-third of primary cancers and almost all of metastatic lesions. This suggests that in prostate cancer, different individual genes in the pathway may be targeted to activate or suppress a common pathway lesion (Fig. 96.2). The sections below focus on those pathways where prostate cancer is most validated.

Androgen Receptor Pathway

It has been 70 years since Higgins and Hodges made the seminal observation that prostate cancers regress after surgical orchiectomy or suppression of androgen production by administration of exogenous estrogens.[22] These observations proved that prostate cancer is an androgen-dependent malignancy, and androgen deprivation therapy became the first targeted therapy in oncology—leading to a Nobel Prize for Charles Huggins in 1966.

Androgens exert their cellular actions through the AR, a 110 kb steroid receptor transcription factor, located on Xq12.[23,24] Upon binding androgen, AR mediates transcription of a number of genes involved in survival and differentiation of prostate epithelial cells. AR activity is required for development of both normal and malignant prostate tissue as men

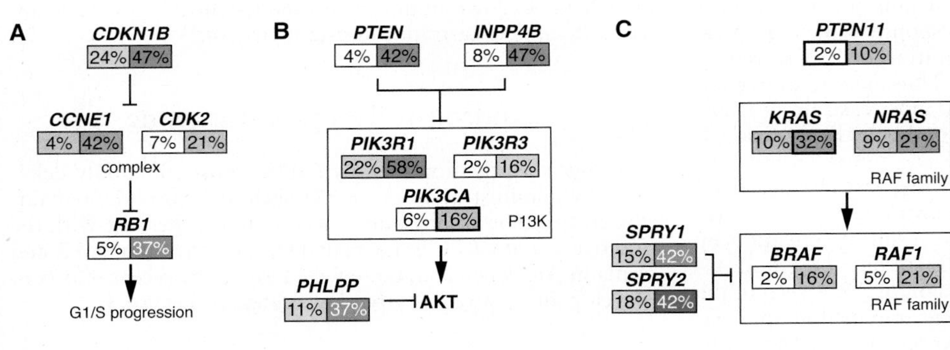

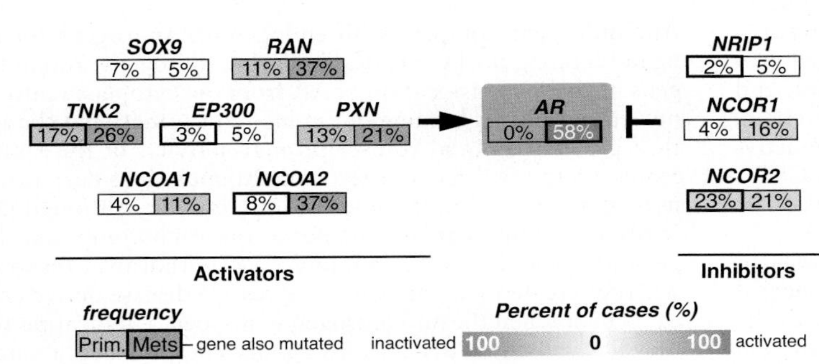

FIGURE 96.2 Alterations in the retinoblastoma (A), phosphatidylinositol 3-kinase (PI3K) (B), RAS/MAP kinase (C), and androgen receptor (AR) (D) pathways in prostate cancer. Alteration frequencies are shown for individual genes and for the entire pathway in primary and metastatic tumors. Alterations are defined as those having significant up- or down-regulation compared with normal prostate samples, or by somatic mutations, and are interpreted as activation (*red*) or inactivation (*blue*) of protein function. (From ref. 21 with permission.)

with germline AR inactivating mutations or men orchiectomized at a young age do not develop a prostate gland. AR plays a critical role in early pathogenesis as well as progression to advanced disease, and drugs that inhibit AR function remain the primary treatment for advanced prostate cancer.

Early Pathogenesis

Several lines of evidence suggest that enhanced AR signaling may play a causative role in prostate cancer initiation. Polymorphisms of three genes in the AR pathway, *AR* itself, *CYP17*, and *SRD5A2*, are low penetrant risk factors for prostate cancer development in some but not all studies.[6] Overexpression of AR in both mouse and human primary prostate cells confers tumor forming ability when injected orthotopically into mice.[25,26] In rat models of carcinogen-induced prostate cancer, implantation of testosterone pellets results in an increased number of tumors.[27] Transgenic mice that overexpress AR in the prostate develop prostatic intraepithelial neoplasia (PIN).[28]

Pathway analysis from a recent large-scale prostate cancer genomic project found AR pathway alterations in 60% of primary tumors. The most commonly altered AR pathway member was *NCOA2* (also called *SRC2*), an AR coactivator that potentiates AR transcriptional output. Copy gains or somatic mutations of the *NCOA2* gene were found in approximately 20% of primary tumors. In addition, several other AR coactivators showed increased expression, while AR corepressors were down-regulated (Fig. 96.2D).

Cancer Progression and Castration-Resistant Growth

Because of the dependence of the prostate lineage on AR function, chemical castration through suppression of testicular function has become the mainstay in systemic treatment of prostate cancer. In normal prostate tissue, castration results in atrophy and cessation of PSA production indefinitely until restoration of testosterone levels. However, prostate cancers progress to the lethal castration-resistant prostate cancer (CRPC) after a variable duration of response. Cancer progression is usually accompanied by restoration of PSA secretion, indicating reactivation of AR activity. Thus, instead of bypassing the requirement for AR function, most castrate-resistant tumors have reactivation of the AR pathway, likely through multiple mechanisms.[23]

Alterations of AR itself represent the best characterized mechanism of castration resistance. Mutations of AR are detected in up to 10% of CRPCs and result in activation by other hormone ligands such as corticosteroids or, paradoxically, by antiandrogens.[29] Overexpression of AR is seen in the majority of CRPCs, and the *AR* gene is amplified in approximately 30% of cases.[30–32] AR overexpression is sufficient to activate AR in the milieu of castrate levels of androgens and to convert the antiandrogen, bicalutamide, into a weak agonist.[33] Alternative splicing of *AR* mRNA can lead to a truncated protein containing the N-terminal transcriptional activation and DNA binding domains but missing the ligand binding domain. Some of these variants have constitutive transcriptional activity in the absence of androgens and can be detected in CRPC samples. Overexpression of at least two variants can confer castration resistance in preclinical models.[34–36]

Alterations in AR pathway genes are found in 100% of metastases and may enhance AR activity in the presence of castrate androgen levels. *NCOA2*, for example, increases the magnitude of AR signaling across a broad range of androgen concentrations. Several other androgen receptor coactivators, including *NCOA1*, *TNK2*, and *EP300*, are up-regulated in metastatic disease, while AR corepressors, including *NRIP1*, *NCOR1*, and *NCOR2*, are down-regulated (Fig. 96.2D).

Intratumoral androgens are not completely eliminated by castration and may be increased in CRPC.[37] Direct measurements of intratumoral androgens by mass spectrometry showed that castration-resistant metastatic tumors in men treated with gonadotropin-releasing hormone (GnRH) agonists such as leuprolide have higher levels of testosterone than primary tumors in untreated men.[38] There is some evidence that CRPC may synthesize androgens to activate AR in an autocrine loop. Two expression profiling studies that compared metastatic CRPC with primary tumors have shown that enzymes involved in androgen synthesis are up-regulated in CRPC. Holzbeierlein et al.[32] found overexpression of enzymes involved in synthesis of cholesterol, the common steroid precursor, from acetyl-CoA, and Stanbrough et al.[39] found overexpression of enzymes involved in synthesis of testosterone and the more potent androgen dihydrotestosterone (DHT) from cholesterol. A third study of patient samples at all stages of disease found an abundance of the enzymes AKR1C3 and SRD5A1 necessary for conversion of androstenedione to DHT. However, the samples lacked high expression of enzymes necessary for *de novo* steroidogenesis.[40] These data suggest that autocrine androgen synthesis may allow tumors to grow despite low serum androgen levels, but that this process may in part be dependent on adrenal precursors (Fig. 96.3).

Multiple kinase signaling pathways have been implicated in CRPC—most notably the HER2 and AKT pathways—with evidence that they exert their effects, in part, through modulation of AR activity. The HER2 receptor tyrosine kinase is progressively overexpressed in more advanced CRPC, though it is seldom amplified as seen in breast cancer. In experimental systems, forced overexpression of HER2 results in castration resistance, while pharmacologic inhibition or protein knockdown results in growth suppression.[41] Loss of PTEN and activation of the AKT pathway, commonly seen in CRPC (Fig. 96.2B), can contribute to castration resistance. Primary tumors with loss of PTEN have lower response rates to neoadjuvant bicalutamide.[42] Prostate cancer in mice with genetically engineered loss of *PTEN* rapidly develop castration resistance, and *PTEN* knockdown in murine hormone-sensitive prostate cancer cells confers castration-resistant growth.[43,44]

Androgen Receptor Targeting

Androgen deprivation therapy (ADT), most commonly delivered by administration of GnRH such as leuprolide, remains the cornerstone of prostate cancer systemic therapy. With the discovery that CRPC is associated with reactivation of AR and remains AR dependent, there have been many recent efforts to develop alternative AR targeting strategies (Fig. 96.3).

Antiandrogens

Antiandrogens compete with endogenous androgens for the ligand binding pocket of AR. Similar to androgens, antiandrogens promote translocation of AR from the cytoplasm into the nucleus and DNA binding but induce conformational changes that prevent optimal transcriptional activity. In the United States, there are three nonsteroidal antiandrogens currently in use—flutamide, bicalutamide, and nilutamide. Although generally active upon treatment initiation, each compound has been associated with the antiandrogen withdrawal response, whereby treated patients with progressive disease derive clinical benefit when the antiandrogen is stopped,[45] indicating that they have potential to act as AR agonists despite their intended

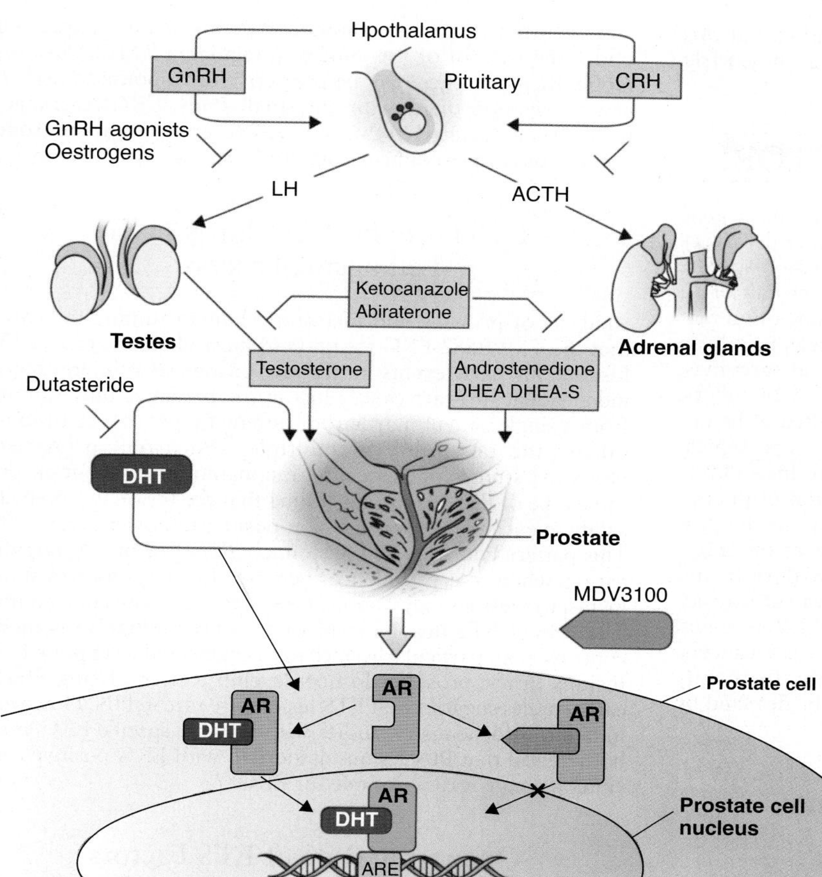

FIGURE 96.3 The androgen-signaling axis and its inhibitors. Testicular androgen synthesis is regulated by the gonadotropin-releasing hormone–luteinizing hormone (GnRH–LH) axis, whereas adrenal androgen synthesis is regulated by the corticotrophin-releasing hormone (CRH)-adrenocorticotropic hormone (ACTH) axis. GnRH agonists and corticosteroids inhibit stimulation of the testes and adrenals, respectively. Abiraterone inhibits CYP17, a critical enzyme in androgen synthesis. MDV3100 competitively inhibits the binding of androgens to androgen receptors. DHEA, dehydroepiandrosterone; DHEA-S, dehydroepiandrosterone sulphate; DHT, dihydrotestosterone; AR, androgen receptor; ARE, androgen-response element. (From ref. 98 with permission.)

role as antagonists. Indeed, overexpression of AR can convert bicalutamide from an antagonist into an agonist.[33]

Novel antiandrogens that have no agonistic properties would likely be clinically superior, and several efforts to identify such compounds are ongoing. Currently, the most promising compound, MDV3100, binds to AR with high affinity and prevents AR binding to DNA. MDV3100 is highly active in preclinical models of castration resistance where bicalutamide functions as an agonist.[46] In a phase 1/2 trial of MDV3100 in 140 CRPC patients previously treated with bicalutamide, the clinical response rate was greater than 50% as measured by a sustained, greater than 50% decline in serum PSA and radiographic evidence of partial response or stable disease. Among those who where chemotherapy naive, PSA response rate was 62% and time to progression was 41 weeks—both compare favorably to docetaxel chemotherapy. Among the more advanced patients refractory to docetaxel, PSA response rate was 51% and time to progression was 21 weeks.[47] A phase 3 trial of MDV3100 in men with chemotherapy-refractory CRPC is ongoing.

Androgen Lowering Therapies

The most commonly used form of ADT, leuprolide, inhibits testicular androgen synthesis but does not impact other sources of androgen sources such as the adrenal glands and the purported autocrine androgen synthesis by tumor cells. Second-line ADT agents such as aminoglutethimide and ketoconazole inhibit adrenal androgen synthesis and have modest activity in CRPC, but their clinical utility is limited by side effects due to off target activities that preclude dose escalation.

CYP17 is a key P450 enzyme in the androgen biosynthesis pathway that functions in the testes and adrenal glands to catalyze the conversion of pregnenolone and progesterone into the weak androgens dehydroepiandrosterone (DHEA) and androstenedione, respectively. These weak androgens are further converted into testosterone and DHT, which may occur in peripheral tissues and in prostate tumor cells. Therefore, specific inhibition of CYP17 should decrease androgen synthesis without affecting the production of other essential steroids. The experimental drug abiraterone acetate is a pregnenolone derivative that is a selective, high affinity (half maximal inhibitory concentration [IC50] = 2 nM), irreversible inhibitor of CYP17. In phase 2 studies, two-thirds of chemotherapy-naive and half of postdocetaxel patients had PSA responses.[48–50] One potentially undesirable consequence of abiraterone treatment is increased production of adrenal progestins (generated by enzymes upstream of the CPY17 block). These progestins may have agonist activity in CRPC patients whose tumors have a highly sensitized AR pathway. Indeed, addition of dexamethasone to suppress this adrenal activity (and to rescue from potential adrenal insufficiency) reversed abiraterone resistance in one-third of patients (Fig. 96.3).[48] Phase 3 trials of abiraterone in men with CRPC are ongoing.

Indirect Approaches

AR activity requires the cooperation of numerous other proteins, some of which can be pharmacologically targeted. AR is stabilized by binding to the molecular chaperone, heat shock protein 90 (HSP90). Indeed, HSP90 inhibitors emerged as hits in a broad screen for chemical compounds that inhibit AR signaling. The clinical HSP90 inhibitor 17-AAG destabilizes AR and causes regression of prostate cancer in preclinical models.[51,52] To activate transcription, AR requires coordinated activity of chromatin remodeling enzymes, including histone deacetylases (HDAC). HDAC inhibitors suppress AR activity and prostate cancer growth in preclinical models.[53,54] Despite these promising preclinical results, clinical trials of HSP90 and

HDAC inhibitors in CRPC have been disappointing, but this may be due to limitations in dose and schedule of these early generation inhibitors.[55]

ETS TRANSCRIPTION FACTORS

In 2005, using bioinformatic analysis of prostate cancer gene expression data, Tomlins et al.[56] made the seminal discovery that one of several members of the E26 transformation-specific (ETS) transcription factors are translocated in over half of all prostate cancers. This discovery also led to the recognition that recurrent genomic translocations, which had previously been observed only in hematopoietic malignancies and sarcomas, can occur commonly in solid tumors. Four ETS members, *ERG*, *ETV1*, *ETV4*, and *ETV5*, have been reported to be targeted by translocations in prostate cancer.[56–58] The typical translocation does not result in a fusion protein. Instead, the translocation usually results in aberrant expression of the targeted ETS factor in the prostate by juxtaposition to the promoter of highly expressed prostate gene—similar to the translocations of *MYC* and *BCL2* to *IgG* locus in Burkitt and follicular lymphomas (Fig. 96.4). The most prevalent translocation is between the androgen-regulated *TMPRSS2* gene and *ERG*, occurring in approximately 50% of all prostate cancers. Both genes are located on 21q22, and the fusion frequently occurs due to an interstitial deletion, which can be detected by high-density CGH approaches.[21]

ETS Fusions as Prognostic and Predictive Factors

The discovery of the ETS translocations immediately raised questions about their prognostic value, which are still under debate. Just prior to the discovery of the translocation, one study noted *ERG* mRNA overexpression in a large subset of prostate cancers (almost certainly a consequence of the TMPRSS2-ERG translocation) reported a favorable prognosis.[59] Yet, presence of the *TMPRSS2-ERG* fusion (detected by fluorescence *in situ* hybridization [FISH]) strongly predicted for increased disease-specific mortality in a watchful waiting cohort from Sweden.[60] Larger studies (of U.S. populations) have found no prognostic role of *ERG* translocation.[61,62] It has been more difficult to assess the effect of the other, non-ERG ETS factors on prognosis due to the much smaller number of affected patients, although several reports consistently report that *ETV1* overexpression is associated with poor prognostic features.[61,63,64]

Given that the most common ETS fusions are expressed under the control of the androgen-regulated *TMPRSS2* promoter, their presence may be predictive of response to androgen deprivation therapy. In one small study, *ERG* rearrangement was associated with improved response to abiraterone acetate, but larger confirmatory studies are needed.[65]

ETS Fusions Occur Early in the Pathogenic Process

Analysis of primary and metastatic human tumors indicates that the TMPRSS2-ERG fusion (and most likely the rarer ETV fusions) are early events in prostate oncogenesis. Interestingly, independent prostate cancer loci in the prostatectomy sample from a single patient may harbor different types of ETS fusions, raising the possibility of multiple, concurrent primaries. However, studies of metastatic lesions uniformly contain the same type of ETS fusion, suggesting that the fusion is a premetastatic event and that not all fusion-positive tumors progress.[66–68] This pattern contrasts with genomic *PTEN* loss or *AR* amplification where the prevalence increases in castration-resistant metastatic lesions, suggesting these may represent later events. The role of ETS fusions in prostate cancer initiation is more controversial, particularly since mice engineered to express ETS fusions in the prostate do not develop cancers. Using FISH, early studies suggests that ETS fusions are rare in PIN. However, immunohistochemistry studies with a highly specific ERG antibody reveal that PIN lesions associated with ERG-positive carcinoma are generally positive for ERG.[69]

Oncogenic Role of ETS Factors

ETS factors are atypical oncogenes in that they can be highly expressed in some normal tissues (e.g., *ERG* in endothelial cells and *ETV1* in neurons). Furthermore, forced ETS overexpression in cells in culture is usually not transforming. Like many transcription factors, aberrant expression under specific contexts is likely required for oncogenesis. In the prostate, activation of the PTEN/AKT pathway provides one context for ETS-mediated tumorigenesis. In mouse models, overexpression of *ERG* or *ETV1* alone in the prostate has only modest effects.[56,70,71] Yet, in the context of PTEN loss or AKT activation, *ERG* overexpression is oncogenic. Indeed, in human prostate cancers, there is a strong correlation between *ERG* overexpression and loss of PTEN.[72–74]

The transcriptional program governed by aberrantly overexpressed ETS in prostate cancer is currently not well understood.

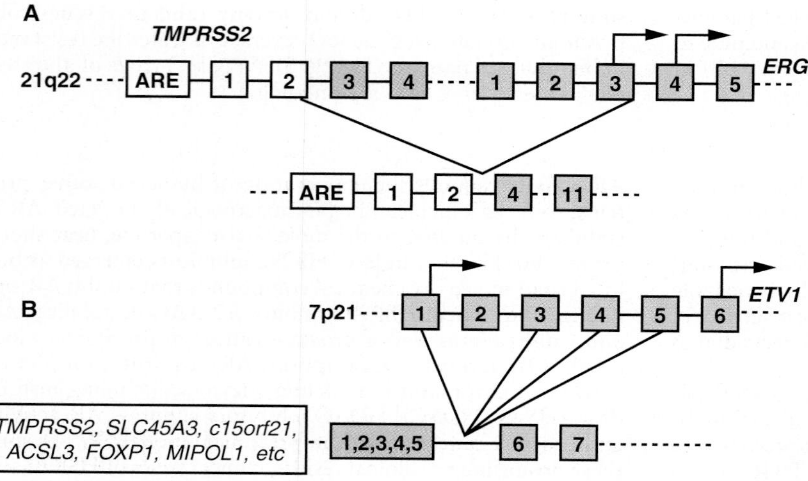

FIGURE 96.4 Schematic of *TMPRSS2-ERG* and *ETV1* fusions. **A:** *TMPRSS2* and *ERG* are separated by 3Mb on 21q22. *TMPRSS2-ERG* fusion is usually formed by interstitial deletion resulting in exon 2 of TMPRSS2 juxtaposed to exon 4 of ERG. Fusion results in slightly truncated protein starting from exon 4. **B:** *ETV1* located on 7p21, can be fused to a number of genomic loci, some of which are shown. Many fusions result in a truncated protein starting in exon 6 but full length protein is also observed. Arrow indicates ATG translation initiation sites.

To address this question, the genomic binding sites of ERG have recently been mapped in prostate cancer. Surprisingly, there is an extraordinarily high overlap between ERG and AR binding sites—suggesting that ERG can modulate AR activity.[75] Since AR can promote both cellular growth and differentiation, one hypothesis is that ERG expression modulates AR function away from differentiation and toward proliferation.

The PTEN/AKT Pathway

The PTEN (*p*hosphatase and *ten*sin homolog deleted on chromosome 10) tumor suppressor gene, originally identified through studies in breast cancer and glioblastoma, is lost in a significant fraction of prostate cancers through deletion, mutation, or epigenetic silencing.[76] Studies using high-density SNP arrays show that *PTEN* is the only gene in the overlapping chromosomal regions lost in a large set of prostate cancers displaying deletion of 10q23.[77] Examination of nine prostate cancer xenografts with neither *PTEN* loss of heterozygosity (LOH) nor mutations showed that five had epigenetic silencing.[78] Three independently generated mouse models with prostate-specific homozygous deletions of *Pten* all developed prostate cancer with progression from PIN to adenocarcinoma to metastasis similar to human disease.[79–81] These data unambiguously implicate *PTEN* as a critical lesion in prostate cancer pathogenesis. Whether *PTEN* loss occurs early or late in prostate tumorigenesis is not clear. Complete genomic loss of *PTEN* is seen in greater than 50% of metastatic lesions but in only approximately 20% of localized lesions. Within the same patient, *PTEN* loss can be observed in metastatic but not primary lesions,[68] suggesting that genomic *PTEN* loss is involved in disease progression but not initiation. However, heterozygous *PTEN* loss or decreased PTEN protein expression by immunohistochemistry has been reported in approximately 25% of PIN and greater than 50% of primary cancers, suggesting that PTEN may be a haploinsufficient tumor suppressor. Partial loss could be important for early tumorigenesis, with progression to complete loss at metastasis.[82] Mouse models have confirmed a dosage effect of *Pten* in prostate cancer progression.

PTEN is the major negative regulator of the PI3K/AKT pathway (Fig. 96.5). PI3K, which can be activated by many growth factors, phosphorylates PIP2 into PIP3 at the plasma membrane and PIP3 recruits pleckstrin homology (PH) domain–containing proteins, including AKT. As a lipid phosphatase, PTEN converts PIP3 back to PIP2 thereby limiting normal activity of the pathway. PI3K also activates mammalian target of rapamycin (mTOR) C2 complex (which contains the kinase mTOR complexed with distinct regulatory factors), which directly phosphorylates and activates AKT. Activated AKT phosphorylates a number of crucial substrates implicated in cell growth and survival, including downstream activation of the other mTOR complex, mTORC1 (Fig. 96.5).

The PTEN→AKT→mTOR pathway has garnered special attention due to the large number of mutations in the genes in this pathway, including PTEN, PI3K, AKT, as well as upstream kinases. Mouse models of prostate cancer suggest that both AKT and mTORC2 are essential mediators of PTEN-loss–mediated tumorigenesis—prostate-specific deletions of either gene abolish the tumor phenotype of Pten loss prostate.[83,84] This pathway is also amenable to pharmaceutical inhibition using approved drugs such as rapamycin, and its analogues, which inhibit mTORC1; investigational kinase inhibitors targeting PI3K, mTORC1 and mTORC2, and AKT are in clinical development (Fig. 96.5). Preclinical data provide strong rationale for their trials in prostate cancer. In addition to AKT, PTEN loss likely has other crucial targets, evidenced by the observation that overexpression of active AKT in mice causes PIN that does not progress into cancer while *Pten*$^{(-/-)}$ mice develop invasive cancer. One candidate pathway involves CDC42 and JNK.[85]

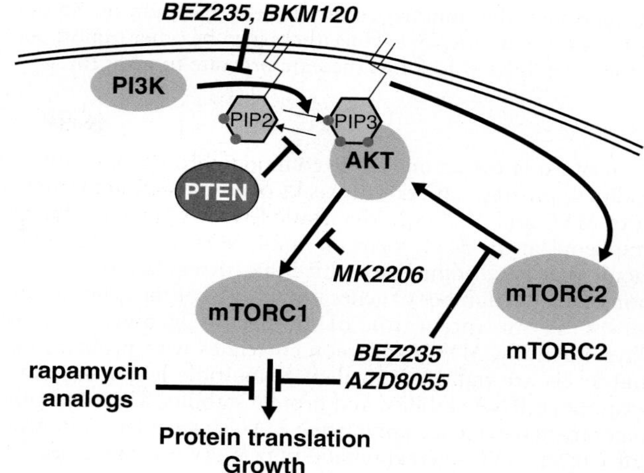

FIGURE 96.5 Schematic of the phosphatidylinositol 3-kinase (PK3K) pathway and inhibitors. PI3K phosphorylates PIP2 into PIP3, while the PTEN phosphatase catalyzes the opposite reaction. PIP3 activates AKT by recruitment to the membrane, activation of mammalian target of rapamycin complex 2 (mTORC2) and pyruvate dehydrogenase kinase (PDK) kinases. AKT activates many growth pathways include mTORC1. BEZ235 is a dual-specificity kinase inhibitor that inhibits both PI3K and mTOR, the common kinase component of mTROC1 and mTORC2 complexes. BKM120 and AZD8055 are kinase inhibitors that inhibit PI3K and mTOR, respectively. Rapamycin analogues (e.g., sirolimus, temsirolimus, everolimus) specifically inhibit assembly of the mTORC1 complex. MK2206 is a new generation allosteric inhibitor of AKT.

Chromosome 8p Loss and 8q Gain

NKX3.1

Heterozygous loss of 8p21 is the most frequent chromosomal aberration in prostate cancer, affecting 60% of PIN and 85% of prostate cancers.[86] The most studied candidate tumor suppressor gene mapping to this region is the AR regulated, prostate specific homeobox transcription factor *NKX3.1*. However, unlike classic tumor suppressor genes, the remaining *NKX3.1* allele is not mutated or deleted, leading to the hypothesis that *NKX3.1* haploinsufficiency is sufficient for oncogenesis. Prostate development in mice with targeted deletion of *Nkx3.1* proceeds normally, albeit with subtle defects in prostate morphogenesis.[86] Mechanistic studies suggest NKX3.1 facilitates terminal differentiation. In castrated mice, introduction of testosterone results in an early intense proliferative response to reconstitute the gland followed by differentiation and quiescence. In *Nkx3.1*$^{(+/-)}$ and *Nkx3.1*$^{(-/-)}$ mice, there is a delay in differentiation, resulting in hypertrophy.[87,88] When crossed into *Pten*$^{(+/-)}$ mice, loss of *Nkx3.1* is reported to accelerate prostate neoplasia. Furthermore, prostate tumors that develop in two genetically engineered mouse models caused by distinct initiating lesions (transgenic expression of *Myc* and conditional *Pten* deletion) both show reduced *Nkx3.1* expression.[79,89] In the case of *Pten* loss, the decline in *Nkx3.1* expression is most likely explained by crosstalk between *Pten* and *Nkx3.1* rather than selection for *Nkx3.1* loss as a progression event.[90]

Other evidence argues against *NKX3.1* as the 8p tumor suppressor. Despite monoallelic loss, mRNA expression is still quite high in prostate tumors. In fact, tumors that harbor single copy loss of *NKX3.1* do not have lower levels of *NKX3.1* transcript.

Furthermore, the minimal common deleted region on 8p does not always span *NKX3.1*. Thus, there may be other tumors suppressors in 8p21 whose loss mediate prostate tumorigenesis.

MYC

Gain of 8q is the second most common chromosomal abnormality in prostate cancer with peaks of amplification located at both *MYC* and *NCOA2*. Metastatic lesions often have further amplicons at the *MYC* locus on 8q24. MYC is a transcription factor that heterodimerizes with Max to regulate the expression of a large number of genes (up to 15% of the genome) and serves as an integrator of numerous growth signals. Physiologically, *MYC* expression correlates with proliferation, and levels are tightly controlled at multiple levels—by transcription, mRNA stability, and protein stability. There is strong experimental evidence implicating *MYC* dysregulation in prostate cancer. *MYC* overexpression in primary prostate epithelial cells leads to transformation,[25] and transgenic mice expressing *MYC* in the prostate develop PIN followed by adenocarcinoma,[89] which histologically represents the closest mimic of human prostate cancer among current mouse models.[91]

Epigenetic Changes

In addition to genetic alternations, a number of epigenetic changes have been implicated in prostate cancer progression, such as altered DNA methylation and histone modifications, that lead to changes in gene expression.[92] One early change in prostate cancer is silencing of the π-class glutathione *S*-transferase (*GSTP*) gene through DNA methylation at CpG islands in transcriptional regulatory regions. *GSTP* is frequently overexpressed in many cancers, perhaps due to oncogenic and chemotherapy stress. Unexpectedly, GSTπ expression is silenced in the vast majority of prostate cancers and PIN lesions through methylation of the GSTπ promoter.[93]

DNA is packaged around the core histone proteins H2A, H2B, H3, and H4 to form chromatin. The amino termini of histones, particularly H3 and H4, are subject to posttranslational modification through lysine acetylation or methylation and arginine methylation, all of which influence gene expression. Altered histone modifications, such as H3K4 methylation and H4R3 methylation, have been reported to correlate with reduced risk of recurrence in surgically resected prostate cancer.[94] Changes in expression of the proteins responsible for these histone modifications have been implicated in prostate cancer. For example, EZH2 (enhancer of Zeste homolog 2) is a polycomb group protein overexpressed in high-grade localized as well as castrate-resistant metastatic prostate cancer.[95] EZH2 is part of a larger suppressive complex that recruits DNA methyltransferases to CpG islands. EZH2 methylates lysine 27 of histone H3 and forms a bridge between suppressive histone and DNA methylation.[96] High levels of EZH2 may be oncogenic through suppression of gene expression due to H3K27 methylation of critical target genes such as the RasGAP family member DAB2IP.[97]

Selected References

The full list of references for this chapter appears in the online version.

6. Nelson WG, De Marzo AM, Isaacs WB. Prostate cancer. *N Engl J Med* 2003;349:366.
7. De Marzo AM, Platz EA, Sutcliffe S, et al. Inflammation in prostate carcinogenesis. *Nat Rev Cancer* 2007;7:256.
8. Schroder FH, Hugosson J, Roobol MJ, et al. Screening and prostate-cancer mortality in a randomized European study. *N Engl J Med* 2009;360:1320.
9. Andriole GL, Crawford ED, Grubb RL 3rd, et al. Mortality results from a randomized prostate-cancer screening trial. *N Engl J Med* 2009;360:1310.
11. Amundadottir LT, Sulem P, Gudmundsson J, et al. A common variant associated with prostate cancer in European and African populations. *Nat Genet* 2006;38:652.
12. Gudmundsson J, Sulem P, Manolescu A, et al. Genome-wide association study identifies a second prostate cancer susceptibility variant at 8q24. *Nat Genet* 2007;39:631.
13. Haiman CA, Patterson N, Freedman ML, et al. Multiple regions within 8q24 independently affect risk for prostate cancer. *Nat Genet* 2007;39:638.
14. Yeager M, Orr N, Hayes RB, et al. Genome-wide association study of prostate cancer identifies a second risk locus at 8q24. *Nat Genet* 2007;39:645.
15. Al Olama AA, Kote-Jarai Z, Giles GG, et al. Multiple loci on 8q24 associated with prostate cancer susceptibility. *Nat Genet* 2009;41:1058.
16. Ahmadiyeh N, Pomerantz MM, Grisanzio C, et al. 8q24 prostate, breast, and colon cancer risk loci show tissue-specific long-range interaction with MYC. *Proc Natl Acad Sci U S A* 2010;107:9742.
17. Eeles RA, Kote-Jarai Z, Giles GG, et al. Multiple newly identified loci associated with prostate cancer susceptibility. *Nat Genet* 2008;40:316.
18. Thomas G, Jacobs KB, Yeager M, et al. Multiple loci identified in a genome-wide association study of prostate cancer. *Nat Genet* 2008;40:310.
19. Zheng SL, Sun J, Wiklund F, et al. Cumulative association of five genetic variants with prostate cancer. *N Engl J Med* 2008;358:910.
21. Taylor BS, Schultz N, Hieronymus H, et al. Integrative genomic profiling of human prostate cancer. *Cancer Cell* 2010;18:11.
22. Huggins C, Hodges CV. Studies on prostatic cancer. I. The effect of castration, of estrogen and of androgen injection on serum phosphatases in metastatic carcinoma of the prostate. *Cancer Res* 1941;1:293.
24. Chen Y, Sawyers CL, Scher HI. Targeting the androgen receptor pathway in prostate cancer. *Curr Opin Pharmacol* 2008;8:440.
25. Berger R, Febbo PG, Majumder PK, et al. Androgen-induced differentiation and tumorigenicity of human prostate epithelial cells. *Cancer Res* 2004;64:8867.
30. Visakorpi T, Hyytinen E, Koivisto P, et al. In vivo amplification of the androgen receptor gene and progression of human prostate cancer. *Nat Genet* 1995;9:401.
32. Holzbeierlein J, Lal P, LaTulippe E, et al. Gene expression analysis of human prostate carcinoma during hormonal therapy identifies androgen-responsive genes and mechanisms of therapy resistance. *Am J Pathol* 2004;164:217.
33. Chen CD, Welsbie DS, Tran C, et al. Molecular determinants of resistance to antiandrogen therapy. *Nat Med* 2004;10:33.
36. Sun S, Sprenger CC, Vessella RL, et al. Castration resistance in human prostate cancer is conferred by a frequently occurring androgen receptor splice variant. *J Clin Invest* 2010;120:2715.
38. Montgomery RB, Mostaghel EA, Vessella R, et al. Maintenance of intratumoral androgens in metastatic prostate cancer: a mechanism for castration-resistant tumor growth. *Cancer Res* 2008;68:4447.
39. Stanbrough M, Bubley GJ, Ross K, et al. Increased expression of genes converting adrenal androgens to testosterone in androgen-independent prostate cancer. *Cancer Res* 2006;66:2815.
41. Mellinghoff IK, Vivanco I, Kwon A, et al. HER2/neu kinase-dependent modulation of androgen receptor function through effects on DNA binding and stability. *Cancer Cell* 2004;6:517.
45. Kelly WK, Scher HI. Prostate specific antigen decline after antiandrogen withdrawal: the flutamide withdrawal syndrome. *J Urol* 1993;149:607.
46. Tran C, Ouk S, Clegg NJ, et al. Development of a second-generation antiandrogen for treatment of advanced prostate cancer. *Science* 2009;324:787.
47. Scher HI, Beer TM, Higano CS, et al. Antitumour activity of MDV3100 in castration-resistant prostate cancer: a phase 1-2 study. *Lancet* 2010;375:1437.
49. Danila DC, Morris MJ, de Bono JS, et al. Phase II multicenter study of abiraterone acetate plus prednisone therapy in patients with docetaxel-treated castration-resistant prostate cancer. *J Clin Oncol* 2010;28:1496.
52. Hieronymus H, Lamb J, Ross KN, et al. Gene expression signature-based chemical genomic prediction identifies a novel class of HSP90 pathway modulators. *Cancer Cell* 2006;10:321.
54. Welsbie DS, Xu J, Chen Y, et al. Histone deacetylases are required for androgen receptor function in hormone-sensitive and castrate-resistant prostate cancer. *Cancer Res* 2009;69:958.
56. Tomlins SA, Laxman B, Dhanasekaran SM, et al. Distinct classes of chromosomal rearrangements create oncogenic ETS gene fusions in prostate cancer. *Nature* 2007;448:595.
58. Tomlins SA, Rhodes DR, Perner S, et al. Recurrent fusion of TMPRSS2 and ETS transcription factor genes in prostate cancer. *Science* 2005;310:644.

60. Demichelis F, Fall K, Perner S, et al. TMPRSS2:ERG gene fusion associated with lethal prostate cancer in a watchful waiting cohort. *Oncogene* 2007;26:4596.
62. Gopalan A, Leversha MA, Satagopan JM, et al. TMPRSS2-ERG gene fusion is not associated with outcome in patients treated by prostatectomy. *Cancer Res* 2009;69:1400.
72. Carver BS, Tran J, Gopalan A, et al. Aberrant ERG expression cooperates with loss of PTEN to promote cancer progression in the prostate. *Nat Genet* 2009;41:619.
73. King JC, Xu J, Wongvipat J, et al. Cooperativity of TMPRSS2-ERG with PI3-kinase pathway activation in prostate oncogenesis. *Nat Genet* 2009;41:524.
74. Zong Y, Xin L, Goldstein AS, et al. ETS family transcription factors collaborate with alternative signaling pathways to induce carcinoma from adult murine prostate cells. *Proc Natl Acad Sci U S A* 2009;106:12465.
75. Yu J, Mani RS, Cao Q, et al. An integrated network of androgen receptor, polycomb, and TMPRSS2-ERG gene fusions in prostate cancer progression. *Cancer Cell* 2010;17:443.
78. Whang YE, Wu X, Suzuki H, et al. Inactivation of the tumor suppressor PTEN/MMAC1 in advanced human prostate cancer through loss of expression. *Proc Natl Acad Sci U S A* 1998;95:5246.
79. Wang S, Gao J, Lei Q, et al. Prostate-specific deletion of the murine Pten tumor suppressor gene leads to metastatic prostate cancer. *Cancer Cell* 2003;4:209.
83. Chen ML, Xu PZ, Peng XD, et al. The deficiency of Akt1 is sufficient to suppress tumor development in Pten+/− mice. *Genes Dev* 2006;20:1569.
84. Guertin DA, Stevens DM, Saitoh M, et al. mTOR complex 2 is required for the development of prostate cancer induced by Pten loss in mice. *Cancer Cell* 2009;15:148.
85. Vivanco I, Palaskas N, Tran C, et al. Identification of the JNK signaling pathway as a functional target of the tumor suppressor PTEN. *Cancer Cell* 2007;11:555.
87. Kim MJ, Bhatia-Gaur R, Banach-Petrosky WA, et al. Nkx3.1 mutant mice recapitulate early stages of prostate carcinogenesis. *Cancer Res* 2002;62:2999.
88. Magee JA, Abdulkadir SA, Milbrandt J. Haploinsufficiency at the Nkx3.1 locus. A paradigm for stochastic, dosage-sensitive gene regulation during tumor initiation. *Cancer Cell* 2003;3:273.
89. Ellwood-Yen K, Graeber TG, Wongvipat J, et al. Myc-driven murine prostate cancer shares molecular features with human prostate tumors. *Cancer Cell* 2003;4:223.
90. Lei Q, Jiao J, Xin L, et al. NKX3.1 stabilizes p53, inhibits AKT activation, and blocks prostate cancer initiation caused by PTEN loss. *Cancer Cell* 2006;9:367.
94. Seligson DB, Horvath S, Shi T, et al. Global histone modification patterns predict risk of prostate cancer recurrence. *Nature* 2005;435:1262.
95. Varambally S, Dhanasekaran SM, Zhou M, et al. The polycomb group protein EZH2 is involved in progression of prostate cancer. *Nature* 2002;419:624.
98. Chen Y, Clegg NJ, Scher HI. Anti-androgens and androgen-depleting therapies in prostate cancer: new agents for an established target. *Lancet Oncol* 2009;10:981.

CHAPTER 97 CANCER OF THE PROSTATE

MICHAEL J. ZELEFSKY, JAMES A. EASTHAM, AND A. OLIVER SARTOR

ANATOMY OF THE PROSTATE

The prostate is an exocrine organ measuring approximately 25 cm^3. It consists of lobular tubuloalveolar glands that secrete fluid through ducts that empty into the prostatic urethra. The fluid comprises the bulk of seminal emissions and is rich in prostate-specific antigen (PSA). The prostate is located deep in the pelvis between the bladder and the external urinary sphincter, anterior to the rectum and below the pubis. Because of the placement of the gland at this critical juncture, cancers of the prostate, and the treatment of such cancers, put urinary, sexual, and bowel function at risk.

Most cancers arise in the peripheral zone near the capsule of the prostate. The disease is generally multifocal, and tumors are often present throughout the gland. Dissemination of cancer may occur by local extension through defects in the capsule where the neurovascular structures and the ejaculatory ducts enter the gland, or in the region of the bladder neck. Local invasion can progress to involve the seminal vesicles, the rectum, the bladder neck, or the levator muscles. Systemic spread can occur via the lymphatics to involve the external iliac, hypogastric, obturator, and presacral nodes or hematogenously to involve bone, lung, or liver. Prostate cancer has a predilection for bone, in part owing to a unique bidirectional interaction between tumor cells and the surrounding bone stroma.

PROSTATE ZONAL ANATOMY

In younger men, four zones can be defined within the prostate: peripheral, central, transition, and anterior fibromuscular stroma (McNeal 1981; McLaughlin et al. 2005) (Fig. 97.1). The peripheral zone makes up the bulk of the normal gland. Posteriorly, the peripheral zone lies against the rectum and is the area palpable by digital rectal examination (DRE). The central zone surrounds the ejaculatory ducts. The anterior fibromuscular stroma is an anterior band of fibromuscular tissue contiguous with the bladder smooth muscle and the external sphincter. The transition zone is located centrally and surrounds the urethra. These zonal boundaries are indistinct in the gland of a normal, postpubescent male, but as men age the transition zone enlarges from nonmalignant growth (benign prostatic hyperplasia [BPH]) to become the dominant zone of the prostate. With hypertrophy, all other zones are compressed and the central zone can no longer be defined as distinct from the peripheral zone (Fig. 97.1). The frequency of malignancy in the different zones is disproportionate to the glandular tissue present. Most cancers originate in the peripheral zone. Only 15% of cancers originate in the transition zone, and very few originate in the central zone.

HISTOPATHOLOGY

Normal prostatic epithelium contains a heterogeneous group of cells representing several distinct levels of differentiation. Epithelial layers are more readily observed in organs such as the skin or colon but are nevertheless present in the normal prostate as well. Secretory luminal cells are well-differentiated epithelial cells that produce PSA and are positive for androgen receptors (ARs). The secretory cells are derived from basal cells through an intermediate proliferating group of cells that are variable in AR and PSA expression. More mature cells in the intermediate pool are positive for AR and PSA, whereas less mature cells in this pool are not. The PSA-producing secretory luminal cells are terminally differentiated and incapable of proliferation (Wang, Hayward et al. 2001; Signoretti and Loda 2006). Rare neuroendocrine cells are also present in normal prostatic epithelium.[1]

More than 95% of malignancies in the prostate are adenocarcinomas that arise in acinar and proximal ductal epithelium. Most tumors arise in the peripheral zone of the prostate but transitional zone tumors are well described.[2,3] Other tumors developing in the prostate include intralobular acinar carcinomas, ductal carcinomas, small cell or scirrhous pattern tumors, a rare clear cell variant resembling renal cell carcinomas, and mucinous carcinoma. Small cell tumors of the prostate have neuroendocrine features and are composed of small, round, undifferentiated cells.[4] Ductal and small cell tumors are prone to early metastases. Urothelial and rectal cancers may invade the prostate and are occasionally diagnosed during a prostate biopsy as a consequence of DRE abnormalities and/or elevations in PSA. The typical adenocarcinoma of the prostate can be distinguished from other neoplasms using PSA immunohistochemistry. Neuroendocrine differentiation can be assessed by markers such as neuron-specific enolase, synaptophysin, and chromogranin A.

Prostate biopsy specimens occasionally contain proliferative foci of small atypical acini that display some features, but not all, diagnostic of adenocarcinoma, referred to as *atypical small acinar proliferation* (ASAP). Prostate cancer has been identified in specimens from subsequent biopsies in up to 60% of cases of ASAP, indicating that this finding is a significant predictor of cancer on subsequent prostate biopsy.[5,6] Identification of ASAP warrants repeat biopsy for concurrent or subsequent invasive carcinoma. Prostate biopsy specimens may also demonstrate intraductal proliferation, termed *prostatic intraepithelial neoplasia* (PIN).[5,7] PIN is defined by the presence of cytologically atypical epithelial cells within architecturally benign-appearing acini and is subdivided into low and high grades.[7] An atrophic but highly proliferative condition associated with chronic inflammation, proliferative inflammatory atrophy (PIA), may in fact be the first histologic

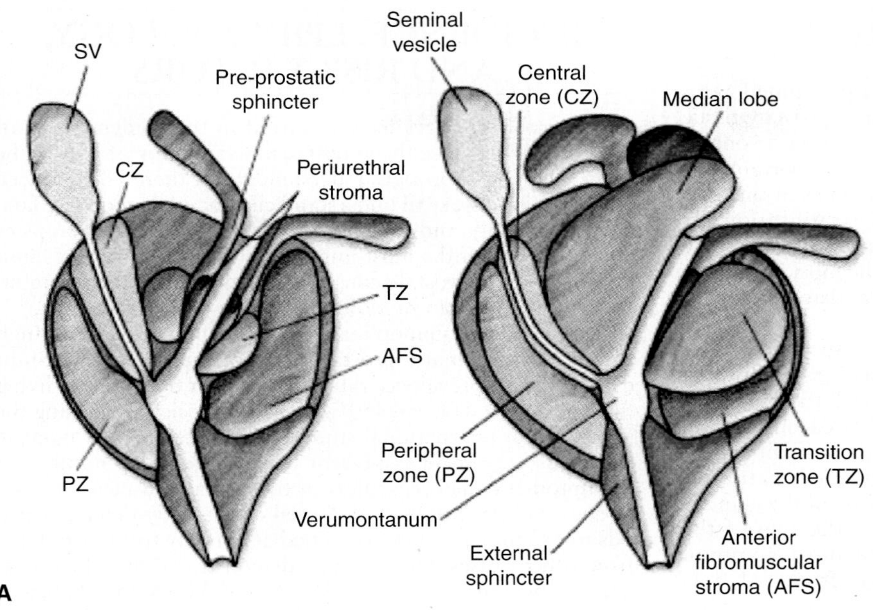

FIGURE 97.1 Zonal anatomy of the prostate. **A:** Young male with minimal transition zone hypertrophy. Note that preprostatic sphincter and periejaculatory duct zone (central zone of McLean) are clearly defined. **B:** Older male with transition zone hypertrophy, which effaces the preprostatic sphincter and compresses the periejaculatory duct zone. SV, seminal vesicle; CZ, central zone; PZ, peripheral zone; TZ, transition zone; AFS, anterior fibromuscular stroma. (From ref. 398, with permission.)

step in the carcinogenic process (Fig. 97.2).[6,8] The epithelial cells in PIA appear to be cycling rapidly based on increased expression of Ki-67 and decreased expression of p27/kip1. Morphologic transitions have been identified between PIA and high-grade PIN in a substantial number of cases, suggesting a causal link between these two entities. Weak expression of PSA and AR, high levels of selected cytokeratins (K8/18), and lack of p63 identify the epithelial cells in PIA as intermediate between the basal and secretory cell phenotype.[9]

Prostatic adenocarcinomas are often multifocal and heterogeneous, a factor that complicates both prognostication and attempts to develop focal therapy. Studies of step-sectioned radical prostatectomy (RP) specimens indicate that most cancers contain multiple grades arranged in heterogeneous and unpredictable interrelationships. Patients not only have multifocal tumors but also an average of 2.7 different grades of cancer in each specimen; only 10% of index cancers in RP specimens are composed of a single histologic grade. Thus, any diagnostic method short of whole-gland sampling is inevitably subject to sampling error. This is a major issue for surveillance protocols. Careful genetic studies indicate that multifocality is typically a function of separately arising tumors rather than intraprostatic tumor spread.[10] Adenocarcinomas typically stain negative for basal cell markers such as basal-specific cytokeratins and p63, and positive for α-methylacyl-coenzyme A racemase, which is up-regulated in adenocarcinoma cells.

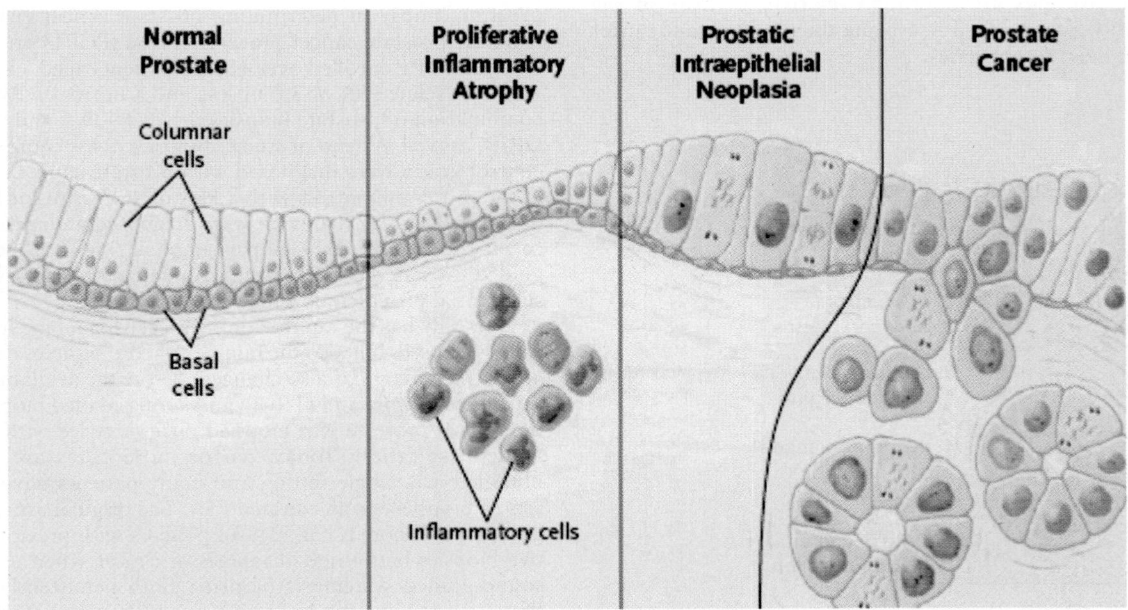

FIGURE 97.2 Proliferative inflammatory atrophy is hypothesized to be a precursor to prostatic intraepithelial neoplasia, which in turn is the precursor of prostate cancer. (From ref. 8, with permission.)

GLEASON SCORE

The contributions of Gleason[11,12] are unquestioned with regard to prognosis. Microscopic evaluation of prostate tissue and careful histologic grading, via Gleason scoring or one of several similar alternatives, is one of the most important factors in understanding clinically relevant outcomes in this heterogeneous disease. Every method of risk stratification for patients with localized prostate cancer incorporates histologic grading (Gleason score or proxy) as one of the most important variables in determining prognosis. Molecular determinants of Gleason are an area of active study.[13]

Gleason grading evaluates the architectural details of individual cancer glands under low-to-medium magnification. Five distinct patterns of growth from well to poorly differentiated were described in the original Gleason grading scale (Fig. 97.3).[11] Pattern 1 tumors are the most differentiated, with discrete glandular formation, whereas pattern 5 lesions are the most undifferentiated, with loss of the glandular architecture. The final Gleason score is the sum of the grades of the most common and second most common growth patterns; the Gleason score can range from 2 (1 + 1) to 10 (5 + 5).

The prognostic importance of Gleason's scoring system has been difficult to improve on; however, some data suggest that the overall prognosis is driven preferentially by the high-grade components of the tumor. Two notable variations of the original Gleason score have consequently evolved. First, for those cancers that have minor but significant high-grade components, a tertiary Gleason score can be reported (i.e., 3 + 4 = 7 with tertiary 5) and this carries significant prognostic information.[14] Second, some investigators have advocated that the percentage of Gleason grade 4/5 cancer be reported as the percentage of high grade is not clearly described by conventional Gleason sums.[15] This is clearly of importance in patients with a Gleason score of 7. It is established that Gleason 3 + 4 = 7 tumors vary from Gleason 4 + 3 = 7 cancers with respect to outcomes after various treatments.[16]

The full Gleason spectrum is rarely used today. Low-grade tumors (Gleason score of 5 or less) are rarely reported in contemporary series. Re-reading of older prostate cancer specimens in a controlled fashion suggests that contemporary pathologic readings are upgraded relative to those in the past,[17] with Gleason 3 + 3 = 6 being the predominant cancer detected in most recent series.

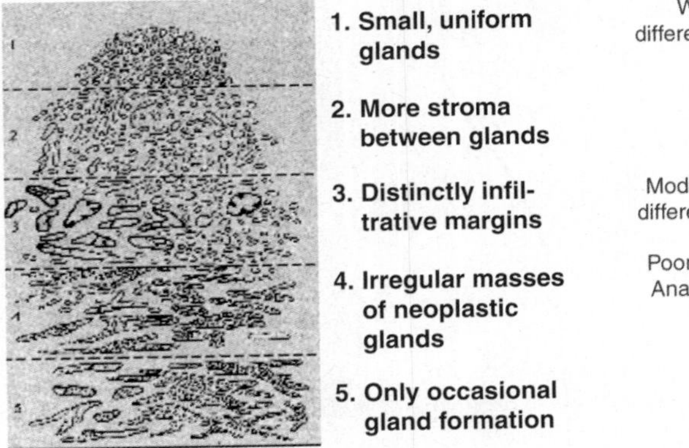

FIGURE 97.3 Gleason histologic grading of prostate cancer demonstrating progressive loss of glandular formation with increasing score. (Adapted from ref. 12.)

INCIDENCE, EPIDEMIOLOGY, AND RISK FACTORS

Considerable changes have occurred in the epidemiology of prostate cancer since the widespread availability of PSA in the early 1990s. A thorough understanding of these PSA-induced changes is necessary to understand current epidemiologic data, both nationally and internationally, as PSA-driven biopsies constitute one of the most important risk factors for the clinical diagnosis of prostate cancer, as recently and clearly demonstrated by European randomized studies of PSA screening.[18]

Unlike other common malignancies, aging men have a high rate of asymptomatic prostate cancer. Autopsy studies indicated a cancer prevalence rate quite distinct from that of living men, although widespread PSA-driven biopsies are closing the gap. Careful international studies in the pre-PSA era indicate that prostate cancer is present in a considerable number of asymptomatic men regardless of their locale. In men 50 years of age or older, Yatani et al.[19] used consistently defined methods to examine prostates obtained at autopsy from men dying from other causes. These studies demonstrated that the prevalence of prostate cancer was 36.9% and 34.6% in U.S. blacks and whites, respectively, 31.5% in Colombians, and 20.5% in Japanese men living in Japan. In a more recent study of men dying from unrelated causes in Detroit, Michigan, men in their third, fourth, fifth, sixth, and eighth decades had a prevalence of prostate cancer of 2%, 29%, 32%, 55%, and 64%, respectively.[20] Taken together, these studies clearly indicate that prostate cancer is extremely prevalent among asymptomatic men both in the United States and throughout the world.

A clinical diagnosis of prostate cancer is highly dependent on the frequency and extent of prostate tissue sampling. Because of this ascertainment bias, understanding the epidemiology of prostate cancer incidence is considerably more complex than other cancers. Dramatic changes in prostate cancer incidence have taken place since the PSA became commercially available, as an increasing number of asymptomatic men have been biopsied. Other issues have also changed in recent years; these include the threshold for PSA-driven biopsies, the number of core biopsy samples obtained when biopsies are performed, and the number of repetitive biopsies in men with a prior negative biopsy. As an example of the importance of prostate biopsy in determining prostate cancer risk, lessons from the prostate cancer prevention trial (PCPT) are noteworthy. The PCPT enrolled over 18,000 patients aged 55 and older with a baseline PSA of 3.0 or less and a normal DRE. Using a combination of prostate biopsies driven by PSA and suspicious DREs, as well as "end of study" biopsies, 24.4% of men in the control group were diagnosed with prostate cancer.[21] Of note, in the subset of controls with a PSA of 4.0 ng/mL or less and a normal DRE, 15.2% of men were diagnosed with prostate cancer at the end of study biopsy, emphasizing that ultrasound-guided prostate needle biopsies can detect prostate cancer in a substantial proportion of men.

Not only has the number of men receiving a biopsy dramatically increased, but also the number of core samples obtained in any given patient has also changed. Before the availability of the transrectal ultrasound (TRUS) and spring-loaded biopsy device, the typical prostate was biopsied once or twice with a digital-guided aspiration. Today, ten or more cores are routinely obtained at a single setting and many patients have repeated sets of biopsies for an elevated PSA. The original article on sextant biopsy[22] noted that 53% of patients with previously negative biopsies had a new diagnosis of cancer when using ultrasound-guided systematic biopsies. Both persistently elevated PSAs and atypical findings on prior biopsy reports (high PIN or ASAP) drive additional ultrasound-guided biopsies. Ascertainment biases are often incompletely acknowledged in the literature and data from international comparisons in particular have potential for misinterpretation. Given that the rate of PSA testing and prostate biopsy varies from country to country, comparison of international incidence rates should be cautiously interpreted. Further, comparison of rates among migrant populations should be cautiously interpreted unless PSA and prostate biopsy rates are understood and comparable between the populations of interest.

INCIDENCE AND MORTALITY OF PROSTATE CANCER

More than 192,000 men were diagnosed with prostate cancer in 2009, and about 27,300 died of the disease.[23] Men in the United States have about a 16% chance of eventually being diagnosed with prostate cancer and about a 3% chance of eventually dying of it. Those who undergo regular PSA testing have a higher likelihood of undergoing prostate biopsy and being diagnosed with prostate cancer compared with men who do not undergo PSA testing. There is no question that prostate cancer and its management is a significant public health issue.

Prostate cancer currently has an exceptionally high incidence/mortality ratio in the United States compared to the other leading causes of cancer death in the United States.[23] The current incidence/mortality ratio is 7.1. In contrast, the other leading causes of cancer death in the United States—pancreas, lung, female breast, and colon cancer—have incidence/mortality ratios of approximately 1.2, 1.4, 4.8, and 2.1, respectively.[23] It should be emphasized, however, that the number of men dying from prostate cancer is substantial, and that a significant subset of men are diagnosed with prostate cancer that poses considerable risk to their well-being. The National Cancer Institute Surveillance, Epidemiology and End Results (SEER) program, has recently estimated that the current risk of prostate cancer in U.S. men during their lifetime is nearly 16%; however, the lifetime risk of dying from prostate cancer is estimated to be 2.8% (http://seer.cancer.gov/csr/1975_2006/results_single/sect_23_table.09_2pgs.pdf).

As previously noted, the incidence of prostate cancer has changed dramatically over the past several decades in the United States, increasing from less than 100 cases per age-adjusted 100,000 population in 1975, rising to a peak of 240 cases per 100,000 in 1992, and then declining to a relatively constant level of 158 cases per 100,000 in recent years.[23] Although it is difficult to determine accurately the percentage of men in the U.S. general population receiving PSA testing, in 1996 83% of prostate cancer diagnoses in whites and 77% in blacks were preceded by a PSA test.[24] Mortality rates from prostate cancer have trended downward sharply in U.S. men during the last decade, yet prostate cancer remains the second leading cause of cancer death in U.S. men. Reasons for the decline are debated; PSA screening may be causal. However, other countries with less active screening have also had declining mortality rates; thus, other explanations are also plausible.

Although geographic variations in the incidence of prostate cancer are susceptible to ascertainment biases, statistical reporting differences, and variations in population age, U.S. statistics are distinct from Asian countries such as Korea and Japan, which report age-adjusted mortality rates of 8 to 9 per 100,000, with Sweden and the United States reporting 60 to 80 per 100,000[25] (Table 97.1). Mortality rates are more reliable estimates of the impact of prostate cancer from population to population. Mortality rates are clearly different among countries with excellent health statistics; for instance, Korea, Japan, and Singapore have age-adjusted prostate cancer mortality rates of 2.5 to 3.6 per 100,000 and the United States and Sweden have rates of 7.1 to 12.0 per 100,000, respectively (Table 97.1). Data from sub-Saharan African countries and the Caribbean may not be as reliable as those from more developed countries, but World Health Organization estimates for prostate age-adjusted mortality rates per 100,000 are much higher than for the United States or Western Europe. For instance, these rates are 33.4 in Antigua and Barbuda, 24.7 for Barbados, 28.7 in Sierra Leone, 23.1 in Swaziland, and 30.8 in Uganda.[25] Hypotheses to explain these discrepancies vary and are controversial.

TABLE 97.1

INCIDENCE AND MORTALITY ESTIMATES PER 100,000 AGE-NORMALIZED POPULATIONS USING WORLD HEALTH ORGANIZATION (WHO) STANDARDIZED POPULATIONS AND DATA FROM 2002[a]

Country	Incidence	Mortality
Antigua and Barbuda	104	33
Argentina	37	9
Australia	64	9
Austria	42	7
Barbados	103	25
Brazil	36	11
Canada	85	8
Congo	52	15
Egypt	8	2
France	42	8
Germany	43	7
Grenada	100	32
India	9	3
Israel	36	7
Italy	29	6
Japan	20	3
Kuwait	10	3
Malaysia	13	6
Mexico	23	7
Norway	69	13
Republic of Korea	9	2
Sierra Leone	92	29
Singapore	12	4
Swaziland	55	23
Sweden	61	12
Uganda	100	31
United Kingdom	44	9
United States	80	7

[a]Note that U.S. age-normalized populations are older than WHO-normalized populations, thus explaining discrepancies between U.S. and WHO data sources.
(From ref. 25, with permission.)

CLINICAL RISK FACTORS FOR PROSTATE CANCER

As previously noted, the overall risk of a clinical diagnosis of prostate cancer in the United States is unequivocally associated with the frequency and extent of prostatic tissue sampling. Thus, PSA testing followed by PSA-driven prostate biopsies may be considered among the most important risk factors for prostate cancer. A variety of other hereditary and environmental risk factors have been hypothesized; however, some degree of controversy surrounds most of these issues. Age, ethnicity, and family history are exceptions; there is general agreement that these factors are important in prostate cancer risk.

Age

Other than male sex, age is the most important risk for prostate cancer. Among adult malignancies, no other cancer is as age-related as prostate cancer. Prostate cancer rarely occurs before the age of 40, but the incidence rises rapidly thereafter. Data from the National Cancer Institute's SEER program show that the incidence of new cases of prostate cancer in white men in 2000 to 2006 was 9, 136, 567, 958, and 786 per 100,000 in men aged 40 to 44, 50 to 54, 60 to 64, 70 to 74, or 80 to 84 years, respectively.[26] Decreases in incidence that occur at advanced age are probably attributable to ascertainment biases. At some point, as a consequence of advanced age and/or significant comorbidities, prostate biopsies are performed at a less frequent rate.

Ethnicity

Black men within the United States have one of the highest incidences of prostate cancer in the world, with striking differences in mortality relative to white men. The incidence of new cases of prostate cancer in black men in 2000 to 2004 was 23, 253, 935, 1,323, and 1,028 per 100,000 in men aged 40 to 44, 50 to 54, 60 to 64, 70 to 74, or 80 to 84 years or older, respectively.[26] Black men are not only diagnosed at a younger age but have higher tumor burdens within each stage category,[27] a 1.5-fold higher frequency of metastatic disease at presentation, and lower survival rates.[26] Ascertainment biases are not explanatory for these findings, as similar findings have been reported in the pre-PSA era and black men have lower PSA screening rates as compared with other ethnic groups.[28] Studies in African and Caribbean men suggest that sub-Saharan ancestry may be more relevant than geographic location. Asian men have lower prostate cancer incidence rates both in the United States and in Asia. It is uncertain whether the reason for populations having a higher incidence of clinical cancers is genetic susceptibility or exposure to causative environmental factors. There is evidence for both.

Family History

A familial component of prostate cancer risk has been definitively identified. Men with a brother or father diagnosed with prostate cancer at age 50 have an approximately twofold increased risk of prostate cancer,[29] and those with two or more first-degree relatives with prostate cancer have approximately a seven- to eightfold increased risk compared with the general population.[29] Older age of cancer diagnosis in the familial member clearly confers less risk than younger ages at cancer diagnosis.

In Swedish twin studies analyzing data from the pre-PSA era, monozygotic twins had a relative risk 6.3-fold higher as compared with dizygotic twins.[30] A large Scandinavian twin study concluded that hereditable factors contributed substantially more to the risk of prostate cancer than either breast or colorectal cancer.[31] In this study, 42% of the risk of prostate cancer was explained by heritable factors.

Diet and Lifestyle

Studies of various environmental factors in the absence of controlling for frequency of prostate biopsies are problematic for the reasons previously noted. Various observational studies have shown increased risk for various dietary intakes including high-saturated fats, red meats, low fruits, low vegetables, low tomato products, low fish, and/or low soy. Defined chemical entities including medications/supplements/toxins have been linked to altered incidence.[32–36] Vitamin D, calcium, lycopene, zinc, omega-3 fatty and α-linoleic fatty acids, selenium, vitamin E, statins, and nonsteroidal anti-inflammatory medications have all been implicated in various observational studies but it is not clear in these types of studies whether PSA modulatory effects may interfere with ascertainment of prostate cancer risk. Various lifestyle, anthropomorphic feature, and activity factors have also been linked to prostate cancer risk.[32–36] Endogenous hormonal levels have been the subject of considerable yet controversial findings.[37,38] Although it seems obvious that androgens influence prostate cancer risk, many conflicting studies have been reported. Higher circulating insulinlike growth factor-I levels may confer higher risk.[39] Ejaculatory frequency may be protective[40] but number of sexual partners may be a risk factor.[41] Obesity relationship to risk is controversial, but obesity is associated with higher-grade cancers,[42] possibly as a consequence of lower testosterone and higher estrogens.

GENETIC ALTERATIONS AND RISK

Prostate cancers are thought to develop from an accumulation of critical genetic alterations that result in an increase in cell proliferation relative to cell death, and which confer the ability to invade and metastasize. Despite evidence that prostate cancer has a strong hereditary component, identifying genetic risk factors has proven challenging. Until recently, widely agreed on susceptibility loci have been difficult to identify. Most studies have relied on linkage analysis to implicate susceptibility loci and multiple chromosomal regions including areas on chromosomes 1q36, 1q24-35, 1q42.2-43, 8q24, 16q23, 17p, 20q13, and Xq27-28. Certain genes of interest have been localized to these regions; RNaseL, macrophage scavenger receptor-1, and *ELAC2/HPC2* have been implicated in carcinogenesis but results have not always been consistent across studies.

Of these putative risk regions, the 8q24 risk allele is by far the most important in the general population. Several independent studies have demonstrated that a region on chromosome 8q24 confers a strong risk of developing sporadic prostate cancer.[43,44] The initially identified risk allele is not within a known gene coding region but is the first genetic risk locus associated with an appreciable fraction of sporadic prostate cancer cases in the general population. The frequency of the risk allele varies according to the population under study. At this time the exact genetic mechanism whereby the 8q24 risk allele confers increased risk is unknown, but given that it is chromosomally adjacent to the *myc* locus, speculation has implicated some aspect of *myc* dysregulation. Germ line studies now implicate a variety of other single nucleotide polymorphisms in the genesis of prostate cancer (Xu group) but the ability of these single-nucleotide polymorphisms to provide insights into the risk of prostate cancer beyond that provided by clinical factors (age, ethnic group, PSA, DRE results, and prior biopsy) are yet to be ascertained.

Certain novel retroviruses (XMRV) have been implicated in some but not all studies as a prostate cancer risk factor, but various techniques and laboratories have failed to yield consistent results.[45]

PROSTATE CANCER PREVENTION

Hormonal Manipulation

There is strong evidence indicating an association between androgens and the risk of prostate cancer. Testosterone, which is converted to the more potent androgen dihydrotestosterone (DHT) within prostate cells by the enzyme 5α-reductase, plays a crucial role in the development of the prostate gland. Normal development of the prostate and male external genitalia requires appropriate androgenic stimulation. Individuals with a hereditary deficiency of 5α-reductase fail to produce enough DHT for proper development of the prostate and external genitalia and present with external genitalia of varying degrees of ambiguity.[46] These individuals have a rudimentary prostate, undetectable serum PSA levels as adults, and no evidence of prostatic epithelium, and develop neither BPH nor prostate cancer.[47] Japanese men have lower levels of 5α-reductase activity compared with their higher-risk counterparts.[48]

Advances in molecular biology have facilitated identification of various genetic polymorphisms associated with an increased risk for prostate cancer. A number of these relate to androgen activity, suggesting that genetic alterations directly related to androgen metabolism may affect the risk of prostate cancer. These findings provide a rationale for hormonal manipulation as a chemopreventive strategy. Finasteride is a competitive inhibitor of type II 5α-reductase (type-2 isoform) that blocks the conversion of testosterone to DHT within prostatic cells. Clinical data suggest a potential role for finasteride in the chemoprevention of prostate cancer. The Southwest Oncology Group completed the PCPT, the first phase 3 trial conducted for the prevention of prostate cancer.[21] In this study, 18,882 men aged 55 years or older with a normal DRE and a PSA level 3.0 ng/mL or less were randomized to receive finasteride 5 mg daily or placebo. Participants remained on the study drug for 7 years. A prostate biopsy was recommended if participants were found to have an abnormal DRE and/or a PSA level more than 4.0 ng/mL after adjusting for finasteride's effect on PSA levels. In addition, and controversially, a prostate biopsy was recommended at the end of the study period for all participants who had not been found to have prostate cancer. This trial demonstrated an overall 24.8% reduction in the prevalence of prostate cancer during the 7-year period in men who received finasteride compared with men treated with placebo. Men on the finasteride arm of the study were slightly more likely to report sexual side effects but less likely to have lower urinary tract symptoms or to need transurethral resection of the prostate. Of concern, however, was the higher proportion of high-grade cancers (Gleason score 7 or more) observed in the finasteride group prostate needle biopsies. Subsequent studies of RP specimens obtained from men on the trial indicate that the prostate needle biopsy Gleason scores were upgraded more often in the placebo than the finasteride group. In fact, in the surgically obtained specimens there were no differences in Gleason score for the placebo and finasteride groups. Based on these and other data, the American Society of Clinical Oncology/American Urological Association issued guidelines in 2008 suggesting that asymptomatic men who are regularly screened with PSA or are anticipating undergoing annual PSA screening for early detection of prostate cancer may benefit from a discussion of both the risks and benefits of 5α-reductase inhibitors.

A recent report[49] in a randomized trial used dutasteride, a type I and II 5α-reductase inhibitor, in 8,231 men with a PSA between 2.5 and 10 ng/mL and a negative 6–12 core prostate biopsy within the prior 6 months. Patients were randomized between placebo or dutasteride 0.5 mg/day. Repeat biopsies were planned at 2 and 4 years after randomization or "for cause" when they were clinically indicated. To maintain a blinded study, the PSAs reported to investigators were doubled in the dutasteride group because of the drug-induced PSA reductions. Over the 4-year course of the study, dutasteride reduced the detection of cancer by 22.8%. Importantly, and unlike in the PCPT, there were no increases in Gleason 7–10 cancers in the dutasteride-treated patients over the 4-year course of the study. Erectile dysfunction was noted in 9.0% and 5.7% of men in the dutasteride and placebo groups, respectively. Decreased libido was also more common in the dutasteride group than in the placebo group (3.3% vs. 1.6%).

Antioxidants

Reactive oxygen species have been implicated in the onset and progression of various malignancies, including prostate cancer; however, large randomized trials using antioxidants have failed to demonstrate benefit. Based on these findings, investigators undertook the Selenium and Vitamin E Cancer Prevention Trial (SELECT), a phase 3, randomized, double-blind, placebo-controlled trial to determine the efficacy of selenium (200 mcg daily) and vitamin E (400 IU daily), either alone or in combination, in the prevention of prostate cancer. The study accrued more than 35,000 men with a normal DRE and a PSA level less than 4 ng/mL. The primary end point of this study was the clinical incidence of prostate cancer, determined by DRE and PSA screening according to current clinical recommendations. The study reported at a median follow-up of 5.46 years and no differences were noted in any of the randomized subgroups.[50]

Multiple other dietary factors are currently being investigated as possible agents to prevent prostate cancer and/or inhibit its progression. Dietary fat intake, dietary soy protein, and carotenoids, among others, have all been associated with prostate cancer risk. Migration studies of Japanese men moving to Los Angeles County provide widely quoted evidence that environmental factors are significant contributors to the progression of prostate cancer; however, unless frequency of prostate biopsies are carefully controlled, such migration studies should be viewed cautiously.[51] Additionally, epidemiologic studies suggest that the incidence of prostate cancer in a given population is associated with per capita fat consumption.[52] Additional studies suggest an increased mortality rate in obese men.[53] Although the precise mechanism is not certain, these studies suggest but do not prove that reduced fat intake and weight loss may reduce the risk of prostate cancer.

Carotenoids have received considerable attention for cancer prevention. In spite of initial epidemiologic studies suggesting that the carotenoid β-carotene had a cancer-preventive effect, subsequent randomized trials demonstrated an increased incidence and mortality from prostate cancer among men receiving β-carotene supplementation.[54]

Taken together, the data to date suggest that men should regard with caution information derived from nonrandomized trials. Given that PSA-driven prostate biopsies represent one of the largest risk factors for prostate cancer diagnosis, findings from studies that fail to control for this critical variable should be confirmed using appropriate controls.

Early Detection/Screening

Early detection refers to the use of diagnostic tests for men who seek an evaluation after being informed of the issues surrounding evaluation. Screening refers to the use of diagnostic procedures for a general population. Serum PSA screening was introduced into clinical use in the late 1980s and it has since outperformed DRE in early prostate cancer detection. Not surprisingly, this has resulted in a remarkable increase in the reported incidence of prostate cancer in many countries, especially the United States. Those who undergo regular PSA testing have a higher likelihood of undergoing prostate biopsy and being diagnosed with prostate cancer than men who do not undergo routine PSA testing. Recent large randomized PSA screening trials have been published that allow additional insights into these issues. One of these trials, performed in the United States, had a high contamination rate for PSA testing in the control group both before and during the trial, rendering conclusions circumspect. The other trial, reported after a median of 9 years follow-up and performed in Europe, evaluated PSA testing every 4 years as compared with no PSA testing. Over the trial period of follow-up, 8.2% of the men with PSA testing were diagnosed with prostate cancer as compared with 4.8% of men in the control group. The primary end point of the study was the ratio of prostate cancer deaths in the screened versus nonscreened populations during the course of study. This ratio was 0.80 (95%; however, the absolute difference was only 0.71 death per 1,000 men). Overall this meant that 1,410 men would need to be screened and 48 additional cases of prostate cancer would need to be treated to prevent one death from prostate cancer. Unless surveillance of low-risk prostate cancer becomes more prevalent, the most common adverse event of screening may be the overdiagnosis and overtreatment of clinically irrelevant prostate cancers.

It is now considered indisputable that the widespread use of PSA screening has had a massive impact in Western countries. This screening strategy has resulted in significantly increased numbers of diagnosed cancer cases, as well as identification of cancer predominantly in its early stages. Moreover, since 1991, an annual percentage drop of 4.3% in prostate cancer mortality rates has been observed in the United States.[55] Simultaneously, a reversal in the prostate cancer mortality rate has been reported for some European countries, with a significant decrease between 1979 and 1997, especially in the age group 40 to 69 years.[56] These trends were significantly associated with a parallel decline of locally advanced or metastatic disease. However, a parallel fall in the prostate cancer mortality rate was also demonstrated in England and Wales despite considerably less widespread PSA testing.[57] Thus, the beneficial survival effect of PSA screening in prostate cancer remains somewhat controversial.

Currently the true benefits of prostate cancer screening are unclear despite the recently published results from two randomized trials investigating whether prostate cancer screening with PSA testing saves lives.[18,58] Schroder et al.[18] reported outcomes from the European Randomized Study of Screening for Prostate Cancer evaluating the effect of screening with PSA testing on death rates from prostate cancer. Men were randomly assigned to a group that was offered PSA screening at an average of once every 4 years or to a control group that did not receive such screening. The predefined core age group for this study included 162,243 men between the ages of 55 and 69 years. During a median follow-up of 9 years, the cumulative incidence of prostate cancer was 8.2% in the PSA-screening group and 4.8% in the control group. The cumulative incidence of local prostate cancer was higher in the PSA-screening group than in the control group. For example, there was a 41% reduction in the likelihood of having positive results on a bone scan (or a PSA value of more than 100 ng/mL in those without bone scan results) in the PSA-screening group than in the control group ($P < .001$). The proportions of men who had a Gleason score of 6 or less were 72.2% in the PSA-screening group and 54.8% in the control group. The rate ratio for death from prostate cancer in the PSA screening group, as compared with the control group, was 0.80 (95%, 0.65 to 0.98; adjusted $P = .04$). The absolute risk difference was 0.71 deaths per 1,000 men. This means that 1,410 men would need to be screened and 48 additional cases of prostate cancer would need to be treated to prevent one death from prostate cancer. The investigators concluded that PSA-based screening reduced the rate of death from prostate cancer by 20% but was associated with a high risk of overdiagnosis. In contrast, the U.S. trial (the Prostate, Lung, Colorectal, and Ovarian Cancer Screening Trial [PLCO]), did not find differences in death from prostate cancer.[58] The likely explanation for this apparent discrepancy is that approximately half of the men in the control arm of the PLCO had undergone PSA screening before randomization, and many in the control arm received a PSA test as the trial progressed.

The American Cancer Society has recently published guidelines for the early detection of prostate cancer.[59] Their recommendation is that "asymptomatic men who have at least a 10-year life expectancy should have an opportunity to make an informed decision with their health care provider about screening for prostate cancer after they receive information about the uncertainties, risks, and potential benefits associated with prostate cancer screening. Prostate cancer screening should not occur without an informed decision-making process. Men at average risk should receive this information beginning at age 50 years. Men in higher-risk groups should receive this information before age 50 years. Men should either receive this information directly from their health care providers or be referred to reliable and culturally appropriate sources."

Certainly not all men diagnosed with prostate cancer will die of this disease. Therefore, if screening with PSA testing is performed, many men who are diagnosed with prostate cancer may not benefit from immediate treatment, and deferred treatment (active surveillance with selective delayed intervention [AS]) is an option for many men regardless of age. Most experts believe, however, that the introduction of early-detection programs such as DRE and the serum PSA test has played a critical role in the downward stage migration of prostate cancer seen over the past decade. Currently, 80% to 90% of prostate cancers are clinically organ-confined at diagnosis. Multiple studies have unequivocally shown that prostate cancer cases detected through screening are more often confined to the prostate than those detected solely by an abnormal DRE. In addition, the recent decline in prostate cancer mortality within the United States may be attributable, in part, to prostate cancer early detection.

Total PSA Thresholds

Numerous studies have demonstrated that a PSA level more than 4 ng/mL increases the likelihood of detecting prostate cancer at prostate biopsy to approximately 30% to 35%. Large programs for the early detection of prostate cancer have shown that nearly 70% of cancer cases can be detected using a PSA cutoff level of 4 ng/mL.[60] Men with serum PSA values over this level (regardless of their DRE results, percent-free PSA, or PSA velocity values) are recommended to undergo a TRUS-guided biopsy of the prostate. False-negative findings should be discussed clearly with the patient, and a repeat biopsy should be considered if total PSA values continue to remain in the high-risk category.

Overall, appropriate use of PSA alone can provide a diagnostic lead time of nearly 5 to 10 years compared with DRE alone. Historically, about 80% of PSA-detected cancers appear biologically significant based on tumor volume and Gleason grade. Detection of prostate cancer by PSA examination results in the diagnosis of earlier, organ-confined disease.

Potential Pitfalls of PSA Screening

There is no PSA level below which there is no risk of having a biopsy yield positive findings for prostate cancer. Results from the control arm of the PCPT provided prostate biopsy results from 9,423 men with a serum PSA less than 4.0 ng/mL and a normal DRE, a group of men traditionally not recommended for prostate biopsy.[61] As summarized in Table 97.2, 15% of men had prostate cancer and 15% of these men

TABLE 97.2

RELATIONSHIP OF THE PROSTATE-SPECIFIC ANTIGEN (PSA) LEVEL TO THE PREVALENCE OF PROSTATE CANCER AND HIGH-GRADE DISEASE

PSA Level (ng/mL)	No. Men (n = 2,950)	Men with Prostate Cancer (n = 449)	Men with High-Grade Prostate Cancer (n = 67)
≤0.5	486	32 (6.6%)	4/32 (12.5%)
0.6–1.0	791	80 (10.1%)	8/80 (10.0%)
1.1–2.0	998	170 (17.0%)	20/170 (11.8%)
2.1–3.0	482	115 (23.9%)	22/115 (19.1%)
3.1–4.0	193	52 (26.9%)	13/52 (25.0%)

From ref. 61, with permission.

had high-grade prostate cancer. As such, PSA level simply reflects a range of risk.

PSA Velocity

PSA velocity is the change in PSA values over time. Studies suggest that PSA velocity provides useful information and increases the specificity of a single PSA measurement for early cancer detection. A cutoff of 0.75 ng/mL per year increased the sensitivity of PSA testing alone. Current recommendations for the use of PSA velocity include collection of PSA levels over no less than 18 months and the use of a minimum of three values to calculate PSA velocity.

PSA velocity has been best used in younger men who have elected to begin early-detection programs before age 50. These men have predominantly lower (normal) serum PSA levels and face the prospect of having their PSA levels followed over many years. The PSA velocity test was designed to better select men to undergo prostate biopsy. Patients and physicians electing to monitor prostate disease by measuring PSA velocity should be cautioned that fluctuations between measurements can occur as a result of either laboratory variability or individual biologic variability.

Age-Specific PSA Reference Ranges

Age-specific PSA reference ranges were introduced as a method to increase cancer detection (improve sensitivity) in younger men by lowering PSA cutoff values and to decrease unnecessary biopsies (improve specificity) in older men by increasing PSA cutoffs. Age-specific PSA cutoffs are shown in Table 97.3.[62]

TABLE 97.3

AGE-SPECIFIC PROSTATE-SPECIFIC ANTIGEN (PSA) LEVELS

Patient Age (years)	Normal PSA (ng/mL)
Up to age 49	0–2.4
50–59	0–3.4
60–69	0–5.4
Age 70 and older	0–6.4

From ref. 399, with permission.

TABLE 97.4

PROBABILITY OF CANCER BASED ON PROSTATE-SPECIFIC ANTIGEN (PSA) AND PERCENT-FREE PSA

PSA (ng/mL)	Probability of Cancer (%)	Percent-Free PSA	Probability of Cancer (%)
1–3	—	<20	11
4–10	25	0–10	56
		10–15	28
		15–20	20
		20–25	16
		>25	8

From ref. 65, with permission.

These age-specific ranges have been investigated by several groups with controversial results.

Percent-Free PSA

Free PSA, expressed as a ratio with total PSA, has emerged as a clinically useful molecular form of PSA with the potential to provide improvements in the early detection of prostate cancer. Several molecular forms of PSA are known to circulate in the blood. In most men, the majority (60% to 90%) of circulating PSA is bound to endogenous protease inhibitors. Numerous studies have suggested that the percentage of free PSA is significantly lower in men who have prostate cancer compared with men who do not. The U.S. Food and Drug Administration (FDA) approved the use of percent-free PSA for the early detection of prostate cancer in men with PSA levels between 4 and 10 ng/mL. The multi-institution study that characterized the clinical utility of this assay showed that a 25% free PSA cutoff detected 95% of prostate cancers while avoiding 20% of unnecessary prostate biopsies. Testing for percent-free PSA has gained widespread clinical acceptance in the United States, primarily for men with a normal DREs who have previously undergone prostate biopsy because they had a total PSA level between 4 and 10 ng/mL (Table 97.4).

DISEASE PRESENTATION AND DIAGNOSIS

The need to pursue a prostate cancer diagnosis is most often based on an abnormal screening test, either an abnormal DRE or more commonly an abnormal PSA level. Any palpable abnormality should be pursued, but only 25% to 50% of men with an abnormal DRE prove to have prostate cancer. Similarly, a normal DRE does not exclude the presence of cancer. The likelihood of a cancer diagnosis based on the results of the DRE and serum PSA level are summarized in Table 97.5.[63]

Symptoms from prostate are rarely present at the time of diagnosis. Local symptoms from prostate cancer usually do not manifest until invasion of the periprostatic tissue has occurred, at which point curative therapy is usually not possible. Therefore, the opportunity to cure prostate cancer depends on detection prior to onset of symptoms. The most common symptom of prostatic disease in men older than 50 years is bladder outlet obstruction, including hesitancy, nocturia, incomplete emptying, and a diminished urinary stream. Their occurrence, although more commonly related to BPH, should prompt a careful DRE and PSA determination. Today, men rarely present with symptoms of metastatic disease such as

TABLE 97.5

PROBABILITY OF A POSITIVE PROSTATE BIOPSY BASED ON THE RESULTS OF THE DIGITAL RECTAL EXAMINATION (DRE) AND SERUM PROSTATE-SPECIFIC ANTIGEN (PSA) LEVEL

	PSA (ng/mL)			
DRE Status[a] (%)	0–2	2–4	4–10	>10
DRE–	1	15	25	>50
DRE+	5	20	45	>75

[a]DRE–, normal findings on the digital rectal examination; DRE+, findings on digital rectal examination suspicious for prostate cancer.
(From ref. 61, with permission.)

TABLE 97.6

PRIMARY TUMOR STAGE FOR PROSTATE CANCER: AMERICAN JOINT COMMITTEE ON CANCER STAGING SYSTEM

TX	Primary tumor cannot be assessed
T0	No evidence of primary tumor
T1	Clinically inapparent tumor neither palpable nor visible by imaging
T1a	Tumor incidental histologic finding in 5% or less of tissue resected
T1b	Tumor incidental histologic finding in more than 5% of tissue resected
T1c	Tumor identified by needle biopsy (e.g., because of elevated PSA)
T2	Tumor confined within prostate[a]
pT2	Organ confined
T2a	Tumor involves one-half of one lobe or less
pT2a	Unilateral, one-half of one side or less
T2b	Tumor involves more than one-half of one lobe but not both lobes
pT2b	Unilateral, involving more than one-half of side but not both sides
T2c	Tumor involves both lobes
pT2c	Bilateral disease
T3	Tumor extends through the prostate capsule[b]
pT3	Extraprostatic extension
T3a	Extracapsular extension (unilateral or bilateral)
pT3a	Extraprostatic extension or microscopic invasion of bladder neck[c]
T3b	Tumor invades seminal vesicle(s)
pT3b	Seminal vesicle invasion
T4	Tumor is fixed or invades adjacent structures other than seminal vesicles: such as external sphincter, rectum, bladder, levator muscles, and/or pelvic wall
pT4	Invasion of rectum, levator muscles and/or pelvic wall

PSA, prostate-specific antigen.
Note: There is no pathologic T1 classification.
[a]Tumor found in one or both lobes by needle biopsy, but not palpable or reliably visible by imaging, is classified as T1c.
[b]Invasion into the prostatic apex or into (but not beyond) the prostatic capsule is classified not as T3 but as T2.
[c]Positive surgical margin should be indicated by an R1 descriptor (residual microscopic disease).

bone pain, anemia, or pancytopenia from bone marrow replacement, involvement, or disseminated intravascular coagulation.

The diagnosis is established by a TRUS-guided transrectal needle biopsy. TRUS is most useful to target sites for needle biopsy in the prostate and to determine prostate volume. TRUS is not used for routine screening for prostate cancer, but in a man undergoing an evaluation of an elevated PSA and/or an abnormal DRE, TRUS findings can help direct where biopsies are taken. Cancers are typically hypoechoic relative to the normal peripheral zone, although there is no pathognomonic imaging finding that predicts cancer with certainty.

The needle biopsy procedure is performed transrectally with an 18-gauge needle mounted on a spring-loaded gun directed by ultrasound. Any palpable abnormality on DRE should be targeted for biopsy using finger guidance. In addition, abnormal areas visible on TRUS should be sampled, along with a total of at least ten systematic biopsies of the prostate taken from the left and right apex, middle, and base of the peripheral zone. Each core should be identified separately as to location and orientation so that the pathologist can report the extent and grade of cancer in each core and the presence of any perineural invasion or extraprostatic extension.

STAGING WORKUP

Clinical Stage and DRE

The DRE is critical to establishing the clinical stage of the cancer (Table 97.6).[64] An assessment of the location, size, and extent of the primary cancer provides prognostic information and is essential for treatment planning. Although not uniformly accurate, DRE provides some evidence of the cancer's size and pathologic stage and correlates to some degree with prognosis.

The overwhelming majority of men diagnosed with prostate cancer today do not present with metastases that can be detected by imaging studies. Patients with clinically localized cancer (T1-T2) have a low probability of metastases detectable by current diagnostic tests, such as bone scan, computed tomography (CT), or magnetic resonance imaging (MRI), unless the serum PSA level and/or the biopsy Gleason sum are high. Consequently, most patients diagnosed with a clinically localized prostate cancer need no further studies to rule out metastases. Patients with very aggressive tumors (PSA >20 ng/mL and biopsy Gleason score >7), advanced local lesions (T3-4), or symptoms suggestive of metastatic disease should have imaging studies, including a bone scan.

Imaging in Prostate Cancer

Transrectal Ultrasound

Ultrasound is the standard imaging tool used by urologists to initially assess the prostate and assist in the guidance of needles for directed tissue biopsies to establish a diagnosis. The sensitivity of TRUS-guided biopsies is reported to be 70% to 80%.[65] Cancers appear hypoechoic on TRUS compared with the normal-appearing peripheral zones of the prostate.

In addition to its function to establish tissue diagnosis, TRUS is also useful in assessing the volume of the prostate and calculating the PSA density. The latter is calculated by dividing the PSA value in nanograms per milliliter by the volume in cubic centimeters obtained on TRUS. Limitations of this imaging modality include the difficulty characterizing the integrity of prostatic capsule and visualizing early extraprostatic extension (EPE) or seminal vesicle involvement. Color duplex and power Doppler have been used to further improve the specificity of TRUS by enhancing regions within the prostate with associated hypervascularity that often corresponds to tumor activity.

Computerized Tomography

Computerized tomography (CT) scans of the pelvis are commonly used by many practitioners in the workup of prostate cancer, but they possess limited capabilities in the detection of intraprostatic disease and quantification of EPE and seminal vesicle involvement (SVI). CT scans are more helpful to detect lymph node metastases within the pelvis, yet there has been a wide range of reported sensitivities and specificities for nodal detection with CT scanning.

Magnetic Resonance Imaging

With current magnet strengths of 1.5 Tesla, the endorectal coil together with a pelvic array coil provides the most optimal imaging to appreciate the prostate anatomy. On T1-weighted images the prostate is homogenous in intensity and tumors are difficult to appreciate. On T2-weighted images prostate tumors have decreased signal intensity relative to the higher signal intensity characteristic of the normal-appearing peripheral zone.

There are varying opinions as to the value of magnetic resonance imaging (MRI) in routine staging and imaging of the prostate, and broad variations in the specificity and sensitivity for the detection for EPE and SVI have been reported. In general, MRI permits better visualization of the prostatic capsule to assess for evidence of EPE or SVI, taking advantage of transverse, sagittal, and coronal images for providing greater anatomic detail (Fig. 97.4).

Magnetic resonance spectroscopy uses *in vivo* proton spectroscopy of the prostate to detect the relative concentrations of choline, creatine, and citrate within defined regions of the prostate. Normal prostate tissue displays citrate while prostate cancer, because of greater cell membrane degradation, contains higher levels of choline and lesser concentrations of citrate. The greater choline-to-citrate ratios observed in tumors have been shown to correlate as well with a higher likelihood of the presence of high-grade cancer. The addition of spectroscopy to MRI appears to improve the ability to localize disease more precisely and reduces the degree of interobserver variability, but this form of imaging has yet to become the standard of care. Diffusion-weighted imaging is a promising functioning imaging modality that takes advantage of the known variability of random movements of water molecules observed between normal tissues and tumors. The rate of diffusion of water molecules is more restricted within tumors than in normal tissues and allows for an important metric known as the *apparent diffusion coefficient*. In one study comparing MRI with combined MRI and diffusion-weighted MRI, the sensitivity and specificity were 86% and 84%, respectively.[66] Dynamic contrast-enhancement MRI may provide further diagnostic information regarding presence of disease, as various quantitative parameters can be derived from contrast-time curves that have been shown by some to correlate with presence of cancerous tissue.[67] In one study, the combination of T2-weighted imaging in conjunction with dynamic contrast-enhancement MRI finding had sensitivity and specificity rates of 77% and 91% for detecting tumor foci that measured 0.2 cm^3, but these values improved to 90% and 88%, respectively, when detecting tumors greater than 0.5 cm^3.[68]

Bone Scan

Radionuclide bone scan is the standard imaging study to assess for the presence of osseous metastases.[69] Because of the low yield in low-risk patients (baseline PSA levels <10 ng/mL), bone scan is unnecessary and not recommended. It has been noted that for patients with PSA levels of less than 10, the incidence of a positive bone scan is less than 1%, while for patients with PSA levels between 10 and 50 and greater than 50 ng/mL, the incidence of positive bone scans is 10% and 50%, respectively.[70] Bone scanning is frequently used to assess the response of hormonal therapy and chemotherapy for those with metastatic disease.

ProstaScint Scanning

Radioimmunoconjugates using monoclonal antibodies are currently undergoing intense investigation for imaging tumor in both soft tissue and bone. The commercially available ProstaScint scan (Capromab; CYTOGEN, Princeton, NJ) is used most frequently in patients with rising PSA levels after primary therapy to help determine whether relapse is local or systemic. Although ProstaScint is helpful in some cases, nonspecific localization to the gastrointestinal (GI) tract may be interpreted incorrectly as metastatic disease. In addition, the interpretation of the scan is subject to interobserver variability, and the results

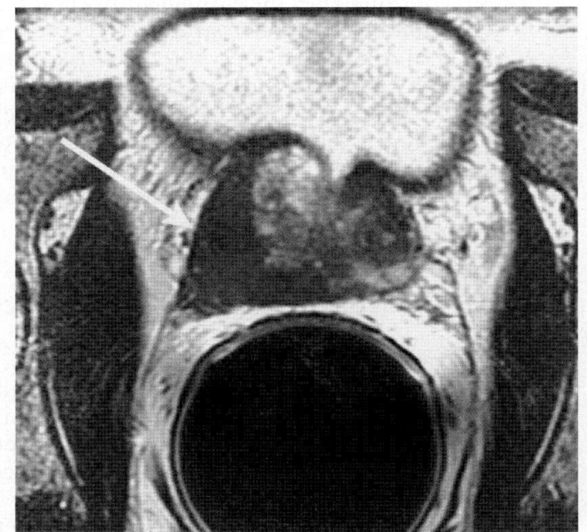

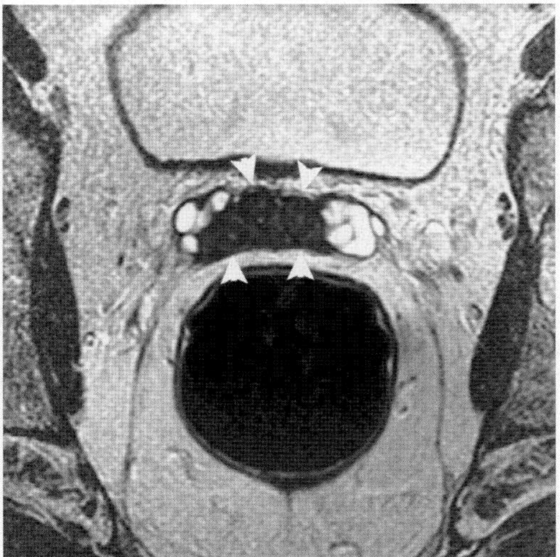

FIGURE 97.4 Clinical stage T2a prostate cancer. On the transverse image (A) the patient was noted to have a dominant tumor at the right base with loss of normal contour and irregular bulging consistent with extracapsular extension (*arrow*). Image (B) indicates the evidence of seminal vesicle involvement (*arrowheads*) demonstrating mild enlargement of the seminal vesicles and low signal intensity tissue replacing normal thin walls and obliterating the lumen. (From ref. 69, with permission of the Radiolgical Society of North America.)

must be used cautiously. ProstaScint scans are rarely indicated in newly diagnosed, previously untreated patients unless the suspicion of metastases is very high (PSA >20 ng/mL and Gleason grade >7 or cT3) and the bone scan is negative.

Positron Emission Tomography

Fluorine 18 fluorodeoxyglucose has been the most commonly used radioisotope for imaging of prostate cancer. In most studies to date, the sensitivity for prostate imaging in patients with localized disease has been poor.[71] Positron-emitting tomography–CT imaging has significantly improved the ability to discern intraprostatic disease and lymph node metastases. Newer tracers including carbon 11 methionine, C11 acetate, and C11 choline may be more valuable for imaging and will require prospective clinical evaluation.

PROGNOSTIC FACTORS AND THE ASSESSMENT OF RISK

Clinical Prognostic Factors (Stage, Grade, and PSA)

The ability of imaging and physical examination (DRE) to determine pathologic stage accurately is limited. As such, Partin et al.[72] developed a nomogram (Partin tables) using clinical tumor stage, biopsy Gleason grade, and PSA to predict pathologic stage. The prediction of pathologic stage can help guide a physician's management of a patient's tumor, but a more important consideration is the probability of cure or long-term cancer control, defined as an undetectable or low, stable PSA level.[73,74] The prognosis or probability of recurrence after definitive therapy of an apparently localized prostate cancer depends on the clinical stage and grade of the cancer, as well as the PSA level before treatment. Prognosis of localized cancers can be estimated more accurately by combining these three factors into a preoperative nomogram[74] that calculates the probability of being progression-free 5 years after surgery. Nomograms have proved highly useful in clinical practice and have been developed for external-beam radiation therapy (EBRT)[75] and brachytherapy as well.[76] These nomograms may provide clues about the relative efficacy of different modalities in patients with comparable tumors. All of these nomograms are available at www.nomograms.com.

An alternative strategy to assess the risk that a cancer poses to the individual patient is to *stratify the risk* on the basis of the key prognostic factors (clinical stage, Gleason grade, and PSA).[77] D'Amico et al.,[77] for example, assign patients to one of three logical (rather than empirical) risk groups according to their clinical T stage, Gleason grade, and PSA. Although it is easy to group patients into such logical risk-group categories, each such group actually contains a heterogeneous population. Predictions are much more accurate when nomograms are used to combine individual prognostic factors into a single prognostic score assigned to each patient. Consequent comparisons of the results of different treatments are also more accurate when patients are more precisely matched.

Pathologic Stage

Several other indices have been developed that improve the biological characterization of a given tumor. Pathologic stage, determined by examining the RP specimen, predicts recurrence much more accurately than clinical stage. The independent prognostic factors include the level of invasion of the cancer into or through the capsule of the prostate, SVI, lymph node metastases, and positive surgical margins, as well as the Gleason sum in the RP specimen and the preoperative serum PSA level. Some investigators have considered tumor volume an important prognostic factor, but others have found it has no independent prognostic significance. Stephenson et al.[78] combined these independent prognostic factors into a postoperative nomogram that is more accurate than the preoperative nomogram because it incorporates the final Gleason grade and pathologic stage as well as preoperative PSA.

Molecular Markers

Other parameters that have been reported to predict outcomes include the apoptotic index (rate of programmed cell death, measured by immunohistochemistry), proliferation rate measured by Ki67, p53, p27, E-cadherin, microvessel density, DNA ploidy, KAI1 expression, p16, bcl-2, bax, and measures of relative nuclear roundness, among others. However, none of these markers has yet been validated, and at this time they should not be considered necessary for evaluation of a patient with localized disease.

PSA Velocity to Assess Patient Risk

Recent studies have suggested that changes in PSA levels before the diagnosis of prostate cancer have prognostic implications for men treated with either RP or EBRT. To assess the prognostic value of PSA velocity during the year before diagnosis, D'Amico et al.[79] evaluated 1,095 men with clinically localized prostate cancer who underwent RP. An annual PSA rise of more than 2.0 ng/mL (approximately 25% of their study population) was associated with a significantly shorter time to biochemical recurrence, death from any cause, and death from prostate cancer. A higher PSA level at diagnosis, a biopsy Gleason score of 8 to 10, and clinical stage T2 cancer also predicted a shorter time to death. The authors conclude that men whose PSA level increases by more than 2.0 ng/mL during the year before the diagnosis of prostate cancer are at high risk for cancer-specific death, even if they have other favorable clinical parameters (such as a PSA level at diagnosis of <10 ng/mL) and undergo RP.[79] For these men, watchful waiting may not be an appropriate option; their increased risk also makes them candidates for enrollment in clinical trials examining multimodal treatment strategies. These findings were confirmed in a group of men with low-risk prostate cancer treated with radiation therapy (RT).[80] These investigators concluded that men with an increase in PSA level more than 2.0 ng/mL during the year before diagnosis who are planning to undergo RT should be considered for RT combined with androgen-suppression therapy because this approach improves survival in men with higher-risk prostate cancer.

Prostate Cancer Disease States

A clinical framework for prognostic assessments, therapeutic objectives, and outcomes assessment are provided by considering prostate cancer as a series of easily recognized disease states.[81] Judgments about the need for and the type of therapy can best be made by understanding prostate cancer as a continuum from diagnosis to death and not on the basis of the clinical stage of the disease. A patient's state is determined by the clinical assessment, physical examination, imaging studies, and whether the level of testosterone in the blood is in the noncastrate or castrate range. As shown in Figure 97.5, the states are initial prostate evaluation, no cancer diagnosis; clinically localized disease; rising PSA, noncastrate; rising PSA,

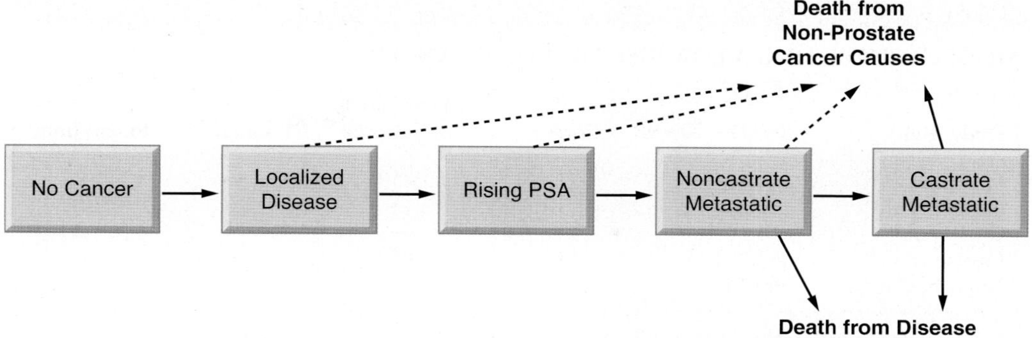

FIGURE 97.5 Synthesis and function of prostaglandins (PG) and leukotrienes (LT) from long chain fatty acids, arachidonic acid (AA), and eicosapentaenoic acid (EPA). PG and LT are synthesized in response to a cell stimulus that activates cytosolic (c) phospholipase A2 (PLA2). Conversion of AA to the prostaglandin endoperoxide PGH_2 by prostaglandin-H synthase (PGHS)-1 and -2 is followed by isomerization of PGH_2 to a "2-series" product—PGD_2, PGE_2, $PGF_{2\alpha}$, PGI_2, or thromboxane A_2 (TxA_2) by specific synthases. LT pathways involve conversion of AA to LTA_4 by 5-lipoxygenase (5-LO) and hydrolysis of LTA_4 to LTB_4 or conjugation of LTA_4 with glutathione to yield the cysteinyl (cys) LT, LTC_4, which along with its cleavage product LTD_4, comprise the bioactive cysLTs. Newly formed PGs and LTs exit cells and function primarily through G-protein—coupled receptors on neighboring or parent cells to elicit responses. EPA can also serve as a substrate for PG formation generating "3-series" PG products, including PGD_3, PGE_3, $PGF_{3\alpha}$, PGI_3, and TxA_3. In comparison to the 2-series PG products, little is known of the biologic effects of the 3-series PGs.[95,96] $sPLA_2$, secretory PLA_2; COX, cyclooxygenase; DP, EP, FP, IP, TP, BLT, CysLT, receptors for PGD, PGE, PGF, PGI, TxA/PGH, LTB, cysteinyl LTs, respectively; LTAH, LTA hydrolase; LTCS, LTC synthase; γ-GGL, γ-glutamyl leukotrienases; mDP, membrane-bound dipeptidase. (Figure provided by Dr. William L. Smith, Department of Biochemistry, University of Michigan.)

PRACTICE OF ONCOLOGY

castrate; clinical metastases, noncastrate; and clinical metastases, castrate. At any one time, a patient resides in only one state. Once the patient's state is identified, a prognostic assessment is made for a specific therapeutic objective, treatment options are considered, and a decision is made as to whether or not to offer an intervention. Certain factors, such as Gleason score and PSA doubling time, predict for the rate at which transition from one state to another occurs and can also influence clinical decision making. A patient who undergoes treatment after having reached a given state remains in that state until he has progressed to the next state. Patients do not go backward.

TREATING CLINICALLY LOCALIZED PROSTATE CANCER

The clinical course of newly diagnosed prostate cancer is difficult to predict. Men with similar clinical stage, serum PSA levels, and biopsy features can have markedly different outcomes. Although prostate cancer is unequivocally lethal in some patients, most men do indeed die with, rather than of, their cancer. The challenge to physicians today is to identify the minority of men with aggressive, localized prostate cancer with a natural history that can be altered by definitive local therapy, while sparing the remainder the morbidity of unnecessary treatment.

Identifying Low-Risk Prostate Cancer

Many physicians and patients consider AS for selected low-risk prostate cancers; the difficulty is defining "low risk." Initial clinical staging (DRE), PSA, and diagnostic biopsy results have limited potential for accurately characterizing localized prostate cancers, although systematic needle biopsies, serial PSA determinations, and modern imaging are promising tools for more accurately assessing the size, grade, and extent of the cancer.

In an attempt to identify patients with low-risk cancers, Epstein et al.[82] examined preoperative clinical and biopsy features in 157 men with clinical stage T1c prostate cancer who underwent RP to find features that could predict insignificant tumors—defined as organ-confined cancers with a total tumor volume less than 0.2 cm^3 and a pathologic Gleason sum 6 or less in the RP specimen. Their model for predicting an insignificant cancer included no Gleason grade of 4 or 5 in the biopsy specimen and either:

- PSA density of 0.1 ng/mL per gram or less, fewer than three biopsy cores involved with cancer (minimum of six cores obtained), and no core with more then 50% involvement, or
- PSA density of 0.15 ng/mL per gram or less and on only one (of six or more) biopsy core with cancer smaller than 3 mm.

As a test for insignificant disease, this model had a negative predictive value of 95% and a positive predictive value of 66% in their own data set. Most physicians use some modification of the previously mentioned "Epstein criteria" to identify potential candidates for AS. Since this initial report, a number of investigators have developed algorithms for predicting low-risk prostate cancer (Table 97.7).[82–86]

Because patient selection for AS is critically dependent on the results of the prostate biopsy (Gleason grade and amount of cancer), some investigators have suggested more extensive biopsy strategies to better assess the true extent of cancer within the prostate. TRUS-guided prostate biopsy has been shown to poorly reflect the grade and extent of a patient's cancer when compared with the RP specimens. Crawford et al.,[87] using computer simulations on 106 autopsy and RP specimens, suggested that transperineal prostate biopsies using a

TABLE 97.7

MODELS PREDICTING A LOW-RISK PROSTATE CANCER

Study (Ref.)	PSAD	No. of + Cores	Maximum % of + Cores	Grade	Extent (mm)
Epstein et al.[82]	<0.10	<3	<50	≤6	—
Bastian et al.[83]	<0.15	1	—	≤6	<3
Goto et al.[85]	<0.10	1	—	≤6	<2
Epstein et al.[84]	F/T >0.15	<3	<50	≤6	—
Noguchi et al.[86]	<0.15	1	—	≤6	<3

PSAD, prostate-specific antigen density; F/T, free-to-total PSA ratio.

brachytherapy template, spaced at 5-mm intervals throughout the volume of the prostate, could determine grade and detect significant cancers with greater sensitivity. Onik and Barzell[88] used a transperineal three-dimensional (3D) mapping method to restage 110 patients, all of whom had had unilateral prostate cancer diagnosed by TRUS biopsies. The median number of cores taken was 46 (SD ± 19). Bilateral cancer was found in 60 patients (55%) and the Gleason score was increased in 25 (23%). Complications were self-limited and included nine patients (8%) who required short-term catheterization and two (2%) with hematuria. Although this study was primarily designed to assess the role of transperineal biopsy in selecting men for focal therapy, the investigators hypothesized that 75% of patients thought to have low-risk cancers eligible for AS were found to have larger, higher-grade tumors better treated with definitive therapy. Although extensive biopsy strategies provide more information than a standard TRUS-guided biopsy does, their role in routinely evaluating a patient for AS is unclear. None of the commonly used guidelines for identifying candidates for AS have relied on extended prostate biopsy. Further information is needed before a routine recommendation for this procedure is embraced.

Active Surveillance with Selective Delayed Intervention

Traditionally, watchful waiting has meant no active treatment until a patient develops evidence of symptomatic disease progression, at which time androgen-deprivation therapy (ADT) is initiated. The goal of this approach is to limit morbidity from the disease and therapy, not to administer potentially curative treatment. The assumption is that definitive local therapy provides little or no benefit to the majority of patients in terms of both quantity and quality of life. A more recent concept is to delay curative local therapy until the natural history and threat posed by the cancer can be more accurately characterized. This approach, termed *active surveillance with selective delayed intervention* (AS) assumes that the risk posed by a given cancer can be assessed with some degree of certainty and that delayed treatment will be as curative as immediate treatment. With active surveillance, we attempt to avoid overtreatment in the majority of patients, but also to administer curative therapy to selected cases.

To recommend AS for a healthy man with a life expectancy longer than 10 years, one must balance the risk that a currently curable cancer becomes metastatic with the risks posed by treatment of an insignificant cancer. As the initial evaluation might seriously underestimate the grade and extent of the present cancer, most men should undergo repeat testing prior to being considered a candidate for AS. Long-term follow-up from watchful waiting studies suggest that the risk of progression *accelerates* over time. Hence, AS patients must accept frequent, regular, detailed evaluations of the status of their cancer for as long as they are healthy and young enough to be candidates for definitive therapy.

For AS candidates who have been diagnosed with what appears to be a low-risk cancer, a complete re-evaluation at baseline is recommended, including a DRE, free and total PSA, imaging study of the prostate (preferably endorectal MRI with spectroscopy), and ultrasound-guided systematic needle biopsy. If these studies confirm a low-risk cancer, and the patient chooses AS, we recommend a checkup every 6 months with DRE and PSA indefinitely, with repeat imaging and biopsy 12 to 18 months after the baseline evaluation, then every 2 to 3 years. The goal is to detect progression of the cancer while cure is still possible.

Outcomes of Active Surveillance with Selective Delayed Intervention

There are as yet few reports of outcomes of deferred definitive therapy for localized prostate cancer. The University of Toronto conducted a prospective phase 2 study of AS, incorporating selective delayed intervention for the subset of patients with short PSA-doubling time or grade progression on repeat biopsy.[89,90] The eligibility criteria for this study included patients with clinical stage T1c or T2a cancer, biopsy Gleason score of 6 or lower, and a serum PSA of 10 ng/mL or less. For patients above the age of 70 years, these eligibility criteria were relaxed to include biopsy Gleason score 7 (3 + 4) or lower and/or PSA of 15 ng/mL or less. The core prospective cohort of 331 patients had a median follow-up of 8 years (range, 2 to 11 years). Patients were observed until they met one of three specific criteria defining rapid or clinically significant progression:

1. PSA progression, defined as a PSA doubling time (PSADT) of 3 years or less, based on multiple serum PSA determinations at 3-month intervals, calculated using a general linear mixed model, which corrects for baseline PSA, grade, and age. This model is freely available at http://psakinetics.sunnybrook.ca.
2. Clinical progression, defined by meeting any of four conditions: more than a doubling of the product of the maximum perpendicular diameters of the primary lesion as measured by DRE, local progression of prostate cancer requiring transurethral resection of the prostate, development of ureteral obstruction, or radiologic or clinical evidence of distant metastasis.
3. Histologic progression, that is, Gleason sum 4 + 3 or higher on repeat biopsy of the prostate. Patients who had progression were offered radical intervention; those without progression were closely monitored. Biopsies were performed for cause at 1 year, then every 4 to 5 years. The

median PSADT was 7 years; 42% had a PSADT longer than 10 years, suggesting an indolent course of disease in these patients. Twenty-two percent of patients had a PSADT of less than 3 years. With a median follow-up of 72 months, 34% of the patients had received radical treatment. Fifteen percent were treated because of a PSADT of less than 3 years, 7% because of histologic or clinical progression, and 12% because of patient preference. Ten percent have been treated with RP and 36% of these had cancer outside of the prostate. The remainder have not required local or systemic therapy. Overall survival is 85% and disease-specific and metastasis-free survival is 99% at 8 years.

In a prospective, longitudinal surveillance program, Carter et al.[91] observed a cohort of 407 men with clinical stage T1c prostate cancer suspected of harboring small-volume cancer based on needle biopsy findings and PSA density.[82,91] Median age was 65.7 years (range, 45.8–81.5 years) and median follow-up was 2.8 years (range, 0.4–12.5 years). Semiannual measurements of total and free PSA, a semiannual DRE, and an annual surveillance prostate biopsy examination were performed. Treatment was recommended if there were findings of adverse pathologic features on an annual surveillance biopsy examination (any Gleason pattern 4 or 5, more than two cores that were positive for cancer, or more than 50% of any one core that was involved with cancer) or if a patient requested a change in management. Of 407 men, 239 (59%) remained on AS; 103 (25%) were treated definitively at a median of 2.2 years after diagnosis (range, 0.96–7.39 years), and 65 (16%) were either lost to follow-up (12), withdrew from the program (45), or died of causes other than prostate cancer.[91] Of the 103 treated men, 53 (51%) underwent RP. Twenty percent of these men were considered to have noncurable disease, defined as pathologic stage T2 if Gleason score was 4 + 3 or greater; positive surgical margins any grade; stage pT3aN0 (extraprostatic extension) if Gleason sum was 7 or greater and/or surgical margins were positive; any stage higher than pT3a regardless of grade or margin status; or any N+ stage. The investigators concluded that a program of careful selection and monitoring of older men who are likely to harbor small-volume, low-grade disease may be a rational alternative to immediate radical therapy for all.

These series (and others) confirm that in appropriately selected men, AS is associated with an extremely low rate of progression to metastatic disease and/or death, and that the majority of patients do not require intervention. Further follow-up is necessary to determine the long-term risk of progression.

Radical Prostatectomy

RP is recommended only for patients with clinically localized prostate cancer (cT1–T3a, N0 or Nx, M0 or Mx) and a life expectancy of 10 or more years. Because of the risk inherent in major surgery, it should be reserved for patients with little or no systemic comorbidity. Although the risk of recurrence after RP rises with higher clinical stage, Gleason grade, and serum PSA level, no absolute cutoff values exclude a patient as a candidate.

Perhaps the most compelling evidence that selected patients with prostate cancer benefit from active treatment compared to watchful waiting comes from a Scandinavian trial that randomized 695 men with clinically localized prostate cancer to either RP or watchful waiting with systemic treatment deferred until the development of symptomatic progression.[92] The primary end point of this study was death from prostate cancer. During a median follow-up of 8.2 years, 50 of the 348 men assigned to watchful waiting died from prostate cancer, compared with 30 of the 347 men assigned to RP (relative hazard, 0.56; 95% confidence interval [CI]: 0.36–0.88; P = .01). The men assigned to surgery had a lower relative risk of distant metastases than the men assigned to watchful waiting (relative hazard, 0.60; 95% CI: 0.42–0.86). For men who were managed conservatively, the cumulative probability of developing metastatic disease 10 years after diagnosis was 25% and the cancer-specific mortality rate was 15%. Most importantly, there was an absolute and statistically significant increase in overall survival at 10 years for patients in the surgery arm. This elegant study firmly documents the overall benefit of RP in patients with clinically localized prostate cancer diagnosed in the absence of systematic screening.[92] The relevance of this study to cancers detected by screening, which may be much earlier in their natural history, is uncertain.

Surgical Technique. The goals of modern RP are to remove the entire cancer with negative surgical margins, minimal blood loss, no serious perioperative complications, and complete recovery of continence and potency. Achieving these goals requires careful surgical planning. As no single test provides a reliable estimate of the size, location, and extent of the cancer, we rely on the results of DRE, serum PSA levels, and a detailed analysis of the amount and grade of cancer in each individually labeled biopsy core, along with the results of the TRUS or the endorectal coil MRI. The results are used to plan the steps necessary to remove the cancer completely and to assess the likelihood that one or both of the neurovascular bundles will have to be resected partially or fully to minimize the risk of a positive surgical margin. The retropubic procedure is performed through either a suprapubic incision (open RP) or using a minimally invasive (laparoscopic or robot-assisted laparoscopic) approach.

Selecting Patients for Pelvic Lymph Node Dissection

Without exception, men whose cancer has spread to the pelvic nodes have a significantly worse prognosis than men with negative pelvic lymph nodes. Even so, controversy persists concerning the role of pelvic lymph node dissection (PLND) in treating patients with locally advanced disease. A number of investigations have found the incidence of lymph node metastasis in patients considered to have low-risk prostate cancer (clinical stage T1c, preoperative PSA values $<$10 ng/mL, and a prostate biopsy Gleason score $\leq$6) to be as low as less than 5%.[93,94] Thus, some surgeons consider PLND unnecessary in these low-risk patients. However, these reports may underestimate the true likelihood of lymph node metastases because they generally are based on a limited lymph node dissection (external iliac nodes only). In men undergoing RP with full extended PLND who have a PSA less than 10 ng/mL, the rate of nodal involvement ranges from 11% to 17%.[95–98] This incidence increases with increasing Gleason score. Schumacher et al.[94] reported that patients with Gleason score of 7 or more on surgical pathology had a 25% chance of positive nodes, whereas only 3% with a Gleason score of 6 or less were node-positive. These relatively high rates of lymph node metastasis stand in contrast to other published series, probably because of the extent of PLND performed, the diligence of the pathologist in reviewing the surgical specimen, and more advanced stage of cancers in the European series where screening was less intense than in the United States. Surgical studies have confirmed that nodal metastases in 15% to 30% of patients may be detected exclusively in areas outside the boundaries of a limited dissection.[94,96–98] Our current practice is to restrict PLND at the time of RP to men with a 2% or more risk of positive nodes according to a contemporary nomogram.

Limited versus Extended PLND

There have been no prospective studies demonstrating the appropriate anatomic limits of a PLND for prostate cancer. However, lymphatic drainage of the prostate is known to be highly variable and involves regions not sampled during an external iliac-only PLND. Some surgeons resect only the external iliac lymph nodes unless imaging suggests abnormal lymph nodes in other regions, while other surgeons routinely perform a more extensive dissection that includes the obturator, external iliac, and hypogastric areas. When such an extended PLND is performed, not only are more nodes retrieved, but the lymph nodes from most of the potential landing zones are removed—significantly increasing the number of patients found to have lymph node invasion.[94] The extended dissection yields a higher lymph node count and detects more positive lymph nodes than a lymphadenectomy that is limited to the nodal tissue between the external iliac vein and top of the obturator nerve (external iliac area).[96–98] A properly performed PLND that includes the external iliac, hypogastric, and obturator node packets has been shown to be feasible in both open and minimally invasive RP.

Potential for Therapeutic Benefit of PLND

Evidence from several surgical series of patients undergoing RP demonstrates a potential therapeutic benefit from extended PLND, particularly in men with a low burden of cancer in the

TABLE 97.8

ACTUARIAL 5-, 10-, AND 15-YEAR (PROSTATE-SPECIFIC ANTIGEN [PSA]-BASED) NONPROGRESSION RATES (%) AFTER RADICAL RETROPUBIC PROSTATECTOMY FOR CLINICALLY LOCALIZED PROSTATE CANCER ACCORDING TO PREOPERATIVE AND PATHOLOGIC FACTORS

	Johns Hopkins University[a]			MSKCC SPORE in Prostate Cancer Database[b]		
	5-Year	10-Year	15-Year	5-Year	10-Year	15-Year
No. of Patients	2,404	2,404	2,404	4,037	4,037	4,037
BCR[b]	412	412	412	630	630	630
BCR-free (%)[b]	84	74	66	82	75	73
PREOPERATIVE SERUM PSA (ng/mL)						
≤4	94 (92–96)	91 (87–93)	67 (34–86)	92 (89–95)	89 (85–93)	86 (80–92)
>4 & <10	89 (86–91)	79 (74–83)	75 (69–80)	87 (85–89)	80 (77–83)	78 (74–81)
≥10 & ≤20	73 (68–78)	57 (48–64)	54* (44–63)	75 (72–78)	68 (64–71)	66 (62–70)
>20	60 (49–69)	48 (36–59)	48 (36–59)	58 (54–62)	52 (47–57)	50 (43–56)
CLINICAL STAGE						
cT1ab	90 (83–95)	85 (76–91)	75 (58–86)	90 (85–95)	85 (79–92)	83 (76–90)
cT1c	91 (88–93)	76 (48–90)	76* (48–90)	88 (86–90)	79 (73–85)	NA
cT2a	86 (83–88)	75 (71–79)	66 (59–72)	85 (82–88)	77 (81–73)	75 (70–80)
cT2b	75 (70–79)	62 (56–68)	50 (41–58)	74 (70–79)	69 (64–75)	69 (64–75)
cT2c	71 (61–79)	57 (45–68)	57 (45–68)	71 (68–75)	64 (59–68)	62 (57–67)
cT3	60 (45–72)	49 (34–63)	NA	54 (44–64)	51 (40–62)	NA
SPECIMEN GLEASON SUM						
2–4	100	100	100	100	100	100
5	98 (96–99)	94 (90–96)	86 (78–92)	92 (90–94)	89 (86–92)	88 (84–92)
6	95 (93–97)	88 (83–92)	73 (59–82)	91 (89–93)	83 (80–86)	81 (78–85)
7	73 (69–76)	54 (48–59)	48 (41–56)	77 (75–79)	70 (66–74)	67 (63–72)
3 + 4	81 (77–84)	60 (53–67)	59 (51–65)	82 (79–84)	74 (69–79)	72 (62–82)
4 + 3	53 (44–61)	33 (22–43)	33 (22–43)	60 (50–70)	53 (44–64)	53 (44–64)
8–10	44 (36–52)	29 (22–37)	15 (5–28)	41 (35–47)	33 (24–42)	NA
PATHOLOGIC STAGE						
Organ Confined	97 (95–98)	93 (90–95)	84 (77–90)	93 (92–94)	89 (87–91)	87 (85–89)
EPE +, GS <7, SM −	97 (94–98)	93 (89–96)	84 (70–92)	92 (89–94)	89 (84–94)	86 (79–92)
EPE +, GS <7, SM +	89 (80–94)	73 (61–82)	58 (41–71)	74 (64–84)	65 (54–76)	65 (54–76)
EPE +, GS ≥7, SM −	80 (75–85)	61 (52–68)	59 (50–67)	76 (66–86)	68 (61–75)	65 (56–74)
EPE +, GS ≥7, SM +	58 (49–66)	42 (32–52)	33 (23–44)	60 (53–67)	55 (44–66)	55 (44–66)
SV +, LN −	48 (38–58)	30 (19–41)	17 (5–35)	44 (38–50)	31 (24–38)	28 (19–37)
LN +	26 (19–35)	10 (5–18)	0	25 (18–32)	15 (5–25)	0
Negative Margins	NA	NA	NA	87 (86–88)	81 (79–83)	79 (76–82)
Positive Margins	NA	NA	NA	66 (63–69)	56 (52–60)	54 (49–59)

MSKCC SPORE, Memorial Sloan-Kettering Cancer Center Specialized Programs of Research Excellence; BCR, biochemical recurrence; EPE, extraprostatic extension; GS, Gleason sum; SM, surgical margin; SV, seminal vesicles; LN, lymph node; NA, not applicable.
*BCR, biochemical recurrence; EPE, extraprostatic extension; GS, Gleason sum; SM, surgical margin; SV, seminal vesicles; LN, lymph node; NA, not applicable.
[a]Single surgeon series (ref. 113).
Minimally invasive refers to laparoscopic radical prostatectomy with or without robotic assistance.
a Includes 1,092 radical prostatectomies performed by a single surgeon (ref. 114).
b BCR, postsurgery PSA relapse.
PSAD, prostate-specific antigen density.

TABLE 97.9

ADVANTAGES AND DISADVANTAGES OF VARIOUS SURGICAL APPROACHES TO RADICAL PROSTATECTOMY

CLAIMS BY MINIMALLY INVASIVE SURGEONS	REBUTTAL BY OPEN SURGEONS
Magnification improves visualization	Magnification achieved with surgical loupes
Less blood loss	Transfusion rates are similar
Improved visualization permits more precise dissection of the prostatic apex and neurovascular bundles	Outcomes fail to demonstrate any advantage in terms of continence and potency.
Less pain and quicker recovery	Postoperative pain and recovery are comparable
Watertight anastomosis allows earlier catheter removal	No difference noted in most large series
CLAIMS BY OPEN SURGEONS	**REBUTTAL BY MINIMALLY INVASIVE SURGEONS**
Lack of proprioception compromises cancer control	Positive margin rates are equivalent
Complication rates are lower with open surgery	Complication rates with laparoscopic surgery decrease with experience
Mobilization of the neurovascular bundles with electrocautery compromises potency	Potency rates are similar
Significant learning curve	Proctoring reduces learning curve
Longer operative time	No rebuttal
Increased cost	No rebuttal

(From 100, with permission.)
14-year data.

pelvic lymph nodes.[95–97] In a series of patients with positive lymph nodes treated at the Johns Hopkins Hospital, men undergoing an extended PLND had an overall 5-year biochemical progression-free rate of 43% compared with 10% of men undergoing a limited PLND, when lymph node–positive disease involved less than 15% of extracted nodes.[95] Furthermore, 10% to 15% of patients with positive lymph nodes remain free of biochemical recurrence up to a decade later with no adjuvant therapy (Table 97.8).

Radical Prostatectomy

RP is one of the most complex operations performed by urologists. It challenges surgeons to obtain results that are exquisitely sensitive to fine details in surgical technique. The elusive goals of RP are to remove the cancer completely with negative surgical margins, minimal blood loss, no serious perioperative complications, and complete recovery of continence and potency. No surgeon achieves such results uniformly. Technical refinements have resulted in lower rates of urinary incontinence and higher rates of recovery of erectile function, less blood loss and fewer transfusions, shorter hospital stays, and lower rates of positive surgical margins. A thorough understanding of periprostatic anatomy and vascular control by contemporary surgeons further increases the probability of a successful RP with reduced morbidity.

Open Radical Prostatectomy

Acute Postoperative Complications. With refinements in anesthesia, perioperative care and surgical technique, blood loss, length of hospital stay, complications, and mortality after open surgery have decreased over time.[99] The mortality rate ranges from 0.16% to 0.66% in modern series, rising with increasing age and comorbidity. Deep venous thrombosis and pulmonary embolism occur in approximately 2% of cases, with little evidence that anticoagulants or sequential pneumatic compression are preventive. Early ambulation, a short hospital stay, and use of epidural anesthesia are probably responsible for the lower rate of thromboembolic events. Rectal injuries are uncommon. Standardized treatment pathways have been shown to decrease the cost of radical retropubic prostatectomy without compromising quality of care. Hospital stays now average less than 3 days for open RP and 1 to 2 days for laparoscopic RP (LRP), with or without robotic assistance.

Laparoscopic RP with or without Robotic Assistance

Surgeons have demonstrated that LRP with or without robotic assistance (RALP) can be performed with excellent results. The initial enthusiasm for LRP was based on the idea that less bleeding and a magnified surgical image would markedly improve patient outcomes. To date, this promise has not been realized. Open RP, LRP, and RALP each have a number of theoretical advantages and disadvantages (Table 97.9).[100] No prospective randomized trials have yet compared the two techniques, and it is unlikely that such a study will be performed. Hu et al.[101] used US SEER-Medicare–linked data from 2003 through 2007 to compare men with prostate cancer treated with either minimally invasive RP (MIRP; n = 1,938) or open retropubic RP (RRP; n = 6,899). Postoperative 30-day complications, anastomotic stricture 31 to 365 days postoperatively, long-term incontinence and erectile dysfunction more than 18 months postoperatively, and postoperative use of additional cancer therapies were examined. Use of MIRP increased from 9.2% (95% CI: 8.1%–10.5%) in 2003 to 43.2% (95% CI: 39.6%–46.9%) in 2006 to 2007. MIRP versus RRP was associated with shorter length of stay (median, 2.0 vs. 3.0 days; $P < .001$) and lower rates of blood transfusions (2.7% vs. 20.8%; $P < .001$), postoperative respiratory complications (4.3% vs. 6.6%; $P = .004$), miscellaneous surgical complications (4.3% vs. 5.6%; $P = .03$), and anastomotic stricture (5.8% vs. 14.0%; $P < .001$). However, MIRP versus RRP was associated with an increased risk of genitourinary (GU) complications (4.7% vs. 2.1%; $P = .001$) and diagnoses of incontinence (15.9 vs. 12.2 per 100 person-years; $P = .02$) and erectile dysfunction (26.8 vs. 19.2 per 100 person-years; $P = .009$). Rates of use of additional cancer therapies did not differ by surgical procedure (8.2 vs. 6.9 per 100 person-years; $P = .35$). The investigators suggested that the rapid increase in the utilization of MIRP despite insufficient data demonstrating superiority over an established gold standard may be a reflection of a society and health care system enamored with new technology that increased direct and indirect health care costs but had yet to uniformly realize marketed or potential benefits during early adoption.[101] As with open surgical techniques, LRP and RALP outcomes, including surgical margin status, continence, and potency, reflect surgical technique (what the surgeon does) more than surgical approach. Current data suggest that the best way to improve outcomes after RP is to have the procedure performed by a skilled surgeon regardless of the approach he or she uses.

Cancer Control with Radical Prostatectomy. Progression rates after RP depend on the clinical stage, biopsy Gleason score, and serum PSA level before surgery as well as pathologic findings in the surgical specimen. Further, after a patient has undergone RP his serum PSA levels should become undetectable. Several major institutions have reported remarkably similar progression-free probabilities at 5 and 10 years, respectively, after surgery (Table 97.10).[102–106] Of 10,523 patients treated with RP between 1966 and 2003, 69% to 84% were free of progression at 5 years, and at 10 years progression-free probabilities ranged from 47% to 78%.

Fifteen-year outcomes have been reported after RP based on preoperative and pathologic factors (Table 97.8).[107,108] Bianco et al.[108] calculated the risk of recurrence in 1,743 consecutive patients with clinical stage T1-T3 N0 or X, M0 cancer treated with RP and followed with serum PSA levels for a mean of 72 months (range, 1-240 months). Failure after RP was defined as a rising serum PSA greater than 0.2 ng/mL, clinical evidence of local or distant recurrence, or the initiation of adjuvant radiotherapy or hormonal treatment. At 5 years 84%, at 10 years 78%, and at 15 years 73% were free of progression (Table 97.10).

Of particular interest are patients with high-grade cancers (Gleason sum 7–10). Of patients with Gleason 3 + 4 = 7 cancers in the RP specimen, 68% were free of progression at 15 years. When the tumor was Gleason 4 + 3 = 7, 51% were free of progression at 15 years.[108] Even patients with Gleason sum 8 to 10 cancers fared well, with 27% free of progression at 10 years. These progression rates are substantially lower than the 15-year cancer mortality rates reported for patients with Gleason sum 7 to 10 cancers managed with watchful waiting.[109]

Once the prostate is removed, the most powerful prognostic factor is the pathologic stage (Table 97.8). When the cancer is confined to the prostate (defined as cancer not extending into the periprostatic soft tissue), 92% to 98% of patients remain free of progression at 5 years and 88% to 96% remain free 10 years after RP.[102] Focal penetration through the capsule into the periprostatic soft tissue alone, in the absence of SVI, results in a 73% 10-year nonprogression rate. Established (extensive) penetration through the prostatitic capsule into the periprostatic soft tissue, in the absence of SVI, results in a 42% 10-year nonprogression rate. Even some patients with SVI (pT3cN0) can be cured with surgery, with 30% being free of disease recurrence at 10 years (Table 97.8).

The slow clinical progression of prostate cancer after RP has necessitated the use of PSA recurrence as the primary end point for evaluating treatment outcome. However, PSA recurrence has a highly variable natural history and poses a limited threat to the longevity of many patients. Reports of long-term, prostate cancer–specific survival rates after RP have clearly shown that many such patients live out their lives free of cancer.[102–104,107,108] Long-term risk of prostate cancer–specific mortality (PCSM) after RP for patients treated in the era of widespread PSA screening has recently been estimated based on a multi-institutional cohort of 12,677 patients treated with RP between 1987 and 2005.[110] Fifteen-year PCSM and all-cause mortality were 12% and 38%, respectively. The estimated PCSM ranged from 5% to 38% for patients in the lowest and highest quartiles of nomogram-predicted risk of PSA-defined recurrence (Table 97.11). Only 4% of contemporary patients had a predicted 15-year PCSM of greater than 5%.

Clearly, few patients will die from prostate cancer within 15 years of RP, despite the presence of adverse clinical features. Whether this favorable prognosis is related to the effectiveness of RP (with or without secondary therapy) or the low lethality of cancers detected by early screening is unknown. Although year of surgery, biopsy Gleason grade, and PSA level are associated with a risk of PCSM, an individual patient's risk cannot be predicted on the basis of clinical features alone. Further research is needed to identify novel markers specifically associated with the biology of lethal prostate cancer.

High-Risk Prostate Cancer. Monotherapy is often believed to be inadequate for high-risk cancers, and some clinicians are reluctant to consider RP in high-risk patients. However, there are no standardized criteria to define high risk before definitive treatment. Among 4,708 patients undergoing RP, high-risk patients were identified based on eight existing definitions, and their pathologic characteristics and PSA outcomes were examined (Table 97.12).[100] Depending on the definition used, high-risk patients composed 3% to 38% of the study population. Among patients defined as high risk, 22% to 63% of tumors proved to be confined to the prostate pathologically.

TABLE 97.10

FREEDOM FROM PROGRESSION AFTER RADICAL RETROPUBIC PROSTATECTOMY, BASED ON PROSTATE-SPECIFIC ANTIGEN (PSA)

				PSA nonprogression (%)		
Group (Ref.)	No. of Patients	Clinical Stage	Years of RP	5-Year	10-Year	15-Year
Han et al.[103]	2,404[a]	T1-2NX	1982–1999	84	72	61
Trapasso et al.[105]	425[b]	T1-2NX	1987–1992	69	47	—
Zinke et al.[104]	3,170[a]	T1-2NX	1966–1991	70	52	40
Catalona and Smith[106]	1,778[c]	T1-2NX	1983–1993	78	65	—
Hull et al.[102]	1,000[b]	T1-2NX	1983–1998	78	75	—
Bianco et al.[108]	1,743[a]	T1-3NX	1983–2003	84	78	73

RP, radical prostatectomy.
[a]Progression defined as a serum PSA >0.2 ng/mL.
[b]Progression defined as a serum PSA >0.4 ng/mL.
[c]Progression defined as a serum PSA >0.3 ng/mL.

TABLE 97.11

RISK OF PROSTATE CANCER–SPECIFIC MORTALITY AT 10 AND 15 YEARS AFTER RADICAL PROSTATECTOMY[a]

Variable	Patients*		Events*		10-Year PCSM		15-PCSM	
	No.	%	No.	%	%	95% CI	%	95% CI
Nomogram-predicted 5-year PFP (%)								
76–99	8,555	73	51	26	1.8	1.2–2.4	5	3–7
51–75	2,228	19	75	38	6	4–7	15	10–21
26–50	656	6	40	21	9	6–12	16	9–22
1–25	209	2	29	15	15	9–22	38	19–56
Risk Group								
PSA <10, Gleason score 6, T1c or T2a	5,200	46	14	7	0.9	0.3–1.5	2	0.3–4
PSA 10–20, Gleason score 7, T2B	4,184	37	64	32	4	2–5	10	6–14
PSA >20, Gleason score 8–10, T2c-T3	1,962	17	121	61	8	7–10	19	14–24
Pretreatment PSA (ng/mL)								
<4	2,285	18	18	9	2	1–4	4	1–7
4–10	7,574	61	75	37	3	2–4	9	5–12
10.1–20	1,874	15	50	24	4	3–6	11	6–15
20.1–50	726	6	62	30	10	7–12	22	15–30
1992 TNM Clinical Stage								
T1ab	174	2	4	2	2	0–4	6	0–12
T1c	6,413	56	28	14	2	1–3	6	5–7
T2a	2,520	22	42	21	3	2–4	7	4–10
T2b	1,461	13	57	29	5	3–7	14	9–19
T2c	714	6	38	19	7	4–9	12	8–17
T3	254	2	28	14	15	9–21	38	22–54
Biopsy Gleason Score								
2–6	7,454	65	78	40	2	1–3	6	4–8
7	3,292	29	55	28	5	3–7	17	8–26
8–10	702	6	61	32	16	11–20	34	23–46

PCSM, prostate cancer–specific mortality; CI, confidence interval; PFP, progression-free probability; PSA, prostate-specific antigen
[a]Note. Values were based on a previously validated nomogram, risks groups, clinical stage, pretreatment PSA, and biopsy Gleason score.
[b]Percentages refer to proportion of total in each category.
(From ref. 110, with permission.)

Although high-risk patients had a 1.8-fold to 4.8-fold increased hazard of PSA relapse, their 10-year relapse-free probability after RP alone was 41% to 74% (Table 97.12). Disease-specific survival at 12 years was between 78% and 94% (Table 97.13). Of the high-risk patients who relapsed, 25% (across all definitions) relapsed more than 2 years after surgery, and in 26% to 39% the PSADT at recurrence was 10 months or more. These results suggest that patients diagnosed with high-risk cancers by current definitions do not have a uniformly poor prognosis after RP.

TABLE 97.12

ESTIMATES OF 5- AND 10-YEAR PROGRESSION-FREE PROBABILITY (PFP) IN MEN UNDERGOING RADICAL PROSTATECTOMY FOR HIGH-RISK PROSTATE CANCER

High-Risk Definition	BCR/No. of Patients	5-year PFP* (95% CI)	10-year PFP* (95% CI)
Biopsy Gleason 8–10	109/274	53 (46,60)	42 (38,56)
Preoperative PSA ≥20	121/275	56 (50,62)	47 (40,54)
1992 TNM stage T3	62/144	49 (39,58)	41 (29,53)
PSA ≥20 or ≥T2c or GS ≥8	299/957	68 (65,71)	59 (55,63)
Nomo 5-y PFP ≤50%	180/391	53 (47,57)	43 (36,49)
PSA ≥20 or ≥T3 or GS ≥8	234/605	57 (53,62)	50 (44,55)
PSA ≥15 or ≥T2b or GS ≥8	466/1,752	73 (71,75)	65 (62,68)
PSA velocity >2 ng/mL/y	161/952	80 (77,83)	74 (70,78)

BCR, biochemical relapse; CI, confidence interval; PSA, prostate-specific antigen; GS, Gleason score.
(From ref. 100, with permission.)

PRACTICE OF ONCOLOGY

TABLE 97.13

ESTIMATED 12-YEAR DISEASE-SPECIFIC SURVIVAL (DSS) AFTER RADICAL PROSTATECTOMY

High-Risk Definition	12-Year DSS (95% CI)
Biopsy Gleason 8–10	80 (69, 91)
Preoperative PSA ≥20	86 (76, 96)
1992 TNM stage T3	78 (69, 89)
PSA ≥20 or ≥T2c or GS ≥8	93 (89, 97)
Nomogram 5-y PFP ≤50%	90 (84, 96)
PSA ≥20 or ≥T3 or GS ≥8	91 (86, 96)
PSA ≥15 or ≥T2b or GS ≥8	94 (92, 96)
PSA velocity >2 ng/mL/y	94 (90, 98)

CI, confidence interval; PSA, prostate-specific antigen; GS, Gleason score; PFP, progression-free probability.
(From ref. 400, with permission.)

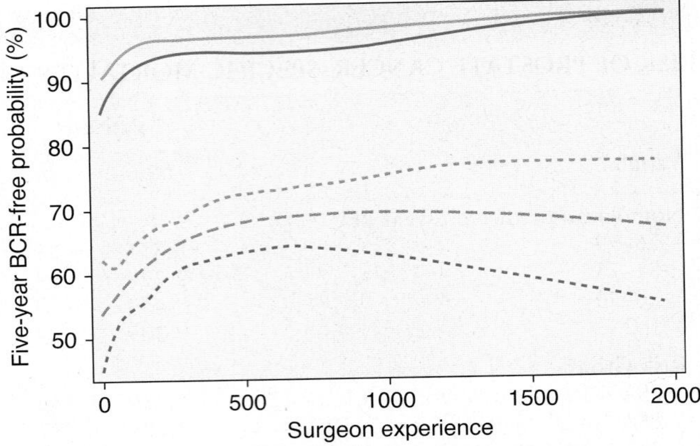

FIGURE 97.6 Biochemical recurrence-free probability by surgeon experience. *Solid lines:* organ-confined; *dashed lines:* non–organ-confined; *grey lines:* 95% confidence interval (Reprinted from ref. 112, with permission.)

Impact of the Surgeon on Outcomes after RP. Recent research has focused on how surgical volume and the individual surgeon influence results after RP. Begg et al.[111] used the SEER-Medicare–linked database to evaluate health-related outcomes after RP. The rates of postoperative complications, late urinary complications (strictures or fistulas 31–365 days after the procedure), and long-term incontinence (>1 year after the procedure) were inferred from the Medicare claims records of 11,522 patients who underwent RP between 1992 and 1996. These rates were analyzed in relation to hospital volume and surgeon volume (the number of procedures performed at individual hospitals and by individual surgeons, respectively). Neither hospital volume nor surgeon volume was significantly associated with surgery-related death. Significant trends in the relation between volume and outcome were observed with respect to postoperative complications and late urinary complications. Postoperative morbidity was lower in very high-volume hospitals than in low-volume hospitals (27% vs. 32%; $P = .03$) and was also lower when the prostatectomy was performed by very high-volume surgeons than when it was performed by low-volume surgeons (26% vs. 32%; $P < .001$). The rates of late urinary complications followed a similar pattern. Results for long-term preservation of continence were less clear-cut. In a detailed analysis of the 159 surgeons who had a high or very high volume of procedures, wide surgeon-to-surgeon variations in these clinical outcomes were observed, and they were much greater than would be predicted on the basis of chance or observed variations in the case mix. These findings suggest that, in general, high-volume surgeons have superior results than low-volume surgeons in terms of early postoperative morbidity and urinary complications after RP. However, the much greater than anticipated outcomes among the highest-volume surgeons suggest that individual surgical technique also influenced these same outcomes.

Individual patient data from four institutions was used to study the association between a surgeon's prior experience and biochemical recurrence after RP (the principal reason that patients visit an oncologic surgeon).[112] This relationship has often been termed the *learning curve* and likely reflects differences in surgical skill. A retrospective cohort study of consecutive patients treated from 1987 to 2003 was conducted at four academic, tertiary referral centers in the United States. There were 7,850 patients with localized prostate cancer who received no neoadjuvant therapy and who underwent open radical retropubic prostatectomy by one of 73 different surgeons.[108] For each patient, surgeon experience was coded as the total number of RPs conducted by the surgeon prior to the incident case, and cancer control was defined as a corroborated rising PSA level more than 0.4 ng/mL. This study demonstrated that cancer control improved with increasing surgeon experience (Fig. 97.6).[112] This relationship remained highly significant ($P < .001$) after adjustment for tumor characteristics and year of surgery. The learning curve for cancer control after radical retropubic prostatectomy was steep but did not start to plateau until a surgeon had completed approximately 250 prior operations. Five-year probability of biochemical recurrence was 17.8% for patients treated by surgeons in the early phase of their career (10 prior operations) compared to 10.9% when surgeons had performed 250 operations (absolute risk difference, 6.9%; 95% CI: 4.3%–9.5%). We saw no evidence that patient risk attenuates the learning curve: there was a statistically significant association between biochemical recurrence and surgeon experience in all analyses. The relative risk for a patient receiving treatment from a surgeon with 10 rather than 250 prior radical prostatectomies was 2.5, 1.8, and 1.3 for low-, medium-, and high-risk patients.

EXTERNAL-BEAM RADIOTHERAPY

Conformal and Intensity-Modulated Radiation Therapy and Image-Guided Techniques

With the advent of 3D conformal radiotherapy (3D-CRT) in the late 1980s, the precision of radiotherapy significantly improved compared with standard conventional techniques. With 3D-CRT, CT-based images referenced to a patient immobilized in the treatment position are used to localize the prostate and surrounding normal tissue structures to generate high-resolution 3D reconstructions of the anatomy. These approaches facilitated the ability to deliver safely higher radiation doses to the prostate, paving the way for critical dose-escalation studies. Intensity-modulated radiotherapy (IMRT) can be considered as second-generation 3D-CRT, which takes advantage of sophisticated computer-aided optimization algorithms to produce dose distributions that conform even more precisely to the tumor target.[113,114] Although 3D-CRT relies on trial-and-error forward-planning techniques to create a treatment plan, IMRT takes advantage of inverse-planning methods used for optimization of the dose distribution. Inverse planning is part of a mathematical optimization algorithm that creates a treatment plan based on predefined desired dose-distribution parameters for the target and dose constraints imposed on the normal tissues. The highly conformal radiation beam is produced with the ability of IMRT to vary the intensities of the x-rays from each treatment field over the entire cross-section of the beam. Tomotherapy is another approach used to achieve varying intensity beam profiles using x-rays directed over a full 360-degree range, modulated by a slit, bimodal multileaf collimation.

Definition of Target Volume

The multifocal nature of prostate cancer and the well-documented risk of microscopic ECE even for patients with early clinical stages of disease are important considerations that influence the design of the target volume for radiation treatment planning. The clinical target volume (CTV) will include the entire prostate gland and immediate periprostatic tissues, as well as the seminal vesicles, as visualized on CT. In general, for patients with low-risk disease with unremarkable imaging studies, the CTV may exclude the seminal vesicles because of the low likelihood of disease involvement. The planning target volume (PTV) places an additional margin around the CTV to take into account patient setup uncertainties and organ motion. This margin is usually 1 cm around the CTV except at the prostate-rectal interface where a tighter margin (5–7 mm) is used. With the current availability of image-guided IMRT-based techniques that can more effectively account for the variability of the prostate position during treatment, tighter margins, in particular for hypofractionated regimens, are being used with circumferential margins of 5 mm along with even more constricted margins at the prostate-rectal interface (3 mm).

The inclusion of pelvic lymph nodes in the CTV appears to be beneficial for selected high-risk patients. The Radiation Therapy Oncology Group (RTOG) conducted a four-arm trial[115] in which patients with a more than 15% estimated risk of pelvic lymph node involvement were randomized to receive (1) whole pelvic radiotherapy with a boost to the prostate plus neoadjuvant and concurrent ADT, (2) radiotherapy to the prostate only plus neoadjuvant and concurrent ADT, (3) whole pelvic radiotherapy with a boost to the prostate plus adjuvant androgen deprivation, or (4) radiotherapy to the prostate only plus adjuvant androgen deprivation.[115] The 4-year progression-free survival rates were 60%, 44%, 49%, and 50%, respectively ($P = .008$), suggesting an advantage to pelvic irradiation when neoadjuvant and concomitant ADT are administered in this subset of patients. In a recent update of this study with a median follow-up of 6.6 years, a trend for difference ($P = .066$) was observed for progression-free survival in favor of whole pelvic radiotherapy combined with neoadjuvant ADT compared with the other treatment arms.[116] Outcome differences for other parameters such as distant metastases-free survival and overall survival were similar among the treatment groups. Other studies, albeit retrospective in nature, using higher radiation doses with high-dose-rate brachytherapy in combination with EBRT have not observed significant improvements in disease-free progression rates with the addition of pelvic lymph node irradiation. Longer follow-up will still be necessary to confirm the trends observed thus far in the aforementioned RTOG study, yet it would appear to be appropriate to incorporate pelvic lymph node irradiation as part of the radiotherapeutic management of high-risk patients.

Treatment Delivery and Organ-Motion Concerns

Movement of the prostate during treatment or between treatment fractions has long been a concern for prostate radiotherapy. Many reports have investigated the extent of inter- and intrafractional motion of the prostate and seminal vesicles.[117–118] Although the reported magnitude of prostate motion varies during a fractionated course of radiotherapy, relatively minimal motion occurs in the lateral directions and potentially significant movement is noted in the anterior-posterior and superior-inferior directions. Many studies have also observed a correlation between prostate and seminal vesicle motion and rectal or bladder filling.[117,119] To compensate for such motion, treatment volumes are routinely expanded with a safety margin to ensure adequate dose coverage of the CTV.

The emergence of image-guided radiotherapy has now resulted in the incorporation of several methods into the treatment-delivery process to reduce uncertainty due to interfractional organ motion, thereby improving the precision of treatment delivery. Image-guided radiotherapy takes advantage of various approaches for online image guidance and positional correction, including the use of computer-assisted transabdominal ultrasonography, radio-opaque marker tracking, or CT image guidance. New developments in image-guided radiotherapy now provide the opportunity of acquiring pre- or posttreatment megavoltage or kilovoltage CT images directly on the linear accelerator with the patient in the treatment position. Such approaches can be used to correct positional errors of the target immediately prior to or during treatment delivery. The verification of the accurate treatment position in conjunction with detailed anatomic information before every fraction can be essential for the outcome of the treatment. Linac-based kilovoltage image-guidance systems have recently become commercially available. These systems are composed of a kilovoltage x-ray tube mounted 90 degrees from the accelerator head and a kilovoltage imaging plate mounted 90 degrees from the standard megavoltage imaging device. They possess capabilities for kilovoltage two-dimensional projection imaging (radiographs), fluoroscopy, and 3D cone beam CT and are thus ideally suited for monitoring of inter- and intrafractional motion. In a commercially available system (Calypso Medical Technologies Inc., Seattle, Washington), transponders are placed transrectally into the prostate serving as fiducial markers. These markers emit an electromagnetic signal when excited and the signal is detected by an alternating current magnetic array that localizes the transponders in real time. With this information of intrafraction motion for each individual patient, the radiation beam could be temporarily interrupted should the target deviate from its set-up location or beyond a preset motion constraint. With image-guided radiotherapy and enhanced target localization, safety margins potentially can be further reduced and ultra hypofractionated regimens can be used with less potential morbidity. Whether these more precise delivery methods will translate into improved tumor control outcomes or reduced morbidity outcomes will require careful evaluation in formal prospective studies.

The Role of Dose Escalation in Patients with Clinically Localized Disease

Several randomized phase 3 trials[120–123] and the long-term results of single-institution studies[124–128] now demonstrate a significant improvement in treatment outcomes for higher radiation dose in patients with clinically localized disease. In a phase 3 trial conducted at M. D. Anderson Hospital,[120] patients with T1-T3 prostate cancer were randomized to receive 70 Gy and 78 Gy. A significant advantage was observed among patients with pretreatment PSA levels more than 10 ng/mL treated to higher doses. In this subset of patients, the 5-year PSA control rates for the 78- and 70-Gy arms were 62% and 43%, respectively (P = .01). However, among patients with PSA levels less than 10 ng/mL, there was no apparent advantage escalating the radiation dose. In a recent update of the trial, with a median follow-up of 9 years, patients with pretreatment PSA levels more than 10 ng/mL or those with high-risk disease (including Gleason 9–10 disease) treated to 78 Gy experienced superior distant metastases-free and cause-specific survival outcomes compared with similar patients treated to lower doses. The data from this update was also noteworthy for improved PSA-relapse-free survival outcomes even among low-risk patients who were treated with 78 Gy compared to 70 Gy (90% vs. 81%).[129]

Zietman et al.[121] recently updated the results of a randomized trial of patients with the overwhelming majority comprising low- and intermediate-risk disease. Patients received either EBRT 70.2-Gy equivalent or 79.2-Gy equivalent using a combination of protons and photons. With a median follow-up of 8.9 years, the 10-year PSA relapse-free survival outcomes were superior for the higher-dose arm compared with the lower dose (87% vs. 68%; P < .001). The predominant biochemical control benefit was observed in the low-risk patient cohort (93% vs. 72%; P <.001) and a strong trend was observed for improvement among intermediate-risk patients (70% vs. 58%; P = .06). No differences in overall survival were observed between the treatment arms (Fig. 97.7).[130] Peeters et al.[122] from The Netherlands Cancer Institute reported the results of a randomized trial comparing 78 Gy with 68 Gy. It is important to note that neoadjuvant ADT in this trial was used in 21% of the enrolled patients based on the preference of the treating physician. Six hundred sixty-nine patients were eligible and stratified by the use of neoadjuvant ADT, age, and treatment group. The 5-year PSA relapse-free survival outcome was superior for the 78-Gy arm compared with the 68-Gy arm (64% vs. 54%; P = .02). A significant advantage in PSA

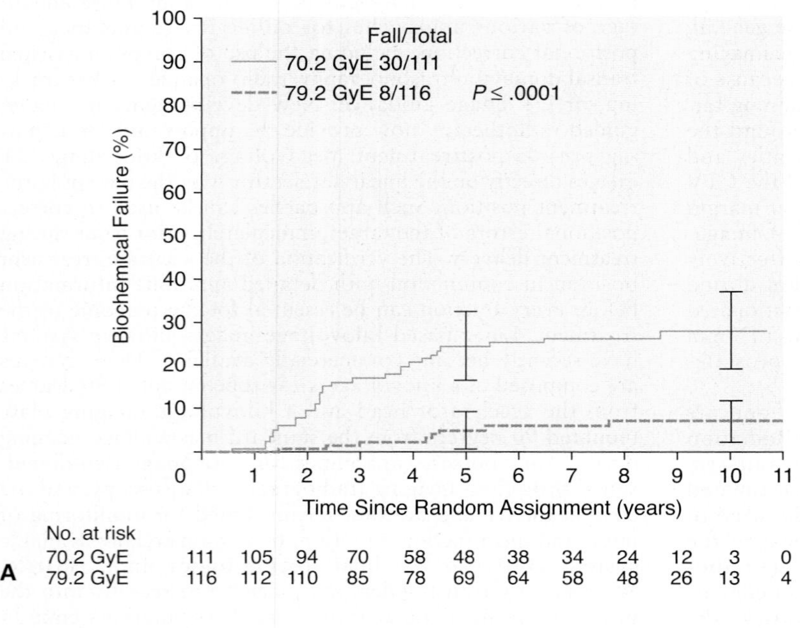

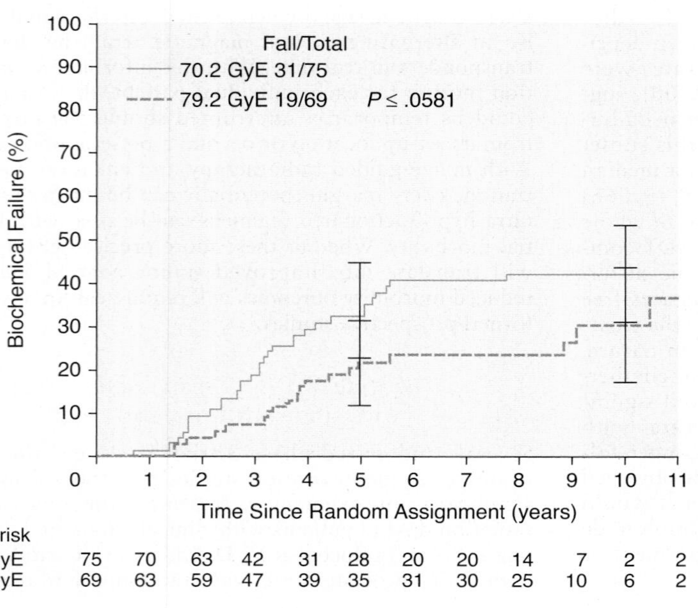

FIGURE 97.7 Prostate-specific antigen (PSA)-relapse-free survival outcomes after high-dose conformal radiation therapy versus conventional dose according to the American Society for Therapeutic Radiology and Oncology PSA consensus definition. **A:** Control rates for low-risk patients. **B:** PSA control rates for intermediate-risk patients.

TABLE 97.14

PHASE 3 EXTERNAL-BEAM RADIOTHERAPY DOSE ESCALATION STUDIES

Study (Ref.)	No. of Patients	Median Follow-Up (mo)	Treatment Arms	5-Year PSA Relapse-Free Survival Outcome	*P* Value
Pollack et al.[120]	301	60	78 vs. 70 Gy (no ADT given)	70% high dose 64% low dose	.03
				PSA >10 ng/mL High dose, 62% Low dose, 43%	.01
Zietman et al.[121]	393	66	79.2 Gy equivalent vs. 70.2 Gy equivalent (dose delivered with combination of protons/photons)	Low risk High dose, 80% Low dose, 60%	<.001
				Intermediate–high-risk High dose, 78% Low dose, 65%	<.001
Peeters et al.[122]	664	51	78 vs. 68 Gy (neoadjuvant short-term and long-term ADT used in two participating institutions for high-risk patients)	Benefit observed for intermediate–high-risk patients: 66% (high dose) 53% (low dose)	<.01
Dearnaley MRC-RT01[123]	843	63	74 vs. 64 Gy 30-CRT (3–6 months neoadjuvant + concurrent ADT administered)	Low risk High dose, 85% Low dose, 79% Intermediate risk High dose, 79% Low dose, 70% High risk High dose, 57% Low dose, 43%	

ADT, androgen deprivation therapy; CRT, conformal radiotherapy.

relapse-free survival was noted in particular among those patients with intermediate-risk disease who received 78 Gy.

Recently the results of Medical Research Council (MRC)-RT01,[123] which randomized 843 patients with clinically localized prostate cancer to 74 Gy and 64 Gy, were reported. In both arms of the study neoadjuvant ADT ranging from 3 to 6 months and concomitant therapy were administered. Higher radiation doses were associated with improved biochemical relapse-free survival outcomes at 5 years for those patients with low-, intermediate-, and high-risk disease. The 5-year PSA control rates for higher versus lower doses for low-risk patients was 85% versus 79%. For intermediate-risk patients the corresponding rates of biochemical control were 79% and 70%, and for high-risk patients 57% and 43% for high versus low dose. These differences between the risk groups were all significant. This study also suggests that even in the setting of ADT, higher radiation doses offer an incremental benefit for improved outcomes compared with lower doses.

The RTOG is completing a phase 3 dose-escalation trial (RTOG 0126) that randomizes eligible patients to 70.2 Gy or 79.2 Gy. In this study, treatment with ADT is not allowed. In contrast to the previously mentioned Dutch trial, the dose is prescribed to the margin of the PTV, and the edge of the PTV is not truncated at the prostate-rectal interface. This technical aspect would ensure a reasonable dose delivery to the posterior aspects of the prostate with the prescription dose. The RTOG 0126 study is powered to test for an overall survival end point, and planned accrual is for 1,520 patients. In addition, a sizable percentage of patients on this trial will be treated with IMRT, potentially reducing the risk of complications for the high-dose arm.[124] Table 97.14 is a summary of the salient findings from the four published randomized dose-escalation trials.

Long-Term Results of Single-Institution Studies

The dose-escalation experience from the Memorial Sloan-Kettering Cancer Center (MSKCC) was reported by Zelefsky et al.[131] A total of 2,047 patients with T1-T3 prostate cancer were treated with 3D-CRT/IMRT. The radiation dose was systematically increased from 64.8 to 86.4 Gy by increments of 5.4 Gy in consecutive groups of patients. The 7-year PSA control outcomes were 90%, 72%, and 54% for low-, intermediate-, and high- risk patients, respectively ($P < .0001$). The radiation dose significantly influenced PSA relapse-free survival outcomes. When patients were stratified according to risk groups, no differences were observed for low-risk patient among the various dose groups. However, higher radiation doses were associated with significant improvements in long-term PSA outcomes for intermediate-risk patients (>75.6 vs. 70.2 Gy) and among high-risk patients (81 vs. <75.6 Gy). In addition, higher radiation doses were associated with improved distant metastases-free survival outcomes among intermediate- and high-risk patients.

Other institutional experiences have corroborated the association of higher radiation doses with concomitant improvements in long-term PSA-relapse-free survival and distant metastases-free survival outcomes. Eade et al.[126] reported the outcomes of 1,531 patients treated with dose escalation using 3D-CRT at the Fox Chase Cancer Center. Patients were retrospectively divided into dose groups included less than 70 Gy, 70 to 74.9 Gy, 75 to 79.9 Gy, and more than 80 Gy. Multivariate analysis demonstrated that higher radiation doses were an independent predictor for biochemical control and improved distant metastases-free survival in addition to the T stage, Gleason score, and initial PSA level. Similar findings demonstrating reduced incidence of distant metastases with dose escalation have been reported by Kupelian et al.[132] in a cohort of 919 patients treated to doses of 68.4 to 83 Gy.

The ability to constrain the dose to normal tissues such as the bladder and the rectum has paved the way for using ultra high-dose IMRT in the treatment of patients with localized disease. Cahlon et al.[133] reported on 478 patients treated to 86.4 Gy using a five- to seven-field IMRT technique. With a median follow-up of 53 months, the 5-year PSA relapse-free survival rates were 98%, 85%, and 70%, respectively, for low-, intermediate-, and high-risk patients. Despite the application of these high-dose levels, the incidence of grade 3 rectal and urinary toxicities were less than 1% and less than 3%, respectively.

Hypofractionated External Beam Radiotherapy

Because of the potential radiobiologic advantages of delivering larger doses for each treatment fraction (hypofractionated radiotherapy), several reports have assessed the feasibility and preliminary outcomes using such regimens. In one study from the Cleveland Clinic,[134] 100 patients were treated to 70 Gy using 2.5 Gy per fraction via IMRT. With a median follow-up of 66 months, the PSA relapse-free survival outcomes (according to the nadir +2 failure definition) at 5 years were 97%, 93%, and 75% for patients with low-, intermediate-, and high-risk disease, respectively. The actuarial late grade 3 rectal and urinary toxicities at 5 years were 3% and 1%, respectively. Higgins et al.[135] from the Edinburgh Cancer Center reported on 300 patients treated with a hypofractionated regimen of 52.5 Gy in 20 fractions in combination with neoadjuvant ADT. With a median follow-up of 58 months, the biochemical control rates at 5 years for patients with low-, intermediate-, and high-risk disease were 75%, 55%, and 35% ($P < .001$). Taken together, these data suggest that hypofractionated regimens can be safely delivered, in particular with CRT, and hypofractionated regimens using higher doses are more likely to be associated with improved long-term outcomes.

Di Staso et al.[136] retrospectively compared the outcomes of patients treated with a hypofractionated regimen (15 fractions of 3.62 Gy delivered three times per week to a total dose of 54.3 Gy) compared with conventional fractionated radiotherapy to 78 Gy. As the majority of these patients had intermediate-risk disease, both treatment groups received short-course ADT prior to and concomitant with their radiotherapy. The 5-year PSA-relapse-free survival outcomes were similar in the two treatment groups (78% and 75% for the hypofractionated and standard-fractionation groups, respectively). Investigators from McGill University Health Centre in Canada reported on 129 patients with favorable-risk disease treated to a dose of 66 Gy in 22 fractions. In this study, no patient received ADT. With a median follow-up of 51 months, the 5-year PSA-relapse-free survival outcome was 98%.[137]

The efficacy and role of stereotactic body radiosurgery is less established at this time. King et al. reported on 41 low-risk prostate cancer patients treated with five fractions of 7.25 for a total dose of 36.25 Gy. At a median follow-up of 33 months, no PSA failure had been observed. More recently, Katz et al.[138] reported on 304 patients, the majority of whom were treated to 36.25 Gy in 7.25-Gy fractions using an image-guided stereotactic radiosurgery technique. Nineteen percent of the patients were treated with neoadjuvant or concurrent ADT. PSA control rates were not reported in that study, yet at 2 years the percentage of patients reaching nadir values of 1.0 and 0.5 ng/mL was 81% and 66%, respectively.

The Role of Proton Therapy for Localized Prostate Cancer

There has been recent increasing interest in the use of proton therapy for clinically localized disease. Because of the known physical advantages of this charged particle, namely, the Bragg peak, the majority of the energy of the proton beam is deposited at the end of its track, creating a rapid fall-off of dose beyond the target. This effectively eliminates exit dose beyond the target volume and could achieve greater normal tissue sparing, making this form of therapy ideal for dose escalation. In addition, this physical advantage of the proton beam may translate into reduced risk of second malignancies due to the reduced exposure of the normal tissue to the radiation beam compared with photon therapy. Investigators from the Massachusetts General Hospital in Boston reported the results of a randomized trial comparing high-dose 75.6 cobalt Gray equivalents (CGE) using a conformal proton boost compared with standard photon irradiation delivering a dose of 67 Gy for patients with locally advanced prostate cancer. Improved local control (based on DRE and in selected cases prostate biopsies) was noted among patients with poorly differentiated tumors who received the higher proton doses.[139] Slater et al.[140] from Loma Linda University Medical Center reported on 1,277 patients treated with proton therapy to a dose of 74 CGE and noted PSA control outcomes and toxicity profiles that appear to be comparable to what has been achieved with standard conformal photon radiotherapy. In that report, the 5-year PSA control rates for patients with pretreatment PSA levels of 0 to 4 ng/mL, 4 to 10 ng/mL, and 10 to 20 ng/mL were 90%, 84%, and 65%, respectively.

The recent update from Zietman et al.[130] demonstrated a 93% 7-year PSA-relapse-free survival for high-dose proton in low-risk patients that appears to be comparable with what has been obtained with high-dose IMRT regimens. A phase 1/2 pilot study using high-dose protons alone to 82 CGE was associated with acceptable toxicity profiles but increased grade 2 and 3 urinary and rectal toxicities compared with reported toxicities observed with high-dose IMRT. Future improvements with intensity-modulated proton therapy will likely further improve the conformality of the proton beam and achieve fewer complications with proton dose escalation. In the meantime, there is no established evidence to date that proton therapy provides superior tumor control outcomes or is associated with fewer complications compared with well-delivered high-dose IMRT/image-guided radiotherapy in the treatment of prostate cancer.

Sequelae of Conventional EBRT

General Management of Symptoms

Complication rates vary as a function of the dose, the volume of normal tissue irradiation to particular dose levels, and the treatment field. Acute symptoms typically appear during the third week of treatment and resolve within days to weeks after its completion. Acute intestinal symptoms, especially those associated with whole pelvic irradiation, are most commonly relieved with dietary manipulations. Otherwise, medications, such as loperamide hydrochloride (Imodium) or diphenoxylate hydrochloride and atropine sulphate (Lomotil), are appropriate to relieve symptoms. Internal and external hemorrhoids may become inflamed during a course of therapy. These symptoms are often best treated with sitz baths and hydrocortisone suppositories. Patients also may experience changes in the consistency of their bowel movements or more mucous discharge. Acute urinary symptoms are treated with phenazopyridine hydrochloride (Pyridium), nonsteroidal anti-inflammatory agents, or alpha-blockers such as tamsulosin hydrochloride (Flomax). Alpha-blockers have been reported to be significantly more effective than nonsteroidal anti-inflammatory agents, resulting in significant resolution of urinary symptoms in 66% and moderate improvement in 22% of patients.[141]

Most late rectal toxicities attributed to radiotherapy manifest initially 12 to 18 months after completion of treatment and may persist for several years thereafter. The development of rectal complications after 5 years is rare. Late rectal toxicities may include rectal bleeding, mucous discharge, and mild incontinence of stool. The more severe toxicities, which include ulcer development and fistula formation, are observed in 1% or fewer patients. Grade 2 rectal bleeding can be effectively treated with steroid suppositories, sitz baths, and an increase in dietary fiber. Deep rectal biopsies and cauterization procedures should be avoided unless absolutely necessary because of the increased risk of further trauma to the rectal mucosa and risk for fistula formation. For radiation-induced proctitis not responsive to conservative measures, argon-beam plasma laser coagulation can decrease the frequency of rectal bleeding episodes.[142] Hyperbaric oxygen treatments at a pressure of 2.4 atmospheres for a median of 36 sessions (90 minutes per session) may be helpful; in one study they were associated with a complete resolution of rectal bleeding in 48% and reduction in bleeding episodes in 28% of patients.[143] It is assumed that hyperbaric oxygen improves the delivery of oxygen to ischemic rectal mucosa, promoting angiogenesis, and improves mucosal healing and fibroblast proliferation.

Late urinary toxicities include chromic urethritis in approximately 10% to 15% of patients, and urethral strictures in 2% to 3%. The risk of hemorrhagic cystitis is uncommon with conformal radiation techniques, which reduce the dose to the bladder. Current treatment approaches for hemorrhagic cystitis include intravesical formalin therapy and selective embolization of the hypogastric arteries. For patients refractory to such measures, hyperbaric oxygen therapy can be considered for radiation-induced hemorrhagic cystitis. In one report, of 57 patients treated 49 (86%) experienced complete resolution or marked improvement of hematuria following hyperbaric oxygen treatment.[144]

Incidence of Predictors of Toxicity

Michalski et al.[145] reported the toxicity outcomes of various risk groups enrolled on RTOG 9406, a phase 1 dose-escalation study. The dose levels evaluated in this report included patients treated to the initial two dose levels of the study, 68.4 Gy and 73.8 Gy. The median follow-up times in these subgroups ranged from 2.2 to 3.4 years. The acute grade 2 bowel/rectal toxicity rates ranged from 16% to 25%. The crude incidence of late bowel/rectal toxicities ranged from 2% to 8%. With a median follow-up of 2.5 years, the crude late grade 2 and 3 GI toxicities for those patients treated to 78 Gy (2-Gy fractions) was 22% and 2%, respectively.

The tolerance of high-dose 3D-CRT and IMRT for 1,571 patients treated at MSKCC has been updated.[146] With a median follow-up of 7 years, the overall incidence of grade 2 and grade 3 or higher rectal toxicities at 10 years were 8% and 1%, respectively. The use of short-term neoadjuvant ADT did not impact significantly on the incidence of long-term rectal toxicities. The overall incidence of grade 2 and grade 3 or higher urinary toxicities at 10 years were 12% and 4%, respectively. Similarly, the use of short-term neoadjuvant ADT had no demonstrable impact on the incidence of long-term urinary toxicities. Higher radiation dose levels were associated with an increase in grade 2 urinary toxicities. However, despite the application of higher doses, the incidence of rectal toxicities did not significantly increase, which is attributed to the use of IMRT. Investigators from the Princess Margaret Hospital in Toronto recently reported on the long-term tolerance of high-dose image-guided 3D-CRT or IMRT (median dose 79.8 Gy in 42 fractions) with a median follow-up of 5 years. The 5-year incidence of late GI and GU grade 2 to 3 toxicities were 14% and 12%, respectively. The incidence of grade 3 rectal toxicity was noted to be 3.5% and the use of androgen deprivation in conjunction with radiotherapy was associated with a significant increase in rectal toxicity.[147]

Peeters et al.[148] reported on the incidence of acute and late complications in a multicenter randomized trial comparing 68 Gy with 78 Gy using 3D-CRT. The median follow-up was 31 months. The 3-year incidence of grade 2 and higher GI and GU toxicities for the 68-Gy dose arm was 23% and 28.5%, respectively. The 3-year incidence of grade 2 and higher GI and GU toxicities for the 78-Gy dose arm was 26.5% and 30%, respectively. The differences were not significant. However, the authors did note a significant increase in grade 3 rectal toxicity requiring laser cauterization for the higher-dose arm. For patients treated to 78 Gy, the incidence of grade 3 rectal bleeding at 3 years was 10% compared with 2% for those treated to 68 Gy. The following variables were found to be predictive of late GI toxicity: a history of abdominal surgery (P <.001) and the presence of pretreatment GI symptoms (P = .001). The following variables were predictive of late GU toxicity: pretreatment urinary symptoms (P <.001), the use of neoadjuvant ADT (P <.001), and prior transurethral resection of the prostate (P = .006).

In an attempt to further improve the conformality of the high-dose therapy plans and decrease the rate of grade 2 toxicity, an IMRT approach was introduced for the treatment of clinically localized disease. Comparison of long-term rectal bleeding rates in the initial cohort of patients treated to 81 Gy with IMRT compared with conventional 3D-CRT demonstrated a significant reduction in the incidence of toxicity in favor of IMRT (Fig. 97.8). In a recent update of 561 patients treated with IMRT to 81 Gy at MSKCC,[149] the 8-year actuarial likelihood of developing grade 2 rectal bleeding was 1.6%. Three patients (0.1%) experienced grade 3 rectal toxicity requiring either one or more transfusions or a laser cauterization procedure. No grade 4 rectal complications have been observed. The 8-year likelihood of developing late grade 2 and

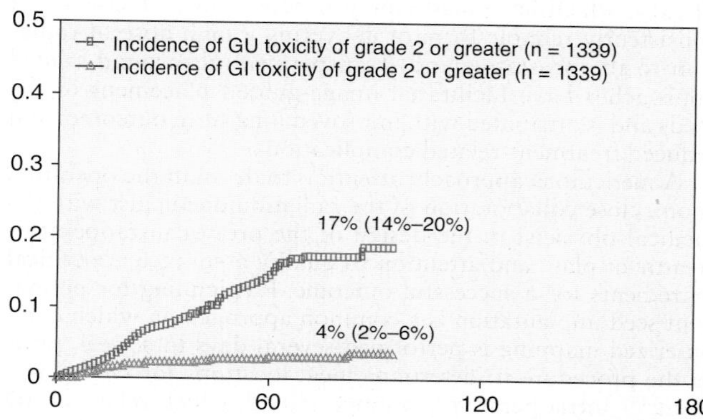

FIGURE 97.8 Incidence of grade 2 or greater genitourinary (GU) and gastrointestinal (GI) toxicities for patients receiving intensity-modulated radiation therapy only for patients treated at Memorial Sloan-Kettering Cancer Center. X-axis represents months from completion of treatment. Y-axis represents the percentage incidence of toxicity.

PRACTICE OF ONCOLOGY

3 (urethral strictures) urinary toxicities were 9% and 3%, respectively. Among patients who were potent prior to IMRT, 49% developed erectile dysfunction.[149]

Potency Preservation with EBRT

The reported rates of impotence at 3 years or thereafter following EBRT range from 36% to 68%.[150] Aside from erectile dysfunction, other aspects of sexual dysfunction after radiotherapy include decreased volume of ejaculate, absence of ejaculate, decreased intensity of orgasm, and decreased libido.

There is a wide range of reported erectile dysfunction rates after EBRT, which reflects the enormous variation of methods as recorded in the literature that have been used to assess this end point. The great deal of heterogeneity in the EBRT patient population contributes to a large extent to variability of reported ranges of erectile dysfunction in the patient population. One must also consider variables that impact this elderly population, especially when comparing the incidence of erectile dysfunction for different treatment modalities. Additional factors include the presence of medical comorbidities such as coronary artery disease, diabetes, and antihypertensive medications, all of which can have a profound effect on erectile function.

Trus-Guided Prostate Brachytherapy

Excellent long-term tumor control can be achieved with brachytherapy, and this approach is considered a standard treatment intervention associated with comparable outcomes to prostatectomy and EBRT for patients with clinically localized disease.[151–156] In general, for patients with low-risk disease, seed implantation alone (i.e., monotherapy) achieves high rates of biochemical tumor control and cause-specific survival outcomes. For those with intermediate risk and selected high-risk disease, a combination of brachytherapy (low-dose-rate permanent interstitial implantation, or high-dose-rate brachytherapy via after-loading catheters) with EBRT is commonly used. Whether the addition of EBRT is necessary in all patients with intermediate-risk prostate cancer is currently being studied in a phase 3 randomized trial (RTOG-0232).

Technical Aspects of Prostate Brachytherapy

During the last 15 to 20 years there have been significant improvements in the technical aspects of delivery of brachytherapy, which have made the procedure more precise and a consistently reliable form of delivering a high dose of radiation to the prostate gland. Transperineal ultrasound-guided approaches have facilitated image-guided placement of the seeds and is attributed with improved long-term outcomes and reduced treatment-related complications.

A meticulous approach, attention to detail in the operating room, close collaboration of the radiation oncologist with the medical physicist in the design of the pre- or intraoperative treatment plan, and attention to quality assurance are critical ingredients for a successful outcome. Preplanning for permanent seed implantation is a common approach, in which computerized mapping is performed several days to a week prior to the procedure to determine ideal locations for seed placement.[151] Intraoperative planning is used, which relies on 3D anatomic reconstruction of the prostate in real time and incorporation of similar inverse planning and sophisticated optimization algorithms used for IMRT to rapidly create a plan in the operating room.[157–162] These approaches have further improved accuracy and consistency of the dose delivery to the target with a concomitant reduction of dose to the urethra and rectum.[157,158]

Recent advances have included the use of adjunctive intraoperative CT scanning to verify the actual deposited seed coordinates for intraoperative evaluation of the implant quality. This approach may eliminate the need for postimplantation assessments and allow for opportunities if necessary to correct suboptimal implanted regions within the gland before the reversal of anesthesia.[163]

The two most commonly used radioisotopes for permanent seed brachytherapy are iodine-125 (^{125}I) and palladium-103 (^{103}Pd). There are clear physical differences between these two isotopes. The half-life of ^{125}I is 60 days with a mean photon energy of 27 KeV and an initial dose rate of 0.07 Gy/hour. In contrast, the half-life of ^{103}Pd is 17 days with a mean photon energy of 21 KeV and an initial dose rate of 0.19 cGy/hour. As five half-lives is considered to represent the life of the implant, the active time periods for ^{125}I and ^{103}Pd are 10 and 3 months, respectively. When ^{125}I is used, the typical prescription dose is 144 Gy, and 125 Gy is routinely used for ^{103}Pd. Based on radiobiologic considerations, it has been suggested, because of its initial lower dose rate, that ^{125}I may be more appropriate for low-grade tumors associated with a slower proliferating tumor cell population. On the other hand, ^{103}Pd, given its higher initial dose rate, may be the more appropriate isotope for more rapidly proliferating tumors (i.e., higher Gleason scores).[164] Comparative dosimetric analyses of treatment plans performed with ^{125}I or ^{103}Pd have not revealed significant differences between these isotopes.[165] Preliminary results of a randomized prospective trial to date have not shown any significant toxicity or tumor-control differences between these isotopes.[166]

The quality of the implant and dose distributions are routinely evaluated using CT scans obtained on the day of the implant or 30 days later. The latter time point may be preferable when prostate edema is less significant after the procedure and would less likely underestimate the prostate coverage with the prescription dose. On the other hand, earlier assessments could provide opportunities for earlier evaluation of the implant quality, which in some cases may require corrective action such as the addition of seeds or EBRT to treat possible underdosed regions of the prostate. Based on the postimplantation CT scans, dose-volume histograms are generated that provide detailed analysis of the radiation dose distribution relative to the prostate and surrounding normal tissues. Dosimetric parameters accounted for in this evaluation include V100 for the target (volume of the prostate receiving 100% of the prescription dose), D90 of the target (dose delivered to 90% of the prostate), and the average and maximum rectal and urethral doses.[167]

Several reports have demonstrated that higher radiation doses delivered to the prostate based on the postimplantation D90 evaluation were associated with improved biochemical control outcomes.[154,156,168–170] Investigators from Mt. Sinai Medical School[169] reported on 279 patients with stages T1-T2 prostate cancer who were treated with seed implantation and followed for a median of 6 years. In a multivariate analysis, independent predictors for long-term biochemical control included the prognostic risk group and the D90 dose based on the postimplantation evaluation. Among patients with D90 dose levels less than 140 Gy and less than 120 Gy, threefold and 5.5-fold increased risks, respectively, of biochemical relapse were observed. The D90 dose was also associated with local tumor control based on postimplantation biopsies performed 2 years or more after treatment. In that report, the incidence of a positive posttreatment biopsy for patients who had D90 doses more than 140 Gy was 4.8% compared with 20.5% for those who received lower dose levels. Further corroboration of a dose-response was noted based on the results of a multi-institutional analysis comprising of 2,693 patients treated with brachytherapy alone.[154] In that report, when D90 doses exceeded 130 Gy, the 7-year PSA relapse-free survival was 93% compared with 76% for those with lower D90 dose levels.

Henry et al.[171] reported on 1,298 patients treated with ^{125}I interstitial implantation and noted 5-year biochemical tumor control in 86%, 77%, and 61% for low-, intermediate-, and high-risk patients, respectively. Among patients with D90 dose levels that exceeded 140 Gy, biochemical control rates were 88% compared with 78% for patients with lower D90 dose levels (P <.01). Taira et al.[172] recently reported on 463 patients treated with ^{125}I or ^{103}Pd seed implantation used as monotherapy. A dose response was noted for both low-risk and intermediate-risk patients. Among low-risk patients with a biologic equivalent dose delivered of more than 116 Gy, the PSA-relapse-free survival at 10 years was 99% versus 92% with lower biologic equivalent dose; similarly for intermediate-risk patients the PSA-relapse-free survival at 10 years was 98% versus 86% for those who received higher than 116 Gy versus dose levels. These data in general indicate that the quality of the dose distribution is important for optimal tumor control and low D90 levels appear to represent a variable that may effectively identify patients who received subquality implants.

Biochemical and Disease Control Outcomes with Low-Dose-Rate Brachytherapy

Table 97.15 summarizes the published biochemical control outcomes after low-dose-rate interstitial seed implantation according to prognostic risk groups. In general these studies have demonstrated for low-risk patients biochemical control rates of 90% and 80% at 5 and 10 years, respectively, after treatment. Grimm et al.[151] reported the outcome of 125 patients treated between 1988 and 1990 with permanent seed implantation using ^{125}I and followed for a median of 81 months. A PSA relapse in that report was defined as three consecutive PSA elevations above the nadir PSA level. Among patients defined as having low-risk disease (PSA <10, Gleason score <7, and clinical stage T2b or lower), the 10-year PSA relapse-free survival outcome was 87%. In another article[173] these investigators reported on a cohort of patients treated with a combined-modality therapy and followed for a median of 9.4 years. The PSA relapse-free survival rates at 10 years for low-, intermediate-, and high-risk patients were 86%, 80%, and 68%, respectively.

Zelefsky et al.[154] reported the results of a multi-institutional analysis that was restricted to patients treated with interstitial seed implantation without hormonal therapy. The median follow-up in the study was 63 months. The 7-year PSA relapse-free survival for low-, intermediate-, and high-risk patients were 82%, 70%, and 48%, respectively (P <.001). A multivariable analysis identified tumor stage (P = .002), Gleason score (P <.001), pretreatment PSA level (P <.001), treatment year (P = .001), and the isotope used (P = .004) as pretreatment and treatment variables associated with biochemical control. When restricted to patients with available postimplantation dosimetric information, D90 emerged as a significant predictor of biochemical outcome (P = .01), and isotope was not significant (Fig. 97.9). The 7-year PSA relapse-free survival was 92%, 86%, 79%, and 67%, respectively, for patients with PSA nadir values of 0 to 0.49, 0.5 to 0.99, 1.0 to 1.99, and more than 2.0 ng/mL (P <.001). Among patients free of biochemical relapse at 7 years, the median nadir level

TABLE 97.15

PROSTATE-SPECIFIC ANTIGEN (PSA) RELAPSE-FREE SURVIVAL OUTCOMES FOR LOW-DOSE-RATE BRACHYTHERAPY

Study (Ref.)	No. of Patients	Median Follow-Up (y)	Treatment	5-Year Biochemical Outcome According to Risk Group	Comments
Stock et al.[174]	1,377	4.2	MT/CMT	Low, 94% Intermediate, 89.5% High, 78%	Interactive real-time planning
Zelefsky et al.[154]	2,693	5.2	MT	Low, 82% Intermediate, 70% High, 48%	D90 ≥130 Gy 8 year PSA control, –93% D90 <130 Gy 8-year PSA control, –76%
Guedea et al.[401]	1,050	2.5	MT	Low, 93% Intermediate, 88% High, 80%	—
Khaksar et al.[402]	300	4	MT	Low, 96% Intermediate, 89% High, 93%	—
Zelefsky et al.[403]	367	5.3	MT	Low, 96% Intermediate, 89%	Real-time intraoperative planned implants
Sylvester et al.[173]	232	9.4	CMT	Low, 86% Intermediate, 80% Unfavorable, 68%	—
Potters et al.[156]	1,449	7	MT/CMT	Low, 89% Intermediate, 78% Unfavorable, 63%	—

MT, monotherapy; CMT, combined-modality therapy (implant + external beam); PSA, prostate-specific antigen.

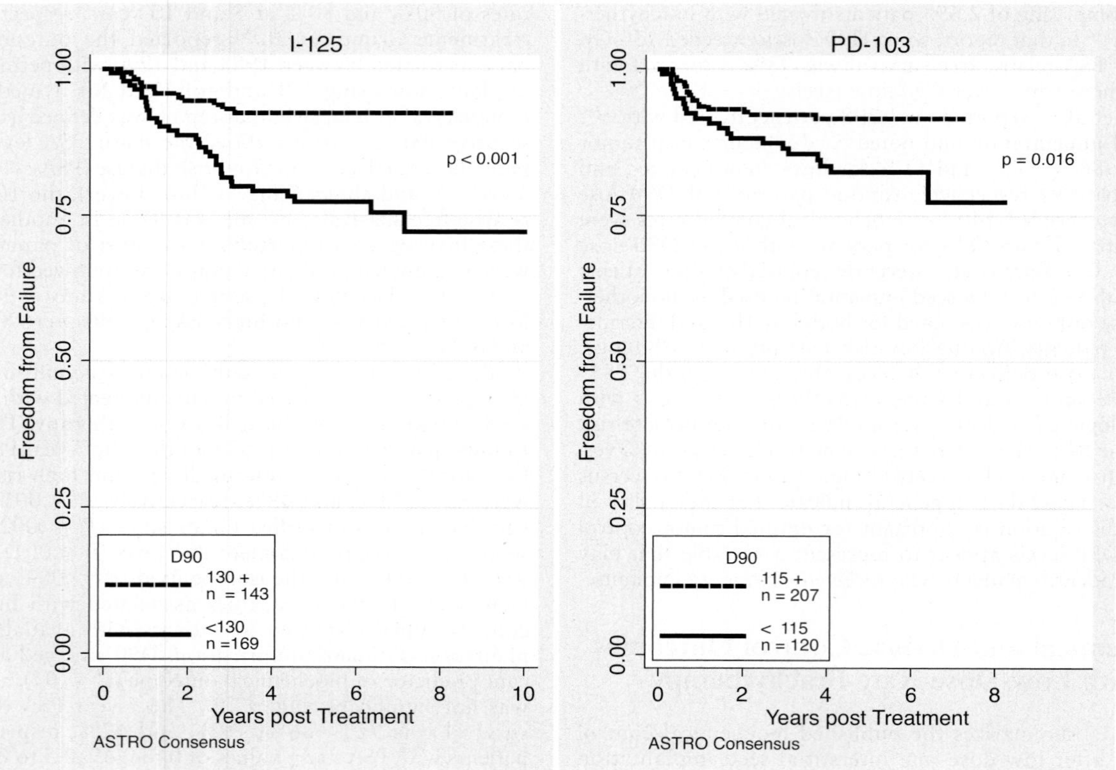

FIGURE 97.9 Multi-institutional analysis of patients treated with prostate brachytherapy using iodine-125 (I-125) or palladium-103 (PD-103). A dose-response for improved prostate-specific antigen (PSA) relapse-free survival outcomes was demonstrated for those patients who received D90 dose levels of 130 Gy or more for I-125–treated patients and 115 Gy or higher for patients treated with PD-103. The PSA failure definition used was the American Society of Therapeutic Radiation Oncology (ASTRO) Consensus Definition. (From ref. 154, with permission.)

was 0.1 ng/mL, and 90% of these patients achieved a nadir PSA level less than 0.6 ng/mL.

Assessment of local control based on posttreatment biopsies was performed in 508 patients who underwent prostate brachytherapy at the Mt. Sinai Medical Center in New York.[174] In 8% of these patients the biopsies were positive for adenocarcinoma. Predictors for a positive biopsy on multivariate analysis were low D90 dose level (P <.0001) and no hormonal therapy (P = .004). Among patients who had negative biopsies, 80% were free of PSA relapse at 10 years compared with 27% with a positive biopsy (P <.001). In this report, 44% of the positive biopsies at 2 years reversed to negative on subsequent postimplantation biopsies. These results further emphasize the importance of achieving a good-quality implant that would deliver an optimal dose distribution to the prostate to achieve tumor control.

Selection Criteria for Seed Implantation

Ideal patients for permanent interstitial implantation as monotherapy are those with favorable risk prognostic features who have a high likelihood of organ-confined disease. This group includes those with PSA levels 10 ng/mL or less, Gleason scores less than 7, and clinical stages T1c- T2a. Prior to treatment, MRI of the prostate with endorectal coil can be helpful in assessing the integrity of the prostatic capsule as well as the geometry of the gland. Such information is invaluable in the planning aspects of seed implantation as well as determining whether a patient is a candidate for the procedure. For patients with imaging findings consistent with gross ECE or SVI not detected on DRE, monotherapy would not be sufficient and supplemental EBRT should be considered.

For seed implantation, the prostate gland size preferably should be less than 60 cm^3 and optimally less than 50 cm^3. With larger gland sizes, the pubic arch may interfere with needle placement reaching the anterolateral portions of the gland, resulting in inadequate dose coverage of the target volume. In addition, larger glands require more seeds and activity to achieve coverage of the gland with the prescription dose, which may result in a concomitant increase in the central urethral doses and potentially increase the risk of urinary morbidity.[157,175,176] The size of the prostate can be effectively treated with combined androgen-blockade therapy. An approximate 30% volume reduction is commonly observed after 3 months of androgen deprivation.

Patients with a significant degree of urinary obstructive symptoms are more prone to develop prolonged morbidity after brachytherapy.[176–179] Such patients often have elevated baseline international prostate symptom assessment scores and would be better suited for other treatment interventions. A prior transurethral resection of the prostate (TURP) may increase the risks of urinary morbidity after seed implantation,[178,179] and brachytherapy should therefore be performed with caution in such patients. Wallner et al.[180] observed a 3-year actuarial incidence of incontinence of 6% among patients who underwent TURP prior to seed implantation. Others[181] reported a 16% incidence of superficial urethral necrosis among similar patients. Careful attention to dose-volume considerations to the periurethral region and area of the TURP defect should reduce the likelihood of long-term morbidities.

Patients with relative contraindications for receiving EBRT may be more suitable candidates for seed implantation. These include patients with bilateral hip replacements where CT-based treatment planning is technically difficult because of the substantial artifact created by the prostheses precluding adequate visualization of the target volume. Ultrasound-based seed implantation would be an appropriate alternative for such patients, as artifacts would not pose a difficulty with this imaging modality. In most cases, patients with hip prosthesis are able to tolerate extended dorsal lithotomy position for adequate perineal exposure during seed implantation. Patients with small bowel in close proximity to the prostate volume are not ideal candidates for high-dose EBRT and are better suited for brachytherapy because of the lower doses to the bowel expected with the latter treatment intervention. In addition, brachytherapy may be safe for patients with a history of inflammatory bowel disease, a condition that represents a relative contraindication for EBRT. One recent study[182] demonstrated that in 24 patients with a history of inflammatory bowel disease who were treated with brachytherapy, none experienced grade 3 or higher toxicities (median follow-up, 4 years). Yet the incidence of grade 2 rectal bleeding (19%) was significantly higher than what is observed with implantation without an antecedent history of inflammatory bowel disease.

Sequelae of Low-Dose-Rate Brachytherapy: Acute and Late Toxicity

Acute urinary retention (AUR) is a known complication that can occur immediately after prostate brachytherapy, and the incidence of AUR generally is in the range of 6% to 15%.[183,184] Keyes et al.[184] reported on the predictors of urinary retention after prostate brachytherapy in 805 patients. With greater experience and improved selection criteria, the incidence of retention declined in their initial experience from 17% to 6% in more recent years. Factors predicting for "prolonged" catheterization (>20 days) on multivariate analysis included higher international prostate symptom assessment scores ($P < .01$), increased number of needles used for the procedure ($P < .001$), and patients with diabetes mellitus ($P = .048$). These data in combination with the lack of correlation of AUR with dose delivered to the urethra or prostate suggest that the etiology of AUR is most likely related to trauma to the prostate gland.

Transient urinary morbidity related to radiation-induced urethritis or prostatitis represents the most common side effects after seed implantation. Symptoms include urinary frequency, urgency, and dysuria. These symptoms usually peak 1 to 3 months after the implant procedure and gradually resolve over the subsequent months. Most patients benefit significantly from the use of an alpha-blocker, which ameliorates such symptoms in 60% to 70% of patients. In general, the incidence of urinary symptoms persisting after 1 year is 15% to 25%. The risk of urethral strictures ranges from 1% to 12%. Otherwise, the incidence of grade 3 and 4 rectal or urinary toxicities including urinary or rectal incontinence are reported to be 1% or less (Table 97.16).

Grade 2 rectal toxicity after prostate brachytherapy ranges in the literature from 2% to 12%.[185,186] The incidence of grade 3 or 4 rectal toxicity is unusual (<2%). Some[187] have also observed a correlation between the volume of the rectum irradiated to the prescription dose and late rectal toxicity after

TABLE 97.16

LATE TOXICITY OUTCOMES AFTER PROSTATE BRACHYTHERAPY

Study (Ref.)	No. of Patients	Median Follow-Up (y)	Genitourinary	Gastrointestinal
Stock et al.[174]	325 Incontinence, 1%	7	Grade 3, 2% (urethral stricture)	Grade ≤2, 24% Grade 3–4, 0%
Waterman and Dicker[185]	98	3		Grade 2, 10%
Merrick et al.[186]	1,186	4.3	Grade 3, 3.6% Urethral stricture	
Gelblum et al.[404,405]	825	4	Grade 3, 4.7% 17% post TURP developed incontinence	Grade 1, 9% Grade 2, 6.6% Grade 3, 0.5%
Bottomley et al.[406]	667	2.5	Acute retention, 14.5% Late retention, 1% Urethritis @ 6 months, 13.5% Urethritis @ 24 months, 2.5%	Grade 4, <1%
Lee et al.[194] (RTOG 0019)	138	4	Late ≥ grade 3 GI/GU, 15% (combined-modality therapy)	
Shah et al.[160]	135	3.5		Diarrhea, 7.3% Urgency, 6.5% Bleeding, 7.3%
Keyes et al.[184]	805	3.3	AUR: IPSS 0–5, 8% IPSS 10–15, 15% IPSS >16, 21%	
Albert et al.[192]	201	2.8	Radiation-cystitis Monotherapy, 0% Combined-modality therapy, 5%	Grade 3 Monotherapy, 8% Combined-modality therapy, 30%
Zelefsky et al.[403]	367	5.2	Grade 2, 19% Grade 3, 4%	Grade 2, 7% Grade 3, 1%

TURP, transurethral resection of the prostate; GI, gastrointestinal; GU, genitourinary; AUR, acute urinary retention; IPSS, international prostate symptom score.

prostate brachytherapy. The 5-year likelihood of rectal toxicity was noted in 18% of patients in whom more than 1.3 cm^3 of rectal tissue was exposed to 160 Gy or higher compared with a 5% incidence among patients in whom less than 1.3 cm^3 of the rectum was exposed to these dose levels. The incidence of rectal toxicity correlated with the volume irradiated: 0% for 0.8 cm^3, 7% for 0.8 to 1.8 cm^3, and 25% for more than 1.8 cm^3. In a dosimetric analysis of 562 patients treated with intraoperative real-time conformal planning,[188] a correlation was also noted between the absolute volume of rectum exposed to higher doses and grade 2 rectal bleeding. Among patients in whom 2.5 cm^3 or more of the rectum was exposed to the prescription dose, the incidence of late grade 2 toxicity rectal toxicity was 9% compared with 4% for smaller volumes of the rectum exposed to similar doses (P = .003). Meticulous attention to needle and seed placement in the operating room as well as to the intraoperative dose-volume histogram data of normal tissue should reduce rectal doses and risks of toxicity to minimal levels.

Erectile Function after Brachytherapy

Impotence rates are likely underestimated in the literature. With longer follow-up, observations and responses based on patient surveys indicate that approximately 40% to 50% maintain erectile function after prostate brachytherapy.[188–190] Using a patient-administered questionnaire, Merrick et al.[190] evaluated sexual function in 132 potent men who underwent prostate brachytherapy. With median follow-up of 29 months, the 3-year actuarial rate of potency preservation was 50%. In a multivariate analysis the preimplant erectile-function score and the dose to 50% of the proximal crura of the penis were significant predictors for erectile dysfunction.

Excellent responses have been observed with sildenafil citrate in the treatment of posttreatment impotence after brachytherapy.[190,191] In one report 80% of patients responded well to the medication.[190] Investigators from the Cleveland Clinic[191] noted in 74% of their patients a continued favorable response to sildenafil after 4 years. With long-term follow-up, 37% of patients discontinued use of the medication. In these patients who discontinued the medication, 67% did so because of observed lack of efficacy while others discontinued secondary to experienced side effects or spontaneous return of natural erections.

Combined EBRT with Brachytherapy

Combination of brachytherapy and EBRT is generally considered a more suitable treatment option than implantation alone for patients with higher-risk disease. The combined approach effectively delivers an escalated dose of radiation that has been estimated to have a biologic equivalent that well exceeds 100-Gy equivalent of EBRT.[174,192] Combination approaches have been delivered in various ways and treatment schemes. In general, 45 to 50 Gy of EBRT is delivered using conventional or conformal-based techniques to the prostate and periprostatic tissues. If a low-dose-rate boost is used, the brachytherapy prescription dose has been 90 to 100 Gy for ^{103}Pd implants and 110 Gy for ^{125}I implants. In the absence of clinical trials comparing high-dose-rate (HDR) brachytherapy boosts versus low-dose-rate boosts, or the optimal sequence of therapy (brachytherapy boost preceding EBRT or vice versa), or the preferred isotope to be used for combined-modality therapy, there is no definitive evidence demonstrating the superiority of a particular treatment strategy over another.

A phase 3 trial, RTOG 0232, compares permanent-source brachytherapy as monotherapy to the combination of external-beam treatment followed by brachytherapy for patients with intermediate-risk prostate cancer. The primary end point of this study is survival outcome, and secondary end points include PSA relapse-free survival, distant metastases-free survival, and quality of life. Eligibility criteria for this study include clinical stage T1c-T2b, Gleason score less than 7 with PSA 10 to 20 ng/mL, or Gleason score 7 with a PSA less than 10 ng/mL. The American Urological Association voiding symptom score should be 15 or less and prostate volume less than 60 g.

Several series have reported a somewhat increased morbidity following combined treatment using conventional brachytherapy and EBRT techniques.[192–194] The RTOG conducted a phase 2 study (RTOG P-0019) to assess the acute and late toxicity for patients with intermediate-risk, clinically localized prostate cancer.[194] One hundred thirty-eight patients from 20 institutions were entered on this study. All patients were treated with EBRT (45 Gy in 25 fractions) followed 2 to 6 weeks later by an interstitial implant using ^{125}I to deliver an additional 108 Gy. Acute grade 3 toxicity was documented in 8%; however, higher toxicity levels were not observed. The 4-year estimate of late grade 3 GU/GI toxicity was 15%. These data suggest that, compared with brachytherapy alone, the acute and late morbidity observed in this multi-institutional, cooperative group study may be associated with increased morbidity. Yet, reduced morbidity with combination therapy has been demonstrated by institutions using intraoperative planning with strict dose constraints imposed on the rectum and urethra as well as the use of carefully planned IMRT for supplemental external beam radiotherapy.[195]

High-Dose-Rate Brachytherapy

HDR brachytherapy has been used as the brachytherapy component in combination with EBRT for the treatment of prostate cancer.[196–203] For this approach patients undergo transperineal placement of afterloading catheters in the prostate under ultrasound guidance. After CT-based treatment planning, several high-dose fractions, ranging from 4 to 6 Gy each, are administered during an interval of 24 to 36 hours using ^{192}Ir. This treatment is followed by supplemental EBRT directed to the prostate and periprostatic tissues to a dose of 45 to 50.4 Gy using conventional fractionation. Recently Hoskin et al.[202] reported the results of a randomized trial comparing hypofractionated EBRT delivering 55 Gy in 20 fractions with 35.75 Gy in 13 fractions of EBRT followed by a HDR brachytherapy boost of 17 Gy in 2 fractions delivered over 24 hours. Two hundred twenty patients were randomized and the median follow-up was 30 months. The 3-year likelihood of biochemical control in the combined-modality group versus EBRT alone was 80% versus 63%, respectively (P = .03). Table 97.17 summarizes the clinical outcomes of patients treated with combination HDR brachytherapy and EBRT.

Investigators from Beaumont Medical Center have used HDR brachytherapy as monotherapy without the addition of EBRT. The fractionation regimen was 38 Gy delivered in 4 fractions, two times daily during 2 days; early tolerance and tumor control outcomes have been promising.[204] Yoshioka et al.[205] also reported on the biochemical control outcomes of HDR brachytherapy used as monotherapy. The 3-year PSA relapse-free survival outcomes for low-, intermediate-, and high-risk patients treated with this intervention were 100%, 89%, and 77%, respectively.

HDR brachytherapy offers several potential advantages over other techniques. Taking advantage of an afterloading approach, the radiation oncologist and physicist can more easily optimize the delivery of radiotherapy to the prostate, reducing the potential for underdosage ("cold spots"). Further, this

TABLE 97.17

BIOCHEMICAL OUTCOMES AFTER COMBINED HIGH-DOSE-RATE (HDR) BRACHYTHERAPY AND EXTERNAL-BEAM RADIOTHERAPY (EBRT)

Study (Ref.) Series	No. of Patients	Median Follow-Up (mo)	Treatment Regimen	PSA Outcome According to Prognostic Risk Grouping
Vargas et al.[201]	560	51	Median HDR, 23 Gy Median EBRT, 42 Gy	High risk with ADT, 84% High risk without ADT, 81%
Galalae et al.[196]	611	60	Seattle, 3-4 Gy × 4 Kiel, 9 Gy × 2 Beaumont, 5.5–11 Gy × 2	Low, 96% Intermediate, 88% High, 69%
Demanes et al.[196]	209	87	6 Gy × 4, HDR + 36 Gy EBRT	Low, 90% Intermediate, 87% High, 69%
Yamada et al.[199]	105	44	5.5–6.5 Gy × 3, HDR + 50.4 Gy IMRT	Low, 100% Intermediate, 98% High, 92%
Phan et al.[200]	309	59	8 Gy × 4, HDR 39.6–45 Gy EBRT	Low, 98% Intermediate, 90% High, 78%
Hoskin et al.[202]	109	30	8.5 Gy × 2, HDR 37.5 Gy EBRT	Low, 100% Intermediate, 90% High, 81%
Deger et al.[198]	442	60	10 Gy × 2 40 Gy EBRT	Low, 80% Intermediate, 65% High, 58%
Pellizzon et al.[203]	119	41	4 Gy × 4–5, HDR 45 Gy EBRT	Low risk, 78% High risk, 76%

PSA, prostate-specific antigen; ADT, androgen deprivation therapy; IMRT, intensity-modulated radiation therapy.

technique reduces radiation exposure to the radiation oncologist and others involved in the procedure compared with permanent interstitial implantation. Finally, HDR brachytherapy boosts may be radiobiologically more efficacious in terms of tumor cell kill for patients with increased tumor bulk or adverse prognostic features compared with low-dose-rate boosts such as ^{125}I or ^{103}Pd.

Morbidity of HDR Temporary Prostate Brachytherapy

The acute and late morbidity reported following HDR is summarized in Table 97.18. The most common late GU morbidity is the development of urethral stricture. Most series have observed that urethral strictures are more common in men with a history of previous TURP. In most cases the strictures can be managed with dilation in the office or in the outpatient surgical setting. Late GI morbidity can take the form of rectal bleeding, rectal ulcer, or (in rare cases) prostatorectal fistulae.

ANDROGEN DEPRIVATION AND RADIATION THERAPY

ADT in conjunction with radiotherapy is routinely recommended for patients with locally advanced prostate cancer. Randomized trials have demonstrated improved outcomes, including an overall survival benefit compared with radiotherapy alone. In addition, studies have demonstrated that ADT can improve local eradication of the locally advanced tumors by reducing the size of the mass or the concurrent elimination of tumor clonogens inherently resistant to radiotherapy, or both. ADT can effectively reduce the size of larger prostate volumes by 30% to 40%, thereby improving the ability to deliver maximal radiation dose levels without exceeding the tolerance of the surrounding normal tissues. This section will outline the putative mechanisms of benefit for ADT with radiotherapy, summarize the results of published randomized trials, and highlight the indications for its use in clinical practice.

Randomized Trials

Randomized trials have demonstrated improved outcomes when ADT is combined with EBRT delivered at dose levels of 70 Gy (Table 97.19). Several trials have employed adjuvant hormonal therapy for various durations after EBRT and demonstrated long-term disease-free survival benefits. RTOG 85-31 randomized patients with clinical stage T3 as well as patients with T1-T2 disease with lymphadenopathy. In this trial, ADT was administered during the last week of radiotherapy and continued indefinitely. With a median follow-up of 7.6 years, a survival benefit was noted for patients treated with long-term ADT compared with radiotherapy alone.[1] Note that the radiation-only arm was treated with hormonal therapy at the time of clinical evidence of relapse. It appeared that the survival benefit was derived in particular from patients with higher grades of disease (Gleason score ≥8). It should be noted that while the intent in the ADT cohort was for the therapy to continue indefinitely, the median duration of ADT usage was 2.2 years (range, 1 day to 13.5 years). Patients who remained on ADT for 5 or more years experienced improved

TABLE 97.18

LATE TOXICITY OUTCOMES AFTER COMBINED HIGH-DOSE-RATE (HDR) BRACHYTHERAPY AND EXTERNAL-BEAM RADIOTHERAPY

Study (Ref.) Series	No. of Patients	Median Follow-Up (y)	Late Genitourinary Toxicity	Late Gastrointestinal Toxicity
Galalae et al.[196]	144	8	Grade 2, 4% Grade 3, 2% Incontinence, 6% (8 of 9 had TURP before or after HDR)	Grade 2, 7% Grade 3, 4%
Deger et al.[198]	442	5	Grade 3, 9% (urethral strictures) Urinary incontinence, 2% Grade 4, 1%	—
Martinez et al.[407]	207	4.4	Grade 3, 8% (urethral strictures) Grade 4, 0	Grade 3, 0.5% Grade 4, 0.5%
Pellizzon et al.[203]	119	3.4	Grade ≤2, 4.6% Grade 3–4, 0	Grade ≤2, 12% Grade 3–4, 0%
Yamada et al.[199]	105	4	Grade 2, 2% Grade 3, 2% (urethral strictures) Grade 4, 0	Grade 1–2, 7% Grade 3–4, 0%
Phan et al.[200]	309	5	Grade 2, 15% Grade 3, 4% (urethral strictures)	Grade 1–2, 4% Grade 4, <1%
Demanes et al.[197]	209	7.25	Grade 2, 8% Grade 3, 7% (urethral strictures) Grade 4, 1%	Grade 1–2, 2% Grade 3–4, 0

TURP, transurethral resection of the prostate.

overall survival and disease-free survival outcomes compared with those patients with shorter ADT duration times.[206]

Another important randomized trial, European Organisation for Research and Treatment of Cancer (EORTC) 22863, assessed the role of adjuvant ADT among node-negative patients with clinical stage T3 disease or T1-T2 patients with high-grade disease. Adjuvant ADT was initiated on the first day of radiotherapy and continued for 3 years. In an update of the outcome, with a median follow-up of 66 months, improved outcomes in all parameters, including absolute survival, were observed.[207]

Neoadjuvant and concurrent ADT in conjunction with EBRT has been shown to improve outcomes in RTOG 86-10. In that study, patients with bulky, locally advanced tumors were randomized to 2 months of ADT prior to radiotherapy and 2 months during treatment compared with radiotherapy alone. The 10-year long-term outcomes including cause-specific mortality, distant-metastases-free survival, and biochemical failure outcomes were significantly improved with ADT.[208]

The use of short-term ADT appeared to effectively delay the onset of distant metastases in these high-risk patients. Among patients treated with EBRT alone, 40% of patients developed bone metastases at 5 years after therapy, while among patients treated with combined ADT and radiotherapy it took 13 years for the development of bone metastases for the same percentage of patients. No differences in cardiac related events were observed in the treatment arms.

The optimal duration of adjuvant ADT was evaluated in RTOG 92-02, the first ADT trial performed with baseline PSA information available. In this study, patients with clinical T2-T4 with PSA baseline levels less than 150 ng/mL were randomized to neoadjuvant and concurrent ADT (4 months) and the same therapy in addition to 24 months of adjuvant ADT. With a median follow-up of 5.8 years, patients treated with the longer course of ADT experienced improvement for all end points compared with overall survival. However, in a subset analysis, a 10% overall survival advantage was observed for those patients with Gleason scores 8 to 10 treated with longer-course ADT compared with short-course neoadjuvant and concurrent ADT.[209]

RTOG 94-13 also evaluated two different sequencing regimens of adjuvant ADT as well as the role of pelvic radiotherapy in the setting of treatment with ADT. Eligible patients included those patients with T2c-T4 disease or those with an estimated lymph node risk of 15% or greater. The risk of lymph nodes was estimated using the equation [2/3]PSA + (Gleason score 6) × 10. Patients were randomized to be treated with 4 months of ADT before and during radiotherapy or as adjuvant therapy at the completion of EBRT. Patients were also randomized to whole-pelvic radiotherapy versus treatment directed to the prostate only. The treatment arm associated with the highest progression-free survival outcome was noted for patients treated with neoadjuvant/concurrent ADT in conjunction with whole-pelvic radiotherapy.[115]

Although the previously mentioned studies focused on patients with high-grade disease with advanced clinical stages, more recent studies have explored the role of ADT for patients with earlier stages of disease. D'Amico et al.[210] reported the results of a randomized trial comparing 70 Gy of 3D-CRT alone or similar radiotherapy in combination with 6 months of ADT in which androgen deprivation was initiated 2 months prior to radiotherapy. Of note, patients included in this study were mostly those with intermediate-risk disease, namely pretreatment PSA 10 to 40 ng/mL or Gleason scores more than 7 with T1-T2 disease. With a median follow-up of 4.5 years, an overall 5-year survival advantage was demonstrated for the combination-therapy regimen compared with radiotherapy alone (88% vs. 78%; $P = .04$).

The duration of neoadjuvant ADT was addressed in a multi-institutional phase Canadian study.[211] The 378 accrued patients were randomized to receive 3 months versus 8 months

TABLE 97.19

RANDOMIZED TRIALS INVOLVING HORMONE THERAPY (HT) AND RADIATION THERAPY (RT) FOR LOCALLY ADVANCED PROSTATE CANCER

Trial	Eligibility	Arms	LF (%)	DM (%)	bNED (%)	DFS (%)	OS (%)
RTOG 85-31	T3 (15%) or T1-2, N+ or path T3 and (+) margin or (+) SV	RT (HT @ failure) vs. RT + AHT indefinite	10-y 38 vs. 23 (*P* <.0001)	10-y 39 vs.24 (*P* <.0001)	10-y 9 vs. 31 (*P* <.0001)	10-y 23 vs. 37 (*P* <.0001)	10-y 39 vs. 49 (*P* = .002)
EORTC 22863	T3-4 (89%) or T1-2 WHO 3	RT vs. RT + CAHT 3 y	5-y 16.4 vs. 1.7 (*P* <.0001)	5-y 29.2 vs. 9.8 (*P* <.0001)	5-y 45 vs. 76 (*P* <.0001)	5-y 40 vs. 74 (*P* <.0001)	5-y 62 vs.78 (*P* = .0002)
RTOG 86-10	Bulky T2b, T3-4, N+ allowed	RT vs. RT + NHT (TAB) 3.7 mo	8-y 42 vs. 30 (*P* = .016)	8-y 45 vs. 34 (*P* = .04)	8-y 3 vs. 16 (*P* <.0001)	8-y 69 vs. 77 (*P* = .05)	8-y 44 vs. 53 (*P* = .10)
RTOG 92-02	T2c-4 w/PSA <150, N+ allowed	RT + NHT (TAB) 4 mo vs. RT + NHT + AHT × 28 mo	5-y 12.3 vs. 6.4 (*P* = .0001)	5-y 17 vs. 11.5 (*P* = .0035)	5-y 45.5 vs. 72 (*P* <.0001)	5-y 28.1 vs. 46.4 (*P* <.0001)	5-y 78.5 vs. 80 (*P* = .73)
RTOG 94-13	T2c-4 w/Gleason ≥6, or >15% risk of N+	WP + NHT WP + AHT PO + NHT PO + AHT	4-y 9.1 WP vs. 8.0 PO (*P* = .78)	4-y 8.2 WP vs. 6.6 PO (*P* = .54)	4-y 69.7 63.3 57.2 63.5 (*P* = .048)	4-y 59.6 48.9 44.3 49.8 (*P* = .008)	4-y 84.7 vs.84.3 (*P* = .94)
Brigham and Women's Hospital	PSA ≥10 Gleason ≥7 T1-T2B	RT 70 Gy 30-CRT vs. RT + 6 months	NS	NS		5-y 82% vs. 57% (*P* = .002)	5-y 88% vs.78% (*P* = .04)

LF, local failure; DM, distant metastasis; bNED, biochemical failure-free survival; DFS, disease-free survival; OS, overall survival; RTOG, Radiation Therapy Oncology Group; SV, seminal vesicle; AHT, adjuvant HT; EORTC, European Organisation for Research and Treatment of Cancer; WHO, World Health Organization; CAHT, concurrent adjuvant HT; NHT, neoadjuvant HT; PSA, prostate-specific antigen; TAB, total androgen blockade; WP, whole pelvis; PO, prostate only; CRT, conformal RT.
(Adapted from ref. 408.)

of total androgen blockade. Conventional radiotherapy delivering 66 Gy was initiated within 2 weeks of completion of the ADT regimen. In that trial, 31% of the patients were considered high risk and the remaining patients had low- or intermediate-risk disease. No differences in any of the end points, including biochemical relapse-free survival, were observed.

The various trials have used different sequencing of delivery of ADT and the eligibility criteria were not consistent throughout all the studies. Nevertheless, some broad conclusions can be drawn regarding the optimal integration of ADT with radiotherapy. It would appear that for patients with high-risk cancers, and in particular high-grade cancers, ADT is indicated and longer courses of hormonal therapy appear to provide more benefit. Preliminary results of EORTC phase 3 trial 22961 have been reported.[212] In this study, 970 patients with locally advanced prostate cancer were randomized to receive 6 months versus 3 years of ADT in conjunction with 70 Gy of EBRT. Biochemical control and disease progression-free survival were shorter for patients treated with the 6-month ADT regimen compared with the longer hormonal therapy course. No survival differences have been noted so far between the two treatment arms. These data suggest that, for high-risk patients, longer courses of ADT may be important in the setting of standard-dose EBRT. For patients with lower Gleason scores but with larger-volume disease, or in select patients with intermediate-risk disease, a shorter course of 6 months may be sufficient to provide a significant clinical benefit.

As all the previously mentioned trials used only doses of radiotherapy of 70 Gy or less, the role of ADT in the setting of an escalated dose of radiotherapy of more than 75.6 Gy remains uncertain. Although a component of benefit of ADT can be the control of low-volume micrometastatic disease, a significant aspect can be related to the improved local tumor eradication radiotherapy in conjunction with ADT functioning as a radiosensitizer. Higher doses of radiotherapy have been shown to improve local tumor control, and such doses may obviate the need for ADT. Nevertheless, in the absence of a randomized trial, total avoidance of ADT in high-risk patients is uncertain. Additional unanswered questions include the optimal duration of adjuvant and neoadjuvant therapy and the necessity of total androgen blockage versus the use of a luteinizing hormone-releasing hormone (LHRH) analogue alone.

Finally, there is increasing awareness of a possible association between the use of ADT and the subsequent risk of congestive heart failure or myocardial infarction. Although in many of the previously mentioned randomized trials there have been no reports of increased cardiac related events, in the Dana Farber study a loss of survival benefit with ADT in unfavorable-risk prostate cancer was observed among patients with moderate to severe medical/cardiac-related comorbidities. In a recent report of 5,077 men treated with brachytherapy, the use of a 4-month course of ADT was associated with an increased risk of all-cause mortality among those with a history of coronary artery disease–induced heart failure of myocardial infarction. The impact of longer courses of ADT among patients with moderate or severe comorbidities is unclear. In addition, these data suggest that the use of ADT in favorable-risk patients, in whom its oncologic benefit is unproven, should be carefully considered, in particular among patients with severe cardiac comorbidities because of its potential morbidity.[213] Future well-designed prospective studies will be needed to elucidate these issues.

The role of ADT in combination with brachytherapy is uncertain and its advantage has been justified based on extrapolations from randomized trials of patients treated with EBRT. Several reports[201,214,215] have suggested that in the setting of brachytherapy (low-dose-rate or HDR brachytherapy boosts), the incremental advantage of ADT to further improve outcomes may be less important compared with EBRT, while others[168] have suggested a benefit for higher-risk patients. It is possible that the primary advantage of ADT is to act as a radiosensitizer with EBRT when lower radiation doses such as 70 Gy are used as the standard dose in the randomized trials. When higher radiation doses have been used or with incorporation of brachytherapy boosts, several retrospective reports could not find a benefit for hormones except in high-grade, high-risk patients. In the absence of randomized trials, it would therefore be reasonable to recommend the use of ADT in high-risk patients even when higher radiation doses are employed.

ADJUVANT RADIATION THERAPY FOR HIGH-RISK PATIENTS AFTER RADICAL PROSTATECTOMY

Adjuvant Radiotherapy

Randomized Studies

The long-term results of Southwest Oncology Group (SWOG) trial 8794 have demonstrated a survival benefit for the use of adjuvant radiotherapy in high-risk patients after RP. This study included 425 patients with high-risk localized disease who were randomized to receive 60 to 64 Gy to the prostatic fossa versus only observation.[216]

Among patients treated with adjuvant radiotherapy, the 10-year distant-metastases-free survival outcomes and overall survival outcomes were 71% and 74% compared with 61% and 66% for the observation arm (P = .01; hazard ratio, 0.71 and 0.72, respectively). The median follow-up time for this report was 14 years. It is interesting to note that the differences between the treatment groups were detected only after 10 years, highlighting the importance of long-term follow-up in these patients (Fig. 97.10).

The EORTC Trial 22911 included 1,005 patients with positive surgical margins or pT3 (ECE and SVI) disease and randomized them to adjuvant EBRT (50 Gy to the prostatic fossa and periprostatic tissue plus a 10- to 14-Gy boost to the prostatic fossa only) versus no immediate treatment.[217] With the use of adjuvant irradiation, 5-year biochemical progression-free survival improved from 52.6% to 74% (P <.0001). Clinical progression-free survival was also significantly improved from 78% to 85% (P = .0009). The cumulative rate of locoregional failure was significantly lower in the irradiated

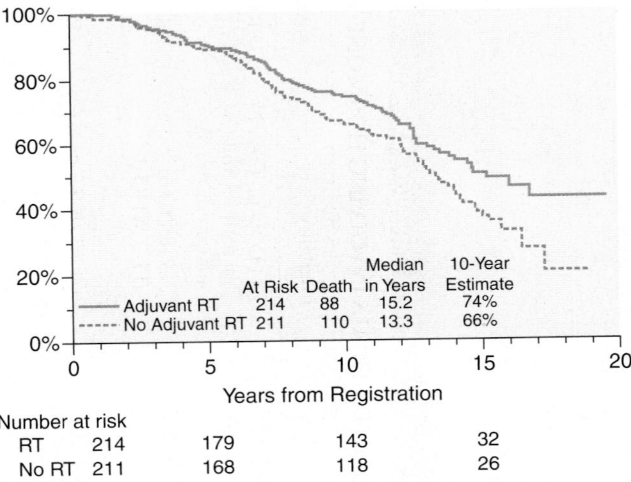

FIGURE 97.10 Overall survival advantage demonstrated for high-risk postoperative patients receiving adjuvant radiation therapy versus observation in the SWOG 8794 trial. (From ref. 130, with permission.)

group (P <.0001). Similar results were observed in a phase 3 German trial (ARO 96-02) that randomized pathologic T3 prostate with postoperative undetectable PSA levels to adjuvant radiotherapy or observation.[218] The 5-year PSA relapse-free survival outcomes for those who received adjuvant radiotherapy was 72% compared to 54% for the observation arm (P = .0015). No survival benefits have been observed in these latter two trials, yet the follow-up times were 5 years or less and may not be long enough to observe such differences.

These trials provide evidence that adjuvant postprostatectomy irradiation reduces the risk of tumor recurrence and distant metastases, and in one trial improved survival was demonstrated. It still remains uncertain whether administration of radiation to patients on immediate detectability of the PSA could provide equally effective long-term outcomes to patients receiving adjuvant therapy while sparing such patients from unnecessary irradiation. To address this issue, the RADICALS trial is currently randomizing patients to immediate radiotherapy versus salvage radiotherapy on detectability of the PSA during follow-up observations.

Role of ADT in Combination with Adjuvant Radiotherapy

To date, limited information is available concerning the role of ADT in combination with adjuvant radiotherapy in the postprostatectomy setting. In study RTOG 85-31, a subset analysis of postprostatectomy patients revealed a better biochemical failure-free survival for patients treated with immediate LHRH analogue, without, however, an impact on survival.[219] RTOG-0534 is currently accruing patients with a rising PSA after prostatectomy to radiotherapy alone to the prostate bed, radiotherapy to the prostate bed plus 4 to 6 months of ADT, and radiotherapy to the pelvis and prostate bed in combination with 6 months of ADT. In addition, the previously mentioned RADICALS study incorporates a second randomization of all patients that would explore the role of ADT in the setting of salvage or adjuvant therapy. Randomized patients who are to be treated with immediate radiotherapy versus delayed salvage therapy would be further randomized to radiotherapy alone, radiotherapy plus 6 months of ADT, or radiotherapy plus adjuvant ADT for 2 years. The results from these studies should help clarify these important issues.

Optimal Radiation Dose

To date there is no established consensus regarding the optimal prescription dose for adjuvant radiotherapy in the postprostatectomy setting. Petrovich et al.[220,221] have indicated that even low doses in the range of 45 to 50 Gy are beneficial in terms of local control and disease-free survival. The positive findings of the EORTC study have been obtained with a prescription dose of 60 Gy with conventional irradiation over 6 weeks.[222]

Based on American Society of Therapeutic Radiation Oncology recommendations, a dose of 64 Gy or higher (with conventional fractionation) should be prescribed.[222] Valicenti et al.[223] have demonstrated evidence of improved biochemical outcomes using higher radiation doses. Despite higher doses, in fact, treatment is generally well tolerated with minimal late severe toxicity.[224]

MANAGEMENT OF THE RISING PSA AFTER DEFINITIVE LOCAL THERAPY

Given the advent of PSA detecting, a substantial number of patients have PSA progression as an only manifestation of relapse after definitive local therapies. Patients failing RP may be candidates for potentially curative salvage radiation[225] and this approach should be strongly considered for patients with an undetectable PSA postsurgery followed by a PSA rise (see "Salvage Radiotherapy after Radical Prostatectomy"). Patients failing radiation may be candidates for salvage radical prostatectomies, salvage cryotherapy, or brachytherapy. Those who are not candidates for definitive salvage therapies might be considered for surveillance or ADT. No randomized trials have been conducted in this setting; thus, treatment options are based on less-than-optimal information.

Prognosis

For the patient with a rising PSA post-RP, studies from Johns Hopkins University have indicated that the consequences of a rising PSA may be less harmful than anticipated for most patients. In studies conducted in patients without androgen deprivation, median time to metastatic disease was 8 years and median survival was 13 years.[225] Importantly, these and other studies have linked survival to several factors, the most important of which is PSADT.[226,227] PSADTs of more than 15 months are rarely associated with prostate-cancer specific mortality whereas PSADTs of less than 3 months are almost invariably associated with death from prostate cancer, with a median survival of 5 to 6 years (Fig. 97.10). Using PSADT as a stratification variable, one can make reasonable but imperfect prognostications for patients with various rates of PSA rise. The majority of deaths from prostate cancer in this setting are associated with PSADTs of less than 9 months. For PSADTs of greater than 15 months, non–prostate cancer deaths vastly predominate.[227] Gleason score and time of recurrence are covariates in some but not all studies evaluating PSADT. Higher Gleason scores and shorter time to recurrence after definitive therapies are associated with worse prognosis. PSADT has also been shown to be of fundamental importance in the prognosis of patients initially treated with radiation as well as RP.[228] To avoid overtreatment, risk stratification by PSADT should be performed prior to ADT and consideration may be given to avoiding the side effects of treatment for patients with slower PSADT, especially those with comorbidities or who are older.

Many factors need to be taken into consideration prior to determining a reliable PSADT. These factors include prior/current treatments, the absolute PSA level, the number of PSA determinations, the timing of the PSA determinations, consistency of assays, and (in nonsurgically treated patients) noncancerous factors capable of influencing PSA levels. Patients treated with surgery have different expected posttreatment PSA levels than those treated with other modalities. Radiation therapies, particularly brachytherapy, may be associated with PSA "bounces" that do not represent cancerous relapse.[229] Because PSAs are influenced by testosterone levels as a consequence of an androgen response element in the PSA promoter,[230] measurement of circulating testosterone is recommended for those having received prior ADT.

PSADTs are not reliable unless stable testosterones are present and drugs that influence the androgen axis (5α-reductase inhibitors, antiandrogens) are discontinued and their influences abated. Reliability of PSADT may also be compromised in patients with PSA levels of less than 0.2 ng/mL, those using more than one assay to determine PSA levels (interassay variations can be problematic), and those with short follow-up. A minimum of three PSA determinations over 3 months or more is suggested to assess doubling times in most patients. PSADT is typically calculated as the natural logarithm of 2 divided by the slope obtained from fitting a linear regression of the natural log of PSA on time. PSADT calculators are available on readily accessible Websites such as http://www.mskcc.org/mskcc/applications/nomograms/PSADoublingTime.aspx.

Most patients with a PSA less than 10 ng/mL postsurgery will have negative bone and CT scans. In fact, when examining postsurgically treated patients, investigators have reported the probability of a positive bone scan as being less than 5% until PSA increased to 40 to 45 ng/mL.[231,232] Nomograms have been constructed to predict probability of metastatic disease for patients in the recurrent PSA setting after surgery. PSA velocity, PSA slope, and PSA value at the time of the scan are several variables implicated in predicting bone scan positivity during this disease state.

Treatment

Salvage Radiotherapy after Radical Prostatectomy

Numerous nonrandomized studies have shown favorable outcomes with salvage EBRT.[224,233–238] Surgical Gleason score, SVI, absolute pre-RT PSA level, and pre-RT PSADT have all been shown to increase the likelihood of subsequent biochemical failure and disease progression.[237] These factors should be considered for the appropriate choice of salvage therapy (i.e., local only, local and systemic, or systemic only). In general, better results with salvage radiotherapy have been achieved when pre-RT PSA values are less than 0.5 ng/mL and, likely, as soon as relapse is indicated by a PSA elevation.[224,235–236]

Katz et al.[224] analyzed 115 patients who received salvage radiotherapy for a rising PSA following RP in search of predictors of subsequent PSA failure. The 4-year progression-free survival was 46%. Multivariate analysis, which was limited to 70 patients without neoadjuvant hormonal manipulation, showed that negative margins (P = .03), absence of ECE (P <.01), and presence of SVI (P <.01) were independent predictors of PSA relapse following RT. Among patients with positive margins and no poor prognostic features, 77% achieved PSA control after salvage 3D-CRT.

Stephenson et al.[236] reported on a large retrospective analysis of salvage irradiation of 501 patients from 5 institutions. At a median follow-up of 45 months, approximately 50% of patients treated had disease progression. The 4-year progression-free probability was 45%. Better outcomes were achieved among patients with favorable risk features, which included positive surgical margins, Gleason scores less than 8, and PSADTs less than 10 months. In such patients, PSA relapse-free survival outcomes were in the range of 70% to 80% at 5 years. Ongoing trials in RTOG are now assessing the role of ADT in combination with radiation in the salvage setting.

The efficacy of salvage EBRT alone for clinically palpable local disease is suboptimal given the greater tumor volume that requires treatment.[237,238] It may be prudent to consider neoadjuvant and concurrent ADT in such patients, extrapolating from randomized trials showing the benefit of ADT in patients treated with the prostate intact. Further studies are needed in this setting.

Salvage Surgery after Radiotherapy Failure

Salvage RP is technically challenging. Reported short-term and long-term complication rates exceed those of standard RP, but with appropriate patient selection and surgical expertise, this procedure has become less hazardous for the patient. Overall, mean estimated blood loss and operative time do not differ significantly from the values for standard RP.

The MSKCC group has performed more than 120 salvage RPs. Salvage surgery can be safely performed after failed EBRT, brachytherapy (open or ultrasound-guided), or combinations of these techniques. Most of these patients (90%) were treated with a retropubic approach, although early in the series we combined abdominoperineal approach for selected patients (10%) who had had open brachytherapy and pelvic lymphadenectomy. Early in our series (before 1995), the mean estimated blood loss, transfusion requirements, and average hospital stay were greater than for standard RP. This is attributable to both the relative inexperience with the surgical approach at that time as well as the fact that most of these patients had undergone prior open pelvic surgery. In the past 10 years, however, the morbidity of the operation has improved substantially. Rectal injuries occurred in 12% of patients we treated before 1995 at MSKCC, but are now rare. With full bowel preparation before the operation, rectal injuries can be repaired primarily without altering postoperative recovery. Using current surgical techniques, salvage RP is technically feasible, with intraoperative and immediate postoperative outcomes similar to those with standard RP.

Despite these improvements in results of salvage RP, long-term complications remain high. Bladder neck contractures have continued to be problematic. Approximately 20% of contemporary patients in our series have developed an anastomotic stricture. Although risk factors for urinary incontinence have not been specifically examined after salvage surgery, the development of an anastomotic stricture is a risk factor for urinary incontinence after standard RP.[239] Careful attention to surgical detail, with a mucosa-to-mucosa anastomosis, is critical to preventing an anastomotic stricture.

In addition, the risk of urinary incontinence remains high. For the entire series of patients undergoing salvage RP at MSKCC, the overall rate (95% CIs) of recovery of urinary control was 62% (49%–75%). For the period before 1995, 57% (39%–75%) of patients recovered urinary control, while after 1995 the rate of recovery improved to 74% (54%–94%). This likely reflects not only an improvement in surgical technique, but better targeted radiation therapies leading to better preservation of the sphincteric mechanism. An artificial urinary sphincter and/or sling procedure has been performed in 20% of patients.

Cancer control outcomes from several salvage RP series are summarized in Table 97.20. For patients treated with salvage RP, the 15-year nonprogression rate was 29% and the 15-year cancer-specific survival rate was 64%. The 5-year actuarial

TABLE 97.20

OUTCOMES AFTER SALVAGE RADICAL PROSTATECTOMY

Study (Ref.)	No. of Patients	Clinical Stage	Nonprogression Rate (%)		Clinical Nonprogression Rate (%)		Cancer-Specific Survival Rate (%)	
			5-Year	10-Year	5-Year	10-Year	5-Year	10-Year
Rogers et al.	38	T1-3N0MX	55	33	83	67	95	87
Amling et al.[409]	108	T1b-N+	70	44	—	42	90	60
Gheiler et al.[410]	40	T2-3N0	47	—	88	—	—	—
Bianco et al.[411]	106	T1-3 N0NX	61	43	90	81	99	94

nonprogression rate was 86% for patients with organ-confined cancer (pT2N0), 61% for those with ECE, and 48% for those with SVI.

Alternative Salvage Therapies

Concerns regarding the risk of urinary incontinence and anastomotic stricture after salvage RP have prompted the search for less invasive salvage therapies. The primary goal of any salvage local therapy for radiation-recurrent prostate cancer is to provide a durable cure; the prevention of symptomatic local and systemic progression is a secondary objective. As such, the oncologic efficacy of any treatment is judged by the ability of that treatment to accomplish these goals. It is difficult to assess the outcomes of most currently available salvage therapies because of a lack of long-term outcome data and/or the small sample sizes reported in published series.[240] Although each of these ablative salvage therapies (high-intensity focused ultrasound [HIFU],[241,242] brachytherapy,[243–245] and cryotherapy[246–250]) can be safely delivered, information regarding the benefit they provide in terms of cancer control is limited.

Salvage Brachytherapy

Initial efforts to use brachytherapy in the salvage setting were restricted because of concerns for treatment-related complications. More recently, however, improvements in imaging, dosimetry, and approaches (including HDR brachytherapy) have significantly lowered the risks of treatment-related complications to an acceptable level.[251] Similar to other salvage therapies, patients undergoing salvage treatment should have histologically confirmed local recurrence, no clinical or radiologic evidence of distant disease, adequate urinary function, age and overall health indicative of more than a 5- to 10-year life expectancy, prolonged disease-free interval (>2 years) from primary radiotherapy, and long PSADT (>6 to 9 months) at the time of recurrence. Additionally, it is suggested that salvage brachytherapy should be avoided in patients with evidence of SVI recurrence and extracapsular disease as these patients are poorly treated in the conventional setting.[251] There is emerging evidence to suggest that salvage HDR brachytherapy, however, may be effective in higher-risk patients.[245]

Permanent interstitial seed implantation has been used in the salvage setting after primary radiotherapy failure[243,251–253] and have reported 5- to 10-year PSA relapse-free survival outcomes that have ranged from 10% to 53%. Recently, investigators from Mt. Sinai Medical Center reported on 37 patients who were treated for local failure after prostate radiotherapy. With a median follow-up of 86 months, the 10-year PSA-relapse-free survival and cause-specific survival outcomes were 54% and 96%, respectively. Multivariate analysis demonstrated that pre-salvage PSA levels of less than 6 ng/mL were associated with improved biochemical tumor control.[254]

Preliminary results have been reported with HDR brachytherapy in the salvage setting. Lee et al.[245] reported on 21 patients with biopsy-proven prostate recurrence after radiotherapy treated with HDR brachytherapy delivering 36 Gy in six fractions using two TRUS-guided HDR prostate implants, separated by 1 week. The 2-year PSA relapse-free survival outcome was 89%. With a median follow-up of 19 months, no patient developed a local or distant recurrence. Both patients with biochemical failure had PSA nadirs 1 ng/mL or more.[245]

Caution and meticulous care in treatment planning is necessary when considering repeat irradiation, especially in the setting of prior high-dose EBRT. In one report, the incidence of complications included urinary retention (14%), hematuria (4%), dysuria (6%), rectal ulcers (4%), and rectal bleeding (2%). Beyer[251,252] reported a 24% rate of incontinence at 5 years following salvage brachytherapy and Wong et al.[255] noted that 8 of the 17 (47%) patients developed grade 3 or 4 GU complications, highlighting the potential side effect profile associated with this treatment. In the previously mentioned salvage HDR series, 14% of patients had grade 3 GU toxicities and 10% had grade 3 sexual dysfunction following HDR brachytherapy. No patients developed grade 3 GI toxicities or any grade 4 toxicities.[245]

Salvage Cryotherapy

With the development of second- and third-generation probes, real-time TRUS for intraoperative monitoring, thermocouplers, and urethral warmers, cryotherapy is potentially less toxic and a feasible alternative as a salvage local therapy after radiation failure. Ideally, prostate volumes for salvage cryotherapy should be 20 to 30 g. Prostate glands more than 60 g and those patients with history of TURP are at an increased risk for urethral sloughing and urinary retention, and should therefore be avoided. Current published cryotherapy series report biochemical disease-free survival rates ranging from 34% to 98%.[256–261]

As expected, cryotherapy in the salvage setting carries a higher morbidity than primary cryotherapy. In early series, treatment-associated complications were significant: urinary incontinence (73%), obstructive symptoms (67%), impotence (72%), and severe perineal pain (8%).[259] Many of the refinements in technique have reduced the morbidity from the procedure. Rectourethral fistulas, the most serious complication following cryotherapy, are relatively uncommon (0% to 4%). Currently reported long-term complications following salvage cryotherapy include erectile dysfunction (77%–100%), rectal pain (10%–40%), urinary incontinence (4%–20%), urinary retention (0%–7%), and urethral sloughing (0%–5%).[256–259,261]

Longer-term outcomes with salvage cryotherapy have recently been reported. Ng et al.[246] assessed the efficacy of salvage cryotherapy in 187 patients with locally recurrent prostate cancer after radiotherapy. Approximately three-quarters of these patients received 3 or more months of neoadjuvant ADT. The mean follow-up period was 39 months. Biochemical recurrence was defined as nadir PSA level plus 2 ng/mL (Phoenix definition). Patients with precryotherapy PSA levels of less than 4 ng/mL had 5- and 8-year biochemical recurrence-free survival rates of 56% and 37%, respectively. In contrast, patients with precryotherapy PSA levels of 10 or more ng/mL had 5- and 8-year biochemical recurrence-free survival rates of only 1% and 7%, respectively. The four-quadrant positive prostate biopsy rate after salvage cryotherapy was 17%. Serum PSA level immediately prior to salvage cryotherapy was a predictive factor for biochemical recurrence, according to multivariate analyses. The investigators recommended that salvage cryotherapy should be performed when serum PSA level is still relatively low because the procedure may potentially be curative in these patients.

Pisters et al.[247] retrospectively compared treatment outcomes between 42 patients undergoing salvage RP and 56 patients receiving salvage cryotherapy at two large cancer centers. Eligibility criteria were locally recurrent prostate cancer after radiotherapy, PSA less than 10 ng/mL, post-RT biopsy Gleason score 8 or less, and prior radiotherapy alone (i.e., no presalvage or postsalvage hormonal therapy). Biochemical failure was assessed using two criteria: (1) PSA more than 0.4 ng/mL and (2) two increases above the postsalvage therapy nadir PSA. Mean follow-up was 7.8 years for the salvage RP group and 5.5 years for the salvage cryotherapy group. Compared with salvage cryotherapy, salvage RP resulted in superior biochemical disease-free survival at 5 years by both definitions of biochemical failure (PSA >0.4 ng/mL, salvage cryotherapy 21% vs. salvage RP 61%, $P < .001$; two increases above nadir, salvage cryotherapy 42% vs. salvage RP 66%, $P = .002$). Salvage RP also resulted in superior overall survival at 5 years (salvage cryotherapy 85% vs. salvage RP 95%, $P = .001$). After adjusting for post-RT biopsy Gleason sum and presalvage treatment PSA, on multivariate analysis salvage RP remained superior to salvage cryotherapy for the end points of any increase in PSA more than 0.4 ng/mL (hazard ratio [HR], 0.24; $P < .0001$), two increases in PSA (HR, 0.47; $P = .02$), and overall survival (HR, 0.21; $P = .01$). The authors suggest that young, healthy patients with recurrent prostate cancer after radiotherapy should consider salvage RP because it offers superior biochemical disease-free survival and may potentially offer the best chance of cure. Further studies are required to appropriately select candidates for salvage ablative therapies and to determine the long-term oncologic efficacy of these treatments.

Salvage High-Intensity Focused Ultrasound

HIFU is a local ablative technology that causes tissue damage through focused ultrasound generating intense heat in targeted areas. Although HIFU was originally designed to treat BPH, HIFU is now being used in Europe for the treatment of both primary and salvage prostate cancers.[242,262,263] Prolonged urinary retention secondary to edema and/or urethral sloughing has been the most common complications following primary HIFU treatment. Therefore, many of the current HIFU techniques include a preprocedural TURP. Additional adaptations that have reduced morbidity include the use of thermocouplers and higher frequency transducers, preservation of a 5-mm apical margin to prevent stress urinary incontinence, and rectal cooling devices that prevent rectourethral fistulas, the most devastating of all treatment-related complications. Reported long-term complications following salvage HIFU include rectourethral fistulas (6%), incontinence (35%), rectal or perineal pain (3%), and bladder neck contractures or urethral strictures (17%).[242]

Zacharakis et al.[241] reviewed 31 patients treated with post-RT salvage HIFU between 2005 and 2007. Side effects included stricture or necrotic tissue in 11 of the 31 patients (36%), urinary tract infection or dysuria syndrome in 8 (26%), and urinary incontinence in 2 (7%). Prostate-rectal fistula occurred in two patients (7%). After a mean follow-up of 7.4 months (range, 3–24 months), half of the patients had PSA levels of less than 0.2 ng/mL and 71% had no evidence of disease. The investigators concluded that salvage HIFU is a minimally invasive outpatient procedure that can achieve low PSA nadirs and good cancer control in the short term, with morbidity comparable to other forms of salvage treatment. Gelet et al.[242] reported their experience treating 71 patients with salvage HIFU after EBRT. Mean follow-up was 14.8 months (range, 6–86 months). Efficacy was assessed by posttreatment biopsy; 57 patients (80%) had a negative biopsy. A nadir PSA level of less than 0.5 ng/mL was achieved in 43 of 71 patients (61%) within 3 months. At the last follow-up, 31 patients (44%) had no evidence of disease progression. Whether the results of salvage HIFU are durable awaits further follow-up, but these short-term oncologic outcomes seem inferior to salvage RP.

ADT for PSA Relapse

Other than definitive local salvage therapies, treatment in the ADT-naive patient with a rising PSA and no metastatic disease is one of the most controversial events in prostate cancer. This controversy arises from lack of data and the more recent understanding of ADT-associated toxicities; no randomized ADT trials are available in this setting.

Retrospective series preliminarily indicate that time to castrate-refractory disease may be quite prolonged for those individuals treated for a rising PSA with ADT. Data from a retrospective series of 355 surgically treated patients treated with ADT for PSA recurrence indicate that median time to development of metastases was 12.4 years after starting ADT.[264] Prospective data for this population are not available. Although median time to prostate cancer–specific mortality has not been determined, PSADT of less than 3 months, PSA nadir of 0.2 ng/mL or more, and PSA prior to initiation of ADT were factors associated with higher risk of prostate cancer death.[265]

Additional retrospective data to support the importance of PSA nadir post-ADT are derived from patients with a PSA rise post-RP, or radiation and no radiologic evidence of metastases. In this population, a PSA nadir of more than 0.2 ng/mL within 8 months of androgen suppression is associated with a 20-fold greater risk of prostate cancer–specific mortality as compared with those patients with a PSA nadir of 0.2 ng/mL or less.[266] This observation has interested clinical trialists, who now have an early prognostic marker to identify those individuals with an increased risk for prostate cancer death.

Data from another large series of patients with PSA recurrence after surgery (n = 1,352) indicated that patients with a PSADT of less than 12 months or a Gleason sum of more than 7 are less likely to develop bone metastatic disease if initially treated with ADT while PSAs are less than 5 ng/mL.[266] The analysis examined various PSA cutpoints and found that initiating treatment when PSAs are less than 1, less than 2, less than 3, or less than 4 ng/mL did not result in differences in time to bone metastasis as compared with those patients with PSAs higher; however, the investigators did report that initiating ADT when PSA cutpoints were less than 5 or less than 10 ng/mL did have a statistically improved time to bone metastasis. Of note, if the data were analyzed to look at all 1,352 patients in a similar manner, no differences in outcome were reported with earlier versus later ADT. Thus, just the subset of men with a post-RP Gleason score of 8 or higher or PSADT less than 12 months had better outcomes with earlier ADT. This study is subject to many biases associated with retrospective studies, and bone scans were not performed at regular intervals during these studies.

For patients with adverse prognostic findings and a rising PSA after definitive therapy, chemotherapy has been safely used in conjunction with ADT[267] but the best chemotherapeutic approaches, timing in relation to ADT (before, during, or after), and benefits are conjectural at this point. Intermittent, as opposed to continuous, hormonal therapy may be a way to diminish morbidity of ADT in this setting (as previously discussed), but the benefits of no therapy until metastatic disease versus early ADT remains a larger issue for most patients. Future clinical trials will need to risk-stratify patients with regard to important prognostic variables such as PSADT. Although it is conjectural to state that early treatment of patients with a very rapid PSADT leads to benefit, it can be more assuredly stated that treatment of patients with a very prolonged natural history, as evidenced by PSADTs more than 15 months, is unlikely to have a survival benefit; this is particularly true for those patients whose lifespan is limited because of age or comorbidities.

Timing of ADT as Initial Therapy in Asymptomatic Patients

Although considerable controversy and lack of randomized trials have surrounded the issue of ADT timing in patients with a rising PSA after initial treatment with surgery or radiation, a number of randomized trials have examined the issue of ADT as a primary therapy for asymptomatic patients, many of whom had nonmetastatic disease at the time ADT was begun.

The Veterans Administration Research Service Cooperative Urological Research Group (VACURG)[268,269] was the first to perform a randomized study of immediate versus deferred therapy for asymptomatic patients in the pre-PSA era. More than 1,900 patients were evaluated in a randomized trial comparing placebo, placebo plus orchiectomy, diethylstilbestrol at 5 mg/day, or a combination of orchiectomy plus diethylstilbestrol in patients with locally advanced or metastatic disease. In locally advanced disease, estrogen-treated patients fared worse in terms of overall survival, as a consequence of cardiovascular complications. These data, with other VACURG studies, confirmed the toxicity of diethylstilbestrol. For patients with metastatic disease, no differences in overall survival were detected between the groups after 9 years of follow-up.[269]

In a trial offering T2-T4NXMO patients either orchiectomy, radiation, or a combination of both, 277 patients were accrued between 1980 and 1985, and both the orchiectomy-alone and orchiectomy-plus-radiation arms were superior to the radiation-alone arm with respect to metastases-free survival.[270] No treatment differences were detected in either local disease control or overall survival between the various arms in long-term follow-up for this relatively small study.

In a trial conducted between 1988 and 1992 (SAKK 08/88), asymptomatic (except for voiding symptoms) patients deemed unsuitable for local therapies were randomized between immediate versus deferred ADT.[271] One hundred ninety-seven patients were randomized; for the immediate and deferred treatment arms, respectively, median age was 76 and 77 years, and median PSA was 46 and 52. No differences in overall survival or the overall pain-free interval were detected; however, a composite time-to-progression end point comprising time to new metastases, time to ureteric obstruction, and/or time to first pain favored those receiving immediate treatment. Prostate cancer–specific survival was not significantly different between the two arms and 42% of the patients in the deferred treatment arm never required any tumor-specific treatments.

The MRC PR03 trial compared immediate versus deferred treatment for patients with either locally advanced or M1 prostate cancer. Although initially reported as being positive,[272] a more mature analysis demonstrated no overall survival differences between the groups.[272] In the deferred arm, treatment was planned at the time of "clinically significant progression." In the trial, deferred treatment was initiated for local progression almost as frequently as for metastatic disease. Time to death from prostate cancer was improved with immediate treatments but overall patients did not live longer. There may be multiple explanations for these findings. This trial has been criticized because the follow-up was left to the discretion of the treating physicians and consequently was irregular, and at times ADT was begun in the deferred arm quite late, with 29 patients dying from prostate cancer without having received ADT. Benefits of immediate ADT were seen in terms of less frequent TURPs and fewer cases of ureteral obstruction, pathologic fracture, and spinal cord compression. Each of these complications was roughly twice as common in the deferred-treatment arm.[272]

A recent large trial (n = 985) has addressed the question of early versus deferred ADT, specifically in M0 patients.[271] At a median follow-up of 7.8 years, 541 patients had died, mostly from prostate cancer (n = 193) or cardiovascular disease (n = 185). Surprisingly, there was an overall survival benefit from immediate treatment but the prostate cancer–specific mortality was not distinct. Non–prostate cancer deaths were fewer, although of borderline statistical significance ($P = .06$), in the early ADT arm. These findings were unexpected, as benefits of other trials have tended to show cancer-specific but not overall survival improvements. Reasons for the reported findings are not clear, although difficulties in accurate attributions of death cannot be excluded. Of note, after 7 years, only 49.7% of the patients in the deferred arm had begun anticancer therapy, indicating that indiscriminate ADT use in this subset of patients leads to some degree of overtreatment. Although the trial had 7.8 years of follow-up, only 18.8% of patients had died from prostate cancer, again emphasizing the relatively slow progression rates in the setting of M0 disease for many patients (Fig. 97.11).

An important international trial (MRC PR07) comparing ADT plus or minus radiation in patients with T3-T4NOMO disease at diagnosis completed accrual of 1,205 patients in 2002. After a median follow-up of 7.6 years, 79 men in the ADT group and 37 men in the ADT/radiation group died from prostate cancer. At 10 years, the prostate cancer–specific mortality was 23.9% in the endocrine-alone group and 11.9% in the endocrine-plus-RT group, yielding a relative risk of 0.44 (95% CI: 0.30–0.66). At 10 years, the overall mortality was 39.4% in the ADT group and 29.6% in the ADT/radiation group, for a relative risk of 0.68 (95% CI: 0.52–0.89). Urinary, rectal, and sexual problems were slightly more frequent in the group receiving radiation. This trial definitively proved the added value of radiation for men with locally advanced pros-

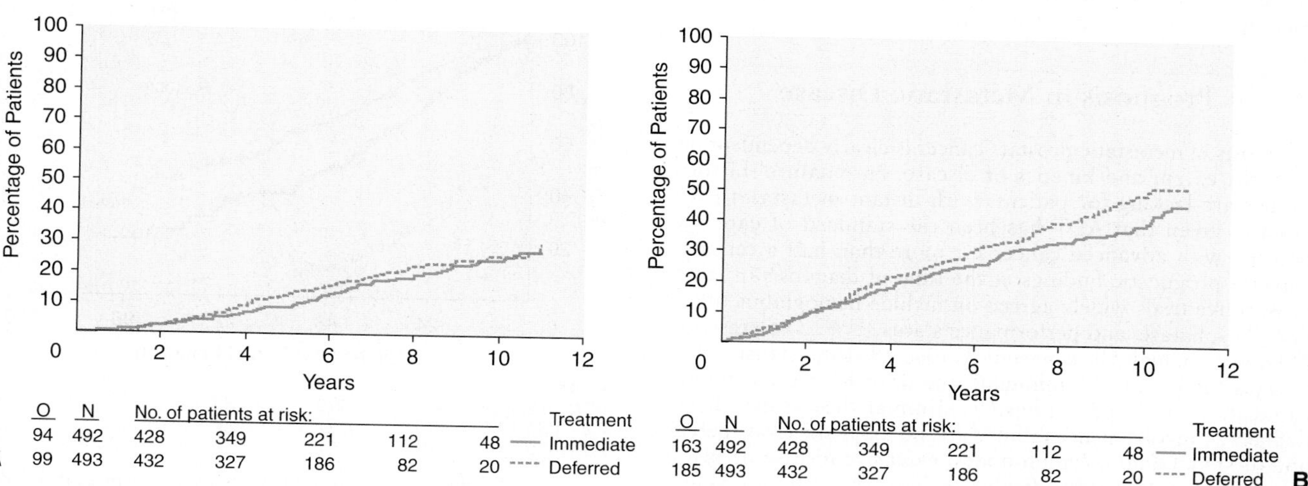

FIGURE 97.11 Immediate versus deferred hormonal therapy in patients with M0 prostate cancer who either refused local therapy or were deemed unsuitable for local therapy. **A:** Prostate cancer-specific survival. **B:** Overall survival. (From ref. 271, with permission.)

tate cancer.[273] Taken together, the question of early versus deferred ADT (until symptoms) remains a valid question using nonestrogenic therapies. One can conclude on the basis of controlled studies that any benefit seen by early ADT is relatively small and that the risks and potential benefits of ADT need to be weighed in individual patients. Several salient points are made by these trials. Men with progressive prostate cancer should be monitored closely, regardless of treatment, as significant complications can develop in a substantial subset of patients. Despite this fact, some men will never develop symptomatic prostate cancer despite having been diagnosed with locally advanced disease. Competing causes of death remain an issue and cardiovascular disease remains a significant issue for men's health throughout the broad spectrum of prostate cancer.

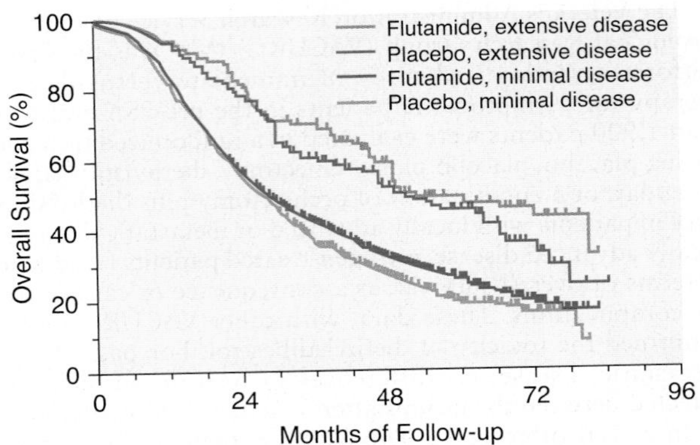

FIGURE 97.12 Overall survival for metastatic prostate cancer patients after treatment by surgical orchiectomy with or without flutamide. Patients are stratified by extensive or minimal disease prior to initiation of therapy. (From ref. 282, with permission.)

MANAGEMENT OF METASTATIC PROSTATE CANCER

Management of metastatic prostate cancer today depends on the same fundamental principles first articulated by Charles Huggins in 1941.[274] At that time, Huggins demonstrated that orchiectomy or estrogens could induce dramatic remissions in patients with advanced prostate cancers and that serum markers could be used to monitor response. These fundamental insights into prostate cancer led to a shared portion of the Nobel Prize in 1966. Toxicities of estrogens, particularly thromboembolic complications at higher doses, were discovered as a consequence of prospective randomized trials performed in the 1960s by the VACURG.[268,269]

Orchiectomy or lower dosages of estrogens were the basic therapies used for most patients with advanced prostate cancer until LHRH agonists were introduced in the 1980s. This advance was enabled by the Nobel Prize–winning work of Andrew Schally,[274] who discovered and characterized LHRH, the hypothalamic peptide responsible for stimulating LH secretion from the pituitary. Shortly thereafter, experiments indicated that sustained LHRH administration led to a paradoxical down-regulation of LH secretion and dramatic testosterone declines. Potent LHRH agonists were developed[275] and, compared with estrogens, LHRH agonists had fewer serious side effects but similar efficacy.[276] Once sustained-release formulations were developed for LHRH, these agents became the preferred choice for treating prostate cancer, as men clearly preferred injections to orchiectomy[277] and the safety profile was superior as compared with estrogens.

Prognosis in Metastatic Disease

Prognosis in metastatic prostate cancer is clearly dependent on both the extent and kinetics of disease. Pure natural history studies are lacking for patients with distant metastases (M1 disease) given that ADT has been the standard of care for patients with advanced cancer for more than half a century. Adverse prognostic findings at the time of diagnosis in large prospective trials widely agreed on include hemoglobin, alkaline phosphatase, and performance status.[278–280] The presence of bone pain, high Gleason sum (Gleason 8–10), extensive disease (as compared with minimal), and prior RP are also implicated in some large studies.[281] Minimal disease has been defined as involvement confined to the axial skeleton (pelvis and/or spine) and/or lymph nodes; extensive disease involves the viscera and/or appendicular skeleton (long bones, skull, ribs plus or minus axial skeleton).

Median progression-free survival (excluding PSA rises as progression) in an overall analysis of orchiectomy-treated M1 patients at the beginning of the PSA era was estimated to be approximately 18.6 months; overall survival was 30 months (Fig. 97.12). For those with minimal disease, median progression-free survival was 46 months and overall survival was 51 months. For those with extensive disease, median progression-free survival was 16 months and overall survival was 27.5 months.[282]

For patients with pelvic node positivity (TXN1MO), studies are available for patients having pathologic confirmation post-RP and "deferred" hormonal therapy. In this setting, without early ADT intervention, about 75% of patients will eventually relapse by 10 years of follow-up.[283,284] Median survival in these patients is greater than 11 years. (See the discussion of adjuvant therapy after RP.)

PSA nadir after ADT has long been known to be a prognostic factor for patients with metastatic disease[285] but a large study in 1,345 patients[286] has quantified this finding and led to a greater appreciation of its importance (Fig. 97.13). For patients initially treated with ADT, failure to achieve a PSA nadir of 4 ng/mL or less within 7 months after initiation of therapy is associated with a very poor prognosis (median survival,

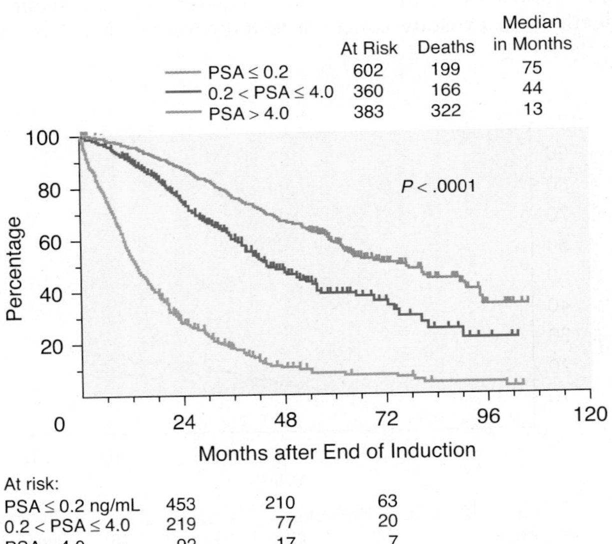

FIGURE 97.13 Percentage of patients with metastatic prostate cancer alive as a function of time stratified by the nadir prostate-specific antigen (PSA) after 7 months of androgen-deprivation therapy. (From ref. 286, with permission.)

approximately 13 months), whereas those patients with a PSA nadir of 0.2 ng/mL or less have a much better prognosis (median survival, 75 months). Patients with a nadir of more than 0.2 and less than 4.0 had an intermediate prognosis (median survival, 44 months). These data clearly support the prognostic importance of the value of the PSA nadir post–androgen suppression in the metastatic patient and suggest that careful PSA monitoring after initiation of hormonal therapy can effectively identify those patients at high risk for early onset of castrate-refractory disease.

The timing of the PSA nadir also conveys prognostic significance in multivariate analyses. In a study examining the time to PSA nadir, those with a PSA nadir occurring less than 6 months post-ADT had a median survival of 4.5 years versus 7.8 years for those with a PSA nadir occurring more than 6 months after ADT initiation.[287]

Hormonal Agents

Two major classes of agents are approved and currently in use in advanced prostate cancer. These include the LHRH analogues and the antiandrogens. Both LHRH agonists and antagonists have been approved by the FDA but the sole approved antagonist is not commercially available; thus, discussion will focus on the agonists alone. We note that bilateral orchiectomy remains a viable option and, although it does not represent the preference of most men, this surgical procedure is relatively inexpensive and extremely reliable in terms of testosterone to the "castrate" range.

Six sustained-release LHRH agonist formulations are currently available in the United States. Three of these products use the same LHRH agonists (leuprolide acetate) but with different methods for achieving sustained release: goserelin acetate, triptorelin pamoate, and histrelin acetate are also FDA-approved in various formulations. Each approved product has demonstrated that levels of less than 50 ng/dL testosterone can be achieved and maintained. No comparative trials have been published with regard to various LHRH agonists but there is no reason to suspect that one agent might be distinct from another in terms of either testosterone or cancer control. One LHRH antagonist is now available and that agent achieves a more rapid rate of testosterone decline,[288] but the clinical consequences of this in most patients is unclear.

Because the LHRH agonists bind and activate the LHRH receptor prior to their sustained effects leading to a receptor down-regulation, the use of all LHRH agonists is associated with an initial transient rise in testosterone that lasts up to 1 week. In patients with advanced metastatic cancer and/or near obstructive lesions, this "flare" may have adverse clinical consequences. Otherwise, for most patients starting treatment today, this transient testosterone rise has no consequences.[285]

Three antiandrogens are available in the United States: flutamide, bicalutamide, and nilutamide. Each binds to the AR and serves as a competitive antagonist for ligands that might otherwise bind and activate the ligand-dependent transcriptional activity of AR. Used as monotherapy, as a consequence of blocking AR at the hypothalamic and pituitary level, circulating testosterone levels rise.[289] None of the antiandrogens are approved as monotherapy. Comparative trials between various antiandrogens are limited. One trial comparing bicalutamide and flutamide demonstrated less GI toxicity and better overall tolerability with bicalutamide.[290]

Schellhammer et al.[290] and Labrie et al.[291] were the first to advocate use of antiandrogens. A large number of controlled clinical trials have subsequently been conducted, some positive and some not. Multiple reviews and meta-analyses regarding this topic are available.[292–294] It is apparent from meta-analyses that the addition of antiandrogens may confer a small benefit in metastatic prostate cancer also treated with a LHRH agonist. Large controlled trials in orchiectomized patients did not demonstrate benefit.[282] A randomized trial with a non–FDA-approved dose of bicalutamide (80 mg) demonstrated a survival benefit in Japanese men.[295] Attempts to add to the effectiveness of ADT by using 5α-reductase inhibitors have not been assessed in randomized trials.

Antiandrogens have several toxicities distinct from LHRH analogues. Hepatic toxicities, typically elevations in liver enzymes such as aspartate aminotransferase and alanine aminotransferase, are associated with all antiandrogens. Rarely, hepatic toxicities can be severe, and monitoring of liver-function tests is recommended when using these agents. GI adverse events are potentially problematic with all antiandrogens, especially flutamide.[290] Pulmonary complications including fibrosis are a rare class effect of antiandrogens[296] but nilutamide has the highest rate of pulmonary-associated side effects.

Toxicities of ADT

In the pre-PSA era, ADT use was primarily administered in metastatic disease; in the post-PSA era, ADT has progressively been used in patients with longer life expectancies, often to achieve PSA control. Thus, in the post-PSA era, ADT has been used for longer durations and in healthier patients. Although ADT has long been associated with sexual side effects and hot flashes, more recently a significant number of adverse events have become better appreciated (Table 97.21), in part because of longer ADT durations and in part because of greater use in nonmetastatic patients whose concerns extend beyond short-term survival.

Hot flashes, libido loss, and erectile dysfunction affect most patients and have each been recognized as adverse effects of ADT since its inception. Despite this, much is not known. Hot flashes are poorly understood mechanistically, and often difficult to quantify as the duration, intensity, and frequency varies tremendously. Loss of libido is an expected complication of ADT. Loss of erectile function is an expectation for patients treated with ADT. The effects of prostate cancer on marital relationships should not be underestimated.[297]

In recent years, ADT-induced changes in weight, hair, muscle, bone, fat, testicular size, penile length, and gynecomastia have become better appreciated.[298–300] In part, the effects are duration-dependent. Postpubertal changes are often reversed by ADT; thus, facial and body hair are decreased but male-pattern baldness may partially reverse. Penile and testicular size may also be diminished. Weight gain is common, primarily a consequence of gain in adipose tissue. Muscle loss occurs with weight gain, and exercise tolerance/strength is decreased. Osteopenia and osteoporosis are well documented.[301] ADT increases markers of bone turnover.[302] In a review of more than 50,000 men in a Medicare/SEER database, fracture rates are substantially increased in men receiving ADT (Fig. 97.14), an effect that clearly increases as a function of ADT duration.[303] Gynecomastia and/or breast tenderness may develop; at times, however, excess adipose tissue may be confused with excess breast tissue.

Laboratory values are also altered by ADT. Declines in hemoglobin and frank anemia may be problematic at times. Hyperlipidemia and hyperglycemia are well documented.[304,305] Incident diabetes is increased[304] in LHRH-treated patients by approximately 44%, a consequence of insulin resistance. Whether glucose intolerance is due to increase in weight gain, increase in adiposity, decrease in exercise tolerance, a combination of these factors, or additional as yet-unidentified factors is not clear.

Cardiovascular issues are a potential concern with ADT therapies. Given that a multiplicity of cardiac risk factors

TABLE 97.21

ADVERSE EFFECTS OF ANDROGEN DEPRIVATION, APPROXIMATE FREQUENCY, AND POTENTIAL THERAPEUTIC OPTIONS FOR AMELIORATION[a]

Effect	Approximate Frequency	Potential Corrective Actions
Libido loss	Universal	None known
Erectile dysfunction	Universal	None known
Hot flashes	50%–80%	Venlafaxine, estrogens, progestins
Muscle loss	Common, duration-dependent	Exercise
Weight gain	Common	Exercise/diet
Facial/body hair loss	Very common	None known
Fatigue	Not defined	Exercise
Emotional lability	Not defined	None known
Depression	0%–30%	Various antidepressants
Cognitive dysfunction	Not defined	None known
Gynecomastia	Up to 20%	Pre-emptive radiation
Breast tenderness	Not defined	Aromatase inhibitors
Osteoporosis	Common, duration-dependent	Exercise/bisphosphonates
Anemia	5%–13%	Erythropoietin not recommended
Hyperlipidemia	10%	Diet, statins
Diabetes	0.8%/year increase	Exercise, oral agents
Myocardial infarction	0.25%/year increase	Treatment of risk factors
Coronary heart disease	1%/year increase	Treatment of risk factors

[a]A number of events are poorly defined in frequency as a consequence of a lack of controlled studies, quantitative assessments, and/or agreed on definitions.

are worsened by ADT (weight gain, increased adipose tissue, decreased exercise tolerance, hyperlipidemia, decreased insulin sensitivity, and glucose intolerance), perhaps it is not surprising that cardiac events would be increased in ADT agonist-treated patients. However, a review of the literature reveals inconsistent results on the issue of ADT and cardiovascular mortality. A recent advisory panel from the American Heart Association concluded that links between ADT use and cardiovascular mortality remain controversial and that studies on this issue should continue. Further, it was concluded that there is no reason at present to initiate specific cardiac testing in patients with cardiovascular disease before ADT initiation.[306] A variety of ADT-treated patients report fatigue, depression, and emotional lability.[307] These effects are not dissimilar to postmenopausal women and are probably underestimated by treating physicians and underreported in clinical trials. Specific psychological tests for cognitive dysfunction in some but not all studies indicate that certain aspects of spatial reasoning and spatial ability,[298,308] memory, attention, and executive function[309] can be impaired by ADT.

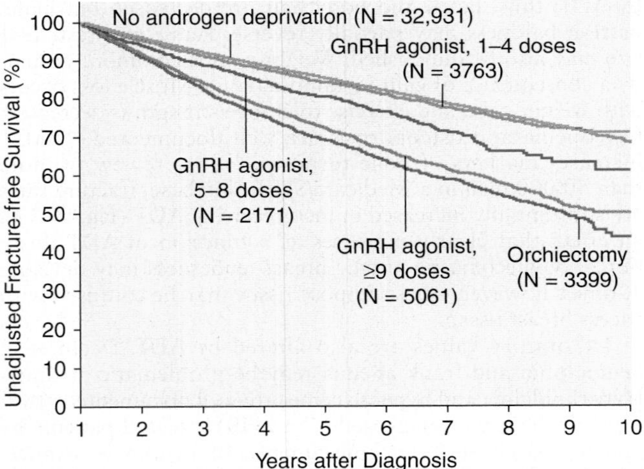

FIGURE 97.14 Fracture rate as a function of time after androgen-deprivation therapy in men older than age 65 in the United States. Luteinizing hormone-releasing hormone agonists (GnRH) monthly doses in the first 12 months after prostate cancer diagnosis. Note that the baseline in the graph begins 1 year after diagnosis. (From ref. 303, with permission.)

Helping patients to understand and recognize anticipated ADT effects prior to starting therapy is appropriate; managing expectations can alleviate anxiety and facilitate management. Various therapeutic options have been used to minimize ADT-induced side effects (Table 97.22). Estrogens have long been used to treat hot flashes, and doses used in postmenopausal women are often effective in men as well.[310] Monitoring of bone density is suggested for those with ongoing ADT. Although the duration of ADT that should trigger monitoring is debated, there is little increased risk of fracture unless ADT is continued for more than a year.[303] Osteopenia and osteoporosis can be effectively prevented or treated with bisphosphonates.[309,311] Calcium and vitamin D are used but data supporting their use are minimal. Prospective trials have demonstrated improvements in both fractures and bone mineral density.[312] Denosumab is a monoclonal antibody binding to RANK-Ligand, thereby inhibiting osteoclast differentiation, and toremifene is a selective estrogen receptor modulator. Denosumab is currently being considered by the FDA for approval for ADT-associated fractures. Although ADT-induced anemia is responsive to erythropoietins, the safety of this approach is not established and it is not recommended. Exercise is potentially helpful in the management of a variety of ADT-induced issues (e.g., bone strength, adiposity).[313,314] Attention to hypertension, glucose intolerance, hyperlipidemias, and other cardiac risk factors is appropriate, and patients with these conditions while on ADT should be followed by a primary care physician.[306]

TABLE 97.22

SELECTED MULTICENTER PROSPECTIVE CLINICAL TRIALS AND MEDIAN SURVIVAL IN FIRST-LINE THERAPY FOR METASTATIC CASTRATION-RESISTANT PROSTATE CANCER

Study	Sponsor	Agent	Year Trial Started	N	Median PSA at Entry	Median Survival (y)	Reference
NCI-Canada	NCI-Canada	Mitoxantrone/prednisone	1990	81	158	10.8	Tannock et al.[343]
		Prednisone		80	209	10.8	
CALGB 9182	CALGB	Mitoxantrone/hydrocortisone	1992	119	150	12.3	Kantoff[385]
		Hydrocortisone		123	141	12.6	
Sm-153 study	Cytogen	Samarium-153 EDTMP	1993	101	140	7.0	Sartor[338]
		Placebo		51	234	7.0	
Suramin	Parke-Davis	Suramin/hydrocortisone	1994	228	162	9.4	Small et al.[412]
		Hydrocortisone		230	186	9.2	
SWOG 9426	SWOG	Antiandrogen withdrawal	1995	164	28	20.0	Sartor et al.[413]
CALGB 9583	CALGB	Ketoconazole/AAW	1996	128	58	15.3	Small et al.[371]
		Antiandrogen withdrawal		132	58	16.7	
Zolendronate	Novartis	Zolendronate 4	1998	214	81	17.9	Saad et al.[376]
		Zolendronate 8/4		221	88	13.4	
		Placebo		208	61	15.3	
Estramustine	BMS	Paclitaxel/estramustine	1998	81	136	16.1*	Berry et al.[414]
		Paclitaxel		85	137	13.1	
SWOG 9916	SWOG	Docetaxel/estramustine	1999	338	84	17.5*	Petrylak et al.[384]
		Mitoxantrone/prednisone		336	90	15.6	
TAX327	Aventis	Docetaxel/prednisone q 3 weeks	2000	335	114	18.9*	Tannock et al.[326]
		Docetaxel/prednisone weekly		334	108	17.4	
		Mitoxantrone/prednisone		337	123	16.5	
D9901	Dendreon	Sipuleucel-T	2000	82	46	25.9*	Small et al.[415]
		Placebo		45	48	21.4	
Atrasentan	Abbot	Atrasentan	2001	408	70	20.5	Carducci et al.[416]
		Placebo		401	80	20.3	
IMPACT	Dendreon	Sipuleucel-T	2003	341	52	25.8*	Kantoff et al.[417]
		Placebo		171	47	21.7	
EPOC**	AstraZenca	ZD4054 15 mg	2004	98	94	23.5*	James et al.[418]
		ZD4054 10 mg		107	106	24.5*	
		Placebo		107	105	17.4	
90401	CALGB	Docetaxel/prednisone/ bevacizumab	2005	524	Not stated	22.6	Kelly et al.[419]
		Docetaxel/prednisone		526	Not stated	21.5	
ASCENT II	Novacea	Docetaxel weekly/Vitamin D_3	2006	477	Not stated	16.8	Scher et al.[420]
		Docetaxel q 3 weeks		476	Not stated	19.9*	
VITAL-1	Cell Genesys	GVAX	2007	311	Not stated	20.7	Higano et al.[421]
		Docetaxel/prednisone		310		21.7	

*Statistically distinct from control group.
PSA, prostate-specific antigen.

Intermittent ADT

Initial interest in intermittent ADT was promoted by experiments in animal models that suggested the possibility that using intermittent therapy might be superior to continuous therapy in terms of time-to-castrate-refractory disease.[315] Clinical data are not supportive of this concept, but interest in intermittent therapy is attractive as a strategy to diminish the adverse effects of hormonal therapies.

Randomized trials of intermittent therapy have been progressively maturing. Data to date indicate that time-to-castrate-refractory disease is not appreciably altered.[316–318] A large phase 3 trial indicated that overall survival after intermittent therapy was similar to that of continuous ADT.[319] In this trial, a slight increase in cancer-related deaths in the intermittent arm was counterbalanced by an increase in cardiovascular deaths in the continuous arm. Tolerability of intermittent therapy is high and costs are lowered; this approach is now commonly employed in the setting of a rising PSA in compliant patients. The time off therapy after initial ADT treatments predicts both time to castrate-resistant disease and death.[316] Intermittent therapy trials in the metastatic populations are ongoing.[286] Continuous ADT is the current standard of care for those with metastatic disease.

Adjuvant ADT after Local Definitive Therapy

Although a variety of nonrandomized data suggest that patients may benefit from androgen deprivation after RP, only one prospective randomized trial has provided clear benefit in terms of both overall and disease-specific survival.[283,284] Because of the importance of this trial, one of the few trials demonstrating a survival benefit with ADT as monotherapy, it will be covered in detail. A total of 100 patients with pathologically proven lymph node metastases at the time of RP were randomized to "early" versus "late" ADT between 1988 and 1993. Early ADT was initiated within 12 weeks of surgery and late ADT was designed to be instituted after the onset of symptoms or on diagnosis of metastatic disease.

The trial was conducted at the beginning of the PSA era, and PSAs were not obtained postoperatively as part of the trial design. Postoperative PSAs were, however, available for the majority of patients and were undetectable in approximately 80% of patients. At baseline, the majority of patients had Gleason score 7 or higher disease, most patients had either margin positivity or SVI, and the median number of positive lymph nodes was two. RT was not used. Baseline CT was done in 80 of the randomized patients; none had radiographic evidence of nodal metastases. ADT was administered continuously; in the early-treatment arm, 13 patients had orchiectomy and 33 had goserelin acetate. End points included disease-specific survival and overall survival. The last study update included patients with a median follow-up of 11.9 years, and at that time the median overall survival had not yet been reached for the early-treatment group as compared with 11.3 years in the late-treatment arm (HR, 1.84). Median prostate cancer-specific survival had not been reached in the early arm but was 12.3 years for the late-treated patients (HR, 4.09). Progression-free survival, which included PSA progression, was 13.9 years in the early group and 2.4 years in the late group (HR, 3.42). In this trial, the definition of "late" ADT did not include the possibility of treating a rising PSA; thus, it is conjectural how results in this trial might have differed had the control group received ADT on PSA rise. Extrapolation of these findings to other treatment groups, including those with rising PSA, is problematic. Surgically treated patients are typically younger and healthier as compared with various other populations, an important consideration given that risks and benefits of ADT must be balanced. Postsurgical patients have also had significant cytoreduction prior to therapy initiation. In some patients the disease burden postoperatively was extremely low; 26% of the patients randomized to late ADT therapy had not relapsed after 10 years of follow-up.

ADT in combination with radiation is standard of care for those with locally advanced disease. ADT and radiation is an extensive and important topic; it is reviewed elsewhere in this chapter.

CASTRATION-RESISTANT PROSTATE CANCER

The appropriate nomenclature for patients with *hormone-refractory*, *androgen-independent*, or *castration-resistant prostate cancer* (CRPC) continues to elicit discussion, but at this time CRPC is the best accepted term because it is now generally accepted that these patients continue to be responsive to secondary hormonal manipulations. CRPC is simply defined as progressive prostate cancer despite castrate serum testosterone levels (<50 ng/dL). Prior to 1990, CRPC patients typically presented with symptoms of pain or weight loss and multiple metastatic lesions. Today, when PSA testing is used to follow patients, virtually all CRPC patients are asymptomatic and manifest progression simply as a rising PSA.

In analysis of studies and trials for CRPC patients, it is essential to interpret the results of these investigations in the context of when these trials were performed. Both the types of pretreatments administered and the extent of disease are critical, and randomized trials are necessary to make conclusive statements.

Natural History and Prognosis

Prognosis for patients with CRPC has clearly changed during the PSA era. In a review of patients at the beginning of the PSA era, most with metastatic disease at diagnosis, a PSA rise preceded death by approximately 12 months.[320] Today data are quite distinct. In patients initiating hormonal treatment without radiographic evidence of disease in the PSA era,[321] survival after PSA rise has been reported to be 40 versus 68 months, respectively. Another retrospective data set review indicated that survival post-PSA rise in the nonmetastatic setting is 63 months.[322] Taken together, these data help to clarify the importance of differentiating patients with metastatic versus nonmetastatic disease when assessing outcomes in CRPC, and suggest a median survival of approximately 5 years once a PSA begins to rise after the initial ADT for patients with nonmetastatic disease.

Attempts to better understand the natural history of nonmetastatic (M0) CRPC prostate cancer are evolving. Time to progression of bone metastases has been studied in several prospective clinical trials.[323,324] In the placebo arm of a randomized trial of zoledronate, both higher baseline PSA levels and faster PSADTs independently predicted shorter time to first bone metastasis. Baseline PSA and PSA velocity also independently predicted overall survival. In one study, after 2 years of follow-up, only one-third of patients had developed radiographic evidence of metastatic disease.[323] In another trial of M0 patients treated with placebo for PSA-progressive CRPC, median time to radiographic metastatic disease was 22 months.[324] Both of these trials had similar entry criteria (rising PSA required) and similar median PSA levels at enrollment (13–14 ng/mL). These data help to define expected time to metastatic disease in the patient with PSA-progressive M0 (nonmetastatic) CRPC and suggest that approximately one-third to one-half of patients with a rising PSA will progress to bone scan–positive metastatic disease after approximately 2 years if the baseline PSA is 10 to 15 ng/mL. Those with a more rapid PSADT are at higher risk for early metastatic disease.

For CRPC patients with metastatic disease, analyses of prospective randomized trials over the past 15 years gives excellent insights into the patient's survival over time (Table 97.22). Prognosis of patients in the Cancer and Leukemia Group B have demonstrated that PSA, lactate dehydrogenase, alkaline phosphatase, Gleason score, performance status, hemoglobin, and the presence of visceral disease are predictive of survival. These variables have been incorporated into a comprehensive nomogram.[325] These nomograms provide an excellent basis for clinical trial design and can contribute to clinical decision making as well.

Patterns of Metastases

Prostate cancer is a remarkably bone-tropic disease and most patients with CRPC and radiographic evidence of metastases (mCRPC) have lesions demonstrable on bone scan. Osteoblastic lesions are far more common than osteolytic lesions but both are described (as are mixed blastic/lytic lesions). Studies requiring mCRPC for trial entry indicate that approximately 85% to 90% of patients will have bone scan–evidence metastatic disease and only 10% to 15% will not.[326,327] This bone tropism presents a potential therapeutic opportunity as well as providing insights into the metastatic process. Measurable soft tissue disease is present in approximately 20% to 40% of mCRPC patients in first-line chemotherapy trials, most commonly in pelvic or intra-abdominal lymph nodes. Liver or lung lesions are found in approximately 5% to 10% of these patients. Other sites of metastatic disease (e.g., adrenal, omental, renal, pancreas, and brain) are rarely detected. These data are contrasted with recent second-line chemotherapy trials; in these trials, lymph node disease and visceral disease were detected in 45% and 25% of patients. In the past, clinical evidence of brain metastases occurred in less than 0.1% of patients,[328] but this may now be more common.

A variant of the CRPC has been identified in which visceral metastases are predominant. In these cases the levels of PSA are often much lower than expected for the tumor burden documented on imaging studies. This variant is termed a *neuroendocrine* variant.[329] This constellation of findings (visceral metastases and very low PSA) may be important to recognize, as platinum-based regimens may be appropriate in this setting.[330] Additional studies are needed to confirm the importance of platinum-based therapies, as current data are minimal.

Serum and Cellular Markers in CRPC

Two types of serum markers can be readily assessed in CRPC patients. The first category includes circulating markers directly derived from cancer cells such as PSA, prostatic acid phosphatase, lactate dehydrogenase (LDH), and chromogranin A. In addition, markers can be derived from noncancerous tissues and reflect the burden of the cancer on normal tissues (e.g., hemoglobin, alkaline phosphatase, acute phase reactants). Use of multiple markers can provide more complete information with regard to the overall status of a patient as each provides distinct information.

PSA is the most commonly available tumor marker in patients with CRPC but caution is necessary in assessing PSA changes after pharmacologic interventions. PSA expression is under control of an androgen-sensitive promoter[331] and PSA changes may be altered by AR modulation in a way that may or may not be reflective of tumor volume. Thus, when assessing PSA changes after therapeutic intervention, it is critical to understand the mechanism of drug action. PSA changes after an antiandrogenic intervention and similar PSA changes after a chemotherapeutic agent may not convey similar prognostic information. It is clearly necessary to understand PSA changes in the context of each class of therapeutic agent rather than to simply equate PSA changes in individual disease states.

PSA declines have not been a perfect surrogate for survival but do predict outcomes. Analyses of PSA decline data for chemotherapy-treated patients suggest that PSA reductions of 30% or more may represent a better surrogate for survival as compared with declines of 50% or more.[332] Data from another chemotherapeutic trial (TAX327) confirm this finding.[333]

Otto Warburg discovered in the 1920s that cancer cells convert glucose to lactate despite adequate oxygen.[334] Pyruvate is the pivotal entity in this pathway and may be shunted to the lactate or to mitochondrial oxidative phosphorylation. LDH is the enzymatic catalyst for the conversion of pyruvate to lactate and is up-regulated in a variety of cancers. LDH levels contribute substantially to CRPC prognosis and, from a multivariate perspective, LDH is the single most important laboratory factor.[325] Alkaline phosphatase and hemoglobin are included in virtually all prognostic models of mCRPC. Alkaline phosphatase may be derived from either bone or liver, and at times fractionation is needed to determine the source of origin. Neither of these proteins is tumor-derived but rather reflects the impact of the cancer on osteoblasts or hematopoietic tissue, which in turn are factors of critical prognostic importance. Some authors have hypothesized that prostate tumor cells inhibit hematopoiesis via production of various cytokines.[335]

The anemia of CRPC is multifactorial and includes factors such as androgen deprivation, nutrition, marrow invasion, and/or red cell destruction via disseminated intravascular coagulation. Not uncommonly, radiation or chemotherapeutic interventions may adversely influence hemoglobin as well. Various acute-phase reactants such as C-reactive protein, fibrinogen, ferritin, and haptoglobin are also elevated in patients with advanced prostate cancer.[327,336–338] Substantial elevations in acute-phase reactants are in general a poor prognostic finding that occurs relatively late in the disease process.

Circulating tumor cells have recently been studied in prostate cancer as well as a variety of other malignant conditions, and the FDA has approved testing from a specific manufacturer (Veridex). Most analyses have used dichotomous testing (four or fewer, five or more cells per 7.5 mL) and found significance in prognosis both at baseline testing and in changes in posttherapeutic intervention.[339] Newer technologies are considerably more sensitive, but more studies are needed to assess clinical utility.

End Points in CRPC Trials

Effectiveness of therapy has been evaluated using a variety of end points in patients with CRPC but the most important of these are how a patient feels, functions, or survives. Biochemical and radiographic end points are commonly embedded into trials as secondary and supportive end points, but overall survival is the only end point generally accepted by regulatory agencies throughout the world.

End points may include either response rates or progression-free survival rates for biochemical end points such as PSA, patient-reported outcomes such as pain, or radiographic end points such as bidimensionally measured disease. Evaluation of PSA may include both response rates and/or progression-free survival analyses; however, no treatments have been FDA-approved as a consequence of PSA changes. Radiographic end points have been accepted as valid in a variety of cancers, especially in patients undergoing adjuvant treatments in which appearance of radiographic lesions precede both treatment changes and the onset of symptomatic disease. Soft tissue response and/or progression rates are often reported in CRPC clinical trials, but only a minority of patients will have measurable disease. Bone lesions are common in mCRPC but because bone scan–detectable lesions rarely improve in CRPC, measuring responses in bone is problematic. Bone scans using ^{99m}Tc-methylene diphosphonate do not detect cancer cells but instead target stromal-induced cancer changes via binding to hydrodroxyapatite. Progression-free analyses of bone lesions have been commonly used in clinical trial settings, but interpretation of bone scan progression can be problematic given variability in reader interpretation and the clear necessity of timing assessments similarly between arms of a study. Further, new lesions early in the course of a trial may represent disease "flare" and not represent failure of a newly instituted therapy.[340] Highly active therapies are commonly associated with bone scan "flares," which in turn are associated with healing bone lesions and initial alkaline-phosphatase elevations. Because increases in bone scan–detectable lesions may

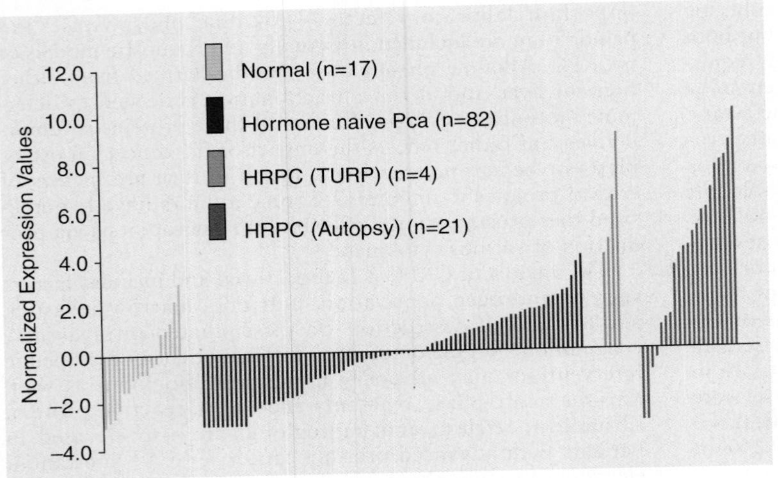

FIGURE 97.15 Quantitative assessment of androgen receptor splice variants in normal, hormonally naïve, castrate-resistant transurethral resection of the prostate specimens, or castrate-resistant metastatic specimens obtained at autopsy. (From ref. 351 with permission.)

result from either disease worsening or flare, "progressive disease" in most trials today requires progressive worsening of repetitive scans rather than reliance on a single scan.[341] Because progressive disease can have diverse manifestations, composite end points of progression-free survival may represent the best approach to capture all clinically relevant events. Circulating tumor cells have been proposed as an intermediate end point, but additional large phase 3 trials are needed to assess this end point before conclusions can be ascertained.`

Clinical benefit from a therapeutic intervention can be shown by improvements in pain, reductions in opiate usage, and/or health-related quality of life. Improvements in pain without concomitant increases in opioid analgesics were instrumental in FDA approval of bone-seeking radiopharmaceuticals[338,342] and in the chemotherapeutic trials with mitoxantrone.[343] Time to new painful sites has been used as a key end point in a pivotal trial combining EBRT and a radiopharmaceutical trial.[344]

Mechanisms of CRPC

Geller et al.[345] noted more than 2 decades ago that concentrations of dihydrotestosterone may not be fully suppressed in patients postorchiectomy. More recent data confirm and extend this initial observation using sensitive and specific techniques.[344] These data indicate that sufficient quantity of prostatic tissue androgens may be present to stimulate the AR, even in orchiectomized patient. Up-regulation in the androgen-synthesis pathway enzymes are clearly demonstrated in various prostate model systems after castration[376] and the concept of androgen synthesis directly occurring in CRPC cells is clearly plausible (but remains to be proved).

Several lines of evidence suggest that the AR continues to play a critical role in pathogenesis of CRPC (see the previous discussion of AR for a more complete discussion). For instance, both increased expression and amplification[346,347] of the androgen receptor (*AR*) gene has been demonstrated in prostate tissue derived from CRPC patients. These AR alterations are associated with a new "set point" for androgen sensitivity. There is little question that many CRPC patients are exquisitely sensitive to rises in androgen concentrations, possibly because of altered coregulator status.[348] Further, data from trials with newer testosterone synthesis inhibitors or AR antagonists both demonstrate that dramatic PSA responses can occur in men despite castrate levels of testosterone.[349,350] These data indicate that castrate levels of serum testosterone are a poor predictor of responsiveness to hormonal agents. Newer data implicate the presence of AR splice variants retaining the DNA-binding domain but deleting the ligand-binding domain. Assessments during the various stages of disease progression indicate that these variants are more prevalent in patients with advanced disease and may function as ligand-independent regulators of AR target genes[351,352] (Fig. 97.15).

Although the AR remains critical in many cellular models of CRPC, it is also important to recognize that a variety of non–AR-dependent pathways may also contribute to prostate cancer growth in the absence of androgens.[353] Both genetic and epigenetic changes have been implicated in current investigations[354]; similar pathways are known to be involved in the progression of a wide variety of non-hormone-dependent epithelial cancers.

Patient Management

From the standpoint of patient management or CRPC, the first issue in treating a patient who has progressed on ADT is to determine if serum testosterone is castrate level or not. Castrate level has been arbitrarily set at less than 50 ng/dL. In rare cases, approximately 1% in prospective trials, LHRH analogues are not effective and will have noncastrate testosterone levels despite LHRH agonist therapy.[355] Patients with progressive cancer after initial treatment with an antiandrogen alone, or those treated with an antiandrogen in combination with a 5α-reductase inhibitor, are likely to respond to castration.[356]

Patients with progressive prostate cancer despite castrate levels of testosterone should continue to have LHRH agonist therapies. One retrospective analysis, but not another,[357,358] demonstrated improved survival in association with continued LHRH agonist administration. No prospective randomized trials have examined this issue, but increases in testosterone are typically associated with more rapid progression.

A wide variety of additional treatment options are available for patients with CRPC and referral to a medical oncologist practiced in this art should be considered for patients failing initial hormonal therapies (Table 97.23). Newer options such as autologous cellular immunotherapies may be considered in those with asymptomatic or minimally symptomatic metastatic CRPC. A listing of the FDA-approved therapies and the year approved are available in Table 97.24.

TABLE 97.23

TREATMENT OPTIONS FOR PATIENTS WITH CASTRATION-RESISTANT PROSTATE CANCER

Secondary hormonal therapies
- Antiandrogen and other withdrawals (e.g., antiandrogens, megestrol acetate)
- Antiandrogen administration (flutamide, bicalutamide, nilutamide)
- Adrenal suppressants (ketoconazole, aminoglutethimide)
- Glucocorticoids (e.g., dexamethasone, prednisone)
- Estrogens (e.g., diethylstilbestrol, fosfestrol, estramustine.)

Bisphosphonates (zoledronate)
External-beam radiation therapy
Bone-seeking radiopharmaceuticals (samarium-153-EDTMP, strontium-89)
Chemotherapies (e.g., mitoxantrone, docetaxel, cabazitaxel.)
Immunotherapies (e.g., sipuleucel-T)

The sequencing of therapeutic options for patients with CRPC typically involves using secondary hormonal manipulations for as long as they are found to be effective in halting disease progression. Such hormonal manipulations may be longer in the future if promising new hormonal therapies such as abiraterone are FDA-approved. Attempts to prospectively assess the effects of secondary hormonal treatments as compared with earlier chemotherapy use failed consequent to poor accrual. Most secondary hormonal manipulations are reasonably well tolerated, particularly as compared with chemotherapy. Newer immune therapies will probably be most commonly used in the prechemotherapy space.

For the CRPC patient with bone metastases, a distinct series of options emerge, including bisphosphonates/denosumab to decrease rates of skeletal related events (*vide infra*) and/or bone-seeking radiopharmaceuticals for palliation.

Optimal strategies for combining focal therapies such as EBRT and systemic therapies such as chemotherapy require an ongoing assessment of patient's symptoms and disease status. For those patients with rapid progression, delays in systemic therapies can be problematic. For patients with vertebral metastases, spinal cord compression represents a potentially problematic issue and clinicians are urged to be vigilant in assessments for this complication. Once neurologic deterioration occurs, the possibility of recovery is diminished.

Secondary Hormonal Therapies

As previously noted, patients with castrate levels of testosterone and progressive prostate cancer are typically responsive to secondary hormonal manipulations such as antiandrogen withdrawal, ketoconazole, glucocorticoids, or estrogens. In general, studies show that PSA declines after most of the currently used second-line hormone therapy last for a median duration of 3 to 5 months. Longer durations may be expected for those with nonmetastatic CRPC and for those with lower PSAs at treatment initiation. There are, however, clear reports of patients who show sustained benefit despite metastatic lesions. Attempts to manage CRPC with secondary and/or tertiary hormonal manipulations are commonly employed despite the absence of randomized prospective trials demonstrating a survival benefit. Newer agents such as abiraterone and MDV3100 are in clinical trials now and these newer agents have promising phase 1/2 results[349,350] with randomized phase 3 trials currently underway.

Withdrawal Responses in CRPC

Patients previously treated with antiandrogens should be evaluated first for the possibility of an antiandrogen withdrawal response. This clinical entity was first recognized in 1993.[383,384] Potential signs of benefit included improvement in cancer-related anemia, pain palliation, PSA declines, and (rarely) regression of measurable disease. Agents to which withdrawal responses have been documented include the antiandrogens flutamide, nilutamide, and bicalutamide; megestrol acetate; diethylstilbestrol; estramustine; and others. It is important to recognize that withdrawal of even low doses of megestrol acetate used in the treatment of hot flashes may elicit PSA responses.[385] In general, withdrawal responses (should they occur) begin within a few weeks after the medication has been discontinued. Bicalutamide is an exception; this agent has a long terminal serum half-life and withdrawal response may not be observed for 6 to 8 weeks after discontinuation.[359]

Glucocorticoids

Glucocorticoids are known to be active agents in this disease state and may provide palliative as well as PSA responses. Tannock et al.[360] showed improvement in symptoms of 33% of cases treated with low-dose prednisone

TABLE 97.24

TIMELINE AND INDICATIONS FOR FOOD AND DRUG ADMINISTRATION (FDA)-APPROVED TREATMENTS FOR METASTATIC CASTRATE-RESISTANT PROSTATE CANCER

Year	FDA-Approved Treatment	Primary End Point Leading to Approval in Metastatic CRPC
1981	Estramustine	"Objective responses" using older criteria
1993	Strontium[89]	Reduction in onset of new painful bone lesions after XRT + isotope vs. XRT alone
1996	Mitoxantrone + prednisone	Reduction in pain compared to prednisone
1997	Samarium[153]-EDTMP	Reduction in bone pain compared to placebo
2002	Zoledronic acid	Reduction in skeletal-related events compared to placebo
2004	Docetaxel + prednisone	Prolonged overall survival compared to mitoxantrone + prednisone
2010	Sipuleucel-T	Prolonged overall survival compared to nonactivated antigen presenting cells
2010	Cabazitaxel + prednisone	Prolonged overall survival compared to mitoxantrone + prednisone in patients previously treated with a docetaxel regimen

CRPC, castration-resistant prostate cancer; XRT, radiation therapy.

PRACTICE OF ONCOLOGY

(10 mg/day). Dexamethasone has had PSA declines of more than 50% reported in up to 59% of patients.[361] Even low-dose hydrocortisone may be associated with transient small declines in PSA.[362] Dose-response curves for steroids have been poorly explored and optimal agents and dosing regimens are not clear. Prednisone has been used at oral dosages of 10 to 20 mg/day and dexamethasone in oral doses of 0.5 to 2 mg/day. These agents are commonly used in palliation of patients as well.

Estrogens

Estrogens have long been known to have palliative effects on patients with hormone-refractory disease, although difficulties with thromboembolic events have limited their use. Diethylstilbestrol at oral doses of 1 to 3 mg/day is associated with PSA declines in approximately 24% to 42% of patients.[363,364] Premarin at higher doses has a similar response rate.[365] Estramustine has estrogenic actions and some portion of its activity in CRPC is probably attributable to estrogenic action rather than interference with microtubular function. Estramustine has not shown activity in nonestrogen responsive malignancies, bringing to question its putative antimicrotubular mechanism of action.

The mechanism of action of estrogens in CRPC remains elusive, although further suppression of total and serum-free testosterone, elevations in sex hormone–binding globulin, and reduction in serum dehydroepiandrosterone sulfate have all been documented.[366] The toxicities of estrogens are well described and include gynecomastia, breast tenderness, and thromboembolic events such as deep vein thrombosis, pulmonary embolism, myocardial infarction, and stroke. Attempts to reduce thromboembolic risk by using transdermal estrogen delivery systems have been made; however, efficacy in these trials has generally been less than anticipated.[367]

Androgen Synthesis Inhibitors

Ketoconazole has been used for patients with CRPC for more than 2 decades. Studies indicate that ketoconazole (600–1,200 mg/day) plus low-dose glucocorticoids may reduce PSA by 50% or more in up to 71% of patients.[322,368–370] Those patients with higher androstenedione are more likely to respond.[369] Cancer progression is associated with rises in androstenedione and dehydroepiandrosterone sulfate,[371] implying that steroidogenic compensatory mechanisms contribute to escape from ketoconazole.

Because cortisol responses are blunted in patients treated with ketoconazole, low doses of glucocorticoids are often used. The mechanism of ketoconazole action is almost certainly further inhibition of androgen synthesis. In the castrate patient, the adrenal glands may continue to serve as a source of androgens and, as previously noted, data suggest that prostate cancer cells themselves may be capable of synthesizing potent androgens. Ketoconazole inhibits several enzymatic steps in the androgen synthetic pathway, most notably 17-hydroxylase/17,20-desmolase (CYP17), and 11-hydroxylase (CYP11B1). It is also important to recognize that ketoconazole absorption requires an acidic gastric environment. Drugs such as proton-pump inhibitors and H_2 antagonists potentially interfere with ketoconazole absorption. Caution is urged with ketoconazole use as it is a potent inhibitor of CYP3A4. This enzyme is responsible for a significant number of clinically relevant drug degradations. Hence, potentially adverse drug interactions are common and should be checked prior to administration.

Caution is urged with ketoconazole use as it is a potent inhibitor of CYP3A4. This enzyme is responsible for a significant number of clinically relevant drug degradations. Hence, potentially adverse drug interactions are common and should be checked prior to administration.

Newer CYP17 inhibitors such as abiraterone are now in phase 3 clinical trials after promising phase 1/2 data. These agents inhibit the synthesis of androgens and substantially decrease serum testosterone, estradiol, dehydroepiandrostenedione, and androstenedione. Responses to abiraterone are clearly documented even in postdocetaxel patients and duration of response depends on the extent of disease. Most patients will have PSA declines; in a recent phase 2 postdocetaxel mCRPC trial conducted in predominately ketoconazole-naïve patients, 45% of patients had PSA declines of 50% or more, lasting for 4 or more weeks. Median time to PSA progression was 5.5 months. Among the subset of men with measurable disease, 27% had partial responses as assessed by Response Evaluation Criteria In Solid Tumors (RECIST). Prior treatment with ketoconazole diminishes the response rate of abiraterone and the phase 3 clinical trials with this novel agent have been conducted in patients without ketoconazole pretreatment. Although no data have been published, the abiraterone phase 3 interim results from the sponsor indicate a prolongation in survival in patients with metastatic CRPC no longer responding to docetaxel.

Antiandrogens

Antiandrogens may be effective in selected men whose cancer has progressed after initial ADT.[372–375] These data are predominantly limited to reductions in PSA. All three of the antiandrogens commercially available in the United States (flutamide, bicalutamide, and nilutamide) have been used in this setting with variable degrees of success, but the most promising agent is a newer antiandrogen (MDV3100) now in a phase 3 trial. This agent was developed with an aim toward developing an antiandrogen with both a high affinity and no partial agonism on AR binding. Assays in preclinical models indicated that MDV3100 has substantial activity in castrate mice xenografts, system in which bicalutamide has little activity. In phase 1/2 clinical trials, performed in a heterogenous group of mCRPC patients with various doses, MDV3100 PSA response rates with PSA declines of more than 50% for 4 or more weeks were not reported, but PSA declines of more than 50% were recorded in 71% and 37% of patients who were ketoconazole-naïve or previously ketoconazole-exposed, respectively. PSA progression-free survival for all patients treated in this trial was 7.3 months.[350]

Bisphosphonates

Zoledronate is the only FDA-approved bisphosphonate for CRPC with bone metastases. Randomized trials of zoledronate demonstrate that 4 mg intravenously every 3 to 4 weeks reduces skeletal-related events (defined as pathologic fractures, radiation to bone, spinal cord compression, and/or surgery to bone) by 25%; however, subset analyses indicate that only fracture rates are appreciably decreased.[376] There is no clinical evidence that this agent or any other bisphosphonate appreciably decreases the rate at which bone metastases develop. Newer phase 3 trials have compared denosumab with zoledronate and found improved rates of skeletal-related events, but these trials have yet to appear in the peer-reviewed literature. Denosumab is also being tested in metastases prevention, but data are yet to mature.

Bisphosphonates and denosumab are associated with osteonecrosis of the jaw. This relatively rare but serious side effect seems associated with bisphosphonate use in combination with dental disease, dental surgery (e.g., tooth extraction), oral trauma, periodontitis, poor dental hygiene, glucocorticoid, and/or chemotherapy use.[377] For bisphosphonates, modifications in dose are essential in renal dysfunction.

Bone-Seeking Radioisotopes

Three radiopharmaceuticals are currently FDA-approved for the palliative treatment of painful bone metastases; phosphorus-32, strontium-89, and samarium-153-EDTMP. The half-life of strontium-89 is 50.5 days, the half-life of phosphorus-32 is 14 days, and the half-life of samarium-153 is 1.9 days (46 hours). Bone-seeking radioisotopes have the potential to palliate multiple metastatic sites in the skeleton, and FDA approval was based on randomized trials demonstrating efficacy in this setting. The pivotal trial for strontium-89 randomized CRPC patients with bone pain to EBRT plus or minus isotope and demonstrated that patients treated with strontium were less likely to have pain in new metastatic sites.[342] The pivotal trial for samarium-153-EDTMP demonstrated a reduction in both opioid analgesic consumption and patient-reported pain scores.[338] Myelosuppression is the predominate toxicity associated with all of the bone-seeking radioisotopes; however, the shorter-lived isotopes with lower beta-energy such as samarium-153 have less suppression and faster recovery after administration. Pain flare, an increase in bone pain occurring hours to days after administration, may also occur. Newer agents such as the alpha-emitter radium-223 are in advanced clinical trials after provocative results in phase 2 trials that suggested a survival benefit.[378]

External-Beam Radiation

For a painful lesion(s) that can be encompassed by a single or regional radiation port, EBRT offers excellent palliation. Randomized trials indicate equivalency for 8 Gy in one treatment fraction as compared with 30 Gy in ten treatment fractions for palliative treatment of bone lesions[379,380]; however, patients treated with 30 Gy are less likely to require repeat treatment (18% vs. 9%). A limitation of EBRT for patients with CRPC is that patients commonly have multiple lesions and, unless the disease process is controlled by systemic therapies, pain progression in other sites commonly occurs after a short interval. Short courses of low-dose hemibody radiation (3 Gy/day × 5 days) have also been used with effective results[381] but may be associated with significant transient toxicity.

Immunotherapy

Immunotherapy of prostate cancer has recently taken a substantial step forward with the FDA approval of sipuleucel-T, an autologous active cellular immunotherapy. This agent requires that a patient's mononuclear cells be obtained by pheresis and that the antigen-presenting cells be isolated and exposed to a granulocyte-macrophage colony-stimulating factor (GM-CSF)/prostatic acid phosphatase fusion protein *ex vivo* (prior to reinfusing the immunized cells back to the patient). In the pivotal trial with sipuleucel-T, 512 patients with asymptomatic or minimally symptomatic mCRCPC were randomized to three doses of the immunotherapy or cells that had been treated similarly but not exposed to the GM-CSF/prostatic acid phosphatase fusion protein. Overall survival was improved from 21.7 months in the control arm to 25.8 months in the sipuleucel-T arm (HR, 0.775; $P = .032$). Adverse reactions were primarily related to the infusion of the activated cells and included chills (53%), fatigue (41%), fever (31%), back pain (30%), nausea (21%), joint aches (20%), and headaches (18%). Most of these reactions had resolved within 2 days of infusion. Grade 3–4 events were less than 3% for each of these conditions. No improvement in progression-free survival or response rate was seen in the large randomized trial, suggesting either that these parameters were not accurately measured or that slower kinetics of the disease were manifest after progression was initially measured.[382,383] The FDA approval was granted in April 2010.

First-Line Chemotherapy

Although chemotherapy has long been used in patients with advanced prostate cancer, only recently has a survival benefit been shown in CRPC patients. Docetaxel is the only agent that prolongs survival in this setting. Two pivotal randomized trials demonstrate this effect, one with a combination of docetaxel/prednisone[326] and the other with a combination of docetaxel/estramustine.[384] In each study, docetaxel was administered every 3 weeks and comparison was made to mitoxantrone/prednisone. Additional details follow. Discussion is limited to agents with proven benefit; a wide variety of chemotherapy trials with cyclophosphamide, anthracyclines, etoposide, 5-fluorouracil, various platins, various vinca alkaloids, and so forth have been executed but none of these agents either alone or in combination have become a standard of care.

Identifying the patient who benefits from chemotherapy is a point of discussion. Both pivotal trials using docetaxel required radiographic evidence of metastatic disease, a castrate level of testosterone, and evidence of progressive disease prior to trial entry. In the current clinical environment it is not uncommon for patients to exhaust nonchemotherapeutic options prior to developing metastatic disease; however, chemotherapy is controversial in the nonmetastatic setting as the pivotal clinical trials excluded men without metastatic disease. For patients with Karnofsky performance status less than 60, there are few data to support the use of chemotherapy.

Results with Specific Chemotherapy Agents

Mitoxantrone

Mitoxantrone has palliative activity as a single agent and was the first chemotherapy shown to confer clinical benefit in randomized trials for patients with mCRPC. Two pivotal randomized trials, comparing mitoxantrone (12–14 mg/m^2 intravenously every 3 weeks) plus a glucocorticoid versus glucocorticoid alone, demonstrated superiority of the combination with respect to palliation of pain.[343,385] In the initial pivotal trial, pain palliation was the primary end point.[343] Palliation was assessed by using a patient-reported scale and measuring daily analgesic consumption. A higher proportion of mitoxantrone patients had a decrease in pain (29% vs. 12%) and overall palliative response (38% vs. 21%). Duration of pain relief among mitoxantrone responders was 43 weeks versus 18 weeks for the control group. Survival was not improved. Common toxicities with mitoxantrone at doses of 12 mg/m^2 every 3 weeks included nausea (61%), fatigue (39%), alopecia (29%), and anorexia (25%). From these and other studies, grade 3–4 neutropenia is reported in approximately 20% of patients but febrile neutropenia is relatively unusual (2% of patients). Cardiac function is a concern; decreased cardiac function was reported in 5% to 7% of patients. The combination of mitoxantrone plus prednisone

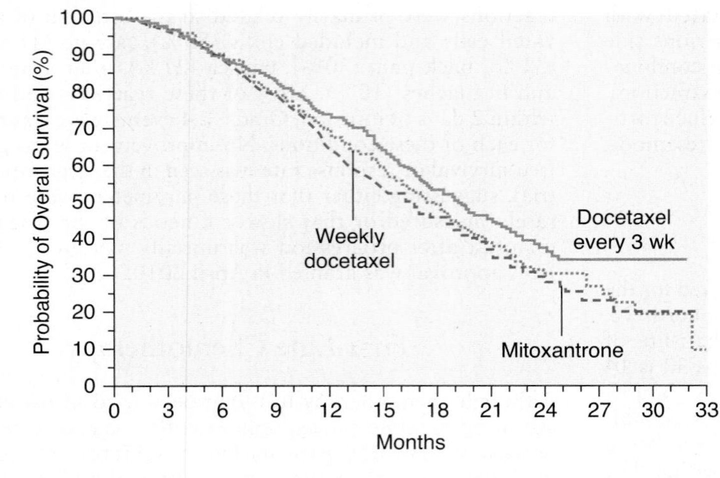

No. at Risk						
Docetaxel every 3 wk	335	296	217	104	37	5
Weekly docetaxel	334	297	200	105	29	4
Mitoxantrone	337	297	192	95	29	3

FIGURE 97.16 Overall survival for patients treated with metastatic castrate-refractory prostate cancer treated with docetaxel weekly or every 3 weeks as compared with mitoxantrone every 3 weeks. (From ref. 326, with permission.)

was approved by the FDA in 1996 for the treatment of mCRPC patients. This regimen became not only the first standard chemotherapy in mCRPC, but also the standard against which newer approaches would subsequently be compared.

Docetaxel

Two phase 3 studies have examined docetaxel in the setting of mCRPC.[326,384] In the TAX327 pivotal trial, Tannock et al. compared three groups: docetaxel 75 mg/m^2 every 3 weeks for up to ten cycles (group 1); docetaxel 30 mg/m^2 weekly for five cycles (group 2); or mitoxantrone 12 mg/m^2 every 3 weeks for ten cycles (group 3). Prednisone (10 mg daily) was added to all regimens. Cross-over was allowed on disease progression. Survival was the primary end point; secondary end points included pain, PSA levels, and quality of life. All patients had metastases on radiographs, castrate serum testosterone, and disease progression prior to entry. Results of TAX327 demonstrated prolongation of survival (Fig. 97.16) in the group receiving docetaxel/prednisone every 3 weeks as compared with the mitoxantrone/prednisone-treated patients (HR, 0.76) and median survival was prolonged by approximately 2.5 months (18.9 vs. 16.5 months, respectively).

The survival advantage of the every 3 weeks docetaxel regimen was detected in various subsets but when given once weekly (as compared with mitoxantrone) survival was not distinct (HR, 0.91; median, 17.4 vs. 16.5 months, respectively). No statistical comparisons were made between the two schedules of docetaxel. Surprisingly, progression-free survival was not reported. PSA reductions of 50% or greater and pain reductions were significantly more common among men in the docetaxel-treated arms. Quality of life was evaluated using the Functional Assessment of Cancer Therapy-Prostate (FACT-P) questionnaire. Patients in both the docetaxel groups reported improvement in quality of life as compared with the mitoxantrone group, with greatest improvements in the domains assessing weight loss, appetite, pain, physical comfort, and bowel and GU function. Toxicities in the group receiving docetaxel every 3 weeks included alopecia (65%), nausea or vomiting (42%), diarrhea (32%), nail changes (30%), sensory neuropathies (30%), and changes in taste (18%). Grade 3–4 neutropenia was detected in 32% of patients; however, febrile neutropenia was relatively rare (3%). Weekly docetaxel was comparable in terms of toxicities except that grade 3–4 neutropenia was only 2%. Treatment-related death was reported in 0.3% of patients in each of the docetaxel arms.

In the second pivotal study of docetaxel (SWOG 9916), Petrylak et al.[384] randomized 770 patients with progressive mCRPC to receive estramustine at a dose of 280 mg orally three times daily days 1 through 5 plus docetaxel at a dose of 60 mg/m^2 every 3 weeks versus mitoxantrone 12 mg/m^2 every 3 weeks plus prednisone 5 mg twice daily. Treatment was planned until disease progression or unacceptable toxicity occurred, or until a maximum of 12 cycles of docetaxel and estramustine or 144 mg/m^2 mitoxantrone had been administered. The primary end point was overall survival. Secondary end points included progression-free survival, objective response rates, and PSA decline rates. Cross-over was not allowed. Study results showed a 20% reduction in mortality (HR, 0.8) in the docetaxel/estramustine group compared with the mitoxantrone/prednisone group. Median overall survival was approximately 2 months longer in the docetaxel/estramustine group (17.5 months) compared with the mitoxantrone/prednisone group (15.6 months). Median time to progression was also significantly superior in the docetaxel/estramustine group (6.3 vs. 3.2 months, respectively). PSA declines of at least 50% occurred in 50% of docetaxel/estramustine-treated patients as compared with 27% of mitoxantrone/prednisone-treated patients. Although docetaxel/estramustine therapy was generally reasonably well tolerated, there was a higher incidence of grade 3–4 neutropenic fevers, nausea and vomiting, and cardiovascular events among patients receiving docetaxel/estramustine as compared with those receiving mitoxantrone/prednisone.

The results of the SWOG 9916 and TAX 327 studies are not easily compared because of the different cross-over patterns, differences in estramustine use, and different doses of docetaxel, as well as different study entry criteria. The use of estramustine has decreased since the TAX327 study demonstrated it was not necessary to achieve survival benefit.

Investigational Docetaxel-Based Combination Regimens

Frontline phase 2 trials of docetaxel in combination with various agents including atrasentan,[386] bevacizumab,[387] bortezomid,[386] capecitabine,[388] calcitriol,[389] thalidomide,[390] and thalidomide/bevacizumab[390] have been completed. Many more combination trials are underway but appropriately designed, large-scale, randomized phase 3 trials are necessary to determine if any of these combinations might confer clinical benefit. A randomized phase 2 trial of thalidomide/docetaxel strongly trended toward a survival benefit but was underpowered, preventing firm conclusions.[390] Docetaxel, prednisone, bevacizumab, thalidomide has substantial activity but the thrombosis rate is high and further data are needed to confirm safety.[391] Other recent phase 3 trials found to be negative for survival benefit as compared with every- 3-week docetaxel/prednisone include docetaxel/prednisone/calcitriol, docetaxel/prednisone/bevacizumab, and docetaxel/GM-CSF-transduced prostate cancer cell lines. Phase 3 trials are ongoing with docetaxel/atrasentan, docetaxel/lenalidomide, docetaxel/anti-clusterin, docetaxel/dasatinib, docetaxel/aflibercept, and docetaxel/zibotentan. These trials will mature over the next several years and have the capacity to change standards of practice.

Second-Line Chemotherapy

The concept of second-line chemotherapy is new in prostate cancer, as frontline chemotherapy has only recently been widely accepted as a treatment alternative. Most reports are composed of small, nonrandomized trials.[392–394] Two significant phase 3 trials have been reported to date. One trial of an oral platin (satraplatin) compared a combination of prednisone and satraplatin to prednisone alone and demonstrated no differences in survival (14.1 months in each arm) in a 950-patient phase 3 trial.[395]

Recently cabazitaxel, a novel taxane, was compared with mitoxantrone in patients with progressive mCRPC postdocetaxel. Each drug was administered every 3 weeks. The median patient had received approximately 550 mg/m^2 prior to docetaxel (slightly over seven cycles at the FDA-approved dose of 75 mg/m^2) and 25% of patients had radiographically measurable visceral disease at baseline. Overall survival was improved in the cabazitaxel arm, 15.1 versus 12.7 months (HR, 0.70; P <.0001). Progression-free survival using a composite end point was improved by cabazitaxel from 1.4 to 2.8 months (P <.0001). Adverse events included febrile neutropenia (7.5%), diarrhea (47%), fatigue (37%), asthenia (20%), back pain (16%), nausea (34%), and vomiting (23%). Grade 3–4 adverse events were similar but varied from 1.9% to 7.5% for the aforementioned issues. The FDA approved this agent in June 2010 for patients previously treated with a docetaxel-containing regimen.[396]

Experimental Agents

A large number of experimental agents have entered clinical trials for CRPC. Although an extensive discussion of experimental agents is not warranted in this context, it is appropriate to say that a variety of specific strategies including both small molecules and antibodies are being explored. The success of agents such as imatinib in both leukemia and certain solid tumors has spurred the development of various small-molecule kinase inhibitors. Both receptor and nonreceptor kinases have been targeted with agents such as dasatinib and sunitinib. Antibodies to cell-surface molecules such as prostate-specific membrane antigen, prostate stem cell antigen, and gastrin-releasing peptide receptors are in current clinical development. "Naked" antibodies, toxin conjugates, and radiolabeled antibodies are all being developed. A variety of novel approaches to angiogenesis are being considered, targeting ligand production, ligands themselves, selected receptors, and specific signal transduction pathways. Perhaps the future of anti-CRPC therapy will use a combination of cancer cell-targeted therapies, stromal targeted therapies, and immune-system modulators.[418]

Investigational Immunologic Therapies

Immune-based therapies have long been sought as cancer treatments but few products are FDA-approved. Recently, GM-CSF–based therapies have demonstrated potential activity in patients with CRPC. GM-CSF alone has demonstrated PSA modulatory activities in patients with androgen-sensitive disease but studies of GM-CSF monotherapy in CRPC are limited. An anti–CTLA-4 antibody is in clinical trial development with occasional substantial toxicities and responses being recorded.[397] A novel vaccine, PROSTVAC-VF Tricom has reported provocative randomized phase 2 data and further studies will ensue.[382]

Complementary and Alternative Therapies

The issue of complementary and alternative therapies is a major one in prostate cancer management. Unique to prostate cancer is the anecdotal reports of PSA declines, which may or may not be related to the product in question. Because most of these putative therapies are not subject to FDA review, details of the formulation, standardization, safety, interactions, and appropriate use are not available. A once-popular herbal product (PC-SPES) was found to contain both an estrogen and an anticoagulant when carefully analyzed.[363] Given that extensive testing in clinical trials is typically dependent on substantial funding and that self-interested parties typically require intellectual property protection before investment, one might anticipate that most claims related to these therapies will not be tested with scientific rigor.

Selected References

The full list of references for this chapter appears in the online version.

11. Gleason DF, Mellinger GT. Prediction of prognosis for prostatic adenocarcinoma by combined histological grading and clinical staging. *J Urol* 1974;111(1):58.
13. True L, Coleman I, Hawley S, et al. A molecular correlate to the Gleason grading system for prostate adenocarcinoma. *Proc Natl Acad Sci U S A* 2006;103(29):10991.
15. Stamey TA, McNeal JE, Yemoto CM, Sigal BM, Johnstone IM. Biological determinants of cancer progression in men with prostate cancer. *JAMA* 1999;281(15):1395.
18. Schroder FH, Hugosson J, Roobol MJ, et al. Screening and prostate-cancer mortality in a randomized European study. *N Engl J Med* 2009; 360(13):1320.
20. Sakr WA, Grignon DJ, Crissman JD, et al. High grade prostatic intraepithelial neoplasia (HGPIN) and prostatic adenocarcinoma between the ages of 20-69: an autopsy study of 249 cases. *In Vivo* 1994;8(3):439.
21. Thompson IM, Goodman PJ, Tangen CM, et al. The influence of finasteride on the development of prostate cancer. *N Engl J Med* 2003;349(3): 215.
31. Lichtenstein P, Holm NV, Verkasalo PK, et al. Environmental and heritable factors in the causation of cancer—analyses of cohorts of twins from Sweden, Denmark, and Finland. *N Engl J Med* 2000;343(2):78.
49. Andriole GL, Bostwick DG, Brawley OW, et al. Effect of dutasteride on the risk of prostate cancer. *N Engl J Med* 2010;362(13):1192.
50. Lippman SM, Klein EA, Goodman PJ, et al. Effect of selenium and vitamin E on risk of prostate cancer and other cancers: the Selenium and Vitamin E Cancer Prevention Trial (SELECT). *JAMA* 2009;301(1):39.

58. Andriole GL, Crawford ED, Grubb RL 3rd, et al. Mortality results from a randomized prostate-cancer screening trial. *N Engl J Med* 2009;360(13):1310.
59. Wolf AM, Wender RC, Etzioni RB, et al. American Cancer Society guideline for the early detection of prostate cancer: update 2010. *CA Cancer J Clin* 2010;60(2):70.
61. Thompson IM, Pauler DK, Goodman PJ, et al. Prevalence of prostate cancer among men with a prostate-specific antigen level < or =4.0 ng per milliliter. *N Engl J Med* 2004;350(22):2239.
78. Stephenson AJ, Scardino PT, Bianco FJ Jr, DiBlasio CJ, Fearn PA, Eastham JA. Morbidity and functional outcomes of salvage radical prostatectomy for locally recurrent prostate cancer after radiation therapy. *J Urol* 2004;172(6 Pt 1):2239.
79. D'Amico AV, Chen MH, Roehl KA, Catalona WJ. Preoperative PSA velocity and the risk of death from prostate cancer after radical prostatectomy. *N Engl J Med* 2004;351(2):125.
90. Klotz L. Active surveillance for prostate cancer: trials and tribulations. *World J Urol* 2008;26(5):437.
91. Carter HB, Kettermann A, Warlick C, et al. Expectant management of prostate cancer with curative intent: an update of the Johns Hopkins experience. *J Urol* 2007;178(6):2359.
92. Bill-Axelson A, Holmberg L, Ruutu M, et al. Radical prostatectomy versus watchful waiting in early prostate cancer. *N Engl J Med* 2005;352(19):1977.
96. Bader P, Burkhard FC, Markwalder R, Studer UE. Is a limited lymph node dissection an adequate staging procedure for prostate cancer? *J Urol* 2002;168(2):514.
101. Hu JC, Gu X, Lipsitz SR, et al. Comparative effectiveness of minimally invasive vs open radical prostatectomy. *JAMA* 2009;302(14):1557.
111. Begg CB, Riedel ER, Bach PB, et al. Variations in morbidity after radical prostatectomy. *N Engl J Med* 2002;346(15):1138.
112. Vickers AJ, Bianco FJ, Serio AM, et al. The surgical learning curve for prostate cancer control after radical prostatectomy. *J Natl Cancer Inst* 2007;99(15):1171.
115. Roach M 3rd, DeSilvio M, Lawton C, et al. Phase III trial comparing whole-pelvic versus prostate-only radiotherapy and neoadjuvant versus adjuvant combined androgen suppression: Radiation Therapy Oncology Group 9413. *J Clin Oncol* 2003;21(10):1904.
116. Lawton CA, DeSilvio M, Roach M 3rd, et al. An update of the phase III trial comparing whole pelvic to prostate only radiotherapy and neoadjuvant to adjuvant total androgen suppression: updated analysis of RTOG 94-13, with emphasis on unexpected hormone/radiation interactions. *Int J Radiat Oncol Biol Phys* 2007;69(3):646.
120. Pollack A, Zagars GK, Starkschall G, et al. Prostate cancer radiation dose response: results of the M. D. Anderson phase III randomized trial. *Int J Radiat Oncol Biol Phys* 2002;53(5):1097.
121. Zietman AL, DeSilvio ML, Slater JD, et al. Comparison of conventional-dose vs high-dose conformal radiation therapy in clinically localized adenocarcinoma of the prostate: a randomized controlled trial. *JAMA* 2005;294(10):1233.
122. Peeters ST, Heemsbergen WD, Koper PC, et al. Dose-response in radiotherapy for localized prostate cancer: results of the Dutch multicenter randomized phase III trial comparing 68 Gy of radiotherapy with 78 Gy. *J Clin Oncol* 2006;24(13):1990.
123. Dearnaley DP, Sydes MR, Graham JD, et al. Escalated-dose versus standard-dose conformal radiotherapy in prostate cancer: first results from the MRC RT01 randomised controlled trial. *Lancet Oncol* 2007;8(6):475.
125. Zelefsky MJ, Fuks Z, Hunt M, et al. High dose radiation delivered by intensity modulated conformal radiotherapy improves the outcome of localized prostate cancer. *J Urol* 2001;166(3):876.
129. Kuban DA, Levy LB, Cheung MR, et al. Long-term Failure Patterns and Survival in a Randomized Dose-Escalation Trial for Prostate Cancer. Who Dies of Disease? *Int J Radiat Oncol Biol Phys* 2010.
130. Zietman AL, Bae K, Slater JD, et al. Randomized trial comparing conventional-dose with high-dose conformal radiation therapy in early-stage adenocarcinoma of the prostate: long-term results from Proton Radiation Oncology Group/American College of Radiology 95-09. *J Clin Oncol* 2010;28(7):1106.
131. Zelefsky MJ, Yamada Y, Fuks Z, et al. Long-term results of conformal radiotherapy for prostate cancer: impact of dose escalation on biochemical tumor control and distant metastases-free survival outcomes. *Int J Radiat Oncol Biol Phys* 2008;71(4):1028.
132. Kupelian PA, Ciezki J, Reddy CA, Klein EA, Mahadevan A. Effect of increasing radiation doses on local and distant failures in patients with localized prostate cancer. *Int J Radiat Oncol Biol Phys* 2008;71(1):16.
133. Cahlon O, Zelefsky MJ, Shippy A, et al. Ultra-high dose (86.4 Gy) IMRT for localized prostate cancer: toxicity and biochemical outcomes. *Int J Radiat Oncol Biol Phys* 2008;71(2):330.
136. Di Staso M, Bonfili P, Gravina GL, et al. Late morbidity and oncological outcome after radical hypofractionated radiotherapy in men with prostate cancer. *BJU Int* 2010.
137. Rene N, Faria S, Cury F, et al. Hypofractionated radiotherapy for favorable risk prostate cancer. *Int J Radiat Oncol Biol Phys* 2010;77(3):805.
138. Katz AJ, Santoro M, Ashley R, Diblasio F, Witten M. Stereotactic body radiotherapy for organ-confined prostate cancer. *BMC Urol* 2010;10:1.
145. Michalski JM, Winter K, Purdy JA, et al. Toxicity after three-dimensional radiotherapy for prostate cancer on RTOG 9406 dose Level V. *Int J Radiat Oncol Biol Phys* 2005;62(3):706.
146. Zelefsky MJ, Levin EJ, Hunt M, et al. Incidence of late rectal and urinary toxicities after three-dimensional conformal radiotherapy and intensity-modulated radiotherapy for localized prostate cancer. *Int J Radiat Oncol Biol Phys* 2008;70(4):1124.
147. Martin JM, Bayley A, Bristow R, et al. Image guided dose escalated prostate radiotherapy: still room to improve. *Radiat Oncol* 2009;4:50.
148. Peeters ST, Heemsbergen WD, van Putten WL, et al. Acute and late complications after radiotherapy for prostate cancer: results of a multicenter randomized trial comparing 68 Gy to 78 Gy. *Int J Radiat Oncol Biol Phys* 2005;61(4):1019.
149. Zelefsky MJ, Chan H, Hunt M, Yamada Y, Shippy AM, Amols H. Long-term outcome of high dose intensity modulated radiation therapy for patients with clinically localized prostate cancer. *J Urol* 2006;176(4 Pt 1):1415.
150. van der Wielen GJ, Mulhall JP, Incrocci L. Erectile dysfunction after radiotherapy for prostate cancer and radiation dose to the penile structures: a critical review. *Radiother Oncol* 2007;84(2):107.
154. Zelefsky MJ, Kuban DA, Levy LB, et al. Multi-institutional analysis of long-term outcome for stages T1-T2 prostate cancer treated with permanent seed implantation. *Int J Radiat Oncol Biol Phys* 2007;67(2):327.
157. Zelefsky MJ, Yamada Y, Marion C, et al. Improved conformality and decreased toxicity with intraoperative computer-optimized transperineal ultrasound-guided prostate brachytherapy. *Int J Radiat Oncol Biol Phys* 2003;55(4):956.
163. Zelefsky MJ, Worman M, Cohen GN, et al. Real-time intraoperative computed tomography assessment of quality of permanent interstitial seed implantation for prostate cancer. *Urology* 2010;76(5):1138.
167. Nag S, Bice W, DeWyngaert K, Prestidge B, Stock R, Yu Y. The American Brachytherapy Society recommendations for permanent prostate brachytherapy postimplant dosimetric analysis. *Int J Radiat Oncol Biol Phys* 2000;46(1):221.
171. Henry AM, Al-Qaisieh B, Gould K, et al. Outcomes following iodine-125 monotherapy for localized prostate cancer: the results of leeds 10-year single-center brachytherapy experience. *Int J Radiat Oncol Biol Phys* 2010;76(1):50.
172. Taira AV, Merrick GS, Butler WM, et al. Long-term Outcome for Clinically Localized Prostate Cancer Treated With Permanent Interstitial Brachytherapy. *Int J Radiat Oncol Biol Phys* 2010.
173. Sylvester JE, Grimm PD, Blasko JC, et al. 15-Year biochemical relapse free survival in clinical Stage T1-T3 prostate cancer following combined external beam radiotherapy and brachytherapy; Seattle experience. *Int J Radiat Oncol Biol Phys* 2007;67(1):57.
176. Keyes M, Miller S, Mirvan V, et al. Acute and late urinary toxicity in 606 prostate brachytherapy patients—The BC Cancer Agency experience. *Brachytherapy* 2007;6(2):91.
195. Zelefsky MJ, Nedelka MA, Arican ZL, et al. Combined brachytherapy with external beam radiotherapy for localized prostate cancer: reduced morbidity with an intraoperative brachytherapy planning technique and supplemental intensity-modulated radiation therapy. *Brachytherapy* 2008;7(1):1.
196. Galalae RM, Martinez A, Mate T, et al. Long-term outcome by risk factors using conformal high-dose-rate brachytherapy (HDR-BT) boost with or without neoadjuvant androgen suppression for localized prostate cancer. *Int J Radiat Oncol Biol Phys* 2004;58(4):1048.
199. Yamada Y, Bhatia S, Zaider M, et al. Favorable clinical outcomes of three-dimensional computer-optimized high-dose-rate prostate brachytherapy in the management of localized prostate cancer. *Brachytherapy* 2006;5(3):157.
202. Hoskin PJ, Motohashi K, Bownes P, Bryant L, Ostler P. High dose rate brachytherapy in combination with external beam radiotherapy in the radical treatment of prostate cancer: initial results of a randomised phase three trial. *Radiother Oncol* 2007;84(2):114.
206. Souhami L, Bae K, Pilepich M, Sandler H. Impact of the duration of adjuvant hormonal therapy in patients with locally advanced prostate cancer treated with radiotherapy: a secondary analysis of RTOG 85-31. *J Clin Oncol* 2009;27(13):2137.
207. Bolla M, Collette L, Blank L, et al. Long-term results with immediate androgen suppression and external irradiation in patients with locally advanced prostate cancer (an EORTC study): a phase III randomised trial. *Lancet* 2002;360(9327):103.
208. Roach M 3rd, Bae K, Speight J, et al. Short-term neoadjuvant androgen deprivation therapy and external-beam radiotherapy for locally advanced prostate cancer: long-term results of RTOG 8610. *J Clin Oncol* 2008;26(4):585.
209. Hanks GE, Pajak TF, Porter A, et al. Phase III trial of long-term adjuvant androgen deprivation after neoadjuvant hormonal cytoreduction and radiotherapy in locally advanced carcinoma of the prostate: the Radiation Therapy Oncology Group Protocol 92-02. *J Clin Oncol* 2003;21(21):3972.
210. D'Amico AV, Manola J, Loffredo M, Renshaw AA, DellaCroce A, Kantoff PW. 6-month androgen suppression plus radiation therapy vs radiation therapy alone for patients with clinically localized prostate cancer: a randomized controlled trial. *JAMA* 2004;292(7):821.

211. Crook J, Ludgate C, Malone S, et al. Report of a multicenter Canadian phase III randomized trial of 3 months vs. 8 months neoadjuvant androgen deprivation before standard-dose radiotherapy for clinically localized prostate cancer. *Int J Radiat Oncol Biol Phys* 2004;60(1):15.
212. Bolla M, van Tienhoven G, de Reijke T, et al. Concomitant and adjuvant androgen deprivation (ADT) with external beam irradiation (RT) for locally advanced prostate cancer: 6 months versus 3 years ADT—Results of the randomized EORTC Phase III trial 22961 (abstract). *J Clin Oncol* 2007;25:5014.
213. Nanda A, Chen MH, Braccioforte MH, Moran BJ, D'Amico AV. Hormonal therapy use for prostate cancer and mortality in men with coronary artery disease-induced congestive heart failure or myocardial infarction. *JAMA* 2009;302(8):866.
216. Thompson IM, Tangen CM, Paradelo J, et al. Adjuvant radiotherapy for pathological T3N0M0 prostate cancer significantly reduces risk of metastases and improves survival: long-term followup of a randomized clinical trial. *J Urol* 2009;181(3):956.
217. Bolla M, van Poppel H, Collette L, et al. Postoperative radiotherapy after radical prostatectomy: a randomised controlled trial (EORTC trial 22911). *Lancet* 2005;366(9485):572.
218. Wiegel T, Bottke D, Steiner U, et al. Phase III postoperative adjuvant radiotherapy after radical prostatectomy compared with radical prostatectomy alone in pT3 prostate cancer with postoperative undetectable prostate-specific antigen: ARO 96-02/AUO AP 09/95. *J Clin Oncol* 2009;27(18):2924.
225. Pound CR, Partin AW, Eisenberger MA, Chan DW, Pearson JD, Walsh PC. Natural history of progression after PSA elevation following radical prostatectomy. *JAMA* 1999;281(17):1591.
226. Freedland SJ, Humphreys EB, Mangold LA, et al. Risk of prostate cancer-specific mortality following biochemical recurrence after radical prostatectomy. *JAMA* 2005;294(4):433.
227. Freedland SJ, Humphreys EB, Mangold LA, et al. Death in patients with recurrent prostate cancer after radical prostatectomy: prostate-specific antigen doubling time subgroups and their associated contributions to all-cause mortality. *J Clin Oncol* 2007;25(13):1765.
236. Stephenson AJ, Shariat SF, Zelefsky MJ, et al. Salvage radiotherapy for recurrent prostate cancer after radical prostatectomy. *JAMA* 2004;291(11):1325.
237. Choo R, Hruby G, Hong J, et al. (IN)-efficacy of Salvage radiotherapy for rising PSA or clinically isolated local recurrence after radical prostatectomy. *Int J Radiat Oncol Biol Phys* 2002;53(2):269–276.
247. Pisters LL, Leibovici D, Blute M, et al. Locally recurrent prostate cancer after initial radiation therapy: a comparison of salvage radical prostatectomy versus cryotherapy. *J Urol* 2009;182(2):517.
254. Burri RJ, Stone NN, Unger P, Stock RG. Long-term outcome and toxicity of salvage brachytherapy for local failure after initial radiotherapy for prostate cancer. *Int J Radiat Oncol Biol Phys* 2010;77(5):1338.
256. Chin JL, Pautler SE, Mouraviev V, Touma N, Moore K, Downey DB. Results of salvage cryoablation of the prostate after radiation: identifying predictors of treatment failure and complications. *J Urol* 2001;165(6 Pt 1):1937.
273. Widmark A, Klepp O, Solberg A, et al. Endocrine treatment, with or without radiotherapy, in locally advanced prostate cancer (SPCG-7/SFUO-3): an open randomised phase III trial. *Lancet* 2009;373(9660):301.
282. Eisenberger MA, Blumenstein BA, Crawford ED, et al. Bilateral orchiectomy with or without flutamide for metastatic prostate cancer. *N Engl J Med* 1998;339(15):1036.
283. Messing EM, Manola J, Sarosdy M, Wilding G, Crawford ED, Trump D. Immediate hormonal therapy compared with observation after radical prostatectomy and pelvic lymphadenectomy in men with node-positive prostate cancer. *N Engl J Med* 1999;341(24):1781.
303. Shahinian VB, Kuo YF, Freeman JL, Goodwin JS. Risk of fracture after androgen deprivation for prostate cancer. *N Engl J Med* 2005;352(2):154.
306. Levine GN, D'Amico AV, Berger P, et al. Androgen-deprivation therapy in prostate cancer and cardiovascular risk: a science advisory from the American Heart Association, American Cancer Society, and American Urological Association: endorsed by the American Society for Radiation Oncology. *CA Cancer J Clin* 2010;60(3):194.
319. Calais da Silva FE, Bono AV, Whelan P, et al. Intermittent androgen deprivation for locally advanced and metastatic prostate cancer: results from a randomised phase 3 study of the South European Uroncological Group. *Eur Urol* 2009;55(6):1269.
323. Smith MR, Kabbinavar F, Saad F, et al. Natural history of rising serum prostate-specific antigen in men with castrate nonmetastatic prostate cancer. *J Clin Oncol* 2005;23(13):2918.
325. Halabi S, Small EJ, Kantoff PW, et al. Prognostic model for predicting survival in men with hormone-refractory metastatic prostate cancer. *J Clin Oncol* 2003;21(7):1232.
332. Petrylak DP, Ankerst DP, Jiang CS, et al. Evaluation of prostate-specific antigen declines for surrogacy in patients treated on SWOG 99-16. *J Natl Cancer Inst* 2006;98(8):516.
338. Sartor O, Reid RH, Hoskin PJ, et al. Samarium-153-Lexidronam complex for treatment of painful bone metastases in hormone-refractory prostate cancer. *Urology* 2004;63(5):940.
343. Tannock IF, Osoba D, Stockler MR, et al. Chemotherapy with mitoxantrone plus prednisone or prednisone alone for symptomatic hormone-resistant prostate cancer: a Canadian randomized trial with palliative end points. *J Clin Oncol* 1996;14(6):1756.
344. Titus MA, Schell MJ, Lih FB, Tomer KB, Mohler JL. Testosterone and dihydrotestosterone tissue levels in recurrent prostate cancer. *Clin Cancer Res* 2005;11(13):4653.
376. Saad F, Gleason DM, Murray R, et al. A randomized, placebo-controlled trial of zoledronic acid in patients with hormone-refractory metastatic prostate carcinoma. *J Natl Cancer Inst* 2002;94(19):1458.
383. Kantoff PW, Higano CS, Shore ND, et al. Sipuleucel-T immunotherapy for castration-resistant prostate cancer. *N Engl J Med* 2010;363:411.
384. Petrylak DP, Tangen CM, Hussain MH, et al. Docetaxel and estramustine compared with mitoxantrone and prednisone for advanced refractory prostate cancer. *N Engl J Med* 2004;351(15):1513.
396. Sartor A, Oudard S, Ozguroglu M, et al. Cabazitaxel or mitoxantrone with prednisone in patients with metastatic castration-resistant prostate cancer (mCRPC) previously treated with docetaxel: Final results of a multinational phase III trial (TROPIC). ASCO GU Cancer Symposi, Abstract 9, 2010.
411. Bianco FJ Jr, Scardino PT, Stephenson AJ, Diblasio CJ, Fearn PA, Eastham JA. Long-term oncologic results of salvage radical prostatectomy for locally recurrent prostate cancer after radiotherapy. *Int J Radiat Oncol Biol Phys* 2005;62(2):448.

CHAPTER 98 CANCER OF THE URETHRA AND PENIS

EDOUARD J. TRABULSI AND LEONARD G. GOMELLA

Penile and urethral carcinomas are uncommon malignancies, with a peak incidence in the sixth decade of life. Often overshadowed by more common genitourinary cancers, penile and urethral cancers represent difficult challenges for the treating physician. Squamous cell carcinoma is the most frequent type of cancer in the penis and the urethra. Carcinoma of the penis is a slow-growing tumor with a usually well-defined pattern of dissemination. This orderly spread allows definitive locoregional management of the primary tumor in most cases. In contradistinction, urethral carcinoma in men and women tends to invade locally and metastasize to regional nodes early. Depending on the site of the urethra involved and disease extent, a multimodal treatment approach may be required to treat this aggressive tumor.[1]

CANCER OF THE MALE URETHRA

Carcinoma of the male urethra is uncommon. Chronic irritation and infection are the strongest risk factors. The incidence of urethral stricture in men with development of urethral cancer ranges from 24% to 76%, and most of these strictures involve the bulbomembranous urethra, also the most frequent site of cancer.[2] Human papillomavirus-16 (HPV-16) likely has a causative role in the development of squamous cell carcinoma of the urethra.[3] No racial predisposition has been noted.

The onset of malignancy in a patient with a long-standing urethral stricture disease is often insidious, and a high index of suspicion is needed to diagnose these tumors early. The new onset of urethrorrhagia or urethral stricture in a man without a history of trauma or venereal disease should raise the possibility of urethral carcinoma. A palpable urethral mass associated with obstructive voiding symptoms is the most common presenting symptom.[4] Pain associated with a periurethral abscess or urethral fistula may be the harbinger of a male urethral cancer.

Pathology

Overall, 80% of male urethral cancers are squamous cell, 15% are transitional cell, and approximately 5% are adenocarcinomas or undifferentiated tumors.[5] The anatomic location of urethral cancer largely determines the histologic type. Carcinomas of the prostatic urethra are transitional cell in 90% and squamous in 10%; conversely, carcinomas of the penile urethra are squamous in 90% and transitional in 10%. Adenocarcinomas of the urethra arise from metaplasia of mucosa or from periurethral glands, but direct invasion of rectal adenocarcinoma must be ruled out. Adenocarcinoma has the same prognosis, stage for stage, as the other histologies.[4]

The bulbomembranous urethra is most commonly involved (60%), followed by the penile urethra (30%) and the prostatic urethra (10%).[4] The incidence of urethral involvement associated with carcinoma of the bladder has been estimated to be approximately 6%,[6] and urethral recurrences after radical cystectomy occur in 4% to 17%.[7]

Male urethral cancer may spread locally to involve the corpus spongiosum or may metastasize to regional nodes. The lymphatics of the anterior urethra drain into the superficial and deep inguinal lymph nodes and occasionally to the external iliac nodes. The lymphatics from the posterior urethra drain into the external iliac, obturator, and hypogastric nodes. Palpable inguinal nodes are found in approximately 20% and almost always suggest metastatic disease, in contrast to penile cancer, where 50% of palpable nodes are inflammatory. Bulbomembranous urethral cancer in particular spreads to the urogenital diaphragm, prostate, perineum, and scrotum. Hematogenous spread is rare except in advanced disease and in primary transitional cell carcinoma of the prostatic urethra.

Evaluation and Staging

The American Joint Committee on Cancer (AJCC) tumor, node, metastasis (TNM) staging system (seventh edition, 2010)[8] is based on the depth of invasion of the primary tumor and the presence or absence of regional lymph node involvement and distant metastasis (Table 98.1). The 2010 AJCC system subdivides T1 lesions into T1a (no lymphovascular invasion [LVI] or poorly differentiated tumors) and T1b (the presence of LVI or poorly differentiated histology); prostatic invasion is now reclassified as T4 disease (previously T3). Examination under anesthesia is useful to evaluate the local extent of disease. Cystoscopy and transurethral or needle biopsy of the lesion, and of the prostate if indicated, are also performed at the time of examination under anesthesia. A complete blood count and serum chemistry analysis coupled with urine culture and cytology are routinely obtained. Cytology is particularly helpful in patients with transitional cell carcinoma. A computed tomography (CT) scan with contrast is useful in local staging with magnetic resonance imaging (MRI) scan with gadolinium the ideal staging modality for evaluating local soft tissue, lymph node, and bone involvement.[9]

Treatment

Surgery is the mainstay of treatment of carcinoma of the male urethra. In general, anterior urethral cancers are more amenable to surgical extirpation, and the prognosis is better than that of posterior urethral tumors, which are more often associated with extensive local invasion and distant metastasis.[10] Radiation therapy is reserved for early-stage lesions of the anterior urethra who refuse surgery. Although it preserves the penis, radiation may cause urethral stricture or chronic penile edema and may

TABLE 98.1

AMERICAN JOINT COMMITTEE ON CANCER TUMOR, NODE, METASTASIS CLASSIFICATION SYSTEM FOR URETHRAL CANCER

Stage Grouping			
0a	Ta	N0	M0
0is	Tis	N0	M0
	Tis (prostatic urethra)	N0	M0
	Tis (prostatic ducts)	N0	M0
I	T1	N0	M0
II	T2	N0	M0
III	T1	N1	M0
	T2	N1	M0
	T3	N0	M0
	T4	N1	M0
IV	T4	N0	M0
	T4	N1	M0
	Any T	N2	M0
	Any T	Any N	M1

From ref. 8, with permission.

not prevent new tumor occurrence. Multimodal treatment combining chemotherapy and radiation therapy with surgical excision for locally advanced urethral carcinomas has yielded promising results (disease-free survival 60% in one series).[11] The median survival without treatment or with palliation is approximately 3 months.

Site-Specific Treatment

Carcinoma of the Distal Urethra. Superficial tumors (Ta, Tis, and T1) are usually treated with transurethral resection and fulguration with close follow-up. Tumors invading the corpus spongiosum (T2) and localized to the distal half of the penis are best treated with a partial penile amputation with a 2-cm margin proximal to the visible or palpable tumor. If infiltrating tumor is confined to the proximal penile urethra or involves the entire urethra, total penectomy is indicated. Isolated reports of penile-sparing surgery (urethrectomy with corpora cavernosa sparing) have a high incidence of failure.[12] Ilioinguinal node dissection is indicated only in the presence of palpable adenopathy. Prophylactic groin dissection has no proven role in this site.

Carcinoma of the Bulbomembranous Urethra. Early superficial tumors (Ta, Tis, and T1) can be treated with transurethral fulguration or segmental resection with end-to-end anastomosis; however, such cases are rare. Invasive tumors (T2, T3) are best treated with radical cystoprostatectomy with *en bloc* penectomy and pelvic lymphadenectomy. In spite of this aggressive approach, the prognosis remains dismal, with a 5-year disease-free survival of 26% in patients with invasive bulbomembranous carcinomas.[13] Isolated reports of penile preservation surgery for invasive bulbomembranous cancers have used adjuvant radiation therapy (45 Gy) and concurrent chemotherapy with 5-fluorouracil (5-FU) and mitomycin C with acceptable results.[14]

Carcinoma of the Prostatic Urethra. Primary carcinoma arising from the prostatic urethra is rare. Adenocarcinomas and transitional cell carcinomas are found. Although superficial lesions (Tis-pu, Tis-pd, T1) can be managed by transurethral resection, such tumors are rare. Invasive transitional cell carcinoma of the prostatic stroma (T2) carries a poor prognosis despite aggressive surgical therapy. Extravesical extension of disease has a worse prognosis than intraurethral disease, with a higher chance of nodal involvement and a 5-year survival rate of only 32%.[15]

Advanced carcinoma (T3-4N1 to N3) of the prostatic urethra is best treated with a combination of neoadjuvant chemotherapy (methotrexate sodium, vinblastine sulfate, doxorubicin hydrochloride [adriamycin], and cisplatin [MVAC]) with consolidative surgery or irradiation. One series of five patients (with T2-4N0M0 lesions) treated with neoadjuvant MVAC chemotherapy had a complete response rate of 60%.[16] MVAC chemotherapy preoperatively was ineffective against nontransitional cell carcinoma.

Radiation and Multimodal Therapy

Radiation therapy alone has poor results in male urethral carcinoma. Patients who receive radiation therapy followed by salvage surgery seem to fare worse than with surgery in an integrated fashion. The most common approach has been external-beam radiotherapy of 50 to 60 Gy with best results for *distal* urethral lesions. Multimodal therapy with chemoradiation has shown the efficacy of 5-FU, mitomycin C, and cisplatin with radiation for squamous cell carcinoma of the urethra.[17,18]

CARCINOMA OF THE FEMALE URETHRA

Carcinoma of the urethra is the only genitourinary neoplasm that is more common in women than in men (four-to-one ratio). The peak incidence is in the sixth decade, more commonly in white women. Chronic irritation, recurrent urinary tract infections, and a host of proliferative lesions (caruncles, papillomas, polyps) are predisposing factors, and HPV may play a role. Leukoplakia of the urethra is considered a premalignant condition. In females the urethra is approximately 4 cm long, mostly buried in the anterior vaginal wall, and divided into the distal one-third (anterior urethra) and the proximal two-thirds (posterior urethra). The most common presenting symptom (greater than 50%) is urethrorrhagia. Urinary frequency, obstructive voiding, a foul-smelling discharge, and a palpable urethral mass are other modes of presentation. Initially it may be difficult to distinguish fungating tumors of the urethra from those of the vagina or vulva.

Spread of urethral carcinoma follows the anatomic subdivision: lymphatics of the anterior urethra drain into the superficial and deep inguinal nodes and the posterior urethra into the external iliac, hypogastric, and obturator nodes. At presentation, one-third of patients have inguinal lymph node metastases and 20% have pelvic node involvement. Palpable inguinal nodes in patients with urethral cancer invariably contain metastatic carcinoma. The most common sites of distant spread are the lungs, liver, and bone.[19]

Pathology

Stratified squamous epithelium lines the distal two-thirds of the female urethra, and transitional epithelium lines the proximal one-third. The majority (60%) of neoplasms of the female urethra are squamous cell carcinomas. Less common types are transitional cell carcinoma (20%), adenocarcinoma (10%), undifferentiated tumors (8%), and melanoma (2%). Clear cell carcinoma is a distinctive clinical entity that has generated considerable interest with respect to its prognosis and relationship to urethral diverticulae.[20] Histology does not affect the prognosis, and all are treated similarly. In general, anterior urethral carcinomas are low grade and stage; carcinomas involving the proximal or entire urethra are of a higher grade and stage.

Evaluation and Staging

The workup for women with suspected urethral carcinoma includes a pelvic examination under anesthesia, cystourethroscopy, and biopsy. Radiographic evaluation includes a chest x-ray and CT of the pelvis and abdomen. MRI is particularly useful for staging of female urethral carcinoma. Although the AJCC (seventh edition) TNM staging includes female urethral cancer,[8] the practical usefulness is limited. Clinically it is more useful to stage, treat, and prognosticate female urethral cancers by stratifying patients based on anatomic location (anterior vs. posterior urethra vs. entire urethra) and clinical stage (low stage vs. high stage).[21]

Treatment

The anatomic location and stage of the tumor are the most significant prognostic factors predicting local control and survival. Treatment is based on the stage at the time of initial presentation, with low-stage distal urethral tumors having a better prognosis than high-stage proximal urethral tumors. In one series the 5-year disease-specific survival was 46%, with 89% survival for low-stage tumors and 33% for high-stage disease.[22]

Local surgical excision is often sufficient in selected patients with low-stage distal urethra carcinoma. With proximal urethra and for bulky locally advanced tumors, more aggressive treatment with an anterior pelvic exenteration is often needed (*en bloc* total urethrectomy, cystectomy, pelvic lymphadenectomy, hysterectomy with salpingectomy, removal of the anterior vaginal wall). Bulky proximal urethral tumors that invade the pubic symphysis may require resection of the pubic symphysis and inferior rami. Anterior exenteration alone has been reported to produce a 5-year survival rate of less than 20% in patients with invasive carcinoma of the female urethra.[23]

Radiation therapy (brachytherapy alone or with external-beam radiation) is an alternative to surgery in low-stage urethral carcinoma with cure rates up to 75%. The reported doses have ranged from 50 to 60 Gy for brachytherapy alone and 40 to 45 Gy external-beam radiation to the whole pelvis followed by a brachytherapy boost of 20 to 25 Gy over 2 to 3 days. Proximal urethral tumors with bladder neck invasion and bulky tumors require combined external-beam and brachytherapy. Large primary tumor bulk and treatment with external radiation alone (no brachytherapy) were independent adverse prognostic factors. Brachytherapy reduced the risk of local recurrence, possibly as a result of the higher radiation dose.[24] Complications from radiation therapy occur in about 20% and include urethral strictures and stenosis, urethrovaginal fistulas, incontinence, and bowel obstruction.

Combined modality treatment with neoadjuvant chemotherapy and preoperative radiation therapy, followed by surgery, is recommended for advanced female urethral carcinoma. A 55% survival rate has been reported with advanced urethral carcinoma treated with radiotherapy plus surgery, as compared with a rate of 34% with radiation alone.[25] Although long-term results from multimodal therapy are not yet available, combination chemotherapy, radiation, and surgery is believed essential for local control and cure with larger or locally advanced urethral cancer.[22] The prognosis for women with carcinoma of the urethra is poor, regardless of the treatment modality used, and the median time to local recurrence for invasive carcinoma is 13 months.

Distal Urethral Carcinoma

Small superficial (Ta, Tis, and T1) tumors of the distal female urethra can be removed surgically with little risk of urinary incontinence. Spatulation of the urethra and approximation to the adjacent vagina preserve urinary continence and prevent meatal stenosis. For small invasive tumors of the distal urethra (T2), brachytherapy alone is an excellent therapeutic option.

Proximal Urethral Carcinoma

Proximal female urethral carcinomas tend to be more aggressive and bulky. For advanced (T3 and T4) lesions, a multimodal approach is preferred. Surgery consists of a radical cystourethrectomy or an anterior exenteration, depending on the extent of the disease. Radiation therapy with a combination of brachytherapy and external-beam irradiation is usually required. Neoadjuvant chemotherapy with 5-FU and mitomycin C has been noted to enhance the therapeutic ratio of radiation therapy.

CANCER OF THE PENIS

Carcinoma of the penis is an uncommon malignancy in Western countries, representing 0.4% of male malignancies and 3.0% of all genitourinary cancers. Penile cancer constitutes a major health problem in many countries in Asia, Africa, and South America, where it may comprise up to 10% of all malignancies. The incidence of penile cancer has been declining in many countries, partly because of increased attention to personal hygiene.[26] It most commonly presents in the sixth decade but may occur in men younger than 40 years. Analysis of the Surveillance, Epidemiology, and End Results (SEER) data shows no racial difference in the incidence of penile cancer among African American men and white men, but significant disparities exist in the mortality of invasive penile carcinoma in the United States.[27] Significantly lower rates of invasive penile cancer are seen in Asian American men and significantly higher rates are seen in Hispanic American men. Regional and socioeconomic differences are also noted, with higher rates in the southern area of the United States and in lower socioeconomic populations.

Etiology

Penile cancer is associated with phimosis and poor local hygiene, with phimosis found in more than half the patients. The irritative effect of smegma, a byproduct of bacterial action on desquamated epithelial cells in the preputial sac, is well known, although definitive evidence of its role in carcinogenesis is lacking. Neonatal circumcision as practiced by religious groups virtually eliminates the occurrence of penile carcinoma. Delaying circumcision until puberty or adult circumcision does not have the same benefit.[28]

HPV infection, particularly HPV-16, has been implicated in the development of invasive penile cancer, as has the number of sexual partners.[28] HPV infection accounts for about half of penile cancers, with HPV-16 and -18 the predominant subtypes.[29,30] The use of tobacco products is an independent risk factor.[31] Thus, avoidance of tobacco products and HPV infection, penile hygiene, and neonatal circumcision represent important preventive strategies against penile cancer.

Symptoms

Local symptoms and signs often draw attention to penile cancer. The clinical spectrum of penile cancer is varied: subtle areas of erythema or induration to a frankly ulcerated, fungating, foul-smelling mass. Penile cancer is commonly associated with concomitant infection, with infection playing an important role in the pathogenesis and ultimately in the presentation of the disease. Pain usually is not a prominent feature and is not proportional to the extent of local destruction. The lesion primarily involves the prepuce and glans, often under a tight phimotic ring. In late stages, involvement and destruction of the shaft of the penis or urethra are seen. Urethral obstruction is rare. Instead, erosion of the urethra with multiple fistulas ("watering-can perineum") may be seen. Rarely, inguinal ulceration may be the presenting symptom, with the primary tumor concealed within a phimotic preputial sac.

Patients with penile cancer, more than with other types of cancer, delay seeking medical attention. Historically, up to 50% of patients delayed more than 1 year in seeking medical help; contemporary series, especially from the United States, fail to show such a trend.

Pathology

More than 95% of penile carcinomas are squamous cell. Non–squamous cell carcinomas consist of melanomas, basal cell carcinomas, lymphomas, and sarcomas. Nearly 18% of patients with acquired immunodeficiency syndrome–related Kaposi's sarcoma have penile involvement.[32]

Squamous cell carcinomas are graded using Broders' classification. Low-grade tumors (grades I and II), typically confined to the prepuce and glans penis, constitute nearly 80% of penile cancers. Most lesions that involve the shaft of the penis are high grade (grade III), with grade and stage often correlated. The incidence of lymph node metastases from squamous cell carcinoma of the penis is related to histologic grade. Verrucous carcinoma, a particularly exuberant variant of squamous cell carcinoma, has low potential for lymph node spread and a good prognosis. Another important predictor of lymph node metastases and, hence, prognosis is the presence of vascular invasion.[33]

Premalignant Lesions

The description of early and premalignant lesions has been complicated by the rarity of the disease and a proliferation of eponyms.

Leukoplakia

Leukoplakia is characterized by the presence of solitary or multiple whitish plaques involving the glans or prepuce in the setting of chronic or recurrent balanoposthitis. Surgical excision in the form of circumcision or local wedge resection is usually curative.

Balanitis Xerotica Obliterans

Balanitis xerotica obliterans (BXO) is an inflammatory condition of the glans and prepuce of unknown cause. BXO is a scaly, indurated, whitish plaque that produces significant phimosis and meatal stenosis. Although selected reports suggest an association with penile cancer, treatment remains controversial and consists of topical steroids and surgical excision. Meatoplasty may be required, with early circumcision the most effective treatment for BXO.[34]

Buschke-Löwenstein Tumor

The Buschke-Löwenstein tumor is a large exophytic mass involving the glans penis and prepuce; it is a giant condyloma acuminatum that has a good prognosis and does not metastasize. Except for unrestrained local growth, this lesion has malignant features. A viral etiology has been proposed, with identification of HPV-6 and -11 in some tumors. Treatment consists of local conservative resection. Recurrence is common. Systemic interferon-alfa therapy combined with neodymium: yttrium aluminum garnet (Nd:YAG) laser therapy is successful in some cases. Radiation therapy is contraindicated because rapid malignant degeneration has been described.

TABLE 98.2

AMERICAN JOINT COMMITTEE ON CANCER TUMOR, NODE, METASTASIS CLASSIFICATION SYSTEM FOR PENILE CANCER

Stage Grouping			
0	Tis	N0	M0
	Ta	N0	M0
I	T1a	N0	M0
II	T1b	N0	M0
	T2	N0	M0
	T3	N0	M0
IIIa	T1-3	N1	M0
IIIb	T1-3	N2	M0
IV	T4	Any N	M0
	Any T	N3	M0
	Any T	Any N	M1

From ref. 8, with permission.

Diagnosis and Staging

The workup for penile cancer begins with physical examination of the genitalia and inguinal nodes to ascertain local extent of the lesion and the presence of inguinal adenopathy. Nodal status is the most significant prognostic variable predicting survival. Approximately 50% of patients with penile cancer present with palpable inguinal nodes. Only half of these patients will have metastatic disease, with the remainder having inflammatory adenopathy secondary to infection of the primary lesion. Conversely, 20% of patients with clinically negative groin examination are found to have metastases on prophylactic node dissection. The most common distant metastatic sites are the lung, bone, and liver. The AJCC system (seventh edition) for staging penile cancer uses the TNM classification to determine the stage of the primary tumor and the extent of nodal metastases (Table 98.2).[8]

After biopsy confirmation of the lesion, no further radiologic workup is generally needed in patients with early-stage disease and the absence of inguinal adenopathy on examination or other worrisome symptoms. Ultrasound and gadolinium-enhanced MRI are recommended for high-grade and high-stage lesions suspected of involving the corporal bodies, especially if partial penectomy is contemplated. Abdominal and pelvic CT scanning is recommended in obese patients to evaluate the inguinal nodes. In patients with known inguinal metastases, CT-guided biopsy of enlarged pelvic nodes, if positive, may be an indication for neoadjuvant chemotherapy. The role of positron emission tomography (PET) scan in the staging of penile cancer is unclear, with conflicting data.[35–37]

Treatment

Treatment of penile carcinoma depends on the local extent of the primary neoplasm and the regional lymph node status. For the primary lesion, a 2-cm proximal margin of resection is recommended. If an adequate margin can be obtained, a partial penectomy offers excellent local control. Leaving the patient with adequate penile length for hygienic upright micturition and sexual intercourse is the goal. Thus, depending on the extent of the primary tumor, resection may include a partial or total penectomy, with local recurrence rare.[38]

In advanced cases (T4), more aggressive resections (emasculation, hemipelvectomy, hemicorpectomy) have been reported. Although surgery is the mainstay for treatment of the primary lesion, radiation therapy can be considered for a select group of patients. Radiation therapy allows preservation of the penis, obviating the psychosocial and physical morbidity caused by partial or total penectomy. External-beam and brachytherapy techniques have been used for treatment of the primary cancer. Circumcision is generally recommended before radiation therapy is initiated. This allows for further evaluation of the tumor extent and reduces morbidity associated with radiation (swelling, maceration, secondary infection), all of which may eventually result in secondary phimosis. Although radiation can control early (T1 and T2) lesions with a 65% to 80% success rate, treatment of more advanced T-stage penile cancers is fraught with local recurrences (20% to 40%) and risk of tumor progression to nodal and systemic disease.[39] Thus, radiation therapy, although cosmetically attractive, has disadvantages, and the number of patients for whom this treatment is appropriate is small.

Of paramount importance in treatment is consideration of the lymphatic drainage of the penis. The inguinal lymph nodes constitute the first echelon of drainage. Superficial and deep inguinal nodes are involved in a stepwise manner. Bilateral drainage occurs as a result of free anastomoses and crossover at the base of the penis. Therefore, the pattern of nodal metastasis is not limited to one side. The superficial inguinal nodes are located in the deep portion of Camper's fascia above the deep fascia of the thigh (fascia lata). The superficial lymphatics drain into the deep inguinal lymphatics, which surround the femoral vessels deep to the fascia lata. Secondary drainage is to the iliac nodes, although direct drainage to these nodes (skip metastases) can occur rarely.

Five-year disease-free survival rates for palpably negative adenopathy (cN0) or low volume palpable groin disease (cN1) are similar and favorable at 93% and 84%, respectively, with a markedly worse survival for palpably bulky disease (cN2 or cN3) of 32% and 0%, respectively.[40] When stratified by pathologic stage, low volume nodal involvement (pN1) had favorable and similar 5-year disease-free survival rates when compared to pathologically negative nodes (pN0) at 93% and 90%, respectively. Pathologically confirmed bulky adenopathy (pN2 and pN3) had very poor long-term outcomes with 5-year disease-free survival rates of 31% and 0%, respectively.

Based on the rarity of advanced penile carcinoma in the Western world, there is growing awareness that these men may receive better outcomes if they are directed to tertiary care centers with expertise in penile carcinoma and inguinal lymphadenectomy. In the United Kingdom, the National Institute for Clinical Excellence (NICE) published guidelines in 2002 that included the treatment of penile carcinoma and advocated the creation of regional multidisciplinary teams.[41] These guidelines have increased the rate of penis-preserving procedures and inguinal lymphadenectomy, with decreased mortality.[42]

Treatment of Primary Lesion

Surgery for penile carcinoma ranges from circumcision, conservative local resection, laser ablation, and Mohs micrographic surgery to partial and total penectomy. Radiation therapy can be used in selected patients with early superficial lesions.

Carcinoma In Situ *(Tis).* Penile squamous cell carcinoma *in situ*, also known as erythroplasia of Queyrat, is a red, velvety, well-marginated lesion of the glans penis or the prepuce of uncircumcised men. After confirmatory biopsy, a conservative approach that spares penile anatomy and function is preferred. Preputial lesions are adequately treated with circumcision. Topical 5-FU cream has been used with excellent cosmetic results for glandular and meatal lesions. A prospective study of carbon dioxide and Nd:YAG lasers has shown good local tumor control and satisfactory cosmetic results.[43] Mohs micrographic surgery has been described as a less-deforming alternative, with local control rates up to 86% in selected patients with early penile cancer.[44] Radiation therapy can often eradicate these lesions with minimal morbidity.

Verrucous Carcinoma (Ta). Penile verrucous carcinoma is characterized by aggressive local growth and a low metastatic potential. Partial or total penectomy is usually overtreatment, and conservative therapeutic approaches are favored. Laser ablation or Mohs micrographic surgical technique has yielded acceptable results. Intra-aortic infusion with methotrexate has been reported with reasonable results.[45] Radiation therapy is contraindicated as it has been shown to cause subsequent rapid malignant degeneration and metastases.

Invasive Penile Cancer (T1, T2, T3, and N1). Distal penile lesions, in which a serviceable penis for upright micturition and sexual function can be achieved, are best treated with a partial penectomy. Extensive lesions that approach the base of the penis usually require total penectomy with corporal body excision and perineal urethrostomy. Local recurrence after a partial penectomy in properly selected cases is rare. Most relapses occur within the first 12 to 18 months after penectomy, and salvage surgery is beneficial.

The effectiveness of radiation therapy in the treatment of penile cancer is hindered by a lack of uniformity of radiation treatment in terms of type of delivery and doses. Radiation therapy is effective for local control of small, 2- to 4-cm, T1 and T2 lesions but also for more advanced T-stage tumors. Local recurrence is higher in those with T3 and T4 tumors, but a significant percentage can be salvaged by adjuvant surgical resection.[46] Before treatment, patients should have a circumcision to allow direct inspection and staging of the tumor and to facilitate management of the acute side effects of radiation. External-beam and brachytherapy techniques have been used. External-beam radiotherapy can be delivered by a direct field method that uses a low-energy photon beam or an electron beam applied directly to the tumor, with a safety margin of 2 cm beyond the visible and palpable extent of the tumor. This approach is suitable only for very superficial tumors (Tis and T1). For T2 and T3 lesions, a parallel opposed field method is used. Using this approach the entire thickness of the penis can be irradiated by encasing the lesion in a wax mold to ensure uniform dosage and to negate the skin-sparing effects of supervoltage beams with a total dose of 60 Gy recommended. A 65% to 80% local success rate has been reported with radiation therapy for small T1 and T2 tumors.[47] Brachytherapy involves placement of radioactive material (usually iridium-192 wire) within the tumor (interstitial brachytherapy) or molded around the tumor (plesiobrachytherapy) and is limited to T1 and T2 tumors. This form of therapy is not suitable for patients with bulky tumors, deeply infiltrating tumors, and obese patients with a short penis. Radiation therapy as primary treatment for invasive penile carcinoma has significant disadvantages: acute effects of skin edema, maceration, and dysuria may persist for 6 to 8 weeks. Telangiectasia and fibrosis are found in more than 90% of cases. The most serious late effects are urethral fistula, meatal stenosis, and penile necrosis. Postradiation fibrosis, scar, and necrosis may be difficult to distinguish from recurrent cancer. Infection is very often associated with penile cancer and reduces the therapeutic efficacy of radiation while increasing the risk of penile necrosis. Thus, in summary, radiation therapy for primary penile cancer should be considered only in a select group of patients: young patients with small (2 to 4 cm) superficial lesions of the distal penis who wish to maintain penile integrity, patients who refuse surgery, and patients with inoperable cancer or those unsuitable for major surgery.

Advanced Penile Cancer (T4, N2-3, and M1). Large proximal shaft tumors require a total penectomy with a perineal urethrostomy. For extensive, proximal tumors with invasion of adjacent structures, total emasculation (total penectomy, scrotectomy, and orchiectomy) is recommended. In extreme cases, a hemipelvectomy or even a hemicorporectomy has been described. Multimodal therapy with chemoradiation and salvage surgery has also been used in this setting.

Management of Regional Lymph Nodes

The presence and extent of inguinal lymph node metastases are the most important prognostic factors in penile cancer. Although 50% of patients with a penile lesion have clinically palpable inguinal nodes at presentation, in more than half of these the adenopathy is inflammatory. A 4- to 6-week course of antibiotics (e.g., first- or second-generation cephalosporin) after treatment of the primary lesion is recommended. Persistent palpable adenopathy after antibiotic therapy should be biopsied. Unlike many other genitourinary malignancies that require systemic chemotherapy, once lymph node metastases are discovered, inguinal metastases from penile cancer are potentially curable by lymphadenectomy alone. Inguinal lymphadenectomy therefore should be performed at the earliest suspicion of metastases.

Clinical Node Negative (N0). Although there is no controversy in the literature regarding management of the patient with clinically positive inguinal lymph nodes after a course of antibiotics, considerable controversy surrounds the management of the clinically N0 patient. Approximately 20% of these clinically negative groins harbor occult lymphatic metastases on prophylactic lymph node dissection. Stated another way, approximately 80% of patients with clinically negative groins would be subjected to the morbidity of inguinal lymph node dissection without benefit. To resolve this dilemma, a risk-based approach to management of the clinically negative groin has been recommended in most contemporary series. Analysis of histopathologic data from the primary penile cancer allows stratification of patients into high- and low-risk groups for lymph node metastases.[48]

Low-Risk Group. Patients with carcinoma *in situ* (Tis), verrucous carcinoma (Ta), and T1 tumors who have grade 1 or 2 tumor histology have a less than 10% chance of developing lymph node metastases and are best served by surveillance and a low incidence of lymphovascular invasion, a risk for nodal metastasis.[33]

High-Risk Group. Patients with invasive penile cancer (T2 and T3) with grade 3 tumors and the presence of vascular invasion have a greater than 50% incidence of inguinal lymph node metastases in various series. Vascular invasion is strongly correlated with lymph node metastases. In pT2 patients the incidence of lymph node metastases was found to be 75% in the presence of vascular invasion and only 25% when vascular invasion was absent.[48] In this cohort of patients, a prophylactic lymphadenectomy is reasonable.

The timing of surgery in the clinically negative groin has been debated in the past. Most contemporary series favor *early adjunctive* lymphadenectomy, especially in the high-risk group, over surveillance and *delayed therapeutic* lymphadenectomy. Sentinel lymph node biopsy, originally described by Cabanas,[49] is no longer recommended in view of the high false-negative rate. Intraoperative lymphatic mapping using dynamic scintigraphy with technetium-labeled sulfur colloid have decreased the false-negative rate considerably.[47] Other approaches that use sentinel lymph node biopsy have also been advocated, including measurement of the size of the micrometastatic sentinel lymph node to determine whether to perform lymphadenectomy.[50] Sentinel node biopsy remains controversial, with recent studies demonstrating a much lower false negative rate,[51,52] but further data are required.[53] Lymphotropic nanoparticle-enhanced MRI has been investigated to detect micrometastasis but awaits validation.[54]

Inguinal lymph node dissection superficial to the fascia lata has been found to be adequate for the N0 patient. Superficial inguinal lymph node dissection should include a frozen section, and if positive, a modified complete dissection should be carried out. Creation of thicker skin flaps, control of infection, and preservation of the areolar fat superficial to the Scarpa fascia have greatly decreased the complications of flap necrosis, scrotal and extremity edema, lymphocele, and lymphorrhea.

Prediction Models. Ficarra et al.[55] and Kattan et al.[56] have developed predictive nomograms to help determine an individual patient's risk of nodal involvement and cancer-specific survival. One nomogram to predict the probability of lymph node involvement uses eight clinical and pathologic variables (tumor thickness, growth pattern, grade, lymphovascular invasion, corpora cavernosal involvement, spongiosal involvement, urethral involvement, palpable lymph nodes). Not surprisingly, clinically suspicious inguinal lymph nodes are a powerful predictor of pathologic nodal involvement. For cancer-specific survival of patients who undergo surgery for squamous cell carcinoma of the penis, two separate nomograms were created, depending on whether clinical or pathologic staging of inguinal lymph nodes was used. These nomograms may guide patients and clinicians alike on the appropriate treatment and can potentially avoid the risks of lymph node dissection in low-risk patients.

Clinical Node Positive (N1, N2, or N3). The modified inguinal lymph node dissection as described by Catalona[57] has replaced the standard complete inguinal lymphadenectomy as the procedure of choice with clinically persistent nodes after antibiotics. It involves a smaller incision, limited field of inguinal dissection, and preservation of the saphenous vein in an effort to reduce the morbidity of the standard procedure while adhering to standard oncologic principles. Unlike superficial dissection, the deep nodes within the fossa ovalis are also removed. In the face of synchronous unilateral N+ disease, it is standard practice to proceed with a bilateral lymph node dissection in view of the high incidence of bilateral drainage. The exception to this rule is the patient with a clinically negative groin in whom metachronous unilateral inguinal lymphadenopathy develops some time after treatment of the primary tumor. In these patients a unilateral dissection of the clinically positive groin usually suffices. The value of pelvic lymphadenectomy in the presence of positive inguinal lymph nodes is for the purposes of staging and identifying patients who would be candidates for adjuvant chemotherapy and had little therapeutic efficacy (5-year survival with pelvic lymph node metastases is less than 5%).

Patients with advanced nodal disease or bulky fixed inguinal nodes (N3) may require neoadjuvant radiation or chemotherapy before any surgery. The groin lymph nodes adherent to the skin or fungating through the skin require wide excision with myocutaneous flaps to cover the skin defect. The published literature unequivocally favors surgical resection as superior to radiation therapy for the treatment of inguinal lymph nodes. Clinical evaluation of the groin is difficult because of postradiation tissue changes, and the inguinal area tolerates radiation rather poorly. Radiation therapy can be used as a palliative measure in patients with fixed inoperable inguinal nodes or in those with advanced unresectable penile cancer in which the primary and the ilioinguinal region can be treated with radiation therapy.

Role of Chemotherapy and Multimodality Therapy

The role of chemotherapy in the management of penile carcinoma is evolving, and the exact role of chemotherapy has not been established. Data suggest that penile cancer is sensitive to chemotherapy.[58] Besides the use of 5-FU in the treatment of superficial penile cancer, single-agent chemotherapy with cisplatin, methotrexate, and bleomycin has modest activity in advanced penile cancer. The combination of methotrexate, bleomycin, and cisplatin (MBP) is more active than cisplatin alone but is associated with marked toxicity.

The Southwest Oncology Group reported on the largest prospective clinical trial in patients with penile cancer.[59] In 40 evaluable patients treated with a combination of MBP, an overall response of 32.5% and a complete response of 12.5% were observed. The median response duration was 16 weeks, and the median survival was 28 weeks. Toxicity was formidable, with 11% treatment-related mortality, and 17% of the remaining patients experiencing life-threatening toxicity. Multimodality therapy, using a combination of chemotherapy and surgery or chemotherapy and radiation, has been used in isolated reports of advanced penile cancer. Small series in men with fixed, unresectable inguinal nodes had neoadjuvant vincristine, bleomycin, and methotrexate (VBM) before surgery with some long-term responses.[60] Another small series of patients who underwent surgical resection after neoadjuvant chemotherapy for unresectable penile squamous cell were treated with several different chemotherapy combinations, including BMP (bleomycin, methotrexate, cisplatin), ITP (ifosfamide, paclitaxel, cisplatin), or paclitaxel/carboplatin with some responses.[6]

Selected References

The full list of references for this chapter appears in the online version.

1. Tefilli MV, Gheiler EL, Shekarriz B, et al. Primary adenocarcinoma of the urethra with metastasis to the glans penis: successful treatment with chemotherapy and radiation therapy. *Urology* 1998;52:517.
3. Wiener JS, Liu ET, Walther PJ. Oncogenic human papillomavirus type 16 is associated with squamous cell cancer of the male urethra. *Cancer Res* 1992;52:5018.
5. Grabstald H. Proceedings: tumors of the urethra in men and women. *Cancer* 1973;32:1236.
6. Erckert M, Stenzl A, Falk M, et al. Incidence of urethral tumor involvement in 910 men with bladder cancer. *World J Urol* 1996;14:3.
7. Sherwood JB, Sagalowsky AI. The diagnosis and treatment of urethral recurrence after radical cystectomy. *Urol Oncol* 2006;24:356.
8. Edge SB, Byrd DR, Compton CC, et al., eds. *AJCC cancer staging manual.* 7th ed. New York: Springer-Verlag, 2010.
9. Ryu J, Kim B. MR imaging of the male and female urethra. *Radiographics* 2001;21:1169.
11. Gheiler EL, Tefilli MV, Tiguert R, et al. Management of primary urethral cancer. *Urology* 1998;52:487.
12. Davis JW, Schellhammer PF, Schlossberg SM. Conservative surgical therapy for penile and urethral carcinoma. *Urology* 1999;53:386.
13. Dalbagni G, Zhang ZF, Lacombe L, et al. Male urethral carcinoma: analysis of treatment outcome. *Urology* 1999;53:1126.
14. Christopher N, Arya M, Brown RS, et al. Penile preservation in squamous cell carcinoma of the bulbomembranous urethra. *BJU Int* 2002;89:464.
15. Shen SS, Lerner SP, Muezzinoglu B, et al. Prostatic involvement by transitional cell carcinoma in patients with bladder cancer and its prognostic significance. *Hum Pathol* 2006;37:726.
16. Scher HI, Yagoda A, Herr HW, et al. Neoadjuvant M-VAC (methotrexate, vinblastine, doxorubicin and cisplatin) for extravesical urinary tract tumors. *J Urol* 1988;139:475.
17. Oberfield RA, Zinman LN, Leibenhaut M, et al. Management of invasive squamous cell carcinoma of the bulbomembranous male urethra with coordinated chemo-radiotherapy and genital preservation. *Br J Urol* 1996;78:573.
18. Licht MR, Klein EA, Bukowski R, et al. Combination radiation and chemotherapy for the treatment of squamous cell carcinoma of the male and female urethra. *J Urol* 1995;153:1918.
19. Srinivas V, Khan SA. Female urethral cancer—an overview. *Int Urol Nephrol* 1987;19:423.
21. Sailer SL, Shipley WU, Wang CC. Carcinoma of the female urethra: a review of results with radiation therapy. *J Urol* 1988;140:1.
22. Dalbagni G, Zhang ZF, Lacombe L, et al. Female urethral carcinoma: an analysis of treatment outcome and a plea for a standardized management strategy. *Br J Urol* 1998;82:835.
23. Grabstald H, Hilaris B, Henschke U, et al. Cancer of the female urethra. *JAMA* 1966;197:835.
24. Milosevic MF, Warde PR, Banerjee D, et al. Urethral carcinoma in women: results of treatment with primary radiotherapy. *Radiother Oncol* 2000;56:29.
25. Narayan P, Konety B. Surgical treatment of female urethral carcinoma. *Urol Clin North Am* 1992;19:373.
26. Yeole BB, Jussawalla DJ. Descriptive epidemiology of the cancers of male genital organs in greater Bombay. *Indian J Cancer* 1997;34:30.
27. Hernandez BY, Barnholtz-Sloan J, German RR, et al. Burden of invasive squamous cell carcinoma of the penis in the United States, 1998–2003. *Cancer* 2008;113:2883.
28. Maden C, Sherman KJ, Beckmann AM, et al. History of circumcision, medical conditions, and sexual activity and risk of penile cancer. *J Natl Cancer Inst* 1993;85:19.
29. Miralles-Guri C, Bruni L, Cubilla AL, et al. Human papillomavirus prevalence and type distribution in penile carcinoma. *J Clin Pathol* 2009;62:870.
30. Backes DM, Kurman RJ, Pimenta JM, et al. Systematic review of human papillomavirus prevalence in invasive penile cancer. *Cancer Causes Control* 2009;20:449.
31. Harish K, Ravi R. The role of tobacco in penile carcinoma. *Br J Urol* 1995;75:375.
32. Grossman HB. Premalignant and early carcinomas of the penis and scrotum. *Urol Clin North Am* 1992;19:221.
33. Lopes A, Hidalgo GS, Kowalski LP, et al. Prognostic factors in carcinoma of the penis: multivariate analysis of 145 patients treated with amputation and lymphadenectomy. *J Urol* 1996;156:1637.
34. Depasquale I, Park AJ, Bracka A. The treatment of balanitis xerotica obliterans. *BJU Int* 2000;86:459.
35. Scher B, Seitz M, Reiser M, et al. 18F-FDG PET/CT for staging of penile cancer. *J Nucl Med* 2005;46:1460.
36. Graafland NM, Leijte JA, Valdes Olmos RA, et al. Scanning with 18F-FDG-PET/CT for detection of pelvic nodal involvement in inguinal node-positive penile carcinoma. *Eur Urol* 2009;56:339.
37. Leijte JA, Graafland NM, Valdes Olmos RA, et al. Prospective evaluation of hybrid 18F-fluorodeoxyglucose positron emission tomography/computed tomography in staging clinically node-negative patients with penile carcinoma. *BJU Int* 2009;104:640.
38. Korets R, Koppie TM, Snyder ME, et al. Partial penectomy for patients with squamous cell carcinoma of the penis: the Memorial Sloan-Kettering experience. *Ann Surg Oncol* 2007;14:3614.
39. Crook J, Esche B, Grimard L, et al. Interstitial brachytherapy for penile carcinoma: an alternative to amputation. *Can J Urol* 1995;2:150.
40. Marconnet L, Rigaud J, Bouchot O. Long-term follow-up of penile carcinoma with high risk for lymph node invasion treated with inguinal lymphadenectomy. *J Urol* 2010;183:2227.
42. Bayles AC, Sethia KK. The impact of improving outcomes guidance on the management and outcomes of patients with carcinoma of the penis. *Ann R Coll Surg Engl* 2010;92:44.
43. Windahl T, Andersson SO. Combined laser treatment for penile carcinoma: results after long-term follow-up. *J Urol* 2003;169:2118.
44. Mohs FE, Snow SN, Larson PO. Mohs micrographic surgery for penile tumors. *Urol Clin North Am* 1992;19:291.
45. Sheen MC, Sheu HM, Huang CH, et al. Penile verrucous carcinoma successfully treated by intra-aortic infusion with methotrexate. *Urology* 2003;61:1216.
47. Jakub JW, Pendas S, Reintgen DS. Current status of sentinel lymph node mapping and biopsy: facts and controversies. *Oncologist* 2003;8:59.
48. Slaton JW, Morgenstern N, Levy DA, et al. Tumor stage, vascular invasion and the percentage of poorly differentiated cancer: independent prognosticators

for inguinal lymph node metastasis in penile squamous cancer. *J Urol* 2001; 165:1138.
49. Cabanas RM. An approach for the treatment of penile carcinoma. *Cancer* 1977;39:456.
50. Kroon BK, Nieweg OE, van Boven H, et al. Size of metastasis in the sentinel node predicts additional nodal involvement in penile carcinoma. *J Urol* 2006;176:105.
51. Leijte JA, Hughes B, Graafland NM, et al. Two-center evaluation of dynamic sentinel node biopsy for squamous cell carcinoma of the penis. *J Clin Oncol* 2009;27:3325.
52. Jensen JB, Jensen KM, Ulhoi BP, et al. Sentinel lymph-node biopsy in patients with squamous cell carcinoma of the penis. *BJU Int* 2009;103:1199.
54. Tabatabaei S, Harisinghani M, McDougal WS. Regional lymph node staging using lymphotropic nanoparticle enhanced magnetic resonance imaging with ferumoxtran-10 in patients with penile cancer. *J Urol* 2005;174:923.
55. Ficarra V, Zattoni F, Artibani W, et al. Nomogram predictive of pathological inguinal lymph node involvement in patients with squamous cell carcinoma of the penis. *J Urol* 2006;175:1700.
56. Kattan MW, Ficarra V, Artibani W, et al. Nomogram predictive of cancer specific survival in patients undergoing partial or total amputation for squamous cell carcinoma of the penis. *J Urol* 2006;175:2103.
57. Catalona WJ. Modified inguinal lymphadenectomy for carcinoma of the penis with preservation of saphenous veins: technique and preliminary results. *J Urol* 1988;140:306.
58. Trabulsi EJ, Hoffman-Censits J. Chemotherapy for penile and urethral carcinoma. *Urol Clin North Am* 2010;37:467.
59. Haas GP, Blumenstein BA, Gagliano RG, et al. Cisplatin, methotrexate and bleomycin for the treatment of carcinoma of the penis: a Southwest Oncology Group study. *J Urol* 1999;161:1823.
60. Pizzocaro G, Piva L. Adjuvant and neoadjuvant vincristine, bleomycin, and methotrexate for inguinal metastases from squamous cell carcinoma of the penis. *Acta Oncol* 1988;27:823.
61. Bermejo C, Busby JE, Spiess PE, et al. Neoadjuvant chemotherapy followed by aggressive surgical consolidation for metastatic penile squamous cell carcinoma. *J Urol* 2007;177:1335.

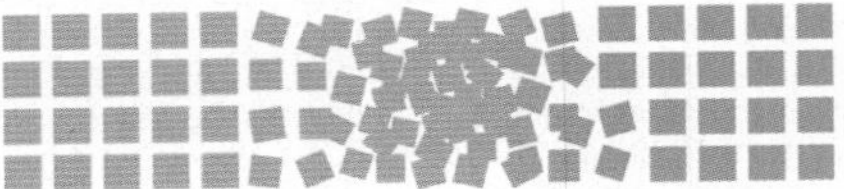

CHAPTER 99 CANCER OF THE TESTIS

GEORGE J. BOSL, DARREN R. FELDMAN, DEAN F. BAJORIN, JOEL SHEINFELD, ROBERT J. MOTZER, VICTOR E. REUTER, MARISA A. KOLLMEIER, AND RAJU S. K. CHAGANTI

Cancers of the testis comprise a diverse group of neoplasms, most of which are germ cell tumors (GCTs). Approximately 90% of GCTs originate in the testis, and 10% are extragonadal. This chapter discusses management of both testicular and extragonadal GCT (mediastinal and retroperitoneal).

BACKGROUND: INCIDENCE

GCTs are the most common solid tumors in men between the ages of 15 and 35 years.[1] In a man age 50 or older, a solid testicular mass is usually a lymphoma. The incidence of testis cancer varies significantly according to geographic area and is increasing,[2] with the highest reported incidence in Scandinavia, Switzerland, and Germany; intermediate in the United States and Great Britain; lowest in Africa and Asia. Approximately 8,480 new cases and 350 deaths from testicular cancer were anticipated in the United States in 2010.[3]

EPIDEMIOLOGY

GCTs are seen principally in young white men and less commonly in African Americans. Familial clustering has been observed, particularly among siblings. A recent study suggested that genetic variants were associated with GCT susceptibility.[4] No convincing association exists between vasectomy, diethylstilbestrol exposure, trauma, or viral infection (including human immunodeficiency virus), and the incidence of GCT.[5]

RISK FACTORS

Cryptorchidism

About 2% of inguinal cryptorchid testes will develop GCT, 5% to 10% in the normally descended testis. It is questionable whether an abdominal cryptorchid testis is more likely to develop GCT than an inguinal cryptorchid testis.[6] For orchiopexy to reduce the likelihood of GCT, it should be performed prior to puberty. If the cryptorchid testis is inguinal, hormonally functioning, and easily examined, surveillance is recommended. If the cryptorchid testis cannot be adequately examined or is nonfunctioning, orchiectomy is recommended.

Klinefelter Syndrome

Characterized by testicular atrophy, absence of spermatogenesis, a eunuchoid habitus, and gynecomastia, Klinefelter syndrome is diagnosed by a 47,XXY karyotype. Patients with Klinefelter syndrome are at increased risk for mediastinal GCT.

INITIAL PRESENTATION AND MANAGEMENT

Symptoms and Signs

A pathognomonic painless testicular mass occurs in a minority of patients. Most patients present with symptoms that mimic epididymitis and/or orchitis, and a trial of antibiotic therapy is sometimes necessary. If the testis does not revert to normal within 2 to 4 weeks, a testicular ultrasound is indicated. Acute testicular pain, simulating testicular torsion, occurs less frequently. On ultrasound, the typical testicular tumor is intratesticular and appears as one or more hypoechoic masses. Although testicular microlithiasis has been reported more frequently in men with GCT and their unaffected male relatives, its association with GCT is poorly defined and requires no special intervention or screening.[7,8] If microlithiasis is bilateral and found in a subfertile male, or is present in the contralateral testis of a patient with GCT, then a higher likelihood of in situ GCT exists, and regular self-examination is recommended.[6] Higher stage at presentation has been associated with delay in diagnosis,[9] and patients treated at experienced treatment units have a better chance of survival.[10]

Diagnosis

A radical inguinal orchiectomy with early, high ligation of the spermatic cord at the deep inguinal ring is the only acceptable diagnostic and therapeutic procedure. The stump is pushed into the retroperitoneal space to facilitate removal of the gonadal vessels at the time of retroperitoneal lymph node dissection (RPLND). The testis and spermatic cord are removed *en bloc,* minimizing local tumor recurrence and aberrant lymphatic spread. A transscrotal orchiectomy is contraindicated because alternate lymphatic drainage to the inguinal and pelvic lymph nodes may develop, and the spermatic cord from the external to the internal ring remains intact. In the rare situation in which the diagnosis of a testicular tumor is in question, an inguinal incision is required. The testis can then be examined *in situ* in a sterile field, and an appropriate biopsy taken with minimal risk of scrotal or inguinal contamination.

Extragonadal GCT, comprising fewer than 10% of GCTs, occurs most frequently in the mediastinum and requires a testicular ultrasound to rule out an occult primary tumor. Pineal tumors, found most often in children, are usually GCT. Because

TABLE 99.1

WORLD HEALTH ORGANIZATION HISTOLOGIC CLASSIFICATION OF TESTIS TUMORS

Germ cell tumors (intratubular germ cell neoplasia, unclassified)
Other types
Tumors of one histological type (pure forms)
Seminoma
Seminoma with syncytiotrophoblastic cells
Spermatocytic seminoma
Spermatocytic seminoma with sarcoma
Embryonal carcinoma
Yolk sac tumors
Trophoblastic tumors
Choriocarcinoma
Trophoblastic neoplasms other than choriocarcinoma
Monophasic choriocarcinoma
Placental site trophoblastic tumors
Teratoma
Dermoid cyst
Monodermal teratoma
Teratoma with somatic type malignancies
Tumors of more than one histologic type (mixed forms)
Mixed embryonal carcinoma and teratoma
Mixed teratoma and seminoma
Choriocarcinoma and teratoma/embryonal carcinoma
Others

From ref. 11.

of its unique access to the meninges, pineal GCT may metastasize to intradural sites, and is less frequently systemic. Very rarely, primary GCT has been found in sites such as the sacrum, thyroid, paranasal sinuses, and soft tissues of the head and neck. The management of extragonadal and testicular GCT is the same, and primary site is an independent factor in risk classification.

HISTOLOGY

GCT is classified into two major subgroups: seminoma and nonseminoma. The classification of the World Health Organization (WHO), derived from Mostofi and Sesterhenn's adaptation of the Dixon/Moore classification, is the system most commonly used in North America and Europe (Table 99.1).[11] The British Tumor Panel's modification of the Pugh classification is used in Great Britain and Australia.

Intratubular Germ Cell Neoplasia

Intratubular germ cell neoplasia, unclassified (IGCNU), precedes invasive testicular GCT in all cases of adult GCT. IGCNU is frequently present in retroperitoneal presentations, but rarely in mediastinal presentations or in tumors arising in prepubertal patients.[5] Cytologically, the IGCNU preceding both seminoma and nonseminoma is identical, although intratubular embryonal carcinoma may infrequently be seen. The median time for progression of IGCNU to invasive disease is approximately 5 years.[12] In the general population, the incidence of IGCNU is low. The incidence of IGCNU in men with impaired fertility is about 0.5%, and 2% to 5% in the cryptorchid and contralateral testis in patients with documented prior testicular GCT. Some European investigators suggest low-dose radiation therapy (RT) as management of biopsy-proven IGCNU, but this is not standard treatment in the United States.

Seminoma

Seminoma accounts for approximately 45% of GCTs, and most frequently appears in the fourth decade of life. Classic seminoma consists of large-cell sheets with abundant cytoplasm, and round, hyperchromatic nuclei with prominent nucleoli. A lymphocytic infiltrate (and/or granulomatous reaction with giant cells) is often present. Trophoblastic giant cells that produce human chorionic gonadotropin (hCG) are seen in a minority of tumors, but do *not* influence prognosis or treatment. *Anaplastic* seminoma, a term used when three or more mitotic figures are seen per high-powered field, has no clinical importance.

Atypical seminoma cytologically resembles seminoma, but lymphocytic infiltrate and granulomatous reaction are absent, necrosis is more common, and the nuclear-cytoplasmic ratio is higher. It may show a greater degree of cytoplasmic expression of low-molecular-weight keratin; typical seminoma stains negative or shows occasional cells with dotlike positivity.[13] Electron microscopy may show individual tumor cells with cytoplasmic cytokeratin-intermediate filaments, suggesting epithelial differentiation. Atypical seminoma has not been associated with an adverse prognosis; its management is the same as any other seminoma. The diagnosis should trigger consideration of solid variants of embryonal carcinoma and yolk sac tumor.

Spermatocytic seminoma is rare and seen generally in older men. Its relation to other GCTs is not clear. It is not associated with IGCNU or bilaterality, does not express placental alkaline phosphatase or OCT3/4 (see "Immunohistochemical Markers"), and has not shown the same genetic abnormalities as other GCTs. Metastatic potential is minimal.

Nonseminomatous Germ Cell Tumors

Nonseminomatous GCT (NSGCT) comprises approximately 55% of GCTs. It most frequently presents in the third decade of life. Most tumors are mixed, consisting of two or more cell types, including seminoma. A testicular tumor with any NSGCT cell type (other than syncytiotrophoblasts) has the same prognosis and management as NSGCT.

Embryonal Carcinoma

Embryonal carcinoma is undifferentiated and pluripotent. Individual cells are epithelioid in appearance, and may be arranged in glandular or tubular nests and cords or as solid sheets of cells. Tumor necrosis and hemorrhage are frequently observed.

Choriocarcinoma

Choriocarcinoma, by definition, consists of both cytotrophoblasts and syncytiotrophoblasts. If cytotrophoblasts are not present, the diagnosis of choriocarcinoma cannot be made. Elements of choriocarcinoma in a mixed tumor have no prognostic importance. Syncytiotrophoblastic giant cells may be a component in any GCT (including pure seminoma), but impart no prognostic value. Pure choriocarcinoma is rare, usually associated with widespread hematogenous metastases and high levels of hCG. Severe spontaneous hemorrhage occasionally occurs at a metastatic site. Other trophoblastic neoplasms are very rare.

Yolk Sac Tumor

Yolk sac tumor (endodermal sinus tumor) mimics the yolk sac of the embryo, produces α-fetoprotein (AFP), and may be confused with a glandular form of embryonal carcinoma. The cells may have a papillary, glandular, microcystic, or solid appearance, and may be associated with Schiller-Duval bodies, which are perivascular arrangements of epithelial cells with an intervening extracellular space. Rarely, embryoid bodies resembling the early embryo may be seen. A pure yolk sac histology is uncommon in the adult testis, but accounts for a significant percentage of primary mediastinal NSGCT. Refractory yolk sac tumor occurring postchemotherapy or as a late recurrence may exhibit unusual histologic features.

Teratoma

Teratoma is composed of somatic cell types from two or more germ layers (ectoderm, mesoderm, or endoderm), and is derived from a pluripotent, malignant precursor (embryonal carcinoma or yolk sac tumor). A primary testicular tumor in a postpubertal male that displays only teratoma is a fully malignant GCT. Management should proceed as if malignant components are present since metastasis may eventually develop, reflecting its evolution from a pluripotent malignant cell (i.e., embryonal carcinoma).[14] It is not unusual to see a parenchymal scar adjacent to an otherwise pure testicular teratoma, thought to be secondary to partial regression of the tumor. Nonteratomatous elements may be seen at metastatic sites, with or without teratoma. *Mature teratoma* consists of adult-type differentiated elements such as cartilage, glandular epithelium, or nerve tissue. *Immature teratoma* generally refers to a tumor with partial somatic differentiation, similar to that seen in a fetus. Secondary somatic malignancy arising in teratoma, previously called *teratoma with malignant transformation,* is a form of teratoma in which one teratomatous component grows independently, taking on the appearance of a non-GCT somatic cancer. These somatic cancers include, but are not limited to, acute nonlymphocytic leukemia (seen almost exclusively in the context of mediastinal NSGCT), sarcomas (e.g., rhabdomyosarcoma), carcinoma (e.g., enteric adenocarcinoma), or primitive neuroectodermal tumors. A somatic malignancy arising in a teratoma behaves like cancer arising at its usual *de novo* site, and treatment should be directed at the transformed histology.[15,16]

BIOLOGY

Adult human male GCTs comprise a unique system for studying the transformation mechanism of a pluripotent germ cell and its ability to elicit embryonal-like lineage differentiation. The pluripotentiality of GCTs manifests as histologic differentiation into germ cell-like undifferentiated (seminoma), primitive zygotic (embryonal carcinoma), somatically differentiated (teratoma), and extraembryonal differentiated (choriocarcinoma and yolk sac tumor) phenotypes. Understanding of this unique GCT histopathology has expanded with gene-expression profiling studies.[17–20] Those genes most highly overexpressed in IGCNU—compared with a normal testis—carry markers of primordial germ cell and/or embryonic stem cell phenotypes such as *POU5F1 (OCT3/4)*, *NANOG*, *XBP1*, *XIST*, *LIN28*, *TFAP2C*, *PDPN*, *PRDM1*, *SOX17*, and *TCL1A*. Also elevated in IGCNU are genes with known oncogenic potential such as *MYCN* and *PIM2*. On invasion, two key genes associated with stem cell pluripotency, (*POU5F1* (*OCT3/4*) and *NANOG*), are expressed by both seminoma and embryonal carcinoma, while the third, *SOX2*, is expressed mainly in embryonal carcinomas.[21] This differential expression of genes known to play functional roles in self-renewal and pluripotency may account for the lack of differentiation potential usually displayed by seminoma. Because seminoma, but not embryonal carcinoma, retains the expression of *KIT*, *TCL1A*, *PDPN*, *XIST*, and *SOX17*, some have suggested that seminoma represents the "default" invasive histologic component, while embryonal carcinoma arises from selective activation/inactivation of key regulators of development, accompanied by a loss of a primordial germ cell phenotype. Further initiation of lineage differentiation in embryonal carcinoma may lead to teratoma, yolk sac tumor, and choriocarcinoma development, each with a unique gene expression signature.[22]

Mechanism of Germ Cell Transformation

Genetic analysis has shown that nearly 100% of male GCTs show an increased 12p copy number. This chromosomal marker, manifested as one or more copies of i(12p) or as tandem duplications of 12p, *in situ* or transposed elsewhere in the genome, has been observed as early as IGCNU, suggesting that it is among the earliest, if not the earliest, genetic change associated with the origin of these tumors (Fig. 99.1).[22] Recent gene-expression profiling studies aimed at identifying genes mapped to 12p and overexpressed in IGCNU and GCTs relative to a normal testis have revealed several candidates with roles in cell growth (the oncogene *CCND2*, the glucose transporter *GLUT3*, and the glycolytic enzymes *GAPDH* and *TPI1*), and/or in self-renewal and pluripotency (*NANOG*, *DPPA3*, and *GDF3*).[20,21] On differentiation into nonseminomatous subtypes, the expression of these genes (either as individuals or as clusters) is subject to transcriptional controls that may normally function in lineage specification during development. One cluster of coordinately regulated genes on 12p was identified as a 200 kbp region comprising *NANOG*,

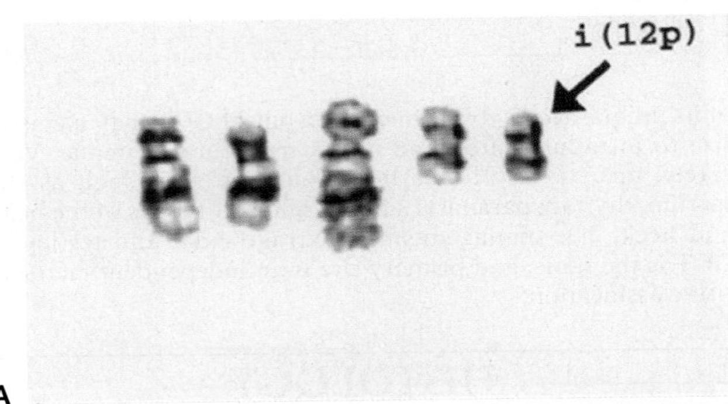

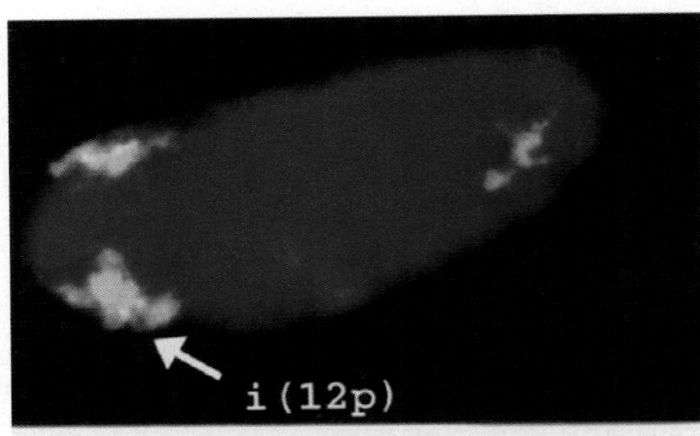

FIGURE 99.1 **A:** Partial karyotype showing four copies of chromosome 12 in a germ cell tumor (GCT) with the i(12p) chromosome (*arrow*) at metaphase. **B:** Fluorescence *in situ* hybridization (FISH) of a GCT cell showing three signals for 12p (turquoise) and three attached signals for chromosome 12 centromere (*pink*), indicating increased copy number of the 12p chromosomal arm. The large turquoise signal represents i(12p) (*arrow*), and the two small turquoise signals represent the normal chromosomes 12p. The probe used for 12p was derived from microdissection of 12pDNA from a chromosome preparation. The FISH test is now routinely used for GCT diagnosis in biopsy specimens.

DPPA3, *GDF3*, and other transcripts, which are also regulated as a cluster in human embryonic stem cells.[20] Thus, gain of 12p is multifunctional and linked to transformation, self-renewal, and maintenance of pluripotency. Epigenetic changes and microRNAs (miRNAs) contribute to the control of gene expression in GCT.[23,24]

Although IGCNU is considered to be the precursor of all GCTs, the stage in germ cell development at which transformation occurs is not known. One model proposed by Skakkebaek et al.[25] suggests that fetal gonocytes that have escaped normal development into spermatogonia may undergo abnormal cell division mediated by a kit receptor/kit ligand (stem cell factor) paracrine loop, leading to uncontrolled proliferation of gonocytes. Subsequent invasive growth may be mediated by postnatal and pubertal gonadotrophin stimulation. A second model proposed by Chaganti et al.[26] suggests that aberrant chromatid exchange events during meiotic crossing-over may lead to increased 12p copy number and overexpression of cyclin D2 (*CCND2*). In a cell containing unrepaired DNA breaks (recombination-associated), overexpressed cyclin D2 may block a p53-dependent apoptotic response and lead to reinitiation of cell cycle and genomic instability. In germ cells that have reentered the cell cycle, downstream events such as loss of tumor suppressor genes brought about by genomic instability may lead to neoplastic progression. Genetic screens ranging from standard karyotypic analysis to array-based comparative genomic hybridization have identified multiple genetic lesions associated with GCT histology, malignant transformation, and progression.[21] Although copy number changes are common, kinase gene mutations are rare, implying little role for mutation in GCT development.[27]

Pluripotency and Embryonal-like Differentiation in GCT

The restoration of self-renewal by IGCNU through 12p gain (up-regulation of *NANOG*) culminates in the acquisition of pluripotency by embryonal carcinoma, in which lineage differentiation takes place as a result of multiple pathways of gene expression. Thus, GCTs display patterns of differentiation that mimic stages normally undergone by the developing zygote. Embryonal carcinoma is the key component in this process, and has often been suggested as the transformed counterpart of embryonic stem cells. Embryonal carcinoma and embryonic stem cells share pluripotency and many key genetic features such as the expression of the core pluripotency-regulating transcription factors *POU5F1-NANOG-SOX2* triad.[28,29] Embryonal carcinoma thus is a complex biological system of malignant transformation, pluripotency, self renewal, and lineage differentiation wherein developmental lineages are laid down in the transformed pluripotent cells. Studies over the past decade have identified a multilevel regulatory circuitry that controls embryonic stem cell identity and differentiation relevant to embryonal carcinoma.[28,29] Central to this network is the *POU5F1*, *NANOG*, and *SOX2* autoregulatory loop. This canonical triad regulates two sets of protein-coding genes, one that is actively expressed in pluripotent cells (for maintenance of pluripotency) and another that is silenced in pluripotent cells by polycomb group proteins, whose later expression facilitates establishment or maintenance of differentiated states.[28,29] The *POU5F1-NANOG-SOX2* triad also occupies promoters of two sets of miRNAs that perform a similar function as the protein-coding genes in maintenance of pluripotency and differentiation. In addition, many protein-coding genes that regulate differentiation pathways are direct targets of multiple miRNAs.

Gene-expression profiling has identified expression patterns associated with distinct histologic subtypes. Lineage differentiation can also be studied using embryonal carcinoma-derived cell lines. Considered to be the malignant counterparts of embryonic stem cells, they share expression signature and DNA methylation patterns. Using these cell lines, temporal changes in gene-expression profiles associated with specific lineage induction were mapped. These studies identified transcriptional networks that led to initiation and development of several lineages (neuronal, epidermal, and endodermal).[30,31] Because GCTs arise from imprint-erased germ cells, epigenetic modifications may be important in the origin and development of transformed germ cells. Overall, seminoma exhibits a lower level of promoter methylation than NSGCT. Investigation of this aspect of GCT biology is expected to inform decision-making as technologies of global assessment of sequence-specific methylation patterns are applied.

Cisplatin Sensitivity and Acquired Resistance of Adult GCT

Molecular genetic studies of GCTs that are clinically resistant to cisplatin-based chemotherapy have identified a subset that harbors *TP53* gene mutations,[32] a molecular alteration not normally associated with GCT. Evaluation of the cellular response to cisplatin in one GCT-derived cell line with a *TP53* gene mutation indicated a relative resistance to cisplatin, in contrast to the extreme sensitivity of another GCT-derived cell line with wild type *TP53*.[32] Presumably, the cisplatin resistance of this subset of GCTs is rooted in its inability to mount an apoptotic response after drug exposure because of an inactivating *TP53* gene mutation. On the whole, GCTs display higher than normal levels of wild type p53,[33] with somewhat lower levels in mature teratomas.[34] Thus, somatic differentiation associated with a decline in p53 levels may comprise a cellular setting with selective pressure for *TP53* gene mutation. Mutations in *BRAF* have been associated with a poor outcome, but validation is required.[35]

Finally, amplified DNA sequences, a genetic abnormality often associated with tumor progression and resistance to therapy, have been reported in cisplatin-resistant GCTs. High-level amplification (other than 12p) was detected in five resistant tumors, but none in the sensitive group.[36] Once the identity and the function of the amplified genes are determined, they may become relevant to understanding the chemotherapy resistance of GCTs.

Male GCTs offer a system to study cellular factors portending exquisite sensitivity to chemotherapy. Some studies have described a reduced ability of GCT cell lines to repair DNA lesions induced by cisplatin.[37] The biochemical link between the induction of physical damage in DNA and the cellular response is unclear. However, cells respond to drug-induced DNA damage either with cell-cycle delay at the G1/S phase boundary, or apoptosis, both of which are thought to be mediated by p53. A high ratio of the proapoptotic BAX protein to the antiapoptotic BCL2 protein has been reported in cell lines to explain the rapid response of GCT, but needs further investigation *in vivo*.[38,39] Other data suggest a failure of response and/or caspase activation as a contributor to cisplatin resistance.[40] A much attenuated apoptotic response to cisplatin has been observed in somatically differentiated GCT cell lines, reflecting the relative resistance of teratoma elements in GCT specimens.[41] This finding is consistent with reports of an association between the expression of genes associated with differentiation (particularly neuronal) and cisplatin resistence.[42] Thus, the molecular basis for the sensitivity of GCT to chemotherapy is probably multifactorial, partly residing in the inherent biologic features of germ cells involved in cell growth, cell death, and differentiation pathways, and partly in the genetic makeup of the tumors.[43]

Molecular Signatures and Clinical Outcome

High throughput methods of genome scanning at the level of gene expression and DNA copy number changes may identify genetic signatures that predict clinical outcome. Such studies have identified predictive signatures in breast, lung, and other tumors. A recent study from one clinical center, using array-based gene-expression profiling and array-based DNA copy analysis,[42] identified 101 gene-probe sets, with a twofold change in expression between tumors having the alteration versus those without the alteration. A prognostic model built to predict 5-year disease-free survival, based on the expression of these genes, correctly classified patients independent of the clinically based International Germ Cell Cancer Collaborative Group (IGCCCG) risk system.[42] These results need to be validated in larger multicenter-based cohorts.

IMMUNOHISTOCHEMICAL MARKERS

Seminoma displays neither differentiation *in vitro* or *in vivo*, nor expresses markers of somatic differentiation. Both seminomas and embryonal carcinoma express OCT3/4. Seminoma expresses CD117 (the kit receptor), while embryonal carcinomas, but not seminoma, express SOX2 and CD30 antigens.[44,45] Loss of KIT expression in seminoma may be associated with a clinically more aggressive phenotype.[13] Embryonal carcinoma and yolk sac tumor display somatic differentiation and surface expression of low-molecular-weight keratins. Vimentin expression is limited to mesenchymal components of mature teratoma and interstitial and other support cells. In tumors of uncertain histogenesis, CD117, OCT3/4, SOX2, CD30, and low-molecular-weight keratins may be useful in distinguishing GCT from tumors of other origin. It should be remembered that cytokeratins are expressed by all epithelial tumors. Two novel markers expressed in GCTs include SALL4 and glypican-3. Used in combination with other markers, they may help identify yolk sac tumors, particularly as AFP is a relatively unreliable immunohistochemical marker.[46–48] Placental alkaline phosphatase immunoreactivity is present in other tumor types and is less useful in the diagnosis of GCT.

STAGING

Physical examination; determination of serum levels of AFP, hCG, and lactate dehydrogenase (LDH); pathology; and radiographic studies are required to define extent of disease and appropriate treatment.

Anatomic Considerations

The initial route of metastasis is lymphatic drainage to retroperitoneal lymph nodes (Fig. 99.2). Lymphatic vessels emerge from the mediastinum testis and accompany the gonadal vessels in the spermatic cord. Where the spermatic vessels cross ventral to the ureter, some lymphatics diverge and drain into the retroperitoneal lymph node chain, while others follow the spermatic vessels to their origin. Lymph nodes located lateral or anterior to the inferior vena cava are paracaval or precaval nodes (Fig. 99.2A). Interaortocaval nodes are located between the inferior vena cava and the aorta. Nodes anterior or lateral to the aorta are preaortic or para-aortic nodes, respectively. The primary landing zone for a *right* testicular tumor lies in the interaortocaval nodes inferior to the renal vessels, and the ipsilateral distribution includes the paracaval, precaval, and right common iliac nodes (Fig. 99.2B). The primary landing zone for a *left* testicular tumor lies in the true para-aortic nodes inferior to the left renal vessels (Fig. 99.2C), and the ipsilateral distribution includes the para-aortic, preaortic, and left common iliac nodes. External iliac lymph node metastasis is usually secondary to a large volume of disease with retrograde spread except in the setting of a prior herniorrhaphy, vasectomy, or other transscrotal procedure. Contralateral retroperitoneal metastasis implies involvement of nodes usually associated with a tumor from the opposite side. For example, para-aortic lymphadenopathy in the presence of a right-sided primary tumor is considered contralateral. Contralateral spread is more common with right-sided tumors, rare with left-sided primaries, and usually occurs in the setting of large-volume disease.

Retroperitoneal lymphatics continue cephalad and empty into the cisterna chyli via the right and left lumbar trunks. Hence, lymphatic metastasis above the retroperitoneal nodes may occur in the retrocrural nodes. Supradiaphragmatic spread occurs via the thoracic duct, leading to posterior mediastinal and left supraclavicular lymph node involvement. The anterior mediastinum is not part of this usual nodal hierarchy.

Tumor Imaging

Computed and Positron Emission Tomography

Computed tomography (CT) is used to identify metastatic involvement above and below the diaphragm. A chest CT might detect very small pulmonary lesions that may be benign, and their clinical importance requires careful clinical judgment. CT scan with oral and intravenous contrast is the best technique for identifying retroperitoneal lymphadenopathy. The abdominal CT scan is normal in 70% of newly diagnosed seminoma and at least one-third of newly diagnosed NSGCT. Because GCTs may grow rapidly, treatment decisions should generally be made within approximately 4 weeks of the last abdominal CT scan. Lymph nodes measuring 10 to 20 mm in a primary landing zone are involved by GCT approximately 70% of the time, and those measuring 4 to 10 mm are involved approximately 50% of the time.[49,50] Oral contrast to opacify the duodenum and proximal jejunum is often helpful to distinguish bowel, tumor, and the great vessels. A normal postchemotherapy CT scan does not mean the absence of disease, because viable tumor, teratoma, and/or necrosis/fibrosis may exist in otherwise normal-size nodes. A plain chest radiograph is indicated in all patients with GCT.

Studies comparing positron emission tomography (PET) with CT in NSGCT have found no improvement in clinical staging and no value in postchemotherapy management of NSGCT with PET.[51,52] PET is useful in detecting residual viable seminoma in masses larger than 3 cm in diameter after chemotherapy.[53,54] Reports have started to call attention to the theoretical cancer risks from CT and PET radiation exposure.[55–59]

Magnetic Resonance Imaging

Although MRI occasionally provides valuable information regarding vascular anatomy or liver disease, it adds little to the management of most patients with GCT. Neither MRI nor CT detects viable GCT after chemotherapy. Studies comparing MRI with CT are needed.[60]

Serum Tumor Markers

α-Fetoprotein

AFP is determined by a two-site immunoenzymatic assay using WHO standard code 72/225, in which 1.0 IU AFP corresponds to 1.21 ng. The normal adult serum concentration is usually less than 15 ng/mL. The serum half-life of AFP is 5 to 7 days. Approximately 10% to 20% of clinical stage (CS) I, 20% to 40% of low-volume CS-II, and 40% to 60% of advanced

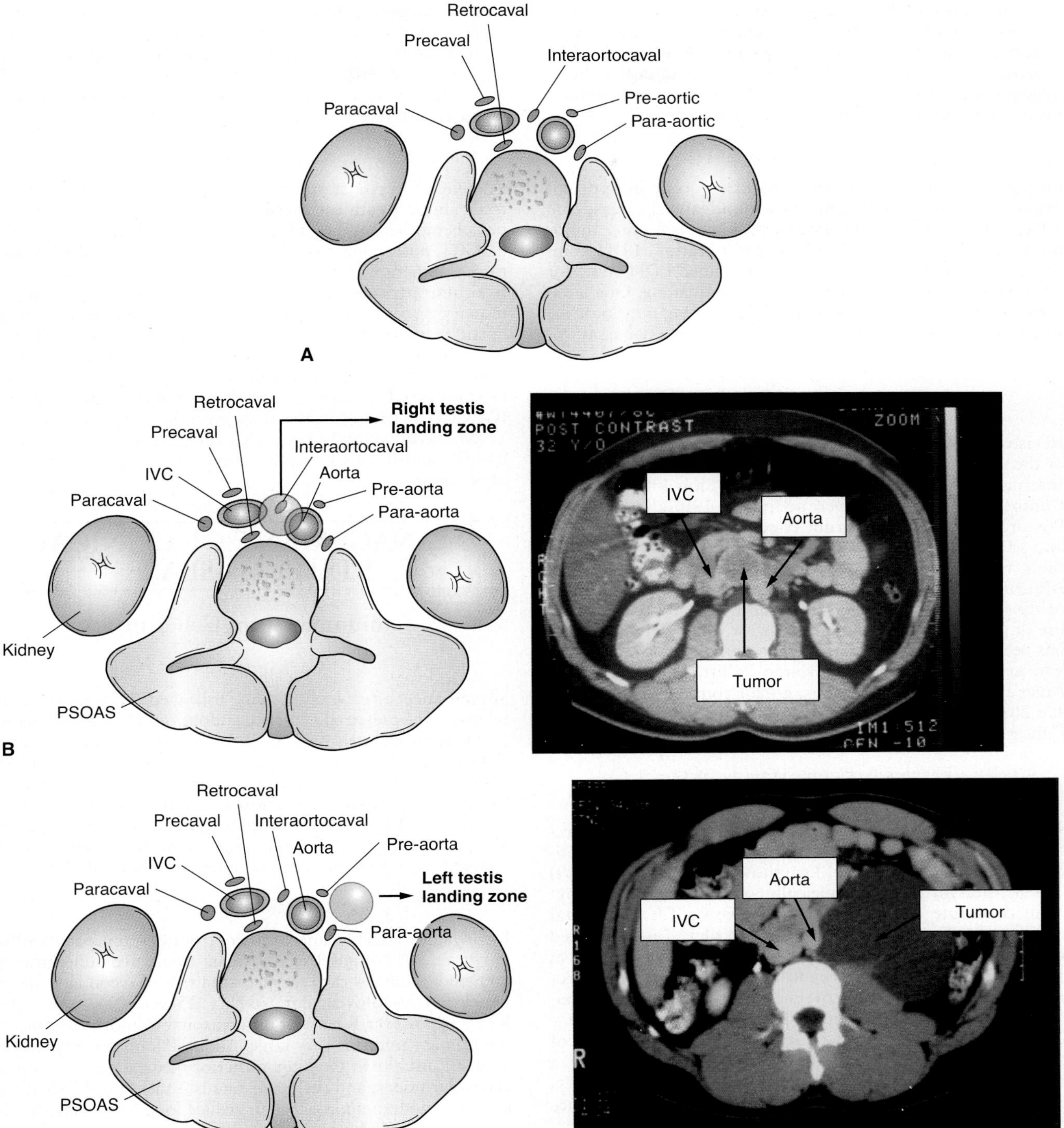

FIGURE 99.2 **A:** Retroperitoneal lymph nodes. **B:** Primary landing site for a right testicular tumor. **C:** Primary landing site for a left testicular tumor.

NSGCT will have increased AFP levels. Pure seminoma never secretes AFP.

Human Chorionic Gonadotropin

hCG, composed of an α and β subunit, is produced by syncytiotrophoblasts. The α subunit is shared by luteinizing hormone (LH), follicle-stimulating hormone (FSH), and thyroid-stimulating hormone. The β subunits of hCG, LH, FSH, and thyroid-stimulating hormone are homologous but have distinct amino acid sequences. Most commercial methods have adopted the WHO Third International Standard (code 75/537), resulting in some immunoassay uniformity. The serum half-life of hCG β is 18 to 36 hours. Approximately 10% to 20% of patients with CS-I, 20% to 30% with low-volume CS-II, and 40% with advanced NSGCT present with elevated serum concentrations of hCG. Approximately 15% to 20% of patients with advanced pure seminoma have increased serum concentrations of hCG.[61] False elevations of hCG secondary to cross-reactivity of the antibody with LH, treatment-induced hypogonadism (which may resolve with testosterone replacement), or heterophile antibodies may be seen.[62]

Lactate Dehydrogenase

Increased serum concentrations of LDH occur in approximately 60% of NSGCT patients with advanced disease and 80% of patients with advanced seminoma, reflecting tumor burden, growth rate, and cellular proliferation. LDH comprises multiple isoenzymes, but the combined LDH value for all isoenzymes is used for clinical decision making. One laboratory may be compared with another by using a ratio of the value to the upper limit of normal for the individual assay.

Staging Classifications

Revised TNM (tumor, node, metastasis) and stage groupings of the American Joint Committee on Cancer (AJCC) and the International Union Against Cancer (Union Internationale Contre le Cancer [UICC]) were adopted in 1997 (Table 99.2).[63] Postorchiectomy nadir serum concentrations of AFP, hCG, and LDH are incorporated into an "S" category because of their independent prognostic significance (see "Factors Affecting Outcome in Advanced Disease"). The seventh edition of the AJCC *Cancer Staging Manual* incorrectly refers to the use of preorchiectomy marker levels for staging, an error that has been corrected on the AJCC web page (cancerstaging.org) and in subsequent editions (Karen Pollitt, Manager, AJCC, American College of Surgeons, e-mail communication, May 17, 2010).[63] The guidelines of the National Comprehensive Cancer Network correctly refer to postorchiectomy status.[64]

Factors Affecting Staging of the Primary Tumor (T Stage)

The T stage of the primary lesion, histology, and postorchiectomy serum tumor marker concentrations predict the likelihood of metastatic disease. Lymphovascular invasion (LVI) and invasion through the tunica albuginea into the tunica vaginalis constitute T2, spermatic cord invasion T3, and scrotal invasion T4. For NSGCT, the presence of LVI is associated with an approximately 50% likelihood of retroperitoneal metastasis. In seminoma, prognostic factors predicting retroperitoneal disease are controversial. In some studies of seminoma surveillance, T2/3 tumors have a higher relapse rate.[65] In other studies, LVI is not an independent predictor of outcome.[66,67] Rete testis invasion has not been validated as a risk factor.[67] Persistently elevated levels of AFP and/or hCG after orchiectomy imply metastasis even if no other evidence of disease is found (CS-IS).

Factors Affecting Staging of Regional (Retroperitoneal) Nodes (N Stage)

Pathologic Staging. The number and size of retroperitoneal lymph nodes found at RPLND have prognostic importance in patients with NSGCT. If fewer than six nodes are involved with tumor, *and* the largest node is no larger than 2 cm, *and* no extranodal tumor extension is evident, then most retrospective studies report a low frequency (10%–15%) of disease relapse. A recent study questioned the importance of extranodal extension.[68] However, the presence of any of these features is generally associated with a relapse rate of 50% or more. Once lymph node involvement is demonstrated, neither primary tumor histology nor LVI adds prognostic value.

Clinical Staging. The transverse diameter of the largest lymph node is used to subcategorize CS-II disease. For seminoma, relapse rates after definitive RT increase progressively to approximately 40% to 60% for nodes greater than 5 cm. In NSGCT, treatment decisions are based on lymph node size, location, and serum tumor marker concentrations.

Factors Affecting Outcome in Advanced Disease

The IGCCCG risk status criteria should be used in all clinical trials and in treatment decisions for patients who require initial chemotherapy for advanced disease (Table 99.3).[69] For NSGCT, postorchiectomy levels of LDH, hCG, and AFP prior to chemotherapy, primary tumor site (i.e., mediastinal vs. testis or retroperitoneal), and the presence or absence of nonpulmonary visceral metastasis are validated independent prognostic factors for progression-free survival.[69,70] In seminoma, nonpulmonary visceral metastasis is the only significant prognostic factor. Good-, intermediate-, and poor-prognosis strata exist for NSGCT, but no poor-risk stratum exists in seminoma. IGCCCG marker cutoff values were incorporated into the TNM classification.[63] Data also suggest that tumor marker half-life and IGCCCG classification are independent markers of outcome.[71]

MANAGEMENT OF CLINICAL STAGE I DISEASE

Seminoma Germ Cell Tumors

Observation

Surveillance after orchiectomy followed by treatment on relapse is the preferred management option. The overall relapse rate is approximately 15% to 20%; the median time to relapse is 12 to 15 months and longer than that of NSGCT; approximately 30% of relapses occur 2 or more years after orchiectomy, and approximately 5% occur more than 5 years after diagnosis.[66] A recent study failed to validate rete testis invasion as a risk factor for relapse.[67] Size alone is associated with relapse.[66,72,73] Relapses have been reported beyond 10 years.[65]

Radiation Therapy

RT is highly effective and local control rates approach 100%. However, 80% of unselected patients are treated unnecessarily, and studies have shown an increased risk of secondary malignancy and cardiovascular toxicity 25 years or more after RT.[74–76] However, RT might be a reasonable informed choice if the primary tumor is very large. About 4% of patients relapse after RT, usually in the lung, posterior mediastinum, or supraclavicular nodes, and the death rate is under 2%.[77–80] If RT is selected, modern approaches to reduce long-term risks should be used. A randomized trial of treatment with either a dog-leg (top of T11 through L5, plus ipsilateral iliac nodes to the midobturator foramen) or para-aortic port (top of T11 to L5, only) showed equal survival with less toxicity in the para-aortic arm. More pelvic relapses occur after a para-aortic port, implying that post-RT surveillance is required, and the advantage is uncertain.[77] Typical doses range from 20 Gy to 30 Gy delivered in daily doses of 1.5 to 2.0 Gy. Outcomes after 30 Gy and 20 Gy are equivalent.[80–82] Prophylactic RT to the mediastinum is contraindicated. Shielding of the contralateral testis results in typical exposures of less than 1% of the prescription dose.

Chemotherapy

Carboplatin in CS-I seminoma has been studied in Europe, but is controversial in the United States. The Medical Research

TABLE 99.2

TUMOR, NODE, METASTASIS STAGING OF TESTIS TUMORS: AMERICAN JOINT COMMITTEE ON CANCER

TNM Category	Description
PRIMARY TUMOR (T)	
pTX	Primary tumor cannot be assessed
pT0	No evidence of primary tumor (e.g., histologic scar in testis)
pTis	Intratubular germ cell neoplasia (carcinoma *in situ*)
pT1	Tumor limited to the testis and epididymis without vascular/lymphatic invasion. Tumor may invade into the tunica albuginea but not the tunica vaginalis
pT2	Tumor limited to the testis and epididymis with vascular/lymphatic invasion or tumor extending through the tunica albuginea with involvement of the tunica vaginalis
pT3	Tumor invades the spermatic cord with or without vascular/lymphatic invasion
pT4	Tumor invades the scrotum with or without vascular/lymphatic invasion.
*Note: Except for pTis and pT4, extent of primary tumor is classified by radical orchiectomy. TX may be used for other categories in the absence of radical orchiectomy.	
REGIONAL LYMPH NODES (N)	
Clinical	
NX	Regional lymph nodes cannot be assessed
N0	No regional lymph node metastasis
N1	Metastasis with a lymph node mass ≥2 cm in greatest dimension; or multiple lymph nodes, none >2 cm in greatest dimension
N2	Metastasis with a lymph node mass >2 cm but not >5 cm in greatest dimension; or multiple lymph nodes, any one mass >2 cm but >5 cm in greatest dimension
N3	Metastasis with a lymph node mass >5 cm in greatest dimension
Pathologic (pN)	
pNX	Regional lymph nodes cannot be assessed
pN0	No regional lymph node metastasis
pN1	Metastasis with a lymph node mass ≥2 cm in greatest dimension and ≤5 nodes positive, none >2 cm in greatest dimension
pN2	Metastasis with a lymph node mass >2 cm but not >5 cm in greatest dimension; or >5 nodes positive, none >5 cm; or evidence of extranodal extension of tumor
pN3	Metastasis with a lymph node mass >5 cm in greatest dimension
Distant Metastases (M)	
M0	No distant metastasis
M1	Distant metastasis
M1a	Nonregional nodal or pulmonary metastases
M1b	Distant metastasis other than to nonregional lymph nodes and lungs

SERUM TUMOR MARKERS

*Note: Except for pTis and pT4, etc.

	LDH[a]	hCG (mIU/mL)	AFP (ng/mL)
S0	Markers within normal limits		
S1	<1.5 × N	<5,000	<1,000
S2	1.5–10 × N	5,000–50,000	1,000–10,000
S3	>10 × N	>50,000	>10,000

(*continued*)

Council (MRC) and European Organization for the Research and Treatment of Cancer (EORTC) compared a single dose of carboplatin after orchiectomy with external beam RT.[72,83] The trial design hypothesized a less than 3% increase in 2-year relapse-free rate (from 4% to 7%) with carboplatin to declare noninferiority (not the same as equivalence). Although the upper limit of the 90% confidence interval (CI) for the difference between the 2-year relapse rates was less than the 3% boundary, the 5-year difference in the relapse-free rate between arms was 1.34% (90% CI, −0.7% to 3.5%) in favor of RT (hazard ratio, 1.27),[72] showing that relapses continue to appear and that a 5-year rate is more revealing than the 2-year rate. Retroperitoneal relapses predominated in the carboplatin arm, a pattern observed in surveillance and requiring CT follow-up.

A risk-adapted approach with two cycles of carboplatin has also been studied, with patients selected on the basis of one or two risk factors (tumor >4 cm, presence of rete testis invasion).[84] This study reported a 3.3% relapse rate (also retroperitoneal), with a short median follow-up of 34 months. Concerns regarding the use of carboplatin in CS-I seminoma include limitations of the trial design comparing it to RT; questions about the design; the inferiority of standard-dose carboplatin compared with cisplatin in metastatic GCT (including seminoma); the observation that most relapses occur in the retroperitoneum, requiring abdomen and pelvis CT monitoring; and relatively short follow-up resulting in an inability to assess the late toxicity of carboplatin. North American investigators generally endorse surveillance in most CS-I seminoma.[81,85]

TABLE 99.2

(CONTINUED)

TNM Category	Description			
ANATOMIC STAGE/PROGNOSTIC GROUPS				
Group	**T**	**N**	**M**	**S**
Stage 0	pTis	N0	M0	S0
Stage I	pT1–4	N0	M0	SX
IA	pT1	N0	M0	S0
IB	pT2	N0	M0	S0
	pT3	N0	M0	S0
	pT4	N0	M0	S0
IS	Any pT/Tx	N0	M0	S1–3[b]
Stage II	Any pT/Tx	N1–3	M0	SX
IIA	Any pT/Tx	N1	M0	S0
	Any pT/Tx	N1	M0	S1
IIB	Any pT/Tx	N2	M0	S0
	Any pT/Tx	N2	M0	S1
IIC	Any pT/Tx	N3	M0	S0
	Any pT/Tx	N3	M0	S1
Stage III	Any pT/Tx	Any N	M1	SX
IIIA	Any pT/Tx	Any N	M1a	S0
	Any pT/Tx	Any N	M1a	S1
IIIB	Any pT/Tx	N1–3	M0	[b] S2
	Any pT/Tx	Any N	M1a	S2
IIIC	Any pT/Tx	N1–3	M0	S3
	Any pT/Tx	Any N	M1a	S3
	Any pT/Tx	Any N	M1b	Any S

TNM, tumor, node, metastasis; AFP, α-fetoprotein; hCG, human chorionic gonadotropin; LDH, lactate dehydrogenase; S, serum tumor markers.
[a]N indicates upper limit of normal for the LDH assay.
[b]Measured after orchiectomy
(Adapted from ref. 63.)

TABLE 99.3

GERM CELL TUMOR RISK CLASSIFICATION: INTERNATIONAL CONSENSUS

Risk Group	Seminoma	Nonseminoma
Good	Any hCG Any LDH Nonpulmonary visceral metastases absent Any primary site	AFP <1,000 ng/mL hCG <5,000 mIU/mL LDH <1.5 × ULN Nonpulmonary visceral metastases absent Gonadal or retroperitoneal primary tumor
Intermediate	Nonpulmonary visceral metastases present Any hCG Any LDH Any primary site	AFP 1,000–10,000 ng/mL hCG 5000–50,000 mIU/mL LDH 1.5–10.0 × ULN Nonpulmonary visceral metastases absent Gonadal or retroperitoneal primary site
Poor	Does not exist	Mediastinal primary site Nonpulmonary visceral metastases present (e.g., bone, liver, brain) AFP 10,000 ng/mL hCG 50,000 mIU/mL LDH 10 × ULN

hCG, human chorionic gonadotropin; AFP, α-fetoprotein; LDH, lactate dehydrogenase; ULN, upper limit of normal.
(From ref. 69.)

Nonseminomatous Germ Cell Tumors

Histologic features and serum tumor marker concentrations determine management of CS-I NSGCT. RT does not have a role in CS-I NSGCT.

Observation

Observation studies in CS-I NSGCT were driven by (1) infertility from retrograde ejaculation after RPLND; (2) frequent absence of therapeutic benefits from RPLND; that is, orchiectomy was curative or systemic disease occurred in the absence of retroperitoneal disease; and (3) ability of cisplatin-based chemotherapy to cure systemic disease. With surveillance in unselected CS-I NSGCT, the retroperitoneum accounts for about two-thirds of relapses and the lungs or increasing markers about one-third. Nonpulmonary visceral relapse alone is rare. About 50% of T2–T4 tumors relapse, compared with 15% of T1 tumors. Fewer than 10% of relapses occur more than 2 years after orchiectomy,[86] compared with about 30% after surveillance for seminoma.[66] Some studies suggest that a high percentage of embryonal carcinoma predicts a higher likelihood of relapse. However, correlation with LVI is high, and the TNM classification does not include embryonal carcinoma as an element in T staging.

Compliant patients with CS-IA NSGCT (T1 primary tumor, normal radiographs and physical examination, and serum tumor markers that are normal or declining at half-life) may be offered either observation or nerve-sparing RPLND. Because 75% to 85% of CS-IA patients will not relapse, surveillance is usually chosen, thereby avoiding a possibly unnecessary RPLND. If RPLND is chosen, a nerve-sparing operation will preserve ejaculatory capacity in more than 90% of patients. Limiting serial CT imaging is relevant, given emerging concern over possible long-term toxicity from CT radiation exposure.[55–57] Routine CT scans of the abdomen are unnecessary after a bilateral RPLND. One study reported an increased incidence of second malignancies after surveillance compared with RPLND.[58] However, no systematic data document an increase in cancer risk after CT scans. Observation is preferred by some investigators for CS-IB NSGCT, but 50% of patients will relapse, usually requiring both chemotherapy and bilateral RPLND (which may not be amenable to a nerve-sparing operation), resulting in a greater overall treatment burden. Hence, the risks and benefits must be carefully weighed in this highly curable disease.

Retroperitoneal Lymph Node Dissection

RPLND provides critical staging information and must be performed with curative intent. Bilateral infrahilar RPLND is the standard against which therapeutic alternatives are judged.[87,88] Because chylous ascites and other complications are more frequent and suprahilar metastasis is rare in low-stage NSGCT, suprahilar dissection is reserved for residual hilar or suprahilar masses following chemotherapy for advanced NSGCT.[87] A bilateral infrahilar RPLND includes the precaval, retrocaval, paracaval, interaortocaval, retroaortic, preaortic, para-aortic, and common iliac lymph nodes (Fig. 99.3). The gonadal vessel

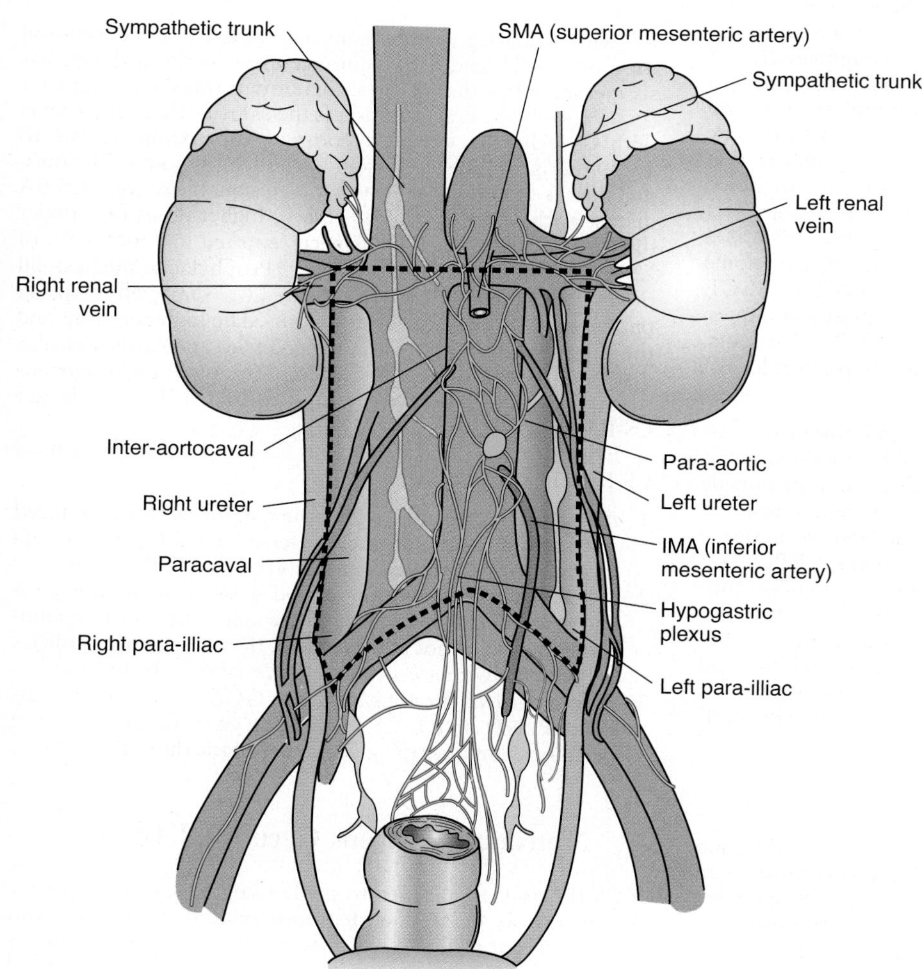

FIGURE 99.3 Standard modified bilateral retroperitoneal lymph node dissection.

itself may harbor disease, but the ipsilateral gonadal vein and surrounding fibroadipose tissue from its insertion to the internal ring must be completely excised to minimize the possibility of a late paracolic recurrence.[89] Mortality is less than 1%, and major complications such as hemorrhage, ureteral injury, bowel obstruction, pulmonary embolus, and wound dehiscence are rare. Minor complications include lymphocele, atelectasis, wound infection, and prolonged ileus.

The most consistent long-term morbidity of a standard bilateral RPLND is retrograde ejaculation and infertility related to sympathetic nerve fiber damage and the extent of the retroperitoneal dissection. Antegrade ejaculation requires coordination of three separate events: (1) closure of the bladder neck, (2) seminal emission, and (3) ejaculation. The sympathetic nerves that mediate seminal emission emanate primarily from the T12 to L3 thoracolumbar spine. After leaving the sympathetic trunk, the postganglionic sympathetic fibers, which are critical in the preservation of antegrade ejaculation, converge to form the hypogastric plexus near the aortic bifurcation, and then travel via pelvic nerves to innervate the vas deferens, seminal vesicles, prostate, and bladder neck. Sympathetic stimulation tightens the bladder neck, and pudendal somatic innervation from S2 to S4 relaxes the external urethral sphincter causing rhythmic contraction of bulbourethral and perineal muscles.

Two general types of nerve-sparing RPLND exist. Margins of resection should not be compromised in an attempt to preserve ejaculation.

1. *Modified RPLND templates* maximize rates of ejaculation by limiting dissection in areas thought to be at reduced risk for metastatic spread based on surgical mapping studies. These templates do *not* identify specific nerve fibers, but should include resection of all interaortocaval and ipsilateral lymph nodes between the level of the renal vessels and the bifurcation of the common iliac artery. This approach reduces trauma to the hypogastric plexus and contralateral postganglionic sympathetic fibers. Emerging data on late relapse and reoperative retroperitoneal surgery suggest that the mapping studies on which modified templates are based may underestimate the extent of retroperitoneal disease.[87,90]
2. *Nerve-dissection bilateral RPLND* prospectively identifies and preserves both sympathetic chains, the postganglionic sympathetic fibers, and hypogastric plexus. In CS-I NSGCT, with prospective nerve-dissecting preservation techniques, antegrade ejaculation is preserved in over 95% of patients. Therefore, the original value of templates to prevent loss of ejaculatory function is diminished.

Comparing standard nerve-dissection and modified bilateral templates, disease outside the modified bilateral templates was observed in 3% to 23% of patients. The histology outside templates did not differ from that within the templates, and teratoma was present in 21% to 30% of positive nodes.[90] Similar findings were observed in postchemotherapy RPLND.[91] Absence of postoperative follow-up, administration of postoperative chemotherapy, and surgical variability in multicenter studies limit the data on relapse. Because teratoma and malignant transformation are overrepresented in late relapse and reoperative surgery, complete resection at first operation is important.[92] Chemotherapy does not compensate for suboptimal initial surgery.[93]

Chemotherapy for Stage I NSGCT

Studies of one to two cycles of BEP (bleomycin, etoposide, and cisplatin) for CS-I, T2-4N0M0S0, NSGCT report fewer than 5% relapses and about 1% deaths from GCT.[94] Proponents argue that the substitution of a brief course of chemotherapy avoids RPLND. However, all of these patients are exposed to transient (e.g., myelosuppression), permanent (e.g., neuropathy), and delayed (i.e., cardiac events, Raynaud phenomenon, acute leukemia) chemotherapy toxicity.[95] Late relapse is rare, but does occur.[96] Because etoposide causes myelosuppression and rarely secondary leukemia, the MRC conducted a trial using two courses of bleomycin, vincristine, and cisplatin. The 5-year relapse-free rate was 98%, but neurotoxicity was worse than that observed in patients treated with three cycles of BEP for advanced disease.[97] Two European studies evaluated a single cycle of BEP in patients with T1–4N0M0S0 NSGCT and reported relapse rates less than 4%.[98,99] An unusually high number of scrotal and infield relapses in patients undergoing RPLND limits interpretation. Because of acute, delayed, and persistent chemotherapy-related toxicity and the lack of long-term follow-up, chemotherapy as initial treatment in patients with T2–4 N0M0S0 NSGCT is not standard in the United States.

Systemic chemotherapy is the treatment of choice when persistently elevated or rising serum concentrations of AFP and/or hCG are observed following orchiectomy without disease on examination or radiography (CS-IS), and disease is usually not limited to the retroperitoneum.[100] Small-volume retroperitoneal teratoma exists in these patients at a frequency similar to CS-II disease.[101] RPLND is required if reevaluation after chemotherapy demonstrates new disease, which usually represents growing teratoma.

MANAGEMENT OF CLINICAL STAGE II (LOW TUMOR BURDEN)

Seminoma

RT with a dog-leg port remains a standard treatment option for most CS-IIA and -IIB seminoma if retroperitoneal metastasis measures less than 3 cm in maximum transverse diameter (Fig. 99.4).[102–104] Fractionation is the same as that for patients with CS-I disease, except a boost of approximately 500 to 1,000 rad is administered to involved lymph nodes. The optimal dose is unknown; however, it is reasonable to treat CS-IIA disease with 25 to 30 Gy and reserve higher doses for bulkier disease. Relapse after RT has been reported in about 10% of CS-IIA and 20% of CS-IIB cases.[105] Prophylactic mediastinal or supraclavicular RT is not indicated.[106] Nearly all relapsing patients are cured with chemotherapy. The high cure rate and the risk for second non-GCT malignancies and cardiovascular disease after RT or RT plus chemotherapy[107] make chemotherapy a consideration for multifocal CS-IIA and larger CS-IIB disease.

Exceptions to the use of RT in CS-I and nonbulky clinical CS-II seminoma include:

1. *Horseshoe kidney.* Because of the risk for radiation-induced renal failure, observation is preferred in CS-I; primary chemotherapy is the treatment of choice for CS-II disease.
2. *Inflammatory bowel disease.* A discussion with an experienced radiation oncologist is indicated under such circumstances. If RT is not administered, the management policies for patients with a *horseshoe kidney* should be followed.
3. *A second metachronous testicular GCT.* After a prior bilateral RPLND or RT, CS-I disease is generally observed, or primary chemotherapy given if metastatic disease is present.

Nonseminomatous Germ Cell Tumors

If CS-II NSGCT is limited to the landing zone of the primary tumor, not associated with tumor-related back pain, and serum levels of AFP and hCG are normal, then solitary nodes less than 2 cm may be managed by nerve-sparing bilateral

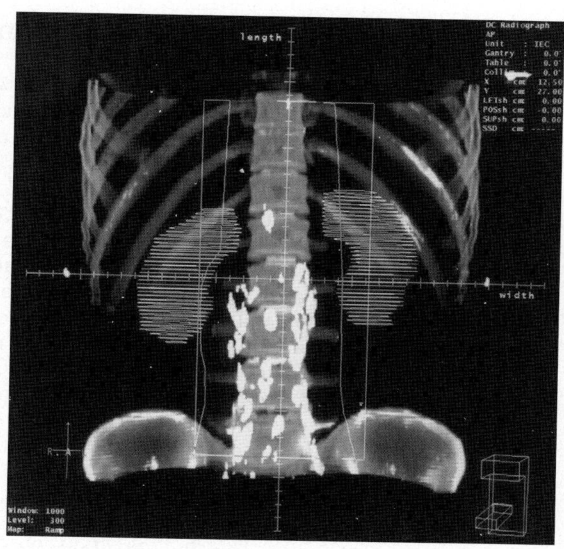

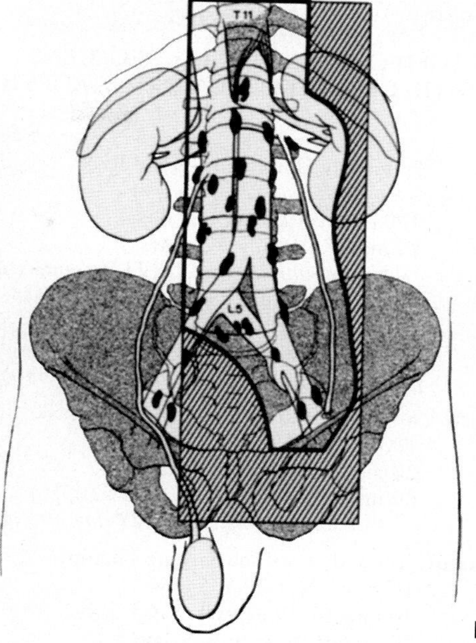

FIGURE 99.4 **A:** Para-aortic portal for clinical stage I seminoma. **B:** Contoured anterior and posterior radiation treatment fields for men with clinical stage II or IIA left testicular cancer. The diagonally shaded area is an individually made, 8-cm thick Cerrobend block.

RPLND. Multifocal, suprahilar or retrocrural, bilateral or contralateral retroperitoneal nodes (even if the ipsilateral lymph nodes do not appear to be involved), the presence of back pain, large nodal size (even if solitary), or increased AFP and/or hCG levels after orchiectomy not declining at half-life, all imply a high likelihood of unresectable disease or metastatic disease, and initial chemotherapy is preferred.[108–110]

Retroperitoneal Lymph Node Dissection

RPLND has been a standard approach in patients with normal serum levels of AFP and hCG, and CS-IIA or smaller solitary CS-IIB disease. Infield recurrence is rare following a definitive therapeutic operation. Nerve-sparing dissection may be possible, depending on the location and volume of disease, but margins should not be compromised to maintain ejaculatory function.

Management of Pathologic Stage II Disease after RPLND

Surveillance is a treatment choice for compliant patients with fewer than six involved nodes and none greater than 2 cm (pN1). Approximately 10% to 20% of such patients relapse. Poor patient compliance, psychological factors, occupation, geography, or other issues may make adjuvant chemotherapy the preferred choice in selected patients. Adjuvant chemotherapy is a strong consideration when six or more nodes are involved, any node is larger than 2 cm, or there is extranodal extension (pN2/N3). One study has questioned the significance of extranodal extension.[68] Both BEP and EP (etoposide and cisplatin) may be used in this highly curable patient population.[111,112] Observation with standard treatment at relapse and two cycles of adjuvant chemotherapy have shown equivalent survival. Patients who relapse during surveillance will require three to four cycles of cisplatin-based therapy according to their disease status at that time.

Identification of Relapse

After dog-leg RT for seminoma, surveillance includes a chest radiograph, measurement of AFP, hCG, and LDH, and a physical examination every 6 weeks to 3 months in the first year, every 3 to 4 months in the second year, and less frequently thereafter. An abdominal CT scan should be done at the conclusion of RT, but none is required thereafter. The need for additional scans should be considered after a para-aortic port because of the higher pelvic relapse rate.

During surveillance for CS-I NSGCT, a physical examination, chest radiograph, and determinations of AFP, LDH, and hCG levels are required at 1- to 2-month intervals in the first year, 2- to 3-month intervals in the second year, and less frequently thereafter. An abdominal CT scan is suggested quarterly in the first year, every 4 months in the second year, and every 6 to 12 months thereafter. A pelvic CT is required only if there is a prior scrotal incision (e.g., vasectomy).

Following RPLND for CS-II NSGCT without adjuvant chemotherapy, a chest radiograph, measurement of AFP, hCG, and LDH, and a physical examination are required approximately every 1 to 3 months in the first year, every 2 to 4 months in the second year, and less frequently in the third year and beyond. In all settings, annual visits are sufficient to detect late relapse and second primary tumors after the fifth year. With adequate follow-up, relapse is nearly always "low volume" (good risk), and can be cured with chemotherapy.[64,94]

MANAGEMENT OF STAGE II AND STAGE III DISEASE (HIGH TUMOR BURDEN)

Cisplatin-based chemotherapy (Table 99.4) will cure 70% to 80% of unselected GCT patients with retroperitoneal, supradiaphragmatic nodal, or visceral metastases. Postchemotherapy

TABLE 99.4

COMMONLY USED CHEMOTHERAPY REGIMENS FOR METASTATIC GERM CELL TUMORS (STAGES II AND III)

Regimen	Previously Untreated—Good Risk
Etoposide	100 mg/m² IV daily × 5 days
Cisplatin	20 mg/m² IV daily × 5 days
	4 cycles administered at 21-day intervals
Etoposide	100 mg/m² IV daily × 5 day
Cisplatin	20 mg/m² IV daily × 5 day
Bleomycin	30 units IV weekly (e.g., days 2, 9, 16)
	3 cycles administered at 21-day intervals
Previously Untreated—Intermediate and Poor Risk	
Etoposide	100 mg/m² IV daily × 5 days
Cisplatin	20 mg/m² IV daily × 5 days
Bleomycin	30 units IV weekly (e.g., days 2, 9, 16)
	4 cycles administered at 21-day intervals
Previously Treated—1st-Line Salvage Therapy	
Ifosfamide	1.2 g/m² IV daily × 5 days
Mesna	400 mg/m² IV every 8 h × 5 days
Cisplatin	20 mg/m² IV daily × 5 days
Vinblastine	0.11 mg/kg IV days 1 and 2
	4 cycles administered at 21-day intervals
Paclitaxel	250 mg/m² IV by continuous infusion over 24 h day 1
Ifosfamide	1.5 g/m² IV daily—days 2–5
Cisplatin	25 mg/m² IV daily—days 2–5
Mesna	500 mg/m² IV every 8 h—on days 2–5
	4 cycles administered at 21-day intervals

IV, intravenously.

surgery in NSGCT is often essential to achieving a disease-free state.

Good-Prognosis Germ Cell Tumors

Complete response (CR) rates range from 88% to 95% in IGCCCG good-risk patients. Greatest efficacy with least toxicity is the goal. Therefore, clinical trials have focused on reducing bleomycin and cisplatin toxicity.[113–120] Three cycles of BEP and four cycles of EP are the only widely used regimens.[116–119] CR rates are greater than 90%, about 5% relapse, and long-term follow-up reports overall survival at 90% to 95%.[116–120] The substitution of carboplatin for cisplatin resulted in an inferior event-free and overall survival in NSGCT and seminoma (Table 99.5).[121–123] Etoposide 360 mg/m² per cycle is associated with a higher relapse rate and inferior survival when compared with etoposide 500 mg/m² per cycle.[124] Neither carboplatin nor low-dose etoposide should be used in previously untreated GCT patients unless a contraindication exists.

One randomized trial compared three cycles of BEP (BEP ×3) and four cycles of EP (EP ×4) using etoposide 500 mg/m² per cycle. At the primary end point of favorable response rate, the regimens were equivalent ($P = .34$) (Table 99.5).[119] Although the 4-year event-free and overall survival of EP ×4 were slightly lower than BEP ×4, the rates were not significantly different ($P = .135$ and $P = .096$, respectively). The results of this trial are inconclusive for several reasons. (1) Dose reductions for both cisplatin and etoposide were stipulated by the protocol. Only 77% of patients in the EP arm received 90% or more of the planned cisplatin dose, and 79% received 90% or more of the planned etoposide dose. In the BEP arm, 83% and 86% received greater than 90% of the planned cisplatin and etoposide doses, respectively.[119] Randomized trials previously demonstrated the superiority of higher-dose etoposide[124] and higher-dose cisplatin

TABLE 99.5

GOOD-RISK CHEMOTHERAPY TRIALS

Study (Ref.)	No. of Patients	Regimen	% CR	% Rel	≥90% Etoposide	>90% Cisplatin
Einhorn et al. (116)	96	$BE_{500}P \times 4$	97	6	NS[a]	100
	88	$B\ E_{500}P \times 3$	NS	NS	NS	NS
Kondagunta et al. (117)	289	$E_{500}P \times 4$	98	6	NS[b]	100
deWit et al. (118)	406	$B\ E_{500}P \times 3$[a]	90	14	84	84
	406	$B\ E_{500}P \times 3/EP \times 1$[a]	89	6	79	84
Culine et al. (119)	132	$B\ E_{500}P \times 3$[a]	92	4	83	86
	130	$E_{500}P \times 4$[a]	91	10	79	77
Bajorin et al. (121)	134	EP	90	6	67	95
	131	EC	88	7	68	95
Horwich et al. (122)	260	$BE_{360}C \times 4$	87	NS	NS	NS
	268	$BE_{360}P \times 4$	94	NS	NS	NS
Toner et al. (124)	83	$BE_{360}P \times 3$[a]	88	6	67	95
	83	$BE_{360}P \times 4$[a]	87	7	68	95

CR, complete response; Rel, relapse; B, bleomycin; E_{500}, etoposide 500 mg/m² per cycle; P, cisplatin; NS, not stated; C, carboplatin; E_{360}, etoposide 360 mg/m² per cycle.
[a]Indiana University dose modification guideline: No standard dose modification for platelet count or renal function. If white blood cell (WBC) count <2.5 on day 22, then delete etoposide dose on day 22.[120]
[b]Memorial Sloan Kettering Cancer Center dose-modification guideline. No standard dose modification for platelet count or renal function. If WBC<2.5 on day 22, then delay treatment for 1 week.[117,124]

TABLE 99.6

RANDOMIZED TRIALS IN PATIENTS WITH INTERMEDIATE- OR POOR-RISK GERM CELL TUMORS

Study (Ref.)	Poor-Risk Criteria	Regimen	No. of Patients	Responses % Complete	Responses % Durable	Benefit Over Standard Arm
Motzer et al. (71)	IGCCCG	BEP	111	46	48	No
		BEP + HD CEC	108	48	52	
de Wit et al. (128)	EORTC	PEB	102	74	NS	No
		PEB/PVB	102	75	NS	
Nichols et al. (129)	Indiana	PEB	77	73	61	No
		P(200)EB	76	68	63	
Kaye et al. (130)	EORTC/MRC	BEP/EP	185	57	55	No
		BOP/VIP-B	186	54	53	
Hinton et al. (131)	Indiana	PEB	141	60	57	No
		VIP	145	63	56	
Daugaard et al. (132)	EORTC	BEP	66	33	45[a]	No
		VIP → HD-VIP × 3	65	45	58[a]	

IGCCCG, International Germ Cell Cancer Collaborative Group Classification; B, bleomycin; E, etoposide; P, cisplatin 100 mg/m^2; HD, high dose; CEC, carboplatin, etoposide, and cyclophosphamide; EORTC, European Organization for the Research and Treatment of Cancer; NS, not stated; V, vinblastine; P(200), cisplatin 200 mg/m^2; MRC, Medical Research Council; O, vincristine; I, ifosfamide.
[a]Two-year failure-free survival.

compared with lower doses.[125] (2) Protocol-prescribed surgery after chemotherapy was omitted in 40% of patients with residual masses. (3) Although neutropenia occurred less frequently in BEP ×3 (72%) compared with EP ×3 (90%), febrile neutropenia (7% vs. 5%, respectively) and growth factor use (36% vs. 29%, respectively) were equivalent. (4) Neurologic (16% vs. 5%, respectively) and dermatologic toxicity, including Raynaud phenomenon (29% vs. 8%, respectively), occurred significantly more often in BEP ×3 than EP ×4.[119] (5) Good-risk status by IGCCCG status was retrospectively assigned.

Given long-term follow-up data, standard therapy for good-risk GCT patients can be either four cycles of EP or three cycles of BEP in which the cumulative dose per cycle of treatment is 100 mg/m^2 for cisplatin and 500 mg/m^2 for etoposide. The choice of one regimen over the other is based on toxicity, balancing the need for one additional weekly cycle in EP against the greater neurologic and dermatologic toxicity (including Raynaud phenomenon), and rare but possible pulmonary toxicity from BEP.[126] Because of the steep dose-response curve for both etoposide and cisplatin in GCT, dose reductions because of toxicity should be rare and limited and they should parallel published recommendations (Table 99.5).[116,120,127]

Intermediate- and Poor-Risk Germ Cell Tumors

Intermediate- and poor-risk GCT account for approximately 25% and 15% of GCT, respectively, and about 75% and 45% survive after treatment. Therefore, an improved cure rate remains a priority. Patients in these risk subgroups should be treated in a clinical trial if possible.

In randomized studies (Table 99.6),[71,128–132] cisplatin at 200 mg/m^2, complicated alternating regimens, and the substitution of ifosfamide for bleomycin (VIP [etoposide, ifosfamide, and cisplatin]) were not superior to the standard regimen of BEP ×4, and neurologic and hematologic toxicity were more severe.[128–131] VIP with hematopoietic growth factor support can be an alternative in treating intermediate- or poor-risk patients with pre-existing conditions that preclude bleomycin.

The success of high-dose, carboplatin-containing chemotherapy in the treatment of patients with refractory disease led to its study as part of initial therapy.[133,134] Clinical trials were designed to determine whether the burden of toxicity associated with high-dose therapy was balanced by improved long-term survival. One trial compared BEP ×4 with BEP ×2 followed by two cycles of high-dose carboplatin, etoposide, and cyclophosphamide with stem cell support in 219 patients with poor- and intermediate-risk GCT.[71] Routine inclusion of high-dose chemotherapy in first-line treatment of patients with intermediate- and poor-prognostic GCT did not improve outcome (Table 99.6). A German phase 1/2 trial provided the rationale for a high-dose VIP arm in a European poor-risk trial.[134] Phase 1/2 studies incorporating paclitaxel reported tolerable toxicity.[135] However, BEP ×4 remains the standard regimen to which all investigational regimens should be compared.

An association between prolonged serum marker decline and a worse CR rate and survival has been observed in retrospective and prospective studies.[71] Compared with a satisfactory decline, a slow serum tumor marker decline (half-life of hCG >3 days, AFP >7 days) during the first two cycles of BEP was associated with a shorter progression-free and overall survival after completing four cycles of BEP, but was not observed in patients whose treatment was switched to high-dose therapy, implying that the rate of marker decline might be an indication to change therapy.[71] The additional toxicity and the number of patients who are cured without treatment change have made it difficult to incorporate marker decline into standard management.

Management of Residual Disease

Resection of all sites of residual disease after chemotherapy and normalization of serum tumor markers an integral part of GCT management. Increased levels of AFP and/or hCG after chemotherapy generally imply residual, viable GCT, and salvage chemotherapy is usually recommended for these patients. One exception is the postchemotherapy cystic retroperitoneal mass. The fluid in those cysts sometimes contains elevated levels of hCG and/or AFP, leading to serum marker elevation that normalizes after surgery.[136]

TABLE 99.7

INFLUENCE OF TERATOMA, RESIDUAL SIZE, AND PERCENT SHRINKAGE ON HISTOLOGY OF RESIDUAL RETROPERITONEAL DISEASE AT POSTCHEMOTHERAPY RETROPERITONEAL LYMPH NODE DISSECTION

Predictive Factor (Ref)	Parameter	*N*	% Necrosis	% Teratoma	% Viable GCT ± Teratoma
Primary tumor (137)	No teratoma	262	59	30	11
	Teratoma	293	32	54	14
Total	—	555	45	42	13
Nodal size after chemotherapy, mm (137,138)	<5	21	80	10	10
	<10	370	72	22	6
	11–20	229	56	37	5
	21–50	306	30	50	20
	>50	222	17	59	24
	>100	54	19	46	35
Shrinkage, % (137)	≥70	155	74	21	8
	50–69	138	52	37	11
	30–49	62	45	42	13
	0–29	120	22	58	21
	Growth	46	0	83	17

GCT, germ cell tumor.

Retroperitoneum

Nonseminomatous Germ Cell Tumors. After chemotherapy, necrosis/fibrosis will be found in approximately 45% of specimens, teratoma in 40%, and viable GCT in 15%.[137–139] Although teratoma in the primary site and/or the size of a postchemotherapy mass are associated with the likelihood of either teratoma or viable disease (Table 99.7), no single criterion can distinguish viable tumor or teratoma from necrosis. Teratoma will be found in about 30% of unselected retroperitoneal tumors despite its absence in the testis.[140] Teratoma or viable GCT was found in 29% of postchemotherapy retroperitoneal nodes less than 10 mm in diameter and in 20% of those less than 5 mm (Table 99.7).[137–139] Occasionally, tumor growth with declining markers occurs during chemotherapy (growing teratoma syndrome) (Fig. 99.5), requiring early surgical intervention and completion of chemotherapy after surgery. PET scans are usually not useful after chemotherapy for NSGCT, because small tumor size and teratoma result in false-negative findings.[51,141] Four factors influence the decision to perform a postchemotherapy RPLND.

1. *Presence of retroperitoneal disease* before *chemotherapy.* A postchemotherapy RPLND should be considered if retroperitoneal disease is present before chemotherapy.[142] In patients who present with stage III disease without retroperitoneal involvement (e.g., pulmonary nodules only), a RPLND is not needed. In patients who present with CS-IS, there is no standard RPLND recommendation. However, retroperitoneal disease does exist in this group, and growing teratoma can occur. Judicious CT follow-up is recommended.[101]
2. *Likelihood of viable NSGCT.* The likelihood of viable NSGCT is associated with residual tumor size. If a tumor shrinks by less than 70% or the residual tumor mass measures more than 1 cm, then the likelihood of viable NSGCT increases to 20% to 30% (Table 99.7). However, viable

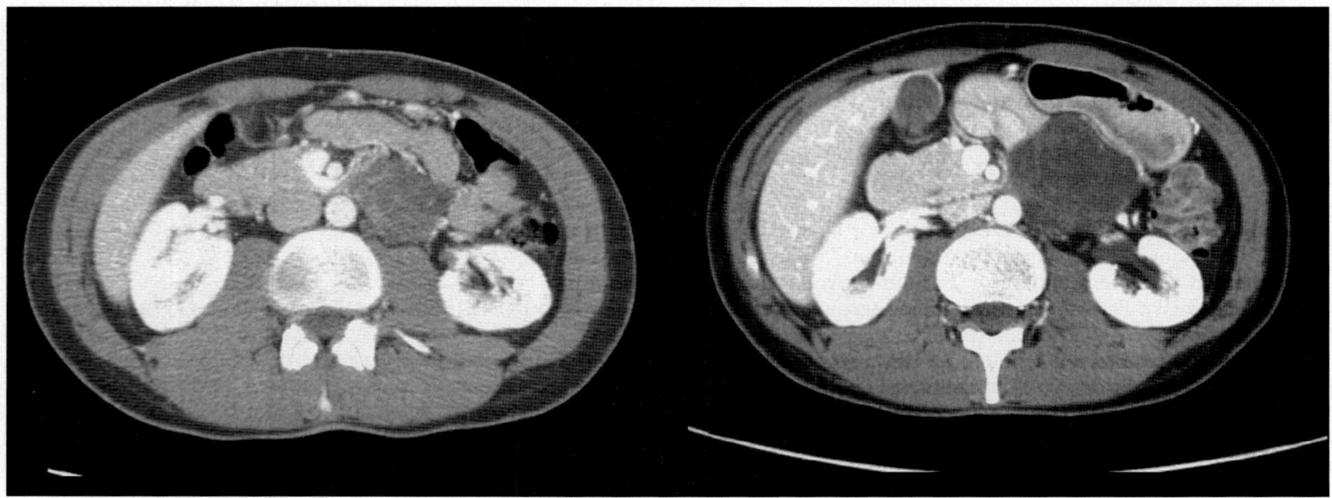

FIGURE 99.5 Growing teratoma syndrome. Patient presented with new back and abdominal pain despite rapidly declining markers after two cycles of cisplatin-based chemotherapy. Retroperitoneal node dissection was performed, showing only mature teratoma.

NSGCT may be found in 5% to 10% of cases with the greatest tumor shrinkage (>90%) and smallest residual size (<5 mm).[137–139] Resection of viable residual GCT, which is at least partially drug resistant, can minimize the risks of unnecessary salvage chemotherapy.

3. *Likelihood of teratoma.* If teratoma is absent in the primary site, about 25% to 45% of nodes will have teratoma. If teratoma is present in the primary site, at least 60% of cases will have residual teratoma in metastatic nodes, even if these nodes are less than 10 mm in diameter (Table 99.7). The likelihood of teratoma increases to 80% or more with a large residual mass, minimal shrinkage, or growth. Unresected teratoma may cause obstruction, or develop somatic malignant transformation (e.g., sarcoma or carcinoma).[143] Late relapse (a relapse occurring >2 years after therapy) is associated with teratoma and viable GCT, chemotherapy resistance, more frequently harbors somatic malignant transformation, and is associated with poor survival.[143,144]
4. *Morbidity of RPLND.* Retrograde ejaculation is the primary postoperative consequence, but nerve-sparing techniques have reduced its likelihood. The complication rate of RPLND following chemotherapy is generally higher than that of primary RPLND, but contemporary studies have reported a decrease in the incidence of both major and minor complications.[145,146] Postchemotherapy desmoplastic reaction, exposure to bleomycin, and more extensive retroperitoneal dissection because of large-volume residual disease increase the technical demands of the procedure. Monitoring of intraoperative and postoperative oxygen concentration (particularly in patients who have received bleomycin), meticulous fluid management, and an emphasis on colloid rather than crystalloid have reduced pulmonary toxicity and nearly eliminated perioperative death.

Residual Nodal Size Less than 1 cm. Surveillance and RPLND are standard options for patients with NSGCT who achieve CR in the retroperitoneum. Two studies reported surveillance after chemotherapy in 302 mostly IGCCCG good-risk patients who achieved a clinical CR (residual mass <1 cm). Among 22 patients with relapses (7%), 15 (68%) occurred in the retroperitoneum, and 2 patients died of disease.[147,148] The discrepancy between relapse rate in these two studies and the pathologic findings (Table 99.7) suggest that small-volume teratoma is unlikely or very slow to progress. However, these studies included a small but unknown number of patients who either did not have retroperitoneal disease at diagnosis or who had CS-IS disease, two groups for which RPLND is not standard practice. Because these young patients may live for decades after treatment, decision making must account for both short-term and long-term risks.

The proponents of surveillance stress the fewer surgeries, reduced risk of retrograde ejaculation, and lesser need for expert surgeons. The proponents of RPLND note that surveillance requires long-term follow-up and some serial imaging that is not necessary after RPLND; near elimination of the retroperitoneum as a site for the infrequent (late) relapse; rare potential malignant transformation; and less frequent exposure to salvage chemotherapy in the minority that relapse.[142] In the context of these considerations, postchemotherapy surveillance is an option for the good-risk patient whose retroperitoneal disease has disappeared (residual disease <1 cm), remembering the impact of the infrequent-to-rare relapse.

Residual Mass Greater than 1 cm. A postchemotherapy RPLND is necessary when residual retroperitoneal disease measures more than 1 cm. Viable GCT and teratoma becomes more frequent, and increasing tumor size is associated with surgical complexity.[142]

Once a decision is made to perform a postchemotherapy RPLND, a bilateral dissection is the standard operation. Less extensive templates leave disease behind in 7% to 32% of cases with histologic subtypes similar to that within the bilateral template.[91] A unilateral template is not an acceptable alternative. The number of resected nodes has been linked with outcome.[149] A reoperation for relapse is associated with a higher postoperative complication rate and worse-than-expected outcome.[150] *En bloc* nephrectomy, bowel resection, and/or *en bloc* resection of a great vessel is sometimes necessary to assure complete resection. Depending on the size and location of adenopathy, individual sympathetic nerves may be identified and antegrade ejaculation maintained.[151,152] The likelihood of retrograde ejaculation increases with the size of the residual disease. These patients will benefit from RPLND by surgeons at tertiary centers with extensive experience in postchemotherapy dissection.

The risk for relapse ranges from 5% to 10% when necrosis or teratoma is present in the retroperitoneal specimen. Therefore, no additional chemotherapy is needed.[153,154] Viable GCT is associated with a high risk for relapse and decreased disease-free survival.[154] One retrospective study reported that additional chemotherapy appeared to benefit only those with complete resection or less than 10% viable malignant cells.[155] This hypothesis has not been tested prospectively, and two additional cycles of chemotherapy following complete resection of viable GCT after first chemotherapy remains a common standard of care, with a cure rate of about 70%.[154]

Seminoma. Two important features distinguish a postchemotherapy seminoma residual mass from those observed with NSGCT. First, teratoma in the residual mass is rare. Seminoma with elevated AFP before chemotherapy has operative findings similar to NSGCT, and RPLND is indicated.[156] Second, a complete RPLND is often not technically feasible, secondary to severe desmoplastic reaction and obliteration of tissue planes. Consequently, perioperative morbidity has been reported as higher for seminoma than for NSGCT. RT does not reduce the likelihood of recurrence.[157] The need for RPLND when residual seminoma exceeds 3 cm in diameter has been clarified.[158] An (18)fluoro-deoxy-D-glucose (FDG)-PET scan study in 52 patients with residual masses following chemotherapy for bulky seminoma reported that all 8 positive scans and 42 of 44 (95%) negative scans were accurate.[53] One study validated these findings, although false-positive findings were observed.[54] Hence, if a residual mass measures 3 cm or larger and an FDG-PET scan is positive, resection may be needed. Size, site, comorbidity, and the possibility of false-positive PET scans should be considered.[54,151,159,160] A residual mass less than 3 cm may be observed without FDG-PET.

Lung and Mediastinal Resections

In the lung, teratoma and viable GCT are not clearly associated with residual tumor size.[161,162] Similar frequencies of teratoma (25%–30%) and viable GCT (about 20%) were observed with tumor size both less than 10 mm and greater than 50 mm, and greater than 70% and less than 70% shrinkage. The histology at RPLND and in the lung are often the same. Nonetheless, even with necrosis at RPLND, about 10% of lung resections harbored teratoma or viable GCT. Viable GCT at RPLND was associated with residual cancer in the lung in almost 50% of cases. Tumor growth, like its counterpart in the retroperitoneum, was associated with a high likelihood of teratoma.[162] Different histologies may be present in each lung. The highest likelihood of viable disease or teratoma is observed in the mediastinum, probably because mediastinal residual disease is usually associated with primary mediastinal NSGCT. Therefore, residual intrathoracic disease should be resected.[161]

Other Procedures

A small percentage of patients require operation to remove disease in the liver or neck.[163,164] The histology of a residual liver or neck mass cannot be predicted based on histology at another site. Multiple procedures may be required, but simultaneous resection of retroperitoneal and other sites is possible in selected cases. If a primary testis tumor is present and an orchiectomy is not performed *prior* to chemotherapy, then it is generally performed *after* chemotherapy, as that testis may harbor viable residual disease.[165] Studies repeatedly confirm that all residual disease should be resected, as histologic findings vary at different sites.

MANAGEMENT OF RELAPSE AND REFRACTORY DISEASE

Twenty percent to 30% of patients with advanced GCT relapse or fail to achieve a CR to cisplatin-based chemotherapy. Effective second- and third-line treatment options exist.

Prognostic Factors: Salvage Chemotherapy

Patients who relapse or fail to achieve CR to initial (B)EP comprise a heterogeneous group with reported cure rates ranging from 0% to 70%. Patients with a testis primary site *and* a CR to initial chemotherapy have a 3-year survival of 35% to 40% with vinblastine + ifosfamide + cisplatin (VeIP) salvage therapy.[166] An incomplete response to initial therapy or a relapsing extragonadal (usually mediastinal) NSGCT portends a 3-year survival of less than 10% with VeIP.[166] In these circumstances, a dose-intensive program or clinical trial should be considered.

Conventional-Dose Salvage Therapy

VeIP is a standard regimen in patients who relapse from CR, and about 25% of patients will achieve a durable CR.[167,168] Gastrointestinal, renal, and severe marrow toxicity are common. When paclitaxel (250 mg/m^2 [TIP]) was substituted for vinblastine,[169] 29 of 46 patients, (63%) were continuously disease-free at nearly 6 years of follow-up, and gastrointestinal toxicity was avoided.[169] Two lower-dose paclitaxel (175 mg/m^2) regimens reported about 40% CR rates, and the authors questioned whether the lower paclitaxel dose led to the inferior results.[170,171]

High-Dose Therapy

Early high-dose trials were conducted in patients with refractory GCT who had received at least two prior regimens. About 20% of patients who received carboplatin and etoposide with or without cyclophosphamide or ifosfamide remained alive and disease-free with long-term follow-up. The major toxicities were hematologic and infectious, and mortality was high. Hematopoietic growth factors and peripheral blood-derived stem cells have decreased the duration of neutropenia and hospitalization, and reduced treatment-related mortality to less than 5% in most studies. Although no randomized trial compared one versus two or three cycles of high-dose therapy, data imply that two or three cycles of high-dose therapy improve the likelihood of cure.

First Salvage

The use of high-dose chemotherapy as first salvage for *all* patients who relapse following a CR or fail to achieve CR to (B)EP is controversial. Standard-dose regimens have resulted in a 35% to 70% CR rate without the use of high-dose therapy, and many investigators believe standard-dose regimens should be used first if the patient has had a prior CR.[169–173] One randomized trial compared a standard salvage ifosfamide regimen with and without a single cycle of high-dose chemotherapy.[172] Another randomized trial compared a standard salvage ifosfamide regimen with either three cycles of high-dose carboplatin plus etoposide or one cycle of carboplatin plus etoposide plus cyclophosphamide.[173] Neither trial demonstrated an advantage of one arm over the other. Hence, in Europe, high-dose therapy is generally administered as second salvage and standard ifosfamide regimens as first salvage therapy.

In contrast, two large series reported benefit when high-dose salvage chemotherapy was administered as first salvage therapy. In a retrospective study at Indiana University, 135 of 186 patients (73%) received one to two cycles of standard VeIP followed by two cycles of high-dose carboplatin plus etoposide as first salvage. At a median follow-up of 4 years, 94 of 135 (70%) of those who had received only one prior cycle of chemotherapy remained continuously disease-free.[174] This study included 61 patients who relapsed from CR, but *excluded* mediastinal NSGCT, late relapses, and other nongonadal primary sites.

In the second study, a prospective trial from Memorial Sloan-Kettering Cancer Center (MSKCC), 81 of 107 patients (76%) received one to two cycles of paclitaxel plus ifosfamide followed by three cycles of high-dose carboplatin plus etoposide (TI-CE) as first salvage. At a median of 5 years, 56% remained free of disease. This study *excluded* patients with a testicular primary tumor who either had a prior CR to first chemotherapy of any duration or a PR with negative markers ("favorable features"), but *included* patients with mediastinal NSGCT, late relapse, and other nongonadal primary sites.[175]

Comparison of disease-free rates is difficult because of major differences in pretreatment eligibility criteria. No patient with "favorable" features"[169] was enrolled in the MSKCC study, compared with 61 in the Indiana study (Table 99.8).[173,174] When comparing only first salvage therapy in patients with gonadal primary tumors who failed to achieve CR to initial therapy, 41 of 70 (59%) patients at MSKCC and 45 of 74 (61%) at Indiana achieved a durable CR (Table 99.8). In the United States, high-dose chemotherapy is considered a standard of care as first salvage in patients with testicular or retroperitoneal primary tumors who have not achieved a CR to first therapy.[174,175] Either the standard-dose or high-dose approach is a reasonable choice for testicular cancer patients who fit the "favorable" disease category.

Second Salvage

High-dose therapy is the standard of care as second salvage. About 20% to 40% of eligible patients will be cured. Patients with high hCG, cisplatin-refractory disease, and mediastinal NSGCT are poor candidates for second-line salvage high-dose therapy, and referral to a center of excellence for a clinical trial is recommended.

Late Relapse, Mediastinal, Other Nongonadal Sites, and Seminoma

The management of late relapse and primary mediastinal NSGCT is evolving. Some studies exclude these presentations[174] while others include them (Table 99.8).[169,173,175,176] Durable CR was reported for 5 of 21 primary mediastinal NSGCT (24%), 2 of 7 late relapses (29%), and 1 of 3 (33%) pineal GCTs with TI-CE, 7 of 14 (50%) late relapses with TIP after CR from first-line chemotherapy, and 11 of 41 (27%) late relapses unselected on the basis of initial response from the

TABLE 99.8

HIGH-DOSE SALVAGE CHEMOTHERAPY STUDIES IN GERM CELL TUMORS

	Trials							
	Feldman[175] TI-CE		Einhorn[174] VeIP × 1 → HD-CE × 2		Lorch Arm A[173] VIP ×1 → HD-CE × 3		Lorch Arm B[173] VIP × 3 → HD-CEC × 1	
Patient Characteristics	N	% NED	N	% NED	N	% NED	N	% NED
Histology								
Seminoma	13	54	35	74	24	71	17	71
NSGCT	94	47	149	60	84	44	84	36
Unknown	0	—	0	—	0	—	2	—
Total	107	48	184	63	108	50	103	49
Primary site								
Testis/retroperitoneal	77	56	184	63	105	51	100	44
Mediastinal	21	24	0	—	2	0	3	0
Other	9	33	0	—	1	0	0	—
Prior chemotherapy								
1 regimen	81	56	135	70	93	53[a]	88	45[a]
≥2 regimens	26	23	49	45	15	33[a]	15	20[a]
Late relapse (>2 years)	7	28	0	—	20	25[a]	21	28[a]
G/R (male) and relapse <2 years	70[b]	59	184	63	85[a]	58[a]	79[a]	47[a]
Beyer score 1[218]	15	73	136	66	56[a]	66[a]	50[a]	54[a]
Beyer score ≥2	55	55	48	58	29[a]	41[a]	29[a]	35[a]
Favorable[c] prognosis[169,174]	0	0	61	80	15[a]	67[a]	21[a]	62[a]
Unfavorable[d] prognosis[169,174]	59	63	74	61	70[a]	56[a]	58[a]	41[a]

[a]A. Lorch, MD, e-mail communications August 23, 2010, and September 20, 2010.
[b]11 had ≥2 prior regimens.
[c]Favorable: Testicular cancer primary tumor with either CR of any duration or PR with negative markers.
[d]Unfavorable: Retroperitoneal or mediastinal primary tumor with a prior CR or PR with negative markers, or any patient with gonadal or extragonadal GCT who failed to achieve favorable status to first-line cisplatin-based chemotherapy (incomplete response).
N, number of patients; NED, no evidence of disease; TI-CE, paclitaxel + ifosfamide followed by high-dose carboplatin + etoposide; VeIP, vinblastine + ifosfamide + cisplatin; VIP, etoposide + ifosfamide + cisplatin; HD, high dose; CE, carboplatin + etoposide; CEC, carboplatin + etoposide + cyclophosphamide; NSGCT, nonseminomatous germ cell tumor; G, gonadal; R, retroperitoneal

German Testicular Cancer Study Group.[169,173,175] Thus, patients with late-relapse or primary mediastinal NSGCT have potentially curable disease, although the cure rate is lower than that reported in other settings. Treatment decisions should be based on disease characteristics and the patient's comorbidity. Whether paclitaxel is necessary is unknown, but the high durable CR rate in patients who achieved a prior CR suggests value. Retroperitoneal primary NSGCT may be treated the same as a gonadal primary tumor. Recurrent seminoma in the salvage setting has an outcome similar to, and should be managed like, NSGCT.[177]

New Agents

Several single-agent trials in refractory GCT have antitumor activity.[178–180] Gemcitabine plus paclitaxel with or without paclitaxel are active, and a report of the three-drug combination had a 15% durable CR in a small group of patients with refractory GCT, including several patients who relapsed from prior CR to high-dose chemotherapy.[181–183] Major responses were reported in a phase 1 trial of flavopiridol plus FOLFOX (folinic acid plus fluorouracil plus oxaliplatin).[184] Responses in refractory teratoma were reported in a trial of an inhibitor of cyclin-dependent kinase 4/6.[185] Oral etoposide continues to play a palliative role in the management of refractory GCT. Participation in a clinical trial is strongly recommended.

Role of Surgery after Salvage Chemotherapy

Surgery is critical in achieving a durable CR.[154] Viable tumor is present in approximately 50% of specimens, teratoma in about 30%, and necrosis in only 20%. After taxane-based salvage chemotherapy, fibrosis was reported in 51%, viable GCT in 28%, and teratoma in 21% of specimens.[186] If viable NSGCT exists after *salvage* chemotherapy, additional standard-dose chemotherapy confers no survival benefit.

Most patients with persistently elevated serum tumor marker levels and chemotherapy-refractory disease are not surgical candidates. However, a highly select group of patients with increased marker levels and chemotherapy-refractory disease remained free of disease after "desperation" surgery.[187–189] The presence of a solitary retroperitoneal mass and increased AFP was associated with the best outcome.[190]

PRACTICE OF ONCOLOGY

Technically difficult, this surgery should be performed at a tertiary center.

TREATMENT SEQUELAE

Chemotherapy

Control of nausea and vomiting is necessary to maintain adequate hydration. Concurrent administration of a 5-HT_3 antagonist, dexamethasone, and aprepitant is superior to a 5-HT_3 antagonist and dexamethasone alone when cisplatin is administered in a single bolus. The role of aprepitant with 5 days of cisplatin is uncertain.[191] Because cisplatin causes delayed emesis, oral antiemetics are administered for 2 to 4 days after therapy. If severe nausea and vomiting develop during chemotherapy, hospitalization may be necessary to protect renal function.

Nephrotoxicity

Cisplatin-related nephrotoxicity occurs to some extent in all patients. Progressive reduction in glomerular filtration, hypomagnesemia, and an increase in serum creatinine from baseline may occur, particularly after ifosfamide-based salvage chemotherapy. Nephrotoxicity may be severe in patients receiving high-dose chemotherapy, but does not appear to influence response rate or hematologic recovery.

Myelosuppression

In first-line therapy, myelosuppression is common. Hematopoietic growth factors are recommended prophylactically after neutropenic fever, but do not improve survival. Anemia occurs in virtually all patients, but red blood cell transfusions are seldom necessary in previously untreated patients. A platelet count of less than 50,000 is rare during first cisplatin-based therapy, but frequent during salvage chemotherapy. Severe anemia, neutropenia and neutropenic fever, and thrombocytopenia often accompany salvage therapy; hematopoietic growth factor support should be used prophylactically from the beginning of salvage therapy.

Peripheral Neuropathy

Cisplatin-induced neuropathy may persist for years.[192] Although less common than peripheral neuropathy, auditory toxicity manifested by reduced high-tone hearing and/or tinnitus may also persist for years.

Pulmonary Toxicity

Pulmonary toxicity from bleomycin is rare in good-risk patients treated with BEP ×3,[116] but caused death in 1% to 2% of patients treated with BEP ×4.[193] The use of pulmonary function tests (vital capacity and diffusion capacity of carbon monoxide) to monitor bleomycin administration is recommended by some,[113] but their ability to predict clinically significant bleomycin-induced lung damage is controversial.

Vascular Toxicity and Metabolic Syndrome

Vascular toxicity is probably the most significant delayed toxicity of GCT chemotherapy. The risk of cardiac events after GCT chemotherapy is increased two- to sevenfold over the general population.[194,195] Raynaud phenomenon, reported in 6% to 24% of patients receiving bleomycin by weekly bolus, only occurs after bleomycin,[114] and does not improve.[192] Cardiac risk factors and the metabolic syndrome, including hypercholesterolemia, increased low-density and decreased high-density lipoprotein levels, excessive weight gain, and increased systolic and diastolic blood pressure were also more common in treated patients.[194–196] Early management of hypertension and hyperlipidemia is warranted. Erectile dysfunction may be a sign of microvascular angiopathy. Recent data suggest that changes in a variety of cardiovascular parameters (e.g., intima media thickness of the carotid artery) may be associated with chemotherapy-induced cardiovascular changes.[197,198] Acute vascular events in large arteries have been reported and require urgent management—further use of cisplatin should be avoided in these rare cases.[199,200]

Hypogonadism and Infertility

A substantial proportion of newly diagnosed patients are subfertile or infertile at diagnosis, with reduced spermatogenesis and higher FSH levels compared with healthy men. Scatter-dose RT for seminoma can affect the sperm count, but less with a para-aortic field.[201] Chemotherapy may affect the germinal epithelium directly, and persistent oligospermia and abnormal forms and motility have been reported.[202] Paternity was successful in 71% of unselected GCT patients at 15 years, decreasing progressively from 81% with surveillance, to 77% after RPLND, 65% after RT, 62% after chemotherapy, and 38% after salvage high-dose chemotherapy.[202] There may be a relationship between the number of cycles of cisplatin and infertility, although the number of cases studied who received fewer than four cycles is small.[203] Cryopreservation of semen should be offered to all patients undergoing RT, RPLND, or chemotherapy.

Second Malignancies

A second primary GCT appears in the contralateral testis in about 2% of testicular GCT patients, is managed as a separate primary tumor, and has excellent survival.[204] After the second orchiectomy, replacement testosterone is required. Etoposide causes secondary leukemia characterized by translocations involving chromosome 11q in about 0.03% of patients receiving etoposide doses of 1,000 mg/m^2 (equal to two cycles of etoposide), about 0.1% of patients receiving total doses of about 2,000 mg/m^2 (equivalent to four cycles of etoposide), and as many as 6% of patients receiving total etoposide doses of greater than 3,000 mg/m^2.[205–208] These data suggest that there is no lower boundary to etoposide-related leukemia risk.[56] The latent period is short, averaging 2 to 4 years. An increased risk of solid tumors occurs after RT, and is particularly apparent in patients who receive both RT and chemotherapy.[74,107]

A new concern, particularly in young patients with a long life expectancy, is the effect of cumulative radiation exposure from CT imaging.[55] Each CT scan of the abdomen and pelvis delivers approximately 14 mSv, and the dose increases to 21 mSv with inclusion of the chest. A diagnostic PET-CT of the chest, abdomen and pelvis delivers about 34 mSv.[142] Considerable variation exists between institutions.[56,57] Few data exist on actual cancer incidence after CT scans,[58,59] and the concern is largely theoretical at this time. However, in atomic bomb survivors, the incidence of secondary malignancies significantly increased when cumulative exposure exceeded 100 mSv.[142] Studies comparing MRI and CT are needed.[60] Unnecessary PET scans should be avoided.[52,57] Risks must always be balanced by potential benefits, which are substantial when following patients with a high likelihood of cure.

Sarcoidosis

Sarcoidosis appears more frequently in GCT patients[209] both before and after GCT diagnosis. Bilateral hilar adenopathy with paratracheal adenopathy and pulmonary nodules without retroperitoneal adenopathy, particularly in seminoma, should raise the question of sarcoidosis.

LONG-TERM FOLLOW-UP

Long-term follow-up is needed to detect early and late relapse; manage treatment-related side effects including hyperlipidemia, hypertension, metabolic syndrome, cardiovascular disease; and to screen for and identify second non-GCT malignancies. Good general health maintenance policies are necessary as these patients age, and the oncologist and internist are important partners.

MIDLINE TUMORS OF UNCERTAIN HISTOGENESIS

Some young patients with midline, poorly differentiated carcinoma of unknown histogenesis and primary site without increased serum concentrations of either AFP or hCG achieve a CR to cisplatin-based chemotherapy. Cisplatin sensitivity, predominant midline tumor distribution, and occurrence in relatively young patients suggest an unrecognized extragonadal GCT. Molecular cytogenetic analysis for excess 12p copy number has permitted a definitive diagnosis of GCT in some.[210] Genetic analyses may identify lymphoma, primitive neuroectodermal tumors, or other tumors, indicating that this group has a heterogeneous histogenesis.

OTHER TESTICULAR TUMORS

Gonadal Stromal Tumors: Leydig and Sertoli Cell Tumors

Leydig cell (interstitial cell) tumors (LCTs) comprise approximately 2% of testicular tumors. Approximately 75% appear in adults; the remainder are in children. The presentation is indistinguishable from GCT. A minority of patients have gynecomastia or decreased libido.[211] A testicular mass associated with virilization in a prepubertal patient is an LCT until proven otherwise. No association has been found between LCT and cryptorchidism. Characteristic intracytoplasmic inclusion bodies (Reinke crystals) are seen in approximately 25% to 40% of cases. A radical inguinal orchiectomy is required, and clinical staging includes a chest radiograph and CT scan of the abdomen and pelvis. Measurement of urinary and serum steroids is reasonable in patients with symptoms of steroid excess but not useful as a tumor marker.

Metastasis, the only reliable criterion of malignancy, is most frequently retroperitoneal, followed by lung, liver, and bone, and is radioresistant and chemoresistant.[212] Vascular invasion, cellular atypia, tumor necrosis, infiltrative margins, increased mitotic rate, tumor size more than 5 cm, and older age at presentation have been associated with greater malignant potential, as have an increased proliferation index and aneuploidy. RPLND is reasonable in selected cases with adverse features. For metastatic disease (particularly those secreting steroids), ortho-para-DDD (Mitotane), a potent inhibitor of steroidogenesis, has produced anecdotal responses.

Sertoli cell tumors (SCTs), subclassified as classic, sclerosing, and large cell calcifying (LCCSCT), account for fewer than 1% of primary testicular neoplasms.[213] The presentation is indistinguishable from that of GCT. LCCSCTs are noted for multifocality, familial tendency, bilaterality, and precocious puberty in boys. An association has been reported between LCCSCT, pituitary adenoma, adrenocortical hyperplasia, cardiac myxoma, and pigmented skin and mucosal lesions (Carney complex), and with Peutz-Jeghers syndrome in boys with gynecomastia.[214] Most SCTs are benign, and morphologic criteria associated with adverse outcome are similar to those described for LCTs. Metastasis, the only reliable indicator of malignancy, may occur in the retroperitoneal lymph nodes, mediastinal nodes, lungs, liver, and bone.[211] RT and chemotherapy are ineffective.

Granulosa Cell Tumors

Granulosa cell tumors histologically are extremely rare and resemble adult-type granulosa cell tumors of the ovary. Gynecomastia and increased estrogen secretion are common. Metastatic disease is anecdotal; responses to antiangiogenesis therapy have been reported.[215] Radical orchiectomy is required. Juvenile granulosa cell tumor is the most common testicular neoplasm in neonates, and is associated with chromosomal and phenotypic abnormalities.

Gonadoblastoma

Gonadoblastoma is composed of sex cord elements admixed with germ cells. Often bilateral, it occurs in men with chromosome abnormalities and those with dysgenetic gonads. Metastasis from the GCT element may occur.

Mesothelioma

Mesothelioma of the tunica vaginalis may invade the testis, and frequently extends to the internal ring. Surgical intervention consists of radical orchiectomy and complete excision of the spermatic cord and hemiscrotum. Retroperitoneal or inguinal metastasis may occur if the testis is invaded or if LVI is present. Aggressive surgery, including RPLND, is the only known curative therapy.[216]

Adenocarcinoma of the Rete Testis

Adenocarcinoma of the rete testis is a rare neoplasm that arises from the collecting system of the testis.[211,217] Many patients develop metastatic disease; 30% to 50% die within 1 year. After radical orchiectomy, RPLND should be considered, and may be curative in some patients with minimal retroperitoneal involvement. Neither RT nor chemotherapy is effective.

Epidermoid Cyst

Epidermoid cysts of the testis usually present between the second and fourth decades, are often asymptomatic, and are discovered incidentally. These tumors are round, firm, and sharply demarcated on gross examination. Microscopically, the cyst is lined with stratified squamous epithelium. The adjacent testicular parenchyma is benign, and IGCNU is not present. The histogenesis of these tumors is uncertain; their clinical behavior is uniformly benign. Testicular ultrasound may be diagnostic, in which case enucleation of the mass is sufficient treatment. Nevertheless, thorough histologic sampling must be performed to rule out a mature teratoma.

Lymphoma

Lymphoma is the most common secondary tumor of the testis. It most frequently occurs in men over the age of 50. Painless testicular enlargement is common. Bilateral involvement occurs in approximately one-third of patients. Radical orchiectomy establishes the diagnosis. Most cases are associated with systemic disease and present with systemic symptoms; central nervous system as well as bone marrow disease is common. Management of lymphoma is discussed in Chapter 125.

Metastatic Carcinoma

Metastatic carcinoma to the testis is rare. It is associated with diffuse systemic disease. Treatment may include radical orchiectomy, with further therapy dictated by the primary tumor.

Selected References

The full list of references for this chapter appears in the online version.

3. Jemal A, Siegel R, Xu J, et al. Cancer Statistics 2010. *CA Cancer J Clin* 2010;60(5):277.
15. Donadio AC, Motzer RJ, Bajorin DF, et al. Chemotherapy for teratoma with malignant transformation. *J Clin Oncol* 2003;21:4285.
22. Feldman DR. Biology and genetics of adult male germ cell tumors. In: Volgelzang NJ, Scardino PT, Linehan WM, et al., eds. *Comprehensive textbook of genitourinary oncology*, 4th ed. Philadelphia, Lippincott Williams & Wilkins, 2011.
27. Bignell G, Smith R, Hunter C, et al. Sequence analysis of the protein kinase gene family in human testicular germ-cell tumors of adolescents and adults. *Genes Chromosomes Cancer* 2006;45:42.
43. Korkola JE, Houldsworth J, Bosl GJ, et al. Molecular events in germ cell tumours: linking chromosome-12 gain, acquisition of pluripotency and response to cisplatin. *BJU Int* 2009;104:1334.
44. Reuter VE. Origins and molecular biology of testicular germ cell tumors. *Mod Pathol* 2005;18:S51.
48. Wang F, Liu A, Peng Y, et al. Diagnostic utility of SALL4 in extragonadal yolk sac tumors: an immunohistochemical study of 59 cases with comparison to placental-like alkaline phosphatase, alpha-fetoprotein, and glypican-3. *Am J Surg Pathol* 2009;33:1529.
49. Leibovitch L, Foster RS, Kopecky K, et al. Improved accuracy of computerized tomography based clinical staging in low stage nonseminomatous germ cell cancer using size criteria of retroperitoneal lymph nodes. *J Urol* 1995;154:1759.
52. Oechsle K, Hartmann M, Brenner W, et al. [18F]Fluorodeoxyglucose positron emission tomography in nonseminomatous germ cell tumors after chemotherapy: the German multicenter positron emission tomography study group. *J Clin Oncol* 2008;26:5930.
53. De Santis M, Becherer A, Bokemeyer C, et al. 2-^{18}fluoro-deoxy-D-glucose positron emission tomography is a reliable predictor for viable tumor in postchemotherapy seminoma: an update of the prospective multicentric SEMPET trial. *J Clin Oncol* 2004;22:1034.
56. Berrington de Gonzalez A, Mahesh M, Kim K-P, et al. Projected cancer risks from computed tomographic scans performed in the United States in 2007. *Arch Intern Med* 2009;169:2071.
64. National Comprehensive Cancer Network. *NCCN clinical practice guidelines in oncology*, 2009.
69. IGCCCG. International germ cell consensus classification: a prognostic factor-based staging system for metastatic germ cell cancers. *J Clin Oncol* 1997;15:594.
77. Fossa SD, Horwich A, Russell JM, et al. Optimal planning target volume for stage I testicular seminoma: a Medical Research Council randomized trial. *J Clin Oncol* 1999;17:1146.
78. Jones WG, Fossa SD, Mead GM, et al. Randomized trial of 30 versus 20 Gy in the adjuvant treatment of stage I testicular seminoma: a report on Medical Research Council trial TE18, European Organisation for the Research and Treatment of Cancer trial 30942 (ISRCTN18525328). *J Clin Oncol* 2005;23:1200.
81. Feldman DR, Bosl GJ. Treatment of stage I seminoma: is it time to change your practice? *J Hematol Oncol* 2008;1:22.
83. Oliver R, Mason M, Mead G, et al. Radiotherapy versus single-dose carboplatin in adjuvant treatment of stage I seminoma: a randomised trial. *Lancet* 2005;366:293.
85. Warde P, Gospodarowicz M. Evolving concepts in stage I seminoma. *BJU Int* 2009;104:1357.
89. Chang SS, Mohse HF, Leon A, et al. Paracolic recurrence: the importance of wide excision of the spermatic cord at retroperitoneal lymph node dissection (RPLND). *J Urol* 2002;167:94.
90. Eggener SE, Carver BS, Sharp DS, et al. Incidence of disease outside modified retroperitoneal lymph node dissection templates in clinical stage I or IIA nonseminomatous germ cell testicular cancer. *J Urol* 2007;177:937.
91. Carver BS, Shayegan B, Eggener S, et al. Incidence of metastatic nonseminomatous germ cell tumor outside the boundaries of a modified postchemotherapy retroperitoneal lymph node dissection. *J Clin Oncol* 2007;25:4365.
95. Bosl GJ. Surveillance and survivorship in men with germ cell tumors: Should it change what the physician does? *Am Soc Clin Oncol Ed Book* 2010;182.
99. Tandstad T, Dahl O, Cohn-Cedermark G, et al. Risk-adapted treatment in clinical stage I nonseminomatous germ cell testicular cancer: the SWENOTECA management program. *J Clin Oncol* 2009;27:2122.
100. Davis BE, Herr HW, Fair WR, et al. The management of patients with nonseminomatous germ cell tumors of the testis with serologic disease only after orchiectomy. *J Urol* 1994;152:111.
103. Chung PW, Warde PR, Panzarella T, et al. Appropriate radiation volume for stage IIA/B testicular seminoma. *Int J Radiat Oncol Biol Phys* 2003;56:746.
107. van den Belt-Dusebout AW, de Wit R, Gietema JA, et al. Treatment-specific risks of second malignancies and cardiovascular disease in 5-year survivors of testicular cancer. *J Clin Oncol* 2007;25:4370.
109. Stephenson AJ, Bosl GJ, Motzer RJ, et al. Retroperitoneal lymph node dissection for nonseminomatous germ cell testicular cancer: impact of patient selection factors on outcome. *J Clin Oncol* 2005;23:2781.
111. Behnia M, Foster RS, Einhorn LH, et al. Adjuvant bleomycin, etoposide and cisplatin in pathological stage II non-seminomatous testicular cancer. *Eur J Cancer* 2000;36:472.
112. Kondagunta G, Sheinfeld J, Mazumdar M, et al. Relapse-free and overall survival in patients with pathologic stage II nonseminomatous germ cell cancer treated with etoposide and cisplatin adjuvant chemotherapy. *J Clin Oncol* 2004;22:464.
117. Kondagunta GV, Bacik J, Bajorin D, et al. Etoposide and cisplatin chemotherapy for metastatic good-risk germ cell tumors. *J Clin Oncol* 2005;23:9290.
119. Culine S, Kerbrat P, Kramar A, et al. Refining the optimal chemotherapy regimen for good-risk metastatic nonseminomatous germ-cell tumors: a randomized trial of the Genito-Urinary Group of the French Federation of Cancer Centers (GETUG T93BP). *Ann Oncol* 2007;18:917.
120. Saxman SB, Finch D, Gonin R, et al. Long-term follow-up of a phase III study of three versus four cycles of bleomycin, etoposide, and cisplatin in favorable-prognosis germ-cell tumors: the Indiana University experience. *J Clin Oncol* 1998;16:702.
121. Bajorin DF, Sarosdy MF, Pfister DG, et al. Randomized trial of etoposide and cisplatin versus etoposide and carboplatin in patients with good-risk germ cell tumors: a multi-institutional study. *J Clin Oncol* 1993;11:598.
122. Horwich A, Sleijfer D, Fossa S, et al. Randomized trial of bleomycin, etoposide, and cisplatin compared with bleomycin, etoposide, and carboplatin in good-prognosis metastatic nonseminomatous germ cell cancer: a multi-institutional medical research council/European Organization for Research and Treatment of Cancer trial. *J Clin Oncol* 1997;15:1844.
123. Bokemeyer C, Kollmannsberger C, Stenning S, et al. Metastatic seminoma treated with either single agent carboplatin or cisplatin-based combination chemotherapy: a pooled analysis of two randomised trials. *Br J Cancer* 2004;91:683.
124. Grimison PS, Stockler MR, Thomson DB, et al. Comparison of two standard chemotherapy regimens for good-prognosis germ cell tumors: updated analysis of a randomized trial. *J Natl Cancer Inst* 2010;102:1253.
126. de Wit R. Refining the optimal chemotherapy regimen in good prognosis germ cell cancer: interpretation of the current body of knowledge. *J Clin* Oncol 2007;25:4346.
127. Motzer RJ, Geller NL, Bosl GJ. The effect of a 7-day delay in chemotherapy cycles on complete response and event-free survival in good-risk disseminated germ cell tumor patients. *Cancer* 1990;66:857.
140. Beck SD, Foster RS, Bihrle R, et al. Teratoma in the orchiectomy specimen and volume of metastasis are predictors of retroperitoneal teratoma in post-chemotherapy nonseminomatous testis cancer. *J Urol* 2002;168:1402.
142. Bosl GJ, Motzer RJ. Weighing risks and benefits of postchemotherapy retroperitoneal lymph node dissection: not so easy. *J Clin Oncol* 2010;28:519.
143. Lutke Holzik MF, Hoekstra HJ, Mulder NH, et al. Non-germ cell malignancy in residual or recurrent mass after chemotherapy for nonseminomatous testicular germ cell tumor. *Ann Surg Oncol* 2003;10:131.
144. George DW, Foster RS, Hromas RA, et al. Update on late relapse of germ cell tumor: a clinical and molecular analysis. *J Clin Oncol* 2003;21:113.
147. Ehrlich Y, Brames MJ, Beck SD, et al. Long-term follow-up of cisplatin combination chemotherapy in patients with disseminated nonseminomatous germ cell tumors: is a postchemotherapy retroperitoneal lymph node dissection needed after complete remission? *J Clin Oncol* 2010;28:531.

148. Kollmansberger C, Daneshman S, So A, et al. Management of disseminated nonseminomatous germ cell tumors with risk-based chemotherapy followed by response-guided postchemotherapy surgery. *J Clin Oncol* 2010;281:537.
152. Heidenreich A, Pfister D, Witthuhn R, et al. Postchemotherapy retroperitoneal lymph node dissection in advanced testicular cancer: radical or modified template resection. *Eur Urol* 2009;55:217.
156. Peterson M, Beck S, Bihrle R, et al. Results of retroperitoneal lymph node dissection after chemotherapy in patients with pure seminoma in the orchidectomy specimen but elevated serum alpha-fetoprotein. *BJU Int* 2009;104:176.
162. Steyerberg EW, Keizer HJ, Messemer JE, et al. Residual pulmonary masses after chemotherapy for metastatic nonseminomatous germ cell tumor: prediction of histology. ReHiT Study Group. *Cancer* 1997;79:345.
163. van Vledder MG, van der hage JA, Kirkels SJ, et al. Cervical lymph node dissection for metastatic testicular cancer [published online ahead of print March 24, 2010]. *Ann Surg Oncol* 2010;17(16):1682.
164. You YN, Leibovitch BC, Que FG. Hepatic metastasectomy for testicular germ cell tumors: is it worth it? *J Gastrointest Surg* 2009;13:595.
165. Geldart TR, Simmonds PD, Mead GM. Orchidectomy after chemotherapy for patients with metastatic testicular germ cell cancer. *BJU Int* 2002; 90:451.
169. Kondagunta GV, Bacik J, Donadio A, et al. Combination of paclitaxel, ifosfamide, and cisplatin is an effective second-line therapy for patients with relapsed testicular germ cell tumors. *J Clin Oncol* 2005;23:6549.
173. Lorch A, Kollmannsberger C, Hartmann JT, et al. Single versus sequential high-dose chemotherapy in patients with relapsed or refractory germ-cell tumors—a prospective randomized multicenter trial of the German Testicular Cancer Study Group. *J Clin Oncol* 2007;25:2778.
174. Einhorn LH, Williams SD, Chamness A, et al. High-dose chemotherapy and stem-cell rescue for metastatic germ-cell tumors. *N Engl J Med* 2007;357:340.
175. Feldman DR, Sheinfeld J, Bajorin DF, et al. TI-CE High-dose chemotherapy for patients with previously treated germ cell tumors: results and prognostic factor analysis. *J Clin Oncol* 2010;28:1706.
178. Einhorn L, Stender M, Williams S. Phase II trial of gemcitabine in refractory germ cell tumors. *J Clin Oncol* 1999;17:509.
182. Bokemeyer C, Oechsle K, Honecker F, et al. Combination chemotherapy with gemcitabine, oxaliplatin, and paclitaxel in patients with cisplatin-refractory or multiply relapsed germ-cell tumors: a study of the German Testicular Cancer Study Group. *Ann Oncol* 2008;19:448.
186. Eggener SE, Carver BS, Loeb S, et al. Pathologic findings and clinical outcome of patients undergoing retroperitoneal lymph node dissection after multiple chemotherapy regimens for metastatic testicular germ cell tumors. *Cancer* 2007;109:528.
190. Ong TA, Winkler MH, Savage PM, et al. Retroperitoneal lymph node dissection after chemotherapy in patients with elevated tumour markers: indications, histopathology and outcome. *BJU Int* 2008;102:198.
192. Brydoy M, Oldenburg J, Klepp O, et al. Observational study of prevalence of long-term Raynaud-like phenomena and neurological side effects in testicular cancer survivors. *J Natl Cancer Inst* 2009;101:1682.
193. Williams SD, Birch R, Einhorn LH, et al. Treatment of disseminated germ cell tumors with cisplatinum, bleomycin and either vinblastine or etoposide. *N Engl J Med* 1987;316:1435.
194. Meinardi MT, Gietma JA, van der Graaf WTA, et al. Cardiovascular morbidity in long-term survivors of metastatic testicular cancer. *J Clin Oncol* 2000;18:1725.
195. Huddart RA, Norman A, Shahidi M, et al. Cardiovascular disease as a long-term complication of treatment for testicular cancer. *J Clin Oncol* 2003;21:1513.
196. Vaughn DJ, Palmer SC, Carver JR, et al. Cardiovascular risk in long-term survivors of testicular cancer. *Cancer* 2008;112:1949.
197. Nuver J, Smit AJ, van der Meer J, et al. Acute chemotherapy-induced cardiovascular changes in patients with testicular cancer. *J Clin Oncol* 2005;23:9130.
198. Steingart R. Mechanisms of late cardiovascular toxicity from cancer chemotherapy. *J Clin Oncol* 2005;23:9051.
202. Brydoy M, Fossa SD, Klepp O, et al. Paternity following treatment for testicular cancer. *J Natl Cancer Inst* 2005;97:1580.
204. Fossa SD, Chen J, Schonfeld SJ, et al. Risk of contralateral testicular cancer: a population-based study of 29,515 U.S. men. *J Natl Cancer Inst* 2005;97:1056.
208. Schneider DT, Hilgenfeld E, Schwabe D, et al. Acute myelogenous leukemia after treatment for malignant germ cell tumors in children. *J Clin Oncol* 1999;17:3226.
209. Paparel P, Devonec M, Perrin P, et al. Association between sarcoidosis and testicular carcinoma: a diagnostic pitfall. *Sarcoidosis Vasc Diffuse Lung Dis* 2007;24:95.
210. Motzer RJ, Rodriguez E, Reuter VE, et al. Molecular and cytogenetic studies in the diagnosis of patients with poorly differentiated carcinomas of unknown primary site. *J Clin Oncol* 1995;13:274.
211. Amin MB. Selected other problematic testicular and paratesticular lesions: rete testis neoplasms and pseudotumors, mesothelial lesions and secondary tumors. *Mod Pathol* 2005;18:S131.
212. Di Tonno F, Tavolini IM, Belmonte P, et al. Lessons from 52 patients with leydig cell tumor of the testis: the GUONE (North-Eastern Uro-Oncological Group, Italy) experience. *Urol Int* 2009;82:152.
216. Plas E, Riedl CR, Pflüger H. Malignant mesothelioma of the tunica vaginalis testis: review of the literature and assessment of prognostic parameters. *Cancer* 1998;83:2437.

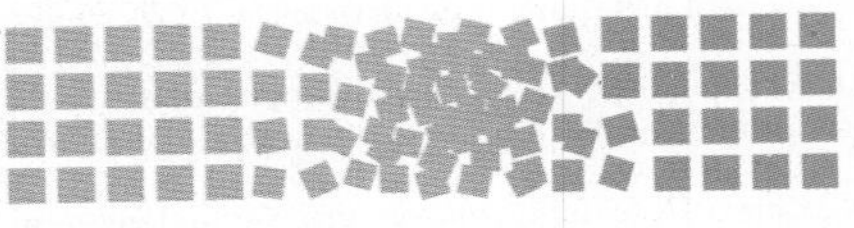

CHAPTER 100 MOLECULAR BIOLOGY OF GYNECOLOGIC CANCERS

KUNLE ODUNSI, TANJA PEJOVIC, AND MATTHEW L. ANDERSON

Gynecologic cancer research has mirrored all cancer research programs in that it has focused largely on molecular defects in oncogenes, tumor-suppressor genes, and DNA repair mechanisms. Several research groups have also channeled their resources into various carcinogenic phenomena such as apoptotic pathway defects, growth signaling, angiogenesis, tissue invasion, or metastasis. These efforts have led to a broad understanding of the chromosomal and molecular abnormalities that underlie malignancies of the female genital tract (vulva, vagina, cervix, uterus, ovaries, and fallopian tubes). It is clear that an improvement in outcome of these malignancies can only be achieved if (1) early diagnosis is achieved, (2) there is accurate prediction of progression and response, and (3) new treatment options reflecting the molecular pathogenesis and progression are developed. This requires detailed disease-specific understanding of the diverse molecular changes in gynecologic malignancies that ultimately lead cells to develop the following hallmarks of cancer: abnormalities in self-sufficiency of growth signals, evasion of apoptosis, insensitivity to antigrowth signals, limitless replicative potential, sustained angiogenesis, and tissue invasion and metastases. Moreover, there is growing evidence for the concept of cancer immunosurveillance and immunoediting based on (1) protection against development of spontaneous and chemically induced tumors in animal systems and (2) identification of targets for immune recognition of human cancer.[1] This concept is supported by several studies in gynecologic cancers and has opened new avenues for the development of novel biomarkers and therapeutic targets. It is the purpose of this chapter to highlight and summarize some of the recent basic findings in gynecologic malignancies, with an emphasis on clinically applicable developments.

OVARIAN CANCER

Origins of Epithelial Ovarian Cancer

Epithelial ovarian cancer (EOC) arises primarily from the ovarian surface epithelium (OSE), with a subset possibly originating in the adjacent fimbria.[2,3] The OSE forms a monolayer surrounding the ovary, but is composed of relatively few cuboidal cells (107 cells per ovary, or 0.05% of the entire organ). Developmentally it derives from the celomic epithelium, which also gives rise to the peritoneal mesothelium and oviductal epithelium.[4] The OSE appears generally stable, uniform, and quiescent, though it can undergo proliferation *in vivo*.[5] Despite the small number of cells within the OSE and their apparent inactivity, the risk for EOC is nearly 2%, suggesting a high malignant potential. The basis for such a high potential is poorly understood. No physiological role for the primate OSE has been established,[6] and the lack of any obvious function could contribute to the asymptomatic nature of early stage EOC.

In other organs, such as colon, distinct premalignant lesions have been identified and found to accumulate genetic defects that ultimately result in malignancy. However, the search to identify similar epithelial precursors in the human ovary has proven only partially fruitful, in large part because normal ovaries are only rarely biopsied or examined. Histologic findings consistent with a preinvasive lesion for ovarian cancer have been described by a number of studies where ovaries were removed from women who eventually developed peritoneal carcinomas, ovaries from high-risk women who were undergoing prophylactic oophorectomy, and in areas of ovarian epithelium adjacent to early-stage ovarian cancers that demonstrate a transition from normal to malignant cells.[7] The hypothesis that these lesions are premalignant is strengthened by observations that regions of epithelial irregularity express levels of p53 and Ki-67 intermediate between those found in normal ovarian epithelium and ovarian cancers.

Each of these observations is consistent with the hypothesis that, similar to cancers originating in other organs, ovarian cancer evolves from an intraepithelial precursor. If so, improved means to detect and/or eradicate these lesions may prove fruitful for preventing ovarian cancer.

Molecular Pathways to Ovarian Cancer

Inherited Syndromes of Ovarian Cancers

Linkage analysis of familial breast and ovarian cancers provided some of the first insights into the molecular basis of ovarian cancer. These efforts ultimately identified two gene products, *BRCA1* and *BRCA2*, each clearly associated with an increased incidence of ovarian cancer. Although only a minority (8% to 10%) of diagnosed ovarian cancers are familial, most (76% to 92%) familial ovarian cancers are associated with mutations at the *BRCA1* locus, located on 17q21. Hundreds of mutations in *BRCA1* have now been identified, most commonly loss of function nonsense or frameshift mutations. Two specific mutations, 185delAG and 5382insC, are found in 1% and 0.1% of Ashkenazi Jewish women.

Functionally, *BRCA1* regulates *p53*, an oncogene frequently implicated in ovarian cancer. Thus, loss of *BRCA1* allows DNA damage to accumulate via a loss of its activation of *p53*.

However, mutations in *BRCA1* also likely contribute to ovarian cancer by mechanisms other than its interactions with *p53*. These include its ability to specifically regulate X chromosome gene expression mediated by an association of Xist with the inactive X chromosome.[8] Consistent with this observation, site-specific dysregulation of X-linked gene expression in *BRCA1*-associated epithelial ovarian malignancies have been described.

Although mutations in *BRCA1* or *BRCA2* are only rarely observed in sporadic, nonfamilial ovarian cancers, it is possible that the mutations in pathways by which *BRCA1* regulates X-chromosome gene expression do, in fact, contribute to this disease. Characterization of genome-wide patterns of gene expression in sporadic breast cancers has allowed investigators to classify these tumors as either BRCA1-like or BRCA2-like in the patterns of their gene expression. This observation implicates the contribution of alterations in other components of the BRCA1 or BRCA2 regulated pathways to sporadic breast cancers and, possibly, ovarian cancer. Any understanding of the role of *BRCA1* in ovarian cancer is further complicated by reports of women with high-risk mutations in *BRCA1* who fail to develop ovarian cancer. These observations speak clearly to the role of genetic modifiers in determining whether *BRCA1* or *BRCA2* mutations ultimately lead to malignancy. For example, CAG repeat polymorphism in the androgen receptor has been shown to modify the subsequent risk of ovarian cancer in women with known mutations in *BRCA1*.

Genomic Instability

Genomic instability, manifested as a cell's ability to tolerate DNA damage, is a hallmark of all cancer, including epithelial ovarian cancers. Tolerance to DNA damage can be achieved by alterations in any of the six major DNA repair pathways: base excision repair, mismatch repair, nucleotide excision repair, homologous recombination, nonhomologous recombination, and translesion DNA synthesis. The specific DNA pathway affected often predicts the specific type of mutations observed in particular cancers, its sensitivity to drugs, as well as clinical outcome of affected patients.

Fanconi Anemia DNA Repair Pathway

Studies on the pathogenesis of rare inherited DNA repair disorders, such as Fanconi anemia (FA), have helped define the molecular basis of defective DNA damage responses linked to cancer risk. FA is a rare genetic disorder characterized by skeletal anomalies, progressive bone marrow failure, cancer susceptibility, and cellular hypersensitivity to DNA cross-linking agents. To date, 13 FA genes have been cloned: *FANCA*, *-B*, *-C*, *-D1*, *-D2*, *-E*, *-F*, *-G*, *-J*, *-L*, *-M*, *-N*, and *-I*. Of these, *FANCA*, *FANCB*, *FANCC*, *FANCE*, *FANCF*, *FANCG*, *FANCL*, and *FANCM* form a nuclear core complex. Although the functional scope of this complex has not been fully defined, it is clear that it must be completely intact to facilitate monoubiquitination of the downstream FANCD2 and FANCI proteins, a change that allows FANCD2 and FANCI to colocalize with *BRCA1*, *BRCA2* (and presumably FANCJ and FANCN), and *RAD51* in damage-induced nuclear foci.[9]

Four lines of evidence link the FA pathway with ovarian carcinogenesis. First, *BRCA2* has been identified as the FA gene *FANCD1*. As a result, heterozygotes for *BRCA2* mutations have a high risk of tissue-specific epithelial cancers, while homozygotes develop FA. Second, an increased prevalence of epithelial cancers, including ovarian malignancies, has been observed in FANCD2 nullizygous mice. Functionally significant silencing of *FANCF* in ovarian cancer through promoter hypermethylation has also been described. Lastly, low levels of FANCD2 protein are found in ovarian surface epithelia from women at risk for ovarian cancer. Taken together, these data suggest that the FA pathway is important in defining predisposition to ovarian (and breast) cancer, and that aberrations of FA genes may account for some familial ovarian cancer cases not accounted for by *BRCA1* and *BRCA2* mutations.

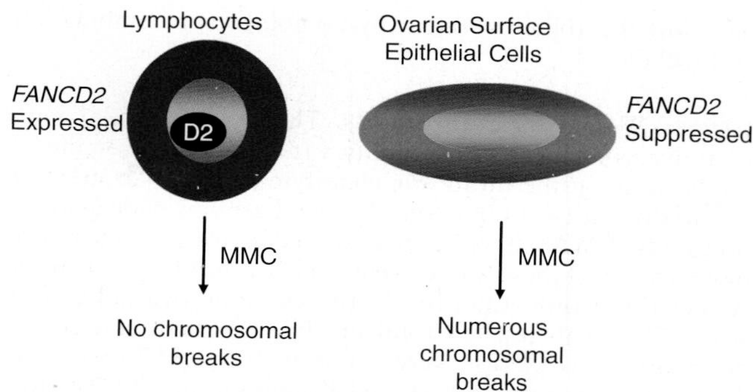

FIGURE 100.1 Tissue-restricted genetic instability in ovarian epithelial cells from women at risk for ovarian cancer with no BRCA mutations. Mitomycin C–induced chromosomal breakage is high and FANCD2 levels are low in ovarian epithelial cells but normal in peripheral blood lymphocytes and may antedate the onset of overt carcinoma. (We thank Dr. Grover Bagby for helping to create this figure.)

In sporadic ovarian cancers, the epigenetic silencing of FA pathway through methylation of the FA gene promoter region is one of the frequent mechanisms of inactivation. One study found that 4 of 19 primary ovarian carcinomas had *FANCF* methylation, although a larger study of 106 ovarian tumors did not identify loss of FANCF expression. Loss of *BRCA2* mRNA and protein has been reported in 13% of ovarian carcinomas, and in contrast to other FA genes, methylation is not a cause of the protein loss. Epigenetic silencing of *BRCA1* through methylation was found in 23% of advanced ovarian carcinomas (Fig. 100.1).

Interestingly, tumors with inactivated BRCA2 are responsive to cisplatin. However, due to their low accuracy of DNA repair, these cells accumulate secondary genetic modifications that can lead to reversal of BRCA2 mutation, allowing these cells to acquire resistance to crosslinking agents.[10]

Other DNA Repair Pathways

Similar to the FA/BRCA pathway, disruptions of other DNA repair pathways have been observed in ovarian cancer. These disruptions account, at least in part, for the specific drug sensitivity of the tumors. Recent studies indicate translesion DNA synthesis defect in ovarian cancer is a consequence of elevation in activity of POLB, an error-prone polymerase. Inhibition of POLB in these cells results in resensitization to cisplatin.[11] Overall it is believed that although inactivation of one DNA repair pathway may confer advantage to tumors, cancer cells may rely more on other repair pathways. Therefore, inactivation of the second pathway would be deleterious for these cells, causing synthetic lethality. An RNA interference screen identified the ataxia-telangiectasia mutated (ATM) pathway to be synthetically lethal with FA.[12] Similarly a strategy for synthetic lethality is under investigation, using base excision repair poly(adenosine diphosphate-ribose) polymerase 1 (PARP1) inhibitors in the treatment of homologous recombination deficient ovarian cancer.[13,14] PARP inhibition has been shown to be up to 1,000 times selectively more toxic to cancer cells than to wild type cells. PARP inhibitors act by exploiting a tumor cell's defect in homologous recombination, a type of DNA repair. This is because following PARP inhibition, cells require homologous recombination to repair common types of DNA damage. Although normal cells can use homologous recombination for repair of this damage and survive, certain types of tumors (e.g., those with BRCA1 or BRCA2 defects) have lost the ability to repair by homologous recombination and will die.

Genome Wide Association Studies. The identification of common ovarian cancer susceptibility variants may have clinical implications in the future for identifying patients at greatest risk of the disease. In this regard, several genome wide association study (GWAS) have been performed in ovarian cancer. The most striking of these was a recent study by the Ovarian Cancer Association Consortium to identify common ovarian cancer susceptibility alleles.[15] A total of 507,094 single nucleotide polymorphisms (SNPs) were genotyped in 1,817 cases and 2,353 controls from the United Kingdom; and 22,790 top ranked SNPs were also genotyped in 4,274 cases and 4,809 controls of European ancestry from Europe, the United States, and Australia. Twelve SNPs were identified at 9p22 associated with disease risk ($P < 10^{-8}$). The most significant SNP (rs3814113; $P = 2.5 \times 10^{-17}$) was genotyped in a further 2,670 ovarian cancer cases and 4,668 controls, confirming its association (combined data odds ratio [OR] = 0.82 95% confidence interval [CI], 0.79 to 0.86; $P_{trend} = 5.1 \times 10^{-19}$). The association was strongest for serous ovarian cancers (OR 0.77; 95% CI, 0.73 to 0.81; $P_{trend} = 4.1 \times 10^{-21}$).

Transcriptional Profiling of Ovarian Cancer Histologic Subtypes

Several gene expression studies using cDNA microarrays have been performed in ovarian cancer. Additionally, several studies have focused on the alterations demonstrated in the DNA copy number.[16–18] Array-based technology has shown that the different histological subtypes of ovarian carcinoma are distinguishable based on their overall genetic expression profiles. A common finding among several studies is the ability to distinguish low-grade serous ovarian carcinoma from high-grade carcinoma based on their gene expression profiles.[17,19–23] A number of genes shown to be differentially expressed in EOC are known to be involved in many important cellular mechanisms, including cell cycle regulation, apoptosis, tumor invasion, and control of local immunity.[20,24,25]

Increased mutagenic signaling by receptor tyrosine kinases plays a major role in ovarian carcinogenesis (Table 100.1). Overexpression of epidermal growth factor receptor (*EGFR*) (*ERBB1*), *ERBB2/HER2/neu*, and *c-FMS* has been reported repeatedly in ovarian cancer. One of the major downstream mediators of signaling initiated by these receptors is the phosphatidylinositol 3-kinase (PI3K)–AKT pathway. Aberrations in this pathway including increased *AKT1* kinase activity, *AKT2* and *PI3K* amplification, and *PI3KR1* mutations may provide opportunities for therapeutic intervention.

It has been reported that more than 75% of ovarian carcinomas are resistant to transforming growth factor-beta (TGF-*β*),[26] and the loss of TGF-*β* responsiveness may play an important role in the pathogenesis or progression of ovarian cancer. In addition, it has been shown that TGF-β_1, the TGF-*β* receptors (T*β*R-II and T*β*R-I), and the TGF-*β* signaling component Smad2 are altered in ovarian cancer. Alterations in *TβR-II* have been identified in 25% of ovarian carcinomas, whereas mutations in *TβR-I* were reported in 33% of such cancers.[27] Protooncogene transformation might lead either to an overexpression of mitogenic molecules or an inactivation of those with inhibitory action, thus contributing to neoplastic transformation and development. The most important protooncogenes of the first group are undoubtedly constituted by *FMS* and *HER2/neu*. The first one encodes a transmembrane tyrosine kinase receptor, which binds *MCSF*. It is possible that *FMS-MCSF* both stimulates epithelial cell proliferation and induces a chemical attraction for macrophages that, in turn, can produce mitogenic stimulating factor. Elevated plasma concentrations of MCSF are present in the sera of 70% of patients with ovarian cancer.[28] The second protooncogene, *HER2/neu*, encodes another tyrosine kinase, which is similar to EGFR. Its action may consist of amplification of mitogenic action in target cells; this oncogene is overexpressed in 30% to 35% of ovarian cancer and is associated with a poor prognosis.[29]

TABLE 100.1

GENETIC ALTERATIONS IN OVARIAN CANCER

Gene	Alteration	Frequency (%)
DNA REPAIR GENES		
BRCA1	Nonsense	5
BRCA2	Frame-shift mutation	3
MLH1	Mutation	1
ONCOGENES		
EGFR	Amplification/ overexpression	20
ERBB2 (Her2/neu)	Amplification/ overexpression	30
FMS	Coexpression with CSF-1	50
PI3K3	Mutation/amplification	12–20
AKT2	Mutation/amplification	20
TGF-β	Mutation/overexpression	12
TβR I	Mutation	33
TβR II	Mutation	25
TUMOR SUPPRESSOR GENES		
p53	Mutation/overexpression	20–50
km23	Mutation	42

Metastasis of Ovarian Cancers

Metastasis is the functional hallmark of all cancer. In general, metastasis involves the invasion of transformed epithelial cells across their basement membrane, through the underlying stroma, and into blood vessels and lymphatic channels, which subsequent disseminate them to distant sites. Only a tiny fraction of cells released into circulation by a tumor ever results in metastasis; understanding the mechanisms by which those cells can land and grow is a priority for cancer researchers. Given the unique need to accommodate the survival of exfoliated cells as well as their subsequent attachment and growth, it seems reasonable to assume that expression and functional organization of molecular pathways important for promoting the metastasis of ovarian cancers will differ from breast and other cancers that depend on hematogenous or lymphatic dissemination. Nonetheless, a wide variety of gene products implicated in the metastasis of other cancers have also been implicated in the metastasis of ovarian cancer. These include growth factor receptors such as EGFR, insulinlike growth factor receptors (IGFRs), and kinases, such as *jak/stat*, focal adhesion kinase, PI3K, and c-met. Comparisons of primary and metastatic ovarian cancers by transcriptional profiling have failed to reveal significant differences in the expression of gene products likely related to the metastatic process.

Particular attention has recently focused on the role of lysophosphatidic acid (LPA) in promoting the metastasis of ovarian cancers. LPA is constitutively produced by mesothelial cells lining the peritoneal cavity; its levels are increased in the ascites of women with both early- and late-stage ovarian cancers.[30] When applied to ovarian cancer cell lines *in vitro*, LPA promotes both the migration of these cells in a manner dependent on Ras MEK kinase-1 as well as their invasion across artificial barriers analogous to a basement membrane. At a molecular level, exogenous LPA enhances ovarian cancer invasiveness both by activating matrix metalloproteinase-2 via membrane-type-1-matrix metalloproteinase (MT1-MMP) and down-regulating the expression of specific tissue inhibitors of metalloproteinases (TIMP-2 and -3).[31] Its application to cultured ovarian cancer cells has also been shown to promote disassembly of intracellular stress fibers and focal adhesions,[32] observations consistent with the idea that LPA promotes dissemination of ovarian cancer by loss of cell adhesion. However, LPA has also been shown to promote the invasiveness of ovarian cancers by additional mechanisms dependent on interleukin-8. The G12/13-RhoA and cyclooxygenase pathways have also been implicated in the LPA-induced migration of ovarian cancers. These mechanisms appear to be independent of the ability of LPA to induce changes in *MMP2* expression. Lastly, it should be noted that LPA appears to promote ovarian cancer metastasis by stimulating *fas*-ligand expression and the shedding of *fas*-ligand–containing microvesicles, potentially leading to an evasion of tumor immunity.

Until recently, the metastasis of ovarian cancer has been almost exclusively studied as a process involving individual cells. However, multicellular clusters of self-adherent cells, known as *spheroids*, can be isolated from the ascitic fluid of women with ovarian cancer. Spheroids readily adhere to both extracellular matrix proteins, such as collagen IV, and mesothelial cells in monolayer culture using beta-1 integrins. Once adherent, the cells contained in spheroids disaggregate, allowing them to invade underlying mesothelial cells and create invasive foci.[33] These observations are consistent with the hypothesis that ovarian cancer spheroids play an important role in the metastatic potential of ovarian cancer. Recent evidence has shown that a loss of circulating gonadotropins results in a dose-dependent decrease in the expression of vascular endothelial growth factor (VEGF) in the outer, proliferating cells of ovarian cancer spheroids,[34] indicating that these cell clusters remain responsive to signals in their microenvironment that may promote metastasis.

The presence of spheroids in ascites may also help to explain the frequent persistence and frequent recurrence of ovarian cancer after treatment. Spheroids express high levels of p27 and P-glycoprotein that contribute, at least in part, to their relative resistance to the cytotoxic effects of paclitaxel when compared with ovarian cancer cells in monolayer culture. Ovarian cancer spheroids have also been shown to be relatively resistant to the cytotoxic effects of radiation.[35] These observations are consistent with *in vitro* studies that demonstrate that the signals generated by adhesion to specific components of the extracellular matrix, such as collagen IV, can modify the sensitivity of ovarian cancers to chemotherapy. However, the mechanisms by which the aggregation of malignant cells promote or enhance cell survival remain unclear. It is also unclear how the aggregation of these malignant cells might promote or enhance the migration, attachment, or invasion of ovarian cancer cells. Insight into these questions is likely to come from genetic models, such as the migration of the border cell cluster in *Drosophila*. Analyses of border cell migration indicate that specific shifts in epithelial polarity, known as the *epithelial-mesenchymal transition* (EMT), and changes in the patterns of signals arising at junctional complexes are necessary for the invasion and migration of epithelial clusters.[36] Signals arising from these junctional proteins appear to be integrated by a specific steroid receptor coactivator, known as AIB1 (Amplified in Breast Cancer 1; SRC3). Ironically, overexpression of AIB1 is a frequent feature of ovarian cancers, suggesting that the pathways regulated by this transcriptional coactivator may also play a critical role in promoting ovarian cancer metastasis. Other proteins first identified in *Drosophila*, such as *Snail*, also appear to play an important role in regulating the EMT of transformed ovarian epithelia, further lending credence to the utility of this genetic model.

Angiogenesis

Growth of both primary ovarian cancers and their metastases requires the formation of new blood vessels to support adequate perfusion. This process, known as *angiogenesis*, mechanistically involves both the branching of new capillaries as well as the remodeling of larger vessels. Other processes, such as vasculogenic mimicry, have also been implicated in tumor angiogenesis.

Angiogenesis is tightly regulated by a balance of pro- and antiangiogenic factors. These include growth factors, such as TGF-β, VEGF, and platelet-derived growth factor; prostaglandins, such as prostaglandin E2; cytokines, such as interleukin 8; and other factors, such as the angiopoietins (Ang-1, Ang-2), and hypoxia-inducible factor-1α (HIF-1α). Many of these angiogenic factors have been implicated in ovarian cancer. For example, VEGF is a family of secreted polypeptides with critical roles in both normal development and human disease. Many cancers, including ovarian carcinomas, release VEGF in response to the hypoxic or acidic conditions typical in solid tumors. Near universal, albeit variable, levels of VEGF expression have been reported in ovarian cancers, in which higher levels correlate with advanced disease and poor clinical prognosis.[37] Circulating levels of VEGF have also been reported to be higher in the serum of women with ovarian cancers when compared with those with benign tumors. Expression of HIF-1 correlates well with microvessel density in ovarian cancers and has been proposed to up-regulate VEGF expression.[38] Culturing ovarian cancer cell lines under hypoxic conditions stimulates the expression of both HIF-1α and VEGF expression in ovarian cancer cell lines; addition of prostaglandin E2 potentiates the ability of hypoxia to induce the expression of both proangiogenic factors.[39]

Ironically, many of the molecules implicated in regulating angiogenesis in cancer, such as c-met, also regulate other processes critical for cancer metastasis, such as cell migration and invasiveness. Inhibition of PI3K decreases transcription of VEGF in ovarian cancer cells, an effect that is reversed by the forced expression of AKT. Such observations are consistent with reports that hypoxia not only induces angiogenesis, but also increases the invasiveness of ovarian cancer cells.[40] Likewise, an acidic environment induces increased interleukin-8 expression in ovarian cancer in a manner dependent on transcription factors AP-1 and nuclear factor-κB–like factor, suggesting that feedback between these pathways may also determine how tumors interact with their external environment. Undoubtedly, better insight into these interactions will help to define the suitability of these molecules as therapeutic targets.

Epigenetics

It has become increasingly apparent that epigenetic events can lead to cancer as frequently as loss of gene function due to mutations or loss of heterozygosity. The overall level of genomic methylation is reduced in cancer (global hypomethylation), but hypermethylation of promoter regions of specific genes is a common event that is often associated with transcriptional inactivation of specific genes.[41] This is critical because the silenced genes are often tumor suppressor genes, and their loss of function can be evident in early stages of cancer but can also drive neoplastic progression and metastasis. Epigenetic gene silencing is a complex series of events that includes DNA hypermethylation of CpG islands within gene-promoter regions, histone deacetylation, methylation or phosphorylation, or histone demethylation. Global hypermethylation of CpG islands appears to be prevalent but highly variable in ovarian cancer tissue.[42] Multiple genes are abnormally methylated in ovarian cancer compared with normal ovarian tissue, including p16, RAR-β, H-cadherin, *GSTP1*, *MGMT*, *RASSF1A*, leukotriene B4 receptor, *MTHFR*, progesterone receptor, *CDH1*, *IGSF4*, *BRCA1*, *TMS1*, estrogen receptor-α, the putative tumor suppressor *km23* (TGFB component), and others.[43] The degree of DNA methylation and the demethylation activity of chemotherapeutic drugs and the sensitive relations of histone acetylation and the specificity of demethylation of select genes are important to ensure the success of treatment and prevent disease recurrence.

Role of Specific Immune Responses

The novel observation by William Coley in the 1890s that severe bacterial infections could induce an antitumor response in patients with partially resected tumors has evolved into an understanding that the immune system can recognize tumor-associated antigens and direct a targeted response. The concept of "cancer immunoediting" suggests that the immune system not only protects the host against the development of primary cancers but also dynamically sculpts tumor immunogenicity.[44] In epithelial ovarian cancer, support for the role of immune surveillance of tumors comes from recent observations that the presence of infiltrating T lymphocytes (TILS) in tumors is associated with improved survival of patients with the disease.[45,46] In one study, there was improved survival of patients with higher frequencies of intraepithelial CD8+ TIL (55 months vs. 26 months; hazard ratio [HR] 0.33; 95% CI, 0.18 to 0.60; $P = .0003$).[46] In addition, the subgroups with a high versus low intraepithelial CD8+/CD4+ TIL ratio had a median survival of 74 versus 25 months (HR 0.30; 95% CI, 0.16 to 0.55; $P = .0001$). This unfavorable effect of CD4+ T cells on prognosis was found to be due to CD25+ Forkhead box P3+ regulatory cells (T_{reg}, suppressor T cells), as indicated by survival in patients with high versus low CD8+/T_{reg} ratios (median, 58 months vs. 23 months; HR 0.31; 95% CI, 0.17 to 0.58; $P = .0002$).[46]

Finally, advanced-stage ovarian cancer patients can have detectable tumor-specific cytotoxic T cell and antibody immunity. This was illustrated in a recent study that indicated that immunity to p53 predicted improved overall survival in patients with advanced-stage disease.[47] All of these observations support clinical trials of immunotherapy for epithelial ovarian cancer in an effort to elicit effective antitumor responses. Major obstacles include the identification of tumor-restricted immunogenic targets, generation of a sufficient immune response to cause tumor rejection, and approaches to overcome tumor evasion of immune attack.

Ovarian Cancer-Specific Antigens

The development of approaches for analyzing humoral and cellular immune reactivity to cancer in the context of the autologous host has led to the molecular characterization of tumor antigens recognized by autologous CD8+ T cells or antibodies. As a consequence of these advances, human tumor antigens defined to date can be classified into one or more of the following categories: (1) differentiation antigens, such as tyrosinase, Melan-A/MART-1, and gp 100; (2) mutational antigens, such as CDK4, β-catenin, caspase-8, and P53; (3) amplification antigens, such as Her2/neu and p53; (4) splice variant antigens, such as NY-CO-37/PDZ-45 and ING1; (5) viral antigens, such as human papillomavirus (HPV) and Epstein-Barr virus; and (6) cancer-testis antigens, such as MAGE, NY-ESO-1, and LAGE-1. Thus, it is clear that some antigens may play a crucial role in progression of tumor cells (e.g., Her2/neu) and could be useful as biomarkers of disease progression and targets of therapy. On the other hand, in considering an antigenic target for ovarian cancer immunotherapy, an ideal candidate antigen should not only demonstrate high-frequency expression in the tumor tissues and restricted expression in normal tissues, but also provide evidence for inherent immunogenicity. In this regard, the cancer-testis antigens are a distinct and unique class of differentiation antigens with high levels of expression in adult male germ cells, but generally not in other normal adult tissues, and aberrant expression in a variable proportion of a wide range of different cancer types. Among cancer-testis antigens, NY-ESO-1, initially defined by serologic analysis of recombinant cDNA expression (SEREX) libraries in esophageal cancer, is particularly immunogenic, eliciting both cellular and humoral immune responses in a high proportion of patients with advanced NY-ESO-1 expressing ovarian cancer.[48]

The reasons for the aberrant expression of cancer-testis antigens in cancer are currently unknown. Nevertheless, the fact that the expression of these antigens is restricted to cancers, gametes, and trophoblast suggests a link between cancer and gametogenesis. Although possible mechanisms include global demethylation and histone deacetylation, the induction of a "gametogenic" program in cancer has also been proposed.[49] Although several lines of evidence have shown that spontaneous or vaccine-induced tumor-antigen–specific T cells can recognize ovarian cancer targets, prolongation of survival in patients treated with immunization has only rarely been observed. This is probably a reflection of several *in vivo* immunosuppressive mechanisms in tumor-bearing hosts. A recently described mechanism in ovarian cancer is the expression of inhibitory molecules such as programmed death-1 (PD-1) and lymphocyte activation gene-3 (LAG-3).[50] Together, these molecules render ovarian tumor infiltrating CD8+ T cells "hyporesponsive," wherein effector function is most impaired in antigen-specific LAG-3+PD-1+CD8+ TILs

ENDOMETRIAL CANCER

The current concept of endometrial cancer integrates histopathology with molecular genetic mechanisms of cancer development. Two major pathogenetic variants of endometrial carcinoma, type I (endometrioid) and type II (serous), evolve via divergent pathways and different precursor lesions, different genetic abnormalities, and ultimately different clinical outcomes parallel their distinct histology.

Type I Cancers

More than 90% of uterine cancers arise in the self-renewing glandular epithelium that lines the uterine cavity. The endometrium epithelium responds to steroid hormones with well-characterized patterns of growth and maturation critical for its role in normal reproduction. Estrogen is a well-recognized growth factor for the endometrium, promoting glandular proliferation. Subsequent exposure to the progestin-rich environment that follows ovulation results in an arrest of endometrial proliferation accompanied by glandular luteinization. Several decades of epidemiologic evidence has convincingly demonstrated that continued, unopposed exposure to estrogen is associated with an increased risk of developing endometrial cancer. These risks are particularly notable among postmenopausal women treated with estrogen-only hormone replacement. Following the introduction of hormone replacement therapy, the incidence of endometrial cancer among women in the United States rose steadily. An association between the growth-promoting effects of estrogen and endometrial carcinomas is thought to underlie the epidemiologic associations found for endometrial cancers, medical conditions such as anovulation, obesity, and other epidemiologically defined risk factors, including early age at menarche and nulliparity.

The estrogen-related endometrioid adenocarcinomas account for 80% of endometrial cancer, demonstrate large number of genetic changes, and appear to arise via a progression pathway. Common genetic changes in this type of endometrial carcinoma include microsatellite instability (MSI), or specific mutations of *PTEN*, *K-ras*, and *βB*-catenin genes.

Microsatellite Instability

Microsatellites are short segments of repetitive DNA found predominately in noncoding DNA and scattered through the genome. The MSI phenotype is expressed in the cells with changes in the number of repeat elements as compared with normal tissue because of DNA repair error during replication. Approximately 20% of type I endometrial cancers demonstrate MSI phenotype, while MSI in type II cancers is very rare, present in less than 5% of the cases.[51] MSI is due to inactivation of any of the mismatch repair genes and proteins: *MLH1*, *MSH2*, *MSH3*, and *MSH6*. The most common mechanism of MSI in the endometrium is inactivation of *MLH1* by epigenetic silencing of its promoter through hypermethylation of CpG islands, followed by *MSH6* mutation and *MSH3* frame shift mutations. In contrast, the MSI present in colon cancer is predominantly due to mutations in *MSH2*, followed by *MLH1* and *MSH6* mutations. MSI is an early event in type I cancers and it has been described in precancerous lesions. Once established, MSI may specifically target or inactivate genes with susceptible repeat elements, such as TGF-β1 receptors and IGFIIR, resulting in new subclones with altered capacity to invade and metastasize.

PTEN

Inactivation of *PTEN* (phosphatase and tensin homolog) tumor suppressor gene located at 10q23 is the most common genetic defect in type I endometrial cancers, and it is present in more than 80% of tumors that are preceded by histologically distinct premalignant phase.[52] The predominant *PTEN* activity is a lipid phosphatase that converts inositol triphosphates into inositol biphosphate, thus inhibiting survival and proliferative pathways that are activated by inositol triphosphatase. PTEN protein functions in maintaining G_1 arrest and enabling apoptosis via an AKT-dependent mechanism. *PTEN* inactivation is caused by various mechanisms. The most common *PTEN* defect in endometrial cancer is its complete loss of function through inactivation of both alleles. Mutations or deletions that result in loss of heterozygosity at *PTEN* locus are also observed with high frequency. The *PTEN* mutations pattern is different in microsatellite stable and MSI cancers. MSI tumors have a higher frequency of deletions, involving three or more base pairs, as compared with the microsatellite-stable tumors. In addition, the mutations in MSI tumors only rarely involve the polyadenine repeat of exon 8, which is the expected target.

KRAS

KRAS mutations have been found in up to 30% of type I endometrial cancers. The frequency of KRAS mutations is particularly high in MSI-positive tumors.[53]

β-catenin

β-catenin (3p21) is a component of the E-cadherin–catenin complex essential for cell differentiation and maintenance of normal tissue architecture, and it also plays a role in signal transduction. The APC protein down-regulates *β*-catenin levels, inducing phosphorylation of serine-threonine residues coded in exon 3 of the *β*-catenin and its degradation via ubiquitin-proteosome pathway. Gain of function mutations in *β*-catenin exon 3 are seen in 25% to 38% of type I cancers.[54] These mutations result in protein stabilization, accumulation, and transcriptional activation. *β*-catenin mutations have been found also in premalignant endometrial lesions. *β*-catenin changes may characterize pathways of endometrial cancer separate from PTEN mutations and are characterized by squamous differentiation. Several genes may be targets of dysregulated *β*-catenin pathway. Although in colon cancer elevated *β*-catenin levels trigger cyclin D1 expression and uncontrolled progression of tumor cells into the cell cycle, in type I endometrial cancers, *β*-catenin may regulate expression of MMP-7, which has a role in the establishment of microenvironment necessary for maintenance of tumor growth.

Type II Endometrial Cancer

The more aggressive, non–estrogen-related, nonendometrioid cancers (predominantly serous and clear cell carcinomas) are characterized by p53 mutations and Her2/neu amplification and bcl-2 changes. These high-grade tumors are known to be associated in some cases with an identifiable intraepithelial neoplasia component. The same pattern of genetic changes is seen in the preneoplastic atrophic endometrium, suggesting that these are early events in type II tumors carcinogenesis[55] (Table 100.2).

CERVIX, VAGINAL, AND VULVAR CANCERS

Role of Human Papillomavirus

Persistent infections with specific high-risk HPV genotypes (e.g., HPV-16, HPV-18, HPV-31, HPV-33, and HPV-45) have been identified as an essential, although not sufficient, factor in the pathogenesis of majority of cancers of the cervix, vagina, and vulva.[56] The existence of papilloma viruses was first demonstrated by Shope in the 1930s using an ultrafiltrate of warts from rabbits.[57] Since then, papilloma viruses with an epithelial tropism have been demonstrated in nearly every mammalian species, including humans. The HPVs are encapsulated DNA viruses containing a double-stranded DNA genome of approximately 7,800 base pairs. After infecting a suitable epithelium, viral DNA replication takes place in the basal cells of the epidermis, where the HPV genome is stably retained in multiple copies, guaranteeing its persistence in the epithelium's proliferative cells. This occurs early in preneoplastic lesions, when the viral genome still persists in an episomal state. In most invasive cancers and also in a few high-grade dysplastic lesions, however, integration of high-risk HPV genomes into the host genome is observed. Integration seems to be a direct consequence of chromosomal instability and an important molecular event in the progression of preneoplastic lesions. In a review of more than 190 reported integration loci, HPV integration sites are found to be randomly distributed over the whole genome with a clear predilection for genomic fragile

TABLE 100.2

GENETIC ALTERATIONS IN ENDOMETRIAL CANCER

Gene	Class	Alteration	Frequency (%)	Type
MSI				
MLH1	DNA repair	Promoter hypermethylation	20 (all repair gene alterations together)	I
MSH6	DNA repair	Frame-shift mutation		
MSH3	DNA repair	Frame-shift mutation		
ONCOGENES				
KRAS	G protein	Mutation	20	II
β-catenin	Transcription factor	Mutation	25–38	I
Her2/neu	Tyrosine kinase	Amplification/overexpression	10	I
BCL2	Antioxidant, prevents apoptosis	Amplification/overexpression		II
TUMOR SUPPRESSOR GENES				
p53	Transcription factor	Mutation/overexpression	20	II
PTEN	Tyrosine phosphatase	Mutation, biallelic loss of function	80	I

MSI, microsatellite instability.

sites. No evidence for targeted disruption or functional alteration of critical cellular genes by the integrated viral sequences could be found.[58]

The ability of high-risk HPVs to transform human epithelia relates to the transcription of specific viral gene products. Transcription from the HPV genome occurs in two waves: an early phase with seven to eight gene products and a late phase with two gene products (L1, L2). Early-phase gene products play a critical role in viral DNA replication (E1, E8) and regulation of transcription (E2, E8). In contrast, the L1 and L2 genes code for the capsid's primary and secondary proteins, respectively. The ability of different high-risk HPVs to transform human epithelia has been primarily associated with the expression of two specific viral gene products, E6 and E7. Transformation of human genital tract epithelium likely requires the expression of both E6 and E7; transfection of human keratinocytes *in vitro* with either is insufficient to accomplish this phenomenon.

At a molecular level, E6 and E7 interfere with important control mechanisms of the cell cycle, apoptosis, and maintenance of chromosomal stability by directly interacting with p53 and pRB, respectively. Moreover, recent studies demonstrated that the two viral oncoproteins cooperatively disturb the mechanisms of chromosome duplication and segregation during mitosis and thereby induce severe chromosomal instability associated with centrosome aberrations, anaphase bridges, chromosome lagging, and breaking.[59] They have also been shown to interact with a number of other cellular proteins whose role in epithelial transformation remains unclear, including transcriptional coactivators, such as p300, and components of junctional complexes, such as hDlg1. Altered expression of hDlg1 has been observed in high-grade cervical dysplasias, consistent with the hypothesis that these gene products play an early role in the HPV-induced progression to cervical cancer. Specific sequence differences have been associated with different levels of risk for ultimately developing cervical cancers. For example, recent evidence demonstrates that the sequence of E6 found in Ashkenazi populations confers a protective advantage against developing cervical cancer, previously attributed to the practice of circumcision. Although much less understood, other early genes, such as E2, have also been implicated in the transformation.

Immune Evasion By Human Papillomavirus

HPV infection has a transitory pattern, whereby most individuals (70% to 90%) eliminate the virus 12 to 24 months after initial diagnosis.[60] HPV has evolved several strategies to evade immune attack. Most obviously, papillomaviruses do not infect and replicate in antigen-presenting cells that are located in the epithelium, nor do they lyse keratinocytes, so there is no opportunity for antigen-presenting cells to engulf virions and present virion-derived antigens to the immune system. Furthermore, there is no blood-borne phase of infection, so the immune system outside the epithelium has little opportunity to detect the virus. Additionally, HPVs have exploited the redundancy of the genetic code to keep the levels of "late" proteins low.[61] Papillomavirus capsid protein production in mammalian cells is markedly up-regulated if the "viral" codons are replaced by the ones that are used by mammals, thereby limiting opportunities for the host to mount an effective immune attack. Following viral integration and subsequent malignant change, the local tumor environment at the cervical lesion is immunosuppressive. Thus, antigen-loaded dendritic cells (DCs) fail to mature, and immature DCs transmit a tolerogenic, rather than an immunogenic, signal to T cells bearing antigen-directed T-cell receptors in draining lymph nodes.

Human Papillomavirus Vaccines

The aim of prophylactic vaccination is to generate neutralizing antibodies against the HPV L1 and L2 capsid proteins. Prophylactic vaccine development against HPV has focused on the ability of the L1 and L2 virion structural proteins to assemble into viruslike particles (VLPs). VLPs mimic the natural structure of the virion and generate a potent immune response. Because the VLPs are devoid of DNA, they are not infectious or harmful. HPV VLPs can be generated by expressing the HPV capsid protein L1 in baculovirus or yeast. They consist of five L1 subunits that multimerize into immunogenic pentamers. Seventy-one L1 pentamers, in turn, multimerize into an HPV VLP. Initial studies have shown that VLPs are capable of inducing high titers of neutralizing antibodies to L1 and L2 epitopes.[62] Furthermore, VLPs have proven effective in generating HPV type-specific protection from viral challenge in animal papillomavirus models.

With the approval of preventive HPV vaccines that encompass HPV-16, -18, -6, and -11, large prevention clinical trials targeting the most prevalent HPV types in different regions of the world are warranted. Questions such as the necessity of repeat vaccinations and longevity of protection from HPV infection remain to be determined. It is estimated that if women were vaccinated against all high-risk types of HPV before they become sexually active, there should be a reduction of at least 85% in the risk of cervical cancer, and a decline of 44% to 70% in the frequency of abnormal Papanicolaou (Pap) smears attributable to HPV.[63] Unfortunately, even after vaccination is implemented, a reduction in the incidence of cervical cancer could not be expected to become apparent for at least a decade.[64] Therefore, therapeutic vaccines are still very much needed to reduce the morbidity and mortality associated with cervical cancer.

The therapeutic approach to patients with preinvasive and invasive cervical cancers is to develop vaccine strategies that induce specific CD8+ cytotoxic T lymphocyte (CTL) responses aimed at eliminating virus-infected or transformed cells. The majority of cervical cancers express the HPV-16-derived E6 and E7 oncoproteins, which are thus attractive targets for T-cell–mediated immunotherapy. Several HPV vaccine strategies have successfully elicited immune responses against HPV E6 and E7 epitopes and have prevented tumor growth on challenge with HPV-16-positive tumor cells in mice. Early-phase human trials using therapeutic vaccines have shown that they are safe, as no serious adverse effects have been reported. Other approaches currently undergoing preclinical development include the use of recombinant alpha viruses such as Venezuelan equine encephalitis virus, Semliki Forest virus, and naked DNA vaccination.

GESTATIONAL TROPHOBLASTIC DISEASE

Gestational trophoblastic disease (GTD) encompasses a diverse group of diseases with unique cytogenetic and molecular pathogenesis. The current concept implies that the abnormal trophoblastic tissue in GTD recapitulates the trophoblast present in the early developing placenta and the implantation site. Complete mole is diploid, usually 46, XX is androgenetic in origin, resulting from duplication of a haploid paternal genome (23X). More than 90% of complete moles contain this DNA content, and the remaining group are also androgenetic except 46, XY, and formed by dispermy. Partial moles are triploid, and diandric, usually XXY (58%), XXX (40%), and XYY (2%). Predominance of paternal chromosomes is therefore characteristics of molar pregnancy. Synergistic up-regulation of *CMYC*, *ERBB2*, *CFMS*, and *BCL2* has been suggested in pathogenesis of complete mole,[65] and similar findings have been confirmed in choriocarcinoma, while mutational analysis of *p53* and *KRAS* failed to show mutations in either complete mole or choriocarcinoma. The other genes involved in the development of choriocarcinoma include *DOC-2*, a candidate tumor-suppressor gene and a putative tumor suppressor at 7p12-7q11.23,[66] and the RAS guanosine triphosphate hydrolase (GTPase) activating protein. It has been postulated that GTD develops by a mechanism of monoallelic contribution, when the gene susceptible to inactivation would be affected by one-hit kinetics. Alternatively, uniparental transmission of genes that are parentally imprinted would impair their regulation.

Placental-site trophoblastic tumor (PSTT) represents neoplastic transformation of implantation site intermediate trophoblast. Placental-site trophoblastic tumor is characterized by aberrant expression of cyclins and p53. Further efforts are needed for better understanding of persistent trophoblastic disease.

Selected References

The full list of references for this chapter appears in the online version.

1. Dunn GP, Old LJ, Schreiber RD. The immunobiology of cancer immunosurveillance and immunoediting. *Immunity* 2004;21(2):137.
3. Levanon K, Crum C, Drapkin R. New insights into the pathogenesis of serous ovarian cancer and its clinical impact. *J Clin Oncol* 2008;26:5284.
5. Wright JW, Pejovic T, Fanton J, Stouffer RL. Induction of proliferation in the primate ovarian surface epithelium in vivo. *Hum Reprod* 2008;23:129.
6. Wright JW, Pejovic T, Lawson M, et al. Ovulation in the absence of the ovarian surface epithelium in the primate. *Biol Reprod* 2010;82:599.
8. Ganesan S, Richardson AL, Wang ZC, et al. Abnormalities of the inactive X chromosome are a common feature of BRCA1 mutant and sporadic basal-like breast cancer. *Cold Spring Harb Symp Quant Biol* 2005;70:93.
9. Garcia-Higuera I, Taniguchi T, Ganesan S, et al. Interaction of the Fanconi anemia proteins and BRCA1 in a common pathway. *Mol Cell* 2001;7(2):249.
10. Sakai W, Swisher EM, Karlan BY, et al. Secondary mutations as a mechanism of cisplatin resistance in BRCA2-mutated cancers. *Nature* 2008;451:1116.
11. Boudsocq F, Benaim P, Canitrot Y, et al. Modulation of cellular response to cisplatin by a novel inhibitor of DNA polymerase beta. *Mol Pharmacol* 2005;67(5):1485.
12. Kennedy RD, Chen CC, Stuckert P, et al. Fanconi anemia pathway-deficient tumor cells are hypersensitive to inhibition of ataxia telangiectasia mutated. *J Clin Invest* 2007;117:1440.
13. Bryant HE, Schultz N, Thomas HD, et al. Specific killing of BRCA2-deficient tumours with inhibitors of poly(ADP-ribose) polymerase. *Nature* 2005;434:913.
14. Farmer H, McCabe N, Lord CJ, et al. Targeting the DNA repair defect in BRCA mutant cells as a therapeutic strategy. *Nature* 2005;434:917.
15. Song H, Ramus SJ, Tyrer J, et al. A genome-wide association study identifies a new ovarian cancer susceptibility locus on 9p22.2. *Nat Genet* 2009;41:996.
17. Meinhold-Heerlein I, Bauerschlag D, Hilpert F, et al. Molecular and prognostic distinction between serous ovarian carcinomas of varying grade and malignant potential. *Oncogene* 2005;24:1053.
24. Landen CN Jr, Birrer MJ, Sood AK. Early events in the pathogenesis of epithelial ovarian cancer. *J Clin Oncol* 2008;26:995.
25. Berchuck A, Iversen ES, Lancaster JM, et al. Prediction of optimal versus suboptimal cytoreduction of advanced-stage serous ovarian cancer with the use of microarrays. *Am J Obstet Gynecol* 2004;190:910.
26. Hu W, Wu W, Nash MA, et al. Anomalies of the TGF-beta postreceptor signaling pathway in ovarian cancer cell lines. *Anticancer Res* 2000;20(2A):729.
28. van Haaften-Day C, Shen Y, Xu F, et al. OVX1, macrophage-colony stimulating factor, and CA-125-II as tumor markers for epithelial ovarian carcinoma: a critical appraisal. *Cancer* 2001;92(11):2837.
30. Ren J, Xiao YJ, Singh LS, et al. Lysophosphatidic acid is constitutively produced by human peritoneal mesothelial cells and enhances adhesion, migration, and invasion of ovarian cancer cells. *Cancer Res* 2006;66(6):3006.
31. Sengupta S, Kim KS, Berk MP, et al. Lysophosphatidic acid down-regulates tissue inhibitor of metalloproteinases, which are negatively involved in lysophosphatidic acid-induced cell invasion. *Oncogene* 2007;26:2894.
32. Do TV, Symowicz JC, Berman DM, et al. Lysophosphatidic acid down-regulates stress fibers and up-regulates pro-matrix metalloproteinase-2 activation in ovarian cancer cells. *Mol Cancer Res* 2007;5(2):121.
33. Burleson KM, Hansen LK, Skubitz AP. Ovarian carcinoma spheroids disaggregate on type I collagen and invade live human mesothelial cell monolayers. *Clin Exp Metastasis* 2004;21(8):685.
34. Schiffenbauer YS, Abramovitch R, Meir G, et al. Loss of ovarian function promotes angiogenesis in human ovarian carcinoma. *Proc Natl Acad Sci U S A* 1997;94(24):13203.
36. Szafranski P, Goode S. A Fasciclin 2 morphogenetic switch organizes epithelial cell cluster polarity and motility. *Development* 2004;131(9):2023.
37. Kassim SK, El-Salahy EM, Fayed ST, et al. Vascular endothelial growth factor and interleukin-8 are associated with poor prognosis in epithelial ovarian cancer patients. *Clin Biochem* 2004;37(5):363.

41. Baylin SB, Ohm JE. Epigenetic gene silencing in cancer—a mechanism for early oncogenic pathway addiction? *Nat Rev Cancer* 2006;6(2):107.
42. Wei SH, Chen CM, Strathdee G, et al. Methylation microarray analysis of late-stage ovarian carcinomas distinguishes progression-free survival in patients and identifies candidate epigenetic markers. *Clin Cancer Res* 2002;8(7):2246.
44. Smyth MJ, Dunn GP, Schreiber RD. Cancer immunosurveillance and immunoediting: the roles of immunity in suppressing tumor development and shaping tumor immunogenicity. *Adv Immunol* 2006;90:1.
45. Zhang L, Conejo-Garcia JR, Katsaros D, et al. Intratumoral T cells, recurrence, and survival in epithelial ovarian cancer. *N Engl J Med* 2003;348 (3):203.
46. Sato E, Olson SH, Ahn J, et al. Intraepithelial CD8+ tumor-infiltrating lymphocytes and a high CD8+/regulatory T cell ratio are associated with favorable prognosis in ovarian cancer. *Proc Natl Acad Sci U S A* 2005;102(51): 18538.
47. Goodell V, Salazar LG, Urban N, et al. Antibody immunity to the p53 oncogenic protein is a prognostic indicator in ovarian cancer. *J Clin Oncol* 2006; 24(5):762.
48. Odunsi K, Jungbluth AA, Stockert E, et al. NY-ESO-1 and LAGE-1 cancer-testis antigens are potential targets for immunotherapy in epithelial ovarian cancer. *Cancer Res* 2003;63(18):6076.
49. Old LJ. Cancer/testis (CT) antigens—a new link between gametogenesis and cancer. *Cancer Immunity* 2001;1:1.
50. Matsuzaki J, Gnjatic S, Mhawech-Fauceglia P, et al. Tumor-infiltrating NY-ESO-1-specific CD8+ T cells are negatively regulated by LAG-3 and PD-1 in human ovarian cancer. *Proc Natl Acad Sci U S A* 2010;107:7875.
51. Mutter GL, Boynton KA, Faquin WC, Ruiz RE, Jovanovic AS. Allelotype mapping of unstable microsatellites establishes direct lineage continuity between endometrial precancers and cancer. *Cancer Res* 1996;56(19):4483.
52. Mutter GL, Lin MC, Fitzgerald JT, et al. Altered PTEN expression as a diagnostic marker for the earliest endometrial precancers. *J Natl Cancer Inst* 2000;92(11):924.
54. Mirabelli-Primdahl L, Gryfe R, Kim H, et al. Beta-catenin mutations are specific for colorectal carcinomas with microsatellite instability but occur in endometrial carcinomas irrespective of mutator pathway. *Cancer Res* 1999; 59(14):3346.
56. zur Hausen H. Papillomaviruses causing cancer: evasion from host-cell control in early events in carcinogenesis. *J Natl Cancer Inst* 2000;92(9):690.
58. Wentzensen N, Vinokurova S, von Knebel Doeberitz M. Systematic review of genomic integration sites of human papillomavirus genomes in epithelial dysplasia and invasive cancer of the female lower genital tract. *Cancer Res* 2004;64(11):3878.
60. Ho GY, Bierman R, Beardsley L, Chang CJ, Burk RD. Natural history of cervicovaginal papillomavirus infection in young women. *N Engl J Med* 1998;338(7):423.
62. Koutsky LA, Ault KA, Wheeler CM, et al. A controlled trial of a human papillomavirus type 16 vaccine. *N Engl J Med* 2002;347(21):1645.
63. Walboomers JM, Jacobs MV, Manos MM, et al. Human papillomavirus is a necessary cause of invasive cervical cancer worldwide. *J Pathol* 1999;189 (1):12.
66. Matsuda T, Sasaki M, Kato H, et al. Human chromosome 7 carries a putative tumor suppressor gene(s) involved in choriocarcinoma. *Oncogene* 1997;15(23):2773.

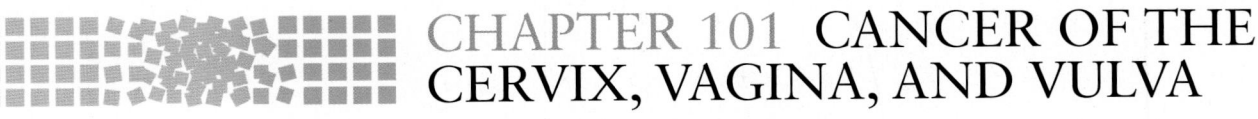

CHAPTER 101 CANCER OF THE CERVIX, VAGINA, AND VULVA

PATRICIA J. EIFEL, JONATHAN S. BEREK, AND MAURIE A. MARKMAN

CARCINOMA OF THE CERVIX

Epidemiology

The American Cancer Society estimated that in the United States in 2010, 12,200 new cases of invasive cervical cancer would be diagnosed and there would be 4,210 deaths due to cervical cancer, representing approximately 1.5% of all cancer deaths in women.[1] In the United States and other developed countries, age-adjusted death rates from cervical cancer have declined steadily since the 1930s. Although this improvement is primarily the result of the adoption of routine screening programs, the death rates from cervical cancer had begun to decrease before the implementation of Papanicolaou (Pap) screening, suggesting that other, unknown factors may have played some role.[2]

International incidences of cervical cancer tend to reflect differences in cultural attitudes toward sexual promiscuity and differences in the penetration of mass screening programs. The highest incidences tend to occur in populations that have low screening rates combined with a high background prevalence of human papillomavirus (HPV) infection and relatively liberal attitudes toward sexual behavior.[3] Rates of invasive cervical cancer are particularly high in Latin America, southern and eastern Africa, India, and Polynesia; in many of these developing countries, cervical cancer is the leading cause of cancer deaths among women. Differences in age-specific incidences between developed and medically underserved countries illustrate the probable impact of mass screening on the development of invasive disease. For example, a comparison between data from Brazil and the United Kingdom showed similar rates of cervical cancer in young women, suggesting similar levels of exposure to HPV, but rapidly diverging rates in older women, probably reflecting differences in the availability of mass screening in the two countries (Fig. 101.1).

Although the overall incidence of cervical cancer is low in the United States, the incidence in black Americans is about 30% higher than the incidence in white Americans, and the incidence in Hispanic women is about twice the incidence in white Americans.[4] Barriers to cervical cancer screening, including lack of insurance, low income, and cultural factors, probably contribute to higher incidences and mortality rates in black and Hispanic women.[5]

Molecular and human epidemiologic studies have demonstrated a strong relationship between HPV, cervical intraepithelial neoplasia (CIN), and invasive carcinoma of the cervix; HPV can be identified in more than 99% of cervical cancers, and infection with HPV is now accepted as a necessary cause of most cervical cancers.[3] It appears that most of the covariables historically associated with an increased risk of cervical cancer are surrogates for sexually transmitted HPV infection. Women who have coitus at a young age, who have multiple sexual partners, or who bear children at a young age are at increased risk. Promiscuous sexual behavior in male partners is also a risk factor. Castellsague et al.[6] have reported that circumcised males have a lower incidence of HPV infection than uncircumcised males and a correspondingly lower incidence of cervical cancer in their female partners.

The strong correlation between high-risk HPV types and cervical carcinoma has led to the suggestion that HPV detection and typing be incorporated into mass screening programs and has led to the recent development of prophylactic HPV vaccines that have proven highly effective in randomized trials.[7] On June 8, 2006, the U.S. Food and Drug Administration approved a prophylactic HPV vaccine for women between the ages of 9 and 26 years; this quadrivalent vaccine has been demonstrated to be highly effective in preventing benign warts and neoplasia caused by the most common HPV types (6, 11, 16, and 18). This subject is discussed in greater detail in Chapter 100.

A number of studies suggest that the incidence of one subtype of cervical cancer, cervical adenocarcinoma, has been increasing, particularly among women in their 20s and 30s.[8,9] In a study based on Surveillance, Epidemiology, and End Results program data, Smith et al.[8] found that the age-adjusted incidence of cervical adenocarcinoma in the United States increased by 29.1% during a period (1973–1996) when the overall incidence of cervical cancer decreased by 41.9%. Several investigators have reported a correlation between cervical adenocarcinoma and prolonged oral contraceptive use.[10] However, this relationship may not be causative, given the many potential confounding risk factors and possible changes in diagnostic criteria over time.[8,11] Another possible explanation for the increase in incidence of cervical adenocarcinoma is that cytologic screening methods may be less effective in detecting preinvasive adenocarcinomas than they are in detecting preinvasive squamous lesions, resulting in a less dramatic reduction in the incidence of invasive adenocarcinomas.

In 1993, the Centers for Disease Control and Prevention added cervical cancer to the list of AIDS-defining neoplasms.[12] However, the relationship between immunosuppression (particularly human immunodeficiency virus [HIV]-related immunosuppression) and the risk of HPV-related disease is complex and incompletely understood.[13,14] Current data strongly suggest that HIV-infected women have an increased incidence and are more likely to have persistence of cervical HPV infection, even when studies are corrected for confounding risk factors; HIV-positive women also tend to have a faster rate of progression to high-grade CIN.[13,14] Iatrogenic immunosuppression in organ transplant recipients is also associated with an increased prevalence of CIN.[15] Although less definitive, evidence linking HIV infection with invasive cervical cancer has also been increasing.[14] Some investigators[16] have suggested that cervical

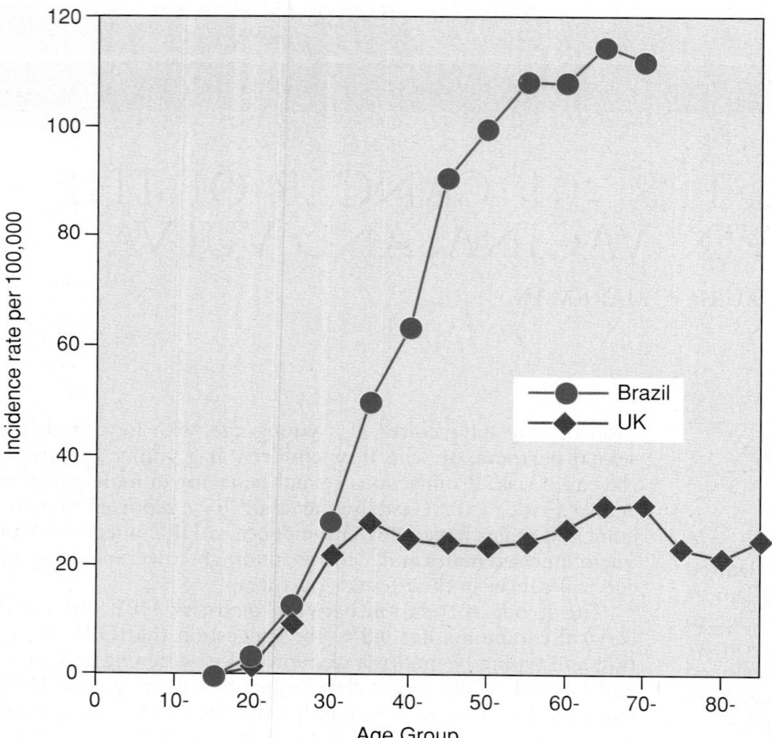

FIGURE 101.1 Age-specific incidences of invasive cervical cancer in Brazil and in the United Kingdom (UK). (From ref. 3, with permission.)

cancer is a more aggressive disease in immunosuppressed patients, but other studies have failed to reveal an independent linkage.[13,14] In most cases, antiretroviral therapy does not appear to affect HPV levels, nor does it appear to decrease the risks of high-grade squamous intraepithelial lesions (HSILs) or invasive cancer.[14] Because of the increased risk of HPV infection in HIV-positive women, vigilant surveillance with Pap smears, pelvic examinations, and colposcopy (when indicated) should be part of the routine care of these women.

Natural History and Pattern of Spread

Most cervical carcinomas arise at the junction between the primarily columnar epithelium of the endocervix and the squamous epithelium of the ectocervix. This junction is a site of continuous metaplastic change, which is greatest *in utero*, at puberty, and during first pregnancy, and declines after menopause. Long before the relationship between HPV and cervical cancer was known, Richart and Barron[17] demonstrated that invasive squamous cell cancer of the cervix was the end result of progressive intraepithelial dysplastic changes within metaplastic epithelium of the transformation zone.[17] The greatest risk of neoplastic transformation of virally induced atypical squamous metaplasia coincides with periods of greatest metaplastic activity. The approximately 15-year difference in the mean ages of women with CIN and women with invasive cervical cancer indicates a generally slow progression of CIN to invasive carcinoma.[18]

Once tumor has broken through the basement membrane, it may penetrate the cervical stroma directly or through vascular channels. Invasive tumors may develop as exophytic growths protruding from the cervix into the vagina or as endocervical lesions that can cause massive expansion of the cervix despite a relatively normal-appearing ectocervix. From the cervix, tumor may extend superiorly to the lower uterine segment, inferiorly to the vagina, laterally to the broad ligaments (where it may cause ureteral obstruction), or posterolaterally to the uterosacral ligaments. Large tumors may appear fixed on pelvic examination, although true invasion of the pelvic wall musculature is probably uncommon. Although the cervix is separated from the bladder by only a thin layer of fascia and cellular connective tissue, extensive bladder involvement is uncommon, occurring in fewer than 5% of cases. Tumor may also extend posteriorly to the rectum, although rectal mucosal involvement is a rare finding at initial presentation.

The cervix has a rich supply of lymphatics that drain the mucosal, muscularis, and serosal layers. The lymphatics of the cervix anastomose extensively with those of the lower uterine segment.[19] The most important lymphatic collecting trunks exit laterally from the uterine isthmus in three groups (Fig. 101.2).[19] The upper branches, which originate in the anterior and lateral cervix, follow the uterine artery, are sometimes interrupted by a node as they cross the ureter, and terminate in the uppermost hypogastric nodes. The middle branches drain to deeper hypogastric (obturator) nodes. The lowest branches follow a posterior course to the inferior and superior gluteal, common iliac, presacral, and subaortic nodes. Additional posterior lymphatic channels arising from the posterior cervical wall may drain to superior rectal nodes or may continue upward in the retrorectal space to the subaortic nodes overlying the sacral promontory. Anterior collecting trunks pass between the cervix and bladder along the superior vesical artery and terminate in the internal iliac nodes.

The incidence of pelvic and para-aortic node involvement is correlated with tumor stage, size, histologic subtype, depth of invasion, and presence of lymph-vascular space invasion (LVSI). Reported rates of regional metastasis, which come primarily from series of patients who underwent lymphadenectomy as part of radical surgical treatment or before radiotherapy, vary widely. For patients with stage I disease treated with radical hysterectomy, most investigators report an incidence of positive pelvic nodes of 15% to 20% and an incidence of positive para-aortic nodes of 1% to 5%. For patients with stage I disease treated with radiation, reported rates of positive para-aortic nodes tend to be higher—usually 10% to 25%—reflecting

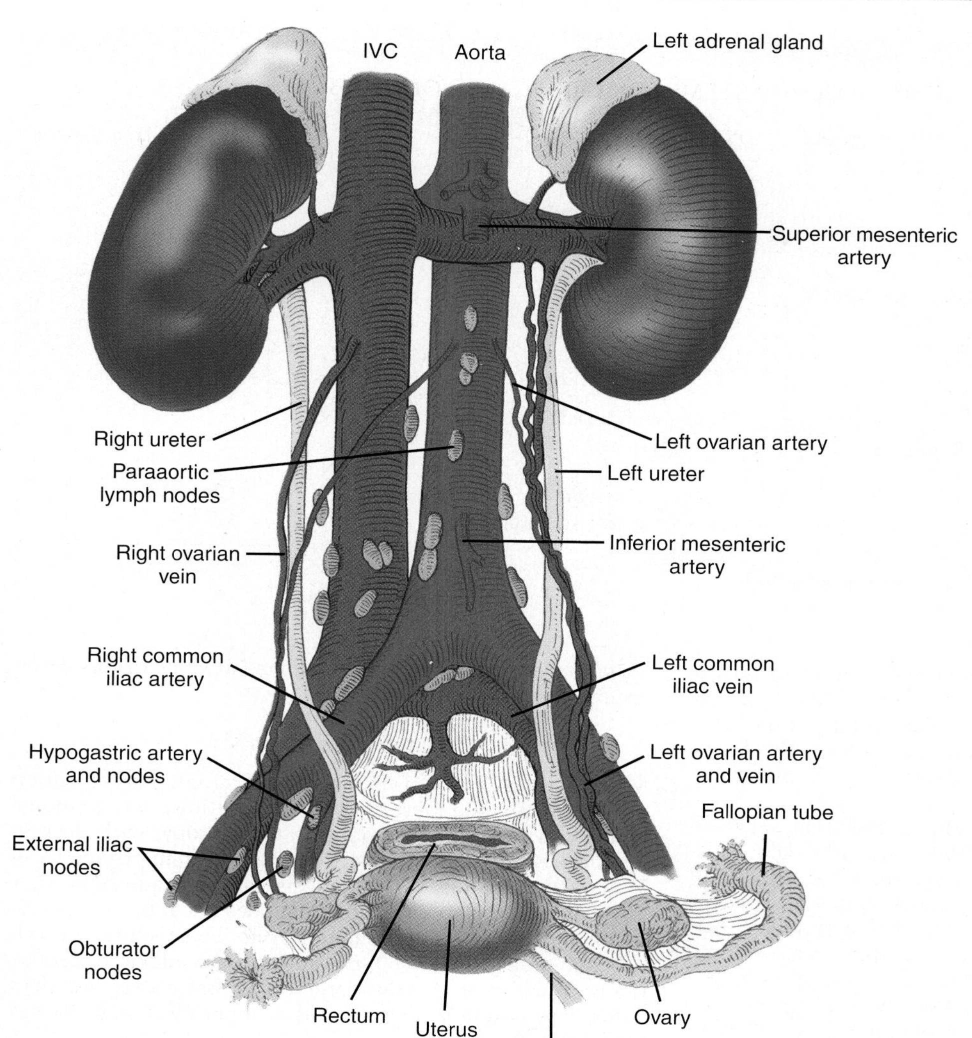

FIGURE 101.2 The pelvic and para-aortic lymph nodes and their relationship to the major retroperitoneal vessels.

the fact that stage I tumors selected for treatment with radiation are usually more advanced. Variations in the completeness of lymphadenectomies and histologic processing may lead to underestimates of the true incidence of regional spread from carcinomas of the cervix.[20]

Cervical cancer usually follows a relatively orderly pattern of metastatic progression, initially to primary-echelon nodes in the pelvis and then to para-aortic nodes and distant sites. Even patients with locoregionally advanced disease rarely have detectable hematogenous metastases at initial diagnosis of cervical cancer. The most frequent sites of distant recurrence are lung, extrapelvic nodes, liver, and bone.

Pathology

Cervical Intraepithelial Neoplasia

Several systems have been developed for classifying cervical cytologic findings (Table 101.1). Although criteria for the diagnosis of CIN and degree of neoplasia vary somewhat between pathologists, the important features of CIN are cellular immaturity, cellular disorganization, nuclear abnormalities, and increased mitotic activity. If mitoses and immature cells are present only in the lower third of the epithelium, the lesion is usually designated *CIN 1*. Lesions involving only the lower and middle thirds are designated *CIN 2*, and those involving the upper third are designated *CIN 3*.

The term *cervical intraepithelial neoplasia*, as proposed by Richart,[21] refers only to a lesion that may progress to invasive carcinoma. Although CIN 1 and CIN 2 are sometimes referred to as *mild-to-moderate dysplasia*, the term *CIN* is now preferred over *dysplasia*.

Following a 1988 National Cancer Institute Consensus Conference, the Bethesda system of classification was developed in an effort to further standardize reporting.[22] This system defines squamous intraepithelial lesions (SILs) as including all squamous alterations in the cervical transformation zone that are induced by HPV; SILs include all lesions that were classified in previous systems as condyloma, dysplasia, or CIN. The Bethesda system divides SILs into two groups, low grade and high grade. Low-grade SILs (LSILs) have nuclear crowding or atypia without frequent mitoses, parabasal cell anisokaryosis, or coarse chromatin; these lesions are usually associated with low-risk HPV types and have a low likelihood of progressing to invasive cancers. These are to be distinguished from HSILs, which have nuclear atypia in lower and upper epithelial layers, abnormal mitoses, coarse chromatin, and loss of polarity. HSILs are usually associated with high-risk HPV types and have a higher likelihood of progressing to invasive cancer. The Bethesda system was meant to replace the Papanicolaou system and is now widely used in the United

TABLE 101.1

COMPARISON OF CYTOLOGY CLASSIFICATION SYSTEMS FOR CERVICAL NEOPLASMS

Bethesda System	Dysplasia/CIN System		Papanicolaou System
Within normal limits	Normal		Class I
Infection (specify organism)	Inflammatory atypia (organism)		Class II
Reactive and reparative changes	—		—
Squamous cell abnormalities	—		—
Atypical squamous cells of undetermined significance	Squamous atypia		Class IIR
	HPV atypia		
Low-grade squamous intraepithelial lesion	Mild dysplasia	CIN 1	Class III
—	Moderate dysplasia	CIN 2	
High-grade squamous intraepithelial lesion	Severe dysplasia	CIN 3	
	Carcinoma *in situ*		Class IV
Invasive squamous carcinoma	Invasive squamous carcinoma		Class V

CIN, cervical intraepithelial neoplasia; HPV, human papillomavirus.

States. However, its use is still controversial. Some groups[23] argue that the new nomenclature has failed to improve diagnostic accuracy and believe that with dichotomization of the spectrum of atypical lesions, lesions that were formerly classified as CIN 2 (now HSIL) may be overtreated despite their relatively low risk of progression.

The Bethesda system also introduced the term *atypical squamous cells of undetermined significance* (ASC-US). This uncertain diagnosis is now the most common abnormal Pap smear result in United States laboratories,[24] with 1.6% to 9% of Pap smears reported as having ASC-US. Although most cases of ASC-US reflect a benign process, about 5% to 10% are associated with an underlying HSIL, and one-third or more of HSILs are heralded by a finding of ASC-US on a Pap smear.[25] There has been considerable controversy about the evaluation and management of ASC-US, leading the National Cancer Institute to initiate the ASC-US-LSIL Triage Study (ALTS).[26] This multicenter, randomized trial compared three methods of management—immediate colposcopy, cytologic follow-up, and triage by HPV DNA testing—in 5,060 patients who were recruited to the study following a community-based Pap smear report of ASC-US or LSIL. Preliminary analyses of this study[26] demonstrated that in patients with LSIL, the prevalence of high-risk HPV was too high to permit useful triage based on HPV DNA testing, but that in the 3,488 patients with ASC-US, HPV DNA testing had a sensitivity in the detection of HSIL similar to that of immediate colposcopy and reduced the number of referrals for colposcopy by 50%. After exclusion of patients who had a diagnosis of CIN 2 or 3 at initial colposcopy, the cumulative risk of subsequent progression to CIN 2 or 3 was equivalent for women with LSIL (27.6%) or high-risk HPV-positive ASC-US (26.7%).[27]

Adenocarcinoma *in Situ*

Adenocarcinoma *in situ* is diagnosed when normal endocervical gland cells are replaced by tall, irregular columnar cells with stratified, hyperchromatic nuclei and increased mitotic activity but the normal branching pattern of the endocervical glands is maintained and there is no obvious stromal invasion. About 20% to 50% of women with cervical adenocarcinoma *in situ* also have squamous CIN.[28] Because adenocarcinoma *in situ* is frequently multifocal, cone biopsy margins are unreliable.[29] Although some investigators have described a possible precursor lesion termed *endocervical glandular dysplasia*, the reproducibility and clinical value of this designation are uncertain.[30]

Microinvasive Carcinoma

Microinvasive carcinoma is defined by International Federation of Gynecology and Obstetrics (FIGO) as "invasive carcinoma which can be diagnosed only by microscopy, with deepest invasion ≤5 mm and largest extension ≥7 mm" (stage IA in Table 101.2). Thus, this diagnosis can be made only after examination of a specimen that includes the entire neoplastic lesion and cervical transformation zone. This requires a cervical cone biopsy. Following the advent of cytologic screening, the proportion of invasive carcinomas that invade less than 5 mm increased more than tenfold to about 20% in the United States.[31]

The earliest invasion appears as a blurring of the stromoepithelial junction with a protrusion of cells into the stroma; these cells are less well differentiated than the adjacent noninvasive cells; have abundant pink-staining cytoplasm, hyperchromatic nuclei, and prominent nucleoli; they also exhibit a loss of polarity at the stromoepithelial junction.[31] Early microinvasion is usually characterized by a desmoplastic response in adjacent stroma with scalloping or duplication of the neoplastic epithelium or formation of pseudoglands (nests of invasive carcinoma that can mimic crypt involvement). In a study of cone specimens, Reich et al.[32] reported that 12% of microinvasive carcinomas were multifocal. The depth of invasion should be measured with a micrometer from the base of the epithelium to the deepest point of invasion. Lesions that have invaded less than 3 mm (FIGO stage IA1) are rarely associated with metastases; 5% to 10% of tumors that have invaded 3 to 5 mm (FIGO stage IA2) are associated with positive pelvic lymph nodes.[33] Until FIGO refined its definition of microinvasive carcinoma (Table 101.2), most clinicians in the United States used a different definition of microinvasive carcinoma formulated by the Society of Gynecologic Oncologists: cancers that invaded less than 3 mm with no evidence of LVSI. The importance of LVSI remains somewhat controversial; the risk of metastatic regional disease appears to be exceedingly low for any tumor that invades less than 3 mm, even in the presence of LVSI.[31] Although most clinicians have adopted the FIGO definitions, many think that the risk of regional spread from tumors that have invaded 3 to 5 mm is sufficiently high to warrant treatment of the parametria and regional nodes.

TABLE 101.2

INTERNATIONAL FEDERATION OF GYNECOLOGY AND OBSTETRICS STAGING OF CARCINOMA OF THE CERVIX (2009)

Stage	Description
I	The carcinoma is strictly confined to the cervix (*extension to the corpus should be disregarded*).
IA	Invasive carcinoma which can be diagnosed only by microscopy, with deepest invasion ≤5 mm and largest extension ≥7 mm.
IA1	Measured stromal invasion of ≤3.0 mm in depth and extension of ≤7.0 mm.
IA2	Measured stromal invasion >3.0 mm and not >5.0 mm in depth with an extension of not >7.0 mm.
IB	Clinically visible lesions limited to the cervix uteri or pre-clinical cancers greater than stage IA.[a]
IB1	Clinically visible lesion ≤4 cm in greatest dimension.
IB2	Clinically visible lesion >4 cm in greatest dimension.
II	Cervical carcinoma invades beyond the uterus, but not to the pelvic wall or to the lower third of the vagina.
IIA	Without parametrial invasion.
IIA1	Clinically visible lesion ≤4 cm in greatest dimension.
IIA2	Clinically visible lesion >4 cm in greatest dimension.
IIB	With obvious parametrial invasion.
III	The tumor extends to the pelvic wall and/or involves the lower third of the vagina and/or causes hydronephrosis or non-functioning kidney.[b]
IIIA	Tumor involves lower third of the vagina, with no extension to the pelvic wall.
IIIB	Extension to the pelvic wall and/or hydronephrosis or nonfunctioning kidney.
IV	The carcinoma has extended beyond the true pelvis or has involved (biopsy-proven) the mucosa of the bladder or rectum. A bullous edema, as such, does not permit a case to be allotted to stage IV.
IVA	Spread of the growth to adjacent organs.
IVB	Spread to distant organs.

[a]All macroscopically visible lesions—even with superficial invasion—are allotted to stage IB carcinomas. Invasion is limited to a measured stromal invasion with a maximal depth of 5.0 mm and a horizontal extension of not >7.0 mm. Depth of invasion should not be >5.0 mm taken from the base of the epithelium of the original tissue—superficial or glandular. The depth of invasion should always be reported in millimeters, even in those cases with "early (minimal) stromal invasion" (~1 mm). The involvement of vascular/lymphatic spaces should not change the stage allotment.
[b]On rectal examination, there is no cancer-free space between the tumor and the pelvic wall. All cases with hydronephrosis or nonfunctioning kidney are included, unless they are known to be the result of another cause.
(Data from ref. 59.)

For adenocarcinoma, in particular, measuring the depth of invasion can be difficult. Because invasive adenocarcinomas may originate anywhere along the profile of architecturally complex glands that course through the cervical stroma, no reproducible method has been found for measuring the depth of invasion of these tumors. Some authors have measured the extent of invasion from the basement membrane or from the nearest abnormal glandular epithelium; others have defined early adenocarcinomas according to the volume of tumor (in cubic millimeters).[30] Despite these differences in measurement method, it is apparent that a subset of patients with very small adenocarcinomas have a low likelihood of lymph node metastasis or recurrence.[30]

Invasive Squamous Cell Carcinoma

Between 80% and 90% of cervical carcinomas are squamous cell carcinomas. Although squamous neoplasms are often subclassified as large cell keratinizing, large cell nonkeratinizing, or small cell carcinomas, these designations do not correlate well with prognosis.[34] Small cell squamous carcinomas have small to medium-sized nuclei, open chromatin, small or large nucleoli, and abundant cytoplasm and are believed by most authorities to have a somewhat poorer prognosis than large cell neoplasms with or without keratin. However, small cell squamous carcinomas should not be confused with the much more aggressive anaplastic small cell neuroendocrine carcinomas discussed later. Papillary variants of squamous carcinoma may be well differentiated (occasionally confused with immature condylomata) or very poorly differentiated (resembling high-grade transitional carcinoma).[31] Verrucous carcinoma is a very rare warty-appearing variant of squamous carcinoma that may be difficult to differentiate from benign condyloma without multiple biopsies or hysterectomy.[35] Sarcomatoid squamous carcinoma is another very rare variant, demonstrating areas of spindle-cell carcinomatous tumor confluent with poorly differentiated squamous cell carcinoma; immunohistochemistry demonstrates expression of cytokeratin as well as vimentin. The natural history of this uncommon tumor is not well understood.[36]

Adenocarcinoma

Invasive adenocarcinoma may be pure or mixed with squamous cell carcinoma (adenosquamous carcinoma). About 80% of cervical adenocarcinomas are endocervical-type adenocarcinomas, which are composed predominantly of cells with eosinophilic cytoplasm, brisk mitotic activity, and frequent apoptotic bodies, although many other patterns and cell types have also been observed. Endocervical-type adenocarcinomas are frequently referred to as *mucinous*; however, although some have abundant intracytoplasmic mucin, most have little or none.[37]

Minimal-deviation adenocarcinoma (adenoma malignum) is a rare, extremely well-differentiated adenocarcinoma that is sometimes associated with Peutz-Jeghers syndrome.[38] Because the branching glandular pattern strongly resembles normal endocervical glands and the mucin-rich cells can be deceptively benign-appearing, minimal-deviation adenocarcinoma may not be recognized as malignant in small biopsy specimens.[37] Earlier studies reported a poor outcome for women with this tumor, but more recently, patients have been reported to have a favorable prognosis if the disease is detected early.[38]

Glassy cell carcinoma[37] is a variant of poorly differentiated adenosquamous carcinoma characterized by cells with abundant eosinophilic, granular, ground-glass cytoplasm with large round to oval nuclei and prominent nucleoli. Adenoid basal carcinoma is a well-differentiated tumor that histologically resembles basal cell carcinoma of the skin and tends to have a favorable prognosis.[39] Adenoid cystic carcinoma consists of basaloid cells in a cribriform or cylindromatous pattern; metastases are frequent, although the natural history of these tumors may be long.[39] Rarely, primary carcinomas of the cervix are composed of endometrioid, serous, or clear cells; mixtures of these cell types may be seen, and histologically, some of these tumors are indistinguishable from those arising elsewhere in the endometrium or ovary. In a study of 17 cases, Zhou et al.[40] found that serous carcinomas of the cervix have an aggressive course, similar to that of high-grade serous tumors originating in the other müllerian sites.

Anaplastic Small Cell/Neuroendocrine Carcinoma

Anaplastic small cell carcinomas resemble oat cell carcinomas of the lung and are made up of small tumor cells that have scanty cytoplasm, small round to oval nuclei, and high mitotic activity; they frequently display neuroendocrine features.[41] Anaplastic small cell carcinomas behave more aggressively than poorly differentiated small cell squamous carcinomas; most investigators report survival rates of less than 50% even for patients with early stage I disease, although recent studies of aggressive multimodality treatments have been somewhat more encouraging.[42–44] Widespread hematogenous metastases are frequent, but brain metastases are rare unless preceded by pulmonary involvement.[44]

Other Rare Neoplasms

A variety of neoplasms may infiltrate the cervix from adjacent sites, and this makes differential diagnosis difficult. In particular, it may be difficult or impossible to determine the origin of adenocarcinomas involving the endocervix and uterine isthmus. Although endometrioid histology suggests endometrial origin and mucinous tumors in young patients are most often of endocervical origin, both histologic types can arise in either site.[45] Metastatic tumors from the colon, breast, or other sites may involve the cervix secondarily. Malignant mixed müllerian tumors, adenosarcomas, and leiomyosarcomas occasionally arise in the cervix but more often involve it secondarily. Primary lymphomas and melanomas of the cervix are extremely rare.

Clinical Manifestations

Preinvasive disease is usually detected during routine cervical cytologic screening. Early invasive disease may not be associated with any symptoms and is also usually detected during screening examinations. The earliest symptom of invasive cervical cancer is usually abnormal vaginal bleeding, often following coitus or vaginal douching. This may be associated with a clear or foul-smelling vaginal discharge. Pelvic pain may result from locoregionally invasive disease or from coexistent pelvic inflammatory disease. Flank pain may be a symptom of hydronephrosis, often complicated by pyelonephritis. Patients with very advanced tumors may have hematuria or incontinence from a vesicovaginal fistula caused by direct extension of tumor to the bladder. External compression of the rectum by a massive primary tumor may cause constipation, but the rectal mucosa is rarely involved at initial diagnosis.

Diagnosis, Clinical Evaluation, and Staging

Diagnosis

The long preinvasive stage of cervical cancer, the relatively high prevalence of the disease in unscreened populations, and the sensitivity of cytologic screening make cervical carcinoma an ideal target for cancer screening. In the United States, screening with cervical cytologic examination and pelvic examination has led to a decrease of more than 50% in the incidence of cervical cancer since 1975.[46] Only nations with well-developed screening programs have experienced substantial decreases in cervical cancer incidence.

Citing a large body of data on screening effectiveness, the American College of Obstetrics and Gynecology recently updated their guidelines for cervical cancer screening.[46] The guidelines are as follows: screening is recommended every 2 years to begin at age 21 years; screening should be avoided before this age because screening at younger ages may lead to unnecessary and harmful evaluation and treatment in women at very low risk of cancer. After age 30 years, the screening interval can be extended to 3 years for women who have no history of CIN 2 or CIN 3, who are not HIV-infected or otherwise immunocompromised, and who were not exposed to diethylstilbestrol (DES) *in utero*. Women who have had a total hysterectomy for benign conditions and who have no history of high-grade CIN may discontinue routine screening. It is also reasonable to discontinue screening for women older than 65 to 70 years who have three or more consecutive negative studies and have had no abnormal test results in the past 10 years. Women previously treated for high-grade CIN or for cancer should continue to have annual screening for at least 20 years and periodic screening indefinitely. Annual gynecologic examination might still be appropriate even if cytologic screening is not performed.[46]

Accurate calculation of false-negative rates for the Pap test is difficult; estimates range from less than 5% to 20% or more.[47] The sensitivity of individual tests may be improved by ensuring adequate sampling of the squamocolumnar junction and the endocervical canal; smears without endocervical or metaplastic cells are inadequate, and in such cases the test must be repeated. The sensitivity of a screening program is increased by repeated testing; studies of the test frequency required to optimize the sensitivity of screening formed the basis of the American College of Obstetrics and Gynecology recommendations.[46]

Most United States gynecologists currently prefer newer liquid-based screening methods to conventional Pap tests. However, the authors of a recent meta-analysis of available data concluded that "liquid-based cervical cytology is neither more sensitive nor more specific for detection of high-grade CIN compared with the conventional Pap."[48] Liquid-based tests are more costly but have the potential advantage that additional studies, such as HPV typing, can be performed on the fluid remaining after cytologic examination. HPV testing of ASC-US smears followed by colposcopy in patients with HPV-positive lesions has been shown to be a highly accurate and cost-effective means of detecting HSIL in cases of equivocal smears and may also be used to triage postmenopausal women with LSIL.[48,49]

Patients with abnormal findings on cytologic examination who do not have a gross cervical lesion must be evaluated with colposcopy and directed biopsies. Following application of a 3% acetic-acid solution, the cervix is examined under 10- to 15-fold magnification with a bright, filtered light that enhances the acetowhitening and vascular patterns characteristic of dysplasia or carcinoma. The skilled colposcopist can accurately distinguish between low- and high-grade dysplasia,[50] but microinvasive disease cannot consistently be distinguished from intraepithelial lesions on colposcopy.[51]

In patients with a high-grade Pap smear finding, if no abnormalities are found on colposcopic examination or if the entire squamocolumnar junction cannot be visualized, an additional endocervical sample should be collected. Although some authorities advocate the routine addition of endocervical curettage to colposcopic examination, it is probably reasonable to omit this step in previously untreated women if the entire squamocolumnar junction is visible with a complete ring of unaltered columnar epithelium in the lower canal.[52] The rate of detection of endocervical lesions may be higher when specimens are collected using a cytobrush rather than by curettage.[53]

Cervical cone biopsy is used to diagnose occult endocervical lesions and is an essential step in the diagnosis and management of microinvasive carcinoma of the cervix. Cervical cone biopsy yields an accurate diagnosis and decreases the incidence of inappropriate therapy when (1) the squamocolumnar junction is poorly visualized on colposcopy and a high-grade lesion is suspected, (2) high-grade dysplastic epithelium extends into the endocervical canal, (3) the cytologic findings suggest high-grade dysplasia or carcinoma *in situ*, (4) a microinvasive carcinoma is found on directed biopsy, (5) the endocervical curettage specimens show high-grade CIN, or (6) the cytologic findings are suggestive of adenocarcinoma *in situ*.[54]

Clinical Evaluation of Patients with Invasive Carcinoma

All patients with invasive cervical cancer should be evaluated with a detailed history and physical examination, with particular attention paid to inspection and palpation of the pelvic organs with bimanual and rectovaginal examinations. Standard laboratory studies should include a complete blood cell count and renal function and liver function tests. All patients should have chest radiography to rule out lung metastases; additional imaging of the abdomen and pelvis should be performed for all patients who have stage IB2 or greater disease. Cystoscopy and either a proctoscopy or a barium enema study should be considered in patients with bulky tumors, particularly for those with computed tomography (CT) or magnetic resonance imaging (MRI) findings suggestive of organ involvement.

Many clinicians obtain CT or MRI scans to evaluate regional lymph nodes, but these studies have suboptimal accuracy because they fail to detect small metastases and because patients with bulky necrotic tumors often have enlarged reactive lymph nodes that may be free of metastasis.[55,56] In a large Gynecologic Oncology Group (GOG) study that compared the results of radiographic studies with subsequent histologic findings, Heller et al.[56] found that the sensitivity of CT in the detection of positive para-aortic nodes was only 34%. Positron emission tomography appears to be a more sensitive, noninvasive method of evaluating the regional nodes of patients with cervical cancer and a useful method for following response to treatment.[57] MRI provides more accurate information than CT about the distribution of tumor in the cervix and paracervical tissues but still has a significant error rate compared with histologic findings.[55]

Clinical Staging

The FIGO staging system is the most widely accepted staging system for carcinomas of the cervix.[58,59] The latest (2009) update of this system is summarized in Table 101.2.[58] Since the earliest versions of the cervical cancer staging system, there have been numerous changes: the designation of preinvasive disease as a separate category (1950), designation and changes in the definition of microinvasive disease (1962, 1985, and 1994), and subdivisions of the stage I and II categories according to tumor or cervical diameter (1994 and 2009). Although these changes have gradually improved the discriminatory value of the staging system, the many fluctuations in the definitions of stages IA and IB have complicated efforts to compare the outcomes of patients whose tumors were staged and treated during different periods.[60]

FIGO stage is based primarily on careful clinical examination. The use of diagnostic imaging techniques to assess tumor size and local extent is encouraged but not mandatory in the 2009 staging system. However, FIGO still does not incorporate evidence of lymph node metastasis gained by surgical staging or advanced imaging studies in the 2009 staging system. Some form of imaging must be performed to evaluate the presence or absence of hydronephrosis, but intravenous pyelography is no longer required. Cystoscopy, sigmoidoscopy, and examination under anesthesia are also optional. However, suspected bladder or rectal involvement must be confirmed by biopsy. Stage should be assigned before any definitive therapy is administered. The clinical stage should never be changed on the basis of subsequent findings. When the stage to which a particular case should be allotted is in doubt, the case should be assigned to the earlier stage.

Although surgically treated patients are sometimes classified according to a TNM pathologic staging system, this practice has not been widely accepted because it cannot be applied to patients who are treated with primary radiotherapy.[61]

Surgical Evaluation of Regional Spread

Lymphadenectomy is performed as part of the surgical treatment of most patients with early carcinomas of the cervix. Early studies of diagnostic preradiotherapy lymph node staging were discouraging because of the high complication rates observed when transperitoneal lymph node dissections were combined with large radiation fields. In 1989, Weiser et al.[62] reported that the proportion of patients with postradiotherapy bowel complications was reduced to less than 5% if lymphadenectomy was performed using a retroperitoneal approach. Today, laparoscopic methods are often used to reduce the perioperative morbidity and hospitalization times associated with surgical staging.[63–65] The rate of late complications from radiotherapy following laparoscopic lymphadenectomy is probably less than with transperitoneal surgery but has not yet been fully evaluated. The role of sentinel node evaluation in cervical cancer is just beginning to be explored, but sentinel node evaluation may improve the sensitivity of lymph node staging, particularly for patients with early cervical cancer.[66,67]

Although the indications for surgical staging are controversial, advocates argue that the procedure identifies patients with microscopic para-aortic or common iliac node involvement who can benefit from extended-field irradiation. Some investigators have also suggested, on the basis of first principles and encouraging results with regard to control of pelvic disease, that debulking of large pelvic nodes before radiotherapy may improve outcome.[68,69] Because patients with radiographically positive pelvic nodes are at greatest risk for occult metastasis to para-aortic nodes, these patients may have the greatest chance of benefiting from surgical staging.

Prognostic Factors

Prognosis is strongly influenced by a number of tumor characteristics that are not included in the staging system. Although FIGO now subdivides the stage IB and IIA categories according to size greater or less than 4 cm (Table 101.2), specific information about clinical tumor diameter remains an important prognostic indicator even within these stage categories (Fig. 101.3).[70] Although FIGO stage is correlated with outcome, assessment by clinical examination tends to be inaccurate, and operative findings often do not agree with clinical estimates of parametrial or pelvic wall involvement.[71,72] Furthermore, some authors have found that the predictive power of stage diminishes or is lost when comparisons are corrected for differences in clinical tumor diameter.[70,73]

Lymph node metastasis is one of the most important predictors of prognosis. In the past, survival rates for patients

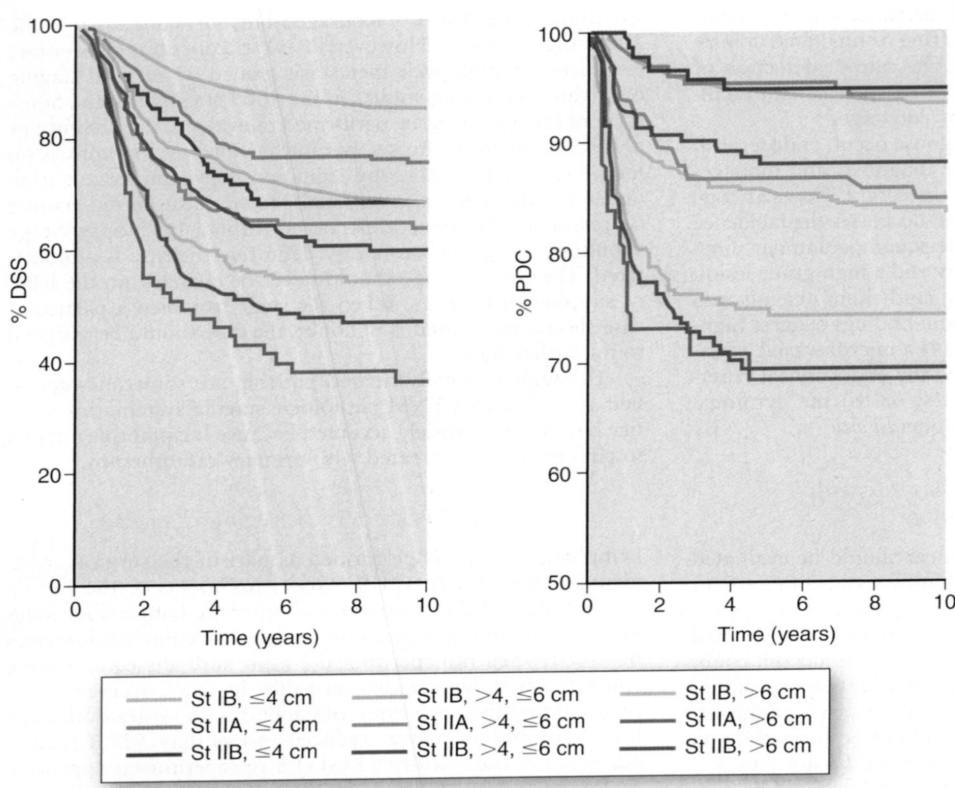

FIGURE 101.3 Disease-specific survival (DSS) and pelvic disease control (PDC) rates for 4,490 patients with stage I or II carcinomas of the cervix divided according to clinical tumor diameter and International Federation of Gynecology and Obstetrics (1988) stage. (From ref. 70, with permission.)

treated with radical hysterectomy with or without postoperative radiotherapy for stage IB disease were usually reported as 85% to 95% for patients with negative nodes and 45% to 55% for those with lymph node metastases.[74,75] However, a randomized trial reported by Peters et al.[76] in 2000 demonstrated that administration of chemotherapy concurrent with and following radical hysterectomy significantly improved the outcome of patients with high-risk disease features; in that trial, the 4-year survival rate was 81% for those in the chemoradiation arm, 87% of whom had positive lymph nodes discovered at hysterectomy.

Survival has also been correlated with the size of the largest lymph node and with the number of involved pelvic lymph nodes.[75,77,78] Survival rates for patients with positive para-aortic nodes treated with extended-field radiotherapy range from 10% to 50% depending on the extent of pelvic disease and para-aortic lymph node involvement.

For patients treated with radical hysterectomy, other histologic parameters that have been associated with a poor prognosis are LVSI, deep stromal invasion (10 or more mm or more than 70% invasion), and parametrial extension.[78–83] Roman et al.[81] reported a correlation between the percentage of histopathologic sections containing LVSI and the incidence of lymph node metastases. Uterine-body involvement has been associated with an increased rate of distant metastases.[84] A strong inflammatory response in the cervical stroma tends to predict a good outcome.[85]

Although some investigators have reported no difference in outcome between patients with squamous carcinomas and those with adenocarcinomas of the cervix, most investigators have concluded that adenocarcinomas confer a poorer prognosis.[86–95] The evidence for a poorer prognosis is particularly strong for patients whose tumors are stage IB2 or greater. In a multivariate analysis of 1,767 patients treated with radiation for stage IB disease, Eifel et al.[88] found that the relative risk of death from cancer for 106 patients with adenocarcinomas 4 cm or more in diameter was 1.9 times that for patients with squamous tumors of the same size ($P < .01$). Pelvic disease control rates were not correlated with histology, but the incidence of distant metastases was significantly higher in patients with adenocarcinomas. For patients with adenocarcinoma of the cervix, outcome appears to be correlated with the degree of tumor differentiation.[86,87,90]

In patients with squamous carcinomas, the serum concentration of squamous cell carcinoma antigen appears to correlate with stage and tumor size, the presence of lymph node metastases, and the presence of recurrent disease; however, the value of this antigen as an independent predictor of prognosis and the cost-effectiveness of measurement of this antigen as a screening modality have been disputed.[96,97]

Many studies have demonstrated a relationship between hemoglobin level and prognosis in patients with locally advanced cervical cancer, although the independent influence of hemoglobin on outcome can be difficult to estimate because of numerous confounding prognostic factors.[98] The strongest evidence that anemia plays a causative role in pelvic recurrence comes from a small 1978 randomized study conducted at the Princess Margaret Hospital; in that study, anemic patients who were transfused to a hemoglobin level of at least 12.5 g/dL had a lower rate of locoregional recurrence than those who were maintained at a hemoglobin level of at least 10 g/dL.[99] Studies aimed at overcoming the theoretical radiobiologic consequences of intratumoral hypoxia with hypoxic cell sensitizers,[100,101] hyperbaric oxygen breathing,[102] or neutron therapy[103] have not been successful. Several investigators have correlated low intratumoral oxygen tension levels with a high rate of regional and distant metastasis and poor survival.[104,105] A recent GOG study designed to test the value of erythropoietin-induced hemoglobin elevation was closed early because of erythropoietin-related thrombotic events; however, overall survival rates of 74% and 60%, respectively, for patients receiving chemoradiation alone or with erythropoietin were not encouraging.[106]

Other clinical and biologic features that have been investigated for their predictive power, with variable results, include patient age,[75,107] peritoneal cytology,[108] platelet count,[109] tumor vascularity,[110] DNA ploidy or S phase,[111] cyclooxygenase-2 expression,[112] and growth factor receptor expression.[113,114] Several investigators have found the presence of HPV DNA in histologically cancer-free lymph nodes to be correlated with poor outcome.[115,116]

Treatment

A number of factors may influence the choice of local treatment for cervical cancer, including tumor size, stage, histologic features, evidence of lymph node metastasis, risk factors for complications of surgery or radiotherapy, and patient preference. However, as a rule, HSILs are managed with a loop electroexcision procedure (LEEP); microinvasive cancers invading less than 3 mm (stage IA1) are managed with conservative surgery (excisional conization or extrafascial hysterectomy); early invasive cancers (stage IA2 and IB1 and some small stage IIA tumors) are managed with radical or modified radical hysterectomy, radical trachelectomy (if fertility preservation is desired), or radiotherapy; and locally advanced cancers (stages IB2 through IVA) are managed with combined chemotherapy and radiotherapy. Selected patients with centrally recurrent disease after maximum radiotherapy may be treated with radical exenterative surgery; isolated pelvic recurrence after hysterectomy is treated with irradiation.

Preinvasive Disease

LEEP is the preferred treatment for HSIL.[117] With this technique, a charged electrode is used to excise the entire transformation zone and distal canal. Although control rates are similar to those achieved with cryotherapy or laser ablation, LEEP is more easily learned, is less expensive than laser ablation, and preserves the excised lesion and transformation zone for histologic evaluation.[117,118] LEEP is an outpatient procedure that preserves fertility. LEEP conization or excisional conization with a scalpel should be performed when microinvasive or invasive cancer is suspected and in patients with adenocarcinoma *in situ*. Although recurrence rates are low (1% to 5%) and progression to invasion rare (less than 1% in most series), patients treated with LEEP require careful post-LEEP surveillance.

Treatment with total hysterectomy currently is reserved for women who have other gynecologic conditions that justify the procedure; invasive cancer still must be excluded before surgery to rule out the need for a more extensive operative procedure.

Microinvasive Carcinoma (Stage IA)

The standard treatment for patients with stage IA1 disease is cervical conization or total (type I) hysterectomy. Because the risk of pelvic lymph node metastases from these minimally invasive tumors is less than 1%,[79,119] pelvic lymphadenectomy is not usually recommended.

Patients who have FIGO stage IA1 disease without LVSI and who wish to maintain fertility may be adequately treated with a therapeutic cervical conization if the margins of the cone are negative. Although reports suggest that recurrences are infrequent,[120,121] patients who have this conservative treatment must be followed very closely with periodic cytologic evaluation, colposcopy, and endocervical curettage.

The likelihood of residual invasive disease after cone biopsy is correlated with the status of the internal cone margin and the results of an endocervical curettage performed after cone biopsy.[122,123] Roman et al.[123] reported the surgical findings in 87 patients who underwent a conization that showed microinvasive squamous carcinoma, followed by either a repeat conization or hysterectomy. Residual invasive disease was present in only 4% of patients whose cone margins were free of CIN and who had no disease detected on endocervical curettage. However, residual invasive disease was present in 13% of women who had either CIN in cone margins or positive endocervical curettage findings and 33% of women who had both of these features ($P < .015$), suggesting the need for a second procedure in any patient who has one of these findings. The authors did not find any correlation between the depth of invasion or the number of invasive foci and residual invasive disease.

Therapeutic conization for microinvasive disease is usually performed with a scalpel while the patient is under general or spinal anesthesia. Because an accurate assessment of the maximum depth of invasion is critical, the entire specimen must be sectioned and carefully handled to maintain its original orientation for microscopic assessment. Complications occur in 2% to 12% of patients, are related to the depth of the cone, and include hemorrhage, sepsis, infertility, stenosis, and cervical incompetence.[124] The width and depth of the cone should be tailored to produce the least amount of injury while providing clear surgical margins.

For patients whose tumors invade 3 to 5 mm into the stroma (FIGO stage IA2), the risk of nodal metastases is approximately 5%.[33,80,119] Therefore, in such patients, bilateral pelvic lymphadenectomy should be performed in conjunction with modified radical (type II) hysterectomy. Modified radical hysterectomy is a less extensive procedure than classic radical (type III) hysterectomy (Fig. 101.4). The uterus, cervix, upper vagina, and paracervical tissues are removed after careful dissection of the ureters to the point of their entry to the bladder. The medial halves of the cardinal ligament and the uterosacral ligaments are also removed. With this treatment, significant urinary tract complications are rare, and cure rates exceed 95%.[125]

Although surgical treatment is standard for *in situ* and microinvasive cancer, patients with severe medical problems or other contraindications to surgical treatment can be successfully treated with radiotherapy. Depending on the depth of invasion, these early lesions are treated with brachytherapy alone or brachytherapy combined with external-beam irradiation, and cure rates exceed 95%.[126,127]

Stage IB and IIA Disease

Early-stage IB cervical carcinomas can be treated effectively with combined external-beam irradiation and brachytherapy or with radical hysterectomy and bilateral pelvic lymphadenectomy. The goal of both treatments is to destroy malignant cells in the cervix, paracervical tissues, and regional lymph nodes. Patients who are treated with radical hysterectomy whose tumors are found to have high-risk disease features may benefit from postoperative radiotherapy or chemoradiation.[76,128]

Disease-specific survival rates for patients with stage IB cervical cancer treated with surgery or radiation usually range between 80% and 90%, suggesting that the two treatments are equally effective.[71,129–131] However, biases introduced by patient selection, variations in the definition of stage IA disease, and variable indications for postoperative radiotherapy, concurrent chemotherapy, or adjuvant hysterectomy confound comparisons of efficacy between radiotherapy and surgery. Because young women with small, clinically node negative tumors tend to be favored candidates for surgery and because tumor diameter and nodal status are inconsistently described in published series, it is difficult to compare the results reported for patients treated with surgery and those treated with radiotherapy.

In 1997, Landoni et al.[132] reported results from the only prospective trial comparing radical surgery with radiotherapy alone for cervical cancer. In their study, 343 patients with stage IB or IIA disease were randomly assigned to treatment with radical (type III) hysterectomy or a combination of external-beam and

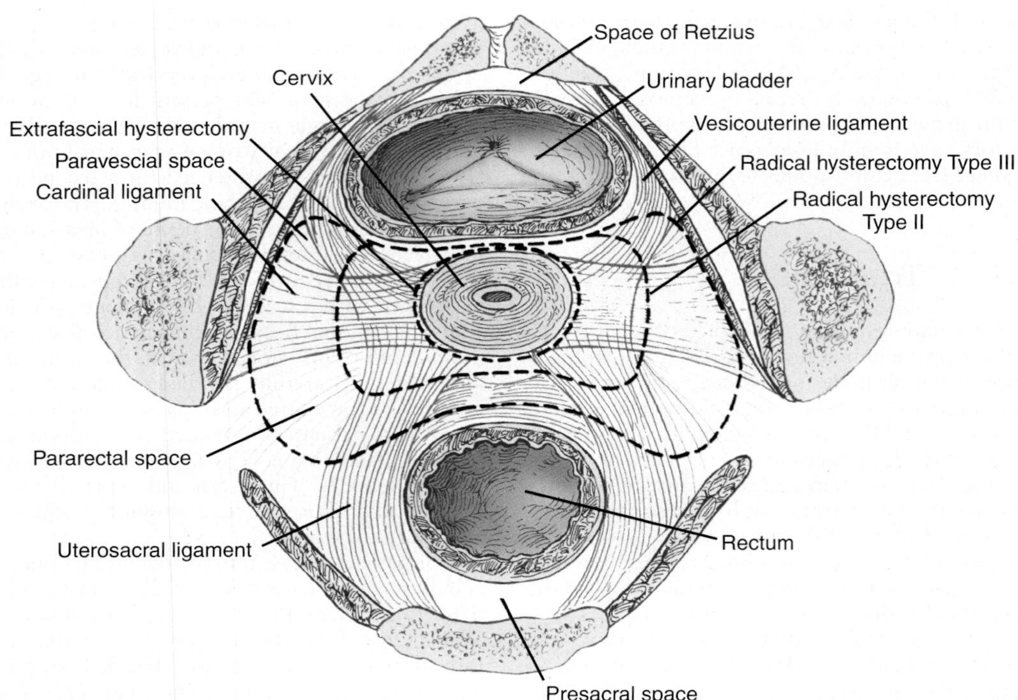

FIGURE 101.4 The pelvic ligaments and spaces. *Dotted lines* indicate the tissues removed with a modified radical (type II) or radical (type III) hysterectomy. (From ref. 354, with permission.)

low-dose-rate (LDR) intracavitary brachytherapy. In the surgery arm, findings of parametrial involvement, positive margins, deep stromal invasion, or positive nodes led to the use of postoperative pelvic irradiation in 54% of patients with tumors 4 cm or smaller in diameter and in 84% of patients with larger tumors. Patients in the radiotherapy arm received a relatively low median dose to point A of 76 Gy. With a median follow-up of 87 months, the 5-year actuarial disease-free survival rates for patients in the surgery and radiotherapy groups were 80% and 82%, respectively, for patients with tumors that were 4 cm or smaller and 63% and 57%, respectively, for patients with larger tumors. The authors reported a significantly higher rate of complications in the patients treated with initial surgery, and they attributed this finding to the frequent use of combined-modality treatment in this group.

For patients with stage IB1 squamous carcinomas, the choice of treatment is based primarily on patient preference, anesthetic and surgical risks, physician preference, and an understanding of the nature and incidence of complications with hysterectomy and radiotherapy. For patients with similar tumors, the overall rate of major complications is similar with surgery and radiotherapy, although urinary tract complications tend to be more common after surgical treatment and bowel complications are more common after radiotherapy. Surgical treatment tends to be preferred for young women with small tumors because it permits preservation of ovarian function and may cause less vaginal shortening. Radiotherapy is often selected for older, postmenopausal women to avoid the morbidity of a major surgical procedure.

For patients with stage IB2 (bulky) tumors, some surgeons have advocated the use of radical hysterectomy as initial treatment.[133–135] However, patients who have tumors measuring more than 4 cm in diameter usually have deep stromal invasion and are at high risk for lymph node involvement and parametrial extension. Because patients with these risk factors have an increased rate of pelvic disease recurrence, surgical treatment is usually followed by postoperative irradiation or chemoradiation, increasing the overall length of treatment and side effects of treatment. Consequently, many gynecologic and radiation oncologists believe that patients with stage IB2 carcinomas are better treated with primary chemoradiation.

Two prospective randomized trials[136,137] demonstrated that patients who are treated with radiation for bulky stage I cancers benefit from concurrent administration of cisplatin-containing chemotherapy. A third study suggested that patients who require postoperative radiotherapy because of findings of lymph node metastasis or involved surgical margins also benefit from concurrent chemoradiation.[76] Patients who have stage IB1 cancers without evidence of regional involvement have excellent pelvic control rates with radiotherapy alone (about 97% at 5 years) and probably do not require chemotherapy when they are treated with primary radiotherapy.[130,131]

Radical and Modified Radical Hysterectomy. The standard surgical treatment for stage IB and IIA cervical carcinomas is radical (type III) hysterectomy and bilateral pelvic lymphadenectomy. This procedure involves *en bloc* removal of the uterus, cervix, and paracervical, parametrial, and paravaginal tissues to the pelvic sidewalls bilaterally, with removal of as much of the uterosacral ligaments as possible (Fig. 101.4). The uterine vessels are ligated at their origin, and the proximal third of the vagina and the paracolpium are resected. Modified radical (type II) hysterectomy may be used for IA2 and selected small (<2 cm in diameter) stage IB lesions; with this procedure, the parametrial and paracervical tissue is removed medial to the ureter, the uterosacral ligaments are partially resected, and only the proximal 1 to 2 cm of the vagina are removed. The decision whether or not to remove the ovaries should be individualized and based on the patient's age, menopausal status, and other factors. Ovarian metastases are rare in the absence of metastases to lymph nodes or other sites. If intraoperative findings suggest a need for postoperative pelvic irradiation, the ovaries may be transposed out of the pelvis.

Radical hysterectomy is increasingly being performed using a laparoscopic approach with or without robotic assistance.[138–140] In experienced hands, these methods may result in reduced blood loss and quicker postoperative recovery times, although operative times may be somewhat longer. Preliminary results suggest that outcomes of laparoscopic radical hysterectomy are similar to those achieved with radical hysterectomy performed using the traditional abdominal approach.

Intraoperative and immediate postoperative complications of radical abdominal hysterectomy include blood loss, ureterovaginal fistula (1% to 2% of patients), vesicovaginal fistula (<1%), pulmonary embolus (1% to 2%), small bowel obstruction (1% to 2%), and postoperative fever secondary to deep vein thrombosis, pulmonary infection, pelvic cellulitis, urinary tract infection, or wound infection (25% to 50%).[141] Subacute complications include lymphocyst formation and lower extremity edema, the risk of which is related to the extent of the node dissection.[142] Lymphocysts may obstruct a ureter, but hydronephrosis usually improves with drainage of the lymphocyst.[143] The risk of complications, particularly small bowel obstruction, may be increased in patients who undergo preoperative or postoperative irradiation.[132]

Most patients have transient decreased bladder sensation after radical hysterectomy. Severe long-term bladder complications are infrequent and are related to the extent of the parametrial and paravaginal dissection but not to the type of surgical approach (abdominal or laparoscopic).[144,145] Even with careful postoperative bladder drainage, chronic bladder hypotonia or atony occurs in approximately 3% to 5% of patients.[144,146,147] Radical hysterectomy may be complicated by stress incontinence, but reported incidences vary widely and may be influenced by the addition of postoperative radiotherapy.[146,147] Patients may also experience constipation and, rarely, chronic obstipation after radical hysterectomy.

Radical Trachelectomy. In 1994, Dargent et al.[148] pioneered the use of radical trachelectomy and laparoscopic pelvic lymphadenectomy as a means of sparing fertility in young women with early cervical cancer. Since then, it has been demonstrated that when these procedures are performed by experienced surgeons, the cure rates are high and many women are able to carry subsequent pregnancies to viability.[149] Successful pregnancies have also been reported after radical abdominal trachelectomy.[150] In order to keep the residual uterine segment intact, a nonabsorbable cervical cerclage is placed around the uterine isthmus at the time of the trachelectomy. Alexander-Sefre et al.[151] reported that radical trachelectomy was associated with shorter operative times and hospital stays, less blood loss, and a lower incidence of bladder hypotony than radical hysterectomy. However, patients who had radical trachelectomy had more problems with dysmenorrhea, irregular menstruation, and vaginal discharge; in addition, 14% had cervical suture problems, 10% had isthmic stenosis, and 7% had prolonged amenorrhea.

The use of radical vaginal or abdominal trachelectomy and laparoscopic lymphadenectomy may be indicated in carefully selected women with small IB1 (≤2 cm) lesions who are eager to preserve fertility. Patients with extensive endocervical extension are poor candidates for fertility-sparing surgery. Preoperative MRI is a relatively sensitive and specific method to evaluate the possibility of tumor extension beyond the internal os.[152] A recent review of 504 women who underwent radical trachelectomy summarized the outcome of 200 pregnancies.[153] Although 84 of 200 pregnancies (42%) produced full-term viable infants, 37% of third-trimester deliveries were preterm, indicating that these women are at high risk for complicated pregnancies.

Radiotherapy After Radical Hysterectomy. Retrospective and prospective studies clearly demonstrate that irradiation decreases the risk of pelvic recurrence after radical hysterectomy in patients with high-risk disease features (lymph node metastasis, deep stromal invasion, positive or close operative margins, or parametrial involvement).[128,154] However, because the patients who received postoperative radiotherapy in most studies were selected because they had high-risk features, it has been difficult to determine the impact of adjuvant irradiation on survival.

GOG-92, a randomized trial first reported in 1999 and updated in 2006,[128,154] tested the benefit of adjuvant pelvic irradiation in patients with an intermediate risk of recurrence after radical hysterectomy for stage IB carcinoma. Patients were eligible for this study if they had at least two of the following risk factors: greater than one-third stromal invasion, LVSI, or clinical tumor diameter of at least 4 cm. Patients with involvement of the pelvic lymph nodes, parametria, or surgical margins were excluded. Patients who received adjuvant radiotherapy experienced a 46% reduction in the risk of recurrence ($P = .007$). Although there was a 30% reduction in the risk of death for patients who received radiotherapy, this difference was not statistically significant ($P = .07$). A subset analysis suggested that the benefit of postoperative radiotherapy was particularly striking for patients who had adenocarcinomas or adenosquamous carcinomas.[128,154]

Although pelvic irradiation reduces the risk of recurrence for patients with pelvic lymph node metastases or parametrial involvement, the risk of pelvic and distant recurrence remains high for these women after radiotherapy. In an attempt to improve the results of combined-modality treatment, the Southwest Oncology Group conducted a prospective trial comparing postoperative pelvic radiotherapy alone versus administration of cisplatin and 5-fluorouracil (5-FU) during and after postoperative pelvic radiotherapy for patients with lymph node metastases, parametrial involvement, or involved surgical margins. Initial results of this trial, published in 2000, demonstrated significantly improved rates of pelvic disease control and survival for patients who received chemotherapy (Table 101.3).[76]

The use of adjuvant radiotherapy undoubtedly increases the rate of posttreatment small bowel and genitourinary complications in patients who have had radical hysterectomy; however, inconsistencies in the methods of analysis, selection biases, and the relatively small number of patients in most series make studies of this subject difficult to interpret.[132,154,155]

Radical Radiotherapy. Radiotherapy alone also achieves excellent survival and pelvic disease control rates in patients with stage IB cervical cancer.[70,130,156] Eifel et al.[130] reported 5-year disease-specific survival and pelvic control rates of 90% and 98%, respectively, for 701 patients treated with radiation alone for stage IB1 disease. Although outcomes are poorer for patients with larger tumors, even these are frequently curable with a combination of external-beam irradiation and brachytherapy. However, patients with stage IB2 and bulky stage IIA cancers are usually treated with concurrent cisplatin-based chemoradiation, which has been demonstrated in randomized trials to yield better outcomes than radiotherapy alone.[137,157]

As with radical surgery, the goal of radical radiotherapy is to sterilize disease in the cervix, paracervical tissues, and regional lymph nodes in the pelvis. Patients are usually treated with a combination of external-beam irradiation to the pelvis and brachytherapy. Even relatively small tumors that involve multiple quadrants of the cervix are usually treated with total doses of 80 to 85 Gy to point A. The dose may be reduced by 5% to 10% for very small superficial tumors. Although patients with small tumors may be treated with somewhat smaller fields than patients with more advanced locoregional disease, care must still be taken to adequately cover the obturator, external iliac, low common iliac, and presacral nodes. Radiation technique, which is similar for patients who have bulky stage I or

TABLE 101.3

PROSPECTIVE RANDOMIZED TRIALS THAT INVESTIGATED THE ROLE OF CONCURRENT RADIOTHERAPY AND CHEMOTHERAPY FOR PATIENTS WITH LOCOREGIONALLY ADVANCED CERVICAL CANCER

Study (Ref.)	Protocol Designation	No. of Patients	Eligibility	Chemotherapy in Investigational Arm	Chemotherapy in Control Arm	Relative Risk of Recurrence (95% CI)	*P* Value
Rose et al. (208)	GOG-120	526	FIGO IIB–IVA, PA nodes negative (dissection)	Cisplatin 40 mg/m^2 (wk 1–6)	Hydroxyurea 3 g/m^2 (twice weekly, wk 1–6)	0.57 (0.42–0.78)	<.001
				Cisplatin 50 mg/m^2 (days 1 and 29) 5-FU 4 g/m^2 (96-hr infusion days 1, 29)	Hydroxyurea 3 g/m^2 (twice weekly, wk 1–6)	0.55 (0.40–0.75)	<.001
				Hydroxyurea 2 g/m^2 (twice weekly, wk 1–6)			
Eifel (214)	RTOG 90-01	403	FIGO IB–IIA (≥5 cm), IIB–IVA, or pelvic lymph nodes positive PA nodes negative (dissection or lymphangiogram)	Cisplatin 75 mg/m^2 (days 1 and 22 and with second brachytherapy) 5-FU 4 g/m^2 (96-hr infusion days 1 and 22 and with second brachytherapy)	None[a]	0.51 (0.36–0.66)	<.001
Keys et al. (137)	GOG-123	369	FIGO IB (≥4 cm) PA nodes negative (CT or lymphangiogram)	Cisplatin 40 mg/m^2 (wk 1–6)[b]	None[b]	0.51 (0.34–0.75)	.001
Whitney et al. (212)	GOG-85	368	FIGO IIB–IVA, PA nodes negative (dissection)	Cisplatin 50 mg/m^2 days 1 and 29) 5-FU 4 g/m^2 (96-hr infusion days 1 and 29)	Hydroxyurea 80 mg/kg (twice weekly during external-beam radiotherapy)	0.79 (0.62–0.99)	.03
Peters et al. (76)	SWOG 87–97	268	FIGO I–IIA after radical hysterectomy with findings of pelvic lymph node metastases and/or positive margins and/or parametrial involvement PA nodes negative	Cisplatin 70 mg/m^2 5-FU 4 g/m^2 (96-hr infusion) Every 21 days for 4 cycles beginning on day 1 of radiation therapy	None	0.50 (0.29–0.84)	.01
Pearcey et al. (215)	NCI Canada	259	FIGO IB–IIA (≥5 cm), IIB–IVA, or pelvic lymph nodes positive	Cisplatin 40 mg/m^2 (wk 1–6)	None	0.91 (0.62–1.35)	.33
Wong et al. (218)		220	FIGO IB–IIA (>4 cm), IIB–III	Epirubicin 60 mg/m^2 then 90 mg/m^2 every 4 wk for five more cycles[c]	None	Not stated	.02
Thomas et al. (216)		234	FIGO IB–IIA (≥5 cm), IIB–IVA	5-FU 4 g/m^2/96 hr × 2	None[d]	Not stated	Not significant
Lorvidhaya et al. (219)		926	FIGO IIB–IVA	Mitomycin 10 mg/m^2 and oral 5-FU 300 mg/m^2/d × 14 days (2 cycles); ± adjuvant 5-FU	None or adjuvant 5-FU only	Not stated	.0001
Lanciano et al. (217)	GOG-165	316	FIGO IIB–IVA	5-FU 225 mg/m^2/d for 5 days per week (protracted venous infusion)	Cisplatin 40 mg/m^2 (wk 1–6)	1.29 (0.93–1.8)	Not stated

CI, confidence interval; GOG, Gynecologic Oncology Group; FIGO, International Federation of Gynecology and Obstetrics; PA, para-aortic; 5-FU, 5-fluorouracil; RTOG, Radiation Therapy Oncology Group; CT, computed tomography; SWOG, Southwest Oncology Group.

[a]Patients in the control arm had prophylactic para-aortic irradiation.

[b]All patients had extrafascial hysterectomy after radiotherapy.

[c]Chemotherapy was begun on day 1 and continued every 4 weeks during and after radiotherapy.

[d]Patients were also randomly assigned to receive standard or hyperfractionated radiotherapy in a four-arm trial.

more advanced cancers, is discussed further in "Stage IIB, III, and IVA Disease."

Irradiation Followed by Hysterectomy. Although early studies from M.D. Anderson Cancer Center suggested that local recurrence rates for patients with bulky stage IB cancers were decreased when radiotherapy was followed by adjuvant hysterectomy, subsequent retrospective studies were less convincing and suggested that selection bias may have been responsible for the observed differences.[158,159] In a study of 1,526 patients with stage IB squamous carcinomas, Eifel et al.[130] reported central tumor recurrence rates of less than 10% for tumors as large as 7 to 7.9 cm treated with radiation alone, suggesting that the margin for possible improvement with adjuvant hysterectomy is small.

In 2003, the GOG reported results of a prospective randomized trial of irradiation with or without adjuvant extrafascial hysterectomy in patients with stage IB tumors 4 cm or more in diameter[160]; the study demonstrated no significant improvement in the survival rate among patients who had adjuvant hysterectomy (relative risk of death, 0.89; 95% confidence interval [CI]: 0.65–1.21).

These results, combined with those of more recent studies demonstrating low pelvic recurrence rates after concurrent treatment with chemotherapy and radiation,[157] suggest that there is little role for routine treatment with adjuvant hysterectomy. However, adjuvant hysterectomy may still play a role in selected cases in which uterine fibroids or other anatomic variations limit the dose of radiation deliverable with brachytherapy and in patients who have involvement of the uterine fundus with cancer. In these cases, extrafascial (type I) hysterectomy is usually performed, in which the uterus, cervix, adjacent tissues, and a small cuff of the upper vagina in a plane outside the pubocervical fascia are removed. Radical hysterectomy is avoided after high-dose irradiation because of an increased risk of fistula and other complications.

Chemotherapy Followed by Radical Surgery. A number of researchers have investigated the use of neoadjuvant chemotherapy followed by radical hysterectomy to treat patients with bulky stage IB or stage II cervical carcinoma. Neoadjuvant regimens have usually included cisplatin and bleomycin plus one or two other drugs.

In an early trial of this approach, Sardi et al.[161] reported better projected 4-year disease-free survival rates when neoadjuvant chemotherapy was added to radical hysterectomy plus postoperative radiotherapy in patients whose tumors were larger than 4 cm. However, in a subsequent randomized trial,[162] the GOG reported no significant difference in recurrence rates (relative risk, 0.998) or death rates (relative risk, 1.008) for patients who did or did not receive neoadjuvant chemotherapy before radical hysterectomy. In their trial, patients who underwent hysterectomy were treated with postoperative irradiation if they had high-risk disease features; the proportion requiring postoperative irradiation was similar in the two arms (45% for those who did and 52% for those who did not receive neoadjuvant chemotherapy). Several trials have compared radiotherapy alone versus neoadjuvant chemotherapy followed by hysterectomy plus or minus postoperative radiotherapy with conflicting results.[163,164] However, these trials, conceived before 1999, did not include concurrent chemotherapy in the radiotherapy arms.

Ultimately, the cost and morbidity of triple-modality treatment can only be justified if it proves to be more effective than treatment with the current standard of concurrent chemotherapy and radiotherapy. Studies comparing these approaches are currently under way.

Stage IIB, III, and IVA Disease

Radiotherapy is the primary local treatment for most patients with locoregionally advanced cervical carcinoma. The success of radiotherapy depends on a careful balance between external-beam radiotherapy and brachytherapy, optimizing the dose to tumor and normal tissues and the overall duration of treatment. For patients treated with radiotherapy alone for stage IIB, IIIB, and IV disease, 5-year survival rates of 65% to 75%, 35% to 50%, and 15% to 20%, respectively, have been reported.[70,165–167] Results of major clinical trials reported at the end of the 1990s indicate that, barring medical contraindications, most patients with locally advanced tumors should also receive concurrent chemotherapy along with radiotherapy. With appropriate chemoradiotherapy, even patients with massive locoregional disease have a significant chance for cure.

External-beam irradiation is used to deliver a homogeneous dose to the primary cervical tumor and to potential sites of regional spread and may also improve the efficacy of subsequent intracavitary brachytherapy by shrinking bulky tumor and bringing it within the range of the high-dose portion of the brachytherapy dose distribution. To facilitate brachytherapy, patients with locally advanced disease usually begin with a course of external-beam treatment with concurrent chemotherapy. Subsequent brachytherapy exploits the inverse square law to deliver a high dose to the cervix and paracervical tissues while minimizing the dose to adjacent normal tissues.

Although intracavitary treatment may be delayed until pelvic irradiation has caused some initial tumor regression, breaks during or between external-beam and intracavitary therapy should be discouraged, and every effort should be made to complete the entire radiation treatment in less than 7 to 8 weeks. Several studies have suggested that treatment courses longer than 8 weeks are associated with decreased pelvic disease control and survival rates.[168–170]

External-Beam Radiotherapy Technique. High-energy photons (15 to 18 MV) are usually preferred for pelvic treatment because they spare superficial tissues that are unlikely to be involved with tumor. At these energies, the pelvis can be treated either with four fields (anterior, posterior, and lateral fields) or with anterior and posterior fields alone (Fig. 101.5). When high-energy beams are not available, four fields are usually used because less-penetrating 4- to 6-mV photons often deliver an unacceptably high dose to superficial tissues when only two fields are used.

CT simulation is recommended to confirm adequate coverage of the iliac lymph nodes. Information gained from radiologic studies such as MRI, CT, and positron emission tomography can improve estimates of disease extent and assist in localization of regional nodes and paracervical tissues that may contain microscopic disease. The caudad extent of disease can be determined by inserting radiopaque markers in the cervix or at the lowest extent of vaginal disease. Potential internal organ motion must be taken into account; prospective studies have revealed that the positions of the uterus and cervix can vary by as much as 4 cm from day to day.[171] For this reason, it is usually wise to cover the entire presacrococcygeal region when locally advanced cancers are treated.

Tumor response should be evaluated with periodic pelvic examinations. Some practitioners prefer to maximize the brachytherapy component of treatment and begin it as soon as the tumor has responded enough to permit a good placement of the brachytherapy applicators, delivering subsequent pelvic irradiation with a central shield. This technique may reduce the volume of normal tissue treated to a high dose but can also result in overdoses to medial structures such as the ureters or underdosage of posterior uterosacral disease.[172] For these reasons, many clinicians prefer to give an initial dose of 40 to 45 Gy to the whole pelvis, believing that the ability to deliver a homogeneous distribution to the entire region at risk for microscopic disease outweighs other considerations. External-beam doses of more than 40 to 45 Gy to the central pelvis

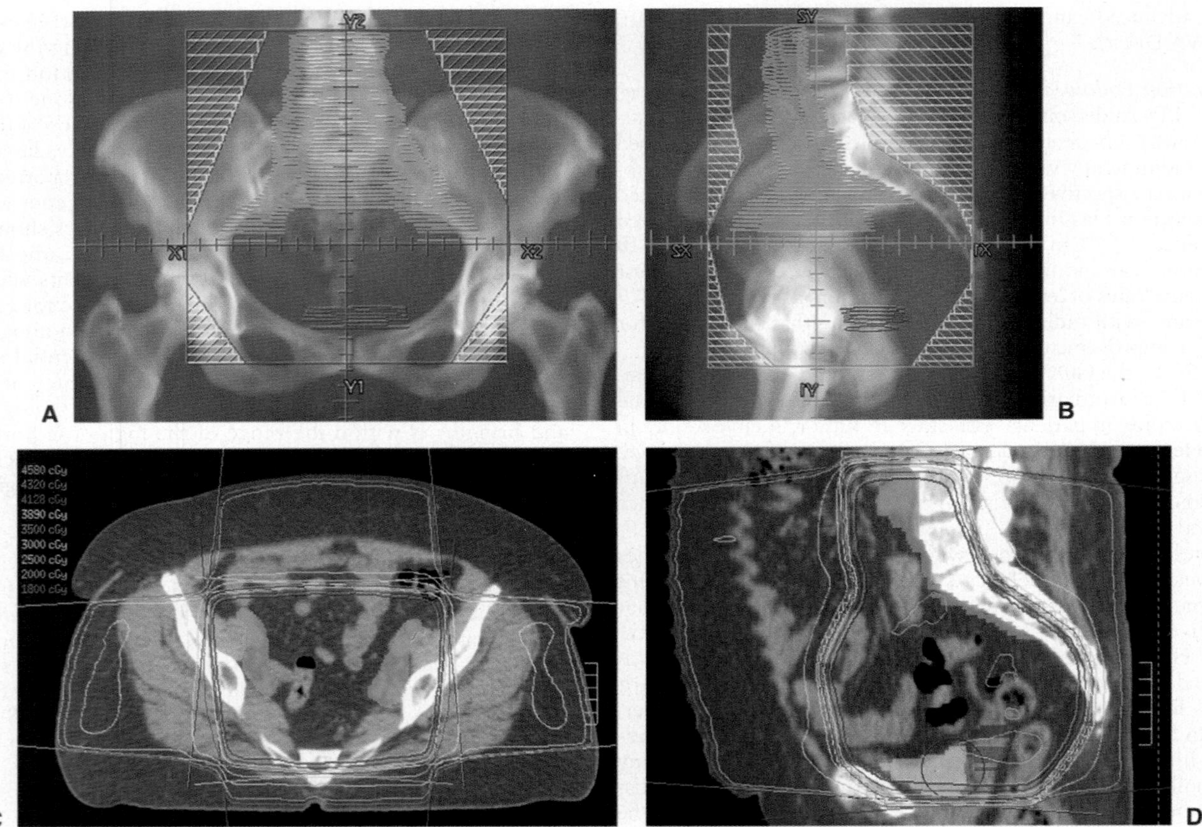

FIGURE 101.5 Typical anterior (**A**) and lateral (**B**) fields used to treat the pelvis with a four-field technique. When lateral fields are used to treat intact cervical cancers, particular care must be taken to adequately encompass the primary tumor and potential sites of regional spread in the radiation fields. Representative axial and sagittal dose distributions obtained with this technique are shown in panels **C** and **D**, respectively.

tend to compromise the dose deliverable to paracentral tissues and increase the risk of late complications.[167]

A total dose (external-beam and intracavitary) of 45 to 55 Gy appears to be sufficient to sterilize microscopic disease in the pelvic nodes in most patients. It is customary to treat lymph nodes known to contain gross disease and heavily involved parametria to a total dose of 60 to 65 Gy (including the contribution from brachytherapy treatments).

Intensity-Modulated Radiotherapy. There has been a recent surge of interest in possible applications of intensity-modulated radiotherapy (IMRT) and other forms of highly conformal radiotherapy in patients with gynecologic tumors.[173–175] Unlike standard two-field and four-field techniques, IMRT makes it possible to deliver a lower daily dose to the intrapelvic contents than to surrounding pelvic lymph nodes (Fig. 101.6). Some of the most intriguing uses of IMRT involve treatment of gross regional disease. With standard techniques, the close proximity of bowel has made it difficult to sterilize disease in nodes larger than 2 cm; IMRT allows delivery of doses exceeding 60 Gy to regional nodes with relative sparing of adjacent critical structures.

However, the highly conformal dose distributions achievable with IMRT also increase the potential for error and require considerable experience and attention to detail on the part of the radiation oncologist. In particular, great attention must be paid to the influence of internal organ motion and intratreatment tumor response on the doses to tumor and critical structures. Although some investigators have begun to explore the use of IMRT to treat patients with intact cervical cancers, large inter- and intratreatment variations in the position and size of the target volume raise serious concerns about the risk of missing tumor with these highly conforming treatments; if very ample margins are used to account for variability in the target, the gain relative to simpler treatments may not justify such complex treatment.[171,176] There is no evidence that IMRT can safely be used as an alternative to brachytherapy for routine treatment of intact cervical cancer. Although IMRT achieves very conformal dose distributions, it cannot accurately reproduce the high-dose gradients produced with intracavitary brachytherapy. More importantly, the large, unpredictable variations that occur in the positions of the bladder, rectum, and target mandate the use of large treatment margins that inevitably encompass adjacent critical structures and reduce the dose deliverable to tumor.

Role of Para-Aortic Irradiation. Two prospective randomized trials conducted during the 1980s addressed the role of prophylactic para-aortic irradiation in patients without known para-aortic node involvement.[177,178] In a Radiation Therapy Oncology Group study of 367 patients, Rotman et al.[179] demonstrated a significantly better survival rate for patients treated with extended fields than for those treated with standard pelvic radiotherapy (67% vs. 55% at 5 years; $P = .02$). A second trial, from the European Organization for Research and Treatment of Cancer,[177] involved a similar randomization but included patients with somewhat more advanced disease; in that study, 4-year disease-free survival rates for patients treated with pelvic radiotherapy and those treated with extended fields were not significantly different, although the rate of para-aortic node recurrence was significantly higher in the pelvic-field group. Both studies revealed an increased rate of enteric complications in patients treated with extended fields.

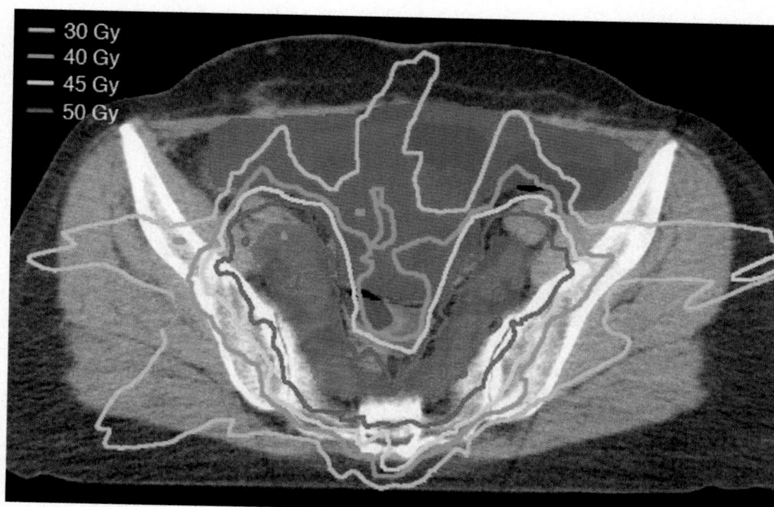

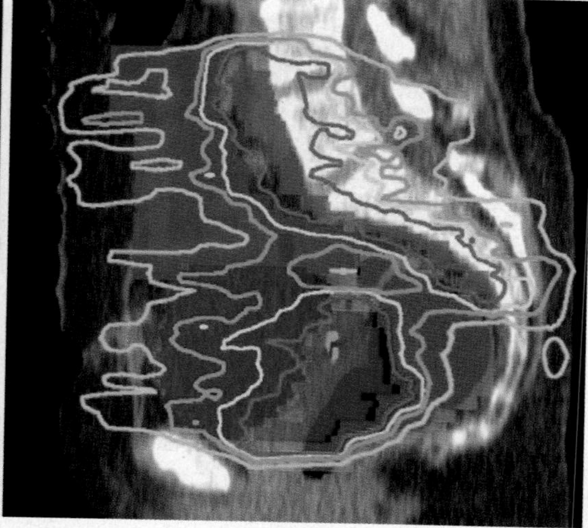

FIGURE 101.6 Axial and midline sagittal views of an intensity-modulated radiation therapy plan for postoperative pelvic radiotherapy in a patient who was at high risk for bowel complications because of a history of peritonitis. With this technique, the central pelvis was protected from receiving the highest doses of radiation; with a more standard two- or four-field technique, bowel in the central pelvis would have received the same dose as the clinical target volume (i.e., 50 Gy).

Numerous small series of patients with documented para-aortic node involvement suggest that 25% to 50% enjoy long-term survival after extended-field irradiation. Survival is correlated with the bulk of central disease and the extent and size of involved lymph nodes. Cunningham et al.[180] reported a 48% 5-year survival rate in patients who had para-aortic node involvement discovered at exploration for radical hysterectomy that was then aborted. This experience with patients who had relatively small primary disease demonstrates that extensive regional spread can occur without distant metastases and that patients with para-aortic node metastases can often be cured if their primary disease can be sterilized.

Although patients with extensive regional disease can often be cured if their locoregional disease can be sterilized, the side effects of extended-field radiotherapy, particularly when combined with concurrent chemotherapy,[181,182] are substantial. Clearly, the addition of concurrent chemotherapy to extended-field radiotherapy for many patients with locally advanced disease increases the importance of careful selection of patients for large-field irradiation. Although studies such as positron emission tomography and minimally invasive surgery add to the expense of treatment and are still infrequently performed in patients with locally advanced cervical cancer, these methods may provide better means of identifying patients with regional metastases who can benefit from extended regional irradiation.

Brachytherapy. Brachytherapy was first used to treat cervical cancers in the early 20th century and continues to play a central role in their curative management. The goal of brachytherapy is to deliver a high dose to disease in the cervix and paracervical tissues while preserving function of adjacent critical structures.

The uterine cavity provides an ideal receptacle for radioactive sources, which are positioned using specially designed applicator systems that capitalize on the distinctive anatomy of the distal female genital tract and the physical advantages of the inverse square law. Most applicator systems consist of an angled or curved intrauterine tandem with some form of intravaginal applicator; vaginal applicators used in various clinical settings include several versions of the Fletcher-Suit afterloading colpostats, vaginal rings, French molds, vaginal cylinders, and others.[183,184] Vaginal packing is used to hold the applicator in place and to maximize the distance between the sources and the bladder and rectum. Radiographs should be obtained at the time of insertion to verify accurate placement, and the system should be repositioned if radiographs indicate that positioning can be improved.

Treatments may be delivered over several days at a continuous LDR or with frequent pulses (pulsed dose rate; PDR); alternatively, treatment may be administered in several fractions of radiation delivered at a high dose rate (HDR). For LDR treatments, cesium-137 sources are usually loaded manually after applicator placement has been optimized. In contrast, the remote afterloading units commonly used for HDR or PDR treatments employ a single "stepping" source of iridium-192 (^{192}Ir) that travels through the applicator tubes, pausing for varying times in a series of "dwell" positions to deliver the desired dose to adjacent tissues. The activity of sources used for HDR is approximately 10 Ci; the activity of sources used for PDR is approximately 0.5 to 1 Ci. However, because a computer controls insertion of the source, exposure to personnel is negligible with these methods. Although the nominal dose of radiation needs to be adjusted for treatment delivered at different dose rates, the applicator systems and rules of optimal brachytherapy placement are similar for LDR, HDR, and PDR treatment. The importance of radiation dose rate and fraction size is discussed in more detail later in this section.

Brachytherapy dose. The paracentral dose from intracavitary brachytherapy is most frequently expressed at a single reference point, usually designated *point A*. Although point A has been specified in a number of different ways, the most widely accepted definition is a point 2 cm lateral to the cervical collar and 2 cm above the top of the colpostats, measured at their intersection with the tandem midpoint on the lateral radiograph (Fig. 101.7).[185] Point A usually lies approximately at the crossing of the ureter and the uterine artery, but it bears no consistent relationship to the tumor or target volume. Originally developed as part of the Manchester treatment system, point A was meant to be used in the context of a detailed set of rules governing the placement and loading of the intracavitary system and was intended to be used primarily as a means of reporting treatment intensity, not as the sole parameter for treatment prescription. Today, this context is often lost.

Other measures have been used to describe the intensity of intracavitary treatment. "Mg-hr" or "mgRaEq-hr" are proportional to the dose of radiation at relatively distant points from

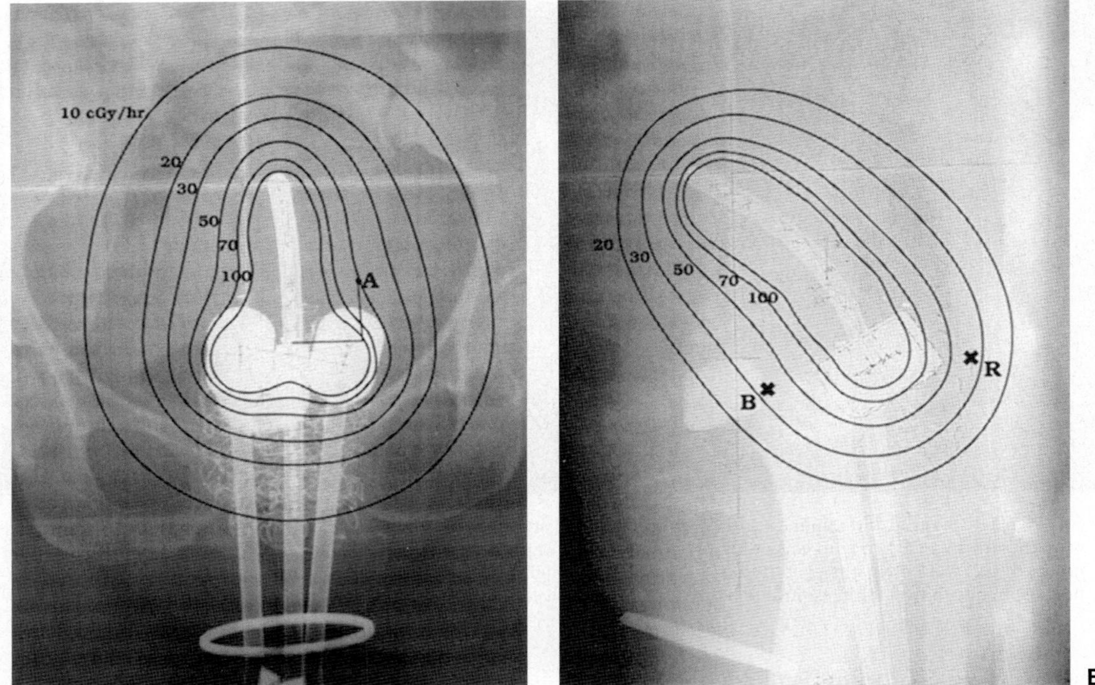

FIGURE 101.7 Posterior-anterior and lateral views of a Fletcher-Suit-Delclos applicator system in a patient with invasive carcinoma of the cervix. Units on the isodose contours are centigray per hour. A, point A; B, bladder reference point; R, rectal reference point.

the system and therefore give a sense of the dose to the whole pelvis. Total reference air kerma—expressed in micrograys at 1 meter—is an alternative measure that allows for the use of various radionuclides.[186] Reference points have also been used to estimate the doses to the bladder and rectum. Although normal tissue reference points provide useful information about the dose to a portion of normal tissue, volumetric studies have demonstrated that they consistently underestimate the maximum dose to normal tissue.[187] Recently, clinicians have increasingly begun to explore the use of volumetric image-guided dose specification for tumor and normal tissue doses.[188] Although the guidelines for these methods are not fully developed, the use of volumetric measurements promises to yield much more accurate information about the relationships between dose, treatment volume, and outcome than has been possible with traditional methods.

Whatever system of dose specification is used, emphasis should always be placed on optimizing the relationship between the intracavitary applicators and the cervical tumor and other pelvic tissues. Source strengths and positions should be carefully chosen to provide optimal tumor coverage without exceeding normal tissue tolerance limits. However, optimized source placement can rarely correct for a poorly positioned applicator.

A detailed description of the characteristics of an ideal intracavitary system and of the considerations that influence source strength and position are beyond the scope of this chapter but can be found elsewhere.[186,189] In brief, an effort should always be made to deliver a dose to point A of at least 85 Gy (with LDR brachytherapy) or its biologic equivalent (with HDR brachytherapy) for patients with bulky central disease. If the intracavitary placement has been optimized, this can usually be accomplished without exceeding a dose of 75 Gy to the bladder reference point or 70 Gy to the rectal reference point, doses that are usually associated with an acceptably low risk of major complications. The dose to the surface of the lateral wall of the apical vagina should not usually exceed 120 to 140 Gy. Suboptimal placements occasionally force compromises in the dose to tumor or normal tissues. To choose a treatment that optimizes the therapeutic ratio in these circumstances requires experience and a detailed understanding of factors that influence tumor control and normal tissue complications.

Brachytherapy dose rate. Traditionally, cervical brachytherapy has been performed with sources that yield a dose rate at point A of approximately 0.4 to 0.5 Gy/hr. These low dose rates permit repair of sublethal cellular injury with preferential sparing of normal tissues. In a randomized trial, Haie-Meder et al.[190] reported a significant increase in complications when the dose rate was doubled from 0.4 to 0.8 Gy/hr, indicating that the total dose must be reduced and the therapeutic ratio of treatment may be compromised with higher dose rates. Differences in the magnitude of the dose-rate effect between tumor and normal tissues may partly reflect differences in the half-times for repair of sublethal radiation damage.[191]

During the past 2 decades, computer technology has made it possible to deliver brachytherapy at very high dose rates (more than 1 Gy/min) using a high-activity ^{192}Ir source and remote afterloading.[184,192,193] Clinicians have found HDR brachytherapy attractive because it usually does not require that patients be hospitalized and may be more convenient for patients and physicians. However, unless it is heavily fractionated, HDR brachytherapy may lose the radiobiologic advantage of LDR treatment, potentially narrowing the therapeutic window for complication-free cure, particularly for patients with unfavorable anatomy.[194,195] Advocates of HDR treatment disagree about the number of fractions and total dose that should be delivered.[183,192] Published experiences suggest that survival rates are roughly similar to those achieved with traditional LDR treatment, although these experiences are difficult to compare because of the same potential problems of selection bias that confound other nonrandomized comparisons.[192,194] Prospective trials[196–198] suggest that LDR and HDR treatment produce similar results, but these trials have been criticized for methodologic flaws. However, logistical advantages, including increasingly scarce availability of cesium for LDR brachytherapy, have contributed to a steady increase in the proportion of patients treated using HDR techniques. Today, HDR brachytherapy is a widely used and accepted method of treatment for cervical cancer. HDR is probably similar to LDR brachytherapy in terms of therapeutic efficacy and side effects when the patient's anatomy permits displacement of the bladder, rectosigmoid, and other critical structures away from intrauterine and intravaginal radiation sources, making it possible to prevent exposure of these tissues to high fractional doses.

As with LDR treatment, successful HDR brachytherapy depends on optimized applicator position, balanced use of external-beam therapy and brachytherapy, compact overall treatment duration, and delivery of an adequate dose to tumor with respect for normal tissue tolerance limits.[199] The advent of image-guided treatment planning may contribute to further improvements in the safety of high-dose-per-fraction intracavitary brachytherapy by providing more realistic assessments of the fractional doses delivered to critical structures. New CT- or MRI-based volumetric treatment planning methods should permit more accurate delineation of target and normal tissues and improve optimization models, although the validity of these treatment planning methods can be determined only through careful analyses of outcome in treated patients.[188]

Interstitial brachytherapy. Several groups have advocated the use of interstitial brachytherapy for patients whose anatomy or tumor distribution makes it difficult to obtain an ideal intracavitary placement. Interstitial implants are usually placed transperineally, guided by a Lucite template that encourages parallel placement of hollow needles that penetrate the cervix and paracervical spaces; needles are usually loaded with ^{192}Ir. Advocates of the procedure describe the relatively homogeneous dose distribution achieved with this method, the ease of inserting implants in patients in whom the uterus is difficult to probe, and the ability to place sources directly into the parametrium. Authors of early reports were enthusiastic, describing high initial local control rates and encouraging projected survival rates.[200,201]

However, more mature survival results from these groups were disappointing. In a 1995 review of the combined experiences of Stanford University and the Joint Center for Radiation Therapy,[202] the 3-year disease-free survival rates for patients with stage IIB and IIIB disease were only 36% and 18%, respectively; local control rates were 22% and 44%, respectively; and the rate of complications requiring surgical intervention was high. A 1997 report from the University of California, Irvine, described 5-year survival rates of only 21% and 29%, respectively, for patients with stage IIB and IIIB disease, again with a high rate of major complications.

More recently, several groups have explored the use of laparoscopic or image-guided techniques to improve local control and complication rates with interstitial brachytherapy.[203,204] However, outside of an investigational setting, interstitial treatment of primary cervical cancers should probably be limited to patients who cannot accommodate intrauterine brachytherapy and patients with distal vaginal disease that requires a boost with interstitial brachytherapy.

Complications of Radical Radiotherapy. During pelvic radiotherapy, most patients have mild fatigue and mild-to-moderate diarrhea that usually is controllable with antidiarrheal medications; some patients have mild bladder irritation. When extended fields are treated, patients may have nausea, gastric irritation, and depression of peripheral blood cell counts. Hematologic and gastrointestinal complications are significantly increased in patients receiving concurrent chemotherapy. Unless the ovaries have been transposed, all premenopausal patients who receive pelvic radiotherapy experience ovarian failure by the completion of treatment.

Perioperative complications of intracavitary brachytherapy include uterine perforation, fever, and the usual risks of anesthesia. Thromboembolisms are rare. In a review of 4,043 patients who had 7,662 intracavitary applications for cervical cancer, Jhingran and Eifel[205] reported 11 patients (0.3%) with thromboembolisms, 4 of whom—all with pulmonary embolisms—died. All four fatal pulmonary embolisms were in patients with advanced pelvic wall disease.

Estimates of the risk of late complications of radical radiotherapy vary according to the grading system, duration of follow-up, method of calculation, treatment method, and prevalence of risk factors in the study population. However, most reports quote an overall risk of major complications (requiring transfusion, hospitalization, or surgical intervention) of 5% to 15%.[157,190,206–208] In a study of 1,784 patients with stage IB disease, Eifel et al.[206] reported an overall actuarial risk of major complications of 7.7% at 5 years. Although the actuarial risk was greatest during the first 3 years of follow-up, there was a continuing risk to surviving patients of approximately 0.3% per year, resulting in an overall actuarial risk of 14% at 20 years.

During the first 3 years after treatment, rectal complications are most common and include bleeding, stricture, ulceration, and fistula. In the study by Eifel et al.,[206] the risk of major rectosigmoid complications was 2.3% at 5 years. Major gastrointestinal complications were rare 3 years or more after treatment, but a constant low risk of urinary tract complications persisted for many years (Fig. 101.8). The actuarial risk of developing a fistula of any type was 1.7% at 5 years.

Small bowel obstruction is an infrequent complication of standard radiotherapy for patients without special risk factors. The risk of small bowel obstruction is increased dramatically in patients who have undergone transperitoneal lymph node dissection.[62,209] However, there appears to be little increase in risk if the operation is performed with a retroperitoneal approach.[62] Other factors that can increase the risk of small bowel complications in patients treated for cervical cancer

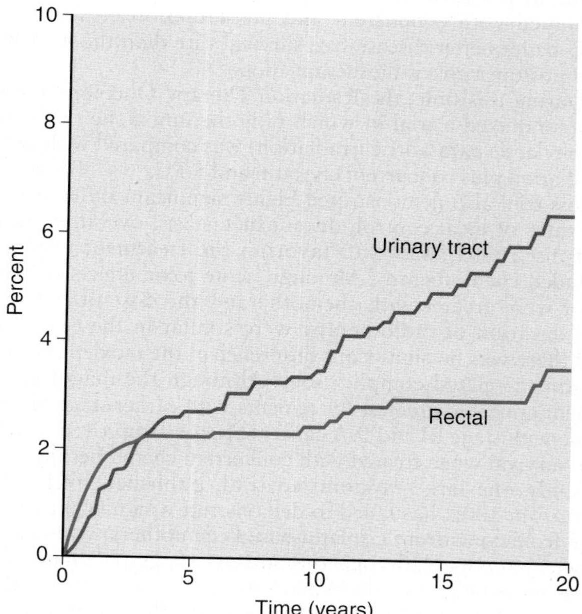

FIGURE 101.8 Rates of major rectal and urinary tract complications in 1,784 patients with stage IB carcinomas of the cervix treated with radiotherapy. Complication rates were calculated actuarially, and patients who died without experiencing a major complication were censored at the time of death. (From ref. 206, with permission.)

PRACTICE OF ONCOLOGY

include pelvic inflammatory disease, thin body habitus, heavy smoking, and the use of high doses or large volumes for external-beam irradiation, particularly with low-energy treatment beams and large daily fraction sizes.[209]

Most patients treated with radical radiotherapy have some agglutination and telangiectasia of the apical vagina. More significant vaginal shortening can occur, particularly in elderly, postmenopausal women and those with extensive tumors treated with a high dose of radiation.[206,210] Vaginal function can be optimized with appropriate estrogen support and vaginal dilatation.

Concurrent Chemoradiation. At the end of the 1990s, publication of a series of prospective randomized trials provided compelling evidence that the addition of concurrent cisplatin-containing chemotherapy to standard radiotherapy reduces the risk of disease recurrence by as much as 50% (Table 101.3).[76,137,157,208,211–213]

Some of the earliest trials of chemoradiation studied the concurrent use of hydroxyurea with radiation; although the validity of these small trials has since been questioned, encouraging results led to the use of hydroxyurea-containing regimens as controls in two subsequent GOG trials.[208,212,214] In these trials,[208,212] the GOG randomly assigned patients with stage IIB–IVA disease to receive either hydroxyurea or cisplatin-containing chemotherapy during external-beam irradiation. All three of the cisplatin-containing regimens produced local control and survival rates superior to those for the control arms (hydroxyurea and radiation). In a third study,[137] patients with stage IB tumors measuring at least 4 cm in diameter were randomly assigned to receive radiation alone or radiation plus weekly cisplatin before extrafascial hysterectomy. Patients who received cisplatin were more likely to have a complete histologic response and were more likely to be disease-free at the time of preliminary analysis. A fourth study, cosponsored by the Southwest Oncology Group and the GOG,[76] included patients who were treated with radical hysterectomy and were found to have pelvic lymph node metastases, positive margins, or parametrial involvement. In this study, patients who were randomly assigned to receive postoperative pelvic irradiation combined with concurrent and postradiation cisplatin and 5-FU had a better disease-free survival rate than those treated with postoperative radiotherapy alone.

During this time, the Radiation Therapy Oncology Group also conducted a trial in which radiotherapy alone (including prophylactic para-aortic irradiation) was compared with pelvic irradiation plus concurrent cisplatin and 5-FU.[157,211] The results of this trial also demonstrated highly significant differences in the rates of local control, distant metastasis, overall survival, and disease-free survival, favoring the treatment arm that included chemotherapy. Although acute toxic effects of treatment were greater with chemotherapy, the dose of radiation and duration of radiotherapy were similar in the two arms, and there was no significant difference in the incidence of late treatment-related complications. Although the magnitude of benefit appeared greatest for patients with earlier-stage disease, those with stage III and IVA cancers also had improved disease-free survival when treated with concurrent chemotherapy.[157,211]

Only one large randomized trial, published by Pearcey et al.[215] in 2002, has failed to demonstrate a significant advantage from concurrent cisplatin-based chemotherapy in cervical cancer patients. Although the authors suggested that differences in technique could explain the difference between their results and the results of the earlier trials, the survival rate in their control arm indicated that the margin for improvement was similar to that in the earlier trials. This trial also was the smallest of the six, resulting in relatively large confidence intervals, which may have contributed to the lack of significant difference between the treatment arms.

These studies raise interesting questions that will undoubtedly be the subjects of future studies. Of four different cisplatin-containing regimens, only two were compared directly. It is unclear from the results which regimen achieves the most favorable therapeutic ratio and whether the inclusion of 5-FU in several of the studies contributed importantly to the results. Although an early trial suggested that 5-FU delivered by protracted venous infusion with radiation might be of benefit,[216] a subsequent GOG trial showed no benefit of 5-FU over a control treatment of weekly cisplatin plus radiation.[217] Although North American studies have emphasized cisplatin-containing regimens, investigators in Southeast Asia have reported improved outcome when radiation was combined with epirubicin[218] or mitomycin and 5-FU.[219] Preliminary results of a recently reported phase 3 trial suggest that a regimen consisting of radiation with concurrent and adjuvant cisplatin and gemcitabine may have greater benefit than chemoradiation with weekly cisplatin alone; however, concerns have been raised about the toxicity of this regimen.[220] Other drugs that are being studied for their radiosensitizing effects in patients with advanced disease are paclitaxel,[221] carboplatin,[222] and several biologic response modifiers.

Taken together, the randomized trials provide strong evidence that the addition of concurrent chemotherapy to pelvic radiotherapy benefits selected patients with locoregionally advanced cervical cancer. A meta-analysis of randomized trials confirmed the benefit of concurrent chemoradiation, showing an advantage for both cisplatin- and non–cisplatin-containing regimens.[223] However, most trials have explicitly excluded patients with evidence of para-aortic lymph node metastases, poor performance status, or impaired renal function. In the future, clinicians will be challenged to determine whether favorable results can be generalized to patients with cervical cancer who differ from those included in the prospective trials because of serious medical or social problems. A large Canadian population-based study that demonstrated a significant improvement in survival of women with cervical cancer after the 1999 adoption of chemoradiation as a standard did indicate that the benefits of chemoradiation can be generalized beyond the trial setting.[224]

Neoadjuvant Chemotherapy with Radiotherapy. Although investigators were initially encouraged by high response rates of untreated cervical cancer to multiple-agent, cisplatin-containing chemotherapy regimens, these results have not translated to a clear advantage when neoadjuvant chemotherapy is given before radiotherapy. Of seven phase 3 trials of this approach, five[225–229] demonstrated no benefit from neoadjuvant therapy and two[230] demonstrated a significantly better survival rate with radiotherapy alone. Combinations of neoadjuvant followed by concurrent chemoradiotherapy have not yet been tested in large randomized trials. Such combinations should probably be avoided outside an investigational setting because neoadjuvant chemotherapy could compromise patients' tolerance of subsequent chemoradiation.

Stage IVB Disease

Patients who present with disease in distant organs are almost always incurable. The care of these patients must emphasize palliation of symptoms with use of appropriate pain medications and localized radiotherapy. Tumors may respond to chemotherapy, but responses are usually brief.

Single-Agent Chemotherapy. Cisplatin has been studied in a variety of doses and schedules in the management of recurrent or metastatic cervical cancer and is considered the most active agent against this malignancy.[231,232] Although a number of other agents (e.g., ifosfamide, carboplatin, irinotecan, and paclitaxel) have exhibited a modest level of biologic activity in cervical cancer (producing response rates of 10% to 15%),[233] the clinical utility of these drugs in patients who have not responded to cisplatin or who have experienced recurrence or progression after chemoradiation is uncertain. Further, it is well recognized that the objective rate of response to chemotherapy is lower in previously irradiated areas (e.g., pelvis) than in nonirradiated sites (e.g., lung).[234]

Combination Chemotherapy. Most reports of combination chemotherapy for carcinoma of the cervix have described small, uncontrolled phase 2 trials of drug combinations. The results of two phase 3 randomized trials, published in 2004 and 2005, have provided the first solid evidence that combination chemotherapy can improve both progression-free survival (cisplatin plus paclitaxel vs. single-agent cisplatin,[235] cisplatin plus topotecan vs. single-agent cisplatin [236]) and overall survival (cisplatin plus topotecan vs. single-agent cisplatin[236]) when it is administered for recurrent or metastatic carcinoma of the cervix. However, a recently reported phase 3 trial comparing combinations of cisplatin with either topotecan, paclitaxel, gemcitabine, or vinorelbine revealed no significant differences in outcome between patients treated with the four cisplatin-based regimens.[237]

Palliative Radiotherapy. Localized radiotherapy can provide effective relief of pain caused by metastases in bone, brain, lymph nodes, or other sites. A rapid course of pelvic radiotherapy can also provide excellent relief of pain and bleeding for patients who present with incurable disseminated disease.

Special Treatment Problems

Treatment of Locally Recurrent Carcinoma of the Cervix. Patients should be evaluated for possible recurrent disease if a new mass develops; if, in irradiated patients, the cervix remains bulky or nodular or cervical cytologic findings are abnormal 3 months or more after irradiation; or if symptoms of leg edema, pain, or bleeding develop after initial treatment. The diagnosis must be confirmed with a tissue biopsy, and the extent of disease should be evaluated with appropriate radiographic studies, cystoscopy, proctoscopy, and serum chemistry studies before treatment is administered.

After radical surgery. The treatment of choice for patients who have an isolated pelvic recurrence after initial treatment with radical hysterectomy alone is aggressive radiotherapy. Treatment using external-beam radiotherapy with or without brachytherapy is similar to that for patients with a primary carcinoma of the vagina. Pelvic wall recurrences are often treated with external-beam irradiation alone, although surgery and intraoperative radiotherapy may contribute to local control in selected patients.[238] Patients with vaginal recurrence usually have a better prognosis than those with pelvic wall recurrence. Ijaz et al.[239] reported a survival rate of 69% 5 years after radical radiotherapy for 16 patients who had isolated vaginal recurrences that did not involve the pelvic wall. Only 18% of patients who had recurrences that were fixed to the pelvic wall or that involved pelvic lymph nodes survived 5 years. Several authors have reported significantly lower rates of successful salvage therapy for patients with locally recurrent adenocarcinoma.[239,240] Thomas et al.[241] reported encouraging results in a group of patients with recurrent cervical carcinoma treated with radiation and concurrent chemotherapy, but further studies will be needed to determine whether this approach is superior to radiotherapy alone.

After definitive irradiation. Some patients who have an isolated central recurrence after radiotherapy can be cured with surgical treatment. Because the extent of disease may be difficult to evaluate and the risk of serious urinary tract complications of pelvic surgery is high after high-dose radiotherapy, surgical salvage treatment usually requires a pelvic exenteration, most often an anterior exenteration. Less extensive operations, such as radical hysterectomy, are reserved for selected patients with small tumors confined to the cervix or lesions that do not encroach on the rectum.[242,243]

In all cases, preparation for total pelvic exenteration must involve a detailed medical and imaging evaluation as well as careful counseling of the patient and family regarding the extent of surgery and postoperative expectations. Tumor involvement of the pelvic sidewall is a contraindication for exenteration but may be difficult to assess if there is extensive radiation fibrosis. Although advanced age may be a contraindication to pelvic exenteration, studies have suggested that, with careful selection, good outcomes can be achieved with pelvic exenteration even in women aged 65 years or older.[244]

The operation begins with a thorough inspection of the abdomen for evidence of intraperitoneal spread, lymph node metastases, or pelvic sidewall infiltration. Despite careful preoperative evaluation, about 30% of operations are aborted intraoperatively.[245] Frozen section biopsies are done of suspicious areas. If the biopsy findings are negative, the surgeon proceeds to remove the bladder, rectum, vagina, uterus, ovaries, fallopian tubes, and all other supporting tissues in the true pelvis. A urinary conduit, a transverse or sigmoid colostomy, and a neovagina are created.

Postoperative recuperation may take as long as 3 months. The surgical mortality rate is less than 10%, with most postoperative complications and deaths related to sepsis, pulmonary thromboembolism, and intestinal complications such as small bowel obstruction and fistula formation.[246,247] The rate of gastrointestinal complications may be reduced by using unirradiated segments of bowel and by closing pelvic floor defects with omentum, rectosigmoid colon, or myocutaneous flaps.[246] Advances in low colorectal anastomosis and techniques for creating continent urinary reservoirs have improved the quality of life for selected patients.[245,248]

Several investigators have studied the quality of patients' lives after surgical salvage treatment for recurrent cervical cancer.[245,249,250] In the first years after exenteration, patients' quality of life is heavily influenced by worries about the progression of tumor.[249] Most investigators report that the most common problems for survivors relate to their adjustment to urostomy or colostomy. Women with vaginal reconstruction tend to report fewer sexual problems and better quality of life than those without reconstruction.[245,249] However, vaginal dryness and discharge still may interfere with intercourse.[250] In a retrospective study of 75 exenterations, Berek et al.[245] found that the approach that produced the best outcome included the creation of a neovagina using a pedicled transverse rectus abdominis myocutaneous flap, the creation of a continent urinary conduit using a clonic (Miami) pouch, and the performance of a primary colon reanastomosis or the creation of a rectal J-pouch. All of these findings indicate the importance of adequate counseling following the exenterative surgery.

The 5-year survival rate for patients who undergo anterior pelvic exenteration is 33% to 60%; the 5-year survival rate for those who undergo total pelvic exenteration is 20% to 46%.[245,249,250]

For patients who have unresectable recurrent disease after definitive irradiation, treatment options are limited. Several groups are exploring the role of intraoperative irradiation in the treatment of selected patients with recurrent disease that involves the pelvic wall.[251] However, most patients who have unresectable pelvic recurrences after radiotherapy are treated with chemotherapy alone; response rates and prognosis are generally poor.

Treatment After Simple Hysterectomy that Reveals Unsuspected Invasive Cancer. Every patient who undergoes a planned hysterectomy should be carefully screened before the procedure to rule out invasive cervical cancer. When unexpected invasive cancer is detected in a hysterectomy specimen, the patient should be referred for consideration of additional treatment.[252] Patients with invasion of less than 3 mm without LVSI usually require no treatment after simple hysterectomy. However, patients with more extensive disease should undergo treatment of the paracolpal tissues and nodes.

Patients who have negative margins usually are treated with pelvic radiotherapy to 45 or 50 Gy. Most clinicians follow this with vaginal intracavitary brachytherapy, delivering an additional vaginal surface dose of 30 to 50 Gy. Patients with positive margins may benefit from a somewhat higher dose of external-beam irradiation through reduced fields designed to include the region at highest risk (e.g., parametria and posterior bladder wall).[252,253] In a report of the results of radiotherapy in 123 patients in whom hysterectomy revealed unsuspected invasive cancer, Roman et al.[252] reported 5-year survival rates of 79% for patients with negative margins and 59% for those with microscopically positive margins. In contrast, the 5-year survival rate for 30 patients with gross residual disease was only 41% (P = .0001). Results of studies of treatment for high-risk cervical cancer after radical hysterectomy suggest that concurrent treatment with chemotherapy and radiation should probably be considered for patients who have positive margins or gross residual disease.

Carcinoma of the Cervical Stump. Supracervical hysterectomy was once a popular treatment for benign uterine conditions. Although enthusiasm for the procedure declined after the 1950s, its use has increased somewhat in recent years. The natural history, staging, and workup for cervical stump carcinomas are the same as those for carcinomas of the intact uterus.

Patients with stage IA1 disease may be treated with simple trachelectomy, and selected patients with stage IA2 or small stage IB tumors may be treated with radical trachelectomy and pelvic lymph node dissection. However, most patients are treated with irradiation alone using a combination of external-beam therapy and brachytherapy. The altered geometry and short uterine canal in these patients complicate treatment planning. MRI may be an important aid to treatment planning in these patients. However, in most cases, the endocervical canal is 2 cm or longer, and after a course of external-beam irradiation, patients can be adequately treated with intracavitary therapy. If the endocervical canal cannot accommodate any sources, a boost dose may be delivered to the tumor with interstitial therapy or transvaginal irradiation. Vaginal ovoids alone rarely deliver an adequate dose to the cervix. If brachytherapy is impossible, some patients can be cured using external-beam irradiation with reduced fields. However, brachytherapy should be used whenever possible. Barillot et al.[254] reported a survival rate of 81.5% for patients treated with combined brachytherapy and external-beam irradiation versus 38.5% for those treated with external-beam irradiation alone. When brachytherapy is used, most investigators have reported survival rates similar to those for patients with carcinomas of the intact cervix.[254,255]

Carcinoma of the Cervix During Pregnancy. Estimates of the incidence of invasive cervical cancer during pregnancy range from 0.02% to 0.9%.[256,257] Estimates of the incidence of pregnancy in patients with invasive cervical cancer usually range between 0.5% and 5%. Hacker et al.[256] reported an incidence of cervical carcinoma *in situ* of 0.013% in pregnant women.

Any suspicious cervical lesion observed during pregnancy should be biopsied. If the Pap smear is positive for malignant cells and the diagnosis of invasive cancer cannot be made with colposcopy and biopsy, a diagnostic conization may be necessary. Because conization subjects the mother and fetus to complications, it should be performed only in the second trimester and only in patients with inadequate colposcopy findings and strong cytologic evidence of invasive cancer. Conization in the first trimester of pregnancy is associated with an abortion rate of up to 33%.[256] Conservative conization under colposcopic guidance may reduce this risk.[258]

It appears to be safe to delay definitive treatment of patients with carcinoma *in situ* or stage IA disease until the fetus has matured.[256–258] Patients whose disease invades less than 5 mm may be followed to term. The infant may be delivered by a cesarean section, which is followed immediately by modified radical hysterectomy or radical trachelectomy and pelvic lymph node dissection.

Treatment of patients with more advanced cancers depends on the stage of gestation and the wishes of the patient. Modern neonatal care affords a very high survival rates for infants delivered at more than 28 weeks of gestational age. Fetal pulmonary maturity can be determined by amniocentesis, and, when pulmonary maturity is documented, the infant can be delivered and prompt treatment of the mother can be instituted. It is probably wise to avoid delays in therapy of more than 4 weeks whenever possible, although this guideline is controversial.[257,259] For most women with stage IB1 tumors, the recommended approach is classic cesarean section followed by radical hysterectomy with pelvic lymph node dissection. There should be a thorough discussion of the risks and options with both parents before any treatment is undertaken.

Patients with stage II–IV tumors and some patients with bulky stage IB cervical cancers will require radiotherapy to treat their cancer. If the fetus is viable at the time of diagnosis, it is delivered by classic cesarean section and radiotherapy is begun postoperatively. If the pregnancy is in the first trimester, external-beam irradiation can be started with the expectation that spontaneous abortion will occur before the delivery of 40 Gy. In the second trimester, a delay of therapy may be entertained to improve the chances of fetal survival. If the patient wishes to delay therapy, it is important to ensure fetal pulmonary maturity before delivery is undertaken.

Compared with other cervical cancer patients, those with cervical cancer during pregnancy have slightly better overall survival because an increased proportion have stage I disease. Although studies differ in their conclusions about whether pregnancy has an independent influence on the prognosis of patients with cervical cancer, case-matched studies have suggested similar survival rates for pregnant and nonpregnant patients.[260]

Patients who are diagnosed with invasive cervical cancer shortly after a vaginal delivery and who had an episiotomy appear to be at risk for recurrence at the site of their episiotomy. At least 13 cases demonstrating this unusual pattern of failure have been reported.[261]

CARCINOMA OF THE VAGINA

Carcinomas of the vagina are rare, accounting for only about 2% of gynecologic malignancies. According to FIGO, cases should be classified as vaginal carcinomas only when "the primary site of the growth is in the vagina."[262] Any tumor that has extended to the cervical portio and has reached the area of the external os should be classified as a cervical carcinoma, and a tumor that has extended from the vulva to involve the vagina should be classified as a primary vulvar cancer.[262] In patients with an intact uterus, it is probable that many tumors that originate in the apical vagina are classified as cervical cancers because they have reached the area of the external os by the time of diagnosis. This may explain why a large percentage (30% to 50%) of patients diagnosed with vaginal carcinoma have previously undergone hysterectomy, which prevents classification of tumors as primary cervical cancers.[263,264]

More commonly, the vagina is a site of metastasis, direct extension, or recurrence of tumors originating in other genital sites, such as the cervix or endometrium, or from extragenital sites, including the rectum and bladder.

Epidemiology

Vaginal intraepithelial neoplasia (VAIN) often accompanies CIN and is thought to have a similar etiology.[265] Kalogirou et al.[266] found 41 cases of VAIN in 993 patients followed with cytologic examination and colposcopy after hysterectomy for CIN. Most VAIN lesions were in the upper vagina, particularly in the vault angles of the suture line.

Investigators have reported an HPV infection rate of 60% to 65% in women with vaginal carcinoma.[267] Population-based studies indicate that the prevalence of HPV infection is similar in the vaginas of women who have undergone hysterectomy and the cervixes of women who still have their uterus.[268] The much lower rate of carcinoma in the vagina is thought to reflect the fact that the vagina does not have a transformation zone of immature epithelial cells susceptible to transformation; HPV-induced vaginal lesions are thought to arise in areas of squamous metaplasia that develop during healing of mucosal abrasions caused by coitus, tampon use, chronic pessary use, or other trauma.[265] Most vaginal cancers arising in patients who used pessaries are located in the posterior wall.[269] Pelvic irradiation might be a predisposing factor in some cases of vaginal cancer.[270] However, viral and other non–treatment-related factors probably play a role in the etiology of vaginal cancers that arise after treatment of another malignancy.

Primary invasive carcinoma of the vagina is predominantly a disease of elderly women; 70% to 80% of cases are diagnosed in women older than 60 years.[271] Except for clear cell carcinomas, which are associated with maternal DES exposure, invasive vaginal carcinomas are extremely rare in women younger than 40 years.[262,271]

In 1971, Herbst et al.[272] first reported a highly significant association between clear cell carcinoma of the vagina and maternal ingestion of DES during pregnancy. The peak number of DES-associated cases occurred in 1975, when 33 cases were reported to a U.S. registry.[272] The peak risk period for exposed women in the United States was between the ages of 15 and 22 years; few cases were diagnosed after the age of 40 years. Obesity, oral contraceptive use, and pregnancy were suggested as possible risk factors for development of clear cell carcinoma in DES-exposed women, but larger case-matched studies generally failed to confirm these associations.[273] Infection with HPV may be a cofactor in some cases. Among 14 cases of clear cell carcinoma studied by Waggoner et al.,[274] 3 contained HPV-31 DNA; 10 of the remaining HPV-negative tumors had p53 protein detected by immunohistochemistry, suggesting a mutation of *p53*.

DES-related clear cell carcinomas appear to have a better prognosis with less likelihood of distant metastasis than other vaginal adenocarcinomas. Because many DES-exposed women with clear cell carcinoma were young at the time of diagnosis, treatment of early lesions has emphasized preservation of vaginal and ovarian function. Senekjian et al.[275] reported successful treatment of early lesions with excision or local radiotherapy only. However, retroperitoneal lymphadenectomy may be indicated when local treatment is considered for stage I lesions, which are reported to have an overall rate of pelvic lymph node metastases of 15% to 20%.[276]

There is as yet no evidence that DES-exposed women are at risk for genital tract malignancies other than clear cell carcinoma,[277] although recent studies suggest that they may have an increased risk of developing breast cancer after the age of 40 years.[278]

Natural History and Pattern of Spread

Approximately 50% of vaginal cancers arise in the upper third of the vagina, and there is a fairly even distribution of lesions arising on the anterior, posterior, and lateral walls. Tumors may exhibit an exophytic or ulcerative, infiltrating pattern of growth.

Tumors may invade directly to involve adjacent structures such as the urethra, bladder, and rectum, although fewer than 10% of vaginal cancers are found to be stage IVA (spread to adjacent organs and/or direct extension beyond the true pelvis) at presentation.[264,279,280] Vaginal cancers may also spread laterally to the paravaginal space and pelvic wall. Although tumors arising in the vagina undoubtedly can spread superiorly to involve the cervix and uterus, such tumors are usually classified as cervical cancers according to FIGO criteria.

The vagina is supplied with a fine anastomosing network of lymphatics in the mucosa and submucosa. Despite the continuity of lymphatic vessels within the vagina, Plentl and Friedman[281] found a regular pattern of regional drainage from specific regions of the vagina. The lymphatics of the vaginal vault communicate with those of the lower cervix, draining laterally to the obturator and hypogastric nodes. The lymphatics of the posterior wall anastomose with those of the anterior rectal wall, draining to the superior and inferior gluteal nodes. The lymphatics of the lower third of the vagina communicate with those of the vulva and drain either to the pelvic nodes or to the inguinofemoral lymph nodes.

Few data are available concerning the incidence of spread of vaginal cancer to the pelvic lymph nodes. However, studies suggest that the incidence of positive pelvic nodes in patients with stage II disease is at least 25% to 30%, emphasizing the importance of regional treatment for these patients.[282]

The most frequent site of hematogenous metastasis is the lung. Less frequently, vaginal cancers may metastasize to liver, bone, or other sites.[262,264]

Pathology

Eighty to ninety percent of primary vaginal malignancies are squamous cell carcinomas.[283] Grossly, these tumors may be nodular, ulcerative, exophytic, or form plaques. Histologically, they are similar to squamous tumors at other sites. Approximately one-third of vaginal squamous cell carcinomas are keratinizing, and more than half are nonkeratinizing, moderately differentiated lesions.

Approximately 5% to 10% of primary vaginal neoplasms are adenocarcinomas.[283,284] The differential diagnosis of adenocarcinoma occurring in the vagina is often difficult, as it must be distinguished from metastatic tumors originating at other sites. Histologic patterns include clear cell, mucinous, adenosquamous, papillary, and undifferentiated. During the 1970s and 1980s, clear cell carcinomas of the vagina were sometimes seen in young women in association with maternal DES exposure. Today, these are extremely rare, and most adenocarcinomas occur in postmenopausal women. The prognosis of patients with adenocarcinoma appears to be poorer than that of patients with squamous carcinoma of the vagina.[284]

Primary small cell carcinomas of the vagina are very rare, with fewer than 30 cases reported in the literature.[285] They are histologically indistinguishable from neuroendocrine small cell carcinomas of the lung or cervix and, like these tumors, may coexist with squamous or adenocarcinoma elements.

Primary vaginal melanomas represent about 3% of primary vaginal cancers and fewer than 20% of genital melanomas.[283] Primary vaginal melanomas are thought to arise from melanocytes in areas of melanosis or atypical melanocytic hyperplasia. They usually originate in the distal third of the vagina and occur at a mean age of 55 years. Vaginal melanomas tend to be associated with a poorer prognosis than vulvar melanomas; 5-year survival rates are 15% to 20% after treatment with surgery, radiation, or both.[286]

About 3% of vaginal cancers are sarcomas; about two-thirds of these are leiomyosarcomas, but endometrial stromal sarcomas, malignant mixed müllerian tumors, and other types have been reported.[287] Embryonal rhabdomyosarcoma (sarcoma botryoides) is a highly malignant sarcoma that occurs in girls, usually before 6 years of age. This tumor usually forms soft nodules that fill and protrude from the vagina. The prognosis for children with this tumor has improved with the use of appropriate multimodality therapy.[288]

TABLE 101.4

INTERNATIONAL FEDERATION OF GYNECOLOGY AND OBSTETRICS CLINICAL STAGING OF CARCINOMA OF THE VAGINA

Stage	Description
0	Carcinoma *in situ*, intraepithelial carcinoma.
I	The carcinoma is limited to the vaginal wall.
II	The carcinoma has involved the subvaginal tissues but has not extended onto the pelvic wall.
III	The carcinoma has extended onto the pelvic wall.
IV	The carcinoma has extended beyond the true pelvis or has clinically involved the mucosa of the bladder or rectum. Bullous edema as such does not permit a case to be allotted to stage IV.
IVA	Spread of the growth to adjacent organs and/or direct extension beyond the true pelvis.
IVB	Spread to distant organs.

Diagnosis, Clinical Evaluation, and Staging

Most patients with VAIN and about 10% to 20% of patients with invasive vaginal carcinoma are asymptomatic at presentation; in these cases, carcinoma is usually diagnosed during investigation of an abnormal Pap smear finding. Colposcopic evaluation in the case of abnormal cytologic findings should always include a detailed examination of the entire vagina and cervix, even when there is an obvious cervical lesion, because patients can present with multiple areas of abnormality. Women who have persistent positive Pap smear findings after treatment of CIN should be examined carefully for VAIN.

About 50% to 60% of patients with invasive vaginal cancer present with abnormal vaginal bleeding. Patients may also present with complaints of vaginal discharge, a palpable mass, dyspareunia, or pain in the perineum or pelvis.[264,279,289]

The initial workup of patients with vaginal cancer should include a careful pelvic examination including thorough visualization of the entire vagina. All patients should have chest radiography, a complete blood cell count, and a biochemical profile. CT is useful to evaluate for possible regional spread and to evaluate the kidneys but usually does not provide accurate information about the extent of primary disease. MRI provides much more detailed information about the extent of paravaginal infiltration but frequently underestimates the extent of superficial vaginal involvement, which is often better appreciated on pelvic examination. If involvement of adjacent structures is suspected on physical examination or imaging, further evaluation with cystoscopy, ureteroscopy, and/or proctoscopy is recommended.

The FIGO stage categories for vaginal cancers are listed in Table 101.4.[262] Because this is a clinical staging system, the classification of lesions as stage I or II tends to be somewhat subjective. In general, thin (<0.5 cm), relatively exophytic tumors tend to be classified as stage I, and thicker, infiltrating tumors and those with obvious paravaginal nodularity tend to be classified as stage II.

The FIGO recommendations for staging of disease associated with positive lymph nodes are somewhat ambiguous.[262,290] Although clinical staging is recommended, with rules similar to those used for cervical cancer (e.g., disallowing use of imaging or surgical information about lymph node involvement in assignment of stage), the most recent FIGO manual quoted stage groupings based on nodal involvement. A more specific method of nodal evaluation is elaborated in the American Joint Committee on Cancer staging manual,[290] which suggests options for pathologic or clinical TNM staging. According to the American Joint Committee on Cancer, results of biopsy or fine-needle aspiration of lymph nodes may be included in the clinical staging[290]; FIGO states that such results can be used for treatment planning only.[262] Although the FIGO system could be interpreted to assign patients who have clinically evident inguinal involvement to stage IV, patients with inguinal metastases are sometimes cured with locoregional treatment; Kucera and Vavra[289] reported uncorrected 5-year survival rates of 29% for patients with clinically suspicious inguinal nodes and 44% for patients with clinically negative groins.

Prognostic Factors

The rates of local control, distant metastasis, and survival in vaginal carcinoma are all correlated strongly with FIGO stage (Table 101.5).[264,279,280,289] Tumor size also is an important predictor of outcome.[264,279,291]

Most investigators have been unable to find a correlation between tumor site and outcome.[279,280,292] However, tumors that involve the entire vagina tend to be associated with a poorer prognosis, probably reflecting the larger size of these lesions. Exophytic tumors may be associated with a better prognosis than infiltrating or necrotic lesions.[280]

Frank et al.[284] reported significantly poorer survival and pelvic disease control rates for patients with non–DES-related adenocarcinomas than for patients with squamous cell carcinomas; at 5 years, the overall survival and pelvic disease control rates were 34% and 39%, respectively, for patients with adenocarcinomas versus 58% and 81%, respectively, for patients with squamous carcinomas of the vagina. Although other investigators[279,293] found no difference in outcome between patients with squamous carcinoma and those with adenocarcinoma, this may reflect inclusion of DES-related clear cell carcinomas, which appear to be associated with a better prognosis than other adenocarcinomas.[275]

Treatment

Technical aspects of the treatment of vaginal cancer are highly specialized and vary widely according to the site, size, and distribution of tumor within the vagina and adjacent structures. To achieve the best results for patients with these rare cancers, treatment should be delivered at a center that has a strong multidisciplinary team, including a radiation oncologist well versed in the specialized brachytherapy and external-beam techniques used to treat these cancers.

TABLE 101.5

CARCINOMA OF THE VAGINA: SURVIVAL RATES ACCORDING TO CLINICAL STAGE

Study (Ref.)	Stage I No. of Patients	Stage I Survival (%)	Stage II No. of Patients	Stage II Survival (%)	Stage III No. of Patients	Stage III Survival (%)	Stage IV No. of Patients	Stage IV Survival (%)	Calculation Method
Perez et al. (280)	59	80	64 (IIa)[a] 34 (IIb)	55 35	20	38	15	0	10-yr, actuarial, disease free
Davis et al. (282)	44	82	45	53					5-yr, actuarial, uncorrected
Eddy et al. (263)	25	73	39	39	15	38	12	25	5-yr, actuarial, corrected
Kucera and Vavra (289)	73	77	110	45	174	31	77	14	5-yr, crude, uncorrected
Kirkbride et al. (279)	40	77	38	78	42	60	19	41	5-yr, actuarial, cause-specific
Chyle et al. (293)	59	55	104	51	55	37	16	40	10-yr, actuarial, uncorrected
		76		69		47		27	10-yr freedom from relapse
Stock et al. (291)	23	67	58	53	9	0	10	15	5-yr, actuarial, disease-free
Frank et al. (264)	50	85	97	78	46[b]	58[b]			5-yr, actuarial, disease-specific

[a]IIa, paravaginal submucosal extension only; IIb, parametrial involvement.
[b]Stages III and IVA combined.

VAIN

Patients with only HPV infection, or VAIN 1, do not require treatment. These lesions often regress spontaneously, are frequently multifocal, and recur quickly after attempts at ablative therapy. VAIN 2 may be treated with observation or topical estrogen. The malignant potential of VAIN 1–2 is uncertain. However, VAIN 3 may progress to an invasive lesion. Thus, when VAIN 3 is found, a careful evaluation should be done to rule out the presence of occult invasive disease.

VAIN 3 lesions that have been adequately sampled to rule out invasion can be treated with laser ablation. Cryosurgery should not be used in the vagina because the depth of injury cannot be controlled and inadvertent injury to the bladder or rectum may occur. Superficial fulguration with electrosurgical ball cautery may be used under careful colposcopic control. Local excision is an excellent method of treatment for small upper vaginal lesions. Intravaginal 5-FU has been used to treat patients who have persistent disease after resection.

Most authors report that about 5% to 10% of patients who undergo excision of VAIN develop subsequent invasive cancers[294,295] and Hoffman et al.[265] reported finding occult invasive disease in upper vaginectomy specimens from 9 of 32 patients (28%) who had surgery for VAIN 3. These risks are sufficient to warrant close follow-up of patients treated for VAIN.

VAIN can also be treated effectively with intracavitary brachytherapy,[279,280,293] but this treatment is usually reserved for patients with multifocal, multiply recurrent disease or high operative risk. Although most experiences have been with LDR brachytherapy, MacLeod et al.[296] reported a high control rate without major complications using HDR intracavitary brachytherapy; the vaginal surface was treated with a total dose of 34 to 45 Gy in 4 to 10 fractions. In contrast, Ogino et al.[297] reported adhesive vaginitis and rectal bleeding in two patients treated to the entire vagina with a less conservative HDR fractionation schedule.

Stage I Disease

Radiotherapy is often the treatment of choice for stage I disease because if surgery is used, total vaginectomy or even exenteration may be needed to obtain satisfactory resection margins. However, surgery has a definite role in selected cases.[282,291] Early tumors that involve the upper posterior vagina can be removed with a radical hysterectomy and partial (proximal) vaginectomy if the uterus is intact or with a radical upper (proximal) vaginectomy if the patient has previously undergone hysterectomy; in both situations, bilateral pelvic lymphadenectomy is also performed. For patients with a prior history of pelvic irradiation, radical surgery (usually pelvic exenteration) is indicated and is often curative.

Disease-specific survival rates for patients with stage I disease treated with definitive irradiation range from 75% to 95%.[264,280,289,298] Although some authors have suggested that selected patients with small, very superficial tumors may be treated with brachytherapy alone,[280] others have noted unacceptable rates of paravaginal recurrence after treatment with brachytherapy alone and suggest that external-beam irradiation should be used to treat at least the distal pelvis.[264] Thicker stage I tumors always should be treated with a combination of external-beam irradiation and brachytherapy with an aim to deliver 40 to 50 Gy to the pelvic nodes and 70 to 75 Gy to the tumor.

Stage II Disease

Because investigators rarely define their criteria for distinguishing stage I from stage II vaginal carcinoma or for selecting patients for various treatments, different institutional experiences cannot easily be compared. Reported disease-specific survival rates for patients with stage II disease range from 50% to 80%. To control possible regional disease, patients with stage II disease should receive 40 to 50 Gy to the whole pelvis delivered using external-beam irradiation; this should be followed by additional irradiation of sites of initial gross disease.[264] In most cases, brachytherapy is used to supplement the dose to the primary vaginal tumor site. Perez et al.[280] achieved pelvic tumor control in only 4 of 11 patients (36%) with stage II tumors treated with brachytherapy alone, compared with 54 of 81 patients (67%) treated with a combination of external-beam irradiation and brachytherapy.[280]

Brachytherapy should be tailored to the volume and distribution of the tumor and its response to external-beam irradiation. For apical tumors that flatten to less than 5 mm in thickness, the dose to the vagina may be boosted using intracavitary sources in a vaginal cylinder, although interstitial brachytherapy or conformal external-beam techniques may still be useful in selected cases. Examination under anesthesia, transvaginal sonography, or MRI may be helpful in evaluation of disease extent for treatment planning. Larger tumors usually require a boost with interstitial brachytherapy or with additional external-beam irradiation (taking into account the influence of internal organ motion on external-beam radiation doses). Most authors emphasize the importance of brachytherapy in the treatment of vaginal cancer.[280,298] However, brachytherapy must be designed to treat the entire vaginal tumor. Frank et al.[264] argue that tumors that cannot be covered adequately with brachytherapy can often be cured with external-beam irradiation alone using carefully designed conformal fields.

Selected patients with stage II disease may be cured with radical surgery.[291] However, total radical vaginectomy or pelvic exenteration is often required to remove the tumor, and results with radical surgery do not appear to be better than those with radiotherapy alone. Primary radical surgery is usually indicated for patients who have previously had pelvic radiotherapy.

Stage III and IVA Disease

Reported 5-year disease-specific survival rates range from 30% to 60% for patients with stage III disease and from 15% to 40% for patients with stage IVA disease.[264,279,280,289] Stage III and IVA tumors are usually bulky, highly infiltrative lesions involving most or all of the vagina as well as the pelvic wall, bladder, or rectum. The extent of these tumors and the proximity of critical normal tissue structures make their management a formidable technical challenge. Pelvic recurrence rates are high in many series; the risk of distant metastasis is also relatively high, although distant relapse is often accompanied by locoregional recurrence.

All patients require treatment with external-beam irradiation. Most authors advocate the use of brachytherapy whenever possible. However, Frank et al.[264] reported a high disease-specific survival rate (58% at 5 years) in a series of patients with stage III and IVA disease in which the majority of patients (31 of 46) were treated with external-beam irradiation alone. Brachytherapy is undoubtedly an important part of disease management in some patients. However, in certain cases, interstitial brachytherapy does not provide adequate coverage of tumors that are very large and intimately associated with critical structures. In these cases, it may be appropriate to place greater emphasis on external-beam treatment. Conformal radiotherapy techniques such as IMRT may help to increase the dose to tumor while limiting the dose to critical structures.

For selected patients with relatively small, mobile stage IVA cancers who are in otherwise good medical condition, pelvic exenteration with vaginal reconstruction using a gracilis myocutaneous flap or rectus abdominis myocutaneous flap may be the treatment of choice, particularly if a rectovaginal or vesicovaginal fistula is present.[299] Radical radiotherapy is also curative in some cases; Frank et al.[264] reported an 86% pelvic control rate in seven patients treated with radiotherapy for stage IVA disease.

Radiotherapy Technique. Pelvic external-beam fields must be individualized according to the primary tumor site and potential sites of regional spread. Radiopaque markers placed at the distal edge of the tumor help to define the lower border and facilitate studies of internal organ motion. Treating the patient in an open ("frog-leg") position can often reduce the severity of vulvar cutaneous reactions when coverage of distal lesions necessitates inclusion of the introitus in the radiation field.

When tumors involve the distal third of the vagina, pelvic fields should be designed to include at least the medial inguinal-femoral lymph nodes. When four fields are used to treat the pelvis, care must be taken to cover all the draining lymph nodes. Lateral fields should adequately cover posterior perirectal nodes, particularly when the primary lesion involves the posterior vaginal wall.

Intracavitary brachytherapy is of limited value in the treatment of locally advanced vaginal cancer because the dose falls off very rapidly from the surface of a vaginal cylinder. In general, the dose at a 5-mm depth is only 60% to 70% of the dose at the vaginal surface. Interstitial brachytherapy can provide better coverage of thick vaginal tumors. Vaginal implants can be inserted freehand. Successful use of this technique requires experience, but direct palpation during needle insertion permits excellent control of the position of sources with respect to the vaginal surface and rectal mucosa (Fig. 101.9). Vaginal implants may also be positioned using a perineal template. This technique provides a more homogeneous dose distribution because it facilitates parallel positioning of sources, but the template interferes somewhat with the ability of the brachytherapist to monitor the placement of needles with respect to the rectal and vaginal mucosa. When tumors involve the vaginal apex in patients who have had a hysterectomy, laparoscopic or laparotomy guidance may be needed to ensure accurate needle placement.

Efforts to correlate radiation dose with tumor control have yielded inconsistent results and may be misleading because the total dose of radiation prescribed for a vaginal tumor is often influenced by the tumor's size, extent, and initial response to irradiation, all of which determine the feasibility of delivering high-dose brachytherapy.[264,280,298] When good brachytherapy coverage of the tumor can be accomplished, an effort should be made to treat the tumor to a dose of 75 to 85 Gy. When brachytherapy is not possible, some patients may be cured with external-beam irradiation alone using shrinking pelvic fields or IMRT to deliver a tumor dose of 60 to 70 Gy. Treatment can usually be completed in less than 6 to 7 weeks and should not be protracted unnecessarily. Lee et al.[300] reported a significantly lower pelvic recurrence rate in patients whose entire treatment course was completed in 9 weeks or less.

Complications of Radiotherapy. The close proximity of the bladder and rectum to the vagina makes them vulnerable to damage when invasive vaginal cancers are treated with radiotherapy. In their review of 193 patients treated with definitive irradiation, Frank et al.[264] reported a 10% actuarial incidence of serious complications at 5 years. The most frequent complications were proctitis, hemorrhagic cystitis, and fistulae. Complication rates were significantly correlated with FIGO stage and with a history of smoking; major complications rates were 4%, 9%, and 21% for patients with stage I, II, or III–IVA disease, respectively. Other authors have reported similar major complication rates.[279,280,289] There have been no comprehensive studies of vaginal function in women with vaginal cancer treated with radiotherapy, although some degree of vaginal stenosis or shortening is common.[279] The severity of vaginal morbidity is probably related to the damage to vaginal mucosa and submucosa from tumor infiltration, ulceration, and infection; the age and menopausal status of the patient; and the radiation dose and the amount of vaginal tissue treated to high doses.

Role of Chemotherapy. Because primary vaginal carcinomas are rare, few reports have specifically addressed the role of

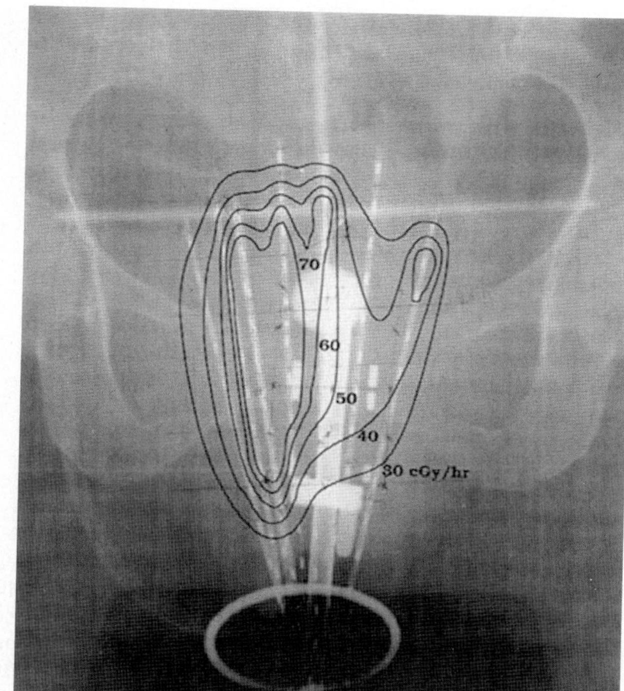

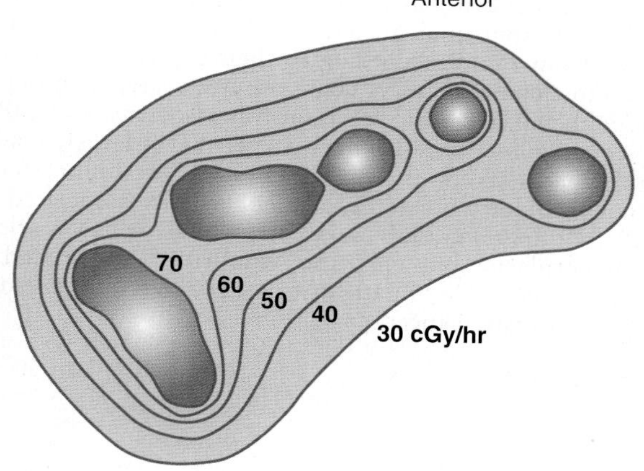

FIGURE 101.9 Interstitial implant of a squamous carcinoma involving the anterior and right lateral walls of the vagina. The brachytherapist placed needles transperineally while monitoring the position of the needles by direct palpation with fingers in the vagina and rectum. A plastic cylinder in the vagina displaced uninvolved tissues away from the needles, which were loaded with ^{192}Ir sources. Needles were placed and sources were selected to deliver a somewhat higher dose to the thickest portion of the tumor on the right lateral wall of the vagina. Isodose contours represent the dose rates (in centigray per hour [cGy/hr]) delivered to tissues in a coronal plane at the approximate center of the implant (**A**) and in a transverse plane through the center of the implant (**B**).

chemotherapy in the treatment of this disease. Chemotherapeutic management is usually based on extrapolations from experience with the treatment of carcinomas of the cervix. For this reason, patients who have metastatic or recurrent vaginal carcinoma that is no longer amenable to locoregional treatment are sometimes treated with cisplatin-based chemotherapy even though the efficacy of this treatment is not well documented in the literature. Thigpen et al.[301] noted several responses among 16 patients with vaginal cancers treated with cisplatin (50 mg/m² every 3 weeks).

Because vaginal carcinoma resembles cervical carcinoma in its location, pattern of spread, histologic appearance, relationship to HPV infection, and response to radiotherapy, it may be reasonable to extrapolate from randomized trials demonstrating a benefit from concurrent chemoradiation in patients with locally advanced cervical cancer to justify a similar approach in selected patients with high-risk invasive vaginal cancer.[136,302]

CARCINOMA OF THE VULVA

Epidemiology

Invasive vulvar carcinoma is a rare disease that accounts for about 4% of gynecologic cancers.[303,304] The median age at diagnosis of patients with invasive vulvar cancer is about 65 to 70 years. In contrast, vulvar intraepithelial neoplasia (VIN) tends to occur in younger women; the median age at diagnosis of women with VIN is 45 to 50 years. The incidence of VIN has more than doubled since the early 1970s.[303,304] This increase has been particularly marked in women younger than 55 years. In the past, the incidence of invasive vulvar cancer was thought to be stable; however, recent data suggest that the median age of women presenting with invasive vulvar cancer may be decreasing, probably reflecting an increase in HPV-related vulvar cancers in young women.[305] This change has also been associated with an increase in the proportion of vulvar cancers involving the periurethral and clitoral region rather than the labia.[305]

Only 30% to 50% of invasive vulvar carcinomas are associated with evidence of HPV infection.[306,307] However, 80% to 90% of VIN lesions contain HPV-16 or other HPV types. On the basis of these statistics, it has been estimated that HPV vaccination could prevent about half of the vulvar carcinomas in young women and about two-thirds of the VIN lesions.

HPV-positive vulvar cancers are usually basaloid or warty carcinomas with little keratin formation, are often associated with VIN, are frequently multifocal, and tend to occur in younger women (35 to 55 years).[305,306,308] Patients with HPV-positive tumors are also more likely to have CIN and to have risk factors typically associated with cervical cancer.[308] In contrast, HPV-negative tumors usually occur in older women (55 to 85 years), are often associated with vulvar inflammation or lichen sclerosis (but rarely with VIN), are generally unifocal, and are usually well differentiated with exuberant keratin formation.[309,310] Although a number of investigators have reported this distinct grouping of patients with vulvar cancer, others have found greater overlap.[311]

Several investigators have reported a high incidence of *p53* mutations in HPV-negative tumors.[312,313] Lee et al.[312] found missense mutations of *p53* in 4 of 9 (44%) HPV-negative tumors but in only 1 of 12 (8%) HPV-positive tumors. They postulated that alteration in *p53* activity, either through point mutations or through E6-mediated loss of *p53* function in HPV-infected cells, could be important in the development of vulvar neoplasms.

Natural History and Pattern of Spread

The vulva includes the mons pubis, labia majora, labia minora, clitoris, vestibular bulb, vestibular glands (including Bartholin glands), and vestibule of the vagina. The region between the posterior commissure of the labia and the anus is termed the *gynecologic perineum*. About 70% of vulvar squamous carcinomas involve the labia majora or minora, most frequently the labia majora. Vulvar tumors may extend locally to invade adjacent structures, including the vagina,

TABLE 101.6

RELATIONSHIP BETWEEN DEPTH OF STROMAL INVASION AND INGUINAL LYMPH NODE METASTASES IN PATIENTS WITH SQUAMOUS CELL CARCINOMA OF THE VULVA

	No. of Patients with Positive Lymph Nodes/Total No. of Patients by Depth of Invasion (mm)				
Study (Ref.)	≤1.0	1.1–2.0	2.1–3.0	3.1–5.0	>5
Binder et al. (315)	0/7	0/23	3/14	6/25	15/31
Ross and Ehrmann (318)	0/17	1/9	1/13	4/15	0/1
Hoffman et al. (317)	0/24	0/19	2/17	8/15	7/13
Hacker et al. (316)	0/34	2/19	2/17	1/7	3/7
Andreasson and Nyboe (314)	0/8	1/13	3/12	5/32	19/57
Total	0/90	4/83 (5%)	11/73 (15%)	24/94 (26%)	44/109 (40%)

urethra, and anus; advanced vulvar tumors may invade adjacent pelvic bones.

A rich network of anastomosing lymphatics that frequently cross the midline drains the vulva. Even minimally invasive vulvar tumors may spread to regional lymph nodes (Table 101.6).[314–318] For most lesions, initial regional metastasis is to the inguinal lymph nodes that are superficial to Camper fascia; tumors may then metastasize secondarily to deeper femoral lymph nodes and to the pelvic lymph nodes (Fig. 101.10). However, some lesions, particularly those involving the clitoris and other medial structures, metastasize directly to medial femoral lymph nodes that lie in the region of the fossa ovalis, a gap in the cribriform fascia.[319] Theoretically, tumors involving the clitoris can spread directly to the obturator nodes through lymphatics that follow the dorsal vein of the clitoris, although evidence of this route is rarely seen in practice. Despite the extensive anastomosis of lymphatics in the region, metastasis of vulvar carcinoma to contralateral lymph nodes is uncommon in patients with well-lateralized T1 lesions.

The lungs are the most common sites of hematogenous metastasis.

Pathology

As classified by the International Society for the Study of Vulvar Disease, nonneoplastic epithelial disorders of the vulva (previously termed *vulvar dystrophies*) include lichen sclerosis, squamous hyperplasia, and other dermatoses.[320] About 10% of these lesions have cellular atypia and are termed *vulvar intraepithelial neoplasia*. Histologically, VIN is characterized by disruption of the normal epithelial architecture, varying degrees of cytoplasmic and nuclear maturation, and giant cells with abnormal nuclei.[306] VIN lesions are assigned a grade from 1 to 3 according to their degree of maturation. The most common VINs contain nuclear atypia throughout the epithelial layers and are frequently associated with HPV.[306] A second subset of VINs have atypia that is largely confined to the basal layers of the epithelium. These lesions tend to occur in older women and are not usually associated with HPV but are commonly adjacent to areas of lichen sclerosis or hyperplasia. Buscema and Woodruff[321] estimated that approximately 4% of patients treated for VIN develop a subsequent invasive cancer.

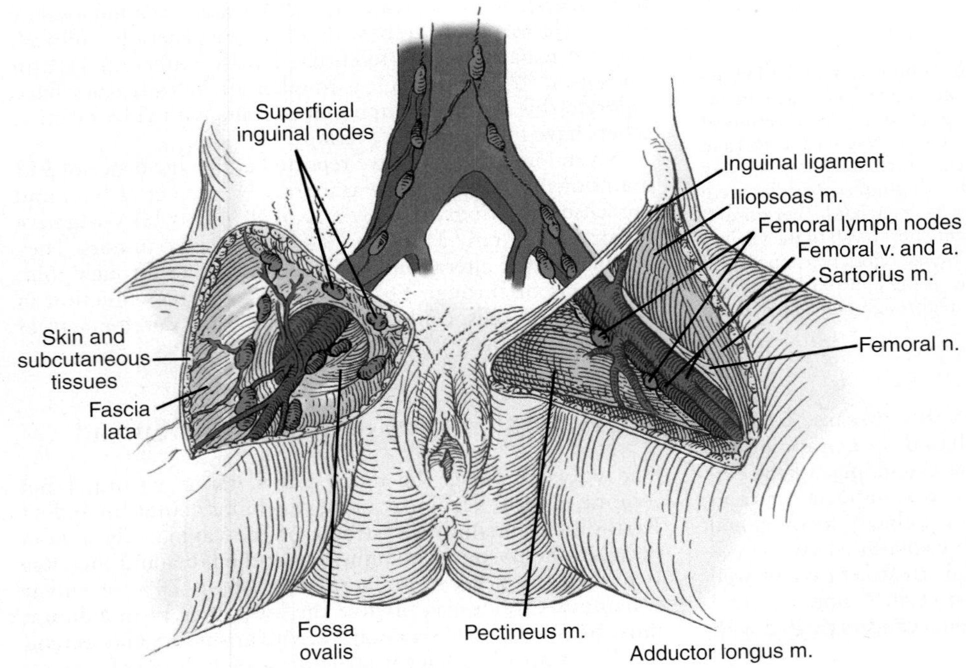

FIGURE 101.10 Inguinal-femoral lymph nodes.

Paget disease of the vulva, a rare intraepithelial lesion located in the epidermis and skin adnexa, accounts for 1% to 5% of vulvar neoplasms. Histologically, vulvar Paget disease is characterized by large, pale, mucopolysaccharide-rich cells that are positive for periodic acid-Schiff. The lesions are usually negative for HPV.[322] Electron microscopic studies have suggested that Paget cells derive from apocrine cells in the stratum germinativum of the epidermis.[323] Paget disease usually occurs in postmenopausal women, who often present with symptoms of vulvar pruritus and discomfort.[324] Grossly, Paget lesions appear eczematoid or, when extensive, may be raised and velvety with persistent weeping. About 5% to 10% of newly diagnosed Paget lesions are associated with underlying adenocarcinoma arising locally in a vulvar vestibular gland or skin appendage or from a distant site such as the breast or rectum.[324]

The term *microinvasive carcinoma of the vulva* should be used with caution. Stromal invasion by vulvar carcinomas is not measured in a uniform manner, and strict criteria for the diagnosis of microinvasive vulvar cancer have not been defined. VIN is not routinely seen adjacent to invasive vulvar cancer, and the transition from normal tissue to invasive cancer can be abrupt. Elongated rete pegs may extend 6 mm or more from the basement membrane and are sometimes misconstrued as invasive cancer. The International Society of Gynecologic Pathologists recommends that the depth of stromal invasion be measured vertically from the most superficial basement membrane to the deepest extent of tumor. Tumor thickness is defined as the distance between the granular layer of the epidermis and the deepest extent of tumor. Lymph node metastases from tumors less than 1 mm in depth or thickness are extremely rare (Table 101.6). For this reason, FIGO now includes in its vulvar carcinoma staging system a stage IA subcategory for tumors that invade no more than 1 mm (Table 101.7).[58] However, the risk of inguinal lymph node metastasis rises steeply as the depth of invasion exceeds 1 mm.

More than 90% of invasive vulvar cancers are squamous cell carcinomas. Atypical keratinization is the hallmark of invasive vulvar cancer. Most squamous cell carcinomas are well differentiated, but mitoses may be noted. About 5% of vulvar cancers are anaplastic carcinomas, which may consist of large immature cells, spindle sarcomatoid cells, or small cells. Vulvar carcinomas consisting of small cells may resemble small cell anaplastic carcinomas of the lung or Merkel cell tumors, and have demonstrated an aggressive biologic behavior in the few reported cases.[325]

The diagnosis of Bartholin gland carcinoma is based on clinical findings of a tumor arising in the anatomic location of Bartholin glands and on the histologic appearance. Biopsy of a tumor arising from a Bartholin gland usually reveals adenocarcinoma, but squamous cell carcinomas, transitional cell carcinomas (arising from the duct and histologically indistinguishable from transitional cell carcinoma of the bladder), and adenoid cystic carcinomas have also been reported.

Rare cases of primary mammary adenocarcinoma of the vulva have been reported, presumably arising in aberrant mammary tissue occurring along the embryonic milk line.[326] Other rare carcinomas that may occur in the vulva include basal cell carcinomas,[327] verrucous carcinomas,[328] and sebaceous carcinomas.[329]

Malignant melanomas of the vulva account for approximately 2% to 4% of primary vulvar malignancies and 1% to 3% of melanomas arising in women.[330] Vulvar melanoma occurs most frequently in women older than 60 years of age, but 10% to 20% of vulvar melanomas occur in women younger than 40 years. In a large Swedish series,[331] 57% of vulvar melanomas were of the mucosal lentiginous type, 22% were nodular, and 16% were superficial spreading or lentiginous. Most investigators have reported a correlation between higher depth of invasion or Breslow thickness and poorer outcome.[331,332] However, because the vulvar epithelium sometimes lacks a well-developed papillary dermis, which makes it difficult to assign Clark's levels of invasion, a modification of the Clark system is often used to categorize patients with vulvar melanoma.[333] Other factors that have been associated with a poorer prognosis are ulceration, clinical amelanosis, and older age.[331]

Vulvar sarcomas constitute 1% to 2% of vulvar malignancies and include leiomyosarcomas, rhabdomyosarcomas, angiosarcomas, neurofibrosarcomas, and epithelioid sarcomas. The prognosis appears to depend on three main determinants: lesion size, tumor contour, and mitotic activity. Lesions greater than 5 cm in diameter with infiltrating margins, extensive necrosis, and more than five mitotic figures per 10 high-power fields are the most likely to recur after surgical resection.[334,335]

TABLE 101.7

INTERNATIONAL FEDERATION OF GYNECOLOGY AND OBSTETRICS (FIGO) STAGING OF CARCINOMA OF THE VULVA (2009)

Stage	Description
I	Tumor confined to the vulva.
IA	Lesions ≤2 cm in size, confined to the vulva or perineum and with stromal invasion ≤1 mm,[a] no nodal metastasis.
IB	Lesions >2 cm or less in size or with stromal invasion >1.0 mm,[a] confined to the vulva or perineum, with negative nodes.
II	Tumor of any size with extension to adjacent perineal structures (1/3 lower urethra, 1/3 lower vagina, anus) with negative nodes.
III	Tumor of any size with or without extension to adjacent perineal structures (1/3 lower urethra, 1/3 lower vagina, anus) with positive inguinofemoral lymph nodes.
IIIA	(i) With 1 lymph node metastasis ≥5 mm), or (ii) 1–2 lymph node metastasis(es) (<5 mm).
IIIB	(i) With 2 or more lymph node metastases (≥5 mm), or (ii) 3 or more lymph node metastases (<5 mm).
IIIC	With positive nodes with extracapsular spread.
IV	Tumor invades other regional (2/3 upper urethra, 2/3 upper vagina) or other distant structures.
IVA	Tumor invades any of the following (i) Upper urethral and/or vaginal mucosa, bladder mucosa, rectal mucosa, or fixed to pelvic bone, or (ii) Fixed or ulcerated inguinofemoral nodes.
IVB	Any distant metastasis including pelvic lymph nodes.

[a] The depth of invasion is defined as the measurement of the tumor from the epithelial-stromal junction of the adjacent most superficial dermal papilla to the deepest point of invasion.

Diagnosis, Clinical Evaluation, and Staging

Patients with VIN may complain of vulvar pruritus, irritation, or a mass, but many are asymptomatic at the time of diagnosis. Patients with invasive vulvar cancer usually complain of a vulvar mass and chronic vulvar pruritus. Advanced lesions may bleed and are often exquisitely tender.

Because VIN can have many manifestations, any new vulvar lesion should be biopsied. Once a diagnosis of high-grade VIN has been established, the entire vulva, cervix, and vagina should be carefully examined because patients often have multifocal or multicentric involvement.[336] Colposcopic examination may help to define the extent of disease.

Diagnosis of invasive vulvar lesions requires a wedge biopsy of the lesion with surrounding skin and with underlying dermis and connective tissue so that the pathologist can adequately evaluate the depth of stromal invasion. This procedure can usually be performed in the physician's office under local anesthesia. Excisional biopsy is preferred for lesions smaller than 1 cm in diameter.

All patients with invasive disease require a careful physical examination including a detailed pelvic examination, chest radiography, and a biochemical profile. Cystoscopy and proctoscopy should be performed in patients with tumors that are near the urethra or anus, respectively. CT or MRI scans can be obtained to evaluate deep inguinal and pelvic lymph nodes and possible local extension of disease to adjacent structures. The role of positron emission tomography is unclear but preliminary studies suggest that this study has relatively poor sensitivity but high specificity in the prediction of lymph node metastases.[337]

The correlation between clinical assessment of the inguinal lymph nodes and pathologic findings is poor.[338] Homesley et al.[338] reported that 24% of patients with clinically negative nodes had inguinal lymph node metastases and 24% of patients with suspicious but mobile nodes had negative findings at lymphadenectomy. For this reason, in 1988, the FIGO staging system was changed from a clinical staging system to one that incorporates the more accurate information gained from surgical assessment of regional lymph nodes; a subsequent amendment provided a definition of minimally invasive vulvar cancer.[339]

Studies also suggest that, when corrected for the number of involved lymph nodes, lymph node bilaterality and local factors such as tumor size and early involvement of adjacent structures have little impact on survival.[340,341] However, extracapsular nodal extension was found to be a powerful prognostic indicator.[342,343] In 2009, to incorporate these findings and to improve the prognostic accuracy of the FIGO staging system, another major revision was implemented.[340] In this revision, the role of tumor diameter was diminished; distal urethral, vaginal, and anal involvement were removed as indications for upstaging; and stage III was subdivided to include more detailed information about the number of positive lymph nodes and the presence of extracapsular nodal extension (Table 101.7).[58]

Prognostic Factors

Our understanding of the importance of various prognostic indicators in vulvar carcinoma has shifted with the increased use of adjuvant radiotherapy and the accumulation of outcome data. In a 1991 retrospective review of 586 patients entered in GOG trials between 1977 and 1984, the presence and number of lymph nodes and tumor diameter were the only independent predictors of survival.[341] Five-year survival rates were 91% for patients with negative inguinal lymph nodes and 75%, 36%, and 24%, respectively, for patients with one or two, three or four, or five or six positive nodes. Using these data, the authors suggested a classification system that categorized patients according to tumor size and number of involved lymph nodes (Table 101.8). Although treatment details were not given, postoperative radiotherapy was not standard in the years of this study, and it is likely that most patients did not receive radiotherapy; more recent reviews suggest that modern adjuvant radiotherapy may reduce the influence of tumor size and number of positive nodes on outcome (Table 101.8).[344] Nevertheless, the GOG risk classification was a major influence on recent modifications of the FIGO staging system. In addition to the number of lymph nodes, the presence of extracapsular extension has been found to be an important predictor of outcome.[344,345] However, in a review of patients treated with radiation after lymphadenectomy, Katz et al.[346] found no correlation between extracapsular extension and inguinal node recurrence if the dose of radiation was 56 Gy or greater.

The presence of pelvic lymph node metastases is generally considered to be a predictor of very poor prognosis.[347] However, this impression comes largely from decades-old studies of outcome in patients who had pelvic lymph node dissection without adjuvant radiotherapy. The generalizability of these data to current practice, in which most patients who have nodal involvement receive radiotherapy, is uncertain.

Other factors that have consistently been correlated with lymph node metastasis and outcome include depth of invasion, tumor thickness, and the presence or absence of LVSI.[338,341,348] More than 75% of patients with LVSI have positive inguinal nodes.[338] Studies of the relationship between tumor grade and outcome have supported various conclusions, possibly reflecting the inconsistent criteria used to grade vulvar tumors.[338,345,349] Other factors that have been associated with poorer prognosis include high mitotic rate, aneuploidy, an infiltrative growth pattern, and a basaloid histologic pattern.[349–351] Several authors have reported that tumors containing HPV DNA have a poorer prognosis than HPV-negative tumors.[310,352] Some investigators have reported a worse prognosis for patients age 70 years or older, whereas others have found no correlation between prognosis and age.[338,349]

Studying the relationship between surgical margins and tumor recurrence, Heaps et al.[348] reported no local failures in

TABLE 101.8

RELATIONSHIP BETWEEN INTERNATIONAL FEDERATION OF GYNECOLOGY AND OBSTETRICS (GOG) RISK GROUPS AND OUTCOME IN PATIENTS WITH INVASIVE VULVAR CANCER

Risk Group	Surgical Findings	5-year Survival Rate (No. of Patients)	
		GOG 36[a]	Landrum et al.[b]
Minimal	Tumor ≤2 cm in diameter and negative lymph nodes	97.9%, n = 154	100%, n = 89
Low	Tumor 2.1–8 cm in diameter and negative lymph nodes or Tumor ≤2 cm in diameter and one positive lymph node	87.4%, n = 232	97.1%, n = 69
Intermediate	Tumor >8 cm in diameter and negative lymph nodes or Tumor >2 cm in diameter and one positive lymph node or Tumor ≤8 cm in diameter and two unilaterally positive lymph nodes	74.8%, n = 104	81.8%, n = 11
High	Tumor >8 cm in diameter and two unilaterally positive lymph nodes	29%, n = 87	100%, n = 6

[a]From ref. 341.
[b]From ref. 344.

91 patients whose narrowest tumor margin (deep or at the skin surface) was 8 mm or more in the fixed specimen. Ten of 23 patients (43%) with margins of 4.8 mm or less experienced a local recurrence, as did 8 of 13 patients (62%) with margins between 4.8 and 8 mm. The risk of recurrence in patients with narrow margins may be diminished when postoperative radiotherapy is given.[353]

Treatment

During the last 30 years, the treatment of vulvar cancer has evolved away from radical *en bloc* surgical resection, which was standard before the 1980s, toward a multidisciplinary approach that emphasizes tissue-sparing operations and selective use of radiotherapy or chemoradiation to optimize locoregional control, survival, and organ function.

High-Grade VIN

After invasive carcinoma has been excluded by a sufficient number of excisional biopsies, the treatment of high-grade VIN (VIN 3) should be as conservative as possible. Focal lesions can be simply excised. Multiple lesions can be excised separately or, if confluent, with a larger single excision. This approach is generally well tolerated and provides material for histologic assessment. When there is more extensive high-grade VIN, the lesions can be vaporized with a CO_2 laser. This method may provide an alternative to more extensive operations but does not yield a specimen for histologic inspection.

Extensive, diffuse VIN 3 may necessitate a wider excision, particularly if the lesion involves the perianal skin. These lesions are sometimes treated with a partial vulvectomy of the superficial skin ("skinning vulvectomy"). Whenever possible, the vulvar skin should be sutured primarily, but a split-thickness skin graft is sometimes needed to close the defect.

VIN 3 often recurs at or near the margins of resection, even when the histopathologic analysis demonstrates that the initial lesions were completely resected. Presumably this phenomenon reflects the multifocal nature of the condition.[336] VIN 3 can also recur within the donor skin from split-thickness grafts.[354]

Invasive Disease

The optimal treatment of invasive disease requires careful consideration of the potential benefits of various local and regional treatment options to find an overall treatment strategy that will maximize locoregional disease control with as little acute and long-term morbidity as possible.

Treatment of the Vulva. Most small lesions (approximately <4 cm) that do not involve the urethra, anus, or other adjacent structures can be controlled locally with a radical local excision. A wide and deep excision of the lesion is performed, with the incision extended down to the inferior fascia of the urogenital diaphragm. An effort should be made to remove the lesion with a 1-cm margin of normal tissue in all directions unless this would require compromise of the anus or urethra. Small lesions that invade 1 mm or less can be managed with local resection alone because the risk of regional spread is very small. Patients with more invasive tumors must also have surgical or radiation treatment of the inguinal nodes as discussed in the next section.

Primary tumors that involve the anus, rectum, rectovaginal septum, or urethra pose a difficult problem because adequate surgical clearance can often be obtained only by sacrificing organ function. Some patients who have tumors that minimally involve the external urethra or anus can undergo initial vulvectomy without sacrifice of major organ function if close margins are accepted near critical structures. Postoperative radiotherapy can then be delivered to prevent local recurrence.[355] Although local recurrences are frequently successfully controlled with additional surgery, Faul et al.[356] reported an overall 5-year survival rate of only 40% after the first local recurrence and emphasized the importance of achieving local control. These authors reported a significant reduction in the local failure rate (from 58% to 16%) when tumors that were within 8 mm of the operative margins were treated with radiotherapy after surgery.[356] Although some patients with more extensive organ involvement may be cured with ultraradical operations, in some cases with pelvic exenteration, the risks of acute and long-term complications of these procedures are substantial.[357,358] For this reason, a number of investigators have explored the use of radiotherapy with or without surgery and chemotherapy to spare critical structures in patients with locally advanced disease.

In the 1980s, several investigators[359–361] reported results of preoperative radiotherapy in small series of patients with locally advanced disease. These reports indicated that modest doses of radiation (45 to 55 Gy) produced dramatic tumor responses in some patients with locally advanced disease, permitting organ-sparing surgery without sacrifice of tumor control. Hacker et al.[361] reported that four of eight patients with T3 or T4 tumors treated preoperatively with 44 to 54 Gy had no residual tumor in the vulvectomy specimen and that seven of these eight had local control of their disease. More recently, investigators have emphasized the use of concurrent chemoradiation, as discussed later in this section.

Treatment of Regional Disease. Effective treatment of regional disease is the single most important element in the curative management of early vulvar cancer. Although patients with vulvar recurrences may have their disease successfully controlled with additional local treatment, patients who suffer inguinal recurrences are rarely curable.

All patients with primary tumors that invade more than 1 mm must have their inguinal lymph nodes treated. In the past, this treatment usually included a bilateral radical inguinal-femoral lymphadenectomy, which initially was combined with vulvectomy using a single incision and, more recently, was performed through separate groin incisions. At one time, pelvic lymphadenectomy was also performed in most patients with invasive vulvar cancer. When subsequent studies demonstrated that pelvic node metastases were found only in patients with positive inguinal nodes, use of the procedure was limited to patients found intraoperatively to have inguinal node metastases.

Then, in 1986, Homesley et al.[347] published results of a prospective randomized study that compared pelvic lymphadenectomy with inguinal and pelvic irradiation in patients with inguinal node metastases from carcinoma of the vulva. All patients were initially treated with radical vulvectomy and inguinal-femoral lymphadenectomy. Patient randomization was done intraoperatively after frozen-section evaluation of the inguinal-femoral lymph nodes. This trial was closed prematurely, after 114 eligible patients had been entered, when interim analysis revealed a survival advantage for the radiotherapy arm (P = .03; Fig. 101.11). The difference was most marked for patients with clinically positive or multiple histologically positive groin nodes. The initial preliminary report was finally updated in 2009,[362] confirming marked reductions in the risks of recurrence and cancer-related death in patients who had radiotherapy. There were three inguinal recurrences in the radiation arm versus 13 in the control arm. Although no differences were seen in the number of pelvic recurrences, competing risks and the lack of high-quality tomographic imaging in this early study may have led to underestimates of the risks of pelvic recurrence. In the updated report, the relative risk of disease progression with radiation was 39% (95% CI: 0.17-0.88; P = .02); the relative risk of death was less impressive, with a hazard ratio of 0.61 (95% CI: 0.3–1.3; P = .18), apparently because of a

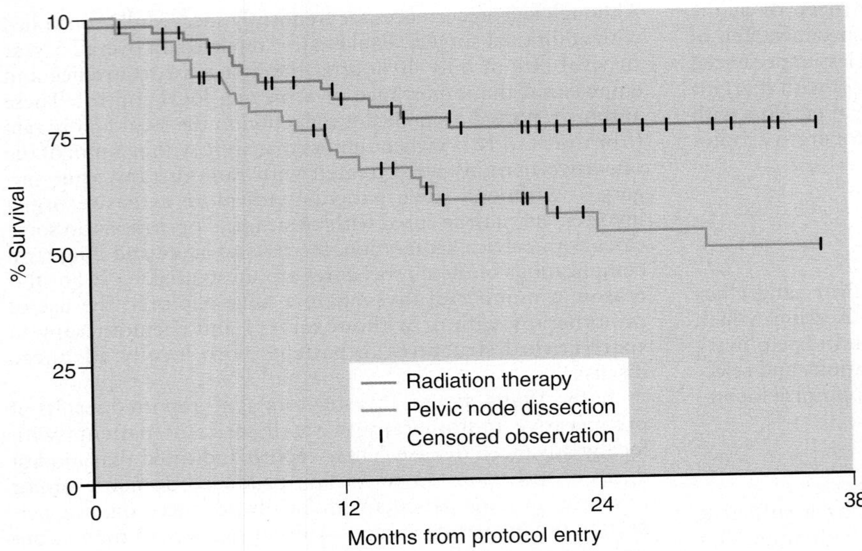

FIGURE 101.11 Survival rates of 114 patients with invasive squamous cell carcinoma of the vulva who were entered on a Gynecologic Oncology Group protocol in which patients with positive groin nodes after radical vulvectomy and bilateral inguinal lymphadenectomies were randomly assigned to undergo pelvic lymph node dissection or postoperative irradiation of the pelvis and inguinal nodes ($P = .004$). (From ref. 347, with permission.)

marked difference in the rate of deaths from other causes: 14 in the radiation arm versus 2 in the control arm. With the 1986 publication of this study, most practitioners abandoned routine pelvic lymphadenectomy, and postoperative radiotherapy became standard for most patients with inguinal lymph node metastases.

Although radical inguinal-femoral lymphadenectomy was historically considered the treatment of choice for regional management of invasive vulvar carcinoma, a number of groups have investigated the possibility that regional radiotherapy may be an effective and less morbid way of preventing recurrence in patients with clinically negative groins.[346,363–365]

In 1992, the GOG reported the results of a trial that randomly assigned patients with clinically negative inguinal nodes to receive inguinal lymph node irradiation or inguinal-femoral lymphadenectomy (followed by inguinopelvic irradiation in patients with positive lymph nodes) after resection of the primary tumor.[365] The study was closed after entry of only 58 patients, when an interim analysis demonstrated a significantly higher rate of inguinal recurrence and death in the radiotherapy group. The authors concluded that lymphadenectomy was the superior treatment, although the morbidity rate of lymphadenectomy was greater than that of groin irradiation. However, the radiotherapy techniques used in this study have since been criticized. Preirradiation CT scans were not consistently obtained to verify the position and size of inguinal nodes. Patients were treated with anterior appositional fields, the dose was prescribed at a depth of 3 cm, and the use of electrons (usually 12 MeV) was emphasized. This method of treatment can lead to significant underdosage of the inguinal-femoral nodes, which frequently extend to a depth of more than 5 to 8 cm.[366]

In contrast, retrospective studies have indicated that patients who have negative inguinal nodes (by tomographic imaging) and careful radiotherapy treatment planning rarely experience a regional recurrence after inguinal-pelvic irradiation to 40 to 50 Gy.[346,363,364] Katz et al.[346] emphasized the importance of careful technique. They reported 3 recurrences in 29 patients treated with radiotherapy alone for clinically negative inguinal nodes; 2 of these recurrences occurred adjacent to radiation fields that had not fully encompassed the lateral inguinal nodes. It appears that, with careful radiotherapy technique, microscopic disease in the inguinal lymph nodes can be readily controlled with radiation alone. Radiation alone appears to be a reasonable treatment to prevent inguinal recurrence, particularly for patients who have clinically and radiographically negative groins but require radiation for locally advanced disease.

Some surgeons have tried to reduce the incidence and severity of surgical complications by reducing the extent of lymph node dissections. In the 1990s, several groups reported the use of a more limited "superficial" inguinal lymphadenectomy for patients with early disease; patients who had positive lymph nodes were referred for radiotherapy. Although many of the complications usually associated with radical lymphadenectomy were avoided, inguinal recurrence rates were higher than expected, ranging from 7% to 16% in patients who had negative dissections.[346,367] It has been suggested that the procedure used in these studies did not remove medial inguinal-femoral nodes, which may be the primary site of drainage of some vulvar cancers[368,369]; for this reason, many gynecologic oncologists now recommend removal of at least the superficial and medial inguinofemoral nodes.

During the last decade, a number of investigators have explored the use of intraoperative lymphatic mapping to identify a "sentinel" node that would predict the presence or absence of regional metastases. A number of studies have evaluated the results from sentinel lymph node biopsy followed by regional lymphadenectomy. From the pooled results for 383 patients entered in 10 trials, the authors concluded that the negative predictive value of sentinel node biopsy was 99.3% and the false-negative rate was 2.4%.[370] In 2008, Van der Zee et al.[371] reported the results of a European cooperative trial that assessed the efficacy of sentinel lymph node evaluation alone in patients with invasive vulvar cancers less than 4 cm in diameter. Of 402 patients registered in this trial, 231 patients with negative sentinel nodes did not undergo lymphadenectomy; at the time of the analysis, groin recurrences had been observed in 9 (3.9%) of these 231 patients, and 7 patients (3.0%) had died. The authors were encouraged by this low recurrence rate. However, long-term follow-up of these patients will be needed to determine whether the sentinel node procedure can effectively supplant lymphadenectomy in selected cases. A large GOG trial designed to estimate the sensitivity of sentinel lymph node biopsy in a community-based setting has completed accrual and should be published soon. Participants in a 2008 expert panel at an International Sentinel Node Society Meeting concluded that sentinel lymph node biopsy "is a reasonable alternative to complete inguinal lymphadenectomy when [it] is performed by a skilled multidisciplinary team in well-selected patients."[370] They concluded that patients who have tumors that invade more than 1 mm, no obvious metastatic disease, and a tumor diameter of less than 4 cm are good candidates for the procedure.

Radiotherapy Technique. Comprehensive regional radiotherapy for vulvar cancer requires adequate coverage of at least the inguinofemoral and distal pelvic lymph nodes. Patients who have extensive inguinal or pelvic disease may require larger fields that encompass the common iliac nodes. If the vulvar cancer has been excised with widely negative margins, some clinicians choose to shield the primary site with a narrow midline block. Several techniques have been used to reduce the dose given to the femoral head and neck during treatment of the groin. One approach is to use a combination of photons and electrons; this technique requires careful image-based planning to assure that the treatment is delivering an adequate dose to the superficial and deep inguinal lymph nodes. Recently, investigators have begun to explore the use of IMRT to treat vulvar cancers.[372] This approach may permit some sparing of bowel and other critical structures, but the technique is technically challenging and requires a sound understanding of the locoregional anatomy.

Patients who have local risk factors for recurrence but negative lymph nodes may be treated with local radiation alone using conformal photon fields or, in selected cases, appositional electron-beam techniques. Whenever photons are used to treat the vulvar surface, tissue-equivalent materials may need to be applied to ensure that the surface dose is adequate.

Chemoradiation in Locoregionally Advanced Disease. To reduce the need for morbid ultraradical surgery and to improve locoregional control rates, a number of investigators have explored combinations of chemotherapy with radiation and surgery in patients with locally advanced vulvar carcinoma.[373–380] Most studies have used combinations of cisplatin, 5-FU, and mitomycin-C (Table 101.9), extrapolating from the high response rates observed with such combinations for locally advanced carcinomas of the cervix and head and neck and from studies that have demonstrated the efficacy of these drugs as radiosensitizers in the treatment of carcinomas of the anus. Although studies have usually included small numbers of patients with very advanced local or regional disease, most investigators have observed impressive responses that often appear to be better than would be expected with radiation alone. Randomized trials have not been done and may be difficult to perform because of the small number of patients with locally advanced vulvar cancer. However, results of trials in other types of cancer are encouraging: trials that demonstrated improved local control and survival when concurrent cisplatin-containing chemotherapy was added to radiation treatment of cervical cancers[157,208] and improved colostomy-free survival when mitomycin-C and 5-FU were added to radiation treatment of anal cancer[381] suggest that this approach may be also be useful in the treatment of women with vulvar cancer.

Several investigators have explored the use of neoadjuvant chemotherapy for locally advanced vulvar cancer.[382,383] Although partial responses to multiagent chemotherapy have been observed, response rates appear to be lower than for cervical cancers, and survival rates have been discouraging.

Caution is warranted in designing aggressive treatment protocols for patients with vulvar cancers, as these patients typically are elderly and often have concurrent medical problems. Serious pulmonary damage has been observed in a number of patients treated on studies that included bleomycin.[379] In the largest published series of patients treated with mitomycin-C and 5-FU, hematologic tolerance was acceptable, but the administered dose of mitomycin-C was somewhat lower than that generally used in the treatment of anal cancers.[380] Although chemotherapy may improve control rates, radiation alone can produce impressive responses and should be considered in patients who are poor surgical candidates and who cannot tolerate chemotherapy.

Complications of Locoregional Treatment

Most of the serious acute and subacute complications of radical vulvectomy are related to the lymphadenectomy, although these risks have decreased somewhat with the use of separate groin incisions. Acute complications include wound seroma, disruption, or infection in up to 50% to 75% of cases, chronic lymphedema in 20% to 50%, and perioperative death in 2% to 5%.[364,367,384,385] Other acute complications include urinary tract infection, wound cellulitis, temporary anterior thigh anesthesia from femoral nerve injury, thrombophlebitis, and, rarely, pulmonary embolus.[347,384–386] The risk of chronic leg edema decreased from approximately 30% to 15% with the use of separate groin incisions and is rare after sentinel lymph node dissection only.[371,387] Other chronic complications include genital prolapse, urinary stress incontinence, temporary weakness of the quadriceps muscle, and introital stenosis. These risks are

PRACTICE OF ONCOLOGY

TABLE 101.9

CONCURRENT CHEMORADIOTHERAPY IN THE MANAGEMENT OF LOCALLY ADVANCED OR RECURRENT CARCINOMA OF THE VULVA (SERIES INCLUDING 20 OR MORE PATIENTS)

Study (Ref.)	No. of Patients	Chemotherapy	Radiotherapy Dose (Gy)	No. (%) with Recurrent or Persistent Local Disease after RT ± Surgery	Follow-Up (Months)
Moore et al. (377)	71	5-FU + CDDP	47.6	11 (16)	22–72
Landoni et al. (374)	58	5-FU + Mito	54	13 (22)	4–48
Lupi et al. (376)	31	5-FU + Mito	54	7 (23)	22–73
Koh et al. (373)	20	5-FU ± CDDP or Mito	30–54	9 (45)	1–75
Russell et al. (378)	25	5-FU ± CDDP	47–72	6 (24)	4–52
Scheistroen and Trope (379)	42	Bleomycin	45	39 (93)	7–60
Thomas et al. (380)	24	5-FU ± Mito	44–60	10 (42)	5–43
Landrum et al. (375)	33	CDDP ± 5-FU	37–63	4 (12)	NS

RT, radiotherapy; 5-FU, 5-fluorouracil; CDDP, cisplatin; Mito, mitomycin-C; NS, not stated.

less when radical local excision of the primary lesion is done instead of radical vulvectomy.[125,388] Patients who undergo vulvectomy without inguinal lymphadenectomy have significantly shorter hospital stays and fewer complications.[364,367]

The most prominent acute complication of radical radiotherapy for vulvar carcinoma is radiation dermatitis. Moist desquamation is commonly seen in the final weeks of treatment but resolves within 2 to 3 weeks after completion; sitz baths and appropriate use of pain medications are helpful during the acute phase. Skin reactions that occur in the first 2 to 4 weeks of treatment are frequently due to superinfection with *Candida albicans* and should be treated presumptively with antifungal agents. Other acute side effects of radiation include diarrhea, dysuria, and painful defecation. Late complications result from a combination of radiation, surgery, and tissue destruction from locally advanced tumors. Introital or vaginal stenosis, tissue atrophy, and other effects of combined therapy may cause sexual dysfunction. Vulvar edema, tissue atrophy, hyperpigmentation, fibrosis, and telangiectasia may occur and are related to the dose of radiation and the volume of tissue irradiated. Combined effects of treatment may also cause bladder or rectal incontinence, urethral or anal stenosis, ulceration, or fistula.

Treatment of Metastatic Disease

Unfortunately, reports of chemotherapy activity in the treatment of metastatic or recurrent squamous cell carcinoma of the vulva are largely anecdotal. In the absence of reliable data specific to this cancer, clinicians often use single agents and combination regimens that have had some activity in the treatment of cervical cancer. However, there are, as yet, few data to indicate that chemotherapy can provide effective palliation for patients with metastatic or recurrent vulvar carcinomas that are not amendable to locoregional treatments.

Selected References

The full list of references for this chapter appears in the online version.

4. American Cancer Society. *Cancer Facts and Figures 2009*. Atlanta: American Cancer Society; 2009.
7. Roden R, Wu TC. How will HPV vaccines affect cervical cancer? *Nat Rev Cancer* 2006;6:753.
9. Vizcaino AP, Moreno V, Bosch FX, et al. International trends in the incidence of cervical cancer: I. Adenocarcinoma and adenosquamous cell carcinomas. *Int J Cancer* 1998;75:536.
12. Buehler JW, Ward JW. A new definition for AIDS surveillance. *Ann Intern Med* 1993;118:390.
13. Chirenje ZM. HIV and cancer of the cervix. *Best Pract Res Clin Obstet Gynaecol* 2005;19:269.
22. Crum CP. Should the Bethesda System terminology be used in diagnostic surgical pathology?: Point. *Int J Gynecol Pathol* 2003;22:5.
26. Schiffman M, Solomon D. Findings to date from the ASCUS-LSIL Triage Study (ALTS). *Arch Pathol Lab Med* 2003;127:946.
27. Cox JT, Schiffman M, Solomon D. Prospective follow-up suggests similar risk of subsequent cervical intraepithelial neoplasia grade 2 or 3 among women with cervical intraepithelial neoplasia grade 1 or negative colposcopy and directed biopsy. *Am J Obstet Gynecol* 2003;188:1406.
29. Wolf JK, Levenback C, Malpica A, et al. Adenocarcinoma in situ of the cervix: significance of cone biopsy margins. *Obstet Gynecol* 1996;88:82.
33. Creasman WT, Zaino RJ, Major FJ, et al. Early invasive carcinoma of the cervix (3 to 5 mm invasion): risk factors and prognosis. A Gynecologic Oncology Group study. *Am J Obstet Gynecol* 1998;178:62.
41. Albores-Saavedra J, Gersell D, Gilks CB, et al. Terminology of endocrine tumors of the uterine cervix: results of a workshop sponsored by the College of American Pathologists and the National Cancer Institute. *Arch Pathol Lab Med* 1997;121:34.
44. Viswanathan AN, Deavers MT, Jhingran A, et al. Small cell neuroendocrine carcinoma of the cervix: outcome and patterns of recurrence. *Gynecol Oncol* 2004;93:27.
46. ACOG Practice Bulletin no. 109: Cervical cytology screening. *Obstet Gynecol* 2009;114:1409.
48. Arbyn M, Bergeron C, Klinkhamer P, et al. Liquid compared with conventional cervical cytology: a systematic review and meta-analysis. *Obstet Gynecol* 2008;111:167.
54. Nanda K, McCrory DC, Myers ER, et al. Accuracy of the Papanicolaou test in screening for and follow-up of cervical cytologic abnormalities: a systematic review. *Ann Intern Med* 2000;132:810.
57. Grigsby PW. PET/CT imaging to guide cervical cancer therapy. *Future Oncol* 2009;5:953.
58. Pecorelli S. Revised FIGO staging for carcinoma of the vulva, cervix, and endometrium. *Int J Gynaecol Obstet* 2009;105:103.
59. Pecorelli S, Zigliani L, Odicino F. Revised FIGO staging for carcinoma of the cervix. *Int J Gynaecol Obstet* 2009;105:107.
62. Weiser EB, Bundy BN, Hoskins WJ, et al. Extraperitoneal versus transperitoneal selective paraaortic lymphadenectomy in the pretreatment surgical staging of advanced cervical carcinoma (a Gynecologic Oncology Group study). *Gynecol Oncol* 1989;33:283.
63. Schlaerth J, Spiritos N, Carson LF, et al. Laparoscopic retroperitoneal lymphadenectomy followed by immediate laparotomy in women with cervical cancer: a Gynecologic Oncology Group study. *Gynecol Oncol* 2002; 85:81.
67. Gortzak-Uzan L, Jimenez W, Nofech-Mozes S, et al. Sentinel lymph node biopsy vs. pelvic lymphadenectomy in early stage cervical cancer: is it time to change the gold standard? *Gynecol Oncol* 2010;116:28.
70. Eifel PJ, Jhingran A, Levenback CF, et al. Predictive value of a proposed subclassification of stages I and II cervical cancer based on clinical tumor diameter. *Int J Gynecol Cancer* 2009;19:2.
75. Delgado G, Bundy B, Zaino R, et al. Prospective surgical-pathological study of disease-free interval in patients with stage IB squamous cell carcinoma of the cervix: a Gynecologic Oncology Group study. *Gynecol Oncol* 1990;38:352.
76. Peters WA III, Liu PY, Barrett RJ II, et al. Concurrent chemotherapy and pelvic radiation therapy compared with pelvic radiation therapy alone as adjuvant therapy after radical surgery in high-risk early-stage cancer of the cervix. *J Clin Oncol* 2000;18:1606.
81. Roman LD, Felix JC, Muderspach LI, et al. Influence of quantity of lymph-vascular space invasion on the risk of nodal metastases in women with early-stage squamous cancer of the cervix [see comments]. *Gynecol Oncol* 1998;68:220.
88. Eifel PJ, Burke TW, Morris M, et al. Adenocarcinoma as an independent risk factor for disease recurrence in patients with stage IB cervical carcinoma. *Gynecol Oncol* 1995;59:38.
96. Chan YM, Ng TY, Ngan HY, et al. Monitoring of serum squamous cell carcinoma antigen levels in invasive cervical cancer: is it cost-effective? *Gynecol Oncol* 2002;84:7.
97. Zanagnolo V, Minig LA, Gadducci A, et al. Surveillance procedures for patients for cervical carcinoma: a review of the literature. *Int J Gynecol Cancer* 2009;19:306.
106. Thomas G, Ali S, Hoebers FJ, et al. Phase III trial to evaluate the efficacy of maintaining hemoglobin levels above 12.0 g/dL with erythropoietin vs above 10.0 g/dL without erythropoietin in anemic patients receiving concurrent radiation and cisplatin for cervical cancer. *Gynecol Oncol* 2008; 108:317.
115. Pilch H, Gunzel S, Schaffer U, et al. Human papillomavirus (HPV) DNA in primary cervical cancer and in cancer free pelvic lymph nodes–correlation with clinico-pathological parameters and prognostic significance. *Zentralbl Gynakol* 2001;123:91.
117. Alvarez RD, Helm CW, Edwards R, et al. Prospective randomized trial of LLETZ versus laser ablation in patients with cervical intraepithelial neoplasia. *Gynecol Oncol* 1994;52:175.
118. Mitchell MF, Tortolero-Luna G, Cook E, et al. A randomized clinical trial of cryotherapy, laser vaporization, and loop electrosurgical excision for treatment of squamous intraepithelial lesions of the cervix. *Obstet Gynecol* 1998;92:737.
119. Kolstad P. Follow-up study of 232 patients with stage Ia1 and 411 patients with stage Ia2 squamous cell carcinoma of the cervix (microinvasive carcinoma). *Gynecol Oncol* 1989;33:265.
125. Magrina JF, Goodrich MA, Weaver AL, et al. Modified radical hysterectomy: morbidity and mortality. *Gynecol Oncol* 1995;59:277.
128. Rotman M, Sedlis A, Piedmonte MR, et al. A phase III randomized trial of postoperative pelvic irradiation in Stage IB cervical carcinoma with poor prognostic features: follow-up of a Gynecologic Oncology Group study. *Int J Radiat Oncol Biol Phys* 2006;65:169.
132. Landoni F, Maneo A, Colombo A, et al. Randomised study of radical surgery versus radiotherapy for stage Ib–IIa cervical cancer. *Lancet* 1997; 350:535.
137. Keys HM, Bundy BN, Stehman FB, et al. Cisplatin, radiation, and adjuvant hysterectomy for bulky stage IB cervical carcinoma. *N Engl J Med* 1999;340:1154.
138. Pellegrino A, Vizza E, Fruscio R, et al. Total laparoscopic radical hysterectomy and pelvic lymphadenectomy in patients with Ib1 stage cervical cancer: analysis of surgical and oncological outcome. *Eur J Surg Oncol* 2009;35:98.

139. Ramirez PT, Soliman PT, Schmeler KM, et al. Laparoscopic and robotic techniques for radical hysterectomy in patients with early-stage cervical cancer. *Gynecol Oncol* 2008;110:S21.
142. Bergmark K, Avall-Lundqvist E, Dickman PW, et al. Lymphedema and bladder-emptying difficulties after radical hysterectomy for early cervical cancer and among population controls. *Int J Gynecol Cancer* 2006;16:1130.
144. Landoni F, Maneo A, Cormio G, et al. Class II versus class III radical hysterectomy in stage IB-IIA cervical cancer: a prospective randomized study. *Gynecol Oncol* 2001;80:3.
145. Uccella S, Laterza R, Ciravolo G, et al. A comparison of urinary complications following total laparoscopic radical hysterectomy and laparoscopic pelvic lymphadenectomy to open abdominal surgery. *Gynecol Oncol* 2007;107:S147.
148. Dargent D, Brun JL, Roy M, et al. Pregnancies following radical trachelechtomy for invasive cervical cancer. *Gynecol Oncol* 1994;52:105 (abstract).
149. Covens A, Shaw P, Murphy J, et al. Is radical trachelectomy a safe alternative to radical hysterectomy for patients with stage IA-B carcinoma of the cervix? *Cancer* 1999;86:2273.
157. Eifel PJ, Winter K, Morris M, et al. Pelvic irradiation with concurrent chemotherapy versus pelvic and para-aortic irradiation for high-risk cervical cancer: an update of Radiation Therapy Oncology Group trial (RTOG) 90-01. *J Clin Oncol* 2004;22:872.
160. Keys HM, Bundy BN, Stehman FB, et al. Radiation therapy with and without extrafascial hysterectomy for bulky stage IB cervical carcinoma: a randomized trial of the Gynecologic Oncology Group. *Gynecol Oncol* 2003; 89:343.
167. Logsdon MD, Eifel PJ. FIGO IIIB squamous cell carcinoma of the cervix: an analysis of prognostic factors emphasizing the balance between external beam and intracavitary radiation therapy. *Int J Radiat Oncol Biol Phys* 1999;43:763.
168. Fyles A, Keane TJ, Barton M, et al. The effect of treatment duration in the local control of cervix cancer. *Radiother Oncol* 1992;25:273.
171. Beadle BM, Jhingran A, Salehpour M, et al. Cervix regression and motion during the course of external beam chemoradiation for cervical cancer. *Int J Radiat Oncol Biol Phys* 2009;73:235.
175. Small W, Jr., Mell LK, Anderson P, et al. Consensus guidelines for delineation of clinical target volume for intensity-modulated pelvic radiotherapy in postoperative treatment of endometrial and cervical cancer. *Int J Radiat Oncol Biol Phys* 2008;71:428.
177. Haie C, Pejovic MH, Gerbaulet A, et al. Is prophylactic para-aortic irradiation worthwhile in the treatment of advanced cervical carcinoma? Results of a controlled clinical trial of the EORTC radiotherapy group. *Radiother Oncol* 1988;11:101.
184. Eifel PJ, Moughan J, Erickson B, et al. Patterns of radiotherapy practice for patients with carcinoma of the uterine cervix: a patterns of care study. *Int J Radiat Oncol Biol Phys* 2004;60:1144.
188. Potter R, Haie-Meder C, Van Limbergen E, et al. Recommendations from gynaecological (GYN) GEC ESTRO working group (II): concepts and terms in 3D image-based treatment planning in cervix cancer brachytherapy-3D dose volume parameters and aspects of 3D image-based anatomy, radiation physics, radiobiology. *Radiother Oncol* 2006;78:67.
190. Haie-Meder C, Kramar A, Lambin P, et al. Analysis of complications in a prospective randomized trial comparing two brachytherapy low dose rates in cervical carcinoma. *Int J Radiat Oncol Biol Phys* 1994;29:1195.
192. Petereit DG, Pearcey R. Literature analysis of high dose rate brachytherapy fractionation schedules in the treatment of cervical cancer: is there an optimal fractionation schedule? *Int J Radiat Oncol Biol Phys* 1999;43:359.
196. Hareyama M, Sakata K, Oouchi A, et al. High-dose-rate versus low-dose-rate intracavitary therapy for carcinoma of the uterine cervix: a randomized trial. *Cancer* 2002;94:117.
197. Patel FD, Rai B, Mallick I, et al. High-dose-rate brachytherapy in uterine cervical carcinoma. *Int J Radiat Oncol Biol Phys* 2005;62:125.
198. Shigematsu Y, Nishiyama K, Masaki N, et al. Treatment of carcinoma of the uterine cervix by remotely controlled afterloading intracavitary radiotherapy with high-dose rate: a comparative study with a low-dose rate system. *Int J Radiat Oncol Biol Phys* 1983;9:351.
202. Hughes-Davies L, Silver B, Kapp D. Parametrial interstitial brachytherapy for advanced or recurrent pelvic malignancy: The Harvard/Stanford experience. *Gynecol Oncol* 1995;58:24.
204. Erickson B, Gillin MT. Interstitial implantation of gynecologic malignancies. *J Surg Oncol* 1997;66:285.
206. Eifel PJ, Levenback C, Wharton JT, et al. Time course and incidence of late complications in patients treated with radiation therapy for FIGO stage IB carcinoma of the uterine cervix. *Int J Radiat Oncol Biol Phys* 1995;32: 1289.
208. Rose PG, Bundy BN, Watkins J, et al. Concurrent cisplatin-based chemotherapy and radiotherapy for locally advanced cervical cancer. *N Engl J Med* 1999;340:1144.
209. Eifel PJ, Jhingran A, Bodurka DC, et al. Correlation of smoking history and other patient characteristics with major complications of pelvic radiation therapy for cervical cancer. *J Clin Oncol* 2002;20:3651.
211. Morris M, Eifel PJ, Lu J, et al. Pelvic radiation with concurrent chemotherapy compared with pelvic and para-aortic radiation for high-risk cervical cancer. *N Engl J Med* 1999;340:1137.
212. Whitney CW, Sause W, Bundy BN, et al. A randomized comparison of fluorouracil plus cisplatin versus hydroxyurea as an adjunct to radiation therapy in stages IIB–IVA carcinoma of the cervix with negative para-aortic lymph nodes: A Gynecologic Oncology Group and Southwest Oncology Group study. *J Clin Oncol* 1999;17:1339.
215. Pearcey R, Brundage M, Drouin P, et al. Phase III trial comparing radical radiotherapy with and without cisplatin chemotherapy in patients with advanced squamous cell cancer of the cervix. *J Clin Oncol* 2002;20:966.
216. Thomas G, Dembo A, Ackerman I, et al. A randomized trial of standard versus partially hyperfractionated radiation with or without concurrent 5-fluorouracil in locally advanced cervical cancer. *Gynecol Oncol* 1998;69:137.
217. Lanciano R, Calkins A, Bundy BN, et al. Randomized comparison of weekly cisplatin or protracted venous infusion of fluorouracil in combination with pelvic radiation in advanced cervix cancer: a gynecologic oncology group study. *J Clin Oncol* 2005;23:8289.
219. Lorvidhaya V, Chitapanarux I, Sangruchi S, et al. Concurrent mitomycin C, 5-fluorouracil, and radiotherapy in the treatment of locally advanced carcinoma of the cervix: a randomized trial. *Int J Radiat Oncol Biol Phys* 2003;55:1226.
220. Dueñas-González A, Zarba JJ, Alcedo JC, et al. A phase III study comparing concurrent gemcitabine plus cisplatin and radiation followed by adjuvant Gem plus Cis versus Concurrent Cis and radiation in patients with stage IIB to IVA carcinoma of the cervix. *J Clin Oncol* 2009;27:18s.
223. Chemoradiotherapy for Cervical Cancer Meta-Analysis Collaboration. Reducing uncertainties about the effects of chemoradiotherapy for cervical cancer: a systematic review and meta-analysis of individual patient data from 18 randomized trials. *J Clin Oncol* 2008;26:5802.
224. Pearcey R, Miao Q, Kong W, et al. Impact of adoption of chemoradiotherapy on the outcome of cervical cancer in Ontario: results of a population-based cohort study. *J Clin Oncol* 2007;25:2383.
245. Berek JS, Howe C, Lagasse LD, et al. Pelvic exenteration for recurrent gynecologic malignancy: survival and morbidity analysis of the 45-year experience at UCLA. *Gynecol Oncol* 2005;99:153.
262. Shepherd J, Sideri M, Benedet J, et al. Carcinoma of the vagina. *J Epidemiol Biostat* 1998;3:103.
264. Frank SJ, Jhingran A, Levenback C, et al. Definitive radiation therapy for squamous cell carcinoma of the vagina. *Int J Radiat Oncol Biol Phys* 2005;62:138.
267. International Agency for Research on Cancer (IARC). Monographs on the evaluation of carcinogenic risks to humans. Human papillomaviruses. Vol 64. Lyon (France): IARC; 1995.
273. Palmer JR, Anderson D, Helmrich SP, et al. Risk factors for diethylstilbestrol-associated clear cell adenocarcinoma. *Obstet Gynecol* 2000;95:814.
279. Kirkbride P, Fyles A, Rawlings GA, et al. Carcinoma of the vagina—experience at the Princess Margaret Hospital (1974–1989). *Gynecol Oncol* 1995;56:435.
283. Creasman WT, Phillips JL, Menck HR. The National Cancer Data Base report on cancer of the vagina. *Cancer* 1998;83:1033.
284. Frank SJ, Deavers MT, Jhingran A, et al. Primary adenocarcinoma of the vagina not associated with diethylstilbestrol (DES) exposure. *Gynecol Oncol* 2007;105:470.
292. Kucera H, Mock U, Knocke TH, et al. Radiotherapy alone for invasive vaginal cancer: outcome with intracavitary high dose rate brachytherapy versus conventional low dose rate brachytherapy. *Acta Obstet Gynecol Scand* 2001;80:355.
303. Beller U, Quinn M, Benedet J, et al. Carcinoma of the vulva. *Int J Gynaecol Obstet* 2006;95 Suppl 1:S7.
305. Hampl M, Deckers-Figiel S, Hampl JA, et al. New aspects of vulvar cancer: changes in localization and age of onset. *Gynecol Oncol* 2008;109:340.
307. Hampl M, Sarajuuri H, Wentzensen N, et al. Effect of human papillomavirus vaccines on vulvar, vaginal, and anal intraepithelial lesions and vulvar cancer. *Obstet Gynecol* 2006;108:1361.
312. Lee YY, Wilczanski SP, Chumakov A, et al. Carcinoma of the vulva: HPV and p53 mutations. *Oncogene* 1994;9:1655.
338. Homesley HD, Bundy BN, Sedlis A, et al. Prognostic factors for groin node metastasis in squamous cell carcinoma of the vulva (a Gynecologic Oncology Group study). *Gynecol Oncol* 1993;49:279.
339. International Federation of Gynecology and Obstetrics. Staging announcement. FIGO staging of gynecologic cancers; cervical and vulva. *Int J Gynecol Cancer* 1995;5:319.
340. Hacker NF. Revised FIGO staging for carcinoma of the vulva. *Int J Gynaecol Obstet* 2009;105:105.
341. Homesley HD, Bundy BN, Sedlis A, et al. Assessment of current International Federation of Gynecology and Obstetrics staging of vulvar carcinoma relative to prognostic factors for survival (a Gynecologic Oncology Group study). *Am J Obstet Gynecol* 1991;164:997.
344. Landrum LM, Lanneau GS, Skaggs VJ, et al. Gynecologic Oncology Group risk groups for vulvar carcinoma: improvement in survival in the modern era. *Gynecol Oncol* 2007;106:521.
346. Katz A, Eifel PJ, Jhingran A, et al. The role of radiation therapy in preventing regional recurrences of invasive squamous cell carcinoma of the vulva. *Int J Radiat Oncol Biol Phys* 2003;57:409.
347. Homesley HD, Bundy BN, Sedlis A, et al. Radiation therapy versus pelvic node resection for carcinoma of the vulva with positive groin nodes. *Obstet Gynecol* 1986;68:733.

348. Heaps JM, Fu YS, Montz FJ, et al. Surgical-pathologic variables predictive of local recurrence in squamous cell carcinoma of the vulva. *Gynecol Oncol* 1990;38:309.
353. Faul C, Miramow D, Gerszten K, et al. Isolated local recurrence in carcinoma of the vulva: prognosis and implications for treatment. *Int J Gynecol Cancer* 1998;8:409.
354. Berek JS, Hacker NF. *Practical Gynecologic Oncology*. Philadelphia, PA: Lippincott Williams & Wilkins; 2005.
356. Faul CM, Mirmow D, Huang Q, et al. Adjuvant radiation for vulvar carcinoma: improved local control. *Int J Radiat Oncol Biol Phys* 1997;38:381.
362. Kunos C, Simpkins F, Gibbons H, et al. Radiation therapy compared with pelvic node resection for node-positive vulvar cancer: a randomized controlled trial. *Obstet Gynecol* 2009;114:537.
368. Levenback C, Morris M, Burke TW, et al. Groin dissection practices among gynecologic oncologists treating early vulvar cancer. *Gynecol Oncol* 1996;62:73.
370. Levenback CF, van der Zee AG, Rob L, et al. Sentinel lymph node biopsy in patients with gynecologic cancers Expert panel statement from the International Sentinel Node Society Meeting, February 21, 2008. *Gynecol Oncol* 2009;114:151.
371. Van der Zee AG, Oonk MH, De Hullu JA, et al. Sentinel node dissection is safe in the treatment of early-stage vulvar cancer. *J Clin Oncol* 2008;26:884.
377. Moore DH, Thomas GM, Montana GS, et al. Preoperative chemoradiation for advanced vulvar cancer: a phase II study of the Gynecologic Oncology Group. *Int J Radiat Oncol Biol Phys* 1998;42:79.

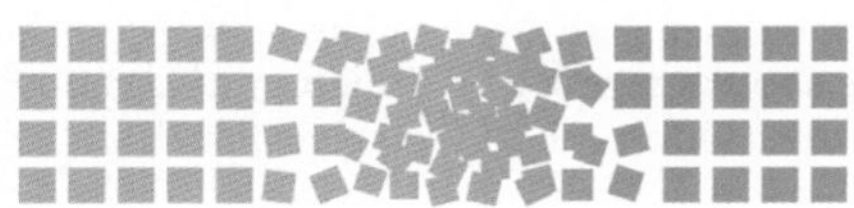

CHAPTER 102 CANCERS OF THE UTERINE BODY

PEDRO T. RAMIREZ, ARNO J. MUNDT, AND FRANCO M. MUGGIA

ENDOMETRIAL CARCINOMA

Clinical Overview

Endometrial cancer is the most common gynecologic malignancy in the United States. The American Cancer Society estimates there will be 42,160 new cases and 7,780 deaths in 2009.[1] The median age of diagnosis for endometrial cancer is 61 years, with most women presenting between the ages of 50 and 60 years. Overall, 90% of cases occur in women over the age of 50 years. About 20% are diagnosed before menopause, including 5% who develop the disease before age 40.

Nearly 75% of women with endometrial cancer present with early stage disease, with over 90% experiencing abnormal uterine bleeding. Approximately 72% of endometrial cancers are stage I, 12% are stage II, 13% stage III, and 3% stage IV.[2] Overall, endometrial cancer is a disease characterized by early onset of symptoms and well-established diagnostic guidelines. Nevertheless, women with high-risk or advanced disease have a poor prognosis and account for most uterine cancer deaths.

A general classification of uterine fundal cancers is provided in Table 102.1. Endometrioid is the most common histologic type. In 90% of instances, tumors arise within the epithelium of the uterine lining and are categorized as endometrial carcinomas with the majority consisting of typical endometrioid adenocarcinomas.[3] These typical endometrial carcinomas are further subdivided into three architectural grades based on the percentage of solid tumor growth: grade 1 cancers have identifiable endometrial glands and are well differentiated, whereas grade 3 tumors demonstrate a solid growth pattern and are poorly differentiated. Rare cell types, including papillary serous carcinoma, clear cell carcinoma, papillary endometrioid carcinoma, and mucinous carcinoma, account for the remaining 10% of cases. Adenosquamous carcinomas are now classified as typical endometrial adenocarcinomas with squamous differentiation. In general, all of these uncommon cell types are associated with a later age of onset, greater risk for extrauterine metastases, and poorer prognosis when compared with typical grade 1 adenocarcinomas.[4–7]

Endometrial cancers fall into two categories according to epidemiologic and clinical features. Type I tumors are most common: they are estrogen related and usually occur in younger, obese, or perimenopausal women, often preceded by endometrial hyperplasia, and are generally low grade. Type II tumors are associated with high-grade disease, as well as more aggressive histologic subtypes such as uterine papillary serous or clear cell carcinoma. These tumors are more commonly seen in older patients and women of African American descent.

Epidemiology

The normal endometrium is a hormonally responsive tissue. Estrogenic stimulation produces cellular growth and glandular proliferation, which is cyclically balanced by the maturational effects of progesterone.[8] Abnormal proliferation and neoplastic transformation of the endometrium have been associated with chronic unopposed exposure to estrogenic stimulation.

The development of endometrial carcinoma can be traced to chronic estrogen exposure, including oral intake of exogenous estrogen (without progestins), estrogen-secreting tumors, low parity, extended periods of anovulation, early menarche, and late menopause.[9–11] Because menarche and menopause are commonly associated with absent or irregular ovulation, women who experience early-onset or late cessation of ovarian function are more likely to have additional estrogenic exposure.[12] Morbidly obese women are at greatest risk of endometrial cancer, presumably because their adipocytes are able to convert androstenedione of adrenal origin to estrone, a weak circulating estrogen. Approximately 70% of women with early-stage endometrial cancer are obese.[13] Women with a body mass index over 30 have two to three times the risk of developing disease.[2] A recent prospective study showed that with increasing body mass index the relative risk of death for endometrial cancer becomes greater.[14] Moreover, those obese women who survived endometrial cancer had a higher relative risk of death when stratified by weight than did women diagnosed and treated for other cancers.

Epidemiologic studies have consistently identified diabetes mellitus and hypertension as risk factors for endometrial carcinoma. Nulliparity and diabetes are associated with a two- to threefold increased incidence of disease, whereas hypertension is related to obesity and diabetes and is not an independent risk factor. As noted earlier, continuous estrogen exposure, either endogenous or exogenous, estrogen-producing granulosa cell tumors, and unopposed estrogen replacement in menopause are all associated with an increased risk of endometrial cancer. Use of vaginal estrogen creams thus far has not been implicated as a risk for developing endometrial cancer. Patients with liver cirrhosis, because of higher circulating free estrogens, may also be at a higher risk of developing this disease. Epidemiologic risk factors for endometrial cancer are listed in Table 102.2.

The potential connection between long-term tamoxifen use as adjuvant therapy for breast cancer and the development of endometrial cancers has been attributed to its estrogen agonist properties. This observation has raised concerns about the safety of such therapy in therapeutic and breast cancer prevention trials.[15–17] On the basis of current information, it seems reasonable to conclude that (1) despite an association between tamoxifen and endometrial carcinoma, the overall risk is small compared with the risk of recurrent breast cancer, and (2)

TABLE 102.1

CLASSIFICATION OF UTERINE FUNDAL CANCER

Tumor Type	Approximate Frequency (%)
Epithelial tumors (endometrioid, papillary endometrioid, papillary serous, clear cell, mucinous)	90
Mesenchymal tumors (endometrial stromal sarcoma, leiomyosarcoma, other nonspecific sarcomas)	5
Mixed tumors (carcinosarcoma, adenosarcoma)	3
Secondary tumors (metastasis, direct local extension: cervix, ovary, colon)	2

women receiving long-term tamoxifen therapy should be monitored carefully for uterine abnormalities. Any woman with abnormal vaginal bleeding should be evaluated promptly by biopsy. Exposure to tamoxifen for prevention should be limited to 5 years. The development and use of new selective estrogen-receptor modulators that do not have stimulatory effects on the endometrium appear to eliminate this risk for women who would potentially benefit from antiestrogen therapy.[18]

Endometrial hyperplasia is the precursor lesion of the most common endometrial cancer, endometrioid adenocarcinoma. This phase is characterized by increases in gland number and complexity as well as cytologic atypia. The World Health Organization classifies endometrial hyperplasia into four subtypes: simple hyperplasia, complex hyperplasia, simple atypical hyperplasia, and complex atypical hyperplasia.[19] A landmark retrospective study showed that complex hyperplasia with atypia had a 30% likelihood of progressing to endometrial cancer if untreated.[20] Atypical endometrial hyperplasia is often found to coexist with low-grade endometrioid adenocarcinoma. The prevalence of underlying cancer in patients diagnosed with atypical complex hyperplasia has been studied prospectively in 306 women with this diagnosis on preoperative biopsy. Following an immediate hysterectomy the findings revealed that 42% of women had an invasive cancer, with some of these patients showing evidence of high-grade lesions and deep myometrial invasion.[21]

TABLE 102.2

EPIDEMIOLOGIC RISK FACTORS FOR ENDOMETRIAL CARCINOMA

Factors	Relative Risk
CHRONIC ESTROGENIC STIMULATION	
Estrogen replacement (no progestin)	2–12
Early menarche/late menopause	1.6–4.0
Nulliparity	2–3
Anovulation	ND
Estrogen-producing tumors	ND
DEMOGRAPHIC CHARACTERISTICS	
Increasing age	4–8
White race	2
High socioeconomic status	1.3
European/North American country	2–3
Family history of endometrial cancer	2
ASSOCIATED MEDICAL ILLNESS	
Diabetes mellitus	3
Gallbladder disease	3.7
Obesity	2–4
Hypertension	1.5
Prior pelvic radiotherapy	8

ND, no data.

Hereditary Syndromes

Endometrial cancer is not typically a hereditary disorder; however, a genetic predisposition is seen in up to 10% of patients, 5% of these associated with a Lynch syndrome, underscoring the need to obtain a thorough family history. Identifying women with Lynch syndrome provides them with appropriate screening, prophylactic surgery, and counseling.

Lynch syndrome, or hereditary nonpolyposis colorectal cancer (HNPCC), is an autosomal dominant inherited cancer susceptibility syndrome caused by a germline mutation in one of the DNA mismatch repair genes (*MSH2*, *MLH1*, *MSH6*, *PMS2*).[22–25] It is associated with early age at cancer diagnosis and the development of multiple cancer types, particularly colon and endometrial cancers. Until recently, the majority of attention and research related to Lynch syndrome has focused on colorectal cancer. However, women with Lynch syndrome have a 40% to 60% risk of endometrial cancer, which equals or exceeds their risk of colorectal cancer.

The mean age at endometrial cancer diagnosis in women with Lynch syndrome has been reported to be 46 to 54 years, compared with a mean age of 60 years in the general population,[26–29] and approximately 18% of women with Lynch syndrome-associated endometrial cancer are diagnosed under the age of 40 years.[28] Women with *MSH6* mutations have been reported to have a higher mean age at endometrial cancer diagnosis compared with women with *MLH1* and *MSH2* mutation carriers.[30,31]

Similar to sporadic endometrial cancer, the majority of Lynch syndrome–associated endometrial cancers are of endometrioid histology. However, nonendometrioid subtypes, including uterine papillary serous carcinoma, clear cell carcinoma, and uterine malignant mixed mullerian tumors (MMMT) have been reported in women with Lynch syndrome.[32]

Given that women with known Lynch syndrome can develop colon cancer before age 50 years and disease may be commonly found in the proximal colon, colonoscopy should be performed every other year starting at the age 20 years and annually after age 35. Annual evaluation, including transvaginal ultrasound, CA 125 examination, and pelvic examination, should start at age 30 years. Endometrial biopsy should be performed if symptoms of irregular bleeding or menorrhagia develop.[2]

Natural History and Routes of Spread

All endometrial lesions originate in the glandular component of the uterine lining. Their initial growth forms a polypoid mass within the uterine cavity (Fig. 102.1). This tumor mass often becomes friable and contains areas of superficial necrosis. Consequently, postmenopausal bleeding is the hallmark symptom for more than 90% of patients. Because most women and their physicians recognize that this is an ominous finding, prompt diagnosis is common.

The primary tumor may extend to involve a greater proportion of the endometrial surface and ultimately reach the lower uterine segment and cervix. Invasion into the myometrium occurs simultaneously. The uterus has a rich and complex

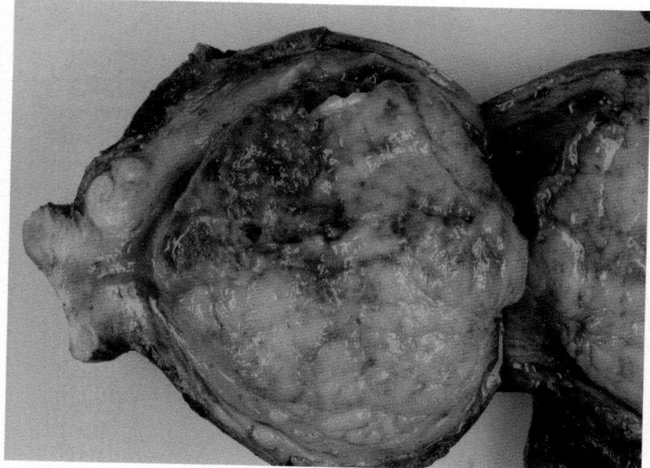

FIGURE 102.1 Endometrial cancers develop as polypoid lesions and gradually expand to fill the uterine cavity. This tumor involves the anterior and the posterior uterine walls throughout the entire fundus. Areas of necrosis give rise to the hallmark symptom of postmenopausal bleeding.

lymphatic network. Channels draining the superior portion of the fundus parallel the ovarian vessels and empty into the para-aortic lymph nodes in the upper abdomen. Lymphatics from the middle and lower portions of the uterus travel through the broad ligaments to the pelvic nodes. A few small lymphatic vessels course through the round ligaments to the superficial inguinal nodes. As a result of this extensive network, nodal metastases can occur at any level and in any combination.[33]

Tumors that break through to the uterine serosa may directly invade adjacent tissues, such as the bladder, colon, or adnexa, or they may exfoliate into the abdominal cavity to form implant metastases. Small tumor fragments may also gain access to the peritoneal cavity by traversing the fallopian tubes. However, the clinical importance of this potential mechanism of spread is uncertain. Hematogenous dissemination is observed but uncommon. Sites of distant spread include lung, liver, bone, and brain.

Diagnosis and Pretherapy Evaluation

Women older than 40 years with abnormal uterine bleeding should also have an endometrial biopsy. Any patient over the age of 35 with evidence of atypical glandular cells on Papanicolaou (Pap) smear should undergo an endometrial biopsy. However, fewer than 50% of women with known endometrial cancer have an abnormal Pap smear.[34] Although a formal dilatation and curettage (D&C) has been the standard technique for diagnosis, outpatient endometrial biopsy has replaced it in most situations.[35]

Dilatation and curettage should be performed in the setting where complex hyperplasia with atypia is diagnosed. In patients in whom the symptoms of abnormal bleeding continue and cannot be explained by the office biopsy, a hysteroscopy is indicated. In order to confirm a diagnosis of endometrial cancer, a tissue diagnosis is required and it must not be substituted by imaging studies such as ultrasonography. However, ultrasonography may be a useful imaging modality, particularly in patients who are medically compromised in whom obtaining a tissue sample is not feasible. It has been previously shown that 96% of women with cancer have an endometrial thickness greater than 5 mm.[36,37]

Preoperative Evaluation

Endometrial carcinoma is both a surgically treated and staged tumor. The only requirements in the preoperative evaluation of patients with endometrial cancer (type I tumors) is a physical examination, a chest radiograph, and electrocardiogram. The use of computed tomography (CT) or magnetic resonance imaging (MRI) is not indicated unless there is suspicion of extrauterine disease or in patients with high-risk histologic subtypes (type II tumors) such as papillary serous carcinoma, clear cell carcinoma, or sarcomas. The utility of CT imaging in changing the management of patients with endometrial cancer has been evaluated prospectively.[38] When patients have a preoperative diagnosis of endometrial hyperplasia or endometrioid low grade carcinoma, CT scan imaging changed the planned treatment only 4% of the time. By contrast, in patients with higher grade histology and high-risk histologic subtypes such as papillary serous or clear cell carcinoma, CT scan imaging changed treatment in 11% of the time.

In patients with suspected cervical involvement, preoperative MRI may facilitate determining if the uterine tumor involves the lower uterine segment or if there is true extension into the cervix. A cervical biopsy or an endocervical curettage should also be performed, since patients with known cervical involvement should undergo a radical hysterectomy. Serum CA 125 levels may be a predictor of extrauterine disease.[39] In a study of 214 endometrial cancer patients, serum CA 125 was found to be an independent risk factor for pelvic and para-aortic lymph node metastasis.[40] Elevated levels of CA 125 may also assist in predicting treatment response or in posttreatment surveillance.[41]

Risk Factors

Histopathologic risk factors in endometrial cancer patients have been extensively evaluated since the late 1970s.[42,43] Major prognostic factors associated with the uterine component of the tumor are grade or cell type, depth of myometrial invasion, and tumor extension to the cervix. Less important are extent of uterine cavity involvement,[44] lymph–vascular space invasion,[45] and tumor vascularity. Obviously, women whose tumors have spread beyond the uterus have a poorer prognosis and are beyond cure from surgery alone. The major extrauterine risk factors are adnexal metastases, pelvic or para-aortic lymph node spread, positive peritoneal cytology, peritoneal implant metastases, and distant organ metastases.

A detailed risk analysis of nearly 1,000 patients by the Gynecologic Oncology Group (GOG) is summarized in Table 102.3.[43] The risk for development of recurrent disease was greatest in women whose tumors had metastasized to pelvic or para-aortic lymph nodes, demonstrated gross intraperitoneal spread, or contained unequivocal lymph–vascular space invasion. An exceptionally high incidence of recurrence was noted in patients with two or more risk factors. Based on the findings of this and other surgical staging trials, the International Federation of Gynecology and Obstetrics (FIGO) adopted a surgical staging system for uterine fundal cancers in 1988, replacing the previous clinical staging.

Staging

In 2009 the FIGO Committee on Gynecologic Oncology revised the 1988 staging for endometrial cancer (Table 102.4). Comprehensive surgical staging includes hysterectomy, bilateral salpingo-oophorectomy, and pelvic and para-aortic lymphadenectomy. Because endometrial cancer originates in

TABLE 102.3

FREQUENCY OF RECURRENCE IN PATIENTS WITH POSITIVE RISK FACTORS

	Frequency of Recurrence[a]			
Positive Risk Factor	Radiation Therapy	No Radiation Therapy	Total (%)	Comment
SPECIFIC FACTOR				
Pelvic node	4/16 (1P)	1/2 (1P)	5/18 (27.7)	—
Aortic node	0/2	2/3	2/5 (40.0)	—
Adnexa	1/5	0/2	1/7 (14.3)	—
Gross disease	1/2	0/2	1/4 (25.0)	—
Cytology	5/18 (1P)	1/14	6/32 (18.8)	2/4 With implants only
CSI	8/30	1/4	9/34 (26.5)	0/2 With implants only
Isthmus/cervix	8/65 (2P, 3V)	7/29 (4P, 1V)	15/94 (16.0)	0/8 With implants only
TOTAL[b]				
One factor	27/138 (19.6%)	12/56 (21.4%)	39/194 (20.1)	2/140 With implants only
Two factors	25/58 (4P, 1V)	6/14 (1P, 1V)	31/72 (20.1)	0/2 With implants only
Three or more factors	24/42 (5P, 1V)	13/18 (5P, 2V)	38/60 (63.3)	—

CSI, capillarylike space involvement; P, pelvic recurrence; V, vaginal recurrence.
[a]Number of cases with recurrence/total number in group.
[b]Twenty-eight patients with one positive factor did not have sufficient follow-up. Eighteen patients with two or more positive factors did not have sufficient follow-up.
From ref. 43, with permission.

the fundus, adequate surgical margins can usually be achieved by simple extrafascial hysterectomy. The more extensive radical hysterectomy has been recommended for selected patients with gross tumor involvement of the cervix.[46–51] Salpingo-oophorectomy is recommended since the ovary is a relatively common site of occult metastasis and because most women are already postmenopausal and no longer have hormonal function from the organ. The status of pelvic cytology is no longer part of the staging; however, the revised staging system requires that cytology be obtained and be reported separately without changing the stage.

TABLE 102.4

REVISED INTERNATIONAL FEDERATION OF GYNECOLOGY AND OBSTETRICS STAGING FOR ENDOMETRIAL CANCER

Stage I[a]	Tumor confined to the corpus uteri
IA[a]	No or less than half myometrial invasion
IB[a]	Invasion equal to or more than half of the myometrium
Stage II[a]	Tumor invades cervical stroma, but does not extend beyond the uterus[b]
Stage III[a,c]	Local and/or regional spread of the tumor
IIIA[a]	Tumor invades the serosa of the corpus uteri and/or adnexae[a]
IIIB[a]	Vaginal and/or parametrial involvement[a]
IIIC[a]	Metastases to pelvic and/or para-aortic lymph nodes[a]
IIIC1	Positive pelvic nodes
IIIC2	Positive para-aortic lymph nodes with or without positive pelvic nodes
Stage IV[a]	Tumor invades bladder and/or bowel mucosa, and/or distant metastases
IVA[a]	Tumor invasion of bladder and/or bowel mucosa
IVB[a]	Distant metastases, including intra-abdominal metastases and/or inguinal lymph nodes

[a]Either G1, G2, or G3.
[b]Endocervical glandular involvement only should be considered as stage I and no longer as stage II.
[c]Positive cytology has to be reported separately without changing the stage.
(From Revised FIGO staging for carcinoma of the vulva, cervix, and endometrium. FIGO Committee on Gynocologic Oncology. *Int J Gynecol Obstet* 2009;105:103–104.)

Surgical staging indications remain a subject of controversy. Proponents of surgical staging propose that it should be performed on all patients regardless of tumor grade or depth of invasion. Opponents argue that there is no indication for staging in patients with clinical early stage disease since they have a low likelihood of lymph node metastases and the risks of a lymphadenectomy outweigh the potential benefits of having the information gained from staging. A third group proposes that surgical staging is indicated in a select group of women at highest risk for extrauterine disease; however, the precise definition of a high-risk patient remains elusive.

Two randomized trials published since 2009 have generated considerable debate on the role of lymphadenectomy in early-stage endometrial cancer. The first study was a randomized trial in clinical stage I patients comparing systematic lymphadenectomy versus no lymphadenectomy (control group).[52] A total of 514 patients were accrued from 31 centers in two countries over a 10-year period. A systematic pelvic lymphadenectomy was required in the lymphadenectomy arm, while aortic dissection was left to the individual surgeon's discretion. After 49 months median follow-up, the adjusted hazard ratio for relapse (HR 1.20; 95% confidence interval [CI], 0.75 to 1.91) and death (HR 1.16; 95% CI, 0.67 to 2.02) were similar. Both early and late postoperative complications occurred more frequently in patients who had undergone a pelvic lymphadenectomy (13.3% vs. 3.2%; $P < .001$). Of note, more patients received adjuvant treatment in the control group compared to the lymphadenectomy group (25% vs. 17%; $P = .03$). The 5-year disease-free and overall survival rates were similar between the two groups (81% and 86% in the lymphadenectomy arm and 82% and 90% in the no-lymphadenectomy arm, respectively).

The second trial is commonly referred to as the ASTEC (A Study in the Treatment of Endometrial Cancer) trial.[53] Its objective was to determine if lymphadenectomy increases survival independent of adjuvant irradiation. This trial included 85 centers in four countries and accrued patients over 7 years. A total of 1,408 women with endometrial cancer were randomly allocated to standard surgery (hysterectomy, bilateral salpingo-oophorectomy, peritoneal washings, and palpation of para-aortic nodes; n = 704) or standard surgery plus lymphadenectomy (n = 704). The primary outcome measure was overall survival. Women with intermediate and high-risk features (FIGO stage IA or IB with high-grade pathology [G3, papillary serous or clear cell], IC, or IIA classification prior to the FIGO 2009 revision) were randomized (independent of lymph node status) to receive radiation versus no further therapy. After adjusting for baseline characteristics and pathology details, the hazard ratio for overall survival was 1.04 (95% CI, 0.74 to 1.45; P = .83) and for recurrence-free survival was 1.25 (95% CI, 0.93 to 1.66; P = .14). The authors concluded that there was no evidence of a benefit in terms of overall survival or recurrence-free survival for pelvic lymphadenectomy in women with early endometrial cancer.

These two trials have been criticized extensively due to multiple flaws in design and to numerous study deviations, leaving many questions still unanswered regarding the role of lymphadenectomy in early stage, intermediate, or high-risk endometrial cancer patients. In addition, these two studies were limited by the short duration of follow-up, use of small-scale and selective lymphadenectomy, and the absence of para-aortic lymphadenectomy.

A retrospective study was aimed to help determine whether complete, systematic lymphadenectomy, including the para-aortic lymph nodes, should be part of surgical therapy for patients at intermediate and high risk of recurrence.[54] A total of 671 endometrial cancer patients who had undergone either systematic pelvic lymphadenectomy or combined pelvic and para-aortic lymphadenectomy at two tertiary centers were analyzed. The primary outcome measure was overall survival. The authors found that the overall survival was significantly longer in the pelvic and para-aortic lymphadenectomy group than in the pelvic lymphadenectomy alone group (HR 0.53; 95% CI, 0.38 to 0.76; P = .0005). These findings were evident in patients with intermediate or high risk of recurrence but not in low-risk patients. In addition, combined pelvic and para-aortic lymphadenectomy reduced the risk of death compared with pelvic lymphadenectomy alone. For intermediate or high-risk patients, 77% in the pelvic and para-aortic lymphadenectomy group and 84% in the pelvic lymphadenectomy group received adjuvant therapy (P = .10).

Using the Surveillance, Epidemiology and End Results (SEER) database, Chan et al.[55] evaluated a total of 39,396 patients with endometrioid uterine cancers. Patients who underwent surgical staging procedures that included a lymphadenectomy were compared with those who did not undergo a lymphadenectomy. During the 14-year study period, the percentage of patients who underwent lymphadenectomy increased steadily from 21%, 36%, to 43% for the time intervals 1988 to 1991, 1992 to 1996, and 1999 to 2001, respectively (P <.001). In stage I grade 3 patients, those who underwent lymphadenectomy had a better 5-year disease-specific survival than those without lymphadenectomy (90% vs. 85%; P = .0001); however, no benefit for lymphadenectomy was seen for patients with stage I grade 1 (P = .26) and grade 2 (P = .14). Additional studies are needed in order to determine the role of lymphadenectomy, the extent of lymphadenectomy, and the indications for surgical staging in patients with endometrial cancer.

Lymphatic Mapping

Lymphatic mapping and sentinel lymph node biopsy have been studied as alternatives to complete pelvic and para-aortic lymphadenectomies for endometrial cancer staging. Unlike women with vulvar, vaginal, or cervical cancers, in whom the tumor mass is easily accessible for injection of mapping material, women with endometrial cancer have tumors that are difficult to visualize and inject. As a substitute for direct peritumoral injection, many investigators have injected mapping material into the cervix or the fundus, with varying success.[56] In a recent study of lymphatic mapping for endometrial cancer with injection of mapping material into the fundus, the investigators showed that the sentinel lymph node only detected 45% of women who underwent mapping.[57]

Lymphatic mapping for endometrial cancer, which is performed by injecting dyes into the cervix or the fundus, maps the lymphatic drainage of the organ but not the tumor. Many investigators are focusing on cervical injection, arguing that the cervical lymphatic channels are reasonable substitutes for direct peritumoral injection. Perrone et al.[58] injected the cervix only in 23 women with endometrial cancer and found sentinel nodes in the pelvis only. Then they performed hysteroscopic peritumoral injection of mapping material and found direct drainage to the para-aortic region in over 10% of the patients.

Other investigators have also explored direct peritumoral injection of mapping dyes using hysteroscopic visualization of the tumor.[59,60] They too have found direct lymphatic drainage of the tumor to nodal basins outside the pelvis, along the aorta and vena cava, as would be expected on the basis of anatomical studies. Unfortunately, hysteroscopic injection remains technically challenging, and its applicability outside the few centers using it routinely remains to be determined.

Surgical Approaches

At present, surgery represents the cornerstone for treatment of endometrial cancer. For many years, the standard approach in these patients has been an exploratory laparotomy in order to perform the hysterectomy and bilateral salpingo-oophorectomy when indicated. Frequently, endometrial cancer patients present with preexisting comorbidities, including severe obesity, diabetes mellitus, and cardiovascular diseases, increasing the risk of postoperative complications and mortality.

In an effort to minimize surgical morbidity, minimally invasive surgery has now become a viable option, providing equivalent cure rates. Laparoscopic surgery and, more recently, robotic-assisted surgery allow patients to have the same procedure as they would via laparotomy while offering a number of benefits, including less blood loss, decreased transfusion rates, shorter length of hospitalization, and a faster return to daily activities.

The benefits of laparoscopic surgery have been published in a large series of retrospective studies and in several series of smaller prospective studies. The largest prospective randomized trial conducted by the GOG was published in 2010.[61] The objective of that study was to compare laparoscopy versus laparotomy for comprehensive surgical staging of uterine cancer. Clinical stage I to IIA patients were randomly assigned to laparoscopy or open laparotomy, including hysterectomy, salpingo-oophorectomy, pelvic cytology, and pelvic and para-aortic lymphadenectomy. The main study end points were 6-week morbidity and mortality, hospital length of stay, conversion from laparoscopy to laparotomy, recurrence-free survival, site of recurrence, and patient-reported quality-of-life outcomes. Laparoscopy was initiated in 1,682 patients and completed without conversion in 1,248 patients (74.2%). Laparoscopy had fewer moderate to severe postoperative adverse events than laparotomy (14% vs. 21%; P <.0001) but similar rates of intraoperative complications. The length of hospitalization was shorter in the laparoscopy group. The authors concluded that laparoscopic surgical staging for uterine cancer is feasible and safe in terms of short-term outcomes and results in fewer complications and shorter hospital stays. At the time of publication, data were not yet mature to determine whether surgical technique impacts patterns of recurrence or disease-free survival.

In 2005 the U.S. Food and Drug Administration approved the daVinci robotic system for gynecologic procedures. Since then, numerous centers worldwide have adopted this technology for the surgical management of endometrial cancer. The advantages of the robotic system over standard laparoscopy include high-definition three-dimensional vision, wristed instrumentation that allow more surgical precision and dexterity, improved ergonomics for the surgeon, and improved teaching capabilities for trainees.

Lowe et al.[62] reported a multi-institutional experience with robotic-assisted hysterectomy with staging for endometrial cancer. A total of 405 patients were identified who underwent robotic surgery. Final pathologic analysis demonstrated that 90% of all patients had stage I and II disease. Mean operative time was 170.5 minutes and mean estimated blood loss was 87.5 mL. The mean hospital stay in this cohort of patients was 1.8 days. Intraoperative complications occurred in 3.5% of the patients, and conversion to laparotomy occurred in 7%. The rate of postoperative complications was 14.6%. To date, there are no prospective trials comparing laparotomy versus laparoscopy versus robotic surgery in the management of patients with endometrial cancer.

An ideal treatment regimen has yet to be established in the management of women with metastatic disease, and the majority of advanced-stage cancer patients will recur. A number of retrospective studies have investigated the role of surgical cytoreduction in this setting. The existing literature to investigate cytoreductive surgery for advanced or recurrent endometrial cancer is confined to small, nonrandomized, retrospective studies.

A recent meta-analysis of 14 retrospective studies of patients with advanced or recurrent endometrial cancer totaling 672 patients was published by Barlin et al.[63] In that study, the authors sought to determine the relative effect and to quantify the impact of multiple prognostic variables on median overall survival time among cohorts of patients with advanced or recurrent endometrial cancer undergoing cytoreductive surgery. Clinical variables associated with median overall survival were the proportion of patients undergoing complete surgical cytoreduction, adjuvant radiation, or adjuvant chemotherapy. Median overall survival was positively associated with an increased proportion of patients undergoing complete surgical cytoreduction (each 10% increase improving survival by 9.3 months; $P = .04$) and receiving postoperative radiation therapy (each 10% increase improving survival by 11.0 months; $P = .004$), while an increasing proportion of patients who received chemotherapy was negatively associated with survival (each 10% increase decreasing survival by 10.4 months; $P = .007$). The authors also concluded that optimal cytoreduction, although variably defined, was achievable in 52% to 75% of patients with advanced or recurrent disease, and complete cytoreduction was possible in 18% to 75% of cases. Complete cytoreduction was associated with a statistically significant improvement in median overall survival, such that each 10% increase in cytoreduction to no gross evidence of disease was associated with a 9.3-month increase in survival.

Surgical staging identifies retroperitoneal lymph node metastases in 7% to 18% of patients with endometrial cancer.[65,66] Bristow et al.[65–67] evaluated the survival benefit of debulking macroscopic adenopathy in patients with node-positive endometrial carcinoma. They found that patients with completely resected macroscopic lymphadenopathy had a significantly longer median disease-specific survival (37.5 months) compared to those with gross residual nodal disease (8.8 months). On multivariate analysis, independent predictors of disease-specific survival were gross residual nodal disease, age 65 years or older, and the administration of adjuvant chemotherapy.

Studies to evaluate the efficacy of radiation therapy have shown that patients with nodal disease who initiated treatment with small-volume residual disease experience superior local control and survival rates compared to patients with unresected bulky adenopathy.[68]

Stage IV disease constitutes 3% to 13% of all the cases of endometrial cancer, with a 5-year survival of 10% to 20%.[69] The impact of cytoreductive surgery in advanced stage endometrial cancer has been previously evaluated. Chi et al.[70] evaluated the importance of cytoreductive surgery by stratifying patients into three categories according to the surgical results as optimal cytoreduction, suboptimal cytoreduction, and unresectable tumors with median survival rates of 31 months, 12 months, and 8 months, respectively ($P < .01$). In a subsequent study, Bristow et al.[71] defined the optimal cytoreduction as a residual tumor 1 cm or less in maximal diameter. Optimal cytoreduction was associated with a median survival of 34 months compared to 11 months in patients who had a suboptimal cytoreduction ($P < .001$).

Radiation Therapy

In the early years of the 20th century, radiation was not commonly used in the treatment of endometrial cancer. Increasing interest became focused on radiation following the publication in 1935 by Heyman[72] of the "Stockholm method" of radium packing. The 5-year survival rate of 58.2% in early-stage patients treated with this approach compared favorably to contemporary surgical series, demonstrating for the first time the curative potential of radiation in endometrial cancer. Radiation soon became commonplace, predominantly delivered preoperatively.[73–75] Today it is delivered almost exclusively following surgery in women with adverse pathologic features. An exception to this rule is a patient with medically inoperable disease in whom definitive irradiation is the treatment of choice.[76–78]

Radiation therapy is typically administered using external beam or brachytherapy. The most common external beam approach is whole pelvic radiotherapy. More comprehensive volumes, namely pelvic para-aortic and whole abdominal radiotherapy, have been used in select locally advanced patients. Brachytherapy is used following surgery or as definitive treatment. Brachytherapy has traditionally been delivered using low-dose-rate (LDR) techniques.

Several novel external beam and brachytherapy techniques have been introduced, improving the quality and delivery of treatment. The first was high-dose-rate (HDR) brachytherapy, which allowed treatment to be delivered over a few minutes as an outpatient, obviating the need for hospitalization and prolonged bedrest.[79]

More recently, attention has been focused on intensity modulated radiotherapy (IMRT), an advanced form of three-dimensional conformal radiotherapy.[80,81] IMRT conforms the prescription dose to the shape of the target, thereby improving the sparing of the surrounding normal tissues and thus reducing the risk of side effects. Unlike conventional approaches, IMRT is an inverse process, whereby the target and normal tissues are first delineated on a planning CT scan. Dose-volume constraints are entered into a computerized optimization program that generates the treatment plan that best satisfies these goals. During this process, each beam is divided into small "beamlets" whose intensity is varied individually. When cast into the patient, the modulated beams result in highly conformal dose distributions with rapid-dose gradients, allowing considerable sparing of normal tissues.

Endometrial cancer is an ideal application for IMRT. Conventional fields result in the irradiation of a considerable volume of normal tissues, exposing patients to a variety of acute and chronic sequelae.[82,83] Improved normal tissue sparing may also allow the delivery of higher than conventional doses, a strategy that could enhance tumor control and patient outcome.

Multiple investigators have reported the superiority of IMRT planning over conventional techniques in gynecology patients undergoing pelvic,[84–86] extended field,[87] and whole abdominal[88] irradiation. In these patients, IMRT has been shown to significantly reduce the dose to various normal tissues, including the small bowel, bladder, rectum, and bone marrow. Preliminary outcome studies have suggested that these dosimetric benefits translate to clinical ones, with patients undergoing IMRT experiencing less acute[89] and chronic[90] sequelae. Of note, bone marrow–sparing IMRT has been shown to reduce hematologic toxicity in cervical cancer patients who undergo chemoradiotherapy, reducing the number of chemotherapy cycles held.[91] Given the growing interest in combined modality regimens in endometrial cancer, such an approach may prove beneficial in these patients as well.

Several groups have reported favorable outcomes of endometrial cancer patients treated with IMRT.[92–95] The largest experience to date is from the University of Pittsburgh.[92] Forty-seven patients underwent pelvic IMRT (eight received extended field) following surgery; all received vaginal HDR brachytherapy. At a median follow-up of 20 months, the 3-year disease-free and overall survivals were 84% and 90%, respectively. The 3-year rate of grade 2 or higher toxicity was 3.3%, with only one patient developing a grade 3 small bowel toxicity. Adjuvant pelvic IMRT for endometrial and cervical cancer patients is currently being evaluated in a multi-institutional trial performed by the Radiation Therapy Oncology Group (RTOG), and consensus guidelines have been developed to aid in the planning of these patients.[96]

Another novel technique is image-guided radiotherapy (IGRT). IGRT comprises myriad sophisticated imaging technologies used to augment the delineation of the target during treatment planning as well as to optimize patient setup and target localization during therapy. The former techniques are currently being explored to improve brachytherapy in patients with recurrent disease.[97] The latter consist of a variety of in-room imaging technologies, including electronic portal imaging, kilovoltage planar, and, most recently, megavoltage and kilovoltage cone-beam CT. Such techniques not only improve the accuracy of treatment delivery, but also open the door to novel approaches such as stereotactic body radiotherapy (SBRT) in which very high dose per fraction regimens are delivered. Initial experience using image-guided SBRT has been promising.[98,99]

Systemic Treatment and Agents

Hormone Therapy

Progesterone treatment is a primary modality for complex atypical hyperplasia and low-grade endometrial cancers diagnosed in women who are still considering child-bearing. Such intervention, however, must be confined to well-sampled grade I cancers with no evidence of extrauterine disease or myometrial invasion.[100,101] Withholding hysterectomy requires counseling regarding risks, subsequent sampling to assess response, and urging not to defer pregnancy, as continued risks for later recurrences exist. The presence of estrogen and progesterone receptors in tumors correlates with well-differentiated cancers and with response to progestogens.[8]

Cytotoxic Chemotherapy

Since the 1970s, chemotherapy based on doxorubicin played a role in the treatment of recurrent disease. During the past two decades, the taxanes (particularly paclitaxel [Taxol]) and platinums (carboplatin or cisplatin) have been tested in large randomized trials (see "Treatment of Recurrent Disease") and are being integrated into the treatment of all high-risk stages of disease together with surgery and radiotherapy.

Nonhormonal Targeted Therapy

Antiangiogenic agents directed against vascular endothelium growth factors (VEGF) and their receptor, such as the antibody directed against VEGF-A, bevacizumab, or treatment directed against epidermal growth factor receptors including HER2, and other tyrosine-kinase pathways including mammalian target of rapamycin (mTOR), are in full clinical testing, as detailed in the next section.

Biologic and Pharmacologic Considerations in Systemic Therapies

The presence of estrogen and progesterone receptors in uterine tumors has been shown to correlate with well-differentiated cancers and with response to progestogens.[8] Sequentially alternating tamoxifen and medroxyprogesterone acetate (MPA) or megestrol acetate regimens are based on the concept of up-regulation of progesterone receptors by the antiestrogen.[102] Other laboratory studies indicate the presence of specific binding sites for luteinizing hormone–releasing hormone and for androgen receptors.[103] The rational selection of specific hormonal manipulations from laboratory findings may become more feasible with the wider applicability of molecular immunohistochemical probes. The potent inhibitors of steroid genesis effective in prostate cancer and other endocrine interventions used in breast cancer need to be tested against endometrial cancer. The role of systemic chemotherapy in relation to various known biologic factors needs to be defined in an analogous way.

Preliminary evidence for activity exists for bevacizumab, anti-HER2 signaling, and mTOR inhibitors. Temsirolimus is being tested as part of a randomized phase 2 study (GOG-248) for hormonally dependent disease. A randomized phase 2 study (GOG-0086P) is also evaluating the addition of bevacizumab or temsirolimus to a carboplatin/paclitaxel backbone, and the addition of bevacizumab to a carboplatin/ixabepilone backbone.

The epidermal growth factor receptor and HER-2/neu are also important in determining chemosensitivity and outcome.[104,105] Papillary serous cancers of uterine origin are more likely to show overexpression of HER2 in comparison to their ovarian counterparts.[106] In addition, the association of endometrial carcinoma with Lynch syndrome[107] has as a consequence microsatellite instability that provides a rationale for testing poly(adenosine diphosphate-ribose) polymerase (PARP) inhibitors, and is also associated with activating mutations of fibroblast growth factor receptor 2 (FGFR2) in 15%.[108] Trials with the tyrosine kinase inhibitor brivanib, which encompasses inhibition of FGFR2, are ongoing within the GOG.

Adjuvant Therapy: Stage I or II Disease

The cornerstone of adjuvant therapy in early stage endometrial cancer is radiation. Most investigators recommend adjuvant irradiation in the setting of adverse pathologic features, notably deep myometrial invasion, high-grade disease, or cervical involvement. Over the years, numerous outcome series have been reported that focus on early-stage patients treated with adjuvant irradiation (Table 102.5).[109–122] These series vary greatly, with some including only low-grade, minimally invasive tumors; whereas others focus on patients with high-grade disease, deep myometrial invasion, or cervical involvement. In

PRACTICE OF ONCOLOGY

TABLE 102.5

SURGERY AND POSTOPERATIVE IRRADIATION STAGE I TO II ENDOMETRIAL CARCINOMA OUTCOME SERIES

Study (Ref.)	No. of Patients (n)	Stage[a]	Radiotherapy	Recurrence (%) Vagina	Recurrence (%) Pelvis	5-Year Survival (%)
Alektiar et al. (109)	233	IBg1–2	VB	—	4	94
Boz et al. (110)	125	IAg3–IC	P	—	4	88
Chadha et al. (111)	124	IBg3–IC	VB	—	0	93
Greven et al. (112)	294	IA–IIB	±VB, VB	3.7	0.7	86
Irwin et al. (113)	314	IA–IC	VB, P ± VB	—	5–6	79–82
MacLeod et al. (114)	143	IA–IIB	VB	1.4	—	86–94
Mayr et al. (115)	115	I–II	P ± VB, VB	—	2.5	65–86
Nori et al. (116)	300	I–II	VB ± P	—	2	96.6
Petereit et al. (117)	191	IBg1–IC[b]	VB	0	—	95 (4-y)
Pitson et al. (118)	143	IIA–IIB	P ± VB, VB	—	5.6	77[c]
Roper et al. (119)	138	I–II[d]	VB	0.8	4.8	92.4 (10-y) (CSS)
Solhjem et al. (120)	100	IA–IC	VB	0	0	97.9 (3-y)
Weiss et al. (121)	159	I–II	P + VB	—	0	77–92 (DFS)
Weiss et al. (122)	61	IC	P	0	1.6	86.7 (DFS)

DFS, disease-free survival; CSS, cause-specific survival; E, extended-field radiotherapy; g, grade; MI, myometrial invasion; NS, not stated; P, pelvic radiotherapy; VB, vaginal brachytherapy.

[a]Based on the 1988 International Federation of Gynecology and Obstetrics surgical staging system.

[b]Majority of patients had stage IBg1 to 2 disease.

[c]Includes some nonirradiated patients.

[d]Includes four IIIA patients.

some, vaginal brachytherapy is used; in others, only pelvic irradiation. Despite such differences, pelvic or vaginal control rates exceed 95% in most reports, with high rates of survival particularly in stage I disease.

To evaluate the impact of adjuvant radiotherapy in early-stage disease, multiple prospective randomized trials have been conducted. The first was performed in Norway and published in 1980.[123] Eligible women had clinical stage I disease and underwent primary surgery without lymph node sampling. Overall, 540 patients received postoperative vaginal brachytherapy and were randomized to no further therapy or pelvic radiotherapy. No difference was seen in the 5-year survival rates between the two groups. However, pelvic irradiation reduced the risk of vaginal or pelvic recurrence in women with deep myometrial invasion and high-grade disease. Chronic toxicities were seen in 1.2% and 0.8% of patients with and without pelvic irradiation, respectively.

The GOG-99 trial included 448 stage IB, IC, and occult II patients (by the staging system preceding 1988) treated with surgery plus pelvic and para-aortic lymph node sampling and randomized to either pelvic radiotherapy or no further therapy.[124] At a median follow-up of 56 months, irradiated patients had a superior 2-year relapse-free survival (96% vs. 88%; $P = .004$). The 2-year pelvic relapse of patients with and without adjuvant irradiation were 2% and 12%, respectively ($P = .001$). Although irradiated patients had a higher 3-year survival (96% vs. 89%), this difference did not reach statistical significance ($P = .09$).

Creutzberg et al.[125] reported the results of the first PORTEC (Post-Operative Radiation Therapy in Endometrial Carcinoma) trial (PORTEC-1). All patients underwent surgery without routine lymphadenectomy. Eligible women had grade 1 tumors with greater than 50% myometrial invasion, grade 2 tumors, and grade 3 tumors with less than 50% invasion. A total of 715 women were randomized to receive pelvic irradiation or no further therapy. At a median follow-up of 52 months, irradiated patients had a superior 5-year pelvic control (96% vs. 86%; $P < .001$). However, no difference was noted in survival.

More recently, the combined Medical Research Council (MRC), ASTEC, and National Cancer Institute of Canada (NCIC) EN.5 trial evaluated adjuvant pelvic irradiation in women with early-stage disease with intermediate or high-risk features.[126] A total of 905 patients were randomized to pelvic irradiation or no further therapy following surgery. However, approximately one-half of the "no further therapy" patients underwent brachytherapy. The percentages of women in the pelvic radiotherapy and surgery alone groups who developed an isolated vaginal recurrence were 1.5% and 4%, respectively. Corresponding percentages of isolated pelvic recurrences were 1.1% and 2.6%. At a median follow-up of 58 months, no difference was seen in 5-year overall survival between the two groups.

Taken together, these trials demonstrate that adjuvant radiotherapy reduces the risk of pelvic recurrence in early stage patients with adverse pathologic features. It remains unclear, however, whether it improves patient survival. The problem is that these trials were not ideally suited to answer this question. Many of the women in the ASTEC/EN.5 trial and all patients in the Norwegian trial received adjuvant radiotherapy. Moreover, while GOG-99 and PORTEC-1 did include a nonradiotherapy arm, the GOG trial *included* many low-risk patients (58% stage I less than 50% myometrial invasion, 82% grade 1 to 2), whereas PORTEC-1 *excluded* high-risk ones (stage I grade 3 with greater than 50% invasion, stage II).

The impact of adjuvant irradiation on survival in early-stage disease was analyzed in two large SEER analyses.[127,128] The first included 21,249 stage I patients, of which 4,080 received adjuvant irradiation.[127] Postoperative radiotherapy was associated with an improved survival in women with greater than 50% myometrial invasion and either grade 1 ($P < .001$) or high-grade ($P < .001$) disease. The second study analyzed 1,577 stage II patients.[128] Overall, patients who did not receive adjuvant irradiation had a higher likelihood of death compared to those treated with surgery plus adjuvant irradiation.

In early-stage patients who undergo adjuvant radiotherapy, the optimal approach is a matter of debate. Previously, pelvic radiotherapy with or without vaginal brachytherapy was delivered. More recently, interest has turned to the use of vaginal brachytherapy alone, particularly in women undergoing surgical staging. Barakat et al.[129] reviewed the management of early-stage patients at the Memorial Sloan-Kettering Cancer Center between 1993 and 2004. An increasing rate of lymph node dissection and decreasing rate of pelvic radiotherapy were noted over time. A Society of Gynecologic Oncologists survey also noted an increase in surgical staging and a decrease in pelvic radiation since 1999.[130]

Multiple series of early stage patients report excellent outcomes using vaginal brachytherapy alone following surgery.[109,111,114,117,120,131] Solhjem et al.[120] noted no pelvic or vaginal failures in 100 stage I patients (40% greater than 50% myometrial invasion, 35% grade 3 disease) treated with adjuvant brachytherapy alone. All patients underwent pelvic node dissection and 42% underwent para-aortic lymph node dissection. The median number of pelvic nodes dissected was 29.5 (range, 1 to 67), with greater than 10 nodes removed in 84% of patients. Investigators at the Roswell Park Cancer Institute reported the outcome of 87 stage I or II patients with high-risk features according to the GOG-99, PORTEC-1, or Norwegian trials who received adjuvant vaginal brachytherapy alone.[131] Forty underwent pelvic lymph node dissection. At a median follow-up of 52 months, only three patients developed a locoregional recurrence.

The growing trend that favors adjuvant vaginal brachytherapy alone is supported by the recently published PORTEC-2 trial, which included 427 high to intermediate risk stage I or II patients (age older than 60 years and stage I grade 1 or 2 tumors with invasion to the outer half of the myometrium, stage I grade 3 tumors with 50% or less myometrial invasion, and patients with glandular cervical involvement [apart from grade 3 tumors with greater than 50% invasion]). Patients were randomized to pelvic radiotherapy or vaginal brachytherapy. At a median follow-up of 45 months, the 5-year actuarial risk of vaginal recurrence in the pelvic radiotherapy and brachytherapy groups were 1.6% and 1.8%, respectively ($P = .74$). Corresponding 5-year locoregional recurrence rates were 2.1% and 5.1% ($P = .17$). No differences were seen in overall or disease-free survival. The percentages of women with chronic grade 3 gastrointestinal toxicity in the pelvic radiotherapy and brachytherapy groups were 2% and less than 1%, respectively. Of note, a higher rate of vaginal mucosal atrophy was noted with brachytherapy. A separate quality-of-life analysis found a higher rate of significant gastrointestinal toxicity in women who received pelvic radiotherapy, which translated to greater restrictions in their daily activities and poorer social functioning.[132,133]

Increasing interest has been focused on adjuvant chemotherapy in early stage disease. The GOG and others have proposed randomized trials comparing radiotherapy and chemotherapy in high-risk patients.[134,135] GOG-156 was designed to assess pelvic irradiation versus doxorubicin (Adriamycin)-cisplatin (AP); however, it closed due to poor accrual. The Japanese Gynecologic Oncology Group (JGOG) randomized stage I to IIIC patients (all with greater than 50% myometrial invasion) to pelvic radiotherapy versus chemotherapy (cyclophosphamide, doxorubicin, and cisplatin [Platinol] [CAP]).[134] No differences in progression-free or overall survivals were seen at 5 years. Maggi et al.[135] performed a similar randomization in women with stage IC (grade 3), stage II (greater than 50% myometrial invasion, grade 3) and stage III disease. No differences were seen in terms of 5-year progression and overall survivals. However, radiotherapy was found to delay pelvic recurrences and chemotherapy delayed distant recurrences.

Multiple investigators have explored combining chemotherapy and radiation in high-risk early-stage patients and have reported promising results.[136–138] The RTOG evaluated chemoradiotherapy in a prospective phase 2 trial (RTOG-9708).[139] Patients with grade 2 or 3 endometrial carcinoma with either greater than 50% myometrial invasion, cervical stromal invasion, or pelvic-confined extrauterine disease underwent pelvic irradiation with concomitant cisplatin, followed by vaginal brachytherapy and additional chemotherapy (cisplatin and paclitaxel). At a median follow-up of 4.3 years, 4-year actuarial pelvic, regional, and distant recurrence rates were 2%, 2%, and 19%, respectively. Four-year disease-free and overall survivals were 81% and 85%, respectively. Grade 3 or higher toxicity was seen in 21% of patients. While promising, efforts at testing this regimen in a phase 3 randomized trial were unsuccessful due to poor accrual.

Several randomized trials have been performed to compare adjuvant radiotherapy and chemoradiotherapy in high-risk early-stage endometrial cancer. The first, GOG-34, randomized 224 stage I or II patients with one or more of the following high-risk features—50% or more myometrial invasion, pelvic or para-aortic nodal involvement, occult cervical invasion, or adnexal metastases—to observation or single-agent doxorubicin following adjuvant radiotherapy.[140] No differences were seen in overall or progression-free survival.

The Nordic Society of Gynecologic Oncology (NSGO) and the European Organisation for Research and Treatment of Cancer (EORTC) study randomized 382 women with stage I or IIIA (peritoneal cytology only) or IIIC (positive pelvic nodes only) to either pelvic radiotherapy versus chemoradiotherapy (cisplatin/doxorubicin) following primary surgery.[141] After August 2004, the trial was amended to allow several chemotherapy regimens including doxorubicin/cisplatin, paclitaxel/epirubicin/carboplatin, and paclitaxel/carboplatin. At a median follow-up of 4.3 years, a significant improvement in 5-year survival was seen favoring chemoradiotherapy. Disease progression was seen in 22% of the radiotherapy patients versus 12% of the chemoradiotherapy patients.

Several phase 3 trials evaluating chemoradiotherapy in high-risk early-stage endometrial cancer are ongoing. PORTEC-3 compares pelvic irradiation versus pelvic irradiation plus concomitant and maintenance chemotherapy. GOG-0249 randomizes patients to pelvic radiotherapy following surgery versus vaginal brachytherapy plus adjuvant chemotherapy. The results of these trials will help determine the optimal adjuvant approach in high-risk early-stage patients.

Adjuvant Therapy: Stage III or IV Disease

Adjuvant therapy in stage III or IV endometrial cancer has traditionally been radiotherapy. Women with disease limited to the pelvis received pelvic irradiation with and without vaginal brachytherapy, while those with more extensive disease were treated with more comprehensive volumes. Table 102.6 summarizes the results of adjuvant radiotherapy studies in stage III to IV disease.[64–66,142–149] These studies span the entire spectrum of locally advanced disease and radiotherapeutic approaches used over the years, including phosphorus-32, extended-field, and whole abdominal radiotherapy. Outcomes vary widely, with the best results seen in stage IIIA disease. The least favorable outcomes are seen in patients with involvement of multiple extrauterine sites or residual disease.

The subset of locally advanced patients most likely to receive radiation has traditionally been those with nodal involvement. Multiple authors have reported long-term cures in women with para-aortic nodes after extended field irradiation.[142,147] Patients with pelvic nodal involvement alone represent a favorable group. Nelson et al.[65] treated 17 stage IIIC patients who had positive pelvic (and negative para-aortic) nodes with pelvic or whole abdominal radiotherapy. Five-year

PRACTICE OF ONCOLOGY

TABLE 102.6

SURGERY AND POSTOPERATIVE RADIOTHERAPY STAGE III TO IV ENDOMETRIAL CARCINOMA OUTCOME SERIES

Study (Ref.)	No. of Patients (n)	Stage[a]	Extrauterine Site(s)[b]	Radiation Therapy	5-Y Survival (%)
Connell et al. (64)	12	IIIA	Adnexa only	P ± VB	70.9 (DFS)
Corn et al. (142)	26	IIIC	PA nodes	E	46 (DFS)[c]
Greven et al. (143)	74	III	Various	P ± VB	54
	42	IIIA	Adnexa only	P ± VB	60
	8	IIIA	Cytology only	P ± VB	60
	5	IIIC	Pelvic nodes only	P ± VB	50
Greven et al. (144)	105	III	Various	P/E ± VB	70
	70	IIIA	Various	P ± VB	68 (DFS)
	3	IIIB	Vagina	P ± VB	50 (DFS)
	32	IIIC	Pelvic/PA nodes	P/E ± VB	56 (DFS)
Klopp et al. (145)	50	IIIC	Pelvic/PA nodes	P/E ± VB	73
Lee et al. (146)	11	IV	Various	W ± VB	45.4 (DFS)[d]
Mundt et al. (66)	30	IIIC	Pelvic/PA nodes	P/E/W ± VB	55.8
Nelson et al. (65)	17	IIIC	Pelvic nodes	P/W ± VB	72
Onda et al. (147)	30	IIIC	Pelvic/PA nodes	P/E	84
Schorge et al. (148)	35	IIIA–B	Various	P ± VB[e]	40
	22	IIIC	Pelvic/PA nodes	P/E ± VB	50
Smith et al. (149)	22	III–IV	Various	W ± VB	89 (3-y)

DFS, disease-free survival; E, extended-field radiotherapy; MS, median survival; P, pelvic radiotherapy; PA, para-aortic radiotherapy; VB, vaginal brachytherapy; W, whole abdominal radiotherapy.
[a]Based on the 1988 International Federation of Gynecology and Obstetrics staging system.
[b]Predominant site of involvement (designated as solitary if specified by the author).
[c]Includes some patients with radiographic-positive involved para-aortic lymph nodes.
[d]Crude result.
[e]Some patients received a portion of the treatment before surgery.

disease-free and overall survivals were 81% and 72%, respectively. Others have reported comparable favorable results.[66,145]

Concerns over abdominal relapse in stage III or IV patients have led many investigators to use whole abdominal irradiation.[146,147,149,150] The GOG conducted a phase 2 trial (GOG-94) of whole abdominal irradiation in stage III to IV disease.[151] After optimal debulking, 77 stage III to IV patients received adjuvant whole abdominal irradiation. Three-year recurrence-free survivals for patients with adenocarcinoma and serous and clear cell tumors were 29% and 27%, respectively. Corresponding 3-year overall survivals were 31% and 35%, respectively. A separate GOG trial evaluated the utility of whole abdominal irradiation in early stage papillary serous or clear cell patients.[152]

Today, interest has shifted away from whole abdominal irradiation. Undoubtedly, this is due to the publication of the results of the GOG-122 trial, which demonstrated the superiority of systemic therapy over whole abdominal irradiation in locally advanced patients.[153] This trial compared whole abdominal radiotherapy versus doxorubicin and cisplatin in 396 patients. At a median follow-up of 74 months, chemotherapy patients had a significantly better 5-year progression-free survival (50% vs. 38%; HR 0.71; 95% CI, 0.55 to 0.91) and death hazard ratio (HR 0.68; 95% CI, 0.52 to 0.89) compared to whole abdominal irradiation patients, with 5-year overall survivals of 53% versus 42%. Recurrences were predominantly in the pelvis and abdomen in both groups.

Based on these results, some investigators have questioned whether radiation should continue to be used in stage III or IV disease. However, analyses of the failure patterns and outcomes in patients undergoing chemotherapy alone have supported its continued use, particularly in patients with node-positive disease or cervical involvement.[145,154] Single institution reviews that compare chemotherapy versus chemoradiotherapy have also favored the combined approach.[155,156]

Although a series of GOG studies have explored chemotherapy combined with whole abdominal irradiation,[157,158] when radiotherapy is administered today in stage III or IV patients in conjunction with systemic therapies, limited volumes are favored, with treatment focused on the pelvis with or without vaginal brachytherapy. Extended field treatment is restricted to women with documented para-aortic nodal involvement. Such an approach is frequently referred to as "tumor volume–directed" irradiation; it has been used in some trials (e.g., GOG-209) as an option to both arms of chemotherapy-based questions. Other trials have mandated volume-directed irradiation, randomizing patients to different chemotherapy regimens. In GOG-184, all patients underwent volume-directed radiotherapy prior to being randomized to doxorubin/cisplatin (DC) versus doxorubicin/cisplatin/paclitaxel (DCP).[159] This study sought to define whether paclitaxel could add to treatment with doxorubicin plus cisplatin; only in the subset with gross residual disease did paclitaxel (in DCP) result in a better outcome. Otherwise, the percentage of patients alive and recurrence free at 3 years was similar: 62% and 64% for DC and DCP, respectively.

As discussed in the earlier, several randomized trials have included stage III disease, randomizing patients to either radiotherapy versus chemotherapy[134,135] or radiotherapy versus chemoradiotherapy.[140,141] However, attention today is focused on GOG-258, which randomizes optimally debulked, advanced stage patients to cisplatin concurrently with tumor volume–directed irradiation followed by carboplatin and paclitaxel in one arm versus carboplatin and paclitaxel alone in the other arm. The outcome of this important trial will help determine the optimal adjuvant approach in locally advanced disease.

Treatment of Recurrent Disease

Local and Regional Recurrences

Approximately 50% of women with endometrial cancer who relapse after surgery have failure in the pelvis, 50% of which recur in the vaginal vault. Patients with local recurrence should be evaluated for surgical resection or radiotherapy. Local recurrence should be further subdivided into recurrent disease within a previously irradiated field versus recurrence in a nonirradiated area. Five-year survival rates between 10% and 43% have been reported in patients with a vaginal relapse in a prior irradiated area versus 65% in patients without prior radiotherapy.[160]

Surgery. Patients with recurrent disease in an irradiated area should be considered for cytoreductive surgery. However, there are no well-defined surgical indications and criteria for patient selection for cytoreductive surgery in the recurrent setting. Previous studies have shown that patients who underwent a complete resection of recurrent endometrial cancer had a median survival of 39 months and those who had gross residual disease had a median survival of 13 months.[161]

Pelvic exenteration may be considered in women with isolated central pelvic recurrences, particularly in patients with tumor involving the bladder or rectum. Five-year survival rates after pelvic exenteration in these patients range between 17% and 62%.[162] Poor prognostic factors include age greater than 69 years, recurrence within 3 years of prior treatment, and positive resection margins.[163] A study by Barakat et al.[164] showed that the complication rate in 44 patients undergoing pelvic exenteration for recurrent endometrial cancer is 80% and the 5-year survival rate was only 20%.

Surgical resection is often the best option for patients with a recurrence within a previously irradiated field. In these women, the most favorable results are usually noted in patients with an isolated recurrence site. The amount of residual disease seems to be a major prognostic factor in these patients.

A study by Scarabelli et al.[165] showed that they were able to optimally (less than 1 cm residual) cytoreduce 75% of patients and demonstrated that patients who underwent optimal debulking had a significantly improved survival compared with those in whom it was not possible. Of note, 36% of optimally cytoreduced patients were alive at 5 years compared with none who were suboptimally cytoreduced. In a similar study, Awtrey et al.[166] evaluated recurrent endometrial cancer patients who underwent nonexenterative surgery and found that patients with residual disease 2 cm or less had a median disease-specific survival of 43 months compared with 10 months for those with greater than 2-cm residual.

Radiation Therapy. Radiotherapy is commonly used in patients with locally recurrent disease (Table 102.7).[167–175] Survival rates in published series vary considerably, ranging from 24.1% to 96%. Patients with isolated vaginal recurrences represent a particularly favorable group. Pai et al.[169] evaluated the outcome of 20 patients with isolated vaginal involvement treated with salvage radiotherapy. The 10-year actuarial local control and cause-specific survival were 74% and 71%, respectively. In contrast, others have reported poor survivals in patients with isolated vaginal recurrences. Favorable prognostic factors include long disease-free intervals, low-grade disease, adenocarcinoma histology, and no prior radiotherapy. Particularly poor outcomes have been reported in women with high-grade disease even when the recurrence is limited to the vagina.[174]

Local control is achieved in 65% to 100% of patients treated with salvage radiotherapy, with the majority of series reporting rates between 40% and 70%. A major determinant of local control is tumor size. Wylie et al.[172] reported 5-year local control rates of 80% and 54% in tumors 2 cm or less and greater than 2 cm, respectively ($P = .02$). In a review of 26 locally recurrent patients, Hoekstra et al.[176] noted local-regional relapse in 6% of tumors of 4 cm or less versus 33% in tumors greater than 4 cm.

The optimal radiotherapeutic approach in patients with locally recurrent disease is a combination of pelvic irradiation and brachytherapy. Select small volume tumors can be treated with brachytherapy alone following excision. Brachytherapy alone is used in women with prior pelvic radiotherapy. Although intracavitary approaches are typically used, interstitial brachytherapy is associated with excellent control rates and is preferable in bulky recurrences.[168,170] High doses are required, and severe complications may occur, primarily related to the gastrointestinal tract and vaginal mucosa.[175] Patients with a history of prior radiation therapy are at high risk. Limited experience exists using radiotherapy in the salvage of noncentral pelvic recurrences.

Combined Modality Therapy. Many patients with locoregional disease recurrence are now entered in trials that combine chemotherapy with radiation with or without surgery, or chemotherapy

PRACTICE OF ONCOLOGY

TABLE 102.7

SALVAGE RADIOTHERAPY, LOCALLY RECURRENT ENDOMETRIAL CANCER

Study (Ref.)	Year	No. of Patients (n)	Local Control (%)	5-Y Survival (%)
Aalders et al. (167)	1984	29	NS	24.1
Nag et al. (168)	1997	15	66.6	42.3
Pai et al. (169)	1997	20	74	71 (10-y)
Charra et al. (170)	1998	78	70.4[a]	56[a]
Hart et al. (171)	1998	26	65	53
Wylie et al. (172)	2000	58	65	53
Jhingran et al. (173)	2003	91	75	43
Lin et al. (174)	2005	50	80	55
Petignat et al. (175)	2006	22	100	96

NS, not stated.
[a]Includes 37 patients with locally recurrent cervical cancer.

TABLE 102.8

SELECTED SERIES OF HORMONALLY BASED THERAPY IN WOMEN WITH ADVANCED ENDOMETRIAL CANCER

Study (Ref.)	Drug	No. of Patients (n)	Response Rate (%)	Comment
Reifenstein (179)	HPC	314	30	20-mo median survival
Thigpen et al. (181) (GOG-81)	MPA, 200 mg vs.	145	25	Median PFS, 3.2; survival, 11.1 mo
	MPA, 1,000 mg	144	15	Median PFS, 2.5; survival, 7 mo
Thigpen et al. (182) (GOG-81F)	Tamoxifen	68	10	Median PFS, 1.9; survival, 8.8 mo
Whitney et al. (183) (GOG-119)	MPA alt with tamoxifen	60	33	Median PFS 4.0; survival, 12.0 mo
Fiorica et al. (184) (GOG-153)	Tamoxifen alt with MA	56	27	Median PFS, 2.7; survival, 14 mo

GOG, Gynecologic Oncology Group; HPC, hydroxyprogesterone caproate; MA, megestrol acetate; MPA, medroxy progesterone acetate; PFS, progression-free survival; alt, alternating.

alone with or without surgery, depending on the degree of resectability. Smaniotto et al.[177] conducted a phase 2 trial of concurrent 5-fluorouracil, mitomycin C, and pelvic radiation with or without brachytherapy in 30 locally recurrent patients. At a median follow-up of 27 months, the 3-year overall and progression-free survival rates were 46.8% and 35.2%, respectively. Three-year local progression-free survival was 41.2%. Treatment was well tolerated, with only three (10%) patients developing severe vaginal stenosis. The GOG is currently conducting a phase 3 randomized trial (GOG-238) in women with pelvic only recurrences to compare radiation only versus chemoradiotherapy consisting of weekly cisplatin.

Distant Recurrences

Hormone Therapy. Progestogens have been used in the management of recurrent endometrial cancer after the original report by Kelley and Baker[178] in 1961 used the parenterally administered hydroxyprogesterone caproate.[179,180] and subsequently replaced by MPA or megestrol acetate (MA, Megace), which allowed daily oral administration at high doses (Table 102.8).[179,181–184]

Beneficial results from these trials were mostly confined to an unusual subset of patients with well-differentiated tumor, metastases to the lung, and a long disease-free interval. Accordingly, the more recent trials have been performed in better-selected patients, including limiting therapy in receptor-positive cases.[180,181] Tamoxifen was tested with results inferior to those obtained with progestogens.[182] Sequentially alternating tamoxifen and MPA or MA regimens—based on the concept of up-regulation of progesterone receptors by the antiestrogen—were not clearly superior but may have the advantage of less progestogen-induced weight gain. Overall, fewer than 30% of women (even limiting entry to receptor-positive patients) show objective responses, and the median survival of patients with metastatic disease is disappointingly short. Nevertheless, some patients may continue to have pulmonary metastases controlled for several years while on treatment.

Aromatase inhibitors have not been subject to formal studies but responses have been reported.[185] The presence of specific binding sites for luteinizing hormone–releasing hormone and for androgen receptors have not been pursued clinically.[103]

Cytotoxic Chemotherapy. Most women with recurrent or stage IV endometrial cancers should be assessed for treatment with cytotoxic chemotherapy. Doxorubicin and its analogue epirubicin have shown reproducible antitumor activity in phase 2 and 3 trials.[186] Phase 3 studies indicated little benefit from adding cyclophosphamide or progestogens[186,187]; the potential contribution of ifosfamide has not been pursued in phase 3 studies.[188]

With cisplatin and carboplatin showing consistent antitumor activity in previously chemotherapy-untreated patients,[189,190] cisplatin with doxorubicin, and then adding paclitaxel (active in previously treated patients —see below) to form the triplet paclitaxel/doxorubicin/cisplatin (TAP) became the standard treatment of the GOG (Table 102.9).[186,187,191–194] However, TAP requires G-CSF support. Considerable experience has also been obtained with the less toxic carboplatin and paclitaxel,[195] setting the stage for a large comparative versus TAP (GOG-209, unpublished to date) study.

With the expanding use of the above mentioned chemotherapies, trials of other drugs in previously treated disease have been published. Modest activity has been seen with paclitaxel, topotecan, and ixabepilone, as well as analogues or formulations of active drugs such as the pegylated liposomal doxorubicin, docetaxel, and oxaliplatin.[196–200]

Palliative Therapy

Both surgery and radiation therapy have been used as palliative therapy. Palliative surgery is largely limited to women with intra-abdominal recurrences, causing bowel obstruction or pain. Candidates for palliative operations must have realistic expectations as to the goals of surgery, and the planned procedure should have a reasonable chance of achieving the desired goal. The patient's life expectancy and clinical status should be adequate for the proposed procedure and the anticipated recovery. The operation performed should be the minimum procedure with the lowest risk capable of correcting the problem. Heroic operations attempted in patients with no chance for long-term survival are pointless.

Palliative radiotherapy is effective in endometrial cancer patients with bone or brain metastases. Palliation can also be achieved with hypofractionated approaches in women with symptomatic locally advanced disease. Onsrud et al.[201] administered one to three fractions of 10 Gy to the pelvis over 4 weeks in 64 patients with locally advanced disease (42% endometrial cancer). A benefit was achieved, with cessation of bleeding noted in 90% of patients. Overall, 56% experienced no significant toxicities. Serious chronic sequelae developed in 6%; however, all appeared 9 to 10 months after treatment.

UTERINE SARCOMAS

Tumor Types

Tumors with a malignant mesenchymal component account for approximately 10% of uterine fundal neoplasms. Pure uterine

TABLE 102.9

RANDOMIZED TRIALS OF CYTOTOXIC DRUGS IN WOMEN WITH ADVANCED OR RECURRENT ENDOMETRIAL CARCINOMA

Study (Ref.)	Drug(s)/Doses (mg/m²)	No. of Patients (n)	Response Rate (%)	Major End Points
Horton et al. (187)	Dox, 40 vs.	56	27	Median survival, 27 wk
	CAF, 250/30/300	58	22[a]	Median survival, 27 wk
Thigpen et al. (186) (GOG-48)	Dox, 60 vs.	132	22	PFS, 3.2; survival, 6.9 mo
	AC, 60/500 every 3 wk	144	30	PFS, 3.9; survival, 7.3 mo
Aapro et al. (191) (EORTC-55872)	Dox, 60 vs.	87	17	Median survival, 7 mo
	AP, 60/50 every 4 wk	90	43	Median survival, 9 mo
Thigpen et al. (192) (GOG-107)	Dox, 60 vs.	137	27	PFS, 3.4; survival, 9.2 mo
	AP, 60/50 every 3 wk	155	46[b]	PFS, 5.4[b]; survival, 8.8 mo
Fleming et al. (193) (GOG-163)	AP, 60/50 vs.	160	40	PFS, 7.2; survival, 12.4 mo
	AT,[c] 50/150	168	44	PFS, 6.0; survival, 13.6 mo
Fleming et al. (194) (GOG-177)	AP, 60/50 vs.	131	33	PFS, 5.3; survival, 12.1 mo
	TAP,[c] 160/45/50	130	57[b]	PFS, 8.3; survival, 15.3 mo[b]
(GOG-209)	carboT, AUC6/175 vs. TAP (as in GOG-177)	662 654	Not yet available	Not yet available

AC, adriamycin/cyclophosphamide; AP, adriamycin/cisplatin; AT, adriamycin/taxol; CAF, cyclophosphamide/adriamycin/fluorouracil; dox, doxorubicin; GOG, Gynecologic Oncology Group; PFS, progression-free survival; TAP, taxol/adriamycin/cisplatin.
[a]Chemotherapy was combined with medroxyprogesterone acetate in this arm.
[b]Statistically significant difference from other arm.
[c]Regimen requires filgrastim beginning on days 3 through 12 after administration.

sarcomas of the homologous type arise from native elements, as is seen in endometrial stromal sarcoma, leiomyosarcoma, and sarcomas of nonspecific supporting tissues (fibrous tissue, vessels, lymphatics). Heterologous sarcomas may contain elements with nonnative differentiation, such as skeletal muscle, bone, and cartilage.[202]

The malignant mixed mullerian tumor is a combination of carcinoma and sarcoma and is now termed *carcinosarcoma*. Although any combination is possible, serous carcinoma admixed with endometrial stromal sarcoma is the most common histologic type. Carcinosarcomas are extremely aggressive tumors with a 5-year overall survival of approximately 30% and for those with stage I disease approximately 50%.[203]

Leiomyosarcoma has become the most common subtype of uterine sarcomas, even if comprising only 1% to 2% of all uterine malignancies.[204] Pathologic diagnosis relies on the extent of tumor cell necrosis, cytologic atypia, and mitotic activity.[205] These tumors arise most often as a single intramyometrial mass and are usually aggressive even when diagnosed at an early stage, with recurrence rates ranging from 53% to 71%.[206] Patients with disease limited to the uterus have a poor prognosis, with a 5-year overall survival of 51% for stage I and 25% for stage II disease.[207]

Endometrial stromal sarcomas account for less than 10% of all uterine sarcomas.[208] These tumors are indolent and have a favorable prognosis.[209] Only about one-third of patients develop recurrent disease, most commonly in the pelvis and abdomen, and less frequently in the lung and vagina.[210] Adenosarcoma is a rare mixed tumor in which a benign epithelial component is mixed with a sarcomatous element.

To be considered in the differential diagnosis of pelvic masses and mesenchymal uterine tumors, particularly in patients with tuberous sclerosis and lymphangiomyomatosis, are the perivascular epithelial cell tumors (PEComas).[211–213] These tumors are smooth muscle actin, HMB-45 (a melanogenesis-related marker) and CD1a positive, only rarely displaying malignant characteristics but often including diffuse pulmonary involvement (clear cell "sugar" tumors in the lungs).[214,215] In a xenograft model estrogens enhanced the growth of these otherwise mostly biologically benign neoplasms.[216]

Clinical Presentation

Uterine sarcomas exhibit the typical gross features of similar tumors at other sites—firm, fleshy growth with areas of hemorrhage and necrosis. The initial growth phase of most sarcomas is within the fundal portion of the uterus. If the tumor involves the endometrial cavity, postmenopausal or abnormal vaginal bleeding is common. Tumors that have a polypoid growth configuration may prolapse through the cervix to present as an upper vaginal mass. This presentation is most often seen with carcinosarcoma in an adult and with rhabdomyosarcomas (sarcoma botryoides) in childhood.

Extensive local growth is another common clinical presentation. Once the tumor has penetrated the uterine serosa, it can rapidly attach to adjacent pelvic structures or loops of bowel positioned in the pelvis (Fig. 102.2). Such a presentation is typical of leiomyosarcoma and leads to symptoms related to an expanding pelvic mass (fullness, pressure, pain, urinary frequency) or to entrapment and destruction of adjacent organs (hematuria, tenesmus, rectal bleeding, bowel obstruction, fistula).

As is seen for epithelial uterine tumors, distant spread from uterine sarcomas may occur by a variety of mechanisms. Intra-abdominal and retroperitoneal nodal metastases are frequently associated with carcinosarcoma.[217] This is not surprising because the epithelial component is usually papillary serous carcinoma and predominates within metastatic sites. Consequently, women with advanced disease follow a clinical pattern similar to those with epithelial ovarian cancer. All uterine sarcomas have a propensity for hematogenous dissemination. Pulmonary metastases are most frequently observed. Other sites include liver, bone, and brain. Women with distant spread at diagnosis have symptoms and examination findings based on the location of their disease.

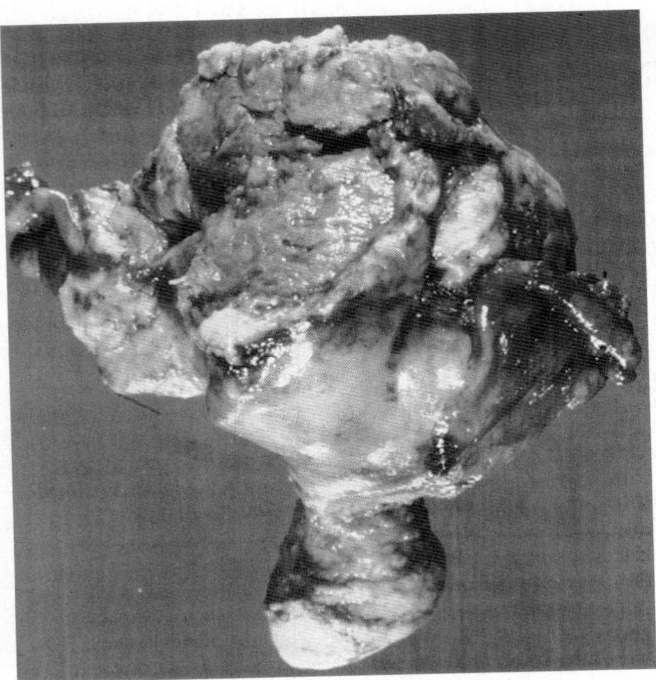

FIGURE 102.2 Uterine sarcomas tend to present as large, fleshy central pelvic tumors. This leiomyosarcoma has replaced most of the uterine fundus and penetrated the serosa to engulf the adnexa and directly contact intraperitoneal structures.

Pretreatment Evaluation

Uterine sarcoma should be suspected in any postmenopausal woman with an enlarging central pelvic mass. If the tumor projects into the uterine cavity or has partially prolapsed through the cervix, an endometrial or direct biopsy should provide a tissue diagnosis. Evaluation by an experienced pathologist is critical because these tumors are rare and the biopsy material is often fragmented or necrotic. Tumors originating within the uterine wall require exploratory laparotomy and hysterectomy to establish a diagnosis. Because primary therapy usually includes hysterectomy, the preoperative evaluation should focus on a search for disease at common metastatic sites and assessment of operative risk.

When the diagnosis of sarcoma is known or suspected, the pretreatment evaluation should include a careful history and physical examination, chest radiograph, and laboratory studies. The CA 125 level may be elevated in some cases, particularly in carcinosarcoma tumors with peritoneal spread. Other markers have not been consistently useful. Abdominal and pelvic CT imaging may be helpful in identifying occult extrauterine disease. At present, national guidelines recommend a CT scan or MRI during the initial evaluation only if extrauterine disease is suspected or if the patient is symptomatic.[218]

A recent study by Nugent et al.[219] explored the yield and impact of perioperative imaging on the management of uterine sarcoma patients. Perioperative imaging was obtained in 84 (91%) cases, including chest x-ray in 66 (72%), CT of the abdomen and pelvis in 59 (64%), chest CT in 33 (36%), positron emission tomography (PET) in 8 (9%), and CT of the head, pelvic MRI, or bone scan in a total of 2 (2.2%). Imaging identified abnormalities concerning metastases in 30 (32%) studies. Of note, imaging contributed to a change in surgical and postsurgical treatment decisions in eight (9%) patients. The authors concluded that pretreatment imaging studies change management in a minority of patients with newly diagnosed uterine sarcomas. Cystoscopy, proctosigmoidoscopy, and barium enema should be performed in advanced pelvic disease patients. Brain, bone, or liver imaging should be considered in patients with abnormal physical or laboratory findings.

Treatment

Surgery

Surgery is the principal treatment modality for all uterine sarcomas, primarily total abdominal hysterectomy and bilateral salpingo-oophorectomy. However, differences exist in the surgical approach used in the various sarcoma histologies.

Treatment of leiomyosarcomas includes total abdominal hysterectomy and debulking of tumor if there is extrauterine disease. Removal of the ovaries and lymph nodes remains a topic of debate as metastases to these organs occur in a small percentage of patients.[220] Leitao et al.[221] evaluated the incidence of lymph node and ovarian metastases in newly diagnosed uterine leiomyosarcoma. A total of 275 consecutive patients were studied. The authors found that no stage I or II disease patients had positive lymph nodes. Only the presence or absence of gross extrauterine disease correlated with lymph node metastases. It was felt that lymph node dissection in uterine leiomyosarcoma patients should be reserved for patients with clinically suspicious nodes. In combining their results with those from other published studies, the authors noted that in 101 patients evaluated, the rate of lymph node metastasis was 5%, and the rate of ovarian metastasis was 3.1%. When disease appeared grossly confined to the uterus. The removal of grossly normal ovaries in premenopausal women with uterine leiomyosarcoma may not be necessary.

Up to 70% of leiomyosarcoma patients confined to the uterus and nearly all with extrauterine disease at initial diagnosis will eventually recur. The impact of surgical resection on long-term survival in these patients has been previously addressed. In a study of 41 patients who underwent surgical resection of recurrent leiomyosarcoma, the authors found that time to first recurrence and optimal resection were significantly associated with longer overall survival.[222] Some women have obtained long-term survival and apparent cure after resection of an isolated pulmonary metastasis.[223]

Appropriate treatment in patients with carcinosarcoma includes total abdominal hysterectomy with bilateral salpingo-oophorectomy, removal of pelvic and aortic lymph nodes, omentectomy, and peritoneal cytology. The role of lymphadenectomy in these patients was studied by Nemani et al.[224] A total of 1,855 patients with stage I or III disease who underwent primary surgical treatment were evaluated. Fifty-seven percent of patients underwent a lymph node dissection. Five-year overall survival, disease-free survival, and median survivals were significantly improved for patients receiving lymph node dissection, irrespective of adjuvant radiotherapy.

The treatment of endometrial stromal sarcomas is primarily total abdominal hysterectomy and bilateral salpingo-oophorectomy. The role of surgical staging in low-grade patients remains unclear. Shah et al.[225] evaluated the impact on overall survival of lymphadenectomy and ovarian preservation in 970 endometrial stromal sarcoma patients. Of these, 384 women had low-grade disease. Among these, the incidence of extrauterine disease and lymph node metastases were 25% and 7%, respectively. Univariate and multivariate analyses demonstrated lymph node metastasis and ovarian preservation were not correlated with survival. Li et al.[226] performed a case-control study of 37 patients with low-grade endometrial stromal sarcoma and found that ovarian preservation had no effect on recurrences or overall survival.

In more extensive disease cases, resection or debulking of the central tumor can provide important palliation of bleeding and pain. Tumor reduction may enhance the ability of postoperative adjunctive therapy to extend survival, but this concept is not as well established as in epithelial ovarian tumors. The aggressiveness of the surgical approach must include a balance between the desire to remove as much tumor as possible and the risks of additional operative procedures. Women with widespread or bulky unresectable disease should not be subjected to high-risk operations under the guise of cytoreduction.

Occasionally, surgical intervention is indicated in patients with advanced or recurrent disease, but such situations are clinically uncommon. Exploration to palliate bowel obstruction or fistula is appropriate in selected refractory disease patients who have a good performance status and reasonable projected survival time. Potentially morbid palliative operations in women with terminal disease should be avoided whenever possible.

Radiation Therapy

Radiotherapy has long been used in uterine sarcomas. Controversy exists, however, over its benefit, which subtypes should be treated, and how it should be performed. Many studies that group the various sarcoma histologies together have reported improved pelvic control with the addition of adjuvant irradiation; some, but not all, have noted improved survival.[227,228] Ferrer et al.[228] analyzed the outcome of 103 uterine sarcoma patients (43 leiomyosarcoma, 40 carcinosarcoma, 17 endometrial stroma sarcoma, 3 other). Radiation remained correlated with improved pelvic control and survival on multivariate analysis. Hornback et al.[229] evaluated the impact of pelvic irradiation in uterine sarcoma patients enrolled on the GOG-20 trial. Of 109 stage I and II patients (87% carcinosarcoma), the pelvis was the first site of failure in 10% and 23% of irradiated and nonirradiated patients, respectively. In a separate clinicopathologic study, irradiated stage I to II patients had a lower rate of first relapse in the pelvis.[206]

Most studies that have focused on the role of radiation in carcinosarcoma have found better pelvic control in irradiated patients, particularly in stage I and II disease.[230,231] Impact on survival has been mixed, however, with a benefit seen in some, but not all, reports. Gerszten et al.[230] noted pelvic recurrences in 55% of stage I or II carcinosarcoma after surgery alone. In contrast, only 3% of irradiated patients had a pelvic recurrence. Isolated pelvic failures occurred in 0% and 22% of irradiated and nonirradiated patients, respectively. Irradiated patients also had a better 5-year survival.

Two SEER studies have evaluated the impact of adjuvant irradiation in uterine sarcomas.[232,233] Wright et al.[232] reviewed the outcomes of 2,907 patients (1,819 carcinosarcomas, 1,088 leiomyosarcomas). On multivariate analysis, carcinosarcoma patients undergoing radiotherapy had a 21% reduction in risk of death compared to those treated with surgery alone; no benefit was seen in leiomyosarcomas. Smith et al.[233] reported on 2,461 carcinosarcoma patients, of which 890 received adjuvant irradiation. Radiation improved both overall and cause-specific survivals. On multivariate analysis, irradiated stage I to III patients had a significantly improved overall survival, while irradiated stage IV patients experienced improved overall and cause-specific survivals.

The EORTC Gynecological Cancer Group conducted a randomized trial in stage I and II disease.[234] Patients underwent surgery with assessment of peritoneal cytology; nodal sampling was optional. A total of 224 women were then randomized to adjuvant pelvic radiotherapy or observation. Irradiated patients were found to have a lower rate of local recurrence compared to those treated with surgery alone (14% vs. 24%; $P = .004$); however, no significant differences were seen in progression-free or overall survival. Pelvic control benefits were limited to carcinosarcoma patients.

The optimal radiotherapy approach in uterine sarcoma remains controversial. For many years, considerable interest focused on whole abdominal irradiation. However, with the publication of a randomized trial of whole abdominal irradiation versus chemotherapy (GOG-150), noting a nonsignificant trend favoring chemotherapy in terms of survival,[235] interest in wide-field irradiation no longer exists. When radiation is administered today, the most common approach is pelvic irradiation. Of note, promising initial results combining pelvic irradiation with systemic chemotherapy have been reported.[236,237]

Systemic Therapy

Endocrine therapy has been widely applied in the treatment of uterine sarcomas, but because of the rarity of these tumors, reports are mostly anecdotal. For cytotoxic chemotherapy, initial trials across various histologies noted the antitumor activity of cisplatin, doxorubicin, taxanes, and ifosfamide.

Doxorubicin was the first drug to be shown effective against uterine leiomyosarcomas. Drug combinations were claimed to improve outcomes in childhood and adult sarcomas of extrauterine origin, but the addition of dacarbazine to doxorubicin did not improve the survival of patients with metastatic uterine sarcomas beyond that obtained with doxorubicin alone.[238] Nevertheless, dacarbazine and temozolomide have been part of combinations purported to have some antitumor activity: a combination of hydroxyurea, etoposide, and dacarbazine had antitumor activity without major toxicities.[239] A randomized GOG trial failed to show that the addition of cyclophosphamide in modest doses was advantageous over doxorubicin by itself.[240] The alkylating agent ifosfamide has modest activity[241] but does not add substantially to the therapeutic efficacy of doxorubicin.[242] Other drugs, such as cisplatin,[243] etoposide,[244] and paclitaxel,[245] have also been evaluated and shown to have modest to minimal activity. The combination of gemcitabine and docetaxel has been reported to have substantial activity and be superior to gemcitabine alone[246,247]; it is now being evaluated together with bevacizumab and as an adjuvant to surgery (Table 102.10).[239–246,248–256] The growth of benign leiomyomas is under estrogenic and progestogenic control.[257] Therefore, the presence of hormone receptors in a high percentage of these tumors has prompted interest in endocrine therapies. Recent case series have reported useful, albeit modest, therapeutic effects of aromatase inhibitors and antiestrogens,[258,259] leading to an ongoing randomized study of letrozole versus expectative management. Further molecular characterization of these tumors has stimulated studies of targeted therapies.[253,260]

The sensitivity of carcinosarcomas to chemotherapy often parallels that of epithelial endometrial and ovarian cancers, suggesting that the sarcomatous component may be a further dedifferentiated portion of the epithelial malignancy. As opposed to leiomyosarcoma, where previously untreated patients had a 17.2% partial response rate to ifosfamide, response rates to this drug are substantially higher in carcinosarcomas patients; and complete responses are not unusual in these patients. In fact, both ifosfamide[261,262] and cisplatin[243] have been shown to have greater antitumor activity than doxorubicin.[240,248] Accordingly, the two drugs in combination were studied in all stages and compared with ifosfamide alone in advanced, persistent, or recurrent disease.[262] The results indicate an advantage for the combination in terms of responses and progression-free survival, but nearly equivalent median survival is achieved at a cost of increased toxicity.

TABLE 102.10

SELECTED CYTOTOXIC DRUG TRIALS IN UTERINE LEIOMYOSARCOMAS

Study (Ref.)	Drug	No. of Patients (n)	Response Rate (% CR + PR)	Comment
SINGLE AGENTS				
Omura et al. (248) (GOG-21)	Doxorubicin	28	25	Includes all uterine sarcomas; addition of dacarbazine did not improve outcome
Muss et al. (240) (GOG-42)	Doxorubicin	38	8	Includes all uterine sarcomas; addition of cyclophosphamide did not improve outcome
Thigpen et al. (243) (GOG-26C)	Cisplatin	50	—	First-line only; response duration, 3.4 mo; survival, 7.8 mo
Sutton et al. (241) (GOG-26U)	Ifosfamide	35	17	Response duration, 3.8 mo; survival, 6 mo
Slayton et al. (249) (GOG-26D)	Etoposide	28	11	IV d 1, 3, 5 every 3 wk
Thigpen et al. (244) (GOG-87D)	Etoposide	—	—	IV d 1, 3, 5 every 3 wk
Rose et al. (250) (GOG 131B)[a]	Etoposide	29	7	PO d 1–21 every 4 wk
Sutton et al. (245) (GOG-87G)	Paclitaxel	33	10	IV 3-h infusion every 3 wk
Gallup et al. (251) (GOG-131C)[a]	Paclitaxel	53	—	IV 3-h infusion every 3 wk
Look et al. (252)	Gemcitabine	42	21	IV d 1, 8, 15 every 3 wk—all prior treatment
Hensley et al. (253) (GOG-231C)	Sunitinib	23	9	2 PR, progression-free survival 1.5 mo
COMBINATION CHEMOTHERAPY				
Sutton et al. (242)	Ifosfamide + doxorubicin	33	30	Response duration, 4.1 mo; survival, 9.6 mo
Currie et al. (239) (GOG-87C)	Hydroxyurea, dacarbazine, etoposide	38	18	Response duration, 12 mo; survival, 15 mo
Edmondson et al. (254)	Mitomycin, doxorubicin, cisplatin	36	22	GOG pilot study
Hensley et al. (246)	Gemcitabine + docetaxel (GD)	34	53	Uterine primaries in 29; 16 had prior doxorubicin ± doxorubicin ± ifosfamide; survival, 18 mo
Hensley et al. (255) (GOG-131G)	GD	48	27	3 CR, 15 PR—all prior treatment
Hensley et al. (253) (GOG-87L)	GD	42	36	2 CR, 13 PR—previously untreated
Hensley et al. (256)	GD	23	NA	Post resection: 10 progression-free at 2 y
Hensley et al. (GOG-250)	GD + bevacizumab vs. GD + placebo		—	Begun accrual in 2009

GOG, Gynecologic Oncology Group; CR, complete response; PR, partial response; NA, not applicable
[a]Previously treated with chemotherapy series.

In resected stage I and II uterine carcinosarcomas, adjuvant ifosfamide plus cisplatin was compared to postoperative radiation, with a trend in favor of chemotherapy.[235] Subsequently, taxanes such as paclitaxel were found active,[263] and in a randomized study, the addition of paclitaxel to ifosfamide demonstrated an improvement in response rates and survival over ifosfamide alone.[264] Paclitaxel has formed part of active combinations with the pegylated liposomal doxorubicin[265] or carboplatin.[268] Minimal activity has been noted for topotecan and etoposide[249,266]; trabectedin is under study (Table 102.11).[238,240,243,248,249,262–264,266–269]

A search is ongoing to characterize whether molecular targets, including hormone receptors, may have therapeutic implications. The delineation of the phenomenon of epithelial to mesenchymal transition (EMT) not only supports a common cell of origin for carcinosarcomas, but also raises the possibility of a number of therapeutic targets. Molecular findings have suggested that the carcinoma and sarcoma elements of these tumors are related.[270] As clinical trials have evolved, carcinosarcomas are increasingly treated in an analogous way to cancers of epithelial origin. Antiangiogenic strategies are undergoing testing in all sarcomas of the uterus.[271]

Receptors have been studied in endometrial stromal sarcomas[272] and justify exploration of inhibition or depletion of hormonal mediators in the management of these tumors. The tumor's relative rarity does not support the conduct of clinical trials and usually relies on reports from individual institutions.[273,274] Low-grade (fewer than 10 mitoses per high-power field) tumors, yield to hormonal therapy.[258,260,275] However, high-grade tumors are usually receptor negative, and chemotherapy rather than hormonal therapy has been the modality used when the disease is disseminated. These high-grade sarcomas are no longer referred as pertaining to "endometrial stromal" sarcomas, unless they are shown to arise in the context of an existing low-grade endometrial stromal sarcoma.[205]

TABLE 102.11

SELECTED PHASE 2 AND RANDOMIZED STUDIES IN UTERINE CARCINOSARCOMAS (MIXED MULLERIAN TUMORS)

Study (Ref.)	Treatment	No. of Patients (n)	Response Rate (%); [PFS]	Comment
Omura et al. (248) (GOG-21)	Doxorubicin	41	10	Includes all uterine sarcomas; addition of dacarbazine did not improve outcome
Muss et al. (240) (GOG-42)	Doxorubicin	51	10	Includes all uterine sarcomas; addition of cyclophosphamide did not improve outcome
Thigpen et al. (243) (GOG-26C)	Cisplatin	50	19 (5 CR)	First-line only; response duration, 9.3 mo; survival, 7 mo
Sutton et al. (262)	Ifosfamide vs.	102	36 [4 mo]	Survival, 7.8 mo
	Ifosfamide + cisplatin	92	54 [6 mo]	Survival, 9.4 mo
Homesley et al. (264)	Ifosfamide vs.	91	29 [3.6 mo]	Survival 8.4 mo
	Ifosfamide + paclitaxel	88	45 [5.8 mo]	Survival 13.5 mo; hazard for death 0.69 ($P = .03$)
Powell et al. (GOG-261)	Carboplatin paclitaxel versus Ifosfamide + paclitaxel	—	—	Ongoing study not yet reported by GOG
Ang et al. (267)	Carboplatin/ doxorubicin → carboplatin/ paclitaxel	11	67	Included one ovarian; only 9 evaluable for response
Slayton et al. (249) (GOG-26D, GOG-87B)	Etoposide	31	6	IV d 1, 3, 5 every 3 wk
Curtin et al. (263) (GOG-130B)	Paclitaxel	53	18.2 (4 CR)	IV 3-h infusion every 3 wk
Miller et al. (266) (GOG-130D)	Topotecan	48	10 (5 CR)	Daily × 5 schedule; response duration 8.3 m (all complete)
Powell et al. (268) (GOG-232B)	Carboplatin + paclitaxel	46	54 (6 CR)	59% completed 6 or more cycles To be studied in phase 3
Miller et al. (269) (GOG-130E)	Gemcitabine + docetaxel	24		Closed after one stage
Currie et al. (238) (GOG-87C)	Hydroxyurea, dacarbazine, etoposide	32	16	Response duration, 6.3 mo
Monk (GOG-87M)	Trabectedin			Study not yet reported by GOG

GOG, Gynecologic Oncology Group; CR, complete response; PFS, progression-free survival; IV, intravenous.

PRACTICE OF ONCOLOGY

Selected References

The full list of reference for this chapter apprears in the online version.

1. American Cancer Society. Cancer facts and figures, 2009. World Wide Web URL: http://www.cancer.org/Research/CancerFactsFigures/cancer-facts-figures-2009.
2. Sorosky JI. Endometrial cancer. *Obstet Gynecol* 2008;111:436.
19. ACOG Practice Bulletin: management of endometrial cancer. *Obstet Gynecol* 2005;106:413.
20. Kurman RJ, Kaminski PF, Norris HJ. The behavior of endometrial hyperplasia: a long-term study of "untreated" hyperplasia in 170 patients. *Cancer* 1985;56:403.
28. Schmeler KM, Lynch HT, Chen LM, et al. Prophylactic surgery to reduce the risk of gynecologic cancers in the Lynch syndrome. *N Engl J Med* 2006;354:261.
29. Hampel H, Frankel W, Panescu J, et al. A. Screening for Lynch syndrome (hereditary nonpolyposis colorectal cancer) among endometrial cancer patients. *Cancer Res* 2006;66:7810.
38. Bansal N, Herzog TJ, Brunner-Brown A, et al. The utility and cost effectiveness of preoperative computed tomography for patients with uterine malignancies. *Gynecol Oncol* 2008;111:208.
52. Panici PB, Stefano S, Maneschi F, et al. Systematic pelvic lymphadenectomy vs no lymphadenectomy in early-stage endometrial carcinoma: randomized clinical trial. *J Natl Cancer Inst* 2008;100:1707.
53. The writing committee on behalf of the ASTEC study group. Efficacy of systematic pelvic lymphadenectomy in endometrial cancer (MRC ASTEC trial): a randomized study. *Lancet* 2009;373:125.
54. Todo Y, Kato H, Kaneuchi M, et al. Survival effect of para-aortic lymphadenectomy in endometrial cancer (SEPAL study): a retrospective cohort analysis. *Lancet* 2010;375:1165.
55. Chan JK, Wu H, Cheung MK, et al. The outcomes of 27,063 women with unstaged endometrioid uterine cancer. *Gynecol Oncol* 2007;106:282.
57. Frumovitz M, Bodurka DC, Broaddus RR, et al. Lymphatic mapping and sentinel node biopsy in women with high-risk endometrial cancer. *Gynecol Oncol* 2007;104:100.
61. Walker JL, Piedmonte MR, Spirtos NM, et al. Laparoscopy compared with laparotomy for comprehensive surgical staging of uterine cancer: Gynecologic Oncology Group study LAP2. *J Clin Oncol* 2009;27:5331.
62. Lowe MP, Johnson PR, Kamelle SA. A multi-institutional experience with robotic-assisted hysterectomy with staging for endometrial cancer. *Obstet Gynecol* 2009;114:236.
63. Barlin JN, Puri I, Bristow RE. Cytoreductive surgery for advanced or recurrent endometrial cancer: a meta-analysis. *Gynecol Oncol* 2010;118:14.
89. Mundt AJ, Mell LK, Roeske JC. Intensity-modulated whole pelvic radiotherapy in women with gynecologic malignancies. *Int J Radiat Oncol Biol Phys* 2002;52:1330.

96. Small W Jr, Mell LK, Anderson P, et al. Consensus guidelines for delineation of clinical target volume for intensity-modulated pelvic radiotherapy in postoperative treatment of endometrial and cervical cancer. *Int J Radiat Oncol Biol Phys* 2008;71:428.
100. Ramirez PT, Frumovitz M, Bodurka DC, et al. Hormonal therapy for the management of grade 1 endometrial adenocarcinoma: a literature review. *Gynecol Oncol* 2004;95:133.
101. Duska LR. Primary hormonal therapy of endometrial cancer. In: Muggia F, Oliva E, eds. *Uterine cancer: current clinical oncology*. New York: Humana Press, 2009:143.
123. Aalders J, Abeler V, Kolstad P, et al. Postoperative external irradiation and prognostic parameters in stage I endometrial carcinoma. *Obstet Gynecol* 1980;56:419.
124. Keys HM, Roberts JA, Brunetto VL, et al. A phase III trial of surgery with or without adjunctive external pelvic radiation therapy in intermediate risk endometrial adenocarcinoma: a Gynecologic Oncology Group study. *Gynecol Oncol* 2004;92:744.
125. Creutzberg CL, van Putten WL, Koper PC, et al. Surgery and postoperative radiotherapy vs surgery alone for patients with stage-1 endometrial carcinoma: multicentre randomized trial. PORTEC Study Group, Post Operative Radiation Therapy in Endometrial Carcinoma. *Lancet* 2000;355:1404.
126. ASTEC/EN.5 Study Group, Blake P, Swart AM, et al. Adjuvant external beam radiotherapy in the treatment of endometrial cancer (MRC ASTEC and NCIC CTG EN.5 randomized trials): pooled trial results, systematic review and meta-analysis. *Lancet* 2009;373:137.
127. Lee CM, Szabo A, Shrieve DC, et al. Frequency and effect of adjuvant radiation therapy among women with stage I endometrial adenocarcinoma. *JAMA* 2006;295:389.
132. Nout RA, Smit VT, Putter H, et al. Vaginal brachytherapy versus pelvic external beam radiotherapy for patients with endometrial cancer of high-intermediate risk (PORTEC-2): an open-label, non-inferiority randomised trial. *Lancet* 2010;375:816.
140. Morrow CP, Bundy BN, Homesley HD, et al. Doxorubicin as an adjuvant following surgery and radiation therapy in patients with high-risk endometrial carcinoma, stage I and occult stage II: a Gynecologic Oncology Group study. *Gynecol Oncol* 1990;36:166.
153. Randall ME, Filiaci VL, Muss H, et al. Randomized phase III trial of whole-abdominal irradiation versus doxorubicin and cisplatin chemotherapy in advanced endometrial carcinoma: a Gynecologic Oncology Group study. *J Clin Oncol* 2006;24:36.
159. Homesley HD, Filiaci V, Gibbons SK, et al. A randomized phase III trial in advanced endometrial carcinoma of surgery and volume directed radiation followed by cisplatin and doxorubicin with or without paclitaxel: a Gynecologic Oncology Group study. *Gynecol Oncol* 2009;112:543.
162. Berek JS, Howe C, Lagasse LD, et al. Pelvic exenteration for recurrent gynecologic malignancy: survival and morbidity analysis of the 45-year experience at UCLA. *Gynecol Oncol* 2005;99:152.
178. Kelley RM, Baker W. Progestational agents in the treatment of carcinoma of the endometrium. *N Engl J Med* 1961;264:216.
181. Thigpen JT, Brady M, Alvarez RD, et al. Oral medroxy-progesterone acetate in the treatment of advanced or recurrent endometrial carcinoma: a dose-response study by the Gynecologic Oncology Group. *J Clin Oncol* 1999;17:1736.
184. Fiorica JV, Brunetto VL, Hanjani P, et al. Phase II trial of alternating courses of megestrol acetate and tamoxifen in advanced endometrial carcinoma: Gynecologic Oncology Group study. *Gynecol Oncol* 2004;92:10.
192. Thigpen T, Brady MF, Homesley H, et al. Phase III trial of doxorubicin with or without cisplatin in advanced endometrial carcinoma: a Gynecologic Oncology Group study. *J Clin Oncol* 2004;22:3902.
194. Fleming GF, Filiaci VL, Cella D, et al. Randomized trial of doxorubicin plus cisplatin with or without paclitaxel plus filgrastim in advanced endometrial carcinoma: a Gynecologic Oncology Group study. *J Clin Oncol* 2004;22:2159.
195. Hoskins PJ. The role of platins in newly diagnosed endometrial cancer. In: Bonetti A., et al., eds. *Platinum and other heavy metal compounds in cancer chemotherapy*. New York: Humana Press, 2009:307.
208. Jemal A, Siegel R, Ward E, et al. Cancer statistics, 2008. *CA Cancer J Clin* 2008;58:71.
212. Vang R, Kempson RL. Perivascular epithelioid cell tumor (PEComa) of the uterus: a subset of HMB-45-positive epithelioid mesenchymal neoplasms with uncertain relationship to pure smooth muscle tumors. *Am J Surg Path* 2002;26:1.
234. Reed NS, Mangioni C, Malmstrom H, et al. Phase III randomized study to evaluate the role of adjuvant pelvic radiotherapy in the treatment of uterine sarcomas stages I and II: an European Organization for Research and Treatment of Cancer Gynaecological Cancer Group Study (protocol 55874). *Eur J Cancer* 2008;44:808.
235. Wolfson AH, Brady MF, Rocereto T, et al. A Gynecologic Oncology Group randomized phase III trial of whole abdominal irradiation (WAI) vs cisplatin-ifosfamide and mesna (CIM) as post-surgical therapy in stage I-IV carcinosarcoma (CS) of the uterus. *Gynecol Oncol* 2007;107:177.
246. Hensley ML, Maki R, Venkrataman E, et al. Gemcitabine and docetaxel in patients with unresectable leiomyosarcomas: results of a phase II trial. *J Clin Oncol* 2002;20:2824.
247. Maki RG, Wathen JK, Patel SR, et al. Randomized phase II study of gemcitabine and docetaxel compared with gemcitabine alone in patients with metastatic soft tissue sarcomas: results of sarcoma alliance for research through collaboration study 002. *J Clin Oncol* 2007;25:2755.
258. Ioffe YJ, Walsh CS, Karlan BY, et al. Hormone receptor expression in uterine sarcomas: prognostic and therapeutic roles. *Gynecol Oncol* 2009;115:466.
259. O'Cearbhaill R, Zhou Q, Iasonos A, et al. Treatment of advanced uterine leiomyosarcoma with aromatase inhibitors. *Gynecol Oncol* 2010;116:424.
260. Amant F, Cooemans A, Debiec-Rychter M, et al. Clinical management of uterine sarcomas. *Lancet Oncol* 2009;10:1188.

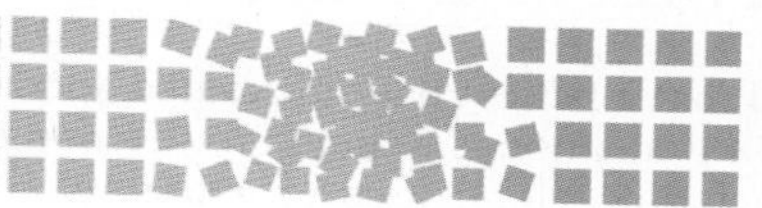

CHAPTER 103 GESTATIONAL TROPHOBLASTIC NEOPLASMS

DONALD P. GOLDSTEIN AND ROSS S. BERKOWITZ

Gestational trophoblastic neoplasms (GTNs) comprise a group of interrelated conditions that arise from an abnormal fertilization, and consist of five distinct clinicopathologic entities: complete hydatidiform mole (CHM), partial hydatidiform mole (PHM), invasive mole (IM), choriocarcinoma (CCA), and placental site trophoblastic tumors (PSTT). Although these tumors represent fewer than 1% of gynecologic malignancies, it is important that medical oncologists understand their natural history and management because of their life-threatening potential in reproductive-age females and their high curability with preservation of reproductive potential if treated early and according to well-established guidelines.

EPIDEMIOLOGY

GTN arises most commonly after a molar pregnancy, but can also occur after normal or ectopic pregnancies and spontaneous or induced abortions. Approximately 20% of women with CHM develop either IM or metastatic disease.[1] There appears to be a greater risk of developing GTN in patients with a history of molar pregnancy.[2] The incidence of GTN after spontaneous miscarriage is estimated at 1:15,000, while the incidence after a term pregnancy is 1:150,000. The overall incidence of GTN following all types of pregnancies is estimated at 1:40,000.[3]

PATHOLOGY AND NATURAL HISTORY

CHM is characterized by clusters of hydropic villi and trophoblastic hyperplasia and atypia. CHMs are diploid and have a chromosomal pattern of either 46XX or 46XY. All chromosomes are androgenetic, that is, from paternal origin and arise from fertilization of an empty ovum by a haploid sperm that then undergoes duplication. Occasionally, CHMs arise from fertilization of an empty ovum by two sperm. Maternally transcribed nuclear genome is lost, although one can identify maternal mitochondrial DNA.[4] PHM shows a variable amount of abnormal villous development and focal trophoblastic hyperplasia in association with identifiable fetal or embryonic tissue. PHM contains both maternal and paternal chromosomes and are triploid, typically XXY, which occurs by fertilization of a normal ovum by two sperm.[5] IM occurs when molar tissue invades the myometrial wall. Deep myometrial invasion can lead to uterine rupture and severe intraperitoneal hemorrhage. IM develops in approximately 15% of patients with CHM and about 5% of patients with PHM.[6] Most IMs remain localized to the uterus, but metastases to distant sites have been reported. CCA consists of invasive, highly vascular, and anaplastic trophoblastic tissue made up of cytotrophoblasts and syncytiotrophoblasts without villi. CCA metastasizes hematogenously and can follow any type of pregnancy, but most commonly develops after CHM. Approximately 50% of cases follow a molar pregnancy, 25% follow a spontaneous or ectopic pregnancy, and 25% follow a term delivery. The most common metastatic site is the lungs, which are involved in over 80% of patients. Vaginal metastases are noted in 30% of patients. Distant sites such as the liver, brain, kidney, gastrointestinal tract, and spleen occur in about 10% of patients and constitute the highest risk of death. Metastatic disease is most commonly encountered in postpartum patients in whom early diagnosis is frequently delayed.[7]

PSTTs are derived from intermediate trophoblastic cells. Microscopically these tumors show no chorionic villi and are characterized by a proliferation of cells with oval nuclei and abundant eosinophilic cytoplasm. They are seen more commonly after a nonmolar abortion or term pregnancy, but can occur after a mole. They are slow-growing and tend to locally infiltrate the myometrium, at which point they metastasize both via the hematogenous and lymphatic systems. Endocrinologically they differ from CCA in that they secrete placental lactogen in greater amounts than human chorionic gonadotropin (hCG). PSTTs are also characterized by high levels of free β-hCG.[8] Therefore, a large tumor burden may be present before the disease is diagnosed. These tumors tend to remain localized in the uterus for long periods before metastasizing to regional lymph nodes or metastatic sites.[9]

INDICATIONS FOR TREATMENT

Following a Molar Pregnancy

The early diagnosis of molar pregnancy with ultrasound has led to changes in the histologic characteristics of CHM without changing the potential for developing persistent disease.[10] Following molar evacuation, the diagnosis of GTN is based on the following International Federation of Gynecologists and Obstetricians (FIGO) guidelines[11]:

1. A plateau in β-hCG of four values plus or minus 10% over 3 weeks,
2. A 10% or greater rise in β-hCG levels for three or more values over at least 2 weeks,
3. Persistence of β-hCG levels for more than 6 months after molar evacuation, or
4. Histologic evidence of choriocarcinoma.

Following a Nonmolar Pregnancy

Patients who develop rising hCG titers following a nonmolar pregnancy have CCA until proven otherwise. Serum hCG levels are not routinely obtained after nonmolar pregnancies (except in following ectopic pregnancies), unless the woman has had a previous molar pregnancy when it becomes the standard of care because of the increased risk of developing GTN. *However, any woman in the reproductive age group who presents with abnormal bleeding or evidence of metastatic disease should undergo hCG screening to rule out choriocarcinoma.* At this point a thorough clinical and radiologic evaluation of the patient should be carried out to determine the extent of disease. Rapid growth, widespread dissemination, and a high propensity for hemorrhage make this tumor a medical emergency. Metastases are found in the lungs (80%), vagina (30%), pelvis (20%), brain (10%), and liver (10%), as well as other sites (<5%).[12]

MEASUREMENT OF hCG

The serial quantitative measurement of serum or urinary hCG is essential for the diagnosis, monitoring the efficacy of treatment, and follow-up of patients with molar pregnancy and GTN. hCG is a glycoprotein that consists of an *a*-subunit common to other glycoproteins, and a *b*-subunit that is hormone-specific. Therefore, the measurement of hCG in patients with GTN should be performed by assays that measure the *β*-subunit only.[13] hCG is synthesized by syncytiotrophoblastic cells of the developing placenta and hydatidiform moles. In contrast, the hyperglycosylated form of hCG (hCG-h) is produced by the cytotrophoblastic cells of the developing placenta during the first 2 weeks of gestation, and by malignant GTN (i.e., invasive moles and CCA).[14] After evacuation of a molar pregnancy, *β*-hCG levels usually disappear in 8 to 10 weeks. After normal delivery or non-molar miscarriage, hCG levels become undetectable within 3-6 weeks. Persistence of hCG levels indicate local or metastatic disease, which allows for early detection and timely intervention. During treatment, *β*-hCG response is used as a guide to determine whether to continue treatment with an agent or switch to another agent. *β*-hCG monitoring after treatment allows for identification of patients who relapse and require additional treatment.

Hyperglycosylated hCG is now believed to be the marker for malignant GTN, and its presence is associated with response to chemotherapy.[14] Some patients treated for molar pregnancy or GTN will have persistent (weeks or months) low levels (<200 mIU/mL) of real hCG, but low or absent concentrations of hCG-h. Characteristically, these women have no radiographic or clinical evidence of active disease, and do not appear to respond to chemotherapy. This condition of persistent low-level nonhyperglycosylated hCG is called *quiescent GTN*.[15] Careful follow-up is necessary because 6% to 10% of these patients will ultimately relapse with evidence of active disease and rising hCG levels with a high concentration (>30%) of hCG-h, at which point chemotherapy becomes effective.

PHANTOM hCG

False-positive findings on hCG tests can occur with the presence of heterophile antibodies that interfere with the immunoassay. Although a rare occurrence, false-positive hCG tests can be confusing to clinicians when attempting to diagnose disorders of pregnancy such as ectopic and GTN. Misinterpretations of false-positive tests have led to inappropriate treatment, including surgery and chemotherapy, when based only on the persistently elevated serum *β*-hCG levels. A false-positive hCG result should be suspected if the clinical picture and the laboratory results are discordant, if there is no identifiable antecedent pregnancy, or if patients under treatment with persistent low levels do not respond appropriately. In rare instances, particularly in women approaching menopause, the source of the hCG is the pituitary gland.[16] When a false-positive hCG test is suspected, a urinary assay should be performed because heterophile antibodies do not cross the renal tubules.

PRETREATMENT EVALUATION

Once it is determined that a patient has an elevated and rising hCG level, a thorough evaluation is required to determine the extent of disease, including blood tests to assess renal and hepatic function, peripheral blood counts, and baseline serum hCG levels. A speculum examination should be performed to identify the presence of vaginal metastases, which may cause sudden heavy vaginal bleeding. Radiologic evaluation should include a pelvic ultrasound, both to look for evidence of retained trophoblastic tissue and to evaluate the pelvis for local spread. Chest imaging is also required as the lungs are the most common site of metastatic disease. Pulmonary metastases can be detected by chest computed tomography in up to 40% of patients with a negative finding on chest radiography.[17] However, chest computed tomography is not mandatory, particularly if detection of overt pulmonary metastases will not alter the treatment plans. In the absence of pulmonary and vaginal involvement, brain and liver metastases are rare; therefore, we frequently omit further imaging of the brain. However, magnetic resonance imaging of the brain with contrast is mandatory in women with metastatic disease and in all patients with a pathologic diagnosis of CCA. It is usually not necessary to obtain histologic confirmation of the diagnosis because of the highly vascular nature of the tumor and the risk of hemorrhage. Positron emission tomography scanning is sometimes indicated to identify sites of active disease and to confirm sites of active disease found on conventional imaging.[18]

STAGING AND PROGNOSTIC SCORE

Table 103.1 summarizes the staging of GTN, which follows the FIGO guidelines. In addition to anatomic staging, a prognostic scoring system has been developed to help determine the appropriate chemotherapy regimen that affords the patient optimal management by reducing the risk of developing resistance to chemotherapy.[19] Patients with a score less than 7 are considered at low risk of developing resistance and generally achieve remission with single-agent therapy. Patients with scores of 7 or greater are at high risk of developing resistance to single-agent therapy and should be treated primarily with multiple-agent regimens. All patients with stage IV disease are considered high risk.

TREATMENT

Chemotherapy is highly effective in most patients with GTN. Cure rates of 100% in low-risk disease, and 80% to 90% in high-risk cases are reported from a number of treatment centers.[20] Despite the success of chemotherapy, the role of other modalities such as surgery and radiation therapy should not be overlooked. The best results are achieved when patients are treated under the auspices of a multidisciplinary team.

Low-Risk Disease

Methotrexate (MTX) and actinomycin D (ACTD), used sequentially, are the most widely used single agents for treating low-risk GTN.[21,22] A number of different regimens are currently in use

TABLE 103.1

INTERNATIONAL FEDERATION OF GYNECOLOGISTS AND OBSTETRICIANS STAGING OF GESTATIONAL TROPHOBLASTIC NEOPLASIA AND WORLD HEALTH ORGANIZATION SCORING SYSTEM BASED ON PROGNOSTIC FACTORS

Stage I	Disease confined to the uterus
Stage II	GTN extends outside of the uterus, but is limited to the genital structures
Stage III	GTN extends to the lungs, with or without genital tract involvement
Stage IV	All other metastatic sites

A risk factor score (see below) should be assigned to each patient.
The stage should be followed by the sum of the risk factor score (e.g., II:4)

	Score			
Prognostic Factors	0	1	2	4
Age in years	<40	≥40	—	—
Antecedent pregnancy	Mole	Abortion	Term	—
Interval (months)[a]	<4	≥4 but <7	≥7 but <13	≥13
Pretreatment serum hCG (mIU/mL)	<1,000	1,000 to <10,000	10,000 to <100,000	≥100,000
Largest tumor, including uterine	—	3 to <5 cm	≥5 cm	—
Site of Metastases	**Lung**	**Spleen, Kidney**	**GI Tract**	**Brain, Liver**
Number of metastases	—	1–4	5–8	>8
Prior failed chemotherapy	—	—	Single drug	2 or more drugs

GTN, gestational trophoblastic neoplasm; hCG, human chorionic gonadotropin; GI, gastrointestinal.
[a]Interval (in months) between end of antecedent pregnancy and start of chemotherapy.

PRACTICE OF ONCOLOGY

(Table 103.2). MTX with calcium leucovorin rescue (also called folinic acid) is the initial choice at the New England Trophoblastic Disease Center because it has the least toxicity. After completion of the first course, hCG levels should be followed weekly. A second course, which is required in 10% to 30% of patients, should be administered if the serum hCG level does not fall by 1 log (tenfold) within 18 days, or if the hCG test plateaus for more than 3 weeks or if it re-elevates. Subsequent courses are administered on the basis of the hCG regression curve. After a second course, if the patient's hCG level declines by less than 1 log, she is considered to be resistant to that drug and an alternate agent is substituted. ACTD is used when the patient develops resistance to MTX or if there is evidence of abnormal liver function tests as MTX is hepatotoxic. Remission is achieved when the hCG level becomes undetectable for 3 consecutive weeks.

At this point the patient should be followed with monthly hCG levels for 12 months. During this time effective contraception is mandatory. Pregnancy may be undertaken after 1 year of normal hCG titers. Hysterectomy with ovarian preservation should also be considered as primary therapy in stage I patients who have completed their family. Adjunctive chemotherapy should be administered at the time of surgery because of the risk of occult disease.

TABLE 103.2

SINGLE-AGENT REGIMENS FOR LOW-RISK GESTATIONAL TROPHOBLASTIC NEOPLASMS

MTX
- MTX 0.4–0.5 mg/kg IV or IM daily for 5 days (not to exceed 25 mg/d)
- Pulse MTX 50 mg/m² IM weekly

MTX/FA
- MTX 1 mg/kg IM or IV on days 1, 3, 5, 7
- FA 0.1 mg/kg PO on days 2, 4, 6, 8

High-dose MTX/FA
- MTX 100 mg/m² IV bolus
- MTX 200 mg/m² 12-h infusion
- FA 15 mg q 12 h in 4 doses IM or PO beginning 24 h after starting MTX

Actinomycin regimens
- ACTD 10–12 mcg/kg IV push daily for 5 days (not to exceed 1000 mcg/d)
- ACTD 1.25 mg/m² IV push q 2 weeks

MTX, methotrexate; IV, intravenous; IM, intramuscular; FA, folinic acid (calcium leucovorin); PO, by mouth; ACTD, actinomycin-D (Cosmegan).

High-Risk Disease

Multiple-agent chemotherapy should be used primarily in all patients with prognostic scores of 7 or greater. Table 103.3 summarizes the most widely used regimens including etoposide, MTX, ACTD, and cyclophosphamide and vincristine (EMA/CO) with cure rates ranging from 70% to 90%.[23] A similar regimen containing cisplatin (EMA/EP) can be used as salvage therapy for patients who develop resistance to EMA/CO.[24] Treatment should be dose-intensive every 2 to 3 weeks, toxicity permitting. The use of recombinant hematopoietic growth factors such as granulocyte colony-stimulating factor and, when absolutely necessary, platelet transfusions are important to maintain adequate dose-intensity and to prevent unnecessary dose reduction. Treatment should be continued until the hCG level becomes undetectable and remains undetectable for 3 consecutive weeks. It is recommended that three courses of the remission regimen be administered after the

TABLE 103.3

PROTOCOLS FOR EMA/CO AND EMA/EP REGIMENS

Day	Drug	Dose
		Protocol for EMA/CO Regimen
1	Etoposide	100 mg/m^2 by infusion in 200 mL saline over 30 min
	ACTD	0.5 mg IV push
	MTX	100 mg/m^2 IV push
		200 mg/m^2 by infusion over 12 h
2	Etoposide	100 mg/m^2 by infusion in 200 mL saline over 30 min
	ACTD	0.5 mg IV push
	Folinic acid	15 mg q 12 h × 4 doses IM or PO beginning 24 h after starting MTX
8	Cyclophosphamide	600 mg/m^2 by infusion in saline over 30 min
	Vincristine	1.0 mg/m^2 IV push
		Protocol for EMA/EP Regimen
1	Etoposide	100 mg/m^2 by infusion in 200 mL saline over 30 min
	ACTD	0.5 mg IV push
	MTX	100 mg/m^2 IV push
		200 mg/m^2 by infusion over 12 h
2	Etoposide	100 mg/m^2 by infusion in 200 mL saline over 30 min
	ACTD	0.5 mg IV push
	Folinic acid	15 mg q 12 h × 4 doses IM or PO beginning 24 h after starting MTX
8	Cisplatin	60 mg/m^2 with prehydration
	Etoposide	100 mg/m^2 by infusion in 200 mL saline over 30 min

EMA/CO, etoposide, methotrexate, and dactinomycin alternating with cyclophosphamide and vincristine; EMA/EP, etoposide/methotrexate/actinomycin-D/etoposide/cisplatin; ACTD, actinomycin-D (Cosmegan); IV intravenous; IM, intramuscular; PO, by mouth; MTX, methotrexate.

patient achieves remission. Death occurs in patients who present with widespread disease frequently the result of delayed diagnosis, from life-threatening complications such as respiratory failure and central nervous system hemorrhage, from the development of drug resistance, or from inadequate treatment. The use of radiation therapy in patients with GTN is limited to the treatment of brain metastases. The use of whole head or localized radiation therapy in conjunction with chemotherapy can prevent a life-threatening or debilitating hemorrhage and should be initiated promptly. Solitary superficial cerebral lesions are best treated surgically. Surgery should also be considered as an important adjunct in the management of high-risk patients.[26] Hysterectomy in patients with heavy bleeding, large bulky intrauterine disease, or in the presence of significant pelvic sepsis should be performed regardless of the patient's parity. Removal of tumor masses in the bowel should also be performed because of the risk of hemorrhage. Unresponsive masses in the liver, kidneys, and spleen should be removed, although embolization has been used with some success in controlling liver metastases. After completion of chemotherapy, patients with high-risk disease should be followed for 24 months before pregnancy is attempted.

PLACENTAL SITE TROPHOBLASTIC TUMORS

The primary treatment of patients with PSTT is surgical because of their relative resistance to chemotherapy. Because the disease infiltrates deeply into the myometrium, lymph node sampling is recommended at the time of hysterectomy. Excellent results have been obtained with EMA/EP in patients with lymphatic spread or extrauterine disease.[9]

SUBSEQUENT PREGNANCY

Patients treated successfully with chemotherapy can expect normal reproductive function. A total of 2,657 subsequent pregnancies have been reported, which resulted in 77% full-term deliveries, 5% premature births, 1% stillbirths, and 14% spontaneous miscarriages.[27] Despite the use of potentially teratogenic drugs, no increase in congenital malformations have been reported, nor was there a difference in either the conception rate or pregnancy outcome in patients treated with single- or multiple-agent protocols. Subsequent pregnancy data from our Center are confirmatory.[28]

PSYCHOSOCIAL ISSUES

Women who develop GTN can experience significant mood disturbance, marital and sexual problems, and concerns over future fertility.[29] Because GTN is a consequence of pregnancy, patients and their partners must confront the loss of a pregnancy at the same time they face concerns regarding malignancy. Patients can experience clinically significant levels of anxiety, fatigue, anger, confusion, sexual problems, and concern for future pregnancy that last for protracted periods of time. Patients with metastatic disease, in particular, are at risk of psychological disturbances; these patients need assessments and interventions both during treatment and after remission is attained.

Selected References

1. Goldstein DP, Berkowitz RS. The diagnosis and management of molar pregnancy. In: Friedman EA, ed. *Gestational trophoblastic neoplasms: clinical principles of diagnosis and management*. Philadelphia: WB Saunders; 1982:143.
2. Parazzinni F, Mangili G, Belloni C, et al. The problem of identification of prognostic factors for persistent trophoblastic neoplasia. *Gynecol Oncol* 1988;34:383.
3. Hertig AT, Sheldon H. Hydatidiform mole: a pathologic-clinical correlation of 200 cases. *Am J Obstet Gynecol* 1947;53:1.
4. Fisher RA. Genetics. In: Hancock BW, Newlands ES, Berkowitz RS, eds. *Gestational trophoblastic disease*. London: Chapman and Hall; 1997:5.
5. McFadden DE, Kalousek DK. Two different phenotypes of fetuses with chromosome triploidy: correlation with parental origin of the extra haploid set. *Am J Med Genet* 1991;38:555.
6. Feltmate CM, Growden WB, Wolfberg AJ, et al. Clinical characteristics of persistent gestational trophoblastic neoplasia after a partial hydatidiform molar pregnancy. *J Reprod Med* 2006;51:902.
7. Dubeshter B, Berkowitz RS, Goldstein DP, et al. Metastatic gestational trophoblastic disease: experience of the New England Trophoblastic Disease Center 1965–1985. *Obstet Gynecol* 1987;69:390.
8. Cole LA, Khanlian SA, Muller CY, et al. Gestational trophoblastic diseases: 3. Human chorionic gonadotropin-free β-subunit, a reliable marker of placental site trophoblastic tumors. *Gynecol Oncol* 2006;102:160.
9. Hassaida A, Gillespie A, Tidy J. Placental site trophoblastic tumor: clinical features and management. *Gynecol Oncol* 2005;99:603.
10. Berkowitz RS, Goldstein DP. Molar pregnancy. *N Engl J Med* 2009;360:1639.
11. Kohorn EI. The new FIGO 2000 staging system and risk factor scoring system for gestational trophoblastic disease: description and critical assessment. *Int J Gynaecol Cancer* 2001;11:73.
12. Berkowitz RS, Goldstein DP. Current management of gestational trophoblastic disease. *Gynecol Oncol* 2009;112:654-62.
13. Hancock BW. hCG measurement in gestational trophoblastic neoplasia. A critical appraisal. *J Reprod Med* 2006;51:859.
14. Cole LA, Butler SA. Hyperglycosylated human chorionic gonadotropin and human chorionic gonadotropin free *B*-subunit: tumor markers and tumor promoters. *J Reprod Med* 2008;53:499.
15. Khanlian SA, Cole LA. Management of gestational trophoblastic disease and other cases with low serum levels of human chorionic gonadotropin. *J Reprod Med* 2006;51:812.
16. Muller CY, Cole LA. The quadmire of hCG and hCG testing in gynecologic oncology. *Gynecol Oncol* 2009;112:663.
17. Garner EI, Garrett A, Goldstein DP, et al. Significance of chest computed tomography findings in the evaluation and treatment of persistent gestational trophoblastic neoplasms. *J Reprod Med* 2004;49:411.
18. Dhillon T, Palmieri C, Sebire NJ, et al. Value of whole body 18 FDG-PET to identify the active site of gestational trophoblastic neoplasia. *J Reprod Med* 2006;51:879.
19. Kohorn EI. Negotiating a staging and risk factor scoring system for gestational trophoblastic neoplasia: a progress report. *J Reprod Med* 2002;47:445.
20. ACOG Practice Bulletin 53. Diagnosis and treatment of gestational trophoblastic neoplasms. *Obstet Gynecol* 2004;103:1365.
21. Hoekstra AV, Lurain JR, Rademaker AW, Schink JC. Gestational trophoblastic neoplasia: treatment and outcomes. *Obstet Gynecol* 2008;112:251.
22. Growdon WB, Wolfberg AJ, Goldstein DP, et al. Evaluating methotrexate treatment in patients with low-risk postmolar gestational trophoblastic neoplasia. *Gynecol Oncol* 2009;112:353.
23. Bower M, Newlands ES, Holden L, et al. EMA/CO for high –risk gestational trophoblastic tumors: results from a cohort of 272 patients. *J Clin Oncol* 1997;15:2636.
24. Xiang Y, Sun Z, Wan X, et al. EMA/EP chemotherapy for chemorefractory gestational trophoblastic tumors. *J Reprod Med* 2004;49:443.
25. Newlands ES, Holden L, Seckl MJ, et al. Management of brain metastases in patients with high-risk gestational trophoblastic tumors. *J Reprod Med* 2002;47:465.
26. Lurain JR, Singh DK, Schink JC. Primary treatment of metastatic high-risk gestational trophoblastic neoplasia with EMA-CO chemotherapy. *J Reprod Med* 2006;51:767.
27. Woolas RP, Bower M, Newlands ES, et al. Influence of chemotherapy for gestational trophoblastic disease on subsequent pregnancy outcome. *Br J Obstet Gynaecol* 1998;105:1032.
28. Garner EIO, Lipson E, Bernstein MR, et al. Subsequent pregnancy experience in patients with molar pregnancy and gestational trophoblastic tumors. *J Reprod Med* 2002;47:380.
29. Wenzel LB, Berkowitz RS, Habbal R, et al. Predictors of quality of life among long-term survivors of gestational trophoblastic disease. *J Reprod Med* 2004;49:589.

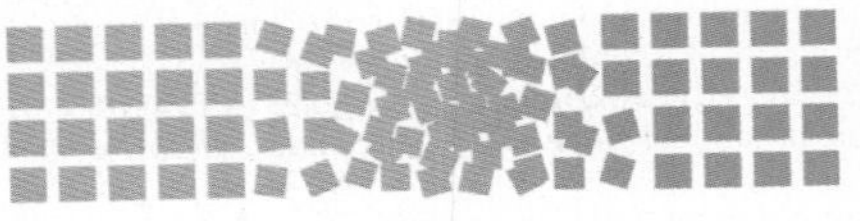

CHAPTER 104 OVARIAN CANCER, FALLOPIAN TUBE CARCINOMA, AND PERITONEAL CARCINOMA

STEPHEN A. CANNISTRA, DAVID M. GERSHENSON, AND ABRAM RECHT

Ovarian cancer is not a single entity but instead represents tumors of epithelial, germ cell, or sex cord–stromal origin. Epithelial ovarian cancer typically occurs in postmenopausal women, most germ cell tumors present in younger women, and sex cord–stromal tumors may occur at any age. Approximately 90% of ovarian cancer is epithelial in origin and poses significant therapeutic challenges due to the advanced stage of most patients with this disease. In contrast, other types of ovarian cancer such as germ cell and sex cord–stromal tumors are often localized in distribution, more amenable to surgical resection, and have a more favorable prognosis. Although primary peritoneal serous carcinoma and fallopian tube carcinoma do not originate in the ovary, they are discussed in this chapter because their clinical and management considerations are similar to those of epithelial ovarian cancer.

EPITHELIAL OVARIAN CANCER

Epidemiology

Epithelial ovarian cancer is expected to occur in 21,550 women and cause 14,600 deaths in the United States in 2009, which makes this tumor the leading cause of gynecologic cancer mortality.[1] The lifetime risk of developing sporadic epithelial ovarian cancer is approximately 1.7%, although patients with a familial predisposition have a much higher lifetime risk, in the range of 10% to 40%.[2] The median age at diagnosis for sporadic disease is 60 years, although patients with a genetic predisposition may develop this tumor earlier, often in their fifth decade. The age-specific incidence of sporadic disease increases with age, from 15 to 16 per 100,000 in the 40- to 44-year-old age group to a peak rate of 57 per 100,000 in the 70- to 74-year-old age group.[1] There has been a statistically significant improvement in 5-year survival over the past decades, with a rate of 36% in 1977, 39% in 1986, and 45% in 2002.[1] This improvement in survival is likely the result of more effective chemotherapy options and surgical techniques for tumor debulking. African American women in the United States have a lower incidence of ovarian cancer (10.3 per 100,000 women) compared to white women, but both have a similar stage distribution and overall survival rate.[1] A higher risk for developing epithelial ovarian cancer is observed for nulliparous women and a lower risk for those who have had children, who have breastfed, who have undergone tubal ligation, or who have taken oral contraceptives.[3]

Pathogenesis and Patterns of Metastases

Some epithelial ovarian neoplasms are thought to arise from the surface epithelium covering the ovary, which is contiguous with peritoneal mesothelium. In some cases, malignant transformation appears to occur within epithelium that becomes trapped within ovarian inclusion cysts during ovulation, where it can develop into a variety of mullerian-type histologies.[4] However, emerging evidence suggests that a subset of epithelial ovarian cancers may instead originate in the fallopian tube fimbria, subsequently spreading to the ovary or peritoneal cavity.[5] Germ cell tumors most likely originate in cells derived from the primitive streak that ultimately migrated to the gonads. The ovarian stroma consists of granulosa cells, theca cells, and fibroblasts, which give rise to the sex cord–stromal tumors.

Several molecular abnormalities have been identified in patients with epithelial ovarian cancer, although their contribution to early malignant transformation is poorly understood. Cytogenetic analysis may reveal complex abnormalities, including deletions of 3p, 6q, 8p, and 10q, and loss of heterozygosity is commonly observed on 11p, 13q, 16q, 17p, and 17q.[6] Mutation in the *p53* protooncogene occurs in over 50% of cases, predominantly involving tumors in patients with advanced stage and high-grade serous histology.[6] In contrast, mutations in B-*raf*, K-*ras*, *PTEN*, or β-catenin may be seen in endometrioid, mucinous, or low-grade histologies.[5] Amplification of the *HER2/neu* gene is observed in only approximately 8% of patients and confers a poorer prognosis.[7] Overexpression of pro-apoptotic genes such as *BAX* is associated with chemoresponsiveness and a more favorable prognosis, although the role of *BAX* in the pathogenesis of this tumor has not been well studied.[8] Surface adhesion proteins such as CD44H and β-1 integrins have been shown to mediate transperitoneal spread of this tumor by promoting the attachment of cancer cells to the peritoneal mesothelial lining.[9] Expression of angiogenic cytokines such as the vascular endothelial growth factor (VEGF) is frequently observed in epithelial ovarian cancer, with high serum levels conferring a worse prognosis.[10]

The ability of tumor cells to exfoliate from the ovarian surface and to spread in an asymptomatic fashion impedes the development of successful screening approaches that would allow for early diagnosis. The tumor typically spreads to the omentum and to peritoneal surfaces such as the underside of the diaphragm, paracolic gutters, and bowel serosa (Fig. 104.1). The lymphatic drainage of the ovary follows its blood supply through the infundibulopelvic ligament to nodes in the para-aortic region. Lymphatic drainage through the broad ligament and parametrial channels can also result in involvement of pelvic sidewall lymphatics, including the external iliac, obturator, and hypogastric chains. Spread may rarely occur along the course of the round ligament, resulting in involvement of inguinal lymph nodes. Approximately 10% to 15% of patients with ovarian cancer that appears to be localized to the ovaries have metastases to para-aortic lymph nodes, and retroperitoneal lymph node involvement is found in over 50% of patients with advanced disease.[2]

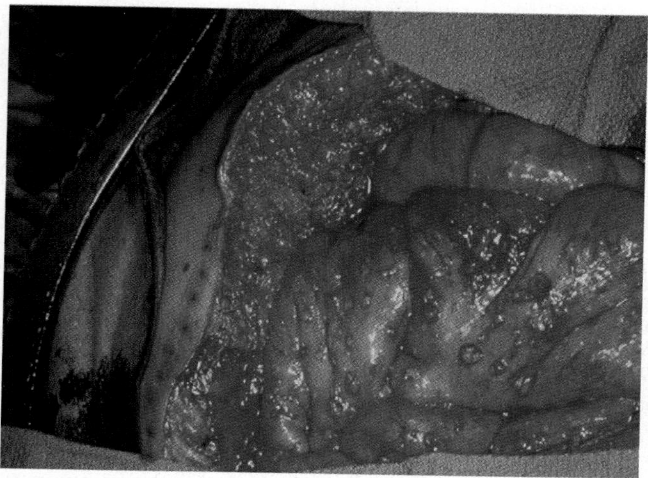

FIGURE 104.1 Intraoperative appearance of advanced epithelial ovarian cancer, with multiple tumor implants involving the peritoneal surface of the upper abdomen. (Courtesy of Dr. Jonathan Niloff, Beth Israel Deaconess Medical Center, Boston.)

Although epithelial ovarian cancer typically spreads in a locoregional fashion to involve the peritoneal cavity and retroperitoneal nodes, it can be found outside the abdomen as well. The most common site of extra-abdominal spread is the pleural space (thought to occur via transdiaphragmatic lymphatics), where it causes a malignant pleural effusion in some patients. Hematogenous metastases to the liver, spleen, or lung can also occur during the course of the disease, but are relatively uncommon at presentation. Bone or central nervous system metastases may rarely be observed in patients who have lived for many years after initial diagnosis, during which unusual patterns of disease spread may occur.

Histologic Classification of Epithelial Tumors

Table 104.1 outlines the classification of common epithelial tumors that has been accepted by the World Health Organization (WHO) and the International Federation of Gynecology and Obstetrics (FIGO).[4] The nomenclature for these tumors reflects the cell type, location of the tumor, and degree of malignancy, ranging from benign lesions to tumors of low malignant potential (LMP) to invasive carcinomas.

Tumors of LMP (borderline tumors) have an excellent prognosis compared with invasive carcinomas.[11,12] They are characterized by epithelial papillae with atypical cell clusters, cellular stratification, nuclear atypia, and increased mitotic activity. In contrast to epithelial ovarian carcinoma, borderline tumors lack stromal invasion.[12]

Epithelial carcinomas are characterized by histologic cell type and degree of differentiation (tumor grade). The histologic cell type has limited prognostic significance independent

TABLE 104.1

WORLD HEALTH ORGANIZATION CLASSIFICATION OF MALIGNANT OVARIAN TUMORS

COMMON EPITHELIAL TUMORS	**Androblastoma: Sertoli-Leydig Cell Tumor**
Malignant Serous Tumor	Well differentiated
Adenocarcinoma, papillary adenocarcinoma, papillary cystadenocarcinoma	Tubular androblastoma, Sertoli cell tumor (tubular adenoma of Pick)
Surface papillary carcinoma	Tubular androblastoma with lipid storage, Sertoli cell tumor with lipid storage
Malignant adenofibroma, cystadenofibroma	Sertoli-Leydig cell tumor (tubular adenoma with Leydig cells)
Malignant Mucinous Tumor	Leydig cell tumor, hilus cell tumor
Adenocarcinoma, cystadenocarcinoma	Of intermediate differentiation
Malignant adenofibroma, cystadenofibroma	Poorly differentiated (sarcomatoid)
Malignant Endometrioid Tumor	With heterologous elements
Carcinoma	Gynandroblastoma
Adenocarcinoma	Lipid (lipoid) cell tumors
Adenoacanthoma	Unclassified
Malignant adenofibroma, cystadenofibroma	
Endometrioid stromal sarcoma	**GERM CELL TUMOR**
Mesodermal (mullerian) mixed tumor: homologous and heterologous	Dysgerminoma
Other	Endodermal sinus tumor
Clear cell (mesonephroid) tumor, malignant	Embryonal carcinoma
Carcinoma and adenocarcinoma	Polyembryoma
Brenner tumor, malignant	Choriocarcinoma
Mixed epithelial tumor, malignant	Immature teratoma
Undifferentiated carcinoma	Mature dermoid cyst with malignant transformation
Unclassified	Monodermal and highly specialized
	Struma ovarii
SEX CORD–STROMAL TUMORS	Carcinoid
Granulosa–Stromal Cell Tumor	Struma ovarii and carcinoid
Granulosa cell tumor	Others
Tumor in the thecoma-fibroma group	Mixed forms
Fibroma	
Unclassified	**GONADOBLASTOMA**
	Pure
	Mixed with dysgerminoma or other form of germ cell tumor

(From ref. 4.)

PRACTICE OF ONCOLOGY

TABLE 104.2

COMMON HISTOLOGIC TYPES OF EPITHELIAL OVARIAN CANCER

Histology	Features
Papillary serous	The most common type of epithelial ovarian cancer. May contain psammoma bodies (Fig. 104.3) and is often associated with CA 125 elevation. Identical histology is observed for primary peritoneal serous cancer (PPSC).
Endometrioid	Sometimes associated with endometriosis or an independent uterine cancer of similar histology. May occur with early stage disease in younger patients, although advanced disease is also possible.
Mucinous	May rarely be associated with pseudomyxoma peritoneii. CA 125 levels may not be markedly elevated. Relatively chemoresistant. Differential diagnosis of a mucinous ovarian tumor includes metastatic disease from an appendiceal primary.
Clear cell	The most chemoresistant type of ovarian cancer. Often contains "hobnail" cells with cleared out cytoplasm due to glycogen. Sometimes associated with endometriosis or humorally mediated hypercalcemia.

of clinical stage, although patients with clear cell and mucinous types of epithelial ovarian cancer fare less well due to the relative chemoresistance of these histologies.[13] Conversely, low-grade serous carcinoma is associated with a better prognosis despite relative chemoresistance.[14,15] High tumor grade appears to be an important prognostic factor, especially in patients with early stage epithelial tumors.

Certain pathologic and clinical features are characteristic of distinct histologic subtypes of epithelial carcinoma (Table 104.2). For instance, concentric rings of calcification called psammoma bodies (Fig. 104.2) are often observed in the papillary serous variety of epithelial ovarian cancer, although they are not pathognomonic for this disease and may also be seen (for example) in breast, lung, and papillary thyroid cancers. The endometrioid variant of ovarian cancer is associated with endometriosis in about 20% to 30% of cases, with a separate endometrioid uterine cancer (often stage I and low grade) simultaneously present in 15% of cases.[16] Likewise, clear cell histology may also be associated with endometriosis, as well as humorally mediated hypercalcemia (which can also be observed with the rare small cell variant of ovarian cancer). Clear cell cancers are relatively resistant to chemotherapy compared to their more common papillary serous counterparts. Finally, primary mucinous ovarian cancers are also relatively chemoresistant, are sometimes associated with pseudomyxoma peritonei, and may not be associated with dramatic elevations of the cancer antigen 125 (CA 125) serum tumor marker.

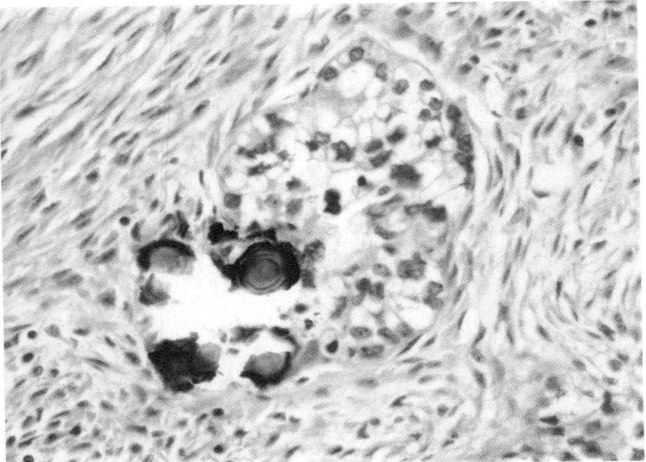

FIGURE 104.2 Photomicrograph of a hematoxylin and eosin-stained section of papillary serous ovarian cancer, showing psammoma bodies. (Courtesy of Dr. Jonathan Hecht, Beth Israel Deaconess Medical Center, Boston.)

Gastric, breast (especially infiltrating lobular carcinoma), mesothelioma, and colorectal cancers may occasionally present with diffuse peritoneal implants, ascites, and ovarian metastases that mimic primary ovarian cancer. It is usually possible to distinguish between these possibilities on routine light microscopic histologic evaluation, although immunohistochemistry can be most helpful when the histologic diagnosis is ambiguous. Staining for cytokeratin CK7 is positive and CK20 is negative in most cases of primary serous ovarian cancer, whereas the reverse staining pattern is typically observed for colorectal cancer. Staining for gross cystic disease fluid protein (GCDFP) may be positive in up to 50% of patients with breast cancer, whereas this marker should be negative in patients with gastric, colorectal, or ovarian cancer. Finally, calretinin is usually expressed in mesothelioma but is typically negative in epithelial ovarian cancer.

Diagnosis

Most patients with epithelial ovarian cancer experience no signs or symptoms of the disease until it spreads to the upper abdomen. Approximately 70% of patients with this tumor present with advanced disease (stage III or IV, Table 104.3), whereas the majority of patients with borderline, germ cell, and sex cord–stromal tumors present with early stage disease limited to the pelvis.[2] Occasionally, patients with epithelial ovarian cancer will be diagnosed with early stage disease due to discovery of a mass on routine pelvic examination or because of pelvic pain caused by ovarian torsion. Unlike epithelial cancers, which are generally asymptomatic at an early stage, ovarian germ cell malignancies tend to stretch and twist the infundibulopelvic ligament, causing severe pain while the disease is still confined to the ovary.

Abdominal discomfort, bloating, and early satiety are the most common symptoms experienced by women with epithelial ovarian cancer. Patients presenting with such nonspecific complaints may be found to have ascites and a pelvic mass on physical examination. Occasionally an umbilical lymph node metastasis will be present (Sister Mary Joseph's node) or a pleural effusion will be found. The mass on pelvic examination is frequently firm and fixed, with multiple nodularities palpable in the cul-de-sac.

The CA 125 serum level is elevated in more than 80% of serous epithelial ovarian cancers.[17] However, it is not a reliable diagnostic test, since it can also be elevated in a variety of benign gynecologic conditions (such as endometriosis, pelvic inflammatory disease, or pregnancy) and nongynecologic malignancies (such as breast, lung, and gastrointestinal cancers). Furthermore, the CA 125 level is elevated in only approximately 50% of patients with early stage epithelial

TABLE 104.3

INTERNATIONAL FEDERATION OF GYNECOLOGY AND OBSTETRICS STAGING SYSTEM FOR EPITHELIAL OVARIAN CANCER

STAGE I	*Tumor limited to ovary or ovaries*[a]
IA	One ovary, without malignant ascites. No malignant cell in ascites or peritoneal washings.
IB	Both ovaries, without malignant ascites. No malignant cell in ascites or peritoneal washings.
IC	Limited to one or both ovaries, with surface involvement, rupture, or malignant cells in ascites or peritoneal washings.
STAGE II	*Ovarian tumor with pelvic extension*[a]
IIA	Involvement of the uterus or fallopian tubes.
IIB	Involvement of other pelvic organs (e.g., bladder, rectum, or pelvic sidewall).
IIC	Pelvic extension, plus findings indicated for IC.
STAGE III	*Tumor involving the upper abdomen or lymph nodes*
IIIA	Microscopic disease outside of the pelvis, typically involving the omentum.
IIIB	Gross deposits less than or equal to 2 cm in diameter.[b]
IIIC	Gross deposits greater than 2 cm in diameter, or nodal involvement.[b]
STAGE IV	*Distant organ involvement, including pleural space*[c] *or hepatic/splenic parenchyma.*

[a]Patients with disease that appears to be confined to the ovaries or pelvis require nodal biopsy for complete staging, in order to exclude the possibility of occult stage IIIC.
[b]Disease measurements for staging purposes are made before debulking has been attempted.
[c]Pleural effusion must be cytologically proven to be malignant if used to define stage IV disease.

ovarian cancer, which also limits its value as a screening test.[17] Other tumor markers, such as CA 19-9, which is elevated in some mucinous ovarian carcinomas, and carcinoembryonic antigen (CEA) are less frequently useful. It is typical for a patient with epithelial ovarian cancer to have a normal CEA level in the setting of a significantly elevated CA 125 level. Postoperatively, the CA 125 level provides a sensitive way to monitor treatment response and development of disease recurrence. Because relapsed epithelial ovarian cancer is usually incurable, however, there is currently no evidence that early detection of recurrence through CA 125 surveillance confers either a quality of life or a survival advantage in this disease.[18]

Transvaginal ultrasonography (TVU) is an important diagnostic tool in the evaluation of patients with a pelvic mass. TVU is more sensitive at detecting ovarian tumors compared to other tests such as computed tomography (CT), and it can provide qualitative information about the mass that might suggest malignancy. The classic sonographic finding of malignancy is a "complex" cyst, defined as containing both solid and cystic components, sometimes with septations and internal echogenicity (Fig. 104.3). Finding a complex cyst on sonography, especially in the presence of signs and symptoms consistent with ovarian cancer, often requires surgery for further evaluation. It is best to avoid percutaneous biopsy during the initial evaluation, which can result in cyst rupture and spillage of malignant cells into the peritoneal cavity. Bilateral ovarian involvement and ascites are sometimes detected by sonography as well. Color Doppler imaging evaluates blood flow to an ovarian mass and can potentially identify a malignant process based on the presence of abnormal neovascularization.[19]

In contrast to complex cysts, "simple" cysts are defined as being thin-walled, fluid-filled, without a mass component, septations, or internal echogenicity on TVU examination. Simple cysts are most often benign in nature and may be found in 5% to 10% of asymptomatic postmenopausal women during TVU examination, especially in the first decade after menopause. Simple cysts do not always require surgical evaluation if they are associated with normal CA 125 levels, although management must be individualized.[20] Postmenopausal women with simple cysts in association with elevated serum CA 125 levels, simple cysts that exceed 5 to 10 cm in diameter, or simple cysts in association with abnormal color Doppler flow studies are often referred for surgery.

In premenopausal women, simple cysts detected on TVU examination may be functional (i.e., a corpus luteum cyst) or represent a benign process such as a serous cystadenoma. Such cysts may generally be followed through several menstrual cycles, during which they often resolve. Functional cysts may also disappear when oral contraceptives are used. However, premenopausal women with simple cysts that are persistent or enlarging, especially in the setting of a rising CA 125 level, are reasonable candidates for surgical evaluation to exclude malignancy.[20] As previously mentioned, several benign conditions in premenopausal women may also be associated with elevated CA 125 levels, such as pregnancy or endometriosis, and there is no absolute CA 125 cutoff to distinguish benign from malignant pathologies.[21]

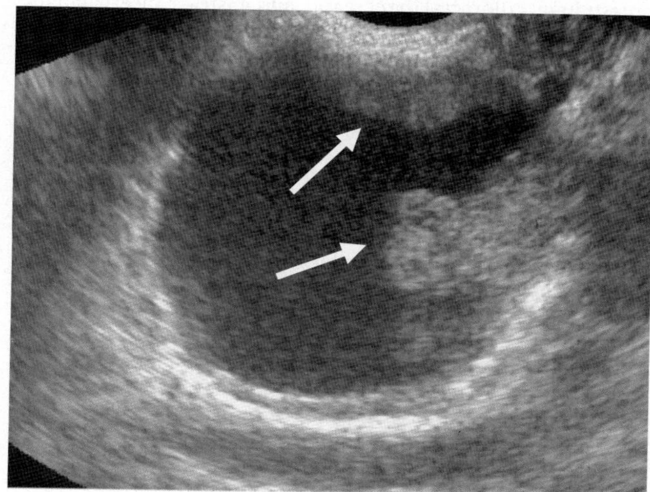

FIGURE 104.3 Transvaginal ultrasound of a complex cyst, containing both solid (*arrows*) and fluid components. (Courtesy of Dr. Ann McNamara, Beth Israel Deaconess Medical Center, Boston.)

PRACTICE OF ONCOLOGY

CT or magnetic resonance imaging (MRI) may sometimes be helpful in defining the extent of peritoneal disease in patients with suspected ovarian cancer. However, for the patient with a complex ovarian cyst and clinical signs and symptoms to suggest ovarian cancer, these studies generally do not obviate the need for surgical exploration. Occasionally, CT may sometimes be helpful in distinguishing a gynecologic malignancy from a metastatic pancreatic neoplasm, for instance, for which an exploratory laparotomy may not be warranted. In selected patients, CT may also assist in surgical planning by locating the site of suspected bowel obstruction. MRI has not been shown to have a clear advantage over CT in patients with an ovarian mass, except for pregnant patients when ultrasonography is inconclusive and there is a desire to avoid radiation exposure. Positron emission tomography (PET) is a form of functional imaging that most frequently uses the positron-emitting glucose analogue fluorodeoxyglucose (^{18}F). Tumor masses are imaged based on their relatively increased glucose metabolism compared to normal tissues. However, there is currently no proven role for PET in the diagnosis or subsequent follow-up of patients with ovarian cancer.[22] Chest radiographs may sometimes be performed to evaluate the presence of pleural effusions, which occur in 10% of patients with epithelial ovarian cancer at diagnosis.

Screening and Early Detection

A successful screening test for ovarian cancer should be capable of identifying the majority of patients with precancerous lesions or early disease. Because a positive screening test for ovarian cancer would result in major surgery with associated morbidity, costs, and even mortality, the false-positive rate of such a screening test must be low, and its positive predictive value (PPV) relatively high (at least 10%). At present, there are no screening tests for epithelial ovarian cancer that convincingly meet these criteria.

Ovarian palpation has not been established as a useful screening procedure, and most screening studies have used either serum tumor marker levels or ultrasonography or both. The CA 125 serum level is not a useful screening test when used alone, since elevations are not specific for ovarian cancer and may be observed in cirrhosis, peritonitis, pleuritis, pancreatitis, endometriosis, uterine leiomyomata, benign ovarian cysts, and pelvic inflammatory disease. In addition, CA 125 serum levels may be elevated in other malignancies such as breast, lung, colorectal, pancreatic, and gastric cancers. Finally, although the CA 125 level is elevated in the majority of patients with advanced epithelial ovarian cancer, it is abnormal in only half of patients with early stage disease.[17] Therefore, by itself this test would fail to detect a sizable fraction of patients with curable disease. More recently, a number of candidate markers have been discovered that show promise for enhancing the accuracy of CA 125 levels, such as HE4 (human epididymis 4), osteopontin, mesothelin, and osteoblast-stimulating factor-2. Algorithms that define the behavior of these markers have also been developed, incorporating biologic characteristics of tumor growth and marker behavior.[23] Levels of OVX-1 and macrophage colony-stimulating factor have been found to be elevated in patients with clinically evident ovarian cancer but normal CA 125 levels, which suggests that these markers may be complementary to CA 125.[24] Lysophosphatidic acid level has also been reported to discriminate ovarian cancer patients from controls, including cases with early stage disease.[25] None of these tests has been proven to have sufficient sensitivity and specificity for routine screening at the current time.

Measurement of the CA 125 level has been combined with performance of TVU in an attempt to improve screening.[19,26,27] Early studies of TVU suggested a sensitivity of close to 100% but a specificity of 98%, which is insufficient to achieve a PPV of 10%. More recent reports suggest that use of color Doppler imaging improves the specificity of TVU, but it is uncertain whether this will achieve the desired PPV. Investigators at the University of Kentucky improved the specificity of TVU by using a morphologic index. They screened 6,470 women, including high-risk premenopausal women and average-risk postmenopausal women.[27] Of 90 women who underwent surgery, 6 were found to have an ovarian malignancy, for a PPV of 6.7%. One interval cancer was found at prophylactic oophorectomy 11 months after screening, for a sensitivity of 86%. All but one of these cancers were stage I, and no deaths due to ovarian cancer were noted in this group.

Two randomized controlled trials are currently under way to evaluate a multimodal screening approach using both CA 125 and TVU. In the United States, the Prostate, Lung, Colorectal, Ovarian Cancer Screening Trial uses measurement of CA 125 level (single threshold elevation of more than 35 U/mL) and TVU together, performed annually, as a first-line screen.[28] If either test is positive, the woman is referred for surgical consultation. In this two-arm, randomized controlled trial, 74,000 women aged 55 to 74 years have been randomly assigned to the screening arm or to a standard-care control arm. Ten centers are collaborating in this 14-year trial, which will require an average of 10 years of follow-up.

The second randomized screening trial is currently being conducted in the United Kingdom and uses CA 125 levels (or rate of rise of CA 125) as a trigger for performing TVU. This trial is based on an earlier study by Jacobs et al.[29] in which 21,935 average-risk postmenopausal women were assigned to undergo three annual screenings or no screening. The screening protocol used CA 125 level as a first-line screen and referred the patient for TVU if the CA 125 level was above 30 U/mL. If the TVU revealed an ovarian mass, then the patient was referred for surgical consultation. Findings from this trial support the notion that this stepwise approach can yield high specificity and an acceptable PPV.[29] Specifically, when the decision rule for surgical referral requires that results of both tests be positive, the PPV is 20%. Furthermore, there were one-half as many deaths in the screened group as there were among controls, and there was a statistically significant improvement in survival. Individuals with index cancers survived an average of 72.9 months in the screening group and 41.8 months in the control group. However, the multimodal screening strategy originally described by Jacobs et al. is limited by the sensitivity of the CA 125 level, which serves as a trigger for performing ultrasound. Accordingly, these investigators are exploring ways to improve on these results by detecting changes in CA 125 levels over time. Skates et al.[30] suggested fitting an exponential model that uses data from several prior CA 125 screens, with an exponential rise triggering a callback for additional ultrasound testing. This screening strategy forms the basis of the three-arm randomized trial currently being conducted in the United Kingdom.

Hereditary Ovarian Carcinoma

Approximately 5% to 10% of patients with epithelial ovarian carcinoma carry a germline mutation that places them at substantially increased risk of developing this disease. The breast–ovarian cancer syndrome accounts for approximately 90% of hereditary ovarian cancer and is often suspected whenever the pedigree reveals multiple affected family members with ovarian cancer, bilateral or early onset breast cancer, both breast and ovarian cancer in the same individual, or a male relative with breast cancer.[31,32] Fallopian tube cancer and primary peritoneal serous cancer (PPSC) are also recognized to be part of this syndrome.[33] The high incidence of breast and ovarian cancers in these families is due to inherited germline mutations in the *BRCA1* or *BRCA2* genes, which may be transferred by either parent, meaning that both maternal and paternal family histories must be obtained to determine risk.[34] The *BRCA1* gene, located on chromosome band 17q12-21, and the *BRCA2* gene, located on chromosome band 13q12-13, were identified and linked to hereditary breast and ovarian cancers in the 1990s. Emerging evidence suggests that these genes act as tumor suppressors and play a critical role in the repair of double-stranded DNA breaks.[34]

Many mutations have been described throughout the *BRCA1* and *BRCA2* genes, with nonsense and frameshift mutations being predominant.[34] Nonsense mutations occur when a nucleotide substitution results in a stop codon, and frameshift mutations occur when one or more nucleotides are deleted to produce a downstream stop codon. Certain ethnic groups have higher frequencies of distinctive *BRCA* mutations, thought to be due to a founder effect in which certain mutations are preserved within a genetically isolated population. Three such founder mutations (185delAG *BRCA1*, 5382insC *BRCA1*, and 6174delT *BRCA2*) are carried by 2% to 2.4% of the Ashkenazic Jewish population.[35] Furthermore, up to 40% of epithelial ovarian cancer patients of Jewish descent may carry one of these mutations (regardless of their family histories).[35] This is compared to a carrier frequency of approximately 5% among non-Jewish women with ovarian cancer.

The lifetime risk of ovarian cancer is approximately 20% to 40% for patients with *BRCA1* mutations, and 10% to 20% for *BRCA2* mutation carriers.[36] Ovarian cancer associated with germline mutations of *BRCA1* appears to present with distinct clinical and pathologic features compared with sporadic ovarian cancer.[37] The majority of *BRCA1*-associated cancers are serous adenocarcinomas, with an average age at diagnosis of 48 years, whereas the mean age for *BRCA2*-associated ovarian cancers is 60 years.[38] Other histologies may also occur, including endometrioid and clear cell tumors, although mucinous ovarian cancer appears to be underrepresented in these genetic syndromes. Furthermore, *BRCA*-associated cancers may have a more favorable course than sporadic ovarian cancer. In a study by Rubin et al.[37] the median survival of 43 patients with advanced *BRCA1*-associated disease was 77 months, compared with 29 months for matched controls. Cass et al.[39] noted a similar survival advantage for carriers in their matched cohort study and suggested that this was a result of having an improved response to platinum-based chemotherapy compared to women with sporadic disease. This increased chemosensitivity may be partly due to the inability of tumor cells to repair platinum-induced DNA damage in the setting of a *BRCA1* or *BRCA2* mutation.[34] The more favorable survival of patients with *BRCA1* or *BRCA2* mutations when compared to their sporadic counterparts is not necessarily related to a higher rate of cure, but may also be related to a longer duration of responsiveness to chemotherapy agents used in the relapsed setting. The Gynecologic Oncology Group (GOG) is conducting a prospective study to better compare the clinical course of sporadic ovarian cancer with that associated with *BRCA1* and *BRCA2* mutations.

The hereditary nonpolyposis colorectal cancer (HNPCC) syndrome accounts for approximately 5% to 10% of all hereditary ovarian cancer cases.[16] It is an autosomal dominant genetic syndrome characterized by nonpolyposis colon cancer, often involving the right colon, as well as an increased risk of developing endometrial, ovarian, hepatobiliary, upper gastrointestinal, and genitourinary cancers.[40] Colorectal and uterine cancers comprise the majority of tumors developing in affected families. The risk of endometrial cancer among women in HNPCC syndrome families is estimated to be 40% to 60% by age 70, compared to 1.5% in the general population. Limited studies have reported a 3.5-fold increase in the risk of ovarian cancer in members of these families.[40] A germline mutation in one of five genes involved in DNA mismatch repair is responsible for the HNPCC phenotype: *hMSH2* (chromosome arm 2p), *hMLH1* (chromosome arm 3p), *hPMS1* (chromosome arm 2q), *hPMS2* (chromosome arm 7p), and *hMSH6* (chromosome arm 2p).[34] The majority of affected patients are found to have defects in either *hMSH2* or *hMLH1*. Patients with HNPCC due to germline mutation of *hMSH6* may be particularly predisposed to uterine cancer. In addition, HNPCC may account for approximately 7% of cases with synchronous uterine and ovarian cancers, which are often low grade and of endometrioid histology.[16]

Patients at high risk of having a hereditary cancer typically undergo genetic counseling, so that the ramifications of genetic testing can be discussed. Multidisciplinary services available in such a setting often include pretest and posttest counseling, screening, treatment, and psychosocial counseling.[41] The most direct approach to determine whether a cancer-associated mutation is present is to test the patient affected with the disease (the proband), because he or she is the most likely to carry a deleterious mutation. The first family member to be tested will often require comprehensive gene sequencing. Other individuals can then be tested for the identified mutation, which may be unique to this particular family. In the Ashkenazic Jewish population, genetic testing for the three founder mutations is required because the carrier frequency in this population is high, and individuals may occasionally harbor germline mutations in both *BRCA1* and *BRCA2*.

Test results may reveal an identifiable mutation, no identifiable mutation, or a polymorphism of indeterminate clinical significance. If the proband has tested positive for a recognized mutation, then a relative with a negative result has likely not inherited the deleterious mutation, and her cancer risk approximates that of the general population. However, if no identifiable mutation is found in the proband, it is still possible that a cancer-associated mutation exists that is not detectable with current testing methods. This is especially the case for probands with a highly suggestive family history of breast, ovarian, or both cancers. In this regard, it has been shown that approximately 12% of probands who test negative for a germline mutation using standard gene sequencing techniques are found to have a clinically significant mutation in *BRCA1* or *BRCA2* when tested by the technique of multiplex ligation dependent probe amplification (MLPA).[42] Finally, a minority of test results represent genetic variants or polymorphisms in *BRCA1* or *BRCA2* that are of indeterminate clinical significance. Further study of these genetic variants and associated cancer risks in large populations will help reduce the number of reports of indeterminate findings.

The management of patients with an inherited genetic predisposition to ovarian cancer is complex due to the variable penetrance of genetic alterations and the lack of effective early detection methods for ovarian cancer. Although annual pelvic examinations, serum CA 125 determinations, and TVU are sometimes considered in affected individuals, there is currently no conclusive evidence that ovarian cancer mortality is reduced as a result of these interventions.[26] In contrast, the efficacy of prophylactic, risk reduction bilateral salpingo-oophorectomy (RRSO) for patients with the hereditary breast–ovarian cancer syndrome has been more convincingly demonstrated.[43,44] One study of 259 patients who underwent RRSO found a 96% decrease in ovarian cancers and an approximately 50% reduction in subsequent breast cancer compared to age-matched controls.[43] Even after RRSO, *BRCA* mutation carriers are still at small risk for developing primary peritoneal serous cancer, which is histologically and clinically similar to epithelial ovarian cancer. Such cancers represent malignant transformation of the peritoneal mesothelium, which is contiguous with ovarian surface epithelium.

RRSO is generally considered for patients at high risk for developing ovarian cancer and who have completed childbearing, especially if they are at least 35 years of age.[26,45] A laparoscopic approach is frequently possible, but the surgical options must be individualized, as must the decision for concomitant hysterectomy (which is an especially relevant consideration for patients with HNPCC undergoing this procedure). It is important to remove the fallopian tubes as part of prophylactic surgery, since the tubal epithelium may harbor dysplasia or may develop *in situ* cancers in this setting.[46] The surgical pathologist must perform a careful examination of the surgical specimens, as occult ovarian and tubal carcinoma have been found in 2% to 10% of RRSO specimens.[47] Some patients with occult disease discovered after careful pathological evaluation may require a second operation to complete surgical staging in order to determine the need for postoperative treatment, as described later in the chapter. Significant issues regarding RRSO remain unresolved, such as the physiologic adjustments to premature surgical menopause and the safety of hormone replacement therapy in this group, especially in those at high risk for breast cancer.[48]

It has been suggested that chemoprophylaxis with oral contraceptives for 5 years might decrease ovarian cancer risk by 50% in both the general population and in high-risk women. For example, a case-controlled study of 207 known *BRCA* mutation carriers and their sister controls found a 60% reduction of ovarian cancer risk with oral contraceptive use.[49] Other risk-reducing strategies such as tubal ligation and hysterectomy have also been associated with a reduced incidence of ovarian cancer among high-risk women.[3] Nonetheless, RRSO is currently the most effective preventative strategy to reduce ovarian cancer risk in patients with *BRCA* mutations.

Staging

Exploratory laparotomy serves three main purposes in the management of patients with suspected ovarian cancer. First, laparotomy permits histologic confirmation of disease, since a complex cyst may not only represent primary ovarian cancer, but may also be caused by metastatic gastric cancer to the ovary (Krukenberg tumor), metastatic disease to the ovary from a gastrointestinal or breast primary (especially infiltrating lobular breast cancer), or benign conditions such as endometriosis.[50] Surgery is also necessary to determine the extent of disease (staging), which is critical in determining whether postoperative treatment will be necessary, as well as to assess prognosis. Finally, exploratory laparotomy is necessary to permit debulking of as much tumor as possible, since patients who are optimally cytoreduced (defined as having less than or equal to 1-cm diameter residual tumor) have a better prognosis compared to those with greater amounts of residual disease.[51]

The staging system for ovarian cancer is defined by FIGO and is based on the findings at exploratory laparotomy (Table 104.3).[52] Proper surgical staging via exploratory laparotomy requires a midline incision large enough to permit inspection of the peritoneal cavity, including the upper abdomen, as well as evaluation of the retroperitoneal spaces and lymph nodes.[53] When the peritoneal cavity is entered, ascitic fluid is aspirated and the peritoneal surfaces are irrigated, with the samples sent for cytologic evaluation. The pelvis and paracolic spaces should be irrigated and the fluid sent for cytologic examination. If intraperitoneal carcinomatosis is absent, it may be most appropriate to first resect the ovarian tumor and then to proceed with surgical staging to avoid rupturing the mass. The grossly normal, opposite ovary may undergo biopsy, or any visible benign-appearing cysts may be excised. Pelvic and para-aortic retroperitoneal lymph nodes are generally evaluated in patients whose tumors do not grossly extend outside the ovary, since approximately 10% to 15% of patients with otherwise stage I disease will have occult nodal involvement that places them in the stage III category.[53] Any enlarged pelvic retroperitoneal lymph nodes should be removed if technically feasible in order to achieve optimal cytoreduction.

It is frequently necessary to extend the vertical incision above the umbilicus in order to fully inspect the upper abdomen. If gross disease is not present in the omentum, an infracolic omentectomy is usually sufficient for diagnostic purposes. When the omentum demonstrates diffuse infiltration by tumor (an omental cake), it should be excised from the greater curvature of the stomach as completely as possible. The upper abdominal evaluation continues with a careful inspection of the right hemidiaphragm, liver serosa, and liver parenchyma. The spleen is then carefully inspected, as is the left diaphragm. A splenectomy could be considered if this procedure would lead to an optimal surgical cytoreduction. The paracolic spaces and large bowel are then carefully inspected. The small intestine and mesentery are evaluated, and any tumor implants are removed as much as possible. If luminal narrowing is present, especially in the area of the terminal ileum, a small bowel resection and reanastomosis are performed. Similarly, if tumor appears to invade the large bowel, a resection may be required if the mass is large enough to pose a threat for bowel obstruction. Lymphadenectomy is considered if this procedure is technically feasible and would lead to a maximally cytoreductive result. In postmenopausal women or in women in whom fertility is no longer desired, a bilateral salpingo-oophorectomy and total abdominal hysterectomy are typically performed.

For women who wish to preserve fertility, which is sometimes possible when the tumor is limited to one ovary, staging may be performed without removal of the contralateral ovary and tube and without hysterectomy.[54] In that regard, patients with endometrioid ovarian cancer may have a synchronous endometrioid uterine cancer in up to 15% of cases, which may not always be appreciated preoperatively.[16] In such cases, the tumor is often minimally invasive and low grade, and the prognosis is often favorable. Therefore, for patients with early stage, endometrioid ovarian cancer in whom a fertility sparing operation is considered, it is reasonable to perform an endometrial biopsy to exclude the presence of a separate uterine cancer that would alter the surgical approach.

On occasion, the initial surgical staging is incomplete due to lack of lymph node or upper abdominal evaluation in a patient with presumptive stage I disease. In this situation, it is reasonable to consider completing the surgical staging if the findings would alter postoperative management. For instance, if a patient has stage IA, grade 1 or 2 disease (Table 104.3) after complete surgical staging, no further postoperative treatment would generally be indicated.[55] However, if a patient is already known to have at least stage IC or stage II disease, or if the tumor is grade 3, then postoperative chemotherapy is generally required, and the impact of additional staging procedures might be less important (except perhaps for the patient who is discovered to have stage III disease on re-exploration, in which case intraperitoneal chemotherapy might play a role if she is optimally cytoreduced, as noted below). Laparoscopic techniques may allow para-aortic lymph node dissections and omentectomies to be performed with less morbidity, which is an important consideration in a patient who might have undergone recent, albeit incomplete, surgical evaluation. If this is not possible or practical, an alternative is to obtain a CT scan in an attempt to identify the presence of any subclinical bulky disease that might be amenable to surgical resection. However, CT is not capable of detecting small volume or microscopic disease that could affect decisions regarding the need for postoperative chemotherapy.

Prognostic Factors for Epithelial Ovarian Cancer

Clinicopathologic findings of prognostic value include FIGO stage, volume of residual disease after cytoreductive surgery, histologic subtype, histologic grade, age, and malignant ascites.[13] Tumor stage remains the most important prognostic factor, although only 30% of patients have early stage disease (defined as having stage I or stage II tumors). Stage IA disease is completely encapsulated, without involvement of the ovarian surface, without rupture, malignant ascites, or positive washings (Table 104.3). The 5-year survival of patients with stage IA disease and grade 1 or 2 histology is greater than 90% after surgery alone, and several investigators include patients with stage IB, grade 1 or 2 disease, in this good prognostic group.[55] However, the relapse rate without postoperative adjuvant treatment is 30% to 40% for patients with stage IC disease (defined by the presence of rupture, surface involvement, malignant ascites, or positive washings), those with stage I, grade 3 disease, or those with stage II tumors. These patients comprise a high-risk group of early stage tumors and experience a 5-year survival rate of approximately 80% after receiving postoperative adjuvant therapy.[55] It should be noted that the prognostic significance of rupture as the sole criterion for stage IC disease is somewhat controversial, as some investigators report that rupture alone does not appear to confer a worse prognosis if it occurred intraoperatively, as opposed to preoperatively.[56]

The majority of patients with epithelial ovarian cancer present with advanced disease (stage III or IV). After postoperative treatment, the 5-year survival rate of patients with stage III optimally debulked, gross residual disease (less than or equal to 1-cm diameter residual tumor) is approximately 20% to 30%, and this decreases to less than 10% for patients with suboptimally debulked stage III disease or those with stage IV tumors.[57,58] Patients who have stage IIIA disease on the basis of microscopic upper abdominal involvement (usually detected on omental biopsy) have survivals in the range of 50% after postoperative adjuvant therapy.[59] Patients with advanced-stage disease who have mucinous or clear cell histologic also have a worse prognosis, which appears to be related to the relative chemoresistance of these histologies. In a GOG study, no patient with advanced clear cell or mucinous histology achieved a pathologic complete response after chemotherapy, as defined by performance of second-look laparotomy.[13]

Preoperative serum CA 125 levels frequently reflect the volume of disease and do not appear to have an independent effect on survival, after correcting for stage and debulking status. However, postoperative CA 125 levels, both during and after completion of first-line chemotherapy, have prognostic value.[60,61] Some investigators have demonstrated that normalization of the serum CA 125 levels after three cycles of chemotherapy is associated with more favorable outcome, as well as achievement of a CA 125 nadir of less than or equal to 10 U/mL upon completion of treatment.[60,61] Although this information has prognostic significance, it has limited therapeutic value in the absence of effective salvage regimens with curative potential.

Several molecular prognostic factors have been investigated in ovarian cancer. These include markers of proliferation or drug resistance, levels of serum cytokines or growth factor receptors, and expression of genes associated with metastases.[62] More recently it has been possible to use microarray analysis, which provides a global snapshot of gene expression, to assess prognosis and response to therapy in this disease. At least two profiles have been defined, referred to as the Ovarian Cancer Prognostic Profile (OCPP) and the Chemo Response Profile (CRP), that provide information of independent prognostic and predictive value for patients with advanced disease.[63,64] However, it remains to be determined how best to incorporate such new techniques into the management of patients with this tumor. In the future, it is hoped that gene expression profiling will be capable of identifying patients who might benefit from novel forms of treatment (such as antiangiogenic therapy) or those with poor prognosis who might be appropriate for clinical trial participation.

Management of Early Stage Disease

Postoperative Chemotherapy

The results of two randomized European trials (International Collaborative Ovarian Neoplasm Trial 1 [ICON-1] and Adjuvant ChemoTherapy in Ovarian Neoplasm Trial [ACTION]) suggest that adjuvant chemotherapy can improve both progression-free and overall survival in patients with high-risk, early stage ovarian cancer.[65] Such patients include those with stage I, grade 3, stage IC, or any stage II disease. These two studies collectively enrolled 925 patients, although they differed in eligibility criteria, requirements for surgical staging and the specific adjuvant chemotherapy program used. Overall survival was superior for platinum-based adjuvant therapy in the entire patient cohort, although subset analysis revealed that the benefit appeared to be restricted to those patients who did not undergo adequate surgical staging. This observation suggested that the observed survival benefit might be due to unintentional enrollment of a subset of patients who actually had occult stage III disease. Nonetheless, caution must be used when interpreting the results of an unplanned subset analysis, and most physicians feel that these data support the use of adjuvant chemotherapy for patients with high-risk, early stage disease.[66]

A study performed by the GOG compared three cycles of carboplatin and paclitaxel to six cycles of this regimen in patients with high-risk, early stage ovarian cancer in order to determine whether a shorter duration of treatment is equally effective and less toxic.[67] The relapse rate and progression-free survival were not statistically different between these two treatment arms, which led some investigators to conclude that administering three cycles of adjuvant chemotherapy was as effective as six cycles in this setting. However, a recent subset analysis of this trial involving patients with serous histology showed that the 5-year recurrence-free survival for patients who received six cycles was 83%, compared with 60% for those who received three cycles ($P = .007$).[68] In addition, this study was not sufficiently powered to determine whether three cycles was equivalent to six cycles in terms of an overall survival benefit. In view of these issues, administration of six cycles of adjuvant carboplatin plus paclitaxel chemotherapy can still be considered a reasonable approach for high-risk, early stage patients, unless more definitive data supporting lesser amounts of chemotherapy become available.[69] The rationale for choosing carboplatin and paclitaxel is based on the experience gained from management of advanced disease, which will be described in detail later in the chapter.

Postoperative Radiation Therapy

The role of radiation therapy in the treatment of patients with primary ovarian cancer has changed markedly over time. For several decades it was used as the sole modality of treatment. As experience with chemotherapy grew, randomized trials were conducted to compare different chemotherapy regimens to whole abdominal radiotherapy (WAR) or to intraperitoneal (IP) administration of radioactive phosphorus (^{32}P). Most are now of only historical interest, as the chemotherapy regimens used did not contain platinum compounds, and they will not be reviewed here. In general, these studies showed that WAR and ^{32}P had similar efficacy compared to prolonged courses of melphalan or chlorambucil, given with or without pelvic irradiation.

The first trial to compare radiation therapy to a platinum-based regimen was conducted from 1981 to 1987 in Birmingham, England. This trial randomized 40 patients with stages IC to III ovarian cancer with no macroscopic residual disease following surgery to either WAR using a moving-strip technique or to cisplatin (100 mg/m^2, given every 3 weeks for five cycles). With a median follow-up of 84 months, the 5-year survival rates in the two groups were 58% and 62%, respectively.[70]

A trial conducted in Genoa, Italy, from 1985 to 1989 included 70 patients with high-risk stage I or II ovarian carcinoma.[71] They received either WAR using an open-field technique (24 fractions delivering 43.2 Gy to the pelvis and 30.2 Gy to the upper abdomen) or cisplatin (50 mg/m^2) plus cyclophosphamide (600 mg/m^2), given every 4 weeks for six cycles. Eight patients randomized to WAR received chemotherapy because of their own or their physicians' preference. Since protocol compliance was poor and accrual low, the study was prematurely closed. At a median follow-up of 60 months, the 5-year overall survival rates in the radiation and chemotherapy arms were 53% and 71%, respectively (P = .16); relapse-free survival rates were 50% and 74%, respectively (P = .07). Of note, late bowel obstruction requiring surgery occurred in only one patient.

From 1982 to 1988, 340 eligible patients with stages I through III ovarian carcinoma without residual disease after surgery seen at the Norwegian Radium Hospital in Oslo were randomized to receive either IP radioactive chromic phosphate (7 to 10 mCi, or 260 to 370 MBq) or six cycles of intravenous (IV) cisplatin (50 mg/m^2) given every 3 weeks.[72] Twenty-eight patients with peritoneal adhesions who were randomized to IP ^{32}P were treated instead with WAR. The 5-year overall survival rates in the two arms were 83% and 81%; disease-free survival rates were 81% and 75%, respectively. Patients with stage II or III tumors had superior survival when treated with cisplatin, although the difference was not statistically significant. The long-term risk of bowel obstruction without recurrence in radiation and chemotherapy arms was 11% and 2%, respectively.

Finally, a trial conducted between 1986 and 1994 by the GOG randomly allocated 229 eligible patients with stage IA-B grade 3 or stage II tumors without macroscopic residual disease after surgery to either IP ^{32}P (15 mCi) or three cycles every 3 weeks of cyclophosphamide (1,000 mg/m^2) and cisplatin (100 mg/m^2).[73] With a median follow-up of nearly 10 years in survivors, the 10-year relapse rates in the radiation and chemotherapy arms were 35% and 28%, respectively, which was not statistically significant. There was a relative reduction of 17% in the overall death rate in the chemotherapy arm, which was not statistically significant. The incidence of nonhematologic grade 3 or 4 toxicities was similar in both arms.

In summary, these randomized trials generally found WAR or IP ^{32}P was less effective or more toxic than platinum-containing regimens. Hence, adjuvant radiation therapy has fallen out of use as the primary treatment for patients with high-risk, early stage ovarian cancer.

Management of Advanced-Stage Disease

Primary Cytoreductive Surgery

The theoretical benefits of cytoreductive surgery include removal of large, necrotic tumors with poor blood supply that might lead to impaired chemotherapy delivery. It has also been postulated that tumor debulking may permit residual tumor to proliferate more rapidly and thereby enhance sensitivity to postoperative chemotherapy. Although neither of these mechanisms has been proven, the association between successful cytoreduction and more favorable outcome has been demonstrated in many surgical series.[13,51,59]

The definition of *optimal cytoreduction* has varied through the years, but residual disease of 1 cm or smaller in maximum individual diameter is most widely accepted. *Primary cytoreduction* refers to performance of debulking surgery prior to administration of first-line chemotherapy and is the standard approach for managing most patients with suspected epithelial ovarian cancer.

Despite the importance of primary cytoreductive surgery, some patients with a poor performance status due to extensive tumor or comorbid disease may not be appropriate candidates for this procedure. In these cases, initiating neoadjuvant chemotherapy is a reasonable approach, followed by an interval attempt at surgical cytoreduction in responding patients after three cycles of chemotherapy have been administered. In this instance, surgery is referred to as an *interval cytoreduction*. Patients with stage IV disease due to extensive parenchymal liver or lung involvement may not be ideal candidates for optimal cytoreductive surgery. Although it is sometimes possible to resect tumor in these sites, many of these patients are left with a suboptimal result, and thus neoadjuvant chemotherapy has often been recommended.[74,75] Theoretical advantages of neoadjuvant chemotherapy in this setting are a more rapid improvement in quality of life, and, if interval debulking surgery is ultimately performed, a technically more feasible operation with shorter hospitalization and less morbidity. Prospective randomized trials incorporating neoadjuvant chemotherapy in the management of advanced-stage ovarian cancer are under way to better define the value of this strategy.

Postoperative Chemotherapy for Epithelial Ovarian Cancer

Advanced-stage epithelial ovarian cancer is a chemoresponsive disease in the majority of cases, although relapse often occurs and resistance eventually develops to most forms of treatment. The platinum compounds remain the single most active drugs in the treatment of this disease. Cisplatin was the most frequently used platinum compound in the late 1970s and early 1980s, although it was soon recognized that the use of carboplatin instead of cisplatin conferred an equivalent survival advantage, but with less neuropathy, nephropathy, and emesis.[76]

Although numerous combination chemotherapy regimens have been studied over the past three decades, the combination of an intravenous platinum compound and a taxane such as paclitaxel is now accepted as an appropriate first-line, postoperative option for many patients. The response rate of this combination is as high as 70% for patients with suboptimally debulked disease, and over 80% for patients who are optimally cytoreduced.[57,58] Platinum agents exert their effects by forming intrastrand DNA adducts with guanosine bases, whereas taxanes mediate cytotoxicity by binding to and stabilizing the tubulin polymer, thereby preventing physiologic dissociation of the mitotic spindle at the completion of M phase. Given these nonoverlapping mechanisms of action, it was not surprising to find that taxanes were active agents in the treatment of some patients with relapsed, platinum-resistant ovarian cancer.[77] These observations formed the basis for investigating the platinum and taxane combination in the first-line setting.

Two phase 3 randomized trials begun in the early 1990s compared a cisplatin and paclitaxel combination to a cisplatin and cyclophosphamide regimen (Table 104.4). In the GOG study, patients with suboptimally resected stage III or IV ovarian cancer were randomized to receive six cycles of either cisplatin and cyclophosphamide or the experimental arm of cisplatin and paclitaxel.[58] Women treated with the paclitaxel-containing program experienced a statistically significant improvement in response rate (73% vs. 60%; P <.01), median progression-free survival (18 vs. 13 months; P <.001), and median overall survival (38 vs. 24 months; P <.001).

These results were confirmed in a trial conducted in Europe and Canada that used a similar but not identical study design.[76] In this trial, paclitaxel was delivered as a 3-hour infusion of 175 mg/m^2, whereas in the GOG study a dose of 135 mg/m^2

TABLE 104.4

RANDOMIZED TRIALS OF PACLITAXEL VERSUS NONPACLITAXEL FIRST-LINE THERAPY IN ADVANCED EPITHELIAL OVARIAN CANCER

Trial and Randomization	Patient Number	Stage	CCR (%)	Median PFS (months)	Median OS (months)
GOG-111 (ref. 58)	386	III, IV			
Paclitaxel (135 mg/m²) Cisplatin (75 mg/m²)			51	18	38
				P <.001	*P* <.001
Cyclosphosphamide (750 mg/m²) Cisplatin (75 mg/m²)			31	13	24
OV10 (ref. 76)	668	IIB–IV			
Paclitaxel (175 mg/m²) Cisplatin (75 mg/m²)			40.7	15.5	35.6
				P = .0005	*P* = .0016
Cyclophosphamide (750 mg/m²) Cisplatin (75 mg/m²)			27.3	12	25.8
ICON-3 (ref. 80)	2074	I–IV			
Paclitaxel (175 mg/m²) Carboplatin (AUC 5 to 6)			NA	17.3	36.1
				P = .16	*P* = .74
Carboplatin (AUC 5 to 6)					
Cisplatin (50 mg/m²) Doxorubicin (50 mg/m²) Cyclophosphamide (500 mg/m²)			NA	16.1	35.4[a]
GOG-132 (ref. 79)	614	III–IV			
Paclitaxel (135 mg/m²) Cisplatin (75 mg/m²)			NA	16	35[b]
Cisplatin (100 mg/m²)			NA	16.4	30.2
Paclitaxel (200 mg/m²)			NA	10.8	25.9

AUC, area under the curve; CCR, clinical complete remission; GOG, Gynecologic Oncology Group; ICON-3, International Collaborative Ovarian Neoplasm trial 3; NA, not available; OS, overall survival; PFS, progression-free survival.
[a]For ICON-3, patients in the control arms could receive either carboplatin alone, or cisplatin, doxorubicin, and cyclophosphamide.
[b]There was no significant difference in overall survival between any of the three treatment arms of GOG132 (*P* = .31).

was administered over 24 hours. In addition, a much larger percentage of patients in the control arm of the European-Canadian study received paclitaxel as second-line therapy after relapse, compared to the control arm of the GOG trial. Despite these differences, this study also revealed a statistically significant improvement in both progression-free and overall survival associated with the paclitaxel-containing regimen (Table 104.4).

Neither the GOG nor the European-Canadian trials was able to address whether the survival benefit observed with the platinum-taxane doublet was related to the use of combination chemotherapy or whether it could also be achieved through the use of sequential monotherapy. In an attempt to address this issue, the GOG conducted a randomized trial in which patients with suboptimally debulked advanced disease received either single-agent cisplatin (100 mg/m²), single-agent paclitaxel (200 mg/m² administered over 24 hours), or the combination of cisplatin (75 mg/m²) and paclitaxel (135 mg/m² administered over 24 hours).[79] Survival was similar between the three study arms, despite a superior objective response rate to both platinum-containing regimens (67%), compared to single-agent paclitaxel (42%). This result is likely explained by the fact that approximately 50% of patients in the single-agent arms were switched to the alternative agent before documented disease progression. These results support the concept that sequential treatment with a platinum agent, followed by paclitaxel, may be therapeutically equivalent to combination therapy with both agents in advanced ovarian cancer. However, since crossover to the alternative agent was not a formal part of this study's design, this interpretation should be viewed with caution, and combination first-line chemotherapy with a taxane and platinum compound remains the standard of care.

A third European randomized trial (ICON-3) compared a nonpaclitaxel, platinum-based control regimen (either single-agent carboplatin or the combination of cisplatin, doxorubicin, and cyclophosphamide), to an experimental arm of carboplatin and paclitaxel.[80] Surprisingly, this study failed to reveal a difference in survival between either control arm and the paclitaxel-containing experimental arm. Perhaps the most likely explanation for this observation is that one third of the patients in the control arms of ICON-3 ultimately received paclitaxel at some point in their disease course.[81] Thus, as in the previously mentioned three-arm GOG study,[79] this outcome provides circumstantial evidence to suggest that the sequential administration of these two active agents may be therapeutically equivalent to combination drug delivery in this setting.

Three randomized trials have directly compared a carboplatin and paclitaxel combination to cisplatin and paclitaxel (Table 104.5).[57,82,83] These studies found equivalent progression-free and overall survivals for either carboplatin- or cisplatin-containing regimens, but with a more favorable toxicity profile associated with carboplatin-based treatment.

TABLE 104.5

RANDOMIZED TRIALS OF CARBOPLATIN AND PACLITAXEL VERSUS CISPLATIN AND PACLITAXEL IN ADVANCED EPITHELIAL OVARIAN CANCER

Trial and Randomization[a]	Patient Number	Stage	Median PFS (months)	Median OS (months)
GOG-158 (ref. 57)	792	III[b]		
Paclitaxel (175 mg/m²) Carboplatin (AUC 7.5)			20.7	57.4
			0.88 (0.75–1.03)[c]	0.84 (0.70–1.02)
Paclitaxel (135 mg/m²) Cisplatin (75 mg/m²)			19.4	48.7
AGO (ref. 82)	798	IIB–IV		
Paclitaxel (185 mg/m²) Carboplatin (AUC 6)			17.2	43.3
			1.05 (0.89–1.23)	1.05 (0.87–1.26)
Paclitaxel (185 mg/m²) Cisplatin (75 mg/m²)			19.1	44.1
Netherlands-Denmark (ref. 83)	208	IIB–IV		
Paclitaxel (175 mg/m²) Carboplatin (AUC 5)			16	31[d]
Paclitaxel (175 mg/m²) Cisplatin (75 mg/m²)				

AUC, area under the curve; GOG, Gynecologic Oncology Group; AGO, Arbeitsgemeinschaft Gynaekologische Onkologie; NA, not available; OS, overall survival; PFS, progression-free survival.
[a]Six cycles of chemotherapy were administered in each trial unless otherwise stated.
[b]Patients enrolled in GOG-158 were required to have an optimal cytoreduction, as defined as residual disease less than or equal to 1 cm in greatest diameter.
[c]Hazard ratio followed by 95% confidence interval in parentheses.
[d]The Netherlands-Denmark trial was not sufficiently powered to assess noninferiority. Therefore, the survival data shown reflect the entire patient cohort, as opposed to the individual treatment groups.

Thus, the carboplatin-based combination (carboplatin, area under the curve [AUC] = 5 to 6 and paclitaxel, 175 mg/m² administered over 3 hours) is preferred when systemic chemotherapy is indicated, due to reduced toxicity and the ability to give paclitaxel over a shorter infusion time. For individuals who may have difficulty tolerating a combination regimen (e.g., those with marginal performance status or significant comorbid medical conditions), it is reasonable to initiate treatment with intravenous single-agent carboplatin and later add intravenous paclitaxel to the regimen or deliver the drugs as sequential single agents. For appropriate patients with stage III disease who are optimally cytoreduced, *intraperitoneal* chemotherapy is an important new option, which will be described in detail below.

The optimal choice of taxane has also been investigated in the first-line setting. A randomized trial comparing intravenous carboplatin (AUC = 5) plus paclitaxel (175 mg/m²) to intravenous carboplatin (AUC = 5) and docetaxel (75 mg/m²) has shown equivalent response rates and progression-free and overall survival for the two programs, although their toxicity profiles differed.[84] More grade 4 neutropenia occurred with the docetaxel-containing regimen, and a greater incidence of grade 2 or 3 neuropathy was observed with the paclitaxel-containing program. These data indicate that a carboplatin and docetaxel combination is an acceptable first-line regimen for patients with advanced ovarian cancer, especially in the setting of pre-existing neuropathy (where paclitaxel may be difficult to tolerate).

There appears to be no value in extending platinum-based first-line therapy beyond 6 cycles.[85,86] Furthermore, there is no convincing evidence to suggest a benefit to the addition of cytotoxic drugs such as liposomal doxorubicin, epirubicin, topotecan, or gemcitabine to the platinum and taxane doublet.[87] A recent randomized trial performed by the Japanese GOG demonstrated a progression-free and overall survival advantage for the use of weekly paclitaxel (in conjunction with day 1 carboplatin) in newly diagnosed patients with ovarian cancer, and confirmatory trials are under way.[88] Given the activity of bevacizumab in the relapsed setting (see below), there is interest in investigating the value of this agent in patients with newly diagnosed disease. The GOG is currently conducting a three-arm, placebo-controlled randomized trial investigating the role of bevacizumab in newly diagnosed patients with stage III or IV disease, with a subsequent randomization to maintenance single-agent bevacizumab or placebo for up to 1 year (GOG 218). Progression-free survival is the primary end point of this trial, and preliminary results are expected in mid-2010. A similar question is being addressed in a two-arm European trial (ICON-7) for newly diagnosed patients with either optimally or suboptimally debulked disease.

Intraperitoneal Chemotherapy

Epithelial ovarian cancer is largely confined to the peritoneal space during most of its natural history.[2] Given this relatively localized distribution, efforts to instill chemotherapy directly into the peritoneal cavity have received a great deal of attention over the past two decades. The rationale for this approach is based on the observation that many active drugs such as cisplatin and paclitaxel have favorable peritoneal-to-plasma concentrations, on the order of 20 to 1 and 1,000 to 1, respectively.[89] The ability to deliver high local concentrations of active drugs, with generally acceptable systemic side effects, suggested that it may be possible to achieve more effective cytoreduction of disease that is present at the peritoneal surface. Given the rather limited penetration of such drugs into peritoneal tumor, to a depth of only a few millimeters, patients

TABLE 104.6

SELECTED RANDOMIZED TRIALS OF INTRAPERITONEAL FIRST-LINE THERAPY IN OPTIMALLY DEBULKED, STAGE III OVARIAN CANCER

Trial and Randomization[a]	Patient Number	Median PFS (months)	Median OS (months)	Hazard Ratio (95% CI, P value)
GOG-104/SWOG-8501 (ref. 90)[b]	546			
Cisplatin IP (100 mg/m^2) Cyclophosphamide IV (600 mg/m^2)		NA	49	0.76 (0.61–0.96; *P* = .02)
Cisplatin IV (100 mg/m^2) Cyclophosphamide IV (600 mg/m^2)		NA	41	
GOG-114 (ref. 91)	462			
Carboplatin (AUC 9 for 2 cycles) Paclitaxel IV (135 mg/m^2) Cisplatin IP (100 mg/m^2)		28	63	0.81 (0.65–1.0; *P* = .056)[c]
Paclitaxel IV (135 mg/m^2) Cisplatin IV (75 mg/m^2)		22	52	
GOG-172 (ref. 92)	429			
Paclitaxel IV Day 1 (135 mg/m^2) Cisplatin IP Day 2 (100 mg/m^2) Paclitaxel IP Day 8 (60 mg/m^2)		23.8	65.6	0.75 (0.58–0.97; *P* = .03)
Paclitaxel IV (135 mg/m^2) Cisplatin IV (75 mg/m^2)		18.3	49.7	

AUC, area under the curve; GOG, Gynecologic Oncology Group; SWOG, Southwest Oncology Group; IP, intraperitoneal; IV, intravenous; NA, not available; OS, overall survival; PFS, progression-free survival.
[a]Six cycles of chemotherapy were administered in each trial unless otherwise stated.
[b]Optimal cytoreduction in GOG-104/SWOG-8501 was defined as less than or equal to 2-cm diameter residual disease, whereas a 1-cm cut-off was used for GOG-114 and GOG-172.
[c]*P* value determined using a one-sided *t* test.

with optimally cytoreduced disease are theoretically most likely to benefit from this approach.

Three randomized trials have addressed the role of IP chemotherapy in the first-line management of patients with optimally debulked stage III disease (Table 104.6). Two of these trials showed a statistically significant improvement in both progression-free and overall survival rates for patients treated with IP chemotherapy, and the other demonstrated improvement in progression-free survival only (although a nonsignificant trend for improved overall survival in the IP arm was noted). The first of these was an intergroup trial performed in 546 optimally debulked stage III patients with less than or equal to 2-cm residual disease.[90] Note that this definition of "optimally debulked" was widely accepted at the time, although subsequently a 1-cm cutoff has been adopted. Patients were randomized to receive either IP cisplatin or IV cisplatin, in combination with IV cyclophosphamide, every 3 weeks for six cycles (note that paclitaxel was not an approved drug at the time of this study's design). The median survival of all eligible patients was 49 months for the IP cisplatin arm compared to 41 months for the IV cisplatin group (*P* = .02; hazard ratio [HR] 0.76). There was also a trend toward a higher likelihood of pathologic complete remission (PCR) in the IP arm compared to IV treatment (47% vs. 36%, respectively). However, the positive results of this study were overshadowed by the emerging value of the IV paclitaxel and platinum combination in the first-line setting,[58] and the added benefit of the IP route remained uncertain. Specifically, it was argued that perhaps the use of IV paclitaxel might negate the benefit of IP therapy, and this issue led to a second randomized IP trial that included paclitaxel.

The second study was performed by the GOG and involved optimally debulked patients with stage III disease (less than or equal to 1-cm diameter residual) who were randomized to receive either IV paclitaxel (135 mg/m^2 over 24 hours) and IV cisplatin (75 mg/m^2) for six cycles, or IV carboplatin (AUC = 9) for two cycles followed by IV paclitaxel (135 mg/m^2 administered over 24 hours) and IP cisplatin (100 mg/m^2) for six cycles.[91] The median progression-free survivals for the IP and IV arms were 28 months and 22 months, respectively (*P* = .01; one-sided *t* test). However, there was only a borderline significant trend in overall survival in favor of the IP treatment arm (63.2 months vs. 52.5 months, respectively; *P* = .05, one-sided *t* test), but with substantial toxicity partly due to the use of high-dose, single-agent carboplatin in the experimental arm. The significant toxicity of this regimen, coupled with only a borderline significant survival difference, did not provide convincing enough evidence to adopt this regimen for widespread use.

A third GOG study eliminated the use of high-dose carboplatin and introduced a second dose of paclitaxel, administered via the IP route, on day 8.[92] Patients with optimally debulked disease (less than or equal to 1-cm diameter residual) were randomized to receive either a control arm of IV paclitaxel (135 mg/m^2 administered over 24 hours) and IV cisplatin (75 mg/m^2) for six cycles, or IV paclitaxel on day 1 (135 mg/m^2 administered over 24 hours), IP cisplatin on day 2 (100 mg/m^2), and IP paclitaxel on day 8 (60 mg/m^2), for six cycles. The median overall-survival was 65.6 months for the IP arm and 49.7 months for the IV arm (HR 0.75; 95% CI [confidence interval], 0.58 to 0.97; *P* = .03). This significant prolongation of median overall survival was associated with several toxicities, including a higher incidence of neutropenia, infection, catheter blockage, neuropathy, abdominal pain, renal dysfunction, and electrolyte abnormalities. Due to this toxicity, only 42% of patients were able to complete all six cycles of planned IP chemotherapy, and approximately 40% could only receive two or fewer cycles. Thus, while 83% of patients assigned to the IP arm eventually completed six cycles of a taxane and platinum combination, the majority required a switch from IP to IV drug administration at some point during the planned IP treatment course. Patients who required bowel resection during their initial surgical debulking procedure appeared to have a higher incidence of postoperative complications that prevented subsequent use of IP therapy.[93] The fact that a survival advantage was observed despite failure of most patients to complete six cycles of IP treatment suggested that the benefits of IP treatment may occur early in the treatment course, although this issue was not formally addressed in this trial.[94]

In addition to the three randomized trials described earlier, four other trials have addressed the value of IP chemotherapy in the first-line setting, and one additional trial has examined the role of IP cisplatin as consolidation therapy after achievement of a complete remission.[95] A meta-analysis of these eight trials showed that IP chemotherapy was associated with a 21.6% reduction in risk of death (HR 0.79; 95% CI, 0.7 to 0.89).[95] Although some investigators still feel that IP chemotherapy should remain experimental, others feel that these data offer strong support for the IP approach.[94,96–98] At present, IP therapy has not been shown to be superior to IV treatment in patients with stage IV disease, suboptimally debulked residual disease, or relapsed disease. It should also be avoided in patients with comorbid conditions such as renal insufficiency, significant baseline neuropathy, or extensive intra-abdominal adhesions.

A number of potential ways to improve the tolerability of IP therapy could be considered, including reduction of the day-2 IP cisplatin dose, administration of day-1 IV paclitaxel over 3 hours instead of 24 hours, or omitting day-8 IP paclitaxel until patient tolerance to the first cycle of IP cisplatin can be assessed. It is unknown whether such modifications will reduce toxicity while still preserving the benefits of the IP approach.[94] There is also interest in the use of IP carboplatin instead of IP cisplatin in an attempt to reduce toxicity.[99] Although the pharmacologic advantage of IP carboplatin appears to be favorable, it is not yet known whether carboplatin is as effective as cisplatin when administered via the IP route. The value of IP carboplatin in newly diagnosed, optimally debulked ovarian cancer is currently being studied in a randomized trial conducted by the GOG (GOG 252).

Technical Aspects of Intraperitoneal Chemotherapy Administration

IP administration of either cisplatin or paclitaxel requires placement of a catheter with a subcutaneous access port in the anterior chest wall region, just below the breast, which then tunnels subcutaneously downward to the midabdomen, where it enters the peritoneal cavity.[100] IP catheter insertion can be performed at the time of primary cytoreductive surgery or afterward by laparoscopy. Makhija et al.[101] reported a reduction in complication rate from 17.6% to 10% by delaying IP catheter insertion in patients undergoing intestinal resection at the time of primary cytoreduction. Walker et al.[93] found that rectosigmoid or descending colon resection, but not other types of bowel resections or colostomy, at the time of primary surgery was associated with a higher risk of failing to start IP chemotherapy. Based on the available data, colon resection with fecal contamination or left colon resection would appear to represent relative contraindications to placement of an IP catheter at the time of primary cytoreduction.

In the past, the Tenckhoff catheter was a very popular device for administering IP chemotherapy. However, this catheter was associated with adhesion formation within the peritoneal catheter related to the development of a fibrous sheath surrounding the catheter fenestrations and intestinal obstruction due to the Dacron sheath migrating into the peritoneal cavity. Using a single-lumen silicone catheter with an implantable port designed for IV injection may be preferable, as this device appears to cause fewer such complications (Fig. 104.4*A*).[102] Catheter insertion typically involves the following steps:

1. A separate 5 to 6 cm transverse incision is made two to three fingerbreadths above the left inferior costal margin in the midclavicular line and is carried down to the fascia.
2. A subcutaneous pocket is created to house the implantable port (Fig. 104.4*B*).
3. The port is sutured to the fascia at the four corners using 2-0 polyprolene or nylon suture.
4. A tonsil clamp or similar instrument is tunneled subcutaneously above the fascia for approximately 10 cm from the port. At a point about 6 cm lateral to the umbilicus, a small aperture is made in the peritoneum.
5. The proximal end of the catheter is grasped with the clamp and brought through from the peritoneal cavity, through the subcutaneous tunnel, to the port.
6. The catheter is connected to the port, and it is trimmed to allow approximately 10 cm of catheter within the peritoneal cavity (Fig. 104.4C).
7. The catheter is flushed with heparinized saline to check patency.
8. The transverse skin incision is closed.

Intraperitoneal instillation of an agent such as cisplatin or paclitaxel is typically performed by mixing the drug in a volume of 1 L, prewarmed so as to minimize discomfort during the infusion, and allowed to infuse under gravity drip over 1 to 2 hours.[100] If the infusion rate is slow, repositioning the patient may be beneficial in an attempt to move the catheter tip away from bowel loops or a pocket caused by adhesions. However, there is no role for applying pressure to the infusion bag, and failure of the solution to infuse over a reasonable period of time may indicate the presence of adhesions that preclude further administration of the IP agent. Once the first liter of fluid has been infused IP, a second prewarmed liter of fluid, which does not contain drug, is then infused IP to further promote homogeneous drug distribution. If the patient becomes uncomfortable due to abdominal distention while receiving the second liter of IP fluid, the infusion may be discontinued. The strategy of mixing the drug with the first liter of IP fluid, followed by a second liter of IP fluid without drug, increases the chance that the patient will receive the intended dose of chemotherapy. Standard premedications for cisplatin and paclitaxel are administered, as well as aggressive attention to IV hydration before and after IP cisplatin administration to prevent nephropathy. Careful monitoring of serum potassium and magnesium levels is required in view of the potential for electrolyte wasting with IP cisplatin.

Interval Cytoreductive Surgery

Interval cytoreduction is defined as a debulking procedure performed after several cycles of chemotherapy have been administered, typically in those patients who had a suboptimal cytoreduction at the time of initial surgery. The European Organisation for Research and Treatment of Cancer (EORTC) investigated this strategy in a randomized trial involving 319 patients with suboptimally debulked stage III or IV disease (defined as greater than 1-cm diameter).[74] All patients initially received three cycles of cyclophosphamide and cisplatin, and patients with responsive or stable disease were then randomized to either interval surgery or continued chemotherapy without interval debulking surgery. After interval surgery, patients received an additional

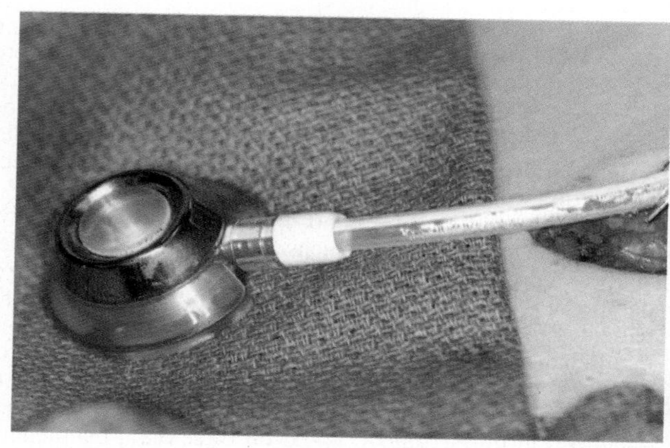
A

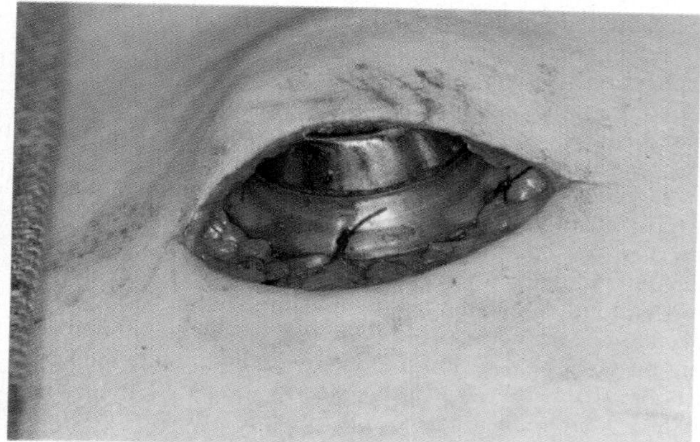
B

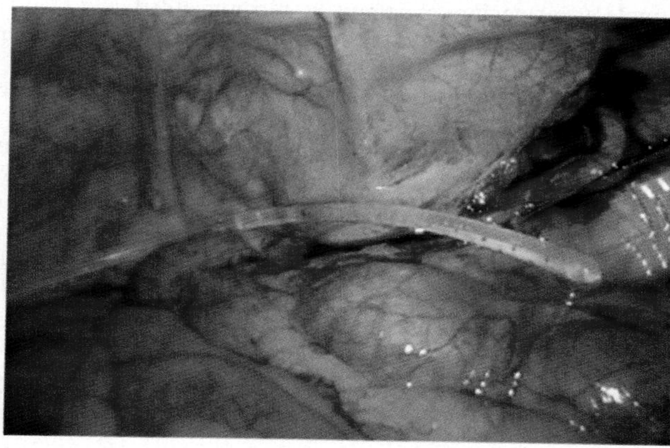
C

FIGURE 104.4 Peritoneal catheter for administration of intraperitoneal chemotherapy. **A:** Catheter port, which is placed subcutaneously in the midclavicular line under the breast. **B:** Appearance of the subcutaneous pocket containing the catheter port, prior to skin closure. **C:** Laparoscopic appearance of the catheter within the peritoneal cavity. (Courtesy of Dr. Douglas Levine, Memorial Sloan Kettering Cancer Center, New York, and Dr. Christopher Awtrey, Beth Israel Deaconess Medical Center, Boston.)

three cycles of chemotherapy, so that all patients received a total of six chemotherapy cycles, regardless of treatment arm. A total of 278 patients were eligible for randomization (140 in the interval surgery group and 138 in the control arm). Patients in the interval cytoreduction group experienced a 6-month improvement in median overall survival (*P* = .01), suggesting a role for this strategy in suboptimally debulked patients who are responding to first-line chemotherapy.

In contrast, a similar study performed by the GOG failed to show an advantage for the use of interval cytoreduction.[103] Five hundred fifty eligible patients with residual disease greater than 1 cm in diameter after initial surgery (performed by a gynecologic oncologist familiar with debulking techniques) were reassessed after three cycles of paclitaxel and cisplatin. Those with stable or responding disease were randomized to either interval cytoreduction followed by three additional cycles of chemotherapy or to three additional cycles of chemotherapy (without interval surgery). This study found no difference in either median progression-free survival (11 months) or median overall survival (32 months) between the two groups.

It is possible that the negative results of the GOG study are partly due to a more rigorous definition of suboptimally debulked disease than in the EORTC trial, related to performance of initial surgery by a gynecologic oncologist, rather than a general surgeon or gynecologist. In addition, the use of the more effective paclitaxel and cisplatin regimen in the GOG trial (compared to cyclophosphamide and cisplatin in the EORTC trial) may have negated any added value of interval cytoreduction. Thus, patients who are deemed to be suboptimally debulked after a cytoreductive effort performed by a surgeon skilled in this procedure, who then receive first-line paclitaxel- and platinum-based chemotherapy, are not likely to benefit from interval cytoreduction. For those patients who did not undergo a technically adequate attempt at initial cytoreduction (due to being a poor operative candidate or due to lack of surgical expertise), the EORTC study suggests that an attempt at interval cytoreduction is reasonable if disease control can be achieved during the first three cycles of chemotherapy.

Radiotherapy After First-Line Chemotherapy

Several randomized trials have examined whether radiation therapy administered after chemotherapy is beneficial. A trial performed in Graz, Austria, from 1985 to 1992 randomized 64 patients (54 of whom had stage III disease) who were clinically disease-free (assessed by examination, CT, and CA 125 level) after six cycles of carboplatin, epirubicin, and prednimustine to observation or WAR (30 Gy in 1.5-Gy fractions, using 12 to 18 MeV photons), followed by pelvic and para-aortic and partial diaphragm boosts (total doses to these regions, 51.6 Gy and 42.6 Gy, respectively).[104] The 5-year relapse-free survival and overall survival rates in the observation arm were 26% and 33%, respectively, compared to rates of 49% and 59% in the WAR arm. One patient in the WAR arm developed a small bowel obstruction.

A trial conducted by the GOG and North Central Cancer Treatment Group from 1987 to 1996 enrolled 202 patients with initial stage III disease in complete clinical remission following chemotherapy (almost all had received a platinum-containing agent, and 39% also received paclitaxel), who then had a second-look laparotomy that found no gross residual disease.[105] They were either observed or treated with IP chromic phosphate (15 mCi). Of note, 15% of patients assigned to the ^{32}P arm did not receive it for various reasons. With a median follow-up time of 63 months, the 5-year relapse-free survival rates in the two arms were 36% and 42%, and the 5-year overall survival rates were 63% and 67%, respectively. These differences were not statistically significant. Results were not analyzed according to whether the patient had microscopic or no pathologic evidence of disease at second-look surgery. Two of 98 patients in the control arm and 3 of 104 in the ^{32}P arm developed long-term grade 3 or 4 gastrointestinal complications.

A trial conducted in Sweden and Norway from 1988 to 1993 enrolled patients with initial stage III ovarian carcinoma who had no evidence of disease after initial surgery or who responded to induction chemotherapy (four courses of cisplatin 50 mg/m^2 with either doxorubicin or epirubicin) who then underwent second-look laparotomy.[106] Ninety-eight patients with no gross or microscopic residual disease were randomly allocated to observation, six further cycles of the same chemotherapy, or WAR (20 Gy in 1-Gy fractions using an open field technique) followed by an extended pelvic boost (from the L3-4 interspace to the pelvic floor, 20.4 Gy in 1.7-Gy fractions using opposed anterior-posterior fields). Seventy-four patients with microscopic residual disease were randomized to the same chemotherapy or WAR. The length of follow-up was not stated, but data were collected up to early 2002. The 5-year progression-free survival rates in the patients with no residual microscopic disease were 36%, 36%, and 56% in the observation, chemotherapy, and WAR arms, respectively; the difference was statistically significant. However, the 5-year overall survival rates were 65%, 57%, and 69%, respectively, and these differences were not statistically significant. In patients with microscopic residual disease, the 5-year progression-free survival rates in the chemotherapy and WAR arms were 25% and 16%; the 10-year rates were 22% and 5%, respectively. The 5-year overall survival rates were 41% for the chemotherapy arm and 32% for the WAR arm; 10-year rates were 23% and 10%, respectively. None of these differences was statistically significant. Four of 69 patients receiving WAR (6%) required bowel diversion due to bowel obstruction or adhesions, compared to no such complications occurring in the chemotherapy or observation group.

Finally, an international trial conducted from 1998 to 2003 enrolled 447 patients with a negative second-look laparotomy following initial treatment with surgery and platinum-based chemotherapy. Patients were randomly assigned to receive or not to receive a single IP injection of a radiolabeled monoclonal antibody directed against the MUC1 antigen using yttrium-90 (18 mCi, or 666 MBq/m^2).[107] Two-thirds of patients had stage III disease; 90% had no microscopic residual disease at second-look. With a median follow-up of 3.5 years, there was no difference in relapse or survival rates between the arms.

In conclusion, the value of radiation therapy as consolidation therapy following chemotherapy for patients with ovarian cancer is uncertain. The available randomized studies have conflicting results, especially in the subgroup of patients with no detectable residual disease after platinum-based chemotherapy. However, these studies were relatively small, with heterogeneous patient characteristics and treatments, and hence their statistical power to show clinically meaningful differences was limited. Further, no trials have been conducted for patients treated initially with both platinum compounds and paclitaxel. However, it seems likely that any benefits of WAR or IP ^{32}P are quite small in this setting, and these must be weighed against their potential toxicity. Hence, routine use of consolidation radiotherapy after chemotherapy is not generally recommended.

Maintenance Therapy

Several investigators have explored the value of maintenance or consolidation approaches after achievement of a clinical complete remission in patients with advanced epithelial ovarian cancer. In a randomized trial conducted by the Southwest Oncology Group and the GOG, women with advanced disease who experienced a clinically defined complete response were randomly assigned to receive either 3 cycles or 12 cycles of single-agent paclitaxel (175 mg/m^2 over 3 hours) administered every 28 days.[108] The study was stopped early when an interim analysis revealed a 50% reduction in the risk of recurrence associated with the 12-month maintenance strategy (median progression-free survival for the 12-month and 3-month paclitaxel arms was 28 months and 21 months, respectively; P = .0023). However, there was no difference in overall survival between the two regimens, which was also true in a subsequent analysis with longer follow-up. Interpretation of long-term data from this study will be confounded by crossover, whereby patients randomized to the three-cycle arm received additional maintenance paclitaxel after study closure. Likewise, a more recent randomized trial conducted in Europe showed no survival benefit to the use of six cycles of maintenance single-agent paclitaxel in this setting.[109] Based on these data, maintenance single-agent paclitaxel cannot be recommended as a standard approach in patients who achieve a complete clinical remission after a platinum-based first-line chemotherapy.

Two randomized trials have investigated the role of consolidation therapy with topotecan after the completion of first-line therapy, with neither study demonstrating a survival benefit to this approach.[110,111] There is currently great interest in studying the value of antiangiogenic agents such as bevacizumab, which is a humanized monoclonal antibody that neutralizes VEGF in the maintenance setting. Two previously mentioned trials, GOG 218 and ICON-7, are addressing this question.

Surveillance After First-Line Chemotherapy

Over 50% of newly diagnosed patients with advanced-stage epithelial ovarian cancer will achieve a clinical complete remission after platinum and taxane induction chemotherapy.[2] Clinical complete remission is defined as no evidence of disease on physical examination, a normal CA 125 level, and normal radiographic studies such as CT. Patients with advanced-stage disease who achieve a clinical complete remission have a high chance of relapse and are typically followed with serial physician visits, including pelvic examinations and CA 125 determinations. The value of routine CA 125 surveillance after completion of first-line chemotherapy has recently been challenged by the OV05 randomized trial.[18] Patients who underwent CA 125 surveillance, with early institution of cytotoxic chemotherapy for serologic relapse, did not experience improved quality of life or survival compared with those followed solely on the basis of physical examination and symptoms. Despite these negative results, it is possible that CA 125 surveillance may prove to be valuable once more effective salvage therapies become available or for those settings in which clinical trials might be available for patients with early relapse. In addition, CA 125 surveillance may still play an important role in well-informed patients who may feel empowered by knowing their CA 125 levels. Thus, the use of this test for surveillance purposes should be individualized. Routine performance of CT in the absence of symptoms, findings on physical examination, or an elevated CA 125 level has no proven value in the management of patients with this disease. This is partly due to the lack of sensitivity of CT compared to serologic testing with CA 125, which is currently the most sensitive method for detection of early relapse. Thus, CT is typically reserved for further evaluation of signs, symptoms, or serologic evidence of relapse. Likewise, there is currently no proven benefit for routine surveillance with other radiographic tests such as PET scans in the posttreatment setting.[22] Although performance of a second-look laparotomy after completion of first-line therapy will reveal residual disease in over half of all patients with advanced ovarian cancer who have achieved a complete clinical remission, this procedure does not appear to confer a survival advantage.[57] This is due to the current lack of curative treatment options for patients with disease that persists after platinum-based, first-line therapy. In addition, a negative second-look laparotomy does not guarantee against the development of disease relapse, which occurs in 50% of patients with advanced stage disease who have a negative second-look procedure.[2] For these reasons, second-look laparotomy is no longer considered a standard procedure in the assessment of patients after completion of first-line therapy, although it is sometimes used as an investigation tool in the context of clinical trials.

Management of Recurrent Disease

Hormonal Therapy

Most patients with advanced ovarian cancer will recur after first-line chemotherapy.[2] Recurrence is often manifested by a rising CA 125 in the absence of symptoms or objective evidence of disease as assessed by examination or CT (marker-only relapse). Unfortunately, the majority of patients with recurrent ovarian cancer are destined to die of their tumors, regardless of the second-line treatment modality used. Patients who demonstrate marker-only evidence of relapse, without symptoms or findings on examination or CT, are often initially managed with a drug like tamoxifen or an aromatase inhibitor. These drugs are potentially active in ovarian cancer[112,113] and are generally well tolerated. The response to hormonal agents is typically slow and may require approximately 2 to 3 months before a reduction in the CA 125 level is evident.

Chemotherapy

Chemotherapy for recurrent disease is usually indicated for the development of tumor-related symptoms, objective evidence of significant disease on examination or CT, or failure of hormonal therapy. Platinum is the most active agent in the management of patients with epithelial ovarian cancer, and retreatment with this drug may produce valuable responses that translate into improvement in quality of life. However, the likelihood of benefit depends on the interval between the last dose of platinum and the time of relapse (i.e., the platinum-free interval, PFI). Patients with a PFI of less than 6 months are less likely to respond to second-line platinum and are often managed with an alternative agent, as described below.[114] Such patients are referred to as platinum resistant, although a small percentage may still derive benefit from platinum rechallenge. Patients with a PFI of between 6 and 24 months have an approximately 30% chance of benefit from second-line platinum used at the time of relapse. In patients with a very prolonged PFI (e.g., greater than 2 years), the response rate with second-line platinum may be as high as 60% to 70%.[114] Patients with a PFI of greater than 6 months are referred to as potentially platinum sensitive and are often treated with either single-agent platinum or a combination of platinum with another agent such as paclitaxel, gemcitabine, or liposomal doxorubicin.

Three randomized trials have investigated the value of combination chemotherapy in the setting of potentially platinum-sensitive relapse (PFI greater than 6 months). The ICON-4 trial compared combination chemotherapy with paclitaxel and platinum to single-agent platinum in patients with potentially platinum-sensitive disease, with most patients having a PFI of 12 months or greater.[115] This study demonstrated a statistically significant improvement in overall survival for the combination regimen, with an absolute difference at 2 years of 7% (P = .023). However, 58% of patients in the single-agent platinum arm never received a taxane as part of first-line therapy, and 69% of patients in the single-agent platinum arm never received a taxane as part of relapse management (i.e., after progression on single-agent platinum). Thus, 40% of patients in the single-agent platinum arm never received a taxane at any point during the course of their disease. Given the proven survival benefit of taxanes in this disease, the imbalance in the use of taxanes between these two treatment arms makes the results of ICON-4 difficult to interpret.

The second trial performed by the Arbeitsgemeinschaft Gynaekologische Onkologie (AGO) from Germany randomized patients with potentially platinum-sensitive relapse to either gemcitabine and carboplatin or carboplatin alone.[116] Progression-free survival was 8.6 months for the combination versus 5.8 months for single-agent carboplatin (P = .0038), although overall survival was not improved in the combination chemotherapy arm. Quality of life appeared to be equivalent between the two arms, despite a higher incidence of thrombocytopenia, neutropenia, and anemia with combination chemotherapy.

The third trial compared paclitaxel and carboplatin with liposomal doxorubicin and carboplatin in patients with platinum-sensitive relapse.[117] There was a statistically significant improvement in median PFS (11.3 months vs. 9.4 months; P = .005), with a lower incidence of severe hypersensitivity reactions (5% vs. 18%), in favor of the liposomal doxorubicin-containing arm. No difference in overall survival was noted at the time of this report.

Since the primary goal of relapse management is palliation of symptoms, the decision to use combinations in this setting should be based on a number of factors, including patient age, amount of disease, kinetics of relapse, and patient preference after a discussion of the issues.[118] For older patients who require chemotherapy for asymptomatic, minimal volume, potentially platinum-sensitive relapse, it is still reasonable to use single-agent carboplatin as a first step. As described below, liposomal doxorubicin is a generally well-tolerated alternative if there is a contraindication to the use of carboplatin, if carboplatin fails to induce a response, or if an allergic reaction develops to carboplatin that precludes further administration. With either single-agent carboplatin or liposomal doxorubicin, patients have minimal problems with alopecia or myelosuppression, and their quality of life is generally well preserved. For younger patients who wish to adopt an aggressive approach to the management of potentially platinum-sensitive relapse, combination chemotherapy with either paclitaxel and carboplatin, gemcitabine and carboplatin, or liposomal doxorubicin and carboplatin is reasonable. This is especially the case for the symptomatic patient with kinetically brisk relapse or the patient who has undergone a successful secondary cytoreduction after a very long PFI.[118] There are currently no data supporting a role for combination chemotherapy regimens in the management of patients with platinum-resistant relapse.

Patients who are platinum resistant, as defined by a short PFI of less than 6 months or progression during platinum-based chemotherapy, or those who tolerate second-line platinum poorly are typically treated with a variety of single agents. Potentially non–cross-resistant drugs with activity in the platinum-resistant setting include liposomal doxorubicin, paclitaxel, docetaxel, topotecan, gemcitabine, pemetrexed, or oral etoposide.[119] Liposomal doxorubicin is often well tolerated in doses of 40 mg/m^2 given every 4 weeks, although the development of palmer-planar erythrodysesthesia (hand-foot syndrome) or mucositis may require dose reductions and treatment delays.[120] Topotecan may cause significant myelosuppression and fatigue, although this agent is generally well tolerated through the use of weekly dosing schedules.[121] Unfortunately, the likelihood of obtaining a response to any of these agents in the platinum-resistant setting is less than 20%, responses are generally short lived (median PFS in the range of 4 to 6 months), and they tend to become progressively shorter with each subsequent regimen.[118]

Several investigational agents are being studied in the relapsed setting. Bevacizumab is a humanized antibody that recognizes and neutralizes VEGF, an angiogenic factor that is often secreted by ovarian cancer cells. Randomized data in metastatic colorectal, breast, and lung cancers have shown a survival advantage for the use of this drug in combination with chemotherapy.[122–124] As a single agent, bevacizumab has been shown by the GOG to induce responses in 18% of patients with relapsed ovarian cancer (either platinum sensitive or platinum resistant, treated with less than or equal to two prior regimens), with 39% of patients progression-free at 6 months.[125] A recent multi-institutional nationwide study restricted to platinum-resistant patients reported a response rate of 16%, with 27% of patients progression free at 6 months.[126] However, there was an 11% incidence of potentially life-threatening bowel perforation, prompting early closure of this study. Compared to the GOG study, all patients in this trial were platinum resistant and heavily pretreated, with 50% having received three prior regimens. It has been suggested that the risk of bowel perforation with bevacizumab in the recurrent ovarian cancer setting might be related to a higher number of prior treatment regimens, radiographic evidence of bowel wall involvement by tumor, or the presence of bowel obstruction.[126] These and other possible risk factors for this complication will require further evaluation.

Other investigational agents with reported activity in platinum-sensitive (and, to a lesser degree, platinum-resistant) disease include ET743 (trabectedin), halichondrin B, pertuzumab, and epothilones.[127] Receptor tyrosine kinase inhibitors that target the VEGF receptor such as AZD2171 (cediranib) appear to have activity and are being studied in combination with platinum-based chemotherapy.[128] In contrast, epidermal growth factor–receptor inhibitors such as gefitinib appear to have low activity in the recurrent disease setting. An exciting new class of agents that inhibit poly-adenosine diphosphate[ADP]-ribose polymerase (PARP) is demonstrating important activity in patients with recurrent disease, especially those who harbor a germline mutation in *BRCA1* or *BRCA2*.[129] At present, none of these agents is currently approved by the U.S. Food and Drug Administration for treating patients with relapsed ovarian cancer, and their ultimate value needs to be better defined.

Surgery

Secondary cytoreductive surgery refers to an attempt at surgical debulking of disease at the time of relapse and is performed in selected patients prior to the administration of second-line chemotherapy. The ability to perform a successful secondary cytoreduction, as generally defined by having no gross residual disease greater than 1 cm in diameter, is associated with a median survival advantage in retrospective studies.[130] However, it is possible that the *ability* to perform a successful secondary cytoreduction may simply identify those patients with biologically less aggressive disease or those with a lower tumor burden at the time of relapse. The only way to determine whether secondary cytoreduction has intrinsic therapeutic value is to conduct a randomized trial of this procedure, which has not yet been performed.

Patients who relapse within 6 to 12 months after completion of first-line therapy, especially if they have ascites, are generally not candidates for this procedure.[130] Occasional patients with late relapses (i.e., greater than 2 to 3 years after finishing chemotherapy) or those with apparently isolated relapses may experience a prolonged disease-free interval after successful secondary cytoreduction followed by additional chemotherapy. The value of secondary cytoreduction is currently being investigated in two prospective, randomized trials, GOG 213 and the AGO Desktop III study.

Palliative surgery may be of benefit for patients with recurrent ovarian cancer. Common operations performed in this setting include colostomy for relief of a large bowel obstruction, lysis of adhesions, and management of small bowel obstruction. The decision to perform surgery to relieve small bowel obstruction should take into account the time elapsed from the original diagnosis to the development of obstruction, as well as the likelihood for continued responsiveness to chemotherapy postoperatively. Women who develop small bowel obstruction during first-line chemotherapy have biologically aggressive tumors that are usually not amenable to surgical intervention. A palliative gastrostomy tube may be most appropriate in this situation, and frequently this can be inserted endoscopically or under CT guidance. In contrast, women who have had prolonged periods of freedom from disease, usually lasting more than 1 year from the original diagnosis, may benefit from small bowel surgery to relieve obstruction. Surgery generally plays no role in management of patients with a pseudo-obstructive pattern due to intra-abdominal carcinomatosis, with infiltration of the myoenteric plexus of the small bowel. Metoclopramide, which improves motility of the upper gastrointestinal tract without stimulating gastric, biliary, or pancreatic secretions, may at times be helpful for this condition. Large bowel obstruction (particularly sigmoid colon obstruction) is often relieved by performing a colostomy, which can provide significant prolongation of survival and improved quality of life in appropriate patients.

Radiation Therapy

A minority of patients with localized recurrences may experience prolonged survival after WAR or limited-field irradiation.[131,132] For example, a study from the Medical College of Wisconsin in Milwaukee included 16 patients treated with various combinations of surgery, chemotherapy, external-beam pelvic irradiation, and intravaginal brachytherapy for recurrent or persistent ovarian carcinoma involving the vagina or rectum without extrapelvic disease.[131] Their survival rate at 1 year after recurrence was 81% and at 2 years 56%. Four patients were alive without disease at the time of last follow-up (one of whom received WAR). In a series from Loyola University Medical Center in Chicago, 20 patients received irradiation for localized extraperitoneal recurrences.[132] With a median follow-up after radiation therapy of 29 months, the 3-year rate of freedom from recurrence within the radiation field was 89% for patients who underwent gross total excision of their recurrence, compared to 42% for nine patients with unresectable or gross residual disease. The respective 3-year disease-free survival rates in these two groups were 72% and 22%; overall survival rates were 50% and 19%, respectively. However, the small number of highly selected patients in these series and the use of multiple concurrent treatment modalities make it difficult to adequately assess whether radiation therapy truly improves long-term outcome in this setting.

Although rarely curative, radiation therapy can play a role in the palliation of some patients with recurrent ovarian cancer. Symptoms from a growing pelvic mass can cause pain, bleeding, and rectal narrowing. Palliative pelvic radiotherapy can provide rapid relief and, in some cases, may prevent or delay the need for diverting colostomy. Doses of 8 to 10 Gy in a single fraction, 20 Gy in five fractions, 30 Gy in ten fractions, or higher total doses given in smaller fractions have produced acceptable short-term results, with serious complications in 5% or fewer patients. Finally, patients with epithelial ovarian cancer may rarely develop isolated cerebral or bone metastases that can sometimes be successfully palliated with radiotherapy.

BORDERLINE TUMORS

Definition and Clinical Features

Ovarian borderline tumors are epithelial neoplasms that are histologically distinguished from ovarian carcinomas by the absence of stromal invasion. These neoplasms are also referred to as tumors of low malignant potential (LMP), which reflects their indolent natural history.[133] Although borderline tumors generally do not exhibit stromal invasion within the ovary, cells from the primary tumor mass can be shed into the peritoneal cavity and eventually form serosal implants that involve the bowel, omentum, and upper abdomen. Nonetheless, the majority of patients with borderline tumors present with early stage disease.[11]

The median age of women developing borderline tumors is 40 years, approximately 20 years younger than the median age for women with epithelial ovarian cancer. Women may be diagnosed with an asymptomatic mass on routine pelvic examination or may come to medical attention due to pelvic pain. Nonspecific gastrointestinal symptoms such as abdominal bloating or early satiety may rarely occur.

As with epithelial cancers of the ovary, borderline tumors may exhibit serous or mucinous features. Serous borderline tumors are more common and may be bilateral in 10% to 20% of cases.[133] Mucinous borderline tumors tend to be larger than their serous counterparts, are infrequently bilateral, and are occasionally associated with pseudomyxoma peritonei. Pseudomyxoma peritonei is characterized by a hypocellular, gelatinous material secreted by an intra-abdominal tumor, eventually filling the peritoneal cavity and encasing abdominal contents such as bowel. This condition may be associated with mucinous borderline ovarian tumor, mucinous ovarian carcinoma, or gastrointestinal tumors such as appendiceal mucinous cystadenocarcinoma. The latter diagnosis may occur synchronously with a primary ovarian mucinous neoplasm or may mimic a primary ovarian tumor by metastasizing to the ovary (often right sided, reflecting the proximity of the appendix to the right ovary). The mainstay of treatment for pseudomyxoma peritonei is intermittent surgery to remove the gelatinous material, although this is not curative in the majority of cases, and repeated debulking attempts are associated with increased potential for adhesions and complications such as bowel obstruction.

The distinctive pathologic and biologic behaviors of these tumors were recognized by the WHO in 1973 (Table 104.1).[4] Borderline malignant potential tumors are distinguished from benign cystadenomas by the presence of epithelial budding, multilayering of the epithelium, increased mitotic activity, and nuclear atypia. They are distinguished from epithelial carcinomas by the absence of stromal invasion. In the spectrum of aggressiveness between epithelial ovarian carcinoma and benign ovarian tumors such as cystadenoma, borderline tumors are closer to benign ovarian tumors in their clinical behavior. However, they are accorded their own classification based on distinctive histologic features, their potential to occasionally spread beyond the ovary, and their ability to recur and lead to death in a minority of patients.

Since the absence of stromal invasion is a criterion for making this diagnosis, careful examination of the tissue blocks is necessary to exclude a component of invasive carcinoma. In this regard, approximately 20% of ovarian tumors diagnosed as borderline on frozen-section analysis prove to be carcinomas on review of the permanent section. The presence of microinvasion (as opposed to deep stromal invasion) is sometimes observed in a borderline tumor, in association with more typical histologic features. In such cases, the microinvasive component is typically no greater than 3 mm in depth, in which case it most likely does not impact on prognosis.[134] Mucinous borderline tumors are characterized by multiloculated cystic masses, with smooth outer surfaces and areas of papulations and solid thickening on the inner surface. Microscopically, the epithelial lining of cysts within a mucinous borderline tumor consists of tall, columnar, mucin-secreting cells, resembling the epithelium of the endocervix or intestine. Although mucinous borderline tumors lack stromal invasion, they are sometimes difficult to distinguish from their invasive mucinous carcinoma counterparts. Most mucinous borderline tumors have less than four layers of stratified mucinous cells and lack invasion, whereas mucinous carcinomas often demonstrate an infiltrative or expansile pattern of stromal involvement.[135]

Greater than 90% of patients with early stage borderline tumors are alive at 10 years, and more than 50% of patients with advanced disease experience long-term survival.[11] The fact that survival does not appear to be improved by postoperative adjuvant treatment with either chemotherapy or radiation attests to the slow growth rate of this tumor, which confers indolent behavior but at the same time results in resistance to modalities that target actively dividing cells. Nevertheless, a small fraction of patients with borderline tumors exhibits a more aggressive course, and attempts have been made to identify histologic correlates that might predict for worse outcome. Some investigators have proposed that borderline serous tumors may behave more aggressively if they are associated with micropapillary features or invasive implants elsewhere in the peritoneal cavity.[12,136,137] Micropapillary serous carcinoma is characterized by thin, elongated micropapillae with minimal or no fibrovascular support. Patients with invasive implants in the setting of a primary borderline tumor typically have a desmoplastic reaction within the implant, associated with an irregular, infiltrative border that invades underlying structures and replaces the fatty tissue of the underlying omentum.[137] An implant that simply shows desmoplasia, without these other features, should be referred to as a desmoplastic *noninvasive* implant and does not appear to predict a worse outcome, in contrast to its invasive counterpart. Patients with serous borderline tumors without invasive implants have expected 10-year survival rates of greater than 95%, whereas those with serous borderline tumors and invasive implants have survival rates of approximately 60% to 70% at 10 years.[138] Of interest, the majority of patients with invasive implants, or those with recurrences that progressed to invasive carcinoma, have been found to have micropapillary features within the primary ovarian tumor on careful sectioning. Thus, it is possible that micropapillary features portend a poorer prognosis because of their association with invasive implants, although this is still an area of controversy.

Surgical Management

Surgery for patients with borderline tumors who have completed childbearing is identical to that recommended for epithelial ovarian cancer, including a total abdominal hysterectomy, bilateral salpingo-oophorectomy, tumor debulking, and full staging. Although unusual, patients with borderline tumors may sometimes have retroperitoneal nodal involvement that can benefit from debulking. In such cases, the tumor typically involves the sinusoidal nodal spaces, as opposed to nodal parenchyma. An appendectomy is considered in patients with suspected mucinous borderline tumors because of its occasional association with a primary appendiceal carcinoma.

In younger patients with early stage borderline tumor who wish to preserve fertility, conservative surgery with preservation of the uterus, the contralateral ovary and fallopian tube, and in some cases the ipsilateral ovary (i.e., cystectomy) may be appropriate treatment. Several studies have reported excellent outcomes with conservative management of such patients. One of the largest studies found a 12% recurrence rate for patients treated conservatively with either unilateral salpingo-oophorectomy (n = 110) or ovarian cystectomy (n = 74), compared to 2.5% for patients treated with hysterectomy and bilateral salpingo-oophorectomy.[139] Recurrences or progression to carcinoma (1.5%) were more common among patients with invasive implants or advanced-stage disease.

Borderline ovarian tumors have also been diagnosed during pregnancy. Conservative surgery is usually performed, and pregnancy does not appear to affect the prognosis. Most patients go on to deliver at full term without any complications.

Postoperative Management

There is currently no convincing evidence that postoperative adjuvant chemotherapy or radiation confers a survival advantage for patients with borderline tumors of any stage.[11] In the absence of effective postoperative adjuvant therapy, in a disease where long-term survival is generally excellent, simple observation with serial examinations is reasonable, with radiographic studies as needed to investigate new symptoms or findings on examination. Late relapses may occur and reveal persistent borderline histology, although transformation to low-grade invasive serous cancer is a more common occurrence in this setting.[140] Surgery is the mainstay of treating recurrent disease and can lead to long-term survival. Some patients who recur with borderline histology may respond to a hormonal option such as tamoxifen.[141] However, for patients with borderline tumors who recur with low-grade invasive serous cancer, surgical debulking followed by platinum-based chemotherapy is often recommended.

GERM CELL TUMORS OF THE OVARY

Definition and Clinical Features

Germ cell tumors of the ovary are much less common than epithelial ovarian neoplasms, accounting for 2% to 3% of all ovarian cancers in Western countries and usually occurring in younger women, with a peak incidence in women in their early 20s. An increased incidence of germ cell tumors is found in Asian and black societies, where these tumors may represent as many as 15% of all ovarian cancers. It is often possible to cure these malignancies while preserving fertility, which is an especially important consideration given the young age of most patients.

The WHO classification for germ cell tumors of the ovary is shown in Table 104.1.[4] These tumors are often divided into dysgerminoma, which is the female counterpart of male seminoma, and nondysgerminoma. Abdominal pain, distention, pelvic fullness, and urinary symptoms are common in patients with germ cell tumors of the ovary. In a minority of patients, abdominal pain can be severe, usually the result of hemorrhage, rupture, or ovarian torsion.

The rapid growth of most ovarian germ cell tumors causes pain due to stretching of the ovarian capsule, often prompting the patient to seek medical attention while the tumor is still confined to the ovary. Patients frequently have a palpable adnexal mass that is typically evaluated by transvaginal ultrasound, which may show a complex cyst comprised of solid and cystic regions. Serum levels of α-fetoprotein (AFP) and β–human chorionic gonadotropin (HCG) are often helpful in recognizing the presence of an endodermal sinus tumor (AFP elevation only), embryonal carcinoma (both AFP and HCG elevation), or choriocarcinoma (HCG elevation only). Patients with pure immature teratoma of the ovary typically have normal levels of AFP and HCG, although the AFP may be elevated in 30% of cases. Patients with mature cystic teratoma (dermoid cyst), which is a benign germ cell tumor, usually have normal levels of AFP and HCG. Measurement of AFP and HCG levels is also useful to gauge the effectiveness of postoperative therapy and in monitoring for disease recurrence.

Occasional patients with choriocarcinoma have extreme elevation of the β-HCG that results in hyperthyroidism due to homology between β-HCG and thyroid-stimulating hormone (TSH). Patients with mature cystic teratoma may also present with hyperthyroidism related to tumor-derived secretion of thyroxine, produced by mature thyroid tissue present within the tumor itself (struma ovarii). Rare patients with mature cystic teratoma will experience a Coomb's positive hemolytic anemia that resolves after surgical resection of the mass.

In contrast to epithelial tumors, 60% to 70% of germ cell tumors are stage I at diagnosis. Stages II and IV tumors are relatively uncommon, and stage III disease accounts for about 25% to 30% of tumors. Bilateral ovarian involvement in most germ cell histologies is uncommon, although dysgerminoma and mature cystic teratoma may be bilateral in 10% to 15% of cases. More advanced disease may involve retroperitoneal lymph nodes and multiple peritoneal surfaces, although ascites is infrequent. Hematogenous spread to the liver, lung, and brain can be observed, especially with choriocarcinoma.

Surgical Management

The principles for surgical management of germ cell tumors are similar to those described for epithelial tumors, with the important caveat that in most patients with germ cell cancer, fertility can be preserved by sparing the contralateral ovary and fallopian tube and the uterus. Even in dysgerminoma, in which bilaterality is more common, bilateral oophorectomy is not routinely necessary because postoperative chemotherapy is often capable of eradicating disease that could not be entirely removed at the time of initial surgery. In cases in which the contralateral ovary is grossly abnormal, cystectomy or biopsy can be performed, and bilateral salpingo-oophorectomy can be undertaken in the case of a dysgenetic gonad.

Once the peritoneal cavity is opened, peritoneal washings are obtained, and all fluids are sent for histological examination. If disease is grossly confined to the pelvis, random biopsies are often performed as in the surgical staging of early stage epithelial ovarian carcinomas. Particular attention is paid to para-aortic and pelvic lymph node enlargement, because these sites are frequently involved in patients with advanced ovarian germ cell tumors. Although lymph node sampling is often performed for staging, no evidence suggests that lymphadenectomy is beneficial. Cytoreductive surgery is recommended as for epithelial tumors of the ovary.

There is no role for routine second-look operations in patients with germ cell tumors who are clinically free of disease after chemotherapy. In particular, if the primary tumor is completely resected and does not contain teratomatous elements, second-look procedures after chemotherapy are of no established benefit. In some patients whose tumor contains teratomatous elements, however, a second-look procedure may be beneficial. Such patients may have residual mature teratoma, which is chemotherapy insensitive, making it reasonable to consider a second-look procedure in selected cases for resection of such residual disease if technically possible. The rationale for this is derived from the experience with testicular germ cell cancer, in which residual teratoma has been known to enlarge and cause local complications or rarely transform to an undifferentiated sarcoma or carcinoma. However, the extent to which residual teratoma may transform to a more aggressive histology in patients with ovarian germ cell tumors has not been well studied.

Postoperative Management of Dysgerminoma

Dysgerminoma is the most common malignant germ cell tumor of the ovary. In contrast to nondysgerminomatous tumors (which contain embryonal, yolk sac, or choriocarcinoma elements), dysgerminomas are more frequently stage I, may involve both ovaries, more often spread to retroperitoneal lymph nodes, and are markedly sensitive to radiotherapy. Because these tumors are also exquisitely sensitive to cisplatin-based chemotherapy, the role of curative radiation therapy has significantly decreased, especially in view of its propensity to cause sterility.

The majority of patients with dysgerminomas are diagnosed with early stage disease. Because preservation of fertility is an important issue for most patients, those with stage IA disease can be observed without further postoperative treatment. Approximately 15% to 25% of such patients will experience recurrence, although salvage chemotherapy is almost always successful.[142] Dysgerminoma in patients with higher than stage IA disease is typically treated with platinum-based chemotherapy. In the early 1980s, ovarian germ cell tumors were treated with the cisplatin-vinblastine-bleomycin (PVB) regimen, similar to the regimens used in the treatment of testicular cancer. The M. D. Anderson Cancer Center group began to use the bleomycin, etoposide, and cisplatin (BEP) combination for patients with metastatic dysgerminoma in 1984 and subsequently reported their findings, with all 14 BEP-treated patients disease free at a median follow-up of 22.4 months.[143] The GOG also reported their experience of 20 patients with incompletely resected dysgerminoma who received either PVB or BEP followed by the combination of vincristine, dactinomycin, and cyclophosphamide.[142] With a median follow-up of 26 months, 19 of the 20 patients were disease free.

In an update of the M. D. Anderson series, Brewer et al.[144] reported 26 patients with ovarian dysgerminoma who received BEP chemotherapy, with all patients being disease free at the time of the report. Of the 14 evaluable patients who underwent fertility-sparing surgery, 93% had normal menstrual function, with five pregnancies reported. In an attempt to identify a less-toxic regimen, the GOG conducted a clinical trial in which 39 eligible patients with completely resected, stages IB through III ovarian dysgerminoma received the combination of etoposide and carboplatin; all 39 patients were in sustained remission (median follow-up 7.8 years), with myelosuppression being the most severe toxicity.[145] Nonetheless, BEP is still considered the preferred regimen for use in this setting, with the etoposide and carboplatin combination being reserved for those patients with completely resected, stages IB through III dysgerminoma who have a contraindication to BEP (such as significant neuropathy or renal dysfunction).

Postoperative Management of Nondysgerminoma

Nondysgerminomas include tumors that contain embryonal, yolk sac, choriocarcinoma, and immature teratoma elements. The vast majority of these histologic subtypes require treatment with surgery followed by combination chemotherapy, as even patients with early stage nondysgerminomas have a significant risk of relapse that can be reduced by postoperative adjuvant therapy. The current regimen of choice is BEP. The GOG reported that 89 of 93 patients with stages I, II, and III disease whose tumors were completely resected remained disease free after three courses of this regimen.[146] Toxicities of BEP include the risk of bleomycin-induced pulmonary damage, etoposide-induced leukemia, and platinum-induced neuropathy and nephropathy. Many patients who receive the BEP regimen will regain fertility after completion of treatment. Several series have reported that at least 80% of patients with germ cell tumors of the ovary who were treated with fertility-sparing surgery and postoperative chemotherapy regained normal menstrual function, and there are several documented normal pregnancies.[147] However, patients are known to be at increased risk for development of premature menopause following chemotherapy.[148]

Although most patients with nondysgerminomatous germ cell cancer will require postoperative chemotherapy, a subset of patients with pure immature teratoma of the ovary has an excellent prognosis after surgery alone. Specifically, patients with stage IA, grade 1 immature teratoma experience 5-year survivals higher than 90%, and there is no evidence to suggest that chemotherapy improves outcome. Patients with stage IA, grades 2 and 3 immature teratoma have a higher relapse rate, which generally warrants consideration of postoperative chemotherapy.

Several investigators have examined the feasibility of surgery followed by close surveillance in a much broader group of patients. Dark et al.[149] reported 24 patients with stage IA germ cell tumors of the ovary who underwent postoperative surveillance. Fifteen of these had nondysgerminomas, with nine immature teratomas and six yolk sac tumors. Three of these 15 (20%) patients relapsed. The two patients with yolk sac tumor each relapsed at 4 months, and both were salvaged with combination chemotherapy. The third patient became pregnant; she presented with ascites and hepatic metastases during the third trimester, 13 months after diagnosis, and died of a pulmonary embolus 4 weeks after starting chemotherapy.

Cushing et al.[150] reported 44 patients with completely resected ovarian immature teratoma, grades 1 through 3 (31 pure and 13 with yolk sac tumor elements). Ten of 12 patients had elevated levels of serum AFP. The 4-year event-free and overall survival rates for the two groups was 97.7% and 100%, respectively. One patient with a mixed tumor relapsed 18 weeks after primary surgery with a rising AFP level; she was treated with four cycles of BEP and was disease free 57 months after completing chemotherapy. Two other studies reported a total of 39 patients with stage I disease who were treated with surgery alone.[151,152] The overall survival for the combined studies was 97.4%; 13 patients relapsed, and 12 were salvaged with chemotherapy.

The Children's Oncology Group (COG) is currently studying the approach of surgery followed by surveillance in patients with stage I germ cell tumors of the ovary. Although this strategy appears to be potentially promising, further study, particularly in adult patients, is warranted to ensure its safety and efficacy.

SEX CORD–STROMAL TUMORS

Definition and Clinical Features

Ovarian sex cord–stromal tumors represent approximately 5% of all ovarian cancers.[52] Patients often present with stage I disease, which has an excellent prognosis. However, the potential for late relapse, sometimes occurring more than 10 years after diagnosis, mandates long-term follow-up. Granulosa cell tumors are the most common type of sex cord–stromal malignancy. Such tumors typically present as a solid mass with

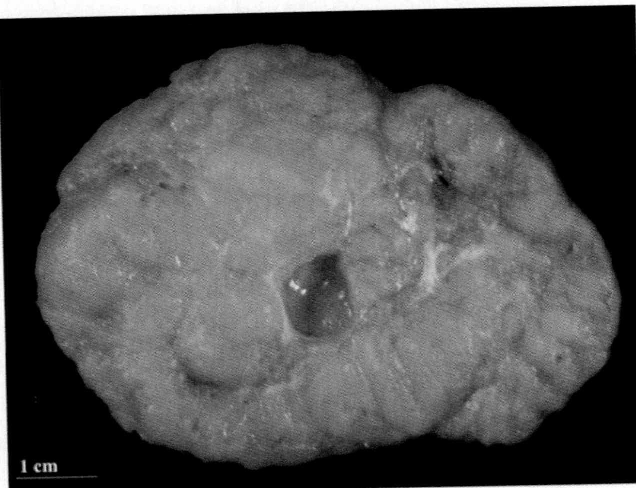

FIGURE 104.5 Cross-section of a granulosa cell tumor, showing the tan-yellow appearance characteristic of steroid production. (Courtesy of Dr. Marisa Nucci, Brigham and Women's Hospital, Boston.)

occasional cystic features, which is often yellow on cross-section due to the presence of cholesterol (Fig. 104.5). In addition, the cells of granulosa cell tumors are characterized by a longitudinal cleft that resembles a coffee bean (Fig. 104.6), and they may be organized into fluid-filled spherical structures known as Call-Exner bodies. These tumors may produce estrogenic or, less commonly, androgenic steroids. The estradiol in such cases is due to production of androstenedione by normal theca cells within the ovarian stroma, which is then converted to estradiol under the influence of aromatase present in the granulosa cell tumor.[52] In addition to estradiol, sex cord–stromal tumors such as granulosa cell tumors may secrete other factors such as inhibin and mullerian inhibitory substance, which can sometimes be useful as tumor markers during the surveillance phase of management.[52,153]

The hormonal manifestations of sex cord–stromal neoplasms such as granulosa cell tumors vary depending on the age of the patient. Thus, granulosa cell tumors occurring in premenarchal girls may present with precocious puberty, whereas women in the reproductive years may present with amenorrhea or abnormal menses or may occasionally develop intra-abdominal hemorrhage that mimics an ectopic pregnancy. Postmenopausal women with granulosa cell tumor may present with postmenopausal bleeding due to endometrial hyperplasia (or a separate uterine carcinoma), resulting from tumor-derived estrogen. Sertoli-Leydig cell tumors may present with symptoms of virilization, but none of these hormonal effects is a reliable diagnostic criterion, and many patients with sex cord–stromal tumors have no hormonal manifestations of their disease. The tumor may present as a mass discovered on routine pelvic examination or during the evaluation of pelvic pain due to ovarian torsion.

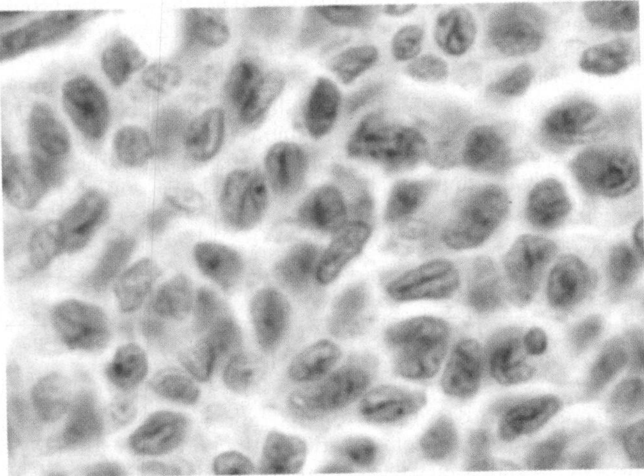

FIGURE 104.6 Photomicrograph of a hematoxylin and eosin-stained section of granulosa cell tumor, showing characteristic nuclear grooves (coffee bean nuclei). (Courtesy of Dr. Jonathan Hecht, Beth Israel Deaconess Medical Center, Boston.)

Surgical Management

Surgical staging of sex cord–stromal tumors is the same as that for epithelial ovarian cancer. Surgical management of sex cord–stromal tumors is based on the stage of the tumor as well as the age of the patient. Since the tumor is rarely bilateral, premenarchal women or patients presenting in the reproductive years with stage I disease are often managed with unilateral salpingo-oophorectomy in an attempt to preserve fertility. In women who have completed childbearing, initial surgery for sex cord–stromal tumors typically consists of bilateral salpingo-oophorectomy and total abdominal hysterectomy, along with standard surgical staging.

Postoperative Management

Stage is the most important prognostic factor, with 10-year survivals of over 85% for stage I tumors, decreasing to 50% to 65% for stage II disease, and to 17% to 33% for stages III and IV.[52] Based on these considerations, patients with stages II to IV sex cord–stromal tumors are reasonable candidates for additional therapy after initial surgery, although the survival benefit of such therapy has not been proven due to the rarity of this tumor and resultant lack of randomized trials. Approximately 30% to 50% of patients will respond to platinum-based chemotherapy, and some patients may be rendered into a clinical and pathologic complete response at the time of second-look laparotomy (usually performed in the context of a clinical trial).[52,154] The most commonly studied platinum combinations are cyclophosphamide, doxorubicin, and cisplatin (CAP), PVB, and BEP. The single-agent activity of drugs such as bleomycin or etoposide has not been well established in this disease, and combinations such as PVB or BEP have been used by analogy with germ cell cancer (which derives from a completely different cell lineage). Although randomized comparisons are lacking, the highest response rates and the best tolerance among these three regimens has been observed with BEP, which is often used for sex cord–stromal tumors that require chemotherapy.[154] However, the BEP regimen is still associated with the potential for serious toxicity, including bleomycin-induced lung damage, etoposide-induced leukemia, renal dysfunction, hypertension, and Raynaud's phenomenon. Furthermore, the added benefit of BEP when compared to EP (without bleomycin) or even single-agent platinum has not been formally demonstrated. Thus, there may be circumstances in which the clinician may choose other platinum-based regimens in this disease, as opposed to BEP, especially in the older patient who cannot tolerate bleomycin due to underlying pulmonary disease, or in the young patient who is not willing to accept the small chance of etoposide-induced leukemia. In this regard, it has been shown that combined paclitaxel and carboplatin has significant activity in patients with sex cord–stromal tumors, with generally improved tolerance compared to BEP.[155] Whether paclitaxel and carboplatin will eventually become the preferred regimen for this disease will require additional study, although it is a consideration in patients who wish to avoid the toxicity of BEP or those who cannot tolerate BEP due to side effects. A randomized trial comparing paclitaxel and carboplatin with BEP in patients with newly diagnosed, advanced stage sex cord–stromal tumors of the ovary is currently under way (GOG 264).

Selected patients with stage I disease may be at higher risk of relapse due to the presence of features such as large tumor size (greater than 10 to 15 cm in diameter) and high mitotic count (greater than 4 to 10 mitoses per 10 high-power fields).[52] Based on the retrospective nature and small size of most series, it is difficult to know whether the prognostic value of tumor size and mitotic rate is independent of stage. The prognostic value of rupture, surface involvement, or age is even less certain. Nonetheless, it is reasonable to consider some form of adjuvant, platinum-based therapy for selected patients with stage I disease who have high-risk features, although the data to support a survival benefit to this approach are lacking at the present time. In such cases, the uncertain benefits of treatment must be weighed against the potential for side effects.

Sex cord–stromal tumors may recur several years after the original diagnosis. Relapses may be associated with abdominal or pelvic discomfort, a mass on pelvic examination, or an asymptomatic rise in serum tumor markers such as estradiol or inhibin. Such recurrences are often limited to the abdomen or pelvis, although may occasionally present with hematogenous spread to the liver, lung, or bone. Locoregional recurrences are treated with surgical resection followed by postoperative therapy such as platinum-based treatment or radiotherapy. In cases in which the recurrence is isolated and can be encompassed in a radiation field, older literature suggests that radiation therapy may be of value for granulosa cell histology. Eventually, patients become resistant to platinum-based chemotherapy, in which case single-agent paclitaxel, or the use of progestational agents or leuprolide, may be considered.[52]

PRIMARY PERITONEAL SEROUS CARCINOMA

PPSC is histologically identical to serous carcinoma of ovarian origin, but typically presents with diffuse peritoneal implants in the absence of a dominant ovarian mass. This entity is thought to represent malignant transformation of peritoneal surface epithelium, which, like ovarian surface epithelium, is derived from coelomic mesoderm.[2] Another possibility is that PPSC represents secondary seeding of the peritoneal cavity from an occult primary lesion residing in the fallopian tube fimbria.[5] Initial reports of PPSC involved patients who underwent a prophylactic oophorectomy for a family history of ovarian cancer, but who later developed diffuse intra-abdominal carcinomatosis that resembled ovarian cancer.[156] In other patients with intact ovaries, diffuse carcinomatosis developed that histologically resembled papillary serous ovarian cancer, but without a dominant ovarian mass. In such cases, it is not unusual to observe small tumor implants involving the ovarian surface, although these are the result of generalized peritoneal seeding from a primary tumor mass in the omentum or deep within the pelvis. These two types of clinical presentations eventually led to the recognition that PPSC is a distinct clinical entity that resembles ovarian cancer histologically, clinically, and in its response to treatment.

Some investigators using molecular markers of clonality have proposed that PPSC is more likely to develop in a multifocal fashion, as opposed to most cases of ovarian cancer, which are clonal in origin.[157] Cases of PPSC that are multifocal may reflect a field defect within the peritoneal mesothelial lining. PPSC occurs at a higher incidence in patients with germline mutations in *BRCA1* and *BRCA2*.[33]

The differential diagnosis for PPSC is similar to that of epithelial ovarian carcinoma. On occasion, poorly differentiated PPSC may be difficult to distinguish from other entities such as metastatic breast cancer to the abdominal cavity. In such cases, expression of GCDFP may be helpful, since this marker is highly specific for breast and salivary gland tumors and is usually negative for mullerian origin tumors such as PPSC or ovarian primaries. The utility of GCDFP as a marker for breast cancer is limited by rather low sensitivity, being positive in only about 50% of cases. Other entities that may rarely be confused with PPSC include peritoneal mesothelioma, gastric or pancreatic cancers, and hepatobiliary tumors.

Patients with PPSC present in a similar fashion to those with epithelial ovarian cancer, although they may not have an adnexal mass on ultrasound or pelvic examination. The abdominal examination may reveal ascites and an omental mass. The stool does not contain blood, and the hematocrit usually does not suggest an iron deficiency anemia (features that would be more suggestive of a gastrointestinal primary site).

In appropriate surgical candidates, an exploratory laparotomy is usually necessary to establish the histologic diagnosis and to perform tumor cytoreduction. Given the more diffuse nature of this entity, almost all patients with PPSC present with stage III or IV disease. The principles of treatment are the same as those for epithelial ovarian cancer. Primary surgical cytoreduction should be performed, followed by combination chemotherapy with paclitaxel and carboplatin. The prognosis of patients with PPSC is likely to be the same, when corrected for stage and debulking status, as for epithelial ovarian cancer.

Since PPSC may sometimes be associated with germline mutations in *BRCA1* and *BRCA2*, a careful family history is important in patients with this entity. In addition, individuals with germline *BRCA1* or *BRCA2* mutations who have undergone prophylactic bilateral salpingo-oophorectomy should be informed that there is a risk for developing PPSC, sometimes many years after the prophylactic procedure has been performed. In a series reported by Piver et al.,[158] 6 of 324 women developed PPSC from 1 to 27 years after prophylactic surgery. There is currently no effective screening procedure that enables early detection of PPSC in this clinical setting.

FALLOPIAN TUBE CANCER

Fallopian tube cancer is a rare disease, with only a few hundred new cases diagnosed annually in the United States.[1] Most tubal carcinomas represent papillary serous adenocarcinoma arising within the lumen of the tube, although other mullerian histologies such as endometrioid tumors may occur. A minority of fallopian tube carcinomas are bilateral at the time of diagnosis. In contrast to patients with ovarian cancer, the majority of patients with tubal carcinoma are diagnosed with disease confined to the tubes and pelvic structures. However, fallopian tube cancer appears to have a higher propensity for retroperitoneal lymph node spread compared to epithelial ovarian cancer. Advanced stage disease may occur with a pattern of intraperitoneal dissemination similar to that observed for epithelial ovarian cancer.

Postmenopausal vaginal bleeding may bring patients with fallopian tube cancer to medical attention. Hydrops tubae profluens, characterized by colicky lower abdominal pain relieved by profuse serous yellow intermittent vaginal discharge, occurs in a minority of cases, but intermittent abdominal pain and leucorrhea are common presentations. Tubal distention produces more intense pain than is usually reported by patients with ovarian cancer. Occasionally, a Papanicolaou (Pap) smear revealing abnormal glandular cells with negative cervical or endometrial findings may lead to the diagnosis of fallopian tube carcinoma. As for ovarian cancer and PPSC, fallopian tube cancer occurs at higher frequency in patients with germline mutations of *BRCA1* and *BRCA2*, thus requiring a careful family history in affected individuals.[46]

Differentiation of a primary fallopian tube cancer from metastatic ovarian carcinoma can sometimes be difficult. Apart from a dominant mass arising within the fallopian tube lumen, the main criterion used to establish the diagnosis of a primary fallopian tube carcinoma is histologic evidence of a transition between *in situ* carcinoma and invasive malignancy within the fallopian tube epithelium. In cases where it is impossible to determine whether the tumor began in the fallopian tube and spread to the ovary, or began in the ovary and spread to the lumen of the fallopian tube, the tumors are referred to as *tubo-ovarian carcinoma*.

Survival is partly dependent on the depth of invasion of the primary lesion.[150] For intramucosal lesions, the 5-year survival is 91%, compared with 53% for tumors that invade the muscular wall, and less than 25% for tumors that have penetrated the tubal serosa. Histologic differentiation and lymphatic capillary space involvement may also have prognostic significance.[159]

The surgical management and staging system of fallopian tube carcinoma is identical to that of patients with epithelial ovarian cancer. Patients rendered into a minimal residual disease state after cytoreductive surgery appear to have an improved prognosis. Postoperatively, it is reasonable to use combination chemotherapy with paclitaxel and carboplatin in patients with fallopian tube carcinoma that has spread beyond the tube. In addition, patients with disease limited to the tubal lumen may also be reasonable candidates for postoperative adjuvant treatment, based on features such as muscle wall invasion, serosal extension, or high-grade histology. However, the survival benefit of platinum-based adjuvant therapy for early stage fallopian tube cancer has not been formally demonstrated in randomized trials due to the rarity of this disease.

Selected References

The full list of references for this chapter appears in the online version.

1. Jemal A, Siegel R, Ward E, et al. Cancer statistics, 2009. *CA Cancer J Clin* 2009;59:225.
2. Cannistra SA. Cancer of the ovary. *N Engl J Med* 2004;351:2519.
3. Hankinson SE, Hunter DJ, Colditz GA, et al. Tubal ligation, hysterectomy, and risk of ovarian cancer. A prospective study [comment]. *JAMA* 1993; 270:2813.
13. Omura GA, Brady MF, Homesley HD, et al. Long-term follow-up and prognostic factor analysis in advanced ovarian carcinoma: the Gynecologic Oncology Group experience. *J Clin Oncol* 1991;9:1138.
15. Gershenson DM, Sun CC, Bodurka D, et al. Recurrent low-grade serous ovarian carcinoma is relatively chemoresistant. *Gynecol Oncol* 2009; 114:48.
16. Soliman PT, Slomovitz BM, Broaddus RR, et al. Synchronous primary cancers of the endometrium and ovary: a single institution review of 84 cases. *Gynecol Oncol* 2004;94:456.
17. Bast RC Jr, Knapp RC. Use of the CA 125 antigen in diagnosis and monitoring of ovarian carcinoma. *Euro J Obstet Gynecol Reprod Biol* 1985; 19:354.
18. Rustin GJ, van der Burg ME. A randomized trial in ovarian cancer (OC) of early treatment of relapse based on CA125 level alone versus delayed treatment based on conventional clinical indicators (MRC OV05/EORTC 55955 trials). *Proc Am Soc Clin Oncol* 2009;27(18s): (abstr 1).
26. National Institutes of Health Consensus Development Conference Statement Ovarian cancer: screening, treatment, and follow-up. *Gynecol Oncol* 1994;55:S4.
27. van Nagell JR Jr, DePriest PD, Reedy MB, et al. The efficacy of transvaginal sonographic screening in asymptomatic women at risk for ovarian cancer. *Gynecol Oncol* 2000;77:350.
29. Jacobs IJ, Skates SJ, MacDonald N, et al. Screening for ovarian cancer: a pilot randomised controlled trial. *Lancet* 1999;353:1207.
30. Skates SJ, Xu FJ, Yu YH, et al. Toward an optimal algorithm for ovarian cancer screening with longitudinal tumor markers. *Cancer* 1995;76:2004.
33. Levine DA, Argenta PA, Yee CJ, et al. Fallopian tube and primary peritoneal carcinomas associated with *BRCA* mutations. *J Clin Oncol* 2003;21:4222.
34. Boyd J, Rubin SC. Hereditary ovarian cancer: molecular genetics and clinical implications. *Gynecol Oncol* 1997;64:196.
35. Tonin P, Weber B, Offit K, et al. Frequency of recurrent BRCA1 and BRCA2 mutations in Ashkenazi Jewish breast cancer families [comment]. *Nat Med* 1996;2:1179.
36. Struewing JP, Hartge P, Wacholder S, et al. The risk of cancer associated with specific mutations of BRCA1 and BRCA2 among Ashkenazi Jews. *N Engl J Med* 1997;336:1401.
37. Rubin SC, Benjamin I, Behbakht K, et al. Clinical and pathological features of ovarian cancer in women with germ-line mutations of BRCA1 [see comment]. *N Engl J Med* 1996;335:1413.
41. American Society of Clinical Oncology policy statement update: genetic testing for cancer susceptibility. *J Clin Oncol* 2003;21:2397.
43. Rebbeck TR, Lynch HT, Neuhausen SL, et al. Prophylactic oophorectomy in carriers of BRCA1 or BRCA2 mutations. *N Engl J Med* 2002;346:1616.
44. Kauff ND, Satagopan JM, Robson ME, et al. Risk-reducing salpingo-oophorectomy in women with a BRCA1 or BRCA2 mutation [comment]. *N Engl J Med* 2002;346:1609.
45. Burke W, Daly M, Garber J, et al. Recommendations for follow-up care of individuals with an inherited predisposition to cancer. II. BRCA1 and BRCA2. Cancer Genetics Studies Consortium [comment]. *JAMA* 1997;277:997.
47. Lu KH, Garber JE, Cramer DW, et al. Occult ovarian tumors in women with BRCA1 or BRCA2 mutations undergoing prophylactic oophorectomy. *J Clin Oncol* 2000;18:2728.
49. Narod SA, Dube MP, Klijn J, et al. Oral contraceptives and the risk of breast cancer in BRCA1 and BRCA2 mutation carriers. *J Natl Cancer Inst* 2002;94:1773.
51. Bristow RE, Tomacruz RS, Armstrong DK, Trimble EL, Montz FJ. Survival effect of maximal cytoreductive surgery for advanced ovarian carcinoma during the platinum era: a meta-analysis. *J Clin Oncol* 2002;20:1248.
52. Schumer ST, Cannistra SA. Granulosa cell tumor of the ovary. *J Clin Oncol* 2003;21:1180.
53. Young RC, Decker DG, Wharton JT, et al. Staging laparotomy in early ovarian cancer. *JAMA* 1983;250:3072.
55. Young RC, Walton LA, Ellenberg SS, et al. Adjuvant therapy in stage I and stage II epithelial ovarian cancer. Results of two prospective randomized trials [comment]. *N Engl J Med* 1990;322:1021.
57. Ozols RF, Bundy BN, Greer BE, et al. Phase III trial of carboplatin and paclitaxel compared with cisplatin and paclitaxel in patients with optimally resected stage III ovarian cancer: a Gynecologic Oncology Group study [comment]. *J Clin Oncol* 2003;21:3194.
58. McGuire WP, Hoskins WJ, Brady MF, et al. Cyclophosphamide and cisplatin compared with paclitaxel and cisplatin in patients with stage III and stage IV ovarian cancer [comment]. *N Engl J Med* 1996;334:1.
59. Hoskins WJ, Bundy BN, Thigpen JT, Omura GA. The influence of cytoreductive surgery on recurrence-free interval and survival in small-volume stage III epithelial ovarian cancer: a Gynecologic Oncology Group study. *Gynecol Oncol* 1992;47:159.
60. Lavin PT, Knapp RC, Malkasian G, et al. CA 125 for the monitoring of ovarian carcinoma during primary therapy. *Obstet Gynecol* 1987;69:223.
63. Spentzos D, Levine DA, Ramoni MF, et al. Gene expression signature with independent prognostic significance in epithelial ovarian cancer. *J Clin Oncol* 2004;22:4700.
64. Spentzos D, Levine DA, Kolia S, et al. Unique gene expression profile based on pathologic response in epithelial ovarian cancer. *J Clin Oncol* 2005; 23:7911.
65. Trimbos JB, Parmar M, Vergote I, et al. International Collaborative Ovarian Neoplasm trial 1 and Adjuvant ChemoTherapy in Ovarian Neoplasm trial: two parallel randomized phase III trials of adjuvant chemotherapy in patients with early-stage ovarian carcinoma [comment]. *J Natl Cancer Inst* 2003;95:105.
74. van der Burg ME, van Lent M, Buyse M, et al. The effect of debulking surgery after induction chemotherapy on the prognosis in advanced epithelial ovarian cancer. Gynecological Cancer Cooperative Group of the European Organization for Research and Treatment of Cancer [comment]. *N Engl J Med* 1995;332:629.
78. Piccart MJ, Bertelsen K, James K, et al. Randomized intergroup trial of cisplatin-paclitaxel versus cisplatin-cyclophosphamide in women with advanced epithelial ovarian cancer: three-year results [comment]. *J Natl Cancer Inst* 2000;92:699.
79. Muggia FM, Braly PS, Brady MF, et al. Phase III randomized study of cisplatin versus paclitaxel versus cisplatin and paclitaxel in patients with suboptimal stage III or IV ovarian cancer: a gynecologic oncology group study [see comment]. *J Clin Oncol* 2000;18:106.
80. Paclitaxel plus carboplatin versus standard chemotherapy with either single-agent carboplatin or cyclophosphamide, doxorubicin, and cisplatin in women with ovarian cancer: the ICON3 randomised trial. *Lancet* 2002; 360:505.

84. Vasey PA, Jayson GC, Gordon A, et al. Phase III randomized trial of docetaxel-carboplatin versus paclitaxel-carboplatin as first-line chemotherapy for ovarian carcinoma. *J Natl Cancer Inst* 2004;96:1682.
87. Bookman MA, Brady MF, McGuire WP, et al. Evaluation of new platinum-based treatment regimens in advanced-stage ovarian cancer: a phase III trial of the Gynecologic Cancer InterGroup. *J Clin Oncol* 2009;27:1419.
88. Katsumata N, Yasuda M, Takahashi F, et al. Dose-dense paclitaxel once a week in combination with carboplatin every 3 weeks for advanced ovarian cancer: a phase 3, open-label, randomised controlled trial. *Lancet* 2009;374:1331.
90. Alberts DS, Liu PY, Hannigan EV, et al. Intraperitoneal cisplatin plus intravenous cyclophosphamide versus intravenous cisplatin plus intravenous cyclophosphamide for stage III ovarian cancer [comment]. *N Engl J Med* 1996;335:1950.
91. Markman M, Bundy BN, Alberts DS, et al. Phase III trial of standard-dose intravenous cisplatin plus paclitaxel versus moderately high-dose carboplatin followed by intravenous paclitaxel and intraperitoneal cisplatin in small-volume stage III ovarian carcinoma: an intergroup study of the Gynecologic Oncology Group, Southwestern Oncology Group, and Eastern Cooperative Oncology Group [comment]. *J Clin Oncol* 2001;19:1001.
92. Armstrong DK, Bundy B, Wenzel L, et al. Intraperitoneal cisplatin and paclitaxel in ovarian cancer. *N Engl J Med* 2006;354:34.
93. Walker JL, Armstrong DK, Huang HQ, et al. Intraperitoneal catheter outcomes in a phase III trial of intravenous versus intraperitoneal chemotherapy in optimal stage III ovarian and primary peritoneal cancer: a Gynecologic Oncology Group Study. *Gynecol Oncol* 2006;100:27.
94. Cannistra SA. Intraperitoneal chemotherapy comes of age. *N Engl J Med* 2006;354:77.
100. Markman M, Walker JL, Armstrong DK, et al. Intraperitoneal chemotherapy of ovarian cancer: a review, with a focus on practical aspects of treatment. *J Clin Oncol* 2006;24:988.
101. Makhija S, Leitao M, Sabbatini P, et al. Complications associated with intraperitoneal chemotherapy catheters. *Gynecol Oncol* 2001;81:77.
103. Rose PG, Nerenstone S, Brady MF, et al. A randomized trial of secondary surgical cytoreduction in advanced ovarian carcinoma: a Gynecologic Oncology Group study. *N Engl J Med* 2004;351:2489.
108. Markman M, Liu PY, Wilczynski S, et al. Phase III randomized trial of 12 versus 3 months of maintenance paclitaxel in patients with advanced ovarian cancer after complete response to platinum and paclitaxel-based chemotherapy: a Southwest Oncology Group and Gynecologic Oncology Group trial [comment]. *J Clin Oncol* 2003;21:2460.
109. Pecorelli S, Favalli G, Gadducci A, et al. Phase III trial of observation versus six courses of paclitaxel in patients with advanced epithelial ovarian cancer in complete response after six courses of paclitaxel/platinum-based chemotherapy: final results of the After-6 Protocol. *J Clin Oncol* 2009;27:4642.
110. Pfisterer J, Weber B, Reuss A, et al. Randomized phase III trial of topotecan following carboplatin and paclitaxel in first-line treatment of advanced ovarian cancer: a gynecologic cancer intergroup trial of the AGO-OVAR and GINECO. *J Natl Cancer Inst* 2006;98:1036.
114. Markman M, Rothman R, Hakes T, et al. Second-line platinum therapy in patients with ovarian cancer previously treated with cisplatin. *J Clin Oncol* 1991;9:389.
117. Pujade-Lauraine E, Mahner S, Kaern J, et al. A randomized, phase III study of carboplatin and pegylated liposomal doxorubicin versus carboplatin and paclitaxel in relapsed platinum-sensitive ovarian cancer (OC): CALYPSO study of the Gynecologic Cancer Intergroup (GCIG). Proc Am Soc Clin Oncol 2009;27: (abstr LBA5509).
119. Miller DS, Blessing JA, Krasner CN, et al. Phase II evaluation of pemetrexed in the treatment of recurrent or persistent platinum-resistant ovarian or primary peritoneal carcinoma: a study of the Gynecologic Oncology Group. *J Clin Oncol* 2009;27:2686.
125. Burger RA, Sill MW, Monk BJ, Greer BE, Sorosky JI. Phase II trial of bevacizumab in persistent or recurrent epithelial ovarian cancer or primary peritoneal cancer: a Gynecologic Oncology Group Study. *J Clin Oncol* 2007;25:5165.
126. Cannistra SA, Matulonis UA, Penson RT, et al. Phase II study of bevacizumab in patients with platinum-resistant ovarian cancer or peritoneal serous cancer. *J Clin Oncol* 2007;25:5180.
127. ten Bokkel Huinink WW, Sufliarsky J, Smit WM, et al. Safety and efficacy of patupilone in patients with advanced ovarian, primary fallopian, or primary peritoneal cancer: a phase I, open-label, dose-escalation study. *J Clin Oncol* 2009;27:3097.
128. Matulonis UA, Berlin S, Ivy P, et al. Cediranib, an oral inhibitor of vascular endothelial growth factor receptor kinases, is an active drug in recurrent epithelial ovarian, fallopian tube, and peritoneal cancer. *J Clin Oncol* 2009;27:5601.
129. Fong PC, Boss DS, Yap TA, et al. Inhibition of poly(ADP-ribose) polymerase in tumors from BRCA mutation carriers. *N Engl J Med* 2009;361:123.
137. Bell DA, Weinstock MA, Scully RE. Peritoneal implants of ovarian serous borderline tumors. Histologic features and prognosis. *Cancer* 1988;62:2212.
138. Seidman JD, Kurman RJ. Ovarian serous borderline tumors: a critical review of the literature with emphasis on prognostic indicators. *Hum Pathol* 2000;31:539.
139. Trope C, Kaern J, Vergote IB, Kristensen G, Abeler V. Are borderline tumors of the ovary overtreated both surgically and systemically? A review of four prospective randomized trials including 253 patients with borderline tumors. *Gynecol Oncol* 1993;51:236.
140. Silva EG, Gershenson DM, Malpica A, Deavers M. The recurrence and the overall survival rates of ovarian serous borderline neoplasms with noninvasive implants is time dependent. *Am J Surg Pathol* 2006;30:1367.
142. Williams SD, Blessing JA, Hatch KD, Homesley HD. Chemotherapy of advanced dysgerminoma: trials of the Gynecologic Oncology Group. *J Clin Oncol* 1991;9:1950.
143. Gershenson DM, Morris M, Cangir A, et al. Treatment of malignant germ cell tumors of the ovary with bleomycin, etoposide, and cisplatin. *J Clin Oncol* 1990;8:715.
144. Brewer M, Gershenson DM, Herzog CE, et al. Outcome and reproductive function after chemotherapy for ovarian dysgerminoma. *J Clin Oncol* 1999;17:2670.
146. Williams S, Blessing JA, Liao SY, Ball H, Hanjani P. Adjuvant therapy of ovarian germ cell tumors with cisplatin, etoposide, and bleomycin: a trial of the Gynecologic Oncology Group. *J Clin Oncol* 1994;12:701.
147. Gershenson DM, Miller AM, Champion VL, et al. Reproductive and sexual function after platinum-based chemotherapy in long-term ovarian germ cell tumor survivors: a Gynecologic Oncology Group study. *J Clin Oncol* 2007;25:2792.
153. Healy DL, Burger HG, Mamers P, et al. Elevated serum inhibin concentrations in postmenopausal women with ovarian tumors. *N Engl J Med* 1993;329:1539.
154. Homesley HD, Bundy BN, Hurteau JA, Roth LM. Bleomycin, etoposide, and cisplatin combination therapy of ovarian granulosa cell tumors and other stromal malignancies: a Gynecologic Oncology Group study [comment]. *Gynecol Oncol* 1999;72:131.
156. Tobacman JK, Greene MH, Tucker MA, et al. Intra-abdominal carcinomatosis after prophylactic oophorectomy in ovarian-cancer-prone families. *Lancet* 1982;2:795.
157. Muto MG, Welch WR, Mok SC, et al. Evidence for a multifocal origin of papillary serous carcinoma of the peritoneum. *Cancer Res* 1995;55:490.
158. Piver MS, Jishi MF, Tsukada Y, Nava G. Primary peritoneal carcinoma after prophylactic oophorectomy in women with a family history of ovarian cancer. A report of the Gilda Radner Familial Ovarian Cancer Registry. *Cancer* 1993;71:2751.

SECTION 6: CANCER OF THE BREAST

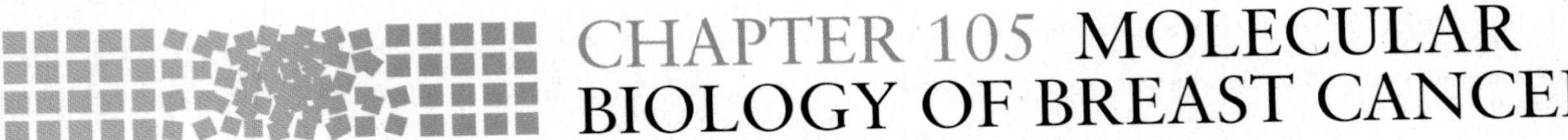

CHAPTER 105 MOLECULAR BIOLOGY OF BREAST CANCER

ERIN WYSONG HOFSTATTER, GINA G. CHUNG, AND LYNDSAY N. HARRIS

It has been said that cancer is a genetic disease and can be best understood by studying the DNA alterations that lead to the development of cancer. However, a deeper understanding of carcinogenesis requires insight into how these genetic changes alter cellular programs that lead to growth, invasion, and metastasis. This chapter is presented following the logical progression of DNA to RNA to protein, and it describes, at each step, the lesions that contribute to breast cancer carcinogenesis. The chapter also introduces new concepts in epigenetics, microRNAs, and gene expression analyses that illustrate how new biologic discoveries, and novel technologies, have profoundly affected our understanding of breast cancer pathogenesis within the past decade.

GENETICS OF BREAST CANCER

Breast cancer is a heterogeneous disease fundamentally caused by progressive accumulation of genetic aberrations, including point mutations, chromosomal amplifications, deletions, rearrangements, translocations, and duplications.[1,2] Germline mutations account for only about 10% of all breast cancers, while the vast majority of breast cancers appear to occur sporadically and are attributed to somatic genetic alterations (Fig. 105.1).[3]

HEREDITARY BREAST CANCER

One of the most important risk factors for breast cancer is family history. Though familial forms comprise nearly 20% of all breast cancers, most of the genes responsible for familial breast cancer have yet to be identified. Breast cancer susceptibility genes can be categorized into three classes according to their frequency and level of risk they confer: rare high-penetrance genes, rare intermediate-penetrance genes, and common low-penetrance genes and loci[4] (Table 105.1).

High-Penetrance, Low-Frequency Breast Cancer Predisposition Genes

BRCA1 and BRCA2

BRCA1 and *BRCA2* mutations account for approximately half of all dominantly inherited hereditary breast cancers. These mutations confer a relative risk of breast cancer 10 to 30 times that of women in the general population, resulting in a nearly 85% lifetime risk of breast cancer development.[5] *BRCA1* and *BRCA2* mutation carriers are quite rare among the general population, however, the prevalence is substantially higher in certain founder populations, most notably in the Ashkenazi Jewish population, where the carrier frequency is 1 in 40.

More than a thousand germline mutations have been identified in *BRCA1* and *BRCA2*. Pathogenic mutations most often result in truncated protein products, although mutations that interfere with protein function also exist.[4,5] Interestingly, penetrance of pathogenic *BRCA1* and *BRCA2* mutations and age of cancer onset appear to vary both within and among family members. Specific BRCA mutations as well as gene–gene and gene–environment interactions as potential modifiers of *BRCA*-related cancer risk are areas of active investigation.[6,7]

BRCA1-related breast cancers are characterized by features that distinguish them from both *BRCA2*-related and sporadic breast cancers.[4] *BRCA1*-related tumors typically occur in younger women and have more aggressive features, with high histologic grade, high proliferative rate, aneuploidy, and absence of estrogen and progesterone receptors and human epidermal growth factor receptor 2 (HER2). This "triple-negative" phenotype of *BRCA1*-related breast cancers is further characterized by a "basal-like" gene expression profile of cytokeratins 5/6, 14, and 17, epidermal growth factor and P-cadherin.[8]

Though *BRCA1* and *BRCA2* genes encode large proteins with multiple functions, they primarily act as classic tumor suppressor genes that function to maintain genomic stability by facilitating double-strand DNA repair through homologous recombination.[8,9] When loss of heterozygosity (LOH) occurs via loss, mutation, or silencing of the wild type *BRCA1* or *BRCA2* allele, the resultant defective DNA repair leads to rapid acquisition of additional mutations, particularly during DNA replication, and ultimately sets the stage for cancer development.

The integral role of BRCA1 and BRCA2 in double-strand DNA repair holds potential as a therapeutic target for *BRCA*-related breast cancers. For example, platinum agents cause interstrand crosslinks, thereby blocking DNA replication and leading to stalled replication forks. Poly(adenosine diphosphate-ribose) polymerase-1 (PARP1) inhibitors additionally show promise as specific therapy for *BRCA*-related tumors. PARP1 is a cellular enzyme that functions in single-strand DNA repair through base excision and represents a major alternative DNA repair pathway in the cell.[10,11] When PARP inhibition is applied to a background deficient in double-strand DNA repair, as is the case in *BRCA*-related tumor cells, the cells are left without adequate DNA repair mechanisms and ultimately undergo cell cycle arrest, chromosome instability, and cell death.[4] Given their phenotypic similarities to *BRCA1*-related breast cancers, sporadic basal-like breast tumors may display sensitivity to PARP inhibition as well.[11] Phase 2 studies are currently under way to

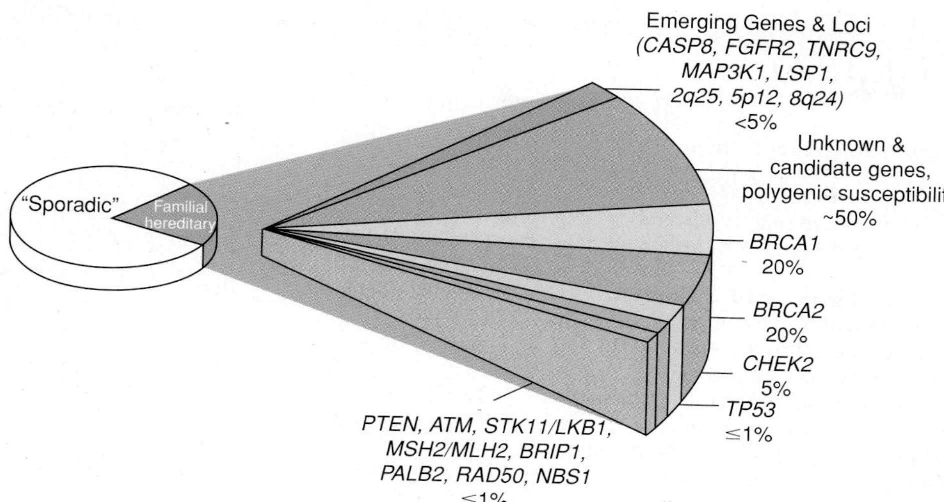

FIGURE 105.1 Genetic susceptibility to breast cancer. Familial breast cancer comprises approximately 20% to 30% of all breast cancers. *BRCA1* and *BRCA2* are two major high-penetrance genes associated with hereditary breast and ovarian cancer syndrome, which together account for nearly half of inherited breast cancers. Other rare breast cancer susceptibility genes have been identified, such as *CHEK2*, *TP53*, *PTEN*, and *STK11*. Several emerging low-penetrance genes and loci recently discovered by genomewide association studies account for a small proportion of familial breast cancers (<5%). To date, about half of familial breast cancers remain unexplained but are likely attributable to as yet unknown genes and/or polygenic susceptibility. (From Olopade O, et al. Advances in breast cancer: pathways to personalized medicine. *Clin Cancer Res* 2008;14(24): Fig 1.)

explore the use of PARP inhibitors in both *BRCA*- and basal-like, non-*BRCA*-related breast tumors.

Other High-Penetrance Genes

A small number of other high-risk, low frequency breast cancer susceptibility genes exist, and they include *TP53, PTEN, STK11/LKB1*, and *CDH1*.[4–6] These high-penetrance genes confer an eight- to tenfold increase in risk of breast cancer as compared to noncarriers, but they collectively account for less than 1% of cases of breast cancer. Like *BRCA1* and *BRCA2*, these genes are inherited in an autosomal dominant fashion and function as tumor suppressors.[12] The hereditary cancer syndromes associated with each gene are usually characterized by multiple cancers in addition to breast cancer, as summarized in Table 105.1.

Moderate-Penetrance, Low Frequency Breast Cancer Predisposition Genes

Four genes have been identified that confer an elevated but moderate risk of developing breast cancer, namely *CHEK2, ATM, BRIP1*, and *PALB2* (Table 105.1). Each of these genes confers approximately a two- to threefold relative risk of breast cancer in mutation carriers, though this risk may be higher in select clinical settings.[5] Mutation frequencies in the general population are rare, on the order of 0.1% to 1%, though some founder mutations have been identified. Together, these genes account for approximately 2.3% of inherited breast cancer. The moderate relative risk of breast cancer of these genes in conjunction with the low population frequency renders this class of genes very difficult to detect with typical association studies. However, these genes were specifically selected for study as candidate breast cancer genes based on their known roles in signal transduction and DNA repair in close association with BRCA1 and BRCA2.[6]

Low-Penetrance, High Frequency Breast Cancer Predisposition Genes and Loci

Both candidate gene and genome-wide association studies (GWAS) have identified a low-risk panel of approximately ten different alleles and loci in 15% to 40% of women with breast cancer[5] (Table 105.1). Despite their frequency, the relative risk of breast cancer conferred by any one of these genetic variants alone is minimal, on the order of less than 1.5.[4] Nevertheless, these alleles and loci may become clinically relevant in their suggestion of interactions with other high-, moderate-, and low-risk genes; these additive or multiplicative relationships could account for a measurable fraction of population risk. For example, association studies of FGFR2 and MAP3K1 within *BRCA* families showed that these single nucleotide polymorphisms (SNPs) conferred an increased risk in the presence of *BRCA2* mutations.

Recent studies suggest that microRNA (miRNA) SNPs may also contribute to breast cancer susceptibility, and miRNAs appear to regulate many tumor suppressor genes (TSGs) and oncogenes via degradation of target mRNAs or repression of their translation. Thus, genetic variations in miRNA genes or miRNA binding sites could affect expression of TSGs or oncogenes and, thereby, cancer risk. For example, specific SNPs located within pre-miR-27a and miR-196a-2 genes have been associated with reduced breast cancer risk.[13]

SOMATIC CHANGES IN BREAST CANCER

The vast majority of breast cancers are sporadic in origin, ultimately caused by accumulation of numerous somatic genetic alterations.[1] Recent data suggest that a typical individual breast cancer harbors anywhere from 50 to 80 different somatic mutations.[2] Many of these mutations occur as a result of erroneous DNA replication; others may occur through exposure to exogenous and endogenous mutagens. To date, hundreds of candidate somatic breast cancer genes have been identified through GWAS.[14,15] Yet the full range of somatic mutations will not be clear until hundreds more breast tumor samples are sequenced. To this end, international efforts are currently underway to produce a comprehensive catalog of these genetic alterations.

Determining the role of each identified mutation in the development of breast cancer remains a substantial challenge. Data suggest that the vast majority of identified somatic DNA mutations in a given tumor are "passenger" mutations, representing harmless, biologically neutral changes that do not contribute to oncogenesis.[1,2] Conversely, "driver" mutations confer a growth advantage on the cell in which they occur and appear to be implicated in cancer development. By definition, driver mutations are found in candidate cancer genes (CAN).[15]

Although the catalog of somatic mutations and CAN genes is still incomplete, it is comprehensive enough that various structural features are starting to emerge. When specific driver

TABLE 105.1

BREAST CANCER SUSCEPTIBILITY GENES AND LOCI

Gene/Locus	Associated Syndrome/Clinical Features	Breast Cancer Risk	Mutation/Minor Allele Frequency
HIGH PENETRANCE GENES			
BRCA1 (17q21)	**Hereditary breast/ovarian cancer:** bilateral/multifocal breast tumor, prostate, colon, liver, bone cancers	60%–85% (lifetime); 15%–40% risk of ovarian cancer	1/400
BRCA2 (13q12.3)	**Hereditary breast/ovarian cancer:** male breast cancer, pancreas, gall bladder, pharynx, stomach, melanoma, prostate cancer. Also causes D1 Fanconi anemia (biallelic mutations)	60%–85% (lifetime); 15%–40% risk of ovarian cancer	1/400
TP53 (17p13.1)	**Li-Fraumeni syndrome:** breast cancer, soft tissue sarcoma, central nervous system tumors, adrenocortical cancer, leukemia, prostate cancer	50%–89% (by age 50); 90% in Li-Fraumeni survivors	<1/10,000
PTEN (10q23.3)	**Cowden syndrome:** breast cancer, hamartoma, thyroid, oral mucosa, endometrial, brain tumor	25%–50% (lifetime)	<1/10,000
CDH1 (16q22.1)	**Familial diffuse gastric cancer:** lobular breast cancer, gastric cancer	RR 6.6	<1/10,000
STK11/LKB1 (19p13.3)	**Peutz-Jeghers syndrome:** breast, ovary, testis, pancreas, cervix, uterine, colon cancers; melanocytic macules of lips/digits; gastrointestinal hamartomatous polyps	30%–50% (by age 70)	<1/10,000
MODERATE PENETRANCE GENES			
CHEK2(22q12.1)	**Li-Fraumeni 2 syndrome(?):** breast, prostate, colorectal, and brain tumors, sarcomas	OR 2.6 (for 1100delC mutation)	1/100–200 (in certain populations)
BRIP1 (17q22)	**Breast cancer:** also causes FA-J Fanconi anemia(biallelic mutations)	RR 2.0	<1/1000
ATM (11q22.3)	**Ataxia-telangiectasia:** breast, ovarian, leukemia, lymphoma, possible stomach/pancreas/bladder cancers; immunodeficiency	RR 2.37	1/33–333
PALB2 (16p12)	**Breast, pancreatic, prostate cancers:** also causes FA-N Fanconi anemia(biallelic mutations)	RR 2.3	<1/1000
LOW PENETRANCE GENES AND LOCI			
FGFR2 (10q26)	Breast cancer	OR 1.26	0.38
TOX3 (16q12.1)	Breast cancer	OR 1.14	0.46
LSP1 (11p15.5)	Breast cancer	OR 1.06	0.3
TGFB1 (19q13.1)	Breast cancer	OR 1.07	0.68
MAP3K1 (5q11.2)	Breast cancer	OR 1.13	0.28
CASP8 (2q33-34)	Breast cancer (protective)	OR 0.89	0.13
6q22.33	Breast cancer	OR 1.41	0.21 (in Ashkenazi Jewish)
2q35	Breast cancer	OR 1.11	0.11–0.52
8q24	Breast cancer	OR 1.06	0.4
5p12	Breast cancer	OR 1.19	0.2–0.31

OR, overall risk; RR, relative risk.

mutations are cataloged among several different breast tumors, a bimodal cancer "genomic landscape" appears, comprising a small number of commonly mutated gene "mountains" among hundreds of infrequently mutated gene "hills."[1,2] Gene mountains correspond to the most frequently mutated genes found within breast tumors, such as *TP53*, *CDH1*, phosphatidylinositol 3-kinase (*PI3K*), cyclin D, *PTEN*, and *AKT*.[6] Each individual gene hill, on the other hand, is typically found in less than 5% of breast tumors.[1,16] This substantial heterogeneity of DNA mutations among breast tumors may explain the wide variations in phenotypes, both in terms of tumor behavior as well as responsiveness to therapy.

Historically, the focus of genetic research has been on the gene mountains, in part because they were the only mutations that available technology could identify. However emerging data suggest that it is actually the gene hills that play a much more pivotal role in breast cancer, consistent with the idea that having a large number of mutations, each associated with a small survival advantage, drives tumor progression. Recent studies have shown that a substantial number of these infrequent somatic mutations sort out among a much smaller number of biologic groups and cell signaling pathways that are known to be pathogenic in breast cancer, thereby vastly reducing the complexity of the genomic landscape. Examples of such pathways include interferon signaling, cell cycle checkpoint, BRCA1/2-related DNA repair, p53, AKT, transforming growth factor-β (TGF-β) signaling, Notch, epidermal growth factor receptor (EGFR), FGF, ERBB2, RAS, and PI3K. In short,

TABLE 105.2

RECURRENT AMPLIFICATIONS IN BREAST CANCER CELL LINES AND HUMAN TUMORS

Cell Line	8q24	11q13	17q12	17q22	20q13
BT-474		11q13-q14	17q12	17q22-24 (avg 49 copies)	20q13 (avg 37 copies)
SKBR-3	8q23.2-q24.21		17q12	17q24	20q13
MCF-7		11q13		17q21-q22, 17q23	20q13.1, 20q13.2-q13.31
MCF-10A			No amplification		
UACC-893		11q13-q14	17q12-q21.2	17q22-24	
UACC-812			17q12	17q23	20q13
MDA-MB361		11q13.4-q14.1	17q12-q21.1	17q23.2-q24.1	
SUM-190		11q13.4-q14.1			
ZR-75-1		11q13.2-q13.4			
ZR-75-30	8q24.22, 8q24.3		17q12-q21.2	17q23.2-q24.2	

it appears that common pathways, rather than individual gene mutations, govern the course of breast cancer development.[16]

Although recurrent point mutations are less common in breast cancer than other solid tumors, emerging data show that particular regions of the genome are commonly amplified and these regions contain genes that drive cancer progression (Table 105.2). The best example of an important amplified region is the 17q12 amplicon that harbors the *HER2* oncogene. This amplicon leads to a more aggressive tumor phenotype, now the target of a highly successful antibody therapy, trastuzumab (Herceptin). It has been observed that RNAi knockdown of coamplified genes within the 17q12 amplicon results in decreased cell proliferation and increased apoptosis.[17] Thus, the 17q12 amplicon appears to encode a concerted genetic program that contributes to the oncogenesis.

There are several other amplicons, in addition to 17q12 (*HER2*), that seem to drive the cancer phenotype and have prognostic significance in breast cancers, for example, 11q13 (*CCDN1*) and 8q24 (*MYC*), 20q13.[18] These regions contain gene sets that are important in DNA metabolism and maintenance of chromosomal integrity, suggesting that response to DNA damaging agents used as anticancer therapy might be modulated by the presence of particular amplicons. Indeed, these coamplicons are frequent in *HER2* amplified tumors and may modify tumor behavior and patient outcome.[19,20] The contribution of these genomic alterations to functional consequences, may lie not in the overexpression of individual genes, but of gene cassettes on the amplicon.

Direct clinical translation of the growing catalog of somatic alterations in breast cancer has yet to evolve. However, with advancing technology and further identification and categorization of genetic mutations, new opportunities for individualized diagnosis and treatment options are likely to emerge.

GENE EXPRESSION PATTERNS IN BREAST CANCER

The cellular programs that are encoded by DNA are enacted by transcription into messenger RNA (mRNA) and translated into protein. Not surprisingly, the DNA alterations described above lead to either under- or overexpression of their associated mRNAs; consequently abnormal gene expression patterns are a common finding in breast tumors. Gene expression profiling has been introduced into the clinical literature during the past decade as research suggests that assessing the expression of multiple genes in a tumor sample may reflect programs turned on by DNA alternations and predict tumor behavior. So-called molecular signatures hold promise for improving diagnosis, prediction of recurrence, and selection of therapies for individual patients.

Several technologies have been developed to generate molecular signatures, including cDNA and oligonucleotide arrays and multiplex polymerase chain reaction (PCR) technologies. These technologies and newly developed statistical methodologies now allow evaluation of hundreds and even thousands of mRNAs simultaneously with grouping of samples based on coexpressed genes.

Molecular Classification of Breast Cancer

The seminal work by Perou et al.[21] and Sorlie et al.[22] suggests a classification of breast cancer subtypes based on gene expression patterns they termed "molecular portraits" of breast cancer. Among the categories they defined were the luminal A and B tumor types (typically estrogen receptor [ER] or progesterone receptor [PR] positive), *HER2* gene-amplified tumors, and a newly recognized class termed "basal-like" due to the expression of basal keratins. Basal tumors typically lack ER, PR, and *HER2*, and are often referred to as triple negative, although not all basal-like tumors are triple negative and the reverse. Although the exact definition of molecular subtypes is an area of active debate, it is clear that these subtypes are reproducible in multiple, unrelated data sets, and their prognostic impact has been validated in these settings.[21,23,24] As a result, clinical trials are now being designed to subdivide patients by ER/PR and *HER2* status to validate claims that therapeutic approaches should address these groups rather than the population of breast cancer patients as a whole.

Prognostic Signatures

Around the same time period, van't Veer et al.[24] and van de Vijver et al.[25] were the first to apply gene expression analysis to define a subgroup of breast cancer patients with increased likelihood of metastasis. The estimated hazard ratio for distant metastases in the group with a poor prognosis signature, as compared with the group with the good prognosis signature, was 5.1 (95% confidence interval, 2.9 to 9.0; $P < .001$). The European Organisation for Research and Treatment of Cancer (EORTC) and the Breast International Group (BIG) are currently conducting a prospective clinical trial to validate the utility of this assay for sparing patients from systemic chemotherapy (the MINDACT study).[26] In a preliminary analysis, the 70-gene profile signature was strongly prognostic, outperforming classic prognostic criteria such as those used by the

St. Gallen consensus panel[27]; however, the magnitude of effect was much less than previously reported with hazard ratios for time to distant metastases of 1.85 (1.14 to 3.0) and for overall survival of 2.5 (1.4 to 4.5). The 70-gene signature is now commercialized as the MammaPrint and has received clearance by the U.S. Food and Drug Administration (FDA) as a class 2, 510(k) product.

Other groups have developed prognostic gene expression signatures, including the 76-gene Rotterdam signature, which identifies a high-risk group of node-negative patients, and the Genomic Grade Index (GGI), which distinguishes poor and good prognosis groups in breast tumors of intermediate histologic grade.[28] The potential value of these signatures has yet to be clearly defined, but it emphasizes the role of gene expression profiling at distinguishing prognostic groups not otherwise recognizable by standard histologic or clinical parameters.

Predictive Signatures

Endocrine Therapy

Several groups have applied gene expression profiling analysis to better define the likelihood of benefit from therapy. Such predictive signatures may have particular value as they help oncologists counsel patients about appropriate choices for treatment. Genomics Health Inc (Redwood City, California) developed the Oncotype DX® assay as a predictor of benefit from antiestrogen therapy using multiple real-time reverse transcriptase polymerase chain reaction (RT-PCR) assays in formalin fixed paraffin-embedded tissue. The assay was developed from 250 candidate genes selected from published literature, genomic databases, and in-house experiments performed on frozen tissue. From these data, a panel of 16 cancer-related genes and 5 reference genes were used to develop an algorithm to compute a recurrence score, ranging from 0 to 100, that can be used to estimate the odds of recurrence over 10 years from diagnosis.[29] Paik et al.[29] reported an analysis of two randomized controlled trials: National Surgical Adjuvant Breast and Bowel Project NSABP-B14, in which node-negative patients with ER-positive tumors were randomly assigned to tamoxifen or nil; and NSABP-B20, in which node-negative patients with ER-positive tumors were randomly assigned to tamoxifen alone or with cyclophosphamide, methotrexate, and fluorouracil (CMF) chemotherapy. Using the tissue samples from NSABP-B20, patients were categorized into three recurrence score groups: low risk (recurrence score less than 18), intermediate risk (recurrence score 18 to 30), and high risk (recurrence score 31 to 100). Samples from NSABP-B14 were then analyzed and found to be 6.8% (4.0% to 9.6%), 14.3% (8.3% to 20.3%) and 30.5% (23.6% to 37.4%). Paik et al. further analyzed the performance of the Oncotype DX assay to include patients in the other arms of NSABP-B14 and NSABP-B20 and found that the Oncotype DX assay was a strong predictor of benefit from CMF in NSABP-B20, with little or no benefit from chemotherapy for patients with low or intermediate recurrence scores but substantial benefit for those with high recurrence scores. Conversely, in NSABP-B14, the benefit from tamoxifen versus observation was confined to the low and intermediate risk categories (*P* value for interaction of .001). These data suggest that in patients who have an apparent favorable prognosis based on clinical features (negative nodes, positive ER), the Oncotype DX assay helps determine those most likely to benefit from tamoxifen only (low recurrence scores) versus those most likely not to benefit from tamoxifen but likely to benefit from chemotherapy (high recurrence scores). The benefits of chemotherapy in the 25% of patients who have intermediate recurrence scores remains uncertain and are the basis of an ongoing prospective randomized trial (Tailor Rx) where those with high recurrence scores will receive endocrine therapy and chemotherapy, those with low recurrence scores will receive endocrine therapy alone, and intermediate recurrence scores are randomly assigned to endocrine therapy versus endocrine and chemotherapy. A recent study by Albain et al.[30] suggests that a low recurrence score predicts a lack of benefit of fluorouracil (5-FU), Adriamycin (doxorubicin), and cyclophosphamide (FAC) chemotherapy in node-positive breast cancer patients treated on Southwest Oncology Group SWOG-8814. Although these provocative data suggest a similar utility for Oncotype DX in node-positive patients, they do not include the use of taxanes and require additional validation with modern-day regimens. The value of the Oncotype DX assay in predicting benefit from hormonal therapy in patients treated with aromatase inhibitor therapy has recently been published, demonstrating that the assay performs equally similarly with both tamoxifen and anastrazole but does not distinguish benefit of one over the other.[31]

Additional predictors for ER-positive breast cancer include the Breast Cancer 2-Gene Expression Ratio (AvariaDx Inc, Carlsbad, California), a quantitative RT-PCR–based assay that measures the ratio of the *HOXB6* and *IL17BR* genes, and is marketed as a marker of recurrence risk in untreated ER-positive/node-negative patients.[32,33] The Breast Cancer Gene Expression Ratio is significantly and independently associated with poorer disease-free survival in two studies of lymph node–negative, ER-positive, tamoxifen-treated patients with breast cancer. In these two studies, patients who were low risk by the two-gene expression ratio had average 10-year recurrence rates of approximately 17% to 25%. Further validation is awaited.

Chemotherapy

Defining predictors of response to chemotherapy and targeted therapies has been more challenging. Ayers et al.[34] from the M. D. Anderson Cancer Center were the first to report that multigene analysis of fine needle aspiration specimens predicts response to neoadjuvant T-FAC chemotherapy. These results require validation and are the subject of a prospective trial of chemotherapy with randomization based on the predictor (F. Symmans, personal communication). Another approach to the development of predictive signatures was pioneered by the group at Duke Center for Health Policy and Informatics where gene signatures were defined in model systems and applied to human data sets. While initially tested in lung cancer, these signatures are now the subject of several prospective randomized trials in breast cancer, and other tumor types.[35] Validation of gene signatures is of utmost importance in the future to determine the value of these expression profiles at predicting treatment response, and clinical outcome, in breast cancer patients. National organizations such as the American Society of Clinical Oncology, National Comprehensive Cancer Network, and College of American Pathologists have ongoing efforts to interpret the data from the burgeoning field of multigene biomarker tests to help the practicing clinician interpret their clinical utility.[36]

EPIGENETICS OF BREAST CANCER

Cells maintain their stable identity and phenotype over many generations without external stimuli or signaling events. This cellular memory is encoded in the epigenome, a collection of heritable information that exists alongside the genomic sequence. DNA methylation and chromatin modification are major epigenetic mechanisms in higher eukaryotes and are tightly coupled to basic genetic processes, such as DNA replication, transcription, and repair. DNA methylation at the promoter proximal CpG sequences is associated with gene silencing. Similarly, specific histone modifications control transcriptional status or capacity of the underlying sequence by regulating the activity of chromatin domains in an active or inactive state. Euchromatin or active chromatin is enriched with acetylated histones H3, H4, and H2A and histone H3 methylated at lysine residues K4, K40, and K36.[37] In contrast, heterochromatin or silent chromatin is depleted of histone acetylation while enriched in histone H3 methylated at lysine resides K9, K27, and K79. It is well documented that cancers, including breast cancer, have altered patterns of DNA methylation and histone acetylation, leading to alterations in transcription that appear to be oncogenic.[37,38] Hence, epigenetic therapies have received intense interest from a large number of clinical and basic cancer studies.

Major epigenetic cancer drugs include DNA methyltransferase (DNMT) and histone deacetylase (HDAC) inhibitors. Preclinical studies show promise that HDAC inhibitors may have activity in breast cancer cells, and many clinical phase 1 and 2 studies are in progress.[39,40]

MicroRNAs: A Newly Discovered Class of Molecules that Regulate Gene Expression

miRNAs are small noncoding RNAs that belong to a novel class of regulatory molecules that control expression of hundreds of target mRNA transcripts. miRNAs are generated from large RNA precursors (termed pre-miRNAs) that are processed in the nucleus into approximately 70 nucleotide pre-miRNAs, which fold into imperfect stem-loop structures.[41] The pre-miRNAs undergo an additional processing step within the cytoplasm, and mature miRNAs of 18 to 25 nucleotides in length are excised from one side of the pre-miRNA hairpin by Dicer. miRNAs regulate gene expression in two ways. First, miRNAs that bind to protein-coding mRNA sequences that are exactly complementary to the miRNA induce the RNA-mediated interference (RNAi) pathway. Messenger RNA targets are then cleaved by ribonucleases in the RNA-induced silencing complex (RISC). Second, miRNAs bind to imperfect complementary sites within the 3′-untranslated regions (3′UTRs) of their target protein-coding mRNAs and repress the expression of these genes at the level of translation.[42]

miRNAs are known to be associated with breast cancer in both cell lines and clinical samples. For example, *miR-21*, *miR-155*, *miR-7*, and *miR-210* are overexpressed in aggressive human breast cancers,[43,44] while *let-7* and *miR-125a* have been shown to be down-regulated in breast cancers.[45] It has also been shown that *miR-125a* may function as a tumor suppressor by inhibiting ERBB2 and ERBB3.

MicroRNAs Predict Response to Cancer Treatment

Soon after they were discovered to be misregulated in cancer, miRNA misexpression patterns were found to be associated with cancer outcome and response to treatment, including radiation and chemotherapy. Certain miRNAs associated with hypoxia, such as *miR-210*, have been shown to be biomarkers of poor outcome in breast cancer.[43] Furthermore, *in vitro* data show that certain miRNAs are associated with resistance to doxorubicin[46] or tamoxifen.[47] In patient samples, an association of miRNA's tumor subtypes have specific miRNA patterns and this is associated with poor outcome. Defining the role of miRNAs as biomarkers for prognosis and prediction, as well as their potential as targeted therapies, is an active area of research in breast cancer.

PROTEIN/PATHWAY ALTERATIONS

The molecular mechanisms that lead to cancer have been characterized as the hallmarks of cancer, as proposed by Hanahan and Weinberg.[48] They include self-sufficiency in growth signals, insensitivity to antigrowth factor signals, evasion of apoptosis, infinite replicative potential, invasion and metastasis, and sustained angiogenesis. The effectors of genetic and epigenetic abnormalities are in most cases reflected in the abnormal levels, functions, and interactions of proteins and signaling pathways. Undoubtedly, numerous alterations coordinate to result in the malignant phenotype; however, a number of key proteins and their pathways have emerged as critical drivers of breast cancer development and growth as well as potential therapeutic targets.

Therapeutic Targets in Breast Cancer

Estrogen Signaling

Most breast cancers are intimately linked with exposure to estrogen and alterations in the estrogen receptor signaling pathway. Estrogen is a steroid hormone that exerts its actions by binding to the nuclear ER. Upon activation by its ligand, ER binds in a coordinated fashion with a number of coregulatory proteins to estrogen response elements in the promoter region of estrogen-responsive genes. This in turn directs the transcription of numerous growth-promoting genes, including PR. Although ER is overexpressed in as many as 70% of invasive breast cancers, the precise mechanism by which this occurs is unclear. Amplification of the gene appears to be one mechanism; however, it was present in only approximately 50% of cases with ER overexpression in one study, suggesting that transcriptional deregulation and posttranscriptional modifications (such as alteration of mRNA levels by miRNAs) may also play a role. The level of ER expression is not only of biologic interest, but it is a highly effective predictor for response to antiestrogens, which is a recommended treatment for all ER-expressing tumors.

Estrogen exerts its actions through both genomic (described above) and nongenomic mechanisms. In contrast to the genomic actions of ER, nongenomic actions of ER are extremely rapid (within seconds to minutes of estrogen exposure) and are believed to result from the hormone-dependent activation of membrane-bound or cytosolic ERs. These nonnuclear ER actions result in rapid phosphorylation and activation of important growth regulatory kinases including EGFRs, insulinlike growth factor-1R (IGF-1R), c-Src, Shc, and the p85α regulatory subunit of PI3K.[5] This "crosstalk" between ER and growth factor receptors is bidirectional: constitutive HER2, for example, can increase ER signaling to the point where it is unresponsive to antiestrogen treatments. These findings suggest a role for HER2/IGF-1R/EGFR activation in both acquired and *de novo* resistance to treatment with antiestrogens.[49]

The ER pathway has proven to be an invaluable target for therapeutic treatments in breast cancer. A number of agents have been developed over the prior decades that can inhibit this pathway by either binding to the receptor itself (e.g., selective ER modulators such as tamoxifen) or by decreasing the production of endogenous estrogen (e.g., aromatase inhibitors and ovarian ablation). Although these agents are highly effective and have made a significant impact on breast cancer morbidity and mortality, unfortunately, *de novo* and acquired resistance is also quite common.

As described above, the Oncotype DX assay adds additional insight into the behavior of ER-positive tumors and provides useful information for treatment decision making.

Growth Factor Receptor Pathways

Growth factor receptor pathways, and in particular tyrosine kinase receptors, play an essential role in initiating both proliferative and cell survival pathways in tissue and are normally tightly regulated. In breast cancer biology, the ErbB family has been studied most extensively, but an expanding number of other growth factors, such as insulinlike growth factor receptors, have also been the subject of intense scrutiny in hopes of identifying effective therapeutic targets.[50] These receptors have an extracellular ligand-binding region, a transmembrane region, and a cytoplasmic tyrosine kinase–containing domain that can activate downstream signaling cascades. These growth factor receptor pathways can be constitutively activated by a number of mechanisms, including excessive ligand levels, gain-of-function mutations, overexpression with or without gene amplification, and gene rearrangements and resultant fusion proteins with oncogenic potential. This can ultimately lead to inappropriate kinase activity and growth promoting second messenger activation (Fig. 105.2).

Human Epidermal Growth Factor Receptor 2

HER2 (EGFR2 or ErbB2) is a member of a family of receptor tyrosine kinases that also includes EGFR (HER1, ErbB1), ErbB3, and ErbB4. Ligand binding to the extracellular domains

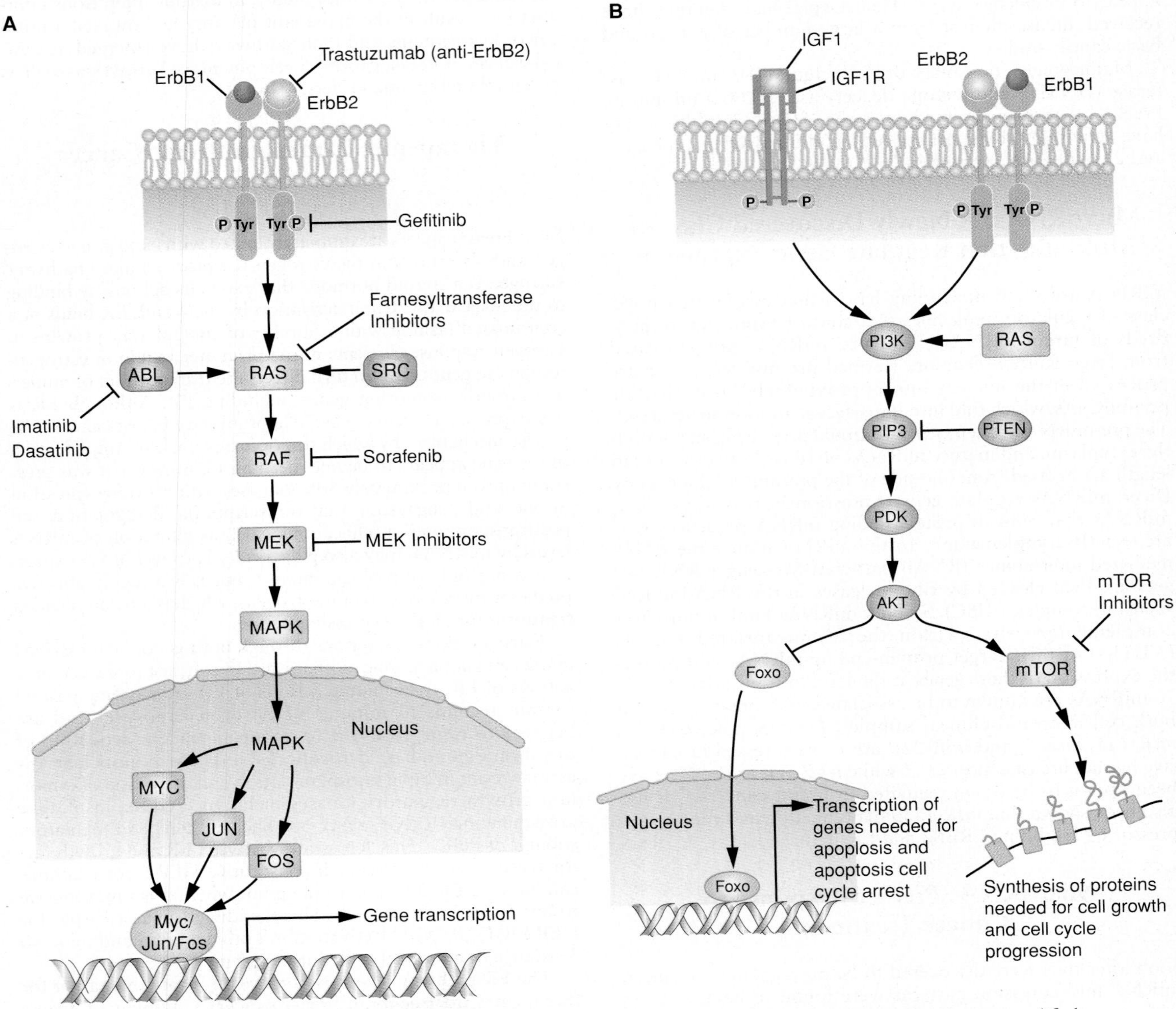

FIGURE 105.2 **A:** The ras/raf/MEK/MAPK pathway is activated by multiple growth factor receptors (here exemplified by ErbB1 and ErbB2) as well as several intracellular tyrosine kinases such as SRC and ABL. Activated RAS stimulates a sequence of phosphorylation events mediated by RAF, MEK, and ERK (MAP) kinases. Activated MAP kinase (MAPK) translocates to the nucleus and activates proteins such as MYC, JUN, and FOS that promote the transcription of numerous genes involved in tumor growth. **B:** The phosphatidylinositol 3-kinase (PI3K)pathway is activated by RAS and by a number of growth factor receptors (here exemplified IGF1R and the ErbB1/ErbB2 heterodimer). Activated PI3K generates phosphatidylinositol-3,4,5-triphosphate (PIP3), which activates phosphoinositide-dependent kinase-1 (PDK). In turn, PDK phosphorylates AKT. PTEN is an endogenous inhibitor of AKT activation. Phosphorylated AKT transduces multiple downstream signals, including activation of the mammalian target of rapamycin (mTOR) and inhibition of the FOXO family of transcription factors. mTOR activation promotes the synthesis of proteins required for cell growth and cell cycle progression. (Redrawn from Golan DE, Tashjian AH, Armstrong EJ. *Principles of pharmacology: the pathophysiologic basis of drug therapy.* 2nd ed. Baltimore: Wolters Kluwer Health, 2008.)

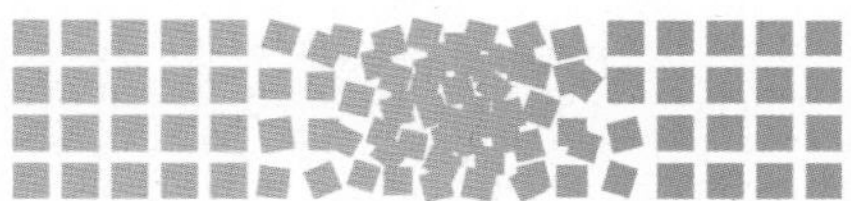

CHAPTER 106 MALIGNANT TUMORS OF THE BREAST

HAROLD J. BURSTEIN, JAY R. HARRIS, AND MONICA MORROW

Breast cancer is a major public health problem for women throughout the world. In the United States, breast cancer remains the most frequent cancer in women and the second most frequent cause of cancer death. In 2009 it is estimated that breast cancer accounted for 27% of cancer cases and 15% of cancer deaths, which translates to 192,370 new cases and 40,170 deaths.[1] Breast cancer was also the most common form of cancer seen in Europe in 2006, with 429,900 new cases, representing 13.5% of all new cancers.[2] Since 1990, the death rate from breast cancer has decreased in the United States by 24% and similar reductions have been observed in other countries.[3,4] Mathematical models suggest that both the adoption of screening mammography and the availability of adjuvant chemotherapy and tamoxifen have contributed approximately equally to this improvement.[5] Although breast cancer has traditionally been less common in nonindustrialized nations, its incidence in these areas is increasing. Industrialization in developing countries is associated with rapid increases in breast cancer risk.[6]

This chapter examines the salient features of breast cancer, stressing practical information of importance to clinicians and the results of prospective randomized trials that guide therapeutic decisions.

ANATOMY OF THE BREAST

The adult female breast lies between the second and sixth ribs and between the sternal edge and the midaxillary line. The breast is composed of skin, subcutaneous tissue, and breast tissue, with the breast tissue including both epithelial and stromal elements. Epithelial elements make up 10% to 15% of the breast mass, with the remainder being stroma. Each breast consists of 15 to 20 lobes of glandular tissue supported by fibrous connective tissue. The space between lobes is filled with adipose tissue, and differences in the amount of adipose tissue are responsible for changes in breast size. The blood supply of the breast is derived from the internal mammary and lateral thoracic arteries. The breast lymphatic drainage occurs through a superficial and deep lymphatic plexus, and more than 95% of the lymphatic drainage of the breast is through the axillary lymph nodes, with the remainder via the internal mammary nodes. The axillary nodes are variable in number and have traditionally been divided into three levels based on their relationship to the pectoralis minor muscle, as illustrated in Figure 106.1. The internal mammary nodes are located in the first six intercostal spaces within 3 cm of the sternal edge, with the highest concentration of internal mammary nodes in the first three intercostal spaces.

RISK FACTORS FOR BREAST CANCER

Multiple factors are associated with an increased risk of developing breast cancer, including increasing age, family history, exposure to female reproductive hormones (both endogenous and exogenous), dietary factors, benign breast disease, reproductive history, and environmental factors. The majority of these factors convey a small to moderate increase in risk for any individual woman. It has been estimated that approximately 50% of women who develop breast cancer have no identifiable risk factor beyond increasing age and female gender. The importance of age as a breast cancer risk factor is sometimes overlooked. In 2009 it was estimated that 18,640 invasive breast cancers and 2,820 breast cancer deaths occurred in U.S. women under age 45 compared with 173,730 cancers and 37,350 deaths in women aged 45 years and older.[1]

Familial Factors

A family history of breast cancer has long been recognized as a risk factor for the disease. The majority of women diagnosed with breast cancer do not have a family member with the disease, and only 5% to 10% have a true hereditary predisposition to breast cancer. Many women with a positive family history overestimate their risk of developing breast cancer, and women considering genetic testing have been shown to overestimate their chance of having a mutation. Overall, the risk of developing breast cancer is increased 1.5-fold to threefold if a woman has a mother or sister with breast cancer. Family history, however, is a heterogeneous risk factor with different implications depending on the number of relatives with breast cancer, the exact relationship, the age at diagnosis, and the number of unaffected relatives. For example, there may be a minimal elevation in breast cancer risk for a woman whose mother was diagnosed with breast cancer at an advanced age and who has no other family history of the disease. In contrast, a woman who has multiple family members diagnosed with early-onset breast cancer is at a much higher risk of developing the disease. Even in the absence of a known inherited predisposition, women with a family history of breast cancer face some level of increased risk, likely from some combination of shared environmental exposures, unexplained genetic factors, or both.

Inherited Predisposition to Breast Cancer

Mutations in the breast cancer susceptibility genes *BRCA1* and *BRCA2* are associated with a significant increase in the risk of breast and ovarian carcinoma and account for 5% to 10% of all breast cancers. These mutations are inherited in an autosomal dominant fashion and have varying penetrance. As a result, the estimated lifetime risk of breast cancer development in mutation carriers ranges from 26% to 85%, and the risk of ovarian cancer from 16% to 63% and 10% to 27%, respectively, in carriers of *BRCA1* and *BRCA2*.[7] More than 700 different mutations of *BRCA1* and 300 different mutations of

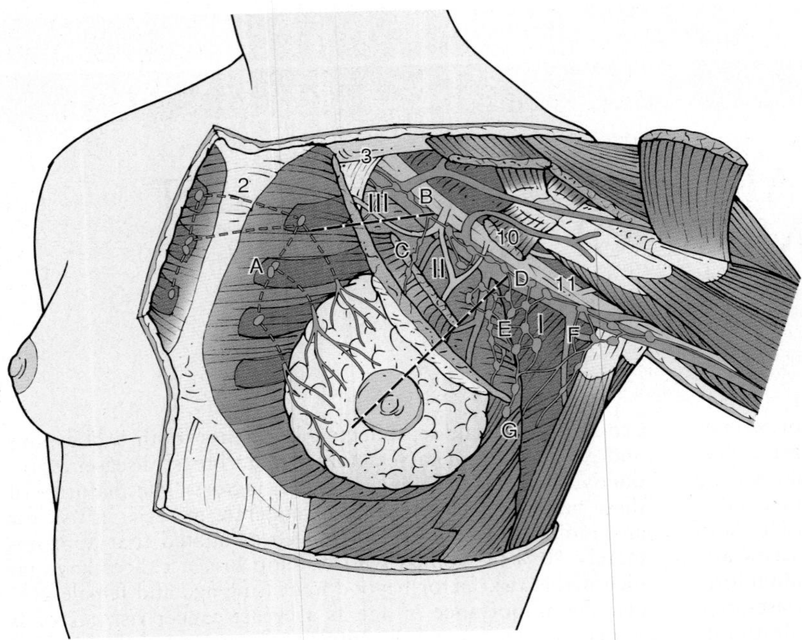

FIGURE 106.1 Lymphatic drainage of the breast showing lymph node groups and levels. 1, Internal mammary artery and vein; 2, substernal cross-drainage to contralateral internal mammary lymphatic chain; 3, subclavius muscle and Halsted ligament; 4, lateral pectoral nerve (from the lateral cord); 5, pectoral branch from thoracoacromial vein; 6, pectoralis minor muscle; 7, pectoralis major muscle; 8, lateral thoracic vein; 9, medial pectoral nerve (from the medial cord); 10, pectoralis minor muscle; 11, median nerve; 12, subscapular vein; 13, thoracodorsal vein. Internal mammary lymph nodes (**A**); apical lymph nodes (**B**); interpectoral (Rotter) lymph nodes (**C**); axillary vein lymph nodes (**D**); central lymph nodes (**E**); scapular lymph nodes (**F**); external mammary lymph nodes (**G**). Level I lymph nodes: lateral to lateral border of pectoralis minor muscle; level II lymph nodes: behind pectoralis minor muscle; level III lymph nodes: medial to medial border of pectoralis minor muscle.

BRCA2 have been described, and the position of the mutation within the gene has been shown to influence the risk of both breast and ovarian cancers, with an increased risk of ovarian carcinoma among *BRCA1* carriers with mutations in the 5′ two-thirds of the gene and an increased risk of ovarian carcinoma among *BRCA2* carriers with mutations between nucleotides 4075–6503.

Other cancers associated with *BRCA1* or *BRCA2* mutations include male breast cancer, fallopian tube cancer, and prostate cancer. Carriers of *BRCA2* may also have an elevated risk of melanoma and gastric cancer. Management strategies available for risk reduction in *BRCA1/2* mutation carriers include intensive surveillance, chemoprevention with selective estrogen receptor modulators (SERMs), and prophylactic (breast and salpino-ovarian) surgery, and these are discussed in a later section. There is a great interest in the role of environmental and lifestyle factors in the modification of cancer risk among *BRCA1* or *BRCA2* carriers; at present, however, the available data are inconsistent. It is worth noting that women with a significant family history of breast cancer (i.e., two or more breast cancers under the age of 50 years, or three or more breast cancers at any age), but who test negative for *BRCA* mutations have approximately a fourfold risk of breast cancer and that women in these families may be candidates for tamoxifen chemoprevention and/or intensified breast screening.[8]

The histologic features of cancers arising in women with *BRCA1* mutations differ from those occurring sporadically, with a higher incidence of medullary features and a higher proportion of grade 3 tumors. The proportion of *BRCA1* cancers expressing the estrogen receptor (ER) or progesterone receptor (PR) is lower than is seen in sporadic cancers, and *HER2* overexpression is infrequent.[9] This triple-negative pattern is consistent with the basal cell phenotype. In contrast, it is not clear that the phenotype of *BRCA2* cancers differs from that seen in sporadic cancers, although some studies have suggested an excess of tubular and lobular carcinomas.

The presence of a *BRCA1* or *BRCA2* mutation may be suggested by the family history on either the maternal or paternal side of the family. The features considered by the 2005 U.S. Preventive Services Task Force[10] are listed in Table 106.1. Less rigorous criteria for referral for genetic counseling are used for individuals of Ashkenazi Jewish ancestry because the carrier frequency of specific *BRCA1* (187delAG, 5385 ins C) and *BRCA2* (6174delT) mutations in this group is 1:40 compared with 1:500 in the general population. These guidelines are particularly useful for individuals not affected with breast cancer. In the newly diagnosed breast cancer patient, young age at diagnosis (40 years or less), bilateral breast cancer, Ashkenazi ancestry, or a malignancy consistent with the *BRCA1* phenotype all constitute reasons for referral to a genetic counselor, particularly in the woman with a small number of female relatives. Genetic testing should be preceded by a careful evaluation of an individual's personal cancer history and family history. Models are available to estimate the likelihood of a *BRCA1* or *BRCA2* mutation based on family history. The implications of genetic testing for both individuals and their family members are considerable, and these issues should be discussed prior to undertaking genetic testing.

TABLE 106.1

FACTORS SUGGESTIVE OF *BRCA1* OR *BRCA2* MUTATION

Non-Ashkenazic Jewish women
Two first-degree relatives[a] with breast cancer, one diagnosed ≤50 years
Three or more first- or second-degree relatives with breast cancer, any age
Breast and ovarian cancer among first- and second-degree relatives
First-degree relative with bilateral breast cancer
Breast cancer in a male relative
Two or more first- or second-degree relatives with ovarian cancer
Ashkenazic Jewish women
First-degree relative with breast or ovarian cancer
Two second-degree relatives with breast or ovarian cancer

[a]Relatives on the same side of the family.

Other genetic mutations have been associated with breast cancer risk, although to a much lesser extent than *BRCA1* and *BRCA2*. *TP53* and *PTEN* each account for less than 1% of cases. Mutations in low-penetrance genes are thought to account for a significant number of non–*BRCA1* or *BRCA2* breast cancers. A specific mutation of the checkpoint kinase 2 (*CHEK2*) gene was found in 11.4% of families with three or more cases of breast cancer diagnosed before age 60,[11] but in a large study of 10,860 unselected breast cancer patients from five countries the *CHEK2* mutation was identified in only 1.9% of cases[12] and 0.7% of controls (odds ratio, 2.34). At this time, because of the low penetrance of this gene, genetic counseling and testing for *CHEK2* is considered premature.[13]

Hormonal Factors

The development of breast cancer in many women appears to be related to female reproductive hormones. Epidemiologic studies have consistently identified a number of breast cancer risk factors associated with increased exposure to endogenous estrogens. Early age at menarche, nulliparity or late age at first full-term pregnancy, and late age at menopause increase the risk of developing breast cancer. In postmenopausal women, obesity and postmenopausal hormone replacement therapy (HRT), both of which are positively correlated with plasma estrogen levels and plasma estradiol levels, are associated with increased breast cancer risk. Furthermore, *in utero* exposure to high concentrations of estrogen may also increase breast cancer risk. Most hormonal risk factors have a relative risk of 2.0 or less for breast cancer development.

The age-specific incidence of breast cancer increases steeply with age until menopause. After menopause, although the incidence continues to increase, the rate of increase decreases to approximately one-sixth of that seen in the premenopausal period. The dramatic slowing of the rate of increase in the age-specific incidence curve suggests that ovarian activity plays a major role in the etiology of breast cancer. There is substantial evidence that estrogen deprivation via iatrogenic premature menopause can reduce breast cancer risk. Epidemiologic studies have shown that premenopausal women who undergo oophorectomy without hormone replacement have a markedly reduced risk of breast cancer later in life. Oophorectomy before age 50 decreases breast cancer risk, with an increasing magnitude of risk reduction as the age at oophorectomy decreases.[14] Data from women with *BRCA1* and *BRCA2* mutations suggest that early oophorectomy has a substantial protective effect on breast cancer risk in this population as well.[15]

Age at menarche and the establishment of regular ovulatory cycles are strongly linked to breast cancer risk. Earlier age at menarche is associated with an increased risk of breast cancer; there appears to be a 20% decrease in breast cancer risk for each year that menarche is delayed. Of note, hormone levels through the reproductive years in women who experience early menarche may be higher than in women who undergo a later menarche.[16] Additionally, late onset of menarche results in a delay in the establishment of regular ovulatory cycles, although there is some controversy over whether this delay confers any additional protective effect. From these data regarding menarche and menopause, it seems likely that the total duration of exposure to endogenous estrogen is an important factor in breast cancer risk.

The relationship between pregnancy and breast cancer risk appears more complicated. Based on epidemiologic studies, women whose first full-term pregnancy occurs after age 30 have a two- to fivefold increase in breast cancer risk in comparison with women who have a first full-term pregnancy before approximately age 18.[16,17] Nulliparous women are at greater risk for the development of breast cancer than parous women, with a relative risk of about 1.4. Breast cancer risk increases transiently after a pregnancy. The increased risk, which lasts approximately 10 years, is then associated with a more durable protective effect.[17] The reason for the increased risk may be the increased proliferation that precedes terminal differentiation before lactation. Alternatively, risk may increase secondarily to the effect of high levels of hormones on subclinical cancers. Abortion, whether spontaneous or induced, does not appear to increase breast cancer risk.[18] Breastfeeding, particularly for longer duration, lowers the risk of breast cancer diagnosis. The combined effects of reproductive history and breastfeeding may account for substantial fractions of the difference in breast cancer risk between developed and developing nations.

The use of combined estrogen and progestin HRT also increases breast cancer risk. In the Women's Health Initiative, 16,688 postmenopausal women aged 50 to 79 years with an intact uterus were randomly assigned to receive conjugated equine estrogen (0.625 mg) and medroxyprogesterone acetate (2.5 mg) daily or placebo. When compared with placebo, the use of HRT was associated with a hazard ratio of 1.24 ($P < .001$) for breast cancer development.[19] The effects of HRT were noted after a relatively short duration of use. An excess of abnormal mammograms was observed after 1 year of HRT use and persisted throughout the study, and an increase in breast cancer incidence was noted after 2 years. The cancers occurring in HRT users were larger and more likely to have nodal or distant metastases than those occurring in the placebo group (25.4% vs. 16%; $P = .04$), although they were of similar histology and grade.[19] The findings of the Women's Health Initiative are supported by the results of the Million Women Study, an observational study of 1,084,110 women in the United Kingdom. In this study, current use of HRT was associated with a relative risk of breast cancer development of 1.66 ($P < .001$) and a relative risk of breast cancer death of 1.22 ($P = .05$).[20]

Dietary and Lifestyle Factors

There is substantial interest in whether dietary or lifestyle factors modify breast cancer risk. Observational studies suggested that high-fat diets were associated with higher rates of breast cancer than low-fat diets. However, meta-analysis of eight prospective epidemiologic studies failed to identify an association between fat intake and breast cancer risk in adult women in developed countries.[21] There may be a moderate protective effect from high vegetable consumption, but results for fruit, fiber, and meat consumption are inconclusive. In contrast, there appears to be a positive association between alcohol and breast cancer risk, with risk increasing linearly with the amount of alcohol consumed.[22] Decreased intake of nutrients such as vitamin C, folate, and β-carotene may enhance the risk related to alcohol consumption.

Obesity is associated with both an increased risk of breast cancer development in postmenopausal women and increased breast cancer mortality. In the placebo arm of the Women's Health Initiative study, women with a body mass index of 31.1 or higher had a 2.5-fold greater risk of developing breast cancer than those with a body mass index of 22.6 or lower.[19] Weight and weight gain appears to play an important but complex role in breast cancer risk. During childhood, rapid growth rates decrease the age of menarche, an established risk factor, and result in greater attained stature, which has been consistently associated with increased risk. During early adult life, overweight is associated with a lower incidence of breast cancer before menopause, but no reduction in breast mortality. Weight gain after age 18 is associated with a graded and substantial increase in postmenopausal breast cancer, particularly in the absence of HRT.[23]

BENIGN BREAST DISEASE

Benign breast lesions are classified as proliferative or nonproliferative. Nonproliferative disease is not associated with an increased risk of breast cancer, whereas proliferative disease without atypia results in a small increase in risk (relative risk [RR], 1.5 to 2.0). Proliferative disease with atypical hyperplasia is associated with a greater risk of cancer development (RR, 4.0 to 5.0).[24] Dupont and Page[25] found a marked interaction between atypia and a family history of a first-degree relative with breast cancer. This subgroup of patients had a risk 11-fold that of women with nonproliferative breast disease. The absolute risk of breast cancer development in women with a positive family history and atypical hyperplasia was 20% at 15 years, compared with 8% in women with atypical hyperplasia and a negative family history of breast carcinoma. Proliferative breast disease appears to be more common in women with a significant family history of breast cancer than in controls, further supporting its significance as a risk factor. Of note, however, the majority of breast biopsies done for clinical indications demonstrate nonproliferative disease. In the study of 10,000 breast biopsies by Dupont and Page,[25] 69% had nonproliferative changes and only 3.6% demonstrated atypical hyperplasia. No increased risk of breast cancer development has been observed in women with a diagnosis of proliferative disease who have used estrogens after breast biopsies.

BREAST DENSITY

Mammographic breast density has emerged as an important predictor of breast cancer risk, in addition to making the detection of cancer more difficult. A significant component of breast density is genetically determined, although density has also been shown to vary with the initiation and discontinuation of postmenopausal HRT. In a case control study of 1,112 case-control pairs undergoing screening mammography, women with more than 75% breast density had a 4.7-fold increase in the odds of breast cancer development compared with those with less than 10% breast density (95% confidence interval [CI], 2.0–6.2).[26] The risk was apparent even after adjustment for other risk factors.

ENVIRONMENTAL FACTORS

Exposure to ionizing radiation increases breast cancer risk, and the increase is particularly marked for exposure at a young age. This pattern has been observed in survivors of the atomic bombings, those undergoing multiple diagnostic x-ray examinations, and in women receiving therapeutic irradiation. A markedly increased risk of breast cancer development has been reported in women who received mantle irradiation for the treatment of Hodgkin lymphoma before age 15 years.[27] Other environmental factors, including exposure to electromagnetic fields and organochlorine pesticides, have been suggested to increase breast cancer risk, but convincing documentation from well-conducted studies is lacking. A summary of the magnitude of risk associated with known breast cancer risk factors is provided in Table 106.2.

MANAGEMENT OF THE HIGH-RISK PATIENT

A woman's risk of developing breast cancer is influenced by a number of factors. There is no formal definition of what constitutes *high risk*. Without question, women who carry mutations in either *BRCA1* or *BRCA2* or who have a family history consistent with genetically transmitted breast cancer are considered to be at higher risk than those in the general population. A second and much less common group of high-risk women consists of those individuals who have received mantle irradiation, usually for treatment of Hodgkin lymphoma. Women with lobular carcinoma *in situ* (LCIS) or atypical hyperplasia on breast biopsy are also considered at high risk. Although a variety of hormonal factors (e.g., early menarche, late age at first full-term pregnancy) affect breast cancer risk on a population basis, these conditions have a relatively small effect on risk for any individual woman.

In approaching women concerned about breast cancer risk, it is important to recognize that many women overestimate their risk of developing breast cancer. Providing women with an accurate assessment of breast cancer risk may have a number of benefits, including allaying anxiety and facilitating management decisions. The first step in determining a woman's risk of developing breast cancer is to take a thorough history, evaluating for the presence of known risk factors. Of these, family history, age, and the presence of a premalignant lesion on previous breast biopsy are probably the most significant. Because of the substantially higher risk of identifying a *BRCA1* or *BRCA2* mutation in women of Ashkenazic Jewish descent, ethnic background should also be established. It can be helpful to provide women who are concerned about their breast cancer risk with a numeric risk estimate. A number of models for risk assessment are available, of which the Gail et al.[28] model and a model developed by Claus et al.[29] from the Cancer and Steroid Hormone Study are the most frequently used. The Gail et al. model, which calculates a woman's risk of developing breast cancer based on age at menarche, age at first live birth, number of previous breast biopsies, the presence or absence of atypical hyperplasia, and the number of first-degree female

TABLE 106.2

MAGNITUDE OF RISK OF KNOWN BREAST CANCER RISK FACTORS

Relative Risk <2	Relative Risk 2–4	Relative Risk >4
Early menarche	One first-degree relative with breast cancer	Mutation *BRCA1* or *BRCA2*
Late menopause	*CHEK2* mutation	LCIS
Nulliparity	Age >35 y for first birth	Atypical hyperplasia
Estrogen plus progesterone	Proliferative breast disease	Radiation exposure before 30
HRT	Mammographic breast density	
Alcohol use		
Postmenopausal obesity		

LCIS, lobular carcinoma *in situ;* HRT, hormone replacement therapy.

TABLE 106.3

AMERICAN CANCER SOCIETY GUIDELINES FOR MAGNETIC RESONANCE IMAGING (MRI) SCREENING

Annual MRI recommended based on evidence
- *BRCA* mutation
- Untested first-degree relative of *BRCA* carrier
- Lifetime risk of breast cancer 20% to 25%

Annual MRI recommended based on expert opinion
- Radiation to chest between age 10 and 30 y
- Li-Fraumeni syndrome and first-degree relatives
- Cowden and Bannayan-Riley-Ruvalcaba syndromes and first-degree relatives

Insufficient evidence to recommend for or against MRI
- Lifetime breast cancer risk 15% to 20%
- Lobular carcinoma *in situ*
- Atypical hyperplasia (lobular or ductal)
- Extremely or heterogeneously dense breasts on mammogram
- Personal history of breast cancer, including ductal carcinoma *in situ*

relatives with breast cancer, has been used in the National Surgical Adjuvant Breast and Bowel Project (NSABP) breast cancer prevention trials. Efforts to validate the Gail et al. model in different settings have produced variable results. In the Nurses' Health Study cohort, the Gail et al. model was found to overestimate breast cancer risk, although in other settings it has proven to be more accurate. In the NSABP P1 prevention trial,[30] the Gail et al. model performed extremely well, with a ratio of observed to predicted cancers in study participants of 1.03 (95% CI, 0.88–1.22). In general, the Gail et al.[28] model is thought to underestimate risk in women with strong family histories, at least in part because it only incorporates a family history in first-degree relatives and does not include ovarian carcinoma.

The Claus et al.[29] model, on the other hand, takes into account both first- and second-degree relatives, although it does not include other risk factors. Models are also available to predict the likelihood of a *BRCA1* or *BRCA2* mutation based on family history, although they do not assess the risk of cancer development. Although limitations of these models must be discussed with women undergoing risk assessment, they provide a useful starting point for discussions regarding genetic testing and the potential benefits of strategies to reduce breast cancer risk.

Management strategies available for risk reduction in the high-risk woman include intensive surveillance, chemoprevention with SERMs, and prophylactic surgery. Surveillance, consisting of monthly breast self-examination, annual screening mammography, and clinical breast examinations once or twice yearly, does not clearly result in early detection in high-risk women. In the placebo arm of the NSABP P1 prevention trial where this strategy was employed, 29% of the women who developed breast cancer had axillary node metastases at diagnosis.[30] In the population of women at risk as a result of known or suspected *BRCA1* or *BRCA2* mutations, an increasing body of evidence indicates that screening with magnetic resonance imaging (MRI) results in earlier detection of breast cancer than conventional surveillance strategies. Warner et al.[31] performed a meta-analysis that included 11 studies comparing screening mammography and MRI in high-risk women. The sensitivity of MRI was 75% compared with 32% for mammography, and combining the examinations resulted in a sensitivity of 84%. The specificity of MRI was 96%. Although these studies have not demonstrated a mortality reduction with MRI screening of *BRCA* mutation carriers, the observation that the cancers detected in the MRI group were smaller and less likely to be associated with nodal positivity suggests that a survival benefit is likely to be present. In contrast, a study examining the benefit of MRI screening in women at risk on the basis of atypical hyperplasia or LCIS failed to find clear evidence of benefit.[32] An expert panel convened by the American Cancer Society in 2007 to develop guidelines for MRI screening recommended the use of MRI in addition to mammography for a small group of women at very high risk of breast cancer development (Table 106.3). For women with less than a 15% risk of breast cancer development, the American Cancer Society recommended against the use of MRI screening.[33] In the remainder, they thought that the evidence was insufficient to recommend for or against MRI screening.

Chemoprevention is an option in addition to surveillance strategies. Two SERMs, tamoxifen and raloxifene, have been shown to reduce the incidence of ER-positive breast cancer. Four prospective, randomized trials have examined the effect of tamoxifen on breast cancer incidence. These studies and their outcomes are summarized in Tables 106.4 and 106.5.[30,34–36] There is considerable heterogeneity in outcome among the trials, much of which can be attributed to differences in the populations studied. An Italian trial required women to have undergone a hysterectomy, but did not require an increase

PRACTICE OF ONCOLOGY

TABLE 106.4

A COMPARISON OF TAMOXIFEN CHEMOPREVENTION STUDIES

Study (Ref.)	Age Range (y)	Family History (%)	HRT Use (%)	Lost to Follow-Up (%)
Royal Marsden (34) N = 2,471	30–70, median 47	100	26	11
NSABP P-1 (30) N = 13,388	>35, median NS	76	0	1.6
Italian (35) N = 5,408	35–70, median 51	21	24.7	0.8
IBIS (36) N = 7,152	35–70, median 50.8	97	39.7	NS

HRT, hormone replacement therapy; NSABP, National Surgical Adjuvant Breast and Bowel Project; NS, not stated; IBIS, International Breast Cancer Intervention Study.

TABLE 106.5

OUTCOME OF TAMOXIFEN CHEMOPREVENTION STUDIES

Study (Ref.)	Median Follow-Up (mo)	Total Cancers	Breast Cancer Rate (per 1,000 women-years)		RR (95% CI)
			Placebo	Tamoxifen	
Royal Marsden (34)	70	70	5.0	4.7	0.94 (0.59–1.43)
NSABP P-1 (30)	54.6	368	6.8	3.4	0.51 (0.39–0.66)
Italian (35)	81.2	79	2.3	2.1	0.87 (0.62–2.14)
IBIS (36)	96	337	6.8	5.0	0.73 (0.58–0.91)

RR, relative risk tamoxifen to placebo; CI, confidence interval; NSABP, National Surgical Adjuvant Breast and Bowel Project; IBIS, International Breast Cancer Intervention Study.

in breast cancer risk,[35] while the Royal Marsden study used a family history of breast cancer as the determinant of risk status.[34] In an overview of the four studies, tamoxifen produced a 38% reduction in breast cancer incidence (95% CI, 8%–46%; P <.001), and a 48% reduction in the incidence of ER-positive breast cancers.[37] No effect on the incidence of ER-negative cancers was seen in any of the trials, and the cancers occurring in women taking tamoxifen were not found to have had more positive nodes or to be larger in size than those in the placebo arm, providing reassurance that tamoxifen chemoprevention does not result in the occurrence of biologically more aggressive cancers.

In the largest of these studies, the NSABP P1 trial, a 49% risk reduction was seen with tamoxifen, with 43.4 cancers per 1,000 women occurring in the placebo arm compared with 22.0 per 1,000 in the tamoxifen arm.[30] The benefits of tamoxifen were observed for both invasive and noninvasive carcinoma and were seen in women of all ages. A particular benefit was seen in those at risk because of atypical hyperplasia, with an 84% reduction in cancer incidence in this group. The risk reductions were similar in those at risk on the basis of a family history of breast cancer and those at risk from other factors. Controversy exists over the benefit of tamoxifen in *BRCA* mutation carriers. Only 19 of 288 women who developed breast cancer in the NSABP P1 study were found to have a *BRCA1* or *BRCA2* mutation. No evidence of tamoxifen benefit was seen in the eight *BRCA1* carriers who received the drug. In contrast, a nonsignificant trend toward tamoxifen benefit was seen in *BRCA2* carriers.[38] These findings are consistent with observations that ER-positive cancers are more common in *BRCA2* mutation carriers than *BRCA1* mutation carriers, but the small sample size limits any conclusions. In a retrospective, case-controlled study of *BRCA* carriers who received tamoxifen for treatment of their initial carcinoma, Narod et al.[39] reported a 50% reduction in the incidence of contralateral cancer. Benefit was seen in both *BRCA1* and *BRCA2* mutation carriers. These findings suggest that it is the likelihood of expressing the ER that determines the efficacy of tamoxifen as a chemopreventive agent rather than the presence of a *BRCA* mutation.

The side effects of tamoxifen were well known from its use as a cancer treatment and were again observed in the prevention trials. In the combined analysis of the four studies, the relative risk of thromboembolic events in tamoxifen users was 1.9 (95% CI, 1.4–2.6; P <.0001) and the relative risk of endometrial cancer was 2.4 (95% CI, 1.5–4.0; P = .0005).[37] Significant elevation in endometrial cancer and thromboembolic events was limited to postmenopausal women. Using this information, populations of women likely to have the most favorable risk-benefit ratio for tamoxifen can be identified. These include premenopausal women, younger postmenopausal women without a uterus, and those at risk on the basis of atypical hyperplasia or LCIS. In spite of this, use of tamoxifen for chemoprevention has been limited because of concerns about side effects.

Raloxifene is another SERM that was initially approved for the treatment and prevention of osteoporosis by the U.S. Food and Drug Administration (FDA). Studies of raloxifene in osteoporotic women demonstrated a reduction in the incidence of breast cancer, a secondary end point. Like tamoxifen, raloxifene reduces the incidence of ER-positive breast cancer and has no effect on the incidence of ER-negative breast cancer. The NSABP P2 trial, the Study of Tamoxifen and Raloxifene (STAR) directly compared the chemopreventive actions and side effects of tamoxifen and raloxifene in 19,747 postmenopausal women at increased risk of breast cancer development.[40] After a mean follow-up of 3.9 years, no difference in the incidence of invasive cancer was seen between women taking tamoxifen and those taking raloxifene (RR 1.02; 95% CI, 0.82–1.28). More cases of noninvasive cancer were noted in the raloxifene group (RR, 1.40; 95% CI, 0.98-2.00), with a cumulative incidence of 11.7 per 1,000 compared with 8.1 per 1,000 in the tamoxifen group at 6 years (P = .052). A more favorable side effect profile was seen for raloxifene, with an 84% reduction in endometrial hyperplasia and a statistically significant reduction in the number of hysterectomies compared with tamoxifen. The number of endometrial cancers was also reduced in the raloxifene group (RR, 0.62; 95% CI, 0.35–1.08), although the difference did not reach statistical significance. Significantly fewer thromboembolic events and cataracts occurred with raloxifene. The results of this study indicate that raloxifene is a viable alternative to tamoxifen for the chemoprevention of breast cancer in postmenopausal women at increased risk for the disease. In addition, the use of raloxifene in women with osteoporosis has the potential to lower breast cancer incidence in a group of women not considered at high risk. Trials of aromatase inhibitors (AIs) for breast cancer prevention are ongoing based on the findings from adjuvant therapy trials (discussed later in this chapter) that show that AIs produce a greater reduction in contralateral breast cancer incidence than is seen with tamoxifen treatment. The reduction in cancer incidence seen with AIs is also limited to ER-positive cancers. At present, there are no chemopreventive agents that have been proven to be effective in reducing the incidence of ER-negative breast cancer.

Prophylactic surgery, in the form of bilateral mastectomy or bilateral salpingo-oophorectomy, is another option for breast cancer risk reduction. The efficacy of prophylactic mastectomy has never been studied in a prospective, randomized trial. Data on the benefits of the procedure are derived from retrospective reviews and case-control studies. Hartmann et al.[41] identified 639 women with a family history of breast cancer who had undergone bilateral prophylactic mastectomy

TABLE 106.6

OUTCOME OF BILATERAL PROPHYLACTIC MASTECTOMY IN HIGH-RISK WOMEN

Author (Ref.)	Population	No. of Women	Follow-Up (y)	Risk Reduction (5)
Hartmann et al. (41)	Women with a family history of breast cancer	639	14 (median)	90–94
Meijers-Heijboer et al. (42)	*BRCA1/2* mutation carriers	139	3 (mean)	100
Rebbeck et al. (43)	*BRCA1/2* mutation carriers	105	6.4 (mean)	90–95

between 1960 and 1993. Women were characterized as high risk if their family history was suggestive of an autosomal dominant predisposition to breast cancer. The expected incidence of cancer in this group was estimated using the age-specific incidence of breast cancer in their sisters. The remaining 425 women were classified as moderate risk, and the predicted incidence of breast cancer was derived from the Gail et al.[28] model. A 90% to 94% reduction in breast cancer incidence (95% CI, 71%–99%) and an 81% to 100% reduction in breast cancer mortality were observed with prophylactic mastectomy. In a prospective study of 139 *BRCA* mutation carriers with a mean follow-up of 3 years, Meijers-Heijboer et al.[42] observed no breast cancers in the group undergoing prophylactic mastectomy compared with a 2.5% per year incidence in those opting for surveillance. Rebbeck et al.[43] reported a mixed retrospective and prospective study of 483 *BRCA* mutation carriers. In this study, prophylactic mastectomy reduced breast cancer incidence by 90% to 95%. Studies of prophylactic mastectomy are summarized in Table 106.6.

Although bilateral prophylactic mastectomy is an effective form of breast cancer risk reduction, even in women at risk because of *BRCA* mutations, it is an intervention that is unacceptable to many women. Prophylactic bilateral salpingo-oophorectomy is an alternative risk-reduction strategy in women at risk on the basis of *BRCA* mutations, which has the added benefit of reducing the risk of ovarian carcinoma, a disease for which effective screening is not available. In a prospective study of the benefits of prophylactic salpingo-oophorectomy in 170 *BRCA* mutation carriers, Kauff et al.[15] observed that the hazard ratio for breast cancer was reduced to 0.32 (95% CI, 0.08–1.20) and that for gynecologic cancer to 0.25 (95% CI, 0.08–0.74) at a mean follow-up of 24 months. Rebbeck et al.[44] performed a meta-analysis of risk-reduction estimates associated with risk-reducing salpingo-oophorectomy in BRCA1 or BRCA2 mutation carriers and found that risk-reducing salpingo-oophorectomy was associated with statistically significant reductions in breast cancer (hazard ratio [HR], 0.49; 95% CI, 0.37–0.65 with similar risk reductions in *BRCA1* and *BRCA2* mutation carriers) and in the risk of *BRCA1/2*-associated ovarian or fallopian tube cancer (HR, 0.21; 95% CI, 0.12–0.39).

DIAGNOSIS AND BIOPSY

The presence or absence of carcinoma in a suspicious clinically or mammographically detected abnormality can only be reliably determined by tissue sampling. The high sensitivity of MRI for cancer detection raised the possibility that this technique could replace biopsy in the evaluation of suspicious breast lesions. In a multi-institutional prospective study of 821 patients referred for breast biopsy, the sensitivity of MRI was 88.1% (95% CI, 84.6%–91.1%) and the specificity was 67.7% (95% CI, 62.7%–71.9%), indicating that an abnormal MRI does not reliably indicate the presence of cancer, and a nonworrisome MRI does not reliably exclude carcinoma.[45]

A biopsy remains the standard technique for diagnosing both palpable and nonpalpable breast abnormalities. The available biopsy techniques for the diagnosis of palpable breast masses are fine-needle aspiration (FNA), core-cutting needle biopsy, and excisional biopsy. The advantages and disadvantages of each are listed in Table 106.7.

Both FNA and core biopsy are office procedures. FNA is easily performed, but requires a trained cytopathologist for accurate specimen interpretation. The sensitivity of FNA ranges from 80% to 95%, and false-positive aspirates are seen in less than 1% of cases in most series. False-negative results are seen in 4% to 10% of cases and are most common in fibrotic or well-differentiated tumors.[46] Although an FNA diagnosis of malignant cells is sufficient to proceed with definitive treatment, FNA does not reliably distinguish invasive

TABLE 106.7

BIOPSY TECHNIQUES FOR BREAST LESIONS

Technique	Advantages	Disadvantages
Fine-needle aspiration cytology	Rapid, painless, inexpensive. No incision prior to selection of local therapy.	Does not distinguish invasive from *in situ* cancer. Markers (ER, PR, *HER2*) not routinely available. Requires experienced cytopathologist. False-negative results and insufficient specimens occur.
Core-cutting needle biopsy	Rapid, relatively painless, inexpensive. No incision. Can be read by any pathologist, markers routinely available.	False-negative results, incomplete lesion characterization can occur.
Excisional biopsy	False-negative results rare. Complete histology before treatment decisions. May serve as definitive lumpectomy.	Expensive, more painful. Creates an incision to be incorporated into definitive surgery. Unnecessary surgery with potential for cosmetic deformity in patients with benign abnormalities.

ER, estrogen receptor; PR, progesterone receptor.

PRACTICE OF ONCOLOGY

cancer from ductal carcinoma *in situ* (DCIS), potentially leading to the overtreatment of gross DCIS.

Core-cutting needle biopsy has many of the advantages of FNA, but provides a histologic specimen suitable for interpretation by any pathologist. In addition, ER and PR status and the presence of *HER2* overexpression can be routinely determined from core biopsy specimens, making core needle biopsy the diagnostic technique of choice for patients who will receive preoperative systemic therapy. False-negative results from sampling error may also occur with core-cutting needle biopsy. If concordance between the core biopsy diagnosis and the clinical and imaging findings is not present, additional tissue should be obtained, usually by excisional biopsy.

When excisional biopsy is performed for diagnosis, a small margin of grossly normal breast should be excised around the tumor, orienting sutures should be placed, and the specimen should be inked to allow margin evaluation. This procedure allows an assessment of the completeness of the excision if carcinoma is found, sparing patients with negative margins further breast surgery and allowing re-excision to be limited to the involved margin surface(s). However, diagnosis by needle biopsy is the preferred initial method of evaluating almost all breast masses. A needle biopsy diagnosis permits a complete discussion of treatment options prior to the placement of an incision on the breast and allows the breast procedure and the axillary surgery to take place at a single operation. In addition, needle biopsy is a more cost-effective method of diagnosing benign lesions than surgical excision.

Nonpalpable lesions can be biopsied with image-guided core needle biopsy or surgical excision after wire localization. Ultrasound guidance is used for lesions that are visualized with this modality; most calcifications require stereotactic mammographic guidance for biopsy. There is little role for FNA in the diagnosis of lesions detected by screening because of the high prevalence of *in situ* lesions. Concerns about the false-negative rate of image-guided core biopsy have been resolved with the availability of large, vacuum-assisted biopsy devices that increase the extent of lesion sampling, coupled with the development of clearly defined indications for follow-up surgical biopsy. In a study of 318 patients with mammographic abnormalities diagnosed by core biopsy between September 1997 and December 2001, the false-negative rate was 3.3%. For radiologists who had done more than 15 biopsies, the false-negative rate was 0.6%. All of the false negatives were recognized at the time, with no delay in the diagnosis of cancer.[47] Indications for surgical biopsy following core biopsy are listed in Table 106.8. Although the finding of atypical ductal hyperplasia on a core biopsy is uniformly accepted as an indication for surgical biopsy, the need for surgical excision of all lesions showing atypical lobular hyperplasia or LCIS remains controversial (discussed in the section "Lobular Carcinoma *in situ*").

TABLE 106.8

INDICATIONS FOR SURGICAL BIOPSY AFTER CORE NEEDLE BIOPSY

Failure to sample calcifications
Diagnosis of atypical ductal hyperplasia
Diagnosis of atypical lobular hyperplasia or lobular carcinoma *in situ*[a]
Lack of concordance between imaging findings and histologic diagnosis
Radial scar
Papillary lesions

[a]See text for details.

Papillary carcinoma *in situ* cannot always be readily distinguished from benign papillary lesions on a core biopsy, and radial scar may be difficult to distinguish from tubular carcinoma without complete removal of the lesion.

The use of core biopsy for the diagnosis of mammographic abnormalities is cost-effective and increases the likelihood that the patient will be able to undergo a single surgical procedure for definitive cancer treatment. In a prospective study of 1,550 consecutive patients undergoing biopsy for mammographic abnormalities, core biopsy reduced the number of surgical procedures needed for cancers presenting as both masses and calcifications as well as in patients requiring axillary staging and those treated by mastectomy.[48] In a cost analysis using patients from this data set, core biopsy resulted in cost savings for all clinical scenarios. In spite of this, in a study of 5.5 million mammograms performed in two U.S. government–sponsored screening programs and the U.K. National Health Service between 1996 and 1999, 51% of the biopsies performed in the United States were surgical, compared with 23% in the United Kingdom.[49]

LOBULAR CARCINOMA *IN SITU*

In 1941 Foote and Stewart[49a] published their landmark study of LCIS, describing a relatively uncommon entity characterized by an "alteration of lobular cytology." Foote and Stewart chose the name to emphasize the morphologic similarities between the cells of LCIS and those of invasive lobular carcinoma (ILC). They hypothesized that LCIS represented a precursor lesion of invasive cancer, and, based on this, mastectomy was initially recommended. Subsequent studies, discussed later, have shown that the risk of subsequent breast cancer is bilateral. More recently, the term *atypical lobular hyperplasia* (ALH) has been introduced to describe morphologically similar, but less well-developed lesions. Some centers use the term *lobular neoplasia* (LN) to cover both ALH and LCIS. Morphologically, LN is defined as "a proliferation of generally small and often loosely cohesive cells originating in the terminal duct-lobular unit, with or without pagetoid involvement of terminal ducts."[50]

In the past, LCIS was most frequently diagnosed in women aged 40 to 50, a decade earlier than DCIS, but recent literature indicates that the incidence in postmenopausal women is increasing.[51] Determining the true incidence of LCIS is difficult as there are no specific clinical or mammographic abnormalities associated with the lesion. LCIS is typically not associated with microcalcifications on mammography. The diagnosis of LCIS is therefore often made as an incidental, microscopic finding in a breast biopsy performed for other indications. The prevalence of LN in an otherwise benign breast biopsy has been reported as between 0.5% and 4.3%.[52] LCIS is both multifocal and bilateral in a large percentage of cases.

In an analysis of nine separate studies evaluating outcome following a diagnosis of LCIS, 172 patients who were treated by biopsy alone were identified. On follow-up averaging about 10 years, 15% of these patients had invasive carcinoma diagnosed in the ipsilateral breast and 9.3% had invasive carcinoma in the contralateral breast.[53] This corresponds to an increased rate of development of invasive carcinoma of about 1% to 2% per year, with a lifetime risk of 30% to 40%. In this study (conducted prior to effective breast imaging), 5.7% of the patients developed metastatic breast cancer. Subsequent cancers are more often invasive ductal carcinoma than ILC, but the incidence of subsequent ILC is substantially increased compared with women without LCIS. Although the risk for development of breast cancer is bilateral, subsequent ipsilateral carcinoma is more likely than contralateral breast, supporting the view that ALH and LCIS act both as precursor lesions and as risk indicators. The relative risk for development of subsequent breast cancer is lower in women diagnosed with ALH compared with LCIS. Therefore, although LN is a helpful term for collectively describing this group of lesions, specific classification into ALH and LCIS is preferable in terms of risk assessment and management.

LCIS is typically positive for ER and PR staining by immunohistochemistry (IHC) and negative for *HER2/neu* staining. LN (and ILC) characteristically lacks expression of E-cadherin, an epithelial cell membrane molecule involved in cell-cell adhesion. E-cadherin negativity serves as a fairly reliable means of distinguishing ductal from lobular disease, both *in situ* and invasive. Pleomorphic LCIS is a relatively uncommon variant of LCIS characterized by medium to large pleomorphic cells containing eccentric nuclei, prominent nucleoli, and eosinophilic cytoplasm. As with classic LCIS, it is usually ER-positive and negative for E-cadherin; it also tests positive by IHC for gross cystic disease fluid protein-15. Pleomorphic LCIS can be associated with central necrosis and may be associated with mammographic microcalcifications. It is not clear at this time whether pleomorphic LCIS has a different natural history than classic LCIS.

Genetic changes in LN have been evaluated in a number of studies using comparative genomic hybridization. In one study ALH showed gain at 2p11.2 and loss at 7p11-p11.1 and 22q11.1, and LCIS showed gain at 20q13.13 and loss at 19q13.2-q13.31.[54] In both ALH and LCIS, there was loss at 16q21-q23.1, an altered region previously identified in invasive carcinoma. This genomic signature, common to LN and ILC, further suggests that LN is a precursor lesion in some women.

Management of LN must address the bilateral risk, and options therefore include surveillance, chemoprevention, and prophylactic bilateral mastectomy. Surveillance is the strategy selected by most patients. Mammographic screening is the standard breast imaging for patients selecting surveillance. Breast MRI has been used, but there is no firm evidence supporting its efficacy; its value is being tested in a randomized clinical trial in Europe. Prophylactic mastectomy reduces breast cancer risk among high-risk women by approximately 90%. Chemoprevention with tamoxifen in patients with LCIS has been evaluated as part of the NSABP P1 study.[30] In this prospective, placebo-controlled clinical trial, with a median follow-up of 54.6 months, tamoxifen reduced the incidence of breast cancer by 49% (P <.00001). Eight hundred twenty-six of the participants had a history of LCIS, and breast cancers were detected in 18 women randomized to placebo and eight to tamoxifen, consistent with the overall reduction in breast cancer risk seen with tamoxifen. However, with the small number of events, this difference was not statistically significant. In the NSABP P2 (STAR) trial comparing tamoxifen and raloxifene, comparable efficacy in risk reduction was observed.[40] In this study, 893 participants gave a history of LCIS, and their rates of subsequent breast cancer were similar with tamoxifen and raloxifene. This benefit with tamoxifen or raloxifene needs to be weighed against the possible side effects of treatment.

Although the data are conflicting, it is generally recommended to perform an excisional biopsy after detection of LN on a core needle biopsy to rule out coexisting DCIS or invasive cancer. Some have advocated a more selective approach to LCIS on core biopsy based on whether or not there is concordance between the pathology and imaging findings. With LCIS, most reported cases of malignant findings on subsequent excision occur in the setting of either a suspicious mass lesion or calcifications that prompted the biopsy initially. The recent recognition that in some cases LCIS may be a precursor lesion has led to confusion as to whether it should be treated like DCIS (i.e., excised to negative margins and irradiated). At this time, there are no data indicating that the incidence of subsequent cancer is reduced with this approach. When LCIS is seen on an excised tissue, it is not necessary to obtain negative margins of resection, and there is no established role for radiation therapy in patients with LN.

DUCTAL CARCINOMA *IN SITU*

DCIS is defined as the proliferation of malignant-appearing mammary ductal epithelial cells without evidence of invasion beyond the basement membrane. Prior to the widespread use of screening mammography, fewer than 5% of mammary cancers were DCIS. At present 15% to 30% of the cancers detected in mammography screening programs are DCIS, and the greatest increase in the incidence of DCIS has been seen in women aged 49 to 69 years. DCIS can present as a palpable mass, Paget disease of the nipple, an incidental finding at biopsy, or a mammographically detected mass or calcifications, with calcifications being the most common presentation.

A central problem in the management of DCIS is the lack of understanding of its natural history and the inability to determine which DCIS will progress to invasive carcinoma during a woman's lifetime. The concordance between risk factors for DCIS and invasive carcinoma suggests that they are part of the same disease process.[55] Attempts to better characterize the natural history of DCIS on the basis of pathologic features have not been particularly successful. The traditional morphologic classification into comedo, papillary, micropapillary, solid, and cribriform types is confounded by the observation that as many as 30% to 60% of DCIS lesions display more than one histologic pattern. To overcome this difficulty, a number of classifications based on nuclear grade and the presence or absence of necrosis have been developed. No single classification scheme has been widely adopted, and most importantly, none of the classification systems have been prospectively demonstrated to predict the risk of development of invasive carcinoma. Molecular profiling studies in DCIS have been limited by the need for histologic examination of the entire lesion to reliably exclude the presence of invasive carcinoma. The available data indicate that DCIS lesions share many of the genetic alterations of invasive carcinoma, but predictors of progression to invasion remain to be identified.

TREATMENT OF THE BREAST

Cancer-specific survival for the woman diagnosed with DCIS exceeds 95%, regardless of the type of local therapy employed.[56,57] Mastectomy, excision and radiotherapy (RT), and excision alone have all been proposed as management strategies for DCIS. The appropriate therapy for the woman with DCIS depends on the extent of the DCIS lesion, the risk of local recurrence with each form of treatment, and the patient's attitude toward the risks and benefits of a particular therapy.

Total or simple mastectomy is a treatment for which all women with DCIS are eligible, and it is curative in approximately 98% of patients regardless of age, DCIS presentation, size, or grade.[58] The primary medical indication for mastectomy in DCIS is a lesion too large to be excised to negative margins with a cosmetically acceptable outcome.[59] The extent of DCIS is most accurately estimated preoperatively with the use of magnification mammography. Conventional two-view mammography underestimates the extent of the lesion, particularly for well-differentiated DCIS.[60] Initial studies indicate that MRI both overestimates and underestimates the size of DCIS lesions and does not improve surgical planning when compared with diagnostic mammography.

For women with localized DCIS, management by excision alone and excision plus RT have both been employed. Four prospective, randomized trials have directly compared these two approaches in more than 4,500 patients.[56,57,61,62] In all

TABLE 106.9

RANDOMIZED TRIALS OF EXCISION WITH OR WITHOUT RADIOTHERAPY IN DUCTAL CARCINOMA *IN SITU*

		Ipsilateral Local Recurrence				Overall Survival		
Trial (Ref.)	No. of Patients	Without RT	With RT	Risk Reduction	*P* Value	Without RT	With RT	*P* Value
NSABP B-17 (56) 12-y results	813	31.7	15.7	50	<.00005	86	87	.8
EORTC 10853 (57) 10.5-y results	1,010	26	15	47	<.0001	95	95	.53
UK/ANZ (61) Med FU = 12.7-y crude incidence	1,030	21	8	68	<.0001	Differences were not statistically different		
Swedish (62) 8 y = mean FU; 10-y cum incidence	1,067	29	13	60	<.0001	Differences were not statistically different		

RT, radiotherapy; NSABP, National Surgical Adjuvant Breast and Bowel Project; EORTC, European Organisation for Research and Treatment of Cancer; UK/ANZ, United Kingdom/Australia New Zealand; FU, follow-up; cum, cumulative.

four trials, the majority of participants had mammographically detected DCIS, and in all but the Swedish trial,[62] negative margins, defined as tumor-filled ducts not touching an inked surface, were required. A dose of 50 Gy of radiation was delivered to the whole breast in 25 fractions, and a boost dose to the tumor bed was not required. A tumor bed boost was employed in 9% and 5% of patients in the NSABP B-17[56] and European Organisation for Research and Treatment of Cancer (EORTC) 10853[57] studies, respectively. The UK/ANZ (United Kingdom/Australia New Zealand) study has a two-by-two randomization that randomized patients to RT versus none and tamoxifen versus none, and institutions and patients could select to participate in one or both randomizations, creating imbalances between the four arms.[61] The other studies did not allow tamoxifen. The results of these trials are summarized in Table 106.9. No differences in overall survival were seen between treatment arms. In all four studies, the use of RT resulted in a highly significant reduction in the risk of an ipsilateral breast tumor recurrence, with proportional risk reductions ranging from 47% in the EORTC study[57] to 68% in the UK/ANZ study.[61] Consistent with observations from many retrospective studies, approximately 50% of the recurrences in both the irradiated and the nonirradiated groups were invasive carcinoma, and a benefit for RT was seen in the reduction of both invasive and noninvasive recurrences.

Subset analyses in these trials failed to identify any patient subgroups not benefiting from RT, but emphasize that the magnitude of the benefit of RT varies with the risk of local recurrence.[57] Patient age has been consistently identified as an important predictor of local recurrence after excision and RT. In the NSABP B-17 trial local recurrence rates ranged from 15% in women age 49 years or less to 9% in those 60 years or older.[56,57] The EORTC trial reported a relative risk of recurrence of 1.89 (95% CI, 1.12–3.19; $P = .026$) for women aged 40 and younger in multivariate analysis.[57] The increased incidence of local recurrence in younger women was confirmed in the NSABP B-24 trial.[56] Clinical presentations of DCIS were associated with a higher rate of local recurrence than mammographic ones in both the EORTC trial[57] and the NSABP B-24 study[56]; and both the NSABP B-17 trial and the EORTC 10853 trials found high- and intermediate-grade DCIS to be more commonly associated with local recurrence than low-grade DCIS.[56,57]

In spite of the clear benefit of RT seen in these four trials, considerable interest in identifying patients who could be spared the cost and inconvenience of RT has persisted. In a retrospective review, Silverstein et al.[63] reported the outcome of patients with DCIS treated with and without RT and suggested that if a negative margin width of 1 cm or greater was obtained, RT was not beneficial in reducing local recurrence, regardless of the characteristics of the DCIS lesion. Wong et al.[64] attempted to duplicate these findings in a prospective study of 158 patients with predominantly grade 1 and 2 DCIS who underwent excision to a negative margin greater than 1 cm. The 5-year local recurrence rate was 12%, and 31% of the recurrences were invasive, resulting in premature closure of the study prior to its planned accrual of 200 patients. The Eastern Cooperative Oncology Group (ECOG) conducted a prospective, single-arm study of the outcome of excision alone in selected patients with DCIS, which involved routine detailed pathologic assessment with sequential sectioning and embedding of the complete specimen.[65] Eligible patients included those with DCIS larger than 3 mm in size excised to a negative margin width of 3 mm or more. For patients with low- or intermediate-grade DCIS, the upper limit of lesion size was 2.5 cm or less, and for those with high-grade lesions the upper size limit was 1 cm or less. There were 579 patients with low- or intermediate-grade DCIS, with a median tumor size of 6 mm; 67% were excised to a margin of 5 mm or greater and 46% to a margin of 1 cm or greater. At a median follow-up of 6.7 years, the 5-year rate of an ipsilateral breast event (local recurrence) was 15.3% (95% CI, 8.2%–22.5%) for the 105 eligible patients with high-grade DCIS, and with a median follow-up of 6.2 years, the 5-year rate of an ipsilateral breast event (local recurrence) was 6.1% (95% CI, 4.1%–8.2%) for the 565 eligible patients with low- and intermediate-grade DCIS. The 101 patients with high-grade DCIS had a median tumor size of 7 mm. Seventy-five percent were excised to a margin of 5 mm or greater, and 48% had a margin of 1 cm or more. In considering the results of excision alone in the low- and intermediate-grade group, it is worth noting that older studies that examined the 5-year results of the treatment of DCIS with excision and RT observed a significantly higher rate of local recurrence for high-grade DCIS compared with low- and intermediate-grade DCIS, but after 10 years of follow-up no differences in the rate of local recurrence on the basis of grade were seen.[66] Additional follow-up of the ECOG study will be important in determining the risks of treatment with excision alone for low- and intermediate-grade DCIS.

Based on the information discussed previously, guidelines for breast-conserving surgery in DCIS developed by a joint committee of the American College of Surgeons, American College of Radiology, and College of American Pathologists recommend mastectomy for multicentric DCIS when there are diffuse malignant calcifications in the breast and when negative margins cannot be obtained.[59] Breast-conserving surgery with radiation is recommended for those with localized DCIS excised to clear margins. Although the value of a "boost" has not been formally tested in patients with DCIS, it is generally recommended, particularly for young patients, based on trial results testing the value of a boost in patients with invasive breast cancer. The committee acknowledged that low local recurrence rates after wide excision of low-grade DCIS have been reported, but thought that the maximum size DCIS lesion for which RT could be safely omitted was unknown. They concluded that these cases must be evaluated individually, with the patients' attitude toward risks and benefits playing a major role in the decision to omit RT.[59]

TREATMENT OF THE AXILLA

In situ carcinoma by definition does not metastasize, so theoretically axillary staging should be unnecessary in the patient with DCIS. Many studies of axillary dissection in patients with DCIS have demonstrated axillary nodal metastases in only 1% to 2% of patients, presumably due to unrecognized microinvasion. The availability of sentinel node biopsy as a low-morbidity method of axillary staging has caused the issue of axillary staging of DCIS to be revisited. Data from the NSABP B-17 and B-24 studies confirm that the risk of isolated axillary recurrence with no axillary surgery is less than 0.1%, regardless of whether RT and tamoxifen are administered.[67] These low rates of axillary recurrence do not provide justification for the routine use of sentinel lymph node biopsy in DCIS. Most investigators agree that selective use of sentinel node biopsy in patients with DCIS who are at significant risk of having coexistent invasive carcinoma is appropriate. Patients diagnosed as having DCIS with large vacuum-assisted biopsy devices are found to have invasive cancer in approximately 5% to 18% of cases after complete excision of the lesion. In patients requiring mastectomy, the opportunity for sentinel node biopsy is lost if it is not performed at the time of mastectomy, and the performance of a mastectomy is an indication for sentinel node biopsy. The diagnosis of DCIS in a palpable breast mass and pathologic interpretation of a core biopsy specimen as suspicious, but not diagnostic of microinvasion, are also circumstances in which invasive cancer is frequently found when the lesion is completely examined and sentinel node biopsy should be considered.

ENDOCRINE THERAPY

The ER is present in about 80% of DCIS lesions and is more frequent in noncomedo than comedo DCIS.[68] Endocrine therapy has two potential benefits in women with DCIS: a reduction in local recurrence after breast-conserving therapy (BCT) and the prevention of the development of new primary breast cancers in the contralateral breast. Although most of the attention in DCIS has focused on local recurrence, Solin et al.[69] have demonstrated that the 15-year risk of new ipsilateral and contralateral cancers in women with DCIS is equal to the risk of true local recurrence at the primary tumor site.

Two trials have examined the use of tamoxifen in women with DCIS with somewhat conflicting results. In the NSABP B-24 trial,[56] 1,804 patients with DCIS were treated with excision and RT and randomized to tamoxifen 20 mg daily or a placebo for 5 years. At a median follow-up of 83 months, patients in the tamoxifen arm had an 28.2% incidence of all breast cancer events compared with 17.7% in the placebo group (P = .0003). Tamoxifen reduced the risk of ipsilateral invasive recurrences by 47% and reduced the risk of contralateral invasive and noninvasive cancers by 47%. Allred et al.[68] reported a subset analysis of 628 patients in the study who had an ER determination. In women with ER-positive breast cancer, tamoxifen reduced the risk of any breast cancer event by 59% (RR, 0.41; 95% CI, 0.25–0.65; P = .0002). In women with ER-negative tumors, no significant benefit was seen. In contrast, little or no benefit for tamoxifen (largely given in the absence of irradiation) in reducing ipsilateral events was demonstrated in the UK/ANZ trial.[60] With 1,575 patients randomized to tamoxifen or to no tamoxifen and with a median follow-up of 12.7 years, tamoxifen marginally reduced ipsilateral events (HR, 0.78; 95% CI, 0.62–0.99), but significantly reduced contralateral events (HR, 0.44; 95% CI, 0.25–0.77) as seen in the NSABP B-24 trial. Taken together, these two trials suggest that tamoxifen adds to the benefit of RT in reducing ipsilateral events, but has little benefit in the absence of RT. In either case, tamoxifen substantially reduced contralateral events. The addition of tamoxifen to RT is particularly attractive in young patients with ER-positive DCIS, in whom the risk of local recurrence is higher and the toxicity of tamoxifen is less than in older patients.

Evidence that the AIs reduce the incidence of contralateral breast cancer to a greater extent than tamoxifen has led to interest in their use in DCIS. Several randomized trials directly comparing tamoxifen with an AI are ongoing and will provide important information about whether the increased benefit in reducing contralateral carcinoma seen with the AIs is outweighed by the increased risk of osteoporosis associated with this drug group.

In summary, patients with localized DCIS have treatment options ranging from simple excision to mastectomy, all of which have high survival rates but different risks of local recurrence. Patient preference plays a major role in treatment selection, but available evidence indicates that patients have limited understanding of the nature of DCIS. In one study, women with DCIS estimated their risk of breast cancer death to be 39%.[70] Perhaps related to this, Katz et al.[71] found that although patients reported that their surgeon infrequently recommended mastectomy for DCIS, greater involvement of patients in the decision-making process was associated with higher rates of mastectomy.

STAGING

The staging system for breast cancer was last updated in 2010.[72] The major changes in this edition were the inclusion of a new classification system for patients after neoadjuvant therapy and the creation of a new M0(i+) category for patients found to have circulating tumor cells, tumor in the bone marrow, or incidentally detected tumor deposits in other tissues not exceeding 0.2 mm in size. Patients in this category are staged according to T and N and are not classified as stage IV.

Tumor, Node, and Metastases Definitions

Definitions for classifying the primary tumor (T) are the same for clinical and for pathologic classification. If the measurement is made by physical examination, the examiner will use the major headings (T1, T2, or T3). If other measurements are used, such as mammographic or pathologic measurements, the subsets of T1 can be used. Tumors should be measured to the nearest 0.1 cm increment. The American Joint Committee on Cancer (AJCC) TNM staging system is illustrated in Table 106.10. Stage IIIC breast cancer includes patients with any T stage who have pN3 disease. Patients with pN3a and pN3b disease are considered operable and are managed as described in the section on stage I, II, IIIA, and operable IIIC breast cancer. Patients with pN3c disease are considered inoperable and are managed as described in the section on inoperable stage IIIB or IIIC or inflammatory breast cancer.[73] Pathologic stage after neoadjuvant therapy is designated with the prefix "yp." Complete response is defined as the absence of invasive carcinoma in the breast and axillary nodes.

TABLE 106.10

AMERICAN JOINT COMMITTEE ON CANCER STAGING

Primary Tumor (T)

TX: Primary tumor cannot be assessed
T0: No evidence of primary tumor
Tis: Carcinoma *in situ*
Tis: DCIS
Tis: LCIS
Tis (Paget): Paget disease of the nipple NOT associated with invasive carcinoma and/or carcinoma *in situ* (DCIS and/or LCIS) in the underlying breast parenchyma. Carcinomas in the breast parenchyma associated with Paget disease are categorized based on the size and characteristics of the parenchymal disease, although the presence of Paget disease should still be noted.
T1: Tumor ≤20 mm in greatest dimension
T1mi: Tumor ≤1 mm in greatest dimension
T1a: Tumor >1 mm but ≤5 mm in greatest dimension
T1b: Tumor >5 mm but ≤10 mm in greatest dimension
T1c: Tumor >10 mm but ≤20 mm in greatest dimension
T2: Tumor >20 mm but ≤50 mm in greatest dimension
T3: Tumor >50 mm in greatest dimension
T4: Tumor of any size with direct extension to the chest wall and/or to skin (ulceration or skin nodules).
[Note: Invasion of the dermis alone does not qualify as T4]
T4a: Extension to chest wall, not including only pectoralis muscle adherence/invasion
T4b: Ulceration and/or ipsilateral satellite nodules and/or edema (including peau d'orange) of the skin, which do not meet the criteria for inflammatory carcinoma
T4c: Both T4a and T4b
T4d: Inflammatory carcinoma

Regional Lymph Nodes (N)

NX: Regional lymph nodes cannot be assessed (e.g., previously removed)
N0: No regional lymph node metastases
N1: Metastases to movable ipsilateral level I, II axillary lymph node(s)
N2: Metastases in ipsilateral level I, II axillary lymph nodes that are clinically fixed or matted; or in clinically detected[a] ipsilateral internal mammary nodes in the *absence* of clinically evident lymph node metastases
N2a: Metastases in ipsilateral level I, II axillary lymph nodes fixed to one another (matted) or to other structures.
N2b: Metastases only in clinically detected[a] ipsilateral internal mammary nodes and in the *absence* of clinically evident level I, II axillary lymph node metastases
N3: Metastases in ipsilateral infraclavicular (level III axillary) lymph node(s) with or without level I, II axillary lymph node involvement; or in clinically detected[a] ipsilateral internal mammary lymph node(s) with clinically evident level I, II axillary lymph node metastases; or metastases in ipsilateral supraclavicular lymph node(s) with or without axillary or internal mammary lymph node involvement
N3a: Metastases in ipsilateral infraclavicular lymph node(s)
N3b: Metastases in ipsilateral internal mammary lymph node(s) and axillary lymph node(s)
N3c: Metastases in ipsilateral supraclavicular lymph node(s)

Pathologic (pN)[b]

pNX: Regional lymph nodes cannot be assessed (e.g., previously removed, or not removed for pathologic study)
pN0: No regional lymph node metastasis identified histologically
[Note: ITC clusters are defined as small clusters of cells not greater than 0.2 mm, or single tumor cells, or a cluster of fewer than 200 cells in a single histologic cross-section. ITCs may be detected by routine histology or by IHC methods. Nodes containing only ITCs are excluded from the total positive node count for purposes of N classification but should be included in the total number of nodes evaluated.]
pN0(i–): No regional lymph node metastases histologically, negative IHC
pN0(i+): Malignant cells in regional lymph node(s) no greater than 0.2 mm (detected by H&E or IHC including ITC)
pN0(mol–): No regional lymph node metastases histologically, negative molecular findings (RT-PCR)
pN0(mol+): Positive molecular findings (RT-PCR), but no regional lymph node metastases detected by histology or IHC
pN1: Micrometastases; or metastases in 1 to 3 axillary lymph nodes; and/or in internal mammary nodes with metastases detected by SLNB but not clinically detected[c]
pN1mi: Micrometastases (>0.2 mm and/or more than 200 cells, but none >2.0 mm)
pN1a: Metastases in 1 to 3 axillary lymph nodes, at least one metastasis >2.0 mm
pN1b: Metastases in internal mammary nodes with micrometastases or macrometastases detected by SLNB but not clinically detected[c]
pN1c: Metastases in 1 to 3 axillary lymph nodes and in internal mammary lymph nodes with micrometastases or macrometastases detected by SLNB but not clinically detected.
pN2: Metastases in 4 to 9 axillary lymph nodes; or in clinically detected[d] internal mammary lymph nodes in the *absence* of axillary lymph node metastases
pN2a: Metastases in 4 to 9 axillary lymph nodes (at least one tumor deposit >2.0 mm)
pN2b: Metastases in clinically detected[d] internal mammary lymph nodes in the *absence* of axillary lymph node metastases

TABLE 106.10

(CONTINUED)

pN3: Metastases in ten or more axillary lymph nodes; or in infraclavicular (level III axillary) lymph nodes; or in clinically detected[d] ipsilateral internal mammary lymph nodes in the *presence* of one or more positive level I, II axillary lymph node(s); or in more than 3 axillary lymph nodes and in internal mammary lymph nodes with micrometastases or macrometastases detected by SLNB but not clinically detected[c]; or in ipsilateral supraclavicular lymph nodes

pN3a: Metastases in ten or more axillary lymph nodes (at least one tumor deposit >2.0 mm); or metastases to the infraclavicular (level III axillary) lymph nodes

pN3b: Metastases in clinically detected[d] ipsilateral internal mammary lymph nodes in the *presence* of one or more positive axillary lymph nodes; or in more than 3 axillary lymph nodes and in internal mammary lymph nodes with micrometastases or macrometastases detected by sentinel lymph node biopsy but not clinically detected[c]

pN3c: Metastases in ipsilateral supraclavicular lymph nodes

Distant Metastases (M)

M0: No clinical or radiographic evidence of distant metastases

cM0(i+): No clinical or radiographic evidence of distant metastases, but deposits of molecularly or microscopically detected tumor cells in circulating blood, bone marrow, or other nonregional nodal tissue that are no larger than 0.2 mm in a patient without symptoms or signs of metastases

M1: Distant detectable metastases as determined by classic clinical and radiographic means and/or histologically proven larger than 0.2 mm

Anatomic Stage/Prognostic Groups

Stage 0
Tis, N0, M0

Stage IA
T1[e], N0, M0

Stage IB
T0, N1mi, M0
T1[e], N1mi, M0

Stage IIA
T0, N1[f],M0
T1[e], N1[f], M0
T2, N0, M0

Stage IIB
T2, N1, M0
T3, N0, M0

Stage IIIA
T0, N2, M0
T1[e], N2, M0
T2, N2, M0
T3, N1, M0
T3, N2, M0

Stage IIIB
T4, N0, M0
T4, N1, M0
T4, N2, M0

Stage IIIC
Any T, N3, M0

Stage IV
Any T, Any N, M1

DCIS, ductal carcinoma *in situ;* LCIS, lobular carcinoma *in situ;* ITC, isolated tumor cells; IHC, immunohistochemical; H&E, hematoxylin and eosin stain; RT-PCR, reverse transcriptase-polymerase chain reaction; SLNB, sentinel lymph node biopsy

[a]Clinically detected is defined as detected by imaging studies (excluding lymphoscintigraphy) or by clinical examination and having characteristics highly suspicious for malignancy or a presumed pathologic macrometastasis based on fine-needle aspiration biopsy with cytologic examination. Confirmation of clinically detected metastatic disease by fine-needle aspiration without excision biopsy is designated with an (f) suffix, for example, cN3a(f). Excisional biopsy of a lymph node or biopsy of a sentinel node, in the absence of assignment of a pT, is classified as a clinical N, for example, cN1. Information regarding the confirmation of the nodal status will be designated in site-specific factors as clinical, fine-needle aspiration, core biopsy, or SLNB. Pathologic classification (pN) is used for excision or SLNB only in connection with a pathologic T assignment.

[b]Classification is based on axillary lymph node dissection with or without SLNB. Classification based solely on SLNB without subsequent axillary lymph node dissection is designated (sn) for "sentinel node," for example, pN0(sn).

[c]"Not clinically detected" is defined as not detected by imaging studies (excluding lymphoscintigraphy) or by clinical examination.

[d]"Clinically detected" is defined as detected by imaging studies (excluding lymphoscintigraphy) or by clinical examination and having characteristics highly suspicious for malignancy or a presumed pathologic macrometastasis based on fine-needle aspiration biopsy with cytologic examination.

[e]T1 includes T1mi.

[f]T0 and T1 tumors with nodal micrometastases only are excluded from stage IIA and are classified as stage IB.

(From ref. 72, with permission.)

PATHOLOGY OF BREAST CANCER

Invasive breast cancers constitute a heterogeneous group of lesions that differ with regard to their clinical presentation, radiographic characteristics, pathologic features, and biologic behavior. Historically, classification of invasive breast cancers has been based on the morphologic appearance of the cancer as seen by light microscopy.[74] The most widely used such classification is that of the World Health Organization (2nd edition).[50] This classification scheme is based on the growth pattern and cytologic features of the invasive tumor cells and, as currently used, is not meant to imply site of origin in the breast. Although the classification system recognizes invasive "ductal" and "lobular" carcinomas, this is not meant to indicate that the former originates in the ducts and the latter in the lobules of the breast. Most invasive breast cancers are thought to arise in the terminal duct lobular unit, regardless of histologic type.

The most common histologic type of invasive breast cancer is invasive (infiltrating) ductal carcinoma. The diagnosis of invasive ductal carcinoma is a diagnosis by exclusion (i.e., this tumor type is defined as a type of cancer not classified into any of the other special categories of invasive mammary carcinoma, such as invasive lobular, tubular, mucinous, medullary, and other special types). To emphasize this point, most classification systems use the term *infiltrating ductal carcinoma, not otherwise specified* (NOS) or *infiltrating carcinoma of no special type* (NST). In practice, the terms invasive ductal carcinoma, infiltrating ductal carcinoma, and infiltrating or invasive carcinoma of no special type are used interchangeably.

Infiltrating or invasive ductal cancer is the most common breast cancer histologic type and comprises 70% to 80% of cases. Special types of cancers comprise approximately 20% to 30% of invasive carcinomas, and at least 90% of a tumor should demonstrate the defining histologic characteristics of a special type of cancer to be designated as that histologic type.

The following is a list of breast cancer histologic classifications.

- Ductal
- Invasive, NOS
- Invasive with predominant intraductal component
- Intraductal (*in situ*)
- Comedo
- Inflammatory
- Medullary with lymphocytic infiltrate
- Mucinous (colloid)
- Papillary
- Scirrhous
- Tubular
- Other
- Lobular
- *In situ*
- Invasive with predominant *in situ* component
- Invasive
- Nipple
- Paget disease, NOS
- Paget disease with intraductal carcinoma
- Paget disease with invasive ductal carcinoma
- Other
- Undifferentiated carcinoma

The following are tumor subtypes that occur in the breast, but are not considered to be typical breast cancers:

- Cystosarcoma phyllodes
- Angiosarcoma
- Primary lymphoma

Recognizing that invasive ductal carcinomas are histologically diverse with variable biologic behavior, many investigators have attempted to subclassify them based on microscopic features. The most common method to subclassify invasive ductal carcinomas has been grading, which can be based solely on nuclear features (nuclear grading) or on a combination of architectural and nuclear characteristics (histologic grading). In nuclear grading, the appearance of the tumor cell nuclei is compared with those of normal breast epithelial cells, and the tumor nuclei are classified as well differentiated, intermediately differentiated, or poorly differentiated. In current practice, histologic grading is the most commonly used method of grading. In histologic grading, breast carcinomas are categorized based on the evaluation of (1) tubule formation, (2) nuclear pleomorphism, and (3) mitotic activity. The most widely used histologic grading is that proposed by Elston and Ellis[75] and is a modification of the grading system proposed by Bloom and Richardson in 1957. Tubule formation (>75%, 10% to 75%, and <10%), nuclear pleomorphism (small and uniform, moderate variation in size and shape, and marked nuclear pleomorphism), and mitotic activity (per field area) are each scored on a scale of 1 to 3. The sum of the scores for these three parameters is the overall histologic grade. Tumors with a sum of the scores of 3 to 5 are designated grade 1 (well differentiated), those with sums of 6 and 7 are designated grade 2 (moderately differentiated), and those with sums of 8 and 9 are designated grade 3 (poorly differentiated). Histologic grading has been shown to have prognostic significance and is discussed in the section "Prognostic and Predictive Factors." In addition, breast cancers with pure tubular, mucinous papillary, or cribriform features are recognized to have a more favorable outcome than the more common types of breast cancer.[74]

LOCAL MANAGEMENT OF INVASIVE CANCER

The evaluation of the patient newly diagnosed with breast cancer begins with a determination of operability. The presence of distant metastases at diagnosis has traditionally been considered a contraindication to surgery. Some retrospective studies have suggested a survival benefit for surgery of the primary tumor in the patient presenting with metastatic disease,[76,77] but systemic therapy remains the initial therapeutic approach. Extensive evaluations to look for metastatic disease are not warranted in asymptomatic patients with stage I and II cancer because of the low likelihood of identifying metastatic disease. A review of the detection rate of staging studies in women with stage I cancer reported a 0.5% incidence of metastases found on bone scan and a 0.1% incidence on chest radiograph. For stage II disease these figures were 2.4% and 0.2%, respectively.[78] The detection rate of occult metastases by computed tomography (CT) scans and positron emission tomography scans is also low, and the routine use of these tests is neither medically appropriate nor cost-effective. In patients with stage III disease, occult metastases are more frequent, often estimated at 20% of cases, and staging studies are recommended.[78]

Patients with T4 tumors and those with N2 nodal disease are also not candidates for surgery as the first therapeutic approach and should be treated with systemic therapy initially. Current management strategies for this group of women are discussed in the section "Locally Advanced and Inflammatory Cancer." In the patient with clinical stage I, II, and T3N1 disease, the initial management is usually surgical. In these patients, the evaluation consists of a determination of their suitability for BCT and a discussion of the options of mastectomy with and without reconstruction. Initial systemic therapy may be used to shrink the primary tumor to allow BCT in a woman who would otherwise require mastectomy but is not mandatory, as it is for women with locally advanced and inflammatory carcinoma. The current status of management approaches for primary operable breast cancer is discussed in detail in the following sections.

BREAST-CONSERVING THERAPY

The goal of BCT using conservative surgery (CS) and RT is to provide survival equivalent to mastectomy with preservation of the cosmetic appearance and a low rate of recurrence in the treated breast. Because of the wide acceptance of the Halstedian dogma, a relatively large number of randomized clinical trials were conducted comparing mastectomy and BCT, and they demonstrated equivalent survival. The long-term stability of this equivalence was confirmed by the 20-year follow-up reports of the two largest studies, the Milan I and NSABP B-06 trials.[79,80] An overview of all the trials has also demonstrated comparable survival,[81] indicating that survival for most breast cancer patients does not depend on the choice of mastectomy versus BCT.

In addition to the results of these trials, retrospective reports from centers in Europe and North America on the use of CS and RT with long follow-up have helped to document the time course and pattern of recurrence in the breast, factors associated with an increased risk of recurrence in the breast, and information regarding cosmetic outcomes after BCT. This information has been useful in determining the optimal approach to CS and RT, in providing guidelines for patient selection, and in providing patients treated with CS and RT with important information on their expected outcome.

Despite the consistency of the evidence, the use of BCT in the United States has shown relatively slow acceptance, with considerable geographic variation.[82] Potential explanations for the continued use of mastectomy in significant numbers of women include (1) large numbers of patients with contraindications to BCT, (2) patient preference for mastectomy, and (3) use of inappropriate selection criteria by physicians. Medical contraindications are not the major factor responsible for underuse of BCT. In a population-based study of 1984 patients with DCIS, stage I and II breast cancer, only 13.4% were advised by their surgeon that mastectomy was medically necessary.[83] In the 1,459 women in whom BCT was attempted, conversion to mastectomy occurred in 12%, and re-excision was not attempted in the majority. Thus, the available data indicate that a minority of patients have contraindications to BCT, and these are readily identified with standard clinical tools. Patient participation in the surgical decision-making process is an important factor in mastectomy use.

Contrary to expectation, in a population-based study of patients diagnosed with breast cancer in 2002 in two large metropolitan areas (Los Angeles and Detroit), more patient involvement in decision making was associated with a *greater* likelihood of undergoing mastectomy.[84] Among white women, only 5% of patients whose surgeon made the decision underwent mastectomy compared with 17% of women who shared the decision and 27% of women who made the decision ($P < .001$, adjusted for other factors). This association was less pronounced among black women. Among women who perceived having a choice between surgical treatments, approximately 40% were greatly concerned about recurrence, approximately 18% about recovery, approximately 15% about RT, and approximately 10% about body/sexuality issues. Patients who were greatly concerned about recurrence and about RT were significantly more likely to undergo mastectomy, while patients who were greatly concerned about body/sexuality issues were significantly less likely to undergo mastectomy. This population-based study also found that similar patients get different treatment depending on their surgeon,[85] and that the most important aspect for satisfaction with decision making is the match between the patients' preferences for decision making and their experiences regarding participation.

Retrospective studies have helped to establish the incidence of local recurrence and its time course. In the 1980s and 1990s, 10-year local recurrence rates ranging from 8% to 19% were commonly reported. These rates are similar to the local recurrence rates seen in the randomized trials of CS and RT from the same era. More recent studies report lower rates of local recurrence, with 10-year actuarial rates of recurrence ranging from 2% to 7% in patients excised to negative margins. Table 106.11 shows the 10-year rates of local recurrence in recent node-negative NSABP trials.[86] This decrease in local recurrence rates is the result of a combination of improved mammographic and pathologic evaluation and the more frequent use of adjuvant systemic therapy (discussed in detail in the section "Treatment Factors and Local Recurrence"). In contrast, rates of local recurrence after mastectomy have remained stable over the same time period.

Recurrences in the breast are typically classified by their location in relation to the original tumor. Recurrences at or near the primary site (presumably representing a recurrence of the original tumor) are classified as either a *true recurrence* (within the boosted region) or a *marginal miss* (adjacent to the boosted region) or *elsewhere* in the breast (occurring at a distance from the original tumor and presumably representing a new primary). The time course to local recurrence in the patient undergoing BCT is prolonged. In one study, the annual incidence rate for a true recurrence/marginal miss recurrence was between 1.3% and 1.8% for years 2 through 7 after treatment and then decreased to 0.4% by 10 years after treatment. The annual incidence rate for recurrence elsewhere in the breast increased slowly to a rate of approximately 0.7% per year at 8 years and remained stable. (These results have been contrasted to those seen after mastectomy, in which most local recurrences occur in the first 3 to 5 years after surgery.) In the Milan I trial after 20 years of follow-up, the risk of any type of recurrence in the treated breast was 0.63 per 100 woman-years compared with a risk of 0.66 per 100 woman-years for contralateral cancer.[80] This suggests that although whole-breast irradiation is effective at eradicating subclinical multicentric foci of breast carcinoma present at the time of diagnosis, it does not prevent the subsequent development of new cancers. Thus, patients who elect BCT require lifelong follow-up to screen for the development of new cancers in both the treated and the contralateral breast.

TABLE 106.11

10-YEAR LOCAL RECURRENCE RATES IN RECENT NATIONAL SURGICAL ADJUVANT BREAST AND BOWEL PROJECT TRIALS

Trial	Systemic Therapy	ER Status	10-Year LR (%)
B-13	No chemo	–	13.3
	Chemo	–	3.5
B-14	No tamoxifen	+	11.0
	Tamoxifen	+	3.6
B-19	Chemo	–	6.5
B-20	Tamoxifen	+	4.7
B-23	Chemo	–	4.3

ER, estrogen receptor; LR, local recurrence; chemo, chemotherapy.
(From ref. 86.)

Risk Factors for Local Recurrence Following Conservative Surgery and Radiation Therapy

Risk factors for recurrence after CS and RT can be subdivided into patient, tumor, and treatment factors. Only those factors that are currently considered important are reviewed here.

Patient Risk Factors

The two important patient risk factors are patient age and inherited susceptibility.

Patient age (less than 35 or 40) has consistently been observed to be associated with an increased risk of local recurrence after BCT. Young patient age is associated with an increased frequency of various adverse pathologic features such as lymphatic vessel invasion, grade 3 histology, absence of ER/presence of *HER2*, and the presence of an extensive intraductal component (EIC). However, even when correction is done for the differing incidence of the pathologic features of the primary tumor between the age groups, young age is still associated with an increased likelihood of recurrence in the breast.[87]

An *inherited susceptibility* to breast and ovarian cancer and other cancers has been mainly linked to germ line mutations in *BRCA1* and *BRCA2*. Breast cancer patients with a mutation have a substantial risk of contralateral and late ipsilateral breast cancers. In a retrospective study, outcome following CS and RT was compared for 160 stage I or II breast cancer patients with germ line *BRCA1* or *BRCA2* mutations and 445 age- and stage-matched control patients without a mutation.[88] With a follow-up time of about 7 years, there was no evidence of increased radiation sensitivity or sequelae in patients with a mutation, and actuarial rates of ipsilateral breast cancer recurrence and survival were similar at 10 years. Patients with a mutation, however, were at greater risk of contralateral breast cancer. The 10-year actuarial rate of contralateral breast cancer was 26% for patients with a mutation compared with only 3% for control patients; however, tamoxifen use significantly reduced the risk of contralateral breast cancer in mutation carriers. In addition, the time course to and the location of ipsilateral breast cancer recurrence was prolonged in carriers with many recurrences located away from the primary tumor site, suggesting a new primary.

In a separate study of 491 patients with stage I or II breast cancer with a known *BRCA1* or *BRCA2* mutation in the family, the 10-year risk of a contralateral breast cancer was 43% in *BRCA1* carriers and 35% for *BRCA2* carriers; however, both the use of tamoxifen and bilateral oophorectomy (especially prior to age 49 years) was associated with reduced risk of contralateral breast cancer.[89] In carriers treated with both tamoxifen and bilateral oophorectomy, the risk of contralateral breast cancer was reduced by about 90%. It is important to consider genetic testing in a patient with newly diagnosed breast cancer with a personal and family history suggestive of a *BRCA1* or *BRCA2* germ line mutation. In patients with a mutation, the option of bilateral mastectomy should be strongly considered to avoid the long-term risk of a second breast cancer in either breast. Breast cancer patients most likely to benefit from bilateral mastectomy are those who are young and have early-stage disease. Given the high risk of a contralateral breast cancer, unilateral mastectomy is generally not performed in a patient who is a candidate for BCT.

The most important *tumor risk factor* is the *margin of resection*. Prior to the routine assessment of margins and detailed mammographic imaging, the presence of an EIC was shown to be a risk factor; however, in patients with negative margins of resection and resection of all suspicious mammographic calcifications, EIC is no longer a risk factor. Tumor size and nodal involvement are not prognostic factors for local recurrence after BCT but are prognostic factors for distant recurrence. In current practice, microscopic margins of resection are the major selection factor for BCT. A negative margin is defined by absence of cancer cells at inked surfaces, but there are variations in the definitions of a close margin, with different groups using 1, 2, or 3 mm as the cutoff. The amount of cancer close to the margin is also important. Margins need to be interpreted in conjunction with the operative findings. A positive deep margin is not significant if the breast resection was carried down to the pectoral fascia; the same is true for a positive anterior margin if the resection extended to the deep dermal surface. Patients with negative margins of excision have low rates of local recurrence after treatment with CS and RT.[90] The outcome of patients with close margins of resection is less clear.[90] In part, this reflects variability in the definition of close margins. It seems prudent in patients with close margins to consider other factors, such as young age, involvement close to a margin along a broad front, or the presence of an EIC, in judging the need for re-excision. Close margins may also be a concern when patients receive initial chemotherapy. However, it is not clear that more widely negative margins than tumor not touching ink reduce the risk of local recurrence when RT is given.

Tumor-Based Risk Factors

An increasing body of evidence suggests that the underlying molecular subtype of the tumor may be the significant determinant of both the likelihood and the time course of local recurrence after BCT and mastectomy, particularly among those treated in the modern era with surgery to achieve negative margins.[91–93]

There is interest in identifying molecular predictors of the risk of local recurrence. One study from the Netherlands found that gene expression profiling using various gene signatures appeared to identify a subgroup of patients at increased risk for local recurrence; however, in multivariate Cox regression analysis with known clinical variables and the 111-gene signature, young age was the only independent predictor of local recurrence, again illustrating the as-yet-unexplained prognostic importance of young age on local recurrence after BCT.[94] Recent data from the NSABP also showed a relationship between the results of recurrence scores from Onco*type* DX (Genomic Health, Redwood City, California) and the risk of local recurrence.[95] In 895 node-negative, ER-positive, tamoxifen-treated patients from NSABP B-14 and NSABP B-20, the 21-gene recurrence score was found to be significantly associated with local-regional recurrence. Three hundred-ninety of the patients were treated with BCT, and 505 were treated with mastectomy. The 10-year local recurrence rate was 4.3% for patients with a low recurrence score (<18), 7.2% for those with an intermediate recurrence score (18–30), and 15.8% for those with a high recurrence score (>30). After adjusting for age, clinical tumor size, type of initial treatment, and tumor grade, recurrence score (as a continuous variable relative to an increment in the recurrence score of 50 units) was associated with a hazard ratio of 2.16 (CI, 1.26–3.68; $P = 0.005$). For the 390 patients who underwent BCT, the 10-year local recurrence rate was 6.8% in the low recurrence score group, 10.8% in the intermediate recurrence score group, and 14.6% in the high recurrence score group. Overall, this study suggests a significant association between the 21-gene recurrence score and the risk for local-regional recurrence in node-negative and ER-positive breast cancer, perhaps reflecting the intrinsic biology of the tumor.

In addition to the extent of breast resection, important *treatment risk factors* are the use of a boost and the use of adjuvant systemic therapy. A *boost* or supplementary irradiation to the area of the primary site is generally used. It is standard in RT after lumpectomy for patients to receive 45 to 50 Gy of whole-breast irradiation followed by a 10 to 16 Gy boost to the region of the tumor bed (Fig. 106.2). The rationale for this treatment approach is that the vast majority of recurrences that develop after lumpectomy (with or without adjuvant RT) are in the immediate area of the excision cavity and that a boost can be delivered safely without significantly affecting the cosmetic result. The use of a boost is supported by the large EORTC trial in which 5,318 patients with negative margins were randomized to a boost of 16 Gy or no boost following 45 Gy to the whole breast.[96] With a median follow-up of 10.8 years, the cumulative incidence of ipsilateral breast recurrence was 10.2% without a boost and 6.2% with a boost ($P < .0001$). This 41% proportional reduction in local recurrence was similar in all age groups; however, the absolute benefit of the boost was greatest in young patients aged 40 years or less (24% decreased to 14%) and was smallest in patients over age 60 (7% decreased to 4%). Severe fibrosis was increased from 2% to 4% with the boost. Survival at 10 years was the same in both arms. A clinicopathologic study was performed on 1,616 patients in the EORTC trial. In multivariate analysis, high-grade invasive ductal carcinoma was associated with an increased risk of local recurrence (HR, 1.67: $P = .026$) and the boost was effective in reducing local recurrence in this subgroup.[97]

The use of *adjuvant systemic therapy* is an important factor associated with recurrence in the treated breast in conjunction with CS and RT. This effect is clearly demonstrated in three randomized clinical trials. In NSABP B-14 trial, node-negative, ER-positive patients were randomized to receive tamoxifen or to a placebo. Among the 1,062 patients treated with CS and RT,

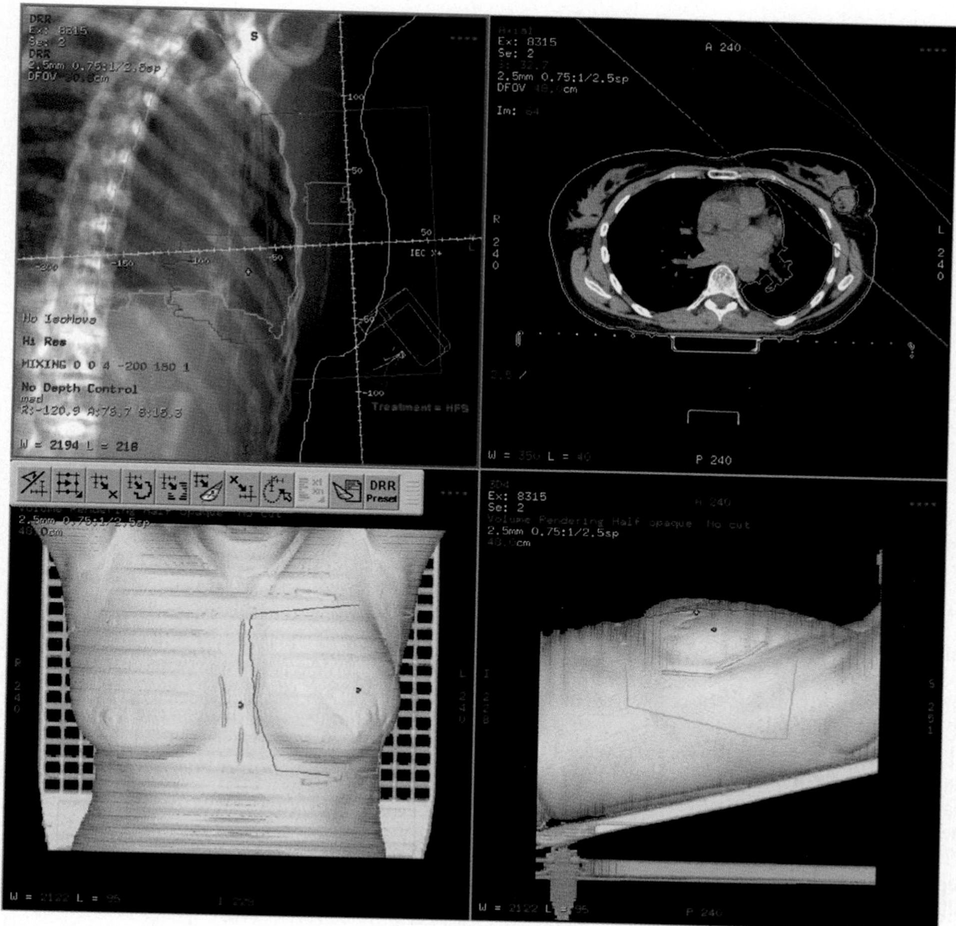

FIGURE 106.2 Computed tomography simulation for a left-sided breast cancer with medial and lateral tangential fields. Left upper is the beam's eye view with the large rectangle being the treatment field. The area of the primary in the upper outer quadrant is contoured in magenta and the heart is contoured in red. Note that for the actual treatment a block was used to block irradiation of her heart, which also blocked out some breast tissue well away from the primary cancer. Right upper is an axial view of the treatment fields in the center of the treatment fields. Left lower shows (in red) the medial tangent borders on the patient's skin. Right lower shows (in green) the lateral tangent borders on the patient's skin.

the 10-year rate of recurrence in the ipsilateral breast was 14.7% without tamoxifen and only 4.3% with tamoxifen.[98] A similar result was seen in the Stockholm Breast Cancer Study Group among node-negative patients randomized to receive tamoxifen or to a placebo. Among the 432 patients treated with CS and RT, the 10-year rate of recurrence in the ipsilateral breast was 12% without tamoxifen and only 3% with tamoxifen.[99] In the NSABP B- 21 trial, patients with node-negative breast cancer measuring 1 cm or less treated with lumpectomy were randomized to tamoxifen alone, RT, or RT and tamoxifen. With a mean follow-up of 87 months, the 8-year rate of ipsilateral local recurrence was 9.3% in the patients treated with RT and 2.8% in the patients treated with RT and tamoxifen.[100] Of note in these trials is that tamoxifen was given concurrently with RT; however, retrospective comparisons of concurrent versus sequential tamoxifen and RT have shown similar recurrence and survival rates. At this time, it seems that either concurrent or sequential administration of tamoxifen and RT is reasonable.

Similar results are seen with adjuvant chemotherapy, but the relationship is more complex, perhaps related to sequencing. In the NSABP B-13 trial, node-negative, ER-negative patients were randomized to chemotherapy or to a no-treatment control group. Among the 235 patients treated with CS and RT, the 8-year rate of recurrence in the ipsilateral breast was 13.4% without chemotherapy and only 2.6% with chemotherapy given concurrently with the RT.[101] Concurrent RT and chemotherapy also has the virtue of abbreviating the overall time for the course of treatment, but there is reluctance to use concurrent RT and an anthracycline. In a French phase III trial comparing concurrent versus sequential RT and chemotherapy with mitoxantrone and cyclophosphamide, local control was improved with concurrent administration, but concurrent treatment was also associated with an increased incidence of grade 2 or greater late side effects.[102] The results of a prospective study of concurrent cyclophosphamide, methotrexate, and fluorouracil (CMF) chemotherapy and *lower-dose* breast RT showed a low rate of local recurrence with acceptable cosmetic results and few complications.[103] However, an attempt to employ concurrent RT and weekly taxol following 4 doses of doxorubicin and cyclophosphamide (AC) resulted in excessive pulmonary toxicity.[103] Thus, the use of concurrent breast RT and chemotherapy has appeal, but is currently not standard with RT and anthracyclines or taxanes.

Updated results of the Dana-Farber/Harvard small randomized clinical trial address the question of sequencing following lumpectomy.[104] In this trial 244 patients were randomized following conservative breast surgery to receive 12 weeks of CAMFP (cyclophosphamide, doxorubicin, methotrexate, fluorouracil, and prednisone) chemotherapy before radiation (CT first), or following radiation (RT first). In the updated results, the median follow-up for surviving patients was 135 months. There were no significant differences between the CT-first and RT-first arms in time to any failure, distant metastasis, or death. Sites of first failure were also not significantly different ($P = .41$). However, the same trends toward greater local recurrence in the CT-first group and greater distant recurrence in the RT-group were seen. In an interaction model, there was a significant interaction between margin status and treatment sequence ($P < .05$). Patients with negative margins had a low rate of local recurrence as a site of first failure with either sequence; patients with positive margins had a high rate of local recurrence with both regimens. Of note, however,

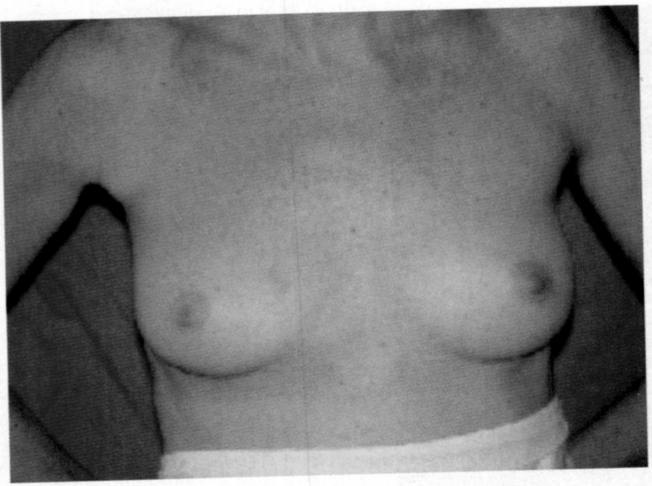

FIGURE 106.3 Cosmetic outcome of breast-conserving therapy. Other than the surgical scar, there is minimal difference between the treated and the untreated breast.

patients with close margins had local recurrence rate of 32% with CT first and 4% with RT first.

Until safe and effective methods of concurrent anthracycline or taxol-based chemotherapy and RT are established, the standard approach is to use sequential chemotherapy and RT. Given the primary importance of preventing systemic relapse, it has been the convention to use initial chemotherapy followed by RT. Although concerns have been expressed about an increased rate of local recurrence with this approach, the results of clinical trials in patients with negative margins have not shown this to be a problem even following four cycles of AC followed by four cycles of taxol, both given every 3 weeks.[105]

A major goal of BCT is the preservation of a cosmetically acceptable breast. When modern treatment techniques are used, an acceptable cosmetic outcome can be achieved in almost all patients (without compromise of local tumor control) (Fig. 106.3). Although treatment-related changes in the treated breast stabilize at approximately 3 years, other factors that primarily affect the untreated breast, such as change in size because of weight gain and the normal ptosis seen with aging, continue to affect the symmetry between a patient's breasts. The major factor determining the cosmetic result is the extent of surgical resection.[106] A variety of factors must be considered together (the size of the patient's breast, the size of the tumor, the depth of the tumor within the breast, and the quadrant of the breast in which the tumor is located) to judge the feasibility of a cosmetically acceptable resection. For example, although the removal of a large tumor in the lower portion of the breast often results in distortion of the breast contour, this is only apparent with the arms raised and is acceptable to most women. A similar distortion in the upper inner quadrant of the breast, which is visible in most types of clothing, might not be as acceptable. Techniques such as latissimus dorsi muscle reconstruction of the defect may be appropriate in selected patients to improve the cosmetic appearance after large resections, and the use of preoperative chemotherapy or endocrine therapy may allow resection of a smaller volume of tissue.

Guidelines for Patient Selection

Because of the potential options for treatment of early-stage breast cancer, careful patient selection and a multidisciplinary approach are necessary. The four critical elements in patient selection for BCT are (1) history and physical examination, (2) mammographic evaluation, (3) histologic assessment of the resected breast specimen, and (4) assessment of the patient's needs and expectations.

Recent (i.e., usually within 3 months) preoperative mammographic evaluation is necessary to determine a patient's eligibility for BCT. Mammographic evaluation defines the extent of a patient's disease, the presence or absence of multicentricity, and other factors that might influence the treatment decision, and evaluates the contralateral breast. If the mass is associated with microcalcifications, an assessment of the extent of the calcifications within and outside the mass should be made using magnification views.

Advances in breast imaging have led some to question whether MRI should be part of the standard preoperative evaluation of the breast cancer patient; however, a prospective randomized trial showed no decrease in unexpected conversion to mastectomy and no increase in the rate of negative margins with the addition of MRI to mammography,[107] and several studies have shown an association between MRI use and greater, but unwarranted, use of mastectomy.[108,109] MRI frequently identifies additional areas of involvement in the breast, but long-term clinical experience has demonstrated that the majority of this disease is controlled with RT. In addition, MRI has a substantial false-positive rate. Ideally, prospective trials demonstrating a clinical benefit in patients selected for BCT with MRI are needed before these examinations are routinely used for patient selection.

The patient and her physician must discuss the benefits and risks of mastectomy compared with those of BCT in her individual case. The following factors should be discussed:

1. The absence of a long-term survival difference between treatments
2. The possibility and consequences of local recurrence with both approaches
3. Psychological adjustment (including the fear of cancer recurrence), cosmetic outcome, sexual adaptation, and functional competence

Psychological research comparing patient adaptation after mastectomy with that after BCT shows no significant differences in global measures of emotional distress. However, women whose breasts are preserved have more positive attitudes about their body image and experience fewer changes in their frequency of breast stimulation and feelings of sexual desirability. In addition, patients treated with BCT have better physical functioning compared with patients treated with mastectomy at the end of primary treatment.[110]

Absolute and Relative Contraindications to Breast-Conserving Therapy

In the selection of patients for BCT, there are some absolute and relative contraindications.[59]

Absolute Contraindications

1. Pregnancy is an absolute contraindication to the use of breast irradiation. However, in many cases, it may be possible to perform BCT in the third trimester and treat the patient with irradiation after delivery.
2. Women with two or more primary tumors in separate quadrants of the breast or with diffuse malignant-appearing microcalcifications are not considered candidates for breast-conservation treatment.
3. A history of prior therapeutic irradiation to the breast region that would require retreatment to an excessively high total radiation dose to a significant volume is another absolute contraindication.

4. Persistent positive margins after reasonable surgical attempts at breast-conserving surgery warrant mastecomy. The importance of a single focally positive microscopic margin needs further study and may not be an absolute contraindication.

Relative Contraindications

1. A history of collagen vascular disease is a relative contraindication to breast-conservation treatment because published reports indicate that such patients tolerate irradiation poorly. Most radiation oncologists will not treat patients with scleroderma or active lupus erythematosus, considering these absolute contraindications. In contrast, rheumatoid arthritis is not a relative or an absolute contraindication.
2. Tumor size is not an absolute contraindication to breast-conservation treatment, although there is little published experience in treating patients with tumor sizes greater than 4 to 5 cm. However, a relative contraindication is the presence of a large tumor in a small breast in which an adequate resection would result in significant cosmetic alteration. In this circumstance, preoperative chemotherapy should be considered.
3. Breast size can be a relative contraindication. Treatment by irradiation of women with large or pendulous breasts is feasible if reproducibility of patient setup can be ensured and the technical capability exists for 6 MV or greater photon beam irradiation to obtain adequate dose homogeneity.

Nonmitigating Factors

There are certain clinical and pathologic features that should not prevent patients from being candidates for breast-conservation treatment. These features include the presence of clinically suspicious and mobile axillary lymph nodes or microscopic tumor involvement in axillary nodes. In addition, it is important to emphasize that it is feasible to evaluate the breast for local recurrence. The changes associated with recurrence can be detected at an early stage through the use of physical examination and mammography. The delivery of irradiation in this setting does not result in a meaningful risk of second tumors in the treated area or in the untreated breast. Tumor location is not a factor in treatment choice. Tumors in a superficial subareolar location may occasionally require the resection of the nipple/areolar complex to achieve negative margins, but this does not have an impact on outcome. Whether this is preferable to mastectomy needs to be assessed by the patient and her physician. A high risk of systemic relapse is not a contraindication for breast conservation, but rather a determinant of the need for adjuvant therapy.

Preoperative Systemic Therapy for Operable Cancer

Women who desire BCT but are not candidates for the procedure because of a large tumor relative to the size of the breast should be considered for preoperative or neoadjuvant therapy. This approach is not appropriate for patients with multicentric carcinoma, those with an EIC that precludes a cosmetic resection, or those who prefer treatment by mastectomy. Patients most likely to benefit from neoadjuvant chemotherapy are those with unicentric, higher-grade, ER-negative cancers.

Prospective, randomized trials of patients with operable breast cancer have demonstrated that clinical response rates to neoadjuvant chemotherapy are high, ranging from 49% in the EORTC study of fluorouracil, epirubicin and cyclophosphamide (FEC)[111] to 79% in the NSABP B-18 study of doxorubicin (A) and cyclophosphamide (C)[112] to 91% in the NSABP B-27 trial examining the addition of docetaxel (T) to AC.[113] Pathologic complete responses in the breast were seen in 4%, 13%, and 19% of patients, respectively, in these trials. In spite of these high response rates, only 25% to 30% of patients who were not candidates for BCT at presentation were able to undergo the procedure after preoperative therapy.[111,112] This is a reflection of both the difficulty of assessing the extent of residual viable tumor after preoperative chemotherapy and the often patchy nature of cancer cell death in response to chemotherapy. This type of response significantly decreases the total number of viable tumor cells, but viable tumor remains scattered throughout the same volume of breast tissue, precluding BCT. MRI shows promise compared with mammography and ultrasound in evaluating the extent of viable tumor and its distribution, but may both underestimate and overestimate the extent of residual disease.

In patients who overexpress human epidermal growth factor receptor-2 (*HER2*), the preoperative administration of trastuzumab in combination with chemotherapy has been associated with high rates of pathologic complete response. In a randomized study of 42 patients treated with four cycles of paclitaxel followed by four cycles of FEC or the same chemotherapy with simultaneous weekly trastuzumab for 24 weeks, the pathologic complete response rate was increased from 26% to 65% with the addition of trastuzumab.[114] In 22 additional patients assigned to chemotherapy plus trastuzumab, the pathologic complete response rate was 54.5%. A significant improvement in disease-free survival was also noted for trastuzumab-treated patients after a median follow-up of 36.1 months. To date, no increase in cardiac dysfunction has been observed in the trastuzumab group.[114] Subsequent clinical trials have confirmed that adding trastuzumab to chemotherapy improves the pathologic complete response rate among women with *HER2*-positive breast cancer receiving neoadjuvant therapy, consistent with the survival benefit observed for trastuzumab when given with chemotherapy in the adjuvant setting, suggesting that this approach may increase the rate of BCT in the population of patients overexpressing *HER2*.

A meta-analysis of nine randomized trials of preoperative chemotherapy demonstrated no increase, or decrease, in survival with preoperative compared with postoperative treatment,[115] but an elevated risk of local-regional recurrence (RR, 1.22; 95% CI, 1.04–1.45) was noted. Some of the increase in local recurrence was due to the inclusion of studies in the meta-analysis in which patients who had a clinical complete response did not have surgery. The majority of patients with a clinical complete response do not have a pathologic complete response, and the elevated risk of local recurrence seen in the meta-analysis emphasizes the importance of surgery to minimize the residual tumor burden in the breast. Even in patients undergoing surgery, an elevated risk of local recurrence has been observed. In the NSABP B-18 study[112] local recurrence rates were 15% in patients who required chemotherapy to undergo BCT compared with only 7% in those who were initially candidates for BCT. The increased rates of local recurrence after neoadjuvant therapy may reflect differences in the meaning of a negative excision margin in a situation in which, by definition, the volume of tissue resected is smaller than the volume originally occupied by the cancer. In this setting a negative margin may still be associated with a clinically significant residual tumor burden that is unlikely to be controlled by RT. Thus, an evaluation of both surgical margins and the extent of viable tumor elsewhere in the specimen is essential and may dictate resection of additional breast tissue even when margins are apparently tumor-free. Percutaneous placement of marker clips within the primary tumor prior to the initiation of chemotherapy will provide a landmark for localization and excision should a clinical and radiographic complete response occur. The lack of a survival benefit for neoadjuvant therapy and the increased complexity in determining the appropriate extent of

TABLE 106.12

EFFECTS OF RADIOTHERAPY (RT) AFTER BREAST-CONSERVING SURGERY (BCS)

	5-Y Gain in Local Control (%)	15-Y Gain, Breast Cancer Mortality (%)	15-Y Gain, Overall Mortality (%)
BCS ± RT: Node-negative	16.1	5.1	4.6
BCS ± RT: Node-positive	30.1	7.1	8.2
MRM ± RT: Node-negative	4.0	−3.6	−4.2
MRM ± RT: Node-positive	17	5.4	4.4

MRM, modified radical mastectomy.
(From ref. 119.)

resection suggest that for women who are candidates for breast conservation at presentation, neoadjuvant therapy outside the context of a clinical trial offers little benefit.

Neoadjuvant endocrine therapy has also been used to increase rates of BCT, although there is less experience with this approach than with chemotherapy. In a randomized trial of 337 hormone-receptor–positive postmenopausal women who were not considered candidates for BCT at presentation, 35% of those who received 4 months of tamoxifen 20 mg daily and 45% of those who received letrozole 2.5 mg daily were able to undergo BCT.[116] A subsequent analysis suggested that a higher response rate to letrozole was particularly likely in patients whose tumors overexpressed *HER1* or *HER2*.[117] In a similar study comparing 3 months of tamoxifen, 20 mg daily, with anastrozole, 1 mg daily, or the combination of the two drugs, 44% of those treated with anastrozole who were thought to require mastectomy at presentation had BCT compared with 31% of those treated with tamoxifen and 24% who received the combination (P = .23).[118] These studies indicate that in postmenopausal women with hormone-receptor–positive tumors, the preoperative use of an AI significantly increases the likelihood of breast conservation. However, in spite of the proven survival benefit seen with endocrine therapy in the adjuvant setting, pathologic complete response is rare with the short duration of treatment used in the neoadjuvant setting. The degree of pathologic response does not appear to have the same prognostic significance as it does when neoadjuvant chemotherapy is used, and failure to achieve complete response should not be interpreted as evidence of resistance to endocrine therapy.

Overall, both neoadjuvant chemotherapy and endocrine therapy are effective strategies for increasing the rate of BCT. Because neoadjuvant therapy may necessitate changes from traditional surgical and RT approaches to treatment of the breast, coupled with the more complex issues of nodal management discussed later in this chapter, this approach is best used as part of a coordinated multidisciplinary treatment effort.

Conservative Surgery without Radiation Therapy

An unresolved question is whether RT is necessary in all patients with invasive breast cancer after CS. It is well known that RT after CS reduces local recurrence by about 70%, but there has been uncertainty about whether this improvement in local recurrence is important to survival and whether there is a subgroup of patients with a low risk of local recurrence following CS alone. The impact of improving local control on overall long-term survival was greatly clarified with the findings of the 2005 Early Breasts Cancer Trialists Group (EBCTCG) meta-analysis.[119] This study found that improvements in 5-year local control resulted in statistically significant improvements in breast cancer–specific mortality and overall survival at 15 years (Table 106.12). The addition of RT to CS in node-negative patients improved 5-year local control by 16.1%, 15-year breast cancer mortality by 5.1%, and 15-year overall survival by 4.6%. The addition of RT to CS in node-positive patients improved 5-year local control by 30%, 15-year breast cancer mortality by 7.1%, and 15-year overall survival by 8.2%. These data provide compelling evidence that RT after CS is not only important for local control but also for survival.

Attempts have been made to identify a subgroup of patients (based on various clinical and histologic features) who have a low risk of local recurrence after CS alone. It was not possible to identify such a subgroup within the available clinical trials. Local recurrence rates are generally lower in trials that use more extensive surgery than in those using lumpectomy, and in older patients than in younger patients. The Joint Center for Radiation Therapy in Boston attempted to identify a suitable subgroup for wide excision alone in a prospective single-arm trial in which patients with a very favorable prognosis were offered the option of CS alone. The criteria for entry onto this protocol were tumor size of 2 cm or less, histologically negative axillary nodes, absence of either lymphatic vessel invasion or an EIC in the cancer, and no cancer cells visualized within 1 cm of inked margins.[120] All but one patient had a completely negative re-excision. The median age of patients in this trial was 66 years, 75% of cancers were detected by mammography alone, and the median pathologic size of the cancers was 9 mm. None of the patients received adjuvant endocrine therapy or chemotherapy. This trial was stopped shortly before it reached its accrual goal of 90 patients because of stopping rules ensuring against an excessively high local recurrence rate. With a median follow-up time of 86 months among the 81 eligible patients, the crude rate of local recurrence was 23%. The average local recurrence rate was 2.8% per year. Of note, of the six patients with a tubular cancer, three had a local recurrence. Examination of subsets of patients by age and tumor size did not find any statistically significant differences. Similar results were seen in a small randomized clinical trial from Finland. Based on the results of these prospective studies, it was concluded that even a highly selected group of breast cancer patients (based on patient and tumor characteristics) have a substantial risk of early local recurrence after treatment with wide excision alone. Newer markers are needed to more reliably identify patients who can be safely treated with wide excision alone.

More recently, there have been four trials that have compared tamoxifen with and without RT after BCS (largely in ER-positive patients) and their details are shown in Table 106.13.[100,121–123] The 5-year local recurrence rates for these trials are shown in Table 106.14. The 5-year results seem reasonable, but the rate of local recurrence appears increased after 5 years. In the Canadian Trial,[121] local recurrence is 7.7%

TABLE 106.13

TRIALS OF TAMOXIFEN WITH OR WITHOUT RADIOTHERAPY AFTER BREAST-CONSERVING THERAPY

Study (Ref.)	No. of Patients: Selection	FU (median months)
NSABP B-21 (100)	1,009: ≤1 cm; pN0	87
Canadian (121)	769: >50, T1,2; pN0	67
Scottish (122)	427: <70, T1,2; pN0	67
CALGB (123)	636: >70, T1; pN0	60

FU, follow-up; NSABP, National Surgical Adjuvant Breast and Bowel Project; CALGB, Cancer and Leukemia Group B.

at 5 years, but 17.6% at 8 years. This raises the question whether tamoxifen is merely delaying local recurrence. As previously discussed, the combination of tamoxifen and RT provides a very low rate of local recurrence. Tamoxifen alone has its greatest appeal in older patients (older than 70 years) where competing risks of other illnesses are substantial. In elderly patients, it is critical for the clinician to assess the patient's particular cancer characteristics as well as her comorbid illnesses and individual value system in determining the advisability of adding RT.

Accelerated Whole-Breast and Partial-Breast Irradiation

There have been a growing number of studies attempting to decrease the overall treatment time for RT after lumpectomy through the administration of larger daily doses (fraction sizes) of RT delivered to the whole breast or only to the portion of the breast containing the primary tumor.

The 10-year results of a randomized clinical trial of accelerated whole-breast irradiation have been recently published.[124] Women with invasive breast cancer who had undergone breast-conserving surgery and in whom resection margins were clear and axillary lymph nodes were negative were randomly assigned to receive whole-breast irradiation either at a standard dose of 50.0 Gy in 25 fractions over a period of 35 days (the control group) or at a dose of 42.5 Gy in 16 fractions over a period of 22 days (the hypofractionated-radiation group). The risk of local recurrence at 10 years was 6.7% among the 612 women assigned to standard irradiation as compared with 6.2% among the 622 women assigned to the hypofractionated regimen (absolute difference, 0.5 percentage points; 95% CI, –2.5 to 3.5). At 10 years, 71.3% of women in the control group as compared with 69.8% of the women in the hypofractionated-radiation group had a good or excellent cosmetic outcome (absolute difference, 1.5 percentage points; 95% CI, −6.9 to 9.8). In a subset analysis, conventional fractionation had better results in patients with high-grade cancers. This trial was initiated before the value of a boost was established, and it is not clear how best to give a boost in patients treated with hypofractionated whole-breast irradiation. As noted previously, the value of a boost is very small in patients aged 60 years and greater, so at a minimum it seems reasonable to treat patients aged 60 and greater with grade 1 or 2 node-negative breast cancer with accelerated whole-breast irradiation without a boost. Additional trials of hypofractionated whole-breast irradiation have been conducted in the United Kingdom, but they have shorter follow-up.

TABLE 106.14

FIVE-YEAR RATES OF LOCAL RECURRENCE IN TAMOXIFEN WITH OR WITHOUT RADIOTHERAPY TRIALS

Study (Ref.)	Tamoxifen (%)	Tamoxifen + RT (%)	End Point
NSABP B-21 (100)	8.4	1.1	LR
Canadian (121)	7.7	0.6	LR
Canadian (121)	13.2	1.1	L-RR
Scottish (122)	25.0	3.1	L-RR
CALGB (123)	4	1	L-RR

RT, radiotherapy; NSABP, National Surgical Adjuvant Breast and Bowel Project; LR, local recurrence; L-RR, local-regional recurrence; CALGB, Cancer and Leukemia Group B.

There are several potential benefits for accelerated partial-breast irradiation (APBI) and a compelling rationale for its use. Potential benefits include (1) the quality of life of patients could be improved by relieving patients of the necessity of daily treatments for 5 to 6 weeks, (2) the underutilization of BCT could be reduced by making it more feasible for patients to receive RT, (3) the integration of local and systemic therapies could be simplified, and (4) long-term complications of RT could be decreased by limiting the volume of critical structures irradiated to high dose. The scientific rationale for the delivery of whole-breast RT after lumpectomy is that many patients harbor areas of occult, residual microscopic disease in the breast after tumor excision (even with negative margins). To this end, RT has been delivered to the whole breast and the lumpectomy bed in an effort to *sterilize* these residual foci of cancer. However, patterns of recurrence after standard whole-breast RT and after excision alone demonstrate that the large majority of recurrences are in the immediate vicinity of the tumor bed.[90] In addition, pathologic studies on the distribution of tumor cells in relation to the primary tumor demonstrate that for the large majority of patients the majority of tumor cells in the breast are found quite close to the primary tumor.[125] This suggests that postlumpectomy RT exerts its maximal effect on eradicating residual disease in the region of the tumor bed, and that areas of occult disease in the remainder of the breast may be of little practical significance. If this hypothesis is correct, it would only be necessary to deliver RT to the region of the lumpectomy bed. By restricting the volume of tissue that requires RT, it may be possible to reduce the overall treatment time by increasing the daily dose (fraction size) of RT. These hypotheses provide the basis for the use of APBI.

These are a number of different APBI techniques and these include interstitial brachytherapy, limited external-beam irradiation, intracavitary brachytherapy, and intraoperative limited RT. The field of APBI is a rapidly moving field, but there are few long-term data, especially from randomized clinical trials. Patient selection for this approach is still controversial. Successful application of this approach requires technical expertise. There is an ongoing NSABP/RTOG phase III trial comparing conventional RT versus APBI (allowing implant or external-beam techniques), and accrual to the trial has been excellent. To provide some direction during this time of uncertainty, the American Society for Radiation Oncology convened a panel of breast cancer experts to provide guidance. Based on the available evidence, the panel identified a "suitable" group, for whom APBI outside a clinical trial is acceptable.[126] Patients meeting all of the following criteria were considered suitable: age 60 years or greater, *BRCA1/2* mutation not present, unicentric invasive ductal carcinoma measuring 2 cm or less, margins negative by at least 2 mm, without lymphatic vessel invasion or an EIC, ERs present, and path node-negative. The panel also identified "cautionary" and "unsuitable" groups.

MASTECTOMY

Mastectomy, with or without immediate breast reconstruction, is the surgical approach for the patient with breast cancer who has contraindications to BCT or who prefers treatment with mastectomy. The mastectomy used today is a total or complete mastectomy, with removal of the breast tissue from the clavicle to the rectus abdominous and between the sternal edge and the latissimus dorsi muscles. A total mastectomy also removes the nipple-areolar complex (NAC), the excess skin of the breast, and the fascia of the pectoralis major muscle. When accompanied by an axillary dissection, the procedure is termed a *modified radical mastectomy*. Mastectomy is an extremely safe operation. The 30-day mortality in women of all ages is less than 1%. Major complications after surgery are infrequent, but there is loss of sensation on the chest wall in 100% of patients. In a population-based study of 1,884 women treated for breast cancer in 2002, 30% underwent mastectomy. This was because of contraindications to BCT in approximately half and patient choice in the remainder.[84]

Advances in plastic surgical technique have made immediate reconstruction an option for most patients who undergo mastectomy. Potential concerns about immediate reconstruction have included the possibility of an increased incidence of local failure, delay in the diagnosis of local failure, or delay in the administration of adjuvant therapy related to wound healing issues. More recently as indications for postmastectomy RT have expanded, the impact of RT on reconstruction has also become an issue. Immediate reconstruction can negatively impact the technical delivery of RT, possibly resulting in greater irradiation of the heart (in left-sided cancers) and lung and undercoverage of the chest wall.[127] There have been no prospective trials comparing mastectomy alone with mastectomy with immediate reconstruction, but the available retrospective data do not support concerns about the incidence or detection of local recurrence in the reconstructed patient. The majority of postmastectomy recurrences occur in the skin or subcutaneous fat of the chest wall and present as palpable masses in the skin flap, so detection is not affected by the presence of the reconstruction.[128]

More recently, skin-sparing mastectomy in which skin excision is limited to the NAC and the excisional biopsy scar (if present) have been used to preserve the skin envelope of the breast and facilitate reconstruction. The reported rates of local recurrence after skin-sparing mastectomy are comparable to those of patients treated with conventional mastectomy.[90] This finding is consistent with prior observations that the extent of skin removal in patients treated with mastectomy alone is not a major determinant of the risk of chest wall recurrence.

Traditionally, skin-sparing mastectomy has included resection of the NAC. The rationale for this approach is the risk of leaving behind malignancy with nipple preservation due to the extension of ductal tissue into the nipple and the need to leave breast tissue on the NAC to provide a blood supply. Recently, however, investigators have begun to explore the safety of nipple-sparing mastectomy (NSM) in selected patients. The reported incidence of occult involvement of the NAC in patients with known breast cancer ranges from 0% to 58%.[129] This wide range is because of differences in tumor stage and in the number of sections taken to evaluate the NAC specimen in different studies. Gerber et al.[130] selected potential candidates for NSM who had peripherally located tumors 2 cm or less in size, no clinical evidence of nipple involvement, and clinically negative axillary nodes. In spite of this, frozen-section analysis demonstrated microscopic tumor in the subareolar tissue in 46% of 112 patients. Of the 61 patients treated by NSM, only one experienced a local recurrence in the NAC with a mean follow-up of 59 months.[130] In a multi-institutional study of 123 patients undergoing NSM for treatment or prophylaxis, no local recurrences in the NAC were observed after a median follow-up of 24.6 months.[131] Necrosis of the nipple was seen in 11% of cases and involved less than one-third of the nipple in 13 of 22 patients. Another approach to the problem of cancer recurrence in the preserved NAC has been to deliver a dose of intraoperative RT to the NAC.

These studies indicate that NSM may be a viable option in highly selected women, specifically patients with small, peripherally located, node-negative tumors with favorable histologic features. Most women in this category, however, are candidates for conventional BCT. The eligible population for NSM is further limited by the requirement that the nipple be in the appropriate position on the reconstructed breast. This is rarely the case for women with large, ptotic breasts, further limiting the application of this procedure.

In summary, immediate reconstruction with preservation of the skin envelope of the breast has not been shown to alter the outcome of mastectomy or to delay the administration of systemic therapy. Immediate reconstruction has the advantages of avoiding the need for a second major operative procedure and the psychological morbidity of the loss of the breast. The two major reconstructive techniques involve the use of implants and/or tissue expanders or the use of myocutaneous tissue flaps to create a new breast mound. The advantages and disadvantages of the techniques are summarized in Table 106.15. Implant reconstructions are best suited for women with small to moderate sized breasts with minimal ptosis, while flap reconstructions allow more flexibility in the size and shape of the reconstructed breast (Fig. 106.4). In the past, most breast implants were filled with silicone gel. However, after reports from uncontrolled studies suggested an increased incidence of connective tissue disease in women with silicone implants, the FDA declared a moratorium on their use. Since

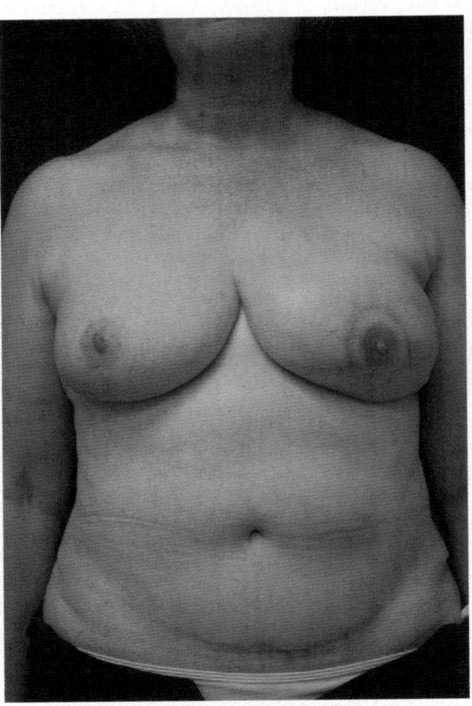

FIGURE 106.4 Cosmetic outcome of transrectus abdominis muscle flap reconstruction after skin-sparing mastectomy.

TABLE 106.15

COMMON RECONSTRUCTIVE OPTIONS AFTER MASTECTOMY

Type	Advantages	Disadvantages
Implant	One-stage procedure, minimal prolongation, hospitalization, or recovery Low cost	Poor symmetry if skin removed or in large ptotic breasts Capsular contracture, leakage, rupture possible
Tissue expander	Short operative time Hospitalization, recovery not prolonged Low cost	Multiple physician visits postop. Poor symmetry large or ptotic breasts Capsular contracture, leakage rupture possible
Latissimus dorsi flap	Very low risk of flap loss Natural contour with autogenous tissue	Donor site scar Usually requires an implant Moderate prolongation hospitalization and recovery
TRAM flap	Natural contour. Good match for large or ptotic breasts Abdominoplasty	Donor site scar Fat necrosis, flap loss possible Abdominal wall weakness plus hernia Significant prolongation hospitalization plus recovery
DIEP flap	Natural contour Muscle-sparing Abdominoplasty	Donor site scar Need for microsurgeon Flap loss possible Moderate prolongation hospitalization plus recovery
Superior gluteal artery perforator flap	Natural contour Alternative donor site	Donor site scar Need for microsurgeon Flap loss possible Moderate prolongation hospitalization plus recovery

Postop, postoperatively; TRAM, transverse rectus abdominous myocutaneous; DIEP, deep inferior epigastric perforator.

PRACTICE OF ONCOLOGY

that time, several epidemiologic studies have failed to demonstrate an increased incidence of connective tissue disorders in women with implants compared with matched control populations. Silicone implants are again available for use in breast cancer patients, but many patients opt for saline implants or flap reconstructions as a result of the adverse publicity surrounding silicone implants.

Reconstructive choices may be influenced by the possible need for postmastectomy RT. As noted previously, immediate reconstruction can result in greater irradiation of heart (in left-sided cancers) and lung and undercoverage of the chest wall. There are a variety of strategies that have been proposed for selecting the type of reconstruction for a patient with a significant likelihood of requiring postmastectomy RT. There is considerable variability in outcome reported in the medical literature for the same approaches and there are no prospective studies reported to date. The use of RT in patients who have been reconstructed with implants is associated with a higher risk of encapsulation and implant loss than in nonirradiated patients. In one study, however, Cordeiro et al.[132] reported that after a mean follow-up of 34 months in 68 patients reconstructed with tissue expanders or implants who received RT, 80% had good to excellent aesthetic results and 72% would have chosen the same form of reconstruction again. The figures for nonirradiated patients were 88% (P = NS) and 85%, respectively. Implant loss occurred in 11% of patients with irradiated implants and 6% of nonirradiated patients. The finding in this study that the majority of patients who require RT after implant reconstruction have good cosmesis and are satisfied with their reconstruction choice has led some to advocate insertion of an expander at the time of mastectomy, which is inflated during chemotherapy and exchanged for a permanent implant prior to RT. In patients who are satisfied with the cosmetic outcome after RT, no further surgery is required. In patients with significant cosmetic deformity, a secondary flap reconstruction is performed. This approach has the advantage of allowing preservation of the breast skin and providing the patient with a breast mound during what may be a prolonged course of postoperative cancer therapy. However, additional favorable experience with irradiation of expanders or implants at other institutions is needed.

A primary flap reconstruction is another alternative for the patient who may require postmastectomy RT. Variable outcomes have been reported for patients who receive RT after transverse rectus myocutaneous flap or latissimus dorsi flap reconstruction. Complete flap loss is rare, but fat necrosis, fibrosis, and volume loss can occur. As in the native breast, the full cosmetic impact may not be evident until 3 years posttreatment. In one study, the 5-year incidence of major complications after transverse rectus myocutaneous reconstruction was 0% ($n = 35$) and 5% after tissue expander/implant ($n = 50$) reconstruction followed by RT.[133] In contrast, 4 of 27 (9%) patients reconstructed with flaps and 6 of 15 (40%) implant patients underwent major corrective surgery a median of 8 months after RT in another series.[134] The extreme variability in reported results emphasizes the need for prospective studies in this area. An alternative approach is to perform sentinel node biopsy prior to mastectomy to identify patients with nodal involvement at highest risk for requiring postmastectomy RT and delay reconstruction in this subset of women until after the completion of oncologic therapy. This is an area that continues to evolve, and multidisciplinary consultation between the oncologic surgeon, reconstructive surgeon, and radiation oncologist will help to ensure optimal patient outcomes.

MANAGEMENT OF THE AXILLA

For many years, standard management of the axilla for patients with invasive breast carcinoma consisted of a complete axillary dissection. Initially, this was thought to be a critical component of the surgical cure of breast cancer. This changed when studies such as the NSABP B-04 trial, in which clinically node-negative patients were randomized to radical mastectomy, total mastectomy with RT to the regional lymphatics, or total mastectomy with observation of the axillary nodes and delayed axillary dissection if nodal metastases developed, showed no survival benefit for the axillary surgery.[135] Axillary dissection came to be regarded as a staging procedure that provided prognostic information and maintained local control in the axilla. However, the observation that 25% to 30% of long-term survivors treated with radical mastectomy alone had positive nodes,[136] coupled with the decreased survival observed after inadequate axillary treatment in the Guys Hospital trial,[137] suggested that axillary dissection was therapeutic for some patients with axillary nodal metastases.

The technique of lymphatic mapping and sentinel node biopsy reliably identifies patients with axillary node involvement with a low morbidity operation, allowing axillary dissection to be limited to patients with nodal metastases who have the potential to benefit from the procedure. The American College of Surgeons Oncology Group (ACOSOG) Z10 trial and the NSABP B-32 trial, involving 5,327 and 5,210 clinically node-negative patients, respectively, demonstrated that a sentinel node could be identified in 98.6% and 97% of patients.[138] In the ACOSOG Z10 trial participating surgeons chose the method of lymphatic mapping, and no significant differences were seen in the rate of sentinel node identification with the use of blue dye alone, radiocolloid alone, or the combination of the two.[138] Increasing body mass index, increasing age, and fewer than 50 patients accrued to the trial were all associated with a significant decrease in sentinel node identification rate, but a sentinel node was successfully identified in more than 95% of patients in all groups. Tumor size, histologic type, tumor location, and breast biopsy type (needle vs. surgical) were not associated with the sentinel node identification rate.

Complications of sentinel node biopsy are infrequent, with anaphylaxis to Lymphazurin blue dye observed in 0.1% of patients in the ACOSOG Z10 trial[139] and axillary paresthesias 6 months postoperatively in 8.6%. Lymphedema does occur after sentinel node biopsy, but at a much lower rate than after axillary dissection. In the randomized Axillary Lymphatic Mapping Against Nodal Axillary Clearance (ALMANAC) trial, the absolute incidence of lymphedema in the sentinel node biopsy group was 5% at 12 months, a relative risk of 0.37 (95% CI, 0.23–0.60) compared with the axillary clearance group in an intention to treat analysis.[140]

The majority of patients with stage I and II cancer are candidates for sentinel node biopsy. Contraindications to the procedure include pregnancy, lactation, and locally advanced breast cancer. Care should be taken to excise any palpably abnormal nodes intraoperatively because lymph nodes that contain a heavy tumor burden may not take up the mapping agent. In the patient with clinically positive nodes, confirmation of metastases preoperatively with FNA allows an immediate axillary dissection. Caution should be used in proceeding directly to dissection without cytologic confirmation because the false-positive rate of physical examination is approximately 20%. The presence of multicentric carcinoma or a T3 primary tumor were initially thought to be contraindications to lymphatic mapping, but studies have shown that sentinel node biopsy is accurate in these circumstances.[141]

Controversy continues over the appropriate timing of sentinel node biopsy in patients receiving neoadjuvant chemotherapy. A retrospective analysis of 428 of 2,365 patients in the NSABP B-27 trial who received chemotherapy followed by sentinel node biopsy and an axillary dissection demonstrated an 85% sentinel node identification rate and a false-negative rate of 11%. These results are similar to those observed in patients undergoing an initial sentinel node biopsy during the same time period.[142] Sentinel node biopsy after neoadjuvant therapy offers the patient the potential benefit of axillary downstaging and avoidance of axillary dissection. Further follow-up on axillary failure rates with this approach is needed. In some circumstances, knowledge of the patient's histologic nodal status prior to chemotherapy may be useful for planning RT, in which case consideration should be given to performing the sentinel node biopsy prior to the initiation of chemotherapy. The accuracy of sentinel node biopsy in patients with clinically evident axillary nodal metastases at presentation who receive neoadjuvant therapy with resolution of clinically apparent adenopathy remains uncertain. In a recent study of 61 patients with nodal metastases documented prior to chemotherapy by FNA, a 25% false-negative rate for sentinel node biopsy was observed.[143] These findings suggest that axillary dissection should remain the standard approach for patients presenting with nodal involvement.

A major concern about sentinel node biopsy has been the false-negative rate of the procedure. In most large, multi-institutional studies, false-negative rates of approximately 10%, determined by completing an axillary dissection after the sentinel node(s) were removed, have been observed even when training requirements for participating surgeons and a standard technique of lymphatic mapping were used.[144] However, three randomized studies directly comparing the identification of axillary metastases with axillary dissection and sentinel node biopsy found no difference in the likelihood of identifying nodal disease.[140,145,146] In the NSABP B-32 trial, 30% of the patients undergoing sentinel node biopsy followed by axillary dissection were found to have nodal metastases compared with 28% of those having sentinel node biopsy only if the sentinel node was negative ($P = .31$). Follow-up studies of patients treated by sentinel node biopsy alone demonstrate that the rate of local recurrence in the axilla is extremely low. In one study with a median follow-up of 31 months, isolated axillary first failure was seen in only 3 of 4,008 patients (0.07%) who had a sentinel node biopsy.[147]

The ability to perform a more detailed examination of the sentinel node has significantly increased the identification of small tumor deposits in the axillary nodes. Registry studies have demonstrated an approximately 10% increase in the proportion of patients with positive axillary nodes, after adjustment for other factors, in the time period since the introduction of sentinel node biopsy.[148] The prognostic significance of isolated tumor cells (<0.2 mm deposits) and very small metastatic deposits (>0.2 mm, <2.0 mm) is uncertain, with retrospective studies providing contradictory results. The initial results from the ACOSOG Z10 trial, a prospective study of the prognostic significance of IHC detected metastases in the sentinel nodes and the bone marrow in 5,539 clinically node-negative women with T1and 2 cancers have been reported. In multivariable analysis, IHC status of the sentinel node was not a predictor of 5-year overall survival, but positive bone marrow IHC status was associated with significantly decreased survival, in spite of the fact that 10.5% of patients had IHC sentinel node metastases and only 3.0% had IHC bone marrow metastasis.[149]

Axillary dissection has been the standard approach to patients with axillary nodal metastases. Studies comparing sentinel node biopsy with axillary dissection have provided important information on the morbidity of the procedure. In the ALMANAC trial, moderate to severe lymphedema was reported by 13% of patients 12 months after axillary dissection as well as sensory loss in 31%.[140] Decreases in shoulder flexion and abduction were present 1 month after surgery but resolved rapidly after that time. Axillary dissection provides excellent long-term local control, with only 1.4% of patients treated by radical mastectomy in the NSABP B-04 trial[135] having an isolated axillary recurrence at 10-year follow-up. The use of axillary irradiation as an alternative to axillary dissection was studied in the presentinel node era in a randomized trial in clinically node-negative patients performed at the Institute Curie. After 15 years of follow-up, the axillary failure rate was 3% in the radiated group and 1% in the surgical group (P = .03),[149] indicating that this is an acceptable alternative in patients with contraindications to axillary surgery or those who refuse the procedure. The ACOSOG Z11 trial was a prospective randomized study to address the need for axillary dissection in clinically node-negative women found to have macrometastases in one to three sentinel nodes. The study was designed to identify a 5% difference in survival between patients undergoing a completion axillary dissection and those treated with sentinel node biopsy alone. It closed prematurely because of a low event rate, but 891 patients were randomized. After a median follow-up of 6.2 years, the 5-year nodal recurrence rate was 0.5% in the dissection arm and 0.9% in the sentinel node biopsy alone arm (P = .11). No difference in 5-year disease-free or overall survival was seen between groups, and no evidence of a trend toward a survival benefit for dissection, which might have been evident with a larger sample size, was observed. All patients in this study were treated with BCT, 97% received some type of systemic therapy, and irradiation of an axillary field was not permitted, but it is likely that the low rate of axillary failure in the sentinel node biopsy alone group is at least in part related to irradiation of the low axilla with the breast tangents. These findings do not apply to women with clinically positive nodes or extensive nodal involvement, but do call into question the need for routine axillary dissection in those with limited disease who will receive RT, and strongly suggest that dissection is not necessary for IHC-positive nodes.

LOCAL-REGIONAL THERAPY AND SURVIVAL

The impact of local-regional therapy on the survival of patients with breast cancer has been debated for decades. Three viewpoints based on different hypotheses concerning the biology of breast cancer have been proposed. The Halstedian theory proposed that breast cancer is strictly a local disease, and that tumor cells spread over time in a contiguous manner away from the primary site by way of lymphatics, even to distant organs. The Halstedian theory dictated that aggressive local-regional therapy (i.e., control of disease in the breast, chest wall, and regional lymph nodes) would have a substantial impact on survival and provided justification for even more radical breast cancer surgery. As it became clear that many breast cancer patients developed distant metastases despite having their disease controlled locally, the "systemic" view arose in reaction to the Halstedian theory. Bernard Fisher and colleagues promulgated the view that breast cancer was a systemic disease, and that it could be divided into two distinct groups: those cancers that have the ability to metastasize to distant sites and those that lack this ability. According to this view, which prevailed in the last half of the 20th century, if distant metastases were destined to develop, this had already occurred at the time of the diagnosis of the cancer in the breast. This theory predicted that treatments that improved local-regional control would have little or no effect on overall survival. Randomized trials from the NSABP that studied the effect of improving local control by increasing the extent of surgery or adding RT after total mastectomy (NSABP B-04)[135] or breast-conserving surgery (NSABP B-06)[79] demonstrated comparable survival for the different treatment arms despite substantial improvement in local-regional control with additional surgery and RT. The results from these trials were widely interpreted as providing strong evidence for the systemic theory. However, in these trials there were insufficient events (in this case, deaths) to detect small but clinically important differences in overall mortality.

A third hypothesis synthesized aspects of these two opposing views.[151] This theory holds that, for many breast cancers, there is a time when tumor cells have not metastasized to distant sites, but it is generally not known whether this time has passed at the point of diagnosis for any individual patient. According to this view, failure to achieve initial local control will allow some tumors to disseminate later to distant sites, reducing a patient's chance of long-term survival.

Recent evidence has cast doubt on the validity of the systemic theory. First, there is strong evidence that mammographic screening reduces breast cancer mortality. The findings from a meta-analysis of randomized studies of mammographic screening demonstrate that in screened populations, the relative risk of death from breast cancer was significantly reduced (RR, 0.85; 95% CI, 0.73–0.99) compared with unscreened populations.[152] Thus, in some patients, earlier diagnosis (with screening) can prevent the development of distant metastases. That screening decreases mortality implies that at least some breast cancers develop the propensity to spread distantly over time.

Second, there is mounting evidence from randomized clinical trials supporting a link between local control and overall survival in breast cancer. A study published in 2005 from the EBCTCG presented the findings from 78 randomized clinical trials evaluating the extent of surgery and the use of RT.[119] This report analyzed data from 42,000 breast cancer patients treated on trials that began by 1995 and examined more extensive versus less extensive surgery, RT versus no RT, and extensive surgery versus RT.

The most striking finding from the EBCTCG study was that improved local control at 5 years resulted in a highly statistically significant improvement in both breast cancer survival and overall survival at 15 years. Further, the absolute reduction in the 5-year rate of local-regional recurrence between treatment arms was proportional to the absolute reduction in 15-year breast cancer mortality. The absolute breast cancer mortality benefit was similar for a given reduction in local-regional recurrence, regardless of the method of achieving the reduction (i.e., by more extensive surgery or by the addition of RT). For the trials in this EBCTCG meta-analysis that studied RT, the addition of RT significantly improved 15-year *absolute* overall survival after breast conservation surgery by 5.3% (P = .005) (Fig. 106.5) and after mastectomy by 4.4% (P = .001). The survival benefits of achieving local-regional control documented in the EBCTCG meta-analysis are of similar magnitude to that for adjuvant systemic therapy, yet they have received considerably less attention.

The impact of local therapy on survival must be considered in the context of systemic therapy. Adjuvant systemic therapy itself reduces the likelihood of both local and distant recurrence. A subset analysis in the EBCTCG meta-analysis of local therapy revealed that the use of RT after mastectomy in node-positive patients only improved 15-year survival in patients who also received adjuvant systemic therapy and not in patients who were treated with mastectomy alone. In those patients at high risk of distant metastases, such as women with positive lymph nodes, RT in the absence of systemic therapy can only improve survival in the rare patient with residual local-regional disease who has no distant dissemination. In contrast, in node-positive patients treated with mastectomy and adjuvant systemic therapy, RT will potentially contribute to survival in patients in whom systemic therapy eradicates microscopic metastases, but not residual local-regional disease. Current systemic therapy is primarily effective against micrometastatic involvement. As systemic therapies are developed that can eradicate clinically evident disease, the influence of local therapy on mortality will be reduced and possibly eliminated.

These results underscore the need to routinely employ prudent measures to achieve local control and to identify more

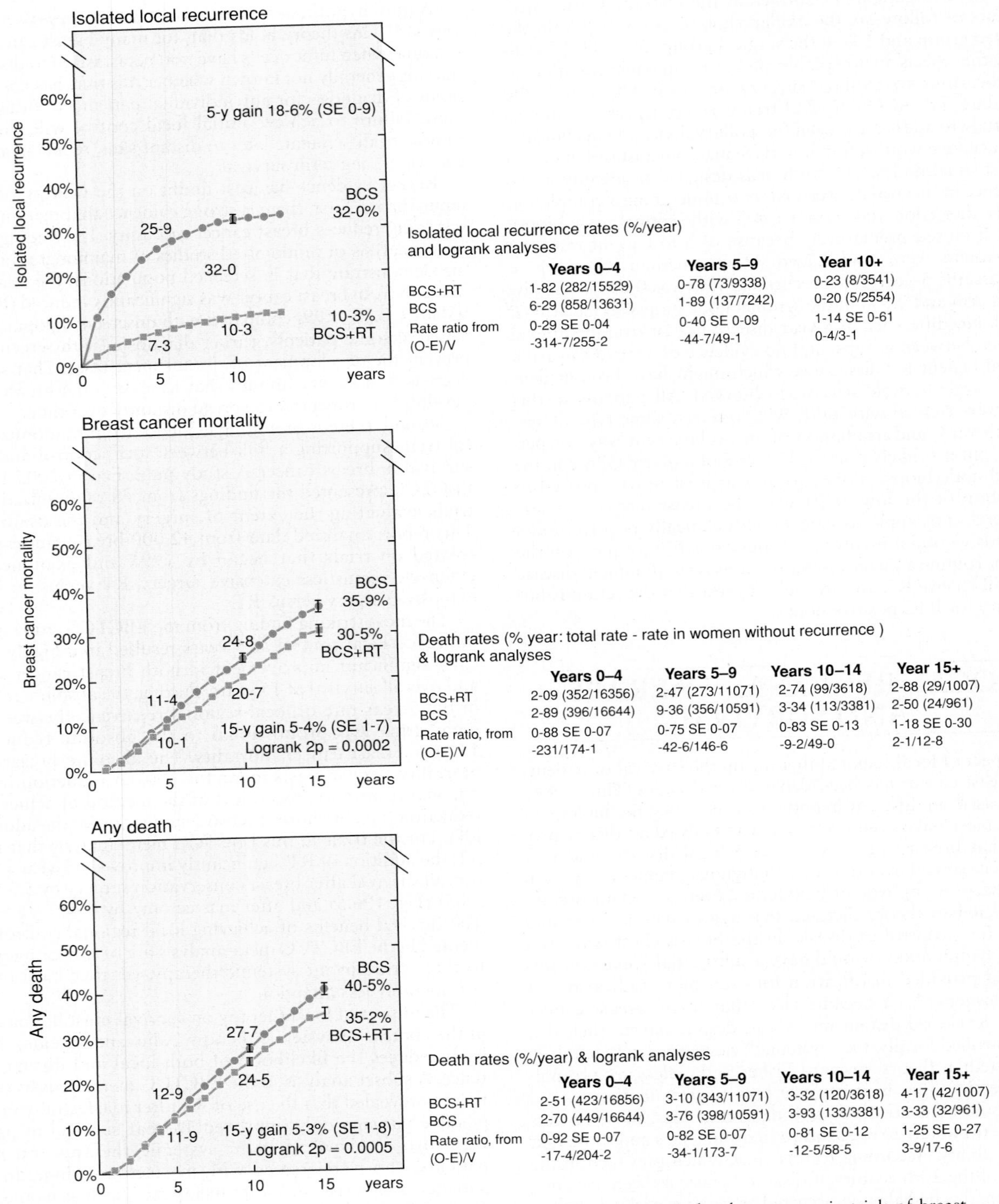

FIGURE 106.5 The Oxford overview analysis of the impact of the reduction in local recurrence in trials of breast-conserving therapy with and without radiotherapy on breast cancer mortality and death from all causes is illustrated. For every four local-regional recurrences avoided, one breast cancer death is prevented.

robust predictors of local recurrence. For example, clinicians should practice careful patient selection for BCT, excision to negative margins, and the use of boost doses of RT, particularly in patients younger than 35 years who are known to have a higher risk of local recurrence. Gene expression analyses have been used to identify patients at increased risk of distance recurrence and, as previously discussed, there is preliminary evidence that such molecular techniques will be helpful in identifying patients at greater risk of local recurrence. There is a need to gain a better understanding of the interplay between tumor biology, the anatomic extent of disease, the use of systemic therapy, and the risk of local-regional recurrence.

PROGNOSTIC AND PREDICTIVE FACTORS

A *prognostic factor* is defined as a measurement taken at the time of diagnosis or surgery that is associated with outcome (e.g., overall survival, disease-free survival, or local control).

Prognostic factors generally refer to a patient's anticipated outcome at the time of diagnosis in the absence of systemic therapy; however, they are sometimes useful to estimate outcome following a specific systemic therapy. Mathematically, a prognostic factor is demonstrated as a statistically (and clinically) significant separation of curves of outcome that are based on the presence or absence of the factor, in a Cox proportional hazards regression. A *predictive factor* is a measurement that predicts response or lack of response to a specific treatment. Mathematically, a predictive factor is modeled as an interaction between a factor and a treatment in a Cox regression. This interaction is best demonstrated in a clinical trial of treatment versus no treatment. In practice, some factors are both prognostic and predictive. Establishing the validity of a prognostic factor (biomarker) requires that the factor have biological relevance, that the methods for determining the factor be validated and reproducible (i.e., confirmed in a second independent data set) with optimal cutoff values, and that the factor be studied with adequate sample sizes without population bias. Guidelines for the evaluation and reporting of such biomarkers have been established.[153]

The AJCC staging system reviewed elsewhere in this chapter[72] is based on established clinical and pathologic prognostic factors, and stage itself remains a major prognostic factor. The *extent of axillary lymph node involvement* by breast cancer is the most established and reliable prognostic factor for subsequent metastatic disease and survival. This is not surprising as it reflects evidence of actual metastatic potential. Axillary nodal involvement has generally been stratified as the *number* of positive lymph nodes (e.g., 0, 1 to 3, 4 to 9, and 10 or more), although more recent analyses have stressed the *percentage* of positive lymph nodes, given the variability in the extent of axillary dissection between surgeons. Tumor size and histologic grading also have established prognostic significance. *Tumor size* is typically given as the microscopic size of the invasive cancer. *Histologic grade* is best determined by an established methodology, such as the Nottingham combined histologic grading system. A criticism of the value of histologic grade has been the lack of concordance among pathologists; however, this is improved by the use of an established methodology.

Estrogen and progesterone receptor expression are the most important and useful predictive factors currently available. Patients with invasive breast cancer whose tumors are totally lacking in ER and PR do not derive benefit from hormonal treatment either in the metastatic or adjuvant setting. Current assays for ER and PR are performed using IHC techniques, which have the advantages of not being confounded by endogenous estrogens, can be correlated with histologic findings to eliminate the possibility that the assessment was done on noncancerous tissue, can be performed on paraffin-embedded tissues, and do not have tumor size as a limiting factor. Laboratories need to adhere to well-described techniques to ensure accurate determination of ER and PR. A recent report from ASCO and the College of American Pathology has highlighted the importance of high-quality ER and PR testing as a centerpiece of breast cancer care.[154] Because ER/PR status is critical to current management guidelines, some centers repeat the assay if the initial determination is ER-negative or PR-negative, particularly if there is any reason to question the result, such as in a patient with a low-grade cancer. Although there are convincing data that patients whose tumors have even as few as 1% of cells staining positively for hormone receptors derive benefit from adjuvant hormonal therapy, it is still controversial whether laboratories can reproducibly report the percentage of positive ER and PR staining.[155] ER/PR status also has some prognostic value. Patients with ER-/PR-positive tumors have improved disease-free survival compared with similarly staged patients with ER-/PR-negative tumors at 5 years, but this difference is less apparent at 10 years.

Using tumor size and grade, ER status, and the number of involved axillary nodes, it is possible to estimate online the prognosis of an individual patient. One such online service that is widely used and has been validated is Adjuvant Online (www.adjuvantonline.com).[156]

Patient age has also consistently been shown to be a prognostic factor. Very young breast cancer patients (35 years or less) have a poorer prognosis than older patients. The cancers in these patients tend to be higher grade, less often ER-/PR-positive, and more likely to have lymphovascular invasion than cancers in older patients. It is not clear whether these differences in pathologic features fully explain the worse outcome in very young patients.[157,158]

Approximately 20% of breast cancer patients have *HER2/neu gene amplification*, which results in glycoprotein overexpression. Approximately 5% of patients have overexpression without gene amplification, but otherwise gene amplification and expression are highly correlated. *HER2* amplification or overexpression has been associated with higher tumor grade, lack of ER receptors, higher levels of tumor proliferation, and poorer prognosis. *HER2* status is the major predictive factor for benefit from trastuzumab (Herceptin), which is discussed later in this chapter. There is some evidence that suggests that *HER2* status is predictive for benefit from anthracycline-based chemotherapy, although this relationship is not certain, particularly with the availability of trastuzumab.[159] Measurements of *HER2* can be performed by either IHC or fluorescent *in situ* hybridization. Similar to ER, laboratories need to adhere to well-described techniques to ensure accurate determination of *HER2*. A recent guideline for *HER2* testing describes these techniques and defines a positive result as IHC staining of 3+, of greater than 30% of invasive cancer cells, a fluorescent *in situ* hybridization result of more than six copies per nucleus, or a fluorescent *in situ* hybridization ratio of more than 2.2.[160]

Involvement of lymphovascular spaces is associated with a greater likelihood of lymph node metastases and is an independent adverse prognostic factor in both node-negative and node-positive patients. Rigid pathologic criteria are required for this factor to be reliable, and this includes assurance that the cancer cells are present in an area outlined by endothelium and present away from the main tumor mass. These findings allow lymphovascular invasion to be distinguished from retraction artifact. In some centers, IHC stains for endothelial cells are used.

OTHER FACTORS

Numerous other prognostic and predictive factors have been evaluated in patients with early breast cancer, but have not been widely adopted in routine clinical use in the United States, and include (1) markers of *proliferation*, such as S-phase fraction, the percentage of cells labeling with thymidine or bromodeoxyuridine or cellular expression of Ki-67 or MIB-1 (which measure the percentage of cells in the G_1 phase of the cell cycle), and mitotic index; (2) measures of the *plasminogen activator system*, such as the concentrations of urokinase plasminogen activator and its inhibitor, plasminogen activator inhibitor-1; (3) measurements of *tumor angiogenesis*, such as counting the number of capillaries with IHC methods that use labeled antibodies against factor VIII in vascular endothelium; and (4) the detection of *occult micrometastases* in the bone marrow using IHC techniques.[161] Sources are available for a more detailed discussion of these and other factors.[162]

MOLECULAR AND GENOMIC FACTORS

Breast cancer is a heterogeneous disease, and it has long been appreciated that tumors with different biological features have different clinical outcomes and responses to therapy. At present, prognosis and treatment selection in breast cancer are based on characterization of tumor growth factor receptor status—ER, PR, and *HER2*. These markers can be used to define four functional groups of tumors: hormone receptor-positive, *HER2*-negative; hormone receptor-negative, *HER2*-negative ("triple negative" tumors), and *HER2* overexpressing tumors with or without hormone receptor expression.

Recent advances in molecular biology have resulted in further refinement of these breast cancer subsets. In particular, multigene arrays and expression analyses have provided a molecular taxonomy for breast tumors, which emphasizes the underlying biological differences between tumors and provides detailed prognostic and treatment outcome–based information. Sorlie et al.[163] and Perou et al.[164] were able to classify breast cancers into tumor subtypes that had different prognoses using complementary DNA microarrays. These studies used hierarchical clustering analysis to identify tumor subtypes with distinct gene expression patterns. The differences in gene expression patterns among these subtypes reflect basic differences in the cell biology of the tumors and are manifest in differences in clinical outcome, and clinicians are increasingly viewing these molecular subtypes as separable diseases. The subtypes are luminal A, luminal B, *HER2/neu* and basal-like (or basaloid, or triple negative). The subtypes are commonly approximated using routine tumor markers, such as luminal A: ER- and/or PR-positive/*HER2*-negative; luminal B: ER- and/or PR-positive/*HER2*-positive; *HER2*-positive: ER-negative/PR-negative/*HER2*-positive; and basal-like ER-negative/PR-negative/*HER2*-negative and/or CK5/6 positive and/or epidermal growth factor (EGFR)-positive. Differences in gene expression pattern affecting hundreds of genes are found between the various subgroups; these differences appear to persist through the natural life history of the breast cancer,[165] and neoadjuvant treatment of breast tumors appears to have little bearing on the gene expression patterns that contribute to the intrinsic tumor subtype.[164,166]

In addition to defining biological tumor subsets, gene expression profiling has been used to stratify tumors as having good-risk or poor-risk prognostic signatures.[167,168] One of these, MammaPrint (Agendia Br, Amsterdam, The Netherlands), a 70-gene signature developed in the Netherlands,[167] was given FDA approval in February 2007. Since then, several additional "poor prognosis" gene expression profiles have been developed using different phenotypic characteristics of aggressive cancer biology, such as wound-response and hypoxia-response. Retrospective analyses suggest that these gene signatures contribute independent prognostic information above and beyond that achieved with use of traditional pathologic markers such as tumor size, nodal status, grade, lymphovascular invasion, and hormone receptor status. An attempt to combine three gene expression signatures did not improve the prognostic accuracy.[169]

One molecular test that has been shown to be of use clinically is the Onco*type* DX recurrence score. The recurrence score is based on a quantitative assessment of 21 genes thought to be relevant to breast cancer biology, including hormone receptors and *HER2*, among others. In contrast to gene expression profiles that classify tumors into specific subsets or dichotomize tumors into good/poor prognostic groups, the recurrence score calculates a continuous, numeric result that correlates with distant metastatic recurrence in tamoxifen-treated patients with node-negative breast cancer,[170] and more recently has been shown as a prognostic marker in postmenopausal women with node-negative or node-positive tumors receiving either tamoxifen or an AI.[171] Although the recurrence score tends to correlate with features like tumor grade, size, nodal status, and quantitative levels of hormone receptor expression, multivariate analyses demonstrate that the score provides significant independent prognostic information. Unlike most other microarray analyses that require freshly frozen or prepared tissues, the recurrence score can be determined on paraffin-embedded tissue, allowing linkage of outcomes from clinical treatment trials to recurrence score measurements. Onco*type* DX has been applied to a common clinical question: whether a node-negative, ER-positive patient should receive chemotherapy in addition to hormonal therapy. Retrospective analyses from NSABP B-20—a trial of tamoxifen alone versus tamoxifen plus chemotherapy for ER-positive, node-negative patients—demonstrated that the recurrence score was a predictive factor for benefit from chemotherapy. Patients with tumors that had a low recurrence score had a very favorable overall prognosis that was not meaningfully improved by chemotherapy, while patients with high recurrence scores derived a substantial benefit from chemotherapy.[172] Qualitatively similar findings have now been reported from the SWOG 8814 study, a randomized trial of tamoxifen alone or tamoxifen plus CAF (cyclophosphamide/doxorubicin/5-fluorouracil) chemotherapy for postmenopausal women with ER-positive, node-positive breast cancer, although the overall prognosis in this node-positive cohort was less favorable than in node-negative cases.[173] Trials of preoperative chemotherapy have confirmed that a major response to treatment is more common among patients with high recurrence scores.[174]

Collectively, these molecular tools have led to the evolution of specific treatment algorithms based on subtype classification, and clinical trials are increasingly designed for specific tumor types. In addition, gene expression assays appear to allow for a more individualized assessment of risk based on the intrinsic biological properties of the cancer cells, with the promise of tailoring treatment programs for individual women.

ADJUVANT SYSTEMIC THERAPY

The goal of adjuvant systemic therapy is to prevent the recurrence of breast cancer by eradicating micrometastatic deposits of tumor that are present at the time of diagnosis. The rationale for adjuvant treatment stems from the systemic hypothesis of breast tumorigenesis, which argues that in the early stages of breast cancer development, tumor cells are disseminated throughout the body (discussed in detail in the section "Local-Regional Therapy and Survival"). Thus, in addition to appropriate local therapy, improvements in breast cancer outcome hinge on effective systemic treatments that prevent disease recurrence as distant metastasis. To a large extent, this hypothesis has been validated through decades of clinical investigation, and approximately half of the recent decline in breast cancer mortality in the United States and Western Europe has been attributed to the widespread use of adjuvant therapy.[5]

In current practice, three systemic treatment modalities are widely used as adjuvant therapy for early-stage breast cancer. These modalities are (1) endocrine treatments such as tamoxifen, AIs, or ovarian suppression; (2) anti-*HER2* therapy with the humanized monoclonal antibody, trastuzumab; and (3) chemotherapy. Selection of adjuvant treatment is determined by the biological features of the breast cancer (Table 106.16). Patients with tumors that are hormone receptor positive (either for ER, PR, or both) are candidates for adjuvant endocrine therapy; patients with tumors that are *HER2* overexpressing are candidates for trastuzumab. Chemotherapy is used irrespective of tumor hormone receptor status or *HER2* status, based largely on features such as tumor size, nodal status, and the patient's other health considerations.

Adjuvant Endocrine Therapy

Tamoxifen is the historic standard for adjuvant endocrine therapy for breast cancer. The Early Breast Cancer Trialists' Group

TABLE 106.16

OVERVIEW OF ADJUVANT TREATMENT APPROACHES IN BREAST CANCER

Tumor HER Status	Tumor Hormone Receptor Status	
	Positive	Negative
HER2-negative/normal	Endocrine therapy ± chemotherapy	Chemotherapy
HER2-positive/overexpressed	Endocrine therapy + chemotherapy + trastuzumab	Chemotherapy + trastuzumab

has performed an overview of the randomized trials of adjuvant tamoxifen therapy.[175] These results reflect data with 15 years of follow-up, from over 60 adjuvant trials including more than 80,000 women. Tamoxifen administered for 5 years results in a 41% reduction in the annual rate of breast cancer recurrence (HR, 0.59) and a 34% reduction in the annual death rate (HR, 0.66) for women with ER-positive breast cancer. The gains associated with tamoxifen are achieved independent of patient age or menopausal status, with and without the use of adjuvant chemotherapy, and are durable, contributing to improved survival through at least 15 years of follow-up. Shorter durations of tamoxifen therapy are also beneficial, but appear to have less impact than 5-year treatment duration. The optimal duration of tamoxifen therapy appears to be 5 years; extending tamoxifen therapy beyond 5 years in patients with no evidence of tumor recurrence has not led to further improvements in disease-free or overall survival.[176] Consistent with its activity as a SERM, tamoxifen is not effective in preventing recurrence of hormone receptor–negative breast cancer.[177,178]

Based on these collective data, the National Institutes of Health Consensus Development Conference on Adjuvant Therapy for Breast Cancer in 2000 recommended the use of adjuvant tamoxifen for 5 years as adjuvant hormonal therapy for all women with hormone receptor–positive breast cancer irrespective of age, menopausal status, tumor size, or nodal status.[179]

In the past 5 years, multiple clinical trials have examined the role of AIs as adjuvant endocrine therapy for early breast cancer. Although tamoxifen works by binding to the estrogen receptor, AIs function through inhibition of the aromatase enzyme that converts androgens into estrogens.[180] The result is profound estrogen depletion in postmenopausal women. AIs are not appropriate for premenopausal patients, as residual ovarian function can lead to enhanced production of aromatase and thus overcome the effects of AIs. In postmenopausal patients, where only baseline levels of aromatase activity are present, AIs effectively lower estrogen levels by 90% to nearly undetectable levels.[181]

A variety of clinical trials have addressed the question of whether the incorporation of an AI improves the results seen with 5 years of tamoxifen in postmenopausal women with hormone receptor–positive breast cancer. Table 106.17 summarizes the major trials of adjuvant AI therapy. AI treatment has been explored as primary or up-front therapy instead of tamoxifen,[182–184] as sequential therapy after 2 or 3 years of tamoxifen,[185,186] and as extended therapy after 5 years of tamoxifen.[187–189] In each instance, the use of an AI at some point in the treatment program improved outcomes compared with the control arm, which consisted of 5 years of tamoxifen therapy. The use of an AI has led to modest improvements in disease-free survival in all of these trials as a result of a lower risk of both distant metastasis and of in-breast recurrences and contralateral tumors. To date, significant survival differences with the use of an AI have not been reported, although in the MA17 trial of letrozole after 5 years of tamoxifen, the addition of letrozole produced a statistically significant survival benefit in the subset of node-positive women (HR, 0.61; 95% CI, 0.38–0.98; P = .04).[188] Two trials, BIG 1-98[190] and the TEAM study,[191] have compared up-front use of an AI against a sequential treatment with tamoxifen followed by an AI. These studies demonstrate equal rates of tumor recurrence with either 5 years of an AI or 2 to 3 years of tamoxifen followed by 2 to 3 years of an AI for a total of 5 years of therapy.

TABLE 106.17

MAJOR STUDIES COMPARING ADJUVANT THERAPY INCORPORATING AROMATASE INHIBITORS WITH 5 YEARS OF TAMOXIFEN

Timing/Setting	Trial (Ref.)	AI	No. of Patients	Hazard Ratio for Disease-Free Survival	Absolute Difference in Disease-Free Survival (%)
Upfront; y 0	ATAC (174)	ANA	9,366	0.87[a]	2.8 @ 5 y
	BIG 1–98 (175)	LET	8,010	0.81	2.6 @ 5 y
Sequential; after 2–3 y of TAM	IES (177)	EXE	4,742	0.68	4.7 @ 3 y
	ARNO/ABCSG (176)	ANA	3,224	0.60	3.1 @ 3 y
Extended; after 5 y of TAM	MA17 (179)	LET	5,187	0.58	4.6 @ 4 y
	NSABP B-33 (180)	EXE	1,598	0.68	2.0 @ 4 y

AI, aromatase inhibitor; ATAC, Arimidex, tamoxifen, alone or in combination; ANA, anastrozole; BIG, Breast International Group; LET, letrozole; TAM, tamoxifen; IES, Intergroup Exemestane Study EXE, exemestane; ARNO/ABCSG, Arimidex-Nolvadex/Austrian Breast and Colorectal Cancer Study Group; MA, National Cancer Institute of Canada MA; NSABP, National Surgical Adjuvant Breast and Bowel Project.
[a]Comparison for ANA versus TAM. The third arm of the trial, combined therapy with ANA plus TAM, yielded outcomes similar to those of TAM alone.

Collectively, these data argue for use of an AI in most postmenopausal women with early-stage, hormone receptor–positive breast cancer, but they leave open many critical questions about the optimal use of these agents.[192] The option of starting with either an AI or tamoxifen appears reasonable for any patient. The appropriate duration of AI treatment is not clear. The up-front trials[183,184] limited treatment to a total of 5 years' duration, and the sequential trials[185,186] used AI therapy for only 2 or 3 years as part of a total of 5 years of adjuvant endocrine treatment. The studies of extended endocrine therapy beyond 5 years[188,189] underscore the long natural history of hormone receptor–positive breast cancer and demonstrate that antiestrogen treatments have ongoing benefits well beyond 5 years after diagnosis. For women who begin taking an AI at the time of diagnosis, the appropriate duration of endocrine treatment is unknown, although at present, a maximum of 5 years is the only duration for which safety and efficacy data exist. Studies are ongoing to address this question.

The recently updated ASCO guidelines on adjuvant endocrine therapy recommend that postmenopausal women consider an AI at some point in their treatment program as either initial therapy or as sequential therapy after several years of tamoxifen[193] (Table 106.18). The ASCO guideline also underscore differences in side effect profiles between tamoxifen and AI therapy, which may inform treatment selection. Tamoxifen is associated with rare risks of thromboembolism and uterine cancer.[176,183,184] AI treatment is associated with accelerated osteoporosis and an arthralgia syndrome[194]; patients receiving AI therapy require serial monitoring of bone mineral density.[195] Both treatments are associated with menopausal symptoms such as hot flashes, night sweats, and genitourinary symptoms including sexual dysfunction. Symptomatically, patients may tolerate one class of agent better than another; those intolerant of either tamoxifen or AI therapy should be offered the alternative type of treatment. Because AI therapy is only effective in postmenopausal women, tamoxifen remains

TABLE 106.18

ADJUVANT TRIALS OF AROMATASE INHIBITORS

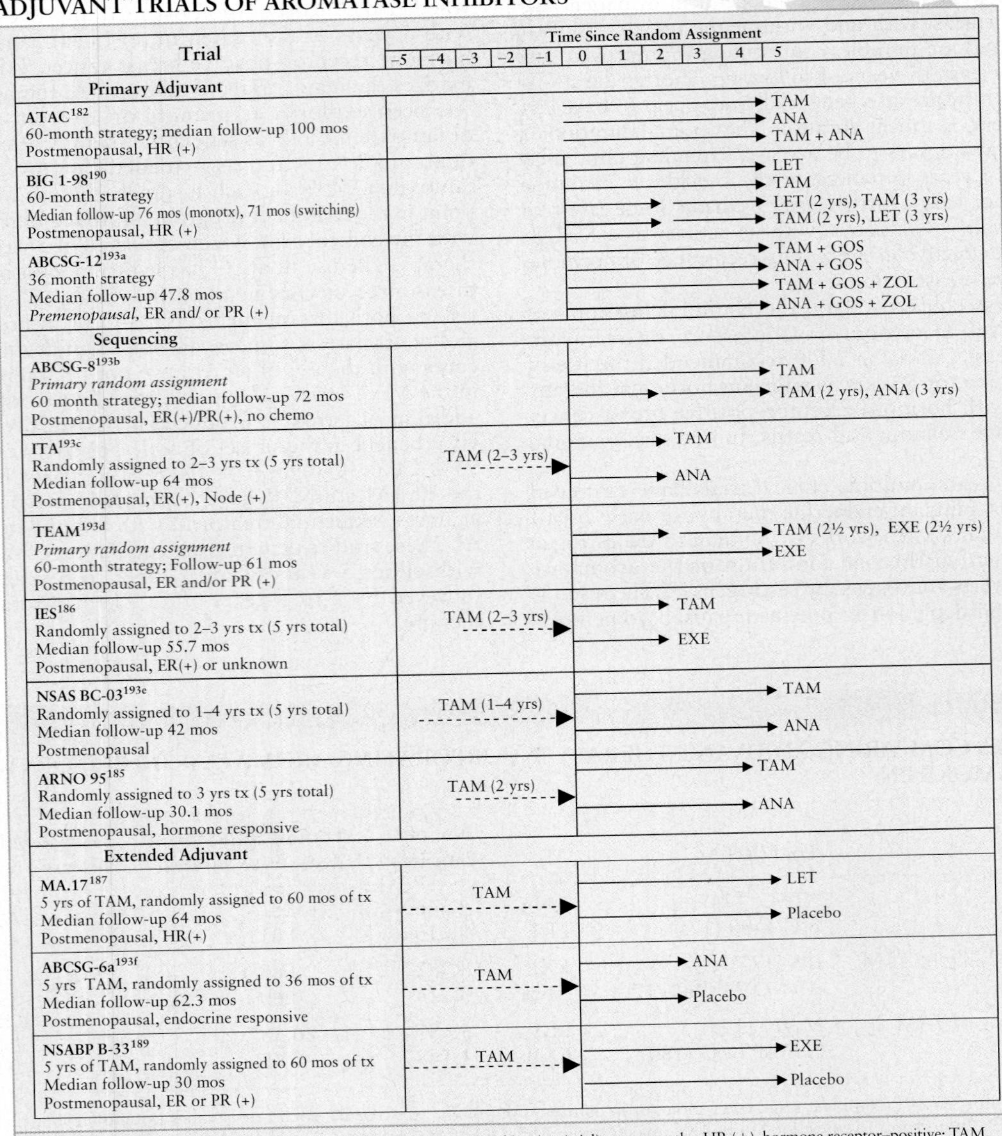

Trial	Time Since Random Assignment (−5 to 5)
Primary Adjuvant	
ATAC[182] 60-month strategy; median follow-up 100 mos Postmenopausal, HR (+)	→ TAM → ANA → TAM + ANA
BIG 1-98[190] 60-month strategy Median follow-up 76 mos (monotx), 71 mos (switching) Postmenopausal, HR (+)	→ LET → TAM → → LET (2 yrs), TAM (3 yrs) → → TAM (2 yrs), LET (3 yrs)
ABCSG-12[193a] 36 month strategy Median follow-up 47.8 mos *Premenopausal,* ER and/ or PR (+)	→ TAM + GOS → ANA + GOS → TAM + GOS + ZOL → ANA + GOS + ZOL
Sequencing	
ABCSG-8[193b] *Primary random assignment* 60 month strategy; median follow-up 72 mos Postmenopausal, ER(+)/PR(+), no chemo	→ TAM → → TAM (2 yrs), ANA (3 yrs)
ITA[193c] Randomly assigned to 2–3 yrs tx (5 yrs total) Median follow-up 64 mos Postmenopausal, ER(+), Node (+)	TAM (2–3 yrs) ▶ → TAM → ANA
TEAM[193d] *Primary random assignment* 60-month strategy; Follow-up 61 mos Postmenopausal, ER and/or PR (+)	→ → TAM (2½ yrs), EXE (2½ yrs) → EXE
IES[186] Randomly assigned to 2–3 yrs tx (5 yrs total) Median follow-up 55.7 mos Postmenopausal, ER(+) or unknown	TAM (2–3 yrs) ▶ → TAM → EXE
NSAS BC-03[193e] Randomly assigned to 1–4 yrs tx (5 yrs total) Median follow-up 42 mos Postmenopausal	TAM (1–4 yrs) ▶ → TAM → ANA
ARNO 95[185] Randomly assigned to 3 yrs tx (5 yrs total) Median follow-up 30.1 mos Postmenopausal, hormone responsive	TAM (2 yrs) ▶ → TAM → ANA
Extended Adjuvant	
MA.17[187] 5 yrs of TAM, randomly assigned to 60 mos of tx Median follow-up 64 mos Postmenopausal, HR(+)	TAM ▶ → LET → Placebo
ABCSG-6a[193f] 5 yrs TAM, randomly assigned to 36 mos of tx Median follow-up 62.3 mos Postmenopausal, endocrine responsive	TAM ▶ → ANA → Placebo
NSABP B-33[189] 5 yrs of TAM, randomly assigned to 60 mos of tx Median follow-up 30 mos Postmenopausal, ER or PR (+)	TAM ▶ → EXE → Placebo

Schema of included trials. ATAC, Arimidex, Tamoxifen, Alone or in Combination (trial); mos, months; HR (+), hormone receptor–positive; TAM, tamoxifen; ANA, anastrozole; BIG, Breast International Group; FU, follow-up; monotx, monotherapy; LET, letrozole; yrs, years; ABCSG, Austrian Breast and Colorectal Cancer Study Group; ER (+), estrogen receptor–positive; PR (+), progesterone receptor–positive; GOS, goserelin; ZOL, zoledronic acid; ABCSG, Austrian Breast and Colorectal Cancer Study Group; Chemo, chemotherapy; ITA, Italian Tamoxifen Anastrozole (trial); tx, therapy; TEAM, Tamoxifen Exemestane Adjuvant Multinational (trial); EXE, exemestane; IES, Intergroup Exemestane Study; Unk, unknown; N-SAS, National Surgical Adjuvant Study (Group); ARNO, Arimidex-Nolvadex (trial); NSABP, National Surgical Adjuvant Breast and Bowel Project.
From ref. 193.

the treatment of choice in women who are pre- or perimenopausal or in whom there is question of residual ovarian function. In particular, women with chemotherapy-induced amenorrhea may have recovery of ovarian function and are not suitable candidates for AI treatment.[196]

Despite long-standing interest in ovarian suppression as adjuvant therapy, its role in addition to tamoxifen or chemotherapy remains unclear. Early studies of ovarian suppression were not limited to patients with hormone receptor–positive tumors, meaning that these trials were often conducted in patients unlikely to benefit from endocrine treatment. In addition, many studies of ovarian suppression in the 1980s and 1990s failed to incorporate tamoxifen, as it was not appreciated that tamoxifen was beneficial in premenopausal women, so the benefits of ovarian suppression in addition to tamoxifen are not well understood. Finally, clinical trials that included chemotherapy for younger women were confounded by the high incidence of chemotherapy-induced menopause.[197] Thus, despite the fact that multiple randomized trials have demonstrated that ovarian suppression can be effective adjuvant therapy for premenopausal women[175] and have demonstrated that ovarian suppression is frequently at least as effective as adjuvant chemotherapy in preventing breast cancer recurrence,[198] there remains little consensus on whether ovarian suppression adds meaningfully to results seen with tamoxifen with or without adjuvant chemotherapy.

Recent observations suggest that ovarian suppression is a critical question for younger women with hormone receptor–positive breast cancer. Very young women—typically those less than age 35 years—who do not routinely experience amenorrhea with adjuvant chemotherapy appear to have a substantially worse prognosis than patients who do enter menopause with chemotherapy.[199] A randomized trial has compared chemotherapy alone, chemotherapy plus ovarian suppression and chemotherapy, and ovarian suppression plus tamoxifen as adjuvant treatment. The addition of tamoxifen clearly improved results compared to chemotherapy with or without ovarian suppression. In subset analyses, younger women (less than age 40 years) who were less likely to experience chemotherapy-induced amenorrhea did appear to benefit from ovarian suppression in addition to chemotherapy.[200] However, the study design does not directly address whether ovarian suppression would substantially add to tamoxifen-based treatment. The Adjuvant Breast Cancer Ovarian Ablation or Suppression Trial compared tamoxifen alone versus tamoxifen with ovarian suppression in premenopausal women and did not show a substantial improvement in disease-free survival with the addition of ovarian suppression.[201] However, in this study, only 40% of patients were known to have ER-positive breast cancer, and 80% of patients additionally received adjuvant chemotherapy, profoundly limiting the interpretation of the results. Ongoing trials are specifically testing the role of ovarian suppression in addition to tamoxifen for premenopausal patients.

Tamoxifen is metabolized by the cytochrome P-450 system into biologically active metabolites. Recent data have suggested that pharmacogenomic variation in P-450 alleles or the concurrent use of tamoxifen and P-450 inhibitors might affect tamoxifen metabolism, with clinically significant effects. Retrospective analyses of small adjuvant treatment have suggested that patients with inefficient tamoxifen metabolism owing to mutations in CYP2D6 enzyme, part of the P-450 complex, might derive less benefit from adjuvant tamoxifen than others.[202–204] Patients receiving certain medicines known to inhibit P-450, such as the selective serotonin reuptake inhibitors paroxetine and fluoxetine, also generate fewer active tamoxifen metabolites, which may interfere with clinical outcomes.[205,206] Neither the full significance of pharmacogenomic allelic variation nor the adequacy of testing for such variation is well characterized at present. Patients receiving tamoxifen should probably avoid the aforementioned selective serotonin reuptake inhibitors in light of the potential pharmacologic interaction.

Adjuvant Chemotherapy

Adjuvant chemotherapy consisting of multiple cycles of polychemotherapy is well established as an important strategy for lowering the risk of breast cancer recurrence and improving survival. Initial studies of adjuvant chemotherapy were conducted in women with higher risk, lymph node–positive breast cancer. Subsequent trials have extended the benefits of adjuvant chemotherapy into lower risk, node-negative patient populations.[175]

Long-term follow-up from the Oxford overview demonstrated benefit from chemotherapy for women irrespective of age, tumor ER status, or whether patients also receive adjuvant endocrine therapy.[175] In addition, the overview suggests that there are advantages for multiple cycles (four to eight) of chemotherapy compared with single-cycle regimens. The overview also supports the findings of multiple individual trials showing superiority of anthracycline-based chemotherapy compared with CMF-based, nonanthracycline regimens.

Based on this collective experience, multiple cycles of adjuvant chemotherapy, typically including anthracycline-based regimens, are recommended for the majority of patients with node-positive and higher risk node-negative tumors.[207,208] The current challenges in adjuvant chemotherapy treatment are to select subsets of patients that might preferentially benefit from chemotherapy or conversely be spared adjuvant chemotherapy and to optimize the dosing and scheduling of chemotherapy to achieve the best clinical results and improve the side effect profile of treatment.

The introduction of taxanes into early-stage breast cancer treatment constitutes an important advance over the historic experience with alkylator and anthracycline-based chemotherapy. The first report on adjuvant taxane therapy was Cancer and Leukemia Group B (CALGB) 9344, a randomized study of doxorubicin dose escalation and the incorporation of sequential paclitaxel therapy for women receiving four cycles of cyclophosphamide-doxorubicin (AC) chemotherapy.[209] CALGB 9344 demonstrated that sequential paclitaxel therapy improved both disease-free and overall survival among women with node-positive breast cancer. Since that time, nearly one dozen studies have reported on breast cancer outcomes with the incorporation of taxanes—either paclitaxel or docetaxel—either as substitutes or sequential additions to anthracycline-based regimens (Table 106.19). Collectively, these data suggest that the use of taxanes can contribute to significant improvement in outcomes, especially among women with node-positive breast cancer, in whom the vast majority of these trials have been conducted. A randomized comparison of AC followed by either docetaxel or paclitaxel, with taxanes given either every 3 weeks or on a weekly schedule, did not show significant differences between the taxanes with respect to breast cancer recurrence.[210] Ongoing studies seeking to define the best taxane regimen are comparing the three-drug regimen TAC (docetaxel/doxorubicin/5-fluorouracil) with sequential treatment with AC followed by paclitaxel given on an every 2-week schedule.

Chemotherapy dose and schedule considerations remain a major area of clinical investigation. Multiple studies have failed to demonstrate that dose escalation of cyclophosphamide[211] or doxorubicin[209] results in a lower risk of recurrence. Administration of either paclitaxel or docetaxel on an every 3-week schedule has been compared with weekly taxane administration following AC chemotherapy without contributing to statistically significant differences, although modest absolute advantages were seen with weekly paclitaxel and

PRACTICE OF ONCOLOGY

TABLE 106.19

TRIALS OF ADJUVANT TAXANE THERAPY

Trial	No. of Patients	Design	Hazard Ratio—DFS	Hazard Ratio—OS
		Paclitaxel		
M. D. Anderson	524	FAC × 8 vs. P × 4 → FAC × 8	0.7	NR
CALGB 9344	3,121	AC × 4 vs. AC × 4 → P × 4	0.83	0.82
ECTO	1,355	A → CMF vs. AP → CMF	0.65	0.71
GEICAM 9906	1,248	FEC × 6 vs. FEC × 4 → P × 8	0.63	0.74
HeCOG	595	E × 4 → CMF vs. E × 3 → P × 3 → CMF × 3	0.86	0.41
NSABP B-28	3,059	AC × 4 vs. AC × 4 → P × 4	0.83	0.93
		Docetaxel		
BCIRG 001	1,491	FAC × 6 vs. DAC × 6	0.72	0.70
ECOG 2197	2,885	AC × 4 vs. AD × 4	0.92	0.92
BIG 2–98	2,887	A ± C × 4 → CMF × 3 vs. A × 3 → D × 3 → CMF × 3 vs. AD × 4 → CMF × 3	0.86	0.92
NSABP B-27	2,411	AC × 4 vs. AC × 4 → D × 4	0.90	1.07
PACS 01	1,999	FEC × 6 vs. FEC × 3 → D × 3	0.83	0.73
TAXIT 216	972	E → CMF vs. E → D → CMF	0.79	0.72
U.S. Oncology	1,016	AC × 4 vs. DC × 4	0.67	0.76

DFS, disease-free survival; OS, overall survival; NR, not reported. Trials: CALGB, Cancer and Leukemia Group B; ECTO, European Cooperative Trial in Operable breast cancer; GEICAM, Grupo Español de Investigación en Cáncer de Mama; HeCOG, Hellenic Cooperative Oncology Group; NSABP, National Surgical Adjuvant Breast and Bowel Project; BCIRG, Breast Cancer International Research Group; ECOG, Eastern Cooperative Oncology Group; BIG, Breast International Group; PACS. Drugs in design column: F, 5-fluorouracil; A, doxorubicin; C, cyclophosphamide; P, paclitaxel; M, methotrexate; D, docetaxel; E, epirubicin (From ref. 193, with permission).

every 3-week docetaxel compared with the other treatment schedules.[210] A neoadjuvant study reported that paclitaxel given weekly yielded superior rates of pathologic complete response compared with every 3-week paclitaxel.[212] The CALGB 9741 trial compared AC followed by paclitaxel given either every 3 weeks or every 2 weeks at the same doses and schedules.[213] Accelerated, every 2-week treatment led to lower risk of recurrence and improved survival. The same study also compared concurrent therapy, giving cyclophosphamide and doxorubicin together followed by paclitaxel, or sequential chemotherapy treatment consisting of doxorubicin/paclitaxel cyclophosphamide, and showed that there was no difference between concurrent or sequential therapy. These trials suggest that chemotherapy schedule, particularly with taxanes, may have an impact on antitumor efficacy.

There is growing interest in adjuvant chemotherapy regimens that might spare patients exposure to anthracycline-based chemotherapy. Historical options include CMF chemotherapy, which was shown to be equivalent to doxorubicin/cyclophosphamide.[214] More recently, the two-drug combination regimen of docetaxel plus cyclophosphamide (TC) has been compared with doxorubicin/cyclophosphamide, each regimen given for a total of four cycles.[215] This trial of 1,016 women with node-negative or one to three positive lymph nodes demonstrated improvement in disease-free survival and overall survival with TC, establishing TC as an option for these intermediate-risk patients. Among higher risk patients, it is unclear that anthracyclines can be safely omitted. NSABP B-30 compared AC followed by docetaxel with four cycles of docetaxel/doxorubicin/cyclophosphamide with four cycles of doxorubicin/docetaxel in node-positive breast cancer.[216] In this study, sequential AC followed by docetaxel was superior to four cycles of docetaxel/doxorubicin/cyclophosphamide, arguing by inference that four cycles of docetaxel/cyclophosphamide might not be sufficient for higher risk node-positive breast cancer patients.

Clinical studies have shown that chemotherapy can be of benefit to women with node-positive and node-negative breast cancers, with tumors that are either hormone receptor–positive or –negative, regardless of age or menopausal status. Retrospective analyses have even shown that chemotherapy can be beneficial to women with tumors as small as 1 cm or less, including both ER-positive and ER-negative tumors.[217] Nonetheless, there is great interest in trying to determine whether specific regimens should be employed in certain groups of patients defined by clinical features or by tumor biology, and whether staging information or pathobiological tumor characteristics can identify groups of women who do not need adjuvant chemotherapy. This interest stems from several considerations. First, although the addition of chemotherapy often leads to statistically significant gains in relative risk

reduction, these often translate into very small differences in the absolute risk of recurrence for patients, especially patients with earlier stage disease[218] or in patients where adjuvant endocrine therapy improves outcome. Second, many chemotherapy trials, particularly those involving women with hormone receptor–positive tumors, are confounded by the endocrine effects of chemotherapy-induced amenorrhea. Third, most clinical trial results do not take into account the existence of molecularly defined breast cancer subsets. Trials that are the benchmarks in the literature generally included patients with tumors that were not necessarily defined by hormone receptor status, or more recently, *HER2* status. There is a concern that these "all comers" trials may overestimate the benefits of chemotherapy in certain subtypes of breast cancer, while underestimating the benefits in others. Finally, for patients in whom the absolute advantages of chemotherapy are modest, efforts to weigh patient preferences and directly quantify chemotherapy benefits for specific patients, as opposed to large cohorts in clinical trials, have led to further individualization of chemotherapy choices.

Hormone receptor status may be an important predictor of benefit from chemotherapy. Retrospective analyses among patients with node-negative breast cancer suggest that tumors that are low or nonexpressors of ER derive substantial benefit from the addition of chemotherapy to tamoxifen; by contrast, tumors with high quantitative levels of ER do not appear to gain substantially from adding chemotherapy to endocrine therapy.[178] A retrospective review of CALGB trials for node-positive breast cancer patients evaluated the gains associated with chemotherapy using a variety of anthracycline- and taxane-based treatments as a function of tumor ER status.[219] Improvements in outcome from changes in chemotherapy schedule and dosing, including the addition of taxane-based therapy, were most noticeable among patients with ER-negative tumors, while patients with ER-positive tumors derived more limited benefit from newer adjuvant chemotherapy regimens. However, not all retrospective studies have shown a clear relationship between ER status and the benefit of chemotherapy,[220] and precise thresholds of ER expression and likely chemotherapy benefit are not well established.

HER2 is also a marker that has been widely studied as a predictor of benefit from adjuvant chemotherapy. Multiple retrospective analyses have suggested that *HER2* overexpression is associated with a relative benefit from anthracycline-based chemotherapy,[221] and that *HER2*-negative tumors do not selectively benefit from anthracyclines, as opposed to CMF-type, chemotherapy treatments. Other retrospective work based on characterizing both *HER2* status and ER status of tumors suggests that chemotherapy with taxanes may be especially critical in tumors that either lack ER expression or express *HER2*.[222] However, the reported interactions between *HER2* status and type of chemotherapy are not uniform across all trials and are largely derived from unplanned, retrospective analyses. More critically, these chemotherapy trials all predate the widespread use of adjuvant trastuzumab, which may render moot the details of chemotherapy selection for *HER2*-positive tumors.

New molecular assays that integrate larger numbers of biomarkers may further clarify the potential role of chemotherapeutic agents in adjuvant treatment. The 21-gene recurrence score (Onco*type* DX, discussed in the section "Prognostic and Predictive Factors"), which incorporates hormone receptor measurement and *HER2* expression into its numeric algorithm, has been used to predict outcome for ER-positive, node-negative breast cancers treated with tamoxifen[170] or tamoxifen plus chemotherapy in node-negative[171] and node-positive[173] patients. Patients with tumors with higher recurrence scores derive substantial benefit from the addition of chemotherapy to endocrine treatment, while patients with low recurrence scores have both a more favorable overall prognosis and do not appear to benefit meaningfully from the addition of chemotherapy. Investigational work with the 21-gene recurrence score and other gene expression–based arrays suggests that pathologic features such as low or no expression of hormone receptors, expression of *HER2*, and high tumor grade all tend to be predictors of likely sensitivity of tumors to chemotherapy.[169,223] Tumors at the other end of the molecular spectrum—low grade, high levels of hormone receptors, lack of *HER2* expression—tend to be more sensitive to endocrine therapies and less sensitive to adjuvant chemotherapy. It is widely expected that within several years, sufficient clinical data will be available to allow a more precise characterization of tumor features that suggest whether or not patients should receive adjuvant chemotherapy.

Critical components of decision making for adjuvant chemotherapy are a consideration of the realistic benefits and likely side effects for a given patient and involvement of the patient in the treatment-selection process. Various chemotherapy regimens have distinctive side effect profiles that can inform regimen selection for an individual patient. For example, anthracyclines are associated with a low but finite risk of cardiomyopathy and may not be appropriate for patients with previous anthracycline exposure or pre-existing cardiac disease. Taxane-based treatments are associated with neuropathy that may be worse in patients with pre-existing peripheral neuropathy.

Patients and doctors may attempt to gauge the absolute gains associated with chemotherapy by considering rigorously the tumor stage, comorbid conditions, age of the patient, and the biological features of the tumor. One tool that allows for such refinement is Adjuvant!, an online program that quantifies the benefits of adjuvant treatment.[156,224] Adjuvant! integrates tumor size and biomarker information, patient age and health status, and the relative benefits of chemotherapy as measured in clinical trials, and reports in bar graph format the absolute benefits that the given patient is likely to achieve with adjuvant chemotherapy. This information, although based on computer simulation and modeling, provides quantitative estimates that may assist patients in making choices about treatment. Patient surveys, inevitably performed after patients have endured adjuvant chemotherapy, suggest that many women would prefer adjuvant chemotherapy for extraordinarily small gains (1% improvement in outcome), and most women would accept chemotherapy for modest differences on the order of a 3% to 5% improvement in chance of recurrence.[225] Nonetheless, a careful and honest appraisal of the likelihood of benefit from chemotherapy should be a part of any decision to recommend adjuvant chemotherapy treatment.

Adjuvant Trastuzumab Therapy for *HER2* Overexpressing Breast Cancer

HER2 expression has historically been considered an adverse prognostic factor associated with a higher risk of recurrence, an early risk of recurrence, and relative resistance to established therapies such as CMF-based chemotherapy.[226] *HER2*-expressing tumors tend to express lower levels of hormone receptors than *HER2*-negative tumors, contributing to relative resistance to adjuvant endocrine therapies even when hormone receptors are present.[208,227] For these reasons, patients with *HER2*-positive tumors have been a clinical challenge, contributing to a large fraction of cancer-related events in adjuvant breast cancer trials, and have been a high-priority population for targeted clinical trials.

In 2005 reports became available from five randomized clinical trials that examined the addition of trastuzumab, the humanized monoclonal antibody against the Her-2 protein, to chemotherapy as adjuvant treatment for *HER2* overexpressing breast cancer (Table 106.20).[228–232] Although these trials used a

TABLE 106.20

ADJUVANT TRIALS OF TRASTUZUMAB

Trial (Ref.)	No. of Patients	Chemotherapy Regimen	Trastuzumab Regimen	Hazard Ratio—DFS	Hazard Ratio—OS
NSABP B-31 (228)/ NCCTG N9831	3,351	AC → P	One year beginning concurrently with P	0.48	0.67
HERA (229)	3,401	Various	One year beginning sequentially after chemotherapy	0.64	0.63
FinHER (230)	232	V or D → FEC	9 weeks beginning concurrently with V or D	0.42	0.41
BCIRG 006 (231)	3,222	AC → D	One year beginning concurrently with D	0.61	0.59
		CbD[a]	One year beginning concurrently with CbD	0.67	0.66

DFS, disease-free survival; OS, overall survival; NSABP, National Surgical Adjuvant Breast and Bowel Project; NCCTG, North Central Cancer Treatment Group; A, doxorubicin; C, cyclophosphamide; P, paclitaxel; HERA, Herceptin Adjuvant; FinHER, Finland Herceptin; V, vinorelbine; D, docetaxel; BCIRG, Breast Cancer International Research Group; Cb, carboplatin.
[a]In comparison to AC → D chemotherapy.

variety of different adjuvant chemotherapy regimens and employed trastuzumab in different schedules and sequences, they all showed significant improvements in disease-free survival (reduction in risk of 50% on average) and in overall survival even after a short duration of follow-up. Subset analyses demonstrated comparable relative risk reduction regardless of tumor size, nodal status, or hormone receptor status, resulting in the rapid incorporation of trastuzumab into standard treatment recommendations for women with *HER2*-positive breast cancer.

Cardiomyopathy is a novel side effect of trastuzumab therapy.[233] Cardiac dysfunction is more pronounced in patients receiving anthracycline-based adjuvant chemotherapy (incidence approximately 2%) than in patients who receive nonanthracycline adjuvant chemotherapy (incidence approximately 1%) in addition to trastuzumab. Other risk factors for cardiac dysfunction with adjuvant trastuzumab include pre-existing cardiac disease such as borderline normal left ventricular ejection fraction or hypertension and age greater than 65 years. Because of the possibility of cardiac toxicity, all patients being considered for adjuvant trastuzumab require baseline determination of left ventricular ejection fraction and serial monitoring of cardiac function.

Despite the rapidly emerging data on adjuvant trastuzumab, there remain several key questions regarding optimal use. Successful determination of the *HER2* status of a tumor is a cornerstone of treatment selection as trastuzumab has been shown to be effective only in tumors with aberrant expression of *HER2*.[160] The duration of trastuzumab therapy is conventionally 1 year, although that length of treatment was arbitrarily chosen in the major adjuvant trials. The FinHER (Finland Herceptin) study[230] used only 9 weeks of trastuzumab given concurrently with chemotherapy and showed benefit for trastuzumab despite the short treatment exposure; the HERA (Herceptin Adjuvant) trial is comparing 1 year versus 2 years of therapy, although data are not as yet available from that comparison.[229] It remains unclear whether trastuzumab should be delivered sequentially after chemotherapy (as done in the HERA trial[229]) or concurrently with chemotherapy (as done in the NSABP B-31/NCCTG [North Central Cancer Treatment Group] N9831,[228] and BCIRG [Breast Cancer International Research Group] trials[231]). Limited direct comparisons in NCCTG N9831 suggest that for women receiving anthracycline- and taxane-based chemotherapy, concurrent administration of trastuzumab during the taxane phase of treatment yielded superior results compared with sequential therapy.[234] All of the adjuvant clinical trials employed chemotherapy with or without trastuzumab; there are no data on whether trastuzumab would be effective as adjuvant treatment in the absence of chemotherapy administration. The optimal chemotherapy backbone for trastuzumab-based adjuvant treatment is uncertain. Most patients treated on the extant clinical trials received sequential anthracyclines and taxane-based treatment, with concurrent use of trastuzumab during taxane treatment. The preliminary results from BCIRG 006 suggest that the nonanthracycline trastuzumab/docetaxel/carboplatin regimen is superior to chemotherapy given without trastuzumab.[231] However, the study was not powered to adequately compare TCH against the AC/TH treatment arms, and numerically, the anthracycline-based regimen followed by trastuzumab was associated with a lower risk of cancer recurrence.[235] TCH is an important treatment option, particularly in patients with contraindications to anthracycline-based treatment. Concomitant RT and maintenance trastuzumab were delivered in most of the adjuvant trials. In short-term follow-up, combination therapy does not appear to alter the risks associated with either treatment modality.

Finally, most of the patients entered onto the major trastuzumab trials had node-positive or high-risk, node-negative breast cancers. The role of trastuzumab treatment for women with smaller, node-negative tumors, particularly tumors less than 1 cm, remains undetermined. Recent studies have suggested that these smaller, *HER2*-positive breast cancers still carried a substantial risk of tumor recurrence (on the order of 15% to 20% through 5 to 10 years of therapy). This risk seems sufficient to warrant consideration of trastuzumab plus chemotherapy for women with *HER2* tumors larger than 5 mm, although the benefits of trastuzumab in such cases are not proven.[236]

INTEGRATION OF MULTIMODALITY PRIMARY THERAPY

Current consensus recommendations for adjuvant therapy are summarized in Table 106.21. The majority of women with breast cancer receive some form of adjuvant therapy, which requires integration of systemic treatments with local therapy including surgery and RT. As discussed in the section "Risk Factors for Local Recurrence Following Conservative Surgery and Radiation Therapy," in patients with negative margins of resection, low rates of local recurrence are seen regardless of

TABLE 106.21

ASCO RECOMMENDATIONS FOR ADJUVANT CHEMOTHERAPY

	St. Gallen Consensus Conference 2005–2007	National Comprehensive Cancer Network 2007
HER2-positive tumors	Adjuvant chemotherapy (no specific size threshold)	Adjuvant chemotherapy tumors >0.5 cm and/or node-positive
HER2-negative tumors	ER-negative: ■ Adjuvant chemotherapy (no specific size threshold) ER-positive: ■ Adjuvant chemotherapy if four or more lymph nodes are positive ■ Consider if tumor >2 cm, or grade 2–3, or age <35, or lymphovascular invasion is present	ER-negative: ■ Adjuvant chemotherapy for tumors ≥1.0 cm and/or node-positive; ■ Consider for tumors 0.5 to 1.0 cm if adverse prognostic factors (lymphovascular invasion, high-grade features) are present ER-positive: ■ Adjuvant chemotherapy if node-positive ■ Consider if tumor >1 cm, or if tumor 0.6 to 1.0 cm and lymphovascular invasion or grade 2–3 features are present

ER, estrogen receptor.

the sequence of RT and chemotherapy.[104] A nonsignificant trend toward a greater risk of distant recurrence in patients receiving RT first was seen in one study,[104] and because of the primary importance of preventing distant relapse, the convention has been to administer chemotherapy first. Tamoxifen therapy should not be given concurrently with chemotherapy because in one randomized study concurrent tamoxifen chemotherapy was associated with greater risk of recurrence than sequential treatment of chemotherapy followed by tamoxifen.[237] There are no compelling data that the concurrent administration of tamoxifen and RT has deleterious consequences, nor that it has particular advantages.[238] It is not known how this observation relates to use of AIs with concurrent chemotherapy or RT; by extrapolation, it is probably best to avoid concurrent use of chemotherapy and any adjuvant endocrine treatment. As discussed in the section "Preoperative Systemic Therapy for Operable Cancer," the timing of surgery either before or after (neo)adjuvant chemotherapy does not alter long-term survival for women with breast cancer.[115] Thus, patients may comfortably proceed in a linear fashion of treatment, receiving one therapeutic modality (surgery, RT, chemotherapy, biological therapy) after another, as they receive definitive treatment for early-stage breast cancer.

FOLLOW-UP FOR BREAST CANCER SURVIVORS

Following initial treatment for breast cancer, patients require surveillance for local-regional tumor recurrence, contralateral breast cancer, and the development of distant metastatic disease. In addition, medical follow-up allows clinicians to monitor for late effects of chemotherapy, RT, or surgery, to gauge ongoing side effects from cancer treatments such as antiestrogen therapies, and to facilitate opportunities to update patients on new developments that may affect their treatment plan.[239] Although the greatest risk of recurrence is in the first 5 years after breast cancer diagnosis, women remain at risk for many years after their treatment, especially those with hormone receptor–positive breast cancer. These experiences justify ongoing follow-up with breast cancer specialists, although particularly in later years, follow-up is often shared with primary care physicians.

Because local recurrence after BCT and contralateral primary tumors can be treated with curative intent, screening for these types of recurrences is a high priority and women should undergo regular breast examinations and annual mammography, with supplemental breast imaging as clinically indicated. By contrast, it is not clear that early detection of distant metastatic disease contributes to substantial improvement in clinically important end points. Most distant recurrences are detected following patient-reported symptoms such as bone discomfort, lymphadenopathy, chest wall/breast changes, or respiratory symptoms; asymptomatic detection through screening laboratory tests or radiology studies occurs in only a modest fraction of patients, even with intensive surveillance.[240] Two randomized trials have compared vigorous surveillance with radiological imaging (chest radiography, bone scanning, and liver ultrasound) and laboratory testing (blood counts, liver function tests, and serum tumor markers) against standard care consisting of regular physical examination and mammography, with more intensive testing performed only if indicated by symptoms or physical examination.[241,242] More intensive surveillance achieved modest gains in early detection of metastatic breast cancer, with a small increase in the fraction of patients diagnosed while asymptomatic, but no improvement in overall survival was noted.

Based on these data, the American Society of Clinical Oncology (ASCO) has issued surveillance guidelines for women with early-stage breast cancer,[243] which are summarized in Table 106.22. These guidelines emphasize the importance of a careful history and examination to elicit symptoms or signs of recurrent breast cancer, but minimize the role of routine imaging studies including plain films and CT scans and do not recommend routine laboratory testing in the absence of symptoms. Patients should be encouraged to perform breast self-examination and to contact their physicians if they develop symptoms possibly suggestive of breast cancer recurrence. Understandably, patients often request additional testing to provide reassurance and to "catch" early recurrences. Clinical experience suggests, however, that patients respond well to discussions regarding optimal testing strategies, the role of surveillance for breast cancer recurrence, the challenges of false-positive and false-negative test results, and the limited need for testing in the absence of symptoms or physical examination findings.[244]

TABLE 106.22

BREAST CANCER FOLLOW-UP

Recommended for Routine Surveillance	
History/physical examination	Every 3 to 6 months for the first 3 years, every 6 to 12 months years 4 and 5, annually thereafter
Mammography	Annually, beginning no earlier than 6 months after radiation therapy
Breast self-examination	All women should be counseled to perform monthly
Pelvic examination	Annually
Coordination of care	Continuity of care with breast cancer specialist and appropriate other health care providers
Not Recommended for Routine Surveillance	
Routine blood tests	Complete blood cell count and liver function tests are not recommended
Imaging studies	Chest radiograph, bone scans, liver ultrasound, computed tomography scans, fluorodeoxyglucose-positron emission tomography scans, and breast magnetic resonance imaging are not recommended for routine breast cancer surveillance
Tumor markers	Cancer antigen 15-3, 27.29, and carcinoembryonic antigen are not recommended

Adapted from ref. 243.

SPECIAL THERAPEUTIC PROBLEMS

Paget Disease

Paget disease of the breast is uncommon, accounting for about 1% of all breast malignancies. Pathologically, Paget disease represents *in situ* carcinoma in the nipple epidermis. The classic pathologic finding is the presence of Paget cells (large cells with clear cytoplasm and atypical nuclei) within the epidermis of the nipple. The clinical manifestations of Paget disease include eczematoid changes, crusting, redness, irritation, erosion, discharge, retraction, and inversion. Rarely, Paget disease is bilateral or occurs in a male patient.

Paget disease may occur in the nipple (1) in conjunction with an underlying invasive cancer (staged by the invasive cancer), (2) with underlying DCIS (staged Tis), or (3) alone without any underlying invasive breast carcinoma or DCIS (also staged Tis). The associated underlying cancer may be located centrally in the breast adjacent to the nipple or it may be located peripherally. It is uncertain whether the origin of Paget disease is primarily an *in situ* intraepidermal malignancy with secondary extension to adjacent structures (intraepidermal theory) or migration of tumor cells into the nipple epidermis from an underlying carcinoma of the breast (epidermotropic theory).

The age-adjusted incidence rates of female Paget disease peaked in 1985 and have decreased yearly thereafter through 2002. From 1988 to 2002, incidence rates decreased by 45%, while the incidence of invasive cancer and DCIS increased. This decreasing incidence was greatest for Paget disease associated with invasive cancer or DCIS.[245] The explanation for this is not certain but can be interpreted as earlier detection of these lesions at a point in their evolution prior to the development of pagetoid changes consistent with the epidermotropic theory.

The workup for the patient with Paget disease includes mammography and physical examination of the breast, in particular to rule out an underlying invasive cancer or DCIS. In a recent series of 40 patients with Paget disease with a negative physical examination and mammogram reported from the Mayo Clinic, 68% had DCIS that extended beyond the nipple and only 5% (two patients) had an underlying invasive cancer.[246] In patients with negative findings on physical examination and mammogram, breast MRI should be considered for patients who are candidates for BCT.

Historically, Paget disease has been treated with mastectomy. Prognosis is determined by the stage of the underlying malignancy, if present. Several studies have focused on the potential for BCT with breast irradiation. The rationale for BCT of Paget disease includes the success of BCT for DCIS and the earlier detection of Paget disease with lower disease burden at presentation. Bijker et al.[247] reported on the results of a prospective trial of 61 patients treated with excision followed by RT. The 5-year local recurrence rate was 5.2%. Four patients had local failure; three were instances of invasive cancer and one was DCIS only. Other small studies of BCT with excision and RT have been reported with similar results.[248] In the Surveillance, Epidemiology, and End Results (SEER) data, 15-year breast cancer–specific survival is similar for patients treated with mastectomy and with BCT. BCT with RT appears to be a reasonable alternative to mastectomy, albeit with the caveats that no randomized trial has been performed and only small series of published cases are of patients who have been so treated.

Local excision alone, without RT, has been used to treat a small number of patients. In one of the largest series, Polgar et al.[249] reported on the results of a prospective study of 33 patients treated with local excision alone. The local recurrence rate was 33% (11 of 33). Of the 11 local recurrences, 10 (91%) were invasive carcinoma and 1 was DCIS. Six of ten patients with invasive local recurrence developed subsequent distant metastatic disease. Based on these findings, the authors recommended the addition of RT after breast-conservation surgery. Because of the small numbers of patients treated without RT and the high rate of local failure, such treatment must be considered as nonstandard at the present time.

For patients treated with BCT, surgery should include excision of the full NAC with at least a 2-cm cone of retroareolar tissue and complete excision of any tissue with abnormal retroareolar radiologic findings. For patients with positive margins after central lumpectomy, additional surgery is indicated. Patients with negative surgical margins should undergo irradiation. The decision for axillary node surgery should be based on the presence of an invasive breast cancer; sentinel node biopsy has been used successfully in this setting. Recommendations for adjuvant systemic therapy are based on the final pathology.

Occult Primary with Axillary Metastases

Axillary metastases in the absence of a clinically or mammographically detectable breast tumor are an uncommon presentation of breast carcinoma, seen in less than 1% of cases. The initial evaluation should include a detailed history and physical examination, bilateral mammogram, ipsilateral breast MRI (if the mammogram is unrevealing), and a chest radiograph. At the time of the lymph node biopsy, the pathologist should be alerted to the lack of a known primary tumor so that immunohistochemical stains can be performed if needed. The presence of ER, PR, or *HER2* overexpression is strongly suggestive of metastatic breast carcinoma, although their absence does not exclude a primary breast tumor.

An increasing body of evidence suggests that MRI identifies the primary tumor in the breast in a significant number of patients with a normal mammogram and breast examination. In one series of 69 patients with occult primary breast cancer seen between 1995 and 2001, MRI identified the primary breast tumor in 62%.[250] Cancer was found in 3 of the 12 patients who did not have a tumor identified by MRI and who underwent mastectomy. This experience is typical of multiple small studies of the use of MRI in this clinical circumstance. The identification of the primary tumor within the breast simplifies local management, allowing these patients to be treated with BCT or mastectomy according to standard guidelines.

In cases in which a primary tumor cannot be identified, treatment has traditionally been with mastectomy. This strategy was based on the observation that approximately 50% of patients who do not receive therapy to the breast will develop clinically evident disease in the breast. In addition, prior to the era of modern mammography and the availability of MRI, the occult cancers found in the breast at mastectomy were sometimes quite large.[251] More recently, RT to the whole breast has been used in these patients. Fourquet et al.[251] treated 54 patients with RT to the whole breast without removal of the primary tumor. The 5- and 10-year rates of ipsilateral breast tumor recurrence were 7.5% and 20%, respectively. Other small studies antedating the use of MRI confirm that although rates of local recurrence after BCT are higher than in patients treated with excision of a known primary tumor and a boost dose of RT to the tumor bed, whole-breast irradiation with a dose of about 50 Gy is an acceptable alternative to mastectomy in this patient population.

Regardless of the management approach chosen for the breast, axillary dissection should be carried out because of the limited ability of radiation to control gross axillary disease. Overall survival for women with occult primary tumors is similar to that of patients with comparable axillary involvement and a known primary tumor, and some investigators have suggested that survival is actually superior for those with occult primary tumors.[252] Because of the small size of most studies of occult primary cancer, the heterogeneous treatments employed, and the variable durations of follow-up, this claim is difficult to substantiate. Systemic treatment for patients with occult primary breast cancer and axillary involvement should follow the current guidelines for patients with node-positive breast cancer.

Breast Cancer and Pregnancy

Breast carcinoma is one of the most commonly diagnosed malignancies during pregnancy. Older studies estimated that breast cancer developed in 2.2 in 10,000 pregnancies[253]; however, the trend toward later age at first childbirth has increased the number of breast cancer cases coexistent with pregnancy, and breast cancer is now estimated to occur in 1 in 1,000 pregnancies.[254] Delay in diagnosis remains a problem in women presenting with breast cancer during pregnancy. The nodularity of the breast in a pregnant woman may obscure small masses, and the presence of a breast mass may be inappropriately attributed to normal physiologic changes. Dominant breast masses developing during pregnancy require biopsy before assuming that they are benign. This can be readily accomplished with a core-cutting needle biopsy in the majority of women. If excisional biopsy is necessary, it should be undertaken; concerns about the development of a milk fistula appear to be overstated.[255] Mammography is not as useful in pregnant patients as in those who are not pregnant because of the increased density in the breast parenchyma associated with pregnancy. Ultrasound may be helpful in confirming the presence of a dominant mass but, as in the nonpregnant patient, normal imaging studies should not lead to a decision to forgo biopsy in the patient with a dominant breast mass.

After a diagnosis is made, the initial evaluation should include an assessment of the extent of the disease. CT and bone scans are not recommended during pregnancy because of concerns about radiation exposure to the fetus. In patients with symptoms suggestive of metastases, MRI without contrast can be used to evaluate bony sites and the intra-abdominal viscera.[255]

Breast cancers occurring during pregnancy are usually high-grade infiltrating ductal carcinomas. In a prospective study of 38 pregnant women who developed breast cancer, only 28% had ER-positive tumors and 24% had PR-positive tumors.[256] In general, the characteristics of cancers occurring during pregnancy are similar to those of nonpregnant women of the same age. Data from retrospective case-control series suggest that after adjusting for age and disease stage, the prognosis of women with breast cancer occurring during pregnancy differs little from that of nonpregnant patients.[255]

For women diagnosed in the first or second trimester, the question of pregnancy termination is inevitably raised. Although some treatment approaches are feasible during pregnancy, others are contraindicated. Depending on the patient's specific situation, continuing the pregnancy may or may not compromise the breast cancer treatment. Even when deviations from standard treatment are required, it is unclear to what extent such changes or delays affect a woman's odds of remaining free from recurrent breast cancer. The concerns about compromising care must be balanced by the woman, her family, and her physicians, with the desire to continue the pregnancy. The woman facing these issues must also consider the possibility that if she receives chemotherapy, her ability to conceive another child could be compromised.[197] There is no clear evidence that pregnancy termination changes overall survival.[257]

Breast surgery can be safely performed during any trimester of pregnancy. Mastectomy is the treatment that has traditionally been undertaken because of the inability to safely deliver RT to the breast without excessive fetal exposure during any trimester. The effect of delaying RT on local recurrence, in the absence of systemic therapy, is unknown and is of concern. Guidelines developed by the American College of Surgeons, American College of Radiology, and College of American Pathologists[59] consider this an appropriate approach for cancers diagnosed in the third trimester and one that must be considered on a case-by-case basis for cancers diagnosed earlier in pregnancy. In the woman who will receive systemic chemotherapy, the delay in the delivery of RT is often no greater than in the nonpregnant patient. The success rate of lymphatic mapping and sentinel node biopsy in the pregnant woman is unknown. Isosulfan blue dye is not approved by the FDA for use during pregnancy. The radiation exposure to the fetus from the use of technetium has been estimated to be low, and it has been suggested that mapping with technetium alone could be discussed with patients as an appropriate management strategy.[258] In the absence of definitive data on the safety and accuracy of sentinel node biopsy in the pregnant woman, axillary dissection remains the standard management strategy.

The risk of congenital malformation from cytotoxic chemotherapy varies with the fetal age at exposure and the agent used. Exposure in the first trimester is associated with risks of 10% to 20%, which decline to less than 2% with exposure in the second and third trimesters.[259] For this reason, chemotherapy in the first trimester should be avoided. Growth retardation may also occur, and the long-term consequences of intrauterine exposure to cytotoxic agents remain uncertain. In a prospective study of 24 pregnant women treated with fluorouracil, doxorubicin, and cyclophosphamide during the second and third trimesters of pregnancy, no complications were observed for the fetus or infant.[260] Experience with the taxanes in pregnancy is very limited, but to date fetal toxicity has not been described.[261] A case report of the use of trastuzumab in pregnancy documented reversible anhydramnois,[262] and more information on the safety of this agent in pregnancy is needed. Methotrexate should be avoided during pregnancy because of the risk of abortion and severe fetal malformation. Similarly, tamoxifen should be withheld until after delivery because its safety is uncertain. When chemotherapy or tamoxifen is given postpartum, breast-feeding should be avoided as these agents may be excreted in the breast milk.

The management of breast cancer during pregnancy is difficult as there is often a conflict between optimal therapy for the mother and the fetus. Multidisciplinary management by a team including medical, surgical, and radiation oncologists, an obstetrician, a maternal-fetal medicine specialist, and a psychologist will facilitate the development of a strategy that optimizes the outcome for both mother and child.

Male Breast Cancer

The incidence of male breast cancer varies on a worldwide basis by geographic location, with the highest rates in some sub-Saharan countries. In the United States, it is estimated that in 2007, 2,030 men will be diagnosed with breast cancer (1.1% of the total for both genders) and that 450 men will die of it (1.1% of both genders).[1] The risk of male breast cancer is related to an increased lifelong exposure to estrogen (as with female breast cancer) or to reduced androgen. The strongest association is in men with Klinefelter syndrome (XXY); they have a 14- to 50-fold increased risk of developing male breast cancer and account for about 3% of all male breast cancer cases. Also, men who carry a *BRCA1*, or particularly a *BRCA2* mutation, have an increased risk of developing breast cancer. The following conditions have been reported to be associated with an increased risk of breast cancer in men: chronic liver disorders, such as cirrhosis, chronic alcoholism, schistosomiasis; a history of mumps orchitis, undescended testes, or testicular injury; and feminization, genetically or by environmental exposure. In contrast, gynecomastia alone does not appear to be a risk factor.[263]

The clinical presentation of male breast cancer is similar to that of female breast cancer, but the median age of onset is later than in women (60 vs. 53 years). Because the diagnosis of breast cancer is often not considered as promptly in men and screening mammography is not used, men often present with more advanced stage than do women. All known histopathologic types of breast cancer have been described in men, with infiltrating ductal carcinoma accounting for at least 70% of cases. However, ILC in men is rare. A majority of male breast cancers are ER-/PR-positive, and the percentage positive is greater than for female breast cancer. As for women, stage is the predominant prognostic indicator, and most studies report that stage for stage, men with breast cancer have the same outcome following treatment as women with breast cancer. A recent study, however, from the Veterans Affairs reports a worse prognosis for men than women in early-stage breast cancer.[264] There appears to be a substantial negative disparity in outcome for blacks with male breast cancer compared with whites.[265]

Primary local treatment is typically total mastectomy. In some patients with early disease, BCT can be considered. However, the subareolar location of most male breast cancers and the small amount of breast tissue present in most men limits eligibility for BCT. The same considerations regarding nodal surgery pertain for men as for women, with sentinel node biopsy the preferred treatment in clinically node-negative patients. The use of postmastectomy RT follows the same guidelines as for female breast cancer. Similarly, the use of systemic therapy follows the same guidelines as for women with postmenopausal breast cancer. Adjuvant systemic chemotherapy is used in men, although no controlled trials have confirmed its value.[266] Tamoxifen is the mainstay for adjuvant systemic therapy in ER-positive male breast cancer; there are no data on the efficacy of AIs as adjuvant treatment for male breast cancer. Metastatic breast cancer in men is treated identically to metastatic disease in women.

Phyllodes Tumor

The term *phyllodes tumor* includes a group of lesions of varying malignant potential, ranging from completely benign tumors to fully malignant sarcomas. Clinically, phyllodes tumors are smooth, rounded, usually painless multinodular lesions that may be indistinguishable from fibroadenomas. The average age at diagnosis is in the fourth decade. Skin ulceration may be seen with large tumors, but this is usually due to pressure necrosis rather than invasion of the skin by malignant cells. Histologically, phyllodes tumor, like fibroadenoma, is composed of epithelial elements and a connective tissue stroma.

Phyllodes tumors are classified as benign, borderline, or malignant on the basis of the nature of the tumor margins (pushing or infiltrative) and presence of cellular atypia, mitotic activity, and overgrowth in the stroma. There is disagreement about which of these criteria is most important, although most experts favor stromal overgrowth. The percentage of phyllodes tumors classified as malignant ranges from 23% to 50%. Local excision to negative margins is an appropriate management strategy for both benign and malignant phyllodes tumors if this can be accomplished with a satisfactory cosmetic outcome. The optimal margin width is not known, but wider excisions appear to reduce the risk of local recurrence. Approximately 20% of phyllodes tumors recur locally if excised with no margin or a margin of a few millimeters of normal breast tissue, regardless of whether they are benign or malignant.[267] In a review of 821 patients with nonmetastatic malignant phyllodes tumors reported to the SEER registry between 1983 and 2002, 52% were treated with mastectomy and the remainder with local excision. The 10-year cause-specific survival was 89%, and no survival benefit for mastectomy was observed.[267]

The role of RT and systemic therapy in phyllodes tumor is unclear. RT is not used for benign or borderline lesions but has been combined with wide excision in the management of malignant phyllodes tumors. When phyllodes tumors metastasize they tend to behave like sarcomas, with lung as the most common site. Axillary metastases are seen in fewer than 5% of cases, and axillary surgery is not indicated unless worrisome nodes are clinically evident. When systemic therapy is used for malignant phyllodes tumors, treatment is based on the guidelines for treating sarcomas.

Locally Advanced and Inflammatory Breast Cancer

Locally advanced breast cancer (LABC) and inflammatory breast cancer (IBC) refer to a heterogeneous group of breast cancers without evidence of distant metastases (M0) and represents only 2% to 5% of all breast cancers in the United States. Patients with these cancers include those with (1) operable disease at presentation (clinical stage T3N1), (2) inoperable disease at presentation (clinical stage T4 and/or N2-3), and (3) IBC (clinical stage T4dN0-3). (All stages refer to the *AJCC Cancer Staging Manual*, 7th edition, 2010.[72]) Subdividing patients into these three broad groups facilitates clinical management.

Comparison of studies of LABC and IBC is problematic for a number of reasons. First, these patients have a high degree of heterogeneity in T and N classification, and the number of patients in each subgroup is typically small and variable between studies. Second, the definition of LABC according to AJCC staging criteria has varied over time.[72] Some studies have included T3N0M0 (now stage IIB) cancers and even large T2 lesions (e.g., lesions 3 cm or larger) as LABC. Also, supraclavicular lymphadenopathy is now classified as N3 disease, although it was previously classified as M1 and therefore excluded from many studies.[269] Third, the subgroups of patients included in studies vary widely. For example, patients with IBC or operable disease at presentation may or may not be combined with patients with LABC. Fourth, studies vary in the extent of diagnostic evaluation prior to treatment. Some centers, for example, have routinely employed ultrasound evaluation of axillary and supraclavicular regions with FNA of suspected involvement; such improved staging will improve the outcome in all stages.

IBC accounts for 1% to 5% of all cases of breast cancer in the United States and is an aggressive variant of LABC. IBC is a clinicopathologic entity characterized by diffuse erythema and edema (peau d'orange) of the breast often without an underlying palpable mass. The clinical findings should involve most of the skin of the breast. IBC typically has a rapid onset and is often initially mistaken as infection and treated with antibiotics before the diagnosis is established. The clinical presentation results from tumor emboli in the dermal lymphatics. According to the AJCC staging rules,[72] IBC is primarily a clinical diagnosis. Involvement of dermal lymphatics in the absence of clinical findings does not indicate IBC. A skin biopsy may be performed to confirm the clinical impression of IBC, but the absence of dermal lymphatic involvement should not affect staging.

As with all cases of breast cancer, the determination of ER, PR, and *HER2* status is critical in the management of LABC and IBC. IBCs are more likely to be high-grade, *HER2*-overexpressing, and lacking in hormone receptor expression compared with other presentations of breast cancer. Because both LABC and IBC are associated with substantial risk of metastatic disease, patients with these cancers should undergo full workup for distant metastases prior to initiation of therapy.

Patients with LABC or IBC should be evaluated by a multidisciplinary team (ideally around the time of diagnosis). Treatment typically includes neoadjuvant chemotherapy, surgery, and RT. Prior to the use of neoadjuvant chemotherapy, long-term survival was uncommon. Long-term survival has been greatly improved with aggressive trimodality treatment. As with early-stage breast cancer, biological tumor markers should affect treatment selection: patients with *HER2*-positive cancers should receive trastuzumab-based therapy, and patients with hormone receptor–positive cancers should receive adjuvant endocrine therapy. The response to neoadjuvant chemotherapy has been assessed in various studies using physical examination, mammography, ultrasonography, and MRI, but none of these methods has proven highly predictive of pathologic response.

Anthracycline- and taxane-based chemotherapy regimens are appropriate as induction chemotherapy for women with LABC or IBC. The vast majority of patients will have clinical response to therapy, and roughly 15% to 25% will experience a complete pathologic response. The addition of paclitaxel to anthracycline-based therapy appears to improve long-term disease outcomes for women with LABC and IBC.[270] There are no studies of trastuzumab specifically for LABC/IBC; however, by extrapolation of results using trastuzumab for early-stage breast cancer, it should be incorporated into the treatment of women with *HER2*-positive LABC or IBC. As with other experiences using neoadjuvant chemotherapy, complete pathologic eradication of the tumor predicts superior outcomes among women with LABC or IBC.[271] However, even among patients with pathologic complete response to neoadjuvant chemotherapy, those with LABC or IBC at baseline have a higher risk of recurrence than patients with lower-stage breast cancer at baseline.[272] Patients with LABC or IBC should be routinely treated with postmastectomy RT, despite a pathologic complete response to neoadjuvant chemotherapy.[273]

Some women with LABC may be candidates for BCT following neoadjuvant chemotherapy. In one series, local-regional control following this approach appeared to be excellent except in patients with one or more of the following features: (1) clinical N2-3 disease, (2) lymphovascular invasion, (3) residual primary pathologic size greater than 2 cm, and (4) multifocal residual disease.[274] However, there is still limited experience with this approach. In a small study of 13 patients with IBC treated with preoperative chemotherapy and BCT, 7 of 13 experienced local recurrence.[275] This coupled with the diffuse nature of IBC indicates that BCT is contraindicated in women with this diagnosis.

Although most women have a clinical response to neoadjuvant chemotherapy, some patients will experience tumor progression or remain inoperable. Such patients may be candidates for noncross-resistant chemotherapy or novel treatments. Surgery is contraindicated in IBC unless there is complete resolution of the inflammatory skin changes. In modern studies, 85% to 90% of patients become operable after initial chemotherapy.[276] RT may facilitate conversion of inoperable to operable disease. In spite of modern multimodality therapy, approximately 20% of IBC patients treated with chemotherapy, surgery, and RT will experience local-regional recurrence.[276] Patients with chest wall recurrence after chemotherapy, surgery, and RT are at high risk for both extensive local-regional tumor spread and for developing metastatic disease to visceral organ sites, and are treated according to guidelines for metastatic breast cancer.

METASTATIC DISEASE

Metastatic (stage IV) breast cancer is defined by tumor spread beyond the breast, chest wall, and regional lymph nodes. Tumor dissemination can occur through blood and lymphatic vessels and via direct extension through the chest wall. The most common sites for breast cancer metastasis include the bone, lung, liver, lymph nodes, chest wall, and brain. However, case reports have documented breast cancer dissemination to almost every organ in the body. Hormone receptor–positive tumors are more likely to spread to bone as the initial site of metastasis; hormone receptor–negative and/or *HER2*-positive tumors are more likely to recur initially in viscera.[277] Lobular (as opposed to ductal) cancers are more often associated with serosal metastases to the pleura and abdomen. Most women with metastatic disease will have been initially diagnosed with early-stage breast cancer, treated with curative intent, and then experience metastatic recurrence. Only about 10% of newly diagnosed breast cancer patients in the United States have metastatic disease at presentation; this proportion is far higher in areas where screening programs are not available.

Symptoms of metastatic breast cancer are related to the location and extent of the tumor. Common symptoms or physical examination findings include bone discomfort, lymphadenopathy, skin changes, cough or shortness of breath, and fatigue. These clinical findings are all nonspecific, and appropriate evaluation is warranted in breast cancer patients with new or evolving symptoms. In some cases, physical examination or radiologic findings will demonstrate unequivocal evidence of metastatic breast cancer. In instances when radiologic or clinical

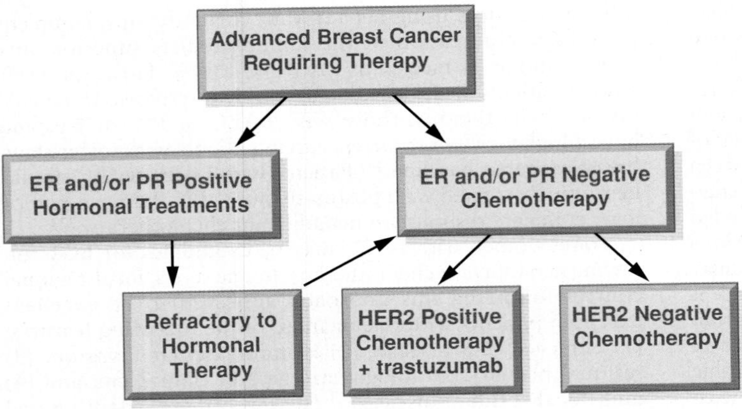

FIGURE 106.6 Algorithm for treatment of the patient with metastatic breast cancer based on hormone receptor status and the presence of *HER2* overexpression. ER, estrogen receptor; PR, progesterone receptor.

findings are equivocal, tissue biopsy is imperative. If a biopsy is performed, ER, PR, and *HER2* should be redetermined.

The treatment goals in women with advanced breast cancer include prolongation of life, control of tumor burden, reduction in cancer-related symptoms or complications, and maintenance of quality of life and function. Therapy is not generally considered curative. A small fraction of patients, often those with limited sites of metastatic disease or bearing tumors with exquisite sensitivity to treatment, may experience very long periods of remission and tumor control. Treatment of advanced breast cancer, like treatment of early-stage breast cancer, is based on consideration of tumor biology and clinical history. Thus, characterization of tumor ER, PR, and *HER2* status is critical for all patients, and a detailed assessment of past treatment including timing of therapies as well as patient symptoms and functional assessment is essential. An overview of treatment for advanced breast cancer is shown in Figure 106.6. Patients with endocrine-sensitive tumors, particularly those with minimal symptoms and limited visceral involvement, are candidates for initial treatment with endocrine therapy alone; initial treatment using combined chemoendocrine therapy has not been shown to improve survival compared with sequential treatment programs. Patients with hormone receptor–negative tumors or those with hormone receptor–positive tumors progressing despite the use of endocrine therapy are candidates for chemotherapy. If the tumor is *HER2*-positive, then trastuzumab treatment is employed in combination with chemotherapy.

Well-established clinical factors can inform the likelihood of response to therapy and long-term outcomes in women with metastatic breast cancer (Table 106.23). Patients who have received less therapy, have a longer disease-free interval since initial diagnosis, soft tissue or bone metastases, fewer symptoms and better performance status, and tumors that are hormone receptor–positive are likely to experience longer survival with metastatic disease than more heavily treated patients with shorter intervals since treatment, visceral metastases, and greater symptoms.

In clinical trials, the measured end points for defining efficacy of therapy for metastatic breast cancer are response rate, time to tumor progression, and overall survival. These landmarks are important for guiding clinical practice as well, although formal measures of response/progression are often difficult to apply owing to inconsistencies in imaging studies, the prevalence of nonmeasurable disease such as bone lesions, subcentimeter tumor deposits, and pleural effusions or ascites. The art of treating patients with metastatic breast cancer involves careful, thoughtful repetition of a process of treatment initiation, evaluation including assessment of patient functional status and symptom profile and by serial measurement of tumor burden and response to therapy, and discontinuation through multiple lines of therapy. Clinical guidelines for the management of metastatic carcinoma[207] are often quite open-ended, acknowledging the multiple treatment pathways that might be legitimately pursued, arguing for judicious use of clinical decision making and treatment selection based on tumor biology, and focusing clinicians on the continuous considerations of patient preference and illness experience.

Endocrine Therapy for Metastatic Breast Cancer

Endocrine treatment is a key intervention for women with hormone receptor–positive, metastatic breast cancer. The first therapy for advanced breast cancer was oophorectomy, and in the 100 years since the advent of that treatment, there has been steady progress in the development of hormonal therapy for metastatic disease. Table 106.24 lists available

TABLE 106.23

PROGNOSTIC FACTORS IN ADVANCED BREAST CANCER

Tumor biology (grade, estrogen receptor status, *HER2* status)
Performance status
Cancer-related symptoms
Sites of recurrence
Number of sites of recurrence
Prior adjuvant therapy
Disease-free interval
Prior therapy for metastatic disease
Response/duration of treatment with prior therapy for metastatic disease

TABLE 106.24

ENDOCRINE THERAPIES FOR METASTATIC BREAST CANCER

Ovarian suppression/ablation (premenopausal women)
Selective estrogen receptor modulators (tamoxifen, toremifene)
Aromatase inhibitors (anastrozole, letrozole, exemestane; postmenopausal women)
Antiestrogens (fulvestrant; postmenopausal women)
Progestins (megestrol and medroxyprogesterone)
Other steroid hormones (high-dose estrogens, androgens; principally of historical interest)

endocrine drugs for treating advanced breast cancer. A variety of well-tolerated commercially available agents are now used to treat advanced breast cancer, including tamoxifen, AIs, fulvestrant, and progestins. Single-agent therapy is the standard approach; combining endocrine agents has not been shown to improve outcomes. Many women will be candidates for multiple types of endocrine therapy to control metastatic breast cancer. On average, first-line treatment is associated with 8 to 12 months of tumor control, and second-line treatment with 4 to 6 months. Individual patients may experience substantially longer time to progression. Sequential single-agent second- and third-line endocrine treatments are often effective, although typically for shorter durations than initial therapy. Patients with either overt tumor shrinkage or stabilization of disease in response to endocrine treatment can have equivalent long-term tumor control. Endocrine therapy can cause regression of soft tissue and bone and visceral metastases.

Eventually most women with hormone receptor–positive metastatic breast cancer will progress despite first-line endocrine therapy. Resistance to treatment does not seem to be associated with loss of hormone receptor expression by the tumor cells. Indications for chemotherapy include symptomatic tumor progression, pending visceral crisis, or resistance to multiple endocrine therapies. Patients presenting with extensive visceral metastases or profound symptoms from breast cancer may benefit from induction chemotherapy, which should then be followed with endocrine therapy.

Tamoxifen was the historic standard as treatment for ER-positive metastatic breast cancer, associated with a 50% response rate and median duration of response of 12 to 18 months among treatment-naive patients. A "tamoxifen flare" reaction, typically characterized by intensification of bone pain, transient tumor progression, and hypercalcemia, can arise in 5% to 10% of patients within the first days or weeks of tamoxifen treatment. Flare reactions are often harbingers of exquisite tumor sensitivity to endocrine manipulation, but must be distinguished from overt tumor progression. Flare reactions are not frequently seen with other endocrine therapies.

In premenopausal women with metastatic breast cancer, combined endocrine therapy with ovarian suppression and tamoxifen can improve survival compared with treatment with either tamoxifen or ovarian suppression alone.[279] Thus, the first intervention for premenopausal women with breast cancer recurrence is ovarian suppression or ablation, with initiation of tamoxifen treatment. Premenopausal women with metastatic tumor despite tamoxifen use are candidates for ovarian suppression/ablation and AI therapy.

Owing to a combination of the demographics of breast cancer, the duration of time between initial tumor diagnosis and metastatic recurrence and chemotherapy-induced amenorrhea, most women with recurrent breast cancer will be postmenopausal. Postmenopausal women are candidates for either tamoxifen, AIs, fulvestrant or progestational agents as palliation for metastatic breast cancer. Aromatase inhibitors appear to be the preferred initial agents for women who received prior tamoxifen treatment in the adjuvant setting.[279,280] For postmenopausal women who are naive to antiestrogens, AIs may have modest clinical advantages over tamoxifen as initial treatment for metastatic disease.[281,282] Fulvestrant appears to have comparable activity to AIs in women previously treated with tamoxifen.[283]

The optimal sequencing of endocrine therapy for postmenopausal women treated with adjuvant AIs is not clear, as few trials have rigorously explored different treatments among such patients. Tamoxifen, fulvestrant, progestins, and possibly different AIs are all reasonable options among such patients.

Chemotherapy for Metastatic Breast Cancer

Cytotoxic chemotherapy remains a mainstay of treatment for women with metastatic breast cancer, irrespective of hormone receptor status, and is the backbone of many novel treatments incorporating biological therapy.[284] Chemotherapy has substantial side effects, including fatigue, nausea, vomiting, myelosuppression, neuropathy, diarrhea, and alopecia. For this reason, chemotherapy treatment of women for advanced breast cancer involves tradeoffs between cancer palliation and toxicities of therapy. Chemotherapy is used in patients with hormone-refractory or hormone-insensitive tumors (Fig. 106.6).

Clinical trials have addressed a number of important treatment principles for use of chemotherapy in women with metastatic breast cancer. Tumor response to chemotherapy is a surrogate for longer cancer control and survival.[285,286] First-line treatment is associated with higher response rates and longer tumor control than second-line, and so forth. There are relatively few studies of fourth or higher lines of chemotherapy, although patients often receive many lines of treatment. Trials have demonstrated palliative benefits of chemotherapy in patients with refractory tumors receiving third-line or subsequent chemotherapy treatment, but the magnitude of such gains must be realistically weighed against the side effects of treatment. Chemotherapy treatment can be interrupted in patients who have had significant response or palliation following initiation of therapy and reintroduced when there is tumor progression or recrudescence of patient symptoms.

Since the advent of chemotherapy administration for metastatic breast cancer, it has been debated whether single-agent sequential treatment or combination treatment with multiple agents is the best strategy. Randomized studies have suggested that combination chemotherapy may be associated with higher response rates and improved time to progression compared with single-agent therapy. However, studies that have specifically planned for crossover treatment with second-line sequential therapy have not shown that combination treatment improves ultimate time to progression or survival compared with a sequential treatment program.[287] Patients with extensive visceral disease or pending visceral crisis may preferentially require initiation of combination chemotherapy, but this has not been demonstrated in prospective studies. Because single-agent chemotherapy facilitates better understanding of which drugs are contributing to benefit or side effects, allowing appropriate treatment modification, and is generally associated with less toxicity, it remains the preferred approach for most women with metastatic breast cancer.

A large number of chemotherapy agents and combinations are effective in treatment of metastatic breast cancer (Table 106.25).[207] A variety of specific drugs and combinations are considered preferred based on a large historical experience, results from randomized trials, and consideration of toxicity profiles. Efforts have been made to demonstrate that one chemotherapy regimen or sequence is superior to another. For the most part, the literature does not support the idea that there is one path or algorithm for treating patients, particularly given the variety of agents and multiple lines of therapy ultimately used during the course of treating metastatic disease. Although anthracycline- and taxane-based treatments are generally considered to be among the most active in treatment of metastatic breast cancer, their utility has led to their incorporation into adjuvant chemotherapy regimens. Thus, many women with metastatic breast cancer will already have been treated with anthracyclines and/or taxanes, diminishing the utility of these agents in the palliation of metastatic disease.

Recent advances in chemotherapy for metastatic breast cancer are related to the development of new agents and schedules

TABLE 106.25

PREFERRED CHEMOTHERAPY AGENTS AND COMBINATIONS FOR ADVANCED BREAST CANCER

Single Agents	Combination Regimens
Anthracyclines (doxorubicin, epirubicin, pegylated liposomal doxorubicin)	Cyclophosphamide/anthracycline ± 5-fluorouracil regimens (such as AC, EC, CEF, CAF, FEC, FAC)
Taxanes (paclitaxel, docetaxel, albumin nano-particle bound paclitaxel)	CMF
5-fluorouracil (continuous-infusion 5-fluorouracil, capecitabine)	Anthracyclines/taxanes (such as doxorubicin/paclitaxel or doxorubicin/docetaxel)
Vinca alkaloids (vinorelbine, vinblastine)	Docetaxel/capecitabine
Gemcitabine	Gemcitabine/paclitaxel
Platinum salts (cisplatin, carboplatin)	Taxane/platinum regimens (such as paclitaxel/carboplatin or docetaxel/carboplatin)
Ixabepilone	Ixabepilone / capecitabine
Cyclophosphamide	
Etoposide	

A, doxorubicin; C, cyclophosphamide; E, epirubicin; F, 5-fluorouracil; M, methotrexate.
(Adapted from ref. 207, with permission.)

for treatment. Capecitabine is an orally available fluoropyrimidine, metabolized in tissues into 5-fluorouracil. Capecitabine has clinical activity in anthracycline- and taxane-resistant breast cancer[289] and improves response and survival as first-line treatment when added to single-agent docetaxel.[289] The antimetabolite gemcitabine similarly yields higher response rates and survival when paired with paclitaxel compared with paclitaxel therapy alone.[290] Ixabepilone, an epothilone chemotherapy agent, has substantial activity as a single agent or in combination with capecitabine in patients previously treated with anthracyclines and taxanes.[291,292]

Dose escalation of taxane therapy with paclitaxel has not been shown to result in clinically important improvements.[192] However, weekly administration of paclitaxel therapy does appear to improve response rate and time to progression compared with less frequent, every 3-week administration.[293,294]

As a strategy to overcome chemotherapy resistance, many investigators in the 1990s explored high-dose chemotherapy with autologous bone marrow or stem cell support as treatment for breast cancer. Preliminary studies suggested favorable clinical outcomes, prompting both widespread use of high-dose chemotherapy in clinical practice and randomized trials for patients with either metastatic or high-risk, node-positive breast cancer. Despite initial hopes, randomized trials did not demonstrate clinical improvement with use of high-dose chemotherapy compared with conventional chemotherapy dosing. In a randomized trial of patients with metastatic breast cancer, women received induction chemotherapy with four to six cycles of standard agents, followed by treatment with either one cycle of high-dose chemotherapy and autologous stem cell rescue or maintenance chemotherapy at conventional doses.[295] There were no differences in either progression-free or overall survival.

Multiple randomized trials explored high-dose chemotherapy in the adjuvant setting. Among patients with ten or more positive axillary lymph nodes, six cycles of CAF chemotherapy was compared with CAF followed by one cycle of intensification with high-dose chemotherapy and autologous stem cell support.[296] Stem cell transplant yielded small gains in relapse-free survival, no gains in overall survival, and was associated with greater risk of short- and long-term treatment-associated mortality. A related trial of FEC with or without the addition of high-dose chemotherapy, open to women with four or more positive axillary lymph nodes, identified a subset of patients with ten or more positive nodes that showed improvement in disease-free survival with use of high-dose chemotherapy but did not suggest significant overall advantage.[297] Another study compared doxorubicin followed by CMF chemotherapy with doxorubicin followed by intensified cyclophosphamide and one cycle of high-dose chemotherapy and bone marrow transplant, showing no difference in relapse-free or overall survival.[298] Trials of moderately intensified adjuvant chemotherapy compared with standard chemotherapy followed by high-dose chemotherapy with autologous stem cell support disclosed no long-term clinical advantages for high-dose chemotherapy.[299,300] Collectively, these studies have been interpreted as showing negligible, if any, benefit for use of high-dose chemotherapy in either the adjuvant or metastatic treatment setting. At present, there is no role for high-dose chemotherapy outside a clinical trial, and it remains unclear which groups of patients—defined by either clinical history or tumor biology—might be most suitable as candidates for such studies.

Anti-*HER2* Therapy for Metastatic Breast Cancer

Patients with *HER2*-overexpressing breast cancer should receive trastuzumab therapy as part of their treatment program. When added to first-line chemotherapy for *HER2*-positive metastatic breast cancer, trastuzumab improved response rates, time to progression, and overall survival in two randomized trials.[301,302] Cardiomyopathy is a known side effect of trastuzumab therapy, and serial determinations of left ventricular ejection fraction should be performed to screen for changes related to trastuzumab.[303] For this reason, concurrent administration of trastuzumab with anthracyclines should be avoided. Neither the optimal timing for initiation of trastuzumab nor the optimal chemotherapy backbone is well characterized. Trastuzumab is generally started with chemotherapy based on data from randomized trials. In some settings, trastuzumab may be considered as single-agent therapy[304] or in combination with endocrine therapy. However, it is not clear how to select patients who are suitable candidates for initial use of trastuzumab without concurrent chemotherapy administration. A variety of chemotherapy agents have shown clinical activity and safety when paired with trastuzumab, including taxanes, vinorelbine, and platinum analogs. The role of combination chemotherapy plus trastuzumab for metastatic disease remains controversial. The results of randomized studies examining the addition of platinum chemotherapy to taxanes plus trastuzumab are conflicting.[305,306] The role of trastuzumab therapy for treatment beyond progression in the metastatic setting has not been studied in randomized trials. However, recent data suggest that ongoing anti-*HER2* treatment may be important for patients with tumor progression on trastuzumab.

Lapatinib is a novel dual-kinase inhibitor that targets both the *HER2* and EGFR tyrosine kinase signaling pathways. Lapatinib has been studied as second-line anti-*HER2* therapy for patients progressing after chemotherapy and trastuzumab.[307] In comparison with the administration of capecitabine chemotherapy alone, the combination of lapatinib plus capecitabine was associated with a longer period of tumor control and improvement in response rate, but not survival. Several trials have examined the role of second or subsequent lines of trastuzumab therapy after initial tumor progression in patients receiving trastuzumab. These studies have demonstrated that continuation of trastuzumab treatment beyond progression is associated with improvements in time to progression.[308,309] These observations justify the practice of continued anti-*HER2* blockade in association with multiple lines of treatment for *HER2*-positive metastatic breast cancer.

Antiangiogenesis Therapy for Advanced Breast Cancer

Drugs that target proteins involved in tumor angiogenesis such as vascular endothelial growth factor (VEGF), VEGF-receptor, and other receptors on tumor and endothelial cells are emerging as important agents for palliating metastatic cancer. VEGF-targeted therapies are approved for use in advanced colorectal, non–small cell, and renal carcinomas. Experience to date suggests that similar principles hold for patients with metastatic breast cancer. Bevacizumab, the humanized monoclonal antibody that neutralizes VEGF, is the most studied antiangiogenic agent in breast cancer. In an initial randomized trial open to patients with prior anthracycline- and taxane-based chemotherapy treatment, the addition of bevacizumab to capecitabine was not associated with improvement in time to tumor progression or survival, but did enhance response rate modestly.[310] In ECOG E2100, a randomized trial of paclitaxel with or without the addition of bevacizumab as first-line treatment for metastatic breast cancer, bevacizumab did lead to clinically meaningful improvements in response rate and time to progression.[311] Unique side effects of bevacizumab include hypertension, impaired wound healing, and a slightly increased risk of thromboembolism. The initial encouraging efficacy and tolerability data have led to exploration of bevacizumab as therapy for early-stage breast cancer.

Multiple other antiangiogenesis agents are now in clinical development for metastatic breast cancer. To date there are no specific markers that identify tumors or patients likely to benefit from antiangiogenic therapy. It is not clear how the various agents in development compare with one another with respect to safety or utility, nor whether chemotherapy is an obligate modality for achieving benefit with these agents.

Emerging Agents in Advanced Breast Cancer

A novel class of therapeutics, drugs that inhibit the poly(adenosine diphosphate-ribose) polymerase (PARP) enzyme, are emerging as potentially valuable drugs in treatment of advanced breast cancer. In a proof of principle open-label phase 2 study, the PARP inhibitor olaparib was studied in patients with *BRCA1*- or *BRCA2*-associated cancers. This select group of patients was chosen because of preclinical data suggested that tumors with *BRCA* deficiency might be particularly dependent on the DNA repair function of the PARP enzyme complex, and thus suitable targets for PARP inhibition. Initial observations have suggested robust responses among *BRCA*-associated breast cancers when patients are given single-agent therapy with olaparib.[312] Additional evidence for a role for PARP inhibitors comes from a randomized phase 2 trial of patients with metastatic, triple-negative breast cancers.[313] In this trial, patients were treated with a combination chemotherapy regimen of gemcitabine plus carboplatin, with or without the PARP inhibitor BSI-201. In comparison with treatment with chemotherapy alone, the addition of the PARP inhibitor improved response rates, times to progression, and overall survival. Confirmatory phase 3 data are anticipated shortly.

In addition to PARP inhibitors, several other novel classes of anti-*HER2* drugs are emerging. These include the anti-*HER2* antibodies pertuzumab, which binds to *HER2* and the related protein, HER3,[314] which has shown activity in combination with trastuzumab in trastuzumab-resistant patients. The chemotherapy-conjugate trastuzumab-DM1, a derivative of trastuzumab created by chemical linkage with the maytansine chemotherapy moiety, has also been shown to achieve responses in trastuzumab-resistant breast cancer.[315] Other tyrosine-kinase–targeted drugs are also emerging, including neratinib, a dual-kinase inhibitor that targets both the HER2 and EGFR proteins, and has activity in both trastuzumab-treated and trastuzumab-naïve *HER2*-positive breast cancer.[316]

Treatment of Special Metastatic Sites in Patients with Breast Cancer

Specialized treatment options are available for breast cancer patients with metastases to selective anatomic sites. Patients with lytic bone metastases should receive intravenous bisphosphonate therapy such as pamidronate or zoledronic acid. These agents lessen the pain associated with bone lesions and prevent complications of skeletal metastases including fracture and hypercalcemia.[317] Extended bisphosphonate therapy can be associated with osteonecrosis of the jaw, so patients should be monitored for atypical oral lesions. It is not known if the intermittent administration of bisphosphonates would compromise their efficacy or minimize the risk of osteonecrosis. Patients with focal pain at sites of skeletal metastases, pending fracture, or pathologic fracture may also benefit from external-beam RT at selected tumor sites, and when necessary, surgical stabilization or repair of the bone or joint.

Improvements in survival in metastatic cancer seen with better chemotherapy and trastuzumab-based treatment have led to an increase in the incidence of central nervous system disease among breast cancer patients, especially those with *HER2*-overexpressing or hormone receptor–negative tumors.[318] This is likely a consequence of at least two clinical factors. First, the brain appears to be a relative "sanctuary site" for such tumors from chemotherapy and biological therapy. Second, the improved longevity of these patients who might previously have succumbed to pulmonary or hepatic metastases places them at greater jeopardy for late complications of cancer such as central nervous system metastases. Therapy for brain metastases remains inadequate, but generally includes whole-brain irradiation. Patients with isolated lesions, dominant masses, or recurrence after whole-brain radiation may additionally be candidates for surgical resection or stereotactic RT to specific lesions. Patients with leptomeningeal disease may achieve symptomatic improvement with whole-brain irradiation, or in some cases, intrathecal chemotherapy with methotrexate or cytarabine. Very limited clinical experience suggests that some systemic therapies, including endocrine treatments, chemotherapy agents including anthracyclines, alkylators, and capecitabine, and lapatinib, may have antitumor activity in the brain.[319] However, none of these is "standard of care" or a substitute for local therapy to the brain.

Some breast cancer patients will have limited sites of metastatic disease, such as isolated pulmonary nodules, isolated lymph node recurrence outside the axilla, or bone lesions. Single-institutional experience from the M. D. Anderson Cancer Center suggests that a fraction of such patients may be treated "aggressively" with curative intent, with favorable long-term results.[320] Investigators identified cohorts of patients who had received definitive surgical treatment to the breast, had not received adjuvant anthracycline-based therapy, and who developed isolated metastatic disease that could be definitively treated with local therapy. Local therapy included surgical excision if possible, or in the case of bone lesions or other unresectable tumor sites, irradiation of the affected site. These patients were considered to be "stage IV–NED (no evidence of disease)." Such stage IV–NED patients were treated with adjuvant-type anthracycline chemotherapy and, where appropriate, endocrine therapy. Many of these patients had long periods of freedom from tumor recurrence, and 25% to 30% remained free of further recurrence through 10 years of follow-up.[320]

The treatment of the primary tumor in the breast in women who present with metastatic disease is another area of controversy. Historically, surgery or RT to the breast was limited to patients with local tumor complications such as pain or skin erosion, and systemic drug therapy was the primary form of treatment. An analysis of 16,023 patients presenting with stage IV disease and an intact primary tumor compared outcomes between patients having surgery of the primary tumor to negative margins or no surgery. In a multivariate analysis adjusting for known prognostic factors, surgery reduced the hazard ratio for death to 0.61 (95% CI, 0.58–0.65).[76] A retrospective population-based study of 300 women reported similar findings.[77] In the absence of a randomized trial it is impossible to exclude unrecognized selection bias as the cause of the benefit observed for surgery. However, improvements in survival for patients with metastatic breast cancer seen even prior to the era of trastuzumab[77] coupled with the stage shift that is occurring by the use of imaging technologies capable of identifying very small metastatic deposits suggest that it may be time to re-examine the role of local therapy in the patient presenting with stage IV disease and an intact primary tumor or limited metastatic disease. At present, it is not known precisely how or when to integrate such surgical management into standard medical therapy for metastatic breast cancer or which patients in particular are most likely to benefit from such treatment. Local therapy should not be used as an initial approach to the patient with metastatic disease, but may be considered in a highly selected group of patients with a good response to systemic therapy and a limited number of metastatic sites.

Selected References

The full list of references for this chapter appears in the online version.

5. Berry DA, Cronin KA, Plevritis SK, et al. Effect of screening and adjuvant therapy on mortality from breast cancer. *N Engl J Med* 2005;353(17):1784.
8. Metcalfe KA, Finch A, Poll A, et al. Breast cancer risks in women with a family history of breast or ovarian cancer who have tested negative for a BRCA1 or BRCA2 mutation. *Br J Cancer* 2009;100(2):421.
10. U.S. Preventive Services Task Force. Genetic risk assessment and *BRCA* mutation testing for breast and ovarian cancer susceptibility: recommendation statement. *Ann Intern Med* 2005;143(5):355.
12. The *CHEK2* Breast Cancer Case Control Consortium. *CHEK2* 1100delC and susceptibility to breast cancer: a collaborative analysis involving 10,860 breast cancer cases and 9,065 controls from 10 studies. *Am J Hum Genet* 2004;74(6):1175.
15. Kauff ND, Satagopan JM, Robson ME, et al. Risk-reducing salpingo-oophorectomy in women with a *BRCA1* or *BRCA2* mutation. *N Engl J Med* 2002;346(21):1609.
19. Chlebowski RT, Hendrix SL, Langer RD, et al. Influence of estrogen plus progestin on breast cancer and mammography in healthy postmenopausal women: the Women's Health Initiative Randomized Trial. *JAMA* 2003;289(24):3243.
20. Beral V. Breast cancer and hormone-replacement therapy in the Million Women Study. *Lancet* 2003;362(9382):419.
21. Alexander DD, Morimoto LM, Mink PJ, et al. Summary and meta-analysis of prospective studies of animal fat intake and breast cancer. *Nutr Res Rev* 2010;25:1.
22. Singletary KW, Gapstur SM. Alcohol and breast cancer: review of epidemiologic and experimental evidence and potential mechanisms. *JAMA* 2001;286(17):2143.
25. Dupont WD, Page DL. Risk factors for breast cancer in women with proliferative breast disease. *N Engl J Med* 1985;312(3):146.
26. Boyd NF, Guo H, Martin LJ, et al. Mammographic density and the risk and detection of breast cancer. *N Engl J Med* 2007;356(3):227.
27. De Bruin ML, Sparidans J, van't Veer MB. Breast cancer risk in female survivors of Hodgkin's lymphoma: lower risk after smaller radiation volumes. *J Clin Oncol* 2009;27(26):4239.
28. Gail MH, Brinton LA, Byar DP, et al. Projecting individualized probabilities of developing breast cancer for white females who are being examined annually. *J Natl Cancer Inst* 1989;81(24):1879.
30. Fisher B, Costantino JP, Wickerham DL, et al. Tamoxifen for prevention of breast cancer: report of the National Surgical Adjuvant Breast and Bowel Project P-1 Study. *J Natl Cancer Inst* 1998;90(18):1371.
31. Warner E, Messersmith H, Causer P. Systematic review: using magnetic resonance imaging to screen women at high risk for breast cancer. *Ann Intern Med* 2008;148(9):671.
33. Saslow D, Boetes C, Burke W, et al. American cancer society guidelines for breast screening with MRI as an adjunct to mammography. *CA Cancer J Clin* 2007;57(2):75.
37. Cuzick J, Powles T, Veronesi U, et al. Overview of the main outcomes in breast-cancer prevention trials. *Lancet* 2003;361(9354):296.
39. Narod SA, Brunet JS, Ghadirian P, et al. Tamoxifen and risk of contralateral breast cancer in *BRCA1* and *BRCA2* mutation carriers: a case-control study. Hereditary Breast Cancer Clinical Study Group. *Lancet* 2000;356(9245):1876.
40. Vogel VG, Costantino JP, Wickerham DL, et al. Effects of tamoxifen vs raloxifene on the risk of developing invasive breast cancer and other disease outcomes: the NSABP Study of Tamoxifen and Raloxifene (STAR) P-2 trial. *JAMA* 2006;295(23):2727.
44. Rebbeck TR, Kauff ND, Domchek SM, et al. Meta-analysis of risk reduction estimates associated with risk-reducing salpingo-oophorectomy in BRCA1 or BRCA2 mutation carriers. *J Natl Cancer Inst* 2009;101:80.
45. Bluemke DA, Gatsonis CA, Chen MH, et al. Magnetic resonance imaging of the breast prior to biopsy. *JAMA* 2004;292(22):2735.
48. Morrow M, Venta L, Stinson T, et al. Prospective comparison of stereotactic core biopsy and surgical excision as diagnostic procedures for breast cancer patients. *Ann Surg* 2001;233(4):537.
56. Fisher B, Land S, Mamounas E, et al. Prevention of invasive breast cancer in women with ductal carcinoma *in situ*: an update of the National Surgical Adjuvant Breast and Bowel Project experience. *Semin Oncol* 2001;28(4):400.
57. Bijker N, Meijnen P, Peterse JL, et al. Breast-conserving treatment with or without radiotherapy in ductal carcinoma-in-situ: ten-year results of European Organisation for Research and Treatment of Cancer randomized phase III trial 10853—a study by the EORTC Breast Cancer Cooperative Group and EORTC Radiotherapy Group. *J Clin Oncol* 2006;24(21):3381.
59. Morrow M, Harris JR. Practice guideline for breast conservation therapy in the management of ductal carcinoma *in situ*. 2006 Practice Guidelines and Technical Standards, American College of Radiology World Wide Web URL: www.acr.org/Secondarymainmenucategories/quality_safety/guidelines/breast/dcis.aspx. Accessed February 17, 2011.
61. Cuzick J, Sestak I, Pinder SE, et al. Beneficial effect of tamoxifen for women with DCIS: Long-Term Results from the UK/ANZ DCIS Trial in Women with Locally Excised DCIS. *Cancer Res* 2009;69:34.
65. Hughes LL, Wang M, Page DL, et al. Local excision alone without irradiation for ductal carcinoma in situ of the breast: a trial of the Eastern Cooperative Oncology Group. *J Clin Oncol* 2009;27(32):5319.
67. Julian TB, Land S, Haile S, et al. Is sentinel node biopsy in DCIS necessary? *Ann Surg Oncol* 2006;135:11.
76. Khan SA, Stewart AK, Morrow M. Does aggressive local therapy improve survival in metastatic breast cancer? *Surgery* 2002;132(4):620; discussion 626.

79. Fisher B, Anderson S, Bryant J, et al. Twenty-year follow-up of a randomized trial comparing total mastectomy, lumpectomy, and lumpectomy plus irradiation for the treatment of invasive breast cancer. *N Engl J Med* 2002; 347(16):1233.
80. Veronesi U, Cascinelli N, Mariani L, et al. Twenty-year follow-up of a randomized study comparing breast-conserving surgery with radical mastectomy for early breast cancer. *N Engl J Med* 2002;347(16):1227.
81. Early Breast Cancer Trialist Group. Favourable and unfavourable effects on long-term survival of radiotherapy for early breast cancer: an overview of the randomised trials. Early Breast Cancer Trialists' Collaborative Group. *Lancet* 2000;355(9217):1757.
83. Morrow M, Jagsi R, Alderman AK, et al. Surgeon recommendations and receipt of mastectomy for treatment of breast cancer. *JAMA* 2009;302(14): 1551.
84. Katz SJ, Lantz PM, Janz NK, et al. Patient involvement in surgery treatment decisions for breast cancer. *J Clin Oncol* 2005;23(24):5526.
86. Anderson SJ, Wapnir I, Dignam JJ, et al. Prognosis After Ipsilateral Breast Tumor Recurrence and Locoregional Recurrences in Patients Treated by Breast-Conserving Therapy in Five National Surgical Adjuvant Breast and Bowel Project Protocols of Node-Negative Breast Cancer. *J Clin Oncol* 2009;15:2466.
88. Pierce LJ, Levin AM, Rebbeck TR, et al. Ten-year multi-institutional results of breast-conserving surgery and radiotherapy in *BRCA1/2*-associated stage I/II breast cancer. *J Clin Oncol* 2006;24(16):2437.
91. Nguyen PL, Taghian AG, Katz MS, et al. Breast cancer subtype approximated by estrogen receptor, progesterone receptor, and HER-2 is associated with local and distant recurrence after breast-conserving therapy. *J Clin Oncol* 2008;26:2373.
92. Millar EK, Graham PH, O'Toole SA, et al. Prediction of local recurrence, distant metastases, and death after breast-conserving therapy in early-stage invasive breast cancer using a five-biomarker panel. *J Clin Oncol* 2009;27:4701.
95. Mamounas EP, Tang G, Fisher B, et al. Association between the 21-Gene recurrence score assay and risk of locoregional recurrence in node-negative, Estrogen receptor-positive breast cancer: results from NSABP B-14 and NSABP B-20. *J Clin Oncol* 2010;28:1677.
96. Bartelink H, Horiot J-C, Poortmans PM, et al. Impact of a higher radiation dose on local control and survival in breast conserving therapy of early breast cancer: 10-year results of the randomized EORTC "Boost versus no Boost" trial 22881-10882. *J Clin Oncol* 2007;25:3259.
98. Fisher B, Dignam J, Bryant J, et al. Five versus more than five years of tamoxifen therapy for breast cancer patients with negative lymph nodes and estrogen receptor-positive tumors. *J Natl Cancer Inst* 1996;88(21):1529.
100. Fisher B, Bryant J, Dignam JJ, et al. Tamoxifen, radiation therapy, or both for prevention of ipsilateral breast tumor recurrence after lumpectomy in women with invasive breast cancers of one centimeter or less. *J Clin Oncol* 2002;20(20):4141.
102. Toledano A, Garaud P, Serin D, et al. Concurrent administration of adjuvant chemotherapy and radiotherapy after breast-conserving surgery enhances late toxicities: long-term results of the ARCOSEIN multicenter randomized study. *Int J Radiat Oncol Biol Phys* 2006;65(2):324.
104. Bellon JR, Come SE, Gelman RS, et al. Sequencing of chemotherapy and radiation therapy in early-stage breast cancer: updated results of a prospective randomized trial. *J Clin Oncol* 2005;23(9):1934.
105. Sartor CI, Peterson BL, Woolf S, et al. Effect of addition of adjuvant paclitaxel on radiotherapy delivery and locoregional control of node-positive breast cancer: cancer and leukemia group B 9344. *J Clin Oncol* 2005;23 (1):30.
107. Turnbull LW, Brown SR, Olivier C, et al. Multicentre randomised controlled trial examining the cost-effectiveness of contrast-enhanced high field magnetic resonance imaging in women with primary breast cancer scheduled for wide local excision (COMICE). *Health Technol Assess* 2010; 14(1):1.
111. van der Hage JA, van de Velde CJ, Julien JP, et al. Preoperative chemotherapy in primary operable breast cancer: results from the european organization for research and treatment of cancer trial 10902. *J Clin Oncol* 2001;19(22):4224.
112. Fisher B, Bryant J, Wolmark N, et al. Effect of preoperative chemotherapy on the outcome of women with operable breast cancer. *J Clin Oncol* 1988; 16(8):2672.
113. Bear HD, Anderson S, Smith RE, et al. Sequential preoperative or postoperative docetaxel added to preoperative doxorubicin plus cyclophosphamide for operable breast cancer: national surgical adjuvant breast and bowel project protocol B-27. *J Clin Oncol* 2006;24(13):2019.
114. Buzdar AU, Valero V, Ibrahim NK, et al. Neoadjuvant therapy with paclitaxel followed by 5-fluorouracil, epirubicin, and cyclophosphamide chemotherapy and concurrent trastuzumab in human epidermal growth factor receptor 2-positive operable breast cancer: an update of the initial randomized study population and data of additional patients treated with the same regimen. *Clin Cancer Res* 2007;13(1):228.
115. Mauri D, Pavlidis N, Ioannidis JP. Neoadjuvant versus adjuvant systemic treatment in breast cancer: a meta-analysis. *J Natl Cancer Inst* 2005;97(3): 188.
118. Smith IE, Dowsett M, Ebbs SR, et al. Neoadjuvant treatment of postmenopausal breast cancer with anastrozole, tamoxifen, or both in combination: the Immediate Preoperative Anastrozole, Tamoxifen, or Combined with Tamoxifen (IMPACT) multicenter double-blind randomized trial. *J Clin Oncol* 2005;23(22):5108.
119. Clarke M, Collins R, Darby S, et al. Effects of radiotherapy and of differences in the extent of surgery for early breast cancer on local recurrence and 15-year survival: an overview of the randomised trials. *Lancet* 2005; 366(9503):2087.
121. Fyles AW, McCready DR, Manchul LA, et al. Tamoxifen with or without breast irradiation in women 50 years of age or older with early breast cancer. *N Engl J Med* 2004;351(10):963.
123. Hughes KS, Schnaper LA, Berry D, et al. Lumpectomy plus tamoxifen with or without irradiation in women 70 years of age or older with early breast cancer. *N Engl J Med* 2004;351(10):971.
124. Whelan TJ, Pignol JP, Levine MN, et al. Long-term results of hypofractionated radiation therapy for breast cancer. *N Engl J Med* 2010;362(6):513.
125. Holland R, Veling SH, Mravunac M, Hendriks JH. Histologic multifocality of Tis, T1-2 breast carcinomas. Implications for clinical trials of breast-conserving surgery. *Cancer* 1985;56(5):979.
126. Smith BD, Arthur DW, Buchholz TA, et al. Accelerated partial breast irradiation consensus statement from the American Society for Radiation Oncology (ASTRO). *Int J Radiat Oncol Biol Phys* 2009;74(4):987.
127. Motwani SB, Strom EA, Schechter NR, et al. The impact of immediate breast reconstruction on the technical delivery of postmastectomy radiotherapy. *Int J Radiat Oncol Biol Phys* 2006;66(1):76.
130. Gerber B, Krause A, Reimer T, et al. Skin-sparing mastectomy with conservation of the nipple-areola complex and autologous reconstruction is an oncologically safe procedure. *Ann Surg* 2003;238(1):120.
135. Fisher B, Jeong JH, Anderson S, et al. Twenty-five-year follow-up of a randomized trial comparing radical mastectomy, total mastectomy, and total mastectomy followed by irradiation. *N Engl J Med* 2002;347(8):567.
136. Quiet CA, Ferguson DJ, Weichselbaum RR, Hellman S. Natural history of node-positive breast cancer: the curability of small cancers with a limited number of positive nodes. *J Clin Oncol* 1996;14(12):3105.
139. Wilke LG, McCall LM, Posther KE, et al. Surgical complications associated with sentinel lymph node biopsy: results from a prospective international cooperative group trial. *Ann Surg Oncol* 2006;13(4):491.
140. Mansel RE, Fallowfield L, Kissin M, et al. Randomized multicenter trial of sentinel node biopsy versus standard axillary treatment in operable breast cancer: the ALMANAC trial. *J Natl Cancer Inst* 2006;98(9):599.
145. Veronesi U, Paganelli G, Viale G, et al. Sentinel-lymph-node biopsy as a staging procedure in breast cancer: update of a randomised controlled study. *Lancet Oncol* 2006;7(12):983.
147. Naik AM, Fey J, Gemignani M, et al. The risk of axillary relapse after sentinel lymph node biopsy for breast cancer is comparable with that of axillary lymph node dissection: a follow-up study of 4008 procedures. *Ann Surg* 2004;240(3):462; discussion 468.
150. Louis-Sylvestre C, Clough K, Asselain B, et al. Axillary treatment in conservative management of operable breast cancer: dissection or radiotherapy? Results of a randomized study with 15 years of follow-up. *J Clin Oncol* 2004;22(1):97.
154. Hammond ME, Hayes DF, Dowsett M, et al. American Society of Clinical Oncology/College of American Pathologists Guideline Recommendations for Immunohistochemical Testing of Estrogen and Progesterone Receptors in Breast Cancer. *J Clin Oncol*. 2010; 28(16):2784–2795.
156. Olivotto IA, Bajdik CD, Ravdin PM, et al. Population-based validation of the prognostic model ADJUVANT! for early breast cancer. *J Clin Oncol* 2005;23(12):2716.
160. Wolff AC, Hammond ME, Schwartz JN, et al. American society of clinical oncology/college of American pathologists guideline recommendations for human epidermal growth factor receptor 2 testing in breast cancer. *J Clin Oncol* 2007;25(1):118.
161. Braun S, Vogl FD, Naume B, et al. A pooled analysis of bone marrow micrometastasis in breast cancer. *N Engl J Med* 2005;353(8):793.
163. Sorlie T, Tibshirani R, Parker J, et al. Repeated observation of breast tumor subtypes in independent gene expression data sets. *Proc Natl Acad Sci U S A* 2003;100(14):8418.
164. Perou CM, Sorlie T, Eisen MB, et al. Molecular portraits of human breast tumours. *Nature* 2000;406(6797):747.
167. van de Vijver MJ, He YD, van't Veer LJ, et al. A gene-expression signature as a predictor of survival in breast cancer. *N Engl J Med* 2002;347(25):1999.
170. Paik S, Shak S, Tang G, et al. A multigene assay to predict recurrence of tamoxifen-treated, node-negative breast cancer. *N Engl J Med* 2004;351 (27):2817.
171. Dowsett M, Cuzick J, Wale C, et al. Prediction of risk of distant recurrence using the 21-gene recurrence score in node-negative and node-positive postmenopausal patients with breast cancer treated with anastrozole or tamoxifen: a TransATAC study. *J Clin Oncol* 2010;28(11):1829.
173. Albain KS, Barlow WE, Shak S, et al. Prognostic and predictive value of the 21-gene recurrence score assay in postmenopausal women with node-positive, oestrogen-receptor-positive breast cancer on chemotherapy: a retrospective analysis of a randomised trial. *Lancet Oncol* 2010;11(1):55.
175. Early Breast Cancer Trialists Group. Effects of chemotherapy and hormonal therapy for early breast cancer on recurrence and 15-year survival: an overview of the randomised trials. *Lancet* 2005;365(9472):1687.
177. Fisher B, Anderson S, Tan-Chiu E, et al. Tamoxifen and chemotherapy for axillary node-negative, estrogen receptor-negative breast cancer: findings

from National Surgical Adjuvant Breast and Bowel Project B-23. *J Clin Oncol* 2001;19(4):931.
178. IBCSG. Endocrine responsiveness and tailoring adjuvant therapy for postmenopausal lymph node-negative breast cancer: a randomized trial. *J Natl Cancer Inst* 2002;94(14):1054.
182. Baum M, Budzar AU, Cuzick J, et al. Anastrozole alone or in combination with tamoxifen versus tamoxifen alone for adjuvant treatment of postmenopausal women with early breast cancer: first results of the ATAC randomised trial. *Lancet* 2002;359(9324):2131.
185. Jakesz R, Jonat W, Gnant M, et al. Switching of postmenopausal women with endocrine-responsive early breast cancer to anastrozole after 2 years' adjuvant tamoxifen: combined results of ABCSG trial 8 and ARNO 95 trial. *Lancet* 2005;366(9484):455.
186. Coombes RC, Hall E, Gibson LJ, et al. A randomized trial of exemestane after two to three years of tamoxifen therapy in postmenopausal women with primary breast cancer. *N Engl J Med* 2004;350(11):1081.
187. Goss PE, Ingle JN, Martino S, et al. A randomized trial of letrozole in postmenopausal women after five years of tamoxifen therapy for early-stage breast cancer. *N Engl J Med* 2003;349(19):1793.
190. BIG 1-98 Collaborative Group, Mouridsen H, Giobbie-Hurder A, et al. Letrozole therapy alone or in sequence with tamoxifen in women with breast cancer. *N Engl J Med* 2009;361(8):766.
192. Winer EP, Berry DA, Woolf S, et al. Failure of higher-dose paclitaxel to improve outcome in patients with metastatic breast cancer: cancer and leukemia group B trial 9342. *J Clin Oncol* 2004;22(11):2061.
196. Smith IE, Dowsett M, Yap YS, et al. Adjuvant aromatase inhibitors for early breast cancer after chemotherapy-induced amenorrhoea: caution and suggested guidelines. *J Clin Oncol* 2006;24(16):2444.
197. Bines J, Oleske DM, Cobleigh MA. Ovarian function in premenopausal women treated with adjuvant chemotherapy for breast cancer. *J Clin Oncol* 1996;14(5):1718.
201. The Adjuvant Breast Cancer Trialists Group. Ovarian ablation or suppression in premenopausal early breast cancer: results from the International Adjuvant Breast Cancer Ovarian Ablation or Suppression Randomized Trial. *J Natl Cancer Inst* 2007;99(7):516.
204. Schroth W, Goetz MP, Hamann U, et al. Association between CYP2D6 polymorphisms and outcomes among women with early stage breast cancer treated with tamoxifen. *JAMA* 2009;302(13):1429.
209. Henderson IC, Berry DA, Demetri GD, et al. Improved outcomes from adding sequential paclitaxel but not from escalating doxorubicin dose in an adjuvant chemotherapy regimen for patients with node-positive primary breast cancer. *J Clin Oncol* 2003;21(6):976.
213. Citron ML, Berry DA, Cirrincione C, et al. Randomized trial of dose-dense versus conventionally scheduled and sequential versus concurrent combination chemotherapy as postoperative adjuvant treatment of node-positive primary breast cancer: first report of Intergroup Trial C9741/Cancer and Leukemia Group B Trial 9741. *J Clin Oncol* 2003;21(8):1431.
214. Fisher B, Jeong JH, Anderson S, et al. Treatment of axillary lymph node-negative, estrogen receptor-negative breast cancer: updated findings from National Surgical Adjuvant Breast and Bowel Project clinical trials. *J Natl Cancer Inst* 2004;96(24):1823.
215. Jones S, Holmes FA, O'Shaughnessy J, et al. Docetaxel with cyclophosphamide is associated with an overall survival benefit compared with doxorubicin and cyclophosphamide: 7-Year follow-up of US Oncology Research Trial 9735. *J Clin Oncol* 2009;27(8):1177.
216. Swain SM, Jeong JH, Geyer CE, et al. NSABP B-30: definitive analysis of patient outcome from a randomized trial evaluating different schedules and combinations of adjuvant therapy containing doxorubicin, docetaxel and cyclophosphamide in women with operable, node-positive breast cancer. *Cancer Res* 2009;69:81s.
217. Fisher B, Dignam J, Tan-Chiu E, et al. Prognosis and treatment of patients with breast tumors of one centimeter or less and negative axillary lymph nodes. *J Natl Cancer Inst* 2001;93(2):112.
219. Berry DA, Cirrincione C, Henderson IC, et al. Estrogen-receptor status and outcomes of modern chemotherapy for patients with node-positive breast cancer. *JAMA* 2006;295(14):1658.
222. Hayes DF, Thor A, Dressler L, et al. HER2 predicts benefit from adjuvant paclitaxel after AC in node-positive breast cancer. *J Clin Oncol* 2006;24(18 suppl):5S (abst 510).
223. Sotiriou C, Wirapati P, Loi S, et al. Gene expression profiling in breast cancer: understanding the molecular basis of histologic grade to improve prognosis. *J Natl Cancer Inst* 2006;98(4):262.
224. Ravdin PM, Siminoff LA, Davis GJ, et al. Computer program to assist in making decisions about adjuvant therapy for women with early breast cancer. *J Clin Oncol* 2001;19(4):980.

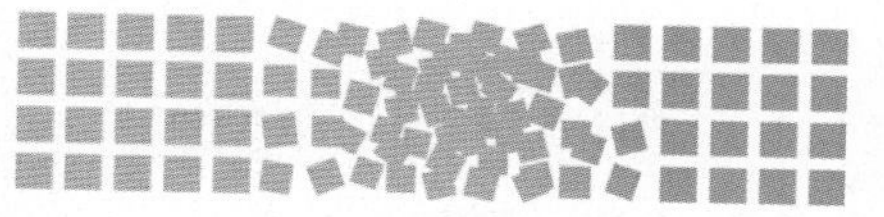

CHAPTER 107 MOLECULAR BIOLOGY OF ENDOCRINE TUMORS

SAMUEL A. WELLS, Jr.

Over the past two decades, the remarkable advances in endocrine oncology have been enhanced by powerful and sophisticated molecular technology. In this regard studies of hereditary endocrine tumors have been especially fruitful, not only in defining the molecular genetic basis of these complex diseases, but in understanding the pathogenesis of the individual component tumor of the syndromes as well as their sporadic counterparts.

THE MULTIPLE ENDOCRINE NEOPLASIA SYNDROMES

Most endocrine tumors involve a single endocrine gland, are usually benign, and occur sporadically. Rarely, endocrine tumors occur in a familial pattern where they are multiple, involving more than one endocrine gland. Over the past 50 years at least six multiple endocrine neoplasia (MEN) syndromes have been described, including MEN-1, MEN-2, von Hippel-Lindau (VHL) disease, neurofibromatosis type 1, Carney complex (CNC), and the McCune-Albright syndrome (MAS). The genetic mutation causing each of these six MEN syndromes has been identified, in many cases leading to improved diagnosis and treatment of patients with a specific syndrome. It is not possible to address each of these syndromes in detail in this chapter, accordingly, the most common ones will be addressed.

Multiple Endocrine Neoplasia Type 1

Clinical Features

In 1954 Wermer[1] described a family with hyperparathyroidism and tumors of the pancreatic islet cells and the pituitary gland. This hereditary syndrome has since been named multiple endocrine neoplasia (MEN) type 1 (MEN-1) (Mendelian Inheritance in Man [MIM] 13001) and over 20 separate endocrine or nonendocrine tumors may occur in patients with this disease. The prevalence of MEN-1 is 2 to 3 per 100,000, and males and females are equally affected. MEN-1 is characterized by high penetrance but variable expressivity. Virtually all patients develop parathyroid hyperplasia by age 40, 50% develop malignant pancreatic islet cell tumors (usually gastrinomas, less often insulinomas, and rarely glucagonomas, or vasoactive intestinal polypeptide secreting tumors [VIPomas]), and 25% develop pituitary tumors (usually prolactinomas). The diagnosis of MEN-1 is established either when a previously unaffected member of a family with MEN-1 develops a single characteristic endocrine tumor, or when a patient with hyperparathyroidism develops a pituitary tumor or a pancreatic islet cell tumor.

Molecular Genetics

Chandrasekharappa et al.[2] discovered the genetic mutation for MEN-1. The *MEN1* gene spans a 9.8 kb segment of chromosome 11q13 and consists of 10 exons with a 1,830 base pair region that encodes transcripts of 2.7 and 3.1 kb. The transcripts, expressed in almost all tissues, encode a novel, highly conserved 610 amino acid, 67 kDa protein, menin.[3] *MEN1*, a putative tumor suppressor gene, mainly resides in the nucleus but is also found in the cytoplasm. The amino acid sequence of menin does not have homologies in the genome, thus clues to its mechanism of action have primarily come from identification of menin partnering to proteins or chromatin. Approximately 25 protein partners for menin have been identified, the first of which was junD, followed by others, such as MLL-containing complex, SMAD3, PEM, NM23, and nuclear factor B; however, at present no one menin partner has been shown convincingly to be critical to MEN-1 tumogenesis. The crystal structure of menin is unknown, and there is no direct evidence that menin binds directly to DNA; however, the protein appears to play a critical role in the regulation of gene transcription, apoptosis, and genome stability. Homozygous mice null for *Men1* die during embryogenesis, while heterologous mice, *Men1*$^{+/}$, develop a pattern of endocrine tumors very similar to that of patients with MEN-1.

The first "hit" in the *MEN1* gene that leads to tumorigenesis involves small mutations in one or several bases, broadly distributed across the *MEN1* open reading frame, such that half of newly diagnosed index cases are found to have novel mutations.[4,5] The second "hit" is a chromosomal mutation in somatic tissue that causes frameshift (deletions, insertions, or splice site defects) and nonsense mutations, including a portion or all of the *MEN1* gene. Approximately 75% of kindreds with MEN-1 will be found to have *MEN1* mutations, however, in patients who demonstrate hyperparathyroidism and pituitary tumors, the incidence of *MEN1* mutations is approximately 10%, suggesting another genetic cause of this MEN-1 variant. To date approximately 400 unique germline or somatic mutations of *MEN1* have been described (Fig. 107.1).[6] There is little correlation between genotype and phenotype, and presymptomatic diagnosis by direct DNA testing is useful only in identifying family members and then monitoring them for the development of specific endocrine tumors associated with MEN-1. There is no rationale for prophylactic removal of the parathyroid glands, the pancreas, or the pituitary gland in asymptomatic patients who have inherited a mutated *MEN1* allele.

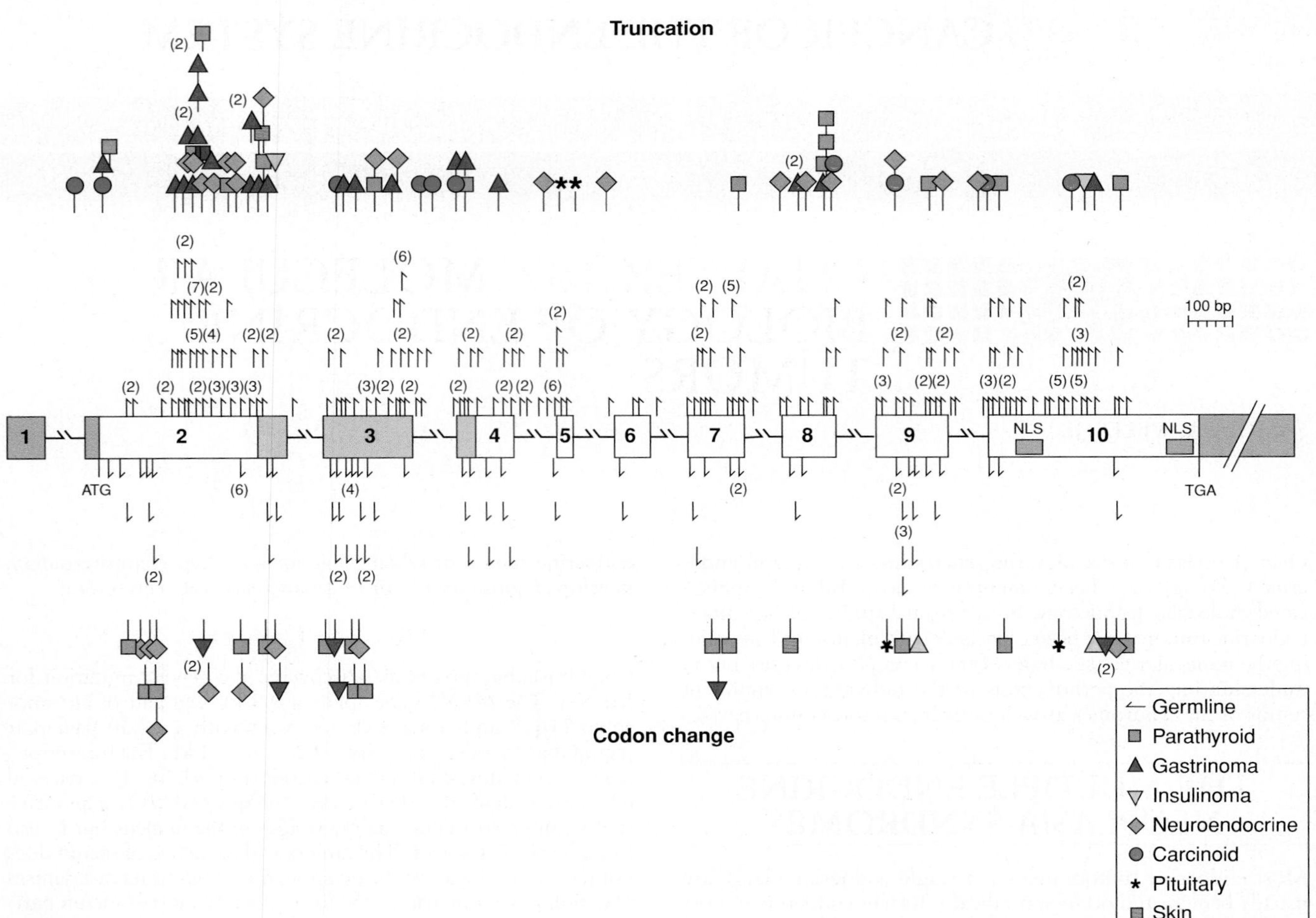

FIGURE 107.1 A schematic diagram of the genomic organization of the gene responsible for multiple endocrine neoplasia type 1 (MEN-1), including MEN-1 germline and somatic mutations. The gene contains ten exons (the first of which remains untranslated) and extends across 9 kb. It encodes a 610 amino acid protein, menin. Mutations shown above the exons cause menin truncation; those shown below the exons cause an amino acid or codon change. All unique mutations are represented; numbers in parentheses represent multiple reports of the same mutation in apparently unrelated individuals. The green-shaded areas indicate the untranslated regions. The location of the two nuclear localization signals (NLS), at codons 479–497 and 588–608, are indicated. Missense mutations in a region of menin (amino acids 139–242, identified by blue shading) prevented interaction with the AP1 transcription factor JunD. (From ref. 6, with permission.)

The endocrine tumors characteristic of MEN-1 occur more commonly in a sporadic setting, where 25% of gastrinomas, 10% to 20% of insulinomas, 50% of VIPomas, 25% to 35% of bronchial carcinoids, and 20% of parathyroid adenomas express somatic *MEN1* mutations. Conversely, somatic *MEN1* mutations rarely if ever occur in sporadic adrenocortical tumors, pituitary tumors, or thyroid tumors.[6]

Other Hereditary Endocrinopathies Involving the Parathyroid and Pituitary Glands

The Parathyroid Gland

While familial hyperparathyroidism is most commonly a component of MEN-1, it can occur in other settings, the most notable being familial (benign) hypocalciuric hypercalcemia (FHH), the hyperparathyroidism jaw-tumor (HPT-JT) syndrome, familial isolated hyperparathyroidism (FIHP), and MEN-2A.

Familial Hypocalciuric Hypercalcemia (FHH, MIM 145980). The calcium-sensing receptor (CASR), a critical regulator of extracellular calcium homeostasis, is a seven-transmembrane-spanning G-protein–coupled receptor, which is expressed in cells of the parathyroid gland and the kidney tubule. The discovery of the CASR was a surprise, since previously no small cation had been shown capable of acting as a ligand for a G-protein–coupled receptor.[7] The human CASR, encoded by six exons of the gene located on chromosome 3q113.3-q21, is sensitive to changes in the ambient calcium concentration and when activated it inhibits parathyroid hormone (PTH) secretion and the renal reabsorption of calcium. With heterogenous inactivating mutations of the *CASR* gene the parathyroid cell fails to sense properly an increased serum calcium concentration, and the resulting increase in PTH secretion causes FHH, an autosomal dominant disease characterized by hypocalciuria, hypercalcemia, and parathyroid hyperplasia. It is important for clinicians to recognize this relatively mild form of familial hyperparathyroidism; although parathyroidectomy reduces the serum calcium level, it is only temporary. With inactivating mutations in both alleles of the *CASR* gene, neonatal severe hyperparathyroidism ([NSHPT] MIM 239200) develops with serum calcium levels in the range of 15 to 20 mg/dL. This disease represents a life-threatening emergency and urgent parathyroidectomy is indicated.[8] Conversely, activating mutations of the *CASR* gene cause the parathyroid cells to sense that serum calcium is "elevated" when it is actually normal. There is a resulting decrease in the blood calcium level expressed as the syndrome of autosomal dominant hypoparathyroidism ([ADH] MIM 168468).[9] To date approximately 115 mutations (60% inactivating and 40% activating) have been described in the *CASR* gene, and most are missense mutations clustered in exons 3, 4, and 7.

Hyperparathyroidism-Jaw Tumor Syndrome (HPT-JT, MIM 145001). HPT-JT is characterized by the autosomal dominant occurrence of hyperparathyroidism, ossifying fibromas of the mandible or maxilla, renal cysts or solid tumors, and uterine fibromas.[10] Approximately 50 families with HPT-JT have been reported and 80% of patients have hyperparathyroidism, and in 15% of cases the parathyroid tumors are malignant. It is noteworthy that the age-related penetrance of HPT-JT is approximately 40% by age 40 in contrast to MEN-1 where the age-related penetrance is 98% by age 40.[11] Members of kindreds with this disease need lifelong surveillance by physical examination and biochemical evaluation. It has even been suggested that serial ultrasound examination of the neck should be performed as parathyroid carcinoma has been reported in normocalcemic kindred members.[12]

The cause of HPT-JT appears to be a tumor suppressor gene, *HRPT2*, which is located on chromosome 1q25-q31. The *HPRT2* gene consists of 17 exons and the mutations are scattered throughout the 1593 coding region, with the majority resulting in functional loss through premature truncation.[13] Approximately 16 activating mutations of *HRPT2*, most of which are frameshift, have been identified. The *HPRT2* gene encodes a 531 amino acid protein, parafibromin (named for parathyroid tumors and jaw fibromas).[14] The function of parafibromin is unknown but it is thought to regulate posttranscriptional events and histone modification. There is recent evidence that parafibromin has pro-apoptotic activity, important as a tumor suppressor function.[15] Germline mutations in *HPRT2* have been identified in approximately half of HPT-JT families, and even in some families with MEN-2A.

Besides the evidence of germline mutations in patients with the HPT-JT somatic *HRPT2* mutations have been detected in the majority of patients with sporadic parathyroid carcinoma.[16,17] It is important to note that mutations in *HRPT2* are rarely if ever seen in sporadic parathyroid adenomas, an important diagnostic finding distinguishing benign from malignant parathyroid tumors.[15,18]

Familial Isolated Hyperparathyroidism (FIHP, MIM 145000). The syndrome of FIHP is a heterogenous condition, and some kindreds thought to have this disease have been shown to have germline mutations of *MEN1*, *CASR*, or *HRP-JT*, suggesting that the disease represents incompletely expressed forms of MEN1, FHH, or HPT-JT.[19] Over 100 families with FIHP have been reported and in most cases the causative genetic mutation is unknown, although there are convincing data that it resides on chromosome 2p13.3-14.[20]

The Pituitary Gland

There is no relationship between genotype and phenotype in patients with MEN-1, thus there is no way to predict the presence or behavior of pancreatic islet cell tumors or pituitary tumors. There are, however, important genetic mutations associated with other hereditary and sporadic pituitary tumors.

Carney Complex (CNC, MIM 160980). Pituitary adenomas can occur as a component of CNC, a familial disease characterized by hypersomatotropenemia, cardiac or cutaneous myxomas, spotty skin pigmentation, primary pigmented nodular adrenal disease, and testicular tumors.[21] About 75% of patients exhibit subclinical increases in growth hormone (GH), insulinlike growth factor-1 (IGF-1), and prolactin. Acromegaly occurs in about 10% of patients. Genetic linkage analysis has shown two loci for CNC, one on chromosome 2p16 (*CNC2*), and the other on chromosome 17q22-24 (*CNC1*). Neither locus is associated with a specific phenotype. In more than 50% of cases the CNC has been linked to an inactivating mutation in the gene coding for the protein kinase A (PKA) type 1α subunit, *PRKAR1A*, at 17q24. The 2p16 locus is uncharacterized.

Familial Isolated Pituitary Adenomas (FIPA, MIM 102200). Pituitary adenomas can also occur as FIPA. Daly et al.[22] evaluated 64 families with FIPA, residing in Belgium, France, Italy, and the Netherlands. Of the 138 affected family members, 55 had prolactinomas, 47 had somatotropinomas, 28 had nonsecreting adenomas, and 8 had adrenocorticotropic hormone–secreting tumors. The incidences of a homogenous (single tumor) phenotype and a heterogeneous tumors phenotype were approximately equal. Affected patients were found to have no mutations in either the *MEN1* or *PRKRA1A* genes.

Recently, Vierimaa et al.,[23] in a study of cases of low penetrance familial pituitary adenoma in Northern Finland identified loss of mutation functions in the aryl hydrocarbon receptor interacting protein (*AIP*) gene. *AIP* forms a complex with the aryl hydrocarbon receptor (AHR) and two 90-kD heat-shock proteins (HSP90). AHR is a ligand-activated transcription factor and also participates in cellular signaling pathways.

Expression profiling in two families resulted in the identification of *AIP* as one of the candidate genes, and a nonsense mutation (Gln14X) was also identified and found to segregate with the GH-secreting adenomas.[23] Daly et al.[24] studied 73 FIPA families with 156 individuals and found that 11 of them harbored 10 *AIP* germline mutations. Kindred members with *AIP* mutations, compared to those without mutations, were younger and had larger tumors. Growth hormone producing tumors predominated among family members with *AIP* mutations.

Multiple Endocrine Neoplasia Type 2

Clinical Features

In 1968 Steiner et al.[25] described a large family with medullary thyroid carcinoma (MTC), pheochromocytomas, hyperparathyroidism, and Cushing's syndrome. The disease was named multiple endocrine neoplasia type 2, and it is now recognized that there are three related syndromes characterized by hereditary MTC: MEN-2A (MIM 171400), MEN-2B (MIM 162300), and familial medullary thyroid carcinoma (FMTC) (MIM 155240). There is near complete penetrance but variable expressivity, as virtually all patients with MEN-2A develop MTC, approximately half develop pheochromocytomas, and 30% develop hyperparathyroidism. Less often MEN-2A is associated with cutaneous lichen amyloidosis (CLA), which develops on the upper back and serves as a precocious marker of the disorder, or Hirschsprung's disease (HD), which is characterized by loss of ganglion cells in variable segments of the large bowel. Patients with MEN-2B develop MTC and pheochromocytomas with the same frequency as patients with MEN-2A, but rather than hyperparathyroidism, they express a generalized gastrointestinal neuromatosis and a characteristic physical appearance. Patients with FMTC develop only MTC. Of patients with hereditary MTC, 80% have MEN-2A, 15% have FMTC, and 5% have MEN-2B.

Medullary thyroid carcinoma originates from C cells, which are derived from the neural crest. The C cells have great biosynthetic capability and secrete the polypeptide hormone calcitonin (CTN) and the glycoprotein carcinoembryonic antigen (CEA). Plasma CTN serves as an excellent marker for MTC, and presently its main use is in detecting persistent or residual MTC following thyroidectomy.

The MTC is the most common cause of death in patients with MEN-2A, MEN-2B, and FMTC, and the only effective therapy is timely thyroidectomy as standard chemotherapy and external beam radiotherapy are not useful.

Molecular Genetics

In 1985 Takahashi et al.[26] discovered the *RET* (*RE*arranged during *T*ransfection) protooncogene. The gene is located in the pericentromeric region of chromosome 10q11.2 and includes 21 exons. *RET* encodes a receptor tyrosine kinase, which is expressed in neuroendocrine cells (including thyroid C cells and adrenal medullary cells), neural cells (including parasympathetic and sympathetic ganglion cells), urogenital tract cells, and the branchial arch cells.

The *RET* gene has an extracellular portion, which contains four cadherin-like repeats, a calcium binding site and a cysteine-rich region, a transmembrane portion, and an intracellular portion, which contains two tyrosine kinase domains. Alternate splicing of *RET* produces three isoforms with either 9, 43, or 51 amino acids at the C terminus, referred to as *RET9*, *RET43*, and *RET51*.[27,28] Mice lacking *RET51* are normal, however, mice lacking *RET9* have renal malformation and defects in innervation of the gut.[29]

RET is essential for the development, survival, and regeneration of many neuronal cells in the gut, the kidney, and the nervous system. A tripartite complex is necessary for *RET* signaling. One of four glial-derived neurotrophic factors (GDNF) family ligands (GFLs)—GDNF, neurturin, persephin, or artemin–binds *RET* in conjunction with one of four glycosylphosphatidylinositol-anchored coreceptors, designated GDNF family receptors (GFR): GFR-α1, GFR-α2, GFR-α3, or GFR-α4.[30–32] The GFL-GFR complex causes dimerization of two *RET* molecules with activation of autophosphorylation and intracellular signaling. The C-terminal of *RET* contains 16 tyrosine residues, among which Y905 is a binding site for Grb7/10 adaptors, Y1015 a binding site for phospholipase Cγ, Y981 a binding site for c-Src, and Y1096 a binding site for Grb2. Tyrosine 1072 is a multidocking binding site for such proteins as SHC, SHCC, IRS1/2, FRS2, DOK1/4/5/, and Enigma. The *RET* receptor may activate various signaling pathways through Y1072, which thereby serves as a prerequisite for initiating transformation of *RET*-derived oncogenes in cell cultures and transgenic animals.[33] The structure of the RET receptor complex and the molecular pathways activated when there is ligand binding or constitutive activation are shown in Figure 107.2.[34]

Recently, the biochemical characterization and structure of the human *RET* tyrosine kinase domain was reported showing that both the phosphorylated and nonphosphorylated forms adopt the same active kinase conformation necessary to bind adenosine triphosphate and substrate and have a preorganized activation loop conformation.[35]

In 1993 and 1994 it was shown that point mutations in the *RET* protooncogene cause MEN-2A, MEN-2B, and FMTC.[36,37] The *RET* mutations are generally of two types and affect either the extracellular ligand binding site or the tyrosine kinase domain.

MEN-2A is associated with mutations involving the extracellular cysteine codons 609, 611, 618, 620 (exon 10) 630, or 634 (exon 11). The mutations associated with FMTC involve a broad range of codons, including those associated with MEN-2A, particularly 609, 618, and 620, as well as others: 768, 790, and 791 (exon 13), 804 and 844 (exon 14), or 891 (exon 15). One must be careful in making a diagnosis of FMTC, especially in small families, which span only one or two generations.

Ninety-five percent of patients with MEN-2B have a point mutation, codon M918T (exon 16), within the intracellular domain of *RET*. A few patients with MEN-2B have a mutation in codon A883F (exon 15). Rarely, compound heterozygous mutations in V804M with either Y806C or S904C occur in patients with a phenotype resembling MEN-2B.[38] In a study of 25 patients with *de novo* MEN-2B, Carlson et al.[39] found that the new mutation was of paternal origin in all cases. The investigators also observed a distortion of the sex ratio in both *de novo* MEN-2B patients and the affected offspring of MEN-2B transmitting males, suggesting a possible role for imprinting.

In patients with MEN-2A there is a clear correlation between genotype and phenotype, concerning both the pattern of clinical expression and the severity of disease.[28,37,40] Over 85% of patients with MEN-2A have a 634 codon mutation, and a C634R substitution is most often associated with hyperparathyroidism.[41,42] Patients with MEN-2A and CLA also have mutations at codon 634. Pheochromocytomas are associated with several codon mutations, most frequently 634, 618, 620, and 791.[43] Patients with the relatively rare association of MEN-2A and Hirschsprung's disease have mutations in exon 10, particularly codons 609, 618, and 620. Recently, the American Thyroid Association published guidelines for the diagnosis and treatment of MTC, including a list of the *RET* mutations so far described in patients with MEN-2A, MEN-2B, and FMTC.[44]

The medullary thyroid carcinoma has an early onset and a very aggressive clinical course in patients with MEN-2B, and it is moderately aggressive in patients with MEN-2A, particularly in patients with *RET* mutations in codons 634, 611, 618, and 620. The MTC is least aggressive in patients with FMTC. A schematic structure of the *RET* protooncogene with the most common codon mutations is shown in Figure 107.3.

It is important to note that approximately half of the patients with sporadic MTC have somatic M918T mutations in the MTC cells, and it has been suggested that the genotype is associated with a more aggressive phenotype, although this is controversial.[45]

The molecular basis for the genotype–phenotype correlations remains poorly understood; however, Iwashita et al.[46] introduced specific *RET* codon mutations into the short and long isoforms of *RET* cDNA and transfected the mutants into NIH3T3 cells. High levels of transforming activity of the mutant *RET* genes M918T and A833F correlated with the aggressive clinical phenotypes, MEN-2B, while low levels of transforming activity of the mutant *RET* genes E768D, V804L, and S891A correlated with the less aggressive FMTC phenotype. A similar study evaluating not only transforming ability of *RET* mutants but apoptosis, anchorage-independent growth, and signaling confirmed the findings of Iwashita et al. and also demonstrated that M918T and A883F mutants significantly enhanced the suppression of apoptosis.[47] It is of interest that mutations at codons 609, 618, and 620 markedly decrease the cell surface expression of *RET*, compared to codon 634 mutants, indicating that the former mutations impair transport of *RET* to the plasma membrane. One would expect this relationship considering the centrality of these *RET* mutations in association with MEN-2A and FMTC with Hirschsprung's disease.

Recently, gene expression studies relating to MEN-2A and MEN-2B have been reported by two groups. Myers and Mulligan[48] used cDNA microarray analysis of cell lines that expressed either the RET9 or the RET51 protein isoform to study *RET*-mediated gene expression patterns. They found that cells expressing *RET* have altered intercellular interactions correlated with increased expression of a number of cell surface molecules. The most striking expression pattern observed, however, was the up-regulation of stress response genes, specifically heat shock protein's (HSP) 70 family members: HSPA1A, HSPA1B, and HSPA1L. Additionally, other members of several HSP families associated with stress response were up-regulated. The increased expression of HSPs, particularly of the HSP70 and HSP90 families, has been documented in breast cancer, gastrointestinal cancer, and endometrial cancer and is associated with a poor prognosis. Conversely, the expression of HSP70 levels in osteosarcomas and renal cell

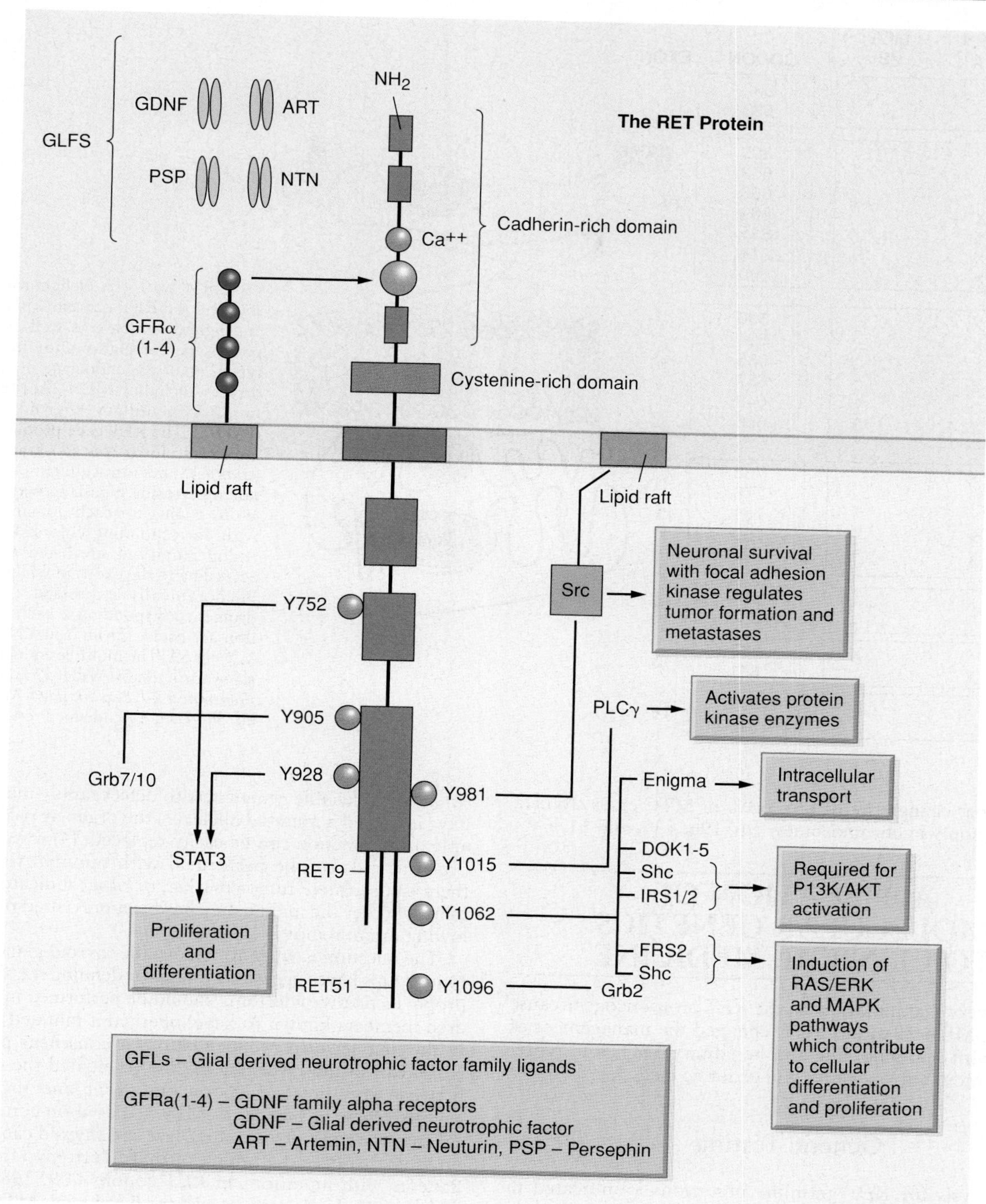

FIGURE 107.2 The RET structure and signaling network. The structure of the RET protein and the signaling network, showing docking sites and targets. RET, rearranged during transfection; GFLS, glial derived neurotrophic factor (GDNF) family ligands; ART, artemin; NTN, neurturin; PSP, persephin; GFRα, GDNF-family α receptors; Ca++, calcium ion. (From ref. 34, with permission.)

carcinomas is associated with an improved prognosis and a positive response to chemotherapy.[49]

Jain et al.[50] performed microarray expression analysis from pheochromocytomas and MTCs in 34 patients with MEN-2A, MEN-2B, and sporadic MTC. They found 118 probe sets that were differentially regulated in MEN-2B tumors compared to MEN-2A tumors (20 were up-regulated in MTCs from patients with MEN-2A and 98 were up-regulated in MTCs from patients with MEN-2B). Five genes were most discriminating by significance analysis microarray and correctly classified all of the cases of MTC associated with either MEN-2A or MEN-2B. The investigators found that genes involved in the process of epithelial to mesenchymal transition, many associated with the tumor growth factor β pathway, were up-regulated in MEN-2B MTCs. Also chondromodulin-1 mRNA and protein expression were localized to the malignant C cells, and its high expression correlated with the presence of skeletal deformities in MEN-2B patients.

Several groups have studied copy number imbalance in patients with MTC. One study of 37 patients with MTC, 29 with sporadic tumors, detected altered amplifications or deletions in chromosomal regions that housed genes likely to influence tumor pathogenesis.[51] Additional studies showed

PRACTICE OF ONCOLOGY

FMTC	MEN 2A	MEN 2B	CODON	EXON
X			532	8
X			533	
X			600	10
X			603	
X			606	
X	X		609	
X	X		611	
X	X		618	
X	X		620	
X	X		630	11
X	X		634	
	X		635	
	X		637	
X			649	
	X		666	
X	X		768	13
X			778	
X			781	
X	X		790	
X	X		791	
X	X		804	14
X			852	
		X	883	15
X	X		891	
X			912	16
		X	918	

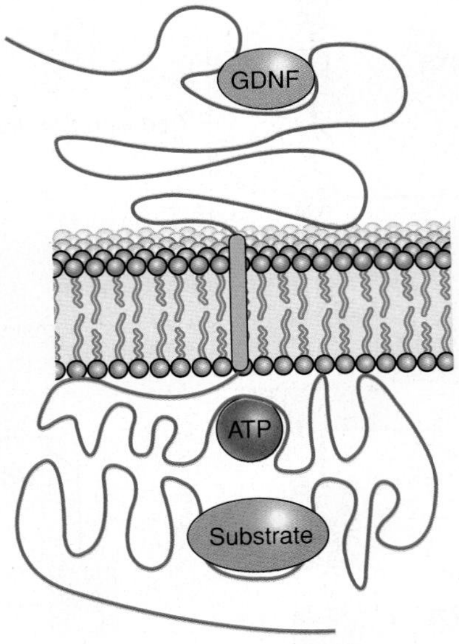

GDNF
ATP
Substrate

FIGURE 107.3 A schematic diagram showing the RET tyrosine kinase receptor and ligand complex as well as genotype-phenotype correlations for patients with type 2 multiple endocrine neoplasia syndromes, including MEN-2A, MEN-2B, and familial medullary thyroid carcinoma (FMTC). The RET gene product is divided into intracellular (*purple*), transmembrane (*orange*), and intracellular domains containing tyrosine kinase activity (*blue*). The exons coding for each domain are shown with corresponding colors. Known *RET* codon mutations are listed and grouped according to the exons in which they occur. Phenotypically expressed clinical syndromes corresponding to each codon mutation are listed. (From You YNY, Lankhani V, Wells SA. The multiple endocrine neoplasia syndromes. In: Willard H, Ginsburg LS. *Genomic and Personalized Medicine*. 1st ed. San Diego: Academic Press; 2009:936.)

copy number changes in 50% to 60% of MTC cases studied, most commonly in chromosomes 19p, 19q, 13q, and 11.[52,53]

APPLICATION OF MOLECULAR GENETICS TO CLINICAL MEDICINE

The discovery that mutations in the *RET* protooncogene cause MEN-2A, MEN-2B, and FMTC changed the management of patients with both sporadic and hereditary MTC and represents a paradigm for personalized genomic medicine.

Genetic Testing

DNA analysis for *RET* germline mutations is indicated in patients with presumably sporadic MTC, as approximately 5% of them will be found to have hereditary disease. It is imperative to screen the family members of patients with newly found germline *RET* mutations, since they are at risk for MTC and approximately half of them will be affected.[54]

Prophylactic Surgery

In patients with MEN-2A, MEN-2B, and FMTC who are shown to have inherited a mutated *RET* allele it is important to remove the thyroid before MTC develops or while it is still confined to the gland.[55] Thus, considering patients with familial cancer syndromes, hereditary MTC fulfills each of the criteria necessary for prophylactic removal of the organ at risk: (1) near complete penetrance, such that virtually all patients who have inherited a mutated allele will develop the malignancy, (2) a highly reliable genetic test to detect family members who have inherited a mutated allele, (3) the organ at risk is expendable or its function can be easily replaced, (4) resection of the organ at risk can be performed with minimal risk, and (5) there is a sensitive tumor marker, or other indicator, to determine whether the malignancy has been prevented or cured following organ removal.

The question is when to remove the thyroid gland. Recently, four groups have suggested criteria for defining the age at which prophylactic thyroidectomy should be performed in young kindred members known to have inherited a mutated *RET* allele. In the first set of recommendations a consensus panel at the MEN Consortium Meeting in 2000 evaluated the relationship between specific *RET* codon mutations and the biological aggressiveness of hereditary MTC.[40] Based on combined clinical data the panel defined three levels of thyroid cancer severity, on which to base the timing of thyroidectomy (Table 107.1). Patients with mutations in *RET* codons 609, 768, 790, 791, 804, or 891 (level 1) are at risk for developing MTC; however, their tumors are generally more indolent and develop at a later age than is the case in patients with other *RET* codon mutations. Recommendation for thyroidectomy in this group is controversial, and many clinicians base their advice for thyroidectomy on plasma calcitonin levels. In patients with mutations in RET codons 611, 618, 620, or 634 (level 2) thyroidectomy is recommended at or before 5 years of age. Patients with MEN-2B and mutations in *RET* codons 883 or 918 (level 3) have the most severe form of MTC, and thyroidectomy is recommended within the first 6 months of life. Subsequently, consensus panels of the British Thyroid Association, the National Comprehensive Cancer Network, and the American Thyroid Association have addressed this topic with largely confirmatory, and in some cases expanded, recommendations.[44,56,57]

Although these recommendations seem reasonable, it is known that there are certain factors that modify the severity

TABLE 107.1

RECOMMENDATIONS FOR PROPHYLACTIC THYROIDECTOMY BASED ON *RET* CODON MUTATION

Risk Level for MTC	1 High	2 Higher	3 Highest
Codons	609, 768, 790, 791, 804, 891	611, 618, 620, 634	883, 918, or known MEN-2B
Thyroidectomy (age)	No consensus: By 5 to 10 years; or at first abnormal stimulated calcitonin	By 5 years	By 6 months; preferably within first month of life

MTC, medullary thyroid carcinoma; MEN, multiple endocrine neoplasia.
(Modified from ref. 40, with permission.)

of the MTC, even within individual families. For example, it has been shown in some kindreds with codon 804 *RET* mutations (generally associated with a nonaggressive form of MTC) that a concomitant somatic 918 codon mutation in MTC cells confers a highly malignant phenotype.[58] Furthermore, it has been proposed that certain specific single-nucleotide polymorphisms (SNPs) influence the clinical behavior of the MTC, however, at present this relationship is unclear.

Realizing the criticalness of removing the thyroid gland while the MTC is curable, and understanding that it is impractical to establish strict guidelines for the timing of thyroidectomy based on the various *RET* codon mutations, clinicians should err on the side of advising thyroidectomy too early rather than too late. This approach is strengthened by the fact that once the MTC has spread beyond the thyroid gland it is virtually incurable, as no chemotherapy or radiotherapy regimen has proven effective.

SPORADIC THYROID CANCERS

Papillary Thyroid Carcinoma

Malignant tumors of the thyroid gland have a great range of biological behavior, ranging from the slow growing to highly aggressive. Over the past two decades the genetic mutations and chromosomal translocations that cause most histological types of thyroid cancer have been identified and have defined potential targets of small molecule therapeutics. The first of these observations came in 1985 with the discovery of the *RET* protooncogene.[26] In 1987 Fusco et al.[59] demonstrated in papillary thyroid carcinoma (PTC) the fusion of the C-terminal *RET* tyrosine kinase-encoding domain to the promoter and N-terminal portion of unrelated genes. The creation of these heterologous partners resulted in the illegitimate expression of a constitutively active chimeric oncogene termed *RET/PTC*. Subsequently, more than 15 molecular fusion oncogenes in PTCs have been identified, all of which differ according to the 5′-terminal region of the heterologous gene (Fig. 107.4). The most common of these chimeric oncogenes are *H4(CCDC6)-RET*, also known as *RET/PTC1* (60% to 70%), and *ELE1-RET*, also known as *RET/PTC3* (20% to 30%). The prevalence of *RET/PTC* in the thyroid cancers of children is greater than 50%, and in youngsters in Kiev and Belarus who developed PTC following exposure to radiation from the Chernobyl accident the prevalence of such rearrangements is 67% to 87%.[60–62] Analysis of components of the chimeric oncogenes showed a physical proximity of the chromatin distribution of follicular epithelial cells, supporting radiation as a cause of the induced fusion.[63] Similar *RET/PTC* rearrangements also occur in Hürthle cell carcinomas and trabecular adenomas, but they have not been described in patients with follicular carcinoma or anaplastic carcinomas.

The reported incidence of these hybrid genes in sporadic PTCs varies widely, from less than 5% to almost 70%, depending on tumor heterogeneity, geographic location, and the techniques used to detect *RET/PTC* rearrangements. In a study of 65 papillary thyroid carcinomas, five techniques (standard-sensitivity reverse transcription-polymerase chain reaction [RT-PCR], high-sensitivity RT-PCR, real-time LightCycler RT-PCR, Southern blot analysis, and fluorescence *in situ* hybridization) were used to detect *RET/PTC1* and *RET/PTC3* rearrangements. Three patterns of detection were evident. When a significant proportion of tumor cells (35% to 86%) contained *RET/PTC* rearrangements (clonal pattern), the translocations were detected by all five techniques. When 17% to 24% of tumor cells (subclonal), or less than 9% of tumor cells (nonclonal), contained *RET/PTC* rearrangements, less than five techniques were able to detect the translocations. Also, in contrast to clonal tumors, where neither *BRAF* nor *ras* mutations were identified, such mutations were found in 40% to 60% of subclonal or nonclonal tumors. *RET/PTC* oncogenes, found in PTC, like the *RET* mutations in the MEN-2 syndromes, potentiate the intrinsic tyrosine kinase activity of *RET* and thereby the downstream signaling events. There does not appear to be any relationship between *RET/PTC* rearrangements and the clinical behavior of PTC.

A much less frequent chromosomal rearrangement associated with PTC involves the neurotrophic receptor–tyrosine kinase *NTRK1* (also known as *TRK* and *TRKA*). Chimeric oncogenes result from the fusion of *NTRK1* and various activating genes: *TRK*, which contains sequences from the *TPM3* gene on chromosome 1q22-23; *TRK-T1* and *TRK-T2*, which contain different sequences of the *TPR* gene on chromosome 1q25; and *TRK-T3*, which combines with sequences of *TFG* on chromosome 3q11-12.[64]

The most common mutation in PTC is the $BRAF^{T17699A}$ mutation (V600E), which occurs in 35% to 65% of tumors.[65] There is virtually no overlap between the presence of *BRAF* mutations and *RET/PTC* gene rearrangements. Compared to the *RET/PTC* rearrangements, the *BRAF* mutations are reportedly associated with a more aggressive form of papillary carcinomas, characterized by extrathyroidal invasion, lymph node metastases, advanced tumor stage, and tumor recurrence. However, this point is controversial.

Follicular Thyroid Carcinoma

The peroxisome proliferators-activated receptor-γ (PPAR-γ), a member of the steroid-nuclear hormone receptor superfamily, is encoded by *PPARG* located on 3p25. Rearrangements involving the thyroid specific transcription factor, paired-box gene 8 (*PAX8*)

PRACTICE OF ONCOLOGY

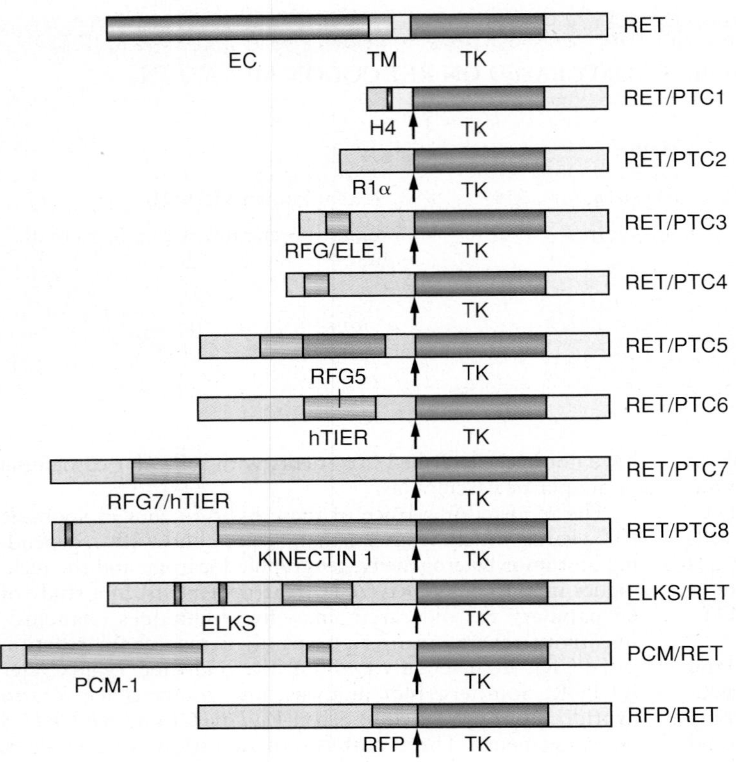

FIGURE 107.4 A schematic showing chimeric forms of the RET receptor formed by the joining of the C-terminus of RET to the promoter and N-terminus of unrelated genes. These chimeric oncogenes result in constitutive activation of RET and have been identified in patients with papillary thyroid carcinoma. EC, extracellular domain of RET; TM, transmembrane domain of RET; TK, tyrosine kinase domain of RET. H4, R1α, RFG/ELE1, RFG5, hTIF1, RFG7/hTIFR, KINECTIN1, ELKS, PCM-1, RFP represent the promoter and N-terminus of unrelated genes. (Modified from Santoro M, Melillo RM, Carlomagno F, Fusco A, Vecchio G. Molecular mechanisms of RET activation in human cancer. *Ann N Y Acad Sci* 2002;963: 116, with permission.)

with the peroxisome proliferators-activated receptor-γ (*PPAR-γ*) were first identified in follicular thyroid carcinoma (FTC) as a cytogenetically detectable translocation t(2,3)(q13; p25).[66] The *PAX8–PPARγ* appears to be confined to atypical follicular adenomas and FTC and has not been detected in PTC or either poorly differentiated or undifferentiated (anaplastic) thyroid carcinomas. In an evaluation of 88 conventional follicular and Hürthle cell tumors analyzed for *ras* mutations and *PAX8-PPARγ* rearrangements, 49% of FTCs had *ras* mutations, 36% had *PAX8-PPARγ* rearrangements, and one had both. *Ras* mutations occurred in almost half of the follicular adenomas, and *PAX8-PPARγ* translocations were present in only 4%. Overt tumor invasiveness was associated with *PAX8-PPARγ* translocations and not *ras* mutations. *PAX8-PPARγ* rearrangements or *ras* mutations were found infrequently in Hürthle cell tumors.[67]

The *H-*, *K-*, and *N-ras* protooncogenes belong to the superfamily of membrane-associated GTP-binding proteins, which play an important role in the transduction of mitogenic signals from growth factor receptors on the cell surface. Activated *ras* phosphorylates *Raf*, which ultimately leads to activation of mitogen-activated protein kinases. Although specific patterns of *ras* mutations appear to be the rule in other tumors (*H-ras* in bladder cancer, *K-ras* in colon and pancreatic cancer, and *N-ras* in hematologic malignancies), mutations of all three *ras* genes have been reported in thyroid tumors.[68] Most often mutations of codon 61 of *H-ras* or *N-ras* are found in thyroid

TABLE 107.2

GENETIC MUTATIONS ASSOCIATED WITH THYROID CANCERS DERIVED FROM FOLLICULAR CELLS

	Well-Differentiated Thyroid Carcinoma				
Genetic Alteration	Papillary Thyroid Carcinoma	Follicular Thyroid Carcinoma	Poorly Differentiated Thyroid Carcinoma	Undifferentiated Thyroid Carcinoma	Post-Chernobyl Childhood Thyroid Cancer
RET rearrangement	13–43%	0%	0–13%	0%	50–90%
BRAF mutation	29–69%	0%	0–13%	10–35%	0–12%
BRAF rearrangement	1%	Unknown	Unknown	Unknown	11%
NTRK1 rearrangement	5–13%	Unknown	Unknown	Unknown	3%
Ras mutation	0–21%	40–53%	18–27%	20–60%	0%
PPARG rearrangement	0%	25–63%	0%	0%	Unknown
CTNNB1 mutation	0%	0%	0–25%	66%	Unknown
TP53 mutation	0–5%	0–9%	17–38%	67–88%	Unknown

CTNNB1, β-catenin; NTRK1, neurotrophic tyrosine kinase receptor type 1; PPARG, peroxisome-proliferator-activated receptor-γ. (Modified from Kondo T, Essat S, Asa SL. *Nat Rev Cancer* 2006;6:292, with permission.)

neoplasms, although the incidence of the mutations varies widely, perhaps due to the various techniques used by different investigators. Garcia-Rostand et al.[69] used PCR and single-strand conformational analysis to detect *H-*, *K-*, or *N-ras* mutations in 125 thyroid carcinomas. Mutations were present in 8.2% of 49 well-differentiated carcinomas (approximate equal frequencies in PTC and FTC), and in 50% to 55% of patients with poorly differentiated or anaplastic thyroid carcinomas (ATC). Furthermore, the mortality rate was two- to threefold higher in patients whose thyroid tumors had *ras* mutations, compared with those absent *ras* mutations.

Anaplastic thyroid carcinoma accounts for less than 2% of all thyroid cancers, but causes half of all thyroid cancer deaths. The tumor arises from follicular cells, and there is good evidence that it is a continuum of PTC or FTC. The tumors are relatively insensitive to standard chemotherapeutic regimens and are not responsive to external beam radiotherapy. The tumors are characterized by substantial chromosomal instability, characterized by *BRAF* or *ras* point mutations, which occur also in well-differentiated thyroid carcinomas and β-catenin (*CTNNB1*) and *p53* mutations, which occur in overt ATC but not in PTC or FTC. Mutations of *p53* have been described in over half of ATCs and represent a potential therapeutic target. The serine/threonine kinases of the *aurora* family play a central role in the regulation of the cell cycle, and the expression of Aurora B is 10- to 20-fold higher in ATC compared to normal thyroid tissue and well-differentiated thyroid carcinoma.[70] A summation of the genetic mutations of thyroid cancers derived from follicular cells is shown in Table 107.2.

FUTURE DIRECTIONS

Advances in molecular genetics have elucidated the oncogenic event(s) of many solid tumors, and this is nowhere more evident than in endocrine tumors. The discovery of the mutations causing MEN-1 and MEN-2 has been important because it has led to an understanding of the pathogenesis, not only of the component hereditary tumors but their sporadic counterparts as well. These discoveries have already been of great benefit in the diagnosis and treatment of patients with endocrine tumors, as evidenced most clearly in families with hereditary MTC.

Another therapeutic benefit of the molecular research has been the identification of molecular targets for small molecule therapy. Already, clinical trials are under way to evaluate agents that have shown promise in preclinical studies, and some have shown significant activity.

Selected References

The full list of references for this chapter appears in the online version.

1. Wermer P. Genetic aspects of adenomatosis of endocrine glands. *Am J Med* 1954;16:363.
2. Chandrasekharappa SC, Guru SC, Manickam P, et al. Positional cloning of the gene for multiple endocrine neoplasia-type 1. *Science* 1997;276:404.
4. Agarwal SK, Debelenko LV, Kester MB, et al/ Analysis of recurrent germline mutations in the MEN1 gene encountered in apparently unrelated families. *Hum Mutat* 1998;12:75.
5. Owens M, Ellard S, Vaidya B. Analysis of gross deletions in the MEN1 gene in patients with multiple endocrine neoplasia type 1. *Clin Endocrinol (Oxf)* 2008;68:350.
6. Schussheim DH, Skarulis MC, Agarwal SK, et al. Multiple endocrine neoplasia type 1: new clinical and basic findings. *Trends Endocrinol Metab* 2001;12:173.
7. Brown EM, Gamba G, Riccardi D, et al. Cloning and characterization of an extracellular Ca(2+)-sensing receptor from bovine parathyroid. *Nature* 1993;366:575.
8. Pollak MR, Brown EM, Chou YH, et al. Mutations in the human Ca(2+)-sensing receptor gene cause familial hypocalciuric hypercalcemia and neonatal severe hyperparathyroidism. *Cell* 1993;75:1297.
10. Jackson CE, Norum RA, Boyd SB, et al. Hereditary hyperparathyroidism and multiple ossifying jaw fibromas: a clinically and genetically distinct syndrome. *Surgery* 1990;108:1006; discussion 1012.
12. Guarnieri V, Scillitani A, Muscarella LA, et al. Diagnosis of parathyroid tumors in familial isolated hyperparathyroidism with HRPT2 mutation: implications for cancer surveillance. *J Clin Endocrinol Metab* 2006;91:2827.
13. Bradley KJ, Cavaco BM, Bowl MR, et al. Parafibromin mutations in hereditary hyperparathyroidism syndromes and parathyroid tumours. *Clin Endocrinol (Oxf)* 2006;64:299.
16. Howell VM, Haven CJ, Kahnoski K, et al. HRPT2 mutations are associated with malignancy in sporadic parathyroid tumours. *J Med Genet* 2003; 40:657.
17. Shattuck TM, Valimaki S, Obara T, et al. Somatic and germ-line mutations of the HRPT2 gene in sporadic parathyroid carcinoma. *N Engl J Med* 2003; 349:1722.
19. Warner J, Epstein M, Sweet A, et al. Genetic testing in familial isolated hyperparathyroidism: unexpected results and their implications. *J Med Genet* 2004;41:155.
20. Warner JV, Nyholt DR, Busfield F, et al. Familial isolated hyperparathyroidism is linked to a 1.7 Mb region on chromosome 2p13.3-14. *J Med Genet* 2006;43:e12.
21. Carney JA, Gordon H, Carpenter PC, Shenoy BV, Go VL. The complex of myxomas, spotty pigmentation, and endocrine overactivity. *Medicine (Baltimore)* 1985;64:270.
22. Daly AF, Jaffrain-Rea ML, Ciccarelli A, et al. Clinical characterization of familial isolated pituitary adenomas. *J Clin Endocrinol Metab* 2006;91:3316.
23. Vierimaa O, Georgitsi M, Lehtonen R, et al. Pituitary adenoma predisposition caused by germline mutations in the AIP gene. *Science* 2006;312: 1228.
24. Daly AF, Vanbellinghen JF, Khoo SK, et al. Aryl hydrocarbon receptor interacting protein gene mutations in familial isolated pituitary adenomas: analysis in 73 families. *J Clin Endocrinol Metab* 2007;92(5):1891.
25. Steiner AL, Goodman AD, Powers SR. Study of a kindred with pheochromocytoma, medullary thyroid carcinoma, hyperparathyroidism and Cushing's disease: multiple endocrine neoplasia, type 2. *Medicine (Baltimore)* 1968; 47:371.
26. Takahashi M, Ritz J, Cooper GM. Activation of a novel human transforming gene, ret, by DNA rearrangement. *Cell* 1985;42:581.
27. Tahira T, Ishizaka Y, Itoh F, Sugimura T, Nagao M. Characterization of ret proto-oncogene mRNAs encoding two isoforms of the protein product in a human neuroblastoma cell line. *Oncogene* 1990;5:97.
28. Myers SM, Eng C, Ponder BA, Mulligan LM. Characterization of RET proto-oncogene 3′ splicing variants and polyadenylation sites: a novel C-terminus for RET. *Oncogene* 1995;11:2039.
29. de Graaff E, Srinivas S, Kilkenny C, et al. Differential activities of the RET tyrosine kinase receptor isoforms during mammalian embryogenesis. *Genes Dev* 2001;15:2433.
33. Ichihara M, Murakumo Y, Takahashi M. RET and neuroendocrine tumors. *Cancer Lett* 2004;204:197.
34. Wells SA Jr, Santoro M. Targeting the RET pathway in thyroid cancer. *Clin Cancer Res* 2009;15:7119.
35. Knowles PP, Murray-Rust J, Kjaer S, et al. Structure and chemical inhibition of the RET tyrosine kinase domain. *J Biol Chem* 2006;281:33577.
36. Donis-Keller H, Dou S, Chi D, et al. Mutations in the RET proto-oncogene are associated with MEN2A and FMTC. *Hum Mol Genet* 1993;2:851.
37. Mulligan LM, Kwok JB, Healey CS, et al. Germ-line mutations of the RET proto-oncogene in multiple endocrine neoplasia type 2A. *Nature* 1993;363: 458.
38. Miyauchi A, Futami H, Hai N, et al. Two germline missense mutations at codons 804 and 806 of the RET proto-oncogene in the same allele in a patient with multiple endocrine neoplasia type 2B without codon 918 mutation. *Jpn J Cancer Res* 1999;90:1.
39. Carlson KM, Bracamontes J, Jackson CE, et al. Parent-of-origin effects in multiple endocrine neoplasia type 2B. *Am J Hum Genet* 1994;55:1076.
40. Brandi ML, Gagel RF, Angeli A, et al. Guidelines for diagnosis and therapy of MEN type 1 and type 2. *J Clin Endocrinol Metab* 2001;86:5658.
41. Eng C, Clayton D, Schuffenecker I, et al. The relationship between specific RET proto-oncogene mutations and disease phenotype in multiple endocrine neoplasia type 2. International RET mutation consortium analysis. *JAMA* 1996;276:1575.
42. Mulligan LM, Eng C, Healey CS, et al. Specific mutations of the RET proto-oncogene are related to disease phenotype in MEN 2A and FMTC. *Nat Genet* 1994;6:70.

43. Machens A, Brauckhoff M, Holzhausen HJ, et al. Codon-specific development of pheochromocytoma in multiple endocrine neoplasia type 2. *J Clin Endocrinol Metab* 2005;90:3999.
44. Kloos RT, Eng C, Evans DB, et al. Medullary thyroid cancer: management guidelines of the American Thyroid Association. *Thyroid* 2009;19:565.
45. Eng C, Mulligan LM, Smith DP, et al. Mutation of the RET protooncogene in sporadic medullary thyroid carcinoma. *Genes Chromosomes Cancer* 1995;12:209.
46. Iwashita T, Kato M, Murakami H, et al. Biological and biochemical properties of Ret with kinase domain mutations identified in multiple endocrine neoplasia type 2B and familial medullary thyroid carcinoma. *Oncogene* 1999;18:3919.
47. Mise N, Drosten M, Racek T, Tannapfel A, Putzer BM. Evaluation of potential mechanisms underlying genotype-phenotype correlations in multiple endocrine neoplasia type 2. *Oncogene* 2006;25:6637.
48. Myers SM, Mulligan LM. The RET receptor is linked to stress response pathways. *Cancer Res* 2004;64:4453.
49. Jaattela M. Heat shock proteins as cellular lifeguards. *Ann Med* 1999;31:261.
50. Jain S, Watson MA, DeBenedetti MK, et al. Expression profiles provide insights into early malignant potential and skeletal abnormalities in multiple endocrine neoplasia type 2B syndrome tumors. *Cancer Res* 2004;64:3907.
54. Elisei R, Romei C, Cosci B, et al. RET genetic screening in patients with medullary thyroid cancer and their relatives: experience with 807 individuals at one center. *J Clin Endocrinol Metab* 2007;92:4725.
55. Skinner MA, Moley JA, Dilley WG, et al. Prophylactic thyroidectomy in multiple endocrine neoplasia type 2A. *N Engl J Med* 2005;353:1105.
56. Sherman SI, Angelos P, Ball DW, et al. Thyroid carcinoma. *J Natl Compr Canc Netw* 2007;5:568.
57. Kendall-Taylor P. Guidelines for the management of thyroid cancer. *Clin Endocrinol (Oxf)* 2003;58:400.
59. Fusco A, Grieco M, Santoro M, et al. A new oncogene in human thyroid papillary carcinomas and their lymph-nodal metastases. *Nature* 1987;328:170.
60. Klugbauer S, Lengfelder E, Demidchik EP, Rabes HM. High prevalence of RET rearrangement in thyroid tumors of children from Belarus after the Chernobyl reactor accident. *Oncogene* 1995;11:2459.
61. Nikiforov YE, Rowland JM, Bove KE, Monforte-Munoz H, Fagin JA. Distinct pattern of ret oncogene rearrangements in morphological variants of radiation-induced and sporadic thyroid papillary carcinomas in children. *Cancer Res* 1997;57:1690.
63. Nikiforova MN, Stringer JR, Blough R, et al. Proximity of chromosomal loci that participate in radiation-induced rearrangements in human cells. *Science* 2000;290:138.
65. Kimura ET, Nikiforova MN, Zhu Z, et al. High prevalence of BRAF mutations in thyroid cancer: genetic evidence for constitutive activation of the RET/PTC-RAS-BRAF signaling pathway in papillary thyroid carcinoma. *Cancer Res* 2003;63:1454.

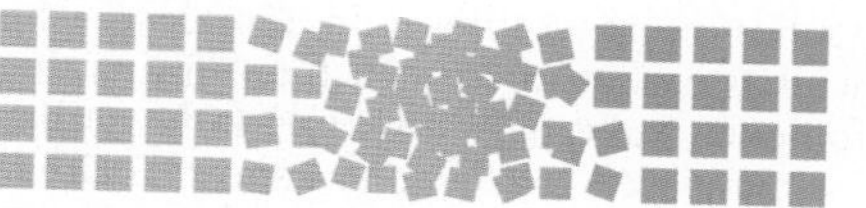

CHAPTER 108 THYROID TUMORS

TOBIAS CARLING AND ROBERT UDELSMAN

Goiter, or enlargement of the thyroid gland, has plagued humans since antiquity and was previously referred to as a *bronchocele* (tracheal outpouch).[1] The modern name of the gland was introduced in 1656 when Thomas Wharton called it the thyroid gland, after the Greek for "shield-shaped," because of the configuration of the nearby thyroid cartilage. Theodor Kocher, professor in 1871 at Berne, markedly enhanced the surgical treatment for disorders of the thyroid gland and was awarded the Nobel Prize 1909 for his work on thyroid physiology, pathology, and surgery. Charles H. Mayo had a major interest in goiter as noted in a publication from 1904: "My first incursion into the field of thyroid surgery began on December 13, 1889, when a big Norwegian came in with an enormous goiter."[2] Charles H. Mayo was not only joined in Rochester by Henry Plummer, who defined toxic multinodular goiter and was instrumental in the growth of the Mayo Clinic, but also by Edward Kendall, who succeeded in isolating bioactive crystalline material from the thyroid on Christmas Day in 1914.[2] He and his associate, A. E. Osterberg, named it *thyroxin*. At Johns Hopkins University Hospital, William S. Halsted revolutionized surgical treatment and education and made enormous contributions to the operative treatment of both the thyroid and parathyroid glands. Since then a number of important advances have been made in the diagnosis and management of patients with thyroid tumors, including the development of antithyroid drugs, fine-needle aspiration (FNA) biopsy, radioiodine treatment, and various imaging modalities. The anatomy of the thyroid gland and its arterial blood supply is depicted in Figure 108.1.

THYROID TUMOR CLASSIFICATION AND STAGING SYSTEMS

The normal thyroid is composed histologically of two main parenchymal cell types. Follicular cells line the colloid follicles, concentrate iodine, and produce thyroid hormones. These cells give rise to both well-differentiated cancers and anaplastic thyroid cancer. The second cell type, the C or parafollicular cell, produces the hormone calcitonin and is the cell of origin for medullary thyroid carcinoma. Immune cells and stromal cells of the thyroid are responsible for lymphoma and sarcoma, respectively. Of the 37,200 new cases of thyroid cancer each year in the United States,[3] approximately 90% are well-differentiated cancers, 5% to 9% are medullary, 1% to 2% are anaplastic, 1% to 3% are lymphoma, and fewer than 1% are sarcomas or other rare tumors.

Within the category of well-differentiated thyroid cancers various histologic subtypes have evolved due to an improved understanding of their biology. Initial categories included papillary, follicular, and mixed tumor with variable areas of both papillary and follicular histology. Recent studies have established that these mixed tumors with areas of papillary features have a similar natural history and prognosis as papillary thyroid cancer without follicular features.[4] Accordingly, mixed papillary and follicular carcinoma are now grouped with papillary carcinoma. Also, the follicular variant of papillary carcinoma has cytologic characteristics of a papillary carcinoma, but appears histologically to have a follicular architecture and behaves biologically as well-differentiated papillary carcinoma. The major cytologic feature shared by all members of this papillary group, regardless of the histologic pattern, is the characteristic nucleus containing Orphan-Annie nuclei, nuclear grooves, and intranuclear pseudoinclusions. Follicular carcinomas lack these cytologic characteristics but do demonstrate capsular or vascular invasion on histopathological examination. A third category of lesions grouped with differentiated thyroid carcinoma is Hürthle cell or oncocytic carcinoma. The distribution of well-differentiated thyroid cancer subgroups in some reports reveals that 80% to 85% are papillary, 10% to 15% are follicular, and 3% to 5% are Hürthle cell carcinomas.[4] This distribution may not reflect adequate pathologic recognition of the recently appreciated follicular variant of papillary carcinoma. True follicular carcinoma now appears to represent 5% or fewer cases of well-differentiated thyroid cancers in countries with iodine-sufficient diets.

Thyroid carcinoma can be categorized by increasing clinical aggressiveness. The least aggressive are well-differentiated (papillary carcinoma, follicular carcinoma), followed by intermediate forms (medullary thyroid carcinoma, Hürthle cell carcinoma, some rare variants of papillary carcinoma, including the tall cell variant, columnar cell variant, diffuse sclerosing variant, and insular carcinoma or poorly differentiated),[5] and the frequently incurable undifferentiated (anaplastic carcinoma). Since medullary thyroid carcinoma has unique inheritance, growth, and treatment options, it is reviewed in an independent section of this chapter (see "Medullary Thyroid Carcinoma").

At least eight systems have been proposed and to a lesser or greater extent validated for staging thyroid cancer (Table 108.1). None has been universally adopted, and the lack of a common staging system has impeded the development of multicenter trials and cross-institutional comparisons of outcomes. In the absence of a universally accepted system, it is recommended that the TNM (tumor-node-metastasis) staging system, introduced by the International Union Against Cancer (UICC) and promoted by the American Joint Committee on Cancer (AJCC), the American Cancer Society (ACS), the National Cooperative Cancer Network (NCCN), and the American College of Surgeons (ACS), be adopted as the international staging system. The TNM (or AJCC) classification system (seventh edition) is outlined in Table 108.2.[6]

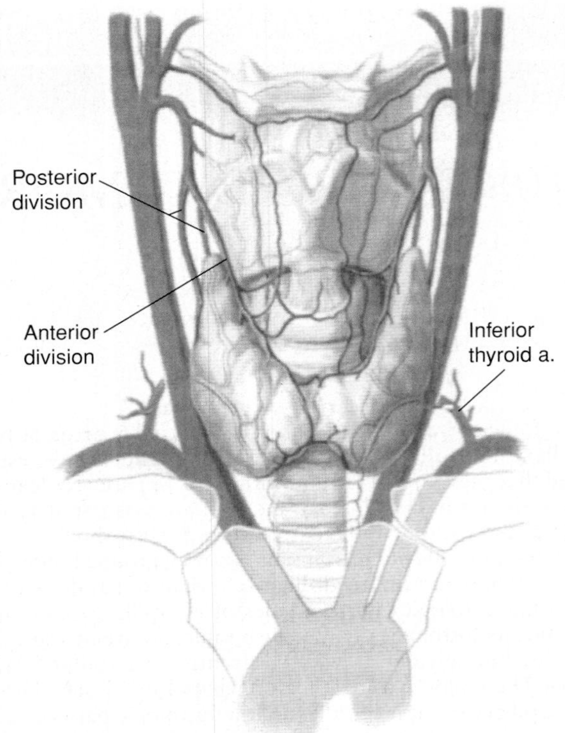

FIGURE 108.1 The thyroid gland and its arterial supply. (Drs. L. J. Rizzolo and W. B. Stewart, Section of Anatomy. Department of Surgery, Yale University School of Medicine, New Haven, CT are acknowledged for providing the figure. With permission from Springer, Berlin-Heidelberg-New York.)

EPIDEMIOLOGY AND DEMOGRAPHICS

Thyroid cancer is one of the fastest growing cancers in the United States, with a 240% increased incidence over the past three decades.[7] Although the majority of newly diagnosed thyroid cancers are small papillary thyroid carcinomas, all sizes and stages of papillary thyroid carcinomas in both genders and in all ethnic groups exhibit an increased incidence.[8] It is the most common endocrine malignancy, accounting for 94.6% of the total new endocrine cancers, and 66.0% of the deaths due to endocrine cancers. Based on cancer statistics, 37,200 new cases of thyroid cancer will be diagnosed in 2010 with a total of 1,630 deaths due to the disease.[3] The discrepancy between the total number of cases of all endocrine cancers arising in the thyroid (94.6%) and the total proportion of endocrine cancer deaths (66.0%) reflects the relatively indolent nature and long-term survival associated with thyroid malignancies.

Both papillary and follicular thyroid carcinomas are approximately 2.5 times more common in females.[9] The median age at diagnosis is earlier in women than in men for both papillary and follicular subtypes and tends to be earlier for papillary cancer as compared to follicular cancer in either gender. Specifically, the median age at diagnosis in white women is between 40 and 41 years, whereas for white men, it is 44 to 45 years for papillary carcinoma. For follicular thyroid carcinoma, the median age at diagnosis is 48 for white women as compared to 53 for white men. Well-differentiated thyroid cancer has a greater incidence in whites than in blacks of both genders. The relative proportion of age-adjusted incidence rates is slightly more than twofold higher for whites. One significant difference in the incidence in terms of race is that the proportion of well-differentiated thyroid carcinomas that are follicular is increased greatly in blacks as compared to whites.

ETIOLOGY AND RISK FACTORS

Radiation exposure to the thyroid gland in childhood, age, female sex, and family history are risk factors known to increase the incidence of well-differentiated thyroid cancer. Exposure of radiation to the thyroid may occur either from external sources or from ingestion of radioactive material.

Several studies have shown an inverse relationship between increased risk of thyroid cancer and age of exposure to radiation. Relative risk is also linearly related to exposure dose, starting as low as 0.1 Gy, and at least up to 30 Gy.[10] The latency period after childhood exposure is at least 3 to 5 years, and there is no apparent drop off in the increased risk even 40 years after the radiation exposure.[10] The majority of cases occur between 20 and 40 years after exposure. However, even after 40 years, the relative risk as compared to a nonirradiated population is still increased. For these reasons, the large cohort of patients who underwent childhood irradiation for benign medical conditions such as thymic enlargement and acne between 1920 and 1960 are now between the ages of 50 and 90 years of age have an increased risk of developing thyroid carcinoma.

Although the use of radiation for benign conditions has not been practiced since the 1960s, there is increased use of radiation treatments for neoplastic conditions, in infants, children, and young adults. The majority of this population have either Hodgkin's or non-Hodgkin's lymphoma but also includes long-term survivors of Wilms' tumor or neuroblastoma in

TABLE 108.1

COMPARISON OF SEVEN DIFFERENT PROGNOSTIC CLASSIFICATION SYSTEMS IN WELL-DIFFERENTIATED THYROID CARCINOMA

System	Criteria	Ref.
AGES	Age, grade of tumor, extent, size	29
AMES	Age, metastases, extent, size	26
MACIS	Metastases, age, completeness of resection, invasion, size	65
Ohio State	Size, cervical metastases, multiplicity, invasion, distant metastases	25
Sloan-Kettering	Age, histology, size, extension, metastases	66
NTCTS	Size, multifocality, invasion, differentiation, cervical metastases, extracervical metastases	30
TNM	Size, extension, nodal metastases, distant metastases	Table 108.2

NTCTS, National Thyroid Cancer Treatment Cooperative Society; TNM, tumor-node-metastasis.

TABLE 108.2

AMERICAN JOINT COMMITTEE ON CANCER (AJCC) CLASSIFICATION OF THYROID CANCER, SEVENTH EDITION (2010)

Primary Tumor (T)[a]

TX	Primary tumor cannot be assessed	
T0	No evidence of primary tumor	
T1	Tumor ≤2 cm confined to the thyroid	
	T1a	Tumor ≤1 cm confined to the thyroid
	T1b	Tumor 1–2 cm confined to the thyroid
T2	Tumor >2 cm and <4 cm confined to the thyroid	
T3	Tumor >4 cm confined to the thyroid *or* tumor of any size with minimal extrathyroid extension	
T4a	Moderately advanced disease. Tumor of any size extending beyond the thyroid capsule to invade subcutaneous soft tissues, larynx, trachea, esophagus, or recurrent laryngeal nerve *or* Intrathyroidal anaplastic carcinoma[b]	
T4b	Very advanced disease. Tumor invades prevertebral fascia or encases carotid artery or mediastinal vessels *or* Extrathyroidal anaplastic carcinoma[b]	

Regional Lymph Nodes (N) (Central Compartment, Lateral Cervical and Upper Mediastinal)

NX	Regional lymph nodes cannot be assessed	
N0	No regional lymph node metastasis	
N1	Regional lymph node metastasis	
	N1a	Metastasis to level VI (pretracheal, paratracheal, and prelaryngeal/Delphian lymph nodes)
	N1b	Metastasis to unilateral, bilateral, or contralateral cervical (levels I, II, III, IV or V) *or* retropharyngeal or superior mediastinal lymph nodes (level VII)

Distant Metastasis (M)

MX	Distant metastasis cannot be assessed
M0	No distant metastasis
M1	Distant metastasis

Stage Groupings

PAPILLARY AND FOLLICULAR

Under 45 years of age			
Stage I	Any T	Any N	M0
Stage II	Any T	Any N	M1
45 years of age and over			
Stage I	T1	N0	M0
Stage II	T2	N0	M0
Stage III	T3	N0	M0
	T1	N1a	M0
	T2	N1a	M0
	T3	N1a	M0
Stage IVA	T4a	N0	M0
	T4a	N1a	M0
	T1	N1b	M0
	T2	N1b	M0
	T3	N1b	M0
	T4a	N1b	M0
	T4a	N1b	M0
Stage IVB	T4b	Any N	M0
Stage IVC	Any T	Any N	M1

Medullary carcinoma			
Stage I	T1	N0	M0
Stage II	T2	N0	M0
	T3	N0	M0
Stage III	T1	N1a	M0
	T2	N1a	M0
	T3	N1a	M0
Stage IVA	T4a	N0	M0
	T4a	N1a	M0
	T1	N1b	M0
	T2	N1b	M0
	T3	N1b	M0
	T4a	N1b	M0
Stage IVB	T4b	Any N	M0
Stage IVC	Any T	Any N	M1
Anaplastic carcinoma			
Stage IVA	T4a	Any N	M0
Stage IVB	T4b	Any N	M0
Stage IVC	Any T	Any N	M1

[a]All categories may be subdivided; (a) solitary tumor, (b) multifocal tumor (the largest determines the classification).
[b]All anaplastic carcinomas are considered T4 tumors.
(Adapted from ref. 6.)

which there is some scatter to the thyroid gland.[11,12] The young age at treatment for neuroblastoma and Wilms' tumor (mean age, 2 and 3 years, respectively) and the relatively high dose of thyroid exposure has led to a dramatic increase in relative risk to 350 for neuroblastoma patients and 132 for survivors of Wilms' tumors for the development of thyroid cancer.[12] Relative risks between 16 and 80 have been reported in this patient population of adolescents and young adults treated for lymphoma.[11] In the adult patient population treated with therapeutic radiation for malignancies, there is a drop off in risk, reflecting the importance of age at exposure.

Radiation exposure to the thyroid gland may also be due to ^{131}I administered for diagnostic thyroid scans. However, in a nationwide, population-based cohort study in Sweden including all 36,792 individuals who received ^{131}I for diagnostic purposes between 1952 and 1969, there was no evidence that the

TABLE 108.3

CLINICAL AND GENETIC CHARACTERISTICS OF FAMILIAL THYROID FOLLICULAR CELL CARCINOMA SUSCEPTIBILITY SYNDROMES

Syndrome	Chromosome Linkage/Gene	Characteristics
Papillary thyroid carcinoma with papillary renal neoplasia (PTC-PRN)	1q21/?	Associated with papillary renal neoplasia Autosomal dominant with partial penetrance
Familial nonmedullary thyroid carcinoma (fNMTC)	2q21/? and 19p13/?	Two genetic loci identified Autosomal dominant with partial penetrance
Familial thyroid tumors with cell oxyphilia (TCO)	19p13.2/?	Characteristic oxyphilic cells Autosomal dominant with partial penetrance
Familial adenomatous polyposis (FAP)	5q21–22/*APC*	Papillary thyroid carcinoma with ~10x increased prevalence Colorectal carcinoma, ampullary carcinoma, hepatoblastoma, medulloblastoma Autosomal dominant
Cowden disease (multiple hamartoma syndrome)	10q23.3/*PTEN*	Follicular and papillary thyroid carcinoma Multiple hamartomas, breast and endometrial cancer Autosomal dominant
Carney complex 1	17q/*PRKAR1A*	Follicular and papillary thyroid carcinoma Skin pigmentation, and cardiac, endocrine, cutaneous, and neural myxomatous tumors Autosomal dominant

diagnostic scans increased the risk of thyroid cancer.[13] Additionally, therapeutic ^{131}I administered for ablation of thyroid tissue to treat hyperthyroidism seems to be associated with, at most, a very modest increased risk of thyroid cancer.[14]

A more harmful type of ingestion of radioisotopes of iodine comes from exposure to nuclear fallout. Data on the effect on thyroid cancer incidence come from populations exposed from the nuclear power station accident at Chernobyl and the results of atomic bomb development and testing at Hanford (Washington), the Nevada test site, and the Marshall Islands.[14] Within the first decade after the Chernobyl accident some regions of Belarus showed a 100-fold increase in thyroid cancer in individuals below the age of 15 at the time of exposure.[14] Essentially all of these radiation-induced tumors were shown to be papillary thyroid cancer, associated with more aggressive growth, a higher likelihood of local invasion, and spread to regional lymph nodes, as well as a higher incidence of ret/PTC translocation (see Chapter 107). These data reflect the importance of age at exposure in the development of radiation-associated thyroid cancer.[15]

Factors other than radiation exposure, including dietary influence, sex hormones, environmental exposures, or genetic susceptibility, have been studied, with mixed results and no clear associations. Dietary influences have primarily focused on the level of iodine in the diet. Iodine-deficient diets or diets that include a large intake of vegetables from the crucifer family (which block iodine uptake) may lead to increased thyroid-stimulating hormone (TSH) levels and are considered goitrogenic. Increased iodine intake due to shellfish occurs in the geographic areas with the highest incidence of predominantly papillary thyroid cancer, such as Iceland, Norway, and Hawaii. However, more recent data suggest that relatively elevated levels of fish consumption do not appreciably increase thyroid cancer risk.[16]

Epidemiologic studies have demonstrated a four- to tenfold increased risk of well-differentiated thyroid cancer in first-degree relatives of subjects with this neoplasia.[17] In contrast to the well-described molecular pathology associated with medullary thyroid carcinoma, the molecular and clinical genetics of follicular cell-derived thyroid cancer have only recently been unveiled. Well-differentiated thyroid cancer can both be inherited in an autosomal dominant fashion as the main feature in some syndromes as well as have an increased incidence in other tumor susceptibility syndromes.[18] The clinical and genetic characteristics of familial thyroid follicular cell carcinoma susceptibility syndromes are outlined in Table 108.3.[18] For details related to the molecular biology of these disorders, see Chapter 107.

EVALUATION OF THE THYROID NODULE

The vast majority of thyroid cancers present as thyroid nodules detected either by the patient, clinician by physical examination, or with imaging techniques of the neck for other disorders. As only a minority of thyroid nodules are malignant, a general review of the incidence, evaluation, and management of thyroid nodules precedes a detailed description of specific thyroid neoplasias (Fig. 108.2).

In iodine-replete areas, thyroid nodules are clinically detectable by physical examination in at least 4% to 7% of the general population. However, the prevalence of thyroid nodules depends on the population under study; gender, age, and history of exposure to ionizing radiation strongly influence the results of various large studies, as does the method by which nodules are detected, physical examination, intraoperative palpation, imaging techniques, histopathologically, or at autopsy. Thus, nodules are approximately ten times more frequent when examined at autopsy, during surgery, or by ultrasonography as compared to physical examination. There is an age-dependent increase in thyroid nodules and in one histopathologic study, up to 90% of women older than 70 years and 60% of men older than 80 years had nodular goiter. All studies show that women develop nodules more frequently than men, although reports of the female to male ratio vary from 1.2:1 to 4.3:1.[15] An increased tendency to develop thyroid nodules is demonstrated in groups exposed to ionizing radiation, especially during childhood (see "Etiology and Risk Factors," earlier in this chapter).

By obtaining information from the history and physical examination, the risk of malignancy in that individual can to a certain extent be assessed. In general, there is an approximately 5% to 10% chance of malignancy in all thyroid nodules for the

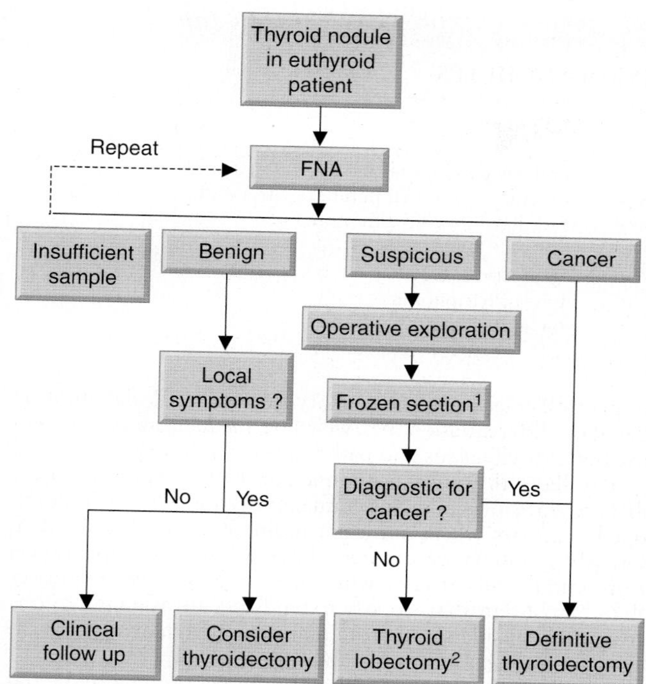

FIGURE 108.2 Flow diagram for the evaluation of thyroid nodule based on the results of fine-needle aspiration biopsy. See text for special considerations in follicular, Hürthle cell, and medullary thyroid carcinoma. **1:** Consider touch preparation, **2:** Consider total thyroidectomy for large, nodular, or bilateral lesion, as well as in patients with a history of radiation exposure in childhood.

total population, but men and patients at the extremes of age are at higher risk for malignancy.[15] Nodules found in a patient with a history of childhood neck irradiation carry a 33% to 37% chance of malignancy.[10] The presence of a solitary nodule is of greater concern than a thyroid with multiple nodules, but a dominant nodule or a nodule that grows in the setting of a multinodular goiter should be investigated to exclude carcinoma. Patients with Graves' disease who develop a nodule may have a higher risk of cancer.[9] However, the occurrence of carcinoma in autonomously functioning nodules is extremely rare.[9]

A history of rapid increase in size, dyspnea, dysphagia, hoarseness, or the development of Horner syndrome, albeit not specific for malignancy, are worrisome findings. Tender nodules are more often associated with thyroiditis and are likely to be benign. A family history of thyroid cancer or history, signs, and symptoms consistent with any of the tumor susceptibility syndromes outlined in Tables 108.3 and 108.4 should prompt an extended investigation. For details see "Etiology and Risk Factors" and "Medullary Thyroid Carcinoma" in this section, and Chapter 107. On examination of the neck, attention to the firmness, mobility, and size of the nodules, their adherence to surrounding structures, and the presence of lymphadenopathy are important clues to the presence of carcinoma. However, these features lack specificity for malignancy. Routine indirect or direct laryngoscopy is important not only in the preoperative evaluation but also in the assessment of a thyroid nodule. Vocal cord paralysis is generally associated with advanced thyroid malignancy.

Thyroid function testing should be performed to identify underlying thyroid pathology and not to differentiate benign from malignant nodules.[15] Subclinical hyperthyroidism, with a suppressed TSH may be secondary to an autonomously functioning nodule. In this case, one can determine whether the nodule is functional with a radionuclide uptake scan. The majority of both benign and malignant thyroid nodules are hypofunctional when compared to normal thyroid tissue; thus, the finding of a "cold nodule" on ^{123}I or ^{99}Tc scan is nonspecific. Routine thyroid scans in the initial evaluation of the thyroid nodule is not advocated since it is less cost effective, specific, and sensitive compared to FNA biopsy. Routine measurement of serum calcitonin has been advocated by some authors to identify patients with medullary carcinoma of the thyroid preoperatively, which seems cost effective.[19] Certainly, serum calcitonin levels should be determined in all patients with a thyroid nodule when either sporadic or familial medullary thyroid carcinoma is suspected.[20]

High-resolution ultrasonography is a useful adjunct to the clinical examination for size assessment of nodules, for the detection of multiple nodules not discerned by palpation, and for assisting in FNA. Several studies have aimed at identifying sonographic criteria in distinguishing between benign from malignant thyroid nodules. Presence of microcalcification, irregular margins, spotty intranodular flow, as well as hypervascularity are suggestive but not diagnostic of malignancy. Ultrasonography can identify whether a lesion is cystic or solid, and the vast majority of purely cystic lesions are benign.

FNA has revolutionized the management of thyroid nodules, providing an extremely sensitive and cost-effective method of detecting thyroid malignancies. The impact this procedure has had on clinical practice is reflected by a reduction of the total number of thyroid surgeries performed, a greater proportion of malignancies removed at surgery, and an overall reduction in the cost of managing patients with thyroid nodules. The accuracy of cytologic diagnosis from FNA ranges from 70% to 97% and is highly dependent on both the skill of the individual performing the biopsy and the cytopathologist interpreting it.[15] If an adequate sample is obtained, the results of FNA are most commonly divided into the categories outlined in Table 108.5. Approximately 70% are classified as benign (range, 53% to 90%), 4.0% as malignant (range, 1% to 10%), 10% as suspicious or indeterminate (range, 5% to 23%), and 17% demonstrate an insufficient sample (range, 15% to 20%).[15] The insufficient sample rate can be improved by performing on-site cytologic assessment of the adequacy of the sample.

TABLE 108.4

CLINICAL AND GENETIC CHARACTERISTICS OF FAMILIAL MEDULLARY THYROID CANCER SYNDROMES

Syndrome	Characteristic Features
FMTC	MTC
MEN-2A	MTC Adrenal medulla (pheochromocytoma) Parathyroid hyperplasia
MEN-2A with cutaneous lichen amyloidosis	MEN-2A and a pruritic cutaneous lesion located over the upper back
MEN-2A or FMTC with Hirschsprung disease	MEN-2A or FMTC with Hirschsprung disease
MEN-2B	MTC Adrenal medulla (pheochromocytoma) Intestinal and mucosal ganglioneuromatosis Characteristic Marfanoid habitus

FMTC, familial medullary thyroid cancer; MEN, multiple endocrine neoplasia; MTC, medullary thyroid carcinoma.

TABLE 108.5

FINE-NEEDLE ASPIRATION DIAGNOSES IN THYROID NODULES

Benign	Suspicious	Malignant
Acute suppurative thyroiditis Subacute thyroiditis Hashimoto (lymphocytic) thyroiditis Nodular goiter Adenomatoid nodule Colloid nodule	Follicular neoplasm Hürthle cell neoplasm Suspicious for papillary carcinoma	Papillary carcinoma Follicular-variant of papillary carcinoma Medullary thyroid carcinoma Anaplastic carcinoma Thyroid lymphoma Metastatic carcinoma

The malignant potential of follicular neoplasms can rarely be determined by cytologic evaluation; thus, the biopsies from such lesions are generally classified as suspicious or indeterminate, and most come to surgical resection. The cells from follicular adenomas and follicular carcinomas appear cytologically identical; only by identifying capsular or vascular invasion on histologic specimens can cancer be diagnosed. Specimens with predominantly Hürthle cells are treated in the same fashion; however, extensive Hürthle cell changes can be seen in Hashimoto thyroiditis. Malignancy is found in approximately 20% of follicular and Hürthle cell nodules that are classified as indeterminate on FNA.

A variety of molecular markers have been assessed in FNA specimens in an attempt to develop more discriminating cytologic subclassifications to improve the yield of malignancy found at surgery. *BRAF* mutational analysis and to a lesser extent analysis of ET/PTC rearrangement and RAS mutations have recently been extensively evaluated in cytological specimens.[21,22] At select institutions, analysis of such biomarkers in FNA samples has become clinical routine in order to improve the accuracy of the preoperative diagnosis.[15]

Biopsies classified as benign or negative are safely followed nonoperatively, with the caveat that false-negative results occur in 1% to 6% of cases. Clinical judgment should dictate the course of action in these cases; if a large, hard nodule is fixed to surrounding tissue, surgery should be performed despite a negative aspirate. Sampling error can occur during biopsy of large, cystic hemorrhagic nodules or due to sampling error. False-positive results for malignancy should not exceed 1% to 2% of all biopsies. The cytologic features of Hashimoto thyroiditis occasionally lead to these false-positive interpretations, but can be greatly reduced with experienced cytopathologists.

Benign thyroid nodules must be followed carefully by routine physical examination or, more precisely, by ultrasonography and do not generally require repeat biopsy.[15] Thyroxine suppression therapy has been widely used in the past, although its efficacy is controversial. Multiple randomized controlled trials and meta-analyses show some decrement in nodule size in relatively iodine-replete populations, but seem to be of no or little value in the iodine-sufficient population. These findings in conjunction with the morbidities of exogenous thyroid hormone administration, including osteoporosis and cardiac side effects, suggest that routine suppression therapy for benign thyroid nodules is not warranted.[15]

WELL-DIFFERENTIATED THYROID CARCINOMA

Pathology

Thyroid malignancies are derived from either follicular cells (papillary, follicular, Hürthle cell, and anaplastic carcinomas) or parafollicular C cells (medullary carcinoma). A classification based on differentiation (i.e., well, intermediate, and poor) is of use both for clinicians and pathologists (Table 108.6).

Papillary thyroid carcinoma constitutes approximately 80% to 85% of malignant epithelial thyroid tumors in developed countries where sufficient iodine is present in the diet. Grossly papillary carcinomas have a variable appearance, from minute subcapsular white scars to large tumors greater than 5 to 6 cm that grossly extend and invade contiguous structures outside the thyroid gland. Cystic change, calcification, and even ossification may be identified.

Microscopically, papillary carcinomas are characterized by the presence of papillae, but some variants contain no papillary areas, are totally follicular in pattern, and are identified as a follicular variant. Biologically, all these tumors, independent of their degree of follicular pattern, show similar clinical characteristics. The nuclei of papillary carcinoma are enlarged and ovoid and contain thick nuclear membranes, small nucleoli often pressed against the nuclear membrane, intranuclear grooves, and intranuclear cytoplasmic inclusions. Because the nuclei are enlarged, they frequently overlap one another, which is a helpful clue in both the cytologic preparations and histologic slides. Papillary carcinoma has a propensity to invade lymphatic spaces and, therefore, leads to microscopic multimodal lesions in the gland as well as a high incidence of regional lymph node metastases. The latter may be the presenting symptom of a thyroid papillary carcinoma as, in some cases, a primary tumor is very small. Papillary thyroid carcinomas less than 1 cm are often referred to as microcarcinomas.

TABLE 108.6

CLASSIFICATION OF THYROID FOLLICULAR AND PARAFOLLICULAR CELL CARCINOMA, BASED ON DIFFERENTIATION (FROM WELL TO POOR DIFFERENTIATION)

Well Differentiated (Low-Grade Malignancy)
Usual papillary thyroid carcinoma (PTC)
Microcarcinoma (lesions <1 cm)
Cystic
Follicular variant of PTC (FVPTC)
Usual follicular thyroid carcinoma (FTC)
Hürthle cell (oxyphilic; oncocytic) carcinomas (HCC)
Intermediate Differentiation
Medullary thyroid carcinoma (MTC)
Diffuse sclerosing variant of papillary carcinoma (DSV)
Columnar cell variant of papillary carcinoma (CCV)
Insular carcinoma (IC)
Tall cell variant of papillary carcinoma (TCV)
Poorly Differentiated (High-Grade Malignancy)
Anaplastic (undifferentiated) carcinoma

True follicular thyroid carcinoma is an unusual tumor comprising approximately 5% to 10% of thyroid malignancies in nonendemic goiter areas of the world.[23] Prior to the introduction of iodinated salt, follicular carcinoma was much more frequently diagnosed. In addition, the pathologic dictum—that any tumor with a pattern that is 50% or more characteristic of follicular carcinoma should be diagnostically placed in a follicular carcinoma category—has been shown to be incorrect. Indeed, most of the follicular pattern of thyroid malignancies represent the follicular variant of papillary carcinoma and share the biological features, natural history, and prognosis of papillary thyroid carcinoma.[24] Follicular thyroid carcinoma is unifocal and thickly encapsulated and shows invasion of the capsule or vessels. Because of the diagnostic confusion, statistical data about the survival rate or the metastatic potential of true follicular carcinoma are not easily obtained. Most studies show that if capsular, but not vascular, invasion is present, the prognosis is excellent, with 85% to 100% of patients surviving at least 10 years of follow-up.[24]

Natural History and Prognosis

The natural history and prognosis of well-differentiated thyroid cancer has been intensively studied since the 1980s. A clear definition of risk factors associated with poor outcome has allowed more selective and less aggressive treatment recommendations. In general, well-differentiated thyroid cancer is one of the least morbid solid carcinomas, with favorable long-term survival. However, a small proportion of patients with papillary cancer and a slightly larger proportion of patients with follicular thyroid cancer die from disease-related causes. As opposed to other solid neoplasms, one major difference is that regional lymph node metastases appear not to have a strong correlation with overall survival in most series, but do consistently correlate to local recurrence.[25]

At presentation, approximately two-thirds of patients have gross disease localized to the thyroid. The median size of tumors is between 2.0 and 2.5 cm in most large series.[25,26] Patients with papillary carcinomas smaller than 1.0 cm are considered to have minimal or occult papillary thyroid cancer (papillary microcarcinoma). In North American studies, the incidence of occult papillary tumors ranges between 0.5% and 14.0%, with a greater proportional incidence in older age groups. It has been shown that a majority of such occult microcarcinomas are unlikely to ever lead to clinically significant disease.[27] For this reason, standard practice is not to investigate or submit to biopsy nodules that are small (less than 10 mm), except in the setting of familial thyroid carcinoma, history of neck irradiation, or otherwise concerning sonographic features.[15]

Regional lymph node metastases are present at the time of primary diagnosis in 20% to 90% of patients with papillary thyroid cancer (PTC) and to a lesser extent in other histiotypes.[5] The wide range depends not only on the actual pathological stage of the tumor, but also on which diagnostic modalities are employed to assess the potential metastases. Factors associated with lymph node metastasis in PTC patients include tumor size, extracapsular invasion, and multifocality. Micrometastases (defined as the presence of metastatic deposits within a lymph node of less than 2 mm in diameter) are common. There is a lack of distinction, however, between macro- and micrometastatic disease in both the scientific literature as well as in tumor staging, complicating the estimation of the true incidence of micro- versus macrometastatic spread. Comprehensive preoperative cervical ultrasonography is the standard of care in evaluating both central and lateral lymph nodes for metastases. It identifies cervical adenopathy in 20% to 31% of the cases.[28]

Only a small minority of patients have distant metastatic hematogenous disease at the time of diagnosis. In a large series, 1% to 2% of papillary thyroid cancer patients and 2% to 5% of follicular thyroid cancer patients had metastases outside the neck or mediastinum at the time of diagnosis.[25] Having distant metastases at the time of presentation is a strong predictor of very poor outcome as 43% to 90% of these patients die secondary to their thyroid malignancy.[25]

In the overall population with papillary thyroid cancer, there is a 90% to 95% long-term survival and a 70% to 80% long-term survival for patients with follicular cancers. The 20% of patients in this group who develop recurrent disease include a majority with local cervical recurrences either in lymph nodes or the thyroid bed, and a minority of patients have distant metastases to the lung, bone, and liver.[4,25]

Several databases define prognostic risk factors for well-differentiated thyroid cancer.[25,26,29] The two dominant factors in both series are the age at diagnosis and the presence of distant metastases. All systems also include some measurement of the size of the lesion and other factors, such as local invasion or grade of the tumor, which have an impact on outcome. In general, younger patients do well with well-differentiated thyroid cancer. Cady and Rossi[26] defined low-risk age categories as men younger than 40 and women younger than 50 years.

Patients who have distant metastatic disease either at presentation or at the time of recurrence do much worse.[25] Similarly, patients with local invasion or high-grade lesions have a poorer prognosis. The risk categorization schema called AMES incorporated these components (*a*ge, *m*etastatic disease, *e*xtrathyroidal extension, *s*ize).[26] Using this system, low-risk patients can be identified who have a long-term overall survival of 98% and overall disease-free survival of 95% as compared to 54% and 45%, respectively, for high-risk patients. The initial system developed by the Mayo Clinic group carried the acronym AGES (*a*ge, tumor grade, tumor *e*xtent, tumor *s*ize). A mathematical formula based on weighted risk factors was developed to yield a prognostic score. The scoring system showed that patients with a prognostic score of less than 4 had a 99% 20-year survival, whereas patients with a prognostic score greater than 6 had a 13% 20-year survival, with graded categories in between.[29] Clearly, if subgroups of patients with 99% 20-year survivals can be prospectively identified, aggressive therapy with potential lifelong complications are difficult to justify in this subpopulation.

The importance of age, extrathyroidal extension, and distant metastases plays important roles in the AJCC staging of thyroid cancer. There is no large database that has verified this adaptation of the other staging system into the AJCC/UICC TNM classification. However, a very similar staging system was developed by the National Thyroid Cancer Treatment Cooperative Study registry, which initiated collection of data in 1987. A report of more than 1,500 patients analyzed by this staging system showed that 5-year disease-specific survivals for papillary thyroid cancer in stage I and II were 100%, 93.8% for stage III, and 78.5% for stage IV.[30] The disease-free survival similarly showed a high correlation with stages I through IV papillary carcinoma, with survivals of 94.4%, 92.5%, 82.7%, and 30.0%, respectively. Additionally, one recent study compared the fifth versus the sixth edition of the AJCC/UICC TNM classification, and concluded that the sixth edition more accurately predicts outcomes in patients with extrathyroidal extension.[31] In 2010 the revised seventh edition of the AJCC/UICC TNM classification for thyroid cancer was published (Table 108.2).[6]

Apart from clinical indicators of prognosis, several molecular genetic alterations have been studied as putative predictive markers in thyroid cancer. Genes, encoding effectors in the mitogen-activated protein kinase (MAPK) pathway, have been of particular interest. Mutations in one such gene, *BRAF*, has been shown in some, but not all, studies to be associated with increased likelihood of extrathyroidal extension, lymph node metastasis, and recurrence.[22] For further discussion on the clinical and molecular genetics of endocrine tumorigenesis, see Chapter 107.

Intermediately Differentiated Thyroid Tumors

Within the category of papillary and follicular thyroid cancer various histological subtypes have evolved due to an improved understanding of their biology. In contrast to the overall indolent behavior of the classical well-differentiated thyroid carcinomas, subtypes of these tumors have been identified as being more aggressive and thus have been labeled thyroid cancers with intermediate differentiation. These tumors comprise approximately 10% to 15% of all thyroid cancers.[5] These include Hürthle cell (oncocytic, oxyphilic) carcinomas (HCC) as well as variants of papillary thyroid cancer such as the tall cell variant (TCV), columnar cell variant (CCV), diffuse sclerosing variant (DSV), and insular carcinoma (IC; Table 108.6).

The Hürthle cell neoplasm is considered a variant of follicular neoplasms. Historically, all such lesions, despite the histologic features, were considered to be malignant; hence, it was recommended that they all be treated aggressively. However, many studies have evaluated the clinical pathologic features of thyroid Hürthle cell tumors and have shown that, on average, only 20% to 33% show histologic evidence of malignancy or invasive growth and may metastasize.[24] However, the size of the lesion is related to the risk of malignancy, and 65% of tumors over 4 cm are found to be malignant.[24] Hürthle cell tumors that do not demonstrate invasion microscopically behave as adenomas and may be treated conservatively.

The variants of papillary thyroid cancer, such as TCV, CCV, DSV, and IC all exhibit unique histopathological features. However, these variants do share some commonalities, such as a high rate of extrathyroidal extension and nodal metastasis at diagnosis, as well as locoregional recurrence and development of synchronous and metachronous metastasis.[5] The TCV is characterized by tumor cells being twice as tall as they are wide that need to be present in greater than 50% of the lesion to make the diagnosis. In contrast to usual PTC, the TCV often demonstrates strong immunoreactivity for antibodies against Leu M1 antigen. In a recent review of all reported cases until 2004, extrathyroidal extension of tumor at diagnosis was found in 67% and cervical adenopathy in 57%.[32] During a mean follow-up period of 61 months, average rates of locoregional recurrence, distant metastasis, and tumor related mortality were 25%, 22%, and 16%, respectively. The CCV is a rare tumor, accounting for only 0.15% to 0.2% of all PTCs.[33] The cell height in CCV is usually at least twice the width, greater than that seen in the TCV, and the presence of prominent nuclear stratification is the most distinctive histological feature. Overall, CCV is associated with a poor prognosis. During a mean follow-up period of 43 months, average rates of locoregional recurrence, distant metastasis, and tumor related mortality were 33%, 36%, and 29%, respectively.[5] However, CCV on its own is not an independently poor prognostic factor. When the tumor is encapsulated or minimally infiltrative, all patients described in the literature remained free of disease at a mean follow-up of 5 years.[33,34] Histologically, DSV is made up of numerous papillae, alternating with areas of solid foci, with squamous metaplasia being a constant feature. Approximately two-thirds of cases with DSV have been described in the adults, whereas the remaining one-third were diagnosed in the pediatric population of Ukraine and Belarus following the Chernobyl nuclear disaster.[32] DSV tends to occur in younger patients, with a mean age of diagnosis at 27 years, and cervical adenopathy is present in approximately 70% of cases. IC displays small uniform neoplastic cells in a characteristic nesting pattern. In a review of more than 200 cases, extrathyroidal extension of tumor at diagnosis was found in 44% and cervical adenopathy in 51%.[32] During a mean follow-up period of 72 months, average rates of locoregional recurrence or distant metastasis and tumor related mortality were 64% and 32%, respectively. In summary, these variants of thyroid follicular cell carcinoma appear to exhibit an aggressive biology and are associated with significant mortality at 5 years, ranging between 25% and 90%.[5]

TREATMENT OF WELL AND INTERMEDIATELY DIFFERENTIATED THYROID CARCINOMA

Surgery

The key decisions in the surgical management of thyroid nodules or cancers (or both) are whom to operate on and how extensive a resection to perform. Before the development and widespread use of preoperative FNA of thyroid nodules, surgeons frequently relied on intraoperative frozen-section analyses to guide the extent of resection. The utility of frozen-section diagnosis for thyroid nodules is limited. The situations in which intraoperative frozen section may be useful is for patients who have suspicious but nondiagnostic FNA results in the setting of papillary thyroid cancer. The quality of both the cytologic specimen and its interpretation is paramount to modern thyroid surgery.[15] If a high-quality FNA specimen is diagnostic of malignancy, a definitive procedure can be performed in the absence of intraoperative frozen-section analysis. If the FNA is highly suggestive but not diagnostic of papillary thyroid carcinoma, frozen-section evaluation can be beneficial especially when touch preparation techniques are employed to assess cytologic features. Most of the lesions in the indeterminate FNA category are follicular neoplasms, the majority of which are benign. Capsular and vascular invasion determine malignancy, and the ability to render an accurate interpretation on frozen-section analysis is very limited. A randomized controlled trial demonstrated a very limited role of frozen-section analysis for the vast majority of patients with follicular neoplasms. Thus, the recommended approach in this group of patients is to perform excision of the thyroid lobe, harboring the nodule, and then waiting for definitive pathologic analyses on paraffin-embedded histology. If the lesion turns out to be a follicular carcinoma with characteristics that place a patient at high risk, such as significant capsular invasion or angioinvasion, a completion total or near total thyroidectomy is performed during a second operation to remove the contralateral thyroid lobe.[24] In cases suspicious for the follicular variant of papillary carcinoma, the presence of specific nuclear features that define papillary thyroid cancer may be identifiable by employing touch preparations in addition to frozen-section analysis. For this reason, patients with FNA results that are read as follicular neoplasm with some features of papillary nuclei should undergo lobectomy and intraoperative assessment (frozen section, touch preparation) in an attempt to identify follicular variant of papillary thyroid cancer.

A long-standing controversy among endocrine surgeons has existed regarding the extent of surgical resection for well-differentiated thyroid cancer. It is becoming accepted that the completeness of surgical resection is associated with less recurrence and improved survival,[35] and thus most surgeons advocate total thyroidectomy over thyroid lobectomy. The difference in procedures relates to the management of the contralateral lobe and how this choice affects both the outcome and operative morbidity. In a thyroid lobectomy, the contralateral lobe is not dissected but is simply examined for abnormalities by palpation. A near-total thyroidectomy leaves a much smaller amount of normal tissue (less than 1 g) immediately adjacent to the ligament of

TABLE 108.7

ARGUMENTS FOR TOTAL THYROIDECTOMY IN WELL-DIFFERENTIATED THYROID CARCINOMA

Higher Survival Rate for Lesions > 1.5 cm in Diameter

- Lowest recurrence rate in all patients
- Prevention of recurrence in the contralateral lobe
- Reduces the risk of developing pulmonary metastasis
- Can be performed with the same morbidity and mortality as thyroid lobectomy
- Improved sensitivity of serum thyroglobulin as a marker for persistent or recurrent disease
- Radioactive iodine can be used to detect and treat persistent or recurrent disease
- Reduces possibility of residual tumor in contralateral lobe undergoing transformation to anaplastic carcinoma

Berry. Both procedures may offer some protection to the recurrent laryngeal nerve, but a near-total thyroidectomy offers minimal benefit in terms of preserving the blood supply of the upper parathyroid. A total extracapsular thyroidectomy implies that every effort is made to excise all thyroid tissue, leaving no macroscopic residual thyroid in either lobe. The difference between a total thyroidectomy and a near-total thyroidectomy usually depends on the particular anatomy of the thyroid in any given patient. A small ledge of thyroid tissue, called the *tubercle of Zuckerkandl*, frequently exist near the ligament of Berry that often lies immediately superficial to the recurrent nerve. Some surgeons routinely leave this small remnant of normal thyroid tissue *in situ*.

The increased risk of performing a total thyroidectomy versus a lesser resection may be in the long-term incidence of hypocalcemia. Virtually all experienced surgeons should be able to perform total thyroidectomies with less than 1% recurrent nerve injuries, with the long-term risk of hypoparathyroidism of 2% to 9%. It should be mentioned, however, that surgeon experience is strongly related to lower complication rates, especially in total thyroidectomy, and when operating on malignant versus benign disease.[36] The authors advocate for a more aggressive treatment (i.e., total thyroidectomy) for the vast majority of patients with well-differentiated thyroid carcinoma, and the reasons are outlined in Table 108.7. This recommendation is also shared with the recent American Thyroid Association Guidelines.[15]

The most compelling argument for performing a unilateral lobectomy in a subset of thyroid cancer patients is from the data that show a 20-year survival of 99% with a 20-year disease-free survival of more than 95% in low-risk patients.[26] However, careful medical surveillance for cancer in the contralateral lobe as well as recurrence must be maintained. Furthermore, in situations in which a small thyroid remnant is left, the true morbidity of treating this patient with ablative doses of ^{131}I (if indicated) is relatively minimal. In fact, it is typical for patients with a surgical report of a "total thyroidectomy" to detect normal residual thyroid tissue within the bed of the thyroid identified on the postresection diagnostic scan. This small thyroid remnant is readily ablated with postoperative ^{131}I treatments, whereas successful ablation of an intact thyroid lobe is associated with considerably more difficulty.

For patients in a high-risk category, there is much less disagreement regarding the extent of surgery. Due to the effectiveness of adjuvant postoperative radioiodine treatments and ease of follow-up with serum thyroglobulin (Tg) measurements, the vast majority of investigators agree that a total or near-total thyroidectomy is indicated for high-risk patients.[15] For patients with extrathyroidal extension, *en bloc* resection of invaded structures should be performed. If the tumor is on the anterior thyroid, this causes minimal morbidity, as resection of the overlying strap muscles causes no symptoms postoperatively. For posterior tumors, the margins are either the trachea or esophagus. For the majority of well-differentiated thyroid cancers, tracheal or esophageal resection is not indicated. However, for gross involvement of either of these structures, resection with reconstruction may be appropriate.[37]

Some investigators have noted a correlation of lymph node metastases and worse outcome and have argued for more routine formal dissections. Tisell et al.,[38] who have widely promoted microdissection of all cervical lymphatic tissue for medullary thyroid carcinoma, reported their results applying the same technique to papillary thyroid cancer. More recent large-scale population-based studies have shown that regional lymph node metastases among patients with thyroid cancer impact both local recurrence and cause-specific mortality.[39] The recent American Thyroid Association Guidelines suggest prophylactic central-compartment neck dissection (ipsilateral or bilateral) may be performed in patients with papillary thyroid carcinoma with clinically uninvolved central neck lymph nodes, especially for advanced primary tumors.[15] The arguments for and against prophylactic central lymph node dissection (CLND) in well-differentiated thyroid carcinoma are outlined in Table 108.8.

TABLE 108.8

SUMMARY OF ARGUMENTS FOR AND AGAINST PROPHYLACTIC CENTRAL LYMPH NODE DISSECTION IN WELL-DIFFERENTIATED THYROID CARCINOMA

For	Against
Presence of lymph node metastasis has a negative effect on patient outcome	May lead to higher rates of hypoparathyroidism
Presence of lymph node metastasis in the central neck cannot reliably be identified preoperatively or at operation	May lead to higher rates of recurrent laryngeal nerve injury
Improves accuracy in staging	Absence of level I data that it would lead to lower recurrence and mortality rates
Decreases postoperative thyroglobulin levels	Majority of thyroidectomies in the United States is performed by low-volume surgeons
Can be performed as safely as total thyroidectomy alone, at least in experienced hands	
Leads to avoidance of reoperations in the central neck which is associated with increased morbidity	
May lead to lower recurrence rates and mortality rates	

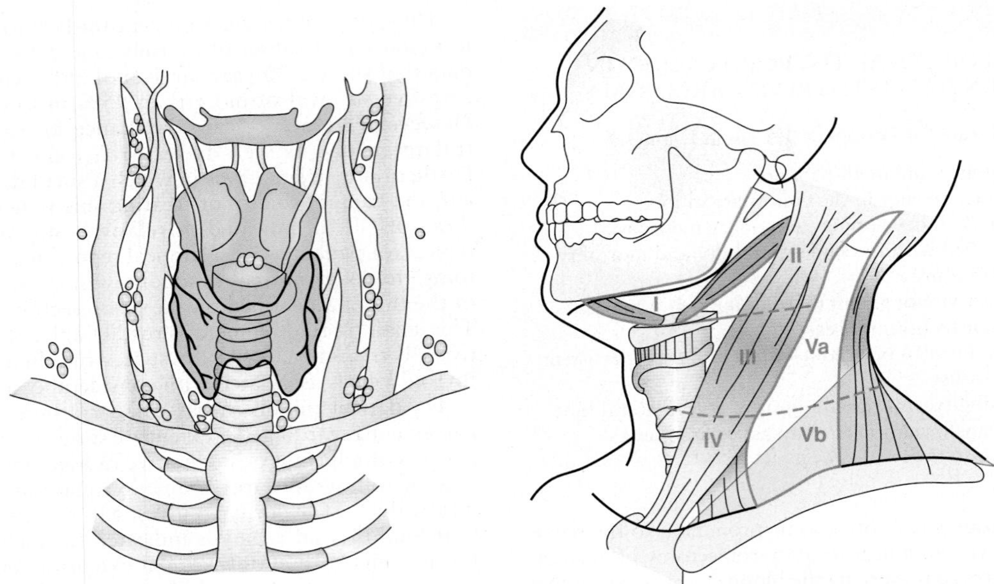

FIGURE 108.3 The thyroid gland and lymphatic node basins. **A:** Schematic representation of the lymphatic node basins of the neck. The lateral neck lymph node compartments (levels II–V) and the central neck compartment (level IV). (Modified from ref. 64.) **B:** Schematic illustration of the anatomical boarders of the central neck compartment (level VI). The superior margin is at the level of the hyoid bone, the inferior margin is at the level of the brachiocephalic vessels, and the lateral margins are at the medial aspect of the common carotid arteries (**A**). The central neck (level VI) contains the precricoid (Delphian), pretracheal, paratracheal, and perithyroidal nodes, including those along the recurrent laryngeal nerves (RLN), and the external branch of the superior laryngeal nerve (ebSLN). The parathyroid glands are also normally located in the central neck (**B**). (Modified from Rubin Pand Hansen, JT: TNM staging Atlas with 3D Oncoanatomy, 2nd edition. Philadelphia, Lippincott Williams & Wilkins, 2011.)

Gross lateral cervical metastatic disease is treated by modified radical neck dissection, preserving the internal jugular vein, sternocleidomastoid muscle, and the accessory nerve, which results in excellent local control and minimal morbidity. The lymph nodes typically involved are the level VI (central compartment) lymph nodes and the level II, III, and IV lymph nodes along the internal jugular vein corresponding to the upper, mid-, and lower neck, and level V (posterior neck; Fig. 108.3*A* and 108.3*B*). During any thyroid resection, these lymph node areas should be palpated. Lymph nodes that are abnormal because they are firm or large should be subjected to biopsy with frozen-section pathologic evaluation. If positive for metastatic cancer, these lymph node areas should be completely dissected.[15]

Radioiodine Therapy

Postoperative radioiodine ablation is increasingly being used in well-differentiated thyroid cancer. The lack of well-designed, randomized controlled studies and the low probability that any large multicenter treatment studies will ever come to fruition force the clinician to rely on retrospective studies, surveys of practice habits, and guidelines.[15] The goals of the treatment are to destroy any residual thyroid tissue to prevent locoregional recurrence and to facilitate long-term surveillance with whole-body iodine scans or stimulated thyroglobulin measurements.

Several large retrospective studies demonstrate reductions in both recurrence and cause specific mortality after ^{131}I ablation.[15,40] It should be noted, however, that other large studies fail to show such a relationship, especially in "low-risk" patients.[40] In studies showing a benefit with ^{131}I ablation, patients with larger tumors (greater than 1.5 cm), multifocality, residual disease, and nodal metastasis seem to gain from the treatment. Thus, the recent American Thyroid Association Guidelines recommend radioiodine ablation for patients with stage III or IV disease, all patients with stage II disease younger than 45 years and most of those older than 45 years, and selected patients with stage I disease, especially those with larger tumors (greater than 1.5 cm), multifocality, residual disease, nodal metastasis, vascular invasion, and intermediately differentiated histology.[15]

The dosing of ^{131}I for ablation is somewhat controversial. Some recommend low-dose ablation with less than 30 mCi administered on an outpatient basis. This approach should be reserved for low-risk young patients who may benefit from an overall lower radiation exposure and who accept the fact that several low radioiodine doses may be necessary before successful ablation. Activities between 30 and 100 mCi show similar rates of successful ablation, although there is a trend toward improved success rates with higher activities.[15] Thus, higher ablative doses ranging from 100 to 200 mCi should be used preferentially for older, high-risk patients, particularly those known to have an incomplete resection of the primary tumor, an invasive primary tumor, tumors of intermediate differentiation, or metastases. Some authors advocate use of dosimetry with the goal to derive the dose of ^{131}I that will deliver no more than 2 Gy to the blood, with no more than 120 mCi retained at 48 hours or 80 mCi in the presence of pulmonary metastases.

Postoperative ablation is typically performed approximately 6 weeks after near-total or total thyroidectomy. Most, but not all, centers perform a pretherapy whole-body iodine scan. Just as there is lack of consensus regarding ablation and therapeutic doses of ^{131}I, the diagnostic scanning dose is also controversial.[15] The ideal dose achieves high sensitivity in detecting residual thyroid tissue, thyroid cancer, and metastatic foci and reduces the potential for sublethal radiation "stunning" of thyroid tissue that prevents optimal uptake of future ^{131}I therapy.

Stunning is defined as a reduction in uptake of the ^{131}I therapy dose induced by a pretreatment diagnostic dose. Some authors suggest that diagnostic scanning with ^{123}I may prevent the stunning effect. If performed, a pretherapy scan should use a low dose of ^{131}I (1 to 3 mCi) or ^{123}I. To optimize uptake by both normal residual thyroid and thyroid cancer, patients are rendered hypothyroid with a goal of increasing serum TSH. To accomplish this, thyroid replacement after thyroidectomy is often performed with the administration of triiodothyronine (T_3), as it has a much shorter half-life than thyroxine (T_4), and it is discontinued 2 weeks before treatment. In response to this hypothyroid state, TSH must achieve levels of greater than 30 mU/L to obtain optimal uptake of radioiodine. It is also recommended that a serum thyroglobulin level is obtained during this period of hypothyroid state (see "Surveillance"). A low-iodine diet is recommended 1 to 2 weeks before scanning or ablative ^{131}I therapy to enhance the uptake and retention of radioiodine.[15] Alternatively, imaging and treatment employing TSH stimulation with recombinant human TSH (rhTSH; Thyrogen) in order to detect and treat residual normal thyroid tissue as well as thyroid cancer is performed with increased frequency. Posttherapy whole-body iodine scanning is typically performed 1 week after ^{131}I treatment to identify metastases. Follow-up diagnostic scanning is performed at outlined in Figure 108.4.

Most but not all studies have demonstrated a role for TSH suppression therapy in the medical management of thyroid cancer after therapy. A recent meta-analysis supported the efficacy of TSH suppression in preventing adverse clinical effects.[41] However, such a benefit has not been substantiated in low-risk patients. Thus, it is recommended that high-risk patients are maintained at a serum TSH level below 0.1 mU/L, while TSH levels at or slightly below the normal range (0.1 to 0.5 mU/L) seem appropriate for low-risk patients. It should be noted, however, that the degree of thyroid suppression is dictated by balancing the risk of recurrent thyroid cancer and the risks associated with subclinical thyrotoxicosis, particularly the cardiovascular risks.

The most common side effects from radioiodine therapy include sialadenitis, nausea, and temporary bone marrow suppression. Women undergoing ^{131}I treatment should be advised to avoid pregnancy during and 6 to 12 months after treatment due to risk of miscarriage and fetal malformation. Temporary amenorrhea or oligomenorrhea occurs in about 25% of cases and typically lasts for 4 to 10 months. In men, testicular function and spermatogenesis may be transiently impaired but appear to recover with time. There is a weak, but dose-dependent relationship between ^{131}I therapy and the development of second malignancies, such as bone and soft tissue tumors, colorectal cancer, salivary tumors, and leukemia.[42]

Surveillance

The goal of long-term follow-up is to identify recurrence in patients thought to be free of disease. Tg, an important serum tumor marker in the surveillance of thyroid cancer patients, is the protein that provides a matrix for thyroid hormone synthesis within thyroid follicles and is critical in the storage of thyroid hormone within the thyroid gland. After successful thyroidectomy and ablation of residual normal or malignant thyroid tissue by radioiodine, the Tg should be in the athyreotic range. Levels above the athyreotic range are indicative of persistent, functioning thyroid tissue or carcinoma. Thyroxine may suppress Tg in patients with metastatic disease; therefore, the test is more sensitive in the setting of thyroid hormone–suppressive therapy withdrawal and frank hypothyroidism documented by an elevated TSH.[15]

At the time of thyroid hormone withdrawal or recombinant human TSH rhTSH stimulation for both initial postoperative scans and for subsequent follow-up scans, Tg is measured in conjunction with the diagnostic whole-body scan and may be more sensitive than the scan in detecting cancer.[43] There is good evidence that a Tg cutoff level above 2 ng/mL after TSH stimulation (either after thyroid hormone withdrawal or 72 hours after rhTSH administration) is highly sensitive in detecting patients with persistent or recurrent tumor.[43] Serum Tg levels should be measured every 6 to 12 months after definitive therapy, as outlined in Figure 108.4. The presence of autoantibodies

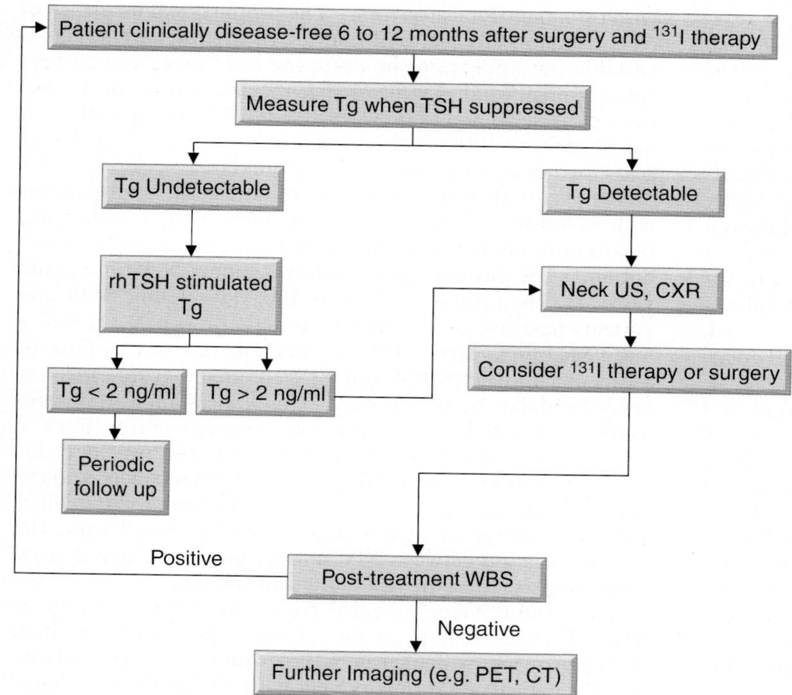

FIGURE 108.4 Flow diagram for follow up after definitive thyroidectomy and remnant ablation for well-differentiated thyroid carcinoma. Certain aggressive variants of well-differentiated carcinoma may not be amenable to this algorithm. Undetectable Tg assumes that there are no Tg autoantibodies interfering with the assay. Tg, thyroglobulin; rhTSH, recombinant human thyroid stimulating hormone; US, ultrasound; CXR, chest x-ray; WBS, whole-body scan; PET, positron emission tomography; CT, computed tomography. (Modified from figure 1, ref. 43.)

to Tg, which occurs in 25% of thyroid cancer patients and 10% of the general population, will falsely lower serum Tg levels. Thus, such antibodies should quantitatively be determined at every measurement of serum Tg levels. Routine use of diagnostic whole-body scanning in the follow-up management of low-risk patients with negative TSH stimulated Tg and neck ultrasound is discouraged. When indicated, a scan should use low dose ^{131}I (1 to 3 mCi) or ^{123}I. Cervical ultrasonography, however, has become increasingly used in the follow-up management of patients with differentiated thyroid cancer. Cervical metastases may occasionally be detected by ultrasonography even when TSH-stimulated Tg levels are negative. Thus, recent recommendations suggest that neck ultrasound should be performed 6 and 12 months after surgery, and then annually for 3 to 5 years, depending on the patients risk for recurrence and Tg status.[15] There has been a great deal of debate regarding the optimal management of patients who are Tg positive but negative on whole-body iodine scans and ultrasonography. Computed tomography (CT), ^{18}F-FDG positron emission tomography (PET) scans and ^{18}F-2-deoxyglucose (^{18}F-FDG) PET/CT fusion imaging has been increasingly used in the surveillance and treatment planning of these patients with iodine-negative, differentiated thyroid carcinoma. Although, ^{18}F-FDG PET/CT show both false-negative and -positive results, its accuracy in selected patients may be as high as 93%.[44]

Management of Local Recurrence and Distant Metastasis

Metastases discovered during surveillance are likely to be manifestations of persistent disease that survived ^{131}I therapy and thus are often incurable by additional such treatment. However, a reduction of the tumor burden with additional treatment may offer survival or palliative benefit. The preferred treatment, in hierarchical order, are surgical excision of locoregional disease in potentially curable patients, ^{131}I therapy, external beam irradiation, close surveillance in asymptomatic patients, and experimental chemotherapy trials.[15]

Patients with nodal locoregional recurrence in the neck should undergo modified radical neck dissection or central compartment (level VI) neck dissection, depending on the location of the recurrence. More aggressive surgery may be warranted in selected patients with invasion into the aerodigestive tract.[37] Tracheal stents and tracheotomy can be used as palliative measures. For regional lymph node metastasis not amenable to surgical therapy or distant metastasis detected with whole-body iodine scan, ^{131}I therapy is usually employed, especially in lesions that are radioiodine avid. Similar to the discussion of initial treatment, no consensus exists regarding dosing of ^{131}I, although most authors use a high dose ranging between 150 to 300 mCi. Pulmonary metastases are frequently detected exclusively on radioiodine scanning and tend to respond to ^{131}I treatment. Treatment can be performed every 6 to 12 months as long as the disease continues to respond. It should be noted, however, that pulmonary fibrosis may limit further ^{131}I treatment.[45] For select patients with incurable pulmonary disease, palliative treatments using metastasectomy, laser ablation, and external beam radiation therapy (EBRT) may be considered. Complete surgical resection of isolated symptomatic bone metastases and ^{131}I treatment for radioiodine avid, widespread disease have both been associated with an increased survival and are recommended especially in younger patients.[45] A combination of treatments may be considered for symptomatic bone lesions when surgery or ^{131}I treatment is not possible or effective.[15] Similarly, complete surgical resection of central nervous system (CNS) metastasis seem to be the most efficacious treatment, whereas EBRT may be considered in those not candidates for surgery.

Role of External Beam Radiation Therapy and Chemotherapy

The role of EBRT and chemotherapy in thyroid cancer is limited. EBRT should be considered in patients with unresectable gross residual cervical disease, painful bone metastases, and for metastases in critical locations that are not amenable to surgery and that would likely result in fracture or neurological or compressive symptoms (such as metastases in the CNS, vertebral bodies, selected mediastinal lymph nodes and pelvis). The single chemotherapeutic agent most commonly used for thyroid cancer is doxorubicin (Adriamycin) with partial response rates of 30% and up to 45% in some series. Combination therapy with doxorubicin and cisplatin has produced disappointing results that were no better than single-agent trials, and the toxicity was worse. For surgically unresectable local disease that has not responded to radioiodine, the best treatment may be a combination of hyperfractionated radiation treatments plus doxorubicin. Response rates of more than 80% have been reported using this regimen, although even in this situation, complete responses are rare and limited in duration.[15]

The management of patients with well-differentiated thyroid cancer that progresses despite current therapies represents a great challenge. During the past decade, biologic discoveries have sparked trials testing novel, biologically targeted therapies for advanced thyroid carcinomas, and several novel agents are currently being tested *in vitro* and in clinical studies.[46] Most clinical trials so far has focused on various tyrosine kinase inhibitors (TKIs) and active clinical trials for advanced thyroid cancer can be found on the Internet.

POORLY DIFFERENTIATED THYROID CARCINOMA

Anaplastic thyroid carcinoma (ATC) is one of the most aggressive and difficult human malignancies to treat and is one of the most lethal. As opposed to the excellent long-term survival for well-differentiated thyroid carcinoma, ATC in most series has a median survival of 4 to 5 months from the time of diagnosis, with rare long-term survivors.[47] The proportional incidence of ATC compared to the total number of thyroid carcinomas is variable but appears to be declining over time, and current epidemiologic studies indicate that this lethal form of thyroid cancer has decreased to between 1% and 3% of the total number of cases. Institutional reviews over a distinct period suggest a real decrease in the incidence of ATC.[47]

Patients with ATC differ epidemiologically from patients with well-differentiated thyroid carcinoma, with a median age two to three decades older and with a more equal gender distribution.[47] The median age at diagnosis ranges between 63 and 74 years. The largest series from the Mayo Clinic with 134 patients demonstrated a female-to-male ratio of 1.5:1 and a mean age of 67 years.[47] ATC is commonly related to a prior or a concurrent diagnosis of well-differentiated thyroid cancer or benign nodular thyroid disease.[47] This association of ATC with well-differentiated thyroid carcinoma suggests two features of the biology of this tumor. First, ATC may arise via the dedifferentiation of prior well-differentiated thyroid cancer, and the aggressive growth pattern of this anaplastic tumor may replace all previous evidence of well-differentiated tumor. Second, the close association between ATC and well-differentiated thyroid cancer suggests that the risk factors are similar.

The natural history, clinical presentation, and outcome of ATC reflect the biology of this tumor as an undifferentiated, rapidly growing malignant neoplasm with invasive characteristics. The patients uniformly present with a palpable mass that is rapidly increasing in size. The median tumor size in patients with ATC was 8 to 9 cm, with a range of 3 to 20 cm as compared to the usual size of 2 to 3 cm for well-differentiated thyroid cancer. Invasion into the trachea, larynx, or recurrent laryngeal nerve leads to obstructive symptoms, hemoptysis, dysphagia, and hoarseness, which are often present at diagnosis.

The majority of patients with ATC die from aggressive local-regional disease, primarily with upper airway respiratory failure. It is usually the local growth and obliteration of the airway that cause the patient's demise. For this reason, aggressive local therapy is indicated in all patients who can tolerate it and for those in whom it is technically possible. As opposed to well-differentiated thyroid cancer, ^{131}I plays no role in the treatment of recurrent or metastatic disease for this tumor. Therefore, total or near-total thyroidectomy is not as important in ATC, except as needed to obtain local control.[47]

Survival after the diagnosis of ATC is very poor. The median survival in most series is less than 5 months from the time of diagnosis. The majority of patients die due to local recurrence, although distant metastases occur primarily in lung, bone, and liver. External radiation has been used with limited success to treat locally recurrent ATC. Doxorubicin is the single most effective chemotherapeutic for ATC, and it has been shown that doxorubicin plus platinum is more effective than doxorubicin alone. Early diagnosis with aggressive surgical therapy supplemented by external-beam radiation therapy and doxorubicin-based chemotherapy is regarded by many as the most appropriate treatment. However, a prospective phase 2 clinical trial demonstrated 1 complete response and 9 partial responses in 19 patients after treatment with paclitaxel, suggesting its potential role in the treatment of anaplastic thyroid carcinoma.[48]

MEDULLARY THYROID CARCINOMA

Pathology

Medullary thyroid carcinoma (MTC) was recognized in the 1950s by Hazard et al.[49] as a distinct clinicopathologic entity. Over the next 10 years, investigators identified and described the parafollicular C cell that produces calcitonin and give rise to MTC. During the decade of the 1970s, Wells et al.[50] extended the measurement of calcitonin by defining a provocative test that rendered this hormonal tumor marker one of the most sensitive and specific in all of oncology. Understanding of the familial associations of MTC with corollary genetic studies reported in the 1980s and early 1990s have defined molecular changes responsible for familial forms of inherited MTC and with implications for sporadic MTC as well. The familial forms of MTC are outlined in Table 108.4. More recent research has identified genotype–phenotype relationships and has led to more individualized treatment of patients with inherited MTC.[51] For details on molecular pathogenesis of MTC see Chapter 107.

MTC constitutes between 3% to 12% of most institutional series of detectible thyroid cancers.[23] As opposed to well-differentiated thyroid cancer, MTC is not associated with radiation exposure, but it does occur in distinct familial syndromes. Sporadic or nonfamilial MTC accounts for 60% to 70% of cases, with three distinct familial syndromes accounting for the remainder. MTC is the most prominent clinical diagnosis in multiple endocrine neoplasia (MEN)-2A and MEN-2B. In 1986, familial MTC in the absence of the associated features of MEN-2A or MEN-2B was described. Appreciation of this syndrome has shifted the percentage of sporadic MTC as a function of the total number of cases from 80% to 60% and even lower in some series. In addition to the presence or absence of other associated endocrine abnormalities, each of these familial forms of MTC has a unique natural history and prognosis.[52]

Parafollicular, or C cells, arise embryologically from the neural crest and are located primarily in the upper and middle thirds of the thyroid lobes, with a particular concentration posteriorly. This feature is important to surgical therapy, as this is in direct proximity to where the recurrent laryngeal nerve passes under the ligament of Berry and enters the larynx. Accordingly, performance of a near-total thyroidectomy is likely to leave remnant neoplastic disease in this location.

Grossly, MTC may be circumscribed or infiltrative and is usually white-yellow. Histologically, this tumor demonstrates a wide variety of patterns, including glandular, solid, spindle-cell, oncocytic, clear cell, papillary, small cell, and giant cell. The nuclei of MTC resemble those of neuroendocrine tumors in other areas of the body. They are usually round and have a stippled "pepper-and-salt" chromatin. Pathologic features associated with a poor prognosis include the presence of necrosis, a squamous pattern, oxyphil cells in the tumor and absence of cells with intermediate cytoplasm, and less than 50% calcitonin immunoreactivity.

Clinical Presentation and Diagnosis

The clinical symptoms at the time of presentation vary. Patients with familial MTC who are identified by screening with stimulation tests or with molecular analysis (detection of *RET* gene mutation) are usually identified before the development of macroscopic disease. Patients with sporadic disease typically present with an asymptomatic thyroid mass. Patients with bulky disease, local or metastatic, with extremely high levels of calcitonin may have severe secretory diarrhea as a principal symptom. Before the availability of genetic testing for familial MTC, basal and stimulated serum calcitonin levels were used to screen patients. Sequential calcitonin and carcinoembryonic antigen (CEA) measurements are still important as a tumor marker for surveillance of patients with MTC.[20]

Various nuclear imaging studies have been evaluated in patients with MTC to identify gross and occult metastases. ^{131}I thyroid scans are of no utility since MTC does not concentrate iodine. Similarly, thallium as well as technetium scans have been used with minimal efficacy. Several studies have used somatostatin receptor scintigraphy in the setting of MTC.[52] The results are promising for this imaging technique, but occult lesions smaller than 1 cm as well as liver lesions are still missed with this technique. Although not specific, ultrasound, magnetic resonance imaging (MRI), CT, PET, and PET/CT imaging are increasingly being used in the management of patients with MTC.[52]

Treatment

Chemotherapy and EBRT are, for the most part, ineffective against MTC, rendering surgical resection the only definitive therapy. For patients with sporadic MTC who are not identified by biochemical or genetic screening, the appropriate operation in most cases is total thyroidectomy, central node dissection, and ipsilateral modified radical neck dissection. Total thyroidectomy is indicated in this sporadic setting because a small proportion of lesions may be bilateral and because it may not be clear at the time of operation, whether a patient is an index case of familial disease or the disorder is a true sporadic case. Because all familial syndromes have a high propensity for bilateral tumors, total extracapsular thyroidectomy is always indicated. Combined with thyroid resection, a central lymph node dissection should generally be performed, removing lymphoid tissue from the level of the hyoid bone superiorly to the innominate vessels inferiorly and laterally to the jugular veins. Because of the high incidence of ipsilateral nodal metastasis at presentation, formal modified radical neck "microdissections" are ideally combined with the initial exploration.[20]

The incidence of positive lymph nodes correlates with the size of the primary lesion at the time of diagnosis. It has been reported that for lesions smaller than 1 cm, there is an 11% incidence of nodal disease, whereas in patients with tumors larger than 2 cm, 60% will have positive cervical lymph nodes.[52] The incidence of distant metastases at the time of diagnosis varies with the clinical setting. Patients with familial non-MEN MTC tend to have even a less aggressive clinical course, and approximately 2% of these patients present with distant metastases. Unfortunately, patients with sporadic disease are often explored without a clear diagnosis or by surgeons without experience in managing this malignancy. FNA specimens suggestive of MTC should be stained for calcitonin, which if positive is highly suggestive of MTC. In addition, a serum calcitonin and CEA levels in this setting are almost always elevated, thereby confirming the diagnosis. It is important to screen for catecholamine excess prior to surgical exploration as an apparent sporadic patient with MTC may in fact have a familial syndrome with an occult pheochromocytoma.

The outcome of treatment of patients with sporadic MTC has improved. Recent studies show a 5-year survival between 80% and 90% and 10-year survival between 70% and 80% for combined series of familial and sporadic MTC.[53] The natural history and prognosis for the various subtypes of MTC correlate with described genetic changes. The introduction of genetic testing and prophylactic surgery has improved the prognosis in cases of familial disease (see "Treatment of Familial Medullary Thyroid Carcinoma").

One challenge in the surgical management of patients with MTC is the proper approach to patients who have persistently elevated basal or stimulated calcitonin after resection of all gross disease.[20,52] In many of these cases, imaging studies fail to demonstrate areas of disease. Excision attempts generally do not produce normalization of calcitonin levels. Tisell et al.[54] has advocated meticulous 12-hour neck dissections, often removing 40 to 60 additional cervical lymph nodes in patients with occult MTC. In a series of 11 patients, 4 demonstrated normalization of calcitonin levels, with another 4 who had dramatic improvement in their calcitonin levels. However, even these improvements in the calcitonin levels do not necessarily translate into improved survival.

For patients with metastatic MTC, surgical resection may still offer the best chance of survival as well as long-term palliation.[20] In the setting of persistent hypercalcitonemia and negative imaging studies, remedial surgery with formal neck dissection is often indicated. However, prior to such an operation it is recommended to perform a laparoscopic evaluation of the liver to rule out superficial hepatic metastases.[52] If present, the enthusiasm for remedial neck dissection, especially in an asymptomatic patient, is markedly reduced.[20]

The results of MTC treatment with EBRT or chemotherapeutic agents are disappointing. Chemotherapeutic agents used in the treatment of MTC include doxorubicin, dacarbazine, streptozocin, and 5-fluorouracil. Single-agent response rates are poor, with aggressive doxorubicin regimens producing 20% to 30% objective responses, and combinations of chemotherapy have so far not been promising. The poor outcome of treatment of metastatic disease validates the treatment recommendation to diagnose patients with MTC early and treat with initial aggressive surgery.[20] Biologic discoveries have sparked trials testing novel, biologically targeted therapies for advanced thyroid carcinomas, and several novel agents are currently being tested in clinical studies.[46] Most clinical trials so far have focused on various TKIs,[55] and active clinical trials for metastatic MTC can be found in the Internet.

TREATMENT OF FAMILIAL MEDULLARY THYROID CARCINOMA

An increasing number of patients are identified in one of the three familial settings of MTC that are diagnosed using biochemical or genetic screening for *RET* gene mutations. Routine use of screening to diagnose MTC led to significant decreases in both the age of diagnosis and the incidence of lymph node metastases, as well as a significant increase in the number of patients cured biochemically at these earlier operations. Wells et al.[56] used a molecular genetic screening technique to identify patients who are carriers of the MEN-2A mutation as infants or young children. Before any abnormality in basal or stimulated calcitonin, these patients undergo a total thyroidectomy and central neck dissection. Pathologic evaluation of these children's thyroid glands identified C-cell hyperplasia, microscopic, or macroscopic MTC. In the initial trial, no patients treated with this strategy had evidence of lymph node metastases, and this surgical strategy should be curative.[56]

The genetic test for the mutations in the *RET* gene are commercially available, and many individuals are reporting series based on early operations for patients identified by RET mutation screening. A recent review noted that in a total of 209 patients treated in this manner, 3.4% had normal thyroid glands with no evidence of C-cell hyperplasia or MTC. It has also been noted in these patients undergoing prophylactic operations that there was an 8.6% incidence of lymph node metastases.[57] Based on these results, it is thought that a prophylactic central neck dissection should be performed at the time of prophylactic thyroidectomy, based on genetic testing. Since different mutations in the *RET* gene are associated with variable disease aggressiveness, more recent research has attempted to correlate a certain mutation (genotype) with the patients clinical course (phenotype) in order to provide genotype-specific recommendations for treatment.[51] Thus, individuals with *RET* gene mutations associated with MEN-2A and familial medullary thyroid carcinoma (FMTC) are advised to undergo prophylactic thyroidectomy at age 5 to 6 years, whereas affected individuals in kindreds with MEN-2B should undergo thyroidectomy during infancy due to the aggressiveness and earlier age at onset of MTC in these patients.[52] At the M. D. Anderson Cancer Center, 86 patients with inherited MTC were stratified into three *RET* gene mutation risk groups; level 1, low risk for MTC (mutations in codons 609, 768, 790, 791, 804, and 891); level 2, intermediate risk (mutations in codons 611, 618, 620, and 634); and level 3, highest risk (mutations in codons 883 and 918).[20] All patients in the level 3 group (all with MEN-2B) had MTC present at initial thyroidectomy performed at a median age of 13.5 years. Similar, but not identical, findings were identified by the large European Multiple Endocrine Neoplasia (EUROMEN) study group.[51] With increased knowledge of genotype–phenotype correlations, more individualized management can be used in the treatment of familial variants of MTC.[20]

THYROID LYMPHOMA

Thyroid lymphoma is a relatively rare disease, constituting fewer than 1% of all lymphomas and accounting for 2% of extranodal non-Hodgkin's lymphoma.[58] Almost all of these thyroid lymphomas are non-Hodgkin's lymphoma, with the majority (70% to 90%) being intermediate grade and the remainder being high grade (see Chapter 127). Many are considered mucosa-associated lymphoid tissue lymphomas (MALTomas), show plasmacytic differentiation, and may be associated with similar lesions in extranodal sites, especially in the gastrointestinal tract.

The majority of patients with thyroid lymphoma have disease on one side of the diaphragm with a proportion confined to the thyroid (stage IE). The majority have thyroid disease plus cervical or mediastinal lymph nodes (stage IIE).[58] The incidence of this disease may be changing, primarily due to improved recognition and diagnosis of thyroid lymphoma. One hypothesis to explain the incidence increase is that these patients were previously diagnosed as having anaplastic thyroid carcinoma and, with better understanding and more sophisticated diagnostic tools, such as immunohistochemistry, these patients are now being correctly categorized as having thyroid lymphoma.

In most series, there is a strong female predominance, ranging from 3:1 up to 8:1. The median age in most series at diagnosis places patients in the seventh decade of life, similar to what is seen for ATC and much older than patients with well-differentiated thyroid cancer. Between 10% and 30% of patients report a symptom or combination of symptoms relating to local invasion, including hoarseness, dyspnea with stridor, or dysphagia. Patients with thyroid lymphoma virtually never have hyperthyroidism but frequently have hypothyroidism. These hypothyroid patients have evidence of autoimmune thyroiditis or Hashimoto thyroiditis, either by FNA or from the pathologic specimen.

The optimal treatment for thyroid lymphoma has evolved with the success of combination chemotherapy used in the treatment of non-Hodgkin's lymphoma and with the ability to obtain an accurate diagnosis without invasive surgery by large-needle or core-needle biopsy. Some argue that the role of surgery in this disease is simply to obtain adequate tissue for diagnosis, and that the primary treatment should be external-beam radiation combined with a chemotherapy regimen based on the histopathological subtype of lymphoma.[59] Patients with extrathyroidal disease, either by direct extension or lymph node involvement, should be considered to have systemic disease. Although some surgeons argue that attempts to clear the trachea to avoid airway obstruction should be performed if at all possible in all patients, others report that the rapid use of radiation therapy (starting the day after the diagnostic biopsy procedure) produces the same beneficial results. All would agree that the efficacy and long-term survival achieved using a combination of radiation therapy and chemotherapy render aggressive surgical resection with sacrifice of the recurrent laryngeal nerve or possibly resulting in hypoparathyroidism contraindicated for thyroid lymphoma.

METASTATIC DISEASE OF THE THYROID

Clinically significant involvement of the thyroid gland by metastases from other sites is rare, accounting for fewer than 1% of thyroid malignancies in most series involving surgical resection or FNA biopsies.[60] On the other hand, the incidence of thyroid metastases identified in autopsy series is greater and can range between 2% and 26%, depending on the thoroughness of the examination by the pathologists.[61] From these autopsy series, the most predominant malignancies metastatic to the thyroid are breast and lung, each accounting for 25% of the total.[61] Melanoma, renal cell carcinoma, and gastrointestinal tract malignancies each account for approximately 10% of these secondary malignancies from autopsy studies. A variety of other miscellaneous diagnoses account for the remainder.

For the more clinically relevant situation in which the thyroid metastasis is detected premortem, the most common primary site is renal cell carcinoma, accounting for 23% of 111 such cases combined from the literature.[60] The next most common sites are breast (16%), lung (15%), melanoma (5%), and colon and larynx (4.5% each). Occasionally, thyroid metastasis may be the initial presentation of an occult primary from a gastrointestinal source or renal primary. Because FNA biopsy is the diagnostic tool used to evaluate thyroid nodules as the initial step, awareness of the potential of secondary metastases is important for interpretation of these biopsy results.

Dependent on the clinical situation, some of these patients may need thyroidectomy for palliation of local symptoms. Thyroid metastases may grow at a rapid rate and can cause airway obstruction.

CHILDREN WITH THYROID CARCINOMA

Well-Differentiated Thyroid Carcinoma

Well-differentiated thyroid carcinoma comprises only 1.4% of all newly diagnosed childhood carcinomas in the United States reported from 1975 to 1995.[62] Current treatment strategies for pediatric patients with well-differentiated thyroid carcinoma are derived from single-institution clinical cohorts, reports of extensive personal experience, and extrapolation of several common therapeutic practices in adults. Children with well-differentiated thyroid carcinoma more often than their adult counterparts have a history of external irradiation to the head and neck, although the majority present without such a history.[63] At presentation, pediatric patients tend to have a higher incidence of palpable cervical adenopathy, local infiltration of the primary cancer, and pulmonary metastases. The incidence of cervical nodal metastases in a series from the University of Michigan remained 88% from 1936 to 1990,[63] and the long-term mortality rate was 2.2%. Despite presenting with more advanced disease compared to adults, children tend to have a better prognosis.[62] Even in children with distant metastases, the survival rates are remarkably good.

Most authors agree that aggressive initial management with total thyroidectomy and cervical lymph node dissection should be performed in most children with well-differentiated thyroid carcinoma. This is commonly followed by administration of radioiodine therapy to destroy any residual normal thyroid remnant.[62] Finally, and importantly, because the duration of follow-up is lifelong, the care of children with prior diagnosis of well-differentiated thyroid carcinoma should be transferred to an adult endocrinologist after they reach adulthood, even if they have no evidence of disease by that time. Due to the limited experience in the management of thyroid cancer in the pediatric population, consideration should be made for referral to centers with experience in managing these challenging cases.

Medullary Thyroid Carcinoma

With the introduction of genetic screening for *RET* gene mutations, an increasing number of patients are diagnosed with inherited forms of MTC during childhood or even infancy. Depending on genotype, the current recommendations advise that individuals with *RET* gene mutations associated with MEN-2A and FMTC undergo prophylactic thyroidectomy between ages 5 to 6 years, whereas affected individuals in kindreds with MEN-2B should undergo thyroidectomy during infancy due to the aggressiveness and earlier age at onset of MTC in these patients.[20] As more information about genotype–phenotype correlations are gathered, these recommendations may be altered, and thus more individual recommendations based on specific genetic information can be made.[51]

References

The full list of references for this chapter appears in the online version.

3. Jemal A, Siegel R, Ward E, et al. Cancer statistics, 2009. *CA Cancer J Clin* 2009;59:225.
5. Carling T, Ocal IT, Udelsman R. Special variants of differentiated thyroid cancer: does it alter the extent of surgery versus well-differentiated thyroid cancer? *World J Surg* 2007;31:916.
6. Edge S, Byrd D, Compton C, et al. *Thyroid tumors*. 7th ed. New York: Springer, 2010.
7. Davies L, Welch HG. Increasing incidence of thyroid cancer in the United States, 1973–2002. *JAMA* 2006;295:2164.
8. Zhu C, Zheng T, Kilfoy BA, et al. A birth cohort analysis of the incidence of papillary thyroid cancer in the United States, 1973–2004. *Thyroid* 2009;19:1061.
11. Hancock SL, Cox RS, McDougall IR. Thyroid diseases after treatment of Hodgkin's disease. *N Engl J Med* 1991;325:599.
12. Tucker MA, Jones PH, Boice JD Jr, et al. Therapeutic radiation at a young age is linked to secondary thyroid cancer. The Late Effects Study Group. *Cancer Res* 1991;51:2885.
13. Dickman PW, Holm LE, Lundell G, Boice JD Jr, Hall P. Thyroid cancer risk after thyroid examination with ^{131}I: a population-based cohort study in Sweden. *Int J Cancer* 2003;106:580.
14. Robbins J, Schneider AB. Thyroid cancer following exposure to radioactive iodine. *Rev Endocr Metab Disord* 2000;1:197.
15. Cooper DS, Doherty GM, Haugen BR, et al. Revised American Thyroid Association management guidelines for patients with thyroid nodules and differentiated thyroid cancer. *Thyroid* 2009;19:1167.
18. Malchoff CD, Malchoff DM. Familial nonmedullary thyroid carcinoma. *Cancer Control* 2006;13:106.
19. Cheung K, Roman SA, Wang TS, Walker HD, Sosa JA. Calcitonin measurement in the evaluation of thyroid nodules in the United States: a cost-effectiveness and decision analysis. *J Clin Endocrinol Metab* 2008;93:2173.
20. Kloos RT, Eng C, Evans DB, et al. Medullary thyroid cancer: management guidelines of the American Thyroid Association. *Thyroid* 2009;19:565.
21. Nikiforov YE, Steward DL, Robinson-Smith TM, et al. Molecular testing for mutations in improving the fine-needle aspiration diagnosis of thyroid nodules. *J Clin Endocrinol Metab* 2009;94:2092.
22. Xing M, Clark D, Guan H, et al. BRAF mutation testing of thyroid fine-needle aspiration biopsy specimens for preoperative risk stratification in papillary thyroid cancer. *J Clin Oncol* 2009;27:2977.
24. Carling T, Udelsman R. Follicular neoplasms of the thyroid: what to recommend. *Thyroid* 2005;6:583.
27. Ito Y, Miyauchi A, Inoue H, et al. An observational trial for papillary thyroid microcarcinoma in Japanese patients. *World J Surg* 2010;34:28.
28. Leboulleux S, Girard E, Rose M, et al. Ultrasound criteria of malignancy for cervical lymph nodes in patients followed up for differentiated thyroid cancer. *J Clin Endocrinol Metab* 2007;92:3590.
31. Wada N, Nakayama H, Suganuma N, et al. Prognostic value of the sixth edition AJCC/UICC TNM classification for differentiated thyroid carcinoma with extrathyroid extension. *J Clin Endocrinol Metab* 2007;92:215.
33. Wenig B, Thompson L, Adair C, Shmookler B, Heffess C. Thyroid papillary carcinoma of columnar cell type: a clinicopathologic study of 16 cases. *Cancer* 1998;4:740.
35. Bilimoria KY, Bentrem DJ, Ko CY, et al. Extent of surgery affects survival for papillary thyroid cancer. *Ann Surg* 2007;246:375.
36. Sosa JA, Bowman HM, Tielsch JM, et al. The importance of surgeon experience for clinical and economic outcomes from thyroidectomy. *Ann Surg* 1998;228:320.
37. Brauckhoff M, Meinicke A, Bilkenroth U, et al. Long-term results and functional outcome after cervical evisceration in patients with thyroid cancer. *Surgery* 2006;140:953.
38. Tisell LE, Nilsson B, Molne J, et al. Improved survival of patients with papillary thyroid cancer after surgical microdissection. *World J Surg* 1996;20:854.
39. Lundgren CI, Hall P, Dickman PW, Zedenius J. Influence of surgical and postoperative treatment on survival in differentiated thyroid cancer. *Br J Surg* 2007;94:571.
40. Sawka AM, Thephamongkhol K, Brouwers M, et al. Clinical review 170: A systematic review and metaanalysis of the effectiveness of radioactive iodine remnant ablation for well-differentiated thyroid cancer. *J Clin Endocrinol Metab* 2004;89:3668.
41. McGriff NJ, Csako G, Gourgiotis L, et al. Effects of thyroid hormone suppression therapy on adverse clinical outcomes in thyroid cancer. *Ann Med* 2002;34:554.
42. Rubino C, de Vathaire F, Dottorini ME, et al. Second primary malignancies in thyroid cancer patients. *Br J Cancer* 2003;89:1638.
43. Mazzaferri EL, Robbins RJ, Spencer CA, et al. A consensus report of the role of serum thyroglobulin as a monitoring method for low-risk patients with papillary thyroid carcinoma. *J Clin Endocrinol Metab* 2003;88:1433.
44. Palmedo H, Bucerius J, Joe A, et al. Integrated PET/CT in differentiated thyroid cancer: diagnostic accuracy and impact on patient management. *J Nucl Med* 2006;47:616.
45. Durante C, Haddy N, Baudin E, et al. Long-term outcome of 444 patients with distant metastases from papillary and follicular thyroid carcinoma: benefits and limits of radioiodine therapy. *J Clin Endocrinol Metab* 2006;91:2892.
46. Sherman SI. Targeted therapy of thyroid cancer. *Biochem Pharmacol* 2010;80:592.
47. McIver B, Hay ID, Giuffrida DF, et al. Anaplastic thyroid carcinoma: a 50-year experience at a single institution. *Surgery* 2001;130:1028.
48. Ain KB, Egorin MJ, DeSimone PA. Treatment of anaplastic thyroid carcinoma with paclitaxel: phase 2 trial using ninety-six-hour infusion. Collaborative Anaplastic Thyroid Cancer Health Intervention Trials (CATCHIT) Group. *Thyroid* 2000;10:587.
49. Hazard J, Hawk W, Crile G. Medullary (solid) carcinoma of the thyroid: a clinicopathologic entity. *J Clin Endocrinol Metab* 1959;19:152.
50. Wells SA Jr, Baylin SB, Linehan WM, et al. Provocative agents and the diagnosis of medullary carcinoma of the thyroid gland. *Ann Surg* 1978;188:139.
51. Machens A, Niccoli-Sire P, Hoegel J, et al. Early malignant progression of hereditary medullary thyroid cancer. *N Engl J Med* 2003;349:1517.
52. Moley JF. Medullary thyroid carcinoma. *Curr Treat Options Oncol* 2003;4:339.
54. Tisell LE, Hansson G, Jansson S, Salander H. Reoperation in the treatment of asymptomatic metastasizing medullary thyroid carcinoma. *Surgery* 1986;99:60.
55. Wells SA Jr, Gosnell JE, Gagel RF, et al. Vandetanib for the treatment of patients with locally advanced or metastatic hereditary medullary thyroid cancer. *J Clin Oncol* 2010;28:767.
56. Wells SA Jr, Chi DD, Toshima K, et al. Predictive DNA testing and prophylactic thyroidectomy in patients at risk for multiple endocrine neoplasia type 2A. *Ann Surg* 1994;220:237.
58. Friedberg MH, Coburn MC, Monchik JM. Role of surgery in stage IE non-Hodgkin's lymphoma of the thyroid. *Surgery* 1994;116:1061.
59. Green LD, Mack L, Pasieka JL. Anaplastic thyroid cancer and primary thyroid lymphoma: a review of these rare thyroid malignancies. *J Surg Oncol* 2006;94:725.
60. Chen H, Nicol TL, Udelsman R. Clinically significant, isolated metastatic disease to the thyroid gland. *World J Surg* 1999;23:177.
61. Rosen IB, Walfish PG, Bain J, Bedard YC. Secondary malignancy of the thyroid gland and its management. *Ann Surg Oncol* 1995;2:252.
62. Hung W, Sarlis NJ. Current controversies in the management of pediatric patients with well-differentiated nonmedullary thyroid cancer: a review. *Thyroid* 2002;12:683.
63. Harness JK, Thompson NW, McLeod MK, Pasieka JL, Fukuuchi A. Differentiated thyroid carcinoma in children and adolescents. *World J Surg* 1992;16:547.
64. Carty SE, Cooper DS, Doherty GM, et al. Consensus statement on the terminology and classification of central neck dissection for thyroid cancer. *Thyroid* 2009;19:1153.
65. Hay ID, Bergstralh EJ, Goellner JR, Ebersold JR, Grant CS. Predicting outcome in papillary thyroid carcinoma: development of a reliable prognostic scoring system in a cohort of 1779 patients surgically treated at one institution during 1940 through 1989. *Surgery* 1993;114:1050.
66. Shah JP, Loree TR, Dharker D, et al. Prognostic factors in differentiated carcinoma of the thyroid gland. *Am J Surg* 1992;164:658.

CHAPTER 109 PARATHYROID TUMORS

REZA RAHBARI AND ELECTRON KEBEBEW

Parathyroid tumors are one of the most common endocrine neoplasms. Parathyroid tumors commonly cause hyperparathyroidism. Hyperparathyroidism is characterized by hypersecretion of parathyroid hormone. Hyperparathyroidism may be primary, secondary, or rarely, tertiary. Primary hyperparathyroidism is the most common form of hyperparathyroidism and occurs as a result of inappropriate parathyroid hormone secretion from an enlarged parathyroid gland(s). Primary hyperparathyroidism is caused by a parathyroid adenoma (85%), parathyroid hyperplasia involving four glands (10%), double parathyroid adenomas (2%–5%), parathyroid cancer (<1%), or rarely, parathyromatosis.[1] Secondary hyperparathyroidism occurs as a response usually from low serum calcium levels, which is usually associated with renal failure. In tertiary hyperparathyroidism, once the secondary cause of hyperparathyroidism is resolved, there is continued autonomous hypersecretion of parathyroid hormone from enlarged parathyroid gland(s). Some parathyroid tumors in primary hyperparathyroidism are associated with inherited familial cancer syndromes: multiple endocrine neoplasia (MEN) type 1 and type 2A, familial isolated hyperparathyroidism, and hyperparathyroidism-jaw tumor syndrome (HPT-JT).[2,3]

Parathyroid cancer is a rare cause of primary hyperparathyroidism and has been reported in some cases of secondary hyperparathyroidism. Most patients with parathyroid cancer present with severe hypercalcemia and metabolic complications of primary hyperparathyroidism (bone and renal disease). The clinical behavior of parathyroid cancer is variable but most patients develop locoregional recurrence; distant metastasis to the lung, bone, and liver occur late. Most patients with parathyroid cancer succumb to uncontrollable hypercalcemia, and not due to direct tumor effect. This chapter will describe the epidemiology, clinical manifestations, diagnosis, molecular biology, treatment, and prognosis of parathyroid cancer in the context of primary hyperparathyroidism.

EPIDEMIOLOGY

Primary hyperparathyroidism is a common clinical disorder with approximately 100,000 new cases diagnosed each year in the United States. It is more common in women (1 in 500 women) than in men (1 in 5,000) and occurs in approximately 0.3% of the general population. Primary hyperparathyroidism occurs most commonly in perimenopausal or postmenopausal women and is rare in children. Parathyroid cancer is a relatively rare endocrine malignancy. The precise incidence of parathyroid cancer is not well established in the United States. Parathyroid cancer, however, accounted for 0.005% of cancer registrants in the National Cancer Data Base[4] and the estimated annual incidence using the Surveillance, Epidemiology and End Results cancer registry data is 5.73 per 10,000 million persons.[5] Parathyroid cancer is often reported in the context of primary hyperparathyroidism, but in rare instances it has been reported to occur in secondary hyperparathyroidism and may be nonfunctioning.

The prevalence of parathyroid cancer in primary hyperparathyroidism is less than 1% of all cases.[6–10] Some investigators have reported higher rates of parathyroid cancer (2.8%–5.2%) in study cohorts from Japan and Italy.[11,12] Variable rates in parathyroid cancer are likely the result of most studies being done at tertiary referral centers where rare diagnoses are more likely to be encountered, and the difficulty in establishing a histologic diagnosis of parathyroid cancer may lead to both over- and underdiagnosis of the disease. Hundahl et al.,[4] in their review of the National Cancer Data Base, reported 286 cases of parathyroid cancer between the years 1985 and 1995. Lee et al.,[5] who used the Surveillance, Epidemiology and End Results cancer registry database for years 1988 through 2003, reported 224 cases of parathyroid cancer. Based on these studies, which capture approximately 60% to 80% of all cancer diagnoses in the United States, between 30 and 50 cases of parathyroid cancers occur annually in the United States.

Parathyroid cancer has an equal gender distribution, unlike benign parathyroid tumors, which have a female predominance in primary hyperparathyroidism (Table 109.1).[4,5] Although there are no differences in gender distribution, male gender is associated with worse overall survival. The age at diagnosis of parathyroid cancer ranges from 23 to 90 years old, with nearly 75% of the patients presenting after the age of 45; the median age at diagnosis is 55 years old.[4,5] No ethnic or racial disparity in the incidence of parathyroid cancer has been observed, unlike benign parathyroid tumors in primary hyperparathyroidism, which are most common in whites.[4,5]

There are very few well-established risk factors associated with parathyroid cancer. Chronic hypercalcemia in the setting of renal failure, secondary hyperparathyroidism, has been reported as a risk factor by some investigators because parathyroid cancer cases developed in patients with end-stage renal disease.[13] It has been proposed that asymmetric nodular parathyroid growth seen in secondary hyperparathyroidism may result in clonal expansion of cells within the polyclonal parathyroid hyperplasia that progress to parathyroid cancer.[14] There have also been some case reports of parathyroid cancer occurring in patients with a history of head and neck irradiation.[3,15] However, unlike benign parathyroid tumors, which develop after head and neck radiation exposure, with a latency period of approximately 30 to 40 years, there is very little clinical evidence to support the association of parathyroid cancer with radiation exposure.[16]

Parathyroid cancer has been observed in some familial cancer syndromes including MEN 1,[17] and to a lesser extent in MEN 2A, but benign parathyroid tumors are much more common in these syndromes.[2,3,18] The familial cancer syndrome associated with the highest risk of developing parathyroid cancer is HPT-JS. Approximately, 75% of affected individuals

TABLE 109.1

DEMOGRAPHICS AND CLINICAL CHARACTERISTICS OF PRIMARY HYPERPARATHYROIDISM DUE TO PARATHYROID CANCER

Institution	Years	Total Cases							
		Cancer	PHPT	% Cancer	M:F Ratio	Mean Age at Presentation (Range)	Mean Tumor Size (cm)	in Tumor Weight (gra)	Mean Serum Calcium (mg/dL)
Mayo	1928–1977	12	2,013	0.6	4:8	51 (29–72)	—	6.8	14.5
Cleveland Clinic	1938–1988	6	1,200	0.47	4:3	47 (20–61)	—	—	15.3
Lahey Clinic	1942–1984	9	0.00	3	3:6	48 (19–64)	3.5	—	14.0
MGH	1948–1983	28	1,200	2.3	14:14	45 (28–72)	3.0	6.7	13.7
MSKCC	1955–1991	14	—	—	7:7	48 (27–81)	3.3	12.0	14.8
Rochester	1958–1990	11	197	5.6	1:10	54 (—)	—	—	15.2
Emory	1960–1982	3	360	0.8	2:1	57 (43–69)	2.9	—	16.1
M.D. Anderson	1968–1982	14	—	—	7:7	— (27–61)	—	16.8	
Michigan	1973–1990	5	1,650	0.37	2:3	46 (35–61)	—	—	17.5
Wake Forest	1975–2004	23	—	—	9:14	54 (26–81)	—	2.7	12.9
Wake Forest	1996–2004	4	586	0.68	—	— (-)	—	—	—
NCD	1985–1995	286	—	—	1:1	54 (14–88)	3.3	—	—
Brazil	1970–1995	10	—	—	2:1	51 (27–74)	—	—	14.3
Italy	1980–1996	19	404	4.7	—	60 (30–78)	3.1	—	15.4
M.D. Anderson	1980–2002	27	—	—	16:11	47 (16–75)	3.0	—	13.4
Dusselorf	1986–1999	4	972	0.4	1:3	41 (13–62)	4.5	—	—
SEER	1988–2003	224	—	—	1:1	56 (23–90)	—	—	—
London	1991–2002	7	—	—	5:2	44 (25–70)	—	—	13.5

PHPT, primary hyperparathyroidism; MGH, Massachusetts General Hospital; MSKCC, Memorial Sloan-Kettering Cancer Center; NCD, National Cancer Data Base; SEER, Surveillance, Epidemiology and End Results Registry.
(Data from refs. 4, 6–10, 35, 36, 40, 54–60.)

develop primary hyperparathyroidism due to parathyroid cancer.[19,20] The predisposing tumor suppressor gene is *HRPT2*. An inactivating germ line mutation of the *HRPT2* gene (*CDC73*) leads to decreased levels of parafibromin.[20] Inactivating somatic mutations of the *HRPT2* gene have also been detected in sporadic cases of parathyroid cancer.

PATHOLOGY

It is often difficult to distinguish parathyroid cancer from what could be an atypical parathyroid adenoma. At the time of the neck exploration, parathyroid cancer is often large (usually larger than 3 cm), hard, and whitish-gray and invades or adheres to the adjacent tissue.[21] For unequivocal diagnosis of parathyroid cancer at the time of neck exploration, there needs to be presence of gross local invasion, lymph node or distant (lung, liver or bone) metastasis, or local recurrence after complete resection (not as a result of tumor spillage at the initial resection). However, distinguishing benign parathyroid tumors (parathyroid adenoma) from parathyroid cancer is difficult, and a diagnosis of parathyroid cancer in most patients is made after disease recurrence.

There is a significant overlap between the histologic appearance of parathyroid adenoma and parathyroid cancer. The most commonly used histologic criteria today were established by Schantz and Castleman[22] in 1973. They reviewed 70 cases of parathyroid cancer and determined microscopic features that distinguished parathyroid cancer from parathyroid adenoma. These microscopic features were trabecular pattern, mitotic figures, nuclear pleomorphism, thick fibrous bands, and capsular and vascular invasion. Most of these criteria, however, are subjective and can also be observed in a spectrum of benign parathyroid tumors (adenoma, atypical adenoma, parathyromatosis, and hyperplasia). Even vascular and capsular invasion may be observed in benign, hemorrhagic, large parathyroid adenoma or as a result of surgical disruption of the capsule during resection of the tumor. Overall, there is no one histopathologic sign that can distinguish between parathyroid cancer and benign disease; definitive diagnosis can be made only with the presence of locoregional invasion or distant metastasis.[2,18]

Because of the difficulty in distinguishing parathyroid cancer from parathyroid adenoma several markers of malignancy have been studied as adjunct to routine hematoxylin and eosin histology. DNA ploidy analysis suggests that parathyroid cancers are more likely to be aneuploid than parathyroid adenomas (60% vs. 9%, respectively).[23] However, variable rates of DNA ploidy have been observed in parathyroid adenoma, making it an unuseful diagnostic adjunct to histology. DNA aneuploidy in parathyroid cancer may be associated with a worse prognosis.[24] Analysis of human telomerase expression in parathyroid tumors may be a helpful adjunct to histology as 100% of parathyroid cancers are positive on immunohistochemistry examination as compared with 6% of parathyroid adenomas (6%).[25]

Another marker of parathyroid cancer that is overexpressed is gelatinase A, but 31% of benign parathyroid tumors are also positive.[26] Immunohistochemistry analysis for increased Ki-67 and galectin 3 expression, and absent parafibromin expression are promising markers for distinguishing parathyroid cancer from benign parathyroid tumors (atypical adenoma, adenoma, parathyromatosis).[14] When used in combination (Ki-67, galectin 3, parafibromin), 15 of 16 parathyroid cancers were correctly identified with only a 3% false-positive rate.[27]

MOLECULAR GENETICS

Our understanding of the genetics of parathyroid tumors has resulted mainly from the clinical and molecular genetic characterization of inherited disorders of primary hyperparathyroidism, including especially HPT-JT. Patients with HPT-JT have ossifying fibromas of the maxilla and mandible, less frequently hamartomas and renal cysts, and develop parathyroid tumors that are mostly parathyroid cancer.[19] The *HRPT2* gene is located on chromosome 1q25-q32 and has been identified to play a key role in development of familial parathyroid cancer and sporadic parathyroid cancer.[19,20,28] *HRPT2* encodes for the tumor suppressor protein parafibromin that is normally expressed in parathyroid tissue. This gene consists of 17 exons but most inactivating germ line mutations occur in exon 1. This germ line inactivation in HPT-JT patients has been linked to the increased risk of parathyroid cancer.[19] Shattuck et al.[20] also reported somatic and germ line mutation in 10 of 15 patients with sporadic parathyroid cancers.

Cyclin D1 has also been implicated in parathyroid tumorigensis. Overexpression of cyclin D1 has been observed in parathyroid adenoma. Vasef et al.[29] showed overexpression of cyclin D1 in 11 of 12 parathyroid cancers. Although cyclin D1 overexpression has been seen in parathyroid cancer, it appears that the increase in expression may be related to increased proliferation and not to pathogenesis of parathyroid cancer.[3] Furthermore, it appears that parafibromin regulates cyclin D1 and thus may be a downstream effector of parafibromin. *In vitro* studies have shown that up-regulation in parafibromin leads to a reduction in cyclin D1 expression.[30] Genomic loss on chromosome 13 has been implicated in parathyroid cancer.[31] Tumor suppressor genes retinoblastoma (*Rb1*) and *BRCA2* are located on chromosome 13. However, analysis of parathyroid cancers has shown no chromosomal loss in the region of these genes.[32]

CLINICAL MANIFESTATIONS

Almost all parathyroid cancers are biochemically active. Nonfunctional parathyroid cancer is extremely rare.[33] The majority of patients with parathyroid cancer have profound clinical manifestations of primary hyperparathyroidism and present with severe hypercalcemia. Nearly 70% of patients with parathyroid cancer have serum total calcium values greater than 14 mg/dL (normal range, 8.0–10.2 mg/dL) and parathyroid hormone levels more than 5 to 10 times greater than normal (Table 109.1).[21] Patients with parathyroid cancer exhibit profound symptoms and signs of hypercalcemia including polydipsia, polyuria, nausea, anorexia, constipation, muscle weakness, fatigue, depression, peptic ulcers, acute pancreatitis, and even parathyrotoxicosis (hypercalcemic crisis).[21] The rate of metabolic complications associated with primary hyperparathyroidism is also much higher in patients with parathyroid cancer than patients with benign parathyroid tumors. Renal disease can manifest itself as nephrolithiasis, nephrocalcinosis, and or renal colic, and can lead to chronic renal insufficiency.[34,35] Hyperparathyroidism bone disease manifestations include osteitis fibrosa cystica, subperiosteal bone resorption, "salt and pepper" skull, diffuse osteopenia, osteoporosis, bone pain, or pathologic fractures, and is present in 22% to 91% of patients with parathyroid cancer at the time of diagnosis.[27,35–40] Up to 50% of patients with parathyroid cancer present with both bone and renal disease; with benign causes of primary hyperparathyroidism, less than 5% of patients present with bone and renal disease.[41]

Parathyroid cancer may be detected on physical examination (Table 109.2). In some series, up to 45% of patients have a palpable fixed neck mass at the time of diagnosis.[11] A palpable parathyroid gland greater than 3 cm is suspicious for cancer.[4] Parathyroid cancer may also cause local symptoms such as dysphagia, dyspnea, dysphonia, odynophagia, and/or ear pain from local invasion.[35] A preoperative laryngoscopy should be performed in patients with voice change, as a vocal cord paralysis may be present from tumor invasion of the recurrent laryngeal nerve and should be recognized before operative intervention. Most commonly, parathyroid cancer invades the adjacent thyroid lobe, but invasion into the esophagus, trachea, carotid sheet, strap muscles, and mediastinum is not uncommon.[21,40] Some patients may present with central or lateral neck lymphadenopathy from regional lymph node metastasis, which occurs in 4% to 8% of patients.[4,5,9] In the Surveillance, Epidemiology and End Results database, distant metastasis was present in 4.5% of cases. Common sites of distant metastasis are lung, bone, and liver.

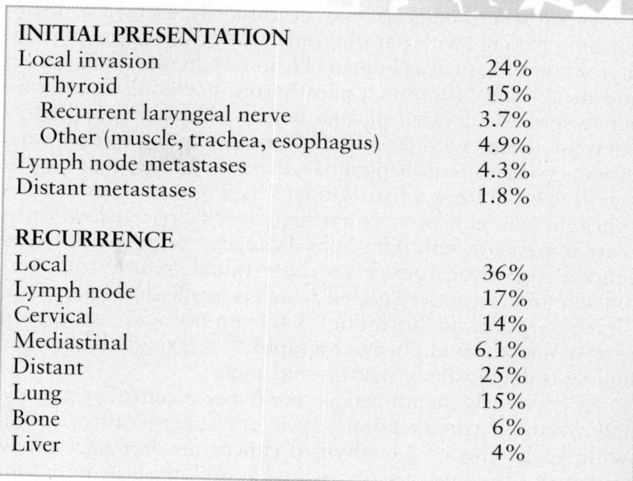

TABLE 109.2

SITES OF PARATHYROID CANCER AT PRESENTATION AND AT RECURRENCE

INITIAL PRESENTATION	
Local invasion	24%
Thyroid	15%
Recurrent laryngeal nerve	3.7%
Other (muscle, trachea, esophagus)	4.9%
Lymph node metastases	4.3%
Distant metastases	1.8%
RECURRENCE	
Local	36%
Lymph node	17%
Cervical	14%
Mediastinal	6.1%
Distant	25%
Lung	15%
Bone	6%
Liver	4%

DIAGNOSIS

The diagnosis of primary hyperparathyroidism can be accurately established by simultaneous biochemical testing for total serum and ionized calcium and intact parathyroid hormone in most cases. In patients with hypercalcemia and normal or high-normal intact parathyroid hormone levels, it is important to exclude benign familial hypercalcemia hypocalciuria by measuring 24 urinary calcium levels. In patients with normal total serum calcium but elevated parathyroid hormone levels and no evidence of renal insufficiency, vitamin D deficiency should be excluded by measuring serum 25-dihyrdoxylvitamin D.

Once the diagnosis of primary hyperparathyroidism is confirmed, making a preoperative diagnosis of parathyroid cancer as the cause is often difficult. No single laboratory finding is diagnostic of parathyroid cancer, but certain findings may suggest the diagnosis. The mean serum calcium in parathyroid cancer patients is 14.6 to 15.0 mg/dL.[27,35,38] and about 60% to 65% of patients present with a calcium level greater than 14 mg/dL.[27,35,38] Only a very small subset of patients with functional parathyroid cancers have normal serum calcium levels despite elevated parathyroid hormone levels at diagnosis.[42] Although intact parathyroid hormone levels in parathyroid cancer are 5 to 10 times the upper limit of the normal range,[27,35,36,38,43] there is no reliable threshold level for malignancy because large benign parathyroid tumors can be associated with high levels and are much more common than parathyroid cancer. Patients with parathyroid cancer often have elevated alkaline phosphatase and low serum phosphorus levels.

Several serum markers may be clinically useful for distinguishing patients with parathyroid cancer from a benign parathyroid tumors, such as human chorionic gonadotropin (serum and urine) and N-terminal parathyroid hormone immunoreactive species. Elevated plasma human chorionic gonadotropin is associated with parathyroid cancer[44] but can be elevated in some patients with benign parathyroid tumors, causing primary hyperparathyroidism. Urinary hyperglycosylated human chorionic gonadotropin G has high specificity but low sensitivity in patients with parathyroid cancer.[45] Some parathyroid cancers also overproduce the N-terminal parathyroid hormone immunoreactive species, which is less hydrophobic than intact parathyroid hormone (1-84 amino acid length) on reverse-phase liquid chromatography.[46] No single laboratory finding is diagnostic of parathyroid cancer.

As previously mentioned, severe hypercalcemia, symptoms and metabolic complication of primary hyperparathyroidism, while suggestive of parathyroid cancer are not necessarily diagnostic. The presence of a palpable neck mass is more suggestive parathyroid cancer, and some preoperative localizing studies may be helpful. Preoperative imaging is frequently helpful for parathyroid tumor localization, but in the evaluation of primary hyperparathyroidism it cannot reliably distinguish between parathyroid cancer and benign parathyroid tumors causing primary hyperparathyroidism. Some investigators have identified several ultrasound features associated with parathyroid cancer, which include heterogeneity, hypoechogenicity, and irregular tumor borders,[47] but such characteristics are not always present in parathyroid cancers.[48] Fine-needle aspiration of a parathyroid tumor should be avoided in patients with suspected parathyroid cancer because of the documented risk of cutaneous or subcutaneous seeding along the needle track, and because cytologic examination is not accurate for the diagnosis of parathyroid cancer.[49,50]

The diagnosis of parathyroid cancer can sometimes be difficult to make clinically or on histologic examination. Like most endocrine malignancies, there are no definitive histologic diagnostic criteria for parathyroid cancer.[2] The diagnosis can be made only in a patient who has either locoregional or distant metastasis at the time of initial neck exploration. If a patient has severe symptoms and metabolic complications associated with their primary hyperparathyroidism, a palpable and large parathyroid tumor, a serum calcium level greater than 14 mg/dL, and parathyroid hormone levels 5 to 10 times greater than the upper limit of normal, then the diagnosis of a parathyroid cancer should be suspected.[21]

MANAGEMENT OF PARATHYROID CANCER

Surgical resection is the only curative therapy for parathyroid cancer. The most critical and yet the most difficult aspect of treating parathyroid cancer is the preoperative or intraoperative diagnosis of parathyroid cancer that will enable the surgeon to perform the appropriate operation. An *en bloc* resection of the tumor and the involved structure(s) has been associated with decreased risk of recurrent disease. At the very least, the surgical resection should include *en bloc* removal of the tumor and ipsilateral thyroid lobectomy. Systemic chemotherapy and external-beam radiation are not effective in patients with parathyroid cancer.

Patients with parathyroid cancer can present with severe or uncontrollable hypercalcemia. Correction of the electrolyte imbalance is critical as it could lead to irreversible cardiac and renal complication. Rehydration with normal saline and repletion of electrolytes such as magnesium can aid with renal function and stabilize the cardiac function.[21] The addition of loop diuretics after adequate hydration can improve the urinary excretion of calcium. Osteoclast inhibitors such as calcitonin and plicamycin can be used in patients with hypercalcemic crisis. Bisphosphonates can also be used to the lower calcium level. However, the effects of bisphosphonates decrease over time. Amifostine, an agent that inhibits parathyroid hormone release, has also been used but its use has been limited because of its side effect profile.[51] In most patients with severe hypercalcemia, vigorous hydration and the use of a loop diuretic are able to make them eucalcemic. In patients with chronic hypercalcemia as a result of unresectable parathyroid cancer, second- generation calcimimetic therapy may helpful.[21]

Surgical Treatment

If parathyroid cancer is suspected at the initial operation, an *en bloc* resection of the tumor should be performed.[21,24] If a patient presents with a hoarse voice, invasion of the recurrent laryngeal nerve should be suspected and direct laryngoscopy should be performed preoperatively to confirm the paralysis. In symptomatic patients and in patients with nerve involvement, it is appropriate to resect the nerve because the risk of recurrence outweighs the benefit of preserving the nerve. Care must be taken to remove the tumor without any capsular disruption, as rupture of the capsule of even benign parathyroid tumor can lead to parathyromatosis (diffuse seeding of the neck and mediastinum with parathyroid cells that implant and grow).[52] Frozen section biopsy of suspicious gland is not recommended as it could also lead to tumor spread and is not accurate for diagnosing parathyroid cancer. The adjacent thyroid lobe is usually involved and removed with isthmusectomy. Such an *en bloc* resection is associated with improved outcome.[21,53]

Parathyroid cancer can also invade the overlaying strap muscles, trachea, esophagus, and recurrent laryngeal nerve. All invaded tissue must be removed and appropriate reconstruction should be done at the time of the initial operation. Lymph node metastasis occurs in up to 8% of patients with parathyroid cancer.[4,5,24] The ipsilateral central neck compartment should be explored and any suspicious lymph nodes should be removed and evaluated by frozen section analysis.[21,38] If there are any clinically involved lymph nodes, a formal dissection of the central and lateral neck compartment should be done. Wide local excision and prophylactic neck dissection do not appear to improve prognosis.[41] In the immediate postoperative period, electrolyte levels should be monitored diligently as the patient is at high risk for severe hypocalcemia secondary to hungry bone syndrome.[34] Phosphate and magnesium levels should be monitored also because calcium supplementation may affect their levels.

Radiotherapy

Parathyroid cancer is generally not radiosensitive, and radiation treatment as primary therapy has not been demonstrated to have a significant effect in either the neck or at sites of distant metastases. Some case reports, however, have suggested that adjuvant radiation treatment after surgical resection may decrease the risk of local recurrence.[35] Patients with parathyroid cancer have been treated with 66 to 70 Gy and showed no evidence of recurrence at 53 to 66 months of follow-up. In one study, negative operative margins were documented for three patients; thus, apparent curative treatment might not be attributable solely to the adjuvant radiation therapy.[54] The possibility that parathyroid cancer might be responsive to radiation was suggested because of six patients with microscopic residual disease at the time of surgery who were found to have no recurrence at mean follow-up of 62 months.[55] In another study, only one of a series of six patients with locally invasive parathyroid cancer treated with postoperative radiation developed a recurrence.[40] However, two of the patients in the study were treated with simple parathyroidectomy, not *en bloc* resection, and neither patient had developed a recurrence at 84 and 228 months of follow-up.[40]

It is difficult to know the efficacy of radiotherapy for decreasing risk of local recurrence given that the level of clinical evidence constitutes only small case series because parathyroid cancer is a rare diagnosis. Moreover, the clinical behavior of parathyroid cancer, with respect to disease recurrence, is variable, and the diagnosis may not always be accurately established to ascertain the effect of adjuvant radiotherapy after resection. Adjuvant radiation therapy does not affect the survival of patients with parathyroid cancer.

Chemotherapy

As previously mentioned, chemotherapy is not effective for parathyroid cancer. In patients with metastatic parathyroid cancer, short-term, partial responses have been reported with dacarbazine alone and with combination regimens of fluorouracil, cyclophosphamide, and dacarbazine.[56] In one patient with metastatic nonfunctioning disease, treatment with methotrexate, Adriamycin, cyclophosphamide, and 1-(2-chloroethyl)-3-cyclohexyl-1-nitrosourea resulted in response of a large anterior mediastinal mass over an 18-month period.[57] There is no clear survival benefit associated with chemotherapy in patients with parathyroid cancer.

Other Treatment Modalities of Parathyroid Cancer

Because the major morbidity and ultimate cause of death in most patients with parathyroid cancer is complications from severe hypercalcemia, medical management has focused on controlling calcium levels in patients with persistent or recurrent disease. Unresectable disease due to diffuse metastases in the lung has been treated with multiple sessions of radiofrequency ablation in a patient with parathyroid cancer.[58] Transcatheter arterial embolization with radiofrequency ablation has been also used to treat multiple metastatic lesions in the liver in one patient.[59] In these case reports, improved control in both serum calcium and parathyroid hormone levels was observed after treatment. Recurrent disease in the neck that was unresectable has been treated with ultrasound-guided percutaneous alcohol injection, and short-term improvements in serum calcium and parathyroid hormone levels have been reported.[60]

As previously mentioned, acute hypercalcemia is treated with standard therapies such as intravenous hydration, furosemide, calcitonin, glucocorticoids, mithramycin, and hemodialysis, but these treatments are ineffective for long-term management. Short-term decreases in serum calcium, on the order of months, have been demonstrated with the intravenous bisphosphonate pamidronate,[61] and long-term remission rarely has been achieved.[62] Similarly, treatment of hypercalcemia with intravenous zoledronate has also been described.[63] Initial treatment appears to be clinically significant in some patients, but the effect generally diminishes with subsequent infusions. Oral bisphosphonates have not been reported to be effective in the management of hypercalcemia that is related to parathyroid cancer. Octreotide may decrease parathyroid hormone secretion,[64] but there is no evidence it improves the hypercalcemia of parathyroid cancer.[65]

Calcimimetic therapy has emerged as a more effective solution to mitigate the hypercalcemia of parathyroid cancer. A second-generation calcimimetic, cinacalcet, was shown to decrease serum calcium by 1 mg/dL in 62% of patients with parathyroid cancer.[66] Patients tolerated total daily doses up to 360 mg. In responders, the magnitude of decrease in calcium levels was greatest in those with the highest baseline calcium levels. Interestingly, decreases in serum calcium were achieved despite no significant decrease in serum parathyroid hormone.[67]

Although modalities such as surgery, adjuvant radiation, radiofrequency ablation, and calcimimetic therapy have demonstrated responses in clinical parameters, insufficient information is available to determine the effects of these therapies on survival.

FOLLOW-UP AND NATURAL HISTORY

Lifelong follow-up is required for patients with parathyroid cancer as locoregional and distant metastasis may occur up to 35 years after initial treatment. Over 50% of patients with parathyroid cancer develop recurrent disease, with the neck being the most common site of recurrence (80%).[54] The mean time to recurrence has been reported to be slightly over 33 months, but recurrence over a long period of time has also been reported.[34] As mentioned earlier, rate of recurrence is much higher when the diagnosis of parathyroid cancer was not known at initial operation and *en bloc* parathyroidectomy was not performed. Disruption of the parathyroid capsule also plays a large role in recurrence. Complete *en bloc* resection is associated with an 8% local recurrence rate.[53] Biochemical monitoring for parathyroid hormone and calcium levels is a very sensitive and accurate method to detect persistent or recurrent disease. If there is biochemical evidence of persistent or recurrent disease, a high-resolution ultrasound of the neck is a fast and noninvasive diagnostic test with a sensitivity of 69%.[43] Distant metastasis is best detected with whole-body sestamibi scan and computed tomography or magnetic resonance imaging scan of the chest, neck, and abdomen because the lung, bone, and mediastinum, which are the most common sites for distant metastasis. The sensitivity of magnetic resonance imaging, sestamibi scan, and computed tomography has been reported to be 93%, 79%, and 67%, respectively.[43]

Once biochemical recurrence has been documented, it is important to distinguish between local and distant recurrence. Noninvasive localizing studies are used to rule out lung and bone metastasis (Fig. 109.1). If noninvasive studies are nondiagnostic, selective venous sampling for parathyroid hormone is done to locate the site of recurrence. If localized sites of distant metastasis are present, resection of this site of disease could be helpful in achieving good biochemical and symptom control. For local recurrence, reoperation is indicated with resection of any cervical and/or mediastinal recurrences. A reduction in tumor burden improves symptoms and may normalize parathyroid hormone and serum calcium levels in up to 75% of patients.[43,68] However, in patients with disseminated disease, reoperation is not likely to provide any symptomatic relief.

In patients with widespread metastatic disease, medical management is the only remaining option. Bisphosphonates are fairly effective but dose escalation may be required as their effectiveness diminishes over time.[34] Recently, cinacalcet, a calcimimetic agent, has been shown to be effective in parathyroid cancer.[63,67] Cinacalcet targets the calcium-sensing receptor on the surface of the chief cells and acts as an allosteric modulator of the calcium-sensing receptor and decreases parathyroid response to any of these regimens will need to have steroid replacement with prednisone or hydrocortisone for adrenal insufficiency and to reduce the risk of Addisonian crisis.

Radiation

Various adjunct treatment methods have been used to improve survival in patients with ACC. Radiation therapy, though beneficial for some malignancies, has been ineffective at increasing survival in patients with ACC. Local irradiation to the tumor bed has been suggested to reduce the rate of local recurrence.[6,73,74] Though the results are variable, radiation therapy is currently reserved as palliative therapy for patients with symptomatic bone metastases.[6,73]

Prognosis

Due to the lack of effective systemic therapy and the late stage of presentation of most patients with ACC, the prognosis for ACC is poor. The overall 5-year survival ranges between 16% to 38%.[13,70,75,76] Prognosis depends on the tumor stage, and based on the new ENSAT staging system, 5-year survival rates were 84% for stage I, 63% for stage II, 51% for stage III, and 15% for stage IV.

PEDIATRIC ADRENOCORTICAL CARCINOMA

As mentioned previously, the incidence of adrenocortical carcinoma has a bimodal distribution with a smaller peak between birth and 10 years old.[9,10] Unlike in adults, the majority of pediatric ACCs are functional and present with symptoms related to excess hormone production and virilization symptoms. There is also a slight female predominance, and just like adult ACC, the mainstay of treatment is a complete surgical resection. As opposed to adult ACC, up to 50% of pediatric ACCs are associated with genetic alterations and associated with syndromes such as Li-Fraumeni syndrome (tumor suppressor gene p53) and Beckwith-Wiedemann syndrome (11p15).[77]

PHEOCHROMOCYTOMA

Pheochromocytomas are neuroendocrine tumors that arise from the chromaffin cells of the adrenal medulla or can arise from the extra-adrenal sympathetic ganglia. Their name is derived from the Greek word *pheos* (dusky or gray brown), which describes the color that they stain when they are exposed to chromium salts. Pheochromocytoma was first described by Frankel in 1886, where he described an 18-year-old patient with a 1-year history of palpitations, headaches, and dizziness. The patient suddenly collapsed and died and at autopsy was found to have bilateral adrenal nodules.[78] Discovery of vasoactive hormones in the 1920s facilitated development of assay to detect such agents, most notably epinephrine. Unlike ACC, virtually all adrenal pheochromocytomas are functional, and their clinical manifestations are secondary to excess catecholamines. Paragangliomas are pheochromocytomas that arise from extra-adrenal chromaffin cells, and they can be found along the paravertebral and para-aortic axes.[79,80] Due to their hormonally functional status, urinary catecholamines, normetanephrine, and metanephrine have been reliable for the diagnosis and screening for this condition. Although measurement of fractionated plasma catecholamines, normetanephrine, and metanephrine levels, which is less cumbersome than measuring 24-hour urinary catecholamines, normetanephrine, and metanephrine, is becoming more widely available and implemented, these tests should be considered to be complementary to increase both sensitivity and specificity rather than mutually exclusive tests.[79,81,82] Both pheochromocytomas and paragangliomas may be malignant in approximately 10% of cases.

Epidemiology

Pheochromocytoma is a rare condition, with an annual incidence of 1 to 8 cases per million persons.[80,83] It is estimated that 0.1% to 0.6% of adults with hypertension and 4% to 5% of those with adrenal incidentaloma harbor pheochromocytoma.[80,83–85] Approximately 25% of pheochromocytomas are discovered incidentally.[86] There is a classic teaching called "the Rule of Tens," which describes the natural history of pheochromocytoma. This rule implies that 10% of pheochromocytomas are malignant, 10% are bilateral, 10% are familial, and 10% are extra-adrenal. To this day, most series concur with this description, with the exception of a few studies that indicate a certain degree of inaccuracy to this rule.[87–89] With the recent advancement in molecular genetics, the cases that were previously described as sporadic are now being identified to have somatic and/or germline mutations associated with familial predisposition in up to 30% of cases.[89] The rate of malignancy is approximately 10% with a range of 3% to 50%.[90] The rate of bilateral tumors varies greatly depending on the patient's germline mutational status; although in sporadic cases the rule still holds to be approximately 10%.[87] As many as 25% of pheochromocytomas are found in an extra-adrenal location.[87] Extra-adrenal pheochromocytomas (paragangliomas) have a slightly higher rate of malignancy, approximately 40%.[91]

Clinical Presentation

The clinical manifestations of pheochromocytomas are commonly related to the production of excess catecholamines. The clinical presentation of benign and malignant pheochromocytomas is similar.[90] The classic triad of symptoms associated with pheochromocytoma (tachycardia with diaphoresis and cephalalgia) is present in 40% to 80% of patients and is highly sensitive and specific for patients with presumptive diagnosis of pheochromocytoma.[79] Although hypertension is present in most patients with pheochromocytoma, it may be paroxysmal and is nonspecific for the diagnosis. Other symptoms associated with pheochromocytomas are tremors, palpitations, and anxiety. Some patients present with an adrenal incidentaloma and no obvious symptoms.

Diagnosis

The combination of free fractionated plasma normetanephrine and metanephrine or 24-hour urinary normetanephrine and metanephrine is an accurate method for making the diagnosis of pheochromocytoma, with a sensitivity ranging from 96% to 100% and 92% to 99%, and a specificity of 87% to 92% and 64% and 72%, respectively.[79]

Although both CT and MRI scans are helpful for localizing pheochromocytoma with similar sensitivity and specificity, MRI is the preferred imaging modality as the intravenous contrast used for CT is known to cause catecholamine release, and pheochromocytoma have a pathognomonic hyperintense characteristic on T2-weighted MRI with gadolinium (Fig. 110.2).[83] Most pheochromocytomas are functional; therefore the diagnosis is based on biochemical analysis rather than on radiography. Imaging studies, however, are still crucial in order to localize the tumor(s) and distinguish between adrenal versus extra-adrenal pheochromocytomas, to assess for any evidence

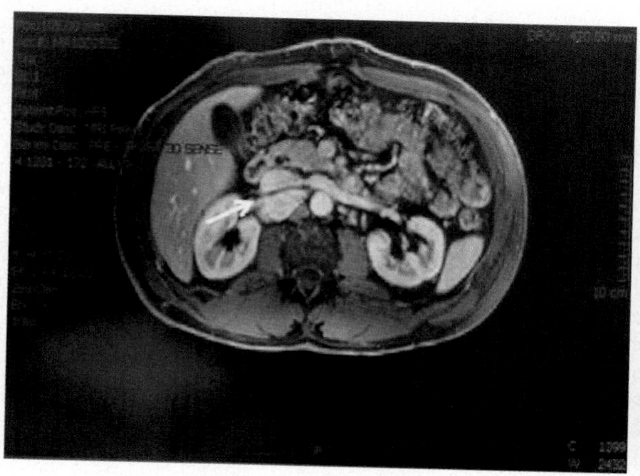

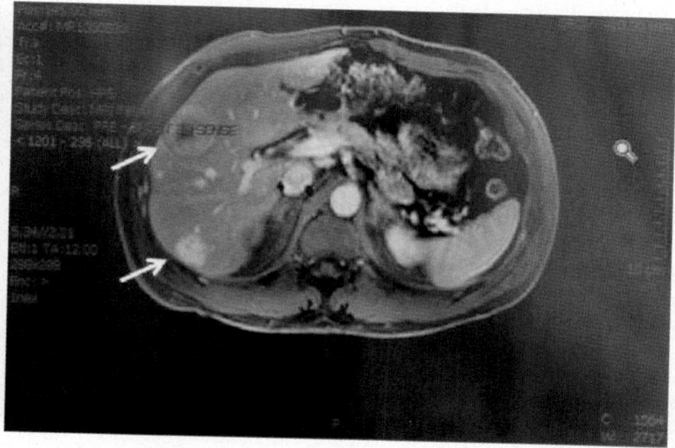

FIGURE 110.2 Magnetic resonance T2-weighted image with gadolinium showing metastatic pheochromocytoma. **A:** In the right adrenal bed extending inferiorly and encompassing the renal vein (*arrow*) and **B:** in segments 7 and 8 of the liver (*arrow*).

of metastatic disease, and to determine resectability. Generally, pheochromocytomas appear homogenous on CT scans and are larger when malignant.[24,92] If there is a clinical suspicion of pheochromocytoma with normal appearing adrenal glands, CT scan should be performed from the level of the diaphragm down to the pelvis to look for extra-adrenal pheochromocytomas or paragangliomas.[23] Iodine-131-meta-iodobenzylguanidine (^{131}I MIBG) is helpful for locating multiple and extra-adrenal pheochromocytomas or paragangliomas. More recent studies have indicated that fluorodeoxyglucose (^{18}F)-DOPA positron emission tomography (PET) and ^{18}F-fluorodopamine (FDA) PET/CT are effective in localizing both adrenal and extra-adrenal pheochromocytomas and should be considered for second-line imaging studies if other studies are nonlocalizing.[93–95]

Molecular Genetics

Much of the understanding of the genetic changes involved in malignant pheochromocytoma is based on studies of inherited familial cancer syndromes associated with pheochromocytoma. Approximately 10% to 25% of pheochromocytoma are associated with autosomal dominant hereditary cancer syndromes such as MEN-2A or MEN-2B, von Hippel-Lindau syndrome (VHL), paraganglioma syndrome type 1, 3, and 4 (PGL-1 [SDHD]; PGL-3 [SDHC]; PGL-4 [SDHB]), and neurofibromatosis 1 (NF-1).[96] At some medical centers, mutation testing is routinely performed for *RET, VHL, SDHB,* and *SDHD,* and germline mutations have been detected in 20% to 30% of all pheochromocytomas, demonstrating a familial predisposition that is higher than the 10% of tumors previously thought to be hereditary.[89,97] Mutations in *SDHB, SDHD, SDH5,* and rarely *SDHC* are associated with relatively high rates of extra-adrenal compared to adrenal tumors, and the presence of *SDHB* mutations is associated with more aggressive tumor behavior and a higher rate of malignancy (38% to 83%).[89,97–101]

Pathology

It is difficult to accurately distinguish benign from malignant pheochromocytomas based solely on histology. However, some features such as local or vascular invasion, tumor necrosis, tumor size greater than 5 cm, and DNA ploidy may be suggestive of malignancy but are not highly accurate.[78] Thompson[102] proposed the pheochromocytomas of the adrenal gland scaled score (PASS) to distinguish benign from malignant tumors based on histomorphologic features. These features included growth pattern, necrosis, cellularity and cellular monotony, tumor cell spindling, mitotic court and atypical mitotic figures, invasion, nuclear pleomorphism, and hyperchromasia. A score of 4 or greater was associated with a significantly higher risk of malignancy compared with a PASS score of less than 4. However, many of the criteria may be subjective, no indeterminate category of lesion with uncertain malignant potential was included, and no follow-up studies by other investigators have validated the scoring system.

Because of the limitations in accurately distinguishing between benign and malignant pheochromocytoma, several investigators have evaluated adjunct molecular markers to improve diagnostic accuracy. Increased Ki-67 expression by immunohistochemistry is associated with malignant pheochromocytoma if 6% or more of the tumor stains positive.[103] Also, increased telomerase expression may be a helpful adjunct diagnostic marker, as 67% of malignant tumors are positive compared to only 9.5% of benign tumors.[104]

Treatment

The only curative treatment for pheochromocytoma is surgical resection. Patients with pheochromocytoma need preoperative blockade with selective or nonselective alpha-1 blockers (prazosin, doxazosin, phenoxybenzamine) and beta-blockers, with or without calcium channel blockers, angiotensin-converting enzyme (ACE) inhibitors, or drugs such as metyrosine (Demser) that blocks synthesis of catecholamines. All these preoperative interventions reduce perioperative morbidity and mortality by reducing perioperative hemodynamic instability.[79,83] Laparoscopic adrenalectomy has become the surgical intervention of choice for pheochromocytoma.[79,105] Some series advocate cortex-sparing adrenalectomy, especially in patients with benign familial pheochromocytoma that require bilateral adrenalectomy.[83,106] Although one can prevent the need for lifelong steroid replacement therapy with cortex-sparing adrenalectomy, a relatively high risk of local disease recurrence has been reported with this procedure.[83]

In malignant pheochromocytoma and functional paraganglioma, resection of the primary lesion and or debulking of metastatic sites may serve to reduce the morbidity associated with the excess hormonal effect, in particular, adverse effect on the cardiovascular system. Palliative surgery may also be applicable when a tumor is located in critical anatomical location.[107] However, there are no data to show that cytoreductive surgery has an impact on survival or even on objective improvement of symptoms.[90] A transabdominal open surgical approach is the preferred method for malignant pheochromocytoma rather than a laparoscopic approach, which is best for small benign pheochromocytomas. Malignant pheochromocytomas are often larger than their benign counterparts, and an open approach enables the surgeon to access the tumor, resection the locoregional lymph nodes, and locate and resect extra-adrenal lesions not detected on preoperative imaging.[90]

After the resection of malignant pheochromocytoma, adjuvant ^{131}I-MIBG is recommended in patients with metastatic disease. The concept of using ^{131}I-MIBG is similar to the use of ^{131}I in well-differentiated thyroid cancer, where selective uptake of the radioactive isotope is intended to ablate mainly the malignant tissue with acceptable systemic toxicity. The use of ^{131}I-MIBG for malignant pheochromocytoma was first used at the University of Michigan in 1984, and there have been multiple studies using this agent since; however, there has been no standardization of the procedure and the dose of ^{131}I used.[108,109] However, complete response rates of up to 25% and partial response rates of up to 35% have been observed using 492 to 1,160 mCu of ^{131}I-MIBG.[110,111]

Several chemotherapeutic regimens have been studied for treatment of malignant pheochromocytoma; however, the small number of patients has made the establishment of standardized cytotoxic regimen difficult. Alkylating agents such as cyclophosphamide have been used in most centers, and the most effective regimen that has been described is the combination of cyclophosphamide, vincristine, and dacarbazine (CVD protocol), first introduced in 1985 by Keiser et al.[112] In some of the most recent studies, the complete response rate ranges between 0% to 33% and the partial response rate is between 0% to 57%.[113]

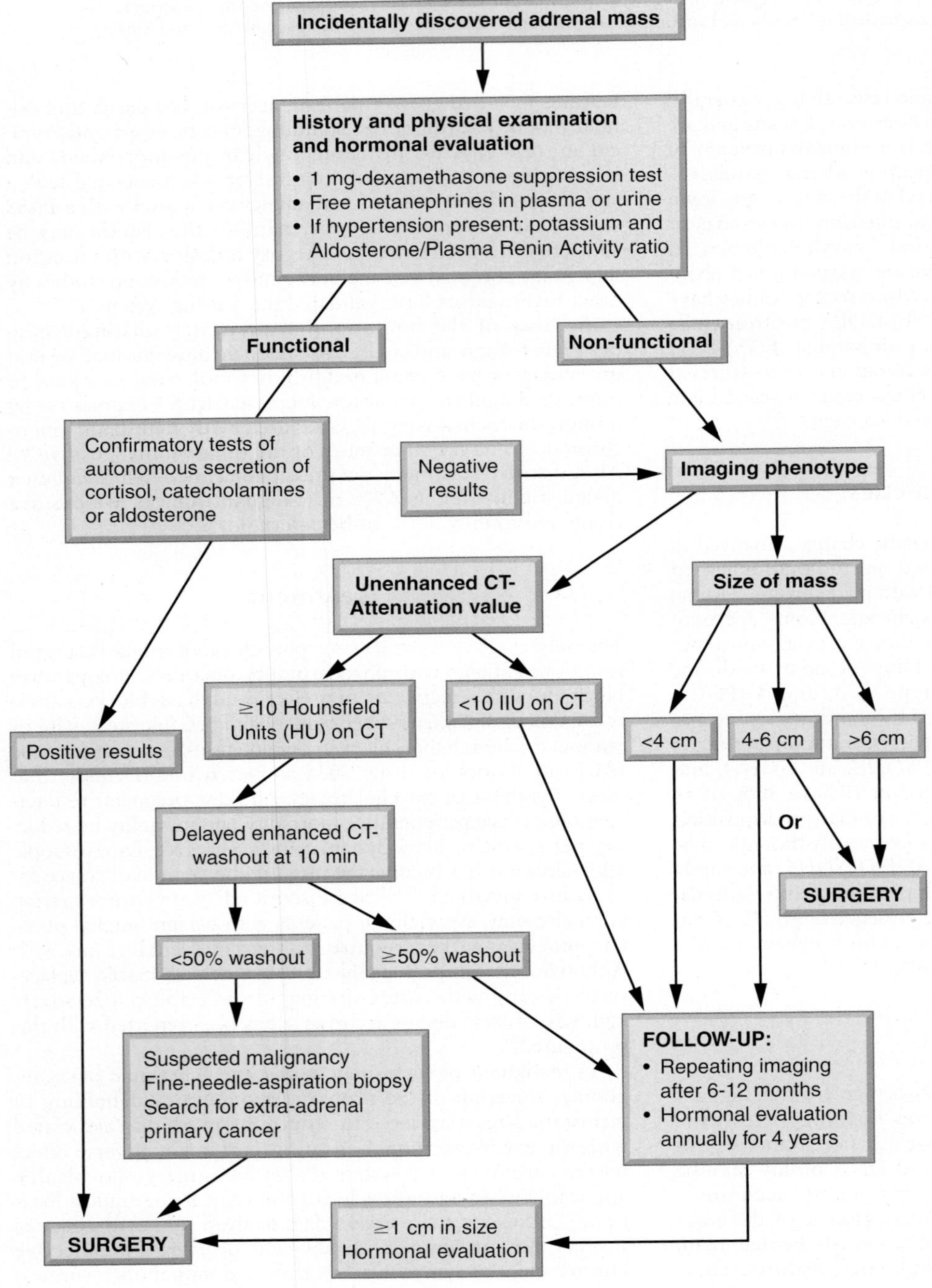

FIGURE 110.3 Algorithm for management of patients with adrenal incidentalomas.

Prognosis

Patients who have malignant pheochromocytoma have more than a 50% mortality rate at 5 years' follow-up.[114] Recurrent disease may develop within 2 to 5 years but could be variable with some patients developing disease recurrence 20 years after initial treatment. There is no American Joint Commission on Cancer staging system for malignant pheochromocytoma.

ADRENAL INCIDENTALOMA

Adrenal incidentalomas (AI) are tumors of the adrenal gland discovered incidentally on imaging studies performed for other indications. The prevalence of adrenal incidentaloma on CT and MRI scans ranges between 0.6% to 4%[1,2] and 1% to 15% at autopsy.[2,115] The prevalence of AI also depends on the age of the study cohort because it is as low as 0.2% in patients less than 30 years of age, whereas patients older than 70 have an adrenal tumor detect in 6% to 15% of cases.[1,115] The rate of AI is also higher in patients with a known history of other malignancy, but some would not consider such a finding as incidental as follow-up imaging studies are performed to detect sites of possible metastasis and disease recurrence.

Adrenal incidentaloma may either be functioning or nonfunctioning, benign adrenocortical adenoma, adrenocortical carcinoma, pheochromocytoma, or a metastatic lesion (Table 110.1). The intervention would depend on the nature of the lesion. It is important to determine the functional status of the tumor as well as to distinguish between benign versus malignant. A thorough history and physical examination, with assessment for the potential for malignancy based on several criteria, are important in the evaluation of patients with AI (Fig. 110.3). All patients with AI should undergo biochemical testing to check the functional status of the tumor, as approximately 15% to 20% hypersecrete hormones at the time of their discovery.[2] Biochemical testing should include plasma aldosterone, plasma renin, plasma fractionated normetanephrine and metanephrine levels, and 24-hour urinary cortisol.

The treatment for virtually all functional AIs is adrenalectomy. For those patients with nonfunctioning AIs, the risk of malignancy should be determined (primary malignancy or metastatic lesion to the adrenal gland). Frequency of malignancy in AI is approximately 1% to 5%, although the number varies greatly depending on the tumor size.[53,116] There are several radiographic characteristics that are also suggestive of malignancy but they are not always accurate, such as irregular margins, heterogeneous appearance, tumor size greater than 6 cm, and high attenuation on CT scan with intravenous contrast.[2] Patients with history of a primary malignancy should have a full work-up with imaging studies, including PET, to accurately determine if the adrenal tumor is a solitary synchronous or metachronous site of disease. This may be a rare instance when a fine-needle aspiration is indicated for tissue diagnosis, although some will argue that simple adrenalectomy should be offered for patients with metastasis confined to the adrenal gland because adrenal metastasis is usually well circumscribed within the capsule.[117] Laparoscopic resection of a metastatic lesion can be performed safely without any increased rate for port-site recurrence.[117,118] For those patients with nonfunctioning tumor without a history of prior primary malignancy and suspicion of primary ACC, the decision to intervene is based on the size of the lesion. The current recommendation is to resect lesions that are suspicious or known ACC, pheochromocytoma, functioning adenoma, and tumors greater than 4 cm.[3] There is also a controversy surrounding the management of subclinical Cushing syndrome (SCS) in adrenal incidentalomas, and there is no standard management for this condition, although some would advocate early surgical resection due to association with cardiovascular morbidity.[1] There is no gold standard for follow-up of adrenal incidentalomas that are not resected, and according to the National Institutes of Health State of the Science, they should be followed with imaging studies every 6 to 12 months. Hormone excess may develop in 20% of these lesions, and further follow-up is not indicated in patients whose lesions do not change in size over time.

PRACTICE OF ONCOLOGY

Selected References

The full list of references for this chapter appears in the online version.

1. Anagnostis P, Karagiannis A, Tziomalos K, et al. Adrenal incidentaloma: a diagnostic challenge. *Hormones* 2009;(3):163.
2. Singh PK, Buch HN. Adrenal incidentaloma: evaluation and management. *J Clin Pathol* 2008;61(11):1168.
3. Terzolo M, Bovio S, Pia A, Reimondo G, Angeli A. Management of adrenal incidentaloma. *Best Prac Res Clin Endocrinol Metab* 2009;23(2):233.
4. Golden SH, Robinson KA, Saldanha I, Anton B, Ladenson PW. Prevalence and incidence of endocrine and metabolic disorders in the United States: a comprehensive review. *J Clin Endocrinol Metab* 2009;94(6):1853.
5. Kebebew E, Reiff E, Duh QY, Clark O, McMillan A. Extent of disease at presentation and outcome for adrenocortical carcinoma: have we made progress? *World J Surg* 2006;30(5):872.
10. Ribeiro RC, Figueiredo B. Childhood adrenocortical tumours. *Eur J Cancer* 2004;40(8):1117.
13. Icard P, Goudet P, Charpenay C, et al. Adrenocortical carcinomas: surgical trends and results of a 253-patient series from the French Association of Endocrine Surgeons study group. *World J Surg* 2001;25(7):891.
15. Kendrick ML, Curlee K, Lloyd R, et al. Aldosterone-secreting adrenocortical carcinomas are associated with unique operative risks and outcomes. *Surgery* 2002;132(6):1008.
20. Halefoglu AM, Yasar A, Bas N, et al. Comparison of computed tomography histogram analysis and chemical-shift magnetic resonance imaging for adrenal mass characterization. *Acta Radiol* 2009;50(9):1071.
22. Ilias I, Sahdev A, Reznek RH, Grossman AB, Pacak K. The optimal imaging of adrenal tumours: a comparison of different methods. *Endocr Relat Cancer* 2007;14(3):587.
23. Johnson PT, Horton KM, Fishman EK. Adrenal Imaging with multidetector CT: evidence-based protocol optimization and interpretative practice. *Radiographics* 2009;29(5):1319.
24. Johnson PT, Horton KM, Fishman EK. Adrenal mass imaging with multidetector CT: pathologic conditions, pearls, and pitfalls. *Radiographics* 2009;29(5):1333.
25. Miller FH, Wang Y, McCarthy RJ, et al. Utility of diffusion-weighted MRI in characterization of adrenal lesions. *Am J Roentgenol* 2010;194(2):W179.
26. Blake MA, Holalkere NS, Boland GW. Imaging techniques for adrenal lesion characterization. *Radiol Clin North Am* 2008;46(1):65.
28. Mazzaglia PJ, Monchik JM. Limited value of adrenal biopsy in the evaluation of adrenal neoplasm: a decade of experience. *Arch Surg* 2009;144(5): 465.
29. de Reynies A, Assie G, Rickman DS, et al. Gene expression profiling reveals a new classification of adrenocortical tumors and identifies molecular predictors of malignancy and survival. *J Clin Oncol* 2009;27(7):1108.
30. Zhao J, Speel EJM, Muletta-Feurer S, et al. Analysis of genomic alterations in sporadic adrenocortical lesions: gain of chromosome 17 is an early event in adrenocortical tumorigenesis. *Am J Pathol* 1999;155(4):1039.
31. Dohna M, Reincke M, Antoaneta MA, et al. Adrenocortical carcinoma is characterized by a high frequency of chromosomal gains and high-level amplifications. *Genes Chromosomes Cancer* 2000;28:145.
32. Kjellman M, Kallioniemi OP, Karhu R, et al. Genetic aberrations in adrenocortical tumors detected using comparative genomic hybridization correlate with tumor size and malignancy. *Cancer Res* 1996;56(18):4219.
33. Sidhu S, Marsh DJ, Theodosopoulos G, et al. Comparative genomic hybridization analysis of adrenocortical tumors. *J Clin Endocrinol Metab* 2002;87(7):3467.

35. Soon PSH, Gill AJ, Benn DE, et al. Microarray gene expression and immunohistochemistry analyses of adrenocortical tumors identify IGF2 and Ki-67 as useful in differentiating carcinomas from adenomas. *Endocr Relat Cancer* 2009;16(2):573.
36. Barlaskar F, Hammer G. The molecular genetics of adrenocortical carcinoma. *Rev Endocr Metab Disord* 2007;8(4):343.
37. de Fraipont F, El Atifi M, Cherradi N, et al. Gene expression profiling of human adrenocortical tumors using complementary deoxyribonucleic acid microarrays identifies several candidate genes as markers of malignancy. *J Clin Endocrinol Metab* 2005;90(3):1819.
38. Fernandez-Ranvier GG, Weng J, Yeh RF, et al. Identification of biomarkers of adrenocortical carcinoma using genomewide gene expression profiling. *Arch Surg* 2008;143(9):841.
39. Giordano TJ, Thomas DG, Kuick R, et al. Distinct transcriptional profiles of adrenocortical tumors uncovered by dna microarray analysis. *Am J Pathol* 2003;162(2):521.
40. Slater EP, Diehl SM, Langer P, et al. Analysis by cDNA microarrays of gene expression patterns of human adrenocortical tumors. *Eur J Endocrinol* 2006;154(4):587.
41. Velazquez-Fernandez D, Laurell C, Geli J, et al. Expression profiling of adrenocortical neoplasms suggests a molecular signature of malignancy. *Surgery* 2005;138(6):1087.
42. West AN, Neale GA, Pounds S, et al. Gene expression profiling of childhood adrenocortical tumors. *Cancer Res* 2007;67(2):600.
43. Almeida MQ, Fragoso MCBV, Lotfi CFP, et al. Expression of insulin-like growth factor-II and its receptor in pediatric and adult adrenocortical tumors. *J Clin Endocrinol Metab* 2008;93(9):3524.
44. Barlaskar FM, Spalding AC, Heaton JH, et al. Preclinical targeting of the type I insulin-like growth factor receptor in adrenocortical carcinoma. *J Clin Endocrinol Metab* 2009;94(1):204.
49. Karl YB, Wen TS, Dina E, et al. Adrenocortical carcinoma in the United States. *Cancer* 2008;113:3130.
50. Stephan EA, Chung TH, Grant CS, et al. Adrenocortical carcinoma survival rates correlated to genomic copy number variants. *Mol Cancer Ther* 2008;7(2):425.
51. Giordano TJ, Kuick R, Else T, et al. Molecular classification and prognostication of adrenocortical tumors by transcriptome profiling. *Clin Cancer Res* 2009;15(2):668.
52. Soon PSH, Tacon LJ, Gill AJ, et al. miR-195 and miR-483-5p identified as predictors of poor prognosis in adrenocortical cancer. *Clin Cancer Res* 2009;15(24):7684.
53. Sturgeon C, Shen WT, Clark OH, Duh QY, Kebebew E. Risk assessment in 457 adrenal cortical carcinomas: how much does tumor size predict the likelihood of malignancy? *J Am Coll Surg* 2006;202(3):423.
54. Ctvrtlík F, Herman M, Student V, Tichá V, Minarík J. Differential diagnosis of incidentally detected adrenal masses revealed on routine abdominal CT. *Eur J Radiol* 2009;69(2):243.
55. Park SH, Kim MJ, Kim JH, Lim JS, Kim KW. Differentiation of adrenal adenoma and nonadenoma in unenhanced CT: new optimal threshold value and the usefulness of size criteria for differentiation. *Korean J Radiol* 2007;8(4):328.
56. Weiss LM, Medeiros LJ, Vickery ALJ. Pathologic features of prognostic significance in adrenocortical carcinoma. *Am J Surg Pathol* 1989;13(3):202.
57. Soon PSH, McDonald KL, Robinson BG, Sidhu SB. Molecular markers and the pathogenesis of adrenocortical cancer. *Oncologist* 2008;13(5):548.
58. Volante M, Bollito E, Sperone P, et al. Clinicopathological study of a series of 92 adrenocortical carcinomas: from a proposal of simplified diagnostic algorithm to prognostic stratification. *Histopathology* 2009;55:535.
79. Ilias I, Pacak K. A clinical overview of pheochromocytomas/paragangliomas and carcinoid tumors. *Nucl Med Biol* 2008;35(Suppl 1):S27.
80. Zelinka T, Eisenhofer G, Pacak K. Pheochromocytoma as a catecholamine producing tumor: implications for clinical practice. *Stress Int J Biol Stress* 2007;10(2):195.
81. Eisenhofer G, Goldstein DS, Walther MM, et al. Biochemical diagnosis of pheochromocytoma: how to distinguish true- from false-positive test results. *J Clin Endocrinol Metab* 2003;88(6):2656.

CHAPTER 111 PANCREATIC NEUROENDOCRINE TUMORS

JAMES C. YAO, GUIDO RINDI, AND DOUGLAS B. EVANS

Pancreatic neuroendocrine tumors (pNETs) are low- to intermediate-grade neoplasms that are thought to arise from the pancreatic islets. Also known as pancreatic endocrine tumors, islet cell carcinoma, or pancreatic carcinoid, pNETs account for a minority of pancreatic neoplasms and can be either functional or nonfunctional. The functional status of pNETs is generally influenced by several factors, including disease bulk, stage, secretory status, and whether the peptide secreted is intact and causes distinct clinical symptoms. pNETs are generally considered functional if they are associated with a hormonal syndrome. Whether staining for the presence of various hormones by immunohistochemistry (IHC), those pNETs not causing a clinical hormonal syndrome are considered nonfunctional. It is also recognized that the functional status of these tumors may change over time or with treatment. Moreover, some of these tumors can produce multiple hormones simultaneously, although symptoms related to one of these hormones often will dominate.

pNETs are usually more indolent than the more common forms of pancreatic cancer are. Management of pNETs generally can be categorized into management of the problems caused by secreted hormone(s) and oncologic issues related to tumor growth and management of metastasis. The organization of this chapter parallels this paradigm. Following discussions of the epidemiology, pathology, and molecular genetics of these tumors, the oncologic issues common to the diagnosis and management of pNETs are discussed in the section on nonfunctional tumors. This is followed by discussions of issues unique to each functional "endocrinoma." Next is a section on "Additional Clinical Considerations," which includes hereditary cancer syndromes, pathology pitfalls, surgical pitfalls, and high-grade NETs. The chapter concludes with a look at emerging therapeutic options. The goal for this chapter is to provide a systemic, up-to-date, and practical approach to pNETs.

EPIDEMIOLOGY

pNETs are reputed to be relatively rare neoplasms, but their exact incidence and prevalence are somewhat elusive. This is in part because most registries, including the Surveillance, Epidemiology, and End Results (SEER) program, only include neoplasms that are deemed malignant. For pNETs, the definition of malignant behavior is complex. In the absence of malignant behavior such as direct invasion of adjacent organs or metastases to regional lymph nodes or distant sites, size is typically used to classify pNETs' malignant potential. The annual age-adjusted incidence of pNETs between 2000 and 2004 was 0.32 per 100,000.[1] Malignant pNETs accounts for approximately 1% of pancreatic cancers by incidence and 10% of pancreatic cancers by prevalence.[2]

The incidence of smaller pNETs in the general population, however, is likely to be much higher. In an analysis of 11,472 autopsies performed at a Hong Kong hospital, pNETs were found in 0.1% of all cases.[3] This suggest that the prevalence of small asymptomatic islet cell tumors, many of which are never diagnosed, may be 100-fold more common than the data suggested by SEER registries.

pNETs are slightly more common among men (53%) than women (47%).[2] The median age at diagnosis was 60 years.[1,2] At diagnosis, 14% had localized disease, 22% had regional disease, and 64% had distant disease. The survival of patients with pNETs has improved over time.[2,4] Among patients diagnosed from 1988 through 2004, the 5-year survival rates for patients with localized, regional, and distant pNETs were 79%, 62%, and 27%, respectively (Fig. 111.1*A*).[1] Older patients generally had shorter survival (Fig. 111.1*B*; $P < .001$).[2]

CLASSIFICATION, HISTOPATHOLOGY, AND MOLECULAR GENETICS

Criteria for Pathologic Diagnosis

A larger fraction of endocrine cells in the pancreas are insulin-producing B and glucagon-producing A cells. Relatively minor populations of cells produce somatostatin (D), and pancreatic polypeptide (PP). Rare cells also produce serotonin (EC) and ghrelin (P/D_1).[5] These endocrine cells are believed to be the source of pNETs. It is a matter of debate if tumors arise from islets or ducts. Transgenic mice that express potent oncogenes in endocrine cells[6] and multiple endocrine neoplasia-1 (MEN-1) knockout mice[7,8] point to an islet origin of tumors consistent with the autorenewal properties of islet cells[9] and observation in MEN-1 patients.[10] Conversely, molecular evidence from islet microdissection in MEN-1 patients indicate a duct cell origin.[11] No matter where the truth lies, endocrine tumor cells largely display the same phenotype as their normal endocrine counterpart.

Endocrine tumors are classified on the basis of tumor cell differentiation as well-differentiated tumors/carcinomas (WDET/C) and poorly differentiated carcinomas (PDEC).[12] WDET/C are characterized by bland features: trabecular, glandular, acinar, or mixed structures; the stroma is generally fine and rich in well-developed blood vessels, sometimes with hyalinized deposits of amyloid; tumor cells are monomorph with abundant, variably eosinophilic cytoplasm, low cytological atypia, and low mitotic index. Necrosis is usually absent or may be seen as spotty, limited areas in histologically more aggressive neoplasms. On the contrary, PDECs are characterized by a prevalent solid structure with abundant necrosis, often a central, round tumor cell of small to medium size with severe cellular atypia and high mitotic index.

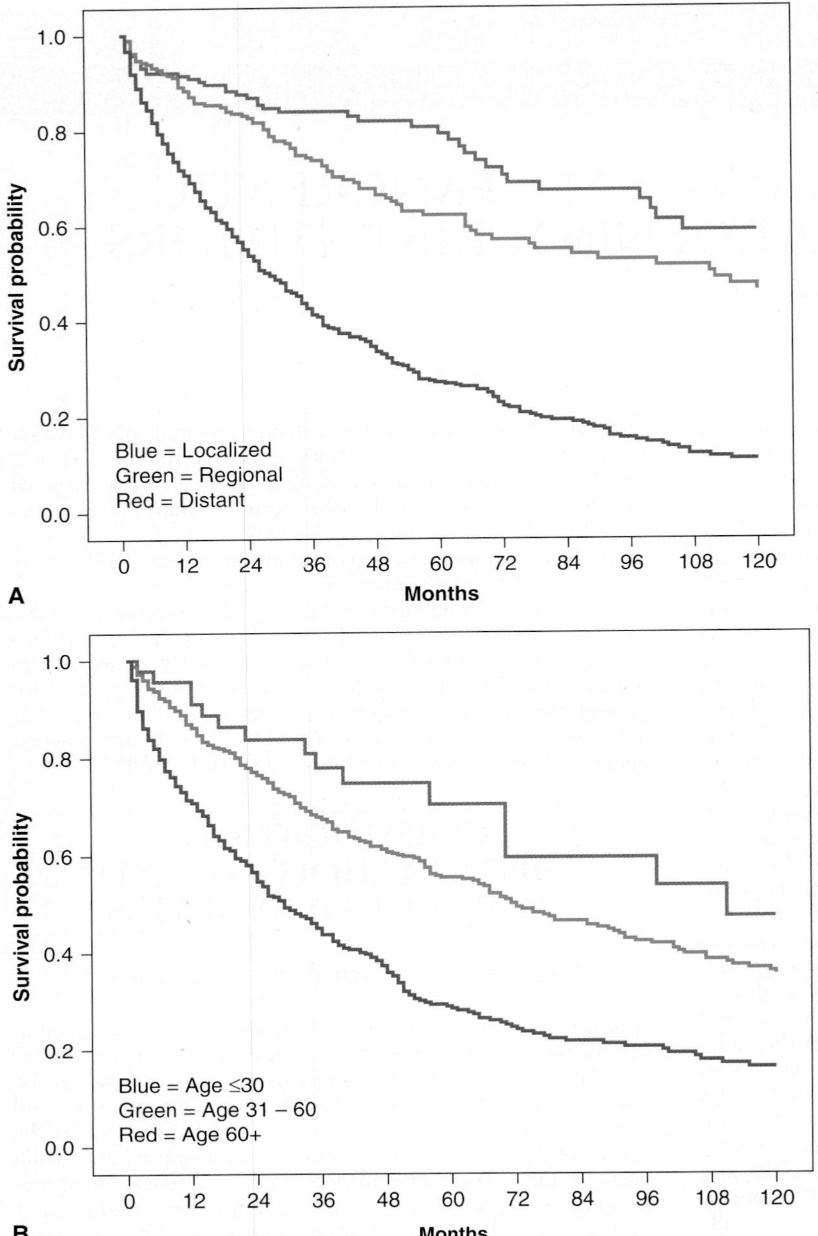

FIGURE 111.1 Survival durations from diagnosis of patient with low to intermediate grade pNETs diagnosed from 1988 to 2004. **A:** Median survival duration of patients with localized, regional, and distant disease were not reached for those with localized disease, 111 (95% CI, 73–149) months for those with regional disease, and 27 (95% CI 23–31) months for those with distant disease (P < 0.001). **B:** Median survival durations of patients by age group were 110 (CI not calculated due to small numbers) months for those age ≤30, 71 (95% CI, 58–84) months for those age 31 to 60, and 28 (95% CI, 23–33) months for those age ≥61 (P < 0.001).

Surveillance, Epidemiology, and End Results (SEER) Program: SEER 17 Regs Nov 2006 sub (1973–2004), ed. released April 2007: National Cancer Institute, DCCPS, Surveillance Research Program, Cancer Statistic Branch, 2007.

Fine-Needle Aspiration versus Core Needle Biopsy

The diagnosis of endocrine tumor entails (1) meeting the above-defined histological and cytological criteria; (2) assessing the status of endocrine differentiation; and (3) evaluating prognostic markers. Fine-needle aspiration biopsy (FNAB) is an effective technique in expert hands, allowing the cytological diagnosis of isolated or grouped cells with little information on tumor structure. The advantages of this methodology are several, including its simplicity, low invasiveness, and cost. The disadvantages are mainly its operator-dependent efficacy, limited option for further examinations, and impossible assessment of prognostic variables.

Conversely, the core needle biopsy (ideally 2 mm in diameter) produces a reasonably sized tumor sample, potentially allowing a cyto- or histological diagnosis complete with all known prognostic parameters. Besides the easier diagnostic approach intrinsic to histology, its major advantage is certainly the potential for further examinations. Disadvantages are the major invasiveness of the procedure(s) and the relatively higher costs.

The choice of the biopsy method ultimately depends on the specificity of each patient or case and the diagnostic environment (i.e., the access to specific pathological expertise and dedicated structure). However, considering the above pros and cons and in view of the usually long, expensive, and difficult route to the diagnosis for patients with endocrine tumor or cancer, the core needle biopsy for histology is recommended when possible. The authors typically recommend core needle when biopsying liver metastases, and FNA when biopsying the pancreas.

Minimum Immunohistochemistry Markers

A large number of antigens, commonly defined as neuroendocrine markers, are expressed in tumor cells.[5] They comprise markers dispersed in the cytosol, such as neuron specific enolase (NSE) and protein gene product 9.5 (PGP 9.5), and markers of the secretory compartment, either associated with electron-dense granules, large-dense-core vesicles (LDCV), such as chromogranins and related fragments (the most popular being chromogranin A, CgA), or associated with small synapticlike vesicles (SSV), such as synaptophysin (Syn). These antigens are defined as *general markers*, since they are widely expressed in cells of the diffuse endocrine system. Hormones and amines are produced by specific cell types and thus defined as *specific markers*. The positive identification of the endocrine cell product(s) in tissue sections is obtained by IHC.

A minimal IHC histology panel aims toward the following: (1) positively identify the degree of endocrine differentiation in tumor cells and (2) determine the proliferation activity status. Determining the proliferation status is achieved by Ki-67 IHC using the MIB-1 antibody or expressed as mitoses per 10 high power microscopic fields (or 2 mm^2). It is recommended to assess positive nuclei at sites of higher labeling (identified at lower magnification survey of the specimen) in percentages of 2,000 cells whenever possible.[13]

Other Immunohistochemistry Markers

The other general neuroendocrine markers mentioned above may be of practical use for difficult diagnosis as well as to overcome poor antigen preservation. In addition, and according to the current World Health Organization (WHO) 2004 indications, assessment of the most represented cell type with hormone IHC may be required on specific clinical grounds. A single endocrine tumor is usually composed of several different endocrine cell types in different proportions.[12] IHC for hormones and amines should be pursued according to the clinical picture and almost exclusively in functioning tumors based on the clinician's request. IHC for the somatostatin receptor 2A (SSR2A) may be performed as grounds for targeted therapy and as an effective and low-cost alternative when *in vivo* receptor scintigraphy is unavailable. The information obtained by SSR2A IHC is intrinsically limited when compared to *in vivo* methods, though good correlation with scintigraphy has been confirmed by independent groups.[14,15]

Grade versus Differentiation: World Health Organization

Three categories are defined by the current WHO 2004 classification:

1.1. WDET of benign behavior, size less than 2 cm, confined to the pancreas, nonangioinvasive, nonfunctioning, or, if functioning, insulinoma only;
1.2. WDET of uncertain behavior, confined to the pancreas, greater than 2 cm in size or angioinvasive, nonfunctioning or functioning (any type);
2. WDEC, low grade, with synchronous metastasis and/or gross local invasion (duodenal wall, fat, spleen), nonfunctioning or functioning (any type);
3. PDEC, high grade.

This classification proved effective and of practical utility; however, it leaves most cases under the vague "uncertain behavior" 1.2 category. No histological grading is provided by WHO 2004. Recently the European Neuroendocrine Tumors Society (ENETS) proposed a simple, three-step grading system for foregut endocrine tumors, implying increased malignancy risk at increased mitotic count and Ki-67 index (Table 111.1) together with a site-specific TNM (tumor, necrosis, metastasis) staging system (Table 111.2).[13] The predicting power of this grading proposal was demonstrated by three retrospective studies,[16–18] and the efficacy of its principles were proven in two large prospective multicenter series.[19,20] This grading system is now supported by the American Joint Committee on Cancer (AJCC) classification system.[21]

TABLE 111.1

GRADING PROPOSAL FOR PANCREATIC NEUROENDOCRINE TUMORS

Grade	Mitotic Count (10 HPF)[a]	Ki-67 Index (%)[b]
G1	<2	≤2
G2	2–20	3–20
G3	>20	>20

[a]10 HPF (high power field) = 2 mm^2, at least 40 fields (at 40× magnification) evaluated in areas of highest mitotic density.
[b]MIB1 antibody; percentage of 2,000 tumor cells in areas of highest nuclear labeling.
(From ref. 13.)

Tumor, Node, Metastasis Staging

The recent ENETS proposal of TNM for endocrine tumors of the pancreas is based on criteria previously identified by the WHO 2004 classification and implies a malignant potential for any tumor type.[13] The practical utility of this system was demonstrated in six independent studies.[16–20,22] In 2010 a TNM system was officially provided by AJCC and the International Union Against Cancer (UICC).[21] The recommendation was to apply to endocrine pancreatic tumors the TNM devised for exocrine pancreatic cancer (Table 111.2). The AJCC-UICC TNM scheme is based on a paper that reported on an investigation of a large tumor registry database series.[23] The current recommendations from AJCC require the use of both grading and staging parameters to classify tumors.[22]

Genetic Profile of Low to Intermediate Neuroendocrine Tumors

No definitive data indicate a precise genetic path leading to tumor formation. Neither has a specific gene(s) responsible for endocrine pancreatic tumorigenesis been identified. In the past decade, relatively abundant information on somatic tumor DNA was generated by a variety of methods with different sensitivity and resolution capacity, so caution is warranted in their analysis. Overall available information points to a complex multigene condition in which deletion or loss of somatic DNA and gain in copy number are both frequent at multiple sites. Loss of heterozygosity (LOH) at chromosome 11q13 region including *MEN-1* gene locus is found in about half of investigated cases.[24] This is confirmed by comparative genomic hybridization (CGH) and high-resolution allelotyping.[25–29] Complex abnormalities that involve losses at chromosome 1, 3p, 6q, 9q, 10p, 11pq, 21, 22q or gains at 4pq, 5, 7qp, 12q, 14q, 17pq have been reported by locus-specific investigation, genome-wide allelotyping, or CGH.[25,26,30–34] Notably, abnormalities of the *p53* gene are rarely observed in well-differentiated tumors, although they are the genetic signature of PDEC.[35,36] This complex picture indicates an unexpected degree of genetic instability. The accumulation of genetic defects appears to be the phenomenon responsible for malignancy progression and the best predictor of metastatic disease in insulinoma.[29] Similarly, in nonfunctioning tumors elevated occurrence of genetic abnormality is associated with malignancy,[26,37,38] and,

TABLE 111.2

AMERICAN JOINT COMMITTEE ON CANCER AND EUROPEAN NEUROENDOCRINE TUMORS SOCIETY PROPOSED TUMOR, NECROSIS, METASTASIS STAGING SYSTEMS FOR PANCREATIC NEUROENDOCRINE TUMORS

American Joint Committee on Cancer				European Neuroendocrine Tumors Society			
PRIMARY TUMOR (T)				**PRIMARY TUMOR (T)**			
TX	Primary tumor cannot be assessed			TX	Primary tumor cannot be assessed		
T0	No evidence of primary tumor			T0	No evidence of primary tumor		
T1	Tumor limited to the pancreas, 2 cm or less			T1	Tumor limited to the pancreas and size <2 cm		
T2	Tumor limited to the pancreas, more than 2 cm			T2	Tumor limited to the pancreas and size 2–4 cm		
T3	Tumor extends beyond the pancreas but without involvement of the celiac axis or the superior mesenteric artery			T3	Tumor limited to the pancreas and size >4 cm or invading duodenum or bile duct		
T4	Tumor involves the celiac axis or the superior mesenteric artery (unresectable primary tumor)			T4	Tumor invading adjacent organs (stomach, spleen, colon, adrenal gland) or the wall of large vessels (celiac axis or superior mesenteric artery)		
REGIONAL LYMPH NODES (N)				**REGIONAL LYMPH NODES (N)**			
NX	Regional lymph nodes cannot be assessed			NX	Regional lymph node cannot be assessed		
N0	No regional lymph node metastasis			N0	No regional lymph node metastasis		
N1	Regional lymph node metastasis			N1	Regional lymph node metastasis		
DISTANT METASTASES (M)				**DISTANT METASTASES (M)**			
—				MX	Distant metastasis cannot be assessed		
M0	No distant metastasis			M0	No distant metastases		
M1	Distant metastasis			M1[a]	Distant metastasis		
STAGE	**T**	**N**	**M**	**STAGE**	**T**	**N**	**M**
				—	—	—	—
0	Tis	N0	M0	I	T1	N0	M0
IA	T1	N0	M0	IIA	T2	N0	M0
IB	T2	N0	M0	IIB	T3	N0	M0
IIA	T3	N0	M0	IIIA	T4	N0	M0
IIB	T1, T2, T3	N1	M0	IIIB	Any T	N1	M0
III	T4	Any N	M0	IV	Any T	Any N	M1
IV	Any T	Any N	M1				

(From ref. 13.)
[a]M1 specific sites defined according to Sobin and Wittekind (ref. 155).

analog to insulinoma, accumulation of genetic changes would mark malignancy progression with likely involvement of genes guarding chromosomal stability.[28] Other mechanisms of abnormal or negative gene regulation were also demonstrated, including DNA silencing by gene promoter methylation[39,40] and specific messanger RNA aberrant hyperexpression.[41] Finally, information on tumor messenger RNA (mRNA) expression profiling provided a large set of data in relatively few, recent reports; however, different genes were identified as abnormal depending on different platform used by different groups.[42–46]

DIAGNOSIS AND MANAGEMENT OF PANCREATIC ENDOCRINE TUMORS

Nonfunctional Tumors

Symptoms and Diagnosis

Nonfunctioning pNETs and PPomas do not cause a clinical syndrome. Rarely, cases have been reported of PPomas associated with watery diarrhea,[47–49] diabetes mellitus, ulcer diathesis,[50] or an erythematous pruritic skin rash different from that seen in patients with glucagonomas.[51] Until the tumor causes obstruction of the biliary or gastric outlet, the patient is usually asymptomatic unless the tumor bulk results in pain. Jaundice may be the presenting symptom in patients with tumors to the right of the superior mesenteric artery (SMA) and superior mesenteric vein (SMV); these tumors originate in the pancreatic head or uncinate process, which may cause obstruction of the intrapancreatic portion of the common bile duct.[52,53] Tumors in this location may also cause gastric outlet obstruction or pain due to invasion of the autonomic mesenteric plexus. Pain may also be secondary to tumor extension into the celiac ganglion (most commonly seen with tumors arising in the body of the pancreas) or to liver metastases that invade the liver capsule or extend to the parietal peritoneum. Occasionally patients may experience gastrointestinal hemorrhage secondary to tumor erosion into the duodenum or splenic vein occlusion, causing gastroesophageal varices, which can intermittently bleed. Nonfunctioning pNETs can sometimes grow to an enormous size without producing jaundice or other symptoms. pNETs arising to the left of the SMA and SMV may cause vague, poorly localized upper abdominal pain or dyspepsia, but such tumors are usually asymptomatic until they reach a considerable size. In contrast to patients with adenocarcinoma of the pancreas, patients with pNETs may not experience

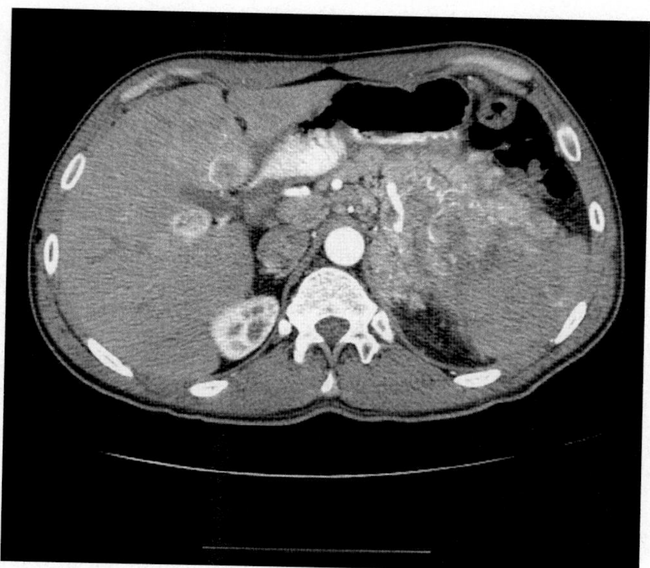

FIGURE 111.2 Axial contrast-enhanced computed tomography image of a hypervascular neuroendocrine carcinoma of the pancreas with liver metastases.

significant weight loss, cachexia, or back pain or show other signs of advanced disease.[52,53] In the absence of a large tumor or metastatic disease, pNETs are often detected incidentally on abdominal imaging studies.

On contrast-enhanced multidetector computed tomography (CT), pNETs characteristically appear hyperdense, as they are hypervascular (Fig. 111.2). Therefore, imaging of the pancreas during the arterial phase is critical to detect these lesions and their hypervascular liver metastases. However, similar to pancreatic adenocarcinomas, pNETs may occasionally appear hypodense compared with adjacent pancreatic parenchyma, and they may contain cystic components or microcalcifications. Importantly, intrapancreatic accessory splenic tissue can present as an asymptomatic, hypervascular mass that involves the distal pancreatic tail, thus mimicking a pNET.

The current practice at the authors' institutions is to obtain high-quality multidetector (multislice) CT images of the pancreatic tumor. The authors use objective CT criteria to determine a tumor's resectability based on the relationship of the pancreatic tumor to the SMA and celiac axis.[54–56] Encasement (greater than 180° involvement of the vessel by tumor) of the celiac axis or the SMA or occlusion of the superior mesenteric-portal venous (SMPV) confluence without the technical option of venous reconstruction are considered criteria for a tumor's unresectability. Similar to the authors' philosophy on local-regional management of pancreatic adenocarcinomas,[57] they do not perform incomplete resection (debulking) of nonfunctioning pNETs. Some investigators have suggested that palliative, incomplete resection of the pancreatic tumor may provide relief of local tumor-related symptoms and improve survival, but most of these reports included patients with syndromes of hormone excess; no accurately reported data are available to support debulking in patients with unresectable nonfunctioning pNETs.[58,59] Magnetic resonance imaging (MRI) is preferred over CT for patients with a history of allergy to iodine contrast material or for those with renal insufficiency. Moreover, MRI may be more sensitive than CT is for the detection of small liver metastases.[60,61] Endoscopic ultrasound (EUS) is currently considered the most sensitive modality for identifying small pNETs and is thus used for preoperative tumor localization in patients with MEN-1, in which multifocal disease is common.

In the absence of an inherited endocrine syndrome associated with multifocal disease, the role of EUS is limited to FNAB of the tumor. In the current era of invasive gastroenterology, EUS is safe and is becoming more widely available.

Accurate preoperative diagnosis and staging of the primary tumor is necessary to ensure correct treatment. The oncologic (surgical *and* medical) approach to a pNET is different from that for pancreatic adenocarcinoma. Because the poor prognosis associated with pancreatic adenocarcinoma is well known, patients with pNETs who are incorrectly thought to have large, locally invasive, or metastatic adenocarcinomas may not undergo surgery when it is indicated and also may receive incorrect chemotherapy. At the authors' institutions a liberal approach to the use of pretreatment EUS-FNA biopsy is followed, especially for those patients in whom the clinical history, physical examination, and radiographic images are not consistent with straightforward pancreatic ductal adenocarcinoma.

Serum Tumor Markers

Several circulating tumor markers have been evaluated for the diagnosis and follow-up management of pNETs. Although these can be very useful for follow-up, isolated elevation of marker levels is generally not sufficient for diagnosis. These markers usually can be divided into those associated with specific endocrine syndromes and those more general markers that may be present in functional as well as nonfunctional tumors. The most important of these markers, CgA, is a 49-kDa acidic polypeptide that is widely present in the secretory granules of neuroendocrine cells. CgA is elevated in a majority of patients with either functioning or nonfunctioning pNETs.[62–65] In a study where patients with advanced pNETs were treated with streptozocin-based chemotherapy, 79% of patients had elevation of CgA at baseline.[66] In addition, response to therapy was associated with a 30% decrease of serum CgA.[66] This concept was also tested in the RADIANT-1 (RAD001 In Advanced Neuroendocrine Tumors) study that treated patients with progressive pNETs after cytotoxic chemotherapy with mammalian target of rapamycin (mTOR) inhibitor, everolimus. In this study, a 30% decrease in CgA 4-weeks after initiation of therapy was associated with significantly longer progression-free survival.[67] Care should, however, be taken in measuring CgA and interpreting the results. For example, since somatostatin analogues are known to affect blood levels of CgA, serial CgA levels should be measured at approximately the same interval from injection in patients receiving long-acting somatostatin analogues. Spuriously elevated levels of CgA have also been reported in patients using proton-pump inhibitors, in patients with renal or liver failure, or in those with chronic gastritis.

Another general neuroendocrine marker, neuron specific enolase (NSE), is a dimmer of the glycolytic enzyme enolase. NSE is present in the cytoplasmic compartment of the cell, and its serum level is thought to be unrelated to the secretory activity of the tumor.[65] Although less specific as a diagnostic marker, it may be helpful in the follow-up of patients with unresectable disease. In the RADIANT-1 study, 30% decrease in CgA at week 4 was also associated with significantly longer progression-free survival.[67]

PP levels also are frequently elevated in patients with pNETs. Elevation of PP is not associated with a distinct hormonal syndrome and is only considered significant when the PP level is at least three times the age-matched normal basal level obtained in a fasting state.[68] A variety of other secreted amines can also be measured. These include other chromogranins such as chromogranins B and C, pancreastatin, substance P, neurotensin, neurokinin A, gastrin, glucagon, vasoactive intestinal peptide, insulin, proinsulin, and c-peptide. In general, blood markers should be drawn in fasting state.

It is recognized that NETs sometimes can change which (if any) hormones and biomarkers are produced. The general principle of biomarker measurement is to evaluate a large panel of markers at key points of the disease, such as diagnosis or relapse, in order to identify a few biomarkers that are elevated in the particular patient in question and follow these over time. It is generally not necessary to check every biomarker at every visit.

Surgical Treatment

The majority of pNETs are malignant, with the exception of insulinomas, which are benign in 95% of patients. It is probably best to assume that if left untreated, all noninsulinoma pNETs have the biologic ability for uncontrolled local growth and metastasis to distant organs. pNETs frequently metastasize to regional lymph nodes, and the frequency of lymph node metastases depends on the extent of surgery and on the degree and accuracy of the pathologist's examination of the surgical specimen.

Based on the authors' published experience, they have developed general guidelines for the surgical management of patients with nonfunctioning pNETs:

1. The authors establish the diagnosis with needle biopsy (EUS-guided FNA of the pancreas or image-guided core needle biopsy of the liver metastases is preferred if present) and decompress the biliary tree with an endobiliary stent when necessary.
2. The authors resect localized, nonmetastatic disease confined to the pancreas if a gross complete resection can be performed. If radiographically occult liver metastases are found at the time of the operation, they are removed if possible. If the liver metastases are of small volume but diffuse, the primary tumor is usually removed due to the potential for major morbidity from the primary, which is a possibility because of the relatively long anticipated survival of the patient.
3. In the setting of known metastatic disease or a large, borderline resectable primary tumor, the authors would first initiate systemic therapy.
4. The degree to which surgery is applied to the primary pancreatic tumor is based on the presence or extent of distant disease and the presence or absence of symptoms (bleeding, obstruction) from the primary tumor. For example, resection of an asymptomatic primary in the distal pancreas has a limited role, if any, in the presence of unresectable moderate-to-large volume extrapancreatic metastatic disease. As treatments for metastatic disease become more effective, the rationale for aggressive management of the primary tumor, despite the presence of extrapancreatic disease, may become more compelling. However, treatment sequencing will likely emphasize a surgery-last strategy (after induction systemic therapy) to identify those patients most likely to benefit from large, multiorgan resections.
5. When dealing with a resectable primary tumor and resectable liver metastases, the authors usually remove the pancreatic tumor first; if that procedure goes well, they then consider resecting the liver under the same induction anesthesia. However, they often use a two-stage procedure.

The goals of surgery are to maximize local disease control and to increase the quality and length of patient survival. These goals must be tempered by the potential operative morbidity and the long-term complications of insulin dependence and gastrointestinal dysfunction. The authors previously reported survival data for 163 patients with nonfunctioning pNETs treated at their institution.[69] As expected, patients with localized or regional disease at diagnosis had a significantly superior median survival compared with those who had metastatic disease (7.1 years vs. 2.2 years; $P < .0001$). Among patients with localized disease, those who underwent complete resection of the primary tumor demonstrated an additional survival advantage over those with locally advanced, unresectable tumors (median survivals of 7.1 years for patients with localized, resectable disease vs. 5.2 years for patients with locally advanced, unresectable tumors).[69] However, only 48% of the 42 patients with localized, nonmetastatic disease who underwent resection of the primary tumor were alive and without evidence of recurrent disease at a median follow-up of 2.7 years (range, 1 to 8 years) from diagnosis. It is thus inappropriate to assume that complete resection of the primary tumor in the absence of metastatic disease corresponds to long-term cure.[69]

Occasionally, extended surgery is required to achieve complete tumor resection of nonfunctioning pNETs. Data from the authors' institution have demonstrated the safety of segmental resection of the SMV or SMPV confluence when necessary to allow complete tumor resection.[49,70] Arterial resection is occasionally performed but usually is limited to cases of isolated tumor involvement of the hepatic artery at the level of the gastroduodenal artery origin. Typically, large tumors of the neck and body of the pancreas involve the celiac axis, and resection of these tumors would require upper abdominal exenteration, with removal of the stomach and spleen in addition to total pancreaticoduodenectomy. The major long-term complication encountered is nutritional. The combination of total pancreaticoduodenectomy plus total gastrectomy leads to long-term gastrointestinal dysfunction, especially when combined with an extensive retroperitoneal dissection and removal of the celiac and mesenteric neural plexus.[71,72] For these reasons, such resections are rarely performed. At present, the authors are highly selective in the use of extended pancreaticoduodenectomy when total gastrectomy or hepatic artery (HA) revascularization may be necessary.

In the absence of extrapancreatic metastatic disease, the appropriate management of patients with locally advanced, surgically unresectable neuroendocrine carcinoma of the pancreas remains a difficult therapeutic dilemma. The median survival duration for patients with unresectable, nonmetastatic, nonfunctioning pNETs is approximately 5 years. As survival time without operation increases, and as potential operative morbidity and mortality increase, the authors are less accepting of the upfront risks of surgery and less inclined to recommend it in this setting. Occasionally, locally advanced tumors of the pancreatic head or uncinate process are associated with significant patient morbidity due to complications such as biliary obstruction, gastric outlet obstruction, or gastrointestinal hemorrhage.[69] In contrast to the management of patients with pancreatic adenocarcinoma (where endoscopic stenting of the bile duct and, occasionally, the duodenum are fairly routine in the setting of locally advanced or metastatic disease), the authors would rarely use a duodenal stent in a patient with neuroendocrine carcinoma and would utilize endobiliary stents only for short-term (months, not years) biliary decompression. Because of the longer survival times of patients with pNET (even advanced disease), the authors favor operative bypass of the bile duct and duodenum in most cases.

Management of Advanced Disease

Advanced, unresectable pNETs generally are not curable. The goals of treatment for nonfunctional tumors include palliation or prevention of symptoms and cytoreduction of bulky tumors in an effort to prolong survival. Although low- to intermediate-grade pNETs have a reputation of being indolent, median patient survival in the setting of advanced disease remains around 2 years.[69] Indeed, most patients with advanced pNETs will not survive the disease; thus, aggressive treatment in the setting of progressive disease is warranted.

Management of patients with advanced pNETs requires an understanding of the disease process and of a multimodality approach. Treatment options include cytotoxic chemotherapy, mTOR inhibitors, vascular endothelial growth factor (VEGF) inhibitors, somatostatin analogues, interferon, and ablative approaches, such as hepatic artery embolization and radiofrequency ablation. Occasionally, systemic therapy may also convert cases of unresectable tumors into cases wherein surgery may render the patients disease free. In such cases, the authors recommend that surgical options in a multidisciplinary setting be considered. Much of what is discussed here for nonfunctional tumors also holds true for managing the growth of functional tumors.

Cytotoxic Chemotherapy

Systemic chemotherapy for advanced pNETs has been studied in many clinical trials over the past three decades. Despite the multitude of publications, the role of cytotoxic chemotherapy continues to be debated. Several issues plague the interpretation of older studies in this area. Because pNETs are relatively rare, patients with carcinoids and those with pNETs were grouped together in many of these trials. Further, older studies often used criteria that are not accepted today to measure outcome. Finally, no study has attempted to document improvements in progression-free survival or overall survival against best supportive care.[73,74]

Single-Agent Chemotherapy. Streptozocin was originally isolated from streptomyces achromogenes in the 1950s. Its antitumor activity in pNETs was first reported in 1973 in a study that included 52 patients, where a response rate of 50% was reported.[75] This led to the only U.S. Food and Drug Administration approval of a drug for the treatment of pNETs. Streptozocin's single-agent activity was subsequently confirmed in a study that compared that agent alone with streptozocin plus fluorouracil (5-FU) for islet cell carcinoma.[73]

Another drug that has demonstrated single-agent activity in pNETs is doxorubicin. It too was studied in a small phase 2 trial that reported responses in 4 of 20 patients.[76] Dacarbazine has also been studied in pNETs. In a phase 2 study that included 42 patients with measurable disease, a response rate of 33% was observed.[77] Fluorouracil has often been included in combination chemotherapy regimens for pNETs, yet its activity as a single agent has not been studied. Evidence of 5-FU's activity may be inferred from a clinical trial that showed a higher response rate for 5-FU plus streptozocin than for streptozocin alone.[73] Etoposide and carboplatin have also been studied as single agents in phase 2 settings. Clinical activity was not observed.[78]

Combination Chemotherapy. With several agents showing moderate clinical activity, investigators have examined a number of drug combinations to build upon earlier successes. Among the various combinations, 5-FU plus streptozocin is the most tested regimen. In four separate studies that included 7, 43, 33, and 31 patients, response rates of 29%, 63%, 45%, and 54% were observed, respectively.[73,79–81] The Eastern Cooperative Oncology Group subsequently compared this combination to streptozocin plus doxorubicin and reported a significantly higher response rate (69% vs. 45%), time to progression (median, 20 vs. 7 months), and overall survival (median, 2.2 vs. 1.4 years) for streptozocin plus doxorubicin than for streptozocin plus 5-FU.[74] Based on these data, combination chemotherapy with streptozocin-based regimens is considered the standard of care by many.

Two small retrospective series, however, have recently cast doubt on the value of streptozocin-based chemotherapy. Each of these studies examined only 16 patients. Both reported a disappointing radiologic response rate of 6%.[82,83] This tenfold difference in response rates has aroused considerable controversy as to the role of chemotherapy in treating islet cell carcinoma. Some differences may be accounted for by differences in response criteria. For example, in a study reported by Eriksson et al.,[84] the response rates, based on either decreased biochemical parameters or decreased tumor measurement, were 36% for streptozocin plus doxorubicin and 58% for streptozocin plus 5-FU. When only radiologic response was counted, the respective response rates were 8% and 32%.

A chemotherapeutic combination of 5-FU, streptozocin, and doxorubicin was studied in two small trials with 10 and 12 patients, and response rates were 40% and 55%, respectively.[66] In light of the continuing controversy regarding the role of chemotherapy in the management of pNETs, a larger retrospective study examined the outcome of 84 consecutive patients treated with the 5-FU-doxorubicin-streptozocin combination and observed a response rate of 39%.[66] The median progression-free survival in that series was 18 months, and median overall survival was 37 months. Data also showed that in some cases, the response may take time to develop. The median time to response among responders was 4 months. The authors generally advocate that patients be treated to best response and that treatment be continued for at least 4 months in absence of disease progression. Consideration should be given to adding dexrazoxane or to stopping the doxorubicin component of therapy based on cumulative exposure to doxorubicin.

Temozolomide is an oral alkylating agent that metabolizes to the same active metabolite as dacarbazine, 5-(3-methyltriazeno) imidazole-4-carboxamide. There has been recent development of temozolomide-based regimens for pNETs. Recent prospective and retrospective studies have suggested that temozolomide in combination with thalidomide, bevacizumab, or capecitabine is also active in pNETs.[18–20] In one large series, 18 of 53 (34%) patients with pNETs had objected response following temozolomide-based chemotherapy.[85] However, the activity of temozolomide as a single agent has never been prospectively examined. Therefore, it is unclear which chemotherapy combination is best or whether a combination is needed at all. Although temozolomide-based therapy is generally well tolerated, absolute lymphopenia occurs frequently and has been associated with opportunistic infections.[86] These studies suggest that temozolomide may have activity in pNETs. A definitive randomized study is needed.

Cytotoxic chemotherapy continues to play an important role in the management of pNETs. Selected regimens are summarized in Table 111.3.

Biologic Therapy

Interferon. Interferon also has been extensively studied in low-grade NETs. However, most of the studies have included a variety of NETs and only a small number of pNETs. In larger series using interferon-α at doses of 5 to 6 MU given three to five times per week, radiological responses have been reported in 12% of patients with pNETs.[87]

The exact mechanism of interferon's action in pNETs is not clear. Possible mechanisms include direct inhibition of cell proliferation, immune cell-mediated cytotoxicity, and induction of differentiation. A possible immune-mediated mechanism is suggested by the expression of tumor testis antigens as well as by reports of antitumor activity by other immunotherapeutic approaches such as interleukin-2 and dendritic cell vaccination.[88,89]

Somatostatin Analogues. Somatostatin is a hormone that binds to specific high-affinity membrane receptors on target tissues. To date, five subtypes of somatostatin receptors (SSTR) have been identified. When activated, these receptors trigger differing biologic activity. The somatostatin analogues octreotide and lanreotide both bind with high affinity to SSTR-2

TABLE 111.3

SELECTED CYTOTOXIC CHEMOTHERAPY FOR PANCREATIC NEUROENDOCRINE TUMORS

Cytotoxic Chemotherapy	Response Rates (Ref.)
Fluorouracil, streptozocin, and doxorubicin—28-day cycle 5-FU 400 mg/m²/day IV bolus on days 1–5 Streptozocin 400 mg/m²/d IV on days 1–5 Doxorubicin 40 mg/m² on day 1 only	39% (66)
Fluorouracil and streptozocin—42-day cycle 5-FU 400 mg/m²/d IV bolus on days 1–5 Streptozocin 500 mg/m²/d IV on days 1–5	32%–45% (74,84)
Streptozocin and doxorubicin—42-day cycle Streptozocin 500 mg/m²/day IV on days 1–4 Doxorubicin 50 mg/m² on days 1 and 22	6%–69% (74,84)

and with slightly lower affinity to SSTR-5. Pasireotide is a novel cyclohexapeptide in development that binds to SSRT-1, -2, -3, and -5.[90]

Somatostatin analogues are effective in controlling symptoms of hormonal hypersecretion in NETs. Somatostatin analogues have also been reported to stabilize the growth of NETs.[91,92] Recently, PROMID (*P*lacebo-controlled prospective *R*andomized study on the antiproliferative efficacy of *O*ctreotide LAR in patients with metastatic neuroendocrine *MID*gut tumors) study reported significant benefit in time to progression for midgut NET patients treated with octreotide long-acting release (LAR) compared to placebo.[93] Similar data supporting an antiproliferative effect in pNETs is, however, lacking.

Liver-Directed Therapy

Because the liver is the most common and sometimes the only site of metastasis, the development of liver-directed therapeutic approaches for pNETs is of interest. These treatment approaches are generally palliative. In the absence of a hormonal syndrome, typical indications include right upper quadrant pain, early satiety due to gastric compression by an enlarged left hepatic lobe, and the need to control slowly progressive but bulky disease.

Hepatic Artery Embolization and Chemoembolization. Hepatic artery embolization takes advantage of the liver's dual blood supply. The normal liver derives most of its blood supply from the portal circulation. pNET metastases, however, receive most of their blood supply from the hepatic artery. Thus, interruption of the blood supply from the hepatic artery preferentially causes ischemic necrosis of the metastases while sparing most of the normal liver. Currently, most procedures for occlusion of the hepatic artery involve the percutaneous infusion of small particles. The choice of embolic material varies by center and may include lipiodol or ethiodized oil, small plastic particles, and gelatin foam particles. Comparative studies of various embolic materials are lacking. In hepatic artery chemoembolization, cytotoxic agents are administered intra-arterially before the vessels are blocked, as this approach has the potential to enable delivery of a higher chemotherapy dose to liver metastases.

Most published studies of hepatic artery embolization or chemoembolization have included a mix of carcinoids and pNETs. Studies have reported a wide range of response rates ranging from 8% to more than 60% using heterogenous response criteria.[94,95] In a retrospective study from M. D. Anderson Cancer Center, where outcomes of pNET patients were separately examined, the objective tumor response rate was 35%. When the blend embolization group was compared with the chemoembolization group, a trend toward improved response rate with the addition of chemotherapy was observed (50% vs. 25%; $P = .06$).[94] In a similar retrospective study of 67 patients with NETs (19 with pNETs) who underwent chemoembolization in France, investigators compared doxorubicin with streptozocin during embolization and reported a higher response rate with streptozocin-based chemoembolization according to multivariate analyses.[96]

Based on these findings, the authors recommend hepatic artery chemoembolization in select pNET patients with liver metastases. The procedure should be carried out in a hospital setting because treatment-related toxic effects are common and may be severe. A constellation of transient symptoms and laboratory abnormalities, sometimes referred to as *postembolization syndrome,* occurs in most patients. These findings include abdominal pain, nausea, fever, fatigue, and elevated liver enzymes. Crises related to massive release of hormone(s) may occur in the presence of functional tumors; prophylactic administration of somatostatin analogues should be considered in this setting. Major complications (even deaths) have been reported in clinical trials. To minimize the risk of hepatic insufficiency, embolization should be carried out in one liver lobe at a time. In patients with bulky disease or poor liver function, more limited embolization of liver segments should be considered.

More recently, radioactive microsphere embolization has emerged as a well-tolerated outpatient procedure, providing symptom relief and varying response rates.[97–99] However, prospective studies in NETs generally and pNETs specifically are lacking.

Hepatic Metastasectomy and Transplantation. Because of the relatively indolent behavior of the disease, aggressive surgical resection has a role in the management of metastatic islet cell carcinoma. The largest published experience with pNETs involving liver resection was included in a series of 170 NET patients at the Mayo Clinic.[100] A total of 52 pNETs were included in this study. A separate analysis of pNETs was not performed, but the overall survival rate for all 170 patients was reported to be 61% and 35% at 5 and 10 years, respectively. It is, however, also clear from this study that liver resection is not curative in most of these cases; the disease recurrence rate was 85% at 5 years.[100]

The authors encourage resection for patients with a solitary metastasis. For patients with more extensive but still resectable disease, the authors advocate resection for those tumors with favorable biologic characteristics. Liver resection should be avoided in patients with a high-grade histologic subtype. A period of systemic chemotherapy may be used as part of a test-of-time approach to select patients whose disease is less likely to progress rapidly and who are therefore more likely to benefit from aggressive surgical intervention.

For those with clearly unresectable liver metastases, there has been some experience, although limited, with hepatic transplantation. However, following liver transplantation, survival of patients with pNETs was found to be inferior to that of patients who had carcinoid tumors (3-year survivals of 8% vs. 80%).[101] Given the upfront operative risk and, as yet, the lack of data supporting a survival benefit, hepatic transplantation for the management of pNETs should be considered investigational.

Radiofrequency Ablation and Cryoablation. Given the natural history of nonfunctional pNETs, most patients are diagnosed with extensive disease. Those with unresectable disease often have diffuse liver involvement or have the primary tumor intact. The majority of these patients should receive systemic therapy or chemoembolization. Occasionally, patients may have liver metastases that are unresectable but still small and few enough to allow for an ablative approach. Radiofrequency ablation (RFA) can be carried out during laparoscopy, laparotomy, or via a percutaneous approach. Although RFA has not been systematically compared with other treatment modalities, an anecdotal description of RFA's clinical benefit has been reported. In one series of 34 patients, including 9 with pNETs who underwent laparoscopic RFA, 79% of patients with symptoms at baseline reported either complete resolution or a significant reduction of tumor-related symptoms.[102]

Functional Tumors

Gastrinoma

Diagnosis and Management of Localized Disease. Gastrinoma, or Zollinger-Ellison syndrome (ZES), is a rare disease caused by a NET (gastrinoma) in the pancreas or duodenum. The hypersecretion of gastrin results in uncontrolled stimulation of parietal cells and production of gastric acid, causing refractory peptic ulcer disease. Consequently, most patients have a long history of ulcers, abdominal pain, diarrhea, severe gastroesophageal reflux, and prolonged use of acid-suppressive medication or a history of gastric or duodenal surgery. Nevertheless, diagnosis of ZES is becoming more difficult due to the frequent use of proton-pump inhibitors (PPIs), which usually control the symptoms of excess acid while using the medication. Importantly, the vast majority of patients who are found to have an elevated level of serum gastrin do not have a gastrinoma. Hypergastrinemia is most commonly caused by acid-suppressive medications, especially PPIs. If serum gastrin level is still elevated 1 week after the patient has stopped acid-suppressive therapy, it is then important to measure gastric pH. Basal gastric acid output analysis is not available in most centers, and gastric pH is rarely measured at the time of upper endoscopy (although at that time, the patient is usually tested for infection with *Helicobacter pylori*, which can also cause hypergastrinemia). Thus, the easiest way to measure gastric pH is to simply place a nasogastric tube and aspirate the gastric contents. These contents can be placed on litmus paper and the pH estimated; patients with ZES should have a gastric pH of less than 2. Elevated serum gastrin level and elevated gastric pH suggest a normal response of the gastric G cells (which produce gastrin) to parietal cell dysfunction associated with achlorhydria, atrophic gastritis, and pernicious anemia.

Patients with sporadic ZES usually have a fasting gastrin level of over 600 pg/mL, and virtually all patients have a gastrin level of more than 100 pg/mL.[103] A serum gastrin of 1,000 pg/mL or more and a gastric pH of 2 or less secure the diagnosis of ZES. In patients with gastrin levels between 100 pg/mL and 1,000 pg/mL and a gastric pH 2 or less, a secretin or calcium stimulation test should be performed. A positive secretin test is associated with a postinjection serum gastrin level increase of greater than 200 pg/mL, and a positive calcium stimulation test, with a postinjection serum gastrin level increase of greater than 395 pg/mL.[103]

Gastrinomas may reside in the duodenum (most often in the proximal duodenum) or pancreas, with duodenal location the most common. Duodenal tumors are usually small (often less than 1 cm in diameter) and rarely associated with liver metastases. When located in the pancreas, gastrinomas are usually found in the pancreatic head or uncinate process in the pancreas, which is to the right of the superior mesenteric vessels. There seems to be an association between tumor size and serum gastrin level, as pancreatic tumors, especially those 3 cm in diameter or larger, have been associated with higher serum gastrin levels.[103] Serum gastrin levels correlate with the extent of disease and are highest in those patients with locally advanced or metastatic disease.

Patients suspected to have ZES should be managed at a referral center experienced in the diagnosis and management of this disease. Once the diagnosis is established biochemically, tumor localization studies should be performed as part of the preoperative evaluation; these include upper endoscopy with EUS of the pancreatic head and duodenum, multidetector CT, and somatostatin receptor scintingraphy.[104] Because of the delay in diagnosing ZES in most patients and because of the improvements in imaging studies and EUS, gastrinomas seen today are usually successfully localized. When all tumor localization studies are negative, the tumor is most likely in the duodenum, which must be opened surgically (duodenotomy) to successfully locate and remove a duodenal gastrinoma. For pancreatic gastrinomas, the operation is based on the anatomy of the tumor and may consist of enucleation or pancreaticoduodenectomy. Consistent with the operative management of most neuroendocrine carcinomas, regional lymphadenectomy is critically important. If the entire pancreatic head and duodenum are removed, regional lymphadenectomy is fairly easy to accomplish; if a less radical resection is performed, the lymph nodes located in the peripancreatic region, adjacent to the hepatic artery, and within the porta hepatis should be removed at the time of operation.

Management of Advanced Disease. As with other functional NETs, the management of malignant gastrinoma has two foci: management of gastrin hypersecretion and its sequelae and management of the malignant proliferation similar to nonfunctional pNETs. This section will focus on issues unique to gastrinomas.

Prior to effective therapy for the control of gastric acid secretion, the principal therapy for ZES is gastrectomy to prevent gastric ulceration. Left unchecked, excessive acid secretion in ZES would frequently lead to massive hemorrhage or gastric perforation. Early medical therapy for ZES included the use of histamine-2 receptor blockers such as cimetidine, ranitidine, and famotidine. These agents were commonly used in combination with anticholinergic agents such as propantheline or isopropamide. However, the failure rates associated with these agents were high in some reported series.[105]

The introduction of proton-pump inhibitors brought significant advances in the management of ZES. Omeprazole, lansoprazole, and pantoprazole have largely replaced H2 blockers in the management of ZES. The dose of proton-pump inhibitors required to manage ZES is significantly higher than those typically used in idiopathic peptic ulcer disease. For example, the usual starting dose of omeprazole for ZES is between 40 and 60 mg/d; however, omeprazole doses greater than 200 mg/d are required in some cases for ZES.[106] Lansoprazole at 30 to 120 mg/d is given to manage ZES.[107] Although proton-pump inhibitors are adequate for the control of symptoms from gastrinoma in most cases, about 5% to 10% of patients will eventually fail standard therapy. In these cases, somatostatin analogues such as octreotide may be effective and may be used in combination with proton-pump inhibitors to control symptoms.[108]

Another aspect that deserves special attention in patients with advanced gastrinoma is the development of type II gastric carcinoids in the setting of MEN-1 and ZES. These gastric carcinoids are often small, multifocal, and of low malignant potential. Occasionally, they can also become large, involve the stomach diffusely, and cause symptoms. When few in number, they can often be excised endoscopically. Regression of these gastric carcinoids has been described in cases where somatostatin analogues or other treatment targeting the gastrinoma successfully reduced gastrin levels in a sustained manner.[109]

Insulinoma

Diagnosis and Management of Localized Disease. Insulinomas are seldom malignant and represent the most common functioning NET of the pancreas. If metastatic disease is not found at the time of initial diagnosis, it is unlikely to develop in the future.[110] It is unknown whether this unique feature of insulinomas results from underlying tumor biology or simply because, owing to their profound symptom complex, these tumors are virtually always surgically excised early, when they are small. As with all functioning and nonfunctioning tumors of the pancreas, insulinoma may occur either as a unifocal sporadic event in a patient or as part of MEN-1. The uncontrolled secretion of insulin results in hyperglycemia, manifested by neuroglycopenic symptoms such as blurred vision, confusion, and abnormal behavior, which may progress to loss of consciousness and seizure. In response to hypoglycemia, the body releases catecholamines, which elicit perspiration, anxiety, palpitations, and hunger. Most insulinoma patients associate the intake of food with the resolution of these symptoms very early in the disease process; this likely accounts for the weight gain experienced by most insulinoma patients.

The diagnosis of insulinoma syndrome is established by supervised fasting of the patient, to include a laboratory workup and observation. Serum levels of plasma glucose, C-peptide, proinsulin, insulin, and sulfonylurea are measured at intervals of 6 to 8 hours and at the point when symptoms develop. Patients with insulinoma have an insulin level greater than 3 mcIU/mL (usually greater than 6 mcIU/mL) when blood glucose is less than 40 to 45 mg/dL and an insulin-to-glucose ratio of 0.3 or less, reflecting the inappropriate secretion of insulin at the time of hypoglycemia. During the body's production of insulin, C-peptide is cleaved from proinsulin and, thus, both are elevated in patients with insulinoma. In contrast, exogenous insulin does not contain C-peptide; therefore, an elevated insulin level combined with no detectable C-peptide would indicate administration of exogenous insulin. Detectable levels of sulfonylurea would indicate the administration of oral medications to induce hypoglycemia. When the patient is under observation as part of a supervised fast, symptomatic hypoglycemia and a serum glucose level less than 45 mg/dL should be treated with 1 mg of glucagon intravenously; if the hypoglycemia is insulin mediated, this will cause the release of glucose from the liver, resulting in an elevation of serum glucose (usually by about 20 mg/dL) and the rapid resolution of symptoms.

In contrast to gastrinomas, which usually occur in the duodenum, pancreatic head, or uncinate process, insulinomas do not develop in the duodenum and may occur anywhere throughout the pancreas. In the absence of MEN-1, insulinomas, similar to gastrinomas, are unifocal. Once the biochemical diagnosis is established, localization studies performed as part of the preoperative evaluation include upper endoscopy with EUS of the pancreas and duodenum and multidetector CT. In the authors' practice, these studies will localize the overwhelming majority of sporadic insulinomas. For the very rare patient in whom tumor localization is not successful, the authors proceed with a regionalization study to determine whether the tumor is located to the right or left of the mesenteric vessels. Regionalization of an insulinoma is performed with selective arterial calcium stimulation and hepatic vein sampling.[111] Calcium is used as a secretagogue for insulin and is injected into the gastroduodenal artery (GDA), SMA, and splenic artery; a serum sample for insulin measurement is obtained from the right hepatic vein. An elevation of insulin obtained from serum in the hepatic vein following selective arterial injection regionalizes the insulinoma to that portion of the pancreas injected with calcium. It is therefore possible to determine whether the insulinoma is in the pancreatic head or uncinate process (elevation of hepatic vein insulin following calcium infusion of the GDA or SMA) or in the body or tail of the pancreas (elevation of insulin following calcium infusion into the splenic artery). Because tumor localization with a combination of multidetector CT and EUS is so successful, when these methods fail to localize the tumor in a patient presumed to have insulinoma syndrome, the authors carefully doublecheck the diagnostic evaluation and then proceed with selective arterial calcium stimulation and hepatic vein sampling to minimize the potential for an unsuccessful operation.

Because nonmetastatic insulinomas are thought to be benign (or at least to have a very low malignant potential), the standard treatment is enucleation. It is important to remove the tumor with the tumor capsule completely and not to leave a portion of the tumor behind, as local recurrence can occur.[112] If enucleation is not possible due to the location of the tumor within the pancreas, segmental resection of the pancreas, distal pancreatectomy, or pancreaticoduodenectomy may be necessary. In the authors' experience over the past 15 years, they have only performed two pancreaticoduodenectomies for sporadic insulinoma. Large defects in the pancreas that result from enucleation are usually treated with a Roux-en-Y pancreaticojejunostomy to prevent a pancreatic leak at the enucleation site. Metachronous distant metastases are very rare but have been reported in the absence of local recurrence.[113] It is interesting to hypothesize that the biology of the disease may change to a more aggressive phenotype in the setting of incomplete surgical excision and local recurrence. In contrast to the findings of a few reports in the literature,[113] the authors have not seen a patient with a surgically excised nonmetastatic isolated insulinoma develop metachronous tumor recurrence in a distant organ. The patients with metastatic insulinoma seen by these authors had liver metastases with or without bone metastases at the time of diagnosis.

Management of Advanced Disease. In rare cases, insulinomas can be metastatic at diagnosis. These cases are challenging to manage because of the often refractory hypoglycemia. There are no data to suggest that insulinomas respond differently to systemic or liver-directed therapy. Thus, the previously discussed strategies outlined for nonfunctional tumors can be applied. This section will focus on the aspects of malignant insulinoma that require special attention.

Glycemic control is a key aspect of managing malignant insulinomas. Mild symptoms sometimes can be controlled by diet. Patients may need to eat frequently; family members or caregivers may need to wake the patient at midnight for a snack to avoid early morning hypoglycemia. In select cases, enteral feeding tubes may be required to provide continuous nocturnal caloric support. Medical therapy may include diazoxide, glucocorticoids, verapamil, and phenytoin. Diazoxide, an antihypertensive known to increase blood sugar, is the best studied of these agents. It is typically administered in doses of 50 to 300 mg/d. Side effects include edema, weight gain, renal impairment, and hirsutism. Glucagon may also have a role in the management of insulinomas. A glucagon pen may be given to the patient's family or caregiver to be used in emergent cases. Not all insulinomas respond well to glucagon, however. The authors suggest that a test dose be given under supervision during a hypoglycemic episode before the drug is prescribed. Although all of the aforementioned drugs may help control symptoms, eventual resistance may develop. These drugs are perhaps best used to maintain glycemic control while other therapeutic strategies are being applied.

Somatostatin analogues such as octreotide may be helpful for the control of insulin release, but they can also suppress counter-regulatory hormones such as growth hormones, glucagons, and catecholamines. In this situation, somatostatin analogues can lead to worsening of hypoglycemia.[114] Therefore, the authors recommend that short-acting somatostatin analogues should be initiated under direct medical supervision. Glucose and insulin levels should be checked before and after the injection to assess the analogue's effect on hormonal production before committing the patient to long-term outpatient therapy.

Despite these measures, refractory hypoglycemia frequently occurs and can be difficult to manage. It has been recently observed that such patients may respond to the mTOR inhibitor everolimus. Data suggest that insulin triggers its own production and release via the insulin receptor.[115,116] mTOR mediates signal transduction downstream of the insulin receptor and mTOR inhibitors block insulin-stimulated synthesis, release, and proliferation.[115,116] In a series of four consecutive patients with malignant hypoglycemia treated with everolimus, all four patients experienced dramatic improvements in glycemic control.[117]

Finally, aggressive therapy targeting the tumor is needed to debulk the disease present. As malignant insulinomas can often be indolent in terms of tumor growth, surgical resection, hepatic artery chemoembolization, and RFA can be considered whenever possible. Streptozocin-based chemotherapy should also be considered. Data suggest that streptozocin is toxic to insulin-producing cells. In addition to its cytotoxic effect, streptozocin can decrease insulin production in β cells. Indeed, the authors' experience with some patients indicates that streptozocin may "turn off" the production of insulin for years, even in the absence of tumor shrinkage. Chemotherapy, however, may require intensive supportive care because the nausea, vomiting, and anorexia associated with treatment may transiently worsen hypoglycemia.

Rare Functional Endocrine Tumors

In addition to gastrinomas and insulinomas, several other less common functional tumors deserve special consideration. These include vasoactive intestinal peptide (VIP)omas, glucagonomas, somatostatinomas, corticotropinomas, and parathyroid hormone–related peptide secreting tumors. Similar to other functional tumors, the bulk of these rare tumors are well differentiated. For the most part, the workup and management of these tumors are similar to those of nonfunctional tumors. Thus, only the unique aspects of these tumors will be discussed here.

Vasoactive Intestinal Peptide Tumors

VIPomas are the cause of the classic Verner-Morrison syndrome.[118] These endocrine tumors secrete vasoactive intestinal peptide, which can cause watery diarrhea, hypokalemia, and achlorhydria (WDHA). Diarrhea in patients with VIPomas is often insidious at onset but extreme by the time of diagnosis. Patients can have more than 20 bowel movements a day, with a daily stool volume exceeding 3 L. Thus, fluid and electrolyte replacement is often needed at the time of diagnosis. In adults, most VIPomas arise from the pancreas. In children, however, most VIP-secreting tumors arise from an extrapancreatic location.

Control of diarrhea is an important part of management. These tumors are often quite sensitive, at least initially, to somatostatin analogues[119]; octreotide can promptly control diarrhea in 80% to 90% of cases. However, over time many patients will escape from control. Dose escalation can be helpful in some cases. With short-acting octreotide, a dose of 50 to 400 mcg/d is typically used. With depot formulation, octreotide LAR doses exceeding 30 mg every 3 weeks have been advocated by some. Somatostatin analogues at high doses, however, can cause exocrine pancreatic insufficiency, leading to malabsorptive diarrhea; pancrelipase can be used concurrently to control these symptoms.

Interferon can also be helpful for symptom control.[120] Because of its toxicity, interferon is rarely used in the frontline setting, but it may have a role in cases refractory to somatostatin analogues. In general, measures aimed at cytoreduction should be initiated (see "Nonfunctional Tumors").

Glucagonoma

Glucagon is a 29-amino acid peptide that causes glycogenolysis, gluconeogenesis, ketogenesis, lipolysis, and catecholamine secretion. Patients typically present with a syndrome that includes diabetes and a characteristic rash known as necrolytic migratory erythema. Weight loss, diarrhea, glossitis, and angular stomatitis have also been reported.[53] These patients typically also have amino acid depletion due to the high level of glucagons. Somatostatin analogues may have a role in the management of the hormonal syndrome in patients with unresectable tumors.[121] Oral hypoglycemic agents and insulin can be used to control the diabetes. Necrolytic migratory erythema is thought to be related at least in part to amino acid depletion.[122] Thus, amino acid and zinc supplementation may also be helpful.[123]

Somatostatinoma

Somatostatinomas are very rare functional endocrine tumors that can arise from the pancreas or the duodenum. Because of the insidious and nonspecific nature of the symptoms, most somatostatinomas are diagnosed at an advanced stage. Patients typically present with symptoms including diabetes, diarrhea, and jaundice due to biliary obstruction. Somatostatinomas may be associated with von Recklinghausen's disease; those tumors so associated are mostly duodenal or ampullary in origin and less likely to be associated with a hormonal syndrome or metastatic at the time of diagnosis.[124] The principles of management for somatostatinomas parallel those of nonfunctional pNETs.

Corticotropinoma

Corticotropin-secreting tumors are also among the rare functional tumors of the pancreas. Patients with corticotropinomas often present with florid Cushing syndrome due to ectopic production of corticotropin. Induction chemotherapy in these patients is fraught with difficulties due to the patient's immunosuppression and often debilitated state. Initial management should be aimed at controlling corticosteroid production. Metyrapone, ketoconazole, and mitotane tend to be more effective in this setting than for adrenal cortical carcinoma and can be used to suppress excess cortisol production. In some cases, bilateral adrenalectomy may be needed.

ADDITIONAL CLINICAL CONSIDERATIONS

Hereditary Syndromes

It is known that pNETs can occur in the setting of several genetic syndromes. These include MEN-1, tuberous sclerosis, neurofibromatosis, and von Hippel-Lindau (vHL) disease. MEN-1 is discussed in greater detail elsewhere in this book. Here, the discussion is limited to special considerations involved in the surgical management of MEN-1-related pNETs. In addition, the aspects of tuberous sclerosis, neurofibromatosis, and vHL disease as they relate to pNETs will be discussed. As in all genetic cancer syndromes, genetic counseling and cancer screening are recommended.

Multiple Endocrine Neoplasia Type 1

Only recently have surgeons considered the oncologic aspects of pancreatic neoplasia in regard to MEN-1 patients who have nonfunctioning pNETs.[125,126] Due to the characteristic multifocality of the pNETs in patients with MEN-1 and to the desire to avoid total pancreatectomy, some investigators have discouraged early surgery in patients with MEN-1.[62] It has been suggested that surgery for nonfunctioning pNETs should be limited to those tumors larger than 2 to 3 cm in diameter.[62,111,127–132] In a single institution series, a trend was shown for larger tumors to be associated with the presence of synchronous distant metastases at the time of diagnosis. In one study none of the 19 pNETs 2.5 cm or smaller in maximum dimension had distant metastases at the time of diagnosis compared with 5 (23%) of the 22 pNETs larger than 2.5 cm ($p = .05$).[66] However, tumor size may not be a completely reliable predictor of malignant behavior, as metastatic disease may be present in MEN-1 patients even when the primary tumors are small.[133]

Thompson et al.[125,134,135] were first to advocate a specific surgical procedure in MEN-1 patients with nonfunctioning pNETs greater than 1 cm in diameter. The operation of these investigators included distal subtotal pancreatectomy, enucleation of any identified lesions in the pancreatic head or uncinate process, and regional lymphadenectomy.

The authors currently operate on all MEN-1 patients who have evidence of a pNET(s) on CT imaging that is 1.5 to 2 cm in size or larger or who has demonstrated an increase in size on serial imaging. The authors concur that the Thompson procedure is often the most appropriate operation for these patients, as it removes all visible tumors and decreases the volume of the remaining at-risk pancreas. This procedure clearly represents a compromise, as it leaves islet cell mass in the pancreatic head, which carries the risk of metachronous neoplasms, while usually preventing the complications of insulin-dependant diabetes associated with total pancreatectomy. The goal of this operation is to delay the need for total pancreatectomy (assuming that some patients may develop metachronous neoplasms in the remaining pancreas and require completion total pancreatectomy) and thereby avoid the long-term complications of type 1 diabetes, especially in young patients. Very long-term follow-up will be necessary to determine the efficacy of this approach. In patients with large tumors within the head of the pancreas that are not amenable to enucleation, pancreaticoduodenectomy (with preservation of a portion of the pancreatic body and tail when possible) is an appropriate alternative.

Von Hippel-Lindau Syndrome

Von Hippel-Lindau syndrome is an autosomal dominant, inherited familial cancer syndrome that was initially discovered in 1927.[136] It is associated with a variety of neoplasms, frequently including retinal, cerebellar, and spinal hemangioblastoma; renal cell carcinoma; pheochromocytoma; and pNETs. The vHL gene is located on chromosome 3p26–p25. Tumors that arise in the setting of vHL disease are often vascular. This is likely due to the role of the vHL gene in regulating angiogenesis.

pNETs occur in about 12% of patients with the vHL syndrome.[137,138] However, the vHL gene may be involved in sporadic cases of pNETs. Allelic deletion at chromosome 3p, the site of vHL gene, has also been described to occur frequently in sporadic pNETs.[26,38]

Tuberous Sclerosis and Neurofibromatosis

Tuberous sclerosis and neurofibromatosis are two other hereditary cancer syndromes associated with the development of pNETs. The genes responsible for tuberous sclerosis, *TSC-1* and *TSC-2*, are located on chromosomes 9q34 and 16p13.3, respectively, and code the proteins hamartin and tuberin. TSC1/2 complex is an inhibitor of mTOR, which is a key regulator of cellular proliferation and survival and of protein production. TSC1/2 are normally expressed in neuroendocrine cells.[139] Although benign hamartomas are the most common manifestation of this expression, patients with defects in the *TSC2* gene have tuberous sclerosis and are known to develop islet cell carcinoma.[140]

Neurofibromatosis type I, also known as Von Recklinghausen disease, is an autosomal dominant disease associated with the development of cutaneous neurofibromas and skin lesions known as café-au-lait spots. The gene responsible for neurofibromatosis 1 (*NF1*) codes for the protein neurofibromin 1 and is located on chromosome 17. It has recently been discovered that NF1 regulates the activity of TSC2. The loss of NF1 in neurofibromatosis leads to constitutive mTOR activation and tumor formation.[141] Neurofibromatosis type I is associated with the development of NETs in the region of the duodenum and ampulla of Vater.[140] Many of the endocrine tumors that arise from Von Recklinghausen disease are somatostatinomas.

High-Grade Neuroendocrine Carcinoma

High-grade neuroendocrine carcinomas (also known as poorly differentiated neuroendocrine carcinomas)[12] rarely arise from the pancreas. These aggressive tumors are characterized by early systemic dissemination and rapid growth. Sometimes also described as small cell carcinomas or large cell NETs, high-grade neuroendocrine carcinomas share a similar pattern of clinical behavior with small cell carcinomas of the lung. Although the diagnosis of poorly differentiated carcinoma is usually straightforward, when the diagnosis is made by FNA, the grade of the tumor may not be specified.

Owing to the rarity of these tumors, few prospective data are available to guide their management. Much of the current practice has been based on experience with small cell lung carcinoma. High-grade NETs of the pancreas are often diagnosed at advanced stages. The authors recommend induction chemotherapy even for potentially resectable cases due to the aggressive nature of this disease and the high rate of relapse.

These rare but aggressive tumors are initially chemosensitive. Treatment generally parallels the therapy developed for small cell lung cancer. Platinum-based chemotherapy is recommended in the front-line setting. Two-drug combinations such as etoposide plus cisplatin or irinotecan plus cisplatin have shown activity.[142,143]

SURGERY PITFALLS

For functioning tumors, it remains critically important to separate the diagnostic and the tumor localization phases of the evaluation. It is tempting to proceed with localization studies before the diagnosis of ZES or insulinoma is firmly established. In such cases, an incidental finding on cross-sectional imaging (now quite common due to the sensitivity of the technology) may prompt an ill-advised surgical procedure. If the diagnosis is biochemically confirmed but localization studies are negative, one should consider referring the patient to a specialty center and an experienced endocrine surgeon.

When dealing with a large, borderline resectable primary tumor, the authors frequently consider preoperative induction chemotherapy. In the newly diagnosed patient with both a pancreatic pNET and liver metastases, determining the patient's candidacy for surgery has become very complex. For example, the authors may follow induction chemotherapy with a two-staged surgical approach if imaging studies suggest that an adequate portion of the liver is uninvolved (or minimally involved) with disease. At the first operation, the primary tumor is removed, and the liver bisegment (or lobe) that is to remain in place is cleared of disease. This may then be followed by portal vein embolization of the hepatic lobe to be removed, with a second surgery planned for liver resection.[144] Such multidisciplinary management requires a dedicated group of physicians and an infrastructure that can assist patients with treatment-related complications such as biliary stent occlusion, nutritional depletion, gastrointestinal and hematologic toxicity, and surgery-related morbidity.

Finally, all physicians must remember that pNETs usually grow slowly and, therefore, if patients have a good performance status, they will usually survive longer than anticipated, despite the presence of locally advanced or metastatic disease. Because of this, treatment-related mortality (especially surgery induced) should be avoided. An ill-advised operation with a bad outcome in an otherwise healthy patient (of any age and especially those of young age where the temptation to operate is often great) should be considered an act of poor judgment rather than heroism.

EMERGING THERAPEUTIC OPTIONS

Peptide Receptor Radiotherapy

The presence of somatostatin receptors in high density on tumor cells has led to the development of peptide receptor radiotherapy (PPRT) for NETs. Early studies with ^{111}In-, ^{90}Y-, or ^{177}Lu-labeled somatostatin analogues have reported promising results in the control of hormonally related symptoms.[145] The earliest studies were carried out with [^{111}In-DTPA^{0}] octreotide. Although symptomatic improvements were reported, objective tumor responses were rarely observed. Subsequently, ^{90}Y was linked to octreotide to create [^{90}Y-DOTA^{0},Tyr^{3}] octreotide. Several studies were carried out in patients with NETs and produced response rates of 10% to 30%.[145] In the largest prospective study that treated 90 patients with NETs, only a modest response rate of 4% was observed.[146]

Finally, a number of European centers are now using octreotate, which substitutes the C-terminal threoninol with threonine. Octreotate is linked to ^{177}Lu to create [^{177}Lu-DOTA0,Tyr3] octreotate. In the largest series, 504 patients with NETs were treated. Authors reported a response rate of 30% among a subset of 310 patients. However, if intent-to-treat analysis was performed, the objective response would be approximately 18%.[147] In general, expected toxicities with peptide receptor radiotherapy include nausea, vomiting, abdominal pain, cytopenia, and hair loss. More serious side effects, including renal failure, leukemia, and myelodysplastic syndrome, have also been reported. Large-scale random assignment trials are needed to define its role in the management of pNETs.

Therapy Targeting Vascular Endothelial Growth Factor

pNETs are vascular tumors known to express VEGF. Recent studies have demonstrated the expression of VEGFR-FLK and VEGFR-FLT1 on tumor cells.[148] In a recent study, the authors investigated VEGF expression patterns by IHC in patients with resected low-grade NETs and found that tumor expression of VEGF correlated with metastases and with a decrease in progression-free survival duration.[149]

Sunitinib is a novel tyrosine kinase inhibitor with activity against VEGFR, c-Kit, and platelet-derived growth factor (PDGFR). In a multicenter phase 2 study, investigators treated carcinoid and pNETs patients in separate strata and also observed evidence of clinical activity in patients with NETs. Interestedly, in this study, the tumor response rate appeared to be higher among patients with pNETs than in patients with carcinoids (17% vs. 2%).[150] A subsequent phase 3 study compared sunitinib to placebo in pNETs (Table 111.4). Results of an early unplanned analysis showed improved progression-free survival by investigator review (5.5 months vs. 11.4 months).[151] Although the study showed clinically meaningful benefit, the small number of events and the unplanned nature of the analyses call into question the validity of hypothesis testing.

Therapy Targeting Mammalian Target of Rapamycin

mTOR is an intracellular protein that has a central role in cellular function. It acts as a nutrient sensor and mediates signaling downstream of key receptor tyrosine kinases such as insulinlike growth factor (IGF), VEGF, and epidermal growth factor (EGF) receptors. It is also involved in the control of cell growth, protein synthesis, autophagy, and angiogenesis. The association between aberrant mTOR pathway signaling and the pathogenesis of pNETs is suggested by the development of pNETs in patients with inherited genetic mutations in *TSC2*, *NF1*, and *vHL* genes. pNETs have also been described to coexpress both IGF-1 and IGF-1R.[152] In the BON-1 line, established from lymph node metastases in a patient with pNET, exogenous IGF has been shown to activate mTOR and to increase cellular proliferation. In this model, rapamycin inhibited both mTOR activation and tumor growth.[152]

Phase 2 studies of mTOR inhibitors, such as everolimus, have reported evidence of clinical activity.[67,153] In the first study, the combination of octreotide LAR and everolimus was studied in

PRACTICE OF ONCOLOGY

TABLE 111.4

PHASE 3 STUDIES OF TARGETED AGENTS IN PANCREATIC NEUROENDOCRINE TUMORS

Regimen (Ref.)	No. of Patients	Median PFS (mo)	Hazard Ratio	*P*
Everolimus 10 mg daily (154) Placebo	204 203	11 4.6	0.35 (95% CI, 0.27–0.45)	<.0001
Sunitinib 37.5 mg daily (151) Placebo	86 85	11.4 5.5	0.42 (95% CI, 0.26–0.66)	.0001

PFS, progression-free survival; CI, confidence interval.

60 patients with NETs.[153] The intent-to-treat overall response rate was 20%. The response rate among 30 patients with pNET was 27%. In a subsequent multinational phase 2 study (RADIANT-1) in advanced pNETs with progression following chemotherapy, 160 patients were treated in two strata, with everolimus (N = 115) or everolimus (N = 45) plus octreotide based on whether patients were on octreotide at study entry.[67] By central radiology review, the response rate was lower at 9.6%. Durable disease stabilizations were, however, observed among patients with progression at study entry. The median progression-free survival for patients receiving everolimus or everolimus plus octreotide were 9.7 months and 16.7 months, respectively. A large confirmatory phase 3 study in pNETs (RADIANT-3) enrolled 410 patients and compared everolimus versus placebo among patients with advanced progressive pNETs. The study showed clinically and statistically significant benefit in PFS among patients receiving everolimus (Table 111.4).[154] Everolimus prolongs median progression-free survival from 4.6 months to 11 months, leading to a 65% risk reduction for progression compared to placebo (hazard ratio 0.35; 95% confidence interval, 0.27 to 0.45; $P < .0001$). Everolimus should be considered a standard of care treatment option for advanced pNETs.

Selected References

The full list of references for this chapter appears in the online version.

1. Yao JC, Hassan M, Phan A, et al. One hundred years after "carcinoid": epidemiology of and prognostic factors for neuroendocrine tumors in 35,825 cases in the United States. *J Clin Oncol* 2008;26:3063.
3. Lam KY, Lo CY. Pancreatic endocrine tumour: a 22-year clinico-pathological experience with morphological, immunohistochemical observation and a review of the literature. *Eur J Surg Oncol* 1997;23:36.
6. Hanahan D. Heritable formation of pancreatic beta-cell tumours in transgenic mice expressing recombinant insulin/simian virus 40 oncogenes. *Nature* 1985;315:115.
7. Crabtree JS, Scacheri PC, Ward JM, et al. A mouse model of multiple endocrine neoplasia, type 1, develops multiple endocrine tumors. *Proc Natl Acad Sci U S A* 2001;98:1118.
13. Rindi G, Kloppel G, Alhman H, et al. TNM staging of foregut (neuro) endocrine tumors: a consensus proposal including a grading system. *Virchows Arch* 2006;449:395.
17. Ekeblad S, Skogseid B, Dunder K, et al. Prognostic factors and survival in 324 patients with pancreatic endocrine tumor treated at a single institution. *Clin Cancer Res* 2008;14:7798.
33. Chung DC, Smith AP, Louis DN, et al. A novel pancreatic endocrine tumor suppressor gene locus on chromosome 3p with clinical prognostic implications. *J Clin Invest* 1997;100:404.
34. Barghorn A, Komminoth P, Bachmann D, et al. Deletion at 3p25.3–p23 is frequently encountered in endocrine pancreatic tumours and is associated with metastatic progression. *J Pathol* 2001;194:451.
62. Norton JA, Fraker DL, Alexander HR, et al. Surgery to cure the Zollinger-Ellison syndrome. *N Engl J Med* 1999;341:635.
65. Bajetta E, Ferrari L, Martinetti A, et al. Chromogranin A, neuron specific enolase, carcinoembryonic antigen, and hydroxyindole acetic acid evaluation in patients with neuroendocrine tumors. *Cancer* 1999;86:858.
66. Kouvaraki MA, Ajani JA, Hoff P, et al. Fluorouracil, doxorubicin, and streptozocin in the treatment of patients with locally advanced and metastatic pancreatic endocrine carcinomas. *J Clin Oncol* 2004;22:4762.
67. Yao JC, Lombard-Bohas C, Baudin E, et al. Daily oral everolimus activity in patients with metastatic pancreatic neuroendocrine tumors after failure of cytotoxic chemotherapy: a phase II trial. *J Clin Oncol* 2010;28:69.
69. Solorzano CC, Lee JE, Pisters PW, et al. Nonfunctioning islet cell carcinoma of the pancreas: survival results in a contemporary series of 163 patients. *Surgery* 2001;130:1078.
73. Moertel CG, Hanley JA, Johnson LA: Streptozocin alone compared with streptozocin plus fluorouracil in the treatment of advanced islet-cell carcinoma. *N Engl J Med* 1980;303:1189.
74. Moertel CG, Lefkopoulo M, Lipsitz S, et al. Streptozocin-doxorubicin, streptozocin-fluorouracil or chlorozotocin in the treatment of advanced islet-cell carcinoma. *N Engl J Med* 1992;326:519.
75. Broder LE, Carter SK. Pancreatic islet cell carcinoma. II. Results of therapy with streptozotocin in 52 patients. *Ann Intern Med* 1973;79:108.
76. Moertel CG, Lavin PT, Hahn RG. Phase II trial of doxorubicin therapy for advanced islet cell carcinoma. *Cancer Treat Rep* 1982;66:1567.
77. Ramanathan RK, Cnaan A, Hahn RG, et al. Phase II trial of dacarbazine (DTIC) in advanced pancreatic islet cell carcinoma. Study of the Eastern Cooperative Oncology Group-E6282. *Ann Oncol* 2001;12:1139.
81. Eriksson B, Oberg K. An update of the medical treatment of malignant endocrine pancreatic tumors. *Acta Oncol* 1993;32:203.
82. Cheng PN, Saltz LB. Failure to confirm major objective antitumor activity for streptozocin and doxorubicin in the treatment of patients with advanced islet cell carcinoma. *Cancer* 1999;86:944.
84. Eriksson B, Skogseid B, Lundqvist G, et al. Medical treatment and long-term survival in a prospective study of 84 patients with endocrine pancreatic tumors. *Cancer* 1990;65:1883.
85. Kulke M, Hornick J, Frauenhoffer C, et al. O6-methylguanine DNA methyltransferase deficiency and response to temozolomide-based therapy in patients with neuroendocrine tumors. *Clin Cancer Res* 2009;15:338.
86. Kulke MH, Stuart K, Enzinger PC, et al. Phase II study of temozolomide and thalidomide in patients with metastatic neuroendocrine tumors. *J Clin Oncol* 2006;24:401.
94. Gupta S, Johnson MM, Murthy R, et al. Hepatic arterial embolization and chemoembolization for the treatment of patients with metastatic neuroendocrine tumors. *Cancer* 2005;104:1590.
98. Kennedy AS, Dezarn WA, McNeillie P, et al. Radioembolization for unresectable neuroendocrine hepatic metastases using resin 90Y-microspheres: early results in 148 patients. *Am J Clin Oncol* 2008;31:271.
117. Kulke MH, Bergsland EK, Yao JC. Glycemic control in patients with insulinoma treated with everolimus. *N Engl J Med* 2009;360:195.
132. Ruszniewski P, Rougier P, Roche A, et al. Hepatic arterial chemoembolization in patients with liver metastases of endocrine tumors. A prospective phase II study in 24 patients. *Cancer* 1993;71:2624.
146. Bushnell DL Jr, O'Dorisio TM, O'Dorisio MS, et al. 90Y-edotreotide for metastatic carcinoid refractory to octreotide. *J Clin Oncol* 2010;28:1652.
147. Kwekkeboom DJ, de Herder WW, Kam BL, et al. Treatment with the radiolabeled somatostatin analog [177 Lu-DOTA 0,Tyr3] octreotate: toxicity, efficacy, and survival. *J Clin Oncol* 2008;26:2124
150. Kulke MH, Lenz HJ, Meropol NJ, et al. Activity of sunitinib in patients with advanced neuroendocrine tumors. *J Clin Oncol* 2008;26:3403.
151. Raymond E, Raoul J, Niccoli P, et al. Phase III, randomized, double-blind trial of sunitinib versus placebo in patients with progressive well-differentiated pancreatic islet cell tumours. *Ann Oncol* 2009;20:vii11.
153. Yao JC, Phan AT, Chang DZ, et al. Efficacy of RAD001 (everolimus) and octreotide LAR in advanced low- to intermediate-grade neuroendocrine tumors: results of a phase II study. *J Clin Oncol* 2008;26:4311.
154. Yao JC, Shah MH, Ito T, et al. Everolimus versus placebo in patients with advanced pancreatic neuroendocrine tumors (pNET) (RADIANT-3). *Ann Oncol* 2010; (in press).

CHAPTER 112 NEUROENDOCRINE (CARCINOID) TUMORS AND THE CARCINOID SYNDROME

GERARD M. DOHERTY

PATHOLOGY AND TUMOR HISTOLOGY

Neuroendocrine tumors (NETs) are derived from the diffuse neuroendocrine system, which is made up of peptide- and amine-producing cells with different hormonal profiles depending on their site of origin. Carcinoid tumors are classified as NETs and share cytochemical features with melanomas, pheochromocytomas, medullary carcinomas of the thyroid, and pancreatic endocrine tumors.[1] Carcinoid tumors are composed of monotonous sheets of small round cells with uniform nuclei and cytoplasm, and mitotic figures are rare. Pathologists cannot differentiate benign from malignant carcinoid tumors based on histologic analysis, nor can they histologically differentiate pancreatic endocrine tumors from carcinoid tumors. Malignancy can only be determined by local invasion or distant metastases. Ultrastructurally, carcinoid tumors possess electron-dense neurosecretory granules and they contain small clear vesicles that correspond to the synaptic vesicles of neurons. Carcinoid tumors synthesize bioactive amines and peptides, including neuron-specific enolase (NSE), 5-hydroxytryptamine serotonin (5-HT), 5-hydroxytryptophan (5-HTP), synaptophysin, and chromogranin A and C, and other peptides like insulin, growth hormone, neurotensin, adrenocorticotropic hormone (ACTH), β-melanocyte-stimulating hormone, gastrin, pancreatic polypeptide, calcitonin, substance P, other various tachykinins (neuropeptide-K), growth hormone–releasing hormone, bombesin, and various growth factors such as transforming growth factor-β, platelet-derived growth factor, and fibroblast growth factor-β.[1,2]

Most carcinoid tumors are tentatively identified on routine histologic analysis. However, these tumors are characterized by their histologic staining patterns. Historically, one of the most important was their staining with silver. Characteristically, carcinoid tumors either take up and reduce silver (argentaffin reaction) or take it up but do not reduce it (argyrophilic reaction). The identification of chromogranin, synaptophysin, or NSE is now generally used.[1–3] The chromogranins (A, B, and C) are acidic polypeptides that are the major component of the secretory granules of many neuroendocrine cells. In general, chromogranin A immunoreactivity is more specific than the argyrophilic reaction because the latter also identifies other intracellular proteins such as melanin. NSE, the γ-γ dimer of the glycolytic enzyme enolase, occurs in the cytoplasm of most neuroendocrine cells and is found in most carcinoid tumors as well as other APUDomas (amine precursor uptake decarboxylase). The advantage of NSE as a marker is that its reactivity is unrelated to secretory granule content. However, NSE occasionally can be misleading, because some tumors not considered neuroendocrine, such as fibroadenomas of the breast, carcinomas, and certain lymphomas, may contain a considerable amount of NSE activity. Synaptophysin is a calcium-binding vesicle membrane glycoprotein that is expressed independently of other neuroendocrine proteins.[2]

In addition to the general histologic NET markers, specific markers for carcinoid tumors may identify the tumor as a carcinoid. Serotonin can be identified by various methods, including the use of the argentaffin reaction of Masson or the use of antibodies to 5-HT. In general, the argentaffin reaction of Masson is usually positive, and the 5-HT antibody localization is frequently weak or negative in midgut carcinoid tumors, whereas in foregut and hindgut carcinoid tumors, 5-HT immunoreactivity is detected more often than is the argentaffin reaction.[1]

Carcinoid tumors can be classified according to their site of origin because carcinoid tumors with similar sites of origin frequently share functional manifestations, histochemistry, and secretory products (Table 112.1). Foregut carcinoid tumors generally have a low 5-HT content, are argentaffin-negative but argyrophilic, occasionally secrete 5-HTP or ACTH, can be associated with an atypical carcinoid syndrome, are often multihormonal, and may metastasize to bone. Although many foregut carcinoid tumors synthesize peptides, clinical syndromes are rarely produced, and elevated plasma hormone levels are generally not detected. Midgut carcinoid tumors are argentaffin-positive, have a high 5-HT content, have smaller numbers of endocrine cells than foregut tumors, most frequently cause the classic carcinoid syndrome when they metastasize, release 5-HT and tachykinins (substance P, neuropeptide K, substance K), rarely secrete 5-HTP or ACTH, and uncommonly metastasize to bone (Table 112.1). Hindgut carcinoid tumors are argentaffin-negative, often argyrophilic, rarely contain 5-HT, rarely cause the carcinoid syndrome, contain numerous gastrointestinal (GI) hormones, rarely secrete 5-HTP or ACTH, and may metastasize to bone (Table 112.1).

Carcinoid tumors within the same site of origin such as lung, thymus, and pancreas can differ significantly in characteristics and behavior. Therefore, it has been proposed that the term *carcinoid* be replaced by the designation *neuroendocrine tumor*. In this classification tumors are divided according to tissue of origin and subdivided by growth behavior. It is argued that this classification system better reflects the biology of these tumors and provides better guidelines for tumors with similar behaviors in different tissues.[4]

Carcinoid tumors can occur throughout the respiratory or GI tracts, but most originate in one of three sites: bronchus, colon-rectum, and jejunoileum.[5,6] In the past, carcinoid tumors were most frequently reported in the appendix (approximately 40%); however, more recently the bronchus and lung and small intestine are the most common sites

Carcinoid tumors can be classified by their histologic growth patterns: insular, trabecular, glandular, undifferentiated, or mixed. The midgut carcinoid tumors frequently possess the most typical morphology, with insularlike formation of regular tumor cells, surrounded by fibrotic stroma. Most foregut carcinoid tumors show a more mixed growth pattern, with a solid, ribbonlike, trabecular, or acinar pattern. Hindgut carcinoid tumors are frequently solid or trabecular. Histologic types do have prognostic significance.

MOLECULAR PATHOGENESIS

Little is known about the induction of malignant growth or the factors promoting the growth of carcinoid tumors. For some gastric carcinoid tumors, studies show that gastrin is an important growth factor.[13] There is an increased occurrence of gastric carcinoid tumors in disease states that result in hypergastrinemia (pernicious anemia, atrophic gastritis, Zollinger-Ellison syndrome). The hyperplastic effect of hypergastrinemia is restricted to gastric ECL cells. In pernicious anemia and atrophic gastritis, up to 4% to 11% of patients develop gastric carcinoid tumors. Patients with Zollinger-Ellison syndrome also develop gastric carcinoid tumors, although these are much more frequent in the subgroup with MEN-1. In patients with Zollinger-Ellison syndrome with MEN-1 with gastric carcinoid tumors, there is allelic loss at the MEN-1 locus on chromosome band 11q13, and thus fundic gastric carcinoid tumors are now included in the spectrum of MEN-1 tumors. Studies suggest that other important growth factors in some carcinoid tumors are transforming growth factor-α, transforming growth factor-β, insulinlike growth factor-1, trefoil peptides, platelet-derived growth factor, vascular endothelial growth factor, acidic and basic fibroblast growth factor, and epidermal growth factor.[14]

CLINICAL FEATURES OF CARCINOID TUMORS

General Characteristics

The tumors can occur at any age; in the SEER data, the median age at diagnosis was 63 years. The gender occurrence was nearly equal (52% women).

Carcinoid Tumors without Systemic Features

The presentation of carcinoid tumors that do not cause carcinoid syndrome is diverse and related to the site of origin of the tumor as well as the malignant spread of the tumor. In the appendix (Table 112.2), carcinoid tumors are usually found incidentally during operation for suspected appendicitis. For small intestinal carcinoid tumors, the jejunoileum is the most common location for carcinoid tumors of clinical significance. Most small intestinal carcinoid tumors found in autopsy studies have not caused symptoms, but these tumors can lead to fibrosis of the mesentery, which results in kinking of the bowel, intestinal obstruction, and gut infarction or intussusception. The most common presenting symptoms from small intestinal carcinoid tumors are periodic abdominal pain (51%), intestinal obstruction with ileus or invagination (31%), an abdominal tumor (17%), and GI bleeding (11%).[15] Because of the vagueness of the symptoms, the diagnosis is frequently delayed, with a median time from onset from symptoms to diagnosis of approximately 2 years and a range of up to 20 years. Duodenal and gastric carcinoid tumors are usually found incidentally during endoscopy. Rectal carcinoid tumors are frequently found incidentally during endoscopy but can be symptomatic. The most common symptoms include melena and bleeding (39%), constipation (17%), and diarrhea (12%). Bronchial carcinoid tumors are frequently discovered on chest radiograph. The most common symptoms are pneumonia, hemoptysis, and cough. Thymic carcinoid tumors present as anterior mediastinal masses, usually on chest radiograph. Ovarian and testicular carcinoid tumors may present as masses detected by physical examination or ultrasonography. Most carcinoid tumors present as an isolated disease, but there are associations between foregut carcinoid tumors and MEN-1, gastric carcinoid tumors and diseases causing hypergastrinemia, and ampullary somatostatin-rich carcinoid tumors and von Recklinghausen disease. Metastatic carcinoid tumors in the liver, presenting as hepatomegaly, may be the initial presentation in a patient who is fully active and productive with minimal symptoms and normal or near-normal liver function test results.

Carcinoid Tumors with Systemic Features

The most common systemic syndrome caused by carcinoid tumors is the malignant carcinoid syndrome. As described previously (in "Pathology and Tumor Histology"), carcinoid tumors may contain and secrete a number of biologically active substances. Carcinoid tumors may contain ACTH, gastrin, somatostatin, insulin, motilin, growth hormone, gastrin-releasing peptide, 5-HT, calcitonin, neurotensin, β-melanocyte–stimulating hormone, tachykinins (substance P, substance K, neuropeptide K), glucagon, pancreatic polypeptide, vasoactive intestinal peptide, and prostaglandins.[15] These substances may not be released in sufficient amounts to cause symptoms.

Foregut carcinoid tumors are more likely to produce various GI peptides than midgut carcinoid tumors. Ectopic ACTH production with Cushing syndrome is increasingly observed with foregut carcinoid tumors, and in some studies these tumors were the most common cause of the ectopic ACTH syndrome. Acromegaly due to release of growth hormone–releasing factors (GRFoma) can occur with a number of carcinoid tumors. The somatostatinoma syndrome due to somatostatin release can occur with duodenal carcinoid tumors.

CARCINOID SYNDROME

Clinical Features

Flushing attacks occur in 23% to 65% of patients with carcinoid syndrome initially and in 63% to 78% at some time during the disease course (Table 112.3).[16–21] The typical flush is the sudden appearance of a deep red erythema of the upper part of the body, primarily the face and neck. Flushes are often associated with an unpleasant feeling of warmth, occasionally with lacrimation, itching, palpitations, facial or conjunctival edema, and diarrhea. Flushes may be spontaneous or precipitated by stress, alcohol, certain foods such as cheese, or exercise, or pharmacologically by injections of agents such as catecholamines, calcium, or pentagastrin. Flushes may be brief, lasting 2 to 5 minutes, especially initially, or may be prolonged for hours, especially later. They are usually found with carcinoid tumors of midgut origin but can also occur in some patients with foregut tumors. With bronchial carcinoid tumors the flushes can be frequently prolonged, lasting for hours to

TABLE 112.3

CLINICAL CHARACTERISTICS IN PATIENTS WITH MALIGNANT CARCINOID SYNDROME

	At Presentation		During Course of Disease			
	Davis et al. 1973[16]	Norheim et al. 1987[18]	Thorson 1958[19]	Feldman 1987[17]	Norheim et al. 1987[18]	Soga et al. 1999[25]
No. of Patients	91	91	79	111	91	748
SYMPTOM OR SIGN (%)						
Diarrhea	73	32	68	73	84	67
Flushing	65	23	74	63	75	78
Pain	—	10	—	—	—	34
Asthma and wheezing	8	4	18	3	15	10
Pellagra	2	—	5	—	—	—
None	12	—	—	22	—	—
Carcinoid heart disease present	11	—	41	14	33	33
DEMOGRAPHICS						
% Male	59	46	61	—	46	52
Mean age, y	57	59	52	—	—	54.5
Range, y	25–79	ND	18–80	—	—	9–91
TUMOR LOCATION (%)						
Foregut	5	9	2	—	9	33
Midgut	78	87	75	—	87	60
Hindgut	5	1	8	—	1	1
Unknown	11	2	15	—	2	6

ND, no data.

days, reddish, and associated with salivation, lacrimation, diaphoresis, facial swelling, palpitations, deep furrowing of the forehead, diarrhea, and hypotension. The flushing with bronchial carcinoid tumors has a greater tendency to cause diffuse body involvement, and after repeated flushing of this type, patients may develop a constant red or cyanotic coloration. The flush associated with gastric carcinoid tumors is also reddish but is patchy in distribution over the neck and face. It is frequently provoked by food intake or pentagastrin, with erythema associated with blotches and wheals with central clearing, frequently occurring around the root of the neck and on the arms, and the lesions are frequently associated with pruritus.

Diarrhea is present in 32% to 73% of patients initially and in 67% to 84% at some time during the disease course (Table 112.3). Diarrhea usually occurs with flushing (85% of cases), but it may occur alone (15% of cases). The diarrhea is described as watery and less commonly as frothy or the pale bulky stool of steatorrhea; the number of stools ranges from 2 to 30 per day and 60% of patients have output of less than 1 L/d. Steatorrhea is present in 67% and is more than 15 g/d in 46%. Abdominal pain may be present with the diarrhea or independently, and the frequency varies from 10% to 34% (Table 112.3).

Cardiac manifestations occur in 11% to 66% of patients (Table 112.3).[21,22] The cardiac disease is due to fibrosis involving the endocardium, primarily of the right side of the heart, although left-side lesions can also occur.[23,24] The fibrous deposits are diffuse and are found most commonly on the ventricular aspect of the tricuspid valve and the associated chordae and less commonly on the pulmonary valve cusps. These fibrous deposits tend to cause constriction of both the tricuspid and pulmonic valves. At the pulmonic valve, stenosis is usually predominant, whereas at the tricuspid valve the constriction results in the valve's being fixed open, and tricuspid regurgitation is usually predominant. Lesions on the left side are seen in 30% of autopsy studies, are less extensive, and most frequently occur on the mitral valve.

Other clinical manifestations of carcinoid syndrome are wheezing or asthmalike symptoms in 3% to 18% of patients and pellagralike skin lesions with hyperkeratosis and pigmentation in 2% to 5% of cases (Table 112.3). Rarely reported are rheumatoid arthritis, arthralgias, changes in mental state or confusion, and ophthalmic changes during flushing leading to vessel occlusion. A variety of noncardiac problems secondary to increased fibrous tissue have been reported, including retroperitoneal fibrosis leading to ureteral obstruction or Peyronie disease of the penis, intra-abdominal fibrosis, and occlusion of mesenteric arteries or veins. Sexual dysfunction is a common complaint of men with carcinoid syndrome.

Pathobiology

Carcinoid syndrome developed in 8% of 8,876 patients with carcinoid tumors, with an incidence of 1.7% to 18.4% in six different series.[25] Carcinoid syndrome occurs only when sufficient concentrations of the hormonal products released by the tumor reach the systemic circulation. Its occurrence and severity are directly related to tumor size in an area that drains into the systemic circulation. In 91% of cases this only occurs after distant metastases (especially to the liver). Rarely, however, primary GI tumors with nodal metastases with extensive invasion retroperitoneally or drainage into the ovarian veins, pancreatic carcinoid tumors with retroperitoneal lymph nodes, or carcinoid tumors such as those in the lung or ovary with direct access to the systemic circulation can produce carcinoid syndrome without hepatic metastases. All carcinoid tumors do not have the same propensity to metastasize and to produce carcinoid syndrome (Table 112.2). Because midgut tumors are the most

PRACTICE OF ONCOLOGY

common and frequently metastasize, midgut tumors account for 60% to 87% of cases of carcinoid syndrome, foregut tumors for 2% to 33%, hindgut tumors for 1% to 8%, and an unknown primary location for 2% to 15% (Table 112.3).

Symptoms of carcinoid syndrome were originally attributed to secretion of 5-HT by the tumor. In one study of 380 patients with carcinoid tumors, 56% had evidence of 5-HT overproduction; 18% of 500 patients in a second study and 88% of 103 patients with carcinoid tumors in a third study had elevated urinary levels of 5-hydroxyindoleacetic acid (5-HIAA), the major metabolite of 5-HT. In a large review of 748 cases of carcinoid syndrome, 92% had increased 5-HT activity.[25]

Patients may develop either a typical or atypical type of carcinoid syndrome. In patients with the typical carcinoid syndrome, the conversion of tryptophan to 5-HTP is the rate-limiting step. Once formed, the 5-HTP is rapidly converted to 5-HT in the tumor by dopa decarboxylase and either stored in the neurosecretory tumor granules or released into vascular compartments, and most is taken up and stored in the granules of platelets. A small amount remains in the plasma. The majority in the circulation is converted by monoamine oxidase and aldehyde dehydrogenase to 5-HIAA, which appears in large amounts in the urine. This is the typical pattern in argentaffin-positive and argyrophil-positive tumors such as midgut carcinoid tumors. Some carcinoid tumors cause an atypical carcinoid syndrome and are thought to be deficient in the enzyme dopa decarboxylase; thus, they cannot convert 5-HTP to 5-HT, and 5-HTP is secreted into the bloodstream. Plasma 5-HT levels are normal in these patients, but urinary levels are usually elevated because some of the 5-HTP is decarboxylated in the kidney and excreted as 5-HT. Foregut carcinoid tumors are more likely to excrete high levels of 5-HT and 5-HTP in the urine and give the atypical carcinoid syndrome.

The exact role of 5-HT in causing the flushing in carcinoid syndrome remains unclear. Antagonists to 5-HT receptor subtypes or somatostatin receptor agonists typically have no effect on the flushing.[26,27] The exact cause of the flushing in patients with carcinoid syndrome may differ depending on the tumor type. In patients with gastric carcinoid tumors, the red, patchy, pruritic flush is thought to be caused by histamine, because this type of flushing can be prevented by the use of H_1- and H_2-receptor antagonists. In addition to 5-HT, other candidates for mediators of flushing include the tachykinins (substance P, neuropeptide K), various GI peptides, and prostaglandins. However, it appears that prostaglandins are unlikely to be major mediators of the flushing or diarrhea.

Numerous tachykinins are stored in carcinoid tumors and are released during flushing. In some studies, changes in plasma substance P or neuropeptide K levels did not correlate with the occurrence of flushing, which led the authors to conclude that circulating tachykinins have only a minor role, if any, in causing the flushing. Even though various GI peptides have been proposed to be involved in the flushing, no changes in plasma levels of vasoactive intestinal peptide, gastric inhibitory polypeptide, neurotensin, pancreatic polypeptide, motilin, insulin, glucagon, or enteroglucagon have been detected with provocation of the flush.

Patients with carcinoid syndrome have increased colonic motility with a shortened transit time and possibly a secretory or absorptive alteration.[28] Serotonin may be predominantly responsible for the diarrhea in some patients through its effects on gut motility and intestinal electrolyte and fluid secretion. Serotonin receptor antagonists (especially 5-HT_3 receptor antagonists such as ondansetron) relieve the diarrhea.[26] In combination with histamine, 5-HT may be responsible for producing asthma and may be involved in the fibrotic reactions causing carcinoid-associated heart disease, Peyronie disease, and ureteral obstruction. The pathogenetic link between the carcinoid and heart disease remains a subject of controversy. No relationship between the severity of the heart disease and other common manifestations such as flushing, diarrhea, or duration of disease has been established. Patients with heart disease have higher urinary 5-HIAA excretion and higher plasma levels of neurokinin A, substance P, or plasma atrial natriuretic peptide than those without heart disease, and more frequently receive chemotherapy.[29,30] Studies support the role of 5-HT in mediating the cardiac disease.

Diagnosis

Diagnosis of carcinoid syndrome relies on the measurement of urinary or plasma levels of 5-HT or its metabolites (5-HIAA), with the measurement of 5-HIAA in a 24-hour urine sample the most commonly used test. False-positive findings may occur if the patient is eating foods rich in 5-HT, such as bananas, plantains, pineapple, kiwi fruit, walnuts, hickory nuts, pecans, and avocados, which would falsely elevate urinary levels. Medications, including cough medicine containing guaifenesin, acetaminophen, salicylates, and L-dopa, should also be avoided because they may affect urinary 5-HIAA levels. If one properly controls dietary and medicinal intake, the normal range for urinary 5-HIAA excretion is between 2 and 8 mg/24 h. Many patients with 5-HT–secreting carcinoid tumors have urinary 5-HIAA excretion in the range of 8 to 30 mg/24 h. The measurement of urinary 5-HIAA levels is the current method of choice to diagnose carcinoid syndrome.

Most physicians rely totally on the measurement of urinary 5-HIAA for diagnosis. However, urinary and platelet measurement of 5-HT itself may give additional information. In one comparative study of platelet 5-HT levels, urine 5-HIAA levels, and urinary 5-HT levels in 44 consecutively treated carcinoid patients, the sensitivities were 50%, 29%, and 55%, respectively, in 14 patients with foregut carcinoid tumors; 100%, 92%, and 82%, respectively, in 25 patients with midgut carcinoid tumors; and 20%, 0%, and 60%, respectively, in five patients with hindgut carcinoid tumors. The data demonstrate the increased sensitivity of measuring platelet 5-HT levels. Elevations of 5-HIAA can occur in malabsorption states and a number of other conditions. Foregut carcinoid tumors tend to produce an atypical carcinoid syndrome with increases in plasma 5-HTP and not 5-HT, because they lack the appropriate decarboxylase, with the result that urinary 5-HIAA levels may not be markedly increased.

Diagnostic difficulties can arise with patients who flush for reasons other than carcinoid syndrome, patients with carcinoid syndrome in whom flushing is not apparent, patients with certain carcinoid tumors (especially foregut tumors) in whom 5-HIAA levels may be normal or minimally elevated, or the rare patient without metastatic disease who presents with flushing. The differential diagnosis of flushing includes menopausal flushing; reactions to alcohol and glutamate; side effects of drugs like chlorpropamide, calcium channel blockers, and nicotinic acid; and other neoplastic disorders such as chronic myelogenous leukemia and systemic mastocytosis. None of these conditions causes increased urinary 5-HIAA levels, and these disorders can be distinguishable pathologically.

The diagnosis of a carcinoid tumor may be suspected by clinical symptoms suggestive of carcinoid syndrome or by the presence of the other clinical symptoms such as abdominal pain or diarrhea, or it can be made in relatively asymptomatic patients from the pathologic report at surgery or after liver biopsy for hepatomegaly. Ileal carcinoid tumors, which make up more than 25% of all clinically detected carcinoid tumors, should be suspected if a patient presents with bowel obstruction, abdominal pain, flushing, or diarrhea. A number of studies demonstrate that serum chromogranin A levels are elevated in 56% to 100% of patients with carcinoid tumors, and the level correlates with tumor bulk.[31,32] Serum chromogranin A elevations are not specific for carcinoid tumors because increased levels occur with high frequency in patients with pancreatic endocrine tumors and certain other NETs, as well as in patients on gastric acid-suppressing medications such as proton pump inhibitors. The α or β subunit of human chorionic gonadotropin is detected frequently by immunocytochemistry in carcinoid tumors, and elevated plasma levels of human chorionic gonadotropin are reported in 28% of patients with carcinoid tumors and 13% of patients with carcinoid syndrome. NSE is also used as a plasma marker of carcinoid tumors, but it is less sensitive than chromogranin A, being positive in only 17% to 47% of patients.

Localization

A number of techniques, including GI endoscopy, barium radiography, chest radiography, imaging studies (ultrasonography, computed tomography [CT], magnetic resonance imaging, angiography), endoscopic ultrasonography, selective venous sampling for various hormones, positron emission tomography (PET), and various forms of radionuclide scanning (radiolabeled somatostatin receptor scintigraphy [SRS], iodinated metaiodobenzylguanidine [MIBG] scanning) have all been used to determine the location of the primary tumor as well as tumor extent.[33]

Bronchial carcinoid tumors are usually detected by chest radiography, CT, or occasionally bronchoscopy. They appear frequently (37%) as opacities with sharp or often notched margins. They are slow-growing and often induce airway compression with resultant atelectasis. Enlarged hilar lymph nodes from metastasis are rare. Rectal, duodenal, colonic, and gastric carcinoid tumors are almost always detected by GI endoscopy, with barium radiograph results being generally negative. When barium radiograph results are positive, they show dilated loops of small bowel or extrinsic filling defects but rarely detect a mucosal lesion, whereas ileal, cecal, and right colon tumors are often diagnosed on radiographic studies.

The main problem in detection is localizing small bowel carcinoid tumors, which may be very small and are frequently missed by barium studies, and small carcinoid tumors in other GI tissues. Some of these tumors can be localized by angiography, SRS, or CT, but many are not seen with these modalities. Liver metastases are usually detected by CT or, more recently, SRS. CT and SRS at present are the primary diagnostic modalities for tumor staging. CT frequently misses the primary tumor, especially if it is small (<1.5 cm). However, CT is generally helpful in evaluating the presence of liver metastases and retroperitoneal lymphadenopathy.

Carcinoid tumors possess high-affinity receptors for somatostatin in 88% to 100% of cases.[15,33] The somatostatin receptors are present in both the primary tumor and metastases. Five subtypes of somatostatin receptor (numbered sst_1 to sst_5) have been described. Octreotide binds with high affinity to sst_2 and sst_5 and with a lower affinity to sst_3; it has a very low affinity for sst_1 and sst_4. Studies show that almost all carcinoid tumors (90% to 100%) possess sst_2, 50% to 60% have sst_5, 10% to 100% possess sst_3, 70% to 100% show sst_1, and 20% to 100% possess sst_4. Indium 111–diethylenetriamine penta-acetic acid–D-phenyl-alanyl octreotide is standard for localizing carcinoid tumors using radionuclide scanning.[34] SRS images the tumor in 73% to 89% of patients with carcinoid tumors.[33] In one comparative study involving 40 patients, SRS localized tumors in 78% and CT in 82% of patients. SRS detected primary tumors in two patients whose tumors were missed on CT, and in 16% of patients it detected lesions not previously seen. Numerous other studies have demonstrated that SRS has high sensitivity for localizing carcinoid tumors, especially the extent of metastatic spread (Fig. 112.1). Studies demonstrate that SRS identifies additional bone metastases from carcinoid tumors not seen with bone scanning.[35] In general, SRS has excellent specificity, but high densities of somatostatin receptors can exist on a number of other normal and abnormal cells, which can lead to increased uptake and a false-positive response. These include granulomas (sarcoid, tuberculosis), activated lymphocytes (wound infections, lymphomas), thyroid diseases (goiter, thyroiditis), pancreatic endocrine tumors, and other endocrine tumors. Because of its sensitivity and ability to image all body areas, SRS should be

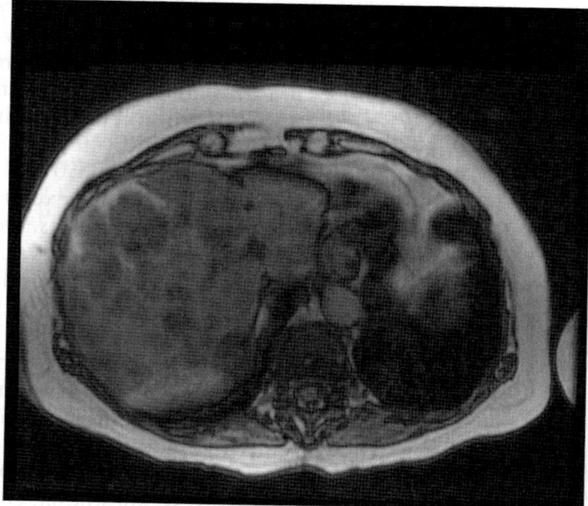

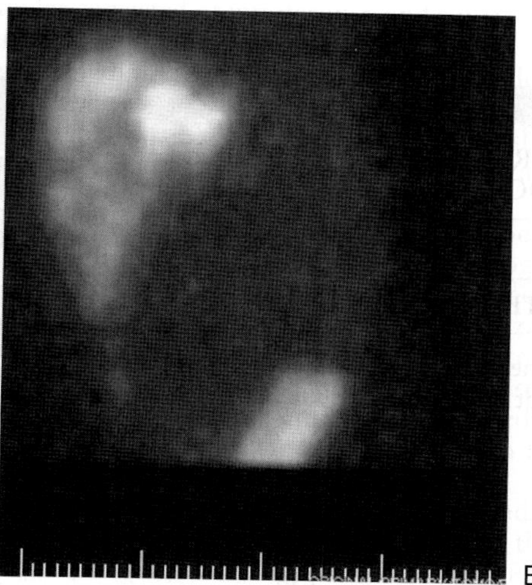

FIGURE 112.1 Demonstration of typical findings of magnetic resonance imaging (MRI) (A) and somatostatin receptor scintigraphy (SRS) (B) to localize hepatic metastases in a patient with carcinoid syndrome and metastatic jejunal carcinoid to the liver. This patient has had a renal allograft, demonstrated in the left lower quadrant on the SRS. The MRI provides detailed anatomic information regarding the location of the tumors in the liver. The SRS is less precise anatomically, but can provide functional and receptor-expression information about lesions also demonstrated on the cross-sectional imaging, and can demonstrate previously unsuspected lesions elsewhere.

sustained-release preparations. If tachyphylaxis develops, the dosage can be increased. If symptoms recur, are severe, and do not respond to an increased octreotide dosage, other 5-HT receptor antagonists such as cyproheptadine or ketanserin should be considered, and if this approach is ineffective then interferon alone or subsequently combined with somatostatin analogs should be considered.

TREATMENT OF THE CARCINOID TUMOR

Resection of local, regional nodal or metastatic disease can result in cure in some patients (Fig. 112.2).[40,41] Because the possibility of metastatic disease is directly related to primary size in most carcinoid tumors, the extent of surgical resection for possible cure should be determined accordingly. In the case of appendiceal tumors smaller than 1 cm without gross metastases, which includes the majority, a simple appendectomy is sufficient. Of 103 such patients treated with a simple appendectomy, all of whom were followed for 5 years and 83 of whom were followed for 10 to 35 years, no patient developed a local recurrence or metastatic disease. With rectal carcinoid tumors smaller than 1 cm, local resection is usually adequate and results in cure. The depth of invasion is also an important prognostic factor, and this should also be assessed in all tumors. If no invasion of the muscularis propria is present for rectal carcinoid tumors smaller than 2 cm, local resection is adequate.

There is not complete agreement of treatment regarding small intestinal carcinoid tumors smaller than 1 cm. In most series 15% to 20% of tumors smaller than 1 cm have metastases. However, in another series 69% of tumors smaller than 0.5 cm were associated with metastases, and in a second series 32% of tumors 0.6 to 1 cm had metastases, which led one group to conclude that with midgut carcinoid tumors malignancy is independent of size.[42] This has led some to recommend a wide *en bloc* resection of the adjacent lymph node–bearing mesentery for all small intestinal carcinoid tumors. If the carcinoid is 2 cm or larger, which is uncommon in the case of carcinoid tumors of the rectum or appendix but occurs in 40% of small bowel carcinoid tumors, a full-scale cancer operation should be done. In the case of carcinoid tumors of the appendix 2 cm or larger, a right hemicolectomy is the operation of choice. For a tumor larger than 2 cm in the rectum or a smaller tumor with invasion through the muscularis propria, an abdominoperineal resection or a low anterior resection with primary anastomosis is recommended by some, but not by others. In two studies involving patients with rectal carcinoid tumors larger than 2 cm, all patients died from or developed metastatic disease to the liver despite abdominoperineal or low anterior resection, and the authors concluded that radical surgery is inappropriate if anorectal carcinoid tumors can be removed by local excision.

In the case of a small intestinal carcinoid of 2 cm or larger, a wide resection is recommended with *en bloc* resection of the adjacent lymph node–bearing mesentery. For carcinoid tumors of the appendix of 1 to 2 cm, simple appendectomy is recommended by some, whereas others favor more aggressive surgery such as a partial cecectomy or formal right hemicolectomy for those lesions located at the base of the appendix to ensure clear margins or in patients with invasion of the mesoappendix or vascular invasion. For carcinoid tumors of the rectum of 1 to 2 cm, it is estimated that 11% to 47% are accompanied by metastases, and thus it is recommended by some that these tumors be locally resected with a wide local full-thickness excision and that those tumors found to invade the muscularis propria be subjected to abdominoperineal or low anterior resection. However, in another study 47% of these patients had metastases and 50% without metastatic disease developed metastases on follow-up, which led the authors to conclude that extensive surgery is not routinely warranted in these patients.

With gastric carcinoid tumors, treatment is generally stratified by whether hypergastrinemia is present (types I and II) or not (type III). Most recommend that in patients with type I or II carcinoid tumors with lesions smaller than 1 cm, the carcinoid tumors be removed endoscopically. In patients with type I or II gastric carcinoid tumors, if the tumor is larger than 2 cm or if there is local invasion, some recommend total gastrectomy, whereas others recommend that the tumor be removed surgically with resection and in type I lesions (pernicious anemia) an antrectomy be performed. For type I or II lesions of 1 to 2 cm, there is no general agreement on treatment, with some recommending that these be treated surgically and others recommending endoscopic treatment. In type III gastric carcinoid tumors not associated with hypergastrinemia, which tend to be larger and more aggressive, if the lesion is larger than 2 cm, excision and regional lymph node clearance is recommended. Some recommend a similar approach for any tumor larger than 1 cm, whereas others recommend that be reserved for

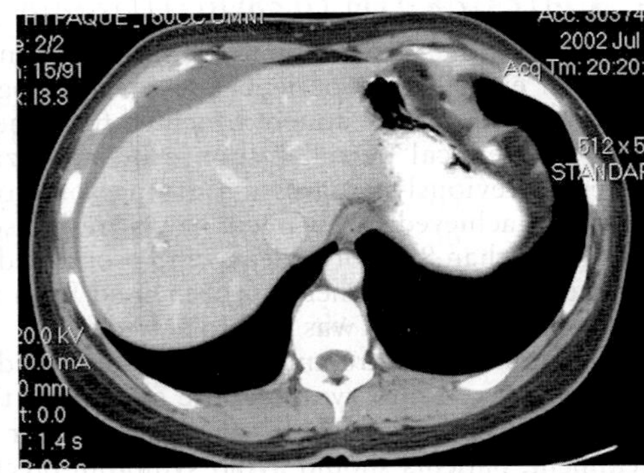

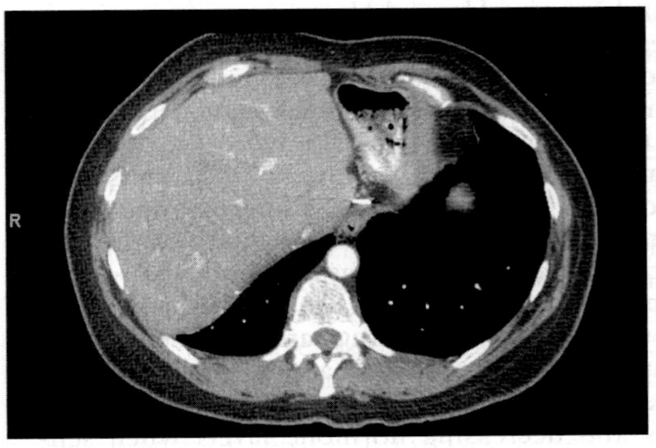

FIGURE 112.2 Management of metastatic carcinoid tumor by liberal resection strategies and systemic somatostatin analog therapy can be very effective in control of disease. **A:** This patient presented with systemic carcinoid syndrome, a jejunal primary lesion, and multiple bilateral liver metastases. Resection of the liver lesions included right hepatic trisegmentectomy, and wedge resection of left lateral segment disease, with concomitant resection of the jejunal primary tumor. **B:** After subsequent resection of a small hepatic recurrence, she has remained free of demonstrable disease, including undetectable chromogranin A for 9 years.

tumors in this size range showing histologic invasion. Most tumors smaller than 1 cm are treated endoscopically.

Resection of isolated hepatic metastases may also be beneficial or curative in select patients.[40,41] In one study, 22% of patients had unilobar disease and could have all tumor resected, whereas in other studies fewer than 10% of patients were surgical candidates because of more disseminated disease. In the 20% with all metastatic disease resected, 5-HIAA levels were normal and 10-year survival was 100%. The role of cytoreductive or debulking surgery in patients in whom all tumor cannot be removed is unclear. There are no prospective randomized trials that have addressed this question. There are a number of retrospective analyses that suggest such an approach should be considered in selected cases. A number of studies recommend debulking of mesenteric metastases and removal of compromised intestinal segments even in the presence of liver metastases. In one study of 314 patients with midgut carcinoid tumors, in those patients subjected to surgery with the principal aim of removing the primary and debulking mesenteric metastases, the authors concluded that this surgery provided considerable symptomatic relief and improved survival. The role of cytoreductive hepatic resection or of cryotherapy for patients with multiple hepatic metastases from carcinoid tumors is also unclear.

In a review of data for 170 patients with metastatic GI NETs to the liver (120 of which were carcinoid tumors) who underwent surgical exploration for possible debulking, 54% had a major hepatectomy (one lobe or more), complication rate was 14%, mortality rate was 1.2%, symptom control occurred in 96% of those undergoing resection, and survival was 61% at 5 years. Resection of hepatic metastases may relieve clinical endocrinopathies and the symptomatic response may last several months. It was recommended that if more than 90% of the imaged tumor could be safely removed, resection should be considered.[34] Local ablative therapies can also be used in the liver to control tumor. Examples include cryotherapy and radiofrequency ablation. Currently, radiofrequency ablation appears more applicable, particularly as it can be performed percutaneously with image guidance.[43]

Because MIBG is frequently taken up by carcinoid tumors and concentrated, the possibility of using radiolabeled MIBG therapeutically has been evaluated in a small number of patients. Iodine-125– or iodine-131–labeled MIBG has been reported to decrease 5-HIAA urine concentrations and control symptomatic metastases in a small number of cases.

Chemotherapy

There is no general agreement on when, or even if, chemotherapy should be started in patients with malignant carcinoid tumors. Some suggest that only patients suffering significant symptoms or disability from malignant disease or syndromes or who have a poor prognosis should undergo chemotherapy. Chemotherapy for metastatic carcinoid tumors has, in general, been disappointing. Single-agent therapy with doxorubicin, 5-fluorouracil, dacarbazine, actinomycin-D, cisplatin, alkylating agents, etoposide, streptozotocin, and carboplatin has provided low tumor response rates of 0% to 30%. In general, the duration of responses is short, usually less than a year. Combination chemotherapy for metastatic carcinoid has not been shown to have any clear advantage compared with single-agent chemotherapy. Two-dose combinations have been used of streptozotocin and 5-fluorouracil, streptozotocin and cyclophosphamide, streptozotocin and doxorubicin, etoposide and cisplatin, dacarbazine and 5-fluorouracil, and CCNU and 5-fluorouracil, with low response rates of 0% to 40% and no apparent significant improvement over the use of single agents alone. Three-drug combinations with 5-fluorouracil, doxorubicin, and cisplatin; dacarbazine, 5-fluorouracil, and epirubicin; and streptozotocin, cyclophosphamide, and 5-fluorouracil; and four-drug combinations with streptozotocin, doxorubicin, cyclophosphamide, and 5-fluorouracil also gave low response rates of 10% to 31% and showed no additional therapeutic advantage over a single agent. Remissions were short-lived, with an average duration of 4 to 7 months. It can be concluded that no combination therapy has clearly had a beneficial effect in the treatment of malignant carcinoid tumors. Given the indolent nature of the tumor, the poor efficacy and undisputed toxicity of chemotherapy, and the availability of excellent symptomatic therapy (octreotide and interferon), currently chemotherapy is usually reserved for advanced tumors with evidence of progression late in the disease course.[44]

Biotherapy

Somatostatin analogs such as octreotide or lanreotide, in addition to controlling symptoms and reducing secretion of 5-HIAA or various peptides, also have been assessed for their antitumor effects, alone and in combination with other agents.[44,45] In general, these analogs have a poor tumoricidal effect, decreasing tumor size in only 0% to 17% of patients. However, both somatostatin analogs have a tumorostatic effect, stabilizing the growth of metastatic disease and, in some studies, prolonging survival. In various studies 30% to 100% of patients with metastatic disease have demonstrated tumor stabilization with treatment with somatostatin analogs. No prospective study has proven that this tumor stabilization results in increased survival.

Numerous studies show that human leukocyte interferon or interferon-α causes a decrease in tumor size in a small number (0% to 20%) of patients with metastatic tumors.[46,47] However, similar to octreotide, interferon appears to have a tumorostatic effect, stopping further tumor growth and stabilizing the extent of metastatic disease, which may lead to prolonged survival. In a number of studies interferon-α therapy demonstrated a reduction in tumor size of more than 50% in fewer than 20% of patients with metastatic NETs, while resulting in stabilization of tumor growth in 30% to 70%. Interferon treatment (3 to 9 mU 3 times per week) was associated with tolerable but significant side effects, including flulike symptoms in 89%, fatigue in 70%, weight loss in 57%, reduction of blood counts in 31% (anemia in 31%, leukopenia in 3%, thrombocytopenia in 14%), increased serum levels of triglycerides in 32%, and increased liver enzyme levels in 31%. Clinical thyroid disease developed in 76% of patients with thyroid antibodies. In 22 patients it was found that the induction of the enzyme 2′,5′-oligoadenylate synthetase with interferon treatment correlated with the development of a clinical response; however, it is unknown if it is predictive of changes in tumor size with interferon treatment. The optimal dosage for long-term treatment seems to be 5 to 10 mU 3 to 5 times per week; subsequently, however, it is important to titrate the dosage individually for each patient.[46,47] It is recommended that the leukocyte count be used as an indication of the antiproliferative effect of interferon-α, with the aim of reducing the leukocytes below 3×10^9/L.

Because of their separate tumorostatic effects and ability to control symptoms, the combination of octreotide and interferon was assessed in small numbers of patients with malignant carcinoid syndrome either alone or in combination with other agents. With octreotide and interferon, interferon-α plus 5-fluorouracil, interferon-α and interferon-β, and streptozotocin with doxorubicin and interferon-α, as with interferon-α alone, only low rates (0% to 10%) of decrease in tumor size occurred.

Embolization and Chemoembolization

Surgical hepatic artery ligation or embolization via interventional radiology has been reported to reduce hepatic tumor bulk either alone, combined with interferon, or as chemoembolization combined with chemotherapy with dacarbazine, cisplatin, doxorubicin, 5-fluorouracil, or streptozotocin.[48] Hepatic artery occlusion with chemotherapy or chemoembolization may be more effective than embolization or hepatic artery occlusion alone. In one large study, the percentage of patients who had tumor regression after hepatic artery ligation alone was similar to that for patients receiving chemoembolization (treatment with dacarbazine and doxorubicin alternating with streptozotocin and 5-fluorouracil; 67% vs. 69%); however, the duration of the response was decreased (4 months vs. 18 months for the combination).

In nine studies involving chemoembolization (embolization combined with doxorubicin in ethiodized oil or with 5-fluorouracil, dacarbazine, doxorubicin, cisplatin, mitomycin-C, or streptozotocin), a decrease in tumor size was seen in 33% to 100% of patients. The average decrease in size in one study was 84%. In one study, 47% of patients survived 2 years (median survival, 17 months), and in another study the median survival time was 15 months. A randomized trial compared the effect of interferon-α in 69 patients with metastatic midgut carcinoid tumors after embolization and surgery. Patients treated with interferon-α and octreotide had a reduced risk of tumor progression (P = .008) compared with those treated with octreotide alone; however, the 5-year survival rate was not significantly different (57% vs. 37%; P = .13).[47]

Liver Transplantation

In contrast to other metastatic tumors to the liver for which liver transplantation has generally given poor results and has been largely abandoned, there is increased interest in liver transplantation in patients with metastatic carcinoid tumors and pancreatic endocrine tumors. In a review of 103 patients with malignant NETs who underwent liver transplantation (43 carcinoid tumors, 48 pancreatic endocrine tumors), the 2- and 5-year survival rates were 60% and 47%, respectively. However, recurrence-free survival was less than 24%.[49] Univariate analysis defined favorable prognostic factors as age younger than 50 years, primary tumor in lung or bowel, and pretransplantation somatostatin therapy. Multivariate analysis identified age older than 50 years and transplantation combined with upper abdominal exenteration or Whipple resection (P <.01) as adverse prognostic factors. It was concluded that liver transplantation might be justified, particularly in young patients with hepatic disease only.

Peptide Receptor Radionuclide Therapy

The discovery that many carcinoid tumors overexpress somatostatin receptors and internalize radiolabeled somatostatin analogs is now being used therapeutically.[50] Indium-111–, yttrium-90–, and lutetium-177–coupled somatostatin analogs are being studied. These results suggest that this novel therapy may be useful, especially in patients with advanced disease, but remain investigational.

Selected References

1. Ferolla P, Faggiano A, Mansueto G, et al. The biological characterization of neuroendocrine tumors: the role of neuroendocrine markers. *J Endocrinolo Invest* 2008;31(3):277.
2. Vinik AI, Silva MP, Woltering G, Go VLW, Warner R, Caplin M. Biochemical testing for neuroendocrine tumors. *Pancreas* 2009;38:876.
3. Helle KB. Chromogranins A and B and secretogranin II as prohormones for regulatory peptides from the diffuse neuroendocrine system. *Results Probl Cell Differ* 2010;50:21.
4. Plockinger U, Rindi G, Arnold R, et al. Guidelines for the diagnosis and treatment of neuroendocrine gastrointestinal tumours: a consensus statement on behalf of the European Neuroendocrine Tumour Society (ENETS). *Neuroendocrinology* 2004;80:394.
5. Modlin IM, Lye KD, Kidd M, Modlin IM, Lye KD, Kidd M. A 5-decade analysis of 13,715 carcinoid tumors. *Cancer* 2003;97:934.
6. Soga J, Soga J. Early-stage carcinoids of the gastrointestinal tract: an analysis of 1914 reported cases. *Cancer* 2005;103:1587.
7. Godwin JD. Carcinoid tumors: an analysis of 2837 cases. *Cancer* 1975;36:560.
8. Modlin IM, Sandor A, Modlin IM, Sandor A. An analysis of 8305 cases of carcinoid tumors. *Cancer* 1997;79:813.
9. Yao JC, Hassan M, Phan A, et al. One hundred years after "carcinoid": epidemiology of and prognostic factors for neuroendocrine tumors in 35,825 cases in the United States. *J Clin Oncol* 2008;26:3063.
10. Soga J, Soga J. Carcinoids of the small intestine: a statistical evaluation of 1102 cases collected from the literature. *J Exp Clin Cancer Res* 1997; 16:353.
11. Burke AO, Sobin LH, Federspiel BH, Shekitka KM, Helwig EB. Carcinoid tumors of the duodenum. *Arch Pathol Lab Med* 1990;114:700.
12. Hage R, de la Riviere AB, Seldenrijk CA, et al. Update in pulmonary carcinoid tumors: a review article. *Ann Surg Oncol* 2003;10:697.
13. Manfredi S, Pagenault M, de Lajarte-Thirouard A-S, Bretagne J-F. Type 1 and 2 gastric carcinoid tumors: long-term follow-up of the efficacy of treatment with a slow-release somatostatin analogue. *Europ J Gastroenterol Hepatol* 2007;19:1021.
14. Oberg K, Oberg K. Carcinoid tumors: molecular genetics, tumor biology, and update of diagnosis and treatment. *Curr Opin Oncol* 2002;14:38.
15. Pasieka JL, McKinnon JG, Kinnear S, et al. Carcinoid syndrome symposium on treatment modalities for gastrointestinal carcinoid tumours: symposium summary. *Can J Surg* 2001;44:25.
16. Davis Z, Moertel CG, McIlrath DC. The malignant carcinoid syndrome. *Surg Gynecol Obstet* 1973;137:637.
17. Feldman JM. Carcinoid tumors and syndrome. *SeminOncol* 1987;14:237.
18. Norheim I, Oberg K, Theodorsson-Norheim E, et al. Malignant carcinoid tumors: an analysis of 103 patients with regard to tumor localization, hormone production, and survival. *Ann Surg* 1987;206:115.
19. Thorson AH. Studies on carcinoid disease. *Acta Med Scand* 1958;334:81.
20. Bendelow J, Apps E, Jones LE, Poston GJ. Carcinoid syndrome. *Eur J Surg Oncol* 2008;34:289.
21. Sippel RS, Chen H. Carcinoid tumors. *Surg Oncol Clin North Am* 2006; 15:463.
22. Dumoulein M, Verslype C, van Cutsem E, et al. Carcinoid heart disease: case and literature review. *Acta Cardiol* 2010;65:261.
23. Quaedvlieg PF, Lamers CB, Taal BG, Quaedvlieg PFHJ, Lamers CBHW, Taal BG. Carcinoid heart disease: an update. *Scand J Gastroenterol* 2002; (Suppl):66.
24. Quaedvlieg PF, Visser O, Lamers CB, et al. Epidemiology and survival in patients with carcinoid disease in The Netherlands: an epidemiological study with 2391 patients. *Ann Oncol* 2001;12:1295.
25. Soga J, Yakuwa Y, Osaka M, Soga J, Yakuwa Y, Osaka M. Carcinoid syndrome: a statistical evaluation of 748 reported cases. *J Exp Clin Cancer Res* 1999;18:133.
26. Wymenga AN, de Vries EG, Leijsma MK, et al. Effects of ondansetron on gastrointestinal symptoms in carcinoid syndrome. *Eur J Cancer* 1998; 34:1293.
27. Wymenga AN, Eriksson B, Salmela PI, et al. Efficacy and safety of prolonged-release lanreotide in patients with gastrointestinal neuroendocrine tumors and hormone-related symptoms. *J Clin Oncol* 1999;17:1111.
28. Makridis C, Theodorsson E, Akerstrom G, et al. Increased intestinal nonsubstance P tachykinin concentrations in malignant midgut carcinoid disease. *J Gastroenterol Hepatol* 1999;14:500.
29. Moller JE, Connolly HM, Rubin J, et al. Factors associated with progression of carcinoid heart disease. *N Engl J Med* 2003;348:1005.
30. Moller JE, Pellikka PA, Bernheim AM, et al. Prognosis of carcinoid heart disease: analysis of 200 cases over two decades. *Circulation* 2005;112:3320.
31. Kolby L, Bernhardt P, Sward C, et al. Chromogranin A as a determinant of midgut carcinoid tumour volume. *Regul Pept* 2004;120:269.
32. Taupenot L, Harper KL, O'Connor DT, Taupenot L, Harper KL, O'Connor DT. The chromogranin-secretogranin family. *N Engl J Med* 2003;348:1134.

33. Gibril F, Jensen RT, Gibril F, Jensen RT. Diagnostic uses of radiolabelled somatostatin receptor analogues in gastroenteropancreatic endocrine tumours. *Dig Liver Dis* 2004;36(Suppl 1):S106.
34. Clark OH, Benson AB 3rd, Berlin JD, et al. NCCN Clinical Practice Guidelines in Oncology: neuroendocrine tumors. *J Natl Compr Cancer Netw* 2009;7:712.
35. Meijer WG, van der Veer E, Jager PL, et al. Bone metastases in carcinoid tumors: clinical features, imaging characteristics, and markers of bone metabolism. *J Nucl Med* 2003;44:184.
36. Koopmans KP, Neels OC, Kema IP, et al. Improved staging of patients with carcinoid and islet cell tumors with 18F-dihydroxy-phenyl-alanine and 11C-5-hydroxy-tryptophan positron emission tomography. *J Clin Oncol* 2008;26:1489.
37. Oberg K, Kvols L, Caplin M, et al. Consensus report on the use of somatostatin analogs for the management of neuroendocrine tumors of the gastroenteropancreatic system. *Ann Oncol* 2004;15:966.
38. Fazio N, de Braud F, Delle Fave G, et al. Interferon-alpha and somatostatin analog in patients with gastroenteropancreatic neuroendocrine carcinoma: single agent or combination? *Ann Oncol* 2007;18:13.
39. Fjallskog ML, Sundin A, Westlin JE, Oberg K, Janson ET, Eriksson B. Treatment of malignant endocrine pancreatic tumors with a combination of alpha-interferon and somatostatin analogs. *Med Oncol* 2002; 19:35.
40. Que FG, Sarmiento JM, Nagorney DM, Que FG, Sarmiento JM, Nagorney DM. Hepatic surgery for metastatic gastrointestinal neuroendocrine tumors. *Adv Exp Med Biol* 2006;574:43.
41. Sarmiento JM, Heywood G, Rubin J, et al. Surgical treatment of neuroendocrine metastases to the liver: a plea for resection to increase survival. *J Am Coll Surg* 2003;197:29.
42. Kerstrom G, Hellman P, Hessman O, Kerstrom G, Hellman P, Hessman O. Midgut carcinoid tumours: surgical treatment and prognosis. *Best Pract Res Clin Gastroenterol* 2005;19(7):717.
43. Eriksson J, Stalberg P, Nilsson A, et al). Surgery and radiofrequency ablation for treatment of liver metastases from midgut and foregut carcinoids and endocrine pancreatic tumors. *World J Surg* 2008;32:930.
44. Bhattacharyya S, Gujral DM, Toumpanakis C, et al. A stepwise approach to the management of metastatic midgut carcinoid tumor. *Nat Rev Clin Oncol* 2009;6:429.
45. Yao JC, Phan AT, Chang DZ, et al. Efficacy of RAD001 (everolimus) and octreotide LAR in advanced low- to intermediate-grade neuroendocrine tumors: results of a phase II study [erratum published in *J Clin Oncol* 2008;26(34)5660.]. *J Clin Oncol* 2008;26:4311.
46. Faiss S, Pape UF, Bohmig M, et al. Prospective, randomized, multicenter trial on the antiproliferative effect of lanreotide, interferon alfa, and their combination for therapy of metastatic neuroendocrine gastroenteropancreatic tumors—the International Lanreotide and Interferon Alfa Study Group. *J Clin Oncol* 2003;21:2689.
47. Kolby L, Persson G, Franzen S, et al. Randomized clinical trial of the effect of interferon alpha on survival in patients with disseminated midgut carcinoid tumours. *Br J Surg* 2003;90:687.
48. Gupta S, Johnson MM, Murthy R, et al. Hepatic arterial embolization and chemoembolization for the treatment of patients with metastatic neuroendocrine tumors: variables affecting response rates and survival. *Cancer* 2005;104:1590.
49. Lehnert T, Lehnert T. Liver transplantation for metastatic neuroendocrine carcinoma: an analysis of 103 patients. *Transplantation* 1998;66:1307.
50. Bushnell D. Treatment of metastatic carcinoid tumors with radiolabeled biologic molecules. *J Natl Compr Cancer Netw* 2009;7:760.

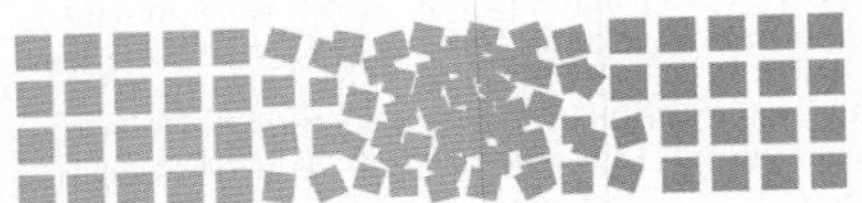

CHAPTER 113 MULTIPLE ENDOCRINE NEOPLASIAS

GERARD M. DOHERTY

Multiple endocrine neoplasia (MEN) syndromes are characterized by tumors of endocrine organs (Table 113.1). MEN-1 affects the parathyroid glands, endocrine pancreas, and pituitary gland, among other organs; MEN-2 affects the thyroid gland, parathyroid glands, and adrenal glands. Because the genetic defects responsible for these syndromes have been identified, genotype–phenotype correlations now guide the timing of interventions for some patients, specifically with MEN-2 and its related *Ret* protooncogene-based syndromes.

MULTIPLE ENDOCRINE NEOPLASIA TYPE 1

MEN-1 is inherited as an autosomal dominant trait. The parathyroid disease always affects multiple glands; the pancreatic endocrine tumors may be malignant; and patients can die from the associated malignancies. Chromosomal linkage studies localized the genetic defect to the long arm of chromosome 11 (q-13 locus), and subsequent studies identified the gene that codes a protein called *menin*.[1] Tumor development follows the two-hit theory of neoplasia of Knudson in which an inherited mutation in one chromosome is unmasked by a somatic deletion or mutation in the other normal chromosome, thereby removing the suppressor effect of the normal gene.

Asymmetric multigland primary hyperparathyroidism is the most frequent feature of MEN-1. Studies have demonstrated that there is a monoclonal abnormality in the enlarged parathyroid glands of patients with MEN-1, suggesting that the process in these glands does not depend on a circulating factor (hyperplasia) but rather occurs through inactivation of the *MEN-1* gene in a precursor cell (neoplasia). The relationship of asymmetry of affected glands to patient age (younger patients have more frequent asymmetric involvement, older patients with involvement of all glands) and the tumor suppressor genetic basis of the syndrome favors the occurrence of multiple adenomas (neoplasia) rather than hyperplasia (Fig. 113.1).[2]

Clinical Presentation

The peak incidence of symptoms in women with MEN-1 is during the third decade of life, whereas the peak incidence in men is during the fourth decade.[3] In individuals from known MEN-1 kindreds, its presence can usually be detected with screening by the age of 18. More than half of patients with MEN-1 have involvement of more than one organ system, and approximately 20% have three affected endocrine glands. The frequency of glandular involvement, in descending order, is parathyroid, pancreas, pituitary, adrenal cortex, and thyroid. Both the adrenal cortex and the thyroid typically have benign, nonfunctioning adenomas. Other clinically important tumors these patients develop include gastric carcinoids, bronchial carcinoids (primarily women), and carcinoid tumors of the thymus (primarily men).[4] The frequency of clinical signs and symptoms, in descending order, is hypercalcemia, nephrolithiasis, peptic ulcer disease, hypoglycemia, headache, visual field loss, hypopituitarism, acromegaly, galactorrhea or amenorrhea, and, rarely, Cushing's syndrome. Patients with MEN-1 have a decreased life expectancy, with a 50% probability of death by age 50. Half of the deaths are due to a malignant tumoral process or a sequela of the disease.[5–7]

Parathyroid Gland Involvement

Primary hyperparathyroidism is the most common abnormality in patients with MEN-1, occurring in 88% to 97% of affected patients. The diagnosis depends on the detection of elevated serum levels of calcium and parathyroid hormone. Primary hyperparathyroidism is usually the initially recognized clinical manifestation of patients with MEN-1, although in prospectively screened patients, other manifestations may be biochemically detected earlier.[8,9] Occasionally patients have clinical manifestations of Zollinger-Ellison syndrome (ZES) before primary hyperparathyroidism. Further, pituitary adenomas or hyperinsulinism may be identified before hypercalcemia. The pathology associated with primary hyperparathyroidism is always multiple gland disease. Although some glands may appear grossly normal, the likelihood of finding normal-weight glands decreases as the age of the patient increases, consistent with the development of multiple parathyroid adenomas.[2] The surgical management requires a strategy that acknowledges that all of the parathyroid glands are, or will be, abnormal, and that the patient is better served by having a smaller amount of abnormal parathyroid tissue than by having none at all. Options include removal of three and a half glands, leaving a part of one gland in the neck, or all four parathyroid glands with immediate autograft of some of the parathyroid tissue into the musculature of the nondominant forearm. Neither strategy yields ideal results. The incidence of recurrent or persistent hyperparathyroidism is 16% to 54%, and the incidence of hypoparathyroidism is between 10% and 25%.[10,11] Repeat operations are frequently necessary, and similar principles should be applied.

Pancreatic Endocrine Tumors

Malignant pancreatic endocrine tumors are the most common MEN-1–related cause of death in MEN-1 kindreds (Table 113.2).[5–7] Pathologic examination of the duodenum and pancreas in patients with MEN-1 demonstrates multiple neuroendocrine tumors.[12,13] Tumors that produce pancreatic polypeptide are the most common pancreatic endocrine tumor in MEN-1 patients, occurring in 80% to 100%. Symptoms of these

TABLE 113.1

MULTIPLE ENDOCRINE NEOPLASIA SYNDROMES AND FAMILIAL MEDULLARY THYROID CANCER

Characteristics	MEN-1	MEN-2A	MEN-2B	Familial Medullary Thyroid Carcinoma
Chromosome	11q12-13	Pericentromeric 10	Pericentromeric 10	Pericentromeric 10
Genetic defect	*MEN-1* mutation	*RET* mutation	*RET* mutation	*RET* mutation
MTC	No	Bilateral	Bilateral	Bilateral
Pheochromocytoma	No	70% bilateral	70% bilateral	No
Parathyroid disease	Hyperplasia	Hyperplasia	No	No
Phenotype	No	No	Bony abnormalities, mucosal neuromas, marfanoid habitus, bumpy lips	No
Mode of inheritance	Autosomal dominant	Autosomal dominant	Autosomal dominant	Autosomal dominant
Course of MTC	No MTC	Variable, frequently indolent	More virulent	Most indolent
Pancreatic endocrine tumors q	Yes: pancreatic polypeptide, 80%–100%; gastrinoma, 50%; insulinoma, 20%; growth hormone–releasing factor, vasoactive intestinal peptide (uncommon)	No	No	No

MEN, multiple endocrine neoplasia; MTC, medullary thyroid carcinoma.

tumors occur only from the tumor mass itself; thus, patients often present when tumor growth is advanced. Many patients develop functional pancreatic endocrine tumors, sometimes coincident with pancreatic polypeptide–producing tumors, of whom most have gastrinoma, approximately 20% have insulinoma, 3% have glucagonoma, and 1% have vasoactive intestinal peptide (VIPoma) (Table 113.1).

A number of studies have suggested that most gastrinomas in patients with ZES and MEN-1 are in the duodenum and not in the pancreas. The ideal treatment of the ZES is surgical excision of the gastrinoma; however, in patients with MEN-1, excision of gastrinoma rarely results in normal serum gastrin levels, although some have suggested that more ablative procedures may be more effective.[13] Because of the low probability of cure and the suggestion that the gastrinoma is less malignant in MEN-1, some have recommended that patients with MEN-1 should not undergo surgery. At present, the best approach is still unclear.

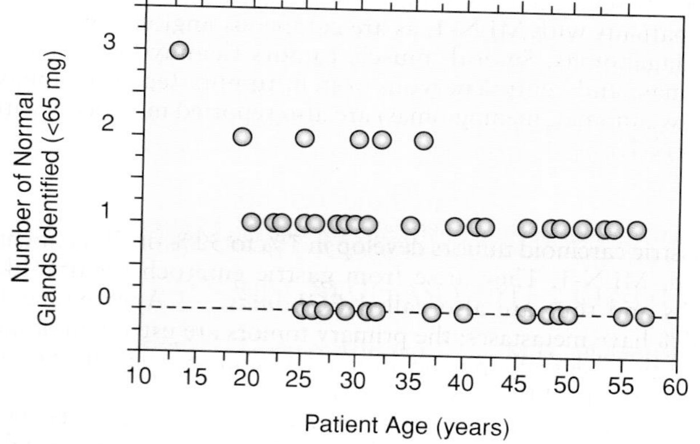

FIGURE 113.1 The number of normal glands identified during 44 initial operations for multiple endocrine neoplasia type 1 (MEN-1) primary hyperparathyroidism. The number of normal glands identified during the operation declined with the age of the patient. No patient of age more than 40 years had more than one gland of normal weight at operation. These data support the concept of multiple parathyroid adenomas in MEN-1, rather than parathyroid hyperplasia. (From ref. 2, with permission.)

To date, there is no definitive evidence that surgical resection of pancreatic neoplasms in MEN-1 is beneficial. One study suggests that surgical resection of primary gastrinomas in patients with and without MEN-1 decreases the probability of the development of liver metastases, which is the most important negative predictor of survival.[14] Somatostatin receptor scintigraphy can be used to rule out distant metastases and to evaluate for other primary sites (Fig. 113.2). Therefore, we currently recommend that all patients with ZES and MEN-1 have extensive localization studies, including somatostatin receptor scintigraphy. Only patients with unequivocally positive imaging studies and no unresectable metastases should undergo surgical exploration with intraoperative ultrasound. Tumors larger than 1 cm identified in the pancreatic head are enucleated, the duodenum is carefully explored by duodenotomy, and solitary or multiple tumors identified are resected; large tumors in the pancreatic body or tail are removed by distal pancreatectomy and splenectomy.[13,15–18]

Complete resection of liver metastases from patients with MEN-1 may also be beneficial. Using this approach, although cure of ZES is unusual, resection should reduce the risk of subsequent metastatic disease. No data conclusively demonstrate that this approach increases survival, although case series are suggestive.[13,17]

MEN-1 is present in 20% of all patients with ZES and 4% of patients with insulinoma. The exact percentage of patients with VIPoma, glucagonoma, or somatostatinoma with MEN-1 is not known, but is estimated to be low (less than 5%) (Table 113.1). The surgical management of insulinoma and VIPoma in MEN-1 patients has had more frequent biochemical cures than resection for gastrinoma. Medical management of the watery diarrhea in VIPoma is effective using either short-acting or depot somatostatin analogues. Hypoglycemia management in

MEN-2A and FMTC and exon 16 (codon 918) for MEN-2B. If a *RET* mutation is detected, each individual (100%) develops MTC. Further, if a *RET* mutation is absent, the individual does not need any additional testing. Virtually all patients with MTC have either elevated basal or stimulated plasma levels of calcitonin. Patients who present with clinically apparent disease usually have basal plasma calcitonin levels exceeding 1 ng/mL. Generally, there is a direct correlation between the tumor mass of MTC and plasma calcitonin levels.

The presence of inherited MTC can be currently diagnosed in individuals from kindreds before detectable elevations in plasma calcitonin levels. Thyroidectomy performed based solely on detection of *RET* mutations always demonstrates MTC or C-cell hyperplasia.[27,28] It is necessary in patients with MEN-2A or MEN-2B to exclude a pheochromocytoma before undertaking surgery for MTC. Pheochromocytomas can be excluded by measuring normal plasma levels of metanephrines. If an elevated level is detected, localization studies to identify the tumor can include abdominal computed tomography and magnetic resonance imaging. The tumors are nearly always within the adrenal glands, rather than in other sites of chromaffin tissue.

Surgical Management

The ability to diagnose MTC in patients at risk allows the physician to treat this malignancy in an early preclinical stage. Should one diagnose MTC in a patient from a MEN-2A kindred, it is absolutely essential that the remainder of the family members at risk be screened. It is in this situation that *RET* testing has the greatest utility. Patients diagnosed by genetic testing typically have surgically curable C-cell hyperplasia or carcinoma confined to the thyroid gland.[29]

MEN-2A or MEN-2B patients with pheochromocytoma have not had extra-adrenal or malignant adrenal medullary tumors. Before surgical exploration, all patients need effective α-adrenergic receptor blockade. Phenoxybenzamine should be administered 1 to 2 weeks before surgery, starting with a dose of 10 mg twice daily and increased to a usual dose of 10 to 20 mg three times daily. The end point is normotension with mild to moderate asymptomatic postural hypotension (15 mm Hg) accompanied by symptoms of a blockade, including nasal stuffiness. β-Adrenergic blockade is usually not required except in patients with persistent sinus tachycardia. The β-blocker should never be administered before the institution of α-adrenergic blockage because this may result in unopposed α-agonism with hypertensive crisis.

Solitary pheochromocytoma should be resected. In the past, some have advocated open exploration and palpation of both adrenal glands to assess for bilateral disease. Modern imaging has made this obsolete, as is the strategy of routinely resecting both adrenal glands. With imaging studies to localize the adrenal tumor, laparoscopic methods are now used to remove the abnormal gland, and careful follow-up is necessary to monitor for the metachronous development of a contralateral pheochromocytoma.[30] Patients with MEN-2A who undergo unilateral adrenalectomy should be followed carefully at 6-month or yearly intervals because a second adrenal tumor may be diagnosed biochemically before it is clinically apparent.

The surgical management of familial MTC is total thyroidectomy with a central lymph node dissection.[3,24] It is essential that a total thyroidectomy be performed because the MTC is always bilateral.

Postoperative Follow-Up

In patients with MEN-2A and MEN-2B, MTC is the disease that is most frequently lethal. The MTC in patients with MEN-2B seems to be more virulent than in patients with MEN-2A (Table 113.1), although a group of children with MTC in the setting of MEN-2B have been reported, some of whom appear to be cured of MTC. Survival of patients with MEN-2A depends on the extent of MTC at initial surgical resection.

With the widespread availability of reliable radioimmunoassays for calcitonin, an individual patient can be easily followed postoperatively. Detection of an elevated basal plasma calcitonin level or the finding of an abnormal response to calcium and pentagastrin indicates recurrent or persistent disease. In patients with metastatic MTC, the best strategy is unclear. Radioactive iodine ablation, thyroid suppression, and radiation therapy have not been helpful. MTC is relatively insensitive to chemotherapy. Because of the indolent nature of the tumor, most have chosen not to aggressively treat metastatic disease but rather to rely on local (surgical and radiation) methods to address symptomatic disease.

The 10-year survival of MTC is 80% to 90%. Aggressive surgical resection has been used to locally control recurrent MTC, and one-third of individuals can be rendered biochemically disease free.[25] However, in patients with MEN-2A, the MTC may be well tolerated. The average life expectancy of patients with MTC and MEN-2A is more than 50 years. The current best therapy for familial MTC is early diagnosis and complete resection of intrathyroidal disease at the initial operation. Ablation of extrathyroidal disease when detected as persistent or recurrent elevations of plasma calcitonin levels following total thyroidectomy requires the development of effective systemic adjuvant treatment.

Selected References

1. Chandrasekharappa SC, Guru P, Manickam S-E, et al. Positional cloning of the gene for multiple endocrine neoplasia-type 1. *Science* 1997;276:404.
2. Doherty GM, Lairmore TC, DeBenedetti MK. Multiple endocrine neoplasia type 1 parathyroid adenoma development over time. *World J Surg* 2004;28:1139.
3. Brandi ML, Gagel RF, Angeli A, et al. Guidelines for diagnosis and therapy of MEN type 1 and type 2 [comment]. *J Clin Endocrinol Metab* 2001;86:5658.
4. Gibril F, Chen YJ, Schrump DS, et al. Prospective study of thymic carcinoids in patients with multiple endocrine neoplasia type 1. *J Clin Endocrinol Metab* 2003;88:1066.
5. Dean PG, van Heerden JA, Farley DR, et al. Are patients with multiple endocrine neoplasia type 1 prone to premature death? *World J Surg* 2000;24:1437.
6. Doherty GM, Olson JA, Frisella MM, et al. Lethality of multiple endocrine neoplasia type I. *World J Surg* 1998;22:581.
7. Wilkinson S, the BT, Davey KR, et al. Cause of death in multiple endocrine neoplasia type 1. *Arch Surg* 1993;128:683.
8. Skogseid B, Oberg K. Experience with multiple endocrine neoplasia type 1 screening. *J Intern Med* 1995;238:255.
9. Skogseid BS, Eriksson B, Lundqvist G, et al. Multiple endocrine neoplasia type 1: a 10-year prospective screening study in four kindreds. *J Clin Endocrinol Metab* 1991;73:281.
10. Hellman P, Skogseid B, ObergK, et al. Primary and reoperative parathyroid operations in hyperparathyroidism of multiple endocrine neoplasia type 1. *Surgery* 1998;124:993.
11. Hubbard JG, Sebag F, Maweja S, et al. Subtotal parathyroidectomy as an adequate treatment for primary hyperparathyroidism in multiple endocrine neoplasia type 1. *Arch Surg* 2006;141:235.
12. Pipeleers-Marichal M, Donow C, Heitz PU, Kloppel G. Pathologic aspects of gastrinomas in patients with Zollinger-Ellison syndrome with and without multiple endocrine neoplasia type I. *World J Surg* 1993;17:481.
13. Tonelli F, Fratini G, Nesi G, et al. Pancreatectomy in multiple endocrine neoplasia type 1-related gastrinomas and pancreatic endocrine neoplasias. *Ann Surg* 2006;244:61.

14. Fraker DL, Norton JA, Alexander HR, Venzon DJ, Jensen RT. Surgery in Zollinger-Ellison syndrome alters the natural history of gastrinoma. *Ann Surg* 1994;220:320.
15. Bartsch DK, Fendrich V, Langer P, et al. Outcome of duodenopancreatic resections in patients with multiple endocrine neoplasia type 1. *Ann Surg* 2005;242:757.
16. Lairmore TC, Chen VY, DeBenedetti MK, et al. Duodenopancreatic resections in patients with multiple endocrine neoplasia type 1. *Ann Surg* 2000; 231:909.
17. Norton JA, Fang TD, Jensen RT, et al. Surgery for gastrinoma and insulinoma in multiple endocrine neoplasia type 1. *J Natl Compr Canc Netw* 2006;4:148.
18. Hausman MS Jr, Thompson NW, Gauger PG, Doherty GM. The surgical management of MEN-1 pancreatoduodenal neuroendocrine disease. *Surgery* 2004;136:1205.
19. Bashir S, Gibril F, Ojeaburu JV, et al. Prospective study of the ability of histamine, serotonin or serum chromogranin A levels to identify gastric carcinoids in patients with gastrinomas. *Aliment Pharmacol Ther* 2002;16:1367.
20. Bordi C, Corleto VD, Azzoni C, et al. The antral mucosa as a new site for endocrine tumors in multiple endocrine neoplasia type 1 and Zollinger-Ellison syndromes. *J Clin Endocrinol Metab* 2001;86:2236.
21. Lim LC, Tan MH, Eng C, et al. Thymic carcinoid in multiple endocrine neoplasia 1: genotype-phenotype correlation and prevention. *J Intern Med* 2006;259:428.
22. Donis-Keller H, Dou S, Chi D, et al. Mutations in the RET proto-oncogene are associated with MEN 2A and FMTC. *Hum Mol Genet* 1993;2:851.
23. Mulligan LM, Kwok JBJ, Healey CS, et al. Germ-line mutation of the RET proto-oncogene in multiple endocrine neoplasia type 2A. *Nature* 1993;363: 458.
24. American Thyroid Association Guidelines Task Force, Kloos RT, Eng C, et al. Medullary thyroid cancer: management guidelines of the American Thyroid Association. *Thyroid* 2009;19:565.
25. Quayle FJ, Moley JF. Medullary thyroid carcinoma: including MEN 2A and MEN 2B syndromes. *J Surg Oncol* 2005;89:122.
26. Yip L, Cote GJ, Shapiro SE, et al. Multiple endocrine neoplasia type 2: evaluation of the genotype-phenotype relationship. *Arch Surg* 2003;138:409.
27. Dralle H, Gimm O, Simon D, et al. Prophylactic thyroidectomy in 75 children and adolescents with hereditary medullary thyroid carcinoma: German and Austrian experience. *World J Surg* 1998;22:744.
28. Piolat C, Dyon JF, Sturm N, et al. Very early prophylactic thyroid surgery for infants with a mutation of the RET proto-oncogene at codon 634: evaluation of the implementation of international guidelines for MEN type 2 in a single centre. *Clin Endocrinol* 2006;65:118.
29. Fialkowski EA, Moley JF, Fialkowski EA, Moley JF. Current approaches to medullary thyroid carcinoma, sporadic and familial. *J Surg Oncol* 2006;94: 737.
30. Brunt LM, Lairmore TC, Doherty GM, et al. Adrenalectomy for familial pheochromocytoma in the laparoscopic era. *Ann Surg* 2002;235:713.

CHAPTER 114 MOLECULAR BIOLOGY OF SOFT TISSUE SARCOMA

SAMUEL SINGER, TORSTEN NIELSEN, AND CRISTINA R. ANTONESCU

Soft tissue sarcomas are life-threatening mesenchymal neoplasms that account for approximately 1% of all human cancer. They pose a significant therapeutic challenge because more than 50% of patients with newly diagnosed sarcoma eventually die of disease. Soft tissue sarcomas also pose significant diagnostic challenges as there are more than 50 histologic subtypes with unique molecular, pathologic, clinical, prognostic, and therapeutic features. Figure 114.1 shows the histologic appearance of the major subtypes.

The expansion in the molecular genetic and cytogenetic characterization of soft tissue sarcoma has improved classification and has divided sarcomas into two broad groups: those with simple karyotypes and those with highly complex karyotypes. Figure 114.2 shows the molecular alterations found in some of the subtypes in each group. The first group consists of sarcomas with simple genetic alterations (translocations or specific activating mutations) and with near-diploid, simple karyotypes. These alterations include translocations in myxoid/round-cell liposarcoma and synovial sarcoma, *APC* or β-catenin mutations in desmoid tumors, and *KIT* or *PDGFRA* activating mutations in gastrointestinal stromal tumors (GIST). Translocation-associated sarcomas typically occur in young adults, with highest incidence in the 30s and 40s. For most translocation-associated sarcomas, oncogenesis results from transcriptional deregulation induced by fusion genes. The second group consists of sarcomas with aberrant, highly complex genomes. Examples include dedifferentiated and pleomorphic liposarcoma, leiomyosarcoma, pleomorphic malignant fibrous histiocytoma, and myxofibrosarcoma. The peak incidence for these complex sarcoma types is in the 50s and 60s. Although these complex sarcoma subtypes commonly have alterations in cell-cycle genes *TP53*, *MDM2*, *RB1*, and *INK4a* and defects in specific growth-factor signaling pathways, the critical subtype-specific molecular alterations that drive sarcomagenesis largely remain to be discovered. This information will be essential for the development of therapeutics that can selectively target the driver genetic alterations required for sarcoma survival. This idea is best illustrated by the development of imatinib, a small molecule that inhibits ABL, KIT, and PDGFRA tyrosine kinases. The discovery of activating mutations in *KIT* and *PDGFRA*, specifically in GIST, led to rapid clinical development of imatinib for GIST, in which it proved to be an effective, low toxicity therapy (see Chapter for a discussion of the molecular biology of GIST). This success illustrates how targeting a sarcoma-specific oncogenic mechanism can lead to dramatic responses.

Table 114.1 outlines the diagnostic histologic characteristics and molecular and cytogenetic abnormalities of the major soft tissue sarcoma subtypes.

TRANSLOCATION-ASSOCIATED SARCOMAS

Myxoid/Round Cell Liposarcoma

Myxoid liposarcoma typically presents in the thigh or other deep soft tissues in adult patients (peak age 30–50 years). The diagnosis can usually be made with confidence based on characteristic morphology: myxoid matrix, plexiform vasculature, and lipoblasts. These features may, however, be partially lost in its high-grade form, termed *round cell liposarcoma*. The great majority of myxoid/round cell liposarcomas carry a balanced translocation, t(12;16)(q13;p11),[1] fusing *FUS* (also known as *TLS*) with *DDIT3* (aka *CHOP*, *GADD153)*.[2] In rare cases, *EWSR1* substitutes for its homologue *FUS*. At least nine *FUS-DDIT3* transcript variants have been reported,[3,4] and several are known to be capable of inducing a sarcoma phenotype in model systems.[5,6] The translocations fuse 5′ exons of *FUS* (encoding transcriptional regulatory domains that interact with the RNA polymerase II complex[7]) to the full coding sequence of *DDIT3*, a leucine-zipper transcription factor with roles in cell cycle control[8] and adipocytic differentiation.[9] The fusion oncoprotein complexes with cofactors including C/EBPβ to deregulate gene expression, although few direct targets have been validated to date.[10,11] The net result is activation of critical pathways including those related to the angiogenic factor interleukin (IL)-8, early adipose differentiation (PPARγ), growth factor signaling (insulinlike growth factor [IGF], the proto-oncoprotein RET), and cell-cycle control (cyclinD-CDK4).[10,12–14]

Clinically, evidence for *FUS-DDIT3* translocations from reverse transcription polymerase chain reaction (RT-PCR)[15] or fluorescence *in situ* hybridization (FISH)[16] can help confirm the diagnosis and may be useful for small biopsies dominated by a round cell component. Fusion subtype, however, appears to have little prognostic value beyond what is known from stage and grade. In general, molecular markers in myxoid liposarcoma have been difficult to test for independent prognostic significance, given the difficulty of assembling large series with long follow-up.[17] Nevertheless, p53, IGF1R/IGF2, and RET overexpression may be adverse factors.[13,18] Such findings support IGF/Akt/mTOR and Ras-Raf-ERK/MAPK pathway inhibitors as potential targeted therapies in myxoid liposarcomas. In addition, mutations in *PIK3CA*, which were found in 18% of myxoid/round cell liposarcomas, were associated with worse outcome.[19]

The dense microvasculature and high levels of IL-8[10] and vascular endothelial growth factor (VEGF)[20] expression seen in this

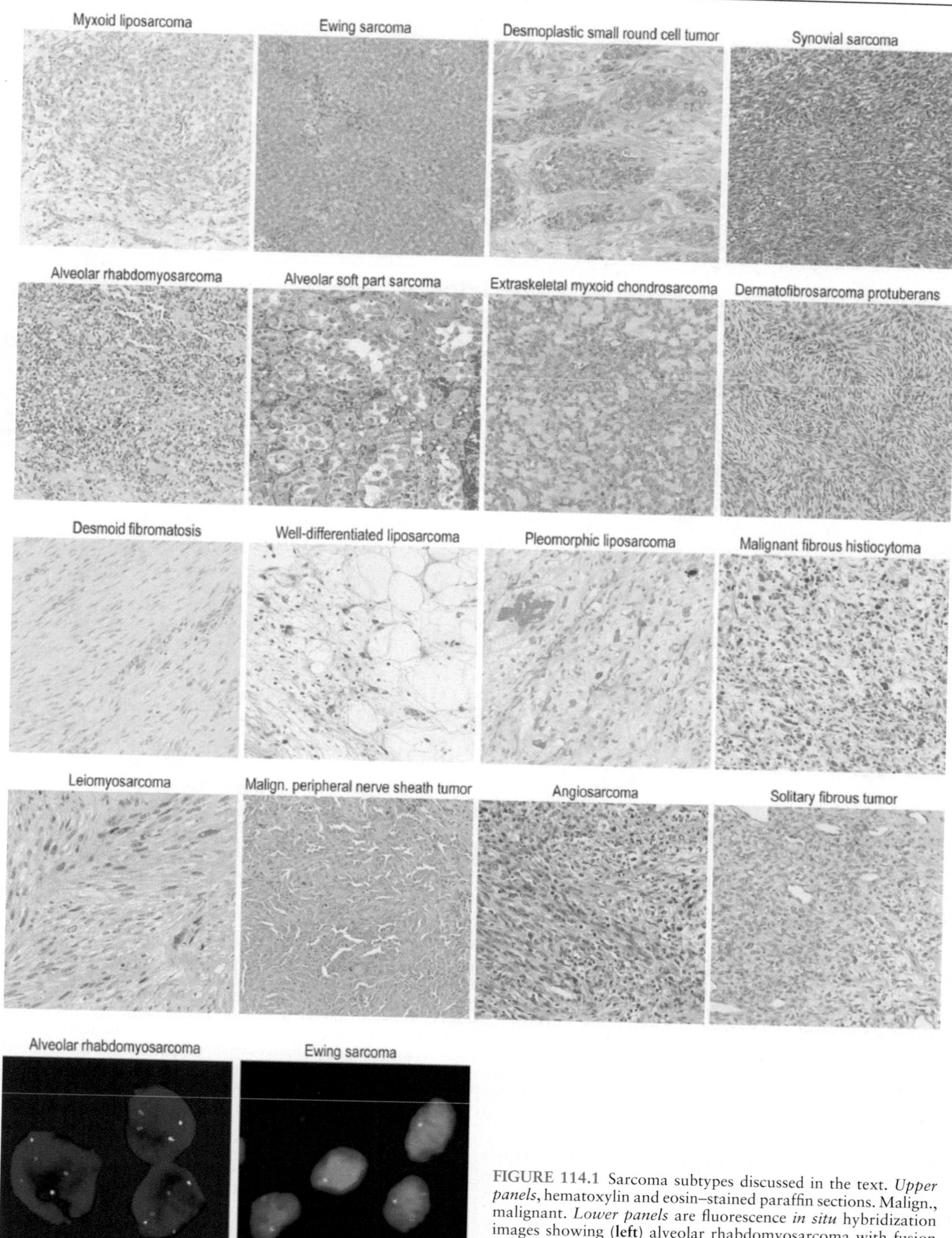

FIGURE 114.1 Sarcoma subtypes discussed in the text. *Upper panels*, hematoxylin and eosin–stained paraffin sections. Malign., malignant. *Lower panels* are fluorescence *in situ* hybridization images showing (**left**) alveolar rhabdomyosarcoma with fusion of probes for *PAX3* (*red*) and *FOXO1* (*green*) and (**right**) Ewing sarcoma with break-apart of probes flanking the EWS breakpoint region, *EWSR1*.

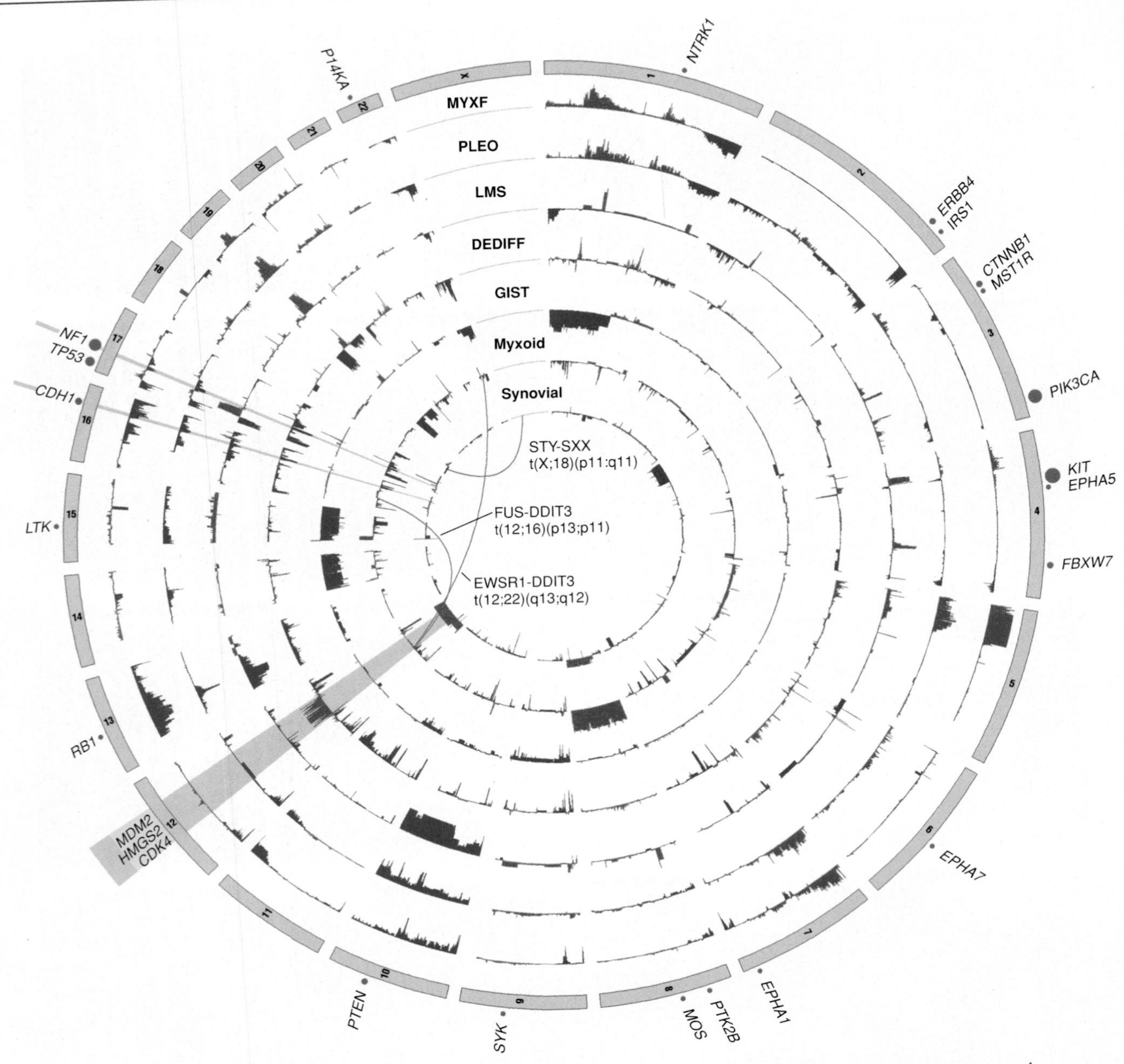

FIGURE 114.2 Nucleotide and copy number alterations in soft tissue sarcoma. The outer ring indicates chromosomal position. The second through fifth rings represent four subtypes with complex karyotypes (as labeled; MYXF, myxofibrosarcoma; PLEO, pleomorphic liposarcoma; LMS, leiomyosarcoma; DEDIFF, dedifferentiated liposarcoma). The three inner rings represent subtypes with simple karyotypes (Myxoid, myxoid/round cell liposarcoma). The plots show the statistical significance of genomic aberrations, with amplification in *red* and deletion in *blue*. *Green* curves indicate the chromosomal breakpoints of pathognomonic translocations in myxoid/round-cell liposarcoma and synovial sarcoma. Genes harboring somatic nucleotide alterations are indicated with *green circles* whose size is proportional to their frequency of occurrence. (Courtesy of Barry S. Taylor, Computational Biology Center, Memorial Sloan-Kettering Cancer. Adapted from ref. 19.)

tumor may underlie its observed sensitivity to radiotherapy[21] and trabectedin,[22] suggesting a value for antiangiogenic therapies. Trabectedin may also function by disrupting the binding of FUS-DDIT3 to target promoters.[11]

Ewing Sarcoma

Ewing family tumors appear most commonly in adolescents and young adults; primary sites can be either bone or soft tissues. A range of aggressive small, blue, round cell tumors with variations in clinical and morphologic features have been subsumed under the general term *Ewing sarcoma family tumor* following the recognition of common pathognomonic chromosomal translocations.[23,24] *EWSR1*, the common 5′ translocation partner, is fused to one of several possible ETS family transcription factor genes (usually *FLI1*). In the fusion protein, EWSR1 provides, at minimum, its 264 amino acid N-terminal transcriptional regulatory domain, and the ETS factor provides its C-terminal DNA-binding domain. In the process, EWSR1 loses its RNA recognition domain, and the ETS factor loses its native transactivation domain. Several direct transcriptional

TABLE 114.1

CYTOGENETIC AND MOLECULAR ABNORMALITIES IN SOFT TISSUE SARCOMAS

Disease	Diagnostic Morphology or Immunohistochemistry	Cytogenetic Event	Molecular Abnormality	Molecular Diagnostic[a]
Myxoid/round cell liposarcoma	Lipoblasts, plexiform vasculature, myxoid atrix	t(12;16)(q13;p11) t(12;22)(q13;q12)	*FUS-DDIT3* (>90%) *EWSR1-DDIT3* (<5%)	*DDIT3* breaks (FISH)[16,187]
Ewing sarcoma family tumor	Small, blue, round cells; CD99 and FLI1 expression; lack of lymphoid biomarker expression	t(11;22)(q24;q12) t(21;22)(q22;q12) Alternative events: fusions of 22q12 with 7p22, 17q22, 2q33; inv 22q12; t(16;21)(p11;q22)	*EWSR1-FLI1* (>80%) *EWSR1-ERG* (10–15%) Other ETS family partners: *ETV1, ETV4, FEV, PATZ1* (~5%) *FUS-ERG* (<1%)	*EWSR1* breaks (FISH)[36] or RT-PCR
Desmoplastic small, round cell tumor	Small, blue, round cell islands in dense stroma; positive for keratin, desmin, vimentin, and WT1	t(11;22)(p13;q12)	*EWSR1-WT1* (>75%)	*EWSR1* breaks (FISH)[36]
Synovial sarcoma	Biphasic histology, positive for TLE1[64]	t(X;18)(p11;q11) (>90%)	*SYT-SSX1* (66%), *SYT-SSX2* (33%), *SYT-SSX4* (<1%)	*SYT* breaks (FISH)[188]
Alveolar rhabdomyosarcoma	Small, blue cells expressing desmin, myogenin, myoD1	t(2;13)(q35;q14) t(1;13)(p36;q14)	*PAX3-FOXO1* (~80%) *PAX7-FOXO1* (~20%) *PAX3-NCOA1* (<1%) *PAX3-NCOA2* (<1%)	*PAX3/7* type-specific FISH or RT-PCR[189]
Alveolar soft-part sarcoma	Nested polygonal cells in vascular network; positive for TFE3[78]	t(X;17)(p11;q25)	*ASPSCR1-TFE3* (>90%)	*ASPSCR1-TFE3* RT-PCR[190]
Dermatofibrosarcoma protuberans	Bland spindle cells, storiform and honeycomb growth in subcutis, positive for CD34	Rings derived from t(17;22) (>75%) t(17;22)(q22; q13.1)[86,87,191] (10%)	*COL1A1-PDGFB*	
Embryonal rhabdomyosarcoma	Spindle cells and rhabdomyoblasts, positive for desmin and myogenin	Trisomies 2q, 8 and 20 (>75%)	LOH at 11p15 (>75%)	
Extraskeletal myxoid chondrosarcoma	Bland epithelioid cells arranged in reticular pattern in myxoid stroma	t(9;22)(q22;q12)	*EWSR1-NR4A3* (75%)	*EWSR1* breaks (FISH); RT-PCR[95–97]
		t(9;17)(q22;q11) t(9;15)(q22;q21) t(3;9)(q12;q22)	*TAF15-NR4A3* (<10%) *TCF12-NR4A3* (<10%) *TFG–NR4A3* (<5%)	RT-PCR[95–97]
Endometrial stromal tumor	Bland spindle cells, positive for CD10 and ER	t(7;17)(p15;q21)	*JAZF1-SUZ12* (30%)	
Clear cell sarcoma	Nested epithelioid cells with clear or amphophilic cytoplasm, positive for S100 and HMB-45	t(12;22)(q13;q12) t(2;22)(q34;q12)	*EWSR1-ATF1* (>75%) *EWSR1-CREB1* (<5%)	*EWSR1* breaks (FISH)[36,192]
Infantile fibrosarcoma	Monomorphic spindle cells, herringbone pattern	t(12;15)(p13;q25)	*ETV6-NTRK3* (>75%)	FISH, RT-PCR
Inflammatory myofibroblastic tumor	Myofibroblastic cells with lymphoplasmacytic infiltrate, positive for ALK	t(1;2)(q25;p23) t(2;19)(p23;p13) t(2;17)(p23;q23)	*ALK-TPM34* *ALK-TPM* *ALK-CLTC*	*ALK* breaks (FISH)

(continued)

TABLE 114.1

(CONTINUED)

Disease	Diagnostic Morphology or Immunohistochemistry	Cytogenetic Event	Molecular Abnormality	Molecular Diagnostic[a]
Gastrointestinal stromal tumor	Spindle (70%), epithelioid (20%) or mixed (10%) morphology, positive for CD117 (KIT), DOG1, and CD34	Monosomies 14 and 22 (>75%) Deletion of 1p (>25)	*KIT* or *PDGFRA* mutation (>90%)[193,194]	PCR mutation analysis
Desmoid fibromatosis	Bland myofibroblastic-type cells, fascicular growth, nuclear positivity for β-catenin	Trisomies 8 and 20 (30%)	*APC* inactivation by mutation/deletion (10%) *CTNNB1* (β-catenin) mutations (85%)	IHC for β-catenin expression
Well-differentiated/ dedifferentiated liposarcoma	Atypical multinucleated stromal cells, lipoblasts, positive for MDM2, CDK4	12q13-15 rings and giant markers	*MDM2* and *CDK4* amplification (>85%)	*MDM2* amplification (FISH)
Pleomorphic liposarcoma	Pleomorphic spindle and giant cells, pleomorphic lipoblasts	Complex[b] (>90%)		None
Myxofibrosarcoma and pleomorphic MFH	Pleomorphic spindle and giant cells, storiform growth, variable myxoid stroma	Complex[b] (>90%)	*SKP2* amplification	None
Leiomyosarcoma	Elongated fusiform cells with eosinophilic cytoplasm, in intersecting fascicles, positive for desmin and smooth muscle actin	Complex[b] (>50%) Deletions of 1p	*RB1* point mutations/ deletions	None
Malignant peripheral nerve sheath tumor	Monomorphic spindle cells, high mitotic count, geographic necrosis	Complex[b] (90%)		None
			NF1 mutation, loss or deletion (>50%)	None

FISH, fluorescence *in situ* hybridization; RT-PCR, reverse transcription polymerase chain reaction; LOH, loss of heterozygosity; IHC, immunohistochemistry; MFH, malignant fibrous histiocytoma.
[a]Refers to molecular tests that can be run on formalin-fixed paraffin-embedded material for molecular confirmation of diagnosis: quantitative RT-PCR of transcripts,[189] or FISH to interphase genomic DNA.[195]
[b]Complex karyotypes containing multiple numerical and structural chromosomal aberrations.

targets for the fusion oncoprotein are supported by strong evidence. Some of these targets are up-regulated (*ID2*,[25] *PTPL1*,[26] *MK-STYX*,[27] *DAX1*[28]) and some repressed (*CIP1*,[29] *TGFBR2*,[30] *IGFBP3*[31]) in Ewing sarcoma, but gene repression events, mediated by cofactors, appear to predominate overall.[32] The net result is activation of pathways driving proliferation and cell survival (including IGF signaling[33]), with concurrent repression of pathways promoting mesenchymal differentiation.[34,35]

Molecular confirmation of an *EWSR1* translocation can be critical for patient management because many of the clinical, morphologic, and immunophenotypic features of Ewing sarcoma are shared with entities such as mesenchymal chondrosarcoma and small cell osteosarcoma. Commercially available *EWSR1* split-apart FISH probes are valuable ancillary diagnostic tools (Fig. 114.1).[36] RT-PCR alternatives are complicated by the need to cover the many alternative gene and exonic fusion sites, but RT-PCR offers the advantage of identifying the specific exon fusion involved, which can have independent prognostic relevance.[37]

Several existing agents (including IGF/mTOR and histone deacetylase inhibitors[38–40]) that target recently identified, translocation-induced mechanisms and pathways are currently being tested in clinical trials for Ewing sarcoma, and novel strategies to directly inhibit the oncoprotein itself are in active development.[41]

Desmoplastic Small Round Cell Tumor

In desmoplastic small round cell tumor, the same 5′ portions of *EWSR1* involved in Ewing sarcomas are fused to *WT1*,[42,43] a tumor suppressor deleted in Wilms tumor.[44] The 56-kDa EWSR1-WT1 chimeric protein includes the last three of the four WT1 DNA-binding zinc finger domains. Despite some similarities to Ewing sarcoma family tumors, desmoplastic small round cell tumors show little response to conventional chemotherapy. Prognosis is dismal, and new therapies are needed.[45] Several transcriptional targets of the EWSR1-WT1 chimeric oncoprotein have been identified.[43] *PDGFA* expression is directly induced by EWSR1-WT1,[46] explaining the desmoplastic background and possibly the recent observation of a partial response to sunitinib.[47] *IL2RB* is also induced, and its downstream JAK/STAT signaling pathway appears active in this tumor,[43,48] representing a potential target for novel treatment approaches.

Synovial Sarcoma

Synovial sarcoma differs from most translocation-associated sarcomas in that the genes involved in its defining translocation, t(X;18)(p11;q11), encode epigenetic regulators, not transcription factors with direct DNA-binding activity.[49] The translocation fuses the widely expressed *SYT* (aka *SS18*) gene with an *SSX* gene normally expressed only in testis.[50] In the fusion oncoprotein, SYT, which interacts with components of the SWI/SNF chromatin remodeling complex,[51] retains all but the last eight amino acids from its C-terminal transcription activation domain. The SSX partner (SSX1, 2 or 4) retains only its C-terminal 78-residue repressor domain, which confers nuclear localization in association with Polycomb group proteins that mediate chromatin condensation and epigenetic gene silencing.[52] The resulting chimeric oncoprotein dysregulates transcription at the level of epigenetic modifications[53] and, when forcibly expressed in a mesenchymal stem cell background[54] or conditionally expressed in mice,[49,55] recapitulates synovial sarcoma. Direct targets of SYT-SSX include the tumor suppressors *COM1*[56] and *EGR1*[57]; both genes are repressed in synovial sarcoma, with the *EGR1* promoter undergoing SYT-SSX-dependent histone methylation.[57] Thus, transcriptional reactivation agents such as histone deacetylase inhibitors are worth investigation in this disease, as they may reactivate mesenchymal differentiation and reverse some effects of the SYT-SSX oncoprotein.[58,59]

The synovial sarcoma oncoprotein may also function by disrupting normal interactions between transcription factors and their DNA-binding sites, such as interactions between SLUG/SNAIL and the E-cadherin promoter, leading to transcriptional activation.[60] Subtle differences in such interactions may underlie the propensity of *SYT-SSX1* translocations, compared to *SYT-SSX2* translocations, to be associated with biphasic histology and poorer outcome, although prognostic differences are controversial.[61,62] The need for diagnostic molecular translocation testing, however, may be obviated by assays for TLE1, a transcriptional corepressor[63] that is highly expressed in synovial sarcoma and serves as a sensitive and specific biomarker.[64] Other oncogenic pathways that are activated, directly or indirectly, in synovial sarcoma include IGF2,[54,65,66] suggesting potential value for IGF/Akt/mTOR inhibitors in this disease.

Alveolar Rhabdomyosarcoma

In alveolar rhabdomyosarcoma, an aggressive cancer of older children and adolescents, the transcriptional activation domain of *FOXO1* (aka *FKHR*) from 13q14 is fused to the DNA-binding domain of paired box transcription factor *PAX3* (2q35) or *PAX7* (1p36).[67,68] Until recently, about 20% of cases were thought to be translocation-negative, but recent work has proven that such tumors in fact represent histologic variants of embryonal rhabdomyosarcoma.[69] Furthermore, those cases with translocations involving *PAX3* have a considerably worse prognosis than those involving *PAX7*.[70] Thus, molecular confirmation of the diagnosis by FISH (Fig. 114.1) and/or RT-PCR is required to optimize patient care.[71] Either translocation results in high-level nuclear expression of a chimeric transcription factor that abnormally activates *PAX* targets, many of which are genes involved in neurogenesis that are not expressed in normal skeletal muscle.[72] In addition, PAX3-FOXO1 directly induces *PDGFRA*; small-molecule (imatinib) and antibody inhibitors of this receptor tyrosine kinase are effective in mouse models.[73] Another probable direct target of PAX3-FOXO1, based on comparison of primary tumor and mouse model expression profiles, is the cell-cycle regulator *SKP2*,[74] perhaps helping explain why alveolar rhabdomyosarcoma is responsive to conventional cytotoxic chemotherapy.

Alveolar Soft-Part Sarcoma

Alveolar soft-part sarcoma has a clinical presentation and pathognomonic molecular event with many similarities to other translocation-associated sarcomas.[75] In this disease, the 5′ half of the widely-expressed *ASPSCR1* (aka *ASPL*) gene on 17q25 is fused to exon 3 or 4 of *TFE3* on Xp11, the latter retaining its transcriptional activation, basic helix-loop-helix, and leucine zipper domains.[76] Interestingly, the same fusion is present in some renal cell carcinomas.[77] Although alveolar soft-part sarcoma has distinctive histology, translocation detection by RT-PCR or by immunohistochemistry for TFE3 can serve as a diagnostic adjunct.[78,79] The disease lacks validated prognostic biomarkers. Direct targets of ASPSCR1-TFE3 are not yet identified, although gene expression profiling and tissue microarray studies have highlighted prominent activation of c-Met signaling and angiogenesis pathways.[80–82] Antiangiogenic targeted therapy is effective in xenograft models[83] and has yielded partial responses in patients with metastatic disease.[84]

Dermatofibrosarcoma Protuberans

The cytogenetic hallmark of dermatofibrosarcoma protuberans (DFSP) is supernumerary ring chromosomes that contain material from chromosomes 17 and 22[85–87] or, less commonly, an unbalanced der(22)t(17;22)(q21-23;q13). The molecular consequence of both types of aberration is the overexpression of the platelet-derived growth factor-beta *(PDGFB)* gene on chromosome 22, through fusion with the collagen gene *COL1A1* on chromosome 17.[88,89] The same fusion gene is also seen in two histologic variants: giant cell fibroblastoma and Bednar tumor (pigmented DFSP). FISH and comparative genomic hybridization (CGH) studies have indicated that increased *COL1A1–PDGFB* copy number is associated with fibrosarcomatous transformation of DFSP, although the copy number increase is not an invariable feature of these cases.[90,91]

The COL1A1-PDGFB fusion product signals through the PDGF receptor in an autocrine loop.[92] This signaling can be blocked using tyrosine kinase inhibitors acting at PDGFR, such as imatinib. A number of clinical studies have shown a high response rate to imatinib therapy in both locally advanced and metastatic DFSP.[85,93,94] These results support the concept that DFSP cells depend on aberrant activation of PDGF signaling for proliferation and survival.

Extraskeletal Myxoid Chondrosarcoma

Most extraskeletal myxoid chondrosarcomas show one of four reciprocal translocations: t(9;22)(q22;q12), t(9;17)(q22;q11), t(9;15)(q22;q21), or t(3;9)(q12;q22), with t(9;22) being the most common. These translocations fuse *NR4A3* in 9q22-q31.1 with either *EWSR1* in 22q12, *TAF15* in 17q11, *TCF12* in 15q21, or *TFG* in 3q12.[95–97] Because these fusion genes have not been described in any other tumor type, they

represent useful diagnostic markers. The four different fusion partners have unknown prognostic significance.

NR4A3 encodes a ubiquitously expressed orphan nuclear receptor also known as NOR-1, TEC, MINOR, or CHN.[98] The t(9;22) fuses the transactivation domain of EWSR1 to the full length of NR4A3. Analogous to EWSR1-ETS fusions, the EWSR1-NR4A3 fusion protein not only displays strong transcriptional activity, but also regulates RNA splicing.[99]

TAF15, like EWSR1 and FUS, belongs to the TET family, and contains a characteristic 87-amino acid RNA recognition motif implicated in protein-RNA binding.[100] The N-terminal regions of EWSR1, FUS, and TAF15 contain degenerate repeats of the SYGQ motif and mediate powerful transcriptional activation when fused to the heterologous DNA-binding domains of a variety of transcription factors.[101]

By gene profiling, **extraskeletal myxoid chondrosarcomas** constitute a distinct genomic entity, showing up-regulation of several genes, including *NMB*, *DKK1*, *DNER*, *CLCN3*.[102] *In situ* hybridization confirmed that *NMB* is highly expressed in **extraskeletal myxoid chondrosarcoma** but not in other sarcoma types, suggesting its potential value as a diagnostic marker. Somewhat surprisingly, the up-regulated genes seen in two different profiling studies had only limited overlap.[96,102]

SIMPLE KARYOTYPE TUMORS ASSOCIATED WITH MUTATIONS

Desmoid Fibromatosis

Desmoid fibromatoses are locally infiltrative, clonal fibroblastic proliferations that arise in the deep soft tissues and never metastasize. Although about 70% result from mutations in *APC* or *CTNNB1*, tumorigenesis may be also be influenced by endocrine and physiologic factors such as pregnancy, trauma, and prior surgery. Desmoids are usually divided into two groups: sporadic desmoids and those in individuals with a heterozygous germline mutation in the adenomatous polyposis coli (*APC*) gene (chromosome 5q). Although germline *APC* mutations also often result in familial adenomatous polyposis,[103] some desmoid patients harboring such a mutation have no polyposis. The desmoids in individuals with a germline *APC* mutation display inactivation of the second copy of *APC*, which usually occurs by point mutation or deletion.[103,104]

Among sporadic desmoids, only a minority display *APC* inactivation. A majority (52%–85%) have an activating point mutation in the β-catenin gene, *CTNNB1*.[105,106] These *CTNNB1* mutations stabilize β-catenin, resulting in its overabundance. β-catenin, a mediator of Wnt signaling, is negatively regulated by APC, so both *APC* inactivation and *CTNNB1* activating mutations result in up-regulation of the Wnt pathway. The specific *CTNNB1* mutation may have prognostic significance; patients with S45F-mutant desmoids were reported to have a 5-year recurrence-free survival of only 23%, compared with 57% for those with T41A-mutant tumors and 65% for those with wild type *CTNNB1*.[106] These results raise the possibility that mutation status might aid in selecting patients for more aggressive therapy.

Based on the findings of *APC* inactivation or activating *CTNNB1* mutations in the majority of patients, the development of small-molecule β-catenin antagonists would be likely to provide significant benefit, particularly for patients with advanced disease in whom surgical resection is not feasible. Although such β-catenin–targeted agents are still in preclinical development, an inhibitor of matrix metalloproteinase, a downstream target of β-catenin, substantially reduced tumor volume and tumor invasion in a transgenic *Apc*+/*Apc*1638N mouse model of aggressive fibromatosis.[107]

Patients with desmoids were found to have elevated levels of PDGF-AA and PDGF-BB, leading to a trial of the tyrosine kinase inhibitor imatinib in patients with advanced desmoid. Three of 19 patients (16%) had a partial response to treatment and four additional patients had stable disease for more than 1 year; overall, the 1-year tumor control rate was 37%.[108] The response in these tumors was thought to be mediated by inhibition of PDGFRB kinase activity.

COMPLEX SARCOMA TYPES

Well-Differentiated and Dedifferentiated Liposarcoma

Well-differentiated and dedifferentiated liposarcomas represent the most common biological group of liposarcoma. This group is characterized by amplification of 12q, including the oncogenes *MDM2*, *HMGA2*, and *CDK4*. The amplifications usually occur in double minutes, ring chromosomes, and large marker chromosomes. In addition, the 12q13.2-q23.1 locus often harbors complex rearrangements (Fig. 114.2).[19,109,110] On the basis of the rearrangements and correlated overexpression results, 12q may contain additional driver genes besides *MDM2*, *HMGA2*, and *CDK4*. The possibilities include *NAV3*, *WIF1*, *MDM1*, *DYRK2*, *ELK3*, *DUSP6*, *YEATS4*, *TBK1*, and *FRS2*, which were found to be amplified in ~14% to 80% of tumors. Some of these genes are known to be involved in liposarcomagenesis, while others were not previously implicated in this disease or in cancer. Aside from 12q aberrations, dedifferentiated liposarcomas have been found to contain significant amplifications of 1p, 1q, 5p, 6q, and 20q.[19,109,110] Amplification of *JUN* (on 1p32) has been suggested as the explanation for the block in adipocyte differentiation in undifferentiated sarcomas.[111] However, more recent studies suggest that *JUN* is amplified or overexpressed in only a subset of dedifferentiated liposarcomas and that other alterations or activated pathways may be required to induce the dedifferentiated phenotype.[19,112]

Microarray analysis of differentially expressed genes in liposarcoma subtypes compared with normal fat has demonstrated activation of cell-cycle and checkpoint pathways, including the up-regulation of CDK4, MDM2, CDK1, CDC7, cyclin B1, cyclin B2, and cyclin E2 in well-differentiated and dedifferentiated liposarcoma, suggesting that these pathways may be useful as therapeutic targets.[113] In fact, nutlin-3a, a selective MDM2 antagonist, induces apoptosis and inhibits proliferation of dedifferentiated liposarcoma cell lines at concentrations that have no phenotypic effects in normal adipose-derived stem cells.[113] Thus, downstream p53 pathway signaling appears to be much more pronounced in dedifferentiated liposarcoma cell lines with overexpressed MDM2 than in adipose-derived stem cells, and MDM2 antagonists might serve as a effective therapeutics for liposarcomas with *MDM2* amplification while having few effects on normal cells. Furthermore, PD0332991, a selective CDK4/CDK6 inhibitor currently in clinical trials, inhibits proliferation of dedifferentiated liposarcoma cells, inducing G1 cell-cycle arrest.[19] These results provide a rationale for use of MDM2 antagonists and CDK4 inhibitors in patients with well-differentiated and dedifferentiated liposarcoma.

Pleomorphic Liposarcoma

Pleomorphic liposarcoma is the least common liposarcoma subtype, accounting for 5% of all liposarcomas. This subtype is characterized by high chromosome counts and complex structural rearrangements, with numerous unidentifiable marker chromosomes, nonclonal alterations, and polyploidy. This complexity has made the detection of specific recurrent rearrangements difficult.

A high-resolution single nucleotide polymorphism (SNP) array analysis has revealed that pleomorphic liposarcoma harbors multiple regions of significant copy number amplification and deletion.[114] The most common alteration, found in approximately 60% of tumors, was a deletion of 13q14.2-q14.3 that includes the *RB1* tumor suppressor. The next most common event was loss of 17p13.1 including *TP53*. Both *RB1* and *TP53* deletions were a mixture of hemizygous loss and less frequent homozygous deletion. Recently, *TP53* point mutations were found in 17% of pleomorphic liposarcomas.[19] Small molecules that reactivate mutant p53, such as PRIMA-1, are presently undergoing phase 1 trials and may have particular utility for pleomorphic liposarcomas harboring deletion or mutation in *TP53*.

A third genetic alteration identified in SNP analysis was frequent deletions of 17q11.2 including the tumor suppressor *NF1* (neurofibromin 1). Among 24 pleomorphic liposarcomas, nine had genomic loss at this locus, eight of which were hemizygous and one was homozygous. In addition, two tumors (8%) had somatic point mutations in *NF1*, and both these tumors also showed deletion of the wild type allele and correspondingly reduced gene expression. These data indicate a diverse pattern of *NF1* aberrations in approximately 38% of pleomorphic liposarcomas[19] and suggest that MEK or mTOR inhibitors may have clinical utility, as loss of NF1 function appears to activate the RAS and mTOR pathways.

Myxofibrosarcoma and Pleomorphic Malignant Fibrous Histiocytoma

Pathologists now regard myxofibrosarcoma as a distinct tumor type with clearly defined criteria for diagnosis.[115–117] Myxofibrosarcoma contains variable degrees of myxoid stroma composed of hyaluronic acid and solid sheets of spindled and pleomorphic (irregularly shaped) tumor cells. Pleomorphic malignant fibrous histiocytoma, however, is less well defined, and it remains controversial whether it represents (1) a pleomorphic sarcoma showing fibroblastic/myofibroblastic differentiation and thus sharing a common set of genomic alterations with myxofibrosarcoma, or (2) an end-stage undifferentiated morphologic pattern with genomic alterations distinct from those of myxofibrosarcoma.

Myxofibrosarcoma

Myxofibrosarcoma, also known as myxoid variant of malignant fibrous histiocytoma, includes a spectrum of malignant fibroblastic lesions with variably myxoid stroma (at least 10%), pleomorphism, and a distinctive curvilinear vascular pattern. At present, little is known about the genetic events specific to myxofibrosarcoma. Cytogenetic data are scarce, with only 49 cases described in the literature.[118] Cytogenetic karyotypes tend to be highly complex, often with multiple numerical and structural rearrangements and with chromosome numbers in the triploid or tetraploid range.[119,120] No specific or consistent chromosomal aberration has emerged, although some chromosomes appear to be more involved than others and ring chromosomes have been reported. In general, karyotype complexity has been greater in high-grade lesions and in recurrences.[120]

In an SNP array analysis of 38 myxofibrosarcomas, approximately 55% of tumors harbored chromosome 5p amplification.[19] This region contains *RICTOR* (the rapamycin-insensitive binding partner of mTOR), *CDH9*, and *LIFR*. Other amplified regions included several discontinuous loci on 1p and 1q spanning *PI4KB*, *ETV3*, and *MCL1*, among others. *MCL1*, an antiapoptotic gene, was concomitantly overexpressed in these tumors. Myxofibrosarcomas also harbored deletions of classic tumor suppressors, including *CDKN2A/CDKN2B*, *RB1*, and *TP53*. These events, in combination with the inactivating mutations detected in *NF1* in 11% and *PTEN* in 3% of myxofibrosarcomas, demonstrate extensive loss of function in several known tumor suppressors.[19]

Pleomorphic Malignant Fibrous Histiocytoma

Over 50% of soft tissue sarcomas occurring in older adults are histologically pleomorphic and high grade. Most have traditionally been classified as malignant fibrous histiocytoma (MFH), which has been regarded as the most common sarcoma in adults.[121,122] MFH was originally defined as a pleomorphic spindle cell malignant neoplasm showing fibroblastic and histiocytic differentiation. More recently, pathologists have accepted that the morphologic pattern known as pleomorphic MFH may be shared by a wide range of malignant neoplasms.[123] Many sarcomas that were previously classified as pleomorphic MFH, on careful immunohistochemical and histopathologic analysis, revealed a specific line of differentiation and could be reclassified as myxofibrosarcoma (30%), myogenic sarcoma (30%), liposarcoma (4%), malignant peripheral nerve sheath tumor (2%), or soft tissue osteosarcoma (3%), and about 30% had no specific line of differentiation or were myofibroblastic.[115] Thus, the term *pleomorphic MFH/sarcoma not otherwise specified* is now reserved for pleomorphic sarcomas that show no definable line of differentiation by current technology.

Because diagnostic criteria have shifted over the years, the genetic aspects of pleomorphic MFH are difficult to evaluate. Among the more than 60 cases in the Mitelman Database of Chromosome Alterations in Cancer published as storiform or pleomorphic MFH or MFH not otherwise specified, the karyotypes are highly complex. The majority of tumors have chromosome numbers in the triploid or tetraploid range, but a few have near-haploid karyotypes.[124–128] No specific aberrations have emerged, but telomeric associations, ring chromosomes, and/or dicentric chromosomes are frequent, although not specific for pleomorphic MFH. Unfortunately many of the cytogenetic and array-based CGH studies to date have included heterogeneous groups of tumors characterized as MFH; these studies typically show loss of 2p24, 2q32, and chromosomes 11, 13, and 16 along with gains of 7p15, 7q32, and 1p31.[129–132] In many of these CGH studies, the copy number profiles of the majority of pleomorphic MFH closely resembled those of leiomyosarcomas[133–135] or pleomorphic or dedifferentiated liposarcomas.[136–138] Mutations and/or deletions of *TP53*, *RB1*, and *INK4a* have been suggested to play a critical role in pleomorphic MFH oncogenesis.[131,133,139–141]

Leiomyosarcoma

Leiomyosarcoma is a malignant tumor composed of cells showing distinct smooth muscle features and typically containing intersecting, sharply marginated groups of spindle cells. Karyotypes tend to be complex, with amplifications, gains, and losses involving multiple chromosomes, and karyotype generally differs between tumors.[142–144] Frequent losses of 1p12-pter, 2p, 13q14-q21 (including the *RB1* tumor suppressor),[145] 10q (including *PTEN*),[146] and 16q and gains of 17p, 8q, and 1q21-31regions have been observed and have been associated with aggressive clinical behavior. In an analysis of copy number alterations in 27 leiomyosarcomas,[19] deletions, which were more common than amplifications, included well-characterized tumor suppressors like *TP53*, *BRCA2*, *RB1*, and *FANCA*. The most prominent changes were chromosome 10 deletions (approximately 50%-70% of cases) (Fig. 114.2). Indeed,

PRACTICE OF ONCOLOGY

75. Fisher C. Soft tissue sarcomas with non-EWS translocations: molecular genetic features and pathologic and clinical correlations. *Virchows Arch* 2010;456:153–166.
82. Stockwin LH, Vistica DT, Kenney S, et al. Gene expression profiling of alveolar soft-part sarcoma (ASPS). *BMC Cancer* 2009;9:22.
84. Stacchiotti S, Tamborini E, Marrari A, et al. Response to sunitinib malate in advanced alveolar soft part sarcoma. *Clin Cancer Res* 2009;15:1096–1104.
85. McArthur GA, Demetri GD, van Oosterom A, et al. Molecular and clinical analysis of locally advanced dermatofibrosarcoma protuberans treated with imatinib: Imatinib Target Exploration Consortium Study B2225. *J Clin Oncol* 2005;23:866–873.
105. Tejpar S, Nollet F, Li C, et al. Predominance of beta-catenin mutations and beta-catenin dysregulation in sporadic aggressive fibromatosis (desmoid tumor). *Oncogene* 1999;18:6615.
106. Lazar AJ, Tuvin D, Hajibashi S, et al. Specific mutations in the beta-catenin gene (CTNNB1) correlate with local recurrence in sporadic desmoid tumors. *Am J Pathol* 2008;173:1518–1527.
108. Heinrich MC, McArthur GA, Demetri GD, et al. Clinical and molecular studies of the effect of imatinib on advanced aggressive fibromatosis (desmoid tumor). *J Clin Oncol* 2006;24:1195–1203.
111. Mariani O, Brennetot C, Coindre JM, et al. JUN oncogene amplification and overexpression block adipocytic differentiation in highly aggressive sarcomas. *Cancer Cell* 2007;11:361–374.
112. Snyder EL, Sandstrom DJ, Law K, et al. c-Jun amplification and overexpression are oncogenic in liposarcoma but not always sufficient to inhibit the adipocytic differentiation programme. *J Pathol* 2009;218:292–300.
113. Singer S, Socci ND, Ambrosini G, et al. Gene expression profiling of liposarcoma identifies distinct biological types/subtypes and potential therapeutic targets in well-differentiated and dedifferentiated liposarcoma. *Cancer Res* 2007;67:6626–6636.
115. Fletcher CD, Gustafson P, Rydholm A, Willen H, Akerman M. Clinicopathologic re-evaluation of 100 malignant fibrous histiocytomas: prognostic relevance of subclassification. *J Clin Oncol* 2001;19:3045–3050.
116. Fletcher CD, Unni KK, Mertens F. Pathology and genetics of tumors of soft tissue and bone. In: Kleihues P, Sobin LH, eds. *World Health Organization Classification of Tumours*. Lyon, France: IARC Press, 2002.
136. Chibon F, Mariani O, Derre J, et al. ASK1 (MAP3K5) as a potential therapeutic target in malignant fibrous histiocytomas with 12q14-q15 and 6q23 amplifications. *Genes Chromosomes Cancer* 2004;40:32–37.
143. Sandberg AA. Updates on the cytogenetics and molecular genetics of bone and soft tissue tumors: leiomyosarcoma. *Cancer Genet Cytogenet* 2005;161:1–19.
144. Yang J, Du X, Chen K, et al. Genetic aberrations in soft tissue leiomyosarcoma. *Cancer Lett* 2009;275:1.
147. Hernando E, Charytonowicz E, Dudas ME, et al. The AKT-mTOR pathway plays a critical role in the development of leiomyosarcomas. *Nat Med* 2007;13:748–753.
149. Kleinerman RA, Tucker MA, Abramson DH, et al. Risk of soft tissue sarcomas by individual subtype in survivors of hereditary retinoblastoma. *J Natl Cancer Inst* 2007;99:24–31.
152. Cichowski K, Jacks T. NF1 tumor suppressor gene function: narrowing the GAP. *Cell* 2001;104:593–604.
154. Mantripragada KK, de Stahl TD, Patridge C, et al. Genome-wide high-resolution analysis of DNA copy number alterations in NF1-associated malignant peripheral nerve sheath tumors using 32K BAC array. *Genes Chromosomes Cancer* 2009;48:897–907.
155. Upadhyaya M, Kluwe L, Spurlock G, et al. Germline and somatic NF1 gene mutation spectrum in NF1-associated malignant peripheral nerve sheath tumors (MPNSTs). *Hum Mutat* 2008;29:74–82.
163. Keizman D, Issakov J, Meller I, et al. Expression and significance of EGFR in malignant peripheral nerve sheath tumor. *J Neurooncol* 2009;94:383–388.
164. Ling BC, Wu J, Miller SJ, et al. Role for the epidermal growth factor receptor in neurofibromatosis-related peripheral nerve tumorigenesis. *Cancer Cell* 2005;7:65–75.
165. Johannessen CM, Reczek EE, James MF, et al. The NF1 tumor suppressor critically regulates TSC2 and mTOR. *Proc Natl Acad Sci U S A* 2005;102:8573–8578.
166. Ambrosini G, Cheema HS, Seelman S, et al. Sorafenib inhibits growth and mitogen-activated protein kinase signaling in malignant peripheral nerve sheath cells. *Mol Cancer Ther* 2008;7:890–896.
167. Maki RG, D'Adamo DR, Keohan ML, et al. Phase II study of sorafenib in patients with metastatic or recurrent sarcomas. *J Clin Oncol* 2009;27:3133–3140.
168. Antonescu CR, Yoshida A, Guo T, et al. KDR activating mutations in human angiosarcomas are sensitive to specific kinase inhibitors. *Cancer Res* 2009;69:7175–7179.
169. Manner J, Radlwimmer B, Hohenberger P, et al. MYC high level gene amplification is a distinctive feature of angiosarcomas after irradiation or chronic lymphedema. *Am J Pathol* 2010;176:34–39.
172. Hadju M, Singer S, Maki RG, et al. IGF2 over-expression in solitary fibrous tumours is independent of anatomical location and is related to loss of imprinting. *J Pathol* 2010;221:300–307.
177. Metzker ML. Sequencing technologies—the next generation. *Nat Rev Genet* 2010;11:31–46.
178. Wang Z, Gerstein M, Snyder M. RNA-Seq: a revolutionary tool for transcriptomics. *Nat Rev Genet* 2009;10:57–63.
180. Mortazavi A, Williams BA, McCue K, Schaeffer L, Wold B. Mapping and quantifying mammalian transcriptomes by RNA-Seq. *Nat Methods* 2008;5:621–628.
182. Strebhardt K, Ullrich A. Paul Ehrlich's magic bullet concept: 100 years of progress. *Nat Rev Cancer* 2008;8:473–480.
185. Oltersdorf T, Elmore SW, Shoemaker AR, et al. An inhibitor of Bcl-2 family proteins induces regression of solid tumours. *Nature* 2005;435:677–681.
186. Schneider G, Fechner U. Computer-based de novo design of drug-like molecules. *Nat Rev Drug Discov* 2005;4:649–663.

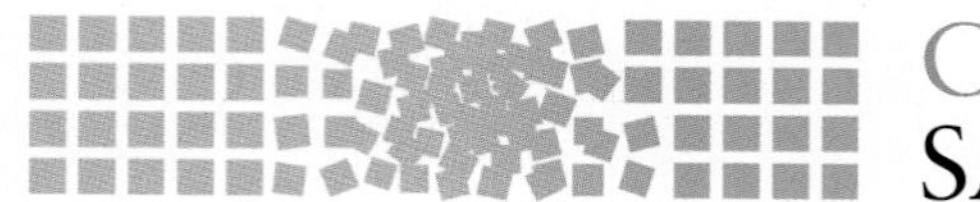

CHAPTER 115 SOFT TISSUE SARCOMA

SAMUEL SINGER, ROBERT G. MAKI, AND BRIAN O'SULLIVAN

Tumors arising in the soft tissue form a diverse and complex group, since they may display varying degrees of mesenchymal differentiation. Most soft tissue tumors are benign and are usually cured with a simple surgical excision. Soft tissue sarcomas account for less than 1% of the overall human burden of malignant tumors but remain life-threatening, and approximately 40% of patients with newly diagnosed soft tissue sarcoma die of the disease, corresponding to approximately 4,000 deaths each year in the United States.[1] The relatively small number of cases and the great diversity in histopathologic features, anatomic sites, and biologic behaviors have made comprehensive understanding of these disease entities difficult. Soft tissue sarcoma, diagnosed at an early stage, is eminently curable. When diagnosed at the time of extensive local or metastatic disease, it is rarely curable. There is an urgent need to develop new treatments.

INCIDENCE AND ETIOLOGY

Incidence and Epidemiology

Benign mesenchymal tumors are 100-fold more common than soft tissue sarcomas.[2] The annual international incidence rates of soft tissue sarcoma range between 1.4 and 5.0 cases per 100,000.[3–7] Incidence patterns vary considerably by histologic type and subtype.[7,8] Incidence for most types of soft tissue sarcoma increases progressively with age from approximately 1 to 2 per 100,000 at age 15, to approximately 6 per 100,000 at age 49, and to as high as approximately 20 per 100,000 at age 80.[7,8] Although several studies have suggested that incidence of soft tissue sarcoma has increased over time,[7,9,10] other studies have not confirmed this,[3,4,6,11] and the true incidence remains difficult to determine.

Etiology and Risk Factors

Most soft tissue sarcomas are believed to be sporadic and have no clearly defined cause. In a small proportion of cases, researchers have identified various associated or predisposing factors, including genetic factors, prior radiation therapy, lymphedema, several carcinogens, and perhaps several other chemical agents and trauma.

Genetic Factors

The genetic syndromes familial adenomatous polyposis, neurofibromatosis 1, Li-Fraumeni syndrome, and retinoblastoma are all associated with the development of soft tissue sarcoma. Desmoid tumors occur in patients with familial adenomatous polyposis (FAP), a disorder caused by germline mutations in the adenomatous polyposis coli (*APC*) gene. The type and site of APC mutation affects β-catenin signaling and may affect the probability that the patient with FAP will develop intra-abdominal desmoid tumors.[12,13] Malignant peripheral nerve sheath tumors (MPNSTs) develop in neurofibromas in patients with germline mutations in the neurofibromatosis 1 (*NF1*) gene. NF1 patients have an estimated annual incidence of MPNST of 1.6 per 1,000, with a lifetime risk of 8% to 13%.[14] Li-Fraumeni syndrome is a rare, highly penetrant familial cancer phenotype usually associated with germline mutations in *TP53*, the gene for tumor suppressor p53.[15] Eighty percent of patients with this syndrome develop cancer by age 45, and the index tumors in 36% of patients are soft tissue or bone sarcomas of diverse histology.[10] Heritable retinoblastoma gene (*RB1*) mutations are associated with an increased risk of bone and soft tissue sarcoma. For instance, patients with RB1 mutations have a 36% cumulative incidence over 50 years of sarcoma in previously irradiated tissue.[16] Most of the excess cancer risk in hereditary retinoblastoma survivors can be prevented by limiting exposure to DNA-damaging agents such as radiotherapy, tobacco, and ultraviolet light,[17] emphasizing the importance of avoiding radiotherapy in sarcoma patients with a known germline mutation in RB1.

Radiation

It has been known since 1922 that radiation exposure can cause soft tissue and bone sarcoma. Soft tissue sarcomas are one of the most common types of radiation-associated tumors, both in the general population[18–21] and in individuals with cancer susceptibility syndromes.[16] They are most often seen in diseases that are commonly treated with radiotherapy and in those in which patient survival is typically long. The prime candidate diseases are breast cancer, lymphomas, genitourinary cancer, and head and neck cancer.[22] Children are at risk due to the time latency involved. In a review of 130 patients with primary radiation-associated sarcoma, the median interval between radiotherapy and development of a radiation-associated sarcoma was 10 years (range, 1.3 to 74.0).[22] This interval varied significantly by histologic type, with the shortest latency observed in liposarcoma (median 4.3 years) and longest in leiomyosarcoma (median 23.5 years). The most common histologic types of radiation-associated sarcomas were pleomorphic malignant fibrous histiocytoma (PMFH) (26%), angiosarcoma (21%), fibrosarcoma (12%), leiomyosarcoma (12%), and MPNST (9%).

The molecular mechanisms and antecedent cause of these lesions is poorly understood. Interestingly, irradiation-induced sarcomas have a reputation for originating close to the penumbra of radiotherapy fields, perhaps because incomplete damage in normal tissues may result in mutagenic responses and disorganized reparative proliferation that can eventually trigger tumor induction. Germline mutations in tumor suppressors and DNA repair genes, accumulated damage to such

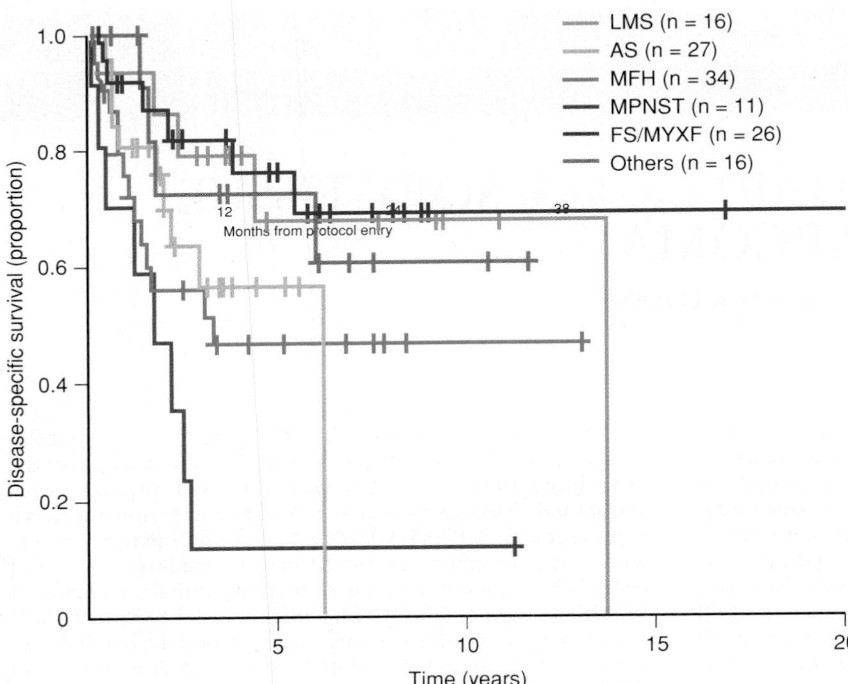

FIGURE 115.1 Histology-specific disease-specific survival for resected primary radiation-associated sarcomas (n = 130). FS/MYXF, fibrosarcoma and myxofibrosarcoma; LMS, leiomyosarcoma; AS, angiosarcoma; MFH, pleomorphic malignant fibrous histiocytoma; MPNST, malignant peripheral nerve sheath tumor. (From ref. 22, with permission.)

genes, or both may lead to neoplasia, but it is unknown whether some individuals with radiation-associated sarcoma have a genetic defect that underpinned the development of both the first cancer and the radiotherapy-induced cancer. If this is the case, then there may be subgroups of individuals at considerably greater risk than is generally appreciated, whereas others may have relatively low risk.

Although uncommon, radiation-induced sarcomas usually have a poor prognosis. Among 130 patients with primary radiation-associated sarcoma, histologic type was a statistically significant predictor of disease-specific survival (P = .004).[22] Disease-specific survival was highest for fibrosarcoma or myxofibrosarcoma (76%), followed by angiosarcoma (57%) and PMFH (47%), and lowest for MPNST (12%) (Fig. 115.1). Independent predictors of disease-specific survival included PMFH (hazard ratio [HR] 4.2; 95% confidence interval [CI], 1.2 to 15.2), and MPNST (HR 7.5; 95% CI, 1.9 to 30.6). A multivariate analysis of the five most common histologic types of primary, high-grade sarcoma showed that radiation-associated sarcoma had a worse disease-specific survival than sporadic soft tissue sarcoma (P = .007; HR 1.7; 95% CI, 1.1 to 2.4). For PMFH—the most common radiation-associated sarcoma type—the 5-year disease-specific survival was 44%, compared to 66% for a matched cohort of sporadic PMFH patients (P = .07). In addition, disease-specific survival was significantly worse in primary radiation-associated MPNSTs than in unmatched sporadic MPNSTs (P = .001). Thus, disease-specific survival in patients with soft tissue sarcoma is significantly worse for primary radiation-associated sarcoma compared to sporadic sarcoma independent of histologic type.[22]

Given the increased use of radiation therapy as a primary treatment for breast cancer, concern has been expressed that the incidence of sarcoma might increase. In one study,[23] all 122,991 women with breast cancer in Sweden from 1958 to 1992 were followed, and 116 soft tissue sarcomas were found: 40 angiosarcomas and 76 other sarcomas. As expected, angiosarcoma was associated with lymphedema (relative risk [RR] 9.5; 95% CI, 3.2 to 28.0), but not with radiation therapy. Other sarcomas showed a dose–response relationship with exposure to radiation therapy.[23] In a retrospective review of data from the SEER database, Huang and Mackillop[19] analyzed the data on 194,798 women treated for breast cancer between 1973 and 1995. Although the follow-up period may have been inadequate to reflect the incidence of radiation-associated sarcoma, they demonstrated a 16-fold increase in angiosarcoma in radiotherapy patients versus controls, and a twofold increase in all soft tissue sarcoma in radiated patients.

Another study cohort included 295,712 patients representing all of the primary cancers of the breast, cervix uteri, corpus uteri, lung, ovary, prostate, and rectum and all of the Hodgkin's and non-Hodgkin's lymphomas registered during 1953 to 2000 in the Finnish Cancer Registry.[24] In total, 147 sarcomas were found versus 88.5 expected. The most-represented prior cancer in the cohort was breast cancer, which therefore had the greatest number of sarcomas: 44 observed for 28.9 expected, an observed-to-expected ratio of 1.5 (95% CI, 1.1 to 2.0). In the total study, soft tissue sarcomas comprised 86% of the sarcomas. After 10 years of follow-up, compared to the national incidence rates, sarcoma risk was increased among patients who had received neither radiotherapy nor chemotherapy (observed to expected ratio 2.0; 95% CI, 1.3 to 3.0) but was higher in patients who had received radiotherapy and in those who had received chemotherapy. For patients who underwent radiotherapy before age 55, the observed-to-expected ratio was 4.2 (95% CI, 2.9 to 5.8). These results confirm that the risk of sarcoma is increased after 10 years in tumors other than retinoblastoma but is also independently related to younger age of exposure to radiation, although the risk is also influenced by chemotherapy.[24]

Lymphedema

Lymphedema has long been established as a factor in the development of lymphangiosarcoma. The best-recognized association is with the postmastectomy, postirradiated lymphedematous arm, described by Stewart and Treves.[25] This is not a radiation-induced sarcoma because lymphangiosarcomas develop both inside and outside the irradiated field. Similar advanced sarcomas have been seen after chronic lymphedema caused by filarial infection.[26] The pathogenic mechanism of this syndrome remains unknown, but one hypothesis, based on the frequent proliferation of lymphatic vessels in the edematous tissue, is that the block of the lymphatics stimulates growth factors and cytokines, leading to proliferation of vessels and lymphatics.[27] Others have postulated that the edematous tissue results in a regional immune deficiency that enables mutant cells to escape recognition by the host's immune surveillance.[28]

Trauma

Whether trauma is a predisposing factor is more controversial. Abdominal desmoid tumors commonly follow parturition. Moreover, desmoid tumors in the extremity, both localized and multifocal, may be associated with antecedent vigorous physical activity.[29] Some authors have speculated that injuries during active sport may predispose to sarcoma, and in turn there has been concern that operative trauma, including arthroplasty surgery, may increase soft tissue sarcoma risk. However, Scandinavian studies on more than 100,000 patients who had undergone total hip or knee arthroplasty showed no increased risk of sarcoma, and there were no cases of sarcoma presenting at the site of operation.[30] An injury may be merely the factor that draws attention to the presence of a mass, without being a causative factor.

Chemical Agents

Chemical agents have been implicated in the etiology of soft tissue sarcoma. Some studies have suggested a link between phenoxy herbicide exposure and development of sarcoma,[31] and soft tissue sarcoma was associated with high occupational exposures in a large industrial cohort.[32,33] However, other studies, including more recent case-control studies, have not confirmed this relationship.[34] Other authors have pointed to the inherent problems in occupational epidemiology in relation to soft tissue sarcoma, among which are possible recall bias in self-reported exposure data; inconsistent classification of soft tissue sarcomas in the International Classification of Diseases, which is organ based; variation in the operational definition of soft tissue sarcomas; and, because of the rarity of soft tissue sarcomas, difficulty in recruiting sufficient patients for case-control studies and the need for extremely large cohorts for cohort studies.

The issue of dioxin as a risk factor also remains controversial. Vietnam veterans who had higher estimated opportunities for exposure to Agent Orange, which contains dioxin, seemed to be at greater risk of soft tissue sarcoma when their counterparts in Vietnam were taken as a reference group. However, this risk was not statistically significant.[35] Moreover, a number of other studies have found no association.[36–38] In fact, one case-control study found that sarcoma risk was highest among those who had the lowest dioxin concentrations.[37,38]

Several chemical carcinogens have an established role in the development of hepatic angiosarcomas: thorotrast, vinyl chloride, and arsenic (including Fowler's 1% arsenic solution).[10]

ANATOMIC AND AGE DISTRIBUTION AND PATHOLOGY

Anatomic and Age Distribution

Soft tissue sarcomas can occur in any site throughout the body. Forty-one percent are located in the extremities, with 29% of all lesions occurring in the lower limb (most commonly in the thigh); 36% are intra-abdominal, divided between visceral (21%) and retroperitoneal (15%) lesions; 10% are truncal; and 5% are head and neck (Fig. 115.2).

Soft tissue sarcomas become more common with increased age, and the median age at diagnosis is 65 years. However, the median age varies significantly by histologic type and subtype. In general, the median age of onset tends to be in the second

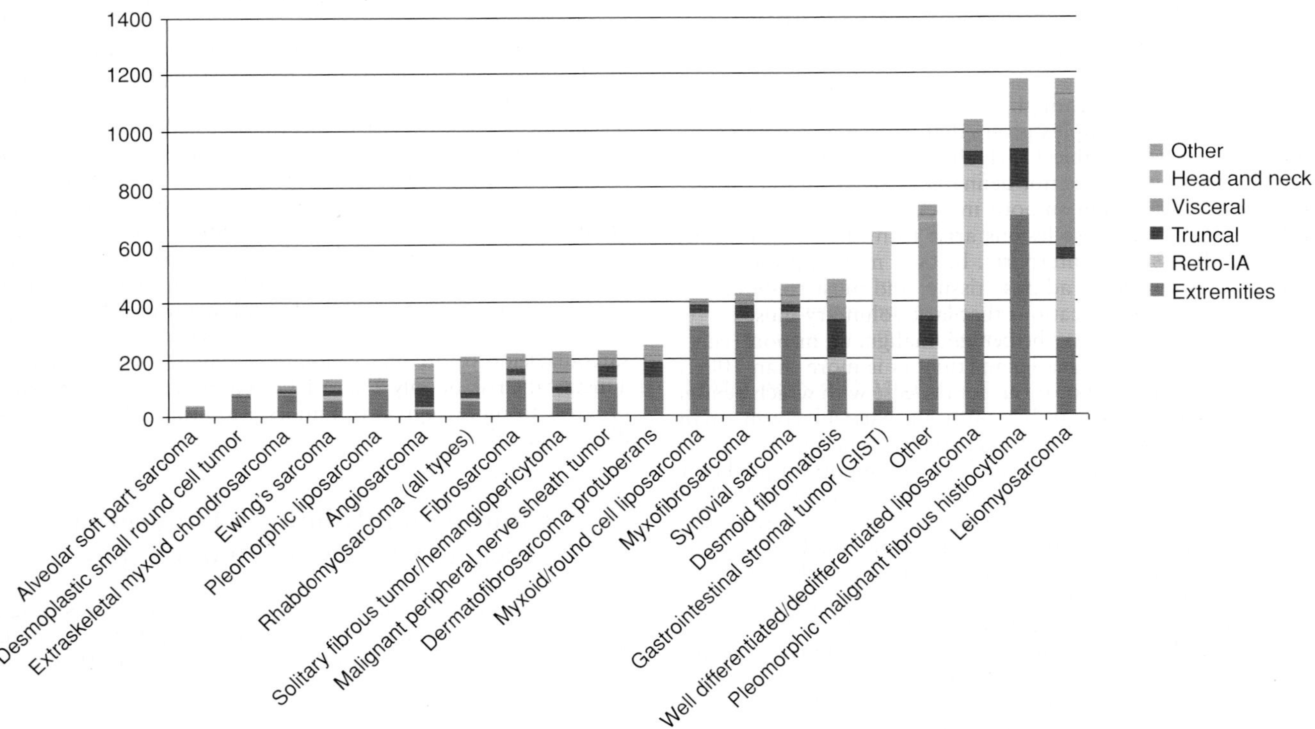

FIGURE 115.2 Distribution by histologic subtype and site of soft tissue sarcomas in 8,328 patients aged 16 years or older admitted to Memorial Sloan-Kettering Cancer Center from 1982 through 2009. The retroperitoneal/abdominal category excludes visceral sarcomas.

TABLE 115.1

(CONTINUED)

Skeletal Muscle Tumors (*continued*)

MALIGNANT TUMORS
Rhabdomyosarcoma
Alveolar rhabdomyosarcoma
Botryoid rhabdomyosarcoma
Embryonal rhabdomyosarcoma
Pleomorphic rhabdomyosarcoma

Vascular Tumors

BENIGN TUMORS
Angiomatosis
Capillary (including juvenile) hemangioma
Cavernous hemangioma
Hemangioma (intramuscular, synovial, perineural)
Epithelioid hemangioma (angiolymphoid hyperplasia, histiocytoid hemangioma)
Lymphangioma
Venous hemangioma

INTERMEDIATE TUMORS
Endovascular papillary angioendothelioma (Dabska tumor)
Papillary intralymphatic angioendothelioma

INTERMEDIATE (LOCALLY AGGRESSIVE) TUMORS
Kaposiform hemangioendothelioma

INTERMEDIATE (RARELY METASTASIZING) TUMORS
Composite hemangioendothelioma
Kaposi sarcoma
Retiform hemangioendothelioma

MALIGNANT TUMORS
Angiosarcoma of soft tissue
Epithelioid hemangioendothelioma

Perivascular Tumors

BENIGN TUMORS
Glomus tumor
Myopericytoma

MALIGNANT TUMORS
Malignant glomus tumor (glomangiosarcoma)

Neural Tumors

BENIGN TUMORS
Ectopic ependymoma
Ectopic meningioma
Ganglioneuroma
Granular cell tumor
Melanotic schwannoma
Morton neuroma
Multiple mucosal neuromas
Nerve sheath ganglion
Neurofibroma (diffuse, plexiform, pacinian, epithelioid)
Neuromuscular hamartoma (benign Triton tumor)
Neurothekeoma (nerve sheath myxoma)
Pigmented neuroectodermal tumor of infancy (retinal anlage tumor, melanotic progonoma)
Schwannoma (cellular, plexiform, degenerated)
Schwannomatosis
Traumatic neuroma

MALIGNANT TUMORS
Malignant granular cell tumor
Malignant peripheral nerve sheath tumor (MPNST) (neurofibrosarcoma)
Epithelioid MPNST
Glandular MPNST
Malignant Triton tumor (MPNST with rhabdomyosarcoma)
Primitive neuroectodermal tumors
Ganglioneuroblastoma
Neuroblastoma

Extraskeletal Chondro-Osseous Tumors

BENIGN TUMORS
Extraskeletal osteoma
Soft tissue chondroma

MALIGNANT TUMORS
Extraskeletal osteosarcoma

Tumors of Uncertain Differentiation

BENIGN TUMORS
Amyloid tumor
Angiomyxoma
Congenital granular cell tumor
Cutaneous myxoma
Intramuscular myxoma
Juxta-articular myxoma
Mesenchymoma
Palisaded myofibroblastoma of lymph node
Pleomorphic hyalinizing angiectatic tumor of soft parts
Tumoral calcinosis

INTERMEDIATE (RARELY METASTASIZING) TUMORS
Angiomatoid fibrous histiocytoma
Myoepithelioma
Ossifying and nonossifying fibromyxoid tumors
Parachordoma

MALIGNANT TUMORS
Alveolar soft part sarcoma
Clear cell sarcoma of soft tissue
Desmoplastic small round cell tumor
Epithelioid sarcoma
Extrarenal rhabdoid tumor
Extraskeletal Ewing sarcoma
Extraskeletal myxoid chondrosarcoma
Follicular dendritic cell tumor/sarcoma
Gastrointestinal stromal tumor
Intimal sarcoma
Lymphangioleiomyomatosis
Malignant extrarenal rhabdoid tumor
Malignant mesenchymoma
Neoplasms with perivascular epithelioid cell differentiation (PEComas)
Synovial sarcoma (biphasic and monophasic)

Unclassified Tumors

MALIGNANT TUMORS
Sarcoma, not otherwise specified

Modified from ref. 39.

contain cells with both fibroblastic and myofibroblastic features. A significant subset of spindle cell and pleomorphic sarcomas are probably myofibroblastic in type but, to date, only low-grade forms have been reproducibly characterized.[39] Recent conceptual changes have recognized the importance of reclassification of tumors formerly labeled myxoid malignant fibrous histiocytoma as myxofibrosarcoma and the clear recognition of solitary fibrous tumor as a fibroblastic or myofibroblastic tumor.

There are a variety of benign tumors and tumorlike lesions of fibrous tissue that must be distinguished from true fibrosarcoma. These lesions are generally composed of fibroblasts and myofibroblasts in varying proportions and may be confused with reactive or reparative processes. A variety of names have been used to designate identical or overlapping entities. In addition, some fibrous proliferations of infancy and childhood resemble lesions in the adult but have a better prognosis. The following sections summarize the features of lesions that may be mistaken for sarcoma, as well as those of fibroblastic and myofibroblastic sarcomas.

Nodular Fasciitis. Nodular fasciitis is a benign lesion usually seen in adults, age 20 to 40 years. The lesions typically grow rapidly over several weeks and reach 1 to 2 cm but rarely more than 5 cm. Pain and tenderness are common. The upper extremity is the most common site, especially the volar aspect of the forearm. Nodular fasciitis generally arises in the subcutaneous fascia or the superficial portions of the deep fascia. However, intra-articular fasciitis has been reported. Histologically the lesions are nodular and nonencapsulated, showing plump mature fibroblasts arranged in short, irregular or intersecting bundles. Some lesions show hyalinization. Because of their high cellular clarity, rapid growth, and high mitotic activity, these lesions are often confused with fibrosarcoma. They are, however, a clinically benign process with a self-limiting course, and recurrence is uncommon after local excision. Computed tomography (CT) and magnetic resonance imaging (MRI) characteristics are not definitive, although they may show either a solid or some partially cystic changes, usually in the subcutaneous tissues.

Myositis Ossificans. Myositis ossificans is usually associated with trauma and appears as a localized self-limiting reparative lesion composed of reactive hypercellular fibrous tissue and bone. Despite its name, myositis ossificans is not necessarily confined to the muscle, nor is inflammation a prominent feature. The condition usually presents in athletic young adults as a tender soft tissue mass. Over a period of weeks, the mass usually becomes firm to hard. Radiographs show calcification several weeks after the lesion appears. Histologically the mass consists of fibroblastic tissue, often with prominent mitotic activity. Nonetheless, this process is benign and may be managed conservatively. It is important to distinguish between myositis ossificans and sarcoma, especially extraskeletal osteogenic sarcoma. The lesions can be very vascular at the time of biopsy, which suggests a more neoplastic process.

Fibroma. Fibroma is a nonspecific term usually applied to a group of poorly defined lesions in the skin or soft tissue. Fibromas should be effectively treated by simple excision. They can be a dense fibrous nodule attached to the tendon sheath with a propensity of recurrence if excision is inadequate. Rarely do they occur in unusual locations such as cardiac ventricle.

Elastofibroma. Elastofibromas are rare, slow-growing benign tumors characteristically arising between the lower portion of the scapula and the chest wall. They may occur bilaterally, and they may grow to large size. Elastofibromas are considered reactive lesions, and they are thought to be associated with repetitive manual tasks. They may occur within families. Histologically they consist of swollen eosinophilic collagen and elastic fibers. If the diagnosis is firm, surgical resection can be reserved for the symptomatic patient.

Superficial Fibromatosis. Superficial fibromatoses arise from the fascia or aponeuroses and generally are small and slow growing. Palmar fibromatosis is associated with flexion contractures (Dupuytren contracture) and is by far the most common form, affecting as many as one in five persons aged 65 years and older. This condition is more common in men than in women and tends to be familial. Although benign, these lesions have a tendency to recur after simple excision. Plantar fibromatosis (Ledderhose disease) tends to occur in a somewhat younger age group but may occur with greater frequency in patients with palmar fibromatosis. Penile fibromatosis (Peyronie disease), which causes pain and curvature of the penis on erection, is much less common. The fibrous mass in Peyronie disease primarily involves fascial structures, the corpus cavernosum, and rarely the corpus spongiosum. Peyronie disease is more common in men with palmar and plantar fibromatosis than in the general population.

Desmoid Tumor. The desmoid (deep) fibromatoses belong to a family of myofibroblastic fibromatoses that are unusual in their bland histology and slow progression. Desmoids arise in the deep soft tissues and are characterized by an infiltrative growth pattern with a propensity for local recurrence, but they never metastasize. They are rare, with an estimated incidence of two to four individuals per million.[45] These clinically diverse neoplasms are usually divided into two main molecular or genetic groups: sporadic and those associated with FAP. In addition, desmoids have been classified by location into three main subsets: extra-abdominal (60% of cases), abdominal wall (25%), and intra-abdominal (15%). As is the case for other sarcomas, site affects management, but it is unclear whether the distinction by site is biologically significant. The term *aggressive fibromatosis,* often applied to these lesions, especially in the retroperitoneum, refers to their potential for invasion and progressive growth. Despite the lack of metastatic potential, some desmoids prove fatal due to local effects (especially in the head and neck region) or as a result of overly aggressive local therapy for small bowel desmoids.[46]

In patients with FAP, abdominal and retroperitoneal desmoids, along with fibromas, osteomas, and epidermoid cysts, are among the extracolonic manifestations that characterize Gardner syndrome.[47] Some FAP patients develop desmoids at multiple sites. Multifocal desmoids of the extremity have been recognized,[29] usually in young women. FAP has been clearly linked to mutations in the *APC* gene.[12] In addition, certain APC germline mutations can result in familial desmoid tumor syndromes in which the polyposis component is not readily apparent or is even absent.[13,48]

Fibrosarcoma. Adult fibrosarcoma is uncommon (approximately 1% of adult sarcomas). It is a malignant or intermediate (rarely metastasizing) tumor, composed of fibroblasts with variable collagen production. In classical cases, fibrosarcoma has a herringbone pattern on light microscopy. Fibrosarcomas usually involve the deep tissues of the extremities, trunk, head, and neck of middle-aged and older adults. Some may arise in the field of previous radiotherapy. Rarely fibrosarcomas can be seen in the ovary and other unusual sites such as the trachea.

Solitary Fibrous Tumor/Hemangiopericytoma. Solitary fibrous tumor/hemangiopericytoma (SFT/HPC) is a ubiquitous mesenchymal tumor of probable fibroblastic type, which shows a prominent hemangiopericytomalike branching vascular pattern. SFT and HPC share histological features and have nearly identical gene expression profiles, so they are now grouped together. SFT/HPC may be found at any location in middle-aged adults (20 to 70 years of age; median 50). Occasional cases may occur in children and adolescents. The adult form is most common in the thorax, pelvis, retroperitoneum, orbit, and lower extremity. The tumors appear as slow growing, well-circumscribed, painless masses and histologically consist of tightly packed cells around thin-walled vascular channels of varying caliber. The cells of SFT/HPC characteristically stain for CD34 but not for factor VIII–related antigen. Many SFT/HPCs are indolent, although some behave like other high-grade sarcomas. Rarely patients present with very large SFT/HPC and hypoglycemia (Doege-Potter syndrome), which is caused by production of a form of insulinlike growth factor 2 (IGF-2) by these tumors.[49–52] SFT/HPCs are highly resistant to standard doxorubicin-based chemotherapy, but sunitinib was recently shown to have activity, possibly through a platelet-derived growth factor receptor beta (PDGFRB)-mediated mechanism.[53]

Inflammatory Myofibroblastic Tumor. The inflammatory myofibroblastic tumor (IMT) or inflammatory pseudotumor is composed of myofibroblastic spindle cells accompanied by an inflammatory infiltrate of plasma cells, lymphocytes, and eosinophils. IMT usually occurs in children or young adults, and it can occur throughout the body, most commonly in the lung, mesentery, and omentum. The site of origin determines the symptoms, with pulmonary IMT presenting with chest pain and shortness of breath, while abdominal IMT may cause intestinal obstruction. About 33% of patients have a syndrome of fever, growth failure, malaise, weight loss, anemia, and thrombocytosis. When the mass is excised the syndrome disappears, and reappearance of the syndrome is typically associated with tumor recurrence. IMT has variable and nonspecific imaging characteristics, with most appearing as a lobulated solid mass that may appear inhomogeneous.[54,55] In the abdomen and retroperitoneum, IMT can often appear much more diffuse and infiltrative, making initial diagnosis difficult if not impossible. Complete nonmutilating surgical resection is the treatment of choice for these locally aggressive lesions. Following complete excision the local recurrence rate is about 23%, with only a small (less than 5%) risk of distant metastasis and a 5-year survival of about 87%.[56] In the absence of complete surgical resection, symptomatic treatment is appropriate, reserving more aggressive chemotherapy and radiation therapy for progression of disease or symptomatic change.

IMT in children and young adults often contains clonal cytogenetic rearrangements that activate the *ALK* receptor tyrosine kinase gene on chromosome 2[57,58] or less commonly contains rearrangements affecting the *HMGA2* gene on chromosome 12.[59] In tumors with rearrangements affecting *ALK*, the constitutive activation and overexpression of *ALK* appears to be restricted to the myofibroblastic component.[60–62] The inflammatory component is normal cytogenetically and does not express detectable ALK protein. In contrast, *ALK* rearrangements are uncommon in IMTs diagnosed in adults over 40 years in age. *ALK* activation has also been found in subsets of patients with large cell anaplastic lymphoma. ALK-positive IMTs may therefore be a good target for ALK inhibitors.[63–65]

Myxofibrosarcoma. Myxofibrosarcoma, also known as a myxoid variant of malignant fibrous histiocytoma, comprises a spectrum of malignant fibroblastic lesions with variably myxoid stroma (at least 10%), pleomorphism, and a distinctive curvilinear vascular pattern. Pathologists now regard myxofibrosarcoma as a reproducibly distinct tumor type with clearly defined diagnostic criteria.[39,44,66] Myxofibrosarcoma is one of the most common sarcomas, usually arising in the limbs of elderly adults (typically in the sixth to eight decades) as a slowly enlarging, painless mass. Local recurrence is common, occurring in up to 50% of cases, and is independent of histologic grade and depth.[67–70] In contrast, metastasis and tumor-associated mortality are much higher in deep-seated and high-grade lesions; metastasis develops in about 35% of high-grade cases. Proliferative activity, the percentage of aneuploid cells, and tumor vascularity are associated with histologic grade, but have no clear relation to clinical outcome.[68,71] Low-grade myxofibrosarcoma may progress to high grade in subsequent local recurrences and thus acquire a higher probability for metastatic spread. The most common sites of metastases are lung, bone, and lymph nodes. The overall 5-year survival is 60% to 70%.[67–70] The 5-year disease-specific survival was 80% for patients presenting to Memorial Sloan-Kettering Cancer Center (MSKCC) with primary myxofibrosarcoma of the extremity and trunk.

So-Called Fibrohistiocytic Tumors

The concept of fibrohistiocytic differentiation has been challenged and is now regarded as a poorly defined morphological descriptor of histiocytic differentiation. The so-called fibrohistiocytic tumors, originally thought to arise from histiocytes that had fibroblastic potential, are almost certainly fibroblastic in origin. Thus, the term *fibrohistiocytic* is merely descriptive of their appearance; virtually none of these lesions show true histiocytic differentiation.[72]

Giant Cell Tumor of Tendon Sheath/Pigmented Villonodular Synovitis. Giant cell tumor of tendon sheath encompasses a variety of benign tumors and tumorlike lesions that most often arise from the synovium of joints. They are usually classified into subtypes by site (intra-articular or extra-articular) and growth pattern (localized or diffuse); growth pattern is predictive of their biological behavior.[73] Nodular tenosynovitis (also termed tenosynovial giant cell tumor or pigmented villonodular synovitis, TGCT/PVNS) is a giant cell tumor that may occur at any age but is most commonly seen between the ages of 30 and 50 years. These tumors are somewhat more common in women. They occur with greatest frequency in the hand but are also seen in the ankles and knees, among other sites. These slow-growing tumors develop as circumscribed lobulated masses and are usually diagnosed when they are smaller than 5 cm in diameter. Because of their location, excision is often done with close margins, and local recurrence is seen in 10% to 20% of patients. A diffuse form occurs in and around joints, most commonly around the knee or ankle. In contrast to most giant cell tumors, this neoplasm grows in expansive sheets without a mature capsule. Treatment is surgical, including arthroscopic resection alone when intra-articular disease has not invaded beyond the joint. A t(1;2) translocation is characteristic of the apparent neoplastic cells of TGCT/PVNS, altering the colony stimulating factor 1 gene (*CSF1*) to encode a form that apparently causes an autocrine loop and causes the characteristic inflammatory infiltrate of this tumor.[74,75] Imatinib, an inhibitor of CSF1 receptor, is active against TGCT/PVNS.[76] Multiple recurrent lesions that threaten limb integrity can be controlled with radiotherapy in both the tendon sheath and intra-articular variants.[77] However, radiotherapy should be reserved for advanced local presentation of diffuse bone disease, neurovascular disease, or extensive soft tissue disease. Malignant giant cell tumors of the tendon sheath are also recognized and should be managed with the same approaches as soft tissue sarcoma elsewhere.

Fibrous Histiocytoma. Fibrous histiocytomas are benign tumors that usually present as solitary, slow-growing nodules, although up to one-third are multiple. Histologically, they consist of fibroblastic and histiocytic cells often arranged in a cartwheel or storiform pattern. When such lesions occur in the skin, they are often called *dermatofibromas* or *sclerosing hemangiomas*. Superficial lesions usually are cured by simple excision. Deeper lesions should be resected with a wider margin of normal tissue to prevent local recurrence.

Xanthoma. *Xanthoma* refers to a collection of lipid-laden histiocytes and is seen in diseases associated with hyperlipidemia. These lesions are generally cutaneous or subcutaneous but may involve deep soft tissues. Presumably, xanthomas are reactive lesions.

Dermatofibrosarcoma Protuberans. Dermatofibrosarcoma protuberans is probably best considered a low-grade sarcoma because it may recur locally but rarely metastasizes. It is a relatively monomorphous, mononuclear, spindle cell lesion involving both dermis and subcutis. This lesion may occur anywhere in the body, but more than 50% occur on the trunk, 20% on the head and neck, and 30% on the extremities. This lesion typically presents in early or midadult life, beginning as a nodular cutaneous mass. Growth is usually slow and persistent, and as the lesion enlarges over many years, it becomes protuberant. Large lesions often are associated with satellite nodules. Dermatofibrosarcoma protuberans is histologically similar to benign fibrous histiocytoma but grows in a more infiltrative pattern, spreading along connective tissue septa and often having unpredictable radial extensions of tumor permeating through the subcutaneous tissue large distances from the primary nodule. The central portion of the tumor consists of uniform plump fibroblasts arranged in a distinct ordered pattern. Unlike fibrous histiocytoma, dermatofibrosarcoma protuberans stains positive for CD34. More than 75% of these tumors carry ring or giant chromosomes, composed of translocated portions of chromosomes 17 and 22, and a consistent gene fusion product has been cloned. This fusion product creates an apparent platelet-derived growth factor autocrine loop, likely explaining the tumor's sensitivity to imatinib, which blocks platelet-derived growth factor receptor action; imatinib is now the U.S. Food and Drug Administration–approved first line of treatment for advanced disease.[78–82]

Up to 50% of these tumors recur after simple excision in some series. With aggressive resection and special attention to radial margins, the local recurrence rate is 5% or less.[83] Cases with positive or close surgical margins in anatomically complex sites (e.g., near the brachial plexus) have an elevated risk of local recurrence that is ameliorated with adjuvant radiotherapy.[84] Postoperative radiotherapy is also indicated in the rare event that a patient has unresectable macroscopic disease. These principles especially apply to recurrent tumors. Occasionally, areas of increased pleomorphism and mitotic activity occur, especially in recurrent lesions. Metastases occur rarely to lung or to lymph nodes and typically only when fibrosarcomatous change is detected in the primary or recurrent lesion.[83,85] Because of their locally aggressive nature, these lesions may invade extensively and ultimately lead to amputation or even death. A variant with melanin pigmentation (Bednar tumor) also is recognized.

High-Grade Undifferentiated Pleomorphic Sarcoma/Pleomorphic Malignant Fibrous Histiocytoma. The term *malignant fibrous histiocytoma* (MFH) was first introduced in 1963 to describe a group of malignant soft tissue tumors with a fibrohistiocytic appearance. This entity has become the most commonly diagnosed extremity sarcoma in some series, but it is falling out of favor in the pathology community as (1) these tumors have no characteristics of histiocytes *per se,* (2) a significant number have features that can be attributed to other histologies such as leiomyosarcoma or dedifferentiated liposarcoma, and (3) a distinct subtype, termed myxofibrosarcoma, has emerged (see "Myxofibrosarcoma," above). Thus, the term pleomorphic MFH (PMFH) is now reserved for a group of undifferentiated pleomorphic sarcomas that by current technology show no definable line of differentiation.[44,66,72] PMFH characteristically is a tumor of later adult life with peak incidence in the seventh decade. PMFH usually presents as a painless, deep-seated mass; the most common site is the lower extremity, followed by the upper extremity. A subset of PMFHs arise at the site of prior radiotherapy[22] and very rare cases arise at the site of chronic ulceration. About 5% of patients present with metastasis, typically to lung. Clinical and pathologic studies have shown a remarkable degree of heterogeneity of morphologic and biologic features, prognosis, and treatment response. PMFH typically has an aggressive clinical course, with many patients developing metastatic disease within 3 years of diagnosis. The 5-year disease-specific survival was 65% for patients presenting to MSKCC with primary PMFH of the extremity and trunk.

Adipocytic Tumors

Lipoma. Lipomas are the most common benign soft tissue neoplasm and they usually arise in the subcutaneous tissue. The most frequent sites are trunk and proximal limbs. Although deep-seated benign lipomas do occur in the mediastinum or retroperitoneum, seemingly mature fatty neoplasms in the retroperitoneum should be regarded with suspicion because most are well-differentiated liposarcoma. Most lipomas are soft, painless, slow-growing, and solitary; however, 2% to 3% of patients have multiple lesions that are occasionally seen in a familial pattern. *Lipomatosis* is a term applied to a poorly circumscribed overgrowth of mature adipose tissue that grows in an infiltrating pattern.

Solitary lipomas are well-circumscribed, lobulated lesions composed of fat cells but are demarcated from surrounding fat by a thin, fibrous capsule. Most subcutaneous, solitary lipomas show reproducible cytogenetic aberrations: translocations involving 12q13–15, rearrangements of 13q, or rearrangements involving 6p21–33.[86] In spindle cell lipoma, mature fat is replaced by collagen-forming spindle cells; this lesion typically arises in the posterior neck and shoulder in men between the ages of 45 and 65 years. Spindle cell lipomas show consistent chromosomal aberrations of 13q and 16q.[87] Pleomorphic lipoma is a closely related lesion. Local excision of lipoma and these variants is generally curative, with a local recurrence after simple excision in no more than 1% to 2% of cases.

Intramuscular lipomas differ from their more superficial counterparts by usually being poorly circumscribed and infiltrative. These typically present in midadult life as slow-growing, deep-seated masses most often located in the thigh or trunk. Approximately 10% of intramuscular lipomas are noninfiltrative and well circumscribed. In a patient with a deep-seated fatty tumor, it is important to exclude atypical lipomatous tumor (see "Liposarcoma"), which tends to be more common than intramuscular lipoma.

Angiolipomas present as subcutaneous nodules, usually in young adults, and in more than 50% of cases are multiple. The most common site is the upper extremity. Angiolipomas rarely reach more than 2 cm in size, but they often are painful, especially during their initial growth period. Microscopically, these tumors consist of adipocytes with interspersed vascular structures. Myxoid and fibroblastic angiolipomas are recognized.

Hibernoma. Hibernoma is a rare, slow-growing, benign neoplasm that resembles the glandular brown fat found in hibernating animals. The literature consists primarily of case reports, and in most of these the tumor arises within the thorax. Lesions of the trunk, retroperitoneum, and extremities are also reported. Excision is generally curative.

presentation is Stewart-Treves syndrome—lymphangiosarcoma in the chronically lymphedematous arms of women who have been treated for breast cancer with radical mastectomy and, often, axillary irradiation.[25] In addition, angiosarcomas are known to occur in sites of prior irradiation without chronic lymphedema—in particular, in the pelvis of women who have received radiation therapy for gynecologic cancers.

The features that have correlated with poor outcome include older age, retroperitoneal location, large size, and high Ki-67 value.[120] Multicentric angiosarcomas on the scalp and face of elderly men typically show unrelenting progression, which can cause severe ulceration and infection and eventually metastasis. Angiosarcoma of the breast is usually an aggressive lesion that recurs locally and may metastasize, primarily to lung; histologic grade has been of prognostic value. Angiosarcomas are relatively sensitive, at least for brief periods of time, to anthracycline-based chemotherapy and taxanes.[122,123]

Considerable concern has been expressed about the possibility of increased incidence of angiosarcoma because of the widespread use of adjuvant radiation and chemotherapy for breast carcinoma or, increasingly, for ductal carcinoma *in situ,* in which there is a greater than 97% cure rate with surgery alone. A particular concern is that patients are now receiving adjuvant therapy for early-stage breast cancer to improve survival by one or two percentage points, meaning that 49 of every 50 patients suffer the consequences of treatment without any benefit. One of the consequences of treatment can be development of angiosarcoma; among breast cancer patients, radiotherapy is associated with a 50-times greater likelihood of subsequent angiosarcoma. A recent study based on the Surveillance, Epidemiology, and End Results (SEER) database found an absolute risk of secondary angiosarcoma of 7 per 100,000 person-years for patients who had surgery and radiotherapy for breast cancer.[124] This should be cause for consideration of the risk-to-benefit ratio of any therapy.[125]

Perivascular Tumors

Glomus Tumor. Glomus tumors are rare mesenchymal tumors composed of cells that closely resemble smooth muscle cells of the normal glomus body, which is a modified arteriovenous anastomosis in the skin involved in thermal regulation. Although benign, glomus tumors can cause considerable pain. They are most commonly found in the distal extremities (subungual region, hand, wrist, and foot) of young adults. Extradigital tumors can occur in multiple sites.[73] Cutaneous glomus tumors are typically small red-blue nodules that are often associated with a long history of pain, particularly when exposed to cold or minor tactile stimulation. The pain usually radiates away from the site of the tumor. Local and complete excision is the appropriate treatment. Multiple lesions may be seen in about 10% of patients. Malignant glomus tumors are exceedingly rare, occurring in less than 1% of patients.[126]

Neural Tumors

Neurofibroma. Solitary neurofibromas are small, slow-growing cutaneous or subcutaneous nodules that usually arise during the third decade of life. Neurofibromas may occur in unidentifiable cutaneous nerves or in larger trunks. Within an identifiable larger nerve, they expand into a fusiform mass and often extend into soft tissue; they are well defined and they may be nodular. Histologically, they show spindle-shaped cells in a myxoid stroma that contains collagen fibers. Multiple neurofibromas may be associated with neurofibromatosis type 1 (NF1, von Recklinghausen disease), a common genetic disorder caused by an autosomal dominant mutation at the 17q11.2 locus and affecting 1 in 3,000 live births. Clinical features of NF1 include café au lait spots, pigmented hamartomas of the iris, and neurofibromas of several types. Cutaneous neurofibromas arise in the skin in all patients with NF1, with sizes varying from millimeters to centimeters, and some may be painful. Plexiform neurofibromas are larger lesions that affect the large segments of a nerve, thickening and distorting the nerve with greater dysesthetic pain. The difficult distinction is neurofibroma versus MPNST, which may develop in patients with NF1. MPNST is usually distinguished based on rapid growth and increasing symptoms and is confirmed by biopsy.

Benign Schwannoma. Benign schwannoma, also called neurilemmoma, occurs most commonly in people between the age of 20 and 50 years. Common sites include the head and neck, the flexor surfaces of the extremities, and the paravertebral area of the retroperitoneum. The lesion grows slowly, and if superficial is usually small at the time of diagnosis, but it can reach large size in the retroperitoneum without symptoms. The tumor is usually encapsulated and consists of two components: an ordered cellular region (Antoni A area) and a loose, myxoid component (Antoni B area). Fortunately, diagnosis can often be made by percutaneous core or needle biopsy in patients with lesions in the retroperitoneum, where morbidity of operation is to be avoided. The cellular variant is the lesion most often seen late in life as a painless vertebral mass.[127] Complete resection is curative in most patients.

Granular Cell Tumor. Granular cell tumor is a rare tumor, probably of neural origin. It typically presents in adults as a small, poorly circumscribed subcutaneous mass, commonly seen in the oral cavity, and it is only rarely malignant. Granular cell tumors have been seen in all parts of the body, including the pancreas and bile duct. They can occur in multiple sites. Metastases have been reported in approximately 2% of cases, although most reports are single cases.

Malignant Peripheral Nerve Sheath Tumors. MPNSTs are highly aggressive soft tissue sarcomas that rarely occur sporadically in the general population. They may, however, occur with a lifetime incidence of 8% to 13% in patients with neurofibromatosis type 1 (NF1), an autosomal dominant tumor predisposition syndrome caused by germline mutations in the *NF1* gene.[14] Most MPNSTs are associated with major nerves of the body wall and extremities and typically affect adults in the third to fifth decades of life. The lower extremity and the retroperitoneum are the most common sites, but MPNSTs can arise anywhere in the body. These tumors originate from the nerve sheath rather than from the nerve itself. There is also an MPNST with rhabdomyosarcomatous elements, termed a triton tumor, suggesting that the Schwann cell may be the source of a variety of heterologous elements in nerve sheath tumors.[128]

Tumor cells are usually elongated, with frequent mitoses, and are arranged in a hypocellular myxoid stroma; pronounced atypia and epithelioid features are also characteristic. The majority of MPNSTs are high grade and characteristically stain for the S-100 protein. Weak S-100 staining in an MPNST is associated with undifferentiated tumors and a fivefold higher risk of distant metastasis.[129] Tumor size and p53 expression remain the most important independent predictors of disease-specific survival.[129,130] Two recent studies have suggested that patients with NF1-associated MPNST have a worse outcome compared to patients with sporadic MPNST,[131,132] and in one study this outcome difference was independent of tumor size.[132]

Complete surgical resection with or without adjuvant radiotherapy remains the most important treatment for those patients with primary disease. The role of neoadjuvant chemotherapy for patients with large primary and locally recurrent MPNSTs remains controversial. The response rate of MPNSTs to standard chemotherapy based on adriamycin and ifosfamide is currently unknown but is undergoing evaluation in a multi-institutional clinical trial. With an increasing understanding of there is a better imaging modality to evaluate metastases of less than 1 cm. Newer techniques, such as FDG-PET, are being used to evaluate distant metastases and, when combined with CT and conventional imaging, may improve the diagnostic accuracy of preoperative staging. However, overstaging remains a problem in 12% of patients, and PET-CT remains limited in evaluating pulmonary metastases of less than 1 cm.[209] FDG-PET lacks specificity in its ability to distinguish between low-grade malignancies and benign entities. An additional concern is that many low-grade sarcoma types and several high-grade types, like round cell liposarcoma, do not reliably show uptake for FDG, further limiting its routine use for staging sarcoma patients.

Biopsy

A biopsy is necessary and appropriate to establish malignancy, to evaluate histologic grade, and to determine histologic type (if possible). Precise knowledge of these features enables the treating physician to tailor the treatment plan to the tumor's predicted pattern of local growth, risk of metastasis, and likely sites of distant spread. Either an incisional biopsy or several Tru-Cut core biopsies are required to obtain enough tissue for definitive diagnosis and accurate grading. The biopsy incision or core track should be placed in a location that can be completely excised at the time of definitive resection with minimal sacrifice of overlying skin. Excisional biopsy should be avoided particularly for lesions greater than 3 cm in size, since such an approach may require a definitive resection to be more extensive due to contamination of surrounding tissue planes.

In general, the important issue with biopsy is the adequacy of the sample. Sufficient viable tissue is required that is both representative of the lesion and available for histopathologic evaluation, immunohistochemistry, and, when necessary, cytogenetics and electron microscopy. As molecular markers become a factor in diagnosis, meticulous attention to the adequacy of biopsy, tissue preservation, and evaluation will be paramount.

Value of Tru-Cut Biopsy

Several studies have examined the value of Tru-Cut biopsy.[210] Its accuracy is lower than for incisional biopsy, though substantially higher than for frozen section, and Tru-Cut biopsy has the advantage that it can be done in an office setting.

Fine-Needle Aspiration Cytology

Fine-needle aspiration (FNA) cytology has been examined by a number of authors but is usually used only for the confirmation of recurrence rather than for the primary diagnosis. Particular problems with FNA are the limited sampling and lack of tissue architecture, which degrade diagnostic accuracy. In addition, the amount of tissue collected usually does not allow for ancillary molecular diagnostic techniques.

Some authors have argued that biopsy itself is not justified if FNA is available. Rydholm[211] suggested that open biopsy is never indicated, with the argument being that open biopsy risks local tumor spread and increases both the magnitude of the subsequent operation and the need for adjuvant radiation therapy. Using FNA, the surgeon proceeds directly to open operation. However, this requires referral before antecedent biopsy, a relatively uncontrollable event in the United States. Other authors suggest that this approach results in the referral of ten patients with benign lesions for every sarcoma patient, certainly an untenable situation under our care system.

The no-biopsy approach presupposes that all that is required is a malignant sarcoma diagnosis and that the type or grade of sarcoma does not determine therapy. The use of FNA in patients with large sarcomas who are candidates for neoadjuvant therapy to improve survival is also problematic due to difficulty in grading and subtyping these tumors accurately from such small samples. However, proponents argue that immunohistochemistry, electron microscopy, DNA cytology, and chromosomal analysis, all of which can be performed on FNA specimens, will ensure the appropriateness of this approach. However, the authors still favor obtaining adequate tissue from several Tru-Cut cores or an incisional biopsy to determine a definitive histologic diagnosis and grade before initiating treatment.

Frozen Section

In some institutions, frozen section is relied on as the diagnostic tool of choice. For diagnosis of malignancy, frozen section is accurate, but for histopathologic subtypes and grade, it is inferior to permanent sections of either Tru-Cut or incisional biopsy.[210]

Sarcoma Staging

The intent of staging systems is to group patients according to their probability of metastasis, disease-specific survival, or overall survival. The major staging used for soft tissue sarcoma is the system developed by the American Joint Committee on Cancer (AJCC). This system, first developed in 1992, has undergone significant changes, based on both histological and clinical information. For example, for the 2002 staging system, changes were made to account for the relative infrequency of high-grade, large, superficial sarcomas[212] and to simplify the category of stage III tumors to represent only large, deep, high-grade sarcomas (Table 115.2).

The current 2010 AJCC TNM (tumor, node, metastasis) system (Table 115.2) incorporates histologic type, histologic grade, tumor size, depth, regional lymph node involvement, and distant metastasis. It accommodates two-, three-, and four-tiered grading systems. It incorporates four major changes compared with the 2002 system. First, it excludes four histologic types: gastrointestinal stromal tumor (GIST), desmoid tumor, Kaposi sarcoma, and infantile fibrosarcoma. Second, it adds the following histologic types: angiosarcoma, extraskeletal Ewing sarcoma, and dermatofibrosarcoma protuberans. Third, it reclassifies N1 disease from stage IV to stage III. Fourth, grading has changed from a four-grade to a three-grade system.[213]

TABLE 115.2

AMERICAN JOINT COMMITTEE ON CANCER STAGING SYSTEM (2010) AND DISEASE-SPECIFIC SURVIVAL BY STAGE

Stage	Grade	Tumor	Nodes	Metastasis
IA	GX–G1	T1a–1b	N0	M0
IB	GX–G1	T2a–2b	N0	M0
IIA	G2–G3	T1a–1b	N0	M0
IIB	G2	T2a–2b	N0	M0
III	G3	T2a–2b	N0	M0
	G any	T any	N1	M0
IV	G any	T any	N any	M1

Adapted from ref. 213.

PRACTICE OF ONCOLOGY

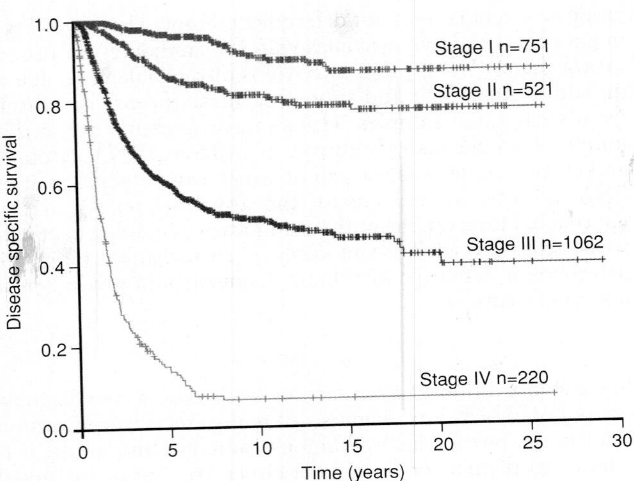

FIGURE 115.4 Disease-specific survival for patients with extremity soft tissue sarcoma according to the 2010 American Joint Committee on Cancer (AJCC) staging system. The data are for 2,554 patients seen at Memorial Sloan-Kettering Cancer Center (MSKCC) from 1982 through 2009.

Analysis of the primary extremity soft tissue sarcomas seen at MSKCC during 1982 to 2009 suggests that the probability of metastasis and disease-specific survival by stage is nicely discriminated in the new AJCC 2010 staging system. Figure 115.4 and Table 115.2 show the excellent discrimination by stage for disease-specific survival and overall survival for patients with extremity disease. Unfortunately, this system still fails to adequately account for sarcomas located in the retroperitoneum. There is as yet no adequate staging system for retroperitoneal or intra-abdominal lesions.

Nomograms

The accuracy of predicting patient outcomes can be increased by integrating multiple clinical and histologic features in a predictive model such as a nomogram. To predict sarcoma-specific survival, MSKCC researchers developed nomograms that integrate information on tumor size, grade (low vs. high), and depth with site, histopathology, and patient age. Nomograms are available for both primary lesions[214] and locally recurrent[215] lesions. These nomograms can be readily transferred to handheld personal organizers for instant calculation of disease-specific survival probability. Because no current grading system performs well for every histologic type of sarcoma, the authors' groups have recently developed histology-specific nomograms in liposarcoma,[40] synovial sarcoma,[216] and GIST.[217] As new molecular and genetic biomarkers are discovered and shown to have prognostic value, they can be incorporated into nomograms along with conventional clinical-pathologic variables to improve assessment of sarcoma prognosis for the individual patient. This would enable the treating physician to design a treatment strategy tailored to an individual patient's risk of relapse and potential for an aggressive clinical course.

Histologic and Prognostic Factors for Primary Extremity and Truncal Sarcoma

Histopathology is related to anatomic site (Fig. 115.2), and the common histologic types in the extremity and truncal location are liposarcoma, PMFH, myxofibrosarcoma, and synovial sarcoma. An analysis of prospective data collected from 1,041 patients older than 16 years with localized soft tissue sarcoma of the extremity[188] determined the clinical and pathologic factors that influence outcome. The 5-year survival rate was 76%, with a median follow-up of 4 years. Factors that increased risk of local recurrence were age, recurrent presentation, positive margin, and fibrosarcoma, MPNST, or leiomyosarcoma histology. Factors that increased the risk of disease-specific death were recurrent presentation, size greater than 5 cm, tumor depth and grade, positive margin, and MPNST or leiomyosarcoma histology.

Factors that increased distant recurrence rates were large tumor size, high histologic grade, deep location, recurrent disease at presentation, and histologic subtype of leiomyosarcoma. Liposarcoma was associated with decreased distant recurrence compared with other histologic types. Disease-specific mortality had the same predictors as did distant recurrence, with the additional adverse factors of histologic type of malignant peripheral nerve tumor and positive histologic margins at resection of the primary. High-grade lesions have a much greater risk of developing a distant metastasis in the first 30 months. Even low-grade lesions, however, have a slow but inexorable increase in risk of metastasis over the long term. Prognostic factors clearly vary with time. Grade is a dominant factor in early metastasis, but in late recurrence initial size becomes equally important.[218] Postmetastasis survival for most patients is independent of factors involved in the primary presentation, although an association has been found with tumor size.

Bone invasion and neurovascular invasion have historically been considered bad prognostic features. Because bone invasion is relatively uncommon in soft tissue sarcoma, it has not been uniformly included in any staging system, but it should be considered as a poor prognostic factor.

Five-year survival does not guarantee cure. An analysis of patients disease-free 5 years after the diagnosis and treatment of extremity lesions showed that 9% would go on to have a recurrence in the next 5 years.[219] Unfortunately, survival has not measurably improved with time when corrected for stage.[220] A review of 1,261 completely resected extremity lesions by 5-year increments for 1982 to 2001 suggested that disease-specific actuarial 5-year survival remained unchanged (approximately 79%) over 20 years. For high-risk patients (those with high-grade, deep tumors of greater than 10 cm), disease-specific survival remains at around 50%.

Site of disease is also a clear determinant of outcome and an important prognostic factor. Patients with extremity and superficial trunk lesions certainly do better than patients with retroperitoneal and visceral sarcomas (Fig. 115.5). Death from local recurrence is uncommon in those with extremity lesions but occurs frequently in patients with retroperitoneal liposarcoma.

Innumerable molecular markers have been defined for soft tissue sarcoma—some with prognostic implications—but they have not been included in staging systems; however, the authors expect them to become increasingly important variables.

Diagnostic and Prognostic Factors for Primary Retroperitoneal/Intra-abdominal Sarcoma

Most patients with retroperitoneal or intra-abdominal sarcoma present with an asymptomatic abdominal mass. On occasion pain is present, and less common symptoms include gastrointestinal bleeding, incomplete obstruction, and neurologic symptoms related to retroperitoneal invasion or pressure on neurovascular structures. In one report, only 27% of patients with retroperitoneal sarcoma had neurologic symptoms, which

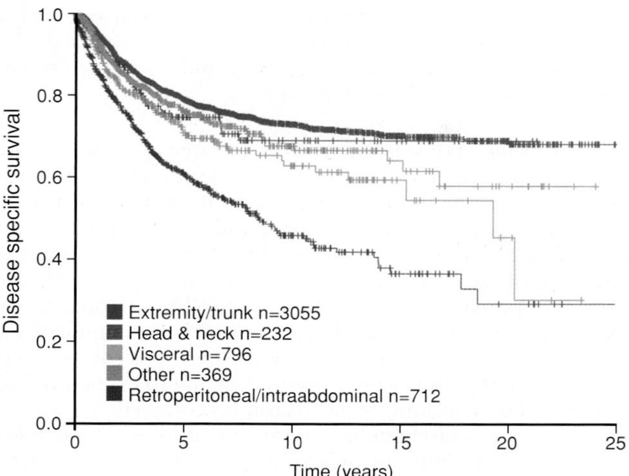

FIGURE 115.5 Disease-specific survival by site of soft tissue sarcoma in 7,049 patients aged 16 years or older admitted to Memorial Sloan-Kettering Cancer Center from 1982 through 2009. Patients with retroperitoneal or visceral sarcomas did worse than patients with extremity lesions.

primarily were related to an expanding retroperitoneal mass.[221] Weight loss is uncommon, and incidental diagnosis is the norm. The diagnosis is usually suspected on finding a soft tissue mass on abdominal CT or MRI. Often the diagnosis is clear without biopsy, and many proceed directly to operative resection in the absence of a clinical trial. FNA biopsy or CT-guided core biopsy has a limited role in the routine diagnostic evaluation of these patients. CT-guided core biopsy is indicated if abdominal lymphoma, germ cell tumor, or carcinoma is strongly suspected as part of the differential diagnosis. Preoperative biopsy is also indicated for patients who present with distant metastasis or advanced local disease that on abdominal or pelvic imaging appears to be difficult to completely remove surgically without substantial morbidity. In most patients, exploratory laparotomy should be performed and the diagnosis made at operation, unless (1) the patient's tumor is clearly unresectable, (2) neoadjuvant chemotherapy or radiotherapy is needed in an attempt to make the tumor more resectable, or (3) the patient will be undergoing preoperative investigational treatment.

CT remains the primary modality for evaluation of retroperitoneal and visceral sarcomas. Because the most likely site of visceral metastasis is the liver followed by lung, a CT scan of the chest, abdomen, and pelvis encompasses the primary lesion and the most likely sites of metastasis in a single examination.

Retroperitoneal or intra-abdominal sarcomas (excluding visceral sarcomas such as GIST) account for approximately 15% of all soft tissue sarcomas. The most common histopathologic types in the retroperitoneum are liposarcoma (47%), leiomyosarcoma (22%), MPNST (2%), and fibrosarcoma (1%). Among primary retroperitoneal liposarcomas (excluding pleomorphic liposarcoma and liposarcoma not otherwise specified), about 50% are low grade, with 46% and 3% classified as well differentiated and myxoid, respectively, and 50% are high grade with 49% and 2% classified as dedifferentiated and round cell liposarcoma, respectively.

An analysis of 278 patients with primary retroperitoneal sarcoma showed that grade and completeness of resection were the most important independent prognostic factors for disease-specific survival, with incompletely resected patients having survival similar to that of patients whose disease was unresectable from the outset. In this same study histology and grade were both significantly associated with local recurrence, with liposarcoma having a 2.6-fold greater risk of local recurrence compared to other histologic types. For patients with retroperitoneal or intra-abdominal sarcomas, similar to patients with extremity sarcomas, the histologic type is an important prognostic factor for disease-specific survival, with this outcome worse for MPNST and leiomyosarcoma patients than for liposarcoma patients ($P < .003$) (Fig. 115.6*A*). Liposarcoma subtype provides additional prognostic information for disease-specific survival (Fig. 115.6*B*). In a multivariate analysis, histologic subtype, completeness of resection, age, and contiguous organ resection were all independent predictors of disease-specific survival, with subtype and completeness of resection having a hazard ratio of 6.0 and 3.8, respectively.[43]

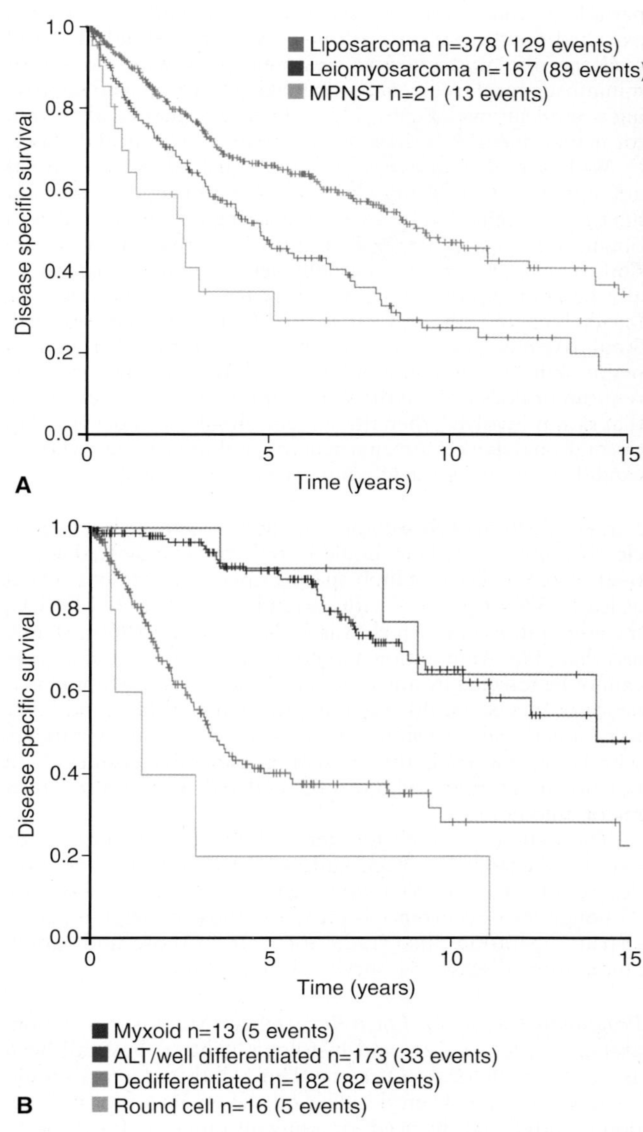

FIGURE 115.6 Disease-specific survival for patients with primary retroperitoneal/intra-abdominal sarcoma, according to histology. **A:** The most common histologic types of retroperitoneal/intra-abdominal sarcoma. Disease-specific survival was significantly longer for patients with liposarcoma than for those with malignant peripheral nerve sheath tumor (MPNST) ($P = .003$) and leiomyosarcoma ($P = .001$). **B:** Liposarcoma subtypes. Disease-specific survival at 5 years was 90% for patients with primary well-differentiated liposarcoma compared with 40% at 5 years for patients with primary dedifferentiated liposarcoma.

MANAGEMENT BY PRESENTATION STATUS, EXTENT OF DISEASE, AND ANATOMIC LOCATION

Management of Extremity and Truncal Sarcoma

Surgical Management of Primary Localized Disease

Although surgery remains the principal therapeutic modality in soft tissue sarcoma, the extent of surgery required, along with the optimum combination of radiotherapy and chemotherapy, remains controversial. The individual patient's clinical and pathologic characteristics—particularly the pattern of spread expected for the patient's histologic subtype—should be used to design the most effective treatment plan, with the aim of minimizing local recurrence, maximizing function, and improving overall survival. Figure 115.7 shows a suggested algorithm for management of patients with extremity or truncal disease.

Wide *en bloc* resection is used most often. Historical attempts to resect all muscle bundles from origin to exertion have been supplanted by an encompassing resection, aiming to obtain a 1- to 2-cm margin of uninvolved tissue in all directions. The limiting factor is usually neurovascular or, occasionally, bony juxtaposition. Because very few soft tissue sarcomas invade bone directly, only rarely does bone need to be resected. Similarly, few soft tissue sarcomas involve the skin, and so major skin resection should be limited. If a primary or recurrent tumor does involve the skin or if the tumor is so extensive that skin is involved, then the surgeon should consider free flap or rotational flap closure, particularly in those patients who are candidates for subsequent adjuvant radiation therapy.

Extent of Surgical Resection. The most extensive resection is clearly amputation. This should be only rarely indicated in soft tissue sarcoma because limb-sparing operations are possible in at least 95% of patients with extremity sarcoma. At MSKCC, the amputation rate, which was 50% in the late 1960s, is now less than 5%. Amputation should be reserved for tumors that cannot be resected by any other means, in patients without evidence of metastatic disease and with potential for good long-term functional rehabilitation. This usually includes patients with large, low-grade tumors with considerable cosmetic and functional deformity, who can be rendered symptom free by a major amputation.

The issue of amputation versus limb-sparing surgery for extremity lesions has been addressed by a prospective, randomized trial at the NCI with well over 10 years' follow-up. Although local recurrence is greater in those undergoing limb-sparing operation plus irradiation than in those undergoing amputation, disease-free survival is not different.[222]

Prognostic Factors for Local Recurrence. Margin of resection, grade, age, lesion size, and histologic subtype have all been associated with local recurrence. Thus, all these factors should be accounted for when deciding on the extent of local resection required and the need for adjuvant radiation for the individual patient. Because size is a prognostic factor for both local recurrence and metastatic disease, the surgical approach can be varied. In patients with small lesions (less than 5 cm), complete surgical excision with margins of more than 1 cm is usually sufficient without the need for any adjuvant therapy. However, neoadjuvant chemotherapy or investigational approaches should be considered for patients with high-grade lesions larger than 10 cm (given the high risk of recurrence and systemic disease) and for those with synovial sarcoma or myxoid/round cell liposarcoma larger than 5 cm (subtypes highly responsive to chemotherapy) (see "Chemotherapy for Primary Localized Extremity/Truncal Sarcoma").

Surgery Alone. For subcutaneous or intramuscular high-grade sarcoma smaller than 5 cm or for low-grade sarcoma of any size, surgery alone should be considered if adequate wide excision with a good 1-cm cuff of surrounding fat and muscle can be achieved. For certain low-grade histologic types, 1-cm margins are not required for excellent local control. For example, atypical lipomas and well-differentiated liposarcoma of the extremities require only complete excision with a minimal surrounding margin, as the majority of these patients will not have recurrence following a limited or microscopic positive margin excision as long as the excision is complete. Thus, radiation therapy is rarely indicated for this histologic type unless there is both a significant sclerosing component and a microscopic positive margin.[96] However, adjuvant radiation therapy should be added to the surgical resection to reduce the probability of local failure for most deep, greater than 5 cm, high-grade sarcomas if the excision margin is close, particularly with extramuscular involvement, or if a local recurrence would necessitate amputation or the sacrifice of a major neurovascular bundle.[223,224] Irrespective of grade, postoperative irradiation is probably used more than is strictly necessary. In fact, several studies have shown that a significant subset of subcutaneous and intramuscular sarcomas can be treated by wide excision alone, with a local recurrence rate of only 8% to 20%.[225–227]

Quality of Life and Functional Outcome. Quality of life is of great significance in patients with soft tissue sarcoma of the extremity who are being treated with conservative surgery to preserve function and potentially improve the overall quality of life. Davis et al.[228] reported a significantly higher level of handicap in amputated patients compared to those treated with conservative surgery. Robinson et al.[229] reported on 54 patients who were disease free for 2 or more years after limb-conserving treatment for soft tissue sarcoma of the leg or pelvic girdle. The extent of surgery was not an independent prognostic factor for limb function, although univariate analysis suggested an association with range of movement ($P < .025$).

Bell et al.[230] showed that neural sacrifice at the time of wide local excision was associated with poorer outcome on both univariate ($P = .002$) and multivariate ($P = .019$) analyses.

Quality-of-life assessment has gained importance in many randomized trials, which are evaluating this issue either as the primary end point or secondary to outcome.

Radiation Therapy for Primary Localized Extremity or Truncal Sarcoma

The goals of adjuvant radiotherapy in the management of soft tissue sarcoma are to enhance local control, preserve function, and achieve acceptable cosmesis by contributing to tissue preservation. Adjuvant radiotherapy is ordinarily used when the surgical margin is of limited size. The alternative, if local control is to be maintained, would be amputation or surgery that leaves structural, functional, or cosmetic deficits. Superficial lesions and smaller contained lesions confined to individual muscles may be managed with surgery alone in expert hands.[203,231] For most other situations, however, evidence strongly suggests that surgery that does not achieve wide clearance through normal tissue has a significantly higher rate of local failure, and even some small lesions may behave adversely.

That adjuvant radiotherapy enhances local control with conservative surgical resection in soft tissue sarcoma overall

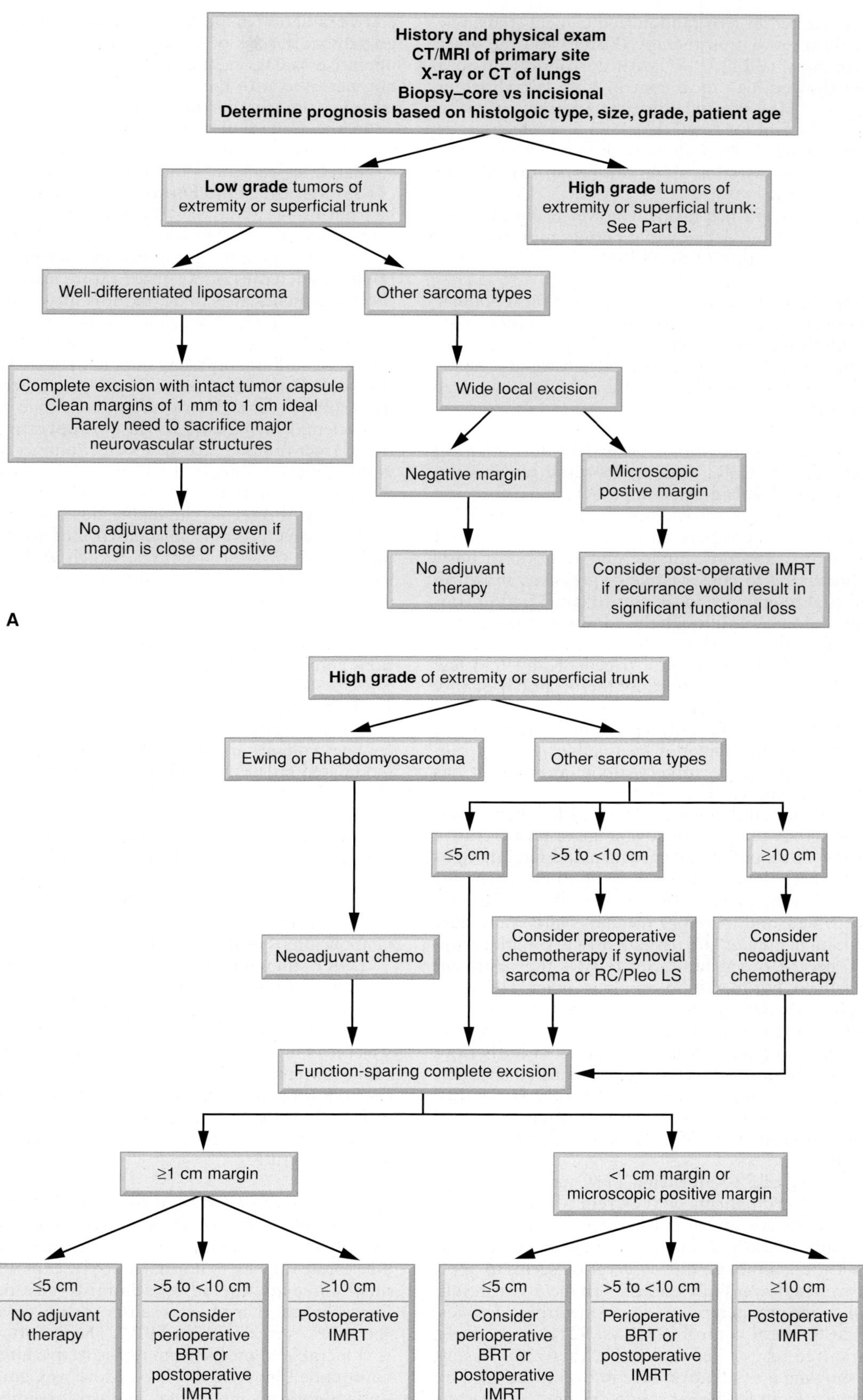

FIGURE 115.7 Management algorithm for extremity and superficial truncal soft tissue sarcoma. **A:** Low-grade sarcomas. **B:** High-grade sarcomas. Note that although postoperative intensity-modulated radiation therapy (IMRT) is mentioned in the algorithm, preoperative IMRT could be used in the same types of patients. BRT, brachytherapy; CT, computed tomography; MRI, magnetic resonance imaging; Rhabdo, rhabdomyosarcoma; RC, round cell; Pleo, pleomorphic; LS, liposarcoma.

has been demonstrated in two randomized clinical trials, one using external beam radiation therapy (EBRT) and the other using brachytherapy (BRT),[223,224] with corroboration in a third trial that showed high local control from two different EBRT strategies.[232] However, whether the addition of radiotherapy confers a benefit for small (less than 5 cm) high-grade lesions is controversial.[233] Radiotherapy should ordinarily not be used when surgical resection alone can be performed with appropriate confidence.

The contemporary era has brought newer techniques for radiotherapy planning and delivery that permit unprecedented accuracy in the use of both BRT and EBRT.

External-Beam Radiation Therapy. EBRT is the most popular adjuvant radiotherapy approach, perhaps because EBRT relies less than does BRT on special technical and operational requirements. Nevertheless, EBRT requires comprehensive and multidisciplinary pretreatment consultation and accurate pathologic and radiologic assessment.

Postoperative versus Preoperative External-Beam Radiation Therapy. Postoperative EBRT was the first and remains the most widely practiced local adjuvant approach, in part because it allows for sterilization of microscopic nests of residual disease without the need to postpone surgery. Its use is supported by numerous single-institution studies, and addition of postoperative radiotherapy to conservative surgery was shown in a randomized trial to enhance local control compared to conservative surgery alone.[224] Although the adjuvant radiotherapy resulted in significantly worse limb strength, edema, and range of motion, these deficits were often transient and had few measurable effects on activities of daily life or global quality of life.[224]

Preoperative EBRT is the only common local adjuvant radiotherapy strategy that has not been subjected to a randomized comparison against surgery alone, although it has been compared to postoperative radiotherapy.

Both preoperative and postoperative EBRT have their advantages and disadvantages. An advantage of postoperative EBRT is that the entire pathology specimen and final margins are available for pathologic analysis, helping to determine the need for further therapy. A major limitation is that the target is less precisely defined, and therefore volume is larger and dose is higher, resulting in greater late tissue morbidity. With preoperative EBRT, on the other hand, not only is the treatment volume well defined, but the blood supply is intact. The intact vascular supply and relative absence of actively proliferating tumor clonogens and radioresistant hypoxic cells may decrease the dose needed compared to postoperative radiotherapy. Confirmation of this principle, however, remains elusive. The major drawback of preoperative radiotherapy, as detailed below, is that irradiation increases the risk of acute wound complications upon surgery. Which approach is superior remains unclear.

In a trial assessing EBRT sequencing, the Canadian Sarcoma Group randomized 190 patients with extremity soft tissue sarcoma to preoperative or postoperative radiotherapy. Preoperative radiotherapy doubled the risk of early acute wound complication, although this observation seems to apply almost exclusively to lower limb lesions.[232] In the 5-year results from this trial,[234] the preoperative and postoperative arms were nearly identical for local control (93% vs. 92%, respectively) and metastatic-free relapse survival (67% vs. 69%). Despite early results showing a small advantage in overall survival for the preoperative arm, in the 5-year results the preoperative and postoperative arms did not differ significantly in overall survival (73% vs. 67%; $P = .5$) or cause-specific survival (78% vs. 73%; $P = .6$). Recently, a meta-analysis of pre- versus postoperative radiation in localized resectable soft tissue sarcoma suggested that the risk of local recurrence may be lower after preoperative radiation, and that the risk of metastatic spread is not increased with the delay in surgical resection necessary to complete preoperative radiotherapy.[235]

In the Canadian randomized trial, functional outcomes were collected prospectively.[236] The trial design specified two validated instruments—the Toronto Extremity Salvage Score (TESS) and the Short Form-36 Health Survey quality-of-life instrument—in addition to the observer-based Musculoskeletal Tumor Society (MSTS) Rating Scale.[236] At 6 weeks after surgery, the preoperative group had inferior function, with worse bodily pain scores on all three rating instruments. However, the assessments at 3 to 12 months after surgery showed no differences between the groups in these rating scores.[236] It can be concluded that, for most of the first posttreatment year, the timing of radiotherapy has minimal effect on the function of soft tissue sarcoma patients. The 2-year function and morbidity results[237] show deteriorating late tissue sequelae (fibrosis and edema) in patients in the postoperative arm, resulting from larger radiotherapy doses and volumes. Of note, patients with significant fibrosis or edema had significantly lower function scores on both the MSTS and TESS measures. In addition, patients who received the higher doses—most of them in the postoperative group—can be expected to eventually have a higher rate of bone fractures, which will mirror the earlier single-institution data from the same authors.[238] These disadvantages of postoperative EBRT may override the higher frequency of acute wound complications with preoperative EBRT, although patients who do experience wound complications continue to experience some impaired function.[239]

Intensity-Modulated Radiation Therapy. The past decade witnessed an unprecedented improvement in delivery of EBRT to complex volumes and shapes. Leading these advances is intensity-modulated radiation therapy (IMRT),[240] which uses computer algorithms for inverse planning and treatment delivery. IMRT may be particularly applicable to complex anatomic volumes such as retroperitoneal sarcoma juxtapositioned to liver or paraspinal lesions, for which conformal avoidance of liver or of kidney and spinal cord is necessary.[241] Avoidance of bone is also possible[242,243] and may reduce the risk of the radiation-induced fracture of weight-bearing bone (see "Serious Complications of Primary Treatment").

IMRT still requires evaluation in soft tissue sarcoma,[241] but the early information suggests that it can enhance normal tissue protection while maintaining oncologic control.[242–244] Notably, the 5-year local control rate for IMRT in one study[245] was very similar to those with conventional EBRT in both arms of the aforementioned Canadian trial that compared preoperative to postoperative radiotherapy.[234] However, any superiority of IMRT over conventional EBRT is likely going to relate to a reduction in late toxicity and especially serious problems such as bone fracture.[244]

Volume Issues in External-Beam Radiation Therapy. Given the generally favorable oncologic results after EBRT (local control rates approximating 90%), it is important to attempt to ameliorate toxicity to normal tissue by exploring reduced treatment intensity, including administered doses or volumes. Nevertheless, there have been no prospective assessments of the volumes irradiated in EBRT. The literature on this subject is vulnerable to problems of retrospective interpretation and is confounded by selection bias. Moreover, guidelines outlining optimal radiotherapy target volumes for either preoperative or postoperative EBRT may now be outdated, and more recent descriptions[246] may soon require modification, because advances in conformal techniques and IMRT make it feasible to consider volumes that are more accurately tailored to the needs of the individual patient.[242,243]

By conventionally accepted principles of treatment, targets are defined differently for preoperative versus postoperative radiotherapy. Preoperative radiotherapy can focus on the extent of definable disease (determined using imaging), and the target is based on the anatomic location, containment by barriers to spread (especially intact fascial planes), and allowance for geometric uncertainty related to potential variation in patient setup and physiologic movement. Special situations must also be considered, such as lesions arising in extracompartmental spaces such as the femoral triangle, antecubital space, and popliteal space, because these lesions have the ability to extend considerable distances proximally and distally with less anatomic restraint. Such lesions may spread to the neurovascular bundle early. The radiotherapy margins should reflect this and include undisturbed tissue planes and barriers to tumor incursion.

In general, coverage for microscopic disease, amounting to 4 cm longitudinally or 2 cm axially in the limb, is used to define a clinical target volume (CTV); this translates into field coverage approximately 5 cm long, allowing for beam penumbra and treatment uncertainties such as patient movement.

Postoperative radiotherapy volumes are significantly larger because they encompass all surgically manipulated tissues, with the recognition that this is impossible in some anatomic sites due to the proximity of critical anatomy. In addition, because surgery has disrupted the anatomic planes and they no longer provide containment barriers to tumor growth, the tumor must be considered high risk for at least the first phase (e.g., an appropriate dose is 50 Gy). Subsequently, the volume is reduced to the immediate area of origin of the tumor. Alternatively, with a single-phase IMRT approach, a higher dose could be delivered to the higher-risk smaller volume while simultaneously treating the more peripheral regions of the CTV to a more moderate dose. This approach is attractive due to the efficiency of creating only one treatment plan, and reports of this approach in patients with durable follow-up are awaited.

Currently, the volume of postoperative radiotherapy is being investigated in a randomized phase 3 trial conducted by the United Kingdom National Cancer Research Network. The trial compares a standard volume (5 cm longitudinal margin to gross tumor volume or 1 cm from the surgical scar, whichever is longer in the cranio–caudal direction and 2 cm axial margin) versus an experimental volume (2 cm longitudinal margin to gross tumor volume and 2 cm axial margin). Patients in both arms of the study will receive 66 Gy over 6.5 weeks; patients in the standard arm, but not the experimental arm, will have a volume reduction after 25 fractions (50 Gy). The goal is to assess if a reduced volume of postoperative radiotherapy will increase limb function without compromising local control.[247]

A final issue concerning choice of irradiation target volume concerns the definition of the areas that may harbor disease and especially whether the risk area should include the peripheral edema that may surround the tumor. A study from the Princess Margaret Hospital correlating MRI characteristics with pathologic features suggests that in some cases the edema does harbor sarcoma cells.[248]

Dose Issues in External-Beam Radiation Therapy. The dose of radiotherapy represents an additional unexplored area. The preoperative dose used in most institutions is approximately 50 Gy in daily fractions of 1.8 to 2.0 Gy over approximately 5 weeks. Generally a postoperative boost is administered only if the surgical margins are positive, and the benefit of this boost is unclear. For example, for patients who had positive surgical margins, Delaney et al.[249] reported that the factors associated with local control included total radiotherapy dose greater than 64 Gy (delivered as pre-, post-, or preoperative with a postoperative boost), with the implication that a boost is beneficial following preoperative radiotherapy. A different conclusion was drawn from a retrospective study at the Princess Margaret Hospital of patients with extremity soft tissue sarcoma and positive surgical margins. All patients had been treated with preoperative radiotherapy (50 Gy); 52 received no other radiotherapy and 41 received a postoperative boost (typically 16 Gy). A common reason for omission of boost was wound complications, which tend to occur in more extensive and adverse cases. Despite this, patients who received a postoperative boost had worse 5-year estimated local-recurrence–free survival (73.8% compared to 90.4% for preoperative radiotherapy only).[250] This is consistent with prior clinical experience, in which patients with extremity sarcoma who could not receive a postoperative boost due to wound healing complications or other contraindications did not seem to be at a higher risk of local recurrence. Consequently at the Princess Margaret Hospital a postoperative boost is not used for patients with microscopically positive resection margins.

Adjuvant Brachytherapy. BRT is an attractive approach because patients usually complete all their treatment in about 2 weeks compared to 6 to 7 weeks with EBRT. The technical aspects of BRT differ from those of EBRT, and specific guidelines for its use and technical delivery have been published. BRT, unlike EBRT, requires a specific collaboration between surgical and radiation oncologists. The rapid dose fall-off with BRT usually spares more normal tissue than EBRT, except when precision techniques such as IMRT are used. With BRT, unlike in postoperative irradiation, no attempts are made to treat large margins or to include the scar and the drainage site, although it is acknowledged that this approach has not been formally compared with EBRT in similar cases.

The efficacy of BRT was compared to that of IMRT among 134 patients with primary high-grade extremity sarcoma in recent data from MSKCC.[245] The BRT and IMRT groups were similar in terms of traditional prognostic factors, although the IMRT group had a significantly greater proportion of patients with positive or close margins, large tumors, and bone or nerve manipulation. The median follow-up was 34 months for the IMRT group and 47 months for the BRT group. The 5-year local control rate was 92% (95% CI, 84 to 99) for the IMRT group compared to 80% (95% CI, 70 to 89) for the BRT group ($P = .03$). On multivariate analysis, IMRT was the only predictor of improved local control ($P = .029$).[245] Earlier evidence from MSKCC suggests that BRT may not provide optimal results in regions unsuited for ideal implant geometry, such as in more proximal regions of the limb.[233]

In patients treated with BRT as the sole radiotherapy, the dose is usually 45 Gy given over 4 to 6 days, and when given as a boost, the dose is usually 15 to 20 Gy from BRT plus 45 to 50 Gy from EBRT. Of importance, the catheters are loaded no sooner than the sixth postoperative day to allow enough time for wound healing.[251] The most commonly used isotope is low–dose-rate ^{192}Ir; however, high-activity ^{125}I is occasionally used in young patients or to protect the gonads. High–dose-rate ^{192}Ir has been advocated to take advantage of its radiation safety and dose-optimization capabilities.

The brachytherapy CTV may be difficult to define, but in general it is represented by the volume of tissue considered at risk for microscopic extension of tumor and includes the tumor bed visualized on radiographic studies and under direct inspection intraoperatively. The results with adjuvant BRT suggest that radiation treatment directed to the tumor bed plus a 2-cm margin is adequate.[252] These guidelines follow those of the American Brachytherapy Society of at least 2- to

5-cm longitudinal margin beyond the CTV and at least 1 cm beyond the lateral edge of the CTV. These guidelines are based on agreement among experts, although there is no consensus on the exact size of the margin beyond the tumor bed. These volumes would seem to approximate for preoperative radiotherapy.

Adjuvant BRT has been evaluated in a randomized trial. Patients who underwent complete gross resection were randomly assigned to receive adjuvant BRT (n = 78) or no further therapy (n = 86). The 10-year actuarial local control rates were 81% in the BRT group and 67% in the no-BRT group (*P* = .03). This improvement in local control, however, was limited to patients with histologically high-grade tumors, whose local control was 89% in the BRT group and 64% in the no-BRT group (*P* = .001).[223] Even though adjuvant BRT did not improve local control in patients with low-grade tumors, the local recurrence rates of 27% (BRT) and 22% (no BRT) indicate the need for adjuvant external radiation in these patients.[253] Rigorous psychofunctional testing of 38 long-term survivors in this trial revealed no significant differences in functional outcome between the BRT group and the no-BRT group. The BRT group did, however, have higher levels of anxiety, depression, and appreciation of illness.[254]

BRT is often used in combination with EBRT, but whether all patients need this combination is unclear.[255] An MSKCC study evaluated 105 patients with primary or locally recurrent high-grade soft tissue sarcomas who were treated with wide local excision and radiotherapy: BRT (87 patients) or BRT and EBRT (18 patients). At a median follow-up of 22 months, the two groups had no statistically significant difference in 2-year actuarial local control rate: 82% in the BRT group and 90% in the BRT plus EBRT group (*P* = .32).[256] However, case selection was such that the two groups are not completely comparable. Notably, patients were selected for EBRT if they had a positive margin (56%) or if anatomic considerations led to concern about the adequacy of dose coverage with BRT.

Brachytherapy is particularly useful when a plan to use surgery alone results in resection margins being close. In this situation, if the surgical and pathologic findings are satisfactory, the unused brachytherapy catheters can be removed. Alternatively, brachytherapy allows early delivery of radiation to a reduced and select volume mapped precisely by the intraoperative findings. The American Brachytherapy Society has recommended that BRT should not be used as a sole treatment modality in several situations: (1) the CTV cannot be adequately encompassed in the implant geometry, (2) the proximity of critical anatomy is expected to prevent administration of a meaningful dose, (3) the resection margins are positive, and (4) the skin is involved with tumor. In such situations EBRT may be used alone or with BRT.

High-dose–rate (HDR) BRT has some potential advantages over low-dose–rate BRT, although the experience with HDR BRT for sarcoma is still limited. A typical HDR dose is approximately 36 Gy in ten fractions using a 6-hour interfraction interval, though some authors have used higher doses.[257] Guided by the more abundant breast cancer experience, a dose of 32 to 34 Gy in twice-daily fractions of 3.4 to 4.0 Gy over 4 to 5 days[258–260] seem useful and safe, though even here there have been reports of fat necrosis in later follow-up.[260] In sarcoma management, authors have observed wound healing complications with HDR BRT.[261,262] In addition, caution should probably be exercised when placing catheters in contact with neurovascular structures, and when such contact cannot be avoided the dose per fraction should probably be curtailed. As yet, no large series evaluating HDR BRT for sarcoma is available, and no studies have directly compared HDR to low-dose–rate BRT. Comparisons are difficult due to nonstandardization of target volumes, dose prescription points, and the delivered dose. However, low-dose–rate BRT may expose the staff caring for patients to radiation, whereas HDR BRT does not. In addition, the HDR approach offers the potential for outpatient delivery.

Intraoperative HDR, a rarely used approach, has been used for the treatment of retroperitoneal sarcoma (see "Retroperitoneal Sarcoma".)

Technical Enhancement of Radiotherapy Delivery. IMRT can now be administered very precisely using reference to the position of external surrogate markers or fiducials to permit the determination of tumor coordinates in all three planes. High-dose, single fraction treatments are often termed stereotactic radiosurgery (SRS), and high-dose, fractionated treatments are variously termed stereotactic radiotherapy or stereotactic body radiotherapy (SBRT). These approaches are used for very adverse presentations of sarcoma, such as primary spinal sarcoma. Levine et al.[263] used SRS to treat 14 patients with primary spine sarcoma. In seven patients the treatment was definitive, and all seven had excellent pain relief and were alive with a mean follow-up of 33 months, although two patients had recurrence of tumor and were retreated. Surgery and adjuvant SRS were used in the other seven patients, of whom five remain free from recurrence at a mean follow-up of 43.5 months. Notably, even though the SRS doses were in the mean range of 30 Gy in three fractions, none of these patients had spinal injury from SRS.

High-dose photon/proton radiotherapy achieved promising results in a phase 2 study of this approach undertaken with or without resection by modern techniques for the management of nonmetastatic spine and paraspinal sarcomas, particularly for primary spine tumors. For 50 patients with a median follow-up of 48 months, the 5-year actuarial rates of local control, recurrence-free survival, and overall survival were 78%, 63%, and 87%, respectively. Three sacral neuropathies appeared after 77.12 to 77.4 Gy equivalents.[264]

Other forms of particle beam radiotherapy are discussed below in the "Definitive Radiation" section.

Small Soft Tissue Sarcomas. The outcome with extremity soft tissue sarcomas that are small is more favorable.[265] Geer et al.[265] reported on 174 patients with primary tumors of 5 cm or smaller. Among the 159 patients with negative margins of resection, adjuvant radiotherapy had no apparent benefit: the 5-year local control rate was 77% in those selected to receive adjuvant radiation, compared to 92% in those undergoing surgery alone (*P* = .08). The policy at MSKCC and Princess Margaret Hospital has been to omit adjuvant irradiation in patients with small primary tumors excised with adequate margins. However, two factors must be considered when deciding whether to omit radiation therapy. The first is the status of the surgical margin of resection. It is the authors' policy to administer radiotherapy to patients with positive margins even if the tumor was 5 cm or smaller. The second factor that should be considered is whether the patient has had a prior unplanned excision (i.e., excision without adequate preoperative staging or consideration of the need to remove normal tissue around tumor). At Princess Margaret Hospital, Noria et al.[266] found a significantly higher rate of local recurrence in patients who were treated after unplanned excision on the outside compared to patients who received their treatment at the institution (22% vs. 7%; *P* = .03). Unplanned excision is very common in community settings when small soft tissue lesions are excised under the presumption that they are benign. In these cases, the authors attempt a re-excision if at all feasible; otherwise, patients are strongly considered for adjuvant irradiation.

Adjuvant Radiation for Positive Surgical Margins. A positive surgical margin is associated with worse outcome. For example, Geer et al.,[265] in their study of small extremity sarcomas, found a 5-year local control rate of only 56% for patients with positive margins, compared to 88% for those with negative margins. Similar findings were reported in a study from M. D. Anderson Cancer Center.[267] For patients with positive microscopic margins the evidence suggests that outcomes can be improved by adjuvant radiotherapy. Data from the Princess Margaret Hospital, Massachusetts General Hospital, and MSKCC have shown that in patients with positive margins, radiotherapy reduces the risk of recurrence compared to no adjuvant treatments, although their 5-year local recurrence rates continue to be higher than those of patients with negative margins.[188,268] In a study at MSKCC, the group that received adjuvant radiation experienced a 5-year local control rate of 75%, compared to 56% for those treated with surgery alone (P = .01). Adjuvant radiation also retained its significance as an independent prognostic factor for local control in multivariate analysis (P = .01).[269] Whether one radiation modality is better than another in such cases is debatable due to the paucity of data and the problems of selection bias. In one study, local control for patients with positive margins was better if BRT was supplemented with EBRT (90% vs. 59%; P = .08).[256] However, others showed no difference in local control between EBRT with or without BRT boost.

Among patients who receive adjuvant radiotherapy for a positive margin, the cause of positive margins influences local control.[270] One cause is an anatomically adverse presentation in which locally advanced disease challenges the goals of conservative resection from the outset and a positive surgical margin is anticipated before surgery. Patients in this class have a low risk of local failure (3.6%). Thus, it seems possible, with appropriate evaluation and anticipation, to resect disease and protect critical juxtapositioned anatomy. This may result in only a minimal microscopic burden in a small area of positive margin that can be eradicated with adjuvant radiotherapy. From a cancer control perspective, it probably does not matter whether radiotherapy is administered as BRT or as EBRT delivered preoperatively or postoperatively. Another cause of positive margins is oncologically inadequate surgery in which positive resection margins may have been avoidable. Patients in this class who have low-grade liposarcomas and microscopically positive surgical margins also have a low risk of local failure (4.2%). However, patients in this class with sarcomas of other histologies have a higher risk (37.5%), as do patients who are referred after unplanned excision and who have positive margins on subsequent re-excision (31.6% risk of local failure).

Definitive Radiation. Surgery remains the main treatment for patients with sarcoma of the extremity, and every effort should be made to attempt resection. However, in some patients with unresectable disease or medical contraindications to operation, definitive radiation can be considered for palliation. In a study of 112 patients treated with definitive irradiation to a median total dose of 64 Gy,[271,272] the 5-year rates of local control and overall survival were 45% and 35%, respectively. Local control at 5 years was 51%, 45%, and 9% for tumors less than 5 cm, 5 to 10 cm, and greater than 10 cm, respectively. Five-year outcomes were worse for patients who received doses of less than 63 Gy than for those receiving higher doses; local control was 22% versus 60%, disease-free survival was 10% versus 36%, and overall survival was 14% versus 52%. Complications, however, were more frequent at doses of 68 Gy or more. Thus, the therapeutic window appears to be 63 to 68 Gy.[271]

Similar findings were reported for 57 patients treated with definitive photon beam irradiation to 44 to 88 Gy. The 5-year local control rate was 28%.[273] An additional 15 patients were treated with neutrons without obvious benefit over photons.

Other investigators have considered neutron radiotherapy either alone or in combination with photon beam irradiation. The attraction of neutrons is their high linear energy transfer (LET) and lower oxygen enhancement ratio compared to x-rays and the consequent possibility of eliminating hypoxic cells. In addition, neutron irradiation results in less repair of sublethal and potentially lethal damage and less variation in radiosensitivity over the phases of the cell cycle. Unfortunately, all of these biologic features also pertain to normal tissue, which implies that late toxicity is likely to be heightened, given the absence of the usual protection afforded by fractionation that occurs with more conventional photon treatment schedules. In a review of the European experience, patients with inoperable tumors or with gross disease after surgery and treated with neutron radiotherapy had a local control rate of 50%, but the rate of severe complications ranged from 6.6% when neutron therapy was used as a boost to 50% when used alone.[274] More recently Schwartz et al.[275] reported a North American experience of fast neutron therapy in a heterogeneous series of bone and in soft tissue sarcomas. Among the 34 patients with unresectable disease, the local relapse-free survival at 1 year was estimated as 62%. Within the entire series of 66 patients, serious chronic radiation-related complications occurred in ten patients (15%), all of whom had had high neutron doses, large radiotherapy fields, or both.

Another high-LET method that has been used for the treatment of unresectable soft tissue sarcoma is carbon ion radiotherapy.[276] The carbon ion beam has substantially better ability to target tissues safely compared to neutrons because of the enormous energy release at the end of its range. In addition, it offers excellent physical dose distribution and higher relative biological effectiveness. Kamada et al.[276] described promising early results for unresectable sarcomas of both bone and soft tissue and suggested that carbon ions may be an alternative to surgery with acceptable morbidity for unresectable sarcomas. Although not widely available, carbon ions and other heavy charged particles have continued to arouse interest. Serizawa et al.[277] recently reported the results of carbon ion radiotherapy for 24 patients with unresectable high-grade retroperitoneal sarcomas, 16 with primary disease and 8 with recurrent disease. The dose ranged from 52.8 to 73.6 Gy equivalents in 16 fixed fractions over 4 weeks. Overall survival rates were 75% at 2 years and 50% at 5 years. Local control rates were favorably 77% and 69% at 2 and 5 years. Notably, toxicities were low, with no gastrointestinal tract complications and no toxicity greater than grade 2.

Spot scanning proton beam therapy has been used in the curative treatment of soft tissue sarcomas located in the vicinity of critical structures such as the spinal cord, optic apparatus, bowel, and kidney, with local control comparable to that with EBRT and with acceptable toxicity.[278,279]

Hyperfractionated photon beam radiation has been combined with intravenous iododeoxyuridine as a radiosensitizer. Among 36 patients treated in this fashion, and with a median follow-up of 4 years, the local control rate was 60%.[280]

Definitive radiation combined with chemotherapy is described below, under "Combined Chemoradiotherapy for Primary Localized Extremity/Truncal Sarcoma."

Chemotherapy for Primary Localized Extremity/ Truncal Sarcoma

Surgery and radiation therapy remain the mainstay for local control of soft tissue sarcoma. Because up to half of patients with primary non-GIST sarcomas and adequate local control of disease will develop distant metastasis, usually to the lungs (extremity sarcomas) or liver (abdominal primary), it was hoped that adjuvant chemotherapy would help to decrease the frequency of distant metastasis and increase overall survival. More than 15 studies of adjuvant therapy for soft tissue sarcoma have been performed. Because anthracyclines are the agents most active against metastatic sarcoma, they have been

TABLE 115.3

ADJUVANT CHEMOTHERAPY STUDIES IN SOFT TISSUE SARCOMA

Study	Regimen	Doxorubicin Dose (mg/m^2)	No. of Evaluable Patients	Extremity Patients	Median Follow-Up (y)	Reported DFS Control (%)	Reported DFS Treated (%)	Reported OS Control (%)	Reported OS Treated (%)	Ref.
NCI extremity	CAM	50–70	65	65	7.1	54[a]	75[a]	60	83	419–421
NCI head and neck, trunk, breast	CAM	50–70	31	0	3.0	49	77	58	68	422
NCI retroperitoneal	CAM	50–70	15	0	2.4	84	50	100	47	423
GOG	Dox	60	156	0	NA	47	59	52	60	424
MDA	VACAR	60	47	43	>10	35[a]	55[a]	57	65	425, 426
Mayo Clinic	VCAct/VAD	50	61	48	5.4	65	83	70	90	290
EORTC	CYVADIC	50	317	216	6.7	43[a]	56[a]	55	63	283
Intergroup	Dox	70–90	78	50	1.7	55	73	70	91	281, 427
ECOG	Dox	70	30	18	>4.9	55	66	52	65	428
Boston	Dox	90	42	25	>3.8	62	67	72	71	429, 430
SSG	Dox	60	181	155	3.3	NA	NA	NA	NA	282
Rizzoli	Dox	75	77	77	NA	45[a,b]	73[a,b]	70[a,b]	91[a,b]	431, 432
UCLA	Dox	90	119	119	2.3	54[b]	58[b]	80[b]	85[b]	433
Fondation Bergonié	CYVADIC	50	59	36	4.4	32[a]	81[a]	54[a]	87[a]	434
RPMI	Dox	60–75	19	0	5.0	46	75	36	63	435
ISSG	I/Epi	Epi at 120	104	104	4.9	37[a]	50[a]	50[a]	69[a]	436
EORTC/NCIC	Dox/I	50	134	123	7.3	52	56	64	65	286
Austria	AI with DTIC (q2wk)	50	59	47	3.4 (mean)	57	77	>80	>80	287
1997 meta-analysis	Any	Various	1,568	904	9.4	44[a]	52[a]	53	57	281

AI, doxorubicin, ifosfamide; CAM, cyclophosphamide, doxorubicin, methotrexate; CYVADIC, cyclophosphamide, vincristine, doxorubicin, dacarbazine; DFS, disease-free survival; Dox, doxorubicin; DTIC, dacarbazine; ECOG, Eastern Cooperative Oncology Group; EORTC, European Organisation for Research and Treatment of Cancer; Epi, epirubicin; GOG, Gynecologic Oncology Group; I, ifosfamide; ISSG, Italian Sarcoma Study Group; MDA, M. D. Anderson Cancer Center; NA, not available; NCI, National Cancer Institute; NCIC, National Cancer Institute of Canada; OS, overall survival; RPMI, Roswell Park Memorial Institute; SSG, Scandinavian Sarcoma Group; UCLA, University of California at Los Angeles; VACAR, vincristine, doxorubicin, cyclophosphamide, dactinomycin; VCAct/VAD, vincristine, cyclophosphamide, dactinomycin alternating with vincristine, doxorubicin, dacarbazine.

Note: DFS and OS are not necessarily indicated at the median follow-up time.

[a]Survival difference reached significance.

[b]Some patients on the control arm received chemotherapy.

universally employed in adjuvant trials, alone or in combination. Unfortunately, most studies have included only small numbers of patients and therefore lack statistical power to detect small changes in overall survival. If there is a benefit to adjuvant or neoadjuvant chemotherapy, it is small, although the results from a few specific studies make adjuvant chemotherapy an attractive option.

The next sections describe in detail selected studies and meta-analyses of neoadjuvant and adjuvant chemotherapy, especially newer randomized studies based on an anthracycline-ifosfamide backbone (Table 115.3). For more details on older studies, see older editions of this text or the Sarcoma Meta-analysis Collaboration paper.[281]

A question that remains unanswered is the timing of chemotherapy with respect to surgery and radiation. Preoperative chemotherapy has been very successful in the management of predominantly pediatric sarcomas such as Ewing sarcoma and osteosarcoma. This approach has been extended to adult soft tissue sarcomas. Preoperative, or neoadjuvant, chemotherapy can make subsequent surgery easier and potentially treats micrometastatic disease early, before acquisition of resistance. In addition, before surgery the primary vasculature is still intact for drug delivery. Preoperative chemotherapy can guide postoperative treatment based on pathologic review of the tissue response after chemotherapy. In experimental models, preoperative chemotherapy eliminates a postoperative surge in growth of metastases noted after resection of primary tumors.[239]

Selected Older Randomized Studies of Adjuvant or Neoadjuvant Chemotherapy. The Scandinavian Sarcoma Group performed the largest study of doxorubicin as single agent used as an adjuvant to local therapy for soft tissue sarcomas.[282] Patients were treated with surgery with the option of adjuvant local radiation. Patients were then randomized to either no chemotherapy or doxorubicin, 60 mg/m^2, every 4 weeks for nine cycles. Chemotherapy was started within 10 weeks of surgery if radiation was used or within 6 weeks if no radiation was used. Of 240 patients enrolled, 181 were evaluable. At a median follow-up of 40 months, there was no difference in local control, disease-free survival, or overall survival for the evaluable patients. There was also no difference in overall or disease-free survival when the entire 240-patient cohort was assessed.

Given the ability to combine agents with somewhat nonoverlapping toxicity in the metastatic setting, combination chemotherapy became an attractive option in the adjuvant setting. The largest single study of adjuvant combination chemotherapy in soft tissue sarcoma was performed by the European Organisation for Research and Treatment of Cancer (EORTC).[283] In total, 468 patients with primary sarcoma (excluding only those with "very low grade" sarcomas) were treated with surgery and with adjuvant radiation if surgical margins were less than 1 cm. Patients were randomly assigned to receive or not to receive combination chemotherapy with cyclophosphamide, vincristine, doxorubicin, and dacarbazine (CYVADIC; Table 115.4), given every 28 days for eight cycles. Disease-free survival and local control were both better in the chemotherapy arm, but overall survival did not

PRACTICE OF ONCOLOGY

TABLE 115.4

COMBINATION CHEMOTHERAPY FOR SARCOMA: A COMPARISON OF FORMULATIONS

Regimen	Dose	Comments
DOXORUBICIN IFOSFAMIDE	60–90 mg/m^2	Bolus or IVCI over 3–4 days q3wk
24-h continuous dosing	5 g/m^2	24-h IVCI with mesna q3–4wk
High dose	2–4 g/m^2/d	Bolus or IVCI with mesna for 4 days q3–4wk
AD		
Doxorubicin	60 mg/m^2	Bolus or IVCI over 3–4 days q3wk
Dacarbazine	750–1,200 mg/m^2	
MAID		
Doxorubicin	60 mg/m^2	Bolus or divided over 3 days by bolus or IVCI q3–4wk
Ifosfamide with mesna	2.0–2.5 g/m^2	Daily × 3 days or IVCI q3–4wk with mesna
Dacarbazine	900–1,200 mg/m^2	Bolus or over 3 days IVCI q3–4 wk
AI OR AIM		
Doxorubicin	50–90 mg/m^2	Bolus or divided over 2–3 days by bolus or IVCI q3–4wk
Ifosfamide (with mesna)	5–10 g/m^2	Daily × 3 days or IVCI q3–4wk with mesna
MAP		
Mitomycin C	8 mg/m^2	Bolus q3wk
Doxorubicin	40 mg/m^2	
Cisplatin	60 mg/m^2	
CYVADIC		
Cyclophosphamide	500 mg/m^2	—
Vincristine	1.5 mg/m^2 days 1 and 5; max 2 mg/dose	—
Doxorubicin	50 mg/m^2	Bolus q3wk
Dacarbazine	250 mg/m^2/d × 5	

IVCI, intravenous continuous infusion; q, every.

differ significantly between the arms. Improvement in local recurrence rates was limited to patients with head, neck, and trunk sarcomas and was not observed for patients with extremity sarcomas. The study has been criticized for long accrual time (11 years), the inability of nearly half of the patients to complete all eight cycles of chemotherapy, and the relatively large number of patients ineligible for analysis, which most commonly was due to inappropriate radiation therapy.

Anthracycline-Ifosfamide Adjuvant or Neoadjuvant Chemotherapy. One of the most important studies of adjuvant chemotherapy for extremity soft tissue sarcomas is that from the Italian Sarcoma Study Group, who examined an anthracycline (epirubicin) and ifosfamide.[284] After surgery with or without local radiation, 104 patients were randomly assigned to receive no chemotherapy or ifosfamide (1.8 g/m^2 on 5 consecutive days) plus epirubicin (60 mg/m^2 on 2 consecutive days), with filgrastim support. The trial concluded early because it had reached its primary end point of improved disease-free survival. At a median follow-up of 36 months, overall survival in the chemotherapy arm was 72%, compared to 55% in the control arm (P = .002). Interpretation of the study was made more difficult by the finding of equal rates of distant or local recurrence or both at 4 years, as well as by subtle imbalances in the distribution of patients on the control and treatment arms. With longer follow-up, overall and disease-free survival no longer reached a statistical significance level (P = .05). Nonetheless, 5-year overall survival was still better with chemotherapy, and this study has been used as a rationale for giving the combination of ifosfamide and an anthracycline as adjuvant therapy. A smaller study of epirubicin alone versus epirubicin plus ifosfamide, which closed due to poor accrual, also showed a nearly statistically significant difference in favor of the combination.[285]

Enthusiasm for adjuvant or neoadjuvant chemotherapy for extremity sarcomas has been tempered by results of three other studies. The first was a randomized, phase 2 study of the EORTC and National Cancer Institute of Canada comparing no adjuvant chemotherapy to neoadjuvant doxorubicin, 50-mg/m^2 bolus, and ifosfamide, 5-g/m^2 24-hour infusion every 3 weeks.[286] There were 134 evaluable patients with "high-risk" soft tissue sarcomas. Overall and disease-free survival rates were not significantly different in the two treatment arms: overall survival was 64% at 5 years with no chemotherapy versus 65% with chemotherapy (±7%). The major criticism of this study is that the dose intensity was lower than that in other studies with a similar combination of drugs.

Second, a dose-intensive schedule of chemotherapy was examined in an Austrian study of 59 patients receiving no chemotherapy or doxorubicin (50 mg/m^2), dacarbazine (total dose 800 mg/m^2), and ifosfamide (6 g/m^2), every 2 weeks, with granulocyte colony-stimulating factor support after surgical resection of the primary sarcoma. Overall and relapse-free survival were not different in the two treatment arms at a mean follow-up of 41 months.[287]

The third and most recent study that tempered enthusiasm for adjuvant chemotherapy for primary soft tissue sarcoma is a comparison of surgery and radiation therapy with or without five cycles of doxorubicin (75 mg/m^2) and a 24-hour infusion of ifosfamide (5 g/m^2), every 21 days, given with supportive mesna and lenograstim.[288] Of the 175 patients randomized to chemotherapy, 163 started chemotherapy and 127 completed five cycles of treatment. The estimated 5-year relapse-free survival was 52% in both arms, and estimated 5-year overall survival was 69% in the observation arm and 64% in the chemotherapy arm. Although there are arguments that the ifosfamide dose was too low to be effective, this remains the largest adjuvant study of chemotherapy with doxorubicin and ifosfamide for soft tissue sarcomas. These data need somewhat more time to mature to confirm these conclusions.

Meta-analyses of Randomized Trials of Adjuvant Chemotherapy. Given the lack of statistical power of the existing randomized trials, it was hoped that combining the data from individual studies of adjuvant chemotherapy for sarcoma would reveal improvement in overall survival that could not be detected in smaller studies. For example, to detect a 10% difference between control group and treatment group with a power of 0.90 would require approximately 1,000 patients to be enrolled in a randomized study.

Several meta-analyses have been performed using data from adjuvant studies on soft tissue sarcoma,[289] the most rigorous of which was published in 1997.[281] This analysis included 14 studies and 1,568 patients. Tumor histology for each patient was recorded, but pathology review was not centralized. Median follow-up was 9.4 years. Disease-free survival at 10 years was improved from 45% for control patients to 55% for chemotherapy patients (P = .0001). Local disease-free survival at 10 years also favored the chemotherapy arm, improving from 75% to 81% (P = .016). However, although overall survival at 10 years improved from 50% to 54%, the difference was not statistically significant (P = .12). The largest difference in overall survival was found in subgroup analysis of the 886 patients with extremity sarcomas: absolute overall survival was shown to increase 7% in the group receiving chemotherapy (P = .029).

Conclusions on Adjuvant and Neoadjuvant Chemotherapy. Despite the promise of the largest positive study of adjuvant chemotherapy for patients with soft tissue sarcoma,[284] the most recent study from the EORTC, the largest undertaken of adjuvant chemotherapy, is negative.[288] The small size of most other adjuvant chemotherapy trials makes interpretation difficult because most studies had no statistical power to detect small (e.g., 10% to 20%) changes in overall survival. Two possible sources of selection bias should be considered. First, in several of the older studies, a significant proportion of patients were ineligible for analysis, raising the question of possible selection bias. Second, patients who enroll in clinical trials are healthier overall and survive longer than nonrandomized patients, as demonstrated in a study from the Mayo Clinic.[290] Historical controls are inadequate for comparison because the continued improvements in diagnosis, specific therapy, and supportive care could affect outcome; for example, the most recent study from EORTC showed that the control group did better than historical controls.[288]

Beyond these general problems with randomized studies, staging and dose intensity also affect the ability to draw conclusions from individual studies. Some of the older trials included a number of patients with low-grade or small tumors. It is increasingly appreciated that sarcomas are indeed heterogeneous in terms of both their biology and their sensitivity to chemotherapy in the metastatic setting. Accordingly, it may be most relevant to move forward with studies of adjuvant therapy for specific subtypes of sarcoma to identify better which might benefit from the use of adjuvant chemotherapy. Adjuvant chemotherapy has been particularly successful in this realm with pediatric sarcomas such as rhabdomyosarcoma and soft tissue Ewing sarcoma, and there is some substantiation of benefit for synovial sarcomas and myxoid–round cell liposarcomas, two subtypes that are sensitive to chemotherapy in the metastatic setting.[41] Conventional chemotherapy has not been shown to affect the functional outcome of patients with extremity sarcoma. Although any impact on overall survival of adjuvant or neoadjuvant chemotherapy appears to be small, the best standard of care that can be offered is a thorough discussion with patients regarding possible options and outcomes.

Intra-arterial Chemotherapy. Several studies have examined intra-arterial chemotherapy for local tumor control, employing doxorubicin, cisplatin, or both. The infusional approach is differentiated from local limb perfusion (see "Hyperthermia and Limb Perfusion"). Intra-arterial chemotherapy has the potential benefit of providing higher doses of chemotherapy to the limb in a first-pass effect. However, pharmacokinetic data have not shown an advantage over intravenous chemotherapy.

Intra-arterial chemotherapy has been used in conjunction with radiation. In a neoadjuvant study at UCLA, patients received 3 days of intra-arterial doxorubicin before administration of 35-Gy external-beam radiation over 10 days or 17.5 Gy administered over 5 days.[291] Patients were then randomly assigned to receive postoperative doxorubicin intravenously or no further chemotherapy. No difference in survival or local control was noted in this study. Thereafter, a randomized trial by the same group examined preoperative intravenous versus intra-arterial chemotherapy before radiation (28 Gy given over 8 days) followed by wide excision. There was no difference in local recurrence or survival between the 45 patients receiving intra-arterial doxorubicin and the 54 patients receiving intravenous doxorubicin.[292]

A number of studies have examined intra-arterial chemotherapy before radiation and surgery: intra-arterial doxorubicin alone[292] or in combination with other drugs such as cisplatin, single-agent intra-arterial cisplatin, or intra-arterial doxorubicin in combination with intravenous doxorubicin or other agents. Doxorubicin with simultaneous radiation has also been examined.[293] In these studies, some patients have been able to avoid amputation.

Infusional chemotherapy has its attendant complications, including arterial thromboembolism, infection, gangrene, and problems with wound healing, requiring amputation. Pathological fractures have been reported in patients who received chemotherapy and relatively large doses of radiation. One study reported ten major complications in 13 patients treated with intra-arterial chemotherapy with simultaneous radiation, which emphasizes the investigational nature of this approach. Although there are situations in which such therapy should be considered, intra-arterial chemotherapy at present has a limited role in the treatment of extremity sarcomas.

Hyperthermia and Limb Perfusion. In contrast to systemic intra-arterial chemotherapy infusion, perfusion of limbs requires isolating the arterial and venous system of the limb by means of a tourniquet and obtaining access to arteries and veins that supply the limb. The arterial and venous supplies of the limb are connected to an extracorporeal circulation system to isolate the limb from the rest of the body. The blood is reoxygenated and recirculated by a heart-lung machine. Care is taken after isolation of the limb to ensure that there is no leakage of the circuit into the systemic circulation; technetium-labeled albumin is injected into the circuit, and a probe is used over the heart to ensure isolation of the bypass circuit. Because mild hyperthermia may make chemotherapy more effective in some clinical settings (as mentioned later in this section), the blood of the circuit is often warmed to 39°C to 40°C.

A number of chemotherapeutic agents have been used for limb perfusion, such as melphalan, nitrogen mustard, dactinomycin, and doxorubicin. The most effective agent has been melphalan when given with tumor necrosis factor (TNF). The greatest experience with this technique is that of Eggermont et al.[293] Two hundred forty-six patients with primary or recurrent sarcomas that would otherwise require amputation or marked loss of function were treated with one and occasionally two isolated limb perfusion sessions. After isolation of the extremity, melphalan (10 to 13 mg/L limb volume) was perfused into the limb with a dose of TNF ten times the lethal dose for humans, under mild hyperthermic conditions. In early studies interferon-α was included in the regimen, but it was later dropped because it did not appear to improve results over melphalan and TNF alone. Both components of the regimen appeared important; the omission of TNF led to a decrease in tissue dose of melphalan, probably because TNF affects the tumor vasculature. Residual tumor was surgically removed 2 to 4 months after limb perfusion. With a median follow-up of 3 years, 71% of patients had successful limb salvage.

Recent efforts, including a randomized trial, have focused on attempts to reduce the dose of TNF to reduce toxicity.[294] Bonvalot et al.[294] performed a four-arm, randomized trial of hyperthermic isolated limb perfusion with melphalan combined with one of four doses of TNF-α: 0.5, 1, 2, and 3 mg (for upper limb) or 4 mg (for lower limb). The objective responses appeared to be equivalent for all dose levels within the trial, but systemic toxicity was significantly correlated with higher TNF-α doses. They concluded that low doses should be used to optimize the safety of this approach. It is difficult to compare this approach to standard chemotherapy, given the heterogeneity of patients in the two types of studies. In aggregate, the response rate does appear to be higher in the perfusion studies than in the infusion studies. However, isolated limb perfusion requires substantial expertise and specialized dedicated equipment. Complications of this technique include shock (from systemic leak of TNF); infection; chronic damage to skin, muscles, and nerve; persistent edema; and arterial or venous thrombosis. Experience has led to a decrease in the incidence and severity of complications. Isolated limb perfusion does appear to hold promise for at least a subset of patients who would otherwise require amputation for local control and has been approved for such patients in Europe. Studies are under way to examine the use of regional limb infusion, which would not require bypass machines, as a simplified means of treating otherwise unresectable extremity sarcomas.

Hyperthermia has been used in other ways to enhance the effects of chemotherapy in patients with locally advanced disease. Whole-body hyperthermia using extracorporeal heating of blood has been combined with ifosfamide and carboplatin intravenous chemotherapy, and responses have been seen in patients with otherwise refractory small cell sarcomas. Regional hyperthermia provided through an external electromagnetic field (phased array) has been examined in combination with ifosfamide and etoposide, as well as other combinations of chemotherapy.[295] In a series of studies over the past 20 years or more, investigators have demonstrated partial and complete responses in patients with locally advanced and metastatic soft tissue sarcoma. The hyperthermia used in these protocols is more aggressive than that used with limb perfusion; higher temperatures have led to a higher rate of local complications.

A study of doxorubicin, ifosfamide, and etoposide chemotherapy with or without regional hyperthermia has recently been completed.[296] The study enrolled 341 patients: 149 had extremity tumors and 192 had nonextremity primary sarcomas. Patients received four cycles of chemotherapy both before and after definitive local therapy; the chemotherapy was administered with or without regional hyperthermia. With median follow-up of 34 months, both local progression-free survival and disease-free survival were superior on the hyperthermia arm. For example, for extremity tumors, the local progression-free survival rate at 4 years was 76% without hyperthermia and 82% with hyperthermia. Although the improved freedom from local progression confirms the hypothesis of the application of such therapy, the molecular mechanisms that account for the improved disease-free survival is unclear. It is hoped that updates of these data will indicate the nature and reasons for differences in both local and distant relapses.

Combined Chemoradiotherapy for Primary Localized Extremity/Truncal Sarcoma

High-risk soft tissue sarcomas (i.e., those of large size, deep location, and high grade) present a significant dual threat: locally and at distant sites. For this reason, researchers at the Massachusetts General Hospital explored a dose-intense chemoradiation strategy in 48 patients with localized, high-grade, large (greater than 8 cm) soft tissue sarcomas of an extremity.[297] The protocol consisted of three courses of doxorubicin, ifosfamide, mesna, and dacarbazine (MAID) interdigitated with two 22-Gy courses of radiation (11 fractions each). Patients with microscopically positive surgical margins received a 16-Gy boost dose (in eight fractions). These patients were compared to an equal number of matched historical controls.

For the chemoradiation group, the 5-year actuarial rates were as follows: local control, 92%; distant metastasis-free survival, 75%, and overall survival, 87%. For the control group, the rates were all significantly lower: 86%, 47%, and 58%, respectively. As expected, toxicities in the chemoradiation group included significant wound-healing complications in the lower limbs (in 29% by the Canadian Sarcoma Group criteria).[298] One patient died from late marrow dysfunction attributed to chemotherapy. Clearly the use of early neoadjuvant chemoradiotherapy delivered in this fashion is appealing for patients at very highest risk. However, the differences in outcome between chemoradiation and control groups could be explained by imbalance between the groups, and the results require confirmation in prospective trials, especially because of the local and systemic toxicity associated with the protocol.[298] A multicenter study that included 64 patients treated according to the same protocol has since also shown significant toxicity, with three patients (5%) having experienced fatal grade 5 toxicities (myelodysplasia in two and sepsis in one). Moreover, another 53 patients (83%) experienced a variety of grade 4 toxicities, and 5 patients required amputation.[299]

Concurrent chemotherapy and definitive radiotherapy has shown evidence of benefit in numerous other cancers, and it should be considered for unresectable soft tissue sarcomas. Local control might be enhanced by dose-intensified chemotherapy regimens with concurrent radiotherapy at higher doses, possibly delivered conformally to protect normal tissues. Preliminary data have been obtained using a concurrent ifosfamide-based protocol. This regimen appears to have acceptable morbidity, although skin toxicity seemed to be enhanced, which makes it important to explore avoidance targeting for the radiotherapy in suitable patients if escalated radiotherapy doses are to be used.

Further evidence on combining systemic agents with radiotherapy to treat unresectable soft tissue sarcoma comes from a randomized trial evaluating the use of the radiation sensitizer razoxane.[300] This trial had a long accrual period (1978 to 1988), a modest number of evaluable cases (130 of 144 accrued), a modest radiation dose, and some imbalance between the treatment arms. Nevertheless, among 82 patients with gross disease, radiotherapy (median dose of 56 to 58 Gy) combined with razoxane (daily oral doses of 150 mg/m^2 throughout radiotherapy) demonstrated an increased response rate compared to radiotherapy alone (74% vs. 49%). The local control rate was also improved (64% vs. 30%; $P < .05$). Acute skin reactions were increased in the sensitizer arm, but late toxicity was not increased.[300]

Multimodal Management of Locally Recurrent Extremity/Truncal Sarcoma

Local recurrence remains a significant factor in long-term morbidity and mortality. Locally recurrent sarcomas are difficult to treat and are more likely to recur, probably as a result of prior contamination of tissue planes as well as intrinsically aggressive tumor biology. Follow-up data confirm that salvage is almost invariably possible, but there is no impact on long-term survival. For patients who undergo resection of their recurrent lesion, important factors in outcome are the size and timing of the recurrence.[301] Patients with a local recurrence of greater than 5 cm in less than 16 months had a 4-year disease-specific survival of 18%, compared to 81% for patients with a local recurrence of 5 cm or less in more than 16 months.

Surgery. Repeat resection is the treatment of choice for locally recurrent soft tissue sarcoma in almost any site that is amenable to low-morbidity surgical resection. Repeat resection usually encompasses all palpable tumor and all potential microscopic foci present in adjacent tissues traversed during previous surgical procedures. When surgical resection can be achieved, then adjuvant radiation therapy should be considered in the vast majority of patients with recurrent disease.

Radiotherapy. Radiotherapy in the recurrent setting should follow the same principles applicable to the treatment of primary tumors. However, the issues are more complex and often dominated by two confounding issues. First, tissue planes will likely have been disrupted from prior interventions and the true anatomic areas at risk are difficult to define, so there is often need to compromise in the choice of target volumes. Second and more problematic is prior radiotherapy, which results in serious concerns about long-term morbidity, especially affecting bone and neurovascular tissues. The substantial rates of serious complications for salvage reoperation and reirradiation[302] indicate that salvage therapy should be performed cautiously with careful monitoring of side effects.

Torres et al.[303] retrospectively reviewed 62 patients who had undergone prior resection and external beam radiotherapy, being treated for an isolated first local recurrence of soft tissue sarcoma arising within a previously irradiated field. Local control rates were similar for patients undergoing reirradiation compared to those who did not undergo reirradiation, but complications that required outpatient or surgical management were more common in reirradiated patients (80% vs. 17%; $P < .001$). The authors have acknowledged that selection for the different treatments may confound interpretation of these results. At the Princess Margaret Hospital, the local control rate among 11 patients treated with conservative surgery and no further irradiation in recurrent disease was only 36%. However, among ten patients treated with further surgery and reirradiation (predominantly using BRT), the local control rate was 100%, with a short median follow-up of 24 months.[304] As a general principle, if radiotherapy is used in a previously irradiated field, brachytherapy is often recommended. However, the possibility of complications is real and these decisions must be approached cautiously.[304–306]

When EBRT is used, various strategies can be considered to ameliorate the risk from reirradiation. First, precision techniques such as IMRT may be used to optimize volume with exclusion of uninvolved tissues. Second, preoperative, rather than postoperative, radiotherapy may be used to reduce dose and volume to the lowest level possible. Third, treatments may involve a smaller dose per fraction to minimize damage to late responding normal tissues; these fractionation approaches normally require treatment more than once per day. Intraoperative radiotherapy (IORT) has also been considered for salvage therapy, and careful dose limitation to major nerves, ureters, and kidneys may reduce related complications in complex anatomic regions.[307,308]

Management of Primary Localized Retroperitoneal Sarcoma

Surgical Management

For retroperitoneal sarcomas, as for extremity or truncal sarcomas, primary surgical resection is the dominant therapeutic modality. A treatment algorithm is shown in Figure 115.8. Preoperative bowel preparation is important, not because of tumor invasion, but because of the frequent technical difficulty of performing resection without encompassing the intestine. Because many tumors involve the retroperitoneum, it is important to evaluate renal function, in particular to establish adequate contralateral renal function, to allow nephrectomy when appropriate.

The major issue in resection of visceral and retroperitoneal lesions is adequate exposure. Thoracoabdominal incisions, rectus-dividing incisions, and incisions extending through the inguinal ligament into the thigh may improve exposure and enhance the ability to achieve a complete resection. The availability of venovenous bypass, adequate and appropriate anesthetic, and blood replacement therapy are all important issues for many of these large lesions.

Although resection of adjacent organs is common,[221] proof that a more extensive resection of adjacent organs

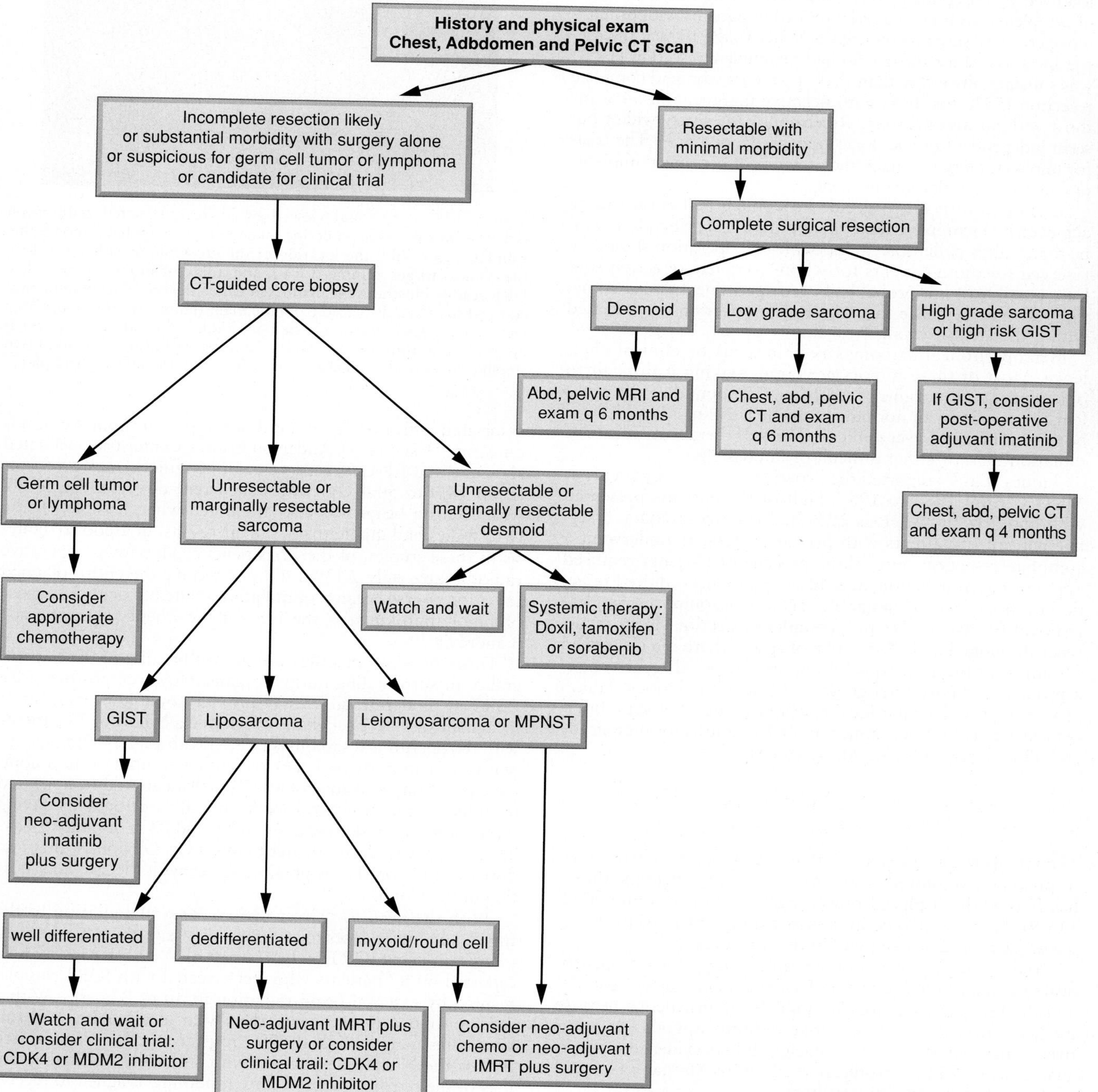

FIGURE 115.8 Algorithm for the management of retroperitoneal and visceral sarcoma.

PRACTICE OF ONCOLOGY

affects long-term survival seems very limited. In two reviews,[221,309] nephrectomy was performed in 46% of cases, but the kidney itself was rarely involved. In the report by Jaques et al.,[221] only 2 of 30 nephrectomy specimens showed true parenchymal invasion. Nevertheless, resection of the kidney is often necessary because of encompassment of the kidney or involvement of the hilar renal vasculature.

The overriding principle is not to be reluctant to resect adjacent organs should they be involved by tumor. Conversely, one should not resect uninvolved organs if they are not the limiting factor for the tumor margin. The resection of a kidney makes little sense when the vena cava is the closest margin. More extended resections do not seem to improve local recurrence or survival.

The primary factor in outcome is complete surgical resection, followed by the grade of the lesion. Illustrating the importance of complete resection, in a series 693 adult patients with primary retroperitoneal sarcoma resected at MSKCC, the 10-year disease-specific survival for those who had incomplete resection (18%) was substantially worse than that of patients who had complete resection (53% for those with negative margins and 54% for those with positive margins). Resectability rates vary widely but seem independent of histologic type, grade, or size.[221] The basis for unresectability is usually the presence of peritoneal implants or extensive vascular involvement.

It is often difficult to decide how much palliation can be achieved by incomplete removal of tumor. The principle should be that, unless palliation can be achieved, operation should be reserved for those patients for whom complete resection is at least possible, if not probable. In retroperitoneal liposarcoma, there is some evidence that incomplete resection is associated with prolonged survival.[310]

Retroperitoneal sarcomas remain a major clinical challenge. Most of these tumors are large, making it difficult to obtain adequate margins of resection. Compounding the problem, the proximity of normal organs such as small bowel, large bowel, kidney, and liver makes delivery of therapeutic doses of radiation therapy either difficult or impossible.

Jaques et al.[221] reported the experience with 114 patients at MSKCC from 1982 to 1987. Half of the patients presented with liposarcoma, whereas 29% had leiomyosarcoma. Sixty-five percent of patients with primary sarcomas underwent a complete resection. Fifty-three percent of patients required adjacent organ resection, and 40% of patients required resection of more than one adjacent organ to accomplish complete removal of disease. Despite complete resection, local recurrence developed in 40% to 50% of cases. There is a clear need for adjuvant local therapy. Of importance, local recurrence is a problem for both high-grade and low-grade lesions. Jaques et al.[221] reported similar local recurrence rates, but very different times to recurrence: a median of 15 months for high-grade and 42 months for low-grade sarcomas.

Radiation Therapy for Primary Localized Retroperitoneal Sarcoma

The retroperitoneum is a site that may be particularly suited to preoperative radiotherapy for sarcoma, because the tumor has frequently displaced bowel from the target volume (Fig. 115.9). Postoperatively, in contrast, loops of bowel are frequently tethered or fixed within the target area.

Trials involving preoperative radiotherapy for retroperitoneal sarcoma conducted at the M. D. Anderson Cancer Center[311] and the Princess Margaret Hospital[312] are instructive because the acute toxicity of preoperative radiotherapy was prospectively separated from overall toxicity, and the evidence supports an excellent tolerance profile. In the Princess Margaret Hospital study, median preoperative radiotherapy doses of 45 Gy in 25 fractions were administered to median radiation volumes exceeding 7 L. BRT, used postoperatively in selected cases, was

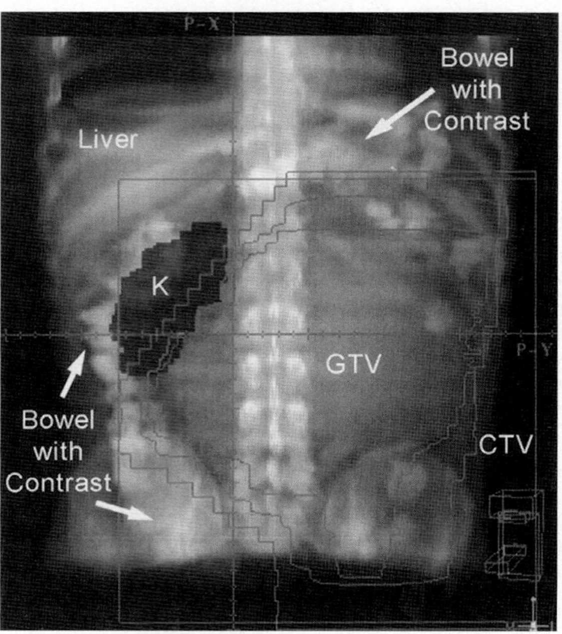

FIGURE 115.9 Coronal view digitally reconstructed radiograph (DRR) with soft tissue rendering taken with a computed tomographic simulator to exhibit the location of the gross tumor volume (GTV), the clinical target volume (CTV), and adjacent organs at risk. The DRR readily illustrates the manner in which the bowel containing oral contrast has been displaced from the main tumor area into more protected areas. Also evident are the right kidney (K) and the liver, which are protected from the high-dose area using multileaf collimation (see steplike edges of the radiation beam) for a traditional two-field plan.

associated with toxicity and did not appear to improve tumor outcome.[312] The M. D. Anderson Cancer Center trial evaluated six sequential 1.8-Gy/fraction escalating radiotherapy protocols (from 18.0 to 50.4 Gy) with concurrent doxorubicin; IORT with electron beam was also attempted when feasible.[311] The two studies had qualitatively similar results. In a pooled analysis of these studies, of the 72 patients eligible for preoperative radiotherapy, only 2 (3%) did not receive the entire planned radiation course because of radiation-related toxicity, 1 because of tumor approximating the liver and the other because of grade 3 anorexia.[313]

Doses of adjuvant EBRT are limited because of the low tolerance of surrounding normal organs. However, postoperative EBRT at moderate doses may provide some improvement in local control.[314] Tepper et al.[315] reviewed a cohort of 23 patients with retroperitoneal sarcomas treated with surgery and postoperative radiation therapy. For patients who underwent a complete resection, local control was 71%. Radiation dose appeared to influence tumor control, with only 30% of patients having local control at doses less than 50 Gy and 83% of patients having control with doses greater than 60 Gy. Obviously, the total dose of radiation that is possible varies with the size and location of the lesion.

With the need to deliver higher doses of radiation to the tumor and lower doses to surrounding tissue, there has been an interest in using IORT.[316] Petersen et al.[317] at the Mayo Clinic reported on 87 patients who were treated with IORT, supplemented by external-beam radiation in 80 of 87 cases. With a median follow-up of 3 years, the 5-year local control and survival rates were 58% and 50%, respectively. In a randomized trial at the NCI,[318] 35 patients with surgically resected sarcomas of the retroperitoneum were randomly assigned to receive IORT (20 Gy) followed by low-dose EBRT (35 to 40 Gy) or to higher-dose EBRT alone (50 to 55 Gy). Local control was significantly better for patients who received IORT, but there was no impact on survival. Patients in the IORT arm, who also received misonidazole, had a higher incidence of peripheral neuropathy than those who received EBRT alone. On the other hand, those who received higher-dose EBRT alone had a higher incidence of radiation enteritis.

At MSKCC, resection was combined with EBRT and high-dose–rate intraoperative BRT (HDR-IOBRT) in an attempt to optimize treatment effect and minimize toxicity to critical anatomy.[319] In this phase 1 and 2 trial, 32 patients with primary and recurrent retroperitoneal sarcoma underwent resection and HDR-IOBRT (12 to 15 Gy). Twenty-five of the patients were treated with EBRT (45.0 to 50.4 Gy) after resection. The high-dose–rate ^{192}Ir was delivered with a Harrison-Anderson-Mick flexible silicone applicator that readily conforms to the tumor bed. The median HDR-IOBRT procedure time was 110 minutes (range, 30 to 240 minutes). Median follow-up was 33 months, and 5-year local recurrence-free survival was 62%. Five-year actuarial rates of local control for primary and recurrent tumors were 74% and 54%, respectively. Treatment-related morbidity was observed in 34% of patients. The most common complication was gastrointestinal obstruction (six patients, 19%: five grade 3, one grade 5), followed by gastrointestinal fistula (three patients, 9%: two grade 3, one grade 5). Peripheral neuropathy, a common complication of IORT, developed in only two patients (6%, both grade 2). Treatment-related mortality was 6% (n = 2). Given the morbidity associated with IORT and its inherent limitations in large tumor beds, IORT is unlikely to be applicable to most primary retroperitoneal sarcomas.

The ideal radiation approach is one that could dose-escalate preoperative radiation. With conventional radiation, preoperative radiation cannot be escalated beyond 50.4 Gy without incurring excessive toxicity. However, dose-painting IMRT allows targeted dose escalation to areas at highest risk. The whole tumor volume can receive 50.4 Gy, thus respecting the tolerance, and at the same time the posterior structures, where there are no intestines, can receive 60 Gy. A report from the University of Alabama showed the feasibility of such an approach.[320] Fourteen patients were treated with preoperative radiation to the whole target volume to 45 Gy, then the area that was judged to be at risk for positive margin was separately boosted with IMRT to bring the total dose to 57.5 Gy. Only one patient experienced grade 3 nausea and vomiting. Eleven patients had complete resection with negative margins. With a median follow-up of 12 months there was no late toxicity related to radiation. Further dosimetric studies showed the technical feasibility of delivering doses as high as 75.2 to 82.8 Gy using this technique.[320]

Another interesting IMRT strategy for retroperitoneal sarcoma is to focus entirely on the posterior tumor attachment without attempting to include the remaining tumor mass in the irradiated target volume. This approach is undergoing prospective assessment in a study that accrued 18 patients over the period 2000 to 2005, with an excellent tolerance profile and promising early evidence of efficacy.[321]

The true benefit of IMRT—or any radiation therapy—for improving local control and hence survival in patients with primary retroperitoneal sarcoma remains to be proven. Until a randomized trial of radiotherapy is performed, surgical resection alone remains the standard of care for patients with retroperitoneal sarcoma.

Chemotherapy for Primary Localized Retroperitoneal Sarcoma

The most common histologic types encountered in the retroperitoneal location (well-differentiated liposarcoma, dedifferentiated liposarcoma, leiomyosarcoma, and MPNST) are typically not very responsive to conventional chemotherapy, and chemotherapy has never been shown to improve survival. Thus, chemotherapy is rarely indicated in the adjuvant setting for patients with completely resected primary retroperitoneal sarcoma. For patients with locally advanced primary retroperitoneal sarcoma that is unresectable or marginally resectable, treatment with neoadjuvant chemotherapy may be indicated based on histologic type as it enables assessment of response in individual patients and occasionally may improve resectability (Fig. 115.8).

Combined Chemoradiotherapy for Primary Localized Retroperitoneal Sarcoma

One of the difficulties in managing retroperitoneal sarcoma relates to the disparate nature of the presenting histological subtypes. Large, low-grade liposarcomas constitute about 50% of lesions and present a prodigious challenge to the surgeon and radiation oncologist because of their potential for late local recurrence, often leading to death. The remaining tumors are of intermediate and high grade, with leiomyosarcoma a frequent histology, and not only recur locally (often rapidly) but have a significant tendency to peritoneal seeding as well as metastasis to liver and other sites. Retroperitoneal sarcomas of all histologies often present as relatively large lesions due to asymptomatic growth within the abdomen. Because of the adverse nature of these sarcomas, a potential strategy is combined chemotherapy and radiotherapy as a neoadjuvant to surgery. However, not many groups have approached this problem specifically, presumably in large part due to the paucity of evidence for a benefit of chemotherapy in these tumors, as outlined above. Another reason is the wish to minimize toxicity in this group of patients already burdened with medical issues related to the treatment of large tumors.

The M. D. Anderson Group has reported results of a prospective trial mentioned earlier in the context of preoperative radiotherapy that included continuous radiosensitization as one of the treatment goals.[311] Eligibility was limited to intermediate- and high-grade tumor. Low-dose infusional doxorubicin was administered for 4 to 5 weeks at a dose of 20 mg/m^2/wk. Radiation was delivered in six escalating dose steps starting with 18.0 Gy total radiation and extending to 50.4 Gy. The protocol also included a 15-Gy electron-beam IORT boost to the bed of the resected tumor using a 9-MeV electron beam prescribed to the 90% isodose line. The maximum preoperative radiation dose of 50.4 Gy, preoperative radiotherapy was well tolerated, with only 2 (18%) of 11 patients having grade 3 or 4 nausea. This very low toxicity profile is attributed to the displacement of bowel from the radiation target volume. These promising feasibility results still remain experimental and ideally should prompt the design of randomized trials to address the efficacies of the different elements of the protocol.

Multimodal Management of Locally Recurrent Retroperitoneal Sarcoma

Surgery. For patients presenting with a second or subsequent recurrence of retroperitoneal sarcoma, complete resection of retroperitoneal sarcoma is usually possible in 60% to 70%. It is clear that, when complete gross resection can be achieved, operation for local recurrence should be attempted and may be combined with neoadjuvant systemic therapy or IMRT dependent on the histologic type or subtype, growth rate or time to local recurrence, and extent of disease. Isolated local recurrence is most common following complete resection of a primary retroperitoneal liposarcoma. Retroperitoneal recurrences are often detected on routine screening with imaging, or patients may present with pain or nonspecific symptoms. After workup to determine the extent of disease, patients with isolated local recurrence should be carefully evaluated for re-resection. As current chemotherapy is ineffective for the majority of patients with liposarcoma and toxicity limits adequate dosing by radiation therapy, complete surgical resection remains the most effective treatment modality. The most difficult decisions in retroperitoneal liposarcoma are selecting those patients most likely to benefit from reoperation and the timing of the reoperation; often a period of monitoring is appropriate. A recent analysis at MSKCC was performed to determine factors that would determine survival after re-resection and would assist with selecting patients most likely to benefit from surgery.[322] Of 105 patients who had at least one local recurrence following complete resection of a primary retroperitoneal liposarcoma, 61 underwent complete resection of their first local recurrence. Local recurrence size, primary histologic variant and grade, and local recurrence growth rate were independent predictors of disease-specific survival. Despite aggressive operative management, patients with a local recurrence growth rate greater than 1 cm per month had poor outcomes that were similar to those of patients who were not treated with resection. Only patients with local recurrence growth rates of less than 0.9 cm per month had improved survival following aggressive resection of the local recurrence. Based on these results, for patients presenting with asymptomatic local recurrence and growth rates equal to or exceeding 1 cm per month, the recommendation now is treatment with systemic chemotherapy or novel targeted therapy trials. Surgery is only considered in this subgroup if they develop symptoms, such as obstruction or bleeding, that do not respond to medical management. If the local recurrence growth rate is less than 1 cm per month, immediate surgery is recommended for all symptomatic patients and for asymptomatic patients whose local recurrence is impinging on critical structures (particularly if further growth may result in the need to sacrifice critical organs) or has a solid appearance on CT scan (suspicious for dedifferentiation). Many asymptomatic patients with a well-differentiated–appearing local recurrence that is well away from critical structures may be safely followed off any therapy and monitored to determine if they develop other sites of disease before recommending complete surgical resection. Such an approach can extend the interval between surgical resections and enables the surgeon to be more confident that all sites of known disease are encompassed with their planned procedure. Debulking, however, has limited overall value in terms of long-term survival of patients with recurrent lesions.

Radiotherapy. Many variables must be considered in deciding whether to use radiotherapy for locally recurrent retroperitoneal sarcoma. If diffuse intra-abdominal recurrence is present, then an accurate delineation of a target volume is unlikely to be feasible. With each successive recurrence, the situation becomes ever more challenging, and the chances of significant acute and chronic complications from reirradiation increase exponentially. Reirradiation is especially associated with increased morbidity due to adhesions from previous procedures. However, when complete gross resection appears technically feasible and the patient is asymptomatic and otherwise well, the authors favor aggressive treatment, preferably combined with preoperative radiotherapy to a conventional volume if the patient has had no prior radiotherapy. If prior radiotherapy has been used, subsequent treatment is much more complicated, and alternative strategies may be considered. These need to be determined case by case, but possibilities include using IMRT to a limited region of the retroperitoneum preoperatively or even postoperatively. In centers with access to them, IORT or proton beam may provide additional options. In all these deliberations, one needs to recognize that the value of radiotherapy remains unproven and the main motivation to use it is the adverse behavior of the tumor. Most important, attempting to eradicate unresectable gross disease using radiotherapy is generally considered futile, and the dose required to attempt this has real potential to damage critical intra-abdominal structures.

Chemotherapy. Intraperitoneal chemotherapy after debulking of peritoneal metastases has been advocated but remains an investigational approach.

Serious Complications of Primary Treatment

Wound Complications

It is well established that radiation and chemotherapy inhibit wound healing. Early studies on the effects of doxorubicin and x-rays on wound healing in animal models demonstrated that the timing and the combination of antineoplastic agents were critical factors.[323] Radiation or chemotherapy used just before, or in close juxtaposition to, the time of wounding significantly impaired wound healing, as demonstrated by wound-breaking strength. This appeared to be due to inhibition of new collagen synthesis as determined by hydroxyproline assays.

The influence of preoperative chemotherapy on the risk of wound complications is a complex topic.[324] Perhaps the most comprehensive study is that reported by the M. D. Anderson Cancer Center.[325] The authors compared morbidity of radical surgery for soft tissue sarcoma in 104 patients who received induction chemotherapy before surgery and in 204 patients who had surgery first. The most common complications were wound infections and other wound complications; more important, however, the incidence of surgical complications was no different for patients who underwent preoperative chemotherapy than for patients who underwent surgery alone, both for those with sarcomas of the limbs (34% vs. 41%) and for those with retroperitoneal or visceral sarcomas (29% vs. 34%). It must be recognized that the data are sparse and entirely retrospective, and the effects of preoperative chemotherapy are often confounded by concomitant use of preoperative radiotherapy (e.g., in the two concurrent radiotherapy MAID studies, discussed earlier in this chapter).[299,326] Preoperative chemotherapy is often delivered by the intra-arterial route, often combined with radiotherapy at the same time, with apparently greater morbidity than when radiotherapy is given alone.[327] Therefore, the risks of intra-arterial preoperative chemotherapy cannot safely be inferred from the results with the "usual" intravenous chemotherapy.

The effects of adjuvant BRT on wound complications have been studied at MSKCC. One finding is that, when radiation delivery via afterloading catheters begins more than 5 days after surgery, the rate of major wound complications approaches that with surgery alone.[251] In the randomized BRT trial,[256] the overall rate of wound complications (wound infection or the need for further operative intervention) in the BRT arm (24%) did not differ significantly from that in the control arm (15%; P = .18). However, the rate of reoperation was higher in the BRT arm (9% vs. 1%; P = .03). The other covariable that contributed to wound reoperation was the width of the excised skin. If the width was more than 4 cm, the reoperation rate was 9%, but if the width was 4 cm or less, the rate was 1% (P = .02).

These types of complications are not unique to BRT but have been shown with external-beam irradiation as well.[224,328] In the Canadian trial discussed earlier,[232] which compared preoperative and postoperative irradiation in 190 patients, wound complication was a primary end point of the study. Wound complications were defined as secondary wound surgery, hospital admission for wound care, or need for deep packing or prolonged dressings within 120 days after tumor resection. Patients undergoing preoperative radiation had a significantly higher rate of wound complications than those undergoing postoperative radiation (35% vs. 17%; $P = .01$).[232] The rates of wound complications in both arms were higher than those in many other studies, most probably because of methods of assessment. In this study, the criteria for an acute wound complication were prospectively applied with a specific requirement for reporting at frequent intervals for the initial 4 months after surgery. In studies using retrospective evaluation, in contrast, complications such as prolonged dressings or packing (often administered to outpatients) may be overlooked.

In situations in which wound complications may be anticipated (because of the magnitude of the wound, extent of the resection, prior radiation, and so on), serious consideration should be given to using fresh vascularized tissue in the form of either transpositional or free grafts to cover the defect before the placement or delivery of radiation therapy. This approach appears to markedly diminish postoperative morbidity, although the point is difficult to prove because of possible selection bias: nonprimary closure is more common for patients expected to have larger tumors and more problematic resections. In the Canadian trial the only significant variables for wound complication in multivariate analysis were the timing of radiotherapy (i.e., preoperative vs. postoperative), the volume of tissue removed at surgery, and the location of the tumor (upper vs. lower extremity). The manner of wound closure, comorbidity, age, smoking history, and treatment center had no apparent influence on the risk.[234] Similar observations were made in the M. D. Anderson Cancer Center study.[329]

These results merit a final comment on the role of anatomic sites in the risk of wound complication. This risk appears to be almost entirely confined to lower-extremity lesions.[232,318,329] This observation implies that, when deciding on the timing of radiotherapy, the risk of wound complications is a less important consideration for sites other than the lower extremities. This may make preoperative radiotherapy advantageous in sites for which restricting radiotherapy dose and volumes may have long-term benefit. Such sites include proximal arm (to protect overlying brachial plexus and lung) and the head and neck (to protect critical anatomy). In the authors' prospective series of patients with head and neck sarcomas treated with preoperative radiotherapy, wound complication rates were relatively low, even in patients specifically selected for preoperative radiotherapy because of adverse anatomic presentations. Frequently these included lesions in the skull base, for which the choice was made based on the wish to avoid the optic apparatus, spine, and brainstem.[330]

Bone Fracture

The impact of adjuvant radiation and chemotherapy on bone fracture has been reported in the literature, but the data are scant. Among 145 patients with soft tissue sarcoma who underwent limb-sparing surgery and postoperative radiation with or without chemotherapy, the fracture rate was 6%.[331] For patients treated with adjuvant BRT in the MSKCC randomized trial, the rate of fracture was 4%, compared to 0% in the control arm, but difference was not statistically significant ($P = .2$).[332] Helmstedter et al.[333] reported a fracture rate of 7% among 285 patients with soft tissue tumors treated by radiation and surgery, and that risk of fracture was not related to the dose, timing, and fractionation of radiation therapy. This series had a high rate of complications, including fracture nonunion (45%) and deep infection (20%). These authors suggested that prophylactic intramedullary fixation of the femur should be considered for patients who undergo resection of large tumors in the anterior compartment of the thigh requiring extensive periosteal stripping and adjuvant radiation therapy.

The factors associated with pathological fracture of the femur were analyzed in a study of 205 patients with soft tissue sarcoma of the thigh treated with adjuvant radiation (115 patients with BRT alone, 59 with EBRT alone, and 31 with both).[334] The 5-year actuarial risk was 8.6%, which on univariate analysis was associated with periosteal stripping, location in the anterior compartment, female gender, the use of chemotherapy, age of 50 years or older, and the use of EBRT instead of BRT (all $P \leq .04$). On multivariate analysis only periosteal stripping retained significance ($P = .01$).[334]

These results can be compared with data from the Princess Margaret Hospital on a long-term prospective series of 364 patients with lower-extremity sarcomas treated with adjuvant EBRT (without adjuvant chemotherapy). The rate of pathological fractures was significantly higher with higher radiotherapy doses (60 or 66 Gy; rate of 10%) than with lower doses (50 Gy; rate of 2%), and was higher with postoperative than with preoperative radiation therapy.[238] Conceivably, the relatively low fracture rate (0% to 4%) in the MSKCC trial of adjuvant BRT may indicate an advantage for BRT, even when accompanied by moderate postoperative EBRT (31 of 205 patients), over conventional full-dose postoperative radiotherapy, which carried the highest risk in the Princess Margaret Hospital study. This advantage in reducing the risk of fracture may result from better dose conformity with BRT and overall lower dose, as is used in preoperative EBRT.

Recently, IMRT dosimetry factors associated with fracture risk were investigated in a case-control study at the Princess Margaret Hospital.[335] The factors that appeared to reduce the risk of radiation-induced fracture were (1) volume of bone irradiated to 40 Gy or more kept below 64%, (2) mean dose to bone less than 37 Gy, (3) maximum dose anywhere along the length of bone less than 59 Gy, and perhaps (4) lower mean radiotherapy volume. Knowledge of these types of volumetric dosimetry data should facilitate the planning of dose objectives for IMRT with the potential to spare vulnerable normal tissue structures such as bone.

Other Complications

The other complication encountered with adjuvant radiation is peripheral nerve damage. In the MSKCC randomized trial of BRT, the rate was 9% in the BRT arm compared to 5% in the control arm ($P = .5$).[256] In a study of 62 patients treated with postoperative radiation, the rate of peripheral nerve damage was 1.6%.[336]

A common concern of practitioners is whether postoperative radiotherapy affects the bone grafts used for musculoskeletal reconstructions. Evidence suggests that postoperative radiotherapy can ordinarily be administered 3 to 4 weeks after grafting without detriment to the graft union.[337] Soft tissue reconstruction (e.g., tissue transfer in the form of pedicle flaps, free flaps, or skin grafts) to repair surgical defects carries a theoretical risk of radiotherapy-related wound breakdown that may require reoperation. This risk has been shown to be very low (5%), and most tissue transfers tolerate subsequent adjuvant radiation therapy well.[338] The authors have observed a higher rate of wound complications that necessitated reoperation in patients who received BRT. It is unclear whether flaps and skin grafts are inherently more susceptible to breakdown in the immediate postoperative period or whether this is a direct result of BRT. When treating foot lesions, practitioners should be aware of the complications that may arise, especially if skin grafts become infected, which may prolong healing.[268]

Evolving results suggest that patients treated with postoperative radiotherapy have worse rates of fibrosis and peripheral edema compared to those receiving preoperative radiotherapy.[237]

Multimodal Management of Advanced Disease

Control of the primary tumor can be achieved in the vast majority of patients with soft tissue sarcoma, but close to one-half of patients with non-GIST sarcomas succumb to metastatic or locally advanced disease. Median survival from the time metastases are recognized is on the order of 12 months, and 20% to 25% of patients with metastatic sarcoma are alive 2 years after diagnosis. Even the most active chemotherapeutic options are of limited value and are associated with serious and potentially life-threatening toxicity. Newer agents offer at least the hope of less toxicity and greater efficacy than anthracyclines and ifosfamide, at least for selected subtypes.

Patients with metastatic sarcoma often feel well at the time that a radiograph or CT reveals metastases and may remain free of symptoms for months or years. Thus, with many patients, alleviation of symptoms is not an immediate concern, although progression is inevitable. Surgical resection can provide selected patients with prolonged periods of freedom from disease, and radiation therapy provides palliation for individual patients who have localized symptomatic metastases. Optimal treatment of patients with unresectable or metastatic soft tissue sarcoma requires an appreciation of the natural history of the disease, close attention to the individual patient, and an understanding of the benefits and limitations of the therapeutic options.

Surgical Resection of Metastatic Disease

Approximately 20% of patients with a soft tissue sarcoma of an extremity or the trunk develop pulmonary metastases, and in the majority, the lung remains the only clinically evident site of metastasis. The histopathology of 1,643 pulmonary metastases has been described.[339] The primary tumors most likely to develop pulmonary metastases are PMFH (23%), synovial sarcoma (19%), and leiomyosarcoma (15%). Most metastases are detected in follow-up because only 30% of all pulmonary metastases present synchronously at the time of diagnosis, although 80% develop within 2 years of diagnosis. In retrospective series, 20% to 30% of patients who undergo metastasectomy are alive 5 years later.

Of 716 patients with primary extremity sarcoma who were treated at MSKCC over a 6-year period, pulmonary-only metastases occurred in 19%, or 135 patients. Of these 135 patients, 58% underwent thoracotomy, and 83% of those had a complete resection of their tumors. In the 65 patients who had a complete resection of their tumors, 69% had recurrence with pulmonary metastases as their only site of disease. Median survival time from complete resection was 19 months, and 3-year survival was 11% among all those presenting with lung metastasis only and 23% among those undergoing complete resection. Patients who did not undergo thoracotomy all died within 3 years.[205] Incomplete resection was no better than no operation. Chemotherapy had no obvious effect on survival in either the patients who did or those who did not undergo thoracotomy. Moreover, at the M. D. Anderson Cancer Center, response to chemotherapy administered before pulmonary resection did not predict improved outcome[340] (in contrast to the experience with chemotherapy for primary sarcoma). After resection of pulmonary metastases with curative intent, 40% to 80% of patients will have recurrence in the lung. Repeat resection is often possible.[341] In a series of 86 patients who underwent repeat resection, predictors of poor survival included more than three lesions, a lesion larger than 2 cm, and high-grade histology. If two or three of these factors were present, disease-specific survival was 10 months.

Histology-Specific Chemotherapy for Advanced Disease

Single Agents. Doxorubicin has been the mainstay of chemotherapy for advanced sarcoma. Whereas early studies suggested an overall response rate of 30%, in more recent trials the response rate was closer to 20%, and it was 11% in one study in which outside review of imaging studies was performed.[342,343] A dose–response relationship was demonstrated in analysis of the subset of patients with soft tissue sarcoma in a large, randomized, phase 2 trial of different dosages of doxorubicin. This relationship has been confirmed in other trials of single-agent doxorubicin and trials with doxorubicin-containing combination therapy.[344] Studies with liposomal doxorubicin showed fewer side effects than those with doxorubicin and similar response rates, despite the fact that the liposomal doxorubicin studies may have had a relatively high proportion of resistant sarcoma subtypes, such as GIST.[345]

Ifosfamide has approximately the same efficacy as doxorubicin. In the past, ifosfamide dosing was limited by severe urothelial toxicity (hemorrhagic cystitis). The uroprotective agent mesna has markedly changed the ability to administer both ifosfamide and cyclophosphamide, and ifosfamide doses as large as 14 to 18 g/m^2 or more over 1 to 2 weeks have been given. There has been a debate as to the relative efficacy of cyclophosphamide versus ifosfamide, in particular, whether ifosfamide truly has a different activity or whether differences in dosing of the two drugs account for the difference in response. The EORTC performed a randomized, phase 2 trial examining the response rates for ifosfamide, 5 g/m^2, and cyclophosphamide, 1.5 g/m^2. Myelosuppression was greater with cyclophosphamide, but response rates were 7.5% for cyclophosphamide and 18% for ifosfamide; although suggestive, this difference did not achieve statistical significance. In addition, some evidence suggests a dose–response relationship for ifosfamide.[346] This is borne out by the results of the many phase 2 trials examining the use of high-dose ifosfamide in metastatic soft tissue sarcoma. Higher doses of ifosfamide occasionally produce responses in patients who do not respond to lower doses of this or other alkylating agents. Note that synovial sarcoma appears to be particularly responsive to ifosfamide.[347]

The response rate is greater for ifosfamide combinations than for regimens without ifosfamide, highlighted in a 2008 meta-analysis.[348] However, 1-year survival was no different with the addition of ifosfamide to other chemotherapy. Thus, any lack of cross-resistance of doxorubicin and ifosfamide, the major rationale for use of chemotherapy combinations for soft tissue sarcomas, appears relevant only to the patient in need of a rapid response to treatment for symptoms, rather than having any effects on that patient's survival. A new, less toxic metabolite of ifosfamide, palifosfamide, is under study in phase 3 for patients with metastatic soft tissue sarcomas. Although data suggest palifosfamide synergizes with doxorubicin *in vitro,* it will be up to the randomized study to help determine whether palifosfamide and doxorubicin truly have clinical activity beyond that observed with combinations of ifosfamide and doxorubicin.

The third drug with modest activity in sarcoma is dacarbazine. Its activity was recognized more than 20 years ago and later confirmed.[349] Dacarbazine has frequently been used in combination chemotherapy with doxorubicin (see "Combination Chemotherapy for Advanced Soft Tissue Sarcoma"). Dacarbazine is given in a variety of schedules, from intravenous continuous infusion as part of the MAID protocol (Table 115.4) to one large bolus. The major side effects of dacarbazine are nausea and vomiting, which have been substantially reduced with the use of serotonin-antagonist antiemetics. Antiemetic use allows for dacarbazine administration in a single treatment rather than in divided doses. Temozolomide, the oral equivalent of dacarbazine, appears to have some activity against leiomyosarcomas as well.

As for other single agents, cisplatin and carboplatin have produced occasional responses in phase 2 trials. However, single-agent vincristine, etoposide, and dactinomycin appear to be inactive in adult sarcomas, unlike in pediatric sarcomas such as Ewing sarcoma and rhabdomyosarcoma. The taxanes also show little activity in sarcomas save for angiosarcoma. More recent data indicate that gemcitabine may have modest activity, dependent on the administration schedule,[350] and more activity when given with docetaxel (see "Combination Chemotherapy for Advanced Soft Tissue Sarcoma"). Few investigational drugs have demonstrated meaningful activity in soft tissue sarcoma, except for epirubicin, a close relative of doxorubicin, now approved for commercial use.

Excluding the remarkable story of the sensitivity of GIST to the tyrosine kinase inhibitor imatinib, the most significant cytotoxic agent in soft tissue sarcomas is probably trabectedin (ecteinascidin, ET-743), with responses in 14 of 189 patients (7%) with a variety of subtypes of sarcoma, in particular myxoid liposarcoma and leiomyosarcoma. When tested as first-, second-, or third-line therapy, a 7% minor response rate was also noted.[351] Trabectedin binds the minor groove of DNA and bends the DNA, interfering with transcription and blocking cell cycle progression. Its potency appears to depend on the cell having an intact nucleotide excision repair system. Its toxicity is largely hematologic and hepatic, with significant posttreatment increases in levels of transaminases and occasionally alkaline phosphatase and bilirubin; these toxicities resolve spontaneously and appear to be mitigated with the use of glucocorticoids. The most exciting recent data regarding trabectedin are its reported activity against myxoid–round cell liposarcoma, the subtype with a characteristic t(12;16) translocation. In this subtype, the radiologic response rate of single-agent trabectedin is on the order of 50% to 60%—activity as great as that of imatinib in GIST.[102–104,352] Responses also appear to be related to translocation subtype. Based on these data, trabectedin was approved for use in Europe in 2007.[351,353,354] Although it was not approved in the United States, as of 2010 it remains available in the United States in an expanded access program.

Immunotherapy for sarcoma, which was used in some of the earliest studies in sarcoma adjuvant chemotherapy, is seeing renewed interest, although without significant success. Cytokines alone appear to be ineffective in sarcoma, as does nonspecific immunotherapy with bacterial cell wall components. Clinical studies at the NCI and elsewhere are beginning to examine vaccines of peptides that represent the fusion proteins observed in specific sarcoma subtypes. Lymphokine-activated killer cell and other T-cell immunotherapy with cytokines was investigated in a very small number of patients at the NCI without any observed responses. Dendritic cell vaccines and other forms of tumor-specific immunotherapy are undergoing investigation and may be relevant to patients with soft tissue sarcoma. The most important development in immunotherapy for soft tissue sarcomas are the anecdotes of responses to a T-cell therapy directed against NY-ESO-1, a "cancer–germ cell" antigen found in the majority of synovial sarcomas. Cytotoxic T cells directed against NY-ESO-1 are generated *in vitro* and used as a therapeutic agent in synovial sarcoma patients in this study, which is ongoing as of May 2010.[355]

Combination Chemotherapy. A variety of chemotherapy combinations have been developed and examined in phase 2 trials. The typical backbone of combination regimens is doxorubicin (or its analogue epirubicin) with an alkylating agent, with or without other agents (Table 115.4). One of the earliest combinations used was doxorubicin and dacarbazine, which has been well studied by the Southwest Oncology Group. Although initial analysis noted a 41% major response rate, a subsequent study of either a bolus or continuous infusion of the same regimen yielded a 17% response rate.[356]

CYVADIC has been widely used for sarcoma therapy in the United States and Europe. Although single-arm studies showed response rates as high as 71%, a randomized trial showed no significant difference in overall survival between patients given CYVADIC and those given doxorubicin as a single agent.[342] The two-drug combinations of ifosfamide with either doxorubicin[342] or epirubicin[357] have consistently given response rates above 25%.

MAID was proven effective in metastatic soft tissue sarcoma in a large phase 2 trial. This randomized trial took place before the routine use of growth factors for aggressive chemotherapeutic regimens and examined MAID versus doxorubicin and dacarbazine. The study showed an increased response rate in the MAID arm (32% vs. 17%; $P < .002$).[358] In results that underscore the increased toxicity of aggressive chemotherapy regimens, there were 8 toxicity-related deaths in the study, 7 among the 170 patients treated with 7.5 g/m^2 of ifosfamide per cycle. This dose was decreased to 6 g/m^2 during the course of the study. All treatment-related deaths occurred in patients older than age 50. In a univariate analysis, the two-drug arm showed a survival advantage (13 months vs. 12 months for MAID); however, this difference was not significant in a multivariate analysis. As noted later in this chapter under "Dose Intensity," with the introduction of growth factors, the dose intensity of this regimen has become better tolerated.

The combination of cisplatin and mitomycin C with doxorubicin (MAP) yielded a 43% response rate in a study at the Mayo Clinic, despite the fact that response rates of metastatic sarcoma to cisplatin are low, and the response rate to mitomycin C was zero in one study. The activity of the MAP regimen has been confirmed in an independent ECOG trial.[290]

A meta-analysis of data from seven large EORTC studies provided a very useful assessment of response rates to doxorubicin- or epirubicin-containing combination chemotherapy in a multi-institutional setting.[359] Data for the 2,185 patients with follow-up were subjected to a univariate and multivariate analysis of survival based on a number of factors, including age, sex, performance status before chemotherapy, presence and site of metastatic disease, histologic subtype, histologic grade, and disease-free interval (time since initial diagnosis of sarcoma). The overall median survival time was 51 weeks. The predictors of overall survival included good performance status, lack of liver involvement, low histopathologic grade, long disease-free interval, and young age ($P < .005$ for all these factors in a multivariate analysis). Although lack of liver involvement, young age, and high histopathologic grade also predicted response to chemotherapy, so did liposarcoma histology (all $P < .01$ in a multivariate analysis); leiomyosarcoma histology was not predictive independent of liver metastasis. Although lesions were not stratified by site, these data provide some of the best evidence that response rate does not necessarily correlate with overall survival. Furthermore, these data were collected before GIST was recognized as a distinct sarcoma subtype, and thus the question of liver metastases as a negative prognostic indicator becomes an open question.

Is combination chemotherapy better than single-agent doxorubicin for overall survival for patients with metastatic soft tissue sarcomas? Again, the concept arises that response rates may be dissociated from overall survival rates. Several phase 3 trials have examined the issue of combination chemotherapy versus single-agent doxorubicin in patients with metastatic disease (Table 115.5), including two trials focused on uterine sarcoma. Several trials had better response rates with combination chemotherapy, but there was no survival advantage over single-agent doxorubicin. Complete responses during these studies were very rare and were not durable. These data argue that single agents are as effective as combination chemotherapy for patients with metastatic disease in terms of overall survival. However, some patients may be eligible for palliative resection

TABLE 115.5

SELECTED RANDOMIZED TRIALS IN ADVANCED DISEASE

Group	Regimen	No. of Patients	Response Rate, % (Complete Response Rate, %)	Median Survival (mo)	Ref.
GOG[a]	A	80	16 (6)	7.7	437
	AD	66	24 (10)	7.3	
GOG[a]	A	50	19 (4)	11.6	438
	ACy	54	19 (8)	10.9	
COG	A	41	17 (2)	8.5	439
	ActL	25	4	8.1	
	ActLV	26	0	11.5	
	ActLCyclo	26	0	5.1	
ECOG	A	54	30 (7)	8.6	440
	CyAV	56	21 (5)	7.9	
	CyActV	58	12 (2)	9.5	
ECOG	A	94	18 (5)	8.0	441
	A	88	17 (3)	8.4	
	ADTIC	92	30 (6)	8.0	
ECOG	A	148	17 (4)	9.4	442
	AVD	143	18 (6)	9.0	
ECOG	A	90	20 (2)	<9	343
	AI	88	34 (3)	11	
	MAP	84	32 (7)	9	
EORTC	A	240	23 (4)	12.0	342
	AI	231	28 (5)	12.6	
	CYVADIC	134	28 (8)	11.7	
CALGB/SWOG	AD	170	17 (2)	13.3	358
	AID	170	32 (2)	11.9	
EORTC	A	112	14 (2)	10.4	443
	Epi	111	15 (3)	10.8	
	Epi	111	14 (3)	10.4	
EORTC meta-analysis	Any anthracycline-based regimen	2,185	26 (NA)	11.8	359

A, doxorubicin; Act, actinomycin D; CALGB, Cancer and Leukemia and Group B; COG, Central Oncology Group; Cy, cyclophosphamide; Cyclo, cycloleucine; D, dacarbazine; DTIC, dacarbazine; Epi, epirubicin; GOG, Gynecologic Oncology Group; I, ifosfamide; L, L-PAM (L-phenylalanine mustard); M, mitomycin C; NA, not available; P, cisplatin; SWOG, Southwest Oncology Group; V, vincristine; VD, vindesine.
[a]Uterine sarcoma only; response rates are only for subset of patients with measurable disease.

of metastatic disease or are symptomatic from their metastases. In these situations, combination chemotherapy, which gives better response rates than single agents, can be considered. A 2008 meta-analysis confirmed the benefit of combination chemotherapy in terms of response rate and the lack of benefit in terms of 1-year survival.[348] These data underscore the need to pursue new directions, including seeking synergistic combinations of chemotherapies or combinations of standard cytotoxic chemotherapy with immunotherapeutic approaches or with newer agents that have (supposedly) more specific targets.

A combination that does appear to confer a survival benefit over single-agent chemotherapy is gemcitabine with docetaxel. Although gemcitabine and docetaxel have only borderline activity in sarcoma, the combination yielded a 53% response rate in patients with leiomyosarcoma, the great majority of whom had a uterine primary tumor.[360] These data have been confirmed in two other phase 2 studies,[361,362] and in a randomized phase 2 study of gemcitabine versus gemcitabine-docetaxel, in which the combination gave a response evaluation criteria in solid tumors a response rate of 16% (vs. 8% for the single agent).[113] Moreover, the combination was associated with improved progression-free and overall survival, which had not been observed in prior studies of combination chemotherapy versus single agents. Although other subtypes may respond to this combination, leiomyosarcoma and MFH were the two subtypes that responded most reproducibly, highlighting the subtype specificity even with standard cytotoxic chemotherapy agents. However, the benefit of the combination of gemcitabine and docetaxel over gemcitabine alone, at least for leiomyosarcoma, has been refuted by a recent study from France of patients with leiomyosarcoma.[363]

Dose Intensity. A central tenet of oncology is that response to chemotherapy is a function of dose intensity. A dose–response effect for doxorubicin and ifosfamide has been suggested in a variety of studies. However, toxicity limits the amount of chemotherapy that can be given in any one cycle, as illustrated by the phase 3 trial of the MAID combination chemotherapy, described previously.[358] If dose could be increased, responses might be better.

Increases in dose intensity can be facilitated by better supportive care. The use of hematopoietic growth factors has allowed the study of higher doses of chemotherapy in sarcoma. Some of the aggressive regimens for treatment of metastatic sarcoma satisfy the American Society of Clinical Oncology guidelines for use of growth factors, given their high rate of associated febrile neutropenia.[364] Granulocyte-macrophage colony-stimulating factor (GM-CSF, sargramostim), the first granulocyte growth factor used, decreased the myelosuppression seen with combinations such as CYVADIC or MAID[364] and high-dose ifosfamide. GM-CSF allowed for escalation of the dose of doxorubicin when given in combination with 5 g/m^2 of ifosfamide, with improvement in response rate.[365] GM-CSF has also been shown to allow increased dose intensity of the MAP combination, allowing addition of ifosfamide.

Similarly, granulocyte colony-stimulating factor (filgrastim) has been widely used to increase dose intensity and decrease myelotoxicity of aggressive chemotherapeutic regimens such as MAID[366] or dose-escalated doxorubicin and ifosfamide. However, with escalated doses (25% increase) in the MAID regimen, response rate does not appear to be significantly increased despite the use of growth factors. There may be other ways to achieve dose intensity. A study of low-dose, long-term (approximately 2-week) ifosfamide treatment showed responses in patients who did not respond to other forms of chemotherapy for sarcoma. As was seen for previous studies, the responsiveness to a particular regimen may not translate into increased survival.

Unfortunately, the cardiac toxicity of doxorubicin and the nephrotoxicity and central nervous system toxicity of ifosfamide prevent much additional dose escalation above the doses used in some studies today. The next logical step is high-dose therapy with stem cell support, which remains investigational for pediatric sarcomas such as rhabdomyosarcoma and Ewing sarcoma. Such treatment has been associated with long-term disease-free survival for a few patients with Ewing sarcoma, osteosarcoma, or rhabdomyosarcoma. Even with these relatively chemotherapy-sensitive tumors, the majority of patients have relapsed rapidly. Given that complete responses (and therefore chemotherapy sensitivity) are rare for metastatic adult soft tissue sarcoma, these rapid relapses are not surprising. High-dose therapy with stem cell rescue should not be considered for patients with metastatic sarcoma outside the setting of a clinical trial. Given the poor results of high-dose therapy, the pursuit of agents with better activity against specific sarcoma subtypes remains a priority for treatment of relapsed disease.

Protein-Targeted Molecular Therapy for Advanced Disease

With the success of imatinib in GIST and chronic myelogenous leukemia, investigators are examining an entire generation of agents that block specific proteins in the cell rather than serving as traditional DNA-damaging agents. Angiogenesis inhibition has emerged as a new frontier for treatment of solid tumors of all types, including sarcoma. However, weak angiogenesis inhibitors such as the interferons have not shown efficacy in sarcoma. Somewhat newer angiogenesis inhibitors such as TNP-470 (AGM-1470) and the vascular endothelial growth factor pathway inhibitor SU5416 have been examined in phase 1 and phase 2 studies,[367] but no partial responses and only one minor response were observed in 31 patients treated in the phase 2 study. The antiangiogenic compound SU6668, an oral drug, was not bioavailable in humans and is no longer under active investigation.

First- and second-generation tyrosine kinase inhibitors have yielded rather disappointing results when employed against non-GIST sarcomas. Imatinib was associated with a very low response rate in a study of ten sarcoma subtypes.[368] Sorafenib, an orally available agent active against B-raf and vascular endothelial growth factor receptor-2, showed only minor activity in patients with soft tissue sarcomas, in particular angiosarcoma.[134] Pazopanib is associated with at least a minor response rate against another subtype, synovial sarcoma.[369]

Newer biologic agents are beginning to be assessed, based on the specific biology of sarcoma subtypes. For example, well-differentiated and dedifferentiated liposarcomas demonstrate amplification of *CDK4* and *MDM2* genes on chromosome 12q. Presumably amplification of these genes is either a permissive or a necessary step in liposarcomagenesis. Drugs are available to block both protein products, for example, flavopiridol for CDK4 and nutlin-3 for MDM2, and show antitumor activity *in vitro*.[370] The issue of whether these drugs are truly useful in people with these largely chemotherapy-unresponsive tumors awaits formal clinical trials.

Other agents with specific targets are under active examination in soft tissue sarcoma patients. Ridaforolimus, despite a less than 3% response rate in metastatic soft tissue sarcomas,[371,372] was tested in a phase 3 trial in patients who have reached maximum benefit from other chemotherapy, in an attempt to increase their time to progression and overall survival. Pazopanib is undergoing phase 3 assessment, again looking for ways to improve at least progression-free survival. The same excitement surrounding imatinib and GIST is being carried over to the studies of newer agents in soft tissue sarcoma subtypes, some of which are discussed below.

Recommendations for Patients with Advanced Disease

Low-grade tumors grow very slowly and may be less responsive to chemotherapy than higher-grade lesions. Accordingly, an asymptomatic patient with stable or only slowly progressive disease can be simply observed. Resection of metastatic disease, in particular lung metastases, provides some patients with long-term survival and can be considered if the lungs are the only site of remaining disease.[205] In patients who present with completely resectable lung metastasis from an extremity primary, perioperative chemotherapy does not appear to be associated with better disease-specific or pulmonary progression-free survival. This suggests that systemic chemotherapy has minimal, if any, long-term impact on the outcome of patients undergoing pulmonary resection for extremity sarcoma metastatic to lung.[373] Histology is of increasing importance in designing effective treatment regimens for patients who present with advanced disease so as to optimize response for the specific soft tissue sarcoma subtype.

Randomized studies have shown that combination chemotherapy can provide a better probability of a response than single-agent doxorubicin. However, overall survival for any combination chemotherapy has not been proven superior to that for single-agent doxorubicin. When a clinical response is needed—for example, before potential surgery for metastases—combinations of agents such as doxorubicin and ifosfamide should be considered, especially for patients with good performance status. For patients with poorer performance status, single-agent doxorubicin remains the standard of care because no other therapy or combination of treatments has proven superior for overall survival. Pegylated liposomal doxorubicin can be considered in patients who would not tolerate the toxicity of doxorubicin, but the response rate may be lower than that of standard doxorubicin.

Single-agent ifosfamide or dacarbazine can be used as a second-line agent if doxorubicin is used alone in first-line therapy; gemcitabine either alone or in combinations appears to be an excellent second-line alternative for leiomyosarcoma (LMS) and PMFH and perhaps other sarcoma subtypes. Ifosfamide is useful against synovial sarcomas and myxoid–round cell and pleomorphic liposarcomas but less effective against leiomyosarcomas. Dacarbazine demonstrates modest activity in soft tissue sarcoma and, with doxorubicin, constitutes a well-studied and well-tolerated combination in metastatic disease. Dacarbazine and temozolomide, an oral version of dacarbazine, show activity against LMS in particular. Patients with angiosarcoma may respond to taxanes, gemcitabine, vinorelbine, pegylated liposomal doxorubicin, sorafenib, as well as standard doxorubicin or ifosfamide chemotherapy. Rhabdomyosarcoma and Ewing sarcoma of soft tissue and bone both respond to single agents and combinations involving topoisomerase 1 inhibitors. Given the paucity of tools to treat patients with advanced sarcomas and the wide variety of newly available kinase-specific agents, such patients are candidates for enrollment in phase 1 and 2 studies of new therapies.

Management of Specific Histologic Subtypes and Sites

Responses of soft tissue sarcoma to chemotherapy differ among the histologic subtypes. Pediatric sarcomas (Ewing sarcoma, osteosarcoma, and rhabdomyosarcoma) are known for their relative sensitivity to chemotherapy. Among adult sarcomas, synovial sarcoma and round cell liposarcoma are generally responsive to chemotherapy. GIST, alveolar soft part sarcoma, and low- to intermediate-grade chondrosarcoma are notorious for their resistance to standard cytotoxic chemotherapy agents. Therefore, an imbalance in the subtypes of sarcoma between patient groups can markedly affect the comparability of the outcomes of those groups.

The site of disease is also an important factor in outcome for patients with soft tissue sarcoma. Patients with large, low-grade liposarcomas of the extremity show lower relapse rates than patients with low-grade liposarcomas of the retroperitoneum; the latter are more difficult to control locally. Similarly, most tumors formerly called leiomyosarcomas of the gastrointestinal tract are now considered GISTs, which are known to be less responsive to standard chemotherapy than leiomyosarcomas of other sites (see "Leiomyosarcoma"), although remarkably sensitive to imatinib. Anatomy of metastatic disease can also affect overall response rates. For example, metastases to liver are less likely to respond to chemotherapy than metastases to another site; however, this may represent the tendency of GISTs to metastasize to the liver. Variations in the site of disease or metastasis pattern may account at least in part for the different responses noted in randomized trials of chemotherapy for soft tissue sarcoma.

The following subsections give examples of specific sites or subtypes of sarcoma and their characteristics.

Leiomyosarcoma

Insight into the differential response of leiomyosarcoma versus other subtypes such as liposarcoma, synovial sarcoma, or PMFH can be obtained from subset analyses from a variety of randomized studies. It should be noted that subset analyses cannot substitute for primary trials of chemotherapy, but they still can be useful in generating hypotheses. Doxorubicin appears to be active against leiomyosarcomas, but ifosfamide appears to add little to the response rate.[343] This finding has been observed in other studies, but again there may be contamination of the leiomyosarcoma group with what would today be classified as GISTs. For uterine leiomyosarcomas, a modest response to ifosfamide was observed in one small study but not in most other studies.

Among the newer agents, trabectedin showed a 6% response rate in a study of leiomyosarcoma and liposarcoma.[374] Gemcitabine and combinations have activity in leiomyosarcomas as well.[105,360,362,375–379] Other targeted agents have been largely disappointing in patients with leiomyosarcoma.

The primary site of leiomyosarcoma can have an equally important effect on survival. In the trials conducted by ECOG and the Southwest Oncology Group,[343,358] only 20% to 25% of uterine leiomyosarcomas responded to chemotherapy, but this was approximately twice as high as the response rate of leiomyosarcomas arising from the gastrointestinal tract (most of which were GIST, in retrospect, although even routine gastrointestinal leiomyosarcomas appear to have a lower response rate to chemotherapy than leiomyosarcomas arising in other sites).

Synovial Sarcoma

Patients with synovial sarcoma have relatively high rates of response to chemotherapy, but this may be due in part to patient factors, not just histologic diagnosis. Patients with synovial sarcoma tend to be younger than patients with other subtypes. Patients with synovial sarcoma are therefore likely to have a better performance status, a positive predictor for response to chemotherapy in the EORTC database.

An analysis of ifosfamide-based chemotherapy in adult patients with primary extremity synovial sarcoma of 5 cm or greater revealed that the 4-year disease-specific survival for the chemotherapy-treated patients was 88%, compared to 67% for those who received no chemotherapy ($P = .01$).[147] Ifosfamide-based chemotherapy was independently associated with improved disease-specific survival (HR 0.3 compared to no chemotherapy, $P = .007$). Adjuvant ifosfamide-based chemotherapy should therefore be considered in the treatment of adult patients with high-risk primary synovial sarcoma of the extremities. A prognostic nomogram specific to synovial sarcoma enables the treating clinician to more precisely assess outcome for the individual patient and to identify those patients who present with primary disease most likely to benefit from adjuvant or neoadjuvant chemotherapy.[216]

In patients with advanced synovial sarcomas, ifosfamide (at a high dose of 14 to 18 g/m^2) appears to be active, with a 100% response rate in one study of 13 patients. In the EORTC meta-analysis of 2,185 patients with metastatic sarcoma patients treated with anthracycline-containing chemotherapy,[359] the 115 evaluable patients with synovial sarcoma had a response rate of 31%. This study was focused on anthracycline-based chemotherapy, and only a portion of patients received ifosfamide (at a maximum dose of 5 g/m^2, a low dose according to some investigators).

Newer protein-directed therapies have shown only modest activity in synovial sarcoma patients. Pazopanib was associated with an approximate 15% response rate,[369] while its cousin sorafenib had a 0% response rate.[134] Sunitinib and other kinase-specific agents, including mTOR inhibitors, are not well examined in synovial sarcoma to date. In the authors' experience, trabectedin, active against myxoid–round cell liposarcoma, also has activity against synovial sarcoma.

Pediatric Sarcomas in Adult Populations

Adults may develop a number of pediatric sarcomas, including Ewing sarcoma (in soft tissue or bone), rhabdomyosarcoma (usually pleomorphic), and osteosarcoma. These diseases differ from typical adult sarcomas in that they are considered systemic diseases even if they appear to be localized at initial presentation. Ewing sarcoma and rhabdomyosarcoma are typically much more sensitive to chemotherapy than are other adult soft tissue sarcomas.[380] For adults with a diagnosis of rhabdomyosarcoma or Ewing sarcoma, the standard of care is adjuvant (or neoadjuvant) chemotherapy. In osteosarcoma, long-term survival has been achieved in pediatric patients with the use of adjuvant chemotherapy. Unfortunately, adults with osteosarcoma are generally more resistant to chemotherapy than are children. Adults with a typical osteosarcoma of bone should receive neoadjuvant or adjuvant chemotherapy in addition to therapy for local control of the tumor. However, extraskeletal osteosarcoma is treated like other soft tissue sarcomas, largely due to the low response rates to chemotherapy observed in patients with metastatic disease.

Typical regimens for small cell pediatric sarcomas, specifically rhabdomyosarcoma and Ewing sarcoma, include the combination of vincristine, doxorubicin, and cyclophosphamide (dactinomycin, in particular, for rhabdomyosarcoma) and the combination of ifosfamide and etoposide. The MAID regimen also shows activity in pediatric sarcomas. There is debate about whether adults do worse than pediatric patients with the same stage of disease. Adults may present with more advanced-stage disease than do children or adolescents. In addition, adults are less likely than children to tolerate the aggressive regimens of chemotherapy used against these diseases. However, one retrospective study showed that older patients with rhabdomyosarcoma tolerated chemotherapy as well as the pediatric population but fared worse overall.[110] In Ewing sarcoma, the role of age in predicting outcome is controversial.[381] A high percentage of patients with pediatric sarcomas are enrolled in randomized trials to examine new therapy. Adults with a sarcoma usually seen in pediatric populations should be included in pediatric protocols whenever feasible to help determine appropriate care for patients with these rare diagnoses.

Insulinlike growth factor 1 receptor (IGF1R) has emerged as a new target for therapy in pediatric sarcomas in adults and children alike, backed by more than 20 years of research confirming the importance of IGF1R in Ewing sarcoma, rhabdomyosarcoma, and osteosarcoma.[382] Unfortunately, response rates for IGF1R antagonists are low, probably well under 20%, for entirely unclear reasons, given that the EWSR1-FLI1 transgene depends upon IGF1R signaling to maintain survival of a Ewing sarcoma cell line.[383] Patients typically have relatively rapid progression after perceived minor benefits, suggesting that parallel pathways are at least in part to blame for the lack of greater activity of IGF1R antagonists as single agents.

Uterine Sarcoma

Uterine sarcomas are very rare, accounting for 3% to 7% of all uterine malignancies. The uterus is unique in that at least three different sarcomatous entities may arise from this organ: (1) leiomyosarcoma, a tumor of the endometrium; (2) endometrial stromal sarcoma, the least common type, which usually has very aggressive behavior; and (3) carcinosarcoma (also known as malignant mixed Müllerian tumor [MMMT]), composed of elements of carcinoma and sarcoma. Other uterine sarcomas such as rhabdomyosarcoma are uncommon.

For localized disease, surgery is the main treatment. The use of adjuvant radiation is controversial. Most studies showed some improvement in local control but not in survival. The efficacy of adjuvant radiation may be a function of disease subtype, because spread beyond the uterus (e.g., to lymph nodes) is common in patients with MMMT but less common in patients with leiomyosarcoma. The literature is well represented by EORTC study 55874, which examined radiation therapy versus surgery alone for 224 patients with International Federation of Gynecology and Obstetrics (FIGO) stage I or II uterine sarcoma.[384] Patients who received radiation had a lower risk of local relapse, a benefit observed for patients with MMMT and not leiomyosarcoma.

Uterine Leiomyosarcoma. After resection of a uterine leiomyosarcoma (LMS), adjuvant radiation therapy is generally not employed unless there is overt pelvic side-wall involvement with sarcoma. This concept is supported by the negative results for LMS in the phase 3 randomized study from EORTC, although this study was relatively small.[384]

Metastatic uterine LMS is responsive to doxorubicin but less sensitive to ifosfamide and to cisplatin. Uterine LMS is particularly responsive to the combination of gemcitabine and docetaxel,[360] apparently due to the synergy of this combination.[385] This combination was superior to gemcitabine alone in a Bayesian adaptive randomized phase 2 study that examined both LMS and non-LMS sarcomas, but the number of LMS patients was relatively small, and the number of uterine LMS smaller still.[386] However, a randomized study from France refutes the synergy of gemcitabine and docetaxel, at least for LMS.[363] Another approach is vinorelbine and gemcitabine in LMS, a combination with at least modest activity, though not yet examined in a randomized fashion. Trabectedin has at least some activity in LMS as well.[352]

Although uterine LMS often shows estrogen- or progesterone-receptor staining, its rate of response to hormone therapy is very low. In a prospective trial of tamoxifen in treatment of uterine sarcomas, none of the 19 patients with leiomyosarcoma responded.[387]

Endometrial Stromal Sarcoma. The pathologic entity endometrial stromal sarcoma (ESS) is divided into low-grade ESS and undifferentiated uterine sarcoma (a high-grade lesion). Although low-grade ESSs carry a t(7;17)(p15;q21) linking JAZF1 and SUZ12 (JJAZ1), it is not known if the same translocation is also in undifferentiated uterine sarcoma.[388]

Low-grade ESS, but not undifferentiated uterine sarcoma, expresses estrogen and progesterone receptors, and responses to hormonal therapy are seen more in this subtype than in perhaps any other form of sarcoma.

For adjuvant therapy in patients with low-grade ESS, estrogen antagonists may be considered based on small clinical trials[389] but are of unproved benefit. There is no clear standard of care for undifferentiated endometrial sarcomas, although some investigators advocate for adjuvant chemotherapy.

In the recurrent setting, estrogen deprivation is an appropriate first-line therapy for low-grade ESS,[389] and surgical debulking can be considered as well since the disease tends to have an indolent course. For metastatic undifferentiated uterine sarcoma (and recurrent low-grade ESS), ifosfamide is active, as may be doxorubicin.[390]

Desmoid Tumor

Surgery remains the treatment of choice for desmoid tumors. They tend to form large infiltrative masses that, if not widely excised, recur repeatedly. However, any attempt at complete wide excision must be balanced by considerations regarding preservation of function, because, as described below, desmoids may often be controlled with systemic therapy,[391–396] and they occasionally regress spontaneously. Local recurrence is frequent after complete surgical excision (25% to 50% at 5 years)[46,397,398] and may be related to the adequacy of resection and the presence and type of mutation in *CTNNB1*, which is mutated in many sporadic desmoids.[397]

The role of adjuvant radiation for completely resected primary desmoid tumor is controversial. Most authors agree that for patients with negative resection margins, postoperative radiation is not recommended.[399] However, for patients with positive microscopic margins the role of adjuvant radiation is more debatable. Spear et al.[399] reported a local control rate of 61% for patients with primary tumors with positive microscopic margins treated with surgery alone. Others, however, have reported lower local control rates. The conclusion from these studies is that residual microscopic tumor from a primary lesion does not invariably lead to treatment failure, and that adjuvant radiation may be omitted as long as local progression would not cause significant morbidity. The usual dose for adjuvant radiation for primary and most recurrent tumors is around 50 Gy.

Although adjuvant radiation is being used less, definitive radiation is emerging as a reasonable alternative to radical surgery. Ballo et al.[400] reported a 5-year local control rate of 69% for patients treated with radiation for gross disease. Others have shown similar findings.[399] The recommended dose for definitive radiation usually ranges from 56 Gy at 2 Gy per fraction to 60 Gy at 1.8 Gy per fraction.

Desmoids classically arise in pregnancy as an abdominal mass independent of the uterus. Desmoids have been examined for hormone receptors, and some have binding sites for estrogens and antiestrogens. There are anecdotal accounts of responses to hormonal manipulation such as tamoxifen, gonadotropin-releasing hormone agonists, or aromatase inhibitors. There are well-documented responses of desmoids to sulindac and other nonsteroidal anti-inflammatory drugs. Responses can take months and continue for years.

Responses have been reported to single-agent doxorubicin and to less toxic liposomal pegylated doxorubicin,[391,401,402] as well as to combination chemotherapy at either standard or relatively low doses.[403] Responses can be slow, with patients needing several months or even 1 to 2 years of therapy to achieve maximum benefit, and therefore therapy should not be abandoned for stable disease, although changes should be made for toxicity. Complete responses are exceptionally rare, and so the timing of discontinuation of therapy in a patient with responding disease remains a difficult question and requires clinical judgment.

Two recent studies indicate that desmoid tumors may occasionally respond to imatinib, although, as with other systemic therapy, it remains somewhat unclear whether some of the responses are truly due to treatment.[404,405] PDGF receptors have been identified in desmoid tumors, providing a possible mechanism of action of imatinib in these tumors. Anecdotally, sorafenib[406] and sunitinib[396] may be more active than imatinib.

In a recent series of 142 patients with primary and locally recurrent desmoids, 83 patients were treated with a "wait and see" policy, whereas 59 were initially offered medical therapy, mainly hormonal therapy and chemotherapy. The 5-year progression-free survival was 49.9% for the "wait and see" group and 58.6% for the medically treated patients. This study suggests that many patients with primary and locally recurrent desmoids tumor can be safely managed by observation and thus can avoid the morbidity of surgery or radiotherapy.[407] In summary, for easily resectable disease, surgery alone appears to be the optimal approach, especially in patients with negative microscopic margins. In advanced cases, a trial of nonsteroidal anti-inflammatory drugs or hormonal therapy can be considered in most patients. A period of close observation is also reasonable because some patients demonstrate regression without any therapy. However, if a patient is symptomatic and not a candidate for surgery, consideration should be given to systemic therapy or occasionally radiation to increase the chance of a response.

Soft Tissue Sarcomas of the Hands and Feet

Wide local excision is the exception rather than the rule for sarcomas of the hands and feet due to the lack of muscular bulk and the proximity to neurovascular structures and bone. The overall prognosis is inferior to that of tumors at other sites in the extremity. At MSKCC, patients with hand tumors, even those 5 cm or smaller, had a survival rate significantly lower than that of patients with tumors at other distal extremity sites (P = .0008).[408]

Although the distal extremities have limited tolerance of radiotherapy, the data suggest that conservative resections with adjuvant radiotherapy should be considered for patients with sarcoma of the hand or foot. Lin et al.[409] reported 115 patients with soft tissue sarcomas of the hand or foot treated between 1980 and 1998. The majority (95%) were referred after surgery elsewhere. Patients treated with definitive wide re-excision had a 10-year local recurrence-free survival rate of 88%, which was significantly better than the 58% for patients who did not have re-excision (P = .05). Radiotherapy improved local control in patients who did not undergo re-excision but did not improve local control in the small number of patients who had definitive re-excision with negative margins. Immediate amputation did not confer a survival benefit. Thus, limb-sparing treatment is possible in many patients with soft tissue sarcomas of the hand and foot. Amputation should be reserved for cases in which the tumor cannot be excised (or re-excised) with adequate margins without sacrifice of functionally significant neurovascular or osseous structures.[409] For patients who undergo adjuvant radiotherapy, special attention needs to be paid to radiation treatment technique to minimize complications and preserve function. Nevertheless, Bray et al.[410] reported good functional outcomes among 20 patients with soft tissue sarcoma of the hand and forearm who received adjuvant radiation. At a mean follow-up of 37 months, the local control rate was 88%. Eighty-eight percent of those who survived and did not require amputation were able to return to work and activities of daily living with minimal or no functional limitation.[410]

PALLIATIVE CARE

Surgery

Surgeons have long employed palliative procedures to relieve surgical emergencies such as obstruction, bleeding, and perforation. More recently, attention has been focused on alleviating the more chronic complaints, such as pain, nausea, vomiting, inability to eat, and anemia. The treating surgeon should not allow attempts to improve survival to overshadow the goals of minimizing morbidity and relieving symptoms, so that a terminal patient may die with dignity and without undue suffering and pain.

A prospective analysis of 1,022 palliative procedures from MSKCC[411] demonstrated initial symptom resolution in 80% of patients, although 25% of them required further intervention for recurrent symptoms and 29% for new symptoms. For those patients who experienced symptomatic improvements, the improvement was noted within 30 days. For patients who underwent repair of a pathological fracture, 87% had resolution of bone pain or instability symptoms; for patients undergoing palliative tumor excision, 83% had resolution of wound or tumor hygiene symptoms. For gastrointestinal (GI) symptoms, upper GI obstruction was resolved in 79% of cases, whereas mid- or lower GI obstruction was resolved in 90% of cases. However, palliative procedures were associated with significant morbidity (40%) and mortality (11%) and with limited overall survival (approximately 6 months). Factors associated with poor palliative outcomes were poor performance status, poor nutrition, weight loss, and no previous cancer therapy. Although this study showed predictable symptom relief following palliative procedures in carefully selected patients, symptom recurrence and development of additional symptoms limits the durability of the symptom relief.[411]

In a retrospective study specific to patients with a diagnosis of intra-abdominal sarcoma who underwent a palliative procedure, 71% of patients had improvement of symptoms at 30 days after the palliative operation, but only 54% of patients remained symptom free after 100 days. For patients with GI tract obstructive symptoms, 54% had symptomatic relief at 30 days, but only 23% of patients remained symptom free at

100 days. The overall operative morbidity was 29%, and postoperative mortality was 12%. Almost 50% of patients who underwent procedures intended to palliate gastrointestinal obstruction encountered significant morbidity.[412]

In summary, decisions regarding the use of surgical procedures for the palliation of symptoms from advanced sarcoma require precise surgical judgment that balances the medical prognosis of the sarcoma, the availability and success of nonsurgical treatments, and the individual patient's quality of life and life expectancy. Palliative decision making needs to be individualized and remain flexible as the sarcoma progresses. Decision making is best optimized through effective and frequent communication between the patient, family members, and the surgeon.

Palliative Radiation

Traditionally, radiotherapy is considered unfruitful in the palliation of soft tissue sarcoma. Exceptions include the expected relatively immediate response of bone pain or cessation of bleeding in fungating tumors. Both are generally regarded as physiological responses, mediated through decrease in osteoclast activity in the case of bone metastasis or by compromising the vascular integrity of bleeding lesions. These effects are independent of histology and seem to apply in the same way to sarcoma as they do to other tumors. They take place following relatively moderate doses of radiotherapy. However, using radiotherapy to address mass effects such as obstruction or compression is more difficult. The tumors involved are often bulky, and generally radiotherapy is considered as sole management only when surgery is not feasible. Radiotherapy has a low likelihood of achieving symptomatic relief from bulky unresectable sarcoma, apart from radiosensitive histologies such as rhabdomyosarcoma, myxoid–round cell liposarcoma, or synovial sarcoma.

Aggressive palliative approaches with radiotherapy have a greatly magnified risk of harm compared to that from the usual use of radiotherapy in sarcoma. This is because the region of concern may already have been irradiated, the doses needed for a useful outcome are higher than the doses for adjuvant radiotherapy, and anatomic issues may present barriers to delivery. As noted earlier, if overt disease is to be controlled with protracted fractionation approaches, relatively high doses are needed, and these are not normally administered for palliation (see "Definitive Radiation" earlier). Palliative radiation is most relevant when a lesion lies in direct proximity to critical anatomy such as spine, small bowel, or base of skull and surgery is either impossible or undesirable. The principles of palliative radiation are similar to those for curative radiotherapy and must include attention to choice of dose and fractionation schedule, the volume that may be treated, and the role of surgery and chemotherapy.

Only limited research has addressed dose fractionation schedules in this area, but promising results have come from a hypofractionation approach that delivered a short and intensive course.[413] Seventeen patients with symptomatic metastases that required rapid palliation were treated with 39 Gy given in 13 fractions of 3 Gy per fraction, 5 times per week. Radiotherapy was the sole treatment for local palliation of 15 sites of metastases, resulting in durable pain control in 12 sites. The protocol was well tolerated.

For patients with limited time remaining and in need of palliative treatment, it appears that reasonably intense regimens that are not overly protracted and inconvenient should be explored further. In addition, such patients may benefit from radiotherapy in combination with surgery, both for metastases and for locally advanced lesions that may themselves be incurable or because of coexisting metastases. This principle is exemplified in a recent report from the University of Miami. Surgery and selected use of local radiotherapy were used to treat selected patients with very advanced fungating tumors, some of whom also had distant metastases. This multimodal approach enhanced both palliative and curative outcomes.[414]

Another approach to palliation in sarcoma is the precision methods stereotactic radiosurgery (SRS) and SBRT, described above. These techniques are being explored especially in the treatment of small volume pulmonary disease as well as for spinal disease. Typical doses for lung lesions are 30 Gy in a single fraction or 60 Gy in three fractions. Early results of SBRT are available for the treatment of lung oligometastases, including a small number of sarcoma metastases, and it appears to be an option in appropriately selected patients unsuited for surgery. However, anatomic selection criteria for SBRT pulmonary oligometastasis are rather similar to those used for surgery. The underlying principles and technical issues have been reviewed recently.[415] The challenges of this location include respiratory motion and the presence of numerous critical structures (e.g., brachial plexus, bronchial tree, liver, ribs) that are relatively resistant to conventional radiotherapy regimens but may be injured by these unusual dose regimens.

Another application for SBRT in sarcoma management is the treatment of spine tumors and spine metastases, where a conformal distribution is created around the complex shape of the vertebral body while creating a steep dose gradient in the immediate region of the spinal cord. Traditional radiotherapy approaches, in contrast, are usually incapable of delivering effective doses for control of overt sarcomatous lesions without significant danger to the spinal cord. Thus Yamada et al.[416] recently reported on a series of patients with spinal metastases that included ten patients with sarcoma. Radiotherapy was delivered with image guidance in a single fraction of 18 to 24 Gy, and only one patient had progression with 12 months' median follow-up. In another study of SRS for sarcomas involving the spine, ten patients with 16 metastases to the spine (four of which had previously been irradiated) were treated with doses of 20 to 30 Gy in one to five fractions. Local control, evaluated by imaging, was achieved in nine of the ten lesions evaluated, although ultimately three lesions showed slight progression. Complete pain relief was achieved in eight lesions, partial relief in seven, and no relief in only one.[263] All these patients succumbed to disease with a mean survival of 11 months, but none suffered a spinal injury from the use of SRS. These results indicate that specialized radiotherapy approaches of this type may benefit patients with very adverse presentations juxtaposed to the spinal cord.

Finally, classical SRS, which was developed for intracranial lesions, has also been applied to the treatment of sarcoma brain metastasis, with promising palliative control.[417] Among 21 patients with 60 brain metastases, the ultimate local control in the brain, when one factors in salvage SRS as well, was 88%. The median survival was 16 months, with a 1-year survival of 61% and progression-free survival of 51%.[417]

The key to realizing useful palliation for sarcoma patients with radiotherapy is to appreciate the clinical setting and the goals of radiotherapy for that situation. Appropriate selection of patients is important, as is judicious use of the various treatments available, including the choice of radiotherapy mode and, where possible, combinations with surgery or systemic treatments when the indications are present. This may allow more benefit to be realized or, alternatively, a lower dose of radiotherapy to be administered. This is especially important when anatomy is unstable from compression or destruction, making surgery a desirable companion to radiotherapy in the palliation of many patients.

Chemotherapy

Sustained complete responses of sarcomas to chemotherapy are quite unusual, seen perhaps in 1% to 3% of patients. As a result, the vast majority of the systemic therapy delivered to patients with metastatic sarcomas is given with palliative intent. Patients with poor performance status are poor candidates for systemic therapy, as they appear to have more adverse events for a given agent or regimen than more fit patients, and appear to benefit less frequently, again with newly diagnosed GIST being perhaps the exception to this rule. When standard chemotherapy agents are exhausted, there are no data that indicate that continuing any sort of systemic therapy is clinically beneficial, with the exception of imatinib in GIST. The means routinely employed to try to relieve symptoms of terminally ill patients include the use of pain medications orally, transdermally, intravenously, or intrathecally; oxygen as needed; and occasionally glucocorticoids. It is also worth emphasizing what is perhaps obvious but often brushed off in the course of a busy day: that even for very ill patients late in the course of their disease, communication with the patient and family will provide a sense of comfort.

FUTURE DIRECTIONS

Although the optimal combination and sequence of surgery, radiation, and chemotherapy remains controversial for sarcoma, optimal treatment increasingly depends on careful stratification of patients by histologic type and subtype and other important prognostic features. New methods for radiation delivery and tumor sensitization as well as continued advances in surgical reconstructive techniques will enable continued improvements in limb preservation and function as well as local control. However, despite these advances, almost 50% of newly diagnosed sarcoma patients will eventually die from their disease. Metastatic sarcoma, whether at the time of disease presentation or after local control of primary disease, remains an extremely difficult problem. The search for effective agents will be the focus of continuing research for patients with advanced disease. Outside a few responsive subtypes, the currently available chemotherapies have not improved survival and are associated with significant toxicity. Thus, there is a pressing need to develop new therapies based on selectively targeting the proteins and signaling pathways that drive the survival of specific sarcoma types and subtypes. There is already a broad movement to identify and test antiangiogenic agents, specific kinase inhibitors, and novel chemotherapeutic agents such as trabectedin in an endeavor to match specific sarcoma subtypes to novel agents. A long effort to understand insulin-like growth factor-1 receptor signaling may pay off in the near future for pediatric sarcomas as well as a number of other cancers. Trials targeting the cell cycle (CDK4-RB1) and MDM2-p53 signaling pathways are currently under way in well-differentiated and dedifferentiated liposarcoma. Biological data and preclinical studies support trials using inhibitors of Wnt/β-catenin in desmoid fibromatosis, inhibitors of histone deacetylase in synovial sarcoma and Ewing sarcoma, and inhibitors of Hedgehog and Notch signaling in several sarcoma types.

In the longer term, some of the results of gene expression arrays, next-generation sequencing, proteomics, tissue arrays, and mouse models of sarcoma may lead to a more comprehensive and precise determination of key molecular genetic alterations that drive sarcomagenesis for specific sarcoma types and subtypes. This knowledge will improve our ability to design new therapeutics for individual patients and to predict response to such therapy based not only on histologic type and subtype but also on pathway activation in the individual patient.

Because sarcoma is a relatively rare disease, it will be particularly important to conduct clinical trials that select patients based on the up-regulation of a particular protein or signaling pathway, since this will increase the chance that the trial will have positive results.

Some biologic interventions may have promise, such as inhibitory RNA interference strategies or immunotherapy with vaccines, monoclonal antibodies, dendritic cells, or T cells. Vaccines of the characteristic fusion proteins of sarcomas (or peptides thereof) will be tested in the near future for their effectiveness in the appropriate subtypes of sarcoma, such as many pediatric sarcomas. Vaccines that incorporate dendritic cells appear to be effective immunogens in preclinical studies. Preparations of the immunogenic glycolipids found in sarcoma cell membranes may also provide interesting agents for therapy.

Another emerging new class of therapeutics for cancer is nanoscale particles. Advances in nanotechnology have enabled the design of nanoparticles (in the size range 1 to 100 nm) that can interact with biomolecules on both the cell surface and within the cell.[418] Overexpressed cell-surface markers in sarcomas could be targeted to establish the presence of even single-cell metastases and to deliver high-potency chemotherapeutic or molecular agents to the cancer cell. Such selective nanoparticles could be used in the future to deliver antisense oligonucleotides or small interfering RNAs against cellular protein targets critical for sarcoma cell survival.

With an increasing number of molecular signaling pathways being actively investigated, the many new systemic treatments on the horizon, and the advances in selective radiation, drug, and nanoparticle delivery to sarcoma cells, outcomes for sarcoma patients are likely to substantially improve in the coming decade.

Selected References

The full list of references for this chapter appears in the online version.

18. Henderson TO, Whitton J, Stovall M, et al. Secondary sarcomas in childhood cancer survivors: a report from the Childhood Cancer Survivor Study. *J Natl Cancer Inst* 2007;99:300.
22. Gladdy RA, Qin LX, Moraco N, et al. Do radiation-associated soft tissue sarcomas have the same prognosis as sporadic soft tissue sarcomas? *J Clin Oncol* 2010;28:2064.
39. Fletcher CD, Unni KK, Mertens F. Pathology and genetics of tumors of soft tissue and bone. In: Kleihues P, Sobin LH, eds. *World Health Organization classification of tumours*. Lyon, France: IARC Press, 2002.
40. Dalal KM, Kattan MW, Antonescu CR, Brennan MF, Singer S. Subtype specific prognostic nomogram for patients with primary liposarcoma of the retroperitoneum, extremity, or trunk. *Ann Surg* 2006;244:381.
41. Eilber FC, Eilber FR, Eckardt J, et al. The impact of chemotherapy on the survival of patients with high-grade primary extremity liposarcoma. *Ann Surg* 2004;240:686.
43. Singer S, Antonescu CR, Riedel E, Brennan MF. Histologic subtype and margin of resection predict pattern of recurrence and survival for retroperitoneal liposarcoma. *Ann Surg* 2003;238:358.
44. Fletcher CD, Gustafson P, Rydholm A, Willen H, Akerman M. Clinicopathologic re-evaluation of 100 malignant fibrous histiocytomas: prognostic relevance of subclassification. *J Clin Oncol* 2001;19:3045.
53. Stacchiotti S, Negri T, Palassini E, et al. Sunitinib malate and figitumumab in solitary fibrous tumor: patterns and molecular bases of tumor response. *Mol Cancer Ther* 2010;9:1286.
92. Bissler JJ, McCormack FX, Young LR, et al. Sirolimus for angiomyolipoma in tuberous sclerosis complex or lymphangioleiomyomatosis. *N Engl J Med* 2008;358:140.

103. Grosso F, Jones RL, Demetri GD, et al. Efficacy of trabectedin (ecteinascidin-743) in advanced pretreated myxoid liposarcomas: a retrospective study. *Lancet Oncol* 2007;8:595.
105. Maki RG, Wathen JK, Patel SR, et al. Randomized phase II study of gemcitabine and docetaxel compared with gemcitabine alone in patients with metastatic soft tissue sarcomas: results of sarcoma alliance for research through collaboration study 002 [corrected]. *J Clin Oncol* 2007;25:2755.
115. Williamson D, Missiaglia E, de Reynies A, et al. Fusion gene-negative alveolar rhabdomyosarcoma is clinically and molecularly indistinguishable from embryonal rhabdomyosarcoma. *J Clin Oncol* 2010;28:2151.
134. Maki RG, D'Adamo DR, Keohan ML, et al. Phase II study of sorafenib in patients with metastatic or recurrent sarcomas. *J Clin Oncol* 2009;27:3133.
141. Wagner AJ, Malinowska-Kolodziej I, Morgan JA, et al. Clinical activity of mTOR inhibition with sirolimus in malignant perivascular epithelioid cell tumors: targeting the pathogenic activation of mTORC1 in tumors. *J Clin Oncol* 2010;28:835.
146. Ladanyi M, Antonescu CR, Leung DH, et al. Impact of SYT-SSX fusion type on the clinical behavior of synovial sarcoma: a multi-institutional retrospective study of 243 patients. *Cancer Res* 2002;62:135.
181. Guillou L, Coindre JM, Bonichon F, et al. Comparative study of the National Cancer Institute and French Federation of Cancer Centers Sarcoma Group grading systems in a population of 410 adult patients with soft tissue sarcoma. *J Clin Oncol* 1997;15:350.
188. Pisters PW, Leung DH, Woodruff J, Shi W, Brennan MF. Analysis of prognostic factors in 1,041 patients with localized soft tissue sarcomas of the extremities. *J Clin Oncol* 1996;14:1679.
214. Kattan MW, Leung DH, Brennan MF. Postoperative nomogram for 12-year sarcoma-specific death. *J Clin Oncol* 2002;20:791.
216. Canter RJ, Qin LX, Maki RG, et al. A synovial sarcoma-specific preoperative nomogram supports a survival benefit to ifosfamide-based chemotherapy and improves risk stratification for patients. *Clin Cancer Res* 2008;14:8191.
222. Rosenberg SA, Tepper J, Glatstein E, et al. The treatment of soft-tissue sarcomas of the extremities: prospective randomized evaluations of (1) limb-sparing surgery plus radiation therapy compared with amputation and (2) the role of adjuvant chemotherapy. *Ann Surg* 1982;196:305.
223. Pisters PW, Harrison LB, Leung DH, et al. Long-term results of a prospective randomized trial of adjuvant brachytherapy in soft tissue sarcoma. *J Clin Oncol* 1996;14:859.
224. Yang JC, Chang AE, Baker AR, et al. Randomized prospective study of the benefit of adjuvant radiation therapy in the treatment of soft tissue sarcomas of the extremity. *J Clin Oncol* 1998;16:197.
227. Pisters PW, Pollock RE, Lewis VO, et al. Long-term results of prospective trial of surgery alone with selective use of radiation for patients with T1 extremity and trunk soft tissue sarcomas. *Ann Surg* 2007;246:675.
232. O'Sullivan B, Davis AM, Turcotte R, et al. Preoperative versus postoperative radiotherapy in soft-tissue sarcoma of the limbs: a randomised trial. *Lancet* 2002;359:2235.
236. Davis AM, O'Sullivan B, Bell RS, et al. Function and health status outcomes in a randomized trial comparing preoperative and postoperative radiotherapy in extremity soft tissue sarcoma. *J Clin Oncol* 2002;20:4472.
244. Alektiar KM, Brennan MF, Healey JH, Singer S. Impact of intensity-modulated radiation therapy on local control in primary soft-tissue sarcoma of the extremity. *J Clin Oncol* 2008;26:3440.
264. DeLaney TF, Liebsch NJ, Pedlow FX, et al. Phase II study of high-dose photon/proton radiotherapy in the management of spine sarcomas. *Int J Radiat Oncol Biol Phys* 2009;74:732.
281. Adjuvant chemotherapy for localised resectable soft-tissue sarcoma of adults: meta-analysis of individual data. Sarcoma Meta-analysis Collaboration. *Lancet* 1997;350:1647.
284. Frustaci S, Gherlinzoni F, De Paoli A, et al. Adjuvant chemotherapy for adult soft tissue sarcomas of the extremities and girdles: results of the Italian randomized cooperative trial. *J Clin Oncol* 2001;19:1238.
293. Eggermont AM, de Wilt JH, ten Hagen TL. Current uses of isolated limb perfusion in the clinic and a model system for new strategies. *Lancet Oncol* 2003;4:429.
296. Issels RD, Lindner LH, Verweij J, et al. Neo-adjuvant chemotherapy alone or with regional hyperthermia for localised high-risk soft-tissue sarcoma: a randomised phase 3 multicentre study. *Lancet Oncol* 2010;11:561.
322. Park JO, Qin LX, Prete FP, et al. Predicting outcome by growth rate of locally recurrent retroperitoneal liposarcoma: the one centimeter per month rule. *Ann Surg* 2009;250:977.
363. Pautier P, Bui Nguyen N, Penel N, et al. Final results of a FNCLCC French Sarcoma Group multicenter randomized phase II study of gemcitabine (G) versus gemcitabine and docetaxel (G+D) in patients with metastatic or relapsed leiomyosarcoma (LMS). *J Clin Oncol* 2009;27: (abst 10527).
374. Demetri GD, Chawla SP, von Mehren M, et al. Efficacy and safety of trabectedin in patients with advanced or metastatic liposarcoma or leiomyosarcoma after failure of prior anthracyclines and ifosfamide: results of a randomized phase II study of two different schedules. *J Clin Oncol* 2009;27:4188.
392. Gega M, Yanagi H, Yoshikawa R, et al. Successful chemotherapeutic modality of doxorubicin plus dacarbazine for the treatment of desmoid tumors in association with familial adenomatous polyposis. *J Clin Oncol* 2006;24:102.
397. Lazar AJ, Tuvin D, Hajibashi S, et al. Specific mutations in the beta-catenin gene (CTNNB1) correlate with local recurrence in sporadic desmoid tumors. *Am J Pathol* 2008;173:1518.

TABLE 116.1

GENERAL CLASSIFICATION OF BONE TUMORS

Histologic Type[a]	Benign	Malignant
Hematopoietic (41.4%)	—	Myeloma
	—	Reticulum cell sarcoma
Chondrogenic (20.9%)	Osteochondroma	Primary chondrosarcoma
	Chondroma	Secondary chondrosarcoma
	Chondroblastoma	Dedifferentiated chondrosarcoma
	Chondromyxoid fibroma	Mesenchymal chondrosarcoma
Osteogenic (19.3%)	Osteoid osteoma	Osteosarcoma
	Benign osteoblastoma	Parosteal osteogenic sarcoma
Unknown origin (9.8%)	Giant cell tumor	Ewing's tumor
	—	Malignant giant cell tumor
		Adamantinoma
	(Fibrous) histiocytoma	(Fibrous) histiocytoma
Fibrogenic (3.8%)	Fibroma	Fibrosarcoma
	Desmoplastic fibroma	—
Notochordal (3.1%)	—	Chordoma
Vascular (1.6%)	Hemangioma	Hemangioendothelioma
	—	Hemangiopericytoma
Lipogenic (<0.5%)	Lipoma	—
Neurogenic (<0.5%)	Neurilemoma	—

[a]Distribution based on Mayo Clinic experience.
(Adapted from ref. 3.)

High-grade sarcomas have a poorly defined reactive zone that may be invaded and destroyed by the tumor. In addition, tumor nodules in tissue may appear to be normal and not continuous with the main tumor. These are termed *skip metastases*. Although low-grade sarcomas regularly demonstrate tumor interdigitation into the reactive zone, they rarely form tumor nodules beyond this area.

Metastasis

Bone tumors, unlike carcinomas, disseminate almost exclusively through the blood; bones lack a lymphatic system. Early lymphatic spread to regional nodes has only rarely been reported. Lymphatic involvement, which has been noted in 10% of cases at autopsy, is a poor prognostic sign. McKenna et al.[46] noted that 6 of 194 patients (3%) with osteosarcoma who underwent amputation demonstrated lymph node involvement. None of these patients survived 5 years. Hematogenous spread is manifested by pulmonary involvement in its early stage and secondarily by bone involvement. Kager et al.,[47] reporting the findings of the Cooperative German-Austrian-Swiss Osteosarcoma Study Group, found that of 1,765 previously untreated newly diagnosed osteosarcoma patients, 202 (11.4%) had proven metastases at the time of diagnosis—9.3% pulmonary and 3.9% in secondary bony sites.

Skip Metastases

A skip metastasis is a tumor nodule that is located within the same bone as the main tumor but not in continuity with it (Fig. 116.2). Transarticular skip metastases are located in the joint adjacent to the main tumor.[48] Skip metastases are most often seen with high-grade sarcomas. They develop by the

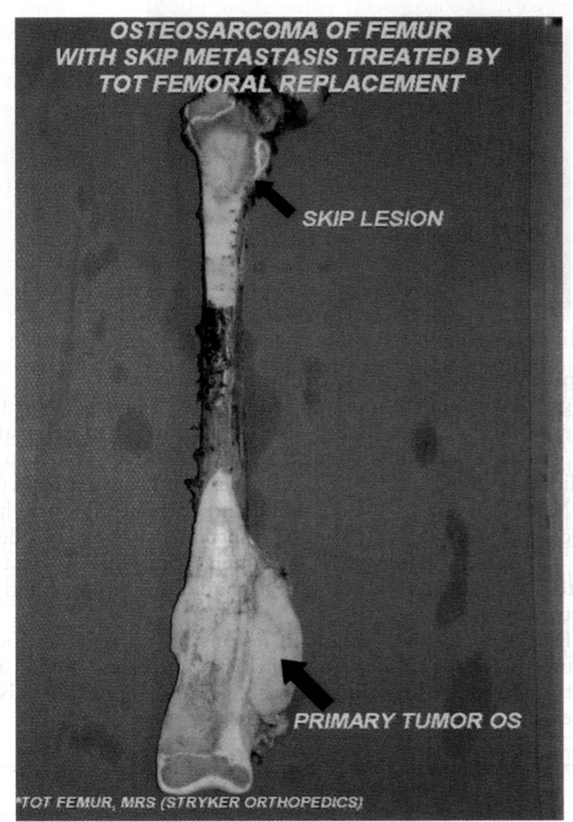

FIGURE 116.2 Gross specimen of a total femur osteosarcoma resection showing the primary tumor (*arrow* in proximal skip lesion). Skip lesions from an osteosarcoma are a poor prognostic finding.

embolization of tumor cells within the marrow sinusoids; in effect, they are local micrometastases that have not passed through the circulation. Transarticular skips are believed to occur via the periarticular venous anastomosis. The clinical incidence of skip metastases is less than 1%. These lesions are a prognosticator of poor survival.[48,49] Wuisman and Enneking[50] reviewed 23 cases with histologically proven skip metastases. Eleven patients received adjuvant chemotherapy. In 22 of the 23 patients, either local recurrence or distant metastases developed within 16 months of surgery. The authors compared the clinical course of these patients with that of 224 individuals without skip lesions. The overall survival rate of patients with skips was comparable to that of those with metastatic (stage III) disease. The authors concluded that patients with skip metastases should be classified as stage III and should be excluded from ongoing therapy trials.

Local Recurrence

Local recurrence of a malignant lesion is due to inadequate removal. Ninety-five percent of all local recurrences, regardless of histology, develop within 24 months of attempted removal. Local recurrence of a high-grade sarcoma was once thought to be independent of overall survival. Today, a local recurrence is believed to represent an inherent biologic aggressiveness and a tendency to metastasize; that is, *tumors that tend to metastasize are those that are likely to recur locally.* Local recurrence in patients who have undergone therapy is associated with an even poorer prognosis.[51]

STAGING BONE TUMORS

Musculoskeletal Tumor Society Classification

Currently there are two staging systems for bone sarcomas. The Musculoskeletal Tumor Society (MSTS) surgical staging system (three tier) and a modification that is recommended by the American Joint Committee on Cancer (AJCC). The AJCC system was modified and created to be consistent with their overall staging (four tier) system for all cancers.

In 1980 the MSTS adopted the first surgical staging system for bone sarcomas. Within their system G represents the histologic grade of a lesion and other clinical data. Grade is further divided into two categories: G1 is low grade, and G2 is high grade. T represents the site of the lesion, which may be intracompartmental (T1) or extracompartmental (T2). Compartment is defined as an anatomic structure or space bounded by natural barriers or tumor extension. The significance of T1 lesions is easier to define clinically, surgically, and radiographically than that of T2 lesions, and the chance is better for adequate removal of the former without amputation. In general, low-grade bone sarcomas are intracompartmental (T1), whereas high-grade sarcomas are extracompartmental (T2).

Lymphatic spread is a sign of widespread dissemination. Regional lymphatic involvement is equated with distal metastases (M1). Absence of any metastasis is designated as M0.

The surgical staging system developed by Enneking et al.[45] for surgical planning and assessment of bone sarcomas is summarized as follows:

- Stage IA (G1, T1, M0): Low-grade intracompartmental lesion, without metastasis
- Stage IB (G1, T2, M0): Low-grade extracompartmental lesion, without metastasis
- Stage IIA (G2, T1, M0): High-grade intracompartmental lesion, without metastasis
- Stage IIB (G2, T2, M0): High-grade extracompartmental lesion, without metastasis
- Stage IIIA (G1 or G2, T1, M1): Intracompartmental lesion, any grade, with metastasis
- Stage IIIB (G1 or G2, T2, M1): Extracompartmental lesion, any grade, with metastasis

Figure 116.3 summarizes 465 patients treated over 30 years with various bone tumors at the University of California–Los Angeles and classified by Enneking's classification system.[52]

American Joint Committee on Cancer Bone Tumor Classification

In 1983 the AJCC Bone Tumor Classification recommended a staging system for the malignant tumors of bone. The 2002 TNM (tumor, node, metastases) classification contains substantial modifications from previous editions (Tables 116.2 and 116.3).

Figure 116.3 shows the long-term survival rates using this new AJCC staging system. It is important to note that there is no significant difference between stage IA and IB and IIA and IIB. There is a significant difference between stage I, II, and III.

The AJCC staging system is applicable to all primary malignant tumors of bone except multiple myeloma, malignant lymphoma (both having different natural history), and juxtacortical osteosarcoma and chondrosarcoma (both with much more favorable prognosis). Most cancer registries will likely use the AJCC system, at the present time most orthopedic oncologists tend to use the MSTS classification. It is necessary to specify which system is being used in discussions and when presenting data.

PREOPERATIVE RADIOGRAPHIC EVALUATION

If the plain radiographs suggest an aggressive or malignant tumor, staging studies should be performed before biopsy. All radiographic studies are influenced by surgical manipulation of the lesion, making interpretation more difficult. More important, the biopsy site may be in a location that is not optimal for subsequent *en bloc* removal or radiotherapy.[53–55] Bone scintigraphy, MRI, CT, angiography, or a combination of these is required to delineate local tumor extent, vascular displacement, and compartmental localization (Fig. 116.4). MRI angiography and CT angiography have more recently obviated the need for traditional angiography (unless embolization is being considered). More recently, positron emission tomography (PET) imaging has been used in both detection of nonpulmonary metastatic sites as well as when attempting to determine the tumor response (percentage of tumor necrosis) following induction or neoadjuvant chemotherapy. Systematic staging includes a three-phase bone scan (looking for bony metastases) and chest CT (to determine the absence or presence of pulmonary metastases). Evaluation of regional lymph nodes, the abdomen, or the pelvis is not necessary.

Bone Scans

Bone scintigraphy helps determine polyostotic involvement and metastatic disease. Malignant bone tumors, although solitary, may in rare cases (less than 5%) present with skeletal metastasis. Skip metastases are rarely detected by bone scan

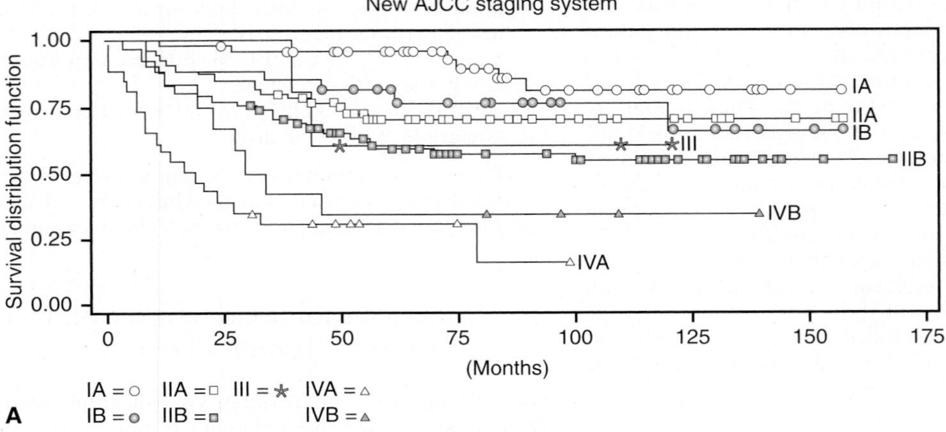

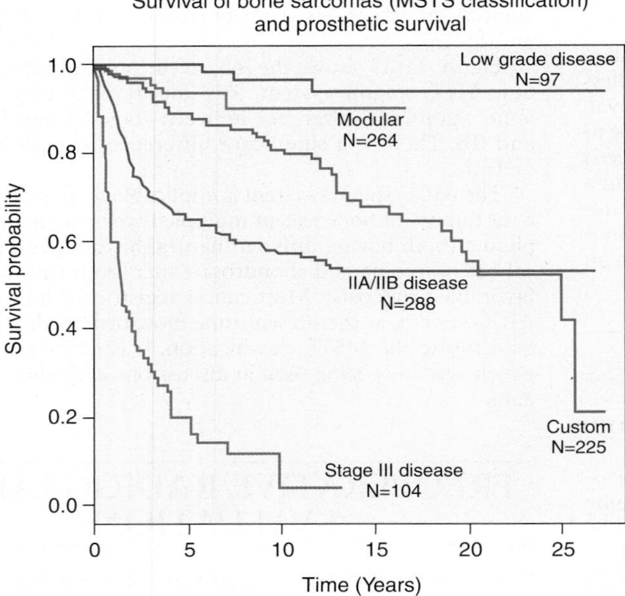

FIGURE 116.3 Long-term survival rates of patients with bone sarcoma according to (**A**) the new AJCC staging system and (**B**) the Musculoskeletal Tumor Society classification system. (From ref. 200.)

because they are small and localized to the fatty marrow and do not excite cortical response.[48,49,56,57]

Three-phase bone scans (flow, pool, and late phase) are necessary to completely evaluate a bony tumor. Pre- and postchemotherapy bone scans can be compared only when identical areas of the scan are evaluated. To eliminate uncontrolled variations in technique, the method of determining the tumor-to-nontumor ratio of uptake is important. This ratio is obtained for each of the three phases. The flow and pool phases indicate tumor vascularity, whereas the late phase is a sign of bone formation (osteoblastic activity).

Computed Tomography

CT allows accurate determination of intra- and extraosseous extension of skeletal neoplasms.[58–61] It accurately depicts the transverse relationship of a tumor. By varying window settings, one can study cortical bone, intramedullary space, adjacent muscles, and extraosseous soft tissue extension. CT should include the entire bone and the adjacent joint. Infusion of intravenous contrast material allows identification of the adjacent large vascular structures. CT evaluation must be individualized. Three-dimensional reconstruction may be useful in surgical planning. Today, CT and MRI are considered complementary studies for bone sarcomas. *Both* studies are recommended for most patients. Pulmonary CT is routinely performed to determine the presence of pulmonary disease; approximately 11% of all newly diagnosed patients with osteosarcoma have pulmonary metastases.[47] CT angiography (noninvasive) has become increasingly popular using the newer and faster CT scanners. CT angiography has replaced the traditional angiography to evaluate the major vessels and anomalies and to determine the vasculature anatomy (e.g., the popliteal trifurcation).

Magnetic Resonance Imaging and Staging

MRI has several advantages in the diagnoses of bone sarcomas. It has better contrast discrimination than any other modality; furthermore, imaging can be performed in any plane. MRI is ideal for imaging the medullary marrow and thus for detection of tumor as well as the extraosseous component. MRIs should be performed in all three planes with and without contrast prior to surgery. It has proven especially helpful in several heretofore

TABLE 116.2

AMERICAN JOINT COMMITTEE ON CANCER STAGING FOR BONE AND SOFT TISSUE SARCOMAS

PRIMARY TUMOR
- T1: ≤5 cm
  - T1a: superficial
  - T1b: deep
- T2: >5 cm
  - T2a: superficial
  - T2b: deep

REGIONAL LYMPH NODES
- N0: no
- N1: yes

DISTANT METASTASES
- M0: none
- M1: yes

GRADE
- AJCC now recommends a three-tier system. The FNCLCC (French) system is the preferred grading system.

STAGE GROUPING
- IA: T1a/b N0 G1—low grade (grade 1), small
- IB: T2a/b N0 G1—low grade (grade 1), large
- IIA: T1a/b N0 G2–G3—moderate/high grade (grade 2–3), small
- IIB: T2a/b N0 G2—moderate grade (grade 2), large
- III: T2a/b G3, or N1—high grade (grade 3), large; or node positive
- IV: M1—metastatic

CHANGES FROM AJCC 6TH EDITION
- Now incorporates a three-tiered grading system. For staging, there is now a distinction between G2 and G3, at least for tumors >5 cm.
- N1 is now stage III instead of stage IV
- Stage I is divided into IA and IB. Stage II is divided into IIA and IIB.
- Deep or superficial location of tumor no longer is a factor in overall stage

Notes
- This staging system does not apply to Kaposi's sarcoma, gastrointestinal stromal tumor (now staged with its own classification), fibromatosis (desmoid tumor), and infantile fibrosarcoma; and does not apply to sarcomas arising in the dura mater or brain, parenchymal organs, and hollow viscera.
- Now includes dermatofibrosarcoma protuberans (which was previously excluded), angiosarcoma, and extraskeletal Ewing's sarcoma
- Superficial—located entirely in the subcutaneous tissues without any degree of involvement of the muscular fascia or underlying muscle

From Edge SB, Byrd DR, Compton CC, et al. eds. *AJCC cancer staging manual*, 7th ed. New York: Springer, 2010.

difficult clinical situations, such as detecting small lesions, evaluating a positive bone scan when the corresponding plain radiograph is negative, determining the extent of infiltrative tumors, and detecting skip metastases.[62–68] Recently, the use of dynamic MRI has been utilized to determine and predict the amount (percentage) of tumor necrosis prior to surgery. There are several proposed algorithms, and this technique remains to be validated by more and larger studies.

TABLE 116.3

NEW MODIFICATIONS TO AMERICAN JOINT COMMITTEE ON CANCER STAGING FOR BONE SARCOMAS

T1 has changed from "Tumor confined within the cortex" to "Tumor 8 cm or less in greatest dimension."

T2 has changed from "Tumor invades beyond the cortex" to "Tumor more than 8 cm in greatest dimension."

T3 designation of skip metastasis is defined as "Discontinuous tumors in the primary bone site." This designation is a Stage III tumor that was not previously defined.

M1 lesions have been divided into M1a and M1b. M1a is lung-only metastases.

M1b is metastases to other distant sites, including lymph nodes. In the stage grouping, stage IVA is M1a, and stage IVB is M1b.

From ref. 200.

Angiography/Computed Tomography, Angiography, and Magnetic Resonance Imaging/Angiography

Traditional angiography has been used to determine the relation of the major vessels to the tumor.[69] Because experience with limb-sparing procedures has increased, it has become essential to determine individual vascular patterns in relationship to the tumor before resection. This is especially crucial for tumors of the proximal tibia, where vascular anomalies are common. CT/angiography and MRI/angiography have largely replaced traditional angiography. They provide accurate vascular anatomic visualization as well as three-dimensional relationship to the tumor in axial, coronal, and sagittal planes. The major advantage of traditional angiography remains its ability to determine residual tumor vascularity, which correlates well with chemotherapy-induced necrosis. This cannot be determined by either CT/- or MRI/angiography (Fig. 116.5).

Positron Emission Tomography

The use of [^{18}F]fluorodeoxy-D-glucose (FDG)-PET (for bony and pulmonary evaluation) is one of the newer techniques to evaluate the local and distal extents of cancers. Today, there has been increasingly positive although conflicting data on the role of PET with respect to diagnosis, imaging, staging, therapy, monitoring, and follow-up for osteosarcomas. These studies show that PET imaging is not accurate in determining pulmonary

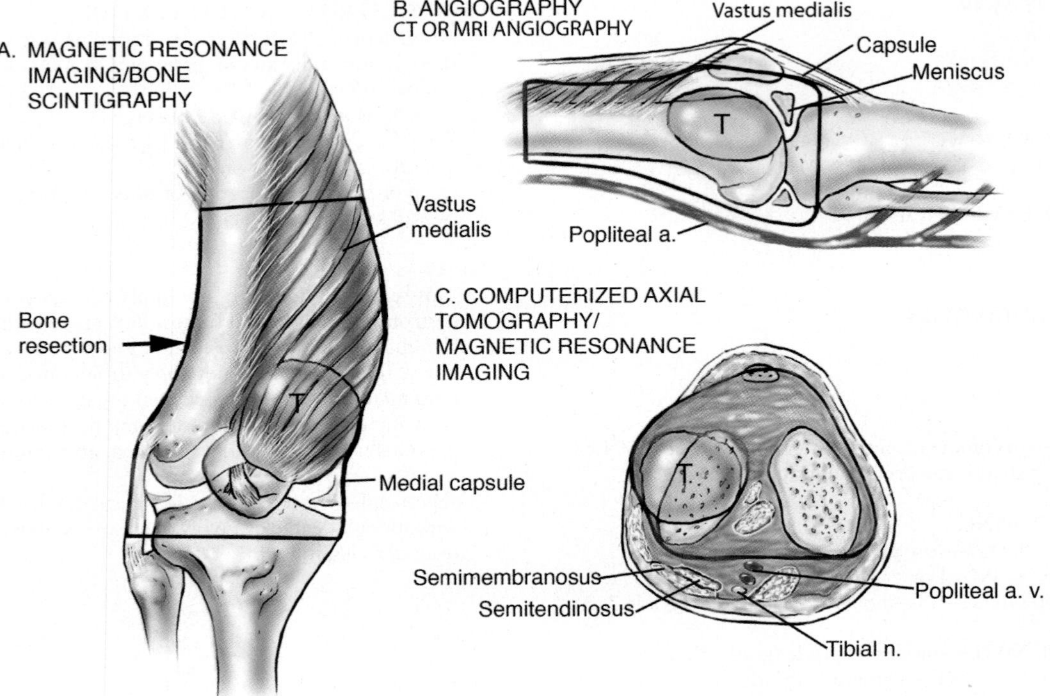

FIGURE 116.4 Schematic of imaging studies. This shows the relationship between computed tomography (CT), magnetic resonance imaging, bone scan, angiography, and three-dimensional CT/angiography for a typical overall survival of the distal femur. All of these studies are necessary in order to determine the anatomical involvement of the tumor (see text for other studies).

metastases. Investigations of the effectiveness of PET imaging in determining tumor response to chemotherapy are under way in several institutions.[70–75]

Franzius et al.[76] evaluated the use of FDG-PET for the detection of osseous metastases from malignant primary tumors, specifically osteosarcoma and Ewing's sarcoma, and compared these findings with bone scintigraphy. PET scans were analyzed with regard to osseous metastasis in comparison to bone scintigraphy. They reported that for osteosarcomas, FDG-PET scans were less reliable than bone scintigraphy; in fact, none of the

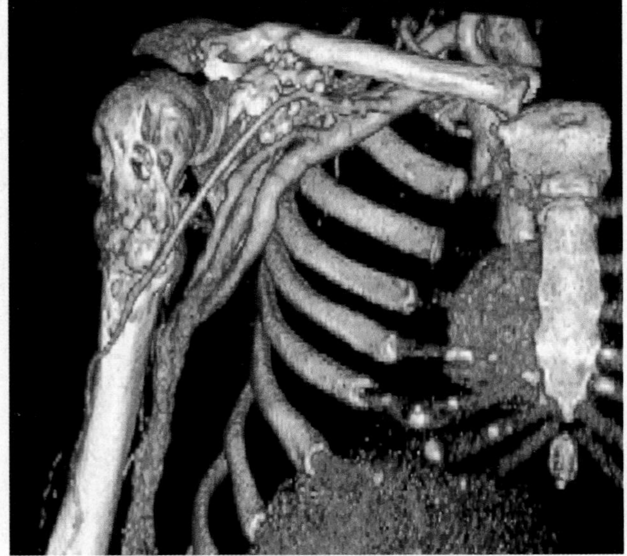

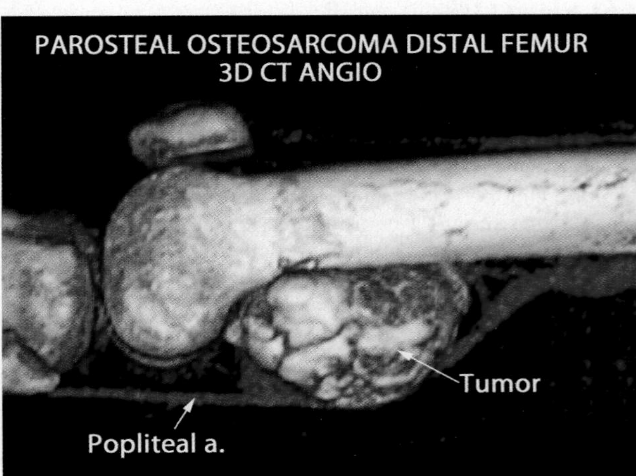

FIGURE 116.5 **A:** Three-dimensional computed tomography/angiogram of distal femur. **B:** Large parosteal osteosarcoma of the distal femur displacing the popliteal artery.

five metastases from osteosarcomas was detected by FDG-PET, although all were true positive on bone scan. In comparison, Ewing's sarcomas were more accurately identified.

Kneisl et al.[72] found only 1 of 38 (2.6%) of patients with osteosarcoma was upstaged with PET alone, although for Ewing's sarcoma 3 of 17 (18%) were upstaged.

BIOPSY TECHNIQUE AND TIMING

The biopsy of a suspected bone tumor must be performed with great care and skill.[54,55] This principle cannot be overemphasized. The consequences of a poorly executed biopsy are often the deciding factor in the choice between a limb-salvage procedure and amputation. Ayala et al.,[77,78] from the M. D. Anderson Cancer Center, determined that only 19% of patients referred to that institution for treatment of primary bone sarcomas had properly placed biopsies. All of these patients had open (incisional) biopsies, whereas 92% of such procedures performed at the M. D. Anderson Cancer Center over the same period were needle biopsies. It is recommended that the biopsy be performed in conjunction with the surgeon who will make the ultimate decision about the operative procedure. Core needle (not fine-needle aspiration) biopsies are performed by an interventional radiologist in conjunction with the orthopedic oncologist. This entails referring some patients who are strongly suspected of having primary bone malignancies to a regional cancer center for the biopsy.

RESTAGING AFTER INDUCTION (PREOPERATIVE) CHEMOTHERAPY

With the advent of induction (preoperative) chemotherapy for osteosarcoma, a need has developed for serial evaluation of the clinical and radiographic response of the tumor before surgery. The staging and preoperative clinical studies previously described are used to evaluate tumor response. These studies have been summarized elsewhere.[79–85] Complete restaging studies should be obtained after the completion of induction chemotherapy. MRI, CT, three-dimensional CT/angiogram, bone scan (three phases), and angiography should be evaluated before a final surgical decision is made. A fusion PET-CT, especially a dynamic study, may be useful.

Clinical Evaluation

Pain often decreases after induction chemotherapy. Alkaline phosphatase (AP) levels also decrease. The tumor shrinks, especially if a significant matrix is not present. Conversely, increase of pain, elevated AP values, and increasing tumor size are signs of tumor progression. Interestingly, Ueda et al.[86] reported that a change in size for bone sarcomas was a valid predictor of response to induction chemotherapy, whereas it was not for soft tissue sarcomas. Similarly, Liu et al.[87] (Peking University) reported in a multivariate analysis that tumor necrosis was related to change in tumor volume and level of AP.

Plain Radiography

A good correlation is found between radiographic response and the amount of necrosis. Smith et al.[84] described the radiographic responses seen on serial radiographs: increased ossification of tumor osteoid, marked thickening and new bone formation of the periosteum and tumor border (giving the tumor a more "benign" appearance), and decreased soft tissue mass. The healing ossification is usually solid, homogeneous, and regular and is easily differentiated from tumor osteoid. Less significant changes take place within the intramedullary component, which may include increased sclerosis and lysis, presumably caused by necrosis and hemorrhage.

Angiography

After chemotherapy, vascularity decreases markedly. Chuang et al.[81] evaluated 53 patients and reported that those with a complete angiographic response had more than 90% necrosis; among those with a partial response, necrosis ranged from 40% to 78%. They concluded that angiographic evaluation was as reliable as pathologic evaluation, and that the angiographic features were the best clinical criteria for the evaluation of tumor response. Carrasco et al.,[82] from the M. D. Anderson Cancer Center, reported on their extensive experience with intraarterial chemotherapy for osteosarcoma (81 patients) and evaluated the angiographic appearance and changes after two and four cycles of preoperative chemotherapy. They developed a simple radiographic system for angiographic changes. They reported that 40% of the histologic responders (more than 90% tumor necrosis) and 91% of nonresponders were identified after two cycles. These authors conclude that the disappearance of tumor vascularity after two courses of chemotherapy was highly suggestive of a good histologic response and was unlikely to occur in the histologic nonresponders.

Computed Tomography

The most consistent finding in patients who respond to therapy is a decrease in soft tissue mass and the development of a rimlike calcification similar to that seen on plain radiographs. Changes in marrow are not helpful in evaluating response.

Tumors with significant matrix, osteoid, or cartilage will not necessarily shrink, although the cellular component will undergo necrosis. Therefore, change in size alone for an osteosarcoma is only significant for the poorly mineralized, soft tissue component—the least differentiated component (Fig. 116.6).

Bone Scintigraphy

Bone scan changes are difficult to evaluate. A decrease in activity generally indicates a favorable response; however, reparative bone formation, signaled by increased activity, may be misleading. Dynamic (quantitative) bone scans, which are based on tumor blood flow and regional plasma clearance by bone and soft tissue, may allow more valid evaluations.[85] Regions that show a greater than 20% decrease in technetium-99m-methylene diphosphonate plasma clearance are reported to be associated with necrotic tumor.

Magnetic Resonance Imaging

Monitoring of neoadjuvant chemotherapy by MRI has become the focus of many studies. Holscher et al.[88] evaluated 57 patients at the University Hospital of Leiden. T1- and T2-weighted images were obtained in longitudinal, coronal or sagittal, and axial planes. The authors conclude that increased tumor volume or increased or unchanged peritumoral edema and inflammation indicated a poor response. Subjective criteria, such as improved tumor demarcation or an increase in size of area of low signal intensity (presumably necrotic tumor), were independent of tumor response. The authors concluded that subjective criteria could not predict the good responders.

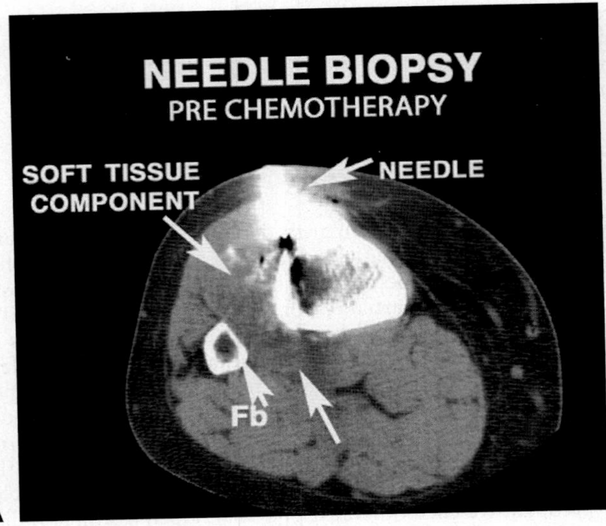

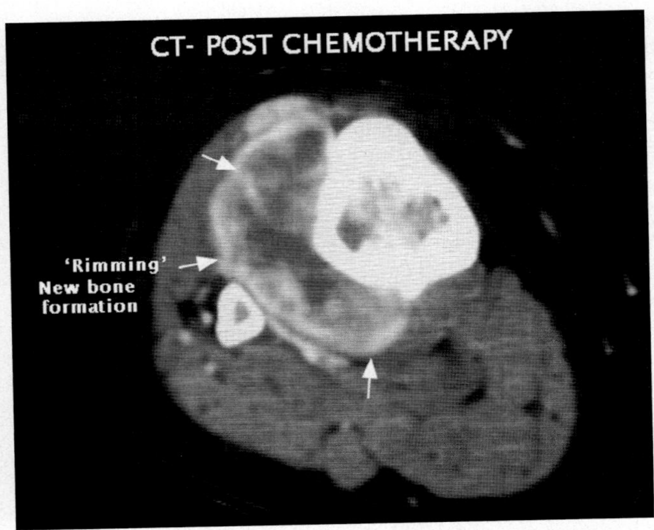

FIGURE 116.6 Pre- and postoperative computed tomography scans of a proximal tibial osteosarcoma. **A:** Prechemotherapy. There is an extraosseous soft tissue mass that has destroyed the underlying lateral cortex of the tibia (*arrows*). **B:** Postchemotherapy. The extraosseous soft tissue component shows reossification and "rimming" of new bone formation. Reossification of an extraosseous mass is a very good prognostic sign of tumor necrosis.

Positron Emission Tomography

PET scans are nuclear medicine scintigraphy techniques that use FDG-PET to measure glycolysis of a tumor. This technique is under investigation. It is hoped that it will be able to metabolically evaluate tumor viability and the percentage of tumor necrosis after chemotherapy. Franzius et al.[89] reported that good responders could be distinguished from poor responders in all cases in which there was a decrease in the tumor-to-nontumor ratio of greater than 30%.

FDG-PET scans are currently being evaluated at many institutions in order to predict, metabolically, which patients are at a higher risk of developing metastatic disease as well as a predictor of response to induction (neoadjuvant) chemotherapy. Cheon et al.,[73] in one of the largest studies to date, evaluated 70 patients with osteosarcoma. Using standard uptake value (SUV) as the guide, SUV1 is the maximum of the tumor prior to receiving chemotherapy and SUV2 is the value following induction chemotherapy. They reported that SUV2 was an independent predictor of tumor response, whereas SUV1 was not. They reported an SUV2 of less than 2 and greater than 5 corresponded to a good and poor response, respectively.

GUIDELINES FOR LIMB-SPARING RESECTION

Limb salvage surgery, in some cases involving the use of cryosurgery[90–94], is a safe operation for appropriately selected patients.[94–96] The surgical guidelines and technique of limb-sparing surgery used by the surgical author (MMM) are as follows (Fig. 116.7):

1. No major neurovascular tumor involvement;
2. Wide resection of the affected bone, with a normal muscle cuff in all directions;
3. *En bloc* removal of all previous biopsy sites and potentially contaminated tissue;
4. Resection of bone 3 to 4 cm beyond abnormal uptake, as determined by CT or MRI and bone scan;
5. Resection of the adjacent joint and capsule;
6. Adequate motor reconstruction, accomplished by regional muscle transfers. Soft tissue coverage should be adequate.

TYPES OF SKELETAL RECONSTRUCTION

Large skeletal defects are reconstructed after tumor resection by several different modalities. Osteoarticular defects are most often reconstructed by segmental, modular prostheses that are fixed to the remaining intramedullary bone by polymethylmethacrylate (PMMA) or press fixation. The newer knee prostheses allow rotation as well as flexion and extension. This mobility decreases the forces on the bone–cement interface and thus reduces the risk of loosening.

Increasing interest has been shown in applying a porous coating to the prosthesis in the hope of obtaining long-term, perhaps even permanent, fixation.[44,97,98] In addition, titanium, an alloy with superior metallurgic properties, has been introduced for prosthesis use. Modular endoprosthetic replacement systems that can be assembled in the operating room are now available and avoid the problem of long delays for custom manufacturing. Alternative methods of segmental replacement include large allografts or osteoarticular allografts that may replace the affected joint.[98,99] Composite allograft (i.e., allograft placed over a prosthesis) has also been used. Today, most large cancer centers in the United States favor the use of endoprosthetic implants for high-grade bone sarcomas. Long-term results of allograft survival in this group of patients have been extremely disappointing.

Contraindications to Limb-Sparing Surgery

Major Neurovascular Involvement

Although vascular grafts can be used, the adjacent nerves are usually at risk, making successful resection less likely. In addition, the magnitude of resection in combination with vascular reconstruction is often prohibitive.

Pathologic Fractures

A fracture through a bone affected by a tumor spreads tumor cells via the hematoma beyond accurately determined limits. The risk of local recurrence increases under such circumstances. If a pathologic fracture heals after neoadjuvant

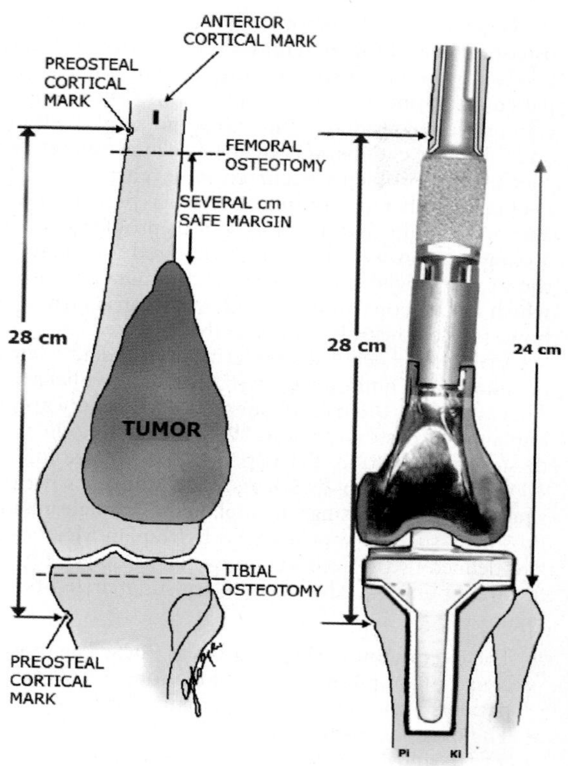

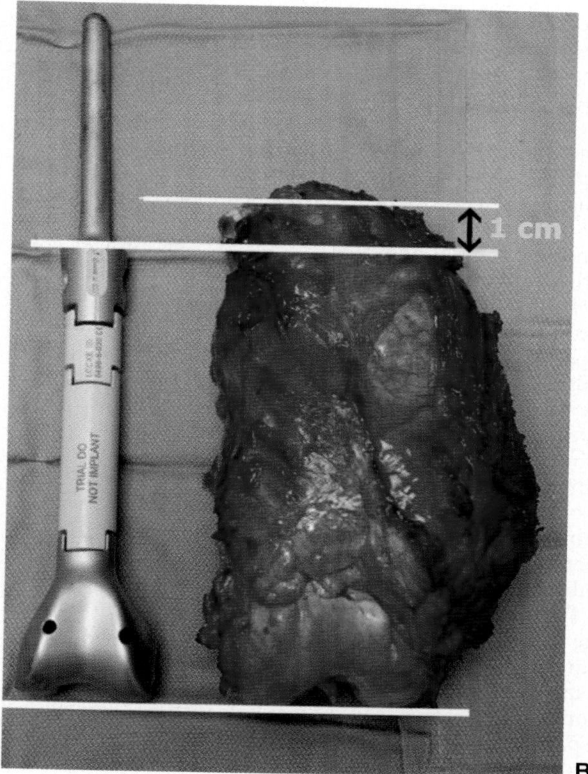

FIGURE 116.7 Resection of a distal femoral osteosarcoma. **A:** Schematic diagram of the distal femoral resection and the corresponding modular prosthetic replacement. **B:** Composite photograph of a modular prosthetic replacement and the resected portion of the distal femur (From ref. 52, with permission.))

chemotherapy, a limb-salvage procedure can be performed successfully.

Inappropriate Biopsy Sites

An inappropriate or poorly planned biopsy jeopardizes local tumor control by contaminating normal tissue planes and compartments.

The risk of infection after implantation of a metallic device or an allograft in an infected area is prohibitive.

The predicted leg-length discrepancy should not be greater than 6 to 8 cm, although expandable prostheses have been used with success in this situation. Upper extremity reconstruction is independent of skeletal maturity.

Enough muscle must remain to reconstruct a functional extremity.

Management Following Inappropriate Surgery for a Benign Tumor

A common problem often seen in major oncology centers is the patient with a sarcoma treated as a benign tumor with an inappropriate surgical procedure. In general, these patients have been treated by an amputation with the assumption that amputation offered the highest survival and local control rate.

Jeon et al.[100] reported their results of 25 patients (22 osteosarcoma) with high-grade primary bone sarcomas who underwent unplanned intralesional procedures and then were treated with adjuvant chemotherapy and limb-sparing surgery. Surprisingly, they showed a 5-year continuous disease-free survival rate of 65% for the 22 osteosarcoma patients. Their indications for limb-sparing procedures included a good response to the induction chemotherapy with attainable negative surgical margins. The relevant contraindications to limb-sparing surgery were cases of pathological fracture and extensive operative procedures.

LIMB-SPARING SURGERY AND PERIOPERATIVE PAIN MANAGEMENT

Pain after extensive limb-sparing resections of bone is severe, and patients require large amounts of narcotics. Pain after amputations in young people is especially difficult to control. Within the past decade, there has been increased interest in managing postoperative pain by various modalities in addition to the standard patient-controlled analgesia (PCA). Patients who have preoperative pain are more difficult to treat adequately and are at a higher risk of postoperative pain syndromes than are those with no preoperative pain.

The aim of postoperative pain management is to eliminate or greatly attenuate pain. The use of multiple modalities is routine. Epidural anesthesia (with or without patient control), an intravenous PCA, and a regional block are ideal.

Quality-of-Life Considerations: Limb-Sparing Surgery versus Amputation

During the 1990s, as the techniques of limb-sparing surgery were being developed, it had been assumed that such surgery was superior to amputation. Nonetheless, when complications occurred, many surgeons thought that an amputation might have been preferable. Despite the extensive literature on the various chemotherapy regimens, surgical techniques, and limb-sparing surgery, few studies have focused on the patients' evaluation of their overall quality of life.

Greenberg et al.[101] from Massachusetts General Hospital and the Children's Hospital/Dana-Farber Cancer Institute evaluated 62 osteosarcoma survivors at a mean of 12 years from diagnosis. These patients responded to a comprehensive battery of psychological questions. In general, most survivors were in good mental and physical health. The authors conclude that attention to the management of depression, treatment of substance abuse, and help with financial difficulties could contribute to the quality of life of patients who undergo limb-sparing surgery or amputation. Pain management, physical and vocational rehabilitation, and sexual counseling may also be beneficial, as may psychotherapeutic counseling.

Christ et al.[102] evaluated the long-term psychosocial effects of limb-sparing surgery and primary amputation for coping capacity and the degree of psychopathology. The overall incidence of emotional disturbance among these patients was no different from that in the general population. Unlike patients in other studies, those in the group with initial amputations had substantial difficulty maintaining an optimal functioning level. Their difficulty was even greater than that of limb-salvage patients with a compromised outcome, including those with late amputation.

Despite good social support scores, the amputees had higher psychopathology scores than did patients who had undergone limb-sparing procedures. The authors conclude that patients undergoing primary amputation need more intensive support than those whose limbs are spared. They recommend an overall approach similar to that for posttraumatic stress disorder.

Clinical Analysis of Limb-Sparing Surgery

Rougraff et al.[103] evaluated 227 patients with nonmetastatic osteosarcoma of the distal femur treated at 26 institutions. They reported 8 local recurrences in 73 patients (11%) with a limb-salvage procedure and 9 local recurrences in 115 patients (8%) who had an above-knee amputation. No local recurrences were reported in the 39 patients who had a hip disarticulation.

Bacci et al.[104] retrospectively evaluated 540 patients treated over 10 years in three multicenter studies with 63 participating institutions. The rate of local recurrence was 8% for patients with a poor histologic response and 3% for those with a good histologic response. A limb-sparing procedure was performed on 84% of the 540 cases evaluated, with a local recurrence rate of 6%. The most important determinant of local recurrence was the type of surgical margin and the response to chemotherapy. Of the 540 patients, 31 had a local recurrence. The overall outcome of this group was extremely poor. All local recurrences were accompanied by metastases, and despite treatment, only one patient remains alive (3%). Local recurrence did not correlate with patient age, gender, histologic type, site and volume, pathologic fracture incidence, chemotherapy, or type of surgical procedure.

Prosthesis Survival, Limb Salvage, and Complications

Prosthetic replacement is commonly used for reconstruction after resection of the proximal humerus, proximal femur, distal femur, and proximal tibia. Several studies have evaluated the long-term results, prosthetic survivorship, and complications associated with prosthetic replacement.

Ruggieri et al.[105] reported on 144 cases of nonmetastatic osteosarcoma of the extremities treated with neoadjuvant chemotherapy and limb-sparing surgery. Sixty-three percent of the patients had one or more complications. Twenty-eight complications were considered minor (i.e., no surgery was required), and 77 complications were major. The infection rate was 6.2%. Mechanical problems occurred in seven patients (5%). The average number of complications per patient was 1.3. The authors thought that the most serious problems resulting from a complication were those that required the delay of chemotherapy or deviation from the recommended dose, either of which could jeopardize survival. Such consequences were not, however, demonstrable statistically.

A recent and detailed long-term survival data study for endoprosthesis and limb-salvage was reported by Shehadeh et al.[106] They analyzed the overall survival and complications of 241 implants (50 custom, prior to 1988) and 191 modular endoprosthesis (after 1988) in 231 patients. The average follow-up was 10 years (range, 5 to 26.8 years). This study was performed at a single institution using an implant by a single manufacturer. Prosthetic survival was analyzed by Kaplan-Meier method and was defined by the need to remove the prosthesis for any reason or an amputation. Their results are summarized below and in Figure 116.8:

- The overall limb-salvage rate was 90%. The most common cause of amputation was infection; 67% (16 of the 24 patients) and one-third (7 patients) for local recurrence.
- The overall prosthetic survival of the modular prosthesis at 5 years and 10 years by anatomic site were distal femur 81% and 70%; proximal tibia 79% and 63%; proximal femur 100% and 100%; and proximal humerus 87% and 78%.
- The overall infection rate was 13% (31 of 241).
- The implant failure rate was 29% (70 of 241 patients). The median implant survival was 189.9 months. Patients undergoing only one procedure was 59% (137 of 231). The remaining 41% (95 patients) had 242 additional procedures.

Cost of Limb-Sparing Surgery versus Amputation

The question of the cost effectiveness of limb-salvage surgery for bone tumors has arisen in the face of managed care, especially within the United States. The only published report on this subject is by Grimer et al.[107] who compared the cost of a limb-sparing procedure in lieu of an amputation at the Royal Orthopaedic Hospital in Birmingham, England. They developed a formula for the cost of the limb-salvage procedure versus an above-knee amputation with subsequent prosthetic replacement over the predicted lifetime of the patient. They concluded the savings for an average patient undergoing a limb-sparing surgery over a 20-year period to be approximately 70,000 British pounds (at 1977 prices), which is approximately six times the cost of the original limb-sparing procedure. This equation can be used for any method of limb-salvage procedure.

The surprising feature of these findings is the considerable cost of amputation. A new prosthesis is required at regular intervals. With the increasing complexity of artificial limbs, it is likely that the maintenance cost following an amputated extremity will increase. There have not been any comparable data from the United States.

AMPUTATIONS

An amputation provides definitive surgical treatment in patients in whom a limb-sparing resection is not a prudent option. Approximately 10% to 15% of patients still require

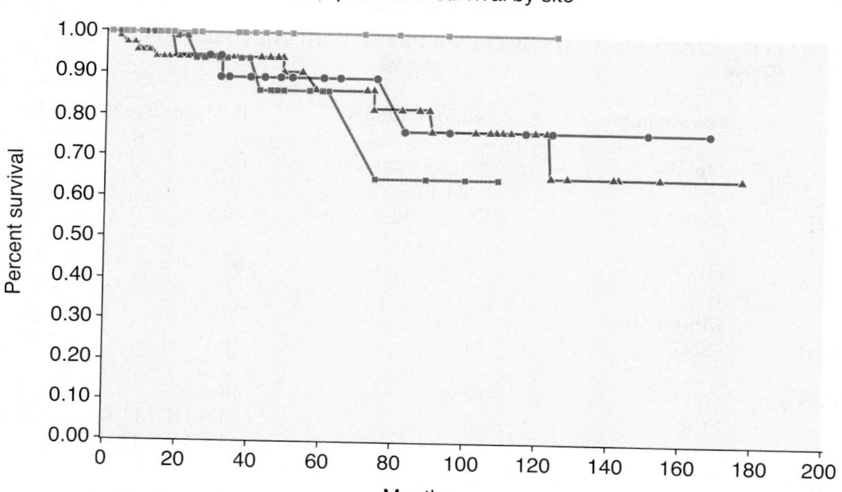

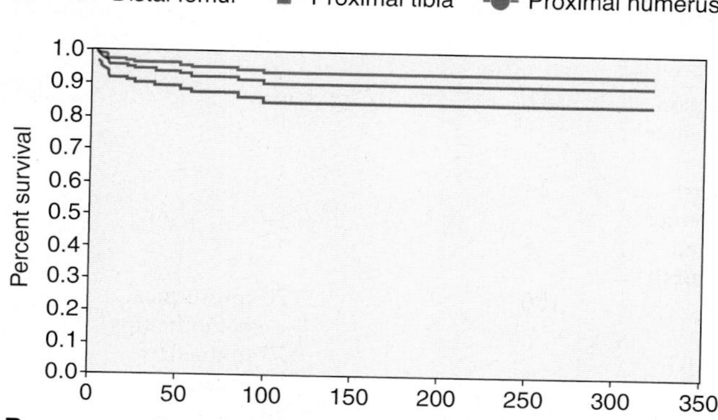

FIGURE 116.8 Kaplan-Meier curves. **A:** Prosthetic survival for all anatomic sites. **B:** Overall limb survival in months for all patients. (From ref. 106.)

amputation, despite the advent of limb-sparing surgery. In contrast to amputations performed for noncancer causes, amputations for cancer tend to be at a more proximal anatomic level, to occur in younger people (reflecting the incidence of bone sarcomas), and to be technically more difficult. The resultant psychological and cosmetic losses are also more substantial.[108]

CHEMOTHERAPY FOR BONE SARCOMAS

Before routine use of systemic chemotherapy for the therapy of osteosarcoma, fewer than 20% of patients survived more than 5 years. Further, recurrent disease developed in 50% of patients, almost exclusively in the lungs, within 6 months of surgical resection. The findings of two randomized clinical studies completed in the 1980s comparing surgery alone to surgery followed by chemotherapy demonstrated conclusively that the addition of systemic chemotherapy improved survival in patients presenting with localized high-grade osteosarcoma (Table 116.4).

The implications of these findings are that the vast majority of patients with apparent localized tumors have the presence of micrometastatic disease, and that available systemic chemotherapy increases the chances of survival by addressing those micrometastases. In the past 20 years, standard treatment has evolved to the routine use of neoadjuvant (presurgical) and adjuvant (postsurgical) chemotherapy. In addition, it is now widely accepted that the four most important drugs used for the treatment of osteosarcoma include high-dose methotrexate (HD-MTX), adriamycin (ADM), cisplatin (CDDP), and ifosfamide (IFOS). However, the optimal use of two-, three-, or four-drug combinations remains somewhat controversial.

Adjuvant versus Neoadjuvant Chemotherapy

Neoadjuvant chemotherapy evolved in concert with the use of limb-salvage surgical approaches. At Memorial Sloan-Kettering Cancer Center, customized endoprosthetic devices in limb-salvage procedures often required several months to manufacture. Rather than delaying treatment, investigators began to administer chemotherapy while waiting for the endoprosthesis to be made. This approach led to suggestions that preoperative chemotherapy improved survival of the patients. In addition, orthopedic oncologists developed their own opinions regarding the advantages and disadvantages of presurgical chemotherapy. These observations ultimately led to a randomized clinical study between 1986 and 1993 by the Pediatric Oncology Group (POG) comparing presurgical chemotherapy to immediate surgery followed by adjuvant chemotherapy to patients less than 30 years of age with nonmetastatic, high-grade tumors (Fig. 116.9). The investigators concluded that there is no benefit to survival whether adjuvant or neoadjuvant therapy is used, and modern-era survival for nonmetastatic osteosarcoma should be at least 65%.

TABLE 116.4

REPORTED RESULTS OF REPRESENTATIVE TRIALS INCORPORATING PRESURGICAL CHEMOTHERAPY FOR OSTEOSARCOMA

Regimen	Investigators	No. of Patients	Relapse-Free (%)	Ref.
HDMTX + VCR + DOX + BCD (T-7 regimen)	MSKCC	54 (younger than 21 y)	74	19, 30, 117
HDMTX + VCR – DOX + BCD ± CDDP (depending on response) (T-10 regimen)	MSKCC	79 (younger than 21 y)	76	30
DOX + HDMTX + (BCD or CDDP) ± interferon (COSS 80)[a]	GPO	116	68	31, 201
HDMTX + DOX + CDDP	Mount Sinai	25	77	202
HDMTX + VCR + DOX + BCD ± CDDP (depending on response) (CCG-782)	CCG	231	56	119
HDMTX + DOX + CDDP + IFOS (COSS 82)	GPO	125	58	32
DOX + CDDP ± HDMTX[b]	EOIS	231	63 (–HDMTX) 48 (1HDMTX)	203
IA CDDP + (HDMTX vs. IDMTX) + DOX ± BCD (depending on response)[c]	Instituto Ortopedico Rizzoli	127	51 (overall) 58 (HDMTX) 42 (IDMTX)	204
HDMTX + DOX + IA CDDP ± etoposide, IFOS (postoperative therapy determined based on response to preoperative therapy)	Instituto Ortopedico Rizzoli	164	63	205
(IA CDDP vs. HDMTX) + DOX (postoperative therapy determined based on response to preoperative therapy) (TIOS I)	M. D. Anderson Cancer Center	43	60	206
IA CDDP + DOX ± CTX (depending on response) (TIOS III)	M. D. Anderson Cancer Center	24	—	—
HDMTX + DOX + IFOS ± CDDP	CCG (selected investigators)	95	82	—
HDMTX + DOX + CDDP BCD (POC 8651)[a]	POG	100	70 (presurgical chemotherapy) 73 (immediate surgery)	—
HDMTX + VCR + DOX + BCD + CDDP vs. DOX + CDDP	EOI	391	44	207
HDMTX + BCD + DOX + CDDP (T-12 regimen)	MSKCC	61	76	208
HDMTX + DOX + CDDP ± IFOS ± MTP-PE[d]	CCG and POG	679	67	—

BCD, bleomycin, cyclophosphamide, and dactinomycin; CCG, Children's Cancer Group; CDDP, cisplatin; COSS, Germany-Austria-Swiss Cooperative Osteosarcoma Study; CTX, cyclophosphamide; DOX, doxorubicin; EOI, European Osteosarcoma Intergroup; EOIS, First European Osteosarcoma Intergroup Study; GPO, German Society for Pediatric Oncology; HDMTX, high-dose methotrexate (12 g/m^2 or more) + leucovorin rescue; IA, intraarterial administration; IDMTX, intermediate-dose methotrexate (750 mg/m^2) + leucovorin rescue; IFOS, ifosfamide; MTP-PE, muramyl-tripeptide phosphatidylethanolamine; MSKCC, Memorial Sloan-Kettering Cancer Center; POG, Pediatric Oncology Group; TIOS, Treatment and Investigation Osteosarcoma Study; VCR, vincristine.

[a]Randomized study; no significant difference in relapse-free survival for patients on each treatment arm of study.

[b]Randomized study; favors treatment without HDMTX (some patients treated only adjuvantly).

[c]Randomized study; difference in results of treatment significant at 7% level.

[d]Randomized study; analysis of results by randomized treatment not yet available.

Assessment of Histologic Responses to Neoadjuvant Chemotherapy

Although the randomized study noted above showed no survival benefit, preoperative chemotherapy has become standard practice at most centers, in large part because of the important survival implications of histologic response to such therapy. Several issues need to be considered when evaluating the predictive value of histologic response on survival. Several related but independent systems have evolved to evaluate histologic response. These include the grading system developed at Memorial Sloan-Kettering Cancer Center by Huvos et al.,[109] the system developed by Salzer-Kuntschik et al.[110] and used by the German-Austrian-Swiss Cooperative Osteosarcoma Study Group (COSS), and the system developed by Picci et al.[111] at the Istituti Ortopedico Rizzoli (IOR) in Bologna. Although each of these grading systems attempts to objectively determine the effect of chemotherapy in tumor necrosis, each has a different scale applied and is subject to observer interpretation (Table 116.5). In addition, the timing of surgery (i.e., the duration of preoperative chemotherapy) would be expected to impact histologic response. However, in spite of these shortcomings, a consensus has emerged that uses greater than 90% necrosis and less than 90% necrosis as separating good and poor responses, respectively. Furthermore, most current studies use 10 to 12 weeks of preoperative chemotherapy (Fig. 116.10).

Using the criteria of greater than 90% as a good response and less than 90% necrosis as a poor response, several studies have reviewed 8- to 18-year experiences. The IOR reviewed

Treatment Plan
Induction Therapy
VP/IFOS + G q 3 weeks × 2
(6 weeks)
Radiologic and Pathologic Assessment
+
Surgery
Continuation Therapy

VP = Etoposide 100 mg/m²/d × 5 days = 500 mg/m²/course × 2 courses = Total 1,000/mg/m²
IFOS = Ifosfamide 3.5 g/m²/d × 5 days = 17.5 g/m²/course × 2 courses = Total 35 g/m²
G = G–CSF 5 μg/kg/d, begin day 6

A

Week	1	2	3	4	5	6	7	8	9	10	11	12	13	14	15	16	17	18
	MTX	MTX	AP			MTX	MTX	I VP G*			MTX	MTX	AP			MTX	MTX	I VP G[a]
Week	**19**	**20**	**21**	**22**	**23**	**24**	**25**	**26**	**27**	**28**	**29**	**30**	**31**	**32**	**33**	**34**		
			AP			I VP G[a]			AP			MTX	MTX	A				

VP = Etoposide 100 mg/m²/d × 5 days: 5 courses = Total 2,500 mg/m²
MTX = Methotrexate, 12 g/m² over 4 hours, plus levcovorin, 15 mg q6h × 10 doses: 10 courses = 120 g/m²
I = Ifosfamide, 2.4 g/m² + mesna/d × 5 days: 3 courses = Total 36 g/m². Total Ifosfomide = 71 g/m²
A = Doxorubicin, 37.5 mg/m²/d × 2 days: 5 courses = Total 375 mg/m²
P = CDDP, 60 mg/m²/d × 2 days: 4 courses = Total 480 mg/m²
[a]G = G–CSF 5 μg/kg/d.

B

FIGURE 116.9 **A:** Treatment plan for induction therapy. Patients received two courses of etoposide and ifosfamide, then radiologic assessment and surgery of primary tumor. The pathologic assessment of tumor necrosis was performed after surgery. **B:** Continuation chemotherapy regimen started 1 to 2 weeks after surgery. CDDP, cisplatin; G-CSF, granulocyte colony-stimulating factor. (From ref. 120, with permission.)

data on localized-extremity osteosarcoma in patients less than 40 years of age over the 19-year period from 1983 to 2002.[112] More than 1,000 patient records were analyzed. Fifty-nine percent of all patients had a good response to chemotherapy, and 41% had a poor response. Patients with a good histologic response to chemotherapy had a 5-year survival of 76%, whereas those with a poor response had a 5-year survival rate of 56%.

The COSS database was similarly reviewed and included 1,700 patients entered on study between 1980 and 1998. This analysis included all sites, ages, and presence or absence of metastases.[113] The data look remarkably similar to those of the Italian study, with 55.6% of patients classified as having a good response to therapy and 44.4% having a poor response. The 5-year survival rate was 77.8% for good responders and 55.5% for poor responders. Of further note, all the patients in both of these analyses received HD-MTX, and the majority also received ADM, CDDP, with or without IFOS. Also, most patients in these two analyses received preoperative chemotherapy, with surgery occurring between weeks 9 and 11 of treatment.

TABLE 116.5

THREE DIFFERENT HISTOLOGIC GRADING SYSTEMS FOR RESPONSE TO INDUCTION CHEMOTHERAPY FOR OSTEOSARCOMA

Salzer-Kuntschik[110]		Picci[111]		Huvos[109]	
I	No viable tumor cells	Total response	No viable tumor	IV	No histologic evidence of viable tumor
II	Single viable tumor cells or cluster <0.5 cm	Good response	90%–99% tumor necrosis	III	Only scattered foci of viable tumor cells
III	Viable tumor <10%	Fair response	60%–89% tumor necrosis	II	Areas of necrosis due to chemotherapy with areas of viable tumor
IV	Viable tumor 10%–50%	Poor response	<60% tumor necrosis	I	Little or no chemotherapy effect
V	Viable tumor >50%				
VI	No effect of chemotherapy				

PRACTICE OF ONCOLOGY

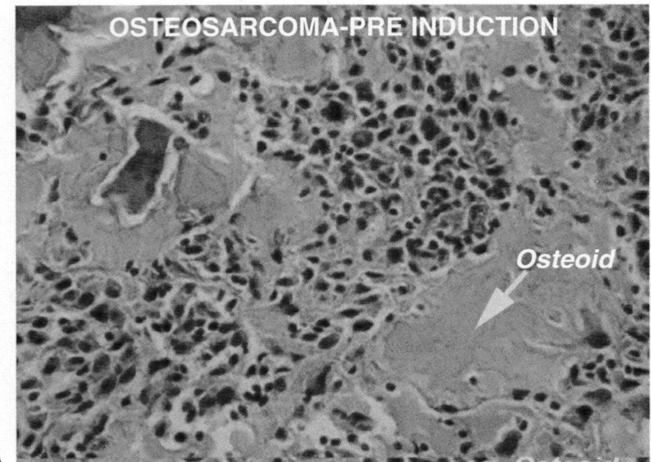

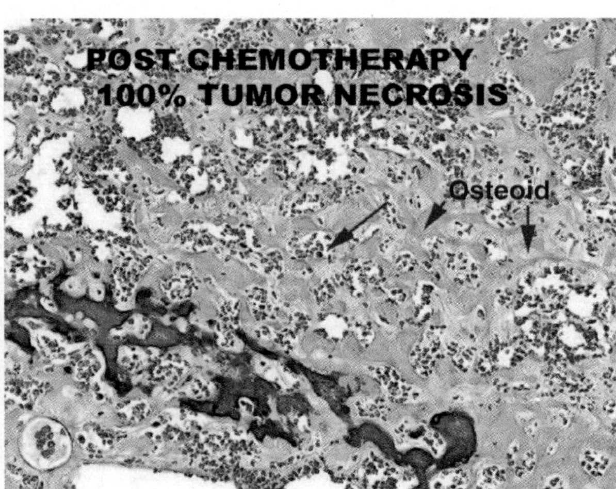

FIGURE 116.10 Pre- and postinduction chemotherapy histology of osteosarcoma. **A:** Tumor prior to induction chemotherapy (hematoxylin and eosin stain, X magnification). This shows viable osteoblast tumor cells forming tumor osteoid. Osteoid formation is the hallmark of an osteosarcoma. **B:** A specimen following induction chemotherapy with complete tumor necrosis. Note the complete absence of osteoblasts and stromal cells. The osteoid remains present and does not resorb. This appearance of a naked lattice of osteoid is characteristic of tumor necrosis. Unlike other tumors, overall survival may not shrink following induction chemotherapy since the matrix (osteoid) always remains.

The European Osteosarcoma Intergroup (EOI) from the European Organisation for Research and Treatment of Cancer, United Kingdom, and International Society of Paediatric Oncology (SIOP) analyzed data for two consecutive studies between 1983 and 1986 and 1986 and 1991.[114] A total of 570 patients were analyzed in the report. This analysis is notable for several differences compared to the COSS and IOR analyses. Only 28% of patients had a good histologic response, whereas 72% of patients had a poor histologic response. Patients with a good histologic response had a 5-year survival of 75%, whereas those with a poor response had a 5-year survival of 45%. Of note, many of the patients included in the analysis did not receive HD-MTX because many were treated on a randomized study comparing two drugs, ADM and CDDP, to more intensive therapy including HD-MTX, similar to the COSS and IOR studies. The large randomized study failed to show an advantage of multiagent therapy compared to ADM and CDDP alone.[115] However, the 5-year survival was 55% overall in this study, which is lower than that of the other studies reported above. Although the findings have continued to stir debate regarding optimal therapy, it suggests that patients who have a poor response to ADM and CDDP therapy alone (the majority of patients) have a much worse 5-year survival than those who have a poor response to three- or four-drug therapy. All three studies together strongly suggest that good responders can be expected to have a 5-year survival of approximately 75%, whereas poor responders have a 5-year survival in the range of 45% to 55%, depending on the treatment. It is important to point out that, although poor responders have a worse outcome than good responders, 45% to 55% 5-year survival is still dramatically improved compared to the less than 20% 5-year survival in the prechemotherapy era.

Another factor that could possibly influence histologic response to therapy and its predictive value on survival is the histologic subtype of the tumor. The clinical and biologic relevance of histologic subtypes has generally been believed to be minimal. In the IOR and the EOI studies discussed above, histology was characterized as osteoblastic or conventional, fibroblastic, chondroblastic, or telangiectatic. In both studies approximately 70% of cases were osteoblastic, whereas approximately 10% of cases were either chondroblastic or fibroblastic, with 6% telangiectatic, a number too small to be analyzed in the EOI study. In both studies, fibroblastic tumors had a higher rate of good histologic response (approximately 80% in the IOR study), whereas chondroblastic tumors had a lower rate of good responders (43% in the IOR study). Perhaps even more important, unlike other histologies, 5-year survival rates were identical for good and for poor responders in chondroblastic histology, at 68%.

To summarize, treatment of patients with nonmetastatic high-grade osteosarcoma with adjuvant chemotherapy including HD-MTX and at least two other drugs among the four most-active drugs in osteosarcoma can be expected to lead to a 75% 5-year survival among good histologic responders (greater than 90% necrosis) and 55% among poor histologic responders (less than 90% necrosis). However, care should be taken when assessing histologic response in patients with chondroblastic histology, as histologic responses may not be as important a predictor of survival in this subgroup.

Adjusting Chemotherapy for Poor Responders

Another hypothetical advantage of determining histologic response to preoperative chemotherapy is the potential to alter therapy in those patients who do not have a good response to preoperative treatment. If this "tailored therapy" approach is successful, one might expect to alter the impact of poor histologic response on survival by treating such patients with different drugs and improving their outcome. This approach has indeed proven to be successful in Hodgkin's lymphoma and leukemia. This approach was initially pioneered in the early 1980s at Memorial Sloan-Kettering Cancer Center, where poor responders had CDDP substituted for HD-MTX in addition to continuing BCD (bleomycin, cyclophosphamide, and dactinomycin) and ADM.[116] Although the initial analysis of this study suggested that there was no longer a difference in survival between good and poor responders, longer follow-up data demonstrated that initial response to preoperative chemotherapy continued to be predictive of survival. Furthermore, patients who had adjustments in their postoperative chemotherapy based on poor initial response did not have improvement in survival compared to those who had no modifications.[117] More recently, the Rizzoli Institute reported long-term follow-up data on a study carried out between 1986 and 1989 on 164 patients less than 40 years of age with nonmetastatic extremity osteosarcoma.[118] Patients with less than 90% necrosis at the time of surgical resection had IFOS and etoposide added to HD-MTX, ADM, and CDDP, whereas patients with greater than 90% necrosis continued to receive only the three drugs. The 10-year event-free survival was 67% for patients with 90% necrosis at the time of surgical resection and 51% for those with less than 90% necrosis. Although this difference in survival did not quite reach statistical significance ($P = .08$), it still favored those patients who had an initial good histologic response to therapy. Several other reports have also failed to demonstrate an ability to rescue poor responders.[32,119] Thus, to date, it has not been possible to improve the outcome of poor responders by altering postoperative chemotherapy.

Chemotherapy for Metastatic Disease

The presence of metastatic disease at presentation continues to be an extremely poor prognostic finding, with most studies showing survival rates in the range of 20%. It is therefore clear that new approaches are needed. The POG reported early data from a small phase 2 study for patients less than 30 years old with newly diagnosed metastatic osteosarcoma.[120] Forty-one patients were treated with two cycles of etoposide and IFOS preoperatively, followed by 32 weeks of postoperative chemotherapy, including three additional cycles of etoposide and IFOS along with standard HD-MTX, ADM, and CDDP (Fig. 116.11). The data are still immature, but the projected 2-year progression-free survival was 43%. In the large analysis of the COSS database that included more than 1,700 consecutively treated patients, the 10-year survival probability was 40% for patients who were able to have all sites of metastatic disease resected.[113] Thus, although there is no accepted standard approach for the treatment of newly diagnosed metastatic patients, available data would suggest that such patients should be treated with currently available aggressive multiagent chemotherapy with complete surgical resection of all sites of disease if at all possible.

Chemotherapy for Relapsed Osteosarcoma

Similar to patients who present with primary metastatic disease, individuals in whom recurrent disease develops have an overall poor prognosis, with 5-year survival rates in the range of 20%. As noted for metastatic disease at presentation, new salvage strategies are needed. Although there is no standard second-line chemotherapy that currently is uniformly applied, several principles have been clearly established. Complete resection of recurrent disease appears to be mandatory for long-term survival. It also is likely that multiagent chemotherapy contributes to successful salvage of some patients. In general, patients should be treated with any of the four most active agents noted earlier if initial therapy did not include one or more of these agents. Patients who have recurrences more than 1 year after completing prior systemic therapy may benefit from reintroduction of at least some of the same drugs in a salvage regimen. The use of high-dose chemotherapy with autologous hematopoietic stem cell rescue has been applied to salvage therapy. However, at least two small pilot studies failed to demonstrate an advantage to standard salvage therapy approaches.[121,122]

Late Effects of Systemic Therapy

The universal application of systemic chemotherapy for all patients with osteosarcoma has led to an increased likelihood of survival, as noted earlier. However, with this increase in survival has come the inevitable increase in late effects secondary to chemotherapy. The most important long-term side effects that have now been well documented are ADM-induced cardiomyopathy, male infertility, and development of second malignant neoplasms. In a long-term follow-up report of 164 patients treated with cumulative doses of 480 mg/m^2 ADM, there were six documented cases of severe cardiomyopathy.[118] It is likely that subclinical cardiac damage may occur and be underestimated.[123] Although earlier reports suggest little effect on infertility, more recent inclusion of IFOS into front-line therapy has likely increased the risk of male infertility after treatment.[124] In the long-term follow-up study from the IOR noted above, 10 of 12 male patients who underwent sperm analysis were noted to have azoospermia. All ten had received chemotherapy at the time of puberty, and nine of ten had received IFOS. As more patients survive their primary osteosarcoma, the development of second malignant neoplasms has become of increasing concern as well. In a long-term follow-up study from St. Jude Children's Research Hospital, there were nine documented cases of second malignant neoplasms among 334 patients treated between 1962 and 1996, for an incidence of 2%. The tumors included two cases of MFH; a chondrosarcoma; carcinomas of

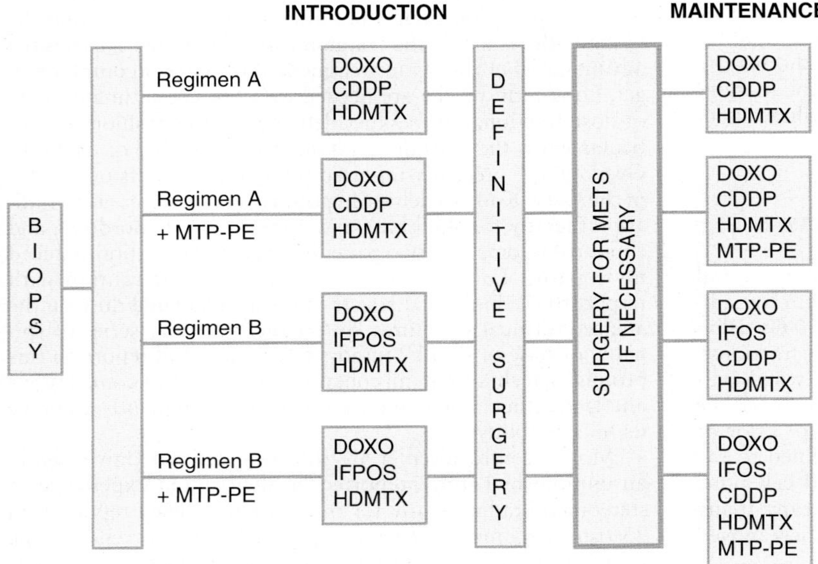

FIGURE 116.11 Typical chemotherapy protocol for pediatric osteosarcoma. CDDP, cisplatin; DOXO, doxorubicin; HDMTX, high-dose methotrexate; IFOS, ifosfamide; MTP-PE, liposomal muramyl tripeptide. (Data from Children's Oncology Group, P. Meyers, personal communication, with permission.)

the rectum, colon, stomach, and breast; a melanoma; and a glioblastoma.[125] Although this incidence is significantly lower than that of survivors of Hodgkin's lymphoma, it is likely that as more patients are cured of osteosarcoma, this problem will continue to increase. Because of these late sequelae of systemic treatment and continued reports of recurrences more than 5 years after treatment, these patients should be followed long term by the centers performing the initial curative treatment.

RADIOTHERAPY FOR OSTEOSARCOMA

Radiation therapy is generally not used in the primary treatment of osteosarcoma, although this may change with the greater implementation of new technologies. Radiation therapy is used for patients who have refused definitive surgery, require palliation, or have lesions in axial locations. Experience with radiotherapy has been greater in the treatment of chondrosarcoma, possibly due to the lesser availability of adjuvant chemotherapy in facilitating the goals of tissue preservation. Radiotherapy assumes greater importance for tumors of the axial skeleton and facial bones where a combination of limited surgery and radiotherapy may be used since function and cosmesis preservation may be paramount. Radiotherapy is more frequently used in Ewing's sarcoma and peripheral primitive neuroectodermal tumors of bone and is discussed in another chapter.

Treatment Planning

Optimal radiotherapy of bone tumors requires careful technical treatment planning and adherence to radiobiologic principles; therefore, all fields should be treated each day to ensure a continuous homogeneous distribution of dose to all areas of the target. Normal tissue should be protected from the high-dose regions wherever possible, and this is achieved using precise, three-dimensional delineation of the target volumes as well as appropriately fractionated courses of radiotherapy. The latter is also necessary to accomplish adequate tumor control by especially exploiting advantages over the tumor such as reoxygenation.

All treatments should implement megavoltage therapy beams to maximize physical reduction in absorbed dose delivered to bone. Radiotherapy is most usually planned volumetrically using computerized CT simulation technologies. Patient immobilization is also essential, especially when very precise delivery is used to avoid irradiating normal tissues.

Patient immobilization is essential to optimal radiotherapy, especially when very precise delivery is used and the margins around the target are less than usual, particularly when avoidance of normal tissues is being undertaken.

Dose and Volume Considerations

Large treatment volumes that include the entire clinical and radiographic extent of tumor plus a generous margin for subclinical extension of disease are needed (e.g., 45 to 50 Gy delivered over a period of approximately 5 weeks in daily fractions). For potential medullary spread (e.g., lymphoma, Ewing's sarcoma), the standard radiation volumes previously included the entire bone, with a boost of radiation to the area of prior or persisting bulky disease. However, radiation confined to the involved area may be sufficient for small, round cell bone tumors that have responded to induction chemotherapy. If any volumes are matched, the junction should be routinely moved every 10 Gy.

The irradiated volume should encompass at least the tissue that would be resected, plus an allowance of approximately 2 cm for microscopic extension with additional allowance for patient movement. A nonirradiated strip of the limb length should be identified and maintained (or at least restricting the maximum dose in such areas to less than 40 Gy) and, wherever possible, overlie the lymphatic drainage pathways located medially in the extremity.

Additional principles involve using multiple beam-shaping devices so that shaped fields can be designed to conform to individual tumor volume and anatomy. When necessary, beam modifiers, such as compensating filters and wedge filters, or beam segmentation with multileaf collimation and intensity-modulated radiotherapy (IMRT) beams are useful aids to optimize the homogeneity of the dose within the target volume while sparing adjacent normal structures and accounting for individual variations in patient thickness.

Precision Technology in Radiotherapy Delivery

Traditional radiotherapy treatment approaches use parallel opposed or relatively standard three- or four-field plans with some beam shaping to reduce the irradiated volume where possible. This may suffice for uncomplicated presentations but for many lesions, more precise targeting with conformal plans or IMRT is necessary. Relatively inaccessible target areas previously only adequately treated with potential and unnecessary toxicity can now be successfully irradiated while avoiding adjacent vulnerable anatomy that may be partially surrounded by the target.

Precision photon methods such as IMRT can be delivered with several forms of delivery platforms. In some situations (e.g., adjacent to the spinal cord or optic chiasm) extremely accurate delivery may demand stereotactic precision for guidance to minimize interfraction differences and ensure safety in tumor coverage and avoidance of critical anatomy. Potential methods include tomotherapy, robotic linear accelerators, and standard linear accelerators modulated by additional collimation controls. A popular robotic system, the CyberKnife (Accuray, Sunnyvale, California) uses a frameless reference system for stereotactic guidance and a robotic delivery system, allowing adaptive beam pointing to account for positional variance.[126] The absence of a frame provides great flexibility and makes it possible to treat extracranial sites with the same or better precision than other systems achieved by fixing the lesion with respect to the cranium using the frame. This has the advantage of efficiency in treatment delivery to a complex target. Long-term results are needed to assess the ultimate safety of dose fractionation regimes delivered in this fashion, in particular when the total dose administered is high. For example, Gwak et al.[127] recently reported preliminary results on the use of the CyberKnife to deliver hypofractionated stereotactic radiation therapy for skull base and upper cervical chordoma and chondrosarcoma, but two patients developed radiation-induced myelopathy. For this reason they advise great caution with respect to the biological effects of the accumulated dose on the adjacent critical structures. So far the first large series of spinal[128] or base of skull[129] tumors to evaluate and report on this promising technology still contains a paucity of sarcoma lesions and lacks clinical outcome from which to confidently embrace its full capability.

Most recently, Eisen et al. from Georgetown University, in an unpublished study, reported on their initial experience of stereotactic radiotherapy for osteosarcoma. They reported on 33 osteosarcomas in 9 patients; 4 for local recurrence at the primary site and 28 metastatic sites. Their metastatic sites were lung (16), distant boney sites (10), and brain (2). The most common fractionation schemes utilized were 7 Gy in five fractions (16 sites) and 15 Gy in three fractions (4 sites). The mean treatment volume was 92.1 cm^3. PET scans were available for 25 cases; responses have been dramatic with near resolution of uptake. In addition, CT of the corresponding lung lesions usually showed significant response. This technique and technology appears to be promising for patients with recurrent local or metastatic disease for palliation.

MALIGNANT BONE TUMORS

Classic Osteosarcoma

Osteosarcoma is a high-grade malignant spindle cell tumor that arises within a bone. Its distinguishing characteristic is the production of "tumor" osteoid or immature bone directly from a malignant spindle cell stroma.[130]

Clinical Characteristics

Osteosarcoma typically occurs during childhood and adolescence. Historically, investigators evaluated 227 patients from 1971 to 1984 and reported the peak incidence to be between 10 and 19 years of age but noted the mean and median values to be 29 and 20 years, respectively.[131] The overall incidence—2.1 cases per million people per year—has not changed. When osteosarcoma occurs in patients older than 40 years, it is usually associated with a pre-existing condition, such as Paget's disease, irradiated bones, multiple hereditary exostosis, or polyostotic fibrous dysplasia.[132,133] Bones of the knee joint and the proximal humerus are the most common sites, accounting for 50% and 25%, respectively, of all osteosarcomas.[134] In general, 80% to 90% of osteosarcomas occur in the long tubular bones,[44,135,136] and the axial skeleton is rarely affected. Fewer than 1% are found in the hands and feet.

With the exception of serum AP (SAP) levels, which are elevated in 45% to 50% of patients, laboratory findings are usually not helpful. Pain is the most common complaint. Night pain gradually develops and becomes a hallmark of skeletal involvement. Physical examination demonstrates a firm, soft mass fixed to the underlying bone with slight tenderness. No effusion is noted in the adjacent joint, and motion is normal. Incidence of pathologic fracture is less than 1%. Systemic symptoms are rare.

Radiographic Characteristics

Typical findings are increased intramedullary radiodensity (due to tumor bone or calcified cartilage), an area of radiolucency (due to nonossified tumor), a pattern of permeating destruction with poorly defined borders, cortical destruction, periosteal elevation, and extraosseous extension with soft tissue ossification. This combination of characteristics is not seen in any other lesion. Six hundred radiographs of osteosarcoma reviewed at the Memorial Sloan-Kettering Cancer Center were classified into three broad categories: sclerotic (32%), osteolytic (22%), and mixed (46%). Although no statistically significant difference was found in overall survival rates among these types, the patterns are important to recognize. The sclerotic and mixed types offer few diagnostic problems. Errors of diagnosis most often occur with pure osteolytic tumors. The differential diagnosis of osteolytic osteosarcoma includes GCT, aneurysmal bone cyst, fibrosarcoma, and MFH.

Clinical and Prognostic Considerations

Before the era of adjuvant chemotherapy, treatment of osteosarcoma consisted of amputation. Metastasis to lungs and other bones generally occurred within 24 months. A large number of series show an overall survival of 5% to 20% at 2 years. Survival in osteosarcomas patients can also correlate with the size and location of the tumor at the time of clinical presentation.[137] This pattern has been altered by adjuvant chemotherapy and aggressive thoracotomy for pulmonary disease.

Marcove et al.,[18] reviewing 145 patients younger than 21 years of age who underwent surgery without adjuvant chemotherapy at Memorial Sloan-Kettering Cancer Center, noted no statistically significant differences with regard to race, gender, or duration of symptoms. Younger patients developed metastases sooner, but this made no difference in overall survival.

Bacci et al.[138] reviewed 789 patients with nonmetastatic osteosarcoma of the extremities treated with neoadjuvant chemotherapy, following them for a minimum of 5 years at the Rizzoli Institute in Bologna, Italy. The significant treatment-related factors were patients' age of 14 years or younger, elevated serum alkaline phosphatase at presentation, tumor volume of 200 mL or more, inadequate surgical margins, and poor histological response to preoperative chemotherapy. Each independently predicted a high risk of systemic recurrence. These are significant findings from an extremely large group of patients treated at an institution devoted to the care of osteosarcoma patients.

Recently, Grimer[139] reported an analysis of size on presentation versus survival for bone and soft tissue sarcomas. The author reviewed 1,460 patients and noted the incidence of metastases at presentation were linearly related to tumor size. For patients without metastases at diagnosis, prognosis became increasingly worse with increasing size, independent of other factors. The author concludes that the smaller the tumor at diagnosis, the better. This finding was consistent with both bone and soft tissue sarcomas.

Alkaline Phosphatase

SAP level is an important biologic marker of tumor activity in patients with osteosarcoma. The early studies of the relationship between AP activity and survival were performed before the introduction of adjuvant chemotherapy (i.e., in patients treated with surgery alone).

Bacci et al.[140] reported on an evaluation of the SAP levels among 560 patients with high-grade osteosarcomas of the extremity who were treated at a single institution. Forty-six percent of these patients had elevated SAP levels before treatment; such levels were most commonly found in males older than 14 years and in patients with tumors greater than 150 mL of the osteoblastic type. Only two factors by a multivariate analysis were independently correlated with 5-year event-free survival: SAP levels ($P = .002$) and grade of chemotherapy-induced tumor necrosis ($P = .0001$). The authors recommend that, in planning randomized trials, patients be stratified according to SAP levels.

Biology and Prognostic Factors

Although the etiology of osteosarcoma remains for the most part unknown, several predisposing conditions have been clearly identified. The most common known risk factor is radiation exposure, and osteosarcoma is the most common histology found in radiation-associated second malignancies. Several hereditary risk factors are known to predispose toward osteosarcoma. Hereditary retinoblastoma associated with germline mutations in the *RB* gene is associated with a 100-fold increase in the risk of osteosarcoma, even in the absence of radiation exposure, which further increases the risk of osteosarcoma development. Li-Fraumeni syndrome is associated with germline mutations in the *p53* gene and also with an increased risk for the development of osteosarcoma. Rothmund-Thomson syndrome is an autosomal recessive disorder known to be associated with an increased risk of osteosarcoma. This syndrome is now known to be associated with mutations in the DNA helicase RECQL4, and a report has demonstrated that all patients with Rothmund-Thomson syndrome in whom osteosarcomas developed had evidence of truncating mutations of the *RECQL4* gene. This is of particular note because alterations in a related RecQ DNA helicase in Werner syndrome are associated with an increased risk of osteosarcoma.

In view of these genetic predisposition syndromes, it is not surprising that RB1 and p53 are frequently found to be altered in patients with osteosarcoma. For p53, numerous studies have found the frequency of p53 mutations to be in the 18% to 30% range. The presence or absence of p53 mutations at diagnosis does not appear to carry prognostic implications. Alterations in the *RB1* gene appear to be even more common than *p53* alterations, with loss of heterozygosity reported in more than 50% of informative cases. The more sensitive technique of allelotyping found high frequencies of RB1 and p53 allelic imbalances, with no association with prognosis. The p53 and RB pathways are regulated by a series of activators and inhibitors, and these can be altered in tumors. In osteosarcomas, the incidence of alterations in either p15ARF or HDM2, positive and negative regulators of p53 function, respectively, is quite low. In contrast, alterations in the positive regulator of RB1 function, p16, Ink4a, was found to be greater than 15%, making overall incidence of RB pathway abnormalities in osteosarcoma likely to be even higher than 50%. No large studies of RECQL4 status in sporadic osteosarcomas have been reported.

Osteosarcomas are genetically characterized by complex karyotypes characteristic of severe disturbances in genomic stability. This virtually invariant presence of a complex karyotype is the cytogenetic hallmark of marked telomere dysfunction. A small, retrospective analysis of 62 patients with osteosarcoma revealed that 11 had no evidence of telomere maintenance. These individuals had significantly increased 5-year survival (90%) compared with the 51 patients with evidence of activation of telomere maintenance, who had a 5-year survival rate of 60%.[141] Although these data require confirmation, they raise the possibility that, although the vast majority of patients with osteosarcoma have activation of telomere maintenance mechanisms, leading to chromosomal instability, a minority may have normal telomere function and may constitute a particularly favorable subset.

Initial enthusiasm was shown in regard to the prognostic significance of expression of the multidrug resistance gene, *MDR1* or P-glycoprotein, in osteosarcoma. The IOR group reported that increased expression of P-glycoprotein was associated with poor prognoses.[142] However, subsequent studies have failed to confirm these observations. In summary, although the overwhelming majority of osteosarcomas occur sporadically, there are several known hereditary risk factors for the development of this tumor. These risk factors have pointed out several key genetic alterations that occur commonly in sporadic osteosarcomas and likely play a major role in the biology of these tumors. The genetic hallmark of osteosarcoma is the presence of complex karyotypes, suggesting that chromosomal instability and mechanisms contributing to this phenotype also contribute to the biology of these tumors.

Changing Pattern of Metastasis

The classic pattern and time frame of metastatic dissemination of osteosarcoma has been modified by the use of adjuvant chemotherapy and thoracotomy. Bacci et al.,[138] in a recent report of 789 nonmetastatic osteosarcoma patients, described the present pattern of metastases, disease-free interval, and overall survival. In the 313 patients who experienced recurrence, the first recurrences were isolated lung metastases in 243 (77.6%) patients, isolated bone metastases in 26 (8.3%), lung and bone metastases in 5 (1.6%), metastases in other sites in 3 (0.9%) (kidney, brain, heart), metastases in more than two sites in 2, isolated local recurrence in 20 (6.4%), local recurrences combined with bone metastases in 8 (2.6%), and local recurrence combined with lung metastases in 6 (1.9%).

Histologic Subtype and Influence on Chemotherapy Response

Within the past decade, as more patients have been treated in cooperative studies and the number of patients treated with induction chemotherapy has increased, the question of the significance of the histologic subtype on the chemotherapy response of an osteosarcoma has begun to be examined. Bacci et al.[143] analyzed the factors that determined the rate of chemotherapy response in the subgroup of patients who attained total (100%) tumor necrosis. Of 510 patients treated between 1983 and 1995, a 100% tumor necrosis was not related to gender, age, tumor site or size, SAP, or route of CDDP administration. The histologic complete response was related to only two factors: the number of drugs used and histologic subtype. According to the drugs used, the percentage of total necrosis was 31% for a four-drug regimen, 18% for a three-drug regimen, and only 1.5% for a two-drug regimen. According to the histologic subtypes, the rates of 100% total necrosis were telangiectatic tumors (41%), fibroblastic tumors (31%), and chondroblastic tumors (3%) (Fig. 116.12).

Limb-Sparing Surgery and Pathologic Fracture

Traditionally, a fracture through an osteosarcoma was treated by amputation. As experience with induction chemotherapy and limb-sparing surgery has increased, however, several centers have attempted limb-sparing surgery in this high-risk patient population. The assumption has been that if the fracture can be immobilized during the induction period and the

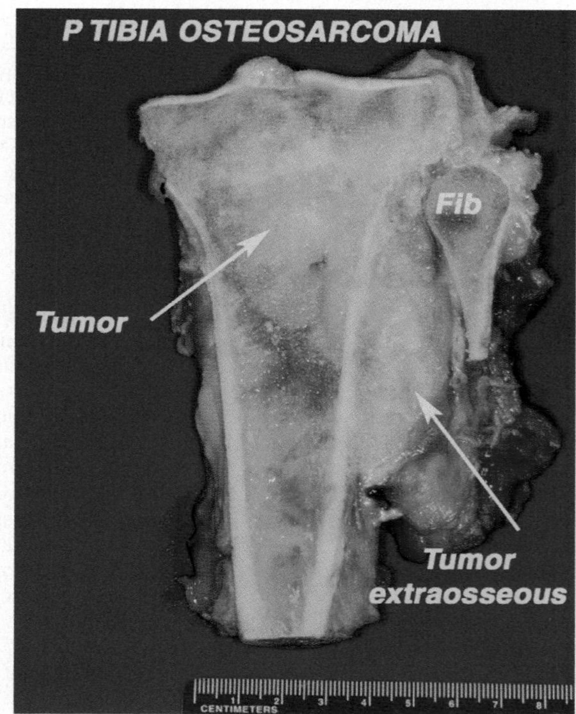

FIGURE 116.12 Pathology of osteosarcoma. Proximal tibia showing intramedullary and extraosseous component. Osteosarcomas typically have a large soft tissue component. Tumors of the proximal tibia often involve the proximal fibula.

tumor shows clear signs of necrosis and secondary fracture healing, an amputation may be avoided.

Steadman et al.[144] evaluated their experience with patients who had osteosarcoma-induced pathologic fractures between 1970 and 1995. Nine primary instances of limb salvage in patients with preoperative chemotherapy and eight primary cases of amputation with postoperative chemotherapy were studied. No significant difference in survival was found. One local recurrence occurred in the limb-salvage group and none in the amputation group. This retrospective analysis, combined with other reported results, makes a convincing case that a pathologic fracture does not indicate the need for an immediate amputation. The strategy today is to immobilize the extremity and proceed with induction chemotherapy. If the fracture heals and the tumor appears to respond to chemotherapy, a limb-sparing operation is warranted.[145] Repeat staging studies after induction chemotherapy and close serial observation during the induction period are essential.

Surgical Resection of Localized-Extremity Osteosarcoma

Rougraff et al.[103] updated a combined study from the MSTS of 227 patients from 26 institutions treated for osteosarcoma of the distal femur; 109 patients (48%) were alive at an average of 11 years after surgery. No differences in local recurrence, overall survival, or duration of disease-free survival were noted between amputation and limb-sparing groups.

Bacci et al.[146] analyzed the type of surgical margin and the responses to chemotherapy compared to local recurrence following induction chemotherapy to a limb-sparing procedure. The differences in outcome were dramatic. The patients with poor necrosis (fewer than 60%) and wide margins had ten times the risk of local recurrence. The worst combination was poor necrosis and less than wide margins. This study emphasizes the need for wide margins following a good response to induction chemotherapy for a safe limb-sparing procedure. This study suggests that large tumors with a poor clinical response and with anticipated close margins are at a very high risk of local recurrence and that a primary amputation may be warranted.

Treatment by Anatomic Site

The unique features of evaluation, management, and resection of tumors of the most common anatomic areas, the shoulder and knee, are described and illustrated in this section.

Shoulder Girdle. A surgical classification for shoulder girdle resections has been described by Malawer et al.[147] This classification is useful for all bony limb-sparing procedures of the shoulder girdle. It is recommended that osteosarcomas arising from the proximal humerus be treated by an extra-articular shoulder resection (type VB) (Fig. 116.13), although small tumors may be treated by an intra-articular resection (type IA). Recently, the choice of intra-articular versus extra-articular resection has been debated. The advantage of an intra-articular procedure is that it is easier and preserves deltoid function, although there is not much difference in function, especially if the axillary nerve cannot be spared. The major disadvantage is the risk of local recurrence.

Most recently, Gupta et al.[148] evaluated their experience from M. D. Anderson Cancer Center with attempted deltoid preservation (intra-articular resection) for osteosarcomas of the proximal humerus following induction chemotherapy. They noted that 3 of 21 (13%) patients developed a local recurrence; 2 of whom had a poor chemotherapy response and the other a positive margin. In addition, 4 of 21 patients had positive margins. Overall 6 of 24 (25%) patients required an extra-articular resection. They concluded that intra-articular resections should *not* be performed routinely but reserved for those who have had a good tumor response and anticipated negative surgical margins (presumably smaller tumors).

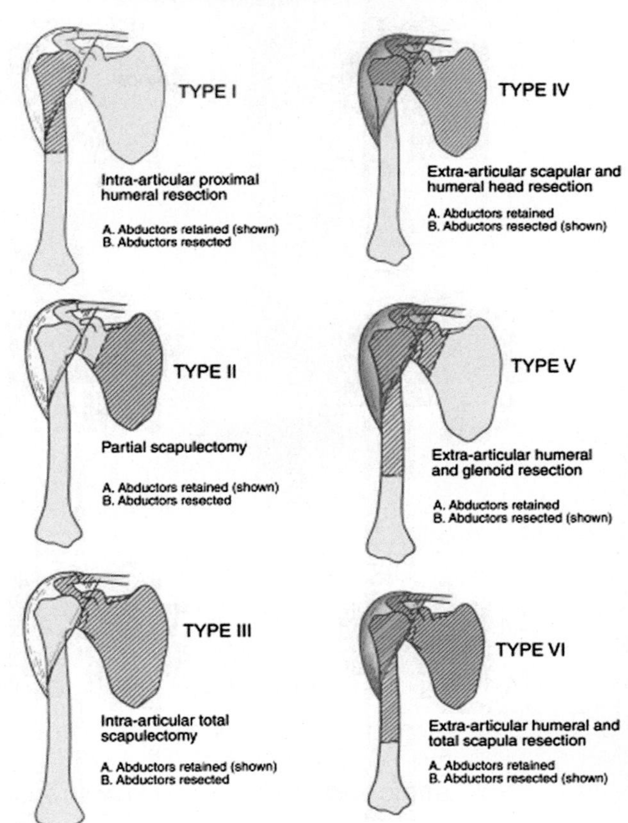

FIGURE 116.13 Surgical classification of shoulder girdle resections. This classification was described in 1991 by Malawer et al. (From ref. 147, with permission.)

Proximal Humerus. The proximal humerus is the third most common site for osteosarcoma. Joint involvement is common in patients with high-grade malignancies of the proximal humerus; for this reason, an extra-articular resection is commonly performed. Intra-articular resections are reserved for small, intraosseous (stage IIA) lesions. The aim of surgery is to create a stable new "shoulder" that allows the placement of the hand in space and enables the patient to retain elbow function (Fig. 116.14). Proximal humeral lesions should not be biopsied through the deltopectoral interval. Biopsy under fluoroscopy or CT guidance through the anterior one-third of the deltoid by a trocar is preferred. Angiography, and more recently CT/angiography, is the most useful in preoperative studies. If the neurovascular bundle is clear, resection is feasible.

CT or MR venography to evaluate the axillary or brachial veins is required for large lesions. Venous occlusion usually denotes major nerve involvement since the infraclavicular nerves run along the same sheath as the major veins. Venous occlusion indicates that the neurovascular bundle must be explored before proceeding with a limb-sparing procedure.

Adequate resection of the proximal humerus requires removal of 15 to 20 cm of the humerus and shoulder joint with the deltoid, rotator cuff, and portions of the biceps and triceps muscles. The procedure involves suspension of the arm, motor reconstruction, and provision of adequate soft tissue coverage.

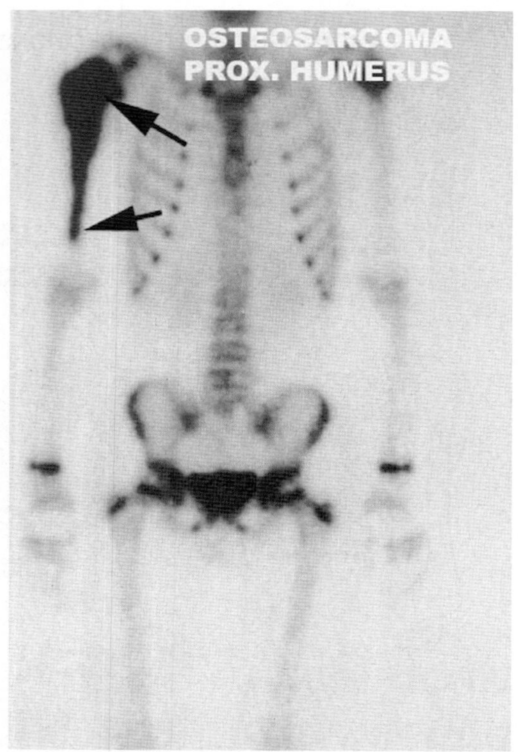

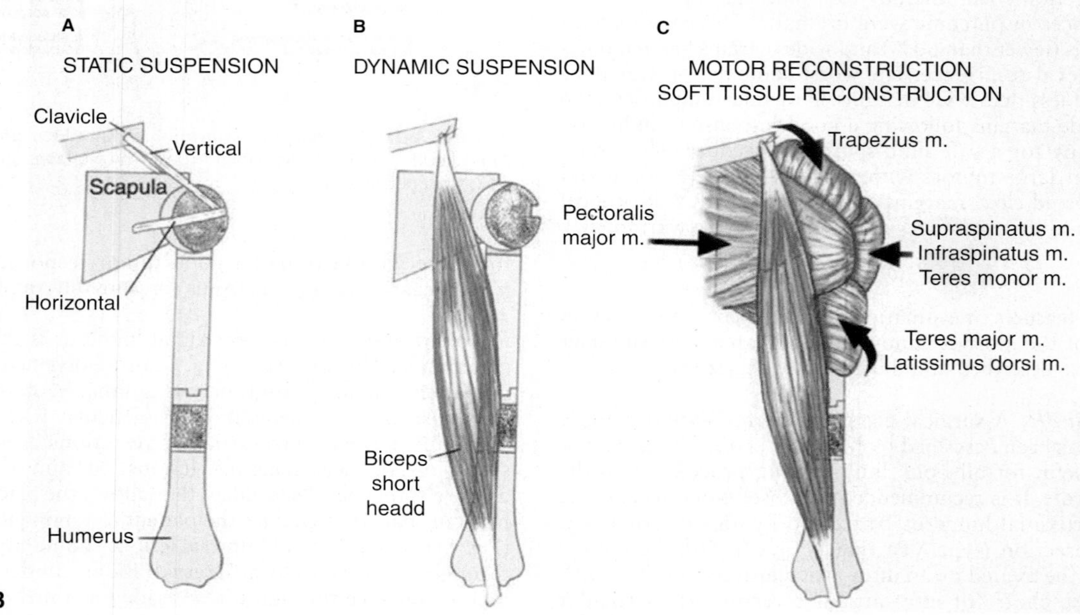

FIGURE 116.14 Osteosarcoma of the proximal humerus. **A:** Bone scan demonstrating the length of the humerus needed to be resected. The ipsilateral glenoid is routinely removed for large tumors. **B:** Schematic of muscle transfers and soft tissue reconstruction following a proximal humeral resection. (From Rubert CK, Malawar MM, Kellar KL. Modular endoprosthetic replacement of the proximal humerus: indications, surgical technique, and results. *Semin Arthroplasy* 10(3):142–153.)

Extra-articular resection of the glenohumeral joint by medial scapulosteotomy is safer than intra-articular resection (Fig. 116.15).

Wittig et al.[149] described the technique of extra-articular resection and reported that of 23 patients with high-grade, stage IIB osteosarcoma of the proximal humerus, 22 were treated by an extra-articular resection; there were no local recurrences. The authors reviewed data regarding intra-articular versus extra-articular resections for osteosarcoma and reported local recurrence rates of 16% and 4%, respectively. A modular endoprosthesis is used for reconstruction. Soft tissue reconstruction and suspension are essential to avoid postoperative pain, instability, and fatigability. Alternatively, resection of the proximal humerus for osteosarcomas can be performed by an intra-articular resection that preserves the glenoid and the adjacent deltoid muscle. The problems associated with this procedure include significant local recurrence and instability of the reconstructed prosthesis or allograft. When the glenoid and deltoid are preserved in this procedure, minimum margins are obtained along the shoulder joint, deltoid muscle, and axillary nerve. Because of this serious drawback, this technique is not recommended by the surgical author (MMM).

Scapula. The scapula is an uncommon site for osteosarcoma (less than 5%); however, it is a common site for round cell tumors (Ewing's sarcoma) and metastatic cancers in adults. A

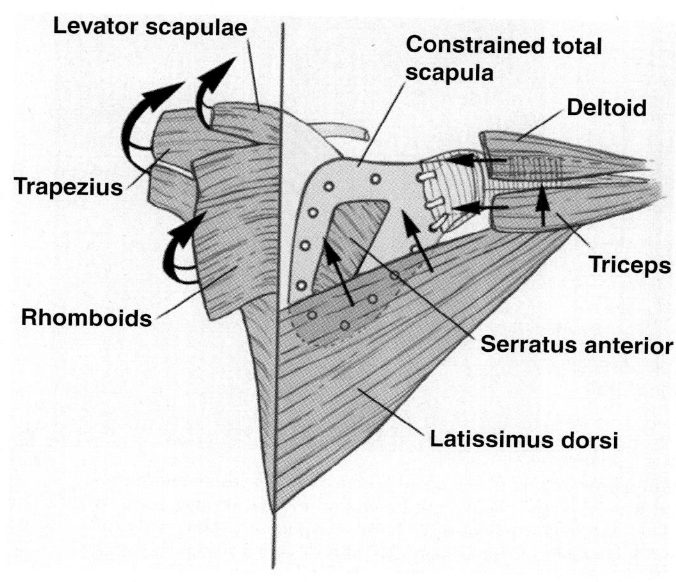

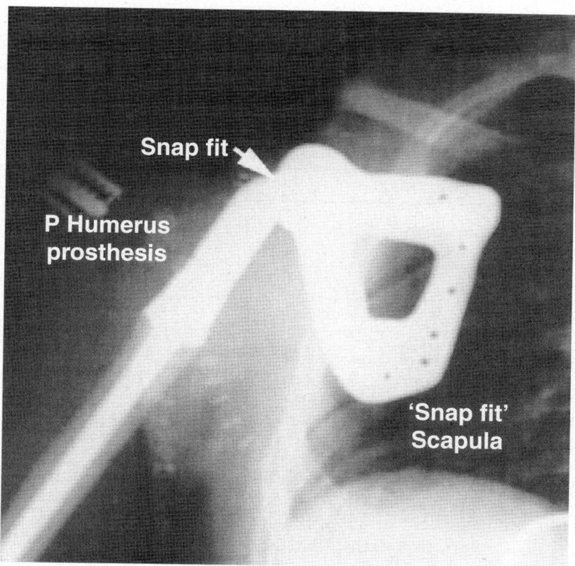

FIGURE 116.15 Tikhoff-Linberg resection of the scapula and proximal humerus. **A:** Schematic drawing of a scapular prosthesis and muscle reconstruction. **B:** Plain radiograph showing a bipolar proximal humeral and scapula replacement postoperatively. The function following a scapula replacement in contrast to a "hanging shoulder" reconstruction is superior.

fair amount of knowledge regarding scapular prosthetic design, indications, and techniques of resection and reconstruction has been developed. Most high-grade sarcomas of the scapula involve the body as well as the glenoid. The glenoid cannot be preserved. The classic operation for high-grade tumors of the scapula has been the Tikhoff-Linberg resection, originally described in 1928 and now identified as Malawer's classification type IVB. The Tikhoff-Linberg resection is a complete (extra-articular) *en bloc* resection of the scapula and the proximal humerus. Reconstruction is by a hanging shoulder and, more recently, by scapular endoprosthetic replacement.

Distal Femur. The distal femur is the most common site of osteosarcoma origination (Fig. 116.16). Adequate *en bloc* resection includes 15 to 20 cm of the distal femur and 1 to 2 cm of the proximal tibia and portions of the adjacent quadriceps around the tumor mass. Angiography (or three-dimensional CT/angiogram or MRI/angiogram) is crucial to determine popliteal vessel involvement. Biopsy must avoid the sartorial canal, popliteal space, and the knee joint. Contraindications to resection are popliteal vessel involvement, massive soft tissue contamination from previous biopsy, and displaced pathologic fracture. Large tumors that require removal of the entire quadriceps or

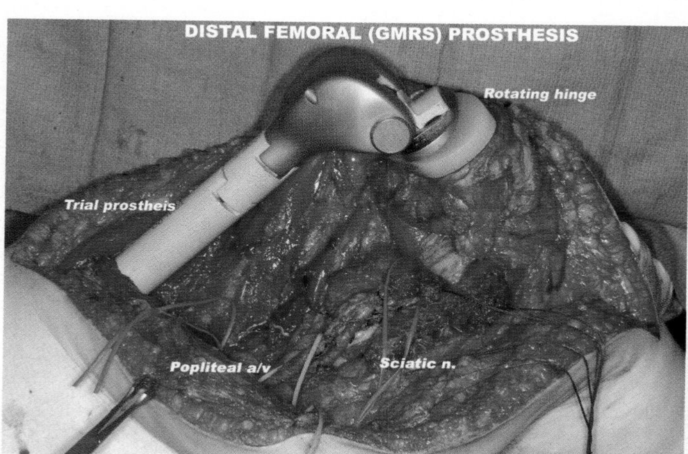

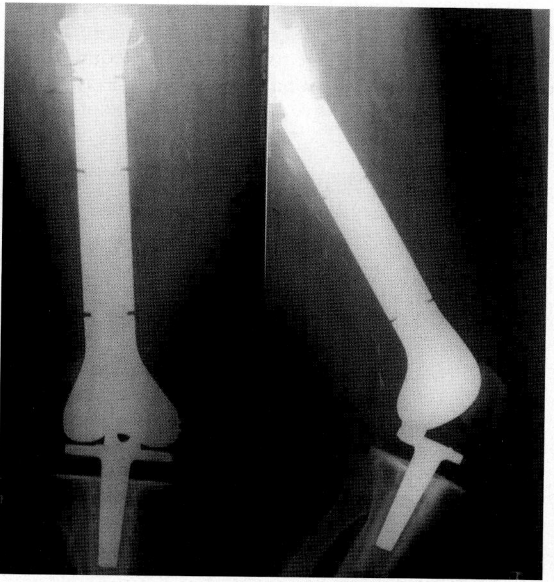

FIGURE 116.16 Distal femoral osteosarcoma resection. **A:** Intraoperative photograph showing a distal femoral modular prosthesis reconstruction following a resection of an osteosarcoma. Note the popliteal artery and vein and sciatic nerve, which must be carefully mobilized prior to resection. **B:** Anteroposterior and lateral radiograph of a distal femoral modular replacement prosthesis. Modularity of body lengths and stem diameters allow the surgeon to customize the fit to each individual patient intraoperatively.

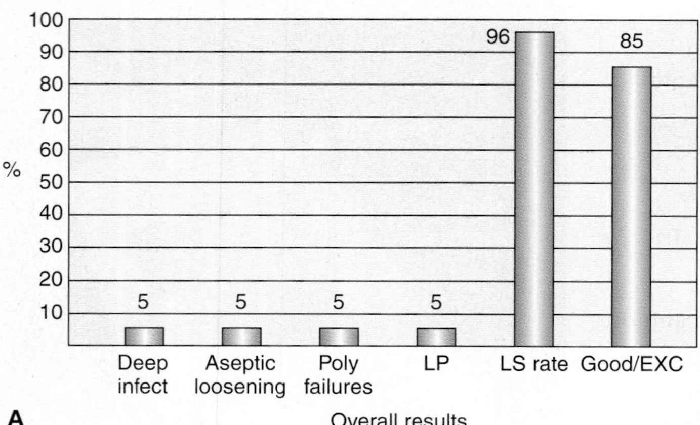

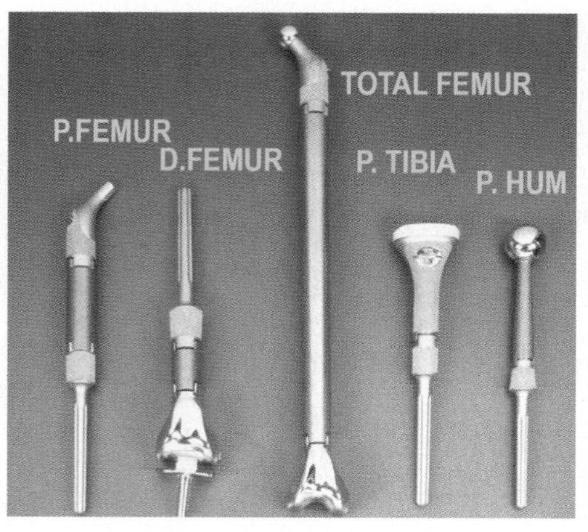

FIGURE 116.17 **A:** Long-term results of 110 patients with osteosarcoma of the distal femur treated with an endoprosthesis replacement. The overall limb-salvage rate reported was 96% and the overall functional evaluation was good to excellent in 85%. **B:** The modular replacement system. This system consists of three basic components: joint, body (of various lengths), and stems (of various diameters). The modular replacement system (MRS) is designed to replace large segments of bone and the adjacent joints: proximal femur, distal femur, total femur, proximal tibia, and proximal humerus (scapula prosthesis not shown). (From Modular Replacement Systems Stryker Orthopedics, Mahwah, New Jersey.)

hamstrings can be adequately reconstructed by an arthrodesis. Segmental endoprostheses are routinely used for the bony reconstruction. The use of large segmental allografts or allograft composite (with an endoprosthesis) has become less frequent within the past decade. Bickels et al.[94] reported a low prosthetic failure in 110 consecutive modular distal femoral endoprostheses. Several surgical techniques were consistently used, including routine cementation of the stem and gastrocnemius rotation flaps for adequate soft tissue coverage when needed. The 5- and 10-year survival rates of persons with distal femoral prostheses were 93% and 88%, respectively (Fig. 116.17). Shehadah et al.[106] from the same institution reported longer term follow-up (average 10 years) of 241 prostheses. A modular rotating-hinge prosthesis with longer median follow-up was successful in 81% and 70% at 5 and 10 years, respectively.

Proximal Tibia. Today, limb-sparing procedures often are feasible for tumors of the proximal tibia after induction chemotherapy. It is more difficult to obtain an adequate margin of resection and a good functional result with lesions of the proximal tibia, which tend to have a higher incidence of local complications than do distal femoral tumors. These problems are directly related to the anatomic constraints: minimal adjacent soft tissue and the normal subcutaneous location of the medial tibial border. It is extremely important that the biopsy be small and that it avoid the knee joint. A core biopsy of medial flare is preferred to avoid contamination of the anterior musculature, patellar tendon, and peroneal nerve (Fig. 116.18). Reconstruction is achieved by endoprosthetic replacement, arthrodesis, or allograft. The medial gastrocnemius is routinely transferred to provide soft tissue coverage of the reconstructed area. The proximal tibia remains the most difficult site in which to perform a limb-sparing resection and reconstruction. As a result of the development of smaller, modular prostheses, which are easier to cover with muscle; the routine use of the medial gastrocnemius flaps for prosthetic coverage; and reconstruction of the extensor mechanism, limb-survival rates have almost doubled from the early 1980s (from 35% to 40% of all cases to 70% to 80%).

Proximal Fibula. Tumors of the proximal fibula require the same evaluation as do proximal tibial lesions. Contraindications

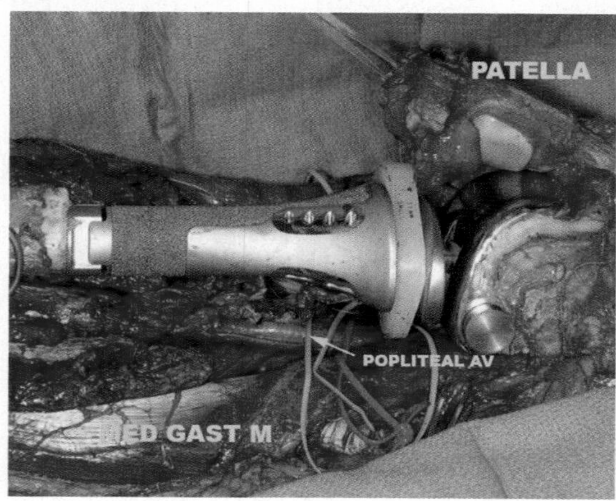

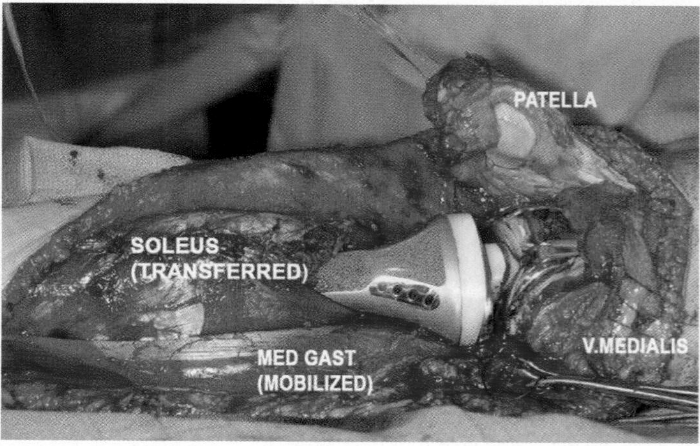

FIGURE 116.18 Limb-sparing resection of the proximal tibia. **A:** Tibia prosthesis following resection of tumor. It is necessary to reconstruct the extensor mechanism and to cover the prosthesis with muscle. **B:** Prosthesis has been partially covered by the soleus muscle. The next step is the medial gastrocnemius muscle transfer. (From Modular Replacement Systems Stryker Orthopedics, Mahwah, New Jersey.)

to resection are direct tibial involvement, an anomalously absent posterior tibial artery, and intra-articular knee joint extension. Adequate resection includes the fibula, the tibiofibular joint, the anterior and lateral muscle compartments. The surgical defect is reconstructed by rotating a lateral gastrocnemius muscle flap. Following resection, the only functional deficit is a foot drop, which is treated by an orthosis. Knee function is normal without any instability.

Osteosarcoma of the Pelvis and Proximal Femur

Osteosarcomas of the pelvis and proximal femur are less common than those occurring at other anatomic areas. They account for 10% and 5%, respectively, of all osteosarcomas.[134] Tumors arising from these structures are often large, involve important structures, and are difficult to resect. Hemipelvectomy is often required for pelvic tumors, whereas modified hemipelvectomy is used for tumors of the proximal femur. The limb-sparing options, when feasible, are all functionally superior to amputation at this level. A poorly planned biopsy often contaminates the extrapelvic structures, typically making a hemipelvectomy the only safe option (Fig. 116.19).

Fahey et al.[150] reviewed 25 patients with osteosarcoma of the pelvis treated at the University of Florida between 1967 and 1990 and described their biologic behavior, growth, and histologic and vascular findings. Common problems included delay in diagnosis, widespread invasion into major pelvic veins, microscopic foci of tumor in otherwise normal tissue, and extension into adjacent (and other) pelvic structures.

The high incidence of venous invasion requires that the iliac vessels be evaluated preoperatively and intraoperatively. Radiographic staging studies should include a thorough evaluation of the iliac vessels. This can best be performed by CT, MRI with contrast, and pelvic venography. Survival for patients with pelvic osteosarcomas is approximately one-half compared to other extremity osteosarcomas.

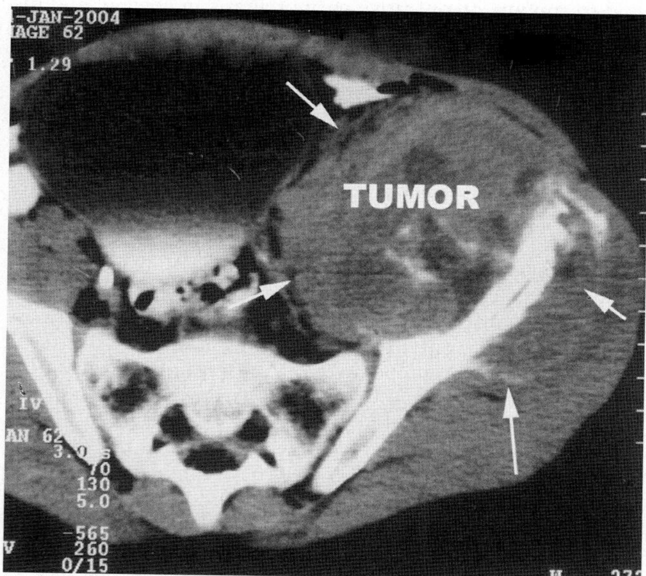

FIGURE 116.19 Osteosarcoma of the pelvis. Computed tomography of a large pelvic osteosarcoma. Pelvic overall survival is often large and may require a hemipelvectomy. The ilium is most commonly involved. Extension to the sciatic joint or hip joint makes a safe resection often difficult. In general, the survival rate of pelvic osteosarcomas is one-half of other appendicular sites. A unique characteristic of pelvic overall survival is the propensity to involve the microvasculature as well as the larger veins of the pelvis.

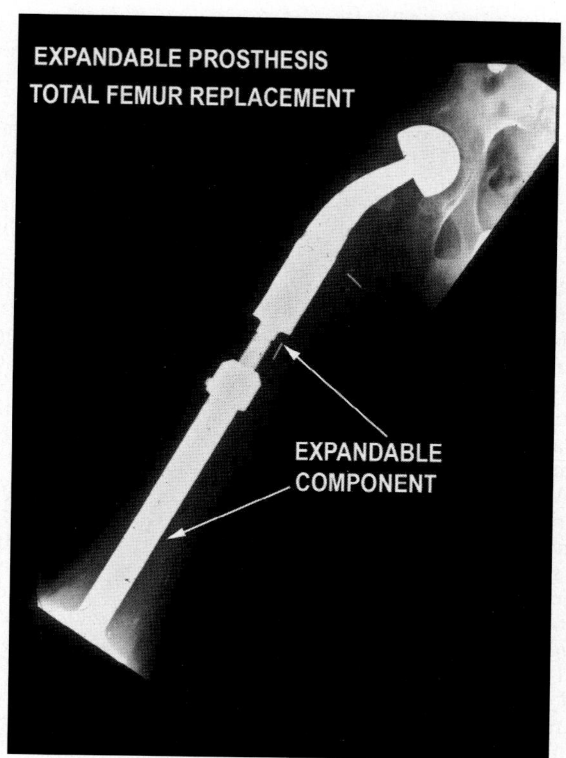

FIGURE 116.20 Total femoral expandable prosthesis. Expandable prostheses are only required in the skeletally immature patients with significant projected growth remaining.

Expandable Prostheses for Young Children

Use of endoprosthetic replacement in young children continues to present problems because of the effect of the procedure on subsequent bone growth. Approximately 70% of the total growth of the lower limb is a result of growth of the distal femoral and proximal tibial growth plates. Grimer et al.[137] has the longest and largest experience of the use of expandable prostheses for over 30 years from the National Health Service (UK). They have treated 176 patients with an expandable prosthesis with various designs over 30 years; 117 patients remain alive and 89 have reached skeletal maturity. The overall limb salvage rate (Kaplan-Meier analysis) was 83.9% at 20 years.

Today, many manufacturers and surgeons are concentrating on designing prostheses that do not require an open or percutaneous surgical procedure for expansion (Fig. 116.20).

Status of Limb-Sparing Surgery in Developing Countries

Since the previous edition of this text, several large studies from the Peoples Republic of China (PRC; University of Peking) and from India (Tata Memorial Hospital) have been reported. Beijing Ji Shui Tan (JST) Hospital is the largest treatment center in the PRC, from which almost all of the large-scale case studies on osteosarcoma treatment are derived. It initiated a nationwide comprehensive treatment program for osteosarcoma in the 1970s. Their treatment protocol was similar to that used in the West—combining preoperative chemotherapy, surgery (either limb-salvage approaches or amputation), and postoperative chemotherapy. Since the 1970s the chemotherapeutic drugs used included HD-MTX, ADR, and DDP, and more recently IFOS (since the 1990s).[151–153]

Niu et al.[154] reported on 189 osteosarcoma patients treated at the University of Peking (Beijing) after 1990 with a survival rate of 78.5% and a local recurrence rate of 16.6% (15 of 90). The functional outcomes of patients undergoing limb sparing surgery using the MSTS system was 85 of 100 with no difference (P = .05) noted from the method of reconstruction.

Recently, the Chinese Osteosarcoma Group of Chinese Anti-Cancer Association[155] organized a multiprosthesis center study to analyze the data of 2,015 patients treated in 17 facilities from 1998 to 2008. They reported an overall survival rate of 64.0%; overall response rate of 86.0%; disease-free survival rate of 56.0%; recurrence-free survival of 60.0%; limb salvage rate of 79%; local recurrence rate of 9.1%; and lung metastasis rate of 24.8%.

Agarwal et al.[156] reported from the Tata Memorial Hospital, Mumbai, India, on an "effective low-cost treatment" for neoadjuvant chemotherapy (without methotrexate) and limb sparing surgery for 135 patients with extremity osteosarcoma, of which 120 patients had follow-up. This was the first large report from India on this subject. They utilized a locally designed and fabricated stainless steel prosthesis and reported a 61% disease-free rate. There were 18 local recurrences (9%), and 17 of these patients developed metastatic disease. These overall results and outcomes are similar to those reported in multiple U.S. and European studies. The main problems emphasized by these authors are the access to medical and specialized care found in other large countries and the lack of financial and insurance coverage. All authors emphasized that the standard of care in their respective countries is chemotherapy combined with limb sparing surgery when possible. Limb-sparing surgery still remains a challenge in the developing countries, but the expertise does exist.

Clinical Presentations of Osteosarcoma and Treatment Considerations

Localized-Extremity Disease. Management of osteosarcoma requires the expertise of a multidisciplinary team familiar with the various management options. CT-guided biopsy is now the most common mode of establishing a diagnosis. Multiple cores should be obtained through one puncture site in line with the potential incision. A pathologist must be present to determine if viable (i.e., readable) material is obtained; touch press and hematoxylin and eosin slides are required.

The patient with a primary tumor of the extremity without evidence of metastases requires surgery to control the primary tumor and chemotherapy to control micrometastatic disease. Routine amputations are no longer performed; all patients should be evaluated for limb-sparing options. Intensive, multiagent chemotherapeutic regimens have provided the best results to date. Almost all patients are treated with induction (preoperative) chemotherapy. Patients who are initially judged unsuitable for limb-sparing surgery often become good candidates following chemotherapy. In making such a decision, the restaging studies (as discussed previously) are important determinants. Those with a good response may become suitable candidates for limb-sparing operations.

Pelvic Tumors and Unresectable Disease. In some pelvic and most vertebral primary tumors, complete resection often is not possible. Most pelvic osteosarcomas can be treated by hemipelvectomy; more centrally located pelvic tumors, especially those involving the sacrum, are unresectable. Only a few pelvic osteosarcomas can be treated by limb-sparing resection (internal hemipelvectomy). Contraindications to resection are unusually large extraosseous extensions with sacral plexus or major vascular involvement. On rare occasions, vertebral and sacral resections have been attempted.[157–159] In general, these tumors cannot be resected with negative margins and are best treated by radiotherapy and chemotherapy. Some success has been achieved with systemic or intra-arterial chemotherapy, which is administered to convert apparently inoperable tumors into lesions that can be ablated surgically.[113] Patients with primary tumors of the axial skeleton usually have a poor outcome because local control is rare. The prognosis for these patients may improve with a more aggressive surgical approach and more effective chemotherapy. Patients whose tumors can be completely resected should be approached with curative intent; radiotherapy may provide significant palliation in individuals with unresectable primary tumors and has been supported in a small series from the COSS database by Ozaki et al.[160] to be associated with improved survival.

Metastatic Pulmonary Disease at Diagnosis

Metastatic disease detected at initial diagnosis does not preclude a curative treatment strategy, although the presence of extrathoracic metastases makes cure extremely unlikely. In general, the surgical principles outlined for the treatment of relapsing patients apply equally to the patient who presents with macroscopic metastases. Newly diagnosed patients have not been exposed to chemotherapy and are, thus, less likely to have drug-resistant tumors. Therefore, several options are available to them. Kager et al.[47] reported that for the patient who presents with resectable disease (i.e., usually fewer than 15 pulmonary nodules and a primary tumor of the extremity), the traditional approach has been resection of all evidence of macroscopic disease by median sternotomy and limb amputation or resection, followed by intensive adjuvant chemotherapy. The tumor burden is thereby reduced to a minimum before the application of adjuvant therapy. Some investigators have favored treatment with chemotherapy, followed weeks or months later by definitive surgery for residual macroscopic disease in primary and metastatic sites.[161] Arguments advanced to justify this approach are similar to those used to support preoperative chemotherapy in general, and the theoretic advantages and disadvantages of this strategy, as discussed above for patients with nonmetastatic osteosarcoma, apply here as well. The risk for the patient with metastases is that growth of tumor nodules in the face of chemotherapy may render small, operable metastases unresectable and prevent cure. Although the timing of the surgery of the primary tumor and metastatic sites has been variable, most modern approaches entail alternating chemotherapy and surgery. The initial treatment is usually a course of chemotherapy, followed by surgical resection of the primary tumor, followed by a second course of chemotherapy and surgical ablation of metastatic sites, followed by the remaining courses of chemotherapy. Patients with tumors that respond to presurgical chemotherapy are more likely to be cured. In those with inoperable metastases, primary treatment with chemotherapy is probably appropriate; metastases may respond sufficiently to allow complete resection. Because these patients usually require surgery for the primary tumor as a palliative procedure, early surgery may be recommended, despite unresectable pulmonary disease. Although improving, the outlook for patients presenting with metastatic disease remains poor.[161,162]

New Systemic Therapeutic Approaches

Over the years, there has been interest in developing immunostimulatory agents that might be of benefit in the treatment of osteosarcoma. A randomized, double-blind study performed in spontaneous canine osteosarcoma in 1989 demonstrated that the macrophage activator muramyl tripeptide (MTP) prolonged survival in dogs after amputation. Subsequent clinical studies in patients with pulmonary metastases at M. D. Anderson Cancer Center showed a median time to relapse of 9 months after metastasectomy and 24 weeks of liposomal MTP (MTP-PE), compared to 4.5 months for historical control patients.[163–165] Based on these promising results, the POG and Children's Cancer Group performed a joint randomized study to determine whether the addition of MTP-PE to chemotherapy would enhance survival in newly diagnosed patients. The study also evaluated whether the addition of IFOS to HD-MTX, ADM, and CDDP improved survival. The results of this study, which accrued almost 800 patients, were somewhat surprising in that the addition of MTP-PE appeared to improve survival only in the patients who received IFOS. The 4-year event-free survival in this group is 70%, compared to 57% for patients receiving IFOS but no MTP-PE. However, patients treated with the standard three-drug combination of HD-MTX, ADM, and CDDP had a 4-year disease-free survival of 65% compared to 62% for those patients who had also received MTP-PE.[166] These results suggest that there may be some modest benefit to patients treated with the macrophage-activating agent MTP. However, there appears to be specific drug interactions because this benefit is only seen in patients receiving IFOS. Longer-term follow-up analysis of 662 nonmetastatic patients has somewhat altered these conclusions, suggesting that the addition of IFOS to HD-MTX, ADM, and CDDP did not enhance overall survival or event-free survival, while the addition of MTP-PE did result in a statistically significant improvement of overall survival (6-year overall survival 78% with MTP-PE vs. 70% without MTP-PE; $P = .03$).[167] Longer-term follow-up of 91 patients with metastatic disease treated with the identical regimens did not demonstrate a statistically improved outcome in any arm of the study, with a 34% overall 5-year event-free survival for all patients.[168]

Data from the Karolinska Hospital has reported that the use of another immunomodulating agent, leukocyte interferon, may enhance survival for high-risk osteosarcoma patients and suggested that this should be studied in more detail in high-risk patients.[169]

Because the overwhelming majority of metastases in osteosarcoma occur in the lung, many investigators have sought to develop therapies that target microscopic and macroscopic disease in the lungs. Toward that end, investigators at the Mayo Clinic have reported the results of early clinical studies using aerosolized granulocyte-macrophage colony-stimulating factor for patients with a variety of tumors and pulmonary metastases. The results of this study were promising and were followed up with a Children's Oncology Group phase 2 study for patients with osteosarcoma and pulmonary metastases. This study has recently been completed, but results are not yet available.

Several groups have recently reported that the expression of the Her-2/neu (ErbB-2) protein occurs in osteosarcoma. In a retrospective study of 26 patients with osteosarcoma treated at the University of Tokyo, 42% of tumors expressed Her-2 protein, and expression was associated with early pulmonary metastases and poor survival.[170] Another retrospective study of 53 patients at Memorial Sloan-Kettering Cancer Center also found Her-2 expression in 42% of tumors at presentation and confirmed that expression was associated with a worse event-free survival.[171] Other groups have reported similar findings. This is of potential therapeutic interest because breast cancers that express Her-2/neu have been shown to respond to the humanized monoclonal antibody trastuzumab directed against Her-2/neu. However, these data have been contradicted by several reports, one finding Her-2/neu expression to be correlated with increased survival in osteosarcoma and another study finding no Her-2/neu membranous staining (that is characteristic of breast cancer) in 66 osteosarcoma samples.[172] It may be of note that none of the studies showing expression of Her-2/neu found clear evidence of gene amplification, which is almost uniformly associated with overexpression in breast cancers. Nonetheless, based on the findings of expression and the promising results of the use of trastuzumab in Her-2-positive breast cancer, the Children's Oncology Group recently completed a study that includes the use of trastuzumab in high-risk osteosarcoma patients with documented expression of Her-2/neu. The results of this study are not yet available.

Vascular endothelial growth factor (VEGF) has been found to play a role in many tumors and led to the development of several agents targeting this pathway, including the approved humanized monoclonal antibody directed against VEGF, bevacizumab, and a variety of kinase inhibitors currently undergoing clinical evaluation. This pathway appears to be operant in osteosarcoma as well.[173] There is also an ongoing study to evaluate the addition of bevacizumab to standard chemotherapy in newly diagnosed patients with osteosarcoma (Helman LJ, personal communication).

Radiation Therapy in the Treatment of Osteosarcoma

Background. Past experience with primary radiotherapy for osteosarcomas has shown that high radiation doses can sterilize some tumors, but it is also associated with significant necrosis of normal tissue. Radiotherapy has, however, been shown to be successful in several distinct clinical situations—facial lesions, palliation, and, possibly, as a postoperative adjuvant.

Radiotherapy in the Radical Setting. As was evident in the local management of patients in randomized trials addressing the role of adjuvant whole lung irradiation, radiotherapy, alone or as a local adjuvant, was used relatively frequently. With the high local control expectation of surgery after induction chemotherapy and pathologic response assessment, the role for radiotherapy in osteosarcoma is now restricted to selected circumstances. For the most part, these are determined by critical and life-threatening locations of primary disease where adequate surgical removal is unlikely. These are represented by lesions in critical areas of the head and neck, spine, and pelvis where surgery has already been attempted or has been deemed not possible.

Palliation

External-Beam and Radiation Sensitizers. Radiation therapy is extremely beneficial in patients requiring palliation of metastatic bony sarcomas; tumors at axial sites, which are unresectable; and advanced, inoperable lesions of the pelvis or extremities.

Bone-Seeking Targeted Radioisotopes. An additional interesting approach is the use of the isotope ^{153}Sm-EDTMP (153-samarium ethylenediaminetetramethylenephosphonate) to target "bone-specific" radiotherapy to osteoblastic osteosarcomas. Originally introduced for palliation of bone pain arising from osteoblastic bone metastasis, preliminary evidence suggests that ^{153}Sm-EDTMP has attractive possibilities to target bone-forming tumors in surgically inaccessible sites and in refractory tumors, possibly in combination with external-beam radiotherapy. The therapeutic effect of this compound comes from its beta-emitting capability derived by neutron capture from ^{153}Sa. The circumstances for the use of this treatment are almost ideal because there is rapid bone uptake and bone surface retention of ^{153}Sm-EDTMP for many months, and unbound compound undergoes rapid urinary excretion. Unfortunately, the beta-emitting property can also result in myeloablation due to marrow tolerance, necessitating autologous peripheral blood stem cell support. Anderson et al.[79] from the Mayo Clinic reported a dose-escalation trial of ^{153}Sm-EDTMP and showed this to be of particular risk with high doses of ^{153}Sm-EDTMP (30 mCi/kg). Of note, however, nonhematologic sequelae are minimal, and reduction or elimination of opiates is a uniform finding in all cases.

Variants of Classic Osteosarcoma

Dahlin and Unni[37] have identified 11 variants of the classic osteosarcoma. These accounted for 268 of 1,021 (26%) cases reviewed at the Mayo Clinic. Excluding tumors arising secondary to Paget's disease, irradiation, or dedifferentiation of a chondrosarcoma, parosteal and periosteal osteosarcomas are the most common variants of classic osteosarcoma arising in the extremities. In contrast to classic osteosarcoma, which arises within a bone, parosteal and periosteal osteosarcomas arise on the surface of the bone (juxtacortical).

The three types of surface osteosarcomas and their respective incidences are parosteal osteosarcoma (4%), periosteal osteosarcoma (1%), and high-grade surface osteosarcoma (less than 1%).[38] The Mayo Clinic reported 518 surface osteosarcomas seen between 1926 and 1996. The incidence was 335 parosteal osteosarcomas (64.7%), 137 periosteal osteosarcomas (26.4%), and 46 high-grade surface osteosarcomas (8.9%). These 518 surface osteosarcomas were from a pool of 4,365 osteosarcoma tumors (i.e., a ratio of 1.0 to 8.4 cases).[174]

Parosteal Osteosarcoma

Clinical Characteristics. Parosteal osteosarcoma is a distinct variant of conventional osteosarcoma that accounts for 4% of all osteosarcomas. It arises from the cortex of a bone and generally occurs in older individuals. It has a better prognosis than classic osteosarcoma. The distal femur is the most common site.[40]

Radiographic Findings. A slight predominance of parosteal osteosarcoma is found in women. The distal posterior femur is involved in 72% of all cases; the proximal humerus and proximal tibia are the next most frequent sites. Parosteal osteosarcoma metastasizes slowly and has an overall survival rate of 75% to 85%. Unni et al.[40] noted that all patients who died of tumor lived longer than 5 years after treatment. The natural history of parosteal osteosarcoma is progressive enlargement and late metastasis. Parosteal osteosarcoma presents as a mass and occasionally is associated with pain. In contrast to conventional osteosarcoma, duration of symptoms varies from months to years. Unni et al.[40] reported that 50 of 79 patients had complaints of longer than 1 year, and one-third of this group had pain for more than 5 years. Tumor size, location, and duration of symptoms did not correlate with survival.

Pathology and Grading. Parosteal osteosarcoma is characterized by well-formed lamellar or woven bone with a mature spindle cell stroma and few signs of malignancy (Fig. 116.21). The cellularity of the spindle cell components varies; generally, it is not anaplastic, with few mitoses. Cortical tumors of the posterior femur should always be suspected of being malignant; this is a rare location for a benign osteochondroma. In contrast to sarcoma, myositis ossificans is rarely attached to the underlying bone. In addition, the periphery is more mature radiographically and histologically. Ahuja et al.[38] reviewed all cases of parosteal osteosarcoma at Memorial Sloan-Kettering Cancer Center from 1934 to 1975 and described three grades: grade I (low grade), grade II (intermediate), and grade III (high grade). They emphasized the importance of evaluating the fibroblastic, cartilaginous, and osseous components independently. Of 24 patients, 8 were grade I, 10 grade II, and 6 grade III. Unni et al.[40] reviewed 79 patients and reported that 18 were grade II (23%) and seven had high-grade foci (9%). The

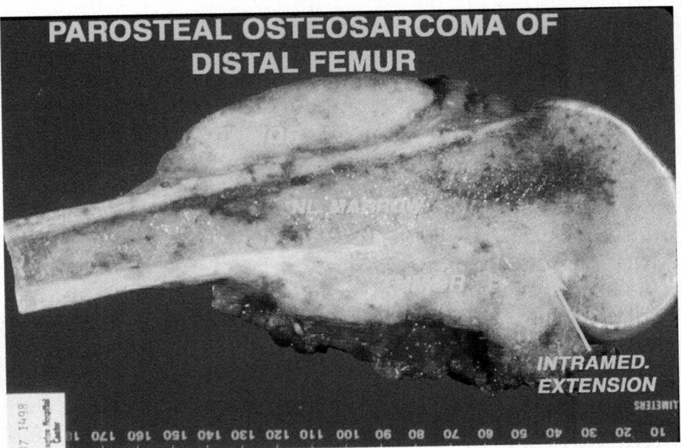

FIGURE 116.21 Parosteal osteosarcoma of the distal femur. Gross specimen following resection of the distal femur. Note the posterior tumor mass, which is characteristic of parosteal osteosarcoma. There is intramedullary extension (*arrow*), which occurs in the majority of these tumors.

survival rate of patients with grade III tumors is similar to that of those with conventional osteosarcoma.

Jelinek et al.[175] reviewed the records of the Armed Forces Institute of Pathology and evaluated 60 patients with parosteal osteosarcomas for tumor size, location, and presence of cleavage plane; intramedullary extension; soft tissue mass; and the presence and pattern of ossification. Tumors were classified as low grade or high grade. A cleavage plane was present in 20 low-grade (62%) and 19 high-grade (68%) lesions. On cross-sectional imaging, intramedullary extension was present in 13 low-grade (41%) and 14 high-grade (50%) lesions. These authors concluded that a poorly defined soft tissue component distinct from the ossified matrix is the most distinctive feature of high-grade parosteal osteosarcoma and may be the optimal site to perform a biopsy.

Treatment. Wide excision of the tumor is the treatment of choice. No experience with preoperative chemotherapy or radiotherapy has been reported. Parosteal osteosarcomas are often amenable to limb preservation due to their distal location, low grade, and lack of local invasiveness. Vascular displacement is not a contraindication for resection. The major surgical decision usually is whether to remove the entire end of the bone and the adjacent joint or to preserve the joint. Small lesions can be resected with joint preservation. If the medullary canal is involved, the joint usually cannot be preserved. A second factor mitigating against joint preservation is extensive cortical involvement. Techniques of resection and reconstruction are similar to those described above for conventional osteosarcoma. The major difference is that only a small amount of soft tissue usually must be resected; consequently, a good functional result is obtained. Grade III parosteal lesions warrant systemic therapy because of the high risk of metastasis.

Dedifferentiated Parosteal Osteosarcoma

Bertoni et al.,[176] in the largest report of dedifferentiated parosteal osteosarcoma (DPOS), described the clinical and radiological features, histological specimens, treatments, and outcomes of 29 patients. They emphasized that the finding of radiographic areas of lucency in an otherwise sclerotic lesion was a clue to the diagnosis of DPOS in 18 of the 29 patients. The histological subtypes of the dedifferentiated components were high-grade osteoblastic osteosarcoma in 14 patients, fibroblastic osteosarcoma in 10 patients, giant cell–rich osteosarcoma in 3 patients, and chondroblastic osteosarcoma in 2 patients. Two-thirds of

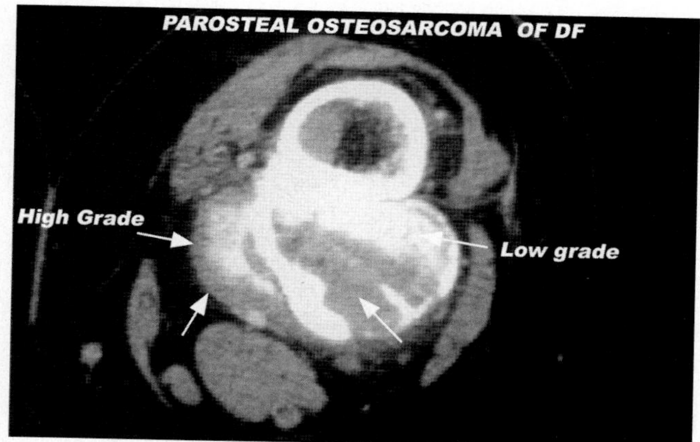

FIGURE 116.22 Computed tomography scan of a dedifferentiated parosteal osteosarcoma of the distal femur. The radiolucent component of this mass represents a high-grade (type 3) dedifferentiation of this tumor. Dedifferentiated parosteal osteosarcomas occur in between 10% to 15% of all parosteal osteosarcomas.

the patients had intramedullary involvement. Twenty of 29 patients (69%) remained disease free at an average follow-up of 107 months. All patients received adjuvant chemotherapy. No conclusion could be made regarding the role of adjuvant chemotherapy for DPOS, although the tendency today is to utilize chemotherapy for all patients with DPOS (Fig. 116.22).

Periosteal Osteosarcoma

Periosteal osteosarcoma is a rare cortical variant of osteosarcoma that arises superficially on the cortex, most often on the tibia shaft. Radiographically, it is a small radiolucent lesion with some evidence of bone spiculation. The cortex is characteristically intact, with a scooped-out appearance and a Codman's triangle. Histologically, periosteal osteosarcomas are relatively high-grade chondroblastic osteosarcomas composed of a malignant cartilage with areas of anaplastic spindle cells and osteoid production (Fig. 116.23). Unni et al.,[39] in a report of 23 cases, found periosteal osteosarcomas to occur one-third as frequently as the parosteal variant. The largest tumor measured 2.5 by 3.5 cm. Four of the 23 patients died of metastatic disease.

One of the largest reported series was by Okada et al.[174] from the Mayo Clinic. They evaluated 46 patients and described their radiographic, clinical, and pathologic evaluation. All the tumors were broad based and attached to the underlying cortex. The authors attempted to evaluate the effectiveness of chemotherapy in this very rare subtype of osteosarcoma. Fifteen of the 21 patients who received systemic treatment showed no response to chemotherapy. Among these 15, only 1 patient remains alive. All six patients who showed a good response to chemotherapy are alive. Medullary involvement did not affect prognosis. The survival rate was 57.5% at 3 years and 46.1% at 5 years. Treatment is similar to that of other high-grade lesions. *En bloc* resection should be performed when feasible; amputation is rarely indicated.

Paget's Sarcoma

In approximately 1% of patients with Paget's disease, a primary bone sarcoma will develop. Greditzer et al.[133] reported 41 sarcomas among 4,415 patients with Paget's disease followed at the Mayo Clinic; 35 were osteosarcomas and 6 were fibrosarcomas. The average patient age was 64 years, and the most common sites were the pelvis, femur, and humerus. One-half of these lesions were osteolytic; the remainder had a mixed pattern. Cortical destruction and a soft tissue component were the most common signs noted; periosteal elevation was rare. The diagnosis is usually made by plain radiography and confirmed by biopsy.

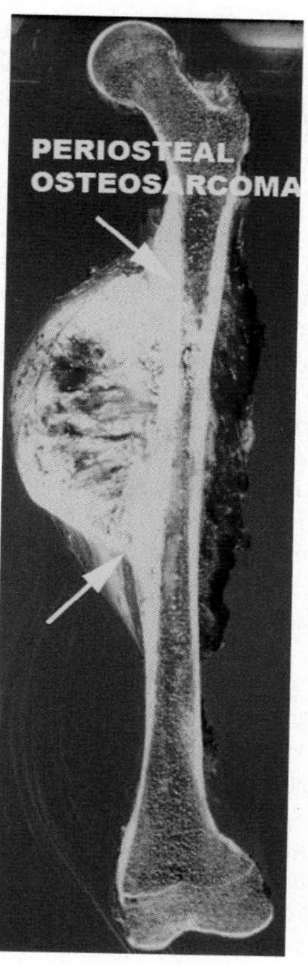

FIGURE 116.23 Periosteal osteosarcoma. Gross specimen of a large periosteal osteosarcoma arising from the cortical diaphysis of the femur (*arrows*).

High-Grade Surface Osteosarcoma

High-grade surface osteosarcoma (peripheral conventional osteosarcoma) is the rarest variant of surface osteosarcoma.[177] The parosteal and periosteal osteosarcomas have a better prognosis, whereas the high-grade surface variant has the same prognosis as the conventional, intramedullary lesion. Schajowicz et al.[177] studied the different surface osteosarcomas. They reported that only 7 of 80 surface osteosarcomas (9%) were considered to be the high-grade variant. Clinically, the median age was 13.5 years (younger than that of patients with other surface lesions), and almost all were located in the diaphyseal region of the bone. Adjuvant chemotherapy is warranted due to the high rate of metastases.

Small Cell Osteosarcoma

The small cell osteosarcoma, a rare variant of osteosarcomas, resembles a Ewing's sarcoma and is often classified as an "atypical" Ewing's sarcoma. Characteristically, areas of osteoid and, on occasion, chondroid formation are present. The differential diagnosis includes Ewing's sarcoma, atypical Ewing's sarcoma, primitive neuroectodermal tumor, mesenchymal chondrosarcoma, lymphoma, and Askin's tumor. Differentiation from Ewing's sarcoma and the typical osteosarcoma is important because the response of small cell osteosarcoma to treatment is poorly defined.[178] The treatment is similar to other high-grade sarcomas. The choice of a "Ewing" protocol or an "osteosarcomas" protocol remains difficult to determine.

Radiation-Induced Osteosarcoma

Radiation-induced osteosarcomas arise in a previously irradiated field and meet the general criteria of a radiation-induced sarcoma (i.e., they appear after a latent period of 5 to 20 years, are documented to be secondary [different from the original one], and occur in a documented irradiated field). Amendola et al.[179] from the University of Michigan reviewed 22,306 patients treated with radiation between 1934 and 1983 and reported 23 patients with radiation-associated sarcoma (prevalence, 0.1%). The median latent period was 13 years (range, 3 to 34 years). The radiation doses ranged from 25 to 72 Gy. The data suggest that intensive chemotherapy may have shortened the latency period.

In two nested case-control studies of 3-year cancer survivors from France and the United Kingdom, the risk of osteosarcoma was found to be a linear function of radiation dose and alkylating agent chemotherapy.[180] The 20-year risk of osteosarcoma among survivors of retinoblastoma (7.2%), Ewing's sarcoma (5.4%), and other bone tumors (2.2%) suggests a genetic influence in the induction of secondary osteosarcoma. However, the risk of developing bone sarcoma within 20 years for the majority of survivors of childhood cancer is less than 0.9%.

The treatment of radiation-associated osteosarcoma is wide resection, when possible, combined with adjuvant chemotherapy. A previously irradiated field presents a unique challenge for the surgeon—choosing the best local option. The likelihood of local complications is greater in such cases. Tabone et al.[181,182] report results from the French Society of Pediatric Oncology that indicate that an intensive approach using chemotherapy and surgery will yield 8-year overall and event-free survival rates of 50% and 41%, respectively.

Chondrosarcoma

Chondrosarcomas are the second most common primary malignant spindle cell tumors of bone. They form a heterogeneous group of tumors whose basic neoplastic tissue is cartilaginous without evidence of direct osteoid formation. Occasionally, bone formation occurs from differentiation of cartilage. If evidence is found of direct osteoid or bone production, the lesion is classified as an osteosarcoma. The five types of chondrosarcomas are central, peripheral, mesenchymal, differentiated, and clear cell. The classic chondrosarcomas are central (arising within a bone) or peripheral (arising from the surface of a bone). The other three are variants and have distinct histologic and clinical characteristics.

Central and peripheral chondrosarcomas can arise as primary tumors or secondary to underlying neoplasm. Seventy-six percent of primary chondrosarcomas arise centrally. Secondary chondrosarcomas most often arise from benign cartilage tumors. The multiple forms of benign osteochondromas or enchondromas have a higher rate of malignant transformation than the corresponding solitary lesions. The treatment of chondrosarcoma is surgical resection, either by a limb-sparing procedure or an amputation (usually reserved for large pelvic chondrosarcomas). In general, there is no role for induction or postoperative chemotherapy. Radiation is required in only a few rare instances.

Central and Peripheral Chondrosarcomas

Clinical Characteristics. One-half of all chondrosarcomas occur in persons older than 40 years of age; only 3.8% develop in those younger than 20 years. Unlike osteosarcomas, the majority of chondrosarcomas arise around the shoulder and pelvic girdles or axial, ribs, and the sacrum. The most common sites are the pelvis (31%), femur (21%), and shoulder girdle (13%). Chondrosarcomas are the most common malignant tumors of the sternum and scapula.

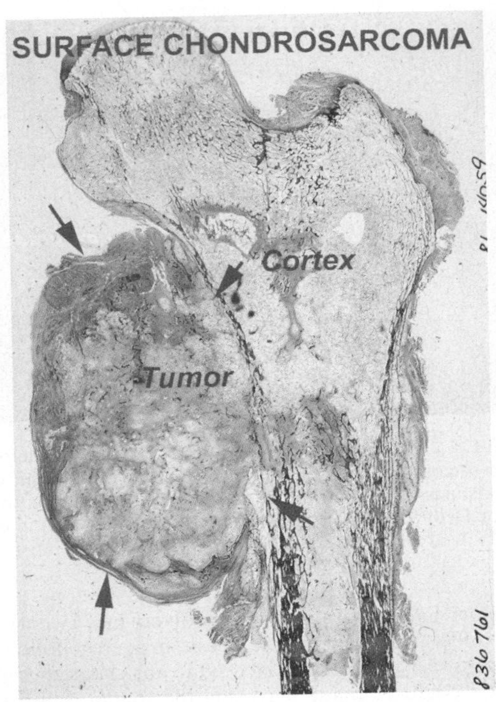

FIGURE 116.24 Surface chondrosarcoma. Whole mount section of the proximal femur showing a large juxtacortical chondrosarcoma.

Histology and Grading. Chondrosarcomas are categorized as grade 1, 2, or 3. The metastatic rate of moderate-grade lesions is 15% to 40% (Fig. 116.24).[183]

Radiographic Diagnosis and Evaluation. Central chondrosarcomas have two distinct radiologic patterns.[184] One is a small, well-defined lytic lesion with a narrow zone of transition and surrounding sclerosis with faint calcification. This is the most common malignant bone tumor, which may appear radiographically benign. The second type has no sclerotic border and is difficult to localize. The key sign of malignancy is endosteal scalloping. It is difficult to diagnose on plain radiographs and may go undetected for a long period. In contrast, peripheral chondrosarcoma is recognized easily as a large, calcified mass protruding from a bone. Proximal or axial location, skeletal maturity, and pain point toward malignancy, even though the cartilage may appear benign.

Prognosis. Metastatic potential tends to correlate with the histologic grade of the lesions. Marcove et al.[185] reported on long-term follow-up of 113 chondrosarcomas of the proximal femur and the pelvis. The survival rates in patients with grade 1, 2, or 3 lesions were 47%, 38%, and 15%, respectively; the overall survival rate was 52%. No significant difference was noted between grades 1 and 2; however, the mortality for grade 3 was significantly higher ($P < .02$) than for the other two. Eleven of 59 deaths occurred after 5 years. The authors emphasized that the meaningful survival interval should be considered 10 or 15 years. No relationship between grade, age, gender, or location was found, and there was no statistical difference between primary and secondary chondrosarcomas. Adequacy of surgical removal was the main determinant of recurrence. In general, peripheral chondrosarcomas have a lower grade than central lesions. Gitelis et al.[12] reported that 43% of peripheral lesions, compared with 13% of central lesions, were grade 1. The 10-year survival rate among those with peripheral lesions was 77%, and among those with central lesions it was 32%. Secondary chondrosarcomas arising from osteochondromas also have a low malignant potential. Eighty-five percent are grade 1. Garrison et al.[35] reported that only 3% of 75 patients with secondary chondrosarcomas from an osteochondroma developed metastases, although 12% died of local recurrence.

Treatment. The treatment of chondrosarcomas is surgical removal. No reports of effective adjuvant chemotherapy have been published. Resection guidelines for high-grade chondrosarcomas are similar to those for osteosarcoma. The shoulder and pelvic girdle are the most common sites for chondrosarcomas. This, combined with the fact that chondrosarcomas tend to be low grade, makes them amenable to limb-sparing procedures. Lesions of the ribs and sternum are treated by wide excision. Cryosurgery, a technique using liquid nitrogen after thorough curettage of the lesion, has been used for central, low-grade chondrosarcomas.[91,92] A few reports have been published of effective radiation therapy for axial chondrosarcomas.

Limb-Sparing Procedures: Specific Anatomic Sites

Pelvis. The pelvis consists of three areas: ilium, periacetabulum, and pubic rami. Each site can be resected independent of the others. Resections are classified as type 1 (iliac wing), type 2 (acetabulum), or type 3 (pubic rami, pelvic floor). Bone scan most accurately determines specific bony involvement, whereas CT and MRI delineate the extraosseous component. Contraindications to resection are vascular (iliac artery and vein), peritoneal, and sacroiliac joint or sarcoplexus involvement, and long-term results of these procedures have been published by Enneking and Dunham[186] who reported that local recurrence was only 4% if adequate margins were obtained. Function was nearly normal if the hip joint was preserved. If the hip joint was removed and fusion was obtained, results were good. A saddle prosthesis has been developed, allowing reconstruction after periacetabular resections. Pelvic allograft combined with hip arthroplasty is an alternative technique of reconstruction. In general, this approach has had a high failure rate as a result of infection, fracture, and dislocation.

Proximal Femur. Chondrosarcoma of the proximal femur can often be treated successfully by resection and prosthetic replacement. A lateral trephine or core biopsy is recommended. A posterior surgical approach should be avoided because of potential contamination of the posterior flap in the event that a hemipelvectomy is required.

Shoulder. The technique of resection of chondrosarcomas of the proximal humerus and scapula is similar to that described for osteosarcomas. In low-grade intracompartmental (stage IA) tumors, preservation of the deltoid, rotator cuff musculature, and glenoid is possible, and alternatives for reconstruction are more variable.[187] Endoprostheses, fibula autografts, and allografts all have a high rate of success but are less common. Wittig et al.[149] have described a technique of intra-articular resection and reconstruction using a GoreTex sleeve as a new capsule. The use of GoreTex capsular reconstruction reduces the incidence of shoulder subluxation or dislocation.

Radiation Therapy in the Treatment of Chondrosarcoma

Although chondrosarcomas have generally been considered radioresistant, data in fact exist from several sources to show that some of these lesions are radiocurable, although it is preferable if it can be combined with surgery. Unresectable or inoperable chondrosarcomas that arise within the axial skeleton and pelvic or shoulder girdle, or both, can be controlled and, in some cases, cured by radiation therapy.

Malignant Fibrous Histiocytoma

MFH is a high-grade bone tumor that is histologically similar to its soft tissue counterpart. It is a disease of adulthood. The most common sites are the metaphyseal ends of long bones, especially around the knee. AP values are normal. Pathologic fracture is common. Huvos[8] emphasized that a lytic metaphyseal lesion with a pathologic fracture in an adult with a normal SAP level suggests a primary MFH rather than an osteosarcoma or fibrosarcoma. MFH disseminates rapidly. Spanier et al.[6] reported that 9 of 11 patients died of their tumors. The average disease-free survival was 6 months. One-third of patients (three of nine) with pulmonary metastasis had lymph node dissemination. The author hypothesized that lymphatic spread was due to the histiocytic component of the tumor.

Radiographic Characteristics

MFH is an osteolytic lesion associated with marked cortical disruption, minimal cortical or periosteal reaction, and no evidence of matrix formation. The extent of the tumor routinely exceeds plain radiographic signs. McCarthy et al.,[7] reporting on 35 patients with MFH, noted that four tumors were multicentric and four were associated with bone infarcts.

Treatment

Today MFH and osteosarcoma of bone are treated in much the same way. Data demonstrate that results of limb-sparing surgery for MFH of bone, as well as responses to chemotherapy among MFH patients, are very similar to those of patients with primary osteosarcoma. Picci et al.[188] evaluated the effects of neoadjuvant chemotherapy of MFH of bone and extremity osteosarcomas. They reported 51 patients treated with high-grade MFH of bone and 390 patients with high-grade osteosarcoma treated with identical regimens of neoadjuvant chemotherapy at the Rizzoli Institute between 1982 and 1994. Rates of limb salvage were approximately the same for MFH (92%) and osteosarcoma (85%), although MFH patients showed a statistically significantly lower rate of good histologic response. Despite this low chemosensitivity, the disease-free survival rates for the two neoplasms were similar (67% vs. 65%). Nevertheless, the two tumors had similar prognoses when treated with chemotherapy regimens based on MTX, CDDP, ADM, and IFOS. The surgical procedures were similar limb-sparing procedures. This study emphasized that induction chemotherapy, followed by limb-sparing surgery and subsequent postoperative chemotherapy, was just as effective for MFH of bone as for the osteosarcomas.

Bacci et al.,[189] again from the Rizzoli Institute, reported on 65 patients treated with MFH of bone in the extremities with neoadjuvant chemotherapy. The limb-salvage rate was 89% (58 patients), and the amputation rate was 11% in seven patients. The histologic response to preoperative chemotherapy was good (90% or more tumor necrosis) in 16 patients (25%) and poor in 49 patients (75%). These authors concluded that a high percentage of patients with MFH of the extremities can be cured with neoadjuvant chemotherapy and that it is usually possible to avoid amputation.

Fibrosarcoma of Bone

Clinical Characteristics

Fibrosarcoma of bone is a rare (1% of all sarcomas) entity characterized by interlacing bundles of collagen fibers (herringbone pattern) without any evidence of tumor bone or osteoid formation. Fibrosarcoma occurs in middle age. The long bones are most affected. Fifteen percent of tumors are found in the bones of the head and neck. Fibrosarcomas occasionally arise in conjunction with an underlying disease, such as fibrous dysplasia, Paget's disease, bone infarcts, osteomyelitis, and postirradiation bone and GCT. Fibrosarcoma may be either central or cortical (periosteal). The histologic grade is a good prognosticator of metastatic potential. Huvos and Higinbotham[4] reported overall survival rates of 27% and 52% for central and peripheral lesions, respectively. Late metastases do occur, and 10- and 15-year survival rates vary. In general, periosteal tumors have a better prognosis than central lesions. Surgical treatment is similar to other high-grade bony sarcomas. Limb-sparing surgery is based on the previous staging and restaging studies. The use of chemotherapy must be individualized considering the older age of these patients.

Radiographic Features

Fibrosarcoma is a radiolucent lesion that shows minimal periosteal and cortical reaction. The radiographic appearance closely correlates with the histologic grade of the tumor. Low-grade tumors are well defined, whereas high-grade lesions demonstrate indistinct margins and bone destruction similar to those of osteolytic osteosarcoma. In general, plain radiographs underestimate the extent of the lesion. Pathologic fracture is common (30%) owing to the lack of matrix formation. Differential diagnosis includes GCT, aneurysmal bone cyst, MFH, and osteolytic osteosarcoma.

Selected References

The full list of references for this chapter appears in the online version.

1. Jaffe H. *Tumors and tumorous conditions of the bone and joints*. 1st ed. Philadelphia: Lea & Febinger, 1958.
2. Lichtenstein L *Bone tumors*. 5th ed. St. Louis: Mosby, 1977.
3. Dahlin DC. *Bone tumors: general aspects and data on 6221 cases*. 3rd ed. Springfield, IL: Charles C Thomas Publisher, 1978.
4. Huvos AG, Higinbotham NL. Primary fibrosarcoma of bone. A clinicopathologic study of 130 patients. *Cancer* 1975;35(3):837.
5. Wilner D. Fibrosarcoma. In: Wilner D, ed. *Radiology of bone tumors and allied disorders*. Philadelphia: WB Saunders, 1983:2291.
6. Spanier SS, Enneking WF, Enriquez P. Primary malignant fibrous histiocytoma of bone. *Cancer* 1975;36(6):2084.
10. Marcove RC. Chodrosarcoma: diagnosis and treatment. *Orthop Clin North Am* 1977;8(4):811.
13. Dahlin DC, Cupps RE, Johnson EW Jr. Giant-cell tumor: a study of 195 cases. *Cancer* 1970;25(5):1061.
14. Hutter V, Worcester JJ, Francis K. Benign and malignant giant cell tumor of bone. A clinicopathological analysis of the natural history of the disease. *Cancer* 1962;15:653.
15. Johnson EJ, Dahlin DC Treatment of giant cell tumor of bone. *J Bone Joint Surg Am* 1959;41:895.
17. Francis K, Worcester JJ. Radical resection for tumors of the shoulder with preservation of a functional extremity. *J Bone Joint Surg Am* 1962;44:1423.
18. Marcove RC, Miké V, Hajek JV, Levin AG, Hutter RV. Osteogenic sarcoma under the age of twenty-one. A review of one hundred and forty-five operative cases. *J Bone Joint Surg Am* 1970;52(3):411.
19. Rosen G, Marcove RC, Caparros B, Nirenberg A, Kosloff C, Huvos AG. Primary osteogenic sarcoma: the rationale for preoperative chemotherapy and delayed surgery. *Cancer* 1979;43(6):2163.
20. Rosen G, Nirenberg A. Chemotherapy for osteogenic sarcoma: an investigative method, not a recipe. *Cancer Treat Rep* 1982;66(9):1687.
21. Muggia F, Catani R, Lee Y. Factor responsible for therapeutic success in osteosarcoma. In: Jones S, Salmon S, eds. *Adjuvant therapy for cancer*. New York: Grune & Stratton, 1979.
22. Cortes EP, Holland JF. Adjuvant chemotherapy for primary osteogenic sarcoma. *Surg Clin North Am* 1981;61(6):1391.
24. Link MP, Goorin AM, Miser AW, et al. The effect of adjuvant chemotherapy on relapse-free survival in patients with osteosarcoma of the extremity. *N Engl J Med* 1986;314(25):1600.
30. Rosen G, Marcove RC, Huvos AG, et al. Primary osteogenic sarcoma: eight-year experience with adjuvant chemotherapy. *J Cancer Res Clin Oncol* 1983;106(Suppl):55.
33. Lichtenstein L. Classification of primary tumors of bone. *Cancer* 1951;4:335.
34. Spjut H, et al. Tumors of bone and cartilage. In: *Atlas of tumor pathology*. Fasc. 5. 2nd series ed. Washington, DC: Armed Forces Institute of Pathology, 1971.
37. Dahlin DC, Unni KK. Osteosarcoma of bone and its important recognizable varieties. *Am J Surg Pathol* 1977;1(1):61.
38. Ahuja SC, Villacin AB, Smith J, Bullough PG, Huvos AG, Marcove RC. Juxtacortical (parosteal) osteogenic sarcoma: histological grading and prognosis. *J Bone Joint Surg Am* 1977;59(5):632.
43. Madewell JE, Ragsdale BD, Sweet DE. Radiologic and pathologic analysis of solitary bone lesions. Part I: internal margins. *Radiol Clin North Am* 1981;19(4):715.
44. Enneking WF. *Musculoskeletal tumor surgery*. Vol. 1. New York: Churchill Livingstone, 1983.
45. Enneking WF, Spanier SS, Goodman MA. A system for the surgical staging of musculoskeletal sarcoma. *Clin Orthop* 1980(153):106.
47. Kager L, Zoubek A, Pötschger U, et al. Primary metastatic osteosarcoma: presentation and outcome of patients treated on neoadjuvant Cooperative Osteosarcoma Study Group protocols. *J Clin Oncol* 2003;21(10):2011.
48. Enneking WF. Intramarrow spread of osteosarcoma. In: Enneking WF, ed. *Management of primary bone and soft tissue tumors*. Chicago: Year Book Medical Publishers, 1976.
49. Malawer MM, Dunham WK. Skip metastases in osteosarcoma: recent experience. *J Surg Oncol* 1983;22(4):236.
51. Campanacci M, Bacci G, Bertoni F, Picci P, Minutillo A, Franceschi C. The treatment of osteosarcoma of the extremities: twenty year's experience at the Istituto Ortopedico Rizzoli. *Cancer* 1981;48(7):1569.
52. Eckardt JJ. Chart of 465 patients treated over 30 years with various bone tumors at UCLA and classified by the MTS (Enneking's) classification. Malawer MM, ed. Accepted at MSTS 2010 meeting, Philadelphia, 2010.
55. Mankin HJ, Lange TA, Spanier SS. The hazards of biopsy in patients with malignant primary bone and soft-tissue tumors. *J Bone Joint Surg Am* 1982;64(8):1121.
56. McKillop JH, Etcubanas E, Goris ML. The indications for and limitations of bone scintigraphy in osteogenic sarcoma: a review of 55 patients. *Cancer* 1981;48(5):1133.
58. deSantos LA, Bernardino ME, Murray JA. Computed tomography in the evaluation of osteosarcoma: experience with 25 cases. *AJR Am J Roentgenol* 1979;132(4):535.
59. Destouet JM, Gilula LA, Murphy WA. Computed tomography of long-bone osteosarcoma. *Radiology* 1979;131(2):439.
62. Bohndorf K, Reiser M, Lochner B, Féaux de Lacroix W, Steinbrich W. Magnetic resonance imaging of primary tumours and tumour-like lesions of bone. *Skeletal Radiol* 1986;15(7):511.
65. Zimmer WD, Berquist TH, McLeod RA, et al. Bone tumors: magnetic resonance imaging versus computed tomography. *Radiology* 1985;155(3):709.
69. Hudson TM, Haas G, Enneking WF, Hawkins IF Jr. Angiography in the management of musculoskeletal tumors. *Surg Gynecol Obstet* 1975;141:21.
71. Benz MR, Tchekmedyian N, Eilber FC, et al. Utilization of positron emission tomography in the management of patients with sarcoma. *Curr Opin Oncol* 2009;21(4):345.
72. Kneisl JS, Patt JC, Johnson JC, Zuger JH. Is PET useful in detecting occult nonpulmonary metastases in pediatric bone sarcomas? *Clin Orthop Rel Res* 2006;450:101.
73. Cheon GJ, Kim MS, Lee JA, et al. Prediction model of chemotherapy response in osteosarcoma by 18F-FDG PET and MRI. *J Nucl Med* 2009;50(9):1435.
74. Hawkins DS, Conrad EU 3rd, Butrynski JE, Schuetze SM, Eary JF. [F-18]-fluorodeoxy-D-glucose-positron emission tomography response is associated with outcome for extremity osteosarcoma in children and young adults. *Cancer* 2009;115(15):3519.
75. Costelloe CM, Macapinlac HA, Madewell JE, et al. 18F-FDG PET/CT as an indicator of progression-free and overall survival in osteosarcoma. *J Nucl Med* 2009;50(3):340.
76. Franzius C, Sciuk J, Daldrup-Link HE, Jürgens H, Schober O. FDG-PET for detection of osseous metastases from malignant primary bone tumours: comparison with bone scintigraphy. *Eur J Nucl Med* 2000;27(9):1305.
79. Mail JT, Cohen MD, Mirkin LD, Provisor AJ. Response of osteosarcoma to preoperative intravenous high-dose methotrexate chemotherapy: CT evaluation. *AJR Am J Roentgenol* 1985;144(1):89.
80. Jaffe N, Knapp J, Chuang VP, et al. Osteosarcoma: intra-arterial treatment of the primary tumor with cis-diammine-dichloroplatinum II (CDP). Angiographic, pathologic, and pharmacologic studies. *Cancer* 1983;51(3):402.

86. Ueda T, Naka N, Araki N, Ishii T, et al. Validation of radiographic response evaluation criteria of preoperative chemotherapy of bone and soft tissue sarcomas: Japanese Orthopaedic Association Committee on Musculoskeletal Tumors Cooperative Study. *J Orthop Sci* 2008;13(4):304.
87. Liu J, Guo W, Yang RL, Tang XD, Yang Y. [Prognostic factors for 72 patients with osteosarcoma of the extremity treated with neoadjuvant chemotherapy]. *Zhonghua Wai Ke Za Zhi* 2008;46(15):1166.
89. Franzius C, Sciuk J, Brinkschmidt C, Jürgens H, Schober O. Evaluation of chemotherapy response in primary bone tumors with F-18 FDG positron emission tomography compared with histologically assessed tumor necrosis. *Clin Nucl Med* 2000;25(11):874.
91. Marcove RC, Stovell PB, Huvos AG, Bullough PG. The use of cryosurgery in the treatment of low and medium grade chondrosarcoma. A preliminary report. *Clin Orthop* 1977(122):147.
92. Marcove RC. A 17-year review of cryosurgery in the treatment of bone tumors. *Clin Orthop* 1982;163:231.
93. Marcove RC, Rosen G. En bloc resections for osteogenic sarcoma. *Cancer* 1980;45(12):3040.
94. Bickels J, Wittig JC, Kollender Y, et al. Distal femur resection with endoprosthetic reconstruction: a long-term follow-up study. *Clin Orthop* 2002; 400:225.
95. Malawer M. Distal femoral osteogenic sarcoma, principles of soft tissue resection and reconstruction in conjunction with prosthetic replacement. In: Chao E, ed. *Design and application of tumor prosthesis for bone and joint reconstruction*. New York: Thieme-Stratton Publisher, 1983:297.
100. Jeon DG, Lee SY, Kim JW. Bone primary sarcomas undergone unplanned intralesional procedures—the possibility of limb salvage and their oncologic results. *J Surg Oncol* 2006;94(7):592.
101. Greenberg DB, Goorin A, Gebhardt MC, et al. Quality of life in osteosarcoma survivors. *Oncology (Huntingt)* 1994;8(11):19.
104. Bacci G, Ferrari S, Mercuri M, et al. Predictive factors for local recurrence in osteosarcoma: 540 patients with extremity tumors followed for minimum 2.5 years after neoadjuvant chemotherapy. *Acta Orthop Scand* 1998; 69(3):230.
106. Shehadeh AM, et al. Long-term results of endoprosthetic reconstruction after segmental bone resection. *J Am Acad Orthop Surg* 2007; (poster 522).
107. Grimer RJ, Carter SR, Pynsent PB. The cost-effectiveness of limb salvage for bone tumours. *J Bone Joint Surg Br* 1997;79(4):558.
111. Picci P, Bacci G, Campanacci M, et al. Histologic evaluation of necrosis in osteosarcoma induced by chemotherapy. Regional mapping of viable and nonviable tumor. *Cancer* 1985;56(7):1515.
112. Bacci G, Bertoni F, Longhi A, et al. Neoadjuvant chemotherapy for high-grade central osteosarcoma of the extremity. Histologic response to preoperative chemotherapy correlates with histologic subtype of the tumor. *Cancer* 2003;97(12):3068.
113. Bielack SS, Nishida Y, Nakashima H, Shimoyama Y, Nakamura S, Ishiguro N. Prognostic factors in high-grade osteosarcoma of the extremities or trunk: an analysis of 1,702 patients treated on neoadjuvant cooperative osteosarcoma study group protocols. *J Clin Oncol* 2002;20(3):776.
114. Hauben EI, Weeden S, Pringle J, Van Marck EA, Hogendoorn PC. Does the histological subtype of high-grade central osteosarcoma influence the response to treatment with chemotherapy and does it affect overall survival? A study on 570 patients of two consecutive trials of the European Osteosarcoma Intergroup. *Eur J Cancer* 2002;38(9):1218.
116. Rosen G, Caparros B, Huvos AG, et al. Preoperative chemotherapy for osteogenic sarcoma: selection of postoperative adjuvant chemotherapy based on the response of the primary tumor to preoperative chemotherapy. *Cancer* 1982;49(6):1221.
117. Meyers PA, Heller G, Healey J, et al. Chemotherapy for nonmetastatic osteogenic sarcoma: the Memorial Sloan-Kettering experience. *J Clin Oncol* 1992;10(1):5.
118. Bacci G, Ferrari S, Bertoni F, et al. Long-term outcome for patients with nonmetastatic osteosarcoma of the extremity treated at the Istituto Ortopedico Rizzoli according to the Istituto Ortopedico Rizzoli/osteosarcoma-2 protocol: an updated report. *J Clin Oncol* 2000;18(24):4016.
120. Goorin AM, Harris MB, Bernstein M, et al. Phase II/III trial of etoposide and high-dose ifosfamide in newly diagnosed metastatic osteosarcoma: a pediatric oncology group trial. *J Clin Oncol* 2002;20(2):426.
127. Gwak HS, Yoo HJ, Youn SM, et al. Hypofractionated stereotactic radiation therapy for skull base and upper cervical chordoma and chondrosarcoma: preliminary results. *Stereotact Funct Neurosurg* 2006;83(5–6):233.
128. Gerszten PC, Ozhasoglu C, Burton SA, et al. CyberKnife frameless stereotactic radiosurgery for spinal lesions: clinical experience in 125 cases. *Neurosurgery* 2004;55(1):89.
130. Dahlin DC, Coventry MB. Osteogenic sarcoma. A study of six hundred cases. *J Bone Joint Surg Am* 1967;49(1):101.
134. Huvos A. *Bone tumors. Diagnosis, treatment, and prognosis*. Philadelphia: WB Saunders, 1979.
135. Francis KC, Kohn H, Malawer M. Osteogenic sarcoma. *J Bone Joint Surg Am* 1976;55:754.
136. Wilner D. Osteogenic sarcoma (osteosarcoma). In: *Radiology of bone tumors and allied disorders*. Philadelphia: WB Saunders, 1982.
140. Bacci G, Longhi A, Ferrari S, et al. Prognostic significance of serum alkaline phosphatase in osteosarcoma of the extremity treated with neoadjuvant chemotherapy: recent experience at Rizzoli Institute. *Oncol Rep* 2002;9(1):171.
143. Bacci G, Ferrari S, Bertoni F, et al. Histologic response of high-grade nonmetastatic osteosarcoma of the extremity to chemotherapy. *Clin Orthop* 2001;386:186.
145. Ebeid WA, Amin S, Abdelmegrid A. Limb salvage management of pathological fractures of primary malignant bone sarcomas. *Cancer Causes Control* 2005;12(1):57.
149. Wittig JC, Bickels J, Kellar-Graney KL, Kim FH, Malawer MM. Osteosarcoma of the proximal humerus: long-term results with limb-sparing surgery. *Clin Orthop* 2002;397:156.
152. Cai Y, Niu XH, Zhang Q. Long-term results of combined therapy for primary osteosarcoma in extremities. *Zhonghua Wai Ka Za Zhi* 2000;38(5):329.
153. Mirabello L, Savage TR. International osteosarcoma incidence patterns in children and adolescents, middle ages and elderly persons. *Int J Cancer* 2009; 125(1):229.
154. Niu X, Cai YB, Zhang Q. Long-term results of combined therapy for primary osteosarcoma in extremities of 189 cases. *Chin J Surg* 2005;43(24):1576.
155. Zhang Q, Xu WP, Niu XH. The current status of the treatment for osteosarcoma in China. *Chin J Bone Tumor Bone* 2009;8(3):129.
156. Agarwal M, Anchan C, Shah M, Puri A, Pai S. Limb salvage surgery for osteosarcoma: effective low-cost treatment. *Clin Orthop Rel Res* 2007;459:82.
162. Meyers PA, Heller G, Healey JH, et al. Osteogenic sarcoma with clinically detectable metastasis at initial presentation. *J Clin Oncol* 1993;11(3):449.
170. Onda M, Matsuda S, Higaki S, et al. ErbB-2 expression is correlated with poor prognosis for patients with osteosarcoma. *Cancer* 1996;77(1):71.
180. Le Vu B, de Vathaire F, Shamsaldin A, et al. Radiation dose, chemotherapy and risk of osteosarcoma after solid tumours during childhood. *Int J Cancer* 1998;77(3):370.
182. Tabone MD, Terrier P, Pacquement H, et al. Outcome of radiation-related osteosarcoma after treatment of childhood and adolescent cancer: a study of 23 cases. *J Clin Oncol* 1999;17(9):2789.
184. Edeiken J. Bone tumors and tumor-like conditions. In: Edeiken J, ed. *Roentgen diagnosis and disease of bone*. Baltimore: Williams & Wilkins, 1981:30.
188. Picci P, Bacci G, Ferrari S, Mercuri M. Neoadjuvant chemotherapy in malignant fibrous histiocytoma of bone and in osteosarcoma located in the extremities: analogies and differences between the two tumors. *Ann Oncol* 1997;8(11):1107.
200. Heck RK, Stacy GS, Flaherty MJ, et al. A comparison study of staging systems for bone sarcomas. *Clin Orthop Rel Res* 2003;415:64.
202. Weiner MA, Harris MB, Lewis M, et al. Neoadjuvant high-dose methotrexate, cisplatin, and doxorubicin for the management of patients with nonmetastatic osteosarcoma. *Cancer Treat Rep* 1986;70(12):1431.
203. Bramwell VH, Burgers M, Sneath R, et al. A comparison of two short intensive adjuvant chemotherapy regimens in operable osteosarcoma of limbs in children and young adults: the first study of the European Osteosarcoma Intergroup. *J Clin Oncol* 1992;10(10):1579.
206. Hudson M, Jaffe MR, Jaffe N, et al. Pediatric osteosarcoma: therapeutic strategies, results, and prognostic factors derived from a 10-year experience. *J Clin Oncol* 1990;8(12):1988.
207. Miser J, Arndt C, Smithson W. Treatment of high grade osteosarcoma with ifosfamide, MESNA, adriamycin, and high dose methotrexate. *Proc Am Soc Clin Oncol* 1991;10:310.
208. Goorin AM, Baker A, Gieser P. No evidence for improved event-free survival with presurgical chemotherapy for nonmetastatic extremity sarcoma: preliminary results of randomised Pediatric Oncology Group trial 8651. *Proc Am Soc Clin Oncol* 1995;14:A1420.

SECTION 9: CANCERS OF THE SKIN

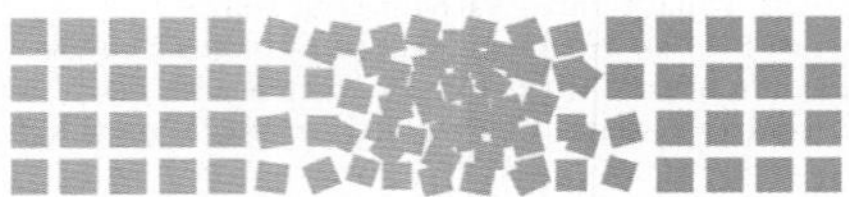

CHAPTER 117 CANCER OF THE SKIN

ANETTA RESZKO, SUMAIRA Z. AASI, LYNN D. WILSON, AND DAVID J. LEFFELL

One in five Americans will develop nonmelanoma skin cancer (NMSC) during his or her lifetime. NMSC is the most common human cancer, with an estimated annual incidence of over 1 million in 2009 in the United States, higher than the incidence of lung cancer, breast cancer, prostate cancer, and colon cancer combined.[1–4] Despite growing public awareness of the harmful effects of sun and ultraviolet (UV) exposure, the incidence continues to rise. The rising frequency of NMSC results from the age shift in the population (incidence of NMSC increases with age), high ambient solar irradiance, and a thinning ozone layer. Prognosis depends of biology and location of the lesion, as well as host characteristics.

Economic implications of NMSC are considerable. In the United States alone, Medicare spends $13 billion each year on skin cancer care treatment. Added to this are costs of treatments of highly prevalent precancerous lesions such as actinic keratoses (AKs).

Prevention strategies aimed at reduction of known risk factors, patient education on the importance of early detection and treatment, and the search for more effective and tissue sparing therapies continues.

NONMELANOMA SKIN CANCER

DIAGNOSIS

Although many NMSCs present with classic clinical findings such as nodularity, tissue friability, and erythema, definitive diagnosis can be established only by tissue biopsy. Adequate tissue samples obtained in an atraumatic fashion is critical to histopathologic diagnosis.

Skin biopsies may be performed by shave, punch, or fusiform excision. The type of biopsy performed should be based on the morphology of the primary lesion and clinical differential diagnosis. A shave biopsy is usually adequate for raised lesions such as nodular basal cell carcinoma (BCC), squamous cell carcinoma (SCC), or tumors of follicular origin. A punch biopsy is appropriate for sampling flat, broad lesions such as Bowen's disease (BD) or SCC *in situ* (SCC*IS*). An excisional biopsy is commonly used to sample deep dermal and subcutaneous tissue. Excision may be required for diagnosis of a dermal nodule when morphologic assessment of overall tumor architecture is crucial for proper diagnostic assessment. An example is distinguishing between a benign dermatofibroma, and a malignant fibrous tumor.

Shave Biopsy

Basic skin biopsy techniques are demonstrated in Figure 117.1A. A shave biopsy is performed under clean conditions. In the authors' opinion, the use of a sterilized razor blade, which can be precisely manipulated by the operator to adjust the depth of the biopsy, is often superior to the use of a No. 15 scalpel. After the procedure, adequate hemostasis is achieved with topical application of aqueous aluminum chloride (20%), ferric subsulfate (Monsel's solution), or electrocautery. Note that ferrous subsulfate may lead to permanent tattooing of the skin so it should not be used on the face unless there is a high likelihood of subsequent definitive surgical treatment.

Punch Biopsy

A punch biopsy is performed under local anesthesia, using a trephine or biopsy punch (Fig. 117.1B). The operator makes a circular incision to the level of the superficial fat, using a rotating or twisting motion of the trephine. Traction applied perpendicularly to the relaxed skin tension lines minimizes redundancy at closure. Hemostasis is achieved by placement of simple, nonabsorbable sutures that can be removed in 7 to 14 days depending on anatomic site. If the punch biopsy is small and not in a cosmetically crucial area, the resulting post-biopsy defect can often heal via second intention.

Excisional Biopsy

After local anesthesia has been achieved under sterile conditions, a scalpel is used to incise a fusiform ellipse to the level of the subcutis. Hemostasis is obtained with cautery as needed, and the wound is closed in a layered fashion using absorbable and nonabsorbable sutures.

GENERAL APPROACH TO MANAGEMENT OF SKIN CANCER

The management of skin cancer is guided by the histologic and biologic nature of the tumor, the anatomic site, the underlying medical status of the patient, and whether the tumor is primary or recurrent. Accurate interpretation of the diagnostic biopsy is essential for appropriate clinical management. Depending on the biologic aggressiveness of the tumor, cancers of the skin may be excised or, in some cases of superficial tumors or precancerous lesions, eliminated in a less invasive fashion. Surgical

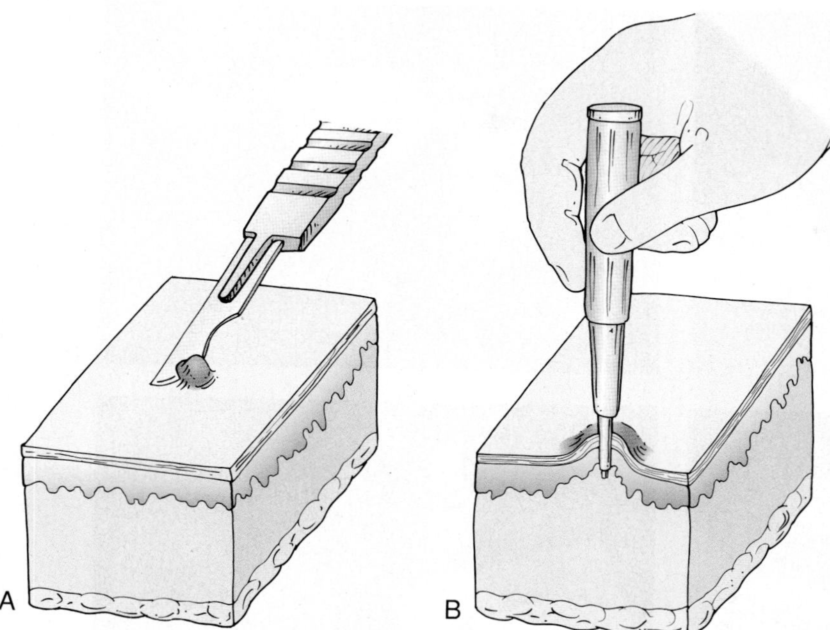

FIGURE 117.1 Biopsy techniques. Local anesthetic (lidocaine 1% with epinephrine, 1:100,000, unless contraindicated) is injected with a 30-gauge needle. A 30-gauge needle minimizes pain and tissue trauma. Unless otherwise specified, postbiopsy care involves daily cleansing with tap water followed by application of an emollient or an antibiotic ointment and a nonadherent dressing. Although popular in the past, the use of hydrogen peroxide is discouraged because of keratinocyte toxicity. Similarly, triple antibiotic ointments that include Neosporin or bacitracin may lead to contact dermatitis. For simple skin wounds, petroleum jelly has been shown to be as effective in facilitating healing as antibiotic ointment. **A:** Shave biopsy. A scalpel blade is manipulated by the operator to adjust the depth of the biopsy. Hemostasis is achieved with topical application of aqueous aluminium chloride, ferrous subsulfate, or electrocautery. **B:** Punch biopsy. The operator makes a circular incision to the level of the superficial fat, using a rotating or twisting motion of the trephine. Traction applied perpendicularly to the relaxed skin tension lines minimizes redundancy at closure. Hemostasis is commonly achieved by placement of sutures.

options include conventional excision and Mohs micrographic surgery (MMS). Destructive modalities include curettage and cautery/electrodessication (C&D), cryosurgery, photodynamic therapy (PDT), laser surgery, and chemotherapy. Other techniques are topical therapy (e.g., imiquimod, 5-fluorouracil [5-FU]), intralesional interferon, chemotherapy, and radiation therapy (RT). None of these latter techniques provide information about the completeness of cancer ablation.

Excision

Excisional surgery involves the removal of the cancer and a margin of clinically uninvolved tissue, followed by layered closure or second intention healing. Frozen or permanent sections interpreted by the pathologist determine adequacy of margins. Margins are assessed from representative sections of the specimen in "bread-loaf" fashion, allowing for sampling of the surgical margin. This sampling may occasionally result in a false-negative assessment of clear margins, especially in cases of infiltrating or aggressive-growth cancers. A similar misdiagnosis may occur when one relies on vertically prepared frozen specimens for intraoperative margin control. Excision, especially when performed in a physician's office rather than in a hospital operating room, is effective and cost-efficient for primary, small (<1 cm) NMSCs, without infiltrative or other high-risk features.

Mohs Micrographic Surgery

MMS facilitates optimal margin control and conservation of normal tissue and it has become the standard of care in a variety of skin cancer subtypes. Individuals trained in the technique perform MMS in the office setting under local anesthesia. After gentle curettage to define the clinical gross margin of the cancer, a 45-degree tangential specimen of tumor with a minimal margin of clinically normal-appearing tissue is excised, precisely mapped in a horizontal fashion, and processed immediately by frozen section for microscopic examination (Fig. 117.2). Optimal margin control is obtained by examination of the entire lateral perimeter of the specimen and contiguous deep margin. Meticulous mapping allows for directed extirpation of any remaining tumor.

A key defining feature of MMS is that the surgeon excises, maps, and reviews the specimen personally, minimizing the chance of error in tissue interpretation and orientation. MMS has gained acceptance as the treatment of choice for recurrent skin cancers, as well as for primary skin cancers located on anatomic sites that require maximal tissue conservation for preservation of function and cosmesis (Fig. 117.3). When long-term costs of various treatment modalities are compared, MMS is a cost-effective treatment compared with surgical excision when considering associated ambulatory surgery center (ASC) facility fee and a subsequent re-excision procedure, and is significantly less expensive than radiotherapy and frozen-section–guided excisional surgery.[5]

Curettage and Cautery/Electrodesiccation

Common methods of treatment of uncomplicated skin cancers on the trunk and extremities and certain facial lesions include C&D and cryotherapy using liquid nitrogen. C&D is performed under clean conditions with local anesthesia. The visible tumor is first removed by curettage, which is extended for a margin of 2 to 4 mm beyond the clinical borders of the cancer. Cautery or electrodesiccation is then performed to destroy another 1 mm of tissue at the lateral and deep margins. C&D can yield satisfactory results after a single cycle of C&D for NMSC tumors smaller than 1 cm, especially if the tumor is of the superficial subtype. Salasche[6] recommended that C&D be performed for three cycles to avoid recurrence. The authors believe, based on extensive clinical experience, that if the tumor requires three cycles of C&D, careful consideration should be given to more definitive approaches such as excision or MMS. Detailed reviews of primary BCC treated by C&D revealed 5-year recurrence rates of 8.6% for lesions located on the neck, trunk, and extremities and between 17.5% and 22% for lesions located on the face.[7]

One potential drawback of the therapy is that recurrent tumors following C&D are often multifocal with more aggressive biological behavior. C&D is thus reserved for small (<1 cm) superficial or nodular BCCs, AKs, and SCC*IS* without follicular involvement located on the trunk or extremities.

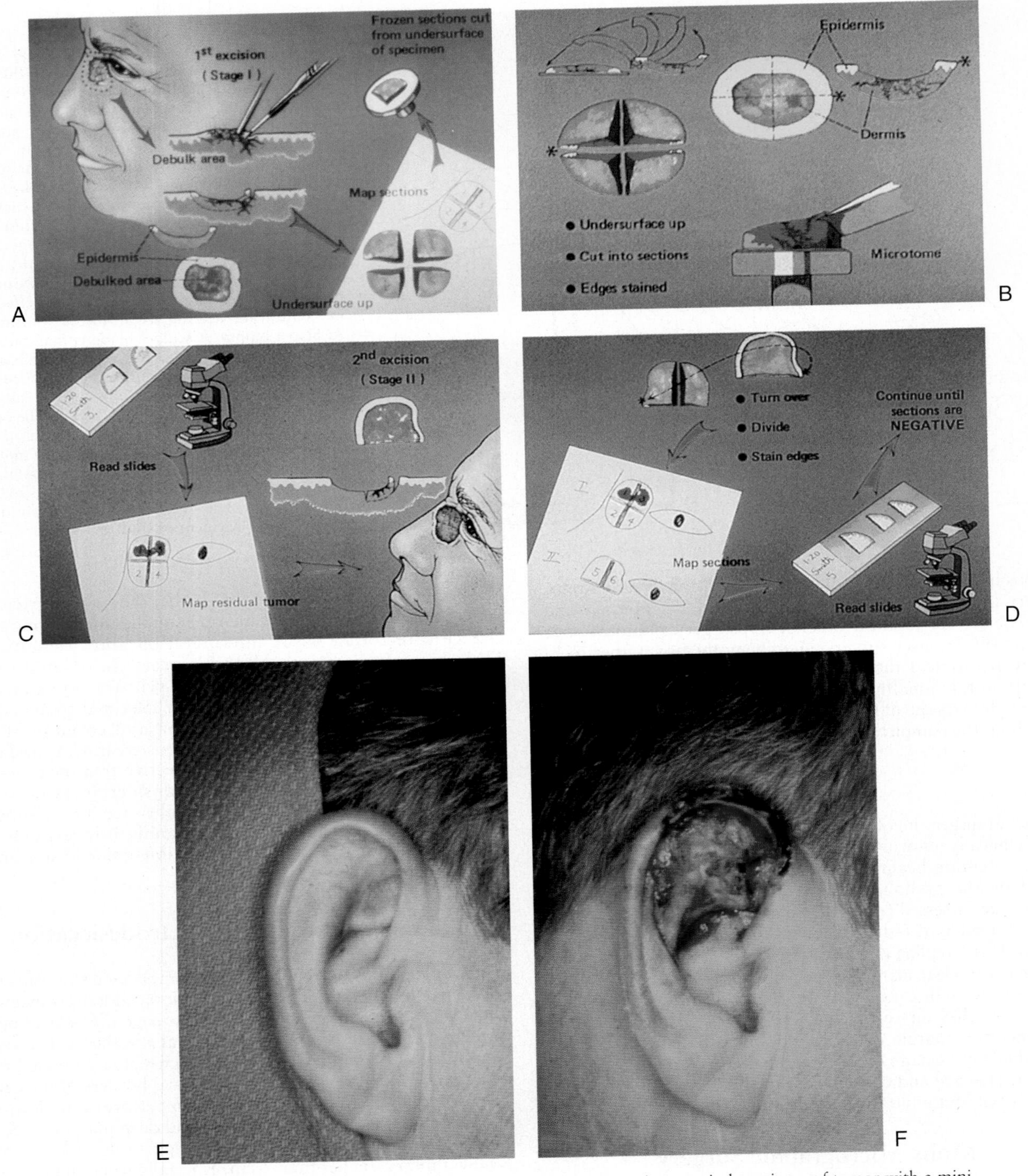

FIGURE 117.2 Mohs micrographic surgery. **A–D:** After gentle curettage. A tangenital specimen of tumor with a minimal margin of clinically normal-appearing tissue is obtained, precisely mapped, nad processed immediately by frozen section for microscopic examination. Superior margin control is obtained through examination of the entire perimeter of the specimen. Percise mapping allows for directed extirpation of any remaining tumor. (Courtesy of Neil A. Swanson, MD.) **E:** Clinical BCC. **F:** Postextirpation of BCC by Mohs micrographic surgery.

Cryosurgery

Cryosurgery exposes precancers and NMSCs to destructive subzero temperatures. Tissue damage is caused initially by direct effects and subsequently by vascular stasis, ice crystal formation, cell membrane disruption, pH changes, hypertonic damage, and finally thermal shock. Successful cryosurgery requires temperatures reaching −50°C to −60°C at the deep and lateral margins of the tumor. The subsequent thaw leads to vascular stasis and impaired local microcirculation. The open-spray technique is used most often and requires pressurized liquid nitrogen spray delivery from a distance of 1 to 3 cm. With the confined-spray technique, liquid nitrogen is delivered through a cone that is open at both ends. With the closed-cone

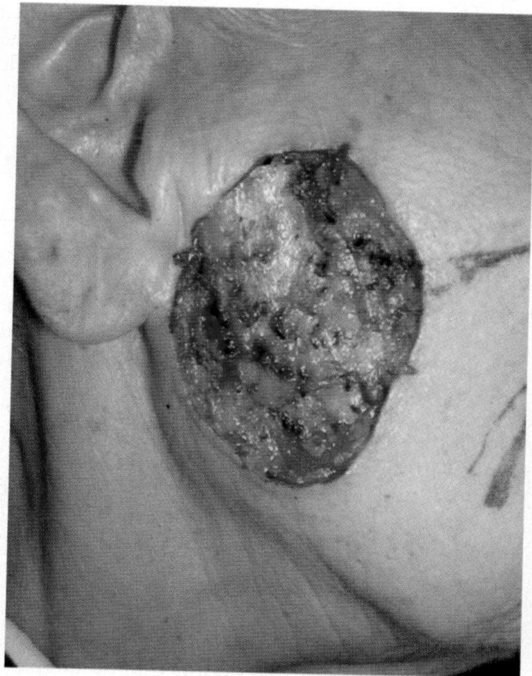

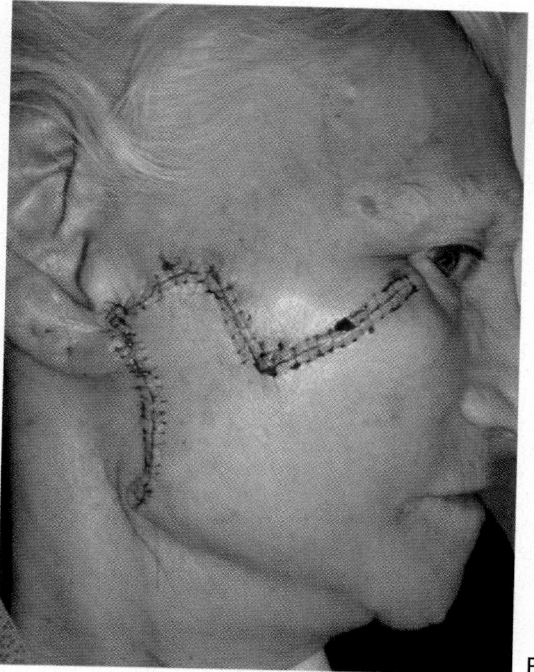

FIGURE 117.3 **A:** Defect resulting from extirpation of basal cell carcinoma by Mohs micrographic surgery. **B:** Defect repaired with rhomboid transposition flap.

technique, one end of the cone is closed and a shorter delivery time is required. With the cryoprobe technique, a prechilled metal probe is applied to the tumor. Delivery time is determined via a depth-dose estimation, which takes into account freeze time, lateral spread, and halo thaw time. Immediately following cryosurgery, local erythema and edema are apparent. An exudative phase ensues in 24 to 72 hours and is followed by sloughing at approximately day 7. Complete healing is usually seen at 2 to 3 weeks for facial lesions and up to 6 weeks for lesions on the trunk and extremities.

Temporary complications may include extensive drainage, edema, bulla formation, and hypertrophic scarring. Delayed hemorrhage can occur suddenly approximately 2 weeks postprocedure, most commonly after treatment of the nose, temple, and forehead. Paresthesia may occur with thermal injury to superficial nerves. Other less common side effects may include headache, syncope, febrile reaction, cold urticaria, pyogenic granuloma, milia formation, or dyschromia (hypo- and hyperpigmentation). Permanent complications may include tissue contraction, hypopigmentation, and scarring.

The clinical usefulness of cryosurgery and C&D is limited by the inability to evaluate treatment margins and therefore thoroughness of tumor eradication. The absence of margin control and a dense postcryosurgery scar, which might obscure recurrence, makes these methods valuable primarily in the care of histologically superficial NMSC.

TOPICAL THERAPY FOR SKIN CANCER

Imiquimod

Imiquimod, an imidazolaquinoline, binds intracellular toll-like receptors 7 and 8 acting as a topical immune-response modifier. Imiquimod promotes cell-mediated immune response through induction of several cytokines particularly interferon-α (INF-α) and interferon-γ (INF-γ) and interleukins (ILs) 6, 8, and 12 by human peripheral blood mononuclear cells including monocytes, macrophages, and toll-like receptor-7 bearing plasmacytoid dendritic cells.[8–11] Keratinocytes exposed to imiquimod produce IL-6, IL-8, and INF-α, resulting in a T-helper type 1–dominant response. INF-α induces cellular immunity by stimulating CD4 T cells to express IL-12 $\beta 2$ receptor. In addition, IL-12 induces INF-γ to stimulate cytotoxic T cells to kill virus-infected and tumor cells. Because suppression of type 1 INF signaling proteins is one of earliest events in development of SCC, imiquimod increased levels of type 1 INF may improve the responsiveness of SCCs to endogenous INF-α.[12,13] The use of imiquimod is approved by the U.S. Food and Drug Administration (FDA) for treatment of AKs and superficial BCCs on the trunk, neck, or extremities. Studies with topical imiquimod for nodular BCC, SCC*IS*, and malignant melanoma *in situ* are currently being conducted.[13–15] Imiquimod appears to be effective as monotherapy in carefully selected cases and may have a role postoperatively to decrease the incidence of recurrence of certain skin cancers. However, long-term data on cure and recurrence remain to be determined. Close careful evaluation of the posttreatment site is essential.

Common imiquimod-related adverse events include application site reactions (i.e., erythema, pain, edema, ulceration, bleeding), fatigue, headache, diarrhea, nausea, rash, and leucopenia.

Retinoids

Both topically applied and systemic retinoids have consistently been shown to be effective in the prevention and management of NMSCs. The effect of topical retinoids is at best mild while oral retinoids have a different efficacy profile and side effects that frequently limit its usefulness for cancer treatment and prevention. Retinoids down-regulate the expression of AP-1 responsive genes, activate transrepression of AP-1, arrest growth, and induce apoptosis and differentiation.[16,17] Retinoids also down-regulate the UV-induced overexpression of cyclooxygenase-2, reducing prostaglandins that are normally elevated in AKs and NMSC.[17,18] Isotretinoin at 0.25 to 0.5 mg/kg/d and acitretin at 10 to 20 mg/d are the most common systemic retinoids used for skin cancer chemoprevention, especially in immunocompromised patients.[19] Routine clinical monitoring for signs of retinoid toxicity and laboratory examinations (fasting lipid profile, liver function tests) are mandatory.

5-Fluorouracil

5-FU, a chemotherapeutic agent that interferes with DNA synthesis by inhibiting thymidylate synthetase, has been used topically since the 1960s for the treatment of AKs. 5-FU is currently approved by the FDA for the treatment of AKs and superficial BCCs. This drug carries a black box warning urging close supervision by a physician experienced with the administration of antimetabolites. Treatment site reactions following topical 5-FU administration include erythema, edema, and pain. In severe cases, ulcerations and bleeding have been reported. Side effects of 5-FU treatment are exacerbated by prolonged UVR. Poor treatment compliance, due to adverse side effects, is associated with significant failure rates.[10,20]

Diclofenac

Diclofenac is a nonsteroidal anti-inflammatory agent that inhibits cyclooxygenase, the rate-limited enzyme in the synthesis of prostaglandins. Diclofenac has high affinity for cyclooxygenase-2-2 that is frequently elevated in AKs, melanoma, and NMSC. In addition, diclofenac inhibits prostaglandin-medicated, UV-induced NMSC by decreasing proinflammatory cytokines such as IL-1, TNF-α, and transforming growth factor-β.[21,22]

Photodynamic Therapy

Topical PDT with 5-aminolevulinic acid (ALA) or methyl- aminolevulinic acid (MAL) is effective in the treatment of certain NMSCs. Following topical application, ALA or MAL accumulates preferentially in malignant and premalignant cells and is metabolized in the intrinsic intracellular heme biosynthesis pathway to protoporphyrin IX. Preferential accumulation of ALA in malignant and premalignant tissues results from the differences in cellular uptake, differential activities of the heme and porphyrin biosynthetic pathways, iron bioavailability, differential properties of stratum corneum, and variable tissue ALA distribution. Protoporphyrin IX is a photoactive intermediate essential for the transfer of singlet oxygen species and the generation of free radicals. The reactive oxygen species induce lipid peroxidation, protein cross-linking, and increased membrane permeability. All these processes contribute to irreversible damage and ultimately cell death of malignant and premalignant cells. Both free radicals and singlet oxygen species have relatively short half-lives, with a radius of action of 0.01 mcm, and thus have low mutagenic potential for normal, nonlocalized DNA damage.[23] Application of the MAL is postulated to lead to a more selective accumulation of protoporphyrin IX in premalignant and malignant cells.[24]

Both lasers and light sources (blue and red light) with wavelengths in a range corresponding to absorption peaks of protoporphyrin IX (from 400 nm to infrared) have been used to activate topically applied ALA and/or MAL.

The use of PDT is currently approved by the FDA for the treatment of AKs. The off-label uses of PDT to treat NMSCs, acne, photodamaged skin, human papillomavirus (HPV)-associated pathologies, lymphocytoma cutis, hidradenitis suppurativa, and other dermatologic conditions are currently under investigation.[25] Scarring and postprocedural dyspigmentation are minimal to nonexisting following PDT. Substantial benefit of PDT is photorejuvenation with softening of the appearance of fine lines, rhytids, and acne scars. The mechanism of photorejuvenation is not fully understood, but may relate to increased type I collagen production.[26]

RADIATION THERAPY FOR SKIN CANCER

RT is a treatment option for certain NMSCs, angiosarcoma, Merkel cell carcinoma (MCC), cutaneous lymphomas, some adnexal carcinomas, and other primary and metastatic cutaneous neoplasms. RT, in properly fractionated doses, is indicated when the patient's overall health status (such as elderly patients who are unwilling or unable to undergo surgery) or size of the tumor precludes surgical extirpation. The procedure is also used as an adjuvant treatment of patients with positive surgical margins, perineural invasion (PNI), or local regional nodal metastasis. The effectiveness of RT, however, is limited by the inability to definitively assess and control the tumor margins. In addition, treatment of an excessively large area of normal skin surrounding the tumor may enhance risk of both postradiation dermatitis and future skin cancers.

Two modes of RT delivery are electrons and superficially penetrating photons (x-rays).[27] Appropriate radiation margins for clinically visible tumors and/or surgical scars should generally be less than 3 cm. A protracted fractionation scheme using 2 to 2.5 Gy fractions to a total of 50 to 66 Gy for NMSCs is commonly used to achieve the best chance of durable local control and acceptable late effects.[28] Nonetheless, treatment may be accelerated to a single large fraction (10–20 Gy) or three to five fractions of 6 to 7 Gy for patients with significant comorbidities with excellent local control but with greater risk of fibrosis, atrophy, telangiectasias, and poor cosmesis. Although a course of RT may be protracted over several weeks, daily treatments last several minutes.

Local control rates for small (<2 cm) BCCs are 90% to 95% with adequate (over 90% rated as excellent or good) cosmesis. For larger tumors with bone or cartilage involvement, local control rates decrease to 50% to 75%. These deeply invasive/destructive lesions are best approached with a combined excision and adjuvant RT. In a randomized trial of patients with incompletely excised recurrent BCCs, adjuvant RT improved the 5-year local control rates from 61% to 91%.[29] The 10-year local control rates were similar for both adjuvant RT and repeat surgery (92% vs. 90%). The local control for SCC is lower by 10% to 15% compared with equivalent-sized BCCs with RT.

The consideration of acute and permanent tissue effects of RT, such as acute and chronic radiation dermatitis, epidermal atrophy, telangiectasias, altered pigmentation, delayed radiation necrosis, alopecia, and secondary cutaneous malignancies, must be anticipated and managed.[30] The late cosmetic effects are more pronounced with a large dose per fraction (over 3-4 Gy), if the total dose is over 55 Gy, following treatment to large fields and/or deeply invasive lesions and with continued unprotected sun exposure. Greater metastatic rates are seen in SCCs arising in an area of previous RT.

RT is commonly used in the head and neck region. RT to lower limb lesions, although not contraindicated, should be considered cautiously as poor vascularization and edema of lower extremities may limit the effectiveness of RT and result in delayed prolonged healing.[29]

ACTINIC KERATOSES

AKs are common cutaneous lesions that occur on sun-exposed areas, particularly in blond or red-haired, fair-skinned individuals with green or blue eyes. They of course can occur in patients who do not possess these phenotypic features, and relate most directly to cumulative sun exposure. AKs represent the initial intraepidermal manifestation of abnormal proliferation of keratinocytes with the possibility of progression to SCC*IS* and invasive SCC.[31]

Clinically, AKs have three possible behavioral patterns: spontaneous regression, persistence, or progression into invasive SCC.[32] The risk of progression of AK to SCC has been calculated to be between 0.025% and 16% per year, and the calculated lifetime risk of malignant transformation for a patient with AKs followed for a period of 10 years ranges from 6.1% to 10.2%.[33] The long-term risk of development of invasive SCC in patients with multiple AKs has been estimated to be as high as 10%. Approximately 60% to 65% of SCCs arise from prior AKs. Spontaneous regression has been reported in as high as 25.9% of AKs over a 12-month period, although a 15% recurrence rate was noted at follow-up.[31]

PATHOGENESIS OF AK

Factors linked to pathogenesis of AKs include (1) exposure to ultraviolet B (UVB) light—UVB causes mutations of the tumor suppressor gene (TSG) *p53*[31]; (2) genetic DNA instability (i.e., xeroderma pigmentosum) or melanin deficiency (albinism); (3) older age; (4) male gender; (5) anatomic location—over 80% of AKs are located on the head and neck, dorsal forearms, and hands; and (6) history of immunosuppression—solid organ transplant patients are at significantly increased risk.

A study of asymptomatic AKs, inflamed AKs, and SCCs showed a stepwise loss of differentiation manifesting as diminishing 27-kD heat-shock protein, an initial increase in lymphocytes suggesting the occurrence of an active inflammatory and immune response, a stepwise increase in the number of cells expressing detectable levels of *p53* suggesting an increase in DNA damage, decreasing levels of Bcl-2, an apoptosis inhibitor, and loss of Fas antigen, suggesting these cells become less sensitive to FasL-mediated apoptosis as they progress.[34] Molecular characterization of the role of the *p53* TSG in AK, and its similar finding in SCC and BCC, suggests that the AKs indeed represent an early stage in the molecular carcinogenesis of NMSC.[35]

CLINICAL FEATURES OF AK

AKs are red, pink, or brown papules with a scaly (hyperkeratotic) surface. They occur on sun-exposed areas and are especially common on the balding scalp, forehead, face, dorsal forearms, and hands. Subclinical (nonvisible) AKs are estimated to occur up to 10 times more often than clinically visible AKs, particularly on sun-exposed skin.[31]

The histologic spectrum of AKs includes hyperplastic, atrophic, Bowenoid, acantholytic, and pigmented subtypes.[36] Each subtype is characterized by disordered, atypical keratinocytes with nuclear atypia. In the hyperplastic variant, pronounced hyperkeratosis coexists with parakeratosis. Epidermal hyperplasia and downward displacement without dermal invasion can be noted. A thin epidermis devoid of rete ridges is characteristic of the atrophic variant. Atypical cells predominate in the basal layer. The Bowenoid AK is virtually indistinguishable from BD SCC*IS*. In the Bowenoid variant, considerable epidermal cell disarray and clumping of nuclei gives a windblown appearance. The presence of suprabasal lacunae is characteristic of acantholytic AK. Excessive melanin is present within the basal layer in the pigmented variant of AK.

TREATMENT OF AK

Prevention of disease is always superior and preferable to the need for treatment. Effective preventative measures include avoidance of excessive sun exposure (use of broad-brimmed hats, sun-protective clothing, and sunscreen), patient education, and regular self-examinations to detect the earliest signs of malignant transformation.

The role of chemoprevention in decreasing the development of new SCC was demonstrated in a randomized, double-blind, controlled trial involving 2,297 patients with a history of moderate to severe AKs. In that trial, daily oral 25,000 IU of vitamin A supplementation significantly decreased (32%) the 5-year probability of generating a new SCC without associated significant systemic toxicity.[37] In a double-blind, randomized clinical trial, 25 patients applied topical all-trans-retinoic acid (tretinoin) 0.05% cream twice daily for 16 weeks, resulting in a 30.3% reduction in the number of AKs compared with baseline.[38]

Because of their low but real potential to develop into invasive SCC, AK therapy is generally recommended. The management options for AKs should be chosen depending on whether a lesion-directed or a field-directed therapy is preferred. Lesion-directed therapy, including ablative and surgical procedures, is reserved for selected cases when only a few clinically visible AKs are present. Field-directed therapy, including ablative, nonablative, and topical treatments, offers the advantage of treating both clinically evident and subclinical lesions that may progress to visible AKs.

Cryotherapy is the most commonly used lesion-directed treatment modality. Clearance rates range from 39% to 98.8%.[31,39] In a large, multicenter Australian study evaluating the efficacy of cryotherapy for the treatment of AKs on the face and scalp, of the 89 patients and 421 lesions in the intended-to-treat population, there was an average of 67.2% lesion response rate per patient.[40] Cryotherapy treatment was associated with "good" and "excellent" cosmetic outcomes in 94% of the lesions.

Other lesion-directed treatment options include C&D and surgical excision. Treatment with C&D may require two or three cycles. High cure rates and good cosmetic outcome have been reported. C&D should be generally avoided in recurrent lesions, punch-biopsied lesions, and hair-bearing sites.[31]

Field-directed treatment modalities include topical pharmacologic therapies including imiquimod, 5-FU, and diclofenac, ablative and nonablative laser resurfacing, PDT, dermabrasion, and deep and medium-depth chemical peels.

Imiquimod (Aldara)

The manufacturer-recommended standard imiquimod treatment protocol for AKs is twice weekly for 16 weeks. Other treatment protocols (3 times a week for 4 weeks followed by a 4-week rest and an additional 4 weeks of treatment if remaining lesions are still present; 2 to 3 times a week for 16 weeks) have been reported.[31] Clearance rates with imiquimod range from 45% to 85%.[41] Reported recurrence rates are 10% and 16% within 1 year and 18 months of treatment, respectively.

Imiquimod is effective and well tolerated for the treatment of AKs in posttransplant, immunosuppressed patients. The safety and efficacy of 5% imiquimod cream for the treatment of AKs in posttransplant patients receiving immunosuppressive therapy within the prior 6 months was evaluated is a multicenter, randomized, placebo-controlled study with reported imiquimod clearance rate of 62.1%.[42] Common reported side effects of imiquimod therapy included site reactions (edema, erythema, vesicles, and erosions/ulcerations), fatigue, headache, diarrhea, nausea, and leucopenia. No serious adverse events were reported.[42]

5-FU

Manufacturer-recommended 5-FU treatment protocol for AKs is twice daily for 2 to 4 weeks. Other protocols proposed in the literature include 5% 5-FU once to twice daily for 2 to 7 weeks; 5% 5-FU once daily, 1 day per week for 12 weeks; and 0.5% 5-FU once or twice daily for 1 to 4 weeks.[31] The literature reports rates of AK resolution with 5-FU that reach 89% with twice-weekly application for 16 weeks, albeit recurrence rates of up to 55% have been reported.[43] In addition, low compliance, because of adverse effects of medication, is associated with significant treatment failure rates.

In a phase 3, double-blind randomized, study of 117 patients with at least five AKs treated with 0.5% 5-FU cream once daily, complete clearance rates at 1, 2, and 4 weeks were 26%, 20%, and 48%, respectively.[44] In a large systematic review of 5-FU randomized clinical trials, treatment with 5% 5-FU resulted in an average reduction of 79.5% in the mean number of lesions with clearance rates of 94% and 98% at 2 and 4 weeks, respectively. In comparison, treatment with 0.5% 5-FU resulted in an average reduction in the mean number of lesions of 86.1%. Higher clearance rates with 0.5% 5-FU may represent increased patient medication compliance from lower side effects profile. In the study comparing 0.5% and 5% 5-FU, 85% of patients preferred 0.5% 5-FU.[31]

A randomized, physician-blinded study compared the efficacy of 5-FU 5% cream applied twice daily for 2 to 4 weeks with imiquimod 5% cream applied twice daily for 16 weeks in 36 patients with AKs on the face and scalp.[45] At week 24 the total AK count was reduced by 94% and 66% with 5-FU and imiquimod, respectively. 5-FU was also found to be more effective in treatment of subclinical AKs. Adverse event profiles were similar for both treatments and included tenderness, burning, erythema, and blistering.

Diclofenac

Efficacy of topically applied 3% diclofenac gel in 2.5% hyaluronic acid vehicle gel versus vehicle was addressed in a multicenter, randomized, double-blind, placebo-controlled study of 195 patients. Treatment with 3% diclofenac gel twice daily for 30 to 90 days resulted in an improvement of 59% compared with 31% with placebo.[46]

PDT with ALA

PDT with ALA activated by either blue or red light showed reported overall clearance values for AKs of 80% and 60%, respectively.[31] Response rates vary with duration of ALA incubation and thickness of AK lesions. In a randomized, blinded, placebo-controlled study, 243 patients with total of 1403 AKs on scalp and face, were treated with ALA (incubation time 14-18 hours) and exposure to blue light.[47] At 8 weeks, 30% of patients with partial response were retreated. At 12 weeks, 91% lesion clearance rate was reported. Discomfort was the most commonly reported adverse event.

A randomized study of 36 patients with at least 4 AKs compared efficacy of two sessions of ALA-PDT or ALA-pulsed dye laser (ALA incubation time, 1 hour) with 0.5% 5-FU cream applied once or twice daily for 4 weeks.[48] At 1 month posttreatment, the overall individual lesion clearance rates for 5-FU, ALA-PDT, and ALA- pulsed dye laser were 70%, 80%, and 50%, respectively. ALA-PDT and ALA- pulsed dye laser were better tolerated than 5-FU.

The efficacy of PDT was compared with that of cryotherapy in an open, randomized, controlled study of 202 patients with 732 AKs.[49] Clearance rates for PDT and cryotherapy were 69% and 75%, respectively. Response rates correlated with the lesion thickness, with thinner lesions having higher response rates. Satisfaction with the cosmetic outcomes for PDT and cryotherapy were 96% and 81%, respectively.

Sustained Clearance

Sustained clearance of AKs at 12 months after the cessation of treatment was assessed by Krawtchenko et al.[50] Sustained clearance was reported in 33% of patients treated with 5% 5-FU, 4% of patients treated with cryotherapy, and in 73% of patients treated with imiquimod.

BASAL CELL CARCINOMA

BCC is a slow-growing neoplasm of nonkeratinizing cells originating from the basal cell layer of the epidermis. BCC is the most common human cancer, accounting for 25% of all human cancers and 75% of skin malignancies diagnosed in the United States.[51] Although BCC rarely metastasizes, it is locally invasive and can result in extensive morbidity through local recurrence and tissue destruction. Typically, BCC develops on sun-exposed areas of lighter-skinned individuals. Approximately 30% of lesions of BCC occur on the nose. Nonetheless, BCC can occur anywhere, including non–sun-exposed areas, and has been reported to occur on the vulva, penis, scrotum, and perianal area. Men are affected slightly more often than are women, and although once rare before the age of 50 years, BCCs are becoming more common in younger individuals.[1,52]

Intermittent recreational sun exposure, exposure to UVR (UVB confers greater risk than UVA) and sun overexposure (i.e., sunburns), especially in childhood and adolescence is a significant risk factor for development of BCC. Other factors involved in the pathogenesis include mutations in regulatory TSG, exposure to ionizing radiation, chemicals (e.g., arsenic, polyaromatic hydrocarbons), psoralen plus UVA (PUVA) therapy, and alterations in immune surveillance (i.e., organ transplantation, underlying hematologic malignancy, immunosuppressive medications, or human immunodeficiency virus [HIV] infection).[1]

BCC can be a feature of inherited conditions. Included among these are the nevoid BCC syndrome (NBCCS), Bazex syndrome (X-linked dominant; characterized clinically by follicular atrophoderma, hypotrichosis, hypohidrosis, milia, epidermoid cysts, and facial BCCs), Rombo syndrome (features similar to those of Bazex syndrome with peripheral vasodilation with cyanosis), xeroderma pigmentosum (autosomal recessive disorder in unscheduled DNA repair, clinically characterized by numerous NMSCs and melanomas), and unilateral basal cell nevus syndrome.

NBCCS is a rare autosomal dominant genetic disorder characterized by a mutation in the human patched (*PTCH*) gene and predisposition to multiple BCC and other tumors, as well as a wide range of developmental defects. Patients with this syndrome may exhibit a broad nasal root, borderline intelligence, odontogenic keratocysts of the jaw, palmar and plantar pits, calcification of the falx cerebri, medulloblastomas, and multiple skeletal abnormalities in addition to a few to thousands of BCCs.[53] Tumor development in patients with NBCCS is related to sun exposure, as BCCs develop most frequently in sun-exposed areas. The clinical course is commonly benign prior to puberty; nonetheless postpuberty individual lesions may progressively enlarge and ulcerate. Individuals with NBCCS are exceedingly sensitive to ionizing radiation.

Hundreds of BCCs were reported in children treated with RT for medulloblastoma.

Genomic analysis of NBCCS patients has elucidated the molecular pathogenesis of BCC. The behavior of neoplasms occurring in NBCCS confirms a classic two-hit model of carcinogenesis—tumors develop in cells sustaining two genetic alterations.[54] The first alteration or hit is inheritance of a mutation in a TSG, and the second is inactivation of the normal homologue by environmental mutagenesis or random genetic rearrangement. Sporadic BCCs would arise in cells that underwent two somatic events, resulting in the inactivation of the NBCCS TSG *PTCH*. Studies of BCC have indicated an association with mutations in the *PTCH* regulatory gene, which maps to chromosome 9q22.3.[55] Loss of heterozygosity at this site is seen in both sporadic and hereditary BCC. Inactivation of the *PTCH* gene is probably a necessary step for BCC formation. The only known function of PTCH protein, part of a receptor complex, is participation in the hedgehog signaling pathway, a key regulator of embryonic development that controls cellular proliferation. The PTCH protein binds in a complex with *Smoothened*, another transmembrane molecule, which together serve as a receptor for the secreted molecule hedgehog. In the absence of hedgehog, *Smoothened*, and *PTCH* form an inactive complex. On hedgehog binding, *Smoothened* is released from the inhibitory effects of *PTCH* and transduces a signal, allowing it to function as an oncogene.[56,57] *PTCH* mutations have also been found in SCC.[57] UV-induced mutations in the *p53* gene, such as cyclobutane pyrimidine dimers (CC → TT) have been reported in up to 60% of BCCs.[58]

CLINICAL BEHAVIOR OF BCC

Some BCCs tend to infiltrate tissues in a three-dimensional fashion through the irregular growth of fingerlike projections.[59] The clinical course of BCC is unpredictable; it may grow extremely slowly, may exhibit periods of rapid growth, or proceed by successive spurts of extension of tumor and partial regression.[60] Biologic behavior of BCC depends on angiogenic factors, stromal conditions, and the propensity for the cancer to follow anatomic paths of least resistance. BCCs can elicit angiogenic factors that account for the clinical presence of telangiectatic vessels on the tumor's surface. Central necrosis is frequently seen as tumors outgrow their blood supply.[61–63]

Tumor stroma is critical for both initiating and maintaining the development of BCC.[63] Transplants of neoplasms devoid of associated stroma are usually unsuccessful. The concept of stromal dependence is supported by the low incidence of metastatic BCC. Invasive BCC can migrate along the perichondrium, periosteum, fascia, or tarsal plate.[62,63] This type of spread accounts for higher recurrence rates in tumors involving the eyelid, nose, and scalp. Embryonic fusion planes likely offer little resistance and can lead to deep invasion and tumor spread, with very high rates of recurrence. The most susceptible areas include the inner canthus, philtrum, middle to lower chin, nasolabial groove, preauricular area, and the retroauricular sulcus.

Batra and Kelley[64] looked at risk factors for extensive subclinical spread of more than 1,000 NMSCs treated by MMS. The most significant predictors were anatomic location on the nose of any type of BCC; morpheaform BCC on the cheek; recurrent BCC in men; any tumor located on the neck in men; any tumor located on the ear helix, eyelid, or temple; and increasing preoperative size.

PNI is infrequent in BCC and occurs most often in recurrent, clinically aggressive lesions. In a case series, Niazi and Lamberty[65] noted PNI in 0.178% of BCC. In all cases, PNI was associated with recurrent tumors that were most often located in the periauricular and malar areas. Clinically, PNI may present with paresthesia, pain, and weakness or, in some cases, paralysis.

Metastatic BCC is rare, with incidence rates varying from 0.0028% to 0.1%.[66] Metastases, when reported, have involved the lung, lymph nodes, esophagus, oral cavity, and skin. Although long-term survival has been reported, the prognosis for metastatic BCC is generally poor, with an average survival of 8 to 10 months following diagnosis. Platinum-based chemotherapy appears to offer some benefit in the treatment of metastatic BCC.[67]

BCC SUBTYPES

Clinical variants of BCC include nodular, micronodular, superficial, infiltrative, morpheaform (also termed *aggressive-growth BCC, desmoplastic BCC, fibrosing BCC, sclerosing BCC*, and *scarlike BCC*), pigmented, cystic BCC, and fibroepithelioma of Pinkus (FEP).[68,69]

Nodular BCC is the most common BCC subtype, accounting for more than 60% of all tumors. Clinically, it presents as a raised, translucent pearly, skin-toned to pink papule or nodule with prominent telangiectasias (Fig. 117.4). Occasionally, the center of the tumor appears depressed or sunken, leaving a rolled, raised border with the classic pearly appearance so-called rodent ulcer. Not infrequently, history of easy bleeding and/or crusting is obtained. Nodular BCC has a propensity for involving sun-exposed areas of the face in individuals over the age of 60. In patients with severe actinic damage, nodular BCCs may appear in the third decade.

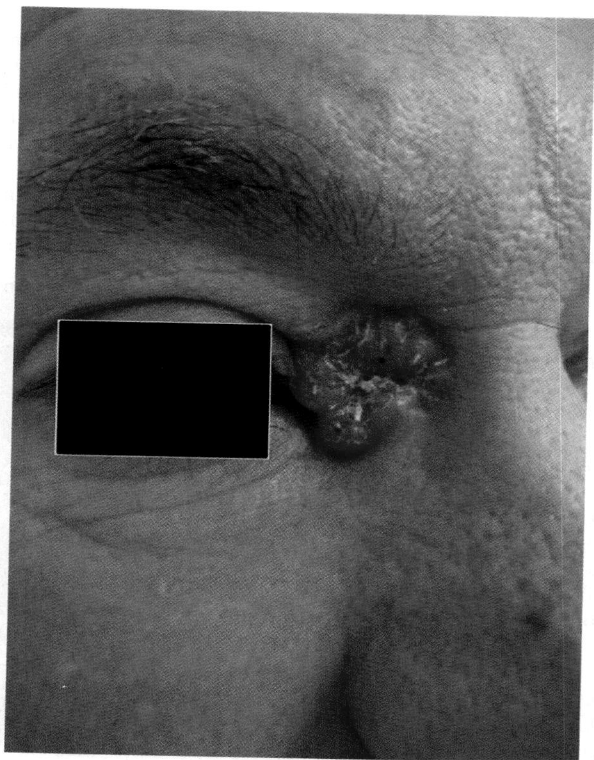

FIGURE 117.4 Nodular basal cell carcinoma (BCC). A slightly erythematous, pearly nodule with rolled borders is a classic presentation of nodular BCC. Central ulceration is a common feature of nodular BCC.

The FDA-approved protocol for treating superficial BCC with topical 5-FU is twice-daily application for 3 to 6 weeks irrespective of tumor size or location. Longer treatment protocols with an average 11 weeks are reported in the peer-reviewed literature. In a study of 31 tumors treated twice daily for an average of 11 weeks, a 90% clearance rate was observed histologically 3 weeks posttreatment.[83]

Topical PDT has also demonstrated efficacy in the treatment of BCC. Clearance rates for BCC using ALA or MAL PDT range from 76% to 97% for superficial to 64% to 92% for nodular BCC after one to three treatments.[23,25,84]

PDT has proven a worthwhile therapy in patients with NBCCS. Average literature reported clearance and recurrence rates in patients with NBCCS are 79% to 90% and 10% to 21%, respectively, at 13 to 34 months of follow-up.[25,85]

It is imperative that patients with a history of BCC receive annual full-body skin examinations. Although most recurrences appear within 1 to 5 years, recurrences decades after initial treatment are reported in the literature. Rowe et al.[86,87] found that 30% of recurrences developed within the first year after therapy, 50% within 2 years, and 66% within 3 years. A separate new primary BCC can present at rates of approximately 40% within 3 years, with 20% to 30% within 1 year of treatment of the original lesion.

SQUAMOUS CELL CARCINOMA

SCC is a neoplasm of keratinizing cells that shows malignant characteristics, including anaplasia, rapid growth, local invasion, and metastatic potential. More than 100,000 cases of SCC are diagnosed in the United States each year, making it the second most common human cancer after BCC. People of Celtic descent, individuals with fair complexions, and those with poor tanning ability and predisposition to sunburn are at increased risk for developing SCC. SCC in blacks arises most often on sites of pre-existing inflammatory conditions such as burn injuries, scars, or trauma.[88] Patients undergoing immunosuppressive therapy following solid-organ transplantation are treated with PUVA and are at increased risk of SCC (see the sections "Immunosuppression" and "Nonmelanoma Skin Cancer").

PATHOGENESIS OF SCC

Major factors involved in the pathogenesis of SCC include cumulative exposure to UVR, genetic mutations, immunosuppression, and viral infections. UVR acts as both a tumor-initiating and a tumor-promoting factor. Both UVA and UVB (UVB more than UVA) contribute to mutagenesis of DNA by inducing UV landmark mutations (two tandem CC:GG to TT:AA and two C:G to T:A transitions at dipyrimidic sites). UV-induced mutations in TSG lead to uncontrolled cell-cycle progression and subsequent transformation of keratinocytes.[89]

Alterations in the TSG *p53* are the most common genetic abnormality found in AK, SCC*IS*, and invasive SCC. Under normal conditions UVR induces *p53* gene activity. The amount of p53 protein rapidly increases in the keratinocytes and drives the expression of downstream genes including *Mdm2, GADD45,* and *p21 CIP/WAF1* and leads to cellular arrest in the G1 phase. The overexpression of p53 protein is associated with *p53* gene inactivation. The percentage of *p53* overexpression in AK and SCC compared with the normal adjacent tissue is 13% and 42%, respectively.[90]

In cases of squamous dysplasia, one allele of *p53* contains a missense point mutation with UV signature, while the remaining *p53* allele is deleted. One possible role for early *p53* mutations in SCC is resistance to apoptosis and subsequent clonal expansion. Other TSGs mutated in SCC include different exons of the CDKN2A locus including p16 and the *PTCH* gene. The frequency of activating mutation in the *ras* oncogene ranges from 10% to 50%.[35,54]

Kanellou et al.[90] studied genomic instability, mutations, and expression analysis of the TSG in the spectrum of dysplastic squamous proliferations ranging from AK to invasive SCC. Authors found new mutations in the genes *p14ARF, p15INK4b,* and *p1616INK4a,* which, combined with the significant frequency of 9p instability found in AK samples, implied that the inactivation not only of both CDKN2A and CDKN2B loci plays a significant role in the progression of AK to SCC. Apart from mutations and loss of heterozygosity at 9p21, the deregulation of the expression profile of the TSGs may play a significant role in AK appearance and the progression of AK to invasive SCC. Furthermore, down-regulation of *p16INK4a* and *p53* mRNA levels was noted in SCC compared with AK, probably leading in collapse of the TSG system.

Compared with BCC, SCC demonstrates widespread loss of heterozygosity with deletions in several chromosomes including 3p, 9p, 9q, 13q, 17p, and 17q. SCC also appears to have a higher degree of genomic instability compared with BCC as 25% to 80% of SCCs are aneuploid.

In addition to direct mutagenesis, exposure to UVB leads to decreased density and antigen-processing capability of Langerhans' cells and may suppress production of the T-helper cell type1 cytokines IL-2 and INF-γ.[91]

Other agents associated with development of SCC include (1) chemical agents (e.g., petroleum, coal tar, soot, arsenic); (2) physical agents (e.g., ionizing radiation); (3) exposure to PUVA, calculated adjusted relative risk for a cumulative exposure of between 100 and 337 treatments is 8.6; (4) HPV, especially important for SCC in the anogenital and periungual regions, in the setting of immunosuppression with HIV and solid-organ transplantation, in patients with epidermodysplasia verruciformis; and (5) smoking. Development of SCC has also been associated with chronic nonhealing wounds, burn scars, and chronic inflammatory dermatoses (discoid lupus, ulcers, osteomyelitis).[92] Certain cervicofacial regions such as the ear and the lower lip are more prone to developing SCC than BCC.

Heritable conditions associated with higher incidence of SCC include xeroderma pigmentosum, dystrophic epidermolysis bullosa, and oculocutaneous albinism. HPV-16 and -18 is frequently implicated in the pathogenesis of subungual and periungual SCC and BD of the digits.

Immunosuppression, including endogenous (underlying lymphoproliferative disorder) and iatrogenic immunosuppression plays a role in pathogenesis of SCC (see the section "Immunosuppression" and "Nonmelanoma Skin Cancer").

BIOLOGIC BEHAVIOR OF SCC

Cutaneous SCC*IS* is a full-thickness intraepidermal carcinoma (Fig. 117.6). Most lesions are indolent and enlarge slowly over years, seldom progressing to invasive carcinoma. The term SCC*IS* includes specific entities such as BD and erythroplasia of Queyrat (SCC*IS* on the glans of penis of uncircumcised male related to HPV infection). Retrospective studies suggest that the risk of progression of BD to invasive SCC is approximately 3% to 5%. The risk of progression into invasive disease for genital erythroplasia of Queyrat is approximately 10%.[93] Bowenoid papulosis classically presents as a reddish brown verrucous papule and is associated with HPV-16 and -18. Bowenoid papulosis usually involves the genitals but may be present elsewhere.

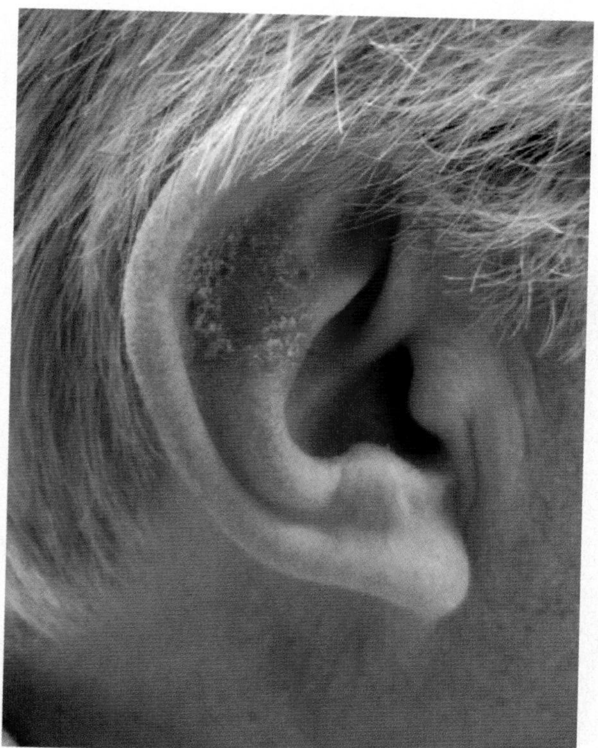

FIGURE 117.6 Squamous cell carcinoma *in situ* presents as an erythematous plaque that can be difficult to differentiate from a benign inflammatory process.

The biologic behavior of invasive SCC is determined by a number of variables including depth of invasion, degree of cellular differentiation (poorly differentiated neoplasms show higher rates of recurrence), known risk factors (see previous discussion), and immune status of the patient. Lesions occurring on sun-exposed skin have better prognosis than those arising on non–sun-exposed skin. Mucosal SCCs have a greater tendency to recur and metastasize than SCCs located on glabrous, sun-exposed skin.

The tendency for regional lymph node metastasis is variable. Tumors arising in areas of chronic inflammation and at mucocutaneous junctions have a 10% to 30% rate of progression to metastatic disease, whereas the incidence of metastasis from SCC arising on sun-exposed skin in the absence of preexisting inflammatory or degenerative conditions varies widely from 0.05% to 16.0%.[86]

Invasive SCC has the potential to demonstrate perineural and neural involvement.[86] SCCs on the midface and lip are especially prone to neural involvement that clinically translates into a lower 10-year survival (23% vs. 88%) and a higher local recurrence rate (47% vs. 7.3%) than do those without perineural or neural involvement. The risk of regional lymph node and distant metastases also increases with PNI. SCCs on the skin of the head and neck may metastasize to cervical lymph nodes and distantly to the central nervous system; the latter occurs either hematogenously or via the perineural space, which directly connects to the subarachnoid space.

CLINICAL FEATURES OF SCC

Clinically, SCC*IS* appears as a discrete solitary, sharply demarcated, scaly pink to red papule or thin plaque (Fig. 117.6). BD presents as a gradually enlarging, well-demarcated erythematous plaque with an irregular border and surface crusting or scaling. Erythroplasia of Queyrat presents as a verrucous or polypoid papule or plaque. Invasive SCC appears as a slightly raised papule plaque or nodule that is skin-colored, pink, or red (Fig. 117.7). The surface of the tumor may be smooth, keratotic, or ulcerated. The lesion may also be exophytic or indurated. Rarely, the tumor is symptomatic with pain or pruritus. Bleeding with minimal trauma is common. It can be clinically difficult to distinguish an invasive SCC from a hypertrophic AK, a benign seborrheic keratosis, or a benign inflammatory lesion. An appropriate biopsy should be performed.

Verrucous carcinoma, a variant of SCC, includes oral florid papillomatosis, giant condyloma of Buschke-Lowenstein, and epithelioma cuniculatum.[94] Verrucous carcinoma is considered a low-grade carcinoma. It grows slowly, rarely metastasizes, but is frequently deeply invasive into underlying tissue and therefore is difficult to eradicate. Following treatment with RT, verrucous carcinoma may become aggressive or even metastasize.

HISTOLOGY

The histologic criteria defining SCC*IS* include involvement of the entire thickness of epidermis with pleomorphic keratinocytes and involvement of the adnexal epithelium. The degree of keratinocytes atypia in SCC*IS* is variable. Marked anaplasia, nuclear crowding, loss of polarity, dysmaturation of the keratinocytes, numerous mitotic figures, including atypical and bizarre forms, and occasional dyskeratotic keratinocytes are seen giving epidermis a "windblown appearance." The epidermis may also be hyperplastic with psoriasiform appearance and broad rete ridges. A pigmented variant of SCC*IS* has abundant melanin accumulated within keratinocytes, and scattered superficial dermal macrophages.

The histologic differential diagnosis of SCC*IS* includes AK, bowenoid papulosis, Paget disease, extramammary Paget disease, and malignant melanoma *in situ*. Immunostaining may be required for proper diagnostic assessment. Bowenoid papulosis is histologically indistinguishable from SCC*IS*.

SCC is characterized histologically by its relatively large cellular size, nuclear hyperchromatism, lack of maturation, nuclear atypia, and the presence of mitotic figures. Presence of dermal invasion separates invasive SCC from SCC*IS*. In well-differentiated SCC, cytoplasmic keratinization is manifested by the presence of keratin pearls (horn cysts) and individual cell dyskeratosis. Invading keratinocytes frequently demonstrate minimal cytologic atypia. In contrast, poorly differentiated or undifferentiated SCC shows decreased evidence of keratinization, higher degree of cytologic atypia, and increased number of mitotic figures.

The histologic classification of cutaneous SCC according to the recent World Health Organization (WHO) classification includes SCC with cutaneous horn formation, spindle cell, acantholytic, SCC arising in BD, verrucous carcinoma, and lymphoepitheliomalike carcinoma. Other subtypes are desmoplastic, adenosquamous (mucin-producing), and cystic SCC.

RECURRENCE AND METASTATIC RISK

In a pivotal review of studies of SCCs from 1940 to 1992, Rowe et al.[86] correlated the risk for local recurrence and metastasis with treatment modality, prior treatment, location, size, depth, histologic differentiation, evidence of perineural involvement, precipitating factors other than UVR, and immunosuppression. The following observations were made: (1) for

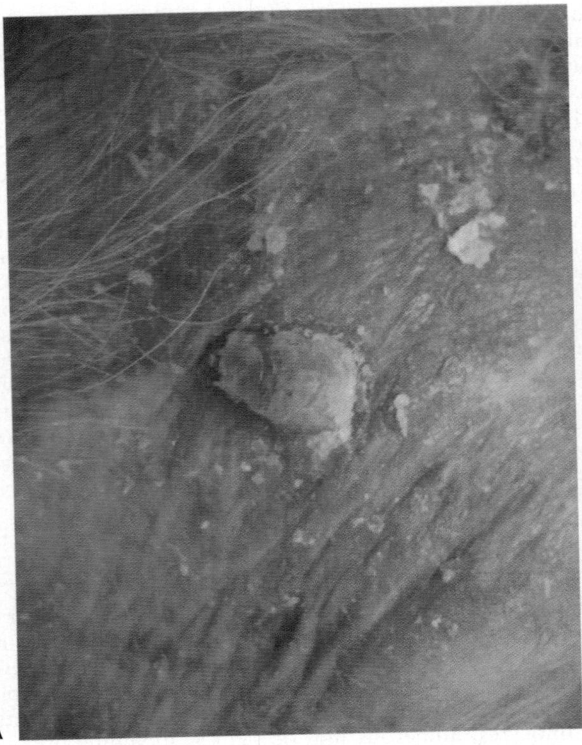

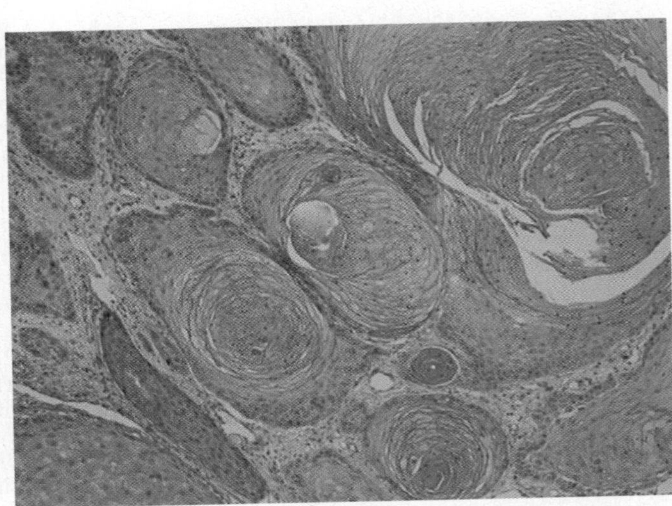

FIGURE 117.7 **A:** Clinical differential diagnosis of cutaneous horn includes squamous cell carcinoma (SCC). Biopsy of the pictured lesion confirmed a clinical diagnosis of SCC. **B:** Histology of well-differentiated SCC.

tumors greater than 2 cm in diameter, recurrence rates double from 7.4% to 15.2%; (2) tumors less than 4 mm in depth are at low risk for metastasis (6.7%) compared with tumors deeper than 4 mm (45.7%).

Locally recurrent SCC shows an overall metastatic rate of 30%, with high rates of metastasis when located on the lip (31.5%) and ear (45%).

The National Comprehensive Cancer Network guidelines of care for NMSC identified the clinical and histologic risk factors for recurrence of NMSC.[95]

Clinical high-risk factors for recurrence of SCC include (1) location and size: trunk and extremities 20 mm or more in diameter; cheeks, forehead, neck and scalp 10 mm or more; and "mask areas" of the face (central face, eyelids, eyebrows, periorbital, nose, lips, chin, mandible, preauricular and postauricular skin, ear, temple), genitalia, hands, and feet 6 mm or more; (2) poorly defined borders; (3) clinical recurrence; (4) immunosuppression; (5) appearance of the tumor at site of prior radiation; (6) presence of tumor at site of chronic inflammatory process; (7) rapid growth; and (8) presence of neurologic symptoms (i.e., pain, paresthesis, numbness, and paralysis).

Histopathologic high-risk factors include (1) presence of perineural involvement; (2) degree of differentiation (moderately or poorly differentiated SCCs have high rate of recurrence); (3) adenoid, adenosquamous, or desmoplastic subtypes; and (4) Clark level of thickness of IV, V, or 4 mm or more.

TREATMENT

Many of the treatments for BCC are also appropriate for SCC. The type of therapy should be selected on the basis of size of the lesion, anatomic location, depth of invasion, degree of cellular differentiation, history of previous treatment, and immune status of the host. There are three general approaches to treatment of SCC: (1) destruction by C&D, (2) removal by excisional surgery or MMS, and (3) radiation therapy.

C&D

C&D is a simple, cost-effective technique for treating low-risk SCCs. Honeycutt and Jansen[96] reported a 99% cure rate for 281 SCCs after a 4-year follow-up. In this study, two recurrences were noted in lesions less than 2 cm in diameter. C&D is frequently used for SCC*IS*; however, as with all forms of destructive therapy, extension of BD down hair follicles and clinically unrecognized foci of invasive tumor are a concern. As such, C&D is not indicated in dense hair-bearing areas, or when tumor extends into the subcutaneous layer.

SCC*IS* may be treated by cryotherapy. As with BCC, two freeze–thaw cycles with a tissue temperature of −50°C are required to destroy the tumor sufficiently. A margin of normal skin also should be frozen to ensure eradication of subclinical disease. Complications include hypertrophic scarring and postinflammatory pigmentary changes both hypo- and hyperpigmentation. Concealment of recurrence within dense scar tissue presents a danger. Imiquimod has demonstrated efficacy in the treatment of SCC*IS*, but is currently not FDA-approved for the treatment of this neoplasm.[10]

Surgical Modalities

Surgical excision is a well-accepted treatment modality for SCC. Brodland and Zitelli[97] have demonstrated that lesions of less than 2 cm in diameter can be safely treated by excision, with a 95% confidence interval using margins of 4 mm and 6 mm for low-risk and high-risk tumors, respectively. These investigators found that certain characteristics were associated with a greater risk of subclinical tumor extension, thus qualifying such tumors as high risk. These included the size of 2 cm or larger, histologic grade higher than 2, invasion of the subcutaneous tissue, and location in high-risk areas.

Carcinomas of the penis, vulva, and anus are usually treated by excision. Surgical excision is the treatment of choice for verrucous carcinoma.

MMS is indicated for high-risk SCCs including invasive, poorly differentiated SCCs, and lesions occurring in high-risk anatomic sites or sites in which conservation of normal tissue is essential for preservation of function and/or cosmesis. MMS is superior to other forms of treatment with regard to local recurrence. Recurrence rates with MMS are superior to those obtained with traditional excisional surgery in primary SCC of the ear (3.1% vs. 10.9%), primary SCC of the lip (5.8% vs. 18.7%), recurrent SCC (10% vs. 23.3%), SCC with PNI (0% vs. 47%), SCC larger than 2 cm (25.2 vs. 41.7%), and poorly differentiated SCC (32.6% vs. 53.6%).[94] MMS has proven useful in SCC involving the nail unit and has been used as a limb-sparing procedure in cases of SCC arising in osteomyelitis.

Radiation Therapy

Indications for RT for patients with SCC are similar to those for patients with BCC. The likelihood of cure for early-stage lesions is similar for both surgery and RT. Therefore, the decision on which modality to employ depends on other factors, including a patient's underlying medical status, the age, cosmesis, cost, and treatment availability.

In young patients, surgical treatment is a preferable because the late effects of irradiation progress gradually with time and, with long-term follow-up, may be associated with a suboptimal cosmetic result compared with surgical resection and reconstruction. In special sites such as lower lip with advanced (over 30%-50% of the lip involved) SCC, RT allows for excellent maintenance of oral competency with cure rates similar to those of surgical modalities.[29]

Advanced cutaneous cancers may be treated with surgery and adjuvant RT. Adjuvant postoperative RT is added in situations in which the possibility of residual disease is high. Babington et al.[98] documented a 37% local recurrence rate in patients who underwent surgery without adjuvant RT compared with a 6% local recurrence rate in patients treated with both treatment modalities in the setting of lip SCC. Indications for postsurgical RT include positive margins, PNI (especially if symptomatic), multiple recurrences, and underlying tissue invasion. Advanced unresectable cancers, such as those with marked PNI or with gross disease in the cavernous sinus, may be treated with RT alone.

Management of Regional Lymph Node Metastases

Treatment of nodal disease may involve local RT, lymph node dissection, or combination of both. Skin cancer metastatic to the parotid nodes is commonly managed with superficial or surgical total parotidectomy followed by adjuvant RT (60 Gy in 30 fractions). Extreme care should be taken to preserve the function of the facial nerve. Nonetheless, in certain cases resection is necessary to achieve a gross total resection. With surgery and adjuvant RT, a 5-year disease-free survival ranges from 70% to 75%. Although the risk of subclinical disease in the clinically negative nodes is 20% or higher, the ipsilateral neck may be electively irradiated when the parotid is treated postoperatively. Preoperative RT is used for patients with borderline resectable metastases. RT alone is used for patients with unresectable disease and for those who are medically inoperable. The likelihood of cure is lower with RT-only treatment compared with RT plus surgery, but nodal regression and good palliation are commonly seen. Treatment and palliative doses should be at least 60 to 66 Gy and 40 Gy, respectively.[29]

Cervical node metastases are managed with neck dissection in patients with a solitary node with no extracapsular extension and postoperative RT in patients with more advanced disease.[99] Depending on the location of the primary tumor, the probability of subclinical disease in the clinically negative parotid may be high and the parotid nodes should be considered for elective treatment.

The probability of local control with RT is higher for primary cancers and is inversely proportional to tumor size. The likelihood of cure for patients with PNI is related to the presence of symptoms and to the radiographic extent of disease. Patients with incidental PNI have a local control rate of 80% to 90% compared with about 50% to 55% for those with clinically evident PNI.[27] Various techniques and fractionation schedules have been proposed, including hyperfractionation (74.4 Gy in 1.2 Gy twice-daily fractions), intensity-modulated RT, or an electron/photon beam.[29] The optimal treatment for patients with clinically positive nodes is surgery and postoperative RT. The likelihood of cure for those with positive parotid nodes reaches 70% to 80%.

Treatment of metastatic SCC may include systemic chemotherapy or treatment with biologic response modifiers. The efficacy of these methods has not been established. Long-term prognosis for metastatic disease is extremely poor. Ten-year survival rates are less than 20% for patients with regional lymph node involvement and less than 10% for patients with distant metastases.[100]

FOLLOW UP

Invasive SCC can be a potentially lethal neoplasm and warrants close follow-up. A critical review and meta-analysis has found that for people with fewer than three previous NMSCs, the risk of developing another NMSC within the following 3 years is 38%. In people with three to nine previous NMSCs, this risk rises to 93%.[101] In another study, approximately 30% of patients with SCC developed a subsequent SCC, with more than half of these occurring within the first year of follow-up.[102] Thus, it is recommended that patients with SCC be examined every 3 months during the first year after treatment, every 6 months during the second year after treatment, and at least annually thereafter. Evaluation should include total-body cutaneous examination and palpation of draining lymph nodes. Currently, radiography, magnetic resonance imaging, and computed tomography (CT) play no role in the routine workup of uncomplicated cutaneous SCC.

IMMUNOSUPPRESSION AND NONMELANOMA SKIN CANCER

The role of the immune system in the pathogenesis of skin cancer is still not completely understood. Immunosuppressed patients with lymphoma or leukemia and patients with depressed cellular immunity secondary to HIV infection develop NMSC at a significantly younger age and show a higher frequency of NMSC than the general population.[103] An Italian linkage study found a threefold increase in the incidence of NMSC over the general population.[104] Incidence of clinically aggressive HPV-related anal SCC is significantly increased in this population, requiring serial examinations and anal cytologies for surveillance.[105]

Solid-organ transplant recipients (e.g., heart, kidney) have a three- to fourfold increased risk over the general population of developing any cancer.[19] These patients experience a marked increase in the incidence of SCCs (40- to 250-fold increase) and BCCs (five- to tenfold increase). In a series of 455 heart transplant patients from Australia, the cumulative incidence of skin cancer was 31% at 5 years and 43% at 10 years with an SCC/BCC ratio of 3:1.[106] Skin cancers in immunosuppressed patients appear primarily on sun-exposed sites. Incidence of NMSC in renal transplant recipients in Australia increases exponentially over time: 3% within the first year, 25% at 5 years, and 44% at 9 or more years posttransplant.[107] Furthermore, the SCCs in organ transplant patients occur at a younger age and tend to be more aggressive. There is an increased risk of local recurrence, regional and distant metastasis, and mortality. In case series of renal transplant patients from the United States and Australian heart transplant recipients, SCC-related mortality rates were 5% and 27%, respectively.[106]

Patients who receive hematopoietic transplants do not experience marked increased in skin cancer incidence, presumably because of the shorter duration of immunosuppression.

Cumulative UV radiation is the primary pathogenic factor for the development of NMSC in solid-organ transplant recipients, but degree, type, and duration of immunosuppression, and age at transplantation are also significant.[106] Rapamycin (sirolimus), a bacterial macrolide and antitumor agent, is a newer immunosuppressive agent that shows promise in decreasing incidence and severity of posttransplant NMSCs.[108] Although organ transplant recipients have an increased incidence of viral warts, the role of HPV in skin cancer is not clearly defined. Prevention, patient education, aggressive sun protection, and timely and aggressive management of skin cancers as well as lowering the degree of immunosuppression whenever possible are crucial to reduce the significant potential of morbidity and mortality. Transplantation immunosuppressive medications that are more selective in impairing recipient immune system activation against the allograft are being developed and may alter the behavior of skin cancer in these patients.

ANGIOSARCOMA

Angiosarcoma (AS; synonyms are malignant hemangioendothelioma, hemangiosarcoma, lymphangiosarcoma) is an uncommon, aggressive, usually fatal neoplasm of vascular endothelium origin accounting for less than 2% of all sarcomas.[109] The overall incidence of this tumor is approximately 0.1 per million per year. Four variants of cutaneous AS currently are recognized and include AS of the "head and neck" (also known as idiopathic AS) accounting for 50% to 60% of all cases, AS in the context of lymphedema (LAS; Stewart-Treves syndrome), radiation-induced AS, and epithelioid AS. Although these variants differ in presentation, they share key features, including clinical appearance of primary lesions, a biologically aggressive nature, and, ultimately, poor outcome.

PATHOGENESIS

Pathogenesis of AS is poorly understood. Approximately 50% of AS express markers of lymphatic differentiation in addition to vascular endothelium-associated antigens. More recently, AS was found to coexpress podoplanin and podocalyxin, markers of lymphatic and vascular endothelium, respectively.[110] HHV-8 etiologic factor in Kaposi sarcoma appears not to be associated with AS. Cumulative sun exposure has not been shown to be a predisposing factor.

CLINICAL PRESENTATION AND PROGNOSIS

Cutaneous AS of the head and scalp usually affects older adults. Approximately 70% of AS occurs in patients over the age of 40 years and the highest incidence of the disease is reported in those over 70 years of age.[109] Men are more commonly affected than women with 1.6 to 3:1 ratio.

Clinically, cutaneous AS presents as a violaceous to red, ill-defined patch on the central face, forehead or scalp, often initially resembling a bruise.[109] Facial swelling and edema may be present. Differential diagnosis at initial presentation may include benign vascular tumor, hematoma secondary to trauma, or even an inflammatory dermatosis. More advanced lesions are violaceous elevated nodules with propensity to bleed easily. Ulceration may also be present. Satellite lesions are common.

The prognosis of cutaneous AS is poor, with a mortality rate of 50% at 15 months after diagnosis, and the survival rates ranging from 10% to 30% over a 5-year period, with median survival 18 to 28 months.[111,112] Metastatic potential of AS is high. Metastases to lung, liver, lymph nodes, spleen, and brain are common. Prognosis for metastatic disease is poor. Although prognosis does not correlate with degree of cellular differentiation, there appears to be a correlation with lesion size at presentation; increased survival has been demonstrated in lesions smaller than 5 cm at time of diagnosis. In a clinical univariate analysis of 69 cases, older age, anatomic site, necrosis, and epithelioid features directly correlated with increased mortality.[113] Other prognostic factors proposed in the literature include depth of invasion greater than 3 mm, mitotic rate, Ki-67 staining, positive surgical margins, and local recurrence.[114]

Lymphedema-associated AS (LAS) accounting for about 10% of all cutaneous AS was first reported by Stewart and Treves[115] in six patients with postmastectomy lymphedema. In each case, AS developed in the ipsilateral arm and occurred several years after mastectomy. Subsequently, LAS was reported after axillary node dissection for melanoma and in the context of congenital lymphedema, filarial lymphedema, and chronic idiopathic lymphedema. The risk for developing LAS 5 years after mastectomy is approximately 5%. The most common site is the medial aspect of the upper arm.

LAS presents as a firm, coalescing violaceous plaque or nodule superimposed on brawny, nonpitting edema. Ulceration may develop rapidly. The duration of lymphedema prior to appearance of AS ranges from 4 to 27 years. The pathogenesis of LAS is incompletely understood and may be related to imbalances in local immune regulation or angiogenesis, leading to proliferation of neoplastic cells. The prognosis is poor, and survival rates are comparable to AS involving the scalp and face. Long-term survival has been reported in isolated cases after amputation of the affected limb.

Radiation-induced AS has been reported to occur after RT for benign or malignant conditions.[109] AS may occur from 4 to 40 years after RT for benign conditions (acne and eczema), or from 4 to 25 years after RT for malignancies. Overall prognosis is poor and comparable to that observed in other forms of AS.

Epithelioid AS is a rare, recently described variant of AS.[116] It tends to involve the lower extremities. On microscopic examination, the tumor may mimic an epithelial neoplasm, with sheets of rounded, epithelioid cells intermingled with irregularly lined vascular channels. Epithelioid AS results in widespread metastases within 1 year of presentation. Prognosis is poor.

HISTOLOGY

Histology of AS, although highly variable in the degree of cellular endothelial differentiation between and within individual tumors, does not vary between individual subtypes.[109] In well-differentiated lesions, an anastomosing network of sinusoidal irregularly dilated vascular channels lined by a single layer of flattened endothelial cells with mild to moderate nuclear atypia is commonly seen. These exhibit a highly infiltrative pattern, splitting collagen bundles and subcutaneous adipose tissue. Less differentiated tumors show proliferation of atypical, polygonal, or spindle-shaped, pleomorphic endothelial cells with increased mitotic activity and anastomosing vascular channels. In poorly differentiated AS, luminal formation may be no longer apparent and mitotic activity is high. Poorly differentiated AS may mimic other high-grade sarcomas, carcinoma, or even melanoma. The state of cellular differentiation, however, has not been shown to correlate with prognosis.[111] Immunohistochemical analysis may be of value in diagnosis of AS, as cells stain positively for *Ulex europaeus* I lectin and factor VIII–related antigen. *Ulex* I is considered to be more sensitive marker for AS. In addition, AS cells express stem cell antigen CD34 and endothelial cell surface antigen CD31. The majority of AS cases stain positively for vimetin, D2-40, and VEGFR-3.

TREATMENT

Because of the clinical aggressiveness, treatment options for AS are limited. Surgical excision with wide margins is the treatment of choice. Nonetheless, the recurrence rates and possibility of metastatic disease are high even with histologically negative margins and may reflect the tendency for multifocality.[117] Amputation with shoulder disarticulation or hemipelvectomy is recommended for tumors involving the extremities. Because AS tends to extend far beyond clinically appreciated margins, complete surgical removal may be challenging. Several cases of AS have been treated by MMS in an attempt to control margins; however, the difference between AS and normal vasculature may be difficult to interpret on frozen sections, even with the use of immunohistochemical stains.[118] RT and electron beam should be considered postoperatively in an effort to enhance local control.

Patients with isolated lymphatic spread treated with taxol-based chemotherapeutic regimens have a favorable outcome. Both chemotherapy and radical radiotherapy are palliative f only or metastatic disease and do not improve overall survival.

DERMATOFIBROSARCOMA PROTUBERANS

Dermatofibrosarcoma protuberans (DFSP) is a rare soft tissue sarcoma with aggressive local but low metastatic potential with an annual incidence of approximately 4 per million. DFSP constitutes approximately 1% of all sarcomas and less than 0.1% of all malignancies.[119] The vast majority, approximately 90% of DFSPs, are low-grade sarcomas, whereas the remainder are classified as intermediate or high grade because of the presence of a high-grade fibrosarcomatous component (DFSP-FS).[120]

DFSP most commonly affects patients in their mid-to-late 30s; however, the disease can occur at any age. Childhood and congenital cases of DFSP have been reported.[121] Blacks have slightly higher incidence than whites. Both men and women are equally affected.[122]

PATHOGENESIS

The pathogenesis of DFSP is incompletely understood but may involve factors as diverse as aberrant TSG or a history of local trauma/scarring.[123] More than 90% of DFSP feature a translocation between chromosomes 17 and 22, resulting in the fusion between the collagen type Iα1 gene (*COL1A1*) and the platelet-derived growth factor (PDGF) β-chain gene (*PDGFB*). Thus, the growth of DFSP is a result of the deregulation of PDGF β-chain expression and activation of PDGF receptor (*PDGFR*) protein tyrosine kinase.[123,124]

DFSP classically presents as a solitary, frequently asymptomatic, plaque with violaceous to blue hue. The tumor exhibits slow growth. Most commonly affected sides include trunk and, less frequently, the extremities, head, and neck but it may occur anywhere.[124] The Bednar tumor is a rare pigmented variant of DFSP.[125] Clinically, it may be difficult to differentiate from a dermatofibroma or a keloid.

HISTOLOGY

Histologically, DFSP arises in the dermis and is composed of monomorphous, dense spindle cells arranged in a storiform pattern and embedded in a sparse to moderately dense fibrous stroma.[126] Irregular projections (tentaclelike) of the tumor are common and may account for the high incidence of local recurrence after excision. The distinction between deep penetrating dermatofibroma (DPDF), which involves the subcutis, and DFSP may be challenging. In most instances, attention to the cytologic constituency of the lesions and the overall architecture is sufficient for differentiation. DPDF is typified by cellular heterogeneity. DPDF includes giant cells and lipidized histiocytes and extends deeply, using the interlobular subcuticular fibrous septa as scaffolds, or is in the form of broad fronts. In contrast, DFSP tends to be monomorphous, surrounding adipocytes diffusely or extending in stratified horizontal plates. This infiltration is characteristically eccentric, often with long, thin extensions in one direction and not another. Immunostaining for factor XIIIa, CD34, and stromelysin 3 may be helpful in distinguishing DPDF from DFSP. Characteristically, DPDF is diffusely factor XIIIa+, CD34−, and stromelysin 3+, whereas DFSP is factor XIIIa−, CD34+, and stromelysin 3−.[127]

TREATMENT

Treatment options for DFSP include WLE and MMS. Most authors advocate WLE with a minimal margin of at least 3 cm of surrounding skin, including the underlying fascia, without elective lymph node dissection.[128] The likelihood of local recurrence is directly proportional to the adequacy of surgical margins. Conservative resection can lead to recurrence rates of 33% to 60%, whereas wider excision margins ($\geq$2.5 cm) have been reported to reduce the recurrence rate to 10%.[129] For well-defined tumors located on trunk or extremities, WLE is likely to achieve tumor clearance with satisfactory cosmetic and functional result. However, extirpation of tumor by MMS, using frozen sections with or without confirmation by examination of paraffin-embedded sections, may be beneficial in sites where maximum conservation of normal tissue is required. Utility of MMS versus WLE was examined in a retrospective review of 48 primary DFSP cases treated at a single institution.[130] Twenty-eight patients underwent WLE and 20 patients underwent MMS. Median WLE margin width was 2 cm. For MMS, the median number of layers required to clear the tumor was two. Positive margins were present in 21.4%

Recommendations about the optimal minimum width and depth of normal tissue margin that should be excised around the primary tumor differ among the various retrospective case series, but this question has not been studied systematically.[150,156,159] No definitive data suggest that extremely wide margins improve overall survival, although some reports suggest that wider margins appear to improve local control.[160]

Recommended management has usually been WLE with 1- to 3-cm margins; however, treatment guidelines are not well defined, owing to the rarity of the tumor, which precludes randomized clinical trials. Recurrence rates after primary therapy for MCC with surgery alone are reported to be within the range of 0% to 50% to 70%. In a single-institution case series of 95 patients with early-stage MCC, a total of 45 (47%) patients relapsed, with 80% of the recurrences occurring within 2 years and 96% within 5 years.[161] Patients with MCC in the head and neck region had a 5-year local-recurrence cumulative incidence of 19% and no distant recurrences, and patients with MCC in the extremity and trunk region had a 5-year local-recurrence cumulative incidence of 2% and a 5-year distant-recurrence cumulative incidence of 22%.[161] MMS has been proposed as being more successful in controlling local disease than WLE, especially in cosmetically sensitive anatomic locations. The relapse rate has been reported to be similar to or better than that of wide excision, but comparatively few cases have been treated in this manner and none in randomized, controlled trials.[159,162,163] In a retrospective review of 38 consecutive patients with MCC of the extremities, WLE and MMS showed similar local recurrence rate.[159]

MCC spreads to regional lymph nodes within 2 years in up to 70% of cases. Because of the propensity for early nodal spread and the significant negative impact that nodal disease has on outcome, regional lymph node dissection or sentinel lymph node (SLN) dissection may be advisable. Surgical nodal staging in clinically negative patients has identified positive nodes in at least 25% to 35% of patients.[156] At present, it is questionable whether lymph node dissection has an impact on survival, but it seems to benefit local and regional control. Clinically or radiographically positive nodes should be resected but it is unclear whether elective lymph node dissection (ELND) provides benefit.

The role of ELND in the absence of clinically positive nodes has not been studied in formal clinical trials. In small case series, ELND has been recommended for larger primary tumors, tumors with more than ten mitoses per high-power field, lymphatic or vascular invasion, and the small cell histologic subtypes.[141,164]

SLN biopsy is a preferred initial alternative to complete ELND for the proper staging of MCC. SLN biopsy is associated with lower morbidity, and in the sites with indeterminate lymphatic drainage, SNL technique can be used to identify the pertinent lymphatic basins.

Several reports support the use of SLN biopsy techniques in MCC staging and management.[165–167] One meta-analysis of ten case series found that SLN positivity strongly predicted a high short-term risk of recurrence and that subsequent therapeutic lymph node dissection was effective in preventing short-term regional nodal recurrence.[167] Another meta-analysis of 12 retrospective case series found that (1) SLN biopsy detected MCC spread in one-third of patients whose tumors would have otherwise been clinically and radiologically understaged, (2) the recurrence rate was three times higher in patients with a positive SLN biopsy than in those with a negative SLN biopsy, and (3) the relapse-free survival rate in patients with positive SLN biopsy who received and those who did not receive additional treatment to the nodes at 3 years was 51% and 0%, respectively.[168]

Based on a small number of retrospective studies, therapeutic dissection of the regional nodes after a positive SLN dissection appears to minimize but not totally eliminate the risk of subsequent regional node recurrence and in-transit metastases.[167] There are, however, no data from prospective randomized trials demonstrating that definitive regional nodal treatment with surgery improves survival.

Nodal basin radiation in contiguity with radiation to the primary site has been considered for patients with larger tumors, locally unresectable tumors, close or positive excision margins that cannot be improved by additional surgery, and those with positive regional nodes (stage II).[141,163] Several small retrospective series have shown that radiation plus adequate surgery improves local-regional control compared with surgery alone,[150,168] whereas other series did not show similar results.[156,162] Adjuvant RT offers a substantial benefit in both time to recurrence and disease-free survival, but a survival benefit is yet to be proven.[169] The controversy regarding the utility of adjuvant RT following excision remains.

Chemotherapy is used for nodal, metastatic, and recurrent MCC, but an optimal treatment regimen is yet to be established. From 1997 to 2001, the Trans-Tasman Radiation Oncology Group performed a phase 2 evaluation of 53 MCC patients with high-risk, local-regional disease. Given the heterogeneity of the population and the nonstandardized surgery, it is difficult to infer a clear treatment benefit of the chemotherapy.[170] Regimens are similar to those used for small cell lung carcinoma. The most commonly used agents are cyclophosphamide, anthracyclines, and cisplatin. In a study by Voog et al.,[171] overall response to first-line chemotherapy for MCC was 61%, with a 57% response in metastatic disease and a 69% response in locally advanced disease. Reported 3-year survival rate was 17% in metastatic disease and 35% in locally advanced disease. Forty-two different regimens were used to treat these 107 reported cases.

PROGNOSIS

The prognosis of MCC is directly correlated with the stage of disease. Reported 5-year survival according to MSKCC classification is 81% for stage I, 67% for stage II, 52% for stage III, and 11% for stage IV.[119] More than 50% of patients experience recurrence with the median time to recurrence of 9 months (range, 2–70 months). Ninety-one percent of recurrences occurred within 2 years of diagnosis.[156] Overall survival of head and neck MCC at 5 years postoperatively ranges between 40% and 68%.[172]

MICROCYSTIC ADNEXAL CARCINOMA

Microcystic adnexal carcinoma (MAC) was first described as a distinct entity in 1982 by Goldstein et al.[173] Synonyms quoted in the literature to describe MAC include sclerosing sweat duct carcinoma, malignant syringoma, sweat gland carcinoma with syringomatous features, aggressive trichofolliculoma, and combined adnexal tumor of the skin. MAC originates from pluripotent adnexal keratinocytes capable of both eccrine and follicular differentiation.

MAC is an aggressive, locally destructive cutaneous appendageal neoplasm with a high rate of local recurrence. It primarily affects white, middle-aged individuals, although it has been reported in children and blacks. Unlike the other primary cutaneous malignancies, MAC has slight female predominance.

PATHOGENESIS

The pathogenesis of MAC is not completely understood but may involve exposure to ionizing and UVR that may precede development of MAC by as long as 40 years.[174] The role of immunosuppression in development of MAC is not yet fully understood. There have been 12 cases of MAC developing in association with other unrelated cancers and 3 cases of MAC reported as occurring in immunosuppressed patients, 2 in organ transplant recipients and 1 in a patient with chronic lymphocytic leukemia.

CLINICAL PRESENTATION

MAC classically presents as a smooth-surfaced, nonulcerated, flesh-colored to yellowish asymptomatic nodule, papule, or plaque (Fig. 117.9A). When symptomatic, common findings include numbness, tenderness, anesthesia, paresthesia, burning, discomfort, and/or rarely pruritus of the affected site. These symptoms can relate to the frequent PNI of the tumor. MAC is locally aggressive with common perineural invasion and extension to muscle, vascular adventitia, perichondrium, periosteum, and bone marrow. To date, seven cases of metastases have been reported for a cumulative metastatic rate of less than 2.1%.

MAC has a clear predilection for the head and neck (86%-88%), particularly the central face (73%). Other sites include eyelid, scalp, breast/chest, axillae, buttocks, vulva, extremities, and tongue. This tumor is often misdiagnosed clinically and histologically.[174,175]

HISTOLOGY

Histologically, MAC is a tumor of pilar and eccrine differentiation. It may be misdiagnosed as a benign adnexal process. The tumor frequently exhibits a stratified appearance with larger keratin horn cysts and epithelial nests, strands, or cords in the superficial dermis and desmoplastic deeper dermis with smaller cysts and more pronounced ductal structures. Horn cysts may contain laminated keratin and/or small vellus hairs. Cysts may be also calcified. Ducts may be well differentiated, with two rows of cuboidal cells, or less differentiated, with single strands without lumina. Lumina may contain eosinophilic secretion, sialomucin. Mitotic figures and cytologic atypia are rare. Histologic differential diagnosis of MAC includes desmoplastic trichoepithelioma, benign syringoma, papillary eccrine adenoma, morpheaform BCC, SCC, and metastatic breast carcinoma. Adequately deep biopsy is crucial for correct diagnostic assessment. Immunohistochemical analysis may be useful in differentiating MAC from desmoplastic trichoepithelioma. Wick et al.[175] reported that MACs were reactive to hard keratin subclasses AE13 and AE14, epithelial membrane antigen (EMA), carcinoembryonic antigen, and LeuM1. Desmoplastic trichoepitheliomas were positive for AE14, EMA, and LeuM1 only focally and were, in contrast, negative for carcinoembryonic antigen.

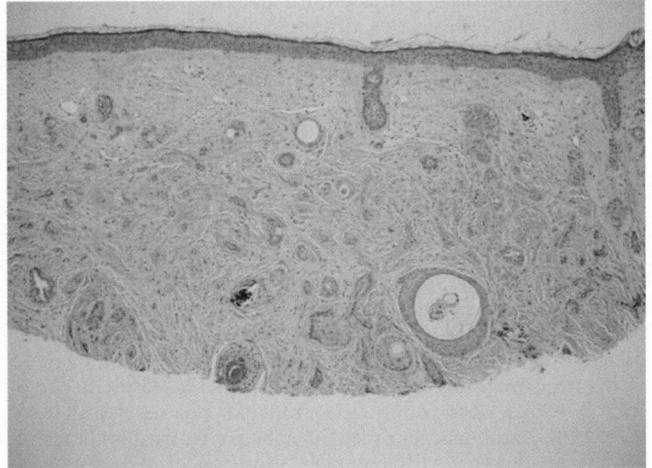

FIGURE 117.9 Histology of microcystic adnexal carcinoma. The tumor frequently exhibits a stratified appearance with larger keratin horn cysts and epithelial nests, strands, or cords in the superficial dermis and desmoplastic deeper dermis with smaller cysts and more pronounced ductal structures. Horn cysts may contain laminated keratin and/or small vellus hairs. Cysts may be also calcified. Ducts may be well differentiated, with two rows of cuboidal cells, or less differentiated, with single strands without lumina.

TREATMENT

Treatment modalities used for MAC include WLE, MMS, RT, and chemotherapy. Current standard of care is to surgically remove the tumor in its entirety whenever feasible. This task can be challenging in clinical practice because the tumor often extends microscopically centimeters beyond the clinically apparent margins. Margins reported in the literature for WLE vary from a few millimeters to 3 to 5 cm. Extirpation of tumor by MMS may prove beneficial in the management of MAC. Recurrence rates vary significantly between the two surgical techniques with rates after WLE and MMS ranging from 40% to 60%[176] and 0 to 12%,[177] respectively. These recurrence rates, however, must be interpreted cautiously because although most recurrences occur within the first 2 to 3 years after treatment, recurrences have been reported up to 30 years after surgical excision.

RT has been used as mono- or adjuvant therapy for MAC in six case reports. Only one of six case reports showed success of RT in the management of MAC on the lower lip, proving tumor's resistance to RT. Bier-Laning et al.[176] reported an unsuccessful trial of chemotherapy (cisplatin and 5-FU) in the management of MAC.

Given these data, surgical removal appears to be the treatment of choice for MAC. Patients must be evaluated regularly for recurrence and for development of MAC and/or other skin cancers. Evaluation should include examination of skin and lymph nodes and, because of the potential for recurrence long after treatment, should continue throughout the patient's life.

SEBACEOUS CARCINOMA

Sebaceous carcinoma (SC) is a malignant adnexal tumor with variable sites of origin, histologic growth patterns, and clinical presentations. About 75% of SCs are periocular in location.[178] Periocular SC may arise from Meibomian glands and, less frequently, from the glands of Zeis. The upper eyelids are most frequently involved. Approximately 25% of cases of SC involve extraocular sites, which may include head and neck, trunk, salivary glands, and external genitalia.[179]

The most frequent clinical presentation is a slowly growing, painless, subcutaneous nodule. Other presentations include diffuse thickening of the skin, pedunculated papules, or an irregular subcutaneous mass. On the eyelid, SC may present as chronic diffuse blepharoconjunctivitis or keratoconjunctivitis, particularly with pagetoid or intraepithelial spread of tumor onto the conjunctival epithelium.[180]

Approximately 50% of SCs are initially incorrectly diagnosed histologically and, in some series, all have been initially misdiagnosed clinically. The most common clinical misdiagnosis is chalazion. SC is the second most common eyelid malignancy after BCC and is the second most lethal after melanoma.[180]

Worldwide, SC affects all races, but Asians are particularly prone to the disease. Women are affected more commonly than men, at a ratio of approximately 2:1. SC classically presents in the seventh to ninth decades.[181] SC is associated with sebaceous adenomas, radiation exposure, BD, and Muir Torre syndrome. SC has been reported after RT for retinoblastoma, eczema, and cosmetic epilation. In addition, recent studies have identified HPV DNA and overexpression of p53 protein in some SCs.[180,182]

SCs have high rates of local recurrence and metastasis. SC can spread by lymphatic or hematogenous routes or by direct extension. Distant metastases are reported in up to 20% of cases and may involve the lungs, liver, brain, bones, and lymph nodes. The parotid gland may be involved secondarily. Ocular SC may spread via the lacrimal secretory and excretory systems.[180]

Mortality of SC ranges from 9% to 50%. Ocular SC has reported recurrence rates ranging from 11% to 30% with distant metastasis occurring in 3% to 25%. Albeit initially considered less aggressive, extraocular SC shows local recurrence rates of 29% and metastatic rate of 21%.

HISTOLOGY

Histologically, SCs are classified as well, moderately, or poorly differentiated. Four histopathologic subtypes of SCs are lobular, comedocarcinoma, papillary, and mixed. Most commonly, lesions have an irregular lobular growth pattern with sebaceous and undifferentiated cells. SC cells exhibit varying degrees of differentiation, nuclear pleomorphism, hyperchromatism, basaloid appearance and high mitotic activity. Local infiltration of the surrounding tissues and neurovascular spaces can be seen. A known feature of the SC is pagetoid spread, the spread of tumor cells into the overlying epithelium. Special stains, including lipid stains as Oil-Red-O or Sudan IV for fresh tissue, and immunohistochemical stains such as EMA or LeuM1 are also helpful.[183]

TREATMENT

Treatment options for SC include WLE with 5- to 6-mm margins and extirpation by MMS. The local recurrence rate after WLE has been reported to be as high as 36% at 5 years and associated 5-year mortality rate of 18%.[184] In one study of 14 cases of SC excised with frozen-section margin control, five recurrences were observed in cases with surgical margins of 1 to 3 mm, whereas no recurrences were seen with margins of 5 mm.[185] Potential difficulties arise because tumors are often multicentric with discontinuous foci of tumor, and pagetoid spread is difficult to determine even on high-quality, paraffin-embedded sections. Extirpation of SC by MMS has yielded varying results. A recent study showed recurrence rates of 11% after MMS. A series of poorly differentiated SC successfully treated with RT has been reported.[186]

Patients with SC should be evaluated by an internist, and routine age-appropriate screening for internal malignancies should be current. A family history for internal malignancy should be sought and family members screened, if indicated, to rule out Muir Torre syndrome. Poor prognostic indicators in SC include a duration of more than 6 months, multicentric origin, poor differentiation, infiltrative pattern, pagetoid spread, vascular invasion, lymphatic channel involvement, previous radiation, and orbital spread.[186] After treatment for SC, patients should be followed for recurrence or progression through regular examination of skin and lymph nodes.

ATYPICAL FIBROXANTHOMA AND MALIGNANT FIBROUS HISTIOCYTOMA

Until recently, atypical fibroxanthoma (AFX) and malignant fibrous histiocytoma (MFH) were thought to be two distinct presentations of the same malignancy with differing clinical courses. AFX was considered a superficial sarcoma of low to intermediate metastatic risk, whereas diagnosis of MFH was reserved for a deeper penetrating tumor of greater metastatic potential.[187] However, following reclassification of soft tissue sarcomas by the WHO in 2002 that mandated identification of cell line origin in classification of tumors, most cases of MFH, as previously considered, were found to be merely a morphologic pattern rather than a defined pathologic entity.[188] In a greater majority of cases, ultrastructural and immunohistochemical examination allowed for reclassification into defined histogenic subtypes of sarcomas. Under the new classification, the term *MFH* is a synonym for undifferentiated pleomorphic sarcoma not otherwise specified. It is likely that with future developments in immunohistophenotyping the term MFH will become obsolete.

ATYPICAL FIBROXANTHOMA

AFX is a spindle cell tumor that occurs on the head and neck of sun-exposed individuals and on the trunk and extremities of younger patients. Tumors of the head and neck characteristically present during the eighth decade, whereas tumors involving the extremities often present during the fourth decade. The ratio of affected men to women appears to be equal. A few cases have been reported in children with xeroderma pigmentosum.

PATHOGENESIS

The pathogenesis of AFX involves exposure to UVR, ionizing radiation, and/or aberrant immune host response. In a series of ten cases of AFX, seven cases showed mutation in TSG *p53*. Of the seven, all showed abnormal single-strand conformation polymorphism, with four showing UVR signature cyclobutane pyrimidine dimmers mutations.[189] Tumors may occur 10 to 15 years after local ionizing radiation. An increased incidence of AFX has been observed in renal transplant patients, and invasive AFX has been reported in a heart transplant patient. Finally, metastatic AFX has been reported in a patient with null cell variant chronic lymphocytic leukemia.

CLINICAL PRESENTATION

AFX usually presents as an asymptomatic, often rapidly growing, dome-shaped papule or nodule covered by thin epidermis on actinically damaged skin of individuals with a fair complexion. Average size at presentation is 1 to 2 cm. Secondary changes such as serosanguinous crust or ulceration may be present. The clinical appearance is not distinctive, and the clinical differential diagnosis of the lesion often includes pyogenic granuloma, SCC, BCC, amelanotic melanoma, MCC, and cutaneous metastasis. AFX may be found in the setting of other NMSCs.

HISTOLOGY

On microscopic examination, AFX is a dermal or partially exophytic nodule composed of a proliferation of atypical spindle-shaped cells with moderate amounts of cytoplasm and large histiocytelike atypical cells with abundant pale-staining vacuolated cytoplasm arranged in haphazard fashion in a collagenous or occasionally myxoid stroma (Fig. 117.9B.).[190] The neoplastic cells have large, pleomorphic, and heterochromatic "bizarre-looking" nuclei, and some of them are multinucleated. There are numerous typical and atypical mitotic figures. Some cells may contain droplets of lipid. The epidermis overlying dermal proliferation in commonly ulcerated.

Both the spindle-shaped and the histiocytelike cells stain positively for vimentin, CD68 staining is weakly positive, whereas stains for HMB-45 and S100 are negative, distinguishing this lesion from spindle cell melanoma.[190,191] In addition, the spindle-shaped cells are positive for muscle-specific actin and the histocytic marker α1-antichymotrypsin. AFX stains negatively for LN2 (CD74), a marker present on B cells, Reed-Sternberg cells, and macrophages, which helps differentiate it from MFH.[192]

TREATMENT

Treatment of AFX is surgical removal by WLE or MMS. In a large retrospective series of 45 patients comparing WLE with MMS, recurrences were observed during a mean follow-up period of 73.6 months in 12% of 25 cases treated by WLE.[193] Metastatic involvement of the parotid gland occurred in one of these patients, for an overall regional metastatic rate of 4%. In contrast, no recurrences or metastases were observed over a mean follow-up period of 29.6 months in patients treated by MMS. Others have reported similarly favorable outcomes after treatment of AFX by MMS.[194,195] The authors favor the use of MMS for AFX because of the superior margin control and conservation of normal tissue.

Although AFX rarely metastasizes, it is a locally aggressive tumor with metastatic potential. Metastases to the parotid gland, lymph nodes, and lung have been reported. Nonetheless, overlap between AFX and MFH may account for the AFX cases with reported metastasis. In a series of eight cases of metastatic AFX, poor prognostic indicators included vascular invasion, recurrence, deep-tissue penetration, necrosis, and impaired host resistance.[195,196] Because AFX is often found in the setting of diffuse actinic damage and other NMSCs, close follow-up after complete tumor extirpation is critical.

MALIGNANT FIBROUS HISTIOCYTOMA

Considering the 2002 WHO soft tissue sarcoma classification, the tumors with a cutaneous presentation are (1) the undifferentiated pleomorphic sarcoma, formerly referred to as pleomorphic and storiform MFH, and (2) the myxofibrosarcoma, formerly myxoid MFH.[186,196] Myxofibrosarcoma represents one of the most common soft tissue sarcoma of the elderly. Both undifferentiated pleomorphic sarcoma and myxofibrosarcoma tend to occur on the limbs (lower extremities affected more commonly than upper extremities) of elderly patients. Approximately 10% to 15% of MFH tumors occur on head and neck region.

CLINICAL PRESENTATION

Clinically, undifferentiated pleomorphic sarcoma and myxofibrosarcoma present as progressively enlarging skin-colored subcutaneous nodules with texture varying from elastic to firm. Lesions are usually solitary but can be multinodular. Clinical differential diagnosis frequently includes SCC, BCC, and amelanotic malignant melanoma.

HISTOLOGY

Histologically, the most common appearance of MFH is that of spindle cells in a storiform pattern.[197] The stroma may be finely fibrillar, myxoid, or densely collagenous. Bizarre epithelioid and giant cells may be present. Numerous bizarre mitotic figures and necrosis are common. Ultrastructurally, the neoplastic cells of both subtypes of MFH show features consistent with fibroblastic, myofibroblastic, and histiocytic differentiation. Histologic differential diagnosis often includes metastatic carcinoma, lymphoma, leiomyosarcoma, and melanoma. Immunohistochemistry is critical for accurate diagnostic assessment.

TREATMENT AND PROGNOSIS

Complete surgical removal of MFH is treatment of choice and offers the best chance for survival.[197] RT plays an important role as an adjuvant to surgery for better local control, particularly in patients with positive surgical margins after wide complete gross excision.

Prognosis of undifferentiated pleomorphic sarcoma is poor. Up to 50% of patients may have distant metastasis at the time of initial presentation, with lung being the most common site. Recurrence rates after surgical removal are high and contribute to 30% to 35% metastatic rates. Low-grade variants, including superficial cutaneous tumors, are less likely to metastasize.

CARCINOMA METASTATIC TO SKIN

The most frequently observed cutaneous metastatic cancers are breast, colon, and melanoma in women and lung, colon, and melanoma in men. Cutaneous involvement is also seen in the leukemias, with a wide variation in the morphology of lesions. The scalp is a common site for cutaneous metastatic disease. The discovery of cutaneous metastatic disease should prompt consultation with an oncologist for staging and management.

Suggested Reading

The full list of references for this chapter appears in the online version.

1. Madan V, Lear JT, Szeimies RM. Non-melanoma skin cancer. *Lancet* 2010;375:673.
2. Stern RS. Prevalence of a history of skin cancer in 2007: results of an incidence-based model. *Arch Dermatol* 2010;146:279–282.
5. Tierney EP, Hanke CW. Cost effectiveness of Mohs micrographic surgery: review of the literature. *J Drugs Dermatol* 2009;8:914–922.
6. Salasche SJ. Status of curettage and desiccation in the treatment of primary basal cell carcinoma. *J Am Acad Dermatol* 1984;10:285–287.
8. Celestin Schartz NE, Chevret S, Paz C, et al. Imiquimod 5% cream for treatment of HIV-negative Kaposi's sarcoma skin lesions: a phase I to II, open-label trial in 17 patients. *J Am Acad Dermatol* 2008;58:585–291.
10. Love WE, Bernhard JD, Bordeaux JS. Topical imiquimod or fluorouracil therapy for basal and squamous cell carcinoma: a systematic review. *Arch Dermatol* 2009;145:1431.
12. Nouri K, O'Connell C, Rivas MP. Imiquimod for the treatment of Bowen's disease and invasive squamous cell carcinoma. *J Drugs Dermatol* 2003;2:669–673.
14. Huber A, Huber JD, Skinner RB Jr, Kuwahara RT, Haque R, Amonette RA. Topical imiquimod treatment for nodular basal cell carcinomas: an open-label series. *Dermatol Surg* 2004;30:429–430.
17. Andersson E, Rosdahl I, Torma H, Vahlquist A. Differential effects of UV irradiation on nuclear retinoid receptor levels in cultured keratinocytes and melanocytes. *Exp Dermatol* 2003;12:563–571.
19. Bath-Hextall F, Leonardi-Bee J, Somchand N, Webster A, Delitt J, Perkins W. Interventions for preventing non-melanoma skin cancers in high-risk groups. *Cochrane Database Syst Rev* 2007;CD005414.
24. Lehmann P. Methyl aminolaevulinate-photodynamic therapy: a review of clinical trials in the treatment of actinic keratoses and nonmelanoma skin cancer. *Br J Dermatol* 2007;156:793–801.
25. Braathen LR, Szeimies RM, Basset-Seguin N, et al. Guidelines on the use of photodynamic therapy for nonmelanoma skin cancer: an international consensus. International Society for Photodynamic Therapy in Dermatology, 2005. *J Am Acad Dermatol* 2007;56:125–143.
31. Berman B, Amini S, Valins W, Block S. Pharmacotherapy of actinic keratosis. *Expert Opin Pharmacother* 2009;10:3015–3031.
33. Salasche SJ. Epidemiology of actinic keratoses and squamous cell carcinoma. *J Am Acad Dermatol* 2000;42:4–7.
34. Berhane T, Halliday GM, Cooke B, Barnetson RS. Inflammation is associated with progression of actinic keratoses to squamous cell carcinomas in humans. *Br J Dermatol* 2002;146:810–815.
35. Brash DE, Ziegler A, Jonason AS, Simon JA, Kunala S, Leffell DJ. Sunlight and sunburn in human skin cancer: p53, apoptosis, and tumor promotion. *J Investig Dermatol Symp Proc* 1996;1:136–142.
39. Lubritz RR, Smolewski SA. Cryosurgery cure rate of actinic keratoses. *J Am Acad Dermatol* 1982;7:631.
42. Ulrich C, Bichel J, Euvrard S, et al. Topical immunomodulation under systemic immunosuppression: results of a multicentre, randomized, placebo-controlled safety and efficacy study of imiquimod 5% cream for the treatment of actinic keratoses in kidney, heart, and liver transplant patients. *Br J Dermatol* 2007;157(suppl 2):25–31.
45. Tanghetti E, Werschler P. Comparison of 5% 5-fluorouracil cream and 5% imiquimod cream in the management of actinic keratoses on the face and scalp. *J Drugs Dermatol* 2007;6:144–147.
47. Piacquadio DJ, Chen DM, Farber HF, et al. Photodynamic therapy with aminolevulinic acid topical solution and visible blue light in the treatment of multiple actinic keratoses of the face and scalp: investigator-blinded, phase 3, multicenter trials. *Arch Dermatol* 2004;140:41–46.
50. Krawtchenko N, Roewert-Huber J, Ulrich M, Mann I, Sterry W, Stockfleth E. A randomised study of topical 5% imiquimod vs. topical 5-fluorouracil vs. cryosurgery in immunocompetent patients with actinic keratoses: a comparison of clinical and histological outcomes including 1-year follow-up. *Br J Dermatol* 2007;157(suppl 2):34–40.
53. Epstein EH. Basal cell carcinomas: attack of the hedgehog. *Nat Rev Cancer* 2008;8:743–754.
57. Lacour JP. Carcinogenesis of basal cell carcinomas: genetics and molecular mechanisms. *Br J Dermatol* 2002;146(Suppl 61):17.
59. Bath-Hextall FJ, Perkins W, Bong J, Williams HC. Interventions for basal cell carcinoma of the skin. *Cochrane Database Syst Rev* 2007;CD003412.
61. Xie J. Molecular biology of basal and squamous cell carcinomas. *Adv Exp Med Biol* 2008;624:241–251.
62. Miller SJ. Biology of basal cell carcinoma (Part II). *J Am Acad Dermatol* 1991;24:161–175.
63. Miller SJ. Biology of basal cell carcinoma (Part I). *J Am Acad Dermatol* 1991;24:1–13.
65. Niazi ZB, Lamberty BG. Perineural infiltration in basal cell carcinomas. *Br J Plast Surg* 1993;46:156–157.
66. Ionescu DN, Arida M, Jukic DM. Metastatic basal cell carcinoma: four case reports, review of literature, and immunohistochemical evaluation. *Arch Pathol Lab Med* 2006;130:45–51.
67. Jefford M, Kiffer JD, Somers G, Daniel FJ, Davis ID. Metastatic basal cell carcinoma: rapid symptomatic response to cisplatin and paclitaxel. *ANZ J Surg* 2004;74:704–745.
68. Raasch BA, Buettner PG, Garbe C. Basal cell carcinoma: histological classification and body-site distribution. *Br J Dermatol* 2006;155:401–407.
69. Saldanha G, Fletcher A, Slater DN. Basal cell carcinoma: a dermatopathological and molecular biological update. *Br J Dermatol* 2003;148:195.
73. Swanson EL, Amdur RJ, Mendenhall WM, Morris CG, Kirwan JM, Flowers F. Radiotherapy for basal cell carcinoma of the medial canthus region. *Laryngoscope* 2009;119:2366–2368.
77. Rowe DE, Carroll RJ, Day CL Jr. Long-term recurrence rates in previously untreated (primary) basal cell carcinoma: implications for patient follow-up. *J Dermatol Surg Oncol* 1989;15:315–328.
82. Vidal D, Matias-Guiu X, Alomar A. Open study of the efficacy and mechanism of action of topical imiquimod in basal cell carcinoma. *Clin Exp Dermatol* 2004;29:518–525.
83. Gross K, Kircik L, Kricorian G. 5% 5-Fluorouracil cream for the treatment of small superficial Basal cell carcinoma: efficacy, tolerability, cosmetic outcome, and patient satisfaction. *Dermatol Surg* 2007;33:433–439.
84. Christensen E, Warloe T, Kroon S, et al. Guidelines for practical use of MAL-PDT in non-melanoma skin cancer. *J Eur Acad Dermatol Venereol* 2009.
86. Rowe DE, Carroll RJ, Day CL Jr. Prognostic factors for local recurrence, metastasis, and survival rates in squamous cell carcinoma of the skin, ear, and lip. Implications for treatment modality selection. *J Am Acad Dermatol* 1992;26:976–990.
88. Gloster HM Jr, Brodland DG. The epidemiology of skin cancer. *Dermatol Surg* 1996;22:217.
90. Kanellou P, Zaravinos A, Zioga M, et al. Genomic instability, mutations and expression analysis of the tumour suppressor genes p14(ARF), p15(INK4b), p16(INK4a) and p53 in actinic keratosis. *Cancer Lett* 2008;264:145–161.
97. Brodland DG, Zitelli JA. Surgical margins for excision of primary cutaneous squamous cell carcinoma. *J Am Acad Dermatol* 1992;27:241–248.
106. Ong CS, Keogh AM, Kossard S, Macdonald PS, Spratt PM. Skin cancer in Australian heart transplant recipients. *J Am Acad Dermatol* 1999;40:27–34.
108. Kovach BT, Stasko T. Skin cancer after transplantation. *Transplant Rev (Orlando)* 2009;23:178.
109. Requena L, Sangueza OP. Cutaneous vascular proliferations. Part III. Malignant neoplasms, other cutaneous neoplasms with significant vascular component, and disorders erroneously considered as vascular neoplasms. *J Am Acad Dermatol* 1998;38:143–175.
112. Mendenhall WM, Mendenhall CM, Werning JW, Reith JD, Mendenhall NP. Cutaneous angiosarcoma. *Am J Clin Oncol* 2006;29:524–528.
114. Morgan MB, Swann M, Somach S, Eng W, Smoller B. Cutaneous angiosarcoma: a case series with prognostic correlation. *J Am Acad Dermatol* 2004;50:867–874.
115. Wysocki WM, Komorowski A. Stewart-Treves syndrome. *J Am Coll Surg* 2007;205:194–195.
118. Bullen R, Larson PO, Landeck AE,, et al. Angiosarcoma of the head and neck managed by a combination of multiple biopsies to determine tumor margin and radiation therapy: report of three cases and review of the literature. *Dermatol Surg* 1998;24:1105.
119. Kampshoff JL, Cogbill TH. Unusual skin tumors: merkel cell carcinoma, eccrine carcinoma, glomus tumors, and dermatofibrosarcoma protuberans. *Surg Clin North Am* 2009;89:727–738.
121. Gu W, Ogose A, Kawashima H, et al. Congenital dermatofibrosarcoma protuberans with fibrosarcomatous and myxoid change. *J Clin Pathol* 2005;58:984–986.
124. Llombart B, Sanmartin O, Lopez-Guerrero JA, et al. Dermatofibrosarcoma protuberans: clinical, pathological, and genetic (COL1A1-PDGFB) study with therapeutic implications. *Histopathology* 2009;54:860–872.
128. Lemm D, Mugge LO, Mentzel T, Hoffken K. Current treatment options in dermatofibrosarcoma protuberans. *J Cancer Res Clin Oncol* 2009;135: 653–665.
141. Haag ML, Glass LF, Fenske NA. Merkel cell carcinoma. Diagnosis and treatment. *Dermatol Surg* 1995;21:669–683.
147. Foulongne V, Dereure O, Kluger N, Moles JP, Guillot B, Segondy M. Merkel cell polyomavirus DNA detection in lesional and nonlesional skin from patients with Merkel cell carcinoma or other skin diseases. *Br J Dermatol* 2009.
150. Goessling W, McKee PH, Mayer RJ. Merkel cell carcinoma. *J Clin Oncol* 2002;20:588–598.
155. Merkel Cell. In: *American Joint Committee on Cancer: AJCC Cancer Staging Manual.* 7th ed. New York: Springer; 2010: 318–319.
156. Allen PJ, Bowne WB, Jaques DP, Brennan MF, Busam K, Coit DG. Merkel cell carcinoma: prognosis and treatment of patients from a single institution. *J Clin Oncol* 2005;23:2300–2309.
160. Miller SJ, Alam M, Andersen J, et al. Merkel cell carcinoma. *J Natl Compr Canc Netw* 2006;4:704–712.

161. Bajetta E, Celio L, Platania M, et al. Single-institution series of early-stage Merkel cell carcinoma: long-term outcomes in 95 patients managed with surgery alone. *Ann Surg Oncol* 2009;16:2985–2993.
162. Boyer JD, Zitelli JA, Brodland DG, D'Angelo G. Local control of primary Merkel cell carcinoma: review of 45 cases treated with Mohs micrographic surgery with and without adjuvant radiation. *J Am Acad Dermatol* 2002;47:885–892.
168. Gupta SG, Wang LC, Penas PF, Gellenthin M, Lee SJ, Nghiem P. Sentinel lymph node biopsy for evaluation and treatment of patients with Merkel cell carcinoma: The Dana-Farber experience and meta-analysis of the literature. *Arch Dermatol* 2006;142:685–690.
169. Wilson LD, Gruber SB. Merkel cell carcinoma and the controversial role of adjuvant radiation therapy: clinical choices in the absence of statistical evidence. *J Am Acad Dermatol* 2004;50:435–437.
174. Leibovitch I, Huilgol SC, Selva D, Lun K, Richards S, Paver R. Microcystic adnexal carcinoma: treatment with Mohs micrographic surgery. *J Am Acad Dermatol* 2005;52:295–300.
175. Yu JB, Blitzblau RC, Patel SC, Decker RH, and Wilson LD. Surveillance, Epidemiology, and End Results (SEER) database analysis of microcystic adnexal carcinoma (aclerosing sweat duct carcinoma) of the skin. *Am J Clin Oncol* 2010;33:125–127.
178. Eisen DB, Michael DJ. Sebaceous lesions and their associated syndromes: part I. *J Am Acad Dermatol* 2009;61:549–560.
188. Fletcher CD. The evolving classification of soft tissue tumours: an update based on the new WHO classification. *Histopathology* 2006;48:3–12.
190. Luzar B, Calonje E. Morphological and immunohistochemical characteristics of atypical fibroxanthoma with a special emphasis on potential diagnostic pitfalls: a review. *J Cutan Pathol* 2009.
193. Davis JL, Randle HW, Zalla MJ, Roenigk RK, Brodland DG. A comparison of Mohs micrographic surgery and wide excision for the treatment of atypical fibroxanthoma. *Dermatol Surg* 1997;23:105–110.
194. Huether MJ, Zitelli JA, Brodland DG. Mohs micrographic surgery for the treatment of spindle cell tumors of the skin. *J Am Acad Dermatol* 2001;44:656–659.
195. Zalla MJ, Randle HW, Brodland DG, Davis JL, Roenigk RK. Mohs surgery vs wide excision for atypical fibroxanthoma: follow-up. *Dermatol Surg* 1997;23:1223–1224.
198. Matushansky I, Charytonowicz E, Mills J, Siddiqi S, Hricik T, Cordon-Cardo C. MFH classification: differentiating undifferentiated pleomorphic sarcoma in the 21st Century. *Expert Rev Anticancer Ther* 2009;9:1135–1144.
199. Nascimento AF, Raut CP. Diagnosis and management of pleomorphic sarcomas (so-called "MFH") in adults. *J Surg Oncol* 2008;97:330–339.

CHAPTER 118 MOLECULAR BIOLOGY OF CUTANEOUS MELANOMA

LEVI A. GARRAWAY AND LYNDA CHIN

Cutaneous melanoma arises from pigment-producing epidermal melanocytes and is the major cause of mortality among skin malignancies. Its incidence has risen steadily at a rate of 3% per year over the past 25 years,[1] with an estimated 68,130 new cases and 8,700 deaths predicted for the United States alone in 2010. Despite a high cure rate for localized primary melanoma (98.3% 5-year survival rate), its aggressive nature results in rapid metastasis to distant sites and a concomitant drop to a 16% 5-year survival rate. Although exposure to ultraviolet (UV) radiation is a known factor contributing to melanoma development, the exact molecular changes that take place in incipient and progressing tumors are still being elucidated.

Currently, vertical tumor (Breslow) thickness (in millimeters) provides the best single indicator of prognosis. This measurement is augmented by additional parameters, including the presence of ulceration, penetration through cutaneous layers, mitotic rate, evidence of "in transit" metastasis, tumor spread to draining lymph nodes, and the presence of distant metastasis. Although melanoma sometimes arises in preexisting nevi, recent data have demonstrated that typical nevi represent senescent lesions that may be irreversibly growth arrested.[2] It is therefore plausible that a substantial fraction of melanomas may alternatively emerge from normal melanocytes via deregulation of oncogenes or tumor suppressors implicated in melanocytic transformation (Fig. 118.1). The myriad genes involved with melanoma genesis and progression have been subjected to varying degrees of validation in humans, in model organisms, and in cell culture (Table 118.1). The identification of these genes and their associated genetic pathways influences diagnosis and prognosis and shows considerable promise in aiding targeted therapeutic implementation.

THE *CDKN2A* LOCUS

As many as 70% of melanomas harbor somatic mutations or deletions affecting the *CDKN2A* locus on chromosome 9p21.[3,4] This observation, together with the initial identification of germline homozygous deletions of *CDKN2A* as susceptibility events in familial melanoma kindreds,[5] indicates a central role for this locus in melanoma pathogenesis. This locus contains an unusual gene organization, which allows for two separate transcripts and corresponding tumor suppressor gene products to be produced: p16^{INK4A} and p19^{ARF} (Fig. 118.2). Loss of p16^{INK4A} results in the suppression of retinoblastoma (RB) tumor suppressor activity via increased activation of the CDK4/6-cyclin D1 complex; loss of ARF (p14^{ARF} in human and p19^{ARF} in mouse) down-modulates p53 activity through increased activation of MDM2. Thus, deletion of the entire locus accomplishes the inactivation of two critical tumor suppressor pathways: RB and p53. Homozygous deletion of exons 2 and 3 of the mouse *Cdkn2a* homolog predisposed to a high incidence of melanomas when combined with an activated H-RAS transgene in melanocytes.[6] Thus, *CDKN2A* lesions may "prime" melanocytic tissue for neoplasia.

THE RETINOBLASTOMA PATHWAY

The RB pathway is responsible for preventing inappropriate cell cycle entry, and germline heterozygous loss of the *RB1* gene triggers retinoblastoma. The tumor-modulating properties of the RB pathway are well established in many solid cancers, and its deregulation in melanoma is evidenced by mutations in *INK4A*, *CDK4*, or occasionally *RB1* itself, as described below.

INK4A

Human intragenic mutations of *INK4A* that do not affect the *ARF* coding region preferentially disrupt the RB pathway and sensitize germline carriers to the development of melanomas.[7] In a mouse model engineered to be deficient only for Ink4a (with intact ARF), melanoma formation was observed in cooperation with an oncogenic initiating event (activated H-RAS), albeit with a longer latency than in mice with deletions affecting the entire locus.[8] Notably, the tumors in these mice were also found to harbor either deletion of ARF or mutation of p53. Therefore, while INK4A is a *bona fide* tumor suppressor, additional genetic dysregulation of the p53 pathway seems obligatory for melanoma genesis, at least in the mouse.

CDK4

CDK4 is a direct target of inhibition by p16^{INK4A} (Fig. 118.2) and is a primary regulator of RB activation. Rare germline mutations of *CDK4* that render the protein insensitive to inhibition by INK4A (e.g., Arg24Cys) have been identified in a melanoma-prone kindred.[9] These tumors retain wild type INK4A function, suggesting that INK4A is epistatic to CDK4 and that RB pathway deregulation is central to melanoma genesis. Somatic focal amplifications of *CDK4* are also observed (albeit rarely) in sporadic melanomas.[10] Carcinogen treatment induced melanomas in the animals without somatic Ink4a inactivation, similar to the mutual exclusivity observed in familial melanoma.[11]

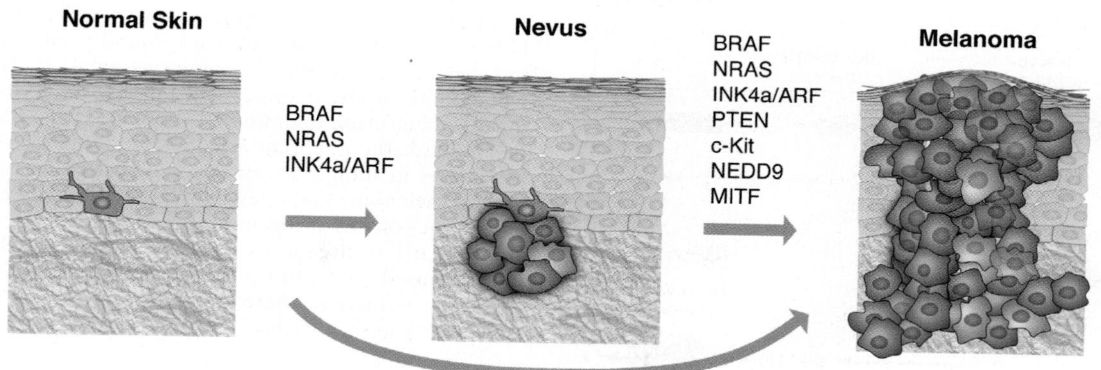

FIGURE 118.1 Validated genes mutated or deregulated in melanoma progression. Progression of normal melanocytes to metastatic melanoma is diagrammed with associated genetic events as a linear process, although in a majority of the cases, melanomas may not arise from a pre-existing nevus. The degree to which the association of each gene has been experimentally validated is shown in Table 118.1.

RB1

Germline mutations in *RB1* confer predisposition to melanoma in patients who have survived bilateral retinoblastoma.[12] These melanomas exhibit loss of heterozygosity (LOH) of the remaining wild type RB1 allele. In such patients, estimates of increased lifetime risk of melanoma range from 4- to 80-fold. Interestingly, the *RB1* gene locus is frequently deleted in primary cutaneous melanomas,[13] and RB1 may be subject to genomic rearrangement in rare instances.[14]

THE p53 PATHWAY

The p53 pathway is critical for maintenance of the normal genome by regulating a multiplicity of mechanisms, including cell cycle checkpoints, DNA damage repair activation, and the appropriate induction of apoptosis. Mutations in the *TP53* gene occur in over 50% of all tumors. Although the *TP53* locus is rarely mutated in human melanomas,[15] this region appears to undergo copy neutral LOH at enhanced frequency, at least in advanced tumors.[4] Furthermore, loss of p53 in mice cooperates with activated H-Ras to induce melanomas.[16] Thus, while *TP53* is rarely deleted in human melanomas, inactivation of its pathway appears critical for melanoma genesis.

ARF

ARF-specific insertions, deletions, and splice donor mutations have been described in human melanomas.[17] However, it remains ambiguous whether the genetic disruption of ARF alone is sufficient for tumorigenesis. In mouse models, *Arf*-specific deletion in conjunction with activated H-RAS leads to a similar melanoma phenotype as the *Ink4a*-specific deletion mouse mentioned above[8]; however, *Arf*-mutant melanomas were enriched for mutations in the RB pathway. Notably, upon UV radiation these mice developed focal amplifications at the *Cdk6* locus,[18] which encodes an orthologue to CDK4. Furthermore, p53 heterozygous mouse melanomas retain Arf, demonstrating their epistatic relationship.[16]

PRACTICE OF ONCOLOGY

TABLE 118.1

SUMMARY OF VALIDATED GENES INVOLVED IN MELANOMA GENESIS AND PROGRESSION

Methods of Discovery	Melanoma Gene	Proposed Gene Product Behavior	Extent of Validation								Ref.
			H	E	I	O	K	X	P	M	
Linkage mapping	INK4A, ARF	Tumor suppressors	•	•	•	•	•	•	•	•	Reviewed in 17
Linkage mapping	NRAS, BRAF	Oncogenes	•	•	•	•	•	•	•	•	Reviewed in 17
Linkage mapping	PTEN	Tumor suppressor	•	•	•	•	•		•	•	Reviewed in 17
Copy number profiling	NEDD9	Metastasis enhancer	•	•	•	•	•	•	•		92
Copy number profiling	MITF	Oncogene	•	•	•	•	•		•		75
Expression profiling	WNT5A	Metastasis enhancer		•	•	•	•		•		86
Copy number profiling	GOLPH3	Oncogene	•	•	•	•	•	•	•		100
Copy number profiling	ETV1	Oncogene	•	•	•	•	•	•	•		79
DNA sequencing	ERBB4	Oncogene	•		•	•	•	•			72
RNAi screening	IGFBP7, GAS1	Tumor suppressor		•	•	•	•	•			101, 102
		Metastasis suppressor		•	•	•	•	•			

H, (human gene aberrations) indicates known mutation, amplification, deletion, or focal loss of heterozygosity (LOH) in patients; E, (expression validation) is achieved by reverse transcription-polymerase chain reaction (RT-PCR), Northern, or Western blots; I, (immunohistocompatibility [IHC] or tissue microarrays) refers to histological protein analysis; O, overexpression; K, (knockdown/dominant negative); X, (xenograft) refers to manipulation of gene expression in cell lines; P, (pathway) indicates studies of interactions with putative pathway members; M, (mouse model of melanoma) indicates validation through genetic engineering in mice.

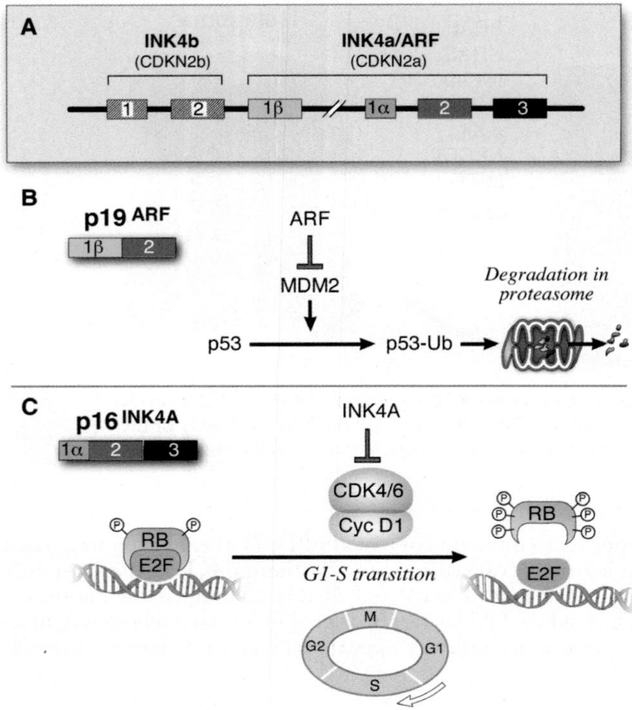

FIGURE 118.2 The unusual genomic structure and products of the *CDKN2A* locus. **A:** INK4A and ARF (p14^{ARF} in human and p19^{ARF} in mouse) initiate in different first exons and share the coding exon 2, but in an alterative reading frame, thus encoding two proteins with no amino acid similarity. The involvement of the neighboring and related *CDKN2B* locus in the pathology of melanoma is unclear, although it is often deleted in conjunction with *CDKN2A*. (From ref. 3.) **B:** ARF participates in the p53 pathway by binding to and sequestering the p53 antagonist, MDM2. The loss of ARF therefore results in the net degradation of p53 by MDM2-mediated ubiquitination. p16^{INK4A} inhibits the action of the CDK4/CDK6-cyclin D1 complex in the retinoblastoma (RB) pathway. The loss of p16^{INK4A} results in the phosphorylation and inactivation of pRB leading to its uncoupling from the transcription factor E2F, allowing for transcription of E2F target genes that are required for cell cycle progression from G_1 to S phase.

THE MAP KINASE PATHWAY

Extensive genetic and mechanistic studies have unearthed a prevalence of activating mitogen-activated protein kinase (MAPK) pathway mutations across many tumor types. The focal point of MAPK activation is the ERK1/2 kinases, which mediate the transcription of many genes governing cell proliferation and survival (Fig. 118.3). In nontransformed cells, key MAPK effectors have also been shown to regulate differentiation and senescence.

THE RAS FAMILY: H-, N-, AND K-RAS

Increasing evidence shows that the three different members of the classical RAS oncogene family exert functionally separable roles. N-RAS is the most frequently targeted in melanoma (33% of primary and 26% of metastatic samples[19]), followed by H-RAS (mainly in Spitz nevi).[20] Despite their high incidence in other cancer types, K-RAS mutations are rarely observed in melanocytic lesions.[21,22] Interestingly, although N-RAS mutations are found in 54% of congenital nevi, they are rare in dysplastic nevi,[23] implying a distinct evolutionary path from dysplastic nevi to melanoma.

In mouse models, overexpression of activated H-RAS or N-RAS on an Ink4a/Arf-null background results in spontaneous melanoma formation.[6,24] However, while H-RAS-induced melanomas rarely, if ever, metastasize, N-RAS tumors frequently metastasize to draining lymph nodes and distal organs, in line with the apparent selection for N-RAS over H-RAS mutations in human melanomas. Knockdown of *NRAS* in human melanoma cell lines inhibits their viability, indicating dependency on this oncogene for tumorigenicity.[25] Furthermore, shutting off transgene expression in an inducible H-RAS model caused regression of melanomas that arose following transgene induction, thereby confirming the RAS oncogene dependency in these tumors.[26]

BRAF

Somatic, activating *BRAF* mutations occur at high frequency in melanoma. These mutations are dominated by a single T→A transversion, resulting in a valine to glutamate amino acid substitution (V600E). Although the T→A transversion is not classically associated with UV-induced damage, BRAF mutations appear to be more common in melanomas arising at sites with intermittent exposure to UV.[13,27] On the other hand, melanomas from chronically sun-damaged skin are typically wild type for *BRAF*.[13] BRAF mutations may be an early preneoplastic event, given their high incidence in benign and dysplastic nevi (Fig. 118.1).[28]

BRAF is an immediate downstream target of RAS (Fig. 118.3) in the MAPK pathway. The BRAF(V600E) mutation confers more than 500-fold induction of kinase activity *in vitro*; this dramatic effect may explain why the V600E mutation dominates in BRAF-mutant melanoma. BRAF(V600E) mutations are often observed in conjunction with PTEN loss (see below), implying that dual modulation of MAPK and phosphatidylinositol 3-kinase (PI3K) pathways may promote a fully transformed phenotype.

Extensive data suggest that wild type BRAF operates on a senescence pathway in benign human nevi. Transgenic expression of BRAF(V600E) targeted to melanocytes in zebrafish produced benign nevuslike lesions, whereas invasive melanomas were produced (after extended latency) when crossed into p53 deficient zebrafish.[29] Inducible expression of BRAF(V600E) alone in murine melanocytes resulted in excessive skin pigmentation and the appearance of nevi containing hallmarks of senescence.[30] Human congenital nevi with activating BRAF mutations were shown to express senescence-associated acidic β-galactosidase (SA-β-Gal), the classical senescence-associated marker.[2] This implied that activated BRAF alone is insufficient to induce tumor progression beyond the nevus stage in patients (Fig. 118.1). Interestingly, immunohistochemical staining of nevoid tissues found heterogeneous patterns of INK4A that only partially overlapped with SA-β-Gal, suggesting the presence of INK4A-independent pathway(s) operative in oncogene-induced senescence.

The high prevalence of activating BRAF and NRAS mutations implied that the MAPK cascade might confer a "drugable" melanoma tumor dependency when such mutations were present. This notion was supported by several lines of preclinical evidence, particularly in BRAF(V600E) melanomas. For example, constitutive ERK activation in BRAF^{V600E} cells was required for their continued proliferation.[31–33] RNAi knockdown of BRAF in this genetic context inhibited ERK activation, blunted cell growth, and in some cases induced apoptosis *in vitro*.[31,32] BRAF silencing also suppressed anchorage-independent growth and tumor formation in BRAF(V600E) melanomas.[34] As noted above, suppression of NRAS expression in *NRAS*-mutant melanomas resulted in similar growth inhibitory effects.[25] Thus, BRAF or NRAS oncogenic mutations appeared to elaborate a

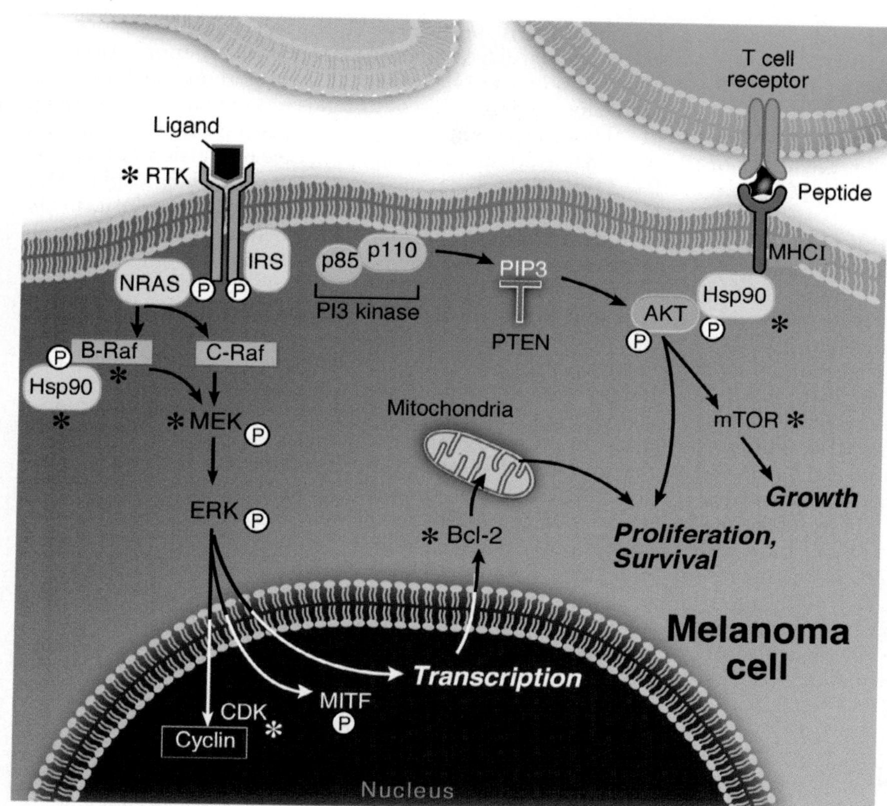

FIGURE 118.3 The melanoma signaling cascades mitogen-activated protein kinase (MAPK) and phosphatidylinositol 3-kinase (PI3K). The MAPK pathway is hyperactivated in melanomas, mainly due to activating mutations in either the NRAS or BRAF genes. The sequential phosphorylations of the downstream MEK and ERK proteins ultimately results in the activation of a number of transcription factors, including MITF, which induce cell proliferation and survival. The PI3K pathway is mainly hyperactivated by loss of the PTEN tumor suppressor, which results in the phosphorylation and activation of the survival gene *AKT* and subsequent stimulation of the mitogenic mammalian target of rapamycin (mTOR) pathway. The relative independence of the MAPK and PI3K pathways is supported by the apparent need for mutations that affect both.

stringent melanoma tumor dependency through aberrant MAPK pathway activation.

In BRAF(V600E) melanomas, the mechanistic basis for oncogene dependency appears to involve both proliferative and apoptotic regulation. Oncogenic *BRAF* inhibits BIM, a pro-apoptotic member of the BCL-2 protein family,[35] and suppression of BRAF activity facilitates translocation of the pro-apoptotic protein BMF to the cytosol in cells harboring the mutation.[36] Moreover, two downstream effectors of RAF signaling—ERK and RSK—were shown to phosphorylate and inhibit the LKB1 tumor suppressor. This results in an inability of LKB1 to activate AMP kinase, which normally down-regulates cell growth under various stress conditions.[37] Thus, activated B-RAF and downstream MAPK effectors appear to augment multiple melanoma cell growth and survival pathways.

The emergence of selective RAF inhibitors has provided an opportunity to evaluate the "drugability" of *BRAF* and *NRAS* oncogene mutations *in vitro* and in the clinical setting. Toward this end, small molecule RAF inhibitors such as PLX4032 potently suppressed the growth of BRAF(V600E) melanoma cells, whereas this inhibitor had little effect on cancer cells lacking this mutation.[38,39] Selective RAF inhibitors also suppressed the formation of BRAF(V600E) tumors in murine xenograft models.[40] These data suggest that stratification of melanomas according to BRAF(V600E) status might be enriched for patients most likely to benefit from small molecule RAF or MEK inhibitors. Recent clinical trial results with selective RAF inhibitors have borne out this prediction. In a phase 1 trial of PLX4032, the overall response rate of BRAF(V600E) melanomas was 90%, with nearly 80% experiencing a partial response by Response Evaluation Criteria in Solid Tumors (RECIST) criteria.[41] NRAS-mutant melanomas did not respond to this agent. Similar results have also been observed with other investigational RAF inhibitors. These initial observations raise the possibility that RAF inhibition may ultimately gain a prominent role in the clinical management of BRAF(V600E) melanomas.

In light of the substantial evidence for "drugable" RAF dependency described above, it was somewhat surprising that selective RAF inhibition showed minimal efficacy against *NRAS*-mutant melanomas both *in vitro* and in early clinical studies. Initial insights into this puzzling discordance emerged from several reports that showed that exposure of RAS-activated cancer cells to selective RAF inhibitors paradoxically increased MAPK signaling, as measured by increased p-MEK and p-ERK levels.[42–44] Biochemical studies revealed that inhibitor-bound BRAF polypeptides retained an ability to form homo- or heterodimers with other (drug-free) RAF molecules, and that this dimerization was associated with MEK phosphorylation in the setting of RAS activation. These provocative results may help explain why some RAF inhibitors fail to inhibit MAPK signaling in cells lacking BRAF(V600E) mutations (e.g., RAS mutant cells). They may also provide a basis for the unexpectedly high incidence (25% to 30%) of keratocanthomas and squamous cell carcinomas that arise in patients treated with selective RAF inhibition.[41]

MEK

Since the MEK1/2 serine-threonine kinases transmit the critical MAPK signal downstream of RAS and RAF, considerable interest has also emerged regarding these kinases in melanoma biology and therapeutics. In contrast to *NRAS* and *BRAF*, MEK1/2 mutations are rare in melanoma (indeed, in cancer in general), although they have occasionally been reported.[45] Nonetheless, pharmacologic MEK inhibition presented another possible therapeutic inroad into *BRAF*- or *NRAS*-mutant melanomas. Robust preclinical evidence favoring this notion derived from a genetic and pharmacologic analysis showing that various MEK inhibitory compounds demonstrated markedly enhanced potency against BRAF(V600E) cancer cells compared to cell lines lacking oncogenic MAPK pathway mutations.[46] In contrast to studies with selective RAF inhibitors, at least some NRAS-mutant melanoma cells were also sensitive to MEK inhibitors, suggesting that the utility of MEK inhibition might extend beyond the BRAF(V600E) context in some cases.[46]

Although initial clinical trial results of MEK inhibition in melanoma were disappointing compared to the RAF inhibitor trials described above, more recent studies have yielded responses in patients with BRAF(V600E) mutations following MEK inhibitor treatment.[47] In addition, molecular analyses have provided an initial glimpse into how mechanisms of resistance might emerge to targeted MAPK pathway inhibition. In one case, a single relapsing focus was resected from a patient who was otherwise responsive to the MEK inhibitor AZD6244[48]; the resistant tumor was found to harbor a somatic *MEK1* mutation capable of conferring resistance to both MEK and BRAF inhibition *in vitro*. These intriguing translational studies have also triggered trials of combined RAF and MEK inhibition as a means to augment the magnitude or duration of clinical responses in BRAF(V600E) melanoma patients. A comprehensive elaboration of resistance to both RAF and MEK inhibition may provide new insights into possible combination therapeutic trials directed against this genetically defined tumor subtype.

THE PHOSPHATIDYLINOSITOL 3-KINASE PATHWAY

The PI3K pathway operates mainly through the downstream activation of the survival kinase AKT (Fig. 118.3), which activates the growth-promoting mammalian target of rapamycin (mTOR) pathway and inhibits proapoptotic effectors such as caspase 9 and BAD. PI3K was capable of replacing N-RAS to induce invasive melanomas in a skin xenograft model.[49] However, unlike the MAPK pathway, genetic alterations specifically targeting components of the PI3K signaling cascade do not occur at high frequency in melanoma.[50]

Several lines of evidence support the cooperative effects of MAPK and PI3K dysregulation in melanoma genesis. For example, transformation of immortalized human melanocytes required the combination of activated BRAF and PI3K, but not BRAF alone, in an artificial skin graft model system.[26] More recently, concomitant expression of oncogenic BRAF together with PTEN silencing in an inducible melanocyte-specific mouse model resulted in robust melanoma development with 100% penetrance.[30,51] These melanomas arose following a short latency and exhibited a high propensity for metastatic dissemination. Together, these data suggest that dysregulated BRAF and PI3K signaling may underpin melanoma genesis in certain subsets of melanomas. Toward this end, a recent study suggested that N-RAS-mutant melanomas may show enhanced reliance on RalGEF signaling,[52] which can be operant downstream of RAS in several contexts.

PTEN

Of the PI3K pathway mutations that do occur, losses of chromosome 10q encompassing PTEN tumor suppressor is the most frequent, the caveat being that additional tumor suppressor(s) may reside in this region (see below). PTEN normally down-regulates phosphorylated AKT via suppression of the second messenger PIP_3 (Fig. 118.3). In various genetically engineered mice bearing solid tumors, PTEN loss can be analogous to p53 inactivation, in that one or the other can be gating for oncogenesis. In melanoma, somatic point mutations and homozygous deletions of PTEN are uncommon. Although allelic loss of PTEN is observed only in about 20% of melanoma, loss of expression of PTEN is reported to be in the range of 40% of melanoma tumors,[53] suggesting other mechanisms of its inactivation. Functionally, ectopic expression of PTEN in PTEN-deficient melanoma cells can abolish phospho-AKT activity, induce apoptosis, and suppress growth, tumorigenicity, and metastasis.[50] Correspondingly, heterozygous germline or homozygous somatic inactivation of *Pten* in the mouse strongly promoted tumor formation in multiple cell lineages, a phenotype that was accelerated by the additional deletion of *Ink4a/Arf*.[54] Significantly, these double mutants developed melanoma at low penetrance, consistent with the hypothesis that PTEN inactivation in human melanoma may require additional genetic events such as the commonly associated BRAF(V600E) mutation. As noted above, this hypothesis was recently borne out in a mouse model of simultaneous PTEN loss and oncogenic BRAF induction in melanocytes.[51] The relevance of PTEN inactivation in NRAS-mutant melanomas is less clear; however, studies in genetically engineered mouse models raise the possibility that RAS and PTEN inactivation may also interact to promote melanoma genesis and metastasis.[55]

Many melanomas harbor chromosome arm level hemizygous deletions involving the *PTEN* locus (10q24), although not all are specific to *PTEN*.[4] Thus, other tumor suppressors may exist in this genomic region. The Myc antagonist *MXI* represents one possibility, as *Myc* is amplified or overexpressed in *RAS*-induced *Trp53*-deficient melanomas in the mouse.[16] Other candidate tumor suppressor genes from chromosome 10q include *CUL2* and *KLF6*; both genes are significantly down-regulated in melanomas harboring 10q deletions,[4] although functional evidence that they exert tumor suppressor roles remains scant.

AKT

Elevated phospho-AKT (indicative of activation) has been adversely associated with patient survival[56] and is common in BRAF(V600E) melanomas.[57] Elevated phospho-AKT was particularly manifest in melanoma brain metastases compared to other metastatic sites.[57] Copy number gains of the *AKT3* locus and rare AKT3 point mutations[58] have been detected in melanomas, suggesting that the AKT signaling point itself may be oncogenic.[59] Interestingly, targeted depletion of AKT3 could trigger apoptosis,[59] while AKT1 behaved as a tumor suppressor in melanoma cell lines,[60] raising the possibility of partially nonredundant functions of AKT isoforms.

RECEPTOR TYROSINE KINASES

Receptor tyrosine kinsases (RTKs) are a diverse family of transmembrane kinases that have been implicated in many neoplasms. Several RTKs map to known regions of recurrent melanoma DNA copy number gain or amplification, with corresponding alterations in their expression levels.

c-KIT

The c-Kit gene plays an essential role in melanocyte development, as does its ligand, stem cell factor. Mutation of either results in pigmentation deficiencies, and injection of c-Kit blocking antibody in mice was used to identify the presence of melanocyte stem cells within hair follicles.[61] Numerous immunohistochemical studies have linked progressive loss of c-KIT expression with the transition from benign to primary and metastatic melanomas.[62–64] Thus, at first glance, KIT appeared to be inactivated during melanoma genesis and progression.

However, KIT is somatically activated by point mutations in a specific subset of melanomas that arise within mucosal, acral, or chronic sun-damaged surfaces of the body.[13] High-resolution amplicon melting analyses followed by direct DNA sequencing revealed that three of these mutations harbored a L576P mutation with selective loss of the normal allele.[65] L576P is a known gastrointestinal stromal tumor–associated mutation that maps to the 5′ juxtamembrane domain where most activating KIT mutations cluster.[66] Importantly, these observations suggest the potential utility of c-KIT targeted kinase inhibitors for this subset of previously incurable melanoma patients. Initial case reports have provided preliminary support for this notion.[67] Clinical trials using imatinib are currently under way to determine whether this discovery may represent a major opportunity for targeted therapy in melanoma as previously shown for gastrointestinal stromal tumors.

EPIDERMAL GROWTH FACTOR RECEPTOR FAMILY

The epidermal growth factor receptor (EGFR) activates both the MAPK and PI3K pathways in many cell types. In melanomas, copy number gain of chromosome 7 (where the *EGFR* gene resides) is linked to overexpression of EGFR, despite the lack of focal amplifications.[68] EGFR activation increased the number of visceral metastases in severe combined immunodeficiency (SCID) mouse xenografts without affecting melanoma growth *in vitro*.[69] In the inducible H-RAS mouse model,[26] transcriptomic analysis revealed upregulation of EGF family ligands including amphiregulin and epiregulin.[70] Furthermore, expression of a dominant negative form of EGFR abolished the tumorigenicity of RAS-driven melanoma cells, indicating that the MAPK pathway is dependent on an uncompromised EGFR signal.[71]

A sequencing-based study of the tyrosine kinome in melanoma found that *ERBB4* mutations may affect as many as 20% of melanomas.[72] Unlike other well-known oncogene mutations, the *ERBB4* mutations identified in this study were mostly nonrecurrent (e.g., the same amino acid or conserved region was rarely affected); however, ERBB4 mutations correlated with increased activation of and dependence on the corresponding protein for viability. If validated by resequencing of large independent sample cohorts, targeted therapeutics against ERBB4 and perhaps other members of the EGFR family may warrant investigation in melanoma.

c-MET

The c-MET gene product and its ligand hepatocyte growth factor/scatter factor (HGF/SF) are known to activate the MAPK pathway, but both have many additional functions. Overexpression of c-MET and HGF is correlated with melanoma progression. Copy gains involving the c-MET locus at 7q33-qter are associated with invasive and metastatic cancers in humans,[73] and elevated MET/HGF expression is correlated with metastatic ability in murine melanoma explants.[47] HGF/SF overexpression in a transgenic mouse model triggered spontaneous melanoma formation after a long latency (up to 2 years); however, time to tumor onset was greatly reduced by exposure to UVB or Ink4a/Arf deficiency.[74] Thus, HGF/MET signaling may play an important role in melanoma genesis and progression. The development of MET inhibitors should allow formal testing of this hypothesis in melanoma patients.

THE MITF PATHWAY

MITF encodes a lineage transcription factor whose function is critical to the survival of normal melanocytes. The identification of *MITF* amplification in melanoma defined this transcription factor as a central modifier of melanoma.[75] In so doing, this discovery identified a novel class of oncogenes termed *lineage survival* oncogenes.[76,77] That is, a tumor may "hijack" extant lineage survival mechanisms in the presence of selective pressures to ensure its own propagation. The elucidation of *MITF* as an oncogene took a cross-tissue approach, wherein the NCI-60 cell line panel representing nine tumor types was subjected to both gene expression and high-density single-nucleotide polymorphism (SNP) array analysis.[75] A recurrent gain of 3p13–14 significantly segregated melanoma from other tumor classes, with MITF as the only gene in the region showing maximal amplification and overexpression. MITF amplification was subsequently detected in 10% of primary cutaneous and 15% to 20% of metastatic melanomas by fluorescence *in situ* hybridization, correlating with decreased survival in Kaplan-Meier analyses of 5-year patient survival. Exogenous MITF, in combination with activated BRAF, showed transforming capabilities in immortalized primary human melanocytes. Additionally, inhibition of MITF in cell lines showing 3p13–14 amplification reduced growth and survival and conferred sensitivity to certain anticancer drugs. MITF gene disruption leads to coat color defects in mice and pigmentation defects in humans, due to diminished viability of melanocytes. This suggested that MITF was essential for the lineage survival of melanocytes, supporting the contention that it is also critical for the survival of melanomas.

The downstream elements of the MITF pathway include both pigment enzyme genes as well as genes involved in proliferation and survival. MITF intersects with a number of established melanoma pathways, including the transcriptional activation of INK4A, c-Met, and CDK2.[17] Moreover, MITF is activated downstream of both c-Kit and MAPK signaling, via ERK-directed phosphorylation (Fig. 118.3).[78] Additionally, activated BRAF is known to target MITF for proteolytic degradation, which may select for refractory cellular variants harboring amplified MITF. Recently, the ETS transcription factor ETV1 was found to positively regulate MITF expression in melanoma, and *ETV1* may function as an amplified melanoma oncogene in its own right.[79] Furthermore, the mouse Bcl2 proapoptotic gene was shown to be a transcriptional target of MITF.[80] Collectively, these observations place MITF in a central role of melanoma signal integration.

THE WNT PATHWAY

WNT signaling has long been implicated in a variety of cancers. Its activation of downstream transcriptional events has been hypothesized to control lineage commitment and differentiation fates as well as self-renewal properties. The WNT pathway has also been linked to major developmental decisions in neural crest derivatives, with a differentiation bias toward the melanocytic lineage.[81] Additionally, the WNT pathway appears to intersect with MITF functionality at several levels, including direct interactions between MITF and the WNT downstream transcriptional coactivator LEF-1.[82] WNT signaling may augment MITF expression, and MITF may mediate at least a portion of WNT functionality in melanoma.[83]

CTNNB1 and WNT5A

Stabilizing *CTTNB1* mutations that render β-catenin resistant to proteolytic degradation promote tumorigenesis. Such

PRACTICE OF ONCOLOGY

mutations are uncommon in patient samples, despite a high incidence in melanoma cell lines.[84] Nevertheless, a significant fraction of clinical melanoma lesions exhibit immunohistochemical evidence of nuclear β-catenin localization,[85] a hallmark of WNT pathway activation. Additional evidence for the importance of the WNT pathway emerged from gene expression studies that identified a β-catenin-independent Wnt5a signaling pathway correlated with higher grades of clinical melanoma samples.[86] Engineered overexpression of Wnt5a enhanced the *in vitro* invasiveness of melanoma cells, a property suppressed by blockade of the Wnt5a receptor Frizzled-5. Mechanistically, Wnt5a was shown to enhance the action of the PKC pathway, which is believed to control cell adhesion and motility.

THE MC1R PATHWAY

Pigmentation exerts a major influence on skin tumor susceptibility, as it is well documented that fair skin is more sensitive to UV radiation and melanoma genesis. The mechanism underlying this observation is partially explained by the protective effects of melanin, which is produced by melanocytes and distributed to interfollicular keratinocytes. Genetically, the red hair color/pale skin (RHC) phenotype is linked to variant alleles of the melanocyte-specific melanocortin 1 receptor gene (MC1R), which is central to melanin synthesis.[87] The ligand for the G-protein–coupled MC1R is the MSH peptide, which activates downstream signaling consisting of a cAMP-CREB/ATF1 cascade, culminating in the induced expression of MITF. Not all individuals carrying RHC alleles have identical melanin production, yet increased risk for melanoma genesis remains notable regardless,[88] implying that melanin-independent mechanisms might impact the susceptibility of RHC carriers. One possible node is cAMP, the MC1R as second messenger, which may activate pathways incompletely understood at present, such as MAPK and PI3K.[89]

Recent data have implicated the MSH/MC1R pathway in the normal UV pigmentation (tanning) response in skin, a response that is linked to skin cancer (and melanoma) risk in humans. A "redhead" mouse model (frameshift mutation in *MC1R*) was used to demonstrate that the UV-tanning response is dependent on MC1R signaling, because keratinocytes respond to UV by strongly up-regulating expression of MSH. The "fairskin" phenotype was rescued by topical administration of a small molecule cAMP agonist.[90] The resulting dark pigmentation in genetically redhead mice was protective against UV-induced skin carcinogenesis. Subsequent analyses revealed that the p53 tumor suppressor protein may function as a "UV sensor" in keratinocytes, translating UV damage into direct transcriptional stimulation of MSH expression.[91]

THE FAK PATHWAY

NEDD9 was recently demonstrated to enhance the metastatic efficiency of both mouse melanomas and human cell lines by activation of the FAK pathway, which enhances cell motility and adhesion.[92] The discovery of these properties of NEDD9 was enabled by the evolutionary conservation of genetic pathways, which highlighted significant genetic changes when mouse tumors were compared to human melanomas. Array comparative genomic hybridization analysis of metastatic and nonmetastatic tumors derived from the *Ink4a/Arf*$^{-/-}$ inducible H-RAS mouse melanoma model[26] pinpointed an 850 kb minimal common region (MCR) of amplification on chromosome 13. Only one gene in this MCR, *Nedd9*, showed a significant up-regulation in metastatic mouse melanomas but not in normal melanocytes or nonmetastatic melanomas. The syntenic human region, 6p24–25, similarly undergoes copy number gain in 36% of human metastatic but not nonmetastatic melanomas.[92] The cross-species comparison allowed the delimitation of a focal region of interest and designation of NEDD9 as a candidate target of 6p gain in humans.

NEDD9 appears to modulate metastasis activity *in vitro* and *in vivo*. In cell-based assays, invasiveness of human melanoma cells was enhanced or inhibited by overexpression or knockdown of *NEDD9*, respectively. Similarly, knockdown of Nedd9 in metastatic melanoma cells with Nedd9 amplification drastically inhibited distal metastasis to various organs from subcutaneous primary tumor sites. Furthermore, inhibition of FAK itself abolished the invasive potential conferred by NEDD9 in Boyden chamber assays, implicating the entire pathway in metastasis.[92] NEDD9 expression was found to be up-regulated in 50% of primary melanomas when compared to benign nevi, raising the possibility that NEDD9 might confer other biological activities during the early stages of melanoma genesis and that elevated NEDD9 expression might predict a risk of future metastasis.

CANCER STEM CELLS AND MELANOMA

Evidence supporting the biological and therapeutic relevance of a precursor tumor stem cell population has been cited in several tumor types; however, the role of cancer stem cells in melanoma remains controversial. Enthusiasm for a melanoma stem cell model was augmented by a study of ABCB5, an adenosine triphosphate–binding cassette transporter whose homologues have been implicated in stem cell multidrug resistance.[93] Cancer cells expressing high ABCB5 were found to correlate significantly with melanocytic lineage and multidrug resistance in the NCI-60 cell line set.[93,94] Mechanistically, ABCB5 was shown to mediate efflux of the anticancer drug doxorubicin and resistance to melanoma cell killing by this agent via modulation of membrane potential. Notably, the tissue distribution of ABCB5 protein partially colocalized with the putative stem cell marker CD133, suggesting that the drug resistance phenotype might be most closely associated with a long-lived, refractory stem cell population.

Evidence challenging the melanoma stem cell model emerged from xenotransplantation studies in immunocompromised mice. Whereas numerous studies in support of cancer stem cells utilized nonobese diabetic/severe combined immunodeficient (NOD/SCID) mice to show that only approximately 1 of 10,000 tumor cells was capable of tumor initiation, a more recent study employed a more severely immunocompromised strain (NOD/SCID interleukin-2 receptor gamma chain null [Il2rg2/2]).[95] In this setting, more than 1 of 4 melanoma cells were capable of tumor initiation; furthermore, neither ABCB5 nor any other stem cell marker expression could stratify the cells based on tumorigenic efficiency.[95] These results suggest that the "classic" tumor stem cell hypothesis may not fully explain melanoma tumorigenesis; on the other hand, it remains unclear which (if any) xenotransplantation context accurately models the tumor stem cell phenotype. Additional studies are therefore needed to determine the extent to which stem cell features modify melanoma biology or chemotherapeutic response.

CANCER GENOMICS AND TRANSLATION

Advances in sequencing technology have made it possible to obtain the complete genome sequence of entire cancer genomes at ever diminishing costs. Together with developments in computational biology, these advances promise to usher in a new understanding of cancer genome alterations and the tumorigenic mechanisms that result. One of the first cancer genomes to be sequenced was that of a cell line (and its paired normal counterpart) derived from a patient with metastatic melanoma.[96] This effort uncovered more than 33,000 somatic base substitutions, of which 187 were nonsynonymous coding mutations. As expected, most base mutations were C→T transitions indicative of ultraviolet exposure. However, the distribution of mutations across the genome was uneven, with a diminished prevalence in "gene footprint" areas.[96] This distribution suggested the presence of transcription-coupled DNA repair in these regions. Thus, the complete sequence of this melanoma genome highlighted the mutational and selection dynamics that gave rise to this tumor.

Other studies have investigated the global transcriptional alterations characteristic of melanoma by deploying similar sequencing technologies to characterize cDNA from melanomas (termed RNA-seq). One recent RNA-seq study of ten melanomas (eight "short-term" cultures and two cell lines) identified multiple gene fusions, chimeric transcripts, splice isoforms, and base mutations not previously described.[14] Whereas the gene fusions derived from structural genomic alterations occurred uniquely, several chimeric "read-through" transcripts (transcripts consisting of exons from two adjacent genes) were recurrently detected in different tumors. One such read-through event involved CDK2, a kinase involved in melanoma cell division that is also a transcriptional target of MITF.[14,97]

The high UV-associated base mutation rate in melanoma suggests that nearly 2% of all genes may harbor nonsynonymous coding mutations in a typical cutaneous melanoma, most of which are likely to be "passenger" events with little biological consequence to melanoma genesis or progression. Thus, cataloging all significant genomic alterations that might represent "driver" events (see below) will require not only sequencing hundreds of tumor specimens but also the principled application of increasingly sophisticated analytical methods for data deconvolution. Several large-scale U.S. (Cancer Genome Atlas) and international efforts (International Cancer Genomic Consortium)[98] have taken on the ambitious goal of comprehensively characterizing the genomes of diverse human tumors including melanomas. Thus, it seems certain that the next decade will witness major breakthroughs in melanoma genome characterization that inform the biology and treatment of this malignancy.

Distinguishing "driver" events that may confer transforming activity or dictate prognosis or response to emerging targeted therapeutics will also require intensive functional validation efforts.[99] An example of this was the recent discovery of *GOLPH3* as an oncogene in melanoma.[100] Intersection of chromosomal copy number variations (CNVs) in melanoma with those observed in other tumors followed by multilevel functional and clinicopathological validation studies led to the identification of the *GOLPH3* gene as a first-in-class Golgi oncogene in a region of recurrent copy number gain.[100] Furthermore, through a broad range of mechanistic and biological studies drawing from model systems as diverse as yeast, mouse, and human, authors showed that GOLPH3 exerts its oncogenic activity in part through regulation of TOR signaling, and that tumor cells with a high level of GOLPH3 exhibited increased sensitivity to mTOR inhibition.[100] In the aggregate, this example highlights the importance of systematic functional validation and detailed biological studies to realize the potential of cancer genomics.

Toward this end, genome-scale functional genetic screens with RNAi have also begun to yield insights in melanoma. For example a systematic RNAi screen found that loss of the secreted protein IGFBP7 could bypass senescence associated with ectopic BRAF(V600E) expression.[101] Moreover, many BRAF(V600E) melanomas showed loss of IGFBP7.[101] In another RNAi study, loss of GAS1 was found to promote melanoma metastases in a murine model, suggesting that GAS1 may function as a metastasis suppressor.[102] While the larger clinical importance of these observations remains to be established, these studies illustrate the power of systematic functional screens to offer new insights into melanoma biology that may ultimately have therapeutic implications.

LOOKING AHEAD

The identification of genetic alterations associated causally or otherwise prominently with melanoma initiation and progression presents the opportunity to exploit the genome for molecular biomarkers of melanoma pathogenesis and progression as well as for targets of therapeutic intervention. The initial success of both targeted therapeutics and immunotherapies that exploit this burgeoning molecular knowledge have paved the way for future rational interventions and in particular therapeutic combinations that may enable more durable clinical responses for many patients with advanced melanoma.

Genome-wide assays for DNA copy number alterations, RNA expression patterns, and increasingly protein activation (phosphorylation) states will continue to inform molecular mechanisms and contribute to melanoma pathogenesis. Within the next several years, many new melanoma cancer genes and effector pathways will likely be discovered through large-scale genome sequencing efforts. Evolving technologies will further uncover additional roles of gene dysregulation, such as epigenetic modification (e.g., methylation) or noncoding RNAs such as microRNAs. The application of sophisticated computational analyses should link these myriad observations so as to allow discovery of cellular networks and modules that exert crucial roles in melanoma genesis, survival, and progression. Finally, application of these types of analyses to relapsing tumor specimens should elaborate the spectrum of mechanisms by which therapeutic resistance emerges, thereby informing additional treatment options. Altogether, the intersection of scientific discovery and therapeutic innovation offers great potential to reduce death and suffering from this malignancy.

Selected References

The full list of references for this chapter appears in the online version.

1. Jemal A, Siegel R, Xu J, Ward E. Cancer statistics, 2010. *CA Cancer J Clin* 2010;60(5):277.
2. Michaloglou C, Vredeveld LC, Soengas MS, et al. BRAFE600-associated senescence-like cell cycle arrest of human naevi. *Nature* 2005;436(7051):720.
4. Lin WM, Baker AC, Beroukhim R, et al. Modeling genomic diversity and tumor dependency in malignant melanoma. *Cancer Res* 2008;68(3):664.
5. Hussussian CJ, Struewing JP, Goldstein AM, et al. Germline p16 mutations in familial melanoma. *Nat Gen* 1994;8(1):15.
6. Chin L, Pomerantz J, Polsky D, et al. Cooperative effects of INK4a and ras in melanoma susceptibility in vivo. *Genes Devel* 1997;11(21):2822.
13. Curtin JA, Fridlyand J, Kageshita T, et al. Distinct sets of genetic alterations in melanoma. *N Engl J Med* 2005;353(20):2135.
14. Berger MF, Levin JZ, Vijayendran K, et al. Integrative analysis of the melanoma transcriptome. *Genome Res* 2010;20(4):413.

15. Chin L. The genetics of malignant melanoma: lessons from mouse and man. *Nat Rev Cancer* 2003;3(8):559.
16. Bardeesy N, Bastian BC, Hezel A, et al. Dual inactivation of RB and p53 pathways in RAS-induced melanomas. *Mol Cell Biol* 2001; 21(6):2144.
17. Chin L, Garraway LA, Fisher DE. Malignant melanoma: genetics and therapeutics in the genomic era. *Genes Dev* 2006;20(16):2149.
22. Thomas RK, Baker AC , Debiasi RM, et al. High-throughput oncogene mutation profiling in human cancer. *Nat Genet* 2007;39(3):347.
24. Ackermann J, Frutschi M, Kaloulis K, et al. Metastasizing melanoma formation caused by expression of activated N-RasQ61K on an INK4a-deficient background. *Cancer Res* 2005;65(10):4005.
26. Chin L, Tam A, Pomerantz J, et al. Essential role for oncogenic Ras in tumour maintenance. *Nature* 1999;400(6743):468.
27. Kabbarah O, Chin L. Revealing the genomic heterogeneity of melanoma. *Cancer Cell* 2005;8(6):439.
30. Dhomen N, Reis-Filho JS, da Rocha Dias S, et al. Oncogenic Braf induces melanocyte senescence and melanoma in mice. *Cancer Cell* 2009;15(4):294.
31. Hingorani SR, Jacobetz MA, Robertson GP, Herlyn M, Tuveson DA. Suppression of BRAF(V599E) in human melanoma abrogates transformation. *Cancer Res* 2003;63(17):5198.
32. Wellbrock C, Ogilvie L, Hedley D, et al. V599EB-RAF is an oncogene in melanocytes. *Cancer Res* 2004;64(7):2338.
33. Karasarides M, Chiloeches A, Hayward R, et al. B-RAF is a therapeutic target in melanoma. *Oncogene* 2004;23(37):6292.
34. Hoeflich KP, Gray DC, Eby MT, et al. Oncogenic BRAF is required for tumor growth and maintenance in melanoma models. *Cancer Res* 2006;66(2):999.
37. Zheng B, Jeong JH, Asara JM, et al. Oncogenic B-RAF negatively regulates the tumor suppressor LKB1 to promote melanoma cell proliferation. *Mol Cell* 2009;33(2):237.
40. Tsai J, Lee JT, Wang W, et al. Discovery of a selective inhibitor of oncogenic B-Raf kinase with potent antimelanoma activity. *Proc Natl Acad Sci U S A* 2008;105(8):3041.
41. Flaherty K, Puzanov I, Kim KB, et al. Inhibition of mutated, activated BRAF in metastatic melanoma. *N Engl J Med* 2010;36(9):809–815.
42. Heidorn SJ, Milagre C, Whittaker S, et al. Kinase-dead BRAF and oncogenic RAS cooperate to drive tumor progression through CRAF. *Cell* 2010;140(2):209.
43. Poulikakos PI, Zhang C, Bollag G, Shokat KM, Rosen N. RAF inhibitors transactivate RAF dimers and ERK signalling in cells with wild-type BRAF. *Nature* 2010;464(7287):427.
44. Hatzivassiliou G, Song K, Yen I, et al. RAF inhibitors prime wild-type RAF to activate the MAPK pathway and enhance growth. *Nature* 2010;464(7287):431.
46. Solit DB, Garraway LA, Pratilas CA, et al. BRAF mutation predicts sensitivity to MEK inhibition. *Nature* 2006;439(7074):358.
48. Emery CM, Vijayendran KG, Zipser MC, et al. MEK1 mutations confer resistance to MEK and B-RAF inhibition. *Proc Natl Acad Sci U S A* 2009;106(48):20411.
49. Chudnovsky Y, Adams AE, Robbins PB, Lin Q, Khavari PA. Use of human tissue to assess the oncogenic activity of melanoma-associated mutations. *Nat Genet* 2005;37(7):745.
51. Dankort D, Curley DP, Cartlidge RA, et al. Braf(V600E) cooperates with Pten loss to induce metastatic melanoma. *Nat Genet* 2009;41(5):544.
57. Davies MA, Stemke-Hale K, Lin E, et al. Integrated molecular and clinical analysis of AKT activation in metastatic melanoma. *Clin Cancer Res* 2009;15(24):7538.
61. Nishimura EK, Jordan SA, Oshima H, et al. Dominant role of the niche in melanocyte stem-cell fate determination. *Nature* 2002;416(6883):854.
67. Hodi FS, Friedlander P, Corless CL, et al. Major response to imatinib mesylate in KIT-mutated melanoma. *J Clin Oncol* 2008;26(12):2046.
70. Bardeesy N, Kim M, Xu J, et al. Role of epidermal growth factor receptor signaling in RAS-driven melanoma. *Mol Cell Biol* 2005;25(10):4176.
71. Sibilia M, Fleischmann A, Behrens A, et al. The EGF receptor provides an essential survival signal for SOS-dependent skin tumor development. *Cell* 2000;102(2):211.
72. Prickett TD, Neena SA, Xiaomu Wei, et al. Analysis of the tyrosine kinome in melanoma reveals recurrent mutations in ERBB4. *Nat Genet* 2009;41(10):1127.
73. Bastian BC, LeBoit PE, Hamm H, Brocker E-B, Pinkel D. Chromosomal gains and losses in primary cutaneous melanomas detected by comparative genomic hybridization. *Cancer Res* 1998;58(10):2170.
75. Garraway LA, Widlund HR, Rubin MA, et al. Integrative genomic analyses identify MITF as a lineage survival oncogene amplified in malignant melanoma. *Nature* 2005;436(7047):117.
76. Garraway LA, Sellers WR. From integrated genomics to tumor lineage dependency. *Cancer Res* 2006;66(5):2506.
77. Garraway LA, Sellers WR. Lineage dependency and lineage-survival oncogenes in human cancer. *Nat Rev Cancer* 2006;6(8):593.
79. Jané-Valbuena J, Widlund HR, Perner S, et al. An oncogenic role for ETV1 in melanoma. *Cancer Res* 2010;70(5):2075.
80. McGill GG, Horstmann M, Widlund HR, et al. Bcl2 regulation by the melanocyte master regulator Mitf modulates lineage survival and melanoma cell viability. *Cell* 2002;109(6):707.
81. Dorsky RI, Moon RT, Raible DW. Control of neural crest cell fate by the Wnt signalling pathway. *Nature* 1998;396(6709):370.
86. Weeraratna AT, Jiang Y, Hostetter G, et al. Wnt5a signaling directly affects cell motility and invasion of metastatic melanoma. *Cancer Cell* 2002;1(3):279.
90. D'Orazio JA, Nobuhisa T, Cui R, et al. Topical drug rescue strategy and skin protection based on the role of Mc1r in UV-induced tanning. *Nature* 2006;443(7109):340.
91. Cui R, Widlund HR, Feige E, et al. Central role of p53 in the suntan response and pathologic hyperpigmentation. *Cell* 2007;128(5):853.
93. Schatton T, Murphy GF, Frank NY, et al. Identification of cells initiating human melanomas. *Nature* 2008;451(7176):345.
96. Pleasance ED, Cheetham RK, Stephens PJ, et al. A comprehensive catalogue of somatic mutations from a human cancer genome. *Nature* 2010;463(7278):191.
100. Scott KL, Kabbarah O, Liang MC, et al. GOLPH3 modulates mTOR signalling and rapamycin sensitivity in cancer. *Nature* 2009;459(7250):1085.
101. Wajapeyee N, Serra RW, Zhu X, Mahalingam M, Green MR. Oncogenic BRAF induces senescence and apoptosis through pathways mediated by the secreted protein IGFBP7. *Cell* 2008;132(3):363.
102. Gobeil S, Zhu X, Doillon CJ, Green MR. A genome-wide shRNA screen identifies GAS1 as a novel melanoma metastasis suppressor gene. *Genes Dev* 2008;22(21):2932.

CHAPTER 119 CUTANEOUS MELANOMA

CRAIG L. SLINGLUFF Jr., KEITH FLAHERTY, STEVEN A. ROSENBERG, AND PAUL W. READ

Melanoma is a neoplastic disorder produced by malignant transformation of the normal melanocyte. Melanocytes are cells responsible for the production of the pigment melanin. During the first trimester of fetal life, precursor melanocytes arise in the neural crest. As the fetus develops, these cells migrate to areas including the skin, meninges, mucous membranes, upper esophagus, and eyes. In each of these locations, melanocytes have demonstrated a potential for malignant transformation, but the site most commonly associated with melanocytic transformation is the skin, where melanocytes reside at the dermal/epidermal junction. When melanoma arises in the skin, it usually arises from melanocytes at the dermal/epidermal junction. In addition, there are alternate presentations, including mucosal melanomas, ocular melanomas, metastatic melanomas from unknown primary sites, and presumed primary visceral melanomas. In the National Cancer Database, 91.2% of melanomas are cutaneous, 5.3% are ocular, 1.3% are mucosal, and 2.2% are of unknown primary site.[1] Each of these types has significant differences in presentation and management. The primary focus of this chapter is on cutaneous melanoma, but summary information is presented for the other forms of melanoma, as well as on the subtypes of cutaneous melanoma. The management of malignant melanoma involves prevention, early diagnosis, surgical extirpation, and combination management of metastatic disease.

CUTANEOUS MELANOMA BIOLOGY

In colon cancer and breast cancer, it has been demonstrated that progression from normal epithelium to an invasive epithelial malignancy is a stepwise process manifested by sequential accumulation of multiple genetic mutations. These are associated with histologic changes along a continuum from normal to invasive malignancy. Similarly, the transition from melanocyte to metastatic melanoma involves several histologic intermediates, including melanocytic atypia, atypical melanocytic hyperplasia, radial growth phase melanoma, vertical growth phase melanoma, and metastatic melanoma. Atypical melanocytes arising in a pre-existing nevus or *de novo* are very common but rarely progress to melanoma. However, some patients develop confluent atypical melanocytic hyperplasia at the dermal/epidermal junction or nests of atypical melanocytes in the epidermis or at the dermal/epidermal junction. As this process progresses, it reaches a point at which it warrants a diagnosis of melanoma. However, early melanomas usually proceed to grow radially, and this is called the *radial growth phase* (RGP) of melanoma, which may continue for years before progressing to the vertical growth phase (VGP). Examples of VGP melanoma arising in pre-existing RGP melanoma are shown in Figure 119.1.

The RGP of a cutaneous melanoma may include either melanoma *in situ* or superficial invasion into the papillary dermis, or both. Melanomas in RGP present clinically as enlarging macules or very minimally raised papular lesions, which are typically (but not always) pigmented. These lesions are rarely symptomatic. This is the ideal time to diagnose melanoma, and the changing nature of these RGP lesions often is adequate for recognition by the patient and by the clinician. However, if not recognized, these lesions typically progress to the VGP, manifest clinically by a nodular growth of the lesion, often described by the patient as a lesion that began to "raise up." This vertical growth usually arises as a nodule within the RGP component and encompassing only part of the RGP (Fig. 119.1A,C). Thus, the VGP appears to represent further steps in the process of malignant transformation due to clonal changes in the cells of the RGP. The radial and vertical growth phases are illustrated well elsewhere.[2]

RGP melanomas have very low metastatic capacity. It has been reported that the risk of subsequent metastasis from RGP lesions is zero,[2] but several case reports illustrate exceptions to that observation.[3] Nonetheless, RGP melanomas are associated with an excellent prognosis and mortality risk at the low end of the 0% to 5% range. There is often a substantial window of time between the appearance of clinically detectable RGP and development of VGP—on the order of months to years—during which there is opportunity for curative discovery and excision of early melanoma.

However, as melanomas develop VGP, they acquire increased metastatic risk. Thus, risk of melanoma progression is most associated with the presence of VGP, the depth of invasion, and other markers of the malignant phenotype in the VGP component of a melanoma. On the other hand, the extent of RGP (e.g., clinically, the diameter of the skin lesion) and multiplicity of RGP lesions are not associated with significant risk of metastasis or melanoma-associated mortality.

Unfortunately, some melanomas are nonpigmented and escape early diagnosis for that reason. Others develop a VGP in the absence of a RGP (nodular melanoma histology), and the time course of progression in these lesions does not afford the same interval for early diagnosis that is observed in melanomas with a preceding RGP component (superficial spreading melanoma, lentigo maligna melanoma, lentiginous melanoma, acral lentiginous melanoma). Finally, some melanomas present as metastatic melanoma in lymph nodes, skin, subcutaneous tissue, or visceral sites without an apparent primary cutaneous site. In some cases, these have been associated with a history of a regressed primary melanocytic lesion. In other cases, such an explanation is less clear. In all of these cases, the prospect of early diagnosis of melanoma is compromised, and the risk of melanoma-associated mortality is increased. Thus, there is still substantial need for more accurate diagnostic methods and more effective screening practices for this difficult disease.

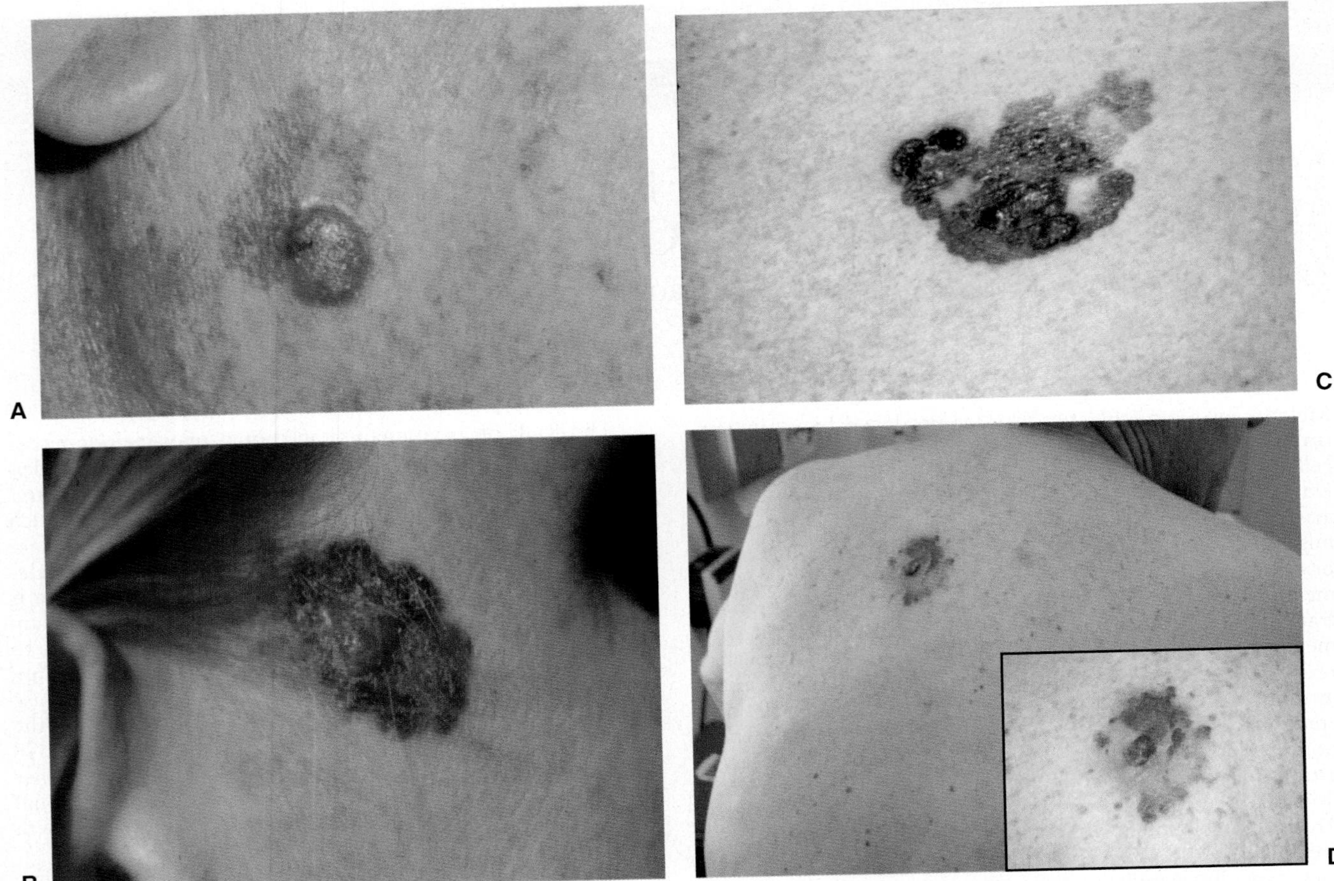

FIGURE 119.1 **A:** A nodule of vertical growth phase melanoma arising from a radial growth phase pigmented macule on the right cheek. **B:** Superficial spreading melanoma, 2.9 mm thick, arising on the temple of a young woman. There were microscopic satellites, and the patient died of disease within several years. **C:** Superficial spreading melanoma (SSM) with all the classic features of the ABCD mnemonic (asymmetry, border irregularity, color variation, and diameter greater than 6 mm). **D:** Large, ulcerated 2.5 mm SSM with regression in elderly man.

EPIDEMIOLOGY

Malignant melanoma is the sixth most common U.S. cancer diagnosis.[4] The actual incidence of melanoma is increasing more rapidly than that of any other malignancy, with 68,130 cases of invasive melanoma and 8,700 melanoma deaths in the United States in 2009,[4] and with 166,900 cases of invasive melanoma annually in developed countries globally.[4a] This amounts to 4% of new cancer diagnoses and 1.5% of cancer deaths. In the early part of the twentieth century, the lifetime risk of a white person developing melanoma was approximately 1 in 1,500. Currently this risk is approximately 1 in 56 for women and 1 in 37 for men.[4] Its incidence is second only to breast cancer for women from birth to age 39 years; similarly, it is the second most common cancer diagnosis for men through age 39 years, slightly less common than leukemia.[4] Despite general physician awareness and excellent public education, this malignancy still has an approximate 14% mortality in the United States, and for patients who present with regional and distant metastases, the 5-year mortality rates are approximately 38% and 85%, respectively.[4] Overall 5-year survival rates for melanoma have increased from 82% in the late 1970s (1975 to 1977) to 91% in the more recent era (2002 to 2006).[4]

This is a disease that disproportionately affects whites over African American, Asian, or other dark-skinned individuals. In the United States, whites account for 98.2% of cutaneous melanomas reported in the National Cancer Database, with African Americans accounting for 0.7% and Hispanics accounting for 1.1%.[1] This is best explained by a combined effect of ultraviolet (UV) sunlight exposure and fair skin. It is most striking that the highest per-capita incidence of melanoma worldwide is in Australia, and that this high incidence afflicts primarily the Australians of Western European descent who have fair skin, and not the darker-skinned aboriginal population. It is also notable that these fair-skinned European descendants who moved to Australia have much higher incidences of melanoma than the Western European populations that remain in the higher latitudes of Europe. In migrant populations, individuals who move during childhood to areas with greater sun exposure develop melanoma at rates higher than those of their country of origin and similar to those of their adopted country.[5,6]

In nonwhite populations, there is a much higher proportion of melanomas in acral (subungual, palmar, plantar) and mucosal locations. However, the incidences of those types of melanoma are similar across races. Their higher relative proportion in Asians and African Americans can be best explained by the disproportionate increase in nonacral cutaneous melanomas in fair-skinned whites rather than by an absolute increase in risk of acral and mucosal melanomas in nonwhite populations.

Ocular and nonacral cutaneous melanomas are 50- to 200-fold more likely in white populations than in nonwhite populations, but melanomas in acral and mucosal sites are within twofold of each other across racial groups. Similarly, the increased incidence of melanoma over the last few decades can

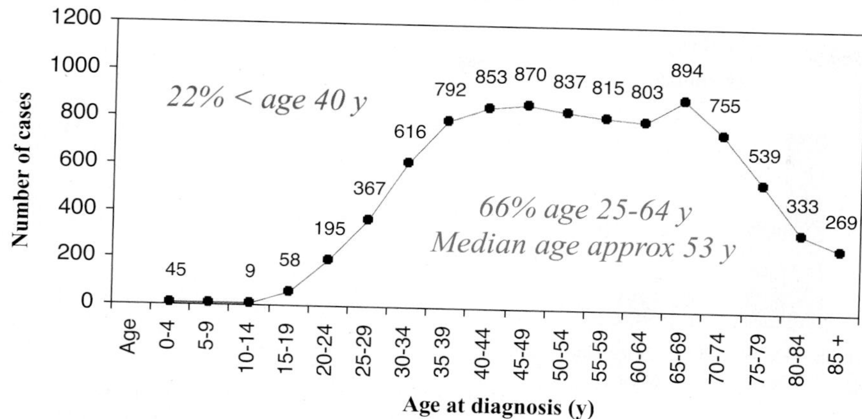

FIGURE 119.2 Age-related incidence of melanoma in Virginia, 1970 to 1996. (From Virginia Cancer Registry, 1999.)

be explained primarily by increased incidence in white populations, not in nonwhite populations.[7] These observations support the hypothesis that most cutaneous melanomas in white populations are etiologically related to sun exposure but that there may be a baseline risk of melanoma in other locations that is unrelated to sun damage. Recent data suggest significant molecular differences between acral melanomas and melanomas arising on the skin associated with chronic sun damage, with *B-RAF* and *N-RAS* mutations in 81% of melanomas on chronically sun-damaged skin, whereas those mutations were uncommon in melanomas from acral or mucosal sites or from skin without chronic sun damage.[8]

CHANGES IN INCIDENCE

Data from the Surveillance, Epidemiology, and End Results program reveal an increase in age-adjusted melanoma incidence rates from 8.2 per 100,000 in the 1970s (1974 to 1978) to 18.7 per 100,000 in more recent years (1999 to 2003).[9] From 1990 to 2003, during which there was a 16% decrease in male cancer deaths overall for all cancers, there was a 2% increase in mortality rate from melanoma. From 1991 to 2003, during which there was an 8% decrease in cancer deaths overall for women, there was only a 4% decrease in mortality rate associated with melanoma.[4]

In Australia, and to a lesser extent in the United States, there has been a substantial increase in awareness about melanoma and the value of screening by total-body skin examinations. There also has been a greater proportion of patients diagnosed at earlier and noninvasive stages of disease. Thus, part of the increase in incidence may be explained by increased early diagnosis of lesions with low metastatic potential. However, there has also been a significant increase in mortality from melanoma over the last few decades. Thus, the increase in incidence represents a real and serious increase as well. The increased awareness in Australia has become so pervasive that it has led to substantially better sun protection practices. Epidemiologic data show slight decreases in melanoma incidence in some Australian populations. Similarly in the United States, the incidence of melanoma is leveling off somewhat in women and younger adults generally. However, especially among older men, the incidence and mortality rate from melanoma continues to increase.[10,11] This may be related in part to well-documented failures of men, more than women, to seek medical attention for changing skin lesions until they become symptomatic.

GENDER AND AGE DISTRIBUTION

In the United States and Australia, the gender ratio of melanoma at diagnosis is approximately 1:1 but is shifting toward a greater proportion of men.[4] The median age of melanoma patients has increased from 51 years in the 1970s (1974 to 1978) to 57 years in a more recent time period (1999 to 2003).[9] Nonetheless, the median age for diagnosis of melanoma is substantially lower than the current median age of diagnosis for the more common solid tumors, including colon (age 73 years), lung (age 70 years), or prostate (age 68 years) cancer.[9] The large majority (approximately 80%) of melanoma patients are diagnosed in the productive years from age 25 to 65 as shown for a representative population from the State of Virginia (Fig. 119.2). Melanoma is common in patients in their 20s and older, but it also is observed in teenagers, and occasionally even in infants and neonates. For women aged 25 to 35 years, melanoma is the leading cause of cancer-related death.

MELANOMA IN CHILDREN, INFANTS, AND NEONATES

Diagnosis and management of melanoma in children, infants, and neonates is complicated by several factors: (1) excisional biopsy of skin lesions often is not feasible under local anesthesia in young children, and (2) pigmented skin lesions with substantial cellular atypia but with structural symmetry may be Spitz nevi, which typically have benign behavior. Thus, some young patients with changing pigmented skin lesions are observed longer than would be advisable because biopsy is more problematic than in most adults. In addition, young patients may undergo incomplete shave biopsy to avoid a full-thickness excision, and information is lost about the architecture of the lesion, leaving a diagnostic dilemma between melanoma and Spitz nevus.

Even in the best of circumstances, some melanocytic tumors are difficult to diagnose with certainty. This has led to a formal definition of melanocytic tumors of uncertain malignant potential.[12] With the advent of sentinel node biopsy techniques, it may be appropriate to perform sentinel node biopsy for melanocytic tumors of uncertain malignant potential because the finding of metastatic tumor in a sentinel node may support a diagnosis of malignant melanoma.

Melanoma deaths in children and young adults have a large effect on total years of life lost because of melanoma.[13] Current recommendations for management of melanoma in children

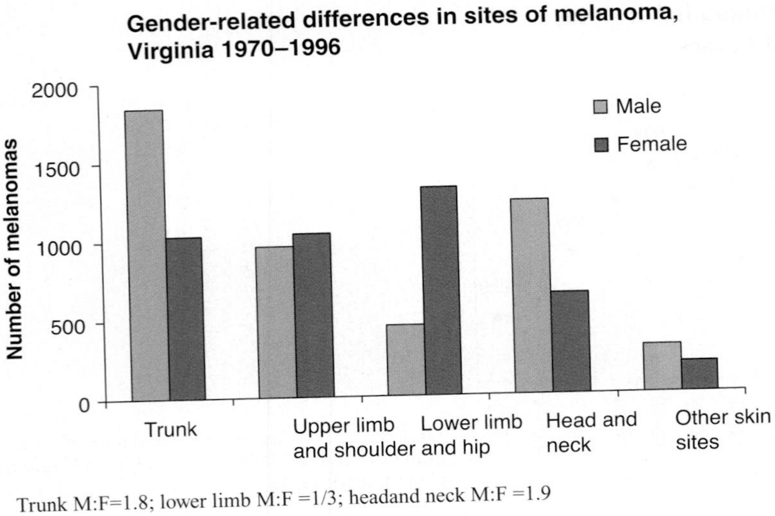

Gender-related differences in sites of melanoma, Virginia 1970–1996

Trunk M:F=1.8; lower limb M:F =1/3; headand neck M:F =1.9

FIGURE 119.3 Incidence of melanoma in Virginia, 1970 to 1996, by gender. (From Virginia Cancer Registry, 1999.)

and infants are the same as for adults, and outcomes are generally believed to be comparable.[14,15]

ANATOMIC DISTRIBUTION

Cutaneous melanoma can occur at any body site. The most common sites in males are on the back and in the head and neck regions. In women, the most common sites are in the lower extremities, commonly below the knee. Data from the Virginia State Cancer Registry are shown SSM in Figure 119.3. Lentigo maligna melanoma (LMM) most commonly arises on sun-damaged surfaces of the head and neck in older patients. Acral lentiginous melanoma (ALM) is most common on subungual and other acral locations.

ETIOLOGY AND RISK FACTORS

The demographic features of melanoma have implicated UV light exposure as a major etiologic factor in the development of melanoma. Multiple studies continue to support an etiologic association between UV irradiation and melanoma.[15–17] Ultraviolet C radiation is generally absorbed by the ozone layer. Ultraviolet-B (UVB) radiation (290 to 320 nm) is associated with sunburn and induction of tanning by melanin pigment production. There are substantial data to support its etiologic role in melanoma.[16,17] There is also some evidence implicating UVA radiation (320 to 400 nm), although UVA is more associated with chronic sun damage changes.[18] However, the relative role of each type of UV irradiation in melanoma etiology is debated. Some animal data suggest that sun exposure early in life increases the risk of melanoma.[19] Human skin grafted on mice will develop nevi and melanomas in the presence of UVB irradiation, further supporting the role of UVB irradiation and melanoma.[20] Burns early in life have been implicated in melanoma incidence.[21] However, chronic sun exposure in individuals who tan may even protect against melanoma.[22] Considering these observations, plus the epidemiology described earlier, suggests that the etiology of many, if not most, cutaneous melanomas appears to be associated with a combination of fair skin that burns easily and high UV/sun exposure. The role of sunlight intensity and frequency is debated, but both chronic and intermittent exposure may be relevant.[15,23] Current data suggest that UV radiation causes melanoma by a combination of DNA damage, inflammation, and immune suppression.[24]

Tanning bed use has been implicated in the etiology of melanoma, with a recent report that any tanning bed use in adolescence or early adulthood is associated with a 1.4-fold increase in melanoma incidence, and that this relative risk increases to 2.0 for individuals with at least ten tanning bed sessions.[25] The association was most significant for the risk of melanoma diagnosed at ages 30 to 39.[25] Tanning bed use has been formally classified as a carcinogen, and increased awareness of the harmful effects of UV exposure promise to control the increase in melanoma incidence. However, this has highlighted another growing health concern, that without sun exposure, there is an increasing rate of vitamin D deficiency. It has been estimated that increasing UVB exposure to allow mean serum 25-hydroxyvitamin D levels to 45 ng/mL would lead to preventing almost 400,000 deaths per year from cardiovascular diseases and cancer, although at the price of increasing melanoma mortality by several thousand deaths per year.[26] Thus, questions remain about the optimal UV exposure and how to optimize vitamin D levels.

Another factor that may increase the risk of melanoma is a heritable predisposition. This may explain a minority of melanomas (e.g., 5% to 10%). Mutations associated with melanoma risk include inactivation of two critical tumor suppression pathways—that mediated through *p16/CDK4* and *CDK6*/retinoblastoma gene, and that mediated through *p14* and *p53*.[27] Mutations of *CDKN2a* have also been identified in 25% to 50% of melanoma kindreds studied.[27]

Other common risk factors include dysplastic nevus syndrome, a history of other skin cancers associated with sun exposure, and a family history of melanoma. Xeroderma pigmentosum also is associated with increased melanoma risk, but it is uncommon. Higher socioeconomic status is also associated with higher risk.

Radiation doses greater than 15 Gy delivered to pediatric oncology patients has been shown to increase the risk of developing malignant melanoma by an odds ratio of 13.[28]

PREGNANCY AND ESTROGEN USE

A large subset of melanoma patients comprises women in their childbearing years. Thus, questions arise frequently about the prognosis and management for patients diagnosed with melanoma during pregnancy, and also about whether it is safe or appropriate for patients to become pregnant after treatment for melanoma. Older literature suggested anecdotally that patients diagnosed with melanoma had a bad outcome. However, multiple systematic and larger studies have shown no evidence of any negative (or positive) impact of prior, concurrent, or subsequent pregnancy on clinical outcome.[29,30] Similarly, there is no clear prognostic relevance for birth control pills or estrogen replacement therapy.[31] The general recommendation for treatment of women with melanoma diagnosed during pregnancy is to manage them in the same fashion as nonpregnant patients. Depending on the time during pregnancy at which a melanoma is diagnosed, there can be circumstances in which radiologic imaging may be limited because of concern for the fetus, and major surgery may be delayed until the fetus is at an age when it can survive independently. However, the excision of a primary melanoma certainly can be done in almost any circumstance, under local anesthesia.

The other related question often asked by patients is whether it is advisable to become pregnant and to bear a child after treatment for melanoma. As just stated, there is no evidence that a subsequent pregnancy adversely impacts outcome. However, the more interesting and challenging question is the more personal or social issue of the potential for premature parental death due to melanoma. Thus, it is helpful for patients to understand their risk of future recurrence and melanoma-related mortality because that translates into the risk that the child will grow up losing a parent. Measures of the risk of future disease progression can be defined based on the initial prognosis and the subsequent elapsed time without recurrence, and such information may help to guide patients with this challenging question.[32]

PREVENTION AND SCREENING

Advanced melanoma has a very poor prognosis. However, melanomas diagnosed and treated during the RGP have an excellent prognosis. Thus, prevention and early diagnosis can have a great impact on decreasing melanoma morbidity and mortality. The apparent leveling off of melanoma-related mortality rates in Australia and the United States likely is the result of better screening and prevention.

Sun Protection

Ultraviolet exposure and sunburns, in particular, appear to be etiologic in most melanomas. Thus, protection from UV light, especially in fair-skinned individuals, is believed to have substantial benefit in preventing melanoma. Although many people tend to think of sunscreens when they think of sun protection, there is no formal proof that sunscreens prevent melanoma.[33] There also are some limitations inherent in sunscreen use. One is that certain body sites are not easily covered with sunscreen, such as the scalp. More important, even "waterproof" sunscreens wash off or become less effective with time. Most people also forget to reapply sunscreens frequently enough and may still get burns.[34] There are also sociological issues, which may differ for different populations and are arguable. However, it is worth considering the provocative findings of a study performed on young adults from Western Europe, who were randomized to receive either sun protection factor (SPF)10 or SPF30 sunscreen. In a blinded fashion, they were asked to report sun exposure times and sunburns. The number of sunburns was the same in both groups, and sun exposure was greater in the SPF30 group, suggesting that some populations may stay in the sun until they get a burn, and that sunscreen simply helps them to stay in the sun longer.[35]

It is safe to say that the best protection from the sun is a building, the next best is protective clothing, and the third best is sunscreen. Patients should be advised to use all three. Avoiding midday sun from about 11 AM to 3 PM by staying indoors is advised, as well as wearing clothing with a thick enough weave that it blocks sunlight, or a formal SPF rating, when possible. Hats are particularly helpful for the face and scalp, which often are highly exposed to sunlight and not so readily covered fully with sunscreen. Otherwise, sunscreen can provide protection to sun-exposed areas when outside.

Screening for Early Diagnosis

Self-Examination

For many patients, they, their spouses, or other family members may be able to screen effectively for new suspicious skin lesions, and this should be encouraged. It is more common for women to detect melanomas than for men to do so, either for themselves or for their partners.[36] In any case, there is value in educating patients about how to detect melanomas if they are at high risk. As many as half of melanomas are identified by the patient or family,[37] and patient self-examination has been associated with diagnosis of thinner melanomas.[38] In a study by Berwick et al.,[38] patients performing self-examination appeared to have melanomas that were detected in an earlier microstage. Teaching aids for patients on how to perform skin self-examination are available from the American Cancer Society and the American Academy of Dermatology. Patients with melanoma or at high risk should be seen regularly by a dermatologist. It is reasonable to suggest that patients perform skin self-examinations more often than their dermatology visits, although there are no proven guidelines. Doing a self-examination once a month may be the easiest for the patient to remember.

Management of the Patient with Numerous Atypical Moles

Some patients have numerous atypical moles. This presentation is commonly described as atypical mole syndrome, dysplastic nevus syndrome, or B-K mole syndrome.[39,40] These patients have a heightened risk of melanoma, and this is commonly a familial feature. When associated with a family history of melanoma, patients with dysplastic nevus syndrome have a risk of melanoma that may approach 100%. These patients deserve particular attention to melanoma prevention through sun protection and to early diagnosis through aggressive screening. However, the optimal approach for screening is not defined. At a minimum, routine skin examinations by a dermatologist are usually recommended, as often as every 3 months. Visual inspection of the atypical nevi may be augmented by routine digital photography to facilitate detection of subtle changes in radial growth or other changes over time. Although these approaches commonly permit identification of melanomas when they are *in situ* or thin, it is not known whether they improve survival. In addition, concern remains that visual inspection alone, even for very experienced dermatologists, is inadequate to diagnose all melanomas when they are still curable.

Thus, substantial effort is in progress to develop more sensitive and specific diagnostic tools than visual inspection alone. One that is employed routinely in many practices is dermoscopy, also known as epiluminescent microscopy. This involves use of a handheld microscope at the bedside to examine skin lesions in an oil immersion setting. This appears to improve diagnostic accuracy in experienced hands, and increasing experience has made its use more feasible in general practice, especially with considerations for standardization.[41–44] When coupled with the use of a digital camera, the images can be stored and compared over time as well. Computer-assisted digital analysis of these images is also being studied but remains investigational.

Evaluation and management of patients with dysplastic nevus syndrome is complicated by the fact that very few dysplastic nevi will develop into melanoma. Estimates range from a risk of 1 per 1,000 nevi examined in a pigmented lesion clinic being melanoma to 1 per 10,000 nevi becoming melanoma per year.[43,45,46] Recommendations for management of dysplastic nevi include those from the Melanoma Working Group in the Netherlands and by a National Institutes of Health Consensus Conference.[47,48]

It is tempting to consider excision of all dysplastic nevi. Although that remains an option, there is no proof that this will decrease risk. Melanomas may arise *de novo* in 30% to 70% of cases, and so it is not clear that removal of all suspicious nevi will lead to a meaningful improvement in survival. However, it is certainly appropriate to biopsy any nevus that is suspicious, especially one that is changing.

DIAGNOSIS OF PRIMARY MELANOMA

Characteristics of Primary Melanoma

The classic appearance of primary cutaneous melanoma is summarized by the mnemonic ABCD for asymmetry, border irregularity, color variation, and diameter greater than 6 mm (Fig. 119.1). Because melanomas arise from melanocytes, which contain the melanin-synthetic pathway, melanomas classically are distinguished by their pigmentation. Melanomas may have shades of brown, black, blue, red, and white. However, there is a wide range in the appearance of melanomas. Some melanomas are pitch black. Others are shades of brown. Some have no visible pigment and appear skin-colored; others have a red color only. When melanomas have all of the classic ABCD features, they are typically easy to diagnose. However, those melanomas that lack some of these features can be difficult to diagnose. In addition, in patients with large numbers of atypical nevi, which may also have ABCD features, this mnemonic is often inadequate to aid in early diagnosis. The other important findings that may aid in early diagnosis are a change in a lesion over time or new development of a lesion. These warrant evaluation, and in high-risk patients there should be a low threshold for biopsy. In addition, some dermatologists recommend considering the "ugly duckling" sign: A lesion that stands out as different from the patient's other nevi should be evaluated and possibly biopsied. This can be particularly helpful in a patient with a large number of clinically atypical nevi. Both of these approaches may help to identify amelanotic (nonpigmented) melanomas, which often do not meet the ABCD criteria. Some melanomas are not diagnosed until they become symptomatic, and whereas awareness of the symptoms of bleeding, itching, pain, and ulceration are worth noting, these usually connote deep vertical growth and are hallmarks of a late diagnosis, not an early one.

Biopsy

Biopsy of a suspicious skin lesion is necessary for an accurate diagnosis and for optimal staging. The correct way to perform such a biopsy is to make a full-thickness biopsy of the entire lesion, with a narrow (1 to 2 mm) margin of grossly normal skin. The depth of excision should include the full thickness of dermis and thus should extend into the subcutaneous tissue, but it does not need to include all of the subcutaneous tissue except in very thin patients or patients with very thick polypoid lesions that may go deep into the subcutis. This allows assessment of the architecture of the lesion, which is critical for differentiation of melanoma from Spitz nevus, and it permits an accurate measure of tumor thickness, which is critical for prognosis and affects the surgical treatment recommendations. Of importance, desmoplastic melanoma often arises from LMM and is difficult to diagnose both clinically and histologically. Shave biopsies of these lesions can often lead to failure to appreciate the desmoplastic melanoma in the dermis and may substantially delay diagnosis.

For some large lesions (e.g., >2 cm diameter) in cosmetically sensitive locations (e.g., face or genitalia), there may be a rationale for an incisional biopsy, but that also should be performed as a full-thickness skin biopsy. Ideally, it should include the most suspicious area of the lesion and also should include, if possible, a portion of the edge of the lesion where it transitions to normal skin to enable assessment of the junctional change. The incisional biopsy may be an elliptical incision or it may be a full-thickness 4- to 6-mm punch biopsy. Punch biopsies are problematic if too small, if they do not include full-thickness skin, if they are crushed during removal, if they are oriented inaccurately in the paraffin block, or if they are too small to include both the edge of the lesion and the most suspicious or most raised part of the lesion.

Orientation of the incision used for an excisional biopsy should be considered in the context of the prospect for the future need for a wider re-excision. On extremities, the incision and scar should be oriented longitudinally rather than transversely, although some exceptions may be considered near joints to avoid crossing a joint. When in doubt about the optimal orientation, it is very reasonable to perform the excisional biopsy as a simple circular excision, leaving the wound open for secondary or delayed primary closure.

Biopsy of subungual lesions is more challenging. The pigmentary changes seen in patients with subungual melanoma usually extend along the length of the nail, but the lesions usually arise at the proximal end of the nail bed. Access to that location often requires removal of all or a large part of the nail. One or more punch biopsies of the base of the nail bed often constitute the most realistic method for obtaining a biopsy of such lesions, and it may need to be repeated to be diagnostic. A punch biopsy tool can remove a circle of the nail, providing access to the nail bed for punch biopsy of the suspicious area.

Melanoma Subtypes: Histologic Growth Patterns

Classically, four main histologic growth patterns are described for melanomas, but two others are also worth mentioning. These are described in the following subsections. All have a RGP prior to the VGP, except for nodular melanomas, which have only a VGP.

Superficial Spreading Melanoma

The most common type is superficial spreading melanoma, which accounts for about 70% of primary cutaneous melanomas (Fig. 119.1C). It is typical for the trunk and extremities, except on acral sites. It is associated with pagetoid growth of atypical melanocytes in the epidermis. Superficial spreading melanoma is commonly associated with sun exposure.

Nodular Melanoma

Nodular melanomas lack an RGP, may be nonpigmented, and commonly are diagnosed when relatively thick. Thus, these carry the worst prognosis of the various subtypes of melanoma. They account for about 20% of cutaneous melanomas. By definition, nodular melanomas are in VGP when recognized.

Acral Lentiginous Melanoma

ALMs account for less than 5% of melanomas.[1,49] They are typically found on acral sites (subungual, palmar, plantar) and on mucosal surfaces (anorectal, nasopharyngeal, female genital tract). ALM occurs across all races and ethnicities. Its etiology is likely independent of UV light exposure. Because other cutaneous melanomas are uncommon in African, Asian, and Hispanic populations, these ALMs on acral sites are proportionately more common in these populations than in fair-skinned whites. ALM is typically associated with a prolonged RGP before vertical growth; however, its locations make it harder to diagnose than other forms of melanoma. Subungual lesions can be detected by linear pigment streaks arising from the base of the nail, but these are not always evident. They can be confused with subungual hematomas, which can lead to diagnostic delay. When there is a question of whether a pigmented subungual lesion may be melanoma or a hematoma, the location of the pigment can be marked and then followed over a short interval (e.g., 3 weeks), during which time a hematoma should move toward the end of the nail, but a melanoma should not.

Subungual melanomas can also present with breakage of the nail or a nonpigmented thickening or drainage, and these are often confused with chronic fungal infections. Any concerning pigmented subungual lesion should be biopsied, but it is sometimes challenging and requires splitting or removing part of the nail. A punch biopsy near the nail bed matrix is often appropriate. In addition, when there is spontaneous chronic inflammation or breakage of the nail, biopsy for melanoma should be considered, even in the absence of pigmentation.

Lentigo Maligna Melanoma

LMMs typically occur in older individuals, in chronically sun-damaged skin, and commonly on the face. They tend to have shades of brown or black, whereas the red and blue colors seen in other melanomas are not typical of LMM. They may also develop areas of regression manifested by depigmentation of part of the lesion. Overall, LMMs account for about 10% to 20% of melanomas in the National Cancer Database experience,[1] 47% of melanomas of the head and neck, and only 2% of melanomas of other regions.[49] LMMs usually have an extensive RGP that extends for many years before developing invasion. When melanoma is just *in situ,* this RGP portion is called *lentigo maligna* or Hutchinson's freckle, as opposed to LMM. These are not to be confused with the benign pigmented macule, lentigo. Lentigo malignas evolve a VGP to become invasive LMMs at a rate estimated to be between 5% and 33%.[50] LMMs are commonly diagnosed as thin lesions. However, more substantial vertical growth can occur, as seen in Figure 119.1A.

Lentiginous Melanoma

Early RGP melanomas sometimes are difficult to classify into the typical patterns of lentigo maligna, superficial spreading melanoma, or ALM. A recent report defined a distinct entity of lentiginous melanoma. Its features include diameter 1 cm or greater, elongated and irregular rete ridges, confluent melanocytic nests and single cells over a broad area of the dermal/epidermal junction, focal pagetoid spread, cytologic atypia, and possible focal dermal fibrosis.[51] Over time, this may represent a growing proportion of melanomas that have traditionally been grouped as superficial spreading melanoma, lentigo maligna, ALM, or unclassified melanomas.

Desmoplastic Melanoma

Desmoplastic melanoma is an uncommon form of melanoma, histologically manifest by dermal melanocytes in a dense stromal response. These lesions are usually nonpigmented and usually have lost the melanin production pathway. They usually stain negative for MART-1/MelanA, gp100, and tyrosinase, but they do stain for S100. The lack of pigmentation and the dense stromal response often interfere with clinical and histologic diagnosis. It occurs most commonly in the head and neck, but it may occur in other body sites.[52] Desmoplastic melanoma may appear *de novo* as a nonpigmented skin papule or as a dermal/VGP component arising from a pre-existing lentigo maligna or other pigmented junctional lesion. Desmoplastic melanomas may have neurotropic features and have been associated with a high rate of local recurrence.[53]

However, recent reports suggest that if adequate margins are taken, the risk of local recurrence is low.

The overall mortality risk for desmoplastic melanomas is comparable to that of other invasive melanomas of similar depth of invasion.[54] However, the risk of lymph node metastasis is lower than for other invasive melanomas. One report from Memorial Sloan-Kettering Cancer Center found that sentinel node biopsies were negative for all of the 22 pure desmoplastic melanomas.[55] The same report found local recurrences in 7% of pure desmoplastic melanomas, compared with only 2% of other cutaneous melanomas. Multiple studies support the contention that desmoplastic melanomas have a significantly lower risk of nodal metastases than other melanomas,[55–59] with only 1.4% sentinel node positivity among 155 patients with pure desmoplastic melanoma, compared with 18.5% in those with mixed desmoplastic melanoma.[54,55,60] On the other hand, nodal metastases have been observed in patients with desmoplastic melanoma, and a recent report from the Sydney Melanoma Unit found no significant difference in these populations but single-digit percentages of sentinel node positivity for pure desmoplastic melanoma and mixed desmoplastic melanoma.[52] Thus, there is debate about whether to abandon histologic staging of regional nodes in patients with desmoplastic melanoma.[56] It may be appropriate at least to have a higher threshold for performing sentinel node biopsy (SNBx) in patients with pure desmoplastic melanoma.

Prognostic Factors for Primary Melanomas

The best predictor of metastatic risk is the depth of invasion, measured with an ocular micrometer, from the granular layer of the skin to the base of the primary lesion. This was originally described by Alexander Breslow[61] and remains an important factor in staging and prognostic stratification. However, many other histologic and clinical features have relevance for estimating the risk of future metastasis and mortality. These include age, angiolymphatic invasion, mitotic rate, gender, and body site.

Depth of Invasion

Clark et al.[62] and Breslow[61] defined the depth of invasion of a primary melanoma as an important histopathologic feature closely associated with risk of metastasis and death from melanoma. Clark et al.[62] defined depth based on the layer of skin to which the melanoma has invaded. Clark level I melanomas are melanomas *in situ,* limited to the epidermis or dermal/epidermal junction. Clark level II melanomas invade into the superficial (papillary) dermis, and these are usually RGP lesions. Clark level III melanomas fill the papillary dermis. Clark level IV

TABLE 119.1

MELANOMA TNM CLASSIFICATION

T Classification	Thickness (mm)	Ulceration Status	Mitotic Rate
T1a	≤1.0	No	Less than 1/mm^2
T1b		Yes	1 or more/mm^2
T2a	1.01–2.0	No	Any
T2b		Yes	Any
T3a	2.01–4.0	No	Any
T3b		Yes	Any
T4a	>4.0	No	Any
T4b		Yes	Any
N Classification	**No. Nodes with Metastasis**	**Presentation**	**Intransit or Satellite Metastasis(es)**
N1a	1	Clinically undetectable[a]	No
N1b	1	Clinically detectable[b]	No
N2a	2–3	Clinically undetectable[a]	No
N2b	2–3	Clinically detectable[b]	No
N2c	0	—	Yes
N3	≥4 or matted		—
N3	1 or more	Any	Yes
M Classification	**Metastatic Site**	**Serum LDH Level**	
M1a	Distant skin, subcutaneous or node	Normal	
M1b	Lung	Normal	
M1c	All other visceral	Normal	
M1c	Any	Elevated	

TNM, tumor, node, metastasis; LDH, lactate dehydrogenase.
[a]Clinically undetectable nodes are those diagnosed only with sentinel node biopsy or elective lymphadenectomy. They are referred to also as micrometastases, but this definition differs from the pathologist's definition of a micrometastasis as one that is <2 mm in diameter.
[b]Clinically detectable nodes are also referred to as macrometastases, but this is a different definition than the pathologist's definition based on a diameter >2 mm.
(Modified from ref. 64.)

melanomas invade into the deep (reticular) dermis and have significant metastatic risk. Clark level V melanomas are uncommon and contain invasion into the subcutaneous fat.

Breslow thickness is the depth of invasion measured from the granular layer of the epidermis to the base of the lesion. Melanoma cells involving adnexal structures are considered junctional and are not included in the Breslow depth. The current melanoma staging system of the American Joint Committee on Cancer (AJCC) identifies tumor (T) stage based on Breslow thickness such that T1 lesions are less than 1 mm thick, T2 lesions are 1 to 2 mm thick, T3 lesions are 2 to 4 mm thick, and T4 lesions are greater than 4 mm thick.[63]

Clark level does not add much additional prognostic value to Breslow thickness and has been removed from the 2010 version of the AJCC staging system.[64] Breslow thickness has an effect on survival, local, regional, and systemic recurrence rates, and that association is continuous, without any apparent breakpoints. Although the staging system requires categorization of thickness ranges, the continuous nature of the risk association should be kept in mind. Thickness is considered in defining the margins of excision for primary melanomas.[65,66]

Ulceration

Ulceration of the primary lesion has been identified as an important negative prognostic feature[65] and is incorporated in the current staging system such that T1a, T2a, T3a, and T4a melanomas are nonulcerated, and T1b, T2b, T3b, and T4b melanomas are ulcerated. In an analysis of prognostic features in a large multicenter database, the prognosis of an ulcerated lesion was comparable to that of a nonulcerated lesion one T level higher. Thus, the overall stage assignment groups ulcerated lesions with nonulcerated lesions one T level higher (e.g., T2b and T3a are both stage IIA). The staging system is summarized in Tables 119.1 and 119.2 and is described in detail elsewhere.[64]

Patient Gender and Skin Location of Primary Melanoma

The incidence of melanoma is similar for women and men; however, there is a slightly greater risk for men. Furthermore, for essentially all patient subgroups, the prognosis is better for women than men. Thus, among patients with stage III and IV melanoma, men outnumber women approximately 1.5:1. Women are more likely to have melanomas on the extremities, whereas men are more likely to have melanomas on the trunk and head and neck. The clinical outcome for patients with melanomas on extremities is better than that for patients with truncal or head-and-neck melanomas; thus, the prognostic impact of gender is difficult to distinguish from the impact of tumor location. There may still be, however, a prognostic benefit for female gender independent of tumor location.[65,67]

TABLE 119.2

PATHOLOGIC STAGE GROUPING FOR CUTANEOUS MELANOMA

Clinical Staging[a]				Pathologic Staging[b]				5-Year Survival (%)	10-Year Survival (%)
0	Tis	N0	M0	0	Tis	N0	M0	>99	>99
IA	T1a	N0	M0	IA	T1a	N0	M0	95	88
IB	T1b	N0	M0	IB	T1b	N0	M0	91	83
T2a	N0	M0		T2a	N0	M0	89	79	
IIA	T2b	N0	M0	IIA	T2b	N0	M0	77	64
T3a	N0	M0		T3a	N0	M0	79	64	
IIB	T3b	N0	M0	IIB	T3b	N0	M0	63	51
T4a	N0	M0		T4a	N0	M0	67	54	
IIC	T4b	N0	M0	IIC	T4b	N0	M0	45	32
III	Any T	Any N	M0	IIIA	T1–T4a	N1a	M0	70	63
				T1–T4a	N2a	M0	63	57	
			IIIB	T1–T4b	N1a	M0	53	38	
				T1–T4b	N2a	M0	50	36	
				T1–T4a	N1b	M0	59	48	
				T1–T4a	N2b	M0	46	39	
				T1–T4a,b	N2c	M0	N/A	N/A	
			IIIC	T1–T4b	N1b	M0	29	24	
				T1–T4b	N2b	M0	24	15	
				Any T	N3	M0	27	18	
IV	Any T	Any N	Any M	IV	Any T	Any N	M1a	19	16
				Any T	Any N	M1b	7	3	
				Any T	*Any N*	*M1c*	*10*	6	

N/A, not available.

[a]Clinical staging includes microstaging of the primary melanoma and clinical-radiologic evaluation for metastases. By convention, it should be done after complete excision of the primary melanoma with clinical assessment for regional and distant metastases.

[b]Pathologic staging includes microstaging of the primary melanoma and pathologic information about the regional lymph nodes after partial or complete lymphadenectomy. Pathologic stage 0 or stage IA tumors are the exception; they do not require pathological evaluation of the lymph nodes.

(Data from refs. 64 and 368.)

In addition, location of tumors has prognostic relevance in that head-and-neck melanomas have poorer prognosis than trunk or extremity melanomas, and melanomas on acral sites have poorer prognosis than other extremity sarcomas.[68] A particular location associated with poor prognosis is the mucosal melanoma. Anorectal, female genital, and head-and-neck melanomas of mucosal origin have a mortality risk of 68% to 89% over 5 years.[1,69,70]

Patient Age

The impact of age on prognosis is confusing. There is a greater risk of lymph node metastasis in young patients at the time of sentinel node biopsy,[71] especially for patients younger than age 35 years, but the melanoma-associated mortality risk increases with age for all thickness ranges.[1,65] This paradox has not been explained. It suggests a possible age-specific curative potential for patients with micrometastatic nodal disease. Alternatively, it is worth considering that the attribution of mortality to melanoma progression is not always straightforward. Older patients have other competing causes for death that could lead to earlier mortality in the presence of metastatic disease. Nonetheless, age does appear to have independent prognostic significance for melanoma patients.

Growth Pattern

Overall, nodular melanomas have the worst prognosis, associated with their diagnosis at a thicker stage. Lesser risk is associated with ALM, superficial spreading melanoma, and LMM, in that order, all associated with decreasing average Breslow thickness. Generally, the histologic growth pattern of melanoma has little prognostic relevance when Breslow thickness is taken into account. The VGP component appears to be the component of melanoma that determines metastatic risk, and these VGP components are similar, independent of the growth phase in the RGP component. LMMs are a possible exception, in that they appear to have a better prognosis than other histologic types, independent of thickness. Desmoplastic melanoma, superficial spreading melanoma, LMM, and ALM have comparable prognosis, for distant metastases and survival, when stratified by thickness.[55,71,72]

Mitotic Rate

It is reasonable to expect that the growth rate of melanomas is linked to the rate of tumor cell division. Accordingly mitotic rate in the dermal component has been identified as a negative prognostic feature, especially with six or more mitoses per square millimeter.[71,73] Similarly, dermal expression of Ki67, a molecular marker of proliferation, is associated with greater risk of metastasis.[74] For thin melanomas, the presence of any mitotic figures has been associated with metastatic risk, whereas the absence of dermal mitoses is associated with an excellent prognosis.[75] The current staging system incorporates mitotic rate in differentiating low-risk thin melanomas (T1a) from higher-risk thin melanomas (T1b), and data used to define the current staging system identify increasing risk with increasing mitotic rate for all thickness.[64]

Other Prognostic Factors

There is also evidence, and biologic rationale, that angiolymphatic invasion has negative prognostic significance[71] and that microscopic satellites are associated with poorer prognosis. Satellitosis is incorporated in the current staging system[64] but will be considered separately because it defines the patient as stage III and thus goes beyond assessment of risk factors of the primary lesion alone.

Unresolved Issues in Melanoma Staging

The current AJCC staging system is substantially improved when compared with the prior version. It is evidence-based and accounts for several important clinical and histopathologic findings that were previously appreciated but not incorporated in staging. However, several clinical settings are not fully addressed by the AJCC staging system. These include the following.

Positive Deep Margin on Biopsy

When a primary melanoma is diagnosed by shave biopsy, and the tumor extends to the deep margin, it is presumed that the melanoma was deeper than the original measured biopsy depth. Sometimes, on wide local excision there is residual melanoma with a greater depth than on the original biopsy. In that setting, it is appropriate to define the T stage based on the latter depth of invasion. However, in many cases, the wide excision does not reveal any more melanoma, or may reveal tumor that is more superficial. It is generally assumed that in those cases, any residual melanoma at the deep margin may have been destroyed by inflammatory changes after the biopsy. One approach for defining T stage in that setting is to call it TX. The other is to use the T stage of the original depth, even though that is incomplete. The latter has the advantage of distinguishing thin melanomas (e.g., a clinically thin melanoma with thickness <1 mm) from a thick melanoma (e.g., a 5-mm melanoma on shave biopsy, with positive deep margin). Thus, use of TX results in substantial loss of information for patients and their clinicians. The best solution is to avoid shave biopsies, but when they occur, it seems reasonable to stage based on the thickness level that is known, when no residual tumor is found on wide excision, while also noting that there was a positive deep margin.

Local Recurrence after Original Incomplete Excision

Some patients present with melanoma after excisional biopsy or destruction (e.g., cryotherapy) of a pigmented skin lesion that was believed to be benign (clinically or histologically) on initial review. When such a lesion recurs and is found to contain melanoma, re-review of the original biopsy is appropriate, if available. Staging of such recurrent melanomas, when the original lesion was not known to be melanoma, is not well addressed.

Skin or Subcutaneous Lesion without Junctional Involvement and without Known Primary Melanoma

This is addressed later in this chapter. Cutaneous or subcutaneous nodules that occur in the absence of junctional melanocytic change, and in the absence of any other known primary are among the most interesting presentations of melanoma. They may be in-transit metastases from primary melanomas that spontaneously regressed (stage IIIB), primary melanomas that arose from dermal nevi or that persisted in the dermis after arising from a partially regressed primary melanoma (stage IIB), or a distant metastasis from an unknown primary melanoma (stage IV, M1a). A review of experience with these lesions at the University of Michigan suggests that they behave more like primary tumors arising in the dermis or subcutaneous tissue.[76] In the current staging system, these are considered stage III.

GENERAL CONSIDERATIONS IN CLINICAL MANAGEMENT OF A NEWLY DIAGNOSED CUTANEOUS MELANOMA (STAGE I–II)

Most melanomas present as clinically localized lesions without clinical or radiologic evidence of metastatic disease. Nonetheless, some of these patients have occult metastases, and the definitive surgical management includes both therapeutic resection and pathologic staging evaluation for regional metastases. The vast majority of primary melanomas are diagnosed on histologic assessment of skin biopsy performed by a dermatologist or a primary care practitioner. The patient then presents to a surgeon or other physician for definitive treatment.

Clinical Evaluation and Radiologic Studies for Patients with Clinical Stage I–II Melanoma

In patients with clinically localized melanoma, there is a wide range of clinical practice in the appropriate radiologic staging studies to be performed. Certainly all patients with such disease should have a complete history and physical examination, with attention to symptoms that may represent metastatic melanoma, including headaches, bone pain, weight loss, gastrointestinal symptoms, and any new physical complaints. Physical examination should carefully assess the site of the primary melanoma for clinical evidence of persistent disease and should evaluate the skin of the entire region (e.g., whole extremity or quadrant of torso, or side of the face) for dermal or subcutaneous nodules that could represent satellite or in-transit metastases. Biopsy should be done for any suspicious lesions and with a very low threshold for biopsy. In addition, physical examination should include thorough evaluation of both the major regional nodal basins (e.g., epitrochlear and axillary for a forearm melanoma) and also any atypical lymph node locations, such as the triangular intermuscular space on the back for upper back primaries.

There is a great deal of uncertainty and debate about appropriate initial staging studies. National Comprehensive Cancer Network guidelines from 2010 recommend no staging radiographs or blood work for melanoma *in situ*, and recommend imaging for low-risk thin melanomas (stage IA) "only to evaluate specific signs or symptoms."[77] For clinical stage IB–IIA, no other imaging is recommended. For stage IIB–IIC melanoma, a chest radiograph (CXR) is suggested but optional, and other imaging is suggested only as clinically indicated.[77] More complete staging studies are suggested for stage III melanoma.[77]

CXR for asymptomatic patients with a new diagnosis of clinically localized melanoma yielded suspicious findings in 15% of patients, of whom only 0.1% had a true unsuspected lung metastasis.[78] In a similar study, the yield of true positive CXR was 0% of 248 patients.[79] In patients with stage IIB melanoma, initial staging computed tomograph (CT) scans identified occult metastasis that changed management in 0.7% of patients.[80] Even in patients with positive sentinel node biopsies, staging positron emission tomography (PET) scan identified no melanoma metastases in 30 patients, even though there were lymph node metastases in 16% of cases.[81] In patients with clinical T1b–T3b melanomas, true positive rates for all imaging studies was 0.3%, and false-positive rates were 50% to 100%

for CXR, 88% for CT and PET-CT scans.[82] Thus, there is a large body of data that argues that CXR, CT, and PET-CT are all of little or no value in initial staging of melanoma stage 0–IIIA. In addition to the data challenging the value of routine CT scans for staging asymptomatic melanomas, recent studies have documented that CT scans increase the risk of future malignancies, and this is appropriate to consider as well.

PET with fluorodeoxyglucose (FDG) has a role in staging patients with advanced melanoma,[1] but its role in earlier-stage disease is less clear both because it is expensive and because it is associated with substantial radiation exposure. In one study, patients with clinically localized melanomas greater than 1 mm thick, with local recurrence, or solitary in-transit metastases, FDG-PET scanning was performed prior to sentinel node biopsy. Sensitivity for detection of sentinel nodes was only 21%, although specificity was high (97%). In addition, 21% of patients had PET evidence of metastases, but none was confirmed by conventional imaging at that time, and the sensitivity for predicting sites of future disease recurrence was only 11%. Overall sensitivity for detecting occult stage IV disease was only 4%, and this is not recommended for initial staging.[83] These findings are similar to other experiences with PET imaging for intermediate-thickness melanomas.[84] The Memorial Sloan-Kettering experience is that in patients with clinically localized melanoma and metastases to sentinel nodes, radiologic staging studies identified distant disease in only 3.7% of patients and also resulted in indeterminate findings in 48% of patients.[85] Those with metastases were all patients who had melanomas at least 4 mm thick and had macrometastases (greater than 2 mm) in the sentinel nodes. That study recommends limiting aggressive staging workup (e.g., CT scans, PET, magnetic resonance imaging [MRI] of the brain) after positive SNBx to those patients with thick melanomas and macrometastases.

Despite the data-driven arguments against aggressive staging studies for melanoma, there still is a wide range of practice patterns in this regard, such that many patients with clinically localized melanomas undergo full staging studies. Patients typically want evidence that there is no metastasis, and this is undoubtedly a driver for these practices. An argument can be made that a CXR provides a lower-cost method for providing comfort to anxious patients that CT or PET-CT scans. Also, baseline CXR (posterior-to-anterior and lateral) may have the dual roles of screening for lung metastases and aiding in preoperative evaluation in the event that general anesthesia is indicated for the primary surgical management.

Also, some clinicians send blood for a complete blood count, for serum chemistries, including liver function tests, and for a lactate dehydrogenase (LDH) level, especially as they may be useful prior to surgery under general anesthesia. These also are of low clinical yield in terms of the melanoma but may detect unappreciated concurrent illness that may affect therapeutic decisions, including preoperative assessment. Specifically, if there is microcytic anemia, it should be worked up, with the differential diagnosis to include gastrointestinal metastasis of melanoma. Elevated LDH should prompt a more extensive staging workup, and elevated liver function tests should prompt a hepatobiliary ultrasound or CT scan unless there is another known explanation.

WIDE LOCAL EXCISION FOR CLINICAL STAGE I–II MELANOMA: GENERAL CONSIDERATIONS

Wide excision of the primary melanoma is performed to provide local control. Multiple randomized, prospective clinical trials support current recommendations for the extent of the margins of resection. The wide excision also provides an opportunity to evaluate the tissue adjacent to the primary lesion for microscopic satellites, which, if present, have clinical and prognostic significance.

There has been considerable debate about the appropriate margins of excision for primary melanomas, and it is helpful to understand the evolution of thought and data about this topic. In the early 1900s, melanoma was a rare disease, and when it was diagnosed, it was often locally advanced. Surgical resection was often associated with recurrence disease, and there were no guidelines for appropriate and successful surgical management of the primary lesion. In 1907, Handley[86] reported a study that involved histologic examination of tissue sections taken at varied distances from the primary melanoma in a human tissue specimen that he obtained from a patient with a large primary melanoma. In that study, he found microscopic evidence of melanoma cells as far as 5 cm from the primary tumor. He recommended wide re-excision of melanomas with a measured margin of 5 cm from the primary lesion. This recommendation became standard management for melanoma for many decades, with patients typically undergoing radical resections requiring skin grafts 10 cm or more in diameter.

As melanoma became a more frequent diagnosis, there was greater awareness of it, and lesions were often diagnosed at an earlier (thinner) stage. In addition, these large re-excisions usually contained no detectable melanoma cells separate from the primary lesion. These observations, and concern for the morbidity of large resections and skin grafts, led to a questioning of the need for 5-cm margins of resection. It is ironic that the origin of this aggressive resection practice was based on data from a single patient in a single study; however, limiting the margins of excision has required multiple large, randomized, prospective trials. These trials are summarized in Table 119.3 and are detailed in the follow sections.

CLINICAL TRIALS TO DEFINE MARGINS OF EXCISION FOR PRIMARY CUTANEOUS MELANOMAS

The World Health Organization (WHO) Melanoma Program Trial No. 10 randomized 612 melanoma patients with melanomas 2 mm or less in thickness to excision margins of 1 cm versus 3 to 5 cm.[87,88] Patients were stratified into two subgroups: Breslow depth less than 1 mm versus 1 to 2 mm. There were no differences in survival rates or in rates of distant recurrences with 1-cm margins versus 3- to 5-cm margins with follow-up beyond 15 years.[89] There were more local recurrences for the group with 1-cm margin (eight vs. three patients), but this was not a significant difference. There were no local recurrences for melanomas less than 1 mm thick treated with 1-cm margins. The lack of local recurrences with thin melanomas (<1 mm) after 1-cm margins of excision support this as a standard excision margin for T1 melanomas. The numerically slightly higher (but statistically insignificant) local recurrence risk with thinner margins for T2 melanomas has left questions about the appropriate margin for thicker lesions.

French and Swedish Cooperative Surgical Trials

The French Cooperative Group randomized 337 patients with melanomas up to 2 mm in thickness to 2- or 5-cm margins.[90] Ten-year disease-free survival rates were 85% and 83%, respectively, and 10-year overall survival rates were 87% and

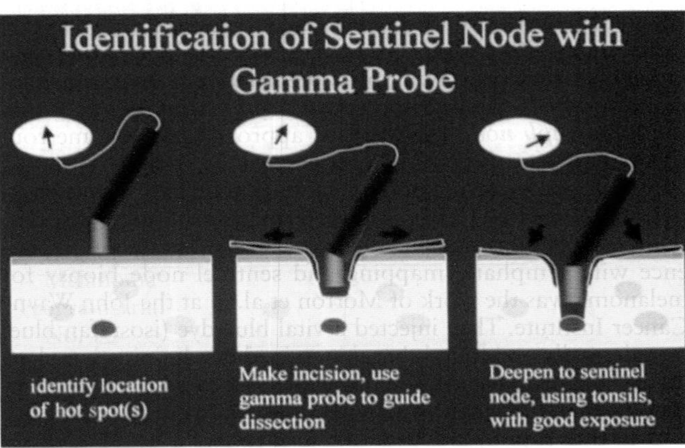

FIGURE 119.5 Schematic of a way to identify and to remove the sentinel node using a handheld gamma camera.

with radiocolloid plus blue dye. There is substantial multicenter and single-center experience with use of radiocolloid alone, which is associated with successful identification of the sentinel node(s) in greater than 99% of patients and with a mean of approximately two sentinel nodes per patient.[112] The effectiveness of blue dye alone is limited because some patients have drainage to lymph node basins that may not be predicted (e.g., drainage from the right upper back to the left axilla) or drainage to atypical nodal basins (e.g., the triangular intermuscular space on the back, epitrochlear or popliteal nodes, or subcutaneous "in-transit" nodes that are outside a traditional nodal basin).[97,113–115] Examples of unusual lymph node locations mapped by lymphoscintigraphy are shown in Figure 119.6. Thus, in the large majority of clinical settings, it is most appropriate to perform radiocolloid lymphoscintigraphy in lymphatic mapping for sentinel node biopsy of melanoma.

In experienced hands, lymphatic mapping should identify a sentinel node in 98% to 100% of cases, and it should be feasible to perform the sentinel node biopsy with minimal morbidity, on an outpatient basis, and in many cases under local anesthesia with sedation. The early reports of sentinel node biopsy stress a long learning curve, but as the technology of gamma probes has improved, the technique is less operator-dependent. In addition, lymphatic mapping has now been performed long enough that surgical residents trained since the mid-1990s typically have had experience with it for melanoma and for breast cancer. The standard evaluation of a sentinel node includes evaluation of multiple sections of the node, often combined with immunohistochemical staining for melanoma markers (e.g., S100, HMB45, tyrosinase, and/or MART-1/MelanA).

Typical results of SNBx reveal that the rate of positive nodes increases with increasing tumor thickness, as would be expected, from less than 5% for the thin melanomas that undergo SNBx (e.g., T1b lesions) to approximately 40% for thick melanomas. Current experience with SNBx in most series supports the prognostic value of SNBx in thick melanomas

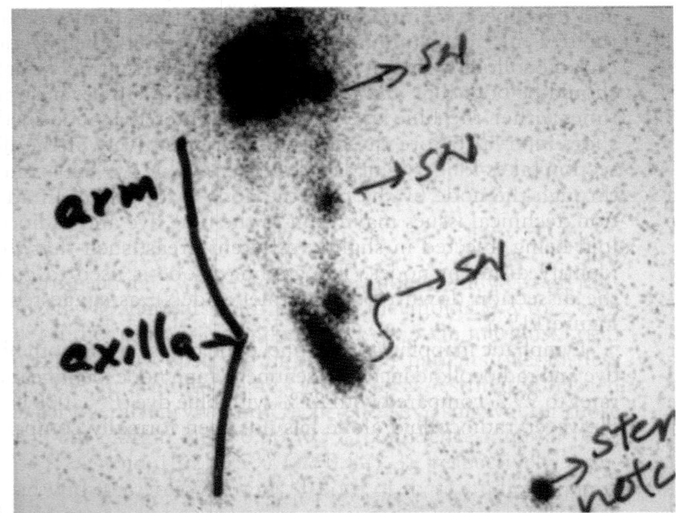

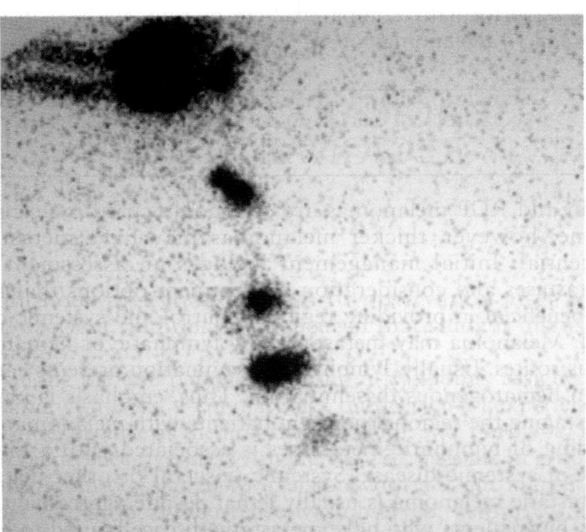

FIGURE 119.6 Lymphatic mapping from near the elbow along two separate lymphatic channels toward the axilla. An early image (**A**) shows the lymphatic channels clearly. A later image (**B**) shows the sentinel nodes clearly, but the channels are much less evident. One of the sentinel nodes is in subcutaneous tissue near the elbow and is almost missed due to proximity to the injection site (no. 4) (**C**). The two nodes near the axilla were actually just distal to the true axillary space. One of them was a true sentinel node (no. 2) and contained tumor (designated by the solid black node), whereas the other node near it was the third node in that lymphatic channel, so that the first node in that channel was truly sentinel (no. 4) and also contained tumor. The other two nodes downstream from no. 4 were both negative for tumor.

(>4 mm)[116] as well as in thinner lesions. When elective lymph node dissection was performed, it was typically recommended only for melanomas 1.5 to 4 mm thick. However, in the Duke experience, the relative risk of distant versus regional metastases is not dramatically higher for thick melanomas, and this supports a clinical approach that includes the potential for curative resection of regional metastases in these cases.[102] In addition, the low morbidity of SNBx supports a threshold for SNBx in thinner melanomas than the 1.5-mm criterion that was used for performance of ELND.

The overall rate of positive SNBx in most series (typically for melanomas >1 mm) is in the range of 15% to 25%. The percentage of patients with false-negative SNBx in experienced hands and with use of radiocolloid and the handheld gamma probe, with or without blue dye, is typically in the range of 1.9% to 4%.[111] The most rigorous definition of false-negative rate is FN/(FN + TP) (FN = false negative, TP = true positive), and 3% FN in the setting of 20% TP represents 13% false-negative rate. False-negative rates have been estimated by seeking nodes containing metastases in the remaining nodal basin after a negative sentinel node biopsy. In other settings, it is done by defining patients who return with clinically evident nodal metastases after a prior negative SNBx in the same node basin. These may or may not be equivalent. Nonetheless, there is a small percentage of patients who have negative SNBx who later return with nodal metastases in the same nodal basin. Although the procedure is very accurate and does identify the large majority of nodal metastases, it is prudent to follow patients for nodal recurrence even after a negative SNBx.

Lymphatic mapping and SNBx has been applied generally for all cutaneous sites and may also be useful for melanomas of mucous membranes.[117,118] A challenging area for SNBx is the head and neck. In particular, melanomas of the scalp and of the face may drain to parotid nodes or periparotid nodes, for which sentinel node biopsy is more complex, more technically challenging, and associated with greater potential morbidity. In addition, false-negative sentinel node biopsies are more common than in trunk and extremity melanomas, occurring in approximately 10% of patients, for a true false-negative rate that may approach 30%. However, in many cases, it can be performed reliably and still has a place in management.

More recent technology that offers promise for improving sentinel node localization are the development of mobile gamma cameras that can replace the single gamma detector of the gamma probe with an array of hundreds of detectors that permit real-time imaging that rivals that of the fixed gamma camera. This approach has the potential to improve identification of nodes in atypical locations and for ensuring adequate clearance of the sentinel nodes.[119,120] Also promising is single photon-emission computed tomographic (SPECT)-CT imaging, which can provide very discrete localization of sentinel nodes, which may be helpful in selected challenging locations.[121] Despite the high accuracy of sentinel node biopsy for nodal staging, the false-negative rate may be as high as 10% to 20%,[122] and these new technologies offer a possibility to reduce that false-negative rate.

In performing SNBx, melanoma metastases are sometimes clinically evident in the operating room as small pigmented spots just under the capsule of the node. When these are present, the hottest part of the node is usually precisely at that location (unpublished clinical observations). This may be particularly relevant for some large nodes, where the pathologist can be guided to the portion most at risk of metastasis for detailed histologic assessment (Fig. 119.7). Morton et al.[123] have formalized a technique that may identify the part of the node that is most likely to contain metastases, based on injecting carbon black dye and isosulfan blue dye. This has not yet become standard, but this or other refinements may further increase the accuracy of staging by this procedure.

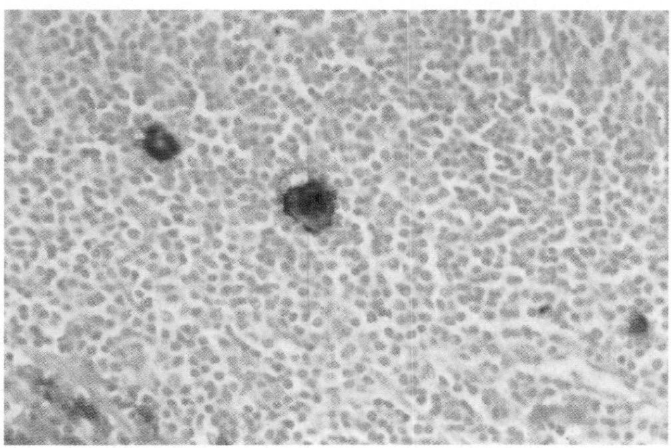

FIGURE 119.7 Immunohistochemical detection of isolated melanoma cells in a sentinel node when stained for the melanoma marker S100.

Another approach under investigation is to perform molecular analysis of sentinel nodes. Reverse transcriptase-polymerase chain reaction (RT-PCR) assay for melanocytic differentiation proteins (e.g., gp100 and tyrosinase) and cancer-testis antigens (e.g., MAGE-A3) permits detection of cells containing those molecules even when they are present below the limit of detection for current histopathologic sampling and immunohistochemistry. Early experience with RT-PCR analysis of sentinel nodes suggested a significant negative prognostic value for RT-PCR–positive, histology-negative nodes, and suggested that patients with RT-PCR–negative, histology-negative nodes have a remarkably high survival rate.[124] However, a larger multicenter experience with RT-PCR molecular staging of sentinel nodes in the Sunbelt Melanoma trial failed to demonstrate a similar benefit.[125] Nonetheless, this technology and other new molecular technologies are very likely to have a major role in the clinical management of patients with melanoma in the future, and such approaches may ultimately revolutionize risk assessment and selection for therapeutic interventions in ways that may well alter the current recommendations for surgical and systemic management. At present, however, such molecular approaches remain experimental.

The Multicenter Sentinel Lymphadenectomy Trial 1 was reported in 2006 as a randomized, prospective trial of 1,269 patients with melanomas 1 to 4 mm thick who were randomized to SNBx or observation in addition to wide local excision of the primary lesion.[109,126] The finding was that there was no difference in 5-year disease-specific survival (87.1% vs. 86.6%).[126]

One important consideration should be kept in mind, which is often overlooked in considering the potential value of SNBx and subsequent complete lymph node dissection (CLND). That consideration is the value to patients of regional control of their tumor, even in the absence of survival benefit. A study evaluating patients' perception of their own utilities for health states suggested that the development of recurrent disease markedly decreases patient perception of their health state, even if it does not impact survival.[127] This study thus suggests that regional tumor control may have value to patients, even in the absence of a survival benefit.

The rationale for performing SNBx for melanoma includes the following:

1. A negative sentinel node biopsy is a good prognostic indicator that may provide comfort to low-risk patients.

2. A positive sentinel node biopsy for patients with T1–T3a clinically N0 melanomas (clinical stage I–IIA) renders them candidates for adjuvant high-dose interferon therapy, which offers some clinical benefit.
3. Patients with T4 melanomas or with microscopic satellites (N2c, stage IIIB) are further upstaged by the finding of a positive sentinel node, which helps these patients in risk assessment and may make them candidates for selected clinical trials.
4. Many clinical trials require surgical staging of regional nodes, and, thus, sentinel node mapping makes patients candidates for trials that may prove to be of benefit.
5. Identification of melanoma in a sentinel node permits selection of patients for CLND to increase the chance of regional tumor control.
6. Excision of the sentinel node may be curative if there is no tumor beyond the node, even if CLND is not feasible. This hypothesis is being explored explicitly in the Multicenter Selective Lymphadenectomy Trial 2 (MSLT2).

Selection of Patients for Sentinel Node Biopsy

Sentinel node biopsy is generally recommended for patients with melanomas at least 1 mm thick. For thinner melanomas, there is debate about the appropriate criteria for performing sentinel node biopsy.[71] A common practice is to offer SNBx for thin melanomas with adverse prognostic features, including ulceration. The 2010 staging system also identifies a mitotic rate of 1 or greater as an adverse prognostic feature, and this is associated with higher risk of sentinel node metastasis.[64] Earlier data also support the relevance of mitotic rate as a prognostic factor in primary melanomas[73] or Clark level IV.[67] There is debate about performing sentinel node biopsy for thin melanomas that are in VGP, that have dermal mitoses, or that occur in young patients.[71,75] Also, there is rationale for offering sentinel node biopsy for melanomas less than 1 mm thick that have a positive deep margin on biopsy and thus are not fully evaluable for depth.

Pure desmoplastic melanomas have a similar overall metastatic and mortality risk as other melanomas, but their risk of regional nodal metastases appears to be lower than that of other melanomas.[54,128,129] Thus, it may be reasonable to limit SNBx for pure desmoplastic melanomas. However, there is limited experience with managing regional nodes in desmoplastic melanoma, and some desmoplastic melanomas can metastasize to regional nodes.[52]

Sentinel Node Biopsy Subsequent to a Prior Wide Local Excision

Sentinel node biopsy should be performed at the same procedure as wide local excision. However, there are some circumstances in which wide local excision may be performed without SNBx, and there is then a question of whether SNBx can be performed reliably after a prior wide local excision. Such circumstances include a thin melanoma on original biopsy, found to be deeper on re-excision or on second-opinion pathology review. A multicenter experience with 76 patients having SNBx performed after a prior wide local excision revealed a 99% success rate in SNBx, a mean yield of 2.0 sentinel nodes per patient, with a 15% overall sentinel node–positive rate, a 4% rate of melanoma recurrence in a negative mapped basin, and only a 1% rate of isolated first recurrence in a node. These and other data support performing SNBx after prior wide local excision, although performing it concurrently with the original wide local excision is preferred.[130,131]

MANAGEMENT OF CLINICALLY LOCALIZED MELANOMA

Management of Melanoma *in situ* (Clinical TISN0M0, Stage 0)

For melanomas confined to the epidermis and epidermal/dermal junction that are diagnosed as melanoma *in situ,* this is a lesion that is curable in the vast majority of cases by wide excision alone. On initial evaluation, the regional nodes should be examined, as should the skin and subcutaneous tissue between the primary site and these regional node basins. Melanoma *in situ* by definition is not invasive or metastatic; however, metastatic melanoma to regional nodes has been observed occasionally from melanoma *in situ* with histologic evidence of regression.[3] Thus, it is prudent to examine the nodes clinically. However, in the absence of clinical evidence of metastasis, there is no need to perform radiologic staging studies. Definitive management involves re-excision with a margin of 5 mm. The standard recommendation is to perform a full-thickness re-excision including underlying subcutaneous tissue, although there are no formal data that a full-thickness skin excision is less adequate for melanoma *in situ*. However, variation in thickness within the original biopsy specimen may lead to occult invasion that is not observed on the evaluated sections. Thus, it is prudent to perform a full-thickness excision of skin and subcutaneous tissue to the underlying deep fascia. A 5-mm margin is the standard recommendation, but melanoma *in situ* can extend beyond its visible extent. Thus, if cosmetically acceptable, it is reasonable to obtain a margin of as much as 1 cm, especially if the original biopsy was incomplete. If the margins are positive or close, re-excision to a widely clear margin is recommended. Sentinel node biopsy is not indicated. No adjuvant therapy is needed if the margins are widely clear.

Clinical Follow-Up after Surgical Treatment of Melanoma *in situ*

Melanomas *in situ* are curable in the vast majority of cases with surgery alone. However, they may very rarely may be associated with metastasis, probably attributable either to an invasive component that was not detected because of sampling error, or to an associated regressed invasive component.[3]

Thus, in accord with the guidelines of the National Comprehensive Cancer Network, it is appropriate to follow these patients for local recurrence, in-transit metastasis, or regional node metastasis on an annual basis. The risk of recurrence is not high enough to require specialty follow-up, but a focused physical examination of the patient by the primary care physician is appropriate. More important, patients with melanoma *in situ* are at increased risk of subsequent primary melanomas, and so close dermatologic follow-up with full-body skin examinations is recommended (Table 119.4).

MANAGEMENT OF THIN PRIMARY MELANOMA (CLINICAL T1A)

The classic definition of a thin melanoma was based on the original report of Breslow[61] of the association between depth of invasion (Breslow thickness) and subsequent risk of metastasis and death. In that report, patients with melanomas less than 0.76 mm thick had no subsequent metastasis. Thus, the definition of a thin melanoma had been a melanoma less than

TABLE 119.4

RECOMMENDATIONS FOR CLINICAL FOLLOW-UP AFTER DEFINITIVE THERAPY OF MELANOMA

Melanoma Stage	Clinical Follow-up[a]	Radiologic and Laboratory Follow-up
0	Annual	None needed
IA	Annual	CXR, CBC, LDH annually; CT scan or other radiologic workup of new findings
IB–IIA	Every 3–6 mo × 3 y, then 4–12 mo × 2 y, then annually	CXR, LDH, and CBC every 6–12 mo; CT scan or other radiologic workup of new findings
IIB–IIIA	Every 3–6 mo × 3 y, then 4–12 mo × 2 y, then annually	CXR, LDH, and CBC every 6–12 mo; CT scan or other radiologic workup of new findings; if lower extremity primary, CT pelvis or PET-CT to evaluate iliac nodes
IIIB–IIIC	Every 3–6 mo × 3 y, then 4–12 mo × 2 y, then annually	CXR, LDH, and CBC every 6–12 mo; CT scan or other radiologic workup of new findings; if inguinal nodes had been involved, get CT pelvis (or PET-CT) every 6–12 mo
IV	Every 2–3 mo × 2 y, then every 3–6 mo × 3 y, then annually	CT or PET-CT, plus MRI brain, LDH, and CBC every 3–6 mo, especially in areas of prior metastases

CXR, chest radiograph; CBC, complete blood count; LDH, lactate dehydrogenase; CT, computed tomography; PET, positron emission tomography; MRI, magnetic resonance imaging.

[a]Physical examination focused on regional skin and lymph nodes, history seeking new symptoms. For all patient subgroups, in addition, a total-body skin examination is recommended at least annually to screen for new primary lesions. Furthermore, self-examination is recommended monthly to include a full skin examination and examination of nodes near the primary melanoma. Follow-up should be for at least 20 y, and probably for life. (Modified and extended from 2005 National Comprehensive Cancer Network guidelines.)[369]

0.76 mm thick. However, subsequent studies have shown a continuous risk association with increasing thickness, without an absolute "cutoff" at 0.76 mm,[61] and melanomas less than 0.76 mm in thickness do have approximately a 5% risk of subsequent metastasis.[132] Additional studies have defined additional histopathologic features that affect the prognosis of thin melanomas. The current AJCC staging system addresses several prognostic features of thin melanomas such that T1a melanomas are those less than 1 mm thick, with less than one mitosis per square millimeter, and without ulceration. In the absence of any clinical evidence of metastasis, these are clinical stage IA melanomas and have a 5-year survival rate of 94%.[63,67]

The patient who presents with a thin melanoma should be examined with a focus on the primary site, the regional nodal basins, and in-transit locations, and a history should elicit any findings that may lead to suspicion of metastases (e.g., weight loss, fatigue, bone pain, headaches, change in appetite). In the absence of any clinical evidence of metastases, patients with thin melanomas (clinical T1a) do not need aggressive radiologic staging studies. A posterior-to-anterior and lateral CXR and an LDH level are adequate and may even be more than is necessary.[48] However, they provide valuable baselines for future follow-up and are of low cost and low morbidity. If there are signs or symptoms to suggest metastatic disease, they should be pursued as clinically indicated.

In most centers, the surgical management of patients with T1a melanomas includes wide excision with a 1-cm margin (including skin and all underlying subcutaneous tissue, to the deep muscle fascia). The margin should be measured from the visible edge of the pigmented lesion or from the biopsy scar, whichever is larger. Excisions of this size can almost always be closed primarily, with exceptions being on the face, palms, and feet, where skin grafts or rotation flaps may be needed.

Surgical Methods in Wide Local Excision (Applies for All Primary Melanoma Thicknesses)

For melanomas of the trunk and proximal extremities, wide local excisions should involve measuring the appropriate margin (usually 1 to 2 cm) around the entire scar from the biopsy, or from the visible edge of residual melanoma, and extending the incision to make an ellipse that is approximately three times as long as it is wide. Ideally, the direction of the scar should be longitudinal on the extremities, occasionally with some modification at joints, and should be along skin lines on the trunk and neck. On the upper back, it is usually best for the scar to run transversely, to minimize tension on it. When the initial biopsy scar is not in the direction that is desired for the final excision, an effective approach is first to mark out the oval shape that is required for the appropriate margins, then rather than extending that to an ellipse that is in the same direction, the ends of that oval can be extended in the desired direction, resulting in a sigmoid-shaped oval, which has two advantages: The closure results in a scar that is more in the desired direction, and the sigmoid shape allows the tension to be distributed in two directions. The excision should include all skin and subcutaneous tissue to the deep fascia, but not including the fascia. When a major cutaneous nerve runs along the deep fascia to innervate distal cutaneous structures, it is appropriate to preserve that nerve. Wide excisions can almost always be performed under local anesthesia, with or without intravenous sedation, in the patient who is thus motivated.

Special Considerations for Sentinel Node Biopsy. Sentinel node biopsy is not usually recommended for histologic staging of the regional nodes for patients with T1a melanomas. However, there is considerable controversy about what features of melanomas less than 1 mm thick may warrant sentinel node biopsy. The negative prognostic impact of ulceration and high mitotic rate support recommendation for sentinel node biopsy for ulcerated thin melanomas or thin melanomas with more than one mitosis per square millimeter. However for T1a lesions, sentinel node biopsy is not routinely recommended.

Clinical Follow-Up for Thin Melanomas (Stage IA)

There are no definitive data showing a survival advantage for close follow-up after surgical management of primary or metastatic melanoma; however, there is an expectation from patients to follow them, and there are treatable recurrences and metastases that can be identified best by physician follow-up. The National Comprehensive Cancer Network has issued useful guidelines for treatment and follow-up of melanoma.[77] The risk of metastasis for thin melanomas is in the 5% to 10% range, and less for RGP lesions. In the uncommon case of recurrent thin melanomas, the recurrences usually occur late, often beyond 5 years from diagnosis; the annual risk of recurrence is fairly constant over a long time,[32] so annual follow-up for many years is recommended rather than frequent follow-up in the first few years. Follow-up suggestions are listed in Table 119.4.

MANAGEMENT OF CLINICAL T2A, T2B MELANOMAS

Melanomas 1 to 2 mm thick, with or without ulceration, should be managed with an initial history and physical examination to elucidate signs or symptoms that could suggest metastatic disease. In the absence of such findings, these patients may be considered for preoperative staging with CXR and LDH. In those patients without evidence of metastasis, definitive management includes wide excision with a 1- to 2-cm margin and sentinel node biopsy. There are definitive data from the Melanoma Intergroup trial that a 2-cm margin is adequate for these patients,[106] and even a 1-cm margin was associated with the same survival as a 3-5 cm margin in long follow-up of the WHO Trial 10 (Table 119.3).[89] However, there has been a slight increase in local recurrence in patients with 1- to 2-mm lesions who had 1-cm margins (vs. 3- to 5-cm margins). This is not statistically significant in the patients studied, but it may signal a slight increase in local recurrence risk. When it is feasible to take a 2-cm margin without a skin graft (trunk and proximal extremities in most cases), this is recommended to minimize the chance of local recurrence. However, when the lesion is located on the face or distal extremities, where such a margin may be difficult to achieve without a skin graft, a 1- to 1.5-cm margin is acceptable. If a skin graft will be necessary even to close a 1-cm margin (rare), it is recommended that a 2-cm margin be taken because the morbidity and cost of the skin graft will already be needed. In addition, for lesions that are barely above 1 mm in depth (e.g., 1.03 mm), it certainly is reasonable to use a 1-cm margin.

Sentinel node biopsy is routinely recommended for patients with melanomas 1 to 2 mm thick. If the sentinel node biopsy is positive, then subsequent management should follow recommendations given later for stage IIIA melanoma (T2a with positive sentinel node biopsy involving one to three nodes) or stage IIIB melanoma (T2b with positive sentinel node biopsy involving one to three nodes). However, if the sentinel node biopsy is negative, then the patient is considered to have been pathologically staged as T2aN0M0 (stage IB) or T2bN0M0 (stage IIA), and no additional surgical management is required and no adjuvant systemic therapy is indicated, other than clinical trials.

MANAGEMENT OF CLINICAL T3A MELANOMAS (CLINICAL STAGE IIA)

Melanomas 2 to 4 mm thick, without ulceration, represent T3a lesions, and in the absence of metastases, these are clinical stage IIA lesions. They should be managed clinically with a history and physical examination as detailed previously and may be considered for a CXR and serum LDH level. Definitive management includes wide excision with a 2-cm margin and sentinel node biopsy for histologic staging of the regional nodes. If the sentinel node biopsy is negative, then no additional surgical or systemic therapy is indicated other than possible clinical trials. If the sentinel node biopsy is positive, then management for stage IIIA melanoma should be followed.

MANAGEMENT OF CLINICAL T3B MELANOMAS (CLINICAL STAGE IIB)

Melanomas 2 to 4 mm thick with ulceration represent T3b lesions and thus are clinical stage IIB melanomas. These are high-risk localized melanomas. Initial management should include a careful history and physical examination and at least a CXR and serum LDH level. Given the higher risk of synchronous metastases that may be detected at diagnosis, more aggressive systemic staging with CT scans of the chest, abdomen, and pelvis (or PET-CT scan) plus MRI scan of the brain may be indicated if there are symptoms or signs suggestive of systemic metastasis.

In the absence of clinical evidence of metastasis, definitive management is wide excision with a 2-cm margin and a sentinel node biopsy. If the nodes are negative, the summary stage is IIB (T3bN0M0). For these patients, no additional surgical therapy is needed. However, high-dose interferon (HDI) therapy has been approved for use as postsurgical adjuvant therapy for patients with resected stage IIB-III melanoma. Thus, these T3b melanoma patients are eligible for HDI. It is worth noting that the randomized clinical trials of adjuvant HDI were performed before the recent revision of the AJCC staging system, when ulceration was not incorporated in the staging system. Thus, the stage IIB patients in whom HDI was tested did not include the current T3bN0 patients. Nonetheless, it is available for such patients, whose risk is comparable to that of patients with nonulcerated thick melanomas (T4aN0). Patients with stage IIB melanoma often are also candidates for some experimental adjuvant systemic therapies. These are discussed later in the section, Adjuvant Systemic Therapy (Stages IIB, IIC, III).

MANAGEMENT OF THICK MELANOMAS (T4A, T4B, GREATER THAN 4 MM THICK)

Thick melanomas have been commonly associated with a risk of metastasis and mortality in the range of 50% over 5 to 10 years. Ulceration increases this risk: T4a melanomas are clinical stage IIB, and T4b melanomas are clinical stage IIC. Initial workup should include a history and physical examination, CXR, and serum LDH plus more aggressive radiologic imaging as indicated by signs and symptoms. For these high-risk patients consideration should be given to more complete staging with CT scans of the chest, abdomen, and pelvis plus MRI of the head. Definitive management includes wide excision with at least a 2-cm margin plus sentinel node biopsy. There are no definitive prospective, randomized data regarding margins for melanomas thicker than 4 mm, but margins of at least 2 cm are recommended. The general experience is that 2-cm margins provide adequate local control for these lesions, suggesting that the strong data supporting the adequacy of 2-cm margins in 1- to 4-mm melanomas may be extrapolated to thicker lesions. The adequacy of 2- to 3-cm margins is supported by retrospective data from M. D. Anderson Cancer Center and Lakeland Regional Cancer Center.[133]

During the era of routine elective lymph node dissection, elective node dissections were recommended for melanomas 1 to 4 mm thick, and thicker lesions were not recommended for elective node dissection because the risk of systemic metastasis was believed to be disproportionately higher for these patients than for those with intermediate-thickness lesions. However, this finding has been challenged by the Duke experience, in which the risks of regional and systemic metastasis increased in parallel as the primary tumor thickness increased.[102] In addition, as sentinel node biopsy has been employed routinely since the early 1990s, most studies show that sentinel node status has independent prognostic value for patients with thick melanomas.[133] Because these patients have a high risk of sentinel node positivity (approximately 35% to 40%), there is a high chance of regional nodal recurrence, and sentinel node biopsy, followed by CLND, offers the prospect of increasing the chance of regional control.

In patients with negative sentinel nodes, adjuvant HDI should be considered because it is approved by the U.S. Food and Drug Administration (FDA) for these patients. This should be discussed in detail with patients. Patients who are not candidates for HDI or who refuse HDI may be candidates for experimental adjuvant therapies.

SPECIAL CONSIDERATIONS IN MANAGEMENT OF PRIMARY MELANOMAS

Primary Melanomas of the Head and Neck

For melanomas on the head and neck, there are important anatomic constraints, and there are times when the optimal margins are not feasible (e.g., a 2-cm margin for a lesion 1 cm below the eye), but to the extent possible, the optimal margins should be obtained and closed with an advancement flap, skin graft, or limited rotation flap. In the unusual circumstance of a large-diameter lentigo maligna on the face that is not amenable to surgical resection because of cosmetic results or comorbid patient conditions, it may be treated with superficial or Grenz x-rays with local control rates reported above 90%.[134] Anecdotal reports of off-label topical treatment with imiquimod ointment have also resulted in effective local control of superficial melanomas.[135,136] This is being used increasingly, with good results in reported experience, but recurrence may occur.[137] Initial experience suggests that imiquimod is not effective at eradicating dysplastic nevi.[138] Desmoplastic melanomas commonly occur in the head and neck region and may have reported local recurrence rates up to 40% to 60% after resection.[139] Other series vary substantially in local recurrence rates of desmoplastic melanomas. One reports local recurrences as first recurrences in 14% of patients, which exceeds that of other histologic types,[56] and another reports no difference in local recurrence rates compared to other melanomas, although the presence of neurotropism was associated with higher risks of local recurrence.[59] An explanation for the high local recurrence rates in some series of desmoplastic melanoma may include inadequate margins of excision because of anatomic constraints in the head and neck. In addition, because desmoplastic melanomas are usually amelanotic, the surgical margins may be underestimated, and the histologic appearance of desmoplastic melanoma can interfere with accurate detection of microscopically positive margins, especially in fibrotic skin. Thus, in patients with desmoplastic melanoma, every effort should be made to obtain adequate margins. If that is not possible, postoperative adjuvant radiation should be considered with 2- to 3-cm margins around the resected lesion because this may reduce subsequent local recurrences.[139]

Neurotropic melanomas of the head and neck have a propensity to recur at the skull base by tracking along cranial nerves, and postoperative adjuvant radiation including the resection bed and the cranial nerve pathway should be considered for this variant.

Primary Melanomas of the Mucous Membranes

Mucosal melanomas of the head and neck, anorectal region, and female genital tract are usually diagnosed when they are thick. They are associated with high risks of distant metastases and death, approaching 100%. They are also associated with high risks of local recurrence and regional nodal metastases. Staging of these lesions is not addressed completely in the AJCC staging system for cutaneous melanomas, but there are general similarities that can be applied to mucosal melanomas. The depth of invasion is difficult to measure because they are often biopsied in a fragmented way, but they usually are deep lesions, with depths often of 1 cm or more. They should be resected with wide margins if possible. Resection of melanomas of the nasopharynx, oropharynx, and sinuses is limited by the bony structures of the skull and the base of the brain. Vulvovaginal melanomas may be widely resected in many cases but may also be constrained by efforts to preserve urinary and sexual function. They may also be associated with extensive radial growth in addition to the invasive lesion, which can lead to multifocal local recurrences. Anorectal melanoma may usually be resected widely by an abdominoperineal resection, but this morbid operation is not associated with higher survival rates than local excision only.[140] Adjuvant local radiation therapy may be of value when widely clear margins are not feasible.[141] However, no randomized, prospective trials of radiation have been performed in this setting. Sentinel node biopsy has been performed for vulvovaginal melanomas, but its impact on ultimate clinical outcome is not known.[118] It may also be performed for anorectal melanomas,[142] but pelvic and systemic metastases are more concerning for ultimate outcome than the risk of groin metastases. Sentinel node biopsy is not generally feasible for mucous membrane melanomas of the head and neck because of technical considerations.

Mucosal melanomas have not specifically been tested for their response to interferon therapy, but they are considered eligible for interferon, which is reasonable to consider after resection of thick mucosal melanomas with or without lymph node involvement. These patients may also be eligible for clinical trials in the adjuvant setting.

Primary Melanomas of the Fingers and Toes

For melanomas of the plantar aspect of the foot, especially on the anterior weight-bearing surface or on the heel, skin grafts are inadequate for bearing the weight of walking. Thus, it is often effective to rotate the skin of the instep of the foot to cover defects in those areas, with skin grafting of the instep area if needed.

For subungual melanomas of any finger or toe, the appropriate management is amputation at the interphalangeal joint of the toe or just proximal to the distal interphalangeal joint of the finger. Even for subungual melanomas *in situ,* such an amputation is indicated. These lesions often are found to contain invasion on the final specimen that is not evident on original biopsy, and it is not feasible to resect the entire nail bed with any margin without taking the bone of the distal phalanx because the two are intimately associated. It is important for amputations of the fingers, especially the thumb, to attach the severed deep flexor tendon to the remaining proximal phalangeal bone, to retain adequate flexor strength after surgery. This can be done by passing a braided multifilament suture through the phalangeal bone and the ligament via holes drilled in the bone in two places. The skin incision for these amputations can be designed by measuring 1 to 2 cm (depending on thickness) from the nail bed and including at least that amount of skin with the amputation. This almost always leaves some skin on the plantar or palmar surface (except when the subungual melanoma has extended well out onto the plantar/palmar surface) that can be used to close the surgical defect and provides a sturdy skin surface.

For melanomas of the proximal toe or finger, the considerations are similar to those for distal and subungual digital melanomas. For melanoma of the toe, amputation of the toe is usually the best choice because the functional morbidity of losing a toe is small. The exception is the great toe, but even amputation of that toe is feasible, although retention of the first metatarsal head is valuable for gait and balance. For small-diameter, thin melanomas proximally located on the fingers, and for toes when appropriate, it occasionally may be feasible to perform a wide excision and skin grafting (rarely primary closure) with preservation of the digit.

Sentinel node biopsies can be performed accurately from these lesions and should usually be performed for melanomas of the fingers or toes if they are at least T1b lesions.

THE ROLE OF RADIATION THERAPY IN THE MANAGEMENT OF PRIMARY MELANOMA LESIONS

The general management of primary melanoma lesions is surgical resection. However, there is a role for definitive or adjuvant radiation therapy in certain histologic variants including lentigo maligna, desmoplastic melanoma, or neurotropic melanoma and for palliation of unresectable primary disease. Lentigo maligna commonly occurs as a large lesion in the head and neck region of elderly patients. If the patient is medically inoperable or if the proposed resection would result in a poor cosmetic outcome, he or she can be treated with superficial or Grenz x-rays with local control rates above 90%.[134] Desmoplastic melanomas also commonly occur in the head and neck region and have high local recurrence rates. Postoperative adjuvant radiation may be delivered with 2- to 3-cm margins around the resected lesion if margins are inadequate, or following resection of a locally recurrent lesion, and thus as this can substantially reduce subsequent local recurrences.[139] Neurotropic melanomas of the head and neck have a propensity to recur at the skull base by tracking along cranial nerves, and postoperative adjuvant radiation including the resection bed and the cranial nerve pathway should be considered for this variant. Large unresectable primary lesions should be considered for palliative radiation therapy or be enrolled onto clinical trials.

Studies to improve locoregional tumor response of melanoma to radiation are ongoing. Duke University reported the results of a single institution randomized trial for patients with superficial melanomas (<3 cm depth) comparing treatment with concurrent hyperthermia and radiation versus radiation alone. One hundred twenty-two patients were randomized, including patients with and without prior radiation. They reported complete response rates for previously untreated patients of 66% and 42% treated with concurrent hyperthermia and radiation versus radiation alone, respectively. Hyperthermia improved the complete response rate of previously irradiated patients to 68% compared with 24% for patients treated with radiation alone.[143] In a small series, intralesional β-interferon injections and concurrent radiation has been reported to result in complete regression of disease in 12 of 17 patients with locoregionally advanced and unresectable melanoma.[144] The concurrent use of interferon-α2b with radiation or its use 1 month following radiation has been reported to cause increased radiation toxicity and should be used cautiously.[145,146]

CLINICAL FOLLOW-UP FOR INTERMEDIATE-THICKNESS AND THICK MELANOMAS (STAGE IB–IIC)

Suggestions for follow-up are listed in Table 119.4. For intermediate-thickness melanomas, history and focused physical examination may be done as often as every 3 months and as infrequently as annually, with CXR, LDH, and complete blood count at least annually, and other scans done as indicated for symptoms. CT or PET-CT is not likely to have much yield if the other studies and clinical examination are all unremarkable. However, there are circumstances in which they may be useful. Especially for the high-risk primary (e.g., T4b) on the lower extremity, pelvic CT scan or PET-CT may be helpful in identifying iliac nodal recurrences that are difficult to detect on examination. In addition, for high-risk melanomas, brain MRI may be helpful in detecting small brain metastases when they are asymptomatic and amenable to treatment with gamma knife radiation therapy.

Most first recurrences will be in local skin, in-transit skin, or lymph nodes, which can be detected on physical examination and can be treated surgically with some chance of cure. The most common first sites of visceral metastasis are lung and liver. Other frequent sites of metastasis include the gastrointestinal tract, brain, bone, distant skin or nodes, and adrenal glands. Clinical follow-up should elicit any information on headaches, weight loss, change in appetite, bone pain, or other symptoms that could be associated with these metastatic sites. There should be a low threshold for performing radiologic studies to work up such symptoms. However, routine extensive scans have not been shown to improve clinical outcome. In a study of follow-up for patients with stage II-III melanoma, melanoma recurrences were detected based on symptoms in 68%, physical examination findings in 26%, and CXR in 6%.[147] In another study of patients with stage I-II melanoma followed with physical examination, blood tests, and CXR, recurrences were detected by physical examination (72%), patient symptoms (17%), and CXR (11%).[148] The diagnostic yield of laboratory tests is low, but elevations of LDH or other liver function tests may signal a liver metastasis or other new metastasis. New microcytic anemia can be a first sign of gastrointestinal blood loss due to a small bowel metastasis.

REGIONALLY METASTATIC MELANOMA (STAGE III): LYMPH NODE METASTASIS, SATELLITE LESIONS, AND IN-TRANSIT METASTASES

Melanoma has a high propensity to regional metastasis in any of several presentations, all presumably via intralymphatic dissemination. These are the most common first metastases. The presence of regional metastasis is a negative prognostic finding; however, there is some chance of long-term disease-free survival and cure for patients with regional metastases, and they should be managed with curative intent whenever feasible.

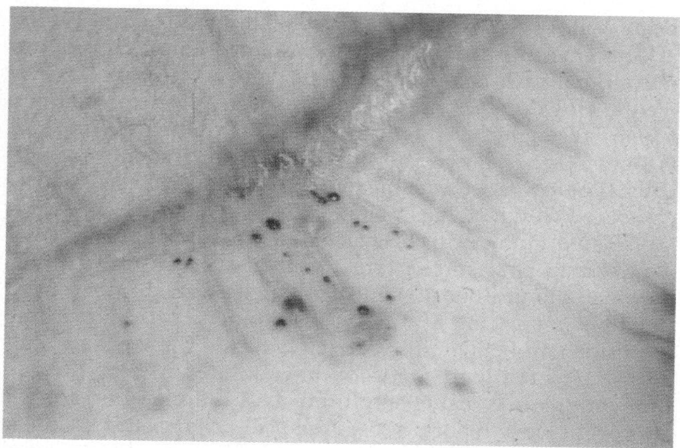

FIGURE 119.8 Local and satellite metastases after wide excision of melanoma on the chest.

There is a wide range of outcomes for patients who develop regional (stage III) metastases. Prognostic features of the primary melanoma have been associated with clinical outcome even after the development of metastases.[149] However, in the assessment of prognosis of stage III melanoma patients performed for the current AJCC staging system, only ulceration of the primary lesion had independent prognostic impact,[63,65] and this has been incorporated in the staging system.

Regional metastases are defined as follows:

- *Local recurrence* is best defined as recurrence of melanoma in the scar from the original excision or at the edge of the skin graft if that was used for closure.
- *Satellites metastases* may occur either simultaneously with the original diagnosis or arise subsequent to original excision. Typically, recurrences that are separate from the scar but within 2 to 5 cm of it are considered satellite metastases (Fig. 119.8)
- Regional recurrences beyond 5 cm of the scar but proximal to regional nodes are considered *in-transit metastases* (Fig. 119.9)
- *Regional node metastases* are typically in a draining nodal basin that is near the lesion.

Thus, for example, melanomas of the forearm usually drain to an axillary node. However, the most proximal regional node may be an epitrochlear node or simply a subcutaneous node in an atypical location. With the use of lymphoscintigraphy and sentinel node biopsy routinely in melanoma, such atypical nodal locations are increasingly defined (Fig. 119.6).[114] It is occasionally difficult to distinguish whether an in-transit metastasis is a regional skin metastasis or a true nodal metastasis.

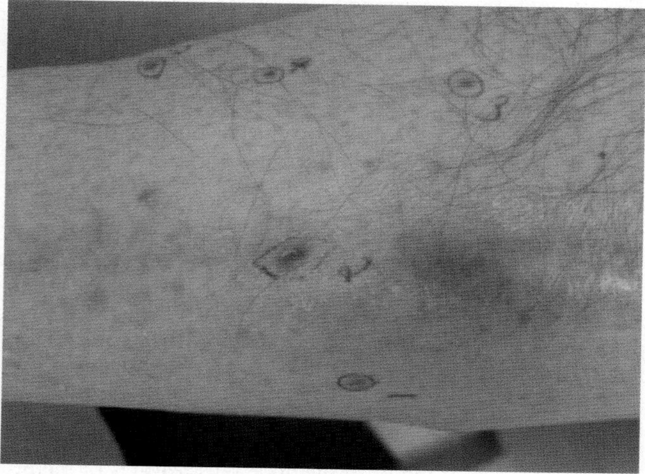

FIGURE 119.9 Close-up view of in-transit metastases involving the dermis, along the skin of the leg.

Management of Local Recurrence

Local recurrence is common after a primary lesion is inadequately excised. This type of local recurrence thus represents a failure of initial surgical management and may not represent the same high risk of distant metastasis and mortality that is associated with local recurrence after what is otherwise considered adequate surgical resection. However, after adequate wide excision, local recurrences are associated with a very poor prognosis. In the Intergroup melanoma trial, local recurrences were associated with 9% to 11% overall 5-year survival rate, as compared with 86% for those without local recurrence.[93]

Despite the bad prognosis associated with local recurrences, some patients either may be cured or may have extended tumor control by surgical resection. It is best to re-resect the entire scar down to the level of fascia, and perhaps including fascia, because there may be more tumor in the scar than is clinically evident, and this type of resection can generally be performed with minimal morbidity. Excision with a 1- to 2-cm margin is reasonable if the recurrences are limited to the scar. In the setting of associated satellite metastases, more extensive resection may be appropriate with a skin graft. In patients with concurrent distant disease, a less aggressive approach to the local recurrence may be justified, and simple excision to a clear margin may be acceptable. In addition, it is appropriate to consider sentinel node biopsy by mapping from the site of the local recurrence.[150] This is usually successful even if there has been a prior sentinel node biopsy or a prior CLND. This may enable regional control in such high-risk patients in whom the sentinel nodes may be positive in up to 50% of cases.[150] Unresectable recurrent lesions should be considered for palliative radiation therapy.

Management of Satellite and In-Transit Metastases

The presence of in-transit or satellite metastases is a negative prognostic feature, with clinical outcomes similar to those observed for patients with palpable nodal metastases. Satellite and in-transit metastases have comparable biologic and prognostic significance to each other.[151–153] When a patient presents with a solitary in-transit metastasis or a localized cluster of in-transit metastases, it is reasonable to perform excision of this along with sentinel node biopsy. The margin of excision should be adequate to obtain free margins. This usually requires a 5- to 10-mm margin. A fairly frequent clinical scenario that is difficult to manage is the patient with multiple in-transit metastases. This most commonly occurs in the lower extremity from primary lesions below the knee, but it may occur in other locations. There is no ideal management for such patients because the natural history almost always involves systemic dissemination of disease, which may occur simultaneously, within a few months, or many years after the in-transit metastases. The large majority of such patients will continue to develop new in-transit metastases over time, and so true control of this process is uncommon. However, there is no reliable systemic therapy for this process; thus, surgery remains the best first option for regional control, when feasible. In some scenarios, surgical management of a symptomatic lesion may be valuable for palliation while addressing the appropriate management of other in-transit disease.

When the number of such metastases is small, it is reasonable to excise them under local anesthesia. Follow-up every 2 to 3 months is usually advisable because new, small, in-transit metastases often occur in that interval and can be excised in the clinic with minimal morbidity. The surgical management of these lesions is limited by the lack of redundant skin in the leg, especially below the knee, and by the frequent appearance of lymphedema in the involved extremity. These factors limit the ability to close excisions done with wide margins. In more advanced cases, it may even be impossible to close the skin after very limited excisions. Options include limited excisions with primary closure, excisions with skin grafting, and excisions followed by leaving the wounds open to granulate in at home. These in-transit metastases can usually be excised with narrow margins, and even with tumor abutting the margin, the patients are more likely to develop new in-transit metastases in different locations on the extremity than to experience recurrence at the same site. Thus, it is reasonable to perform simple excisions with clear margins. For those isolated in-transit metastases, there also is an argument for performing sentinel node biopsy from the site of the metastasis.[150]

Because these patients typically continue to progress with more in-transit metastases and shorter intervals between metastases, other options for management are needed. Radiation therapy may be considered after surgical resection in this setting. Other regional options include intralesional therapy with interferon-α, interleukin-2 (IL-2), or bacillus Calmette-Guérin (BCG) or topical treatment of superficial metastases with imiquimod, all of which can induce responses in the treated lesions and occasionally in untreated lesions.

Thus, the usual recommendations are to perform limited excisions when feasible and to consider isolated limb perfusion or infusion (see later discussion) if that fails and the patient remains free of evidence of systemic metastases. It is tempting in such cases to consider amputation of the extremity, and this may be associated with long-term, disease-free survival in some patients. However, the high likelihood of concurrent occult systemic disease in these patients is a disincentive to such a disabling procedure. Nonetheless, amputation of the extremity may be discussed with a patient, and it may be appropriate in very selected cases. We performed amputation of the leg in one patient who had extensive in-transit recurrences covering most of the skin of the left lower extremity and who also had tumor filling the femoral vein and artery, making her ineligible for isolated limb perfusion. She has remained clinically free of disease without other therapy for almost a decade. We also performed an amputation in a patient with extensive muscle involvement in addition to cutaneous metastases and whose leg was paralyzed from childhood polio; the patient was not disabled significantly by the surgery. However, these are certainly the extreme exceptions.

Isolated Limb Perfusion and Infusion

An option for management of some patients with extensive regional recurrences in an extremity is isolated limb perfusion with melphalan or isolated limb infusion. Isolated limb perfusion can lead to complete responses in 60% to 90% of patients, with complete responses reported in 25% to 69% of patients.[154,155] Some patients will fail to respond and others may have short-duration responses, but a subset of patients may have durable complete responses and long-term survival.[154,156] Retreatment with isolated limb perfusion or infusion is feasible with some benefit. There also is some morbidity associated with isolated limb perfusion, including a low risk of limb loss.[89] Isolated limb perfusion may also shrink an unresectable recurrence, rendering it resectable. Tumor necrosis factor-α has been explored as a regional therapy agent for use in combination with melphalan in isolated limb perfusion for melanoma, with some encouraging findings in initial assessments. However, a randomized, prospective clinical trial performed through the American College of Surgeons Oncology Group, Z0020, showed no improvement in response rates or clinical outcome with melphalan plus tumor necrosis factor-α compared with melphalan alone.[155]

Isolated limb perfusion has also been studied in the adjuvant setting after surgical treatment of a primary melanoma on the extremity, but no benefit was seen with this therapy in the adjuvant setting.[157] Because the toxicity of isolated limb perfusion can be high in some patients and the logistical hurdles to isolated limb perfusion have limited its use, isolated limb infusion is being explored as a simpler but similar approach. Early reports suggest clinical response rates similar to those of isolated limb perfusion, but there has been limited experience and follow-up.[158,159]

Management of Regional Lymph Node Metastases

In patients with metastases to regional nodes, prognosis is related to tumor burden in the nodes and the number of nodes involved with tumor. In numerous studies, the number of metastatic nodes is the dominant prognostic factor in stage III melanoma.[65,160] The extent of lymph node involvement has been studied in various ways. For the current staging system, differentiation was made between clinically occult metastases (sentinel node positive, clinically negative) and clinically positive (palpable) metastatic nodes. This was a significant prognostic distinction.[63,65] Patients with nonulcerated primary melanomas and one positive sentinel node are stage IIIA, and 5-year survival probability is significantly better than 50%. However, a palpable node represents stage IIIB disease. Prognosis also is worse for patients with four or more tumor-involved nodes or with satellite or in-transit metastases in addition to nodal metastases (stage IIIC).

Management of Patients after a Positive Sentinel Node Biopsy (Stage IIIa if Nonulcerated Primary Lesion, One to Three Positive Nodes)

The rationale for performing SNBx, when first developed, was to avoid the morbidity of CLND in the 80% to 85% of patients with negative regional nodes, but simultaneously to stage patients accurately and to select those patients with regional nodal metastasis for CLND. However, experience with SNBx for melanoma has been that most patients with positive sentinel nodes have only one positive node, and only about 15% of patients have melanoma metastases identified in CLND specimens.[161] This finding has prompted consideration of abandoning CLND for some patients after positive SNBx. Review of data from the National Cancer Database showed that only about 50% of patients with positive sentinel nodes in the United State undergo CLND.[162] Thus, there is a wide range of practice without clear consensus. Several studies have identified features of the positive sentinel node that predict a low risk of a positive CLND, with the suggestion that CLND may not be necessary in such situations. Features such as the number of positive sentinel nodes, the tumor burden, and the location of tumor in the node plus features of the primary melanoma all are associated with greater risk of positive non-sentinel nodes.[163]

However, most clinical experience with SNBx and evaluation of non-sentinel nodes is complicated by the fact that sentinel nodes are evaluated by a much more rigorous histopathologic approach than non-sentinel nodes, and thus the incidence of positive non-sentinel nodes may be greater than the reported 15%. One study used multiantigen RT-PCR to evaluate non-sentinel nodes from patients whose formal pathology report was negative for melanoma and found molecular evidence of melanoma metastases in 54% of these patients.[164] This PCR approach is typically more sensitive than standard histology and may detect positive nodes that have such a low tumor burden as to be clinically insignificant. However, the current limited data suggest that the true rate of positive non-sentinel nodes after a positive SNBx may be somewhere between 15% and 50%.

The standard recommendation has been to perform CLND of any lymph node basin with a positive sentinel node for melanoma.[165] However, some patients refuse to have CLND or are not eligible for it because of medical contraindications. A recent article summarized the combined experience from 16 institutions and reported on the clinical outcome of 134 patients who had positive sentinel node biopsies but who did not undergo completion lymph node dissections.[166] Their outcomes were compared with a cohort of patients with positive sentinel nodes who did undergo completion lymph node dissection. At a median follow-up of 20 months, 15% of patients had developed recurrent melanoma in lymph nodes as a component of a first recurrence. This was not significantly different from the outcome in patients who underwent CLND.[166] Thus, there is now justification for reconsidering the best surgical management after positive sentinel node biopsy. Donald Morton has initiated the Multicenter Sentinel Lymphadenectomy Trial 2 (MSLT2), which is randomizing patients with positive SNBx to (1) CLND or (2) close observation with lymph node basin ultrasound.[166a] This trial will take several years to accrue and additional years for mature data. Until then, there will likely be evolution of perspectives about CLND after SNBx. There is support both for CLND and for close observation after positive SNBx, and thus equipoise exists for the MSLT2 trial.

Management of Palpable Metastatic Melanoma in Regional Nodes: Therapeutic or Completion Lymphadenectomy

The other clinical settings for lymphadenectomy include various presentations with clinically evident regional nodes: after a negative sentinel node biopsy, after observation of a nodal basin, or from an unknown primary melanoma. If lymph node recurrence appears after a prior complete dissection in the same basin, the surgical management may include a repeat node dissection, but if there is confidence that the original dissection was thorough, the repeat procedure may be more limited to the site of evident tumor recurrence.

Metastasis to a regional node represents stage III (A, B, or C) disease and is associated with a subsequent risk of distant metastasis in the range of 40% to 80%. Nonetheless, there is a significant chance of cure after complete lymphadenectomy for stage III melanoma,[102,160] with overall 25-year survival rates of 35%.[167] Thus, lymphadenectomy for stage III melanoma is performed with curative intent. However, even if the patient develops distant disease in the future, there is benefit in achieving regional control, which is obtained in about 90% of patients.[102] When regional nodal disease is left in place, it can become extensive, with skin involvement, even ulceration, and with extension to involve major neurovascular structures. An example of extensive axillary recurrence with skin involvement is shown in Figure 119.10. Aggressive surgical management of less extensive disease can avoid these changes in most patients.

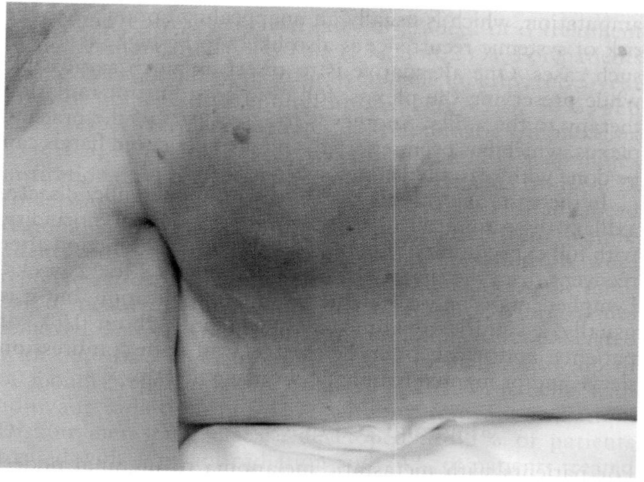

FIGURE 119.10 Extensive axillary adenopathy before resection.

As discussed earlier, aggressive staging studies are of very low yield in patients with micrometastases found on sentinel node biopsy. However, for patients with thick melanomas or with macrometastases or palpable clinical nodes, the yield is higher. Preoperative staging is recommended for those patients, using MRI of the brain and with CT or PET-CT.

There are some specific considerations related to lymph node dissections in different node basins. These are summarized as follows.

Axillary Dissection

Axillary dissection should include all node-bearing tissue in levels I, II, and III. The long thoracic nerve and thoracodorsal neurovascular bundle should be identified and preserved unless involved with tumor. The superior border of dissection should be the axillary vein, anteriorly, which should be skeletonized. However, deep to the axillary vein and plexus, the axillary space extends superiorly and medially substantially above the level of the axillary vein, and that region should be cleared surgically, with careful attention to preservation of the long thoracic nerve, which runs along the chest wall to its origin from spinal nerves. The intercostobrachial nerve and lower intercostal nerves that run through the axillary space may usually be sacrificed. The pectoralis major and minor muscles are usually preserved along with the medial pectoral nerve and vessels, but in reoperative cases or cases with involvement of one or both of these muscles, part of all of them may be sacrificed. It is rare for the long thoracic node to be involved with tumor, and it should be preserved because denervation of the serratus anterior muscle leads to "winged scapula" and can be associated with chronic pain related to destabilization of the shoulder. When there is bulky axillary disease, though, it is not uncommon for the thoracodorsal nerve to be involved, and patients usually tolerate sacrifice of that nerve when necessary. However, the possibility of resection of it should be discussed with patients preoperatively, especially when there is bulky adenopathy. In addition, if there is bulky axillary disease, the tumor often abuts or involves the axillary vein. The axillary vein often actually consists of more than one vessel running in parallel; thus, sacrifice of the lowest limb of the axillary vein often is accomplished without evident morbidity. Even sacrifice of the entire axillary vein (one or several trunks) is usually tolerated well and should be considered in cases of advanced disease. A troublesome finding is tumor involvement of the brachial plexus. Definitive therapy of that may require forequarter

TABLE 119.5

CLINICAL TRIALS ADMINISTERING INTERFERON IN THE ADJUVANT SETTING

Trial	No. of Patients	Interferon Regimen	Control Arm	Eligible Patients (Stage)	Relapse-free Survival (% Improvement by Hazard Ratio)	Overall Survival (% Improvement by Hazard Ratio)
E1684	280	20 million IU/m² IV daily for 5 of 7 days for 4 wk, followed by 10 million IU/m² SC 3 times weekly for 48 wk	Observation	IIB or III	39; $P = .012$[a]	33; $P = .01$[a]
E1690	642	20 million IU/m² IV daily for 5 of 7 days for 4 wk, followed by 10 million IU/m² SC 3 times weekly for 48 wk	Observation	IIB or III	22; $P = .05$ for HD IFN vs. observation	0; $P = .99$ for HD IFN vs. observation
		or 10 million IU/m² SC 3 times weekly for 24 mo			16; $P = .17$ for LD IFN vs. observation	4; $P = .81$ for LD IFN vs. observation
E1694	880	20 million IU/m² IV daily for 5 of 7 days for 4 wk, followed by 10 million IU/m² SC 3 times weekly for 48 wk	Ganglioside vaccine	IIB or III	32; $P = .0015$	34; $P = .009$
E18952	1388	10 million IU daily for 5 of 7 days for 4 wk, followed by 10 million IU SC 3 times weekly for 1 y	Observation	IIB or III	15; $P = .09$ for 2 y vs. observation[b]	15; $P = .12$ for 2 y vs. observation
		or 10 million IU daily for 5 of 7 days for 4 wk, followed by 5 million IU SC 3 times weekly for 2 y			5; $P = .59$ for 1 y vs. observation[b]	3; $P = .73$ for 1 y vs. observation
E18991	1256	Pegylated interferon 6 mcg/kg SC weekly for 8 wk, followed by 3 mcg/kg SC weekly for 5 y	Observation	III	18; $P = .01$	2; $P = .78$

SC, subcutaneously; IV, intravenously; HD, high dose; IFN, interferon; LD, low dose.
[a]After adjustment for other prognostic factors in multivariate model.
[b]Distant metastasis–free survival.

Interferon alpha-2b was evaluated in three single-agent phase 2 trials in metastatic melanoma and was associated with a 22% objective response rate among 96 patients.[184] No randomized trial comparing interferon-α with dacarbazine in metastatic disease has been conducted. On the basis of durable responses in some patients with metastatic disease, an adjuvant therapy trial was initiated in patients with high-risk stage 2 and stage 3 melanoma (Eastern Cooperative Oncology Group trial E1684).[185] Interferon-α was administered by intravenous infusion, 20 million U/m², for 5 consecutive days every 7 days for 4 weeks during the "induction" phase. For a subsequent 48 weeks, 10 million U/m² were administered by subcutaneous injection on alternate days for a total of three doses every 7 days in the "maintenance" phase. The control arm was observation, the standard at the time that the trial was conducted. Two hundred eighty-seven patients were enrolled, 80% of whom had stage III melanoma; 20% had stage IIB melanoma. Pathologic staging was performed with regional lymph node dissection because sentinel lymph node biopsy had not yet been introduced. Overall survival was the primary end point, and the trial was designed to detect a 33% improvement. The protocol-specified analysis in 1996 was performed with median follow-up 6.9 years and revealed a statistically significant 33% improvement by hazard ratio in overall survival compared to the observation arm after adjusting for other prognostic factors in a multivariate model ($P = .012$). Relapse-free survival was also significantly improved (39% improvement by hazard ratio compared to observation after adjusting for other prognostic factors; $P = .001$). This efficacy came at the expense of significant toxicities, with approximately three-fourths of the interferon-treated patients experiencing severe toxicities (defined as grade 3 or 4 by National Cancer Institute Common Toxicity Criteria). The most common severe side effects were fatigue, asthenia, fever, depression, and elevated liver transaminases. A subsequent quality-of-life analysis of this trial population suggested that the toxicity associated with this regimen was largely compensated for by the psychological benefit derived from prevention of disease relapse.[186] On the basis of E1684, interferon-α was approved by the FDA for the treatment of resected stage IIB and stage III melanoma.

Given uncertainty regarding the optimal dose and schedule of interferon and the significant toxicity associated with the high-dose regimen tested in E1684, a second trial was initiated in the year that accrual was completed to E1684 (E1690).[187] In this study, the high-dose regimen from E1694 was compared to a low-dose regimen as well as to observation. In the low-dose arm, interferon-α was administered at 3 million units by subcutaneous injection 3 times weekly for 24 months. Six hundred forty-two patients were assigned in equal proportions to the three groups. This trial was designed to detect a 33% improvement in overall survival. Of note, surgical staging of lymph nodes was not required, allowing for the possibility that stage III disease was present but undetected in some patients. Thus, the extent of disease could have been greater in this population than in E1684. With a median follow-up of 4.3 years, the final analysis revealed no significant improvement in overall survival for either the high-dose or low-dose arms compared to observation (no difference for high-dose interferon vs. observation; 4% improvement for low-dose interferon vs. observation; $P = .99$ for high-dose interferon vs. observation). A relapse-free survival advantage was confirmed for high-dose interferon compared to observation (22% reduction in risk of relapse by hazard ratio; $P = .05$) but not for low-dose interferon. A pooled analysis of E1684 and E1690 with longer follow-up (median, 7.2 years) for both trials revealed a continued, statistically significant effect on relapse-free survival but not overall survival.[188] The patients receiving high-dose interferon had an aggregate reduction in risk of relapse of 23% by hazard ratio ($P = .006$). However, the risk of death from any case was reduced by a statistically insignificant 7%.

Two additional randomized trials were conducted comparing high-dose interferon to vaccination with ganglioside GM2/keyhole-limpet hemocyanin (E1694 and E2696).[189,190] Although these trials did not include an observation control arm, the relative superiority of high-dose interferon to the experimental arm has been marshaled as supportive evidence of the benefit of interferon therapy. E1694, the larger of the two trials, accrued 880 patients and thus represented the largest pool of patients treated with high-dose regimen. This trial was stopped after an interim analysis was performed with a median follow-up of only 16 months. Overall survival was significantly better for the interferon arm (34% reduction in risk by hazard ratio compared to vaccine; $P = .009$). Relapse-free survival was also significantly better for the interferon-treated patients (32% lower risk of relapse by hazard ratio; $P = .0015$). E2696 indirectly evaluated the benefit of high-dose interferon by comparing the combination of high-dose interferon plus ganglioside GM2/keyhole-limpet hemocyanin vaccine (in sequence or simultaneously administered) to vaccine alone. The sequential regimen was associated with a 49% reduction in risk of relapse by hazard ratio compared to vaccine alone ($P = .03$), whereas the simultaneous regimen was associated with a 43% reduction ($P = .016$).

Thus, interferon has been consistently shown to improve relapse-free survival compared to either observation or ganglioside GM2/keyhole-limpet hemocyanin vaccination. The longevity of this benefit has been established with 12.6 years of median follow-up for E1684.[188] With twice the follow-up of the initial protocol-defined analysis, the improvement in relapse-free survival continued to be statistically significant (28% reduction in risk by hazard ratio; $P = .02$). However, with longer follow-up or by pooled analysis of E1684 and E1690, a definitive benefit with high-dose interferon in overall survival is lacking. With long-term follow-up of E1684, high-dose interferon was associated with a statistically insignificant 18% improvement ($P = .18$). The consistency of relapse-free survival data across all trials, in the absence of a consistent or durable survival benefit, has raised speculation that interferon may contribute to causes of death that are unrelated to melanoma recurrence, such as cardiovascular disease. In addition to the negative result for low-dose interferon in E1690, another phase 3 trial evaluated intermediate-dose interferon compared to observation in the adjuvant setting (European Organization for the Research of the Treatment for Cancer [EORTC] 18952).[191] A total of 1,388 patients were randomly assigned to one of three arms: interferon 10 million units daily for 5 days out of 7 repeated for 4 weeks followed by 10 million units 3 times weekly for 1 year; interferon 10 million units daily for 5 days out of 7 repeated for 4 weeks followed by 5 million units 3 times weekly for 2 years; or observation. Neither interferon arm was associated with a significant improvement in the distant metastasis-free interval (7% improvement for higher dose vs. observation; 3% improvement for lower dose vs. observation). Overall survival was slightly better for the higher-dose group (5% improvement compared to observation) but not different for the lower-dose group. As a consequence, such regimens remain investigational.

The EORTC has completed a randomized trial comparing a pegylated form of interferon-α-2b to observation in patients with resected stage II and stage III melanoma.[192]

Pegylation results in substantially slower clearance of interferon after administration. This allows for more stable drug exposure than can be achieved with the shorter-lived conventional interferon-α administered on alternating days by subcutaneous injection. To achieve a similar amount of drug exposure over the course of several days, pegylated interferon can be administered less frequently and at a lower dose per injection. This results in a lower maximum concentration after each dose while increasing the percentage of the dosing interval for which interferon is at biologically active concentrations. Per month of therapy, this regimen is less toxic than the high-dose interferon regimen tested in E1684 and E1690. However, in EORTC 18991, 1,256 patients with resected stage III melanoma were randomized between observation and treatment with pegylated interferon 6 mcg/kg once weekly for 8 weeks by subcutaneous injection followed by maintenance at 3 mcg/kg weekly for 5 years. Given the long duration of therapy, it is not surprising that the cumulative toxicities reported were only marginally less than that observed with 1 year of high-dose therapy. Nonetheless, the dose intensity achieved during the induction phase was 88% of that intended, and for the maintenance phase it was 83%. The primary end points of the trial were distant metastasis–free survival and relapse-free survival. Patients treated with pegylated interferon had significantly reduced risk of relapse (18% improvement by hazard ratio; $P = .01$), but an insignificant improvement of distant metastasis–free survival (12% improvement; $P = .11$). Survival follow-up was immature at the time of the analysis of the primary end points, but no significant difference in survival was observed.

Given the substantially improved tolerability of pegylated interferon, the data supporting an improvement in relapse-free survival is being reviewed by the FDA and European regulatory authorities. Three years of pegylated (100 mcg subcutaneously once weekly) was compared to 18 months of low-dose interferon (3 million units subcutaneously 3 times weekly) in a recently reported randomized trial among 898 patients with primary melanomas greater than 1.5 mm in thickness with or without microscopic involvement of regional lymph nodes. Because sentinel lymph node biopsy or prophylactic axillary node dissection was not routinely performed (only 68% of patients were staged with sentinel node biopsy), the exact stage distribution for this population is not known. Because of a higher rate of grade 3 and 4 toxicities among the pegylated interferon-treated patients, only 28% of patients completed the intended 36 months of therapy. After a median follow-up of 4.7 months, relapse-free survival (9% improvement), distant metastasis-free survival (2% worse outcome), and overall survival (9% worse outcome) were not significantly different between the two arms.[193] Because low-dose interferon has inconsistently been associated with improved relapse-free survival compared to observation, it is not clear how to interpret these findings in relationship to EORTC 18991, which compared pegylated interferon to observation. Taken together, these trials suggest that pegylated interferon administered at these doses and schedules is not substantially superior to more conventional interferon regimens.

Another approach under investigation is a shortened course of high-dose interferon-α, in the ECOG1697 trial, evaluating whether the first month of high-dose interferon improves survival in patients at high risk for recurrence. If this offers clinical benefit with much less morbidity than the full year of interferon, it would have a lower risk-to-benefit profile than the full year. A prospective randomized trial comparing 1 month to 1 year of high-dose interferon revealed no difference in outcome, but was not powered to test equivalence definitively.[194]

Cytotoxic Chemotherapy and Combination Chemotherapies in Adjuvant Therapy of Melanoma

Single-agent chemotherapy or combination chemotherapy regimens have not been comprehensively evaluated for the adjuvant treatment of melanoma. To date, however, they have not been associated with significant improvement in survival compared to observation. Dacarbazine (DTIC) was not effective in the postoperative setting, whether administered alone or combined with BCG.[89] The largest randomized trial compared an intravenously administered regimen of carmustine (BCNU, 80 mg/m^2 every 4 weeks), actinomycin-D (10 mcg/kg), vincristine (1.0 mg/m^2 every 2 weeks) for 6 months, to observation among 173 patients with resected stage III or stage IV melanoma.[195] This trial, small in comparison to interferon trials, demonstrated a significant improvement in relapse-free survival (5-year Kaplan-Meier estimates of relapse-free survival of 29% vs. 9%; $P = .03$). No difference in overall survival was observed. In another study, 192 patients with resected stage II or III melanoma were randomly assigned to receive DTIC, and 185 patients were randomly assigned to observation.[196] The 3-year relapse-free rate was 42% for the DTIC arm compared to 30% for observation but was not statistically significant. The relative improvements in relapse-free survival for these regimens compared to observation are in the range of that observed for high-dose interferon, but given the small size of these trials and the lack of confirmatory results, chemotherapy remains an investigational approach in the adjuvant setting.

A biochemotherapy regimen is being evaluated in the adjuvant setting compared to high-dose interferon (SWOG 0008). Four hundred thirty-two patients were randomized between the treatments, with completion in late 2007. This trial was designed to detect a 30% improvement in overall survival, corresponding to a 21% improvement in the 5-year survival rate. The biochemotherapy regimen employed in S0008 is the same as that evaluated in ECOG 3695, which was found not to be superior to a triplet chemotherapy regimen. Only three cycles of biochemotherapy are administered in this adjuvant trial, and the amount of interferon administered per cycle is only a small fraction of that given in same cycles of high-dose interferon. Similarly, the doses of IL-2 administered are far below the single-agent doses given in the high-dose regimen. The hypothesis being tested in S0008 is whether such doses of interferon and IL-2 augment the activity of full-dose chemotherapy.

Neoadjuvant Therapy for Resectable Stage III or IV Melanoma

Neoadjuvant therapy for resectable stage III or stage IV melanoma remains an investigational approach. Unlike breast and rectal cancer, for which chemotherapy regimens are associated with clinical downstaging and pathologic complete responses, systemic therapies for melanoma are not sufficiently active to support incorporation into neoadjuvant treatment. This setting does provide an excellent opportunity to evaluate novel therapies because the mechanism of action and resistance can be directly studied by analyzing the effect of treatment on tumor cells, the microenvironment, or immune responses. One recent study of neoadjuvant interferon for patients with palpable regional lymph node metastases was associated with an objective tumor response rate of 55%.[197] Further studies of this or other neoadjuvant therapies provide opportunities to investigate tumor biology in the tumor microenvironment and may lead to better understanding of the mechanism of antitumor effects of novel therapies.

Adjuvant Immunotherapy

There is substantial evidence that the immune system responds naturally to melanoma and that immune modulation can be therapeutic for advanced melanoma. Murine studies provide strong support for the immune surveillance hypothesis that the immune system protects against spontaneous malignancy in the normal mammalian host.[198] It is also evident that as melanomas (and other cancers) develop in the otherwise healthy human host, they evolve mechanisms for immune escape, immune dysfunction, or tolerance.[199–202] Furthermore, long-term cancer survivors often have some degree of persistent effective antitumor immunity.[199,203] In the last 20 years, there have been dramatic and durable clinical tumor regressions with high-dose IL-2 therapy, now approved for use in advanced melanoma, and recent experience with antibody to the cytotoxic T-lymphocyte antigen-4 (CTLA-4) molecule and with combination adoptive T-cell therapy reveals the therapeutic efficacy of immunotherapy for treatment of advanced melanoma (presented in more detail later in this chapter). Challenges for development work in immunotherapy include extending the infrequent successes in advanced disease to a larger proportion of patients and also developing effective immunotherapy to prevent melanoma recurrence, for use in the adjuvant setting.

Immunotherapy of cancer has been studied for more than 100 years, most notably with the work of William Coley[204] in the late nineteenth century using bacterial toxins as nonspecific stimuli of the immune system in patients with cancer. This approach was successful in causing tumor regressions in a few percent of his patients, and we now understand that bacterial toxins are potent activators of innate immunity through activation of Toll-like receptors. However, systematic evaluation of bacterial toxins for adjuvant therapy of melanoma has failed to show significant clinical benefit. Studies have included use of the mycobacterium BCG, *Corynebacterium parvum*, and the putative immunotherapy levamisole, all without evidence of clinical benefit.[205] Some of these studies have been performed in conjunction with systemic chemotherapy using dacarbazine. It is illustrative to review the experience of the WHO in this area. The WHO Trial 6 enrolled 761 patients after lymphadenectomy for regional node metastasis and randomized them to a four-arm trial including BCG and DTIC. Those four arms were surgery only (S), surgery + BCG (B), surgery + DTIC + BCG (DB), and surgery + DTIC (D). Overall survival for is equivalent for all four arms ($P \sim .17$), with very mature follow-up out to 15 years.[206]

Specific Immunotherapy

In the wake of negative studies with nonspecific immunotherapy using bacterial toxins, efforts have been made to develop vaccines specifically targeting immune responses against melanoma. Initial efforts have used autologous or allogeneic melanoma cells as immunogens. It is now known that many melanoma antigens are shared by multiple allogeneic melanomas[207] and that there also are unique antigens due to specific mutations in autologous tumors and related malignant transformation.[206] Vaccination strategies using autologous and allogeneic melanoma cells have been studied in phase 2 and phase 3 trials over the last few decades. The vaccine preparations have used live melanoma cells, melanoma cell lysates, molecular isolates from cultured melanoma cells, or heat shock proteins derived from allogeneic or autologous melanoma cells. Studies with these agents continue, but there has been a series of negative randomized, prospective cell-based vaccine trials in the last few years.[208–213] There have been provocative subgroup analyses in some of these trials that suggest potential benefit in patient subsets and deserve further study.[209,211]

Defined Molecular Melanoma Antigens and Vaccines

Ganglioside Antigens and Vaccines

Antibody responses to human melanoma cells have prompted identification of the melanoma cell surface antigens recognized by those antibodies. Among them are the ganglioside antigens GD2, GD3, and GM2. When GM2 is coupled to the keyhole-limpet hemocyanin protein and combined with the adjuvant QS-21, this is very effective at inducing immunoglobulin G (IgG) and IgM antibodies to GM2 in humans.[214] Because of the promising work with this vaccine approach, it has been studied in the adjuvant setting in the phase 3 randomized trial E1694, described earlier in this chapter. However, survival and disease-free survival were not improved over use of high-dose interferon-α-2b.[189]

T-Cell–Defined Antigens and Vaccines

In the late 1980s and early 1990s, the molecular nature of melanoma antigens recognized by T cells was defined: short peptides, derived from endogenous melanoma proteins, presented in association with major histocompatibility complex class I or class II molecules on the melanoma cell surface. The molecular identity of many of these peptide antigens has now been defined.[206] The source proteins include melanocytic differentiation proteins (e.g., MART-1/MelanA, gp100, and tyrosinase) and the cancer-testis antigens (e.g., *MAGE* gene family, NY-ESO-1, and others). These discoveries have launched an era of specific synthetic vaccines using peptides, proteins, and genes (viral or naked DNA) encoding these proteins or peptides and also using these defined antigens to dissect the immune response and to monitor immune responses to vaccines in human trials. Clinical trials using these defined antigens have induced objective clinical tumor regressions in 3% to 6% of patients enrolled in studies worldwide, which is disappointing therapeutically but does suggest a potential benefit of these approaches in a small number of patients, which needs to be exploited further based on better understanding of the biology of the host–tumor relationship and by integration of combined immunotherapies.[215]

The adjuvant setting is commonly considered to be the more appropriate setting for vaccine trials than the setting of advanced melanoma, and so there continues to be substantial investigation of immune therapy and of experimental melanoma vaccines in particular for patients in the adjuvant setting. In most of Europe, there is no standard approved therapy for adjuvant therapy of high-risk melanoma because high-dose interferon is not widely accepted there. In the United States, where high-dose interferon is FDA-approved for the adjuvant therapy of patients with stage IIB-III melanoma, there is no approved therapy for patients with resected stage IV melanoma. In addition, patients who are medically ineligible for, have failed, or choose not to take high-dose interferon have no other FDA-approved option and are good candidates for clinical trials with low anticipated morbidity.

Peptide-based vaccines for melanoma can elicit reactivity against the peptides, sometimes with high percentages of peptide-reactive cells in the circulation.[216,217] T cells generated by vaccination can lyse human melanoma cells expressing the cognate antigens.[218–220] Multiple peptides have been found to be immunogenic and safe in humans, and it is feasible to immunize simultaneously with multipeptide mixtures.[221] However, questions remain about how best to target the T cells to tumor, to ensure that they have appropriate antitumor function *in vivo*, and to ensure long-term immunologic memory.[222,223] Ongoing studies include investigation of combination of vaccines with immune modulators including antibodies to CTLA4, immune modulatory chemotherapy, cytokines, and Toll-like receptor agonists. Development of effective immune therapy for cancer may ultimately benefit from (1) more comprehensive and real-time immune monitoring in various tissue compartments, and (2) patient-specific modulation of immune responses, informed by the real-time monitoring. To characterize the host–tumor relationship and to optimize cancer vaccines, clinical studies using defined antigens offer special opportunities to advance the field and thus have an important place in the ongoing development of effective immune therapy of melanoma. However, a peptide vaccine targeting the melanocytic differentiation protein gp100 was combined with high-dose IL-2 therapy in a randomized phase 3 trial compared to IL-2 alone, whose primary end point was prolongation of progression-free survival: addition of the vaccine significantly increased response rate and prolonged progression-free survival, with a trend toward improved survival.[224]

Granulocyte Macrophage Colony-Stimulating Factor

Granulocyte macrophage colony–stimulating factor (GM-CSF) has attracted attention as a vaccine adjuvant in murine studies.[225,226] Thus, it has been assessed as a vaccine adjuvant in clinical trials. Two recent prospective randomized trials, however, show a negative impact of GM-CSF on immunologic or clinical outcomes.[227,228]

GM-CSF also is being investigated as a potential single-agent therapy for melanoma because of described effects on macrophage and dendritic cell function.[229,230] A single-arm study was performed in high-risk melanoma patients in which GM-CSF was administered subcutaneously daily at 125 mcg/m^2 for 14 days, followed by a 14-day rest period and with repeat of that cycle for 1 year. This has been a well-tolerated regimen. In this study of 48 patients with stage IIIC or IV melanoma, overall 2-year survival was 69%, which exceeded the outcome for matched historical controls.[231] These data led to a placebo-controlled, randomized, prospective trial in high-risk resected melanoma performed through the ECOG E4697. That trial accrued approximately 800 patients and closed to accrual in 2006. Results presented in 2010 showed no significant impact on clinical outcome overall, but leave open some question about potential benefit in the subset of resected stage IV patients.[232]

Clinical Follow-Up for Patients with Regionally Metastatic Melanomas (Stage III)

Suggestions for follow-up are listed in Table 119.4. Regional metastases are associated with increased risk of future systemic metastasis. For patients with microscopic metastases (stage IIIA), the prognosis is good enough that follow-up may reasonably be limited to clinical examination with or without CXR and limited laboratory studies. However, for patients with stage IIIB–IIIC melanomas, annual CXR or CT scans may be indicated as well. In particular, for patients who had prior metastasis to inguinal nodes, there is a high risk of subsequent iliac nodal metastasis, which is not generally evident on physical examination. Thus, CT scans of the pelvis are recommended for such patients. In addition, for high-risk melanomas, brain MRI may be helpful in detecting small brain metastases when they are asymptomatic and amenable to treatment with gamma knife radiation therapy.

MANAGEMENT OF DISTANT METASTASES OF MELANOMA (STAGE IV)

Any patient with distant metastases is considered stage IV. Distant metastases may include skin or soft tissue metastases distant from a known primary site, visceral, bone, or brain metastases. All are associated with a very poor prognosis, with median survivals of 6 to 15 months.[63,65,233,234] The prognosis is better for skin and subcutaneous tissue metastases, which are considered M1a, than for lung metastases (M1b) or other distant metastases (M1c). In addition, an elevated serum LDH in the setting of distant metastases is associated with a poor prognosis and also is considered M1c disease.[64]

Timing of Distant Metastases

It is uncommon for patients with melanoma to present initially with stage IV disease. Most patients who develop distant metastases do so after an interval from their original management for clinically localized disease or after management for regionally metastatic disease. In general, the interval to detection of distant metastases is shorter for patients who initially present with high-stage disease (e.g., stage IIB–III) and is longest for patients who present with clinically localized thin melanomas (e.g., stage IA). Often, metastases become evident within 2 to 3 years of diagnosis, but delayed metastasis is also common, and for melanoma, regional and distant metastases have occurred after disease-free intervals measured in decades.[235]

Patterns of Metastases

Approximately 60% to 80% of first metastases are at local or regional sites including regional nodes. The most common first sites of visceral metastasis are lung and liver (about 10% each), and metastases to distant skin sites are also common. After an initial metastasis, subsequent metastases are more commonly visceral or distant and increasingly become multiple. Common visceral sites of metastasis are lung, liver, brain, gastrointestinal tract (especially small bowel), bone, and adrenal gland.

Prognostic Factors in Distant Metastatic Melanoma (Stage IV)

The prognosis of patients with metastatic melanoma is very poor. The median survival is 6 to 9 months for those who present with visceral metastatic disease beyond the lung and may be as long as 15 months for those who present with skin and lymph node metastases only.[63]

Patients with lung metastases as their only site of visceral organ involvement have an intermediate prognosis. Because 70% of patients with metastatic disease have visceral metastases beyond the lung, the median survival of the entire population of patients with metastatic disease is less than 12 months. Negative prognostic factors in stage IV melanoma also include a large number of metastatic sites, elevated LDH level, and poor performance status.[233,234] No clinical trials have been conducted comparing systemic therapy with best supportive care. However, there is little evidence that the available therapies significantly alter the natural history of melanoma, given that median survival duration on the most recent phase 3 trials has ranged between 8 and 9 months.[236] However, there is substantial promise with new therapies, summarized in this chapter.

Clinical Evaluation of Patients with Distant Metastasis (Stage IV)

When a patient is found to have a distant metastasis, the initial steps are to perform full restaging studies. This typically should include MRI scan of the brain and either total-body PET-CT scan or CT scans of the chest, abdomen, and pelvis. Other scans or imaging studies (bone scan, soft-tissue MRI, ultrasound, or plain films) may be indicated to evaluate known areas of metastasis (e.g., soft-tissue masses in extremities) or to evaluate symptoms (e.g., plain films or bone scans for bony symptoms). PET-CT scans are very helpful in distinguishing tumor from scar in areas of prior surgery, although surgical sites may remain FDG-avid for up to 3 months after surgery. PET is substantially more sensitive for detection of small bowel metastases and lymph node metastases that are borderline in size.[237] PET-CT scan may also be helpful in assessing patients for resectability when there is limited disease on initial assessment.

Histologic or Cytologic Diagnosis

Patients being followed for a history of melanoma may develop new evidence of metastatic disease. In such patients, a new and growing mass in the chest (e.g., abnormal CXR) or abdomen is likely to be metastatic melanoma, but tissue confirmation of metastatic melanoma is usually recommended. New masses can represent new primary lung cancers, lymphoma, sarcoid, inflammatory masses, or other changes, and the management and prognosis of these lesions usually differs dramatically from the management and prognosis of stage IV melanoma.

If the lesion is in an accessible area of the lung and is about 1 cm in diameter or greater, a CT-guided transthoracic needle biopsy is usually feasible and appropriate for making the diagnosis. If there is a solitary lung mass, and especially if the mass is less than 1 cm in diameter, then thoracoscopic resection with preoperative localization can be performed with great success and with low morbidity.[238] In the event that the lesion is malignant, then the biopsy may also have some therapeutic value.

Fine-needle aspiration biopsy of soft-tissue masses or lymph nodes can be rapid and accurate diagnostic approaches either at the bedside or with radiologic localization. Similarly, biopsies of many other tissue lesions can be accomplished by minimally invasive techniques. A fine-needle aspirate will be diagnostic in most cases, but a core-needle biopsy, when feasible, can improve diagnostic accuracy further. Immunohistochemical stains for S100, HMB45, tyrosinase, and MART-1/MelanA can all be helpful in confirming a diagnosis of melanoma.

Surgery for Distant Metastases (Stage IV)

Patient Selection and Prognostic Factors

Selected patients may benefit from surgery for distant metastatic (stage IV) melanoma. The benefit can be palliative in some patients and may be curative in rare cases. There are numerous clinical scenarios in which surgery may be considered, and it is not possible to address all of them here. However, it is useful to consider some of them.

Cases in Which the Benefit of Surgery Is Clear

- Anemia due to occult bleeding from intestinal metastasis
- Bowel obstruction due to small bowel metastasis
- Cutaneous or subcutaneous metastasis with ulceration, pain, or impending ulceration
- Lymph node metastasis with neurologic symptoms
- Symptomatic brain metastasis
- Life-threatening hemorrhage from metastasis

Melanoma frequently metastasizes to the gastrointestinal tract. It usually originates as an intramural lesion but grows into the lumen and through the serosa with time. These usually present as anemia due to occult gastrointestinal bleeding or as intermittent small bowel obstruction due to intussusception (Fig. 119.11). They are difficult to diagnose by CT scan in the absence of symptoms. PET-CT is probably the best study now available. However, it may miss small lesions. Nonetheless, when a patient presents with gastrointestinal blood loss or obstruction associated with a small bowel (or other gastrointestinal) metastasis of melanoma, operation is usually indicated. If the tumor involves the mesenteric nodes and is matted, then it may not be feasible or appropriate to resect the entire tumor, but enteroenteric bypass of the obstruction will be palliative. Resection of most or all small bowel metastases can manage bleeding and obstruction effectively. If there is a single small bowel metastasis, then a simple resection and reanastomosis is appropriate (Fig. 119.12). However, if there are numerous small bowel metastases, then excision of large lesions with reanastomosis is appropriate, but small lesions may be excised by partial-diameter excision and stapled (or sewn) closure. If the patient can be rendered surgically free of disease, then there may be long-term survival greater than 5 years in as many as 25% of patients and mean survival greater than 2 years.[239]

Cutaneous, subcutaneous, and nodal metastases are not usually a cause of death, but they can be a cause of substantial morbidity. As they grow, they develop substantial inflammation in the overlying skin (Fig. 119.10) and without resection may often ulcerate. Because such lesions usually can be resected under local anesthesia with minimal morbidity, it is reasonable to offer resection.

Extensive lymph node metastasis with neurologic symptoms is commonly an issue in the axilla, where tumor growth

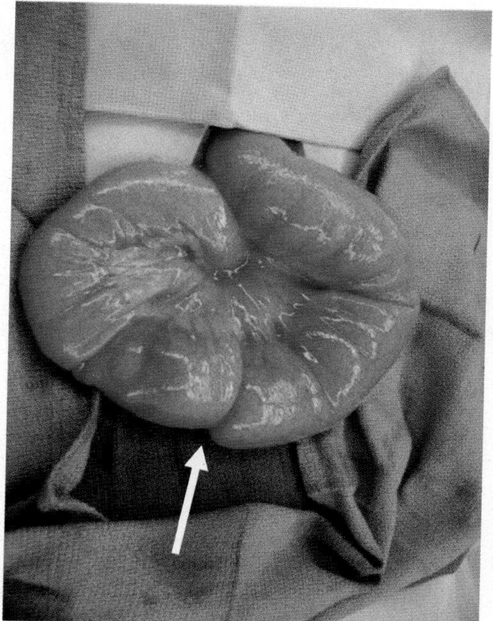
A

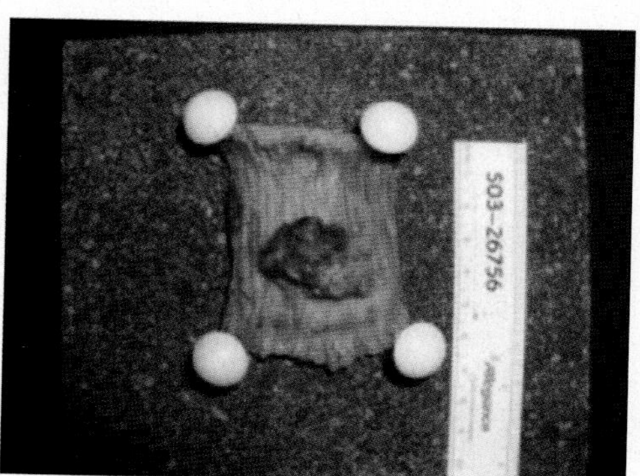

B

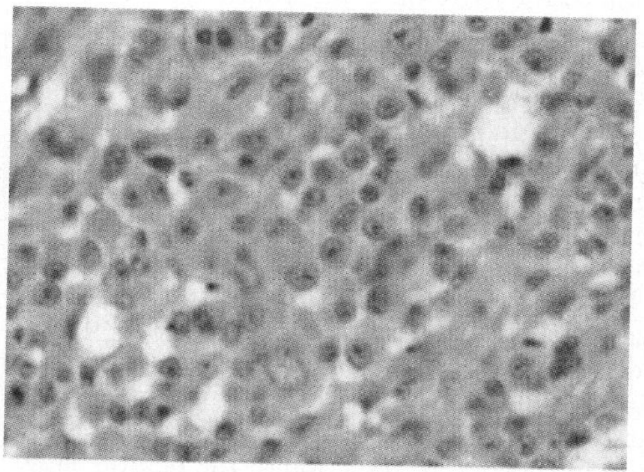
C

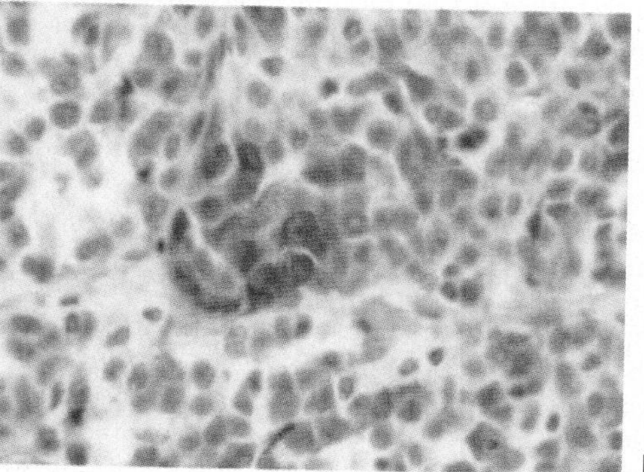
D

FIGURE 119.11 Patient presenting with intussusception due to a small bowel metastasis of melanoma. **A:** The loop of small bowel with intussusception is shown at the time of surgery, prior to enterectomy and reanastomosis. The arrow shows the point of intussusception. **B:** The intraluminal mass is shown with surrounding bowel mucosa. **C:** Hematoxylin-eosin–stained tissue section of the intussuscepting mass shows melanoma. **D:** Immunohistochemical stain for a melanoma marker.

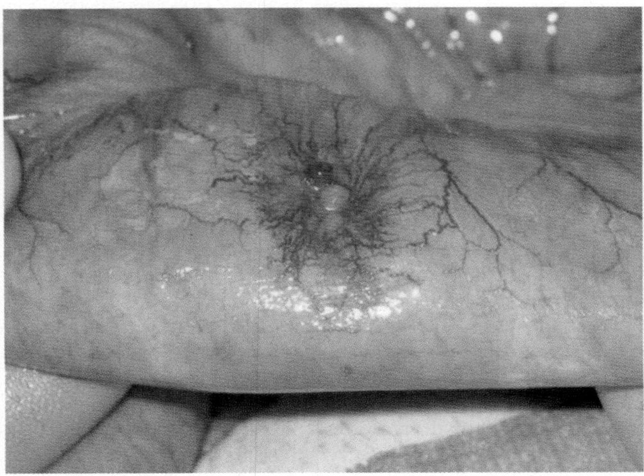

FIGURE 119.12 Small bowel metastasis of melanoma with extension through the bowel wall and with extensive neovascularity.

may compress or invade the brachial plexus, and axillary vein. Patients with extensive axillary recurrence with neurologic symptoms and patients with other nodal disease and neurologic symptoms should be considered for radical resection of the involved nodal basin. The morbidity of surgery usually is much less than the morbidity of the tumor left untreated. Major risks of tumor growth include paralysis or major neurologic dysfunction of the extremity, intractable lymphedema, disabling pain, and unresectability.

Brain metastasis is a particularly ominous sign in terms of future survival, which can usually be measured in months. For patients with symptomatic brain metastases, the presentation with acute cognitive deficits can be dramatic. Steroid therapy should be instituted immediately (4 mg orally every 6 hours per day initially). However, if this fails, or if the presentation is particularly acute with impending herniation, then surgical resection of the brain metastasis can be therapeutic.

Melanoma can metastasize to nodes, adrenal glands, or other sites and then develop spontaneous hemorrhage. Sometimes such bleeding can be trivial, but in some cases, there can be massive hemorrhage into the tissues, with associated hypovolemia. In such cases, resection of the hemorrhagic mass may diminish future risk of bleeding, decrease pain, and delay death.

Cases in Which the Benefit of Surgery Is Likely

- Solitary asymptomatic visceral metastasis resectable with minimal morbidity
- Bony metastasis with pain or joint involvement, unresponsive to radiation
- Solitary brain metastasis without symptoms
- Large, asymptomatic nodal metastasis with concurrent low-volume systemic disease
- Extensive skin and soft tissue metastases in the absence of visceral metastases
- Isolated growing metastasis in the setting of stable or regressing metastases after therapy

In general, in a patient with solitary visceral metastasis, if excision can be accomplished with minimal morbidity, the excision can be both therapeutic and diagnostic. The overall survival for patients with one or several distant metastases resected coupled with experimental melanoma vaccine therapy has been associated with 5-year survival rates in the 40% to 60% range.[212,240] Another reasonable option for the patient with a single (or few) resectable distant and/or visceral metastases is to enroll in an experimental therapeutic trial or to take an approved systemic therapy in the hope of clinical response but with the additional benefit of having about 3 months of observation time to be sure that no other new visceral lesions appear prior to resection of the lesion in question.

Bone metastases can cause pain and fracture. Radiation therapy is usually the first choice for therapeutic intervention if significant pain exists. If patients are at risk of impending fracture, orthopaedic stabilization should be considered before radiation. However, if the lesion does not respond to radiation or is solitary, resection with bone grafting or joint replacement can be considered. Current success rates with such therapy are high, but the period of postoperative recovery can be extended, and so careful patient selection is indicated.

An asymptomatic solitary brain metastasis that is amenable to resection can often be removed surgically with minimal morbidity and often with approximately a 3-day hospital stay. Stereotactic radiosurgery (e.g., gamma knife) is often the first choice for treatment of such lesions, but surgery is another reasonable option and probably will have benefit, especially if the solitary brain lesion is larger than 2 to 3 cm diameter, in which case stereotactic radiosurgery may be less effective and surgery may be a preferred option.

In patients with multiple metastases, systemic therapy may be associated with partial clinical responses with progressive growth of one or more lesions while the remainder are stable or shrinking and asymptomatic. In that case, patients may benefit from resecting the one or several tumor deposits that are progressing. This will not be curative, but it may lead to a more prolonged period of good quality of life, with minimal perioperative morbidity.

Cases in Which Some Patients May Benefit from Surgery But Risk and Benefit Are Closely Balanced

- More than one visceral metastasis, without symptoms
- Multiple lung nodules
- Bilateral adrenal metastases
- Extensive skin and soft tissue metastases in the setting of visceral disease

A more difficult decision is whether to treat patients with surgery when they have multiple asymptomatic visceral metastases, such as multiple lung nodules, bilateral adrenal metastases, or extensive skin metastases in the presence of visceral disease. These are generally situations in which surgery is not recommended as the treatment of choice, but there are anecdotes of such patients enjoying prolonged disease-free survival after such surgery, and so it is worth considering in very selected patients. Situations that may push the patient and the clinician toward such an aggressive surgical approach include (1) prior failure of systemic therapy, (2) a young patient for whom perioperative morbidity is not a major concern, and (3) disease sites that are particularly amenable to surgery through limited surgery (e.g., multiple lung nodules amenable to thoracoscopic lobectomy).

Adjuvant Therapy for Resected Stage IV Melanoma

There is no standard adjuvant therapy after resection of metastatic melanoma (stage IV). Interferon has not been thoroughly evaluated in this setting. Therefore, observation remains the standard management of patients in this setting. Investigational vaccines, GM-CSF, and other experimental therapies are being evaluated for these patients. Recent data from the ECOG 4697 trial, using GM-CSF as an adjuvant therapy for resected stage IIIB-IV melanoma, suggests that there is no impact on survival

TABLE 119.6

SELECTED CHEMOTHERAPY AGENTS EVALUATED IN PHASE 2 AND PHASE 3 TRIALS IN MELANOMA

Chemotherapy	Evaluable Patients (n)	Objective Response Rate (%)	95% Confidence Interval (%)
Alkylating Agents			
Dacarbazine	2,470	18	16–19
Temozolomide	350	15	11–19
Nitrosoureas			
Lomustine	270	13	9–17
Fotemustine	153	24	17–31
Platinum Analogues			
Cisplatin	188	23	17–29
Carboplatin	43	16	5–27
Microtubule-Stabilizing/Destabilizing			
Paclitaxel	85	13	7–22
Docetaxel	105	11	6–19
Vincristine	52	12	3–20
Vinblastine	62	13	5–21
Vindesine	273	14	10–18

overall.[232] A subgroup analysis suggested a possible trend for better outcome in stage IV patients. The impact of that finding is not known at this point, and may be clarified with longer follow-up. Given the limitations of subgroup analyses, these data do not support routine use of GM-CSF for adjuvant therapy for stage IV melanoma, but may warrant follow-up clinical investigation.

Treatment of Unresectable Metastatic (Stage IV) Melanoma

Single-Agent Chemotherapy

Melanoma is regarded as a relatively chemotherapy-refractory tumor. The mechanisms underlying resistance to the same agents that are effective in other solid tumors is incompletely understood but likely derives from the inherent resilience of melanocytes. In particular, DNA repair enzymes as well as the expression of efflux pumps for xenobiotics are more highly expressed in melanoma compared with many other cancers.[241–243] In addition, the activation of cell survival pathways such as the mitogen-activated protein kinase pathway and phosphoinositol-3 kinase pathway likely contributes to the ability to withstand the apoptosis-inducing effects of chemotherapy. In melanoma, these pathways are constitutively turned on by the presence of activating mutations in *NRAS* and *BRAF* and genetic deletion of *PTEN* and amplification of *AKT*. Abrogation of these signaling pathways may potentiate the effects of chemotherapy.

Durable objective responses have been observed in a small minority of patients with metastatic melanoma treated with single-agent chemotherapy. However, long-term complete and partial responses have been observed in the context of large, multicenter clinical trials. In the phase 3 trial comparing temozolomide with dacarbazine as first-line therapy, 3% of patients on either arm experienced complete responses.[244] The underpinning of the unique sensitivity of these patients' tumors has not been elucidated. In the few studies that have reported long-term follow-up, chemotherapy-induced complete responses can be maintained for more than 5 years in a small subpopulation of patients treated with single-agent chemotherapy.[245–248] In patients who have durable partial responses for several years, long-term outcome of reported cases is confounded by the nearly universal conduct of surgery to resect residual disease. Nonetheless, the association of low-toxicity therapy, such as dacarbazine, with such outcomes is probably the most compelling evidence to support their routine clinical application.

The greatest antitumor activity has been observed with alkylating agents, platinum analogues, and microtubule interactive drugs (Table 119.6). Of interest, the percentage of treatment-naïve patients who achieve responses is nearly identical for these classes of therapy. On the basis of preclinical evidence of synergy and the improvement in survival observed with combination chemotherapy regimens in other cancers, combination of these classes of agents has been extensively evaluated in phase 2 trials and, to a lesser extent, in phase 3 trials in melanoma. Antimetabolites, nucleoside analogues, and topoisomerase inhibitors have produced low but detectable activity in single-agent phase 2 trials and have not been further developed in melanoma.

The reference standard to which novel agents and regimens are compared is dacarbazine. This imidazole carboxamide [5-(3,3-dimethyl-l-triazeno)-imidazole-4-carboxamide] is a classic alkylating agent. It was first evaluated in clinical trials in melanoma in the late 1960s and FDA-approved for the treatment of metastatic melanoma in 1974 on the basis of a response rate of greater than 20%, using more liberal criteria than are currently employed in clinical trials.[249] In the majority of trials, dacarbazine was administered intravenously at daily doses of 200 mg/m^2 for 5 days every 3 or 4 weeks; however, 1,000 mg/m^2 given once every 3 or 4 weeks has been the standard regimen in recent trials (Table 119.7). The most common toxicities are myelosuppression and nausea. The severity of myelosuppression rarely requires the use of growth factor support, and the advent of potent antiemetics in recent years has significantly improved the tolerability of this agent.

The largest phase 3 trial in which patients received single-agent dacarbazine (1,000 mg/m^2 intravenously every 28 days) for metastatic melanoma and were evaluated using the currently standard response evaluation criteria in solid tumors

TABLE 119.7

SELECTED RANDOMIZED CHEMOTHERAPY TRIALS IN METASTATIC MELANOMA

Regimen	No. of Patients	Objective Response Rate (%)	Progression-Free Survival (Median)	Overall Survival (Median)
Temozolomide 200 mg/m^2 orally daily for 5 days every 28 days	156	13.5	1.9	7.7
DTIC 250 mg/m^2 IV daily for 5 days every 21 days	149	12.1	1.5	6.4
DTIC 1,000 mg/m^2 IV every 21 days + oblimersen 7 mg/kg/d IV continuous infusion for 5 days	386	13.5[a]	2.6	9.0
DTIC 1,000 mg/m^2 IV every 21 days	385	7.5[a]	1.6	7.8
Dartmouth regimen (DTIC 220 mg/m^2 and cisplatin 25 mg/m^2 days 1–3, carmustine 150 mg/m^2 day 1 every other cycle, and tamoxifen 10 mg orally every 2 days)	119	18.5	—	7.7
DTIC 1,000 mg/m^2 IV every 21 days	121	10.2	—	6.3
DTIC 800 mg/^{2} IV day 1, cisplatin 20 mg/m^2/d IV days 1–4, vinblastine 1.2 mg/m^2 IV days 1–4, IL-2 9 million IU/m^2/d IV continuous infusion for 4 days, interferon 5 million U/^{2} SC days 1–5, 8, 10 and 12 every 21 days	204	16.6	5.0	8.4
DTIC 800 mg/^{2} IV day 1, cisplatin 20 mg/m^2/d IV days 1–4, vinblastine 1.2 mg/m^2 IV days 1–4 every 21 days	201	11.9	3.1	9.1

DTIC, dacarbazine; IV, intravenously; IL-2, interleukin-2; SC, subcutaneously.
[a]$P < .05$ for comparison; all other differences not statistically significant.

(RECIST) revealed an objective response rate (partial and complete responses) of 7% based on investigator assessment and 3.5% based on independent radiology review.[250] Median progression-free survival has been reported to range between 1.5 and 2 months in large, randomized trials.[244,251] Overall survival for dacarbazine-treated patients is 6 to 9 months and is not clearly different than the natural history of metastatic melanoma. Of note, a randomized trial of dacarbazine or any other systemic therapy compared with best supportive care has never been undertaken in melanoma. Given the modest response rate and survival for patients treated with this agent, it serves as a weak standard. There is preclinical evidence suggesting that melanoma cells that survive dacarbazine exposure are capable of more rapid growth *in vivo* than the same cells that are unexposed to dacarbazine.[252] Of interest, these refractory cells produce greater levels of angiogenesis-inducing factors such as vascular endothelial growth factor (VEGF), interleukin-8, and basic fibroblast growth factor.

The diagnosis of brain metastases at the time of initial diagnosis with metastatic melanoma or the emergence of brain metastases early in the course of the disease is a particularly common clinical problem. For that reason, the development of therapies that can equally treat visceral and central nervous system involvement has been a high priority in melanoma. In particular, temozolomide has been the subject of numerous investigations in melanoma. This orally available prodrug is metabolized into the active form MTIC [5-(3-methyltriazen-1-yl) imidazole-4-carboxamide], which is closely related to DTIC.[253] MTIC demonstrates excellent penetration into the cerebrospinal fluid.[254] Because it is an oral therapy, temozolomide is also more amenable to protracted dosing schedules than dacarbazine, particularly an advantage when combined with fractionated radiation therapy. Single-arm phase 2 trials clearly demonstrated activity in patients with metastatic melanoma, but more modest activity was noted for patients with brain metastases treated with this agent.[255,256] A randomized phase 3 trial was conducted comparing temozolomide with dacarbazine in patients with metastatic melanoma without brain metastases.[244] Three hundred five patients were enrolled in the trial, which sought a 50% improvement in overall survival as the primary end point. This study suggested that temozolomide was marginally more active with regard to progression-free survival (1.9-month median for temozolomide vs. 1.5-month median for DTIC) but did not substantially improve objective response rate or overall survival. The observed 18% improvement in survival would require a substantially larger trial to establish that benefit with statistical significance. Each regimen was equally well tolerated. A larger phase 3 trial was conducted by the EORTC, in which a more dose-intense schedule of temozolomide was administered (150 mg/m^2 daily for 7 of every 14 days), compared with dacarbazine (1,000 mg/m^2 intravenously every 28 days). This trial (EORTC 18032) randomized 859 patients and sought a 23% improvement in overall survival as the primary end point. Overall survival was not significantly different between the two arms (hazard ratio, 1.0; $P = 1.0$) Response rate was superior in the temozolomide group (14.4% vs. 9.8%, $P = .05$), but progression-free survival was not (hazard ratio, 0.92 in favor of temozolomide; $P = .092$).[257]

The only other single-agent chemotherapy that has been systematically evaluated in comparison to DTIC is fotemustine. This nitrosourea was administered by intravenous infusion (100 mg/m^2) weekly for 3 weeks followed by a 4- to 5-week break in a phase 2 trial, with continued administration every 3 weeks for stable or responding patients.[258] One hundred fifty-three patients with metastatic disease, including patients with brain metastases, were evaluated for response. The

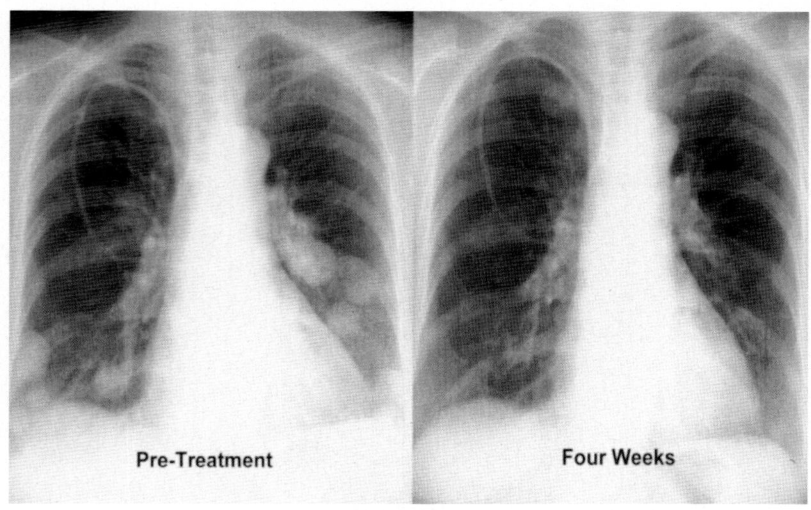

FIGURE 119.13 Complete response of metastatic melanoma in a patient treated with high-dose bolus interleukin-2.

observed response rate among all patients was 24%; it was 30% for the 62 patients with no prior therapy. In a phase 3 trial, fotemustine was administered once every 3 weeks at a dose of 100 mg/m^2 without the weekly induction phase used in the phase 2 trial.[226] Two hundred twenty-nine patients were randomized to fotemustine or DTIC, seeking to demonstrate a 17% absolute difference in objective response rate. The observed difference in response rate (13% for fotemustine vs. 6% for DTIC) was not statistically significant. Median time to progression was similar for the two arms. Overall survival, a secondary end point, was not significantly improved with fotemustine compared to DTIC (median, 7.3 vs. 5.6 months). As with the temozolomide/DTIC phase 3 trial, the small size of the fotemustine phase 3 trial could not detect a smaller but still potentially clinically significant improvement in overall survival.

Immunotherapy for Systemic Treatment of Stage IV Melanoma

Interleukin-2

The intravenous administration of high-dose IL-2 (aldesleukin) represents an effective treatment for patients with metastatic melanoma and the treatment most likely to provide long-term complete responses and cure in these patients. The basic biology and pharmacokinetics of IL-2 are presented in Chapter 45. IL-2 was first described as a T-cell growth factor in 1976.[259] The DNA sequence of the gene coding for IL-2 was determined in 1983,[260] and soon thereafter, the IL-2 gene was expressed in *Escherichia coli*, produced at high concentrations, and purified to homogeneity, and the biologic characteristics of this recombinant IL-2 were determined.[261] Although early studies with IL-2 used material from mammalian sources, all clinical studies of IL-2 since 1985 have used the recombinant material. The administration of IL-2 represented the first demonstration that purely immunotherapeutic maneuvers could mediate the regression of metastatic cancer.[262,263] IL-2 has no direct effect on cancer cells, and all of its antitumor activity is a function of its ability to modulate immunologic responses in the host.

The FDA-approved regimen for the treatment of patients with metastatic melanoma using IL-2 involves the use of an intravenous bolus infusion of 600,000 to 720,000 IU/kg every 8 hours to tolerance using two cycles separated by approximately 10 days (maximum of 15 doses per cycle). Results of this treatment are evaluated at 2 months after the first dose, and if tumor is regressing or stable, a second course is then administered. This regimen was approved by the FDA for the treatment of patients with metastatic melanoma in January 1998 based on the ability of this IL-2 regimen to mediate durable responses.

The hallmark of IL-2 therapy is its ability to mediate durable complete responses in patients with widespread metastatic disease (Fig. 119.13). In a report of the original 270 patients treated at 22 different institutions that was the basis of the approval of IL-2 by the FDA, a 16% objective response rate was obtained, with 17 complete responses (6%) and 26 partial responses (10%).[264] At the last full analysis of these 270 patients, the median duration of response for complete responders had not been reached but exceeded 59 months, and disease progression was not observed in any patient who responded for more than 30 months. An analysis of patients treated from 1988 to 2006 in the Surgery Branch, National Cancer Institute, reported 13 complete responders, only 2 of which had recurred with the remainder ongoing at 1 to 21 years.[265] Thus, IL-2 appears to be one of a very small group of systemic treatments capable of curing patients with a metastatic solid cancer (Fig. 119.14).

Because of the side effects associated with high-dose bolus IL-2 administration, this treatment is generally restricted to patients younger than the age of 70 years with an ECOG performance status of 2 or less and in patients who do not have active systemic infections or other major medical illness of the cardiovascular respiratory or immune system. Because IL-2 often causes transient renal and hepatic toxicity, eligibility criteria generally require normal serum creatinine and serum bilirubin levels. Patients with any history of systemic ischemic heart disease or pulmonary dysfunction should undergo stress testing and pulmonary function tests before initiating therapy, and patients with significant abnormalities should not be included.

The administration of high-dose bolus IL-2 is different than the administration of most cancer therapeutics in that dosing is continued every 8 hours until patients reach grade 3 or 4 toxicity that is not easily reversible by supportive measures.[266] The toxicities of IL-2 administration are transient, with virtually all returning to baseline after IL-2 administration is stopped. Thus, patients are often treated despite creatinine levels that increase to the 2- to 3-mg/dL range because of confidence that renal function will return to normal after cessation

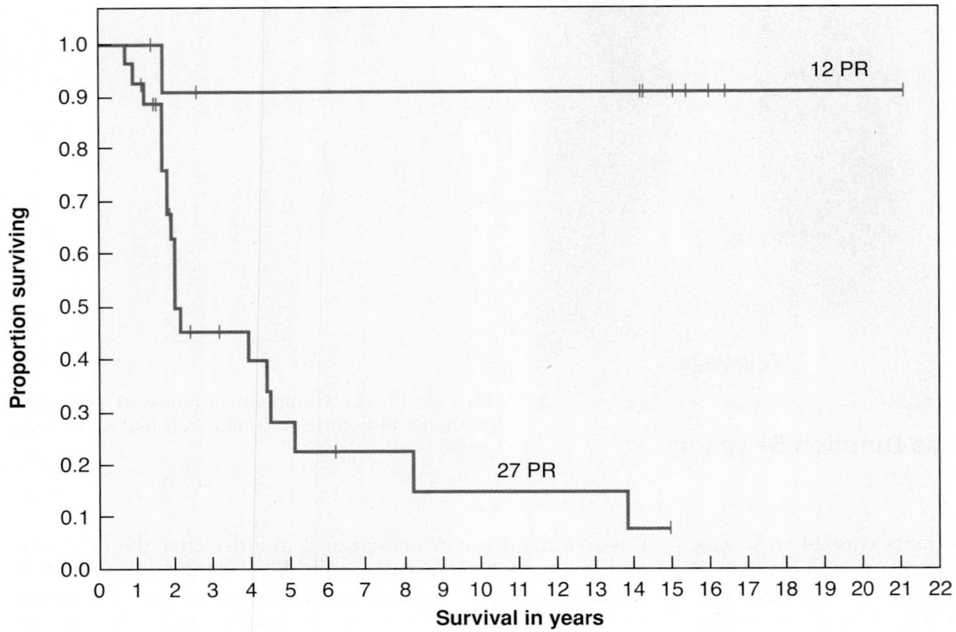

FIGURE 119.14 Kaplan-Meier estimates of survival of patient experiencing a complete response (CR) or partial response (PR) to high-dose interleukin-2 (IL-2) in the Surgery Branch of the National Cancer Institute.

of IL-2 administration. Thus, there are no set doses that patients receive, and there is no correlation between the number of doses seen and the likelihood of achieving a response so long as patients receive dosing to tolerance based on physical findings and laboratory measurements.

A variety of alternative regimens of IL-2 have been described, including the use of subcutaneous administration, continuous infusion, and a variety of lower-dose regimens. Lower doses of IL-2 result in a substantially decreased response rate and are not recommended.

Administration of IL-2 Plus Vaccine

In 1998 Rosenberg et al.[267] reported an increase in objective response to IL-2 when administered in conjunction with a heteroclitic gp100:209–217(210M) melanoma peptide vaccine. An updated analysis showed a response rate of 12.8% to IL-2 alone compared to a 25.0% response rate to IL-2 plus immunization with this peptide (P = .01). A prospective randomized trial in patients with metastatic melanoma of IL-2 alone or in conjunction with this peptide in 185 patients by Schwartzentruber et al.[224] reported response rates of 9.7% and 22.1%, respectively (P = .02), with an increase in progression-free survival in the vaccine arm (P = .008) but not an increase in survival (P = .11).

Toxicities of IL-2 Administration

IL-2 causes a pulmonary capillary leak with extravasation of fluid into soft tissue and visceral organs. A summary of high-dose IL-2 toxicities seen in a multicenter trial is shown in Table 119.8.[264] Supportive measures are often required for patients during treatment, and these are listed in Table 119.9. Although substantial toxicity was seen in early studies using IL-2, the administration of high-dose bolus IL-2 has been shown to be safe in experienced hands. An analysis of the trends in the safety of administering high-dose bolus IL-2 in a consecutive series of 1,241 patients with metastatic cancer treated with 720,000 IU/kg of IL-2 either alone or in conjunction with other treatments showed that the safety of administration of IL-2 increased as experience increased.[268] When comparing the initial group of 155 patients with the final group of 155 patients, line sepsis was shown to be reduced from 18% to 4%, grade 3/4 diarrhea from 92% to 12%, grade 4 neuropsychiatric toxicity from 19% to 8%, pulmonary intubations from 12% to 3%, and grade 4 cardiac ischemia from 3% to 0%. No treatment-related deaths were seen in the final 809 patients reported in this series. Thus, IL-2 can be administered to patients with metastatic melanoma with a treatment-related mortality expected to be less than 0.5%. In this series, the maximum number of administered IL-2 doses during the first cycle of therapy decreased over time from a median of 13 doses to 7 doses without an effect on the overall and complete response rates.

IL-2 mediates a chemotactic defect in neutrophils, and thus bacterial infections occurring in patients receiving IL-2 can be problematic. All patients receiving IL-2 should receive prophylactic oxacillin for line sepsis coverage. In a prospective, randomized trial of 92 patients, oxacillin reduced the incidence of line sepsis from 9.4% to 0 (P = .0001).[269] IL-2 does not cause immunosuppression, and there is no increase in opportunistic infections in patients treated with IL-2.

In summary, although chemotherapy and biochemotherapy regimens can result in objective regression rates that can be comparable to those seen with high-dose bolus IL-2, none of these regimens achieve the level of durable complete responses seen with IL-2. It is thus recommended that patients with metastatic melanoma eligible for this treatment receive high-dose IL-2 as an initial treatment.

COMBINATION CHEMOTHERAPY

Systematic *in vitro* analyses have not been conducted to determine which combination of chemotherapies might be synergistic in melanoma. As with other types of cancer, combinations of agents with some measurable single-agent activity in melanoma have been empirically developed. Clinical

TABLE 119.8

INCIDENCE OF MOST COMMON AND MOST SEVERE ADVERSE EVENTS WITH HIGH-DOSE INTERLEUKIN-2 THERAPY

Event	Grade 3	Incidence (%) Grade 4	All Grades
Cardiovascular			
Hypotension	44	1	64
Tachycardia			
Supraventricular	1	0	17
Ventricular	1	1	1
Myocardial infarction	0	1	1
Myocardial ischemia	2	<1	4
Gastrointestinal			
Nausea	6	0	24
Vomiting	34	3	55
Diarrhea	29	3	54
Stomatitis	1	<1	14
Neurologic			
Confusion	13	0	30
Somnolence	3	0	17
Coma	0	1	1
Pulmonary			
Dyspnea	9	1	31
Adult respiratory distress syndrome, pulmonary edema	5	4	16
Hepatic			
Elevated bilirubin levels	7	2	51
Elevated transaminase levels	6	1	39
Elevated alkaline phosphatase levels	1	<1	13
Renal			
Oliguria	30	9	49
Increased creatinine levels	1	0	35
Anuria	0	8	8
Hematologic			
Thrombocytopenia	16	1	43
Anemia	1	<1	29
Leukopenia	1	<1	21
Skin			
Rash	2	0	27
Exfoliative dermatitis	0	0	15
General			
Fever and/or chills	18	1	47
Malaise	14	0	34
Infection	9	2	15
Sepsis	1	1	2

trials combining chemotherapy have produced promising response rates in single-arm, single-institution studies, but have never demonstrated an improvement in overall survival compared with single-agent chemotherapy in multicenter randomized trials (Table 119.7). Given the increased toxicity associated with such regimens, the modest improvements in progression-free survival and absence of a survival advantage limit their consideration as standard therapies. The most intensively investigated combination chemotherapy regimens are cisplatin, vinblastine, and dacarbazine (CVD) and the Dartmouth regimen (cisplatin, BCNU, dacarbazine, and tamoxifen). CVD was initially reported to be associated with a complete response rate of 4% and partial response rate of 36% among 50 patients treated in a single-arm, phase 2 trial.[270] However, in the context of ECOG 3695, in which CVD was the control-arm therapy for 201 patients with metastatic melanoma, the response rate was 12% and median progression-free survival was 3.1 months.[271] Another three-drug regimen—cisplatin, vinblastine, and bleomycin—was evaluated in a phase 2 trial among 42 patients with metastatic melanoma.[272] An objective response rate of 43% was reported. A randomized trial was conducted among 57 patients comparing this same regimen with single-agent DTIC.[273] The response rate for the combination was 10% versus 14% for DTIC. This negative result precluded further evaluation of the regimen.

The Dartmouth regimen was first reported as an active regimen in two small phase 2 trials among patients with metastatic melanoma. In the first trial, 11 responses were observed among 20 evaluable patients (55% response rate); in the second trial, 10 responses were observed among 20 evaluable patients (50% response rate).[274,275] A phase 3 trial was conducted among

PRACTICE OF ONCOLOGY

TABLE 119.9

EXPECTED INTERLEUKIN-2 TOXICITIES AND THEIR MANAGEMENT

Expected Toxicity	Expected Grade	Supportive Measures	Stop Cycle[a]	Stop Treatment[b]
Chills	3	IV meperidine 25–50 mg, IV q1h, PRN	No	No
Fever	3	Acetaminophen 650 mg, PO, q4h Indomethacin 50–75mg, PO, q8h	No	No
Pruritus	3	Hydroxyzine HCL 10–20 mg, PO, q6h, PRN Diphenhydramine HCL 25–50 mg, PO, q4h, PRN	No	No
Nausea/vomiting/anorexia	3	Ondansetron 10 mg, IV, q8h, PRN Granisetron 0.01 mg/kg, IV, daily, PRN Droperidol 1 mg, IV, q4–6h, PRN Prochlorperazine 25 mg PR, PRN, or 10 mg, IV, q6h, PRN	No	No
Diarrhea	3	Loperamide 2 mg, PO, q3h, PRN Diphenoxylate HCI 2.5 mg and atropine sulfate 25 mcg, PO, q3h, PRN; codeine sulfate 30–60 mg, PO, q4h, PRN	If uncontrolled after 24 h despite all supportive measures	If uncontrolled after 24 h despite all supportive measures
Edema/weight gain	3	Diuretics PRN	No	No
Hypotension	3	Fluid resuscitation, vasopressor support	If uncontrolled despite all supportive measures	If uncontrolled despite all supportive measures
Dyspnea	3 or 4	Oxygen or ventilatory support	If requires ventilatory support	No
Oliguria	3 or 4	Fluid boluses or dopamine at renal doses	If uncontrolled despite all supportive measures	No
Confusion	3	Observation	Yes	No
Somnolence	3 or 4	Intubation for airway protection	Yes	Yes
Arrhythmia	3	Correction of fluid and electrolyte imbalances; chemical conversion or electrical conversion therapy	If uncontrolled despite all supportive measures	No
Bilirubinemia	3 or 4	Observation	For grade 4 without liver metastases	If changes have not improved to baseline by next dose

IV, intravenously; PRN, as needed; PO, orally; PR, per rectum.
[a]Unless the toxicity is not reversed within 12 hours.
[b]Unless the toxicity is not reversed to grade 2 or less by next treatment.

240 patients comparing the Dartmouth regimen with single-agent DTIC with the goal of detecting a 50% improvement in overall survival.[276] The median overall survival was similar between the two arms (7.7 months for Dartmouth vs. 6.3 months for DTIC; $P = .52$), and 1-year survival rates were also very similar (23% for Dartmouth vs. 28% for DTIC; $P = .38$). The response rate was not significantly higher for the combination regimen (17% for Dartmouth vs. 10% for DTIC; $P = .09$) and was substantially lower than the reported response rate in the smaller, single-institution studies. Among the subset of patients with less extensive metastatic disease (M1a and M1b), there was a significant difference in response rate (32% for Dartmouth vs. 14% for DTIC; $P = .05$), but this did not translate into a survival difference even for this subgroup. This observation magnifies the importance of observing activity in patients with M1c disease in the context of phase 2 trials because they constitute the largest subpopulation of patients with metastatic melanoma (59% in the trial of the Dartmouth regimen vs. DTIC). The Dartmouth regimen was associated with significantly more severe neutropenia, anemia, nausea, and vomiting. Twenty-one percent of patients treated with the Dartmouth regimen discontinued treatment because of toxicity, compared with 2% on single-agent DTIC. Although the difference in overall survival that was sought in this trial was large on a percentage basis, the targeted absolute improvement in survival was 4.5 months. A larger trial could have detected a more modest difference in survival, but this design was appropriate, given the far greater toxicity associated with the combination regimen and the need to show a substantial improvement in light of that.

In the absence of an improvement in overall survival, combination chemotherapy regimens cannot be considered as standard therapy for metastatic disease. The toxicity of these combination regimens is considerably greater than that of single-agent chemotherapy. Inpatient treatment is standard for most of these regimens, and the severity of myelosuppression often requires growth factor support not needed for single-agent chemotherapies. Given that the duration of life is not affected and the life expectancy of metastatic melanoma patients is so short, the quality-of-life detriment associated with combination therapy cannot be justified in routine practice.

The Role of Tamoxifen in Combination with Chemotherapy

After multiple anecdotes of tumor regression were reported with the estrogen receptor agonist/antagonist tamoxifen, single-agent phase 2 trials were undertaken administering either conventional or high doses. Very little activity was noted in these prospective studies.[277,278] Preclinical experiments suggested that tamoxifen was cytotoxic to melanoma cells in an estrogen receptor–independent manner and that the efficacy of cisplatin was significantly enhanced.[279,280] Clinical trials were undertaken combining tamoxifen with individual chemotherapy agents or combination regimens. As with other combination chemotherapy trials, single-arm phase 2 trials of regimens containing tamoxifen appeared promising. However, in randomized trials in which the same chemotherapy regimen was administered to all patients and tamoxifen given only to the experimental arm, no evidence of clinical benefit was observed with the addition of tamoxifen. The experience with the Dartmouth regimen, one of several tamoxifen-containing regimens, was described earlier and partly supports the observation that tamoxifen does not improve outcomes when combined with chemotherapy.

The incremental benefit of adding tamoxifen to DTIC was evaluated in a randomized phase 2 trial among 117 patients with metastatic disease.[281] The response rate observed with the combination was significantly greater than with single-agent DTIC (28% vs. 12%; *P* = .03). Median overall survival was also significantly better (11.0 months for DTIC/tamoxifen vs. 6.7 months for DTIC). The majority of the benefit appeared to be among women. Three definitive randomized trials were conducted to evaluate the contribution of tamoxifen to a chemotherapy backbone. Two hundred seventy-one patients were randomized to one of four treatment arms: DTIC alone, DTIC with tamoxifen, DTIC with interferon, or DTIC with tamoxifen and interferon.[251] A 50% improvement in overall survival compared with DTIC alone was targeted. The survival of the 134 patients who received tamoxifen was slightly inferior to that of the 137 patients who did not receive tamoxifen (8.4-month median for regimens containing tamoxifen vs. 9.5 months for regimens without tamoxifen) but not significantly so. Response rate and time to treatment failure were also similar in the arms. Two randomized trials evaluated the benefit of tamoxifen added to three-drug chemotherapy regimens. In both trials, patients with metastatic disease were randomly assigned to receive cisplatin, BCNU, and DTIC with or without tamoxifen.[282,283] The primary end point of the first trial was response rate; 211 patients were required to detect an absolute increase of 20% in objective response rate with the addition of tamoxifen. The observed response rate of 30% for the chemotherapy/tamoxifen arm was not significantly superior to a rate of 21% for the chemotherapy alone. Progression-free and overall survival were no different with the addition of tamoxifen. The primary end points of the second trial were progression-free and overall survival, with 184 patients enrolled. Progression-free survival was slightly superior for the control arm (3.4-month median without tamoxifen vs. 3.1 months with tamoxifen) but not significantly so. Response rate was also slightly superior among those who did not receive tamoxifen (33% vs. 27%). Overall survival was very similar between the groups (6.9-month median with tamoxifen vs. 6.8 months without tamoxifen). Both trials failed to observe evidence of benefit in the subset of women. In aggregate these randomized trials refuted the concept that tamoxifen substantially modulates the efficacy of chemotherapy in metastatic melanoma.

Biologic Agents Combined with Chemotherapy

Interferon-α and IL-2 are standard therapies for the treatment of stage III and stage IV melanoma, respectively. For metastatic melanoma, each agent is associated with response rates that are comparable with those of single-agent chemotherapies. More frequently observed durable complete responses distinguish high-dose IL-2 from interferon and chemotherapeutic agents that have been evaluated in melanoma.[264] The distinct mechanism of action of these biologic agents and evidence of single-agent activity have led investigators to combine these agents with chemotherapy for the treatment of metastatic melanoma. The more recent documentation of secondary immune responses to chemotherapy alone in other cancers lends further rationale to such "biochemotherapy" regimens. Given the toxicity associated with high-dose IL-2, it is not possible to administer chemotherapy safely concurrently with it. However, lower-dose IL-2 regimens can be safely coadministered even with combination chemotherapy. Similarly, the high-dose interferon regimen that is the current standard therapy for adjuvant treatment of stage II and stage III melanoma cannot be easily combined with chemotherapy, whereas modified schedules of interferon can.

The first biochemotherapy regimens tested in phase 2 trials and then subsequently in large, randomized phase 3 trials combined interferon-α with dacarbazine. Several small, single-arm phase 2 trials suggested that the response rate associated with this regimen was modestly superior to that of either single-agent DTIC or interferon.[284,285] A randomized phase 2 trial was conducted among 64 patients with metastatic melanoma.[286] The objective response rate of the combination was significantly higher than that observed with single-agent DTIC (50% vs. 19%). Secondary end points of progression-free and overall survival also appeared to be significantly superior with the combination. Definitive phase 3 trials failed to confirm the benefits suggested by this trial. In one trial, 266 patients were randomized to three treatment groups: DTIC, 800 mg/m^2 intravenously every 3 weeks; DTIC combined with 3 million units 3 times weekly by subcutaneous injection; and DTIC combined with 9 million units 3 times weekly. Overall survival was the primary end point. No differences in survival were observed. The response rates for the DTIC/interferon arms were slightly but not significantly higher than for DTIC alone (28% for DTIC/interferon 3 million units and 23% for DTIC/interferon 9 million units vs. 20% for DTIC).

The previously discussed trial evaluating the contribution of interferon and/or tamoxifen to DTIC was the other pivotal study of the DTIC/interferon regimen. Among 136 patients who received interferon (15 million units daily for 5 days repeated weekly for 3 weeks, followed by 10 million units 3 times weekly by subcutaneous injection), overall survival was not significantly superior compared with the 135 patients who did not receive interferon (9.4-month median with interferon vs. 8.4 months without interferon). Time to treatment failure was also similar (2.7-month median with interferon vs. 2.1 months without interferon), and response rate was not significantly different (20% with interferon vs. 16% without interferon). These large, randomized, multicenter trials definitively ruled out a significant benefit in combining interferon with DTIC.

More intensive regimens combining chemotherapy with biologic agents requiring inpatient administration have been evaluated subsequent to numerous trials failing to show a benefit for combination chemotherapy regimens versus single-agent. A regimen containing cisplatin, vinblastine, and dacarbazine with concurrent interferon and IL-2 was evaluated in a single-institution, single-arm, phase 2 trial.[287] The regimen consisted of cisplatin, 20 mg/m^2 daily for 4 days; vinblastine, 1.6 mg/m^2 daily for 4 days; a single dose of DTIC, 800 mg/m^2; IL-2, 9 million units/m^2 per day for 4 days by continuous infusion; and interferon-α-2b, 5 million units per day for 5 days by subcutaneous injection. This was subsequently referred to as "concurrent" biochemotherapy. Cycles were repeated every 21 days. Fifty-three patients were enrolled. A complete response rate of 21% and a partial response rate of 43% were reported. Median time to progression was 5 months, and median overall survival was 11.8 months. The same center further evaluated a modified, sequential biochemotherapy regimen in a single-center, randomized, phase 3 trial in which 190 patients were randomized between biochemotherapy (with IL-2 and interferon administered following the completion of CVD) and CVD. Response rate was the primary end point, with time to progression and overall survival as secondary end points. The response rate observed for those receiving biochemotherapy was significantly higher than for those receiving CVD (48% vs. 25%; $P = .001$). Time to progression was significantly improved (4.9 months for biochemotherapy vs. 2.4 months for CVD; $P = .008$). Overall survival was not significantly improved, but the difference suggested that a slightly larger trial could detect such an improvement with statistical significance (11.9-month median for biochemotherapy vs. 9.2 months for CVD; $P = .06$). Variations of this regimen have been evaluated in the context of phase 3 trials. Two randomized, phase 3 trials have been conducted evaluating the contribution of biologic therapy to the chemotherapy "backbone" contained in these regimens.

In E3695, the combination of CVD with interferon and IL-2 administered concurrently was compared with CVD in patients with metastatic melanoma.[288] Of note, a modified regimen was selected for this trial out of concern that the original regimen was associated with too much toxicity for the cooperative group setting. The E3695 biochemotherapy regimen was first evaluated among 44 patients with metastatic melanoma.[289] The differences were that vinblastine was administered at 1.2 instead of 1.6 mg/m^2, and interferon was administered for 3 additional days after completion of the inpatient treatment. The response rate observed in this pilot study was comparable to that reported in the previous single-center trial of concurrent biochemotherapy. In E3695, overall survival was the primary end point, and 482 patients were needed to demonstrate a 33% improvement. Accrual was stopped after 416 patients were enrolled because of a preplanned futility analysis. Overall survival was not improved (8.4-month median for biochemotherapy vs. 9.1 months for CVD). Progression-free survival was superior (5.0-month median for biochemotherapy vs. 3.1 months for CVD) but not significantly so. Response rate was not significantly higher in the biochemotherapy arm (17% vs. 12%). Among the 40% of patients who had no prior adjuvant interferon use, progression-free and overall survival appeared better in the biochemotherapy arm. This lends support to the current investigation of biochemotherapy in the adjuvant setting in S0008, a cooperative group phase 3 trial comparing this regimen with high-dose interferon-α among patients with resected stage III melanoma.

In EORTC 18951, cisplatin, dacarbazine, and interferon-α were administered to all patients, with "decrescendo" IL-2 administered only to one cohort.[290] Three hundred sixty-three patients were accrued, with all receiving DTIC, 250 mg/m^2 daily for 3 days; cisplatin, 30 mg/m^2 daily for 3 days; and interferon-α-2b, 10 million units/m^2 daily for 5 days. The experimental arm also received IL-2 for 4 days after completion of the chemotherapy. The dose per day was fixed, but the duration of the infusion was lengthened each day. Survival rate at 2 years was the primary end point, and an improvement from 10% to 20% was sought. The observed difference in 2-year survival (18% for the IL-2–containing arm vs. 13% for the arm without IL-2) was not statistically significant. Progression-free survival and response rates were not significantly different between the two treatments.

Biochemotherapy regimens remain investigational. The toxicity associated with these inpatient treatments has not been justified by demonstration of efficacy in randomized trials. Even in single-center trials, the high response rates are not associated with overall survival that is significantly different than the expected outcome for these patients. This is consistent with the observation that most responses are short lived. For that reason, the biochemotherapy regimens that are being developed contain "maintenance" therapy with agents that are amenable to long-term use, such as GM-CSF and temozolomide.

EXPERIMENTAL AND DEVELOPING IMMUNOLOGIC THERAPIES FOR STAGE IV MELANOMA

Adoptive Cell Therapy

Adoptive cell therapy (ACT) refers to an immunotherapy approach for the treatment of cancer that involves the infusion to the tumor-bearing host of cells with antitumor activity that can recognize cancer antigens and result in the destruction of cancer cells. Although it is still experimental, ACT has emerged as the most effective treatment for patients with metastatic melanoma; from 50% to 70% of patients with metastatic melanoma experience objective cancer regressions by response evaluation criteria in solid tumors (RECIST) when treated with ACT.[291,292]

ACT has a variety of advantages compared with other forms of cancer immunotherapy.[292,293] T lymphocytes, once identified as cancer reactive, can be expanded to large numbers *in vitro* using cytokine growth factors. Thus, patients can be administered very large numbers of cells, often much larger than can be naturally generated *in vivo*. These antitumor lymphocytes can be activated *in vitro* to express appropriate effector functions such as the ability to lyse tumor cells and secrete cytokines. Secreted cytokines can have a variety of secondary antitumor effects at the cancer site such as the destruction of surrounding blood vessels, the direct lysis of tumor cells, and providing chemokine signals to attract additional effector cell types, such as activated macrophages, to the tumor site. Perhaps most important, when using ACT, it is possible to modify the host to enhance the ability of the infused cells to establish, grow, and function *in vivo*. The ability to immunosuppress the host prior to cell infusion is unique to ACT. Immunosuppression can counteract the impact of T-regulatory cells that can suppress cellular immune reactions as well as remove other endogenous lymphocytes that compete with the infused cells for homeostatic cytokines such as IL-7 and IL-15, which are necessary for antitumor T-cell expansion *in vivo*.[292]

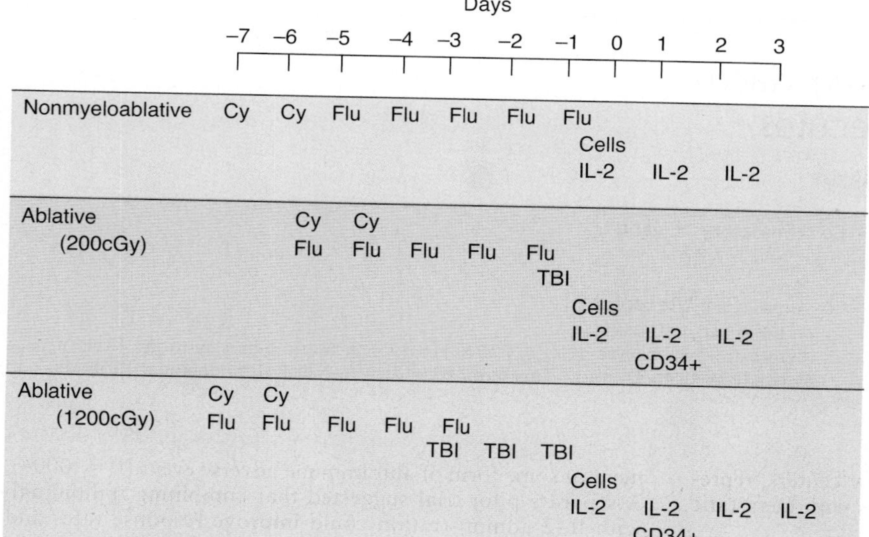

FIGURE 119.15 Adoptive Cell Therapy protocol developed at the Surgery Branch of the National Cancer Institute.

A critical step in the development of effective ACT for human cancer was the demonstration in 1987 that lymphocytes infiltrating into deposits of human metastatic melanoma could be grown in IL-2.[294] Tumor-infiltrating lymphocytes (TIL) with antitumor activity could be generated from approximately 70% of patients with metastatic melanoma.[295] Using these human TIL, over 50 different antigenic epitopes have been identified in patients with melanoma, including antigens such as MART1 and gp100 that are widely shared among melanomas from different individuals.[296] The first report of ACT in humans in 1988,[297] and extending into 1994,[298] used the transfer of autologous TIL followed by the administration of high-dose IL-2. An objective response rate of 34% was seen in 86 consecutive patients with metastatic melanoma.

A major improvement in human ACT occurred when immunosuppressive regimens were administered prior to cell infusions, and this change led to a new generation of ACT clinical protocols.[291,292] A schematic of ACT treatment in humans with metastatic melanoma developed in the Surgery Branch of the National Cancer Institute is shown in Figure 119.15. In this treatment, metastatic melanoma deposits are resected and used to generate cultures of TIL with antitumor activity. When cultures reach from 1 to 5 × 10^{10} cells, they are infused into patients following an immunosuppressive preparative regimen. The first trial of this approach used a nonmyeloablative preparative regimen consisting of 60 mg/kg of cyclophosphamide for 2 days followed by 5 days of fludarabine at 25 mg/m^2. On the day following the last dose of fludarabine the TIL were administered intravenously and IL-2 was then administered for 2 to 3 days at 720,000 IU/kg intravenously every 8 hours. An objective response rate by standard RECIST criteria was seen in 21 of 43 patients (49%)[292] (Fig. 119.16).

Because animal models demonstrated that more profound lymphodepletion was associated with higher antitumor effects, two additional clinical trials were performed in 25 patients each who received this cyclophosphamide–fludarabine chemotherapy plus 2 Gy or 12 Gy of whole-body irradiation (Fig. 119.16). Objective tumor regressions were seen in 13 of 25 (52%) and in 18 of 25 (72%) patients, respectively, including 8 complete regressions (32%) in the latter trial.[292] In these trials only 1 of 16 complete responders has recurred, with the others ongoing at 34 to 82 months. These results, although

Cell Transfer Therapy

Treatment	Total	PR	CR	OR (%)
	Number of patients (duration in months)			
No TBI	43	16 (84, 36, 29, 28, 14, 13, 11, 8, 8, 7, 4, 3, 3, 2, 2, 2)	5 (95+, 82+, 79+, 78+, 64+)	21 (49%)
200 TBI	25	8 (14, 9, 6, 6, 5, 4, 3, 3)	5 (68+, 64+, 60+, 57+, 54+)	13 (52%)
1200 TBI	25	8 (21, 13, 7, 6, 6, 5, 4, 3)	10 (48+, 45+, 44+, 44+, 39+, 38+, 38+, 38+, 37+, 19)	18 (72%)

FIGURE 119.16 Clinical outcomes for each of three preparative regimens used in patients prior to receiving adoptive cell transfer at the Surgery Branch of the National Cancer Institute. Nonmyeloblative chemotherapy is administered over 7 days. When 2 Gy whole-body irradiation is given, the chemotherapy is condensed to a 5-day regimen with the total-body irradiation (TBI) following the last dose of fludarabine and the cells and interleukin 2 (IL-2) a day later. For these patients CD34+ stem cells, harvested from peripheral blood after granulocyte cell stimulating factor administration, are administered on the day after cell administration. Patients receiving 12 Gy whole-body irradiation receive 2 Gy twice a day for 3 days prior to cell administration.

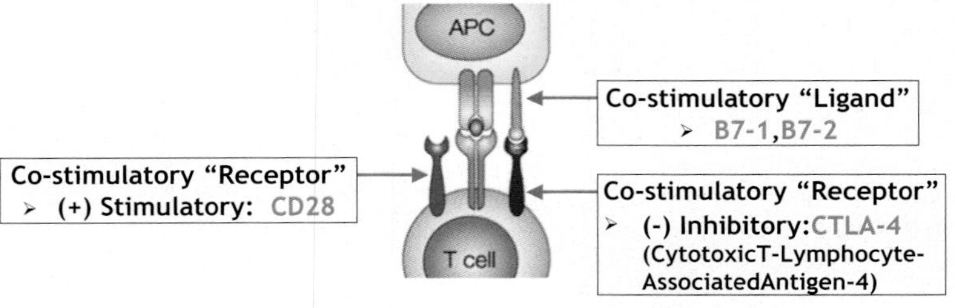

FIGURE 119.17 Schematic representation of the mechanism of action of anti–CTLA-4 monoclonal antibody.

still experimental and available in only a few centers, represent the most effective treatments for patients with metastatic melanoma.

Recent studies using the adoptive transfer of autologous peripheral lymphocytes transduced with genes encoding antitumor T-cell receptors have also shown objective responses in patients with metastatic melanoma and are under vigorous development.[299,300]

Administration of Anti–CTLA-4 Monoclonal Antibody

CTLA-4 monoclonal antibody (ipilimumab) is a molecule expressed on lymphocytes that binds the B7-1 and B7-2 (CD80 and CD86) molecules on the surface of antigen-presenting cells (Fig. 119.17). Engagement of the CTLA-4 molecule can suppress lymphocyte reactivity and interfere with IL-2 secretion and IL-2 receptor expression. The T-regulatory cells are the only lymphocytes in the resting circulation that constitutively expressed CTLA-4 on their surface; however, expression of CTLA-4 is transiently up-regulated after binding of the T-cell receptor. Multiple preclinical murine models have shown that CTLA-4 blockade can enhance immune-mediated tumor rejection when combined with vaccines.

Although the administration of anti–CTLA-4 monoclonal antibody to patients with metastatic melanoma has not been approved by the FDA as of the writing of this chapter, multiple clinical studies have shown that objective clinical responses can be achieved in patients treated with CTLA-4 blockade. In an updated study of 143 consecutive patients with metastatic melanoma treated with varying doses of anti–CTLA-4 either alone or in conjunction with peptide vaccination, an objective response rate of 17% was seen, including 10 patients (7%) with complete response.[301,302] A multi-institutional prospective randomized trial was performed in 676 HLA-A*0201–positive patients with unresectable stage III or IV melanoma who received either (1) ipilimumab, (2) ipilimumab plus a gp100 peptide vaccine, or (3) the vaccine alone.[303] Objective response rates were 11.0%, 5.7%, and 1.5%, respectively. Median overall survival was 10.1, 10.0, and 6.4 months, respectively ($P = .003$ for ipilimumab compared with vaccine). There were 14 (2.1%) study drug–related deaths. About 15% of patients develop autoimmune adverse events, which can include severe diarrhea, hypophysitis, and dermatitis, and rarely patients experience nephritis and hepatitis. Most of these side effects could be abrogated by the administration of steroids. A strong association exists between the probability of achieving an objective antitumor response and the development of some form of autoimmune adverse event ($P = .0004$). A separate pilot trial suggested that combining ipilimumab with IL-2 administration could improve response rates and possibly lessen toxicity, although additional studies are necessary to evaluate this.[304]

In early studies another antibody, directed against programmed death-1, an inhibitory receptor expressed on activated T cells, mediated a partial response in one of ten patients with melanoma.[305]

Melanoma Vaccines

These have been discussed under "Specific Immunotherapy" and "Defined Molecular Melanoma Antigens and Vaccines" sections.

RATIONALE FOR TARGETED THERAPY IN MELANOMA

The elucidation of somatic genetic mutations in melanoma underlying aberrant signal transduction in melanoma cells has provided leads for molecularly targeted therapy. In particular, the mitogen-activated protein (MAP) kinase pathway and the phospho-inositol-3-phosphate (PI3) kinase pathway have been implicated in the pathogenesis of melanoma. Mutation in *BRAF*, a constituent of MAP kinase pathway, is the most common oncogenic event in melanoma.[306]

Among the most common subtypes of melanoma—superficial spreading and nodular histologies—these activating mutations in this kinase domain are found in at least two-thirds of cases.[8] Activating mutations in *NRAS* have also been described in a nonoverlapping subset of cases, 15% of all melanomas.[307] Taken together, *BRAF* and *NRAS* mutations account for activation of the MAP kinase pathway in approximately 80% of melanomas. Of note, these mutations are detected in benign nevi as well as invasive primary melanoma and metastatic disease.[308] Promising investigational molecularly targeted agents are listed in Table 119.10.

The presence of mutations in *NRAS* is sufficient to activate both the MAP kinase and PI3 kinase pathways. Loss of the tumor suppressor gene *PTEN* or amplification of *Akt-3* results in constitutive activation of the PI3 kinase pathway.[309] Deletion or mutation of *PTEN* is found in 40% of melanomas, whereas gene amplification of Akt-3 has been described in 33% of cases.[310] The presence of *NRAS* mutation, *PTEN* deletion, or Akt-3 amplification each appears sufficient to activate the PI3 kinase pathway.

TABLE 119.10

PROMISING INVESTIGATIONAL AGENTS

Target	Drug	Phase of Melanoma Clinical Trials	Single-Agent Response Rate (%)
CTLA-4	Ipilimumab	2 and 3	13
	Ticilimumab	2 and 3	7
BRAF	Sorafenib	3	2
	RAF-265	1	—
	PLX4032	1	—
MEK	PD0325901	2	7
	AZD6244	2	—
mTOR	CCI-779	2	3
VEGF	Bevacizumab	2	—
CDK4	PD332991	1	—

Activating mutations and genetic amplification of *KIT* have been identified in the uncommon clinical subtypes of melanoma: acral-lentiginous and mucosal.[311] To a far lesser extent, LMMs have been found to harbor such aberrations. Overall, approximately 1% of all melanoma patients with advanced melanoma harbor activating mutations in *KIT*. Activating mutations in *KIT* appear to activate the MAP kinase and PI3 kinase pathways and, thus, could serve as the functional equivalent of an *NRAS* mutation or *BRAF* mutation combined with *PTEN* loss.[312] Although a large number of distinct *KIT* mutations have described in melanoma, they largely overlap with those found in gastrointestinal stromal tumors.

Other signal transduction pathways have been implicated in melanoma pathogenesis, but their contribution, independent of the MAP kinase and PI3 kinase pathways, has not been well elucidated. These include NF-κB, Stat3, FAK, β-catenin, and the transcription factor Notch.[313]

Angiogenesis is necessary for the progression of all solid tumors, and increased expression of certain proangiogenic factors have been associated with invasive capacity of primary melanomas but not as consistently with poor prognosis in patients with advanced disease.[314,315] The relative importance of such growth factors as VEGF, platelet-derived growth factor (PDGF), basic fibroblast growth factor (bFGF), and IL-8 is not well understood. Whereas VEGF has been clearly implicated as the primary promoter of angiogenesis in renal cell, colorectal, non–small cell lung, and breast cancers, in melanoma VEGF is overexpressed only in a minority of primary or metastatic tumors.[316] On the other hand, most melanoma cell lines produce some VEGF, and autocrine signaling through VEGFR2 has been identified in a subset of melanomas.[317] bFGF expression is not associated with increasing stage of disease, and the presence of bFGF in tumor blood vessels is paradoxically associated with good prognosis.[318,319] On the other hand, platelet-derived growth factor and IL-8 are overexpressed in the majority of melanomas, are associated with invasiveness, and correlate with poor prognosis.[320–324] Given the clinical benefit associated with inhibition of angiogenesis in other cancers, this strategy is worthy of pursuit in melanoma. It may be that the optimal angiogenesis-inhibiting strategy in melanoma will be different than for other cancers.

Targeted Therapy Trials in Melanoma

Since the identification of *BRAF* mutations in melanoma in 2002, the MAP kinase pathway has been the focus of most clinical investigations. Direct blockade of Raf and indirect inhibition at the level of the immediate downstream signaling mediator, MEK, have been two strategies most extensively investigated in preclinical models and clinical trials. The most extensive clinical investigations have been conducted with sorafenib, a small-molecule inhibitor B-Raf, RAF1 (formerly known as c-Raf), VEGF receptors, and several other kinases. Although this agent has been demonstrated to suppress signaling and cell viability in the cells that harbor a *BRAF* mutation, clinical data do not support the ability to effectively inhibit the MAP kinase pathway in tumors when administered at the maximum tolerated dose.[325,326] In single-agent phase 2 trials in melanoma, objective responses and prolonged disease control were infrequently observed. Biopsies of metastatic lesions performed before and during therapy demonstrated modest inhibition of the MAP kinase pathway after several weeks of treatment.[327]

Highly potent and selective Raf inhibitors have only recently emerged from early-phase clinical trials. PLX4032 and GSK2118436 are the best characterized examples. In cell lines and animal models such selective Raf inhibitors inhibit only the MAP kinase pathway and tumor growth in tumors that harbor *BRAF* mutations. In phase 1 trials, conducted among metastatic melanoma patients who were prospectively screened for *BRAF* mutations, the objective response rate observed with both agents appears very high. Once the phase 2 dose was determined for PLX4032, at the conclusion of dose escalation, 32 patients with *BRAF* mutant melanoma received a dose of 960 mg orally twice daily in a multicenter study.[328] Twenty-one patients experienced a partial response and two had complete responses (81% objective response rate). The median duration of response had not yet been reached, but was approximately 9 months. Both response rate and durability of response appear vastly superior to conventional cytotoxic therapies in this setting, but must be confirmed in larger patient cohorts. Although less mature clinical data are available for GSK2118436, this agent appears similarly promising.[329] These single-agent Raf inhibitors are poised to challenge DTIC as the standard therapy for metastatic melanoma. Less selective Raf inhibitors, XL281 and RAF-265, are also in development, but their efficacy in *BRAF* mutant melanoma is still undefined.

MEK inhibitors have also been of interest in this setting because the leads that have been developed clinically are highly selective for MEK, and B-Raf has no known substrate other than MEK. AZD6244 is an orally available MEK inhibitor with a very short half-life, and when dosed twice daily provides inconsistent inhibition of the MAP kinase pathway.[330] In a randomized phase 2 trial comparing AZD6244 with temozolomide among patients with metastatic melanoma, modest activity was observed. Five objective responses were observed among 45 patients defined, in retrospect, to harbor *BRAF* mutations. When confining outcome analysis to patients with

BRAF mutation, those who received AZD6244 did not have a significantly improved progression-free survival compared with temozolomide (hazard ratio = 0.85). However, an equally selective MEK inhibitor with a substantially longer half-life has recently emerged from phase 1 clinical testing.[331] Once a maximum tolerated dose was defined, GSK1120212 was administered orally daily to patients with metastatic melanoma harboring *BRAF* mutations. Among 20 patients, 6 partial and 2 complete responses were observed (40% response rate; 95% CI: 19%–64%). This preliminary report does not adequately characterize the activity of this agent, but it is clear that responses can be observed with this unique point of intervention in the MAP kinase pathway. A question that remains to be resolved is the potential role of a MEK inhibitor when selective Raf inhibitors appear to have a significantly higher response rate.

Given the validation of *KIT* mutation as a predictor of responsiveness to KIT inhibitors, such imatinib and sunitinib phase 2 trials have been mounted to document responses in these patients. Individual patient reports confirm that objective response can be seen in patients with metastatic melanoma harboring a *KIT* mutation.[332,333] The mature results of phase 2 trials selecting patients on the basis of activating mutation and/or genetic amplification only are awaited.

Combinations of Targeted Therapy with Chemotherapy

Despite limited clinical activity observed with single-agent sorafenib, more promising results were observed for sorafenib in combination with chemotherapy. Randomized trials of sorafenib in combination with chemotherapy proceeded with the hope that inhibition of the VEGF signaling pathway would augment the activity of chemotherapy, as has been observed in numerous other cancer types. However, the results of two small randomized trials did not suggest a significant improvement outcome for patients who receive sorafenib combined with chemotherapy compared with those who receive chemotherapy alone.[334,335] One phase 2 trial combining DTIC with sorafenib was conducted with a single-agent DTIC control arm.[335] One hundred one patients with metastatic melanoma who had not previously received chemotherapy were randomly assigned to treatment with DTIC and placebo or DTIC and sorafenib. Patients treated with DTIC and sorafenib were more likely to achieve an objective response (24% vs. 12%) and more prolonged progression-free survival (median 4.9 vs. 2.7 months). The likelihood of remaining progression-free 6 months after initiation of treatment was significantly more likely for patients receiving the combination compared with those receiving DTIC alone (41% vs. 18%). This small trial suggests a benefit with the addition of sorafenib to DTIC in patients who have not received prior chemotherapy, but it requires validation in a larger, randomized, phase 3 trial.

The combination of sorafenib with carboplatin and paclitaxel has also been evaluated in a randomized trial. In that study, 270 patients whose metastatic melanoma had progressed despite DTIC or temozolomide-containing chemotherapy regimens were randomly assigned to receive carboplatin, paclitaxel, and placebo or carboplatin, paclitaxel, and sorafenib.[336] The objective rate and progression-free survival were not significantly different between the two groups. The objective response rate of 11% and median progression-free survival of 4.1 months for patients treated on the control arm were significantly better than expected for a cohort of patients whose tumors had proven refractory to prior chemotherapy.

A definitive phase 3 trial was conducted among chemotherapy-naïve metastatic melanoma patients, enrolled regardless of *BRAF* mutation status.[337] In this trial, 823 patients were randomly assigned to receive carboplatin and paclitaxel with or without sorafenib. Overall survival, the primary end point, was not improved with the addition of sorafenib to this chemotherapy backbone (hazard ratio of = 1.0). Progression-free survival and response rate were also not significantly better. In particular, phase 2 trials have been completed combining sorafenib with DTIC, temozolomide, and the doublet regimen of carboplatin and paclitaxel. In total, the results of sorafenib in combination with chemotherapy do not support a role for this agent in genetically unselected patients. For patients whose tumors harbor *BRAF* mutation, more active Raf inhibitors have now been identified.

Few trials have been undertaken with agents that target other signal transduction pathways implicated in the pathogenesis of melanoma, such as the PI3 kinase pathway. A phase 2 trial evaluating the mammalian target of the rapamycin (mTOR) inhibitor temsirolimus was conducted among 33 patients with metastatic melanoma.[338] The observation of only one objective response terminated further investigations of single-agent temsirolimus in melanoma. However, preclinical data support a synergistic effect with mTOR inhibition combined with either chemotherapy or a MAP kinase pathway inhibitor such as sorafenib.[339] Similar results have been generated for agents that directly inhibitor PI3 kinase. Combinations of inhibitors that block signaling pathways individually implicated in melanoma pathophysiology are likely to emerge as a theme in melanoma clinical research in the years to come.

Clinical Trials with Inhibitors of Angiogenesis in Melanoma. Inhibition of VEGF signaling has proven to be beneficial as a stand-alone strategy in renal cell carcinoma and in combination with standard cytotoxic chemotherapies in colorectal, non–small cell lung, and breast cancers. Few investigations have been undertaken with this strategy in melanoma, with the exception of the trials with sorafenib cited earlier. Bevacizumab, a monoclonal antibody with specificity for secreted VEGF, has only recently been evaluated in combination with chemotherapy in metastatic melanoma.[340] Among 200 patients randomized to carboplatin (AUC 5) and paclitaxel (225 mg/m^2) given every 3 weeks with or without bevacizumab, 15 mg/kg every 3 weeks, two-thirds of the trial population received bevacizumab. Progression-free survival (hazard ratio = 0.78, P = .14), response rate (25.5% vs. 16.4%, P = .16), and overall survival (hazard ratio = 0.79, P = .19) were all improved, but not with statistical significance. Nonetheless, this exploratory, randomized phase 2 trial suggests that bevacizumab may improve outcomes in combination with chemotherapy and that a definitive phase 3 trial is warranted.

Thalidomide is an agent that has been reported to inhibit tumor angiogenesis in some preclinical models but not others.[341,342] Phase 2 trials with single-agent thalidomide at "low" doses or the individually maximum tolerated dose did not result in objective responses.[343–345]

In combination with temozolomide, objective responses and prolonged disease stabilization were observed in a subset of patients enrolled on single-arm, phase 2 trials.[346–348] One randomized, phase 2 trial was conducted comparing single-agent temozolomide (55 patients) with temozolomide combined with "low-dose" thalidomide (60 patients).[349] The objective response rate was not significantly different (9% for the single-agent temozolomide vs. 15% for the combination), and no difference was observed in progression-free survival. Although the temozolomide/thalidomide arm produced a marginally higher response rate, these data, combined with the results of single-arm trials, have not established the benefit of thalidomide in melanoma.

RADIATION THERAPY FOR METASTATIC MELANOMA (STAGE IV)

Radiation Dose Fractionation Schedules

There is no consensus regarding the optimal dose fractionation schedule for melanoma. Controversy surrounding the radiosensitivity of melanoma began in the early 1970s when cell survival curves for several human melanoma cell lines were published showing a broad shoulder, indicative of high levels of potentially lethal damage repair; this fostered the hypothesis that melanomas were less likely to respond to conventionally fractionated radiation at 2 to 2.5 Gy per fraction and that higher dose per fraction schedules might result in superior clinical outcomes.[170] These studies caused many investigators to adopt high-dose (4 Gy or greater per fraction) fractionation schedules for melanoma, and several investigators published improved clinical outcomes with these large fractional doses compared with conventional fractionation.[171,172] This led the RTOG to initiate RTOG 83-05, a prospective, randomized trial comparing the effectiveness of high dose per fraction radiation and conventionally fractionated radiation in the treatment of melanoma. RTOG 83-05 randomized 126 patients with measurable lesions to 8.0 Gy × 4 fractions (32 Gy total) in 21 days delivered once weekly or 2.5 Gy × 20 fractions (50 Gy total) in 26 to 28 days delivered 5 days a week. The study was closed early when interim statistical analysis suggested that further accrual would not reveal a statistical difference between the arms. The 8.0 Gy × 4–fraction arm had a complete remission of 24.2% and partial remission of 35.5%, and the 2.5 Gy × 20–fraction arm had a complete remission of 23.4% and a partial remission of 34.4%.[350] This randomized trial demonstrated that melanoma is a radioresponsive tumor, and conventional and high dose per fraction schedules are equally effective clinically.

Despite the results of this study, many investigators still report that melanoma is a radioresistant histology, and most current retrospective clinical reports regarding radiation for melanoma use a high dose per fraction schedule. Although high dose per fraction treatments can result in increased risk of late radiation toxicity, there are little data to suggest that high dose per fraction schedules such as 30 Gy in five fractions over 2.5 weeks, which is currently commonly used in the adjuvant treatment of nodal basins after lymph node dissection,[173] results in increased late toxicity compared with conventionally fractionated regimens to 50 to 70 Gy. High-dose fractionation schedules are more convenient for the patient and less expensive, and allow patients to proceed with systemic therapy sooner; they should be considered as a reasonable option unless critical structures are in the irradiated volume that would be treated above their radiation tolerance or the volume has previously been irradiated. They are particularly appropriate for patients with widespread disease and short life expectancies because they can provide rapid palliation in a few fractions, and late radiation toxicity is not a concern for this patient population.

The Role of Radiation Therapy in the Management of Distant Metastatic Disease

In general, patients with one to two sites of metastatic melanoma, good performance status, and long interval from diagnosis of the primary lesion should be considered for surgical resection. Patients with widespread metastatic disease may be managed with systemic chemotherapy or immunotherapy, with palliative radiation to symptomatic areas of progressive disease. From a radiotherapy perspective, patients with distant metastasis of melanoma are generally managed similar to patients with distant metastases of other solid tumors, with the only main area of controversy being the role of whole-brain radiation therapy (WBRT) for patients with melanoma brain metastases. Patients with widespread systemic disease and short life expectancies should be treated with short courses of high dose per fraction radiation.

Radiation Therapy for Brain Metastases

Carella et al.[351] retrospectively analyzed 60 patients from two RTOG studies performed in the 1970s with cerebral metastases from malignant melanoma to determine the response to whole-brain irradiation and reported that the palliative and survival benefit of WBRT for melanoma patients was comparable to those found for all other primary tumors. However, the median survival times for the two studies were short, only 10 and 14 weeks, and response was measured as symptomatic improvement, which may have been at least partially due to corticosteroids given to reduce cerebral edema. In a retrospective study from the M. D. Anderson Cancer Center reporting on 87 patients treated for metastatic melanoma to the brain with WBRT with total doses of at least 30 Gy, it was concluded that the frequent use of corticosteroids made it difficult to assess palliative benefit from the radiation, although some patients may have derived benefit as approximately 50% of patients were able to discontinue corticosteroids on the completion of radiation treatments. However, despite this potential benefit, the median survival was only 19 weeks.[352]

Three more recent prospective clinical trials with objective imaging criteria to assess tumor response have shown that WBRT with 30 to 37.5 Gy in 10 to 15 fractions results in objective responses of only 10% or less when delivered with concurrent chemotherapy in patients with melanoma brain metastases.[256,353,354] The Cytokine Working Group reported on a phase 2 trial that investigated the role of temozolomide and WBRT delivered as 30 Gy in 10 fractions delivered over 2 weeks with response determined by both neurologic examination and gadolinium-contrast MRI imaging.[256] Thirty-one patients were enrolled in the study and there were only two complete responses and one partial response for an overall objective response rate of 9.7%. The median central nervous system progression-free interval was only 2 months, and the authors concluded that WBRT has lower than expected activity in central nervous system metastasis of malignant melanoma. The Cytokine Working Group subsequently reported a phase 2 study of 39 patients treated with WBRT (30 Gy in 10 fractions), temozolomide, and thalidomide that resulted in a response rate of only 7.6%, with a median time to progression of 7 weeks and median overall survival of 4 months.[353] A phase 3 trial randomizing 76 patients with central nervous system metastases from melanoma to fotemustine or fotemustine and WBRT (37.5 Gy in 15 fractions) delivered over 3 weeks revealed an objective response rate of 7.4% in the fotemustine alone arm and 10.0% in the fotemustine and WBRT arm.[354] The authors concluded that although fotemustine and WBRT delayed the time to brain progression of melanoma brain metastases compared with fotemustine alone, there was no significant difference between objective control rates and overall survival between the two arms. Therefore, data from these three small prospective trials suggest that WBRT has limited activity in the treatment of malignant melanoma metastatic to the brain and should be reserved for patients with widespread systemic metastases or diffuse brain metastases that are not amenable to surgical resection or stereotactic radiosurgery.

Stereotactic radiosurgery delivers high doses of radiation in a single fraction to cerebral lesions that are generally less than 3 cm in diameter and do not involve the brainstem. Yu et al.[355] reported one of the largest retrospective studies to date from University of California, Los Angeles, consisting of 122 consecutive patients with 332 intracranial melanoma metastases who underwent gamma knife radiosurgery with a median prescribed dose of 20 Gy (range, 14–24 Gy). One-third of the patients also received WBRT. The overall median survival was 7.0 months from radiosurgery and 9.1 months from the onset of brain metastasis. In multivariate analysis WBRT did not improve survival, and freedom from subsequent brain metastasis depended on intracranial tumor volume. The University of Utah reported a retrospective study of 68 patients with up to five brain metastases from histologies considered radioresistant (melanoma, renal cell carcinoma, or sarcoma) who underwent stereotactic radiosurgery with or without WBRT or surgical resection; all patients had a Karnofsky performance score of more than 70 and stereotactic radiosurgery treatment before initiation of systemic therapy.[356] Their population had a median survival of 14.2 months; they found no benefit to the addition of WBRT, with a median survival of 12.8 months with WBRT and 14.9 months without WBRT. Retrospective studies reporting the survival of patients treated with stereotactic radiosurgery with and without WBRT delivered at the discretion of the treating physicians need to be interpreted cautiously, as generally, patients with multiple or larger lesions receive WBRT and those with smaller and or fewer lesions do not. This may result in a significant patient selection bias favoring the stereotactic radiosurgery only group.

The RTOG trial 9508 was a phase 3 randomized trial that enrolled 333 patients with one to three brain metastases with multiple histologies (4% of patients had melanoma) to receive WBRT to a total dose of 37.5 Gy in 15 fractions over 3 weeks with and without a radiosurgery boost, with the dose depending on the tumor volume (tumors 2 cm or less received 24 Gy, tumors more than 2 cm and 3 cm or less received 18 Gy, and tumors more than 3 cm and 4 cm or less received 15 Gy).[357] Patients with a single brain metastasis had statistically improved survival with a radiosurgical boost compared with those without a boost (6.5 vs. 4.9 months, respectively), and the authors concluded that WBRT and stereotactic radiosurgical boost should be the treatment of choice for patients with solitary unresectable brain metastasis. Given the historic data suggesting limited benefit from WBRT for patients with melanoma brain metastasis, the Eastern Cooperative Oncology Group initiated study E6397, which was a phase 2 trial of radiosurgery for one to three newly diagnosed brain metastases for renal cell carcinoma, melanoma, and sarcoma without WBRT.[358] The dose prescription was based on tumor size and was similar to the RTOG 9508 trial. Thirty-one eligible patients were accrued to this study. The median survival was 8.3 months. The intracranial failure rate in and outside the radiosurgically treated volume at 3 months was 19% and 16%, and at 6 months it was 32% and 32%, respectively. The authors concluded that delaying WBRT may be appropriate for some subgroups of patients with radioresistant tumors, but routine avoidance of WBRT should be approached judiciously given the high intracranial failure rates.

In summary, current data would support the following treatment recommendations for patients with brain metastases from melanoma. All patients with symptomatic cerebral edema should be administered corticosteroids initially. Patients with good performance status and no or minimal systemic disease and a solitary resectable brain lesion should undergo resection. Similar patients with an unresectable brain lesion or up to five small metastatic lesions should be treated with stereotactic radiosurgery, and both groups should be considered for WBRT or close observation with serial imaging. Patients with poor performance status, diffuse systemic disease, and more than five brain lesions have a poor overall prognosis and should be considered for palliative WBRT only.

Radiation Therapy for Vertebral Metastases

Patients with vertebral metastases causing spinal cord compression with a reasonable life expectancy of more than 1 to 2 months should be treated with corticosteroids and surgical decompression if they are operative candidates, with subsequent postoperative radiotherapy as opposed to palliative radiation alone, as this has been shown to result in superior preservation of neurologic function.[359] Patients who are not operative candidates should be considered for radiation therapy. Recent advancements in radiation therapy planning and delivery have led to the development of stereotactic body radiation therapy (SBRT) for lesions in multiple organ sites (lung, liver, and spine). With SBRT, patients are treated with one to five fractions of high-dose and highly conformal radiation isodose distributions.[360] Patients who have limited systemic disease burden who are not considered surgical candidates, or patients with spinal cord compression from disease progression following palliative conventional radiation therapy, should be considered for SBRT. Figure 119.18 shows the highly conformal radiation isodose distributions that are achievable with SBRT techniques for a representative lung and vertebral body lesion.

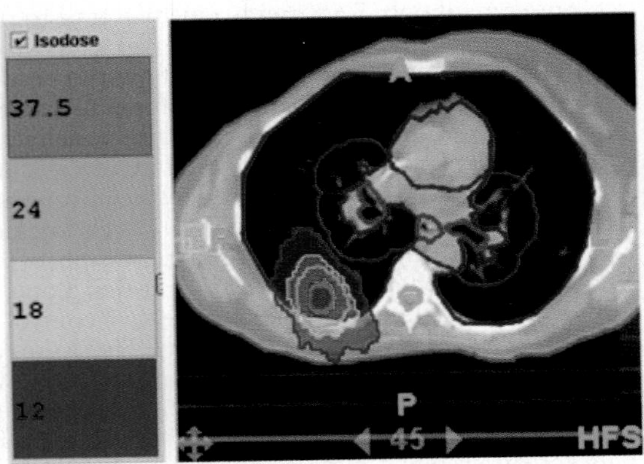

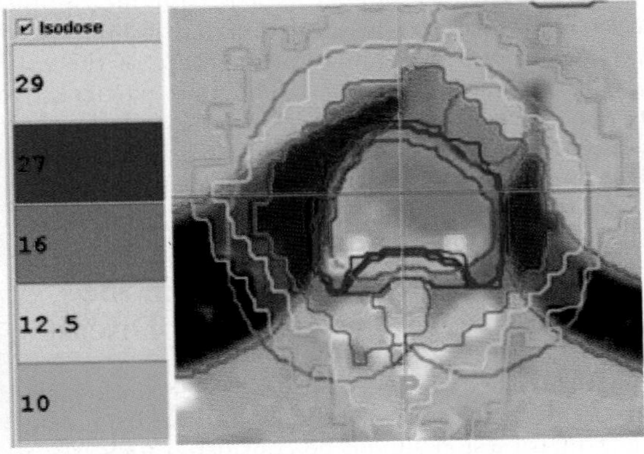

FIGURE 119.18 Radiation isodose distribution in gray of a stereotactic body radiation therapy treatment plan for a lung and vertebral body metastasis.

Current Radiation Research for Melanoma: Interactions with Immune Therapy

Radiation has been reported to have immunomodulatory effects in melanoma animal models thought to be secondary to cell death and inflammation leading to enhanced antigen presentation and antigen-specific cellular immunity, and *in vivo* preclinical and clinical studies suggest that radiation can mediate modulation of tumor-specific immunity.[361,362] The two main strategies of integration of radiation into immune-based treatment strategies include local tumor irradiation resulting in enhanced tumor-antigen presentation and antigen-specific cellular immunity,[361–363] and total-body irradiation–induced host lymphodepletion resulting in enhanced efficacy of adoptive T-cell transfer-based immunotherapy.[364]

Radiation combined with intratumoral injections of bone marrow–derived, unpulsed dendritic cells was reported to induce a potent local and systemic antitumor response in melanoma tumor–bearing mice that was superior to that seen with IL-2 and the same intratumoral injections.[362] Local tumor irradiation reportedly increased the antigen-presenting capability within tumor-draining lymph nodes and increased the numbers of T cells within draining lymph nodes that secreted interferon-α after tumor peptide stimulation in mice compared with treatment without radiation.[361] In humans with metastatic melanoma, a phase 2 trial with 45 patients treated with low-dose total-body irradiation as a potential immunomodulator and subcutaneous IL-2 failed to show increased clinical efficacy compared with historical controls of subcutaneous IL-2 alone.[365] Other investigators have demonstrated the efficacy and feasibility of melanoma-targeted radiopharmaceutical therapies in murine models using either a radiolabeled melanoma-targeted α-melanocyte–stimulating hormone peptide analogue[366] or radiolabeled melanin-binding monoclonal antibody.[367]

PRACTICE OF ONCOLOGY

Selected References

The full list of references for this chapter appears in the online version.

8. Curtin JA, Fridlyand J, Kageshita T, et al. Distinct sets of genetic alterations in melanoma. *N Engl J Med* 2005;353:2135.
9. Hayat MJ, Howlader N, Reichman ME, Edwards BK. Cancer statistics, trends, and multiple primary cancer analyses from the Surveillance, Epidemiolog, and End Results (SEER) Progam. *Oncologist* 2007;12:20.
10. Geller J, Swetter SM, Leyson J, Miller DR, Brooks K, Geller AC. Crafting a melanoma educational campaign to reach middle-aged and older men. *J Cutan Med Surg* 2006;10:259.
24. Garibyan L, Fisher DE. How sunlight causes melanoma. *Curr Oncol Rep* 2010;12:319.
25. Cust AE, Armstrong BK, Goumas C, et al. Sunbed use during adolescence and early adulthood is associated with increased risk of early-onset melanoma. *Int J Cancer* 2010;Epub ahead of print.
26. Grant WB. In defense of the sun: An estimate of changes in mortality rates in the United States if mean serum 25-hydroxyvitamin D levels were raised to 45 ng/mL by solar ultraviolet-B irradiance. *Dermatoendocrinology* 2009;1:207.
39. Clark WH Jr, Reimer RR, Greene M, Ainsworth AM, Mastrangelo MJ. Origin of familial malignant melanomas from heritable melanocytic lesions: 'The B-K mole syndrome'. *Arch Dermatol* 1978;114:732.
51. King R, Page RN, Googe PB, Mihm MC Jr. Lentiginous melanoma: a histologic pattern of melanoma to be distinguished from lentiginous nevus. *Mod Pathol* 2005;18:1397.
52. Murali R, Shaw HM, Lai K, et al. Prognostic factors in cutaneous desmoplastic melanoma: a study of 252 patients. *Cancer* 2010;116(17):4130.
54. George E, McClain SE, Slingluff CL, Polissar NL, Patterson JW. Subclassification of desmoplastic melanoma: pure and mixed variants have significantly different capacities for lymph node metastasis. *J Cutan Pathol* 2009;36:425.
55. Hawkins WG, Busam KJ, Ben-Porat L, et al. Desmoplastic melanoma: a pathologically and clinically distinct form of cutaneous melanoma. *Ann Surg Oncol* 2005;12:207.
61. Breslow A. Thickness, cross-sectional areas and depth of invasion in the prognosis of cutaneous melanoma. *Ann Surg* 1970;172:902.
62. Clark WH, From L, Bernardino EA, Mihm MC. The histogenesis and biologic behavior of primary human malignant melanomas of the skin. *Cancer Res* 1969;29:705.
64. Balch CM, Gershenwald JE, Soong SJ, et al. Final version of 2009 AJCC melanoma staging and classification. *J Clin Oncol* 2009;27:6199.
71. Paek SC, Griffith KA, Johnson TM, et al. The impact of factors beyond Breslow depth on predicting sentinel lymph node positivity in melanoma. *Cancer* 2007;109:100.
73. Azzola M, Shaw HM, Thompson JF, et al. Tumor mitotic rate is a more powerful prognostic indicator than ulceration in patients with primary cutaneous melanoma: an analysis of 3661 patients from a single center. *Cancer* 2003;97:1448.
77. National Comprehensive Cancer Network. *NCCN practice guidelines in oncology* - v.2.2010. Melanoma. 2010. 8-6-2010.
78. Terhune MH, Swanson N, Johnson TM. Use of Chest Radiography in the Initial Evaluation of Patients With Localized Melanoma. *Arch Dermatol* 1998;134:569.
79. Vermeeren L, van der Ent FW, Hulsewe KW. Is there an indication for routine chest x-ray in initial staging of melanoma? *J Surg Res* 2011;166:114–119.
81. Constantinidou A, Hofman M, O'Doherty M, Acland KM, Healy C, Harries M. Routine positron emission tomography and positron emission tomography/computed tomography in melanoma staging with positive sentinel node biopsy is of limited benefit. *Melanoma Res* 2008;18:56.
82. Yancovitz M, Finelt N, Warycha MA, et al. Role of radiologic imaging at the time of initial diagnosis of stage T1b-T3b melanoma. *Cancer* 2007;110:1107.
83. Wagner JD, Schauwecker D, Davidson D, et al. Inefficacy of F-18 fluorodeoxy-D-glucose-positron emission tomography scans for initial evaluation in early stage cutaneous melanoma. *Cancer* 2005;104:570.
84. Clark PB, Soo V, Kraas J, Shen P, Levine EA. Futility of fluorodeoxyglucose F 18 positron emission tomography in initial evaluation of patients with T2 to T4 melanoma. *Arch Surg* 2006;141:284.
86. Handley WS. The pathology of melanotic growths in relation to their operative treatment (II). *Lancet* 1907;1:927.
87. Veronesi U, Cascinelli N. Narrow excision (1-cm margin): a safe procedure for thin cutaneous melanoma. *Arch Surg* 1991;126:438.
92. Balch CM, Urist MM, Karakousis CP, et al. Efficacy of 2-cm surgical margins for intermediate-thickness melanomas (1 to 4 mm). Results of a multi-institutional randomized surgical trial. *Ann Surg* 1993;218:262.
93. Balch C, Soong SJ, Smith T, et al. Long term results of a prospective surgical trial comparing 2 cm. vs 4 cm. incision margins for 740 patients with 1–4 mm melanomas. *Ann Surg Oncol* 2001;8:101.
94. Thomas J, Newton-Bishop JA, A'Hern R, et al. Excision margins in high-risk melanoma. *N Engl J Med* 2004;350:757.
95. Thomas JM, Newton-Bishop J, A'Hern R, et al. Excision margins in high-risk malignant melanoma. *N Engl J Med* 2004;350:757–766.
96. Sappey C. *Description et Iconographie des Vaisseaux Lymphatiques Conside're's Chez L'homme et les Verte'bre's.* Paris, France: Delahaye, 1885.
97. Norman J, Cruse CW, Espinosa C, et al. Redefinition of cutaneous lymphatic drainage with the use of lymphoscintigraphy for malignant melanoma. *Am J Surg* 1991;162:432.
101. Coates AS, Ingvar CI, Petersen-Schaefer K, et al. Elective lymph node dissection in patients with primary melanoma of the trunk and limbs treated at the Sydney Melanoma unit from 1960 to 1991. *J Am Coll Surg* 1995;180:402.
102. Slingluff CL Jr, Stidham KR, Ricci WM, Stanley WE, Seigler HF. Surgical management of regional lymph nodes in patients with melanoma. Experience with 4682 patients [see comments]. Comment in: Ann Surg 1995;221(4):435. *Ann Surg* 1994;219:120.
106. Balch CM, Soong S, Ross MI, et al. Long-term results of a multi-institutional randomized trial comparing prognostic factors and surgical results for intermediate thickness melanomas (1.0 to 4.0 mm.). *Ann Surg Oncol* 2000;7:87.
108. Morton DL, Wen DR, Wong JH, et al. Technical details of intraoperative lymphatic mapping for early stage melanoma. *Arch Surg* 1992;127:392.
110. Reintgen D, Cruse CW, Wells K, et al. The orderly progression of melanoma nodal metastases. *Ann Surg* 1994;220:759.
112. Harlow SP, Krag DN, Ashikaga T, et al. Gamma probe guided biopsy of the sentinel node in malignant melanoma: a multicentre study. *Melanoma Res* 2001;11:45.
114. Thompson JF, Uren RF, Shaw HM, et al. Location of sentinel lymph nodes in patients with cutaneous melanoma: new insights into lymphatic anatomy. *J Am Coll Surg* 1999;189:195.

115. Gershenwald JE, Thompson W, Mansfield PF, et al. Multi-institutional melanoma lymphatic mapping experience: the prognostic value of sentinel lymph node status in 612 stage I or II melanoma patients. *J Clin Oncol* 1999;17:976.
116. Gershenwald JE, Mansfield PF, Lee JE, Ross MI. Role for lymphatic mapping and sentinel lymph node biopsy in patients with thick (> or = 4 mm) primary melanoma. *Ann Surg Oncol* 2000;7:160.
117. Morton DL, Cochran AJ, Thompson JF, et al. Sentinel node biopsy for early-stage melanoma: accuracy and morbidity in MSLT-I, an international multicenter trial. *Ann Surg* 2005;242:302.
126. Morton DL, Thompson JF, Cochran AJ, et al. Sentinel-node biopsy or nodal observation in melanoma. *N Engl J Med* 2006;355:1307.
127. Kilbridge KL, Weeks JC, Sober AJ, et al. Patient preferences for adjuvant interferon alfa-2b treatment. *J Clin Oncol* 2001;19:812.
129. Urist MM, Balch CM, Soong SJ, et al. Head and neck melanoma in 534 clinical stage I patients. A prognostic factors analysis and results of surgical treatment. *Ann Surg* 1984;200:769.
130. Evans HL, Krag DN, Teates CD, et al. Lymphoscintigraphy and sentinel node biopsy accurately stage melanoma in patients presenting after wide local excision. *Ann Surg Oncol* 2003;10:416.
136. Rajpar SF, Marsden JR. Imiquimod in the treatment of lentigo maligna. *Br J Dermatol* 2006;155:653.
139. Vongtama R, Safa A, Gallardo D, et al. Efficacy of radiation therapy in the local control of desmoplastic malignant melanoma. *Head Neck* 2003;25:423.
148. Mooney MM, Michalek AM, Petrelli NJ, Kraybill WG. Life-long screening of patients with intermediate-thickness cutaneous melanoma for asymptomatic pulmonary recurrences detection in stage I and II cutaneous melanoma. *Ann Surg Oncol* 1998;5:54.
154. Sanki A, Kam PCA, Thompson JF. Long-term results with hyperthermic, isolated limb perfusion for melanoma: a reflection of tumor biology. *Ann Surg* 2007;245:591.
155. Cornett WR, McCall LM, Petersen RP, et al. Randomized multicenter trial of hyperthermic isolated limb perfusion with melphalan alone compared with melphalan plus tumor necrosis factor: American College of Surgeons Oncology Group Trial Z0020. *J Clin Oncol* 2006;24:4196.
160. Slingluff CL Jr, Vollmer R, Seigler HF. Stage II malignant melanoma: presentation of a prognostic model and an assessment of specific active immunotherapy in 1,273 patients. *J Surg Oncol* 1988;39:139.
162. Bilimoria KY, Balch CM, Bentrem DJ, et al. Complete lymph node dissection for sentinel node-positive melanoma: assessment of practice patterns in the United States. *Ann Surg Oncol* 2008;15:1566.
166. Wong SL, Morton DL, Thompson JF, et al. Melanoma patients with positive sentinel nodes who did not undergo completion lymphadenectomy: a multi-institutional study. *Ann Surg Oncol* 2006;13:809.
167. Young SE, Martinez SR, Faries MB, Essner R, Wanek LA, Morton DL. Can surgical therapy alone achieve long-term cure of melanoma metastatic to regional nodes? *Cancer J* 2006;12:207.
170. Barranco SC, Romsdahl MM, Humphrey RM. The radiation response of human malignant melanoma cells grown in vitro. *Cancer Res* 1971;31:830.
176. Chang DT, Amdur RJ, Morris CG, et al. Adjuvant radiotherapy for cutaneous melanoma: Comparing hypofractionation to conventional fractionation. *Int J Radiat Oncol Biol Phys* 2006;66:1051.
185. Kirkwood JM, Strawderman MH, Ernstoff MS, Smith TJ, Borden EC, Blum RH. Interferon alfa-2b adjuvant therapy of high-risk resected cutaneous melanoma: the Eastern Cooperative Oncology Group Trial EST 1684. *J Clin Oncol* 1996;14:7.
187. Kirkwood JM, Ibrahim JG, Sondak VK, et al. High- and low-dose interferon alfa-2b in high-risk melanoma: first analysis of intergroup trial E1690/S9111/C9190. *J Clin Oncol* 2000;18:2444.
188. Kirkwood JM, Manola J, Ibrahim J, et al. A pooled analysis of eastern cooperative oncology group and intergroup trials of adjuvant high-dose interferon for melanoma. *Clin Cancer Res* 2004;10:1670.
189. Kirkwood JM, Ibrahim JG, Sosman JA, et al. High-dose interferon alfa-2b significantly prolongs relapse-free and overall survival compared with the GM2-KLH/QS-21 vaccine in patients with resected stage IIB-III melanoma: results of intergroup trial E1694/S9512/C509801. *J Clin Oncol* 2001;19:2370.
192. Eggermont AM, Suciu S, Santinami M, et al. Adjuvant therapy with pegylated interferon alfa-2b versus observation alone in resected stage III melanoma: final results of EORTC 18991, a randomised phase III trial. *Lancet* 2008;372:117–126.
193. Grob JJ, Jouary T, Dreno B, et al. Adjuvant therapy with pegylated interferon alfa-2b (36 months) versus low-dose interferon alfa-2b (18 months) in melanoma patients without macro-metastatic nodes: EADO trial. *J Clin Oncol* 2010;28(18s):Abstract # LBA 8506.
197. Moschos SJ, Edington HD, Land SR, et al. Neoadjuvant treatment of regional stage IIIB melanoma with high-dose interferon alfa-2b induces objective tumor regression in association with modulation of tumor infiltrating host cellular immune responses. *J Clin Oncol* 2006;24:3164.
199. Yamshchikov GV, Mullins DW, Chang CC, et al. Sequential immune escape and shifting of T cell responses in a long-term survivor of melanoma. *J Immunol* 2005;174:6863.
200. Munn DH, Sharma MD, Lee JR, et al. Potential regulatory function of human dendritic cells expressing indoleamine 2,3-dioxygenase. *Science* 2002;297:1867.
212. Morton DL, Mozzillo N, Thompson JF, et al. An international, randomized, phase III trial of bacillus Calmette-Guerin (BCG) plus allogeneic melanoma vaccine (MCV) or placebo after complete resection of melanoma metastatic to regional or distant sites. *J Clin Oncol, 2007 ASCO Annual Meeting Proceedings Part I* 2007;25:abstract 8508.
215. Rosenberg SA, Yang JC, Restifo NP. Cancer immunotherapy: moving beyond current vaccines. *Nat Med* 2004;10:909.
217. Slingluff CL Jr, Chianese-Bullock KA, Bullock TN, et al. Immunity to melanoma antigens: from self-tolerance to immunotherapy. *Adv Immunol* 2006;90:243.
218. Yamshchikov GV, Barnd DL, Eastham S, et al. Evaluation of peptide vaccine immunogenicity in draining lymph nodes and blood of melanoma patients. *Int J Cancer* 2001;92:703.
219. Chianese-Bullock KA, Pressley J, Garbee C, et al. MAGE-A1-, MAGE-A10-, and gp100-derived peptides are immunogenic when combined with granulocyte-macrophage colony-stimulating factor and montanide ISA-51 adjuvant and administered as part of a multipeptide vaccine for melanoma. *J Immunol* 2005;174:3080.
220. Speiser DE, Lienard D, Rufer N, et al. Rapid and strong human CD8+ T cell responses to vaccination with peptide, IFA, and CpG oligodeoxynucleotide 7909. *J Clin Invest* 2005;115:739.
221. Slingluff CL Jr, Petroni GR, Chianese-Bullock KA, et al. Immunologic and clinical outcomes of a randomized phase II trial of two multipeptide vaccines for melanoma in the adjuvant setting. *Clin Cancer Res* 2007; 13:6386.
222. Appay V, Jandus C, Voelter V, et al. New generation vaccine induces effective melanoma-specific CD8+ T cells in the circulation but not in the tumor site. *J Immunol* 2006;177:1670.
223. Le Gal FA, Widmer V, Dutoit V, et al. Tissue homing and persistence of defined antigen-specific CD8 tumor reactive T cell clones in melanoma long-term survivors. *J Invest Dermatol* 2007;127:622.
224. Schwartzentruber DJ, Lawson D, Richards J, et al. A phase III multi-institutional randomized study of immunization with the gp100:209-217(210M) peptide followed by high-dose IL-2 compared with high-dose IL-2 alone in patients with metastatic melanoma. *J Clin Oncol* 2009; 27:abstract CRA9011.
227. Slingluff CL Jr, Petroni GR, Olson WC, et al. Effect of GM-CSF on circulating $CD8^+$ and $CD4^+$ T cell responses to a multipeptide melanoma vaccine: Outcome of a multicenter randomized trial. *Clin Cancer Res* 2009;15:7036.
228. Faries MB, Hsueh EC, Ye X, Hoban M, Morton DL. Effect of granulocyte/macrophage colony-stimulating factor on vaccination with an allogeneic whole-cell melanoma vaccine. *Clin Cancer Res* 2009;15:7029.
232. Lawson DH, Lee SJ, Tarhini AA, Margolin KA, Ernstoff MS, Kirkwood JM. E4697: Phase III cooperative group study of yeast-derived granulocyte macrophage colony-stimulating factor (GM-CSF) versus placebo as adjuvant treatment of patients with completely resected stage III-IV melanoma. *J Clin Oncol* 2010;28(15s):8504.
233. Manola J, Atkins M, Ibrahim J, Kirkwood J. Prognostic factors in metastatic melanoma: a pooled analysis of Eastern Cooperative Oncology Group trials. *J Clin Oncol* 2000;18:3782.
236. Korn EL, Liu PY, Lee SJ, et al. Meta-analysis of phase II cooperative group trials in metastatic stage IV melanoma to determine progression-free and overall survival benchmarks for future phase II trials. *J Clin Oncol* 2009; 26:527.
240. Tagawa ST, Cheung E, Banta W, Gee C, Weber JS. Survival analysis after resection of metastatic disease followed by peptide vaccines in patients with Stage IV melanoma. *Cancer* 2006;106:1353.
241. Bradbury PA, Middleton MR. DNA repair pathways in drug resistance in melanoma. *Anticancer Drugs* 2004;15:421.
248. Durando X, Thivat E, D'Incan M, Sinsard A, Madelmont JC, Chollet P. Long-term disease-free survival in advanced melanomas treated with nitrosoureas: mechanisms and new perspectives. *BMC Cancer* 2005;5:147.
261. Rosenberg SA, Grimm EA, McGrogan M, et al. Biological activity of recombinant human interleukin-2 produced in *E. coli*. *Science* 1984;223: 1412.
263. Lotze MT, Chang AE, Seipp CA, Simpson C, Vetto JT, Rosenberg SA. High dose recombinant interleukin-2 in the treatment of patients with disseminated cancer: Responses, treatment related morbidity and histologic findings. *JAMA* 1986;256:3117.
264. Atkins MB, Lotze MT, Dutcher JP, et al. High-dose recombinant interleukin 2 therapy for patients with metastatic melanoma: analysis of 270 patients treated between 1985 and 1993. *J Clin Oncol* 1999;17:2105.
265. Smith FO, Downey SG, Klapper JA, et al. Treatment of metastatic melanoma using interleukin-2 alone or in conjunction with vaccines. *Clin Cancer Res* 2008;14(17):5610.
270. Legha SS, Ring S, Papadopoulos N, Plager C, Chawla S, Benjamin R. A prospective evaluation of a triple-drug regimen containing cisplatin, vinblastine, and dacarbazine (CVD) for metastatic melanoma. *Cancer* 1989;64:2024.
271. Atkins MB, Lee S, Flaherty LE, Sosman JA, Sondak V, Kirkwood JM. A prospective randomized phase III trial of concurrent biochemotherapy (BCT) with cisplatin, vinblastine, dacarbazine (CVD), IL-2 and interferon alpha-2b (IFN) versus CVD alone in patients with metastatic melanoma (E3695): an ECOG-coordinated intergroup trial. *J Clin Oncol* 2003; 22:2847.

287. Legha SS, Ring S, Eton O, et al. Development of a biochemotherapy regimen with concurrent administration of cisplatin, vinblastine, dacarbazine, interferon alfa, and interleukin-2 for patients with metastatic melanoma. *J Clin Oncol* 1998;16:1752.
290. Keilholz U, Punt CJ, Gore M, et al. Dacarbazine, cisplatin, and interferon-alfa-2b with or without interleukin-2 in metastatic melanoma: a randomized phase III trial (18951) of the European Organisation for Research and Treatment of Cancer Melanoma Group. *J Clin Oncol* 2005;23:6747.
291. Dudley ME, Wunderlich JR, Robbins PF, et al. Cancer regression and autoimmunity in patients after clonal repopulation with antitumor lymphocytes. *Science* 2002;298:850.
292. Rosenberg SA, Dudley ME. Adoptive cell therapy for the treatment of patients with metastatic melanoma. *Curr Opin Immunol* 2009;21:233.
299. Morgan RA, Dudley ME, Wunderlich JR, et al. Cancer regression in patients after transfer of genetically engineered lymphocytes. *Science* 2006; 314:126.
301. Attia P, Phan GQ, Maker AV, et al. Autoimmunity correlates with tumor regression in patients with metastatic melanoma treated with anti-cytotoxic T-lymphocyte antigen-4. *J Clin Oncol* 2005;23:6043.
302. Maker AV, Yang JC, Sherry RM, et al. Intrapatient dose escalation of anti-CTLA-4 antibody in patients with metastatic melanoma. *J Immunother* 2006;29:455.
303. Hodi FS, O'Day SJ, McDermott DF, et al. Improved Survival with Ipilimumab in Patients with Metastatic Melanoma. *N Engl J Med* 2010.
304. Maker AV, Phan GQ, Attia P, et al. Tumor regression and autoimmunity in patients treated with cytotoxic T lymphocyte-associated antigen 4 blockade and interleukin 2: a phase I/II study. *Ann Surg Oncol* 2005;12:1005.
305. Brahmer JR, Drake CG, Wollner I, et al. Phase I study of single-agent anti-programmed death-1 (MDX-1106) in refractory solid tumors: safety, clinical activity, pharmacodynamics, and immunologic correlates. *J Clin Oncol* 2010;28:3167.
306. Davies H, Bignell GR, Cox C, et al. Mutations of the BRAF gene in human cancer. *Nature* 2002;417:949.
307. Tsao H, Zhang X, Fowlkes K, Haluska FG. Relative reciprocity of NRAS and PTEN/MMAC1 alterations in cutaneous melanoma cell lines. *Cancer Res* 2000;60:1800.
311. Curtin JA, Busam K, Pinkel D, Bastian BC. Somatic activation of KIT in distinct subtypes of melanoma. *J Clin Oncol* 2006;24:4340.
312. Jiang X, Zhou J, Yuen NK, et al. Imatinib targeting of KIT-mutant oncoprotein in melanoma. *Clin Cancer Res* 2008;14:7726.
325. Eisen T, Ahmad T, Flaherty KT, et al. Sorafenib in advanced melanoma: a Phase II randomised discontinuation trial analysis. *Br J Cancer* 2006;95 (5):581.
326. Garnett MJ, Marais R. Guilty as charged: B-RAF is a human oncogene. *Cancer Cell* 2004;6:313.
327. Flaherty KT, Redlinger M, Schuchter LM, et al. Phase I/II, pharmacokinetic and pharmacodynamic trial of BAY 43-9006 alone in patients with metastatic melanoma. *J Clin Oncol* 2005;23:3037.
328. Flaherty KT, Kim KB, Ribas A, et al. Inhibition of mutated, activated BRAF in metastatic melanoma. *N Engl J Med* 2010;363(9):809.
329. Kefford R, Arkenau H, Brown MP, et al. Phase I/II study of GSK2118436, a selective inhibitor of oncogenic mutant BRAF kinase, in patients with metastatic melanoma and other solid tumors. *J Clin Oncol* 2010; 28:8503.
331. Infante JR, Fecher LA, Nallapareddy S, et al. Safety and efficacy results from the first-in-human study of the oral MEK 1/2 inhibitor GSK1120212. *J Clin Oncol* 2010;28.
332. Hodi FS, Friedlander P, Corless CL, et al. Major response to imatinib mesylate in KIT-mutated melanoma. *J Clin Oncol* 2008;26:2046.
337. Flaherty KT, Schuchter LM, Flaherty LE, et al. Final results of E2603: A double-blind, randomized phase III trial comparing carboplatin/paclitaxel with or without sorafenib in metastatic melanoma. *J Clin Oncol* 2010; 28(15s):abstract # 8511.
350. Sause WT, Cooper JS, Rush S, et al. Fraction size in external beam radiation therapy in the treatment of melanoma. *Int J Radiat Oncol Biol Phys* 1991;20(3):429.

SECTION 10: NEOPLASMS OF THE CENTRAL NERVOUS SYSTEM

CHAPTER 120 MOLECULAR BIOLOGY OF CENTRAL NERVOUS SYSTEM TUMORS

C. DAVID JAMES, DAVID N. LOUIS, AND WEBSTER K. CAVENEE

Neoplastic transformation in the nervous system is a multistep process in which the normal controls of cell proliferation and cell-cell interaction are suppressed or disabled. This process involves the alteration of several types of genes, including oncogenes, tumor suppressor genes, DNA repair genes, and cell death genes, among others.[1] Our increased knowledge of the molecular genetics that underlie this process has been facilitated by improved methods for detailed and rapid analysis of molecular characteristics of tumors, and information obtained from the application of current technology is beginning to influence the clinical diagnosis and management of CNS cancer. Results from comprehensive analyses of tumor genomes (DNA, DNA modification) and transcriptomes (mRNA, miRNA) are proving especially powerful with regard to applications involving the differential diagnosis of adult malignant gliomas,[2–7] embryonal brain tumors such as medulloblastoma,[8,9] and to the subset of meningiomas that display variable clinical course.[10] In addition to clinical applications, detailed molecular characterizations of CNS tumors continue to help improve our ability to develop increasingly accurate and relevant mouse models of brain tumors,[11] which, in turn, facilitate precise dissection of tumorigenic pathways investigation of therapy-response relationships,[12,13] and improved understanding of the earliest stages of brain tumorigenesis, including the nature of cells that give rise to brain tumors.

NEUROLOGIC TUMOR SYNDROMES

In addition to information obtained through molecular characterizations of sporadically occurring CNS tumors, as well as through cancer stem cell investigations, much of our current understanding of brain tumorigenesis is associated with decades of observation and analysis of inherited cancer predisposition. Neurologic tumor syndromes are accompanied by characteristic panoplies of both neurologic and nonneurologic tumors. A catalog of the major primary brain tumors associated with neurologic tumor syndromes would feature optic nerve gliomas and other astrocytomas in neurofibromatosis type 1 (NF1), ependymomas and meningiomas in neurofibromatosis type 2 (NF2), various malignant gliomas in Li-Fraumeni syndrome, Turcot syndrome and the hereditary glioma pedigrees, and medulloblastomas in Gorlin, Turcot, and Li-Fraumeni syndromes.[14]

Linkage studies that were applied to the initial chromosome regional assignments of the genes associated with these tumor syndromes[15] revealed the *NF1* gene as residing on chromosome 17q, the *NF2* gene on chromosome 22q, and at least one gene for the Turcot syndrome on chromosome 5q (*APC* gene). For the Li-Fraumeni syndrome, mutation analyses identified the *TP53* gene on 17p and the *hCHK2* gene on 22q as being responsible for cancer predisposition. Similarly, germ line mutations of the chromosome 10q-localized *PTEN* gene are responsible for the multicancer Cowden syndrome, and the inactivation of *PTEN* is very common among high malignancy grade astrocytomas in adults.

As has been the case for the examination of tumor DNAs, studies of constitutional DNAs from brain tumor patients for the identification of inherited allelic variants that increase the likelihood of brain tumor occurrence have evolved toward comprehensive investigation, as exemplified by genome-wide association study approaches that have recently revealed possible glioma susceptibility loci. Two recent reports, published simultaneously and independently by multi-institutional consortia, suggested susceptibility loci at 9p21 (CDKN2A-CDKN2B as candidate loci) and 20q13 (RTEL1 as candidate locus reviewed in refs. 16 and 17). Consequently, there appear to be additional CNS tumor predisposing or susceptibility genes, not necessarily associated with definable clinical syndromes, that increase risk for CNS tumor development, and our knowledge of such factors is rapidly expanding from such investigations.

CNS TUMOR HISTOPATHOLOGY AND MOLECULAR CORRELATES

Diffuse, Fibrillary Astrocytomas

Diffuse, fibrillary astrocytomas are the most common type of primary brain tumor in adults. These tumors are divided histopathologically into three grades of malignancy[14]: World Health Organization (WHO) grade II diffuse astrocytoma, WHO grade III anaplastic astrocytoma, and WHO grade IV glioblastoma (GBM) (Fig. 120.1). WHO grade II diffuse astrocytomas are the most indolent of the spectrum. Nonetheless, these tumors are infiltrative (Fig. 120.1A) and have a marked potential for malignant progression.[18]

Alterations of p53, a tumor suppressor encoded by the *TP53* gene on chromosome 17p, play a key role in the development of

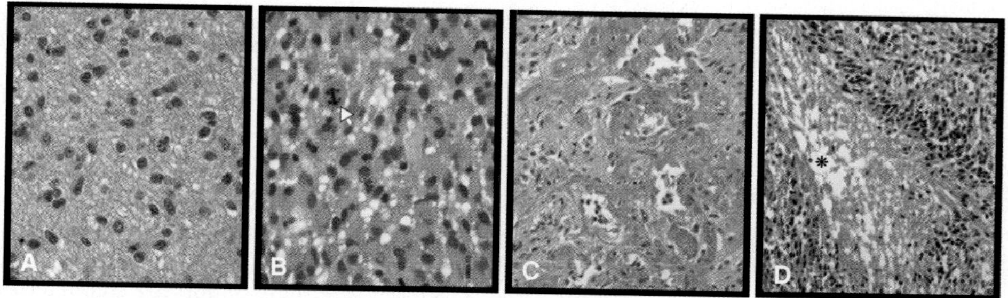

FIGURE 120.1 Examples of grade II (*panel A*), grade III (anaplastic: *panel B*), and grade IV (glioblastoma: *panels C and D*) astrocytoma histopathology. Arrow in panel B shows mitotic figure that is a classification criterion of grade III malignancy. Panels C and D show microvascular proliferation and necrosis with perinecrotic cellular palisading, respectively, which are diagnostic criteria of glioblastoma, grade IV. The asterisk in panel D denotes the necrotic focus.

at least one-third of all three grades of adult astrocytoma.[19,20] In addition, in higher-grade astrocytomas, p53 function may be deregulated by alterations of other genes, including amplification of *MDM2* or *MDM4* and 9p deletions that result in loss of the p14 product of the *CDKN2A* gene (Fig. 120.2). A recent survey of this pathway demonstrated gene alterations that compromise p53 function in 87% of glioblastoma.[21]

Studies revealing frequent alterations of *TP53* in sporadic astrocytoma are complemented by various model system investigations that support the contribution of p53 inactivation in the early stages of astrocytoma formation. For instance, cortical astrocytes from mice without functional p53 appear immortalized when grown *in vitro* and acquire a transformed phenotype with sustained propagation in defined media.[22] Cortical astrocytes from mice with haploid *TP53* status behave more like wild type astrocytes and only show signs of immortalization and transformation after losing their sole wild type copy of *TP53*.[22] Results associated with p53 inactivation in genetically modified mouse models also support the importance of p53 loss of function in promoting astrocytoma initiation, although such demonstrations have been reported in the context of an accompanying, second gene alteration, such as *NF1* gene inactivation.[23] In total, there is ample evidence provided through numerous avenues of investigation that indicate the importance of compromised p53 function to the formation of astrocytoma.

During the 16 months prior to this writing, it has become well established that mutations of the isocitrate dehydrogenase 1 gene (*IDH1*) occur in a large fraction of grade II and grade III gliomas, irrespective of relative astrocytic versus oligodendroglial histology.[24] The possible consequences of this gene alteration are discussed later, but, notably, antibodies specific to the mutant form of the IDH1 protein can now be used reliably for glioma diagnosis on routine tissue sections.[25] Interestingly, both *TP53* and *IDH1* mutations have been positively correlated with tumor MGMT methylation, which, in turn, is thought to accelerate G:C to A:T transition mutations. Others have previously noted that gliomas with MGMT methylation have a higher incidence of such mutations in *TP53*,[26] and MGMT methylation has recently been correlated with *IDH1* mutation in glioma,[27] with the most common *IDH1* alteration also being of the G:C to A:T transition type. Thus, it is possible that epigenetic alteration of low-grade glioma genomes, specifically methylation inhibition of MGMT expression, promotes the mutation of genes whose alteration are well established as occurring frequently in low-grade tumors.

PRACTICE OF ONCOLOGY

Progression to Anaplastic Astrocytoma

The transition from WHO grade II astrocytoma to WHO grade III anaplastic astrocytoma is accompanied by a marked increase in malignant behavior.[14] Although patients with grade II astrocytomas may survive for 5 or more years, patients with anaplastic astrocytomas often die within 2 or 3 years and frequently show progression to GBM. Histologically, the major differences between grade II and grade III tumors are increased

TABLE 120.1

COMMON CENTRAL NERVOUS SYSTEM TUMORS AND CORRESPONDING GENE ALTERATIONS[a]

Common Adult Tumors	Frequent Gene and Chromosomal Alterations
Grade II astrocytoma	*IDH1*, *TP53*
Grade III anaplastic astrocytoma	*IDH1*, *TP53*-***MDM2/4***, *CDKN2A*-***CDK4/6***-*RB*
Grade IV glioblastomas	*TP53*-***MDM2/4***, *CDKN2A*-***CDK4/6***-*RB*, ***EGFR***, *PTEN*, *NF1*
Grade II oligodendroglioma	*IDH1*, chromosome 1p–19q translocations
Grade III oligodendroglioma	*IDH1*, chromosome 1p–19q translocations
Meningioma	*NF2*
Common Pediatric Tumors	**Frequent Gene and Chromosomal Alterations**
Medulloblastoma	*PTCH*, ***MYCC***, ***MYCN***, chromosome 17p deletions
Ependymoma	*NF2* (spinal), chromosome 22 deletions (central)
Pilocytic astrocytoma	***KIAA1549-BRAF*** fusion rearrangements

[a]Oncogene alterations are in bold text; tumor suppressor gene alterations are in plain text; functionally related gene alterations have been grouped (e.g., *TP53*-***MDM2/4***).

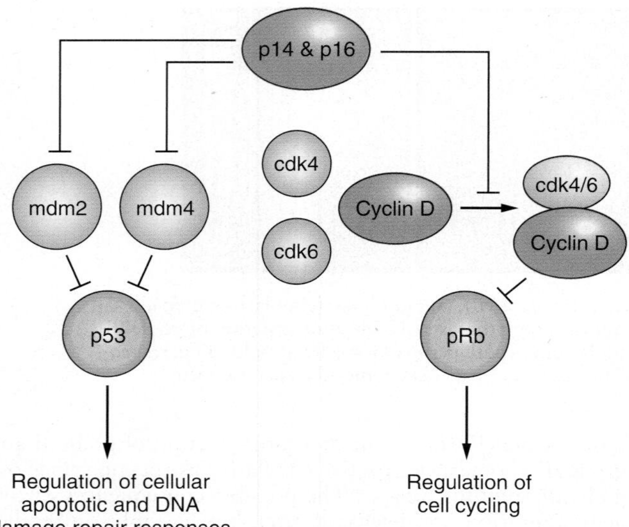

FIGURE 120.2 Regulation of p53 and pRb function. p14 and p16 function is inactivated in approximately half of glioblastoma, as well as in a significant fraction of grade III (anaplastic) astrocytoma, due to homozygous deletion of a DNA sequence at chromosomal location 9p21 that encodes each of these tumor suppressors. The genes encoding mdm 2 and 4, as well as for cdk4 and 6, are amplified in some high-grade astrocytomas, and provide alternative genetic mechanisms to the p14 + p16 gene deletions for achieving suppression of p53 and pRb function. The *TP53* and *RB* genes that encode these tumor suppressor proteins are themselves inactivated in many high-grade astrocytomas, and in such instances the gene alterations affecting upstream regulators are not observed. Proteins indicated in green are oncogenic, whereas those indicated in red act as negative regulators of cell growth (tumor suppressors). Percent values indicate gene alteration frequencies, as defined by The Cancer Genome Atlas project.[21]

cellularity and the presence of mitotic activity (Fig. 120.1B), implying that higher proliferative activity is the hallmark of the progression to anaplastic astrocytoma.

A number of molecular abnormalities have been associated with anaplastic astrocytoma, and several studies indicate that these abnormalities converge on one critical cell-cycle regulatory complex which includes the p16, cyclin-dependent kinase 4 (cdk4), cdk6, cyclin D1, and retinoblastoma (Rb) proteins. The simplest schema suggests that p16 inhibits the cdk6/cyclin D1 and/or cdk4/cyclin D1 complexes, preventing these from phosphorylating Rb, and so ensuring that phospho-Rb (pRb) maintains its brake on the cell cycle (Fig. 120.2).

Chromosome 9p loss occurs in approximately 50% of anaplastic astrocytomas and GBMs, and these 9p alterations target the CDKN2A locus, which encodes the p16 and ARF proteins. The *CDKN2A* gene is inactivated either by homozygous deletion or, less commonly by point mutations or hypermethylation.[28,29] Loss of chromosome 13q occurs in one-third to one-half of high-grade astrocytomas, with the *RB1* gene preferentially inactivated by losses and mutations. *RB1* and *CDKN2A* alterations in primary gliomas are inversely correlated, and rarely occur together in the same tumor. Inactivation of pRb or p16 in mouse astrocytes has been shown to lead to anaplastic astrocytomas.[30] Amplification of the *CDK4* gene, located on chromosome 12q13–14, provides an alternative to subverting cell-cycle control and facilitating progression to GBM in up to 15% of malignant gliomas.[28] Detection of any of the gene alterations known to influence Rb protein function (CDKN2A homozygous deletion, CDK4 amplification, or RB deletion + mutation) is associated with a poor prognosis for anaplastic astrocytoma patients.[31]

Allelic losses on chromosome 19q have been observed in up to 40% of anaplastic astrocytomas and GBMs, indicating a progression-associated glial tumor suppressor gene that maps to 19q13.3, but the gene(s) being targeted for inactivation has is yet to be identified.

Progression to Glioblastoma

GBM is the most malignant grade of astrocytoma, with survival times of substantially less than 2 years for most patients. Histologically, these tumors are characterized by dense cellularity, high proliferation indices, microvascular proliferation (Fig. 120.1C) and focal necrosis (Fig. 120.1D). The highly proliferative nature of these lesions is most likely the result of multiple mitogenic effects. As previously mentioned, at least one such effect is deregulation of the p16-cdk4/6-cyclin D1-pRb pathway of cell-cycle control (Fig. 120.2). The vast majority, if not all, GBM have alterations of this system, whether it involve inactivation of p16 or pRb, or overexpression of cdk4.[9,28,29,32]

Chromosome 10 loss is a frequent finding in GBM, occurring in 60% to 95% of these tumors, and is far less commonly observed in anaplastic astrocytomas. The *PTEN* tumor suppressor gene at 10q23.3 is clearly one target of the chromosome 10 deletions, with *PTEN* mutations of the remaining allele identified in up to 30% of GBM, and a lesser percent of GBM having deletion of all or part of their remaining *PTEN* gene.[21,33] *PTEN* functions as a 3′ phosphoinositol phosphatase that influences cell proliferation through modulation of the PI3-kinase signaling pathway; *PTEN* also has protein tyrosine phosphatase activity. Results from model system studies, involving approaches such as the introduction of wild type *PTEN* into glioma cells with inactivated endogenous *PTEN*, and which results in the suppression of cell growth,[34] or the inactivation of *PTEN* function in genetically modified mice, which accelerates tumor formation,[30,35] support the loss of *PTEN* function as a critical step in the development of high-grade astrocytic malignancy.

In contrast to the deletion of tumor suppressor genes such as *PTEN*, key oncogenes experience increased copy number and/or elevated expression in GBM. A signature example of this is the gene for epidermal growth factor receptor (*EGFR*), which encodes a transmembrane receptor tyrosine kinase, whose ligands include EGF and transforming growth factor-a. GBMs with *EGFR* gene amplification display overexpression of EGFR transcript and protein. *EGFR* amplification is consistently reported in approximately 40% of all GBM,[36] while being amplified at a much lower frequency in anaplastic astrocytomas. GBMs that exhibit *EGFR* gene amplification have, in nearly all instances, lost genetic material on chromosome 10, and often have *CDKN2A* deletions.[37] Approximately one-third of those GBM with *EGFR* gene amplification also have specific *EGFR* gene rearrangements,[38] which produce truncated molecules that are constitutively activated in the absence of ligand and that enhance tumor cell proliferative properties.[39,40] The most common of the *EGFR* mutants, EGFRvIII or ΔEGFR, when expressed in mouse astrocytes lacking p16, causes the formation of intracranial tumors that resemble human GBM.[41]

Much of our existing knowledge, reviewed in the previous sections, regarding gene alterations in GBM, was confirmed by results generated from two ambitious projects that combined detailed genome and transcriptome analyses of large series of histopathologically validated GBM. One of these identified mutation of *IDH1* in 12% of GBM,[32] an observation that was subsequently extended to grade II and grade III gliomas, among which *IDH1* gene alterations are much more common. Our understanding of the roles of mutant IDH proteins in gliomagenesis is at an early stage, but one investigation suggests that these mutations may result in the accumulation of metabolites that activate the hypoxia-induced factor transcription factor,[42] the tumorigenic effects of which are well established.[43]

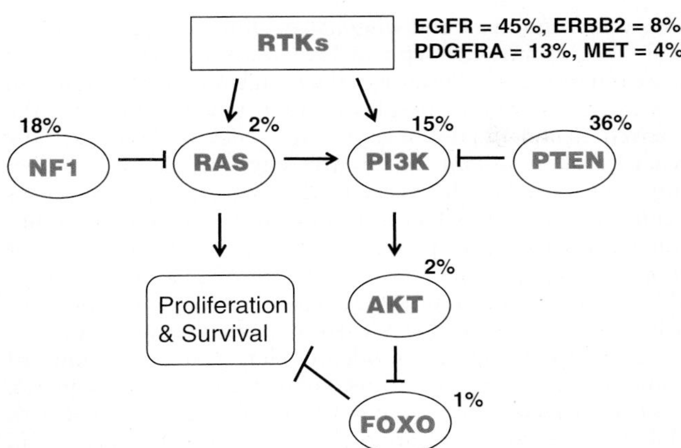

FIGURE 120.3 Alterations of RTK/RAS/PI3K signaling in glioblastoma. The third core signaling pathway, at least one element of which is altered in nearly all GBM, as confirmed by The Cancer Genome Atlas (TCGA) project.[9] Receptor tyrosine kinase (RTK) alterations most frequently involve EGFR, with decreasing involvement of PDGFRA, ERBB2, and MET. Downstream signaling mediators RAS and PI3K can be activated by mutation, but are more frequently deregulated by inactivating alterations of the *NF1* and *PTEN* tumor suppressor genes. Percent values indicate gene alteration frequencies, as defined by the TCGA project.

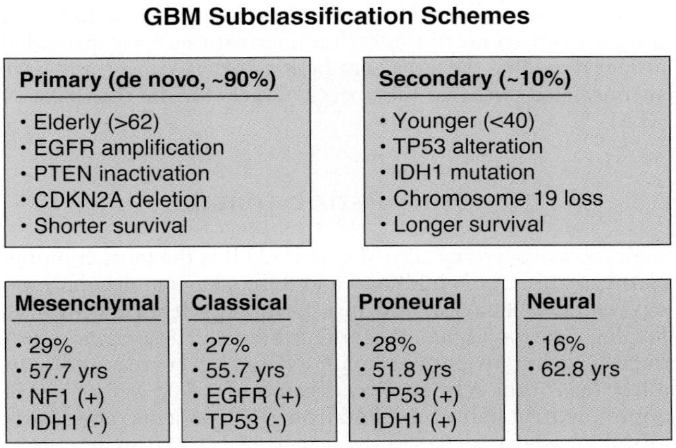

GBM Subclassification Schemes

Primary (de novo, ~90%)	Secondary (~10%)
• Elderly (>62) • EGFR amplification • PTEN inactivation • CDKN2A deletion • Shorter survival	• Younger (<40) • TP53 alteration • IDH1 mutation • Chromosome 19 loss • Longer survival

Mesenchymal	Classical	Proneural	Neural
• 29% • 57.7 yrs • NF1 (+) • IDH1 (-)	• 27% • 55.7 yrs • EGFR (+) • TP53 (-)	• 28% • 51.8 yrs • TP53 (+) • IDH1 (+)	• 16% • 62.8 yrs

FIGURE 120.4 Current schemes for major subgroup classification of glioblastoma. The primary versus secondary classification is based on the presence or absence of clinical history indicating GBM development from a pre-existing glioma of lesser malignancy, with specific gene alterations found to be associated with such clinical history.[81] Descriptive terms for the lower classification scheme are based on tumor molecular profiles suggesting specific stages of neurogenesis.[58] This classification scheme has recently undergone modification in association with The Cancer Genome Atlas project.[80] +, presence of gene alteration; −, absence of gene alteration.

Another suggested that the mutant and wild type IDH1 molecules may combine in a pathway that results in an oncogenic metabolite, 2-hydroxyglutarate.[44]

The second molecular profiling study, from The Cancer Genome Atlas (TCGA) initiative of the National Institutes of Health, confirmed and extended the importance of receptor tyrosine kinases and downstream signaling mediators in GBM by identifying frequent mutation of the *NF1* tumor suppressor gene, PI3 kinase regulatory and catalytic subunits, ERBB2, and amplifications of PDGFRA (Fig. 120.3).[21] Previous GBM involvement of this signaling network, as indicated through frequently occurring gene alterations, had primarily been limited to EGFR and PTEN, although each of the individual alterations had been noted in prior publications. This comprehensive study indicated that as many as 88% of GBM have one or more alterations affecting RTK-RAS-PI3K signaling.

The identification of frequent *NF1* gene alterations by the TCGA consortium merits special commentary. Activating mutations of *RAS*, one of the most common gene alterations in human cancer, have long been known to be infrequent in brain tumors, and, therefore, activated RAS has been generally assumed to not play a significant or frequent role in CNS tumor development. Given the new information from TCGA, indicating that *NF1* gene inactivation occurs in 15% to 20% of all GBMs, elevated Ras activity is now implicated in a subset of these tumors, with particularly high incidence of inactivation noted in the so-called mesenchymal GBM subtype[45] (see "Subsets of Glioblastoma").

Subsets of Glioblastoma

Suggesting that all astrocytomas progress through identifiable genetic stages in a linear fashion is an oversimplification. Indeed, it appears as if there are biologic subsets of astrocytomas that reflect the spectrum of clinical heterogeneity observed in these tumors. For instance, approximately one-third of GBM have TP53/chromosome 17p alterations, one-third have *EGFR* gene amplifications, and one-third have neither change.[46]

GBMs with *TP53* mutations that result from the malignant evolution of a lower malignancy grade astrocytic lesion are referred to as secondary (or progressive) GBM. The recently discovered *IDH1* mutations, seen commonly among grade II and III gliomas, similarly show preferential association with GBM that have evolved from lower malignancy grade precursors.[24] In contrast to secondary GBMs, GBMs with *EGFR* amplification may arise *de novo* or rapidly from a pre-existing tumor, without a clinically evident, lower malignancy grade precursor, and are referred to as primary GBM (Fig. 120.4).

Another genomic alteration that defines a significant subset of GBM is the loss of chromosome 10, and in a study using array comparative genomic hybridization (CGH) to identify tumors with chromosome 10 deletion, the analysis of corresponding expression profile data revealed that a novel gene product, the transcript for YKL-40, is significantly upregulated in tumors with chromosome 10 loss.[47] Whereas the underlying basis of this relationship is yet to be determined, regulation of YKL-40 expression is a matter of interest given the association of elevated YKL-40 with reduced survival for GBM patients.[48]

In contrast to the use of single biomarkers, such as chromosome 10, or EGFR copy number status, or *TP53* and *IDH1* mutation status for the subclassification of GBM, the comprehensive molecular screening techniques, that generate thousands of data points for each tumor specimen analyzed, and various algorithms (often referred to as *hierarchical clustering*) are proving useful and increasingly popular for identifying patterns associated with clinical or biological properties of interest. An example of this approach, which has served as a paradigm for GBM molecular subclassification, showed that gene expression profiling reproducibly identified three prognostically significant subsets of GBM patients.[49] Descriptive terms for GBM subclassification that were introduced by this study have undergone revision as a result of the TCGA initiative, and currently include classical (proliferative), mesenchymal, proneural, and neural subgroups.[21] These subgroups have strong associations with *EGFR*, *NF1*, and *TP53* + *IDH1* gene alterations, respectively, with the neural subgroup mostly lacking a distinct signature (Fig. 120.4).[45]

Taking into consideration the cumulative results of GBM molecular profiling studies to date, comprehensive molecular characterizations are clearly providing approaches for a clinically relevant classification of GBM that is more robust than achieved using conventional histopathology.[3,4,50] Furthermore, results from transcriptome characterizations have provided insight regarding the molecular biology of this cancer, and have also revealed potential therapeutic targets for the treatment of GBM.

Other Astrocytomas

Pilocytic astrocytoma (PA; WHO grade I) is the most common astrocytic tumor of childhood and differs in its molecular biology, clinical behavior, and histopathology from the diffuse, fibrillary astrocytomas that affect adults. These tumors frequently occur in patients with NF1, and correspondingly, allelic loss of the *NF1* gene on chromosome 17q is observed in approximately half of the PAs from NF1 patients, and nearly all NF1-associated PAs show a lack of NF1 protein expression. Observations derived from the analysis of NF1-associated PAs have shown, however, their distinct gene expression signatures relative to sporadic PAs,[51] suggesting distinct molecular etiologies for sporadic PAs. The recent discovery of a gene alteration that is frequent among sporadic PAs has provided important insight regarding the molecular etiology of these tumors. Specifically, the determination of gene rearrangements and fusions between the *BRAF* and *KIAA1549* genes, have been shown in the majority of PAs examined.[52] Alternative genetic alterations involving *RAF1* and *BRAF* have also been demonstrated in PAs.[53] The demonstration of KIAA1549-BRAF fusion proteins having activated BRAF kinase activity establishes these gene alterations as being oncogenic.[52] However, because PAs do not generally progress to high-grade malignancy, *BRAF* oncogenic activation does not apparently mark these tumors for malignant conversion.

Malignant pediatric astrocytic tumors are histologically similar to their adult counterparts (astrocytomas, anaplastic astrocytomas, and GBMs), and share some of the genetic alterations associated with the adult tumors, especially *TP53* alterations.[54] However, *EGFR* and *PTEN* alterations that are commonly observed among adult grade III and IV astrocytomas do not occur at high incidence among the pediatric cases.[55] Consequently, the molecular basis of high-grade malignancy in many pediatric astrocytomas may well be distinct from that of corresponding adult tumors. Such a possibility is supported by results from a recent study in which a common point mutation of *BRAF* was identified in nearly one-fourth of grade II, III, and IV pediatric astrocytomas.[56] *BRAF* missense mutations are uncommon among adult glioblastomas.[57] Pediatric astrocytomas with *BRAF* alterations were shown as having frequent, accompanying *CDNK2A* homozygous deletion, suggesting a cooperativity between these alterations for contributing to the malignant progression of pediatric astrocytoma.

Oligodendrogliomas and Oligoastrocytomas

Oligodendrogliomas and oligoastrocytomas (mixed gliomas) are diffuse, usually cerebral tumors that are clinically and biologically related to the diffuse, fibrillary astrocytomas.[14] These tumors are less common than diffuse astrocytomas and have generally better prognoses. Patients with WHO grade II oligodendrogliomas, for instance, may have mean survival times of 10 years. In addition, oligodendroglial tumors appear to be differentially chemosensitive, when compared with the diffuse astrocytomas.

Microdissection of the oligodendroglial and astrocytic portions of oligoastrocytomas has shown identical genetic alterations in morphologically distinct portions of individual tumors, suggesting a common underlying molecular biology despite an apparent heterogeneous cellular composition. Allelic losses in oligodendrogliomas and oligoastrocytomas occur preferentially on chromosomes 1p and 19q, affecting 40% to 80% of these tumor types.[58] Because of the frequent loss of these loci in low-grade as well as anaplastic tumors, inactivation of the inferred 1p and 19q tumor suppressor genes has been generally regarded as important to the early stages of oligodendroglial tumorigenesis. The discovery of the majority of these losses being caused by unbalanced translocations between chromosomal arms 1p and 19q implies a scenario in which two tumor suppressor genes could be inactivated through a single event,[59] although target loci have yet to be demonstrated. Alternatively, it has been suggested that the 1p–19q translocations reflect a process of chromatin remodeling that exposes regions of homology that are prone to recombination.[59] In this scenario, the loss of DNA from 1p and 19q would be associated with global chromatin methylation changes, and would suggest an underlying molecular biology of the translocations that is not specifically directed at the deletion of 1p and 19q sequences.

In addition to 1p and 19q deletions, oligoastrocytomas may suffer allelic losses of chromosome 17p, although these losses are not consistently associated with *TP53* mutations. Oncogene amplifications are rare in tumors with oligodendroglial composition, and in total, as well as in contrast to malignant astrocytomas, there is relatively little known regarding the genetic etiology of these tumors, with the exception being the frequent occurrence of *IDH1* mutations, which have been demonstrated as occurring in all grade II and III gliomas, including oligodendrogliomas.[24] Potential associations of such mutations with epigenetic alterations were discussed previously, and it may well be that further insight regarding the molecular etiology of low and intermediate malignancy gliomas will be forthcoming with the maturation of methods for characterizing tumor epigenomes.[60]

Anaplastic oligodendrogliomas have proven to be the first brain tumor for which molecular genetic analysis has had practical clinical ramifications: anaplastic oligodendrogliomas with translocation-associated allelic losses of chromosomes 1p and 19q follow different clinical courses from those tumors that do not have this genetic alteration.[59] Tumors with 1p and 19q loss are usually sensitive to procarbazine, CCNU and vincristine chemotherapy, with nearly 50% of the cases demonstrating complete neuroradiologic responses; correspondingly, patients whose tumors have 1p and 19q loss have median survivals of approximately 10 years.[61] These tumors also appear to have better responses to radiation therapy as well as to temozolomide.[62] On the other hand, anaplastic oligodendrogliomas that lack 1p and 19q loss are only vincristine-sensitive about 25% of the time, and only rarely have complete neuroradiologic responses. As a result, patients whose anaplastic oligodendrogliomas lack 1p and 19q loss have median survivals of approximately 2 years.[61] Recent studies have demonstrated intermediate recurrence-free survival times in those anaplastic oligodendrogliomas that have polysomy for chromosomes 1 and 19 in addition to the typical 1p and 19q losses.[63] At the present time, molecular genetic testing is recommended for: patients diagnosed with anaplastic oligodendrogliomas, small cell malignant tumors in which the differential diagnosis is anaplastic oligodendroglioma versus small cell glioblastoma, and for patients with grade II oligodendrogliomas for whom therapeutic decisions might be influenced by additional knowledge of probable tumor behavior.[58] Thus, molecular genetic analysis of 1p/19q allelic status has become a clinically useful test in neuro-oncology.[64,65]

Ependymomas and Choroid Plexus Tumors

Ependymomas are a clinically diverse group of gliomas that vary from aggressive intraventricular tumors of children to benign spinal cord tumors in adults. Chromosome 22q loss is common in ependymomas, and in spinal ependymomas these losses are associated with mutations of the *NF2* gene that resides on chromosome 22.[66] For cerebral ependymomas, the paucity of *NF2* mutations[66] suggests that another, as yet unidentified, chromosome 22q gene is critical to the development of the intracranial form of this cancer.

Choroid plexus tumors are also a varied group of tumors that preferentially occur in the ventricular system, ranging from aggressive supratentorial intraventricular tumors of children to benign cerebellopontine angle tumors of adults. Choroid plexus tumors have been reported occasionally in patients with Li-Fraumeni syndrome and rhabdoid predisposition syndrome, raising the possibility of the involvement of the *TP53* gene on chromosome 17p or the *hSNF5/INI1* gene on chromosome 22q. However, there is no evidence of *hSNF5/INI1* point mutations in patients with choroid plexus papilloma, and the mutational status of *TP53* have not been extensively studied in these tumors.

CGH studies of ependymoma have confirmed frequent deletions of chromosome 22, and have additionally revealed frequent losses of 6q.[67,68] Recently, array CGH was used in identifying 9q33–34 gains as being associated with ependymoma recurrence and malignant progression.[69] Transcriptome analysis has been applied to multiple series of ependymomas, with the results from one such study indicating potential target genes for the 6q and 22q deletions,[70] the latter of which being especially important to tumors having no apparent involvement of *NF2*. Another report has shown increased ependymal tumor expression of genes having defined roles in cell proliferation, and suggests that the expression level of these genes may reliably distinguish between ependymomas of grade II and grade III malignancy.[66–71] As has been the case for other types of CNS cancer, gene expression profiling has been used in attempts to identify clinically distinct subsets of ependymoma, with results identifying transcriptional profiles that could distinguish long vs. short-term survivors.[72]

Medulloblastomas

Medulloblastomas are highly malignant, primitive tumors that arise in the posterior fossa, primarily in children. One-third to one-half of all medulloblastomas have an isochromosome 17q on cytogenetic analysis, and corresponding allelic loss of chromosome 17p has been noted on molecular genetic analysis. *TP53* mutations, however, are less common than 17p deletions in medulloblastoma, with the majority of 17p losses occurring preferentially at regions telomeric to the TP53 locus, implying the presence of a second, more distal chromosome 17p tumor suppressor gene. For the fraction of medulloblastomas with *TP53* mutation, clinical outcomes appear to be unfavorable,[73] thereby supporting determination of medulloblastoma p53 status as an important diagnostic test. In addition to allelic losses on 17p, deletions of chromosome 6q, 8p, 10q, 11, and 16q have also been noted in these tumors. Oncogene amplifications are not common in medulloblastomas, with only *MYCC* and *MYCN* shown to be amplified in significant numbers of cases.[74] Copy number gains of the *OTX2* gene, which encodes a transcriptional regulator of MYCC,[75] occur in a small proportion of medulloblastomas.[75,76] Gene amplifications and copy number increases may be restricted to the more aggressive large cell and anaplastic subclasses of medulloblastoma.

The discovery of genes underlying two hereditary tumor syndromes has directed attention to signaling pathways involved in medulloblastoma tumorigenesis.[77] Gorlin syndrome (also termed *nevoid basal cell carcinoma syndrome*), a condition characterized by multiple basal cell carcinomas, bone cysts, dysmorphic features, and medulloblastomas arises from defects in *PTCH* (a homolog of the Drosophila *patched* gene) on the long arm of chromosome 9. Medulloblastomas, particularly the nodular desmoplastic variants that are characteristic of Gorlin syndrome, can show allelic loss of chromosome 9q and *PTCH* mutations, and mice that have only one functional copy of the murine *Ptch* gene are predisposed to the development of tumors that are histologically identical to medulloblastoma. The protein encoded by PTCH functions in the pathway regulated by the Sonic hedgehog protein (SHH). Other molecules in this pathway include smoothened (SMO), and rare SMO mutations have been documented in sporadic medulloblastomas. Intriguingly, both germ line and somatic mutations, along with allelic loss, have been identified in SUFU, another member of the SHH pathway that maps to 10q.[78] Alterations in various members of the SHH pathway likely account for the majority of desmoplastic medulloblastomas.

Turcot syndrome, a condition characterized by colonic tumors and brain tumors, is also associated with medulloblastoma; patients with the adenomatous polyposis phenotype may develop medulloblastomas and these patients often have mutations of the *APC* gene on chromosome 5q.[77] The Apc protein operates in the Wnt signaling pathway that includes b-catenin and axin-1, and rare mutations of these genes have been found in sporadic medulloblastomas.

In spite of the contribution of human genetics to our understanding of medulloblastoma development, *PTCH* and *APC* gene alterations, as well as alterations of other genes encoding components of their signaling pathways, are associated with less than 15% of sporadic medulloblastomas, suggesting that the genetic etiology of a significant fraction of these tumors has yet to be determined. The question of whether molecular profiling will provide needed information regarding the genetic etiology of these tumors, as well as provide guidance for the management of medulloblastoma patients, has received substantial attention. A recent study evaluated candidate prognostic markers, selected from medulloblastoma expression data, that were immunohistochemically analyzed for their prognostic value using medulloblastoma tissue arrays. Combined expression of three genes, *MYCC, LDHB,* and *CCNB1,* was able to predict survival in medulloblastoma patients.[79]

Collectively, the results from studies of medulloblastoma genome and transcriptome characterizations suggest that these comprehensive approaches are generating information that will be useful in tumor diagnosis and treatment, and for increasing our understanding of the molecular biology of this cancer.

Meningiomas

Meningiomas are common intracranial tumors that arise in the meninges and compress the underlying brain. Meningiomas are usually benign, but some "atypical" meningiomas may recur locally, and some are frankly malignant.[14] Homozygous inactivation of the chromosome 22 localized *NF2* gene is the rule in the meningiomas of NF2 patients, and *NF2* inactivation is observed in the majority of sporadic fibroblastic and transitional meningioma subtypes.[80] Inactivating *NF2* gene alterations primarily involve immediate truncations, splicing abnormalities or altered reading frames, and result in a lack of, or grossly truncated, proteins.

Approximately 40% of meningiomas have neither *NF2* gene mutations nor allelic loss of chromosome 22q. For these tumors, it is likely that alternative tumor suppressor genes are involved, with potential genomic locations of such genes, including chromosomes 1p, 3p, 5p, 5q, 11, 13, and 17p, as suggested by the results of numerous genetic investigations.

Atypical and malignant meningiomas are not as common as benign meningiomas. Atypical meningiomas often show allelic losses for chromosomal arms 1p, 6q, 9q, 10q, 14q, 17p, and 18q, suggesting the presence of progression-associated genes.

Chromosome 10 loss, in particular, has been associated with meningiomas displaying clinically malignant behavior beyond that associated with normal brain invasion alone,[81] which can occur with tumors that are otherwise benign. Chromosome 10 loss as a predictor of meningioma malignancy provides another example of how molecular genetic investigations have clarified grading issues in neuro-oncology. Another study showed a potential correlation between gain of 1q and shorter progression-free survival for patients with atypical meningioma.[10]

Hierarchical clustering of expression profiles has also been used to distinguish high-grade from benign meningiomas.[82,83] Consistent with cytogenetic-based interpretations, the results of such studies have shown that genes on chromosome 1p and 14q are commonly down-regulated in anaplastic meningiomas, and the 14q11.2-localized *NDRG2* gene has been of particular interest because of its decreased expression being associated with meningioma progression.[84] Increased expression of the reverse transcription subunit hTERT (reverse telomerase transcriptase), whose enzymatic activity is critical to chromosome telomere maintenance, may also serve as a potential predictor of meningioma malignancy by its association with tumor recurrence and reduced progression-free survival.

CURRENT BASIS OF CNS TUMOR TREATMENT AND RESPONSE TO THERAPY

Most therapeutic approaches fail to eradicate entire CNS tumors, and tumor cells that evade primary therapies are responsible for "recurrent" cancer. One concept that is relevant to acquired therapeutic resistance involves tumor initiating cells (also referred to as tumor stem cells), which exist as a subpopulation of cells within individual tumors and that are capable of sustained self-renewal, thereby promoting unlimited tumor growth.[85] Therapeutic targeting of these tumor stem cells may be critically important for the development of curative treatment approaches.[86]

An additional perspective that is proving highly influential for the treatment of cancer involves the individualization of therapy based on specific tumor genome alterations: two examples of this approach that involve the treatment of glioblastoma are described here.

The first example involves a landmark study that demonstrated an association between glioblastoma *MGMT* gene methylation status and tumor response to treatment with the DNA alkylating agent temozolomide.[87] The molecular basis of this relationship may be attributable, in part, to methylguanine methyltransferase (MGMT) gene promoter methylation, observed in approximately 40% of GBM, which markedly down-regulates the synthesis of MGMT transcript and protein. Patients whose glioblastomas had methylated MGMT who received combined radiation and temozolomide therapy survived significantly longer than patients with MGMT-methylated tumors receiving radiation only, or patients whose tumors lacked MGMT methylation and received mono or combination therapy. However, it is also clear that a significant number of glioblastomas treated with temozolomide develop mismatch repair gene defects, most commonly *MSH6* mutations or down-regulation, that lead to a hypermutation phenotype and more rapid progression of disease while being treated with temozolomide.[21,88,89]

Other studies have addressed the relationship between a molecular subset of GBM and therapeutic response involved therapy with EGFR kinase inhibitors, implicating EGFR and PTEN status in predicting response to these inhibitors.[90,91] This interpretation is tenuous, however, as subsequent clinical trials have not demonstrated significant therapeutic effects of these inhibitors, potentially because multiple receptor tyrosine kinases are activated in individual tumors, and the inhibition of one receptor tyrosine kinase, such as EGFR, may contribute to the activation of others.[92,93]

Nonetheless, such studies suggest that current approaches should combine individual tumor biomarker status with corresponding therapies directed against specific biomarkers, or against signaling mediators of the biomarkers. The wealth of GBM biomarker information made available through the TCGA initiative[21] will undoubtedly contribute to the further popularization of this conceptual approach to CNS tumor treatment.

Selected References

The full list of references for this chapter appears in the online version.

1. Louis DN, Pomeroy SL, Cairncross JG. Focus on CNS neoplasia. *Cancer Cell* 2002;1: 125.
4. Nutt CL, Mani DR, Betensky RA, et al. Gene expression-based classification of malignant gliomas correlates better with survival than histological classification. *Cancer Res* 2003;63:1602.
9. Pomeroy SL, Tamayo P, Gaasenbeek M, et al. Prediction of central nervous system embryonal tumour outcome based on gene expression. *Nature* 2002; 415:436.
13. Huse JT, Holland EC. Genetically engineered mouse models of brain cancer and the promise of preclinical testing. *Brain Pathol* 2009;19:132.
14. Louis DN, Ohgaki H, Wiestler OD, Cavenee WK, eds. *World Health Organization Histological Classification of Tumours of the Central Nervous System*. Lyon: IARC Press, 2007.
17. Wrensch M, Jenkins RB, Chang JS, et al. Variants in the CDKN2B and TEL1 regions are associated with high-grade glioma susceptibility. *Nat Genet* 2009;41:905.
19. Louis DN, von Deimling A, Chung RY, et al. Comparative study of p53 gene and protein alterations in human astrocytic tumors. *J Neuropathol Exp Neurol* 1993;52:31.
21. Cancer Genome Atlas Research Network. Comprehensive genomic characterization defines human glioblastoma genes and core pathways. *Nature* 2008;455:1061.
22. Bogler O, Huang H-JS, Cavenee WK. Loss of wild-type p53 bestows a growth advantage on primary cortical astrocytes and facilitates their in vitro transformation. *Cancer Res* 1995;55:2746.
23. Reilly KM, Loisel DA, Bronson RT, McLaughlin ME, Jacks T. Nf1;Trp53 mutant mice develop glioblastoma with evidence of strain-specific effects. *Nat Genet* 2000;26:109.
24. Yan H, Parsons DW, Jin G, et al. IDH1 and IDH2 mutations in gliomas. *N Engl J Med* 2009;360:765.
27. Weller M, Felsberg J, Hartmann C, et al. Molecular predictors of progression-free and overall survival in patients with newly diagnosed glioblastoma: a prospective translational study of the German Glioma Network. *J Clin Oncol* 2009;27:5743.
28. Ichimura K, Schmidt EE, Goike HM, and Collins VP. Human glioblastomas with no alterations of the CDKN2A (p16INK4A, MTS1) and CDK4 genes have frequent mutations of the retinoblastoma gene. *Oncogene* 1996;13:1065.
29. Ueki K, Ono Y, Henson JW, Efird JT, von Deimling A, Louis DN. CDKN2/p16 or RB alterations occur in the majority of glioblastomas and are inversely correlated. *Cancer Res* 1996;56:150.
30. Xiao A, Wu H, Pandolfi PP, Louis DN, Van Dyke T. Astrocyte inactivation of the pRb pathway predisposes mice to malignant astrocytoma development that is accelerated by PTEN mutation. *Cancer Cell* 2002;1:157.
32. Parsons DW, Jones S, Zhang X, et al. An integrated genomic analysis of human glioblastoma multiforme. *Science* 2008;321:1807.
34. Furnari FB, Lin H, Huang HS, and Cavenee WK. Growth suppression of glioma cells by PTEN requires a functional phosphatase catalytic domain. *Proc Natl Acad Sci U S A* 1997;94:12479.
35. Kwon CH, Zhao D, Chen J, et al. Pten haploinsufficiency accelerates formation of high-grade astrocytomas. *Cancer Res* 2008;68:3286.

36. Ekstrand AJ, James CD, Cavenee WK, Seliger B, Pettersson RF, Collins VP. Genes for epidermal growth factor receptor, transforming growth factor alpha, and epidermal growth factor and their expression in human gliomas in vivo. *Cancer Res* 1991;51:2164.
37. Hayashi Y, Ueki K, Waha A, Wiestler OD, Louis DN, von Deimling A. Association of EGFR gene amplification and CDKN2 (p16/MTS1) gene deletion in glioblastoma multiforme. *Brain Pathol* 1997;7:871.
38. Ekstrand AJ, Sugawa N, James CD, Collins VP. Amplified and rearranged epidermal growth factor receptor genes in human glioblastomas reveal deletions of sequences encoding portions of the N- and/or C-terminal tails. *Proc Natl Acad Sci U S A* 1992;89:4309.
40. Nishikawa R, Ji XD, Harmon RC, et al. A mutant epidermal growth factor receptor common in human glioma confers enhanced tumorigenicity. *Proc Natl Acad Sci U S A* 1994;91:7727.
41. Holland EC, Hively WP, DePinho RA, Varmus HE. A constitutively active epidermal growth factor receptor cooperates with disruption of G1 cell-cycle arrest pathways to induce glioma-like lesions in mice. *Genes Dev* 1998; 12:3675.
42. Zhao S, Lin Y, Xu W, et al. Glioma-derived mutations in IDH1 dominantly inhibit IDH1 catalytic activity and induce HIF-1alpha. *Science* 2009;324:261.
44. Dang L, White DW, Gross S, et al. Cancer-associated IDH1 mutations produce 2-hydroxyglutarate. *Nature* 2009462:739.
45. Verhaak RG, Hoadley KA, Purdom E, et al; Cancer Genome Atlas Research Network. Integrated genomic analysis identifies clinically relevant subtypes of glioblastoma characterized by abnormalities in PDGFRA, IDH1, EGFR, and NF1. *Cancer Cell* 201017:98.
46. von Deimling A, von Ammon K, Schoenfeld D, Wiestler OD, Seizinger BR, Louis DN. Subsets of glioblastoma multiforme defined by molecular genetic analysis. *Brain Pathol* 1993;3:19.
49. Phillips HS, Kharbanda S, Chen R, et al. Molecular subclasses of high-grade glioma predict prognosis, delineate a pattern of disease progression, and resemble stages in neurogenesis. *Cancer Cell* 2006;9:157.
50. Maher EA, Brennan C, Wen PY, et al. Marked genomic differences characterize primary and secondary glioblastoma subtypes and identify two distinct molecular and clinical secondary glioblastoma entities. *Cancer Res* 2006;66:11502.
52. Jones DT, Kocialkowski S, Liu L, et al. Tandem duplication producing a novel oncogenic BRAF fusion gene defines the majority of pilocytic astrocytomas. *Cancer Res* 2008;68:8673.
54. Pollack IF, Finkelstein SD, Burnham J, et al; Children's Cancer Group. Age and TP53 mutation frerequency in childhood malignant gliomas: results in a multi-institutional cohort. *Cancer Res* 200161:7404.
56. Schiffman JD, Hodgson JG, VandenBerg SR, Flaherty P, Polley MY, Yu M, Fisher PG, Rowitch DH, Ford JM, Berger MS, Ji H, Gutmann DH, James CD. Oncogenic BRAF mutation with CDKN2A inactivation is characteristic of a subset of pediatric malignant astrocytomas. *Cancer Res* 70:512–9, 2010.
58. Reifenberger G, Louis DN. Oligodendroglioma: toward molecular definitions in diagnostic neuro-oncology. *J Neuropathol Exp Neurol* 2003;62:111.
59. Jenkins RB, Blair H, Ballman KV, et al. A t(1;19)(q10;p10) mediates the combined deletions of 1p and 19q and predicts a better prognosis of patients with oligodendroglioma. *Cancer Res* 2006;66:9852.
61. Cairncross JG, Ueki K, Zlatescu MC, et al. Specific chromosomal losses predict chemotherapeutic response and survival in patients with anaplastic oligodendrogliomas. *J Natl Cancer Inst* 1998;90:1473.
64. Ino Y, Betensky RA, Zlatescu MC, et al. Molecular subtypes of anaplastic oligodendroglioma: implications for patient management at diagnosis. *Clin Cancer Res* 2001;7:839.
65. Yip S, Iafrate AJ, Louis DN. Molecular diagnostic testing in malignant gliomas: a practical update on predictive markers. *J Neuropathol Exp Neurol* 2008;67:1.
66. Ebert C, von Haken M, Meyer-Puttlitz B, et al. Molecular genetic analysis of ependymal tumors. NF2 mutations and chromosome 22q loss occur preferentially in intramedullary spinal ependymomas. *Am J Pathol* 1999; 155:627.
71. Korshunov A, Neben K, Wrobel G, et al. Gene expression patterns in ependymomas correlate with tumor location, grade, and patient age. *Am J Pathol* 2003;163:1721.
73. Tabori U, Baskin B, Shago M, et al. Universal poor survival in children with medulloblastoma harboring somatic TP53 mutations. *J Clin Oncol* 2010;28: 1345.
77. Raffel C. Medulloblastoma: molecular genetics and animal models. *Neoplasia* 2004;6:3102004.
79. de Haas T, Hasselt N, Troost D, et al. Molecular risk stratification of medulloblastoma patients based on immunohistochemical analysis of MYC, LDHB, and CCNB1 expression. *Clin Cancer Res* 2008;14:4154.
80. Wellenreuther R, Kraus JA, Lenartz D, et al. Analysis of the neurofibromatosis 2 gene reveals molecular variants of meningioma. *Am J Pathol* 1995; 146:827.
82. Watson MA, Gutmann DH, Peterson K, et al. Molecular characterization of human meningiomas by gene expression profiling using high-density oligonucleotide microarrays. *Am J Pathol* 2002;161:665.
85. Singh SK, Hawkins C, Clarke ID, S et al. Identification of human brain tumour initiating cells. *Nature* 2004;432:396.
86. Bao S, Wu Q, McLendon RE, et al. Glioma stem cells promote radioresistance by preferential activation of the DNA damage response. Nature 2006;444:756.
87. Hegi ME, Diserens AC, Gorlia T, et al. MGMT gene silencing and benefit from temozolomide in glioblastoma. *N Engl J Med* 2005;352:997.
88. Cahill DP, Levine KK, Betensky RA, et al. Loss of the mismatch repair protein MSH6 in human glioblastomas is associated with tumor progression during temozolomide treatment. *Clin Cancer Res* 2007;13:2038.
90. Mellinghoff IK, Wang MY, Vivanco I, et al. Molecular determinants of the response of glioblastomas to EGFR kinase inhibitors. *N Engl J Med* 2005; 353:2012.
93. Stommel JM, Kimmelman AC, Ying H, et al. Coactivation of receptor tyrosine kinases affects the response of tumor cells to targeted therapies. *Science* 2007;318:287.

CHAPTER 121 NEOPLASMS OF THE CENTRAL NERVOUS SYSTEM

MINESH MEHTA, MICHAEL A. VOGELBAUM, SUSAN CHANG, AND NEHA PATEL

EPIDEMIOLOGY OF BRAIN TUMORS

Incidence and Prevalence

The precise incidence and prevalence of brain tumors is imprecisely documented because benign tumors were not required to be reported prior to 2003, and metastatic disease to the brain remains unreported. The major data sources include the Surveillance, Epidemiology, and End Results (SEER) program and the Central Brain Tumor Registry of the United States (CBTRUS).[1,2] The SEER registry reports a primary central nervous system (CNS) tumor incidence of 6.4 cases per 100,000 per year (7.6 per 100,000 men and 5.4 per 100,000 women), translating to an estimated case load of 22,070, with an anticipated 12,920 deaths, and an age-adjusted death rate of 4.4 per 100,000. The median age at diagnosis is 55, and an age-dependent bimodal distribution is observed, with the incidence estimated at 3.1 per 100,000 up to age 4, 1.8 per 100,000 from age 15 to 24 years, and a peak of 18 per 100,000 around age 65 years. The CBTRUS database quotes the estimated incidence of new CNS tumors in the United States at 62,930 cases, primarily because it includes both benign and malignant histologies in the assessment.

In 1993, the World Health Organization (WHO) ratified a new classification, assuming that each tumor results from a specific cell type. Most registries do not contain detailed information regarding the distribution of various CNS tumors, as specified in the WHO classification.[3–5] Many of these tumors are radiographically and clinically diagnosed; examples include infiltrating pontine gliomas, vestibular schwannomas, skull-base meningiomas, and brain metastases. Specific CNS tumor types also differ in incidence based on anatomic location. Figure 121.1 presents a simplified distribution by subtype.

The increased utilization of cranial imaging for headaches, seizures, or trauma has led to an increase in the diagnosis of benign tumors. SEER suggests that between 1975 and 1987 there was a significant increase in the incidence of CNS tumors, which leveled off between 1991 and 2006. Because many patients with CNS tumors survive for several years, the prevalence exceeds the incidence; as of 2004, there were 612,000 Americans alive with CNS tumors, 124,000 with malignant and 488,000 with nonmalignant tumors.

Etiologic Factors

No agent has been definitively implicated in the causation of CNS tumors, and risk factors can be identified only in a minority. Commonly implicated associations described with other malignancies, such as diet, exercise, alcohol, tobacco, and viruses, are generally not considered to be significant for CNS tumors.

Environmental Factors

Farmers and petrochemical workers have been shown to have a higher incidence of primary brain tumors. A variety of chemical exposures have been linked.[6] Ionizing and nonionizing radiation has been implicated, with the clearest association coming from the occurrence of superficial meningiomas, in individuals receiving cranial or scalp irradiation, with the association being stronger for young children receiving low doses of irradiation for benign conditions.[7] Exposure to ionizing radiation is a known risk factor for a small percentage of astrocytomas, sarcomas, and other tumors.[8] There is a 2.3% incidence of primary brain tumors in long-term survivors among children given prophylactic cranial irradiation for acute leukemia, a fourfold increase over the expected rate.[9]

There are conflicting reports regarding nonionizing radiation emitted by cellular telephones.[10] Several investigators have reported meta-analyses of case control studies evaluating cell phone use and the development of a brain tumor. Kan et al.[11] reviewed nine studies (5,259 cases and 12,074 controls) and showed an overall odds ratio (OR) of 0.90 for cellular phone use and brain tumor development; the OR was 1.25 for long-term users. An OR of 0.98 for developing malignant and benign tumors of the brain as well as the head and neck was reported by Myung et al.[12] when collating 23 case control studies (12,544 cases and 25,572 controls). The International Commission for Non-Ionizing Radiation Protection Standing Committee on Epidemiology reviewed the epidemiologic evidence and they concluded that there was not a causal association between mobile phone use and malignant glioma, but for slow-growing tumors, the observation period was too short for conclusive statements.[13] A recent report of the INTERPHONE study, an international, population-based case control study, also did not find an increased risk of glioma or meningioma.[14] Further studies continue.

Viral Associations

Although certain canine and feline CNS tumors may have a viral association, the human evidence remains weak. Specifically, no increase in the risk of developing a brain tumor has been associated with previous polio vaccination, which discredits claims that simian virus 40 that contaminated older polio vaccine preparations caused brain tumors.[15] The exception to this is primary CNS lymphoma, which has been shown to be associated with Epstein-Barr virus.[16] An increase in incidence of primary CNS lymphoma is most likely due to the increasing numbers of immunosuppressed patients in the setting of human immunodeficiency virus and posttransplant use of immunosuppressants.[16,17]

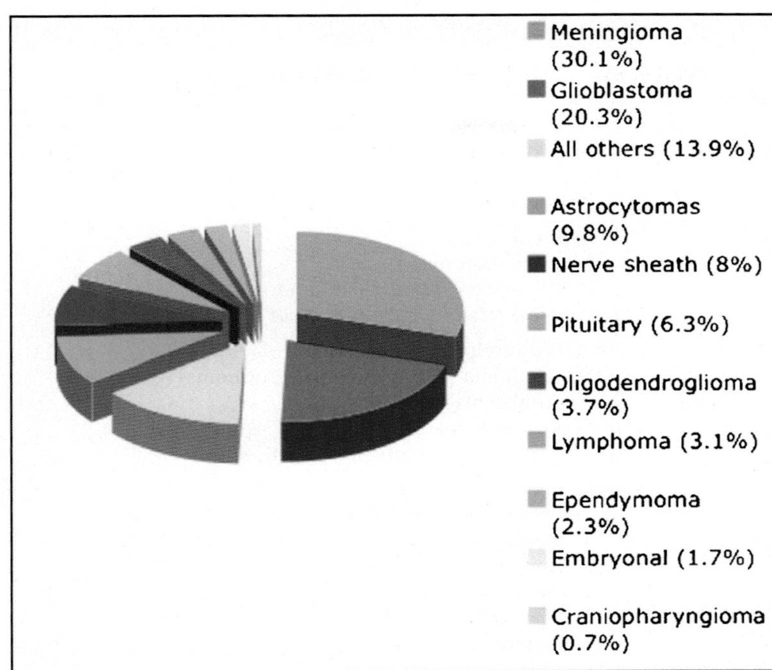

FIGURE 121.1 Proportionate distribution of the incidence of central nervous system neoplasms by histopathologic type, based on the Central Brain Tumor Registry of the United States database.

The association between human cytomegalovirus (HCMV) infection and glioblastoma was first described by Cobbs et al.[18] in 2002. The presence of HCMV was also demonstrated in glioblastoma and in other gliomas.[19] Further work is needed to evaluate the role of this virus.

Hereditary Syndromes

Neurofibromatosis type 1 (NF1) is an autosomal dominant disorder associated with intra- and extracranial Schwann cell tumors. Optic gliomas, astrocytomas, and meningiomas also occur at higher frequency in NF1. NF2 is characterized by bilateral vestibular schwannomas and meningiomas. Systemic schwannomas also occur in NF2. Subependymal giant cell astrocytoma commonly occur in children with tuberous sclerosis, an autosomal dominant disorder caused by mutation in the *TSC1* and *TSC2* genes. Other hereditary tumor syndromes affecting the CNS include Li-Fraumeni syndrome (germ line mutation in one p53 allele; malignant gliomas); von Hippel-Lindau syndrome (germ line mutation of the *VHL* gene; hemangioblastomas), and Turcot's syndrome (germ line mutations of the adenomatous polyposis gene; medulloblastoma).[20] The nevoid basal cell carcinoma syndrome (Gorlin's syndrome) is associated with medulloblastomas (and possibly meningiomas) and represents mutations in the *PTCH* suppressor gene or other members of the Sonic hedgehog pathway.[21,22]

Meningiomas and schwannomas are more common in females; gliomas, medulloblastomas, and most other CNS tumors are more common in males. Meningiomas are more common in African Americans and gliomas and medulloblastomas in whites. It has been suggested that there is a lower incidence of meningiomas and a higher incidence of gliomas and vestibular schwannomas in higher socioeconomic groups.[23–27]

Classification

Primary CNS tumors are of ecto- and mesodermal origin and arise from the brain, cranial nerves, meninges, pituitary, pineal, and vascular elements. The WHO classification lists approximately 100 subtypes of CNS malignancies in seven broad categories (Table 121.1).[3,28,29] A listing of tumors of glial origin is summarized in Table 121.2. In spite of the low proliferation rate within the meninges, meningiomas are among the most common CNS tumors. Astrocytes are among the most mitogenically competent cells, and astrocytomas, also referred to interchangeably as *gliomas*, are among the more common primary CNS tumor. The precise cell of origin of gliomas, however, remains unclear.

The WHO classification can be reduced to a simpler working formulation, categorizing the neoplasms into tumors presumably derived from glia, neurons, or from cells that surround the CNS or form specialized anatomic structures. Glial cells are believed to give rise to astrocytomas, oligodendrogliomas, and ependymomas. Neuronal cells are involved in the development of medulloblastoma and primitive neuroectodermal tumors (PNETs). In PNETs, anatomic location is pivotal; transformation of cortical neuroblasts leads to cortical PNETs; retinal neuroblasts form retinoblastoma; and pineal neuroblasts form pineoblastomas. Specialized anatomic structures within the CNS give rise to pituitary adenomas, pineocytomas, chordomas, hemangioblastomas, germ cell tumors, and choroid plexus papillomas and carcinomas.

This working formulation is speculative, based on scanty phenotypical and immunohistochemical evidence. For example, oligodendrogliomas are diagnosed based on cellular morphology, including prominent nuclei surrounded by a cytoplasmic halo with a characteristic "fried egg" appearance, and many have codeletions of 1p and 19q. However, no definitive markers for oligodendrogliomas currently exist; these tumors can stain both for glial fibrillary acidic protein, an astrocytic marker, and for synaptophysin, a presumptive neuronal marker.[30] A third of all gliomas have morphologic characteristics of both astrocytoma and oligodendroglioma, leading some to separate gliomas based on their molecular and genetic characteristics.[31] Evidence that suggests that some oligodendrocytes derive from a neuronal lineage, whereas some neuron-derived tumors (embryonal tumors) can show significant areas of glial differentiation, highlights the uncertainly.[32,33]

TABLE 121.1

CLASSIFICATION OF TUMORS OF THE CENTRAL NERVOUS SYSTEM: SELECTED FROM THE 2007 WORLD HEALTH ORGANIZATION CLASSIFICATION

1. Neuroepithelial tumors
   Astrocytic tumors
   a. Pilocytic Astrocytoma
   b. Subependymal giant cell astrocytoma
   c. Pleomorphic xanthroastrocytoma
   d. Diffuse astrocytoma
      a. Fibrillary astrocytoma
      b. Gemistocytic astrocytoma
      c. Pro-oplasmic astrocytoma
   e. Anaplastic astrocytoma
   f. Glioblastoma
      a. Giant cell glioblastoma
      b. Gliosarcoma
   g. Gliomatosis cerebri

   Oligodendroglial tumors
   a. Oligodendroglioma
   b. Anaplastic oligodendroglioma

   Ependymal tumors
   a. Subependymoma
   b. Myxopapillary ependymoma
   c. Ependymoma
   d. Anaplastic ependymoma

   Choroid plexus tumors
   a. Choroid plexus papilloma
   b. Atypical choroid plexus papilloma
   c. Choroid plexus carcinoma

   Other neuroepithelial tumors
   a. Astroblastoma
   b. Chordoid glioma of the third ventricle
   c. Angiocentric glioma

   Neuronal and mixed neuronal-glial tumors
   a. Dysplastic gangliocytoma of cerebellum (Lhermitte-Duclos)
   b. Desmoplastic infantile astrocytoma/ganglioglioma
   c. Dysembryoplastic neuroepithelial tumor
   d. Gangliocytoma
   e. Ganglioglioma
   f. Anaplastic ganglioglioma
   g. Central neurocytoma
   h. Extraventricular neurocytoma
   i. Cerebellar liponeurosytoma
   j. Papillary glioneuronal tumor
   k. Rosette-forming glioneuronal tumor of the fourth ventricle
   l. Paraganglioma

   Tumors of the pineal region
   a. Pineocytoma
   b. Pineoblastoma

   Embryonal tumors
   a. Medulloblastoma
   b. Primitive neuroectodermal tumors
   c. Atypical teratoid/rhabdoid tumor

2. Tumors of cranial/spinal nerves
   a. Schwannoma (neurilemmoma, neurinoma)
   b. Neurofibroma
   c. Perineurinoma
   d. Malignant peripheral nerve sheath tumor

3. Tumors of the meninges
   A. Tumors of meningothelial cells
      a. Meningioma
      b. Fibrous
      c. Psammomatous
      d. Clear cell
      e. Atypical
      f. Anaplastic (malignant)

   B. Mesenchymal tumors
      a. Lipoma
      b. Solitary fibrous tumor
      c. Rhabdomyosarcoma
      d. Malignant fibrous histiocytoma
      e. Chondrosarchoma
      f. Osteoma
      g. Hemangioma
      h. Hemangiopericytoma
      i. Kaposi sarcoma

4. Lymphomas and Hematopoietic neoplasms
   a. Malignant lymphomas
   b. Plasmacytoma

5. Germ cell tumors
   a. Germinoma
   b. Yolk-sac tumor
   c. Choriocarcinoma
   d. Teratoma
   e. Mixed-germ cell tumors

6. Sellar tumors
   a. Pituitary adenoma
   b. Craniopharyngioma

7. Metastatic tumors

An alternative hypothesis is that all neuroepithelial cells are derived from a common precursor cell (i.e., a multipotent neural stem cell), and hence all neuroepithelial tumors are derived from neural stem cells or their committed progeny.[34] The recent discovery, isolation, and characterization of cancer stem cells from human brain tumors provides supportive evidence.[35]

Approximately 15% of all primary CNS tumors arise in the spinal cord, where the distribution of tumor types is significantly different from that in the brain (Table 121.3). Tumors of the lining of the spinal cord and nerve roots predominate (50% to 80% of all spinal tumors); schwannomas and meningiomas are most common, followed by ependymomas. Primary gliomas of the spinal cord are uncommon.[4,5]

ANATOMIC LOCATION AND CLINICAL CONSIDERATIONS

Intracranial Tumors

Intracranial tumors produce four categories of symptoms: those arising from increased intracranial pressure (ICP), physiologic deficits specific to location, higher order neurocognitive deficits, and endocrinologic dysfunction. Headache arises from irritation of the dura or intracranial vessels or due to elevated ICP from tumor bulk, edema, or obstruction of a cerebrospinal fluid (CSF) pathway. Slow-growing tumors may grow remarkably

TABLE 121.2

THE VARIETY OF CENTRAL NERVOUS SYSTEM GLIAL TUMORS (BASED ON 2007 WORLD HEALTH ORGANIZATION CLASSIFICATION)

Astrocytic Tumors:
Pilocytic astrocytoma
Pilomyxoid astrocytoma
Subependymal giant cell astrocytoma
Pleomorphic xanthroastrocytoma
Fibrillary astrocytoma
Gemistocytic astrocytoma
Protoplasmic astrocytoma
Glioblastoma
Giant cell glioblastoma
Gliosarcoma
Gliomatosis cerebri

Oligodendroglial Tumors:
Oligodendroglioma
Anaplastic oligodendroglioma

Oligoastrocytic Tumors:
Oligoastrocytoma
Anaplastic oligoastrocytoma

Ependymal Tumors:
Subependymoma
Myxopapillary ependymoma
Ependymoma
Anaplastic ependymoma

Choroid Plexus Tumors:
Choroid plexus papilloma
Choroid plexus carcinoma

Other Neuroepithelial Tumors:
Astroblastoma
Anaplastic astroblastoma
Chordoid glioma of the third ventricle

large without producing headache, whereas rapidly growing tumors can cause headache early in their course. Small tumors can cause headache by growing in an enclosed space that is richly innervated with pain fibers, such as the cavernous sinus, or by causing obstructive hydrocephalus. Nausea and vomiting, gait and balance alterations, personality changes, and slowing of psychomotor function or even somnolence may be present with increased ICP. Because ICP increases with recumbency and hypoventilation during sleep, early-morning headaches that awaken the patient are typical. Sometimes the only presenting symptoms are changes in personality, mood, or mental capacity or slowing of psychomotor activity. Such changes may be confused with depression, especially in older patients. Although fewer than 6% of first seizures result from brain tumors, almost one-half of patients with supratentorial brain tumors present

TABLE 121.3

PRIMARY SPINAL TUMORS

Histology	Sloof et al. (5)[a]	Preston-Martin (4)[a]
Schwannoma	29.0	22.0
Meningioma	25.5	42.0
Ependymoma	12.8	15.1
Sarcomas	11.9	—
Astrocytoma	6.5	11.2
Other gliomas	—	1.9
Vascular tumors	6.2	—
Chordomas	4.0	—
Epidermoids	1.4	—
Other	2.7	5.6

[a]These two references provide data regarding tumor type.

with seizures. An adult with a first seizure that occurs without an obvious precipitating event should undergo magnetic resonance imaging (MRI).

Tumors are sometimes associated with location-specific symptoms. Frontal tumors cause changes in personality, loss of initiative, and abulia (loss of ability to make independent decisions). Posterior frontal tumors can produce contralateral weakness by affecting the motor cortex and expressive aphasia if they involve the dominant (usually left) frontal lobe. Bifrontal disease, seen with "butterfly" gliomas and lymphomas, may cause memory impairment, labile mood, and urinary incontinence.

Temporal tumors might cause symptoms detectable only on careful testing of perception and spatial judgment, but can also impair memory. Homonymous superior quadrantanopsia, auditory hallucinations, and abnormal behavior can occur with tumors in either temporal lobe. Nondominant temporal tumors can cause minor perceptual problems and spatial disorientation. Dominant temporal lobe tumors can present with dysnomia, impaired perception of verbal commands, and ultimately fluent (Wernicke's-like) aphasia. Seizures are more common from tumors in this location.

Parietal tumors affect sensory and perceptual functions. Sensory disorders range from mild sensory extinction or stereognosis, observable only by testing, to a more severe sensory loss such as hemianesthesia. Poor proprioception in the affected limb is common and is sometimes associated with gait instability. Homonymous inferior quadrantanopsia, incongruent hemianopsia, or visual inattention may occur. Nondominant parietal tumors may cause contralateral neglect and, in severe cases, anosognosia and apraxia. Dominant parietal tumors lead to alexia, dysgraphia, and certain types of apraxia. Occipital tumors can produce contralateral homonymous hemianopsia or complex visual aberrations, affecting perception of color, size, or location. Bilateral occipital tumors can produce cortical blindness.

Classic corpus callosum disconnection syndromes are rare in brain tumor patients, even though infiltrative gliomas often cross the corpus callosum in the region of the genu or the splenium. Interruption of the anterior corpus callosum can cause a failure of the left hand to carry out spoken commands. Lesions in the posterior corpus callosum interrupt visual fibers that connect the right occipital lobe to the left angular gyrus, causing an inability to read or name colors.

Thalamic tumors can cause local effects and also obstructive hydrocephalus. Headaches from hydrocephalus or trapping of one lateral ventricular horn are common. Either sensory or motor syndromes or, on the dominant side, aphasia is possible. "Thalamic" pain disorders or motor syndromes from basal ganglia involvement may also occur.

The brainstem, composed of the midbrain, pons, and medulla, has both nuclear groups and traversing axons. The most common brainstem tumor is the pontine glioma, which presents most frequently with cranial nerve VI and VII palsies. Long tract signs usually follow, with hemiplegia, unilateral limb ataxia, gait ataxia, paraplegia, hemisensory syndromes, gaze disorders, and occasionally hiccups.

The midbrain, juxtaposed between the pons and the cerebral hemispheres, encompasses the tectum, the cerebral peduncles, and the cerebral aqueduct. Tectal involvement causes Parinaud syndrome, peduncular lesions cause contralateral motor impairment, and obstruction of the aqueduct causes hydrocephalus.

Tumors in the medulla can have a fulminant course, including dysphagia, dysarthria, and deficits in cranial nerves IX, X, and XII. Involvement of the medullary cardiac and respiratory centers can result in a rapidly fatal course. Fourth ventricular tumors, because of their location, cause symptomatic obstructive hydrocephalus at a relatively small size, with associated disturbances of gait and balance. Rapidly enlarging lesions may end in cerebellar herniation.

Cerebellar tumors have variable localizing presentations. Midline lesions in and around the vermis cause truncal and gait ataxia, whereas more lateral hemispheric lesions lead to unilateral appendicular ataxia, usually worst in the arm. Abnormal head position, with the head tilting back and away from the side of the tumor, is seen often in children but rarely in adults. Bilateral sixth cranial nerve palsies are uncommon and reflect hydrocephalus.

Mass lesions within or abutting the brain or spinal cord can cause displacement of vital neurologic structures. This can lead, in the brain, to herniation syndromes with respiratory arrest and death and, in the spine, to paraplegia or quadriplegia. Subfalcine herniation, usually from a unilateral frontal tumor, is often asymptomatic. In transtentorial (temporal lobe) herniation, the medial temporal lobe shifts into the tentorial notch, compressing cranial nerve III and the ipsilateral cerebral peduncle, resulting in pupillary dilation and lack of response to light. Coma usually follows. In tonsillar herniation, increasing posterior fossa mass effect displaces one or both cerebellar tonsils into the foramen magnum, causing posturing, coma, and respiratory arrest. Both tonsillar and transtentorial herniation are rapidly fatal without prompt intervention.

Hemorrhage into a tumor can also cause acute neurologic deterioration. This is often associated with iatrogenic coagulopathies such as thrombocytopenia due to chemotherapy or anticoagulation therapy for deep venous thrombosis. Primary tumors that most often bleed *de novo* are glioblastoma and oligodendrogliomas; of the metastatic tumors, lung cancer, melanoma, renal cell cancer, thyroid cancer, and choriocarcinoma most often show hemorrhage.

Lumbar puncture should not be performed in any of the acute herniation syndromes or when herniation is imminent. In fact, lumbar puncture should be avoided in the setting of significantly elevated ICP associated with a brain tumor.

Spinal Axis Tumors

For the clinical presentation of tumors of the spinal axis to be understood, the local anatomy must be appreciated (Fig. 121.2). Intracranially, the dura is adherent to the skull, and there is normally no extradural space. In the spinal canal, the extradural space contains fat and blood vessels. Through the intervertebral foramina, the extradural space communicates with the mediastinum and the retroperitoneum. Nearly all extradural tumors are metastases or locally invasive non-CNS neoplasms (e.g., carcinomas, sarcomas), with direct extension from adjacent vertebral bodies or through the foramina.

TABLE 121.4

CLINICAL MANIFESTATIONS OF SPINAL CORD TUMORS

Location	Findings
Foramen magnum	11th and 12th cranial nerve palsies; ipsilateral arm weakness early; cerebellar ataxia; neck pain
Cervical	Ipsilateral arm weakness with leg and opposite arm in time; wasting and fibrillation of ipsilateral neck, shoulder girdle, and arm; decreased pain and temperature sensation in upper cervical regions early; pain in cervical distribution
Thoracic	Weakness of abdominal muscles; sparing of arms; unilateral root pains; sensory level with ipsilateral changes early and bilateral with time
Lumbosacral	Root pain in groin region or sciatic distribution, or both; weakened proximal pelvic muscles; impotence; bladder paralysis; decreased knee jerk, and brisk ankle jerks
Cauda equina	Unilateral pain in back and leg becoming bilateral when the tumor is quite large; bladder and bowel paralysis

Intradural spinal tumors arise from the spinal cord (intramedullary) or from surrounding structures (extramedullary). The two common extramedullary intradural tumors, schwannoma and meningioma, arise from nerve roots and from the dura, respectively. A spinal tumor can produce local (focal) and distal (remote) symptoms, or both. Local effects indicate the tumor's location along the spinal axis, and distal effects reflect involvement of motor and sensory long tracts within the cord. Table 121.4 summarizes the clinical findings useful in localizing a spinal cord tumor.

Distal symptoms and signs are confined to structures innervated below the level of the tumor. Neurologic manifestations often begin unilaterally, with weakness and spasticity, if the tumor lies above the conus medullaris, or weakness and flaccidity if the tumor is at or below the conus. Impairment of sphincter and sexual function occurs later unless the tumor is in the conus. The upper level of impaired long-tract function usually is several segments below the tumor's actual site. Local manifestations may reflect involvement of bone (with axial

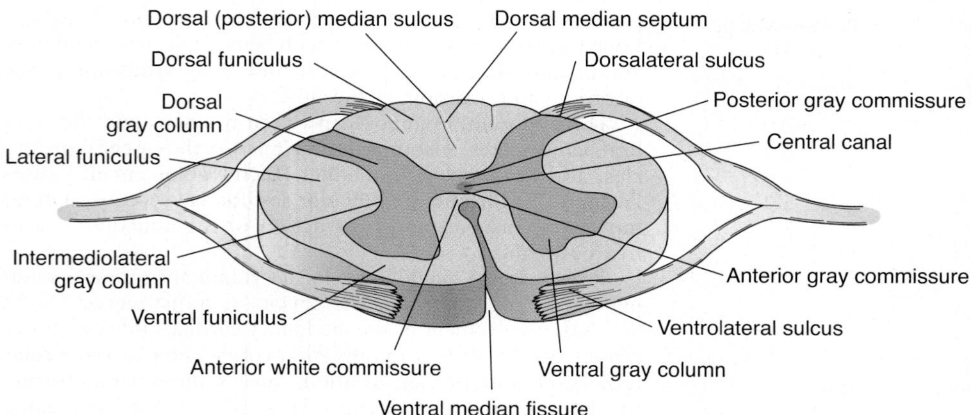

FIGURE 121.2 Cross-section of thoracic spinal cord shows relation of spinal nerves to intraspinal tracts.

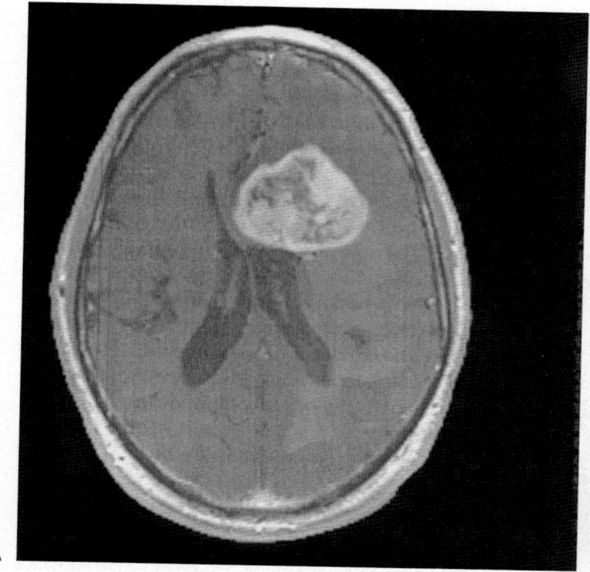

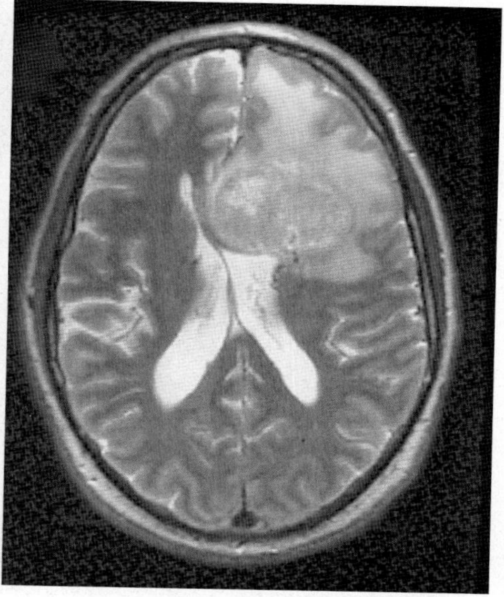

FIGURE 121.3 Magnetic resonance imaging of a patient with a malignant glioma demonstrates a large mass with heterogenous enhancement (**A**) and significant edema (**B**) on the T2-weighted sequences.

pain) or spinal roots, with radicular pain and loss of motor and sensory functions of the root or roots.

NEURODIAGNOSTIC TESTS

Magnetic Resonance Imaging

The imaging modality of choice for most CNS tumors is MRI, which can demonstrate anatomy and pathologic processes in detail.[36] Computed tomography (CT) is generally reserved for those unable (implanted pacemaker, metal fragment, paramagnetic surgical clips) or unwilling (because of claustrophobia) to undergo MRI. Because of the link of nephrogenic systemic fibrosis to the infusion of gadolinium-based contrast agents, there are new preventative guidelines regarding the administration of gadolinium in patients who may be at high risk.[37]

The most useful imaging studies are T1-weighted sagittal images, gadolinium (Gd)-enhanced and unenhanced T1 axial images, and T2-weighted axial images (Fig. 121.3). Contrast-enhanced MRI provides an improved ability to discern tumors from other pathologic entities, one tumor type from another, and putatively higher- from lower-grade malignancies. There are, however, limitations in anatomic MRI to definitively diagnose a mass lesion as a tumor. Other confounding diagnoses include bacterial abscess, tumor refractive demyelination, and acute ischemic disease. It is conventionally believed that most low-grade gliomas (except pilocytic astrocytomas and pleomorphic xanthoastrocytoma) do not enhance, but in reviewing imaging studies of patients enrolled in several clinical trials, it is apparent that this may not be so categorical, in that even low-grade gliomas may frequently contain areas of enhancement, raising the concern that these areas might represent high-grade or malignant transformation (Fig. 121.4).[38]

Neuraxis or Spinal Imaging

In the evaluation of spinal cord tumors, MRI is also the preferred modality, providing superb visualization of the spinal cord contour and (with gadolinium contrast) of most intrinsic tumors (such as ependymomas, astrocytomas, meningiomas, and schwannomas), as well as facilitating the diagnosis of leptomeningeal dissemination. Tumor cysts are readily identified on MRI, and spinal cord tumors can often be distinguished from syringomyelia. Ideally, neuraxis imaging should be performed before surgery. In the immediate postoperative period, spinal MRI scans may be difficult to interpret because arachnoiditis and blood products can mimic leptomeningeal metastasis. Delayed spinal MRI (more than 3 weeks after surgery) combined with an increased dose of gadolinium is a sensitive imaging study for leptomeningeal disease.

Newer Imaging Modalities

Newer MRI techniques include magnetic resonance spectroscopy, dynamic contrast-enhanced MRI, diffusion-perfusion MRI, and functional MRI. In addition, metabolic imaging using positron emission tomography using various tracers is being explored.[38,39] These newer techniques remain to be validated as biomarkers of biological behavior or clinical outcome. Posttreatment metabolic scans may help distinguish recurrence from treatment-related changes, although most modalities have a relatively high false-negative rate. A modification of the standard MRI is quick brain MRI, which uses single-shot fast-spin echo imaging to allow adequate demonstration of ventricular anatomy and appropriate evaluation of shunt function.[40]

Pseudoresponse and Pseudoprogression

In malignant gliomas treated with combined modality therapy, it is speculated that 25% to 40% or even more may experience imaging changes relatively early in the course of therapy, usually within a few months, which appears consistent with radiographic progression. However, with time, and without any therapy, many of these changes actually improve or even resolve, and in patients operated on with a presumptive diagnosis of tumor, the histopathology often reveals large areas of tumor necrosis.[41,42] With the advent of antiangiogenic therapies for malignant glioma, rapid resolution of tumor enhancement is visualized on MRI, sometimes, within days. This is consistent with the traditional definition of response, but in several

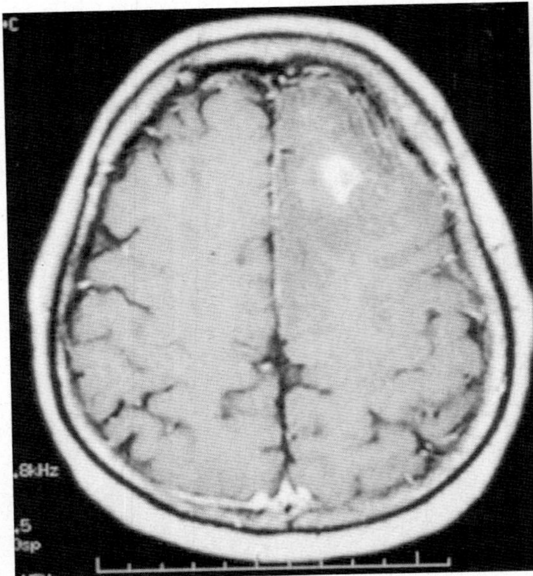

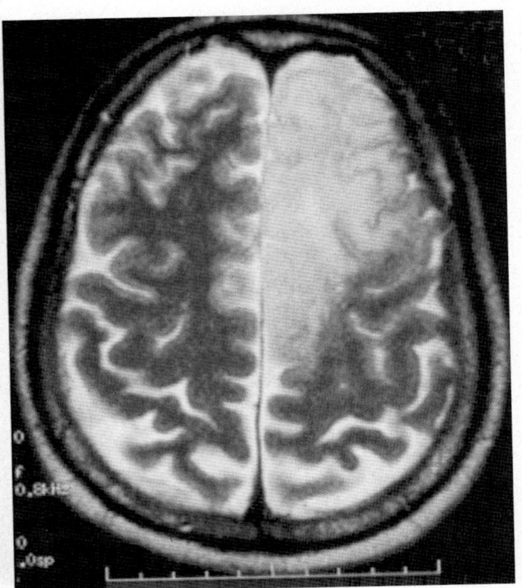

FIGURE 121.4 **A:** Low-grade astrocytomas often do not enhance and contrast-enhanced T1-weighted magnetic resonance sequences considerably underestimate the true infiltrative extent of these neoplasms. **B:** The fluid-attenuated inversion recovery (FLAIR) sequence is considerably more useful in appreciating the true extent of such neoplasms.

instances, especially with time, even in the absence of contrast enhancement, tumor progression and clinical deterioration occurs, which is sometimes appreciated as T2 or fluid-attenuated inversion recovery (FLAIR) changes; this phenomenon is labeled as *pseudoresponse*.[42]

Cerebrospinal Fluid Examination

Typically, medulloblastoma, ependymoma, choroid plexus carcinoma, lymphoma, and some embryonal pineal and suprasellar region tumors have a high enough likelihood of spreading to justify CSF examinations to look for malignant cells (cytology) and specific markers, such as human chorionic gonadotropin-β and α-fetoprotein.

CSF spread of tumor may be associated with several possible findings, including CSF pressure above 150 mm H_2O at the lumbar level in a laterally positioned patient, elevated protein, typically greater than 40 mg/dL, reduced glucose (below 50 mg/mL), and tumor cells by cytologic examination. A high protein concentration with normal glucose levels and normal cytology is also seen with base of skull tumors, such as vestibular schwannoma, and with spinal cord tumors that obstruct the subarachnoid space and produce stasis of the CSF in the caudal lumbar sac. Sampling of the CSF in the immediate postoperative period may lead to false-positive results, however, and is best done before surgery or more than 3 weeks after surgery, as long as there is no uncontrolled raised intracranial pressure.

SURGERY

Preoperative Considerations

The major objectives of surgery are to maximally remove bulk tumor, reduce tumor-associated mass effect and elevated ICP, and provide tissue for pathologic analysis in a manner that minimizes risk to neurological functioning. For some tumors complete resection can be curative. However, most brain tumors are diffusely infiltrative; for these, surgical cure is rarely possible. Surgery can rapidly reduce tumor bulk with potential benefits in terms of mass effect, edema, and hydrocephalus. The requirement for histopathologic confirmation of diagnosis is not necessary in certain well-defined situations, but a tissue diagnosis is still required to determine the appropriate treatment course in most circumstances. As molecularly targeted therapies become useful, tissue removal for molecular analysis will become more necessary to guide therapy. Pseudoprogression may make tissue-based confirmation necessary before changes in therapy are instituted.[43] Technologic advances in surgical approaches, techniques, and instrumentation have rendered most tumors amenable to resection; however, for some tumor types or locations, the risk of open operation supports the choice of biopsy for obtaining diagnostic tissue. Biopsy techniques include stereotactic biopsy (with or without a stereotactic frame) using CT, MRI, or both, to choose the target. Metabolic or spectroscopic imaging can be coregistered with anatomic images to choose targets that may be of higher biologic aggressiveness within a tumor that appears homogeneous on standard imaging. In certain settings, an approach using simple ultrasonic guidance can also be considered for obtaining diagnostic tissue.

Unless lymphoma is being considered, patients are given corticosteroids, usually dexamethasone, immediately preoperatively and often for several days before surgery to reduce cerebral edema and thus minimize secondary brain injury from cerebral retraction. Steroid administration is then continued in the immediate postoperative period and tapered off as quickly as possible. Antibiotics are given just before making the incision to decrease the risk of wound infection.

Anesthesia and Positioning

The routine use of prophylactic anticonvulsants in the perioperative period is less commonly recommended, although practice patterns seem to indicate their widespread use.[44,45] Patients with a history of seizures need to have their anticonvulsants maintained at therapeutic dose levels. Under certain circumstances, such as for awake craniotomies with electrocorticography, the use of anticonvulsants for a short time might be warranted.

Either general endotracheal anesthesia or local anesthesia with sedation can be used for craniotomies. Specific techniques to reduce patient discomfort during surgery are required when local anesthesia is used. Most craniotomies today are performed under general anesthesia. Inhalational agents, such as isoflurane, may be used, but total intravenous anesthesia, with agents such as propofol and dexmedetomidine, is becoming a more widespread practice as there may be a lower risk of producing fluctuations in cardiac function and ICP.

Ordinarily, cranial fixation is used to minimize patient movement during surgery, although rigid fixation may be less desirable during awake procedures. Steps are taken during the procedure to minimize ICP. The patient's head is placed slightly above the level of the heart to increase venous drainage, and jugular vein compression is avoided. Mild hyperventilation is used. These measures, along with the use of image-guided minimal access craniotomies, are generally sufficient to avoid the routine use of mannitol and furosemide. However, should ICP remain elevated, mannitol (between 0.25 and 1.0 g/kg of body weight) can be administered and may be followed by furosemide to potentiate its action.

General Surgical Principles

In the past, localization of the surgical incision and craniotomy were most often performed by a surgeon's understanding of cranial anatomy and interpretation of preoperative imaging. More recently, image-guided navigation systems have been employed to more effectively localize tumor margins, as they project to the cranial surface and thus allow for smaller, precisely positioned craniotomies.[46,47] Once the dura has been opened, the tumor should once again be localized and most tumors are approached through an incision in the crest of an overlying gyrus or through a sulcus. The selection of the cortical entry site is aided by cortical mapping when appropriate, intraoperative ultrasonographic images, and the frameless image-guided stereotactic system, or with intraoperative MRI. If the tumor presents to the surface, its surface margins should be identified and dissection should begin at the margins. If the tumor does not present on the surface, often a fissure or sulcus may be split to gain access to it, reducing the distance through which the brain must be dissected. If this is not possible or desirable, the pia-arachnoid may be coagulated and incised and a transcortical route taken to the tumor. The operating microscope may be used for the approach through the subcortical white matter to the tumor, although use of surgical loupe magnifiers is commonly used for tumors that do not involve vascular structures or are not adjacent to the brainstem. The glistening peritumoral white matter is seen easily through the microscope as each of the tumor's margins is reached, and at this interface the resection is stopped. Hemostasis is sometimes difficult to achieve but must be perfect. Hemispheric tumor cysts can be drained and, when possible, fenestrated into an adjacent ventricle to prevent reaccumulation. For tumors not resectable because of their location or diffuseness, biopsy can be performed stereotactically using frameless or frame-based technique. Tumors that are limited to the cortical surface may be best sampled with an open biopsy, under direct vision, due to the risk of inadvertent injury to a cortical vessel with a more limited, needle-based approach.

Specialized technology can be used to help define the completeness of resection. Image-guided navigation systems are almost always employed, but the guidance may lose accuracy over the course of an operation due to brain shift or cyst decompression. Intraoperative imaging with ultrasound, CT, or MRI may be used to determine the extent of residual tumor and to further localize areas where additional tumor may be removed safely.[48] There has been growing use of 5-aminoleuvilinic acid (5-ALA), a prodrug which is converted by glioma cells into fluorescent porphyrins that can be visualized with an operating microscope equipped with a fluorescent imaging package. The impact of the use of 5-ALA to guide resection of glioblastoma multiforme (GBM) on completeness of surgical resection and progression-free survival has been demonstrated in a phase 3 trial.[49] Its use is limited to tumors that enhance with contrast on MRI (or CT), as low-grade tumors do not appear to convert the prodrug to a fluorescent porphyrin that can be visualized intraoperatively.

Intraoperative cortical-stimulation mapping facilitates resection of tumors in or adjacent to functionally critical areas. Motor functions can be mapped even under general anesthesia; however, anesthetic agents may increase the threshold to response and hence decrease the sensitivity of mapping. Sensory and speech-associated cortex are typically mapped during an awake craniotomy. Often preoperative mapping of functional areas and their connections with MRI-based techniques are used to delineate both cortical areas and important subcortical white matter tracts that subserve speech and motor function.[50]

Reresection of recurrent cerebral astrocytomas can be modestly efficacious.[51] When the initial tumor was low grade, histologic resampling may be necessary to guide further treatment at recurrence. Reoperation offers a chance to implant polymer wafers containing carmustine (BCNU) or to administer experimental agents, such as gene therapy agents or immunotoxins. Smaller volume of disease at initiation of chemotherapy predicts longer survival, thus, reoperation may improve the efficacy of adjuvant treatment as well as relieve mass effect in some patients.[52] An increasingly important aspect of resection is the need for tumor sampling to allow molecular marker analysis, which might provide and aid in assessing of prognosis as well as probability of benefit from both chemotherapeutic and targeted therapies.

Craniotomy for Supratentorial Tumors

The bony opening is designed to be generous enough to facilitate surgery but small enough to avoid possible injury to the surrounding normal brain, particularly if the brain is under pressure, and there is risk of intraoperative herniation into the cranial opening. A frameless stereotactic neuronavigation system is commonly used to design the craniotomy flap, to localize subcortical tumors, and to estimate progress during tumor resection. For this, a preoperative MRI or CT is done with fiducials on the scalp, which are used along with a reference array to register the patient's head and thereby map the images onto the operative area as localized by a handheld probe. The craniotomy is centered over the tumor or positioned to give access to the route of approach. The scalp flap is designed to surround the bone flap fully; the scalp's vascular supply is given careful consideration in the design. After the scalp incision is made and periosteum cleared, burr holes are drilled and connected with an air-powered saw or craniotome. The bone flap can then be removed. The dura is opened and reflected, and the approach to the tumor is made. A peripherally located lesion may be immediately seen. However, when the lesion is subcortical, the exposed field may appear normal. If critical functional cortex is in the field, motor and speech can be mapped intraoperatively using electrical cortical stimulation or somatosensory evoked potential techniques.[53] A preoperative functional MRI scan or magnetoencephalography can serve as a guide. Motor mapping can be done under general anesthesia if muscle relaxants are avoided; however, many anesthetic agents can raise the threshold to electrical response and some surgeons favor awake mapping or monitoring of function. Glioma resections in the dominant hemisphere are often done under local anesthesia to allow speech mapping.

Localization of subcortical tumors can often be accomplished using intraoperative ultrasonography, as well as with frameless image-guided neuronavigation systems.[54] Because preoperative images are used, brain shift that occurs during the operation can cause discrepancy. Intraoperative imaging with ultrasonography, CT, and MRI can now be used to provide an immediate estimate of the progress of the resection and can be used to update the navigation system. Although neuronavigation systems do increase the degree of resection achieved, the impact on patient outcome has not yet been clarified. For contrast-enhancing tumors, there is growing use of 5-ALA and a suitably equipped fluorescent operating microscope.[49] When technically possible, it is preferable to perform a circumferential dissection of the tumor.

Patients are monitored in the specialized care unit overnight after surgery, and an MRI is done within 24 to 48 hours to evaluate the extent of any remaining tumor.

Craniotomy for Posterior Fossa Tumors

Patients may be positioned prone, three-quarters prone, or lateral, depending on lesion location, surgeon preference, and patient body habitus. A linear incision is used for a midline approach, and a paramedian or retromastoid linear incision is used for more laterally located lesions. Bony removal is often performed with a high speed drill, rather than as a bone flap. With larger and more caudal lesions, it is common to open the foramen magnum and even to remove the arch of C1 to allow room for postoperative brain swelling, which otherwise can cause tonsillar herniation through the foramen magnum. A low exposure allows drainage of CSF from the cisterna magna to relax the brain. After resection, the dura is tightly closed. A dural patch is often used, but some dural substitutes may suffice. Some surgeons also replace a craniectomy defect with a methylmethacrylate cranioplasty or with titanium mesh.

Stereotactic Tumor Biopsy

For deeply situated intrinsic tumors, multicentric tumors, or diffuse nonfocal tumors, resection is not practical and stereotactic needle biopsy is used for diagnosis. Open, stereotactically guided biopsy is reserved for unusual situations, such as a lesion abutting a large blood vessel or one that is restricted to the cortical surface.

Many image-guided stereotactic systems are available and frame-based or frameless techniques may be used.[55,56] Typically, the patient undergoes a CT or an MRI with either a rigid array of fiducial bars fixed tightly to the skull to minimize movement or skull-implanted or scalp-applied surface fiducials in the case of frameless stereotaxy. For cooperative adults, local anesthesia may be used; for children, general anesthesia is usually required. The images are loaded into a navigation system that can be used preoperatively to plan an entry point and target combination, which will provide a safe trajectory with the opportunity to sample multiple parts of a lesion along a single path. After the entry point is localized, a scalp incision is made and either a burr hole or a stereotactically guided twist drill craniostomy is made. The dura is perforated and the stereotactic biopsy needle is advanced to the target. A small tissue core is obtained from the target using a side-biting needle. Hemorrhage at the biopsy site, the principal risk of the surgery, occurs in few patients and a CT may be performed to evaluate for the presence of blood. Occasionally, cerebral edema is exacerbated by biopsy.

RADIATION THERAPY

General Concepts

Radiation therapy plays an integral role in the treatment of most malignant and many benign primary CNS tumors. It is often employed postoperatively as adjuvant treatment to decrease local failure, to delay recurrence, and to prolong survival in gliomas, as definitive treatment in more radiosensitive diseases such as PNET and germ cell tumors, or as therapy to halt further tumor growth in schwannomas, meningiomas, pituitary tumors, and craniopharyngiomas, and as ablative therapy to abrogate hormonal overproduction in secretory pituitary adenomas. Radiation therapy is also the primary modality in palliating brain metastases.

Radiobiologic and Toxicity Considerations

Most neoplasms can potentially be cured if the correct radiation dose can be delivered to the entire tumor and its microscopic extensions. This is not always feasible as the maximum radiation dose deliverable is limited by the tolerance of the surrounding normal tissues, and the identification of regions of microscopic extension remains vague. Radiation tolerance of the CNS depends on several factors, including total dose, fraction size, volume irradiated, underlying comorbidities (particularly hypertension and diabetes), and innate sensitivity. Adverse reactions to cranial irradiation differ in pathogenesis and temporal presentation and are not discussed here.

A major radiobiologic consideration revolves around the selection of total dose and the fractionation schedule. Late or long-term toxicities are generally a function of fraction size, and therefore, as the fraction size is increased, such as with radiosurgery, higher late toxicity rates must be anticipated. These late toxicities from larger fraction sizes can be minimized by sharply targeting the dose, which can drastically reduce dose to normal tissues, and by minimizing the volume irradiated, which explains the limited size of tumors treated with radiosurgery. In conventional radiotherapy, fraction sizes of 2 Gy are routinely utilized and may be lowered to 1.8 Gy per fraction in proximity to the visual apparatus or may be increased to 3 Gy per fraction in patients in whom shorter palliative schedules, with lesser concern regarding long-term morbidities, exist. For radiosurgery, doses in the order of 12 to 21 Gy in single fractions are often utilized. In general, the entire target is treated with a relatively uniform dose, but with the advent of newer delivery methods, it is possible to create dose gradients or dose inhomogeneities within the tumor to match the differential radiosensitivity, but this concept of dose painting remains investigational.

Treatment Planning and Delivery Methods

High-resolution MR fusion with CT planning images has allowed more precise delineation of targets, although a significant margin, particularly with gliomas, is still necessary to cover microscopic extension.[57] Patient immobilization devices limit intrafraction motion and provide precision in positioning, decreasing the margin required for setup variability. Image-guided radiotherapy (IGRT), using biplanar orthogonal x-ray imaging systems, cone beam CT, or megavoltage CT, further improves setup reproducibility and allows decreased margins. For the cranium, IGRT localization approaches utilize either external fiducials, such as those mounted on a bite-block system, with in-room monitoring cameras, or imaging, which principally relies on comparing baseline bony anatomy to the anatomy visualized on the images obtained for each treatment fraction. IGRT therefore offers the opportunity to precisely and accurately set the patient up with millimeteric precision (less than 1 to 3 mm) prior to daily treatment, and several systems also allow for continuous monitoring while the patient is being treated. Newer systems in development incorporate MRI on-board.

The primary benefit of incorporating IGRT into treatment delivery is that by improving daily patient setup, it allows a decrease in the margin of delivery error, effectively reducing the total volume irradiated. IGRT can be incorporated with any radiotherapy method, such as fractionated external-beam radiotherapy and stereotactic radiosurgery (SRS), and is practically mandatory for charged-particle therapy, frameless radiosurgery, fractionated stereotactic radiotherapy (FSRT), and intensity-modulated radiotherapy (IMRT). CT-based three-dimensional conformal radiation (3DCRT) in which noncoplanar fields with unique entrance and exit pathways can be mapped on the target has improved normal tissue sparing. This allows avoidance of critical structures, such as the brainstem, optic apparatus, and spinal cord. In IMRT, the photon flux of a beam is modulated in multiple directions during treatment, aimed at mimicking the shape of the target from various viewpoints, thereby producing improved conformality and nonuniform dose distribution. IMRT is increasingly being utilized for CNS tumors, based primarily on dosimetric studies, which suggest superior tumor coverage and reduction in the dose to critical structures (Fig. 121.5).[58] This can be beneficial in specific instances, such as to preserve cochlear function, vision, or pituitary activity. Huang et al.[59] were able to show a reduction in cochlear dose from 54.2 to 36.7 Gy and a reduction of grade 3 or 4 hearing loss from 64% to 13% with the use of IMRT compared to conventional radiation therapy.

In FSRT, the concepts of 3DCRT or IMRT are merged with the accuracy and precision in delivery that characterizes SRS, and, typically, the radiation fraction size is considerably increased, so that the total course of therapy is reduced from the typical 20 to 30 or more fractions to five or fewer fractions. Various FSRT systems have been developed, with reported precision between 1 to 3 mm.[60,61] FSRT is often used for larger lesions (e.g., 4 cm or more) and for lesions located in critical regions where single fraction SRS is disadvantageous because of a higher risk of toxicity, such as larger vestibular schwannomas or meningiomas.

SRS is used to treat a diverse group of lesions. Stereotactic treatments generally reference the target lesion to a reproducible Cartesian coordinate system outside the patient, although frameless systems may utilize fiducials directly on the patient or the bony anatomy itself as a surrogate. The coordinate system is generally affixed to the patient, most commonly in the

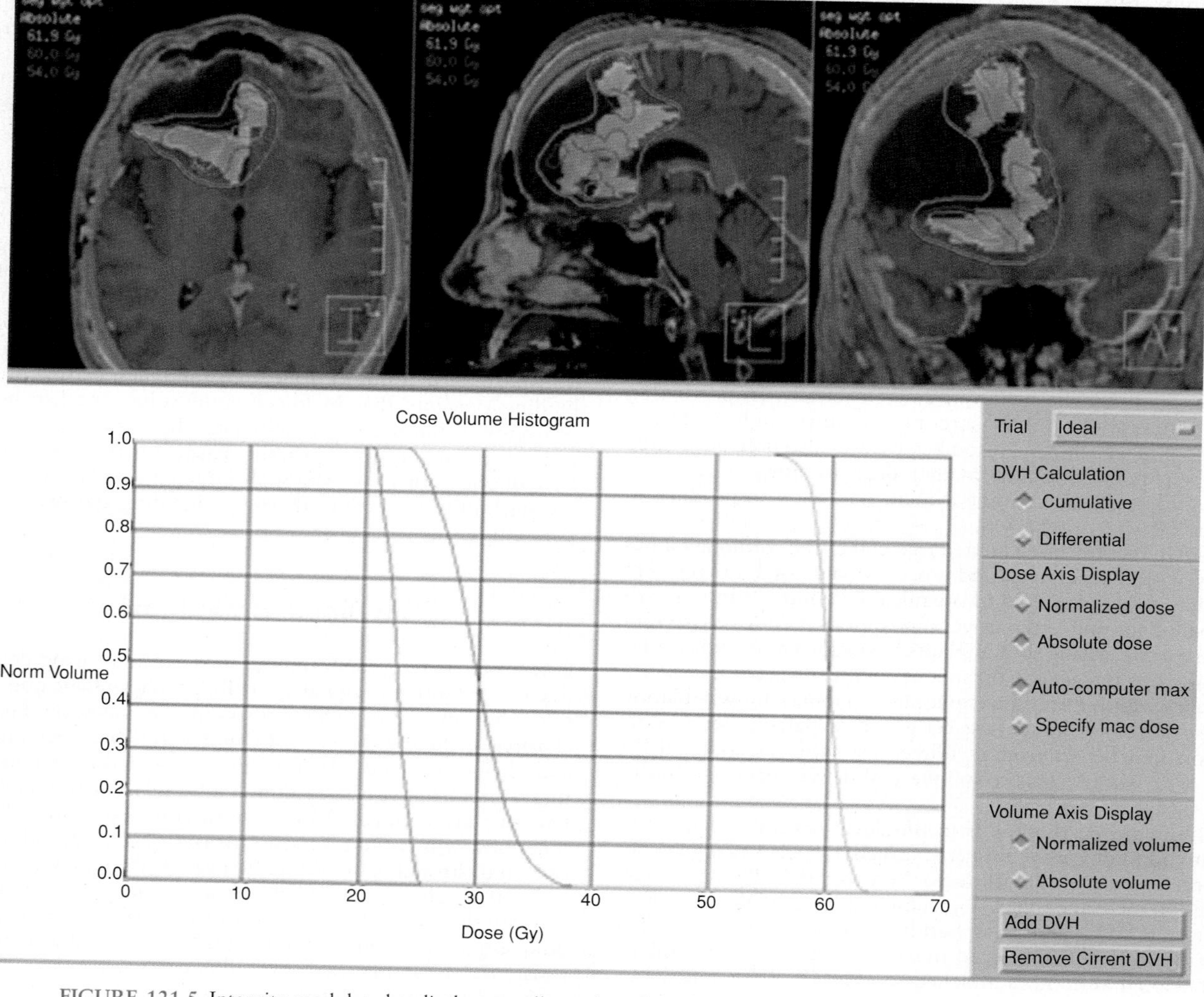

FIGURE 121.5 Intensity-modulated radiotherapy allows dose shaping to avoid critical structures. In this treatment plan of a right frontal oligodendroglioma (*orange*), tight target coverage and excellent conformal avoidance of the optic chiasm (*red*) and pituitary (*purple*) are achieved, as evidenced by the dose-volume histogram (DVH).

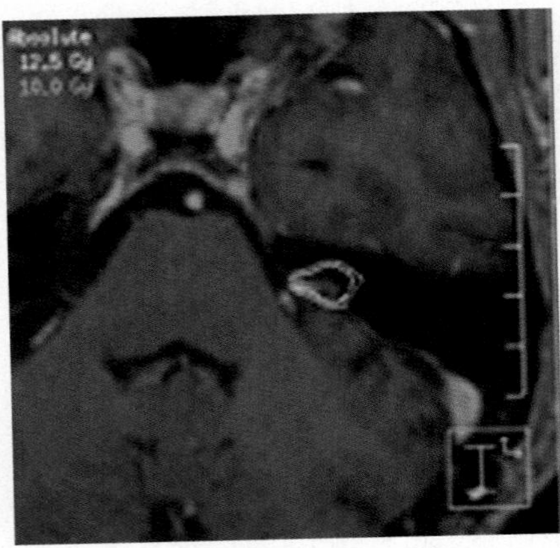

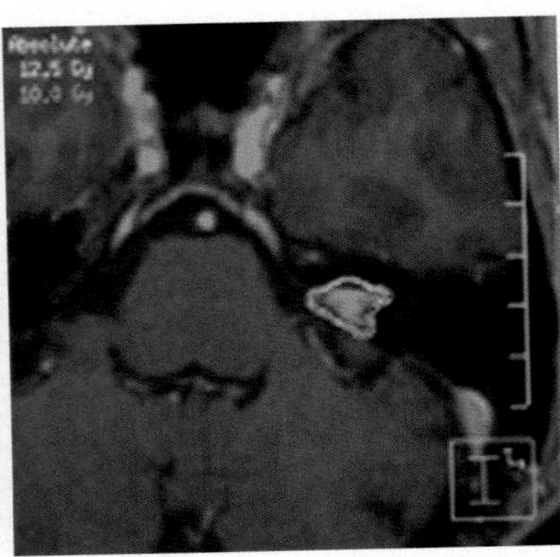

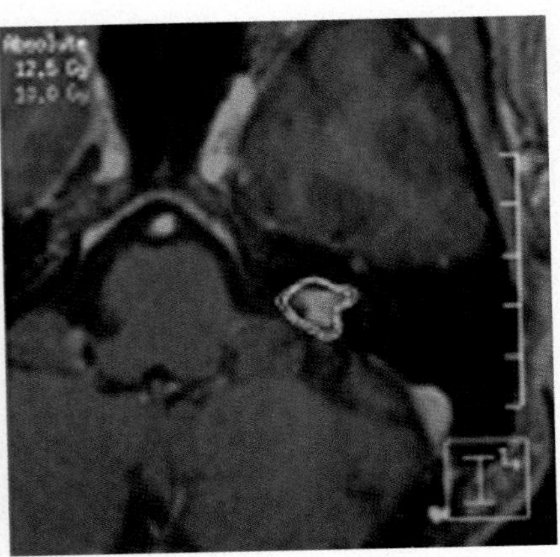

FIGURE 121.6 Example of radiosurgery dose distribution. This schwannoma is being treated with radiosurgery; the 12.5-Gy prescription isodose line very conformally covers the lesion.

form of a head frame. Treatment can be carried out using either a modified or dedicated linear accelerator, cobalt-60 units, or charged particle devices. Several commercial devices have now been developed, each with slightly unique features, including robots that position the linear accelerator at various angles, collimation systems that provide prefixed circular collimators of various sizes, or shaped collimated beams, and even intensity modulated delivery from one or multiple directions, delivered serially, helically, or volumetrically.[62] Radiosurgery plays a dominant role in the treatment of oligometastases to the brain, arteriovenous malformations, schwannomas, and meningiomas and is occasionally used to treat malignant recurrences (Fig. 121.6).

Charged-particle beams deposit the majority of their dose at a depth dependent on the initial energy, avoiding the exit dose of photon therapy. This localized dose is known as the *Bragg peak*. Although pencil-scanning proton beams have narrow Bragg peaks, in order to cover larger volumes, proton beams have traditionally been modified by passive range modulators that disperse the Bragg peak and broaden the dose deposition. Charged-particle radiotherapy has been particularly utilized to treat tumors of the skull base to doses higher than can be achieved conventionally. In particular, chordomas and chondrosarcomas require high radiation doses for local control. Proton beams have also been advocated for the childhood tumors as they decrease integral radiation dose, although concern about incidental neutron production exists.[63,64]

Brachytherapy has a limited role in the CNS, although it has enjoyed some resurgence and is occasionally used for recurrent gliomas. A liquid colloid of organically bound ^{125}I in a spherical balloon is one of the newer innovations.[65] At least two randomized trials using seed implants have failed to demonstrate a survival advantage in malignant glioma. The injection of radioisotopes within the cystic craniopharyngiomas allows ablation of the secretory lining. A select group of patients with cystic tumors may benefit from the direct instillation of colloidal ^{32}P, ^{90}Y, or ^{198}Au.[66,67] This technique will deliver between 200 to 400 Gy to the cyst wall.

Radiolabeled therapy is in the developmental phase. The most commonly used antigenic targets for CNS malignancies are the epidermal growth factor receptor (EGFR), neural cell adhesion molecule (NCAM), tenascin, placental alkaline phosphatase (PLAP), and phosphatidylinositide. Institutions using this technique have utilized murine, chimeric, or humanized monoclonal antibodies attached to ^{131}I, ^{90}Y, ^{188}Re, and ^{211}At. The evolution of the trials has seen the delivery route move from systemic (intra-arterial or intravenous) to local instillation of the agent into a surgically created resection cavity. Even though the blood–brain barrier is often disrupted by a rapidly growing CNS malignancy, 150 kDa antibodies would still not likely cross to a significant degree.[68] Most of the trials to date are of "dose searching pilot" or phase 1 design. Using ^{131}I-81C6 (antitenascin monoclonal antibody), a trend toward significant improvement in median survival was shown for patients receiving 40 to 48 Gy versus less than 40 Gy.[69] Unlike brachytherapy, there appears to be a very low rate of CNS toxicity and a minimal need for surgical intervention for removal of necrotic regions.

CHEMOTHERAPY AND TARGETED AGENTS

Drug therapies alone are effective for only a few types of CNS tumors (i.e., primary CNS lymphoma) but are useful as adjunctive therapy for many CNS tumors. Among the reasons for the poor efficacy of chemotherapeutic and targeted agents is the low concentration of drug penetration to the tumor because of the difficulty of agents to cross the blood–brain barrier, active transport mechanisms of drug efflux, and high plasma protein binding of agents, thereby lowering the volume of distribution of agents in the brain parenchyma.[70] Intrinsic and acquired resistance remains an important reason for the lowered efficacy of chemotherapy. Although targeted agents are in early testing, multiplicity and alternate signaling pathways limit their efficacy.

The Blood–Brain Barrier

Central to treating CNS tumors is the issue of drug delivery, due to the blood–brain barrier (BBB), a physiologic and functional barrier.[71] The CNS microvasculature has several unique features, including the lack of fenestrations between adjacent endothelial cells and relatively fewer pinocytotic and endocytotic endothelial vesicles. Additionally, adjacent BBB endothelial cells are connected by a continuous extension of tight junctions, which limit passive diffusion between endothelial cells and through capillary structures. Tight junctions within the BBB are also enveloped by astrocytic foot processes, which increase the barrier to passive diffusion across the BBB. These unique tight junctions result in a high transendothelial electric resistance and diminished paracellular resistance.[72]

Brain microvasculature selectively transports nutrients through 20 or more active or facilitated carrier transport systems expressed on the endothelial surface.[73] The endothelium is also rich with efflux pumps, including the multidrug resistance (MDR) gene-encoded P-glycoprotein. These and other efflux pumps actively remove substrate molecules that may have passed the BBB.[74] The hydraulic conductivity of brain capillaries, and thus the oncotic pressure driving protein influx across endothelium, is 500, 1,000, and 3,000 times less than in heart, muscle, and intestinal capillaries, respectively.

The coadministration of chemotherapeutic agents with inhibitors of efflux transporters has been performed to increase the BBB permeability of anticancer agents, but to date, the results have largely been disappointing.[75]

The Blood–Tumor Barrier

The microvascular differences between the blood–tumor barrier (BTB) and the normal BBB range from a subtle increase in endothelial fenestrations to a dramatic breakdown of tight junctions, enlargement of the perivascular space, and swelling of the basal lamina.[76] Different tumors display different degrees of disruption of the BTB. Most low-grade gliomas do not enhance with contrast and have BTBs that are similar to the normal BBB. In contrast, highly malignant tumors such as glioblastoma have significant disruption of most barrier functions within the avidly contrast-enhancing portion of the tumor. Even in these tumors, however, drug delivery is not normal because the tumor-induced neovasculature is often poorly perfused or not patent, and there is a relatively long distance between tumor-induced angiogenic vessels and individual tumor cells. Furthermore, even in these highly malignant and angiogenic tumors, the leading front of infiltrating tumor cells is located in normal brain parenchyma with a relatively intact BBB. Several strategies are being explored to improve delivery of anticancer drugs to brain tumors and range from disruption of the BBB to noninvasive or direct delivery of agents into the brain.[77]

Disrupting the Blood–Brain Barrier

Physicochemical characteristics largely determine a drug's ability to cross the BBB. Smaller, ionically neutral, lipophilic drugs, with a high octanol or water coefficient, are more likely to penetrate the BBB and BTB.[78] Unfortunately, most drugs lack these characteristics and are excluded by the barrier. This has led to the development of alternate drug administration techniques. The most widely used method for disrupting the BBB is through an intravascular osmotic load using mannitol, which results in cerebral endothelial shrinkage and disruption of endothelial tight junctions.[79] More refined attempts to disrupt the BBB have focused on specific drugs that selectively target cerebral endothelial cellular signaling pathways, such as the bradykinin pathway, and result in transient BBB disruption.[80] Unfortunately, clinical studies have not demonstrated convincing improvements in patient outcome.

Another strategy to enhance drug delivery to brain tumors while minimizing systemic exposure is intra-arterial administration. After the first pass of the drug through the brain, it becomes diluted into the total-body blood volume. Most clinical experience suggests slightly higher response rates at the expense of significant neurotoxicity.[81] Another drawback of selective arterial drug delivery is that tumors often obtain their vascular supply from multiple arteries. Finally, intra-arterial drug delivery has been associated with significant morbidity, including strokes from arterial dissection and embolism. Thus, there is currently limited enthusiasm for this strategy, with the potential exception of primary CNS lymphomas.

Noninvasive delivery systems using specialized carriers with favorable pharmacokinetic and pharmacodynamic properties are being explored. Use of nanosystems (colloidal carriers) focus on liposomes and polymeric nanoparticles, which allow for sustained, gradual release of drug.[82] Conventional liposomes, however, are rapidly cleared from the circulation by macrophages of the reticuloendothelial system, thereby limiting the potential for drug delivery to the brain. Modification of the liposomes through a decrease in the size or surface modification and use of monoclonal antibodies for specific tumor targeting are some mechanisms used to optimize this technology.[83,84]

Intracranial or Intratumor Drug Delivery

Another strategy to circumvent the BBB is to deliver drugs directly into the brain through local administration. One way to do this is surgical placement of biodegradable synthetic polymers impregnated with a drug. The prototype for this is the Gliadel Wafer (Eisai Inc, Woodcliff Lake, New Jersey), which contains BCNU.[85] BCNU is highly lipid-soluble and crosses the BBB readily in both directions. BCNU that diffuses out of the polymer therefore passes into the local bloodstream, where the BCNU concentration is low. This carries the drug away from the brain, a phenomenon known as the *sink effect*. Another limitation is that drug penetrates the surrounding brain only by passive diffusion, a slow and inefficient process. High concentrations of BCNU are thus found only within a few millimeters of the wafers, which makes it unlikely that cytotoxic drug concentrations will reach distant infiltrating tumor cells.[86] Implantations that contain other chemotherapeutic agents (e.g., paclitaxel and cisplatin) have also been evaluated.[87,88]

Convection-enhanced delivery (CED) is another strategy for local drug delivery. CED requires the implantation of catheters directly into the brain, followed by continuous infusion of the drug under a constant pressure gradient. CED offers several theoretical advantages such as the ability to move very large molecules (i.e., immunoglobulins, liposomes, small virions) through the interstitial space and the ability to achieve homogeneous concentrations of the drug even at the leading edge of the infusate.[89,90] This results in much larger volumes of distribution with CED.[91] CED also theoretically offers the ability to target a specific anatomic zone of cerebral tissue for treatment while sparing other areas. The efficiency of CED depends on the physicochemical characteristics of the administered drug and the volume of distribution of the agent. Because an invasive procedure is required, multiple administrations may be impractical, and the lack of efficacy of some of the initial clinical trials may be explained by these factors. Current research focuses on optimizing convection parameters (i.e., type of agent, volume, infusion rate, pressure), technology (catheters and pumps), and finding methods to allow the imaging of the convected infusate.[92]

Another approach is direct administration of the agent into the CSF. Because the CSF has the pharmacokinetic characteristics of a closed (albeit dynamic) compartment, drugs given directly into the CSF can reach high levels. Because this compartment is separate from systemic circulation, drugs given in this way must be in their active form. Given the high CSF drug levels that can be attained through direct administration, intra-CSF treatment can be highly effective in treating tumor cells that are in the CSF and are lining the leptomeninges. Unfortunately, there is a significant delay in equilibration between the CSF and extracellular space of the brain even for small soluble molecules given directly into the CSF. For larger, less diffusible molecules, equilibrium between the two compartments never occurs. This pharmacologic phenomenon, referred to as the *CSF–brain barrier*, explains why intra-CSF drug administration is an inefficient and ineffective delivery strategy for parenchymal tumors.[93] Additionally, intra-CSF delivery is limited by significant neurologic morbidity. With a few exceptions (i.e., methotrexate, cytarabine, thiotepa), most compounds cause unacceptable neurologic toxicity, including death, when given into the CSF. Because of this, intrathecal chemotherapy is used principally to treat leptomeningeal metastases and for CNS prophylaxis for high-risk leukemia.

Challenges Specific for Targeted Agents

Despite the availability of targeted agents specific to aberrant signaling pathways in high-grade glioma, the results of phase 2 studies of many agents have been disappointing. In addition to the difficulty of delivery of agents across the BBB, there are other challenges that limit the efficacy of these agents. These include accounting for the heterogeneity of tumors, redundancy of pathway interactions, lack of accurate and reproducible biomarkers to select patients for specific therapies, and difficulty in assessing target modulation.[94–96]

Other Systemic Therapy Considerations

Many antiepileptic agents, including phenytoin, carbamazepine, and phenobarbital, induce the hepatic cytochrome P-450 isoenzyme and glucuronidation drug elimination systems. The specific isoenzymes induced by these drugs are often capable of metabolizing many agents. For example, standard paclitaxel doses commonly result in subtherapeutic serum levels in patients also using phenytoin.[97] In fact, the maximally tolerated paclitaxel dose in patients using enzyme-inducing P-450 antiepileptics is nearly threefold higher than in patients not using such agents. Similar observations have been made with regard to 9-aminocampothecin, vincristine, teniposide, irinotecan, and targeted agents.[98–101] In addition to different MTDs being established depending on the use of enzyme-inducing antiepileptics, the side effect profile and dose-limiting toxicities can also differ.[101,102] Most phase 1 clinical trials in brain tumor patients now use separate arms for patients who are or are not taking enzyme-inducing antiepileptic drugs or limit enrollment to patients not taking enzyme-inducing antiepileptic drugs. It may be preferable to change to a non–enzyme-inducing antiepileptic agent (e.g., levetiracetam [Keppra]), although it may take days to make the switch and some time for the P-450 enzyme induction to resolve.

SPECIFIC CENTRAL NERVOUS SYSTEM NEOPLASMS

Cerebral Glioma

Pathologic Classification

The histological subtypes of glioma include tumors of astrocytic, oligodendroglial, ependymal, and neuroepithelial origin. The first widely used classification system was devised by Kernohan et al.[103] Unfortunately, there was little reproducible prognostic significance among the four grades. Recognizing this limitation, Ringertz[104] established a three-tiered system that allowed for easier distinction between low- and high-grade tumors, but the system suffered from significant intraobserver variability. A more useful approach was suggested by Daumas-Duport et al.,[105] who reintroduced a four-tiered system based on a set of objective criteria: nuclear pleomorphism, mitoses, endothelial proliferation, and necrosis. Although the classification initially appeared to demonstrate good separation in survival among patients by grade, it did not provide adequate prognostic differentiation between grades 2 and 3 in a validation study.[106]

To resolve these controversies, the WHO convened an international panel of neuropathologists to define a new classification system, which has since garnered worldwide acceptance.[3] In this revised WHO schema, noninfiltrative glioma are classified as grade I and infiltrating glioma are subsequently categorized from grades II to IV. Infiltrative astrocytic tumors are divided into three categories: astrocytoma (including grade II fibrillary, gemistocytic, and protoplasmic), anaplastic astrocytoma (grade III), and glioblastoma (including grade IV giant cell glioblastoma and gliosarcoma). Oligodendroglioma and ependymoma are either grade II or anaplastic (grade III).

Grade I Astrocytoma

Low-grade astrocytomas (grade I) such as pilocytic astrocytoma, pleomorphic xanthoastrocytoma, and subependymal giant cell astrocytoma are typically circumscribed and indolent tumors. Complete surgical resection, whenever feasible, is the curative mainstay therapy for such tumors. Despite aggressive near total resection, delayed recurrence and eventual malignant transformation are unfortunately common. However, resection of a low-grade glioma can be difficult in locations such as the optic pathway, hypothalamus, and in those involving deep midline structures. In these instances, asymptomatic patients can be observed carefully for a prolonged period of time and undergo a maximally safe resection only at the time of progression.

In patients who have recurrent tumor that are not amenable to further resection or who have residual tumor causing significant morbidity, adjuvant chemotherapy or radiotherapy can improve recurrence-free survival, although the role of chemotherapy in adults remains controversial. Immediate postoperative adjuvant therapies may be appropriate in some cases depending on the location of the tumor, the extent of residual disease, the impracticability of repeated surgical excision, and availability for follow-up. Generally, radiotherapy is the primary adjuvant treatment used in older children and adults with low-grade glioma. In young children with unresectable progressive low-grade glioma, there is a desire to avoid or delay radiotherapy owing to the long-term radiation related sequelae; chemotherapy is often utilized here as the initial therapeutic option.[107–110] Some responses from chemotherapy can last for years, and nearly half of all children treated with chemotherapy ultimately require radiotherapy for tumor progression.

In terms of radiotherapy used with curative intent, in children, the most common situation is with cerebellar and optic-pathway pilocytic astrocytoma, typically after progression on chemotherapy, whereas in adults, this tends to occur most commonly with hypothalamic pilocytic astrocytoma. The typical radiation dose used in this setting is 50.4 to 54.0 Gy, in 1.8 Gy fractions. There is evidence of improved progression-free survival in this situation.[111]

Grade II Infiltrating Low-Grade Glioma

Nonpilocytic or diffusely infiltrating low-grade gliomas are classified as WHO grade II tumors. They may arise from astrocytic, oligodendrocytic, or mixed lineage. Like astrocytomas, oligodendrogliomas display various degrees of clinical aggressiveness. In addition to histology and molecular characteristics, several variables have been found to be of prognostic importance in low-grade glioma. Pignatti et al.[112] performed the most comprehensive of these analyses and developed a scoring system to identify patients at varying level of risk for mortality. Multivariate analysis showed that age 40 or older, astrocytoma histology, maximum diameter 6 cm or greater, tumor crossing the midline, and presence of neurologic deficits negatively impacted survival.

Patients with up to two factors were considered low risk (median survival, 7.7 years) and patients with three or more were considered high risk (median survival, 3.2 years).

Surgery for Low-Grade Glioma

Retrospective analyses have suggested that the extent of resection is a significant prognostic variable. The Radiation Therapy Oncology Group (RTOG) performed a prospective evaluation of the natural history of completely resected low-grade gliomas (RTOG-9802), evaluating the recurrence risk in 111 patients with surgeon-defined gross total resections (GTR) and found that the extent of postoperative residual disease was an important variable for time to first relapse.[113] Five-year recurrence rates were 26% versus 68% for patients with less than 1 cm residual tumors versus 1 to 2 cm residual tumors.

Radiation Therapy

The role of radiotherapy, in particular the timing, remains controversial. Early intervention is indicated for patients with increasing symptoms and radiographic progression. In younger patients (less than 40 years) who have undergone complete resection, observation with imaging is an option. In RTOG-9802 median time to progression in 111 good-risk patients defined as younger than 40 and a gross total tumor resection was 5 years.[113] In those who have undergone a subtotal resection or those with high-risk features, postoperative radiotherapy may be recommended, typically 50.4 Gy in 1.8 Gy fractions.

Three phase 3 trials provide the best evidence with respect to the indications for radiotherapy as well as the dose (Table 121.5). In a study by the European Organisation for Research and Treatment of Cancer (EORTC-22845), 314 patients were randomized to postoperative radiotherapy to 54 Gy (n = 157) or radiotherapy at progression (n = 157).[114] Statistically significant improvement in progression-free survival was associated with early radiotherapy, 5.3 versus 3.4 years ($P < .0001$), without a difference in median survival, 7.4 versus 7.2 years. Malignant transformation occurred in 65% to 72% of patients with no difference between the two groups.

Two other trials investigated the dose question. In EORTC-22844, 379 patients were randomized to 45 Gy versus 59.4 Gy.[115] With a median follow-up of 74 months, overall survival (58% vs. 59%) and progression-free survival (47% vs. 50%) were similar. In an Intergroup study, 203 patients were randomized to 50.4 Gy (n = 101) or 64.8 Gy.[116] There was no significant difference in progression-free or overall survival.

TABLE 121.5

PHASE 3 RADIOTHERAPY TRIALS IN LOW-GRADE GLIOMA

Study	Treatment Arm	No. of Patients	5-Y Survival (%)
EORTC-22845	Observation[a]	157	66
	54 Gy (30 fractions)	157	68
EORTC-22844	45 Gy (25 fractions)	171	58
	59.4 Gy (33 fractions)	172	59
NCCTG	50.4 (28 fractions)	101	72
	64.8 (36 fractions)	102	64

EORTC, European Organisation for Research and Treatment of Cancer; NCCTG, North Central Cancer Treatment Group.
[a]Treatment with reresection, radiotherapy, or both, at progression (for most patients).

Consequently, low-dose radiotherapy, 50.4 to 54.0 Gy in 1.8 Gy fractions, has become an accepted practice for selected patients with low-grade gliomas. The target volume is local, with a margin of 2 cm beyond changes demonstrated on traditional MRI sequences. FLAIR images usually show considerable abnormality beyond any enhancing or nonenhancing tumor and whether a smaller margin may be used for planning if FLAIR sequences are utilized is unknown.

Brown et al.[117] reviewed the results of the Mini-Mental Status Examination for 203 adults irradiated for low-grade gliomas. Most patients maintained stable neurocognitive status after radiotherapy, and patients with abnormal baseline results were more likely to have improvement in cognitive abilities than to deteriorate after therapy; few patients showed cognitive decline. In a more in-depth analysis of formal neurocognitive testing, 20 patients were analyzed before radiotherapy and then every 18 months for 5 years, and cognitive function remained stable; these results suggest that the tumor itself has the most deleterious effect on cognitive function.[118]

Chemotherapy

Low-grade gliomas have historically been considered chemotherapy resistant. With the recent demonstration of the chemotherapy responsiveness of some low-grade astrocytomas and oligodendrogliomas has come renewed interest in investigating chemotherapy for low-grade glioma.[119,120] It has been demonstrated that some low-grade gliomas, especially optic pathway and hypothalamic tumors, can be responsive to chemotherapy.[121,122] In children, various single and multichemotherapeutic and biological agents are effective in controlling the growth of a low-grade glioma in a setting of a newly progressive lesion, multiply recurrent, or unresectable residual tumors.[107–109,110,123,124] Platinum-containing regimens result in radiographic response rates greater than 60%.[123] A national randomized phase 3 trial by the Childrens' Cancer Group (CCG-9952) tested the efficacy of vincristine/carboplatin versus 6-thioguanine, procarbazine, lomustine, vincristine (TPCV) in children less than 10 years of age with unresectable or progressive low-grade gliomas, the results of which are currently not available. In the recently completed pediatric national trial by the Children's Oncology Group (ACNS-0223), temozolomide was added to the vincristine and carboplatin backbone. Vinblastine has also demonstrated substantial activity in recurrent low-grade gliomas and is a commonly used second-line agent after treatment failure with vincristine and carboplatin.[125,126] Other second- and third-line therapies for multiply recurrent tumors include TPCV and temozolomide. Irinotecan and bevacizumab are currently being investigated in a multi-institutional phase 2 trial for the treatment of progressive low-grade gliomas. Rapamycin, an oral immunosuppressive agent, has been effective in reducing the growth of astrocytoma associated with tuberous sclerosis.[127] Most of the chemotherapy responses seen in children with low-grade gliomas are for contrast-enhancing masses that probably represent pilocytic astrocytomas. Nonenhancing, diffusely infiltrating astrocytomas in children appear to be much less responsive to chemotherapy. Some of these responses can last for years, although nearly half of all children treated with chemotherapy ultimately require radiotherapy.

Data on the use of chemotherapy for low-grade glioma in adults are sparse. In a small Southwest Oncology Group trial, adults with incompletely excised low-grade gliomas were randomly assigned to radiation therapy alone or radiation therapy and lomustine (CCNU). There was no difference in survival between the two arms.[128] The role of adjuvant procarbazine, CCNU, and vincristine (PCV) for "high-risk" patients (less than total resection, age older than 40 years) with low-grade obvious, possibly because salvage treatment at recurrence results in equivalent survival. Importantly, both trials confirm the prognostic value of 1p and 19q.

Temozolomide has produced high response rates in patients with anaplastic oligodendroglioma. Chinot et al.[160] treated 48 PCV-failed patients with anaplastic oligodendroglioma/oligoastrocytoma with temozolomide. The objective response rate was 44%. Vogelbaum et al.[161] reported the results of RTOG-0131, a phase 2 trial in which temozolomide was given before radiotherapy to newly diagnosed patients with anaplastic oligodendroglioma/oligoastrocytoma. In 27 patients, the objective response rate was 33%. The 6-month progression rate was 10%. Response to temozolomide has also been shown to be significantly associated with loss of 1p in a small retrospective study.[162]

Chemotherapy for Recurrent Anaplastic Oligodendroglioma

Prospective trials have demonstrated that approximately 50% to 70% of patients with anaplastic oligodendrogliomas that recur after radiotherapy respond to chemotherapy.[129] Although there is no evidence that the sequence of temozolomide and PCV is superior in terms of efficacy, the absence of cumulative myelosuppression with temozolomide argues for its use initially in the setting of recurrent disease.

Ongoing Clinical Trials for Newly Diagnosed Grade 3 Glioma

Two international trials are being conducted in patients with newly diagnosed grade 3 glioma stratified by 1p 19q status rather than histology. Nondeleted patients are randomized to radiation with or without temozolomide; following radiotherapy there is a second randomization to adjuvant temozolomide or not. Codeleted patients are randomized to three arms, a phase 2 temozolomide alone arm, and two phase 3 arms, radiotherapy alone or radiotherapy and concurrent and adjuvant temozolomide.

Grade IV Glioblastoma

Surgery

Gliomas are heterogeneous, and therapy is guided by the most aggressive grade in the specimen. Resection provides the best opportunity to obtain an accurate diagnosis. Studies have shown that more complete resections are more likely to provide a high-grade diagnosis and to detect an oligodendroglial component.[163] Resection relieves mass effect, and more extensive resections are associated with greater neurologic improvement. Response to postoperative radiation therapy is more favorable, and deterioration during treatment is less likely after resection.[164] Finally, it is likely that resection has a modest survival benefit through cytoreduction. Two randomized trials of resection of malignant gliomas have been published. In a study by Vuorinen et al.,[165] survival was twice as long with resection. Stummer et al.[49] reported that patients without residual contrast-enhancing tumor had a higher overall median survival time than did those with residual enhancing tumor (17.9 months vs. 12.9 months, respectively; $P < .001$). Many retrospective studies of both low- and high-grade glioma have shown longer survival with resection, after adjustment for age, performance score, histologic type, and other prognostic factors.[52,166] Although selection bias accounts for some of the difference, most surgeons believe resection is beneficial. Complete resection of an enhancing tumor enhances certain approved or investigational adjuvant therapies (e.g., carmustine wafers, immunotherapy).

Radiotherapy

Randomized trials have demonstrated a survival benefit with radiotherapy.[167] Localized radiation volumes are recommended based on evidence from several sources that GBM typically recur locally, and the bulk of the infiltrative disease is within a few centimeters of the enhancing rim. However, the wide and somewhat unpredictable degree and direction of dissemination, which is not visualized well with any imaging technique, renders radiotherapy field definition difficult. Dandy[168] for example, identified recurrences in the contralateral hemisphere even after hemispherectomy, showing the capability of malignant gliomas to spread along white matter tracts. Such findings as well as autopsy studies that show diffuse dissemination have led to some recommendations that the entire intracranial contents should be irradiated.[169]

However, Hochberg and Pruitt[170] reported that in 35 GBM patients who had a CT scan within 2 months prior to autopsy, 78% of recurrences were within 2 cm of the margin of the initial tumor bed and 56% were within 1 cm or less of the volume outlined by the CT. Halperin et al.[171] reviewed CT scans and multiple pathologic sections of 15 brains of patients with GBM who received minimal or no radiotherapy. If radiation treatment portals had been designed to cover the contrast-enhancing volume and peritumoral edema with a 1 cm margin, the portals would have covered histologically identified tumor in only 6 of 11 cases. On the other hand, treatment of the contrast-enhancing area and all surrounding edema with a 3 cm margin around the edema would have covered histologically identified tumors in all cases.

Standard therapy uses a total dose of 60 Gy in 30 to 33 fractions. Walker et al.[172] reported a dose–response relationship using data from 420 patients treated on Brain Tumor Cooperative Group protocols. Doses ranged from less than 45 to 60 Gy, using daily fractions of 1.7 to 2.0 Gy. A significant improvement in median survival from 28 to 42 weeks was found in the groups treated to 50 to 60 Gy. A Medical Research Council study in 443 patients showed a survival advantage in patients who received 60 compared to 45 Gy (12 months vs. 9 months; $P = .007$).[173] A benefit for doses greater than 60 Gy has not been shown. The RTOG and ECOG randomized 253 patients to either whole-brain irradiation to 60 Gy with or without a 10-Gy boost to a limited volume.[174] There was no benefit shown from the higher dose.

For patients with poor prognostic factors and for those who are not able to tolerate conventional treatment, a shorter course may provide palliation. Older patients (older than 65 years), especially those with poor performance status, have been shown to have limited posttreatment improvement following conventional radiotherapy.[175] Phillips et al.[176] randomized 68 patients to standard radiotherapy to 60 Gy in 30 fractions or a shorter course of 35 Gy in 10 fractions. There was no significant survival difference between the two arms. In another trial, Roa et al.[177] randomized 100 patients older than 60 years of age with GBM to 60 Gy in 30 fractions or 40 Gy in 15 fractions. Overall survival between the two arms was not different. Keime-Guibert et al.[178] randomized 85 patients older than 70 years to radiotherapy or supportive care only, but aborted the trial early because of significantly superior survival in the radiotherapy arm.

Dose Intensification

Dose intensification using 3DCRT or IMRT has not been shown to improve survival. Chan et al.[179] published the results of 34 patients with high-grade gliomas treated using 3DCRT conformal IMRT radiation to 90 Gy. At median follow-up of 11.7 months, 1- and 2-year survivals were 47% and 13%, respectively, not superior to historic expectations.

Several groups have used hyperfractionated or accelerated regimens to escalate dose. In a randomized phase 1 and 2 study,

RTOG-8302 examined escalation using twice-daily fractionation. Hyperfractionated doses were 64.8, 72.0, 76.8, and 81.6 Gy given in 1.2 Gy fractions twice daily and accelerated hyperfractionated regimens were 48.0 and 54.4 Gy given in 1.6 Gy twice-daily fractions. In the final report on 747 patients, there were no survival differences between the arms.[180]

Dose Escalation Using Radiosurgery and Fractionated Stereotactic Radiotherapy

In a prospective randomized trial, Souhami et al.[181] compared conventional radiotherapy and BCNU with or without radiosurgery in 203 patients with GBM. The radiosurgery dose depended on tumor size, ranging from 15 to 24 Gy. No significant improvement in survival was identified. There was also no difference in failure patterns between the groups, and quality of life and cognitive decline were comparable.

The use of a boost using FSRT was tested in RTOG-0023. Seventy-six patients with GBM with postoperative tumor plus cavity less than 60 mm were treated with 50 Gy radiotherapy in daily 2-Gy fractions, plus four FSRT treatments given once weekly. The FSRT dose was either 5 or 7 Gy per fraction for a cumulative dose of 70 or 78 Gy in 29 treatments during 6 weeks. Overall, no survival advantage was seen when compared with the historical database. However, subset analysis showed that patients who had undergone gross total resection had a median survival time of 16.6 compared to 12 months for controls, suggesting that patients with minimal disease may benefit from dose escalation.[182]

Dose Escalation Using Brachytherapy

Laperriere et al.[183] used brachytherapy as a boost to conventional radiotherapy. Patients were randomized to external-beam radiotherapy with or without a temporary ^{125}I implant. Median survival was not different between the two arms (13.8 months vs. 13.2 months). The results of the Brain Tumor Cooperative Group Trial 87-01 reported by Selker et al.[184] mirror these findings.

Radiotherapy delivered by an inflatable balloon is a newer approach. Tatter et al.[185] evaluated the safety and performance of one such device (GliaSite, Proxima Therapeutics, Inc, Alpharetta, Georgia). Twenty-one patients with recurrent malignant glioma underwent resection and device placement. At 1 to 2 weeks following implantation, the balloon was filled with an aqueous solution of organically bound ^{125}I, delivering 40 to 60 Gy during 3 to 6 days. This was well tolerated with no serious adverse effects. Median survival was 12.7 months. Prospective, randomized trials are needed for further evaluation.

Radiosensitizers

Studies using radiation modifiers to overcome the hypoxia present in malignant gliomas have generally yielded disappointing results. Chang[186] reported no benefit in 38 patients treated with hyperbaric oxygen and irradiation using schedules ranging from 36 Gy given in 3 weeks to 60 Gy given in 6 to 7 weeks.

Miralbell et al.[187] reported the results of an EORTC trial examining the addition of carbogen and nicotinamide to overcome the effects of hypoxia. In this phase 1 and 2 trial, 107 patients received radiotherapy with carbogen, breathing during each treatment or a daily oral dose of nicotinamide, or both. Patients who received nicotinamide had higher rates of acute toxicity. Overall survival was similar in all groups (median survival, 10.1 months vs. 9.7 months vs. 11.1 months) and did not differ from historic controls. RSR-13, an agent that specifically delivers oxygen to hypoxic tumor regions, has been evaluated in phase 1 and 2 clinical trials, but due to the limited activity observed, further phase 3 development is not currently being pursued.[188]

Nitroimidazoles such as misonidazole (MISO) are oxygen-mimetic agents. A double-blind randomized trial conducted by the Medical Research Council found no difference in survival between patients treated with radiotherapy to 45 Gy in combination with either MISO or placebo.[189]

Tirapazamine is a bioreductive agent with enhanced toxicity for hypoxic cells. In a phase 2 trial of tirapazamine given with 60 Gy in newly diagnosed GBM (RTOG-9417), patients at two dose levels of tirapazamine were observed to have median survivals of 10.8 and 9.5 months, not superior to historic controls.[190]

Halogenated pyrimidines are incorporated into the DNA of dividing cells due to their biochemical similarity to thymidine. After being incorporated, cells are much more susceptible to single-strand breaks from radiation-induced free radicals and have impaired ability to repair DNA. Early clinical trials focused on intra-arterial BUdR, but later it was determined that prolonged intravenous infusion could achieve equivalent radiosensitization with fewer complications. Phase 1 and 2 studies to evaluate continuous infusion iododeoxyuridine (IUdR) with hyperfractionated radiotherapy reported median survivals of 11 to 15 months. This led to a single-institution trial investigating higher doses of BUdR with hyperfractionated radiotherapy. Median survival was not improved, and significant toxicities were observed.[191] The NCOG later published data comparing survival from pooled data within the NCOG (patients treated with BUdR with radiotherapy) with a similar population of patients from the RTOG database (patients who did not receive BUdR). They reported a median survival of 16.9 months for the NCOG patients (BUdR) compared with 9.8 months for the non-BUdR group ($P < .0001$).[192] However, there were many limitations with this comparison, including wide variations among radiotherapy fractions, total radiotherapy dose, use of chemotherapy, and use of other potential radiosensitizers, severely limiting the interpretation of this data set.

Motexafin gadolinium (MGd) is a redox-active drug that selectively accumulates in tumor cells. It is thought to sensitize tumors through the production of reactive oxygen species that destabilize cellular metabolism. In a phase 1 clinical trial, MGd was shown to be a radiosensitizer for GBM. A phase 2 RTOG trial has been completed, but results are not available to date.[193]

Radiosensitizers and Radiation-Synergistic Cytotoxics. Camptothecins are systemic agents able to effectively penetrate the BBB and are hypothesized to act as radiation sensitizers by preventing DNA repair through inhibition of the topoisomerase-I enzyme. RTOG-9513 evaluated topotecan as a radiosensitizer in GBM, but the median survival of 9.3 months was not significantly different from matched historical controls from the RTOG database.[194]

Preclinical studies with platinum agents have suggested that these drugs are able to inhibit the repair of radiation-induced damage and potentially exert a direct cytotoxic effect on glioma cells. A phase 3 Intergroup trial to evaluate continuous infusion cisplatin in combination with radiotherapy compared with conventional radiotherapy found no significant difference in survival between the groups.[195]

Based on preclinical studies showing paclitaxel as a radiosensitizer in malignant glioma cell lines, the RTOG performed a phase 2 study (RTOG-9602) to evaluate the feasibility and efficacy of conventional radiotherapy and concurrent weekly paclitaxel in newly diagnosed GBM. An objective response was observed in 23% of the patients, with an observed median survival of 9.7 months, not improved compared with historical controls.

Radioimmunotherapy

Radioimmunotherapy, using monoclonal antibodies against EGFR tagged with ^{125}I, has been evaluated. In a phase 2 trial,

25 patients with malignant gliomas were treated with resection or biopsy followed by definitive external-beam radiotherapy and one or multiple doses (35 to 90 mCi per infusion) of ^{125}I-labeled monoclonal antibody-425. The total cumulative dose ranged from 40 to 224 mCi. At 1 year, 60% of patients were alive and the median survival was 15.6 months. In an updated report on 180 patients with a minimum follow-up of 5 years, median survival was 13.4 months.[196]

Radiolabeled antibodies to tenascin have been evaluated in phase 1 and 2 trials showing activity against newly diagnosed and recurrent malignant gliomas. In a phase 2 trial ^{125}I-labeled murine antitenascin monoclonal antibody was injected into the resection cavity in 33 patients with malignant glioma, followed by external-beam radiotherapy and 1 year of chemotherapy. Median survival (87 weeks) was longer than that of historical controls. Only one patient required reoperation for radionecrosis.[197]

Particle Beam Therapy

Alternate radiation modalities used in the treatment of gliomas include neutrons, protons, helium ions, other heavy nuclei, negative pi-mesons, and thermal neutrons in conjunction with boronated compounds (boron neutron capture therapy). To date, most studies have been designed to determine optimal dose scheduling, efficacy, and safety. Despite theoretical advantages with respect to dose distribution and radiobiologic effect, most trials have failed to demonstrate improved survival.

In a pilot study, Griffin et al.[198] did not find a difference in survival in patients treated with fast neutrons to 14 Gy versus external-beam photons to 50 Gy, and in an RTOG study, 166 patients with GBM were randomized to receive a neutron boost or a photon boost after 50 Gy external-beam radiotherapy with no significant difference in median survival (9.8 months vs. 8.6 months). A randomized neutron dose searching study was performed by the RTOG to test the efficacy of neutron boost following whole-brain photon irradiation in patients with malignant glioma. There was no difference in overall survival in the groups tested.[199]

Chemotherapy

In a landmark international trial, patients were randomized to radiotherapy with or without concurrent and adjuvant temozolomide. Median and 2-year survival were increased by 2.5 months and 16.1%, respectively, in patients receiving temozolomide, and long-term follow-up showed a persistent survival benefit.[200] A companion correlative study demonstrated that methylation of the promoter region of the *MGMT* gene in the tumor was associated with superior survival, regardless of treatment received, but the benefit was maximal for methylated patients.[146] MGMT removes the methyl group from the O6 position of guanine, reversing the cytotoxic effects of methylating agents (such as temozolomide), making the tumor resistant to treatment, while methylation of the promoter region of *MGMT* results in inactivation of *MGMT*. *MGMT* status was strongly associated with survival (Fig. 121.8). Recognizing that a different schedule of temozolomide may overcome chemotherapy resistance, there have been several studies of alternative dosing of temozolomide both at the time of recurrence and in the newly diagnosed setting.[201,202] A large phase 3 randomized international study led by the RTOG has completed accrual to standard treatment versus a 21- or 28-day adjuvant temozolomide schedule. Results are pending. Strategies to increase the therapeutic ratio of existing chemotherapies, such as the inhibition of DNA repair enzymes (i.e., poly[ADP-ribose] polymerase [PARP]) are being evaluated. These agents are being combined with radiation and chemotherapy to increase the cytotoxicity of the combination approach.[203–205]

Although nitrosourea-based chemotherapy is modestly effective for patients with GBM, its use has been supplanted by temozolomide. There is evidence that carmustine-impregnated wafers implanted into the brain at the time of resection provide

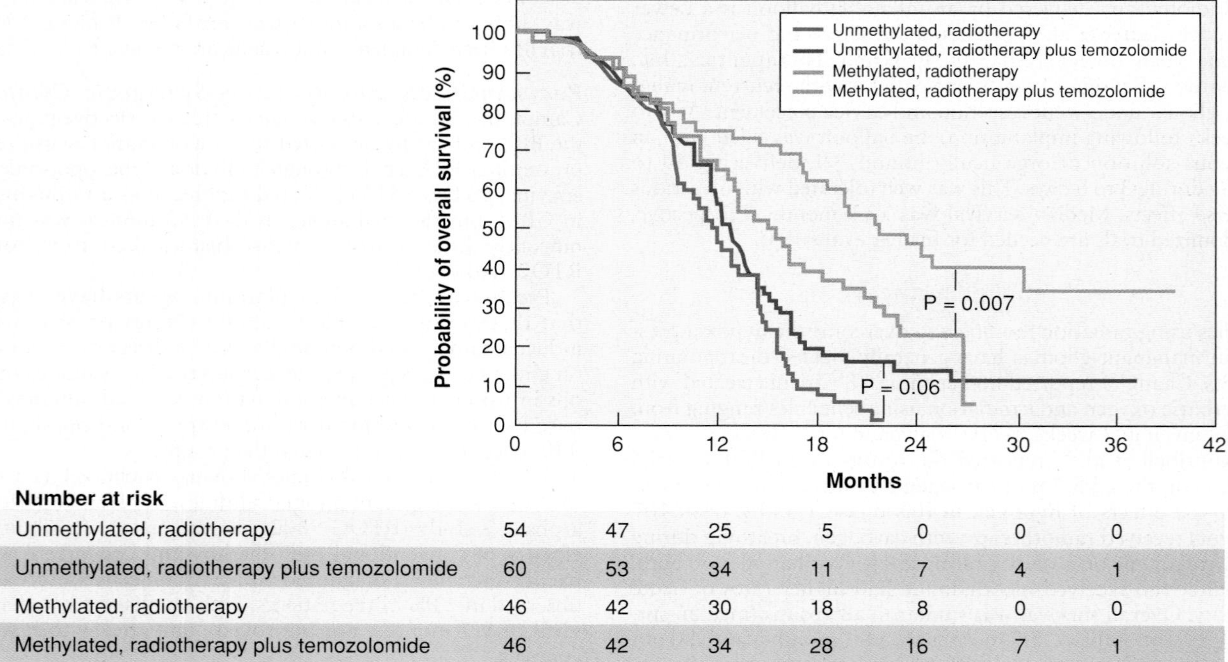

Number at risk							
Unmethylated, radiotherapy	54	47	25	5	0	0	0
Unmethylated, radiotherapy plus temozolomide	60	53	34	11	7	4	1
Methylated, radiotherapy	46	42	30	18	8	0	0
Methylated, radiotherapy plus temozolomide	46	42	34	28	16	7	1

FIGURE 121.8 Kaplan-Meir survival curves for the two arms of the international glioblastoma trial, demonstrating a significant survival benefit from chemoradiotherapy, compared with radiotherapy. The patients are evaluated by methylguanine DNA-methyltransferase (MGMT) gene promoter methylation status, and the maximum survival benefit is seen in the combination arm when the gene promoter is silenced. (From ref. 146, with permission.)

modest improvement in outcomes in selected patients compared with patients who received placebo wafers.[206]

Chemotherapy for Recurrent Glioblastoma. Treatment options for recurrent GBM must be tailored to the individual. Few agents have proven activity. A randomized phase 2 trial of temozolomide versus procarbazine in 225 patients with GBM at first relapse demonstrated that treatment with temozolomide improved median progression-free survival (12.4 weeks vs. 8.3 weeks; $P < .006$).[207] Radiographic responses were disappointing (5.4% vs. 5.3%).

Several agents such as the platinoids, taxanes, 5-fluorouracil (5-FU), and irinotecan have been tested, most demonstrating very little activity. In a review of eight clinical trials with 225 recurrent malignant gliomas, the 6-month survival was 15% versus 31% for GBM versus anaplastic astrocytoma.[208]

Targeted Therapies

As the genetic and molecular pathogenesis of gliomas is better understood, new targets are being identified and inhibitors of associated signaling pathways are being developed. One example is EGFR as a frequently deregulated signaling molecule in GBM, prompting phase 1 and 2 trials of erlotinib and gefitinib for recurrent high-grade gliomas. Both have shown limited activity.[100,209–211] Patients whose tumors demonstrate the variant 3 mutant (EGFRvIII), with resulting constitutive activation of EGFR tyrosine kinase activity, along with intact phosphatase and tensin analogue (PTEN), appear to be more responsive to EGFR inhibitors.[212] There are two reports of the combination of erlotinib with radiation and chemotherapy for newly diagnosed glioblastoma showing modest additional benefit to standard radiochemotherapy, and an additional completed but as yet unreported RTOG trial (0211), none of which show convincing survival improvement.[213,214] Preliminary reports using other targeted agents including the mammalian target of rapamycin (mTOR) inhibitor, temsirolimus, and the farnesyl transferase inhibitor, tipifarnib, have shown objective responses in a few high-grade gliomas.[215–219]

The most promising results have been seen for angiogenic inhibitors. The most important mediator of angiogenesis in GBM is vascular endothelial growth factor (VEGF). Antiangiogenic therapies such as the anti-VEGF monoclonal antibody bevacizumab have produced dramatic radiological responses and prolonged progression-free survival relative to historical controls.[220,221] Based on the results of a randomized phase 2 study of 167 patients who received bevacizumab with or without irinotecan, the U.S. Food and Drug Administration granted accelerated approval to bevacizumab for recurrent glioblastoma in 2009.[152] The progression-free survival at 6 months was 43% for single agent bevacizumab and 50% for the combination arm. The objective response rates were 28% and 38% for the two arms, and median survival times were 9.2 months and 8.7 months, respectively. The most common side effects associated with bevacizumab include fatigue, headache, and hypertension; proteinuria and poor wound healing are also seen. There are several reports of small single-arm phase 2 studies of the combination of bevacizumab with radiation and temozolomide in the newly diagnosed setting and two large randomized placebo-controlled trials are ongoing.[222] Recognizing that tumors ultimately evade the effect of antiangiogenic agents through various mechanisms, other strategies include the evaluation of the combination of bevacizumab with chemotherapeutic and targeted agents, and the investigation of other VEGF targeted agents. Batchelor et al.[223] reported reduction in contrast enhancement and edema in 12 of 16 GBM patients who received cediranib (AZD2171), an orally administered pan-VEGF receptor inhibitor, with median progression-free survival of 3.7 months. VEGF Trap (aflibercept), a recombinantly produced fusion protein that captures circulating VEGF and CT-322 (Angiocept, Adnexus Therapeutics, Waltham, Massachusetts), a pegylated recombinant peptide with a high affinity for VEGF, are currently being tested in both the recurrent and newly diagnosed setting. Other promising antiangiogenic agents under investigation include celengitide (EMD121974),[224,225] an integrin inhibitor; XL184 a multitargeted tyrosine kinase inhibitor that acts on the VEGFR, hepatocyte growth factor receptor (MET) and c-KIT; and enzastaurin, an inhibitor of protein kinase C-beta that targets VEGF as well as the mTOR pathway.[226]

Other mechanisms of cell growth that are being targeted include epigenetic modulation through histone deacetylase inhibitors, the proteasome inhibitor bortezomib, and the glutamate receptor inhibitor talampanel.[227–229]

Convection-Enhanced Delivery

CED is designed to circumvent the BBB and BTB and deliver even large molecules to discrete areas of the brain and spinal cord by direct infusion of an agent into the brain under positive pressure. Proof of principle for CED has been demonstrated in several studies, but unfortunately phase 3 results have been disappointing.[230,231] Significant challenges of optimizing the volume of distribution of the agent to the infiltrating tumor will need to be addressed before the ultimate therapeutic potential of this approach can be realized. The initial experience has demonstrated the need for more reliable delivery technology and methods for demonstrating the success and extent of drug delivery.

Issues in Study Designs for Novel Agents

Several key issues confront the incorporation of new agents in the upfront management of malignant glioma. First, there is the issue of defining the appropriate end point. In recurrent malignant glioma, progression-free survival is frequently employed, but because of insufficient evidence linking this to survival in newly diagnosed malignant glioma, survival remains the gold standard. However, there is considerable heterogeneity in survival outcomes, based on clinical and possibly molecular prognostic variables. An adequate staging system has never been developed. The RTOG has analyzed an extensive database of prospectively treated patients (primarily with surgery, radiotherapy, and alkylating chemotherapy), and, using a statistical method known as recursive portioning analysis, has developed six prognostic groups, referred to as RTOG recursive portioning analysis classes I to VI. Patients can be segmented into classes using eight variables: age, histology, Karnofsky performance score, mental status, neurologic function, symptom duration, extent of resection, and radiotherapy dose. GBM patients fall in classes III through VI, and their median survival ranges from 4.6 months to 17.9 months (Table 121.8).[232]

TABLE 121.8

RADIATION THERAPY ONCOLOGY GROUP RECURSIVE PORTIONING ANALYSIS (RPA) CLASSIFICATION: SURVIVAL BY CLASS

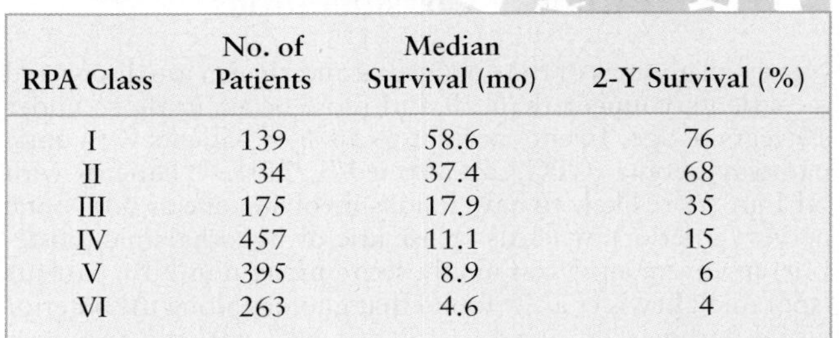

RPA Class	No. of Patients	Median Survival (mo)	2-Y Survival (%)
I	139	58.6	76
II	34	37.4	68
III	175	17.9	35
IV	457	11.1	15
V	395	8.9	6
VI	263	4.6	4

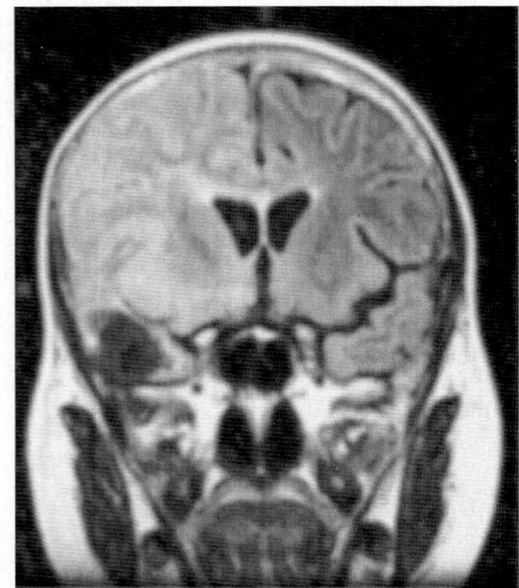

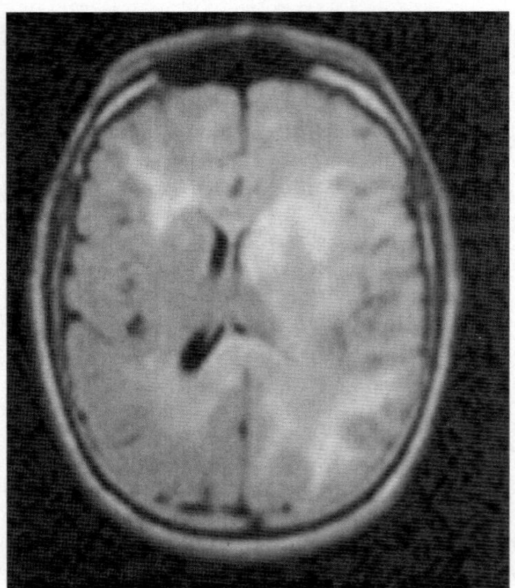

FIGURE 121.9 Two case examples of gliomatosis cerebri. Note the extensive changes visualized on fluid-attenuated inversion recovery (FLAIR) imaging, involving multiple lobes of the brain, and even an entire hemisphere.

GLIOMATOSIS CEREBRI

Gliomatosis cerebri is a rare condition with diffuse involvement of multiple parts of the brain (greater than two lobes). On MRI, there is typically diffuse increased signal on T2-weighted and FLAIR images and low or absent signal in the affected areas on T1-weighted images (Fig. 121.9). Treatment remains undefined. Perkins et al.[233] reviewed the outcomes of 30 patients. Transient improvement or stabilization was achieved in 87% of patients with clinical improvement in 70%. Patients younger than 40 and those with nonglioblastoma histology had better overall survival.

In a French trial, 63 patients were treated with PCV or temozolomide.[234] Objective responses were observed in 26% of patients with no significant difference between the two regimens. Median progression-free and overall survival were 16 months and 29 months, respectively. Patients with an oligodendroglial component had better progression-free and overall survival.

A retrospective review of 296 patients from the literature and the Association des Neuro-Oncologues d'Expression Francaise (ANOCEF) network was recently published.[235] Median survival was 14.5 months. Patients younger than 42, with better Karnofsky performance score, low-grade histology, or oligodendroglial subtype had better outcomes. The impact of radiotherapy on survival remained unclear.

OPTIC, CHIASMAL, AND HYPOTHALAMIC GLIOMAS

Clinical Considerations

Nearly all gliomas of the optic nerve and chiasm are discovered in patients younger than 20 and most occur in those under 10 years of age. Twenty percent to 50% of patients with optic pathway glioma (OPG) are affected by NF1.[236] Patients with NF1 are more likely to have lesions involving one or both optic nerves (anterior), whereas chiasmatic or hypothalamic (posterior) involvement is commonly seen among non-NF1 patients (sporadic). Lewis et al.[236] found that gliomas along the anterior visual pathway occurred in 15% of NF1 patients and were occasionally bilateral; 67% of these were neither suspected clinically nor obvious on ophthalmologic examination. In one series, 25% involved the chiasm alone, 33% the chiasm and hypothalamus, and 42% the chiasm and optic nerves or tracts.[237] Clinically, they cause loss of visual acuity (70%), strabismus and nystagmus (33%), visual field impairment (bitemporal hemianopsia, 8%), developmental delay, macrocephaly, ataxia, hemiparesis, proptosis, and precocious puberty. Funduscopic evaluation demonstrates a range of findings from normal optic discs, to venous engorgement, to disc pallor because of atrophy. Chiasmal tumors often grow to involve the hypothalamus, causing a diencephalic syndrome characterized by emaciation (especially in children between 3 months and 2 years of age), motor overactivity, and euphoria. In general, optic nerve gliomas have a better prognosis than those involving the chiasm, and tumors confined to the anterior chiasm have a better outcome than posterior chiasmal tumors.

The natural history of these tumors ranges from indolent growth or spontaneous regression (with NF1) to rapid progression or dissemination (with hypothalamic lesions).[238–240] Generally, the prognosis of OPG is good with overall 5-year survival rates ranging between 70% and 90%; however, the long-term morbidity is high.[240–243] NF1 and age less than 5 years at diagnosis have better progression-free survival.[240,244]

Pathologic Considerations

Histopathologically, a majority of these tumors are low-grade gliomas, typically pilocytic or fibrillary astrocytomas. They range from primarily piloid and stellate astrocytes (most common), with or without oligodendroglia, through the gamut of malignant astrocytomas to GBM (rarely). Typically, optic gliomas appear as fusiform expansions of any part of the nerve. They may bridge through the optic foramen and expand as dumbbell tumors. The nerve can be infiltrated by tumor originating in the chiasm, the walls of the third ventricle, or the hypothalamus.

Imaging Findings

Diagnosis is best made by MRI, which demonstrates enlargement of the affected optic pathway, often with enhancement.

T2 signal may extend posteriorly along the optic tracts as far as the visual cortex, which may represent tumor infiltration or edema. Cysts and calcification are uncommon, but the hypothalamic component can be cystic.

Treatment Decision Making

In general, children with asymptomatic lesions of the optic pathways found by MRI are not treated unless clinical or radiographic progression is documented. Tumors in children with NF1 tend to be more indolent than sporadic tumors. Only one-third to one-half of children with NF1 with asymptomatic optic pathway tumors found on screening MRIs require treatment for increasing visual symptoms.[245] Most children with sporadic tumors undergo imaging because of symptoms and should be treated. Sporadic tumors often present with advanced findings such as hydrocephalus, decreased visual acuity, and endocrinopathies.[246] Rarely, both sporadic and NF-associated optic pathway gliomas can regress spontaneously.[239]

Surgery

Surgery is indicated only for some optic pathway gliomas. In appropriate patients, surgery may decrease the recurrence rate and increase the time to recurrence. Patients treated with surgery, followed by radiation and chemotherapy, appear to have the highest long-term control.[247] In patients with progressive symptoms (e.g., severe visual loss and proptosis), unilateral anterior tumors that do not involve the optic chiasm may be resected. Biopsy or subtotal resection can be performed for posterior optic pathway gliomas that involve the hypothalamus and optic tract, particularly if they are symptomatic because of local compression and mass effect.

A transcranial approach to orbital tumors allows sparing of the globe and improves the cosmetic result. Initially a craniotomy is performed ipsilateral to known tumor, and the nerve and chiasm are examined directly. If the tumor is limited to the nerve, then the nerve can be sectioned just anterior to the chiasm. The orbit is unroofed, and the remainder of the nerve extending into the globe is resected. Resection of the chiasm is not indicated due to resultant bilateral blindness.

If the tumor involves the chiasm and the MRI raises suspicion of another tumor type, such as an optic nerve sheath meningioma or another parasellar mass, a confirmatory biopsy can be performed. This is rarely needed in patients with NF1, in whom there is a high index of suspicion for an optic nerve glioma. Subtotal resection is indicated if mass effect produces dysfunction of adjacent structures such as the hypothalamus or the nerve itself. Hydrocephalus can be produced by more posteriorly situated tumors and may be alleviated by debulking. If hydrocephalus persists after debulking, CSF shunting (which may need to be biventricular or require fenestration of the septum) becomes necessary.

Radiation Therapy

Untreated optic gliomas, especially those involving the chiasm or extending into the hypothalamus or optic tracts, progress locally or are fatal in 75% of patients. Tenny et al.[248] found that only 21% of patients who were followed after biopsy or exploration survived compared with 64% of those who received radiation therapy.

Routine postoperative irradiation is not indicated for gliomas confined to the optic nerve, which can be completely resected.[249] Radiation therapy can prevent tumor progression, improve disease-free survival, and stabilize or improve vision in patients with chiasmal lesions, for whom postoperative residual is the rule. Wong et al.[250] reported that 86% of chiasmal gliomas not treated with radiation therapy progressed locally, whereas treatment failure occurred in 45% that underwent radiation therapy. Furthermore, control was achieved in 87% of the irradiated patients who received a dose of 50 to 55 Gy compared to 55% of those who received 46 Gy or less.

The prognosis for patients with optic nerve tumors may be better than for those with chiasmal-hypothalamic lesions. In a literature review, local control was found to be achieved for 154 of 189 irradiated anterior chiasmal tumors (81%), whereas 92 of 142 posterior tumors (65%) were controlled. Vision improved in 61 of 210 evaluable patients (29%) and remained stable in 118 of 210 patients (56%).[251] For chiasmal-hypothalamic tumors, radiation therapy produced radiographic shrinkage in 11 of 24 (46%) with a median progression-free survival of 70 months compared with 30 months for patients who did not receive radiation therapy.[252] Age and tumor location were important prognostic factors, with younger children (less than 3 years), and children with lesions posterior to the chiasm faring less well after radiotherapy.

Three-dimensional conformal radiotherapy, IMRT, and stereotactic techniques are used to minimize the dose to adjacent structures. A report by Debus et al.[253] summarized results in patients treated with FSRT (52.2 Gy median dose at 1.8 Gy/d). All patients remained disease free, and no significant complications or marginal failures were seen despite highly conformal radiation fields. Because these tumors are often focal, techniques like FSRT can offer both excellent local control and decreased late effects.

Chemotherapy

In recent years, chemotherapy has played a pivotal role in the management of OPG in young children in order to spare the developing brain from the adverse effects of irradiation.[242,254–257] This is especially important in patients with NF1 who are at significant risk of developing vasculopathy such as moyamoya syndrome and second malignancy after receiving radiotherapy.[256,258] Retrospective series suggest that cognitive function is preserved better in children who receive initial chemotherapy compared with radiation therapy.[242,259] Although the appropriate agents are still evolving, vincristine plus carboplatin remains the most common first-line regimen.[121] Gnekow et al.[260] reported a 5-year progression-free survival of 73% in 55 patients who were treated with this regimen. The randomized Children's Oncology Group A9952 study showed a 5-year progression-free survival of 35% using carboplatin with vincristine and 48% using thioguanine, procarbazine, lomustine, and vincristine regimen in children with newly diagnosed progressive low-grade glioma.[261] Cisplatin-based regimens have shown responses between 50% and 60% and 5-year progression-free survival of 50%.[262–264] Other studies have shown temozolomide to be effective.[265–267] Results from a phase 2 trial of temozolomide for progressive disease showed imaging improvement in 4 of 26 patients, and stable disease in 54% for a median of 34 months.[266] Vinblastine has also been active in these tumors and is generally a second-line agent.[125,126] Collectively, these data suggest that chemotherapy is helpful in delaying tumor progression in a significant portion of children.

Whether chemotherapy alone can improve vision is controversial. Most studies in the literature lack objective data on visual outcome prior and after chemotherapy. Recently Moreno et al.[268] conducted a systematic review of eight reports and found only 14.4% of the children treated with chemotherapy had improvement in their vision. Due to the risk of second malignancy, alkylator-based chemotherapies are generally avoided in patients with NF1. Current studies are evaluating rapamycin, an oral mTOR inhibitor; erlotinib, an EGFR inhibitor; and bevacizumab and irinotecan.[124]

BRAINSTEM GLIOMAS

Clinical and Pathological Considerations

Brainstem gliomas account for 15% of all pediatric brain tumors but are rare in adults. They can be divided into several distinct types. The diffuse intrinsic pontine tumors are generally high-grade astrocytomas, either anaplastic astrocytomas or GBM, and focal, dorsally exophytic or cervicomedullary lesions are usually low grade with a better prognosis. Although rare, ependymomas, PNETs, and atypical teratoid-rhabdoid tumors also occur in the brainstem. Nonneoplastic processes that may be confused with a brainstem tumor include neurofibromatosis, demyelinating diseases, arteriovenous malformations, abscess, and encephalitis.

The diagnosis is usually based on a short history of rapidly developing neurologic findings of multiple cranial nerve palsies (most commonly VI and VII), hemiparesis, and ataxia. The initial manifestations of a brainstem glioma are unilateral palsies of cranial nerves VI and VII in approximately 90% of patients. The classic MRI finding is diffuse enlargement of the pons with poorly marginated T2 signal involving 50% or greater of the pons (Fig. 121.10).[269] Most are nonenhancing; in children, enhancing lesions could have either a pilocytic or malignant component; in adults, enhancement is worrisome for a malignant glioma.[270] Cervicomedullary tumors are nonenhancing, well-circumscribed lesions with an exophytic component. Tectal gliomas are nonenhancing and enlarge the tectal plate, often expanding it into the supracerebellar cistern with associated hydrocephalus. Overall, the prognosis is poor, with 5-year survival varying between 0% and 38% and a median survival of less than 1 year.[271]

Surgery

Complete resection is almost never possible, and even biopsy is restricted because of substantial morbidity and mortality.[272,273] When a biopsy is thought to be necessary because atypical imaging findings or clinical characteristics suggest another diffuse brainstem disorder, stereotactic needle biopsy is used, usually with an entry point on the frontal convexity or over the lateral cerebellar convexity if the lesion is accessible via the middle cerebellar peduncle without crossing pial planes. Resection has no place in the treatment of diffuse pontine gliomas in children or adults. For the rare focal astrocytic lesions of the adult or pediatric brainstem, surgery may play a larger role. Tectal gliomas have a typical imaging appearance, and biopsy is neither necessary nor safe. However, the accompanying noncommunicating hydrocephalus (from compression of the aqueduct of Sylvius) can be treated with CSF diversion, either by third ventriculocisternostomy or by ventriculoperitoneal shunting.[274] Dorsally exophytic astrocytomas within the fourth ventricle or at the cervicomedullary junction are often resectable with low morbidity and excellent long-term results, if a complete removal is achieved.[275] Intrinsic astrocytomas or ependymomas at the cervicomedullary junction can often be completely removed through a posterior midline approach.[276] Kestle et al.[277] treated 28 patients with juvenile pilocytic astrocytoma of the brainstem with resection in 25 cases and biopsy in 3. The 5- and 10-year progression-free survival rates were 74% and 62%, respectively, after gross total resection or resection with linear enhancement and 19% and 19%, respectively, when solid residual tumor was present; thus, long-term survival after resection of these tumors seems to relate to the extent of initial excision.

Radiation Therapy

Radiation therapy, the primary treatment for brainstem tumors, improves survival and can stabilize or reverse neurologic

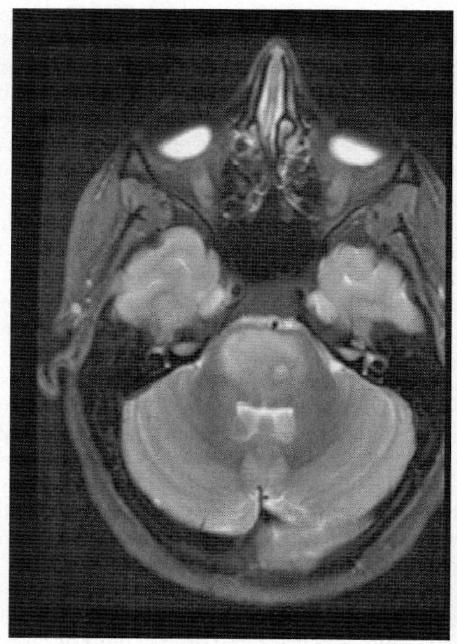

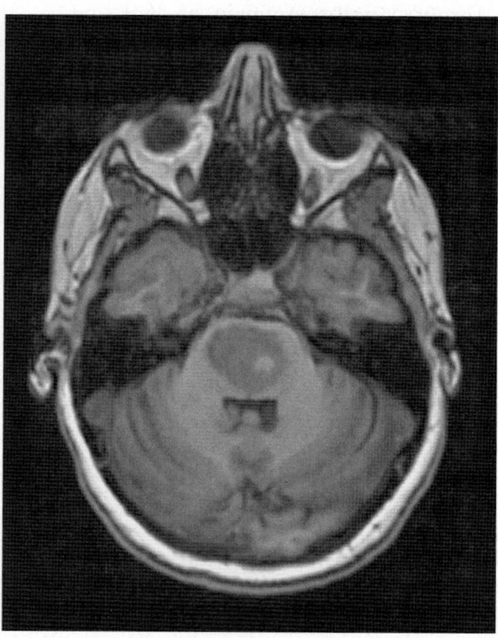

FIGURE 121.10 Typical magnetic resonance appearance of a diffuse pontine glioma. Diffuse enlargement of the pons is visualized on the T2-weighted image (**A**); a small amount of hemorrhage is visualized on the noncontrast T1-weighted image (**B**).

dysfunction in 75% to 90% of patients.[271] The GTV is usually best defined using T2-weighted or FLAIR MRI. A margin of 1.0 to 1.5 cm is added to create a CTV. These lesions should be treated to 54 to 60 Gy using daily fractions of 1.8 to 2.0 Gy. In a multi-institutional survey by Freeman and Suissa,[278] the 1-, 2-, and 5-year survival rates of children treated with conventional radiation therapy techniques were 50%, 29%, and 23%, respectively. Hyperfractionation, designed to deliver higher tumor doses, has been evaluated, without a significant survival advantage (median survival, 8.5 months vs. 8.0 months for conventional vs. hyperfractionated regimens).[279] Several drugs, such as topotecan, and motexafin-gadolinium have been investigated as radiosensitizers, without clear evidence of benefit, and therefore, the role of sensitizers remains investigational.

Fewer data exist with respect to brainstem glioma in adults, but there is some evidence that these tumors may be less aggressive in adults, with overall survival that ranges from 45% to 66% at 2 to 5 years, perhaps because of a greater frequency of more favorable tumor types.[280] In the series from ANOCEF, 48 adult patients with brainstem gliomas were grouped on the basis of their clinical, radiological, and histologic features.[281] Nearly half had nonenhancing, diffusely infiltrative tumors and had symptoms that were present for longer than 3 months. Eleven of these 22 patients underwent biopsy, and 9 had low-grade histology. Nearly all underwent radiotherapy and had a median survival of 7.3 years. A second group of 15 patients who had presented with rapid progression of symptoms and had contrast enhancement on MRI were described. Fourteen of these patients underwent biopsy, and anaplasia was identified in all 14 specimens. Despite radiotherapy, the median survival in this group was 11.2 months, which approximates the survival in pediatric series.

Chemotherapy

In one study, radiation therapy was compared with radiation therapy followed by CCNU, PCV, and prednisone; chemotherapy did not improve survival.[282] Another study by the CCG randomly assigned 32 patients to preradiation chemotherapy with three courses of carboplatin, etoposide, and vincristine; and 31 patients to preradiation cisplatin, etoposide, cyclophosphamide, and vincristine.[283] Response rates and overall survival were not substantially different in either arm. Clinical trials using temozolomide during and after radiation therapy have not shown improvement in the outcome.[284–286] Thus, no agent used either during or after radiation treatment has been shown to have benefit over radiation alone.

Various molecularly targeted therapies such as EGFR antagonists, or antiangiogenic therapies are being explored, but no definitive data support their routine use.

CEREBELLAR ASTROCYTOMAS

Clinical and Pathological Considerations

Cerebellar astrocytomas, which occur most often during the first two decades of life, arise in the vermis or more laterally in a cerebellar hemisphere. They are usually well circumscribed and can be cystic, solid, or some combination of both. It is not uncommon to have a small tumor (mural nodule) associated with a large cystic cavity.

Histologically, most are low-grade juvenile pilocytic astrocytomas that lack anaplastic features. In a series of 451 children, cerebellar astrocytomas accounted for 25% of all posterior fossa tumors, and 89% of the 111 cerebellar astrocytomas were low grade.[287] Approximately 75% of these tumors are located only in the cerebellum, with the remainder involving the brainstem as well. Because these tumors usually arise in the vermis or median cerebellar hemisphere, the clinical presentation is similar to that of medulloblastoma, with truncal ataxia, headache, nausea, and vomiting. In infants, head enlargement from hydrocephalus is seen.

Surgery

Cystic cerebellar astrocytomas are exposed through a posterior fossa craniotomy. The cyst is located with ultrasonography or stereotaxy, cannulated, and then exposed by an incision through the cerebellar folia. With the operating microscope, the cyst is examined and the vascular, firm mural nodule is identified, dissected, and removed. The nonneoplastic cyst wall is not excised. Solid cerebellar astrocytomas are separated carefully from surrounding white matter, again using the improved visualization offered by the operating microscope. Ordinarily, the tumor has a distinctive appearance and is easily separated from surrounding white matter; the only barriers to complete resection are penetration of the tumor into the dentate nucleus, cerebellar peduncles, or brainstem. Gross total resection is tantamount to a cure for these lesions.[288,289]

Radiation Therapy

Most completely resected cerebellar astrocytomas do not require radiation therapy. The management of partially resected pilocytic astrocytomas remains controversial because many remain stable for years without additional treatment. Even when they progress, repeat resection is reasonable if a majority of the tumor can be removed. The overall prognosis for diffuse cerebellar astrocytomas in children tends to be poorer than for pilocytic tumors, with only 30% to 40% of patients free of progression at 5 years.[290] Thus, radiation is often used after surgery for partially resected diffuse cerebellar astrocytomas. Doses of 50 to 60 Gy are delivered, depending on the histologic features and the age of the patient.

Chemotherapy

In general, chemotherapy is not indicated. Based on the experience with optic pathway glioma, several of which have pilocytic features, carboplatin has been used for recurrent tumors.[291,292] There is limited experience with the use of temozolomide in this setting. High-grade gliomas that arise in the cerebellum are treated with regimens identical to their supratentorial counterparts.

GANGLIOGLIOMAS

Clinical and Pathological Considerations

Gangliogliomas, along with pilocytic astrocytomas, pleomorphic xanthoastrocytomas, and subependymal giant cell astrocytomas, are considered "astroglial variant" forms of low-grade glioma.[293] They are more circumscribed than diffuse low-grade gliomas, are classified as grade 1 or 2, and do not typically invade normal brain. Because they do not generally progress to higher-grade lesions, surgery alone is frequently curative. Gangliogliomas are more common in children than adults. They are the most common neoplasms to cause chronic focal epileptic disorders, and they typically arise in the temporal lobe

TABLE 121.9

OUTCOMES FOLLOWING TREATMENT IN PATIENTS WITH GANGLIOGLIOMA

Treatment	No. of Patients	10-Y Local Control Rate (%)	10-Year Survival Rate (%)
Gross total resection	188	89	95
Gross total resection with postoperative radiotherapy	21	90	95
Subtotal resection	113	52	62
Subtotal resection with postoperative radiotherapy	80	65	74

but may also occur in the brainstem, spinal cord, and diencephalon.[294] They may include a cystic component, and the solid portion is free of normal brain parenchyma. Unlike diffuse low-grade gliomas, gangliogliomas enhance on MRI scans. They contain both glial and neuronal elements. The glial elements, which stain for glial fibrillary acidic protein, are almost always astrocytic and often pilocytic, but fibrillary astrocytes are also common. The glial elements dictate whether the lesion is grade 1 or 2. The neurons in the tumor are neoplastic and are characteristically large and relatively mature (i.e., they contain ganglion cells). The presence of neoplastic neurons may be confirmed by immunostaining for neuron-specific enolase and synaptophysin. Grade 2 lesions have rarely been observed to progress to a higher grade.[295,296]

Surgery

Surgical resection is directed at removal of the contrast-enhancing portion of the tumor. Nevertheless, although lesions located within eloquent brain regions are resectable, they may present significant surgical challenges because the boundary between tumor and functional brain may be difficult to define, even with the aid of modern surgical adjuncts (e.g., operating microscope, computer-assisted navigation, functional brain mapping). Although no phase 3 prospective studies have documented the superiority of surgery over other approaches (e.g., radiotherapy), retrospective studies have indicated that complete resection is associated with long-term survival.[295,296] Resection of gangliogangliomas also can result in seizure control.[297] Grade 2 gangliogliomas may recur, and some patients do poorly. The degree of anaplasia determines the prognosis.

Radiation Therapy

Because resection has the potential to cure most of these lesions, radiotherapy is generally reserved for subtotally resected cases or for recurrences.[298] It is also used for lesions in complex locations where further resection may result in significant morbidity. To determine the optimal strategy for ganglioglioma, Rades et al.[299] conducted a literature-based retrospective study of more than 400 patients treated for ganglioglioma. They examined four different treatment strategies (GTR or subtotal resection [STR] with or without radiotherapy) in 402 patients identified from reports published between 1978 and 2007. Surgery was found to be the mainstay of therapy, with 209 patients undergoing GTR and 193 undergoing STR. Adjuvant radiotherapy was used in 101 patients (20 following GTR and 81 following STR). Patients who underwent GTR had higher rates of overall survival and progression-free survival advantage than individuals who underwent STR (Table 121.9). For patients undergoing GTR, the 10-year rates of local control and overall survival were 89% and 95%, respectively, better than the 52% and 62% observed for patients undergoing STR. This indirectly indicates that GTR is the most effective treatment strategy for ganglioglioma. For patients undergoing STR followed by postoperative radiotherapy, the 10-year rate of local control was 62%, better than the 52% for patients undergoing STR without postoperative radiotherapy; although the 10-year survival also improved from 65% to 74% with the use of postoperative radiotherapy in patients with subtotally resected tumors, this did not reach statistical significance. For the 40 patients undergoing STR for whom radiotherapy details were known, local recurrence was observed in 6 of 22 (27%) receiving 54 Gy, compared to 7 of 18 (39%) receiving greater than 54 Gy, implying no specific dose–response relationship.

Chemotherapy

Chemotherapy for gangliogliomas is generally reserved for young children who have undergone subtotal resection and who demonstrate disease progression. In older patients, it is typically used as salvage therapy to treat recurrent tumors after the failure of surgery and radiation therapy. In general, for astroglial variants such as ganglioglioma, no optimal chemotherapeutic regimens have been defined, and most researchers consider disease stabilization (rather than a complete tumor response) to be a successful outcome.

EPENDYMOMA

Clinical and Pathologic Features

Ependymomas arise from the ependymal cells lining the cerebral ventricles and the vestigial central canal of the spinal cord. As a result, they arise in the periventricular area, as intramedullary spinal cord tumors, and in the filum terminale. Approximately 60% of intracranial ependymomas are infratentorial and 40% are supratentorial.[300] The most frequent location is in the fourth ventricle (Fig. 121.11). Tumor extension through the foramina of Luschka or Magendie into the basal cisterns is common. Other locations include the walls of the lateral and third ventricles. Half of supratentorial ependymomas are intraventricular and half are parenchymal, likely arising from embryonic ependymal rests retained within white matter.[3]

Grade 2 or differentiated ependymomas make up the majority. Rosette formation is a hallmark of ependymoma on pathologic examination. Less often, they may have grade 3 anaplastic features. The difference in prognosis between differentiated ependymomas and anaplastic ependymomas is not clear, and histologic features of malignancy do not always imply short survival. Individual ependymomas do not tend to

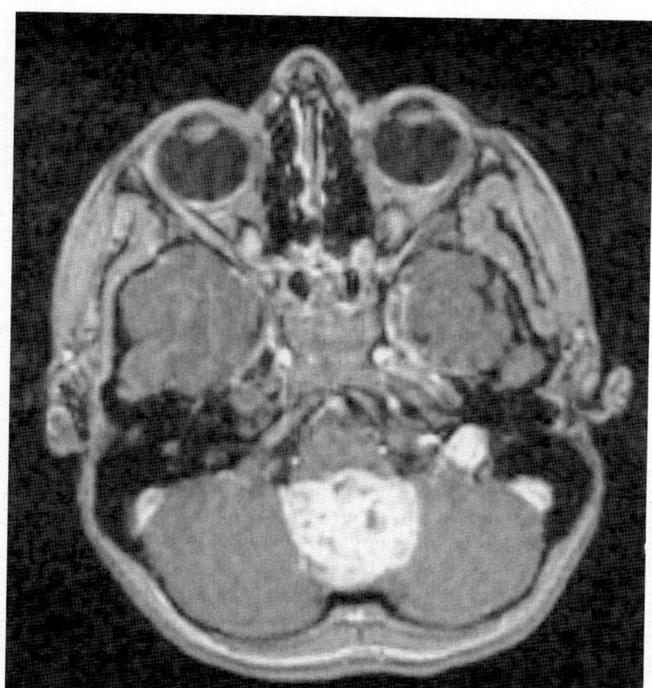

FIGURE 121.11 Typical magnetic resonance appearance of a posterior fossa ependymoma. The tumor arises from the floor of the fourth ventricle and rapidly expands to occupy it, compress the pons/medulla ventrally, and the vermis of the cerebellum dorsally. The enhancement is typically heterogenous.

progress from grade 2 to 3 as do other gliomas.[3] Seeding of CSF pathways has been reported to occur more frequently with anaplastic tumors and heralds a poorer prognosis.[301] Myxopapillary ependymomas generally arise in the conus, cauda equina, or filum terminale; they are considered grade 1, and resection is often curative.

Clinical presentation depends on location. Tumors with ventricular involvement often cause increased ICP and hydrocephalus by obstruction of CSF pathways. Headaches, nausea and vomiting, papilledema, ataxia, and vertigo are frequent. Focal neurologic signs and symptoms are seen with supratentorial ependymomas that involve the parenchyma. The presence of calcification in a fourth ventricular tumor on CT is very suggestive of an ependymoma. Supratentorial parenchymal tumors cannot be readily distinguished from other gliomas by imaging. For anaplastic ependymomas, a staging spinal MRI with gadolinium and CSF cytologic examination are essential.

In a literature review, Vanuytsel and Brada[302] found that the overall incidence of spinal seeding in ependymomas was 6.9%. Infratentorial lesions were more likely to seed (9.7%) than were supratentorial lesions (only 1.6%), and anaplastic ependymomas seeded at a higher rate (8.4%) than low-grade tumors (4.5%). In total, 15.7% of those with high-grade infratentorial tumors developed spinal dissemination, whereas none with supratentorial anaplastic lesions did. For low-grade tumors, 2.7% of supratentorial lesions showed seeding compared with 5.5% of infratentorial lesions. Spinal seeding was directly related to local progression, regardless of tumor grade. The incidence of spinal dissemination was 3.3% in patients with locally controlled primary lesions and 9.5% in those with uncontrolled primary lesions.

Ependymoblastomas, an aggressive subtype of embryonal cell neoplasm, are distinct from anaplastic ependymomas. They tend to disseminate throughout the neuraxis, and inclusion of these tumors in series evaluating leptomeningeal spread of ependymomas tends to overestimate the risk of seeding.[301,303]

Subependymomas are benign tumors with an admixture of fibrillary subependymal astrocytes. They are distinct from subependymal giant cell astrocytomas, which occur in the lateral ventricles in tuberous sclerosis. Subependymomas occur most often in the floor or walls of the fourth ventricle in older men. Most are asymptomatic and slow growing, and treatment is rarely needed except for hydrocephalus or demonstrated growth. They are often incidentally found at autopsy.

Surgery

Several retrospective studies support the relationship between postsurgical residual ependymoma and a poorer outcome, and therefore maximal safe resection is the goal.[304–306] Ependymomas arising from the floor of the fourth ventricle are approached through a bilateral suboccipital craniectomy and laminectomy of C1. The inferior subarachnoid space is occluded to minimize the possibility of CSF dissemination of tumor cells to the spine. The tumor is exposed by retracting the cerebellar tonsils laterally and splitting the inferior vermis or by opening the cerebellomedullary fissure on one or both sides. Often a tongue of tumor is visible over the dorsal aspect of the medulla and upper cervical spinal cord before the tonsils are retracted. The dorsal tumor surface is seen as the vermis is divided, and its attachment to the floor of the fourth ventricle can then be exposed and evaluated. Firm attachment precludes complete removal because the floor of the fourth ventricle must be carefully protected from injury. Tumor is removed to the extent possible using illumination and magnification afforded by the operating microscope. Residual tumor is often simply amputated flush with the floor. These tumors may also extend through the foramen of Luschka, entangling the cranial nerves in the basal cisterns, which also precludes a complete resection. The less common supratentorial tumors are removed as with any glioma. Avoidance of bleeding into the ventricular system is important to prevent postoperative hydrocephalus.

Radiation Therapy

No definitive trials exist to make absolute recommendations regarding postoperative radiotherapy. Postoperative irradiation improves the recurrence-free survival of patients with intracranial ependymomas, and 5-year survival rates with doses of 45 Gy or more range from 40% to 87%.[307]

Historically, for posterior fossa tumors, the entire craniospinal axis and later the entire posterior fossa has been irradiated.[308] Modern series document that local recurrence is the primary pattern of failure and that the incidence of isolated spinal relapses is low even among the highest-risk patients, with the majority of spinal failures associated with local recurrences.[303,309] Paulino[310] has shown that the pattern of failure is predominantly local. In nine patients who received radiation therapy to the tumor bed plus a 2-cm margin, the two failures in this group were within the tumor bed, and there were no failures within the posterior fossa outside the tumor bed. For most patients, a more usual volume now consists of the tumor bed and any residual disease plus an anatomically defined margin of 1 to 1.5 cm to create a CTV. Larger margins may be required in areas of infiltration, and special attention must be paid to areas of spread along the cervical spine since 10% to 30% of fourth ventricular tumors extend down through the foramen magnum to the upper cervical spine.[311,312] Patients with neuraxis spread (positive MRI or positive CSF cytology) should receive craniospinal irradiation (40 to 45 Gy) with boosts to the areas of gross disease and to the primary tumor to total doses of 50 to 54 Gy.

Craniospinal irradiation for low-grade, nondisseminated ependymomas has largely been abandoned in the United States.

In their literature review, Vanuytsel and Brada[302] found that risk of seeding was independent of whether prophylactic spinal irradiation was given. For high-grade lesions, spinal dissemination occurred in 9.4% of patients who received craniospinal axis irradiation (CSI) and in 6.7% of those treated with local radiation therapy only. Similarly, for low-grade tumors, spinal seeding occurred in 9.3% after craniospinal irradiation, whereas 2.2% developed seeding without prophylactic treatment.

The treatment volumes recommended for low-grade supratentorial ependymomas vary from generous local fields to fields encompassing the whole brain, whereas for low-grade infratentorial tumors they include local fields, the whole brain with cervical spine extension, and the craniospinal axis. Wallner et al.[312] reviewed data for 20 patients with supratentorial and infratentorial low-grade ependymomas treated with partial or whole-brain postoperative irradiation. Of 16 patients, only 1, who was eventually found to have a local recurrence, developed spinal dissemination. The 5- and 10-year survival rates for those who received greater than 45 Gy were 67% and 57%, respectively. Because local failure dominated the recurrence patterns, whole-brain treatment was thought unnecessary. Based on this series and others, low-grade supratentorial ependymomas are treated using partial brain fields with a dose of approximately 54 Gy. Low-grade infratentorial ependymomas are also treated using limited fields. The craniospinal axis is irradiated only if pretreatment CSF cytologic studies reveal malignant cells or if radiographic studies show evidence of tumor spread.

Rogers et al.[313] studied outcomes in 45 patients with nondisseminated posterior fossa ependymomas (low grade in 43) who underwent either gross total resection (n = 32) or subtotal resection (n = 13) with or without subsequent radiation therapy (median = 54 Gy). The 10-year actuarial local control rate was 100% for patients who underwent gross total resection and radiotherapy, 50% for those who underwent gross total resection alone, and 36% for those who underwent both subtotal resection and radiotherapy. The 10-year overall survival rate was superior in patients who underwent both gross total resection and radiotherapy: 83% compared with 67% in those who underwent gross total resection alone and 43% in those who underwent both subtotal resection and radiotherapy. In their smaller series, Massimino et al.[314] recommended adjuvant radiotherapy after gross total resection of ependymomas especially with posterior fossa tumors.

Some authors recommend CSI in the treatment of anaplastic ependymomas, whereas others recommend only whole-brain irradiation with a boost to the tumor for supratentorial lesions located away from the CSF pathways.[302,303,308,312] A dose of 54 Gy is given to the primary tumor and 36 Gy to the remainder of the axis if CSI is to be given. If spread within the brain is demonstrated, the entire brain receives 45 to 54 Gy, based on age. Spinal imaging studies are routinely performed, and areas of gross involvement are boosted to 50 Gy. Local recurrence is the primary pattern of failure with high-grade ependymomas.[302,303,308,312] Subarachnoid seeding is uncommon in the absence of local recurrence. Furthermore, the patterns of failure are similar in patients treated with local fields or with CSI, and prophylactic treatment may not prevent spinal metastases. In one series of 28 patients with anaplastic ependymomas, 12 received CSI, 2 received treatment to the whole brain, and 14 received treatment to limited fields.[315] Actuarial 5- and 10-year survival rates were 56% and 38%, respectively. All 19 radiotherapy failures were local, and in one of these cases CSF seeding also developed. A benefit from CSI could not be demonstrated. Based on these and other data, CSI is generally not recommended for patients with anaplastic (high-grade) ependymomas unless CSF seeding is pathologically or radiographically documented. Prophylactic CSI for patients with infratentorial high-grade lesions is still advocated by some.[316]

Clinical trials are examining more aggressive local therapies to improve local control in ependymoma. In a recent trial, 3DCRT was employed in localized ependymoma to reduce treatment volume. Eighty-eight patients were treated to 59.4 Gy, targeting only the resection bed and a modest margin, and the 3-year local failure rate was under 15%. These patients also underwent neurocognitive evaluation, and with 24-month follow-up, no major deficits were identified.[317,318]

Chemotherapy

There is no evidence that chemotherapy improves survival in these cases.[319] The CCG tested carboplatin and found a response plus stable disease rate of 28%.[320] In a CCG evaluation of cisplatin, the overall median time to progression was only 3.8 months.[321] A small trial of etoposide in ten adult patients with recurrent spinal cord ependymoma showed a 20% response rate, a median time to progression of 15 months, and overall survival of 17.5 months.[322] A multicenter trial conducted by the French Society of Pediatric Oncology used alternating courses of three different regimens (procarbazine plus carboplatin, etoposide plus cisplatin, vincristine plus cyclophosphamide) as adjuvant postsurgical treatment in 72 children younger than 5 years of age. Forty percent of patients were spared radiotherapy 2 years after treatment and 23% at 4 years after treatment. Chemotherapy has a potential role in deferring radiotherapy, although patients spared radiation with this strategy might also have been progression free with surgery alone, especially because no chemotherapy responses were seen in patients with measurable disease after surgery.[323] Thus, to date, few if any drugs have shown even modest consistent activity in ependymomas.

Although, a complete removal of the ependymoma has a positive impact on the outcome, a complete resection is achieved in only 40% to 60% of cases.[324,325] Responsiveness to preirradiation chemotherapy was therefore investigated in a Children's Oncology Group (COG) study. Garvin et al.[326] reported an objective response rate of 58% to preirradiation chemotherapy, consisting of cisplatin, etoposide, cyclophosphamide, and vincristine, in children with incompletely resected ependymoma. The 3-year event-free survival in patients assigned to preirradiation chemotherapy because of incomplete resection was 58% and was comparable to those who had a complete resection and were assigned to irradiation alone. However, 15% of the children who received preirradiation chemotherapy experienced progression prior to radiation therapy. Therefore, a subsequent COG study was carried out that aimed to decrease the progression rate prior to radiotherapy by employing a strategy of "second-look" surgery following the preirradiation chemotherapy in children with residual disease. In this study, patients who had a complete resection of a differentiated supratentorial ependymoma were observed without any further therapy. The results of this study are pending. The recently opened randomized COG study is exploring whether maintenance chemotherapy following radiation will improve event-free and overall survival.

The primary application of chemotherapy, therefore, is investigational and it is within the realm of neoadjuvant therapy to improve respectability as primary adjuvant therapy in young children to delay radiotherapy and as possible salvage. In the Baby Pediatric Oncology Group study a 48% response rate was reported to two cycles of vincristine and cyclophosphamide in 25 children younger than 3 years of age with ependymoma, allowing a delay in radiotherapy by 1 year without impacting the outcome.[327] However, the use of chemotherapy to delay radiotherapy has to be approached cautiously. In a trial of 34 patients with anaplastic ependymoma, 25 patients relapsed relatively rapidly and only 3 patients who did not receive radiotherapy survived.[328]

Despite multimodal therapy, 50% of the patients with ependymoma will experience a relapse. The majority of the recurrences are local, and prognosis is poor after relapse.[329] Resection, reirradiation, and chemotherapy are the common treatment modalities for relapsed ependymoma. Various antineoplastic agents such as etoposide, cyclophosphamide, temozolomide, cisplatin, and irinotecan have failed to improve survival in these patients.[286,330,331] Novel therapies to target molecular pathways are currently under investigation. Coexpression of ERBB2 and ERBB4 has been described in over 75% of pediatric ependymoma and impacts prognosis. Consequently, inhibitors of ERBB are being evaluated in both pediatric and adult patients with recurrent ependymoma.[332] As in other malignant glioma, tumor vasculature represents an attractive target.[333] Agents that directly inhibit or indirectly dysregulate this target (bevacizumab, ZD6474, metronomic therapy) are being examined.[334] In a study reported by Kiernan et al.,[335] three of the five patients with recurrent ependymoma were alive at 2.5 years after treatment with a metronomic regimen consisting of oral thalidomide and celecoxib with alternating oral etoposide and cyclophosphamide every 21 days for a 6-month period.

MENINGIOMAS

Clinical and Pathological Considerations

Meningiomas are believed to arise from epithelioid cells on the outer surface of arachnoid villi in the meninges, also known as *arachnoidal cap cells*. The most frequent locations are along the sagittal sinus and over the cerebral convexity (Fig. 121.12). Meningiomas are extra-axial, intracranial, and sometimes intradural, extramedullary spinal tumors that produce symptoms and signs through compression of adjacent brain tissue and cranial nerves. They often also produce hyperostosis; bony invasion does not indicate malignancy. They rarely metastasize except after multiple resections when they may spread to the lung, where growth is typically slow.

The WHO updated its grading criteria recently, categorizing this tumor into three grades.[336] Benign (WHO grade I) meningiomas comprise about 70%to 85% of intracranial primaries. With appropriate treatment, approximately 80% of WHO grade I meningiomas remain progression-free at 10 or more years.[337] Atypical (WHO grade II) meningiomas account for 15% to 25% of patients. These have greater proliferative capacity, and a seven- to eightfold increased recurrence risk within 5 years.[338] Only about 35% patients with WHO grade II meningiomas remain disease-free at 10 years. About 1% to 3% of intracranial meningiomas are anaplastic (WHO grade III). These aggressive malignant tumors have a median overall survival of less than 2 years.[337]

Surgery

The goal is total resection, including a dural margin, because this is often curative for WHO grade I tumors. The risks of resection must be balanced against the advantages of less-aggressive removal because these tumors are typically slow-growing, and the patients are sometimes elderly. Observation is appropriate

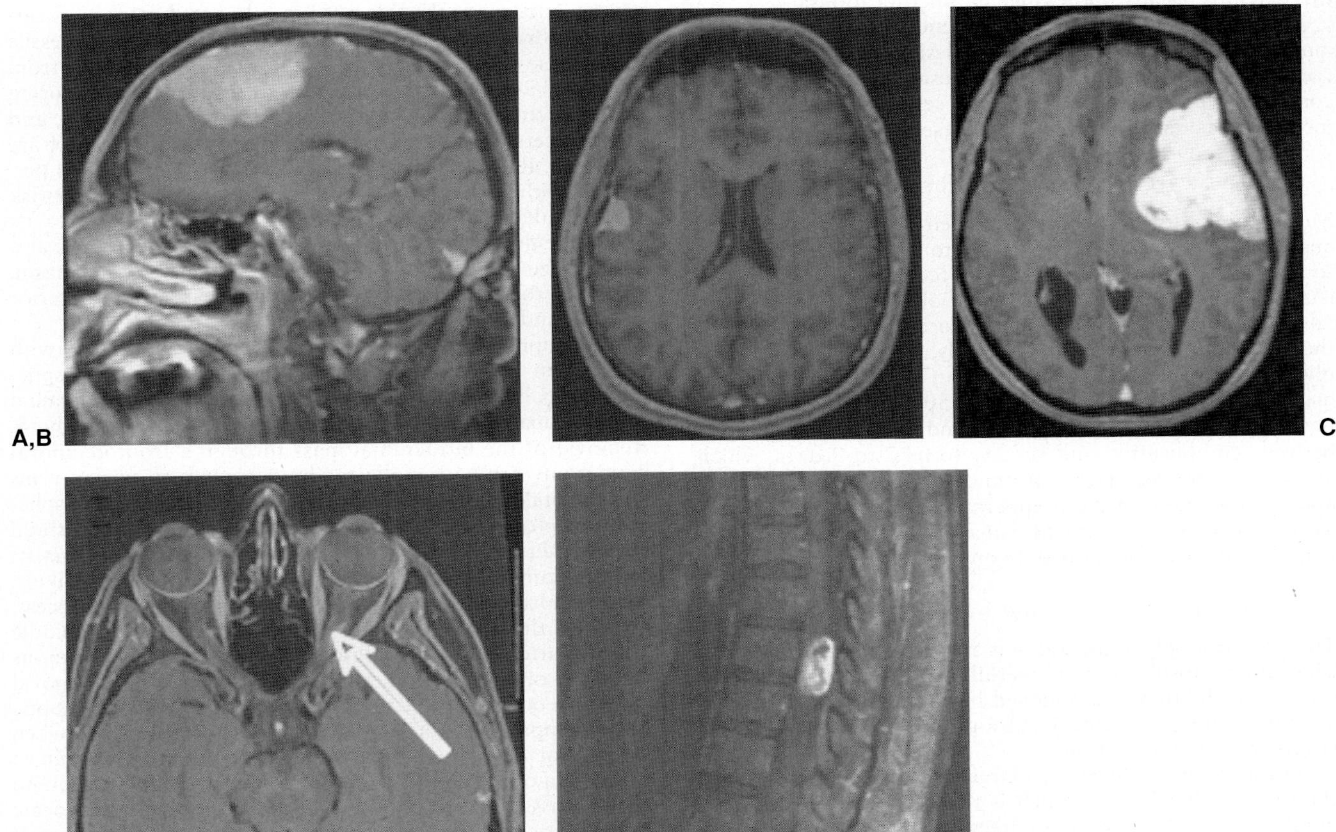

FIGURE 121.12 These five images show various appearances of meningioma. The most common location is parasagittal (**A**). Some meningiomas remain small (**B**), whereas others achieve a massive size with midline shift (**C**). An optic nerve meningioma (*arrow*) is illustrated in (**D**), whereas spinal locations are also possible (**E**).

for some, especially small tumors that are incidentally discovered. In a series of 603 patients who had asymptomatic meningiomas that were treated conservatively, Yano and Kuratsu[339] found that approximately 63% exhibited no growth, and only 6% ultimately experienced symptoms.

Simpson Grades of Resection

The completeness of surgical removal is a crucial prognostic factor, and historically, the definitions provided by Donald Simpson have served as a useful guideline.[340] By following 470 patients during a 26-year span, he described five "grades of resection," based on recurrence. Grade 5 resection refers to a biopsy only and is associated with near-universal progression. A partial tumor resection is labeled Simpson grade 4 and is associated with a recurrence rate of 44%. A Simpson grade 3 resection refers to gross total resection of the tumor, without addressing hyperostotic bone or dural attachments, and is associated with a 29% rate of relapse. A Simpson grade 2 resection includes gross tumor removal, and the dural attachments are either removed or coagulated and the relapse rate drops to 19%; and finally, when hyperostotic bone is also removed for a Simpson grade 1 resection, the relapse rate is 9%.

This definition has subsequently been expanded to include a category referred to as grade 0 resection. Kinjo et al.[341] reported on 37 convexity meningioma patients who underwent gross total resection of the tumor, any hyperostotic bone, and all involved dura with a 2-cm dural margin, and observed no local recurrences, with over half of the patients followed beyond 5 years; this is now widely termed the grade 0 resection. However, apart from convexity primaries, resection to this extent is usually not feasible in other locations.

The likelihood of gross total resection varies considerably among primary sites, with convexity lesions most amenable to complete resection and skull-base lesions least likely to be completely resected. In most surgical series, at least a third of meningiomas reported are not fully resectable.[342]

Preoperative Planning

Meningioma surgery requires a detailed knowledge of surgical anatomy. A preoperative angiogram to assess vascularity and to identify or embolize surgically inaccessible feeding arteries is sometimes indicated. Typically, embolization is done within 24 to 96 hours of surgery so that collateral vascular supply to the tumor does not develop. Normally, only the vascular supply from the external carotid artery can be embolized safely. In meningiomas that receive more than 50% of their blood supply from this artery, Kai et al.[343] found the optimum interval between embolization and surgery to be 7 to 9 days, which allowed the greatest degree of tumor softening. For convexity and parafalcine tumors, preoperative imaging may be performed to allow use of a neuronavigation system to aid in planning the scalp incision and bony opening.

Surgical Principles and Impact of Location

The arterial supply to the tumor is addressed first, if accessible. The tumor capsule is then carefully dissected, as the central portion of the tumor is removed by the use of an ultrasonic aspirator, an electrocautery cutting loop, scissors or bipolar electrocautery, and suction.

At the cerebral convexity, a large bone flap is made around the tumor's dural base, which is then circumscribed with a dural incision. Microdissection frees the tumor from surrounding brain as the tumor is lifted away. Overlying hyperostotic bone, which contains tumor cells, can be replaced with a cranioplasty. This results in a Simpson grade 1 or 0 resection, and these tumors rarely recur.

Parasagittal meningiomas abut the midline. Critical draining veins from adjacent brain, invasion or occlusion of the sagittal sinus by the tumor, and massive overlying bony erosion or hyperostosis are the surgical challenges. Preoperative vascular imaging defines sagittal sinus patency and relations between cerebral veins and the tumor. A patent sagittal sinus cannot be transected except in its anterior one-third. Further posteriorly, the involved sagittal sinus may be opened to remove tumor within, or the involved sinus wall may be resected and replaced by a graft. Sindou and Alvernia[344] achieved gross total resection in 93% of instances in 100 consecutive patients, with meningiomas arising primarily in the superior sagittal sinus. The overall recurrence rate was 4%, with a mean follow-up period of 8 years. Use of sinus reconstruction with wall and lumen invasion led to significantly less clinical deterioration after surgery relative to the subgroup not undergoing venous repair, leading them to conclude that venous flow restoration is justified when not too risky. Because recurrence-free survival after subtotal resection of these lesions can be lengthy and because residual tumor may grow to occlude the sinus completely, which makes complete resection possible later with a lesser risk, subtotal resection is also an option.[342,345] Alternatively, residual tumor within the sagittal sinus can be treated in a delayed manner with the use of stereotactic radiosurgery.[346]

Falx meningiomas do not involve the sagittal sinus but occupy the falx below, often becoming bilateral. Surgical interruption of adjacent cerebral veins can cause cerebral edema and venous infarction. Overzealous retraction of the adjacent brain to provide a surgical access corridor can also cause postoperative neurologic deficits.

Olfactory groove meningiomas typically grow extremely large before personality change or headache leads to their discovery. Anosmia is the rule but is rarely noted. Surgery is carried out through a large bifrontal exposure. The broad sessile tumor base is divided first to interrupt feeding arteries from the skull base. The tumor is then debulked by internal coring and dissection, while the optic nerves, carotid arteries, and anterior cerebral arteries on the tumor's posterior aspect are protected. Reconstruction of the skull-base dura is often performed with a vascularized pericranial graft to reduce the risk of CSF leakage into the frontal and ethmoid sinuses.

Tuberculum sellae meningiomas become symptomatic at a smaller size through compression of optic nerves and chiasm. Attention to the safety of the optic apparatus and the anterior cerebral and carotid arteries is axiomatic.

The approach to sphenoid ridge meningiomas varies with their origin on the lateral, middle, or medial third of the sphenoid bone. Lateral-third tumors can present as an intracranial tumor, as massive temporal bone hyperostosis, or often as both. Removal of the intracranial mass through a frontotemporal craniotomy can be complicated by adherence to sylvian veins and the middle cerebral artery. Bony hyperostosis of the sphenoid wing can cause proptosis, requiring removal and orbital reconstruction. Middle-third tumors grow intracranially. Surgical cure through a frontotemporal craniotomy is likely. Medial-third tumors arise from the anterior clinoid process, compress the optic nerve, and encase the carotid and middle cerebral arteries. They can grow diffusely into the cavernous sinus and optic canal and even the orbit proper. Total removal is feasible only when the tumor presents early, because of optic nerve compression; for larger tumors, the surgeon stops when the risk of further removal exceeds the potential benefit.[347] Many tumors occupy the cavernous sinus with little or no tumor mass in the temporal fossa itself. Few surgeons advocate radical resection for these lesions; they may be observed or, if growing or symptomatic, treated with radiosurgery or FSRT.

Cerebellopontine angle meningiomas arise from the petrous bone and if small and laterally situated are exposed through a posterior fossa craniectomy, with the cerebellum retracted

TABLE 121.10

RECURRENCE AFTER GROSS TOTAL RESECTION ALONE OF MENINGIOMA

Study (Ref.)	No. of Patients	Local Recurrence Rate (%)		
		5-Y	10-Y	15-Y
Mirimanoff et al. (342)	145	7	20	32
Stafford et al. (351)	465	12	25	—
Condra et al. (349)	175	7	20	24
Total	785	7–12	20–25	24–32

medially. Tumors arising more ventrally, from the petroclival junction or clivus, require a combined approach above and below the tentorium, which affords better exposure with less brain retraction.[348] Posterior fossa meningiomas may engulf critical blood vessels and cranial nerves and may adhere to the brainstem, so surgical removal must proceed cautiously.

Recurrence Following Resection

Gross total resection for benign meningiomas remains the preferred treatment and is generally considered definitive. Three large series with extended follow-up are available (Table 121.10). These have remarkably similar rates of local recurrence after gross-total resection: 7% to 12% at 5 years, 20% to 25% at 10 years, and 24% to 32% at 15 years.[342,349–351]

As expected, recurrence following subtotal resection is more frequent. Outcomes following subtotal resection alone, from four single institutions with up to 20 years of follow-up, are available. Collectively, the rates of progression following subtotal resection at 5, 10, and 15 years are 37% to 47%, 55% to 63%, and 74%, respectively.[342,349–351]

Radiation Therapy

Given the long natural history of meningiomas and the relatively late recurrences, radiotherapy has not been routinely adopted in the adjuvant context. Further, there is a paucity of clinical trials on which to base recommendations. However, in almost every retrospective series, cohort comparisons suggest that radiotherapy leads to a decrease in recurrence.

The need for adjunctive radiation therapy is determined by the extent of resection, tumor grade, patient age, and performance status. The risk of recurrence following resection has been outlined previously. In general, it is common practice to not use adjunctive radiotherapy after Simpson grade 0, 1, 2, and sometimes 3 resection for benign histology.

The risk of relapse after subtotal resection is high, as previously mentioned.[342,349–351] Several reports, now numbering more than 50, suggest that postoperative irradiation prolongs the time to recurrence. As an illustrative series, Barbaro et al.[352] compared 54 patients treated with subtotal resection and radiation therapy with 30 patients undergoing subtotal resection alone. The absolute rates of recurrence were 60% versus 32% in favor of radiotherapy, with the median recurrence times being 10.4 years for the irradiated patients and 5.5 years for the nonirradiated group. Goldsmith et al.[353] reported the results for 140 patients (117 with benign and 23 with malignant tumors) treated with subtotal resection and postoperative irradiation. For patients with benign meningiomas, the 5- and 10-year progression-free survival rates were 89% and 77%, respectively. Patients who received at least 52 Gy had a 20-year progression-free survival rate of greater than 90%. The 5-year progression-free survival of patients treated after 1980 was 98%, compared to 77% for those treated prior to 1980. This improvement was attributed to the availability of cross-sectional imaging for tumor localization and 3D treatment planning. Condra et al.[349] found that at 15 years, 70% of their patients had experienced relapse after subtotal excision alone, whereas only 13% of those treated with subtotal excision and postoperative irradiation experienced recurrence. The 15-year cause-specific survival rate was 86% for patients treated with adjuvant radiation, compared to 51% for nonirradiated patients. The actuarial relapse-free survival rates at 5, 10, and 15 years for patients undergoing subtotal resection and irradiation in another series were 78%, 67%, and 56%, respectively.[354]

The size of the residual tumor as well as grade affect the outcome after radiotherapy. Connell et al.[355] showed that for tumors 5 cm or larger, the 5-year progression-free survival rate was 40%, significantly lower than the 93% observed for smaller tumors. Among patients irradiated for unresectable tumors and in those with residual disease, the volume of visible tumor on imaging studies rarely decreases by more than 15% and often only after many years.

Radiation Therapy for Anaplastic and Malignant Meningioma

Atypical and malignant meningiomas behave more aggressively. Chan and Thompson[356] found that the median survival of six patients treated with surgery alone was only 7.2 months, compared with 5.1 years for 12 patients treated with surgery and postoperative irradiation. Six of the nine patients with malignant histology reported by Glaholm et al.[354] died within 5 years. Goldsmith et al.[353] reported a 5-year progression-free survival of 48% for 23 patients treated by subtotal resection and irradiation. The recurrence rate among 53 patients with malignant meningiomas collected from six series in the literature was 49%. The recurrence rates were 33% for patients treated with complete resection alone, 12% for those undergoing complete resection and radiation therapy, 55% for patients treated by subtotal resection and irradiation, and 100% for those treated by subtotal resection alone.[357] These and other data suggest that all patients with atypical and malignant meningiomas should be offered postoperative irradiation, regardless of the extent of resection.[358,359]

Primary Radiotherapy

Radiation therapy has been used as primary treatment following biopsy, or on the basis of imaging findings alone, in several small series. An early report from the Royal Marsden Hospital found 47% disease-free survivorship at 15 years in 32 patients.[354] In a recent series, Debus et al.[360] noted no recurrences in patients treated by radiotherapy alone (n = 59).

Optic nerve sheath meningiomas are rare tumors, generally not resected, but treated with radiotherapy as primary management. Narayan et al.[361] found no radiographic progression in any of 14 optic nerve sheath meningioma patients treated with conformal radiotherapy, with more than 5 years of median follow-up. In a study by Turbin et al.,[362] radiation therapy alone provided more favorable outcome than observation or surgery alone.

Radiation Dose and Volume Considerations

For benign meningiomas, the planning target volume consists of the residual tumor with a modest margin of normal tissue, defined by MRI and modified by the neurosurgeon's description of the site of residual disease. Extensive tumors of the base of the skull and malignant meningiomas require more generous margins, with special attention to dural extensions toward and through skull foramina. The preoperative tumor volume is used for planning for completely resected malignant lesions. A dose of 54 Gy in daily fractions of 1.8 Gy is recommended for benign meningiomas, and 60 Gy or higher for atypical and malignant tumors. Complex 3DCRT treatment planning and delivery techniques and IMRT are used to restrict the dose to normal tissues.

Radiosurgery

Numerous retrospective reports describe the use of radiosurgery for small meningiomas, either residual or progressive after resection, or untreated, skull-base lesions. Local control rates range from 75% to 100% at 5 to 10 years. Kondziolka et al.[363] found that 93% of their patients treated with radiosurgery and followed for 5 or more years required no further therapy. Nearly 85% of patients treated by Hakim et al.[364] were free of progression with a median follow-up of 22.9 months.

Pollock and Stafford[365] treated 49 patients with radiosurgery for cavernous sinus meningiomas. With mean follow-up of 58 months, no tumor enlarged, and event-free survival rates were 98%, 85%, and 80% at 1, 3, and 7 years, respectively. Zachenhofer et al.[366] treated 36 subtotally resected skull-base meningiomas with radiosurgery, and with a mean follow-up period of 8.5 years, the neurologic status improved in 44% of patients, remained stable in 52%, and deteriorated in 4%. In contrast, Couldwell et al.[367] reported 13 cases of skull-base meningiomas that progressed after radiosurgery, with some demonstrating rapid growth immediately after radiosurgery and others progressing up to 14 years later; the denominator for this series is ill-defined. They cautioned that regrowth can be aggressive and suggested careful extended follow-up.

Radiosurgery Complications

Cranial neuropathies, transient neurologic deficits, radiation necrosis, and significant edema have been reported in 6% to 42% of patients treated with radiosurgery.[368,369] Complications are more frequent in patients with large or deep-seated tumors and in those treated with high single doses.[363,370] Fractionated radiotherapy may be preferable for larger tumors.

Chemotherapy

There is currently no defined role for chemotherapy for newly diagnosed or nonirradiated meningiomas. Chemotherapy is generally reserved for recurrent meningioma not amenable to further surgery or radiotherapy. Responses are anecdotal, with no drug or combination yielding consistent responses. Because many meningiomas express estrogen and progesterone receptors, there have been unsuccessful attempts to use agents such as tamoxifen. Grunberg et al.[371] reported the use of mifepristone (RU-486), an antiprogesterone, in 14 patients with recurrent meningiomas. Five of 14 patients showed objective response after 6 or more months; a subsequent Southwest Oncology Group phase 3 trial of mifepristone for meningiomas showed no benefit.[372]

Preliminary data suggest that hydroxyurea may have activity.[373] Mason et al.[374] reported stabilization in 12 patients with unresectable or progressive meningiomas with a median duration of treatment of 122 weeks.

Kaba et al.[375] reported on six patients with either a recurrent malignant or an unresectable meningioma treated with interferon-alfa-2B. Five of six patients exhibited response, with stabilization in four and slight regression in one for 6 or more months. Targeted agents such as STI-571 (imatinib), angiogenesis inhibitors, and EGFR inhibitors have been evaluated, without clear efficacy.[376,377]

PRIMITIVE NEUROECTODERMAL OR EMBRYONAL CENTRAL NERVOUS SYSTEM NEOPLASMS

These tumors of putative embryonal origin predominantly arise in children and include supratentorial primitive neuroectodermal tumors (PNETs), pineoblastoma, medulloblastoma, ependymoblastoma, and atypical teratoid or rhabdoid tumors. They are characterized by sheets of small, round, blue cells with scant cytoplasm. Supratentorial PNETs, medulloblastomas, and pineoblastomas have a similar appearance with differentiation based on location, although there is accumulating evidence of different cytogenetics.[378] Historically, small round cell tumors arising in the posterior fossa were called *medulloblastomas*. Given the cytologic similarity between all these tumors regardless of location, it was suggested in the 1980s that they all be designated as PNETs. Although still controversial, the current WHO classification retains medulloblastoma as a distinct type of PNET within the larger group of "embryonal" tumors that includes medulloepithelioma, neuroblastoma, and ependymoblastoma. Pineoblastoma also retains a separate position within the category of pineal parenchymal tumors. Regardless of formal classification, these tumors are viewed as developmentally aberrant early neural (glial or neuronal or both) progenitor or stem cell neoplasms.

Supratentorial PNETs and medulloblastomas continue to be treated with similar regimens. The embryonal neoplasms are grouped together, given their tendency to spread within the neuraxis, infrequent extracranial dissemination, an aggressive natural history, and a treatment approach that combines aggressive resection, chemotherapy, and both local and craniospinal irradiation in noninfants. Most of the experience has been accumulated with medulloblastoma and extrapolated to the other tumors.

Medulloblastoma

Epidemiology

Medulloblastomas comprise 15% to 30% of CNS tumors in children and an estimated 350 to 400 cases are diagnosed in the United States annually. There is a 1.5:1 male-to-female predominance, and 70% are diagnosed by age 20. Medulloblastomas become progressively more rare with increasing age, with few cases found in those older than 50.[379,380] Gorlin and Turcot syndromes have increased rates of medulloblastoma, but account for only 1% to 2% of medulloblastomas.[21,381]

Pathology

Medulloblastomas classically have Homer-Wright (neuroblastic) rosettes, although these are found in less than 40% of the cases.[382] Mitoses are frequent, representing a high proliferative index. Immunohistochemical analysis is positive for synaptophysin, most prominent in nodules and within the centers of the Homer-Wright rosettes, correlating with a presumed neuronal progenitor origin.[383] According to the WHO classification, medulloblastomas are histologically grade IV and classified into five variants: classical, desmoplastic/nodular, medulloblastoma with extensive nodularity, anaplastic, and large cell.[29] The desmoplastic subtype has collagen bundles interspersed with the densely packed undifferentiated cells of the classic subtype as well as nodular, reticulin-free "pale islands," or follicles.[384] Inactivation mutations of the *PTCH* gene, the underlying genetic anomaly in Gorlin syndrome, are seen in the desmoplastic subtype, which is more common.[385] Medulloblastoma with extensive nodularity is similar to the desmoplastic variant except that the reticulin-free zones are large and rich in neuropillike tissue. Anaplastic medulloblastoma is relatively rare, accounting for approximately 4% of cases, and has marked nuclear pleomorphism, nuclear moulding, cell-cell wrapping, and high mitotic activity, with high degree of atypia. It has a high rate of amplification of the *myc* oncogene, a known negative prognostic factor, and correlates with a worse clinical outcome.[386–388] Gene expression profiles for medulloblastomas have been correlated with outcome independent of clinical factors.[389,390]

Radiographic and Clinical Features

Childhood medulloblastoma typically arises within the vermis, expanding into the fourth ventricle. In older patients, tumors in the lateral cerebellar hemispheres are more common (greater than 50% in adults compared with 10% in children).[379]

Clinical signs and symptoms depend on both age, with infants having less specific symptoms, and the anatomic location within posterior fossa. Midline tumors usually present with symptoms of increased intracranial pressure, including nocturnal or morning headaches, nausea and vomiting, irritability, and lethargy, manifestations of progressive hydrocephalus from fourth ventricle compression. Truncal ataxia may be present because of involvement of the vermis, and sixth nerve palsies are the most common nerve deficit. In younger children, bulging of open fontanelles may occur. Tumors of a lateral origin more frequently have ataxia and unilateral dysmetria. On CT, medulloblastomas are classically discrete vermian masses that are hyperattenuated compared with the adjacent brain and enhance avidly. Imaging variance is common with frequent cyst formation and calcification (59% and 22% of cases, respectively).[391] MRI is the gold standard. Medulloblastomas are typically iso- to hypointense on T1-weighted images, of variable signal intensity on T2-weighted images, and enhance heterogeneously.[392] MRI provides improved evaluation of foraminal extent beyond the fourth ventricle, invasion of the brainstem, and subarachnoid metastases. Diffusion-weighted images exhibit restriction, allowing PNETs to be distinguished from ependymomas.[393,394]

Staging and Risk Groups

A modified version of the Chang staging system is currently used.[395] T stage has been made less relevant than the extent of residual disease due to advances in neurosurgical techniques. M stage remains crucial. M0 represents no tumor dissemination, whereas M1 represents tumor cells in the CSF. M2 represents presence of gross tumor nodules in the intracranial, subarachnoid, or ventricular space, and M3 represents gross tumor nodules in the spinal subarachnoid space. M4 represents systemic metastasis.

Clinical staging requires the assessment of tumor dissemination and includes CSF cytologic examination. This is frequently not performed prior to surgery because of concern for cerebellar herniation from increased pressure within the posterior fossa. Ventricular fluid is not as sensitive as lumbar fluid in detecting dissemination within the neuraxis.[396] Negative CSF cytology does not preclude more advanced leptomeningeal disease.[397] MRI examination of the spine has supplanted conventional myelography. CSF dissemination is identified on MRI scans as diffuse enhancement of the thecal sac, nodular enhancement of the spinal cord or nerve roots, or nerve root clumping, predominantly seen along the posterior aspect of the spinal cord based on CSF circulatory patterns.[392] Spine MRI is ideally performed prior to surgery if medulloblastoma is suspected and the patient is stable; otherwise 10 to 14 days should elapse after surgery to avoid a potential false-positive interpretation from surgical cellular debris and blood products.[398] Metastases outside the CNS are less common and occur in less than 5% of patients and correlate with advanced disease within the neuraxis. Eighty percent of systemic metastases are osseous. A bone scan, chest x-ray, and bilateral marrow biopsies should be routinely performed for M2 and M3 stages.

Patients with medulloblastomas are currently classified as "average" or "high risk" based on age, M stage, extent of residual disease, and pathology. Average-risk patients have M0 stage arising within the posterior fossa, are more than 3 years old, and have less than 1.5-cm tumor residual. Due to the poor prognosis, all patients with anaplastic medulloblastoma are classified as high risk.[388,399] Patients less than 3 years old have particularly poor prognoses.[400] This may represent the presence of more primitive, aggressive tumors, but could also be due to the higher likelihood metastatic disease, subtotal resection, and reduced-dose or withholding of radiotherapy. Between 20% and 30% of patients present with neuraxial dissemination, most commonly along the spinal cord. The presence of metastatic disease is prognostically significant, with 5-year progression-free survival rates of 70% for M0 disease, to 57% for M1, and to 40% for M2 or higher in CCG-921.[400] The disease-free survival of high-risk patients treated with CSI with or without chemotherapy is 25% to 30%.[401] Average-risk patients have historically had a 5-year disease-free survival of 66% to 70%, which has increased to 70% to 80% in recent reports.[400,401]

Surgery

In one study, 3-year survival was reduced by 60% in patients who had incomplete resection of their primary tumor.[402] Although hydrocephalus associated with medulloblastoma obstructing the fourth ventricle can be relieved with a ventriculostomy, ICP may be controlled with corticosteroids, and in most patients aggressive tumor resection is sufficient to relieve hydrocephalus. An occipital burr hole is commonly placed at surgery, before the posterior fossa is exposed, to allow cannulation of the ventricles for drainage of CSF if needed to lower the increased ICP so the dura can be opened safely.

Surgery for medulloblastoma is usually carried out with the patient prone. The incision and bony exposure are usually in the midline, but a paramedian incision and unilateral bony removal are done when the tumor is limited to one hemisphere, particularly in adults. The more common midline craniotomy includes the ring of the foramen magnum, and a laminectomy of C1 (and rarely C2) is performed to decompress herniated cerebellar tonsils or to remove a caudally extending tongue of tumor.

After opening the dura, the cerebellar tonsils are retracted laterally. The tumor is usually first seen in the midline foramen of Magendie. The floor of the fourth ventricle is separated from the tumor by a cottonoid pledget, which is advanced to protect the floor as the tumor is resected. The thinned vermis is incised in the midline as the dorsum of the tumor is exposed. Alternatively, the naturally occurring corridor through the cerebellomedullary fissure between the tonsils and medulla is opened and exploited for exposure on one or both sides. The tumor is usually soft and moderately vascular and is readily removed under the operating microscope with suction or ultrasonic aspirator. Dissection is continued laterally to remove tumor from the cerebellar hemispheres and ventrally to remove tumor from the fourth ventricle.

When the obstructive hydrocephalus has been relieved, CSF can be seen flowing from the aqueduct of Sylvius. Watertight closure is obtained. Following surgery, gradual weaning of the ventriculostomy is attempted, with internalization 7 or more days after surgery, if clamping is untenable. Postoperative shunting for hydrocephalus is necessary in approximately 35% to 40% of patients because of scarring and decreased capacity to resorb CSF.[403] Patients who require long-term shunting are younger and have larger ventricles and more extensive tumor at presentation.[404] Concern has existed that a VP shunt may cause peritoneal seeding, but this has not been upheld.[405]

With advances in neurosurgical technique, the number of patients not undergoing a gross total or near-total resection is dwindling. MRI should be performed to evaluate the extent of residual disease within 48 to 72 hours following surgery to prevent postsurgical changes from influencing interpretation. Patients with either gross total resection or subtotal resection have better 5-year overall survival and posterior fossa local control rates than patients who undergo biopsy alone. Although retrospective data infer that a total resection is prognostically favorable, the majority of trials have found that patients who undergo substantial subtotal resection with minimal residual disease treated with both chemotherapy and radiation do just as well as those who undergo total resection.[406] This justifies opting for a near-total resection, particularly when there is invasion of the floor of the fourth ventricle or envelopment of cranial nerves or the posterior inferior cerebellar artery. It is clear, however, that the extent of resection does not impact survival in patients with disseminated disease.[406]

The value of an aggressive resection must be balanced against surgical complications, interchangeably referred to as *posterior fossa syndrome* or *cerebellar mutism syndrome*. These conditions consist of diminished speech and can include emotional lability, hypotonia, long-tract signs, bulbar dysfunction, decreased respiratory drive, urinary retention, and ataxia. These changes can be seen in up to 25% of patients who have undergone resection of a midline posterior fossa tumor.[407] Although thought to be a temporary, a significant number have persistent deficits.

Radiation Therapy

The aims of radiotherapy are to treat residual posterior fossa disease (or gross deposits of disease anywhere in the craniospinal axis) and treat microscopic disease in the craniospinal axis. Historically, CSI has been delivered to 36 Gy with a posterior fossa boost of 54 Gy using conventional fractionation of 1.8 Gy/d.[408] Radiation is typically initially withheld in patients younger than 3 years of age because of the higher risk of neurocognitive damage. Supratentorial PNETs and other embryonal tumors have been treated with the same CSI regimen, with a boost to the tumor bed and residual disease. Supratentorial PNETs treated with an appropriate dose and volume of radiotherapy were found to have a 49% progression-free survival at 3 years compared with 7% with major violations of radiotherapy.[409]

Various alterations to the radiotherapy regimen have been made endeavoring to limit late toxicities. Hyperfractionation has been examined, with one study showing no improvement in survival and an excess of failures outside the primary site, although this was likely attributable to a reduced craniospinal dose of 30 Gy.[410] A recent trial showed adequate disease-free survival with possible preservation of intellectual function with short follow-up.[411] IMRT has been used to provide radiation to the posterior fossa, with a 32% reduction in dose to the cochlear apparatus, reducing the risk of grade 3 or 4 hearing loss from 64% to 13%.[59] Improved imaging methods have allowed more precise delineation of tumor within the posterior fossa, providing the possibility of avoiding treatment to the entire posterior fossa with the boost dose. Although standard practice has been to boost the entire posterior fossa, retrospective data have shown isolated recurrences outside the tumor bed to be rare.[412,413] Encompassing the tumor bed and a 2-cm margin only for the boost led to less than 5% isolated posterior fossa recurrences.[414]

A combined CCG/Pediatric Oncology Group trial compared standard and reduced dose CSI (36 vs. 23.4 Gy) with a posterior fossa boost to 54 Gy in average-risk patients. All patients received concurrent vincristine during radiation with no adjuvant chemotherapy. Patients who received the lower dose had a higher rate of early relapse, lower 5-year event-free survival (67% vs. 52%), and lower overall survival.[415] Comparison of CSI doses of 35 versus 25 Gy in International Society of Paediatric Oncology (SIOP) II yielded similar results.[416]

Strong advocates for proton therapy have emerged as a result of the sharply diminished exit dose from spinal irradiation and the more conformal treatment of the posterior fossa. Dosimetric analysis that compared photons to protons has demonstrated a decrease in the dose to 50% of the heart volume from 72.2% to 0.5%, and the dose to the cochlea was reduced from 101.2% of the prescribed posterior fossa boost dose to 2.4%.[64] Proton-based radiotherapy also demonstrated decreased radiation dose to normal tissues compared with IMRT. However, this area remains controversial, as some recent analyses contend that the current generation of proton-beam machines might in fact pose a greater risk of second malignancies because of a higher rate of neutron production and contamination, which is more carcinogenic.[63]

Chemotherapy

Chemotherapy has been used in medulloblastoma with the dual goals of reducing radiation dose while maintaining optimal disease-free survival rates in average-risk patients and improving disease-free survival in high-risk patients.

Tait et al.[417] in SIOP I compared radiotherapy alone versus radiotherapy with concurrent vincristine followed by maintenance vincristine and CCNU. Overall, there was no survival benefit from chemotherapy, but unprespecified *post hoc* subgroup analysis identified subgroups that appeared to benefit from chemotherapy, including T3 or T4 disease, and subtotal resection. Similar results were seen in a CCG study.[401] The 5-year disease-free survival rates in the CCG and SIOP studies were 59% and 55%, respectively, for radiation therapy plus chemotherapy, and 50% and 43%, for radiation therapy alone. Based on these results, routine use of chemotherapy for "high"-risk medulloblastoma has become standard.

For "standard"-risk patients, chemotherapy has been postulated to lead to a reduction in the CSI dose necessary to control microscopic disease. A phase 2 trial of CCNU, vincristine, and cisplatin for eight cycles following the reduced CSI prescription of 23.4 Gy had a progression-free survival rate of 86% and 79% at 3 and 5 years, respectively.[415] This was superior to historical controls, and CSI to 23.4 Gy with chemotherapy was adopted as the standard of care and reference dose for further trials.

The most recent COG trial for average-risk patients compared cisplatin and vincristine with either CCNU or cyclophosphamide and 23.4 Gy CSI. No differences in outcome were noted, with a 5-year event-free and overall survival rates of 81% and 86%, respectively. The overall outcomes indirectly validated the use of reduced-dose CSI in conjunction with chemotherapy. The ongoing COG trial for average-risk patients is investigating a CSI dose of 18 Gy in patients between 3 to 7 years of age. The 2 × 2 randomization also compares boosting the entire posterior fossa versus a local boost.

Current approaches for high-risk medulloblastoma focus on chemotherapy dose intensification. Vincristine, CCNU, and prednisone had a 63% 5-year progression-free survival rate, better than an "8-in-1" chemotherapy regimen.[400] High-dose cyclophosphamide with autologous stem cell rescue is feasible and provided a 5-year event-free survival of 70% in patients with high-risk disease.[418] In a pilot study involving 57 children, the COG incorporated carboplatin as a radiosensitizer with CSI to 36 Gy and a posterior fossa boost followed by six cycles of maintenance cyclophosphamide, vincristine, and cisplatin. Four-year overall survival and progression-free survival rates were 81% and 66%, respectively, with an inferior outcome in patients with anaplastic medulloblastoma.[399]

The ongoing COG trial for high-risk medulloblastoma includes a randomization to full dose CSI with and without carboplatin followed by a second randomization to maintenance therapy with or without a proapoptotic agent, isotretinoin.

As the risk of cognitive deficits increases with decreasing patient age, extensive effort has been made to develop regimens that can delay or potentially eliminate the need for radiation in patients younger than 3 years of age. The avoidance of radiation has proved to be more feasible for patients with M0 disease.[419] Addition of intraventricular methotrexate following surgery in a five-drug chemotherapy regimen provided 5-year progression-free and overall survival rates of 58% and 66%, respectively.[402] Although asymptomatic leukoencephalopathy was detected by MRI and mean intelligence quotient (IQ) scores were lower than healthy controls, the mean IQ scores were significantly higher than previous cohorts who had received radiation. A prospective randomized trial of supratentorial PNETs in children younger than 3 years old treated with chemotherapy and omitted or delayed radiation yielded less promising results, with a progression-free and overall survival rates at 3 years of 15% and 17%, respectively. Administration of radiation was the only positive prognostic variable for progression-free and overall survival.[420] The Head Start I trial for young children with localized medulloblastoma consisted of five cycles of cisplatin, vincristine, etoposide, and cyclophosphamide followed by a single high-dose myeloablative chemotherapy regimen of thiotepa, carboplatin, and etoposide.[421] The 5-year survival was 79%. With the addition of methotrexate, children with disseminated disease had a 5-year progression-free survival of 45% and overall survival of 54%.[422]

Recurrent medulloblastomas is essentially an incurable and lethal disease. Although it is responsive to a variety of neoplastic agents, including vincristine, nitrosoureas, procarbazine, cyclophosphamide, etoposide, and cisplatin, with several regimens yielding relatively high response rates, durability is limited. A CCG trial to evaluate carboplatin, thiotepa, and etoposide with peripheral stem cell rescue showed 3-year event-free and overall survival of 34% and 46%, respectively.[418]

Long-term effects from treatment can be categorized as neurocognitive, neuropsychiatric, neuroendocrine, and growth retardation. Hypothalamic and pituitary endocrinopathies such as delayed hypothyroidism and decreased growth hormone secretion may occur. Growth retardation can also be secondary to delayed or reduced bone growth, leading to reduction in sitting height. Neurocognitive deficits have long been recognized secondary to surgery, radiotherapy, and chemotherapy. In one study, 58% of children showed an IQ above 80 at 5 years after treatment, but by 10 years after treatment, only 15% of the patients had an IQ that remained above 80.[423] A prospective study of cognitive function showed an average decline of 14 points in mean IQ, with an average decline of 25 points in patients younger than 7 years.[424] Even with risk-adapted radiation therapy patients had a significant yearly decrease in mean IQ, reading, spelling, and math.[425] Psychologic secondary effects are partially attributable to the diminished cognitive function as well as the social challenges caused by the physical manifestations of CSI (hearing loss, decreased truncal stature, and thin hair) and potential ataxia and abnormal speech patterns. Risk for secondary malignancies also exists. A population-based study tabulated a 5.4-fold increased rate of malignancy when compared with the general population, although this only affected 20 of 1,262 patients at risk.[426]

PINEAL REGION TUMORS AND GERM CELL TUMORS

Clinical and Pathological Considerations

Pineal and germ cell tumors account for less than 1% of intracranial tumors in adults and 3% to 8% of brain tumors in children.[427] Germinomas are the most common type, accounting for 33% to 50% of pineal tumors. The peak incidence of germ cell tumors is in the second decade, and few present after the third decade. Gliomas are the next most common pineal region tumor (approximately 25%). Pineal parenchymal tumors are nearly as common as glial tumors and are called *pineocytomas* if benign and *pineoblastomas* (a variant of PNET) if malignant; a rare intermediate form also exists.

Germ cell tumors commonly involve the two midline sites, suprasellar and pineal regions, and occasionally are found in other areas such as basal ganglia, ventricles, cerebral hemispheres, and spinal cord. Germinomas can occur bifocally or rarely even multifocally; the most common bifocal presentation is synchronous involvement of the suprasellar region and the pineal gland.[428] Based on histology and the presence of tumor markers in the serum or CSF, the WHO classification system divides intracranial germ cell tumors into germinomas and nongerminomatous germ cell tumors.[29] Nongerminomatous germ cell tumors are further divided into embryonal carcinoma, yolk sac tumor, choriocarcinoma, and teratoma (mature, immature or teratoma with malignant transformation). A quarter of the intracranial germ cell tumors have more than one histologic component and are known as mixed germ cell tumors. Alpha-fetoprotein (elevated in yolk sac tumors) and β-human chorionic gonadotropin (elevated in choriocarcinoma, and to a modest extent in germinoma) are generally secreted by these tumors. Mature teratomas do not have elevated tumor markers.

Neurologic signs and symptoms are caused by obstructive hydrocephalus and involvement of ocular pathways. Major symptoms are headache, nausea and vomiting, lethargy, and diplopia. Signs are primarily ocular but can include ataxia and hemiparesis. The major ocular manifestation is paralysis of conjugate upward gaze (Parinaud syndrome), but pupillary and convergence abnormalities are seen, as are skew deviation and papilledema. Some patients with pineal germ cell tumor can present with symptoms of diabetes insipidus (DI) without any radiological evidence of overt suprasellar disease.[429,430]

On CT, these lesions are hyperdense. On MRI the mass is hypointense on T2-weighted sequences (due to the high cellularity of the mass) and shows enhancement with gadolinium. Calcification and fat may be seen in teratomas or mixed malignant germ cell tumors. Germinomas tend to surround a calcified pineal gland, whereas pineal parenchymal tumors tend to disperse the calcification into multiple small foci. The potential for leptomeningeal dissemination requires imaging of the neuraxis before surgery. Determination of histology, tumor markers, and extent of disease is critical for optimal management of pineal region tumors. The prognosis varies depending on the histologic type, the size of the tumor, and the extent of disease at presentation.

Surgery

Because pineal tumors are near the center of the brain, they are among the most difficult brain tumors to remove. The application of modern surgical technology with superb illumination, magnification, surgical guidance, and neuroanesthesia has made this region much more accessible. Surgeons can choose from several approaches depending on preference and the tumor's position and extent.[431] The current recommendation is to obtain tissue when a diagnosis cannot be made from serum tumor markers, CSF tumor markers, cytologic examination, or both. Whenever possible the tumor is completely excised, except when a germinoma is found at open surgery; a biopsy suffices in this situation because germinomas respond well to radiation.[432] Resection is important when tumors are radioresistant or when excision may be curative (teratomas, arachnoid cysts, and pineal parenchymal tumors).

The most commonly used microsurgical approaches are the infratentorial supracerebellar approach, in which the surgical corridor is in the midline between the tentorium above and the superior surface of the cerebellum below, and the occipital transtentorial approach, under the occipital lobe and through an incision in the tentorium to reach the pineal region from above and to the side.[431] Both have been associated with low morbidity and mortality in experienced hands.

The place of stereotactic biopsy in the diagnosis of pineal region tumors is unclear. Although biopsies have been described as safe, particularly for large tumors, some avoid it because of the risk of damaging large veins that flank the pineal gland.[433] In addition, there is a risk that tissue sampling of these heterogeneous tumors may not depict the correct histologic nature of all parts of the tumor. Without an accurate diagnosis, treatment planning may be erroneous or inadequate. In favor of biopsy are the advantages of a rapid tissue diagnosis and shortened hospital stay. Transventricular endoscopic biopsy can also be performed, which reduces the risk of hemorrhage because the trajectory is mostly traversed under direct vision.

In patients with a pineal mass and obstructive hydrocephalus from blockage of the aqueduct of Sylvius, endoscopic surgery can play a special role. Through a frontal burr hole, the endoscope can be passed through the foramen of Monro into the third ventricle. An endoscopic third ventriculostomy is performed by making a fenestration in the floor of the third ventricle, which relieves hydrocephalus, and the mass in the posterior third ventricle can be viewed and biopsied through a flexible endoscope. A rigid endoscope can also be safely used by placing a second burr hole for the biopsy. CSF for cytology and marker studies can also be obtained and the walls of the third ventricle inspected for tumor studding. There is a small risk of intraventricular hemorrhage.[434]

Radiation Therapy

With certain exceptions, such as benign teratomas, radiation therapy has an established role in the curative treatment of pineal germ cell and parenchymal tumors. The location and infiltrative nature of these lesions often does not allow complete resection. In the past, the risk of biopsy or attempted resection often led to the use of radiation therapy without histologic confirmation. In such instances, response to low-dose radiation therapy, measurement of α-fetoprotein and human chorionic gonadotropin-β, and CSF cytology were used to provide diagnostic information. There is a tendency to increase the use of biopsy and resection, and treatment without histology is less common.

Five-year survival rates with radiation therapy range from 44% to 78% and vary with histology, extent of disease, age, radiation volume, and dose to the primary.[307] In a multi-institutional survey by Wara and Evans,[435] the survival of patients with pineal parenchymal cell tumors or malignant teratomas was 21% (3 of 14) compared with 72% (26 of 36) for those with germinomas. Wolden et al.[436] reported 5-year disease-free survival rates of 91% for germinomas, 63% for unbiopsied tumors, and 60% for nongerminomatous germ cell tumors irradiated to 50 to 54 Gy to the local site with or without treatment to the whole brain or ventricular system. Patients younger than 25 to 30 years old have survival rates of 65% to 80% compared with 35% to 40% for older patients. This may reflect the increased incidence of germinomas in younger patients.

Germinomas are infiltrative tumors that tend to spread along the ventricular walls or throughout the leptomeninges. The incidence of CSF seeding ranges from 7% to 12%. For this reason, fields encompassing the entire ventricular system, the whole brain, and even the entire craniospinal axis have been recommended. The appropriate treatment volume for pineal germinomas was evaluated by Haas-Kogan et al.[437] in 93 patients treated at the University of California–San Francisco (UCSF) or at Stanford. The UCSF group favored whole ventricular irradiation; the Stanford group included CSI. Five-year survival for the combined cohort was 93%, with no difference in survival or distant failure regardless of whether CSI or whole ventricular radiation was given. In some institutions, 25.5 Gy (1.5 Gy/d) whole-brain or whole-ventricular radiation is followed by a boost to the primary to 45 to 50 Gy. CSI is reserved for patients with disseminated disease at presentation.

Neoadjuvant chemotherapy and low-dose (30 to 40 Gy) focal irradiation is employed by some.[438,439] Chemotherapy might be useful in the young child to defer irradiation. For disseminated or multiple midline germinomas, systemic chemotherapy or CSI is given. CSI doses of 20 to 35 Gy have been used when CSF cytology results are positive. When response to primary chemotherapy is incomplete or the tumor recurs, salvage radiotherapy yields good results.[440]

Nongerminomatous malignant germ cell tumors, whether localized or disseminated, are treated with chemotherapy followed by restaging. After restaging, localized tumors receive focal radiation therapy to 54 to 60 Gy, and disseminated tumors receive CSI (54 to 60 Gy to the primary, 45 Gy to the ventricular system [controversial], 35 Gy to the spinal cord, and 45 Gy to localized cord lesions).[436] In a German study 63 supratentorial PNETs were treated with chemotherapy before or after radiation (35 Gy CSI with a boost to the primary of 54 Gy).[409] The 3-year survival was 49.3% in those for whom treatment was delivered as prescribed, but only 6.7% in those with major protocol violations. This indicates the importance of CSI in pineoblastoma, analogous to the situation with medulloblastoma.

Tumors that tend not to metastasize to the cord, such as teratomas, pineocytomas, and low-grade gliomas, are treated by resection, with localized radiotherapy reserved for patients with residual disease.[441] For selected patients with small residual disease, radiosurgery has been shown to be effective in terms of local control.

Chemotherapy

Chemotherapy for pineal glial neoplasms is similar to that for gliomas elsewhere. Germinomas are chemosensitive and responsive to cisplatin, carboplatin, ifosfamide, cyclophosphamide, bleomycin, and etoposide. Adjuvant multidrug therapy with radiotherapy has produced encouraging disease-free and overall survival. Newly diagnosed germinomas treated with two courses of high-dose cyclophosphamide showed a complete response rate of 91%.[442] Building on this, Allen et al.[443] reduced the radiation dose and volume. Of the ten patients with a complete response treated with reduced radiation, only 10% failed within 5 years. A comparable approach that used carboplatin produced an 88% response rate, and radiation dose was reduced in five of eight patients. Bouffet et al.[438] reported 3-year event-free survival of 96% in 57 patients with germinoma using four courses of alternating etoposide/carboplatin and etoposide/ifosfamide followed by 40 Gy localized radiation therapy for nondisseminated patients and CSI for those with dissemination. Despite reducing the dose of involved-field radiation to 24 Gy Aoyama et al.[444] achieved a 5-year overall survival of 100% and an event-free survival of 86% in patients with pure germinomas with addition of a few cycles of cisplatin-based induction chemotherapy. Similar results were seen in other trials where lower doses of irradiation (24 to 35 Gy) were combined with chemotherapy.[445,446]

Given the poor outcome of CNS nongerminomatous germ cell tumors after radiotherapy alone, there is significant interest in the use of chemotherapy. Balmaceda et al.[447] reported the results from using four cycles of carboplatin, etoposide, and bleomycin without radiation. Of 71 patients (45 germinoma and 26 nongerminomatous), 68 were assessable for response; after four cycles, the complete response rate was 57%. The 29 patients with less than a complete response received dose-intensified chemotherapy or surgery, and a further 16 achieved a complete response, for an overall complete response rate of 78%. Despite these high response rates, only 28 of 71 (39%) patients were alive and progression free within 31 months. Subsequently, they treated 20 patients with two cycles of cisplatin, etoposide, cyclophosphamide, and bleomycin, and the 16 patients achieving a complete response received two additional cycles of carboplatin, etoposide, and bleomycin.[448] Nine of the 14 survivors received radiation therapy. The chemotherapy response rate was 94%, 5-year overall survival was 75%, and 36% of patients were event free. Although the complete response rate was high, approximately half the patients developed recurrent disease, suggesting that a multimodal therapeutic approach of surgery, chemotherapy, and radiotherapy is necessary to improve the overall outcome of these tumors. Matsutani et al.[449] analyzed 153 germ cell tumors treated with surgery and radiation therapy with or without chemotherapy. The 10-year survival rates for mature and malignant teratoma were 92.9% and 70.7%, respectively. Patients with pure malignant germ cell tumors (embryonal carcinoma, yolk sac tumor, or choriocarcinoma) had a 3-year survival rate of 27.3%. The mixed tumors were divided into three subgroups: (1) mixed germinoma and teratoma; (2) mixed tumors whose predominant characteristics were germinoma or teratoma combined with some elements of pure malignant tumors; and (3) mixed tumors with predominantly pure malignant elements. The 3-year survival rates were 94.1%, 70.0%, and 9.3%, respectively, for the three groups.

High-dose chemotherapy with autologous stem cell rescue has been used for pineoblastoma.[450] Twelve patients were treated with induction chemotherapy followed by CSI with a pineal boost (36 Gy CSI, 59.4 Gy to primary), then with high-dose chemotherapy with stem cell support. Nine of the 12 patients remained disease free, including two infants who never received radiation. The actuarial 4-year progression-free and overall survivals were 69% and 71%, respectively. Although still considered investigational, the survival results are impressive. The use of high-dose chemotherapy and autologous bone marrow support has not been as promising for patients with recurrent tumors, although reported data are few.[450]

PITUITARY ADENOMAS

Clinical and Pathological Considerations

Pituitary tumors are identified incidentally or present through symptoms of local mass effect or as a result of endocrine effects. Pituitary adenomas almost always arise from the anterior pituitary, the adenohypophysis. The tumor initially compresses the gland and, subsequently, the optic chiasm and nerves. Tumors less than 10 mm, microadenomas, rarely compress the optic apparatus. Larger macroadenomas can involve the cavernous sinus bilaterally, the third ventricle (sometimes producing hydrocephalus), and, less commonly, the middle, anterior, or even posterior fossae. The classic ophthalmologic finding is visual loss, typically starting with bitemporal hemianopsia and loss of color discrimination. Automated visual field testing is more sensitive than simple confrontation. Occasionally, extraocular palsies can result from compression or invasion of the nerves in the cavernous sinus. Tumors that present with mass effect are often nonsecreting, but prolactin, growth hormone, thyrotropin, and gonadotropin-producing tumors may also present in this way.

Neuroendocrine abnormalities are usually from tumors that oversecrete hormones but can also result from compression of the pituitary gland and the stalk. The most commonly secreted hormones are prolactin, adrenocorticotropic hormone, or growth hormone. The incidence of the various types of adenoma is variable. In 800 patients operated on at UCSF between 1970 and 1981, 79% were endocrinologically active. Of these, 52% were prolactin secreting, 27% were growth hormone secreting, 20% were corticotropin secreting, and only 0.3% were thyroid-stimulating hormone secreting.[451] Sexual impotence in men and amenorrhea and galactorrhea in women are hallmarks of a prolactin-secreting tumor. Hypogonadism, infertility, and osteopenia are also common.[452] Growth hormone hypersecretion causes acromegaly or, in the rare patient with a tumor occurring before epiphyseal closure, gigantism. The secondary production of insulinlike growth factor-1 (IGF-1; primarily from the liver) or somatomedin C produces skeletal overgrowth changes (e.g., increased hand and foot size, macroglossia, frontal bossing). Soft tissue swelling, peripheral nerve entrapment syndromes, and arthropathies may occur. Hypertension, cardiomyopathy, diabetes, and an increased risk of colon cancer are prevalent with acromegaly. Adrenocorticotropic hormone hypersecretion by a pituitary tumor results in Cushing's disease, with weight gain, hypertension, striae, hyperglycemia, infertility, osteoporosis, increased skin pigmentation, and psychiatric symptoms. Rarely, pituitary adenomas can present acutely with headache, visual loss, and confusion, which can progress to obtundation. This potentially life-threatening condition is termed *pituitary apoplexy*. The etiology of apoplexy is thought to involve tumor infarction due to interruption of its blood supply, but the exact mechanism is not known. Symptomatic pituitary apoplexy is a surgical emergency and patients need to be carefully medically managed with judicious fluid and salt replacement and administration of high-dose corticosteroids. A need for prolonged hormone replacement therapy is often a consequence of apoplexy.

On MRI, pituitary microadenomas are generally seen within the gland according to the distribution of normal cells. For example, prolactinomas tend to be located laterally within the sella. Microadenomas show subtle hypointensity to the normal gland on T1-weighted sequences and are often more difficult to detect on T2 sequences.[453] Immediately after administration of contrast, adenomas show less enhancement than adjacent normal gland (Fig. 121.13). On delayed views, the tumor enhances more than the normal gland. Indentation of the sellar floor, stalk deviation, and mass effect on adjacent structures also provide evidence of the presence of tumor.

Surgery

There are two primary goals of surgery for macroadenomas: to decompress the visual pathways by reducing tumor bulk and, for secreting tumors, to normalize hypersecretion, with preservation of remaining normal pituitary function.

The standard surgical approach for the majority of pituitary tumors is transsphenoidal, which is safer and better tolerated than the transcranial (frontotemporal craniotomy) approach.[454–456] The transsphenoidal approach is used for microadenomas that occupy the sella turcica and for many macroadenomas. Image-guided neuronavigation and intraoperative fluoroscopy are essential to reduce the risk of injury to the carotid arteries. Even when the majority of tumor is actually suprasellar, transsphenoidal resection can be safely accomplished if the tumor consistency is soft (and tumor aspiration and curettage can thus easily be performed) and if the tumor is situated so that it can drop into the sella with progressive resection. Tough, fibrous suprasellar tumors and those that extend laterally into the middle fossa, anteriorly beneath the frontal lobes, or into the posterior fossa may require a craniotomy for

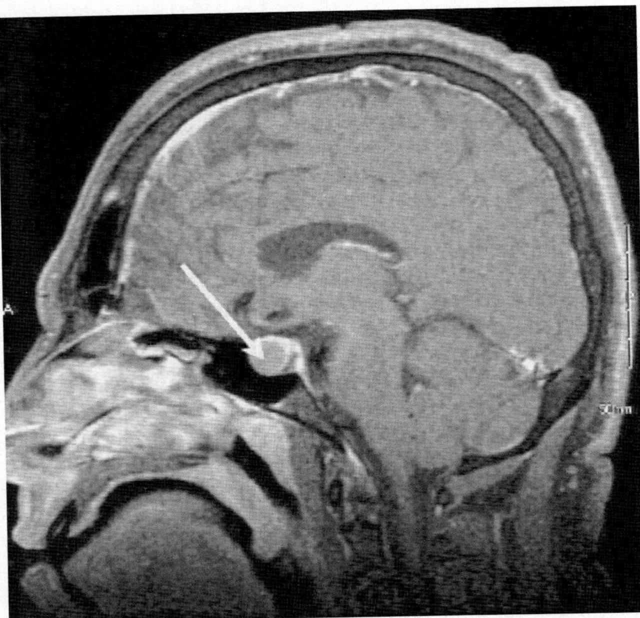

FIGURE 121.13 Pituitary adenomas are usually isointense to the gland on noncontrast T1-weighted magnetic resonance images; on contrast administration, the normal gland enhances early, as visualized on this sagittal image, whereas the adenoma (*arrow*) continues to remain unenhanced. With late imaging, the adenoma enhances.

resection.[457] Tumor that invades the cavernous sinus is generally not removed. The role of endoscopic transsphenoidal surgery for pituitary adenomas is currently being expanded. Potential advantages include a less-invasive surgical approach with a wider field of view and quicker postoperative recovery. Moreover, Cappabianca et al.[457] observed a decreased incidence of complications in a series of 146 consecutively treated patients who underwent an endoscopic endonasal transsphenoidal approach to the sellar region for resection of these tumors, compared with large historical series that employed the traditional microsurgical transsphenoidal approach.

Current surgical cure rates for hormonally active adenomas are 80% to 90% if there is no involvement of the cavernous sinus, suprasellar region, or clivus.[458] Patients with microadenomas have a higher surgical cure rate than patients with macroadenomas.[459] Patients cured of their endocrine disease can expect to have a normal lifespan; however, those with persistent endocrinopathies, and particularly those with acromegaly, may not enjoy a normal lifespan due to the impact of the high hormone levels on multiple organ systems.[458] In patients not biochemically cured with initial surgery, tumor is often found at the time of second surgery just next to the original site. Patients with persistent acromegaly, however, may not be amenable to biochemical cure with a second surgery as the residual growth hormone secreting cells can be difficult to visualize. Growth through the dura into the adjacent cavernous sinus is often found at repeat surgery even when no tumor is seen preoperatively on MRI.[460] Benveniste et al.[461] found that, although repeated transsphenoidal surgery to treat recurrent or residual tumor mass was associated with a 93% rate of clinical remission, its use to treat recurrent or persistent hormone hypersecretion produced only a 57% rate of initial endocrinological remission, with a 37% likelihood of sustaining such remission at a mean of 31 months. Thus, they suggested that for treatment of residual or recurrent adenomas that cause persistent or recurrent hormone hypersecretion, radiosurgery may be a better option.

Radiation Therapy

Radiation therapy may be indicated for hormone-secreting adenomas that are not surgically cured and are refractory to pharmacologic management. After subtotal resection of a macroadenoma, more than 50% of patients demonstrated radiographic evidence of progression during a 5-year period.[462] Younger patients (less than 50 years old) with residual disease have faster tumor regrowth than older counterparts. Ki-67 antigen labeling of more than 1.5% predicts more rapid growth of residual disease.[463] For these patients, immediate postoperative radiotherapy should be considered.

Radiation therapy decreases serum growth hormone concentrations to normal levels in 80% to 85% of acromegalic patients.[464] Growth hormone levels decrease at a rate of 10% to 30% per year, so several years may be required for the levels to normalize.[464] The probability of endocrine cure is highest for tumors with relatively low preradiation therapy growth hormone elevations (30 to 50 ng/mL); response is less reliable for tumors that produce higher growth hormone levels. In contrast, serum IGF-1 levels remain elevated after radiotherapy, and long-term treatment with somatostatin or its analogues may be required.[465,466] Radiation therapy controls hypercortisolism in 50% to 75% of adults and 80% of children with Cushing's disease. Response occurs within 6 to 9 months of treatment.[467]

Pituitary adenomas may be treated using several different techniques. The most commonly used techniques include 3DCRT, IMRT, and stereotactic radiotherapy. Treatment with charged-particle beams and radiosurgery is emerging.[468,469] The total dose used for nonfunctioning lesions is 45 to 50 Gy in 25 to 28 fractions of 1.8 Gy. Slightly higher total doses are recommended for secretory lesions. This controls tumor growth in 90% of cases at 10 years.[470–472] Radiation-induced injury to optic apparatus or adjacent brain with this dose-fractionation scheme is rare, whereas larger fractions or greater total doses lead to a higher incidence of injury. Hypopituitarism may develop, often years after radiation treatment.[472] It is more common in patients who have had both surgery and radiation therapy than in those treated with either modality alone. Hypopituitarism is largely correctable by hormone-replacement therapy, and patients treated for pituitary adenomas should have lifelong endocrine follow-up. One publication suggests that patients treated with surgery and radiation have an elevated risk for late cerebrovascular mortality.[473] Possible contributing factors include hypopituitarism, radiotherapy, and extent of initial surgery. The risk of developing a radiation-induced brain tumor after treatment is 1.3% to 2.7% at 10 years and 2.7% at 30 years.[473–475]

Radiosurgery is increasingly being used for treating small residual adenomas.[469,476] In general, patients are eligible for radiosurgery only if the superior extent of the lesions is more than 3 to 5 mm from the optic chiasm. Doses of more than 10 Gy in a single fraction to the optic pathways can cause visual loss.[477] Radiosurgery results in excellent tumor control and appears to cause more rapid biochemical normalization than is seen with conventional radiation therapy, with the caveat that it is used primarily for smaller tumors.[478] In a comparison of radiosurgery with fractionated radiotherapy, Landolt et al.[479] found the median time to normalize IGF-1 levels in acromegaly was 1.4 years after radiosurgery and 7.1 years after fractionated therapy. In a series of 67 patients treated with radiosurgery for growth hormone–producing pituitary adenomas, Kobayashi et al.[480] found that, although safe and effective tumor control was obtained, normalization of growth hormone and IGF-1 secretion was difficult to achieve in cases with large tumors and low-dose radiation. Losa et al.[481] found that radiosurgery was effective in controlling the growth of residual nonfunctioning pituitary adenomas after prior surgical debulking and that the risk of side effects with radiosurgery, especially of hypopituitarism, was lower compared with fractionated radiotherapy. Cranial nerve injury after radiosurgery is seen in fewer than 5% of the cases treated.[482]

Reirradiation can be considered for patients with recurrent pituitary adenomas when there has been a long interval after the first course of radiotherapy and other therapeutic methods have been unsuccessful. Schoenthaler et al.[483] reported the outcomes of 15 patients who were retreated (median dose, 42 Gy) after a median of 9 years from the initial course of radiation therapy (median dose, 40.8 Gy). At a median follow-up of 10 years, 80% of patients had local control. No visual complications were observed, but all patients developed hypopituitarism and two sustained temporal lobe injury.

Medical Therapy

Medical therapy is very important and effective for patients with secreting pituitary tumors.[484] Dopamine agonists (e.g., bromocriptine or cabergoline) are the most effective therapy for prolactinomas and are often used as primary treatment, with definitive treatment reserved for patients who either cannot tolerate or do not respond to a dopamine agonist. Somatostatin analogues (e.g., octreotide and lanreotide) are effective for patients with acromegaly and are usually reserved when there is persistent growth hormone hypersecretion after resection. Control rates with octreotide are approximately 50%; dopamine agonists can control growth hormone production in 10% to 34%.[485] A recently approved growth hormone receptor antagonist (pegvisomant) can be used for patients for whom somatostatin analogues fail. Rates of IGF-1 level normalization as high as 97% have been reported with this agent, but concerns persist that because it acts at the end-organ receptor level, tumor growth may continue in some patients, and the lifetime cost of the agent is prohibitive.[486] Medical therapy for patients with Cushing's disease is directed at the adrenal glands to reduce cortisol hypersecretion (ketoconazole). Unfortunately, no known drug effectively reduces pituitary corticotropin production.

CRANIOPHARYNGIOMAS

Clinical and Pathological Considerations

Craniopharyngiomas are the most common nonglial brain tumors in children, occurring primarily in the late first and second decades, although they can present at any age.[487] Craniopharyngiomas arise from epithelial cell rests that are remnants of Rathke's pouch at the juncture of the infundibular stalk and the pituitary gland. Most have a significant associated cystic component with only 10% being purely solid (Fig. 121.14). Most craniopharyngiomas become symptomatic because of effects of the combined tumor and cyst on the optic apparatus or hypothalamus or both. They may also compress the pituitary gland or extend superiorly into the third ventricle. Cyst fluid is proteinaceous, and this can be seen on MRI. CT shows calcification in 30% to 50% of cases.

Common presenting symptoms include headache, visual complaints, nausea, vomiting, and intellectual dysfunction (especially memory loss). Specific visual signs include optic atrophy, papilledema, hemianopsia, unilateral or total blindness, and diplopia with associated cranial nerve palsies. Endocrine abnormalities at presentation can include growth retardation, menstrual abnormalities, and disorders of sexual development or regression of secondary sexual characteristics (or both). Diabetes insipidus is uncommon at presentation.[488]

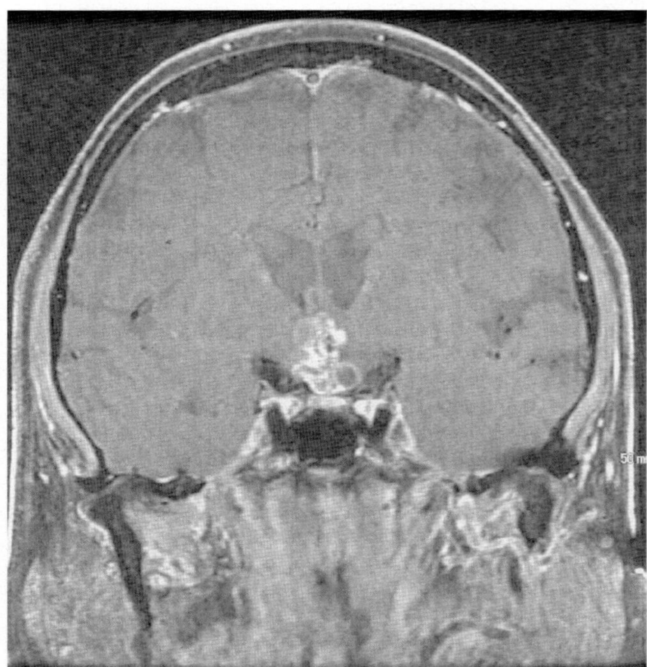

FIGURE 121.14 Craniopharyngiomas usually have both solid and cystic components, with significant suprasellar extension as visualized in this coronal postcontrast T1-weighted magnetic resonance imaging; the tumor shows typical enhancement in the solid portions.

Surgery

Craniopharyngiomas are generally resected using a microsurgical subfrontal or pterional approach. Larger tumors may require bifrontal or skull-base approaches, including supraorbital craniotomy. Endoscopically assisted surgery is sometimes used, although outcome advantages have not yet been clearly shown. In a series of 36 patients treated with radical resection for craniopharyngiomas using a combination of endoscopic-assisted and microsurgical techniques, all 27 patients who had no previous treatment developed diabetes insipidus, among minor neurologic deficits, with or without degrees of panhypopituitarism.[489] Although complete resection remains the optimal surgical goal, the risk of devastating long-term effects on hypothalamic function and quality of life cannot be ignored. In some cases, there is no clearly defined plane between tumor and surrounding hypothalamus, which makes aggressive resection dangerous. Aggressive removal is frequently associated with some injury to the pituitary stalk, with subsequent temporary or permanent diabetes insipidus and elements of hypopituitarism.[490,491] These patients require lifelong replacement hormones and inhaled desmopressin acetate spray for the control of diabetes insipidus. Most patients with preoperative visual loss can expect at least some improvement after surgery. The reported mortality rates for craniopharyngioma resection range from 2% to 43%, with severe morbidity in 12% to 61%.[492] Complications are less likely with experienced surgeons. Alternative approaches include placement of an Ommaya reservoir for largely cystic tumors through which one can instill sclerosing agents (e.g., bleomycin) or radioisotopes. There is also a developing interest in the use of radiosurgery, which may be associated with a lower risk of endocrinologic morbidity.

Radiation Therapy

Radioisotope Therapy

Predominantly cystic craniopharyngiomas can be treated with stereotactic or endoscopic instillation of colloidal therapeutic radioisotopes, particularly yttrium-90 or phosphorus-32.[490,493] The short penetrance of the beta-particles emitted by these isotopes allows the epithelial cells lining the cyst to be treated without significant dose to neighboring structures. Intracystic therapy may have a role in treating cysts that recur after conventional external-beam irradiation, or even as a primary cyst treatment. Although most cysts shrink with intracystic therapy, one-third of patients require further surgery later.

External-Beam Radiation Therapy

Numerous reports demonstrate that subtotal removal and irradiation produce local tumor control and survival rates comparable to those after radical excision.[494–496] The local control rates after complete resection, subtotal resection alone, and subtotal resection with postoperative irradiation are 70%, 26%, and 75%, respectively. A study at Children's Memorial Hospital in Chicago found 32% recurrence after complete resection and none after subtotal resection and adjuvant radiotherapy.[497] Ten-year survival rates range from 24% to 100% for complete resection, 31% to 52% for subtotal resection, 62% to 86% for incomplete resection and irradiation, and 100% after radiotherapy alone.[492,494,495,497,498] Patients who undergo conservative treatment, including biopsy and cyst drainage and irradiation, appear to enjoy a better quality of life and demonstrate less psychosocial impairment than those initially treated with more extensive resections.[494] Furthermore, conservative therapy is associated with less hypothalamic and pituitary dysfunction and a lower incidence of persistent diabetes insipidus than when a total or near-total excision is attempted. More extensive resections, using a subfrontal approach, may be associated with frontal lobe and visual perceptual dysfunction. The negative impact on IQ is greater in patients treated with aggressive resection than in those treated with conservative surgery and postoperative irradiation.[499]

The radiation treatment volume is based on CT and MRI scans, with relatively small margins. Generally, more sophisticated 3DCRT and IMRT approaches and stereotactic radiotherapy techniques are increasingly being used to spare surrounding normal tissues.[498] One report showed excellent tumor control (100%) with minimal late toxicity when FSRT (mean dose, 52.2 Gy in 29 fractions) was used.[500] No significant effect on cognition or visual injury was reported. The total dose is 50 to 55 Gy, given in daily 1.8-Gy increments. One review suggested better local control when doses of 55 Gy or more are delivered.[501]

Radiosurgery

The use of radiosurgery is limited by the proximity of most lesions to the optic chiasm and brainstem. In a long-term analysis by the Karolinska Hospital, 9 of 11 children treated (82%) ultimately experienced recurrence after radiosurgery.[502] This was thought to be due to the required low marginal dose of 6 Gy to parts of the tumor abutting the optic chiasm. These results suggest that radiosurgery plays a limited role in the treatment of most craniopharyngiomas and should be reserved for those uncommon tumors confined to the pituitary fossa and away from the chiasm and hypothalamus.[503]

Kobayashi et al.[504] reviewed long-term results (follow-up of 65.5 months) of radiosurgical treatment for residual or recurrent craniopharyngiomas after microsurgery in 98 consecutive patients and found only a 20.4% tumor progression rate. They used a tumor margin dose of 11.5 Gy at the retrochiasm and ventral stalk area, which decreased the rate of visual and pituitary function loss so that deterioration both in vision and endocrinological functions occurred in only six patients (6.1%). Similarly, Albright et al.[490] used radiosurgery as the initial treatment for the solid component of craniopharyngiomas in five children, limiting radiation to the optic chiasm to 8 Gy, and reported no operative morbidity or mortality, whereas 5 of 27 children who underwent microsurgical tumor resection suffered worsened vision postoperatively.

VESTIBULAR SCHWANNOMAS

Clinical and Pathological Considerations

Schwannomas, also known as *neurilemmomas* or *neurinomas*, are benign neoplasms derived from Schwann cells that show a predilection for sensory nerves. Most intracranial schwannomas arise from the vestibulocochlear nerve, with trigeminal nerves being a distant second in frequency. Previously called *acoustic neuromas*, these neoplasms are more correctly termed *vestibular schwannomas* as they arise from both the superior and inferior portions of the vestibular nerve rather than the cochlear nerve. Vestibular schwannomas are equally common between genders and median age at diagnosis is approximately 50, with an overall increased incidence between 45 and 64 years of age. Vestibular schwannomas account for approximately 6% to 8% of intracranial neoplasms. The incidence of vestibular schwannomas is between 0.8 and 1.7 per 100,000, with an increasing incidence since the early 1980s.[505,506] This increased incidence may represent the discovery of asymptomatic lesions by a rising number of cranial imaging studies, predominantly MRI. The rate of incidental vestibular schwannomas detected on MRI ranges from 0.02% to 0.07%.[507,508] More than 90% of vestibular schwannomas are sporadic and unilateral. Bilateral vestibular schwannoma is virtually pathognomonic for NF2 and is one of the key components of the Manchester criteria for the diagnosis of NF2.[509] When associated with NF2, vestibular schwannomas have a significantly earlier disease manifestation and tend to occur in the second or third decade of life.

Vestibular schwannomas arise along the zone of transition between the central and peripheral myelin located near the medial aperture of the internal auditory canal (IAC). Macroscopically, they are typically lobulated, with the eighth cranial nerve located eccentrically along the surface as these tumors grow in an expansile fashion, displacing rather than invading nerves. Vestibular schwannomas in NF2 tend to embed within the seventh and eighth cranial nerve bundles more frequently.[510] As with peripheral schwannomas, microscopic examination yields Antoni A and B tissue patterns. Vestibular schwannomas are benign, with few case reports of malignant dedifferentiation.

Although vestibular schwannomas arise from the vestibular portion of cranial nerve VIII, cochlear symptoms predominate, with the two most common being hearing loss and tinnitus.[511] Progressive unilateral sensorineural hearing loss is characteristic. Evaluation is typically delayed, with the duration of hypacusis averaging 3.7 years prior to diagnosis. Vertigo and unsteadiness are the most common vestibular symptoms. Facial nerve paresis or spasm may be seen. Large tumors can compress the trigeminal nerve, with paresthesias or neuralgia. Impingement of the brainstem or cerebellum may lead to ataxia and long-tract signs as well as involvement of the lower cranial nerves. Most ominous is the rare patient with nausea and vomiting from fourth ventricular compression and obstructive hydrocephalus.

MRI with thin-section, high-resolution, gadolinium-enhanced T1- and T2-weighted images of the cerebellopontine angle is the study of choice (Fig. 121.6). Vestibular schwannomas typically enhance along the course of the eighth cranial nerve with variable intra- and extracanalicular components. Cystic changes are frequently identified in larger lesions. MRI allows identification of the lesion and potential differentiation from other masses of the cerebellopontine angle such as meningiomas, epidermoid cysts, arachnoid cysts, and, rarely, lipomas. Auditory brainstem response audiometry is less sensitive than MRI.[512] Pure tone and speech audiometry continue to be performed to document hearing loss. Hearing loss is more pronounced at higher frequencies, and the degree of speech discrimination loss is disproportionately worse than the pure tone hearing loss.

Treatment

Treatment revolves around the dual goals of local control and cranial nerve function preservation. Factors that influence treatment choice include tumor size, location, patient age, the presence and degree of symptoms such as tinnitus and vertigo, whether a patient has NF2, the status of contralateral hearing, and patient preference. Consultation with a multidisciplinary team is essential.

Observation

Vestibular schwannomas are typically slow-growing, and various studies have shown an increase in size ranging from 0.35 to 2.2 mm/y (mean, 1.42 mm/y).[513] Chalabi et al.[514] reported that with mean follow-up of 4.2 years, 85% of observed vestibular schwannoma were noted to have exhibited measurable growth. Given the slow growth pattern and the recognition that neither surgery nor radiation therapy restore hearing lost to a vestibular schwannoma, and both pose risks to cranial nerve function, observation is a reasonable choice for some patients. Such an approach requires that the patient be willing to undergo regular annual or semiannual clinical and imaging follow-up. This course may be selected by many patients with small acoustic neuromas, particularly older patients and patients with multiple medical comorbidities. Patients with functional hearing must understand that further hearing loss, including sudden hearing loss, can occur while under observation.

Surgery

Surgery has the unique advantage of removal of the schwannoma, with a low risk of recurrence following complete resection. Microsurgical resection has been the mainstay of treatment for many years and was previously recommended as the standard of care in a 1991 consensus statement.[515] The three standard surgical approaches are translabyrinthine, middle cranial fossa, and retrosigmoid. The translabyrinthine approach uses a retroauricular excision and traverses the mastoid with removal of the petrous bone using a high-speed drill. The facial nerve is best visualized with this approach, being seen in the lateral IAC and separated from the tumor. The dura of the posterior fossa is then exposed and opened to remove the intradural tumor portion. Historically, this approach has sacrificed hearing due to destruction of the labyrinth. More recent techniques have allowed hearing preservation with a partial labyrinthectomy or avoidance of the bony labyrinth altogether.[516,517] The translabyrinthine approach is generally used when patients have significant ipsilateral hearing loss and the chance of maintaining usable hearing is low. A commonly used cutoff is less than 50 db speech reception and 50% speech discrimination.[518] The middle cranial fossa and retrosigmoid approaches both allow hearing preservation but suffer from poor visualization of small segments of the IAC.[519,520] These "blind spots" can be visualized by adding endoscopy to the microsurgical resection. The middle cranial fossa approach starts with a supra-auricular incision and temporal craniotomy. The middle fossa floor is exposed and drilled to reveal the IAC, which is opened for tumor removal. This approach is limited in the size of tumors that can be removed (15 to 20 mm) and retraction of the temporal lobe is also required. The retrosigmoid approach uses a unilateral posterior fossa craniectomy, dural opening, and medial retraction of the cerebellum to expose the cerebellopontine angle. The lower cranial nerves are protected while the IAC is unroofed with a drill. The approach offers the ability to resect all tumor sizes and potential functional preservation of all cranial nerves, including a slightly diminished risk of facial nerve injury compared to the middle cranial fossa approach.[521]

Surgical risks include the inherent risk of general anesthesia, CSF leak, meningitis, headache, hearing loss, and facial nerve paralysis. Hearing preservation is influenced by preoperative hearing acuity, location of the tumor, and size. Loss of facial nerve function is the most significant surgical concern, as well as morbidity. Again, tumor size is a factor, as is the relationship between the facial nerve and tumor. Surgery is made particularly challenging by the increased adherence and infiltration in NF2.[522] The risk of facial nerve injury has decreased since the advent of facial nerve electromyography for intraoperative monitoring. Auditory brainstem response may also be used to evaluate the integrity of the cochlear portion of the eighth cranial nerve intraoperatively, improving the odds of potential avoidance and preservation.

Most modern surgical series achieve complete resection in more than 90% of patients, with some reporting significantly higher rates.[511,523] Subtotal resections are frequently deliberate to preserve hearing or provide emergent, life-saving decompression of the brainstem and fourth ventricle. Results appear to be both surgeon- and volume-dependent, leading to questions of the widespread applicability of results obtained by subspecialty surgeons in academic institutions.[524] There also appears to be a significant learning curve of 20 to 60 patients with new surgical teams.[525,526] An extensive surgical series of 962 patients undergoing 1,000 vestibular schwannoma operations has been compiled by Samii and Matthies,[511] who reported a 98% complete resection rate with fewer than 1% of non-NF2 patients having a recurrence. The facial and cochlear nerves were preserved in 93% and 68% of patients, respectively, and functional preservation was 39% for patients with intact hearing preoperatively. Mortality was 1.1%, although this included several individuals who were disabled with advanced disease prior to surgery. If hearing is to be preserved, the auditory nerve is also identified and preserved; preservation of hearing is more likely in patients lacking severe adhesion in the interface between the cochlear nerve and the tumor.[527] Life-threatening complications of acoustic neuroma resections are rare except in patients with extremely large tumors.[528] The tendency of postoperative CSF leaks to develop in patients (10% to 13%) is independent of the surgical approach employed and tumor size and may stem from factors such as transient postoperative increases in CSF pressure.[529] Postoperative headache was a significant morbidity in a cohort of 1,657 patients who underwent surgery for acoustic neuroma.[530] Patients who underwent tumor resection by the retrosigmoid approach (82.3%) were significantly more likely to report their worst postoperative headache as "severe" than those resected using the translabyrinthine (75.2%) or middle fossa approaches (63.3%). In another quality-of-life study, hearing loss was perceived as the most disabling symptom among 386 patients who underwent acoustic neuroma surgery.[531]

Radiosurgery

The most substantial experience in radiation-based treatment is with SRS. Both Gamma Knife (Elekta Corp, Stockholm) units and SRS-compatible linear accelerators may be used to perform SRS. The University of Pittsburgh published a review of 162 consecutive patients treated with SRS to a mean dose of 16 Gy with a tumor control rate of 98%.[532] Subsequent surgical resection was required in four patients. Normal facial function was preserved in 79% and normal trigeminal function was preserved in 73% of patients. Because of the unacceptable cranial nerve morbidity in this and other series, the prescription dose for radiosurgery was lowered to 12 to 13 Gy. Results from the decreased prescription dose have a similarly low rate of recurrence, with 97% tumor control at a mean dose of 13 Gy.[533] The risk of facial nerve weakness dropped to 1% and hearing preservation improved to 71%. These results were confirmed with longer follow-up.[534] Recently, a prospective cohort study of 82 patients with unilateral vestibular schwannomas smaller than 3 cm compared surgery and SRS and provided level 2 evidence favoring SRS over microscopic surgical resection. Tumor control was not statistically different (100% for surgery vs. 96% for SRS). Normal facial movement and preservation of serviceable hearing was more frequent in the SRS group at all time points, and no quality-of-life decline was seen in the SRS group.[535]

New incomplete trigeminal and facial cranial neuropathies typically develop at approximately 6 or more months after radiosurgery. These tend to be mild and usually improve within a year after onset. Approximately half of patients with useful hearing before radiosurgery maintain their pretreatment hearing level, and hearing lost before treatment is not regained. The risk of treatment-induced cranial neuropathy is directly related to the volume of the lesion, the dose given, and the length of nerve irradiated.

Fractionated Radiation Therapy

Different fractionation regimens have been tried to capitalize on theoretical radiobiologic differences between the neoplastic vestibular schwannoma and surrounding normal tissue. Multiple fractions also allow treatment of lesions that would otherwise not be amenable to treatment with SRS based on size (more than 3 cm) or location (direct compression of the brainstem). Hypofractionation was examined in a series that compared 25 Gy in five fractions and 30 Gy in ten fractions. Actuarial hearing preservation rate was 90% at 2 years, and no recurrence or facial nerve weakness occurred.[536] A nonrandomized prospective trial from the Netherlands, however, had a nonstatistically inferior outcome in hearing preservation when comparing hypofractionation to SRS at 10 to 12 Gy.[537] Comparison of FSRT (50 Gy in 25 fractions) to SRS in a prospective trial showed comparable high control rates and minimal cranial nerve injury, with the exception of retention of useful hearing, which was 81% versus 33% at 1 year (in favor of FSRT) when followed by serial audiometry.[538] Similar rates of tumor control and hearing preservation have been reported by single-institution experiences elsewhere.[539–541] Koh et al.[540] treated 60 acoustic neuromas with FSRT and at a median follow-up of 31.5 months, the 5-year actuarial local tumor control rate was 96.2%, the overall hearing preservation rate was 77.3%, and there were no cases of new cranial nerve toxicity after treatment. FSRT appears to reduce cranial neuropathy rates compared to radiosurgery and allows treatment of larger tumors, but no randomized comparisons have been made.

Several issues confound radiation outcomes assessment for vestibular schwannoma. First, documentation of recurrences can be confounded by inherently slow growth rates and transient postprocedure lesion enlargement.[542,543] Second, ionizing radiation does carry a small inherent risk of inducing secondary neoplasms or malignant transformation of the vestibular schwannoma.[544,545] The risk of a secondary neoplasm can be particularly concerning in tumor-prone genetic conditions such as NF2. However, given the immense number of individuals who have undergone SRS worldwide, the number of presumed radiation-induced malignancies is only a handful and represents at most 1 per 1,000 patients. This is substantially lower than the rate of surgery-related mortality. Malignant transformation can also be seen in resected vestibular schwannoma patients who did not receive radiation.[546] Finally, because of increased adherence of the facial nerve to the tumor, eighth nerve preservation rates are lower when excision is performed for regrowth after radiation when compared to a nonirradiated control group.[547]

Targeted Therapy for Vestibular Schwannoma

There is significant interest in the development of medical therapy for patients with refractory vestibular schwannoma. Aberrant signaling pathways are known to be present, and there are now reports of the use of targeted agents in this disease. In a single patient case report, the EGFR inhibitor erlotinib was associated with radiographic response of the tumor and improved audiologic function.[548] There are also two reports of the use of bevacizumab in the treatment of vestibular schwannoma in the setting of NF1 in patients with a single hearing ear.[549,550] These studies consisted of a small number of patients, but the demonstration of objective regression of tumors and improvement in hearing was impressive, highlighting the need for larger prospective trials of antiangiogenic agents for this disease.

GLOMUS JUGULARE TUMORS

Clinical and Pathological Considerations

Glomus jugulare tumors (paragangliomas) arise from glomus tissue in the adventitia of the jugular bulb (glomus jugulare) or along Jacobson's nerve in the temporal bone, sometimes multifocally. The tumor invades the temporal bone diffusely, but growth is characteristically slow. Sometimes these tumors are endocrine active, with a carcinoid- or pheochromocytomalike syndrome.[551] Because glomus jugulare tumors occur in the jugular foramen, they commonly cause lower cranial nerve palsies and early symptoms of hoarseness and difficulty swallowing. Facial weakness, hearing loss, and atrophy of the tongue from hypoglossal palsy can follow. Pulsating tinnitus also may be a presenting symptom, and a red pulsating mass is often visible behind the eardrum. A presumptive diagnosis of glomus tumor can be made by CT or MRI scanning, with jugular schwannoma and meningioma being the main differential diagnoses. On CT scans, glomus tumors show a characteristic salt-and-pepper appearance in involved bone; MRI often discloses large blood vessels within the mass. Glomus tumors give positive results on octreotide scintigraphy. These tumors incite a tremendous blood supply, particularly by way of the ascending pharyngeal artery. Angiography provides the definitive diagnosis. Because preoperative tumor embolization is essential to surgical removal of glomus tumors, the diagnostic angiogram should be taken just before surgery. Histopathologically, numerous vascular channels are distinctive. The background is composed of clear cells clumped in a fibrous matrix. A small percentage of glomus tumors are malignant. There is a familial form in which the tumors are multiple.

Surgery

The treatment of glomus jugulare tumors is controversial, with advocates for surgery, radiation therapy, radiosurgery, and combined approaches. Although surgery can often provide a cure for these benign tumors, especially for small lesions, radiation therapy and radiosurgery avoid the morbidities that may follow surgical removal (lower cranial nerve and facial palsies). Surgery for glomus tumors is most often jointly performed by a neurosurgeon and an otorhinolaryngologist, after preoperative embolization, which may decrease intraoperative blood loss during resection of these extremely vascular tumors. Because these tumors often have intra- and extracranial components, surgery is usually conducted in two parts. The base of the skull in the region of the jugular foramen is first exposed, and neurovascular structures are identified and mobilized through a high transverse cervical incision. When the incision is extended behind the pinna and a mastoidectomy is completed, the facial nerve can be identified and protected, and the entire tumor bulb, jugular bulb, and internal jugular vein can be seen passing through the base of the skull. Finally, suboccipital craniectomy is performed, which allows the sigmoid sinus above and the jugular vein to be ligated, and the segment between them excised with the attached tumor. Complications of this procedure can include swallowing and aspiration problems, CSF leak, and facial palsy.

Liu et al.[552] have recently described a single-stage transjugular posterior infratemporal fossa approach that allows radical resection of glomus jugulare tumors that are located around the jugular foramen, the lower clivus, and the high cervical region from an anterior direction. This approach allows exposure of the infratemporal carotid artery without transection of the external ear canal, permanent rerouting of the facial nerve, or mandibular translocation, and avoids morbidity from these procedures.

Radiation Therapy

Even though glomus tumors are histologically benign, radiation therapy is effective and has been recommended for symptomatic lesions that cannot be totally resected, even as primary treatment.[553] These tumors regress slowly after irradiation, and the success of radiation therapy is measured by the amelioration of symptoms and the absence of disease progression. A review of the literature demonstrated local control rates with radiation in excess of 90% with or without surgery.[554] A dose of 45 to 50 Gy in 5 weeks is recommended.

Radiosurgery

A literature review by Gottfried et al.[555] showed that the use of SRS to treat glomus jugulare tumors has increased. Compared with conventional radiotherapy, radiosurgery involves a shorter treatment time, precise stereotactic localization, and irradiation of a small volume of normal tissue, which results in a reduced incidence of complications. Among 142 patients treated radiosurgically in eight series reviewed by Gottfried et al., tumors diminished in 36.5%, tumor size was unchanged in 61.3%, and subjective or objective improvements occurred in 39%. Although residual tumor was present in all of these patients, only 2.1% experienced progression, the morbidity rate was 8.5%, and no deaths occurred; however, the incidence of late recurrence is unknown. In another study of eight patients who underwent radiosurgery (median dose of 15 Gy to the tumor margin) for recurrent, residual, or unresectable glomus jugulare tumors, all remained stable without cranial nerve palsies at a median follow-up of 28 months.[556] The authors suggested treatment of small glomus tumors (3 cm or less in average dimension) with radiosurgery and treatment of young patients with large tumors (3 cm or more in average dimension) and patients with symptomatic tumors with surgical resection.

HEMANGIOBLASTOMAS

Clinical and Pathological Considerations

Hemangioblastomas account for 1% to 2% of intracranial tumors, arising most often in the cerebellar hemispheres and vermis. Although usually solitary, these tumors can be multiple and may also occur in the brainstem, spinal cord, and, less often, the cerebrum. Cerebellar hemangioblastoma can be sporadic or occur as part of the autosomal dominant von Hippel-Lindau complex, which is transmitted with more than 90% penetrance.[557] Other entities associated with von Hippel-Lindau disease are retinal angiomatosis, polycystic kidneys, pancreatic cysts, pheochromocytoma, and renal cell carcinoma. Identification of the *VHL* gene on chromosome band 3p25–26 allows individuals who are at risk for the syndrome, or who have some of its components as an apparent sporadic case, to undergo genetic testing with a high degree of accuracy.[558]

Cerebellar hemangioblastomas usually are recognized in the third decade in patients with von Hippel-Lindau disease and in the fourth decade or later in patients with sporadic tumors. These tumors can cause symptoms and signs of cerebellar dysfunction, especially gait disturbance and ataxia, and hydrocephalus from obstruction of CSF pathways. These tumors tend to enlarge slowly, but patients may become symptomatic from tumor cysts, which can grow quickly.[559]

Hemangioblastomas are composed of capillary and sinusoidal channels lined with endothelial cells. Interspersed are groups of polygonal stromal cells with lipid-laden cytoplasm and hyperchromatic nuclei. Immunohistochemical study of these cells shows expression of neuron-specific enolase, vimentin, and S100 protein but not epithelial membrane antigen or glial fibrillary acidic protein.[560] Grossly, the tumor is often cystic, containing proteinaceous, xanthochromic fluid, with an orange-red, vascular, firm mural nodule. The cyst wall is a glial nonneoplastic reaction to fluid secreted by the nodule. Some hemangioblastomas lack cysts, especially in the brainstem and spinal cord, but cystic lesions are more often symptomatic, at least in patients with von Hippel-Lindau disease.[559]

The natural history of spinal hemangioblastomas has been described.[559] The authors reviewed the clinical records and MRIs of 160 consecutively treated patients with 331 spinal hemangioblastomas. Most lesions were located in the posterior cord. Cysts were commonly associated with the lesions, often showing faster growth than the solid portion of the tumor. When symptoms appeared, the mass effect derived more from the cyst than from the tumor. These tumors often have alternating periods of tumor growth and stability, and some remain stable in size for many years. These factors have to be considered in the timing and choice of treatment.

Surgery

Complete resection of a hemangioblastoma is often curative. Patients with preoperative hypertension should be evaluated for the presence of a pheochromocytoma, which can be associated with von Hippel-Lindau disease. Hemangioblastomas are very vascular lesions, and biopsy of a suspected hemangioblastoma, either through an open approach or stereotactically, is usually ill advised because of the high risk of hemorrhage. Surgical resection should be carried out *en bloc* with avoidance of entry into the lesion, which can result in fierce bleeding reminiscent of that of an arteriovenous malformation. Embolization is rarely safe. Fortunately, these lesions can be resected with minimal bleeding if resection is carried out entirely in the gliotic plane that surrounds the mass. This is straightforward in most cerebellar tumors, for which a margin of gliotic tissue can be resected with the lesion with little neurologic risk. In contrast, brainstem hemangioblastomas are immediately adjacent to critical structures. Sometimes, dissection immediately adjacent to the tumor can cause significant bleeding, with a high risk of inducing neurologic deficits. A report of 12 patients with von Hippel-Lindau disease confirmed that brainstem hemangioblastomas can be safely resected in some instances.[561] In another study of 13 pediatric patients, successful surgical treatment of all patients, including 2 with brainstem tumors, was achieved. Morbidity was low and there were no recurrences during the follow-up period (mean, 24.6 months).[562]

These tumors are often associated with significant cysts. Surgery is the optimal treatment for rapid relief of mass effect. The cyst wall is not lined with tumor cells, and drainage, rather than excision of the cyst lining, is required. The mural tumor nodule must be entirely resected to avoid cyst recurrence. Cysts can be drained before opening the dura completely to provide brain relaxation, but great care must be taken not to disturb the tumor nodule during this maneuver to avoid inducing significant bleeding. The risk of hemorrhage during the resection is minimized by coagulating and dividing arterial feeders before tumor removal.

Finally, hemangioblastomas that occur in patients known to have von Hippel-Lindau disease need not be resected or otherwise treated unless they have demonstrated active growth or are symptomatic from mass effect or hydrocephalus. Because many of these patients harbor multiple tumors, other approaches, including radiosurgery, should also be considered, although surgery remains a viable option.

Radiation Therapy

Radiation therapy is recommended for patients with unresectable, incompletely excised, and recurrent hemangioblastomas and for those who are medically inoperable. Smalley et al.[563] reported outcomes of 25 patients treated with radiation therapy. Nineteen patients had gross residual disease after initial surgery or recurrent tumors; six had only microscopic disease. The overall 5-, 10-, and 15-year survival rates were 85%, 58%, and 58% and the recurrence-free survival rates were 76%, 52%, and 42%, respectively. In-field disease control rates were significantly higher in patients who received at least 50 Gy of radiation than in those who received lower doses. Based on these data, doses of at least 50 to 55 Gy in 5.5 to 6 weeks appear to be warranted. Because of the noninvasive nature of these lesions, conformal radiotherapy or radiosurgery is indicated.

Patrice et al.[564] summarized the outcomes for 38 lesions in 22 patients who received radiosurgery as definitive treatment or for recurrent tumors after surgery with or without conventional radiotherapy. The median tumor volume was 0.97 cc and the median radiation dose was 15.4 Gy. With a median follow-up time of 24.5 months, 31 of 36 evaluable tumors (86%), including all tumors treated definitively with radiosurgery, remained locally controlled. The five lesions that relapsed after radiosurgery had all been treated for recurrence after initial surgery. Better control rates were associated with higher doses and smaller tumor volumes. The 3-year actuarial progression-free survival rate was 86%. Of 29 hemangioblastomas treated by Chang et al.,[565] only one (3%) progressed. Jawahar et al.[566] reported treatment of 29 lesions in 27 patients. The actuarial control rate was 84.5% at 2 years and 75.2% at 5 years. In multivariate analysis, smaller tumor volume and higher dose (more than 18 Gy) were favorable. Radiosurgery should be considered for surgically unresectable hemangioblastomas, as adjuvant treatment for incompletely excised tumors, as definitive treatment for multifocal disease, and as salvage therapy for discrete recurrences after surgery.[564,565] Nevertheless, based on a series of 30 hemangioblastomas arising in 14 patients with von Hippel-Lindau disease, Rajamaran et al.[567] concluded that, although radiosurgery offered reasonable local control rates (reaching 83% at 6 years), the greater problem is the tendency for intracranial disease progression, the average time for this being 3 to 4 years (both before and after radiosurgery). To determine the effectiveness of radiosurgery for CNS hemangioblastomas, Asthagiri et al.[568] analyzed long-term results in von Hippel-Lindau disease patients treated with SRS. Patients were enrolled in a prospective von Hippel-Lindau disease natural history study, undergoing SRS treatment of CNS hemangioblastomas. Treatment regimens, serial clinical evaluations, and longitudinal imaging data were analyzed. Twenty von Hippel-Lindau disease patients (10 males and 10 females) underwent SRS treatment of 44 CNS hemangioblastomas (39 cerebellar and 5 brainstem), with a mean dose of 18.9 Gy. At a mean follow-up of 8.5 years, all patients were alive, and local control rates at 2, 5, 10, and 15 years after SRS were 91%, 83%, 61%, and 51%, respectively. Thirty-three percent of SRS-treated small (less than 1.0 cm diameter) asymptomatic tumors progressed over long-term follow-up. There were no long-term adverse radiation effects. Although SRS treatment of hemangioblastomas in von Hippel-Lindau disease has a low risk for adverse radiation effects, it is associated with diminishing control over a long-term follow-up. These results indicate that SRS should not be used to prophylactically treat asymptomatic tumors and should be reserved for the treatment of tumors that are not surgically resectable.

Because stromal cells in hemangioblastomas secrete VEGF, there is much interest in evaluating small-molecule inhibitors of the VEGF-2 (KDR, FLK-1) receptor as medical management for these tumors, especially for patients with von Hippel-Lindau disease, who routinely harbor multiple hemangioblastomas. Unfortunately, the extreme heterogeneity of tumor growth, with periods of spontaneous stability and a slow overall growth rate, makes it extremely difficult to design trials to test rigorously the efficacy of any systemic therapy.

CHORDOMAS AND CHONDROSARCOMAS

Chordomas and chondrosarcomas are rare, locally destructive, slow-growing, malignant bone tumors. Although skull-base chordomas and chondrosarcomas are sometimes pooled together, recent studies have shown important differences between these entities.

Clinical and Pathological Considerations

Chordomas arise within aberrant chordal vestiges along the pathway of the primitive notochord that extends from the tip of the dorsum sellae to the coccyx.[569] One-third of chordomas arise cranially, with this location more common in women and younger individuals.[570] Chordomas are extradural, pseudoencapsulated, multilobulated tumors, with a gelatinous consistency centered in the bone, classically with soft tissue extension. Microscopically, the typical chordoma is characterized by cord-like rows of "physaliferous" cells with multiple round, clear cytoplasmic vacuoles that impart a bubbly appearance to the cytoplasm. Two pathologic variants have been described. The *chondroid chordoma* has areas with cartilaginous features but a genetic profile distinct from chondrosarcomas.[571] The *dedifferentiated chordoma* contains areas of typical chordoma admixed with components that resemble high-grade or poorly differentiated spindle cell sarcoma. In typical chordomas, mitotic figures and atypia are rare; a higher mitotic rate and Ki-67 more than 6% are associated with a shorter doubling time.[572]

Chondrosarcomas are cartilage-producing neoplasm that arise within any of the complex synchondroses in the skull base, with the most common sites of origin being the temporo-occipital synchondrosis (66%), the spheno-occiput synchondrosis (28%), and the sphenoethmoid complex (6%).[573] Thus, chondrosarcomas predominantly originate in more lateral skull-base structures, unlike most chordomas, which originate in the midline. Chondrosarcomas can be difficult to differentiate from chordomas on pathologic examination. Immunohistochemical advances have improved differentiation between chordomas and chondrosarcomas. In one series of 200 chondrosarcomas, 99% stained positive for S100, 0% for keratin, and epithelial membrane antigen was expressed in 8%.[573] These immunohistochemical studies allow a chondrosarcoma to be differentiated from a chordoma, which is reactive for keratin and epithelial membrane antigen. The same series confirmed the low-grade nature of base of skull chondrosarcomas as a majority were grade 1, with no grade 3 tumors identified. Mesenchymal chondrosarcomas may have a separate, more aggressive natural history.[574]

Symptoms that prompt evaluation are typically cranial nerve deficits with the precise deficit dependent on the location and extent of the tumor. In one series, the most common presentation was headaches with intermittent abducens nerve palsy.[575] Additional symptoms can be caused by intracranial extension with compression of the brainstem, pituitary gland, or optic apparatus. Neck pain may develop in lower clival tumors, possibly the result of pathologic fracture or periosteal expansion.

The differential diagnosis of cranial chordoma and chondrosarcoma includes basal meningioma, schwannoma (neurilemoma), nasopharyngeal carcinoma, pituitary adenoma, and craniopharyngioma. Chondrosarcomas and chordomas cannot be reliably distinguished from each other based on imaging features or location alone.[576] High-resolution CT images with bone and soft tissue algorithms show a discrete, expansile soft tissue mass with extensive bony destruction.[577] On MRI scanning, both chordomas and chondrosarcomas are hyperintense on T2-weighted sequences, with variegated enhancement. The location may be useful in distinguishing chordomas (midline clivus) from chondrosarcomas (petrous apex), although there is considerable overlap. Given the low risk of nodal or hematogenous dissemination, imaging beyond the primary site other than a chest x-ray is typically not indicated unless metastatic disease is suspected clinically.[578] A baseline endocrine evaluation and neuro-ophthalmologic examination are both recommended if diagnostic imaging or symptoms suggest involvement.

Surgery

Surgery for cranial chordomas and chondrosarcomas provides the backbone of treatment and is obligatory to obtain diagnostic tissue, to enhance the effectiveness of subsequent radiation therapy, and to improve the patient's clinical condition. An aggressive initial approach may improve overall outcome.[579] Intracranial chordomas occur at the base of the skull, a region relatively remote from surgical access. Approaches to skull-base chordomas and chondrosarcomas often involve teams that include both neurosurgeons and otolaryngologists. For chordomas in the upper clivus that extend into the sella or sphenoid sinus, or both, a transseptal, transsphenoidal approach (as for pituitary tumors) is best. Large, compressive, transdural extensions of these upper clivus tumors into the interpeduncular cistern can be removed using a transcranial, subtemporal, intradural approach. For more lateralized upper clival tumors and some lateralized midclival tumors, an approach through a sphenoethmoidectomy (to which may be added a maxillectomy) is useful. For midline tumors of the midclivus and lower clivus, a transoral resection is often used. The palate or mandible and tongue can be split if upward or downward extension of the approach is necessary. There is developing interest in the use of endoscopy for primary removal of chordomas or to assist in the removal of these tumors via traditional open approaches. Although most series remain small, excellent results have been reported in appropriately selected patients not having extension lateral to the carotid arteries.[580,581] A combination of exposures and procedures can be used for extremely large tumors. One goal of surgery is to remove as much tumor from the optic system and brainstem as possible so that very high doses of radiation can be delivered safely. Optimal treatment of these lesions is complete resection, if possible.

A potentially serious complication of the transsphenoidal, transsphenothmoid, and transoral approaches is CSF leakage into the nose or oropharynx and consequent meningitis. Therefore, every attempt is made to keep the dura intact during these procedures. Because dural invasion by cranial chordomas may occur 50% of the time, dural entry during tumor resection is sometimes unavoidable. Careful intraoperative patching of the leak with fat and muscle grafts followed by postoperative spinal CSF drainage should be undertaken to decrease the risk of infection in these cases. This may be more challenging in the setting of a total endoscopic tumor removal, although some techniques appear to be associated with reasonably low rates of CSF leak. Surgical series have reported gross total resection rates of 43% to 72%, with the most recent series using modern imaging and microsurgical techniques reporting the highest gross total resection rate. In this series there was a 31% recurrence-free survival at 10 years, which was improved for those without previous intervention, and a 35% recurrence after gross total resection.[582,583] Extent of resection correlated with both recurrence rates and survival. Surgical morbidity can be significant, with Gay et al.[584] reporting a significant transient (53%) and permanent (43%) worsening of Karnofsky performance score following surgery.

Approaches for chondrosarcomas are different because of the paramedian location of the tumors. Like chordomas, chondrosarcomas begin as extradural tumors, and maintaining the intact dural barrier is paramount. Most commonly, a variation of the subtemporal middle fossa approach to the upper clivus is used to approach the petroclival synchondrosis. Extradural tumors can be removed through both the middle fossa and presigmoid avenues combined with a presigmoid and retrosigmoid approach. Complete tumor excision, which is paramount in chordoma surgery, is less critical for chondrosarcomas because tumor control rates with adjuvant high-dose radiation are high. Surgery is often tailored to emphasize removal of tumor portions abutting critical structures such as the chiasm or brainstem to allow adequate radiation treatment.

Cranial chordomas often recur after surgery and radiation therapy. In this situation, reoperation directed toward symptomatic improvement is the only treatment option. Reoperations are complicated by surgical scarring and tissue compromise from irradiation, and CSF leaks and other complications are more frequent.

Radiation Therapy

Radical excision with negative margins is often not feasible, and even gross excision is often obtained piecemeal with the risk of persistent microscopic disease. As relentless extension is typical of chordomas and chondrosarcomas and recurrence is a strong predictor of overall survival, adequate local control is paramount in determining outcome. Radiotherapy is a mainstay of treatment in preventing recurrence or progression of tumor.

Local control of chordomas appears to be dose dependent. Conventional radiation at doses of 50 to 55 Gy does not offer satisfactory local control. A median dose of 50 Gy to chordomas of the skull, sacrum, and mobile spine provided only a 27% local control rate with a median time to progression of 35 months.[578] Durable control was worse in base of skull disease, with only 1 of 13 clival chordomas remaining disease free. FSRT to 37 spheno-occipital chordomas to a mean dose of 66.6 Gy provided local control rates of 82% at 2 years and 50% at 5 years. Despite a median tumor volume of 55.6 cc, complications were limited with one patient developing a pontine infarct 25 months posttreatment. No instances of optic neuropathy were identified. Chondrosarcomas treated with the same fractionation scheme had 100% 5-year local control.[585]

Radiosurgery

SRS has been used to treat chordomas and chondrosarcomas of the skull base, although its application is limited because of size constraints and proximity to critical structures. In one series, candidates were limited to less than 3 cm in greatest diameter and 5 mm from the optic chiasm, with a mean treatment volume of 4.6 cc and a maximum volume of 10.3 cc.[586] With a mean margin dose of 18 Gy, more than 50% of patients in this mixed series of chondrosarcomas and chordomas had symptomatic improvement and, at a mean follow-up of 40 months, 20% had recurred locally outside the treatment field. Krishnan et al.[587] reported a similar local control rate (24%) with both in-field and out-of-field recurrences, although no recurrences occurred in patient with chondroid chordoma or chondrosarcomas. The risk of significant radiation-related complication was high at 34%, although complications were seen only in patients who had received prior fractionated radiotherapy.

Particle-Beam Therapy

Charged-particle therapy, because of its innate dose-distribution advantages, has been used for many years to escalate dose to chordomas and chondrosarcomas while minimizing radiation-related side effects. The most extensive experience in treating base of skull chordomas and chondrosarcomas with proton therapy arises from the experience at the Harvard Cyclotron Laboratory. Chordoma relapse-free survival was 59% at 4 years and 44% at 10 years, with similar rates seen in other series.[588–591] Mean dose ranged from 67 to 70.7 CGE (cobalt gray equivalent). Female gender, dose heterogeneity, large tumor size (more than 25 to 75 cc), brainstem invasion, and dose constrained by proximity to critical structures were all associated with higher rates of recurrence.[592] In a study of skull-base chordomas in 73 children and adolescents (mean age, 9.7 years), patients were treated with partial or gross surgical excision and postoperative proton beam irradiation.[589] The mean follow-up period was 7.25 years, and the overall patient survival rate was 81% among 42 patients with conventional chordomas, 17 with chondroid chordomas, and 14 with cellular chordomas, 6 of which were poorly differentiated and highly aggressive.

Chondrosarcomas of the skull base had remarkably high local control rates of 99% and 98% at 5 and 10 years, respectively. Pituitary dysfunction and hearing loss were the most common side effects, with depression, memory loss, temporal necrosis, hearing loss, and blindness being less common. Given the relative lack of morbidity and the suboptimal local control for chordomas, dose escalation has been proposed. Recent radiotherapeutic advances include spot-scanning proton radiation, which creates a near-monoenergetic Bragg peak and improved radiation dose falloff.[593] Carbon ion radiotherapy, charged-particle therapy using a heavier ion, has also been used with good local control with short follow-up and better than expected radiographic responses.[594] Amichetti et al.[595] recently conducted a systematic review of the scientific literature published between 1980 and 2008 on data regarding irradiation of chondrosarcoma of the skull base with proton therapy. From 49 reports retrieved, there were no prospective trials and 9 uncontrolled single-arm studies mainly related to advanced and frequently incompletely resected tumors. According to the inclusion criteria, only four articles, reporting the most recent updated results of the publishing institution, were included in the analysis, providing clinical outcomes for 254 patients. The major findings corroborated the high control rates with low morbidity described above.

CHOROID PLEXUS TUMORS

Clinical and Pathological Considerations

Primary tumors of the choroid plexus (CP) are classified according to the World Health Organization as CP papilloma (CPP, WHO grade I), atypical CPP (grade II), and choroid plexus carcinoma (CPC, grade III).[29] These are rare tumors that occur most often in children younger than 12 years of age. They appear irregular and lobulated, often very red because of underlying vasculature. Histopathologic examination of papilloma often shows apparently normal choroid plexus, with increased cellular crowding and elongation. Rarely, these tumors show malignant features such as increased cellularity, high mitotic activity, loss of typical cellular architecture, and invasion of the brain parenchyma, and are then classified as choroid plexus carcinoma. Bridging the CPP and CPC is the entity called atypical CPP. Histologically atypical CPP retains the architecture of the CPP but has high mitotic activity and an increase probability for recurrence after surgical resection.

CPC is commonly seen in families who carry a germline mutation in either the *TP53* gene (Li-Fraumeni syndrome) or *INI1* gene (rhabdoid predisposition syndrome).[596] However, most patients with CPP and sporadic CPC do not harbor a germ-line TP53 mutations.

In children, choroid plexus papillomas most often occur in the lateral ventricles. In adults, the fourth ventricular papilloma is most common. Third ventricle tumors are exceedingly rare. Because papillomas tend to grow slowly within ventricles, they expand to fill the ventricle and block CSF flow. In addition, papillomas can secrete CSF. Choroid plexus papillomas and carcinomas can produce hydrocephalus secondary to obstruction of the CSF, CSF overproduction by the tumor, or damage to the CSF resorptive bed from recurrent hemorrhages. As a result, increased ICP without focal findings is the most common presentation. Fourth ventricular tumors can also be associated with focal findings of ataxia and nystagmus. Although choroid plexus papillomas rarely seed throughout the CSF spaces, seeding from carcinomas is frequent and often symptomatic.

Choroid plexus tumors are seen easily by MRI. Imaging demonstrates a lobulated, well-circumscribed, enhancing, intraventricular lesion, often with associated hydrocephalus. Calcification is not common. Choroid carcinoma may show areas consistent with necrosis and brain invasion.[597] Staging of the craniospinal axis with brain and spinal MRI and CSF analysis is recommended for patients with choroid tumors with anaplastic features.

Surgery

The treatment of choroid plexus papillomas is total excision. Tumors in the lateral ventricle are approached through the ventricular trigone using a high parietal incision or a low temporal approach, depending on the degree of cortical mantle thinning and the location of the tumor. The predilection of these tumors for the left (usually dominant) side can make the approach worrisome. Hydrocephalus is the rule and simplifies the exposure once the ventricle is opened. Tumor associated branches of the choroidal vessels are coagulated and divided as early as is feasible in the procedure as this greatly reduces hemorrhage. Smaller tumors are removed intact and larger tumors piecemeal. Perioperative CSF drainage is used to prevent subdural hygromas. In half of patients, hydrocephalus is relieved by tumor resection, but persistent hydrocephalus requires shunting. Endoscopy is increasingly used for intraventricular surgery. A review of 75 cases treated between 1985 and 2000 showed 84% survival in patients who had complete resections, compared with 18% survival in those undergoing less than a gross resection.[598] This significant survival difference was seen regardless of adjuvant therapies. Unfortunately, total resection is not possible in many patients. The ability to perform a complete resection depends on histologic type, with nearly a 100% complete resection rate for papillomas versus only a 33% complete resection rate for choroid plexus carcinoma.[599] A meta-analysis of all individual cases of choroid plexus carcinoma reported as of 2004 (347 patients) showed that in the subgroup of incompletely resected carcinomas, 22.6% of patients required a second surgery.[600] The prognosis for these patients appeared better than for those with incomplete resections who did not undergo a second surgery (2-year overall survival times were 69% and 30%, respectively). Often, tumor hypervascularity is the limiting surgical factor, especially in infants, who have small total blood volumes. When carcinoma is suspected before surgery, the tumor can be embolized or neoadjuvant chemotherapy given to shrink it and reduce its vascularity, which facilitates resection.[601]

Radiation Therapy

Because choroid plexus papillomas are often cured by complete resection, radiotherapy is infrequently employed. Further, in a study of 41 patients, Krishnan et al.[602] noted that reoperation for recurrence was required only half the time after initial subtotal resection, suggesting that adjuvant radiotherapy may not be necessary after initial subtotal resection in all patients. Because local control outcome at first relapse was poor after subtotal resection, they concluded that the most reasonable role for radiation therapy is after subtotal resection of a recurrence.

Radiation therapy may be beneficial in some patients with choroid plexus carcinomas even after gross total resection.[603,604] A review of 566 choroid plexus tumors suggested that adjuvant radiotherapy increased survival in patients with choroid plexus carcinoma regardless of the extent of surgery.[605] All of the long-term survivors had complete resection and adjuvant radiation therapy. Another study analysed choroid plexus tumors in 64 patients and found 50% of the CPCs harbored TP53 mutation; 14 of the 16 patients who did not have mutated TP53 were long-term survivors after complete resection and no irradiation. The 5-year survival rate was 0% after resection and irradiation in patients whose tumors showed TP53 immunopositivity.[596]

Because CSF seeding occurs in up to 44% of cases, craniospinal axis irradiation has been proposed, although no significant studies support this practice.[606] Chow et al.[603] recommend that patients with completely excised localized choroid plexus carcinomas be treated with limited field irradiation if their spinal MRI and CSF cytologic study results are negative. They advised CSI for those with incompletely excised tumors or evidence of leptomeningeal spread.

Chemotherapy

Chemotherapy is not used for choroid plexus papillomas, although it has been attempted for choroid plexus carcinomas. As with many of the less-common CNS tumors, there are no firm guidelines. Anecdotal reports have cited moderate responses to the platinum compounds, as well as to alkylating agents, etoposide, methotrexate, and possibly anthracyclines. A Pediatric Oncology Group study of eight infants with choroid plexus carcinoma suggests that radiation can be forestalled by using chemotherapy in some infants with these tumors.[607] In a meta-analysis conducted by Wrede et al.[608] 347 CPCs were analysed; 104 cases with CPC received chemotherapy and had a statistically better survival that those without chemotherapy. Chemotherapy remained beneficial in the subgroup who did not receive irradiation and who had a incomplete resection. There is scarcity of data on optimal chemotherapy. The SIOP is conducting a study for choroid plexus tumors. In the study patients with CPP tumors will be observed while CPC tumors will be randomized to receive maintenance chemotherapy consisting of cyclophosphamide, etoposide, and vincristine versus carboplatin, etoposide, and vincristine. Radiation therapy is recommended for children older than 3 years of age.

SPINAL AXIS TUMORS

Clinical and Pathological Considerations

Most primary spinal axis tumors produce symptoms and signs as a result of cord and nerve root compression rather than parenchymal invasion. The frequency of primary spinal cord tumors is between 10% and 19% of all primary CNS tumors. Parenthetically, the majority of neoplasms that affect the spine are extradural metastases, whereas most primary tumors are intradural. Of the intradural neoplasms, extramedullary schwannomas and meningiomas are the most common. Schwannomas and meningiomas are normally intradural, but occasionally may present as extradural tumors. Other intradural, extramedullary neoplasms include vascular tumors, chordomas, and epidermoids. Intramedullary tumors include ependymomas, comprising approximately 40% of intramedullary tumors; the remainder are astrocytomas, oligodendrogliomas, gangliogliomas, medulloblastomas, and hemangioblastomas.

Approximately half of spinal tumors involve the thoracic spinal canal (the longest spinal segment), 30% involve the lumbosacral spine, and the remainder involve the cervical spine, including the foramen magnum. Schwannomas occur with greatest frequency in the thoracic spine, although they can be found at other levels. They often extend through an intervertebral foramen in a dumbbell configuration. Meningiomas are dural based and arise preferentially at the foramen magnum and in the thoracic spine. Most patients are women. Astrocytomas are distributed throughout the spinal cord, and most ependymomas involve the conus medullaris and the cauda equina. Spinal chordomas are characteristically sacral and only rarely affect the cervical region or the rest of the mobile spine.

Patients may present with a sensorimotor spinal tract syndrome, a painful radicular spinal cord syndrome, or a central syringomyelic syndrome. In the sensorimotor presentation, symptoms and signs reflect compression of the cord (Table 121.4). The onset is gradual during weeks to months, initial presentation is asymmetric, and motor weakness predominates. The level of impairment determines the muscle groups involved. Because of external compression, dorsal column involvement results in paresthesia and abnormalities of pain and temperature on the side contralateral to the motor weakness.

Radicular spinal cord syndromes occur because of external compression and infiltration of spinal roots. The main symptom is sharp, radicular pain in the distribution of a sensory nerve root. The intense pain is often of short duration, with pain that is more aching in nature persisting for longer periods. Pain may be exacerbated by coughing and sneezing or other maneuvers that increase ICP. Local paresthesia and numbness are common, as are weakness and muscle wasting. These findings often precede cord compression by months. Often the pain is difficult for the clinician to differentiate from ordinary musculoskeletal symptoms, which causes diagnostic delay.

Intramedullary tumors in particular can give rise to syringomyelic dysfunction by destruction and cavitation within the central gray matter of the cord. This produces lower motor neuron destruction with associated segmental muscle weakness, atrophy, and hyporeflexia. There is also a dissociated sensory loss of pain and temperature sensation with preservation of touch. As the syrinx increases in size, all sensory modalities are affected.

Surgery

The operating microscope is essential for spinal cord tumor surgery. Ultrasonography can be used to examine the spinal cord through either intact or open dura to find the level of maximum tumor involvement or to differentiate tumor cysts from solid tumors. Intraoperative monitoring of somatosensory evoked potentials is commonly used, although some surgeons think that changes in somatosensory evoked potentials may occur only after irretrievable damage has occurred, and this remains a topic of controversy. Motor-evoked potentials are used in some centers to guide resection and have retrospectively been shown by some to decrease long-term motor deficits.

MRI is invaluable for the diagnosis, localization, and characterization of spinal tumors. For extremely vascular tumors, notably hemangioblastoma, angiography may provide important preoperative delineation of the tumor blood supply. CT scanning is useful for tumors of the bony axis. Determination of the spinal level of the tumor and its exact relation to the cord is important. Corticosteroids are given before, during, and after spinal cord tumor surgery to help control spinal cord edema.

Meningiomas and schwannomas occur in the intradural, extramedullary spinal compartment. Most of these tumors can be completely resected through a laminectomy. They can be easily separated away from the cord, which is displaced but not invaded by tumor. Schwannomas arise most often in the dorsal spinal rootlets, and their removal includes the rootlets involved. They can grow along the nerve root in a dumbbell fashion through a neural foramen. Some of these can be removed by extending the initial laminectomy exposure laterally, whereas others require a separate operation (thoracotomy, costotransversectomy, or a retroperitoneal approach). Strictly anteriorly situated cervical tumors can successfully be removed via an anterior approach using corpectomy of the appropriate vertebral levels, followed by strut grafting after the tumor resection.

The most common intramedullary tumors are ependymoma and astrocytoma. Except for malignant astrocytomas, resection is the principal treatment for these tumors. Intramedullary tumors are approached through a laminectomy. After dural opening, a longitudinal myelotomy is made, usually in the midline or dorsal root entry zone. The incision is deepened several millimeters to the tumor surface. Dissection planes around the tumor are sought microsurgically and, in the case of ependymomas, usually found and extended gradually around the tumor's surface, whereas removal of the central tumor bulk (by carbon dioxide laser or ultrasonic aspirator) causes the tumor to collapse. Such tumors are usually completely removed, with good long-term outcome.[609] Some patients later develop spinal deformity, requiring stabilization procedures.[610] Tumors without clear dissection planes (usually astrocytomas) cannot be removed completely, but bulk reduction can cause long-term palliation. If frozen-section analysis shows a tumor to be a malignant glioma, a less aggressive surgery is typically performed due to increased risk of morbidity with little benefit achieved from an extensive debulking procedure.

Radiation Therapy

Radiation therapy is recommended for unresectable and incompletely resected neoplasms of the spinal axis. In general, doses of 50 to 54 Gy (1.8 Gy/d) are used so that the risk of injury to the cord from radiation is minimized. When lesions involve only the cauda equina or when complete, irreversible myelopathy already has occurred, higher doses are used.

Ependymomas have a longer natural history than astrocytomas. Recurrence of ependymomas may be delayed for as long as 12 years.[611,612] Radiation therapy is not necessary when ependymomas are removed completely in an *en bloc* fashion.[609] All nonirradiated patients with incompletely excised lesions reported by Barone and Elvidge[613] and by Schuman et al.[614] experienced recurrence. Postoperative irradiation appears to improve tumor control for incompletely resected ependymomas. Five- and 10-year survival rates in irradiated patients with localized ependymomas range from 60% to 100% and 68% to 95%, respectively, whereas 10-year relapse-free survival rates vary from 43% to 61%.[615] Tumor grade has a significant effect on outcome. Waldron et al.[612] found that for patients with well-differentiated tumors, the 5-year cause-specific survival was 97% compared with 71% for patients with intermediate or poorly differentiated tumors ($P = .005$). Myxopapillary ependymomas that arise in the conus medullaris and filum terminale have a better prognosis than the cellular ependymomas that arise in the cord.[616] Local recurrence is the predominant pattern of treatment failure, occurring in 25% of irradiated patients.[612]

The 5- and 10-year survival rates for irradiated patients with low-grade astrocytomas of the spinal cord vary from 60% to 90% and 40% to 90%, respectively; 5- and 10-year relapse-free survival rates range from 66% to 83% and 53% to 83%, respectively.[610,612] Fifty percent to 65% of astrocytomas are controlled locally. Good neurologic condition at the time of irradiation, lower histologic grade, and younger age are favorable factors.[617] Patterns of recurrence for malignant astrocytomas of the spine have been analyzed by MRI.[618] Despite surgery and full-dose radiation, spinal or brain dissemination is the predominant mode of failure.

Chemotherapy

There are no significant controlled clinical trials of chemotherapy for primary spinal axis tumors. Drugs active against intracranial tumors logically may be assumed to be equally efficacious against histologically identical tumors in the spinal cord. Temozolomide is being increasingly used in this setting.

Selected References

The full list of references for this chapter appears in the online version.

1. Ries LAG, Melbert D, Krapcho M, et al. *SEER cancer statistics review, 1975–2004*. Bethesda, MD: National Cancer Institute, 2007.
2. Central Brain Tumor Registry of the United States (CBTRUS). Statistical Report: Primary Brain Tumors in the United States, 2004–2006. World Wide Web URL: http://www.CBTURS.org.
3. Kleihues P, Burger PC, Scheithauer BW. The new WHO classification of brain tumours. *Brain Pathol* 1993;3(3):255.
4. Preston-Martin S. Descriptive epidemiology of primary tumors of the spinal cord and spinal meninges in Los Angeles County, 1972–1985. *Neuroepidemiology* 1990;9(2):106.
6. Ohgaki H, Kleihues P. Epidemiology and etiology of gliomas. *Acta Neuropathol (Berl)* 2005;109(1):93.
7. Sadetzki S, Chetrit A, Freedman L, Stovall M, Modan B, Novikov I. Long term follow-up for brain tumor development following childhood exposure to ionizing radiation for tinea capitis. *Radiat Res* 2005;163:424.
12. Myung SK, Woong J, McDowell DD, et al. Mobile phone use and risk of tumors: a meta-analysis. *J Clin Oncol* 2009;27:5565.
16. Cote TR, Manns A, Hardy CR, Yellin FJ, Hartge P. Epidemiology of brain lymphoma among people with or without acquired immunodeficiency syndrome. AIDS/Cancer Study Group. *J Natl Cancer Inst* 1996;88(10):675.
19. Scheurer ME, Bondy ML, Aldape KD, Albrecht T, El-Zein R. Detection of human CMV in different histological types of glioma. *Acta Neuropathol* 2008;116:79.
20. Melean G, Sestini R, Ammannati F, Papi L. Genetic insights into familial tumors of the nervous system. *Am J Med Genet C Semin Med Genet* 2004; 129:74.
25. Inskip PD, Linet MS, Heineman EF. Etiology of brain tumors in adults. *Epidemiol Rev* 1995;17(2):382.
27. Wrensch M, Bondy ML, Wiencke J, Yost M. Environmental risk factors for primary malignant brain tumors: a review. *J Neurooncol* 1993;17(1):47.
28. Kleihues P, Louis DN, Scheithauer BW, et al. The WHO classification of tumors of the nervous system. *J Neuropathol Exp Neurol* 2002;61(3):215.
29. Louis DN, Ohgaki H, Otmar D, et al. The 2007 WHO classification of tumours of the central nervous system. *Acta Neuropathol* 2007;114:97.
35. Dirks PB. Cancer: stem cells and brain tumours. *Nature* 2006;444(7120): 687.
36. Cha S. Neuroimaging in neuro-oncology. *Neurotherapeutics* 2009;6:465.
42. Brandes AA, Franceschi E, Tosoni A, et al. MGMT promoter methylation status can predict the incidence and outcome of pseudoprogression after concomitant radiochemotherapy in newly diagnosed glioblastoma patients. *J Clin Oncol* 2008;26(13):2192.
43. Wen PY, Macdonald DR, Reardon DA, et al. Updated response assessment criteria for high-grade gliomas: response assessment in neuro-oncology working group. *J Clin Oncol* 2010;28(11):1963.
44. Siomin V, Angelov L, Li L, Vogelbaum MA. Results of a survey of neurosurgical practice patterns regarding the prophylactic use of anti-epilepsy drugs in patients with brain tumors. *J Neurooncol* 2005;74(2):211.
48. Hatiboglu MA, Weinberg JS, Suki D, et al. Impact of intraoperative high-field magnetic resonance imaging guidance on glioma surgery: a prospective volumetric analysis. *Neurosurgery* 2009;64(6):1073.
49. Stummer W, Pichlmeier U, Meinel T, et al. Fluorescence-guided surgery with 5-aminolevulinic acid for resection of malignant glioma: a randomised controlled multicentre phase III trial. *Lancet Oncol* 2006;7(5):392.
52. Keles GE, Lamborn KR, Berger MS. Low-grade hemispheric gliomas in adults: a critical review of extent of resection as a factor influencing outcome. *J Neurosurg* 2001;95(5):735.
53. Berger MS, Kincaid J, Ojemann GA, Lettich E. Brain mapping techniques to maximize resection, safety, and seizure control in children with brain tumors. *Neurosurgery* 1989;25(5):786.
57. Kelly PJ, Daumas-Duport C, Scheithauer BW, Kall BA, Kispert DB. Stereotactic histologic correlations of computed tomography- and magnetic resonance imaging-defined abnormalities in patients with glial neoplasms. *Mayo Clin Proc* 1987;62(6):450.
58. Hermanto U, Frija EK, Lii MJ, Chang EL, Mahajan A, Woo SY. Intensity-modulated radiotherapy (IMRT) and conventional three-dimensional conformal radiotherapy for high-grade gliomas: does IMRT increase the integral dose to normal brain? *Int J Radiat Oncol Biol Phys* 2007;67(4):1135.
62. Stieber VW, Bourland JD, Tome WA, Mehta MP. Gentlemen (and ladies), choose your weapons: gamma knife vs. linear accelerator radiosurgery. *Technol Cancer Res Treat* 2003;2:79.
70. Muldoon LL, Soussain C, Jahnke K, et al. Chemotherapy delivery issues in central nervous system malignancies: a reality check. *J Clin Oncol* 2007;25: 2295.
77. Laquintana V, Trapani A, Denora N, Wang F, Gallo JM, Trapani G. New strategies to deliver anticancer drugs to brain tumors. *Exp Opin Drug Deliv* 2009;6:1017.
85. Brem H, Mahaley MS Jr, Vick NA, et al. Interstitial chemotherapy with drug polymer implants for the treatment of recurrent gliomas. *J Neurosurg* 1991;74(3):441.
95. Chang SM, Lamborn KR, Kuhn JG, et al. Neuro-oncology clinical trial design for targeted therapies: lessons learned from the North American Brain Tumor Consortium. *Neuro oncol* 2008;10:631.
96. Huang T, Sakaria SM, Cloughesy TF, et al. Targeted therapy for malignant glioma patients: lessons learned and the road ahead. *Neurotherapeutics* 2009;6:500.
98. Grossman SA, Hochberg F, Fisher J, et al. Increased 9-aminocamptothecin dose requirements in patients on anticonvulsants. NABTT CNS Consortium. The new approaches to brain tumor therapy. *Cancer Chemother Pharmacol* 1998;42(2):118.
103. Kernohan JW et al. A simplified classification of gliomas. *Proc Staff Meet Mayo Clin* 1949;24:71.
104. Ringertz J. Grading of gliomas. *Acta Pathol Microbiol Scand* 1950;27:51.
105. Daumas-Duport C, Scheithauer B, O'Fallon J, Kelly P. Grading of astrocytomas. A simple and reproducible method. *Cancer* 1988;62:2152.
112. Pignatti F, van den Bent M, Curran D, et al. Prognostic factors for survival in adult patients with cerebral low-grade glioma. *J Clin Oncol* 2002;20(8): 2076.
113. Shaw EG, Berkey B, Coons SW, et al. Recurrence following neurosurgeon-determined gross-total resection of adult supratentorial low-grade glioma: results of a prospective clinical trial. *J Neurosurg* 2008; 109(5):835.
114. van den Bent MJ, Afra D, de Witte O, et al. Long-term efficacy of early versus delayed radiotherapy for low-grade astrocytoma and oligodendroglioma in adults: the EORTC 22845 randomised trial. *Lancet* 2005;366 (9490):985.
115. Karim AB, Maat B, Hatlevoll R, et al. A randomized trial on dose-response in radiation therapy of low-grade cerebral glioma: European Organization for Research and Treatment of Cancer (EORTC) Study 22844. *Int J Radiat Oncol Biol Phys* 1996;36(3):549.
116. Shaw E, Arusell R, Scheithauer B, et al. Prospective randomized trial of low- versus high-dose radiation therapy in adults with supratentorial low-grade glioma: initial report of a North Central Cancer Treatment Group/ Radiation Therapy Oncology Group/Eastern Cooperative Oncology Group study. *J Clin Oncol* 2002;20(9):2267.
118. Laack NN, Brown PD, Ivnik RJ, et al. Cognitive function after radiotherapy for supratentorial low-grade glioma: a North Central Cancer Treatment Group prospective study. *Int J Radiat Oncol Biol Phys* 2005;63 (4):1175.
129. van den Bent MJ, Taphoorn MJ, Brandes AA, et al. Phase II study of first line chemotherapy with temozolomide in recurrent oligodendroglial tumors: the European Organization for Research and Treatment of Cancer Brain Tumor Group Study 26971. *J Clin Oncol* 2003;21:2525.
134. Buckner JC, Gesme D Jr, O'Fallon JR, et al. Phase II trial of procarbazine, lomustine, and vincristine as initial therapy for patients with low-grade oligodendroglioma or oligoastrocytoma: efficacy and associations with chromosomal abnormalities. *J Clin Oncol* 2003;21:251.
135. van den Bent MJ, Chinot O, Boogerd W, et al. Second-line chemotherapy with temozolomide in recurrent oligodendroglioma after PCV (procarbazine, lomustine and vincristine) chemotherapy: EORTC Brain Tumor Group phase II study 26972. *Ann Oncol* 2003;14:599.
139. Jenkins RB, Blair H, Ballman KV, et al. A t(1;19)(q10;p10) mediates the combined deletions of 1p and 19q and predicts a better prognosis of patients with oligodendroglioma. *Cancer Res* 2006;66(20):9852.
140. Prados MD, Scott C, Curran WJ Jr, Nelson DF, Leibel S, Kramer S. Procarbazine, lomustine, and vincristine (PCV) chemotherapy for anaplastic astrocytoma: a retrospective review of radiation therapy oncology group protocols comparing survival with carmustine or PCV adjuvant chemotherapy. *J Clin Oncol* 1999;17(11):3389.
142. Prados MD, Seiferheld W, Sandler HM, et al. Phase III randomized study of radiotherapy plus procarbazine, lomustine, and vincristine with or without BUdR for treatment of anaplastic astrocytoma: final report of RTOG 9404. *Int J Radiat Oncol Biol Phys* 2004;58(4):1147.
143. Stewart LA. Chemotherapy in adult high-grade glioma: a systematic review and meta-analysis of individual patient data from 12 randomised trials. *Lancet* 2002;359(9311):1011.
144. Randomized trial of procarbazine, lomustine, and vincristine in the adjuvant treatment of high-grade astrocytoma: a Medical Research Council trial. *J Clin Oncol* 2001;19(2):509.
145. Wick W, Hartmann C, Engel C, et al. NOA-04 randomized phase III trial of sequential radiochemotherapy of anaplastic glioma with procarbazine, lomustine, and vincristine or temozolomide. *J Clin Oncol* 2009;27:5874.
146. Hegi ME, Diserens AC, Gorlia T, et al. MGMT gene silencing and benefit from temozolomide in glioblastoma. *N Engl J Med* 2005;352(10):997.
148. Yan H, Parsons DW, Jin G, et al. IDH1 and IDH2 mutations in gliomas. *N Engl J Med* 2009;360:765.
149. Levin VA, Hess KR, Choucair A, et al. Phase III randomized study of postradiotherapy chemotherapy with combination alpha-difluoromethylornithine-PCV versus PCV for anaplastic gliomas. *Clin Cancer Res* 2003;9(3):981.
150. Yung WK, Prados MD, Yaya-Tur R, et al. Multicenter phase II trial of temozolomide in patients with anaplastic astrocytoma or anaplastic

oligoastrocytoma at first relapse. Temodal Brain Tumor Group. *J Clin Oncol* 1999;17(9):2762.

152. Friedman HS, Prados MD, Wen PY, et al. Bevacizumab alone and in combination with irinotecan in recurrent glioblastoma. *J Clin Oncol* 2009;27:4733.
155. Cairncross G, Macdonald D, Ludwin S, et al. Chemotherapy for anaplastic oligodendroglioma. National Cancer Institute of Canada Clinical Trials Group. *J Clin Oncol* 1994;12(10):2013.
156. Cairncross G, Berkey B, Shaw E, et al. Phase III trial of chemotherapy plus radiotherapy compared with radiotherapy alone for pure and mixed anaplastic oligodendroglioma: Intergroup Radiation Therapy Oncology Group Trial 9402. *J Clin Oncol* 2006;24(18):2707.
157. van den Bent MJ, Carpentier AF, Brandes AA, et al. Adjuvant procarbazine, lomustine, and vincristine improves progression-free survival but not overall survival in newly diagnosed anaplastic oligodendrogliomas and oligoastrocytomas: a randomized European Organisation for Research and Treatment of Cancer phase III trial. *J Clin Oncol* 2006;24(18):2715.
158. van den Bent MJ, Dubbink HJ, Sanson M, et al. MGMT promoter methylation is prognostic but not predictive for outcome to adjuvant PCV chemotherapy in anaplastic oligodendroglial tumors: a report from EORTC Brain Tumor Group Study 26951. *J Clin Oncol* 2009;27:5881.
159. Kouwenhoven MC, Gorlia T, Kros JM, et al. Molecular analysis of anaplastic oligodendroglial tumors in a prospective randomized study: A report from EORTC study 26951. *Neuro oncol* 2009;11:737.
165. Vuorinen V, Hinkka S, Färkkilä M, Jääskeläinen J. Debulking or biopsy of malignant glioma in elderly people—a randomised study. *Acta Neurochir (Wien)* 2003;145(1):5.
168. Dandy WE. Removal of right cerebral hemisphere for certain tumors with hemiplegia. *JAMA* 1928;90:823.
170. Hochberg FH, Pruitt A. Assumptions in the radiotherapy of glioblastoma. *Neurology* 1980;30(9):907.
172. Walker MD, Strike TA, Sheline GE. An analysis of dose–effect relationship in the radiotherapy of malignant gliomas. *Int J Radiat Oncol Biol Phys* 1979;5(10):1725.
173. Bleehen NM, Stenning SP. A Medical Research Council trial of two radiotherapy doses in the treatment of grades 3 and 4 astrocytoma. The Medical Research Council Brain Tumour Working Party. *Br J Cancer* 1991;64(4):769.
177. Roa W, Brasher PM, Bauman G, et al. Abbreviated course of radiation therapy in older patients with glioblastoma multiforme: a prospective randomized clinical trial. *J Clin Oncol* 2004;22(9):1583.
178. Keime-Guibert F, Chinot O, Taillandier L, et al. Radiotherapy for glioblastoma in the elderly. *N Engl J Med* 2007;356(15):1527.
181. Souhami L, Seiferheld W, Brachman D, et al. Randomized comparison of stereotactic radiosurgery followed by conventional radiotherapy with carmustine to conventional radiotherapy with carmustine for patients with glioblastoma multiforme: report of Radiation Therapy Oncology Group 93–05 protocol. *Int J Radiat Oncol Biol Phys* 2004;60(3):853.
183. Laperriere NJ, Leung PM, McKenzie S, et al. Randomized study of brachytherapy in the initial management of patients with malignant astrocytoma. *Int J Radiat Oncol Biol Phys* 1998;41(5):1005.
184. Selker RG, Shapiro WR, Burger P, et al. The Brain Tumor Cooperative Group NIH Trial 87–01: a randomized comparison of surgery, external radiotherapy, and carmustine versus surgery, interstitial radiotherapy boost, external radiation therapy, and carmustine. *Neurosurgery* 2002;51(2):343.
195. Grossman S, O'Neill A, Grunnet M, et al. Phase III study comparing three cycles of infusional BCNU/Cisplatin followed by radiation with radiation and concurrent BCNU for patients with newly diagnosed supratentorial glioblastoma multiforme (ECOG 2394-SWOG 9508). *Proc Am Soc Clin Oncol* 2000; (abst 612).
202. Perry JR, Bélanger K, Mason WP, et al. Phase II trial of continuous dose-intense temozolomide in recurrent malignant glioma: RESCUE study. *J Clin Oncol* 2010;28:2051.
205. Sandhu SK, Yap TA, de Bono JS. Poly(ADP-ribose) polymerase inhibitors in cancer treatment: a clinical perspective. *Eur J Cancer* 2010;46:9.
206. Westphal M, Hilt DC, Bortey E, et al. A phase 3 trial of local chemotherapy with biodegradable carmustine (BCNU) wafers (Gliadel wafers) in patients with primary malignant glioma. *Neuro oncol* 2003;5(2):79.
208. Wong ET, Hess KR, Gleason MJ, et al. Outcomes and prognostic factors in recurrent glioma patients enrolled onto phase II clinical trials. *J Clin Oncol* 1999;17(8):2572.
212. Mellinghoff IK, Wang MY, Vivanco I, et al. Molecular determinants of the response of glioblastomas to EGFR kinase inhibitors. *N Engl J Med* 2005;353(19):2012.
220. Vredenburgh JJ, Desjardins A, Herndon JE 2nd, et al. Phase II trial of bevacizumab and irinotecan in recurrent malignant glioma. *Clin Cancer Res* 2007;13(4):1253.
221. Kreisl TN, Kim L, Moore K, et al. Phase II trial of single-agent bevacizumab followed by bevacizumab plus irinotecan at tumor progression in recurrent glioblastoma. *J Clin Oncol* 2009;27:740.
222. Lai A, Filka E, McGibbon B, et al. Phase II pilot study of bevacizumab in combination with temozolomide and regional radiation therapy for up-front treatment of patients with newly diagnosed glioblastoma multiforme: interim analysis of safety and tolerability. *Int J Radiat Oncol Biol Phys* 2008;71:1372.
225. Stupp R, Hegi ME, Neyns B, et al. Phase I/IIa study of cilengitide and temozolomide with concomitant radiotherapy followed by cilengitide and temozolomide maintenance therapy in patients with newly diagnosed glioblastoma. *J Clin Oncol* 2010;28:2712.
232. Curran WJ Jr, Scott CB, Horton J, et al. Recursive partitioning analysis of prognostic factors in three Radiation Therapy Oncology Group malignant glioma trials. *J Natl Cancer Inst* 1993;85(9):704.
235. Taillibert S, Chodkiewicz C, Laigle-Donadey F, et al. Gliomatosis cerebri: a review of 296 cases from the ANOCEF database and the literature. *J Neurooncol* 2006;76(2):201.
244. Opocher E, Kremer LC, Da Dalt L, et al. Prognostic factors for progression of childhood optic pathway glioma: a systematic review. *Eur J Cancer* 2006;42:1807.
259. Lacaze E, Kieffer V, Streri A, et al. Neuropsychological outcome in children with optic pathway tumours when first-line treatment is chemotherapy. *Br J Cancer* 2003;89(11):2038.
261. Ater J, Holmes E, Zhou T, et al. Results of COG protocol A 9952: a randomized phase 3 study of two chemotherapy regimens for incompletely resected low-grade glioma in young children. *Neuro oncol* 2008;10:451.
268. Moreno L, Bautista F, Ashley S, Duncan C, Zacharoulis S. Does chemotherapy affect the visual outcome in children with optic pathway glioma? A systematic review of the evidence. *Eur J Cancer* 2010;44:2253.
270. Guillamo JS, Monjour A, Taillandier L, et al. Brainstem gliomas in adults: prognostic factors and classification. *Brain* 2001;124:2528.
279. Freeman CR, Krischer JP, Sanford RA, et al. Final results of a study of escalating doses of hyperfractionated radiotherapy in brain stem tumors in children: a Pediatric Oncology Group study. *Int J Radiat Oncol Biol Phys* 1993;27(2):197.
282. Levin VA, Edwards MS, Wright DC, et al. Modified procarbazine, CCNU, and vincristine (PCV 3) combination chemotherapy in the treatment of malignant brain tumors. *Cancer Treat Rep* 1980;64(2–3):237.
283. Jennings MT, Sposto R, Boyett JM, et al. Preradiation chemotherapy in primary high-risk brainstem tumors: phase II study CCG-9941 of the Children's Cancer Group. *J Clin Oncol* 2002;20(16):3431.
284. Broniscer A, Iacono L, Chintagumpala M, et al. Role of temozolomide after radiotherapy for newly diagnosed diffuse brainstem glioma in children: results of a multiinstitutional study (SJHG-98). *Cancer* 2005;103(1):133.
285. Lashford LS, Thiesse P, Jouvet A, et al. Temozolomide in malignant gliomas of childhood: a United Kingdom Children's Cancer Study Group and French Society for Pediatric Oncology Intergroup Study. *J Clin Oncol* 2002;20(24):4684.
286. Nicholson HS, Krestschmar CS, Krailo M, et al. Phase 2 study of temozolomide in children and adolescents with recurrent central nervous system tumors: a report from the Children's Oncology Group. *Cancer* 2007;110(7):1542.
299. Rades D, Schild SE. The role of postoperative radiotherapy for the treatment of gangliogliomas. *Cancer* 2010;116, 432.
303. Goldwein JW, Corn BW, Finlay JL, Packer RJ, Rorke LB, Schut L. Is craniospinal irradiation required to cure children with malignant (anaplastic) intracranial ependymomas? *Cancer* 1991;67(11):2766.
309. Timmermann B, Kortmann RD, Kühl J, et al. Combined postoperative irradiation and chemotherapy for anaplastic ependymomas in childhood: results of the German prospective trials HIT 88–89 and HIT 91. *Int J Radiat Oncol Biol Phys* 2000;46(2):287.
317. Merchant TE, Mulhern RK, Krasin MJ, et al. Preliminary results from a phase II trial of conformal radiation therapy and evaluation of radiation-related CNS effects for pediatric patients with localized ependymoma. *J Clin Oncol* 2004;22(15):3156.
329. Bouffet E, Perilongo G, Canete A, et al. Intracranial ependymomas in children: a critical review of prognostic factors and a plea for cooperation. *Med Pediatr Oncol* 1998;30(6):319.
340. Simpson D. The recurrence of intracranial meningiomas after surgical treatment. *J Neurol Neurosurg Psychiatry* 1957;20(1):22.
346. Kondziolka D, Flickinger JC, Perez B. Judicious resection and/or radiosurgery for parasagittal meningiomas: outcomes from a multicenter review. Gamma Knife Meningioma Study Group. *Neurosurgery* 1998;43(3):405.
353. Goldsmith BJ, Wara WM, Wilson CB, Larson DA. Postoperative irradiation for subtotally resected meningiomas. A retrospective analysis of 140 patients treated from 1967 to 1990. *J Neurosurg* 1994;80(2):195.
356. Chan RC, Thompson GB. Morbidity, mortality, and quality of life following surgery for intracranial meningiomas. A retrospective study in 257 cases. *J Neurosurg* 1984;60(1):52.
395. Chang CH, Housepian EM, Herbert C Jr. An operative staging system and a megavoltage radiotherapeutic technic for cerebellar medulloblastomas. *Radiology* 1969;93(6):1351.
400. Zeltzer PM, Boyett JM, Finlay JL, et al. Metastasis stage, adjuvant treatment, and residual tumor are prognostic factors for medulloblastoma in children: conclusions from the Children's Cancer Group 921 randomized phase III study. *J Clin Oncol* 1999;17(3):832.
401. Evans AE, Jenkin RD, Sposto R, et al. The treatment of medulloblastoma. Results of a prospective randomized trial of radiation therapy with and without CCNU, vincristine, and prednisone. *J Neurosurg* 1990;72(4):572.

409. Timmermann B, Kortmann RD, Kühl J, et al. Role of radiotherapy in the treatment of supratentorial primitive neuroectodermal tumors in childhood: results of the prospective German brain tumor trials HIT 88–89 and 91. *J Clin Oncol* 2002;20(3):842.
414. Gajjar A, Chintagumpala M, Ashley D, et al. Risk-adapted craniospinal radiotherapy followed by high-dose chemotherapy and stem-cell rescue in children with newly diagnosed medulloblastoma (St Jude Medulloblastoma-96): long-term results from a prospective, multicentre trial. *Lancet Oncol* 2006;7 (10):813.
415. Packer RJ, Goldwein J, Nicholson HS, et al. Treatment of children with medulloblastomas with reduced-dose craniospinal radiation therapy and adjuvant chemotherapy: a Children's Cancer Group Study. *J Clin Oncol* 1999;17(7):2127.
416. Bailey CC, Gnekow A, Wellek S, et al. Prospective randomised trial of chemotherapy given before radiotherapy in childhood medulloblastoma. International Society of Paediatric Oncology (SIOP) and the (German) Society of Paediatric Oncology (GPO): SIOP II. *Med Pediatr Oncol* 1995; 25(3):166.
417. Tait DM, Thornton-Jones H, Bloom HJ, Lemerle J, Morris-Jones P. Adjuvant chemotherapy for medulloblastoma: the first multi-centre control trial of the International Society of Paediatric Oncology (SIOP I). *Eur J Cancer* 1990;26(4):464.
420. Timmermann B, Kortmann RD, Kühl J, et al. Role of radiotherapy in supratentorial primitive neuroectodermal tumor in young children: results of the German HIT-SKK87 and HIT-SKK92 trials. *J Clin Oncol* 2006;24 (10):1554.
421. Dhall G, Grodman H, Ji L, et al. Outcome of children less than three years old at diagnosis with non-metastatic medulloblastoma treated with chemotherapy on the "Head Start" I and II protocols. *Pediatr Blood Cancer* 2008;50(6):1169.
438. Bouffet, E, Baranzelli MC, Patte C, et al. Combined treatment modality for intracranial germinomas: results of a multicentre SFOP experience. Societe Francaise d'Oncologie Pediatrique. *Br J Cancer* 1999;79(7–8):1199.
444. Aoyama H, Shirato H, Ikeda J, Fujieda K, Miyasaka K, Sawamura Y. Induction chemotherapy followed by low-dose involved-field radiotherapy for intracranial germ cell tumors. *J Clin Oncol* 2002;20:857.
447. Balmaceda C, Heller G, Rosenblum M, et al. Chemotherapy without irradiation–a novel approach for newly diagnosed CNS germ cell tumors: results of an international cooperative trial. The First International Central Nervous System Germ Cell Tumor Study. *J Clin Oncol* 1996;14(11):2908.
459. Krieger MD, Couldwell WT, Weiss MH. Assessment of long-term remission of acromegaly following surgery. *J Neurosurg* 2003;98(4):719.
474. Breen P, Flickinger JC, Kondziolka D, Martinez AJ. Radiotherapy for nonfunctional pituitary adenoma: analysis of long-term tumor control. *J Neurosurg* 1998;89(6):933.
476. Sheehan JP, Niranjan A, Sheehan JM, et al. Stereotactic radiosurgery for pituitary adenomas: an intermediate review of its safety, efficacy, and role in the neurosurgical treatment armamentarium. *J Neurosurg* 2005;102 (4):678.
486. Parkinson C, Scarlett JA, Trainer PT. Pegvisomant in the treatment of acromegaly. *Adv Drug Deliv Rev* 2003;55(10):1303.
491. Stripp DC, Maity A, Janss AJ, et al. Surgery with or without radiation therapy in the management of craniopharyngiomas in children and young adults. *Int J Radiat Oncol Biol Phys* 2004;58(3):714.
501. Varlotto JM, Flickinger JC, Kondziolka D, Lunsford LD, Deutsch M. External beam irradiation of craniopharyngiomas: long-term analysis of tumor control and morbidity. *Int J Radiat Oncol Biol Phys* 2002;54(2):492.
535. Pollock BE, Driscoll CL, Foote RL, et al. Patient outcomes after vestibular schwannoma management: a prospective comparison of microsurgical resection and stereotactic radiosurgery. *Neurosurgery* 2006;59(1):77.
538. Andrews DW, Suarez O, Goldman HW, et al. Stereotactic radiosurgery and fractionated stereotactic radiotherapy for the treatment of acoustic schwannomas: comparative observations of 125 patients treated at one institution. *Int J Radiat Oncol Biol Phys* 2001;50(5):1265.
550. Mautner VF, Nguyen R, Kutta H, et al. Bevacizumab induces regression of vestibular schwannomas in patients with neurofibromatosis type 2. *Neuro oncol* 2010;12:14.
555. Gottfried ON, Liu JK, Couldwell WT. Comparison of radiosurgery and conventional surgery for the treatment of glomus jugulare tumors. *Neurosurg Focus* 2004;17(2):E4.
562. Vougioukas VI, Gläsker S, Hubbe U, et al. Surgical treatment of hemangioblastomas of the central nervous system in pediatric patients. *Childs Nerv Syst* 2006;22(9):1149.
568. Asthagiri AR, Mehta GU, Zach L, et al. Prospective evaluation of radiosurgery for hemangioblastomas in von Hippel–Lindau disease. *Neuro oncol* 2010;12(1):80.
577. Erdem E, Angtuaco EC, Van Hemert R, Park JS, Al-Mefty O. Comprehensive review of intracranial chordoma. *Radiographics* 2003;23(4):995.
595. Amichetti M, Amelio D, Cianchetti M, Enrici RM, Minniti Get al. A systematic review of proton therapy in the treatment of chondrosarcoma of the skull base. *Neurosurg Rev* 2010;33(2):155.
608. Wrede B, Liu P, Wolff JE, et al. Chemotherapy improves the survival of patients with choroid plexus carcinoma: a meta-analysis of individual cases with choroid plexus tumors. *J Neurooncol* 2007;85(3):345.

SECTION 11: CANCERS OF CHILDHOOD

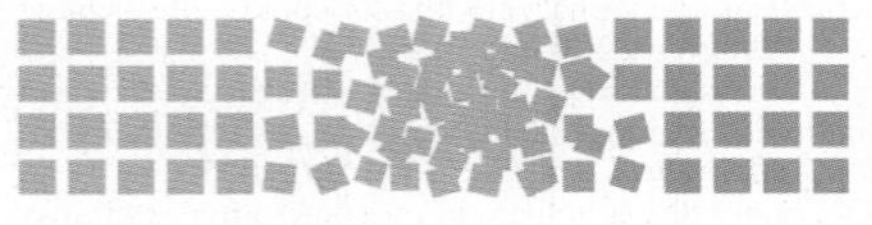

CHAPTER 122 MOLECULAR BIOLOGY OF CHILDHOOD CANCERS

LEE J. HELMAN AND DAVID MALKIN

The biologic nature of tumors of childhood is clinically, histopathologically, and biologically distinct from that of adult-onset malignancies. Childhood cancers tend to have short latency periods, are often rapidly growing and aggressively invasive, are rarely associated with exposure to carcinogens implicated in adult-onset cancers, and are generally more responsive to standard modalities of treatment, in particular chemotherapy. Most childhood tumors occur sporadically in families with at most a weak history of cancer. In at least 10% to 15% of cases, however, a strong familial association is recognized or the child has a congenital or genetic disorder that imparts a higher likelihood of specific cancer types.[1] Examples of genetic disorders that render a child at increased risk of tumor development include xeroderma pigmentosa, Bloom syndrome, or ataxia-telangiectasia, which predispose to skin cancers, leukemias, or lymphoid malignancies, respectively. In all three cases, constitutional gene alterations that disrupt normal mechanisms of genomic DNA repair are blamed for the propensity to cell transformation. Other hereditary disorders, including Beckwith-Wiedemann syndrome (BWS), von Hippel-Lindau disease, Rothmund-Thomson syndrome, and the multiple endocrine neoplasias types 1 and 2, are thought to be associated with their respective tumor spectra through constitutional activation of molecular pathways of deregulated cellular growth and proliferation. The cancers that occur in these syndromes are generally secondary phenotypic manifestations of disorders that have distinctive recognizable physical stigmata. On the other hand, some cancer predisposition syndromes are recognized only by their malignant manifestations, with nonmalignant characteristics being virtually absent. These include hereditary retinoblastoma, Li-Fraumeni syndrome (LFS), familial Wilms tumor, and familial adenomatous polyposis coli. Each of these presents with distinct cancer phenotypes, and the identified molecular defect is unique for each (Table 122.1). Careful attention to detailed cancer family histories continues to lead to the discovery of new cancer predisposition syndromes and the coincident identification of novel cancer genes.[2]

The study of pediatric cancer and rare hereditary cancer syndromes and associations has led to the identification of numerous cancer genes, including dominant oncogenes, DNA repair genes, and tumor suppressor genes. These genes are important not only in hereditary predisposition but also in the normal growth, differentiation, and proliferation pathways of all cells. Alterations of these genes have been consistently found in numerous sporadic tumors of childhood and led to studies of their functional role in carcinogenesis. The numerous properties of transformed malignant cells in culture or *in vivo* can be explained by the complex abnormal interaction of numerous positive and negative growth-regulatory genes. Pediatric cancers offer unique models in which to study these pathways in that they are less likely to be disrupted by nongenetic factors. The embryonic ontogeny of many childhood cancers suggests that better understanding of the nature of the genetic events leading to these cancers will also augment the understanding of normal embryologic growth and development.

This chapter begins with an outline of tumor suppressor genes—the most frequently implicated class of cancer genes in childhood malignancy. This leads into a discussion of molecular features of retinoblastoma, the paradigm of cancer genetics, followed by analysis of the molecular pathways associated with other common pediatric cancers. Evaluations of the importance of molecular alterations in familial cancers, as well as new approaches in molecular therapeutics, are also addressed.

TUMOR SUPPRESSOR GENES

Faulty regulation of cellular growth and differentiation leads to neoplastic transformation and tumor initiation. Many inappropriately activated growth-potentiating genes, or *oncogenes*, have been identified through the study of RNA tumor viruses and the transforming effects of DNA isolated from malignant cells. However, activated dominant oncogenes themselves do not readily explain a variety of phenomena related to transformation and tumor formation. Among these is the suppression of tumorigenicity by fusion of malignant cells with their normal counterparts. If these malignant cells carried an activated dominant oncogene, it would be expected that such a gene would initiate transformation of the normal cells, likely leading to either embryonic or fetal death. The observation is more readily explained by postulating the existence of a factor in the normal cell that acts to suppress growth of the fused malignant cells. Malignant cells commonly exhibit specific chromosomal deletions (Table 122.2). The best example of this occurs in retinoblastoma, a rare pediatric eye tumor in which a small region of the long arm of chromosome 13 is frequently missing. The presumed loss of genes in specific chromosomal regions argues strongly against the concept of a dominantly acting gene being implicated in the development of the tumor. Hereditary forms of cancer are not readily explained by altered growth-potentiating genes. Comparisons between the frequencies of familial tumors and their sporadic counterparts led Knudson[3] to suggest that the familial forms of some tumors could be explained by constitutional mutations in growth-limiting genes. The resulting

TABLE 122.1

HEREDITARY SYNDROMES ASSOCIATED WITH CHILDHOOD CANCER PREDISPOSITION

Syndrome	OMIM Entry[a]	Major Tumor Types	Mode of Inheritance	Genes
HEREDITARY GASTROINTESTINAL MALIGNANCIES				
Adenomatous polyposis of the colon	175100	Colon, thyroid, stomach, intestine, hepatoblastoma	Dominant	*APC*
Juvenile polyposis	174900	Gastrointestinal	Dominant	*SMAD4/DPC4*
Peutz-Jeghers syndrome	175200	Intestinal, ovarian, pancreatic	Dominant	*STK11*
GENODERMATOSES WITH CANCER PREDISPOSITION				
Nevoid basal cell carcinoma syndrome	109400	Skin, medulloblastoma	Dominant	*PTCH*
Neurofibromatosis type 1	162200	Neurofibroma, optic pathway glioma, peripheral nerve sheath tumor	Dominant	*NF1*
Neurofibromatosis type 2	101000	Vestibular schwannoma	Dominant	*NF2*
Tuberous sclerosis	191100	Hamartoma, renal angiomyolipoma, renal cell carcinoma	Dominant	*TSC1/TSC2*
Xeroderma pigmentosum	278730, 278700, 278720, 278760, 278740, 278780, 278750, 133510	Skin, melanoma, leukemia	Recessive	*XPA,B,C,D,E,F,G, POLH*
Rothmund Thomson syndrome	268400	Skin, bone	Recessive	*RECQL4*
LEUKEMIA/LYMPHOMA PREDISPOSITION SYNDROMES				
Bloom syndrome	210900	Leukemia, lymphoma, skin	Recessive	*BLM*
Fanconi anemia	227650	Leukemia, squamous cell carcinoma, gynecological system	Recessive	*FANCA,B,C,D_2, E,F,G*
Shwachman Diamond syndrome	260400	Leukemia/myelodysplasia	Recessive	*SBDS*
Nijmegen breakage syndrome	251260	Lymphoma, medulloblastoma, glioma	Recessive	*NBS1*
Ataxia telangiectasia	208900	Leukemia, lymphoma	Recessive	*ATM*
GENITOURINARY CANCER PREDISPOSITION SYNDROMES				
Simpson-Golabi-Behmel syndrome	312870	Embryonal tumors, Wilms tumor	X-linked	*GPC3*
Von Hippel-Lindau syndrome	193300	Retinal and central nervous hemangioblastoma, pheochromocytoma, renal cell carcinoma	Dominant	*VHL*
Beckwith-Wiedemann syndrome	130650	Wilms tumor, hepatoblastoma, adrenal carcinoma, rhabdomyosarcoma	Dominant	*CDKN1C/NSD1*
Wilms tumor syndrome	194070	Wilms tumor	Dominant	*WT1*
WAGR syndrome	194072	Wilms tumor, gonadoblastoma	Dominant	*WT1*
Costello syndrome	218040	Neuroblastoma, rhabdomyosarcoma, bladder carcinoma	Dominant	*H-Ras*
CENTRAL NERVOUS SYSTEM PREDISPOSITION SYNDROMES				
Retinoblastoma	180200	Retinoblastoma, osteosarcoma	Dominant	*RB1*
Rhabdoid predisposition syndrome	601607	Rhabdoid tumor, medulloblastoma, choroid plexus tumor		*SNF5/INI1*
Medulloblastoma predisposition	607035	Medulloblastoma	Dominant	*SUFU*
SARCOMA/BONE CANCER PREDISPOSITION SYNDROMES				
Li-Fraumeni syndrome	151623	Soft tissue sarcoma, osteosarcoma, breast, adrenocortical carcinoma, leukemia, brain tumor	Dominant	*TP53*
Multiple exostosis	133700, 133701	Chondrosarcoma	Dominant	*EXT1/EXT2*
Werner syndrome	277700	Osteosarcoma, meningioma	Recessive	*WRN*
ENDOCRINE CANCER PREDISPOSITION SYNDROMES				
MEN1	131000	Pancreatic islet cell tumor, pituitary adenoma, parathyroid adenoma	Dominant	*MEN1*
MEN2	171400	Medullary thyroid carcinoma, pheochromocytoma, parathyroid hyperplasia	Dominant	*RET*

WAGR, Wilms tumor, aniridia, genitourinary abnormalities, mental retardation; MEN, multiple endocrine neoplasia.
[a]Online Mendelian Inheritance in Man, http://www.ncbi.nlm.nih.gov/Omim/getmorbid.cgi.
(Adapted from ref. 137.)

TABLE 122.2

COMMON CYTOGENETIC REARRANGEMENTS IN SOLID TUMORS OF CHILDHOOD

Solid Tumor	Cytogenetic Rearrangement	Genes[a]
Ewing sarcoma	t(11;22) (q24;q12), +8	*EWS(22) FLi-1(11)*
Neuroblastoma	del1p32–36, DMs, HSRs, +17q21-qter	*N-MYC*
Retinoblastoma	del13q14	*Rb*
Wilms tumor	del11p13, t(3;17)	*WT1*
Synovial sarcoma	t(X;11) (p11;q11)	*SSX(X) SYT(18)*
Osteogenic sarcoma	del13q14	?
Rhabdomyosarcoma	t(2;13) (q37;q14), t(2;11),3p-,11p-	*PAX3(2) FKHR(13)*
Peripheral neuroepithelioma	t(11;22) (q24;q12), +8	*EWS(22) FLi-1(11)*
Astrocytoma	i(17q)	?
Meningioma	delq22, -22	*MN1, NF2, ?*
Atypical teratoid/rhabdoid tumor	delq22.11	*SNF 5*
Germ cell tumor	i(12p)	

[a]Chromosomal location in parentheses.

inactivation of these genes would facilitate cellular transformation.[4] Such growth-limiting genes were termed *tumor suppressor genes*.

Whereas acquired alterations of dominant oncogenes most commonly occur in somatic cells, mutant tumor suppressor genes may be found either in germ cells or somatic cells. In the former, they may arise *de novo* or be transmitted from generation to generation within a family. The diversity of functions, cellular locations, and tissue-specific expression of the tumor suppressor genes suggest the existence of a complex, yet coordinated, cellular pathway that limits cell growth by linking nuclear processes with the intra- and extracytoplasmic environment. This discussion is limited to those genes for which pediatric tumors are frequently associated.

RETINOBLASTOMA: THE PARADIGM

Retinoblastoma is the prototype cancer caused by mutations of a tumor suppressor gene. It is a malignant tumor of the retina that occurs in infants and young children, with an incidence of approximately 1:20,000.[5] Approximately 40% of retinoblastoma cases are of the heritable form in which the child inherits one mutant allele at the retinoblastoma susceptibility locus (Rb1) through the germ line, and a somatic mutation in a single retinal cell causes loss of function of the remaining normal allele, leading to tumor formation. Tumors are often bilateral and multifocal. The disease is inherited as an autosomal dominant trait, with a penetrance approaching 100%.[6] The remaining 60% of retinoblastoma cases are sporadic (nonheritable), in which both Rb1 alleles in a single retinal cell are inactivated by somatic mutations. As one can imagine, such an event is rare, and these patients usually have only one tumor that presents itself later than in infants with the heritable form. Fifteen percent of unilateral retinoblastoma is heritable[6] but by chance develops in only one eye. Survivors of heritable retinoblastoma have a several 100–fold increased risk of developing mesenchymal tumors such as osteogenic sarcoma, fibrosarcomas, and melanomas later in life.[7] It is thought that several genetic mechanisms may be involved in elimination of the second wild type Rb1 allele in an evolving tumor. These mechanisms include chromosomal duplication or nondisjunction, mitotic recombination, or gene conversion.[8]

The *Rb1* gene was eventually mapped to chromosome 13q14.[9] Using Southern blot analysis, it was then possible to demonstrate that the second target gene that led to disease was actually the second copy of the Rb1 locus. Reduction to homozygosity of the mutant allele (or loss of heterozygosity [LOH] of the wild type allele) would lead to the loss of functional Rb1 and account for tumor development.

Using classic cloning techniques, a 4.7-kb complementary DNA fragment was isolated from retinal cells.[10] This gene, *Rb1*, consisted of 27 exons and encoded a 105-kD nuclear phosphoprotein. As well as being altered in retinoblastoma, this gene and its protein product have been found to be altered in osteosarcomas, small cell lung carcinomas, and bladder, breast, and prostate carcinomas.[10,11] *Rb1* plays a central role in the control of cell-cycle regulation, particularly in determining transition from G_1 through S (DNA synthesis) phase in virtually all cell types.

Although it is clear that *Rb1* and its protein product play some role in growth regulation, the precise nature of this role remains obscure. In the developing retina, inactivation of the *Rb1* gene is necessary and sufficient for tumor formation.[12] It is now clear, however, that these tumors develop as a result of a more complex interplay of aberrant expression of other cell-cycle control genes. In particular, a tumor surveillance pathway mediated by Arf, MDM2, MDMX, and p53 (see later discussion) is activated after loss of *Rb1* during development of the retina. *Rb1*-deficient retinoblasts undergo p53-mediated apoptosis and exit the cell cycle. Subsequently, amplification of the *MDMX* gene and increased expression of MDMX protein are strongly selected for during tumor progression as a mechanism to suppress the p53 response in *Rb1*-deficient retinal cells.[13] Not only do these observations provide a provocative biological mechanism for tumor formation in retinoblastoma, but it also offers potential molecular targets for novel therapeutic approaches to this tumor.[14,15] Although the *Rb1* gene is expressed in virtually all mammalian tissues, only in the retina is its inactivation sufficient for tumor initiation. On the other hand, some *Rb1* mutations appear to lead to an attenuated form of the disease, an observation that highlights the variable penetrance in families.[16,17] Outside the retina, *Rb1* inactivation is often a rate-limiting step in tumorigenesis generated by multiple genetic events. The molecular characteristics and potential functional activities of *Rb1* are outlined in detail elsewhere in this volume.

The patterns of inheritance and presentation of retinoblastoma have been well described and the responsible gene identified. The basic mechanisms by which the gene is inactivated are understood, and provocative evidence indicates that the intricate functional interactions of pRB with its binding partners and other cell cycle targets will provide targets for development of novel small molecule therapies.

WILMS TUMOR: THREE DISTINCT LOCI

Wilms tumor, or nephroblastoma, is an embryonal malignancy that arises from remnants of an immature kidney. It affects approximately 1:10,000 children, usually before the age of 6 years (median age at diagnosis, 3.5 years). Five percent to 10% of children present with either synchronous or metachronous bilateral tumors. A peculiar feature of Wilms tumor is its association with nephrogenic rests, foci of primitive but nonmalignant cells whose persistence suggests a defect in kidney development. These precursor lesions are found within the normal kidney tissue of 30% to 40% of children with Wilms tumor. Nephrogenic rests may persist, regress spontaneously, or grow into a large mass that simulates a true Wilms tumor and presents a difficult diagnostic challenge.[18] Another interesting feature of this neoplasm is its association with specific congenital abnormalities, including genitourinary anomalies, sporadic aniridia, mental retardation, and hemihypertrophy. The *WT1* tumor suppressor gene is reduced to homozygosity, at least in part, in a small but highly informative set of sporadic Wilms tumors. In addition, sporadic and hereditary Wilms tumors have been described in which *WT1* is specifically altered.

A genetic predisposition to Wilms tumor is observed in two distinct disease syndromes with urogenital system malformations: the WAGR (Wilms tumor, aniridia, genitourinary abnormalities, mental retardation) syndrome and the Denys-Drash syndrome (DDS)[19] as well as in BWS, a hereditary overgrowth syndrome characterized by visceromegaly, macroglossia, and hyperinsulinemic hypoglycemia.[20] These congenital disorders have now been linked to abnormalities at specific genetic loci implicated in Wilms tumorigenesis.

The WAGR syndrome has been correlated with constitutional deletions of chromosome 11q13.[21] Whereas it is now known that the WAGR deletion encompasses a number of contiguous genes, including the aniridia gene *Pax6*,[22] the cytogenetic observation in patients with WAGR was also important in the cloning of the *WT1* gene at chromosome 11p13.[23–25] Characterization of *WT1* demonstrated that this gene spans approximately 50 kb of DNA and contains ten exons. The WT1 protein is a transcription factor. However, the identity of the gene(s) targeted by WT1 during normal kidney development is not known.

The second syndrome closely associated with this locus was initially described by Denys in 1967 and recognized as a syndrome by Drash 3 years later.[26,27] DDS is a rare association of Wilms tumor, intersex disorders, and progressive renal failure.[27] It has been demonstrated that virtually all patients with DDS carry *WT1* point mutations in the germ line.[28]

WT1 is altered in only 10% of Wilms tumors. This observation implies the existence of alternative loci in the etiology of this childhood renal malignancy. One such locus also resides on the short arm of chromosome 11, telomeric of *WT1*, at 11p15. This gene, designated *WT2*, is associated with BWS. Patients with BWS are at increased risk of developing Wilms tumor, as well as other embryonic malignancies, including rhabdomyosarcoma (RMS), neuroblastoma, and hepatoblastoma.[29] The putative *BWS* gene maps to chromosome 11p15 and is tightly linked to the Ha-*ras* oncogene homologue *HRAS-I* and the insulinlike growth factor-2 gene (*IGF-2*). Whether the *BWS* gene and *WT2* are one and the same or two distinct yet closely linked genes remains to be determined. Other genes, including *CDKN1C* (p57KIP2), a maternally expressed gene that encodes a cyclin-dependent kinase inhibitor and negatively regulates cell proliferation,[30] show aberrant methylation in tumors that are associated with cell-cycle deregulation. However, *CDKN1C* is rarely mutated in Wilms tumors.[31] Thus, the search for other genes linked to Wilms tumor continues. Using long-oligonucleotide array comparative genomic hybridization (array CGH), a novel gene termed *WTX* was identified on chromosome Xq11.1. *WTX* is inactivated in one-third of Wilms tumors, and tumors with *WTX* mutations lack *WT1* mutations. Whereas autosomal tumor suppressor genes undergo biallelic inactivation, *WTX* is inactivated by a monoallelic "single-hit" event that targets the single X chromosome in Wilms tumors in males and the active X chromosome in tumors from females.[32] This observation suggests a more important role of the X chromosome in human cancers than had previously been appreciated.[33]

Although linkage studies have indicated that the gene for familial Wilms tumor must be distinct from *WT1* and *WT2*, and from the gene that predisposes to BWS, to date, this gene has been neither cytogenetically localized nor isolated. Whether, of course, the gene for familial Wilms tumor interacts with the gene product of either of the two Wilms tumor suppressor genes has yet to be determined.

Finally, loss of the long arm of chromosome 16 has been observed in approximately 20% of Wilms tumor samples.[34] This observation implicates yet another genetic locus in Wilms tumor. Linkage studies have generally also excluded this locus as the "familial" Wilms tumor gene.[35] However, it is plausible that alterations at 16q can initiate tumorigenesis or be implicated in subsequent steps in the progression of malignancy.

Although both tumors represent classic models of the Knudson "two-hit hypothesis" of tumor development, the spectrum of genetic alterations in Wilms tumor is quite different from that in retinoblastoma. In the latter, there is strong evidence that a single gene is involved whose function is mediated through related cell-cycle control pathway genes, whereas a series of genetic alterations, or at least distinct genetic events, is required for Wilms tumorigenesis. Second, the "single-hit" mechanism of *WTX* inactivation suggests a novel basis for Wilms tumorigenesis; and third, unlike retinoblastoma, which is not associated with other developmental anomalies or congenital abnormalities, patients with Wilms tumor commonly exhibit a spectrum of nonmalignant urogenital, skeletal, and cardiac congenital abnormalities that suggest a dual role of the genes involved in both tumor formation and normal embryonic development.

NEUROFIBROMATOSES

The neurofibromatoses (NFs) comprise two similar entities. NF1 is one of the most common autosomal dominantly inherited disorders, affecting approximately 1 in 3,500 people,[36] and half of them arise from new spontaneous mutations. Carriers of mutant *NF1* are predisposed to a variety of tumors, including optic nerve glioma, neurofibroma and neurofibrosarcoma, malignant schwannoma, or malignant peripheral nerve sheath tumor, astrocytoma, and pheochromocytoma.[37] Occurring with less frequency are leukemias, osteosarcoma, RMS, and Wilms tumor and pediatric gastrointestinal stromal tumors.[38]

Using standard linkage analysis, the *NF1* gene was mapped to chromosomal band 17q11.2 and subsequently cloned.[39] The *NF1* gene is composed of 60 exons spanning 350 kb of the genome and is unusual in that it contains three embedded genes—*OMGP*, *EV12A*, and *EV12B*—of unknown function.[40] The *NF1* gene encodes a 2,818-amino acid protein, termed *neurofibromin*, which is ubiquitously expressed. One region of the gene shows extensive structural homology to the guanosine triphosphatase–activating domain of mammalian guanosine triphosphatase–activating proteins: loss of the protein's activity results in failure of hydrolysis of guanosine triphosphate to guanosine diphosphate by the ras oncoprotein. Loss of neurofibromin function usually results from mutations in one allele of the gene, leading to premature truncation of the protein, followed by absence or mutations of the second allele in tumors. More than one mechanism appears to exist whereby malignant tumors develop in patients with NF.

In addition to structural alterations of both alleles of the *NF1* gene, alternative splicing leading to dysregulation at the level of transcription has also been demonstrated. It appears that the two types of resulting protein may modify the modulation of RAS-regulated signal transduction. This loss of function is thought to lead to elevated levels of the guanosine triphosphate–bound RAS protein that transduces signals for cell division. NF1 is now considered to be one of the RASopathies, a class of developmental disorders caused by activation of the RAS-MAPK pathway.[41] Loss of neurofibromin also is associated with activation of mammalian target of rapamycin (mTOR), suggesting a potential therapeutic target for *NF1*-associated tumors.[42] NF type 2 (*NF2*) is much less frequent than *NF1*, occurring in only one in one million persons. Although it is also inherited as an autosomal dominant disorder with high penetrance, the new mutation rate in *NF2* is low.[43] It is clinically characterized by bilateral acoustic neuromas, spinal nerve root tumors, and meningiomas.

The *NF2* locus was mapped to chromosome 22, band q12,[44] and its 69-kD encoded protein, termed *merlin*, has been shown to be expressed in various tissues, including brain, although not as ubiquitously as *NF1*.[45] The mechanism of tumor formation in *NF2* appears to be in concordance with the Knudson two-hit model, although the mechanism of action of the NF2 protein has not yet been elucidated. Merlin is a member of the ERM (ezrin-radixin-moesin) family of proteins that links cell surface proteins to the cytoskeleton.[46] Although ezrin expression has been linked to metastatic behavior,[47] merlin appears to compete with ezrin activation,[43] and merlin deficiency seems to enhance metastases and promote tumorigenesis through destabilization of adherens junctions.[48] Vestibular schwannomas, a hallmark of NF2, have been shown to signal through epidermal growth factor receptor family receptors, suggesting a potential target for medical therapy in these difficult to manage tumors.[49]

NEUROBLASTOMA

Nonrandom chromosomal abnormalities are observed in more than 75% of neuroblastomas,[50] and many of these are also found in neuroblastoma-derived cell lines. The most common of these is deletion or rearrangement of the short arm of chromosome 1, although loss, gain, and rearrangements of chromosomes 10, 11, 14, 17, and 19 have also been reported. The allelic losses indicate loss of function of as yet unknown tumor suppressor genes in these regions. It is believed that a tumor suppressor gene that lies on band p36 of chromosome 1 is critically important in the pathogenesis and aggressive nature of neuroblastoma. It has been shown that the loss of chromosome 1p is a strong prognostic factor in patients with neuroblastoma, independent of age and stage.[51] Although it is as yet unclear which gene(s) in this region may be directly implicated in neuroblastoma development, aberrant expression of one candidate—*p73*—which is a member of the *p53* tumor suppressor family, has been suggested to play a role in the neuroblastoma cell growth as well as chemotherapy resistance.[52] *p73* gives rise to multiple functionally distinct protein isoforms as a result of alternative promoter utilization and alternative mRNA splicing.[53,54] Alternative splicing of the *p73* mRNA results in more than seven protein isoforms that differ in the coding sequences of the COOH terminus (TA-p73 $\alpha, \beta, \gamma, \delta, \varepsilon, \zeta, \eta$).

In addition to these COOH-terminal splice forms, three additional forms, Np73α, ΔNp73β, and ΔNp73γ, are transcribed from an alternative promoter located in intron 3. Their protein products lack the NH2-terminal transactivation domain and are thus called *ΔNp73*. The full-length forms that contain the NH2-terminal transactivation domain are denoted *TA*. Higher levels of ΔNp73 are associated with an overall worse clinical prognosis, presumably because of the "antiapoptotic" properties of ΔNp73 and its ability to inactivate both TAp73 and p53.[55,56]

Two other unique cytogenetic rearrangements are highly characteristic of neuroblastoma.[57] These structures, homogeneous staining regions and double-minute chromosomes, contain regions of gene amplification. The *N-myc* gene, an oncogene with considerable homology to the cellular protooncogene *c-myc*, is amplified within homogeneous staining regions and double-minute chromosomes. Virtually all neuroblastoma tumor cell lines demonstrate amplified and highly expressed *N-myc*,[58] and *N-myc* amplification is thought to be associated with rapid tumor progression. Expression of *N-myc* is increased in undifferentiated tumor cells compared with much lower (or single-copy) levels in more differentiated cells (ganglioneuroblastoma and ganglioneuroma). *N-myc* expression is diminished in association with the *in vitro* differentiation of neuroblastoma cell lines.[59] This observation formed the basis for current therapeutic trials demonstrating a survival advantage to patients treated with *cis*-retinoic acid.[60] Furthermore, a close correlation exists between *N-myc* amplification and advanced clinical stage.[61]

Although it is clear that altered expression of *N-myc* contributes to the development of malignancy, it is not yet apparent which cellular functions are altered. The molecular mechanisms underlying regulation of neuroblastoma differentiation may be explained in part through the contribution of other genes and proteins. This is currently under intense investigation through the use of gene expression profiling of *N-myc*–positive versus –negative tumors.

Neuroblastoma cells that express the high-affinity nerve growth factor receptor trkA[62] can be terminally differentiated by nerve growth factor and may demonstrate morphologic changes typical of ganglionic differentiation. Tumors showing ganglionic differentiation and *trk* gene activation have a favorable prognosis.[62] In contrast, trkB receptor expression is associated with poor-prognosis tumors and appears to mediate resistance to chemotherapy.[63,64] Resistance to multidrug chemotherapeutic regimens (multidrug resistance) is characteristic of aggressive, poorly responsive *N-myc*–amplified neuroblastomas. It is interesting to note that expression of the multidrug resistance–associated protein, found to confer multidrug resistance *in vitro*, is increased in neuroblastomas with *N-myc* amplification and decreased after differentiation of tumor cells *in vitro*.[65] It has been demonstrated that high levels of multidrug resistance–associated protein expression are significantly associated with poor outcome, independent of *N-myc* amplification.[65] Gain of chromosome segment 17q21-qter has been shown to be the most powerful prognostic factor yet.[66] However, no gene has yet been implicated at this site.

A small subset of neuroblastomas is inherited in an autosomal dominant fashion. Until recently, the only gene definitively associated with neuroblastoma risk was *PHOX2B*, also linked to central apnea.[67] *De novo* or inherited missense mutations in the tyrosine kinase domain of the *ALK* (anaplastic lymphoma kinase) gene on chromosome 2p23 have been observed in the majority of hereditary neuroblastoma families, as well as in somatic tumor cells.[68–71] Current phase 1/2 clinical trials with ALK inhibitors substantiate the value of such target identification for novel therapies. The role of other molecular alterations in neuroblastoma continues to be elucidated. In addition to chromosomal loss on chromosome 1p36, unbalanced LOH at 11q23 is independently associated with decreased event-free survival. Alterations at 11q23 occur in almost one-third of neuroblastomas, being most commonly associated with stage 4 disease and age at diagnosis greater than 2.5 years. Both 1p36 LOH and 11q23 LOH were independently associated with decreased progression-free survival in patients with low- and intermediate-risk disease.[72]

Yet another valuable biological marker of clinical significance is telomerase expression and telomere length. In particular, short telomere length is predictive of favorable prognosis, irrespective of disease stage, while long or unchanged telomeres are predictive of poor outcome.[73,74] Telomerase expression, as measured by telomerase reverse transcriptase (hTERT), has been shown to be negative in good-risk neuroblastoma, although it is high in tumors with unfavorable histology.[74] The combined use of these markers—chromosomes 1p and 11q, *N-Myc* amplification, *trkA* and telomerase expression—as prognostic indicators provides a powerful armamentarium with which to develop rational stratified treatment programs for neuroblastoma.

EWING SARCOMA FAMILY OF TUMORS

Ewing sarcoma (ES) is one of the first examples in which the application of molecular diagnostics led to improved tumor classification. ES was first described by James Ewing[75] as a bone tumor characterized by small, blue, round cells and minimal mitotic activity. Turc-Carel et al.[76] identified a recurring reciprocal t(11;22) chromosomal translocation in these tumors in 1983. Investigators subsequently demonstrated a cytogenetically identical t(11;22) in adult neuroblastoma or peripheral primitive neuroectodermal tumor (pPNET), so named because of its histologic similarity to neuroblastoma.[77] Based on the presence of the identical translocation, it was hypothesized that pPNET was related to ES. This translocation breakpoint has been molecularly characterized as an in-frame fusion between a new ES gene, *EWS*, on chromosome 22 and an ETS transcription family member, FLI-1, on chromosome 22.[78–80]

In addition to this fusion transcript being identified in pPNET, other variants, notably the chest-wall Askin tumor and soft tissue ES—previously treated as an RMS because of its location in soft tissue—were also shown to bear the identical fusion transcript. In total, five translocations also have been identified, invariably fusing the *EWS* gene to an ETS family member.[81–84] More than 90% of the ES family of tumors (ESFTs) carry the *EWS-ETS* fusion gene, and a search for *EWS-ETS* by either reverse transcriptase-polymerase chain reaction or fluorescence *in situ* hybridization should be considered standard practice in the diagnostic evaluation of suspected ESFTs. Interestingly, although it was suggested that the specific fusion protein expressed in ESFT has prognostic significance,[85] several prospective studies in the United States and Europe demonstrated no prognostic impact.[86,87] The nature of the novel fusion transcription factor and its downstream targets is currently under intense investigation. One target of the EWS-ETS fusion is repression of the transforming growth factor-β type II receptor,[88] a putative tumor suppressor gene.

Expression profiling analysis has also revealed that p53 is transcriptionally up-regulated by the *EWS-ETS* fusion gene.[89] This is of particular interest because it is now known that expression of *EWS-ETS* can lead to apoptosis, and that additional alterations such as loss of *p53* or *p16* signaling, or both, appear to be necessary components of EWS-ETS–induced transformation.[90] Investigators have now taken advantage of RNA interference technology to inhibit EWS-FLI-1 in Ewing cell lines to identify genes regulated by the fusion in the proper context. Using this approach, *NKX2.2* and *NR0B1* have been found to be a target gene of EWS-FLI-1 that is necessary for oncogenic transformation.[91,92] Recent findings suggest that GGAA microsatellites might mark genes that are up-regulated by EWS-FLI-1 binding.[93]

RHABDOMYOSARCOMA

The two major histologic subtypes of RMS, embryonal and alveolar, have unique histologic appearances as well as distinctive molecular genetic abnormalities, while sharing a common myogenic lineage. Embryonal tumors comprise two-thirds of all RMS and are histologically characterized by a stroma-rich spindle cell appearance. Alveolar tumors comprise approximately one-third of RMS and are histologically characterized by densely packed, small, round cells, often lining a septation reminiscent of a pulmonary alveolus, giving rise to its name. Both histologic subtypes express muscle-specific proteins, including α-actin, myosin, desmin, and MyoD,[94,95] and they virtually always express high levels of *IGF-2*.[96]

At the molecular level, embryonal tumors are characterized by LOH at the 11p15 locus, which is of particular interest because this region harbors the *IGF-2* gene.[97] The LOH at 11p15 occurs by loss of maternal and duplication of paternal chromosomal material.[98] Although LOH is normally associated with loss of tumor suppressor gene activity, in this instance LOH with paternal duplication may result in activation of *IGF-2*. This occurs because *IGF-2* is now known to be normally imprinted; that is, this gene is normally transcriptionally silent at the maternal allele, with only the paternal allele being transcriptionally active.[99] Thus, LOH with paternal duplication potentially leads to a twofold gene-dosage effect of the IGF-2 locus. Furthermore, in alveolar tumors in which LOH does not occur, the normally imprinted maternal allele has been shown to be re-expressed.[100] Thus, LOH and loss of imprinting in this case may lead to the same functional result—namely, biallelic expression of the normally monoallelically expressed *IGF-2*. However, loss of an as yet unidentified tumor suppressor activity due to LOH also remains a possibility. *HRAS* oncogene is also located at 11p15, and germ line mutations of *HRAS* occur in Costello syndrome, another tumor within the RASopathy family. Patients with Costello syndrome have an increased incidence of embryonal RMS.[101] These data suggest the possibility of cooperativity between *HRAS* mutations and UPD at 11p15 in the development of ERMS.[102]

Alveolar RMS is characterized by a t(2;13) (q35;q14) chromosomal translocation.[103] Molecular cloning of this translocation has identified the generation of a fusion transcription factor, fusing the 5′ DNA-binding region of PAX-3 on chromosome 2 to the 3′ transactivation domain region of *FKHR* gene on chromosome 13.[104] A variant t(1;13) (q36;q14) has been identified in a smaller number of alveolar RMS tumors that fuse the 5′ DNA-binding region of the *PAX-7* gene on chromosome 1 with the identical 3′ transactivation domain of the *FKHR* (Foxo 1A) gene.[105] Fluorescence *in situ* hybridization or reverse transcriptase-polymerase chain reaction can be used to identify these PAX-FKHR fusions. In a review of 171 patients entered into the Intergroup Rhabdomyosarcoma Study Group IV study, the gene fusion was found only in alveolar RMS cases. In the 78 alveolar RMS cases, 55% were PAX3-FKHR+, 22% were PAX7-FKHR+, and 23% were fusion-negative.[106] It has now become clear that these fusion-negative alveolar RMS tumors are clinically and molecularly indistinguishable from embryonal RMS, thus making the presence of the PAX-FKHR fusion a diagnostic criteria for alveolar RMS.[107] The nature of this fusion-derived novel transcription factor and its downstream targets is the subject of active investigation. It also has been suggested that, like ESFT, in which the specific expressed fusion transcript has prognostic significance, the PAX-3–FKHR and the PAX-7–FKHR fusions lead to distinct clinicopathologic entities.[108] The critical role of PAX-3-FKHR in the generation of alveolar RMS has now been recapitulated in a mouse PAX-3-FKHR knock-in model, coupled with either p53 or CDKN2a inactivation.[109]

The PAX-3–FKHR fusion is associated with increased expression of *c-met*.[110] Met is the receptor tyrosine kinase for hepatocyte growth factor/scatter factor and is overexpressed in embryonal and alveolar RMS.[111] A mouse model of embryonal RMS has been generated by expressing a hepatocyte growth factor transgene in Ink4a/Arf$^{-/-}$ mice. The tumors appear to arise from hyperplastic satellite cells (myoblastic precursor cells).[112] The putative role of satellite cells in the pathogenesis of embryonal RMS is supported by a report demonstrating high PAX-7 expression in embryonal RMS compared to alveolar RMS and the association of PAX-7 expression with satellite cells.[113] Other frequently reported genetic alterations that may be common to embryonal and alveolar RMS include activated forms of N- and K-RAS,[114] inactivating *p53* mutations,[115] and amplification and overexpression of *MDM2*, *CDK-4*, *N-MYC*,[116] and *FGFR4* activating mutations.[117]

HEREDITARY SYNDROMES ASSOCIATED WITH TUMORS OF CHILDHOOD

Li-Fraumeni Syndrome

A few hereditary cancer syndromes are associated with the occurrence of childhood as well as adult-onset neoplasms. The paradigm LFS cancer was first described in 1969 from an epidemiologic evaluation of more than 600 medical and family history records of patients with childhood sarcoma.[118] The original description of a kindred with a spectrum of tumors that includes soft tissue sarcomas, osteosarcomas, breast cancer, brain tumors, leukemia, and adrenocortical carcinoma (ACC) has been overwhelmingly substantiated by numerous subsequent studies,[119] although other cancers, usually of particularly early age of onset, are also observed.[120] Germ line alterations of the *p53* tumor suppressor gene are associated with LFS.[121,122] These are primarily missense mutations that yield a stabilized mutant protein. The spectrum of mutations of *p53* in the germ line is similar to somatic mutations found in a wide variety of tumors. Carriers are heterozygous for the mutation, and in tumors derived from these individuals, the second (wild type) allele is frequently deleted or mutated, leading to functional inactivation.[123]

Several comprehensive databases document all reported germ line (and somatic) *p53* mutations and are of particular value in evaluating novel mutations as well as phenotype-genotype correlations.[124] Only 60% to 80% of "classic" LFS families have detectable alterations of the gene. It is not yet determined whether the remainder is associated with the presence of modifier genes, promoter defects yielding abnormalities of *p53* expression, or simply the result of weak genotype-phenotype correlations (i.e., the broad clinical definition encompasses families that are not actual members of LFS). Other candidate predisposition genes, such as *p16*, *p15*, *p21*, *BRCA1*, *BRCA2*, and *PTEN*, associated with multisite cancer associations have generally been ruled out as potential targets. The role of the hCHK2 checkpoint kinase as an alternative mechanism for functional inactivation of *p53* in LFS has been suggested,[125] although its place as a major contributor to the phenotype has been controversial.[126]

Germ line *p53* alterations have also been reported in some patients with cancer phenotypes that resemble the classic LFS phenotype. Between 3% and 10% of children with apparently sporadic RMS or osteosarcoma have been shown to carry germ line *p53* mutations.[127,128] These patients tend to be younger than those who harbor wild type *p53*. It appears as well that more than 75% of children with apparently sporadic ACC carry germ line *p53* mutations, although in some of these cases, a family history develops that is not substantially distinct from LFS.[129,130] These important findings indicate a broader spectrum of patients at risk of germ line *p53* mutations, and refined criteria for *p53* mutation analysis.[131,132] A striking genotype-phenotype correlation has been observed in a unique subgroup of ACC patients in Brazil in whom the same germ line *p53* mutation at codon 337 has been observed in 35 unrelated kindred.[133] Other cancers typical of LFS are not observed in these families, and the functional integrity of the mutant protein appears to be regulated by alterations in cellular pH,[134] which suggests potential biologic mechanisms in ACC cells by which the *p53* mutation leads to malignant transformation. All these observations suggest that germ line *p53* alterations may be associated with early-onset development of the childhood component tumors of the syndrome.[135] It is not clear what clinical significance these findings have in that no studies of prognostic significance or potential impact on anticancer treatment modalities are reported. Nevertheless, in light of the critical role played by *p53* in the initiation and potentiation of gamma irradiation or chemotherapy-induced DNA damage repair, studies into the effect of such germ line mutations on the potentiation of tumor development related to therapeutic interventions would be important.

The variability in age of onset and type of cancer among LFS families suggests modifier effects on the underlying mutant *p53* genotype. Analysis of mutant genotype-to-phenotype correlations reveals intriguing observations. Nonsense, frameshift, and splice mutations yield a truncated or nonfunctional protein commonly associated with early-onset cancers, particularly brain tumors. Missense mutation in the *p53* DNA binding domain are frequently observed in the setting of breast and brain tumors, while adrenocortical cancers are the only group that are associated with mutations in the non-DNA binding loops. Age of onset modifiers have also now been established. The protein murine double-minute-2 (MDM2) is a key negative regulator of p53 and targets p53 toward proteasomal degradation. The MDM2 single nucleotide polymorphism 309 increases Sp1 transcription factor binding, leading to increased *MDM2* expression levels. Coinheritance of the MDM2 single nucleotide polymorphism 309 T/G isoform is associated with earlier-onset cancer.[136] The earlier age of onset of cancers with subsequent generations in mutant *p53* LFS families suggests genetic anticipation. This observation can be partially explained by several molecular mechanisms including accelerated telomere attrition from generation to generation, absence of the PIN3 polymorphism, or excessive DNA copy number variation in *p53* mutation carriers, all of which may be useful predictive markers of tumor age of onset.[136–138] Thus, although germ line *p53* mutations establish the baseline risk of tumor development in LFS, a complex interplay of modifying genetic cofactors likely defines the specific phenotypes of individual patients.

Beckwith-Wiedemann Syndrome

BWS occurs with a frequency of 1 in 13,700 births. More than 450 cases have been documented since the original reported associations of exomphalos, macroglossia, gigantism, and other congenital anomalies. With increasing age, phenotypic features of BWS become less pronounced. Laboratory findings may include, at birth, hypoglycemia (extremely common), polycythemia, hypocalcemia, hypertriglyceridemia, hypercholesterolemia, and high serum α-fetoprotein levels. Early diagnosis of the condition is crucial to avoid deleterious neurologic effects of neonatal hypoglycemia and to initiate an appropriate screening protocol for tumor development.[139] The increased risk for tumor formation in BWS patients is estimated at 7.5% and is further increased to 10% if hemihyperplasia is present. Tumors occurring with the highest frequency include Wilms tumor, hepatoblastoma, neuroblastoma, and ACC.[20]

The genetic basis of BWS is complex. Various 11p15 chromosomal or molecular alterations have been associated with the BWS phenotype and its tumors.[140] It is unlikely that a single gene is responsible for the BWS phenotype. Because it appears that abnormalities in the region impact an imprinted domain, it is more likely that normal gene regulation in this part of chromosome 11p15 occurs in a regional manner and may depend on various interdependent factors or genes. These include the paternally expressed genes *IGF-2* and *KCNQ10T1* and the maternally expressed genes *H19*, *CDKN1C*, and *KCNQ1*. BWS children who develop rhabdomyosarcoma or hepatoblastoma have epigenetic changes in domain 1, whereas those with Wilms tumor have domain 2 changes or uniparental disomy.[141]

Chromosomal abnormalities associated with BWS are extremely rare, with only 20 cases having been associated with 11p15 translocations or inversions. The chromosomal breakpoint in each of these cases is always found on the maternally derived chromosome 11. This parent-of-origin dependence in BWS suggests that the chromosome translocations disrupt imprinting of a gene in the 11p15 region. On the other hand, BWS-associated 11p15 duplications (approximately 30 reported cases) are always paternally derived, and the duplication breakpoints are heterogeneous.[142] Paternal uniparental disomy, in which two alleles are inherited from one parent (the father), has been reported in approximately 15% of sporadic BWS patients.[143] It is interesting that the insulin/IGF-2 region is always represented in the uniparental disomy, although the extent of chromosomal involvement is highly variable. Alterations in allele-specific DNA methylation of *IGF-2* and *H19* reflect this paternal imprinting phenomenon.[143] A minority of BWS patients have demonstrable constitutional DNA sequence alterations, the most common of these being *CDKN1C* mutations.[144] Twenty-five percent to 50% of BWS patients exhibit biallelic rather than monoallelic expression of *IGF-2*. Another 50% have epigenetic mutations resulting in loss of imprinting of *KCNQ10T0*. Of interest, epigenetic changes, such as methylation and chromatin modification, occur in many pediatric and adult cancers,[145] indicating the value of the BWS model in understanding the broad scope of molecular changes in cancer. Despite the associated cytogenetic and molecular findings for some patients, no single diagnostic test exists for BWS. This observation is not unlike that described for LFS, or perhaps for other multisite cancer phenotypes, in which the clarity of the phenotype is often weak, making the genetic link cloudy and the likelihood of multiple pathways to tumor formation strong.

Gorlin Syndrome

Nevoid basal cell carcinoma syndrome, or Gorlin syndrome, is a rare autosomal dominant disorder characterized by multiple basal cell carcinomas, developmental defects including bifid ribs and other spine and rib abnormalities, palmar and plantar pits, odontogenic keratocysts, and generalized overgrowth.[146] The Sonic hedgehog (SHH) signaling pathway directs embryonic development of a spectrum of organisms. Gorlin syndrome appears to be caused by germ line mutations of the tumor suppressor gene *PTCH*, a receptor for SHH.[147,148] Medulloblastoma develops in approximately 5% of patients with Gorlin syndrome. Furthermore, approximately 10% of patients diagnosed with medulloblastoma by the age of 2 are found to have other phenotypic features consistent with Gorlin syndrome and also harbor germline *PTCH* mutations.[149] Although Gorlin syndrome develops in individuals with germ line mutations of *PTCH*, a subset of children with medulloblastoma harbor germ line mutations of another gene, *SUFU*, in the SHH pathway, with accompanying LOH in the tumors. Of further note, mice with heterozygous PTC deletions develop RMS.[151] Although RMS is not associated with Gorlin syndrome, the mouse studies suggest a possible link between PTC signaling and RMS.[152]

MALIGNANT RHABDOID TUMORS

Malignant rhabdoid tumors are unusual pediatric tumors that occur as primary renal tumors, but have also been described in lung, liver, soft tissues, and the central nervous system, where they are often termed *atypical* and *teratoid rhabdoid tumors*.[153] Recurrent chromosomal translocations of chromosome 22 involving a breakpoint at 22q11.2, as well as complete or partial monosomy 22, have been observed, strongly suggesting the presence of a tumor suppressor gene in this area. The *hSNF5/INI1* gene has been isolated and has been shown to be the target for biallelic, recurrent inactivating mutations.[154] The encoded gene product is thought to be involved in chromatin remodeling. Studies have not only demonstrated the presence of inactivating mutations in the majority of malignant rhabdoid tumors (renal or extrarenal) but also in chronic myelogenous leukemia,[155] as well as in a wide variety of other childhood and adult-onset malignancies.[156] An intriguing feature in some individuals with malignant rhabdoid tumors is the observation of germ line mutations, suggesting that this family of tumors may occur as a result of a primary inherited defect in one allele of the *INI1* gene.[157] Further studies of the function of this gene will be important in determining its role in tumorigenesis of this wide spectrum of neoplasms.

PREDICTIVE TESTING FOR GERM LINE MUTATIONS AND CHILDHOOD CANCERS

Several important issues have arisen as a result of the identification of germ line mutations of tumor suppressor genes in cancer-prone individuals and families. These include ethical questions of predictive testing in such families and in unaffected relatives and selection of patients to be tested, as well as the development of practical and accurate laboratory techniques, the development of pilot testing programs, and the role of clinical intervention based on test results. This chapter was not meant to discuss these problems in detail, but one would be remiss to ignore their significance.

For several reasons, testing cannot as yet be offered to the general pediatric population, particularly in light of the demonstrably low carrier rate of the abnormal tumor suppressor genes and the general lack of standardized methods of preclinical screening of carriers. Exceptions to these limitations include screening of gene carriers in families with retinoblastoma, BWS, multiple endocrine neoplasia, familial adenomatous polyposis, and von Hippel-Lindau disease. For some of these diseases, clinical surveillance tools are available, whereas for others, risk-reductive surgery has also been shown to be of value.[158,159] In general, it has been demonstrated that genetic testing does not lead to clinical levels of anxiety, depression, or other markers of psychological distress in the children who are tested, or their parents.[160,161] However, certain circumstances or personality traits are associated with a greater likelihood of an individual experiencing psychological distress after a positive result.[160] Parents now routinely discuss the options of prenatal diagnosis and preimplantation genetic diagnosis. Multidisciplinary teams must be engaged to provide parents and families the necessary tools with which to approach these ethically challenging decisions.[162,163] The development of screening programs should address aspects of cost, informed consent (particularly where it affects children), socioeconomic impact on the individual tested, consistency in providing results, and counseling. Concerns of risk of employment, health insurance, or life insurance discrimination exist but may be alleviated by congressional legislation to ban such practices.[164]

MOLECULAR THERAPEUTICS

With the identification of alterations in a variety of molecular signaling pathways, including activated growth factor signaling pathways (e.g., *IGF-2*) and altered tumor suppressor pathways (e.g., retinoblastoma), it has become increasingly apparent that these alterations may potentially represent the "Achilles' heel" for these tumors. New agents targeting the tyrosine kinase enzymes that transduce growth factor signals are at various stages of development in early clinical studies. Several IGF-I receptor (IR) antibodies have been tested in ES and rhabdomyosarcoma, and small-molecule IGF-IR kinase inhibitors are entering clinical trials. Several mTOR inhibitors are now approved for treatment of kidney cancer, and these agents are currently being tested in both NF1 as well as in combinations with IGF-IR inhibitors in pediatric sarcomas.

Fusion proteins derived from tumor-specific translocations may themselves represent targets, either as potential neoantigens that could be targeted by cytotoxic T cells or as targets for novel compounds. It is likely that the molecular characterization of pediatric tumors will lead to novel and perhaps more effective treatment approaches in the near future. It is also likely that some of these innovative approaches will at least initially be integrated into standard therapeutic protocols.

Selected References

The full list of references for this chapter appears in the online version.

3. Knudson AG Jr. Mutation and cancer: statistical study of retinoblastoma. *Proc Natl Acad Sci U S A* 1971;68:820.
8. Cavenee WK, Dryja TP, Phillips RA, et al. Expression of recessive alleles by chromosomal mechanisms in retinoblastoma. *Nature* 1983;305:779.
10. Friend SH, Bernards R, Rogelj S, et al. A human DNA segment with properties of the gene that predisposes to retinoblastoma and osteosarcoma. *Nature* 1986;323:643.
23. Call KM, Glaser T, Ito CY, et al. Isolation and characterization of a zinc finger polypeptide gene at the human chromosome 11 Wilms' tumor locus. *Cell* 1990;60:509
32. Rivera MN, Kim WJ, Driscoll DR, et al. An X chromosome gene, WTX, is commonly inactivated in Wilms tumor. *Science* 2007;315:642.
40. Viskochil D, Buchberg AM, Xu G, et al. Deletions and a translocation interrupt a cloned gene at the neurofibromatosis type 1 locus. *Cell* 1990; 62:187.
41. Tidyman WE, Rauen KA. The RASopathies: developmental syndromes of Ras/MAPK pathway dysregulation. *Curr Opin Genet Dev* 2009;19:230.
49. Ammoun S, Cunliffe CH, Allen JC, et al. ErbB/HER receptor activation and preclinical efficacy of lapatinib in vestibular schwannoma. *Neuro Oncol* 2010;12:834.
50. Brodeur GM, Sekhon G, Goldstein MN. Chromosomal aberrations in human neuroblastomas. *Cancer* 1977;40:2256.
51. Caron H, van Sluis P, de Kraker J, et al. Allelic loss of chromosome 1p as a predictor of unfavorable outcome in patients with neuroblastoma. *N Engl J Med* 1996;334:225.
58. Schwab M, Alitalo K, Klempnauer KH, et al. Amplified DNA with limited homology to myc cellular oncogene is shared by human neuroblastoma cell lines and a neuroblastoma tumour. *Nature* 1983;305:245.
59. Thiele CJ, Reynolds CP, Israel MA. Decreased expression of N-myc precedes retinoic acid-induced morphological differentiation of human neuroblastoma. *Nature* 1985;313:404.
61. Schwab M, Ellison J, Busch M, et al. Enhanced expression of the human gene N-myc consequent to amplification of DNA may contribute to malignant progression of neuroblastoma. *Proc Natl Acad Sci U S A* 1984;81: 4940.
62. Nakagawara A, Arima-Nakagawara M, Scavarda NJ, et al. Association between high levels of expression of the TRK gene and favorable outcome in human neuroblastoma. *N Engl J Med* 1993;328:847.
68. Mosse YP, Laduenslager M, Longo L, et al. Identification of ALK as a major familial neuroblastoma predisposition gene. *Nature* 2008;455:967.
72. Attiyeh EF, London WB, Mosse YP, et al. Chromosome 1p and 11q deletions and outcome in neuroblastoma. *N Engl J Med* 2005;353(21):2243.
74. Ohali A, Avigad S, Ash S, et al. Telomere length is a prognostic factor in neuroblastoma. *Cancer* 2006;107:1391.
77. Whang-Peng J, Triche T, Knutsen T, et al. Chromosome translocation in peripheral neuroepithelioma. *N Engl J Med* 1984;311:584.
78. Delattre O, Zucman J, Ploustagel B, et al. Gene fusion with an ETS DNA binding domain caused by chromosome translocation in human cancers. *Nature* 1992;359:162.
87. van Doorninck JA, Ji L, Schaub B, et al. Current treatment protocols have eliminated the prognostic advantage of type 1 fusions in Ewing sarcoma: a report from the Children's Oncology Group. *J Clin Oncol* 2010;28:1989.
89. Lessnick SL, Dacwag CS, Golub TR. The Ewing's sarcoma oncoprotein EWS/FLI induces a p53-dependent growth arrest in primary human fibroblasts. *Cancer Cell* 2002;1:393.
92. Kinsey M, Smith R, Lessnick SL. NR0B1 is required for the oncogenic phenotype mediated by EWS/FLI in Ewing's sarcoma. *Mol Cancer Res* 2006;4:851.
95. Dias P, Parham DM, Shapiro DN, et al. Myogenic regulatory protein (MyoD1) expression in childhood solid tumors: diagnostic utility in rhabdomyosarcoma. *Am J Pathol* 1990;137:1283.
97. Scrable H, Witte D, Shimada H, et al. Molecular differential pathology of rhabdomyosarcoma. *Genes Chromosomes Cancer* 1989;1:23.
99. Rainier S, Johnson LA, Dobry CJ, et al. Relaxation of imprinted genes in human cancer. *Nature* 1993;362:747.
100. Zhan S, Shapiro DN, Helman LJ. Activation of an imprinted allele of the insulin-like growth factor II gene implicated in rhabdomyosarcoma. *J Clin Invest* 1994;94:445.
101. Gripp KW. Tumor predisposition in Costello syndrome. *Am J Med Genet C Semin Med Genet* 2005;137C:72.
104. Barr FG, Galili N, Holick J, et al. Rearrangement of the PAX3 paired box gene in the paediatric solid tumour alveolar rhabdomyosarcoma. *Nat Genet* 1993;3:113.
106. Sorensen PH, Lynch JC, Qualman SJ, et al. PAX3-FKHR and PAX7-FKHR gene fusions are prognostic indicators in alveolar rhabdomyosarcoma: a report from the Children's Oncology Group. *J Clin Oncol* 2002;20(11): 2672.
109. Keller C, Arenkiel BR, Coffin CM, El-Bardeesy N, DePinho RA, Capecchi MR. Alveolar rhabdomyosarcomas in conditional Pax3:Fkhr mice: cooperativity of Ink4a/ARF and Trp53 loss of function. *Genes Dev* 2004;18: 2614.
117. Taylor JG 6th, Cheuk AT, Tsang PS, et al. Identification of FGFR4-activating mutations in human rhabdomyosarcomas that promote metastasis in xenotransplanted models. *J Clin Invest* 2009;119:3395
118. Li FP, Fraumeni JF Jr. Rhabdomyosarcoma in children: epidemiologic study and identification of a familial cancer syndrome. *J Natl Cancer Inst* 1969;43:1365.
121. Malkin D, Li FP, Strong LC, et al. Germ line p53 mutations in a familial syndrome of breast cancer, sarcomas, and other neoplasms. *Science* 1990; 250:1233.
124. Olivier M, Eeles R, Hollstein M, et al. The IARC TP53 database: new online mutation analysis and recommendations to users. *Hum Mutat* 2002; 19:607.
132. Tinat J, Bougeard G, Baert-Desurmont S, et al. 2009 version of the Chompret criteria for Li-Fraumeni syndrome. *J Clin Oncol* 2009;27 (26):e108.
133. Ribeiro RC, Sandrini F, Figueiredo B, et al. An inherited p53 mutation that contributes in a tissue-specific manner to pediatric adrenal cortical carcinoma. *Proc Natl Acad Sci U S A* 2001;98:9330.

135. Olivier M, Goldgar DE, Sodha N, et al. Li-Fraumeni and related syndromes: correlation between tumor type, family structure, and TP53 genotype. *Cancer Res* 2003;63:6643.
138. Shlien A, Tabori U, Marshall CR, et al. Excessive genomic DNA copy number variation in the Li-Fraumeni cancer predisposition syndrome. *Proc Natl Acad Sci U S A* 2008;105:11264.
142. Henry I, Bonaiti-Pellie C, Chehensse V, et al. Uniparental paternal disomy in a genetic cancer-predisposing syndrome. *Nature* 1991;351:665.
148. Hahn H, Wicking C, Zaphiropoulous PG, et al. Mutations of the human homolog of Drosophila patched in the nevoid basal cell carcinoma syndrome. *Cell* 1996;85:841.
150. Taylor MD, Liu L, Raffel C, et al. Mutations in SUFU predispose to medulloblastoma. *Nat Genet* 2002;31:306.
154. Versteege I, Sevenet N, Lange J, et al. Truncating mutations of hSNF5/INI1 in aggressive paediatric cancer. *Nature* 1998;394:203.
157. Biegel JA, Zhou JY, Rorke LB, et al. Germ-line and acquired mutations of INI1 in atypical teratoid and rhabdoid tumors. *Cancer Res* 1999; 59:74.
162. Lammens C, Bleiker Aaronson N, Aaronson N, et al. Attitudes towards pre-implantation genetic diagnosis for hereditary cancer. *Fam Cancer* 2009;8(4):457.

CHAPTER 123 SOLID TUMORS OF CHILDHOOD

LISA L. WANG, JASON YUSTEIN, CHRYSTAL LOUIS, HEIDI V. RUSSELL, ALBERTO S. PAPPO, ARNOLD PAULINO, JED G. NUCHTERN, AND MURALI CHINTAGUMPALA

Approximately 12,400 children and adolescents younger than 20 years are diagnosed with cancer each year in the United States,[1] and childhood cancer remains the leading cause of disease-related mortality in children.[2] Malignant solid tumors account for approximately 30% of childhood cancers.[1] The predominant histologies of specific solid tumors vary significantly with age.[3] The overall distribution of pediatric solid tumors by histologic subtype is shown in Figure 123.1.

The outcomes of patients with solid tumors has dramatically increased during the past 30 years, and this success can be attributed to several factors, including enrollment of patients into well-designed prospective clinical trials (Fig. 123.2),[4,5] systematic collection of tissue to better define the biology of disease,[6] availability of more effective chemotherapy agents, use of multimodal therapy, better supportive care, and more refined diagnostic imaging methods that accurately define the extent of disease at diagnosis.

THE IMPORTANCE OF MULTIDISCIPLINARY MANAGEMENT TEAMS IN PEDIATRIC SOLID TUMORS

The management of childhood malignant solid tumors is complex and requires an integrated multidisciplinary approach that often involves various treatment modalities such as surgery, radiotherapy, and chemotherapy. Surgery plays a dual role in the management of pediatric solid tumors because it is required for establishing a histologic diagnosis and for resecting the disease when possible. It is important that the surgeon work in a collaborative fashion with the pediatric oncologist and radiation oncologist prior to attempted resection because mutilating or disfiguring surgeries may no longer be indicated in the era of effective chemotherapy and radiotherapy. For the radiation oncologist it is important to evaluate the patient prior to any treatment (resection or chemotherapy) if radiotherapy is likely to be used so that the extent of tumor can be determined by physical examination and imaging studies prior to any intervention.

NEUROBLASTOMA

Neuroblastoma comprises a spectrum of tumors that arise from primitive sympathetic ganglion cells and includes neuroblastoma, ganglioneuroblastoma, and ganglioneuroma. This group of tumors is known for a broad spectrum of clinical behaviors ranging from spontaneous regression to widely disseminated, aggressive disease. Tumors can be subdivided into distinct risk categories based on clinical and biological features. Historically, the intensity of treatment has been determined by stage of disease and risk classification such that the majority of patients with low-risk disease have been treated with surgical resection followed by clinical observation. Conversely, patients with high-risk disease require multimodal treatment with chemotherapy, surgery, radiation, and biologic agents.

Epidemiology

Neuroblastoma is the third most common childhood cancer after leukemia and brain tumors. From 2003 to 2007, the age-adjusted incidence of neuroblastoma was 10.1 per 1 million children aged 0 to 14 years.[1] Of the approximate 650 children diagnosed each year in the United States, the median age is 17.3 months. Neuroblastoma is slightly more common in white versus black infants (1.7 and 1.9 to 1 for male and female infants, respectively), but this difference is not evident in older children.[1]

The majority of neuroblastomas are sporadic. However, a small subset of children may have concomitant neural crest disorders, including neurofibromatosis, Hirschsprung disease, congenital hypoventilation syndrome, or other predisposing conditions such as Turner syndrome and Beckwith-Wiedemann syndrome. About 1% to 2% of cases are associated with a history of neuroblastoma in immediate or extended family members. These cases appear to be inherited in an autosomal dominant pattern, have an earlier age at presentation (9 months vs. 17 months), and have multifocal or bilateral adrenal primaries.[7,8] The recent description of a new familial autosomal dominant disorder with incomplete penetrance, anaplastic lymphoma kinase (ALK)-related neuroblastoma susceptibility syndrome, has led to accelerated clinical testing of small molecule inhibitors targeting ALK tyrosine kinase in patients with neuroblastoma.[8–10]

Pathology

Tumors of neuroblastic origin are classified according to the balance between neural-type cells (primitive neuroblasts, maturing neuroblasts, and ganglion cells) and Schwann-type cells (Schwannian blasts and mature Schwann cells). The three major types of neuroblastic tumors from most to least aggressive are neuroblastoma, ganglioneuroblastoma, and ganglioneuroma (Fig. 123.3), and they can be further subdivided into differentiating, poorly differentiated, or undifferentiated. The International Neuroblastoma Pathology Classification System,[11] proposed in 1999 and revised in 2003,[12] is a modification of the earlier Shimada classification system (Fig. 123.4) whose prognostic significance was confirmed in a retrospective review of two

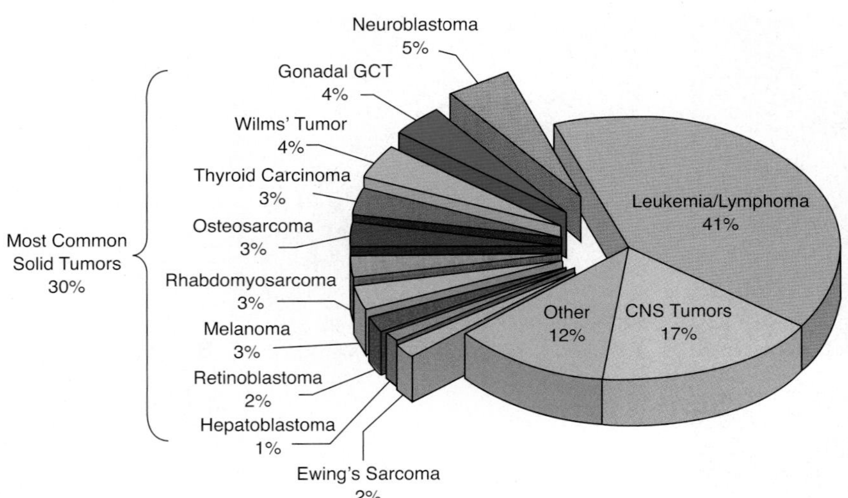

FIGURE 123.1 Distribution by histologic types of the most common pediatric tumors and subtypes of solid tumors in patients under 20 years of age. Surveillance, Epidemiology, and End Results 1986–1995. GCT, granulosa cell tumor.

Children's Cancer Group (CCG) protocols that demonstrated a threefold difference in the 5-year event-free survival (EFS) for patients with favorable versus unfavorable histologic features.[13]

The most undifferentiated neuroblastoma tumors are composed of neuroblasts with very few Schwannian (stromal) cells. Morphologically they appear as monotonous sheets of small, round, blue cells and may be difficult to distinguish from other tumors such as lymphoma, Ewing's sarcoma, and rhabdomyosarcoma that affect bone and soft tissues. Immunohistochemistry may be useful in distinguishing neuroblastoma from these tumors, and immunoreactivity is commonly observed to neuron-specific enolase, synaptophysin, chromogranin, NB84, and S100. As tumors become more differentiated, the ratio of Schwann to neuroblastoma cells increases, and the neuroblasts appear more mature. Ganglioneuroblastoma can be subdivided into either a stroma-rich, intermixed variant, or nodular variant. Ganglioneuroma is predominantly composed of Schwann cells studded with maturing or fully mature ganglion cells and is considered a benign tumor.

Molecular Biology

Risk-based treatment strategies rely heavily on molecular and cytogenetic features of the tumor. A five- to 400-fold amplification of the *MYCN* gene is found in approximately 30% to 40% of advanced stage neuroblastomas. Amplification (increased gene copy number) results in persistently high levels of the MYCN protein, a DNA binding transcription factor known to cause malignant transformation in tumor models. The negative prognostic significance of *MYCN* amplification has been well established and is clearly illustrated in a study of infants with 4S neuroblastoma in whom the 3-year survival was found to be less than 50% for patients with *MYCN*-amplified tumors versus greater than 90% for those with nonamplified tumors.[14]

Chromosomal deletions or gains are frequently identified. Losses at chromosome 1p36 and 11q occur in 23% and 35% of tumors, respectively.[15] Gain of chromosome 17 or 17q is present in 50% to 60% of neuroblastomas and is associated with an aggressive phenotype.[16] Increase in total DNA content (hyperdiploidy, DNA index greater than 1) is associated with local disease, better response to therapy, and overall improved clinical outcome in younger patients. The 2-year EFS for patients with near-triploid neuroblastoma is approximately 94% compared with 45% for patients with diploid tumors without *MYCN* amplification.[17] Trk, a family of neurotropin receptors, is important in the development of normal central and peripheral nervous systems. Elevated expression of TrkA or TrkC is seen in favorable, low-stage tumors. Low expression of TrkA or elevated expression of full-length TrkB is seen in advanced-stage *MCYN*-amplified tumors.[18] Additionally, TrkB expression has been linked to chemotherapeutic resistance.[18,19]

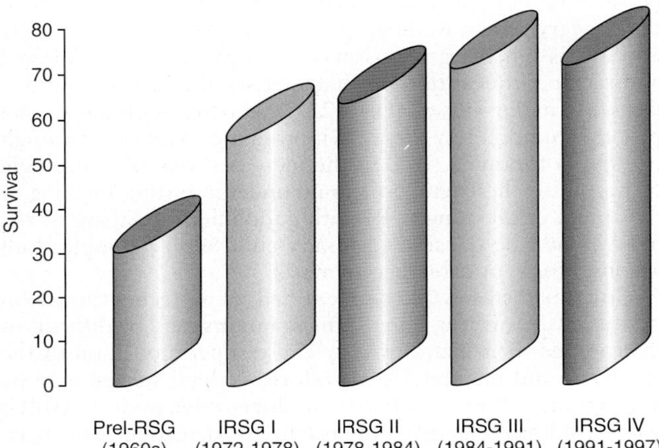

FIGURE 123.2 Overall survival rates for childhood rhabdomyosarcoma according to treatment era. IRSG, Intergroup Rhabdomyosarcoma Study Group.

Clinical Presentation

The age at presentation is an important prognostic factor as infants tend to have tumors with more favorable features, including stage and histology. Multivariate analysis of 3,666 patients enrolled in cooperative group studies demonstrated an 82% 4-year EFS for children less than 18 months versus 42% for those more than 18 months.[20] Adolescents and young adults rarely present with neuroblastoma, but their tumors tend to be indolent and fatal.[21]

Neuroblastoma may arise in any part of the sympathetic nervous system. The most common sites are the adrenal gland (40%), followed by abdominal (25%), thoracic (15%), cervical (5%), and pelvic sympathetic ganglia (5%). Approximately 60% of tumors have spread to the bone, bone marrow, lymph nodes, liver, or skin at presentation.[22] The pattern of metastatic spread varies with age and histology of the tumor. Infants with favorable histologies are more likely to have liver and skin metastases. Unfavorable histology tumors are more likely to spread to the bone marrow and bones.[22]

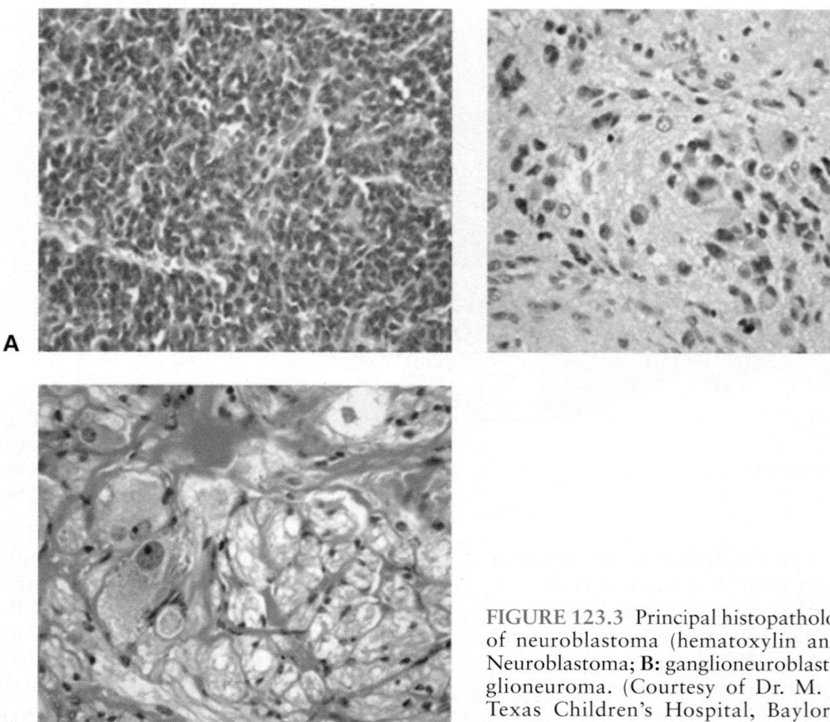

FIGURE 123.3 Principal histopathologic subtypes of neuroblastoma (hematoxylin and eosin). **A:** Neuroblastoma; **B:** ganglioneuroblastoma; **C:** ganglioneuroma. (Courtesy of Dr. M. John Hicks, Texas Children's Hospital, Baylor College of Medicine, Houston, TX.)

At presentation, abdominal tumors can cause increased abdominal girth, a palpable mass, diarrhea, or constipation. Many thoracic tumors are detected incidentally; however, large thoracic or cervical tumors can cause Horner syndrome, superior vena cava syndrome, or mechanical airway obstruction. Children with bone metastases may have a limp, complain of pain, or develop periorbital swelling, ecchymoses, or proptosis. Fever and hypertension are often present.

Two well-described paraneoplastic syndromes are associated with histologically mature tumors. Tumors can secrete vasoactive intestinal polypeptide resulting in intractable diarrhea and abdominal distention that resolves after resection. Opsoclonus-myoclonus-ataxia (OMA) syndrome is seen in up to 3% of children and presents with dancing eye movements, rhythmic jerking, or ataxia. Although thought to be immune mediated, no specific antibody or lymphocyte marker has been identified.[23] Although the movements may resolve over time, most children have persistent neurologic deficits, including speech and cognitive delays.[24]

Spinal cord involvement is found in 7% to 15% of children at the time of diagnosis. Spinal cord compression is considered an oncologic emergency. Although there is no current consensus as to the best treatment, retrospective analysis suggests that chemotherapy and laminectomy provide equivalent outcomes.[25] The current Children's Oncology Group (COG) intermediate risk clinical trial (ANBL 0531) is prospectively collecting data related to this question. At this time, however, recommendations should be made on a case-by-case basis specific to the clinical presentation and short- and long-term risks of either intervention.[26,27]

Clinical Evaluation and Staging

The International Neuroblastoma Staging System, revised in 1993 and shown in Table 123.1, is the current staging system used in North American and European cooperative group trials.[28] The European groups have also incorporated information about the feasibility of surgery based on imaging studies,[29] leading to the development of an International Risk Group classification system. The significance of this system will be tested in future prospective clinical trials.

The evaluation of a child suspected of having neuroblastoma begins with a careful history and physical examination. Attention to neurologic function is critical due to the paraspinal location of many tumors. In infants, examination must include a search for skin and subcutaneous metastases that appear as reddish-purple, raised lesions. Complete blood cell count, liver and renal function tests, serum ferritin, urinalysis, and urine sample for quantitative excretion of vanillylmandelic acid (VMA) and homovanillic acid (HVA) are needed in the assessment of newly diagnosed patients.

Ultrasound is often the initial radiologic study to identify the tumor. However, magnetic resonance imaging (MRI) or computerized tomography (CT) of the chest, abdomen, and pelvis is required to clearly define the location and extent of the primary tumor. Radiographically, neuroblastoma typically appears as a heterogeneous mass with calcifications. Adrenal and retroperitoneal tumors characteristically involve and displace the major vessels (Fig. 123.5). Patients with paraspinal primary tumors may have asymptomatic extension through the spinal foramina. Due to the increased risk of neurologic compromise, these patients should undergo further imaging of the spinal canal using MRI with gadolinium. Imaging of the head should be considered in any child with palpable skull lesions, ptosis, or orbital ecchymosis.

Bone metastases can be identified using technetium-99m bone scans. However, bone scans in infants may be difficult to interpret as their anatomy may cause superimposition of the epiphysis and metaphysis; therefore, skeletal survey may be appropriate.[30] Radiolabeled metaiodobenzylguanidine (MIBG) scans are both sensitive and specific for detecting neuroblastoma. MIBG is a chemical analogue of norepinephrine, whose receptors are selectively concentrated in sympathetic nervous tissue lesions such as neuroblastoma and pheochromocytoma (Fig. 123.5C). Because of its sensitivity and specificity, all

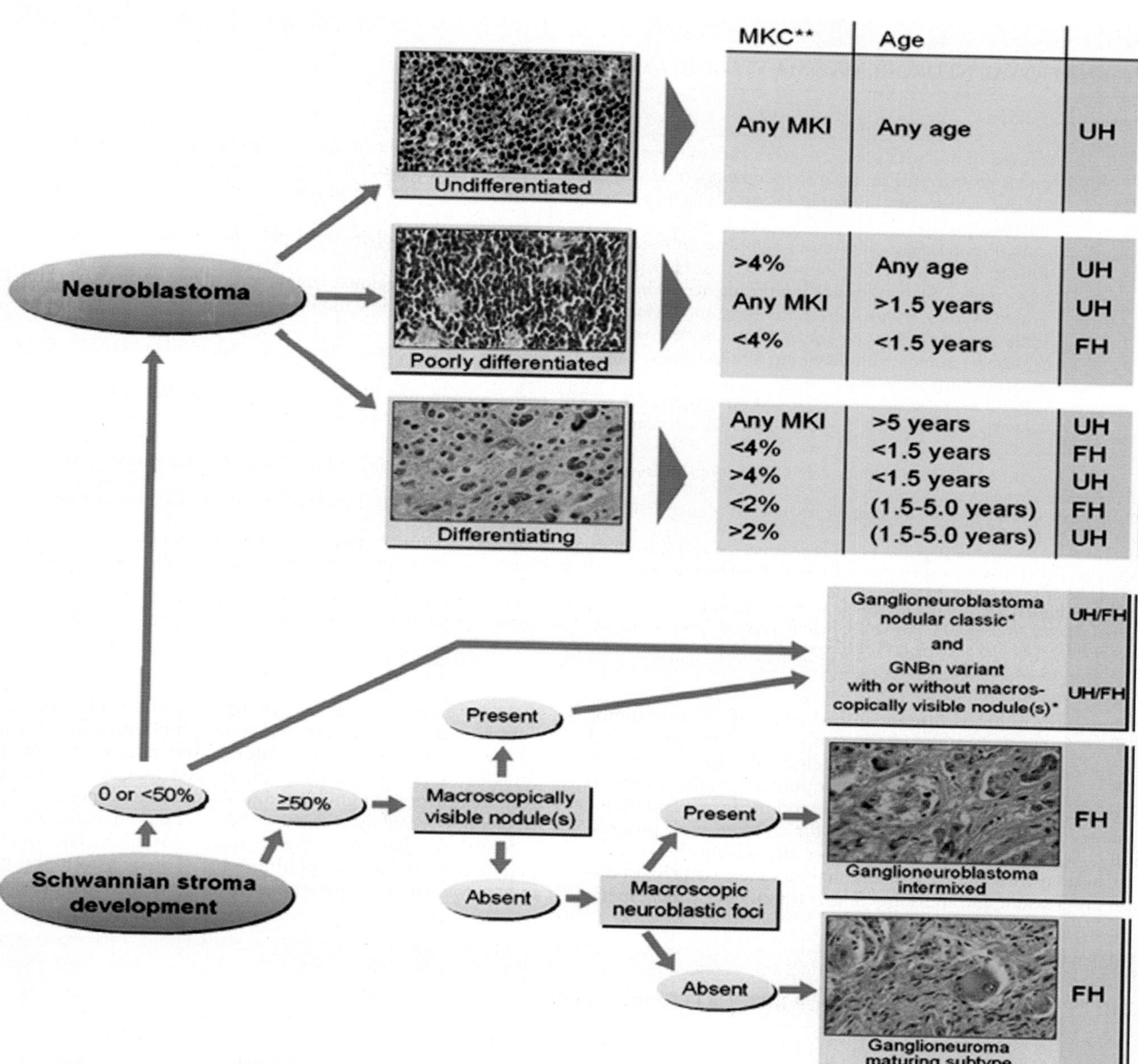

FIGURE 123.4 International Neuroblastoma Pathology Classification Schema. Neuroblastoma tumors are classified into favorable (FH) and unfavorable (UH) histology lesions based on degree of stromal development, morphology, mitosis-karyorrhexis index (MKI), and age. (From ref. 8, with permission.)

patients should undergo MIBG scans at the time of diagnosis and at subsequent intervals after the start of treatment to assess response. Bone marrow disease should be evaluated by bilateral aspiration and biopsy.

Treatment

Current risk categories incorporate the patient's age at presentation, stage of the tumor, histologic appearance, quantitative DNA content, and presence or absence of *MYCN* amplification within the tumor cells (Table 123.2).

Tumors considered "low risk" are generally stage I or II with favorable features (histologic appearance, DNA ploidy, and absence of *MYCN* amplification). Low-risk tumors comprise about 50% of all neuroblastomas. Surgery is the primary treatment, and overall survival rates greater than 90% have been reported for these patients.[31] In the rare event of recurrent tumor growth, further surgery or multimodality chemotherapy is generally successful.

A 4S neuroblastoma is a special entity because the high rate of spontaneous regression allows for a delay or elimination of chemotherapy for 80% of children.[32] Two subsets are more likely to require chemotherapy: those tumors with unfavorable biologic features (i.e., *MYCN* amplification) and tumors in infants younger than 2 months who have extensive liver disease. Untreated, the latter case leads to a higher incidence of mortality, as massive hepatomegaly prevents adequate chest wall expansion.[32] These children should receive chemotherapy or low-dose radiation (4.5 to 6 Gy in three to four fractions) to decrease tumor size.

Intermediate-risk tumors comprise 10% to 15% of new cases. They are generally large, without distant metastatic spread, and have favorable biologic features, or they appear in

TABLE 123.1

INTERNATIONAL NEUROBLASTOMA STAGING SYSTEM CRITERIA

Stage	Definition
1	Localized tumor with complete gross excision, with or without microscopic residual disease; representative ipsilateral lymph nodes negative for tumor microscopically (nodes attached to and removed with the primary tumor may be positive)
2A	Localized tumor with incomplete gross excision; representative ipsilateral nonadherent lymph nodes negative for tumor microscopically
2B	Localized tumor with or without complete gross excision, with ipsilateral nonadherent lymph nodes positive for tumor. Enlarged contralateral lymph nodes must be negative microscopically
3	Unresectable unilateral tumor infiltrating across the midline[a] with or without regional lymph node involvement; or localized unilateral tumor with contralateral regional lymph node involvement; or midline tumor with bilateral extension by infiltration (unresectable) or by lymph node involvement[b]
4	Any primary tumor with dissemination to distant lymph nodes, bone, bone marrow, liver, skin, and/or other organs (except as defined for stage 4S)
4S	Localized primary tumor (as defined for stage 1, 2A, or 2B), with dissemination limited to skin, liver, and/or bone marrow[c] (<10% involvement) (limited to infants <1 year of age)

[a]The midline is defined as the vertebral column. Tumors originating on one side and crossing the midline must infiltrate to or beyond the opposite side of the vertebral column.
[b]Patients are upstaged to International Neuroblastoma Staging System stage 3 if there is proven malignant effusion within the abdominal cavity or bilateral thoracic cavity.
[c]Marrow involvement in stage 4S should be minimal (i.e., <10%) of total nucleated cells identified as malignant on bone marrow biopsy or on marrow aspirate. More extensive marrow involvement would be considered to be stage 4. The metaiodobenzylguanidine (MIBG) scan, if performed, should be negative in the marrow.
Note: Multifocal primary tumors should be staged according to the greatest extent of disease and followed by the subscript "M."
(From ref. 28, Brodeur GM, Prichard J, Berthold F, et al. Revisions of the international criteria for neuroblastoma diagnosis, staging, and response to treatment. *J Clin Oncol* 1993;11(8):1466–1477.)

infants with minimal disease spread and unfavorable tumor biology. Surgery is an important component of treatment, and the addition of moderately intensive chemotherapy (i.e., carboplatin, etoposide, adriamycin, cyclophosphamide) results in 4-year EFS rates of 54% to 100% depending on age and tumor biology.[33] Radiotherapy is reserved for children with progression or who have unresectable tumors after chemotherapy.

Children with high-risk disease have an increased risk of disease progression and mortality. These tumors are widely metastatic, have unfavorable biologic features, and tend to occur in children older than 1 year. Aggressive, multimodality therapy induces remission in most children, but relapse is common (30% to 50% 3-year EFS).[34] Short- and long-term toxicities from treatment are significant and include hematopoietic toxicity, deafness, renal insufficiency, and secondary malignancies.

Standard chemotherapy regimens for high-risk disease include combinations of platinum-based agents, cyclophosphamide, doxorubicin, and etoposide; other active agents such as

TABLE 123.2

CHILDREN'S ONCOLOGY GROUP RISK CATEGORIES FOR NEUROBLASTOMA

INSS Stage	Age	MYCN Status	Pathology Classification	DNA Ploidy	Risk Group Assignment
1	0–21y	Any	Any	Any	Low
2	<365d	Any	Any	Any	Low
	>365d–21y	Non-Amp	Any	—	Low
	>365d–21y	Amp	Fav	—	Low
	>365d–21y	Amp	Unfav	—	High
3	<365d	Non-Amp	Any	Any	Intermediate
	<365d	Amp	Any	Any	High
	>365d–21y	Non-Amp	Fav	—	Intermediate
	>365d–21y	Non-Amp	Unfav	—	High
	>365d–21y	Amp	Any	—	High
4	<365d	Non-Amp	Any	Any	Intermediate
	<365d	Amp	Any	Any	High
	>365d–21y	Any	Any	—	High
4S	<365d	Non-Amp	Fav	>1	Low
	<365d	Non-Amp	Any	= I	Intermediate
	<365d	Non-Amp	Unfav	Any	Intermediate
	<365d	Amp	Any	Any	High

INSS, International Neuroblastoma Staging System.

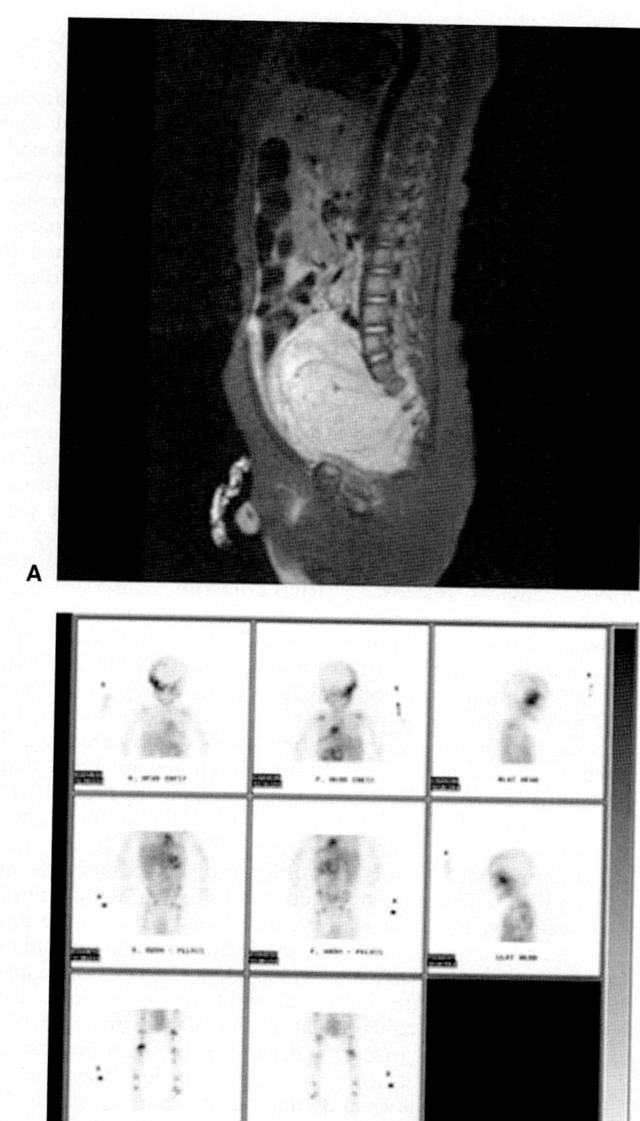

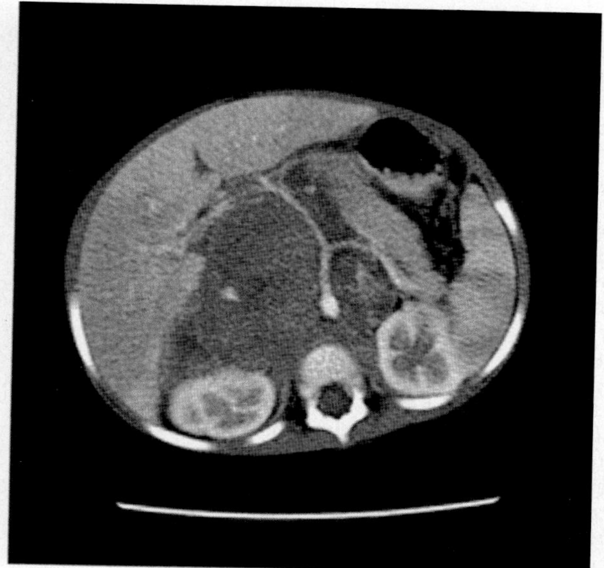

FIGURE 123.5 **A:** Magnetic resonance image of pelvic neuroblastoma with spinal canal invasion. **B:** Computed tomography of an adrenal neuroblastoma demonstrating displacement of the major vessels. **C:** Meta-iodobenzylguanidine scan demonstrating widespread metastatic neuroblastoma.

teniposide, ifosfamide, and topotecan have also been included in some regimens. High-dose chemotherapy with autologous hematopoietic stem cell rescue (HDT/SCR) may improve the disease-free survival once remission is achieved. The CCG randomized 379 children to receive consolidation therapy with chemotherapy or HDT/SCR. The EFS for children receiving HDT/SCR was significantly better than those receiving chemotherapy alone (34% vs. 22%; P = .034).[34] The European Neuroblastoma Study Group performed a randomized study of high-dose melphalan with unpurged SCR versus no further therapy for patients with stage III (n = 15) or IV (n = 50) disease who had achieved a complete or very good response after induction chemotherapy with six to ten cycles of OPEC (vincristine, cyclophosphamide, cisplatin, and etoposide).[35] The median progression-free survival (PFS) was 23 months in the transplanted group versus 6 months for the group with no further treatment, suggesting that consolidation of high-dose therapy with SCR improves PFS. To optimize survival of high-risk neuroblastoma patients, the primary and residual bulky tumors must be controlled locally using both surgery and postoperative radiation. The goal of surgical local control is to remove all visible tumors without jeopardizing vital organs or delaying chemotherapy; however, most primary tumors invade local structures and surround major blood vessels, making resection difficult. Complete removal at the time of diagnosis is possible for less than 20% of patients.[36,37] Resection of invasive tumors is associated with complications, including removal of normal organs, hemorrhage, renal injury,[30] and chronic diarrhea. After treatment with chemotherapy, complete removal becomes possible in 70% to 95% of cases.[36]

The use of radiation therapy to the primary site has led to decreased local failure rates. In the CCG-3891 study, patients were randomized to receive consolidation with chemotherapy alone or with therapy including 10 Gy of total-body irradiation. Patients received either 10 Gy (abdominal or thoracic primary tumors) or 20 Gy (nonaxial primary tumors) to the primary tumor if they had less than a complete surgical resection. Although not statistically significant, patients who received at least 20 Gy to their primary site had the best local control outcomes.[36,38] Doses of radiotherapy have varied from study to study, but current recommendations include 21 to 24 Gy for the primary site, with up to 36 Gy if residual disease remains.[39]

Some studies advocate radiation for all metastatic sites visible at diagnosis,[40] while others use total body irradiation for metastatic control.[41] Tolerability of either approach in heavily treated patients requires consideration; therefore, most centers limit treatment to the primary tumor bed and metastatic sites still visible on MIBG scan after induction chemotherapy. Distant sites of failure have not consistently been reported using this schema, but skull and orbital lesions appear more difficult to control.[38,40,41] In the setting of recurrent or incurable disease, radiotherapy can be used to treat bone and soft tissue metastasis for pain control and to prevent loss of organ function.[42]

Finally, additional treatment with biologics (i.e., 13-*cis*-retinoic acid) in the setting of minimal residual disease appears to improve survival. CCG randomized children after consolidation with high-dose chemotherapy and SCR to receive 6 months of *cis*-retinoic acid. The 3-year EFS was significantly better among those who received *cis*-retinoic acid than those assigned to receive no further therapy (46% vs. 29%, respectively; $P = .027$).[34] Monoclonal antibodies have been the most actively studied among immunotherapies. A recent report from the COG found that administration of a monoclonal antibody directed against GD2 (a ganglioside molecule detected on almost neuroblastoma cells), in combination with interleukin-2 and granulocyte macrophage colony stimulating factor, during maintenance therapy with *cis*-retinoic acid was associated with an improved 2-year event-free and overall survival.[43] Adoptive cellular therapies for neuroblastoma offer potential advantages because it is a nonimmunosuppressive approach.[44] A phase 1 study demonstrated feasibility along with some clinical responses in patients with refractory disease.[45]

WILMS' TUMOR

Wilms' tumor is the most common primary malignant renal tumor of childhood, accounting for 6% of all childhood tumors and an estimated 500 new cases per year in the United States.[1]

Epidemiology and Genetics

Among North American children less than 15 years of age, the incidence of Wilms' tumor is eight cases per 1 million.[1] Wilms' tumor accounts for more than 90% of all renal cancers in patients under the age of 20 years, with a mean age at diagnosis of approximately 40 months for patients with unilateral disease and 30 months for those with bilateral disease.

A variety of syndromes and congenital abnormalities are associated with the development of Wilms' tumor, including WAGR syndrome (Wilms' tumor-aniridia-genitourinary anomalies and mental retardation), Denys-Drash syndrome, and Frasier syndrome.[46,47] All of these syndromes involve mutations in the *WT1* gene at the 11p13 locus. A second Wilms' tumor gene, *WT2*, located at 11p15, has been linked to increased incidence of Wilms' tumor in Beckwith-Wiedemann syndrome, an overgrowth syndrome associated with increased risk of other malignancies such as hepatoblastoma and adrenocortical carcinoma.[46–48] Overexpression, loss of imprinting, hypermethylation, and silencing of one or more genes contained within the *WT2* locus such as *IGF2, H19, p57,* and *LIT1* have been documented.[46,47,49] Other syndromes associated with an increased susceptibility for the development of Wilms' tumor include Simpson-Golabi-Behmel syndrome, Sotos syndrome, and Perlman syndrome. Familial predisposition accounts for 1% to 2% of cases, and putative familial Wilms' tumor genes have been mapped to 17q12-21 (*FWT1*), and 19q13.4 (*FWT2*).[46] Children with hereditary syndromes that predispose to the development of Wilms' tumor such as WAGR or Beckwith-Wiedemann appear to respond to treatment similarly as other children, but they have a higher incidence of bilateral disease, intralobar nephrogenic rests, and end-stage renal disease.[1,50]

Pathology

Most Wilms' tumors are solitary and are composed of varying proportions of blastemal, stromal, and epithelial cells that recapitulate normal kidney development. Anaplasia is characterized by the presence of large nuclei with multipolar mitotic features and is associated with an increased risk of recurrence. Anaplasia can be either "focal" or "diffuse." In focal anaplasia, cells with anaplastic nuclear changes are confined to sharply restricted foci within the primary tumor.[51] A recent analysis has demonstrated that the presence of anaplasia even in stage I disease adversely affects clinical outcome.[1,52]

Wilms' tumor must be distinguished histologically from other pediatric renal tumors, including clear cell sarcoma and rhabdoid tumor of the kidney, as well as neuroblastoma. Clear cell sarcoma is the second most common pediatric renal neoplasm and is associated with a higher rate of relapse and death when compared with favorable histology Wilms' tumor.[53] Rhabdoid tumor of the kidney, previously confused with Wilms' tumor, is a monomorphous tumor similar to clear cell sarcoma of the kidney. The cell of origin for this distinctive tumor remains unknown.[54] Rhabdoid tumor of the kidney tends to metastasize to the lung and brain. Primary rhabdoid tumors of the kidney and brain (atypical teratoid or rhabdoid tumors) share deletions of chromosome band 22q11.2, the site of *INI1*, a putative tumor suppressor gene.[55] Congenital mesoblastic nephroma is important to recognize because it is usually curable by nephrectomy alone. These tumors are typically identified in the first months of life, with a median age at diagnosis of 2 months.[56] They are associated with the t(12;15) translocation that produces the *ETV6-NTRK3* fusion gene product.[57]

Most Wilms' tumors are unilateral, but about 6% are bilateral. The existence of precursor lesions of Wilms' tumor has been recognized for many years.[58] These precursor lesions, or nephrogenic rests, are identified in the renal parenchyma of approximately 30% of Wilms' tumor cases. Nephroblastomatosis describes kidneys with multifocal or diffuse nephrogenic rests. Children with nephroblastomatosis have an increased risk of developing Wilms' tumor and require close monitoring.[59] Biologic prognostic factors such as loss of heterozygosity at chromosomal regions 1p and 16q, found in approximately 5% of favorable histology tumors, are associated with increased risk of relapse and mortality.[60] The current COG trial incorporates these factors prospectively into treatment decisions.

Clinical Presentation and Natural History

Most children with Wilms' tumor come to medical attention because of abdominal swelling or the presence of an abdominal mass. This feature is usually noticed by a caregiver while bathing or dressing the child. Abdominal pain, gross hematuria, and fever may be present at diagnosis. Hypertension is present in approximately 20% of cases.[61]

Clinical Evaluation and Staging

On physical examination, location and size of the abdominal mass and its movement with respiration should be noted. A varicocele may be associated with the presence of a tumor thrombus in the renal vein or inferior vena cava. Signs of Wilms' tumor–associated syndromes such as aniridia, hemihypertrophy, and genitourinary abnormalities should be assessed. Laboratory evaluation should include a complete blood cell count, liver function tests, renal function tests, serum chemistries including calcium, and urinalysis.

Diagnostic Imaging

Imaging studies of the primary tumor should define the extent of the tumor, detect the presence of a tumor thrombus that may extend through the renal vein into the inferior vena cava, and assess the contralateral kidney to rule out bilateral lesions, all of which are important prior to surgery. Imaging of the abdomen and lungs is needed to evaluate distant metastatic spread. Imaging of the brain or skeleton is usually reserved for patients with rhabdoid tumors of the kidney and clear cell sarcoma of the kidney.

The initial radiographic study is often an abdominal ultrasound examination to determine the consistency of the mass and the organ from which it arises, and to assess patency of the inferior vena cava. CT or MRI is appropriate for imaging of the primary tumor to provide adequate visualization of the contralateral kidney, liver, and abdomen to define metachronous and metastatic tumors in the abdomen and pelvis. MRI is superior to other imaging modalities in delineating nephroblastomatosis lesions.

Both plain radiographs of the chest (chest x-ray) and chest CT should be performed to define pulmonary metastases. Although insufficient data are currently available to firmly establish the need for CT of the chest in the initial evaluation of children with Wilms' tumor, the available data suggest that, in many cases, nodules detected by newer, more sensitive CT scans do not necessarily represent metastatic tumor.[62] The current National Wilms' Tumor Study Group (NWTSG) trial will evaluate the feasibility of eliminating radiotherapy in children whose chest CT scans demonstrate complete resolution of pulmonary nodules at week 6 of therapy.

Staging

Staging criteria for Wilms' tumor are based on the anatomic extent of the primary tumor. Two staging systems are currently used: the prechemotherapy staging system developed by the NWTSG (Table 123.3) and the postchemotherapy-based system developed by the International Society of Pediatric Oncology (SIOP). Both systems accurately predict clinical outcome and reflect therapeutic differences between the two cooperative groups. The NWTSG approach allows adequate assessment of the extent of disease and histologic characteristics of the tumor and facilitates the collection of tumor tissue for biologic studies prior to therapy. The SIOP approach uses preoperative chemotherapy, decreasing the volume of tumor and thereby decreasing the perioperative risk of tumor spillage. As a result of these treatment philosophies, children enrolled on NWTSG trials receive radiation therapy more often, whereas patients on the SIOP trials receive more cumulative doses of anthracyclines.

TABLE 123.3

NWTSG STAGING SYSTEM FOR RENAL TUMORS

Stage	Description
I	a. Tumor is limited to the kidney and completely excised b. The tumor was not ruptured before or during removal c. The vessels of the renal sinus are not involved beyond 2 mm d. There is no residual tumor apparent beyond the margins of excision
II	a. Tumor extends beyond the kidney but is completely excised b. No residual tumor is apparent at or beyond the margins of excision c. Tumor thrombus in vessels outside the kidney is stage II if the thrombus is removed en bloc with the tumor
III	Residual tumor confined to the abdomen: a. Lymph nodes in the renal hilum, the periaortic chains, or beyond are found to contain tumor b. Diffuse peritoneal contamination by the tumor c. Implants are found in the peritoneal surfaces d. Tumor extends beyond the surgical margins either microscopically or grossly e. Tumor is not completely resectable because of local infiltration into vital structures
IV	Presence of hematogenous metastases or metastases to distant lymph nodes
V	Bilateral renal involvement at the time of initial diagnosis

NWTSG, National Wilms' Tumor Study Group.
(From ref. 63, with permission.)

Treatment

With current therapies, more than 90% of children with Wilms' tumor are expected to survive 5 years after diagnosis. Tumor stage and histology are the main prognostic indicators that determine the treatment regimen for Wilms' tumor. Patient age at presentation and biologic factors such as loss of heterozygosity at chromosomes 1p and 16q are being tested prospectively.[63] Surgery and chemotherapy are the main components of treatment of all Wilms' tumors, and radiation is added for the more advanced or histologically aggressive tumors.

Surgery

Surgical resection is the primary method for achieving local control in North American studies and is usually performed at the time of initial presentation. Despite the presentation of most Wilms' tumors as a large mass, resection is generally feasible along with sampling of lymph nodes. A transabdominal, transperitoneal approach allows for adequate visualization and removal of the tumor, inspection of the tumor bed, and sampling of lymph nodes. A review of children treated in National Wilms' Tumor Study (NWTS)-4 demonstrated an increased incidence of local recurrence in those cases in which lymph node biopsies were not obtained.[64] Presumably, these children were understaged and thus undertreated. This same review clearly demonstrated that operative rupture, whether localized to the renal fossa or diffuse in the peritoneal cavity, was associated with an increased incidence of local recurrence.[64]

Routine exploration of the contralateral kidney is not necessary if imaging is satisfactory and does not suggest a bilateral process. If the imaging studies are suggestive of a possible contralateral lesion, the contralateral kidney should be formally explored. This should be done prior to nephrectomy. Partial nephrectomy is feasible in less than 5% of children with Wilms' tumor, and nephrectomy alone can cure the majority of children (more than 85%) less than 2 years of age with stage I favorable histology tumors and tumor weight less than 550 g.

Preoperative treatment of Wilms' tumor should be considered in children with a solitary kidney, bilateral renal tumors, tumor in a horseshoe kidney, tumor thrombus in the inferior vena cava above the level of the hepatic veins, and respiratory distress as a result of metastatic disease. In most instances, pretreatment biopsy should be obtained to ensure proper diagnosis. In children with bilateral disease or involvement of a solitary kidney, preoperative chemotherapy is intended to permit maximal conservation of uninvolved renal parenchyma. In the current COG renal tumor protocol, children who present with bilateral renal masses receive two cycles of chemotherapy without biopsy. Biopsy is reserved for those patients whose tumors do not show appropriate volume reduction.

The role of surgery in the treatment of pulmonary relapse has been evaluated by the NWTSG in 211 patients. Although diagnostic confirmation of relapse may be required, there was no therapeutic benefit identified for resection of a solitary pulmonary metastasis in addition to pulmonary radiotherapy and chemotherapy alone.[65] Four-year survival rates were identical in the two groups.

Chemotherapy

Chemotherapy plays a crucial role in the treatment of Wilms' tumor. All patients with Wilms' tumor should receive chemotherapy. Vincristine, dactinomycin, and doxorubicin form the backbone of most combinations for the treatment of Wilms' tumor. The recommended drugs and duration of therapy according to stage and intergroup studies are listed in Table 123.4. The need for chemotherapy in patients less than 2 years of age with stage I favorable histology tumors who weigh less than 550 g will be evaluated in the current trial.

The major conclusions derived from the four NWTSs are: (1) routine, postoperative radiation therapy of the flank is not necessary for children with stage I favorable histology, stage I anaplastic, or stage II favorable histology tumors when postnephrectomy combination chemotherapy consisting of vincristine and dactinomycin is administered; (2) the prognosis for patients with stage III favorable histology is optimized when the treatment program includes either dactinomycin plus vincristine plus doxorubicin plus 10 Gy radiation therapy to the flank, or dactinomycin plus vincristine plus 20 Gy radiation therapy to the flank; (3) the addition of cyclophosphamide to the combination of vincristine plus dactinomycin plus doxorubicin does not improve the outcome of patients with stage IV/favorable histology tumors; and (4) "pulse-intensive" regimens maintain excellent relapse-free survival with less toxicity than previous regimens.[63] The regimens of NWTS-5 are considered standard therapies for children with favorable histology Wilms' tumor (Table 123.4).

Anaplasia, either diffuse or focal, adversely affects the outcome even after the administration of conventional chemotherapy with vincristine, dactinomycin, and doxorubicin. Cyclophosphamide and etoposide, when added to vincristine, dactinomycin, and doxorubicin, improved the survival of patients with stage II through IV diffuse anaplasia.[52,63] In addition, the ongoing trial for these patients incorporates carboplatin in an attempt to improve the clinical outcome. For patients with stage I anaplasia, a more aggressive regimen that incorporates doxorubicin will be used. Patients with stage IV diffuse anaplasia continue to do extremely poorly, with 4-year EFS of less than 35%, and novel investigational combinations including carboplatin, topotecan, and irinotecan are under investigation.

Salvage is particularly successful for patients with low-stage tumors who were initially treated with dactinomycin and vincristine and in patients who had a longer remission. At the time of relapse, the original agents used may again have some benefit, although additional agents such as ifosfamide, carboplatin, and etoposide have significantly improved overall survival after relapse from 30% to around 55%.[66,67]

Radiation Therapy

Successive NWTSG trials have refined the dosages and indications to decrease radiation exposure while maintaining local control and control of metastatic pulmonary lesions (Table 123.4). Patients with stage I and II favorable histology tumors do not require abdominal radiotherapy, while those with stage III favorable histology or stages I to III focal or diffuse anaplastic disease require adjuvant radiotherapy to the flank or abdomen. The tumor and renal beds with a 1- to 2-cm margin are treated in cases of positive resection margins, nodal involvement, or local spillage during surgery. Care must be taken to provide a uniform dosage to the vertebral column to limit risk of scoliosis. Whole abdominal radiotherapy is used for patients with preoperative hemorrhage or rupture, diffuse spill during surgery, or when peritoneal metastasis is present. A dose of 10 Gy is sufficient for local control in stage III favorable histology patients if they also received chemotherapy with vincristine, dactinomycin, and doxorubicin.[68] Most patients receive radiotherapy within 8 to 12 days of nephrectomy without compromise in locoregional control.[69] Currently, it is recommended that radiotherapy start within 14 days of nephrectomy.

TABLE 123.4

TREATMENT REGIMENS FOR WILMS' TUMOR WITH FAVORABLE OR STANDARD HISTOLOGIC FEATURES FROM RECENTLY COMPLETED NWTSG AND SIOP STUDIES

	NWTS-5		SIOP93-01		
			Chemotherapy		
Stage	Chemotherapy	Radiation Therapy	Preoperative	Postoperative	Radiation Therapy
I	VA × 18 weeks	—	VA × 4 weeks	VA × 4 weeks	—
II	VA × 18 weeks	—	VA × 4 weeks	VDA × 27 weeks	Node-negative: none Node-positive: 15 Gy
III	VDA × 24 weeks	10.8 Gy	VA × 4 weeks	VDA × 27 weeks	15 Gy
IV	VDA × 24 weeks	12 Gy lung (if lung metastasis) 10.8 Gy flank (if local stage III)	VDA × 6 weeks	CR after 9 weeks: VCA × 27 weeks	None if lung lesions disappear by week 9, otherwise 12 Gy No CR after 9 weeks: ICED × 34 weeks

NWTS, National Wilms' Tumor Study; SIOP, Society of Pediatric Oncology; V, vincristine; A, dactinomycin; D, doxorubicin; CR, complete remission; I, ifosfamide; C, carboplatin; E, etoposide (From ref. 63, with permission.)

Whole-lung irradiation (12 Gy) has been recommended for patients who present with pulmonary metastases. However, controversy remains over which of these patients will benefit the most. Historically, pulmonary metastases were defined by presence of tumor on chest x-ray, but CT now allows for identification of much smaller lesions. The NWTSG and SIOP have both recommended treatment for tumors seen on chest x-ray but not CT, leaving the final decision in the hands of the treating physician and making outcome measures difficult to interpret. Additionally, SIOP delays the decision to use pulmonary radiation until week 9 of chemotherapy if persistent lung lesions are present. The NWTS-5 identified 129 patients with favorable histology and CT-only pulmonary lesions, and no benefit of lung irradiation was apparent when appropriate chemotherapy was administered.[70] Furthermore, Ehrlich et al.[62] found that in those patients whose pulmonary lesions were biopsied, only 82% of isolated lesions and 69% of multiple pulmonary lesions were actually tumor. A current COG study is investigating the omission of whole-lung radiotherapy in selected patients with pulmonary nodules who achieve a complete response after a 6-week trial of chemotherapy.

RETINOBLASTOMA

Retinoblastoma is the most frequent malignant ocular tumor in pediatric patients and one of the most curable neoplasms affecting young children, with survival rates exceeding 90%.

Epidemiology and Genetics

The incidence rate for the period 1975 to 1995 is estimated at 3.8 cases per million.[1] Approximately 70% to 75% of all cases are unilateral. Among children with unilateral disease, 10% to 15% have hereditary germ line deletions of chromosome 13, band q14, which contains the *RB1* tumor suppressor gene locus. Germline mutations of 13q14 uniformly affect the remaining 25% to 30% of children with bilateral disease. For unilateral disease, the median age at diagnosis is 2 years for boys and 1 year for girls. For bilateral disease, the median age at diagnosis is less than 12 months for both boys and girls.[71]

Whereas the majority of new cases of retinoblastoma arise spontaneously from new somatic mutations in *RB1*, a significant fraction of retinoblastoma cases are hereditary. Retinoblastoma is transmitted as a highly penetrant, autosomal dominant trait, and parents and siblings of all patients should undergo a thorough ophthalmoscopic examination.[72]

Pathology

Retinoblastoma is composed of uniform small, round, or polygonal cells, which have scanty, poorly staining cytoplasm. The sparse cytoplasm is located at one side of the cell, suggesting the appearance of an embryonal retinal cell. The nucleus is large and deeply staining. Three types of cellular arrangements may be identified: the Homer-Wright rosette, the Flexner-Wintersteiner rosette, and the fleurette. Calcification and necrosis are often observed.[73]

Clinical Presentation

Patients with retinoblastoma most frequently come to medical attention because of leukocoria. Strabismus, conjunctival erythema, and decreased visual acuity are other common presenting complaints. Physical examination reveals the presence of a white pupillary reflex. Esotropia or exotropia may be present. The eye may be red and painful because of uveitis after spontaneous necrosis of a retinal tumor or from neovascular glaucoma. Decreased visual acuity may be due to involvement of the macula by the tumor or the presence of cells and debris in the vitreous.[74]

Evaluation

The diagnosis of retinoblastoma is based on clinical history (including family history) and results of examination of both eyes under general anesthesia. In addition to meticulous inspection of both eyes, the staging evaluation of a child with suspected retinoblastoma must include a CT or MRI of the orbit or orbital ultrasonography.[75] MRI is used to define the extent of the intraocular tumor, to assess vitreal seeding, and to determine the presence and extent of extraocular disease. Retinoblastoma may metastasize to the central nervous system, bones, or bone marrow.[76] Lumbar puncture and bone marrow examination should only be performed in patients with involvement of extraocular structures, including the orbit or optic nerve, or when symptoms, signs, or diagnostic imaging studies suggest involvement of distant sites.[77] Radionuclide bone scans should be obtained only for patients with extensive ocular involvement, symptoms suggesting the presence of a bone metastasis, and bone marrow involvement.[78]

Staging

Martin and Reese[79] proposed the first staging system for patients with retinoblastoma in 1942. Several staging systems have since been used that incorporate prognosis and therapy to help guide clinicians. St. Jude Children's Research Hospital developed a staging system defined by the extent of tumor involving the retina and globe, or by the presence of extrachoroidal disease.[80,81] The Reese and Ellsworth[82] grouping was developed to predict the risk of enucleation with external-beam radiotherapy alone (Table 123.5). The clinical value of the Reese-Ellsworth grouping in the era of combined modality therapy is unclear, yet it remains widely used for historical reasons. In 2001, COG incorporated a new classification system for intraocular retinoblastoma for use in clinical trials (Table 123.6). This classification system was originally developed at Childrens Hospital Los Angeles and is now used internationally.[83] Another staging system developed by Chantada et al.[84] provides a common international classification for patients with extraocular retinoblastoma.

Treatment

Surgical Considerations

In view of the excellent response of this tumor to vision-sparing interventions, enucleation of the involved eye must be undertaken very selectively. Given the high percentage of long-term survivors, treatment decisions must carefully weigh the functional outcome and potential long-term sequelae of local and systemic therapies.[85] The indications for enucleation include (1) unilateral retinoblastoma that completely fills the globe or that has damaged and disrupted the retina or vitreous so extensively that restoration of useful vision is not possible; (2) bilateral retinoblastoma in which the previously mentioned conditions exist in only one eye; (3) a tumor present in the anterior chamber; (4) painful glaucoma with loss of vision after rubeosis iridis; (5) extensive bilateral retinoblastoma in which there is no potential for restoration of useful vision; (6) retinoblastoma unresponsive to all other forms of local therapy; and (7)

TABLE 123.5

STAGING SYSTEM FOR RETINOBLASTOMA

Group	Description
GROUP I	
A	Solitary tumor, <4 disc diameters in size, at or behind the equator
B	Multiple tumors, 4–10 disc diameters in size, all at or behind the equator
GROUP II	
A	Solitary tumor, 4–10 disc diameters in size, at or behind the equator
B	Multiple tumors, 4–10 disc diameters in size, behind the equator
GROUP III	
A	Any lesion anterior to the equator
B	Solitary tumors >10 disc diameters behind the equator
GROUP IV	
A	Multiple tumors, some >10 disc diameters
B	Any lesion extending anteriorly to the ora serrata
GROUP V	
A	Massive tumors involving more than one-half the retina
B	Vitreous seeding

Adapted from ref. 82.

cases with permanent vision loss in which extraocular tumor is suspected.

Advanced Unilateral Disease. Patients with suspected retinoblastoma should be referred to a pediatric ophthalmologist experienced in the treatment of retinoblastoma. The standard surgical technique is modified to allow excision of the longest possible segment of optic nerve in continuity with the globe.[86] The globe and optic nerve are inspected for evidence of extraocular extension of the tumor. After the globe is enucleated, a plastic implant is placed in the muscle funnel. Although the presence of the ocular prosthesis may prevent early detection of an orbital recurrence of tumor, the cosmetic result and promotion of normal development of the bony orbit are considerably improved.[87] The survival rate for patients with retinoblastoma confined to one or both globes, treated only with enucleation, is greater than 95%.[82]

Limited Unilateral or Limited Bilateral Disease. Patients with limited unilateral or bilateral residual or focal recurrent disease may benefit from local surgical modalities, including photocoagulation, cryotherapy, or radioactive plaque brachytherapy. Combining chemoreduction with a local modality controls 85% of patients with Reese-Ellsworth groups I to IV disease[88]; with Reese-Ellsworth group V patients, the likelihood of local control without external-beam radiation is much lower.

Laser photocoagulation is reported to have successfully eradicated retinoblastomas in 80% of the patients treated. Small tumor size is closely related to success of this treatment. For this reason, tumors 2.5 mm or less in thickness and 4.5 mm or less in diameter are considered appropriate candidates.[88]

Radioactive plaque brachytherapy is more commonly used for salvage in the setting of localized recurrence.[89] Excellent local control is seen with iodine-125 (^{125}I) radiation plaque brachytherapy when combined with chemoreduction.[90] Shields et al.[91] showed that plaque brachytherapy is most successful as a secondary treatment in those eyes that fail to respond to laser photocoagulation, thermotherapy, cryotherapy, or chemoreduction. Plaque brachytherapy does not appear to have the risk of secondary malignancies seen in external-beam radiation.[91]

Cryotherapy was first used for the treatment of a patient with retinoblastoma in 1967.[92] Subsequent reports that included some patients treated sequentially with local irradiation and cryotherapy suggested that long-term control was possible using this technique. Abramson et al.[93] reported long-term control of retinoblastoma with one cryotherapy session in 80% of patients with previously untreated tumors, 59% of new postirradiation tumors, and 56% of recurrent tumors after irradiation. Tumors arising from the vitreous base were not responsive to cryotherapy. These investigators stated that previously untreated patients with tumors located anterior to the equator and those with recurrent or new tumors after irradiation were candidates for cryotherapy. Cryotherapy is generally effective for tumors up to 2.5 mm in diameter and 1.0 mm thick that are confined to the sensory retina.[94]

Bilateral Disease

Bilateral retinoblastoma is currently treated with initial chemotherapy, with careful assessment of treatment response by examination under anesthesia after each cycle. Assessment of

TABLE 123.6

INTERNATIONAL CLASSIFICATION SYSTEM FOR INTRAOCULAR RETINOBLASTOMA

Group	Description
GROUP A	**Very low risk** Eyes with small discrete tumors away from critical structures. All tumors 3 mm or smaller, confined to the retina, and located 3 mm from the foveola and 1.5 mm from the optic nerve. No vitreous or subretinal seeding.
GROUP B	**Low risk** Eyes with no vitreous or subretinal seeding and discrete retinal tumor of any size or location. Any retinal tumor not in group A. No vitreous or subretinal seeding. A small cuff of subretinal fluid no more than 5 mm from the base of the tumor is allowed.
GROUP C	**Moderate risk** Eyes with focal vitreous or subretinal seeding and discrete retinal tumors of any size or location. Any seeding must be local, fine, and limited. Retinal tumors are discrete and of any size and location. Up to one quadrant of subretinal fluid may be present.
GROUP D	**High risk** Eyes with diffuse vitreous or subretinal seeding and/or massive, nondiscrete endophytic and exophytic disease. Eyes with more extensive seeding than group C. Intraocular disseminated disease may consist of fine or "greasy" vitreous seeding or avascular mass.

Adapted from ref. 83.

which eye is most likely to be capable of functional vision is difficult until response to chemotherapy is determined. The consensus is to use a regimen containing carboplatin, vincristine, and etoposide for six courses with frequent evaluations. This regimen is accompanied by local treatments with cryotherapy and thermotherapy as determined by the ophthalmologist. External beam radiation therapy is indicated for bilateral disease where the eye has advanced disease, has not responded adequately to chemotherapy and local treatments, but has useful vision.

Radiation Therapy

Modern radiotherapy uses megavoltage accelerators and CT- and MRI-based treatment planning to allow for sparing of the lens and bony orbits. Together with daily image guidance for field placement, these techniques may further reduce radiotherapy-related late effects to surrounding structures. Proton therapy can potentially decrease dosage to the surrounding bony orbits by more than 60% and avoid significant dosage to the hypothalamus compared with intensity-modulated radiotherapy, with equivalent target coverage.[95]

The risk of secondary malignancies after external-beam radiation is becoming better defined. Kleinerman et al.[96] published long-term results of 1,601 survivors of retinoblastoma and analyzed dosage distributions based on the technique used to treat specific patients. The cumulative incidence of a second cancer at 50 years was 38.2% and 21.0% for irradiated and nonirradiated patients, respectively. The authors also found the risk of osteosarcomas was higher in patients who received chemotherapy with radiation, compared with radiation alone.

Patients requiring radiation receive doses between 40 and 45 Gy, depending on tumor size, patient age, and the presence of vitreal seeding.[97] The survival rate of the combined series of patients treated with bilateral irradiation was 82%, compared with a survival rate of 71% among a group of patients treated with bilateral enucleation only.[98] Although the risk of a treatment-related second malignant tumor developing in a patient with bilateral retinoblastoma is considerable, the data available suggest the long-term survival of patients treated with bilateral irradiation is not worse than that of patients treated with bilateral enucleation only. The preservation of some useful vision in these patients is an obvious advantage of such a treatment approach, but prolonged follow-up of patients treated in this manner is necessary to thoroughly evaluate the effect of treatment-related second malignant tumors on long-term survival.[99]

Local irradiation, after enucleation, is recommended for all patients with extension of retinoblastoma into the orbit. Presentation with exophthalmos or a palpable mass through the eyelids suggests the presence of orbital extension of the tumor. The identification of an encapsulated or unencapsulated extraocular mass, enlargement of the cut end of the optic nerve at the time of enucleation, or rupture of the globe during removal is associated with orbital contamination with the tumor. These findings are confirmed histologically by the identification of an episcleral mass of tumor tissue or tumor at the margin of the cut end of the optic nerve. Patients with orbital retinoblastoma should receive irradiation to a volume that includes the entire orbit and the optic nerve up to the optic chiasm.

Chemotherapy

The use of adjuvant chemotherapy in treating intraocular and bilateral disease has been prompted by success in salvaging patients with recurrent extraocular disease with chemotherapy-based regimens. Most efforts at chemoreduction have included a platinating agent (cisplatin or carboplatin) in various combinations with vincristine, etoposide, cyclophosphamide, and doxorubicin, with or without cyclosporin A as a multidrug-resistant reversal agent. Although platinum-based regimens appear to have significant activity in retinoblastoma, chemotherapy alone rarely achieves durable disease control.[100]

Because tumor shrinkage may decrease the need for enucleation, the goal of early trials was preservation of vision, primarily in children with bilateral disease. Since the 1990s, there have been a series of studies documenting promising rates of vision-sparing therapy without external-beam radiotherapy in intraocular disease.[90,101,102] The benefits of chemotherapy were most pronounced in patients with Reese-Ellsworth group I to III tumors, allowing globe preservation in more than two-thirds of patients. Friedman et al.[101] demonstrated that group V patients receiving systemic treatment had decreased vitreous seed recurrence, but 75% ultimately required external beam radiation.

One of the recent areas of clinical investigation has been the use of periocular chemotherapy involving injection of carboplatin around the globe to increase drug concentration within the eye. This method of drug delivery when given along with systemic chemotherapy is being evaluated in a COG trial with the goal of improving the outcome of patients with groups C and D disease. Preliminary data suggest that another method of increasing intraocular concentrations of a chemotherapeutic agent could be through cannulating the ophthalmic artery and injecting the drug into the ophthalmic artery.[103–105] Research into the pathways involved in the origin of the tumor is likely to lead to future targeted therapies and thereby not only preserve the globes but also reduce the long-term effects of radiation and chemotherapy.

PEDIATRIC BONE SARCOMAS: OSTEOSARCOMA AND EWING'S SARCOMA

Osteosarcoma (OS) and Ewing's sarcoma, which together account for approximately 6% of all pediatric malignancies,[1,106] are the most common primary malignant tumors of bone in the pediatric and adolescent population. Although the biologic properties of these tumors are distinct, their treatment principles are quite similar.[107] A comprehensive discussion of osteosarcoma is provided in Chapter 116. The main features of OS in the pediatric population, including its unique molecular genetic and cytogenetic features, will be discussed in this section.

Osteosarcoma

Epidemiology

OS, the most common primary bone tumor in children and adolescents, accounts for 4% of all childhood cancers.[1] The majority of cases occur in the second decade of life, with a peak age of incidence of 16 years in males and 12 years in females.[108] OS occurs more frequently in boys than in girls, and the incidence in black children is slightly higher than in white children.[108]

Biology and Molecular Genetics

The majority of osteosarcomas are sporadic. However, certain conditions are known to predispose to the development of OS, such as previous exposure to ionizing radiation[109] and alkylating agents.[110] Approximately 3% of cases are attributable to prior irradiation. OS in patients older than 40 years are almost always attributable to Paget disease.[111]

OS is associated with several cancer predisposition syndromes, including hereditary retinoblastoma, Li-Fraumeni syndrome (LFS), and Rothmund-Thomson syndrome (RTS).

PRACTICE OF ONCOLOGY

Patients with hereditary retinoblastoma have germline mutations in the *RB1* gene and somatic mutations in retinal cells resulting in retinoblastoma. The majority of secondary nonocular malignancies in these patients are sarcomas, and about 50% of these are osteosarcomas.[112,113] LFS is a familial cancer syndrome in which affected family members display a wide spectrum of cancers, including OS.[114] Many of these patients carry germline mutations in the *p53* tumor suppressor gene.[115,116] Screening of a large series of children with OS showed that approximately 3% to 4% carried constitutional germline mutations in *p53*.[117] RTS is an autosomal recessive condition characterized by a distinctive rash (poikiloderma), small stature, skeletal anomalies, sparse hair, and increased risk for OS. In a cross-sectional study of 41 patients with RTS, 13 patients (30%) were found to have OS.[118] Two-thirds of patients had constitutional mutations in the *RECQL4* gene, and presence of mutations correlated with OS risk.[119] Because these genetic conditions have a known predisposition to OS, careful detailing of family history in a patient newly diagnosed with OS is important to identify underlying genetic risk and for genetic counseling of family members.

In view of these genetic predisposition syndromes, it is not surprising that the *RB1* and *p53* genes are frequently altered in sporadic OS tumors. Approximately 70% of primary OS tumors have alterations in the *RB1* gene.[120–122] Regulators of the *RB1* pathway, including cyclin-dependent kinase 4 and 6, cyclin D1, and p16^{INK4a}, have also been found to be altered in some cases of OS.[123–125] Inactivating mutations of the *p53* gene occur in approximately 50% of all sporadic cancers. The overall frequency of *p53* mutations in OS ranges from 15% to 30% depending on the detection methods used.[126] Other members of the *p53* pathway, including p14^{ARF} and MDM2, are altered in some cases of sporadic OS.[127,128] Unlike *p53* and *RB1*, the *RECQL4* gene has not been found to be mutated in cases of sporadic OS.[129]

Clinical Presentation and Natural History

Most patients with OS present with pain in the involved area. Soft tissue swelling may be present, and 5% to 10% of patients may present with a pathologic fracture of the affected bone.[130] Systemic symptoms such as fever, weight loss, and malaise are generally absent. Physical examination usually demonstrates a firm, soft mass with tenderness. Laboratory evaluation is usually normal except for elevated alkaline phosphatase (in approximately 40%),[131] elevated lactate dehydrogenase (in approximately 30%),[132] and elevated erythrocyte sedimentation rate, none of which is specific for OS.

Pediatric OS preferentially involves the metaphyseal region of the long bones, in contrast to Ewing's sarcoma, which typically arises in the diaphyseal region of the long bones. The most common sites of disease in descending order are distal femur, proximal tibia, proximal humerus, middle and proximal femur, and other bones. Unlike Ewing's sarcoma the axial skeleton is less commonly affected.[133] Approximately 20% of OS patients present with clinically detectable metastatic disease, most commonly to the lungs. Although 80% of patients will not have visible metastatic disease at presentation, the use of surgery alone is associated with an 80% risk of disease recurrence.[133] Thus, micrometastatic disease is already present at the time of diagnosis, and systemic chemotherapy is necessary for virtually all patients.

Diagnostic and Staging Evaluation

Initial evaluation of a suspected bone tumor involves obtaining a complete history and physical examination. Radiographic studies allow assessment of anatomic site, extent of local invasion, and the pattern of extension.[134] If the tumor involves an extremity, plain x-rays should encompass both proximal and distal joint regions, and they should be taken in two planes. Characteristic findings on x-ray include a mixed lytic and sclerotic appearance, periosteal new bone formation with lifting of the cortex and formation of Codman's triangle, and ossification of the soft tissue in a radial or "sunburst" pattern.[133] Occasionally, no abnormalities will be evident on plain radiographs; therefore, if clinical suspicion for a bone tumor is high, MRI or CT scans should be obtained. Even if the plain x-rays are classic for OS, further imaging of the primary tumor by MRI or CT is required for evaluation of the extent of the tumor for planning of definitive surgery. While both are equally accurate for local staging of tumor, MRI is preferable for evaluation soft tissue extension and joint and marrow involvement, and it also spares radiation associated with CT.[134]

None of the radiographic features is pathognomonic for OS; therefore, biopsy with pathologic review is still required for diagnosis and for distinguishing OS from other malignant neoplasms of bone, such as Ewing's sarcoma, lymphoma, and metastatic tumor, and from benign bone lesions, such as osteochondroma and giant cell tumor, and nonneoplastic conditions, such as osteomyelitis, eosinophilic granuloma, and aneurysmal bone cyst.

Because patients with metastatic disease at presentation have a significantly worse outcome than patients with localized disease, a thorough search for sites of metastases is imperative. Staging workup for OS includes a technetium-99 bone scan to evaluate involvement of other bones and skip lesions within the same bone, chest x-ray, and chest CT to detect pulmonary metastases. Visible metastases will be present in 15% to 20% of patients at initial diagnosis. CT scans will identify some pulmonary lesions not detected by plain radiographs, although false-positive findings with CT scans may also occur. If a single lesion cannot be defined unequivocally as metastatic disease by CT scan, then histologic confirmation is indicated, particularly if the lesion was not detected on plain films. One or more pulmonary (or pleural) nodules greater or equal to 1 cm *or* three or more nodules greater than or equal to 0.5 cm maximum diameter generally indicates definite pulmonary metastases and may not require biopsy. Fewer or smaller lesions may or may not represent metastatic disease; therefore, confirmation by resection may be indicated.[134] There are no laboratory studies that are diagnostic or prognostic for OS.[135] General laboratory tests such as a complete blood count, electrolytes including calcium, magnesium and phosphorus, liver and renal function tests, alkaline phosphatase, and lactate dehydrogenase (LDH) should be obtained as baseline values.[135]

Biopsy of the tumor is required for diagnosis. The biopsy should be performed by an orthopedic surgeon experienced in the management of patients with OS, ideally by the same surgeon who will perform the definitive surgery. Proper planning of the biopsy with careful consideration of the future definitive surgery is important so as not to jeopardize the subsequent treatment, particularly a limb-salvage procedure.[136]

Pathology

The diagnosis of OS depends on histopathologic criteria with confirmatory radiologic appearance. OS is believed to derive from primitive bone-forming mesenchymal cells.[137] The histologic diagnosis is based on the presence of a malignant sarcomatous stroma associated with the production of "tumor" osteoid or immature bone (Fig. 123.6*A*).[138] Several clinicopathologic variants of OS have been defined based on histologic, clinical, and radiographic features. These include conventional OS, which is the largest group, comprising 80% of all osteosarcomas and the type most frequently encountered in children and adolescents. Conventional OS are further subdivided into osteoblastic (50% of conventional OS), fibroblastic (25%), and chondroblastic (25%) variants depending on the

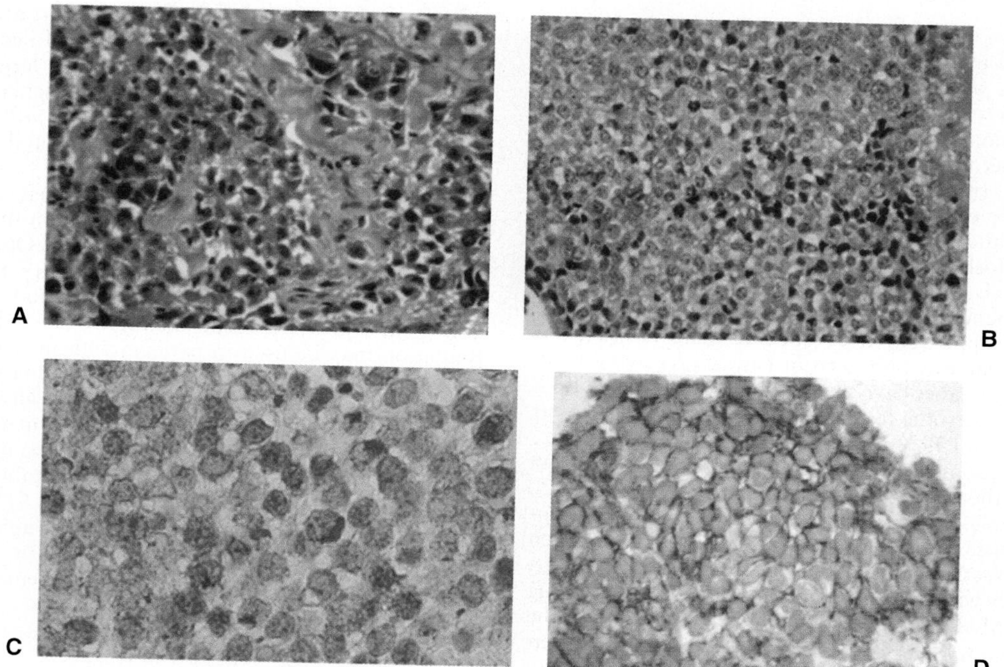

FIGURE 123.6 Staining methods: **A:** Hematoxylin and eosin (H&E), osteosarcoma. **B:** H&E, Ewing's sarcoma. **C:** Periodic acid–Schiff reagent, Ewing's sarcoma. **D:** CD99, Ewing's sarcoma. (Courtesy of Dr. M. John Hicks, Texas Children's Hospital, Baylor College of Medicine, Houston, TX.)

degrees of cellular differentiation.[139] The main feature that distinguishes these tumors from the malignant fibrosarcomas and chondrosarcomas, which also arise from primitive mesenchymal cells, is the production of osteoid, the *sine qua non* for the diagnosis of OS.[138]

Other variants of OS include parosteal (juxtacortical, 4%), telangiectatic (<3%), small cell (1%), periosteal (1%), and multifocal (<1%). Small cell OS can be confused with Ewing's sarcoma by routine hematoxylin-eosin staining; therefore, specific immunohistochemistry and cytogenetic analyses for Ewing's sarcoma may be useful (e.g., CD99 staining and detection of the 11;22 translocation).[140,141] Another distinct variant is OS of the jaw, which tends to occur in older patients, has an indolent course, and is more often associated with local recurrences than with distant metastases. Extraosseous OS, usually of the soft tissues, is rarely encountered and usually occurs after exposure to radiation.[142]

In contrast to other pediatric sarcomas, osteosarcomas do not have any specific translocations or other molecular genetic abnormalities that can serve as diagnostic or tumor-specific markers of disease. Cytogenetically, OS tumors display complex numerical and structural chromosomal abnormalities with significant cell-to-cell variation and heterogeneity, highlighting the complexity and instability of the genetic makeup of OS.[143,144]

Treatment

The mainstays of therapy for OS are surgery and chemotherapy. Unlike Ewing's sarcoma, OS is relatively resistant to radiation; therefore, this modality is not used routinely.[133,145] The outcome of patients with nonmetastatic OS has improved dramatically during the past three to four decades from an EFS of 10% to 20% to 65% to 70%, mostly because of the addition of adjuvant chemotherapy, as well as improvements in surgical and diagnostic imaging techniques.[133,146–148] The care of patients with OS requires a team approach involving oncologists, orthopedic surgeons, oncology nurses, physical therapists, social workers, and child life specialists.

Chemotherapy

Localized Disease. With current combinations of surgery and chemotherapy, long-term disease-free survival and overall survival rates for OS are greater than 60%. The current standard three-drug chemotherapy regimen includes doxorubicin, cisplatin, and high-dose methotrexate. Efforts are ongoing to determine if more aggressive combinations of chemotherapy for poor histologic responders will improve outcome. Current therapy for localized OS involves neoadjuvant chemotherapy for approximately 10 weeks followed by definitive surgery, followed by adjuvant chemotherapy for a total of approximately 40 weeks. The exception to this therapy scheme in localized disease is for the superficial surface juxtacortical osteosarcomas (parosteal and periosteal), which have traditionally been treated with surgery alone if they are low grade and do not invade the medullary cavity.[149]

The benefit of adjuvant chemotherapy in the treatment of OS was clearly demonstrated in two prospective trials that randomly assigned patients to observation or chemotherapy following surgery.[132,147,150] The concept of "neoadjuvant" or "induction" chemotherapy (i.e., chemotherapy given before definitive surgical resection) was prompted by the development of techniques for limb-sparing procedures and the need to control disease while the prosthesis was being constructed.[151] It was observed that the tumors often decreased in size in response to upfront chemotherapy. A prospective randomized trial was conducted by the Pediatric Oncology Group (POG) to compare neoadjuvant chemotherapy, surgery, and maintenance chemotherapy versus primary surgery followed by adjuvant chemotherapy.[152] The outcomes were similar between the two groups with a 5-year EFS of about 60%. Therefore, most centers currently adhere to the strategy of using neoadjuvant chemotherapy, followed by definitive surgery, and then maintenance chemotherapy.

Subsequent trials examining whether intensification or addition of other chemotherapy agents either preoperatively, in order to increase the proportion of good responders, or postoperatively, to improve the outcome for poor responders, have not resulted in substantial improvements in overall survival for patients with OS.[153,154] The use of immunostimulatory agents in the treatment of OS was tested in a joint POG and CCG randomized study. This aim of this study was to determine whether the addition of the macrophage-activating agent MTP-PE (muramyl tripeptide phosphatidylethanolamine) to chemotherapy would enhance survival in newly diagnosed OS patients.[155] The study also evaluated whether the addition of ifosfamide to the standard three-drug regimen improved survival. Initial results suggested that there may be some modest benefit to patients treated with MTP-PE. However, there appeared to be specific drug interactions because this benefit was only seen in patients receiving ifosfamide. Follow-up studies have shown that addition of MTP-PE does appear to have some benefit by improving overall 6-year overall survival from 70% to 78%.[156]

The standard regimen for treating OS remains a combination of high-dose methotrexate, doxorubicin, and cisplatin (MAP). The current active trial, designated EURAMOS (European-American Osteosarcoma), is a cooperative trial between European and North American consortiums. This prospective, randomized study will treat all patients with standard three-drug induction with MAP. Good responders will continue with the same chemotherapy, but will be randomized to receive interferon-α, an immune-modulating cytokine that has been shown in some Scandinavian studies to have activity against OS.[157,158] Patients with poor histologic response will be randomized to receive high-dose ifosfamide and etoposide in addition to the standard three drugs. This trial is continuing to accrue patients.

Metastatic Disease. The presence of metastatic disease at presentation continues to be an extremely poor prognostic finding. The ability to control all foci of macroscopic disease is essential in managing metastatic OS. Patients with pulmonary metastatic disease have a survival rate on the order of 30% to 50%, whereas patients with bone metastases have a worse prognosis. Similarly, patients with multifocal OS have a dismal prognosis.

Multiple studies have demonstrated that removal of all sites of metastatic or recurrent disease (e.g., pulmonary lesions) even after completion of chemotherapy can result in long-term survival.[159–161] In a large analysis of the Cooperative Osteosarcoma Study Group that included more than 1,700 consecutively treated patients, the 10-year survival probability was 40% for metastatic patients who were able to have all sites of metastatic disease resected.[162] However, patients with extrapulmonary metastases (e.g., bone metastases) are less likely to be cured, particularly those with multifocal disease.[163]

Local Control. OS is relatively radioresistant; therefore, surgery alone is the mainstay of local control. The choice of limb salvage versus amputation for extremity tumors depends on the exact location and extent of the tumor, the ability to achieve good surgical margins, and proximity to the joints and neurovascular bundle. The goal of definitive surgery is to remove the tumor completely with disease-free margins. The pathologist will determine the extent of necrosis of the tumor in response to initial chemotherapy. The extent of necrosis has been shown to be prognostically significant in predicting outcome with more than 90% necrosis (grade 3 or 4) being favorable and less than 90% (grade 1 or 2) necrosis less favorable.[164]

Pelvic Tumors and Unresectable Disease. Patients with primary tumors of the axial skeleton in general have poor outcomes because of an inability to achieve adequate local control. In some pelvic and most vertebral primary tumors, complete resection often is not possible. Most pelvic osteosarcomas can be treated by hemipelvectomy; more centrally located pelvic tumors, especially those involving the sacrum, are unresectable. Only a few pelvic osteosarcomas can be treated by limb-sparing resection (internal hemipelvectomy). Contraindications to resection are unusually large extraosseous extensions with sacral plexus or major vascular involvement. In general, these tumors cannot be resected with negative margins and are best treated by chemotherapy and radiotherapy.

Radiation Therapy. Historically, OS has been considered to be relatively radioresistant; therefore, radiation therapy is generally not used in the primary treatment of OS, although this may change with increased multidisciplinary approaches and new radiotherapy technologies. CT simulation ensures that the gross tumor and soft tissue extension is included in the field. Radiation may be used in patients with microscopic positive margins of resection such as in the head and neck region where wide margins of resection are not possible and can be helpful for primary site control in the setting of metastatic disease. Doses of 66 to 70 Gy are typically used. The use of radiotherapy in the setting of metastatic or unresectable osteosarcoma may provide durable response. In one study, 97% had stable or improvement in positron emission tomography (PET)-CT or bone scan after a median dose of 30 Gy in ten fractions to metastatic and unresectable sites. Improvement in pain was seen in 76% of painful sites.[165]

Prognostic Factors

The most important prognostic factor for survival in patients with OS remains the presence of metastatic disease. Other prognostic variables, either characteristics of the patients or the tumors themselves, have been less definitive in predicting outcomes. These include tumor size, tumor location, LDH and alkaline phosphatase levels, and tumor retinoblastoma protein (RB) and Her2 status.[162] Location is important because axial tumors, such as pelvic, skull, or vertebral, fare worse because of the difficulty in achieving a complete surgical resection with disease-free margins. Histologic response of nonmetastatic primary tumors to preoperative chemotherapy has been shown to be an important predictor of disease-free survival.[164] Patients with less than 10% residual viable tumor in the resection specimen have a better prognosis than those with more residual viable cells. Current studies are determining whether more aggressive therapy for those with poor histologic response will improve their survival outcomes.

Ewing's Sarcoma

Epidemiology

Ewing's sarcoma belongs to the Ewing's sarcoma family of tumors (ESFT), which comprises a group of small round cell neoplasms that also includes Askin tumor and peripheral primitive neuroectodermal tumor. ESFT may arise in osseous or nonosseous sites and in multiple locations, including the soft tissues anywhere in the body such as the paravertebral and thoracic areas.[166] Ewing's sarcoma is the second most common primary bone tumor in pediatric patients after OS, accounting for approximately 2% of childhood malignancies.[167] The incidence per year is three cases per 1 million U.S. white persons younger than 21 years, with approximately 225 new cases diagnosed per year in North America.[1,140] Most of these tumors arise in the second decade of life. Only 20% to 30% are diagnosed in the first decade of life, and black and Asian children are rarely affected by this cancer.[1]

Biology and Molecular Genetics

ESFTs have long been considered to originate from neural crest progenitor cells[168]; however, recent genetic profiling and

TABLE 123.7

CHROMOSOMAL TRANSLOCATIONS AND GENE REARRANGEMENTS IN EWING'S SARCOMA/ EWING'S SARCOMA FAMILY OF TUMORS

Translocation	Genes Involved		Chromosome
t(11;22) (q24;q12)	EWS		22
		FLI1	11
t(21;22) (q22;q12)	EWS		22
		ERG	21
t(7;22) (p22;q12)	EWS		22
		ETV1	7
t(17;22) (q12;q12)	EWS		22
		E1AF	17
t(2;22) (q33;q12)	EWS		22
		FEV	2

From ref. 172.

overexpression of EWS-FLI1 in mesenchymal stem cells suggest that Ewing's sarcoma may actually arise from mesenchymal stem cells.[169–171] This family of tumors belongs to the group of sarcomas associated with unique chromosomal translocations that give rise to specific fusion transcripts.[172,173] Eighty-five percent of Ewing's sarcoma are associated with the translocation t(11;22) (q24;q12) resulting in the fusion of the *EWS* and *FLI1* genes. Another 10% to 15% of tumors are associated with the translocation t(21;22) (q22;q12) that generates the *EWS-ERG* fusion gene. In both cases, a portion of the *EWS* gene on chromosome 22 is fused to part of another gene. Both *FLI* (on chromosome 11) and *ERG* (on chromosome 21) are members of the ETS family of transcription factors (Table 123.7). The exact mechanism of tumorigenesis mediated by EWS-FLI1 and other fusion proteins is not totally clear and is an active area of research.

The most common rearrangement, designated type 1, consists of the first seven exons of *EWS* fused to exons six to nine of *FLI1*. This fusion gene accounts for nearly two-thirds of all cases. The type 2 rearrangement, accounting for 25% of cases, fuses *EWS* to exon 5 of *FLI1* and was thought to be associated with a poorer prognosis through retrospective studies.[174–176] However, a recent report of 119 patients with chimeric fusion constructs refutes those findings, as no statistical prognostic difference could be concluded for type 1 versus nontype 1 fusions.[177] As a chimeric transcription factor, EWS-FLI1 is believed to regulate a number of critical downstream target genes that have been implicated in tumor biology, including members of the Sonic-Hedgehog and GLI1 pathways.[178,179]

Recent evidence has shown that direct inhibition of EWS-FLI1 oncogenic activity, through altering its interaction with critical binding partners, such as RNA helicase A (RHA), can cause significant alterations in tumor biology. Through the use of a small-molecule inhibitor that disrupts the EWS-FLI1/RHA interaction, investigators showed decrease xenograft growth and increased tumor cell apoptosis.[180] Additional evidence suggests that several intracellular signal transduction pathways are significantly altered in these tumors, including the dysregulation of the insulin-like growth factor receptor 1 (IGF-1R) and its subsequent activation of the phosphatidylinositol 3 (PI3) kinase-mammalian target of rapamycin (mTOR) pathway.[181] Drugs targeting these pathways are being explored as possible new therapeutic agents for ESFTs, including anti-IGF-1R antibodies and mTOR.[182–185]

Clinical Presentation and Natural History

Patients with osseous Ewing's sarcoma typically present with localized pain and swelling in the affected bone and may have other nonspecific symptoms such as fever, decreased appetite, and weight loss, which are usually seen in advanced disease.[186,187]

The lower extremity is the most common primary site for Ewing's sarcoma, accounting for approximately 40% to 45% of newly diagnosed cases, with about half of these occurring in the femur.[140] The pelvis is the second most common primary site, accounting for an additional 20% to 25% of new cases. Upper extremity sites account for another 10%, with the majority of these cases occurring in the humerus. Chest wall lesions make up 15% to 20% of primary Ewing's sarcomas, representing the most frequent chest wall tumor in children. The remaining osseous tumors originate from the vertebrae, mandible, and skull.

ESFT can affect nonosseous structures as well, and these usually occur in the soft tissues, but can also arise in the gastrointestinal tract, kidney, adrenal gland, lung, and other rare sites.[140] Depending on the location of the tumor, the patient may develop a limp, have pain that increases with respiration, or experience pain that is radicular in nature. Rarely, patients may present with paraplegia secondary to vertebral disease. Metastatic disease is present in approximately 25% of patients at initial diagnosis.[188] The most frequent sites of metastases are the lungs, bones, and bone marrow. Other sites of metastases such as the lymph nodes, liver, or brain are relatively rare, unless in end-stage disease.

There is no specific blood or urine test to diagnose Ewing's sarcoma. Abnormal laboratory findings at the time of diagnosis may include elevated LDH and alkaline phosphatase. LDH is useful as a gauge of tumor burden and usually falls with effective therapy and rises with disease recurrence.[189]

Diagnostic Staging Evaluation

Evaluation of a patient suspected of having Ewing's sarcoma includes radiographic examination of the primary tumor site and documentation of the presence or absence of distant metastases. Biopsy of the tumor and histopathologic examination are required for diagnosis. It is critical for the surgeon performing the diagnostic biopsy to place the incision appropriately to avoid complicating future resection.

Ewing's sarcoma typically spreads via the hematogenous route to the lungs, bone, and bone marrow. Plain x-rays and MRI or CT scan should be obtained initially to characterize and define the local extent of the primary tumor. MRI provides the most precise definition of the local extent of the tumor and the relation to nearby nerves and vessels. Lesions that originate in the long bones characteristically involve the diaphyses, with extension toward the metaphyses. On plain films, a lytic or mixed lytic-sclerotic lesion is usually identified in the bone. Multilamellated periosteal reaction (onion skin appearance) and lifting of the periosteum (Codman's triangle), or less frequently radiating bone spicules, may be present. The lesion is usually poorly marginated and has a permeative and destructive pattern. A soft tissue mass is frequently identified and best characterized on gadolinium-enhanced MRI, which is also useful in delineating the extent of marrow infiltration of the tumor.

CT scan of the chest should be obtained to search for pulmonary metastases. Biopsy of solitary pulmonary nodules should be strongly considered before classifying the disease as metastatic. Whole-body radionuclide bone scan should be obtained to search for bone metastases, which can be identified in approximately 10% of patients with Ewing's sarcoma. A newer modality that has been shown to be highly sensitive in screening for bone metastases is fluorine-18 (^{18}F) fluorodeoxyglucose PET in conjunction with CT (PET-CT),[190,191] as it has shown promise as a predictor of outcome, similar to histologic response, after induction chemotherapy.[192]

Bilateral bone marrow sampling is required to complete the staging of all patients regardless of primary site or tumor size. Microscopically detectable bone marrow metastases occur in less than 10% of patients and are associated with a poor prognosis.[193] Disseminated bone marrow disease may be present even in the absence of radiographically detectable bone metastases. Utilization of flow cytometry in the detection of disease in both the peripheral blood and bone marrow via the detection of CD99+CD45− cells has been reported and could potentially be used in the near future for staging and therapy response assessment.[194] The prognostic relevance of detection of micrometastatic disease detection by reverse transcription-polymerase chain reaction of fusion genes is still under investigation.[195–197]

Pathology

ESFT are grouped with the small round blue cell tumors of childhood. Based on light microscopy features, this grouping includes neuroblastoma, rhabdomyosarcoma, lymphoblastic lymphoma, and, less commonly, histiocytosis and small cell OS. Cells have a high nuclear to cytoplasmic ratio and appear homogenous with uniform round nuclei that contain evenly distributed chromatin and little mitotic activity.[173] The cytoplasm is typically scant and weakly eosinophilic; intracellular accumulation of glycogen may confer a positive acid-Schiff test (Fig. 123.6*B,C,D*). More than 95% of tumors within the Ewing's sarcoma family express the adhesion receptor CD99 (encoded by the *MIC2* gene) on their cell membranes.[140]

Peripheral primitive neuroectodermal tumors are characterized by neuroectodermal differentiation. These tumors typically demonstrate Homer-Wright pseudorosettes on light microscopy and positive immunohistochemical staining for synaptophysin, neuron-specific enolase, S100, and CD57.[173] In contrast, Ewing's sarcomas are poorly differentiated tumors that do not form pseudorosettes and do not typically stain positively for neural markers.[173]

Rapid identification of *EWS* gene rearrangements using reverse transcription-polymerase chain reaction or fluorescence *in situ* hybridization on fresh, frozen, or paraffin-embedded specimens are useful tools for discriminating between the ESFT and other morphologically similar small round cell tumors, expediting the initiation of appropriate therapy.[172]

Treatment

Chemotherapy. During the past three decades, overall improvement in the survival of patients with Ewing's sarcoma has occurred because of the addition of systemic multiagent chemotherapy, in particular anthracycline and alkylating agents, to surgery and radiation therapy, as well as improvements in surgical and radiation techniques and supportive care, including the use of growth factors. Currently, the EFS rates approach 79% for nonmetastatic and 25% for metastatic disease.[188]

Localized Disease. Results of the major treatment trials for Ewing's sarcoma are summarized in Table 123.8.[198–214] In 1973, the Intergroup Ewing Sarcoma Study (IESS) initiated a trial (IESS-I) to evaluate the potential benefit of adding the anthracycline doxorubicin (D) and prophylactic whole-lung irradiation to existing protocol of vincristine, dactinomycin, and cyclophosphamide (VAC) in patients with nonmetastatic disease. Patients treated with the four-drug regimen VACD had superior relapse-free survival (60%) compared with VAC alone (24%), demonstrating the value of doxorubicin.[198] In a subsequent study (IESS-II), the efficacy of administration of high-dose (1,400 mg/m^2) cyclophosphamide every 6 weeks was compared with administration of cyclophosphamide (500 mg/m^2) weekly for 6 weeks. The regimen that included high-dose cyclophosphamide also included a higher dose of doxorubicin (75 mg/m^2) than did the weekly cyclophosphamide schema. The 5-year relapse-free survival was 73% for the high-dose regimen, compared with 56% for the weekly cyclophosphamide regimen (P = .03), demonstrating the value of aggressive early cytoreduction.[199]

The North America cooperative groups, POG and CCG, completed their first intergroup study comparing the combination of vincristine, doxorubicin, cyclophosphamide, and dactinomycin to the combination of these four drugs plus ifosfamide and etoposide (INT-0091, CCG-7881/POG-8850).[200] The 5-year EFS was 69% for those who received the six-drug regimen, compared with 54% for those who received the four-drug regimen (P = .0005), demonstrating the value of adding ifosfamide and etoposide in nonmetastatic patients with Ewing's sarcoma. Similar improvements in survival with the addition of ifosfamide have been reported in studies by the National Cancer Institute and multiple European cooperative groups.[212,215,216] The second intergroup POG-CCG study for nonmetastatic Ewing's sarcoma compared the 48-week, five-drug combination of vincristine, doxorubicin, and cyclophosphamide alternating with ifosfamide and etoposide (VCD-IE) to a dose-intensified 30-week schedule using the same agents (CCG-7942/POG-9354). The experimental arm increased the dosage intensity of alkylating agents by 25%. Statistical analysis of this study revealed no evidence of improved EFS with the dose-intensified 30-week regimen.[201]

Recent cooperative studies in North America through COG (AEWS0031) determined that interval compression of the five-drug standard therapy (VCD-IE) schedule to 30 weeks (chemotherapy every 14 days vs. every 21 days) without changing the doses of drugs led to improved survival rates with 4-year EFS of 79% for the compressed cohort versus 70% for the patients treated every 21 days.[217] This is now the current standard chemotherapy regimen for nonmetastatic disease in North America. The current nonmetastatic COG Ewing's sarcoma trial is examining the efficacy of addition of vincristine, topotecan, and cyclophosphamide to standard therapy. Cyclophosphamide in combination with topotecan has been studied in a pediatric phase 2 study and showed activity in recurrent or refractory solid tumors. Responses were reported in 6 of 17 patients with Ewing's sarcoma. Hematopoietic toxicities were common but only 11% of 307 courses were associated with grade 3 or 4 infection.[218] Recently reported data from Germany confirm a similar response rate in patients with recurrent Ewing's sarcoma.[219]

In Europe, the collaborative study EURO-Ewing 99 is using risk-based stratification to assign patients into three risk groups based on tumor volume, presence and pattern of metastatic disease, and histologic response to chemotherapy.[140,220] This study incorporates six cycles of four-drug induction (vincristine, ifosfamide, doxorubicin, and etoposide [VIDE]) based on results of EICESS 92 and UK ET-2, which demonstrated the importance of ifosfamide in induction. After induction therapy, the study includes two randomized comparisons: for patients with localized disease and a good response (less than 10% viable tumor after VIDE), continuation therapy with either vincristine, dactinomycin, and cyclophosphamide (VAC) versus vincristine, dactinomycin, and ifosfamide (VAI); for patients with large tumors (more than 200 mL) or poor response (more than 10% viable tumor after VIDE), patients receive VAI versus busulfan-melphalan megatherapy. This study is nearing completion of accrual.

Metastatic Disease. In contrast to the improvement in survival for nonmetastatic patients treated with the addition of ifosfamide and etoposide, no comparable benefit has been

TABLE 123.8

TREATMENT RESULTS IN SELECTED CLINICAL STUDIES OF LOCALIZED EWING'S SARCOMA

Study	Authors	Schedule	Patients	5-year EFS	p value[a]	Comments
IESS studies						
IESS-I (1973–1978)	Nesbit et al.[198]	VAC	342	24%	VAC vs VAC + WLI, .001	Value of D
		VAC + WLI		44%	VAC vs VACD, .001	Benefit of WLI?
		VACD		60%	VAC + WLI vs VACD, .05	
IESS-II (1978–1982)	Burgert et al.[199]	VACD-HD	214	68%	.03	Value of aggressive cytoreduction
		VACD-MD		48%		
First POG-CCG INT-0091 (1988–1993)	Grier et al.[200]	VACD	200	54%	.005	Value of combination IE in localized disease, no benefit in metastatic disease
		VACD + IE	198	69%		
Second POG-CCG (1995–1998)	Granowetter et al.[201]	VCD + IE 48 weeks	492	75% (3 yr); 72.1% (5 yr)	.57	No benefit from dose escalation of alkylating agents
		VCD + IE 30 weeks		76% (3 yr); 70.1% (5 yr)		
Memorial Sloan-Kettering Cancer Center Studies						
T2 (1970–1978)	Rosen et al.[202]	VACD (adjuvant)	20	75%		After local therapy only, cumulative dose of D up to 600 mg/m²
P6 (1990–1995)	Kushner et al.[203]	HD-CVD+IE	36	77% (2 yr)		C dose escalation 4.2 g/m² per course
P6 (1991–2001)	Kolb et al.[204]	HD-CVD+ IE	68	Localized, 81% (4 yr); metastatic, 12% (4 yr)		Good results in localized disease, poor outcome in metastatic patients
St. Jude Studies						
ES-79 (1978–1986)	Hayes et al.[205]	VACD	52	82%, <8 cm (3 yr); 64%, ≥8 cm (3 yr)		Tumor size as prognostic factor
ES-87 (1987–1991)	Meyer et al.[206]	Therapeutic window with IE	26	Clinical responses in 96%		Combination IE effective
EW-92 (1992–1996)	Marina et al.[207]	VCD-IE × 3 VCD/IE intensified	34	78% (3 yr)		Tumor size (< or ≥8 cm) loses prognostic relevance with more intensive treatment
ROI, Bologna, Italy						
REN-3 (1991–1997)	Bacci et al.[208]	VDC + VIA + IE	157	71%		Surgery in 78% of patients
SFOP, France						
EW-88 (1988–1991)	Oberlin et al.[209]	VD + VD/VA	141	58%		Histological response better predictor of outcome than tumor volume
SSG, Scandinavia						
SSG IX (1990–1999)	Elomaa et al.[210]	VID + PID	88	58% (metastasis-free survival)		70% overall survival after 5 years

(*continued*)

TABLE 123.8

(CONTINUED)

Study	Authors	Schedule	Patients	5-year EFS	p value[a]	Comments
UKCCSG/MRC Studies						
ET-1 (1978–1986)	Craft et al.[211]	VACD	120	41%: extremity, 52%; axial, 38%; pelvic, 13%		Tumor site as the most important prognostic factor
ET-2 (1987–1993)	Craft et al.[212]	VAID	201	62%: extremity, 73%; axial, 55%; pelvic, 41%		Importance of the administration of high-dose alkylating agents (I)
CESS Studies						
CESS-81 (1981–1985)	Jürgens et al.[213]	VACD	93	<100 mL, 80%; ≥100 mL 31% (both 3 yr) Viable tumor <10%, 79%; >10%, 31% (both 3 yr)		Tumor volume (< or ≥100 mL) and histological response are prognostic factors
CESS-86 (1986–1991)	Paulussen et al.[214]	<100 mL (SR): VACD	301	52% (10 yr)		Intensive treatment with I for high-risk patients. Tumor volume (< or ≥200 mL) and histologic response as prognostic factor ≥100 mL
		≥100 mL (HR): VAID		51% (10 yr)		
EICESS Studies (CESS + UKCCSG)						
EICESS-92 (1992–1999)		SR: VAID vs VACD HR: VAID vs EVAID	155 326	68% vs 61% 51% vs 61%	.8406 .2141	Stage, histologic response, type of local therapy as prognostic factors; randomized comparisons not significant

A, actinomycin D; C, cyclophosphamide; CESS, Cooperative Ewing Sarcoma Studies; D, doxorubicin; E, etoposide; EFS, event-free survival; EICESS, European Intergroup Cooperative Ewing Sarcoma Studies; HD, high dose; HR, high risk; I, ifosfamide; IESS, Intergroup Ewing Sarcoma Study; MD, moderate dose; MRC, Medical Research Council; NA, not available; P, cisplatinum; POG-CCG, Pediatric Oncology Group–Children's Cancer Group; ROI, Rizzoli Orthopaedic Institute; SFOP, French Society of Paediatric Oncology; SSG, Scandinavian Sarcoma Group; SR, standard risk; UKCCSG, United Kingdom Children's Cancer Study Group; V, vincristine; WLI, whole-lung irradiation.

[a]*P* values are given only for trials comparing randomized treatment arms.

(Reprinted and modified from ref. 140, with permission.)

demonstrated for metastatic patients, and the 5-year overall survival rates remain less than 25%.[221] Among patients with metastatic disease, those with extrapulmonary metastases fare worse than those with isolated pulmonary metastases. In the first CCG-POG intergroup study (INT-0091), 120 patients with metastatic disease were evaluated using similar treatment regimens as previously described for nonmetastatic patients. The addition of ifosfamide and etoposide in the metastatic group provided no survival advantage, with an EFS of 20% in both treatment groups.[222] The results of a COG study investigating dose-intensity treatment regimen utilizing alternating cycles of vincristine, doxorubicin (90 mg/m²), and cyclophosphamide (2,200 mg/m²) and ifosfamide (2,800 mg/m²/d for 5 days) and etoposide (100 mg/m²/d for 5 days) showed a 6-year EFS of 28% and an overall survival rate of 29%.[223] Previous studies have demonstrated some improved survival with the addition of radiation to metastatic sites of disease. Patients with hematogenous metastases who were entered on IESS-II were treated with radiation to the primary tumor in addition to whole-lung radiation (18 Gy) for patients with pulmonary metastases and local bone irradiation for bone metastases. This strategy yielded a progression-free survival of 39%.[224]

Recurrent Disease. Overall improvements with current multimodal approach to therapy have led to a decrease in recurrent disease, particularly local recurrence.[225] However, 30% to 40% of patients still experience some form of recurrence, either local, distant, or combined, and the prognosis for these patients is dismal overall, with less than 20% survival.[225] Patients with early relapse (less than 2 years from diagnosis) have poorer prognosis, with less than 10% survival.[225] Twenty percent of patients with primary localized disease will relapse within 4 years, and the risk for relapse is much higher for patients with primary metastatic disease.[140,204] Recurrences of Ewing's sarcoma can occur late, more than 5 years from diagnosis.[226] There is no established salvage regimen for patients with recurrent disease, but in general, patients require surgery for local recurrence and chemotherapy for both local and distant recurrences. Patients with isolated lung nodules may benefit from whole-lung irradiation and appear to have better prognosis particularly if the relapse is late.[227] One retrospective study evaluating the efficacy of the combination of irinotecan and temozolomide in recurrent or progressive Ewing's sarcoma found an overall 63% response rate, with five complete and seven partial responses in 19 evaluable patients.[228] Studies looking at the use of combinations of topotecan and cyclophosphamide as well as gemcitabine and docetaxel, demonstrate that these agents have some activity in relapsed Ewing's sarcoma.[218,229,230] Myeloablative chemotherapy in combination with total body irradiation has been attempted in an effort to improve the prognosis for high-risk or relapsed patients with no improvements in outcome due to increased toxicities.[220,221]

Local Control. Local control with surgical resection or high-dose radiotherapy in addition to chemotherapy is imperative for curative therapy in Ewing's sarcoma. The inclusion of 12 to 15 weeks of systemic chemotherapy before introduction of local control measures has become standard practice, regardless of tumor size, location, or stage, unless the tumor causes an immediate threat to survival, such as spinal cord compression or cardiopulmonary compromise. To date there has been no randomized trial to determine whether surgery or radiotherapy is superior in achieving local control. For decades, radiotherapy was regarded as the standard of local treatment modality, but surgery is now the preferred modality if complete resection is feasible.[231] In prospective but nonrandomized trials, the improved survival in the surgical resection group has been generally attributed to the allocation of larger tumors with correspondingly poorer prognosis to the radiation group. In some situations, particularly in patients who are at high risk for local failure after resection, a combination of surgery and radiation is warranted. Decisions about local control should take into account resectability, functional outcome, long-term morbidity and the risk of late-onset secondary malignancies in tissues exposed to high-dose radiotherapy, and individual preference. Factors that influence the success of local control include initial location of primary tumor, with central disease having a poorer prognosis, as well as initial tumor response to chemotherapy based on the percentage of tumor necrosis.[232]

Surgery. In general, patients with isolated, resectable tumors receive induction chemotherapy followed by definitive surgery alone. Preoperative radiation may help in some cases to render a tumor more resectable. Limb salvage is almost always attempted, but in certain cases in which limb salvage or irradiation would lead to an unsatisfactory orthopedic outcome, amputation is warranted. Central pelvic or spinal lesions are frequently treated with radiation alone as surgery with negative margins is often not feasible. Chest wall lesions often present as large tumors extending into the thoracic cavity. Preoperative chemotherapy can greatly reduce the size, vascularity, and friability of the tumor, facilitating resection and decreasing the risk of intraoperative tumor rupture.[233] Analysis of 53 patients with nonmetastatic chest wall primaries treated on the first IESS demonstrated a decreased incidence of residual tumor in those patients resected after induction chemotherapy, in contrast to those who underwent resection prior to chemotherapy.[234] Because surgical outcome was improved in patients receiving preoperative chemotherapy, they were less likely to require postoperative chest wall radiotherapy with its well-established risks of cardiac and pulmonary damage and the risk of radiation-induced second malignancies.[235]

Radiation Therapy. Radiation responsiveness was one of the cardinal features of the bone tumor first described by Ewing in 1921.[236] Unfortunately, the long-term survival rate of patients after treatment with local radiation alone was only 9%. This finding presaged the routine inclusion of systemic chemotherapy, leading to a marked improvement in survival since the 1970s.

Local control of Ewing's sarcoma with radiation is dose dependent. Although some controversy remains regarding the optimal dose, several recent studies demonstrate excellent local control with dosages between 45 and 60 Gy.[237] Combined chemoradiation strategies have further improved local control. Donaldson[237] analyzed a large cohort of patients and found local control rates with combined chemoradiation ranging from 58% to 93%, while radiation alone achieved rates of 53% to 86%. In general, doses of 45 and 55.8 Gy are given for microscopic and gross disease, respectively. The exception may be in the spine where doses of 45 to 50.4 Gy are typically used for gross disease because of the radiation tolerance of the spinal cord.

The IESS examined the relation of primary tumor site, radiation therapy dose, treatment volume, and adjuvant chemotherapy regimen to local tumor control. Local recurrence occurred in 22.6% of patients with primary tumors in the humerus, 15.3% of those with pelvic primary tumors, 10.3% of tibial primaries, and 6.7% of tumors originating in the femur. A dose-response relationship was not apparent when local control was evaluated in patients who had received treatment to an adequate volume.[238] Other single-institution studies have found a dose response from 40 to 49 Gy in tumors less than 8 cm and 54 Gy in tumors 8 cm or larger.[239,240]

Historically, Ewing's sarcoma was treated with large radiation portals encompassing the entire involved bone. In the era of adjuvant chemotherapy, radiation treatment portals have become smaller with equivalent or improved local control. Local or tailored fields encompassing the primary tumor with a 2- to 5-cm margin, rather than treatment of the entire bone, have been evaluated.[241,242] Marcus et al.[242] reported excellent local control using tailored fields, noting the ability to spare a component of the long bones in tumors less than 8 cm in diameter, whereas frequently requiring whole-bone irradiation to achieve a 4-cm margin around larger tumors.

POG prospectively evaluated whole-bone (conventional) irradiation compared with tailored treatment fields, ultimately collapsing a planned randomized study to a single-arm trial using only tailored fields. A published analysis of this trial supports the efficacy of more limited treatment volume as defined by prechemotherapy tumor extent.[241] There was no difference in local control rates between patients receiving whole-bone versus involved-field radiation. This more tailored field with a 1.5- to 2.0-cm margins has become the standard strategy used in the most recent North American Ewing's sarcoma trials.

The risk of secondary sarcomas arising in irradiated bone is variably reported ranging from 5% to 10% at 20 years from diagnosis. Although no clear therapeutic advantage can be attributed to radiation doses in excess of 60 Gy, analysis of the long-term outcomes in patients treated with doses of 60 Gy or more demonstrated an unacceptable excess risk of secondary bone sarcomas. In marked contrast to the late complications seen in patients receiving very high-dose radiation, the risk of developing a secondary bone tumor in the irradiated field was negligible at doses below 48 Gy.[243]

Ewing's sarcoma is one of few diseases in which radiation therapy is used curatively for metastatic disease. Whole-lung irradiation has proven effective for consolidation of lung metastasis after chemotherapy. Multiple trials have demonstrated superior EFS and overall survival when whole-lung radiation is given.[231] Paulussen et al.[227] analyzed patients in three Cooperative Ewing Sarcoma Studies and found that EFS was significantly higher in patients who received whole-lung irradiation. Whole-lung doses between 15 and 18 Gy are used to treat patients after initial chemotherapy with minimal acute toxicity.

Prognostic Factors

Historically, the prognosis for children and young adults with Ewing's family tumors has been assessed on the basis of metastases, age of onset, tumor size, and location (trunk and pelvic primaries). However, with improvements in chemotherapeutic, surgical, and radiotherapeutic regimens, some of these traditional prognostic factors have been challenged and may hold less significance. The most important prognostic factor for outcome still remains the presence of metastatic disease at diagnosis. Patients with isolated pulmonary metastases do better (about 30% disease-free survival) compared to those with bone or bone marrow metastases (about 20% disease-free survival), but all fare worse than patients with nonmetastatic disease.[200,244,245] Large tumor size and volume and high serum LDH levels at diagnosis have been shown in some studies to correlate with adverse outcome.[188,189,246] Children with nonmetastatic pelvic primary sites have also been shown to have a poorer prognosis than children with extremity primaries, although this difference may be related to the larger size and more difficult resectability of pelvic tumors.[244]

Although not a prognostic factor assessable at the time of diagnosis, histologic response to chemotherapy appears to be a strong predictor of treatment outcome. Poor histologic response (<90% tumor necrosis) correlates with a poor prognosis, whereas complete or near-complete tumor necrosis correlates with good outcome, with a 5-year EFS of 84% to 95%.[247,248]

As understanding of the molecular pathogenesis of Ewing's sarcoma continues to increase, other prognostic markers, such as those derived from genetic expression analyses from primary and metastatic tumors, could potentially identify genetic signatures that may allow stratification of patients into low- and high-risk subgroups.[249,250]

RHABDOMYOSARCOMA

Epidemiology and Genetics

Rhabdomyosarcoma is the most common soft tissue sarcoma in children, accounting for 3% to 4% of all cases of childhood cancer, approximately 350 new cases diagnosed each year in the United States.[1,5] Rhabdomyosarcoma is more common in males and whites, and two-thirds of cases occur in patients under the age of 10 years.[251,252] Since the inception of the Intergroup Rhabdomyosarcoma Study Group (IRSG) in 1972 (now called the Soft Tissue Sarcoma Committee of COG), more than 4,000 patients have been treated in five well-designed multidisciplinary prospective trials for rhabdomyosarcoma that have boosted the survival rates of these patients from 30% to 72% (Fig. 123.2).[253,254]

The majority of cases of rhabdomyosarcoma are sporadic, but genetic and environmental factors have been associated with a predisposition for the development of this disease, including the Li-Fraumeni syndrome, neurofibromatosis type 1, Costello syndrome, Beckwith-Wiedemann syndrome, and parental use of marijuana and cocaine.[254–256] Because rhabdomyosarcoma arises from a primitive mesenchymal cell, it can be found in multiple areas of the body, but the most commonly affected anatomic regions by order of decreasing frequency are the head and neck (including the orbit and parameningeal areas), 35%, genitourinary tract (including the bladder, prostate, vagina, vulva, uterus, and paratesticular area), 22%, and extremities, 18%.[5,256]

Pathology and Molecular Biology

Rhabdomyosarcoma has been traditionally classified into three histologies, consisting of embryonal (including botryoid), alveolar, and pleomorphic subtypes.[6,257] The two major histologic subtypes, embryonal (60%) and alveolar (21%), have unique clinical and genetic features (Fig. 123.7). Embryonal tumors affect younger male patients and most commonly arise in the head, neck, and genitourinary regions.[251,256] The botryoid variant commonly involves hollow organs, and the spindle cell subtype preferentially arises in the paratesticular area, where it is associated with a superior prognosis.[256,257] Embryonal tumors are characterized by loss of heterozygosity at the 11p15 locus,[5] the region of the *IGF-II* gene.[258] Recent studies using comparative genomic hybridization have also documented cytogenetic gains and losses involving chromosomes 1p35, 2, 6, 7, 8, 9q22, 11, 12, 13q21, 14q21, 17, and 20.[259] In contrast, alveolar tumors most commonly affect older patients and arise in the trunk and extremity.[256] They are characterized by the presence of two translocations, t(2;13) (q35;q14) and t(1;13) (p36;q14), in which the *PAX3* gene on the long arm of chromosome 2 or the *PAX7* gene on chromosome 1 is fused with the *FKHR* gene on the long arm of chromosome 13.[260,261] These fusion transcripts can be readily detected using reverse transcriptase-polymerase chain reaction and can aid in the diagnosis and monitoring of the disease.[262] Patients with *PAX7-FHKR* fusion–positive tumors may have an improved outcome in the presence of metastatic disease when compared with patients who have *PAX3-FHKR* fusion–positive disease.[263]

Clinical Presentation and Evaluation

Given the heterogenous location of this tumor, rhabdomyosarcoma can cause a variety of signs and symptoms.[254] For example,

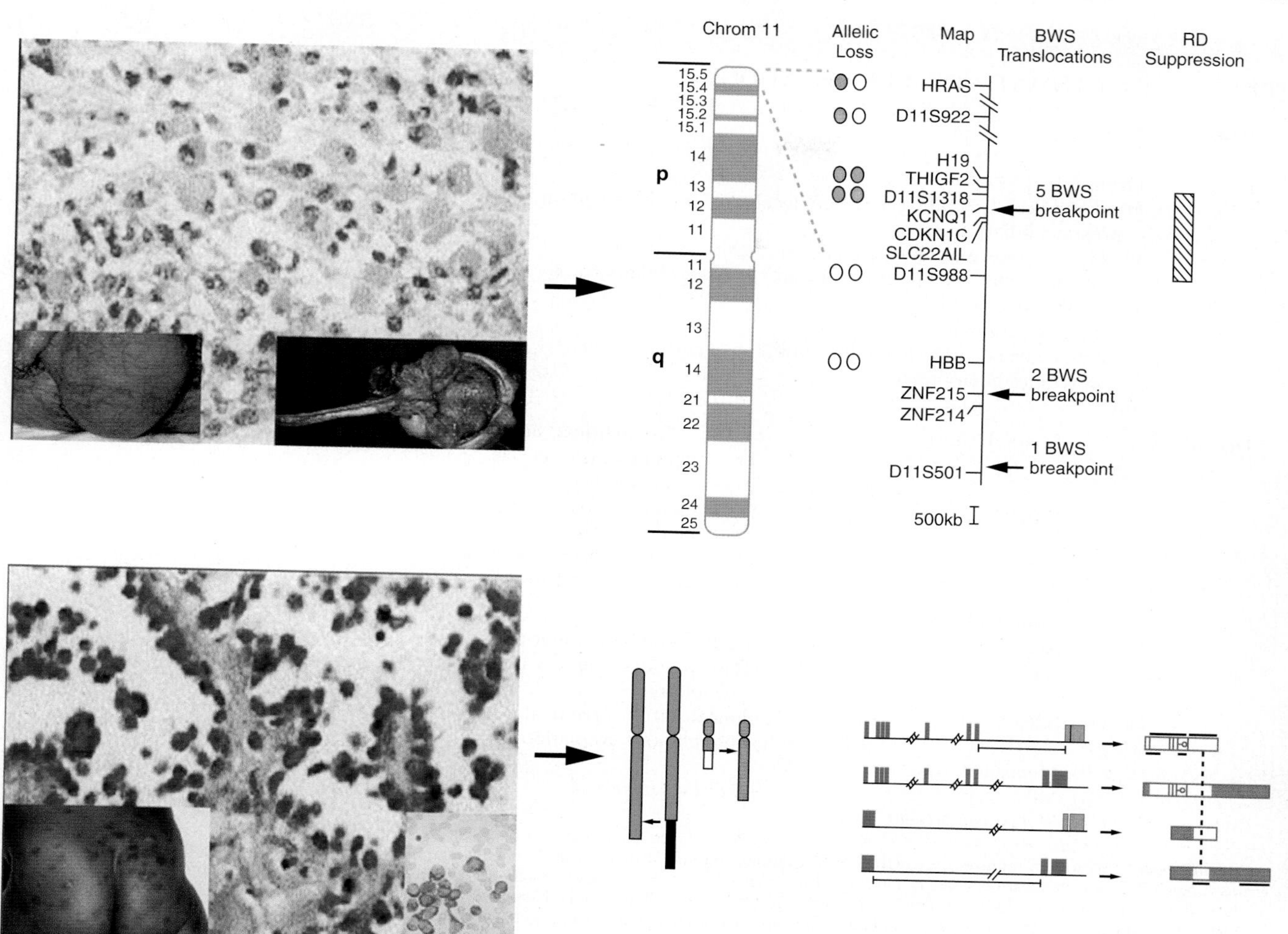

FIGURE 123.7 Embryonal tumors (**top panel**) more commonly affect the head and neck and the genitourinary regions and are associated with loss of heterozygosity at 11p15. Alveolar tumors (**bottom panel**) are more commonly found in the trunk and extremity and often have *PAX3* or *PAX7 FKHR* rearrangements.

head and neck tumors can cause proptosis, ophthalmoplegia, nasal or sinus obstruction, cranial nerve palsy, and painless or progressive enlarging neck masses.[214] Patients with bladder or prostate tumors can present with hematuria, a palpable abdominal mass, constipation, and urinary obstruction.[264] Female genital tract rhabdomyosarcoma can present as a protruding mass or mucosanguineous discharge, whereas paratesticular tumors commonly present with unilateral scrotal enlargement.[264] Tumors in the extremities present with an enlarging mass and evidence of palpable regional adenopathy, and tumors in the trunk, retroperitoneum, and biliary tract can produce symptoms related to direct involvement of the lung, abdominal organs, spine, and obstructive jaundice.

Staging evaluation should include a complete blood count, serum chemistries, bone scan, bilateral bone marrow aspirates and biopsies, and CT of the chest, abdomen, and pelvis.[5] Routine cranial imaging is not indicated unless there is evidence of spinal involvement; cerebrospinal fluid examination should be reserved for those patients who present with parameningeal primaries.[265,266] A biopsy usually establishes the diagnosis in the majority of patients, but further surgical intervention to evaluate regional nodes should be performed in all children with extremity tumors and in those older than 10 years with a paratesticular primary tumor.[267,268] Sentinel node biopsy is emerging as a valid technique to assess nodal involvement in patients with extremity tumors.[269]

Staging

Staging and risk group stratification is performed using the IRSG clinical grouping and staging systems [270,271] (Tables 123.9 and 123.10). Clinical grouping is a surgicopathologic staging system that depends on the surgical resectability of the disease and the presence or absence of metastases. About 16% of patients have group I disease (completely resected), 20% have group II disease, 48% have group III disease (incompletely resected), and 16% have group IV disease (metastatic).[4,5] In addition, all patients should be staged using the pretreatment tumor, necrosis, metastasis (TNM) staging system, which stratifies patients into four different categories based on the site of the primary tumor, tumor size, presence or absence of nodal and distant disease, and invasiveness. Both systems, in addition to histologic subtype, should be used to stage patients with pediatric rhabdomyosarcoma as therapy and outcome are closely dependent on the variables outlined by each of these staging systems (Table 123.11).

TABLE 123.9

PRETREATMENT TNM STAGING CLASSIFICATION

Stage	Sites	T	Size	N	M
1	Orbit Head and neck (excluding parameningeal); GU non-bladder/non-prostate; biliary tract	T1 or T2	a or b	N0 or N1 or NX	M0
2	Bladder/prostate, extremity, cranial parameningeal, other (includes trunk, retroperitoneum, etc.) (excludes biliary tract)	T1 or T2	a	N0 or NX	M0
3	Bladder/prostate Extremity, cranial Parameningeal, other (includes trunk, retroperitoneum, etc.) (excludes biliary tract)	T1 or T2	a b	N1 N0 or N1 or Nx	M0 M0
4	All	T1 or T2	a or b	N0 or N1	M1
Definitions:	Tumor T(site)1	confirmed to anatomic site of origin (a) ≤5 cm in diameter in size (b) >5 cm in diameter in size			
	T(site)2	extension and/or fixative to surrounding tissue (a) ≤5 cm in diameter in size (b) >5 cm in diameter in size			
	Regional Nodes				
	N0	regional nodes not clinically involved			
	N1	regional nodes clinically involved by neoplasm			
	NX	clinical status of regional nodes unknown (especially sites that preclude lymph node evaluation)			
	Metastasis				
	M0	no distant metastasis			
M1	Metastasis present				

Staging prior to treatment requires thorough clinical examination and laboratory and imaging examinations. Biopsy is required to establish the histologic diagnosis. Pretreatment size is determined by external measurement or magnetic resonance imaging or computed tomography (CT) depending on the anatomic location. For less accessible primary sites, CT will be employed as a means of lymph node assessment as well. Metastatic sites will require some form of imaging (but not histologic confirmation, except for bone marrow examination) confirmation.
(Adapted from ref. 270.)

Prognostic Factors

Clinical group, stage, histologic subtype, age, and treatment (Fig. 123.7) are the most important predictors of outcome in childhood rhabdomyosarcoma.[254,272] Patients with stage I group I/IIa or III orbit and stage 2 group I embryonal tumors have an estimated 90% 5-year FFS, which is similar to the 87% seen in patients with embryonal stage 1 group IIb,c, group III nonorbit, stage 2 group II, and stage 3 group I or II patients. Those with stage 2 or 3 group III disease have a 5-year FFS of 73%, and for those with invasive embryonal tumors who were less than 1 year or 10 years or more it was only 56%. Patients with embryonal extremity group III tumors had a 5-year FFS of 43%. Children with alveolar tumors fare worse overall and those with group III N1 disease had a 5-year EFS of 31%, a figure that is comparable to that seen in children with high-risk disease.[272] The survival of patients with rhabdomyosarcoma has increased from 55% in IRSG I, to 63% in IRSG II, to 69% in IRSG III, and to 73% in IRSG IV[5,256] (Fig. 123.2). Despite remarkable improvements in outcome, children with metastatic disease continue to fare poorly, with 5-year survival rates between 20% and 30%.[273] A subset of patients with metastatic rhabdomyosarcoma have a more favorable outcome and include those whose ages range between 1 and 9 years, those who have a favorable primary site, less than three metastatic sites, and do not have bone or bone marrow disease.[274] A recent publication suggests that multivariate gene expression models are highly predictive of clinical outcome and correlate with the current risk classification used by COG.[275]

Treatment

Principles of Therapy

Patients with rhabdomyosarcoma require detailed initial evaluation by a multidisciplinary care team comprised of oncologists, pathologists, surgeons, and radiation therapists. Current risk-based protocols stratify treatment of patients with rhabdomyosarcoma into one of three distinct risk groups (low, intermediate, and high) based on the initial staging, grouping, and histology of the tumor (Table 123.11).

Surgical considerations for the treatment of rhabdomyosarcoma are site specific, and extensive surgeries are not necessary in sites that may produce significant morbidity because rhabdomyosarcoma is a highly chemoresponsive tumor. The role of surgery is therefore often limited to obtaining a biopsy to establish the diagnosis. Re-excision of tumors located in the extremity and trunk to achieve negative margins and debulking of retroperitoneal tumors might offer a survival advantage in selected patients.[276,277] Second-look surgeries in selected sites may help verify the diagnosis and responsiveness of the tumor to chemotherapy and obviate the need for or decrease the dose of radiotherapy.[278,279]

TABLE 123.10

IRS CLINICAL GROUPING CLASSIFICATION

Group I: Localized disease, completely resected
(Regional nodes not involved—lymph node biopsy or dissection is required except for head and neck lesions)
(a) Confined to muscle or organ of origin
(b) Contiguous involvement—infiltration outside the muscle or organ of origin, as through fascial planes.
NOTATION: This includes both gross inspection and microscopic confirmation of complete resection. Any nodes that may be inadvertently taken with the specimen must be negative. If the latter should be involved microscopically, then the patient is placed in group IIb or IIc (see below).

Group II: Total gross resection with evidence of regional spread
(a) Grossly resected tumor with microscopic residual disease (surgeon believes that he has removed all of the tumor, but the pathologist finds tumor at the margin of resection and additional resection to achieve clean margin is not feasible). No evidence of gross residual tumor. No evidence of regional node involvement. Once radiotherapy and/or chemotherapy have been started, re-exploration and removal of the area of microscopic residual does not change the patient's group.
(b) Regional disease with involved nodes, completely resected with no microscopic residual.
NOTATION: Complete resection with microscopic confirmation of no residual disease makes this different from groups IIa and IIc. Additionally, in contrast to group IIa, regional nodes (which are completely resected, however) are involved, but the most distal node is histologically negative.
(c) Regional disease with involved nodes, grossly resected, but with evidence of microscopic residual and/or histologic involvement of the most distal regional node (from the primary site) in the dissection.
NOTATION: The presence of microscopic residual disease makes this group different from group 2b, and nodal involvement makes this group different from group 2a.

Group III: Incomplete resection with gross residual disease
(a) After biopsy only
(b) After gross or major resection of the primary (>50%)

Group IV: Distant metastatic disease present at onset
(Lung, liver, bones, bone marrow, brain, and distant muscle and nodes)
NOTATION: The above excludes regional nodes and adjacent organ infiltration, which places the patient in a more favorable grouping (as noted above under group II).

The presence of positive cytology in CSF, pleural, or abdominal fluids, as well as implants on pleural or peritoneal surfaces are regarded as indications for placing the patient in group IV.

IRS, Intergroup Rhabdomyosarcoma Study.
(Adapted from ref. 271.)

All children with the exception of those with group I embryonal tumors should receive radiotherapy.[280] The recommended doses are 36 Gy for microscopic residual disease and 41.4 Gy for completely resected regional nodal disease. For gross residual tumor, the recommended dose is 45 Gy for orbital and 50.4 Gy for nonorbital primary sites. In a pilot study for group III patients, the use of hyperfractionated radiotherapy was found to provide similar local control and survival rates when compared with conventional dose radiation.[281] The majority of patients with rhabdomyosarcoma can have radiotherapy safely delivered 3 to 12 weeks after starting chemotherapy; however, patients with parameningeal tumors with high-risk features such as intracranial involvement benefit from early institution of radiation and doses that exceed 47.5 Gy.[282] Proton-beam radiotherapy is being investigated by several groups and may offer advantages in decreasing long-term side effects in selected anatomic locations.[283]

TABLE 123.11

RISK SUBGROUPS IN PEDIATRIC RHABDOMYOSARCOMA

Risk Subgroup	Histology	Stage	Group	Proportion of Patients	Therapy	Expected Survival
Low	Embryonal	1–3	I	33%	VA ± C ± RT	95%
	Embryonal	2	I–II			
	Embryonal	3	I–II			
Intermediate	Alveolar	1–2	I–III	48%	VAC ± T or IR + RT	75%
	Embryonal	2,3	III			
High	Alveolar or embryonal	4	IV	19%	VAC ± I,E,D,IR + RT	27%

V, vincristine; A, actinomycin D; C, cyclophosphamide; RT, radiotherapy; T, topotecan; IR, irinotecan; D, doxorubicin; I, ifosfamide; E, etoposide.
(Modified from ref. 256.)

PRACTICE OF ONCOLOGY

Chemotherapy

All children with rhabdomyosarcoma should receive chemotherapy. The most common regimen used in North America consists of vincristine, actinomycin D, and cyclophosphamide (VAC); ifosfamide is preferentially used in the European trials.[284] Other agents such as topotecan, melphalan, methotrexate, ifosfamide, etoposide, irinotecan, and doxorubicin have also proven active, but their addition to VAC regimens failed to improve outcome.[285] Table 123.11 shows the treatment recommendations for patients with low-, intermediate-, and high-risk tumors. For low-risk patients, who account for one-third of all cases of rhabdomyosarcoma, administration of VA or VAC with or without radiotherapy is associated with survival rates in excess of 90%. Because of the excellent prognosis, the current trial for low-risk patients is examining the feasibility of limiting the duration of therapy and the exposure to alkylating agents. Patients with intermediate-risk disease comprise 55% of all patients with rhabdomyosarcoma and their survival—depending on stage, group, and histology—ranges from 59% to 83%. The use of alternating drug combinations with VAC and irinotecan is currently being investigated.[285] Despite marked improvements in survival of nonmetastatic patients, survival for the remaining 16% of high-risk patients who present with metastatic disease has remained unchanged during the past 30 years. End-intensification with high-dose chemotherapy, dose intensification of alkylating agents, and integration of novel agents have failed to improve survival in these patients.[286,287] The Soft Tissue Sarcoma Committee of COG has relied on the preclinical xenograft model to identify potentially active agents and to translate these findings into frontline window studies for children with previously untreated poor-prognosis rhabdomyosarcoma.[288] The current initiative by COG is to use the most active combinations of agents identified in window trials and to incorporate IGF-1R inhibitors to try to improve the outcome of these patients.[289–291]

LIVER TUMORS

Epidemiology and Genetics

Approximately two-thirds of primary liver tumors in children are malignant, and they account for 1.1% of all childhood cancers.[1] Hepatoblastoma is the most common malignant liver tumor in children, accounting for two-thirds of all pediatric liver cancers.[1,292] The incidence rates for hepatoblastoma have steadily increased over time, doubling from 0.8 per million in the 1970s to 1.5 per million in the 1990s and more recently, increasing at a rate of 4.3% annually.[1,293] In contrast, the incidence of hepatocellular carcinoma (HCC) has decreased from 0.6 per million to 0.2 per million.[1]

Hepatoblastoma accounts for over 90% of all malignant liver tumors in children under the age of 5 years, preferentially affecting males and whites.[294,295] The median age at presentation is 16 to 18 months.[1,294,295] In contrast, HCC affects both sexes equally and accounts for 87% of primary hepatic malignancies in patients 15 to 19 years of age.[1,3]

The most common risk factors for the development of hepatoblastoma include low birth weight, familial adenomatous polyposis, Gardner syndrome, Beckwith-Wiedemann syndrome, and hemihypertrophy.[3,296–298] In two studies, up to 10% of patients with sporadic hepatoblastoma had germline mutations of the *APC* gene; thus, routine screening of all children with hepatoblastoma remains controversial.[296,299,300] Prematurity has been increasingly recognized as a risk factor for the development of hepatoblastoma, and in one Japanese study, hepatoblastoma accounted for nearly 60% of all cancers seen in premature babies weighing less than 1,000 g at birth.[301] In another study, a clear correlation between a rising rate in hepatoblastoma and the percentage of low- and very low-birth weight newborns was documented.[302] A case-controlled study is currently being conducted by the COG to better delineate the role of prematurity and other factors in the development of hepatoblastoma.

HCC has commonly been associated with infection by the hepatitis B virus.[3] Several studies have documented nearly a 100% rate of seropositivity for hepatitis B surface antigen in children who develop HCC, and vaccination efforts to reduce the incidence of hepatitis B infection in Taiwan have produced a significant decrease in the risk of developing the disease.[303,304] Hepatitis C has also been linked to the development of HCC, mostly in adults.[3] Other risk factors associated with the development of HCC include tyrosinemia, biliary cirrhosis, Fanconi's anemia, glycogen storage diseases, α_1-antitrypsin deficiency, hemochromatosis, Sotos syndrome, and neurofibromatosis.[3]

Pathology

Hepatoblastomas most commonly have mixtures of epithelial components comprising fetal, embryonal, macrotrabecular, or undifferentiated cells and mesenchymal elements.[305,306] Pure fetal tumors have an excellent prognosis when treated with surgery alone, whereas small undifferentiated tumors have a poor prognosis and may represent a variant of rhabdoid tumors.[306–308] Numeric chromosomal abnormalities are seen in about one-third of hepatoblastomas and commonly involve trisomies of chromosomes 2, 8, and 20. Unbalanced translocations involving 1q12-21 have been reported in 18% of cases.[309] HCC in children has a similar pathologic appearance when compared with the adult counterparts, although the fibrolamellar variant appears to be more common in adolescents and young adults.[310]

Clinical Presentation

Infants and children with hepatoblastoma most commonly present with a palpable asymptomatic abdominal mass. Nausea, vomiting, anorexia, and weight loss are apparent in advanced disease, but jaundice is uncommon. Isosexual precocity can rarely be seen as a consequence of elevations of β-human chorionic gonadotropin (HCG), and hemihypertrophy can be seen in up to 10% of patients.[305,311] The presenting physical findings in children with HCC are similar to those encountered in patients with hepatoblastoma.

Evaluation and Staging

Laboratory evaluation should include a complete blood count, tests of renal and hepatic function, and urinalysis. The serum levels of total bilirubin, alkaline phosphatase, and alanine aminotransferase and aspartate aminotransferase are not generally useful for the differential diagnosis of malignant hepatic tumors in children. Serum levels of α-fetoprotein (AFP) are elevated in approximately 90% of patients with hepatoblastoma and in 78% of adult patients with HCC.[305,311] A very low or high value (<100 ng/L or >1,000,000 ng/L) at diagnosis as well as a low early decline (<1 log) prior to definitive surgery has been associated with a poor prognosis in hepatoblastoma.[312,313] If the diagnosis of HCC is established, testing for hepatitis B surface antigen, hepatitis B antibody, serum iron, total iron-binding capacity, serum ferritin, and α_1-antitrypsin should be performed. Radiographic evaluation should include a CT of the chest to search for metastases and an abdominal CT or MRI. Sonography may be helpful in assessing the anatomic status of the kidneys and the patency of the vena cava.

The grouping system used in therapeutic studies of hepatic tumors conducted by COG segregates patients according to

TABLE 123.12

COG CLINICAL STAGING SYSTEM FOR CHILDHOOD HEPATIC TUMORS

Stage	Description
STAGE I	Completely resected tumor
STAGE II	Microscopic residual disease after surgical resection Resected tumors with preoperative or intraoperative rupture
STAGE III	Gross residual disease or regional lymph node involvement by tumor
STAGE IV	Presence of distant metastases

COG, Children's Oncology Group.
(From Ortega JA, Douglass EC, Feusner JH, et al. Randomize comparison of cisplatin/vincristine/fluorouracil and cisplatin/continuous infusion doxorubicin for treatment of pediatric hepatoblastoma: a report from the Children's Cancer Group and the Pediatric Oncology Group. *J Clin Oncol* 2000;18(14):2665–2675.)

the resectability of the primary tumor and the presence or absence of metastatic disease (Table 123.12).[314] The European SIOP Liver Tumor Study Group (SIOPEL) uses a pretreatment extent of disease (PRETEXT) staging system (Fig. 123.8).[315,316] This preoperative classification scheme identifies four PRETEXT categories reflecting the number of sections of the liver free of tumor and describes extension of disease into portal and hepatic veins, vena cava, or intra-abdominal extrahepatic sites. A recent study comparing both staging systems suggests that the PRETEXT and COG systems can accurately predict survival in patients who might benefit from up-front surgical resection and reduced therapy as well as patients with unresectable disease who are at increased risk of death.[317]

Prognostic Factors

Staging (COG or SIOPEL) and tumor resectability as well as a low AFP value of less than 100 ng/L and small cell undifferentiated histology are the main predictors of outcome in hepatoblastoma.[317]

Treatment

Surgery

Surgical resection is the mainstay of therapy for hepatoblastoma and HCC and is required for cure.[311] Unfortunately, fewer than half of patients with hepatoblastoma and 30% of patients with HCC have resectable disease at the time of diagnosis.[314,318,319] Factors that render a liver tumor unresectable include involvement of both lobes and lymph node involvement in the porta hepatis or mediastinum. Additional features that may preclude resection include direct extension into the inferior vena cava, a central lesion that involves the left and right hepatic arteries or the portal vein, or lesions that involve all branches of the hepatic vein.

Treatment with chemotherapy before definitive surgery has allowed complete tumor resection in more than two-thirds of children whose hepatoblastomas were initially deemed unresectable.[311,314,320] In contrast, HCC is much less responsive to chemotherapy, limiting the effectiveness of preoperative pharmacologic intervention. When feasible, aggressive attempts at initial resection of HCC should be pursued.

Liver transplantation has been used by several centers for children with unresectable hepatoblastoma, with 10-year survival rates in excess of 80% for those who underwent this procedure as "primary" surgical therapy (Fig. 123.9).[321] This approach has also been used for patients with HCC.[322] Cryoablation or radiofrequency ablation of hepatic malignancies has been increasingly used in adults, particularly for metastatic lesions in the liver. Although these techniques have been used for the treatment of recurrent disease, their overall role in treatment of pediatric neoplasms remains to be defined. Arterial chemoembolization has also been recently reported as a therapeutic alternative in a small series of patients.[323]

Radiation Therapy

Traditionally, radiation therapy has had a limited role in the treatment of hepatoblastoma or HCC given the low tolerance for radiation of liver tissue. In the era of image-guided radiotherapy, radiation may be delivered to liver tumors with less hepatotoxicity. Not much information is available in children regarding the use of radiotherapy in hepatoblastoma or HCC. In one report, doses of 25 to 45 Gy were associated with six of eight incompletely resected hepatoblastoma children surviving after multimodality treatment.[324]

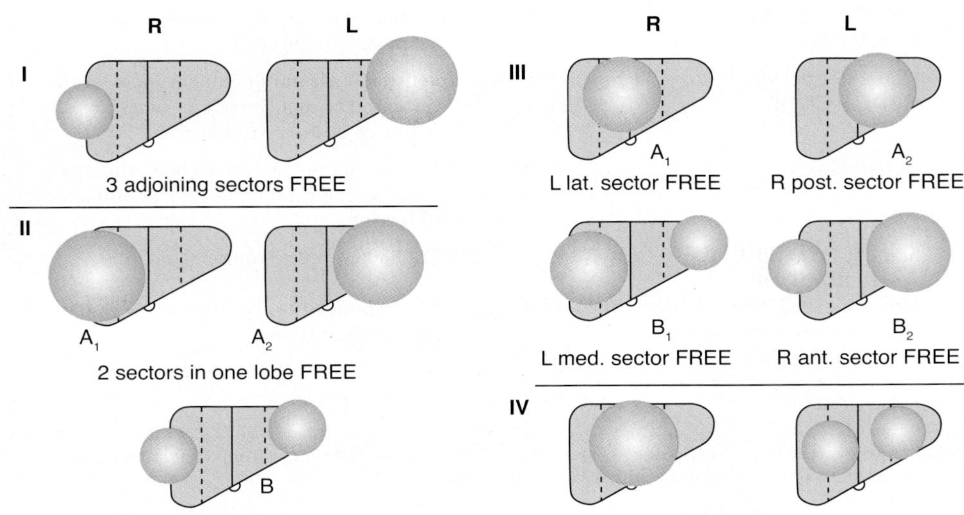

FIGURE 123.8 The International Society of Pediatric Oncology Preoperative Staging System (SIOPEL I). The liver is divided into four sectors. Classification (stage I, II, III, and IV) depends on the number of unaffected sectors (free from tumors). Extrahepatic growth is considered separately. (From ref. 315, with permission of Elsevier.)

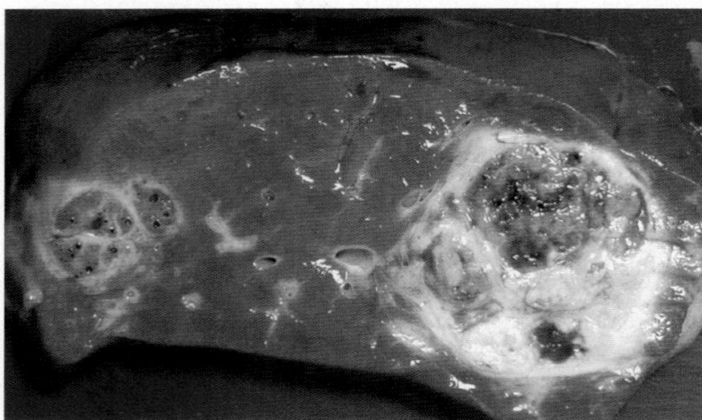

FIGURE 123.9 Liver resection of a patient with pretreatment extent of disease (PRETEXT) stage IV disease who underwent a successful liver transplant. The resected specimen shows multiple areas of viable tumor.

Chemotherapy

The role of chemotherapy in the treatment of hepatoblastoma is well established.[305] In addition to its role in reducing the size of the tumor before attempted resection, chemotherapy has been used as a postoperative adjuvant after complete excision of the primary tumor with improved survival.[325] The most active agents against hepatoblastoma include cisplatin and doxorubicin.[314] A randomized study using cisplatin-based chemotherapy demonstrated that the combination of doxorubicin and cisplatin was equivalent to the combination of cisplatin, vincristine, and 5-fluorouracil (CFV), but the latter triplet was associated with less myelosuppression, toxic deaths, and decreased need for prolonged hyperalimentation.[314] Thus, the latter regimen has become the standard for treating patients in North America. In Europe, SIOPEL preferentially uses a cisplatin-doxorubicin–containing regimen (Table 123.13).[326] A recent SIOPEL prospective randomized trial suggests, however, that patients with localized hepatoblastoma who have three or less liver sectors involved can be successfully treated with single agent cisplatin.[327] Other agents that have been used as part of combination chemotherapy include ifosfamide, cyclophosphamide, and carboplatin.[328,329] A significantly worse outcome was recently reported by investigators of the COG when carboplatin and cisplatin were used in newly diagnosed patients with advanced-stage disease (Table 123.13).[329]

Following administration of neoadjuvant chemotherapy, up to 90% of patients with unresectable disease will experience a response, and about 70% of these patients will be candidates for surgical resection.[330] The overall survival for patients with hepatoblastoma using cisplatin-containing regimens is about 70%, but survival is closely dependent on tumor stage at diagnosis: 85% for stage I, 100% for stage II, 62% for stage III, and 23% for stage IV.[314] Similar results based on PRETEXT staging have been published by SIOPEL investigators: 100%, 83%, 56%, and 46%, respectively, for patients with PRETEXT stages I to IV.[330] Patients with metastatic disease continue to fare poorly regardless of the regimen used, and their survival is less than 30%. Nearly one-third of patients who relapse following therapy with CFV can be salvaged with further surgery and a doxorubicin-based regimen.[331]

HCC is much less responsive to chemotherapy, and the results using these regimens have been disappointing, with an estimated 5-year event-free and overall survival of 19% and 28%, respectively.[319] Targeted therapies such as sorafenib have not been systematically studied in children with hepatocellular carcinoma.[332]

GERM CELL TUMORS

Germ cell tumors can arise in gonadal and extragonadal sites and comprise 3% to 4% of all pediatric malignancies. Although extragonadal germ cell tumors are relatively infrequent in adults, accounting for only 5% to 10% of all cases, they account for nearly two-thirds of all germ cell tumors in children.[1,333,334] The sacrococcygeal region represents the most common site for pediatric tumors (40% of all childhood germ

TABLE 123.13

RESULTS OF INTERGROUP STUDIES (COG AND SIOPEL) FOR THE TREATMENT OF HEPATOBLASTOMA

Study (Ref.)	No. of Patients	Treatment	Outcome	Comments
POG/CCG (314)	173	CDDP-V-5-FU vs CDDP-DOX	5-yr S 69% 5-yr S 72%	Regimen without doxorubicin less toxic with similar survival
COG P 9645 (329)	53 56	CDDP-V-5FU vs CBDCA-CDDP	1-yr EFS 57% 1-yr EFS 37%	Intensified platinum regimens increase the probability of adverse outcomes in children with hepatoblastoma
SIOPEL I (326)	154	CDDP-Dox	5-yr S 75%	138 received preoperative chemotherapy only and of these 72% had a complete resection.
SIOPEL 2 (318)	67 58	Standard risk (PRETEXT I, II, III) CDDP	3-yr S 91%	97% had complete tumor resections
		High risk (PRETEXT IV, metastases, extrahepatic or portal/hepatic involvement) CBDCA/Dox/CDDP	3-yr S 53%	78% responded to therapy and 67% had resection of tumor

COG, Children's Oncology Group; SIOPEL, European SIOP Liver Tumor Study Group; POG/CCG, Pediatric Oncology Group/Children's Cancer Group; CDDP, cisplatin; V, vincristine; 5-FU, 5-fluorouracil; Dox, doxorubicin; CBDCA, carboplatin.

cell tumors and 78% of all extragonadal disease).[335] Less commonly, extragonadal lesions can arise in the mediastinum, retroperitoneum, vagina, and pineal region. The biologic behavior of pediatric germ cell tumors is diverse and highly dependent on the histologic nature of the primary lesion, ranging from benign mature teratomas to highly malignant embryonal carcinomas and choriocarcinomas. The introduction of platinum-based chemotherapy has dramatically improved survival for the majority of children,[336] and because of their high curability, newer trials are focusing on strategies to decrease therapy-related morbidity.

Embryogenesis

Germ cell tumors are thought to arise from a common primordial germ cell. Primordial germ cells arise in the embryonic yolk sac endoderm. These cells migrate through the wall of the midgut to the genital ridge by week 5 of gestation. Arrested migration of germ cells along this pathway has been proposed as an explanation for the near midline location of most extragonadal germ cell tumors, including the sacrococcygeal region, retroperitoneum, mediastinum, and intracranial sites, including the pineal and suprasellar regions.[334]

Pathology and Genetics

Pediatric germ cell tumors comprise a diverse group of histologies. The majority of extragonadal tumors arising in infancy are benign teratomas. Similarly, most ovarian tumors (70%) are of germ cell origin, and the predominant histology is teratoma. In the testis, however, 75% of tumors are of germ cell origin, but most contain a malignant component intermixed with a benign element.[334,337,338]

Teratomas are the most common histologic subtype of pediatric germ cell tumors that arise in extragonadal sites and the ovary.[334] They are composed of elements derived from more than one of the three primary germ layers—ectoderm, mesoderm, and endoderm. Mature teratomas can be cystic or solid, although the cystic presentation predominates in gonadal sites. Immature teratomas are similar to mature teratomas but they contain blastemal or neuroectodermal tissues and are graded according to the amount of immature tissue present. Both low- and high-grade teratomas can be successfully treated with surgical excision alone followed by close observation. In a study of 73 children with immature teratomas, the 3-year EFS for these patients following surgical resection alone was 93%, and in five patients who developed a recurrence and received chemotherapy, the 3-year overall survival was 100%.[339]

Yolk sac (endodermal sinus) tumors are the most common pure malignant germ cell tumor in younger patients and the most common germ cell tumor of the testis.[333] They typically contain hyaline droplets that are composed of AFP as well as other proteins. Teilum et al.[340] suggested that the presence of AFP in these tumors supported the theory that they originated from the yolk sac endoderm.

Embryonal carcinoma is more often a component of mixed malignant germ cell tumors. They are composed of CD30+ cells that resemble epithelial cells arranged in solid sheets. Frequently, small or large acinar, tubular, and papillary structures are formed. Hemorrhage and necrosis are frequently present.

Germinomas, also termed *seminomas* or *dysgerminomas*, depending on whether they arise in the testis or ovary, are the most common pure germ cell tumor of the ovary in children.[334] Typical seminomas are composed of uniform cells supported by a delicate connective tissue stroma. Lymphocytic infiltration is present in most seminomas, with a granulomatous reaction identifiable in approximately half of cases. As is commonly found in adult testicular tumors, isochrome 12p is often identified in adolescent testicular germinomas.[341] This chromosomal abnormality is rarely seen in malignant testicular tumors of infancy in which yolk sac is the predominant histology.

Choriocarcinomas usually arise within the context of a mixed malignant germ cell tumor in adolescents and consists of two distinct cell types: syncytiotrophoblast and cytotrophoblast. The syncytiotrophoblast is a large, multinucleated cell with many hyperchromatic, irregular nuclei whose cytoplasm stains positive for β-HCG. Cytotrophoblast cells are medium sized and closely packed with clear cytoplasm, distinct cell borders, and a single, uniform, moderate-sized vesicular nucleus.

Gonadoblastoma is a rare benign tumor that has the potential of becoming malignant and is almost exclusively seen in patients with intersex disorders.[342] Histologically, they are composed of small and large cells, and the germ cells stain positively for placental alkaline phosphatase. Sex chromosomal disorders increase the risk of developing germ cell tumors in young patients. Patients with intersex disorders, specifically those with androgen insensitivity, mixed gonadal dysgenesis, and selected patients with Turner syndrome, are at increased risk for developing gonadoblastoma, which has the ability to transform into a malignant germ cell tumor, most commonly a dysgerminoma.[334] Patients with Klinefelter syndrome also have an increased risk of developing extragonadal germ cell tumors.[341] Cryptorchidism is another major risk factor for developing testicular cancer.[343]

Laboratory Markers

AFP and the β subunit of human chorionic gonadotropin (β-HCG) are oncofetoproteins that are elevated in the serum of patients with a variety of germ cell tumors. These proteins are clinically useful both as diagnostic tools and in surveillance of children on or off treatment for tumors that secrete these markers. The serum concentration of AFP reaches a maximum value at 13 weeks of gestation. It is readily detectable at birth, and owing to its long serum half-life of 7 days, the level of AFP may remain elevated in healthy infants as old as 6 months.[344] High serum levels of AFP are identified in pediatric patients with testicular, ovarian, presacral, and vaginal primary yolk sac tumors.[333]

β-HCG is a glycoprotein secreted by the placenta. Patients with pure yolk sac tumors do not have detectable serum HCG levels. Patients with choriocarcinoma, seminoma, and germinoma with syncytiotrophoblastic cells and occasionally patients with adult embryonal carcinoma of the ovary or testis have elevated serum HCG levels.[334] HCG has a much shorter serum half-life than AFP, lasting only 24 to 36 hours. Thus, a decline in HCG levels occurs much more rapidly with successful therapeutic intervention than in tumors that secrete AFP.

Clinical Presentation, Staging, and Treatment

The following section briefly summarizes the clinical presentation and treatment recommendations for germ cell tumors in specific anatomic areas. In general, with the use of surgery, either alone or in combination with chemotherapy that contains cisplatin, etoposide, and bleomycin (PEB), more than 90% of children with localized germ cell tumors and more than 80% of children with advanced-stage disease can be cured.[339,345] Risk-based therapeutic approaches based on primary tumor location and stage are summarized in Table 123.14. The use of higher doses of cisplatin might benefit a subset of patients with

TABLE 123.14

THERAPY OF PEDIATRIC GERM CELL TUMORS BASED ON RISK GROUP

Group	Type of Tumor	Treatment	Comments
Low risk	Stage I testicular Stage I ovarian Immature teratomas	Surgical resection and close observation	Surgical observation alone for stage I ovarian tumors is being prospectively tested.
Intermediate risk	Stage II–IV gonadal Stage II extragonadal	Standard-dose PEB	The new trial from the COG is exploring the feasibility of decreasing the number of days and cycles of chemotherapy in these patients.
High risk	Stage III–IV extragonadal	High-dose PEB or standard-dose PEB with an alkylator	The use of high-dose P is associated with significant ototoxicity and the current COG trial is exploring the use of standard-dose PEB with high doses of cyclophosphamide.

COG, Children's Oncology Group; P, cisplatin 20mg/m^2/day × 5 days; High dose P 40 mg/m^2/d for 5 days; E, etoposide 100 mg/m^2/d for 5 days; B, bleomycin 15 U/M^2 day 1.

advanced-stage disease, specifically those with extragonadal tumors.[345]

Sacrococcygeal Tumors

Sacrococcygeal teratoma is the most common germ cell tumor of childhood, accounting for 40% of all cases. Its reported incidence is 1 in 35,000 live births, and 75% of affected patients are female.[334,346] Children with presacral or sacrococcygeal teratomas frequently have congenital anomalies of the vertebrae, genitourinary system, or anorectum. Approximately 80% of these tumors are diagnosed within the first month of life, but the diagnosis can also be made by prenatal ultrasonography.

Four types of sacrococcygeal teratomas have been defined on the basis of the extent of pelvic and abdominal extension and the presence or absence of external extension (Fig. 123.10).[334] The frequency of malignancy is closely associated with the type of teratoma, ranging from 8% in patients with type I to 38% for those with type IV lesions.[334] The most

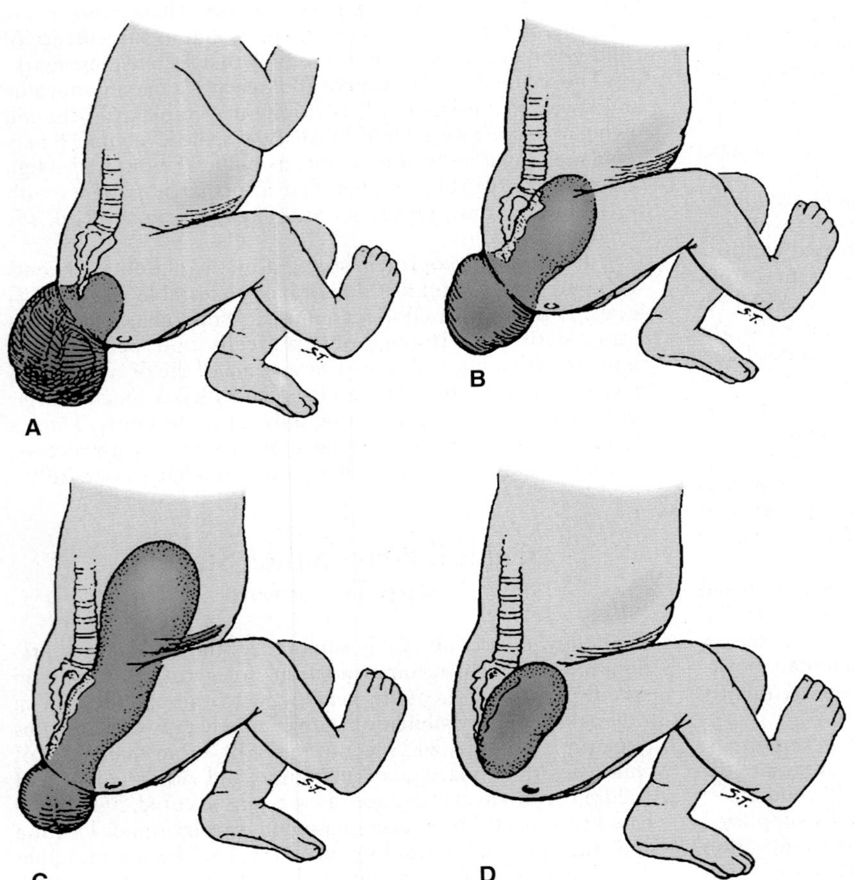

FIGURE 123.10 Types of sacrococcygeal teratoma. **A:** Type I, predominantly external; **B:** type II, external and intrapelvic; **C:** type III, predominantly pelvic; **D:** type IV, presacral. (From ref. 334, with permission from Elsevier.)

common malignant elements in sacrococcygeal teratomas are yolk sac and embryonal carcinomas. Staging should include a complete blood count, serum chemistries, and serum levels of AFP and β-HCG, radionuclide bone scan, and CT of the chest, abdomen, and pelvis.

Surgery is the mainstay of therapy for sacrococcygeal tumors and should include a sacral incision to remove the coccyx. In approximately 10% of infants, a combined perineal and abdominal approach is required. If the tumor is identified in an older child or there is suspicion of malignancy, a preliminary biopsy should be performed, followed by preoperative chemotherapy if malignancy is confirmed.[346] Children with benign sacrococcygeal tumors have an excellent outcome with surgery alone, but close follow-up is mandatory because recurrent disease has been documented in 11% of patients, with mature teratomas most commonly recurring as endodermal sinus tumors.[347] Patients with malignant yolk sac tumors located in the abdomen and pelvis are highly responsive to chemotherapy and have an excellent survival (approximately 90%) when treated with platinum-containing regimens.[348]

Mediastinal Tumors

These tumors are more common in adolescent males. Although the majority are benign teratomas, malignant yolk sac tumor and choriocarcinoma have also been identified. The clinical presentation is characterized by a brief history of cough, dyspnea, and chest pain due to tracheobronchial compression. Routine chest radiographs may demonstrate an incidental anterior mediastinal mass. The diagnosis is established by biopsy of the primary tumor or an involved supraclavicular lymph node. Staging studies should include serum chemistries, complete blood count, tumor marker studies, CT of chest, abdomen, and pelvis, MRI of the brain if clinically symptomatic, and bone scan if metastases are evident at diagnosis in other sites such as the lung.

The use of cisplatin-containing regimens has dramatically improved the outcome of children with malignant mediastinal germ cell tumors; however, patients who are 12 years or older continue to fare poorly, with 5-year survival rates of 50%.[349] The administration of high-dose cisplatin-containing regimens (200 mg/m^2 per cycle) appears to benefit some patients but is associated with a very high incidence of significant hearing loss, which is not improved by the administration of amifostine[349,350] (Table 123.14).

Testicular Tumors

Testicular tumors make up approximately 10% of all pediatric germ cell tumors, and in contrast to adult testicular tumors, 90% of pediatric tumors are localized. Yolk sac tumor is the most common type in prepubertal boys, with a median age at diagnosis of 24 months.[334] Children with primary testicular tumors present with painless testicular enlargement. In the relatively infrequent cases of metastatic disease, patients present with abdominal swelling due to malignant ascites, inguinal lymphadenopathy, or acute abdominal pain. About 20% can be associated with hydroceles or inguinal hernias.

The preoperative evaluation of a child suspected to have a malignant testicular tumor should include a complete blood count, chest radiograph, serum chemistries, including AFP and β-HCG levels. Additional studies, including CT of the abdomen, pelvis, and chest, are not necessary before orchiectomy, although they are ultimately required for complete staging for tumors with malignant elements that can spread to retroperitoneal lymph nodes, liver, and lungs.

All scrotal masses should be explored through an inguinal incision. A transscrotal biopsy contaminates the scrotum and its lymphatic drainage and prevents high ligation of the spermatic cord. If the tumor is clearly malignant, high ligation of the spermatic cord should be performed at the internal ring.[334]

Infants have a predominance of early-stage lesions that are primarily endodermal sinus tumors (yolk sac tumors), in contrast to teenage boys in whom embryonal carcinomas or mixed germ cell tumors predominate. Patients with stage I disease (completely resected tumors) can be treated with radical orchiectomy alone, reserving chemotherapy for relapse. Close monitoring is essential and should include frequent examinations, measurements of AFP, and periodic imaging of the chest and abdomen. The North American Intergroup trial reported a 6-year event-free and overall survival of 78% and 100%, respectively, in 63 patients with testicular germ cell tumors treated with surgery alone.[351] Similar results have also been reported by the United Kingdom CCGStudy.[348] Children with stage II through IV disease (Table 123.15) can be treated with standard doses of cisplatin, etoposide, and bleomycin, with reported 6-year EFS rates of 100% for stage II and III disease and 90% for stage IV disease.[345] Patients older than 15 years fare worse, with an overall 6-year EFS of 84%.

For patients with stage I pure seminoma, adjuvant radiotherapy to the para-aortic or para-aortic and ipsilateral external iliac (dogleg) field to a dose of approximately 25 Gy after inguinal orchiectomy has resulted in greater than 95% cure rates. Other options have included close observation associated with a 5-year PFS of about 82%[352] and single-dose carboplatin, which on short-term follow-up has shown equivalent relapse-free survival rates compared to adjuvant radiotherapy.[353]

Ovarian Tumors

Ovarian tumors account for approximately 25% of all pediatric germ cell tumors.[334] In contrast to adult tumors, malignancies of epithelial or stromal cell origin are uncommon in children. The majority of pediatric ovarian germ cell tumors arise in older patients, with the incidence peaking at 10 years of age. Most tumors are benign mature cystic teratomas, although nearly one-third contain malignant elements. The most common malignant pediatric ovarian neoplasias are dysgerminomas and yolk sac tumors.[334]

Patients with ovarian tumors present with abdominal pain or an abdominal mass. The pain may be severe due to torsion of the ovarian pedicle by the ovary and tumor. Fever is present in 24% of patients at the time of diagnosis. Laboratory studies should include a complete blood count, serum chemistries, including AFP and β-HCG. Preoperative radiographic evaluation should include abdominal ultrasonography and CT of the abdomen and pelvis. Once the tissue diagnosis is established, CT of chest will determine if the tumor has spread to the lungs. Ovarian tumors are staged using the POG/CCG staging system, which represents a simplified version of the International Federation of Gynecology and Obstetrics staging system (Table 123.15).

Surgical exploration of an ovarian mass must allow complete resection of the mass and provide sufficient information to adequately stage the patient. Peritoneal fluid should be aspirated for cytology when present, and if absent, peritoneal washings should be obtained. Any peritoneal seeding should be biopsied and a partial or complete omentectomy performed. Ipsilateral lymph nodes should be examined and, if enlarged, biopsies should be obtained from the iliac, periaortic, and pericaval nodes. The contralateral ovary should be examined closely, and if nodules are present, particularly in dysgerminomas or teratomas, a biopsy should be obtained. With current techniques available for *in vitro* fertilization, efforts are made to preserve the fallopian tube and uterus in cases where both ovaries must be resected. As previously mentioned, mature and immature teratomas can be treated with surgery alone. The presence of implants from immature teratomas in the peritoneal surfaces (gliomatosis peritonei) does not adversely affect clinical outcome.

TABLE 123.15

STAGING OF GERM CELL TUMORS BY ANATOMIC SITE

Stage	Extent of Disease
Testicular Germ Cell Tumors	
I	Limited to testis (testes), completely resected by high inguinal orchiectomy; no clinical, radiographic, or histologic evidence of disease beyond the testes. Patients with normal or unknown tumor markers at diagnosis must have a negative ipsilateral retroperitoneal node sampling to confirm stage I disease if radiographic studies demonstrate lymph nodes >2 cm.
II	Transscrotal biopsy; microscopic disease in scrotum or high in spermatic cord (≤5 cm from proximal end). Failure of tumor markers to normalize or decrease with an appropriate half-life.
III	Retroperitoneal lymph node involvement, but no visceral or extra-abdominal involvement. Lymph nodes >4 cm by CT or >2 cm and <4 cm with biopsy proof.
IV	Distant metastases, including liver.
Ovarian Germ Cell Tumors	
I	Limited to ovary (peritoneal evaluation should be negative). No clinical, radiographic, or histologic evidence of disease beyond the ovaries. (Note: The presence of gliomatosis peritonei does not result in changing stage I disease to a higher stage.)
II	Microscopic residual; peritoneal evaluation negative. (Note: The presence of gliomatosis peritonei does not result in changing stage II disease to a higher stage.) Failure of tumor markers to normalize or decrease with an appropriate half-life.
III	Lymph node involvement (metastatic nodule); gross residual or biopsy only; contiguous visceral involvement (omentum, intestine, bladder); peritoneal evaluation positive for malignancy.
IV	Distant metastases, including liver.
Extragonadal Germ Cell Tumors	
I	Complete resection at any site, coccygectomy for sacrococcygeal site, negative tumor margins.
II	Microscopic residual; lymph nodes negative.
III	Lymph node involvement with metastatic disease. Gross residual or biopsy only; retroperitoneal nodes negative or positive.
IV	Distant metastases, including liver.

CT, computed tomography.

French and German investigators have treated patients with malignant ovarian germ cell tumors with surgical resection alone followed by close observation, and this approach has translated into an EFS of 67% and an overall survival of over 95%.[348] The COG has adopted these recommendations for their front-line therapeutic trial for patients with stage I ovarian tumors. Current pediatric regimens for the treatment of stages II through IV ovarian germ cell tumors use a combination of standard-dose cisplatin, etoposide, and bleomycin with 6-year event-free and overall survival rates in excess of 86% and 93%, respectively[337,345] (Table 123.14).

Selected References

The full list of references for this chapter appears in the online version.

1. Ries LAG, Smith MA, Gurney JG, et al. eds. *Cancer incidence and survival among children and adolescents: United States SEER Program 1975–1995*, National Cancer Institute, SEER Program. NIH Pub. No. 99-4649. Bethesda, MD: National Cancer Institute, 1999.
2. Jemal A, Siegel R, Ward E, et al. Cancer statistics, 2009. *CA Cancer J Clin* 2009;59(4):225–249.
3. Bleyer A, O'Leary M, Barr R, Ries LAG (eds). *Cancer epidemiology in older adolescents and young adults 15 to 29 years of age, including SEER incidence and survival: 1975-2000*. National Cancer Institute, NIH Pub. No. 06-5767. Bethesda, MD 2006.
5. Pappo AS, Shapiro DN, Crist WM, et al. Biology and therapy of pediatric rhabdomyosarcoma. *J Clin Oncol* 1995;13(8):2123.
9. Mosse YP, Laudenslager M, Longo L, et al. Identification of ALK as a major familial neuroblastoma predisposition gene. *Nature* 2008; 455(7215):930.
12. Peuchmaur M, d'Amore ES, Joshi VV, et al. Revision of the International Neuroblastoma Pathology Classification: confirmation of favorable and unfavorable prognostic subsets in ganglioneuroblastoma, nodular. *Cancer* 2003;98(10):2274.
20. London WB, Castleberry RP, Matthay KK, et al. Evidence for an age cutoff greater than 365 days for neuroblastoma risk group stratification in the Children's Oncology Group. *J Clin Oncol* 2005;23(27):6459.
23. Hayward K, Jeremy RJ, Jenkins S, et al. Long-term neurobehavioral outcomes in children with neuroblastoma and opsoclonus-myoclonus-ataxia syndrome: relationship to MRI findings and anti-neuronal antibodies. *J Pediatr* 2001;139(4):552.
25. De Bernardi B, Balwierz W, Bejent J, et al. Epidural compression in neuroblastoma: diagnostic and therapeutic aspects. *Cancer Lett* 2005;228 (1–2):283.
32. Nickerson HJ, Matthay KK, Seeger RC, et al. Favorable biology and outcome of stage IV-S neuroblastoma with supportive care or minimal therapy: a Children's Cancer Group study. *J Clin Oncol* 2000;18(3):477.
34. Matthay KK, Villablanca JG, Seeger RC, et al. Treatment of high-risk neuroblastoma with intensive chemotherapy, radiotherapy, autologous bone marrow transplantation, and 13-cis-retinoic acid. Children's Cancer Group. *N Engl J Med* 1999;341(16):1165.
43. Yu AL, Gilman AL, Ozkaynak MF. A phase III randomized trial of the chimeric anti-GD2 antibody ch14.18 with GM-CSF and IL2 as immunotherapy following dose intensive chemotherapy for high-risk neuroblastoma: Children's Oncology Group (COG) study ANBL0032. *J Clin Oncol* 2009;27: (abstr 10067z).
45. Pule MA, Savoldo B, Myers GD, et al. Virus-specific T cells engineered to coexpress tumor-specific receptors: persistence and antitumor activity in individuals with neuroblastoma. *Nat Med* 2008;14(11):1264.
47. Grundy P, Coppes MJ, Haber D. Molecular genetics of Wilms tumor. *Hematol Oncol Clin North Am* 1995;9(6):1201.

50. Porteus MH, Narkool P, Neuberg D, et al. Characteristics and outcome of children with Beckwith-Wiedemann syndrome and Wilms' tumor: a report from the National Wilms Tumor Study Group. *J Clin Oncol* 2000;18(10): 2026.
52. Dome JS, Cotton CA, Perlman EJ, et al. Treatment of anaplastic histology Wilms' tumor: results from the fifth National Wilms' Tumor Study. *J Clin Oncol* 2006;24(15):2352.
55. Biegel JA, Tan L, Zhang F, et al. Alterations of the hSNF5/INI1 gene in central nervous system atypical teratoid/rhabdoid tumors and renal and extrarenal rhabdoid tumors. *Clin Cancer Res* 2002;8(11):3461.
60. Grundy PE, Breslow NE, Li S, et al. Loss of heterozygosity for chromosomes 1p and 16q is an adverse prognostic factor in favorable-histology Wilms tumor: a report from the National Wilms Tumor Study Group. *J Clin Oncol* 2005;23(29):7312.
62. Ehrlich PF, Hamilton TE, Grundy P, et al. The value of surgery in directing therapy for patients with Wilms' tumor with pulmonary disease. A report from the National Wilms' Tumor Study Group (National Wilms' Tumor Study 5). *J Pediatr Surg* 2006;41(1):162.
63. Metzger ML, Dome JS. Current therapy for Wilms' tumor. *Oncologist* 2005;10(10):815.
68. Thomas PR, Tefft M, Compaan PJ, et al. Results of two radiation therapy randomizations in the third National Wilms' Tumor Study. *Cancer* 1991;68 (8):1703.
76. Freeman CR, Esseltine DL, Whitehead VM, et al. Retinoblastoma: the case for radiotherapy and for adjuvant chemotherapy. *Cancer* 1980;46(9): 1913.
77. Pratt CB, Meyer D, Chenaille P, et al. The use of bone marrow aspirations and lumbar punctures at the time of diagnosis of retinoblastoma. *J Clin Oncol* 1989;7(1):140.
82. Reese AB, Ellsworth RM. Management of retinoblastoma. *Ann N Y Acad Sci* 1964;114(2):958.
83. Linn MA. Intraocular retinoblastoma: the case for a new group classification. *Ophthalmol Clin North Am* 2005;18(1):41.
84. Chantada G, Doz F, Antoneli CB, et al. A proposal for an international retinoblastoma staging system. *Pediatr Blood Cancer* 2006;47(6):801.
85. Shields CL, Honavar SG, Meadows AT, et al. Chemoreduction for unilateral retinoblastoma. *Arch Ophthalmol* 2002;120(12):1653.
90. Shields CL, Honavar SG, Meadows AT, et al. Chemoreduction plus focal therapy for retinoblastoma: factors predictive of need for treatment with external beam radiotherapy or enucleation. *Am J Ophthalmol* 2002;133 (5):657.
96. Kleinerman RA, Tucker MA, Tarone RE, et al. Risk of new cancers after radiotherapy in long-term survivors of retinoblastoma: an extended follow-up. *J Clin Oncol* 2005;23(10):2272.
98. Abramson DH, Ronner HJ, Ellsworth RM. Second tumors in nonirradiated bilateral retinoblastoma. *Am J Ophthalmol* 1979;87(5):624.
103. Yamane T, Kaneko A, Mohri M. The technique of ophthalmic arterial infusion therapy for patients with intraocular retinoblastoma. *Int J Clin Oncol* 2004;9(2):69.
104. Abramson DH, Dunkel IJ, Brodie SE, et al. A phase I/II study of direct intraarterial (ophthalmic artery) chemotherapy with melphalan for intraocular retinoblastoma initial results. *Ophthalmology* 2008;115(8): 1398.
107. Bielack SS, Carrle D, Hardes J, et al. Bone tumors in adolescents and young adults. *Curr Treat Options Oncol* 2008;9(1):67.
108. Mirabello L, Troisi RJ, Savage SA. Osteosarcoma incidence and survival rates from 1973 to 2004: data from the Surveillance, Epidemiology, and End Results Program. *Cancer* 2009;115(7):1531.
111. Mirabello L, Troisi RJ, Savage SA. International osteosarcoma incidence patterns in children and adolescents, middle ages and elderly persons. *Int J Cancer* 2009;125(1):229.
112. Neglia JP, Friedman DL, Yasui Y, et al. Second malignant neoplasms in five-year survivors of childhood cancer: childhood cancer survivor study. *J Natl Cancer Inst* 2001;93(8):618.
115. Malkin D, Li FP, Strong LC, et al. Germ line p53 mutations in a familial syndrome of breast cancer, sarcomas, and other neoplasms. *Science* 1990;250(4985):1233.
130. Bacci G, Ferrari S, Longhi A, et al. Nonmetastatic osteosarcoma of the extremity with pathologic fracture at presentation: local and systemic control by amputation or limb salvage after preoperative chemotherapy. *Acta Orthop Scand* 2003;74(4):449.
132. Link MP, Goorin AM, Horowitz M, et al. Adjuvant chemotherapy of high-grade osteosarcoma of the extremity. Updated results of the Multi-Institutional Osteosarcoma Study. *Clin Orthop Relat Res* 1991;(270):8.
134. Meyer JS, Nadel HR, Marina N, et al. Imaging guidelines for children with Ewing sarcoma and osteosarcoma: a report from the Children's Oncology Group Bone Tumor Committee. *Pediatr Blood Cancer* 2008;51(2):163.
135. Bielack S, Carrle D, Casali PG. Osteosarcoma: ESMO clinical recommendations for diagnosis, treatment and follow-up. *Ann Oncol* 2009; 20(Suppl 4):137.
137. Gorlick R, Khanna C. Osteosarcoma. *J Bone Miner Res* 201025(4):683.
140. Bernstein M, Kovar H, Paulussen M, et al. Ewing's sarcoma family of tumors: current management. *Oncologist* 2006;11(5):503.
147. Link MP, Goorin AM, Miser AW, et al. The effect of adjuvant chemotherapy on relapse-free survival in patients with osteosarcoma of the extremity. *N Engl J Med* 1986;314(25):1600.
152. Goorin AM, Schwartzentruber DJ, Devidas M, et al. Presurgical chemotherapy compared with immediate surgery and adjuvant chemotherapy for nonmetastatic osteosarcoma: Pediatric Oncology Group Study POG-8651. *J Clin Oncol* 2003;21(8):1574.
155. Meyers PA, Schwartz CL, Krailo M, et al. Osteosarcoma: a randomized, prospective trial of the addition of ifosfamide and/or muramyl tripeptide to cisplatin, doxorubicin, and high-dose methotrexate. *J Clin Oncol* 2005; 23(9):2004.
156. Meyers PA, Schwartz CL, Krailo MD, et al. Osteosarcoma: the addition of muramyl tripeptide to chemotherapy improves overall survival—a report from the Children's Oncology Group. *J Clin Oncol* 2008;26(4):633.
160. Harting MT, Blakely ML, Jaffe N, et al. Long-term survival after aggressive resection of pulmonary metastases among children and adolescents with osteosarcoma. *J Pediatr Surg* 2006;41(1):194.
165. Mahajan A, Woo SY, Kornguth DG, et al. Multimodality treatment of osteosarcoma: radiation in a high-risk cohort. *Pediatr Blood Cancer* 2008; 50(5):976.
166. Rodriguez-Galindo C, Navid F, Khoury J. Ewing sarcoma family of tumors. In: Pappo A, ed. *Pediatric bone and soft tissue sarcomas*. New York: Springer, 2006:181.
169. Potikyan G, France KA, Carlson MR, et al. Genetically defined EWS/FLI1 model system suggests mesenchymal origin of Ewing's family tumors. *Lab Invest* 2008;88(12):1291.
171. Tirode F, Laud-Duval K, Prieur A, et al. Mesenchymal stem cell features of Ewing tumors. *Cancer Cell* 2007;11(5):421.
180. Erkizan HV, Kong Y, Merchant M, et al. A small molecule blocking oncogenic protein EWS-FLI1 interaction with RNA helicase A inhibits growth of Ewing's sarcoma. *Nat Med* 2009;15(7):750.
181. Geryk-Hall M, Hughes DP. Critical signaling pathways in bone sarcoma: candidates for therapeutic interventions. *Curr Oncol Rep* 2009;11(6): 446.
182. Kolb EA, Gorlick R. Development of IGF-IR Inhibitors in pediatric sarcomas. *Curr Oncol Rep* 2009;11(4):307.
185. Olmos D, Postel-Vinay S, Molife LR, et al. Safety, pharmacokinetics, and preliminary activity of the anti-IGF-1R antibody figitumumab (CP-751,871) in patients with sarcoma and Ewing's sarcoma: a phase 1 expansion cohort study. *Lancet Oncol* 2010;11(2):129.
188. Rodriguez-Galindo C, Spunt SL, Pappo AS. Treatment of Ewing sarcoma family of tumors: current status and outlook for the future. *Med Pediatr Oncol* 2003;40(5):276.
192. Hawkins DS, Schuetze SM, Butrynski JE, et al. [18F]Fluorodeoxyglucose positron emission tomography predicts outcome for Ewing sarcoma family of tumors. *J Clin Oncol* 2005;23(34):8828.
200. Grier HE, Krailo MD, Tarbell NJ, et al. Addition of ifosfamide and etoposide to standard chemotherapy for Ewing's sarcoma and primitive neuroectodermal tumor of bone. *N Engl J Med* 2003;348(8):694.
204. Kolb EA, Kushner BH, Gorlick R, et al. Long-term event-free survival after intensive chemotherapy for Ewing's family of tumors in children and young adults. *J Clin Oncol* 2003;21(18):3423.
222. Miser JS, Krailo MD, Tarbell NJ, et al. Treatment of metastatic Ewing's sarcoma or primitive neuroectodermal tumor of bone: evaluation of combination ifosfamide and etoposide—a Children's Cancer Group and Pediatric Oncology Group study. *J Clin Oncol* 2004;22(14):2873.
227. Paulussen M, Ahrens S, Craft AW, et al. Ewing's tumors with primary lung metastases: survival analysis of 114 (European Intergroup) Cooperative Ewing's Sarcoma Studies patients. *J Clin Oncol* 1998;16(9):3044.
231. Dunst J, Schuck A. Role of radiotherapy in Ewing tumors. *Pediatr Blood Cancer* 2004;42(5):465.
246. Rodriguez-Galindo C, Navid F, Liu T, et al. Prognostic factors for local and distant control in Ewing sarcoma family of tumors. *Ann Oncol* 2008;19(4):814.
251. Ognjanovic S, Linabery AM, Charbonneau B, et al. Trends in childhood rhabdomyosarcoma incidence and survival in the United States, 1975–2005. *Cancer* 2009;115(18):4218.
252. Sultan I, Qaddoumi I, Yaser S, et al. Comparing adult and pediatric rhabdomyosarcoma in the surveillance, epidemiology and end results program, 1973 to 2005: an analysis of 2,600 patients. *J Clin Oncol* 2009;27(20): 3391.
253. Pappo AS, Shapiro DN, Crist WM. Rhabdomyosarcoma. Biology and treatment. *Pediatr Clin North Am* 1997;44(4):953.
254. Pappo A, Wolden S. Pediatric rhabdomyosarcoma: biology and results of the North American Intergroup Rhabdomyosarcoma trials. In: Pappo AS, ed. *Pediatric bone and soft tissue sarcomas*. Berlin: Springer-Verlag, 2006:103.
257. Qualman SJ, Coffin CM, Newton WA, et al. Intergroup Rhabdomyosarcoma Study: update for pathologists. *Pediatr Dev Pathol* 1998;1(6):550.
260. Fredericks WJ, Galili N, Mukhopadhyay S, et al. The PAX3-FKHR fusion protein created by the t(2;13) translocation in alveolar rhabdomyosarcomas is a more potent transcriptional activator than PAX3. *Mol Cell Biol* 1995;15(3):1522.

262. Barr FG, Chatten J, D'Cruz CM, et al. Molecular assays for chromosomal translocations in the diagnosis of pediatric soft tissue sarcomas. *JAMA* 1995;273(7):553.
271. Maurer HM, Beltangady M, Gehan EA, et al. The Intergroup Rhabdomyosarcoma Study-I. A final report. *Cancer* 1988;61(2):209.
272. Meza JL, Anderson J, Pappo AS, et al. Analysis of prognostic factors in patients with nonmetastatic rhabdomyosarcoma treated on intergroup rhabdomyosarcoma studies III and IV: the Children's Oncology Group. *J Clin Oncol* 2006;24(24):3844.
274. Oberlin O, Rey A, Lyden E, et al. Prognostic factors in metastatic rhabdomyosarcomas: results of a pooled analysis from United States and European cooperative groups. *J Clin Oncol* 2008;26(14):2384.
289. Lager JJ, Lyden ER, Anderson JR, et al. Pooled analysis of phase II window studies in children with contemporary high-risk metastatic rhabdomyosarcoma: a report from the Soft Tissue Sarcoma Committee of the Children's Oncology Group. *J Clin Oncol* 2006;24(21):3415.
294. Darbari A, Sabin KM, Shapiro CN, et al. Epidemiology of primary hepatic malignancies in U.S. children. *Hepatology* 2003;38(3):560.
297. Giardiello FM, Offerhaus GJ, Krush AJ, et al. Risk of hepatoblastoma in familial adenomatous polyposis. *J Pediatr* 1991;119(5):766.
305. Perilongo G, Shafford EA. Liver tumours. *Eur J Cancer* 1999;35(6):953.
314. Ortega JA, Douglass EC, Feusner JH, et al. Randomized comparison of cisplatin/vincristine/fluorouracil and cisplatin/continuous infusion doxorubicin for treatment of pediatric hepatoblastoma: a report from the Children's Cancer Group and the Pediatric Oncology Group. *J Clin Oncol* 2000;18(14):2665.
317. Meyers RL, Rowland JR, Krailo M, et al. Predictive power of pretreatment prognostic factors in children with hepatoblastoma: a report from the Children's Oncology Group. *Pediatr Blood Cancer* 2009;53(6):1016.

CHAPTER 124 LEUKEMIAS AND LYMPHOMAS OF CHILDHOOD

JUDITH F. MARGOLIN, KAREN R. RABIN, AND DAVID G. POPLACK

The cure rates seen in pediatric oncology are some of the best in modern oncology. These are largely related to the remarkable progress in the treatment of leukemias and lymphomas, which represent approximately 50% of all childhood cancer. The cure rates for these diseases have gone from less than 10% in the early 1960s to a range of 60% to 90% (depending on various prognostic factors related to both biologic parameters and clinical presentation features).[1–4] The overall cure rate for pediatric lymphoid cancer is currently 85% to 95%. Cure rates for pediatric myeloid leukemia have lagged behind the lymphoid neoplasms. Pediatric patients with acute myelogenous leukemia (AML) have slightly better results than adults with AML, and are currently reported to have disease-free survival (DFS) rates in the 40% to 66% range using a variety of intensive conventional chemotherapy, radiotherapy, and bone marrow transplant.[5–9] The improvement in outcomes for all of pediatric cancer are the result of the successful implementation of a large number of clinical trials, initially conducted in large single institutions and later through national, and now international, cooperative group mechanisms.[10] Participation in a clinical trial has become the standard of care for pediatric malignancies. Currently, more than two-thirds of children with cancer in the United States are treated on clinical trials. Children consistently demonstrate better outcomes than adults with hematopoietic and lymphatic cancers.[10]

Although there are many similarities in treating children and adults with these diseases, there are also differences that pertain to development and growth, differences in drug metabolism, as well as psychosocial issues that are unique to pediatric oncology. The results are clear: children and adolescents who are treated in pediatric centers on clinical trials have better outcomes than those who are not. Young adults (up to age 30 years) are now eligible for enrollment on some pediatric clinical trials, and work continues to define the biologic differences between the various forms of these diseases in different age groups.[11–13]

LEUKEMIAS

Epidemiology, Histology, and General Outcomes

Acute lymphoblastic leukemia (ALL), the most common malignancy of childhood, accounts for 75% of the leukemia cases, and is curable in 80% to 95% of the patients.[1] Figure 124.1 demonstrates the improvement in survival in pediatric ALL on successive Children's Cancer Group trials between the years 1968 and 2002. Although there are variations with age, sex, and ethnicity, the majority of ALL cases have pre-B immunophenotype and Fab1 histology (80% of cases); 20% are of T-cell origin. The peak incidence of pediatric ALL is between ages 2 and 5 years. ALL is slightly more common in American whites than in blacks, and there is a slightly increased incidence in male patients.[14] Approximately 5,000 children are diagnosed with ALL each year in the United States, with an incidence of 3 to 4 cases per 100,000 white children or 29.2 per million including all U.S. children.[14] Surveillance, Epidemiology, and End Results (SEER) program data from the National Cancer Institute (NCI) show that the incidence of ALL has been climbing slowly. Controversy exists concerning whether outcomes of children with ALL differ between children of different racial groups. When studies using data from the 1990s are carefully matched for known prognostic features, there does appear to be significant outcome differences related to race/ethnicity.[15,16] In general, white children have slightly higher event-free survival (EFS) and DFS than black and Hispanic children. The racial differences in outcomes usually vary by 5% to 10%, but they do meet statistical significance. An issue that often confounds these types of analyses is the fact that black and Hispanic children tend to develop higher-risk forms of ALL at higher rates than white children.[3,15] As ALL treatment protocols become more generally effective, the results related to race, as well as other prognostic variables, need to be periodically re-evaluated.

AML accounts for approximately 15% to 20% of childhood leukemia cases, chronic myelogenous leukemia (CML) accounts for 3% to 4%, and juvenile myelomonocytic leukemia (JMML) and other rarer histologies account for less than 1% of cases. The incidence of AML is currently estimated to be five to seven cases per million in the United States.[17] The ratio of 1:4 AML to ALL cases in children is the opposite of the AML to ALL ratio in older adults (age 50 years and older).[7] With the exception of small peaks in the neonatal and adolescent periods, the incidence of AML rises steadily with age until age 55. After age 55 there is a dramatic increase because of increased incidence secondary to AML (which develops after exposure to chemotherapy or radiotherapy delivered at an earlier time for a different cancer) and myelodysplastic syndrome (MDS).[18] MDS is a relatively rare diagnosis in childhood, generally progresses to AML, and is treated with similar regimens (including bone marrow transplant) as AML.[18,19]

Approximately 1,000 of the 6,500 children per year in the United States who develop leukemia will have one of the eight FAB types of AML outlined in Chapter 131, along with some of the associated cytogenetic, classic staining characteristics, and molecular changes. There are no significant differences between AML incidence in males and females, but there is evidence of variation in incidence by racial and ethnic groups. Black and Hispanic children both have a slightly higher incidence of AML than white children in the United States.[20] There are also racial disparities in pediatric AML outcomes, with blacks and Hispanics demonstrating significantly lower overall survival compared with white patients (35% vs. 48 % in two recent U.S. studies that included 1,600 patients).[21] Because of

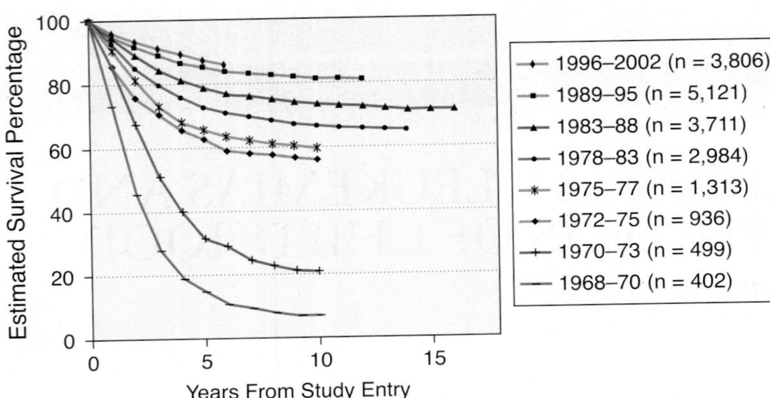

FIGURE 124.1 Improvement in survival of children with acute lymphoblastic leukemia. Curves represent the survival outcomes for patients treated on successive Children's Cancer Group (CCG) clinical trials conducted over the 1968–2002 period. (From H. Sather, personal communication, used with permission.)

intrinsic differences in drug sensitivity between ALL and AML cells, progress in treating AML has been less dramatic than that of ALL. Nevertheless, current cure rates in AML have risen to approximately 45% to 65% with the advent of more intensive conventional chemotherapy and bone marrow transplant (BMT) (Fig. 124.2).[7,22]

Although there is an extensive literature and continued interest in exploring possible relationships between infectious or environmental exposures and increased risk of childhood leukemia, most studies show weak or no correlation of these factors with the incidence of leukemia.[23–25] Electromagnetic fields, usually associated with power lines, are no longer believed by most to be associated with any significant increase in the incidence of pediatric malignancies, although research in this area continues.[26–28] There is an emerging body of evidence from population-based studies of polymorphisms of drug-metabolizing genes, such as *NQO1* and *GST* polymorphisms, that may be associated with an increase or decrease in an individual's risk for developing leukemia based on exposures to particular environmental toxins like benzene and other organic solvents, quinine-containing substances, and flavinoids.[29] Currently, the reason(s) that most patients develop leukemia is unknown.

Genetics

There is significant evidence that genetic factors play a role in the formation of many cases of pediatric leukemia. Within the leukemic blasts themselves, there are characteristic cytogenetic changes (Table 124.5), many of which have prognostic significance (see later discussion). Furthermore, some of the newer therapies are targeted specifically at the proteins that are encoded by the oncogenic fusion transcripts that result from the known chromosomal translocations, or by the biochemical pathways that have been shown to be directly affected by the cytogenetic changes.[1] Many of the genetic changes found in childhood leukemia (especially in younger patients) can be shown to actually be present in a subpopulation of these patient's hemopoietic cells at birth.[30,31] The evidence for this

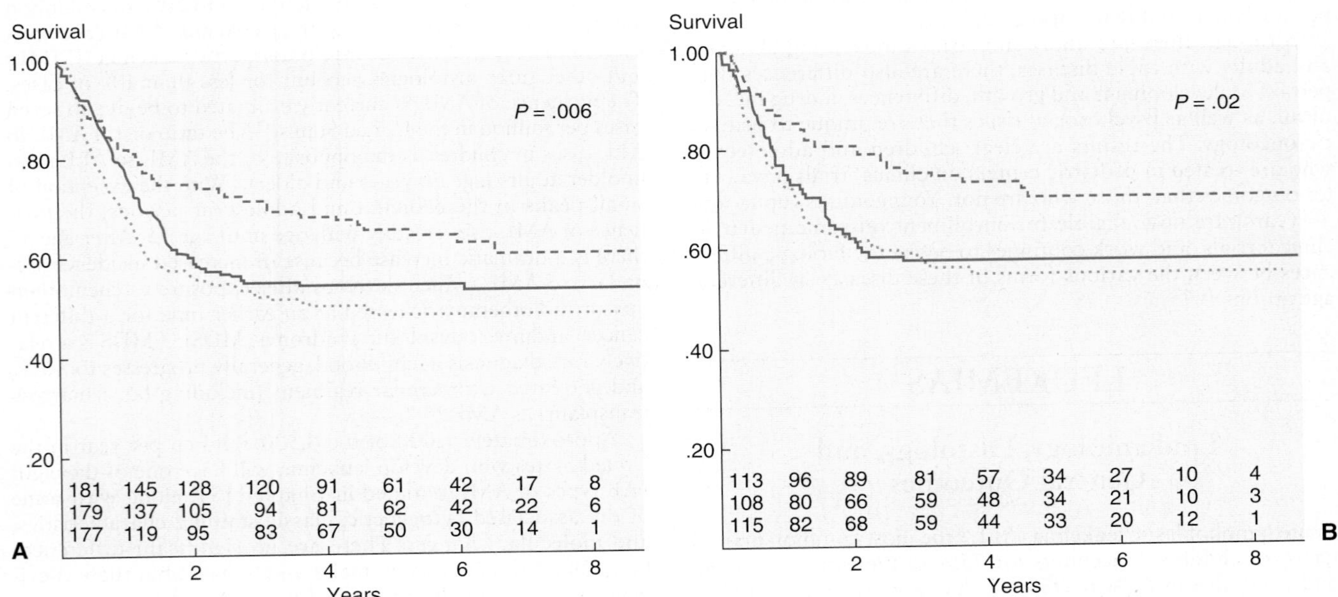

FIGURE 124.2 **A:** Actuarial survival from acute myelogenous leukemia (AML) remission, comparing the three post-remission regimens from Children's Cancer Group (CCG)-2891. Numbers are patients at risk at yearly intervals; rows are the same order as curves. *P* value is for homogeneity. *Dashed line,* allogeneic bone marrow transplant (BMT); *solid line,* intensive nonmarrow ablative chemotherapy; *dotted line,* autologous BMT. **B:** Actuarial survival from AML remission for the CCG-2891 patients who received intensive-timing induction therapy, comparing the three postremission regimens. (From ref. 103, with permission.)

TABLE 124.1

PERCENTAGE DISTRIBUTION OF IMMUNOPHENOTYPES OF ACUTE LYMPHOBLASTIC LEUKEMIA BY AGE GROUP[a]

Immunophenotype	Infants (<1.5 y)	Children (1.5–10.0 y)	Adolescents (>10 y)
Early pre-B	64	68	58
CD10 (CALLA)	49	94	87
Pre-B (cIgM)	26	18	18
T	6	13	23
B	4	1	1

cIgM, cytoplasmic immunoglobulin M.
[a]Numbers shown are weighted means from eight different studies.
Modified from Rivera G, Crist W. Blood: principles and practice of hematology. In: Handin R, Stossel T, Lux S, eds. *Acute Lymphoblastic Leukemia*. Philadelphia: JB Lippincott, 1995:747.

primarily arises from polymerase chain reaction (PCR) studies on the blood spots (formerly known as *Guthrie cards*) that are obtained at birth for disease screening.[32] Other lines of evidence that some preleukemic events happen *in utero* or very early in life include epidemiologic associations with various environmental exposures as well as evidence for leukemia spread by twin-twin transfusion.[33] These findings provide support for the "delayed infection" hypothesis, which holds that children in developed countries are spared the frequent early infections that are necessary for normal development of the immune system. An infection occurring at a later time is then hypothesized to elicit a pathologic, myelosuppressive response, providing a selective growth advantage to the preleukemic clone, which leads to the development of overt leukemia.[34]

In most cases the development of leukemia appears to result from a complex interplay between environmental and genetic factors. Recently, large-scale genome-wide association studies have identified several constitutional genetic variations that cause moderate but statistically significant effects on the relative risk of developing ALL.[35–37] Collectively, variants in *IKZF1, ARID5B, CEBPE,* and *CDKN2A* may account for up to 80% of the attributable risk of developing ALL in European populations.[36]

In addition to somatic and germ line genetic changes associated with leukemia, there are well-described cases of familial leukemia, as well as strong associations between several somatic genetic disorders (most notably Down syndrome [DS]), immunodeficiency, and other genetic disorders (e.g., Bloom, ataxia telangiectasia, Shwachman-Diamond, Sotos, and Noonan syndromes, neurofibromatosis) and an increased incidence of leukemia.[1]

Patients with DS have an increased risk of developing leukemia.[38] The occurrence of leukemia (ALL or AML) in DS patients appears to be unrelated to the other congenital abnormalities and medical problems of DS.[39] For those with somatic trisomy 21, this risk is 15- to 20-fold higher than in normal children. ALL is the predominant form of leukemia in all but the neonatal period in DS patients. Most investigations have reported a lower incidence of common ALL cytogenetic changes in ALL blasts from DS patients.[40–43] Recently several molecular differences between DS ALL and ALL in cytogenetically normal children have been identified including (1) Janus kinase 2 (*JAK2*) activating mutations, which have been found in 20% of DS-ALL, and (2) genetic changes leading to overexpression of cytokine receptor-like factor 2 (*CRLF2*) in up to 50% of DS ALL.[44,45] These aberrations also occur in non-DS ALL, but in a smaller proportion of cases.[46,47] Studies in non-DS ALL suggest an adverse prognosis associated with *JAK2* and *CRLF2* aberrations.[48,49]

In the neonatal period, DS patients have a propensity for developing a nonneoplastic entity known as *transient myeloproliferative disease* (TMD) of DS, which at presentation can appear very similar to AML (very high white blood cell counts with peripheral myeloblasts), but usually resolves spontaneously.[50] TMD may be difficult to distinguish from AML. Although TMD itself is not a form of malignancy or leukemia, approximately 30% of the DS patients with TMD will develop AML later in childhood.[50]

When patients with DS do develop AML (especially those younger than age 2 years), they tend to develop Fab M7, display particular mutations in a hematopoietic transcription factor known as *GATA-1,* and have an excellent prognosis. The DFS for DS patients with *GATA-1+* Fab M7 is more than 90% with regimens that are significantly less intensive than those required for normal children with either Fab M7 or other forms of AML.[51] This represents the highest DFS for any known subgroup of AML patients (adult or pediatric). Despite a large research effort in this area, the reasons behind the increased risk of developing both AML and ALL in children with DS remain unknown. The increased risk for the development of leukemia of any type in DS exists only to age 13.[40] In ALL, in which hyperdiploidy is quite common (see "Prognostic Factors and Treatment of Pediatric Acute Lymphoblastic Leukemia"), extra copies of chromosome 21 are a common finding, but they carry no specific prognostic meaning by themselves.[52]

Clonal Nature of Lymphoid Cancers

Accumulated molecular evidence shows that lymphoid malignancies appear to have derived from an original abnormal progenitor that lost the ability to fully differentiate, continued to divide, and formed a "clone" of leukemic blast cells. ALL blasts are characterized by early lymphoid antigens that can be found in the cytoplasm or on the surface of the cell (detectable by flow cytometry [FACS]), as well as by evidence of incomplete immunoglobulin (Ig) G and T-cell receptor gene rearrangements. This indicates that ALL arises from either precursor T- or precursor B-lymphoid cells.[1] Evidence of preleukemic cells can be seen in the changes found by PCR in neonatal blood samples (discussed previously). The cell of origin for AML is alternatively postulated to be either a multipotent or a committed myeloid progenitor. Except in the case of infant AML with 11q23 abnormalities, most pre-AML clones appear to develop *post utero*. Other subclones probably form under the selective pressure of chemotherapy. The existence of subclinical amounts of the leukemia or lymphoma clones/subclones during or after therapy is called *minimal residual disease* (MRD).[53] The most sensitive assays for MRD use the PCR or reverse transcriptase-PCR (RT-PCR) techniques for detection of IgG, T-cell receptor rearrangements, or chromosomal translocations. Alternatively, multicolor flow cytometry can be used to quantify MRD, as long as the particular patient's leukemia clone displays an antigen pattern that can be distinguished from normal marrow precursors. Each method has its advantages and disadvantages, and measurements of MRD by one of these two methods have been incorporated into most current cooperative group trials in these diseases.[54,55] The results of MRD testing, both qualitatively and quantitatively, must always be interpreted within the context of the specific trials in which it is being evaluated.

Clinical Presentation and Diagnostic Testing

The presenting signs and symptoms of a child with leukemia reflect the impact of bone marrow infiltration, the extent of extramedullary disease spread, and problems related to changes in blood viscosity and chemistry that are related to the size, number, and potential breakdown products of the leukemic blasts (tumor lysis).[3] Leukostasis from high white blood cell (WBC) counts may cause signs and symptoms ranging from mild respiratory symptoms and infiltrates on chest radiographs, to CNS stroke, cranial or peripheral neuropathies, hematuria, renal failure, and various ocular findings.[1] In general, AML blasts are larger, less flexible, and contain granules that can cause local inflammatory and clotting cascade reactions. Thus, high presenting blast counts in AML (i.e., WBC >100,000/mm^3) are more likely to cause serious systemic problems than similar WBC counts in ALL. Specific Fab types of AML (particularly Fab 4 and Fab 5) have a higher tendency to present with localized white cell masses (chloromas), with or without overt bone marrow involvement. Infiltration of the gums (appearing as periodontal disease with mucosal bleeding), orbital, and periorbital soft tissue masses are often seen in patients with AML.[18]

Extramedullary involvement has prognostic implications (see later discussion), but also affects the presenting signs and symptoms. CNS involvement is more common in ALL but is also possible with AML.[56,57] Most CNS involvement is related to meningeal infiltration, but parenchymal and cranial nerve sheath infiltrates are also possible. CNS involvement at initial presentation can be asymptomatic, but it may also manifest as cranial nerve palsies, seizures, or focal neurologic findings. Hepatosplenomegaly is common in both ALL and AML. In small children and infants, this can compromise respiration. Lymphomatous involvement of nodes or extranodal tissue can cause superior mediastinal or superior venacaval syndromes, and bowel wall or lymph node infiltrations can cause intussusceptions or bowel perforations. Although problems with mass effects are more commonly seen in non-Hodgkin's lymphoma (NHL; see later discussion), both ALL and AML can present with large nodal or extranodal masses.

Tables 124.2 and 124.3 summarize the clinical and laboratory findings and differential diagnosis, respectively, for pediatric patients presenting with ALL. All patients newly diagnosed as having leukemia should be regarded as immunocompromised. Fever in such patients should be treated as a medical emergency, and after obtaining appropriate cultures (i.e., blood, urine, and cerebrospinal fluid) and other relevant diagnostic tests, the patient should receive intravenous broad-spectrum antibiotics. In addition to infection, the other major medical emergency that commonly occurs at the time of diagnosis is bleeding. In general, AML patients (particularly those with type Fab M3) have more problems with bleeding at or around the time of diagnosis, but ALL patients can also demonstrate these problems. Regardless of the leukemic histology, patients should be immediately supported with transfusions of packed red blood cells, platelets, and/or plasma, as clinically indicated.

Although peripheral blasts are frequently present, the definitive diagnosis of any form of leukemia requires that the bone marrow has more than 20% to 25% leukemic blasts (blast percentage required for diagnosing leukemia varies somewhat with the pathologic classification system used).[58] Bone marrow aspirate and biopsy morphology using Wright or Romanowsky, acid phosphatase, myeloperoxidase, Sudan black, and the esterase stains are routinely performed. Obtaining cytogenetics is critically important as many cytogenetic findings have prognostic importance. Flow cytometry (see Chapter 131) using standardized panels of antibodies helps define the lineage of the leukemic clone.

Newer diagnostic approaches that have become routine in many centers are extremely helpful. These include multicolor/multilaser extra- and intracellular FACS, molecular cytogenetics by fluorescent *in situ* hybridization (FISH), spectral karyotyping, PCR and RT-PCR (used for diagnosis of particular cytogenetic changes), microarray gene expression profiling (RNA expression arrays), and DNA-based bacterial artificial chromosome arrays (used for expression as well as DNA copy studies).[59–61] Array methods are currently mostly investigational/part of large cooperative group trials, but are proving quite useful for defining new prognostic groupings and uncovering new relationships between genes that may affect response to specific therapies. It is expected that the array methods (and certainly diagnostic tests derived from their findings) will become part of the standard of care for these diseases over the next several years.

TABLE 124.2

CLINICAL AND LABORATORY FEATURES AT DIAGNOSIS IN CHILDREN WITH ACUTE LYMPHOBLASTIC LEUKEMIA

Clinical and Laboratory Features	Percentage of Patients
SYMPTOMS AND PHYSICAL FINDINGS	
Fever	61
Bleeding (e g., petechiae or purpura)	48
Bone pain	23
Lymphadenopathy	50
Splenomegaly	63
Hepatosplenomegaly	68
LABORATORY FEATURES	
Leukocyte count (mm^3)	
<10,000	53
10,000–49,000	30
>50,000	17
Hemoglobin(g/dL)	
<7.0	43
7.0–11.0	45
>11.0	12
Platelet count (mm^3)	
<20,000	28
20,000–99,000	47
>100,000	25
Lymphoblast morphology	
L1	84
L2	15
L3	1

TABLE 124.3

DIFFERENTIAL DIAGNOSIS IN CHILDHOOD ACUTE LYMPHOBLASTIC LEUKEMIA

Nonmalignant conditions
- Juvenile rheumatoid arthritis
- Infectious mononucleosis
- Idiopathic thrombocytopenic purpura
- Pertussis; parapertussis
- Aplastic anemia
- Acute infectious lymphocytosis

Malignancies
- Neuroblastoma
- Retinoblastoma
- Rhabdomyosarcoma

Unusual presentations
- Hypereosinophilic syndrome

Prognostic Factors and Treatment of Pediatric Acute Lymphoblastic Leukemia

As outcomes with modern therapy in pediatric ALL have improved, many factors that had previously been shown to be important for predicting prognosis have lost statistical significance. Five factors that are readily apparent at either initial diagnosis or within the first month of treatment have retained their prognostic significance and constitute the basis on which patients are stratified in most treatment protocols. These factors are (1) age at presentation, (2) WBC at presentation, (3) specific cytogenetic abnormalities, (4) presence or absence of CNS involvement, and (5) rapidity of initial response to chemotherapy.[1] A consensus conference held at the NCI in 1996 led to the publication of the NCI consensus criteria that standardized the recording and use for ALL protocol stratification of three of these prognostic variables (age at presentation, WBC at presentation, and staging of CNS involvement).[62] The use of common criteria for stratification has made it much easier to compare the results of ALL clinical trials conducted by different groups. The cooperative groups differ in how they incorporate the remaining two prognostic features (blast cell cytogenetics and initial response to therapy). In general, modern ALL protocols treat children with low-risk disease with less-intensive chemotherapy in an effort to minimize toxicity while maintaining an excellent (80% to 90%) chance of cure. High-risk ALL patients who are treated with intensive therapies currently have an approximately 60% to 75% chance of cure with most cooperative group regimens.[1]

The age-determined risk groups are age less than 1 year (infant ALL), ages 1.0 to 9.99 years (standard risk ALL), and age 10 years and above (high-risk ALL). The infant group is a very high-risk subcategory of patients who usually demonstrate 11q23 abnormalities, most often the t(4;11) (q21;q23) translocation. These infants generally have high presenting WBCs, large amounts of extramedullary disease, and their leukemic blasts are usually CALLA (CD10)-negative.[63,64] Infants are currently treated on separate, highly intensive protocols of relatively short duration (approximately 1 year, in contrast to standard ALL treatments of 2 to 3 years). The data from the most recent infant protocols are still being reviewed, but it is clear thus far that the cure rate (with intensive treatment) has climbed to approximately 50%, especially for infants who are older (i.e., >6 months) at diagnosis.[65] Results for infants between 3 and 6 months at diagnosis are worse, and results are particularly poor for those under 3 months of age at diagnosis. Adolescents (age 10 years and above) up until young adulthood are the other age group that has traditionally demonstrated lower cure rates, although their survival has been improved significantly with the addition of early intensive postinduction therapy.[3,66]

Presenting WBC count more than 50,000/mcL is associated with a high risk of relapse. Patients with extremely high presenting WBC counts (i.e., several hundred thousand) have a higher risk of ultimate treatment failure. High presenting WBC counts are often associated with other factors (i.e., CALLA-negative infants, as previously explained, and adolescents with T-cell ALL).[3]

Blast cell cytogenetics are currently some of the strongest prognostic factors for assigning risk-based therapy in pediatric ALL. With standard karyotyping methods employed on fresh bone marrow samples combined with FISH, 80% to 100% of ALL blasts can be shown to have chromosomal abnormalities.[52] The most common cytogenetic abnormalities found in ALL are disorders of ploidy (overall DNA content and chromosome number). High hyperdiploidy, defined as chromosome number 50 or higher or DNA index (performed by FACS) of 1.16 or more, is associated with good prognosis (Fig. 124.3).[67]

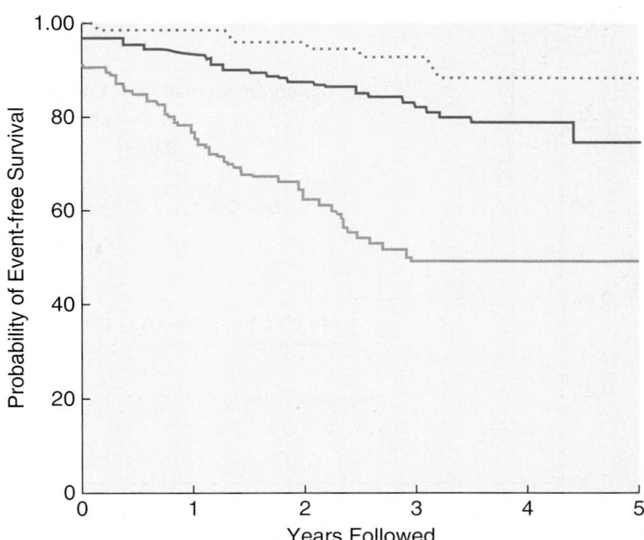

FIGURE 124.3 Ploidy is a prognostic determinant. Results are shown for patients with B precursor acute lymphoblastic leukemia (infants excluded) treated by the Pediatric Oncology Group. Patients (n = 114) with a DNA index greater than 1.16 (i.e., hyperdiploid, *dotted line*) have a better prognosis than those patients (n = 353) with a DNA index less than or equal to 1.16, white blood cell count less than 50,000/mcL, and age younger than 11 years (*bold line*); or DNA index less than 1.16, white blood cell count less than 50,000/mcL and age older than 11 years (*lowest curve*). (From ref. 67, with permission.)

This is particularly true if the leukemic blasts include trisomies of chromosome 4, 10, and 17 (Fig. 124.4), although other chromosomes (i.e., 21, 22, and X) are frequently present in extra copies.[52,68] Hypodiploidy (chromosome number <45) and especially haploidy (23 chromosomes) are associated with a poor prognosis (Fig. 124.5).[52,69]

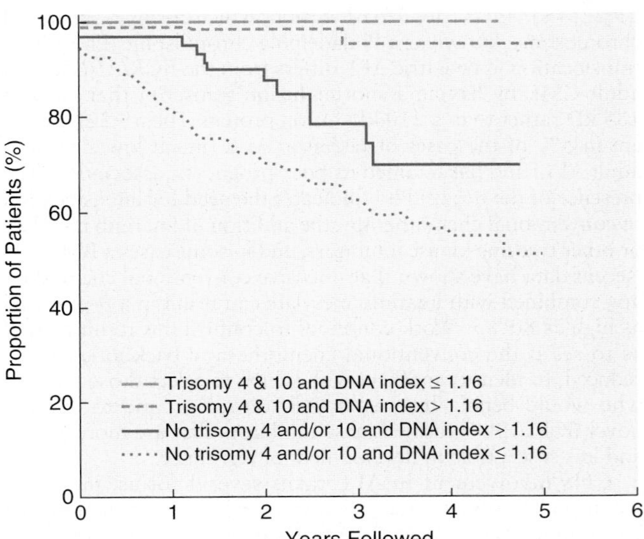

FIGURE 124.4 Prognosis of patients with trisomies of chromosomes 4 and 10. Presence of trisomies of chromosomes 4 and 10 is associated with low risk of treatment failure. Results are shown for patients with B precursor acute lymphoblastic leukemia (infants excluded) treated by the Pediatric Oncology Group. Patients with these trisomies have a better prognosis than those of patients in the good risk (DNA index >1.16) and poor risk (DNA index ≤1.16) groups. (From ref. 68, with permission.)

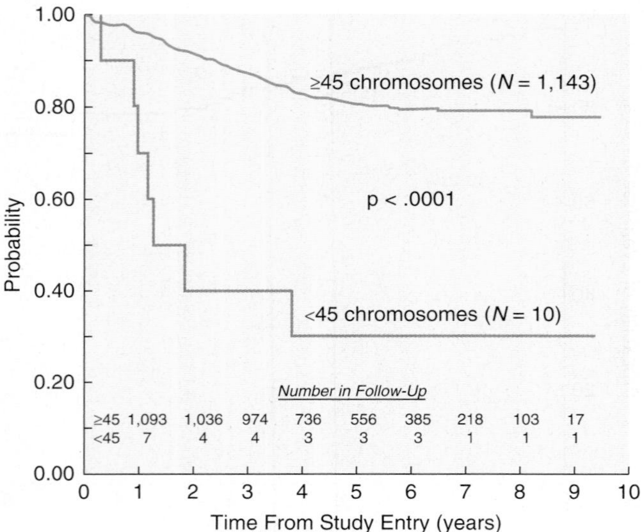

FIGURE 124.5 Event-free survival for patients with fewer than 45 chromosomes in their leukemic blasts. Patients were classified as standard risk by National Cancer Institute criteria (age 1–9 years with leucocyte counts less than 50,000/mcL) (From ref. 69, with permission.)

Many of the prognostically important structural chromosomal abnormalities seen in ALL are translocations. The most common translocation found in pediatric ALL blasts is the t(12;21) (p12;q22), which causes a fusion of the *ETV6* (also known as the *TEL*) gene on chromosome 12 with the *RUNX1* (also known as *AML1*) gene on chromosome 21.[1,70] The t(12;21) is a cryptic translocation (generally only seen by FISH or PCR technologies) that is present in 25% of U.S. pediatric ALL cases, in lower amounts in other geographic and ethnically defined populations, and is a good prognostic indicator.[71,72] Other chromosomal translocations seen in ALL have neutral or less favorable prognostic implications. Perhaps the most significant is the t(9;22) (9q34;q11) *BCR/ABL* fusion, which forms a shortened chromosome, known as a Philadelphia chromosome (Ph+). This translocation in pediatric ALL differs from the *BCR/ABL* seen in adult CML by having a shorter fusion transcript that yields a 185 kD rather than a 210 kD fusion protein. The t(9;22) is present in 5% of the cases of pediatric ALL (much lower than in adult ALL) and has retained its poor prognostic association. The presence of the t(9;22) Ph+ indicates the need for intensification of conventional chemotherapy, the addition of imatinib mesalate or other tyrosine kinase inhibitors, and in some cases a BMT.[73,74] Recent data have shown that intensive conventional chemotherapy combined with imatinib mesylate can result in a 3-year EFS as high as 80%.[74] Work continues to confirm this result as well as to see if the conventional chemotherapy backbone can be reduced, to identify markers with which to select those patients who would benefit from stem cell transplant, and to develop novel BCR/ABL tyrosine kinase inhibitors that are more potent and less susceptible to development of resistance.

CNS involvement in ALL takes several forms, including meningeal involvement, cranial nerve involvement (manifested by cranial nerve palsies), and, occasionally, frank leukemic infiltrates in the parenchyma of the brain.[1] CNS status at diagnosis is of prognostic importance and is graded according to the consensus criteria outlined in Table 124.4. The CNS is considered a sanctuary site because it is difficult to treat effectively and many systemic treatments do not adequately penetrate the blood–brain barrier. Without the administration of appropriate CNS preventive therapy, most patients would eventually relapse in the CNS. For these reasons, CNS involvement at diagnosis is an unfavorable prognostic sign, and therapy is intensified using more intrathecal, higher dose systemic, and in specific circumstances radiation therapy in response to this finding.[57]

TABLE 124.4

DEFINITIONS OF CNS DISEASE STATUS AT DIAGNOSIS OF ACUTE LYMPHOBLASTIC LEUKEMIA BASED ON CEREBROSPINAL FLUID FINDINGS

Status	Cerebrospinal Fluid Findings
CNS-1	No lymphoblasts
CNS-2	<5 WBCs/mcL with definable blasts on cytocentrifuge examination
CNS-3	≥5 WBCs/mcL with blast cells (or cranial nerve palsy)

WBC, white blood cell.

Extramedullary testicular involvement may occur in ALL, manifesting as a painless, palpable mass. A testicular examination should be part of all routine physical examinations for males with leukemia. Both testicular and CNS relapses require a systemic reinduction (as the risk of bone marrow relapse is increased) and site-directed therapy in the form of testicular or CNS radiation.[3,75] Although CNS relapse can be addressed with intensified systemic and intrathecal chemotherapy, radiation is a component of most CNS relapse protocols.[75,76]

Although once considered a poor prognostic sign, children with predominantly lymphoid blasts that express some mixed lineage (myeloid antigens like CD11, 13, or 15 in addition to specific lymphoid antigens such as CD10, 19, 20, and 22) are no longer considered high risk and are stratified onto current protocols on the basis of other presenting features.[1,3] In contrast, biphenotypic leukemias present with evidence of two immunophenotypically separate clones (usually pre-B ALL and AML) with shared cytogenetic changes indicating their origin from a multipotential leukemic stem cell.[77] These rare patients require therapy targeted at both the ALL and AML components of their disease and are quite difficult to cure.

All modern pediatric ALL treatment protocols use the prognostic factors outlined here, in varying ways, to stratify patients into different risk groups that receive treatment of different intensity. ALL treatment is divided into different phases. The first phase of treatment (*induction phase*) lasts 4 to 6 weeks and includes a glucocorticoid (dexamethasone or prednisone), the vinca-alkaloid vincristine (VCR), and one or two other drugs: L-asparaginase and an anthracycline (usually daunomycin).[3] Lower- and standard-risk patients generally do not receive anthracycline, whereas higher-risk patients do.[3] Other variations in induction schedules exist; for example, the Berlin-Frankfurt-Munster group uses a "steroid window" to begin therapy with a cytoreductive test of the sensitivity of each individual patient's disease to glucocorticoids.[78,79] This has prognostic significance in their protocols and does not seem to induce steroid resistance. Some study groups have intensified induction with the addition of other medications, but there is no convincing evidence that this increases the remission induction rate (currently 95% to 98%), and little evidence that it changes overall cure rate. Induction failure (defined as bone marrow blasts more than 25% on day 29 or the end of the scheduled induction period) is rare (2% to 5% of cases) and associated with very poor prognosis.[80] Although remissions can be achieved in these patients, the durability of the remission is usually significantly less than in patients who responded rapidly to induction therapy. As previously noted, rapid response to the induction therapy is an important prognostic variable.[1,81] Clearance of peripheral blasts by day 7 or 8 and bone marrow blasts by day 15 are validated time points that are used in many protocol schemas.[3,82]

Induction protocols are usually followed by a *consolidation phase* in which therapy is primarily aimed at reinforcing the bone marrow remission, and CNS preventive therapy is administered. Consolidation therapies vary but usually contain intensified (often weekly), intrathecal treatments. CNS consolidation can also be provided by using higher-dose systemic methotrexate or ara-C.[57]

Most ALL protocols are based on a strategy of intensive therapy that is delivered within the first 6 to 12 months of treatment, followed by *prolonged maintenance* or *continuation phases* (lasting 2 to 3 years) in which the therapy principally consists of antimetabolite treatments (i.e., methotrexate weekly and 6-mercaptopurine daily). Periodic "pulses" of intravenous VCR and oral glucocorticoid are used in most maintenance protocols, and CNS preventive therapy usually continues with periodic intrathecal treatments. The intensity of treatment given in the first year is varied based on the patient's prognostic "risk category" (degree of risk for relapse) and often includes intensive treatment phases termed *intensification, delayed intensification,* or *reinduction/reconsolidation*.[3,79,83] To minimize and avoid treatment-related mortality, strict supportive care guidelines are employed to prevent treatment-related complications. In general, expected, therapy-related mortality on a frontline pediatric ALL protocol should not exceed 2% to 3%. Cooperative group clinical trials include comprehensive monitoring guidelines to ensure patient safety.

The overall duration of ALL treatment varies with the cooperative group trials but is usually between 2 and 3.5 years. On the current Children's Oncology Group regimens, boys require an additional year of maintenance (bringing their therapy to a little more than 3 years), and girls receive a little more than 2 years of treatment. Other cooperative study groups are no longer seeing any survival difference between boys and girls and have shortened their proposed therapies to approximately 2 years. It is anticipated that future clinical trials will be focused on determining the optimal duration of therapy, as well as on decreasing intensification (and toxicity) of therapy for favorable-risk patients.[1,84,85]

CNS-directed therapy is usually present in all phases of therapy, but is most intensive during the first several months. CNS therapy uses intrathecal chemotherapy, high-dose systemic chemotherapy (principally higher dose methotrexate or cytarabine), and/or cranial radiation.[57,86] Because it is often associated with neurocognitive deficits, endocrine, and growth abnormalities, cranial radiation is reserved only for patients judged to be at highest risk of CNS relapse (i.e., those with very high initial WBC counts or T-cell disease).[87,88] Currently, this includes approximately 5% of newly diagnosed patients. Through the years, the doses of cranial radiation have decreased from the 36 to 24 Gy range, used on early protocols to 18 Gy for treatment and 12 Gy on some CNS preventive therapy regimens.[57]

Therapy for relapsed ALL depends on the location of relapse (i.e., isolated CNS or testicular vs. marrow, or combined marrow and extramedullary relapse) and the duration of the patient's initial remission. Extramedullary ALL relapse cases generally have a better prognosis than bone marrow relapses, but also require localized therapy in addition to a second full course of systemic chemotherapy.[3] For testicular relapse, local therapy involves the removal of the affected testes (later prostheses can be inserted in the scrotal sac), followed by irradiation of the remaining testicle and scrotal area.[3,89] Fertility will be compromised (so postpubertal males should be offered sperm banking), and hormonal supplements should be offered as needed. Prognosis after a testicular relapse remains quite good. For CNS relapse, local therapy involves intensified intrathecal therapy, varying regimens of high-dose systemic therapy, and usually the addition of cranial and/or craniospinal radiation. Prognosis with an isolated CNS relapse depends on the intensity of prior therapy and the timing of the relapse before or after the first 18 months of therapy.[90,91]

Relapses of any type while the patient is receiving primary treatment are particularly difficult to manage. Bone marrow relapses during therapy or within 6 months of completing therapy are worse than those that happen more than 6 months off therapy.[92] Although there are individual patient and treatment protocol differences, isolated CNS relapses that happen less than 18 months on treatment have a worse outcome than those that happen more than 18 months on therapy.[57,91]

Second complete bone marrow remissions in ALL are often achievable.[3] The ease or difficulty with which a second or higher complete remission (CR) can be obtained as well as maintained in relapsed ALL is primarily related to the amount and intensity of prior therapy.[75,93,94] Multiple medications and regimens are being tested for induction in relapsed and refractory leukemia. A complete discussion of this topic is beyond the scope of this chapter, but promising results have been recently obtained with clofarabine and clofarabine-containing regimens.[95–97] Which patients can be effectively treated with chemotherapy alone in CR2 versus which should be treated with a BMT has been controversial. BMT is usually used in cases in which the bone marrow relapse has occurred before or within 6 months of completion of an initial ALL treatment (CR1 <30 months), but the decision of whether to perform a BMT as part of relapse ALL therapy still needs to consider: (1) timing of the relapse, (2) the availability of a suitable donor, (3) the intensity and duration of the original therapy, and (4) overall health of the recipient in terms of the risk of various transplant preparative regimens.[3,98] A BMT for relapsed ALL should not be done unless the patient is in remission (CR2) and, optimally, the patient should receive some conventional consolidative treatment prior to undergoing BMT. Autologous BMT in ALL is no longer recommended, both because of poor results in the past and the fact that results with matched unrelated donor transplants are comparable to those achieved with matched sibling transplants.[99]

Prognostic Factors and Treatment of Pediatric AML

In contrast with ALL, there are very few standard clinical or laboratory-based factors in AML that consistently relate to prognosis. Table 124.5 reviews prognostic factors in both

TABLE 124.5

ACUTE LEUKEMIA: FAVORABLE PROGNOSTIC FACTORS

ACUTE LYMPHOBLASTIC LEUKEMIA
Age, 1–9 y
White blood cell count <50,000/mcL
DNA index >1.16 (trisomies for chromosomes 4, 10, and 17)
Chromosomal translocation t(12;22) or *ETV6-RUNX1*
CNS-1
Rapid response to induction chemotherapy
ACUTE MYELOGENOUS LEUKEMIA
White blood cell count <100,000/mcL
Core binding factor transcription complex, t(8;21) or inv(16)
Acute promyelocytic leukemia t(15;17)
Down syndrome
Complete remission following one chemotherapy cycle

pediatric ALL and AML. Poor prognostic factors that predict lower remission rates and/or decreased EFS include presenting WBC count of more than 100,000/mm^3, blast cytogenetics with monosomy 5 or 7, 5q-, FLT-3ITD, and secondary AML/MDS.[7,100–102] Swift response to induction chemotherapy (i.e., remission after one cycle of chemotherapy), favorable cytogenetics, and DS (with Fab M7) are predictive of better outcomes.[101] Favorable cytogenetics in AML include translocations or inversions involving core binding transcription factors, the t(8;21) (*AML1/ETO* fusion), and inv (16) and the t(15;17) (*PML/RARα* fusion) seen in acute promyelocytic leukemia (APL; Fab M3) (see Chapter 131). Although many findings in AML are similar between adults and children, important biological and therapeutic differences are emerging. An example of this is mutations of the *KIT* receptor tyrosine kinase have a similar frequency in pediatric core binding factor AML (patients with t(8;21) and inv 16 cytogenetics) as those found in adult AML, but they do not seem to convey poor prognosis as they do in the adult patients.[102]

There have been some modest improvements in AML therapy outcomes since the early 1980s when remission rates were approximately 50% and DFS was approximately half that. Improvements in CR rate to 85% to 92% have come through increasing the intensity of induction treatment and improved supportive care.[5,7] Despite the improvement in CR rates, DFS rates are currently reported in the 40% to 66% range, varying by treatment protocol and prognostic subgroup (Fig. 124.2).[7,22,101]

With the exception of DS patients with Fab M7 AML and patients with APL, most pediatric AML induction therapies include two cycles of ara-C and daunomycin, with or without thioguanine and/or etoposide. Studies have shown that the intensity of induction therapy is important for overall survival.[7] In the Children's Cancer Group 2891 protocol, intensively timed induction (starting the second chemotherapy cycle on day 14 regardless of count recovery) did not change the induction (CR1) rate, but it did have a profound effect on eventual cure rate (Fig. 124.2).[103] Although fewer than 5% of pediatric AML patients present with CNS disease, as many as 20% will suffer an isolated CNS relapse.[56] Intrathecal chemotherapy (usually ara-C) has been found by several groups to effectively reduce the risk of CNS relapse.[7]

Conventional postinduction consolidative chemotherapy in pediatric AML usually involves two to three cycles of high-dose ara-C–based combinations, to which (depending on the cooperative group protocol) anthracycline, etoposide, or ifosfamide/cyclophosphamide are added. There is no proven benefit to maintenance chemotherapy, so conventional treatment for AML is rarely more than four to eight chemotherapy cycles lasting 6 to 12 months.[6,7] The indications for BMT in pediatric AML, whether to perform the procedure in CR1 or later, the preparative regimens used, and the type of donor (matched sibling, matched unrelated donor, selectively mismatched donors, or even haploidentical donor marrow)[104,105] are the focus of intensive and ongoing controversy and research. A full discussion of BMT in pediatric AML is beyond the scope of this chapter, but it is clear that many of the lower risk patients (defined by the criteria previously discussed) are being cured without resorting to BMT.[105] The reader is directed to several recent reviews and the results of recent trials.[8,103–105]

Pediatric patients who have APL have some of the highest cure rates in pediatric AML. These patients should receive all-*trans*-retinoic acid (ATRA), which directly binds to the t(15;17) PML/RARα fusion protein, which is causative for this form of AML.[106] They should also receive conventional chemotherapy during both induction and consolidation phases. Patients who respond to this therapy have an 80% to 85% survival rate and should not be subjected to BMT.[107] Similar to adult therapies for APL (see Chapter 131), arsenic trioxide, found to be useful for salvage in patients who became resistant to ATRA, is currently being tested in upfront pediatric APL regimens (both alone and in combination with ATRA and conventional chemotherapy) in an effort to improve DFS in CR1.[108] Despite the remarkable successes with ATRA and arsenic trioxide with and without conventional chemotherapy, there remain patients with APL with relapsed and refractory disease, and many of these can still be cured with BMT.[109]

DS patients with M7 AML (see previous discussion related to DS and leukemia) do well with lower-dose ara-C regimens and standard timing of their induction cycles. Current results in DS M7 AML are the best of any AML subgroup outside APL, with 70% to 85% EFS, with the younger patients (ages 0 to 2 years) showing the best results.[110–112] These good results apply only to the DS patients with M7 AML who tend to be younger (<4 years old at diagnosis) and have *GATA-1* mutations.[113] DS patients also show increased toxicities with BMT and more intensive regimens, thus BMT should not be considered except as a consolidative therapy in CR2 for these patients.[7,110]

The prognosis for pediatric patients who relapse after either conventional or BMT therapy for AML is poor. A second CR can be obtained using similar ara-C and anthracycline-containing regimens in 20% to 70% of patients, but the likelihood of obtaining a cure is approximately half the rate for *de novo* AML.[93] Clofarabine alone and in combination (see ALL relapse discussion) with other chemotherapeutic agents has also been found to be helpful in reinducing relapsed AML.[96,97] BMT in early relapse or CR2 for AML patients who were previously transplanted in CR1 is a strategy that has had some success.[93,114,115] Gemtuzumab ozogamicin, a newer agent consisting of an antibody to CD33 coupled to calicheamicin (a toxic antitumor antibiotic), has shown some promise in inducing a second CR in relapsed patients.[116,117] Unfortunately, this agent has also shown significant toxicity associated with an increased rate of veno-occlusive disease of the liver in patients who receive it before or after a BMT.[118] This complication can be treated, and perhaps effectively prevented, with defibrotide.[119,120] The value of Flt-3 inhibitors in AML is currently being studied.[121]

Rarer Forms of Leukemia in Children

Chronic leukemias, with the exception of CML, do not occur in children. Ph+ CML is rare in childhood (<1% to 2% of all pediatric leukemia cases).[122] When it does occur, it typically presents in adolescents and is in chronic phase. Therapy is similar to that recommended in adults, with imatinib (along with hydroxyurea if the initial counts are high, and/or the patient presents with a high degree of hepatosplenomegaly) as the mainstay of induction and maintenance therapy. The use of alternative tyrosine kinase inhibitors such as dasatinib and nilotinib are being investigated in children as well as adults.[123–125] Because there is no clear end point for when or whether any of these tyrosine kinase inhibitors can be safely discontinued, many pediatric oncologists continue to consider hematopoietic stem cell transplantation in remission.[126,127]

JMML, a myeloproliferative disorder unique to childhood, is characterized by extreme monocytosis, hepatosplenomegaly, thrombocytopenia, and increased fetal hemoglobin.[128,129] Bone marrow morphology is often consistent with myelodysplasia as well as myeloproliferation, and cytogenetics frequently reveals a monosomy 7 clone. Mutations in *PTN11* and other *RAS* pathway genes have also been noted.[129] Although the clinical course can be indolent (requiring only intermittent blood product and antibiotic support), these patients often progress to frank marrow failure. Aggressive AML-type chemotherapy has been occasionally effective, but current trials are exploring the addition of immunomodulatory chemotherapy (fludarabine combined with ara-C) and the use of 13-*cis*-retinoic acid, which has been reported to induce clinical remission in some patients. These responses should be considered transient, and the most definitive therapy in JMML is an allogeneic BMT with either matched sibling or matched unrelated donor.[130] Overall DFS with BMT in JMML has been in the 40% to 55% range, with relapse of the JMML clone the major reason for failure.[131] Recently, aberrant STAT5 activation has been identified in a subset of patients with JMML, and may offer an opportunity for development of novel targeted therapy inhibiting this pathway.[132]

LYMPHOMAS

Lymphomas constitute approximately 10% of cancer in children, and are the third most common pediatric malignancy (behind leukemias and brain tumors).[133] Two-thirds of lymphomas in children are NHL and the other third are Hodgkin's lymphoma (HL). Children demonstrate a different spectrum of histology (especially in NHL) than adults, and there are important differences between the biology and proper treatment of these diseases in children compared with that of adults. Although all forms of lymphoma are quite radiation-sensitive, this modality is avoided in pediatric NHL, and in HL the doses and fields are carefully limited to minimize detrimental effects on growth and development, as well as the formation of second malignancies. Table 124.6 compares the differences in presenting and staging features between pediatric NHL and HL.

Non-Hodgkin's Lymphoma

Similar to the situation in leukemia, children develop a different spectrum of disease than that seen in adults. Follicular center and low-grade B-cell lymphomas (the most common forms of the disease in adults) are rarely seen in children. Using the updated Revised European-American Lymphoma (REAL) version of the World Health Organization classification of lymphomas (outlined in Table 127.5), children are seen to develop four major histologies of NHL: (1) precursor B- and precursor T-lymphoblastic lymphoma (30% of the cases), (2) Burkitt and atypical Burkitt lymphoma (40% to 50%), (3) anaplastic large cell lymphoma (10%), and (4) diffuse large B-cell lymphoma (15%).[133] All of these histologies should be considered high-grade, acute diseases compared with the more indolent forms of NHL seen in adults. Major improvement in the survival of these children has occurred during the past 15 to 20 years, which correlated with the realization that the mainstay of therapy should be systemically delivered multiagent chemotherapy, as opposed to a reliance on localized therapies such as surgery and radiation.

NHL in children is rarely a truly localized disease. The Cotswold revision of the Ann Arbor NHL staging and classification system used in adult NHL (see Chapter 127) has mostly been replaced in pediatrics by the staging system outlined in Table 124.7. Surgical/pathologic staging is no longer carried out in either pediatric NHL or HL cases. Diagnosis generally relies on biopsy and radiologic scans, including a combination of nuclear medicine and conventional plain films, computed tomography, and magnetic resonance imaging scans.[135] The current 5-year EFS rates for early low-stage disease are in the 90% to 95% range, and from 70% to 90% for the higher-stage presentations.[3,133]

Unlike in ALL, there is no sharp age peak for the occurrence of NHL in children, and there is a marked imbalance in the male to female incidence, which approaches a 3:1 ratio.[2,133] With the exception of children with rare, inherited, or acquired immunodeficiency syndromes (e.g., Wiskott-Aldrich, common variable immune deficiency, ataxia-telangiectasia, X-linked lymphoproliferative syndrome, human immunodeficiency virus [HIV]-acquired immunodeficiency disease syndrome, or exposure to immunosuppressive drugs after solid organ or bone marrow transplants), most children who develop NHL have a history of normal health and no known risk factors. The main exception to this concerns the possible etiologic role of the Epstein-Barr virus (EBV). EBV is strongly associated not only with lymphomas in HIV patients and lymphoproliferative diseases found in posttransplant patients, but also with both sporadic and endemic Burkitt lymphoma and many cases of HL (see later discussion) found in otherwise healthy children.

Lymphoblastic lymphomas share many molecular, biologic, and cytogenetic, as well as therapeutic, response characteristics with ALL, and at times have been treated on the same protocols.[2,3] The arbitrariness of the distinction can be seen in the fact that if patients can be shown to have more than 25% lymphoblasts in their bone marrow (despite the existence of a large lymphomatous mass elsewhere in the body), they are designated as having ALL. Morphologically, the cells are indistinguishable, and the FACS profiles generally overlap, with CD10/CALLA showing more variable expression than in ALL.[2,136,137]

The presentation of most children with lymphoblastic lymphoma is that of a patient with rapidly enlarging neck and mediastinal lymphadenopathy. Particular attention needs to be paid to hydration status, kidney function, and whether or

PRACTICE OF ONCOLOGY

TABLE 124.6

COMPARISON OF HODGKIN'S LYMPHOMA AND NON-HODGKIN'S LYMPHOMA IN PEDIATRIC PATIENTS

Feature	Hodgkin's Lymphoma	Non-Hodgkin's Lymphoma
Age	Mostly >10 y	Any age in children
Stage at diagnosis	Mostly localized	Commonly widespread
Constitutional symptoms	Alter prognosis	Do not affect prognosis
CNS involvement	Rare	Occurrence increases with AIDS
Mediastinal involvement	Most common with nodular sclerosing Hodgkin's lymphoma	Most common with lymphoblastic lymphoma
Gastrointestinal involvement	Rare	Occurs
Abdominal nodal involvement	Can be small or large, mesenteric rare	Usually enlarged, mesenteric common
Bone involvement	Rare	Occurs
Marrow involvement	Rare	Common

AIDS, acquired immunodeficiency virus.
(Adapted from ref. 4.)

TABLE 124.7

ST. JUDE CHILDREN'S RESEARCH HOSPITAL STAGING SYSTEM FOR PEDIATRIC NON-HODGKIN'S LYMPHOMA

Stage	Description
I	A single tumor (extranodal) or single anatomic area (nodal), with the exclusion of mediastinum or abdomen
II	A single tumor (extranodal) with regional node involvement Two or more nodal areas on the same side of the diaphragm Two single (extranodal) tumors with or without regional node involvement on the same side of the diaphragm A primary gastrointestinal tract tumor, usually in the ileocecal area, with or without involvement of associated mesenteric nodes only[a]
III	Two single tumors (extranodal) on opposite sides of the diaphragm Two or more nodal areas above and below the diaphragm All the primary intrathoracic tumors (mediastinal, pleural, thymic) All extensive primary intra-abdominal disease[a] All paraspinal or epidural tumors, regardless of other tumor sites
IV	Any of the above with initial central nervous system or bone marrow involvement[b]

[a]Stage II abdominal disease typically is limited to a segment (usually distal ileum) of the gut plus or minus the associated mesenteric nodes only, and the primary tumor can be completely removed grossly by segmental excision. Stage III abdominal disease typically exhibits spread to para-aortic and retroperitoneal areas by implants and plaques in mesentery or peritoneum, or by direct infiltration of structures adjacent to the primary tumor. Ascites may be present, and complete resection of all gross tumor is not possible.
[b]If bone marrow involvement is present at diagnosis, the percentage of blasts or abnormal cells must be 25% or less to be classified as stage IV non-Hodgkin's lymphoma. If there are more than 25% blasts, the patient is classified as having acute leukemia (either precursor B or T acute lymphoblastic leukemia or L3 acute lymphoblastic leukemia).

not the kidneys are directly involved (infiltrated) with the disease. Positron emission tomography (PET), computed tomography, and magnetic resonance imaging scans of the neck, chest, abdomen, and pelvis are helpful for assessing the degree of organ involvement, but care must be taken in requiring children with mediastinal masses to lay supine. Severe medical emergencies can be precipitated with the combination of laying such patients supine (which can compress both central blood vessels and airways) and sedation (which causes vasodilation and decreased blood return to the heart).[138] Histologic diagnosis should be sought in the least-invasive way possible. Prebiopsy steroids or "postage stamp irradiation" (use of a small radiation field to emergently relieve airway compression) can be done, but the steroids may jeopardize obtaining the histologic diagnosis. CNS status should be assessed prior to systemic chemotherapy, and prophylactic intrathecal chemotherapy should be administered early.[2]

Primary therapy for lymphoblastic lymphoma (of either B- or T-cell histology) consists of multiagent chemotherapy without radiation. Stage I and II lymphoblastic cases do very well with short treatments (three to five cycles) of cyclophosphamide, doxorubicin, vincrisitine, and prednisone, the so-called CHOP or similar regimens, and a relatively short (24 weeks vs. 2 to 3 years with ALL) maintenance phase of antimetabolite (6-mercaptopurine daily and weekly oral methotrexate).[2,133] Higher-stage (stages III and IV) lymphoblastic cases require more intensive regimens (alkylators, ara-C, and VP-16 are usually added into the first 6 to 8 months of treatment), and many regimens include maintenance phases similar to those on ALL protocols. Nelarabine is a novel nucleoside analogue with preferential cytotoxicity in T-lineage lymphoid malignancies that is being studied in current protocols.[139] Because activating *NOTCH1* mutations are found in the majority of T-cell leukemias, gamma-secretase inhibitors that block Notch 1 signaling are another class of agents whose role in treatment regimens is being assessed.[140,141]

Relapse in lymphoblastic lymphoma is fortunately an uncommon problem, but when it does occur it happens either during or shortly after completion of therapy. Relapse of low-stage disease can frequently be salvaged using the more intensive chemotherapy designed for high-stage disease.[142] Lymphoblastic lymphoma patients who relapse after higher-stage treatment have a poor prognosis and are candidates for phase 1 agents and/or BMT.[142,143] Radiation to areas of bulk disease and total-body irradiation are incorporated into the transplant regimens, but in general radiation does not have a role in primary treatment or reinduction at relapse.

Burkitt and atypical Burkitt lymphoma are common histologies of NHL seen in 40% to 50% of pediatric NHL cases.[2,133] Endemic Burkitt lymphoma (usually presenting with localized head and neck masses, most frequently the jaw) in Africa is quite common (100 cases per million children), and 95% are associated with EBV. Sporadic Burkitt lymphoma, as seen in the United States, typically presents with an abdominal mass, occurs in 1 to 2 cases per million children, and only 15% are associated with EBV.[144,145] The most common presentation in the United States is of a boy age 5 to 10 years, with a right lower quadrant mass and/or acute abdomen secondary to an ileocecal intussusception. If the tumor is limited to the distal ileum or cecum, it should be completely excised along with its associated mesentery, and the bowel repaired with an end-to-end anastomosis.[146] These children have low-stage disease, require less chemotherapy, and have an excellent outcome. More frequently, the abdominal involvement is much more diffuse. Ascitic fluid can be sent for diagnostic cytology to avoid an invasive abdominal procedure.[145]

Burkitt lymphoma cells have a mature B-cell FACS profile (express cell surface immunoglobulin, usually IgM) and are characterized morphologically by homogeneous round-to-oval nuclei, multiple nucleoli, and intensely basophilic cytoplasm with large vacuolated areas containing fat. Atypical Burkitt lymphoma cells may be difficult to distinguish pathologically from large cell B histologies, but they respond to similar chemotherapy.

The majority of Burkitt lymphoma cases display the t(8;14) (q24;q32) translocation in which *c-myc* from chromosome 8 is translocated to the Ig heavy-chain locus on chromosome 14. In this translocation and in two variants, t(2;8) (p12;q24) and t(8;22) (q24;q11), the *c-myc* oncogene is overexpressed because of the influence of Ig regulatory regions (enhancers).

The diagnosis of Burkitt lymphoma must be done very expeditiously as these tumors grow swiftly and patients are at high risk of intestinal obstruction (from intussusception) and metabolic problems related to tumor lysis syndrome.[147] Tumor lysis often begins even before chemotherapy. Special attention must be paid to serum electrolyte balance (including calcium/phosphate balance), and vigorous intravenous hydration and alkalinization to improve uric acid excretion is essential. Allopurinol or recombinant urate oxidase, rasburicase, is used to block uric acid production.[148,149] Occasionally, the lysis syndrome can be severe enough to cause acute renal failure, and dialysis must be used to maintain fluid and re-establish electrolyte balance.

Children with low-stage, African-endemic Burkitt lymphoma have been successfully treated with single or multiple doses of cyclophosphamide. Short therapies, including one incorporating four low doses of cyclophosphamide along with four doses of intrathecal methotrexate and hydrocortisone given over a 28-day period, have been successfully employed.[150] These strategies result in lower cure rates, but they make it feasible to treat large numbers of children with lower toxic death and complication rates in resource-poor settings.[151,152]

Higher-stage Burkitt lymphoma (stages 3 and 4) requires significantly more intensive chemotherapy, involving much higher doses of cyclophosphamide, and the addition of an anthracycline, high-dose ara-C, methotrexate, and VP-16 to the CHOP schemas. Many current high-stage Burkitt lymphoma protocols use hematopoietic growth factor support to enhance bone marrow recovery in order to allow intensive cycles to be given approximately every 3 weeks. These protocols are intensive, but they are usually of short (6- to 8-month) duration. Recently, there have been some efforts to reduce chemotherapy and to add biologic agents like rituximab (anti-CD20 antibody) to reduce toxicity of treatment in patients who have HIV or other medical problems in which intensive Burkitt lymphoma protocols would be contraindicated.[153,154] The cure rate for pediatric patients with higher-stage (stage III and IV) Burkitt lymphoma is now 80% to 90%.[134]

The management of relapsed Burkitt lymphoma is problematic. Relapses usually occur during therapy or shortly after the cessation of therapy. Low-stage patients can sometimes be effectively treated with using a high-stage primary protocol, but higher-stage relapsed patients should be considered for BMT or phase 1 therapies.[155]

The large cell NHLs of childhood—anaplastic large cell lymphoma (ALCL) and diffuse large B-cell lymphoma (DLBCL)—comprise 25% to 30% of pediatric NHL. The workup and staging of large cell lymphomas are similar to that described for other forms of NHL. ALCL tends to present with involvement of lymph nodes and extranodal sites including skin, lung, other soft tissues, and bone. The majority of ALCL cases have T-cell immunophenotype. ALCL is also known for cytogenetically presenting with the t(2;5) (p23;q35) translocation, which fuses nucleophosmin with a transmembrane tyrosine-specific protein kinase known as anaplastic lymphoma kinase.

DLBCL tends to present with large mediastinal masses, but bone, lymph node, and abdominal presentations have been described. DLBCL of the mediastinum often presents with sclerosis and can be more refractory to treatment. Neither DLBCL nor ALCL has a tendency to spread to either bone marrow or CNS, so stage IV disease with either histology is rare. Both ALCL and DLBCL are generally quite responsive to chemotherapy. Some cooperative groups treat both on uniform protocols with three to five cycles of CHOP or APO (Adriamycin, prednisone, Oncovin/VCR) with EFS that ranges from 70% to 85%.[2,133]

Hodgkin's Lymphoma

The natural history and outcome of treatment in HL is similar in young children and adults, but treatment decisions (and regimens) are different in children based on the need to limit radiation and certain types of chemotherapy.[4,156,157] The goal remains to maximize cure rates (which are already in the 80% to 90% range) while avoiding undue effects on various organs, bones, joints and soft tissue growth, problems with fertility, and secondary malignancies later in life. HL is quite rare below age 5, with the majority of pediatric cases presenting in children older than 11 years.[4,158] Young patients (<10 years) have a 3:1 male to female ratio. This imbalance returns to the approximately equal male to female ratio seen in adult disease as the age of presentation climbs. The age of HL incidence in industrialized countries is bimodal, with the first peak in adults 20 to 30 years of age and the second peak much later in adulthood.[4]

The etiology of HL is unknown, but there does appear to be a causal association with EBV in up to 40% of cases.[159] There are also familial and geographic clusters that suggest an inherited susceptibility, environmental, or infectious contributions to etiology.[159,160] Most children (90%) present with painless adenopathy in the neck, and 60% have involvement of anterior mediastinum, paratracheal, or hilar lymph nodes. The Cotswold modification of the Ann Arbor Staging System (described in Chapter 126) is used for all ages. B symptoms (defined as in adults) include unexplained fever (more than 38°C or 100.4°F), drenching night sweats, and more than 10% weight loss. B symptoms are present in approximately 30% of newly diagnosed pediatric HL cases.[161] The process of clinical staging is similar to that of pediatric NHL, previously discussed, and described in detail for adult patients in Chapter 126. There is no longer any role for staging laparotomy as localized radiation is no longer used as a sole treatment modality in pediatric HL. Although there are problems with expense, availability, and false-positivity with PET scanning, PET and/or gallium are usually required assessments on most cooperative group protocols and can be invaluable later in therapy for assessing whether residual masses contain live tumor.[162,163]

The malignant cells in HL constitute a minority (estimated at 0.1% to 10%) of the cell population of the discernible tumor.[164] Inflammatory cells (histiocytes, plasma cells, lymphocytes, eosinophils, and neutrophils) make up the bulk of the tumor. The malignant cells are actually malignant lymphocytes with specific, characterized immunophenotypes. The standard histologic subtypes classified by the World Health Organization (Table 127.5) are nodular lymphocyte predominant HL (NLPHL) and the four subtypes of classic HL: (1) nodular sclerosing, (2) mixed cellularity, (3) lymphocyte-rich, and (4) lymphocyte-depleted.

NLPHL disease affects 10% to 15% of pediatric patients, is more common among male and younger patients, and is usually clinically localized (low stage). Current cooperative group protocols for low-stage NLPHL in children call for stage I patients to receive surgical resection only (no chemotherapy or radiotherapy) and close follow-up. For stage II/III, most would be treated with several cycles of relatively low-dose chemotherapy (i.e., avoiding the use of alkylators, topoisomerase inhibitors) and radiation therapy. Preliminary evidence suggests that this approach for NLPHL leads to an overall survival close to 100%, and should decrease the late effects of secondary malignancy and infertility.[165] Many current study protocols would forgo even low-dose involved field (IF) for these young patients who achieve a CR to low-dose chemotherapy, but this should still be considered an experimental approach as combination low-dose chemotherapy and IF radiation has been the standard of care, and there are reports of relapse after chemotherapy only treatments.[166]

Both pathologists and oncologists need to be aware of an entity known as *progressive transformation of germinal centers* (PTGC), which can be confused with NLPHL and sometimes is associated with this and other forms of HL.[167] PTGC is a reactive phenomenon usually associated with benign follicular hyperplasia. PTGC can be found in approximately 10% of otherwise benign reactive nodal biopsies in children.[168] The finding of PTGC in a lymph node biopsy is not considered a premalignant finding. No specific or precautionary follow-up plans need to be made for patients with PTGC, beyond what would normally be done for patients with recurrent adenopathy after HL therapy, or normal clinical prudence when reactive nodes are sampled in patients who do not have a history of prior malignancy.

The most common presenting histology in pediatric HL is nodular sclerosing type, which accounts for more than 50% of the cases (40% of the younger patients but 70% of the adolescents).[4] It is characterized by bands of fibrosis and a thickened lymph node capsule that are discernible even in gross pathologic section. These nodes and masses tend to form scars that can lead to residual masses, which appear as opacified lesions on radiologic studies for years after a full clinical response. Mixed cellularity is responsible for approximately 30% of pediatric cases, and tends to occur in children more than 10 years of age. The lymphocyte-depleted form of HL is quite rare, except in children with HIV. This type of classic HL is also often EBV-positive. The lymphocyte-rich variant is quite rare in children (approximately 5% of the cases), has a high incidence of mediastinal masses and stage III disease, but has an older average age of presentation (32 years).[4]

With the exception of NLPHL, the treatment for all of the various HL histologies is the same and is based on staging rather than histology. Therapy in pediatric HL is composed of three to six cycles of combination chemotherapy followed by IF radiation therapy. The composition of the chemotherapy regimens has varied during the years, but combinations of vinca alkaloids, alkylating agents (originally nitrogen mustard but now cyclophosphamide is more commonly used), steroids, procarbazine, anthracyclines, bleomycin, and DTIC have been used. Treatment is currently scaled to the risk of the disease recurrence or primary treatment failure.[158] Current therapies for low-stage HL attempt to dose-reduce or eliminate alkylators, anthracyclines, and bleomycin (to reduce late effects) and to lower or even eliminate the IF radiation doses.[168]

Therapy for higher-stage and less rapidly responding HL currently involves approximately 8 to 12 months of higher-dose combination chemotherapy and IF radiation therapy, with EFS rates currently in the 80% to 90% range.[157] Treatment for relapsed or refractory pediatric HL is beyond the scope of this chapter, but the medications (e.g., gemcitabine and vinorelbine) and approaches (e.g., BMT) are usually similar to those used in adults (see Chapter 126).[170,171]

SUPPORTIVE CARE

There is no question that a large part of the success of modern leukemia and lymphoma treatment is related to the major improvements in supportive care that coincided with improvements in chemotherapy. These advances have included improved blood products, antibiotics, antifungals, and better intensive care unit support of critically ill pediatric patients. Erythropoietin has been used sparingly in pediatric oncology, and is not generally incorporated in front-line therapies for any of the lymphoid cancers. Leukocyte growth factors (granulocyte colony-stimulating factor, granulocyte-macrophage colony-stimulating factor, and PEGylated forms, such as pegfilgrastim) are used sparingly in pediatric leukemia and lymphoma therapies for multiple reasons, including (1) concerns (mostly not substantiated in the literature) that these factors may stimulate the growth of these diseases, (2) multiple studies that show no changes in overall outcome when these factors are used, (3) financial burden, and (4) the addition of needle sticks in small children and/or the increased infection risk from allowing the parents and other caregivers to enter central lines daily to administer these agents. Growth factors (usually granulocyte colony-stimulating factor) are, however, used routinely in many higher-stage HL and NHL and pediatric BMT protocols so that the chemotherapy can be given in a dose-intensive manner (i.e., every 2- to 3-week cycles) and long periods of profound neutropenia can be avoided.

LONG-TERM, PALLIATIVE, AND HOSPICE CARE IN PEDIATRIC ONCOLOGY

The survivors of the lower-risk (less intensively treated) forms of ALL, NHL, and HL in childhood can now expect prolonged DFS, intact fertility, lesser cognitive and social disruption, and an easier integration into standard medical and social environments. Survivors from the use of higher doses and larger radiation fields used in the 1960s and 1970s, as well as from other past and current regimens that involve higher cumulative doses of chemotherapy, continue to have increased risk of important long-term toxicities and disabilities. The problems these survivors encounter include endocrine, growth, fertility, and learning disabilities, along with cardiac, renal, liver, and other end-organ toxicities.[172] Second malignancies are another serious problem that the survivors of pediatric oncology diagnoses encounter. These tumors arise from the combined carcinogenic exposures to chemotherapy and radiotherapy, as well as from possibly an innate propensity to develop cancer in many of these patients.[173] It has been estimated that pediatric cancer survivors will soon represent as many as 1 in 250 adult Americans in the 15- to 45-year-old population. Slightly more than half of these patients will have survived the diseases and treatments discussed in this chapter.[174]

Even with cure rates that reach into the low 90% region, a substantial number of children still die of leukemia and lymphoma. A small number die after failing their first regimens, but many succumb after alternately succeeding and then failing several attempts at cure. Discussion of hospice and palliative care for these children and support for their families is beyond the scope of this chapter, but this is an area of active interest and involvement in most pediatric oncology programs. Hospice and palliative care treatments in pediatrics share some of the same concerns, goals, and methods as programs for adults. However, the unique requirements of psychosocial support in children, and the impact of a possible death of a child on a family, lead most experts to guide these patients to pediatric centers.

Selected References

The full list of references for this chapter appears in the online version.

1. Pui CH, Robison LL, Look AT. Acute lymphoblastic leukaemia. *Lancet* 2008;371:1030.
2. Pinkerton R. Continuing challenges in childhood non-Hodgkin's lymphoma. *Br J Haematol* 2005;130:480.
3. Pui CH, Evans WE. Treatment of acute lymphoblastic leukemia. *N Engl J Med* 2006;354:166.
4. Rademaker J. Hodgkin's and non-Hodgkin's lymphomas. *Radiol Clin North Am* 2007;45:69.
9. Rubnitz JE, Gibson B, Smith FO. Acute myeloid leukemia. *Hematol Oncol Clin North Am* 2010;24:35.

10. Bleyer A, Morgan S, Barr R. Proceedings of a workshop: bridging the gap in care and addressing participation in clinical trials. *Cancer* 2006;107:1656.
12. Faderl S, O'Brien S, Pui CH, et al. Adult acute lymphoblastic leukemia: concepts and strategies. *Cancer* 2010;116:1165.
15. Bhatia S, Sather HN, Heerema NA, Trigg ME, Gaynon PS, Robison LL. Racial and ethnic differences in survival of children with acute lymphoblastic leukemia. *Blood* 2002;100:1957.
35. Trevino LR, Yang W, French D, et al. Germline genomic variants associated with childhood acute lymphoblastic leukemia. *Nat Genet* 2009;41:1001.
38. Zwaan MC, Reinhardt D, Hitzler J, Vyas P. Acute leukemias in children with down syndrome. *Pediatr Clin North Am* 2008;55:53, x.
40. Rabin KR, Whitlock JA. Malignancy in children with trisomy 21. *Oncologist* 2009;14:164.
43. Maloney KW, Carroll WL, Carroll AJ, et al. Down syndrome childhood acute lymphoblastic leukemia has a unique spectrum of sentinel cytogenetic lesions that influences treatment outcome: a report from the Children's Oncology Group. *Blood* 2010;116(7):1045.
53. Pui CH, Campana D. New definition of remission in childhood acute lymphoblastic leukemia. *Leukemia* 2000;14:783.
55. Campana D. Minimal residual disease in acute lymphoblastic leukemia. *Semin Hematol* 2009;46:100.
57. Pui CH, Howard SC. Current management and challenges of malignant disease in the CNS in paediatric leukaemia. *Lancet Oncol* 2008;9:257.
59. Holleman A, Cheok MH, den Boer ML, et al. Gene-expression patterns in drug-resistant acute lymphoblastic leukemia cells and response to treatment. *N Engl J Med* 2004;351:533.
62. Smith M, Arthur D, Camitta B, et al. Uniform approach to risk classification and treatment assignment for children with acute lymphoblastic leukemia. *J Clin Oncol* 1996;14:18.
63. Hilden JM, Dinndorf PA, Meerbaum SO, et al. Analysis of prognostic factors of acute lymphoblastic leukemia in infants: report on CCG 1953 from the Children's Oncology Group. *Blood* 2006;108:441.
66. Nachman JB, La MK, Hunger SP, et al. Young adults with acute lymphoblastic leukemia have an excellent outcome with chemotherapy alone and benefit from intensive postinduction treatment: a report from the Children's Oncology Group. *J Clin Oncol* 2009;27:5189.
71. Rubnitz JE, Wichlan D, Devidas M, et al. Prospective analysis of TEL gene rearrangements in childhood acute lymphoblastic leukemia: a Children's Oncology Group study. *J Clin Oncol* 2008;26:2186.
74. Schultz KR, Bowman WP, Aledo A, et al. Improved early event-free survival with imatinib in Philadelphia chromosome-positive acute lymphoblastic leukemia: a Children's Oncology Group Study. *J Clin Oncol* 2009; 27(31):5175.
80. Silverman LB, Gelber RD, Young ML, Dalton VK, Barr RD, Sallan SE. Induction failure in acute lymphoblastic leukemia of childhood. *Cancer* 1999;85:1395.
81. Borowitz MJ, Devidas M, Hunger SP, et al. Clinical significance of minimal residual disease in childhood acute lymphoblastic leukemia and its relationship to other prognostic factors: a Children's Oncology Group study. *Blood* 2008;111:5477.
84. Chauvenet AR, Martin PL, Devidas M, et al. Antimetabolite therapy for lesser-risk B-lineage acute lymphoblastic leukemia of childhood: a report from Children's Oncology Group Study P9201. *Blood* 2007;110:1105.
85. Pui CH, Evans WE, Relling MV. Are children with lesser-risk B-lineage acute lymphoblastic leukemia curable with antimetabolite therapy? *Nat Clin Pract Oncol* 2008;5:130.
88. Waber DP, Turek J, Catania L, et al. Neuropsychological outcomes from a randomized trial of triple intrathecal chemotherapy compared with 18 Gy cranial radiation as CNS treatment in acute lymphoblastic leukemia: findings from Dana-Farber Cancer Institute ALL Consortium Protocol 95-01. *J Clin Oncol* 2007;25:4914.
90. Barredo JC, Devidas M, Lauer SJ, et al. Isolated CNS relapse of acute lymphoblastic leukemia treated with intensive systemic chemotherapy and delayed CNS radiation: a pediatric oncology group study. *J Clin Oncol* 2006;24:3142.
92. Nguyen K, Devidas M, Cheng SC, et al. Factors influencing survival after relapse from acute lymphoblastic leukemia: a Children's Oncology Group study. *Leukemia* 2008;22:2142.
95. Jeha S. New therapeutic strategies in acute lymphoblastic leukemia. *Semin Hematol* 2009;46:76.
103. Woods WG, Neudorf S, Gold S, et al. A comparison of allogeneic bone marrow transplantation, autologous bone marrow transplantation, and aggressive chemotherapy in children with acute myeloid leukemia in remission. *Blood* 2001;97:56.
104. Bunin NJ, Davies SM, Aplenc R, et al. Unrelated donor bone marrow transplantation for children with acute myeloid leukemia beyond first remission or refractory to chemotherapy. *J Clin Oncol* 2008;26:4326.
105. Horan JT, Alonzo TA, Lyman GH, et al. Impact of disease risk on efficacy of matched related bone marrow transplantation for pediatric acute myeloid leukemia: the Children's Oncology Group. *J Clin Oncol* 2008;26:5797.
107. Ribeiro R. Update on the management of pediatric acute promyelocytic leukemia. *Clin Adv Hematol Oncol* 2006;4:263.
108. Zhou J, Zhang Y, Li J, et al. Single-agent arsenic trioxide in the treatment of children with newly diagnosed acute promyelocytic leukemia. *Blood* 2010;115:1697.
113. Hasle H, Abrahamsson J, Arola M, et al. Myeloid leukemia in children 4 years or older with Down syndrome often lacks GATA1 mutation and cytogenetics and risk of relapse are more akin to sporadic AML. *Leukemia* 2008;22:1428.
126. Belgaumi AF, Al-Shehri A, Ayas M, et al. Clinical characteristics and treatment outcome of pediatric patients with chronic myeloid leukemia. *Haematologica* 2010;95(7):1211.
127. Maziarz RT. Who with chronic myelogenous leukemia to transplant in the era of tyrosine kinase inhibitors? *Curr Opin Hematol* 2008;15:127.
129. Hasle H. Myelodysplastic and myeloproliferative disorders in children. *Curr Opin Pediatr* 2007;19:1.
130. Locatelli F, Nollke P, Zecca M, et al. Hematopoietic stem cell transplantation (HSCT) in children with juvenile myelomonocytic leukemia (JMML): results of the EWOG-MDS/EBMT trial. *Blood* 2005;105:410.
133. Shukla NN, Trippett TM. Non-Hodgkin's lymphoma in children and adolescents. *Curr Oncol Rep* 2006;8:387.
138. Perger L, Lee EY, Shamberger RC. Management of children and adolescents with a critical airway due to compression by an anterior mediastinal mass. *J Pediatr Surg* 2008;43:1990.
139. DeAngelo DJ. Nelarabine for the treatment of patients with relapsed or refractory T-cell acute lymphoblastic leukemia or lymphoblastic lymphoma. *Hematol Oncol Clin North Am* 2009;23:1121, vii–viii.
141. Real PJ, Ferrando AA. NOTCH inhibition and glucocorticoid therapy in T-cell acute lymphoblastic leukemia. *Leukemia* 2009;23:1374.
143. Cohen MH, Johnson JR, Justice R, Pazdur R. FDA drug approval summary: nelarabine (Arranon) for the treatment of T-cell lymphoblastic leukemia/lymphoma. *Oncologist* 2008;13:709.
147. Lowe EJ, Pui CH, Hancock ML, Geiger TL, Khan RB, Sandlund JT. Early complications in children with acute lymphoblastic leukemia presenting with hyperleukocytosis. *Pediatr Blood Cancer* 2005;45:10.
149. Crews KR, Zhou Y, Pauley JL, et al. Effect of allopurinol versus urate oxidase on methotrexate pharmacokinetics in children with newly diagnosed acute lymphoblastic leukemia. *Cancer* 2009;116:227.
150. Hesseling P, Molyneux E, Kamiza S, Israels T, Broadhead R. Endemic Burkitt lymphoma: a 28-day treatment schedule with cyclophosphamide and intrathecal methotrexate. *Ann Trop Paediatr* 2009;29:29.
153. Patte C, Auperin A, Gerrard M, et al. Results of the randomized international FAB/LMB96 trial for intermediate risk B-cell non-Hodgkin lymphoma in children and adolescents: it is possible to reduce treatment for the early responding patients. *Blood* 2007;109:2773.
158. Schwartz CL, Constine LS, Villaluna D, et al. A risk-adapted, response-based approach using ABVE-PC for children and adolescents with intermediate- and high-risk Hodgkin lymphoma: the results of P9425. *Blood* 2009;114:2051.
162. Furth C, Denecke T, Steffen I, et al. Correlative imaging strategies implementing CT, MRI, and PET for staging of childhood Hodgkin disease. *J Pediatr Hematol Oncol* 2006;28:501.
165. Pellegrino B, Terrier-Lacombe MJ, Oberlin O, et al. Lymphocyte-predominant Hodgkin's lymphoma in children: therapeutic abstention after initial lymph node resection—a study of the French Society of Pediatric Oncology. *J Clin Oncol* 2003;21:2948.

CHAPTER 125 MOLECULAR BIOLOGY OF LYMPHOMAS

URBAN NOVAK, LAURA PASQUALUCCI, AND RICCARDO DALLA-FAVERA

The term *lymphoma* identifies a heterogeneous group of biologically and clinically distinct neoplasms that originate from the lymphoid organs and have historically been divided into two distinct categories, namely non–Hodgkin's lymphoma (NHL) and Hodgkin's lymphoma (HL).[1,2] During the past 3 decades, significant progress has been made in elucidating the molecular pathogenesis of lymphoid malignancies as a clonal malignant expansion of B cells (in the majority of cases) or of T cells. The molecular characterization of the most frequent genetic abnormalities associated with lymphoma development has led to the identification of a number of protooncogenes and tumor suppressor genes that are altered in B-cell NHL (B-NHL) and whose abnormal functioning contributes to lymphoma pathogenesis. Relatively less is known about the pathogenesis of T-cell NHL (T-NHL) and HL. This chapter will focus on the molecular pathogenesis of the most common types of lymphoma, including B-NHL, T-NHL, HL, and chronic lymphocytic leukemia/small lymphocytic lymphoma (CLL/SLL), which also derives from mature B cells. Emphasis will be given to the mechanisms of genetic lesion and the nature of the involved genes in relationship to the normal biology of lymphocytes.

THE CELL OF ORIGIN OF LYMPHOMA

Lymphomas originate from mature B cells in approximately 85% of the cases, while the remaining 15% derive from the T-cell lineage. A key concept for the understanding of lymphomagenesis is the relationship between these tumors and the unique DNA modification events that take place in normal lymphocytes in order to enable the production of highly efficient neutralizing antibodies in B cells, and to encode T-cell receptors in T cells.

Normal B-Cell Development and the Dynamics of the Germinal Center Reaction

B lymphocytes are generated from a common pluripotent stem cell in the bone marrow, where precursor B cells first assemble their immunoglobulin heavy chain locus (*IGH*) followed by the light chain loci (*IGL*) through a site-specific process of cleavage and rejoining, known as V(D)J recombination.[3,4] Cells that fail to express a functional (and nonautoreactive) antigen receptor are eliminated within the bone marrow, while B-cell precursors that have successfully rearranged their antibody genes are positively selected to migrate into peripheral lymphoid organs as mature, naive B cells.[5] In most B cells, the subsequent maturation steps are linked to the histologic structure of the germinal center (GC), a highly specialized microenvironment that forms following encounter of naive B cells with a foreign antigen, together with signals from CD4+ T and antigen-presenting cells.[5–7]

The development of the GC can be schematically described as occurring in two stages. First, B cells enter the GC dark zone, which consists of rapidly proliferating centroblasts (CBs) (doubling time <12 hours). In this phase, CBs modify the variable region of their Ig genes (*IgV*) by the process of somatic hypermutation (SHM), which introduces mostly single nucleotide substitutions but also deletions and duplications in order to change their affinity for the antigen.[5,7–10] CBs express elevated levels of BCL6,[11,12] a transcriptional repressor[13] that negatively regulates a broad set of genes, including those involved in (1) B-cell receptor (BCR) and CD40 signaling[14,15]; (2) T-cell mediated B-cell activation[14]; (3) induction of apoptosis[14,16]; (4) response to DNA damage, by modulation of genes involved in the sensing and execution of DNA damage responses[17–20]; (5) multiple cytokine and chemokine signaling pathways, including the ones involved in interferon and transforming growth factor-β responses[14,16]; and (6) plasma cell differentiation, via suppression of the PRDM1/BLIMP1 master regulator.[21–24] This transcriptional program suggests that the BCL6 function is critical to establish the proliferative status of CBs while allowing the execution of DNA modification processes (SHM and class-switch recombination) without eliciting responses to DNA damage, and preventing premature activation and differentiation prior to the selection for the survival of cells producing high affinity antibodies.

In the light zone, CBs are thought to cease proliferation and differentiate into centrocytes (CCs), which are rechallenged by the antigen through the interaction with CD4+ T cells and follicular dendritic cells.[5,6] CCs expressing a BCR with reduced affinity for the antigen are eliminated by apoptosis, while a few cells with high affinity will be stimulated by a variety of signals, including the engagement of their BCR by the antigen itself and the activation of the CD40 receptor by the CD40 ligand present on CD4+ T cells. These signals down-regulate BCL6, allowing the arrest of proliferation and the restoration of DNA damage responses, as well as activation and differentiation capabilities, such that B cells can be selected for survival and differentiation into memory cells and plasma cells.[6,25] In the GC, CCs also undergo class-switch recombination (CSR), a DNA remodeling event that confers distinct effector functions to the antibodies.[26] Both SHM and CSR depend on the activity of the activation-induced cytidine deaminase (AID) enzyme and represent B-cell–specific functions that modify the genome of B cells via mechanisms involving

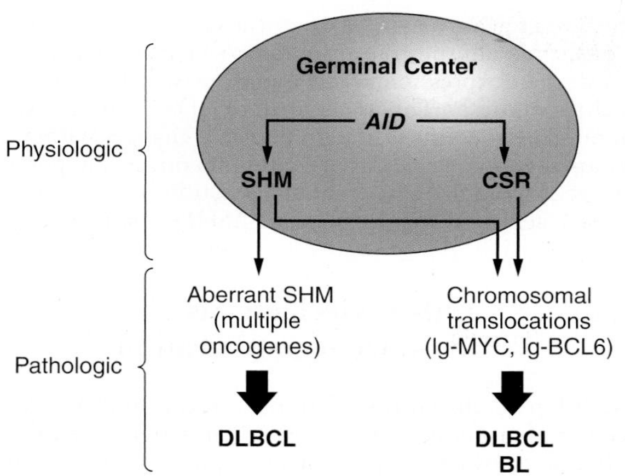

FIGURE 125.1 Model for the generation of genetic lesions during lymphomagenesis. B-NHL–associated genetic lesions appear to be due to mistakes occurring during the physiologic processes of somatic hypermutation and class-switch recombination in the highly proliferative environment of the germinal center (*top*). These include chromosomal translocations, which in most cases juxtapose the *Ig* genes to one of several protooncogenes (e.g., *BCL6* or *MYC*), and aberrant somatic hypermutation of multiple target genes AID, activation-induced cytidine deaminase; SHM, somatic hypermutation; CSR, class-switch recombination.

single- or double-strand breaks,[27–29] a notion that will become important in the understanding of the mechanisms generating genetic alterations in B-NHL.

This schematic description is useful to focus on two key concepts for the understanding of B-NHL pathogenesis. First, the activity of SHM, which introduces irreversible DNA changes in the genome, allowed to conclude that most B-NHL types, with the exception of mantle-cell lymphoma (MCL), derive from GC-experienced B cells, as they contain hypermutated IgV sequences, and that clonal expansion occurred within the GC, because the malignant clones contain largely identical mutations, suggesting the derivation from a single founder cell.[30] Second, the most frequent oncogenic events in B-NHL—namely, chromosomal translocations and aberrant somatic hypermutation (ASHM)—result from mistakes in the machinery that normally diversifies the *Ig* genes during B lymphocyte differentiation, further supporting the GC origin of most B-NHL (Fig. 125.1). Finally, the definition of two distinct phases during GC development reflects stages of B-cell differentiation and function that can to some extent be recognized in different B-NHL subtypes.

Normal T-Cell Development

T-cell development proceeds through sequential stages defined according to the expression of the molecules CD4 and CD8. Committed lymphoid progenitors exit the bone marrow and migrate to the thymus as early T-cell progenitors or double-negative 1 (DN1) cells, which lack expression of CD4 and CD8 as well as of the T-cell receptor (TCR).[31] In the thymic cortex, T cells advance through the double-negative stages DN2, DN3, and DN4, while undergoing specific rearrangements at the TCRβ locus in order to acquire expression of the pre-TCR.[31] Those thymocytes that have successfully recombined the pre-TCR will be selected to further differentiate into double-positive cells (DP; CD4+CD8+), which express a complete surface TCR and can then enter a process of positive and negative selection in the medulla, before exiting the thymus as single positive T cells.[31] The end result of this process is a pool of mature T cells that exhibit coordinated TCR and coreceptor specificities as required for effective immune responses to foreign antigens. Most mature T-NHLs arise from postthymic T cells in the lymphoid organs.

GENERAL MECHANISMS OF GENETIC LESION IN LYMPHOMA

Chromosomal Translocations

Chromosomal translocations are the genetic hallmark of malignancies derived from the hematopoietic system. Lymphoma-associated translocations represent reciprocal and balanced recombination events that occur between two specific chromosomes, are clonally represented in each tumor case, and are often recurrently associated with a given tumor type.

Although the precise molecular mechanisms that are responsible for the generation of translocations remain partially obscure, significant advances have been obtained during the past decade in our understanding of the events that are required for their initiation.[32] It has now been documented that chromosomal translocations occur at least in part as a consequence of mistakes during *Ig* and *TCR* gene rearrangements in B and T cells, respectively. Based on the characteristics of the chromosomal breakpoint, three distinct scenarios can be distinguished: (1) translocations derived from mistakes of the RAG-mediated V(D)J recombination process, as is the case for translocations involving *IGH* and *CCND1* in MCL or *IGH* and *BCL2* in follicular lymphoma (FL)[32–34]; (2) translocations mediated by errors in the AID-dependent CSR process, such as those involving the *Ig* genes and *MYC* in sporadic Burkitt lymphoma (BL)[32]; and (3) translocations occurring as by-products of the AID-mediated SHM mechanism, which also generates DNA breaks, such as those joining the *Ig* and *MYC* loci in endemic BL.[32] Conclusive experimental evidence for the involvement of antibody-associated remodeling events has been recently provided through *in vivo* studies performed in lymphoma-prone mouse models, where the removal of the AID enzyme was sufficient to abrogate the generation of *MYC-IGH* translocations in normal B cells undergoing CSR[35,36] and to prevent the development of GC-derived B-NHL.[37,38]

The common feature of all NHL-associated chromosomal translocations is the presence of a protooncogene in proximity to the chromosomal recombination sites. In most lymphoma types, and in contrast with acute leukemias, the coding domain of the oncogene is not affected by the translocation, but its pattern of expression is altered as a consequence of the juxtaposition of heterologous regulatory sequences derived from the partner chromosome (protooncogene deregulation) (Fig. 125.2). Two distinct types of protooncogene deregulation (i.e., homotopic and heterotopic) can be distinguished. Homotopic deregulation occurs when the protooncogene becomes constitutively expressed in the lymphoma cell, while its expression is tightly regulated in normal lymphoid cells. Conversely, heterotopic deregulation occurs when the protooncogene is not expressed in the normal tumor counterpart and undergoes ectopic expression in the lymphoma. In most types of NHL-associated translocations, the heterologous regulatory sequences responsible for protooncogene deregulation are derived from antigen receptor loci that are expressed at high levels in the target tissue.[32] However, in certain translocations, such as the ones involving BCL6 in diffuse large B-cell lymphoma (DLBCL), different promoter regions from distinct chromosomal sites can be juxtaposed to the protooncogene in individual tumor cases, a concept known as *promiscuous translocations*.[39–46]

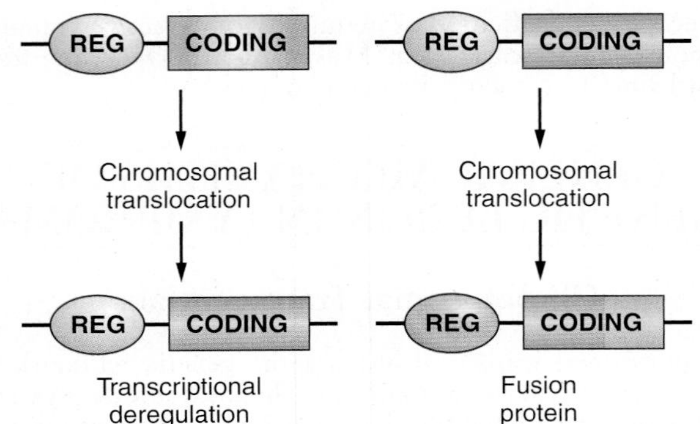

FIGURE 125.2 Molecular consequences of chromosomal translocations. *Top panel*: schematic representation of the two protooncogenes involved in prototypic chromosomal translocations, with their regulatory (REG) and coding sequences. Only one side of the balanced, reciprocal translocations is indicated. *Bottom panel*: two distinct outcomes of chromosomal translocations. In the case of transcriptional deregulation (*left scheme*), the normal regulatory sequences of the protooncogene are substituted with regulatory sequences derived from the partner chromosome, leading to deregulated expression of the protooncogene. In most cases of B-NHL, the heterologous regulatory regions derive from the *Ig* loci. In the case of fusion proteins (*right scheme*), the coding sequences of the two involved genes are joined in frame into a chimeric transcriptional unit that encodes for a fusion protein, characterized by novel biochemical and functional properties.

Less commonly, B-NHL–associated chromosomal translocations juxtapose the coding regions of the two involved genes to form a chimeric unit that encodes for a novel fusion protein, an outcome typically observed in chromosomal translocation associated with acute leukemia (Fig. 125.2). Examples are the t(11;18) of mucosa-associated lymphoid tissue (MALT) lymphoma and the t(2;5) of anaplastic large cell lymphoma (ALCL). The molecular cloning of the genetic loci involved in most recurrent translocations has led to the identification of a number of protooncogenes involved in lymphomagenesis (Table 125.1).

Aberrant Somatic Hypermutation

The term *aberrant somatic hypermutation* (ASHM) defines a recently identified mechanism of genetic lesion that is uniquely associated with B-NHL, particularly DLBCL, leading to the mutation of multiple non-Ig genes.[47] ASHM has been proposed to derive from a malfunction in the physiologic SHM process, although the mechanism involved in this malfunction has not been identified.

In GC B cells, SHM is tightly regulated both spatially and temporally to introduce mutations only in the rearranged *IgV* genes[8] as well as in the 5′ region of a few other genes, including *BCL6* and the *CD79* components of the B-cell receptor,[48–52] although the functional role of the mutations found in these other genes remains obscure. On the contrary, multiple mutational events were found to affect numerous loci in over 50% of DLBCL cases, as well as in a few other lymphoma types, including, among others, AIDS-associated B-NHL, primary central nervous system lymphomas, and posttransplant lymphoproliferative disorders.[53–57] The identified target loci comprise more than 10% of the genes transcribed in B cells and include several well-known protooncogenes such as *PIM1* and *MYC*, one of the most frequently altered human oncogenes.[47] These mutations are typically distributed within ~2 Kb from the transcription initiation site (i.e., the hypermutable domain in the Ig locus)[58] and, depending on the genomic configuration of the target gene, may affect nontranslated as well as coding regions, thus altering the response to factors that normally regulate their expression, or changing key structural and functional properties.[47] This is the case of *MYC*, where a significant number of events lead to amino acid changes with proven functional consequences in activating its oncogenic potential. However, a comprehensive characterization of the potentially extensive genetic damage caused by ASHM is still lacking.

Other Mechanisms of Protooncogene Alteration

In addition to chromosomal translocations and ASHM, the structure of protooncogenes and/or their pattern of expression can be altered by gene copy number amplifications and somatic point mutations. Compared with epithelial cancer, only a few genes have been identified so far as specific targets of chromosomal amplification in B-NHL, as exemplified by *REL* and *BCL2* in DLBCL,[59–62] and PD-1 ligands in primary mediastinal B-cell lymphoma (PMBCL).[63] However, the recent introduction of advanced cytogenetic and high-resolution, genome-wide single nucleotide polymorphism array technologies is likely to reveal a more complex scenario, leading to the identification of additional chromosomal sites of amplification. Somatic point mutations may alter the coding sequence of the target protooncogene and thus the biological properties of its protein product, as observed in *MYC* and *BCL2*.[25,64–66] More recently, a number of genes involved in the activation of the NF-κB transcription complex have also been found to harbor oncogenic point mutations in DLBCL, leading to constitutive activation of NF-κB.[67,68] Mutations of the *RAS* genes, a very frequent protooncogene alteration in human neoplasia, are virtually absent in lymphomas.[69]

Inactivation of Tumor Suppressor Genes

Until recently, the *TP53* gene, possibly the most common target of genetic alteration in human cancer,[70] remained one of few *bona fide* tumor suppressor genes involved in the pathogenesis of NHL, although at generally low frequencies and restricted to specific disease subtypes, such as BL and DLBCL derived from the transformation of FL or CLL.[71–73] The mechanism of *TP53* inactivation in NHL is similar to that detected in human neoplasia in general, entailing point mutation of one allele and chromosomal deletion or mutation of the second allele.[70] In recent years, additional genes have been identified as targets of biallelic inactivation in B-NHL through specific chromosomal deletions and/or mutations. Two such genes lie on the long arm of chromosome 6 (6q), a region long known to be deleted in a large percentage of aggressive lymphomas, and associated with poor prognosis[74,75]: the *PRDM1/BLIMP1* gene on 6q21, which is biallelically inactivated in ~25% of activated B-cell-like (ABC)-DLBCL cases,[76–78] and the gene encoding for the negative NF-κB regulator *INFAIP3* on chromosome 6q23, which is commonly lost in ABC-DLBCL, PMBCL, and subtypes of marginal-zone lymphoma and HL.[67,79–81]

Deletions of chromosome 13q14.3 represent the most frequent lesions in CLL (>50% of cases)[82,83] and encompass three noncoding elements, namely the *DLEU2/mir-15a/16-1* cluster,[84–87] whose deletion in mice promotes the development of CLL,[88] documenting its pathogenetic role. Tumor suppressor inactivation via epigenetic transcriptional silencing was described for *CDKN2A* (*p16/INK4a*) as an infrequent event in various B-NHL.[89,90] More recently, monoallelic inactivating mutations and deletions were found to affect the acetyltransferase genes *CREBBP* and *EP300* in a significant proportion

TABLE 125.1

MOST COMMON GENETIC LESIONS ASSOCIATED WITH NON-HODGKIN'S LYMPHOMA (NHL)

NHL Subtype	Genetic Abnormality	% of Cases Affected	Involved Gene	Functional Consequences	Gene Function
Mantle cell lymphoma	t(11;14)(q13;q32)	95	*CCND1*	Transcriptional deregulation	Cell-cycle regulation
Burkitt lymphoma	t(8;14)(q24;q32)	80	*MYC*	Transcriptional deregulation	Control of proliferation and growth
	t(2;8)(p11;q24)	15	*MYC*	Transcriptional deregulation	
	t(8;22)(q24;q11)	5	*MYC*	Transcriptional deregulation	
Follicular lymphoma	t(14;18)(q32;q21)	90	*BCL2*	Transcriptional deregulation	Antiapoptosis
	t(2;18)(p11;q21)	Rare	*BCL2*	Transcriptional deregulation	
	t(18;22)(q21;q11)	Rare	*BCL2*	Transcriptional deregulation	
Diffuse large B-cell lymphoma (GCB)	t(8;14)(q24;q32)	10	*MYC*	Transcriptional deregulation	Proliferation and growth
	t(14;18)(q32;q21)	30	*BCL2*	Transcriptional deregulation	Antiapoptosis
	t(3;other)(q27;other)	15	*BCL6*	Transcriptional deregulation	DNA damage responses; differentiation
	EZH2 M	20	*EZH2*	Unknown	Chromatin remodeling
Diffuse large B-cell lymphoma (ABC)	t(3;other)(q27;other)	25	*BCL6*	Transcriptional deregulation	DNA damage responses; differentiation
	TNFAIP3 M/D	20	*TNFAIP3*	Loss of function	Negative NF-κB regulator
	PRDM1 M/D	20	*PRDM1*	Loss of function	Terminal B-cell differentiation
	CD79B M	18	*CD79B*	Gain of function	Chronic active BCR signaling
	CARD11 M	9	*CARD11*	Gain of function	Positive NF-κB regulator
	18q21 amplifications	30	*BCL2*	Increased gene dosage	Antiapoptosis
Primary mediastinal B cell lymphoma	9p24.1 amplifications	50	*JAK2*	Increased gene dosage	JAK-STAT pathway regulation
			PDL1, PDL2	Increased gene dosage	Immunomodulatory responses
MALT lymphoma	t(11;18)(q21;q21)	30	*API2-MALT1*	Fusion protein	Positive NF-κB regulator
	t(14;18)(q32;q21)	15–20	*MALT1*	Transcriptional deregulation	Positive NF-κB regulator
	t(3;14)(p13;q32)	10	*FOXP1*	Transcriptional deregulation	Transcription factor
	t(1;14)(p22;q32)	5	*BCL10*	Transcriptional deregulation	Positive NF-κB regulator
Lymphoplasmacytic lymphoma	t(9;14)(p13;q32)	50	PAX5	Transcriptional deregulation	B-cell proliferation and differentiation
Anaplastic large cell lymphoma	t(2;5)(p23;q35)	60[a]	*NPM/ALK*	Fusion protein	Tyrosine kinase
Classic Hodgkin's lymphoma	TNFAIP3 M/D	40[b]	*TNFAIP3*	Loss of function	Negative NF-κB regulator
	SOCS1 M/D	45	*SOCS1*	Loss of function	JAK-STAT pathway regulation
	2p13 amplifications	50	*REL*	Increased gene dosage	Positive NF-κB regulator
	9p24.1 amplifications	50	*JAK2*	Increased gene dosage	JAK-STAT pathway regulation
			PDL1, PDL2	Increased gene dosage	Immunomodulatory responses

GCB, germinal center B-cell-like; ABC, activated B-cell-like; BCR, B-cell receptor; MALT, extranodal marginal zone lymphoma of mucosa-associated lymphoid tissue; M, mutation; D, deletion.
[a]In the adult population; 85% in childhood.
[b]Sixty percent in Epstein-Barr virus–negative cases.

of DLBCL and FL, suggesting a role as haploinsufficient tumor suppressors.[91] Major efforts are currently ongoing to identify the total complement of genetic lesions that are associated with the development of various lymphoma types by taking advantage of recently developed genome-wide technologies.

Infectious Agents

Viral and bacterial infections have both been implicated in the pathogenesis of lymphoma. At least three viruses are associated with specific NHL subtypes: the Epstein-Barr virus (EBV), the human herpesvirus-8 (HHV-8/KSHV), and the human T-cell leukemia virus type 1 (HTLV-1). Other infectious agents, such as human immunodeficiency virus (HIV), hepatitis C virus (HCV), *Helicobacter pylori,* and *Chlamydophila psittaci,* have an indirect role in NHL pathogenesis by either impairing the immune system and/or providing chronic antigenic stimulation.

EBV was initially identified in cases of endemic African BL[92,93] and subsequently detected also in a fraction of sporadic BL, HIV-related lymphomas and primary effusion lymphomas (PELs).[71,94–100] On infection of a B lymphocyte, the EBV genome is transported into the nucleus, where it exists predominantly as an extrachromosomal circular molecule (episome).[101] The formation of circular episomes is mediated by the cohesive terminal repeats, which are represented by a variable number of tandem repeats sequence.[101,102] Because of this termini heterogeneity, the number of tandem repeats sequences enclosed in newly formed episomes may differ considerably, thus representing a clonal marker of a single infected cell.[102] Evidence for a pathogenetic role of the virus in NHL infected by EBV is at least twofold. First, it is well recognized that EBV is able to significantly alter the growth of B cells.[101] Second, EBV-infected lymphomas usually display a single form of fused EBV termini, suggesting that the lymphoma cell population represents the clonally expanded progeny of a single infected cell.[71,94] Nonetheless, the role of EBV in lymphomagenesis is still unclear as the virus infects virtually all humans during their lifetime and its transforming genes are commonly not expressed in the tumor cells of BL.

HHV-8 is a gammaherpesvirus initially identified in tissues of HIV-related Kaposi sarcoma[103] and subsequently found to infect PEL cells as well as a substantial fraction of multicentric Castleman disease.[104–107] Phylogenetic analysis has shown that the closest relative of HHV-8 is herpesvirus saimiri, a gamma-2 herpesvirus of primates associated with T-cell lymphoproliferative disorders.[108] Like other gammaherpesviruses, HHV-8 is also lymphotropic and can be found in lymphocytes both *in vitro* and *in vivo*.[103,106,107] Lymphoma cells naturally infected by HHV-8 harbor the viral genome in its episomal configuration and display a marked restriction of viral gene expression, suggesting a pattern of latent infection.[108]

HTLV-1 is a member of the lentivirus group that can immortalize normal T cells *in vitro* and can cause adult T-cell leukemia/lymphoma (ATLL).[109–112] Unlike acutely transforming retroviruses, the HTLV-1 genome does not encode a viral oncogene. Moreover, this retrovirus does not transform T cells by *cis*-activation of an adjacent cellular protooncogene because the provirus appears to integrate randomly within the host genome.[110–112] Rather, the pathogenetic effect of HTLV-1 seems to be due to viral production of a transregulatory protein (HTLV-1 tax) that activates the transcription of several host genes.[113–119]

An association between B-NHL and infection by HCV, a single-stranded RNA virus of the Flaviviridae family, has been proposed because of the increased risk of developing lymphoproliferative disorders among HCV-positive patients.[120] Although the underlying mechanisms remain unclear, current models suggest that chronic B-cell stimulation by antigens associated with HCV infection may induce nonmalignant B-cell expansion, which subsequently evolves into B-NHL by accumulating additional genetic lesions.

A causal link between antigen stimulation by *H. pylori* and MALT lymphoma originating in the stomach is documented by the observation that *H. pylori* can be found in the vast majority of the lymphoma specimens,[121–123] and long-term complete regression of the disease is achieved in 70% of cases on eradication of infection with antibiotics.[124] However, cases with t(11;18)(q21;21) respond poorly to antibiotic eradication.[125]

C. psittaci, an obligate intracellular bacterium, was recently linked to the development of ocular adnexal marginal zone B-cell lymphoma, although variations in prevalence among different geographic areas remain a major investigational issue.[4,126,127] In this indolent lymphoma, *C. psittaci* causes both local and systemic persistent infection, presumably contributing to lymphomagenesis via its mitogenic activity as well as through its ability to promote polyclonal cell proliferation and to induce resistance to apoptosis in the infected cells *in vivo*. Notably, bacterial eradication with antibiotic therapy is often followed by lymphoma regression.[128]

MOLECULAR PATHOGENESIS OF B-CELL NON-HODGKIN'S LYMPHOMA

The following section will focus on well-characterized genetic lesions that are associated with the most common types of B-NHL, classified according to the World Health Organization classification of lymphoid neoplasia.[2] The molecular pathogenesis of HIV-related NHL will also be addressed, while the pathogenesis of other B-cell NHL types remains far less understood.

Mantle Cell Lymphoma

Cell of Origin

MCL is an aggressive disease representing ~5% of all NHL diagnoses and generally regarded as incurable.[2,89] Based on immunophenotype, gene expression profile, and molecular features, such as the presence of unmutated *IgV* genes in most cases, MCL is thought to derive from naïve, pre-GC peripheral B cells located in the inner mantle zone of secondary follicles (Fig. 125.3).

Genetic Lesions

MCL is typically associated with the t(11;14)(q13;q32) translocation that juxtaposes the *IGH* gene on chromosome 14q32 to a region containing the *CCND1* gene (also known as *BCL1*) on chromosome 11q13 (Table 125.1).[129–131] The translocation consistently leads to homotopic deregulation and overexpression of cyclin D1, a member of the D-type G_1 cyclins that regulates the early phases of the cell cycle and is normally not expressed in resting B cells.[132–134] By deregulating cyclin D1, t(11;14) is thought to contribute to malignant transformation by perturbing the G_1-S phase transition of the cell cycle.[89] In addition to t(11;14), up to 10% of MCLs overexpress aberrant or shorter cyclin D1 transcripts, as a consequence of secondary rearrangements, microdeletions, or point mutations in the gene 3′ untranslated region.[135–137] These alterations may lead to cyclin D1 overexpression through the removal of destabilizing sequences and the consequent increase in mRNA half-life. Typically, this subset of cases is characterized by high proliferative activity and a more aggressive clinical course.[138] The pathogenetic role of cyclin D1 deregulation in

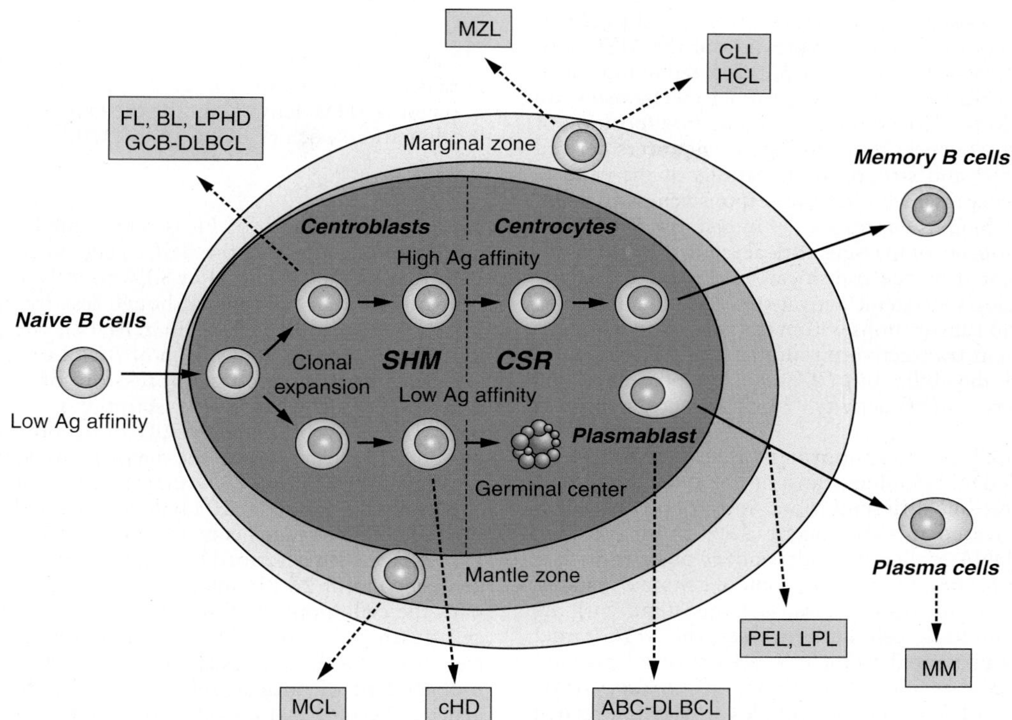

FIGURE 125.3 Normal B-cell development and lymphomagenesis. Schematic representation of a lymphoid follicle, constituted by the germinal center (GC) and the mantle zone, along with the surrounding marginal zone. B cells that have successfully rearranged their *Ig* genes in the bone marrow move to peripheral lymphoid organs as naïve B cells. On encounter with a T-cell–dependent antigen, B cells become proliferating centroblasts in the GC and eventually mature into centrocytes. These events are associated with the activation of somatic hypermutation and class-switch recombination. Only GC B cells with high affinity for the antigen will be positively selected to exit the GC and further differentiate into plasma cells or memory B cells, while low-affinity clones are eliminated by apoptosis. *Dotted arrows* indicate the putative normal counterpart of various lymphoma subtypes, as identified based on the presence of somatically mutated *IgV* genes, as well as on distinctive phenotypic features. MCL, mantle cell lymphoma; FL, follicular lymphoma; BL, Burkitt lymphoma; DLBCL, diffuse large B-cell lymphoma (GCB, germinal center B-cell-like; ABC, activated B-cell-like); CLL, chronic lymphocytic leukemia/ HCL, hairy cell leukemia; MM, multiple myeloma; LPHD, lymphocyte predominance Hodgkin disease; LPL, lympho plasma cytic lymphoma; MZL, marginal zone lymphoma; PEL, primary effusion lymphoma.

human neoplasia is suggested by the ability of the overexpressed protein to transform cells *in vitro* and to promote B-cell lymphomagenesis in transgenic mice,[139–141] although a specific animal model that faithfully recapitulates the features of the human MCL is still lacking. Importantly, the frequency and specificity of this genetic lesion, together with the expression of CCND1 in the tumor cells, provide an excellent marker for MCL diagnosis.[2]

Other genetic alterations involved in MCL include frequent biallelic inactivation of the *ATM* gene by genomic deletions and mutations,[142] loss of the *TP53* gene in 20% of patients, where it represents a marker of poor prognosis,[143] and inactivation of the *CDKN2A* gene by genomic deletion, mutation, or hypermethylation in approximately half of the cases belonging to the MCL variant characterized by a blastoid cell morphology.[144] In a small number of cases, *BMI1* is amplified and/or overexpressed, possibly as an alternative mechanism to the loss of *CDKN2A*.[138,145]

Burkitt Lymphoma

Cell of Origin

BL is an aggressive lymphoma comprising three clinical variants, namely sporadic Burkitt lymphoma (sBL), endemic Burkitt lymphoma (eBL), and HIV-associated BL, often diagnosed as the initial manifestation of AIDS.[2] The presence of highly mutated IgV sequences that carry the hallmark of SHM,[146–149] together with the expression of a distinct gene expression signature,[150,151] indicates the derivation from a GC B cell.

Genetic Lesions

All BL cases, including the leukemic variants, share a virtually obligatory genetic lesion, that is, chromosomal translocations involving the *MYC* gene on region 8q24 and one of the *Ig* loci on the partner chromosome.[152,153] In ~80% of cases, this is represented by the *IGH* locus, leading to t(8;14)(q24;q32), while in the remaining 20% of cases either *IGκ* (2p12) or *IGλ* (22q11) are involved.[152–155] Although fairly homogeneous at the microscopic level, these translocations display a high degree of molecular heterogeneity. The t(8;14) breakpoints are located 5′ and centromeric to *MYC*, whereas they map 3′ to *MYC* in t(2;8) and t(8;22).[152–156] Further molecular heterogeneity derives from the exact breakpoint sites on chromosomes 8 and 14 in t(8;14). Translocations of eBL tend to involve sequences on chromosome 8 at an undefined distance 5′ to *MYC* (>1,000 Kb) and sequences on chromosome 14 within or in proximity to the *Ig* I_H region.[157,158] In sBL, t(8;14) preferentially involves sequences within or immediately 5′ to *MYC* (<3 Kb) on chromosome 8, and sequences within the Ig switch regions on chromosome 14.[157,158]

The common consequence of t(8;14), t(2;8), and t(8;22) is the ectopic and constitutive overexpression of the *MYC* protooncogene,[159–161] which is normally not detected in most proliferating GC B cells.[11] At least two distinct mechanisms are responsible for MYC deregulation, including juxtaposition of the *MYC* coding sequences to heterologous enhancers derived from *Ig* loci,[159–161] and structural alterations of the gene 5′ regulatory sequences, which alter the responsiveness to cellular factors controlling its expression.[162] In fact, the *MYC* exon 1/intron 1 junction, encompassing critical regulatory elements, is either decapitated by the translocation or mutated in the translocated alleles. Oncogenic activation of MYC can also be due to amino acid substitutions within the gene exon 2, encoding for the protein transactivation domain.[64,65] These mutations can abolish the ability of *p107*, a nuclear protein related to *RB1*, to suppress *MYC* activity,[163] or can increase protein stability.[164,165]

MYC is a nuclear phosphoprotein that functions as a sequence specific DNA-binding transcriptional regulator controlling proliferation, differentiation, and apoptosis, all of which are implicated in carcinogenesis.[166,167] In addition, MYC controls DNA replication independent of its transcriptional activity, a property that may promote genomic instability by inducing replication stress.[168] Consistent with its involvement in multiple cellular processes, the MYC target gene network is estimated to include ~15% of all protein-coding genes as well as noncoding RNAs.[167,169] *In vivo,* MYC is found mainly in heterodimeric complexes with the related protein MAX, and such interaction is required for MYC-induced stimulation of transcription and cell proliferation.[170–176] In B-NHL carrying *MYC* translocations, constitutive expression of MYC induces transcription of a subset of target genes that have diverse roles in regulating cell growth by affecting DNA replication, energy metabolism, protein synthesis, and telomere elongation.[167,176,177] In addition, deregulated MYC expression is thought to cause genomic instability, thus contributing to tumor progression by facilitating the occurrence of additional genetic lesions.[178] Dysregulation of MYC expression in a number of transgenic mouse models leads to the development of aggressive B-cell lymphomas with high penetrance and short latency.[165,179,180] These mouse models confirm the pathogenetic role of deregulated MYC in B cells, although the resulting tumors tend to be more immature than the human BL, most likely because of the early activation of the promoter sequences used for expression of the *MYC* transgene.

Cooperating oncogenic events in BL include loss of *TP53* by mutation and/or deletion (30% of both sBL and eBL cases),[72] inactivation of *CDKN2B* by hypermethylation,[181] and deletions of 6q, detected in ~30% of cases, independent of the clinical variant.[74] Additionally, one contributing factor to the development of BL is monoclonal EBV infection, present in virtually all cases of eBL and in ~30% of sBL.[92,94,182,183] The consistent expression of EBER, a class of small RNA molecules, has been proposed to mediate the transforming potential of EBV in BL.[184] However, because EBV infection in BL displays a peculiar latent infection phenotype characterized by negativity of both EBV-transforming antigens LMP1 and EBNA2, the precise pathogenetic role of the virus has remained elusive.[185]

Follicular Lymphoma

FL represents the second most common type of B-NHL, accounting for ~20% of all diagnoses, and the most common low-grade B-NHL.[2] Over time, FL tends to transform into an aggressive lymphoma with a diffuse large cell architecture (Fig. 125.3).[2]

Cell of Origin

FL arises from a GC-derived B cell, as documented by the presence of somatically mutated *Ig* genes that show evidence of ongoing SHM activity, and by the expression of specific GC B-cell markers such as BCL6 and CD10.[1]

Genetic Lesions

The genetic hallmark of FL is represented by chromosomal translocations affecting the *BCL2* gene on chromosome band 18q21, which are detected in 80% to 90% of cases independent of cytologic subtype, although less frequent in grade 3 FL[130,186–189] (Table 125.1). In t(14;18), the rearrangement joins the 3′ untranslated region of *BCL2* to an *Ig* J_H segment, resulting in the ectopic expression of BCL2 in GC B cells,[186,187,190–194] where its transcription is normally repressed by BCL6.[16,25] Approximately 70% of the breakpoints on chromosome 18 cluster within the major breakpoint region, while the remaining 5% to 25% map to the more distant minor cluster region, located ~20 kb downstream of the *BCL2* gene.[186,187,190,191] Rearrangements involving the 5′ flanking region of *BCL2* have been described in a minority of cases.[195] The *BCL2* gene encodes a 26-kD integral membrane protein that controls the cell apoptotic threshold by preventing programmed cell death[196–199]; BCL2 may thus contribute to lymphomagenesis by inducing resistance of tumor cells to apoptosis independent of antigen selection. Nevertheless, additional genetic aberrations are likely required for malignant transformation, a major role being played by chronic antigen stimulation.[200–202]

More recently, somatic mutations of the polycomb-group oncogene *EZH2*, which encodes a histone methyltransferase responsible for the trimethylation of Lys27 of histone H3 (H3K27), were found in 7% of FL patients.[203] These mutations result in the replacement of a single tyrosine (Tyr641) in the SET domain of the EZH2 protein, and were associated with increased levels of H3K27me3 through a mechanism that involves altered substrate catalytic specifity.[203] However, the precise mechanism by which this amino acid change contributes to tumorigenesis remains to be clarified.

Chromosomal translocations of the *BCL6* gene are detected in 6% to 14% of all FL cases, and were shown to have a significantly higher prevalence in the group of patients known to eventually transform into aggressive DLBCL.[204–207] Other genetic lesions are also predominantly observed in FL cases that have undergone histologic progression to a high-grade NHL, and include deletions of chromosome 6 (20% of the cases),[74] *TP53* mutations (25% to 30%),[73,208–210] inactivation of *CDKN2A* through deletion, mutation, and hypermethylation (one-third of patients),[144,211] rearrangements of *MYC* in rare cases,[212] and a variety of copy number aberrations.[213] Overall, the molecular events that lead to the clinical progression of FL remain poorly characterized.

Diffuse Large B-Cell Lymphoma

DLBCL is the most common type of B-NHL, accounting for ~40% of all new diagnoses in adulthood, and includes cases arising *de novo*, as well as cases that derive from the clinical evolution of various, less aggressive B-NHL types (i.e., FL and CLL).[2,214]

Cell of Origin

Over the past decade, the advent of genome-wide gene expression profile technologies has allowed the identification of multiple phenotypic DLBCL subgroups that reflect the derivation from B cells at various differentiation stages. These include at least three well-characterized subtypes: a GC B-cell-like (GCB) DLBCL, which appears to derive from proliferating GC centroblasts; an ABC DLBCL, which shows a transcriptional signature related to plasmablastic B cells presumably blocked during post-GC differentiation; and PMBCL, which is postulated to arise from thymic B cells; the remaining 15% to 30% of cases remain unclassified.[215–218] Stratification according to gene expression profiles has prognostic value, as patients diagnosed with a GCB-DLBCL display a better overall survival compared with ABC-DLBCL,[62] but does not direct differential therapy, and is imperfectly replicated by immunophenotyping or morphology[219,220]; thus, it is not officially incorporated into the World Health Organization classification. A separate classification scheme identified three subsets defined by the expression of genes involved in oxidative phosphorylation, B-cell receptor/proliferation, and tumor microenvironment/host inflammatory response.[221]

Genetic Lesions

The heterogeneity of DLBCL is reflected in the catalogue of genetic lesions that are associated with its pathogenesis. These include balanced reciprocal translocations deregulating the expression of protooncogenes, gene amplifications, chromosomal deletions, single-point mutations, and aberrant somatic hypermutation.[222,223] Notably, most of these abnormalities are preferentially or exclusively associated with individual DLBCL phenotypic subtypes, indicating that GCB- and ABC-DLBCL use distinct oncogenic pathways.[224]

GCB-DLBCL. Genetic lesions that are specific to GCB-DLBCL include the t(14;18) and t(8;14) translocations, which deregulate the *BCL2* and *MYC* oncogenes in 34% and 10% of cases, respectively[25,62,225–227]; mutations affecting an autoregulatory domain within the BCL6 5′untranslated exon 1[228–230]; mutations of the *EZH2* gene[203]; and deletions of the tumor suppressor *PTEN*.[224] In addition, recent studies have identified frequent monoallelic mutations and deletions inactivating the acetyltransferase genes *CREBBP* and *EP300* predominantly in this subtype of DLBCL, where they affect nearly 40% of cases.[91]

Somatic mutations of the BCL6 5′ regulatory sequences are detected in up to 75% of DLBCL cases,[48,231,232] and reflect the activity of the physiologic SHM mechanism that operates in normal GC B cells.[48,49,52] However, functional analysis of numerous mutated *BCL6* alleles revealed that a subset of mutations are specifically associated with DLBCL while being absent in normal GC cells or in other B-cell malignancies.[229] These mutations deregulate *BCL6* transcription by disrupting an autoregulatory circuit through which the BCL6 protein controls its own expression levels via binding to the promoter region of the gene[229,230] or by preventing CD40-induced BCL6 down-regulation in post-GC B cells.[233] Because the full extent of mutations deregulating *BCL6* expression has not been characterized, the fraction of DLBCL cases carrying abnormalities in *BCL6* cannot be determined.

Approximately 50% of all DLBCL are also associated with ASHM.[47] The number and identity of the genes that accumulate mutations in their coding and noncoding regions due to this mechanism varies in different cases and is still largely undefined. However, preferential targeting of individual genes has been observed in the two main COO-defined DLBCL subtypes, with mutations of *MYC* and *BCL2* being found at significantly higher frequencies in GCB-DLBCL, and mutations of *PIM1* almost exclusively observed in ABC-DLBCL. ASHM may therefore contribute to the heterogeneity of DLBCL via the alteration of different cellular pathways in different cases. Mutations and deletions of the *TP53* tumor suppressor gene are mostly detectable in cases originating from the transformation of FL, and are therefore more often associated with chromosomal translocations involving *BCL2* and with a GCB-DLBCL phenotype.[73]

ABC-DLBCL. Several genetic abnormalities are observed almost exclusively in ABC-DLBCL, including amplifications of the *BCL2* locus on 18q24[234,235]; mutations within the NF-κB (*CARD11*, *TNFAIP3/A20*)[67,68] and B-cell receptor signaling (*CD79B*)[236] pathways; inactivating mutations and deletions of *BLIMP1*[76–78]; chromosomal translocations deregulating the *BCL6* oncogene; deletion or lack of expression of the *p16* tumor suppressor gene and, rarely, mutations of the *ATM* gene.[237,238]

Chromosomal translocations affecting band 3q27 cause rearrangements of the *BCL6* gene in up to 35% of all DLBCL cases,[75,205,239] with a twofold higher frequency in the ABC-DLBCL subtype[228] (Table 125.1). These rearrangements juxtapose the intact coding domain of *BCL6* downstream and in the same transcriptional orientation to heterologous sequences derived from the partner chromosome, including *IGH* (14q23), *IGκ* (2p12), *IGλ* (22q11), and at least 20 other chromosomal sites unrelated to the Ig loci.[39–46] The majority of these translocations result in a fusion transcript in which the promoter region and the first noncoding exon of Bcl6 are replaced by sequences derived from the partner gene.[40,240] Because the common denominator of these promoters is a broader spectrum of activity throughout B-cell development, including expression in the post-GC differentiation stage, the translocation prevents the down-regulation of *BCL6* expression that is normally associated with differentiation into post-GC cells. Deregulated expression of a normal *BCL6* gene product may play a critical role by enforcing the proliferative phenotype typical of GC cells while blocking terminal differentiation, as confirmed by a mouse model in which deregulated *BCL6* expression causes DLBCL.[241]

In up to 25% of ABC-DLBCL, the *PRDM1* gene is inactivated by a variety of genetic lesions, including truncating or missense mutations and/or genomic deletions, as well as by transcriptional repression through constitutively active, translocated BCL6 alleles.[76–78] The *PRDM1* gene encodes for a zinc finger transcriptional repressor that is expressed in a subset of GC B cells undergoing plasma cell differentiation and in all plasma cells,[242,243] and is an essential requirement for terminal B-cell differentiation.[244] Thus, *BLIMP1* inactivation may contribute to lymphomagenesis by blocking post-GC B-cell differentiation. Notably, translocations deregulating the *BCL6* gene are virtually never found in *BLIMP1* mutated DLBCLs, suggesting that *BCL6* deregulation and *BLIMP1* inactivation represent alternative oncogenic mechanisms converging on the same pathway (Fig. 125.4).

A predominant feature of ABC-DLBCL is the constitutive activation of the NF-κB signaling pathway, initially evidenced by the selective expression of a signature enriched in NF-κB target genes, and by the requirement of NF-κB for proliferation and survival in ABC-DLBCL cell lines. A number of recent studies have led to the identification of multiple oncogenic alterations affecting positive and negative regulators of NF-κB, specifically in this disease subtype, providing genetic evidence for this phenotypic characteristic. In up to 30% of cases, the *TNFAIP3* gene encoding for the negative regulator A20 is biallelically inactivated by mutations and/or deletions, thus preventing termination of NF-κB responses.[67,79] The tumor suppressor role of A20 was documented by the observation that reconstitution of A20 knockout cell lines with wild type protein induces apoptosis and blocks proliferation, in part due to suppression of NF-κB activity.[67,79] In an additional ~10% of ABC-DLBCL, the *CARD11* gene is targeted by oncogenic mutations clustering in the coiled-coil domain and enhancing its ability to transactivate NF-κB target

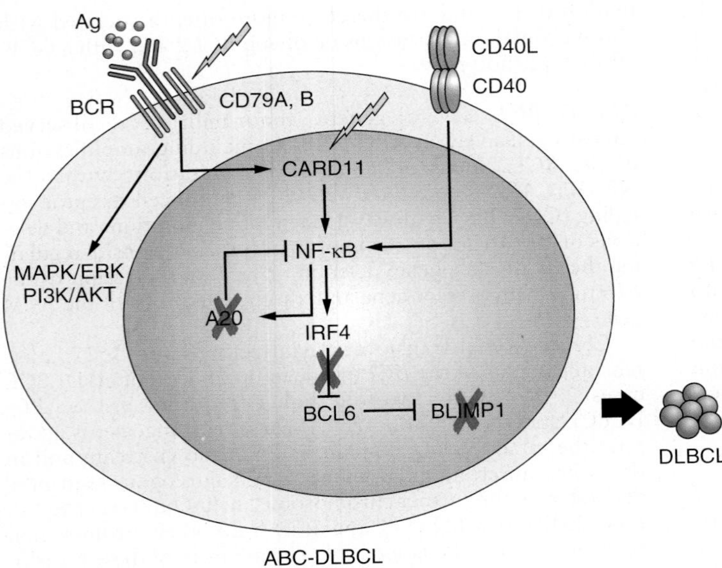

FIGURE 125.4 Pathway lesions in activated B-cell-like diffuse large B-cell lymphoma (ABC-DLBCL). Schematic representation of a germinal center centrocyte, expressing a functional surface B-cell receptor (BCR) and CD40 receptor. In normal B cells, engagement of the BCR by the antigen (spheres) or interaction of the CD40 receptor with the CD40L presented by T cells induce activation of the NF-κB pathway, including its targets IRF4 and A20. IRF4, in turn, down-regulates *BCL6* expression, allowing the release of *BLIMP1* expression, a master plasma cell regulator required for plasma cell differentiation. In ABC-DLBCL, multiple genetic lesions converge on this pathway and disrupt it at multiple levels in different cases (percentages as indicated), presumably contributing to lymphomagenesis by favoring the antiapoptotic and proproliferative function of NF-κB while blocking terminal B-cell differentiation through mutually exclusive deregulation of *BCL6* and inactivation of *BLIMP1*.

genes.[67,68] Less commonly, mutations were found in a variety of other genes encoding for NF-κB components, overall accounting for over half of all ABC-DLBCL[67] and suggesting that yet unidentified lesions may be responsible for the NF-κB activity in the remaining fraction of cases. In addition to constitutive NF-κB activity, ABC-DLBCLs display evidence of chronic active BCR signaling, which is associated with somatic mutations affecting the immunoreceptor tyrosine-based activation motif signaling modules of *CD79B* and *CD79A* in 10% of ABC-DLBCL biopsy samples but rarely in other DLBCLs.[236]

PMBCL. PMBCL is a tumor observed most commonly in young female adults, which involves the mediastinum and displays a distinct gene expression profile, largely similar to a particular type of HL.[217,218] A genetic hallmark of both PMBCL and HL is the amplification of chromosomal region 9q24, detected in nearly 50% of patients.[224,245] This relatively large interval encompasses multiple genes of possible pathogenetic significance, including the gene encoding for the *JAK2* tyrosine kinase or the *PDL1* and *PDL2* genes, which encode for inhibitors of T-cell responses.[63,224,245] Besides contributing to lymphomagenesis, elevated expression levels of these genes may partly explain the unique features of these lymphoma types, which are characterized by a significant inflammatory infiltrate. PMBCL also shares with HL the presence of genetic lesions affecting the NF-κB pathway and the deregulated expression of receptor tyrosine kinases.[81,246–248]

Extranodal Marginal Zone Lymphoma of Mucosa-Associated Lymphoid Tissue

Cell of Origin

MALT lymphoma represents the third most common form of B-NHL,[2] and has steadily risen in incidence over the past 2 decades.[249] The presence of rearranged and somatically mutated *IgV* genes,[30,250] together with the architectural relationship with mucosa-associated lymphoid tissue,[2] indicate the post-GC origin of these tumors, possibly from a marginal zone, memory B cell (Fig. 125.3). A critical role for antigen stimulation, particularly in the pathogenesis of gastric MALT lymphoma, is supported by the observation that (1) this disease is associated with chronic infection of the gastric mucosa by *H. pylori* in virtually all cases,[121–123] (2) eradication of *H. pylori* by antibiotic treatment can lead to tumor regression in ~70% of cases,[124,251] and (3) MALT lymphoma cells express autoreactive BCR, in particular to rheumatoid factors.[252,253]

Whether the development of MALT lymphoma arising in body sites other than the stomach is also dependent on antigen stimulation remains an open question. In this respect, it is remarkable that salivary gland and thyroid MALT lymphoma are generally a sequela of autoimmune processes, namely Sjögren syndrome and Hashimoto thyroiditis, respectively.

Genetic Lesions

Of several structural aberrations that are selectively and recurrently associated with MALT lymphoma, most target the NF-κB signaling pathway, suggesting a critical role in the pathogenesis of the disease. The most common one is the t(11;18)(21;21) translocation, which involves the *API2 (BIRC3)* gene on 11q21 and the *MALT1* gene on 18q21,[254,255] and is observed in 25% to 40% of gastric and pulmonary MALT lymphomas.[256–258] API2, a member of the family of Inhibitor of Apoptosis Proteins, plays an evolutionary conserved role in regulating programmed cell death in diverse species. MALT1, together with BCL10 and CARD11, is a component of the CBM ternary complex and plays a central role in BCR and NF-κB signaling activation.[90] Notably, the wild type proteins encoded by these two genes are incapable of activating NF-κB, as opposed to the API/MALT1 fusion protein, suggesting that the translocation may confer a survival advantage to the tumor by leading to inhibition of apoptosis and constitutive NF-κB activation without the need for upstream signaling.[254,255,259] In an additional 15% to 20% of cases, the *MALT1* gene is translocated to the *IGH* locus in t(14;18)(q32;q21).[260,261]

Recurrent abnormalities of chromosomal band 1p22, generally represented by t(1;14)(p22;q32), occur in ~5% of MALT lymphomas and cause deregulated expression of *BCL10*, a cellular homologue of the equine herpesvirus-2 *E10* gene, which encodes an amino-terminal caspase recruitment domain (CARD) homologous to that found in several apoptotic molecules.[262,263] BCL10, however, does not have proapoptotic activity *in vivo*, where it functions as a positive regulator of antigen-induced activation of NF-κB.[90,264,265] Thus, the translocation may provide both antiapoptotic and proliferative signals mediated via NF-κB transcriptional targets. Trisomy 3 represents a recurrent numerical abnormality in MALT lymphomas; however, the genes involved remain presently unknown.[266,267]

A more recently identified translocation associated with, although not restricted to, MALT lymphoma is t(3;14)(p13;q32),[268,269] which leads to deregulated expression of FOXP1, a member of the Forkhead box family of winged-helix transcription factors involved in regulation of Rag1 and Rag2, and essential for B-cell development.[270] Finally, homozygous or hemizygous loss of *TNFAIP3* due to mutations and/or deletions has been reported in 20% of MALT lymphoma patients, where it is mutually exclusive with other genetic lesions, leading to NF-κB activation.[80] Genetic lesions also involved in other lymphoma types include *BCL6* alterations and *TP53* mutations.[271–273]

Chronic Lymphocytic Leukemia/Small Lymphocytic Lymphoma

Cell of Origin

CLL is a malignancy of mature, resting B lymphocytes, which originates from the oncogenic transformation of a common cellular precursor resembling an antigen-experienced B cell.[274,275] This notion was conclusively demonstrated when gene expression profile studies revealed that, although CLL can express somatically mutated or unmutated *IgV* genes at approximately equal percentages,[276,277] all cases share a homogeneous signature more related to that of CD27+ memory and marginal zone B cells.[278,279] Moreover, analysis of the *Ig* gene repertoire in these patients indicates very similar, at times almost identical, antigen receptors among different individuals.[280–285] This finding, known as *stereotypy*, strongly supports a critical role for the antigen in CLL pathogenesis. The histogenetic heterogeneity of CLL carry prognostic relevance, as cases with mutated *Ig* genes associate with a significantly longer survival.[286,287] Intriguingly, 6% of the normal elderly population develops a monoclonal B-cell lymphocytosis (MBL) that seems to be the precursor to CLL in 1% to 2% of cases.[288]

Genetic Lesions

Different from most mature B-NHLs, and consistent with the derivation from a post-GC or GC-independent B cells, CLL cases are largely devoid of balanced, reciprocal chromosomal translocations.[82,83] On the contrary, CLL is recurrently associated with several numerical abnormalities, including trisomy 12 and monoallelic or biallelic deletion/inactivation of chromosomal regions 17p, 11q, and 13q14 (Table 125.1).[82,83] Of these, deletion of 13q14 represents the most frequent chromosomal aberration, being observed in up to 76% of cases as a monoallelic event, and in 24% of cases as a biallelic event. Interestingly, this same deletion is also found in those with MBL.[288] In all affected cases, the minimal deleted region encompasses a long noncoding RNA (*DLEU2*) and two microRNAs expressed as a cluster, namely miR-15a and miR-16-1.[84,85,87] The causal involvement of 13q14-minimal deleted region–encoded tumor suppressor genes in CLL pathogenesis was recently demonstrated *in vivo* in two animal models that developed clonal lymphoproliferative diseases including MBL, CLL, and DLBCL, at 25% to 40% penetrance.[88] Trisomy 12 is found in approximately 16% of patients evaluated by interphase fluorescent *in situ* hybridization and correlates with a poor survival, but no specific genes have been identified.[289–291] Deletions of chromosomal region 11q22-23 (18% of cases) almost invariably encompass the *ATM* gene and may thus promote genomic instability.[292–294] Because these mutations may occur in the patient germ line, it is thought that they may account, at least in part, for the familial form of the disease. A similar pathogenetic mechanism may be involved in cases with 17p13 genomic deletions (~7%), which include the *TP53* tumor suppressor and are frequently accompanied by mutation of the second allele.[72,295] A higher frequency of *TP53* alterations is observed after transformation of CLL/SLL to Richter syndrome, a highly aggressive lymphoma with a poor clinical outcome.[72]

HIV-Related NHL

The association between an immunodeficiency state and the development of lymphoma has been recognized in several clinical conditions, including congenital (e.g., Wiskott-Aldrich syndrome), iatrogenic (e.g., treatment with immunosuppressor agents), and viral-induced (e.g., AIDS) immunodeficiencies. HIV infection has emerged as a major risk factor for lymphomagenesis, prompting detailed investigations of the molecular pathophysiology of HIV-related NHL, which are primarily classified into three clinicopathologic categories: HIV-related BL, DLBCL, and PEL.[2,296–298] Based on the site of origin, HIV-related NHLs are generally grouped into systemic HIV-related NHL (i.e., DLBCL and BL) and HIV-related PCNSL, which is characterized by a uniform morphology consistent with a diffuse architecture of large cells.[2,296–298]

Cell of Origin

HIV-related NHLs invariably derive from B cells that have experienced the GC reaction, as indicated by the presence of somatically mutated *Ig* and *BCL6* genes, as well as by several phenotypic and genome-wide transcriptional features.[296–298] Based on the presence or absence of immunoblastic features, and on the expression pattern of the BCL6 protein, the EBV-encoded LMP1, and the CD138/syndecan-1 antigen, a proteoglycan associated with the terminal phases of B-cell differentiation, both HIV-related DLBCL and PCNSL can be segregated into two distinct histogenetic categories: cases displaying the BCL6+/CD138−/LMP1− phenotype closely resemble the phenotype of GC B cells; conversely, BCL6−/CD138+/LMP1+ cases are morphologically consistent with immunoblastic lymphoma, plasmacytoid, and reflect a post-GC stage of B-cell differentiation.[296–298] PEL consistently derives from B cells, reflecting a preterminal stage of B-cell differentiation.[105,106,299,300]

Genetic Lesions

The different categories of HIV-related NHL associate with distinctive molecular pathways. Cases of HIV-related BL consistently display activation of MYC by chromosomal translocations that are structurally similar to those found in sporadic BL, while rearrangements of *BCL6* are always absent.[296–298,301] HIV-related BLs also frequently harbor mutations of *TP53* (60%), mutations of the *BCL6 5′* noncoding regions (60%), and, in 30% of cases, infection of the tumor clone by EBV, although the EBV-encoded antigens LMP1 and EBNA2 are not expressed.[302,303] Stimulation and selection by antigens, frequently represented by autoantigens, appear to be a prominent feature of HIV-related BL.[148,304]

Different from BL, the most frequent genetic alteration detected in HIV-related DLBCL is infection by EBV, which occurs in approximately 60% to 70% of the cases and associates frequently, although not always, with expression of *LMP1*.[71,98,303] Also different from HIV-BL, HIV-related DLBCL displays rearrangements of *BCL6* in 20% of cases.[301] Mutations of *BCL6 5′* noncoding regions occur in 70% of cases.[305]

All HIV-related PCNSLs harbor EBV infection.[306] However, only the subset of cases with immunoblastic plasmacytoid morphology expresses the LMP1-transforming protein of EBV.[100] HIV-related PCNSLs display evidence of ASHM[54] and harbor oncogenic mutations in the *CARD11* gene (16% of cases),[307] which may explain in part the presence of constitutive NF-κB activity previously recognized in this lymphoma subtype. Although some reports have suggested that HHV-8 may be related to PCNSL pathogenesis in immunocompromised patients, extensive analysis of HIV-related PCNSL has unequivocally ruled out this hypothesis.[308,309]

The last type of HIV-related NHL that has been characterized at the molecular level is represented by PEL, also known as *body cavity–based lymphoma*.[105,106,299] This lymphoma entity is associated with HHV-8 infection in 100% of cases and clinically presents as effusions in the serosal cavities of the body (pleura, pericardium, and peritoneum) in the absence of solid tumor masses.[105,106,299] In addition to HHV-8, cases of PEL frequently carry coinfection of the tumor clone by EBV.[97,99,105,106,299]

MOLECULAR PATHOGENESIS OF T-CELL NHL

Peripheral T-cell lymphomas (PTCLs) encompass a highly heterogeneous and relatively uncommon group of diseases representing 5% to 10% of all cases of NHL worldwide, with significant geographic variation in both incidence and relative prevalence.[2] PTCLs arise from mature postthymic T cells and, according to the clinical presentation of the disease, are listed as leukemic or disseminated, predominantly extranodal, cutaneous, and predominantly nodal.[2] Although the study of T-cell neoplasms is hampered by the rarity of these diseases and the difficulty of collecting homogeneous sample series, significant advances have been made over the past decades in our understanding of their biology, classification, and prognosis.

Adult T-Cell Lymphoma/Leukemia (HTLV-1–Positive)

Cell of Origin

The term ATLL encompasses a spectrum of lymphoproliferative diseases associated with HTLV-1 infection and mainly restricted to southwestern Japan and the Caribbean basin.[2,310] The United States and Europe are considered low-risk areas as less than 1% of the population are HTLV-1 carriers,[311] and only 2% to 4% of seropositive individuals eventually develop ATLL.[2,110,111] Clonal rearrangement of the TCR is evident in all cases, and clonal integration of the virus has been observed.[312,313]

Genetic Lesions

Compared with other mature T-cell tumors, the molecular pathogenesis of ATLL has been elucidated to a wider extent. Particularly, the role of HTLV-1 has been linked to the production of a transregulatory protein (HTLV-1 tax), which markedly increases expression of all viral gene products and transcriptionally activates the expression of certain host genes, including *IL2, CD25* (the α chain of the IL-2 receptor), *c-sis, c-fos*, and *GM-CSF*.[113–117,242] Indeed, a property of ATLL cells is the constitutive high level expression of IL-2 receptors. The central role of these genes in normal T-cell activation and growth, together with the results of *in vitro* studies, support the notion that tax-mediated activation of these host genes represents an important mechanism by which HTLV-1 initiates T-cell transformation.[113] In addition, tax interferes at multiple sites with DNA damage repair functions and with mitotic checkpoints,[118,119,314] consistent with the fact that ATLL cells harbor a high frequency of karyotypic abnormalities.

The long period of clinical latency that precedes the development of ATLL (usually 10–30 years), the small percentage of infected patients who develop this malignancy, and the observation that leukemic cells from ATLL are monoclonal suggest that HTLV-1 is not sufficient to cause the full malignant phenotype.[110–112] A model for ATLL therefore implies an early period of tax-induced polyclonal T-cell proliferation which, in turn, facilitates the occurrence of additional genetic events, leading to the monoclonal outgrowth of a fully transformed cell. In this respect, a recurrent genetic lesion in ATLL is represented by mutations of the *TP53* tumor suppressor gene, which is inactivated in 40% of cases.[315,316]

Peripheral T-Cell Lymphoma, Not Otherwise Specified

This category represents the largest and most heterogeneous group of PTCLs, and includes all cases that lack specific features allowing classification within another entity. The majority of these cases derive from αβ CD4+ T cells and show aberrant defective expression of one or several T-cell–associated antigens.[317] Based on gene expression profile analysis, PTCL not otherwise specified (NOS) as a group appears to be most closely related to activated T cells than to resting T cells, and can be segregated according to similarities with the transcriptional signature of CD4+ and CD8+ T cells. However, no correlation can be observed between gene expression profile and immunophenotype, likely reflecting the variable detection of T-cell antigens in the disease.

Genetic Lesions

Clonal numerical and structural aberrations are found in most PTCL NOS by conventional cytogenetics and in all cases by more sensitive approaches such as array-based methods. For a few loci, correlation between gene copy number and expression has been confirmed, suggesting a pathogenetic role. Candidate genes targeted by copy number gains include *CDK6* on chromosome 7q, *MYC* on chromosome 8, and the NF-κB regulator *CARD11* at 7p22, while losses of 9p21 are associated with reduced expression of *CDKN2A/B*.[318] Chromosomal translocations involving the TCR loci have been reported in rare cases and remain poorly understood because the identity of the translocation partner has not been identified, with few exceptions: the *BCL3* gene, the poliovirus receptor-related 2 (*PVRL2*) gene, found in the t(14;19)(q11;q13) translocation, and the *IRF4* gene, cloned in two cases.[319–321]

Angioimmunoblastic T-Cell Lymphoma

Cell of Origin

Angioimmunoblastic T-cell lymphoma (AITL) is an aggressive disease of the elderly and accounts for about one-third of all PTCL in Western countries.[322] The tumor cells display a mature CD4+CD8–T-cell phenotype, with frequent aberrant loss of one or several T-cell markers, and coexpression of *BCL6* and CD10 in at least a fraction of cells. Recently, gene expression profile studies allowed the conclusive establishment of the cellular derivation of AITL from follicular T-helper cells,[323] as initially suspected based on expression of single markers.[324]

Genetic Lesions

Clonal aberrations have been reported in up to 90% of AITL patients and are mostly represented by chromosomal imbalances, while chromosomal translocations affecting the TCR loci are extremely rare.[318] However, the scarce number of genetic studies performed so far has failed to provide any significant clues regarding the oncogenic pathways involved in AITL.

Cutaneous T-Cell Lymphoma

Genetic lesions are involved in a limited but significant fraction of primary CTCLs showing molecular markers of clonality.[325] Rearrangements of the *NFKB2* gene at 10q24 encode for a protein that lacks the ankyrin regulatory domain required for regulating the physiological NFKB2 nuclear/cytoplasmic distribution, but retains the rel effector domain and can bind kappa B sequences *in vitro*.[326] The translocation may thus contribute to lymphoma development by causing constitutive activation of the NF-κB pathway.

Anaplastic Large Cell Lymphoma

Cell of Origin

ALCL is a distinct subset of T-NHL (~12% of cases) whose normal cellular counterpart has not yet been established.[2,310] The tumor is composed of large pleomorphic cells that exhibit a unique phenotype characterized by positivity for the CD30 antigen and loss of most T-cell markers.[2,327] Based on the expression of a chimeric protein containing the cytoplasmic portion of anaplastic lymphoma kinase (ALK) as a consequence of translocations involving the *ALK* gene, ALCL may be subdivided into two groups, which display distinct transcriptional signatures[328]: the most common and curable ALK-positive ALCL and the more aggressive ALK-negative ALCL.[2,329–331] However, the identification of a common 30-genes predictor that can discriminate ALCL from other T-NHL, independent of ALK status, suggests that these two subgroups are closely related and may derive from a common precursor.[332]

Genetic Lesions

The genetic hallmark of ALK+ ALCL is chromosomal translocations involving band 2p23 and a variety of chromosomal partners, with t(2;5)(p23;q35) accounting for 70% to 80% of the cases.[2,333] Cloning of the translocation breakpoint in t(2;5) demonstrated the involvement of the *ALK* gene on 2p23 and the nucleophosmin (*NPM1*) gene on 5q35.[334] As a consequence, the aminoterminus of NPM is linked in frame to the catalytic domain of ALK, driving transformation through multiple molecular mechanisms[334]: (1) the *ALK* gene, which is not expressed in normal T lymphocytes, becomes inappropriately expressed in lymphoma cells, conceivably because of its juxtaposition to the promoter sequences of *NPM1*, which are physiologically expressed in T cells; and (2) all translocations involving *ALK* produce proteins with constitutive tyrosine activity, due in most cases to spontaneous dimerization induced by the various fusion partners.[333] Constitutive ALK activity, in turn, results in the activation of several downstream signaling cascades, with the JAK-STAT and PI3K-AKT pathways playing central roles.[335–338] The transforming ability of the chimeric NPM/ALK protein has been proven both *in vitro* and *in vivo* in transgenic mouse model.[339–341]

In a minority of cases, fusions other than NPM-ALK cause the abnormal subcellular localization of the corresponding chimeric ALK proteins and the constitutive activation of ALK. Among these alternative rearrangements, the most frequent involve *TPM3* or *TPM4*, *TRK-fused genes*,[342] *ATIC*,[343,344] *CLTCL1*, and *MSN*. No recurrent cytogenetic abnormality has been described in ALK-negative ALCL, and the molecular events responsible for this disease subtype remain largely unknown.

MOLECULAR PATHOGENESIS OF HL

HL is a B-lymphoid malignancy characterized by the presence of scattered large atypical cells—the mononucleated Hodgkin cells and the multinucleated Reed-Sternberg cells (HRS)—residing in a complex admixture of inflammatory cells.[2,345] Based on the morphology and phenotype of the neoplastic cells, as well as on the composition of the infiltrate, HL is segregated into two major subgroups: nodular lymphocyte-predominant HL (NLPHL; ~5% of cases) and classic HL (cHL), comprising the nodular sclerosis, mixed cellularity, and lymphocyte-depletion and lymphocyte-rich variants. Until recently, molecular studies of HL have been hampered by the paucity of the tumor cells in the biopsy (typically <1%, although occasional cases can present >10% HRS cells). However, the introduction of sophisticated laboratory techniques allowing the isolation and enrichment of neoplastic cells has markedly improved our understanding of HL histogenesis.

Cell of Origin

Despite the HRS of cHL cells having lost expression of nearly all B-cell–specific genes,[346–348] both HL types represent clonal expansions of B cells, as revealed by the presence of clonally rearranged and somatically mutated *Ig* genes.[349,350] In about 25% of cHL cases, nonsense mutations disrupt originally in-frame V_H gene rearrangements (crippling mutations), thereby preventing antigen selection and suggesting that HRS cells of cHL have escaped apoptosis through a mechanism not linked to antigen stimulation.[350]

Genetic Lesions

A number of structural alterations lead to the constitutive activation of NF-κB in cHL. Nearly half of the cases display amplification of *REL*, associated with increased protein expression levels[351,352]; gains or translocations of the positive regulator BCL3 were also reported.[319] More recently, a number of inactivating mutations were found in genes coding for negative regulators of NF-κB, including *NFKBIA* (20% of cases), *NFKBIE* (15%), and *TNFAIP3* (40%).[81,353–355] Notably, *TNFAIP3*-mutated cases are invariably EBV-negative, suggesting that EBV infection may substitute in part for the pathogenetic function of A20 in causing NF-κB constitutive activation.[81,355] Amplification of *JAK2* and inactivating mutations of *SOCS1*, a negative regulator of the JAK-STAT signaling pathway, are often found in NLPHL[245,248]; in an additional large number of cases, constitutive JAK-STAT activity is sustained by autocrine and paracrine signals.[345] BCL6 translocations have been reported in the lymphocytic and histiocytic cells of NLPHD, but only rarely in cHL,[356,357] and translocations of *BCL2* or mutations in positive or negative regulators of apoptosis (e.g., *TP53, FAS, BAD*, and *ATM*) are virtually absent.[345] Finally, an important pathogenetic cofactor in cHL, but not NLPHL, is represented by monoclonal EBV infection, which occurs in approximately 40% of cHL and up to 90% of HIV-related HL, suggesting that infection precedes clonal expansion.[345] Of the viral proteins encoded by the EBV genome, infected HRS cells most commonly express LMP1, LMP2, and EBNA1 but not EBNA2.[345]

Selected References

The full list of references for this chapter appears in the online version.

2. Swerdlow SH, Campo E, Harris NL, et al. *WHO Classification of Tumours of Haematopoietic and Lymphoid Tissues*. Lyon, France: IARC, 2008.
5. Rajewsky K. Clonal selection and learning in the antibody system. *Nature* 1996;381:751–758.
6. Klein U, Dalla-Favera R. Germinal centres: role in B-cell physiology and malignancy. *Nat Rev Immunol* 2008;8:22–33.
17. Phan RT, Dalla-Favera R. The BCL6 proto-oncogene suppresses p53 expression in germinal-centre B cells. *Nature* 2004;432:635–639.
28. Muramatsu M, Kinoshita K, Fagarasan S, et al. Class switch recombination and hypermutation require activation-induced cytidine deaminase (AID), a potential RNA editing enzyme. *Cell* 2000;102:553–563.
29. Revy P, Muto T, Levy Y, et al. Activation-induced cytidine deaminase (AID) deficiency causes the autosomal recessive form of the Hyper-IgM syndrome (HIGM2). *Cell* 2000;102:565–575.
35. Ramiro AR, Jankovic M, Eisenreich T, et al. AID is required for c-myc/IgH chromosome translocations in vivo. *Cell* 2004;118:431–438.
37. Pasqualucci L, Bhagat G, Jankovic M, et al. AID is required for germinal center-derived lymphomagenesis. *Nat Genet* 2008;40:108–112.
41. Ye BH, Lista F, Lo Coco F, et al. Alterations of a zinc finger-encoding gene, BCL-6, in diffuse large-cell lymphoma. *Science* 1993;262:747–750.
47. Pasqualucci L, Neumeister P, Goossens T, et al. Hypermutation of multiple proto-oncogenes in B-cell diffuse large-cell lymphomas. *Nature* 2001;412: 341–346.
48. Pasqualucci L, Migliazza A, Fracchiolla N, et al. BCL-6 mutations in normal germinal center B cells: evidence of somatic hypermutation acting outside Ig loci. *Proc Natl Acad Sci U S A* 1998;95:11816–11821.
49. Shen HM, Peters A, Baron B, Zhu X, Storb U. Mutation of BCL-6 gene in normal B cells by the process of somatic hypermutation of Ig genes. *Science* 1998;280:1750–1752.
67. Compagno M, Lim WK, Grunn A, et al. Mutations of multiple genes cause deregulation of NF-kappaB in diffuse large B-cell lymphoma. *Nature* 2009;459:717–721.
68. Lenz G, Davis RE, Ngo VN, et al. Oncogenic CARD11 mutations in human diffuse large B cell lymphoma. *Science* 2008;319:1676–1679.
69. Neri A, Knowles DM, Greco A, McCormick F, Dalla-Favera R. Analysis of RAS oncogene mutations in human lymphoid malignancies. *Proc Natl Acad Sci U S A* 1988;85:9268–9272.
72. Gaidano G, Ballerini P, Gong JZ, et al. p53 mutations in human lymphoid malignancies: association with Burkitt lymphoma and chronic lymphocytic leukemia. *Proc Natl Acad Sci U S A* 1991;88:5413–5417.
76. Mandelbaum J, Bhagat G, Tang H, et al. BLIMP1 is a tumor suppressor gene frequently disrupted in activated B-cell like diffuse large B-cell lymphoma. *Cancer Cell* 2010;18(6):568.
79. Kato M, Sanada M, Kato I, et al. Frequent inactivation of A20 in B-cell lymphomas. *Nature* 2009;459:712–716.
81. Schmitz R, Hansmann ML, Bohle V, et al. TNFAIP3 (A20) is a tumor suppressor gene in Hodgkin lymphoma and primary mediastinal B cell lymphoma. *J Exp Med* 2009;206:981.
82. Dohner H, Stilgenbauer S, Benner A, et al. Genomic aberrations and survival in chronic lymphocytic leukemia. *N Engl J Med* 2000;343:1910–1916.
84. Calin GA, Dumitru CD, Shimizu M, et al. Frequent deletions and down-regulation of micro-RNA genes miR15 and miR16 at 13q14 in chronic lymphocytic leukemia. *Proc Natl Acad Sci U S A* 2002;99:15524–15529.
88. Klein U, Lia M, Crespo M, et al. The DLEU2/miR-15a/16-1 cluster controls B cell proliferation and its deletion leads to chronic lymphocytic leukemia. *Cancer Cell* 2010;17:28–40.
94. Neri A, Barriga F, Inghirami G, et al. Epstein-Barr virus infection precedes clonal expansion in Burkitt's and acquired immunodeficiency syndrome-associated lymphoma. *Blood* 1991;77:1092–1095.
103. Chang Y, Cesarman E, Pessin MS, et al. Identification of herpesvirus-like DNA sequences in AIDS-associated Kaposi's sarcoma. *Science* 1994; 266:1865–1869.
130. Tsujimoto Y, Yunis J, Onorato-Showe L, et al. Molecular cloning of the chromosomal breakpoint of B-cell lymphomas and leukemias with the t(11;14) chromosome translocation. *Science* 1984;224:1403–1406.
132. Motokura T, Bloom T, Kim HG, et al. A novel cyclin encoded by a bcl1-linked candidate oncogene. *Nature* 1991;350:512–515.
152. Dalla-Favera R, Bregni M, Erikson J, et al. Human c-myc onc gene is located on the region of chromosome 8 that is translocated in Burkitt lymphoma cells. *Proc Natl Acad Sci U S A* 1982;79:7824–7827.
153. Dalla-Favera R, Martinotti S, Gallo RC, Erikson J, Croce CM. Translocation and rearrangements of the c-myc oncogene locus in human undifferentiated B-cell lymphomas. *Science* 1983;219:963–967.
167. Meyer N, Penn LZ. Reflecting on 25 years with MYC. *Nat Rev Cancer* 2008;8:976–990.
168. Dominguez-Sola D, Ying CY, Grandori C, et al. Non-transcriptional control of DNA replication by c-Myc. *Nature* 2007;448:445–451.
169. Eilers M, Eisenman RN. Myc's broad reach. *Genes Dev* 2008;22:2755–2766.
179. Adams JM, Harris AW, Pinkert CA, et al. The c-myc oncogene driven by immunoglobulin enhancers induces lymphoid malignancy in transgenic mice. *Nature* 1985;318:533–538.
188. Cleary ML, Smith SD, Sklar J. Cloning and structural analysis of cDNAs for bcl-2 and a hybrid bcl-2/immunoglobulin transcript resulting from the t(14;18) translocation. *Cell* 1986;47:19–28.
196. Hockenbery D, Nunez G, Milliman C, Schreiber RD, Korsmeyer SJ. Bcl-2 is an inner mitochondrial membrane protein that blocks programmed cell death. *Nature* 1990;348:334–336.
215. Alizadeh AA, Eisen MB, Davis RE, et al. Distinct types of diffuse large B-cell lymphoma identified by gene expression profiling. *Nature* 2000; 403:503–511.
217. Savage KJ, Monti S, Kutok JL, et al. The molecular signature of mediastinal large B-cell lymphoma differs from that of other diffuse large B-cell lymphomas and shares features with classical Hodgkin lymphoma. *Blood* 2003;102:3871–3879.
218. Rosenwald A, Wright G, Leroy K, et al. Molecular diagnosis of primary mediastinal B cell lymphoma identifies a clinically favorable subgroup of diffuse large B cell lymphoma related to Hodgkin lymphoma. *J Exp Med* 2003;198:851–862.
224. Lenz G, Wright GW, Emre NC, et al. Molecular subtypes of diffuse large B-cell lymphoma arise by distinct genetic pathways. *Proc Natl Acad Sci U S A* 2008;105:13520–13525.
229. Pasqualucci L, Migliazza A, Fracchiolla N, et al. Mutations of the BCL6 proto-oncogene disrupt its negative autoregulation in diffuse large B-cell lymphoma. *Blood* 2003;101:2914–2923.
232. Migliazza A, Martinotti S, Chen W, et al. Frequent somatic hypermutation of the 5′ noncoding region of the BCL6 gene in B-cell lymphoma. *Proc Natl Acad Sci U S A* 1995;92:12520–12524.
233. Saito M, Gao J, Basso K, et al. A signaling pathway mediating downregulation of BCL6 in germinal center B cells is blocked by BCL6 gene alterations in B cell lymphoma. *Cancer Cell* 2007;12:280–292.
236. Davis RE, Ngo VN, Lenz G, et al. Chronic active B-cell-receptor signalling in diffuse large B-cell lymphoma. *Nature* 2010;463:88–92.
251. Wotherspoon AC. Gastric lymphoma of mucosa-associated lymphoid tissue and *Helicobacter pylori*. *Annu Rev Med* 1998;49:289.
274. Caligaris-Cappio F, Hamblin TJ. B-cell chronic lymphocytic leukemia: a bird of a different feather. *J Clin Oncol* 1999;17:399–408.
278. Klein U, Tu Y, Stolovitzky GA, et al. Gene expression profiling of B cell chronic lymphocytic leukemia reveals a homogeneous phenotype related to memory B cells. *J Exp Med* 2001;194:1625–1638.
279. Rosenwald A, Alizadeh AA, Widhopf G, et al. Relation of gene expression phenotype to immunoglobulin mutation genotype in B cell chronic lymphocytic leukemia. *J Exp Med* 2001;194:1639–1647.
288. Rawstron AC, Bennett FL, O'Connor SJ, et al. Monoclonal B-cell lymphocytosis and chronic lymphocytic leukemia. *N Engl J Med* 2008;359: 575.
310. de Leval L, Bisig B, Thielen C, Boniver J, Gaulard P. Molecular classification of T-cell lymphomas. *Crit Rev Oncol Hematol* 2009;72:125–143.
333. Chiarle R, Voena C, Ambrogio C, Piva R, Inghirami G. The anaplastic lymphoma kinase in the pathogenesis of cancer. *Nat Rev Cancer* 2008;8:11–23.
334. Morris SW, Kirstein MN, Valentine MB, et al. Fusion of a kinase gene, ALK, to a nucleolar protein gene, NPM, in non-Hodgkin's lymphoma. *Science* 1994;263:1281–1284.
349. Küppers R, Rajewsky K, Zhao M, et al. Hodgkin disease: Hodgkin and Reed-Sternberg cells picked from histological sections show clonal immunoglobulin gene rearrangements and appear to be derived from B cells at various stages of development. *Proc Natl Acad Sci U S A* 1994;91:10962–10966.

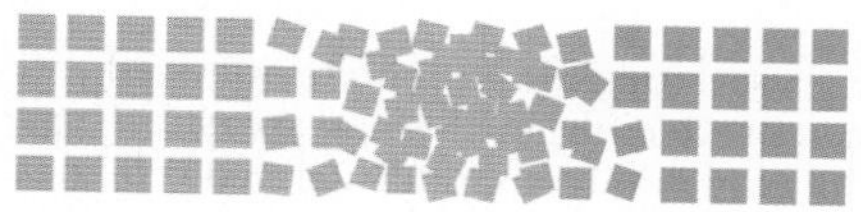

CHAPTER 126 HODGKIN LYMPHOMA

ANDREAS ENGERT, DENNIS A. EICHENAUER, NANCY LEE HARRIS, PETER M. MAUCH, AND VOLKER DIEHL

HISTORY OF HODGKIN LYMPHOMA

A great deal has been written about the life and accomplishments of Thomas Hodgkin.[1] In his historic paper titled "On Some Morbid Appearances of the Exorbant Glands and Spleen" presented to the Medical Chirurgical Society in London on January 10, 1832, Hodgkin described the clinical history and postmortem findings of the massive enlargement of lymph nodes and spleens of six patients studied at Guy's Hospital in London and of a seventh patient who had been seen by Robert Carswell in 1828.[2] Without a microscope, Hodgkin recognized that these patients had suffered from a disease that started in the lymph nodes located along the major vessels in the neck, chest, or abdomen, rather than from an inflammatory condition.

In 1856, Sir Samuel Wilks, a Guy's Hospital pathologist, described ten postmortem cases that had "a peculiar enlargement of the lymphatic glands frequently associated with disease of the spleen." By 1865, Wilks had collected data from 15 cases, which were published in a second article titled "Cases of the Enlargement of the Lymphatic Glands and Spleen (or Hodgkin's Disease) with Remarks." This linked Hodgkin's name permanently to this newly identified disease. Wilks's initial descriptions gave us some of our earliest understanding of Hodgkin disease.[3] He described the disease as a cancer that started and remained in the lymph nodes for a long time, perhaps years, before involving the spleen and then spreading to other organs. He also noted anemia, weight loss, and fevers in some of the patients with this disease.

Although other physicians had provided descriptions of the characteristic giant cells present in the lymph nodes and spleens of patients with Hodgkin disease, W. S. Greenfield in 1878 was the first to contribute drawings of them from a low microscopic magnification of a lymph node specimen.[4] Despite Greenfield's findings, Carl Sternberg in 1898 and Dorothy Reed in 1902 are credited with the first definitive microscopic descriptions of Hodgkin disease.[5,6]

Both Sternberg and Reed, along with many other physicians, believed that Hodgkin disease was caused by an associated infection rather than by a separate malignant process of the lymph nodes. Proponents of the infectious theory cited the frequent association of Hodgkin disease with tuberculosis. Eight of Sternberg's 13 cases of Hodgkin disease had coexistent tuberculosis, and he believed Hodgkin disease to be a variant of tuberculosis. Other physicians believed that Hodgkin disease was a cancer of the lymph nodes. Clinical and pathologic studies, available in the early 20th century, helped to confirm their view.[7] Despite the very strong evidence for the malignant nature of Hodgkin lymphoma during the past century, it was only recently shown that Hodgkin Reed-Sternberg (HRS) cells are clonal, confirming their origin from a single malignant cell.[8]

Hodgkin lymphoma is pathologically and clinically heterogeneous. Two major subtypes are now recognized: classic Hodgkin lymphoma (CHL) and nodular lymphocyte predominant Hodgkin lymphoma (NLPHL). Although they share sufficient distinctive features to warrant separating both from other lymphomas (so-called non-Hodgkin lymphomas), they differ from one another in morphology, normal counterpart, epidemiology, and clinical features and are considered two distinct disease entities.[9]

ETIOLOGY AND EPIDEMIOLOGY

There are approximately 7,500 new cases of Hodgkin lymphoma diagnosed each year in the United States. The cHL comprises 95% of the cases, and NLPHL 5%.[10] Slightly more men than women develop this malignancy (1.4:1). In economically developed countries, there is an age-related bimodal incidence for cHL, with a first peak in the third decade of life and a much smaller peak occurring after the age of 50.[9–11] In contrast, the incidence of NLPHL remains relatively constant from childhood through old age, with the majority of cases occurring between 30 and 50 years of age.[10]

A number of studies have suggested a genetic predisposition for Hodgkin lymphoma. There is an increased incidence in Jews and also among first-degree relatives.[11] Hodgkin lymphoma has also been linked with certain HLA antigens.[12,13]

There is less support for most other potential causes of Hodgkin lymphoma. In contrast to other malignancies, Hodgkin lymphoma is rarely seen as a second malignancy and does not appear to be increased in patients with illness or treatment-related chronic immunosuppression. Although cHL has been noted in patients with acquired immunodeficiency syndrome (AIDS), there remains lack of evidence that there is a direct correlation with the immune suppression associated with AIDS.[14] In the opposite, it seems that under HAART (highly active antiretroviral therapy) the incidence of Hodgkin lymphoma seems to increase with rising numbers of CD4 cells. In contrast, there is some evidence to suggest a viral etiology for Hodgkin lymphoma. In economically developed countries, studies report an association between Hodgkin lymphoma in younger patients and increased maternal education, decreased numbers of siblings and playmates, early birth order, and single-family dwellings in childhood.[15] The association between Hodgkin lymphoma and childhood factors that decrease exposure to infectious agents at an early age has led investigators to propose that the epidemiologic features of Hodgkin lymphoma appear to mimic those of a viral illness that has an age-related host response to infection. Finally, in about 40% of cases of cHL, most often of mixed cellularity type, the neoplastic cells contain Epstein-Barr virus (EBV) genomes and express latency-associated antigens, suggesting a role for EBV in the pathogenesis of at least some cases.[16]

BIOLOGY AND CELL OF ORIGIN

Lineage, Origin, and Clonality of Hodgkin/Reed-Sternberg Cells

Specific Morphologic Features of Hodgkin Lymphoma

Lymph nodes affected by both CHL and NLPHL contain a minority of neoplastic cells in a prominent reactive background, consisting of varying numbers of lymphocytes, histiocytes, eosinophils, plasma cells, fibroblasts, and other cells. The malignant cells of cHL comprise mononuclear cells known as Hodgkin cells and their multinucleated counterparts, the Reed-Sternberg cells; collectively, HRS cells. In NLPHL, the neoplastic cells have been called lymphocytic and histiocytic (L&H) cells (based on earlier classifications in which this subtype was known as "lymphocytic and histiocytic predominance"); the term lymphocyte predominant (LP) cells is now preferred. These cells are also known as popcorn cells, because of their resemblance to popped kernels of corn. While in NLPHL, LP cells consistently express B-cell–specific surface antigens (CD19, CD20), in cHL HRS cells express the activation marker CD30, and in the majority of the cases CD15. They also express the B-lineage antigen Pax-5, but most cases lack or only weakly and variably express B-cell antigens such as CD20.[17]

Cell Lines and Animal Models

The establishment of permanently growing cell lines allowed the biological and genetic characterization of the tumor cell population in numerous human neoplasias. In contrast, outgrowth of a cell line is extremely rare in Hodgkin lymphoma. The first two permanent cell lines (designated L428 and L540) were established in 1979 from patients with advanced-stage Hodgkin lymphoma (clinical stage IVB).[18] These cell lines grew from a pleural effusion and bone marrow. With few exceptions, all subsequently established cell lines were also obtained from body fluids (bone marrow, pleural effusion, peripheral blood) of advanced-stage patients. This observation may reflect an *in vivo* adaptation of the cells to the conditions of suspension culture as prerequisite for *in vitro* outgrowth. So far, only 15 cell lines have been established that may be regarded as Hodgkin lymphoma derived. Analysis of immunophenotype, karyotype, Ig (immunoglobulin), or T-cell receptor (TCR) gene rearrangements of these cell lines revealed heterogeneous results, in analogy to analysis of primary tissue, not allowing any conclusion to be drawn on the cell of origin of Hodgkin lymphoma. In addition, their derivation from primary HRS cells could not be determined unequivocally.[19] An EBV-negative cell line (L1236) was established from peripheral blood mononuclear cells of a patient with end-stage Hodgkin lymphoma of mixed cellularity subtype.[20] Using single-cell polymerase chain reaction (PCR) it could be shown that the genomic sequences of the Ig gene rearrangements of the HRS cells in the patient's bone marrow were identical to those detected in L1236 cells.[21] Thus, the derivation from the primary HRS cells could definitely be proven on the molecular level in this cell line.

Hodgkin lymphoma–derived cell lines were successfully used for the discovery of HRS cell–associated antigens, which include CD30 (Ki-1), CD70, and Ki-27, for cloning the CD30 gene and for studying the CD30 signal transduction pathway.[22–24] They also enabled the *in vitro* testing of new immunotherapeutic modalities such as Ricin A-linked anti-CD30 immunotoxins, Saporin-linked anti-CD30 immunotoxins, anti-CD16/CD30 bispecific antibodies, and CD30 anti-idiotype vaccine.[25–27]

Although none of these Hodgkin lymphoma–derived cell lines could be grown reproducibly in thymus-aplastic T-cell deficient nude mice, the Hodgkin lymphoma–derived cell lines L540, HD-MyZ, L428, and L1236 have been shown to disseminate intralymphatically after inoculation into T- and B-cell–deficient severe combined immune deficiency (SCID) mice.[20,28] The SCID mouse model was also used for the preclinical *in vivo* testing of new experimental therapeutic approaches. Unfortunately, however, no reproducible growth of primary HRS cells has been observed after transplantation of biopsy material.[29]

IMMUNOLOGY OF HODGKIN LYMPHOMA

Cellular Immune Deficiencies

Hodgkin lymphoma is characterized by the predominance of a reactive infiltrate consisting of T cells, B cells, neutrophils, and eosinophils surrounding a few malignant HRS cells. This morphology suggests a major role of the interplay between the tumor and the host immune system. Although HRS cells and the HRS-derived cell lines express several molecules that are necessary for efficient antigen presentation (major histocompatibility complex [MHC] class I or II, CD80, CD86, CD54, CD58),[24,30] an effective immune response is not mounted.[20,31] The T cells, predominantly CD4+, TCRab+, and only very scarce CD8+ cytotoxic T lymphocytes, are characterized by the expression of activation markers like CD38, CD69, CD71, and MHC class II, but lack CD26 and CD25, the interleukin 2 (IL-2) receptor. This may be due to the concerted interplay of various chemokines and cytokines secreted by HRS cells. The predominant secretion of Th2-favoring cytokines and chemokines may especially inhibit an effective cytotoxic Th1 response in favor of a primarily humoral Th2 response.[32] This Th2-biased immune response is further strengthened by the surrounding eosinophils attracted by chemokines like eotaxin.[33] Moreover, secretion of IL-10 and transforming growth factor beta (TGF-β) by the HRS cells in conjunction with the inability of T cells to secrete IL-2 suppresses an effective immune reaction.[34] On the other hand, HRS cells seem to be highly dependent on their specific microenvironment as demonstrated by the difficulty to culture these cells. All established cell lines are derived from patients with advanced stages of Hodgkin lymphoma, where the malignant clone loses its dependence on the surrounding cells and spreads into the blood system, the pleural cavity, or the bone marrow.[20,35] In summary, HRS cells effectively escape the host immune system by modulating the immune response to an impaired Th2 response, which even seems to support the growth of the malignant T cells in cHL.

Pathology and Classification

Two major types of Hodgkin lymphoma are now recognized: NLPHL and cHL.[9,36] Both are defined by the presence of relatively small numbers of neoplastic cells in a characteristic reactive, inflammatory background. The clinical features and responses to treatment of Hodgkin lymphoma differ dramatically from those of most so-called non-Hodgkin lymphomas

(NHLs), suggesting that a specific immunologic reaction is important not only in the definition but also in the clinical behavior of this disease. In NLPHL, the RS cell variants express the full B-cell program, including B-cell–associated antigens such as CD19 and CD20, while those of most cases of nodular sclerosis (NS) and mixed cellularity (MC) Hodgkin lymphoma lack or only partially express these antigens.[37] This difference in immunophenotype, together with the observation that NLPHL had a more indolent clinical course, led to the suggestion that NLPHL was a low-grade B-cell lymphoma and should be removed from the category of Hodgkin lymphoma and placed with the NHLs. However, both immunophenotypic and, molecular genetic studies have shown that both cHL and NLPHL have rearranged immunoglobulin genes and are thus of B-cell lineage.[38,39]

The early classification of Jackson and Parker[40] recognized three categories: paragranuloma, granuloma, and sarcoma. The distinction between the three categories was based on the ratio of neoplastic to normal cells, which increased from paragranuloma to granuloma to sarcoma, and predicted decreasing survival. In 1966 Lukes et al.[41] recognized that the category of "granuloma" could be subdivided into two categories—nodular sclerosis and mixed cellularity—which were characterized by distinctive morphology and clinical features. They also recognized that there were two variants of what they called lymphocytic or histiocytic predominance type (replacing paragranuloma), a nodular and a diffuse variant, which they found differed in prognosis. The Lukes et al. classification was modified and simplified at the Rye Conference in 1966. The Rye classification remained the standard classification for many years.

In 1994 the International Lymphoma Study Group introduced an updated classification, incorporating new immunologic and genetic data, as part of the Revised European-American Lymphoma (REAL) Classification.[42] These concepts were incorporated into the World Health Organization (WHO) classification of hematologic malignancies, a joint effort of the Society for Hematopathology and the European Association of Hematopathologists (Table 126.1).[9]

There are several major differences between the REAL/WHO classification of Hodgkin lymphoma and older classifications. Most important is the recognition, as previously stated, that there are two distinct diseases that have been called Hodgkin lymphoma: "classic" Hodgkin lymphoma, which consists predominantly of nodular sclerosis and mixed cellularity, and nodular lymphocyte predominant Hodgkin lymphoma (Table 126.2). Simply a predominance of lymphocytes in the background is not sufficient to classify a case as NLPHL; cases that have the RS-cell morphology and immunophenotype of classic Hodgkin lymphoma, even if they contain predominantly lymphocytes, are classified as lymphocyte-rich classic Hodgkin lymphoma (LRCHL). A second difference is that, in the Lukes et al. and Rye classifications, mixed cellularity was a heterogeneous category, including both typical cases and all other cases that did not fit into one of the other categories. The REAL/WHO classifications now recommend that mixed cellularity be restricted to typical cases, and that unclassifiable cases be classified as Hodgkin lymphoma unclassifiable. Finally, it is now clear that immunophenotype is important in the subclassification of Hodgkin lymphoma, both in distinguishing NLPHL from classic types and in distinguishing Hodgkin lymphoma from NHL; thus, the immunophenotype is included in the definitions of Hodgkin lymphoma in the REAL/WHO classification.

Nodular Lymphocyte Predominant Hodgkin Lymphoma

Morphologic Features. NLPHL is defined in the WHO Classification as a monoclonal B-cell neoplasm characterized by a nodular or a nodular and a diffuse proliferation of scattered large neoplastic cells known as LP RS cell variants.[43] The LP cells differ from classic HRS cells: they have vesicular, polylobated nuclei and distinct but small, usually peripheral, nucleoli without perinucleolar halos. Although LP cells may be very numerous, usually no classic, diagnostic RS cells are found. In occasional cases, however, the neoplastic cells may resemble classic or lacunar types; in such cases, immunophenotyping may be essential in establishing the diagnosis and excluding LRcHL. The background is predominantly lymphocytes; clusters of epithelioid histiocytes may be numerous; plasma cells, eosinophils, and neutrophils are rarely seen and,

TABLE 126.1

CLASSIFICATIONS OF HODGKIN LYMPHOMA (HL)

Jackson and Parker[a]	Lukes and Butler[b]	Rye Conference[c]	REAL Classification[d]	WHO Classification[e]
Paragranuloma	Lymphocytic or histiocytic, nodular Lymphocytic or histiocytic, diffuse	Lymphocyte predominant	Nodular lymphocyte predominant Lymphocyte-rich CHL	Lymphocyte predominant, nodular Lymphocyte-rich CHL
Granuloma	Nodular sclerosis Mixed cellularity[g]	Nodular sclerosis Mixed cellularity[g]	Nodular sclerosis Mixed cellularity	Nodular sclerosis Mixed cellularity
Sarcoma	Lymphocytic depleted Diffuse fibrosis and reticular	Lymphocyte depleted	Lymphocyte depleted	Lymphocyte depleted Unclassifiable CHL

HL, Hodgkin lymphoma; REAL, Revised European-American Lymphoma; WHO, World Health Organization.
[a]Jackson JH, Parker JF. Hodgkin's disease. General considerations. *N Engl J Med* 1944;230:1.
[b]Lukes RJ, Butler JJ. The pathology and nomenclature of Hodgkin's disease. *Cancer Res* 1966;26:1063.
[c]Lukes RJ, Craver LF, Hall TC, et al. Report of the nomenclature committee. *Cancer Res* 1966;26:1311.
[d]Harris NL, Jaffe ES, Stein H, et al. A revised European-American classification of lymphoid neoplasms: a proposal from the International Lymphoma Study Group. *Blood* 1994;84:1361.
[e]Harris NL, Jaffe ES, Diebold J, et al. The World Health Organization classification of hematological malignancies report of the Clinical Advisory Committee Meeting, Airlie House, Virginia, November 1997. *Mod Pathol* 2000;13:193.
[f]Includes some lymphocytic and/or histiocytic nodular cases.
[g]Includes unclassifiable cases.

TABLE 126.2

MORPHOLOGIC AND IMMUNOPHENOTYPIC FEATURES OF NODULAR LYMPHOCYTE-PREDOMINANT HODGKIN LYMPHOMA AND CLASSIC HODGKIN LYMPHOMA

	CHL	NLPHL
Pattern	Diffuse, interfollicular, nodular	Nodular, at least in part
Tumor cells	Diagnostic RS cells; mononuclear or lacunar cells	LP or popcorn cells
Background	Lymphocytes, histiocytes, eosinophils, plasma cells	Lymphocytes, histiocytes
Fibrosis	Common	Rare
CD15	+	–
CD30	+	–
CD20	–/+	+
CD45	–	+
EMA	–	+
EBV (in RS cells)	+ (approximately 40%)	–
Background lymphocytes	T cells > B cells*	B cells > T cells
CD57+ T cells	P**	+
Ig genes (single-cell PCR)	Rearranged, clonal, mutated, "crippled"	Rearranged, clonal, mutated, ongoing

*In LRCHL with a nodular pattern, B cells may predominate in the background.
**IN LRCHL with a nodular pattern, CD57+ cells may be numerous and surround RS cells.
cHL, classic Hodgkin lymphoma; NLPHL, nodular lymphocyte-predominant Hodgkin lymphoma; RS, Reed-Sternberg; L&H, lymphocytes and histiocytes; +, present; –, absent; EMA, epithelial membrane antigen; EBV, Epstein-Barr virus; Ig, immunoglobulin; PCR, polymerase chain reaction.

if present, are not numerous. Occasionally, sclerosis may cause some cases to resemble nodular sclerosis classic Hodgkin lymphoma (NSCHL).

Progressive Transformation of Germinal Centers. A distinctive type of follicular lymphoid hyperplasia, known as progressive transformation of germinal centers (PTGCs), is seen focally in about 20% of lymph nodes involved by NLPHL and may be seen in the absence of Hodgkin lymphoma in other lymph nodes in the same patient. PTGCs are enlarged follicles that contain numerous small B cells of mantle zone type; these follicles may closely resemble the nodules of NLPHL. This phenomenon has given rise to speculation that NLPHL may arise from PTGCs. PTGCs are usually seen as single or only a few enlarged follicles in a setting of nonspecific reactive follicular lymphoid hyperplasia; however, on occasion, they may be numerous and associated with prominent lymph node enlargement, particularly in adolescents and young adults.[44]

Nodular Lymphocyte Predominance Hodgkin Lymphoma and Diffuse Large B-Cell Lymphoma. Patients with NLPHL have a slightly higher risk of development of NHL than patients with other types of Hodgkin lymphoma.[45] Transformation of NLPHL to diffuse large B-cell lymphoma (DLBCL) is most common, occurring in 2% to 6% of the cases. The DLBCL may consist of typical LP cells, but usually resembles other DLBCLs. In most cases, a clonal relationship between the LP and the DLBCL has been shown by molecular genetic analysis.[46]

One problem that may arise in NLPHL is that in relapsed cases, the pattern may become partly or entirely diffuse, and distinction between diffuse areas of LPHL and T-cell/histiocyte-rich large B-cell lymphoma (THRLBCL) may be impossible. Pathologists vary in their interpretation of this phenomenon; some will make a diagnosis of relapse of NLPHL with a diffuse pattern, while others may make a diagnosis of progression to THRLBCL. In the 2008 WHO classification, it was agreed that the diagnosis of THRLBCL should be restricted to primary cases, and that relapse of NLPHL with a diffuse pattern should be called either diffuse LPHL or as "NLPHL with THRLBCL-like areas."[43]

Immunophenotype of Nodular Lymphocyte Predominance Hodgkin Lymphoma. LP cells are CD45+, express B-cell–associated antigens (CD19, 20, 22, 79a, PAX5, the transcription factors Oct2 and BOB-1, and the germinal-center–associated protein Bcl-6) and epithelial membrane antigen (EMA), and lack CD15 and CD30. Immunoglobulin J-chain and in some cases, light chain mRNA can be detected, often of kappa type. IgD expression has been reported in more than 25% of the cases, occurring predominantly in young males.[47]

The nodules of NLPHL are expanded B-cell follicles that contain small polyclonal B lymphocytes with a mantle zone phenotype (IgM and IgD+), as well as T cells, many of which have a follicular helper phenotype (PD1 [CD274]+, CD57+), similar to the T-cell population in normal and progressively transformed germ cells that surround the neoplastic B-cells, forming rings or rosettes. Nodular meshworks of CD21+ follicular dendritic cells surround the nodules; CD23+ may be less frequent. An unusual population of CD4+CD8+ double-positive T cells is detected by flow cytometry in many cases of NLPHL.[48]

Clinical Features of Nodular Lymphocyte Predominance Hodgkin Lymphoma. NLPHL accounts for about 5% of all Hodgkin lymphoma cases. The median age is in the mid-30s, but both children and older patients can be affected. The male-to-female ratio is 3:1 or greater. NLPHL usually involves peripheral lymph nodes, sparing the mediastinum. About 80% of patients are stage I or II at the time of the diagnosis. Fewer patients present with stage III or IV disease and these may have a poorer prognosis. More than 90% of patients have a complete response to therapy, and 90% are alive at 10-year follow-up. The cause of death is often NHL, other cancers, or complications of treatment, rather than Hodgkin lymphoma.[10,49]

Classic Hodgkin Lymphoma

Classic Hodgkin lymphoma in the WHO classification is defined as a monoclonal lymphoid neoplasm (in most cases deriving from B cells) composed of mononuclear Hodgkin cells and multinucleated RS cells residing in an infiltrate containing a variable mixture of nonneoplastic small lymphocytes, eosinophils, neutrophils, histiocytes, plasma cells, fibroblasts, and collagen fibers.[50] Classic Hodgkin lymphoma includes nodular sclerosis, mixed cellularity, lymphocyte-rich and lymphocyte-depleted types. Because the immunophenotype, genetic features, and postulated normal counterpart are the same for all of the classic types, these will be discussed together at the end of this section.

Nodular Sclerosis Classic Hodgkin Lymphoma

Morphologic Features. NScHL is a subtype of cHL characterized by collagen bands that surround at least one nodule, and HRS cells with lacunar type morphology. The lacunar type RS cell has a multilobated nucleus, small nucleoli, and abundant, pale cytoplasm, which retracts in formalin-fixed sections, producing an empty space, or lacune. Diagnostic RS cells may be rare. The background usually contains lymphocytes, histiocytes, plasma cells, eosinophils, and occasionally neutrophils.[50]

In some cases with characteristic lacunar cells and a nodular or diffuse pattern, fibrous bands may be absent, and the differential diagnosis with NLPHL may be difficult (Table 126.3). These cases have been called the cellular phase of NScHL.[51] Another morphologic variant, syncytial NScHL, has been described, in which there are large sheets of cells resembling lacunar RS cell variants.

NScHL can be stratified according to the number of neoplastic cells or the characteristics of the background infiltrate (proportion of eosinophils), either of which may predict prognosis. However, these grading schemes are not currently used to determine therapy.[52–54]

Clinical Features. NScHL is the most common subtype of Hodgkin lymphoma in developed countries (60% to 80% in most series). It is also most common in adolescents and young adults, but can occur at any age; affected females equal or exceed males. The mediastinum and other supradiaphragmatic sites are commonly involved.

Mixed Cellularity Classic Hodgkin Lymphoma

Morphologic Features. In mixed cellularity classic Hodgkin lymphoma (MCcHL), the infiltrate is usually diffuse or at most vaguely nodular, without band-forming sclerosis, although fine interstitial fibrosis may be present. RS cells are of the classic, diagnostic type and are usually easily identified. Many mononuclear variants are usually also present; rare lacunar cells may be seen. Diagnostic RS cells are large cells with bilobed, double, or multiple nuclei, with a large, eosinophilic, inclusion-like nucleolus in at least two lobes or nuclei. The infiltrate typically contains lymphocytes, epithelioid histiocytes, eosinophils, and plasma cells.

Clinical Features. MCcHL comprises 15% to 30% of Hodgkin lymphoma cases in most series; it may be seen at any age and lacks the early adult peak of NScHL. Involvement of the mediastinum is less common than in NScHL, and abdominal lymph node and splenic involvement are more common.

Lymphocyte-Rich Classic Hodgkin Lymphoma

Morphologic Features. Some cases of Hodgkin lymphoma with RS cells of classic type, both by morphology and immunophenotype, may have a background infiltrate that consists predominantly of lymphocytes, with rare or no eosinophils. The term lymphocyte-rich classic Hodgkin lymphoma (LRcHL) was proposed for these cases in the REAL classification and was adopted by the WHO.[9] Some cases of LRcHL have a nodular pattern, with remnants of regressed germ cells in the nodules, and RS cells and variants located within the mantle zones and interfollicular regions, mimicking NLPHL.

Clinical Features. LRcHL comprises about 5% of cases of Hodgkin lymphoma. The clinical features at presentation of LRcHL seem to be intermediate between those of LPHL and cHL: similar to NLPHL, patients have early-stage disease, lack bulky disease or B-cell symptoms, lack mediastinal disease, and have a predominance in males and a median age higher than that for NScHL. The prognosis appears to be slightly better than that of other subtypes of cHL.[9]

Lymphocyte Depleted Classic Hodgkin Lymphoma

Morphologic Features. Lymphocyte-depleted classic Hodgkin lymphoma (LDcHL) produces a diffuse and often hypocellular

TABLE 126.3

DIFFERENTIAL DIAGNOSIS OF HODGKIN LYMPHOMA

Diagnosis	Morphology (Large Cells)	Immunophenotype (Large Cells)	T-Cell Rings	Genetics (Southern Blot)
NLPHL	LP (popcorn) cells	CD20+, EMA+, CD15–, CD30–	+	Ig polyclonal
Classic HL, lymphocyte-rich	Classic RS cells	CD20−, EMA−, CD15+, CD30+	+	Ig polyclonal
PTGC	Centroblasts	CD20+, EMA−, CD15−, CD30−	–	Ig polyclonal
Follicular lymphoma	Centroblasts	CD20+, EMA– (Ig monoclonal)	–	Ig monoclonal
T-cell, histiocyte-rich large B-cell lymphoma	Centroblasts, immunoblasts, popcorn cells	CD20+, EMA±, CD15−, CD30− (Ig monoclonal±)	–	Ig monoclonal
Anaplastic large-cell lymphoma (T cell)	Horseshoe-shaped nuclei, paranuclear hof	CD20−, EMA±, CD15−, CD30+, T-Ag±, ALK± Pax5−	–	TCR monoclonal
Large B-cell lymphoma, anaplastic subtype	Bizarre, large cells, RS-like cells	CD20+, EMA±, CD15−, CD30+	–	Ig monoclonal

HL, Hodgkin lymphoma; NLPHL, nodular lymphocyte-predominant Hodgkin lymphoma; EMA, epithelial membrane antigen; Ig, immunoglobulin; PTGC, progressive transformation of germinal centers; Ag, antigen; TCR, T-cell receptor; RS, Reed-Sternberg.
Note: EMA may be difficult to detect in formalin-fixed tissues. Classic HL may be CD20+ (15%) or CD15+ (15%).

infiltrate because of the presence of diffuse fibrosis and necrosis; there are large numbers of RS cells and bizarre "sarcomatous" variants, with a paucity of other inflammatory cells. Confluent sheets of RS cells and variants may occur and rarely predominate ("reticular" variant or "Hodgkin sarcoma").[55] Before the availability of immunophenotyping studies, many cases diagnosed as LDcHL were in reality cases of large B-cell lymphoma or T-cell lymphomas, often of the anaplastic large cell type.

Clinical Features. LDcHL is the least common variant of Hodgkin lymphoma, comprising less than 1% of the cases in recent reports. It is most common in older people, in human immunodeficiency virus-positive (HIV+) individuals, and in nonindustrialized countries. LDcHL frequently presents with abdominal lymphadenopathy, spleen, liver, and bone marrow involvement, without peripheral lymphadenopathy.[56] Disease is usually advanced at diagnosis; however, response to treatment is reported not to differ from that of other subtypes of comparable stage.[9]

Immunophenotype of Classic Hodgkin Lymphoma. In most cases of NS, MC, and LDcHL, the tumor cells are CD15+, CD30+, CD45–. The frequency with which CD15 and CD30 is detected varies in reported series, probably because of technical problems. With optimal technique, about 75% to 85% are positive for CD15, and nearly 100% are positive for CD30. Expression of CD20 occurs in up to 40% of cases, usually weakly and not in all of the cells.[57] Expression of CD20 does not exclude a diagnosis of Hodgkin lymphoma if the morphologic features are typical. Other B-cell antigens such as CD79a and the immunoglobulin promoter-associated proteins OCT2 and BOB1 are typically absent; however, expression of PAX5/BSAP, another B-cell antigen, is seen in the majority of the cases, although expression is often fainter than in normal B cells.[50,58] Failure to detect CD15 or expression of a B-cell–associated antigen does not preclude a diagnosis of Hodgkin lymphoma; however, absence of both CD15 and CD30 and expression of CD20 should prompt reexamination of the slides and consideration of either NLPHL or LRcHL. Expression of T-cell antigens is distinctly unusual and should prompt both re-review of the slides and molecular genetic analysis of the T-cell receptor gene.

In addition to CD15 and CD30, classic HRS cells express CD25, HLA-Dr, ICAM-1, CD95 (apo-1/fas), and both CD40 and CD86, molecules associated with B-cell activation and interaction with T cells; T cells surrounding the RS cells express both CD40 ligand and CD28, the ligand for CD86. In contrast to NLPHL, the RS cells of cHL typically lack the nuclear Bcl-6 protein associated with germinal center B cells. In EBV-positive cases, the tumor cells express EBV latent membrane protein (LMP) but not EBNA2.

Several studies have addressed the impact of immunophenotype on the survival of patients with cHL, with varying results. A study from the German Hodgkin Study Group (GHSG) found that cases of cHL that lacked CD15 but expressed CD30 had a significantly worse freedom from relapse and overall survival than CD15+ cases.[59] Coexpression of CD20 with CD15 or CD30 had no impact on outcome, but cases that expressed CD20 alone had much poorer survival. Other studies have addressed the role of the microenvironment, including regulatory and cytotoxic T cells and macrophages.[60,61] Steidl et al.[61,62] recently analyzed fresh-frozen biopsies from 130 patients with cHL and found a correlation between increased numbers of CD68+ macrophages and shorter progression-free survival after adequate standard treatment. This finding was true for patients with both primary diagnosis and relapsed disease. Patients with limited-stage disease and a reduced number of CD68+ cells had a disease-specific survival of 100%. On the basis of these results, the possibility to implement the number of CD68+ macrophages in current strategies for risk stratification in cHL was discussed. However, before using the CD68+ macrophages as a marker for risk stratification in diagnostic lymph node samples routinely, the reported findings require validation[61,62]. As with morphologic prognostic features, these studies do not yet have a role in daily clinical practice in determining treatment.

Association of Classic Hodgkin Lymphoma with Other Lymphomas. Classic Hodgkin lymphoma may be associated with other lymphoma, most often of B-cell type either before, simultaneously with, or after Hodgkin lymphoma. Patients treated for Hodgkin lymphoma are at risk of developing aggressive B-cell lymphomas (DLBCL) and Burkitt's or Burkitt-like lymphoma, which have been presumed to arise in a setting of immune suppression secondary to therapy for Hodgkin lymphoma; the estimated risk ranges from 1% to 5%. Numerous cases of cHL associated with follicular lymphoma or DLBCL have been reported; the Hodgkin lymphoma may precede, follow, or occur simultaneously with the NHL. When studied by single-cell PCR, a common clone was found in the Hodgkin lymphoma and the NHL.[63,64]

Rare cases of B-cell chronic lymphocytic leukemia may contain cells with the morphology and immunophenotype of classic RS cells, while other patients with typical chronic lymphocytic leukemia may go on to develop Hodgkin lymphoma, the so-called Hodgkin lymphoma variant of Richter's syndrome.[65] These cases may be clonally related or unrelated to the chronic lymphocytic leukemia.[66] Finally, cases of mycosis fungoides or lymphomatoid papulosis associated with Hodgkin lymphoma have been reported.[67] In some patients, a single neoplastic B cell can give rise to both Hodgkin lymphoma and NHL, while in others it appears that either immunosuppression or other unknown factors can give rise to two independent malignancies.

B-Cell Lymphoma, Intermediate between Classic Hodgkin Lymphoma and Diffuse Large B-Cell Lymphoma. Recently, it has become apparent that some lymphomas have features of both cHL and DLBCL. These lymphomas are most commonly found in the mediastinum, and the term mediastinal gray-zone lymphoma has been used for these cases.[68] Gene expression profiling data suggest that mediastinal large B-cell lymphoma is more closely related to cHL than to most other large B-cell lymphomas; thus, this phenomenon may reflect true biological overlap between these two diseases.[69,70] The WHO classification in 2008 added a provisional category, B-cell lymphoma, intermediate between DLBCL and cHL.[71] It is defined as a B-lineage lymphoma that demonstrates overlapping clinical, morphological, or immunophenotypic features between cHL and DLBCL, especially primary mediastinal large B-cell lymphoma (PMBL). This category is meant to be used infrequently, and only cases where all information is available can be truly diagnosed as borderline between cHL and DLBCL.

Morphologic Features. The tumors are usually composed of confluent sheets of pleomorphic, large tumor cells, often with fibrosis. The cells are often larger and more pleomorphic than typical DLBCL/PMBL, and may resemble lacunar RS cell variants. There may be variation from one area to another, with some areas resembling PMBL and others NScHL.[71]

Immunophenotype. The immunophenotype is typically borderline between cHL and DLBCL. Tumor cells usually express CD45 and B-cell antigens (CD20, Oct 2, Bob1) as well as CD30 and often CD15. They typically lack immunoglobulin and tumors are typically EBV negative.[71]

Clinical Features. These tumors mainly occur in young men and are clinically more aggressive than either PMBL or NScHL. Optimal treatment is not known, and management must be individualized.[71]

DIAGNOSIS AND STAGING OF HODGKIN LYMPHOMAS

Natural History and Patterns of Spread

The Swiss radiotherapist René Gilbert is credited with first reporting that Hodgkin lymphoma spread by contiguity from one lymph node chain to adjacent chains.[72] His work was extended by Kaplan,[73] Peters,[74] and others,[75] who evaluated the use of prophylactic radiation therapy to lymph nodes adjacent to those involved with disease. The development of new radiographic studies and the routine use of staging laparotomy improved the understanding of the presentation and evolution of Hodgkin lymphoma.[73–75] There is considerable evidence that Hodgkin lymphoma begins in a single group of lymph nodes and then spreads to contiguous lymph nodes. Eventually the malignant cells may become more aggressive, invade blood vessels, and spread to organs in a manner similar to other malignancies. This is more likely to occur in patients with stage III than with stage I or II disease.

One study of more than 700 patients evaluated contiguous nodal involvement from a combination of clinical and surgical stagings.[76] Evidence for contiguous spread was most convincing for patients with NS or MC histology. The mediastinum, left side of the neck, and right side of the neck were each involved in more than 60% of patients with MC or NS histology. These sites were four or more times as common as other nodal sites above or below the diaphragm, suggesting that most cases of NS or MC Hodgkin lymphoma begin in the chest or neck. Significant associations were found between the mediastinum and the right or left neck, the neck and the ipsilateral axilla, the mediastinum and the hilum, and the spleen and abdominal nodal involvement. There was a negative association between the right and left neck if the mediastinum was not involved, suggesting that spread from one neck to the other occurred through the mediastinal nodes. A study evaluating sites of relapse in patients with minimal stage IIIA Hodgkin lymphoma treated with radiation therapy alone provides additional information.[77] It appears that when the spleen is involved with Hodgkin lymphoma, even minimally, there is a high risk of extranodal involvement. This suggests that Hodgkin lymphoma spreads from above the diaphragm to the spleen, perhaps through the vascular system, and that splenic involvement may herald spread to extranodal sites through a similar process.

Most patients with NS or MC Hodgkin lymphoma have a central pattern of lymph node involvement (cervical, mediastinal, para-aortic). In contrast, certain nodal chains (mesenteric, hypogastric, presacral, epitrochlear, popliteal) are seldom involved. The spleen is involved more frequently in patients with adenopathy below the diaphragm, systemic symptoms, and MC histology. Involvement of the liver in an untreated patient is rare and almost always occurs with concomitant splenic involvement. Infiltration of the bone marrow is usually focal and almost invariably associated with extensive disease and systemic symptoms. In the great majority of patients, the initial pattern of spread occurs nonrandomly and predictably via lymphatic channels to contiguous lymph node chains. This important observation, first made more than 50 years ago, continues to form the basis for determination of treatment strategies in patients with apparently localized Hodgkin lymphoma treated with radiation therapy alone and in determining radiation fields in patients who receive combined modality treatment consisting of radiation therapy and chemotherapy.

Staging Classifications

The advent of new imaging modalities and the frequent use of combined-modality treatment have made staging procedures simpler and less invasive in recent years. The latest international staging classification was proposed in 1989 during a meeting held in Cotswolds, England.[78] The Cotswolds classification (Table 126.4) is a modification of the Ann Arbor classification using information from staging and treatment during the past 20 years.

Some of the recommended modifications include adding a criteria for clinical involvement of the spleen and liver, which require evidence of focal defects with two imaging techniques, eliminating consideration of abnormalities of liver function, adding the suffix "X" to designate bulky disease (more than 10 cm maximum dimension), adding a new category of response to therapy, that is, unconfirmed or uncertain complete remission, to accommodate the difficulty of persistent radiologic abnormalities of uncertain significance following primary therapy, and separately classifying certain selected patients with localized extranodal disease (e.g., lung, pleura, chest wall, bone) contiguous to involved nodes as the appropriate lymph node system stage followed by the subscript E. The E designation excludes multiple extranodal deposits or bilateral lung extension, which constitute stage IV disease. Recommended staging procedures are listed in Table 126.5.

An adequate surgical biopsy, possibly of more than one intact lymph node, is required for histopathologic examination.

Radiographic Staging above the Diaphragm

More than 60% of patients with newly diagnosed Hodgkin lymphoma have radiographic evidence of intrathoracic involvement. Frontal and lateral chest radiographs should be routinely ordered, which represents a low cost method for subsequent surveillance.

Computerized tomography (CT) scanning has become the standard thoracic staging examination for patients with Hodgkin lymphoma, both for determination of sites of initial involvement in the chest and for determination of the extent of the mediastinal adenopathy. CT scanning is especially apt at detecting pulmonary disease, pleural or pericardial involvement, apical cardiac nodal enlargement, extension into the chest wall, and in defining the extent of involved axillary lymph nodes. Identification of the extent of thoracic disease will help define the use of combination chemotherapy and the dose, extent, and need for radiation therapy. It also helps to classify early-stage patients as having favorable or unfavorable prognosis disease.

Large mediastinal adenopathy has been defined as the ratio greater than one-third between the largest transverse diameter of the mediastinal mass over the transverse diameter of the thorax at the diaphragm on a standing poster-anterior chest x-ray.[79] Others have defined extensive mediastinal disease as more than 35% of the thoracic diameter at T5 or T6, or as measuring more than 5 to 10 cm in width. These patients make up 20% to 25% of clinical stage I or II patients, generally present with involvement of multiple supradiaphragmatic nodal chains, and may have extension of tumor into the lung, pericardium, or chest wall.[80] Systemic symptoms are frequently present.

TABLE 126.4

COTSWOLDS STAGING CLASSIFICATION FOR HODGKIN LYMPHOMA

Stage	Description
I	Involvement of a single lymph node region or lymphoid structure (e.g., spleen, thymus, Waldeyer's ring) or involvement of a single extralymphatic site (IE).
II	Involvement of two or more lymph node regions on the same side of the diaphragm (hilar nodes, when involved on both sides, constitute stage II disease); localized contiguous involvement of only one extranodal organ or site and lymph node region(s) on the same side of the diaphragm (IIE). The number of anatomic regions involved should be indicated by a subscript (e.g., II_3).
III	Involvement of lymph node regions on both sides of the diaphragm (III), which may also be accompanied by involvement of the spleen (III_S) or by localized contiguous involvement of only one extranodal organ site (IIIE) or both (IIISE).
III_1	With or without involvement of splenic, hilar, celiac, or portal nodes.
III_2	With involvement of para-aortic, iliac, and mesenteric nodes.
IV	Diffuse or disseminated involvement of one or more extranodal organs or tissues, with or without associated lymph node involvement.
Designations Applicable to Any Disease Stage	
A	No symptoms.
B	Fever (temperature, >38°C), drenching night sweats, unexplained loss of >10% body weight within the preceding 6 months.
X	Bulky disease (a widening of the mediastinum by more than one-third or the presence of a nodal mass with a maximal dimension >10 cm).
E	Involvement of a single extranodal site that is contiguous or proximal to the known nodal site.
CS	Clinical stage.
PS	Pathologic stage (as determined by laparotomy).

TABLE 126.5

RECOMMENDED STAGING

Adequate surgical biopsy reviewed by an experienced hemopathologist
Detailed history with attention to the presence or absence of systemic symptoms
Careful physical examination, emphasizing node chains, size of liver and spleen, and Waldeyer's ring inspection
Routine laboratory tests: complete blood cell count, erythrocyte sedimentation rate, and liver function tests
Chest radiograph (posteroanterior and lateral) with measurement of mass-thoracic ratio
Chest and abdominal computed tomography
Evaluation with FDG-positron emission tomography recommended when the results of other conventional diagnostic procedures are not conclusive
Core-needle biopsy of bone marrow from the posterior iliac crest in patients with stages IIB–IV disease
Needle or surgical biopsy of any suspicious extranodal (e.g., hepatic, osseous, pulmonary, cutaneous) lesion(s)
Cytologic examination of any effusion
Staging laparotomy (with splenectomy, needle and wedge biopsy of the liver, and biopsies of para-aortic, mesenteric, portal, and splenic hilar lymph nodes) in rare circumstances in early-stage Hodgkin lymphoma in which the use of limited radiation therapy alone depends on pathologic staging

FDG, [^{18}F]fluorodeoxyglucose.

Following initial chemotherapy, residual abnormalities often remain on thoracic CT scanning. The use of gallium or positron emission tomography (PET) scanning may aid in the management and follow-up of patients in this setting. The gallium scan is a sensitive indicator of disease above the diaphragm, particularly when a dose of 10 mCi and single-photon emission CT (SPECT) techniques are employed. Data obtained in patients who receive both chemotherapy and radiation therapy suggest that a negative gallium scan might have prognostic impact in early-stage patients.

Whole-body PET using ^{18}F-fluorodeoxyglucose (FDG-PET scan) appears to be a more sensitive radiographic modality than gallium scanning and has almost universally replaced it as a staging tool. Many of the early clinical studies using gallium scanning provide the basis for ongoing trials using PET. Increasingly, PET scanning is being used in the initial evaluation and in the staging procedures after having completed treatment.[81,82] However, similar to the gallium scan, PET scanning is not an absolute indicator of cure after chemotherapy alone, and at present, there is only little information supporting the use of these studies to guide whether or not to use adjuvant involved-field radiotherapy (IF-RT) in patients with early-stage disease.

Radiographic Staging below the Diaphragm

CT scanning, lymphangiography, magnetic resonance tomography, and nuclear medicine imaging all have limitations in the radiologic evaluation of the abdominal nodes. No single study is reliable for detecting Hodgkin lymphoma in normal-size nodes, and all studies have a 20% to 25% false-negative rate because of the inability to detect occult Hodgkin lymphoma in the spleen.[83,84] From staging laparotomy studies, 90% of patients who are upstaged have splenic involvement either alone or in addition to other infradiaphragmatic nodal sites.[83] Bipedal lymphangiography has given way to CT scanning and more recently to PET/CT scanning as the radiologic examination of choice for abdominal staging. With the infrequent use of staging laparotomy and splenectomy in the staging of Hodgkin lymphoma, the risk of overstaging based on a single radiographic test of abdominal involvement (false positive) has greater potential consequences. Therefore, the authors strongly recommend that two separate studies (i.e., CT scanning and gallium/PET scanning) should be used to assess abdominal involvement. Positive findings on both tests should be used to confirm abdominal involvement.

Staging Laparotomy

Staging laparotomy was extensively used when radiation therapy was the preferred treatment for early-stage Hodgkin lymphoma and if it was mandatory to define the extent of abdominal disease to help determine whether there was an indication for the initial use of chemotherapy. With the current use of prognostic factors to determine treatment for Hodgkin lymphoma, laparotomy has disappeared as a routine staging procedure.

CLINICAL PRESENTATION OF HODGKIN LYMPHOMAS

In general, Hodgkin lymphoma patients present with peripheral lymphadenopathy. The nodes usually are not tender, and changes in the overlying skin are unusual. Otherwise, tenderness and skin changes are thought to reflect rapid growth with stretching of nodal capsules. In most cases, the nodes are discrete and freely movable. Occult presentation with central (chest and abdomen) lymphadenopathy, visceral involvement, or with systemic symptoms of the disease is more uncommon. The most characteristic clinical presentation of Hodgkin lymphoma is enlarged superficial lymph nodes in young adults, with the most frequent locations being cervical or supraclavicular (60% to 80%), high in the neck, or axillary. Less often it is found in the inguinal and femoral region.

A mediastinal involvement is discovered often by routine staging chest radiography, and even fairly large masses may occur without producing local symptoms. Otherwise, symptoms of retrosternal chest pain, cough, or shortness of breath may be clinical signs of an intrathoracic disease presentation. A bulky mediastinal mass may be associated with small amounts of pericardial and pleural fluid, but malignant effusions, diagnosed by thoracocentesis or pleural biopsy, are rare.

Involvement of the liver in a newly diagnosed patient is uncommon and occurs almost always with concomitant splenic involvement; Hodgkin lymphoma limited to the spleen is also very rare. Patients may present with abdominal swelling secondary to hepato- or splenomegaly or, rarely, with ascites. Infradiaphragmal lymphadenopathy may give rise to discomfort and pain in the retroperitoneum, the paravertebral, or loin regions, particularly in the supine position, by nodular compression of nerves or nerve roots. Advanced intra-abdominal disease may be associated with obstruction of the ureters or compression of the renal vein or ascites.

Bone marrow infiltration is usually focal, and in most cases associated with extensive disease including systemic symptoms. Laboratory findings like leukopenia, anemia, thrombocytopenia, and an elevated alkaline phosphatase level may indicate bone marrow infiltration.

Involvement of the central nervous system is rare, although invasion of the epidural space can occur by nodular extension from the para-aortic region through the intervertebral foramina, presenting neurologic symptoms and pain as leading clinical features.[84,85] Several paraneoplastic neurologic syndromes have been reported in association with Hodgkin lymphoma, but all are very rare.

Complaints from extranodal manifestations of disease may occur, such as cough from pulmonary infiltration, jaundice from hepatic involvement, or abdominal pain from disease adjacent to the bowel. Gastrointestinal involvement is an extremely rare event and might occur as infiltration from mesenteric lymph nodes. Initial symptoms of disease limited to extranodal tissue are more rare in Hodgkin lymphoma than in NHL.

A significant proportion of undiagnosed patients with Hodgkin lymphoma present with systemic symptoms prior to the discovery of enlarged lymph nodes. Typical symptoms are fever, drenching night sweats, and weight loss (so-called B-symptoms, relating to the Ann Arbor classification). This characteristic Hodgkin lymphoma–associated fever occurs intermittently and recurs at variable intervals for several days or weeks. Fever and drenching night sweats are found in up to 25% of all patients at first time of presentation; increasing to 50% in patients with more advanced disease. Other nonspecific symptoms are pruritus, fatigue, and the development of pain shortly after drinking alcohol. This pain is usually transient at the site of nodal involvement and may be severe. Pruritus, although currently not a defined B-symptom, may be an important systemic symptom of disease, but occurs infrequently, in less than 20% of patients. It often occurs months or even a year before the first diagnosis of Hodgkin lymphoma.[86] The underlying pathophysiologic mechanisms that lead to pruritus are unknown but may be due to an autoimmune reaction in which a number of cytokines are activated by tumor lysis.

TREATMENT METHODS FOR HODGKIN LYMPHOMA

Radiotherapy

Principles

The early treatment of Hodgkin lymphoma with crude x-rays in 1901 followed the discoveries of Roentgen, Becquerel, and the Curies at the end of the 18th century. The first reports of x-ray treatments that would dramatically shrink enlarged lymph nodes produced great excitement and premature predictions for the successful treatment of Hodgkin lymphoma.[87] During the first two decades of the 20th century, physicians mainly used two methods to treat Hodgkin lymphoma with radiation. Small doses of radiation were administered to the entire trunk at weekly intervals for many weeks or given as a single massive dose just to the tumor. Neither method controlled the disease, and both caused severe side effects.[72] Enlarged nodes usually shrank with both techniques, but recurrence and spread to previously uninvolved nodes invariably followed. After several courses of radiotherapy, the Hodgkin lymphoma became more resistant to treatment, and very few patients survived 5 years from diagnosis. These multiple recurrences were not attributed to poor radiotherapy techniques but viewed as inherent to the Hodgkin lymphoma itself. Therefore, most physicians stopped using radiation as a means to cure Hodgkin lymphoma by 1920. For the next 40 years, in most centers, treatment was mainly palliative, with the intention to shrink large nodes that were painful or interfered with movement, eating, or breathing.

The development of modern radiation therapy techniques for the treatment of Hodgkin lymphoma began with the work of Gilbert in the 1920s. He began to advocate treatment to apparently uninvolved adjacent lymph node chains that might contain suspected microscopic disease, as well as to the evident sites of lymph node involvement. Peters also adapted this technique at the Princess Margaret Hospital in the late 1930s and early 1940s. In her historic article published in the *American Journal of Roentgenology* in 1950, Peters provided evidence that patients with limited Hodgkin lymphoma could be cured with aggressive radiation therapy that treated involved nodal disease as well as adjacent nodal sites. She did this by identifying a group of patients with limited-stage Hodgkin lymphoma that was cured with high-dose, fractionated radiation therapy. She reported 5- and 10-year survival rates of 88% and 79%, respectively, for patients with disease limited to a single lymph node region, rates that were notably high for a disease in which virtually no one survived 10 years. Nevertheless, the concept that early-stage Hodgkin lymphoma might be curable with radiation therapy using higher doses and larger fields was slow to be accepted. Prior to the 1960s, most patients with limited Hodgkin lymphoma were not treated at all or only with small doses of radiation.

No one deserves more credit than Henry Kaplan for the development of successful modern treatment for Hodgkin lymphoma. His accomplishments are many and include pioneering work on the development of the linear accelerator that defined radiation field sizes and doses for a curative approach for early Hodgkin lymphoma, refining and improving diagnostic staging techniques, developing models for translating laboratory findings into clinical practice, and promoting early randomized clinical trials in the United States.[73]

Techniques

Historically, when treatment of early-stage Hodgkin lymphoma consisted of radiation therapy alone, radiation-fields design attempted to include multiple involved and uninvolved lymph node sites often above and below the diaphragm. These fields should no longer be used today as chemotherapy is almost always an integral part of the initial treatment, and the standard field used in combination with chemotherapy is called the involved field. Even when radiation is used as the only treatment in early-stage NLPHL, the field should be limited to the involved site or to the involved sites and immediately adjacent lymph node groups. Further, even more limited radiation fields restricted to the originally involved lymph node are currently under study by several European groups.

The many terminologies given to radiation field variations in Hodgkin lymphoma have caused significant confusion. Although the final determination of the field may vary from patient to patient and depends on many clinical, anatomic, and normal tissue tolerance considerations, general definitions and guidelines are available and should be followed.

The involved field is limited to the site of the clinically involved lymph node group. The main involved-field nodal regions are the neck (unilateral cervical and supraclavicular nodes), mediastinum (including the hilar and supraclavicular regions bilaterally), axilla (including the supraclavicular and infraclavicular lymph nodes), para-aortic lymph nodes, and inguinal (including the femoral and iliac nodes) nodes. In general, the fields include the involved prechemotherapy sites and volume, except that the postchemotherapy transverse diameter of the mediastinal and para-aortic lymph nodes is treated. In these areas the regression of the lymph nodes is easily depicted by CT imaging, and critical normal tissues are spared by reducing irradiated volumes. Thus, prechemotherapy and postchemotherapy information (both CT and PET) regarding lymph node localization and size is critical and should be available at the time of planning the field.

Chemotherapy

The development of chemotherapy programs for Hodgkin lymphoma is a story of success. Following the discovery of the cytotoxic effects of nitrogen mustard in the 1940s, a number of different drugs, including chlorambucil, cyclophosphamide, procarbazine, vinblastine, and vincristine, were developed and showed efficacy in Hodgkin lymphoma. Response rates were about 50% to 60% with 10% to 30% complete response. However, relapse was seen in almost all cases, but no cure could be achieved.

Based on a murine leukemia cell line, Skipper et al. postulated a model of tumor cell kill based on the logarithmic cell growth and a logarithmic response to cytotoxic agents. From this model, the authors predicted that response to chemotherapy would depend on tumor burden, drug dose, and kinetics of residual tumor cells. It was further postulated that the simultaneous use of several drugs with different modes of action might yield superior results. The combination of drugs might be tolerated if the toxicities were nonoverlapping. Initial attempts with two-drug combinations revealed the potential of this approach.

The important role of this model was realized in 1967, when DeVita et al. reported on a four-drug combination chemotherapy program, MOPP (nitrogen mustard, vincristine, procarbazine, and prednisone). This combination established the curability of more than 50% of patients with stages III and IV disease.

The development of MOPP was a milestone in oncology, demonstrating that advanced-stage Hodgkin lymphoma could be cured. The differences in survival between historical controls and MOPP-treated patients were so dramatic that randomized clinical trials were not needed to validate these results. Further information on chemotherapy is given later in the section on advanced disease.

Combined Modality

In addition to the many factors that affect either chemotherapy or radiation therapy when used alone, there are several issues that arise specifically because of potential interaction and summing of effects when they are combined. It is important to remember that the purpose of adding a second modality is to overcome resistance to the first, and in the case of adding irradiation to chemotherapy for Hodgkin lymphoma, it seemed likely that full-dose irradiation might be needed to overcome primary resistance to chemotherapy. Of particular interest the first two trials by the GHSG in which patients with stage IA+B, IIA+B, and stage IIIA disease with extensive mediastinal or splenic involvement or E lesions were treated with two courses of cyclophosphamide, vincristine, procarbazine, prednisone/doxorubicin, bleomycin, vinblastine, dacarbazine (COPP/ABVD) followed by irradiation.[88] In the first trial (HD1), responders to chemotherapy were then given extended-field irradiation with a dose to nonbulky sites assigned randomly to be either 20 or 40 Gy. In the second trial (HD5), a similar group of patients received 30 Gy to the nonbulky sites. Bulky sites received 40 Gy in each trial. Failure-free survival (FFS) was the same in all groups, strongly implying that after optimal chemotherapy, irradiation dose, at least to nonbulky sites, can be reduced without sacrificing efficacy.

Furthermore, studies of the GHSG in early favorable (HD10) patients showed very similar results for freedom from treatment failure (FFTF) and overall survival (OS) when given 20 or 30 Gy after two or four courses of ABVD chemotherapy. However, there was a significantly poorer tumor control for those receiving 20 Gy as compared to 30 Gy in early unfavorable patients after four courses of ABVD (HD11).[31]

The risk of severe late complications of irradiation may be reduced by lowering the dose applied. Studies of late sequelae of treatment for Hodgkin lymphoma suggest that the risk of second neoplasms, especially breast cancer in women, may be reduced by lower radiation dose.[89,90] The other late toxicity possibly associated with radiation dose is cardiovascular. A study at Stanford University found that a higher dose of irradiation to the mediastinum was associated with increased mortality from cardiac disease.[91]

An alternative approach to reduce toxicity from irradiation when used in combined modality treatment is to reduce not the dose but the extent of the field encompassed. Several trials in patients with limited-stage Hodgkin lymphoma have shown that as good results can be achieved when chemotherapy is combined with IF-RT compared to irradiation alone to an extended field.[92,93] The ability to preserve efficacy while limiting toxicity by reducing the size of the treatment fields is one of the most attractive aspects of using combined modality treatment. The same theoretical considerations that apply to irradiation are also relevant when one considers reduction of the dose of chemotherapy used in combined modality treatment.

In theory, either chemotherapy or radiation therapy could come first in the sequence of combined modality treatment. In practice, it is almost always desirable for chemotherapy to come first. The reason for this includes early effective treatment of disseminated disease, delay in induction of irreversible loss of bone marrow function, and the opportunity to use smaller, potentially less-toxic radiation treatment fields after chemotherapy has induced tumor regression.

High-Dose Chemotherapy Plus Stem Cell Support

Principles

High-dose chemotherapy (HDCT) has been used extensively in patients with relapsed and refractory Hodgkin lymphoma. Implicit in the rationale for this approach is the assumption of a steep dose–response relationship for lymphoma patients subjected to chemoradiotherapy. Although care must be exercised in interpreting clinical results, both animal models and clinical studies support the existence of such a relationship.

The use of autologous bone marrow or peripheral blood stem cells (PBSC) to support intensification of chemotherapy as salvage treatment has changed the options available for relapsed patients. Autologous transplantation involves the replacement of hematopoietic stem cells that have been irreversibly injured by HDCT or radiotherapy. This can be accomplished either with bone marrow cells obtained by multiple aspirations from the posterior iliac crest under anesthesia or with PBSC collected by apheresis. The use of PBSC has surpassed the use of bone marrow, and PBSC are now almost exclusively used. The advantage of using PBSC includes avoiding general anesthesia and more rapid hematopoietic reconstitution.

Conditioning Regimens

Several conditioning regimens have been used and summarized previously.[94] The most commonly used are BEAM (carmustine [BCNU], etoposide, cytarabine, melphalan) or CVB (cyclophosphamide, carmustine [BCNU], etoposide) given in different dose schedules. When BCNU-containing regimens are used, careful clinical monitoring to detect early signs of delayed lung toxicity is important, particularly when BCNU doses of 450 mg/m^2 or more are given. Mucositis and enterocolitis represent the most significant nonhematologic toxicities associated with high-dose melphalan. Total-body irradiation has been used in only a few studies because many Hodgkin patients have already received thoracic irradiation by the time they reach the transplant stage and because of the high treatment-related mortality of patients prepared by total-body irradiation–containing regimens.[95] Although the toxicity profiles differ with these regimens, there is currently no evidence to support the superiority of any particular regimen in Hodgkin lymphoma.

Sequential HDCT had been employed a few years ago in the treatment of solid tumors and lymphoma. Results from phase 2 studies suggest that this approach might offer a safe and effective treatment option. Following initial cytoreduction, few non–cross-resistant agents were given in short time intervals in accordance with the Norton-Simon hypothesis. In general, the transplantation of autologous stem cells and the use of growth factors allow the application of the most effective drugs in highest doses in intervals of 1 to 3 weeks. Sequential HDCT therapy might allow the highest possible dosing in a minimum of time.

More recently, the European intergroup study HDR2 evaluated the impact of sequential HDCT prior to myeloablative therapy with BEAM in patients with histologically confirmed relapsed Hodgkin lymphoma.[96] In the standard arm, patients received two cycles of DHAP (cisplatin, cytarabine, dexamethasone) followed by BEAM and PBSC transplant. Patients in the experimental arm additionally received sequential cyclophosphamide, methotrexate, and etoposide in high doses before BEAM. From a total of 284 patients included, 241 responding patients were randomized after DHAP. Somewhat surprisingly, there were no differences in terms of FFTF (P = .56) and OS (P = .82) between arms at a median observation time of 42 months. FFTF at 3 years was 62% (95% confidence interval [CI], 56% to 68%) and OS was 80% (95% CI, 75% to 85%). Patients with stage IV, early relapse, multiple relapse, anemia, or B-symptoms had a higher risk of recurrence (P <.001). Compared to conventional HDCT, additional sequential HDCT was associated with more side effects and did not improve the prognosis of patients with relapsed Hodgkin lymphoma in this study, thus strongly questioning the sequential HDCT concept.

Incorporating Radiotherapy in High-Dose Chemotherapy Programs

The rationale for incorporating radiotherapy into HDCT programs stems from the observation that disease progression following HDCT often occurred in sites of prior involvement. Several investigators showed that the sites of failure in 65% to 95% were involved immediately prior to HDCT.[95,97] Retrospective analyses suggested that radiation therapy may be incorporated as cytoreductive treatment prior to HDCT or as a consolidative therapy after HDCT.[98,99] However, there has been no prospective clinical trial to answer the question regarding the extent of the radiation field, the timing of treatment, and the appropriate dose to use.

CHOICE OF TREATMENT

Prognostic Factors and Treatment Groups

A prognostic factor is a measurement or classification of an individual patient, performed at or soon after diagnosis, which gives information on the likely outcome of the disease. This information will generally be phrased in terms of probability; for instance, the likelihood of cure for various values of a prognostic factor. It may be used for informing the patient or in the context of clinical trials for defining or describing study populations or adjusting the data analysis; however, for the clinician, the most important role of prognostic factors is to help choose an appropriate treatment strategy.

In Hodgkin lymphoma, patients have been traditionally classified into two or three prognostic groups, chiefly according to stage and B-symptoms but also taking various other factors into consideration. Most basically, patients with advanced stages (i.e., those staged IIIB or IV), have been associated with the poorest prognosis and assigned an intensive chemotherapy protocol, sometimes followed by adjuvant radiotherapy. Further prognostic factors were often used to assign stage IIIA or IIB patients to the advanced-stage group. Among early stages, a favorable and an unfavorable subgroup were defined, depending on clinical risk factors identified in prior clinical trials. For each risk group, typical standard treatment approaches are being defined:

- Early favorable stages: a brief chemotherapy (typically two or three cycles) plus IF-RT
- Early unfavorable stages: moderate amount of chemotherapy (typically four cycles) plus IF-RT
- Advanced stages: extensive chemotherapy (typically eight cycles) with or without consolidation radiotherapy (usually to residual tumors).

These standard-of-care strategies are not uniformly applied, and the investigation of alternatives is continuing, as will be reported in the following sections. In this scheme, two divisions between the three prognostic groups must be defined, each division possibly defined by a different set of factors. Furthermore, the attempt has been made to identify advanced-stage patients with a particularly high risk for failure to potentially intensify therapy in this group; attempts include early HDCT with stem cell support. This approach, however, has not shown any benefit when compared with six to eight courses of conventional chemotherapy, such as ABVD.[100]

The selection of factors and the definition of prognostic groups can vary among collaborative groups and countries, as does the choice of treatment (Table 126.6).

Prognostic factors are rarely the subject of specific clinical studies but are rather discovered and evaluated using data from large cohorts of uniformly treated, well-documented, and reliably followed patients, usually from large clinical trials.[101] The diversity of diagnostic and treatment strategies used for early stages, as well as statistical problems caused by the low rate of treatment failures, has led to the reporting and use of modestly different prognostic factors by different institutions and trial groups.

In the following sections, recognized prognostic factors will be described for early and advanced-stage patients, respectively. Such factors are required to show independent prognostic value in multivariate analyses of a large number of patients. This account refers in general to clinically staged patients, as laparotomy is now rarely performed. The use of these factors to define prognostic groups for treatment purposes, as practiced by various institutions and study groups, will also be described.

The European Organisation for the Research and Treatment of Cancer (EORTC) has, since 1982, defined clinical stages I and II (supradiaphragmatic only) patients as unfavorable if they had any of the following factors: age 50 years or more, asymptomatic with erythrocyte sedimentation rate (ESR) more than 50, B-symptoms with ESR more than 30, and large mediastinal mass (LMM), based on the results of earlier EORTC trials H1 and H2. In previous trials, stage II, mixed cellularity or lymphocyte depletion histology, and number of involved regions had also been counted as adverse factors.

The GHSG has, since 1988, assigned combined-modality treatment to clinical stages I and II patients with any of the following adverse factors: LMM, number of involved regions, ESR, localized extranodal infiltration (so-called E-lesions), or massive splenic involvement[102] Due to the rarity of splenectomy, the latter factor was seldom reported and was abandoned for the more recent trial generations. It can be difficult to distinguish consistently between E-lesions and stage IV disease, and varying assessments of the prognostic value of this feature have been obtained by different investigators. A study at Stanford University began in 1980 to give combined-modality treatment to clinical stages I and II patients with LMM or multiple E-lesions.

The EORTC has investigated the use of localized radiotherapy in a "very favorable" subgroup of early stage patients. Inclusion criteria were stage IA female patients aged less than 40, NS or LP histology, without elevated ESR or LMM. However, a 30% long-term failure rate was observed, and this policy was discontinued.

TABLE 126.6

DEFINITION OF TREATMENT GROUPS BY THREE LARGE STUDY GROUPS

Treatment Group	EORTC/GELA	GHSG	NCIC/ECOG
Early stage favorable	CS I–II without risk factors (supradiaphragmatic)	CS I–II without risk factors	Standard risk group: favorable CS I–II (without risk factors)
Early stage unfavorable (intermediate)	CS I–II with ≥1 risk factors (supradiaphragmatic)	CS I, CSIIA ≥1 risk factors; CS IIB with C/D but without A/B	Standard risk group: unfavorable CS I–II (at least one risk factor)
Advanced stage	CS III–IV	CS IIB with A/B; CS III–IV	High-risk group: CS I or II with bulky disease; intra-abdominal disease; CS III, IV
Risk factors	A: large mediastinal mass B: age ≥50 years C: elevated ESR D: ≥4 involved regions	A: large mediastinal mass B: extranodal disease C: elevated ESR D: ≥3 involved areas	A: ≥40 years B: not NLPHL or NS histology C: ESR ≥50 mm/h D: ≥4 involved nodal regions

EORTC, European Organisation for Research and Treatment of Cancer; GELA, Groupe d'Etude des Lymphomes de l'Adulte; GHSG, German Hodgkin Study Group; ECOG, Eastern Cooperative Oncology Group; NCIC, National Cancer Institute of Canada; CS, clinical stage; NLPHL, nodular lymphocyte predominance Hodgkin lymphoma, NS, nodular sclerosis; ESR, erythrocyte sedimentation rate (≥50 mm/h without or ≥30 mm/h with B-symptoms).

Prognostic Factors for Early Stages (Clinical Stages I and II)

Despite the different mode of action of chemotherapy compared with radiotherapy, similar prognostic factors have emerged from analyses of cohorts treated with radiation and with combined modality either in early or in advanced stages. This similarity of prognostic effects is supported by the observation from a meta-analysis of radiation versus combined modality treatment in early stages, that the size of the difference in FFS between these two treatment strategies was essentially constant over different prognostic groups.

As a consequence, the prognostic factors relevant to the division between early unfavorable and advanced stages, that is, between moderate and extensive chemotherapy, are essentially the same as those used for the division between favorable and unfavorable. However, generally only stage IIB patients are given advanced-stage treatment in case these factors are present.

The EORTC includes in its advanced-stage cohorts stages III and IV only, without regard to other factors, as did the U.S. National Cancer Institute (NCI) and several U.S. cooperative groups.

In the GHSG, all stages III and IV patients plus stage IIB with LMM or E-lesions are included in the advanced group. Earlier trials had also included either all stage IIIA patients or just those without any of the GHSG risk factors in the early unfavorable group. This gradual shift to more use of intensive therapy was based on prognostic factor analyses.

Certain other trial groups include further stages I and II patients in the advanced prognostic group; for instance, stages IB and IIB patients or those with bulky stage II disease.

Prognostic Factors for Advanced Stages

The more uniform treatment modality and the greater frequency of treatment failures has allowed more conclusive and generally applicable results for prognostic factor analyses for the advanced stages. The results of the International Prognostic Factor Project (IPS), while not necessarily including all possible factors, can be taken as reliable (Table 126.7).[103]

All these factors were highly significant in the multivariate analysis of data from 5,141 patients treated in 25 centers, and their prognostic power was confirmed in an independent sample. Note that factors 1, 2, 4, and 5 as listed on Table 126.7 are also prognostic for early-stage patients. All seven factors were associated with similar relative risks of between 1.26 and 1.49. Therefore, Hasenclever and Diehl[103] recommended combining these factors into a single score by simply counting the number of adverse factors, giving an integer prognostic score between 0 and 7. However, even patients with five or more factors (7% of cases) had a 5-year failure-free rate of more than 40%. The best failure-free rate was close to 80% for those with at most one factor (29% of cases), suggesting that a group of advanced-stage patients with a relatively favorable prognosis could be recognized.

A number of other factors have been shown to correlate with prognosis in advanced stages, but their independent importance is not proven because of conflicting results or lack of confirmation in a large data set. These include pathologic grade in nodular sclerosis classic Hodgkin lymphoma, tissue eosinophilia, inguinal involvement, serum lactate dehydrogenase, and β_2-microglobulin.

Factors relevant to advanced-stage patients may be used to identify patients either for treatment intensification or for treatment reduction. Reduction can be achieved by creating a modified protocol or by including these patients in the early-stage group.

Concerning intensification, various investigators have treated a poor prognosis subset of advanced-stage patients who had attained a remission by conventional chemotherapy, with HDCT accompanied by hematologic stem cell support.[104,105] Proctor et al.[106] constructed a continuous numerical index for this purpose as a weighted sum of the variables age, stage, lymphocyte count, hemoglobin, and presence of bulky disease, and included patients with an index of more than 0.5 in the poor prognosis subset.[106] Federico et al.[138] included patients with two or more of the following factors: high lactate dehydrogenase, very large mediastinal mass, two or more extranodal sites, inguinal involvement, low hematocrit, and bone marrow involvement. However, none of these methods could consistently select a subset with a failure rate of less than 40% with conventional therapy. This means that the early high-dose approach is unlikely to show a clinically relevant long-term survival benefit compared with conventional treatment.[107]

In conclusion, the three-level scheme of division into early favorable, early unfavorable, and advanced-stage cases remains valid according to current knowledge. Separation of very favorable early or poor-risk advanced-stage patients for especially mild or intensive therapy, respectively, does not appear justified. Several prognostic factors, other than clinical stage, are employed in the divisions between favorable, unfavorable, and advanced cases, and no universally valid set of factors has been determined. Nevertheless, the list of reliably confirmed, independently prognostic factors encompasses most of the factors used by the major institutions and study groups. For early and advanced stages receiving radiotherapy or chemotherapy or both, the set of relevant factors is fairly similar.

A number of other factors have been shown to correlate with prognosis in advanced stages, but their independent

PRACTICE OF ONCOLOGY

TABLE 126.7

FINAL COX REGRESSION MODEL (INTERNATIONAL PROGNOSTIC FACTORS PROJECT)

Factor	Log Hazard Ratio	*P* Value	Relative Risk
Serum albumin <4 g/dL	0.40 ± 0.10	<.001	1.49
Hemoglobin <10.5 g/dL	0.30 ± 0.11	.006	1.35
Male gender	0.30 ± 0.09	.001	1.35
Stage IV disease	0.23 ± 0.09	.011	1.26
Age >45 y	0.33 ± 0.10	.001	1.39
White blood cell count >15,000/mm³	0.34 ± 0.11	.001	1.41
Lymphocyte count <600/mm³ or <8% of white blood cell count	0.31 ± 0.10	.002	1.38

impact is not proven because of conflicting results or lack of confirmation in a larger data set. Currently, the search for biologically specific factors directly related to tumor activity is ongoing, but thus far no reliable and clinically robust factors have been described.

TREATMENT FOR EARLY FAVORABLE HODGKIN LYMPHOMA

For years, radiotherapy alone had been considered the treatment of choice for patients with early favorable Hodgkin lymphoma. Many patients achieved complete remission, but the relapse rate was common and overall survival not satisfying.[108] In addition, late effects such as secondary solid tumors were increasing since radiation usually was not only delivered to clinically involved but also to adjacent sites. To improve treatment results, combined modality strategies were subsequently introduced, and randomized trials demonstrated this approach to be more effective than radiotherapy alone.[109,110] Thus, there is currently no justification for the use of radiotherapy alone in Hodgkin lymphoma except for patients with stage IA nodular lymphocyte predominant Hodgkin lymphoma presenting without clinical risk factors. In this small subset of patients, analyses by the GHSG and the EORTC revealed no significant outcome differences between patients treated with 30 Gy IF-RT and patients receiving extended-field radiotherapy (EF-RT) or combined modality strategies.[30,111] Consequentially, the least toxic approach, 30 Gy IF-RT, was adopted as standard of care within both study groups.

Combined Modality Approaches

Various randomized trials demonstrated the superiority of combined modality treatment over radiotherapy alone in patients with early favorable Hodgkin lymphoma (Table 126.8). In the HD7 trial conducted by the GHSG, 650 patients were randomized to receive either 30 Gy EF-RT plus 10 Gy to the IF alone or two cycles of ABVD chemotherapy followed by the same radiotherapy. Tumor control was superior in patients treated with the combined modality approach, resulting in a

TABLE 126.8

CLINICAL TRIALS IN FAVORABLE-PROGNOSIS STAGE I AND II HODGKIN LYMPHOMA: TRIALS TO IDENTIFY THE OPTIMAL NUMBER OF CHEMOTHERAPY CYCLES

Trial	Eligibility	Treatment Regimens	No. of Patients	Outcome
GHSG HD7, 1994–1998	CS IA–IIB *without* large mediastinal mass >0.33 m/t ratio); massive splenic involvement; localized extranodal involvement; ESR ≥50 mm/h in A, ≥30 mm/h in B; three or more involved areas	A: EFRT 30 Gy (IFRT 40 Gy) B: 2 ABVD + EFRT 30 Gy (IFRT 40 Gy)	311 316	FFTF (84 mo) 67%; SV (84 mo) 92% FFTF, (84 mo) 88%; SV (84 mo), 94% (FFTF: *P* <.0001; SV: *P* NS)
GHSG HD10, 1998–2003	CS IA–IIB *without* large mediastinal mass >0.33 m/t ratio); localized extranodal involvement; ESR >50 mm/h in A, ≥30 mm/h in B; three or more involved areas	A: 2 ABVD + IFRT (30 Gy) B: 2 ABVD + IFRT (20 Gy) C: 4 ABVD + IFRT (30 Gy) D: 4 ABVD + IFRT (20 Gy)	298 299 295 299	FFTF (96 mo) 86%; SV (96 mo) 94% FFTF (96 mo) 86%; SV (96 mo) 95% FFTF (96 mo) 87%; SV (96 mo) 95% FFTF (96 mo) 90%; SV (96 mo) 95% (FFTF = NS; SV = NS)
SWOG 9133/ CALGB 9391	CS IA–IIA *without* age <16 y; large mediastinal disease; pericardial involvement	A: 3 (doxorubicin + vinblastine) + STLI (S) (36–40 Gy) B: STLI (S) (36–40 Gy)	166 163	FFTF, 94%; SV (3 y), 98% FFTF, 81%; SV (3 y), 96% (FFTF: *P* <.001; SV: *P* = NS)
EORTC/GELA H8F	CS IA–IIB *without* age <50 y; ESR ≥50 mm/h in A, ≥30 mm/h in B; ≥4 sites of disease; large mediastinal disease	A: 3 MOPP/ABV + IFRT (36 Gy) B: STLI (S)	271 272	EFS (10 y), 93%; SV (10 y), 97% EFS (10 y), 68%; SV (10 y), 92% (EFS: *P* <.0001; SV: *P* .0001)
Stanford V for favorable CS IA–IIA HL	CS I–II *without* B-symptoms; age <16 y and >60 y; large mediastinal disease; <2 extranodal sites	Stanford V for 8 wk + modified IFRT (30 Gy)	87	Median follow-up, 5.7 y; FFP (8 y), 96%; SV, 98%

HL, Hodgkin lymphoma; GHSG, German Hodgkin Study Group; CS, clinical stage; ESR, erythrocyte sedimentation rate; EFRT, extended-field radiotherapy; IFRT, involved-field radiation therapy; ABVD, doxorubicin, bleomycin, vinblastine, dacarbazine; FFTF, freedom from treatment failure; NS, not significant; SV, survival; SWOG, Southwest Oncology Group; CALGB, Cancer and Leukemia Group B; STLI (S), subtotal nodal irradiation (splenic irradiation); EORTC, European Organisation for Research and Treatment of Cancer; GELA, Groupe d'Etude des Lymphomes de l'Adulte; MOPP, mechlorethamine, vincristine, procarbazine, prednisone; m/t ratio, mass to thorax ratio; ABV, doxorubicin (Adriamycin), bleomycin, vinblastine; EFS, event-free survival; AVD, doxorubicin, vinblastine, dacarbazine; AV, doxorubicin and vinblastine; Stanford V, mechlorethamine, doxorubicin, vinblastine, prednisone, vincristine, bleomycin, VP-16; FU, follow-up; FFP, freedom from progression.

significantly better 7-year freedom from treatment failure rate (88% vs. 67%; $P < .001$).[110] The final results of the EORTC H8F trial, including 542 patients with early favorable Hodgkin lymphoma, were similar. In this trial, combined modality treatment, consisting of three cycles of MOPP/ABV chemotherapy followed by 36 or 40 Gy IF-RT, was compared with 36 or 40 Gy subtotal nodal irradiation (STNI) alone. With a median follow-up of 92 months, the estimated 5-year event-free survival rates in the combined modality group and in the RT alone group were 98% and 74%, respectively. The estimated 10-year overall survival was 97% in the combined modality group and 94% in the RT alone group.[112]

In the GHSG HD10 study, 1,370 patients were randomly assigned to either receive two or four cycles of ABVD chemotherapy followed by 20 or 30 Gy IF-RT. Aims of the study were to evaluate a reduced number of chemotherapy cycles, to apply a lower radiation dose, or both. In the recently published final analysis with a median follow-up of more than 8 years, no significant differences between treatment arms were observed regarding freedom from treatment failure and overall survival with rates beyond 90%. Less toxicity was seen in patients treated with only two cycles of ABVD chemotherapy and a reduced radiation dose of 20 Gy IF-RT. Thus, treatment with two cycles of ABVD followed by 20 Gy IF-RT can be considered appropriate in patients with early favorable stages.[113]

The GHSG follow-up trial for early favorable disease, HD13, finished recruitment in 2009. The study aimed at decreasing toxicity by deleting drugs from the ABVD backbone. Patients were randomized between two cycles of ABVD, ABV, AVD, or AV chemotherapy followed by 30 Gy IF-RT. A safety analysis performed in 2006 detected a fourfold increase of events in the dacarbazine-deleted arms (ABV and AV), respectively, compared to the ABVD standard arm. This increase could not be explained by chance variation. Hence, the ABV/AV arms were closed. The question whether AVD is equivalent to ABVD will be answered with longer follow-up in future analyses of this trial.

Chemotherapy Alone

Since it is well documented that a number of severe long-term sequelae such as secondary malignancies, pulmonary fibrosis, or hypothyroidism are potentially caused by radiotherapy, several groups initiated trials evaluating the necessity of radiotherapy after adequate chemotherapy.

In a trial conducted by the National Cancer Institute of Canada and the Eastern Cooperative Oncology Group, 399 patients with limited-stage Hodgkin lymphoma (nonbulky clinical stages IA and IIA) were enrolled. They were randomly assigned to either receive four to six cycles of ABVD chemotherapy alone or ABVD combined with STNI. With a median follow-up of 4.2 years, freedom from disease progression was superior in patients who had received combined modality treatment (93% in the combined modality vs. 87% in the chemotherapy alone arm). These findings indicate a better tumor control by consolidating radiation after chemotherapy. There were no significant differences in terms of event-free survival and overall survival rates (88% vs. 86% and 94% vs. 96%, respectively). However, longer observation and documentation of patients included in this trial is required to draw final conclusions since follow-up is still too short to assess particularly radiotherapy-related long-term side effects.[114]

Another study that was conducted at the Memorial Sloan-Kettering Cancer Center led to similar results. A total of 152 patients with nonbulky clinical stages IA, IB, IIA, IIB, and IIIA were prospectively randomized between either six cycles of ABVD chemotherapy alone or six cycles of ABVD followed by radiotherapy. Although no significant differences in terms of complete remission duration, freedom from progression, and overall survival were detected, a tendency toward superior outcome in patients receiving combined modality treatment was observed. At 60 months, 91% of patients who had received combined modality treatment and 87% of patients who had received chemotherapy alone were still in complete remission; 94% of patients in both arms had initially achieved complete remission. Freedom from progression and overall survival rates were 86% and 97%, respectively, for patients treated with chemotherapy plus radiotherapy compared to 81% and 90%, respectively, for patients who received chemotherapy alone.[115]

In the EORTC/GELA (Groupe d'Etude des Lymphomes de l'Adulte) H9F study for patients with early favorable Hodgkin lymphoma, all patients received six cycles of EBVP (epirubicin, bleomycin, vinblastine, prednisone) chemotherapy. Patients who achieved a complete remission or an unconfirmed complete remission were then randomized between 36 Gy IF-RT, 20 Gy IF-RT, and no RT. The trial could not be completed according to plan since the no-RT arm had to be closed prematurely due to an excessive rate of events.[116] However, since EBVP was shown to be less active than ABVD, the current standard chemotherapy protocol in early favorable stages, these results have to be interpreted with care. It is possible the results would have been different if a more active chemotherapy protocol had been used.

A recent publication from the Dana-Faber Cancer Institute reported outcomes of 71 patients with favorable, limited-stage cHL who received six cycles of ABVD without subsequent radiation. All patients achieved complete remission or complete remission unconfirmed and with a median follow-up of at least 60 months, and six patients experienced relapse. However, all relapses could be successfully salvaged so that no patient died during the period of observation.[117]

The results of these trials indicate that omission of radiotherapy after appropriate chemotherapy might be possible in carefully selected patients. Identifying and further reducing toxicity in these patients are the most relevant issues currently addressed in clinical trials in this setting. Since response assessment based on CT scans alone did not reliably distinguish between those patients who were sufficiently treated with chemotherapy alone and those who required additional radiotherapy or even more intensive treatment, ongoing trials mainly focus on a possible stratification based on the results of interim FDG-PET.

Response Adapted Therapy Based on Fluorodeoxyglucose–Position Emission Tomography

As indicated by Danish and Italian groups, early interim FDG-PET might be a good predictor for treatment failure in Hodgkin lymphoma patients.[55,118] Furthermore, the results of the GHSG HD15 trial for patients with advanced Hodgkin lymphoma suggest that FDG-PET is a valuable tool for identifying patients with residual lymphoma after chemotherapy whether they need additional radiotherapy or not. Patients who have residual lymphoma larger than 2.5 cm after chemotherapy were evaluated by PET. Patients with negative scans did not receive additional radiotherapy, while those with a positive PET were irradiated. The negative prognostic value defined as the portion of patients without progression, relapse, or radiotherapy within 12 months was 94%.[119]

A number of ongoing trials in early favorable disease are evaluating the prognostic impact of PET performed early during the course of chemotherapy. In the ongoing EORTC/GELA H10F trial, treatment in the standard arm consists of three cycles of ABVD chemotherapy. Chemotherapy is followed by involved-node radiotherapy (IN-RT), which means a reduction of the radiation field compared to the standard IF-RT technique.[120] In the experimental study arm, treatment is stratified on the basis of the result of a PET scan performed after the second chemotherapy cycle. Patients with negative PET receive two additional cycles of ABVD without subsequent radiotherapy, patients with positive PET receive an intensified treatment consisting of two cycles of escalated BEACOPP (bleomycin, etoposide, doxorubicin, cyclophosphamide, vincristine, procarbazine, prednisone) followed by IN-RT.

In the ongoing GHSG HD16 trial for patients with early favorable Hodgkin lymphoma, all patients receive two cycles of ABVD chemotherapy. A PET scan is then performed. In the experimental arm, patients with a positive PET receive an additionally 20 Gy IF-RT; those with a negative PET do not. In the standard arm, all patients receive 20 Gy IF-RT subsequent to chemotherapy, irrespective of the PET result.

In a large British trial that was initiated in 2003, patients with a negative PET after three cycles of ABVD chemotherapy are being randomized between either no further treatment or IF-RT. Patients with a positive PET receive a fourth cycle of ABVD chemotherapy followed by IF-RT.[121]

Future Strategies and Recommendations

In early favorable Hodgkin lymphoma, standard treatment consists of two cycles of chemotherapy followed by IF-RT. ABVD is the chemotherapy protocol most commonly used and is being considered the standard of care. The possibility of stratifying treatment according to the results of interim PET scans is currently under investigation in several large prospective randomized trials. In these trials, PET-negative patients receive no consolidating radiotherapy, while patients with a positive PET have more intensive treatment including post-chemotherapy radiotherapy or more aggressive chemotherapy. Thus, the current major goal for this group of patients is to reduce the risk of late effects in patients who are sufficiently treated and maintain or even improve the cure rates in patients with positive interim PET.

EARLY UNFAVORABLE HODGKIN LYMPHOMA

Risk Factors Defining Early Unfavorable Hodgkin Lymphoma

The extent of disease in patients with stage I or II Hodgkin lymphoma varies substantially. Thus, risk-adapted treatment is required. In many early-stage patients, disease presents with mediastinal bulk, which has been demonstrated to be correlated with a more unfavorable prognosis. Other poor prognostic clinical factors include higher age, an increased number of affected nodal sites, extranodal involvement and elevated ESR, and optionally accompanied by B-symptoms. Though there are still some minor definition differences between the major cooperative groups, clinical stages I and II Hodgkin lymphoma patients in Europe are generally grouped into an early favorable and an early unfavorable (intermediate stage) subgroups depending on the existence of the risk factors described above. In contrast, most U.S. patients who present with adverse factors (mainly the presence of bulky disease) typically are being treated together with stages III and IV patients in the advanced-stage risk group.

Combined Modality Approaches for Early Unfavorable Hodgkin Lymphoma

Patients with early unfavorable Hodgkin lymphoma are commonly treated with combined modality approaches. However, the optimal chemotherapy regimen and the number of chemotherapy cycles needed were and still are a matter of debate (Table 126.9).

In the EORTC/GELA H8U study, 996 patients were treated with either six cycles of MOPP/ABV plus IF-RT, four cycles of MOPP/ABV plus IF-RT, or four cycles of MOPP/ABV plus STNI. All groups had similar 5-year event-free survival (84% vs. 88% vs. 87%) and 10-year overall survival estimates (88% vs. 85% vs. 84%). Thus, four cycles of chemotherapy followed by IF-RT was proposed as standard treatment for patients with early unfavorable Hodgkin lymphoma.[112]

In the EORTC/GELA follow-up study, H9U, patients were randomized into three treatment arms, consisting of four cycles of ABVD, six cycles of ABVD, or four cycles of BEACOPP baseline each followed by 30 Gy IF-RT. An interim analysis at a median follow-up of 4 years showed no significant differences regarding event-free and overall survival between the treatment arms, while increased toxicity was observed with BEACOPP baseline.[116]

In the GHSG HD11 trial, 1,395 patients were randomized in a two-by-two factorial design to receive either four cycles of ABVD or BEACOPP baseline followed by either 20 or 30 Gy IF-RT.[31] The aims of the study were to investigate whether intensification of chemotherapy from ABVD to BEACOPP baseline resulted in an improvement of freedom from treatment failure and overall survival rates and whether a reduction of the radiation dose is possible without worsening treatment results. The final analysis revealed no differences between four cycles of ABVD plus 30 Gy IF-RT, four cycles of BEACOPP baseline plus 30 Gy, or four cycles of BEACOPP baseline plus 20 Gy arms. In contrast, patients randomized into the four cycles of ABVD plus 20 Gy IF-RT arm tended to have a poorer outcome. When all patients were grouped together, freedom from treatment failure at 5 years was 85% and overall survival 94.5%. Consequently, the standard chemotherapy protocol for patients with early unfavorable Hodgkin lymphoma within the GHSG was not changed to four cycles of BEACOPP baseline since toxicity with this protocol was increased as compared to ABVD (73.8% vs. 51.5 grade 3 or 4 toxicity; $P < .001$). Furthermore, standard radiation dose was left at 30 Gy since the combination of four cycles of ABVD followed by 20 Gy IF-RT appeared to be less effective than the same chemotherapy followed by radiation with a higher dose.[122]

In the GHSG follow-up trial, HD14, patients were randomly assigned to either two cycles of BEACOPP escalated followed by two cycles of ABVD or to four cycles of ABVD chemotherapy. All patients received 30 Gy IF-RT. In 2008, a planned interim analysis of the trial including data from 1,010 patients at a median observation of 3 years was performed. This analysis revealed a significant superiority of the treatment with two cycles of BEACOPP escalated followed by two cycles of ABVD plus 30 Gy IF-RT compared to four cycles of ABVD plus 30 Gy IF-RT in terms of FFTF (96% vs. 90%).[123] Therefore, the study arm consisting of four cycles of ABVD followed by 30 Gy IF-RT was closed and the regimen consisting of two cycles of BEACOPP escalated plus two cycles of ABVD followed by 30 Gy IF-RT was adopted as the new standard for patients with early unfavorable Hodgkin lymphoma within the GHSG. However, taking into consideration the final results of the HD11 trial, it should also be appropriate to use the reduced radiation dose of 20 Gy in this setting after two cycles of BEACOPP escalated followed by two cycles of ABVD.

TABLE 126.9

RANDOMIZED CLINICAL TRIALS IN UNFAVORABLE-PROGNOSIS STAGE I AND II HODGKIN LYMPHOMA: TRIALS TO IDENTIFY THE OPTIMAL CHEMOTHERAPY COMBINATION AND APPROPRIATE RADIATION VOLUME AND DOSAGE

Trial	Treatment Regimens	No. of Patients	Outcomes	
			FFTF (5 y)	*SV (5 y)*
GHSG HD8 (1993–1998)	A: 4 COPP/ABVD + EFRT (30 Gy) + bulk (10 Gy)	532	86%	91%
	B: 4 COPP/ABVD + IFRT (30 Gy) + bulk (10 Gy)	532	84%	92%
			(FFTF = NS)	(FFTF = NS)
			EFS (10 y)	*SV (10 y)*
EORTC/GELA H8U (1993–1998)	A: 6 MOPP/ABV + IFRT (36 Gy)	335	82%	88%
	B: 4 MOPP/ABV + IFRT (36 Gy)	333	80%	85%
	C: 4 MOPP/ABV + STLI	327	80%	84%
		(NS, NS)		
			FFTF (5 y)	*SV (5 y)*
GHSG HD11 (1998–2002)	A: 4 ABVD + IFRT (30 Gy)	327	85%	94%
	B: 4 ABVD + IFRT (20 Gy)	325	81%	94%
	C: 4 BEACOPP + IFRT (30 Gy)	319	87%	95%
	D: 4 BEACOPP + IFRT (20 Gy)	329	87%	95%
			FFTF (4 y)	*SV (4 y)*
EORTC H9U (1998–2002)	A: 6 ABVD + IFRT (30 Gy)	277	94%	96
	B: 4 ABVD + IFRT	276	89%	95
	C: 4 BEACOPP + IFRT	255	91%	93
		(NS, NS)		
			FFTF (3 y)	*SV (3 y)*
GHSG HD14 (2003–2009)	A: 4 ABVD + IFRT (30 Gy)	A total of 1216 in both arms	90%	
	B: 2 BEACOPP escalated + 2 ABVD + IFRT (30 Gy)		96%	

MOPP, mechlorethamine, vincristine, procarbazine, prednisone; STLI, subtotal nodal irradiation; ABVD, doxorubicin, bleomycin, vinblastine, dacarbazine; FFTF, freedom from treatment failure; SV, survival; EORTC, European Organisation for Research and Treatment of Cancer; EFS, event-free survival; EBVP, epirubicin, bleomycin, vinblastine, prednisone; IFRT, involved-field irradiation; ABV, doxorubicin (Adriamycin), bleomycin, vinblastine; EFRT, extended-field radiotherapy; NS, not significant; GHSG, German Hodgkin Study Group; COPP, cyclophosphamide, vincristine, procarbazine, prednisone; BEACOPP, bleomycin, etoposide, doxorubicin, cyclophosphamide, vincristine, procarbazine, prednisone.

Chemotherapy Alone

In patients with early unfavorable Hodgkin lymphoma, a small number of trials that compared combined modality approaches with chemotherapy alone were conducted to date. The GATLA (Grupo Argentine de Tratamiento de la Leucemia Aguda) randomized 104 early unfavorable disease patients between six cycles of CVPP (cyclophosphamide, vinblastine, procarbazine, and prednisone) alone or six cycles of CVPP sandwiched around 30 Gy IF-RT. The 7-year survival rates were 66% and 84%, respectively, the freedom from relapse rates were 34% and 75% ($P < .001$), both favoring the combined modality approach.[124]

Another trial by the National Cancer Institute of Canada and the Eastern Cooperative Oncology Group compared a chemotherapy only approach consisting of up to six cycles of ABVD with a combination of a reduced number of chemotherapy cycles followed by consolidating radiotherapy. However, patients who presented with bulky disease, a risk factor frequently found in early unfavorable disease, were excluded from this study. In the final analysis, freedom from disease progression was inferior in patients who received chemotherapy only, while no significant differences regarding event-free and overall survival were detected.[114] Although these results indicate a tendency toward a worse outcome for patients treated with chemotherapy only, it might be speculated that the reduced freedom from progression rate for the chemotherapy only arm will be outweighed by a reduced rate of long-term toxicities and secondary malignancies with a longer follow-up.

Fluorodeoxyglucose–Positron Emission Tomography–Based Response-Adapted Therapy

Very similar to early favorable disease, FDG-PET holds the promise of predicting which remission is robust and whether residual masses will benefit from additional radiotherapy. Several ongoing studies aim to evaluate the value of PET in the decision of whether consolidating radiotherapy after completed chemotherapy is necessary.

In the EORTC/GELA H10 trial, standard chemotherapy for patients with unfavorable risk profile consists of four cycles of ABVD. Chemotherapy is followed by IN-RT. In the experimental study arms, treatment is stratified on the basis of the result of a PET scan performed after the second chemotherapy cycle. Patients with a negative PET receive four additional cycles of ABVD not followed by consolidating radiation, while patients with a positive PET receive an intensified treatment consisting of two cycles of BEACOPP escalated followed by IN-RT.

In the GHSG HD17 trial for early unfavorable Hodgkin lymphoma, all patients receive two cycles of BEACOPP escalated followed by two cycles of ABVD. A PET scan is then performed in all patients. In the standard arm of the study, all patients receive IF-RT with a radiation dose of 30 Gy. In the experimental arm, only those patients with a positive PET receive 30 Gy IN-RT, while those with a negative PET are not irradiated.

Future Strategies and Recommendations

Similar to early favorable Hodgkin lymphoma, early unfavorable stages are generally treated with combined modality strategies. Four cycles of chemotherapy followed by IF-RT represents the widely accepted treatment of choice. To answer the question whether radiation can be omitted in selected patients is the aim of currently ongoing randomized prospective trials. FDG-PET is regarded the most promising tool to distinguish between patients who do not need radiation and patients who require standard or even more intensive therapy. In patients who require radiation after chemotherapy, a reduction of the radiation field from IF to IN might reduce the radiotherapy-associated long-term sequelae such as secondary solid cancers, hypothyroidism, and pulmonary fibrosis.

ADVANCED STAGES OF HODGKIN LYMPHOMA

Chemotherapy Regimens

Before the introduction of combination chemotherapy, more than 95% of patients with advanced Hodgkin lymphoma succumbed to their disease within 5 years after diagnosis. Thus, remission rates in excess of 50% achieved with MOPP were a major breakthrough in oncology.[125,126] MOPP was successfully introduced almost 40 years ago and used for many years in the treatment of advanced Hodgkin lymphoma, resulting in a long-term remission rate of about 50%[125,127] It was then replaced by ABVD after a series of large multicenter trials had investigated ABVD versus alternating MOPP/ABVD or MOPP alone.[127–129]

Bonnadonna et al.[127] were the first to report on the relevance of ABVD and the impact of anthracyclines in the treatment of advanced Hodgkin lymphoma. Patients were randomly assigned to receive either MOPP or MOPP alternating monthly with ABVD. All 88 evaluable patients had not received prior chemotherapy and 25 had relapsed after primary radiotherapy. The complete remission rate with MOPP/ABVD was 88.9% and 74.4% with MOPP alone. The 8-year results reported that MOPP/ABVD was superior to MOPP in terms of freedom from progression (64.6% vs. 35.9%; $P < .005$), relapse-free (72.6% vs. 45.1%; $P < .01$), and overall survival (83.9% vs. 63.9%; $P < .06$). Thus, this study impressively showed the benefit of ABVD in terms of efficacy when added to MOPP.

Also ABVD alone led to superior results when compared to MOPP. Santoro et al.[129] investigated 3×MOPP+RT+3×MOPP versus 3×ABVD+RT+3×ABVD. In this trial, the 7-year results indicated that ABVD was superior to MOPP in terms of freedom from progression (80.8% vs. 62.8%; $P < .002$), relapse-free survival (87.7% vs. 77.2%; $P = .06$), and most importantly overall survival (77.4% vs. 67.9%; $P = .03$). Another U.S. trial also tested six to eight cycles of ABVD against six to eight cycles of MOPP or MOPP alternating with ABVD for 12 cycles.[130] Of 361 eligible patients, 123 received MOPP, 123 received MOPP alternating with ABVD, and 115 received ABVD alone. The overall response rate was 93%, with an overall complete remission rate of 77%. Among patients who received MOPP, 67% achieved complete remission compared to 82% in the ABVD and 83% in the MOPP/ABVD arm. The rates of failure-free survival at 5 years were 50% for MOPP, 61% for ABVD, and 65% for MOPP/ABVD. Overall survival rates at 5 years were 66% for MOPP, 73% for ABVD, and 75% for MOPP/ABVD ($P = .28$). MOPP was associated with more severe acute hematologic toxicity and also with more late sequelae such as infertility and the development of secondary leukemia. Since ABVD was equally effective and less toxic than MOPP/ABVD, this trial supported the use of ABVD alone as first-line therapy for advanced-stage Hodgkin lymphoma.

Hybrid and Alternating Regimens

A few years later, upfront ABVD was compared with alternating multidrug regimens such as ChlVPP/PABlOE (chlorambucil, vinblastine, procarbazine, prednisolone alternating with prednisolone, doxorubicin, bleomycin, vincristine, etoposide) and ChlVPP/EVA (etoposide, vincristine, doxorubicin) in a study performed in the United Kingdom.[131,132] Radiotherapy was intended for incomplete response or initial bulky disease. At a median follow-up of 52 months, the event-free survival rates at 3 years were 75% (95% CI, 71% to 79%) for ABVD and 75% (95% CI, 70% to 79%) for the multidrug regimens (hazard ratio [HR] = 1.05; 95% CI, 0.8 to 1.37). The 3-year overall survival rates were 90% (95% CI, 87% to 93%) in patients allocated to ABVD and 88% (95% CI, 84% to 91%) in patients receiving one of the multidrug regimens (HR = 1.22; 95% CI, 0.84 to 1.77). Patients treated with either multidrug regimen experienced more grade 3 or 4 side effects, including infection, mucositis, and neuropathy. To conclude, in the absence of significant differences in event-free and overall survival between ABVD and multidrug regimens, ABVD remained the standard for treatment of advanced Hodgkin lymphoma. It should be mentioned that this study reported a better event-free and overall survival for ABVD than other trials. This could be explained by the fact that this trial included patients with stage I or II disease that had systemic symptoms, multiple sites of involvement, or bulky disease. Stages III and IV patients had 5-year event-free and overall survival rates of 65% and 82%, respectively, which were clearly lower.

Taken together, ABVD remained the treatment of choice for advanced-stage Hodgkin lymphoma based on equivalent efficacy and lower toxicity.

Stanford V

Stanford V (doxorubicin, vinblastine, mechlorethamine, vincristine, bleomycin, etoposide, prednisone) was developed as a short-duration, reduced-toxicity program applied weekly over 12 weeks. Consolidation of radiotherapy to sites of initial disease was employed and data were generated in a single center setting including 142 patients who had stage III or IV or extensive mediastinal stage I or II Hodgkin lymphoma.[133] Stanford V chemotherapy was given over 12 weeks followed by 36 Gy RT to initial sites of bulky (greater than or equal to 5 cm) or macroscopic splenic disease. With a median follow-up of 5.4 years, the 5-year freedom from progression rate was 89% and overall survival was 96%. Freedom from progression was significantly inferior among patients who presented with an international prognostic score of 3 and higher (94% vs. 75%; $P = .0001$). One hundred twenty-nine of 142 patients (91%) received additional radiotherapy.

An Italian prospectively randomized multicenter comparison of Stanford V with MOPP/EBV/CAD and ABVD suggested that Stanford V was inferior in terms of response rates (76% vs. 89% vs. 94%) and progression-free survival (73% vs. 85% vs. 94%).[131] These conflicting results were partially explained by the reduced use of radiotherapy in the randomized setting and the better treatment quality in single-center studies. Stanford V was also compared to ABVD in a larger intergroup trial.[134] Patients had clinical stage IIB, III, or IV or stage I to IIA disease with bulk or other adverse features. Radiotherapy was administered in both arms to sites of previous bulk (greater than 5 cm) and to splenic deposits, although this was omitted in the later part of the trial for patients who achieved complete remission in the ABVD arm. Five hundred twenty patients received treatment according to protocol, and radiotherapy was administered to 73% of patients in the Stanford V arm and 53% in the ABVD arm. The overall response rates after completion of treatment were 91% for Stanford V and 92% for ABVD. During a median follow-up of 4.3 years, there was no difference in the projected 5-year progression-free and overall survival rates (76% and 90%, respectively, for ABVD; 74% and 92%, respectively, for Stanford V). Thus, in this large, randomized trial, Stanford V when given in combination with radiotherapy was equally effective as ABVD. However, 20% more patients had to be irradiated in the Stanford V arm, and the 5-year progression-free survival was about 15% lower than reported in the single-center setting.

BEACOPP Escalated Regimen

The BEACOPP regimen was introduced by the GHSG in a baseline and a dose-escalated version, with a substantial increase of dose density and dose intensity as compared to ABVD and hybrid regimens. Although some indications for a role of dose intensity were available in the early 1990s, no prospective randomized trial had been undertaken. In order to obtain an impression of the shape of the essential dose–response characteristics, Hasenclever et al. developed a theoretical model that was used to simulate the effect of dose escalation and changes of schedule and architecture of the COPP/ABVD regimen. On the basis of such simulations, the model predicted that shortening cycle intervals from 4 to 3 weeks should lead to small benefits (about 3% in 5-year tumor control rates), but a moderate average dose escalation by 30% of a standard chemotherapy would lead to a potential benefit of about 10% to 15% in tumor control at 5 years. On the basis of this theoretical model the BEACOPP regimen was designed. Granulocyte colony-stimulating factor (G-CSF) was introduced to compensate the higher myelotoxicity in the escalated version. In an initial phase 2 study, the optimal dose of BEACOPP baseline and BEACOPP escalated were determined.[135] The subsequent HD9 trial of the GHSG then compared eight cycles of COPP/ABVD with BEACOPP baseline and BEACOPP escalated. Results including 1,195 randomized patients showed a clear superiority of BEACOPP escalated over BEACOPP baseline and COPP/ABVD at 5 years.[136] The follow-up data at 10 years confirmed these results: with a median follow-up of 112 months, freedom from treatment failure and overall survival rates were 64% and 75% after COPP/ABVD, 70% and 80% in the BEACOPP baseline group, and 82% and 86% in the BEACOPP escalated group, respectively.[113] The 10-year update of the HD9 study not only confirmed a significant improvement in long-term freedom from treatment failure and overall survival for BEACOPP escalated, but also showed that this advantage was significant for freedom from treatment failure in all risk groups as defined by the International Prognostic Score. Overall survival was also significantly better in the largest cohort (IPS 2-3) (Table 126.10, Figs. 126.1 and 126.2).

However, toxicity of this more aggressive approach remained a concern. The subsequent GHSG HD12 trial thus aimed at deescalating chemo- and radiotherapy by comparing eight courses of BEACOPP escalated with four courses of escalated and four courses of BEACOPP baseline (4 + 4).[137] In addition, the role of radiotherapy was investigated by a second randomization between consolidating radiation to initial bulky and residual disease and no radiotherapy. At 5 years, overall survival in HD12 was 91%, freedom from treatment failure was 85.5%, and progression-free survival 86.2%. However, there was no statistical difference between eight courses of BEACOPP escalated and the 4 + 4 arm in all outcome parameters. There was also no significant difference between the RT or no-RT arms in this study, with the caveat that a number of high-risk patients received RT based on the blinded panel decision in those arms where no RT was intended. More recent analyses suggest that only those patients who present with residual tumor after the end of chemotherapy profit from additional radiotherapy. Since some subgroup analyses in the HD12 trial are pending, the GHSG still considers eight cycles of BEACOPP escalated as standard for advanced-stage Hodgkin lymphoma patients.

What is the standard treatment for advanced Hodgkin lymphoma today? Two strategies are commonly being used:

1. Starting with the less toxic ABVD regimen and accepting a relapse-free survival of 60% to 70% at 5 years, trying to salvage relapsing patients with high-dose chemotherapy and autologous stem cell transplantation (including substantial toxicities for patients undergoing this procedure),[128,130] or

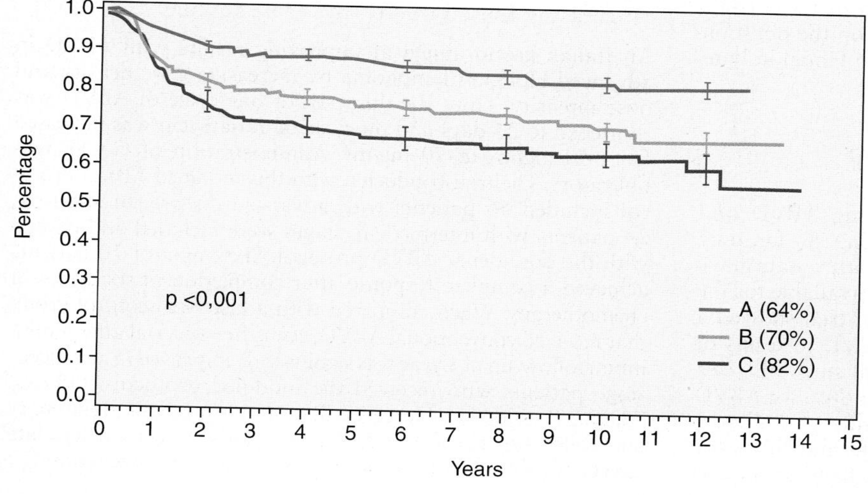

FIGURE 126.1 Treatment of advanced-stage Hodgkin lymphoma (10-year freedom from treatment failure [FFTF], HD9 trial of the German Hodgkin Study Group.) Arm A, COPP/ABVD, cyclophosphamide, vincristine, procarbazine, and prednisone plus doxorubicin, bleomycin, vinblastine, and dacarbazine. Arm B, standard dose BEACOPP, bleomycin, etoposide, doxorubicin, cyclophosphamide, vincristine, procarbazine, and prednisone. Arm C, dose-escalated BEACOPP.

TABLE 126.10

RANDOMIZED CLINICAL TRIALS IN ADVANCED-STAGE HODGKIN LYMPHOMA: MAJOR TRIALS FOR WHICH RESULTS HAVE BEEN PUBLISHED

Trial	Therapy Regimen	No. of Patients	Outcome
Stanford	Stanford V (12 wk) (+ RT to initial mediastinal bulk + hilar + supraclavicle nodes)	108	96% (OS) 89% (FFP) (5 y)
Intergroup Italy	A: ABVD (6 cycles) B: Stanford V (12 wk) C: MEC hybrid (6 courses) (+ RT initial bulk/residual mass)	98 89 88	81% (FFS); 92% (FFP); 95% (OS) 53% (FFS); 76% (FFP); 80% (OS) 87% (FFS); 95% (FFP); 95% (OS) (3 y)
Intergroup GB & Italy	A: ChlVPP/EVA hybrid (6 cycles) B: VAPEC-B (11wk) (+/– RT initial bulk/residual mass)	144 138	82% (FFP); 78% (EFS); 89% (OS) 62% (FFP); 58% (EFS); 79% (OS) (5 y)
GHSG HD9	A: COPP/ABVD (4 cycles) B: BEACOPP baseline (8 cycles) C: BEACOPP escalated (8 cycles)	260 469 466	64% (FFTF); 75% (OS) 70% (FFTF); 80% (OS) 82% (FFTF); 86% (OS) (10 y)
GHSG HD12	A: 8 BEACOPP escalated B: 8 BEACOPP escalated C: 4 BEACOPP escalated + 4 BEACOPP baseline D: 4 BEACOPP escalated + 4 BEACOPP baseline (A + C: + RT bulk/residual mass)	348 345 351 352	87% (FFTF); 91% (OS) 86% (FFTF); 91% (OS) 86% (FFTF); 90% (OS) 83% (FFTF); 89% (OS) (5 y)
HD 2000	A: 6 ABVD B: 4 BEACOPP escalated + 2 BEACOPP baseline C: 6 CEC	99 98 98	65% (FFS); 84% (OS) 78% (FFS); 92% (OS) 71% (FFS); 91% (OS) (5 y)

Stanford V, mechlorethamine, doxorubicin, vinblastine, prednisone, vincristine, bleomycin, etoposide; RT, radiotherapy; OS, overall survival; FFS, failure-free survival; CS, clinical stage; ABVD, doxorubicin, bleomycin, vinblastine, dacarbazine; FFP, freedom from progression; GB, Great Britain; ChlVPP, chlorambucil, vinblastine, procarbazine, and prednisone; EVA, etoposide, vincristine, and doxorubicin; VAPEC-B, doxorubicin, cyclophosphamide, etoposide, vincristine, bleomycin, prednisolone; EFS, event-free survival; GHSG, German Hodgkin Study Group; COPP, cyclophosphamide, vincristine, procarbazine, prednisone; FFTF, freedom from treatment failure; BEACOPP, bleomycin, etoposide, doxorubicin, cyclophosphamide, vincristine, procarbazine, prednisone; CEC, cyclophosphamide, lomustine, vindesine, melphalan, prednisone, epidoxorubicin, vincristine, procarbazine, vinblastine, bleomycin.

2. Starting with the aggressive BEACOPP escalated regimen (generating a freedom from treatment failure of 87% at 5 years) in order to cure as many patients as possible with first-line treatment, accepting an excess of toxicity for those patients who could have been cured with less intensive therapy.[113]

These opposing treatment strategies are being intensively discussed and have resulted in a series of larger international trials that are currently ongoing. The results of these trials will, hopefully, provide the ultimate evidence on the question of the best strategy for patients with advanced Hodgkin lymphoma.

ABVD versus BEACOPP

Three studies have been initiated comparing ABVD and BEACOPP in a prospective randomized setting. So far, only one trial has undergone final analysis, immature data have been reported for the second, and no data are available for the third. The final results of the HD2000 Italian trial showed a significant superiority of BEACOPP over ABVD in terms of freedom from progression but not for overall survival.[138] At 5 years, the freedom from progression rate was 68% for ABVD and 81% for BEACOPP (4 escalated + 2 baseline [4 + 2]); the overall survival rates were 84% for ABVD and 92% for BEACOPP, respectively. However, the lack of significance is likely due to the low power of this study that enrolled 307 patients in three treatment arms. In the IIL-GITIL(Gruppo Italiano Terapie Innovative nei Linfomi)-Michelangelo study, ABVD (six to eight courses) or BEACOPP given in 4 + 4 fashion generated a comparable 3-year outcome.[139] Finally, a large intergroup trial organized by the EORTC is currently ongoing. In this trial, ABVD is compared to BEACOPP 4 + 4. First results from this trial are pending.

Increasing Dose Density and Dose Intensity in ABVD

An Italian group aimed at improving results with ABVD in advanced Hodgkin lymphoma by increasing dose density and dose intensity. Thus, the duration of one cycle of ABVD was shortened to 21 days and the dose of adriamycin was increased from 50 mg/m^2 to 70 mg/m^2. Administration of G-CSF was obligatory. The trial conducted with this modified ABVD protocol included 46 patients with advanced disease. In addition, 24 patients with intermediate stages were included and treated with the dose-dense ABVD protocol. Sixty-nine of 70 patients achieved a complete response after completion of six cycles of chemotherapy. When compared with a historical control group that received conventional ABVD, event-free survival after a minimum follow-up of 1 year was significantly improved in advanced-stage patients who received the modified protocol (93% vs. 73.2%; $P = .0041$). However, these results are still preliminary and follow-up is too short to particularly detect cardiac late effects possibly caused by the increase of the adriamycin dose.[140]

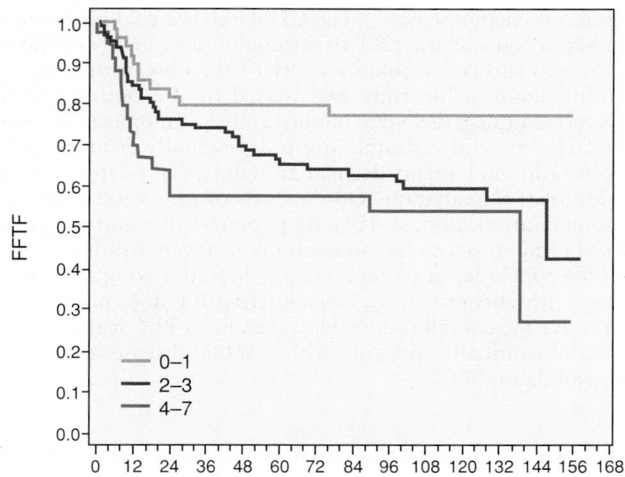

Time [months]

Pts. at Risk								
0–1	49	40	38	35	26	19	4	0
2–3	97	72	64	51	41	27	7	0
4–7	34	21	17	15	11	6	1	0

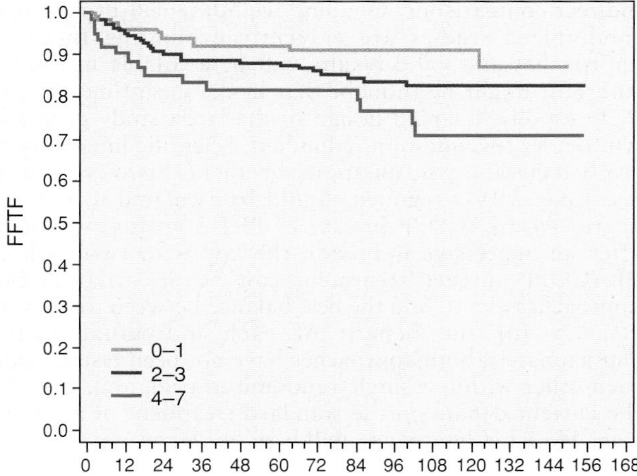

Time [months]

Pts. at Risk								
0–1	104	94	89	77	56	25	3	0
2–3	177	157	147	120	90	33	6	0
4–7	60	50	44	39	26	9	2	0

FIGURE 126.2 Freedom from treatment failure (FFTF) rates according to the IPS score in patients with advanced Hodgkin lymphoma treated with either COPP/ABVD (cyclophosphamide, vincristine, procarbazine, and prednisone plus doxorubicin, bleomycin, vinblastine, and dacarbazine) (*above*) or BEACOPP escalated (bleomycin, etoposide, doxorubicin, cyclophosphamide, vincristine, procarbazine, and prednisone) (*below*). (Adapted from ref. 89.)

Outcome Predictions for Advanced Disease

The International Prognostic Score

Overall, it would be preferable to treat each patient with advanced disease according to his or her individual risk profile in order to better balance efficacy and toxicity. Accordingly, some current concepts also include prognostic factors into the treatment plan and apply the International Prognostic Score (IPS) for risk stratification.[103]

The score was derived from 5,141 patients who had been treated with COPP/ABVD-like regimens given with or without additional radiotherapy. The end point was freedom from progression of disease. Seven factors had similar independent prognostic effects: serum albumin of less than 4 g/dL, hemoglobin level of less than 10.5 g/dL, male sex, age of 45 years or older, stage IV disease (according to the Ann Arbor classification), leukocytosis (white cell count of at least 15,000/mm^3), and lymphocytopenia (lymphocyte count of less than 600/mm^3, or less than 8% of the white cell count, or both). The IPS is currently being used for a risk-adapted therapy in a clinical practice and a number of clinical trials. One example is an Israelian phase 2 study. In this study patients in good prognostic advanced stages (IPS 0-2) are treated with ABVD, and patients with an IPS 3 or higher receive BEACOPP escalated induction therapy. This strategy is supported by the excellent outcome of IPS 0-2 patients after ABVD or BEACOPP. However, a distinct group of patients at very high risk still cannot be identified on the basis of routinely documented demographics and clinical characteristics as used in the IPS.

Positron Emission Tomography

The IPS as the major instrument to tailor risk-adapted treatment is increasingly being challenged by more sophisticated strategies. It has been demonstrated for Hodgkin lymphoma patients whose response to chemotherapy has an impact on the final treatment outcome[141,142] However, response as measured by CT scan might occur with some delay in advanced Hodgkin lymphoma. This is likely due to the fibrotic tissue infiltrating lymph nodes in this disease, which often results in residual masses that remain several months after therapy, especially in cases of bulky disease. For example, in the GHSG HD15 trial, 311 of 817 patients (38%) showed residual disease greater than 2.5 cm as determined by CT scan after completion of chemotherapy.[119] However, 79% (n = 245) of these patients at the same time had a negative FDG-PET scan. These patients did not receive any additional RT and, with a rather short median observation time of 18 months, their outcome was not inferior compared to patients who reached a complete remission after chemotherapy. These data indicate, at least, that the biologic response determined by FDG-PET is superior to the morphologic response in terms of its negative predictive value. The work by Hutchings et al.[55] and Gallamini et al.[118] must also be mentioned in this context. They were able to show that the early PET response (after two cycles of ABVD) overshadows the prognostic value of the IPS and thus is an important tool for planning risk-adapted treatment in advanced Hodgkin lymphoma.

Thus, current concepts include early response evaluation guided by FDG-PET into treatment strategies and will hopefully define a new standard of care in which patients receive a more individualized treatment.

Current Concepts: Response-Adapted Therapy

Deescalating BEACOPP

The GHSG HD15 trial was the first large trial to investigate the negative predictive value of PET in advanced Hodgkin lymphoma, which was used to guide therapy after completion of chemotherapy. Patients were randomized between eight courses of BEACOPP escalated, six courses of BEACOPP escalated, or eight courses of BEACOPP-14 (a time-intensified variant of BEACOPP baseline).[143] As described above, additional radiotherapy was applied only to PET-positive residual lesions greater than 2.5 cm and a high negative predictive value (NPV) for progression or early relapse was found (NPV = 94%). Based on these results and reports from other studies, the GHSG is currently evaluating an interim PET-guided risk-adapted treatment in the current HD18 trial.[55,144] In this study, PET is used to assess early response after two cycles of BEACOPP escalated. Cycle number is reduced to a total of four in PET-negative patients (and compared to the standard of eight cycles). This is a deescalating approach based on the excellent NPV of PET in Hodgkin lymphoma. First results from the Israelian study group have recently supported this approach.[145] Patients with advanced-stage Hodgkin lymphoma and an IPS of 3 or greater received two initial cycles of BEACOPP escalated and were then evaluated by PET/CT. In cases of PET negativity, they were treated with four cycles of ABVD, and in cases of PET positivity, high-dose chemotherapy followed by autologous stem cell transplant was performed. After a median follow-up of 48 months, progression-free survival and overall survival at 4 years were 78% and 95%, respectively. Though the progression-free survival of 78% in this trial published by Avigdor et al.[145] looks disappointing at first glance, this is within the expected range. In the HD9 trial, freedom from treatment failure for patients in the unfavorable risk group (IPS 4 to 7) was 82% at 5 years. Stratified by PET results, the 4-year progression-free survival for early PET-negative patients was 87% (n = 31) and 53% for early PET-positive patients (n = 13), respectively (P = .01). Though the absolute patient number is small, these data seem to suggest that a deescalating approach in early PET-negative patients after two cycles of BEACOPP escalated might be feasible.

Escalating ABVD

Several groups follow an alternative approach of escalating treatment in patients not responding to two cycles of ABVD as defined by PET positivity. These patients have a rather poor outcome with ABVD or ABVD-like therapy. The 2-year progression-free survival was reported as low as 6%.[146] So far only very preliminary data are available from ongoing trials. However, first results of the GITIL trial were published in 2009.[147] In this trial, PET-positive patients receive two cycles of ABVD followed by eight cycles of BEACOPP (4+4). Of 164 enrolled patients, 24 were PET-2-positive and 136 PET-2-negative. The two cohorts of patients were well matched in terms of prognostic factors and an IPS 3 or greater was equally frequent in both arms (29% and 28%; P = .95). Of the 24 PET-positive patients, 15 (62%) were in continuous complete remission after BEACOPP and 9 progressed; the mean duration of complete remission for the responding patients was 18 months (range 11–37). One hundred twenty-seven of 136 PET-negative patients (93.5%) were in continuous complete remission after standard ABVD and 9 progressed or relapsed. The 2-year progression-free survival of PET-positive patients was 56% only and 93% for the PET-negative patients.

The Role of Radiotherapy

The role of consolidating radiotherapy for advanced Hodgkin lymphoma depends on the efficacy of the prior chemotherapy. After MOPP or MOPP-like regimen, there might be a potential advantage of IF-RT as detected by a meta-analysis of 16 randomized studies, whereas this advantage is not evident after ABVD or ABVD-like regimens.[148,149] A randomized EORTC study demonstrated that consolidation with IF-RT did not improve the outcome in patients who achieved complete remission after six to eight courses of alternating MOPP and ABV, but potentially improved the outcome of patients who only achieved partial remission.[150] A randomized GELA trial showed that consolidation with IF-RT after doxorubicin-induced complete remission was not superior to two additional cycles of chemotherapy.[56] The GHSG HD12 trial randomized between consolidating RT to residual disease and observation only and showed a noninferiority of the observation arm.[137] Unfortunately, the study was biased by the central review. Experts in this panel were blinded to the randomization result and recommend radiotherapy independently from the randomization in patients deemed at high risk of relapse without additional radiotherapy. On the basis of the expert panel recommendation, almost 10% of patients who had originally been randomized to the observation arm were irradiated.

To conclude, in patients who achieved a complete remission with chemotherapy, consolidating RT does not seem to improve the overall results. However, FDG-PET scan might be helpful to identify patients with residual disease at need for consolidating RT.[119]

Future Strategies and Recommendations

Advanced Hodgkin lymphoma has become a curable disease for the majority of patients. First-line treatment with six to eight cycles of ABVD is the widely accepted standard. However, the more aggressive BEACOPP escalated regimen induces a clinically relevant superior progression-free survival that translates into an improved overall survival in indirect comparisons. Ongoing well-designed prospectively randomized studies are currently evaluating these two approaches and valid results will be available in the near future. It might be thought that in the meantime the early PET response-adapted design of the latest study generation will render this question redundant. Scientific interest is currently focused on the questions whether (1) two cycles of the less toxic ABVD regimen should be escalated to the more aggressive BEACOPP in case of PET-2 positivity, or (2) if after an aggressive induction therapy with two cycles of BEACOPP further treatment can be deescalated. Both approaches aim to find the best balance between toxicity and efficacy for the benefit of each individual patient. Unfortunately, both approaches have not been tested against each other within a single randomized trial, and, therefore, the current debate on the standard treatment of advanced-stage Hodgkin lymphoma will very likely continue.

PROGRESSIVE AND RELAPSED DISEASE

Diagnosis and Staging at Disease Progression or Relapse

Although very late relapses that occur more than 10 years after primary treatment have been reported, relapses in Hodgkin lymphoma are generally observed within the first 5 years following first-line therapy.[151] At relapse, a new histology should be obtained since secondary tumors—NHL or solid tumors in particular—have to be excluded. Moreover, some NHL patients initially misdiagnosed as Hodgkin lymphoma or composite lymphomas are thus not detected at first diagnosis. In all patients with relapsed or progressive Hodgkin lymphoma, clinical and radiographic restaging is recommended. As relapsed patients will need salvage treatment, correct staging is of therapeutic and also prognostic relevance.

Prognostic Factors

Adverse prognostic factors for patients with treatment failure include the treatment modality used in first-line therapy, age,

TABLE 126.11

POLYCHEMOTHERAPY REGIMENS USED IN HODGKIN LYMPHOMA

Drug	Dose (mg/m^2)	Route	Schedule (days)	Cycle Length (days)
MOPP				21
Mechlorethamine	6	IV	1, 8	
Oncovin (vincristine)	1.4	IV	1, 8	
Procarbazine	100	PO	1–14	
Prednisone	40	PO	1–14	
COPP				28
Cyclophosphamide	650	IV	1, 8	
Oncovin (vincristine)	1.4	IV	1, 8	
Procarbazine	100	PO	1–14	
Prednisone	40	PO	1–14	
ABVD				28
Adriamycin (doxorubicin)	25	IV	1, 15	
Bleomycin	10	IV	1, 15	
Vinblastine	6	IV	1, 15	
Dacarbazine	375	IV	1, 15	
BEACOPP (BASELINE)				21
Bleomycin	10	IV	8	
Etoposide	100	IV	1–3	
Adriamycin (doxorubicin)	25	IV	1	
Cyclophosphamide	650	IV	1	
Oncovin (vincristine)	1.4[a]	IV	8	
Procarbazine	100	PO	1–7	
Prednisone	40	PO	1–14	
BEACOPP ESCALATED				22
Bleomycin	10	IV	8	
Etoposide	200	IV	1–3	
Adriamycin	35	IV	1	
Cyclophosphamide	1,250	IV	1	
Oncovin (vincristine)	1.4[a]	IV	8	
Procarbazine	100	PO	1–7	
Prednisone	40	PO	1–14	
G-CSF	—	SC	From d 8	
STANFORD V				12 wk
Mechlorethamine	6	IV	Wk 1, 5, 9	
Adriamycin (doxorubicin)	25	IV	Wk 1, 3, 5, 7, 9, 11	
Vinblastine	6	IV	Wk 1, 3, 5, 7, 9, 11	
Vincristine	1.4[a]	IV	Wk 2, 4, 6, 8, 10, 12	
Bleomycin	5	IV	Wk 2, 4, 6, 8, 10, 12	
Etoposide	60	IV	Wk 3, 7, 11	
Prednisone	40	IV	Wk 1–10 qod	
G-CSF	—	PO	Dose reduction or delay	
VAPEC-B				11 wk
Vincristine	1.4[a]	IV	Wk 2, 4, 6, 8, 10	
Adriamycin (doxorubicin)	35	IV	Wk 1, 3, 5, 7, 9, 11	
Prednisolone	50	PO	Wk 1–6	
Etoposide	75–100	PO	Wk 3, 7, 11	
Cyclophosphamide	350	IV	Wk 1, 5, 9	
Bleomycin	10	IV	Wk 2, 4, 6, 8, 10	

IV, intravenously; PO, orally; G-CSF, granulocyte colony-stimulating factor; SC, subcutaneously.
[a]Vincristine dose capped at 2 mg.

number of involved areas and organs at relapse, extent of disease, anemia, and presence of systemic symptoms at relapse. In addition, the duration of first remission is a major determinant of a second complete response. On this basis, chemotherapy failures can be divided into three subgroups:

- Primary progressive disease: patients who never achieved a complete remission or relapse within 3 months after the end of first-line treatment.
- Early relapses: relapse occurs 3 to 12 months after the end of first-line treatment.
- Late relapses: relapse after a complete remission lasting at least 12 months.

Primary Progressive Disease

Primary progressive Hodgkin lymphoma is defined as progression of disease or relapse within the first 3 months after completion of first-line treatment. Prognosis of patients with primary progressive disease who are treated with conventional salvage protocols is poor, with an 8-year overall survival of 0% to 8%.[57,152] However, data on this subgroup of patients are rare since they are often excluded from clinical trials. The GHSG retrospectively analyzed 206 patients with primary progressive Hodgkin lymphoma to determine their outcome after salvage therapy and to identify prognostic factors. The 5-year freedom from second failure and overall survival rates for all patients included in the analysis were 17% and 26%, respectively. As mainly reported from transplant centers, the 5-year freedom from second failure and overall survival for patients treated with high-dose chemotherapy followed by autologous stem cell transplant was 31% and 43%, respectively, but only one-third of all patients were treated with this modality.[153] The low percentage of patients who received high-dose chemotherapy was due to rapidly progressing fatal disease or life-threatening severe toxicity after salvage therapy. Other factors that prohibited proceeding to high-dose chemotherapy were insufficient stem cell harvest, poor performance status, and advanced age. In a multivariate analysis, Karnofsky performance score at progress ($P < .0001$), age ($P = .019$), and achieving at least a temporary remission with first-line chemotherapy ($P = .0003$) were significant prognostic factors for survival. Patients presenting with none of these risk factors had a 5-year overall survival of 55% compared with 0% for patients presenting with all three unfavorable prognostic factors. Other analyses also showed that the use of high-dose chemotherapy and autologous stem cell transplant improves the prognosis of patients with primary induction failure. The European Blood and Marrow Transplant (EBMT) Registry reported their analysis on 175 patients with primary progressive disease who received high-dose chemotherapy and autologous stem cell transplant. The 5-year actuarial progression-free survival and overall survival rates were 32% and 36%, respectively.[154] The Autologous Blood and Marrow Transplant Registry (ABMTR) reported a progression-free survival of 38% and an overall survival of 50% at 3 years in 122 patients with primary induction failure.[155] On the basis of these data, Hodgkin lymphoma patients who suffer from primary progressive disease should receive high-dose chemotherapy and autologous stem cell transplant whenever possible.

Treatment of Patients with Early or Late Relapse of Hodgkin Lymphoma

Patients who relapse after initial radiotherapy for localized Hodgkin lymphoma achieve satisfactory results with conventional polychemotherapy and are not considered candidates for high-dose chemotherapy and autologous stem cell transplant. The survival of patients who relapse after radiotherapy for early-stage disease is similar to that of advanced-stage patients who are initially treated with chemotherapy. Overall and disease-free survival ranges from 57% to 71%.[156,157]

In patients who relapse after conventional first-line chemotherapy, high-dose chemotherapy followed by autologous stem cell transplant has been shown to produce long-term disease-free survival rates of 30% to 65% in patients with refractory or relapsed Hodgkin lymphoma.[158,159] In addition, the reduction of early transplant-related mortality ranged from 10% to 25% in earlier studies to less than 3% in more recent studies and led to the widespread acceptance of high-dose chemotherapy and autologous stem cell transplant. Although outcome with high-dose chemotherapy has generally been better when compared to conventional salvage therapy, the validity of these results has been questioned due to the lack of randomized trials. The most compelling evidence for the superiority of high-dose chemotherapy and autologous stem cell transplant in relapsed Hodgkin lymphoma came from two randomized trials: one was conducted by the British National Lymphoma Investigation (BNLI) and the other by the GHSG together with the EBMT. In the BNLI trial, patients with relapsed or refractory Hodgkin lymphoma were treated with a combination of carmustine (BCNU), etoposide, cytarabine, and melphalan at a conventional-dose level (mini-BEAM) or at a high-dose level (BEAM) supported by autologous bone marrow transplantation. The actuarial 3-year event-free survival was significantly better in patients who received high-dose chemotherapy (53% vs. 10%).[160] The second randomized multicenter trial in this setting performed by the GHSG and the EBMT also demonstrated the benefit of high-dose chemotherapy in relapsed Hodgkin lymphoma. Patients who relapsed after polychemotherapy were randomly assigned to either four cycles of Dexa-BEAM (dexamethasone, BCNU, etoposide, Ara-C, and melphalan) or two cycles of Dexa-BEAM followed by high-dose chemotherapy with BEAM and autologous bone marrow or stem cell transplantation. The final analysis of 144 evaluable patients revealed that among the 117 patients who achieved partial or complete remission after two cycles of induction chemotherapy, freedom from treatment failure in the high-dose chemotherapy group was 55% compared with 34% for patients receiving conventional-dose chemotherapy. Overall survival was not significantly different between treatment groups.[161]

A potential alternative to the commonly used multiagent high-dose chemotherapy regimens was seen in the principle of sequential high-dose chemotherapy. This approach has been increasingly employed in the treatment of hematologic and lymphoproliferative malignancies.[162,163] Initial results from phase 1 or 2 studies indicated that this approach was safe and effective. In accordance with the Norton-Simon hypothesis, few noncross-resistant agents were given after initial cytoreduction at short time intervals. In general, the transplantation of stem cells and the use of growth factors allowed application of the putatively most effective drugs at highest doses and shortest possible time intervals.

In 1997 a multicenter phase 2 trial that evaluated a high-dose sequential chemotherapy program followed by a final myeloablative course (BEAM) was evaluated for feasibility and efficacy of this strategy in patients with relapsed Hodgkin lymphoma. Eligibility criteria included histologically proven first relapse or primary progressive Hodgkin lymphoma or second relapse with no prior high-dose chemotherapy. The treatment program consisted of two initial cycles of DHAP before high-dose chemotherapy. Patients who achieved partial or complete remission after DHAP proceeded to sequential high-dose chemotherapy, consisting of cyclophosphamide 4 g/m^2 IV (intravenous), methotrexate 8 g/m^2 IV plus vincristine 1.4 mg/m^2 IV and etoposide 2 g/m^2 IV. The final myeloablative

TABLE 126.12

RECOMMENDATIONS FOR PRIMARY TREATMENT OUTSIDE CLINICAL TRIALS

Group	Stage	Recommendation
Early stages (favorable)	CS I–II A/B no RF	2–3 cycles CT[a] + IFRT (20–30 Gy)
Early stages (unfavorable)	CS I–II A/B + RF	4–6 cycles CT[b] + IFRT (20–36 Gy)
Advanced stages	CS IIB + RF; CS III A/B; CS IV A/B	6–8 cycles CT[c]; addition of RT only if PET positive residual disease is detected after completion of CT.

CS, clinical stage; RF, risk factors; EFRT, extended-field radiotherapy; CT, chemotherapy; IFRT, involved-field radiotherapy; RT, radiotherapy.
[a]ABVD (doxorubicin [Adriamycin], bleomycin, vinblastine, and dacarbazine)
[b]ABVD, Stanford V (mechlorethamine, Adriamycin, vinblastine, vincristine, etoposide, bleomycin, and prednisone), or MOPP/ABV (mechlorethamine, vincristine [Oncovin], procarbazine, and prednisone/Adriamycin, bleomycin, vinblastine).
[c]ABVD or BEACOPP (bleomycin, etoposide, Adriamycin, cyclophosphamide, vincristine, procarbazine, and prednisone) escalated.

course was BEAM followed by autologous stem cell transplant of at least 2 × 10^6 CD34+ cells/kg. At final evaluation, 102 patients were available for analysis. Among those patients, 10 had multiple relapses, 16 progressive disease, 20 early relapse, and 44 late relapse. At a median follow-up of 18 months (range 3–31 months), response at the final evaluation was 80% (72% complete remission, 8% partial remission). Toxicity was tolerable, with no treatment-related deaths. Freedom from treatment failure and overall survival rates were 62% and 81% for patients with early relapse, 65% and 81% for patients with late relapse, 41% and 48% for patients with progressive disease and 39% and 48% for patients with multiple relapses.[164]

Based on these results, an intergroup trial, including the GHSG, EORTC, GEL/TAMO and the EBMT, was initiated to compare a standard high-dose regimen (BEAM) with a sequential high-dose chemotherapy concept. Patients with histologically confirmed early and late relapse as well as patients with second relapse and no prior high-dose chemotherapy, fulfilling the entry criteria, received two cycles of DHAP. Those not progressing after DHAP were centrally randomized to receive either BEAM followed by autologous stem cell transplant (arm A of the study) or high-dose cyclophosphamide followed by high-dose methotrexate plus vincristine followed by high-dose etoposide and a final myeloablative course of BEAM (arm B of the study) prior to autologous stem cell transplant.

A total of 284 patients were included in this trial of whom 241 were randomized. The median follow-up was 42 months. There were no major differences in patient characteristics between treatment arms, with most of the patients presenting with late first relapse. Treatment duration was significantly longer with intensified treatment. There were also more WHO grade IV toxicities before BEAM and more protocol violations ($P < .05$) in this arm. Mortality was nearly identical in both arms (20% vs. 18%), and there were no differences in terms of freedom from treatment failure, progression-free survival, and overall survival. The respective 3-year rates for the standard arm and the intensified arm were freedom from treatment failure 71% versus 65%, progression-free survival 72% versus 67%, and overall survival 87% versus 80%, respectively. Patients with Ann Arbor stage IV, early relapse, or multiple relapses and anemia had a significantly higher risk of recurrence (all single bivariate $P < .05$, combined $P < .001$). In conclusion, both regimens tested showed equally favorable results regarding outcome and survival. Since further intensification did not improve results, two cycles of conventional induction chemotherapy (DHAP) followed by high-dose chemotherapy with BEAM and autologous stem cell transplant is the standard of care for patients with relapsed Hodgkin lymphoma within the GHSG.[96] The question whether DHAP is the best induction regimen in relapsed Hodgkin lymphoma has not been answered in a randomized fashion. Other regimens used that show good antitumor activity in phase 2 trials include ICE (ifosfamide, carboplatin, etoposide) and IGEV (ifosfamide, gemcitabine, prednisolone, vinorelbine).[165,166]

The Role of Allogeneic Stem Cell Transplantation in Hodgkin Lymphoma

Given the high nonrelapse mortality of myeloablative allogeneic stem cell transplantation in Hodgkin lymphoma, the use of reduced intensity nonmyeloablative conditioning regimens represents a possible alternative. The goal of this strategy is to reduce the treatment-related toxicity while providing sufficient immunosuppression to facilitate donor engraftment with a subsequent graft versus lymphoma effect. There are several published regimens, ranging from the truly nonmyeloablative single fraction total body irradiation with a dose of 2 Gy to moderately myelosuppressive chemotherapy-based regimens, which often combine fludarabine with an alkylating agent such as melphalan or busulfan. The marked reduction of upfront toxicity with these regimens theoretically extends the applicability of allogeneic stem cell transplantation to older patients, patients with comorbidities, and particularly to those who had previously failed autologous stem cell transplant.

In recent years, several groups reported on the outcome of patients with relapsed Hodgkin lymphoma treated with reduced-intensity conditioning and allogeneic stem cell transplant. However, these reports are often difficult to interpret due to differences in patient populations and conditioning regimens used. In general, transplant-related mortality was lower as compared to classical myeloablative conditioning regimens. A reduction in transplant-related mortality was shown by the Lymphoma Working Party of the EBMT who retrospectively compared patients who had standard myeloablative conditioning with patients who had received reduced intensity regimens. Transplant-related mortality at 1 year was 46% in the myeloablative group and 23% in the reduced intensity group ($P = .003$).[167]

There is mounting evidence that successful allogeneic transplantation in Hodgkin lymphoma needs a combination of an effective salvage chemotherapy and a moderately intensive pretransplant conditioning regimen to keep the disease under control and to allow the withdrawal of immunosuppression or the use of donor lymphocyte infusions to achieve an effective graft versus lymphoma response.

Another retrospective analysis by the EBMT included a total of 285 patients with relapsed or refractory Hodgkin lymphoma who were treated with reduced intensity allogeneic stem cell transplant. The aim of the study was to identify prognostic factors that predicted long-term outcome. Sixty patients died from nonrelapse mortality at a median of 91 days (ranging from 1 day to 20 months) following transplantation. The cumulative incidence estimates of nonrelapse mortality at 100 days, 1 year, and 3 years after allogeneic transplant were 10.9%, 19.5%, and 21.1%, respectively. In multivariate analysis, nonrelapse mortality was associated with poor performance status, chemorefractory disease, age more than 45 years, and transplantation before 2002. With a median follow-up of 26 months (range 3–94 months), 126 patients were alive and 159 had died. The Kaplan-Meier estimates of overall and progression-free survival at 1, 2, and 3 years were 67% and 52%, 43% and 39%, 29% and 25%, respectively. Refractory disease and poor performance status were identified as risk factors for poor overall and progression-free survival. Patients with none of these risk factors had a 3-year progression-free and overall survival rate of 42% and 56% compared to 8% and 25% for patients who presented with one or two risk factors. In an analysis restricted to patients who had relapsed after a prior autologous stem cell transplant, relapse within the first 6 months after transplant was associated with a significantly worse disease progression rate (RR [relapse rate] = 1.9 (1.2–3.1); $P = .01$) and reduced progression-free survival (RR = 1.9 (1.2–2.9); $P = .003$) after reduced intensity allogeneic stem cell transplant.[168] In summary, reduced intensity allogeneic stem cell transplant may be an effective salvage strategy for selected patients with good risk features who relapse after autologous stem cell transplant. The major limitation of this approach, however, is the poor tumor control reported after reduced intensity conditioning, with relapse rates of 59% at 3 years.[169] Patients with chemorefractory disease or those who present with poor performance status still have a poor overall outcome and are poor candidates for allogeneic stem cell transplant. Further optimization of an allogeneic stem cell transplant approach in Hodgkin lymphoma, particularly related to the optimal reinduction regimen and a better selection of patients who might benefit, is warranted.

Future Directions and Recommendation

In the treatment of primary progressive and relapsed Hodgkin lymphoma, high-dose chemotherapy followed by autologous stem cell transplant is the current standard of care for most patients. After a brief induction therapy with protocols such as DHAP, ICE, or IGEV, high-dose chemotherapy, mostly consisting of high-dose BEAM followed by autologous stem cell support, results in long-term cure of more than 50% of cases (Table 126.13). In patients with multiple relapses, allogeneic stem cell transplantation might be a curative option in selected young patients who achieve a good remission upon reinduction. In the future, PET might become a predictor of outcome in this group of patients. Here, initial reports suggest a positive PET prior to or after high-dose chemotherapy as negative prognostic marker so that intensification of treatment or change of the induction protocol might be possible consequences of a positive transplant-related PET scan.[170]

LYMPHOCYTE-PREDOMINANT HODGKIN LYMPHOMA

NLPHL is a rare Hodgkin lymphoma subtype accounting for about 5% of all cases. Immunophenotype as well as clinical course of NLPHL differ substantially from cHL.[49] However, current standard treatment of NLPHL is not different from cHL standard treatment for most stages, a fact that can be explained by the rarity of the disease and, consequentially, a lack of clinical trials to evaluate novel treatment approaches in NLPHL.

Clinical Presentation

Due to the rarity of this disease, distinct clinical features were not recognized in detail until the European Task Force on Lymphoma (ETFL) conducted an analysis comprising 219 patients with histologically confirmed NLPHL.[49] Another analysis in which characteristics of 394 NLPHL patients were compared with characteristics of 7,904 cHL patients was performed by the GHSG. Both analyses revealed that NLPHL was more often diagnosed in early stages. B-symptoms, bulky

TABLE 126.13

SALVAGE PROTOCOLS USED FOR REINDUCTION IN RELAPSED HODGKIN LYMPHOMA

Drug	Dose	Route	Schedule	Cycle Length
DHAP				14–21 days
Cisplatin	100 mg/m²	IV	1	
Cytarabine (Ara-C)	2,000 mg/m²	IV	12 q on day 2	
Prednisone	40 mg	IV	1–4	
IGEV				21 days
Ifosphamide	2,000 mg/m²	IV	1–4	
Gemcitabine	800 mg/m²	IV	1 and 4	
Vinorelbine	20 mg/m²	IV	1	
Prednisone	100 mg	IV	1–4	
ICE				14 days
Ifosphamide	5,000 mg/m²	IV	2	
Carboplatin	AUC5	IV	2	
Etoposide	100 mg/m²	IV	1–3	

and extranodal disease, elevation of ESR and lactate dehydrogenase, as well as involvement of three or more nodal areas were less frequently found in NLPHL than in cHL.[171]

Treatment Results

In the GHSG analysis mentioned above, freedom from treatment failure (88% vs. 82%) and overall survival (96% vs. 92%) rates tended to be superior in NLPHL patients. This might in partially due to the increased rate of NLPHL patients diagnosed in early stages.[171] Patients with early favorable NLPHL in clinical stage IA have an excellent overall survival that is close to 100%. Different approaches can be applied in these patients. Those include watch and wait, radiotherapy in IF or EF technique, combined modality strategies, and treatment with anti-CD20 antibodies.

The major goal of NLPHL treatment in early stages is to induce as little acute and late toxicity as possible. Particularly in children with NLPHL, treatment strategies focus on avoiding long-term side effects such as secondary malignancies, infertility, growth retardation, hypothyroidism, and damage of heart and lung. In an attempt to postpone treatment, watch-and-wait strategies after diagnostic lymphadenectomy were evaluated in a smaller series of patients. In one study comprising 27 pediatric patients, 13 underwent lymphadenectomy and only 10 were treated with combined modality treatment, 1 patient had IF-RT, and 3 patients received chemotherapy only. At a median follow-up of 70 months, the overall survival for all 27 patients was 100% with an event-free survival rate of 69%. The event-free survival in the watch-and-wait group was 42% compared with 90% in those patients who had additional treatment. Patients with residual lymphoma after the diagnostic operation clearly had an inferior event-free survival when receiving no further treatment.[172] Thus, watch and wait has to be regarded as experimental and cannot be routinely recommended in clinical practice. In addition, more studies such as one currently being conducted by the EORTC are needed to obtain clear and reliable data. In this study, stage IA NLPHL patients with infradiaphragmatic disease are followed by watch and wait after complete tumor resection.

For most NLPHL patients in early favorable stages, radiotherapy is the mainstay of treatment. In a smaller series, including 36 stage I or IIA patients who were either treated with IF-RT or a modified localized radiation, the event-free survival rate was 95% and overall survival was 100% after 5 years.[173] A larger Australian series analyzed 202 stage I or II patients treated with radiotherapy in mantle field technique or reverted Y field. In this group of patients, the progression-free survival was 82%, with an overall survival of 83% at a median follow-up of 15 years.[174] In their studies, the GHSG treated a total of 131 stage IA NLPHL patients with different treatment modalities, including EF-RT (45 patients), IF-RT (45 patients), and combined modality treatment (41 patients). Median follow-up was 78 months for the EF-RT treated group, 17 months for those patients treated with IF-RT, and 40 months for those who received combined modality treatment. Overall, 99% of patients achieved a complete remission. There was no difference in terms of freedom from treatment failure between the treatment modalities applied.[30] Similar results were seen in a recently published large single institution retrospective study by Chen et al.[175] that included 113 patients with stage I or II NLPHL. In this study, the outcome of patients treated with IF-RT, EF-RT, or combined modality treatment was also comparable with a shorter follow-up for patients who received IF-RT only. Although longer follow-up is required for a more comprehensive picture, the efficacy and tolerability of IF-RT has resulted in the recommendation of this treatment modality by the GHSG for patients with stage IA NLPHL without risk factors. The EORTC has also adopted IF-RT as standard of care for stage IA NLPHL.[111] Similarly, the guidelines panel of the U.S. National Cancer Center Network (NCCN) recommends small-field radiotherapy as the treatment of choice for stage IA NLPHL.[176]

In a phase 2 study conducted by the GHSG, 28 NLPHL patients with clinical stage IA without risk factors received four weekly doses of rituximab. Results of this trial are pending but could influence future strategies in the treatment of clinical stage IA NLPHL, especially in pediatric and young adults where the second tumor risk may represent a greater problem than in older patients.

A North American Group conducted a trial that included patients with both first diagnosis of NLPHL and relapsed disease. Patients either received four weekly doses of rituximab without further treatment (limited treatment) or four weekly doses of rituximab followed by repeated rituximab administrations every 6 months (extended treatment). Preliminary results indicate that extended administration of rituximab might prolong freedom from progression. After a median follow-up of 30 months, the median freedom from disease progression was not reached in the extended treatment group and it was 24 months in the limited treatment group.[92]

Treatment of Early Unfavorable and Advanced Stages

The treatment of early unfavorable and advanced NLPHL is usually identical to the treatment of cHL. This is based on larger analyses performed by several groups that revealed similar treatment results of NLPHL and cHL patients when treated with protocols widely accepted in the treatment of Hodgkin lymphoma. The GHSG analysis reported that 86% of patients in early unfavorable and 77% of patients in advanced stages reached complete remission. This compares with rates of 83% and 78%, respectively, in cHL patients. There were only 0.3% of NLPHL patients with progressive disease compared with a rate of 3.9% in cHL patients. Although the overall relapse rate was very similar (NLPHL 8.1% vs. 8.0% in cHL), early relapses were more frequent in patients with cHL (3.2% vs. 0.8% in NLPHL) while late relapses were found more often in NLPHL patients (7.4% vs. 4.7% in cHL). With a median follow-up of 50 months, no significant differences between NLPHL and cHL were observed in terms of overall survival rates (96% in NLPHL vs. 92% in cHL).[177] Similar data were reported by the ETFL. Here, at a median follow-up of 8 years, the overall survival rate was 89% in both NLPHL and cHL.[49]

Treatment of Relapsed Nodular Lymphocyte Predominance Hodgkin Lymphoma

If possible, NLPHL patients with suspected relapse should undergo a renewed biopsy since transformation into aggressive non-Hodgkin lymphoma must be excluded. In the ETFL analysis, 14% of NLPHL relapses were identified as cHL and 10% as NHL. However, patients with NLPHL showed a tendency to more favorable survival after relapse as compared with cHL patients ($P = .05$), but this finding has to be handled with care: more NLPHL patients had been diagnosed in early stages at primary diagnosis and were treated with less intensive first-line treatment than most cHL patients.[1]

With the advent of the anti-CD20 monoclonal antibody rituximab in the treatment of CD20-positive lymphomas, some phase 2 studies that used this antibody were initiated in patients with relapsed or refractory NLPHL. This was based on the fact that in NLPHL not only the reactive background usually stains strongly for CD20 but, importantly, also the malignant LP cells are CD20+. In a study conducted by the GHSG, 14 patients were treated with weekly rituximab at a dose of 375 mg/m^2 for 4 consecutive weeks. Overall response rate was 86%. Eight patients achieved complete remission and four patients partial remission. At a short median follow-up of 12 months, nine patients were in remission.[178] An update analysis on this study, including 15 patients who had reconfirmed NLPHL, reported an overall response rate of 94%. With a median follow-up of 63 months, the median time to progression was 33 months; the median overall survival was not reached.[179] Similar results were reported from at study at Stanford University on 22 less intensively or previously untreated NLPHL patients who received rituximab. Here, the response rate was 100% but nine patients relapsed.[180] However, with excellent response rates even in heavily pretreated patients, anti-CD20 antibodies such as rituximab and novel follow-up products might become an inherent part in future strategies for the treatment of NLPHL, possibly in combination with classical chemotherapy protocols such as ABVD or others.

Transformation into Non-Hodgkin Lymphoma

The possibility of transformation from NLPHL into aggressive NHL is well documented. In one study from the International Database on Hodgkin Lymphoma, a significantly higher risk for secondary NHL was found for NLPHL patients compared with cHL patients.[181] Several smaller NLPHL studies report a secondary NHL rate of 2% to 3%.[87] In contrast, two recent analyses independently indicated higher transformation rates. In one analysis, including 164 patients initially diagnosed with NLPHL, the 10-year cumulative transformation rate was 12%; another analysis, including 95 NLPHL patients, reported an actuarial risk of transformation to aggressive lymphoma of 7% at 10 years and of 30% at 20 years. It is possible that the risk of transformation from NLPHL into NHL, particularly into T-cell rich B-cell lymphoma and diffuse large cell lymphoma, has been underappreciated in the past.[182,183]

Future Strategies and Recommendation

In NLPHL, early favorable patients seem to be sufficiently treated with IF-RT only. Early unfavorable and advanced stages are currently still treated with the same combined modality approaches as cHL. In relapsed NLPHL, remission rates after anti-CD20 antibody treatment are very promising. However, high-dose chemotherapy and autologous stem cell transplantation, possibly supplemented by rituximab or follow-up products, might be necessary in more extensive relapses.

In the future, the use of anti-CD20 antibodies might also become part of the first-line treatment of NLPHL. This might allow a reduction in the dose and number of cycles of conventional chemotherapy needed.

SPECIAL POPULATIONS

Hodgkin Lymphoma in the Elderly Patient

Clinical experience and data from large trials indicate that patients older than 60 years have a higher risk of treatment failure and experience more treatment-related toxicity than younger patients.[184] Regarding the incidence of Hodgkin lymphoma in elderly patients, the most accurate assessments were derived from population-based studies. Two Swedish studies covering the years from 1979 to 1988 and 1973 to 1994 showed a proportion of 31% and 26% of Hodgkin lymphoma patients older than 60 years, respectively.[93,185] The Scotland and Newcastle Lymphoma Group (SNLG) data demonstrated that from 1979 to 2003, 624 (20%) of 3,373 patients registered in the population registry were over 60 years.[94] With 35% of cases, mixed cellularity subtype is more frequent in elderly patients.[184] Also, EBV positivity of HRS cells is more often present in patients aged 50 and above compared with younger patients.[186] This EBV positivity is associated with poorer prognosis, as suggested by an analysis from Stark et al.[187] With respect to the clinical presentation, elderly patients are more often diagnosed in early favorable and advanced stages, and early unfavorable stages are less frequent.[184]

The patient's physical and mental condition, disease history, and the presence of concurrent disorders influence the treatment strategy. Age in general is no contraindication against aggressive treatment; but compared with younger patients, fewer elderly patients receive the intended chemotherapy dose. The survival analysis of one large trial performed by the GHSG showed a significantly poorer treatment outcome for elderly patients in terms of 5-year overall survival (65% vs. 90%) and freedom from treatment failure (60% vs. 80%).[184] However, biologically young patients in good physical and mental condition should be treated in a stage-adapted manner.

ABVD is regarded as standard chemotherapy for most elderly Hodgkin lymphoma patients. In early favorable and unfavorable stages, two to six cycles of ABVD followed by IF-RT represent a widely accepted standard of care. In advanced stages, six to eight cycles of ABVD are usually being given. Unfortunately, no prospectively randomized studies using this chemotherapy regimen in elderly patients have been published so far, and a reliable statement on ABVD toxicity in older patients cannot be given. There is only one currently ongoing study using ABVD as standard treatment, comparing it with VEPEMB (vinblastine, cyclophosphamide, procarbazine, prednisolone, etoposide, mitoxantrone, bleomycin).

Another very well-tolerated regimen, containing an anthracycline, an alkylating agent, and a vinca alkaloid, is the CHOP-21 (cyclophosphamide, doxorubicin, vincristine, prednisone) protocol, which is widely used in the treatment of non-Hodgkin lymphoma. Compared to ABVD, the anthracycline dose density is somewhat higher, and myelotoxicity is not a major problem at least in elderly non-Hodgkin lymphoma patients. In a Norwegian study evaluating CHOP-21 in elderly patients with Hodgkin lymphoma, 18 of 29 patients had advanced disease and received six to eight cycles of CHOP-21 with subsequent radiotherapy in case of any residual mass. Patients with early stages received two to four cycles of chemotherapy followed by radiation. The overall response rate at final staging was 93%, the 3-year overall survival rate was 79% and the 3-year progression-free survival rate was 76%. Twenty-seven (93%) of the included patients completed the planned therapy, and there were two therapy-associated fatal events.[188] However, a larger study to ensure the reliability of the results is warranted before final conclusions can be drawn.

More aggressive regimens should be avoided in elderly patients since they were shown to cause inacceptable toxicity. The GHSG HD9 elderly trial was designed for patients aged 66 to 75 years in stages IIB to IV. Patients were randomized between eight cycles of COPP/ABVD (26 patients) and eight cycles of BEACOPP baseline (42 patients). Eighteen patients with bulky or residual disease after chemotherapy received consolidating radiotherapy. The full number of planned treatment cycles was given to 18 patients (69%) in the COPP/ABVD group and to 23 patients (55%) in the BEACOPP baseline group. The complete remission rate was the same in both treatment arms (76%), and there was also no difference regarding the number of patients with progressive disease (8% for COPP/ABVD and 7% for BEACOPP baseline). The disease-specific freedom from treatment failure at 5 years was better for the more aggressive BEACOPP baseline regimen than for COPP/ABVD (74% vs. 55%; $P = .13$). This did not translate into a superior overall survival at 5 years due to more treatment-related fatal events in the BEACOPP baseline arm (21% vs. 8% for COPP/ABVD).[189]

Since etoposide was thought to contribute to the poorer tolerability of BEACOPP in elderly patients, the GHSG then developed a new BEACOPP variant especially for this patient cohort. This new schedule, BACOPP, contained no etoposide, whereas the dose of adriamycin was increased (from 25 mg/m^2 to 50 mg/m^2). Sixty patients (92%) were eligible for the final analysis of the phase 2 trial to evaluate the regimen. In total, 51 patients showed complete remissions (85%), 2 had partial remissions (3%), and 4 had primary progression of disease (7%). WHO grade III to IV toxicities were documented in 52 patients (87%). With a median observation of 33 months, 18 deaths (30%) have been observed including seven therapy-associated fatal outcomes. Thus, with a therapy-associated death rate beyond 10%, this regimen also requires modification and is not recommended for routine use.[171]

Another phase 2 study by the GHSG investigated the incorporation of gemcitabine into the first-line treatment of older patients. Bleomycin and dacarbazine were replaced from the ABVD backbone by gemcitabine and prednisone, resulting in the PVAG regimen. Fifty patients have been included in the trial, with the final analysis pending.

Since high-dose chemotherapy followed by autologous stem cell transplantation is not possible in most elderly patients, second-line treatment is generally of palliative nature. Several single-agents including gemcitabine and trofosfamide were described to be active in a relevant portion of patients.[190,191] In addition, there is some possibility to treat relapsed elderly Hodgkin lymphoma patients with a second polychemotherapy (e.g., a regimen that has been developed years ago and utilized by the SNLG as palliative therapy) over a prolonged period. The regimen is a well-tolerated all oral schedule consisting of prednisolone, etoposide, chlorambucil, and lomustine (CCNU) (PECC). Recently, an update on the use of the protocol in relapsed Hodgkin lymphoma from the SNLG database demonstrated a complete remission rate of 58% in the 12 included patients who were older than 60 years. This finding suggests that PECC might have a useful role in the treatment of relapsed Hodgkin lymphoma in elderly patients.[192]

Treatment for patients with impairment of lung, liver, heart, or kidney should be adapted individually. Single drugs with organ-specific toxicities (e.g., bleomycin and doxorubicin) may be omitted, replaced, or modified in dose. IF-RT or the use of less aggressive drugs such as gemcitabine and vinorelbine with or without dexamethasone are possible treatment alternatives in case standard treatment is impossible. Of note, a concomitant application of bleomycin and gemcitabine should be avoided since a high incidence of pulmonary toxicity was observed in one trial.[104]

Future Directions and Recommendations for the Treatment of Elderly Patients

Due to a lack of definitive prospective randomized studies, it is currently not possible to provide sound evidence-based recommendations for the treatment of elderly Hodgkin lymphoma patients. Of course, Hodgkin lymphoma should be potentially curable in all age groups but the results for the elderly remain disappointing. The poor clinical outcome in this age group has been related to the fact that there are more patients who present with advanced stages. In addition, most analyses indicate that the delivery of appropriate drugs at an optimal dose intensity and density is compromised in patients over 65 years of age. This fact probably has a major effect on the disappointing clinical outcome. Furthermore, it might be possible that additional chemoresistance mechanisms are operational in a proportion of Hodgkin lymphoma cases in this age group.

From the available data it seems clear that elderly patients with early-stage Hodgkin lymphoma (stages I and II) should be treated with a brief chemotherapy followed by IF-RT. Though ABVD has some toxicity in elderly patients and no prospective studies using ABVD in these patients are available, this regimen is also considered standard of care for older patients. Recent results from the GHSG HD10 trial reveal that the administration of only two cycles of ABVD followed by only 20 Gy IF-RT is sufficient in early favorable Hodgkin lymphoma.[193] In early unfavorable stages, four to six cycles of ABVD followed by 30 Gy IF-RT are appropriate, while in advanced-stage disease six to eight cycles of ABVD are accepted standard of care. Dose density is often unsatisfactory in elderly patients, and the outcome therefore is poor as compared to younger patients. Thus, the best approach would be to include patients into study protocols whenever possible so that clear treatment strategies can be developed and evaluated. Due to the obvious limitations of conventional chemotherapy in elderly Hodgkin lymphoma patients, these protocols should incorporate new therapeutic approaches.

Hodgkin Lymphoma during Pregnancy

The peak incidence of Hodgkin lymphoma occurs within female's reproductive age. Therefore, the association with pregnancy is not uncommon. Hodgkin lymphoma is the fourth most common cancer occurring during pregnancy.[194] One case of Hodgkin lymphoma occurs per 1,000 to 6,000 deliveries. Several studies have shown that pregnancy is not associated with a worse clinical course, and that the 20-year survival rate of pregnant women with Hodgkin lymphoma is not different from that of nonpregnant women.[195]

The clinical presentation of Hodgkin lymphoma is not influenced by pregnancy. However, there are significant limitations regarding staging and treatment of pregnant patients. CT and PET scans should be avoided since limiting radiation exposure to the fetus is essential especially during early stages of gestation. Ultrasound is helpful for assessing the fetal status and detecting tumor lesions in the abdomen of the mother. Magnetic resonance imaging can complete the radiologic staging because it does not seem to be associated with risk to the fetus. Decisions about the need for a chest radiograph should be made on the basis of clinical examination.

If Hodgkin lymphoma is diagnosed during the first trimester and disease requires immediate therapeutic intervention, most experts agree that a therapeutic abortion should be encouraged since the risk to negatively affect the development of the fetus by applying antineoplastic drugs during that period is high. If an immediate start of therapy is indicated and the mother does not want an abortion, low-dose supradiaphragmatic irradiation or application of vinblastine monotherapy may be considered. In cases with no need for an immediate therapeutic intervention, the start of treatment should be deferred.[196]

In the second or third trimester, patients with stage I or II disease may be closely observed, and treatment can be postponed until an early delivery is achieved. If there is any sign of accelerated disease progression, especially supradiaphragmatic lymphadenopathy, radiotherapy alone is recommended. Most studies recommend doses of 10 to 36 Gy applied as mantle field or IF irradiation with abdominal shielding. At this time of fetal development, the risk of adverse sequelae for the child from supradiaphragmatic irradiation is low. Pregnant Hodgkin lymphoma patients in the second or third trimester who present with infradiaphragmatic lymphadenopathy or advanced disease should receive combination chemotherapy. Because most chemotherapeutic agents freely cross the placenta and enter the fetal circulation, the patient and the fetus should be monitored closely. Application of cytotoxic drugs shortly before birth may be particularly hazardous because the placenta is also the primary means of drug elimination, and metabolism and excretion are delayed in the neonate. The current concept is that antimetabolites, especially methotrexate, must not be given since they carry a high risk of teratogenesis, whereas doxorubicin, bleomycin, etoposide, and the vinca alkaloids appear acceptable. Thus, the ABVD regimen may be used when chemotherapy is indicated beyond the first trimester. Because chemotherapeutic agents accumulate in breast milk, mothers are best advised not to breastfeed during treatment.

Hodgkin Lymphoma in Human Immunodeficiency Virus–Positive Patients

Epidemiology and Clinical Presentation

Hodgkin lymphoma is diagnosed more frequently in patients with HIV infection than in the general population. Given the background incidence of Hodgkin lymphoma in the population groups at high risk for HIV infection, epidemiological studies conducted during the first years of the HIV epidemic in North America and Europe had difficulty including Hodgkin lymphoma in the spectrum of HIV-associated cancers. However, with the spread of the epidemic and longer survival of infected people, the impact of Hodgkin lymphoma in HIV-positive patients could be better recognized. All studies available to date strongly support the evidence that those infected with HIV have an approximately tenfold higher risk of developing Hodgkin lymphoma than HIV-negative persons. Such an excess risk is more pronounced in HIV-infected individuals with moderate immune suppression, as found in patients under antiretroviral therapy. In contrast to HIV-negative patients with Hodgkin lymphoma, the mixed cellularity subtype is more frequently found in HIV-positive Hodgkin lymphoma patients and almost all cases are EBV associated, a fact that also contrasts to what is observed in HIV-negative Hodgkin lymphoma patients.[197,198] Here, only 20% to 50% of patients have EBV-associated disease depending on histological type and age at diagnosis.[199]

Regarding clinical presentation, B-symptoms defined as fever, night sweats, or weight loss of more than 10% of the body weight are consistently found among HIV-positive Hodgkin lymphoma patients, with a portion of more than 70% presenting with these symptoms. In addition, the majority of patients have advanced disease and involvement of extranodal sites, particularly of bone marrow, liver, and spleen.[200]

Treatment of Hodgkin Lymphoma in Human Immunodeficiency Virus–Positive Patients

The optimal therapy for Hodgkin lymphoma in HIV-positive patients has not been defined yet. Because most patients present with advanced stages, treatment mostly consists of combination chemotherapy regimens, but the complete remission rates achieved with these regimens remain lower than in patients without HIV infection and overall survival is only about 1.5 years.[105,200,201] Due to the low overall incidence of HIV-related Hodgkin lymphoma, no randomized controlled trials have been conducted in this setting. However, several phase 2 studies have evaluated the feasibility and activity of different regimens. In a prospective trial conducted by an Italian group between 1989 and 1992, 17 previously untreated HIV-positive Hodgkin lymphoma patients received treatment with epirubicin, vinblastine, and bleomycin (EVB) plus antiretroviral medication. Complete remission was achieved in 53% of patients, lasting a median of 20 months. The median overall survival was 11 months.[202] In an attempt to improve these results, a second prospective trial to evaluate full-dose EVB plus prednisone (EVBP) and concomitant antiretroviral therapy was conducted from 1993 until 1997. The results of this trial, including 35 patients, showed a complete remission rate of 74% and a 3-year overall survival of 32%.[203] The AIDS Clinical Trials Group reported the results of a phase 2 study that included 21 patients treated with four to six cycles of ABVD followed by obligatory G-CSF support. Antiretroviral therapy was not used. The complete remission rate was 43% with an objective overall response rate of 62%. Median survival for all patients was 18 months.[204]

The widespread introduction of antiretroviral therapy allowed the use of more aggressive chemotherapeutic regimens such as Stanford V or BEACOPP. From 1997 to 2001, 59 consecutive patients were treated with Stanford V in a prospective phase 2 study. Treatment was well tolerated and 69% of the patients included completed therapy with no dose reduction or delay in chemotherapy administration. The most important dose-limiting side effects were bone marrow toxicity and neurotoxicity. Eighty-one percent of the patients achieved complete remission and with a median follow-up of 17 months, 56% of patients were alive and disease free. The estimated 5-year overall survival was 59%.[205] Within the German group, treatment with BEACOPP in baseline dosage showed promising results in terms of complete remission, toxicity, and median survival. In contrast, it cannot be recommended to use BEACOPP escalated in HIV-positive patients.[206] Recently, the results of a large prospective phase 2 study with ABVD have been published. Within a cooperative network in Spain, 62 HIV-positive patients with Hodgkin lymphoma received standard ABVD plus antiretroviral therapy. The scheduled six to eight ABVD cycles were completed in 82% of cases. Six patients died during induction, 54 (87%) achieved a complete remission, and 2 were resistant. The 5-year overall and event-free survival probabilities were 76% and 71%, respectively. The immunological response to antiretroviral therapy had a positive impact on overall (P = .002) and event-free survival (P = .001).[207]

Because a large portion of HIV-positive patients with Hodgkin lymphoma have disease progress or relapse, the use of high-dose chemotherapy and autologous stem cell transplant in this setting has been evaluated by several groups and the data published so far have demonstrated the feasibility of this approach so that it can be considered standard of care in progressive or relapsed patients.[208,209]

TREATMENT-RELATED LATE SIDE EFFECTS

Pulmonary Complications

Radiation pneumonitis typically occurs 1 to 6 months after completion of radiotherapy. Once it resolves, there usually are no long-term sequelae. A mild nonproductive cough, low-grade fever, and dyspnea on exertion characterize symptomatic radiation pneumonitis. Ten percent to 15% of patients with large mediastinal tumors who receive a combination of chemotherapy and mantle field radiation therapy develop radiation pneumonitis.[75] Radiographically, pneumonitis is characterized by the formation of infiltrates confined to the original radiation fields. Infection rather than pneumonitis is more likely if the infiltrates extend into areas of the lung initially protected from radiation. Severe pneumonitis may require treatment with steroids. However, with modern radiation techniques, the incidence of radiation pneumonitis should decrease.

Cardiac Complications

Chemotherapy-Associated Cardiac Complications

The most relevant cardiotoxic drugs used in the treatment of Hodgkin lymphoma are anthracyclines. Anthracycline-associated toxicity may occur at different intervals after therapy. Cardiotoxicity often presents as electrocardiographic changes, arrhythmias, or as cardiomyopathy, leading to congestive heart failure. Anthracycline-associated cardiotoxicity is caused by direct damage of the myoepithelium and is strongly related to the cumulative dose applied.[210,211] Doses less than 500 mg/m^2 are usually well tolerated. The total dose of anthracyclines used in the first-line therapy of Hodgkin lymphoma is relatively low compared with regimens used in the treatment of breast cancer or pediatric malignancies. The cumulative dose of eight cycles is 400 mg/m^2 for ABVD and 280 mg/m^2 for escalated BEACOPP. However, most patients are treated with less than eight cycles of anthracycline-containing chemotherapy.

Whether cardiac toxicity observed after chemotherapy and radiotherapy is additive or synergistic remains unclear. However, several clinical studies showed that anthracycline-containing therapy may increase the radiation-related risk of congestive heart failure and valvular disorders by two- to threefold compared to radiotherapy alone.[212,213]

Radiotherapy-Associated Cardiac Complications

Radiation-associated heart disease in cancer survivors includes a wide spectrum of cardiac pathologies such as coronary artery disease, myocardial dysfunction, valvular heart disease, pericardial disease, and electrical conduction abnormalities.[212,214] Radiation-associated heart diseases, except for pericarditis, usually present 10 to 15 years after exposure, although nonsymptomatic abnormalities may develop much earlier. The long delay before expression of serious damage probably explains why radiation sensitivity of the heart has previously been underestimated.

Radiation causes both increased mortality and increased morbidity. Epidemiologic studies on Hodgkin lymphoma survivors show relative risk estimates for cardiac deaths in the range of two to seven, depending on the patient's age. An increased risk was observed for patients irradiated at a young age, depending on the radiation technique used and the duration of follow-up.[214–216] In a Dutch study on Hodgkin lymphoma patients treated before the age of 41, three- to fivefold increased standardized incidence ratios for the development of various heart diseases were observed when compared to the general population, even after a follow-up of more than 20 years.[212] The persistence of an increased risk over prolonged follow-up is a major concern because this implies increased absolute excess risks over time, due to the rising incidence of cardiovascular diseases with age.

The heart volume included in the radiation field influences the risk of cardiotoxicity, although there are still many uncertainties regarding dose– and volume–effect relations.[213,217] A reduction in the risk of death from cardiovascular diseases other than myocardial infarction has been reported in Hodgkin lymphoma patients treated after partial shielding of the heart and restriction of the total, fractionated, mediastinal dose to less than 30 Gy.[218] Therefore, the number of radiotherapy-associated cardiac long-term sequelae might decrease in the upcoming years.

Secondary Neoplasia

Radiotherapy and certain chemotherapeutic agents such as nitrogen mustard, procarbazine, cyclophosphamide, and etoposide are well known to have the potential to induce the development of secondary malignancies.

The highest incidence of acute leukemia usually spikes within the first 10 years after initial treatment. Several analyses on incidence and outcome of secondary leukemia were performed. The largest report came from the GHSG who retrospectively assessed 5,411 patients with Hodgkin lymphoma treated within the group`s studies conducted between 1981 and 1998. After a median observation time of 55 months, incidence of secondary acute myeloid leukemia/myelodysplastic syndrome (AML/MDS) was 1%. Most patients were treated with COPP/ABVD, COPP/ABVD-like combinations, or BEACOPP. With a median observation of 24 months, only one patient had not died from secondary AML/MDS.[219]

The classic form of a treatment-related leukemia is characterized by a latency period of 3 to 5 years, a preceding myelodysplastic phase with trilineage bone marrow dysplasia, and abnormalities of chromosome 5 or 7. Topoisomerase II inhibitors, especially the epipodophyllotoxins, have been implicated in the development of a clinically and cytogenetically distinct form of secondary AML. When compared with classic secondary AML induced by alkylating agents, etoposide-related AML typically occurs sooner after exposure, generally lacks a preceding myelodysplastic phase, and is characterized by balanced translocations involving chromosome bands 11q23 and 21q22.[220]

Secondary NHL occurring after Hodgkin lymphoma includes intermediate- or high-grade lymphomas and presents

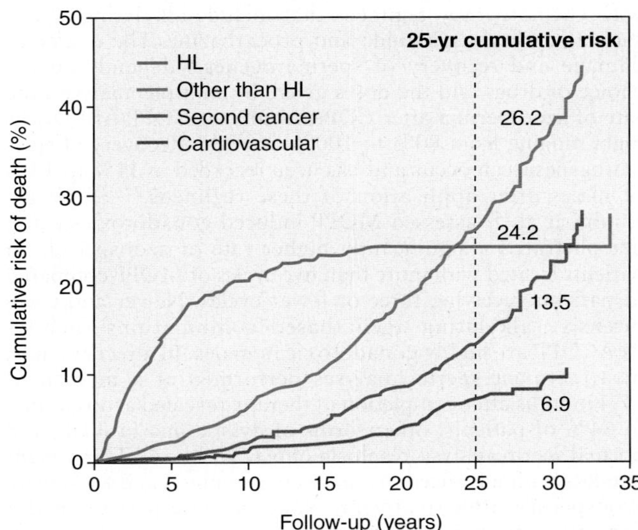

FIGURE 126.3 The 25-year cumulative risk of death from Hodgkin lymphoma or treatment-related late sequelae. (Adapted from ref. 218.)

PRACTICE OF ONCOLOGY

similar to lymphomas seen in patients with chronic suppression of the immune system. There is a cumulative risk of 1.2% to 2.1% at 15 years for the development of these lymphomas. In general, outcome of patients with secondary NHL is worse than that of patients with primary NHL. However, there are patients with secondary NHL who achieve durable remission after adequate chemotherapy.[221,222]

The incidence of solid tumors after Hodgkin lymphoma treatment increases with time and does not reach a plateau, even in the second decade after treatment. The causative role of radiotherapy and chemotherapy is debated, but most epidemiologists tend to place the greatest blame on intensive irradiation with large fields and high doses. The organs at major risk appear to be lung and breast, especially among women who were irradiated at a young age during development of the breast.[89] A retrospective analysis by the GHSG with a median follow-up of 72 months revealed an overall cumulative risk to develop a solid secondary malignancy of 2% with relative risk estimates for secondary malignancies of lung, colon, and breast of 3.8, 3.2, and 1.9, respectively.[223] Other secondary cancers observed after successful treatment for Hodgkin lymphoma include sarcomas, melanomas, and bone tumors.[224,225] However, as indicated by registry-based reports, the portion of patients with secondary solid tumors among Hodgkin lymphoma survivors will further increase with longer follow-up since particularly radiotherapy-related secondary malignancies have a latency of decades from exposure to the carcinogenic noxa to the diagnosis of the secondary cancer.

Gonadal Dysfunction

Seventy-eighty percent of male Hodgkin lymphoma patients in advanced stages have inadequate pretreatment semen quality due to the lymphoma itself.[226–228] The mechanisms involved are still unknown, however, possible factors include damage of the germinal epithelium, disturbances in the hypothalamic–hypophysial axis, immunological processes associated with cancer that impair spermatogenesis, and the dysregulated release of cytokines.[227,229–233] In a recent study by the GHSG, male fertility was assessed in a total of 243 patients. In pretreatment semen analyses, only 20% of patients had normal sperm. Azoospermia was observed in 11% and other dysspermia conditions were found in 69% of patients.[228]

Posttreatment gonadal damage is most often associated with chemotherapy regimens that include alkylating agents such as cyclophosphamide and procarbazine. The degree of damage and recovery of spermatogenesis depends on the choice of drugs and the doses given. In multiple analyses, the rate of azoospermia after COPP, MOPP, or COPP/ABVD was high, ranging from 80% to 100%.[226,234–238] Recovery of spermatogenesis can occur and has been recorded in 11% to 14% of males after application of these regimens.[226,237–239] Da Cunha et al.[240] assessed MOPP-induced gonadotoxicity and demonstrated a significantly higher rate of azoospermia in patients treated with more than five cycles of MOPP compared to patients receiving three or fewer cycles. Newer and more intensive alkylating agent–based combinations such as BEACOPP are highly gonadotoxic in males. In a recent study, posttreatment sperm analyses performed at a median of 17.4 months after completion of therapy revealed azoospermia in 64% of patients, other forms of dysspermia in 30%, and normal sperm analysis results in only 6% cases.[228] Thirty-eight patients with advanced disease were examined and 89% were azoospermic after treatment. None of these patients had a normal sperm status. There was no statistically significant difference in the posttreatment status between a group of patients treated with eight cycles of BEACOPP baseline (with a cumulative cyclophosphamide dose of 5200 mg/m^2) and a group treated with eight cycles of BEACOPP escalated (with a cumulative cyclophosphamide dose of 10.000 mg/m^2).[228] In contrast, ABVD, probably the most widely used regimen in the treatment of Hodgkin lymphoma, is less gonadotoxic, with gonadal damage that might be only transient.[238,241,242] However, due to the gonadotoxic effects of many drugs used in the current treatment of Hodgkin lymphoma, cryoconservation of sperm should be offered to every young male before starting with chemotherapy.

Very similar to male patients, alkylating agents are most commonly involved in treatment-associated gonadal damage in female patients. This is well documented for the treatment with older chemotherapy regimens such as MOPP or MVPP (mustine, vinblastine, procarbazine, prednisolone). In an early study, only 17 of 44 women maintained regular menses when one of these regimens was used.[243] In a similar study, Schilsky et al.[244] investigated ovarian function after treatment with MOPP and documented persistent amenorrhea in 11 of 24 women. Similarly, after treatment with alternating COPP/ABVD for advanced Hodgkin lymphoma, therapy-induced ovarian failure was described in 17 of 22 women.[236] A more recent analysis included a total of 84 female patients with Hodgkin lymphoma and NHL treated with at least three cycles of chemotherapy, including alkylating agents. Premature ovarian failure was defined as persistent amenorrhea for at least 2 years after the end of chemotherapy and elevated follicle-stimulating hormone levels. After a median follow-up of 100 months, 31 (37%) women with preserved fertility achieved natural pregnancy; in 34 women (40.5%), premature ovarian failure was reported.[245] In a retrospective analysis by the GHSG, the menstrual status after Hodgkin lymphoma treatment of 405 female patients younger than 40 years was analyzed. With a median follow-up of 3.2 years, 51.4% of women who had received eight cycles of escalated BEACOPP had continuous amenorrhea. Amenorrhea was significantly less common in women treated with two cycles of ABVD (3.9%), two cycles of alternating COPP/ABVD (6.9%), four cycles of alternating COPP/ABVD (37.5%), or eight cycles of BEACOPP baseline (22.6%). In a multivariate analysis, amenorrhea was most pronounced in women with advanced-stage Hodgkin lymphoma, women older than 30 years of age at treatment, and women who did not take oral contraceptives during chemotherapy.[246]

After ABVD alone, chemotherapy-induced ovarian failure is less likely, especially when women are younger than 30 years at the time of treatment.[241,247–250]

Older women have a significantly lower likelihood of ovarian recovery than those of younger age.[236,243–246,251,252] In the GHSG analysis, 40% of women younger than 30 years of age experienced amenorrhea after treatment with eight cycles of escalated BEACOPP, compared to 70% of women aged 30 or older.[246]

Recent studies suggested that anti-Mullerian hormone (AMH) is the most sensitive marker of gonadal function and can therefore be used for posttreatment assessment of the ovarian reserve. Anti-Mullerian hormone is produced by the granulosa cells of early developing preantral and antral follicles in the ovary. The serum AMH levels can be used as a marker for the number of growing follicles: the levels decrease when the number of follicles declines. The AMH levels are not influenced by the day of the menstrual cycle. They are therefore a potentially convenient and useful marker.[253–255] Recently, AMH has been tested to identify subgroups of childhood cancer survivors at risk for premature ovarian failure.[256]

QUALITY OF LIFE

A review of most randomized clinical trials in Hodgkin lymphoma reveals that quality of life (QoL) has been neglected as a primary or even secondary outcome measure in the past.

However, the number of clinical trials evaluating health-related QoL (HRQoL) assessment is increasing. It has become widely accepted that the multidimensional approach of HRQoL assessment reflects the patient's situation and reveals important information for the process of treatment evaluation. With the constantly growing cohort of long-term survivors that indicates the progress of cancer therapy, there is a need for new approaches in HRQoL assessment that deal with the particular problems of these long-term survivors. Several studies have highlighted the difficulties that survivors may experience long after treatment ends, such as general fatigue, health fragility, and social and financial problems. These findings have been demonstrated in studies where a HRQoL approach has been used. Since the studies mostly used a cross-sectional design, there is a need for new approaches to describe the patients' situation more precisely, to detect reasons for maladaptation, and to identify patients at high risk to develop problems.

Combined comprehensive approaches could help to overcome the difficulties in assessing HRQoL in long-term survivors. Furthermore, this approach can be used with few modifications in the assessment of normal control persons. It seems plausible that many years after treatment the daily living circumstances have a stronger impact on patients' HRQoL. Therefore, it is essential to also have reference data from age- and gender-matched healthy population for the interpretation of HRQoL results. In addition, a more comprehensive approach that accounts for the patients' life situation is necessary to represent the complexity of HRQoL. The results from the studies by the EORTC/GELA and the GHSG within the next few years will reveal whether this approach proves to be successful. QoL assessment should benefit patients by defining relevant issues, even long after initial treatment. Disease- and therapy-independent predisposing factors for long-term HRQoL functions on one hand and those factors associated with the applied therapy or the lymphoma itself on the other hand must be evaluated in well-designed prospective studies.

NEW DRUGS IN HODGKIN LYMPHOMA

Despite the excellent cure rates achieved with current first-line protocols, treatment of relapsed or refractory Hodgkin lymphoma has remained a field of unmet medical need. Relapse after high-dose chemotherapy and autologous stem cell transplant is especially associated with poor prognosis and a median overall survival of less than 3 years.[257] Fortunately, a growing number of signaling pathways misdirected in HRS cells have been discovered in recent years, and a plethora of novel substances that target these pathways or influence the interaction between HRS cells and their microenvironment have become available. Several of these drugs are currently undergoing clinical trials, and some preliminary but promising data have been reported recently. In this section, some of the new drugs, including monoclonal antibodies, immunotoxins, radioimmunoconjugates and small molecules, are briefly introduced.

Anti-CD30 Antibody-Based Approaches

Since it is selectively overexpressed on HRS cells, CD30 is considered a privileged target antigen for antibody-based immunotherapy of cHL. However, despite encouraging preclinical data, results of phase 1 or 2 clinical trials with naked first-generation anti-CD30 antibodies were disappointing. Both first-generation antibodies applied in Hodgkin lymphoma patients, MDX-060 and SGN-30, only showed modest clinical activity when given as single agent. In a phase 1 or 2 trial, a total of 72 patients with CD30+ malignancies, including 63 patients with multiple relapsed Hodgkin lymphoma, were treated with MDX-060, but there were only six patients who achieved an objective response and 25 with stable disease.[258] In another phase 2 trial that used a different monoclonal antibody (SGN-30), none of the 38 Hodgkin lymphoma patients responded.[259] There are several possible reasons that might explain this lack of activity, including poor binding properties *in vivo* and a neutralization of the antibodies by the soluble form of CD30 shed from the target cells.[260] However, second-generation antibodies were developed. One interesting candidate is XmAb2513, which has already undergone phase 1 clinical trial and first data on pharmacokinetics, where immunogenicity and safety were obtained.[261]

The most advanced and promising anti-CD30 construct so far is the antibody-drug conjugate SGN-35 (brentuximab vedotin), consisting of the antibody cAC10 and the synthetic antimitotic agent monomethyl auristatin. In a phase 1 study, 42 patients with relapsed Hodgkin lymphoma, 2 patients with systemic anaplastic large cell lymphoma, and 1 patient with angioimmunoblastic T-cell lymphoma were included. With a median of three prior lines of treatment, 86% of patients showed reductions in target lesion size and 46% achieved partial or complete remission. Side effects were mainly mild and manageable.[262] A pivotal phase 2 trial including 102 Hodgkin lymphoma patients with relapse after high-dose chemotherapy and autologous stem cell transplant finished recruitment at the end of 2009. Results of this trial will be used to seek U.S. Food and Drug Administration approval for the drug.

Antibody-Based Strategies Targeting Other Antigens

CD25 (IL-2 receptor) is expressed on a few normal cells and can consistently be found on malignant T cells in a number of lymphoma entities, including Hodgkin lymphoma. Therefore, there is a rationale to target CD25 with antibodies and antibody-based constructs, respectively. Efficacy and safety of a radioimmunoconjugate consisting of an anti-CD25 antibody (daclizumab) and radioactive yttrium-90 (daclizumab-90Y) were evaluated in a phase 2 trial including 30 heavily pretreated Hodgkin lymphoma patients (one to eight prior lines of treatment). The response rate was promising, with 19 achieving either partial (7 patients) or complete (12 patients) remission. Only six patients progressed. However, since the drug also exhibited relevant toxicity, with seven patients showing an insufficient platelet count recovery and three patients developing myelodysplastic syndromes, the future role for this treatment approach is unclear, despite its clearly proven antilymphoma activity.[263]

Other antibodies that have shown promising preclinical activity and are under evaluation in patients with relapsed Hodgkin lymphoma target antigens such as CD40 or the IL-13/IL-13 receptor. First interim results of these trials should be available soon.

Small Molecules

An increasing number of small molecules have become available in recent years. In the following, the immunomodulatory drug lenalidomide, the histone deacetylase inhibitor panobinostat and the mammalian target of rapamycin (mTOR) inhibitor everolimus will be described in a more detailed way as examples for this group of drugs.

The efficacy of the thalidomide-derivate lenalidomide as single agent in Hodgkin lymphoma patients relapsed after autologous stem cell transplant was independently reported by three groups so far. In an individual patient program conducted by the GHSG, 12 patients with a median of six prior therapies received lenalidomide at doses of 25 mg/d for 21 days of each 28-day cycle. Fifty percent of patients responded to treatment. Hematological and nonhematological side effects were mostly mild and manageable and did not prevent continuation of treatment at the initial dose level.[264]

An interim analysis of a phase 2 trial using the same treatment schedule reported the outcome of 15 patients with relapsed disease of whom 13 had not responded to their prior treatment. Thirty-three percent of evaluable patients achieved partial or complete remission and another 25% had stable disease lasting 6 months or longer. In this trial, treatment was also well tolerated so that lenalidomide appears to be active in a relevant portion of heavily pretreated patients without excessive or treatment-limiting toxicity.[265] Therefore, lenalidomide can also be considered as a possible part of combination therapies with other small molecules, antibodies, or conventional chemotherapy.

Histone deacetylases are a family of enzymes involved in diverse activities, including cell proliferation, survival, angiogenesis, and immunity. In recent years, several histone deacetylase inhibitors were developed for clinical use, including vorinostat, MGCD-0103, and panobinostat.

Panobinostat is an inhibitor of class I and II histone deacetylases. This drug was evaluated in a large phase 2 trial in Hodgkin lymphoma patients who had relapsed after autologous stem cell transplant. Patients received 40 mg three times weekly every week of a 21-day cycle. In an interim analysis of the trial, the disease control rate was 79% (complete remission rate plus partial remission rate plus stable disease rate). Adverse events were manageable, with the main side effect being reversible thrombocytopenia.[266] Currently, the role of panobinostat in maintenance treatment of patients after high-dose chemotherapy is being evaluated in a phase 3 trial.

The PI3K/Akt/mTOR pathway is aberrantly activated in many cancer entities. It was also shown to be dysregulated in HRS cells by several mechanisms including activation of CD30 and CD40 and is therefore considered a possible target pathway for novel treatment approaches. Safety and activity of the mTOR inhibitor everolimus were proven in a phase 2 study, including 19 patients who continuously received 10 mg of the drug. Forty-seven percent of patients responded to treatment with eight achieving partial remission and one achieving a complete remission. No excessive toxicity was observed.[267] Thus, the drug is currently undergoing further clinical studies.

Other signaling pathways dysregulated or aberrantly activated in HRS cells such as Notch or STAT-dependent signal transduction might serve as targets of novel treatment strategies. Drugs inhibiting or modulating these signaling pathways might become available in the near future and may complement the armamentarium for the treatment of relapsed Hodgkin lymphoma.

Selected References

The full list of references for this chapter appears in the online version.

2. Hodgkin T. On some morbid appearances of the absorbent glands and spleen. *Medica Chir Trans* 1832;1832:69.
10. Anagnostopoulos I, Hansmann ML, Franssila K, et al. European Task Force on Lymphoma project on lymphocyte predominance Hodgkin disease: histologic and immunohistologic analysis of submitted cases reveals 2 types of Hodgkin disease with a nodular growth pattern and abundant lymphocytes. *Blood* 2000;96:1889.
16. Hummel M, Anagnostopoulos I, Dallenbach F, et al. EBV infection patterns in Hodgkin's disease and normal lymphoid tissue: expression and cellular localization of EBV gene products. *Br J Haematol* 1992;82:689.
18. Diehl V, Kirchner HH, Burrichter H, et al. Characteristics of Hodgkin's disease-derived cell lines. *Cancer Treat Rep* 1982;66:615.
23. Schwab U, Stein H, Gerdes J, et al. Production of a monoclonal antibody specific for Hodgkin and Sternberg-Reed cells of Hodgkin's disease and a subset of normal lymphoid cells. *Nature* 1982;299:65.
24. Durkop H, Latza U, Hummel M, et al. Molecular cloning and expression of a new member of the nerve growth factor receptor family that is characteristic for Hodgkin's disease. *Cell* 1992;68:421.
25. Engert A, Martin G, Pfreundschuh M, et al. Antitumor effects of ricin A chain immunotoxins prepared from intact antibodies and Fab' fragments on solid human Hodgkin's disease tumors in mice. *Cancer Res* 1990;50:2929.
30. Nogova L, Reineke T, Eich HT, et al. Extended field radiotherapy, combined modality treatment or involved field radiotherapy for patients with stage IA lymphocyte-predominant Hodgkin's lymphoma: a retrospective analysis from the German Hodgkin Study Group (GHSG). *Ann Oncol* 2005;16:1683.
32. Skinnider BF, Mak TW. The role of cytokines in classical Hodgkin lymphoma. *Blood* 2002;99:4283.
35. Drexler HG. Recent results on the biology of Hodgkin and Reed-Sternberg cells. II. Continuous cell lines. *Leuk Lymphoma* 1993;9:1.
39. Kuppers R, Rajewsky K, Zhao M, et al. Hodgkin disease: Hodgkin and Reed-Sternberg cells picked from histological sections show clonal immunoglobulin gene rearrangements and appear to be derived from B cells at various stages of development. *Proc Natl Acad Sci U S A* 1994;91:10962.
43. Poppema S, Delsol G, Pileri SA, et al. Nodular lymphocyte predominant Hodgkin lymphoma. In: Swerdlow SH, Campo E, Harris NL, et al., eds. *WHO classification of tumours of haematopoietic and lymphoid systems*, 4th ed. Lyon: IARC, 2008:323.
50. Stein H, Delsol G, Pileri S, et al. Classical Hodgkin lymphoma: introduction. In: *WHO classification of tumours of haematopoietic and lymphoid systems*, 4th ed. Lyon: IARC, 2008:326.
55. Hutchings M, Loft A, Hansen M, et al. FDG-PET after two cycles of chemotherapy predicts treatment failure and progression-free survival in Hodgkin lymphoma. *Blood* 2006;107:52.
56. Ferme C, Mounier N, Casasnovas O, et al. Long-term results and competing risk analysis of the H89 trial in patients with advanced-stage Hodgkin lymphoma: a study by the Groupe d'Etude des Lymphomes de l'Adulte (GELA). *Blood* 2006;107:4636.
59. von Wasielewski R, Mengel M, Fischer R, et al. Classical Hodgkin's disease. Clinical impact of the immunophenotype. *Am J Pathol* 1997;151:1123.
62. DeVita VT Jr, Costa J. Toward a personalized treatment of Hodgkin's disease. *N Engl J Med* 2010;362:942.
66. Kuppers R, Sousa AB, Baur AS, et al. Common germinal-center B-cell origin of the malignant cells in two composite lymphomas, involving classical Hodgkin's disease and either follicular lymphoma or B-CLL. *Mol Med* 2001;7:285.
70. Savage KJ, Monti S, Kutok JL, et al. The molecular signature of mediastinal large B-cell lymphoma differs from that of other diffuse large B-cell lymphomas and shares features with classical Hodgkin lymphoma. *Blood* 2003;102:3871.
74. Peters MV. Prophylactic treatment of adjacent areas in Hodgkin's disease. *Cancer Res* 1966;26:1232.
77. Marcus KC, Kalish LA, Coleman CN, et al. Improved survival in patients with limited stage IIIA Hodgkin's disease treated with combined radiation therapy and chemotherapy. *J Clin Oncol* 1994;12:2567.
79. Mauch P, Goodman R, Hellman S. The significance of mediastinal involvement in early stage Hodgkin's disease. *Cancer* 1978;42:1039.
80. Hughes-Davies L, Tarbell NJ, Coleman CN, et al. Stage IA-IIB Hodgkin's disease: management and outcome of extensive thoracic involvement. *Int J Radiat Oncol Biol Phys* 1997;39:361.
84. Castellino RA, Dunnick NR, Goffinet DR, Rosenberg SR, Kaplan HS. Predictive value of lymphography for sites of subdiaphragmatic disease encountered at staging laparotomy in newly diagnosed Hodgkin's disease and non-Hodgkin's lymphoma. *J Clin Oncol* 1983;1:532.
89. Bhatia S, Robison LL, Oberlin O, et al. Breast cancer and other second neoplasms after childhood Hodgkin's disease. *N Engl J Med* 1996;334:745.
97. Reece DE, Connors JM, Spinelli JJ, et al. Intensive therapy with cyclophosphamide, carmustine, etoposide +/− cisplatin, and autologous bone marrow transplantation for Hodgkin's disease in first relapse after combination chemotherapy. *Blood* 1994;83:1193.
100. Proctor SJ, Mackie M, Dawson A, et al. A population-based study of intensive multi-agent chemotherapy with or without autotransplant for the highest risk Hodgkin's disease patients identified by the Scotland and Newcastle Lymphoma Group (SNLG) prognostic index. A Scotland and Newcastle Lymphoma Group study (SNLG HD III). *Eur J Cancer* 2002;38:795.
102. Loeffler M, Pfreundschuh M, Ruhl U, et al. Risk factor adapted treatment of Hodgkin's lymphoma: strategies and perspectives. *Recent Results Cancer Res* 1989;117:142.

106. Proctor SJ, Taylor P, Mackie MJ, et al. A numerical prognostic index for clinical use in identification of poor-risk patients with Hodgkin's disease at diagnosis. The Scotland and Newcastle Lymphoma Group (SNLG) Therapy Working Party. *Leuk Lymphoma* 1992;7(Suppl):17.
110. Engert A, Franklin J, Eich HT, et al. Two cycles of doxorubicin, bleomycin, vinblastine, and dacarbazine plus extended-field radiotherapy is superior to radiotherapy alone in early favorable Hodgkin's lymphoma: final results of the GHSG HD7 trial. *J Clin Oncol* 2007;25:3495.
111. Raemaekers J, Kluin-Nelemans H, Teodorovic I, et al. The achievements of the EORTC Lymphoma Group. European Organisation for Research and Treatment of Cancer. *Eur J Cancer* 2002;38(Suppl 4):S107.
113. Engert A, Diehl V, Pluetschow A, et al. Two cycles of ABVD followed by involved-field radiotherapy with 20 Gray (Gy) is the new standard of care in the treatment of patients with early-stage Hodgkin lymphoma: final analysis of the German Hodgkin Study Group (GHSG) HD10 study. ASH Annual Meeting Abstracts. *Blood* 2009;114: (abst 716).
114. Meyer RM, Gospodarowicz MK, Connors JM, et al. Randomized comparison of ABVD chemotherapy with a strategy that includes radiation therapy in patients with limited-stage Hodgkin's lymphoma: National Cancer Institute of Canada Clinical Trials Group and the Eastern Cooperative Oncology Group. *J Clin Oncol* 2005;23:4634.
115. Straus DJ, Portlock CS, Qin J, et al. Results of a prospective randomized clinical trial of doxorubicin, bleomycin, vinblastine, and dacarbazine (ABVD) followed by radiation therapy (RT) versus ABVD alone for stages I, II, and IIIA nonbulky Hodgkin disease. *Blood* 2004;104:3483.
116. Noordijk EM, Thomas J, Fermé C, et al. First results of the EORTC-GELA H9 randomized trials: the H9-F trial (comparing 3 radiation dose levels) and H9-U trial (comparing 3 chemotherapy schemes) in patients with favorable or unfavorable early-stage Hodgkin lymphoma (HL). *J Clin Oncol* 2005;23: (abst 6505).
117. Canellos GP, Abramson JS, Fisher DC, LaCasce AS. Treatment of favorable, limited-stage Hodgkin's lymphoma with chemotherapy without consolidation by radiation therapy. *J Clin Oncol* 2010;28:1611.
118. Gallamini A, Hutchings M, Rigacci L, et al. Early interim 2-[18F]fluoro-2-deoxy-D-glucose positron emission tomography is prognostically superior to international prognostic score in advanced-stage Hodgkin's lymphoma: a report from a joint Italian-Danish study. *J Clin Oncol* 2007;25:3746.
119. Kobe C, Dietlein M, Franklin J, et al. Positron emission tomography has a high negative predictive value for progression or early relapse for patients with residual disease after first-line chemotherapy in advanced-stage Hodgkin lymphoma. *Blood* 2008;112:3989.
120. Girinsky T, van der Maazen R, Specht L, et al. Involved-node radiotherapy (INRT) in patients with early Hodgkin lymphoma: concepts and guidelines. *Radiother Oncol* 2006;79:270.
121. Radford J, O'Doherty M, Barrington S, et al. Results of the 2nd planned interim analysis of the RAPID trial (involved-field radiotherapy vs no further treatment) with clinical stages 1A and 2A Hodgkin lymphoma and a negative FDG-PET scan after 3 cycles ABVD. ASH Annual Meeting Abstracts. *Blood* 2008;112: (abst 369).
123. Borchmann P, Engert A, Pluetschow A, et al. Dose-intensified combined-modality treatment with 2 courses of BEACOPP escalated followed by 2 cycles of ABVD and involved-field radiotherapy (IF-RT) is superior to 4 cycles ABVD plus IF-RT in patients with early unfavorable Hodgkin lymphoma (HL): an analysis of the German Hodgkin Study Group (GHSG) HD14 trial. ASH Annual Meeting Abstracts. *Blood* 2008;112: (abst 367).
124. Pavlovsky S, Maschio M, Santarelli MT, et al. Randomized trial of chemotherapy versus chemotherapy plus radiotherapy for stage I-II Hodgkin's disease. *J Natl Cancer Inst* 1988;80:1466.
125. Longo DL, Young RC, Wesley M, et al. Twenty years of MOPP therapy for Hodgkin's disease. *J Clin Oncol* 1986;4:1295.
127. Bonadonna G, Valagussa P, Santoro A. Alternating non-cross-resistant combination chemotherapy or MOPP in stage IV Hodgkin's disease. A report of 8-year results. *Ann Intern Med* 1986;104:739.
128. Duggan DB, Petroni GR, Johnson JL, et al. Randomized comparison of ABVD and MOPP/ABV hybrid for the treatment of advanced Hodgkin's disease: report of an intergroup trial. *J Clin Oncol* 2003;21:607.
130. Canellos GP, Anderson JR, Propert KJ, et al. Chemotherapy of advanced Hodgkin's disease with MOPP, ABVD, or MOPP alternating with ABVD. *N Engl J Med* 1992;327:1478.
131. Gobbi PG, Levis A, Chisesi T, et al. ABVD versus modified Stanford V versus MOPPEBVCAD with optional and limited radiotherapy in intermediate- and advanced-stage Hodgkin's lymphoma: final results of a multicenter randomized trial by the Intergruppo Italiano Linfomi. *J Clin Oncol* 2005;23:9198.
132. Johnson PW, Radford JA, Cullen MH, et al. Comparison of ABVD and alternating or hybrid multidrug regimens for the treatment of advanced Hodgkin's lymphoma: results of the United Kingdom Lymphoma Group LY09 Trial (ISRCTN97144519). *J Clin Oncol* 2005;23:9208.
133. Horning SJ, Hoppe RT, Breslin S, et al. Stanford V and radiotherapy for locally extensive and advanced Hodgkin's disease: mature results of a prospective clinical trial. *J Clin Oncol* 2002;20:630.
134. Hoskin PJ, Lowry L, Horwich A, et al. Randomized comparison of the Stanford V regimen and ABVD in the treatment of advanced Hodgkin's lymphoma: United Kingdom National Cancer Research Institute Lymphoma Group Study ISRCTN 64141244. *J Clin Oncol* 2009;27:5390.
135. Diehl V. Dose-escalation study for the treatment of Hodgkin's disease. The German Hodgkin Study Group (GHSG). *Ann Hematol* 1993;66:139.
137. Diehl V, Haverkamp H, Mueller RP, et al. Eight cycles of BEACOPP escalated compared with 4 cycles of BEACOPP escalated followed by 4 cycles of BEACOPP baseline with or without radiotherapy in patients in advanced stage Hodgkin lymphoma (HL): final analysis of the randomised HD12 trial of the German Hodgkin Study Group (GHSG). ASH Annual Meeting Abstracts. *Blood* 2008;26: (abst 1558).
138. Federico M, Luminari S, Iannitto E, et al. ABVD compared with BEACOPP compared with CEC for the initial treatment of patients with advanced Hodgkin's lymphoma: results from the HD2000 Gruppo Italiano per lo Studio dei Linfomi Trial. *J Clin Oncol* 2009;27:805.
139. Gianni AM, Rambaldi A, Zinzani PL, et al. Comparable 3-year outcome following ABVD or BEACOPP first-line chemotherapy, plus pre-planned high-dose salvage, in advanced Hodgkin lymphoma: a randomized trial of the Michelangelo, GITIL and IIL cooperative groups. *J Clin Oncol* 2008; 26: (abst 8506).
140. Russo F, Corazzelli G, Lastoria S, et al. Dose-dense (dd) ABVD and dose-dense/dose-intense (dd-di) ABVD in newly diagnosed patients (pts), intermediate- and advanced-stage with classical Hodgkin's lymphoma (cHL): final results. ASH Annual Meeting Abstracts. 2009;114: (abst 715).
141. Carde P, Koscielny S, Franklin J, et al. Early response to chemotherapy: a surrogate for final outcome of Hodgkin's disease patients that should influence initial treatment length and intensity? *Ann Oncol* 2002;13(Suppl 1):86.
144. Dann EJ, Bar-Shalom R, Tamir A, et al. Risk-adapted BEACOPP regimen can reduce the cumulative dose of chemotherapy for standard and high-risk Hodgkin lymphoma with no impairment of outcome. *Blood* 2007; 109:905.
145. Avigdor A, Bulvik S, Levi I, et al. Two cycles of escalated BEACOPP followed by four cycles of ABVD utilizing early-interim PET/CT scan is an effective regimen for advanced high-risk Hodgkin's lymphoma. *Ann Oncol* 2010;21:126.
146. Gallamini A, Rigacci L, Merli F, et al. The predictive value of positron emission tomography scanning performed after two courses of standard therapy on treatment outcome in advanced stage Hodgkin's disease. *Haematologica* 2006;91:475.
147. Gallamini A, Fiore F, Sorasio R, et al. Early chemotherapy intensification with BEACOPP in high-risk, interim-PET positive advanced-stage Hodgkin lymphoma, improves the overall treatment outcome of ABVD: a GITIL Multicenter Clinical Study. 2009 (abst 0502).
154. Sweetenham JW, Carella AM, Taghipour G, et al. High-dose therapy and autologous stem-cell transplantation for adult patients with Hodgkin's disease who do not enter remission after induction chemotherapy: results in 175 patients reported to the European Group for Blood and Marrow Transplantation. Lymphoma Working Party. *J Clin Oncol* 1999;17: 3101.
155. Lazarus HM, Rowlings PA, Zhang MJ, et al. Autotransplants for Hodgkin's disease in patients never achieving remission: a report from the Autologous Blood and Marrow Transplant Registry. *J Clin Oncol* 1999;17:534.
158. Josting A, Katay I, Rueffer U, et al. Favorable outcome of patients with relapsed or refractory Hodgkin's disease treated with high-dose chemotherapy and stem cell rescue at the time of maximal response to conventional salvage therapy (Dex-BEAM). *Ann Oncol* 1998;9:289.
161. Schmitz N, Pfistner B, Sextro M, et al. Aggressive conventional chemotherapy compared with high-dose chemotherapy with autologous haemopoietic stem-cell transplantation for relapsed chemosensitive Hodgkin's disease: a randomised trial. *Lancet* 2002;359:2065.
162. Gianni AM, Siena S, Bregni M, et al. High-dose sequential chemo-radiotherapy with peripheral blood progenitor cell support for relapsed or refractory Hodgkin's disease—a 6-year update. *Ann Oncol* 1993;4:889.
166. Santoro A, Magagnoli M, Spina M, et al. Ifosfamide, gemcitabine, and vinorelbine: a new induction regimen for refractory and relapsed Hodgkin's lymphoma. *Haematologica* 2007;92:35.
167. Sureda A, Robinson S, Canals C, et al. Reduced-intensity conditioning compared with conventional allogeneic stem-cell transplantation in relapsed or refractory Hodgkin's lymphoma: an analysis from the Lymphoma Working Party of the European Group for Blood and Marrow Transplantation. *J Clin Oncol* 2008;26:455.
168. Robinson SP, Sureda A, Canals C, et al. Reduced intensity conditioning allogeneic stem cell transplantation for Hodgkin's lymphoma: identification of prognostic factors predicting outcome. *Haematologica* 2009; 94:230.
169. Sureda A, Canals C, Arranz R, et al. Allogeneic stem cell transplantation after reduced intensity conditioning (RIC-allo) in patients with relapsed or refractory Hodgkin's lymphoma (HL). Final analysis of the HDR-Allo Protocol—a prospective clinical trial by the Grupo Español de Linfomas/Trasplante de Medula Osea (GEL/TAMO) and the Lymphoma Working Party (LWP) of the European Group for Blood and Marrow Transplantation (EBMT). ASH Annual Meeting Abstracts. *Blood* 2009;114:(abst 658).

171. Mueller H, Nogova L, Eichenauer DA, et al. The newly developed modified BEACOPP-regimen (BACOPP) is active and feasible in elderly patients with Hodgkin lymphoma: results of a phase II study of the German Hodgkin Study Group (GHSG). ASH Annual Meeting Abstracts. *Blood* 2008;112: (abst 2600).
176. U.S. National Cancer Center Network. http://www.nccn.org/professionals/physician_gls/f_guidelines.asp.
178. Rehwald U, Schulz H, Reiser M, et al. Treatment of relapsed CD20+ Hodgkin lymphoma with the monoclonal antibody rituximab is effective and well tolerated: results of a phase 2 trial of the German Hodgkin Lymphoma Study Group. *Blood* 2003;101:420.
180. Ekstrand BC, Lucas JB, Horwitz SM, et al. Rituximab in lymphocyte-predominant Hodgkin disease: results of a phase 2 trial. *Blood* 2003; 101:4285.
181. Henry-Amar M. Second cancer after the treatment for Hodgkin's disease: a report from the International Database on Hodgkin's Disease. *Ann Oncol* 1992;3(Suppl 4):117.
185. Enblad G, Glimelius B, Sundstrom C. Treatment outcome in Hodgkin's disease in patients above the age of 60: a population-based study. *Ann Oncol* 1991;2:297.
190. Santoro A, Bredenfeld H, Devizzi L, et al. Gemcitabine in the treatment of refractory Hodgkin's disease: results of a multicenter phase II study. *J Clin Oncol* 2000;18:2615.
191. Helsing MD. Trofosfamide as a salvage treatment with low toxicity in malignant lymphoma. A phase II study. *Eur J Cancer* 1997;33:500.
194. Sadural E, Smith LG Jr. Hematologic malignancies during pregnancy. *Clin Obstet Gynecol* 1995;38:535.
206. Hartmann P, Rehwald U, Salzberger B, et al. BEACOPP therapeutic regimen for patients with Hodgkin's disease and HIV infection. *Ann Oncol* 2003;14:1562.
207. Xicoy B, Ribera JM, Miralles P, et al. Results of treatment with doxorubicin, bleomycin, vinblastine and dacarbazine and highly active antiretroviral therapy in advanced stage, human immunodeficiency virus-related Hodgkin's lymphoma. *Haematologica* 2007;92:191.
208. Re A, Michieli M, Casari S, et al. High-dose therapy and autologous peripheral blood stem cell transplantation as salvage treatment for AIDS-related lymphoma: long-term results of the Italian Cooperative Group on AIDS and Tumors (GICAT) study with analysis of prognostic factors. *Blood* 2009;114:1306.
209. Spitzer TR, Ambinder RF, Lee JY, et al. Dose-reduced busulfan, cyclophosphamide, and autologous stem cell transplantation for human immunodeficiency virus-associated lymphoma: AIDS Malignancy Consortium Study 020. *Biol Blood Marrow Transplant* 2008;14:59.
213. Moser EC, Noordijk EM, van Leeuwen FE, et al. Long-term risk of cardiovascular disease after treatment for aggressive non-Hodgkin lymphoma. *Blood* 2006;107:2912.
216. Boivin JF, Hutchison GB, Lubin JH, Mauch P. Coronary artery disease mortality in patients treated for Hodgkin's disease. *Cancer* 1992;69:1241.
220. Sandoval C, Pui CH, Bowman LC, et al. Secondary acute myeloid leukemia in children previously treated with alkylating agents, intercalating topoisomerase II inhibitors, and irradiation. *J Clin Oncol* 1993;11:1039.
221. Valagussa P. Second neoplasms following treatment of Hodgkin's disease. *Curr Opin Oncol* 1993;5:805.
223. Behringer K, Josting A, Schiller P, et al. Solid tumors in patients treated for Hodgkin's disease: a report from the German Hodgkin Lymphoma Study Group. *Ann Oncol* 2004;15:1079.
224. van Leeuwen FE, Somers R, Taal BG, et al. Increased risk of lung cancer, non-Hodgkin's lymphoma, and leukemia following Hodgkin's disease. *J Clin Oncol* 1989;7:1046.
225. Hancock SL, Hoppe RT. Long-term complications of treatment and causes of mortality after Hodgkin's disease. *Semin Radiat Oncol* 1996;6:225.
228. Sieniawski M, Reineke T, Josting A, et al. Assessment of male fertility in patients with Hodgkin's lymphoma treated in the German Hodgkin Study Group (GHSG) clinical trials. *Ann Oncol* 2008;19:1795.
229. Huleihel M, Lunenfeld E, Levy A, Potashnik G, Glezerman M. Distinct expression levels of cytokines and soluble cytokine receptors in seminal plasma of fertile and infertile men. *Fertil Steril* 1996;66:135.
245. Franchi-Rezgui P, Rousselot P, Espie M, et al. Fertility in young women after chemotherapy with alkylating agents for Hodgkin and non-Hodgkin lymphomas. *Hematol J* 2003;4:116.
247. Bonadonna G. Modern treatment of malignant lymphomas: a multidisciplinary approach? The Kaplan Memorial Lecture. *Ann Oncol* 1994; (5 Suppl 2):5.
251. Horning SJ, Hoppe RT, Kaplan HS, Rosenberg SA. Female reproductive potential after treatment for Hodgkin's disease. *N Engl J Med* 1981; 304:1377.
256. Lie Fong S, Laven JS, Hakvoort-Cammel FG, et al. Assessment of ovarian reserve in adult childhood cancer survivors using anti-Mullerian hormone. *Hum Reprod* 2009;24:982.
261. Younes A, Zalevsky J, Blum KA, et al. Evaluation of pharmacokinetics, immunogenicity and safety of Xm2513Ab in the ongoing study Xm2513Ab-01: a phase I study of every other week XmAb2513 to evaluate the safety, tolerability and pharmacokinetics in patients with Hodgkin lymphoma or anaplastic large cell lymphoma. ASH Annual Meeting Abstracts. *Blood* 2007;112: (abst 5012).
263. O'Mahony D, Janik JE, Carrasquillo JA, et al. Yttrium-90 radiolabeled humanized monoclonal antibody to CD25 in refractory and relapsed Hodgkin's lymphoma. ASH Annual Meeting Abstracts. *Blood* 2008;112: (abst 231).
265. Fehniger TA, Larson S, Trinkaus K, et al. A phase II multicenter study of lenalidomide in relapsed or refractory classical Hodgkin lymphoma. ASH Annual Meeting Abstracts. *Blood* 2008;112: (abst 2595).

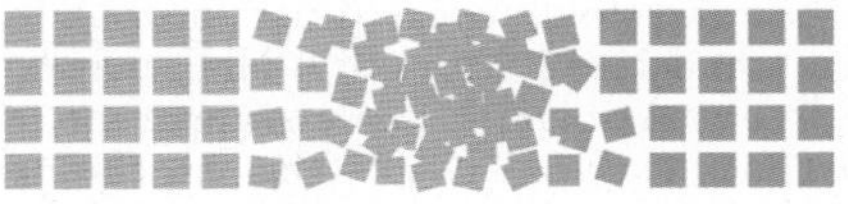

CHAPTER 127 NON-HODGKIN LYMPHOMAS

JONATHAN W. FRIEDBERG, PETER M. MAUCH, LISA RIMSZA, AND RICHARD I. FISHER

It has been known for more than 35 years that some patients with non-Hodgkin lymphoma (NHL) can be cured using chemotherapy. In the past decade, advances in molecular medicine have provided exciting insights into the biology of NHL. The viral and bacterial etiology of certain lymphomas has now been well established. Cell surface antigens have been defined that provide targets for therapy with monoclonal antibodies and radioimmunotherapy. Moreover, knowledge of critical cell signaling pathways and the results of gene expression analyses have revealed the importance of the malignant microenvironment in the neoplastic process and have provided opportunities for targeted therapy with novel small molecules. With these advances, improved survival has been observed in patients with both indolent and aggressive B-cell NHLs.

EPIDEMIOLOGY

The NHLs and Hodgkin lymphoma are the most commonly occurring hematologic malignancies in the United States. They now represent 4% to 5% of all new cancer cases and are the fifth leading cause of cancer death in the United States and the second fastest growing cancer in terms of mortality. International NHL incidence rates vary as much as fivefold. The highest reported incidence rates are in the United States, and also Europe and Australia; the lowest rates have generally been reported in Asia.[1] In 2007, it was estimated that there were 438,325 people alive with a history of NHL diagnosis; the incidence rate was 20.2 per 100,000 Americans that year.[2] Among children, lymphomas are the third most frequent malignancy, representing 15% of pediatric malignancies, with 1,700 new cases each year.

A striking increase in NHL incidence rates has occurred over the past four decades that has been referred to as an *epidemic of NHL*. The reasons for this are not entirely clear. Although there have been increases in most histologies, the largest increases have occurred in patients with aggressive lymphomas. This increase in primary central nervous system (CNS) lymphoma is in part related to the occurrence of primary CNS lymphomas in patients with acquired immunodeficiency syndrome (AIDS),[3] although the increase in incidence began before the AIDS epidemic, and incidence rates have increased in non-AIDS populations.[4] Geographic differences in histologic subtypes of NHL have been noted. Examples include the endemic form of Burkitt lymphoma, which is seen most commonly in children in equatorial Africa.[5] Higher rates of gastric lymphoma have been reported to occur in northern Italy.[6] Other examples include nasal T-cell lymphomas, which are most common in China; certain small intestinal lymphomas, which are most common in the Middle East; and adult T-cell leukemia/lymphoma (ATL), which is most common in southern Japan and the Caribbean. Several reports have shown a lower incidence of follicular lymphomas in Asia and in developing countries.[7] The incidence of follicular lymphomas is lower in Asian immigrants to the United States as compared with later generations, suggesting an environmental influence. Geographic differences in the distribution of mantle cell lymphoma, certain T-cell lymphomas, and the incidence of primary extranodal lymphomas have also been described.[7]

Even when factors such as accuracy and completeness of diagnosis, the effect of human immunodeficiency virus (HIV), and occupational exposures are considered, the reason for most of the increase in NHL incidence is unexplained.[8] Of note, over the past few years, the increased incidence has been less striking, but has continued at least through 2007.[2] Many investigators have postulated that a ubiquitous environmental or toxic exposure may be responsible.[9]

ETIOLOGY

The cause of most cases of NHL is unknown, although several genetic diseases, environmental agents, and infectious agents have been associated with the development of lymphoma. Although the existence of a familial NHL risk is debated, familial aggregations of NHL have been described, and some studies have shown a higher risk of NHL in siblings or first-degree relatives of people with lymphoma or other hematologic malignancies.[8]

Several rare inherited immunodeficiency states are associated with as much as a 25% risk of developing lymphoma.[10] These disorders include severe combined immunodeficiency, hypogammaglobulinemia, common variable immunodeficiency, Wiskott-Aldrich syndrome, and ataxia-telangiectasia. Lymphomas associated with these disorders are often associated with Epstein-Barr virus (EBV) and vary in appearance from initial polyclonal B-cell hyperplasia to monoclonal lymphomas.

In addition to these inherited immunodeficiency states, a number of acquired conditions are associated with an increased risk of NHL. The occurrence of NHL in patients with AIDS and after solid organ transplantation is discussed later in "Special Clinical Situations." Patients with a variety of autoimmune disorders, including rheumatoid arthritis,[11] psoriasis,[12] and Sjögren syndrome,[13] also have an increased risk of developing NHL. For example, the risk of developing NHL in association with Sjögren syndrome is increased approximately 30- to 40-fold; these are usually marginal zone lymphomas that most commonly occur in salivary glands and other extranodal sites such as the stomach and lung.[14] Celiac sprue is associated with poor-prognosis lymphomas that are now classified as enteropathy-type intestinal T-cell lymphomas.[15]

Infectious Agents

EBV DNA is associated with 95% of endemic Burkitt lymphomas and less commonly with sporadic Burkitt lymphoma.[16]

Because EBV is not seen in all cases of Burkitt lymphoma, the actual relationship and the mechanism by which EBV might contribute to the development of Burkitt lymphoma is unknown. It is hypothesized that early EBV infection and environmental factors may increase the numbers of EBV-infected precursors and the risk of genetic error; additionally, the EBV virus may contain tumor survival factors.[17]

EBV is also linked to posttransplant lymphoproliferative disorders (PTLDs), some AIDS-associated lymphomas, and some lymphomas associated with congenital immunodeficiency. Virtually all AIDS-associated primary CNS lymphomas have EBV in the tumor clone, although EBV is associated with other AIDS-associated lymphomas less frequently.[18] After EBV infection, normal host immune responses mediated by T lymphocytes suppress EBV-induced proliferation. In patients with depressed T-cell immunity, clones of EBV-transformed B cells can proliferate, leading to the development of lymphoma. The pattern of EBV-associated nuclear proteins in AIDS-associated Burkitt lymphomas differs from that of large cell lymphomas.[18] *MYC* activation in the absence of EBV infection can occur in AIDS-associated lymphomas.[19] The EBV latent membrane protein 1 is a viral analogue of the tumor necrosis factor receptor. The activity of this protein is similar to activated CD40 and is essential for *in vitro* transformation of B cells by EBV.[20] In EBV-positive AIDS-associated NHL and posttransplant lymphoproliferative disorder (PTLD), it appears that latent membrane protein 1 binds to members of the tumor necrosis factor receptor–associated factor family and activates the NFκB transcription factor, leading to cellular proliferation.[20] EBV is also seen in association with human herpesvirus-8 (HHV-8) in primary effusion lymphomas.

The human T-cell lymphotropic virus type 1 (HTLV-1) was the first human retrovirus associated with a malignancy. HTLV-1 is an RNA virus that is responsible for ATL in addition to HTLV-1–associated myelopathy/tropical spastic paraparesis and other disorders.[21] HTLV-1 is primarily transmitted by means of breastfeeding, sexual contact, and blood transfusion. The latent period between infection and development of ATL is several decades. HTLV-1 seropositivity and ATL are most prevalent in southern Japan, South America, Africa, and the Caribbean,[22] although ATL is sometimes seen in the United States.[23] In endemic areas more than 50% of all NHL cases are ATL, although the risk of developing disease is only approximately 5% in infected patients. The HTLV-1 genome contains the regulatory *tax* gene, whose product is a potent transcriptional activator of several genes and is thought to be responsible for the transforming features of HTLV-1.[24] The receptor-binding domains of HTLV-1 and -2 envelope glycoproteins and inhibit glucose transport by interacting with GLUT-1, the ubiquitous vertebrate glucose transporter.[25] Perturbations in glucose metabolism resulting from interactions of HTLV envelope glycoproteins with GLUT-1 and are likely to contribute to HTLV-associated disorders.

A third virus associated with NHL is HHV-8. This virus was originally discovered in Kaposi sarcoma lesions from AIDS patients and was called *Kaposi's sarcoma–associated herpesvirus*.[26] The virus is also associated with multicentric Castleman disease. An analysis of 193 lymphoma specimens from patients with and without AIDS identified the presence of virus in only eight specimens, all of which were from patients with primary effusion lymphomas.[27] The virus was subsequently shown to be a member of the gamma herpesvirus subfamily and was named *HHV-8*. Subsequent studies have demonstrated that primary effusion lymphomas are EBV associated, lack *MYC* gene rearrangements, and have distinct clinical and phenotypic features.[28] The mechanism of HHV-8 growth stimulation is unknown, although several potential mechanisms have been proposed.[29] It has been suggested that HHV-8 may be necessary for EBV-induced transformation in these patients.

Evidence also links hepatitis C virus (HCV) infection with NHL, especially in Italy. Infection with HCV is strongly associated with essential mixed cryoglobulinemia, which is itself associated with low-grade NHL. Several analyses have demonstrated significantly higher rates of HCV infection when patients with B-cell NHL were compared with controls. In Italy, there appears to be a threefold increased risk for B-NHL in HCV-infected patients, and 1 in 20 cases of B-NHL may be attributable to HCV.[30] This association is less apparent in countries with a lower incidence of HCV.[31] The association appears strongest for patients with monocytoid B-cell lymphoma and lymphoplasmacytoid lymphomas.[32] Neoplastic transformation is probably related to chronic antigen stimulation of B cells by HCV. HCV sequences have been detected in lymph node biopsy specimens from patients with B-cell NHL, and the presence of HCV-associated proteins within lymphoma cells has been demonstrated.

Finally, reports have suggested that simian virus 40 (SV40) may have a role in the development of NHL.[33] SV40, a monkey polyoma virus confirmed as a viable contaminant of the Salk polio vaccine, has demonstrated oncogenic potential in laboratory animals.[34] Although early epidemiologic studies demonstrated no apparent risk of cancer among cohorts likely to be exposed to SV40-contaminated vaccine, reports suggesting that the virus may be transmitted horizontally as well as vertically to nonimmune individuals were disconcerting. Although controversial, several investigations reported the presence of SV40 DNA in more than 40% of NHL tumor specimens examined.[35,36] Studies to further evaluate the role of SV40 in specific subtypes of NHL are ongoing.

Bacterial infections have also been associated with the development of lymphoma. Several lines of evidence link the bacteria *Helicobacter pylori* to gastric mucosa-associated lymphoid tissue (MALT) lymphomas. *H. pylori* can be found in the gastric mucosa of patients with gastric MALT lymphoma, and patients with gastric lymphoma are more likely than controls to have serologic evidence of past *H. pylori* infection.[37] It is hypothesized that development of gastric MALT lymphomas is a multistep process beginning with *H. pylori* colonization. This leads to chronic antigenic stimulation and gastritis and the subsequent development of malignant B-cell clones.[38] Stimulation by *H. pylori*–associated antigens appears to be strain-specific and T-cell mediated. *Campylobacter jejuni* has been found in specimens of patients with immunoproliferative small intestinal disorder (α chain disease).[39] In addition, a relationship between *Borrelia burgdorferi* and primary cutaneous B-cell lymphoma has been confirmed after demonstration of the organism in lesional skin of patients with this lymphoma, presumably implicating chronic antigen stimulation in the skin in response to *B. burgdorferi* infection.[40] Preliminary results suggest that patients with ocular adnexal lymphoma (marginal zone phenotype) display a high prevalence of *Chlamydia psittaci* infection, which is highly specific and does not reflect a subclinical infection widespread among the general population. Unlike the situation with *H. pylori*, sequencing analysis suggests that these lymphoma specimens have variable strains of *C. psittaci*, and similar to the situation with hepatitis C, the association is geographical, highly significant in parts of Europe, but absent in the United States.[40–42] Finally, *C. jejuni* has been found to be associated with alpha chain disease, an uncommon lymphoproliferative disorder.[39]

Environmental and Occupational Exposures

Studies of occupational and environmental NHL risk are frequently inconsistent and contradictory. Difficulties in estimating risk are often related to sample size and other methodologic difficulties in addition to difficulties in quantifying exposure. The risk of NHL is increased in several occupations, including farmers, forestry workers, and agricultural workers.[8] Several studies have shown an increased risk of NHL in relation to herbicide exposure, especially phenoxy herbicides such as 2,4-dichlorophenoxyacetic acid,[43–45] although this is controversial.[46] The development of NHL, particularly indolent types, has also been linked to hair dyes, especially darker and permanent colors used before 1980.[47,48]

Furthermore, NHL has been associated with organic solvents[49] and high levels of nitrates in drinking water.[50]

Diet and Other Exposures

Cohort and case-control studies suggest that the risk of NHL is increased approximately twofold in association with higher intake of meats and dietary fat.[8] Recreational drug use has been associated with increased NHL risk, and tobacco use has been associated with a higher risk in some studies, particularly of follicular lymphoma.[51] The risk of NHL may be increased more than 20-fold after treatment for Hodgkin lymphoma.[52,53] Studies examining the relative risk of combined modality treatment have been inconsistent, although the risk of NHL in association with ionizing radiation is minimal. Solar ultraviolet exposure has been associated with NHL in some studies.[54] Although some analyses have shown that the risk of NHL is increased after blood transfusion, other studies have failed to identify a significantly increased risk.[55] Recent experience has suggested an association between T-cell lymphoma and silicone breast implants.[56,57]

BIOLOGIC BACKGROUND FOR CLASSIFICATION OF LYMPHOID NEOPLASMS

Although the normal counterpart of the neoplastic cell is not known for all types of lymphoid neoplasms, it can be postulated for many of them. Understanding the normal counterpart of neoplastic cells can provide a useful framework for understanding the morphology, immunophenotype, and, to some extent, the clinical behavior of the neoplasms (Fig. 127.1).

Anatomy and Morphology of Normal Lymphoid Tissues

Lymphoid tissues can be divided into two major categories: (1) the central or primary lymphoid tissues, in which lymphoid precursor cells mature to a stage at which they are capable of performing their function in response to antigen, and (2) the peripheral or secondary lymphoid tissue, in which antigen-specific reactions occur.

Primary (Central) Lymphoid Tissues

Bone Marrow (Bursa Equivalent). Many of the early experiments that elucidated the basic biology of the lymphoid system used chickens and other avian species; an organ known as the *bursa of Fabricius* was the source of antibody-producing cells. Thus, these cells were termed *B cells*, for bursa-derived cells. In mammals, the bursa does not exist, and the precursors of antibody-producing cells come from the bone marrow.

Thymus. The thymus is the site at which immature T-cell precursors (prethymocytes), which migrate from the bone marrow, undergo maturation and selection to become mature, naive T cells, which are capable of responding to antigen. The thymus is divided into a cortex and a medulla, each of which is characterized by specialized epithelium and accessory cells, which provide the milieu for T-cell maturation.

Secondary (Peripheral) Lymphoid Tissues

Lymph Nodes. Lymph nodes are strategically placed at sites throughout the body to process antigens present in lymph fluid drained from tissues and organs via the afferent lymphatics. Lymph nodes have a capsule, a cortex, a medulla, and sinuses (subcapsular, cortical, and medullary). The sinuses contain macrophages, which take up antigens and process them into peptides, which are then presented to lymphocytes in the pocket of the major histocompatibility complex class II (class II) molecules. The cortex contains B-cell follicles and paracortical T-cell zones, and the medulla contains medullary cords and sinuses. The paracortex contains high endothelial venules, through which T and B lymphocytes enter the node, and specialized antigen-presenting cells (APCs), the interdigitating dendritic cells, related to the cutaneous Langerhans cell, which present antigen to T cells. The follicles also contain a specific type of accessory cells, follicular dendritic cells (FDCs), which bind antigen-antibody complexes and help regulate the differentiation of B cells in response to antigen. Recently recognized T cells known as follicular T-helper cells, located inside the germinal center, are important in regulating B-cell responses. Memory B cells, plasma cells, and effector T cells generated by immune reactions accumulate in the medullary cords and exit via the medullary sinuses.

Spleen. The spleen has two major compartments: the red pulp and the white pulp. The red pulp is a complex web of sinuses lined by phagocytic cells and functions as a filter for particulate antigens and formed elements of the blood. The white pulp is identical in its compartments to the lymphoid tissue of the lymph node. Follicles and germinal centers are found in the malpighian corpuscles, whereas T cells and interdigitating dendritic cells are found in the adjacent periarteriolar lymphoid sheath.

Mucosa-Associated Lymphoid Tissue. Specialized lymphoid tissue is found in association with certain epithelia, in particular the naso- and oropharynx (Waldeyer's ring: adenoids, tonsils), the gastrointestinal tract (gut-associated lymphoid tissue: Peyer's patches of the distal ileum, mucosal lymphoid aggregates in the colon and rectum), and lung (bronchus-associated lymphoid tissue). Collectively, this is known as MALT. These tissues tend to have prominent B-cell follicles with broad marginal zones but also may have discrete T-cell zones, similar to the paracortex of lymph nodes. MALT is thought to function in response to intraluminal antigens and the generation of mucosal immunity. MALT can also be acquired in other body sites that normally do not have any lymphoid tissue (e.g., stomach, thyroid, or conjunctiva) in response to chronic infection or inflammation.

B- AND T-CELL DIFFERENTIATION

T cells and B cells undergo two major phases of differentiation: antigen independent and antigen dependent. Antigen-independent differentiation occurs in the primary lymphoid organs without exposure to antigen and produces a pool of lymphocytes that are capable of responding to antigen (naive or virgin T and B cells). The early stages of lymphocyte development are called stem cells and lymphoblasts (also known as *precursor T* and *B cells*), which are self-renewing, whereas the later stages are differentiated cells with a finite lifespan ranging from weeks to years. On exposure to antigen, the naive lymphocyte undergoes "blast transformation" and becomes a large, proliferating cell, which gives rise to progeny that are capable of direct

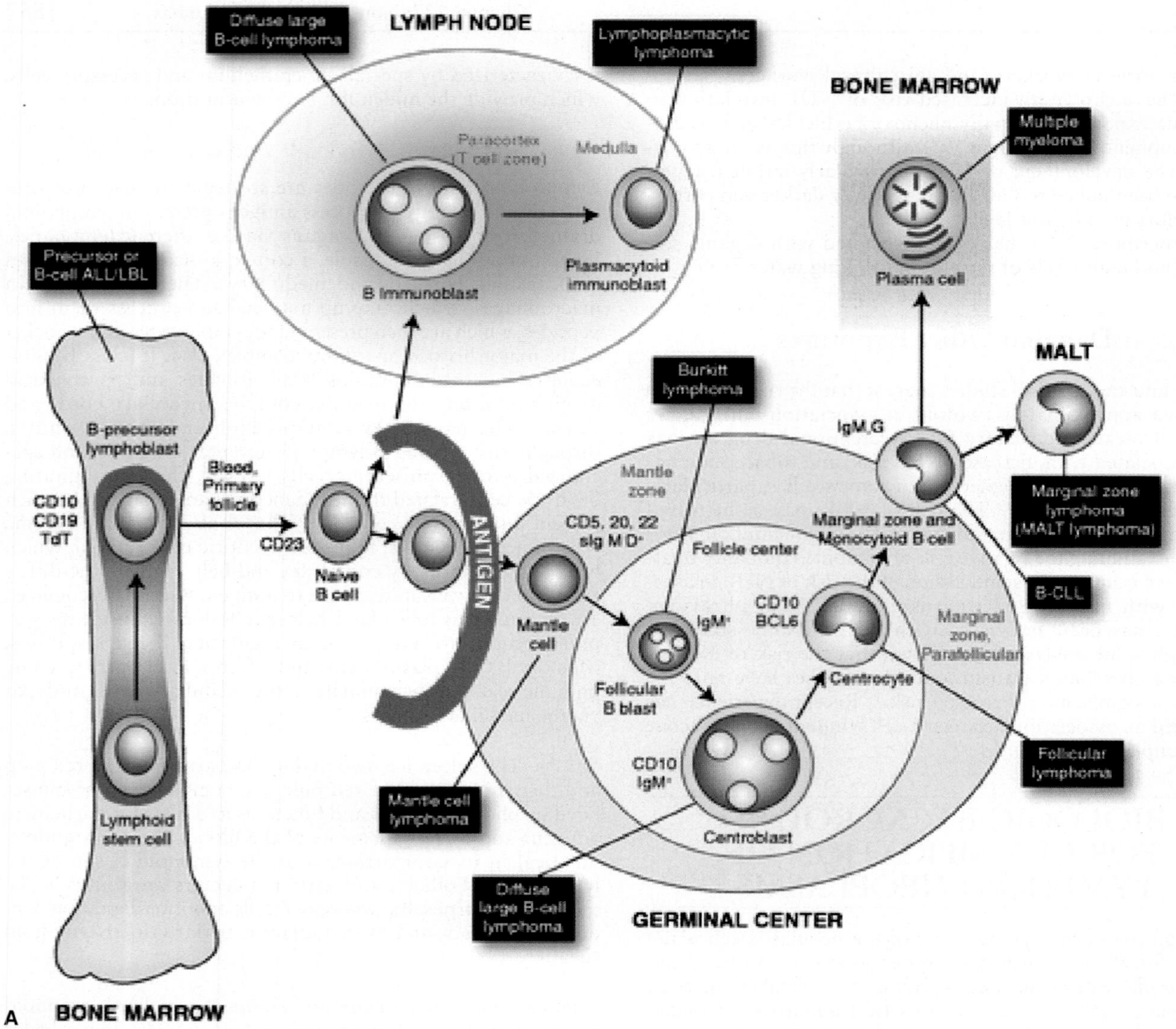

LYMPH NODE

Diffuse large B-cell lymphoma

Lymphoplasmacytic lymphoma

Paracortex (T cell zone)

Medulla

B Immunoblast

Plasmacytoid immunoblast

BONE MARROW

Multiple myeloma

Plasma cell

Precursor or B-cell ALL/LBL

MALT

Burkitt lymphoma

IgM,G

B-precursor lymphoblast

Blood, Primary follicle

CD10
CD19
TdT

CD23

Naive B cell

ANTIGEN

Mantle zone

CD5, 20, 22
sIg M D+

Mantle cell

Follicle center

Marginal zone and Monocytoid B cell

Marginal zone lymphoma (MALT lymphoma)

B-CLL

IgM+

CD10
BCL6

Marginal zone, Parafollicular

Follicular B blast

Centrocyte

Follicular lymphoma

CD10
IgM+

Centroblast

Lymphoid stem cell

Mantle cell lymphoma

Diffuse large B-cell lymphoma

GERMINAL CENTER

A BONE MARROW

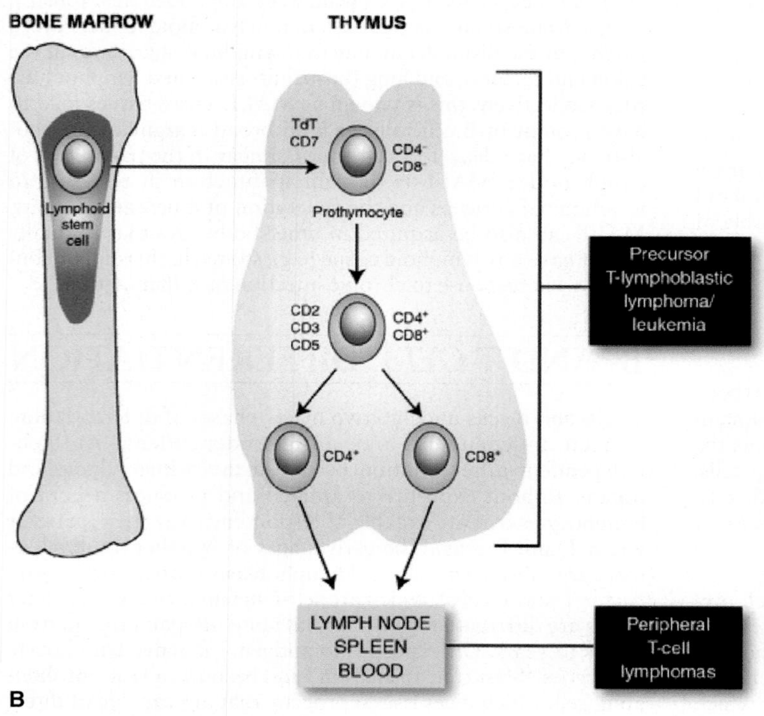

FIGURE 127.1 **A:** Pathway of B-cell differentiation and corresponding B-cell lymphomas. Following the precursor status, B cells mature into naive B lymphocytes. The germinal-center response represents an important turntable for immunoglobulin variable region gene mutations, immunoglobulin (Ig) heavy-chain switch, and differentiation into plasma cells and memory cells. Cluster designation (CD) markers are shown. B-immunoblasts and plasmacytoid immunoblasts reside in the T-cell–rich paracortex and medulla, respectively. Marginal zone B cells home to mucosa-associated lymphoid tissue (MALT) sites and bone marrow. Neoplastic transformation occurs at all phases of B-cell differentiation. ALL/LBL, acute lymphoblastic leukemia/ lymphoma; B-CLL, B-cell chronic lymphocytic leukemia. **B:** Pathways of T-cell development and corresponding lymphomas. TdT, terminal deoxynucleotidyl transferase.

activity against the inciting antigen: antigen-specific effector cells. The early stages of antigen-dependent differentiation are composed of proliferating cells, whereas the fully differentiated effector cells are less mitotically active. Thus, neoplasms that correspond to proliferating stages of either antigen-independent or antigen-dependent differentiation are likely to be aggressive, whereas those that correspond to naive or mature effector stages are likely to be indolent. Neoplasms corresponding to precursor cells tend to be more common in children (lymphoblastic leukemia/lymphoma), whereas those corresponding to mature effector or memory cells tend to be seen more often in adults (lymphoplasmacytic lymphoma, mycosis fungoides).

Antigen-Independent B-Cell Differentiation

Precursor B Cells

B-cell differentiation begins with rearrangements of the genes involved in immunoglobulin (Ig) production.[58] Precursor B cells have rearranged immunoglobulin heavy-chain genes but lack surface immunoglobulin (sIg). Later, they have cytoplasmic μ heavy chain, but no light chain, and still lack surface immunoglobulin. Both types of cells are lymphoblasts, with dispersed chromatin and small nucleoli. They contain the nuclear enzyme, terminal deoxynucleotidyl transferase (TdT), express CD34, a glycoprotein present on immature cells of lymphoid and myeloid lineage, major histocompatibility (MHC) class II antigens (such as HLA-DR), and the common acute lymphoblastic leukemia antigen (CD10).[59] Expression of MHC class II antigens persists throughout the life of the B cell, but is lost at the final plasma cell stage. Pan-B-cell antigens are sequentially expressed on precursor B cells: CD19, CD79a, cytoplasmic CD22 followed by surface CD22, and finally CD20 and surface immunoglobulin (both light and heavy chains). Many of the surface antigens are lost during terminal differentiation into plasma cells; however, high amounts of cytoplasmic immunoglobulin remain.

Fetal early B-cell development occurs in the liver, bone marrow, and spleen, whereas in adults it is restricted to the bone marrow. Benign precursor B cells can be found in normal and regenerating bone marrow, particularly in children, where they correspond to the lymphoid cells known as *hematogones*.[60] Neoplasms of precursor B cells usually involve bone marrow and peripheral blood and are known as *precursor B acute lymphoblastic leukemia*. Rarely, these neoplasms present as solid tumors (precursor B-cell lymphoblastic lymphoma).

Naive B Cells

The end stage of antigen-independent B-cell differentiation is the mature, naive, antigen unexposed B cell, which expresses surface IgM and IgD, lacks TdT and CD10, and is capable of responding to antigen. Naive B cells have rearranged, but unmutated, immunoglobulin genes.[61] In addition to surface immunoglobulin, naive B cells express pan-B-cell antigens (CD19, CD20, CD22, and CD79a), MHC class II molecules, complement receptors (CD21 and CD35), CD44, L-selectin, and CD23; a small subset expresses the pan-T-cell antigen, CD5, whereas most do not.[62] CD5-positive naive B cells have surface immunoglobulin that often has broad specificity (cross-reactive idiotypes) and reactivity with self-antigens (autoantibodies). Resting B cells also express Bcl-2, which promotes survival in the resting state.[63]

Naive B cells are small, resting lymphocytes. In adults, they circulate in the blood and comprise a minor fraction of the B cells in primary lymphoid follicles and follicle mantle zones (so-called recirculating B cells).[64] Studies of single cells picked from the mantle zones of reactive follicles show that they are clonally diverse and contain unmutated immunoglobulin genes, consistent with naive B cells. Two neoplasms may correspond in part to CD5-positive naive B cells: chronic lymphocytic leukemia/small lymphocytic lymphoma (40% of cases) and mantle cell lymphoma (80% of cases).[65]

Antigen-Dependent B-Cell Differentiation

Immunoblastic/Plasma Cell Reaction

On encountering antigen, the naive B cell transforms into a proliferating cell, which ultimately matures into an antibody-secreting plasma cell. In T-cell–independent reactions, and in the early primary immune response, naive B cells transform into IgM+ blast cells (B blasts or immunoblasts) in the T-cell zones, proliferate, and differentiate into IgM-secreting plasma cells, producing the IgM antibody of the primary immune response.[61] Surface IgD is lost during blast transformation, and antigens associated with activation are up-regulated. With maturation to plasma cells, most surface antigens are lost, including pan-B-cell antigens and secretory cytoplasmic IgM accumulates. The immunoblastic reaction occurs in the lymph node paracortex, and IgM-producing plasma cells accumulate in the medullary cords. Lymphoplasmacytic lymphoma, associated with Waldenström's macroglobulinemia, may correspond to the IgM-producing plasma cell. However, these tumors typically show low levels of variable region gene mutation and may thus derive from memory B cells. The activated B-cell subtype of diffuse large B-cell lymphoma may be derived from proliferating B cells of the paracortex that have not passed through the germinal center reaction.

Germinal Center Reaction

Later in the primary immune response (within 3 to 7 days of antigen challenge in experimental animals) and in secondary responses, the T-cell–dependent germinal center reaction occurs. Each germinal center is formed from between three and ten naive B cells and ultimately contains approximately 10,000 to 15,000 B cells.[66] Proliferating IgM-positive B blasts formed from naive B cells that have encountered antigen in the paracortex migrate into the center of the primary follicle and fill the FDC meshwork, forming a germinal center.[67] These B blasts differentiate into centroblasts, which appear at approximately 4 days and accumulate at one pole of the germinal center, forming the "dark zone." Centroblasts are large proliferating cells with vesicular nuclei, one to three peripherally located nucleoli, and a narrow rim of basophilic cytoplasm. They express no or low levels of surface immunoglobulin and also switch off the gene that encodes the bcl-2 protein. Thus, they and their progeny are susceptible to death through apoptosis.[63] Germinal center B cells express nuclear bcl-6 protein, a zinc finger transcription factor that is expressed by centroblasts and centrocytes but not by naive or memory B cells, mantle cells, or plasma cells, making bcl-6 protein specific for germinal center B cells, although it is also expressed by follicular T-helper cells as well.[68,69]

Centroblasts undergo somatic mutation of the immunoglobulin gene variable (V) region, which alters the affinity for antigen of the antibody that will be produced by the cell.[70] The *bcl-6* gene also undergoes somatic mutation of the 5′ noncoding promoter region, at a lower frequency than is seen in the immunoglobulin genes.[71,72] Thus, immunoglobulin gene mutation and *bcl-6* mutation serve as markers of cells that are experiencing or have experienced the germinal center environment.

Centroblasts mature to nonproliferating medium-sized cells with irregular nuclei, inconspicuous nucleoli, and scant cytoplasm, called *centrocytes* (cleaved follicular center cells), which accumulate in the opposite pole of the germinal center, known as the *light zone*, and which also contains a high concentration of FDCs. Centrocytes re-express surface immunoglobulin, which has an altered antibody-combining site, because of the somatic mutations in the variable region. This process results in marked diversity of antibody-combining sites in a population of cells derived from only a few precursors.

Centrocytes whose variable region gene mutations result in an inability to produce complete immunoglobulin molecules or those with *decreased* affinity for antigen, rapidly die by apoptosis. The prominent "starry sky" pattern of phagocytic macrophages seen in germinal centers is a result of the engulfment of apoptotic centrocytes. In contrast, centrocytes whose mutations have resulted in *increased* affinity are able to bind to antigen trapped in antigen-antibody complexes on the processes of the FDCs. The centrocytes present the antigen to T cells in the light zone of the germinal center. The activated T cells express CD40 ligand (CD40L), which engages CD40 on the B cell. Ligation of the antigen receptor by antigen and ligation of CD40 on the surface of germinal center B cells "rescues" the centrocytes from apoptosis.[67,73] Interaction with surface molecules expressed by FDCs, such as CD23, directs differentiation of the centrocytes into plasma cells and stimulates class switching from IgM to IgG or IgA production,[74] whereas interaction with T cells via CD40–CD40 ligand appears to be important in the generation of memory B cells.[66] In addition, antigen receptor ligation and CD40 ligation switch off BCL6 messenger RNA production and bcl-6 protein expression.[75] Through the mechanisms of immunoglobulin variable region mutation and class switching, the germinal center reaction gives rise to the better-fitting IgG or IgA antibody of the late primary or secondary immune response.[76]

Follicular lymphomas are tumors of germinal center B cells, in which centrocytes fail to undergo apoptosis because they have a chromosomal translocation, t(14;18)(q32;q21), that prevents the normal switching off of bcl-2.[63] A significant proportion of diffuse large B-cell lymphomas are composed of cells that at least in part resemble centroblasts and have mutated immunoglobulin V-region genes and are therefore thought to derive from the germinal center stage of differentiation.[77] Finally, it is thought that Burkitt lymphoma corresponds to the early surface IgM+ B blast found in the early germinal center reaction in experimental animals.[78]

Marginal Zone and Monocytoid (Parafollicular) B Cells

When the germinal center polarizes into a dark and a light zone, the mantle zone becomes better defined and eccentric, with the broader portion surrounding the light zone. Antigen-specific B cells generated in the germinal center reaction leave the follicle and reappear in the outer mantle zone to form a "marginal zone." The marginal zone is particularly prominent in mesenteric lymph nodes, Peyer's patches, and the spleen. Marginal zone B cells have slightly irregular nuclei and clear cytoplasm. Marginal zone B cells from spleen and Peyer's patches have mutated immunoglobulin variable region genes, consistent with post–germinal center cells.[79] When rechallenged with antigen, splenic marginal zone B cells rapidly give rise to antigen-specific plasma cells, consistent with their role as memory B cells. Memory B cells are also detectable in the peripheral blood, where they may be IgM+ and even CD5+.[80] Tumors of this population give rise to splenic marginal zone lymphomas.

Monocytoid B lymphocytes are cells that resemble marginal zone B cells but with more nuclear indentation and more abundant cytoplasm. These cells are found in clusters adjacent to subcapsular and cortical sinuses of some reactive lymph nodes. In contrast to marginal zone B cells, monocytoid B cells in reactive lymph nodes have either unmutated variable region genes or show only a small number of randomly distributed mutations that do not suggest selection by antigen in a germinal center reaction.[79] Tumors of this population give rise to nodal marginal zone lymphomas.

Plasma Cells

IgG- and IgA-producing plasma cells accumulate in the lymph node medulla to create the nodal plasma cell population. In addition, the immediate precursors of bone marrow plasma cells leave the node and migrate to the marrow. Bone marrow plasma cells lack surface immunoglobulin and pan-B-cell antigens and contain cytoplasmic IgG as well as expressing CD38 and CD138. The latter may be important in adhesion to bone marrow stroma. Plasma cells have decreased expression of many B-cell antigens and have turned off the germinal center transcription program through down-regulation of *BCL-6* and paired box gene 5 (*PAX5*) as well as activation of BLIMP1, which turns off CIITA and MHC class II expression. These changes in turn activate XBP1 and CD138 for final plasma cell differentiation. Plasma cells have rearranged and mutated immunoglobulin genes but do not have the ongoing mutations seen in follicle center cells. Tumors of plasma cells correspond to plasmacytoma, plasma cell myeloma, monoclonal immunoglobulin-deposition disease, and heavy chain diseases.

Mucosa-Associated Lymphoid Tissue

A subset of B cells, including all the differentiation stages previously listed in "Antigen-Dependent B-Cell Differentiation," is programmed for gut-associated rather than nodal lymphoid tissue. In these tissues (Waldeyer's ring, Peyer's patches, and mesenteric nodes), similar responses occur to antigen, but the intermediate and end-stage B cells that originate in the gut or mesenteric lymph nodes preferentially return there, rather than to lymph nodes at other sites or bone marrow. Thus, the plasma cells generated in gut-associated lymphoid tissue home preferentially to the lamina propria rather than to the bone marrow. MALT is characterized by reactive follicles with germinal centers and prominent marginal zones, as well as numerous plasma cells in the lamina propria. Marginal zone B cells in normal MALT typically infiltrate the overlying epithelium, forming a lymphoepithelium.

Many extranodal B-cell lymphomas are thought to arise from MALT in various locations, which have been termed *extranodal marginal zone lymphoma of MALT type*. MALT-type lymphomas have somatically mutated immunoglobulin genes, consistent with an antigen-selected post–germinal center B-cell stage.

Antigen-Independent T-Cell Differentiation

Cortical Thymocytes

The exact site at which precursor cells become committed to the T lineage is not known because the thymus contains cells that can differentiate into either T cells or natural killer (NK) cells, but not B cells. Cortical thymocytes are lymphoblasts which, like B lymphoblasts, contain the intranuclear enzyme TdT. Within the thymus these cells sequentially acquire CD1a, CD2, CD5, and cytoplasmic CD3 (cyCD3) and both the CD4 "helper" and the CD8 "suppressor" antigens (termed *double-positive cells*). T-cell antigen receptor gene rearrangement occurs during T-cell differentiation. This gene begins with the γ and δ chains, followed by the β and then the α chain genes, whose proteins are then expressed on the cell surface. Surface

CD3 expression appears at the same time as expression of the T-cell antigen receptor β chain, with which it is closely associated, and participates in signal transduction. Cortical thymocytes, like germinal center B cells, lack the antiapoptosis protein bcl-2[63] and are thus susceptible to apoptosis.

In addition to providing a pool of mature T cells through proliferation of precursor cells, the thymus is involved in the selection of T cells, so that the resulting mature T cells recognize self-MHC molecules (positive selection) and do not react to other self-antigens (negative selection). Thymocytes that have anti–self-specificity bind strongly via their T-cell receptor (TCR) complex to self-antigens presented by the MHC on thymic dendritic cells and die by apoptosis. Those that lack anti–self-reactivity but bind strongly to MHC molecules undergo positive selection on thymic epithelial cells; they then express increased levels of surface CD3, lose CD1 and either CD4 or CD8, and express bcl-2, to become mature, naive T cells.[81] The tumor that corresponds to the stages of T-cell differentiation in the thymic cortex is precursor T-lymphoblastic leukemia/lymphoma.

Naive T Cells

Mature, naive T cells are small lymphocytes with a low proliferation fraction that lack TdT and CD1 and express either (but not both) CD4 or CD8, as well as surface CD3, CD2, CD5, CD7, and bcl-2. These cells are found in the thymic medulla, in the circulation, and in the paracortex of lymph nodes. Some cases of T-cell prolymphocytic leukemia and peripheral T-cell lymphoma may correspond to naive T cells.

Antigen-Dependent T-Cell Differentiation

In contrast to B cells, which can recognize unprocessed antigen free in the tissues, T cells can only recognize antigen after it has been processed by phagocytes and presented on the surface of APCs in the "pocket" of the MHC molecule. On the T cell, the CD4 or CD8 molecules bind to MHC class II or class I molecules, respectively, on the APC. The T cell is then activated via CD40–CD40L and binding of CD28 and CTLA4 on the T cell to B7-1 and B7-2 (CD80/86) on the APC.[82]

T Immunoblasts

On encountering antigen, mature T cells transform into immunoblasts, which are large cells with prominent nucleoli and basophilic cytoplasm that are morphologically indistinguishable from B immunoblasts. T immunoblasts, in contrast to T lymphoblasts, are TdT- and CD1a-negative, strongly express pan-T-cell antigens, and continue to express either CD4 or CD8, not both. Antigen-dependent T-cell reactions occur in the paracortex of lymph nodes and the periarteriolar lymphoid sheath of the spleen, as well as at extranodal sites of immunologic reactions. Some mature T-cell lymphomas probably correspond to T immunoblasts.

Effector T Cells

Antigen-specific effector T cells of either CD4 or CD8 type, as well as memory T cells, evolve from the antigen-stimulated T-cell reaction. Effector T cells of the CD4 type typically act as helper cells while those of the CD8 type act as suppressor cells *in vitro*, but both types can be cytotoxic.[83] CD4 cells recognize antigen complexed with MHC class II antigens on antigen-presenting macrophages, dendritic cells, and B cells, whereas CD8 cells recognize MHC class I antigen on infected epithelial cells.[84] Cytotoxic T cells contain cytoplasmic granule-associated proteins that attack target cells (TIA-1, perforin, granzyme B) and that can be used to identify cytotoxic cells in tissue sections. CD4+ helper T cells produce cytokines that affect the function of B cells and APCs and modulate the immune response. Three major types have been described based on the different types of cytokines they produce: T helper 1 (Th1), T helper 2 (Th2), and T helper 17 (Th17). Th1 T cells produce interleukin-2 and interferon-gamma, which activate macrophages and cytotoxic T cells to kill infected cells. In contrast, Th2 cells produce interleukin-4, -5, -6, and -10, which help B cells to produce antibodies.[84] Th17 cells are characterized by elaboration of interleukin (IL)-17 and IL-22.[85] These cells play roles in host defense against bacterial pathogens and allergic and autoimmune diseases. T regulatory cells are another recently defined subset of CD4+ T cells, which dampen the immune response by suppressing helper T-cell function. Regulatory T cells play a role in self-tolerance, autoimmunity, and tumor immunity.[86] Follicular T cells, found within the germinal center, are CD4+. Through expression of CXCR5, they home B-cell follicles which contain high levels of CXCL13. In the germinal centers, follicular T cells stimulate B-cell isotype class switching and immunoglobulin production.[87]

In addition to differences in subset antigen (CD4 vs. CD8 or double-negative) expression, peripheral T cells may differ in their TCR expression ($\gamma\delta$ vs. $\alpha\beta$). It should be noted that although T cells begin with rearrangement of their $\gamma\delta$ genes, most go on to also rearrange their $\alpha\beta$ genes and so express the $\alpha\beta$ type of protein receptor. Thus, the majority of T cells in the circulation and in most lymphoid tissues are $\alpha\beta$+, while $\gamma\delta$+ T cells are more numerous in mucosa and in the spleen.

Some cases of peripheral T-cell lymphomas are thought to correspond to effector T cells. For example, mycosis fungoides corresponds to a mature, effector CD4+ cell, hepatosplenic T-cell lymphoma to $\gamma\delta$ T cells that reside in the spleen, T-cell large granular lymphocytic leukemia (LGL) to a mature effector CD8+ cell, adult T-cell leukemia lymphoma to regulatory T cells, and angioimmunoblastic T-cell lymphoma to follicular T cells. However, the relationship between neoplastic and normal T cells is not nearly as well understood as in the B-cell system. The prominent systemic symptoms, such as fever, skin rashes, and hemophagocytic syndromes associated with some peripheral T-cell lymphomas, may be a consequence of cytokine production by the neoplastic T cells.

Natural Killer Cells

A third line of lymphoid cells, called *NK cells* because they can kill certain targets without sensitization and without MHC restriction, appears to derive from a common progenitor with T cells. NK cells recognize self–class I MHC molecules on the surfaces of cells and kill cells that lack these antigens, such as virally infected and malignant cells. They also have Fc receptors and can kill antibody-coated targets. NK cell activity is influenced by inhibitory and activating membrane receptors on their surface interacting with MHC class I on host cells. These receptors include the c-type lectins and members of the immunoglobulin super family of receptors including killer immunoglobulinlike receptors. These receptors are extremely polymorphous and, together with their ligands, send positive and negative signals to the NK cell.[88]

Immature NK cells have cytoplasmic CD3, but these cells do not rearrange their TCR genes or express TCRs or surface CD3. They are characterized by certain NK cell–associated antigens (CD16, CD56, and CD57), which can also be expressed on some T cells, and express some T-cell–associated antigens as well (CD2, CD7, and CD8) while usually lacking CD5. NK cells appear in the peripheral blood as a small proportion of circulating lymphocytes; they are usually slightly larger than most normal T and B cells, with abundant pale cytoplasm containing azurophilic granules—the so-called LGLs. Extranodal NK/T-cell lymphoma, nasal type, aggressive

NK cell leukemia, and some types of LGL leukemias arise from NK cells.

IMMUNOPHENOTYPING OF LYMPHOID CELLS

Individual B and T lymphoid cells as well as accessory cells of the mononuclear phagocyte system can be recognized by the presence of surface or cytoplasmic molecules (antigens) that can be detected using labeled antibodies. A series of international workshops have developed a standardized nomenclature for many of the antigens detected by more than one monoclonal antibody (Table 127.1). Immunophenotyping with monoclonal antibodies can be done using viable cell suspensions and fluorescently labeled antibodies via flow cytometry on fresh blood, bone marrow, body fluids, or disaggregated tissues. Immunophenotyping is also extensively performed on

TABLE 127.1

CLUSTER DESIGNATIONS (CDS) OF ANTIGENS USEFUL IN THE CLASSIFICATION OF LYMPHOID NEOPLASMS

CD	Expression on Normal Cells	Useful Diagnostic Applications in These Neoplasms
1a	Cortical thymocytes (strong), Langerhans cells	Precursor T-lymphoblastic lymphoma/leukemia, Langerhans cell neoplasms
2	T cells, NK cells	T-cell and NK cell neoplasms
3	T cells (surface and cytoplasmic), NK cells (cytoplasmic epsilon chain only)	T-cell and NK cell neoplasms
4	T subset (MHC class II restricted), monocytes	Some T-cell neoplasms
5	T cells, naive B cells	T-cell neoplasms, CLL/SLL, mantle cell lymphoma
7	T cells, NK cells	T-cell and NK cell neoplasms
8	T subset (MHC class I restricted), NK subset, splenic sinus lining cells	Some T-cell and NK cell neoplasms
10	Precursor B cells, germinal center B cells, granulocytes, fibroblasts, kidney epithelium	Precursor B or T lymphoblastic lymphoma/leukemia, Burkitt lymphoma, follicular lymphoma, diffuse large B-cell lymphoma
11c	Monocytes, granulocytes, activated CD8+ T cells, NK cells, B cell subset	Hairy cell leukemia; CLL/SLL, splenic marginal zone lymphoma
15	Granulocytes, monocytes	Reed-Sternberg cells of classic HL
16	NK cells, granulocytes, macrophages	NK cell neoplasms, some T-cell neoplasms
19	B cells in all stages of maturation	B-cell neoplasms
20	Mature B cells (not plasma cells), T-cell subset	Mature B-cell neoplasms, some classic HL
21	Mature B-cell subset, FDCs	Mature B-cell neoplasms, groups of background FDCs in some lymphomas, FDC neoplasms
22	Nearly all stages of B cells (cytoplasm), B-cell subset (surface)	B-cell neoplasms, especially hairy cell leukemia
23	IgE Fc receptor: activated B cells, monocytes, FDCs	CLL/SLL, other B-cell lymphomas, groups of background FDCs in some lymphomas
25	IL-2 receptor: activated T cells, activated B cells, activated monocytes	Hairy cell leukemia, adult T-cell leukemia/lymphoma, other T-cell neoplasms
30	Activated T, B, and NK cells, monocytes	Reed-Sternberg cells in classic HL, ALCL, primary cutaneous CD30+ LPD
35	Follicular dendritic cells, myeloid cells, B cells, T cells, monocytes, erythroid cells, glomerular podocytes	Follicular dendritic cell sarcoma
38	Activated T and B cells, NK cells	Plasma cell neoplasms, B- and T-cell lymphoma
43	T cells, B subset, NK cells, monocytes, plasma cells, and myeloid cells	T-cell neoplasms, some B-cell neoplasms, myeloid neoplasms
45	Leukocyte common antigen, all leukocytes except plasma cells	Lymphoid and myeloid neoplasms
45RA	B cells, naive T cells, NK cells	B-cell neoplasms, T-cell neoplasms
45RO	T cells (most), granulocytes, monocytes	T-cell neoplasms
56	Neural cell adhesion molecule: NK cells, activated T cells	NK cell neoplasms, T-cell neoplasms, plasma cell neoplasms
57	T cell and NK cell subset, neural tissue	NK-like T-cell neoplasms, T-cell neoplasms, NK cell neoplasms,
68	Monocytes, macrophages, activated T cells	Myeloid and histiocytic neoplasms
79a	B cells, including precursor B and plasma cells	B-cell neoplasms, rare T-lymphoblastic neoplasms, rare classic HL
95	Fas (apoptosis receptor): activated T cells, B cells	Some B- and T-cell neoplasms, HL
99	Cortical thymocytes	Precursor B- and T-cell neoplasms, Ewing sarcoma
103	Mucosal intraepithelial lymphocytes	Hairy cell leukemia; enteropathy-type T-cell lymphoma
138	Syndecan-1 (stromal binding): plasma cells	Plasma cell neoplasms, plasmablastic lymphomas

NK, natural killer; MHC, major histocompatibility complex; CLL, chronic lymphocytic leukemia; SLL, small lymphocytic lymphoma; FDC, follicular dendritic cells; IgE, immunoglobulin E; IL-2, interleukin-2; ALCL, anaplastic large cell lymphoma; LPD, lymphoproliferative disorders; HL, Hodgkin lymphoma.

paraffin-embedded tissue sections using enzymatically tagged antibodies followed by a colorimetric reaction via immunohistochemistry. These techniques have become vital to diagnosis and residual disease monitoring in lymphoid neoplasms.

CHROMOSOMAL TRANSLOCATIONS AND ONCOGENE REARRANGEMENTS

Lymphoid neoplasms frequently have specific chromosomal translocations, which result in activation of oncogenes or inactivation of tumor suppressor genes (Table 127.2). Most translocations in lymphoid neoplasms place a gene that is normally silent in that cell type under the influence of a promoter associated with either an immunoglobulin or TCR, resulting in activation of the gene and giving the cell either a growth or survival advantage. Examples include the t(8;14)(q24;q32) in Burkitt lymphoma, which places the *MYC* gene under the immunoglobulin heavy-chain promoter[89]; the t(14;18)(q32;q32) of follicular lymphoma, which places the *BCL2* gene on chromosome 18 under the immunoglobulin promotor[90]; and the t(11;14)(q13;q32) in mantle cell lymphoma, which places the *CCND1* gene on chromosome 11 under the immunoglobulin promotor.[91]

In some lymphoid neoplasms, a translocation results in a fusion of two genes, resulting in an abnormal protein, which can be activated or inactivated as a consequence of the fusion. Examples include the t(2;5)(p23;q35) and its variants in anaplastic large cell lymphoma (ALCL), which result in activation of the ALK (anaplastic lymphoma kinase) tyrosine kinase[92]

TABLE 127.2

GENETIC ABNORMALITIES IN LYMPHOID NEOPLASMS

Genetic Abnormality	Genes	Lymphoid Neoplasms
TRANSLOCATIONS INVOLVING ACTIVATION OF ANOTHER GENE BY AN ANTIGEN RECEPTOR PROMOTER		
t(8;14)(q23;q32)	*MYC/IgH*	Burkitt lymphoma
t(2;8)(p12;q23)	*MYC/Igκ*	Burkitt lymphoma
t(8;22)(q23;q11)	*MYC/Igλ*	Burkitt lymphoma
t(11;14)(q13;32)	*BCL1(CCND1)/IgH*	Mantle cell lymphoma, plasma cell myeloma[a]
t(14;18)(q32;q21)	*BCL2/IgH*	Follicular lymphoma, diffuse large B-cell lymphoma
t(3;14)(q27;q32) and t(V;3q27)[b]	*BCL6/IgH, variable/BCL6*	Large B-cell lymphoma, follicular lymphoma
t(14;18)(q32;q21)	*MALT1/IgH*	MALT lymphoma (gastric, pulmonary)
t(3;14)(p14;q32)	*FOXP1/IgH*	MALT lymphoma (ocular adnexal, thyroid)
t(1;14)(p22;q32)	*BCL10/IgH*	MALT lymphoma (pulmonary)
t(9;14)(p13;q32)	*PAX5(BSAP)/IgH*	Lymphoplasmacytic lymphoma, plasma cell myeloma
inv(14)(q11;q32) or t(14;14)(q11;q32)	*TCRα/TCL1*	T-Prolymphocytic leukemia
t(X;14)(q28;q11)	*TCRα/MTCP1*	T-Prolymphocytic leukemia
TRANSLOCATIONS PRODUCING FUSION GENES/PROTEINS (ACTIVATION OR INACTIVATION)		
t(11;18)(q21;q21)	*API2/MLT*	MALT lymphoma
t(2;5)(p23;q35)	*NPM/ALK*	ALCL (70%–80%)
t(1;2)(q25;p23)	*TPM3/ALK*	ALCL (10%–20%)
t(2;3)(p23;q35)	*TFG/ALK*	ALCL (2%–5%)
inv(2)(p23;q35)	*ATIC/ALK*	ALCL (2%–5%)
t(2;17)(p23;17q11)	*CLTC/ALK*	ALCL (2%–5%)
CHROMOSOMAL ADDITIONS AND DELETIONS		
i(7q)(q10)	Unknown	Hepatosplenic T-cell lymphoma
+3	Unknown	MALT lymphoma, large B-cell lymphoma, lymphoepithelioid variant of PTCL-unspecified
+3, +5, + X	Unknown	Angioimmunoblastic T-cell lymphoma
6q21-q27	Unknown	B-cell lymphomas including CLL/SLL
7q21-32 deletion	*CDK6*	Splenic marginal zone lymphoma
9p gain	*REL*	Mediastinal large B-cell lymphoma
+8	Unknown	PTCL
11q23 deletion	*ATM*	T-PLL, CLL/SLL
+12	Unknown	CLL/SLL
13q14 deletion	Unknown	CLL/SLL, plasma cell myeloma
17p13 deletion	*TP53*	CLL/SLL, plasma cell myeloma

MALT, mucosa-associated lymphoid tissue; ALCL, anaplastic large cell lymphoma; PTCL, peripheral T-cell lymphoma; CLL, chronic lymphocytic leukemia; SLL, small lymphocytic lymphoma; PLL, prolymphocytic leukemia.
[a]In myeloma, translocation is into switch region of immunoglobulin H (IgH); in mantle cell, into joining region.
[b]Promoters other than IgH activate *BCL6*.
[c]May involve 7q34 (*TCRγ*) instead of 14q11.
[d]Deletions in the 5′ regulatory region of *TAL1* may also be seen.
[e]May involve *RBTN2* at 11p13.

and the t(11;18)(q21;q21) in MALT lymphoma, which produces an API2-MLT fusion protein.[93]

Using polymerase chain reaction (PCR), cells carrying a given translocation can be detected by using probes that span the breakpoint or using a reverse transcriptase technique (RT-PCR) to detect RNA produced by an altered or fused gene. PCR can be used to detect minimal residual disease in patients whose tumors carry a translocation.[94] Both numeric abnormalities of chromosomes and translocations can be detected by cytogenetics of cultured cells or fluorescence *in situ* hybridization on suspended nuclei, imprints, or tissue sections, using probes to specific chromosomes or segments.[95] Finally, many translocations result in abnormal protein expression, which can be detected by immunohistochemistry.[96]

USE OF IMMUNOPHENOTYPING AND GENETIC STUDIES IN THE DIAGNOSIS OF LYMPHOID NEOPLASMS

The lymphoid neoplasms each have a characteristic morphology, which is sometimes sufficient to permit diagnosis and classification if well-prepared, adequately sized sections are available. However, there are many pitfalls in the histologic diagnosis of malignant lymphoma, and since so many categories exist and are well defined using a variety of criteria, immunophenotyping, genetic, laboratory, and radiologic studies end up being extremely useful for resolving differential diagnostic problems. Immunophenotyping and genetic studies are also developing key roles in patient management beyond diagnosis including identification of prognostic molecules, detection of minimal residual disease, and assessment of appropriate molecules for targeted therapy. The major immunophenotypic and genetic features of the more common B- and T-cell neoplasms are listed in Tables 127.3 and 127.4.

PRINCIPLES OF THE WORLD HEALTH ORGANIZATION CLASSIFICATION OF LYMPHOID NEOPLASMS

In the World Health Organization (WHO) approach to classification, all available information—morphology, immunophenotype, genetic features, and clinical features—are used to define a disease entity. The relative importance of each of these features varies among diseases. Morphology is always important, and some diseases are primarily defined by morphology, with immunophenotype as backup in difficult cases. Some diseases have a virtually specific immunophenotype, such that one would hesitate to make the diagnosis in the absence of the immunophenotype. In a few lymphomas a specific genetic abnormality is an important defining criterion, whereas most lack specific genetic abnormalities. Still others require knowledge of clinical features as well, particularly nodal versus extranodal presentations. *Tumours of the Haematopoietic and Lymphoid Tissues* published in 2001 represented the first true international consensus on the classification of hematologic malignancies. This classification was further updated to the fourth edition published in 2008.[97]

Categories of Lymphoid Neoplasms

The WHO classification recognizes five major categories of lymphoid neoplasms based on a combination of cell lineage and stage of differentiation: precursor B- and T-cell neoplasms,

TABLE 127.3

IMMUNOHISTOLOGIC AND GENETIC FEATURES OF COMMON B-CELL NEOPLASMS

Neoplasm	sIg; CIg	CD5	CD10	CD23	CD103	Cyclin D1	Genetic Abnormality	Immunoglobulin Genes
B-CLL/SLL	Weak+; −/+	+	−	+	−	−	+12; del 13q14; del 17p13 del 11q22–23; del 6q21	R, U (50%); M (50%)
Lymphoplasmacytic lymphoma	+; +	−	−	−	−	−	t(9;14)(p13;q32)	R, M
Hairy cell leukemia	+;−	−	−	−	++	+/−	None known	R, M
Splenic marginal zone lymphoma	+; −/+	−	−	−	+	−	del 7q21–32	R, M
Follicular lymphoma	+; −	−	+	−	−	−	t(14;18)(q32;q21)	R, M
Mantle cell lymphoma	+; −	+	−	−	−	+	t(11;14)(q12;q32)	R, U
MALT lymphoma	+; +/−	−	−	−/+	−	−	+3; t(11;18)(q21;q21)	R, M
Diffuse large B-cell lymphoma	+/−; −/+	−	−/+	−/+	NA	−	t(14;18)(q32;q21); t(8;14)(q24;q32); translocations involving 3q27	R, M
Burkitt lymphoma	+; −	−	+	−	NA	−	t(8;14) (q24;q32); t(2;8) (q11;q24), t(8;22) (q24;q11)	R, M

sIg, surface immunoglobulin; CIg, cytoplasmic immunoglobulin; B-CLL/SLL, B-cell chronic lymphocytic leukemia/small lymphocytic lymphoma; R, rearranged; U, unmutated; M, mutated; MALT, mucosa-associated lymphoid tissue; NA, not available.

TABLE 127.4

IMMUNOHISTOLOGIC AND GENETIC FEATURES OF COMMON T-CELL NEOPLASMS

Neoplasm	CD3 S;C	CD5	CD7	CD4	CD8	CD30	TCR	CD16/56	Cytotoxic Granule[a]	EBV	Genetic Abnormality	T-Receptor Genes
T-PLL	+,+	–	+,+	+/–	–/+	–	αβ	–	–	–	inv 14(q11;q32); t(14;14)(q11;q32); trisomy 8q; t(8;8)(p11-12;q12); t(X;14)(q28;q11); del 11q23	R
T-LGL	+,+	–	+,+	–	+	–	αβ	+/– (CD57+)	+	–	None known	R
NK-LGL	–,+	–	+,–	–	+/–	–	–	+	+	+	None known	G
Extranodal NK/T-cell lymphoma	–,+	–	–/+	–	–	–	–	+	+	++	Del(6)(q21;q25)	G
Hepatosplenic T-cell lymphoma	+,+	–	+	–	–	–	γδ	+/–	+	–	Iso 7q	R
Enteropathy-type T-cell lymphoma	+,+	+	+	–	–/+	+/–	αβ>>γδ	–	+	–	HLA DQA1*0501, DQB1*0201 genotype associated with Celiac disease	R
Mycosis fungoides	+,+	+	–	+	–	–	αβ	–	–	–	None known	R
Primary Cutaneous CD30+ LPD	+,+	+/–	+/–	+/–	–	++	αβ	–	–/+	–	None known	R
Subcutaneous panniculitislike T-cell lymphoma	+,+	+	+	–	+	–/+	αβ	–	+	–	None known	R
PTCL-unspecified	+,+	+/–	+/–	+/–	–/+	–/+	αβ>γδ	–/+	–/+	–/+	Complex, +3	R
Angioimmunoblastic	+,+	+	+	+/–	–/+	–	αβ	–	–	–[b]	+3, +5, +X	R
Primary systemic ALCL	–/+	–/+	–/+	–/+	–/+	++	αβ	–/+	+	–	t(2;5)(p23;q35), t(1;2)(q25;p23), t(2;3)(p23;q35), inv(2)(p23;q35), t(2;17)(p23;q11)	R

TCR, T-cell receptor gene; EBV, Epstein-Barr virus; T-PLL, T-cell prolymphocytic leukemia; +, >90% positive; +/–, >50% positive; –/+, <50% positive; –, < 10% positive; R, rearranged; T-LGL, T-cell large granular lymphocytic leukemia; NK, natural killer; G, germ line; LPD, lymphoproliferative disorders; PTCL, peripheral T-cell lymphoma; ALCL, anaplastic large cell lymphoma.

[a]Cytotoxic granule = TIA-1, perforin, and/or granzyme.

[b]Although negative in the T cells, background B cells are often positive

mature B-cell neoplasms, mature T/NK-cell neoplasms, Hodgkin lymphoma, and immunodeficiency-associated lymphoproliferative disorders. Lymphomas and lymphoid leukemias are included because solid and circulating phases are present in many lymphoid neoplasms and distinction between them is artificial. Thus, chronic lymphocytic leukemia (CLL) and small lymphocytic lymphoma (SLL) are grouped together as different manifestations of the same neoplasm, as are lymphoblastic leukemia/lymphoma, and Burkitt lymphoma/leukemia. Although nearly all cases of Hodgkin lymphoma are of B-cell origin, their distinctive histologic and clinical features continue to warrant a separate category.

The 2008 WHO classification of lymphoid neoplasms includes 86 distinct entities plus additional variants (Table 127.5). The term *lymphoma* or *non-Hodgkin lymphoma*, even if categorized into B or T, low, intermediate, or high grade, can no longer be considered as a single disease or an adequate diagnosis. One of the corollaries of defining distinct lymphoma entities is that it is not helpful to sort lymphomas based on histologic grade to denote clinical aggressiveness, as was done in prior classification schemes. For example, although it is true that many lymphomas composed of relatively small cells with a low proliferation fraction generally have an indolent course, at least one entity, mantle cell lymphoma, is rather aggressive. Several lymphomas have within themselves a range of histologic grade (number of large cells or proliferation fraction) and clinical aggressiveness (e.g., follicular lymphoma). Thus, histologic grade is applied within a disease entity, not across

TABLE 127.5

WORLD HEALTH ORGANIZATION CLASSIFICATION OF LYMPHOID NEOPLASMS 2008

PRECURSOR B- AND T-CELL NEOPLASMS	**MATURE T-CELL AND NK CELL NEOPLASMS**
Precursor B-lymphoblastic leukemia/lymphoma	T-cell prolymphocytic leukemia
Precursor T-lymphoblastic leukemia/lymphoma	T-cell large granular lymphocytic leukemia
	Chronic lymphoproliferative disorder of NK cells
MATURE B-CELL NEOPLASMS[a]	Aggressive NK cell leukemia
Chronic lymphocytic leukemia/small lymphocytic lymphoma	EBV-positive T-cell lymphoproliferative diseases of childhood
B-cell prolymphocytic leukemia	Systemic EBV+ T-cell lymphoproliferative disease of childhood
Lymphoplasmacytic lymphoma/Waldenström macroglobulinemia	Hydroa vacciniforme-like lymphoma
Splenic marginal zone B-cell lymphoma	Adult T-cell leukemia/lymphoma
Hairy cell leukemia	Extranodal NK/T-cell lymphoma, nasal type
Splenic B-cell lymphoma/leukemia, unclassifiable	Enteropathy-type T-cell lymphoma
Splenic diffuse red pulp small B-cell lymphoma	Hepatosplenic T-cell lymphoma
Hairy cell leukemia-variant	Subcutaneous panniculitis-like T-cell lymphoma
Plasma cell neoplasms:	Mycosis fungoides
Monoclonal gammopathy of undetermined significance (MGUS)	Sézary syndrome
Plasma cell myeloma	Primary cutaneous CD30-positive T-cell lymphoproliferative disorders:
Solitary plasmacytoma of bone	Primary cutaneous anaplastic large cell lymphoma
Extraosseous plasmacytoma	Lymphomatoid papulosis
Monoclonal immunoglobulin deposition diseases	Primary cutaneous peripheral T-cell lymphomas, rare subtypes
Extranodal marginal zone B-cell lymphoma (MALT lymphoma)	Primary cutaneous gamma-delta T-cell lymphoma
Nodal marginal zone B-cell lymphoma	Primary cutaneous CD8-positive aggressive epidermotrophic cytotoxic T-cell lymphoma
Follicular lymphoma	Primary cutaneous CD4-positive small/medium T-cell lymphoma
Primary cutaneous follicle center lymphoma	Peripheral T-cell lymphoma, not otherwise specified
Mantle cell lymphoma	Angioimmunoblastic T-cell lymphoma
Diffuse large B-cell lymphoma (DLBCL)	Anaplastic large cell lymphoma, ALK-positive
T-cell/histiocyte-rich large B-cell lymphoma	Anaplastic large cell lymphoma, ALK-negative
Primary DLBCL of the central nervous system	
Primary cutaneous DLBCL, leg type	**IMMUNODEFICIENCY-ASSOCIATED LYMPHOPROLIFERATIVE DISORDERS**
EBV-positive DLBCL of the elderly	Lymphoproliferative diseases associated with primary immune disorders
DLBCL associated with chronic inflammation	Lymphomas associated with HIV infection
Lymphomatoid granulomatosis	Posttransplant lymphoproliferative disorders (PTLD)
Primary mediastinal (thymic) large B-cell lymphoma	Plasmacytic hyperplasia and infectious mononucleosis–like PTLD
Intravascular large B-cell lymphoma	Polymorphic PTLD
ALK-positive large B-cell lymphoma	Monomorphic PTLD
Plasmablastic lymphoma	Classic Hodgkin lymphoma type PTLD
Large B-cell lymphoma arising in HHV8-associated multicentric Castleman disease	Other iatrogenic immunodeficiency-associated lymphoproliferative disorders
Burkitt lymphoma/leukemia	
B-cell lymphoma, unclassifiable, with features intermediate between DLBCL and Burkitt lymphoma	
B-cell lymphoma, unclassifiable, with features intermediate between DLBCL and classic Hodgkin lymphoma	

MALT, mucosa-associated lymphoid tissue; ALK, anaplastic lymphoma kinase; HHV8, human herpesvirus-8; NK, natural killer; EBV, Epstein-Barr virus; HIV, human immunodeficiency virus.
[a]B- and T/NK-cell neoplasms are grouped according to major clinical presentations (predominantly disseminated/leukemic, primary extranodal, predominantly nodal).

the whole range of lymphoid neoplasms. In addition, each lymphoma has a distinctive set of presenting features and, often, different treatments. For example, hairy cell leukemia, CLL, and MALT lymphoma, although all indolent, are treated quite differently with different expectancies for survival. Therefore, in practice, treatment of a specific patient is determined not by which broad "prognostic group" the lymphoma falls into but by the specific histologic type of lymphoma, with the addition of grade within the tumor type, if applicable, and clinical features such as stage, age, performance status, and the International Prognostic Index (IPI).[98]

The current WHO classification lists the lymphoid neoplasms first according to differentiation stage (precursor or mature), then lineage (B or T/NK), then specific disease entities according to predominant clinical presentation. Three broad categories of clinical presentation are recognized: predominantly disseminated diseases that often involve bone marrow and may be leukemic, primary extranodal lymphomas, and predominantly nodal diseases that are often disseminated and may also involve extranodal sites.[97] This approach is intended for convenience and ease of learning only, by placing diseases that are likely to resemble one another clinically and histologically in proximity to one another in the list and text.

Impact of High Throughput mRNA, microRNA, DNA Methylation, Genomic, and Single Nucleotide Polymorphism Profiling on Lymphoma Classification

Gene expression profiling is a powerful technique that allows assessment of mRNA expression of thousands of genes simultaneously on a solid platform. One of the first publications using gene expression profiling examined a series of snap-frozen lymph node biopsies from different types of lymphomas and benign tissues. The results demonstrated marked differences in gene expression profiling pattern between lymphoma types as compared with each other and compared with benign tissues.[99] Of particular interest was the identification of at least two subtypes of diffuse large B-cell lymphoma, with different gene expression patterns (activated B-cell and germinal center B-cell subtypes) that also had prognostic significance in cases that were otherwise histologically indistinguishable.[100] Array comparative genomic hybridization, which assesses chromosomal amplifications, gains, and losses, further demonstrated different genomic profiles in these two subtypes of diffuse large B-cell lymphoma (DLBCL).[101] Additional investigation into microRNA expression patterns, DNA methylation patterns, and single nucleotide polymorphism patterns are proceeding rapidly. Details of these findings will be highlighted under particular disease subtypes in the following sections.

PRINCIPLES OF MANAGEMENT OF NON-HODGKIN LYMPHOMA

The phases of patient management include obtaining an adequate biopsy for an accurate diagnosis, a careful history and physical examination, appropriate laboratory studies, imaging studies, and possibly further biopsies to determine an accurate stage and to plan therapy. Finally, taking into account factors related to the patient, type of lymphoma, and stage and pace of disease, a treatment recommendation must be made.

History and Physical Examination

A careful history and physical examination are the basis for subsequent studies to determine the extent of the disease and a key factor in the therapeutic decision. The duration of symptoms and the pace of progression of the illness should be documented. The physician should not discount the possibility that waxing and waning lymphadenopathy could be related to the lymphoma. Especially in follicular lymphomas, spontaneous regressions are not infrequent. The presence of specific symptoms known to have an adverse prognosis in patients with some types of lymphoma should be ascertained. These include fevers, night sweats, and unexplained weight loss. Symptoms referable to a particular organ system, such as pain in the chest, abdomen, or bones, might lead to identification of specific sites of involvement. For example, symptoms of CNS lymphoma include headache, lethargy, focal neurologic symptoms, seizures, or paralysis.

History of a concurrent illness such as diabetes or congestive heart failure might modify therapeutic decisions. A careful physical examination can lead to important observations that will direct subsequent care. Obviously, examination of all lymph node–bearing areas and a search for hepatomegaly or splenomegaly are important. Pharyngeal involvement, a thyroid mass, evidence of pleural effusion, abdominal mass, testicular mass, or cutaneous lesions are all examples of findings that might direct further investigations and subsequent therapy.

Laboratory Evaluation

Laboratory studies should include complete blood count and screening chemistry studies to include renal and hepatic function studies, serum glucose, calcium, albumin, lactate dehydrogenase (LDH), and β_2-microglobulin level. Serum protein electrophoresis is frequently appropriate. The purpose of these studies is to aid in determining the prognosis (e.g., LDH, β_2-microglobulin, albumin) and identifying abnormalities in other organ systems that might complicate therapy (e.g., renal or hepatic dysfunction). As reactivation of hepatitis B has been associated with rituximab use, we recommend obtaining hepatitis B surface antigen and core antibody for any patient in whom rituximab therapy is anticipated.[102] Assessment of HIV risk factors and testing should be offered to all patients with a new diagnosis of NHL.

In addition to the diagnostic biopsy, almost all patients should have a bone marrow aspirate and biopsy performed. The chance of finding bone marrow involvement varies considerably among different subtypes of lymphoma. It is present in approximately 70% of patients with SLL, lymphoplasmacytoid lymphoma, and mantle cell lymphoma. Patients with follicular lymphoma have bone marrow involvement approximately 50% of the time, whereas it is seen in approximately 15% of patients with DLBCL.[103]

In certain situations, cytologic and flow cytometric[104] evaluation of the cerebrospinal fluid is indicated. Patients with paranasal sinus, testicular involvement, epidural lymphoma, and possibly bone marrow involvement with large cells are especially prone to meningeal spread and should have a diagnostic lumbar puncture. In addition, a lumbar puncture is often recommended for highly aggressive histologies and lymphoma in the setting of immunocompromise, including HIV infection.

Imaging Studies

Chest Radiography and Computed Tomography Scans

Chest radiography and computed tomography (CT) scans of the chest, abdomen, and pelvis should be performed at the initial evaluation in almost all patients with NHL. Although the chest radiograph is abnormal in fewer than 50% of patients, identification of hilar or mediastinal adenopathy, parenchymal lesions, or pleural effusions is important and provides an easy method for re-evaluation. CT scanning can identify nodal and extranodal sites of involvement and provides an important approach to monitoring the response to therapy. Involvement of intra-abdominal organs, such as kidney, ovary, spleen, and liver, can be identified on CT scans.

Magnetic Resonance Imaging

The value of magnetic resonance imaging (MRI) in the staging of NHL is limited. MRI is particularly useful in identifying bone and CNS involvement. MRI can suggest leptomeningeal involvement when gadolinium has been used. MRI can also identify bone marrow involvement[105]; however, it is not acceptable as a substitute for bone marrow biopsy.

Nuclear Medicine Studies

Nuclear scintigraphy may improve staging at the time of diagnosis, particularly through the detection of otherwise occult abdominal or splenic disease. Perhaps more important, nuclear scintigraphy may help to characterize a residual mass on anatomic imaging after therapy as either fibrosis or residual active lymphoma. Bone scans can sometimes be useful in patients who present with or develop back pain during the course of their lymphoma, looking for vertebral involvement and potential spinal cord compression.

Positron emission tomography (PET) is a functional imaging technique that can use a glucose analogue (2-fluoro-2-deoxy-D-glucose [FDG]) radiolabeled with the positron emitter fluorine 18 to evaluate glycolytic activity, which is increased in malignancies, including lymphoma.[94] PET provides several inherent advantages compared with other nuclear imaging techniques, and is now a standard part of the evaluation of patients with lymphoma.[106] The short half-life of FDG allows patient convenience and improved imaging characteristics. With modern dedicated PET/CT machines, a resolution of approximately 5 mm can be achieved.

The majority of studies evaluating FDG-PET in NHL include patients with diffuse large cell NHL. Limited data are available on the role of PET in other histologies. A retrospective review of 172 patients with various types of lymphoma who underwent FDG-PET imaging revealed that FDG-PET accurately detected disease in patients with DLBCL NHL, mantle cell lymphoma, and follicular lymphoma.[107] PET was less reliable at detecting marginal zone lymphoma, a finding that has been confirmed by other groups, particularly in the case of extranodal marginal zone lymphomas.[44] Every published study to date has suggested increased sensitivity of PET when compared with other imaging modalities, including gallium, when used for lymphoma staging.[43,108] PET may have particular utility in the evaluation of the spleen.

Persistently positive PET scans during and after chemotherapy have high sensitivity for predicting subsequent relapse of aggressive lymphoma.[45,109] Several studies have suggested that a negative PET scan is more informative than a positive result in the evaluation of a residual mass after therapy for lymphoma because of a high false-positive rate.[110,111] Even among experts, there is often disagreement over what constitutes a "positive" scan during and after therapy.[112] Therefore, persistently positive PET scans at the end of therapy, or in follow-up, warrant close follow-up or additional diagnostic procedures because some of these patients may remain in prolonged remission.

Staging and Prognostic Systems

The goal of the initial evaluation of a patient with lymphoma is to provide information that allows intelligent planning of therapy, imparting the prognosis to the patient, and making possible comparisons between patients in clinical trials. The studies to accomplish these goals can be aimed at identifying sites of involvement, characteristics of the patient (e.g., age, performance status), or characteristic of the lymphoma (e.g., serum LDH, serum β_2-microglobulin, growth fraction) that predict treatment outcome.

TABLE 127.6

ANN ARBOR STAGING SYSTEM

Stage	Description[a]
I	Involvement of a single lymph node region or a single extralymphatic organ or site (IE)
II	Involvement of two or more lymph node regions on the same side of the diaphragm (II) or localized involvement of an extralymphatic organ or site (IIE)
III	Involvement of lymph node regions on both sides of the diaphragm (III) or localized involvement of an extralymphatic organ or site (IIIE) or spleen (IIIS) or both (IIISE)
IV	Diffuse or disseminated involvement of one or more extralymphatic organs with or without associated lymph node involvement. Bone marrow and liver involvement are always stage IV

[a]Identification of the presence or absence of symptoms should be noted with each stage designation: A, asymptomatic; B, fever, sweats, weight loss greater than 10% of body weight.

The Ann Arbor Staging System was developed for patients with Hodgkin lymphoma. This system (Table 127.6)[113] identifies anatomic sites of involvement by lymphoma and assigns patients into four categories based on the extent of disease dissemination. Patients are also subcategorized by the presence of unexplained fevers, night sweats, or weight loss. This system has a significant effect on prognosis and is important in treatment planning.

At present, the most valuable and widely used clinical system to stratify patients with lymphoma is the IPI.[114] It was developed by investigators throughout the world for use in predicting outcome for patients with diffuse aggressive NHLs treated with an anthracycline-containing combination chemotherapy regimen. Five features were found to have approximately an equal and independent effect on survival. These include age greater than 60 years, serum LDH greater than upper limit of normal, performance status greater than 2, advanced-stage disease, and more than two extranodal sites. Because of the approximately equal effect on outcome, the number of abnormalities were simply summed to develop the prognostic index. Thus, patients might have a score of 0 to 5. This system was initially developed only for patients with diffuse aggressive lymphoma. However, it is clear that it applies to patients with almost all subtypes of NHL.[115]

The one area in which the IPI appears less useful is in the follicular lymphomas, where it fails to identify a significant subset of poor-prognosis patients. Other clinical predictive models for indolent lymphoma ("FL-IPI") and mantle cell ("M-IPI") lymphoma have been reported more recently.[116–118]

Restaging

After patients have completed the entire planned treatment regimen, re-evaluation should be done to determine the response to therapy. Achieving a complete remission to therapy is the most important single prognostic factor in patients with NHL. It is particularly true because salvage treatment such as high-dose therapy and autologous or allogeneic bone marrow transplantation can sometimes cure disease in patients who fail to respond to initial therapy.[119]

A restaging evaluation typically involves repeating all previous studies with abnormal results to document their current normal results. However, especially in sites of bulky disease, masses do not always completely regress. This does not necessarily mean that patients will have persisting lymphoma. Correlation with nuclear studies, and possibly rebiopsy under these circumstances, are required to determine whether or not persistent disease is present. An international workshop has established response criteria for use in clinical trials.[120]

SPECIFIC DISEASE ENTITIES

Precursor B- and T-Cell Neoplasms

Precursor B-Lymphoblastic Leukemia/Lymphoma

Precursor B-cell acute lymphoblastic leukemia/lymphomas are neoplasms of lymphoblasts committed to the B-cell lineage, typically composed of small to medium-sized blast cells with scant cytoplasm, moderately condensed to dispersed chromatin and indistinct nucleoli, involving bone marrow and blood (acute lymphoblastic leukemia), and occasionally presenting with primary involvement of nodal or extranodal sites (lymphoblastic lymphoma). This disease most commonly presents as an acute leukemia in children, is divided according to several different recurrent genetic abnormalities, and is described in detail in Chapter 100.

Precursor T-Lymphoblastic Leukemia/Lymphoma

Precursor T-lymphoblastic lymphoma/leukemias are neoplasms of lymphoblasts committed to the T-cell lineage, typically composed of small to medium-sized blast cells with scant cytoplasm, round to indented nuclei with moderately condensed to dispersed chromatin and indistinct nucleoli, variably involving bone marrow and blood (precursor T-cell acute lymphoblastic leukemia), thymus, or lymph nodes (precursor T-lymphoblastic lymphoma). Clinically, a case is defined as lymphoma if there is a mediastinal or other mass and fewer than 25% blasts in the bone marrow and as leukemia if there are more than 25% bone marrow blasts, with or without a mass. The morphology, immunophenotype and genetic features, and therapy are discussed in detail in Chapter 100.

Mature B-Cell Neoplasms

Chronic Lymphocytic Leukemia/Small Lymphocytic Lymphoma

CLL/SLL is a neoplasm of monomorphic, small, round B lymphocytes in the peripheral blood and lymph nodes usually expressing B-cell antigens (often of weak intensity) with coexpression of CD5 and CD23. A minor component of large cells is often admixed (prolymphocytes in the blood or paraimmunoblasts in the lymph nodes). This large cell component can sometimes lead to transformation to a more aggressive lymphoma. SLL is defined as a tissue infiltrate with the morphology and immunophenotype of CLL. Clinically there is lymphadenophathy, no cytopenias because of bone marrow infiltration by CLL/SLL, and less than 5×10^9/L peripheral blood B cells. The morphologic, immunophenotypic, and genetic features of CLL are described in detail in Chapter 106; SLL is handled in more detail here.

Postulated Normal Counterpart. Cases may carry either mutated or unmutated immunoglobulin variable region genes indicating two genetic subgroups, which correlate with better and worse prognosis, respectively. For cases with no little or no somatic mutation of the variable region immunoglobulin genes, CLL/SLL is thought to arise from recirculating, antigen-naive autoreactive B cells. For other cases in which somatic V region gene mutations are present, the cell of origin is thought to be an antigen-experienced, but germinal center-independent B cell.

Clinical Features. In the International Non-Hodgkin's Lymphoma Classification Project, 6.7% of 1,378 cases were diagnosed as B-cell CLL (B-CLL)/SLL. The median age of the patients was 65 years, and 83% had stage IV disease, 73% with bone marrow involvement. Generalized lymphadenopathy, hepatosplenomegaly, and extranodal infiltrates may occur. Sixty-four percent had an IPI score of 2/3. The 5-year overall actuarial survival was 51%, with a failure-free survival of 25%; for those patients with an IPI of 0/1, the overall actuarial survival was 76%, whereas for those with an IPI of 4/5 it was only 38%. Thus, the extent of the disease at the time of the diagnosis is the best predictor of survival; however, chromosomal abnormalities, immunophenotype, and somatic mutation status clearly have prognostic importance, as detailed in Chapter 106.[121,122]

Patients with SLL can present with hypogammaglobulinemia or develop it over the course of the illness. The presence of hypogammaglobulinemia is associated with an increased incidence of infections and can be managed in some patients with intermittent gammaglobulin injections. Polyclonal or monoclonal hypergammaglobulinemia can also be seen. Autoimmune hemolytic anemias can be seen in patients with SLL and are particularly likely to develop in patients treated with fludarabine.[123] Autoimmune thrombocytopenia is not rare. Autoimmune neutropenia and pure red cell aplasia are unusual.

Therapy. Localized SLL is unusual and was seen in only 4% of patients in a large series.[115] The rare patient who presents in this manner could be treated with local radiotherapy. Low to intermediate doses of radiation therapy can be effective in relieving symptoms in patients with SLL/CLL who have a localized problem and who do not require immediate systemic therapy. Radiation therapy can also be effective in relieving chylous effusions of the thorax in patients with SLL/CLL or other low-grade lymphomas (we usually use 15 Gy total dose to the thorax given in 10 fractions). Such patients should have their slides reviewed to make certain they do not have a MALT lymphoma.

Some patients with disseminated SLL/CLL have a slowly progressive or stable disorder that does not require therapy. The majority of patients with documented SLL should be approached as detailed in Chapter 106.

Lymphoplasmacytic Lymphoma (With or Without Waldenström's Macroglobulinemia)

Lymphoplasmacytic lymphoma is a neoplasm of small B lymphocytes, plasmacytoid lymphocytes, and plasma cells involving bone marrow, lymph nodes, and spleen, usually lacking CD5, often with a serum monoclonal protein with hyperviscosity or cryoglobulinemia. Plasmacytoid variants of other neoplasms are excluded.

Morphology

The tumor contains small lymphocytes, plasmacytoid lymphocytes, and plasma cells, with variable numbers of immunoblasts. Cells may contain intranuclear inclusions of immunoglobulin (Dutcher bodies). By definition, features of other lymphomas,

PRACTICE OF ONCOLOGY

particularly marginal zone lymphomas and SLL, that may have plasmacytoid differentiation are absent. The bone marrow infiltrate may be either diffuse or nodular and is often interstitial and rather subtle. Peripheral blood involvement is less prominent than in CLL, and the cells often have a plasmacytoid appearance.

Immunophenotype and Genetic Features

The cells have surface and cytoplasmic (some cells) immunoglobulin, usually of IgM type; usually lack IgD; and strongly express B-cell–associated antigens (CD19, CD20, CD22, CD79a). The cells are CD5–, CD10–, CD23–; CD25 or CD11c may be faintly positive in some cases. Recently, weak expression of CD5 in a minority of cases has been reported using flow cytometry. However, in general, lack of CD5 and CD23, strong surface immunoglobulin and CD20, and the presence of cytoplasmic immunoglobulin are useful in distinction from B-CLL.[124]

Immunoglobulin heavy- and light-chain genes are rearranged, and variable region genes show a small load of somatic mutations, suggesting that these cells arise from a population of B cells that have been exposed to antigen.[125] Translocation t(9;14)(p13;q32) and rearrangement of the *PAX-5* gene are reported in some cases.[126] *PAX-5* encodes a protein, B-cell–specific activator protein, which is important in early B-cell development. Expression of B-cell–specific activator protein is restricted to B cells and is independent of the translocation; however, it is usually absent in plasma cells lacking the translocation.[127]

Postulated Normal Counterpart

The postulated normal counterpart is a postfollicular B cell that differentiates into plasma cells, which has undergone somatic mutation but not heavy-chain class switch.

Clinical Features and Therapy

Lymphoplasmacytic lymphoma made up only 1.2% (16 of 1,378) of the cases in the REAL clinical study.[115] Similar to B-CLL/SLL, the median age of the patients was 63 years; 53% were men; most (73%) had bone marrow involvement. Sixty-nine percent had an IPI of 2/3. Lymph node and splenic involvement are common. A monoclonal serum paraprotein of IgM type, with or without hyperviscosity syndrome (Waldenström's macroglobulinemia), is present in most patients[128]; as with B-CLL, the paraprotein may have autoantibody or cryoglobulin activity.

Most cases of mixed cryoglobulinemia have been shown to be related to HCV infection, even in patients who have demonstrable B-cell lymphoma in the bone marrow.[129] Treatment of patients with HCV and cryoglobulinemia with interferon to reduce viral load has been associated with regression of the lymphoma.[130]

The clinical course of LPL is indolent; in some European series it has been reported to be more aggressive than typical B-CLL,[131] but in the REAL clinical study, 5-year overall actuarial survival (58%) and failure-free survival (25%) were identical to that of CLL/SLL.[115] The traditional therapy for this disorder has been chlorambucil with or without prednisone.[128] Anthracycline-based combination chemotherapy has not been shown to be more effective. However, purine analogues are frequently used as initial therapy for this disorder.[132,133]

The response rate of lymphoplasmacytic lymphoma to rituximab is lower than that of follicular lymphoma, and has the risk of an IgM flare phenomenon[134]; however, combinations of chemotherapy and rituximab are frequently used as both initial therapy and for relapsed disease.[135]

Novel therapeutic agents have demonstrated clinical activity in patients with lymphoplasmacytic lymphoma. These include inhibitors of the mTOR pathway, immunomodulatory agent derivatives, and bortezomib, a proteosome inhibitor.[136–138]

In patients who require therapy, the authors suggest a purine analogue–containing regimen with rituximab as initial therapy for most patients. Young patients with refractory disease should be considered for high-dose therapy with autologous or allogeneic stem cell support.

Extranodal Marginal Zone B-Cell Lymphoma (Low-Grade B-Cell Lymphoma of MALT)

Extranodal marginal zone B-cell lymphoma of MALT is an extranodal lymphoma consisting of heterogeneous small B cells, including marginal zone (centrocytelike) cells, monocytoid cells, and small lymphocytes in varying proportions, and scattered immunoblastlike and centroblastlike cells, with plasma cell differentiation in 40% of the cases. The infiltrate is in the marginal zone of reactive B-cell follicles and extends into the interfollicular region and associated epithelial or mucosal structures.

Morphology

MALT lymphoma reproduces the morphologic features of normal or acquired benign MALT tissue including a polymorphous infiltrate of small lymphocytes, marginal zone (centrocytelike) B cells, monocytoid B cells, and plasma cells, as well as rare centroblastlike or immunoblastlike cells. Reactive follicles are usually present, with the neoplastic cells occupying the marginal zone or the interfollicular region, or both. Occasional follicles may be "colonized" by marginal zone or monocytoid cells. In epithelial tissues, neoplastic cells typically infiltrate the epithelium, forming so-called lymphoepithelial lesions (Fig. 127.2). In the stomach, associated *H. pylori* organisms may be identified. Large B cells with the appearance of centroblasts or immunoblasts are typically present but by definition constitute a minority of cells. In the case of confluent solid sheets of large B cells, a separate diagnosis of DLBCL should be made.

Immunophenotype and Genetic Features

The tumor cells of MALT lymphoma express surface immunoglobulin, usually IgM but occasionally IgG or IgA, and lack

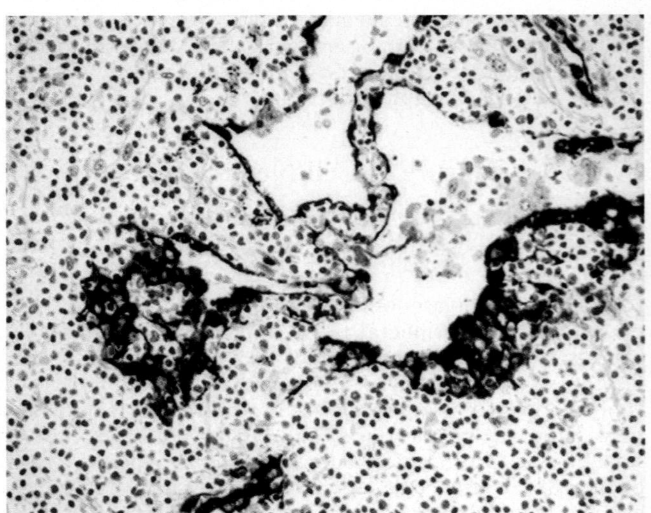

FIGURE 127.2 Mucosa-associated lymphoid tissue (MALT) lymphoma. Pan-keratin immunostain: The brown-stained epithelial cell structures are invaded by the unstained lymphoid cells to form a lymphoepithelial lesion.

IgD, and 40% have monotypic cytoplasmic immunoglobulin, indicating plasmacytoid differentiation. They express B-cell–associated antigens (CD19, CD20, CD22, CD79a) and are usually negative for CD5 and CD10. Immunophenotyping studies are useful in confirming malignancy (light-chain restriction) and in excluding SLL or mantle cell (CD5+), and follicle center (CD10+, BCL6+, usually cytoplasmic immunoglobulin-negative) lymphomas.

Immunoglobulin genes are rearranged, and the variable region has a high degree of somatic mutation, as well as intraclonal diversity consistent with a post–germinal center, memory B cell.[139] Trisomy 3 (60%) and t(11;18)(q21;q21) (25% to 40%) are the most common reported cytogenetic abnormalities.[140] Translocation t(14;18)(q32;q21) involving the immunoglobulin heavy-chain locus and the *MLT1* gene may occur, more often in nongastric locations than in gastric MALT lymphoma.[141] The t(3;14)(p14;q32) places the *FOXP1* gene adjacent to the immunoglobulin heavy-chain promoter leading to overexpression of *FOXP1*. This translocation has been described in MALT lymphomas in the ocular adenexae and thyroid.

Analysis of the t(11;18)(q21;q21) breakpoint has shown fusion of the apoptosis-inhibitor gene *API2* to a novel gene at 18q21, named *MLT*, in cases of MALT lymphoma.[142] A gene involved in a breakpoint in MALT lymphomas with t(1;14)(p22;q21) has been cloned—*BCL10*, which is an apoptosis-promoting gene that in mutated form may cause cellular transformation.[143] Abnormalities in *MALT1* and *BCL10* both appear to be involved in oncogenesis by targeting the NFκB pathway.[144]

The t(11;18)(q21;q21) is found with varying frequency in MALT lymphomas from various sites: 25% to 40% of gastric cases, 40% to 60% of pulmonary cases, and seldom in thyroid, skin, orbital, and cutaneous cases.[145] Patients with gastric MALT lymphoma harboring t(11;18)(q21;q21) do not respond to *H. pylori* eradication and are less likely to transform into DLBCL. Tumors with t(11;18)(q21;q21) tend to have this as their only cytogenetic abnormality, whereas those with trisomy 3 often have complex karyotypes. Therefore, t(11;18)(q21;q21) and trisomy 3 appear to be mutually exclusive,[146] indicating there are likely two pathways of lymphomagenesis in MALT lymphomas: one involving prolonged dependence on *H. pylori* infection, with acquisition of multiple cytogenetic abnormalities and risk of progression to DLBCL, and another involving early t(11;18)(q21;q21), which confers independence from *H. pylori* and has a low risk of other cytogenetic abnormalities or progression.

Postulated Normal Counterpart

The postulated normal counterpart is a post–germinal center memory B cell with capacity to differentiate into marginal zone B cells, monocytoid B cells, and plasma cells.

Clinical Features

Extranodal marginal zone B-cell (MALT) lymphoma accounts for the majority of low-grade gastric lymphomas and almost 50% of all gastric lymphomas[147]; in other sites, such as the ocular adnexa, they make up approximately 40% of the cases, and they account for the majority of low-grade pulmonary lymphomas. Patients are usually older adults, although they may be in their 20s and 30s. A slight female predominance has been reported in some series. The majority of patients present with localized stage I or II extranodal disease involving glandular epithelial tissues of various sites. The stomach is the most frequent site, but most indolent lymphomas presenting in the lung, thyroid, salivary gland, and orbit are of this type; skin and soft tissues may also be the presenting site. Many patients have a history of autoimmune disease, such as Sjögren syndrome or Hashimoto thyroiditis, or of *Helicobacter* gastritis in the case of gastric MALT lymphoma. Acquired MALT secondary to autoimmune disease or infection in these sites is thought to be the substrate for lymphoma development.

Proliferation of the cells of marginal zone lymphoma at certain sites depends on the presence of activated, antigen-driven T cells; in gastric tumors, it has been shown that the T cells are driven by *H. pylori* antigens. Therapy directed at the antigen (*H. pylori* in gastric lymphoma) results in regression of most early lesions.[148] The long-term prognosis of these patients is not known, however, and patients treated with antibiotic therapy require long and careful follow-up. The disease known as *Mediterranean abdominal lymphoma*, a *heavy-chain disease*, and *immunoproliferative small intestinal disease*, which occurs in young adults in eastern Mediterranean countries, is another example of a MALT-type lymphoma that may respond to antibiotic therapy in its early stages and has been shown to be associated with chronic *C. jejuni* infection.[39]

Therapy

The indolent extranodal lymphomas associated with MALT involve the gastrointestinal tract, salivary glands, breast, thyroid, orbit, conjunctiva, skin, lung, and, less commonly, other sites. As these diseases tend to remain localized for long periods of time, local treatment (surgery or radiation therapy [RT]) is effective at long-term control of disease. In particular, low doses of RT (30 Gy) almost always control sites of disease. These doses are somewhat lower than used for patients with localized follicular grade 1 and 2 disease. Retrospective studies provide dose control data for MALT lymphoma.[149,150] Local control rates ranged from 97% to 100%; 5-year progression-free survival (PFS) and overall survival (OS) rates were approximately 75% and 95%, respectively.

One-half or more of patients with gastric NHL have the indolent MALT type. The optimal treatment of gastric MALT lymphoma remains to be determined. Gastric MALT lymphoma is frequently associated with chronic gastritis and *H. pylori* infection. Because it has been postulated that *H. pylori* infection leads to the accumulation of MALT in the stomach and that gastric MALT lymphomas arise within this acquired MALT tissue, promising results have been seen with the use of antibiotics for gastric MALT NHL. In one study from the German MALT Lymphoma Group, 33 patients with low-grade MALT were treated with antibiotics. At 1-year median follow-up more than 70% of patients remained in complete remission (CR). However, in a follow-up study, 22 of 31 patients in continuous complete remission (median follow-up, 16 months) had a monoclonal B-cell population on PCR analysis, leaving open the question of durability of CR after antibiotics.[151] Nonetheless, the standard treatment for patients with gastric MALT who test positive for *H. pylori* is antibiotics and follow-up endoscopy 3 and 6 months later. Patients who have a CR should be followed without further treatment. Patients who have a partial response and remain *H. pylori*-positive should receive a second course of antibiotics before proceeding to more definitive treatment.

Patients who are negative for *H. pylori* are unlikely to respond to antibiotics; initial treatment of *H. pylori*–negative patients should be RT in most instances. For patients who have persistent disease after antibiotics, local regional irradiation therapy is the treatment of choice. Good results have been obtained with total or partial gastrectomy; however, this approach has been associated with long-term morbidity. Local and regional radiation through the three-field approach (anterior and two lateral fields to minimize radiation to the left kidney) provides local control and relief of symptoms in more than 90% of patients.

The use of chemotherapy for MALT lymphomas has received limited attention, as this indolent NHL does not routinely require the use of systemic treatment in patients with early-stage disease. In one study of 24 patients with low-grade MALT treated with daily cyclophosphamide or chlorambucil for 12 to 24 months, the CR rate at 1 year was 75%, and approximately 50% continued to be in remission at the time of the study.[152] Rituximab is another therapeutic option with reasonable activity and low morbidity.[153]

Although these results are favorable, control of limited disease is superior with RT, and the use of chemotherapy should be limited to patients with advanced or recurrent disease. MALT lymphomas can be disseminated and present at an advanced stage in approximately one-third of cases.[154] Dissemination is usually to lymph nodes but can involve other extranodal sites. Patients with widespread MALT lymphoma should be treated with strategies similar to those described for follicular lymphoma. In the setting of disseminated disease, very low radiation therapy (2 consecutive days of 2 Gy per day) can be very effective at reducing nodes and relieving symptoms.[155,156]

Nodal Marginal Zone B-Cell Lymphoma

Nodal marginal zone B-cell lymphoma (NMZL) is a primary nodal lymphoma with features identical to lymph nodes involved by MALT lymphoma. This diagnosis should not be made in patients with extranodal MALT lymphoma or splenic marginal zone lymphoma or in patients with Sjögren syndrome or Hashimoto thyroiditis, in which case the MZL may represent nodal dissemination of an extranodal MALT lymphoma.

Morphology

NMZL shows infiltration by marginal zone (centrocytelike cells), monocytoid B cells (more abundant clear cytoplasm), small B cells, and plasma cells in the paracortical and perifollicular regions. The germinal centers are usually preserved. Mantle zones are also often preserved but may be attenuated. Monocytoid B cell morphology may be prominent.

Immunophenotype and Genetic Features

Most cases are similar to splenic MZL and express pan B-cell antigens, BCL2, and lack CD5, CD23, CD10, BCL6, and cyclin D1. IgD is positive in a minority of cases. The t(11;18)(q21;q21) and trisomy 3 associated with extranodal marginal zone lymphoma are infrequent.

Postulated Normal Counterpart

The postulated normal counterpart is a post–germinal center marginal zone B cell.

Clinical Features and Therapy

NMZL is a rare disorder, accounting for 1% of the cases in the international study of the REAL.[115] The patients presented with isolated or generalized nodal disease; bone marrow was involved in 30%; rarely, peripheral blood may be involved. A retrospective survey of 180 patients with pathologically reviewed extragastric MALT lymphomas from 20 institutions revealed that the median age was 59 years (range, 21 to 92 years). Ann Arbor stage I disease was present in 115 patients (64%) and stage II disease in 16 (9%).[141] Most cases were in the low or low-intermediate risk groups according to the IPI. Patients were treated with a variety of therapeutic strategies, including chemotherapy in 78 cases. The 5-year OS rate was 90%, and the 5-year PFS was 60%. At a median follow-up of 3.4 years, only six patients showed histologic transformation. The optimal therapy for patients with nodal marginal zone lymphoma is not known. Patients are frequently treated with regimens that are used for follicular lymphoma, including combinations of alkylating agents or purine analogues with rituximab.[157]

Splenic Marginal Zone Lymphoma

Splenic marginal zone lymphoma (SMZL) is a neoplasm of small B lymphocytes that surround and replace splenic white pulp germinal centers, merging with an outer marginal zone of larger cells with pale cytoplasm admixed with large transformed centroblasts or immunoblasts. Small and large cells infiltrate red pulp. There may or may not be an associated lymphocytosis of "villous" lymphocytes in the peripheral blood. Splenic hilar lymph nodes and bone marrow are often involved. Diffuse variants of SMZL have been described, but are now thought to be unrelated to true SMZL. These cases currently reside under the disease category splenic diffuse red pulp small B-cell lymphoma.[97]

Morphology

In the spleen, the neoplastic cells of SMZL occupy the mantle and marginal zones of the splenic white pulp, usually with a central residual germinal center, which may be either atrophic or hyperplastic. The cells in the mantle zone are small, with slight nuclear irregularity and scant cytoplasm, whereas those in the marginal zone have more dispersed chromatin and abundant, pale cytoplasm and are admixed with centroblasts and immunoblasts. The red pulp is involved with a diffuse and a micronodular pattern and sinus infiltration. Splenic hilar lymph nodes are often involved; the neoplastic cells form vague nodules, often without a central germinal center, and a marginal zone pattern may or may not be present. The marrow usually contains discrete lymphoid aggregates, often with an accompanying intrasinusoidal component. When tumor cells are present in the peripheral blood, they often have abundant cytoplasm with small, polar, surface "villous" projections (splenic lymphoma with villous lymphocytes). The circulating component may also appear plasmacytoid.

Immunophenotype and Genetic Features

The tumor cells are IgM+, IgD+, CD5–, CD10–, BCL6–, CD23–; express B-cell antigens (CD19, CD20, CD22) and bcl-2; and lack CD11c and CD25. In the majority of cases, lack of CD5 serves to distinguish this disorder from B-CLL, and lack of CD103 and CD25 is useful in distinguishing it from hairy cell leukemia. The cells are cyclin D1-negative by immunohistochemical staining.

Analysis of the immunoglobulin variable region genes indicates a high degree of somatic mutation, consistent with a post–germinal center stage of B-cell development.[158] Ongoing mutations of V region genes, similar to germinal center cells, have been reported. However, a study found somatic mutations in only 50%.[159] Interstitial deletions of 17q31-32 are found in approximately 40%. Studies suggest that there are two subsets of SMZL: those with and some without somatic mutations. Those that lack mutations often have interstitial deletions of 7q and are associated with a worse prognosis.

Postulated Normal Counterpart

The normal counterpart is thought to be roughly divided between a post–germinal center, memory B cell of splenic type or a naive B cell.

Clinical Features and Therapy

SMZL accounts for only 1% to 2% of chronic lymphoid leukemia found on bone marrow examination but up to 25% of low-grade B-cell neoplasms in splenectomy specimens.[160] It may make up the majority of chronic B-cell leukemia and low-grade splenic lymphomas that do not fit the defining criteria of B-CLL, lymphoplasmacytic lymphoma, mantle cell lymphoma, follicular lymphoma, or hairy cell leukemia. Patients typically present with weakness, fatigue, or symptoms related to splenomegaly. In one study, physical examination revealed splenomegaly in almost all patients and hepatomegaly in up to 40% of patients, but lymphadenopathy is rare.[160] Lymphocytosis is a uniform finding, but extreme lymphocytosis is unusual. Anemia and thrombocytopenia are present in a minority of patients. In some series more than half of the patients have been shown to have a monoclonal immunoglobulin. Although most commonly seen in elderly men, the disease can occur in both genders and in young patients. Although SMZL is usually confined to the spleen, bone marrow, and blood, unusual sites of involvement such as leukemic meningitis have been described.

Most patients have an indolent course and require no immediate therapy or respond to splenectomy.[160] For patients in whom splenectomy is inappropriate, splenic radiation or single-agent rituximab can be an alternative.[161] Other systemic treatment options include oral alkylating agents or purine analogues, in combination with rituximab, as for follicular lymphoma.[162]

Follicular Lymphoma

Follicular lymphoma (FL) is defined as a lymphoma of follicle center B cells (centrocytes and centroblasts), which has at least a partially follicular pattern.

Morphology

FL is composed of a mixture of centrocytes (cleaved follicle center cells) and centroblasts (large noncleaved follicle center cells) and by definition has at least a partially follicular pattern. Rare lymphomas with a follicular growth pattern consist almost entirely of centroblasts. The proportion of centroblasts varies from case to case, and the clinical aggressiveness of the tumor increases with increasing numbers of centroblasts. The WHO classification uses the centroblast-counting method of Mann and Berard[162a] to assign cases into grades 1 through 3; in addition, the proportions of follicular and diffuse areas in the lymph node are also reported as summarized in Table 127.7. The bone marrow is frequently involved by lymphoid aggregates that are generally paratrabecular. Variants include pediatric FL, primary intestinal FL, other extranodal FL, and intrafollicular neoplasia/"in situ" FL. Primary cutaneous follicle center lymphoma, formerly considered a variant of nodal FL, is now considered a separate entity in the current WHO 2008 with different immunophenotype, genetics, and clinical course.

TABLE 127.7

FOLLICULAR LYMPHOMAS: GRADING AND VARIANTS

GRADES
1: 0–5 centroblasts per high-power field
2: 6–15 centroblasts per high-power field
3: >15 centroblasts per high-power field
3a: >15 centroblasts, but centrocytes are still present
3b: Centroblasts form solid sheets with no residual centrocytes

PATTERNS
Follicular: >75% of biopsy shows follicular pattern
Follicular and diffuse: 25%–75% of biopsy shows follicular pattern
Focally follicular: <25% of biopsy shows follicular pattern

VARIANTS
Diffuse follicular lymphoma (grade 1 or 2)
"In situ" follicular lymphoma

Immunophenotype and Genetic Features

The tumor cells of FL usually express surface immunoglobulin; approximately 60% are IgG and 40% either IgG or, less often, IgA. The tumor cells express pan-B-cell–associated antigens; most are CD10+, and they are CD5−, and CD23−/+. Tightly organized meshworks of FDCs are present in follicular areas. Most cases are bcl-2+, and nuclear bcl-6 is expressed by at least some of the neoplastic cells[163] (Fig. 127.3). The Ki-67+ fraction is lower than that of reactive follicles.

Immunoglobulin heavy- and light-chain genes are rearranged, with extensive and ongoing somatic mutations, similar to normal germinal center cells. t(14;18)(q32;q21) and *BCL-2* gene rearrangement are present in the majority of the cases.[164] However, a subset of cases may lack this transformation and have subtle differences in gene expression patterns.[165] Abnormalities of 3q27 or *BCL6* rearrangement, or both, are found in approximately 15% of FLs, whereas 5′ mutations of the *BCL6* gene are found in approximately 40%. Translocations

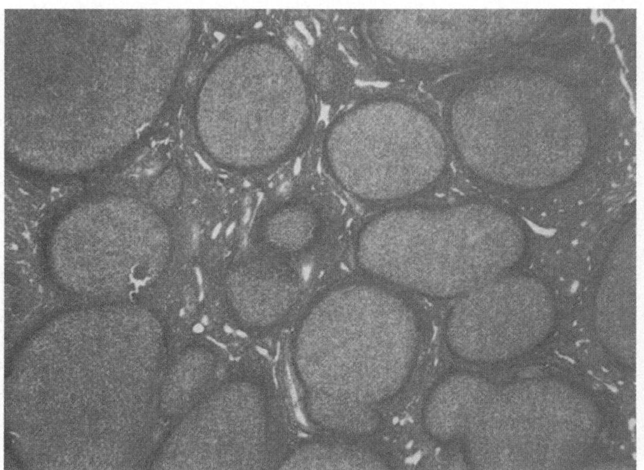

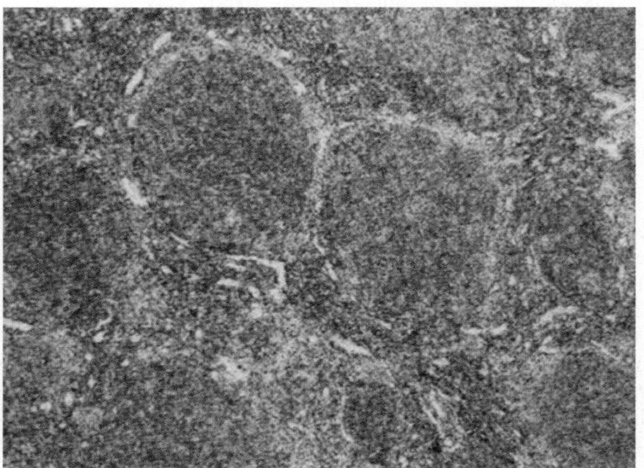

FIGURE 127.3 **A:** Follicular lymphoma. The normal lymph node architecture is replaced by malignant back-to-back lymphoid follicles with attenuated mantle zones. **B:** Follicular lymphoma. Malignant lymph follicles are marked with an antibody against Bcl-2.

PRACTICE OF ONCOLOGY

involving *BCL6* appear to be associated with an increased risk of transformation to DLBCL.[166]

Most cases have complex karyotypes, and t(14;18)(q32;q21) is rarely the sole abnormality.[167] Analysis of cases of the rare grade 3B FL has shown that t(14;18)(q32;q21) and 3q27 translocations are mutually exclusive, suggesting that some cases may be more closely related to FL and others to *de novo* DLBCL.

Gene expression profiling has been applied to the issues of prognosis and transformation of FL. One study looking at patient survival revealed two different gene expression "signatures" (patterns of gene expression) that could be used to calculate an outcome score that successfully split patients into four groups with median survivals ranging from 3.9 to 13.6 years. These signatures consisted largely of genes expressed by cells in the tumor microenvironment, particularly the nonmalignant immune cells. Therefore, it was the inflammatory immune response, not the tumor cells themselves, that predicted patient survival.[167a] Transformation of FL into DLBCL has also been investigated with gene expression profiling. Different groups described at least two distinct gene expression profiling signatures in transformed cases that were related to over- or underexpression of the *MYC* oncogene and/or proliferation, supporting the concept of the existence of more than one genetic mechanism for FL transformation.[168,169] A study of recurrent regions of acquired uniparental disomy has also led to new genetic insights into the transformation process.[169]

Postulated Normal Counterpart

The postulated normal counterpart is a germinal center B cell, both centrocytes and centroblasts.

Clinical Features

FL is the second most common lymphoma in the United States and western Europe, accounting for approximately 30% of all NHLs and up to 70% of low-grade lymphomas reported in American and European clinical trials.[115] Thus, our understanding of the clinical features and response to treatment of indolent lymphoma is essentially that of FL. Follicular lymphoma affects predominantly older adults, with a slight female predominance. Most patients have widespread disease at diagnosis, usually predominantly involving lymph nodes, but also spleen, bone marrow, and occasionally peripheral blood or extranodal sites. Despite the advanced stage, the clinical course is generally indolent, with median survivals in excess of 10 years; however, the disease is not usually curable with available treatment. In the current era of rituximab therapy, the survival of patients with FL has significantly improved.[170]

Therapy of Localized Follicular Lymphoma

RT alone is standard treatment for patients with clinical stage I to II follicular grade 1 to 2 lymphoma. Nine large series (defined as 50 or more patients per study) have reported results of treatment for follicular grade 1 to 2.[171–179] All but one study contains stage I and stage II patients (in approximately equal frequencies). The 10-year freedom from treatment failure in these studies ranges from 41% to 49%. The 10-year OS (all causes) ranges from 43% to 79%, with a median survival of 11.9 to 15.3 years. Nearly all patients were treated with RT alone except for those in the Foundation Bergonie study, in which the majority of patients received some form of systemic treatment.[177] The freedom from treatment failure and OS in this combined RT and chemotherapy study was no better than in the radiation-alone studies. The majority of patients had FL grade 1 and grade 2 histologies; however, FL grade 3 patients were included in some of the series.

Adverse prognostic factors for freedom from treatment failure are analyzed by multivariate analysis in many of the studies. Age was the adverse factor most often reported and was seen in five of the nine studies. Follicular grade 3 histology, extensive clinical stage IIA disease, bulky disease (defined as >2 or 3 cm), and extranodal presentations also were reported, but each of these adverse factors were seen in only one or two of the nine studies. No significant difference appears to be present in outcome between follicular grade 1 versus grade 2 disease.

No large prospective or randomized studies have evaluated the dose and field size of RT for patients with stage I to II follicular grade 1 to 2 lymphoma. The median radiation doses vary from 30 to 40 Gy in eight of the nine series, with the two largest series reporting a median dose of 35 Gy.[173,175] Infield recurrences range from 0% to 11%, with higher percentages occurring in patients with bulky disease or those who receive a radiation dose of less than 30 Gy. Based on these data, the authors recommend 30 to 36 Gy, with a boost to areas of initial involvement to 36 to 40 Gy for early-stage follicular grade I to II lymphoma. Bulky disease should be treated to the upper end of the range; 30 to 36 Gy should suffice for smaller disease. When there is a possibility of significant morbidity from treatment, such as long-term xerostomia from irradiation of the salivary glands in an elderly patient, slightly lower doses should be considered (i.e., 25 to 30 Gy).

The role of combination chemotherapy in the management of early-stage FL is unclear. Randomized studies conducted in the 1970s failed to demonstrate that non–Adriamycin-containing combination chemotherapy regimens plus RT were superior to RT alone.[180,181] A more recent British National Lymphoma Investigation study randomized 148 patients to receive either RT alone or RT plus chlorambucil chemotherapy.[182] No differences were found in freedom from recurrence or survival between the groups. A single-arm study of 91 stage I to II patients treated at the M. D. Anderson Hospital with COP (cyclophosphamide, vincristine, and prednisone) or CHOP-B (cyclophosphamide, doxorubicin, vincristine, prednisone plus bleomycin) chemotherapy in addition to RT demonstrated an improved freedom from recurrence compared with historic controls but there were no OS differences.[183]

The choice of therapy may lie in the careful assessment of prognostic factors. Most patients with Ann Arbor clinical stage I or II follicular grade 1 to 2 lymphoma should have a good prognosis after local-regional RT alone. For patients whose prognosis is less certain, such as those with stage II disease with multiple sites of involvement or bulky nodes, or patients with FL grade 3 histology, chemotherapy followed by involved-field irradiation may provide more durable remissions. Moreover, selected patients may be observed; in a series from Stanford University, the outcome of patients observed without therapy was similar to historical outcomes with radiation therapy.[184]

Therapy of Disseminated Follicular Lymphoma

The optimal treatment strategy for patients with advanced-stage FL is controversial, and a recent registry of patients in the United States suggests that widely disparate therapies are used for this group of patients.[185]

Observation at diagnosis remains a therapeutic option for many asymptomatic patients. The National Cancer Institute initiated a prospective randomized study comparing conservative treatment (no initial therapy) with aggressive combined modality therapy with ProMACE (prednisone, methotrexate-leucovorin, doxorubicin [Adriamycin], cyclophosphamide, etoposide)/MOPP (mechlorethamine [Mustargen], vincristine [Oncovin], procarbazine, prednisone) chemotherapy followed by low-dose (24 Gy) total lymphoid RT.[186] Eighty-nine patients were randomized. The disease-free survival was significantly higher in the combined modality therapy group at 4 years (51% vs. 12%); however, no differences in OS were seen.

When a decision is made to treat a patient with disseminated FL using cytotoxic chemotherapeutic agents, a wide variety of choices are available. In general, CRs occur more rapidly with combination chemotherapy regimens, but it is unclear that the ultimate treatment result is superior with combinations.

Rituximab as Initial Induction Therapy. Because of the toxicity of chemotherapy and interferon, investigators have examined the role of monoclonal antibody therapy as initial treatment for patients with follicular NHL. A phase 2 study treated 50 patients with stage II to IV FL and low tumor burden with single-agent rituximab as first therapy.[187] The overall response rate at 50 days was 73%. Toxicity was minimal.

Hainsworth et al. also used rituximab (375 mg/m^2 intravenously per week for 4 consecutive weeks) as initial therapy in patients with indolent lymphoma. Patients who did not progress received an additional 4-week course of rituximab every 6 months for 2 years. In 62 chemotherapy-naive patients, most of whom had stage III or IV disease, overall response rates at 6 weeks and at maximum response were 47% and 73%, with 7% and 37% complete remissions, respectively. At a median follow-up of 30 months, median PFS was 34 months.

Generally, single-agent rituximab is an option for patients with low disease burden, or patients with comorbidities making chemotherapy unattractive. As outlined later, extended schedules of rituximab may prolong the benefit of this agent with relatively minor toxicity.

Chemotherapy-Biologic Combinations as Initial Induction Therapy. The highest response rates in FL have been observed with the addition of the monoclonal antibody rituximab to chemotherapy combinations as an initial treatment strategy. A small phase 2 study demonstrated a very high response rate (95%) and a median PFS of approximately 5 years after the combination of CHOP chemotherapy with rituximab,[188] which led to widespread use of this regimen. The Southwest Oncology Group has reported similarly favorable results of a phase 2 trial evaluating CHOP chemotherapy followed by rituximab.[189] Since these early reports, four randomized trials have demonstrated the superiority of PFS and ultimately OS when rituximab is combined with initial chemotherapy for FL compared with chemotherapy alone. For example, Marcus et al.,[190] in a randomized phase 3 trial of over 300 patients with previously untreated FL, randomized patients to cyclophosphamide, vincristine, prednisone (CVP) versus rituximab-CVP (R-CVP). A statistically significant improvement in PFS and time to next therapy was noted in the R-CVP group. Additionally, with a median follow-up of 53 months, an impact on 4-year OS (83% vs. 77%) was achieved with R-CVP versus CVP alone.

A German study randomized over 400 patients with FL to R-CHOP versus CHOP alone as an induction therapy component. In this trial, R-CHOP reduced the relative risk for treatment failure by 60% and significantly prolonged the time to treatment failure, with a borderline impact on overall survival.[191] Similar findings have been reported in a trial comparing fludarabine, mitoxantrone, cyclophosphamide, with rituximab to chemotherapy alone.[192]

Based on these observations, when chemotherapy is used as first treatment for indolent lymphoma, rituximab is generally combined with chemotherapy. There are no randomized data to guide the choice of initial chemotherapy regimen. The importance of an anthracycline is debated; in an analysis conducted by the Southwest Oncology Group of 415 patients treated with a variety of chemotherapy regimens without rituximab, doxorubicin-containing treatment did not prolong the overall median survival of indolent lymphoma patients compared with less intensive treatment programs.[193] Long-term follow-up of a Cancer and Lymphoma Group B trial comparing CHOP-bleomycin with oral cyclophosphamide similarly did not demonstrate a survival benefit.[194] Whether these observations are true in the rituximab era is not known. In the United States, the most commonly used chemotherapy regimens for FL are R-CHOP and R-CVP.[185]

Preliminary results of a German randomized trial comparing R-CHOP with bendamustine-rituximab in previously untreated patients with indolent and mantle cell lymphoma have been presented. The bendamustine-rituximab combination was superior to R-CHOP in PFS and had a lower rate of toxicities.[195] We await a definitive article before recommending this regimen as upfront therapy.

Consolidation Options

Autologous Stem Cell Transplantation. Two trials of autologous hematopoietic stem cell transplantation (ASCT) incorporated in the primary therapy of patients with FL have reported high CR rates, but with continued observation it does not appear that this modality is curative for the majority of patients.[196,197] In addition, the incidence of secondary myelodysplasia after these treatments may exceed 15%, tempering the enthusiasm of this approach.[198] ASCT is generally reserved for the relapsed setting.

Interferon. Interferon-α has long been known to be an active drug in the treatment of patients with FL and has an objective response rate of 30% to 55% when used as a single agent with relapsed disease.[199] The value of adding interferon to standard combination chemotherapy regimens has been tested in a number of clinical trials. Several prospective randomized trials have conflicting results, with some suggesting a survival benefit,[200] whereas other larger trials failed to demonstrate it.[201] Because of significant toxicity, and the availability of other options, interferon is rarely used in the United States for patients with NHL.

Rituximab. Rituximab consolidation or maintenance therapy prolongs PFS after single-agent rituximab induction therapy. Hainsworth et al.[202] randomized 114 patients to rituximab "maintenance" (four times weekly every 6 months for 2 years) versus observation after rituximab induction therapy. Final overall and complete response rates were higher in the maintenance group. However, the duration of rituximab benefit was similar in the maintenance and re-treatment groups (31.3 vs. 27.4 months, respectively). This question was the subject of an Eastern Cooperative Oncology Group trial that enrolled over 600 patients ("RESORT"); results are pending as of this writing.

Ghielmini et al.[203] also demonstrated the efficacy of rituximab maintenance (single infusion every 2 months × 4) versus observation after rituximab induction, with a significant failure-free survival benefit to the maintenance strategy. Long-term follow-up of this strategy suggests that up to 45% of patients remain in remission at 8 years in the maintenance group, without significant increased toxicities.[204] Prolonged rituximab maintenance strategies are now under investigation for patients initially treated with rituximab alone.

Rituximab maintenance has also been evaluated after chemotherapy. An Eastern Cooperative Oncology Group clinical trial randomized patients with indolent lymphoma to rituximab maintenance (every 2 months for 2 years) versus observation after CVP chemotherapy. PFS at 3 years was significantly prolonged in the maintenance arm (68% vs. 33%) with a trend toward improved OS in the maintenance arm.[205] Based on these results, rituximab was approved for maintenance following chemotherapy by the U.S. Food and Drug Administration (FDA).

Rituximab maintenance has demonstrated activity following rituximab-containing chemotherapy in the relapsed/refractory setting. Van Oers et al.[206] have published results of a phase 3 trial in the relapsed setting evaluating rituximab maintenance after CHOP and R-CHOP in rituximab-naive patients. PFS benefit was noted in the rituximab maintenance group, with a trend toward overall survival benefit. Based on these data, the international PRIMA trial was conducted, which randomized previously untreated patients following rituximab-containing chemotherapy to rituximab maintenance versus observation. Preliminary results of this trial suggest a substantial benefit in PFS in patients receiving maintenance rituximab. Therefore, patients with FL should be offered maintenance rituximab after rituximab-containing regimens.

Vaccines

Several approaches of vaccination have been used in clinical trials of patients with follicular NHL. The most frequent target of vaccination approaches is the idiotype. In phase 2 clinical trials, anti-idiotype immune responses occur after vaccination in approximately 50% of patients, and these patients had prolonged PFS compared with historic controls.[207]

Three randomized trials have been completed studying idiotype vaccination versus placebo after induction therapy for newly diagnosed follicular NHL. Two trials were negative[208] and one underpowered trial suggested benefit in a selected subgroup of patients.[209] Based on these results, and the significant activity of rituximab in this setting, there is limited enthusiasm for idiotype vaccines at the present time.

Radioimmunotherapy

Finally, use of the radio-labeled monoclonal antibody iodine-131 (^{131}I) tositumomab in previously untreated patients has also been reported to produce a high CR rate. Between 1996 and 1999, 76 patients with previously untreated follicular NHL received ^{131}I tositumomab therapy on a phase 2, single-center study.[210] Fifty-six patients (74%) had a confirmed CR. Forty-five of these patients remained in CR with a follow-up of 30 to 66 months. The Southwest Oncology Group reported the outcome of a novel chemoimmunotherapeutic approach, combining standard induction chemotherapy (CHOP) followed by consolidation with ^{131}I tositumomab. This phase 2 trial included 90 patients with previously untreated advanced-stage follicular NHL.[211] The overall response rate to the entire treatment regimen (chemotherapy + ^{131}I tositumomab) was 90%, including 67% complete remissions. The 2-year PFS was estimated to be 81%, which is better than observed historically with CHOP alone or CHOP with rituximab, and this benefit persisted through 5 years of follow-up.[212] A phase 3 trial comparing this regimen to R-CHOP chemotherapy has been completed, and results are awaited at this writing.

Radioimmunotherapy consolidation has also been studied using ibritumomab tiuxetan. An international study randomized 414 patients in response to chemotherapy (<20% received rituximab combinations) to consolidation with ibritumomab tiuxetan versus observation. Prolonged 2-year PFS and conversion of partial responses to complete responses were noted in the ibritumomab group.[213] This trial resulted in approval of ibritumomab tiuxetan as consolidation following induction chemotherapy for FL by the FDA. Whether or not these results will be similar in a group of patients treated with rituximab-containing induction is not known. The Southwest Oncology Group is currently studying rituximab maintenance following R-CHOP plus ^{131}I tositumomab consolidation.

Summary: Initial Treatment of Follicular Lymphoma

Patients with early-stage FL should be considered for treatment with primary RT. Clearly, many treatment options exist for the majority of patients with newly diagnosed, disseminated FL. Whenever possible, the authors strongly encourage participation in clinical trials. Observation is an option for certain asymptomatic patients; however, this approach has no chance at improving survival for these individuals. Rituximab has activity as a single agent for patients with nonbulky disease. For symptomatic patients, or those with bulky disease requiring a rapid response, combination chemotherapy regimens including alkylating agents or purine analogues with rituximab are appropriate. For many patients, there appears to be a role to consolidate initial response with either radioimmunotherapy or maintenance rituximab. The role of idiotype vaccination or more aggressive approaches, including ASCT as part of initial therapy, remain to be defined.

Therapy for Progressive Disease

Almost all patients with FL, despite CR to initial chemotherapy, relapse and are candidates for salvage treatment. In an asymptomatic patient, particularly if the individual is elderly, observation without treatment can be an acceptable option. Local RT can be used in a palliative manner. In particular, we have been increasingly using the two-dose regimen of 2 Gy each day for 2 consecutive days.[156,214]

A wide variety of second-line chemotherapy regimens have been used in patients with FL. When the initial therapy is repeated, patients with FL often respond. For example, purine analogue–containing chemotherapy regimens are often used in the relapsed setting. Preliminary results of a cooperative German study, in which patients with relapsed or refractory follicular or mantle cell lymphoma after treatment with CHOP were randomly assigned to receive four cycles of chemotherapy with fludarabine, cyclophosphamide, and mitoxantrone (FCM), with or without rituximab, reveal that overall response rates were 89% with FCM-R and 54% with FCM.[215] The highest response rates for relapsed indolent lymphoma have been reported with bendamustine either as a single agent[216] or in combination with rituximab.[217] This drug is now approved by the FDA for this indication. As previously mentioned, rituximab maintenance following chemotherapy appears to prolong PFS in the relapsed setting, at least in a group of rituximab-naive patients.

Radio-labeled antibodies directed against CD20 also have high response rates in patients with relapsed FL.[218,219] A phase 3 randomized study compared yttrium 90 ibritumomab tiuxetan radioimmunotherapy with rituximab in 143 patients with relapsed or refractory low-grade, follicular, or transformed CD20 (+) NHL.[220] The overall response rate was 80% for the yttrium 90 ibritumomab tiuxetan group versus 56% for the rituximab group, which reached statistical significance. However, there was no statistically significant benefit in response duration or survival between the two groups. Iodine-131 tositumomab (Bexxar) has also been approved for the treatment of recurrent indolent and transformed B-cell NHL, with results similar to ibritumomab tiuxetan in the rituximab-refractory patient population.[221]

Novel agents, such as mTOR inhibitors, proteosome inhibitors, antibodies, and immunomodulatory drugs, have also been shown to produce objective responses. Current studies are combining these agents with standard rituximab-containing chemotherapy in the relapsed setting.[222]

Autologous[196,223] and allogeneic[224] hematopoietic stem cell transplantations have been used for patients with relapsed FL. Patients transplanted after multiple treatment failures have a poorer outcome.[225] A single randomized study has been published addressing the role of autologous transplantation.[226] Patients with recurrent FL received three cycles of CHOP chemotherapy. Responding patients with limited bone marrow infiltration were eligible for random assignment to three further cycles of chemotherapy (C), unpurged ASCT (U), or purged ASCT (P). Because of poor accrual, the study was closed prematurely, and only 89 patients in total were randomized. With a median follow-up of 69 months, ASCT significantly improved PFS and OS compared with chemotherapy alone; however, the study was underpowered to address the purging question. Long-term follow-up of two single-institution experiences of purged ASCT using cyclophosphamide and total-body irradiation conditioning demonstrates an apparent plateau on the remission duration curve at 48% at 12 years despite significant treatment-related toxicity.[227]

An International Bone Marrow Transplantation Registry study retrospectively evaluated 904 patients undergoing transplantation for FL. A total of 176 (19%) received allogeneic, 131 (14%) received purged autologous, and 597 (67%) received unpurged autologous transplants.[225] In multivariate analyses, allotransplantation had higher transplant-related mortality and lower disease recurrence. Purged autotransplantation had a 26% lower recurrence risk than unpurged autotransplantation. Five-year probabilities of survival were 51%, 62%, and 55% after allogeneic, purged autotransplantation, and unpurged autotransplantation, respectively. To decrease the transplant-related mortality associated with allogeneic transplantation and foster a graft-versus-lymphoma effect, there has been great interest in the use of nonmyeloablative conditioning regimens for patients with indolent lymphoma.[228] Studies are under way to define appropriate patients to consider for this approach.

Therapy of Transformed Disease

In a patient with FL who progresses with transformation to a DLBCL, treatment is almost always indicated. The clinical manifestations of histologic transformation to DLBCL typically include rapidly progressive lymphadenopathy (i.e., often localized); the development of new symptoms, such as fevers, night sweats, weight loss, and pain; or both. In general, histologic transformation to DLBCL has a poor prognosis and frequently a rapidly fatal outcome. In a series from Stanford, previously untreated patients and patients with limited disease at transformation had improved prognosis.[229] Although the median survival for all patients with transformation was only 22 months, those who achieved a CR to therapy after histologic conversion had an actuarial survival of 75% at 5 years. More recent studies suggest that R-CHOP may improve overall survival for patients with transformed disease.[230]

Patients who have not previously received an anthracycline-containing regimen should be treated with R-CHOP. Other chemotherapy regimens used as salvage treatment for DLBCL (see "Salvage Therapy") are also effective. Young patients who respond to salvage chemotherapy should be considered for consolidation with high-dose therapy and ASCT because selected patients with histologic transformation, particularly those whose transformation occurs early in the course of their disease and who remain chemosensitive, may experience prolonged survival after ASCT.[231] Significant responses, of relatively short duration, have also been observed in patients treated with radioimmunotherapy, particularly ^{131}I tositumomab.[231] Patients who respond to therapy for transformed disease often have recurrences at a later date with indolent FL.

Mantle Cell Lymphoma

Mantle cell lymphoma is a neoplasm of monomorphous small to medium-sized B cells with irregular nuclei and a characteristic translocation resulting in overexpression of the cell cycle protein cyclin D1 in the vast majority of cases.

Morphology

Mantle cell lymphomas may have a diffuse, nodular, mantle zone or mixed pattern in lymph nodes. Most cases are composed of monomorphous small to medium-sized lymphoid cells, with slightly irregular or "cleaved" nuclei. However, the cytology can range from small lymphoid, to large cleaved, to lymphoblastoid. Neoplastic centroblasts, immunoblasts, and pseudofollicles are not seen. Despite the small size and bland appearance of the cells, they are often more proliferative than other small cell B-cell lymphomas and contain scattered mitotic figures. The background cells include "epithelioid" histiocytes and endothelia from hyalinized vessels.

Immunophenotype and Genetic Features

The tumor cells express strong IgM and IgD, which is often of λ light-chain type, and strongly express B-cell–associated antigens; most coexpress CD5, similar to B-CLL/SLL, and are usually, but not always, CD23-negative. A prominent, irregular meshwork of FDC is found even in diffuse cases. Nuclear cyclin D1 protein is present in nearly all cases. However, a very small minority of cases of mantle cell lymphoma (as categorized by morphology, CD5 expression, and gene expression profiling) may lack cyclin D1 overexpression.

Immunoglobulin heavy- and light-chain genes are rearranged and lack somatic mutations in 80% or more of the cases, indicating a pregerminal center stage of differentiation. A t(11;14)(q13;q32) in the majority of the cases results in rearrangement of the *BCL1* locus and overexpression of a cell-cycle–associated protein that is not normally expressed in lymphoid cells. Overexpression of this protein may explain the high proliferation fraction and aggressive clinical course of this histologically low-grade appearing lymphoma. The translocation can best be detected by fluorescence *in situ* hybridization. More than 90% of cases have genetic abnormalities in addition to the t(11;14)(q13;q32).[130]

One large study of gene expression profiling of mantle cell lymphoma demonstrated that a large proportion of genes associated with survival formed a "proliferation" signature. These genes were often associated with cell-cycle progression and DNA synthesis, but not with *MYC*. Other predictive factors included higher expression levels of cyclin D1 transcripts and deletion of the INK4a/ARF locus encoding the p16^{INK4a} and p14^{ARF} tumor suppressor genes, which are also related to cell-cycle progression.[232] Interestingly, approximately 5% of cases had the typical pathologic features and gene expression profiling pattern of mantle cell lymphoma but did not overexpress the mRNA or cyclin D1 protein. However, high levels of cyclin D2 or D3 protein expression were noted, indicating an alternative molecular mechanism of pathogenesis may be operative in the cyclin D1-negative cases.[233]

Postulated Normal Counterpart. Mantle cell lymphoma is thought to arise in most cases from an antigen-naive peripheral B cell of the inner mantle zone.

Clinical Features. Mantle cell lymphoma accounts for approximately 7% of adult cases of NHL in the United States and Europe.[115] In a review of 376 cases of disseminated low-grade lymphoma (Working Formulation categories A through E), mantle cell lymphoma made up 10%.[234] It is a tumor of older adults, with a marked male predominance (75%). The majority (70%) of patients are in stage IV at diagnosis; sites involved include lymph nodes, spleen, Waldeyer's ring, bone marrow (>60%), blood (up to 50%), and extranodal sites, especially the gastrointestinal tract (lymphomatous polyposis).[235] The course is moderately aggressive. The median OS in most series is 3 years, with no plateau in the curve, but OS may be improving in recent series. The blastoid variant is reported in some studies to be more aggressive.[236]

Therapy. Localized mantle cell lymphoma is quite rare, seen in only 13% of unselected patients in one large series.[33] The

PRACTICE OF ONCOLOGY

failure-free survival of patients treated for localized mantle cell lymphoma is quite poor, suggesting that unrecognized dissemination was usually present. The optimal treatment for these patients is not known. Approaches reported in these individuals include involved-field radiation and the combination of R-CHOP chemotherapy and involved-field irradiation.

Most patients present with disseminated disease. A randomized trial comparing CVP and CHOP showed no significant difference in OS (84% vs. 88%) and failure-free survival (41% vs. 58%).[237] A phase 2 study evaluated the combination of CHOP and rituximab for newly diagnosed mantle cell lymphoma and demonstrated an improved response rate, with no evidence of prolongation of PFS.[238] A randomized trial comparing R-CHOP and CHOP demonstrated modest benefit to R-CHOP in failure-free survival, without any plateau on the PFS curve.[239]

A chemotherapy regimen that was originally used for patients with leukemia, called *hyper-CVAD* (cyclophosphamide, vincristine, doxorubicin, dexamethasone alternating with methotrexate and cytarabine), has been used in mantle cell lymphoma and has a high CR rate.[240]

In a historic control study from M. D. Anderson Cancer Center, hyper-CVAD had a superior 3-year event-free survival to CHOP (72% vs. 28%). Sequential phase 2 studies using this regimen have incorporated consolidation with high-dose chemotherapy and ASCT or with rituximab, with similar outcomes. However, when this regimen was studied in a cooperative group setting, half of the patients could not complete the regimen because of toxicity, and results were inferior to those reported by M. D. Anderson.[241]

Because of the poor long-term outlook, patients with mantle cell lymphoma who are sufficiently young and healthy often undergo autologous or allogeneic bone marrow transplantation at best response. The long-term benefits of autologous and allogeneic transplantation are still uncertain,[242] although long-term survivors with both approaches are reported. Aggressive induction regimens incorporating high doses of cytarabine and autologous transplantation offer prolonged PFS, but there is no apparent survival plateau.[243] Whether these aggressive approaches offer any benefit over standard R-CHOP therapy followed by ASCT is not known.[244]

Patients who relapse and are not candidates for transplantation or those who relapse after transplantation can be treated with rituximab or salvage chemotherapy regimens. Two series containing small numbers of patients with mantle cell lymphoma suggest high response rates to the combination of bendamustine and rituximab in the relapsed setting.[217,245] The proteasome inhibitor bortezomib is approved as a single agent in relapsed/refractory mantle cell lymphoma based on a pivotal trial demonstrating a response rate of 33%.[246] A randomized trial comparing the mTOR inhibitor temsirolimus to investigator's choice therapy in relapsed/refractory mantle cell lymphoma demonstrated improved responses of limited duration in the temsirolimus arm.[247] Early studies also suggest promising activity of lenalidomide in this histology.[248]

Given the relatively poor prognosis of patients with mantle cell lymphoma, the authors strongly advocate participation in clinical trials of novel agents. Young patients should be considered for high-dose therapy and autologous or allogeneic stem cell support in first remission. Long-term follow-up of ongoing studies is required to determine the optimal induction chemotherapy regimen.

Diffuse Large B-Cell Lymphoma

As indicated by the name, DLBCL is a neoplasm of large B cells in a diffuse (nonnodular) pattern. The cytologic features differ among cases, and several morphologic and clinical variants exist, many of which are now considered distinct entities. This is a heterogeneous category, likely containing diverse entities. DLBCL as described here is primary, but cases may arise through transformation of small B-cell lymphomas, such as small lymphocytic, lymphoplasmacytic, splenic marginal zone, extranodal marginal zone, or FLs. Currently, there is believed to be at least two different cells of origin, either from germinal center B-cells (GCB type) or activated B-cells (ABC type).

Morphologic Variants and Subtypes

DLBCLs are a heterogeneous group of neoplasms. They are typically composed of large cells (2–3 times the size of normal lymphocytes) that resemble centroblasts or immunoblasts, most often with a mixture of the two. Three morphologic variants of otherwise typical DLBCL can be recognized, but their clinical significance is debated. The usual centroblastic variant (80% of the cases) is composed of cells resembling germinal center centroblasts, with one to three peripheral nucleoli and a narrow rim of basophilic cytoplasm, often with a variable admixture of immunoblasts. Some cases have multilobated centroblasts (Fig. 127.4). The immunoblastic morphologic variant (10% of the cases) has more than 90% immunoblasts with a prominent central nucleolus and abundant, basophilic cytoplasm, often with plasmacytoid differentiation. In the anaplastic morphologic variant, the cells are cytologically similar to those of ALCL, with pleomorphic nuclei, abundant cytoplasm and sinusoidal growth pattern, and CD30 expression. Rare morphologies include spindle cell, signet ring cell, pseudorosette formation, and myxoid or fibrillar background matrix.

In addition to the morphologic variants, currently four different subtypes of DLBCL are recognized. The T-cell–rich/histiocyte-rich variant has a prominent background of reactive T cells and histiocytes.[249] The difficulty with this variant is the differential diagnosis with Hodgkin lymphoma of either the lymphocyte-predominant or classic types. In fact, there may be a spectrum of disease including nodular lymphocyte-predominant Hodgkin lymphoma on one end and T-cell–rich/histiocyte-rich large B cell lymphoma on the other.[250]

Primary DLBCL of the CNS includes primary intracerebral or intraocular lymphomas, excluding lymphomas of the dura and secondary involvement by systemic lymphomas. This category also excludes all immunodeficiency-associated lymphomas. As opposed to CNS lymphomas in the setting of immunodeficiency, EBV is generally not found in primary DLBCL of

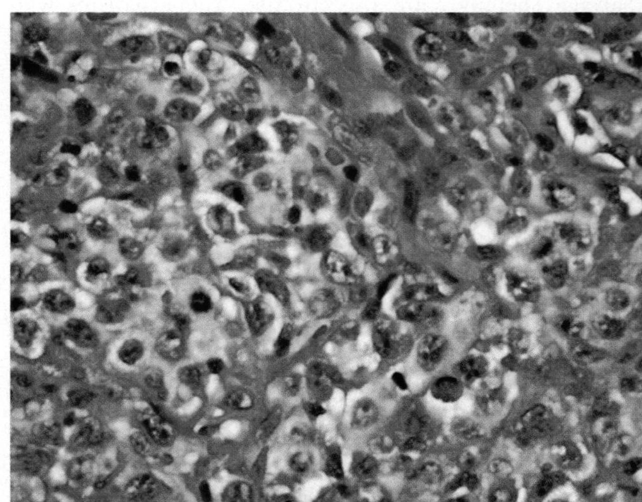

FIGURE 127.4 Diffuse large B-cell lymphoma. Large atypical lymphoid cells with predominantly centroblastic morphology are effacing the tissue architecture.

the CNS in immunocompetent patients. Many cases show loss of MHC class I and II expression through genetic deletions at the 6p21.3 locus, allowing the tumors to escape from tumor immunosurveillance.[250a]

Primary cutaneous DLBCL, leg type typically occurs in elderly women on the lower leg and may be bilateral. The cells are centroblastic and immunoblastic in appearance. By immunohistochemical analysis (IHC), these are often of the ABC subtype, and typically express the bcl-2 protein and MUM1/IRF4. Gene expression profiling shows similarity to the ABC subtype of DLBCL.[251] These are relatively aggressive lymphomas, which may disseminate to extracutaneous sites.

The fourth recognized subtype within the spectrum of DLBCL is termed EBV+ DLBCL of the elderly. This is a new entity in the WHO 2008. First described in Japan, these typically extranodal lymphomas are EBV-positive and are thought to represent a malignancy in the face of senescence of the immune system in older (defined as >50 years of age) patients. Typically, the lymphoma is pleomorphic and may contain Reed-Sternberg–like malignant cells, sometimes with a mixed inflammatory background, and zonal necrosis.[252]

Bone marrow involvement in DLBCL may take two forms. In approximately 10% of the cases, large cell lymphoma is present in the marrow. However, approximately 20% may show so-called discordant marrow involvement consisting of aggregates of small, atypical lymphoid cells consistent with involvement by low-grade lymphoma, particularly FL.[253] Several studies have shown that for discordant marrow involvement, the OS is similar to that of patients of similar stage with negative bone marrows; however, late relapses are more common.[254]

Immunophenotype and Genetic Features

DLBCLs express one or more B-cell–associated antigens (CD19, CD20, CD22, CD79a), as well as CD45 and often surface immunoglobulin. They may coexpress CD5 or CD10, bcl-6, and/or MUM1/IRF4 as well as a variety of other antigens. In various studies, 25% to 80% express bcl-2 protein, and this may be associated with a worse prognosis.[255] However, later studies indicate that the relationship between bcl-2 protein and prognosis is more complex and probably relates to the cell of origin subtype of the DLBCL. In particular, DLBCL cases expressing bcl-2 protein as part of the GCB subtype do not have a worse prognosis, while those overexpressing bcl-2 in the context of an ABC subtype do have a worse outcome.[256]

There are a variety of chromosomal alterations in DLBCL. A common change involves alterations of the *BCL6* gene at the 3q27 locus, which is critical for germinal center formation. *BCL6* can be translocated next to the immunoglobulin heavy chain (IgH) or light chain (Igκ or Igλ) or other genes.[257] Alternatively, *BCL6* function can be altered through point mutations in the 5′ upstream regulatory region. The t(14;18)(q32;q21) translocation characteristic of FL places BCL-2 under the regulation of the IgH promoter leading to increased antiapoptosis signals. This finding is characteristic of the GCB subtype of DLBCL but not the ABC subtype.[258] Cases with a combination of both the t(14;18)(q32;q21) characteristic of FL as well as the t(8;14)(q23;q32) characteristic of Burkitt lymphoma have been described as "double-hit" lymphomas. Presumably the t(8;14)(q23;q32) is a secondary event and is correlated with a particularly aggressive course.[259] Double hits including BCL2 and BCL6 have also been described as well as triple hits including BCL2, BCL6, and MYC. Many of these cases fall into the proposed category of "B-cell lymphoma, unclassifiable with features intermediate between DLBCL and Burkitt lymphoma."[97] The exact criteria and clinical significance of this category are a matter of intense investigation. Many cases of DLBCL have additional abnormalities in addition to the few listed here and can have quite complex karyotypes. Evidence of EBV infection is common in DLBCL cases associated with immunodeficiency and in the elderly.

Gene expression profiling revealed that in otherwise histologically and immunophenotypically similar cases, there were at least two different subtypes of DLBCL called the germinal center B-cell (GCB) and activated B-cell (ABC) subtypes. The GCB cases have a better survival than the ABC subtype. The GCB subtype correlates with the presence of the t(14;18)(q32;q21) translocation supporting the hypothesis that the GCB subtype of DLBCL is of follicular cell origin as it shares the t(14;18)(q32;q21) characteristic of FL.[258,260,261] Additionally, amplification of the mir-17-92 microRNA cluster and deletion of the tumor suppressor *PTEN* are recurrent alterations seen exclusively in the GCB subtype. In contrast, trisomy 3 (possibly leading to overexpression of *FOXP1*), deletion of the *INK4a/ARF* tumor suppressor locus, and chromosome 19q amplifications (possibly leading to *SPIB* overexpression) are present in the ABC subtype, which also has frequent activation of the NF-κB pathway. Cases of GCB and ABC subtypes also have distinct microRNA profiles, further supporting the biological differences between these two subgroups.[262] The prognostic importance of this distinction has recently been confirmed in the current R-CHOP treatment era.[100] On a practical level, a panel of three immunohistochemical stains (CD10, BCL6, and MUM1) was validated for distinction of the GCB and ABC subtypes and more recently refined with the addition of FOXP1 and GCET1 to create an antibody panel for making this distinction in routinely fixed, paraffin-embedded tissue sections.[263,264]

Gene expression profiling studies of prognostic genes in DLBCL initially identified four signatures, which were highly related to patient survival: "germinal center," "major histocompatibility (MHC) class II," "lymph node," and "proliferation." Two of the four signatures, MHC class II and lymph node, contain antigen-presenting molecules, T-cell–associated genes, inflammatory genes, and stromal genes, which directly reflect the critical role of host immunosurveillance on patient outcome independent of the clinical IPI score.[261] Using a different methodology, other investigators identified three different gene expression profiling-defined subgroups called "oxidative-phosphorylation," "B-cell receptor/proliferation," and "host response," which were also associated with favorable outcome,[265] implicating metabolic pathways, alterations of normal B-cell functioning, and host response as important factors. A later study analyzing cases treated with R-CHOP identified "stromal 1" and "stromal 2" signatures related to vasculogenesis and extracellular matrix with inflammatory cells, respectively, as key prognostic signatures.[100] Other investigators have focused on smaller prognostic gene sets, which may be easier to measure,[266] and others have focused on gene expression profiling out of fixed paraffin-embedded tissues.[267] It remains to be seen which morphologic, genetic, phenotypic, or other characteristics will be the most useful for prognostication in the long run.

Postulated Normal Counterpart

DLBCL is most likely a heterogeneous disease with more than one normal counterpart, probably including germinal center B cells and post–germinal center-activated peripheral B cells.

Clinical Features

DLBCL was the most common lymphoma in the international study of the REAL, accounting for 31% of the cases.[115] Patients typically present with a rapidly enlarging symptomatic mass, with B symptoms in one-third of the cases. Localized (stage I or II) extranodal disease occurs in up to 30%; bone marrow involvement was seen in only 16%. Up to 40% of DLBCLs are extranodal; common sites include the gastrointestinal tract, bone, and CNS. The prognosis was highly associated with the

TABLE 127.8

CHEMOTHERAPY VERSUS COMBINED MODALITY THERAPY FOR STAGE I/II INTERMEDIATE- OR HIGH-GRADE LYMPHOMA: PROSPECTIVE RANDOMIZED TRIALS

Study	Patients (n)	Stage	CT	RT Dose (Gy)	% CR or PR	% FFS	% Survival (y)
ECOG[234]	352	CS I (EN/B) and all CS II,	CHOP × 8 (CR)	—	61 (CR)	58	70 (6)
		CS I–II	CHOP × 8 (CR)	30 (IF)	—	73[a]	84 (6)[b]
			CHOP × 8 (PR)	40 (IF)	28 (PR)	60	64 (6)
SWOG[233]	401	CS I/IE (B/NB) and CS II	CHOP × 8	—	73	64	72 (5)
		(NB)	CHOP × 3	40–55	75	77[a]	82 (50)[a]
GELA[235]	518	IPI 0, 1	CHOP × 4	—	—	69	78
		CS I–II	CHOP × 4	40	—	64	70
GELA[236]	631	CS I–II	ACVBP	—	—	83[b]	89[b]
		Low risk	CHOP × 3	30–40	—	74	80

CT, chemotherapy; RT, radiation therapy; CR, complete response; PR, partial response; FFS, failure-free survival; ECOG, Eastern Cooperative Oncology Group; CS, clinical stage; EN, extranodal; B, bulky disease; CHOP, cyclophosphamide, doxorubicin, vincristine, prednisone; IF, involved field; SWOG, Southwest Oncology Group; NB, no bulky disease; GELA, Groupe d'Etude des Lymphomes de l'Adulte; IPI, International Prognostic Index.
[a]Significant difference between RT and no RT; borderline significant difference between RT and no RT, $P = .06$.
[b]Significantly better result with ACVBP (doxorubicin, cyclophosphamide, vindesine, bleomycin, prednisone).

IPI score. Large B-cell lymphoma may occur as a high-grade transformation of several low-grade B-cell lymphomas (B-CLL, lymphoplasmacytic lymphoma, FL, MALT lymphoma, SMZL). DLBCL of certain extranodal sites, such as the CNS, may be clinically distinctive and may have specific treatment protocols.

Therapy of Localized Diffuse Large B-Cell Lymphoma

Four prospective randomized trials have further evaluated the role of RT in patients with early-stage DLBCL (Table 127.8) in the pre-rituximab era. The Southwest Oncology Group trial randomized 401 stage I and nonbulky stage II patients to receive either three cycles of CHOP and involved-field irradiation (40–55 Gy) or eight cycles of CHOP alone.[268] The 5-year PFS (77% vs. 64%; $P = .03$) and OS (82% vs. 72%; $P = .02$) results favored the CHOP and involved-field RT treatment arm, although at 5 to 10 years this survival benefit is less apparent, with late disease recurrences observed in the RT arm. A separate analysis of PFS and OS was performed using a modified IPI. Patients with zero or one risk factor had a higher PFS and OS compared with those with two or three risk factors. As a result of this trial, combination chemotherapy and adjuvant RT became the standard care for patients with stage I to II DLBCL.

The Eastern Cooperative Oncology Group randomized 352 patients with bulky stage I (mediastinal or retroperitoneal involvement or masses >10 cm), stage IE, and stage II to IIE disease to eight cycles of CHOP chemotherapy with or without RT. Patients with no response or progression to chemotherapy were removed from the study. Individuals in complete remission were randomized to 30 Gy involved-field RT or no further treatment.[269]

Patients in partial remission received 40 Gy to the site(s) of pretreatment involvement plus radiation to contiguous uninvolved region(s). In patients randomized after complete remission, the 5-year disease-free survival (73% vs. 58%; $P = .03$), freedom from recurrence (73% vs. 58%; $P = .04$), and survival (84% vs. 70%; $P = .06$) all favored the patients who received adjuvant involved-field irradiation.[63] At 10 years, the disease-free survival continued to favor the addition of RT (57% vs. 46%; $P = .04$), but the survival differences no longer were statistically significant, similar to the aforementioned Southwest Oncology Group trial.

Bonnet et al.[270] compared CHOP × 4 with CHOP × 4 followed by 40 Gy in 518 patients more than 60 years of age who all had an age-adjusted IPI score of zero. With a median follow-up of 7 years, EFS and OS did not differ between the two regimens. There is some concern about the quality control of radiation in this trial. Reyes et al.[236] compared CHOP × 3 followed by 30 to 40 Gy involved-field radiotherapy with the chemotherapy regimen ACVBP (doxorubicin, cyclophosphamide, vindesine, bleomycin, prednisone) followed by consolidation chemotherapy using methotrexate, ifosfamide, etoposide, and cytarabine in 631 patients with low-risk, localized aggressive lymphoma. Event-free survival (CHOP + RT 74% vs. ACVBP 82%) and OS (CHOP + RT 81% vs. ACVBP 90%) was significantly better in the chemotherapy-alone arm. Unfortunately, a significant number of patients in this study had bulky disease, and CHOP × 3 + RT would have been predicted to be inadequate for these individuals.

The aforementioned randomized trials did not include rituximab. The Southwest Oncology Group ran a pilot trial of patients with at least one modified IPI risk factor and early-stage disease of R-CHOP followed by involved-field radiation therapy. Outcomes were excellent, with 4-year PFS at 88% and OS at 92%.[271] The MabThera International Trial randomized patients between six cycles of CHOP and six cycles of R-CHOP, and included radiation for patients with bulky disease or extranodal disease at presentation. Seventy-five percent of patients had early-stage disease in this trial, and significant benefit was demonstrated with the addition of rituximab to chemotherapy.[272] Based on these results, and extrapolating from advanced-stage disease, rituximab should be incorporated into induction treatment regimens for early-stage disease.

In summary, abbreviated R-CHOP chemotherapy plus involved-field RT is excellent therapy for patients with low-risk, nonbulky early-stage DLBCL. Patients with poor prognostic features, such as advanced stage, tumor bulk, or high LDH, may benefit from additional systemic therapy or clinical trials involving novel agents. Current trials are evaluating the role of PET imaging as response-directed therapeutic marker to select patients who may not require radiation therapy after induction chemotherapy.

Therapy of Disseminated Diffuse Large B-Cell Lymphoma

Disseminated DLBCL is a curable disease. More than 40 randomized clinical trials have been reported to identify the best treatment regimen for patients with advanced diffuse aggressive lymphoma. The majority of these trials have not found a significant treatment advantage for any particular regimen. The most widely quoted trial was carried out in the United States comparing CHOP, m-BACOD, ProMACE/CytaBOM, and MACOP-B.[273] This trial was carried out because of enthusiasm generated by single-arm trials showing apparent superiority of m-BACOD, ProMACE/CytaBOM, and MACOP-B over the older CHOP regimen. This study of 899 patients showed no improvement in failure-free survival or OS with the newer regimen but did find increased toxicity with m-BACOD and MACOP-B. The 6-year OS for the four regimens were CHOP, 33%; m-BACOD, 36%; ProMACE/CytaBOM, 34%; and MACOP-B, 32%. The conclusion from the study was that the less complicated and less expensive CHOP regimen should be considered the treatment of choice. This has been widely applied, and today most patients with DLBCL or other aggressive lymphomas receive CHOP-based chemotherapy.

Attempts have been made to improve the response to CHOP by combining it with the monoclonal antibody rituximab. The Groupe d'Etude des Lymphomes de l'Adulte (GELA) group randomized 399 previously untreated patients with DLBCL, 60 to 80 years old, to receive either eight cycles of CHOP every 3 weeks or eight cycles of CHOP plus rituximab given on day 1 of each cycle.[274] With a median follow-up of 2 years, the addition of rituximab to the CHOP regimen increased the CR rate (76% vs. 63%; P = .005) and prolonged event-free survival and OS in these patients, without a clinically significant increase in toxicity.

A larger (n = 632) intergroup United States study randomized a similar population of patients to CHOP versus CHOP with rituximab.[275] Responding patients then were randomized to receive either rituximab maintenance therapy (four doses every 6 months for 2 years) or no maintenance. Three-year failure-free survival rate was 53% for R-CHOP patients and 46% for CHOP patients (P = .04) at a median follow-up time of 3.5 years. There was no effect of maintenance in patients treated initially with R-CHOP. In a secondary analysis excluding maintenance rituximab patients, R-CHOP alone reduced the risks of treatment failure (P = .003) and death (P = .05) compared with CHOP alone.

Based on these results, CHOP with rituximab therapy (all therapy administered on day 1) has emerged to become the standard initial treatment for advanced-stage DLBCL in the United States. Subgroup analyses have suggested that the benefit of rituximab is most present in patients with lymphoma that overexpressed bcl-2 on IHC analysis,[276] in patients that expressed p21,[277] or in patients with bcl-6–negative tumors.[278]

Other attempts to improve the response to CHOP involve adjuvant therapy with high-dose therapy and autologous bone marrow transplantation.[279] Several studies have now concluded that all patients with aggressive lymphoma do not benefit when stem cell transplantation is incorporated into their initial treatment strategy compared with patients who are treated with conventional strategy of initial chemotherapy followed by stem cell transplant at first relapse.[280,281] Thus, there seems to be no indication to add ASCT to the initial combination chemotherapy treatment for *all* patients with aggressive lymphoma.

However, when the IPI[98] was retrospectively applied to the GELA LNH-87 study, a failure-free (59% vs. 39%) and OS benefit (65% vs. 52%) was demonstrated for the high-/intermediate-risk and high-risk groups.[282] A retrospective subset analysis of an Italian trial yielded similar results.[281]

All positive trials have incorporated a standard course of induction therapy (rather than an abbreviated course) before consolidative transplantation and have not included rituximab therapy in induction. An international consensus conference reached the conclusion that autologous high-dose therapy and autotransplantation in patients with high-risk IPI scores seemed to provide benefit,[283] and this is the subject of a completed but not yet analyzed intergroup randomized trial in the United States. At the present time, the authors do not recommend routine use of ASCT as consolidative therapy for newly diagnosed large cell lymphoma outside a clinical trial.

Investigators at the National Cancer Institute have published impressive single-institution and multicenter studies of an infusional version of CHOP given with etoposide ("EPOCH") combined with rituximab.[284–286] Outcomes of this regimen appear particularly favorable compared with historical controls in patients with activated B-cell lymphomas. The Cancer and Lymphoma Group B is currently conducting a randomized trial comparing R-CHOP with EPOCH-R for patients with advanced-stage DLBCL.

The German High-Grade Lymphoma Group has suggested that time-intensive therapy, giving CHOP every 14 days rather than every 21 days, has superior outcomes,[287] and that six cycles of R-CHOP 14 is equivalent to eight cycles.[288] The British and French groups have compared R-CHOP 14 with R-CHOP 21 in randomized trials; preliminary results demonstrate equivalent response rates. At the present time, we recommend R-CHOP 21 as standard induction therapy for advanced-stage DLBCL.

Salvage Therapy

The phrase *salvage therapy* encompasses subsequent treatment administered to patients who failed to achieve an initial remission and the treatment administered to patients who relapse from complete remission. A major prognostic factor for patients receiving any form of salvage therapy relates to the chemotherapy sensitivity of the lymphoma (i.e., those who achieve an initial complete remission and then relapse generally have a better prognosis than patients who are primarily resistant to chemotherapy). Patients with lymphoma that progresses on the previous chemotherapy regimen have a poorer outlook than those who have stable or partially responding disease. Patients who have been in complete remission and then relapse require a rebiopsy before salvage therapy is initiated. Some patients who present with DLBCL are found to have a FL at the time of relapse.

The initial step in planning salvage chemotherapy is to determine the goal of treatment. Some patients who fail to achieve an initial remission or relapse from complete remission can be cured. This is less likely in elderly patients, those with extensive disease, and those with a poor performance status. In such patients less intensive, palliative treatments might be better pursued.

Radiotherapy can frequently be used to alleviate the symptoms at a particular site of involvement in patients with relapsed DLBCL. This can frequently be accomplished with minimal morbidity. However, the chance for cure with salvage RT is extremely small. Palliative chemotherapy approaches include single-agent treatment with vincristine, cytarabine, alkylating agents, or anthracyclines. Responses to single-agent rituximab occur approximately 30% of the time and are generally of brief duration.[289]

Most patients receive second-line combination chemotherapy regimens. These regimens usually incorporate drugs such as cisplatin, ifosfamide, etoposide, and cytarabine, often in combination with rituximab. For example, Memorial Sloan-Kettering Cancer Center has published results of ICE chemotherapy (ifosfamide, carboplatin, and etoposide), in patients with recurrent aggressive NHL.[290] The overall response rate was 66%, with no treatment-related mortality. This was a very effective cytoreduction and mobilization regimen in patients with NHL and has become a widely used salvage option for those who are eligible for subsequent ASCT. Preliminary results from the CORAL study, which randomized patients requiring salvage therapy to R-ICE versus R-DHAP (dexamethasone, cytarabine, and cisplatin), suggested no difference between these regimens, with response rates of 66% in both arms.[291]

A subset of completely responding patients can be long-term survivors, with the overall cure rate for salvage chemotherapy in patients with relapsed DLBCL being approximately 5% to 10%.

An international randomized trial referred to as the *PARMA study* defined the role of bone marrow transplant in relapsed DLBCL prior to rituximab.[119] In this trial, 109 patients who had relapsed from complete remission and responded to two cycles of DHAP were randomly allocated to high-dose chemotherapy using the BEAC regimen (carmustine, etoposide, cytarabine, and cyclophosphamide) or continued treatment with DHAP. Both groups were to receive involved-field RT. Bone marrow transplantation was associated with a superior failure-free survival (51% vs. 12% at 5 years) and OS (53% vs. 32% at 5 years). It is important to remember that the trial enrolled only young patients at first relapse who remained chemosensitive. Although this is the only randomized trial in this patient population, a United States cooperative group phase 2 trial achieved nearly identical results in a similar patient population.[292] Salvage autologous bone marrow transplant (ABMT), as currently used, however (in patients relapsing after rituximab-containing chemotherapy), results in survival of approximately 30% of all patients who actually receive transplants. Attempts at improving outcome of autologous transplant have included the addition of radioimmunotherapy to conditioning regimens,[293] and evaluating novel agents as maintenance posttransplantation. For these patients, however, high-dose therapy and autologous bone marrow transplantation are the treatments of choice.

Allogeneic bone marrow transplantation has been used less frequently for patients with DLBCL. Although occasional patients failing autologous transplantation can have prolonged survival with allogeneic transplantation, overall results from the North American Bone Marrow Transplant Registry have favored autologous transplantation. In a report from the European Bone Marrow Transplantation Registry, recurrence rates after allogeneic transplantation were lower than those after autologous transplantation.[294] However, there was no OS advantage by increased transplant-related mortality after allogeneic transplantation. Ongoing studies in high-risk patients are evaluating "tandem" transplantation (autologous transplant followed by nonmyeloablative allogeneic transplantation), with encouraging preliminary results.

Primary Mediastinal (Thymic) Large B-Cell Lymphoma

Mediastinal (thymic) large B-cell lymphoma, originally a subtype of DLBCL arising in the mediastinum, is now classified as a separate disease entity based in large part on strong gene expression profiling data. These lymphomas are from a putative thymic B-cell origin, with distinctive clinical, immunophenotypic, and genotypic features.

Morphology

Primary mediastinal large B-cell lymphoma usually involves the thymus at presentation. The tumor is composed of large cells with variable nuclear features, resembling centroblasts, large centrocytes, or multilobated cells, often with abundant clear cytoplasm in a background of fine, compartmentalizing sclerosis. The major differential diagnoses are thymoma, germ cell tumor, and Hodgkin lymphoma, and otherwise usual DLBCL involving the mediastinum.

Immunophenotype and Genetic Features

The tumor cells are usually surface immunoglobulin–negative but express B-cell–associated antigens (CD19, CD20, CD22, CD79a) and CD45.[295] Most cases are bcl-6–positive, and approximately 25% are CD10-positive. Immunoglobulin heavy- and light-chain genes are rearranged. The *BCL2* and *BCL6* genes are usually untranslocated. Expression of FIG1, amplification of the *REL* oncogene at chromosome 9p, and overexpression of the *MAL* gene at chromosome 2p13-15 are all characteristic of primary mediastinal B-cell lymphoma and not other DLBCLs.[296] Overexpression of the *JAK2-STAT5* pathway is also characteristic and has been related to deletion of the *SOCS1* gene in cell lines.[297,298]

By gene expression profiling, primary mediastinal large B-cell lymphoma shows an expression signature distinct from nodal DLBCL, including overexpression of the *MAL* and *FIG1* genes. Gene express profiling analysis also discovered similarities to Hodgkin lymphoma. In particular, loss of expression of B-cell receptor signaling genes and activation of both the *JAK-2* and NFκ pathways were noticed, implying overlapping mechanisms of lymphomagenesis. The observation that primary mediastinal large B-cell lymphoma and Hodgkin lymphoma have some similarities in gene expression pattern may also shed light on the rare lymphomas known as *mediastinal gray zone* lymphomas, which have features of both Hodgkin lymphoma and NHL.[299]

Postulated Normal Counterpart

The postulated normal counterpart is a B cell of the thymic medulla.

Clinical Features and Therapy

Primary DLBCL of the mediastinum is a distinct clinicopathologic entity, requiring knowledge of morphology, immunophenotype, and presenting site for the diagnosis.[115] It accounted for 7% of DLBCLs (2.4% of all NHLs) in the international REAL study. It has a female predominance and a median age in the fourth decade; patients present with a locally invasive anterior mediastinal mass originating in the thymus, with frequent airway compromise and superior vena cava syndrome.[300] Relapses tend to be extranodal, including liver, gastrointestinal tract, kidneys, ovaries, and CNS.

Although early studies suggested an unusually aggressive, incurable tumor, others have reported cure rates similar to those for other large cell lymphomas with aggressive therapy, usually combining chemotherapy with mediastinal irradiation. With no evidence to the contrary, the authors recommend treating these patients similarly to other patients with localized diffuse large cell lymphoma (i.e., CHOP + rituximab and involved-field RT for patients presenting with localized disease or bulky disease). The prognosis of patients with localized mediastinal large cell NHL is similar to that of other patients with poor-prognosis, early-stage disease; approximately 50% of patients are alive without disease at 5 years. Individuals with disseminated disease should be treated like other patients with disseminated DLBCL.

In a study by Zinzani et al.,[301] 50 patients with primary mediastinal large B-cell lymphoma were prospectively treated with MACOP-B followed by RT. CT and gallium 67 citrate single-photon emission (GaSPECT) were obtained at diagnosis, at the end of chemotherapy, and at 3 months after RT. Three patients with progressive disease during chemotherapy were excluded from the analysis. After chemotherapy, 31 of 47 (66%) patients had a positive GaSPECT. Among these 31 patients, 22 became GaSPECT-negative after RT. None of the patients with a negative GaSPECT after treatment relapsed at a median follow-up of 39 months.

Other Large B-Cell Lymphomas

Intravascular Large B-Cell Lymphoma

Rare cases of large B-cell lymphoma present with a disseminated intravascular pattern, involving small blood vessels, without an obvious extravascular tumor mass or leukemia. This tumor has also been variously known as *intravascular lymphomatosis*, *angiotropic lymphoma*, and *malignant angioendotheliomatosis*. The neoplastic lymphoid cells are contained within the lumina of small vessels in many organs. The tumor cells may resemble centroblasts or immunoblasts and express B-cell–associated antigens and are usually CD10-negative, IRF4/MUM1-positive by IHC. The cell of origin is thought to be a transformed peripheral B cell. The organs most commonly involved are brain, kidneys, lungs, adrenals, skin, and bone marrow, but virtually any site may be involved. Patients present with a variety of symptoms related to organ dysfunction secondary to vascular occlusion. Because of this, the diagnosis is often not suspected and many reported cases are diagnosed at autopsy. This is an extremely aggressive lymphoma that responds poorly to chemotherapy. However, recent publications have suggested the outcome of this histology has improved with the addition of rituximab.[302,303]

Large B-Cell Lymphoma, Lymphomatoid Granulomatosis Type

The entity described as lymphomatoid granulomatosis has been shown in most cases to be an EBV-positive large B-cell lymphoma with a T-cell–rich background.[304] Patients typically present with extranodal disease, most commonly involving lung, CNS, and/or kidneys. Evidence of past or present immunosuppression may be found. The infiltrates show extensive necrosis, often with only a few atypical large B cells in a background of small T lymphocytes; the infiltrate may be angiocentric as well as angioinvasive. Lymphomatoid granulomatosis is graded according to the number of large B cells. The lower-grade cases are not typically treated as an aggressive lymphoma; grade 3 cases fulfill the criteria for large B-cell lymphoma in a T-cell–rich background and may be clinically aggressive. The cell of origin is thought to be an EBV-transformed B cell. The prognosis for this entity is variable and in general is approached[97] with immunotherapy (rituximab or interferon) for low-grade cases, with standard immunochemotherapy used for disseminated DLBCL in higher grade cases. In addition to combination chemotherapy, responses have been reported using high-dose therapy and autologous stem cell support.[304]

Primary Effusion Lymphoma

Primary effusion lymphoma is a recently recognized disease that occurs most often in immunosuppressed patients, either with HIV or in the posttransplant setting, but occasional cases in nonimmunosuppressed patients have been reported.[28] Patients present with effusions in serous cavities—pleura, pericardium, or peritoneum. Occasionally, infiltration of other tissues may be seen in the absence of an effusion. The tumor cells are large, often pleomorphic cells resembling either bizarre plasma cells or the cells of anaplastic large cell lymphoma. They often lack B-cell–associated antigens such as CD20, CD19, or CD22 and are bcl-6–negative but may be CD79a-positive and CD45-positive, sometimes contain cytoplasmic immunoglobulin, and often express CD30 and the plasma cell–associated antigen CD138. Immunoglobulin genes are clonally rearranged. They typically contain EBV and the Kaposi sarcoma herpesvirus/HHV-8.[305] The cell of origin is thought to be a post–germinal center B cell. The prognosis of this disease is very poor.[97]

DLBCL Associated with Chronic Inflammation

These lymphomas are found in situation of long-term chronic inflammation. Most cases involve body cavities or narrow spaces. The typical situation is pyothorax-associated lymphoma, sometimes from patients with artificial pneumothorax for treatment of pulmonary tuberculosis. Males are predominantly affected. Most cases have been described in Japan. The tumors are typically associated with latent EBV infection and may produce IL-10 in order to escape immunosurveillance. IL-6 is also an autocrine and paracrine growth factor. After the pleural cavity, bone, joint, and periparticular soft tissue are the most common sites of involvement. Most cases have typical centroblastic/immunoblastic morphology and sometimes plasmacytic differentiation. The cell of origin is thought to be an EBV-transformed late germinal center/post–germinal center B cell. This is an aggressive B-cell lymphoma with poor 5-year OS.[97]

Large B-Cell Lymphoma Arising in HHV8-Associated Multicentric Castleman Disease

This is a large B-cell lymphoma arising most often in HIV-positive patients with multicentric Castleman disease. Although the lymph node may show background changes of Castleman disease, the confluent sheets of large B cells effacing the lymph node architecture are key to the diagnosis. The cells are often plasmablastic in appearance and express the HHV8 viral proteins, LANA1 as well as cytoplasmic IgM with variable expression of B cell and plasma cell antigens. EBV is negative. The cell of origin is thought to be an HHV8-infected naïve B cell. Nodal, splenic, extranodal, and blood involvement have been reported. Kaposi sarcoma may be concurrent. This is a highly aggressive lymphoma with a median survival of only a few months.[97]

PRACTICE OF ONCOLOGY

Plasmablastic Lymphoma

Plasmablastic lymphoma (PBL) consists of B cells with the appearance of immunoblasts, which, however, express the immunophenotype of plasma cells (positive for CD38, CD138, and IRF4/MUM1). Originally described in the oral cavity of HIV-positive patients, this disease can be associated with other types of immunodeficiency (autoimmune or therapy-induced). The cells are typically EBV-infected. The cell of origin is thought to be a blastic proliferative B cell that has switched its phenotype to a plasma cell stage of differentiation. Tumors may arise in patients with a previous history of plasma cell myeloma; however, these should be considered plasmablastic transformations of the underlying myeloma rather than a plasmablastic lymphoma.[97]

ALK-Positive Large B-Cell Lymphoma

This is a rare variant of large B-cell lymphomas that expresses the ALK1 protein, but lacks the t(2;5)(p23;35) found in the T/NK cell anaplastic large cell lymphomas. In these B-cell lymphomas, ALK may be full length or may be associated with a Clathrin-ALK fusion protein. The latter results in a distinctive pattern of granular cytoplasmic expression of ALK-1 when examined by IHC analysis. The cell of origin is thought to be a post–germinal center B cell with plasma cell differentiation.[97]

B-Cell Lymphoma, Unclassifiable

Borderline cases of large B-cell lymphoma with features intermediate between diffuse large B-cell lymphoma and Burkitt lymphoma or classic Hodgkin lymphoma are now being described. The former are often associated with double-hit genetics (rearrangements of both the *BCL2* and *MYC* oncogenes). The latter are part of the group of lymphomas known as *grey zone* lymphomas. Whether these evolve into distinct entities or are folded back into variants of DLBCL, Burkitt lymphoma, or Hodgkin lymphoma remains to be determined.[97] Recent studies have suggested these lymphomas have an extremely poor prognosis even with the addition of rituximab to standard CHOP chemotherapy, particularly when both BCL-2 and MYC rearrangements are present.[306,307]

In general, these lymphomas occur in older patients, making dose escalation difficult. These therefore represent a group of lymphomas that should be approached with novel agents in the clinical trials setting.

Burkitt Lymphoma/Leukemia

Burkitt lymphoma is a highly aggressive B-cell neoplasm, often presenting in extranodal sites or as an acute leukemia, composed of monomorphic, medium-sized cells with basophilic cytoplasm and an extremely high proliferation rate. Translocation and deregulation of *MYC* on chromosome 8 is a constant feature. EBV is found in a high proportion of the cases, particularly in the African endemic from. The morphology, immunophenotype, and genetics of Burkitt lymphoma/leukemia are discussed in detail in Chapter 100.

Burkitt lymphoma/leukemia was one of the first malignancies shown to be curable with chemotherapy,[308] and the majority of adult patients should be curable today with aggressive combination chemotherapy regimens. High-dose regimens (such as cyclophosphamide, vincristine, doxorubicin, methotrexate, ifosfamide, mesna, etoposide, cytarabine [CODOX-M-IVAC]) of fairly brief duration are frequently used to treat patients with Burkitt lymphoma/leukemia.[309] Importantly, these regimens include higher doses of alkylating agents than CHOP, and because of the propensity for CNS metastases, treatment regimens for Burkitt lymphoma/leukemia always involve prophylactic therapy to the CNS. Patients with localized disease are cured in approximately 90% of the cases with these intensive regimens, and cure rates in excess of 50% have been reported in patients with extensive disease.[310]

When treated with similar regimens, adults and children have similar outcomes, although the literature has limited information regarding outcome of older patients with this histology.[309,311] The addition of rituximab to hyper-CVAD-methotrexate-cytarabine has improved outcome compared to historical controls, and we recommend that rituximab be incorporated into treatment regimens for Burkitt lymphoma.[312] Salvage therapy for patients with relapsed Burkitt lymphoma/leukemia has generally been unsatisfactory. However, occasionally patients can be cured with autologous bone marrow transplantation.[259]

MATURE T-CELL AND NK CELL NEOPLASMS

Mycosis Fungoides

For a discussion of mycosis fungoides, see Chapter 128.

Adult T-Cell Lymphoma and Leukemia

Adult T-cell lymphoma and leukemia is a peripheral T-cell neoplasm usually composed of highly pleomorphic cells involving lymph nodes and peripheral blood and often skin and extranodal sites. ATL is caused by the human retrovirus HTLV-1 and is found in areas of the world where the virus is endemic.

Morphology

In lymph nodes, the infiltrate is diffuse with architectural effacement. Neoplastic cells are usually medium to large-sized with a high degree of nuclear pleomorphism, which may include giant cells with convoluted or cerebriform nuclei. Rare cases may be composed of small atypical lymphocytes or may resemble ALCL. Cells with hyperlobated nuclei (flower cells) are common in the peripheral blood in leukemic cases.

Immunophenotype and Genetic Features

Tumor cells express T-cell–associated antigens (CD2, CD3, and CD5) but usually lack CD7. Most cases are CD4+, CD8–, and strongly express the activation antigen CD25 (IL-2 receptor). Rare cases are CD4−, CD8+ or CD8+, CD4+.

Clonally integrated HTLV-1 genes are found in all cases. The *TCR* genes are clonally rearranged.[313] Abnormalities of chromosome 14q11, involving the *TCRα* gene, 14q32 involving the *IgH* gene, deletions at 6q, trisomy 3, and monosomy X and Y are common.[314] Complex karyotypes may be associated with a worse prognosis. Several viral genes appear to be involved in lymphomagenesis.

Postulated Normal Counterpart

The proposed normal counterpart is the T-regulatory cell.[315]

Clinical Features

ATL is one manifestation of infection by HTLV-1. Tropical spastic paraparesis and HTLV-1–associated myelopathy appear to be more common manifestations of infection than ATL. The diagnosis is established when a patient with a typical clinical and pathologic syndrome is found to have antibodies to HTLV-1. Most patients are adults, although children are occasionally seen with the disorder if they have received transfusions in infancy. The virus can be acquired by vertical transmission from mother to child, sexual transmission, or via blood products. Most cases occur in Japan or the Caribbean, with sporadic cases found elsewhere in the world.

In the United States, the diagnosis is frequently difficult; ATL is not considered because many clinicians are not acquainted with the syndrome. Several variants have been described depending on the clinical features: acute, lymphomatous, chronic, and smoldering. The most common *acute type* presents with neoplastic cells in the blood, skin rashes, generalized lymphadenopathy, hepatosplenomegaly, and hypercalcemia. The *lymphomatous type* is characterized by prominent lymphadenopathy but no blood involvement. The *chronic type* shows skin lesions and an increased white blood cell count with absolute lymphocytosis but no hypercalcemia. The *smoldering type* shows normal blood lymphocyte counts, with 5% circulating neoplastic cells. Patients frequently have skin or pulmonary lesions, but hypercalcemia is not present. Progression from chronic and smoldering to acute types eventually occurs in up to 25% of the cases. Peripheral blood and bone marrow are the most frequent sites of involvement, but any organ can be involved by the disease, including gastrointestinal tract, liver, lung, and CNS.

Therapy

The treatment of ATL has been unsatisfactory. Patients with the chronic or smoldering syndromes can sometimes be followed without therapy for extended periods of time. When the disease becomes asymptomatic, combination chemotherapy regimens have usually been used. Although patients may respond to the initial combination chemotherapy regimen, the OS remains poor, with fewer than 10% of the patients surviving 5 years after the initiation of therapy. A variety of the new treatment approaches have been studied, including new chemotherapeutic agents, monoclonal antibodies, biologic agents, and allogeneic bone marrow transplantation. In one study, 15 patients with T-cell leukemia/lymphoma, 8 of whom were in partial or complete remission, were treated with interferon-α and zidovudine.[316] Median survival of the nonresponders was 6 months, whereas 55% of the responders were alive at 4 years. Recent consensus recommendations have been issued suggesting a therapeutic strategy based on the clinical subclassification and prognostic factors, with options including watchful waiting approach, chemotherapy, antiviral therapy, allogeneic hematopoietic stem cell transplantation, and targeted therapies.[317]

Peripheral T-Cell Lymphoma, Unspecified

Peripheral T-cell lymphoma, unspecified, comprises a group of nodal and extranodal T-cell lymphomas that do not have consistent immunophenotypic, genetic, or clinical features. Because of their relative rarity and heterogeneity, it has been impossible to arrive at a generally useful classification system for these diseases. However, as additional disease entities are identified and moved into their own categories, this category may eventually become better defined. For the time being, these tumors are simply designated "peripheral T-cell lymphomas, unspecified."

Morphology

Peripheral T-cell lymphomas, not otherwise categorized, typically contain a mixture of small and large atypical cells, which may have irregular, round to oval, and sometimes immunoblastic nuclei. An inflammatory background including admixed eosinophils or epithelioid histiocytes may be numerous. High endothelial venules are often increased (Fig. 127.5). In lymph nodes, peripheral T-cell lymphomas, not otherwise categorized, manifest as paracortical expansions or may completely efface the node. Outside lymph nodes, peripheral T-cell lymphomas, not otherwise categorized, are generally diffuse, may invade epithelium, and may be angiocentric and therefore associated with necrosis.

Three variants are currently recognized: (1) lymphoepithelioid (Lennert lymphoma) for cases rich in epithelioid cells; (2) follicular variant for cases with colonization of the lymphoid follicles suggestive of B-cell FL; and (3) T-zone variant for cases with a perifollicular growth pattern.

Immunophenotype and Genetic Features

T-cell–associated antigens are variably expressed, and aberrant immunophenotypes are common (CD3+/−, CD2+/−, CD5+/−, CD7−/+); CD4 is more often expressed than CD8, and tumors may be CD4− and CD8−. B-cell–associated antigens for the most part are lacking, although rare CD20+ cases have been reported. The *TCR* genes are usually clonally rearranged. Most cases have numeric and structural chromosomal abnormalities. Recurrent chromosomal gains at 7q, 8q, 17q, and 22q; recurrent losses at 4q, 5q, 6q, 9p, 10q, 12q, and 13q have been noted. Complex[318,319] karyotypes are common in cases with larger cells.[320]

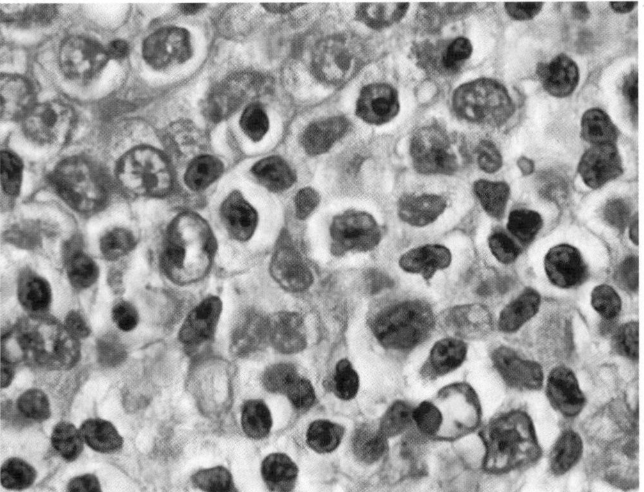

FIGURE 127.5 Peripheral T-cell lymphoma showing a spectrum of intermediate-sized to large atypical lymphocytes with oval to irregular nuclei, many with clear cytoplasm; an eosinophil is present.

Postulated Normal Counterpart

The cell of origin is thought to be an activated mature T cell, usually CD4+ memory type. However, this category is heterogeneous.

Clinical Features

Peripheral T-cell lymphomas accounted for only 6% of lymphomas in the international study of the REAL, reflecting their rarity in American and European populations.[115] The median age of patients was in the seventh decade, and 65% of the patients had stage IV disease. Blood eosinophilia, pruritus, and hemophagocytic syndromes may occur; lymph nodes, skin, liver, spleen, and other viscera may be involved. The clinical course is aggressive, and relapses may be more common than in large B-cell lymphoma. In the international REAL study, this group had one of the lowest overall and failure-free survival rates.

Therapy

Treatment regimens used for peripheral T-cell lymphoma have historically been the same as those used for DLBCL, with the omission of rituximab. Because of the poorer OS in peripheral T-cell lymphoma as compared with DLBCL, bone marrow transplantation is more frequently required, and frequently used to consolidate first remission. Bone marrow transplantation may be as effective in peripheral T-cell lymphoma as in DLBCL.[321] In the setting of recurrent disease, purine analogues, gemcitabine, and Campath-1H (anti-CD52 monoclonal antibody) may have modest activity. Recently a novel antifolate drug, pralatrexate, has been approved as a single agent for the treatment of relapsed/refractory peripheral T-cell lymphoma, with response rates of approximately 30% in a multicenter pivotal trial.[322]

Angioimmunoblastic T-Cell Lymphoma

Angioimmunoblastic T-cell lymphoma is a peripheral T-cell lymphoma characterized by systemic disease, a polymorphous infiltrate involving lymph nodes, and a prominent proliferation of high endothelial venules and FDCs. Associated EBV-positive transformed B cells are often present.

Morphology

The nodal architecture is effaced. Peripheral sinuses are typically open and even dilated, but the abnormal infiltrate often extends beyond the capsule into the perinodal fat. Prominent arborizing high endothelial venules are present, many of which show thickened or hyalinized periodic acid-Schiff–positive walls. Clusters of epithelioid histiocytes and numerous eosinophils and plasma cells may be present. Expanded aggregates of FDCs, visible on immunostained sections, surround the proliferating blood vessels and may have the appearance of "burnt-out" germinal centers. The lymphoid cells are a mixture of small lymphocytes, immunoblasts, plasma cells, and medium-sized cells with round nuclei and clear cytoplasm. B-immunoblasts may be numerous and may occasionally become so numerous and sheetlike as to qualify for a second diagnosis of an associated large B-cell lymphoma.

Immunophenotype and Genetic Features

Tumor cells express T-cell–associated antigens (CD2+, CD3+, CD4+, CD5+, and CD7−) and usually CD4, but many nonneoplastic CD4+ and CD8+ cells are often present; CD4 may be lost on some or all of the cells. CD10 expression on some of the neoplastic T cells has been reported in the majority of the cases, as is expression of the bcl-6 protein, CXCL13, and PD-1, in most cases leading to the interpretation that these are neoplasms of T-follicular helper cells.[323–325] Expanded clusters of CD21+, CD35+, CD23+, and FDCs are present in extrafollicular areas and around proliferated venules. The latter feature is useful in distinguishing this disorder from other T-cell lymphomas. Polyclonal plasma cells and B-immunoblasts may be numerous.

The *TCR* genes are rearranged in 75% and IgH in 10%, corresponding to expanded B-cell clones. EBV genomes are detected in many cases and are usually in the large B cells. Trisomy 3 or 5, or both, is common.[326]

Postulated Normal Counterpart

The normal counterpart is presumed to be a CD4+ follicular helper T cell.

Clinical Features

Angioimmunoblastic T-cell lymphoma is one of the more common peripheral T-cell lymphomas encountered in Western countries. In the Kiel Registry, it accounted for 20% of all T-cell lymphomas and approximately 4% of all lymphomas. Angioimmunoblastic T-cell lymphoma is clinically distinctive: Patients typically have generalized lymphadenopathy, fever, weight loss, skin rash, and polyclonal hypergammaglobulinemia and are susceptible to infections. The course is moderately aggressive, with occasional spontaneous remissions, and is not reliably predicted by the histologic appearance.

Therapy

Approximately 30% of the patients may have initial remission on corticosteroids alone, but most require some form of cytotoxic chemotherapy. Median survivals range from 15 to 24 months, and curability has not been well established. In some patients, a secondary EBV-positive large B-cell lymphoma develops. A prospective but nonrandomized trial compared an anthracycline-based combination chemotherapy regimen with prednisone followed by combination chemotherapy only if the disease progressed. Initial chemotherapy yielded a higher complete remission rate (64% vs. 29%) and median survival (19 vs. 11 months).[327]

Extranodal Natural Killer/T-Cell Lymphoma, Nasal Type

Extranodal NK/T-cell lymphoma, nasal type, is an extranodal lymphoma, usually with an NK-cell phenotype and EBV-positive, with a broad morphologic spectrum and with frequent necrosis and angioinvasion, most commonly presenting in the midfacial region but also in other extranodal sites (palate, skin, soft tissue, gastrointestinal tract, and testis). Although most cases appear to be of NK lineage, it is designated NK/T because some have a cytotoxic T-cell phenotype. Previous synonyms have included malignant midline reticulosis, polymorphic reticulosis, lethal midline granuloma, angiocentric immunoproliferative lesion, and angiocentric T-cell lymphoma.

Morphology

Extranodal NK/T-cell lymphoma is typically characterized by a polymorphous infiltrate composed of a mixture of normal-appearing small lymphocytes and atypical lymphoid cells of varying size, along with plasma cells and occasionally eosinophils and histiocytes. A characteristic feature is invasion of vascular walls and occlusion of lumina by lymphoid cells with varying degrees of cytologic atypia; however, this is not seen in all the cases. Prominent ischemic necrosis of tumor cells and normal tissue is usually present. Because the most characteristic presentation is midfacial and the cells have T- and NK-cell features, the term *extranodal NK/T-cell lymphoma, nasal-type* was chosen by the WHO classification.

Immunophenotype and Genetic Features

The atypical cells in most cases are CD2+, CD56+, surface CD3−, and cytoplasmic CD3+. They are typically CD4− and CD8− but may express CD4 or CD7. Most cases express cytotoxic granule proteins such as granzyme B, perforin, and TIA-1.

The *TCR* and *Ig* genes are usually germ line, indicating an NK cell neoplasm rather than a T-cell neoplasm in most cases. EBV genomes are nearly universally present and clonal. EBV expression is detectable in most cases by *in situ* hybridization for EBV-encoding RNA (EBER)-1.[328] The most common cytogenetic abnormality is del(6)(q21;q25) or i(6)(p10).

Postulated Normal Counterpart

The normal counterpart is an activated NK cell in most cases and a cytotoxic T cell in some cases.

Clinical Features

Nasal-type T/NK lymphoma is a rare disorder in the United States and Europe but is more common in Asia and in native populations in Peru. It may affect children or adults. Extranodal sites are invariably involved, including nose, palate, upper airway, gastrointestinal tract, and skin. The clinical course is typically aggressive, with relapses in other extranodal sites. Hemophagocytic syndromes may occur. Some cases of the aggressive variant of NK cell leukemia and lymphoma may be related to this disorder.

Therapy

Patients with localized NK/T-cell lymphoma in the nasal pharynx can be cured with a combination of chemotherapy and local radiotherapy. With radiotherapy alone, treatment failure is frequent. Patients with disseminated NK/T-cell lymphoma have an extremely poor outlook. Occasional long-term survivors are seen who have been using the CHOP regimen. Recently, a study of concomitant chemotherapy using multidrug resistance–nonrelated agents and etoposide and radiation has demonstrated improved response rates compared with historical controls.[329] Usually intensity-modulated RT is used for planning and treatment so as to avoid a high dose to other crucial organs. Ideally, up to 55 Gy are given; less aggressive regimens have a uniformly poor outcome.

High-dose chemotherapy and autologous bone marrow transplantation can be curative in some patients after relapse from standard therapy. Because of the poor results with standard chemotherapeutic approaches, incorporation of bone marrow transplantation as a primary management of patients with disseminated NK/T-cell lymphoma in the setting of a clinical trial may be appropriate.

Enteropathy-Type T-Cell Lymphoma

Enteropathy-type T-cell lymphoma is a tumor of intraepithelial T lymphocytes, usually involving the small intestine, showing varying degrees of cytologic transformation, and associated with childhood or adult onset of celiac disease, or histologic evidence of the disorder, HLADQA1*0501, DQB1*0201 genotype, and serum antigliadin antibodies. A second type, termed *type II EATL,* is not associated with a particular HLA type or celiac disease.

Morphology

On gross examination, circumferentially oriented jejunal ulcers are present, often multiple and frequently with perforation. A mass may or may not be present. The tumor may involve liver, spleen, lymph nodes, and other viscera, such as the stomach, gallbladder, and skin.

The tumors contain a variable admixture of small, medium/mixed, large, or anaplastic tumor cells, often with a high content of intraepithelial T cells in adjacent mucosa. Rare cases contain small to medium-sized monomorphic cells (usually type II EATL). Large numbers of histiocytes and eosinophils are often present and may obscure the tumor cells.

The adjacent mucosa may or may not show villous atrophy; this varies depending on the segment analyzed because in celiac sprue, villous atrophy is most prominent in the proximal small intestine and may be absent in distal jejunum or ileum. Early lesions may show mucosal ulceration with only scattered atypical cells and numerous reactive histiocytes, without formation of large masses; these lesions are nonetheless clonal. Intraepithelial lymphocytes in adjacent mucosa may also be clonal. Clonal *TCR* gene rearrangements have been found in cases of celiac disease that is unresponsive to a gluten-free diet (refractory sprue), suggesting that these cases represent early T-cell lymphoma.

Immunophenotype and Genetic Features

The tumor cells express pan-T-antigens (CD3+, CD5−, and CD7+), are usually CD4− and CD8−/+, and express the mucosal lymphoid antigen CD103. Expression of cytotoxic T-cell–associated proteins (granzyme B, TIA-1, perforin) is seen in many of the cases. CD30 may be positive in some cells. Type II is more often CD8+ and CD56+. In both types, lymphocytes in adjacent mucosa usually have a phenotype identical to that of the lymphoma.

The *TCRβ* gene is clonally rearranged; no specific cytogenetic abnormality has been described. As noted previously, patients have the HLA DQA1*0501, DQB1*0201 genotype associated with celiac disease. Partial trisomy of chromosome 1q is found in 16% of cases and has been detected in intraepithelial T cells in cases of refractory celiac sprue.[330]

Postulated Normal Counterpart

The normal counterpart is believed to be an intestinal intraepithelial T cell.

Clinical Features and Therapy

Enteropathy-type T-cell lymphoma occurs in adults, typically with a rather brief history of gluten-sensitive enteropathy, as the initial event in a patient found to have villous atrophy in the resected intestine, or without evidence of enteropathy but with either or both antigliadin antibodies or the typical HLA type (DQA1*0501, DQB1*0201) in patients with celiac disease. It is uncommon in most areas of the United States and Europe but is seen with increased frequency in places in which gluten-sensitive enteropathy is common. Treatment of celiac disease with a gluten-free diet effectively prevents the development of lymphoma, so that lymphoma does not usually develop in patients diagnosed with celiac disease early in life, and patients with lymphoma rarely have a long history of celiac disease. Patients present with abdominal pain, often associated with jejunal perforation; stomach or colon is affected less often, and other viscera, skin, or soft tissues may be involved. The course is aggressive, and death usually occurs from multifocal intestinal perforation due to refractory malignant ulcers. A poor response to therapy has been reported. It is probably related to the severe nutritional and immunologic abnormalities found in patients with uncontrolled celiac disease.

Hepatosplenic T-Cell Lymphoma

Hepatosplenic T-cell lymphoma is an extranodal, systemic neoplasm of cytotoxic T cells, usually expressing the $\gamma\delta$ T-cell receptor, but occasionally the $\alpha\beta$, with sinusoidal infiltration of spleen, liver, and bone marrow. A significant minority of cases arise in patients with chronic immune suppression, such as following solid organ transplant. The peak incidence is in young adults with a male predominance.

Morphology

Hepatosplenic T-cell lymphoma produces a sinusoidal infiltrate in liver and spleen, as well as bone marrow, of medium-sized lymphoid cells with round nuclei, moderately condensed chromatin, and moderately abundant, pale cytoplasm. Mitotic activity is generally low. The white pulp is atrophic. Erythrophagocytosis may be prominent in splenic and bone marrow sinuses.

The *TCRγ* and *TCRδ* genes are rearranged; the *TCRβ* gene may be rearranged or germ line. The tumor cells are EBV-negative. Isochromosome 7q is characteristic of both types; trisomy 8 is also common in many cases.

Immunophenotype and Genetic Features

The tumor cells are CD2+ and CD3+, and CD5−, CD4−, and CD8− ("double-negative"), CD16+ and CD56+/−, and most cases lack the $\alpha\beta$TCR protein, expressing instead the $\gamma\delta$ complex. Although there is currently no IHC test for expression of the $\gamma\delta$ protein in formalin-fixed paraffin-embedded tissue sections, lack of the staining for the $\alpha\beta$ receptor using the BF1 antibody, can be used as presumptive evidence of a $\gamma\delta$ phenotype. A number of clinically and histologically similar cases expressing the $\alpha\beta$ receptor have been reported. Cytotoxic granule protein TIA-1 is typically expressed, but granzyme B and perforin are absent, indicating a nonactivated cytotoxic T-cell phenotype.

Postulated Normal Counterpart

The postulated normal counterpart is an immature cytotoxic T cell, usually $\gamma\delta$ but occasionally $\alpha\beta$.

Clinical Features and Therapy

Hepatosplenic T-cell lymphoma is a rare neoplasm, and diagnosis is often difficult. Patients with this disease frequently present as with a multisystem disease, with hepatomegaly, splenomegaly, or both.[295] The absence of lymphadenopathy and the sinusoidal pattern of infiltration of the liver, spleen, and bone marrow make the diagnosis difficult. Frequently, only the demonstration of a T-cell gene rearrangement leads to the correct diagnosis.

A series of 21 patients with hepatosplenic T-cell lymphoma revealed the median age to be 34 years.[295] Patients had splenomegaly (n = 21), hepatomegaly (n = 15), and thrombocytopenia (n = 20). Unusual sites of involvement, such as skin, nasal cavity, gastrointestinal tract, lung, mucosa, and larynx, have also been described. Marrow involvement can be demonstrated by phenotyping in all patients. Isochromosome arm 7q was documented in 9 of 13 patients.

Subcutaneous Panniculitislike T-Cell Lymphoma

Subcutaneous panniculitislike T-cell lymphoma is a cytotoxic $\alpha\beta$ T-cell lymphoma that infiltrates subcutaneous tissues. It is composed of atypical lymphoid cells of varying size, often with necrosis and karyorrhexis, and sometimes associated with a hemophagocytic syndrome. Previously, some cases were included that derived from $\gamma\delta$ T cells, which were often double-negative (expressed neither CD4 nor CD8), had more prominent dermal involvement and possibly poorer outcome. These cases are now recategorized as part of the spectrum of primary cutaneous $\gamma\delta$ T-cell lymphomas.

Morphology

A variable mixture of small, medium, and large atypical cells is present in the subcutis, sparing the dermis, often containing irregular, hyperchromatic nuclei and pale cytoplasm. Apoptosis and karyorrhexis of tumor cells are prominent. Reactive histiocytes with phagocytized nuclear debris or lipid, or both, are numerous. Granulomas may be present. Individual adipocytes are characteristically rimmed by the neoplastic cells.

Immunophenotype and Genetic Features

Most cases express pan-T-antigens and usually CD8, although they may be CD4+ and express cytotoxic granule proteins TIA-1 and perforin and the $\alpha\beta$ TCR. No specific cytogenetic abnormalities have been described.

Postulated Normal Counterpart

The normal counterpart is a mature cytotoxic $\alpha\beta$ T cell.

Clinical Features and Therapy

Patients present with one or more subcutaneous nodules and are often misdiagnosed as having panniculitis. Hemophagocytic syndrome is common. The disease may present in an indolent fashion but typically becomes aggressive. Patients may respond to combination chemotherapy regimens, but the responses are usually transient. These lymphomas are generally radiosensitive, and radiotherapy can be used to control symptoms. However, the long-term outlook with this disorder is poor.

Anaplastic Large Cell Lymphoma, ALK-Negative and Anaplastic Large Cell Lymphoma, ALK-Positive

Anaplastic large T/null cell lymphoma, primary systemic type, is a T-cell lymphoma consisting of large lymphoid cells with pleomorphic, multiple, or horseshoe-shaped nuclei and abundant cytoplasm, a cohesive growth pattern, and sinusoidal spread in lymph nodes. These lymphomas uniformly express CD30, and either T-cell or no lineage-specific antigens. The pattern of disease involvement includes nodal or extranodal sites, but by definition is not limited to the skin, which would warrant a diagnosis of primary cutaneous anaplastic large cell lymphoma. ALK-positive cases and ALK-negative cases are categorized as distinct diseases in the WHO 2008 classification. The two entities are considered together here because of the overlapping morphologic and immunophenotypic features. However, a large clinical and immunophenotypic study demonstrated that although ALK-negative cases had a worse outcome than ALK-positive cases, they had clearly superior survival than peripheral T-cell lymphomas, not otherwise categorized, and should be separated from that more heterogeneous category.[331]

Morphology

The tumor is usually composed of large cells with round or pleomorphic, often horseshoe-shaped or multiple nuclei with multiple or single prominent nucleoli and with abundant cytoplasm, which gives the cells an epithelial or histiocytelike appearance. The so-called hallmark cell has an eccentric nucleus and a prominent, eosinophilic Golgi region. There can be a high degree of pleomorphism or a more monomorphic appearance. The tumor cells grow in a cohesive pattern and often preferentially involve the lymph node sinuses or paracortex. A small cell variant with a perivascular pattern is also recognized. The sinusoidal involvement can sometimes mimic a cohesive cell population such as a carcinoma. Lymphohistiocytic and small cell variants have been described, more commonly in children. Study of cytogenetic and molecular genetic abnormalities as well as clinical features suggests that these cases belong to the same disease entity as the more anaplastic cases.

Immunophenotype and Genetic Features

The tumor cells are CD30+ and usually express CD25 and epithelial membrane antigen; they are typically CD45+ and CD15−. Approximately 60% express one or more T-cell–associated antigens: CD2 and CD4 are most consistently expressed, as is CD43. CD3, CD5, and CD7 are often negative. Cytotoxic granule proteins are expressed by most cases. The ALK protein is detected in 60% to 85% of the cases using the ALK1 monoclonal antibody, showing nuclear and cytoplasmic staining in cases with the t(2;5), because nucleophosmin is a nuclear protein. Membrane or cytoplasmic staining may be seen in cases with variant translocations. ALK-positive cases are more common in children and have a better prognosis than ALK-negative cases.[332]

The majority of the cases have rearranged *TCR* genes; 10% have no rearrangement of *TCR* or *Ig* genes. Primary systemic ALCL often have a t(2;5)(p23;q35), which results in a fusion of the nucleophosmin gene on chromosome 5 to a novel tyrosine kinase gene on chromosome 2, called *ALK*.

In the current WHO 2008 classification, t(2;5)(p23;q35) and ALK protein presence or absence are considered defining features of two separate distinct clinical entities known as ALCL-ALK-positive and ALCL-ALK-negative. Importantly, the positive cases are clinically homogeneous: young patients with a relatively good prognosis; whereas ALK-negative cases are often older adults with more aggressive disease. Array comparative genomic hybridization has distinguished different chromosomal gains or losses between the two entities[333] as well as some similarities. Gene expression profiling studies have further confirmed differences between these ALK-positive and -negative cases.[334]

Postulated Cell of Origin

The postulated normal counterpart is an activated mature cytotoxic T cell.

Clinical Features

ALCL represents approximately 2% of all lymphomas, but approximately 10% of childhood lymphomas and 50% of large cell pediatric lymphomas. Primary systemic ALCL may involve lymph nodes or extranodal sites, including the skin, but is not localized to the skin. Tumors that present with systemic disease (with or without skin involvement) have a bimodal age distribution in children and adults, and are associated with the t(2;5), particularly in children, in 20% to 40% of the cases. Patients may present with isolated lymphadenopathy or extranodal disease in any site, including gastrointestinal tract and bone.[335] In adults the tumor is aggressive but potentially curable, similar to other aggressive lymphomas. Cases with the t(2;5) have a significantly better prognosis than cases that lack the t(2;5).

Therapy

Treatment regimens used for anaplastic cell lymphoma of the primary systemic type are the same as those used in DLBCL, without rituximab therapy. Treatment results have been excellent, with better survival in ALK-positive patients (71% to 93%) than in ALK-negative patients (31% to 37%). Preliminary results of two studies have suggested clinical activity of monoclonal antibodies directed against CD30 in patients with anaplastic T-cell lymphoma.[336]

SPECIAL CLINICAL SITUATIONS

Children

See Chapter 124 for a discussion of lymphomas and leukemias in children.

Elderly Patients

The incidence of NHL increases with age, and more than 50% of patients are beyond 60 years of age at diagnosis. The IPI demonstrated that NHL patients older than 60 years of age had a significantly lower complete remission rate, greater chance of relapsing from remission (relative risk, 1.8), and higher risk of death (relative risk, 1.96).[98] Several explanations may account for the poorer outcome in elderly adults. Some analyses have shown that older patients were more likely to have mortality from chemotherapy-related toxicity than younger patients, despite similar complete remission rates. Other studies have identified higher relapse rates in elderly patients. Still other analyses have shown inferior survival in elderly patients to be a result of increased deaths from cardiovascular disease and other nonrelapse causes. A Non-Hodgkin's Lymphoma Classification Project demonstrated that elderly patients were more likely to have a high IPI than were younger individuals.[337] Older patients are also more likely to have comorbid conditions. These factors have often led to arbitrary dose reductions or use of less aggressive therapy, which may reduce the possibility of cure. This is exemplified by Southwest Oncology Group studies that revealed a complete remission rate of 37% in patients 65 years of age and above who received initial 50% dose reductions of cyclophosphamide and doxorubicin.[338] Complete remission rates were 52%, a rate similar to those of younger patients, when full-dose chemotherapy was used.

Some analyses have shown that less intensive regimens may be associated with diminished mortality and equivalent outcomes when compared with more aggressive regimens in elderly NHL patients. In general, these regimens have used anthracyclines with less cardiotoxicity than doxorubicin, have substituted mitoxantrone for doxorubicin, or have used short-duration weekly therapy.[339] Although these regimens may be well tolerated, selection bias and lack of appropriate comparisons make it difficult to determine whether these novel regimens are superior to standard regimens, and more recent studies suggest that doxorubicin is superior to mitoxantrone in this population.[340]

Elderly patients who participate in clinical trials may be subject to selection bias, although these results suggest that these patients may be able to tolerate aggressive anthracycline-containing regimens. When adverse characteristics such as poor performance status are excluded, elderly NHL patients may have outcomes similar to those of younger patients.[341] The use of colony-stimulating factors may allow elderly patients to receive planned chemotherapy doses, although they may be less effective for the oldest patients and do not entirely prevent neutropenic complications. A randomized trial showed that the routine addition of granulocyte colony-stimulating factor to CHOP did not improve response rates or survival in elderly patients with aggressive lymphoma and that the rate of hospitalization and infection was not different between the two arms.[342] A nationwide study suggested that reduced relative dose intensity was more prevalent in older patients with lymphoma, with 60% of patients older than 60 years receiving relative dose intensity less than 85%.[343]

We initially approach elderly patients with aggressive lymphoma in a similar manner to younger patients, with intent to cure. Supportive care with filgrastim or pegfilgrastim, transfusions, and antibiotic support is often required. These patients may be eligible for ongoing national clinical trials and should be considered for participation whenever possible.

Posttransplant Lymphoproliferative Disorders

The risk of developing lymphoma is markedly increased after solid organ transplantation. PTLDs occur in 0.8% to 20.0% of transplanted patients.[344] Although a mortality of 60% to 80% is frequently reported, more favorable outcomes have been described. Identical disorders are seen after allogeneic bone marrow transplantation, especially in recipients of T-cell–depleted marrow. PTLDs are almost always EBV-related, although cases unrelated to EBV have been described. The development of PTLD results from proliferation of EBV-transformed B-cell clones when patients receive immunosuppressive therapy after transplantation.[345] Occasional cases of Hodgkin lymphoma and T-cell NHL have been reported. Most PTLDs after solid organ transplants are host-derived.

The histologic appearance of PTLD is highly variable. The WHO classification system includes the following categories:

1. Early lesions: reactive plasmacytic hyperplasia, infectious mononucleosislike
2. Polymorphic PTLD: infectious mononucleosislike appearance with architectural effacement and tissue destruction
3. Monomorphic PTLD (classified according to lymphoma classification schemes) including DLBCL, Burkitt/Burkitt-like, multiple myeloma, plasmacytoma, peripheral T-cell–unspecified, other types of T-cell lymphoma
4. Hodgkin and Hodgkin-like

PTLD after solid organ transplantation has several unique features, which differentiates it from NHL in the immunocompetent host. Most patients present with lymphadenopathy or a mass; however, extranodal involvement, a poor prognostic indicator in large cell lymphoma, is often present. In many series, isolated extranodal disease is the most common presentation of PTLD, and, similar to AIDS-related lymphoma, a minority of patients has disease confined to the lymphatic system. CNS involvement occurred in 22% of PTLDs in a registry experience of more than 1,000 patients.[346] Other common extranodal sites include the lung and gastrointestinal tract, which may be associated with a better prognosis. An unusual site of involvement is the allograft, which occurred 22% of the time in a study evaluating heart, lung, and liver transplants. Particularly in lung transplant patients, this phenomenon has been confused with rejection, emphasizing the importance of experienced hematopathology in evaluating questionable biopsies. Diagnosis is made by autopsy in a minority of cases, often when concomitant infection or rejection is present.

The two major risk factors for the development of PTLD after organ transplantation are pretransplant negative recipient EBV serology and the degree of posttransplant immunosuppression. Prophylactic approaches should include elimination, when possible, of these risk factors. Very few prospective trials of PTLD treatment have been performed, and management decisions must be individualized. Initial management should consist of reduction or cessation of immunosuppression. Patients in whom early-onset PTLD develops are most likely to benefit from this approach. Surgical excision or RT may be curative for patients with localized PTLD. Surgery should be considered for patients with isolated PTLD in renal transplants. Responses have also been reported with anti–B-cell monoclonal antibodies, including rituximab.[347] This modality is often considered before the use of chemotherapy, and a recent large series from Chicago suggests that patients who received rituximab-based therapy as part of initial treatment had 3-year PFS of 70% and OS 73% compared with 21% (*P* <.0001) and 33% (*P* = .0001), respectively, without rituximab.[348]

Patients who fail to respond to reduction of immunosuppression or antibody therapy should be treated with anthracycline-based combination chemotherapy combined with rituximab.[349,350] Durable remissions can be seen, although mortality is higher than in nonimmunosuppressed NHL patients. In the now uncommon setting of PTLD after bone marrow transplantation, donor leukocyte infusion is standard therapy and is highly effective.[351]

Human Immunodeficiency Virus–Associated Non-Hodgkin Lymphoma

The risk of developing NHL is markedly increased in patients infected with HIV type 1. Large cell lymphomas, small non–cleaved cell NHL, and primary CNS lymphoma are considered AIDS-defining conditions. AIDS-related lymphomas are nearly always B-cell neoplasms. Virtually all primary CNS lymphomas and approximately 50% of other AIDS-related NHLs are EBV-related. HIV lymphomas are roughly divided into the broad categories of lymphomas that also occur in immunocompetent patients, occurring more specifically in HIV-positive patients, and those also occurring in other immunodeficient states. Most cases are aggressive lymphomas, although the risk of low-grade NHL may also be increased. These latter lymphomas are not considered to be diagnostic of AIDS.

AIDS-associated NHL usually behaves aggressively. Systemic symptoms are common, along with involvement of extranodal sites. Gastrointestinal tract involvement is common, as well as unusual sites such as anus and rectum, skin and soft tissues, and heart. Approximately 15% of cases are primary CNS lymphomas.

Before the highly active antiretroviral therapy era, aggressive chemotherapy regimens were associated with significant toxicity. A randomized trial comparing m-BACOD with reduced-dose m-BACOD demonstrated median survival rates of 31 weeks and 35 weeks, respectively (*P* = .25), with less toxicity in the low-dose arm.[352] The AIDS Malignancy Consortium conducted a randomized trial comparing CHOP and rituximab therapy with standard CHOP chemotherapy. This trial suggested similar CR rates (58% vs. 50%) but a possible increased infection risk associated with rituximab in this setting, limited to the patients with low CD4 counts.[353]

Other investigators have advocated infusional chemotherapy regimens, such as EPOCH (etoposide, doxorubicin, vincristine, cyclophosphamide, prednisone), for these patients; and recently the AIDS Malignancy Consortium published results of a randomized phase 2 trial evaluating concurrent versus sequential EPOCH and rituximab. The outcome of patients treated with concurrent rituximab was superior, although patients with a baseline CD4 count less than 50/mcL had a high infectious death rate in the concurrent arm.[354]

In general, we recommend standard doses of CHOP or EPOCH, with rituximab, for these patients, in combination with highly active antiretroviral therapy. Antiretroviral therapy and prophylactic antibiotics should be continued during therapy. Opinions differ on the use of CNS prophylaxis, although patients with small non–cleaved cell histology and those with sinus or testicular involvement should receive prophylactic intrathecal therapy. For patients with relapsed or refractory disease, there is an evolving literature suggesting tolerability and clinical benefit to high-dose therapy and ASCT in selected settings.[355]

The prognosis for AIDS patients with primary CNS lymphoma is also poor, although the incidence of this has decreased in the era of highly antiretroviral therapy. Standard therapy has historically consisted of whole-brain irradiation, although median survival is 3 to 4 months. Patients may respond to high-dose methotrexate, and the role of combined modality therapy is being investigated. No standardized approaches have been developed for primary effusion lymphoma, and these patients should probably be treated like other patients with AIDS-related NHL.

Extranodal Sites

Primary Central Nervous System Lymphoma

Primary CNS lymphoma is the subject of Chapter 129.

Testicle

Primary testicular NHL accounts for approximately 1% to 9% of all testicular neoplasms frequently associated with involvement of Waldeyer's ring, skin and subcutaneous tissue, lung, and CNS.[356] Involvement of the contralateral testis is common at diagnosis or later in the course of disease. Most tumors are classified as diffuse large B-cell histology (most often the ABC subtype)[357] or immunoblastic lymphoma, although Burkitt lymphoma is common in children, and FLs and other histologic subtypes have been described.

Most series have reported poor outcomes with relatively few long-term survivors. The best results in patients with stage IE and IIE disease have been reported by the Vancouver Group following orchiectomy.[358] Patients were treated with a brief course of doxorubicin-based chemotherapy followed by scrotal radiation for stage IE patients and additional pelvic and para-aortic radiation for patients with stage IIE disease. The 4-year OS and relapse-free survival rates were 93%, as compared with 50% in a historic control group treated with orchiectomy and radiation alone. No relapses in the contralateral testis or CNS were observed, and the routine use of CNS prophylaxis was thought to be unnecessary.

However, other groups have reported CNS relapses and contralateral testis relapse after doxorubicin-based chemotherapy and RT in stage IE patients. High rates of parenchymal CNS relapse after aggressive combination chemotherapy[356] have led the authors to recommend high-dose systemic methotrexate prophylaxis in conjunction with standard CHOP and rituximab therapy. Because of low morbidity and the high rate of contralateral testis recurrence, the authors also recommend prophylactic scrotal radiation after completion of chemotherapy.

Skin

After the gastrointestinal tract, the skin is the second most common extranodal site primarily involved by NHL. As opposed to lymph nodes and most other extranodal sites of presentation of lymphoma, the skin is unusual in that T-cell lymphomas occur more frequently than B-cell lymphomas. The most common cutaneous T-cell lymphoma, mycosis fungoides, is dealt with in Chapter 128. The most common presentation is a new or unusual skin lesion.

Skin lymphomas can be classified using the WHO 2008 classification, which is a synthesis of the prior WHO classification and the European Organisation for Research on the Treatment of Cancer. These two entities held a consensus conference on cutaneous lymphoma classification, which has resulted in new clarity for the field.[359] An important feature of primary cutaneous lymphomas is that the clinical behavior may be different than when the same diagnosis is made in nodal or other extranodal sites. Importantly, full-thickness biopsies and clinical histories are often used for diagnosis. For example, the self-limiting, recurrent lesions of lymphomatoid papulosis are histologically and immunophenotypically similar to the more aggressive primary cutaneous ALCL.

Primary T-cell lymphomas of the skin include mycosis fungoides and its variants (folliculotropic pattern and granulomatous slack skin disease) and the CD30+ T-cell lymphoproliferative disorders (lymphomatoid papulosis and primary cutaneous anaplastic large cell lymphoma). Rare entities include primary cutaneous gamma-delta T-cell lymphoma, primary cutaneous CD4-positive small/medium T-cell lymphoma, and primary cutaneous CD8-postive aggressive epidermotrophic T-cell lymphoma. Mycosis fungoides and its variants are by far the most common lymphomas in the skin; these are addressed in Chapter 128.

Primary B-cell lymphomas in the skin are less common but occur more frequently than previously appreciated. These include extranodal marginal zone lymphoma of MALT type, primary cutaneous FL, and large B-cell lymphoma, leg type. The marginal zone lymphomas of the skin have an excellent survival with local therapy, although local recurrence sometimes occurs. Primary cutaneous FL often occurs on the trunk and tends to behave indolently; it can be managed with local therapy. These are distinct from nodal or system FL in that they do not harbor the t(14;18)(q32;q21), do not express bcl-2 protein, and often do not express CD10. Importantly, these cases progress over time, and while initially nodular with FDC meshworks and background T cells, they may become diffuse, lose FDCs, and develop a predominantly large cell cytology that may include multilobated nuclei, yet still retain their indolent behavior. These more diffuse lesions with frequent large cells can be difficult to distinguish from other large B-cell lymphomas such as typical DLBCL involving the skin or the large cell lymphoma, leg type, which follow a more aggressive course (described under subtypes of DLBCL). Thus, every effort must be made with careful cytologic evaluation and phenotyping to distinguish among large B-cell lymphomas arising in the skin.

PRACTICE OF ONCOLOGY

Selected References

The full list of references for this chapter appears in the online version.

2. Altekruse SF KC, Krapcho M, Neyman N, et al., eds. *SEER Cancer Statistics Review*, 1975–2007. http://seercancergov/csr/1975_2007/. 2010.
7. Anderson JR, Armitage JO, Weisenburger DD. Epidemiology of the non-Hodgkin's lymphomas: distributions of the major subtypes differ by geographic locations. Non-Hodgkin's Lymphoma Classification Project. *Ann Oncol* 1998;9(7):717.
8. Chiu BC, Weisenburger DD. An update of the epidemiology of non-Hodgkin's lymphoma. *Clin Lymphoma* 2003;4(3):161.
17. Kennedy G, Komano J, Sugden B. Epstein-Barr virus provides a survival factor to Burkitt's lymphomas. *Proc Natl Acad Sci U S A* 2003;100(24): 14269.
18. Gaidano G, Carbone A, Dalla-Favera R. Genetic basis of acquired immunodeficiency syndrome-related lymphomagenesis. *J Natl Cancer Inst Monogr* 1998;(23):95.
19. Subar M, Neri A, Inghirami G, Knowles DM, Dalla-Favera R. Frequent c-myc oncogene activation and infrequent presence of Epstein-Barr virus genome in AIDS-associated lymphoma. *Blood* 1988;72(2):667.
20. Liebowitz D. Epstein-Barr virus and a cellular signaling pathway in lymphomas from immunosuppressed patients. *N Engl J Med* 1998;338(20): 1413.
24. Mori N, Fujii M, Ikeda S, et al. Constitutive activation of NF-kappaB in primary adult T-cell leukemia cells. *Blood* 1999;93(7):2360.
27. Cesarman E, Chang Y, Moore PS, Said JW, Knowles DM. Kaposi's sarcoma-associated herpesvirus-like DNA sequences in AIDS-related body-cavity-based lymphomas. *N Engl J Med* 1995;332(18):1186.
28. Nador RG, Cesarman E, Chadburn A, et al. Primary effusion lymphoma: a distinct clinicopathologic entity associated with the Kaposi's sarcoma-associated herpes virus. *Blood* 1996;88(2):645.
35. Vilchez RA, Madden CR, Kozinetz CA, et al. Association between simian virus 40 and non-Hodgkin lymphoma. *Lancet* 2002;359(9309):817.
38. Zucca E, Bertoni F, Roggero E, et al. Molecular analysis of the progression from Helicobacter pylori-associated chronic gastritis to mucosa-associated lymphoid-tissue lymphoma of the stomach. *N Engl J Med* 1998;338(12): 804.
39. Lecuit M, Abachin E, Martin A, et al. Immunoproliferative small intestinal disease associated with Campylobacter jejuni. *N Engl J Med* 2004;350(3): 239.
41. Rosado MF, Byrne GE Jr, Ding F, et al. Ocular adnexal lymphoma: a clinicopathologic study of a large cohort of patients with no evidence for an association with Chlamydia psittaci. *Blood* 2006;107(2):467.
52. Ng AK, Bernardo MP, Weller E, et al. Long-term survival and competing causes of death in patients with early-stage Hodgkin's disease treated at age 50 or younger. *J Clin Oncol* 2002;20(8):2101.
53. Ng AK, Bernardo MV, Weller E, et al. Second malignancy after Hodgkin disease treated with radiation therapy with or without chemotherapy: long-term risks and risk factors. *Blood* 2002;100(6):1989.
56. de Jong D, Vasmel WL, de Boer JP, et al. Anaplastic large-cell lymphoma in women with breast implants. *JAMA* 2008;300(17):2030.
58. Korsmeyer SJ, Hieter PA, Ravetch JV, Poplack DG, Waldmann TA, Leder P. Developmental hierarchy of immunoglobulin gene rearrangements in human leukemic pre-B-cells. *Proc Natl Acad Sci U S A* 1981;78(11):7096.
59. Shipp MA, Richardson NE, Sayre PH, et al. Molecular cloning of the common acute lymphoblastic leukemia antigen (CALLA) identifies a type II integral membrane protein. *Proc Natl Acad Sci U S A* 1988;85(13):4819.
63. Hockenbery DM, Zutter M, Hickey W, Nahm M, Korsmeyer SJ. BCL2 protein is topographically restricted in tissues characterized by apoptotic cell death. *Proc Natl Acad Sci U S A* 1991;88(16):6961.
68. Cattoretti G, Chang CC, Cechova K, et al. BCL-6 protein is expressed in germinal-center B cells. *Blood* 1995;86(1):45.
70. French DL, Laskov R, Scharff MD. The role of somatic hypermutation in the generation of antibody diversity. *Science* 1989;244(4909):1152.
72. Shen HM, Peters A, Baron B, Zhu X, Storb U. Mutation of BCL-6 gene in normal B cells by the process of somatic hypermutation of Ig genes. *Science* 1998;280(5370):1750.
73. Liu YJ, Joshua DE, Williams GT, Smith CA, Gordon J, MacLennan IC. Mechanism of antigen-driven selection in germinal centres. *Nature* 1989; 342(6252):929.
77. Lossos IS, Alizadeh AA, Eisen MB, et al. Ongoing immunoglobulin somatic mutation in germinal center B cell-like but not in activated B cell-like diffuse large cell lymphomas. *Proc Natl Acad Sci U S A* 2000;97 (18):10209.
80. Klein U, Kuppers R, Rajewsky K. Evidence for a large compartment of IgM-expressing memory B cells in humans. *Blood* 1997;89(4):1288.
83. Meuer SC, Schlossman SF, Reinherz EL. Clonal analysis of human cytotoxic T lymphocytes: T4+ and T8+ effector T cells recognize products of different major histocompatibility complex regions. *Proc Natl Acad Sci U S A* 1982;79(14):4395.
92. Downing JR, Shurtleff SA, Zielenska M, et al. Molecular detection of the (2;5) translocation of non-Hodgkin's lymphoma by reverse transcriptase-polymerase chain reaction. *Blood* 1995;85(12):3416.
97. *WHO Classification of Tumours of the Haematopoietic and Lymphoid Tissues*. Lyon, France: IARC Press, 2008.
98. A predictive model for aggressive non-Hodgkin's lymphoma: the International Non-Hodgkin's Lymphoma Prognostic Factors Project. *N Engl J Med* 1993;329(14):987.
99. Alizadeh AA, Eisen MB, Davis RE, et al. Distinct types of diffuse large B-cell lymphoma identified by gene expression profiling. *Nature* 2000;403 (6769):503.

100. Lenz G, Wright G, Dave SS, et al. Stromal gene signatures in large-B-cell lymphomas. *N Engl J Med* 2008;359(22):2313.
102. Yeo W, Chan TC, Leung NW, et al. Hepatitis B virus reactivation in lymphoma patients with prior resolved hepatitis B undergoing anticancer therapy with or without rituximab. *J Clin Oncol* 2009;27(4):605.
103. A clinical evaluation of the International Lymphoma Study Group classification of non-Hodgkin's lymphoma. The Non-Hodgkin's Lymphoma Classification Project. *Blood* 1997;89(11):3909–3918.
104. Hegde U, Filie A, Little RF, et al. High incidence of occult leptomeningeal disease detected by flow cytometry in newly diagnosed aggressive B-cell lymphomas at risk for central nervous system involvement: the role of flow cytometry versus cytology. *Blood* 2005;105(2):496.
106. Juweid ME, Stroobants S, Hoekstra OS, et al. Use of positron emission tomography for response assessment of lymphoma: consensus of the Imaging Subcommittee of International Harmonization Project in Lymphoma. *J Clin Oncol* 2007;25(5):571.
117. Federico M, Vitolo U, Zinzani PL, et al. Prognosis of follicular lymphoma: a predictive model based on a retrospective analysis of 987 cases. Intergruppo Italiano Linfomi. *Blood* 2000;95(3):783.
119. Philip T, Guglielmi C, Hagenbeek A, et al. Autologous bone marrow transplantation as compared with salvage chemotherapy in relapses of chemotherapy-sensitive non-Hodgkin's lymphoma. *N Engl J Med* 1995; 333(23):1540.
121. Dohner H, Stilgenbauer S, Benner A, et al. Genomic aberrations and survival in chronic lymphocytic leukemia. *N Engl J Med* 2000;343(26):1910.
122. Crespo M, Bosch F, Villamor N, et al. ZAP-70 expression as a surrogate for immunoglobulin-variable-region mutations in chronic lymphocytic leukemia. *N Engl J Med* 2003;348(18):1764.
129. Agnello V, Chung RT, Kaplan LM. A role for hepatitis C virus infection in type II cryoglobulinemia. *N Engl J Med* 1992;327(21):1490.
139. Qin Y, Greiner A, Trunk MJ, Schmausser B, Ott MM, Muller-Hermelink HK. Somatic hypermutation in low-grade mucosa-associated lymphoid tissue-type B-cell lymphoma. *Blood* 1995;86(9):3528.
148. Wotherspoon AC, Doglioni C, Diss TC, et al. Regression of primary low-grade B-cell gastric lymphoma of mucosa-associated lymphoid tissue type after eradication of Helicobacter pylori. *Lancet* 1993;342(8871):575.
164. Levy S, Mendel E, Kon S, Avnur Z, Levy R. Mutational hot spots in Ig V region genes of human follicular lymphomas. *J Exp Med* 1988;168(2):475.
166. Akasaka T, Lossos IS, Levy R. BCL6 gene translocation in follicular lymphoma: a harbinger of eventual transformation to diffuse aggressive lymphoma. *Blood* 2003;102(4):1443.
170. Fisher RI, LeBlanc M, Press OW, Maloney DG, Unger JM, Miller TP. New treatment options have changed the survival of patients with follicular lymphoma. *J Clin Oncol* 2005;23(33):8447.
176. Mac Manus MP, Hoppe RT. Is radiotherapy curative for stage I and II low-grade follicular lymphoma? Results of a long-term follow-up study of patients treated at Stanford University. *J Clin Oncol* 1996;14(4):1282.
185. Friedberg JW, Taylor MD, Cerhan JR, et al. Follicular lymphoma in the United States: first report of the national LymphoCare study. *J Clin Oncol* 2009;27(8):1202.
188. Czuczman MS, Weaver R, Alkuzweny B, Berlfein J, Grillo-Lopez AJ. Prolonged clinical and molecular remission in patients with low-grade or follicular non-Hodgkin's lymphoma treated with rituximab plus CHOP chemotherapy: 9-year follow-up. *J Clin Oncol* 2004;22(23):4711.
196. Freedman AS, Neuberg D, Mauch P, et al. Long-term follow-up of autologous bone marrow transplantation in patients with relapsed follicular lymphoma. *Blood* 1999;94(10):3325.
198. Friedberg JW, Neuberg D, Stone RM, et al. Outcome in patients with myelodysplastic syndrome after autologous bone marrow transplantation for non-Hodgkin's lymphoma. *J Clin Oncol* 1999;17(10):3128.
199. Cheson BD. The curious case of the baffling biological. *J Clin Oncol* 2000;18(10):2007.
201. Fisher RI, Dana BW, LeBlanc M, et al. Interferon alpha consolidation after intensive chemotherapy does not prolong the progression-free survival of patients with low-grade non-Hodgkin's lymphoma: results of the Southwest Oncology Group randomized phase III study 8809. *J Clin Oncol* 2000;18(10):2010.
202. Hainsworth JD, Litchy S, Shaffer DW, Lackey VL, Grimaldi M, Greco FA. Maximizing therapeutic benefit of rituximab: maintenance therapy versus re-treatment at progression in patients with indolent non-Hodgkin's lymphoma—a randomized phase II trial of the Minnie Pearl Cancer Research Network. *J Clin Oncol* 2005;23(6):1088.
203. Ghielmini M, Schmitz SF, Cogliatti SB, et al. Prolonged treatment with rituximab in patients with follicular lymphoma significantly increases event-free survival and response duration compared with the standard weekly × 4 schedule. *Blood* 2004;103(12):4416.
206. van Oers MH, Klasa R, Marcus RE, et al. Rituximab maintenance improves clinical outcome of relapsed/resistant follicular non-Hodgkin lymphoma in patients both with and without rituximab during induction: results of a prospective randomized phase 3 intergroup trial. *Blood* 2006;108(10): 3295.
211. Press OW, Unger JM, Braziel RM, et al. A phase 2 trial of CHOP chemotherapy followed by tositumomab/iodine I 131 tositumomab for previously untreated follicular non-Hodgkin lymphoma: Southwest Oncology Group Protocol S9911. *Blood* 2003;102(5):1606.
216. Friedberg JW, Cohen P, Chen L, et al. Bendamustine in patients with rituximab-refractory indolent and transformed non-Hodgkin's lymphoma: results from a phase II multicenter, single-agent study. *J Clin Oncol* 2008; 26(2):204.
221. Kaminski MS, Zelenetz AD, Press OW, et al. Pivotal study of iodine I 131 tositumomab for chemotherapy-refractory low-grade or transformed low-grade B-cell non-Hodgkin's lymphomas. *J Clin Oncol* 2001;19(19):3918.
225. van Besien K, Loberiza FR Jr, Bajorunaite R, et al. Comparison of autologous and allogeneic hematopoietic stem cell transplantation for follicular lymphoma. *Blood* 2003;102(10):3521.
226. Schouten HC, Qian W, Kvaloy S, et al. High-dose therapy improves progression-free survival and survival in relapsed follicular non-Hodgkin's lymphoma: results from the randomized European CUP trial. *J Clin Oncol* 2003;21(21):3918.
228. Khouri IF, Keating M, Korbling M, et al. Transplant-lite: induction of graft-versus-malignancy using fludarabine-based nonablative chemotherapy and allogeneic blood progenitor-cell transplantation as treatment for lymphoid malignancies. *J Clin Oncol* 1998;16(8):2817.
234. Fisher RI, Dahlberg S, Nathwani BN, Banks PM, Miller TP, Grogan TM. A clinical analysis of two indolent lymphoma entities: mantle cell lymphoma and marginal zone lymphoma (including the mucosa-associated lymphoid tissue and monocytoid B-cell subcategories): a Southwest Oncology Group study. *Blood* 1995;85(4):1075.
238. Howard OM, Gribben JG, Neuberg DS, et al. Rituximab and CHOP induction therapy for newly diagnosed mantle-cell lymphoma: molecular complete responses are not predictive of progression-free survival. *J Clin Oncol* 2002;20(5):1288.
239. Lenz G, Dreyling M, Hoster E, et al. Immunochemotherapy with rituximab and cyclophosphamide, doxorubicin, vincristine, and prednisone significantly improves response and time to treatment failure, but not long-term outcome in patients with previously untreated mantle cell lymphoma: results of a prospective randomized trial of the German Low Grade Lymphoma Study Group (GLSG). *J Clin Oncol* 2005; 23(9):1984.
242. Freedman AS, Neuberg D, Gribben JG, et al. High-dose chemoradiotherapy and anti-B-cell monoclonal antibody-purged autologous bone marrow transplantation in mantle-cell lymphoma: no evidence for long-term remission. *J Clin Oncol* 1998;16(1):13.
244. Dreyling M, Lenz G, Hoster E, et al. Early consolidation by myeloablative radiochemotherapy followed by autologous stem cell transplantation in first remission significantly prolongs progression-free survival in mantle-cell lymphoma: results of a prospective randomized trial of the European MCL Network. *Blood* 2005;105(7):2677.
246. Fisher RI, Bernstein SH, Kahl BS, et al. Multicenter phase II study of bortezomib in patients with relapsed or refractory mantle cell lymphoma. *J Clin Oncol* 2006;24(30):4867.
247. Hess G, Herbrecht R, Romaguera J, et al. Phase III study to evaluate temsirolimus compared with investigator's choice therapy for the treatment of relapsed or refractory mantle cell lymphoma. *J Clin Oncol* 2009;27(23): 3822.
263. Hans CP, Weisenburger DD, Greiner TC, et al. Confirmation of the molecular classification of diffuse large B-cell lymphoma by immunohistochemistry using a tissue microarray. *Blood* 2004;103(1):275.
268. Miller TP, Dahlberg S, Cassady JR, et al. Chemotherapy alone compared with chemotherapy plus radiotherapy for localized intermediate- and high-grade non-Hodgkin's lymphoma. *N Engl J Med* 1998;339(1):21.
269. Horning SJ, Weller E, Kim K, et al. Chemotherapy with or without radiotherapy in limited-stage diffuse aggressive non-Hodgkin's lymphoma: Eastern Cooperative Oncology Group study 1484. *J Clin Oncol* 2004;22 (15):3032.
270. Bonnet C, Fillet G, Mounier N, et al. CHOP alone compared with CHOP plus radiotherapy for localized aggressive lymphoma in elderly patients: a study by the Groupe d'Etude des Lymphomes de l'Adulte. *J Clin Oncol* 2007;25(7):787.
271. Persky DO, Unger JM, Spier CM, et al. Phase II study of rituximab plus three cycles of CHOP and involved-field radiotherapy for patients with limited-stage aggressive B-cell lymphoma: Southwest Oncology Group study 0014. *J Clin Oncol* 2008;26(14):2258.
272. Pfreundschuh M, Trumper L, Osterborg A, et al. CHOP-like chemotherapy plus rituximab versus CHOP-like chemotherapy alone in young patients with good-prognosis diffuse large-B-cell lymphoma: a randomised controlled trial by the MabThera International Trial (MInT) Group. *Lancet Oncol* 2006;7(5):379.
273. Fisher RI, Gaynor ER, Dahlberg S, et al. Comparison of a standard regimen (CHOP) with three intensive chemotherapy regimens for advanced non-Hodgkin's lymphoma. *N Engl J Med* 1993;328(14):1002–1006.
275. Habermann TM, Weller EA, Morrison VA, et al. Rituximab-CHOP versus CHOP alone or with maintenance rituximab in older patients with diffuse large B-cell lymphoma. *J Clin Oncol* 2006;24(19):3121.
277. Winter JN, Li S, Aurora V, et al. Expression of p21 protein predicts clinical outcome in DLBCL patients older than 60 years treated with R-CHOP but not CHOP: a prospective ECOG and Southwest Oncology Group correlative study on E4494. *Clin Cancer Res* 2010;16(8):2435.
283. Shipp MA, Abeloff MD, Antman KH, et al. International Consensus Conference on High-Dose Therapy with Hematopoietic Stem Cell

Transplantation in Aggressive Non-Hodgkin's Lymphomas: report of the jury. *J Clin Oncol* 1999;17(1):423.

286. Wilson WH, Dunleavy K, Pittaluga S, et al. Phase II study of dose-adjusted EPOCH and rituximab in untreated diffuse large B-cell lymphoma with analysis of germinal center and post-germinal center biomarkers. *J Clin Oncol* 2008;26(16):2717.
287. Pfreundschuh M, Trumper L, Kloess M, et al. Two-weekly or 3-weekly CHOP chemotherapy with or without etoposide for the treatment of elderly patients with aggressive lymphomas: results of the NHL-B2 trial of the DSHNHL. *Blood* 2004;104(3):634.
288. Pfreundschuh M, Schubert J, Ziepert M, et al. Six versus eight cycles of bi-weekly CHOP-14 with or without rituximab in elderly patients with aggressive CD20+ B-cell lymphomas: a randomised controlled trial (RICOVER-60). *Lancet Oncol* 2008;9(2):105.
304. Wilson WH, Kingma DW, Raffeld M, Wittes RE, Jaffe ES. Association of lymphomatoid granulomatosis with Epstein-Barr viral infection of B lymphocytes and response to interferon-alpha 2b. *Blood* 1996;87(11):4531.
307. Savage KJ, Johnson NA, Ben-Neriah S, et al. MYC gene rearrangements are associated with a poor prognosis in diffuse large B-cell lymphoma patients treated with R-CHOP chemotherapy. *Blood* 2009;114(17):3533.
309. Magrath I, Adde M, Shad A, et al. Adults and children with small non-cleaved-cell lymphoma have a similar excellent outcome when treated with the same chemotherapy regimen. *J Clin Oncol* 1996;14(3):925.
310. Mead GM, Barrans SL, Qian W, et al. A prospective clinicopathologic study of dose-modified CODOX-M/IVAC in patients with sporadic Burkitt lymphoma defined using cytogenetic and immunophenotypic criteria (MRC/NCRI LY10 trial). *Blood* 2008;112(6):2248.
311. Kelly JL, Toothaker SR, Ciminello L, et al. Outcomes of patients with Burkitt lymphoma older than age 40 treated with intensive chemotherapeutic regimens. *Clin Lymphoma Myeloma* 2009;9(4):307.
321. Vose JM, Peterson C, Bierman PJ, et al. Comparison of high-dose therapy and autologous bone marrow transplantation for T-cell and B-cell non-Hodgkin's lymphomas. *Blood* 1990;76(2):424.
322. O'Connor OA, Horwitz S, Hamlin P, et al. Phase II-I-II study of two different doses and schedules of pralatrexate, a high-affinity substrate for the reduced folate carrier, in patients with relapsed or refractory lymphoma reveals marked activity in T-cell malignancies. *J Clin Oncol* 2009;27(26):4357.
331. Savage KJ, Harris NL, Vose JM, et al. ALK- anaplastic large-cell lymphoma is clinically and immunophenotypically different from both ALK+ ALCL and peripheral T-cell lymphoma, not otherwise specified: report from the International Peripheral T-Cell Lymphoma Project. *Blood* 2008;111(12):5496.
335. Sehn LH, Donaldson J, Chhanabhai M, et al. Introduction of combined CHOP plus rituximab therapy dramatically improved outcome of diffuse large B cell lymphoma in British Columbia. *J Clin Oncol* 2005;23(22):5027–5033.
352. Kaplan LD, Straus DJ, Testa MA, et al. Low-dose compared with standard-dose m-BACOD chemotherapy for non-Hodgkin's lymphoma associated with human immunodeficiency virus infection. National Institute of Allergy and Infectious Diseases AIDS Clinical Trials Group. *N Engl J Med* 1997;336(23):1641.

CHAPTER 128 CUTANEOUS LYMPHOMAS

FRANCINE M. FOSS, RICHARD L. EDELSON, AND LYNN D. WILSON

The cutaneous lymphomas comprise a heterogeneous group of malignancies of both T and B lymphocytes that localize to the skin. According to Surveillance, Epidemiology, and End Results (SEER) data, the skin is the second most common site of extranodal non-Hodgkin's lymphoma, with an estimated annual incidence of 1 in 100,000.[1] The Dutch and Austrian Cutaneous Lymphoma registries report that more than 70% of all cutaneous lymphomas are of T-cell origin, and 22% are of B-cell origin.[2] The term *cutaneous T-cell lymphoma* (CTCL) was formally adopted in 1979 at a conference sponsored by the National Cancer Institute to describe a heterogeneous group of malignant T-cell lymphomas with primary manifestations in the skin. This term has fallen out of favor recently with the World Health Organization (WHO) and European Organisation for Research and Treatment of Cancer (EORTC) classification of primary cutaneous lymphomas (Table 128.1), which defines distinct disease entities within the cutaneous T- and B-cell lymphomas.[2]

The WHO-EORTC classification identifies three groups of cutaneous lymphomas: the cutaneous T-cell and natural killer (NK) lymphomas, the cutaneous B-cell lymphomas, and the precursor hematologic neoplasms. In the cutaneous T/NK group are mycosis fungoides (MF) and its subtypes, the Sézary syndrome (SS), which is now defined as a distinct entity, human T-cell leukemia virus 1 (HTLV-1) associated T-cell leukemia/lymphoma, the primary cutaneous CD30+ lymphomas, subcutaneous panniculitislike T-cell lymphoma of the alpha-beta type, extranodal NK/T-cell lymphomas of the nasal type, and peripheral T-cell lymphoma (PTCL) and its subtypes. The B-cell lymphoma group includes a number of entities based on histopathologic and clinical characteristics. These include the cutaneous marginal zone (mucosa-associated lymphoid tissue) type lymphomas, primary cutaneous follicle cell lymphoma, diffuse cutaneous B-cell lymphoma (leg type or other), intravascular large B-cell lymphoma, lymphomatoid granulomatosis, and cutaneous involvement by systemic disorders such as chronic lymphocytic leukemia, mantle cell lymphoma, and Burkitt's lymphoma. The precursor hematopoietic malignancies include the blastic NK cell hematodermic neoplasms, precursor lymphoblastic lymphomas of T- or B-cell origin, and myeloid leukemias that involve the skin.

Further subgrouping based on clinical outcomes has been proposed for the cutaneous T-cell entities.[2,3] The entities with indolent clinical behavior include MF and its variants, the cutaneous CD30+ entities, subcutaneous panniculitislike T-cell lymphoma, and the primary cutaneous CD4+ PTCL. Included in the aggressive group are the SS, the NK/T-cell disorders, CD8+ cutaneous diseases, and primary cutaneous PTCL. A similar classification for the cutaneous B-cell lymphomas has been proposed based on the histology (follicular or large cell type) and site of disease, with favorable outcomes seen in disease of the head or upper trunk and unfavorable prognosis with either disseminated lesions or disease in the lower extremities (Table 128.2).

MYCOSIS FUNGOIDES AND THE SÉZARY SYNDROME

MF, the most frequently observed CTCL, was first reported by Alibert in 1806 as a common epidermotropic lymphoma with an indolent evolution characterized by cutaneous lesions in the forms of patches, plaques, or skin tumors. In 1980, Bunn et al.[4] reported that atypical lymphocytes with hyperconvoluted nuclei (Sézary cells) were present in the blood in a high frequency of patients with MF. It was subsequently noted that patients with high Sézary counts often presented with diffuse erythroderma, thus identifying the SS as the erythrodermic variant of MF with disseminated disease and often involvement of lymph nodes and bone marrow.[5–7] Because many patients with nonerythrodermic MF may have evidence of blood involvement either by the presence of Sézary cells on the smear or by flow cytometry, the International Society of Cutaneous Lymphoma established criteria for diagnosis of SS, which include an absolute Sézary count of at least 1,000 cells/mm^3 in the blood, demonstration of immunophenotypic abnormalities (expanded CD4+ populations or loss of antigens such as CD2, CD3, CD5, or CD4), or presence of a T-cell clone in the blood.[8]

Epidemiology and Etiology

According to SEER data, the incidence of MF-CTCL had increased 3.2-fold between 1973 and 1984. The overall incidence rate is approximately 4 per 1 million, with an incidence of 1,500 cases per year. The actual incidence rate may be an order of magnitude higher, given possible underreporting and the difficulty and confusion in making the diagnosis. The incidence of MF rises with age such that the majority of patients are between 40 and 60. The disease is 2.2 times more common in men than in women, and incidence rates are somewhat higher in African Americans than in whites.

One hypothesis regarding the etiology of MF/SS is that it may possibly represent a clonal evolution from a chronic antigenic stimulus. Associations with exposure to occupational chemicals or pesticides have been proposed but not definitely demonstrated in epidemiologic studies.[5,6] In other studies, an association with *Chlamydia* infection of keratinocytes has been proposed, but data demonstrating *Chlamydia* proteins in affected skin lesions are equivocal.[9,10] The association between human T-cell leukemia virus type 1 infection and adult T-cell leukemia-lymphoma (ATLL) or Epstein-Barr virus in conjunction with nasal NK/T-cell lymphoma is not reflected in the epidemiology of MF-CTCL, but there are reports of detection of HTLV-like viral particles in affected skin lesions and antibodies to HTLV-1 tax protein in patients with MF/SS.[11–14] These results suggest association of perhaps a yet unknown

TABLE 128.1

WORLD HEALTH ORGANIZATION–EUROPEAN ORGANISATION FOR RESEARCH AND TREATMENT OF CANCER CLASSIFICATION OF CUTANEOUS LYMPHOMAS WITH PRIMARY CUTANEOUS MANIFESTATIONS

Cutaneous T-cell and NK-cell lymphomas
Mycosis fungoides
MF variants and subtypes
 Folliculotropic MF
 Pagetoid reticulosis
 Granulomatous slack skin
Sézary syndrome
Adult T-cell leukemia/lymphoma
Primary cutaneous CD30+ lymphoproliferative disorders
 Primary cutaneous anaplastic large cell lymphoma
 Lymphomatoid papulosis
Subcutaneous panniculitislike T-cell lymphoma
Extranodal NK/T-cell lymphoma, nasal type
Primary cutaneous peripheral T-cell lymphoma, unspecified
 Primary cutaneous aggressive epidermotropic CD8+ T-cell lymphoma (provisional)
Cutaneous γ/δ T-cell lymphoma (provisional)
Primary cutaneous CD4+ small/medium-sized pleomorphic T-cell lymphoma (provisional)
Cutaneous B-cell lymphomas
 Primary cutaneous marginal zone B-cell lymphoma
 Primary cutaneous follicle center lymphoma
 Primary cutaneous diffuse large B-cell lymphoma, leg type
 Primary cutaneous diffuse large B-cell lymphoma, other
  Intravascular large B-cell lymphoma
Precursor hematologic neoplasm
 CD4+/CD56+ hematodermic neoplasm (blastic NK-cell lymphoma)

WHO-EORTC, World Health Organization and European Organization for Research and Treatment of Cancer; NK, natural killer; MF, mycosis fungoides.
(Adapted from ref. 2.)

retrovirus in some cases of MF/SS. Although there is no known geographic clustering and no evidence of maternal transmission of the disease, there are reports of multiple cases of MF/SS in a small number of families.

Pathobiology

The immunophenotypic profile of MF is one of clonal mature CD4+ CD45RO+ T cells with a marked homing capacity for the papillary dermis and epidermis. Some CTCL variants are CD8+ and different subtypes have distinct prognoses. Antigen loss is characteristic of the disease, with loss of CD7, CD5, or CD2 and dim staining for CD3. The clinical characteristics of the disease are driven in large part by the cytokine profile of the malignant cells. It has been demonstrated that Sézary cells express a TH2 phenotype, with secretion of interleukin (IL) -4, -5, -6, -10, and -13. The pruritus characteristic of the disease is related to secretion of IL-5 as well as other chemokines. One characteristic of the disease, even at its earliest

TABLE 128.2

CUTANEOUS B-CELL LYMPHOMA PROGNOSTIC INDEX

CBCL-PI Group	Histology	Site	Overall	Relative	HR	95% CL	*P*
IA	Any indolent[a]	Any	81	94	1.0		
IB	Diffuse large B-cell	Favorable[b]	72	86	1.3	0.99 to 1.7	.06
II	Diffuse large B-cell	Unfavorable[c]	48	60	2.1	1.6 to 2.7	<.0001
	Immunoblastic diffuse large B-cell	Favorable					
III	Immunoblastic diffuse large B-cell	Unfavorable	27	34	4.5	2.8 to 7.2	<.0001

HR, hazard ratio; CBCL-PI, cutaneous B-cell lymphoma prognostic index.
Note: Model is adjusted for age, sex, race, year of diagnosis, confirmed B-cell lineage. Surveillance, Epidemiology, and End Results historic stage, and treatment with radiation.
[a]Indolent histologies include follicular, marginal zone, small lymphocyte not otherwise specified, and lymphoplasmacytic.
[b]Favorable skin sites include head/neck and arm.
[c]Unfavorable skin sites include trunk, leg, and disseminated.
(Adapted from ref. 92.)

stages, is profound immunosuppression with aberrant T-cell repertoires, cutaneous anergy, and increased susceptibility to bacterial and opportunistic infections.[15,16]

The homing to skin by CTCL cells appears to be mediated in part by expression of the surface glycoprotein cutaneous lymphoid antigen (CLA), an antigen whose expression is low or absent on normal infiltrating T cells.[17,18] CLA mediates binding to E-selectin on endothelial cells of cutaneous venules, thereby facilitating their exit from the circulation and into the skin. ICLA is the physiologic ligand of endothelial cell E-selectin, a cell adhesion molecule expressed on the surface of endothelial cells of cutaneous venules during chronic inflammation.[19] Interactions between CLA on the cell surface and E-selectin on endothelial cells allow CTCL cells to roll along the walls of cutaneous venules. Chemokine receptor CCR4 expressed by cells binds chemokine CCL17 that has adhered to the luminal side of the endothelium, facilitating T-cell leukocyte function antigen-1 binding to endothelial cell intracellular adhesion molecule-1 and fostering extravasation into the dermis.[4]

One of the most striking features of MF/SS is epidermotropism, or infiltration of the epidermis by malignant T cells. The pathognomic feature of MF is the Pautrier microabscess, a collection of clonal malignant cells within the epidermis. The Pautrier microabscesses may be a consequence of the expression of intracellular adhesion molecule-1 (ICAM) on keratinocytes. ICAM expression is induced by interferon, which is produced by infiltrating T cells and is a ligand for leukocyte function antigen-1.[20,21] Typical Pautrier microabscesses are only seen in 10% of cases of MF/SS. In advanced disease or SS, the keratinocytes lose the ability to express ICAM-1 due to low levels of interferon-γ production, resulting in loss of epidermotropism.[21] Although specimens from early lesions of MF have lymphocytes in both the epidermis and dermis, clonality studies on dissected cells demonstrate that virtually all of the lymphocytes found in the epidermis belong to the malignant clone, whereas the dermis contains a predominance of inflammatory cells and nonmalignant lymphocytes.[22–24]

Although there is no characteristic chromosomal translocation in patients with MF and SS, significant chromosomal instability is noted, and losses on 1p, 10q, 13q, and 17p and gains of 4, 17q, and 18 are commonly observed.[25,26] Recent studies have shown a high prevalence of deletions or translocations involving the gene *NAV3*, at 12q2, which has helicase-like activity and might therefore contribute to genomic instability.[27] Chromosomal amplification of JunB at 19p12 has also been detected in MF/SS and is thought to be contributory to the TH2 cytokine profile characteristic of Sézary cells.[28]

DIAGNOSIS AND STAGING

The diagnosis of MF depends on both clinical and histopathologic criteria. The clinical features of the disease are variable and may be in the form of patches, plaques, erythroderma, cutaneous tumors, or ulcers. In early patch or plaque stage disease, the clinical features are indistinguishable from those of benign dermatoses, including psoriasis, eczema, large plaque parapsoriasis, or drug eruptions. Moreover, MF can appear as a single lesion (unilesional MF) or in several sites. The distribution of the lesions is suggestive, as MF has the propensity to occur in non–sun-exposed areas such as the "bathing trunk" distribution. In some cases in which there is follicular involvement, the disease may appear on the face or scalp. Early diagnosis can be difficult and may rely on multiple biopsies obtained from different lesions over time. The International Society for Cutaneous Lymphoma has developed criteria for the diagnosis of early stage MF that relies on clinical, histopathologic, immunopathologic, and molecular criteria (Table 128.3).[29] The use of T-cell receptor clonality as determined by polymerase chain reaction (PCR) assay solely to distinguish MF from benign dermatoses is inadequate as it has been demonstrated that a number of entities, such as lymphomatoid papulosis and pityriasis lichenoides, may demonstrate clonal dominance, thus giving rise to the term *clonal dermatitis*.[30,31] Long-term follow-up of patients with clonal dermatitis reveals a significant risk of progression to overt MF, suggesting careful follow-up.

TABLE 128.3

INTERNATIONAL SOCIETY FOR CUTANEOUS LYMPHOMAS ALGORITHM FOR THE DIAGNOSIS OF EARLY STAGE MYCOSIS FUNGOIDES

Criteria	Major (2 Points)	Minor (1 Point)
CLINICAL		
Persistent and/or progressive patches and plaques plus	Any 2	Any 1
1. Non–sun-exposed location		
2. Size/shape variation		
3. Poikiloderma		
HISTOPATHOLOGIC		
Superficial lymphoid infiltrate plus	Both	Either
1. Epidermotropism		
2. Atypia		
MOLECULAR/BIOLOGICAL		
Clonal *TCR* gene rearrangement	—	Present
IMMUNOPATHOLOGIC		
1. CD2, 3, 5 <59% of T cells	—	Any 1
2. CD7 <10% of T cells		
3. Epidermal discordance from expression of CD2, 3, 5, and 7 on dermal T cells		

(Adapted from ref. 29.)

The classic MF presentation involves lesions that are persistent or progressive and may evolve from patch or plaque to more infiltrated plaques, and then to more advanced stages (Fig. 128.1). Early in the course of the disease, the lesions are often asymptomatic, scaling erythematous macular eruptions often in sun-shielded areas. A patch is defined as a lesion that is not elevated or indurated and may be hyper- or hypopigmented. A plaque is raised or indurated and may be associated with scaling, crusting, or ulceration. A tumor is a lesion that is more than 1 cm with evidence of depth or vertical growth. Erythroderma is defined as diffuse erythema involving more than 80% of the skin surface with or without scaling.[8]

Painful or pruritic erythroderma may arise *de novo* or during any of the earlier described phases and is not always associated with frank T-cell leukemia (as in SS). Infrequently, MF presents with cutaneous tumor nodules in the absence of patches or plaques (as in *tumor d'emblée*). Patients may also present with or progress to involvement of visceral organs.

Mycosis Fungoides Variants

Although MF may manifest cutaneous lesions of diverse color, morphology, and distribution (e.g., pink to red to violaceous to brown, eczematous to psoriasiform, nummular to oval to annular to linear) and may variably demonstrate tropisms or

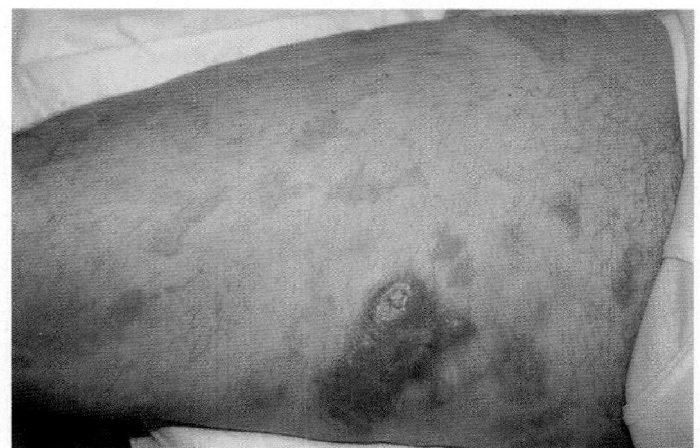

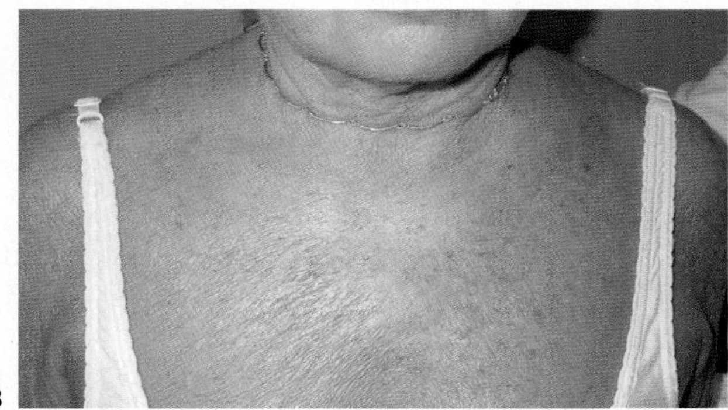

FIGURE 128.1 Mycosis fungoides and the Sézary syndrome. A: Mycosis fungoides patient with cutaneous plaques and a tumor. B: Sézary syndrome patient with diffuse erythroderma.

other findings histologically (e.g., follicular mucinosis, granulomatous inflammation), several variants of MF have been described in which certain clinicopathologic features predominate. Alopecia mucinosa is characterized by follicular papules with hair loss clinically and infiltrative, perifollicular clonal T cells, admixed with other mononuclear cells histologically. The accumulation of acid mucopolysaccharides in the sebaceous glands and root sheaths of hair follicles results in the histologic pattern termed *follicular mucinosis*. Overall, 15% to 30% of alopecia mucinosa–follicular mucinosis patients either have or will develop CTCL. Rarely, the folliculotropic pattern may be seen, with or without mucinosis, manifesting clinically as acneiform or cystic lesions with a predilection for the head and neck regions. Any follicular variant of MF may prove more difficult to treat by skin-directed therapies.

Pagetoid reticulosis, or Woringer-Kolopp disease, typically presents as a solitary cutaneous lesion of long duration, characterized histologically by marked numbers of abnormal CLA+ clonal T cells infiltrating the epidermis. Unilesional disease responds well to local radiotherapy or surgical excision. A disseminated, more aggressive disease that shows a similar histologic pattern of striking epidermal involvement is called the *Ketron-Goodman variant*, which has been characterized by clonal CD8+ cells.

Granulomatous slack skin is a very rare MF variant in which patients develop folds or pendulous bags of lax skin, most commonly in the axillae, neck, breast, or groin areas. Histologically, there is a striking granulomatous inflammation, with multinucleated giant cells admixed with atypical T cells. The lax skin is attributed to a marked destruction of elastin fibers by the granulomatous inflammation. It should be noted that approximately one-third of such cases have been associated with Hodgkin's lymphoma.

The Sézary Syndrome

The SS is defined as diffuse erythroderma with circulating neoplastic Sézary cells and lymphadenopathy and should be distinguished from erythrodermic MF, which is defined as erythroderma that develops in a patient with antecedent MF. The diagnostic criteria for SS have been described previously and are dependent on the presence of a circulating Sézary count of at least 1,000 cells/mm^3. The phenotype is typically that of a mature, memory CD4+ T cell with frequent loss of normal T-cell antigens (CD3, CD5, CD2, CD7, CD26).[8] The CD4/CD8 ratio is elevated, usually more than ten, and a T-cell clone is detected in the blood by PCR. The presence of more than 1,000 Sézary cells/mm^3 is not absolutely diagnostic of SS in the absence of other clinical features of the disease, as these cells may be seen in about 5% of patients with benign dermatoses manifested by erythroderma.[32,33] Histopathologic features in skin biopsies of patients with SS can be nonspecific and there is loss of epidermotropism in up to 70% of cases. Cytogenetic studies demonstrate unbalanced translocations and deletions, often involving 1p, 10q, 14q, and 15q, with evidence of clonal evolution and chromosomal instability over time.[34] Differential diagnosis includes viral or drug-induced exanthems, atopic dermatitis, or psoriasis.

Clinical features of the SS include extensive skin involvement with erythroderma, which may progress to lichenification, palmoplantar hyperkeratosis, and diffuse exfoliation. Skin edema, hypoalbuminemia due to insensible fluid loss related to impaired skin integument, and intense pruritus are frequently observed in patients with advanced disease. Lymphadenopathy, histopathologically effaced nodes, and bone marrow involvement are common. Significant immunosuppression occurs related to impaired T-helper function as well as T-cell repertoire skewing, leading to a high incidence of infections, particularly related to indwelling intravenous catheters. The overall prognosis is poor, with a median survival of 2 to 4 years.[35]

Staging and Prognosis of Mycosis Fungoides and the Sézary Syndrome

Staging systems for MF have been developed based on clinical features of skin involvement as well as infiltration of lymph nodes and viscera. Skin involvement is defined on the basis of the type of lesions and extent. T1 and T2 disease are patches or plaques involving less than or more than 10% of the skin surface, respectively. T3 disease is the presence of at least one cutaneous tumor. T4 disease is erythroderma, which may be flat and patchlike, or may be diffusely infiltrated and associated with a leathery skin appearance or with thickening and fissuring of the skin, particularly on the palms or soles of the feet. Lymph node involvement has been classified based on the degree of infiltration with malignant cells. The dermatopathic node typically demonstrates many atypical lymphocytes in three to six cell clusters (LN2) or larger aggregates of atypical lymphocytes with nodal architecture preserved (LN3) clusters of T cells, often with expansion of the parafollicular zones. LN4 nodes are effaced by tumor cells, and typically such effacement is by atypical lymphocytes or neoplastic cells.[36] T-cell receptor rearrangement (TCRR) is found in half of all patients with LN3 nodes and rarely in those with LN2 histology.[37] Bone marrow involvement has been shown to have prognostic significance based on degree of involvement, with cytologically atypical lymphoid aggregates and infiltrative disease associated with inferior survival.[38] In retrospective studies, bone marrow involvement was associated with blood involvement and advanced lymph node disease.[5,7,39,40]

The initial staging system for MF/SS was proposed by the MF Cooperative Group in 1979 and was based on skin

TABLE 128.4

STAGING SYSTEMS FOR MYCOSIS FUNGOIDES

MF Cooperative Group 1979[a]				ISCL Group 2007[b]				
Stage	T	N	M	Stage	T	N	M	B
IA	1	0	0	IA	1	0	0	0, 1
IB	2	0	0	IB	2	0	0	0, 1
IIA	1–2	1	0	II	1–2	1–2	0	0, 1
IIB	3	0, 1	0	IIB	3	0–2	0	0, 1
III	4	0, 1	0	III	4	0–2	0	0–1
				IIIA	4	0–2	0	0
				IIIB	4	0–2	0	1
IVA	1–4	2–3	0	IVA_1	1–4	0–2	0	2
IVB	1–4	2–3	1	IVA_2	1–4	3	0	0–2
				IVA_3		0–3	1	0–2

MF, mycosis fungoides; ISCL, International Society for Cutaneous Lymphomas; T1 patches or plaques. <10% bovine serum albumin (BSA); T2 patches or plaques, >10% BSA; T3, cutaneous tumors; T4, erythroderma; N1 = LN 0–2; N2 = LN 3; N3 = LN 4; B0, <5% of lymphocytes are atypical; B1, >5% of lymphocytes are atypical; B2, >1,000 Sézary cells/mm^3 with positive clone.

[a](Data derived from ref. 41.)

[b]Proposed modifications to the staging system by the International Society of Cutaneous Lymphoma (ISCL). (From Olsen E, Vonderheid E, Piminelli N, et al. Revisions to the staging and classification of mycosis fungoides and Sézary syndrome: a proposal of the International Society for Cutaneous Lymphomas (ISCL) and the cutaneous lymphoma task force of the European organization of Research and treatment of Cancer (EORTC). *Blood* 2007;110:1713.)

involvement, palpable nodes, and visceral involvement.[41] Recently, the International Society for Cutaneous Lymphoma has proposed a new system that takes into consideration the degree of blood involvement as well as the degree of lymph node infiltration (Table 128.4). In this new system, patients with significant blood involvement are identified in the erythroderma, or stage III group, and patients with stage IVA disease are further categorized based on degree of lymph node and blood infiltration.

Overall outcome in MF/SS is correlated with clinical stage, and retrospective studies have identified skin involvement as well as visceral disease as the most important prognostic factors.[5,7,39] Patients with limited patch or plaque disease covering less than 10% of their skin surface have a prognosis indistinguishable from that of age-, sex-, and race-matched controls.[42] The 10-year disease-specific survival for patients with more extensive skin involvement with patches or plaques is 83%, whereas those with tumors or histologically documented lymph node involvement had survivals of 42% or 20%, respectively.[5] Patients with effaced lymph nodes or the presence of large cell transformation had a uniformly poor prognosis.[43,44]

Human T-Cell Leukemia Virus-1–Associated Adult T-Cell Leukemia

ATLL is associated with the HTLV-1. The virus is endemic in southwest Japan, the Caribbean basin, South America, and parts of the Mediterranean basin and Central Africa and is transmitted primarily through breast milk. Clinical disease in the form of acute leukemia, smouldering leukemia, or lymphoma develops in 1% to 5% of seropositive individuals after a long latency of at least two to four decades. The chronic and smouldering variants can present with skin lesions that are indistinguishable from those of MF with or without circulating leukemia cells. Patients with ATLL present with fevers and B symptoms, high numbers of circulating leukemia cells, lymphadenopathy, organomegaly, hypercalcemia, and skin involvement. Histopathologic features in the skin are similar to MF, and the immunophenotype of the malignant cells is characteristically CD4+ with high expression of the IL-2 receptor, CD25. Clonally integrated HTLV-1 virus is found by real-time PCR in all cases and is useful in distinguishing MF from HTLV-1–associated disease in individuals from endemic areas. The prognosis depends on the clinical subtype, with smoldering variants having a more protracted course. The outcome for acute ATLL is poor, despite novel treatment advances.

CLINICAL EVALUATION OF PATIENTS WITH CUTANEOUS LYMPHOMA

Initial evaluation should include a careful assessment of the number and distribution of each type of skin lesion. A number of skin scoring systems have been developed to quantitate the skin disease burden in cutaneous lymphomas. The Skin Weighted Assessment Tool, a validated assessment tool, divides the body surface into areas that are assigned a value based on the percentage of total body surface area represented.[45] The observer then estimates the percentage of each body area involved with disease based on the estimation that the palm of the hand is 1%. The involvement is weighted based on whether the lesions are patch, plaque, or tumor. The sum is the skin score, which can be recorded and monitored during therapy.

Skin biopsies at multiple sites may be necessary to establish the diagnosis, especially for patients with MF, because lesion morphology varies even for different lesions from the same patient and the quality and quantity of infiltrating cells may be affected by topical therapies, including topical steroids. In addition, most of the cells in the underlying, often much more impressive dermal infiltrate are nonneoplastic reactive CD4+ and CD8+ T lymphocytes. Features of pleomorphism and the presence of large cells should be noted. Transformation to a large cell phenotype in patients with MF/SS is associated with a poor prognosis. Immunophenotyping should be performed on skin biopsies to better define the identity of the benign and neoplastic cell populations present in the cutaneous lesions. PCR-based assays should be performed as part of the initial diagnostic evaluation and are able to detect clonal T-cell populations in

90% of skin biopsies that show diagnostic CTCL pathology. The 10% false-negative rate may reflect the fact that the currently available PCR primer pairs amplify only 90% of gamma chain variable regions.

Laboratory studies should include routine complete blood count, chemistry panel, lactate dehydrogenase, and flow cytometry to detect circulating neoplastic cells. In investigational settings, it is possible to use monoclonal antibodies directed against TCR-Vb families to detect and precisely quantitate the levels of circulating leukemia cells. In most instances, the level of circulating CTCL cells is actually much higher than estimated by less-sensitive techniques such as by evaluation of the peripheral smear for atypical cells.[21] In many patients, the expansion of the neoplastic T-cell clone is accompanied by depression of normal T cells to levels comparable with those observed in advanced acquired immunodeficiency syndrome. Such a *de facto* T-cell deficiency may both explain the susceptibility of erythrodermic CTCL patients to infection by bacterial, viral, and fungal pathogens[22] and contribute to the progression of the disease, which is often held in check by host immune mechanisms.

In the absence of specific anti-CTCL monoclonal antibodies, routine flow can accurately detect and quantitate circulating Sézary cells. Flow cytometry should be performed with antibodies to the CD4, CD8, CD3, CD45R0, and CD26 antigens. The ratio of CD4+ to CD8+ cells is normally 0.5 to 3.5; elevations in this ratio correlate with total leukocyte count and with extent of skin disease in CTCL patients. An elevated ratio of CD4+ to CD8+ cells above 4.5 to 1.0 strongly suggests significant levels of circulating CTCL cells. Dual color staining with CD4 and other antigens can detect low or absent expression of CD3, CD7, or CD26 as a feature of Sézary cells.

The incidence of lymphadenopathy and bone marrow involvement increases with T stage and is associated with a poorer prognosis in patients with MF. Imaging studies (computed tomography scan or magnetic resonance imaging) are recommended at initial evaluation, especially for those with advanced disease, as well as during follow-up, to detect enlargement of thoracic, abdominal, or pelvic nodes. Positron emission tomography has been performed for patients with CTCL, but there is not enough experience to reliably determine the sensitivity and specificity in cutaneous lymphoma.[46,47] Pathologically enlarged lymph nodes should be biopsied at initial staging and subsequently if enlargement is detected on physical examination or imaging studies because a proportion of patients with CTCL may have other lymphomas (B or T cell; e.g., Hodgkin's) concurrently. Bone marrow biopsy should be obtained in patients with advanced disease, including those with SS, as well as in patients with compromised hematologic function. Biopsies of visceral organs such as liver should be dictated based on clinical indication or to confirm findings on imaging studies.

PRINCIPLES OF THERAPY OF MYCOSIS FUNGOIDES AND THE SÉZARY SYNDROME

Treatment approaches for MF/SS depend on the clinical stage of disease. Early stage disease that is localized to the skin (patch or plaque disease) has an excellent chance of cure or long-term control with therapies directed to the skin alone. In contrast, tumor stage disease, extensive plaque stage disease that is refractory to topical therapies, and nodal or visceral disease can be palliated but rarely cured. The many modalities used for the different stages of disease are shown in Table 128.5. Because MF/SS is immunosuppressive and an immunologically responsive disease, initial therapies for many patients involve cutaneous and biological approaches that act directly on CTCL cells (e.g., they are directly cytotoxic) but also have indirect effects (e.g., alter the cutaneous environment) that may play a role in disease control.[48]

Skin-Directed Therapy

Skin-directed modalities include those for localized disease (radiotherapy, bexarotene, carmustine) and those applicable to total skin therapy (topical chemotherapy with nitrogen mustard [NM], phototherapy, and total skin electron-beam therapy [TSEBT]). All skin-directed therapies exert their primary effects on disease confined to the skin. Most are capable of destroying CTCL cells directly, probably by triggering T-lymphocyte apoptosis, and many may interfere with the local production of cytokines by epithelial and stromal cells necessary for neoplastic T-cell survival and proliferation.[49]

Approximately 7% of patients with stage I disease present with a solitary cutaneous lesion or several in proximity. Wilson et al.[50] found that the rate of clinical remission after local external-beam radiotherapy is very high (approximately 95%) in these patients and may be the treatment of choice. In one study, a total of 21 patients were treated with electron-beam radiation to a median dose of 20 Gy. With a median follow-up of 36 months, the actuarial disease-free survival rates at 5 and 10 years were 75% and 64%, respectively, with a local control rate of 83% at 10 years.

Topical Chemotherapies

Topical NM is one of the first treatments for cutaneous manifestations of MF. The NM liquid can be applied to the skin as an aqueous solution of 10 mg/dL or applied in an ointment base. Allergic response in the form of hyperemia, erythema, or skin pain can occur after application. Long-term effects include induction of second cutaneous malignancies (e.g., squamous cell carcinomas) and hyperpigmentation and hypopigmentation. Between 64% and 90% of NM-treated patients with T1 and T2 CTCL can achieve a complete response to therapy. Although many patients appear to be cleared by topical NM therapy, seven of eight patients relapse within 3 years unless a maintenance topical NM regimen has been instituted. Maintenance topical NM can also be used to prevent or delay relapse of cutaneous lesions in patients who have achieved a complete response to TSEBT or to treat minimal patch or plaque recurrences after such therapy.

Another topical chemotherapeutic agent useful in the treatment of CTCL is carmustine. Ointment-based preparations of carmustine are stable. The selection of a concentration of 10 to 30 mg/dL depends on the size of the lesions being treated. Carmustine is absorbed and leads to bone marrow suppression if too high a concentration is used over too large an area. However, given the marked variability in absorption, it is best to use 20 mg/dL for up to 10% of body surface area (BSA) and monitor blood counts weekly. An irritant response may occur, and cutaneous telangiectasias may develop in one-third of patients. A typical course of topical carmustine would extend for 3 to 4 months to induce a remission.

Topical Bexarotene Gel

Bexarotene is a novel RXR retinoid (retinoid X receptor) that has been shown to be effective both systemically and topically for patients with MF/SS. Topical bexarotene gel is applied once or twice daily and often results in an irritant dermatitis. The overall response rate to topical bexarotene in clinical trials was 44%. The drug is not absorbed to any significant level. The irritant dermatitis generally limits the use of the gel to patients with BSA of less than 15% because of discomfort. Typically, bexarotene gel is applied to lesions with a frequency dictated

PRACTICE OF ONCOLOGY

TABLE 128.5

TREATMENTS FOR MYCOSIS FUNGOIDES/SÉZARY SYNDROME

Therapy	Response (%)	Toxicities
TOPICAL AGENTS		
Mechlorethamine or carmustine	CRR Stage I: 76–86 Stage IIA: 55 Stage III: 22–49	Contact dermatitis, secondary cutaneous malignancies
Bexarotene	Stage IA–IIA: 21 CR, 42 PR	Contact dermatitis
PHOTOTHERAPY		
UVB	CRR Stage IA/IB: 75–83	Erythema, pruritus
PUVA	CRR Stage IA: 79–88 Stage IB: 52–59 Stage IIA: 83 Stage III: 46	Nausea, phototoxic reactions, secondary cutaneous malignancies
PUVA plus interferon alpha (1) vs. acitretin plus interferon alpha (2)	CRR Stage I/II: 70 (1) vs. 38 (2)	Flulike symptoms
RADIOTHERAPY		
Total skin electron-beam therapy	CRR Stage IA–IIA: 96 Stage IIB: 36 Stage III: 60	Secondary cutaneous malignancies, pigmentation, anhydrosis, pruritus, alopecia, xerosis, telangiectasia
CYTOTOXIC CHEMOTHERAPY		
EPOCH	ORR Stage IIB–IV: 80	Myelosuppression
Pentostatin	ORR Stage IIB: 75 Stage III: 58 Stage IV: 50	Lymphopenia
Fludarabine plus interferon alpha	ORR Stage IIA–IVA: 58 Stage IVB: 40	Neutropenia
Gemcitabine	ORR Stage IIB/III: 70	Neutropenia
Pegylated liposomal doxorubicin	ORR Stage IA–IV: 88	Infusion-related events
NOVEL TARGETED STRATEGIES		
Bexarotene	ORR Stage IA/IIA: 20–67 Stage IIB–IV: 49	Hypertriglyceridemia hyperlipidemia, hypothyroidism
Vorinostat	ORR 29 Stage IA/IIA: 20–31 Stage IIB–IV: 25–30	Diarrhea, nausea, vomiting, fatigue
Denileukin diftitox	ORR Stage I/IIA: 37 Stage IIB–IV: 24 Stages II–IV (less heavily pretreated) 62	Flulike symptoms, infusion-related events, vascular leak syndrome
Denileukin diftitox + bexarotene	ORR 72	

CRR, complete response rate; CR, complete response; PR, partial response; ORR, overall response rate; UVB, ultraviolet B; PUVA, ultraviolet A light with oral methoxypsoralen; EPOCH, etoposide, vincristine, doxorubicin, cyclophosphamide, and prednisone.

by the irritant response, once or twice a day. The involved areas are kept in an irritated state for 12 weeks; the patient holds off therapy for a month and then is evaluated for persistent disease.[29] In many cases, topical bexarotene gel is used alternating with topical steroids to minimize the irritant effect.

Phototherapy

Phototherapy has been effective for patients with MF/SS because keratinocytes are resistant to ultraviolet (UV) light–induced injuries, whereas lymphocytes are extremely sensitive to light in the form of either UVA (320 to 400 nm), UVB (290 to 320 nm), or narrow-band UVB (311 nm). Currently, narrow-band UVB is used most commonly because of the low risk of secondary skin neoplasms. Patients typically are treated three to four times per week for approximately 30 to 40 treatments to achieve a remission, and then treatment frequency is decreased to a maintenance schedule at weekly intervals. Broad-band UVB has the same treatment schedule.[33]

Photochemotherapy with orally administered PUVA (ultraviolet A light with oral methoxypsoralen) irradiation of the skin therapy requires the ingestion of 0.6 mg/kg of 8-methoxypsoralen 1 to 2 hours before the exposure of the skin surface to UVA light (320 to 400 nm). Alternatively, the drug may be dissolved in bath water and applied to the skin, for minimal absorption, before light exposure. To induce remission, treatments should begin three times per week at doses that are minimally phototoxic. After most of the lesions have cleared, the frequency of PUVA can be decreased to twice weekly until the patient has achieved a remission. However, patients should probably not be considered "cured" until they have remained disease free for at least 5 years after completing therapy. It is recommended that PUVA maintenance be started at once-weekly intervals, eventually extended to once-monthly sessions, subsequent to a complete response, and that maintenance be continued for several years to reduce the risk of early relapse of disease.

Combination Regimens Involving PUVA Photochemotherapy. Several well-conducted trials have assessed the role of PUVA in combination with various systemic agents, notably interferon alfa and retinoids. Phase 1 and 2 studies of PUVA (three times weekly) combined with variable doses of interferon alfa (maximum tolerated dose of 12 MU/m^2 three times weekly) in 39 patients with MF (all stages) and SS have reported an overall response rate of 100%.[51] Complete response rates were 79% in stage IB patients, 80% in stage IIA patients, 33% in stage IIB patients, 63% in stage III patients, and 40% in stage IVA patients. PUVA was continued as a maintenance therapy indefinitely and interferon alfa was continued for 2 years or until disease progression or withdrawal resulting from adverse effects. The median duration of response (DOR) was 28 months, with a median survival of 62 months.

A randomized controlled trial compared PUVA (two to five times weekly) plus interferon alfa (9 MU three times weekly) with interferon alfa plus an RAR retinoid (retinoic acid receptor) acitretin (25 to 50 mg/d) in 98 patients with a maximum duration of treatment in both groups of 48 weeks.[52] In 82 patients with stage I or II disease, complete response rates were 70% in the PUVA/interferon group compared with 38% in the interferon/acitretin group. Time to response was 18.6 weeks in the PUVA/interferon group, compared with 21.8 weeks in the interferon/acitretin group. These studies suggest that combined PUVA and interferon alfa are more effective than a combination of interferon alfa and acitretin in early stage I or II disease.

Total Skin Electron-Beam Therapy

Treatment of the entire cutaneous surface with TSEBT is technically much more challenging than local x-ray therapy and should be attempted only in centers with appropriate equipment and in which a close working relationship has been established between dermatologists and radiation oncologists committed to and experienced in the treatment of patients with CTCL. Several recent publications have detailed the history and evolution of TSEBT, from 1952 to the present, including consideration of physical dosimetry, radiobiology, and all published clinical results.[53] Electrons ranging in energy between 4 and 7 MeV are used to homogeneously treat the epidermis and dermis. Structures below the deep dermis are relatively spared because most of the dose (80%) is typically administered within the first 10 mm of depth and less than 5% beyond 20 mm depth. Generally, doses to skin target are in the range of 30 to 36 Gy. Blood and superficial lymph nodes may receive 20% to 40% of the skin surface dose, and this may be clinically important. Technical factors such as completeness of skin treatment, surface dose, and energy or penetration of the electrons are related to clinical outcomes; more intense TSEBT is associated with a greater rate of complete remission and better progression-free experience, and low dose per fraction is associated with reduced acute and chronic side effects.

TSEBT may be administered as just one in a sequence of treatments for CTCL in a particular patient. For example, TSEBT is an excellent treatment for patients with diffuse involvement with thick plaques or cutaneous tumors and is also suitable for patients with symptomatic erythroderma T4 disease.[54] TSEBT is also an excellent alternative for patients with extensive patches or thin plaques refractory to PUVA or other skin-directed therapies. When used in these ways, TSEBT is typically delayed after diagnosis of CTCL until other topical, and even systemic therapies, have been administered and disease has become progressive or refractory. In contrast, TSEBT may be used as an important component of a radiation-based management strategy to control CTCL. This clinical strategy uses radiation whenever and wherever it seems clinically indicated, with the intent to minimize time spent with disease, treatments and related procedures, and toxicities.[55] From this perspective, TSEBT is offered to patients with early or stage IA disease at the time of initial diagnosis. Supplemental patch radiotherapy fields to regions of skin that are relatively underdosed are required to reduce isolated failures in those regions, which otherwise occur approximately 19% of the time. Further, for patients at high risk for more generalized relapse in skin subsequent to TSEBT, adjuvant therapies are seriously considered to build on the initial effects of TSEBT. Subsequently, TSEBT may be administered to a patient several times using a variety of dose schedules, as clinically required to help control progressive disease.

Clinical complete response rates for patients with T1 or T2 (patch or plaque) disease range from 71% to 98% and are higher in patients with less-extensive disease. Patients with T1 and T2 disease treated with TSEBT have disease-free and overall survivals of 50% to 65% and 80% to 90%, respectively, at 5 years, although patients with antecedent or coexisting lymphomatoid papulosis or alopecia mucinosa–follicular mucinosis appear to have shorter disease-free survival after TSEBT than those who do not. Patients with more advanced T3 and T4 disease fare significantly worse, with 5-year disease-free and overall survivals of approximately 20% and 50%, respectively. However, those T3 patients with less than 10% of the total skin surface involved by CTCL have significantly better disease-free and overall survival after TSEBT than those with more extensive disease. For patients with erythrodermic MF (T4) who are managed with TSEBT alone (32 to 40 Gy), without concomitant or neoadjuvant therapy, the complete response rate is approximately 70%. The 5-year progression-free, cause-specific, and overall survivals are 26%, 52%, and 38%, respectively.[54]

Palliation of adenopathy or visceral involvement in patients with N3 disease can be accomplished by the use of appropriate

PRACTICE OF ONCOLOGY

high-energy orthovoltage or megavoltage photons to doses of 20 to 30 Gy. Even 6 to 8 Gy in three fractions is sufficient (e.g., when combined with TSEBT). Combinations of TSEBT with total nodal radiation have been investigated. Although feasible, such combinations do not appear to prolong survival and may be associated with hematologic toxicities not observed with TSEBT alone.

TSEBT is well tolerated by most patients; acute sequelae either during or within the initial 6 months after treatment may include pruritus, desquamation, alopecia, epilation, hypohidrosis, xerosis, erythema, lower extremity edema, bullae of the feet, and onychoptosis. Chronic changes can include atrophy of the skin, telangiectasia, alopecia, hypohidrosis, and xerosis. Because of the superficial penetration of the electron beam, patients do not experience gastrointestinal nor hematologic toxicities. Second malignancies such as squamous and basal cell carcinomas, as well as malignant melanomas have been observed in patients treated with TSEBT, particularly in patients exposed to multiple therapies that are themselves known to be mutagenic, such as PUVA and mechlorethamine.[55,56] It is interesting that additional x-ray or electron-beam irradiation after TSEBT does not appear to increase the risk of second cutaneous malignancies.[55]

For patients who suffer diffuse cutaneous recurrences after TSEBT not amenable to other skin-directed therapies, a second course of TSEBT is both feasible and worthwhile. At Yale University, a total of 14 patients have received two, and five patients received three, courses of TSEBT. The median total dose after these additional courses was 57 Gy, and 86% of the patients achieved a complete response after the second course, with a median disease-free interval of 11.5 months. Median dose was 36 Gy for the first course, 18 Gy for the second, and 12 Gy for the third.[57] A similar experience was reported from Stanford University, where 15 patients were identified who had been treated with a second course of TSEBT (median dose of 20 Gy), with a complete response rate of 40%.[58] Nine of these patients had a partial response to therapy, and the median total dose for the entire group was 56 Gy. In both series, repeat courses were relatively well tolerated, and sequelae were similar to those observed during and after the first course of therapy.

Combined and Sequential Therapy

The adjuvant use of PUVA after TSEBT in patients with T1 and T2 disease significantly decreased cutaneous relapse. Patients treated with adjuvant PUVA after TSEBT had a 5-year disease-free survival of 85%, compared with 50% for those not receiving PUVA ($P < .02$). The median disease-free survival for the T1 patients receiving adjuvant PUVA was not reached at 103 months versus 66 months for the non-PUVA group ($P < .01$). For those with T2 disease, the disease-free survival figures were 60 and 20 months, respectively ($P < .03$).[59] Adjuvant topical NM also appears able to delay cutaneous recurrence after TSEBT. In 1999, Chinn et al.[60] from Stanford University showed that TSEBT with or without NM provided improved response rates compared with mustard alone for those patients with T2 and T3 level disease (76% vs. 39%; $P < .03$ for T2; 44% vs. 8%; $P < .05$ for T3). For those with patch or plaque (T2), adjuvant mustard offered improved freedom from relapse after TSEBT compared with no adjuvant treatment. No significant survival differences were noted between the groups.

The combination of extracorporeal photochemotherapy (ECP) administered during and after TSEBT appears to improve survival ($P < .06$) for patients with T3 or T4 disease who have achieved a complete response to TSEBT; however, the group of treated patients was small, and the data are retrospective.[61] Wilson et al.[62] identified a significant improvement in cause-specific survival for erythrodermic patients (blood status both B0 and B1) treated with the combination of TSEBT and ECP compared with those not treated with ECP. The 2-year progression-free, cause-specific, and overall survivals for those receiving TSEBT/ECP were 66%, 100%, and 88%, respectively, compared with 36%, 69%, and 63% for those not managed with the combination.

SYSTEMIC THERAPY FOR MYCOSIS FUNGOIDES AND THE SÉZARY SYNDROME

Biological Therapies

Interferon alfa has been demonstrated in a number of studies to be a highly active agent in CTCL, with response rates ranging from 40% to 80%.[63] Doses have ranged from 1 to 18 mU administered subcutaneously on a number of schedules, the most common being three times a week. Interferon gamma has also demonstrated activity but is not as widely used. Constitutional symptoms and bone marrow suppression have limited aggressive and long-term use of interferons for many patients. Early studies with high-dose IL-2 has demonstrated activity in relapsed CTCL but with significant toxicity. In a recent study of intermediate-dose IL-2, 11 patients (median age, 60 years) with advanced or refractory CTCL underwent 8-week cycles of daily subcutaneous injections of 11 MIU, 4 days per week for 6 weeks, followed by 2 weeks off therapy. This dose was well tolerated, and there were four partial responses, three of which were sustained.[64] IL-12 has also demonstrated activity in early and advanced MF. A phase 2 study demonstrated responses in 43% of the patients, with response durations ranging from 3 to 45 weeks.[65]

Photopheresis (Extracorporeal Photochemotherapy)

ECP, or photopheresis, involves a leukapheresis to isolate mononuclear cells that are exposed *ex vivo* to UVA in the presence of methoxypsoralen and then reinfused back into the patient. Methoxypsoralen incorporates into DNA and in the presence of UV light, induces strand breaks and subsequently apoptosis. Circulating T cells and Sézary leukemia cells are more susceptible to UVA-induced apoptosis than are monocytes. The mechanism of action of ECP is believed to be related to the induction of apoptosis in clonal Sézary T cells, leading to uptake and processing of tumor antigens by immature dendritic cells generated from the effects of the ECP process on circulating monocytoid precursors.[66,67] The process of ECP has been shown to induce a cell-mediated antitumor response. Clinical improvement with ECP has been demonstrated in both patients with SS and in patients with tumor and plaque-stage CTCL.

Currently, ECP is frequently used as monotherapy for CTCL, but its combination with other therapies is currently under study. ECP is initially administered on a once-a-month schedule, with therapy continued until maximal clearing is established. An additional 6 months of therapy may be administered to consolidate the clinical response. After the patient's disease has stabilized, the interval between ECP treatments is gradually prolonged by 1 week per cycle every three cycles. After the interval between treatments has reached 8 weeks for three cycles, therapy can be discontinued.

Patients with CTCL in the original cohort treated with ECP have also been carefully studied to determine whether this therapy exerted any adverse effects on host immune response, but none were found. The immunomodulatory effects of ECP have been augmented by the use of cytokines and by the use of transimmunization, an extension of the conventional ECP procedure. Immune adjuvant therapies, including interferon alfa, bexarotene, and granulocyte-macrophage colony-stimulating factor have been combined with ECP and have shortened the time to response.[68] Transimmunization involves the overnight incubation of the ECP-treated cells prior to reinfusion into the patient in order to enhance the uptake of apoptotic Sézary leukemia cells by maturing antigen presenting cells. A phase 1 trial of transimmunization in advanced CTCL has been completed and demonstrated a significant mean reduction of 50.1% in the circulating malignant Sézary cells, as determined with family-specific anti-T-cell receptor Vβ-monoclonal antibodies, after several months of therapy.[69]

Bexarotene (Retinoid Therapy)

Retinoid analogues have been categorized based on their binding patterns with respect to the major classes of retinoid receptors, RAR and RXR. Initial studies demonstrated that the retinoids approved for acne and psoriasis (binding both RAR and RXR) could produce responses in MF-CTCL. Bexarotene is an oral RXR selective retinoid with activity both topically and orally. In a clinical trial of heavily pretreated refractory CTCL, oral monotherapy with bexarotene had a response rate of 54% in early stage and 45% in advanced-stage CTCL patients. The median response duration was 299 days with continuous dosing at a dose of 300 mg/m^2/d, and responses occurred in all groups of patients (57% at stage IIB, 32% at stage III, 44% at stage IVA, and 40% at stage IVB), including those with large cell transformation. Pruritus decreased significantly in the treated patients and led to overall improvement in quality-of-life indices.

The major toxicities of bexarotene included elevations in serum lipids and cholesterol and suppression of thyroid function. Elevations in the lipids occurred rapidly, within 2 to 4 weeks, requiring the use of lipid-lowering agents in the majority of patients. Patients taking bexarotene also developed a dose-dependent central hypothyroidism with low thyroid-stimulating hormone and free thyroxine levels within weeks of starting the medication. Bexarotene has been widely used as a first systemic oral therapy for patients with both early and advanced MF/SS. Therapy is often initiated at a low dose (two to four capsules per day) and titrated to achieve a therapeutic effect. Laboratory studies should be performed weekly until lipid and thyroid functions are stable and then intermittently during therapy.

Histone Deacetylase Inhibitors

Histone deacetylase (HDAC) inhibitors modulate gene expression by inhibiting the deacetylation of histone proteins associated with DNA, thereby allowing expression of a number of genes. HDAC inhibition has been shown to induce histone acetylation, cell cycle arrest, and apoptosis in leukemia and lymphoma cell lines. Depsipeptide was the first HDAC inhibitor tested in clinical trials at the National Cancer Institute, and responses were seen in patients with T-cell lymphomas who received 14 mg/m^2 given intravenously on days 1, 8, and 15 of a 21-day cycle.[70] Two multicenter phase 2 trials of romidepsin have been completed and have led to U.S. Food and Drug Administration (FDA) approval for romidepsin in CTCL.[71] In both studies, the dose was 14 mg/m^2 given by a 4-hour intravenous infusion weekly times three on a 4-week schedule. The overall response rate in 167 patients with advanced or refractory CTCL was 35%, with 6% achieving a clinical complete response. The median response duration was 11 and 14 months in the National Cancer Institute's (NCI) and the sponsor's phase 2 studies, respectively. The most frequent adverse events (all grades) were nausea, constitutional symptoms, and thrombocytopenia. Reversible ST-T segment changes and QT prolongation were seen on electrocardiograms but returned to baseline within 24 hours, and there were no clinically relevant sequelae.

Vorinostat (Zolinza, suberoylanilide hydroxamic acid), an orally bioavailable HDAC inhibitor, was recently approved by the FDA for the treatment of advanced or refractory CTCL. In a phase 2 single-agent study, oral vorinostat was administered at doses of 400 mg daily, 300 mg twice a day for 3 days with 4 days rest, or 300 mg twice daily for 14 days with 7 days rest, followed by 200 mg twice daily.[72] The overall response rate in this heavily pretreated population was 24%. The 400-mg daily schedule had the most favorable response rate and was subsequently evaluated in a phase 2 study that led to the approval of the drug. In this study of 74 patients with refractory CTCL, including 61 with stage IIB or higher disease, the response rate was 29%, with a median time to response of 56 days and a median response duration ranging from 34 to 441+ days.[73] Overall, 32% of patients had relief of pruritus.

The recommended dose of vorinostat is 400 mg/d. The most common side effects are gastrointestinal (diarrhea in 49%, nausea in 43%, anorexia in 26%), fatigue, and mild thrombocytopenia, which is reversible on discontinuation of the drug. Dehydration may occur because of anorexia, and patients should be encouraged to remain well hydrated and to use antiemetics if needed. Because of the propensity of HDAC inhibitors to induce prolongation of the QTC interval, patients and their physicians should be advised to obtain baseline electrocardiograms and to carefully review concomitant medication lists for potential QTC prolonging agents, which should be avoided during vorinostat administration.

Denileukin Diftitox

Denileukin diftitox is a fusion protein consisting of the *IL-2* gene joined to the active and membrane-translocating domains of diphtheria toxin. Denileukin diftitox intoxicates cells that express both intermediate- and high-affinity IL-2 receptors by inhibiting protein synthesis. The expression of the IL-2 receptor on MF/SS cells and on other T- and B-cell lymphomas has been defined by immunohistochemistry in the clinical trials of denileukin diftitox, as eligibility was defined as expression of CD25, the alpha subunit of the receptor, on at least 20% of the tumor cells. About 50% of patients with MF/SS who were screened for entry onto the clinical trials were CD25+ by these criteria. However, the limitations of immunohistochemistry are that low levels of receptor expression (less than 500 receptors per cell) are below the threshold of the assay, and it is difficult to determine in many instances whether the tumor cells or infiltrating normal lymphocytes are positive for CD25. *In vitro* studies have demonstrated that denileukin diftitox is capable of intoxicating cells with less than 500 CD25 receptors. Cells that are CD25− and express the intermediate affinity IL-2R (CD122, CD132) have intermediate susceptibility to the drug.

In the pivotal trial that led to FDA approval of denileukin diftitox, the drug was administered at a dose of either 9 mg/kg or 18 mg/kg, for 5 days every 21 days, in 71 patients with relapsed or refractory CTCL.[74] The median number of prior therapies in this study was five. The overall response rate was similar for both dose groups and was 30% overall, with 10% complete responses (7 patients) and 20% partial responses (14 patients).[73] Most of the responses occurred in the first four cycles of therapy, and the median response duration was approximately 6.9 months. The major toxicities included a reversible elevation of hepatic transaminases, a hypersensitivity syndrome associated with drug infusion, and a mild vascular leak syndrome that occurred in 29% of patients. A subsequent study that combined corticosteroid pretreatment with denileukin diftitox in a less heavily pretreated group of patients demonstrated a response rate of 70% with a significantly reduced incidence of hypersensitivity reactions and clinically significant vascular leak.[75]

A randomized, placebo-controlled phase 3 trial has been completed to compare denileukin diftitox at doses of 9 and 18 mcg/kg daily for 5 days on a 21-day schedule in patients with earlier stage CTCL who have had fewer prior therapies.[76]

Of 144 patients treated, 67% had stage I or IIA disease. The overall response rates were 46%, 37%, and 15% for the 18 mcg, 9 mcg, and placebo arms, respectively. A combination study of bexarotene and denileukin diftitox was initiated based on the observation that bexarotene up-regulates expression of IL-2 receptor on lymphoma cells and enhances the susceptibility of these cells to undergo apoptosis in the presence of denileukin diftitox. Fourteen patients with refractory CTCL received escalating daily doses of bexarotene (75 to 300 mg) and denileukin diftitox (18 mcg/kg for 3 days every 21 days).[77] The overall response rate for all evaluable patients was 70%, with four complete responses (35%) and four partial responses (35%). Four patients developed grade 2 or 3 leukopenia, and two developed grade 4 lymphopenia. This study demonstrated that doses of bexarotene greater than 150 mg/d were capable of *in vivo* up-regulation of CD25 (IL-2) expression and may enhance the efficacy of denileukin diftitox.

Monoclonal Antibodies

Alemtuzumab, a humanized monoclonal antibody that targets the CD52 antigen, has been shown to be active in relapsed or refractory T-cell lymphomas. Because of its profound effects on immune effector cells, alemtuzumab treatment has been associated with significant immunosuppression and a high incidence of opportunistic infections. Recent studies with lower doses of alemtuzumab (10 mg three times per week) have reported responses in six of ten patients, including two complete responses and four partial responses, with minimal immunosuppression.[78,79] Zanolimumab, a high-affinity, fully humanized monoclonal antibody that targets the CD4 receptor, has shown promising results in 49 patients with biopsy-proven CD4+ CTCL, including 23 patients with advanced-stage disease.[80] Patients were initially treated with intravenous zanolimumab at a dose of 280 mg/wk, which was increased to 560 mg/wk in early stage patients and 980 mg/wk in patients with advanced disease. Partial remissions were reported in 16 of 36 (44%) evaluable patients overall, including 3 of 6 with advanced disease at treated with 980 mg/wk.

Cytotoxic Chemotherapy

A number of agents have demonstrated activity in CTCL. These include alkylating therapies, such as cyclophosphamide, chlorambucil and prednisone, etoposide, and methotrexate. Although combination chemotherapy regimens have produced higher responses in patients with advanced refractory CTCL, these responses have not been durable. A study of infusional EPOCH (etoposide, vincristine, doxorubicin, bolus cyclophosphamide, and oral prednisone) in advanced refractory CTCL demonstrated an overall response rate of 80% (12 patients), with 4 (27%) complete responses.[81] However, the median response duration was just 8 months (range, 3 to 22 months) and the median survival was 13.5 months. Treatment-related toxicity was significant, with 61% of the patients experiencing grade 3 or 4 myelosuppression. Because of the high risk of infection and myelosuppression and modest response durations with combination chemotherapy, single-agent therapies are preferred except in patients who are refractory or who present with extensive adenopathy or visceral involvement and require immediate palliation.

Purine Analogues

One class of agents that has demonstrated significant activity is the nucleoside analogues. Overall response rates up to 70% have been reported for single-agent pentostatin in refractory patients. Investigators at the M. D. Anderson Cancer Center reported a response rate of 56% for dose-escalated pentostatin (3 to 5 mg/m^2/d for 3 days on a 21-day schedule) in 42 patients with CTCL.[82] The failure-free survival was 2.1 months. Grade 3 or 4 neutropenia occurred in 21% of patients. The incidence of infectious complications with pentostatin was initially high but was subsequently reduced by prophylactic trimethoprim and antiviral therapies. In a combination study of pentostatin at 4 mg/m^2/d for 3 days with intermediate dose interferon alfa, the overall response rate was similar, but the median progression-free survival was improved to 13.1 months.[83]

Fludarabine and cladribine have demonstrated more modest single-agent activity in MF/SS. The combination of fludarabine with interferon alfa had greater efficacy with an overall response rate of 51% (4 complete responses, 14 partial responses) with a median progression-free survival of 5.9 months and an overall survival of 19.6 months; however, hematologic toxicity was significant, with 62% of patients experiencing grade 3 or 4 neutropenia.[84] Similarly, a combination of fludarabine (18 mg/m^2) and cyclophosphamide (250 mg/m^2) for 3 days monthly was associated with a DOR of 10 months but with significant hematologic toxicity.[85]

Gemcitabine has demonstrated impressive clinical activity in advanced and refractory CTCL, with a 70% response rate when administered on days 1, 8, and 15 of a 28-day schedule at doses of 1,000 to 1,200 mg/m^2.[86,87] The incidence of grade 3 neutropenia was 25%. Median response duration was 8 months. In a study of chemotherapy-naive patients treated with 1,200 mg/m^2, the response rate was 70%, with five complete responders.[88]

Forodesine (BCX-1777) is a novel nucleoside analogue that inhibits purine nucleoside phosphorylase, resulting in accumulation of deoxyguanosine and dGTP and apoptosis in T lymphocytes. A phase 1 and 2 study of intravenous forodesine enrolled 13 patients with CTCL or SS who received at least one course of forodesine.[89] Nine of the 13 patients had a skin improvement or a pharmacodynamic response, as measured by a decrease in the absolute numbers of Sézary cells or a decrease in the CD4/CD8 ratio. A study of oral forodesine is under way in patients with relapsed or refractory CTCL at doses of 40, 80, 160, and 320 mg/d for 28 days. Toxicities associated with forodesine have been mild and include nausea and reversible lymphopenia.[90]

Liposomal Doxorubicin

Pegylated liposomal doxorubicin is an active agent in Kaposi's sarcoma and has been shown to accumulate in involved skin lesions. In patients with advanced MF, response rates of 80% have been reported. In one study at a dose of 20 mg/m^2 every 28 days, there were four complete responses, and in a larger study of 34 patients with CTCL or PTCL who received 20 mg/m^2 every 2 weeks (n = 6), every 2 to 3 weeks (n = 4), or every 4 weeks (n = 23), there were 15 complete responses and 15 partial responses, with a median event-free survival of 12 months. With the exception of infusion related events, liposomal doxorubicin was well tolerated.

Pralatrexate

Pralatrexate is a promising new folate antagonist with activity in patients with T-cell lymphoma and has been approved for patients with aggressive peripheral T-cell lymphoma. A phase 1 study of pralatrexate in advanced and refractory CTCL has demonstrated responses and further studies are under way.

Autologous and Allogeneic Bone Marrow Transplantation

Results with autologous stem cell transplantation have not been promising in patients with MF/SS. One major issue in many studies is eradication of disease prior to transplant, and most patients have undergone extensive prior therapy. Allogeneic stem cell transplantation has been shown to induce complete and durable remissions in a small number of patients with CTCL, with disappearance of the malignant clone from the peripheral blood. Molina et al.[91] reported successful outcomes with donor transplants in six of eight refractory CTCL patients. All achieved a complete remission; however, two died from transplant-related complications. Reduced-intensity allogeneic transplantation has been developed to reduce the toxicity related to induction therapy and to increase graft-versus-lymphoma effect, and it has been shown to induce a graft-versus-host effect in a small number of patients with advanced refractory MF and transformed disease. The use of reduced-intensity conditioning regimens in advanced CTCL patients is still undergoing investigation.

OTHER CUTANEOUS LYMPHOMAS

Primary CD30+ Lymphoproliferative Disorders

The primary CD30+ lymphomas comprise the second most frequent group of cutaneous lymphomas and include cutaneous CD30+ anaplastic large cell lymphoma (C-ALCL) and lymphomatoid papulosis (LyP). These two disorders represent a spectrum of disease, with LyP being a clonal but nonmalignant variant that must be distinguished from MF, which may undergo large cell transformation and express CD30 and also result from benign skin lesions containing CD30+ blastic cells, such as arthropod reactions, viral eruptions, and drug-related rashes. Clinically and histopathologically, LyP and C-ALCL may be indistinguishable. The classic presentation of LyP is papular, papulonodular, or papulonecrotic skin lesions at different stages of development with a waxing and waning course. The lesions often disappear within 12 weeks and often leave a scar. The median patient age is 45, but the disease does occur in children; the ratio of men to women patients is 1.5 to 1.0. Three histologic subtypes have been identified, all demonstrating large CD30+ cells with (type A) or without (type C) infiltrating inflammatory cells.[92] In some cases (type B), there is infiltration of the epidermis, similar to MF. Up to 60% of cases demonstrate clonality for TCR, but the (2:5) (p23;q35) translocation characteristic of alk+ ALCL is not present. Up to 20% of cases may be preceded by or follow another lymphoma, including MF, ALCL, or Hodgkin's lymphoma. For most patients, the prognosis is excellent, and the disease is managed either with no treatment, low doses of oral methotrexate, or PUVA. In a series of 118 isolated cases of LyP, only 4% of patients developed systemic lymphoma.

C-ALCL is similar to systemic ALCL except for the cutaneous presentation and the absence of systemic disease. All patients with C-ALCL should undergo careful staging to rule out systemic involvement before being classified as C-ALCL. Most patients present with solitary nodules, tumors, or ulcerating lesions that may spontaneously regress, but multifocal disease has been observed in up to 20% of patients. The histopathologic features of the disease include the presence of large, anaplastic cells that express CD30 antigen in more than 70% of the tumor cells. The tumor cells demonstrate clonality for TCRR, an activated CD4 phenotype with loss of other T-cell antigens and frequent expression of cytotoxic proteins (granzyme B, TIA-1, perforin). The (2:5) (p23;q35) alk translocation that is frequently seen in systemic ALCL is uncommonly observed in C-ALCL. In addition, the systemic ALCL expresses epithelial membrane antigen, which is absent in C-ALCL. The overall prognosis is excellent, and most patients are treated by surgical excision or local radiotherapy to the lesions. For recurrent disease, low doses of methotrexate or other cytotoxic agents may be used. A new family of humanized anti-CD30 antibodies has been developed and has shown efficacy in both systemic and cutaneous ALCL.

Subcutaneous Panniculitislike T-Cell Lymphoma and Cutaneous Peripheral T-Cell Lymphoma Unspecified

Subcutaneous panniculitislike T-cell lymphoma and cutaneous peripheral T-cell lymphomas (PTL) are disorders of medium-sized or large pleomorphic T cells. These diseases have distinct clinicopathologic features and outcomes. The subcutaneous panniculitislike T-cell lymphomas comprise two subtypes, the alpha/beta and the gamma/delta, and both are characterized by subcutaneous masses or flat plaques that mainly involve the legs but may be generalized. Often patients present with B symptoms such as fever, fatigue, and weight loss. The WHO-EORTC classification has separated these phenotypes because of their disparate outcomes and has included the gamma/delta variant in the category of PTL, gamma/delta type.[2] The alpha/beta SPTL is characterized by subcutaneous infiltrates that spare the epidermis and dermis and rim individual fat cells. In early stages, the tumor cells may lack significant atypia and an inflammatory infiltrate may be present, leading to a diagnosis of inflammatory panniculitis.

The classic phenotype of the malignant lymphocytes is CD3+, CD4–, CD8+ with expression of cytotoxic proteins. The outcome for alpha/beta type of SPCL is excellent, with an 80% 5-year survival. Treatments include corticosteroids, single-agent chemotherapy, and radiotherapy. The cutaneous gamma/delta T-cell lymphomas are characterized by disseminated disease with frequent mucosal and extranodal involvement. The hematophagocytic syndrome may occur. Histopathologic features include involvement of the dermis, epidermis, and fat with rimming of fat globules and angioinvasion. The phenotype of the cells is CD3+, C2+/–, CD8+, CD56+ beta F1– with lack of expression of either CD4 or CD8. Most patients have a poor outcome despite aggressive chemotherapy, with a median survival of 15 months reported in one series of 33 patients.

The cutaneous PTL is characterized by infiltration of the dermis by CD3+ CD4+ or CD3+ CD8+ pleomorphic small and medium-sized cells, in many cases with an admixture of reactive lymphocytes. Most cases demonstrate a loss of T-cell markers and are CD30– and rarely CD56+. The clinical features are plaques or tumors, often on the face, neck, or upper trunk. Outcome is variable and depends on the subtype. The estimated 5-year survival of the CD4+ types is 80% and the preferred treatments are surgery, radiation, or single-agent chemotherapy. The CD8+ variants often express cytotoxic phenotypes (granzyme B+, perforin+, TIA-1+) and are characterized by ulcerative or necrotic tumors or plaques with frequent dissemination to visceral sites but rarely to lymph nodes. Invasion and destruction of adnexastructures are seen on histopathology. The median survival for this group of patients is 32 months, despite aggressive systemic chemotherapy.

The Cutaneous Natural Killer Lymphomas

Extranodal NK/T-cell lymphoma is an Epstein-Barr virus–positive lymphoma with an NK or cytotoxic T-cell phenotype. The skin is the second most common site of involvement after the nasal cavity and sinuses. Skin may be a primary or secondary manifestation of the disease, which is disseminated in most patients. The disease is most common in South America, South Asia, and Central America. The clinical features include ulcerative or necrotic skin lesions characterized histopathologically by angiodestruction and extensive necrosis. Many patients have B symptoms and may manifest the hematophagocytic syndrome. The neoplastic cells express CD2, CD56, and cytotoxic proteins but lack surface CD3. The TCR is often germline and Epstein-Barr virus is almost always expressed. The median survival for disease presenting in the skin alone is 27 months and 5 months for those presenting with other sites of disease.

Another variant of cutaneous NK lymphoma, the blastic NK lymphoma, has been recently reclassified by the WHO-EORTC as CD4+/CD56+ hematodermic neoplasm because recent studies have demonstrated a plasmacytoid dendritic cell derivation. This neoplasm commonly presents in the skin with solitary or multiple tumors or nodules. Most patients who present with skin involvement only rapidly develop widespread disease in multiple visceral sites. The infiltrates are CD4+ CD56+, CD45RA+ cells, which lack CD3 and cytotoxic proteins and express CD123 and TCL-1, which are characteristic of plasmacytoid dendritic cell. The differential diagnosis is myelomonocytic or lymphocytic leukemia cutis, which can be distinguished by staining for myeloperoxidase and CD3, respectively. The skin biopsy is notable for a diffuse nonepidermotropic infiltration of the dermis by intermediate-sized blastlike cells with frequent mitoses. The prognosis is poor, with a median survival of 14 months. Initial therapy is often with acute myeloid leukemia type of regimens, which induce brief initial responses.

Cutaneous B-Cell Lymphoma

The primary cutaneous B-cell lymphomas (PCBCLs) have demonstrated an increase in the incidence rate since 1993, compared with MF, which has been relatively stable. PCBCL is 1.4 times more common in men than women and more common in whites.[93] The etiology of PCBCL is also unclear and the pathogenesis not well understood, but *Borelia* has been identified in a small percentage of patients presenting with PCBCL.

For PCBCL, nodal classification systems have been used, but given the different natural history of such lesions, specific classification and prognostic systems are necessary. Recently, the WHO-EORTC developed a classification system for both T- and B-cell cutaneous lymphomas.[2] Although it does not include immunohistochemistry (as these data are not available in the SEER registry), Smith et al.[94] have developed a clinically useful prognostic index that takes location and histology of the cutaneous lesion into account. Survival outcomes are based on multivariate analysis that accounts for a variety of factors, including the use of radiotherapy.

Types of Primary Cutaneous B-Cell Lymphomas

The histologic subtypes of PCBCL include marginal zone, follicular center cell type, and diffuse large cell (Table 128.1). Mucosa-associated lymphoid tissue can be found in a variety of anatomic locations, and marginal zone lymphoma of the skin is the cutaneous counterpart. Small lymphocytes and reactive germinal centers are frequently appreciated in conjunction with marginal zone cells. Expression of CD20, CD79, and, commonly, bcl-2 but not bcl-6 has been identified in addition to identification of the *IHG* and *MLT* genes of chromosomes 14 and 18, respectively. Follicle center cell cutaneous lymphomas often spare the epidermis and may consist of centrocytes, germinal centers, and reactive T cells. A follicular pattern is common and expression of CD20 and CD79 is often noted. Expression of bcl-2 and MUM-1 is typically absent. The t(14:18) translocation, which is often seen in the nodal counterpart, is absent in the cutaneous presentation.

Cutaneous plasmacytoma consists of a cutaneous infiltrate of plasma cells without bone marrow involvement. This presentation of PCBCL is quite rare and may present as papules, plaques, or tumors or nodules. Typically, the dermis is occupied by mononuclear cells, and amyloid deposition is often identified within the infiltrate. Immunoglobulins are often present and cells may express CD38.

Diffuse large B-cell type is distinguished based on whether it occurs on the leg or whether it is intravascular. Expression of CD20 and CD79 may be seen, and lesions identified on the lower extremity may express bcl-2, bcl-6, and MUM-1. Lesions that are found in other cutaneous locations may also express these markers, but more typically they are found on the lower extremities. Inactivation of p16 suppressor genes, additions for 18q and 7p, and loss of 6q may be noted with cutaneous diffuse large B-cell lymphoma.[95]

Treatment for PCBCL depends on the histopathologic subtype. More indolent forms of PCBCL, such as marginal zone or follicle center cell, tend to be bothersome to the patient but rarely follow an aggressive clinical course. Radiotherapy, surgical excision, and observation are options for such patients. Radiotherapy for PCBCL is very much the same as that described for MF-CTCL, but doses are somewhat higher to a total of 36 to 40 Gy via 2-Gy fractions, for example. The technical aspects of the treatment delivery are quite similar as are the side effects. Patients who present with diffuse large cell–leg type histology are typically treated more aggressively, given the relatively poor outcomes with radiotherapy alone. Combined modality therapy is often considered for this group of patients, and therapeutic courses tend to follow those used in nodal lymphomas of similar histology.

If the histology is diffuse large cell, but not of the leg type, consideration can be given to the use of radiotherapy alone as the sole therapeutic modality. Rituximab has been used in the management of patients with PCBCL and in those with widespread disease, but the evidence regarding efficacy and outcomes is anecdotal and series are small. For patients with localized CBCL, the complete response rates approach 100%, with 5-year disease-free survivals of approximately 50%.[93,96–100]

Selected References

The full list of references for this chapter appears in the online version.

2. Willemze R, Jaffe ES, Burg G, et al. WHO-EORTC classification for cutaneous lymphomas. *Blood* 2005;105:3768.
3. Willemze R, Meijer CJ. Classification of cutaneous T-cell lymphoma: from Alibert to WHO-EORTC. *J Cutan Pathol* 2006;33(Suppl 1):18.
4. Bunn PA Jr, Huberman MS, Whang-Peng J, et al. Prospective staging evaluation of patients with cutaneous T-cell lymphomas. Demonstration of a high frequency of extracutaneous dissemination. *Ann Intern Med* 1980;93: 223.
8. Vonderheid EC, Bernengo MG, Burg G, et al. Update on erythrodermic cutaneous T-cell lymphoma: report of the International Society for Cutaneous Lymphomas. *J Am Acad Dermatol* 2002;46:95.
18. Girardi M, Heald PW, Wilson L. Medical Progress: The pathogenesis of mycosis fungoides. *N Engl J Med* 2004;350:1978.
19. Berg EL, Yoshino T, Rott LS, et al. The cutaneous lymphocyte antigen is a skin lymphocyte homing receptor for the vascular lectin endothelial cell-leukocyte adhesion molecule 1. *J Exp Med* 1991;174:1461.
24. Foss FM, Koc Y, Stetler-Stevenson MA, et al. Costimulation of cutaneous T-cell lymphoma cells by interleukin-7 and interleukin-2: potential autocrine

or paracrine effectors in the Sezary syndrome. *J Clin Oncol* 1994;12:326.
36. Sausville EA, Worsham GF, Matthews MJ, et al. Histologic assessment of lymph nodes in mycosis fungoides/Sezary syndrome (cutaneous T-cell lymphoma): clinical correlations and prognostic import of a new classification system. *Hum Pathol* 1985;16:1098.
37. Lynch JW Jr, Linoilla I, Sausville EA, et al. Prognostic implications of evaluation for lymph node involvement by T-cell antigen receptor gene rearrangement in mycosis fungoides. *Blood* 1992;79:3293.
41. Bunn PA Jr, Lamberg SI. Report of the Committee on Staging and Classification of Cutaneous T-Cell Lymphomas. *Cancer Treat Rep* 1979;63:725.
42. Kim YH, Bishop K, Varghese A, Hoppe RT. Prognostic factors in erythrodermic mycosis fungoides and the Sezary syndrome. *Arch Dermatol* 1995;131:1003.
48. Kim YH, Liu HL, Mraz-Gernhard S, Varghese A, Hoppe RT. Long-term outcome of 525 patients with mycosis fungoides and Sezary syndrome: clinical prognostic factors and risk for disease progression. *Arch Dermatol* 2003;139:857.
50. Wilson LD, Kacinski BM, Jones GW. Local superficial radiotherapy in the management of minimal stage IA cutaneous T-cell lymphoma (Mycosis Fungoides). *Int J Radiat Oncol Biol Phys* 1998;40:109.
51. Kuzel TM, Roenigk HH Jr, Samuelson E, et al. Effectiveness of interferon alfa-2a combined with phototherapy for mycosis fungoides and the Sezary syndrome. *J Clin Oncol* 1995;13:257.
53. Jones GW, Kacinski BM, Wilson LD, et al. Total skin electron radiation in the management of mycosis fungoides: Consensus of the European Organization for Research and Treatment of Cancer (EORTC) Cutaneous Lymphoma Project Group. *J Am Acad Dermatol* 2002;47:364.
54. Jones GW, Rosenthal D, Wilson LD. Total skin electron radiation for patients with erythrodermic cutaneous T-cell lymphoma (mycosis fungoides and the Sezary syndrome). *Cancer* 1999;85:1985.
57. Wilson LD, Quiros PA, Kolenik SA, et al. Additional courses of total skin electron beam therapy in the treatment of patients with recurrent cutaneous T-cell lymphoma. *J Am Acad Dermatol* 1996;35:69.
58. Becker M, Hoppe RT, Knox SJ. Multiple courses of high-dose total skin electron beam therapy in the management of mycosis fungoides. *Int J Radiat Oncol Biol Phys* 1995;32:1445.
59. Quiros PA, Jones GW, Kacinski BM, et al. Total skin electron beam therapy followed by adjuvant psoralen/ultraviolet-A light in the management of patients with T1 and T2 cutaneous T-cell lymphoma (mycosis fungoides). *Int J Radiat Oncol Biol Phys* 1997;38:1027.
60. Chinn DM, Chow S, Kim YH, Hoppe RT. Total skin electron beam therapy with or without adjuvant topical nitrogen mustard or nitrogen mustard alone as initial treatment of T2 and T3 mycosis fungoides. *Int J Radiat Oncol Biol Phys* 1999;43:951.
62. Wilson LD, Jones GW, Kim D, et al. Experience with total skin electron beam therapy in combination with extracorporeal photopheresis in the management of patients with erythrodermic (T4) mycosis fungoides. *J Am Acad Dermatol* 2000;43:54.
64. Foss F, Higgins B. Intermediate dose interleukin-2 demonstrates activity in patients with relapsed or refractory cutaneous T-cell lymphoma. *Blood* 2004;104:2642.
66. Berger CL, Xu AL, Hanlon D, et al. Induction of human tumor-loaded dendritic cells. *Int J Cancer* 2001;91:438.
67. Girardi M, Berger C, Hanlon D, Edelson RL. Efficient tumor antigen loading of dendritic antigen presenting cells by transimmunization. *Technol Cancer Res Treat* 2002;1:65.
69. Girardi M, Berger CL, Wilson LD, et al. Transimmunization for cutaneous T cell lymphoma: a phase I study. *Leuk Lymphoma* 2006;47:1495.
72. Duvic M, Talpur R, Ni X, et al. Phase 2 trial of oral vorinostat (suberoylanilide hydroxamic acid, SAHA) for refractory cutaneous T-cell lymphoma (CTCL). *Blood* 2007;109:31.
74. Olsen E, Duvic M, Frankel A, et al. Pivotal phase III trial of two dose levels of denileukin diftitox for the treatment of cutaneous T-cell lymphoma. *J Clin Oncol* 2001;19:376.
75. Foss FM, Bacha P, Osann KE, et al. Biological correlates of acute hypersensitivity events with DAB(389)IL-2 (denileukin diftitox, ONTAK) in cutaneous T-cell lymphoma: decreased frequency and severity with steroid premedication. *Clin Lymphoma* 2001;1:298.
77. Foss F, Demierre MF, DiVenuti G. A phase-1 trial of bexarotene and denileukin diftitox in patients with relapsed or refractory cutaneous T-cell lymphoma. *Blood* 2005;106:454.
81. Koizumi K, Sawada K, Nishio M, et al. Effective high-dose chemotherapy followed by autologous peripheral blood stem cell transplantation in a patient with the aggressive form of cytophagic histiocytic panniculitis. *Bone Marrow Transplant* 1997;20:171.
83. Foss FM, Ihde DC, Breneman DL, et al. Phase II study of pentostatin and intermittent high-dose recombinant interferon alfa-2a in advanced mycosis fungoides/Sezary syndrome. *J Clin Oncol* 1992;10:1907.
84. Foss FM, Ihde DC, Linnoila IR, et al. Phase II trial of fludarabine phosphate and interferon alfa-2a in advanced mycosis fungoides/Sezary syndrome. *J Clin Oncol* 1994;12:2051.
86. Duvic M, Talpur R, Wen S, et al. Phase II evaluation of gemcitabine monotherapy for cutaneous T-cell lymphoma. *Clin Lymphoma Myeloma* 2006;7:51.
89. Duvic M, Forero-Torres A, Foss, F, et al. Oral forodesine is clinically active in refractory cutaneous T-cell lymphoma: results of a phase I/II Study. *Blood* 2006;108:2467.
91. Molina A, Zain J, Arber DA, et al. Durable clinical, cytogenetic, and molecular remissions after allogeneic hematopoietic cell transplantation for refractory Sezary syndrome and mycosis fungoides. *J Clin Oncol* 2005;23:6163.
93. Smith BD, Glusac EJ, McNiff JM, et al. Primary cutaneous B-cell lymphoma treated with radiotherapy: a comparison of the European Organization for Research and Treatment of Cancer and the WHO classification systems. *J Clin Oncol* 2004;22:634.
94. Smith BD, Smith GL, Cooper DL, Wilson LD. The cutaneous B-cell lymphoma prognostic index: a novel prognostic index derived from a population-based registry. *J Clin Oncol* 2005;23:3390.
100. Rijlaarsdam JU, Toonstra J, Meijer OW, Noordijk EM, Willemze R. Treatment of primary cutaneous B-cell lymphomas of follicle center cell origin: a clinical follow-up study of 55 patients treated with radiotherapy or polychemotherapy. *J Clin Oncol* 1996;14:549.

CHAPTER 129 PRIMARY CENTRAL NERVOUS SYSTEM LYMPHOMA

LISA M. DEANGELIS AND JOACHIM YAHALOM

Primary central nervous system lymphoma (PCNSL) is the term applied to non-Hodgkin lymphoma (NHL) arising in and confined to the central nervous system (CNS). In the past, this tumor was called microglioma, reticulum cell sarcoma, or perivascular sarcoma, but its lymphocytic origin, usually the B-cell, is now well established. How a lymphoma develops within the CNS, which lacks lymph nodes and lymphatics, remains an unanswered question; however, lymphocytes do traffic in and out of the CNS normally, and these lymphocytes are possibly the source of PCNSL.

PCNSL was once a rare tumor, accounting for only 0.5% to 1.2% of intracranial neoplasms, but recent data from the Central Brain Tumor Registry of the United States shows the incidence has risen to 2.4% of all brain tumors diagnosed between 2004 and 2006.[1] This change cannot be attributed to new diagnostic techniques or the adoption of a uniform nosology, but the reason for this marked rise is unknown.

PCNSL occurs with increased frequency in patients with congenital, acquired, or iatrogenic immunodeficiency states such as Wiskott-Aldrich syndrome or renal transplantation. The highest incidence (1.9%–6.0%) was in patients with the acquired immunodeficiency syndrome (AIDS); however, the frequency of AIDS-related PCNSL has fallen dramatically since the institution of highly active antiretroviral therapy (HAART) and improved control of the immune suppression.

CLINICAL FEATURES

General

PCNSL affects all ages, but the median age at diagnosis is about 60 years in immunocompetent patients but younger in immunosuppressed patients.[2] Among apparently immunocompetent individuals, there is a 3:2 male-to-female ratio, but in the AIDS population, more than 90% are men.

By definition, if lymphoma is found outside the CNS using chest, abdominal, and pelvic computed tomography (CT) scans, body positron emission tomography (PET), or bone marrow biopsy in patients suspect for PCNSL, the diagnosis is not PCNSL but rather NHL metastatic to the nervous system. The absence of systemic tumor even at autopsy in virtually all patients confirms this disease is restricted to the nervous system even though the cell of origin is not neuroectodermal.

Brain

Most PCNSLs present with symptoms of an intracranial mass lesion. The specific presenting symptoms and signs reflect the location of the tumor, with focal cerebral deficits occurring in approximately one-half of all patients.[2] Because the frontal lobe is the most frequently involved region of the brain and multiple lesions are often seen, changes in personality and level of alertness are more common presenting symptoms in PCNSL than in other brain tumors. Headaches and symptoms of increased intracranial pressure are also seen frequently. Because PCNSL affects deep brain structures and not cerebral cortex, seizures are less common than in patients with other brain tumors, occurring in about 10% of patients as a presenting sign. PCNSL generally grows more rapidly than malignant gliomas and, thus, symptoms are usually present for only weeks before a diagnosis is made.

PCNSL may be disseminated within the CNS at diagnosis. Brain lesions are multifocal in 40% of immunocompetent patients and almost 100% of AIDS patients. Multiple lesions may cause diagnostic confusion with brain metastases, particularly because 13% of PCNSL patients have a history of a prior systemic malignancy. Furthermore, PCNSL widely infiltrates brain parenchyma, and at autopsy, disease is usually seen microscopically in areas where magnetic resonance images (MRI) were completely normal.[3] Many lesions are periventricular, allowing tumor cells to gain easy access to the cerebrospinal fluid (CSF). At least 42% of patients have demonstrable leptomeningeal seeding on the basis of a positive CSF cytologic examination, leptomeningeal invasion seen on pathologic specimens, or unequivocal radiographic evidence of subarachnoid tumor, but patients rarely have symptoms or signs of leptomeningeal lymphoma. At autopsy, many patients have leptomeningeal tumor either from direct invasion into the ventricular system by periventricular tumor or by local involvement of the leptomeninges overlying a cortical lesion.

Eye

The eye, distinct from the orbit, is a direct extension of the brain, and approximately 20% of PCNSL patients have ocular involvement at diagnosis.[2] Conversely, 80% to 90% of patients with ocular lymphoma eventually develop cerebral lymphoma, usually after a latency of several years.[4] Ocular lymphoma typically involves the vitreous, retina, or choroid, but optic nerve infiltration can also occur.[4] Ocular lymphoma can present with blurred vision or floaters or may be clinically silent; it may begin unilaterally, but most patients eventually develop bilateral, albeit asymmetric, disease. A cellular infiltrate of the vitreous can be visualized only by slit-lamp examination; choroidal or retinal lesions often require indirect ophthalmoscopy. Lymphoma can be identified in vitrectomy specimens of patients with cells in the vitreous; false-negative biopsy may occur when patients have too few vitreal lymphocytes for the pathologist to examine or if the patient has been given corticosteroids to treat a presumed uveitis.[4]

Leptomeninges

Primary leptomeningeal lymphoma in the absence of a parenchymal brain mass is rare, accounting for approximately 7% of the cases of PCNSL.[5] Patients can present with progressive leg weakness, urinary incontinence or retention, cranial neuropathies, increased intracranial pressure, confusion, or a combination of these symptoms. Symptoms are usually present for only 2 to 3 months before diagnosis, but an occasional patient can have symptoms for 1 to 2 years before the diagnosis is made. Diagnosis is established by demonstration of malignant lymphocytes in the CSF or on meningeal biopsy. The CSF invariably shows an elevated protein concentration and a lymphocytic pleocytosis often in excess of 100 cells/mcL; CSF glucose is low in approximately one-third of patients. Gadolinium MRI scan of the head or spine reveals meningeal enhancement, hydrocephalus but no brain tumors, or multiple intradural nodules.

Spinal Cord

Primary spinal cord lymphoma is even less common than primary leptomeningeal lymphoma.[6] Lymphoma in the spinal cord parenchyma can occur in isolation or accompany brain lymphoma. Patients present with painless bilateral limb weakness, usually involving the legs; sensory symptoms and signs may initially follow a radicular pattern, but eventually a sensory level may be found. CSF may be normal or have a mildly elevated protein concentration with a few lymphocytes. Prognosis has been poor, with patients surviving only a few months from the onset of symptoms, but this is often because the diagnosis was not made until autopsy and no appropriate therapy was administered.

DIAGNOSTIC TESTS

Cranial Imaging

MRI should be the standard imaging technique for any patient with a cerebral neoplasm. The MRI of PCNSL may be quite distinctive, and the diagnosis may be suspected on the basis of the radiographic appearance alone. The tumor has an isointense signal on the pregadolinium T1-weighted images, and after contrast administration, there is dense and diffuse enhancement. The lesions often have indistinct borders, and the amount of surrounding edema is quite variable. Unlike brain metastases or malignant gliomas, ring enhancement is rarely seen.

Prominent contrast enhancement is characteristic of PCNSL, occurring in more than 90% of patients; however, nonenhancing lesions may be seen in approximately 10% of patients, particularly at recurrence. Magnetic resonance spectroscopy may provide additional diagnostic information; PCNSL has marked elevation of lipids and a much higher choline-to-creatine ratio than all grades of astrocytoma.[7] In addition, the apparent diffusion coefficient as measured on standard diffusion MR sequences may predict clinical outcome.[8]

The radiographic features of PCNSL may differ in the immunosuppressed patient from the characteristic image seen in immunocompetent individuals. In the AIDS patient, multiple lesions are seen in more than 70% of patients. Ring enhancement is common, reflecting the higher incidence of necrosis seen pathologically in this group. Spontaneous hemorrhage may occur, and nonenhancing lesions may be seen in about 25% of AIDS patients. It is impossible to distinguish PCNSL in the AIDS patient from infections, such as toxoplasmosis, or from other cerebral processes on the basis of MRI alone. PET or single photon emission computed tomography (SPECT) can differentiate between PCNSL and CNS infection with a high degree of reliability.[9] PCNSL is hypermetabolic in comparison to infection, which is usually hypometabolic.

Lumbar Puncture

A lumbar puncture should be part of the diagnostic evaluation of every patient with PCNSL. The protein concentration is elevated in 85% of patients, although rarely above 150 mg/dL. The glucose concentration is usually normal but can be low when florid leptomeningeal tumor is present. A CSF pleocytosis is seen in more than one-half of patients and always consists of lymphocytes, either reactive or malignant (see "Pathology"). Tumor markers, such a β_2-microglobulin, lactate dehydrogenase isoenzymes, and β-glucuronidase, can, when the level is elevated, provide circumstantial evidence for tumor invasion of the leptomeninges. Flow cytometry or polymerase chain reaction (PCR) of immunoglobulin gene rearrangements may detect a monoclonal population of lymphocytes even if they appear cytologically benign.[10,11]

Systemic lymphomas in immunocompromised patients are often associated with the Epstein-Barr virus (EBV), and EBV has been detected in the tumor tissue of most AIDS-related PCNSLs and some non-AIDS patients with this neoplasm. EBV may play an important role in the development of PCNSL in immunosuppressed patients, comparable to the presumed role it plays in systemic polyclonal and monoclonal lymphoid proliferations seen in the immunocompromised host. The prevalence of EBV, particularly in AIDS-related PCNSL, can serve a useful diagnostic function. Using PCR, EBV has been detected in the CSF of AIDS patients with PCNSL but not in the CSF of AIDS patients without PCNSL. This approach may offer a simple, noninvasive diagnostic alternative to brain biopsy in the AIDS population. Identification of EBV DNA in the CSF of an AIDS patient, combined with demonstration of hypermetabolic lesions on PET or SPECT imaging, can diagnose PCNSL and exclude other CNS processes with a high degree of accuracy.[9] Biopsy can be avoided in such patients and definitive treatment for PCNSL can be instituted.

PATHOLOGY

Histologically, PCNSL may be any type of NHL but about 75% are identical to the diffuse large B-cell subtype. T-cell lymphomas are rare but have a comparable response and outcome to treatment as the more common B-cell neoplasms.[12] Low-grade lymphoma subtypes are uncommon but have a better prognosis and may require less vigorous therapy.[13] Lymphomas confined to the dura represent a separate category that are identical to mucosa-associated lymphoid tissue lymphomas elsewhere and are treated in a distinctive fashion.[14]

PCNSL can grow as sheets of cells, but a characteristic vasocentric growth pattern with tumor infiltrating the brain parenchyma between involved blood vessels is found in virtually all cases. In immunocompetent patients, neither necrosis nor hemorrhage is a dominant histologic feature.[3]

More than 98% of PCNSLs are B-cell lymphomas. Immunohistochemistry evaluation to demonstrate monoclonal heavy or light immunoglobulin chain production, or immunoglobulin gene rearrangement, can be useful in some diagnostically difficult cases. Studies of clonality have demonstrated that multifocal PCNSL lesions arise from a single neoplastic clone.[15] A study of adhesion molecules revealed an identical pattern of expression for PCNSL and systemic lymphomas. *Bcl-1* and *bcl-2* rearrangements have not been detected in PCNSL, and no unique molecular marker has been identified that discriminates PCNSL from its systemic counterparts. Recent work suggests that *Bcl-6* expression was associated with longer survival in patients treated with high-dose methotrexate.[16] PCNSL from AIDS and non-AIDS patients has been studied for evidence of human herpesvirus 8 as a potential cause of chronic antigenic stimulation leading to tumor formation, but none has been found.[17] The few T-cell PCNSLs must be distinguished from reactive T-lymphocytes that may infiltrate the more typical B-cell tumor.[18] This is usually straightforward, but in lesions partially treated by corticosteroids, the reactive T-cells may be all that is apparent on a biopsy specimen, making accurate diagnosis difficult (see "Management and Therapy" and "Corticosteroids"). The few data available on gene expression profiling of PCNSL from immunocompetent patients suggests both germinal center and activated B-cell subtypes are observed in addition to an unclassified group.[19] However, further work is necessary to clarify the cell of origin for PCNSL.

MANAGEMENT AND THERAPY

The appropriate management of a patient with PCNSL requires a correct diagnosis. This may be difficult because the clinical presentation of PCNSL is not distinctive, and other primary and secondary brain tumors are much more common; however, the method outlined here and in the "Corticosteroids" section can aid in the approach to a patient who harbors this tumor (Table 129.1).

When an MRI scan reveals an intracranial mass, the radiographic appearance may strongly suggest the diagnosis of PCNSL (e.g., multiple lesions, a deep or periventricular location, diffuse and dense contrast enhancement, poorly defined borders and relatively little edema surrounding the mass). In addition, the clinical setting may suggest the diagnosis (e.g., an immunocompromised patient). If PCNSL is a reasonable diagnostic consideration, corticosteroids should be withheld unless the patient is in immediate danger of herniation, a rare situation. Corticosteroids may alter or even eliminate the ability to establish the diagnosis pathologically. Histologic confirmation is essential, by stereotactic biopsy, by lumbar puncture demonstrating leptomeningeal lymphoma, or by vitreous biopsy demonstrating lymphomatous cells. If the patient requires the immediate use of corticosteroids or if PCNSL was not considered originally and the patient was prescribed corticosteroids, a repeat MRI should be done to evaluate for possible resolution or marked shrinkage of the lesion(s). Biopsy should still be attempted if the lesion(s) is reduced in size but still evident.[20] Steroid-induced resolution of an intracranial mass does not establish the diagnosis of PCNSL because other neoplasms and nonneoplastic contrast-enhancing processes such as multiple sclerosis or sarcoidosis can resolve after steroid administration.

Using the clinical staging criteria developed for systemic lymphomas, PCNSL corresponds to stage IE—that is, disease confined to a single extranodal site. Systemic stage IE disease has a 100% complete response rate and at least a 70% 10-year survival or cure rate with focal radiotherapy (RT). Despite the highly responsive nature of PCNSL to cranial RT, median survival is only 12 to 18 months with a 3% to 4% 5-year survival rate.[2,21] This short survival is the result of tumor recurrence. Relapse occurs primarily in the brain, often in regions remote from the original site but within the prior radiation port, and also occurs in the leptomeninges and eye. Systemic relapse develops in 7% to 10% of patients, and it is unclear if the systemic tumor is a new primary or a systemic metastasis from nervous system tumor.

Regardless of treatment, recent studies clearly indicate the importance of prognostic factors. Several scoring systems have been proposed, all of which include age and performance status. One validated model used a recursive partitioning analysis that segregated patients into one of three classes: class 1 (patient age 50 years or less), class 2 (patient more than age 50 years and KPS [Karnofsky performance status] of 70 or more), and class 3 (patient more than age 50 years and KPS <70).[22] This model significantly distinguished progression-free and overall survival, and can be applied to all trials of PCNSL (Fig. 129.1).

TABLE 129.1

MANAGEMENT OF PRIMARY CENTRAL NERVOUS SYSTEM LYMPHOMA

SURGERY
Avoid corticosteroids before diagnostic biopsy
Biopsy for diagnosis
Resection should be avoided

CHEMOTHERAPY
Should be considered at diagnosis for every patient
Must penetrate the blood–brain barrier
High-dose with central nervous system penetration (e.g., methotrexate)
Lipophilic (e.g., procarbazine)
Must have antilymphoma activity
Should be given before radiotherapy

RADIOTHERAPY
Must be whole brain
Avoid boost
Dose is variable
- 24–45 Gy upfront, depending on response to chemotherapy
- 45 Gy for refractory/relapsed disease
- 36 Gy to eyes, if indicated

May be deferred in patients aged 50 y or older who have a complete response to chemotherapy

Immunologically Normal Patients

Corticosteroids

A unique feature of PCNSL in comparison to other brain tumors is its exquisite sensitivity to corticosteroids. At least 40% of patients have significant shrinkage or disappearance of tumor masses on MRI scan after administration of corticosteroids.[23] This apparent remission is due to a direct cytotoxic effect by the corticosteroids; biopsy after steroid administration often yields normal, necrotic, or nondiagnostic tissue. Clinically, disappearance of PCNSL lesions is accompanied by improvement that may last long after the corticosteroids have been discontinued. There are isolated reports of patients being cured or having prolonged survival after treatment with steroids alone. However, achievement of clinical improvement after the administration of corticosteroids does not require resolution or diminution of tumor, as many patients have amelioration of symptoms without any detectable change in tumor size on CT scan, a situation similar to glioma and probably related to stabilization of the blood–brain barrier. Regardless of apparent tumor regression, steroid-induced

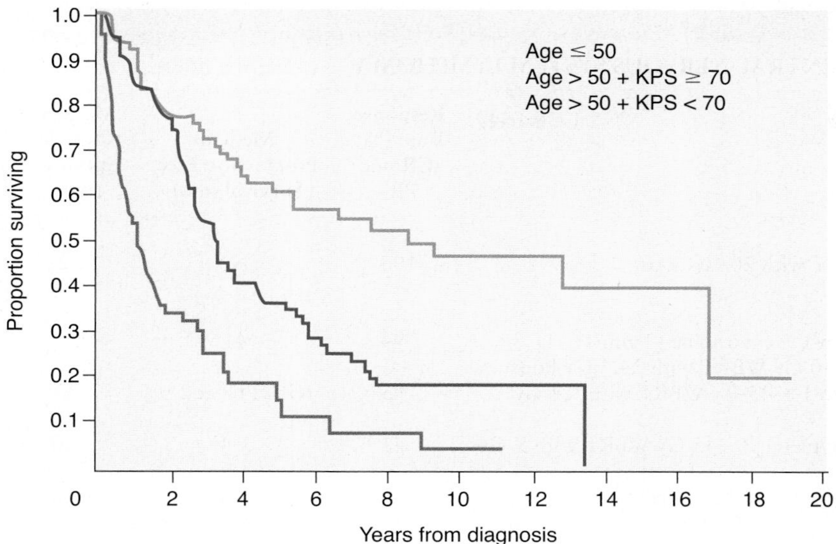

FIGURE 129.1 The Memorial Sloan-Kettering Cancer Center prognostic model for primary central nervous system lymphoma. Kaplan-Meier curve showing overall survival of 282 patients stratified by recursive partitioning analysis classification. KPS, Karnofsky performance status. (From ref. 22, with permission.)

remission is short-lived in most patients and is not definitive treatment.

Surgery

Surgery is important to confirm the histologic diagnosis but has no therapeutic role. The mean survival of patients with PCNSL with supportive care alone is 1 to 3 months. Surgical resection adds little, prolonging the average survival to only 3 to 5 months. Unlike malignant glioma, in which extensive resection is an important component of therapy, surgical extirpation is usually ineffective in PCNSL because of its multifocal and infiltrative nature. Furthermore, the deep location of many PCNSLs leaves the patient susceptible to severe postoperative deficits if a complete resection is attempted. Therefore, stereotactic biopsy is the diagnostic method of choice that also allows for biopsy of deep lesions that cannot be approached safely by conventional surgery.

Radiotherapy

Whole-brain RT (WBRT) combined with corticosteroids had been the conventional treatment for PCNSL, yielding median survivals of 12 to 18 months (Table 129.2). There have been no prospective studies to ascertain the optimal dose or fractionation of WBRT in the treatment of this disease, but retrospective data suggest that 40 to 50 Gy improved survival over lower doses.[2] The Radiation Therapy Oncology Group (RTOG) conducted a prospective study of PCNSL patients treated with 40 Gy WBRT plus a 20 Gy boost to the involved area to assess whether dose intensification improved outcome.[21] Median survival was only 12.2 months, and most recurrences were in the boosted field.

Because of the risk of late neurotoxicity when RT is combined with chemotherapy, attempts have been made to reduce the dose or volume of RT. The RTOG reported a study using a high-dose methotrexate-based regimen in combination with 45 Gy WBRT.[24] During the trial, the protocol was changed such that only 36 Gy WBRT in a hyperfractionated schedule was given to patients who achieved a complete response with the pre-RT chemotherapy. Survival and disease control were identical regardless of WBRT dose, although neurotoxicity was not reduced, suggesting that even lower doses of RT are necessary to decrease the risk of leukoencephalopathy. These data are in contrast to those reported by Bessell et al.,[25] who used a pre-RT regimen of cyclophosphamide, doxorubicin, and vincristine with dexamethasone plus carmustine, vincristine, and cytarabine to reduce the dose of WBRT from 45 Gy to 30.6 Gy in patients who achieved a complete response. No difference in outcome was observed for older patients, but patients younger than 60 years had a significantly better survival (3-year overall survival 92% vs. 60%; $P = .04$) if the full dose of WBRT was used. In contrast, recent preliminary data suggest excellent disease control and survival can be achieved when only 23.4 Gy WBRT is administered after achieving a complete response to a high-dose methotrexate-based regimen.[26]

The need for WBRT has been examined by Shibamoto et al.,[27] who reviewed PCNSL patients treated with focal RT only. Patients treated with RT using margins of less than 4 cm had higher out-field recurrences (83%) compared with those treated with 4 cm or more margins. Collectively, these data suggest that the whole-brain port remains necessary to achieve optimal benefit from RT in PCNSL, but a boost does not improve local control. Furthermore, a reduced dose of WBRT may provide adequate disease control if combined with effective chemotherapy, but this requires additional study.

Treatment of ocular disease is often focal RT of 35 to 45 Gy over 4 to 5 weeks.[4] Because ocular lymphoma is predominately a binocular process, both eyes may need RT even when only monocular disease can be detected on slit-lamp examination. Most patients experience both symptomatic improvement and resolution of cells in the vitreous after RT; however, some have vitreal clearing without improved vision, and others may not respond to RT. The incidence of ocular toxicity from RT in this disease is unknown, but may increase with improved survival because many of the complications are delayed. Conjunctivitis, retinal atrophy, vitreous hemorrhage, and cataract formation have all been reported in PCNSL patients after ocular RT.

Chemotherapy

No large prospective trials have compared chemotherapy plus RT with RT alone, but accumulated data from multiple phase II studies clearly document the chemosensitivity of PCNSL to systemic chemotherapy and superior outcomes with combined modality therapy. It is improbable that a phase III trial will ever be mounted to study this issue given the small number of patients with PCNSL and the extended number of years necessary to complete such a protocol.

TABLE 129.2

TREATMENT REGIMENS FOR PRIMARY CENTRAL NERVOUS SYSTEM LYMPHOMA

Study (Ref.)	Regimen	Response Rate (%) (CR and PR)	Median Progression-Free Survival (mo)	Median Overall Survival (mo)
WBRT ALONE				
Nelson et al., 1992 (21)	40 Gy WBRT with 20-Gy boost	100	NA	12.2
CHEMORADIOTHERAPY				
DeAngelis et al., 1992 (41)	MTX (1 g/m²) + cytarabine (3 g/m²) + IT MTX + 40-Gy WBRT with 14.4-Gy boost	94	41[a]	42.5
O'Brien et al., 2000 (41)	MTX (1 g/m²) + 45-Gy WBRT with 5.4-Gy boost	95	65% PFS at 2 y	33
Ferreri et al., 2009 (31)	MTX (3.5 g/m²) + 36–45 Gy WBRT with 9-Gy boost	41	~4[b]	~10
Ferreri, et al., 2009 (31)	MTX (3.5 g/m²) + cytarabine (2g/m²) + 36–40 Gy WBRT with 9-Gy boost	69	~8[b]	~32
DeAngelis et al., 2002 (24)	MPV (MTX 2.5 g/m²) + IT MTX + 36–45 Gy WBRT	94	24	37
Poortmans et al., 2003 (41)	MTX (3 g/m²)/teniposide/carmustine + IT MTX+ IT cytarabine + 30-Gy WBRT with 10-Gy boost	81	NA	46
Omuro et al., 2005 (30)	MTX (1 g/m²)/thiotepa/procarbazine + IT MTX + 41.4-Gy WBRT with 14.4-Gy boost	88	18	32
Gavrilovic et al., 2006 (29)	MPV (MTX 3.5 g/m²), cytarabine (3 g/m²) T MTX ± 45-Gy WBRT	94	129	51
Shah et al., 2007 (26)	Rituximab, MPV, cytarabine + 23.40-Gy WBRT for CR	93	≥37	40
MULTIDRUG MTX CHEMOTHERAPY WITHOUT WBRT				
Sandor et al., 1998 (41)	MTX (8.4 g/m²)/thiotepa/vincristine + IT cytarabine	100	16.5	NA
Abrey et al., 2000 (41)[c]	MPV (MTX 3.5 g/m²), cytarabine (3 g/m²), IT MTX	NA	NA	33
Pels et al., 2003 (41)	MTX (5 g/m²) + cytarabine (3 g/m²) + ifosfamide/vinca-alkaloids/cyclophosphamide + IT MTX + IT cytarabine	71	21	50
Hoang-Xuan et al., 2003 (41)[c]	MTX (1 g/m²) + lomustine/procarbazine + IT MTX + IT cytarabine	48	6.8	14.3
MTX SINGLE AGENT				
Batchelor et al., 2003 (41)	MTX (8 g/m²)	74	12.8	≥23
Herrlinger et al., 2002 2005 (41)	MTX (8 g/m²)	35	10	25

CR, complete remission; PR, partial remission; WBRT, whole-brain radiotherapy; NA, not available; IT, intrathecal; MTX, methotrexate; MPV, methotrexate, procarbazine, vincristine; PFS, progression-free survival.
[a]Median time to recurrence.
[b]Median failure-free survival.
[c]Patients over age 60 y only.

Most studies have focused on the use of preradiation chemotherapy for two reasons:

1. It permits an assessment of response to treatment. Almost all patients have a complete, albeit short-lived, response to RT; therefore, no measurable disease is present to assess adjuvant chemotherapy. This is particularly important in PCNSL, in which investigators are still trying to identify active agents, as regimens that are effective against comparable systemic NHLs that cannot simply be adopted (see "Systemic Non-Hodgkin Lymphoma Regimens").
2. Giving drugs, particularly methotrexate, before RT may reduce the risk of late neurologic toxicity. Opening of the blood–brain barrier by cranial irradiation may persist for weeks to months after completion of RT. This continued breakdown of the blood–brain barrier permits greater drug concentrations to accumulate in normal brain tissue. Completion of chemotherapy before cranial irradiation should minimize normal brain exposure to potentially neurotoxic chemotherapeutic agents. This enhanced neurotoxic potential of multimodality therapy applies to other agents in addition to methotrexate.

Systemic Non-Hodgkin Lymphoma Regimens

Several investigators have used chemotherapeutic regimens successful in the treatment of systemic NHL for use in PCNSL. The combination of preradiation cyclophosphamide, doxorubicin, vincristine, and prednisone (CHOP) or dexamethasone

(CHOD) has been studied most extensively. Early reports described responses of brain lesions to CHOP, although patients quickly developed florid leptomeningeal tumor or multifocal brain recurrence in sites distant from the original location of disease before chemotherapy could be completed. In contrast to these data, there are isolated patients reported to have prolonged survival with CHOP plus WBRT, although many of these patients also received intrathecal methotrexate. There have now been two multicenter phase II studies and one prospective randomized phase III trial that definitively establish the poor efficacy and high toxicity of CHOP for PCNSL.[25] The RTOG conducted a study in which patients received three cycles of CHOP followed by cranial irradiation. The median survival was only 12.8 months for the 51 patients treated.

A separate multi-institutional trial of preradiation CHOP had 46 evaluable patients, with an estimated median survival of only 9.5 months. Only 54% of patients completed two cycles of CHOP to begin RT; the others had disease progression or toxicity, with 15% mortality. The randomized trial was terminated before completion because of poor accrual, but there was no difference in survival or failure-free survival in patients treated with WBRT alone compared with WBRT and CHOP.[28] Therefore, CHOP or similar regimens have no role in the treatment of PCNSL, and they should not be used; these agents should have excellent activity against PCNSL tumor cells, but they are unable to penetrate an intact blood–brain barrier. Adequate drug concentrations are likely achieved only in areas of bulky disease seen on MRI scan, which accounts for the initial resolution of tumor masses; however, the drugs are unable to reach microscopic disease that persists behind a relatively preserved blood–brain barrier. Although issues of drug delivery may only partially explain the difficulty treating PCNSL, these data strongly argue for the use of drugs that can permeate the blood–brain barrier.

High-Dose Methotrexate

High-dose methotrexate is the single most important agent for the treatment of PCNSL. Originally chosen because of its ability to penetrate the blood–brain barrier and its known activity against lymphoma, methotrexate is now the cornerstone of PCNSL therapy despite the small role it plays in the treatment of comparable systemic lymphomas. Sensitivity to methotrexate may indicate a fundamental biologic difference between PCNSL and NHL.

Methotrexate has been used as a single agent and in combination with other drugs. Doses have ranged from 1 to 8 mg/m^2, without a clear indication that more is necessarily better. However, doses of 3 g/m^2 or more penetrate into the CNS more reliably than lower doses. Several phase II trials using a high-dose methotrexate-based regimen in combination with WBRT have all shown improved survival (median, 33-51 months) over WBRT alone. To date, the best results have been achieved combining high-dose methotrexate with vincristine and procarbazine before WBRT, giving a median survival of 51 months.[29] A large multicenter phase II trial based on this regimen was completed by the RTOG and median survival was 37 months, less than seen in the single-institution experience.[24,29] Part of this difference may have been the reduction in methotrexate dose from 3.5 to 2.5 g/m^2, but other factors, such as unfamiliarity with the administration of high-dose methotrexate, undoubtedly contributed to the decreased outcome observed when the regimen was used in the multicenter setting.

All methotrexate-based regimens, when combined with WBRT, carry a significant risk of severe, irreversible neurotoxicity characterized by dementia, ataxia, and incontinence.[30] Patients aged 60 years and older are most vulnerable to this toxicity. This has led to the development of several regimens using chemotherapy alone. The previous regimen using methotrexate, vincristine, and procarbazine achieved an identical median survival of 29 months in patients 60 years of age or older whether or not WBRT was included. However, patients who received WBRT died of neurotoxicity, whereas those who did not died of recurrent PCNSL. A randomized phase 2 trial of methotrexate with or without high-dose cytarabine demonstrated superior response rate and outcome with combination therapy.[31] These data and others suggest that single-agent methotrexate has limited efficacy and rarely produced sustained disease control.

The high incidence of leptomeningeal involvement by PCNSL led to the incorporation of intrathecal or intra-Ommaya methotrexate into many PCNSL regimens to ensure that therapeutic concentrations of drug were achieved in the CSF. However, the need for intra-Ommaya methotrexate in regimens using frequent administration of high-dose intravenous methotrexate that reliably produces therapeutic CSF levels of drug is unclear. A case-controlled retrospective study examining survival and recurrence in patients receiving systemic methotrexate at a dose of 3.5 g/m^2, with or without intra-Ommaya methotrexate, suggested that intrathecal drug did not improve outcome or reduce the risk of subsequent leptomeningeal relapse.[32] Consequently, intrathecal chemotherapy is usually reserved for those PCNSL patients (~15%) who have tumor cells identified on their initial CSF examination. However, in at least one study, elimination of intraventricular chemotherapy compromised disease control in all patients.[33]

In an effort to circumvent the blood–brain barrier and to deliver multiagent treatment, Angelov et al.[34] used blood–brain barrier disruption followed by intra-arterial methotrexate in combination with systemic cyclophosphamide, procarbazine, and dexamethasone without cranial irradiation. Median survival was 37 months. These results are superior to WBRT alone but are quite comparable to regimens using systemic high-dose methotrexate without requiring the technically complex and potentially complicated procedure of repeated angiography over the course of 1 year.

Ocular lymphoma may be treated with chemotherapy.[4] The most effective agents are high-dose methotrexate and high-dose cytarabine, both of which can achieve therapeutic concentrations in the vitreous. Clinical responses have been observed. Experience is too limited to know if using systemic chemotherapy to treat isolated ocular lymphoma reduces the risk of subsequent CNS relapse. Ocular lymphoma can also be treated with intravitreal methotrexate, which can give a sustained remission.

Transplantation Approaches

High-dose chemotherapy with autologous stem cell transplantation (ASCT) has been successful for some patients with systemic lymphomas, and this approach is under investigation for PCNSL. Using high-dose methotrexate as an induction regimen followed by high-dose chemotherapy with carmustine (BCNU), etoposide, cytarabine, and melphalan (BEAM) and ASCT without cranial RT, only 14 of the 28 patients had an objective response to induction and proceeded to transplant. Overall event-free survival was only 5.6 months for all patients and 9.3 months for the transplanted patients; however, overall survival was not reached, and 6 of the 14 transplanted patients (43%) remained free of disease at last follow-up.[35]

Other ASCT trials for newly diagnosed PCNSL patients also incorporated WBRT after ASCT.[36,37] They all reported high response rates (77% to 100%) and survival rates of 64% to 67% at 3 years, and one had a 5-year overall survival of 87%. Neurotoxicity was not reported, but is likely to be significant when WBRT follows such intensive multiagent chemotherapy. Preliminary data on comparable high-dose chemotherapy regimens without WBRT appear promising and are under further investigation.[38,39]

Recurrent Disease

There is no established second-line therapy for patients with recurrent PCNSL. The choice of treatment depends on the site of relapse (e.g., isolated ocular relapse or leptomeningeal lymphoma) and the patient's prior therapy. However, most relapses occur within the first 2 years of diagnosis, and the overwhelming majority occur in the brain. If the patient did not receive WBRT as part of the initial therapy, it is available at relapse. Most patients respond to WBRT, and some can have a durable response that lasts several years.[40] Ocular RT should be used for recurrent ocular lymphoma if not previously administered.

High-dose methotrexate can be effective at relapse, particularly if the patient had a long disease-free interval after initial treatment incorporating methotrexate. Other drugs that have been reported useful include high-dose cytarabine (3 g/m^2), temozolomide, temozolomide and rituximab, the PCV regimen (procarbazine, lomustine, and vincristine), and thiotepa.[41] Intraventricular rituximab may be effective for patients with relapsed subarachnoid disease and may have activity against parenchymal disease as well.[42]

High-dose chemotherapy and ASCT in patients with relapsed or progressive disease can be effective, particularly in younger patients.[43] Outcome was excellent with 63% of 43 patients proceeding to ASCT; median survival of the entire population was 18.3 months, but was 59 months in those who completed the transplant regimen.

Immunocompromised Patients

AIDS-related PCNSL is treated in the same way as in immunocompetent patients, although generally treatment is less effective and more toxic in immunodeficient patients. The initiation of treatment first requires an accurate diagnosis of PCNSL. In AIDS patients, this diagnosis may be established if both EBV DNA is identified in the CSF by PCR and a hypermetabolic lesion is seen on PET or SPECT imaging.[9] However, if only one of these tests is positive, biopsy is necessary. There is no role for a therapeutic trial with antitoxoplasmosis antibiotics for a cerebral mass lesion in an AIDS patient. This delays accurate diagnosis, usually resulting in clinical deterioration that ultimately compromises outcome.

AIDS-related PCNSL usually occurs in patients with low CD4 counts, often less than 25×10^6 cells/L. Age is not an important prognostic factor in AIDS PCNSL because most patients are young; however, performance status is a critical factor that strongly predicts outcome.

The most important component of PCNSL therapy in the immunosuppressed population is treatment of the underlying immune deficiency. In organ transplant recipients, this may necessitate reduction or elimination of immunosuppressive therapy. In AIDS, it means institution of or a change in HAART. HAART plays a critical role in the successful treatment of AIDS PCNSL regardless of the nature of the tumor-specific therapy.[44] The absolute CD4 count should not be used to determine the choice of PCNSL therapy because co-institution of HAART improves the underlying immune suppression. There are some reports that institution of HAART plus anti-EBV–directed therapy, such as ganciclovir, may be sufficient to eradicate PCNSL in some AIDS patients without any specific antitumor therapy, but this is not typical.[45]

In addition to HAART, corticosteroids and cranial irradiation remain the mainstay of treatment for PCNSL in immunosuppressed patients. Use of corticosteroids should be limited because they can contribute to the underlying immunosuppressive process, but they are still useful for the short-term control of neurologic symptoms and may be necessary during a course of WBRT. AIDS patients with PCNSL respond to cranial irradiation; median survival is a few months for those who receive WBRT without HAART, but survival may exceed a few years for those treated with HAART plus WBRT.[44]

Chemotherapy for PCNSL has been used infrequently in immunodeficient patients. High-dose methotrexate has been successful for some AIDS patients with PCNSL. Jacomet et al.[46] treated 15 patients with 3 g/m^2 of methotrexate as sole therapy. Median survival was 9.7 months, with some patients surviving more than a year. HAART combined with chemotherapy is well tolerated and there is no increase in toxicity. However, chemotherapy should be avoided in patients with active comorbid conditions. Monitoring CSF EBV DNA levels can predict response to chemotherapy and may be a useful adjunct to standard neuroimaging. Although experience with chemotherapy in AIDS patients has been relatively limited, patients in good neurologic condition without active opportunistic infections should be considered for a high-dose methotrexate-based regimen combined with HAART because these patients may have prolonged disease control and survival.

References

1. Central Brain Tumor Registry of the United States. CBTRUS statistical report: Primary Brain and Central Nervous System Tumors Diagnosed in the United States in 2004-2006. www.cbtrus.org, 2010.
2. Gerstner ER, Batchelor TT. Primary central nervous system lymphoma. *Arch Neurol* 2010;67:291.
3. Lai R, Rosenblum MC, DeAngelis LM. Primary CNS lymphoma: a whole brain disease? *Neurology* 2002;59:1557.
4. Grimm SA, Pulido JS, Jahnke K, et al. Primary intraocular lymphoma: an International Primary Central Nervous System Lymphoma Collaborative Group Report. *Ann Oncol* 2007;18:1851.
5. Kim HJ, Ha CK, Jeon BS. Primary leptomeningeal lymphoma with long-term survival: a case report. *J Neurooncol* 2000;48:47.
6. Herrlinger U, Weller M, Kuker W. Primary CNS lymphoma in the spinal cord: clinical manifestations may precede MRI detectability. *Neuroradiology* 2002;44:239.
7. Harting I, Hartmann M, Jost G, et al. Differentiating primary central nervous system lymphoma from glioma in humans using localized proton magnetic resonance spectroscopy. *Neurosci Lett* 2003;342:163.
8. Barajas RF Jr, Rubenstein JL, Chang JS, et al. Diffusion-weighted MR imaging derived apparent diffusion coefficient is predictive of clinical outcome in primary central nervous system lymphoma. *AJNR Am J Neuroradiol* 2010;31:60.
9. Antinori A, DeRossi G, Ammassari A, et al. Value of combined approach with thallium-201 single-photon emission computed tomography and Epstein-Barr virus DNA polymerase chain reaction in CSF for the diagnosis of AIDS-related primary CNS lymphoma. *J Clin Oncol* 1999;17:554.
10. Gleissner B, Siehl J, Korfel A, et al. CSF evaluation in primary CNS lymphoma patients by PCR of the CDR III IgH genes. *Neurology* 2002;58:390.
11. Schinstein M, Filie AC, Wilson W, et al. Detection of malignant hematopoietic cells in cerebral spinal fluid previously diagnosed as atypical or suspicious. *Cancer* 2006;108(3):157.
12. Shenkier TN, Blay JY, O'Neill BP, et al. Primary CNS lymphoma of T-cell origin: a descriptive analysis from the International Primary CNS Lymphoma Collaborative Group. *J Clin Oncol* 2005;23(10):2233.
13. Jahnke K, Korfel A, O'Neill BP, et al. International study on low-grade primary central nervous system lymphoma. *Ann Neurol* 2006;59(5):755.

14. Iwamoto FJ, DeAngelis LM, Abrey LE. Primary dural lymphomas: a clinicopathologic study of treatment and outcome in eight patients. *Neurology* 2006;66(11):1763.
15. Pilozzi E, Talerico C, Uccini S, et al. B cell clonality in multiple localizations of primary central nervous system lymphomas in AIDS patients. *Leuk Lymphoma* 2003;44:963.
16. Levy O, DeAngelis LM, Filippa DA, Panageas KS, Abrey LE. Bcl-6 predicts improved prognosis in primary central nervous system lymphoma. *Cancer* 2008;(1)112:151.
17. Montesinos-Rongen M, Hans VH, Eis-Hubinger AM, et al. Human herpes virus-8 is not associated with primary central nervous system lymphoma in HIV-negative patients. *Acta Neuropathol* 2001;102:489.
18. Gijtenbeek JM, Rosenblum MK, DeAngelis LM. Primary central nervous system T-cell lymphoma. *Neurology* 2001;57:716.
19. Rubenstein JL, Fridlyand J, Shen A, et al. Gene expression and angiotropism in rimary CNS lymphoma. *Blood* 2006;107:3716.
20. Porter AB, Giannini C, Kaufmann T, et al. Primary central nervous system lymphoma can be histologically diagnosed after previous corticosteroid use: a pilot study to determine whether corticosteroids prevent the diagnosis of primary central nervous system lymphoma. *Ann Neurol* 2008;63(5):662.
21. Nelson DF, Martz KL, Bonner H, et al. Non-Hodgkin's lymphoma of the brain: can high dose, large volume radiation therapy improve survival? Report on a prospective trial by the radiation therapy oncology group (RTOG): RTOG 8315. *Int J Radiat Oncol Biol Phys* 1992;23:9.
22. Abrey LE, Ben-Porat L, Panageas KS, et al. Primary central nervous system lymphoma: the Memorial Sloan-Kettering Cancer Center prognostic model. *J Clin Oncol* 2006;24(36):5711.
23. Weller M. Glucocorticoid treatment of primary CNS lymphoma. *J Neurooncol* 1999;43:237.
24. DeAngelis LM, Seiferheld W, Schold SC, Radiation Therapy Oncology Group Study 93–10. Combination chemotherapy and radiotherapy for primary central nervous system lymphoma: Radiation Therapy Oncology Group Study 93–10. *J Clin Oncol* 2002;20:4643.
25. Bessell EM, Lopez-Guillermo A, Villa S, et al. Importance of radiotherapy in the outcome of patients with primary CNS lymphoma: an analysis of the CHOD/BVAM regimen followed by two different radiotherapy treatments. *J Clin Oncol* 2002;20:231.
26. Shah GD, Yahalom J, Correa DD, et al. Combined immunochemotherapy with reduced whole-brain radiotherapy for newly diagnosed primary CNS lymphoma. *J Clin Oncol* 2007;25(30):4730.
27. Shibamoto Y, Hayabuchi N, Hiratsuka J-I, et al. Is whole-brain irradiation necessary for primary central nervous system lymphoma? Patterns of recurrence after partial-brain irradiation. *Cancer* 2003;97:128.
28. Mead GM, Bleehen NM, Gregor A, et al. A medical research council randomized trial in patients with primary central non-Hodgkin lymphoma: cerebral radiotherapy with and without cyclophosphamide, doxorubicin, vincristine, and prednisone chemotherapy. *Cancer* 2000;89:1359.
29. Gavrilovic IT, Hormigo A, Yahalom J, et al. Long-term follow-up of high-dose methotrexate-based therapy with and without whole brain irradiation for newly diagnosed primary CNS lymphoma. *J Clin Oncol* 2006; 24(28):4570.
30. Omuro AM, Ben-Portat LS, Pangeas KS, et al. Delayed neurotoxicity in primary central nervous system lymphoma. *Arch Neurol* 2005;62(10):1595.
31. Ferreri AJ, Reni M, Foppoli M, et al. High-dose cytarabine plus high-dose methotrexate versus high-dose methotrexate alone in patients with primary CNS lymphoma: a randomized phase 2 trial. *Lancet* 2009;374(9700):1512.
32. Khan RB, Shi W, Thaler TH, et al. Is intrathecal methotrexate necessary in the treatment of primary CNS lymphoma? *J Neurooncol* 2002;58:175.
33. Pels H, Juergens A, Glasmacher A, et al. Early relapses in primary CNS lymphoma after response to polychemotherapy without intraventricular treatment: results of a phase II study. *J Neurooncol* 2009;91(3):299.
34. Angelov L, Doolittle ND, Kraemer DF, et al. Blood-brain barrier disruption and intra-arterial methotrexate-based therapy for newly diagnosed primary CNS lymphoma: a multi-institutional experience. *J Clin Oncol* 2009;27 (21):3503.
35. Abrey LE, Moskowitz CH, Mason WP, et al. Intensive methotrexate and cytarabine followed by high-dose chemotherapy with autologous stem cell rescue in patients with newly diagnosed primary CNS lymphoma: an intent-to-treat analysis. *J Clin Oncol* 2003;21:4151.
36. Illerhaus G, Marks R, Ihorst G, et al. High dose chemotherapy with autologous stem cell transplantation and hyperfractionated radiotherapy as first line treatment of primary CNS lymphoma. *J Clin Oncol* 2006;24:3865.
37. Colombat PH, Lemevel A, Bertrand P, et al. High dose chemotherapy with autologous stem cell transplantation as first line therapy for primary CNS lymphoma in patients younger than 60 years: a multicenter phase II study of the GOELAMS group. *Bone Marrow Transplant* 2006;38:417.
38. Illerhaus G, Muller D, Feuerhake F, et al. High-dose chemotherapy and autologous stem-cell transplantation without consolidating radiotherapy as first-line treatment for primary lymphoma of the central nervous system. *Haematologica* 2008;93(1):147.
39. Yoon DH, Lee DH, Choi DR, et al. Feasibility of BU, CY and etoposide (BUCYE), and auto-SCT in patients with newly diagnosed primary CNS lymphoma: a single-center experience [published online ahead of print April 12, 2010]. *Bone Marrow Transplant* doi:10.1038/bmt.2010.71.
40. Hottinger AF, DeAngelis LM, Yahalom J, Abrey LE. Salvage whole brain radiotherapy for recurrent or refractory primary CNS lymphoma. *Neurology* 2007;69(11):1178.
41. Morris PG, Abrey LE. Therapeutic challenges in primary CNS lymphoma. *Lancet Neurol* 2009;8:581.
42. Rubenstein JL, Fridlyand J, Abrey L, et al. Phase I study of intraventricular administration of rituximab in patients with recurrent CNS and intraocular lymphoma. *J Clin Oncol* 2007;25;1350.
43. Soussain C, Hoang-Xuan K, Taillandier L, et al. Intensive chemotherapy followed by hematopoietic stem-cell rescue for refractory and recurrent primary CNS and intraocular lymphoma: Société Francaise de Greffe de Moëlle Osseuse-Therapie Cellulaire. *J Clin Oncol* 2008;20(15):2512.
44. Diamond C, Taylor TH, Im T, et al. Highly active antiretroviral therapy with improved survival among patients with AIDS-related primary central nervous system on non-Hodgkin's lymphoma. *Curr HIV Res* 2006;4 (3):375.
45. Raez L, Cabral L, Cai JP, et al. Treatment of AIDS-related primary central nervous system lymphoma with zidovudine, ganciclovir, and interleukin 2. *AIDS Res Hum Retroviruses* 1999;15:713.
46. Jacomet C, Girard PM, Lebrette MG, et al. Intravenous methotrexate for primary central nervous system non-Hodgkin's lymphoma in AIDS. *AIDS* 1997;11:1725.

SECTION 13: LEUKEMIAS AND PLASMA CELL TUMORS

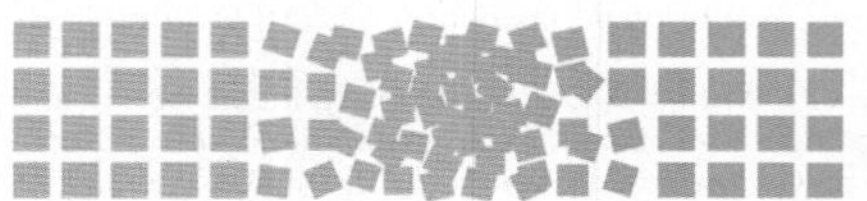

CHAPTER 130 MOLECULAR BIOLOGY OF ACUTE LEUKEMIAS

GLEN D. RAFFEL AND JAN CERNY

Our understanding of the molecular genetics of acute leukemias has improved dramatically over the past decade. Fueled in part by the availability of the complete sequence of the human genome, more than 100 different mutations have been identified that can be causally implicated in the pathogenesis of acute leukemias. At first glance, the plethora of mutations presents a discouraging prospect for the development of molecular targeted therapies. However, far more mutations are identified than there are phenotypes of acute leukemia, and a theme is developed in this chapter that many of these mutations must target similar signal transduction or transcriptional pathways. Thus, it is plausible to consider therapeutic approaches that target these shared pathways of transformation. Although many mutations remain to be identified, those observed thus far have provided critical insights into the pathophysiology of leukemia and the development of novel therapeutic targets.

LEUKEMIC STEM CELL

An important emerging concept in the pathobiology of leukemia is the existence of a "leukemic stem cell." In normal hematopoietic development, there is a rare population of hematopoietic stem cells that have self-renewal capacity and give rise to multipotent hematopoietic progenitors. These multipotent myeloid or lymphoid progenitors do not have self-renewal capacity but mature into normal terminally differentiated cells in the peripheral blood. It is hypothesized that there is a leukemic stem cell that has limitless self-renewal capacity and gives rise to clonogenic leukemic progenitors that do not have self-renewal capacity but are incapable of normal hematopoietic differentiation.

The first convincing evidence in support of the existence of a leukemic stem cell was derived from experiments in which human leukemic cells were injected into immunodeficient NOD-SCID mice (nonobese diabetic mice with severe combined immunodeficiency disease).[1] These data show that the resultant leukemias are derived from as few as 1:1,000 to 1:10,000 cells, indicating that there is a rare population of human leukemic cells that have self-renewal capacity in this assay. These cells have similar immunophenotypes to normal self-renewing hematopoietic progenitors and suggest that the leukemogenic mutation occurs in a hematopoietic stem cell. In support of this hypothesis, clonal cytogenetic abnormalities, such as the t(9;22), have been detected in primitive hematopoietic progenitors such as CD34+/CD38− cells (reviewed in ref. 2).

However, this paradigm has been recently challenged and revised. First, new protocols that enhance engraftment of human leukemia in xenotransplant setting have been described suggesting the importance of homing and the role of microenvironment.[3,4] Data also show that it may be the leukemic oncogenes themselves that confer properties of self-renewal. In a murine system, transduction of the leukemia oncogenes *MLL-ENL* (mixed-lineage leukemia 1-eleven nineteen leukemia), *MOZ-TIF2* (monocytic leukemia zinc finger protein-transcriptional intermediary factor 2), or *MLL-AF9* (mixed-lineage leukemia *ALL1*-fused gene from chromosome 9 protein) can confer properties of self-renewal to purified committed hematopoietic progenitors that have no capacity for self-renewal.[5,6] *MLL-AF9* oncogene-induced leukemia showed that leukemic stem cells account for as high as 25% of the leukemic cells while exhibiting mature myeloid immunophenotype.[7] High frequency of leukemic stem cells have been also described in a murine AML *Sfpi−/−*.[8] *HOX* family and *Notch* genes, frequent mutational targets in acute leukemia, as discussed later in this chapter, are being found to have significant roles in hematopoietic stem cell self-renewal.[9] Secondary mutations may also enable activation of similar self-renewal pathways. For example, analysis of cells from acute myeloid leukemia (AML) blast crisis in chronic myeloid leukemia (CML) shows a shift in the leukemic stem cell to an immunophenotype of a committed myeloid progenitor and concurrent nuclear localization of β-catenin, a process thought to increase stem cell self-renewal.[10] Further investigation will be required to determine to what extent these findings can be extrapolated to other leukemia oncogenes and to human leukemia. One of the major goals is identification of transcriptional programs, genes, and pathways that confer limitless self-renewal and may be targets for therapeutic intervention. In addition, these transcriptional programs may be commandeered to confer properties of self-renewal to adult somatic tissues for therapeutic purposes such as tissue regeneration. For further development of this issue, see Chapter 11.

ELUCIDATION OF GENETIC EVENTS IN ACUTE LEUKEMIA

The search for causative mutations in acute leukemia has accelerated in recent years because of the availability of new means for evaluating genome integrity in leukemic cells. The bulk of known translocations and deletions was found by analyzing conventionally stained chromosomal banding patterns of karyotypes. Classic karyotypic analysis is able to identify lesions with a resolution of 5 to 10 Mb. An improvement on this technique is spectral karyotyping, in which 24 unique dye combinations are used on conjugated probes specific to each chromosome. Mutations can be observed in the resolution of 1 to 2 Mb. This technique is particularly useful in finding otherwise cryptic or complex translocations as chromatin in derivative chromosomes are "painted" to identify their chromosome of origin.

New technologies such as comparative genomic hybridization (CGH) and single nucleotide polymorphism (SNP) arrays allow detailed (<35 kb) mapping of unbalanced insertions or deletions (reviewed in refs. 11 and 12). Array comparative genomic hybridization determines DNA copy gain or loss by comparing the hybridization of sample DNA to a series of clones or oligonucleotides from regions throughout the genome bound to a chip with a normal reference DNA sample. SNP arrays differ in that oligomers of SNP sequences representing known alleles throughout the genome are used in the array to measure changes in expected genotype and copy number. Finally, low-cost, high-throughput sequencing and microarray-based resequencing techniques have allowed identification of new somatic mutations at the single nucleotide level and are making enormous inroads into the pathogenesis, prognosis, and classification of leukemias with "normal" cytogenetics. Sequencing of complete AML genomes has been accomplished and alternative strategies limiting sequencing to the transcriptome or kinase-encoding regions (kinome) to reduce cost and effort are also uncovering new, significant mutations.[13–15] Worldwide initiatives to sequence large numbers of cancer genomes, including leukemia subtypes, are being coordinated and cataloged through the International Cancer Genome Consortium (http://www.icgc.org).[16]

RECURRING CHROMOSOMAL ABNORMALITIES IN ACUTE LEUKEMIA

Nonrandom chromosomal abnormalities can be detected in the majority of cases of acute leukemia using classic high-resolution banding techniques. These include balanced reciprocal chromosomal translocations, such as t(8;21)(q22;q22) or t(15;17)(q22;q21); internal deletions of single chromosomes, such as 5q- or 7q-; gain or loss of whole chromosomes (+8 or −7); or chromosome inversions, such as inv(3), inv(16), or inv(8). Complex chromosomal abnormalities are observed in approximately 15% of *de novo* cases that do not have an antecedent hematologic disorder; this constitutes a clinical group of patients with particularly poor prognoses. Selected recurring cytogenetic abnormalities observed in acute leukemias are annotated in Table 130.1.

Initial insights into the pathobiology of acute leukemias were derived from analysis and molecular cloning of recurring chromosomal translocations.[17] First, it appears that certain genomic loci are associated with specific subtypes of leukemia. For example, more than 40 different recurring translocations target the *MLL* gene locus on chromosome 11q23 and are generally associated with a myelomonocytic or monocytic AML phenotype (FAB M4 or M5). As another example, five different translocations target the retinoic acid receptor alpha locus (RAR-α), including the t(15;17)(q22;q21), which is the most common of these, and are all associated with an acute promyelocytic leukemia (APL) phenotype (FAB M3). Second, it appears that most chromosomal translocations associated with AMLs target transcription factors that are important for normal hematopoietic development. For example, more than a dozen translocations target the core-binding factor (CBF), a heterodimeric transcriptional complex essential for hematopoiesis. The translocations that target *CBF*, such as the t(8;21), result in expression of dominant negative inhibitors of normal CBF function, such as the AML1/ETO fusion. Thus, one consequence of many of these chromosomal translocations in acute leukemias is impaired hematopoietic differentiation. A third general observation has been that fusion genes associated with acute leukemias are necessary but not sufficient to cause acute leukemia.

CHROMOSOMAL TRANSLOCATIONS THAT TARGET CORE-BINDING FACTOR

CBF is targeted by more than a dozen different chromosomal translocations in acute leukemias, including the t(8;21) or inv(16), observed in approximately 20% of AMLs, and the t(12;21), present in approximately 25% of patients with pediatric B-cell acute lymphoblastic leukemia (ALL).[18] As discussed in Chapter 131, adult patients with CBF leukemias have a favorable prognosis and the TEL/AML1 fusion that is expressed as a consequence of t(12;21) in children confers a favorable prognosis among B-cell ALL.[19]

CBF is a heterodimeric transcription factor composed of the AML1 and CBFβ proteins that is critical for normal hematopoietic development. Loss of function of either subunit results in a complete lack of definitive hematopoiesis.[20,21] The AML1 subunit of CBF contacts DNA but only weakly transactivates target genes as a monomer. When bound to its heterodimeric partner CBFβ, which does not contact DNA itself, transactivation of CBF target genes is dramatically enhanced.[19] CBF transactivates a spectrum of target genes that are important in normal myeloid development, including cytokines (e.g., granulocyte-macrophage colony-stimulating factor) and cytokine receptors (such as M-CSF receptor), as well as in lymphoid development, such as the TCRβ enhancer and the immunoglobulin heavy-chain loci. Because CBF targets genes that are important for normal hematopoietic development, a mutation or gene rearrangement that resulted in loss of function of either *AML1* or *CBFβ* might be expected to impair hematopoietic differentiation.[19]

Compelling evidence has been shown that translocations that target CBF result in loss of function through dominant negative inhibition. The *AML1/ETO* fusion associated with t(8;21) and the CBFβ/SMMHC (smooth muscle myosin heavy chain) fusion associated with inv(16) are dominant negative inhibitors of CBF and impair hematopoietic differentiation. Expression of either the *AML1/ETO* or *CBFβ/SMMHCC* fusion genes from their endogenous promoter in mice completely inhibits the function of the residual AML1 or CBFβ alleles, resulting in a lack of definitive hematopoiesis and resultant embryonic lethality.[20,21] The phenotype observed is the same as that seen in *AML1–/–* or *CBFβ–/–* mice, indicating that the AML1/ETO or CBFβ/SMMHC fusions, respectively, act as complete dominant negative inhibitors of the native proteins. Repression of CBF target genes by the AML1/ETO or CBFβ/SMMHC fusions is mediated by aberrant recruitment of the nuclear corepressor complex, as it is for the PML/RAR-α fusion (reviewed in refs. 22 and 23). Thus, it has been suggested that histone deacetylase, a component of the corepressor complex, may be a therapeutic target for leukemias associated with translocations that target CBF.[24]

Although expression of AML1/ETO leads to alterations of gene expression and hematopoietic cell proliferation leukemia and confers the ability to serially replate in methylcellulose culture (a measure of self-renewal potential), this does not result in development of leukemia in an animal model. However coexpression of an alternatively spliced isoform of the *AML1-ETO* transcript, *AML1-ETO9a*, that includes an extra exon, exon 9a, of the *ETO* gene (*AML1-ETO9a* encodes a C terminally truncated AML1-ETO protein of 575 amino acids) leads to a rapid development of leukemia in a mouse retroviral transduction–transplantation model.[25] The presence of *AML1-ETO9a* closely correlates with presence of activating c-Kit

PRACTICE OF ONCOLOGY

TABLE 130.1

SELECTED EXAMPLES OF CYTOGENETIC AND MOLECULAR ABNORMALITIES IN LEUKEMIA

Cytogenetic Abnormality	Genes Involved	Derivation of Abbreviation	Protein Characterization	Disease
FUSIONS INVOLVING THE CORE-BINDING FACTORS (CBFs)				
t(8;21)(q22;q22)	*CBFA2T1/ETO* (8q22)	Eight twenty-one	Zinc finger protein	AML
	CBFA2/AML1 (21q22)	AML 1	α subunit of CBF complex	
inv(16)(p13q22)	*MYH11* (16p13)	Myosin heavy chain 11	Smooth muscle myosin heavy chain	AML
	CBFB/CBFβ (16q22)	CBF-β	β subunit of CBF complex	
t(3;21)(q26;q22)	*EVI1* (3q26)	Ecotropic virus integration site 1	Multiple zinc fingers	MDS, AML
	CBFA2/AML1 (21q22)	AML 1	α subunit of CBF complex	CML-BC
t(12;21)(p13;q22)	*TEL* (12p13)	Translocation ETS leukemia	ETS-related transcription factor	ALL
	CBFA2/AML1 (21q22)	AML 1	α subunit of CBF complex	
FUSIONS INVOLVING *MLL*				
t(4;11)(q21;q23)	*AF4* (4q21)	*ALL1* fused chromosome 4	Transactivator	ALL, AML
	MLL (11q23)	Mixed-lineage leukemia	*Drosophila* trithorax homologue	
t(11;19)(q23;p13.3)	*MLL* (11q23)	Mixed-lineage leukemia	*Drosophila* trithorax homologue	AML, ALL
	ENL (19p13.3)	ENL	Transcription factor	
t(9;11)(p22;q23)	*AF9* (9p22)	*ALL1* fused chromosome 9	Nuclear protein, ENL homology	AML, ALL
	MLL (11q23)	Mixed-lineage leukemia	*Drosophila* trithorax homologue	
t(11;22)(q23;q13)	*MLL* (11q23)	Mixed-lineage leukemia	*Drosophila* trithorax homologue	AML
	P300 (22q13)	Protein 300 kD	Adenoviral E1A-associated protein	
t(1;11)(q21;q23)	*AF1q* (1q21)	*ALL1* fused chromosome 1q	No homology to any known protein	AML
	MLL (11q23)	Mixed-lineage leukemia	*Drosophila* trithorax homologue	
+11 (sole) or normal cytogenetics	*MLL* (11q23)	Mixed-lineage leukemia	*Drosophila* trithorax homologue MLL partial tandem duplication	AML
FUSIONS INVOLVING *RAR-α*				
t(15;17)(q22;q12–21)	*PML* (15q21)	Promyelocytic leukemia	Zinc finger protein	APL
	RAR-α (17q21)	Retinoic acid receptor-α	Retinoic acid receptor-α	
t(11;17)(q23;q21)	*PLZF* (11q23)	Promyelocytic leukemia zinc finger	Zinc finger protein	APL
	RAR-α (17q21)	Retinoic acid receptor-α	Retinoic acid receptor-α	
T(5;17)(q32;q21)	*NPM1*	Nucleophosmin	Chaperone	APL
	RAR-α (17q21)	Retinoic acid receptor-α	Retinoic acid receptor-α	
FUSIONS INVOLVING *E2A*				
t(1;19)(q23;p13.3)	*PBX1* (1q23)	Pre-B transformation 1	Homeodomain	ALL
	E2A (19p13.3)	Early region 2A	bHLH transcription factor	
t(17;19)(q22;p13.3)	*HLF* (17q22)	Hepatic leukemia factor	Leucine zipper	ALL
	E2A (19p13.3)	Early region 2A	bHLH transcription factor	
FUSIONS INVOLVING NUCLEOPORIN GENES AND *HOX* GENES				
t(6;9)(p23;q34)	*DEK* (6p23)	Not relevant to molecule	Transcription factor	AML
	CAN /NUP214 (9q34)	Nuclear pore 214	Nucleoporin	
t(7;11)(p15;p15)	*HOXA9* (7p15)	Homeobox A9	Homeobox protein	AML/ MDS
	NUP98 (11p15)	Nuclear pore 98	Nucleoporin	AML
FUSIONS INVOLVING OTT1 AND MAL				
t(1;22)(p13;q13)	*OTT1* (1p13)*MAL* (22q13)	One twenty-two megakaryocytic acute leukemia	*Spen* homologue unknown Serum response cofactor	AML (M7)

TABLE 130.1

(CONTINUED)

Cytogenetic Abnormality	Genes Involved	Derivation of Abbreviation	Protein Characterization	Disease
TRANSLOCATIONS INVOLVING THE IMMUNOGLOBULIN ENHANCER LOCI				
t(8;14)(q24;q32)	*MYC* (8q24)	Myelocytomatosis virus	bHLH/bZIP transcription factor	ALL
	IGH (14q32)	Ig heavy chain	Ig heavy chain promoter	
t(2;8)(p12;q24)	*IGK* (2p12)	Ig κ-chain	Igκ-chain promoter	ALL
	MYC (8q24)	Myelocytomatosis virus	bHLH/bZIP transcription factor	
t(8;22)(q24;q11)	*MYC* (8q24)	Myelocytomatosis virus	bHLH/bZIP transcription factor	ALL
	IGL (22q11)	Ig λ-chain	Igλ-chain promoter	
TRANSLOCATIONS INVOLVING THE T-CELL RECEPTOR GENES				
t(1;14)(p32;q11)	*TAL1/SCL* (1p33)	T-cell acute leukemia 1/stem cell leukemia	bHLH transcription factor	ALL
	TCRα/δ (14q11)	T-cell receptor-α/δ	T-cell receptor promoter	
t(1;7)(p32;q34)	*TAL1/SCL* (1p32)	T-cell acute leukemia 1/stem cell leukemia	bHLH transcription factor	ALL
	TCRβ (7q34)	T-cell receptor-β	T-cell receptor promoter	
t(7;9)(q34;q34)	*TCRβ* (7q34)	T-cell receptor-β	T-cell receptor promoter	ALL
	TAL2/SCL2 (9q34)	T-cell acute leukemia 2/stem cell leukemia	bHLH transcription factor	
t(7;19)(q34;p13)	*TCRβ* (7q34)	T-cell receptor-β	T-cell receptor promoter	ALL
	LYL1 (19p13)	Lymphoid leukemia 1	bHLH transcription factor	
t(8;14)(q24;q11)	*MYC* (8q24)	Myelocytomatosis virus	bHLH/bZIP transcription factor	ALL
	TCRα/δ (14q11)	T-cell receptor-α/δ	T-cell receptor promoter	
t(11;14)(p15;q11)	*LMO1* (11p15)	LIM only 1	Zinc finger	ALL
	TCRα/δ (14q11)	T-cell receptor-α/δ	T-cell receptor promoter	
t(11;14)(p13;q11)	*LMO2* (11p13)	LIM only 2	Zinc finger	ALL
	TCRα/δ (14q11)	T-cell receptor-α/δ	T-cell receptor promoter	
t(7;10)(q34;q24)	*TCRβ* (7q34)	T-cell receptor-β	T-cell receptor promoter	ALL
	HOX11 (10q24)	Homeobox 11	Homeobox gene	

AML, acute myeloid leukemia; MDS, myelodysplastic syndrome; CML, chronic myeloid leukemia; ETS, E twenty-six retrovirus; ENL, eleven nineteen leukemia; ALL, acute lymphoblastic leukemia; MLL, mixed-lineage leukemia; APL, acute promyelocytic leukemia; bHLH, basic helix-loop-helix; bZIP, basic region/leucine zipper; Ig, immunoglobulin; LIM, Lin-11, Isl-2, Mec-3 homeodomain.

mutations in humans, conferring a poor prognosis.[26] Similarly, expression of CBFβ/SMMHC in adult hematopoietic cells results in leukemia only after a markedly prolonged latency; this latency can be shortened using mutagenesis strategies.[27] Translocations that target *CBF* impair hematopoietic differentiation and confer certain properties of leukemic stem cells, such as the ability to serially replate, but are not sufficient to cause leukemia. In some situations fusion proteins from alternatively spliced isoforms of a chromosomal translocation may work together to induce cancer development.[26]

CHROMOSOMAL TRANSLOCATIONS THAT TARGET THE RETINOIC ACID RECEPTOR ALPHA GENE

The empiric observation that all-*trans*-retinoic acid (ATRA) induces complete responses in patients with APL drove the subsequent cloning of the t(15;17)(q22;q21) fusion gene involving the RAR-α locus. Several groups demonstrated at approximately the same time that the RAR-α (*RARα*) gene on chromosome 17 was fused to a novel partner that was eventually identified as the promyelocytic leukemia (PML) gene.[28–30] Two reciprocal fusion RNA species are produced as a consequence of the translocation, *RARα/PML* and *PML/RARα*. The PML/RAR-α fusion protein contains the zinc finger of PML fused to the DNA- and protein-binding domains of RAR-α. Several other chromosomal translocations associated with an APL phenotype have been cloned and characterized. Each of these targets the *RARα* locus, with fusion to various partners (see Table 130.1). The best studied of these is the PLZF/RAR-α fusion, which also aberrantly recruits the nuclear corepressor complex (Table 130.1). However, in contrast with the PML/RAR-α fusion, ATRA is not able to relieve corepression mediated by the PLZF/RAR-α fusion, and thus is not effective in patients who harbor the t(11;17) associated with this fusion gene.[31]

As with CBF fusions, the PML/RAR-α fusion protein functions as a dominant inhibitory oncogene for RAR-α–interacting proteins, including RXR-α. In addition, the PML/RAR-α fusion interferes with the function of the native PML protein, which is thought to function as a tumor suppressor gene.[32] Collectively, the dominant interfering activities of the PML/RAR-α fusion protein result in a block in differentiation at the promyelocyte stage of development. The clinical response of these patients to ATRA, as discussed in Chapter 131, is explained by the ability of this retinoid to bind to the PML/RAR-α fusion protein and reverse repression of target genes required for normal hematopoietic development. The ability of the PML/RAR-α fusion protein to repress transcription is partly due to the aberrant recruitment of the nuclear corepressor complex, including histone deacetylase, suggesting that pharmacologic agents that inhibit histone deacetylases may be useful in therapy of APL.[24,33]

The transforming properties of the *PML/RARα* fusion gene have been tested in murine models. Expression of *PML/RAR-α* in transgenic mice from promoters that direct expression to the promyelocyte compartment result in an APL-like phenotype.[34–36] However, there is approximately a 6-month lag before the development of leukemia, incomplete penetrance of approximately 15% to 30%, and acquired karyotypic abnormalities, all suggesting that second mutations are required for induction of leukemia. In at least some cases, activating mutations in *FLT3*, as discussed later in "Activating Mutations in *FLT3* and *KIT*," may be the additional mutation required. ATRA is efficacious in leukemic animals, expressing both PML/RAR-α and activated FLT3, and this model has allowed for the preclinical testing of novel agents such as arsenic trioxide.[37]

CHROMOSOMAL TRANSLOCATIONS THAT TARGET HOX FAMILY MEMBERS

The large HOX family of transcription factors is important in patterning in vertebrate development and also plays a critical role in normal hematopoietic development (reviewed in ref. 38). *HOX* genes may also be targeted by chromosomal translocations, with examples including the NUP98/HOXA9 and NUP98/HOXD13 fusions, associated with t(7;11) and t(2;11), respectively (see Table 130.1).[39,40] *HOX* gene expression is tightly regulated during hematopoietic development. HOXA9, for example, is expressed in early hematopoietic progenitor cells but is down-regulated during hematopoietic differentiation and is undetectable in terminally differentiated cells. It has been suggested that unregulated overexpression of the HOXA9 moiety from the constitutively active NUP98 promoter may result in aberrant differentiation. Experimental support for this hypothesis includes the observation that the NUP98/HOXA9 fusion protein can transform 3T3 fibroblasts, an activity that requires the HOXA9 DNA-binding domain.[41]

The contribution of the NUP98 moiety to leukemic transformation is not fully understood. NUP98 is normally a component of the nuclear pore complex and is constitutively and ubiquitously expressed. However, several lines of evidence suggest that NUP98 contributes more than a constitutively activated promoter. For example, NUP98 motifs known as *FG repeats* are essential for transformation and may serve to recruit transcriptional coactivators, such as CBP/p300, to HOXA9 DNA-binding sites.[41] In murine models of leukemia, overexpression of HOXA9 alone is not sufficient to cause AML, but coexpression of HOXA9 with transcriptional cofactors, such as MEIS1, results in efficient induction of AML. Thus, the NUP98 moiety in the context of the NUP98/HOXA9 fusion may serve multiple functions, including provision of an active promoter, and recruitment of transcriptional coactivators such as CBP/p300 that subserve the function of other cofactors such as MEIS1. Epidemiologic evidence that the NUP98 moiety contributes to leukemogenesis includes the observation that there are now a spectrum of fusion proteins involving components of the nuclear pore that are targeted by chromosomal translocations in acute leukemias. These include *NUP98* and *NUP214* fused to a diverse group of partners, including *HOXA9* and *HOXD13*, and the *DDX10*, *PMX1*, *DEK*, and *ABL1* genes, respectively.

It has been hypothesized that dysregulated *HOX* gene expression may be important in leukemias that do not directly target HOX family members. Several proteins that are upstream of HOX expression have been observed as fusion genes associated with AML, the most frequent of these are *MLL* gene rearrangements. More than 40 chromosomal translocations target *MLL* and result in fusions of *MLL* with a broad spectrum of partners. However, a common biologic feature of all of these may be their ability to dysregulate *HOX* gene expression during hematopoietic development. For example, t(12;13) associated with AML results in expression of high levels of CDX2 from the *TEL* locus.[42] CDX2 is a homeotic protein that regulates expression of HOX family members in the colonic epithelium. As in hematopoietic development, *HOX* gene expression is highest in colonic stem cells in the colonic crypts and is down-regulated with maturation. It has been shown that CDX2 and CDX4 can dysregulate HOX expression in hematopoietic progenitors and result in leukemia.[42,43] Evidence to support this includes the ability of CDX2 to induce leukemia in murine retroviral transduction models.[42,43] Although CDX2 is not normally expressed in hematopoietic cells, a family member, CDX4, has been cloned and appears to play a similar role in hematopoietic development as CDX2 does in the gut. Of note, CDX4 in hematopoietic cells appears to either be downstream or epistatic with MLL in regulation of *HOX* gene expression.[44]

Taken together, these data indicate that the NUP98/HOXA9 fusion transforms hematopoietic progenitors in part through dysregulated overexpression and by transactivation mediated through the NUP98 transactivation domain that recruits CBP. However, like other gene rearrangements involving hematopoietic transcription factors, expression of NUP98/HOXA9 alone is not sufficient to cause leukemia. In murine bone marrow transplant models, NUP98/HOXA9 induces AML only after markedly prolonged latencies indicative of a requirement for second mutation.

CHROMOSOMAL TRANSLOCATIONS THAT TARGET THE *MLL* GENE

As noted earlier in "Recurring Chromosomal Abnormalities in Acute Leukemia," the *MLL* locus is involved in more than 40 different chromosomal translocations with a remarkably diverse group of fusion partners,[45,46] and are associated with mostly FAB subtype M4 or M5, and fewer with M2 AML. Patients who have received prior chemotherapy for cancer and develop AML (therapy-related myelodysplastic syndrome [MDS]/AML, t-AML) often have abnormalities in 11q23, especially those patients treated with topoisomerase inhibitors such as etoposide or topotecan. Chromosomal translocations involving band 11q23 result in expression of a fusion gene containing amino-terminal *MLL* sequences fused to a wide variety of partners. There has been no common functional motif or activity ascribed to all partners; however, specific fusions may be associated with specific leukemic phenotypes. The MLL/AF4 fusion associated with t(4;11) is frequently observed in infant leukemias and is associated with an ALL phenotype in more than 90% of cases, whereas the MLL/AF9 fusion associated with the t(9;11) is almost exclusively associated with AML. Certain MLL fusion genes also have prognostic significance. For example, patients with t(9;11)(p22;q23) have a better outcome than those with other translocations involving 11q23.

The *MLL* gene encodes a large, ubiquitously expressed protein. The *Drosophila* protein trithorax, a homologue of *MLL*, regulates patterning and *HOX* gene expression during development. It has been hypothesized, in part based on these observations, that MLL might be required for maintenance of *HOX* gene expression. In support of this hypothesis, mice that lack *Mll* express HoxA7 but are not able to maintain its expression.[47] Mice that have homozygous deficiency for *Mll* have an embryonic lethal phenotype at day 10.5 postconception. Even heterozygous animals have developmental anomalies in the axial skeleton and hematopoietic deficits including anemia.[47] Thus, as for other genes targeted by chromosomal translocations, *MLL* is important for normal hematopoietic development.

The function of *MLL* is not fully understood, but cell culture and murine models have provided some insight into transforming activity of the fusion proteins. The MLL protein of the fusion protein retains the amino terminal AT hooks that facilitate binding to DNA, as well as a methyltransferase domain. With the exception of CBP/p300, the function of the remaining broad spectrum of divergent fusion partners is poorly understood. In fact, the remarkable divergence of partners has suggested that alteration in the *MLL* gene itself is a critical required event for transformation. In support of a central role of *MLL* rearrangement in AML, it has been reported that partial tandem duplications of *MLL* are associated with AML, in particular AML associated with +11.[48] Data demonstrating that MLL is a processed polypeptide provide further support for this hypothesis. MLL is processed by proteolytic cleavage into two component parts by a novel protease called *taspase 1*.[49] Cleavage is required for normal regulation of expression of anterior and posterior *HOX* gene paralogs during development. It has thus been suggested that *MLL* fusion genes, which are not cleavable, may mimic the uncleaved native MLL protein, thereby dysregulating *HOX* gene expression.[50]

MLL fusion genes have transforming properties in serial replating assays in retrovirally transduced hematopoietic progenitors as well as in murine models (reviewed in ref. 45). Although various *MLL* fusions have similar transforming properties *in vitro*, there are distinctive differences in disease penetrance and latency in the murine models, depending on the fusion partner. It is possible that the *MLL* gene rearrangement may be critical for transformation, whereas the fusion partners confer properties related to disease phenotype. The long latency of disease in murine models supports the hypothesis that *MLL* fusions, like the PML/RAR-α and CBF-related fusion proteins, require second mutations to cause leukemia.

As noted in "Leukemic Stem Cell," data indicate that certain *MLL* fusion genes may also confer properties of self-renewal to hematopoietic progenitors. MLL/ENL expression in common myeloid progenitors or granulocyte-monocyte progenitors in a murine system conferred properties of self-renewal, including the ability to serially replate in methylcellulose cultures and to engender a transplantable AML phenotype in recipient animals.[5] Similarly in a mouse model of *MLL-AF9* oncogene-induced leukemia, up to a quarter of the leukemic cells exhibit stem cell behavior.[7] Furthermore the *MLL-AF9*–positive leukemic stem cells are heterogeneous as they give rise to ALL when injected into immunodeficient mice. The same cells cause AML when injected into immunodeficient mice that are transgenic for the human genes *SCF, GM-CSF*, and *IL-3*.[51] These data indicate that leukemogenic mutations may occur in cells that have no intrinsic self-renewal capacity and yet confer these properties by activation of specific transcriptional programs, which may be further modified by clues from microenvironment. These exciting observations provide tools for identification of target genes that confer properties of self-renewal and may have value as therapeutic targets for treatment of leukemia.

CHROMOSOMAL TRANSLOCATIONS THAT INVOLVE TRANSCRIPTIONAL COACTIVATORS AND CHROMATIN REMODELING PROTEINS

Several translocations associated with leukemia involve transcriptional coactivators and chromatin-modifying proteins that have no apparent DNA-binding specificity. These include the MLL/CBP and MOZ/CBP fusions that involve the transcriptional coactivator CBP and the MLL/p300 and MOZ/TIF2 fusions, which involve the coactivators p300 and TIF2, respectively.[52,53] Although TIF2 itself is not known to have histone acetylase transferase (HAT) activity, a hallmark of the coactivators CBP and p300, it has a well-characterized CBP interaction domain that serves to recruit CBP into a complex with MOZ/TIF2.[54] Thus, recruitment of CBP/p300 is a shared theme among this group of fusion genes.

The transcriptional targets and transformation properties of this class of fusion proteins are not fully understood. Transduction of MLL/CBP into primary murine bone marrow cells followed by transplantation results in a long-latency AML, suggesting the need for secondary mutations.[55] MOZ/TIF2 also results in leukemia in a similar model system. MOZ is a HAT protein that contains a nucleosome-binding domain and an acetyl–coenzyme A–binding catalytic domain. Mutational analysis shows that leukemogenic activity requires MOZ nucleosome-binding activity and CBP recruitment activity, but the MOZ HAT activity is dispensable. These data would be consistent with a CBP gain of function in which CBP is recruited to MOZ nucleosome-binding sites.[54] However, it has also been hypothesized that the leukemogenic potential of this class of fusions may be related to dominant negative interference with CBP/p300 or that the translocation leads to simple loss of function of CBP expressed from one allele. In support of this hypothesis, loss of a single allele of CBP/p300 in the human Rubinstein-Taybi syndrome increases predisposition to malignancies including colon cancer, and mice that are heterozygous for CBP that develop hematopoietic tumors.[56]

t(1;22) TRANSLOCATION ASSOCIATED WITH INFANT ACUTE MEGAKARYOBLASTIC LEUKEMIA

Until recently, little was known about the molecular pathogenesis of acute megakaryoblastic leukemias (AMKLs; FAB M7), partly because of the difficulty in obtaining adequate quantities of material for analysis from densely fibrotic bone marrow. The t(1;22) that is associated with the majority of non–Down syndrome AMKL in infants has been cloned. The translocation results in expression of the *OTT1/MAL* fusion gene.[57,58] *OTT1 (RBM15)* contains three amino-terminal RNA recognition motifs and a Spen paralog and ortholog C terminal motif that is conserved in *Drosophila. Ott1* deletion in mice reveals multiple roles in hematopoietic development including megakaryocyte growth.[59] The *MAL* (*MKL1)* gene is a Rho-GTPase-regulated cofactor for serum response factor and controls megakaryocyte development.[60,61] A knock-in mouse model expressing OTT1/MAL is able to recapitulate AMKL and demonstrated that constitutive transcriptional activation from RBPJκ, a downstream Notch effector, is essential for its pathogenesis.[62]

DELETIONS AND NUMERIC ABNORMALITIES IN ACUTE LEUKEMIAS

Deletions of all or part of chromosomes 5 and 7 and trisomy 8 are among the most common chromosomal abnormalities associated with gain or loss of genetic material but are not associated with a specific subtype of AML. They are considerably

PRACTICE OF ONCOLOGY

more frequent in older patients, whereas the frequency of the specific translocations and inversions described previously decreases with age. These same abnormalities (+8, −7, −5/5q-) are more common in patients with an antecedent MDS, therapy-related AML, or exposure to environmental mutagens. Specific translocations or inversions are relatively less common in these patient groups. An exception to this is AML, which develops in patients who have received high doses of etoposide for treatment of a previous malignancy. As noted in "Chromosomal Translocations that Target the *MLL* Gene," translocations involving 11q23 are commonly observed in this setting.

The high frequency of deletions of the long arm of chromosome 5 (5q-) has interest because the genes encoding several hematopoietic growth factors and their receptors are located on this arm, including *GM-CSF* (5q23–31), *IL-3* (5q23–31), and *IL-4* (5q23–31). The *M-CSF* receptor, *c-fms*, and the *PDGFβR* are also on this chromosome, at 5q33. In some 5q- chromosome defects, one or more of these genes may be deleted. An intensive effort has been made to identify putative tumor suppressor genes in several critically deleted regions of chromosome 5q, as well as 7q and 20q (reviewed in ref. 63). In addition, genomic wide loss of heterozygosity screens have identified a spectrum of other smaller recurrent deletions associated with AML.[64]

An RNA-mediated interference (RNAi)-based screen of each gene within the common deleted region led to identification of *RPS14* gene. A partial loss of function of the ribosomal subunit protein RPS14 in normal hematopoietic progenitor cells recapitulated the disease with impaired erythropoiesis and relative preservation of the other lineages. Conversely, a forced expression of *RPS14* rescued the disease phenotype in patient-derived bone marrow cells. In patients with the 5q- syndrome, 1 allele of *RPS14* is deleted, and haploinsufficient expression of *RPS14* has been confirmed in patient samples. These results indicate that the *RPS14* gene is a causal gene in the 5q- syndrome.[65] However, it is conceivable that other genes (on 5q or elsewhere) collaborate with *RPS14* to cause the disease phenotype and eventually to progress to AML. In that regard, the 5q- syndrome region on chromosome 5 should be distinguished from a more centromeric locus on 5q that has been associated with therapy-related and aggressive subtypes of MDS as well as AML, and for which two candidate genes, *CTNNA1* and *EGR1*, have been recently reported.[66,67]

Acquired deletions are a hallmark of cancer and precancerous states. In general, such deletions flag the existence of a tumor suppressor gene conforming to two-hit hypothesis, in which one allele is often deleted and the other allele is inactivated by deletion, mutation, or epigenetic modification. However, the search for the key tumor suppressor gene has been elusive in the 7q or 20q deleted regions in MDS or AML. Several possible explanations can be made for the difficulty in identification of classic tumor suppressors, despite the availability of complete genomic sequence and detailed annotations of expressed sequences in these regions. The residual allele may be affected by epigenetic mutations that interfere with expression, such as promoter or aberrant methylation, or both, but do not affect coding sequence. These types of mutations are more difficult to detect. Alternatively, it is possible that haploinsufficiency for one or more genes in the critically deleted loci is responsible for the MDS/AML phenotype.[68] Haploinsufficiency for the transcription factor AML1 has been reported in a familial leukemia syndrome, and haploid gene dosage is increasingly being identified as a genetic basis for inherited human diseases.[69,70] RNAi-based discovery of the 5q- syndrome gene suggests that haploinsufficient disease genes can be identified with this approach.

CHROMOSOMAL TRANSLOCATIONS THAT RESULT IN OVEREXPRESSION OF OTHERWISE NORMAL GENES

The chromosomal translocations described thus far result in expression of aberrant fusion genes. Chromosomal translocations may also result in overexpression of otherwise normal genes as a result of juxtaposition of a gene not normally expressed in adult hematopoietic tissues adjacent to an active promoter or enhancer. Most of those identified thus far involve the immunoglobulin or T-cell receptor (TCR) enhancer loci, and thus most of these are associated with lymphoid malignancies.

The prototypical example of juxtaposition of an immunoglobulin enhancer locus to an oncogene resulting in B-cell leukemia and lymphoma is the t(8;14)(q24;q32), resulting in overexpression of the *MYC* bHLH/bZIP transcription factor on chromosome 8 because of juxtaposition to the immunoglobulin heavy-chain enhancer on chromosome 14. Similar phenotypes ensue from juxtaposition to other immunoglobulin enhancers in the human genome, such as the Igκ locus on chromosome 2 or the Igλ locus on chromosome 22, and are characterized as B-ALL or lymphoma (Table 130.1). Overexpression of *MYC* from immunoglobulin enhancers in murine models results in B-cell leukemias and lymphomas, confirming a central role for *MYC* overexpression in transformation. However, the mechanism of transformation of *MYC*, and, indeed, a complete understanding of its target genes, is not fully understood. MYC is fully active as a transcription factor when heterodimerized with MAX. MAX is normally a homodimer, or a heterodimer complexed with MAD, which represses transcription. Overexpression of *MYC* is thought to shift the equilibrium in favor of an MYC-MAX homodimer that transactivates genes that confer the leukemic phenotype to B cells.

CHROMOSOMAL TRANSLOCATIONS INVOLVING THE T-CELL RECEPTOR

T-cell leukemias are often associated with overexpression of a number of genes because of juxtaposition to the TCR enhancer loci (*TCRβ* at chromosome 7q34 or *TCRα/δ* at chromosome 14q11). Overexpression is thus associated with T-cell phenotypes, including T-cell ALL and lymphoma. For example, T-cell ALL may be associated with overexpression of bHLH family members that include TAL1/SCL, TAL2/SCL2, LYL1, HOX11, HOX11L2, LMO2, LMO1, and MYC (Table 130.1; reviewed in refs. 71 and 72). In addition to the minority of T-ALL cases with gene rearrangements involving these loci, it has been demonstrated that many patients without evident cytogenetic abnormalities overexpress TAL1, LMO2, HOX11, or HOX11L2.

POINT MUTATIONS IN ACUTE LEUKEMIA

Although intensive effort has focused on chromosomal translocations in leukemia, in part because of their high frequency in various kinds of leukemia, it has become increasingly clear that point mutations play an important role in a spectrum of leukemias (Table 130.2). Ongoing high-throughput sequencing initiatives have identified numerous solitary and recurring

TABLE 130.2

POINT MUTATIONS IN ACUTE LEUKEMIA

Mutation	Frequency in AML (%)
SIGNAL TRANSDUCTION PATHWAYS—ACTIVATING	
FLT3-ITD	~20–25
FLT3 activation loop	~5–10
RAS (N- and K-)	~15–20
KIT (D816V and D816Y)	~5
PTPN11	<5
MPL (W515L and T487A) (more common in AMKL)	<5
JAK2 and *JAK3* (more common in AMKL)	<5
TRANSCRIPTION FACTORS—LOSS OF FUNCTION	
C/EBPα (more common in FAB M2)	8–10
RUNX1 (*AML1*; more common in FAB M2)	<5
GATA-1 (more common in AMKL in Down syndrome)	<5

AML, acute myeloid leukemia.

somatic point mutations within the various leukemic subtypes. The interpretation of these sequencing data requires the identification of "driver" *versus* "passenger" mutations. Driver mutations cause genetic alterations contributing to leukemic pathophysiology, whereas passenger mutations occur in leukemia cells and are propagated but are not etiologic to the disease.[73] It is therefore essential that newly discovered somatic mutations in leukemia through sequencing studies undergo subsequent biologic validation in an experimental model system.

Oncogenic *RAS* Mutations

Activating mutations in *RAS* may be associated with AML and MDS, typically at codons 12, 13, or 61, or *N-* or *K-RAS*. The reported incidence varies widely between studies from 25% to 44% and *RAS* mutations may confer a worse prognosis (reviewed in ref. 74). Considerable effort has been devoted to developing small-molecule inhibitors of RAS activation, with a focus on prenylation inhibitors, including farnesyl transferase and geranyl-geranylation inhibitors that preclude appropriate targeting of activated RAS to the plasma membrane.[75] Specifically targeting activated RAS mutants remains an attractive option, and prenyltransferase inhibitors appear to have activity in AML. However, clinical activity is not correlated with the presence of activating mutations in RAS or even with inhibition of the target farnesyl transferase itself.[75,76] Several possible interpretations can be made of these observations, including the possibility that RAS is activated by mechanisms other than intrinsic point mutations (e.g., constitutively activated tyrosine kinases such as FLT3), or that other proteins that are targets of prenylation are important in leukemia pathogenesis, or that farnesyl transferase inhibitors have off-target effects.

Activating Mutations in Tyrosine Kinases

One of the more exciting recent developments in the pathogenesis of AMLs has been identification and characterization of activating mutations in hematopoietic tyrosine kinases. Substantial evidence has been shown that chromosomal translocations that activate tyrosine kinases can contribute to the pathogenesis of CML syndromes. The most common of these is the *BCR/ABL* gene rearrangement, but other examples include the TEL/ABL, TEL/PDGFβR, TEL/JAK2, H4/PDGFβR, FIP1/PDGFβR, and rabaptin/PDGFβR fusion proteins. However, these fusion genes are only rarely encountered in AMLs. Approximately 1% to 2% of cases of *de novo* AML have the *BCR/ABL* gene rearrangement. In addition, there are very rare cases of disease progression from CML to AML associated with acquisition of second mutations such as the *NUP98/HOXA9*, *AML1/ETO*, or *AML1/EVI1* rearrangement noted in Table 130.1. However, point mutations in the tyrosine kinase activation loop and juxtamembrane (JM) mutations that activate *FLT3* and *c-KIT* have been identified in a significant proportion of AML cases. These findings may have important therapeutic implications with the demonstration of the efficacy of molecular targeting of the ABL kinase in *BCR/ABL*-positive CML and CML blast crisis with imatinib.[77]

Activating mutations in *FLT3* have been reported in approximately 30% to 35% of cases of AML.[78] In 20% to 25% of cases, internal tandem duplications (ITDs) of the JM domain result in constitutive activation of FLT3. These can range in size from a few to more than 50 amino acids and are always in frame. Because of the extensive variability in size and exact position of the repeats within the JM domain, it has been hypothesized that these are loss-of-function domains that impair an autoinhibitory domain, resulting in constitutive kinase activation in the absence of ligand. In support of this, the crystallographic structure of FLT3 demonstrates a 7 amino acid extension of the JM domain that intercalates into the catalytic domain, thereby precluding kinase activation.[79] It is likely that ITD mutations in this region would disrupt structure of the autoinhibitory domain, resulting in kinase activation. In an additional 5% to 10% of cases, so-called activating loop mutations occur near position D835 in the tyrosine kinase.[80] Several large studies have confirmed the frequency of these mutations in adult and pediatric AML populations and the fact that mutations in *FLT3* appear to confer a poor prognosis.[81–83] High-throughput sequencing of AML patient samples lacking known FLT3 mutations revealed nine novel acquired mutations resulting in amino acid changes within the extracellular, JM, and activation domains; however, only four of the nine changes were driver mutations capable of kinase activation and conferring growth factor independence, thus emphasizing the need for biologic validation of sequencing data.[84]

FLT3 mutations may occur in conjunction with known gene rearrangements, such as *AML1/ETO*, *PML/RARα*, CBFβMYH11, or MLL. Analogous activating loop mutations at position D816 have also been reported in *C-KIT* in approximately 5% of cases of AML. Activating mutations in the thrombopoietin receptor, MPLW515L, originally identified in myelofibrosis with myeloid metaplasia, and MPLT487A have been observed in both primary cases of AMKL and those secondary to myeloid metaplasia.[85–87]

The Janus kinase family (JAK1-3) of nonreceptor tyrosine kinases, in addition to involvement in translocation-derived fusions such as TEL/JAK2, have been found to contain activating point mutations. JAK kinases are important signaling intermediaries of multiple hematopoietic cytokine receptors and downstream effectors such as STAT proteins.[88] *JAKV617F*, originally identified as a causative mutation in *polycythemia vera*, is also seen to a minor extent in AML.[89] Additional mutations in *JAK2* and *JAK3* have been isolated in AMKL.[87,90,91] Mutations in *JAK1*, *2*, or *3* are found in approximately 11% of *BCR/ABL*-negative childhood acute lymphoid leukemia and were often concurrent with deletion of the IKAROS lymphoid-specific transcription factor and the CDKN2A/B tumor suppressor.[92] As sequencing efforts continue, it is probable the list of activating kinase mutations will dramatically increase. As kinases are proving to be relatively amenable to targeted therapy, the opportunities for treatment tailored to these activated kinases should likewise expand.

MUTATION IN TUMOR SUPPRESSOR GENES

Wilms' tumor gene was originally described as a tumor suppressor gene in patients with WAGR (Wilms' tumor predisposition-aniridia-genitourinary-mental retardation).[93] *WT1* is found in adult tumors from different origin, and these tumors arise in tissues that normally do not express *WT1*. It has therefore been suggested that expression of *WT1* might play an oncogenic role in these tumors (reviewed in ref. 94). *WT1* is located at the chromosome 11p and encodes for a transcription factor with N-terminal transcriptional regulatory domain and C-terminal zinc finger domain (exon 7 to 10). The expression of *WT1* inversely correlates with the degree of differentiation in the hematopoietic system as it is present in CD34+ cells and absent in mature leukocytes.[94,95] *WT1* functions as a potent transcription regulator of genes important for cell survival and cell differentiation. The disruption of *WT1* function promotes stem cell proliferation and hampers differentiation.[94] Although the precise role of *WT1* in normal and malignant hematopoiesis remains to be further elucidated, it seems to have a dual role in leukemia.[96]

The wild type form of *WT1* is highly (75% to 100%) expressed in a variety of acute leukemias.[97] Consistent with the function of an oncogene is the pattern of *WT1* expression in CML, where low levels are found in the chronic phase but are frequently increased in the accelerated and blast crisis phase.[98] High levels of *WT1* in patients after chemotherapy is associated with poor prognosis.

WT1 can act as a tumor suppressor in mice.[99] Mutation of the *WT1* gene can be detected in approximately 10% of normal karyotype AMLs.[100,101] Mutations that cluster to exon 7 (mostly frameshift mutations resulting from insertions and deletions) and exon 9 (mostly substitutions) are associated with poor clinical outcome.[101–103] These data are examples of *WT1* as a tumor suppressor. On the other hand, a recent study has analyzed mutations within the entire *WT1* coding sequence in a very large cohort of young adults with normal karyotype AML. Contrary to the previous observations,[101–103] *WT1* mutations had no prognostic impact.[104] The different results from these large studies could be explained by the variable biological role of *WT1* in AML, possible differences in therapy, and other patient characteristics. It is therefore desirable that testing for *WT1* mutations becomes part of the risk assessment in future clinical trials to resolve these discrepancies.

TP53 is a tumor suppressor that induces cell-cycle arrest in a response to apoptotic cell death or DNA repair due to genotoxic substances, oncogenes, hypoxia, DNA damage, or ribonucleotide depletion.[105] Inactivation of *TP53* plays an important role during neoplastic transformation in solid tumors and also during progression of hematologic malignancies.[106–108] Animal experiments suggest that the loss of one *TP53* allele could be sufficient for tumorigenesis.[109] This could be relevant for the development of leukemia in patients with single *TP53* deletion. The loss of 17p in AML is often accompanied by a *TP53* mutation resulting in a loss of heterozygosity.[110,111] Another possibility is the inactivation of downstream mediators of *TP53*, which affect not only cell-cycle arrest but also DNA repair and apoptosis. Alternatively, overexpression of genes inhibiting or promoting degradation of TP53 can be considered; for example, *MDM2* gene amplifications have been detected in B-CLL.[112] *TP53* deletion can be present as a loss of 17p as a part of a complex aberrant karyotype or as a single chromosomal aberration, both resulting in a poor clinical outcome.[110,113–115]

The incidence of *TP53* aberrations is high in AML with a complex aberrant karyotype (up to 70%),[110] but relatively rare in other AML groups (2% to 9%),[83,110,116] and *TP53* mutations without cytogenetic alteration are to rare events.[111,117] Low-risk AML t(8;21) or inv(16) is not associated with *TP53* deletion. There is significant positive association between *TP53* deletion and other high-risk chromosomal aberrations such as del(5q), and monosomy 5 and 7.[115,118] Molecular risk factors *FLT3-ITD* and *NPM1* mutation do not seem to cluster with the *TP53* deletion in complex karyotype patients.[115] *TP53*-deleted cells have greater resistance to various conventional antileukemic drugs.[119] Although published data of multidrug-resistance gene expression showed negative influence on therapy response in complex aberrant patients,[120] the association of *TP53* deletion and *MDR1* expression has been confirmed for CML, but not for AML.[121] Hence, an independent mechanism of resistance needs to be considered.[115] Taken together, *TP53* deletion is a high-risk factor conveying a poor outcome, and further studies are necessary to provide and evaluate alternative therapies.

ACTIVATING MUTATIONS OF NOTCH

NOTCH1 is a component of an evolutionarily conserved pathway shown to direct T-cell lineage determination in early and late stages of lymphocyte development as well as play a role in hematopoietic stem cell self-renewal (reviewed in ref. 122). NOTCH1 is a heterodimeric transmembrane receptor. Ligand binding to NOTCH1 allows proteolytic cleavage of the heterodimerization domain (HD) by γ-secretase of the C-terminal intracellular domain (ICN), which then localizes to the nucleus to function as a transactivator. Involvement of NOTCH1 in T-ALL had been observed with the rare t(7;9)(q34;q34.3) in which translocation of TCRβ locus into the *NOTCH1* gene results in the expression of the truncated, transcriptionally active ICN.

Recently, a series of point mutations in NOTCH1 were identified in over half of all T-ALL cases[123] (reviewed in ref. 124). These mutations clustered in two primary locations, the HD and the proline, glutamate, serine, and threonine-rich (PEST) domain. The missense mutations within the HD domain make NOTCH1 more amenable to γ-secretase–mediated cleavage, thus enhancing activation. The PEST domain controls the rate of degradation of the activated ICN. PEST domain mutants are primarily small insertions/deletions into the reading frame causing deletion of all or part of the domain and extending the half-life of the activated ICN. Fortuitously, γ-secretase inhibitors (GSIs) had already undergone significant clinical development from the involvement of γ-secretase in processing the pathogenic β-amyloid peptide associated with Alzheimer dementia. Initial clinical trials of GSIs in T-ALL have shown minimal effects on disease and significant gastrointestinal toxicity.[125] Use of GSIs in combination with agents affecting alternative pathways may provide synergism and improve efficacy. Treatment of a mouse model of T-ALL with GSIs and corticosteroids has demonstrated that GSIs are capable of abrogating corticosteroid resistance in established cell lines as well as limiting GSI-mediated gut toxicity.[126]

MUTATIONS ALTERING LOCALIZATION OF NPM1

NPM1 (*nucleophosmin1*) encodes a protein that acts as a molecular chaperone between the nucleus and cytoplasm. It is involved in multiple cellular processes including regulation of TP53/ARF pathways, ribosome biogenesis, and duplication of centrosomes. *NPM1* had been previously identified in acute leukemias as a translocation fusion partner with *RAR* and *MLF* as well as with *ALK* in anaplastic large cell lymphoma. Aberrant cytoplasmic localization of *NPM1* has been observed in 25% to 30% of adult AML and is associated with point mutations within exon 12, which are hypothesized to enhance a nuclear export motif within the expressed protein.[127] The mechanism by which mutated *NPM1* causes leukemia is not clear; however, the cytoplasmic localization of *NPM1* is thought to be intrinsic to its altered function.[128] *NPM1* mutations are found more frequently in AML with normal karyotypes (50% to 60%) and more apt to have *FLT3-ITD* mutations as well. Among normal cytogenetic AMLs, the presence of cytoplasmic *NPM1* in the absence of the *FLT3-ITD* is associated with a more favorable prognosis.[128]

LOSS-OF-FUNCTION POINT MUTATIONS IN *AML1*, *C/EBPα*, AND *GATA-1*

AML1 (also known as *RUNX1*, *CBFA2*) is a frequent target of translocations in human leukemias. In addition to frequent involvement of *AML1* as a consequence of chromosomal translocations, it has been determined that loss-of-function mutations in *AML1* are responsible for the inherited leukemia syndrome FPD/AML (familial platelet disorder with propensity to develop acute myelogenous leukemia).[69,129] In addition, approximately 3% to 5% of sporadic cases of AML harbor loss-of-function mutations in *AML1*,[69,130] with a higher frequency in M0 AML (25%) and in AML or MDS with trisomy 21. It is not known whether loss-of-function mutations in *AML1* confer the favorable prognosis associated with translocations involving the *AML1* gene.

C/EBPα is a 42-kDa hematopoietic transcription factor that is required for normal myeloid lineage development. Because many translocations associated with AML phenotypes result in loss of function of hematopoietic transcription factors, it has been hypothesized that *C/EBPα* may also be a target for loss-of-function mutations in human leukemia. Two major types of *C/EBPα* point mutations have been described in AML: short frame-shifting mutations in the region encoding the amino-terminus causing expression of a shortened 30-kDa protein with dominant negative activity and in-frame insertions or deletions in the region of the carboxy-terminus that alter the DNA-binding or dimerization domains causing loss of function.[131] Thus, these mutations would be predicted to impair hematopoietic differentiation. Although the bulk of *C/EBPα* occur in patients with normal cytogenetics, overall and progression-free survival is closer to the favorable rather than intermediate prognostic group.[132] Therefore, *C/EBPα* mutational status may provide a more accurate risk assessment for normal cytogenetic AML.

GATA-1 mutations are associated with a subset of AMKLs (FAB M7), in particular leukemias arising in patients with Down syndrome (constitutional trisomy 21). These mutations result in early termination of the full-length GATA-1 protein; however, translation of a short form, GATA-1s, from an alternate initiation codon occurs. GATA-1s is theorized to function as either a hypomorphic or dominant negative allele and dysregulation of GATA-1 pathways is thought to contribute to leukemogenesis.[133,134] *GATA-1* mutations are often seen in a tansient myeloproliferative disorder that precedes Down syndrome–associated AMKL, suggesting that *GATA-1* mutation is an early event.[133] *GATA-1* mutations thus far have only been associated with Down syndrome and have not been observed in other infant AMKLs, including those with the t(1;22) described earlier in "t(1;22) Translocation Associated with Infant Acute Megakaryoblastic Leukemia."

MUTATION OF LYMPHOID DEVELOPMENT GENES IN ALL

Analysis of pediatric acute leukemia samples through a combination of high-resolution SNP arrays and genomic sequencing revealed numerous cryptic translocations, small deletions, and point mutations affecting genes required for B-cell commitment and differentiation.[135] These genes include *PAX5, E2A, EBF1, LEF1, IKAROS,* and *AIOLOS,* and their mutations predominantly produce haploinsufficiency resulting in hypomorphic expression. Forty percent of acute precursor B-cell leukemias possessed mutation of at least one gene required for B-cell development, and 31.7% specifically had mutations within the *PAX5* gene. Because of the requirement of these factors for normal early to late precursor B development, the immunophenotypic stage most closely related to the leukemias, it is hypothesized that loss of normal expression levels leads to a block in differentiation, a critical step in leukemogenesis.[135]

MUTATIONAL COMPLEMENTATION GROUPS IN ACUTE LEUKEMIAS

Several lines of evidence indicate that more than one mutation is necessary for the pathogenesis of acute leukemia. First, there is evidence for acquisition of additional cytogenetic abnormalities with disease progression from CML to AML (i.e., CML blast crisis). Published examples of progression in *BCR/ABL*-positive CML include acquisition of t(3;21) *AML1/EV11*, t(8;21) *AML1/ETO*, or t(7;11) *NUP98/HOXA9* gene rearrangements. Progression of chronic myelomonocytic leukemia to AML in a patient with the *TEL/PDGFβR* gene rearrangement was associated with acquisition of a t(8;21) *AML1/ETO* gene rearrangement.[136] Second, expression of the AML1/ETO or CBFβ/MYH11 fusion proteins in murine models is not sufficient to cause AML.[27,137] Chemical mutagens must be used in these contexts to generate second mutations that cause the AML phenotype. Third, evidence indicates that in some cases the *TEL/AML1* gene rearrangement associated with pediatric ALL may be acquired *in utero*, but ALL does not develop until years later, indicating a requirement for a second mutation.[138] Fourth, AML develops in transgenic mice that express the PML/RAR-α fusion protein only after a long latency of 3 to 6 months, with incomplete penetrance, indicating a need for a second mutation.[34–36]

The genetic epidemiology of AML provides important clues to the nature of the collaborating mutations. One broad complementation group in AML (Fig. 130.1) is composed of mutations that activate signal transduction pathways. These include activating mutations in *FLT3, RAS,* and *KIT* and, more rarely, the *BCR/ABL* and *TEL/PDGFβR* fusion associated with disease progression in CML. These can be viewed as a complementation group because even though they are collectively present in approximately 50% of cases of AML, they rarely, if ever, occur together in the same patient.

A second complementation group, typified by translocations involving hematopoietic transcription factors, includes

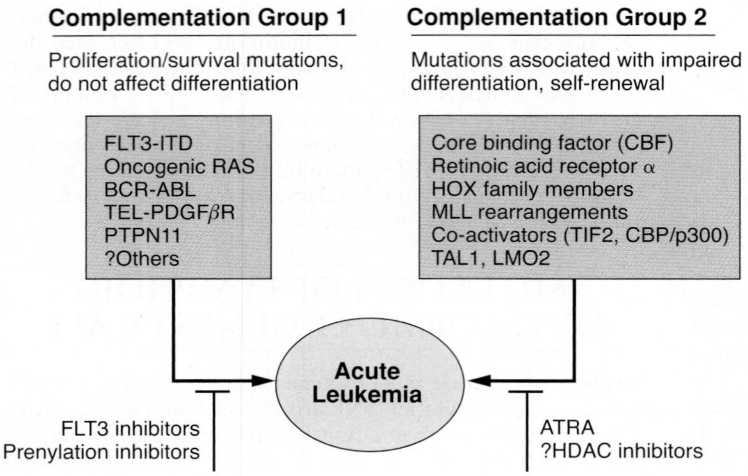

Complementation Group 1

Proliferation/survival mutations, do not affect differentiation

FLT3-ITD
Oncogenic RAS
BCR-ABL
TEL-PDGFβR
PTPN11
?Others

Complementation Group 2

Mutations associated with impaired differentiation, self-renewal

Core binding factor (CBF)
Retinoic acid receptor α
HOX family members
MLL rearrangements
Co-activators (TIF2, CBP/p300)
TAL1, LMO2

Acute Leukemia

FLT3 inhibitors
Prenylation inhibitors

ATRA
?HDAC inhibitors

FIGURE 130.1 Cooperating mutations in acute leukemia. Leukemia is composed of two broad complementation groups, defined by lack of concurrence of any two mutations in the same complementation group in the same patient. One group is characterized by activating mutations in signal transduction pathways, such as FLT3-ITD or oncogenic N-RAS. When expressed alone, these mutations confer a proliferative or survival advantage, or both, but do not affect differentiation. The second group exemplified by AML1/ETO or PML/RAR-α are associated with impaired differentiation and the ability to confer properties of self-renewal to hematopoietic progenitors. Together, the complementation groups collaborate to engender the acute leukemia phenotype. This model has important therapeutic implications in that each of the complementation groups can be potentially targeted for therapeutic intervention, such as small-molecule inhibitors of FLT3 or RAS, or agents that override the block in differentiation, such as all-*trans*-retinoic acid (ATRA) or possibly histone deacetylase (HDAC) inhibitors.

AML1/ETO, CBFβ/SMMHC, PML/RARα, NUP98/HOXA9, and *MLL* gene rearrangements, and *MOZ/TIF2,* and they are never observed together in the same leukemia. In general, this second class of mutations impairs hematopoietic differentiation and may confer properties of self-renewal to the leukemic stem cell but is not sufficient to cause leukemia when expressed alone (see "Recurring Chromosomal Abnormalities in Acute Leukemia"). However, one mutation from each of these two complementation groups often coexists in the same leukemia. For example, activating mutations in *FLT3* or *RAS* have been observed in association with virtually all of the fusion genes in the second class described earlier.[139]

Support has also been given for the hypothesis of collaborating classes of leukemia oncogenes derived from analysis of genotypes of CML patients who progress to AML. Some cases of *BCR/ABL*-positive CML progress to AML associated with acquisition of the t(7;11) translocation associated with expression of the *NUP98/HOXA9* fusion gene discussed earlier. As another example, TEL/PDGFβR-positive chronic myelomonocytic leukemia may progress to AML associated with acquisition of the t(8;21) translocation related to expression of the AML1/ETO fusion. These cases of disease progressions from CML to AML imply that constitutively activated tyrosine kinases cooperate with mutations in hematopoietic transcription factors to cause the AML phenotype.

These findings suggest a hypothesis for the pathogenesis of AML in which there are two broad classes of cooperating mutations (Fig. 130.1).[139] One class, exemplified by activating mutations in *FLT3* or *RAS*, confer either a proliferative or survival advantage, or both, to hematopoietic progenitors but do not affect differentiation. These mutations do not confer self-renewal capacity as assessed in part by the ability to serially replate in culture or to serially transplant disease in murine models.[140,141] A second class of mutations, exemplified by *AML1/ETO, CBFβ/SMMHC, PML/RARα, NUP98/HOXA9,* and *MLL* gene rearrangements, and *MOZ/TIF2* serve primarily to impair hematopoietic differentiation and confer properties of self-renewal. Together, these cooperating mutations induce the AML phenotype characterized by enhanced proliferative and survival advantage, impaired differentiation, and limitless self-renewal capacity. Experimental evidence supports this model of cooperativity in murine models between BCR/ABL and NUP98/HOXA9,[142] TEL/PDGFβR and AML1/ETO,[143] and FLT3/ITD and PML/RAR-α.[144] These findings have important therapeutic implications in that it may be possible to target both classes of mutations. For example, in APL with activating mutations in *FLT3*, it may be possible to target FLT3 with small-molecule inhibitors and PML/RAR-α with ATRA (see Chapter 131 and Fig. 130.1).

CONCLUSION

The quest to elucidate the essential pathophysiologic changes involved in leukemogenesis has been accelerated with the use of newer technologies such as high-resolution mapping and high-throughput sequencing. It is now possible to identify specific molecular pathways complementing known recurrent translocations as well as gain insight into the mechanisms underlying normal karyotype leukemias. Not only can these novel mutations be used for more accurate prognostication, but they also provide an opportunity for drug development, targeting the essential pathways dysregulated in leukemia. As the availability of pathway-targeted therapeutics increases, interrogation of a patient's leukemia for alterations at the genomic level may allow individualized therapy addressing the pathways responsible for leukemic cell survival, proliferation, and differentiation, which ideally would improve treatment efficacy and reduce therapy-related morbidity and mortality.

Selected References

The full list of references for this chapter appears in the online version.

1. Bonnet D, Dick JE. Human acute myeloid leukemia is organized as a hierarchy that originates from a primitive hematopoietic cell. *Nat Med* 1997;3:730.
3. Saito Y, Kitamura H, Hijikata A, et al. Identification of therapeutic targets for quiescent, chemotherapy-resistant human leukemia stem cells. *Sci Transl Med* 2007;2(17):17.
6. Huntly BJ, Shigematsu H, Deguchi K, et al. MOZ-TIF2, but not BCR-ABL, confers properties of leukemic stem cells to committed murine hematopoietic progenitors. *Cancer Cell* 2004;6:587–596.
7. Somervaille TCP, Cleary ML. Identification and characterization of leukemia stem cells in murine MLL-AF9 acute myeloid leukemia. *Cancer Cell* 2006;10:257–268.
9. Huntly BJ, Gilliland DG. Leukaemia stem cells and the evolution of cancer-stem-cell research. *Nat Rev Cancer* 2005;5:311–321.

10. Jamieson CH, Ailles LE, Dylla SJ, et al. Granulocyte-macrophage progenitors as candidate leukemic stem cells in blast-crisis CML. *N Engl J Med* 2004;351:657–667.
13. Ley TJ, Mardis ER, Ding L, et al. DNA sequencing of a cytogenetically normal acute myeloid leukaemia genome. *Nature* 2008;456:66.
14. Loriaux MM, Levine RL, Tyner JW, et al. High-throughput sequence analysis of the tyrosine kinome in acute myeloid leukemia. *Blood* 2008;111:4788.
16. International Cancer Genome Consortium. International network of cancer genome projects. *Nature* 2010;464:993–998.
17. Rowley JD. The role of chromosome translocations in leukemogenesis. *Semin Hematol* 1999;36:59–72.
18. Koschmieder S, Halmos B, Levantini E, Tenen DG. Dysregulation of the C/EBP{alpha} differentiation pathway in human cancer. *J Clin Oncol* 2009;27:619–628.
26. Jiao B, Wu CF, Liang Y, et al. AML1-ETO9a is correlated with C-KIT overexpression/mutations and indicates poor disease outcome in t(8;21) acute myeloid leukemia-M2. *Leukemia* 2009;23:1598.
32. Salomoni P, Pandolfi PP. The role of PML in tumor suppression. *Cell* 2002;108:165–170.
33. Scaglioni PP, Pandolfi PP. The theory of APL revisited. *Curr Top Microbiol Immunol* 2007;313:85–100.
37. Tallman MS, Nabhan C, Feusner JH, Rowe JM. Acute promyelocytic leukemia: evolving therapeutic strategies. *Blood* 2002;99:759–767.
38. Abramovich C, Humphries RK. Hox regulation of normal and leukemic hematopoietic stem cells. *Curr Opin Hematol* 2005;12:210–216.
45. Eguchi M, Eguchi-Ishimae M, Greaves M. Molecular pathogenesis of MLL-associated leukemias. *Int J Hematol* 2005;82:9–20.
46. Slany RK. The molecular biology of mixed lineage leukemia. *Haematologica* 2009;94:984–993.
51. Wei J, Wunderlich M, Fox C, et al. Microenvironment determines lineage fate in a human model of MLL-AF9 leukemia. *Cancer Cell* 2008;13:483.
56. Kung AL, Rebel VI, Bronson RT, et al. Gene dose-dependent control of hematopoiesis and hematologic tumor suppression by CBP. *Genes Dev* 2000;14:272–277.
62. Mercher T, Raffel GD, Moore SA, et al. The OTT-MAL fusion oncogene activates RBPJ-mediated transcription and induces acute megakaryoblastic leukemia in a knockin mouse model. *J Clin Invest* 2009;119:852–864.
64. Sweetser DA, Chen CS, Blomberg AA, et al. Loss of heterozygosity in childhood de novo acute myelogenous leukemia. *Blood* 2001;98:1188.
65. Ebert BL, Pretz J, Bosco J, et al. Identification of RPS14 as a 5q(-) syndrome gene by RNA interference screen. *Nature* 2008;451:335.
69. Song WJ, Sullivan MG, Legare RD, et al. Haploinsufficiency of CBFA2 causes familial thrombocytopenia with propensity to develop acute myelogenous leukaemia. *Nat Genet* 1999;23:166–175.
71. Armstrong SA, Look AT. Molecular genetics of acute lymphoblastic leukemia. *J Clin Oncol* 2005;23:6306–6315.
72. O'Neil J, Look AT. Mechanisms of transcription factor deregulation in lymphoid cell transformation. *Oncogene* 2007;26:6838–6849.
73. Stratton MR, Campbell PJ, Futreal PA. The cancer genome. *Nature* 2009;458:719–724.
75. Lancet JE, Karp JE. Farnesyltransferase inhibitors in hematologic malignancies: new horizons in therapy. *Blood* 2003;102:3880–3889.
76. Braun BS, Shannon K. Targeting Ras in myeloid leukemias. *Clin Cancer Res* 2008;14:2249–2252.
84. Frohling S, Scholl C, Levine RL, et al. Identification of driver and passenger mutations of FLT3 by high-throughput DNA sequence analysis and functional assessment of candidate alleles. *Cancer Cell* 2007;12:501–513.
85. Pardanani AD, Levine RL, Lasho T, et al. MPL515 mutations in myeloproliferative and other myeloid disorders: a study of 1182 patients. *Blood* 2006;108:3472–3476.
86. Hussein K, Bock O, Theophile K, et al. MPLW515L mutation in acute megakaryoblastic leukaemia. *Leukemia* 2009;23:852–855.
88. Baker SJ, Rane SG, Reddy EP. Hematopoietic cytokine receptor signaling. *Oncogene* 2007;26:6724–6737.
91. Walters DK, Mercher T, Gu TL, et al. Activating alleles of JAK3 in acute megakaryoblastic leukemia. *Cancer Cell* 2006;10:65–75.
92. Mullighan CG, Downing JR. Genome-wide profiling of genetic alterations in acute lymphoblastic leukemia: recent insights and future directions. *Leukemia* 2009;23:1209.
94. Hohenstein P, Hastie ND. The many facets of the Wilms' tumour gene, WT1. *Hum Mol Genet* 2006;15:R196.
96. Yang L, Han Y, Saurez Saiz F, Minden MD. A tumor suppressor and oncogene: the WT1 story. *Leukemia* 2007;21:868–876.
97. Miyagi T, Ahuja H, Kubota T, et al. Expression of the candidate Wilm's tumor gene, WT1, in human leukemia cells. *Leukemia* 1993;7:970–977.
101. Summers K, Stevens J, Kakkas I, et al. Wilms' tumour 1 mutations are associated with FLT3-ITD and failure of standard induction chemotherapy in patients with normal karyotype AML. *Leukemia* 2007;21:550–551.
102. Virappane P, Gale R, Hills R, et al. Mutation of the Wilms' tumor 1 gene is a poor prognostic factor associated with chemotherapy resistance in normal karyotype acute myeloid leukemia: the United Kingdom Medical Research Council Adult Leukaemia Working Party. *J Clin Oncol* 2008;26:5429–5435.
103. Paschka P, Marcucci G, Ruppert AS, et al. Wilms' tumor 1 gene mutations independently predict poor outcome in adults with cytogenetically normal acute myeloid leukemia: a Cancer and Leukemia Group B Study. *J Clin Oncol* 2008;26:4595–4602.
105. Vousden KH, Lu X. Live or let die: the cell's response to p53. *Nat Rev Cancer* 2002;2:594.
109. Venkatachalam S, Shi Y-P, Jones SN, et al. Retention of wild-type p53 in tumors from p53 heterozygous mice: reduction of p53 dosage can promote cancer formation. *EMBO J* 1998;17:4657–4667.
110. Haferlach C, Dicker F, Herholz H, et al. Mutations of the TP53 gene in acute myeloid leukemia are strongly associated with a complex aberrant karyotype. *Leukemia* 2008;22:1539–1541.
115. Seifert H, Mohr B, Thiede C, et al. The prognostic impact of 17p (p53) deletion in 2272 adults with acute myeloid leukemia. *Leukemia* 2009; 23:656.
122. Radtke F, Wilson A, MacDonald HR. Notch signaling in hematopoiesis and lymphopoiesis: lessons from *Drosophila*. *Bioessays* 2005;27:1117–1128.
123. Weng AP, Ferrando AA, Lee W, et al. Activating mutations of NOTCH1 in human T cell acute lymphoblastic leukemia. *Science* 2004;306:269–271.
124. Grabher C, von Boehmer H, Look AT. Notch 1 activation in the molecular pathogenesis of T-cell acute lymphoblastic leukaemia. *Nat Rev Cancer* 2006;6:347–359.
125. DeAngelo DJ, Stone JR, Silverman LB, et al. A phase I clinical trial of the Notch inhibitor MK-0752 in patients with T-cell acute lymphoblastic leukemia/lymphoma (T-ALL) and other leukemias. *ASCO Meeting Abstracts* 2006:6585.
126. Real PJ, Tosello V, Palomero T, et al. Gamma-secretase inhibitors reverse glucocorticoid resistance in T cell acute lymphoblastic leukemia. *Nat Med* 2009;15:50–58.
127. Falini B, Mecucci C, Tiacci E, et al. Cytoplasmic nucleophosmin in acute myelogenous leukemia with a normal karyotype. *N Engl J Med* 2005; 352:254.
131. Mueller BU, Pabst T. C/EBPalpha and the pathophysiology of acute myeloid leukemia. *Curr Opin Hematol* 2006;13:7–14.
133. Wechsler J, Greene M, McDevitt MA, et al. Acquired mutations in GATA1 in the megakaryoblastic leukemia of Down syndrome. *Nat Genet* 2002;32:148–152.
134. Malinge S, Izraeli S, Crispino JD. Insights into the manifestations, outcomes, and mechanisms of leukemogenesis in Down syndrome. *Blood* 2009;113:2619–2628.
135. Mullighan CG, Goorha S, Radtke I, et al. Genome-wide analysis of genetic alterations in acute lymphoblastic leukaemia. *Nature* 2007;446:758–764.
144. Kelly LM, Kutok JL, Williams IR, et al. PML/RARalpha and FLT3-ITD induce an APL-like disease in a mouse model. *Proc Natl Acad Sci U S A* 2002;99:8283.

CHAPTER 131 MANAGEMENT OF ACUTE LEUKEMIAS

PARTOW KEBRIAEI, RICHARD CHAMPLIN, MARCOS de LIMA, AND ELIHU ESTEY

Acute leukemias result from malignant transformation of immature hematopoietic cells followed by clonal proliferation and accumulation of the transformed cells. The pathogenesis of leukemia transformation is incompletely defined but is likely to be a multistep process.[1] Acute leukemias are characterized by aberrant differentiation and maturation of the malignant cells, with a maturation arrest and accumulation of leukemic blasts in the bone marrow. Acute leukemias are categorized according to their differentiation along the myeloid or lymphoid lineage. In 10% to 20% of patients, the leukemic cells have characteristics of both myeloid and lymphoid cells.

Hematopoietic cells are derived from stem cells and progenitors giving rise to the myeloid and lymphoid system. Stem cells have the fundamental properties of self-renewal and differentiation into distinct lineages. Hematopoietic stem cells and progenitors are resident in the bone marrow where they are supported and regulated through interactions with the local microenvironment. Leukemia likely develops after transformation of a hematopoietic stem cell or progenitor, which acquires stem cell–like properties of unlimited self-renewal.[2] The malignant stem cells represent a small fraction of the leukemia. The bulk of leukemic cells are the differentiated progeny that undergo limited maturation along the myeloid or lymphoid lineage. Leukemia chemotherapy must eradicate the disease while sparing normal hematopoietic stem cells. Treatments that eradicate the differentiated leukemia cells typically do not eradicate the malignant stem cells; consequently, relapse of the leukemia commonly occurs.[3] High-dose, stem cell toxic therapies may be used if followed by hematopoietic transplantation to restore normal hematopoiesis, and hematopoietic transplantation is an important modality of treatment for acute leukemias. A better understanding of the biology of normal and malignant stem cells and the marrow microenvironment is required for development of more effective therapies.

Although the cause of acute leukemias is unknown, malignant transformation is unlikely to be the result of a single event. Rather, it is likely caused by the culmination of multiple processes that produce genetic damage secondary to physical or chemical exposure in susceptible progenitor cells. Leukemia may occur following exposure to a number of carcinogens, such as benzene or radiation exposure. A clear cause of leukemia can be found in only a minority of patients. Acute leukemias may occur following chemotherapy or radiation therapy given for another malignancy.[4,5] These secondary leukemias typically have a high risk of cytogenetic abnormalities and have a poor prognosis.

Inherited genetic abnormalities that predispose to leukemia include ataxia telangiectasia, Down syndrome, and certain polymorphisms in *MTHFR* (a gene involved in the folate metabolism).[6] Acquired factors include somatic cytogenetic abnormalities, such as secondary leukemias following chemotherapy or radiation therapy. Alkylating agents and topoisomerase II inhibitors are most commonly associated with therapy-related leukemias and typically lead to myeloid leukemias. However, an increasing number of acute lymphoblastic leukemia (ALL) patients are being noted following the use of topoisomerase II inhibitors.[6] Other acquired factors include infectious agents and environmental toxins. Among infectious causes, the Epstein-Barr virus is associated with mature B-cell or Burkitt's ALL. Finally, many environmental toxins have been implicated, but only exposure to nuclear or atomic agents have been clearly demonstrated to be involved in the development of ALL.[7]

The presenting clinical symptoms are a result of bone marrow failure or the effects of tissue infiltration or circulating leukemia cells. Patients commonly complain of fatigue or spontaneous bleeding. Weight loss, fever, night sweats, and lethargy may also be present. Infections related to neutropenia may occur. Central nervous system (CNS) involvement is more common in ALL than in acute myeloid leukemia (AML). Bone and testicular involvement is also more commonly seen in ALL, and most commonly in children rather than adults.[8] On physical examination, pallor and signs associated with thrombocytopenia may be present, such as gingival bleeding, epistaxis, petechiae, ecchymoses, or fundal hemorrhages. Less commonly, generalized lymphadenopathy, hepatosplenomegaly, or dermal involvement by leukemia cutis may be present. T-lineage ALL may commonly present with a mediastinal mass.

The diagnosis of acute leukemias requires morphologic identification of malignant blasts in the blood and bone marrow.[9] This requires evaluation of peripheral blood and bone marrow aspirate smears, phenotypic analysis of the blasts by cytochemical studies and flow cytometry, or immunohistochemistry with an appropriate panel of surface and cytoplasmic markers. Acute leukemias are classified according to their differentiation into the myeloid or lymphoid lineage, although some cases appear biphenotypic. The French American British Group (FAB) described a widely utilized classification system[10] that has been largely replaced by the World Health Organization's (WHO) classification system.[11] Cytospin slides made from cerebrospinal fluid (CSF) are used to diagnose CNS involvement. The current definition of CNS involvement used by the Children's Cancer Group (CCG) is greater than five white blood cells (WBC) per microliter of CSF plus unequivocal blasts identified on the cytospin.[12] However, the risk for CNS relapse and need for additional CNS-directed therapy is controversial when there are less than WBC per microliter of CSF, but blasts are present. Some studies suggest that the presence of blasts, even in the absence of pleocytosis, requires additional CNS-directed therapy,[13] while others do not. A related concern is the prognostic significance of a traumatic lumbar puncture at diagnosis. Most studies concur that the presence of blasts in a traumatic lumbar puncture is associated with an inferior outcome.[14]

TABLE 131.1

CYTOGENETIC CLASSIFICATION SYSTEMS FOR ACUTE MYELOGENOUS LEUKEMIA

Group	NCRI (formerly MRC)	SWOG/ECOG	CALGB
Favorable	inv(16); t(8;21)	inv(16); t(8;21) w/o del (9q) or complex changes	inv(16); t(8;21)
Intermediate	Normal; 11q abnormalities;[a] +8; Others not in favorable or unfavorable groups	Normal; +8; Others not in favorable or unfavorable groups	Normal; t(9;11); +8 (for relapse); del(5q); Loss of 7q
Unfavorable	−5/−7; Complex (≥5 chromosomes involved)	−5/−7; Complex (≥3 chromosomes involved); 11q abnormalities;[a] inv(3q); del(20q); t(6;9); abnormal 17p	Complex (≥3 chromosomes involved); −7; +8 (for survival); inv(3)

NCRI, National Cancer Research Institute; MRC, Medical Research Center; SWOG, Southwest Oncology Group; ECOG, Eastern Cooperative Oncology Group; CALGB, Cancer and Leukemia Group B.
[a]Patients with t(9;11) may fall into the intermediate group and patients with other 11q abnormalities into the unfavorable group.

ACUTE MYELOGENOUS LEUKEMIA

AML is characterized by limited myeloid differentiation of the malignant cells. The malignant cells characteristically undergo maturation arrest at the level of the blast or promyelocyte, although varying proportions of mature hematopoietic cells are leukemia derived. The cells display myeloid specific markers, including Auer rods (aberrant primary granules), cytochemistry (Sudan black, myeloperoxidase, or nonspecific esterase), and cell surface antigens.[10]

AML encompasses a family of hematologic malignancies that can be categorized according to their cytogenetic and associated genetic abnormalities that have major prognostic importance. Favorable, intermediate, and unfavorable prognostic groups can be defined; the classification systems used by the major cooperative groups are summarized in Table 131.1. Increasingly, treatment is being individualized by prognostic group, with a goal of developing treatment tailored to the molecular basis of the patient's malignancy.

Cytogenetics, Molecular Abnormalities, and Prognosis in Acute Myelogenous Leukemia

The core binding factor (CBF)–related AMLs have the most favorable prognosis and constitute 10% to 15% of cases in patients under age 60.[15] CBFs regulate transcription of genes involved in differentiation of normal blasts into mature progeny. CBFs contain a β unit (*CBFB*, located on the long arm of chromosome 16) and an α unit, one of which is known as *RUNX1* (formerly *AML1* and located on chromosome 21). The CBF AMLs result from translocations involving *RUNX1* or *CBFB*. Specifically, in t(8;21) *RUNX1* is fused with *RUNX1T1* (formerly *ETO*) located on chromosome 8, while in inv(16) *CBFB* is linked with the *MYH11* gene located on the short arm of chromosome 16. These abnormal CBFs exert a "dominant negative" effect over normal CBFs, leading to differentiation block and, in the presence of other genetic aberrations that promote survival of the affected stem cells, to AML.

It is important to distinguish deletion of the long arm of chromosome 16(del16q), which does not affect *CBFB*, from translocation between the 2 chromosome 16s, t(16;16), which is quite rare but does disrupt *CBFB* and, unlike del16q, behaves clinically like inv(16). Eighty-five percent of cases of inv(16) or t(8;21) AML are found in those under age 60. Although inv(16) is most frequently associated with FAB subtype M4Eo, 40% of the 145 cases of inv(16) AML seen at the M. D. Anderson Cancer Center over the past 25 years have had less than 5% eosinophils. Similarly, although t(8;21) AML is most often seen in FAB subtype M2, 30% of the 124 cases at M. D. Anderson Cancer Center were seen in association with other FAB subtypes. Inv(16) AML and t(8;21) AML differ in several ways. For example, t(8;21) tends to present with lower WBC counts and is frequently accompanied by loss of a sex chromosome (particularly the Y) or a deletion (del) of the long arm (q) of chromosome 9(del9q) while inv(16) is often accompanied by trisomy (+) 22 (+22), +(8), or +(21). Although both inv(16) and t(8;21) are distinguished by complete remission (CR) rates of approximately 90% and long remissions (probability of being alive in CR at 5 years about 50%), inv(16) AML is more apt to respond once relapse occurs; as a result, patients with inv(16) tend to live longer than those with t(8;21).

Acute Myelogenous Leukemia with Normal Cytogenetics

A normal karyotype is seen in 35% to 40% of AML patients aged 16 to 60 years old. Acute myelogenous leukemia with normal cytogenetics (NC-AML) is associated with greater variation in outcome than any other single cytogenetic group. Recent years have seen the use of molecular biology to dissect this heterogeneity. In particular, aberrations in the FMS-like tyrosine kinase 3 (*FLT3*) gene, mutations in the nucleophosmin (*NPM1*), or CCAAT enhancer binding protein alpha (*CEBPA*) genes, partial tandem duplication of the mixed lineage leukemia (*MLL*) gene, and overexpression of either the brain and acute leukemia cytoplasmic (*BAALC*) gene or the ETS-related gene (*ERG*) each have prognostic significance in patients under age 60 years with NC-AML (Table 131.2).

TABLE 131.2

MOLECULAR ABERRATIONS IN NORMAL CYTOGENETICS ACUTE MYELOGENOUS LEUKEMIA

Abnormality	Approximate Incidence (%)	Effect on Outcome
FLT3 ITD	30	Median RFS and survival 48 months without, 10–12 months with, ITD
FLT3 TKD	10	Inconsistent
NPM mutation	50	Favorable, particularly in patients without FLT3 ITD and (40,41) and with low ERG expression[a]
CEBPA mutation	15	Median remission duration 26 months without, not reached with, mutation
MLL PTD	10	Median remission duration 23 months without, 7 months with, PTD[b]
Overexpression of BAALC	—	Incidence of relapse at 3 years 36% if not, 54% if, overexpressed
Overexpression of ERG	—	Incidence of relapse at 5 years 33% if not, 81% if, overexpressed

FLT3, FMS-like tyrosine kinase 3; TKD, tyrosine kinase domain; ITD, internal tandem duplication; NPM, nucleophosmin; RFS, remission-free survival; ERG, ETS-related gene; BAALC, brain and acute leukemia cytoplasmic; CEBPA, CCAAT enhancer binding protein alpha; MLL, mixed lineage leukemia; DFS, disease-free survival.
[a]Five-year disease-free survival rates: NPM+/FLT3–, 60%; NPM+/FLT3+, 40% to 45%; NPM–/FLT3–, 30% to 35%; NPM–/FLT3+, 30% to 35%. However, high ERG expression may identify NPM+/FLT3– patients who do poorly: DFS at 3 years 14% versus 72% with low ERG expression.

Perhaps the most well-known abnormality in patients with NC-AML involves internal tandem duplication (ITD) of the *FLT3* gene.[16,17] *FLT3* encodes a tyrosine kinase (TK), and the ITD acts to allow constitutive activation of the kinase, imparting a survival advantage to the affected cells. Patients with *FLT3* ITDs tend to present with high WBC and peripheral blast counts. Although it has little impact on CR rate, which is typically 75% to 80% in patients aged 16 to 60 with NC-AML, the presence of an *FLT3* ITD has considerable effect on relapse-free survival and survival after remission induction therapy (Table 131.2). Patients with *FLT3* ITDs can be divided into those who retain one wild type allele and those who lack a wild type allele. The latter have a particularly poor prognosis: Whitman et al.[16] noted a median relapse-free survival of only 4 months and a median survival of only 7 months after high-dose cytarabine (HDAC)–containing postremission therapy. An additional 10% of younger patients with a NC-AML have mutations in the activation loop of the *FLT3* TK. A recent meta-analysis suggests that *FLT3* TK domain mutations also negatively affect relapse-free survival,[17,18] although the British Medical Research Council (MRC) group has recently reported a positive effect.

The most common gene alterations in AML are mutations in the *NPM1* gene. NPM1 protein "shuttles" between the cytoplasm and the nucleus, and *NPM1* mutations result in cytoplasmic localization of the protein, potentially disturbing its tumor suppressor function.[19] *NPM1* mutations occur in approximately 60% of patients with and 40% of patients without *FLT3* ITDs.[20] Patients with an *NPM1* mutation without an *FLT3* ITD (NPM+/FLT3−) constitute about 30% of patients aged 16 to 60 with NC-AML and appear to be a particularly favorable group, although this may only apply to the 75% of such patients who are "low ERG expressors."[21,22] These latter patients appear to have prognoses similar to those seen in better prognosis CBF AML.

C/EBPα is a transcription factor found in myelomonocytic cells; its expression increases during granulocytic differentiation.[23] Frohling et al.[24] reported that mutations in the *CEBPA* gene occurred in 15% of patients aged 16 to 60 with NC-AML and were associated with a favorable outcome (Table 131.2).

AML patients with abnormalities involving 11q often have a poor prognosis (Table 131.2). The *MLL* gene is located at 11q. Perhaps understandably then NC-AML patients with partial tandem duplications involving *MLL* have shorter remissions (but similar CR rates) than other NC-AML patients.[25]

BAALC is a gene thought to play a role in normal hematopoiesis and in development of leukemia. Baldus et al.[26] divided patients aged 16 to 60 with NC-AML into those with concentrations of RNA for *BAALC* above and below the median. The former group had a lower CR rate (62% vs. 73%; $P = .04$) and a higher incidence of relapse (Table 131.2). As with CEBPA, the effect of *BAALC* expression was seen in patients with, as well as without, *FLT3* ITDs. Specifically when patients were divided into four groups according to *BAALC* expression and presence of a *FLT3* ITD (*BAALC* low/no ITD 125 patients, *BAALC* high/no ITD 110 patients, *BAALC* low/ITD 12 patients, and *BAALC* high/ITD 21 patients), the incidences of relapse at 3 years were 28%, 44%, 60%, and 100%, respectively.

The *ERG* gene is frequently overexpressed in patients with AML and complex karyotypes. Since these patients have poor prognoses, the Cancer and Leukemia Group B (CALGB) examined *ERG* expression in NC-AML, dividing the patients aged 16 to 60 into those in the upper 25% and those in the lower 75%.[27] The former had worse outcomes (Table 131.2), even after accounting for the presence of an *MLL* ITD and *FLT3* ITD. Furthermore, *ERG* expression may be useful in further stratifying the favorable *NPM+/FLT3* ITD– subset.[22]

It seems likely that eventually virtually all patients with NC-AML will be found to have one or more molecular aberrations and that more will be learned about their prognostic interactions. Furthermore, genome-wide gene expression profiling based on DNA microarrays is likely both to discover new classes of AML and to provide additional prognostic information. For examples, hierarchical clustering has identified two normal karyotype-predominant classes that differ in survival, and a gene expression predictor has emerged as the strongest prognostic factor in multivariate analysis.[28]

Other Karyotypes

Approximately 50% of patients aged 16 to 60 will have karyotypes other than inv(16), t(8;21), or normal (Fig. 131.1). Among these, the group collectively referred to as "−5/−7" and comprising patients with monosomy (−) of chromosome 5 (−5), −7, del5q, or del7q, has the worst prognosis (Fig. 131.1). There are a few exceptions. Thus, patients with only a single abnormal clone, greater than one residual normal metaphase, and no history of abnormal blood counts before AML are diagnosed with antecedent hematologic disorder (AHD) and have a prognosis equivalent to patients with NC-AML, as may patients with a simple del5q or loss of 7q (Table 131.1). However such favorable −5/−7 patients constitute only 20% of the −5/−7group.

There is some debate as to the placement of patients with other karyotypes. Thus, for example, both the MRC and the Southwest Oncology Group (SWOG) cytogenetic classification systems include patients with +8,−Y in an "intermediate" prognostic group together with NC-AML (Table 131.1).

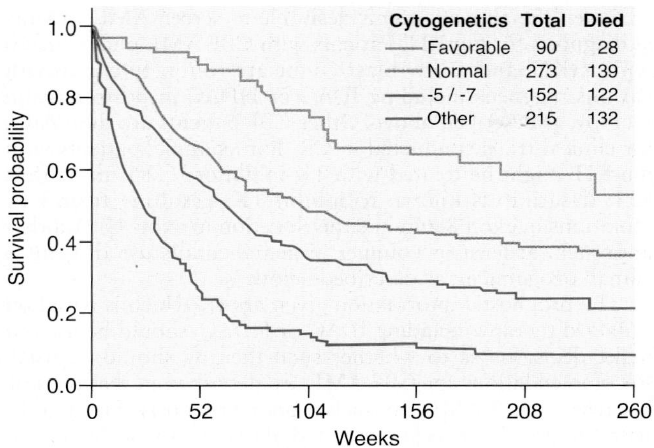

FIGURE 131.1 Influence of cytogenetics in M. D. Anderson Cancer Center patients aged 16 to 60 (1997 to present).

However, while the MRC considers del20q or t(6;9) AML in its intermediate group, the SWOG places these in its "unfavorable" group, and other differences exist (Table 131.1). These differences reflect small sample sizes and heterogeneity within each cytogenetic group. Although abnormalities such as *FLT3* ITD, *NPM1* mutations, and *CEBPA* mutations appear most common in NC-AML, it is likely that other molecular abnormalities (e.g., mutations in the Wilms' tumor gene) together with gene expression studies will shed light on prognosis in this other karyotype group.

Treatment of Newly Diagnosed Acute Myelogenous Leukemia

Treatment of AML requires initial induction chemotherapy with the goal of achieving CR with resolution of morphologically detectable disease and restoration of normal blood counts. This is followed by postremission therapy to eradicate minimal residual disease (MRD). Both chemotherapy and hematopoietic stem cell transplantation (HSCT) have been utilized, and each approach has a major role in the treatment of this disease. Cure of AML occurs in only a minority of patients with available forms of chemotherapy. Stem cell transplantation has a greater antileukemia effect but is associated with a higher risk of treatment-related morbidity and mortality.

There are two obstacles to cure: treatment-related mortality (TRM) and resistance to chemotherapy. Age is a major factor that influences the outcome.[29] Clinical trials usually distinguish between younger and older patients. Although outcome becomes worse with each succeeding year past about age 5 to 10 years, for practical purposes older patients are generally considered to be those aged 60 and above. Older age is strongly associated with poor performance status and abnormal cytogenetics, partially accounting for the poorer prognosis in the elderly.

Regardless of a patient's age, the initial goal in treating AML is to produce a CR, defined as a marrow with less than 5% myeloblasts, a neutrophil count greater than 1,000/mcL, and a platelet count greater than 100,000/mcL.[30] For many years remission induction has relied on use of chemotherapy. When successful, such therapy preferentially targets AML blasts, thus allowing normal blasts to resume control of hematopoiesis. Obtaining CR is critical because, essentially, only patients who do so have a chance of potential cure. However, to be considered potentially cured, patients must stay in CR for 2 to 3 years, after which the risk of relapse declines sharply to less than 10%. Prolongation of the initial CR has traditionally entailed further chemotherapy, typically two to four courses of "consolidation" with or without subsequent prolonged lower dose "maintenance." However, perhaps because such therapy fails to eliminate the AML "stem cell," disease recurs in the majority of even younger patients, with only a small likelihood of potential cure following administration of "salvage" therapy. Stem cell transplantation has been employed to overcome this problem; its role is discussed in a later section of this chapter. This section focuses on strategies with conventional chemotherapy.

Several randomized studies suggest that maintenance chemotherapy, while often prolonging remissions, particularly if little consolidation therapy is given, does not lengthen survival and may shorten it consequent to promotion of resistance to salvage therapy.[31] These results have spurred interest in development of new approaches. In particular, recent years have seen the advent of targeted therapy. Although, as described above, successful chemotherapy is itself selectively toxic to AML blasts, targeted therapy is taken to mean therapy that, while perhaps less toxic to AML blasts than chemotherapy, is much less toxic than chemotherapy to normal blasts and to gastrointestinal epithelium, damage to which can lead to sepsis and death. Thus targeted therapy is of special interest in the treatment of older patients, who are at relatively high risk of TRM. Regardless of the patient's age, however, it is incumbent upon treating physicians to know which patients are likely to do poorly with standard approaches. Such patients then become prime candidates for investigational therapy, preferably given in the context of a clinical trial.

Treatment of Younger Patients

Remission induction for patients under age 60 almost invariably consists of 3 days (days 1 through 3) of drugs, such as daunorubicin or idarubicin, that interact with the enzyme topoisomerase 2 (topo II) and 7 days (days 1 through 7) of the pyrimidine analogue cytarabine (ara-C) at 100 to 200 mg/m^2 daily; such combinations are called "3 + 7." Randomized trials comparing various topo II–reactive drugs have often found greater differences in outcome between the separate studies than between the different topo II–reactive drugs in a given study. As a result, there is a consensus that these drugs are interchangeable, with idarubicin (12 mg/m^2 daily, days 1 through 3) and daunorubicin (45 mg/m^2 daily, days 1 through 3) used most frequently. Similarly, randomized studies have shown equivalence between daily ara-C doses of 100 mg/m^2 and 200 mg/m^2 and have also shown no reproducible benefit from addition of 6-thioguanine or the topo II–reactive drug etoposide to 3 + 7.[32] Recently the Eastern Cooperative Group has demonstrated a survival advantage for patients under age 60 who receive daunorubicin at 90 mg/m^2 daily × 3, rather than 45 mg/m^2 daily × 3, together with ara-C at standard dose.[33] The same has been demonstrated for patients aged 61 to 65. In both cases, however, the improvement seems limited to patients who are likely to respond to standard 3 + 7, for example, those with normal cytogenetics and without *FLT3* ITDs.[34]

A bone marrow aspiration is typically obtained approximately 14 days after initiation of 3 + 7. If the marrow shows less than 10% blasts or is hypocellular, marrows are repeated, usually weekly, until it is clear that either CR has occurred or that there has been reappearance of AML. It is important to note that the first marrow obtained after the hypocellular marrow may show greater than 20% to 30% blasts, which, however, subsequently differentiate until the marrow criterion for CR is met; thus it is often advisable to obtain a second marrow before making a decision to retreat. Such retreatment usually takes the form of either another course of 3 + 7 or administration of high-dose ara-C, with subsequent lack of response mandating a change in treatment. A similar approach is taken in patients whose day 14 marrow is cellular with greater than 10% to 20% blasts.

The past 10 years have seen acceptance of the role of high-dose ara-C (2 to 3 g/m^2 per dose, HDAC) or intermediate-dose ara-C (0.4 to 1.5 g/m^2 per dose, IDAC), rather than conventional dose (as in 3 + 7) ara-C, in postremission therapy of younger patients. A crucial CALGB study randomized patients in CR after 3 + 7 to receive four courses of HDAC (3 g/m^2 every 12 hours on days 1, 3,and 5), IDAC (400 mg/m^2 daily × 5 by continuous infusion), or conventional dose (100 mg/m^2 daily × 5, also by continuous infusion).[35] After a median follow-up of 7 years, outcome varied according to cytogenetic group. Specifically, among 57 patients with pericentric inversion of one of the two chromosome16s [inv(16)] or translocation between chromosome 8 and chromosome 21 [t(8;21)], 78% were still in CR at 5 years if given HDAC versus 57% with IDAC, and 16% with the 100 mg/m^2 dose. HDAC and IDAC were equivalent in the 140 patients with a normal karyotype (40% and 37% of patients in CR at 5 years after HDAC and IDAC, respectively), with both superior to the 100 mg/m^2 dose (20% in CR at 5 years). However, 20% or less of the 88 patients with cytogenetic abnormalities other than inv(16) or t(8;21) were in CR at 5 years, regardless of ara-C dose.

Although the CALGB study was distinctive in relating outcome to both cytogenetics and ara-C dose, many other studies have reported the primary importance of cytogenetics in determining outcome following treatment with 3 + 7 type regimens in younger patients[36] (Table 131.1). Consequently, treatment recommendations in these patients depend on cytogenetic findings, and it is accordingly imperative to obtain cytogenetic information at presentation.

CBF AMLs, both inv(16) and t(8;21), clearly benefit from use of higher doses of ara-C in remission, as made clear by the CALGB results described above.[35] Questions remain as to the number of cycles needed and the dose of ara-C. Subsequent studies by CALGB suggest that three or four consecutive postremission cycles of HDAC (cumulative dose: 54 to 72 g/m^2) are superior to one cycle (18 g/m^2).[37,38] However, since the patients given only one cycle did not receive any other ara-C in remission, the CALGB results speak primarily to the effectiveness of ara-C rather than to the value of three or four postremission cycles of HDAC. Indeed, results of the German AML Intergroup survey suggest that two cycles—in combination with daunorubicin, idarubicin, or mitoxantrone—are as effective as three or four, and that outcome is similar in an ara-C dose range between 20.8 g/m^2 and 56.8 g/m^2.[39] Furthermore, use of only one cycle of IDAC (1 g/m^2 daily × 5) consolidation in the British AML10 study produced results in patients with CBF AML similar to those seen with three or four postremission courses in the CALGB studies.[36]

Several studies have investigated factors other than ara-C dose associated with prognosis in CBF AML (Table 131.2). Older age is probably the biggest predictor of poorer outcome,[29] while in younger patients given IDAC or HDAC, particularly those with t(8;21), a higher peripheral blast percentage is also predictive.[40] The most prevalent factor associated with poorer outcome may be a mutation in the KIT gene (located on chromosome 4).[41] Thirty percent of patients under age 60 with inv(16) AML have been reported to have mutant cKIT (mutKIT), 16% with a mutation in exon 17+/− exon 8 and 13% with a sole mutation in exon 8. Corresponding figures for t(8;21) patients under age 60 are 22%, 18%, and 4%, respectively. Although mutKIT does not affect CR rate, it has a substantial effect on probability of relapse in patients given HDAC, even after accounting for WBC count: in inv(16) AML the 5-year incidence of relapse is 56% in patients with mutKIT, 80% in patients mutKIT in exon 17, and 29% in patients with wild type cKIT (wtKIT), while in t(8;21) AML 5-year relapse rates are 36% with wtKIT and 70% with mutKIT.[41]

Given the above it seems desirable to screen AML patients at diagnosis for mutKIT. Patients with CBF AML under age 60 with wtKIT and a low blast count are routinely cured with various regimens including IDAC or HDAC in postremission therapy, as described above. Other CBF patients are candidates for clinical trials conducted in CR. For example, patients with mutKIT might be treated with TK inhibitors (TKI) that affect KIT: dasatinib is known to inhibit TKs resulting from KIT mutations in exon 8 and in either location in exon 17. Another approach, at least in younger patients, entails use of gemtuzumab ozogamicin, as described below.

The prognostic information given above, which is based on standard therapy including IDAC or HDAC, should be used to make decisions as to whether such therapy should be used. Recommendations for CBF AML are described in that section. Because −5/−7 AML has such a poor prognosis (Fig. 131.1), with the possible exceptions noted above, it should be treated with investigational therapy. Although there is evidence that duration of remission is influenced not only by postremission therapy but also by the induction regimen,[42] no consistent data exist to demonstrate that use of IDAC or HDAC for both phases of treatment alters prognosis in AML[43]; furthermore, the CALGB data indicate a relation between sensitivity to conventional dose ara-C and sensitivity to IDAC or HDAC[35] and suggest that since general benefit is not seen following this strategy, specific benefit for −5/−7 AML is particularly unlikely. NC-AML with a *FLT3* ITD is another group for whom investigational therapy is currently appropriate (drugs that inhibit the aberrant TK associated with the *FLT3* ITD are obvious candidates, see below), and such treatment is also recommended for patients falling into the "unfavorable" cytogenetic group portrayed in Table 131.1. Regardless of other factors, patients who require more than one course to obtain CR tend to have short remissions[44] and are therefore candidates for investigational postremission therapy. The recommendations provided in Table 131.3 are in concert with those of the National Comprehensive Cancer Network, a consortium of academic medical centers.[45] Finally, since in general the effect of cytogenetics following allogeneic stem cell transplant parallels the effect seen after ara-C–containing therapy, it is unclear whether patients for whom Table 131.3 recommends investigational therapy should receive such a transplant in first remission unless the transplant program is itself considered investigational.

An important question is when investigational therapy should begin (at diagnosis or once in CR) in patients for whom such therapy is deemed appropriate, as described above. Given the ability of induction therapy to affect CR duration, it seems that investigational therapy might begin at diagnosis in patients with particularly poor prognoses (e.g., those with −5/−7 or *FLT3* ITDs). One problem is that it may take at least a week for the cytogenetic or *FLT3* results to become available. However, in patients under age 60, there is little to be lost by delaying therapy for this amount of time. Thus, the CALGB awaits *FLT3* results, randomizing patients with ITDs to 3 + 7 with or without the *FLT3* inhibitor PKC412. Exceptions should be made for patients presenting with WBC greater than 50,000, particularly if rapidly rising, since such counts predispose to leukostasis or infiltration of the lung or brain. In such patients investigational therapy would begin once the patient is in CR (Table 131.3).

Treatment of Older Patients

The same cytogenetic classification systems found useful in younger patients (Table 131.1) are also highly relevant prognostically in patients 60 years or older; the CALGB has recently stressed the negative effect of complex karyotypes with at least five abnormalities in older patients.[46] To some extent, the worse outcomes in elderly patients reflect the association of older age

TABLE 131.3

SUGGESTED POSTREMISSION TREATMENT OF NON–CORE BINDING FACTOR ACUTE MYELOGENOUS LEUKEMIA IN PATIENTS AGED 16 TO 60

Karyotype	Group	Postremission Treatment	Comment
−5/−7	Any	Investigational[a]	Exception may be patients with only one abnormal clone, residual normal metaphases, and no AHD or patients with del(5q) or loss of 7q as sole abnormality
Normal	No FLT3 ITD	IDAC- or HDAC-containing	Particularly if NPM mutation present; reconsider if BAALC or EGG expression high or MLL PTD present
Normal	FLT 3 ITD	Investigational[a]	Reconsider if *CEBPA* mutation present
Other Intermediate (Table 131.1)	—	IDAC- or HDAC-containing, or investigational	—
Other unfavorable (Table 131.1)	—	Investigational	—
Any	More than one course to complete remission	Investigational	—

AHD, antecedent hematologic disorder; ITD, internal tandem duplication; NPM, nucleophosmin; IDAC, intermediate-dose ara-C; HDAC, high-dose ara-C; BAALC, brain and acute leukemia cytoplasmic; MLL, mixed-lineage leukemia.
[a]In some patients (e.g., those with white blood cell counts less than 50,000), investigational therapy might begin at diagnosis (see text).

with unfavorable cytogenetics, the presence of an AHD (presumably reflecting a prior myelodysplastic syndrome), or secondary AML (AML arising after administration of chemotherapy for another condition). Older age is also associated with factors predicting TRM such as performance status greater than Zubrod 1, higher serum $\beta 2$ microglobulin levels, and various comorbidities such as infection, elevated bilirubin or creatinine at start of treatment, or chronic lung disease. However, even after accounting for these factors, older patients have worse outcomes than younger patients,[47] although there is less difference in outcome between, for example, a 58-year-old and a 61-year-old than between the same 61-year-old and a 69-year-old, although the 58-year-old would be considered "young" and both the 61-year-old and the 68-year-old would be considered "elderly" in current classification schemes that regard older patients as those aged 60 or older. Although the effect of age undoubtedly reflects the effect of genetic or biologic abnormalities, the incidence of most of the markers described above as associated with poor prognosis in younger patients remains unknown in older patients, although *FLT3* ITDs appear less common. Importantly, the effect of age is not constant throughout a patient's course of treatment. Rather, approximately 1 year after treatment begins the effect of age on prognosis disappears; this reflects the disproportionate influence of age on "early death."

Use of IDAC- or HDAC-containing regimens in older patients produces an increase in TRM that is out of proportion to any increase in efficacy.[48] Standard care in these patients thus implies the use of either 3 + 7 or low-dose ara-C (LDAC, e.g., 10 mg/m^2 every 12 hours for 14 to 21 days without other drugs). The 3 + 7 regimens in older patients often produce CR rates of only about 50%[49] (Table 131.4), making it difficult to recommend standard induction therapy to many older patients, particularly given the 15% to 20% risk of TRM occurring during the approximately 1- to 2-month remission induction period. Reducing the doses or duration of the topo II–reactive drug or of ara-C tends to decrease both TRM and efficacy, resulting in no improvement in survival. For example, in one of the only randomized comparisons of 3 + 7 and LDAC, involving 87 patients older than 65, Tilly et al.[50] found median survivals of 9 months with LDAC and 13 months with 3 + 7; patients given LDAC, however, spent less time in the hospital (median, 28 days vs. 34 days) and required fewer transfusions (median, 7 vs. 10). Addition of granulocyte colony-stimulating factor (G-CSF) or granulocyte-macrophage colony-stimulating factor (GM-CSF) to 3 + 7, substitution of mitoxantrone for daunorubicin, or use of single agent gemtuzumab ozogamicin has also failed to lengthen survival[51] (Table 131.4).

Reported survival data likely overestimate the effectiveness of standard therapy in older patients. This overestimation results from the tendency to treat only very fit older patients. Indeed most elderly patients probably do not receive anti-AML therapy. The characteristics of untreated patients, as a group, are often not known in adequate detail, making outcome without treatment difficult to compare to outcome with standard treatment. In one of the few randomized studies to address the issue,[52] the European Organisation for Research and Treatment of Cancer (EORTC) assigned patients aged older than 65 to immediate 3 + 7 or to observation or supportive care, with use of hydroxyurea or LDAC if blood counts worsened or symptoms developed. Median survival was 21 weeks in the 3 + 7 arm and 10 weeks in the observation arm, and the number of days spent in the hospital was essentially identical. However, the degree to which the enrolled patients represented AML in the elderly is in some doubt since the former were required to have a performance status less than 3, and relatively normal organ function, and since 50% of the patients randomized to observation had to begin therapy within 1 month, suggesting that they were on the verge of progression when randomized; in contrast, it is commonly observed that AML in older patients can have an indolent course for months if not longer. Suffice it to say, however, that regardless of their relative merits, none of 3 + 7, LDAC, or supportive care only is an appealing approach for the majority of older patients with AML. The corollary (i.e., elderly patients with AML are typically candidates for investigational induction therapy) is widely accepted; for example, the National Cooperative Cancer Network explicitly cites "clinical trial" as the preferred option in patients with untreated AML age 60 and above.[45] As discussed below, these trials have emphasized use of targeted therapy as well as new chemotherapeutic agents such as Cloretazine (VNP40101M) and clofarabine.

As implicitly stressed throughout this chapter, the outcome following use of standard therapy for AML is so variable that to speak of an "average" outcome is potentially misleading. It

TABLE 131.4

OUTCOMES IN OLDER PATIENTS GIVEN ANTHRACYCLINE PLUS ARA-C FOR ACUTE MYELOGENOUS LEUKEMIA

Study (Ref.)	No. of Patients	Median Survival (months)	Probability Survival at 2 Years (%)	Complete Remission Rate (%)	Induction Death Rate (%)	Comments
ECOG (49)	234 Age ≥56	7–8	≈20	41	19	Results same with daunorubicin, idarubicin, or mitoxantrone and with or without GM-CSF priming
NCRI (formerly MRC; AML 11) (232)	1314 Age ≥56	≈12	≈25	62	16	Results same with one or four courses post–complete remission and with or without G-CSF starting 8 days after end induction
SWOG (233)	161 Age ≥56	9	19	43	15	Survival worse with mitoxantrone plus etoposide
HOVON (234)	211 Age ≥60	≈10	≈25	48	15	Results same with or without PSC-833
M. D. Anderson (235)	31 Age ≥65	≈12	≈20	48	Not given	Ara-C at 1.5 g/m^2 daily in three doses; survival worse with single-agent gemtuzumab

ECOG, Eastern Cooperative Oncology Group; NCRI, National Cancer Research Institute; MRC, Medical Research Center; AML, acute myelogenous leukemia; SWOG, Southwest Oncology Group; GM-CSF, granulocyte macrophage colony-stimulating factor; G-CSF, granulocyte colony-stimulating factor; HOVON, Dutch-Belgian Hemato-Oncology Cooperative Group.

is useful to attempt to identify groups of older patients for whom standard induction therapy might be reasonable. Performance status and serum bilirubin, creatinine, and β2 microglobulin levels are readily available and can be used to assign patients. M. D. Anderson Cancer Center data over the past 10 years indicate a 27% CR rate and a 62% TRM rate (within the first 8 weeks of beginning therapy) in the 183 patients with either a Zubrod performance status greater than 2, a serum bilirubin greater than 1.9 mg/dL, or a serum creatinine greater than 1.9 mg/dL and who received standard therapy. Intensive therapy is not advisable for such patients. In the (likely) event that they are ineligible for clinical trials of new agents, they should be considered for palliative care. The remaining patients can be divided into two groups: those with a performance status of 0 or 1 and a serum β2 microglobulin level less than 3.0 mg/L and those with either a performance status equal to 2 or with a serum β2 microglobulin level greater than 2.9 mg/L. Over the past decade at M. D. Anderson Cancer Center, the CR rate in the latter is only 45% while the TRM rate is 24% with a median survival of only 6 months (Fig. 131.2). Hence these patients seem to be appropriate candidates for investigational induction treatments. In contrast, patients with performance status less than 2 and serum β2 microglobulin level less than 3 mg/L had a 72% CR rate and only a 9% TRM rate. Nonetheless, their median survival is still only 14 months (Fig. 131.2), reflecting the transient nature of most of these CRs. Given the data that suggest induction therapy can influence CR duration, it seems plausible that some patients in this group might prefer investigational induction therapy and some standard induction therapy, given the possibility that investigational therapy can be worse than standard. Certainly once these patients reach CR, they are candidates for investigational approaches to postremission therapy. This is true even for patients with inv(16) or t(8;21), whose remissions are much shorter than those seen in younger patients with the same abnormalities; eventually decisions about postremission therapy will be based on the detection of MRD, as discussed below. Obviously, the weight given to the recommendation for investigational induction therapy should increase if the patient has an ongoing infection or secondary AML (i.e., AML following a myelodysplastic syndrome or chemotherapy). Table 131.5 summarizes these treatment recommendations. Regardless of specific recommendations, any choice of therapy in older patients must refer to the observations of Sekeres et al.[53] that 74% of older patients estimated that their chances of cure with 3 + 7 were at least 50%; in contrast, 85% of their physicians estimated this chance to be less than 10%. Although the most plausible cause of this discrepancy is a patient's natural tendency to hope for a favorable outcome, there may also be gaps in communication between physicians and patients.

Acute Promyelocytic Leukemia

Acute promyelocytic leukemia (APL) has a unique pathophysiology and requires special considerations for treatment. In more than 95% of cases, APL results from a chromosomal

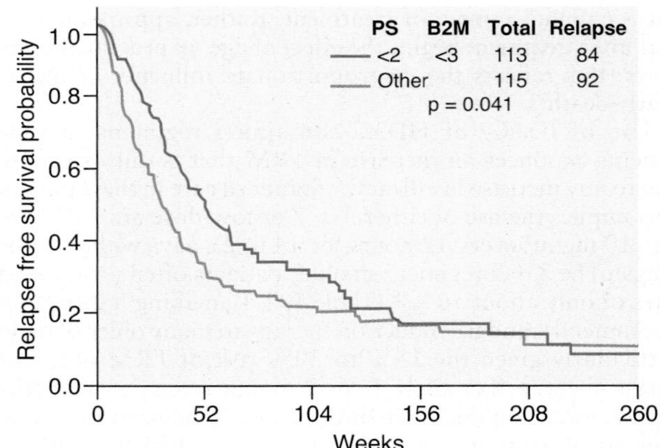

FIGURE 131.2 Survival and relapse-free survival probabilities according to performance status (PS) and serum β2 migroglobulin (B2M) level in patients age 60 and above given standard regimens at M. D. Anderson Cancer Center over the past decade. The data suggest that standard therapy is not sufficient for the worse risk group.

TABLE 131.5

SUGGESTED INDUCTION THERAPY FOR PATIENTS AGE 60 OR MORE

Group	Recommended Treatment	All Patients Age 60 or More (%)	Comments
PS >2, bilirubin >1.9, or creatinine >1.9	Investigational; particularly targeted therapy plus low-dose chemotherapy	15	Often not eligible for investigational trials; if not, prefer palliative to standard therapy, given that TRM rate is higher than complete remission rate with former
PS <2, bilirubin and creatinine each <2 mg/dL, β_2 M <3	Standard[a] or investigational	35	Presence of AML arising after MDS or of infection might favor investigational
Bilirubin and creatinine each <2; PS = 2 or β_2 M >2.9	Investigational	50	

PS, performance status; TRM, treatment-related mortality; AML, acute myelogenous leukemia; MDS, myelodysplastic syndrome; β_2 M, β_2 microglobulin.

[a]As discussed in the text, those patients who receive standard induction therapy (e.g., 3 + 7) are candidates for investigational therapy once in complete remission (e.g., reduced-intensity allogeneic hematopoietic stem cell transplant).

translocation, t(15;17). This translocation results in a fusion protein PML/RARα, the gene for *PML* being located on chromosome 15 and the gene for *RARα* on chromosome 17. The PML-RARα protein, an aberrant form of the normal retinoic acid receptor (RAR), recruits corepressor complexes that inhibit transcription of genes involved in promyelocytic differentiation.[54] APL occurs relatively more frequently than other types of AML in the young, Hispanics, and the obese.[55] Although it typically has a distinctive morphology characterized by abnormal granules and multiple Auer rods, a microgranular variant exists. The possibility of this variant must be borne in mind in patients who present without morphologically typical APL but with the coagulopathy that is the clinical hallmark of the disease. The diagnosis of APL requires proof of the PML-RARα rearrangement. Although this can be obtained by demonstration of the presence of t(15;17), at least 2 to 3 days are required for test results. Immediate confirmation of the diagnosis can be made by using immunohistochemistry to demonstrate an abnormal pattern of anti-PML antibody nuclear staining consequent to formation of PML-RARα (the PML oncogenic domains test).[56] If doubt remains about the diagnosis, all-transretinoic acid (ATRA) should be added to 3 + 7.

APL is very sensitive to daunorubicin or idarubicin[57] and is uniquely sensitive to ATRA. The responsiveness to the anthracyclines may reflect the absence of MDR1 in APL cells, while pharmacologic doses of ATRA release corepressor complexes and lead to degradation of PML-RARα. Standard treatment of APL consists of idarubicin 12 mg/m^2 daily for 4 to 5 days and ATRA 45 mg/m^2 until CR.[58] Use of transfusions to maintain the platelet count above 30,000/uL, serum fibrinogen above 150 mg/mL, and the international normalized ratio (INR) below 1.5 is mandatory. Ten percent to 25% of patients will develop the APL differentiation syndrome (APLDS) characterized by fever, weight gain/edema, pleural effusions, and pulmonary infiltrates; the WBC is often elevated. Steroids (e.g., methylprednisolone 45 mg intravenous daily with subsequent tapering) are effective for treatment of APLDS. The principal prognostic factor in untreated APL is initial WBC. Patients with WBC less than 10,000/mcL will have CR rates greater than 90% with idarubicin plus ATRA, while patients with higher WBC counts will have CR rates of 70% to 85%. Almost all patients who fail to achieve CR die of organ failure, usually related to bleeding before treatment begins or in the first few days thereafter. Once in CR patients typically receive three courses of consolidation with idarubicin 12 mg/m^2 daily × 3 days and ATRA 45 mg/m^2 daily on a 2-week on, 2-week off basis.

A polymerase chain reaction (PCR) test to detect residual PML-RARα transcripts is of considerable value. At least 90% of patients should be PCR negative after completion of consolidation therapy; patients who are not have a 50% chance of relapse versus 25% for patients who are PCR negative.[59] The former should receive arsenic trioxide (ATO) with our without gemtuzumab ozogamicin and an allogeneic stem cell transplant if these measures do not produce PCR negativity. Patients who are PCR positive after completion of consolidation are principally those who presented with WBC greater than 10,000/mcL. There are two approaches to patients who are PCR negative after consolidation. One, of particular use in patients presenting with WBC less than 10,000/mcL, is to discontinue therapy. The second is to give 6 months to 2 years of maintenance therapy with 6 mercaptopurine and methotrexate, while continuing ATRA. There is no consensus as to which approach is superior, although a recent Japanese study suggested that use of maintenance was associated with shorter survival.[60] Although many protocols omit ara-C, allowing administration of higher doses of idarubicin or daunorubicin, a French trial found superior results in patients randomized to receive ara-C in addition to ATRA and daunorubicin.[61] It has been suggested, however, that this outcome reflected use of relatively low doses of daunorubicin.

Perhaps more important than choosing a particular approach is use of the PCR test to detect molecular relapse. Tests should be done every 3 months for 2 years in patients who presented with WBC greater than 10,000/mcL; there is probably much less need for testing in patients presenting with lower WBC counts who are PCR negative after consolidation. There is controversy whether blood can substitute for bone marrow. A positive test should be repeated in 2 to 4 weeks. Molecular relapse (i.e., two consecutive positive tests) is highly specific for subsequent hematologic relapse. The principal problem with the PCR test is a relative lack of sensitivity. Indeed most cases of hematologic relapse occur in patients who were PCR negative. Quantitative PCR testing is being investigated to improve sensitivity while maintaining specificity.[62]

ATO, which degrades PML-RARα, is almost certainly more effective than ATRA in treatment of APL. For example, cure of APL using single-agent ATO occurs much more commonly than cure using single-agent ATRA.[63] Another effective agent is gemtuzumab ozogamicin (GO),[51] perhaps consequent to the large amounts of CD33 expressed on APL cells' surface and the absence of MDR1 in APL. Lo-Coco et al.[64] demonstrated that GO was highly effective in treating molecular relapse and that treating patients at the time of molecular relapse, rather than waiting until hematologic relapse, prolonged survival. Although the latter observation is confounded by the fact that the interval from molecular relapse to death is longer than the interval from hematologic relapse to death even without treatment, it is unlikely that a trial randomizing patients in molecular relapse between immediate treatment and treatment at hematologic relapse will be done. Accordingly, molecular relapse should be treated with ATO or GO.

The future will certainly see the incorporation of ATO, and possibly of GO, into therapy of newly diagnosed APL. It has also been reported that use of ATO plus ATRA in untreated patients presenting with WBC less than 10,000/mcL obviated the need for chemotherapy in the great majority of patients[65]; such a strategy would be particularly useful in older patients, in whom there is a 15% to 20% TRM rate following consolidation with idarubicin or daunorubicin. An Italian cooperative group (GIMEMA) trial is randomizing between ATRA/idarubicin and ATO/ATRA patients age less than 70 years old who have WBC less than 10,000/mcL.

TRM due to drug toxicities and infections remains a substantial problem in older patients, particularly those with poor performance status, abnormal organ function, or high serum $\beta 2$ microglobulin levels. Novel interventions that might decrease mucositis and subsequent translocation of bacteria or fungal infections are of considerable interest.

Newer Therapies for Acute Myelogenous Leukemia

Clofarabine and Cloretazine

Clofarabine[66] and Cloretazine[67] have been investigated in untreated older patients; the former is a nucleoside analogue combining features of fludarabine and cladribine, the latter a new category of alkylating agent (a 1,2–bis(sulfonyl) hydrazine). Both appear to produce CR rates of 25% to 30%, and clofarabine also produces an appreciable rate of responses less than CR; preliminary evidence suggests that, after accounting for the time needed to achieve response, these minor responses improve survival more than an even lesser degrees of response, although not to the same extent as CR. Median survival is quite short with either agent, and it remains to be seen, as in an ongoing Eastern Cooperative Oncology Group (ECOG) trial involving clofarabine, whether they are superior to 3+7. Of note, at least with Cloretazine, the same covariates that predict lower response rates with 3+7 (e.g., secondary AML and abnormal cytogenetics) also predict lower response rates with the newer drug. It is likely that the future of these drugs will lie in combination (e.g., with ara-C), although the myelosuppressive properties of Cloretazine may complicate such combination.

Tipifarnib

Although tipifarnib is referred to as a farnesyltransferase inhibitor, correlations between enzyme inhibition and clinical response have not been obvious. Although the drug produces CR,[68] the U.S. Food and Drug Administration (FDA) did not believe the level of activity was sufficient to warrant approval for older patients with untreated AML. Combinations with etoposide and low-dose ara-C are being investigated in untreated older patients. A two-gene expression signature has recently been proposed to predict response to tipifarnib.

Epigenetic-Acting Agents

Epigenetics refers to changes affecting gene expression without altering the sequence of base pairs in genes. One such change is associated with hypermethylation of CpG-rich "islands" in the genome, which leads to silencing of the involved genes. Since, once present, hypermethylation is permanent, it is functionally equivalent to a genetic mutation.[69] Various putative tumor suppressor genes have been demonstrated to be hypermethylated in myelodysplastic syndrome (MDS),[70] leading to interest in hypomethylating agents (the principal ones in clinical trial are decitabine and azacitidine). A second change involves acetylation or deacetylation of histones, proteins in physical proximity to DNA. Specifically, deacetylation of histones leads to chromatin condensation, a configuration blocking transcription.[71] Accordingly, various histone deacetylase inhibitors (HiDAC) have been developed (e.g., suberoylanilide hydroxamic acid [SAHA]); the antiepileptic drug valproic acid has also been used as an HiDAC. Although decitabine and azacitidine have been used primarily in MDS, Lubbert et al.[72] reported an appreciable CR rate for decitabine in older patients with untreated AML. Combinations of decitabine with HiDACs may provide synergistic epigenetic activity and are the subject of several clinical trials in older untreated patients. Another possible use for these drugs is in patients in remission. Although difficult, it will be important to determine whether response to hypomethylating agents correlates with induced hypomethylation. Demonstration of the same would provide a firmer rationale for epigenetic-acting therapy.

FLT Inhibitors

The adverse effect of *FLT3* ITDs on prognosis (Table 131.2) has encouraged development of drugs that inhibit the *FLT3* kinase. Most experience has been with PKC412[73] and lestaurtinib[74] (formerly CEP701) as single agents in older patients. CR rates have been quite modest, motivating combination with chemotherapy in relapsed AML (lestaurtinib) and untreated patients less than 60 years old (PKC412). The high CR rate was seen in the latter patients who had a *FLT3* ITD, which has led to an ongoing U.S. Intergroup trial randomizing untreated patients under age 60 with *FLT3* ITDs to 3 + 7 with or without PKC412. PKC412 and lestaurtinib are relatively weak inhibitors of *FLT3*. A more potent inhibitor, AC220, appears more active as a single agent in relapsed *FLT 3* positive AML.[75] A multicenter international trial of AC220 in relapsed AML is under way to confirm these results.

Gemtuzumab Ozogamicin

GO is a combination of an antibody directed against CD33, an antigen found on the surface of AML blasts, and calicheamicin, an intercalating agent. When used alone, it, like FLT inhibitors, is not demonstrably better than 3 + 7,[51] except perhaps in patients with APL (see below). Like FLT3 inhibitors it is being combined with chemotherapy. At the GO dose used in these combinations (3 mg/m^2), the risk of veno-occlusive disease of the liver is much reduced compared to the risk seen at the single agent dose (9 mg/m^2). Of most note Burnett et al.[76] randomized untreated patients less than 60 years old to various chemotherapies with or without GO 3 mg/m^2. CR rates were similar. However, although with a median follow-up of 15 months, there was no difference in deaths in CR, and relapse was reduced, resulting in improved disease-free survival (DFS) (P = .008) (Table 131.6). This effect was seen principally in patients with favorable or intermediate cytogenetics (Table 131.1), in whom there was also a trend for longer survival. There was also more mucositis in the GO arm, suggesting that the effect of GO merely reflected administration of "more chemotherapy." Arguing against this possibility, however, the effect of GO was similar with 3 + 7 and with FLAG-ida, a regimen that uses IDAC rather than conventional dose ara-C. The Burnett et al. results are the most striking, yet they were obtained with any new agent in untreated AML. Recently the

TABLE 131.6

EFFECT OF DURATION OF FIRST COMPLETE REMISSION ON COMPLETE REMISSION RATE WITH SALVAGE THERAPY[a]

Weeks First Complete Remission	0[b]	1–26	27–52	>52
No. of Patients	92	73	82	106
Complete Remission	19 (21%)	13 (18%)	18 (26%)	58 (64%)

[a]Patients given intermediate-dose ara-C or high-dose ara-C–containing therapy at M. D. Anderson Cancer Center 1997–2006.
[b]Primary refractory acute myelogenous leukemia.

SWOG has confirmed the benefit of addition of GO to 3 + 7 therapy for patients with CBF AML, although not for patients with other karyotypes.

Antagonists of *BCL-2* and *MDR1*

Large randomized trials in older patients of 3+7 with or without Genasense, a drug thought to enhance chemotherapy-induced apoptosis by antagonizing *BCL-2*,[77] and of 3 + 7 with our without zosuquidar,[78] postulated to overcome the effect of *MDR1*, a protein that promotes extrusion of topo II–reactive drugs, have failed to show a benefit for the experimental arm.

Aurora Kinase Inhibitors

Aurora kinases A, B, and C play an essential role in formation and operation of the mitotic spindle and are overexpressed in many cancers. The aurora kinase inhibitor VX680 has been shown to reduce colony formation by AML blasts taken from patients and to reduce AML development in nude mice. Use of these drugs in AML will be of considerable interest.[79]

Immune System Modulators

As noted in the next section, there has, to date, been a strong relation between response to new drugs and response to standard drugs. This suggests that investigating new agents in remission after standard therapy (i.e., after the latter has been shown to have a modicum of success) might be useful (e.g., in patients predicted to relapse quickly). With agents that modulate the immune system, the remission setting is particularly attractive. For example, after randomizing 320 patients median age 55, 78% of whom were less than 3 months from completion of consolidation therapy and 260 of whom were in first CR, Brune et al.[80] reported that leukemia-free survival was superior in patients assigned histamine dihydrochloride and interleukin-2 rather than no treatment. Although this study can be criticized because less than 10% of patients had unfavorable karyotypes and because survival was unaffected, results were similar to those often seen in studies randomizing patients to maintenance with standard chemotherapy or no maintenance. It is likely that other immune modulators will also be investigated in patients in CR. A promising strategy is vaccination against aberrantly expressed leukemia-related antigens including proteinase-3[81] and WT-1.[82]

Current data suggest targeted agents are most likely to be used in combination with chemotherapy. It is important to remember that clinical trials emphasize the average result. Consequently, it is quite plausible that some patients will benefit from a therapy even when most patients do not, emphasizing the importance of correlative lab studies to identify such patients. Practically speaking, however, it is difficult to continue a trial to identify responsive patients when it is clear the average patient will not respond. Furthermore, future AML trials will be increasingly done in smaller and smaller subgroups, defined by a biologic marker, emphasizing the need to reconsider current statistical methodology, which is based on small probabilities of false-negative and especially false-positive results under the assumption that large numbers of patients will be treated.

Salvage Therapy

Salvage therapy refers to treatment given for relapsed AML or AML that has never gone into CR (*primary refractory*). The principal predictor of response to first salvage therapy is whether the duration of the first CR was longer than 1 year[83] (Table 131.6, Fig. 131.3). This is true not only when first salvage therapy contains HDAC or IDAC, but also when other agents are used; thus, over the past 10 years at M. D. Anderson Cancer Center, the CR rate with drugs other than ara-C or idarubicin or daunorubicin has been 16 of 241 in patients whose first CRs were less than 1 year contrasted with 9 of 32 in patients with longer first CRs. More sophisticated prognostic systems are available.[84] Data presented in the section on transplantation suggest that HSCT should be the first option for patients who require salvage treatment after first CR lasting less than 1 year or after failing initial induction therapy. If stem cell transplant is unavailable or while a search for a donor is ongoing, patients should receive investigational treatments, including or not including IDAC or HDAC.

When given IDAC or HDAC, patients with first CR durations longer than 1 year have a CR rate (60% to 65%) and median survival (13 months) similar to that of patients with untreated AML given similar therapies. Consequently, it is plausible to give such patients IDAC or HDAC. However, if a similar strategy is followed once in CR, the duration of second remission will almost inevitably be shorter than the duration of the first. Accordingly once in second CR consideration should be given to an allogeneic transplant or, at the least, a postremission therapy different from that used in the first CR. Another approach is to combine an investigational agent with IDAC or HDAC as first salvage therapy. Ongoing studies are randomizing patients between HDAC with or without either clofarabine or Cloretazine. Patients who are candidates for second salvage therapy should almost always receive investigational therapies or an allogeneic stem cell transplant.

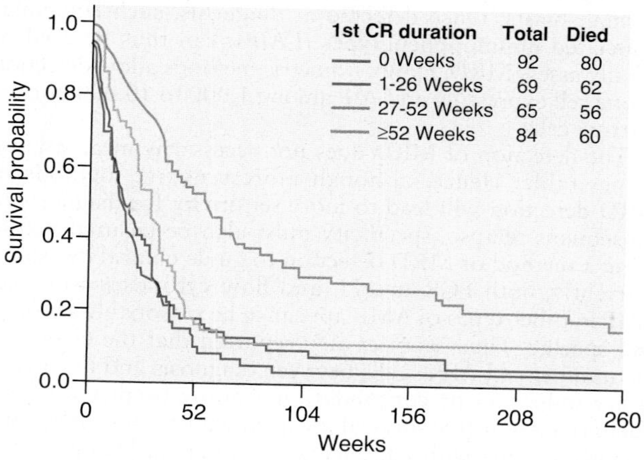

FIGURE 131.3 Survival in M. D. Anderson Cancer Center salvage patients according to duration of first complete remission (CR).

PRACTICE OF ONCOLOGY

New Response Criteria

For many years response to induction therapy for AML was classified as CR or no CR. However, responses less than CR have recently been recognized. An example is CRp (i.e., CR with incomplete platelet recovery). Attaining CRp suggests that a treatment is more "active" than if, despite survival time sufficiently long to observe CR or CRp, neither response had occurred ("resistant"). However, it is also important to assess whether CRp conveys clinical benefit (i.e., lengthens survival relative to resistant). This appears to be the case, and the same appears to be true for hematologic improvement, although little information is available regarding "marrow CR," in which the marrow has less than 5% blasts but blood counts remain low. However, available data suggest that more than 90% of the patients potentially cured of AML have a CR, rather than a CRp, hematologic improvement, or marrow CR with initial induction therapy.

Minimal Residual Disease in Acute Myelogenous Leukemia

Given that AML relapses in most patients, such patients presumably have residual AML (MRD) even in CR. Quantification of MRD would allow broad recommendations for postremission therapy, based on data in a large number of patients to be replaced by more patient-specific recommendations. In particular, patients with low levels of MRD that remain stable or drop might continue on their initial therapy. In contrast, therapy might be changed in patients with high or rising MRD levels. This change might avert subsequent hematologic relapse. Since relapse can only be diagnosed when more than 5% blasts are present in the marrow, the sensitivity of morphologic examination of the marrow for detection of relapse is only 1 in 20. In contrast, if 30 metaphases are examined, cytogenetic examination has a sensitivity of 1 in 30, while fluorescence *in situ* hybridization (FISH) typically has a sensitivity of 1 in 500. PCR techniques allow detection of transcripts of such fusion genes as *RUNX1-CBFA2T1*, *CBFB-MYH11*, or *PML-RARα* at a frequency of 10(−4) or less. Assays for *NPM1* have been proposed as another means of MRD detection.

Although the molecular abnormalities described above are not detectable even at diagnosis in many patients, all patients may have blasts characterized by aberrant surface marker expression; for example, the same blast may display markers characteristic of both an early and a later stage of differentiation. These patterns are quite specific for AML, as opposed to normal, blasts. Once detected at diagnosis, such leukemia-associated immunophenotypes (LAIPs) can thus be used to serially assess MRD. Flow cytometric methods allow detection of one cell expressing an LAIP among 1,000 to 10,000 normal marrow cells.

The detection of MRD does not necessarily mean relapse is inevitable. Hence, although more sensitive methods of MRD detection will lead to more sensitivity for diagnosis of subsequent relapse, specificity must also be ensured before using a method of MRD detection to guide clinical decisions. Currently, both PCR in APL and flow cytometry to detect LAIP in other types of AML appear to be reasonably sensitive and specific. Thus, Kern et al.[85] reported that the change in the number of LAIP+ cells between diagnosis and the end of either induction or consolidation therapy predicted subsequent remission-free survival independent of cytogenetics and in both patients with intermediate or unfavorable cytogenetics. A future challenge is to make this methodology routinely available.

Hematopoietic Stem Cell Transplantation for Acute Myelogenous Leukemia

Stem cell transplantation provides the possibility of cure for a significant fraction of patients with AML. The approach utilizes a preparative regimen of chemotherapy or radiation with the goal of eradicating the leukemia and providing sufficient immunosuppression of the recipient to prevent rejection of the transplant. There is also an allogeneic graft-versus-leukemia effect in which donor T and natural killer (NK) cells act to eradicate malignant cells that survive the preparative regimen.[86] Autologous transplants can be done; patients initially have their own hematopoietic cells collected and cryopreserved; these cells are then reinfused after high-dose therapy to restore hematopoiesis. Improvements in supportive care, histocompatibility and tissue matching, and development of less toxic preparative regimens have all increased the likelihood of success with autologous or allogeneic transplantation. This section reviews the role of HSCT in the treatment of AML in adults.

Prognostic Factors and Indications for Transplant

Outcomes of HSCT are improved if the transplant is performed earlier in the disease course, preferably in CR, due to less chemo refractoriness and lower likelihood of infectious or chemotherapy-related side effects. The major prognosticator is disease status at transplant. Prognostics of patients in CR are significantly better than for those with active disease at the time of HSCT. Similarly, most of the covariates discussed in the previous paragraphs retain their influence in the setting of HSCT, such as cytogenetics and FLT3 mutational status (Figs. 131.4 and 131.5).[87] Therapy-related AML (due to previous exposure to alkylators agents, ionizing irradiation, or topoisomerase II inhibitor use) and AML evolving from MDS are considered high risk and the outcome without allogeneic HSCT is generally poor.[88] A large retrospective registry study investigated outcomes of AML patients transplanted with active disease. The authors found that five adverse pretransplant variables significantly influenced survival: presence of circulating blasts, first CR duration less than 6 months, use of a donor other than an HLA-identical sibling,

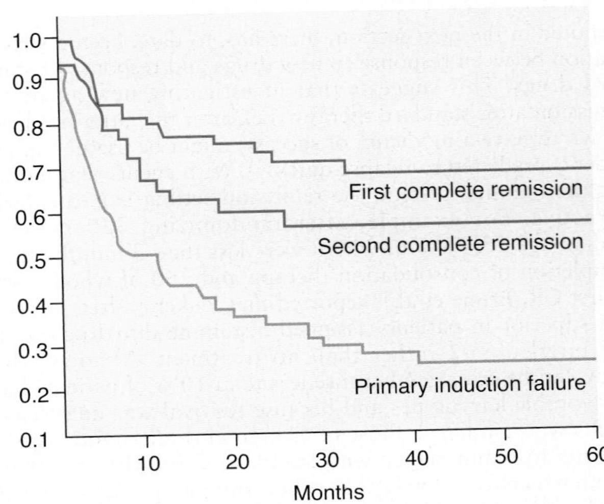

FIGURE 131.4 Disease status at transplantation is the major determinant of survival after allogeneic hematopoietic stem cell transplantation for acute myelogenous leukemia. Overall survival of patients in first or second remission was significantly better than that of patients transplanted after failure of induction therapy. All patients (n = 243) received an unrelated donor transplant at the M. D. Anderson Cancer Center. All patients were transplanted from 2002 to 2009 using myeloablative or reduced-intensity conditioning regimens.

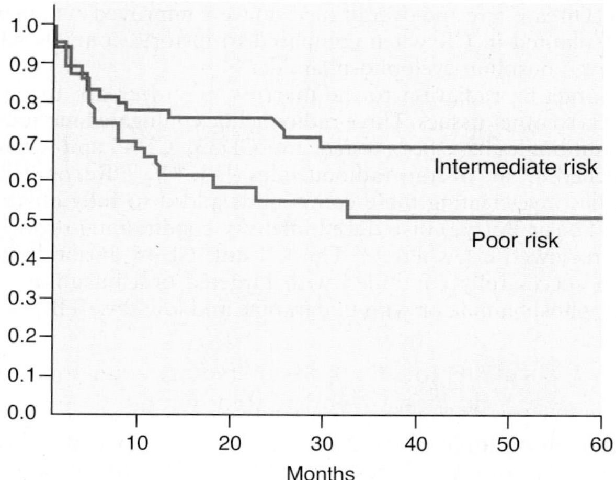

FIGURE 131.5 The influence of cytogenetics on survival is illustrated here. Kaplan-Meier actuarial survival of patients with acute myelogenous leukemia in first, second, or third remission treated with unrelated allogeneic hematopoietic stem cell transplantation at the M. D. Anderson Cancer Center is shown here. Median age was 54 years (n = 127). All patients were transplanted from 2002 to 2009 using myeloablative or reduced-intensity conditioning regimens.

Karnofsky score less than 90, and poor risk cytogenetics.[89] It is generally accepted that fit patients with disease that is primarily refractory to chemotherapy or that has relapsed are eligible for allogeneic or autologous HSCT, as discussed in detail below. There is, however, controversy surrounding HSCT in first CR. Table 131.7 lists indications for allogeneic HSCT in AML.

Preparative Regimens

The preparative regimen (chemo- with or without radiation therapy that precedes the infusion of hematopoietic progenitor cells) provides treatment for AML and the necessary immunosuppression to prevent graft rejection of an allogeneic transplant. Preparative regimens may be chemo- or total body irradiation (TBI)-based. A myeloablative regimen generally causes cessation of normal marrow function to a degree that requires autologous or allogeneic hematopoietic cell transplant. Hematopoietic transplantation allows use of stem cell toxic agents, which eradicate both normal and leukemic stem cells; hematopoiesis is restored by normal stem cells present in the transplant. Recently, reduced intensity regimens have been developed to decrease regimen related toxicity; this approach relies on the immune graft-versus-leukemia effect to eradicate residual disease that would survive the preparative regimen. Conditioning utilizes either a lower dose of alkylating agents or low doses of radiation. The advent of these reduced intensity preparative regimens has allowed the use of hematopoietic transplantation in older patients and those with comorbidities, which would make them ineligible for myeloablative therapy. This has been an important advance, since the peak incidence of AML is in the sixth and seventh decades of life.

Allogeneic HSCT have historically been associated with a high risk of treatment-related mortality, due to toxicity of myeloablative chemotherapy and radiation, graft-versus-host disease (GVHD), and posttransplant immune deficiency. There has been substantial improvement in treatment-related mortality over time related to optimized preparative regimens and improved supportive care.

Autologous Stem Cell Transplantation

With autologous transplantation, patients undergo a collection of hematopoietic cells from the bone marrow or peripheral blood while in CR.[90] They can subsequently receive high-dose myeloablative therapy with reinfusion of the stored cells. This approach has been successful in selected patients in first or second remission. Use of autologous cells avoids the risk of graft rejection and GVHD, but autologous transplants do not benefit from the immune graft-versus-leukemia effect observed with allogeneic transplants. There is also concern that the stored "remission" cells may be contaminated by clonogenic AML cells, which may contribute to relapse.[91] Purging of autologous hematopoietic progenitor cell products *ex vivo* prior to infusion has been investigated and is discussed below.

Myeloablative Preparative Regimens for Transplantation in Acute Myelogenous Leukemia

The most commonly used regimens are cyclophosphamide-TBI (Cy-TBI),[92] busulfan-cyclophosphamide (BuCy),[93] and more recently busulfan and fludarabine.[94] This is a rapidly evolving field, however, and major changes are expected to occur in the coming years.

TABLE 131.7

INDICATIONS FOR ALLOGENEIC TRANSPLANT IN ACUTE MYELOID LEUKEMIA

Disease Stage	Cytogenetics[a]	Mutations
First remission	Diploid: presence of mutations may dictate decision to transplant	FLT3 ITD FLT3 TKD NPM (nucleophosmin gene) with FLT3 or ERG mutation MLL PTD Overexpression of BAALC Overexpression of ERG
First remission	Complex; del 5, del 7	
First remission, age >50–55 years	Diploid cytogenetics: controversial	
First remission, therapy-related or secondary disease[b]	All eligible	All eligible
Primary induction failure	All eligible	All eligible
Second or subsequent remission	All eligible	All eligible
Relapsed, active disease	All eligible	All eligible

ITD, internal tandem duplication; NPM, nucleophosmin; ETS-related gene; FLT3, FMS-like tyrosine kinase 3; TDK, tyrosine kinase domain.
[a]There is variability in the definition of high-risk cytogenetics depending on the classification used. There is also some controversy surrounding the influence of chromosomal abnormalities involving the *MLL* gene located at 11q23, such as in t(9;11), t(6;11), and t(11;19). Some authors will classify patients with these abnormalities as intermediate-risk disease, as opposed to granting them high-risk status. Presence of 9q and 11q abnormalities may also place patients in first complete remission in a higher than desired risk of relapse.
[b]Secondary disease: preceding myelodysplastic syndrome or chemo- or radiation-therapy induced.

In 1977 Thomas et al.[92] reported results of allogeneic HLA-identical sibling transplants in 54 heavily pretreated patients with AML and 46 with ALL. Preparative regimen consisted of cyclophosphamide (120 mg/kg) and TBI (10 Gy). Thirteen patients became long-term leukemia-free survivors. Subsequently, Thomas et al.[92] also investigated TBI-containing preparative regimens using fractionated doses of radiation, which led to less extramedullary toxicity and improved outcomes. HSCT trials for AML in first CR and chronic myelogenous leukemia (CML) in chronic phase demonstrated that increasing TBI dose decreased leukemia relapse at the expense of higher transplant-related mortality and toxicity.[95]

Santos et al.[93] developed the combination of cyclophosphamide and busulfan as a non-TBI–containing preparative regimen for allogeneic HSCT. Busulfan (16 mg/kg) and cyclophosphamide (120 mg/kg; BuCy2)[96] became an alternative to cyclophosphamide and TBI-containing regimens (Cy-TBI) and is currently one of the most used regimens. Oral administration of busulfan, however, is limited by unpredictable absorption of the drug. High plasma levels may cause toxicities, whereas low levels may be associated with increased relapse rates. An intravenous busulfan formulation was developed by Andersson et al.[97] and has overcome the pitfalls associated with oral administration of the drug. Nonrandomized studies indicate a decreased rate of hepatic veno-occlusive disease and other regimen-related toxicities.

The development of BuCy as an alternative to TBI-containing regimens led to ongoing debates as to which conditioning regimen is the best for the treatment of myeloid leukemias with HSCT. Two randomized studies were performed. The Nordic group compared Cy-TBI to BuCy in a heterogeneous group of patients with AML, lymphoid malignancies, and CML receiving allogeneic HSCT.[98] Results indicated improved DFS among advanced stage disease patients treated with Cy-TBI, along with an increased rate of long-term complications for recipients of BuCy. Similarly, Blaise et al.[99] studied young patients with AML in first CR and concluded that Cy-TBI and allogeneic HSCT produced better disease-free and overall survival than BuCy. The major pitfall of these reports is the use of the oral busulfan formulation and the lack of busulfan blood level monitoring and dose adjustment. The Center for International Bone Marrow Transplant Research (CIBMTR) compared the use of BuCy and Cy-TBI in AML patients who received allogeneic transplantation in first remission; there was no difference in leukemia-free or overall survival.[100] A SWOG-sponsored clinical trial investigated a comparison of the preparative regimens etoposide and TBI versus BuCy for the treatment of patients with AML not in first remission and found similar DFS.[101]

Pharmacokinetic-guided oral administration of busulfan or use of the intravenous formulation have markedly decreased the TRM associated with this drug, as well as improved the therapeutic efficacy by minimizing underdosing. Meanwhile, there have been improvements in TBI delivery, making the decision as to which one is the best regimen a matter of institutional and personal experience.

Busulfan and acrolein, a cyclophosphamide metabolite, are both metabolized by glutathione-S-transferase conjugation. Exchanging cyclophosphamide for the nucleoside analogue fludarabine may increase the safety margin of the regimen.[102] Fludarabine appear to increase alkylator-induced cell killing by inhibiting DNA-damage repair and is highly immunosuppressive. A preparative regimen using fludarabine and single daily dosing of intravenous busulfan (130 mg/m^2) has been studied in multiple centers and appears to be effective and potentially less toxic than the commonly used busulfan-cyclophosphamide regimen. Ninety-six patients at the M. D. Anderson Cancer Center with AML or MDS were prepared with this regimen and had a low regimen-related mortality rate of 3% at 1 year, with only two cases of moderate, reversible hepatic veno-occlusive disease. Disease-free and overall survival were improved in patients transplanted in CR when compared to historic controls who received busulfan-cyclophosphamide.[94]

Targeting radiation to the marrow may decrease the side effects to other tissues. Three radionuclide conjugated monoclonal antibodies have been tested, anti-CD33, -CD45 and -CD66, attached to one of four radionuclides (^{131}I, ^{90}Y, ^{188}Re, or ^{213}Bi). Studies investigating these compounds added to fully ablative (Cy-TBI or BuCy2) or reduced intensity conditioning regimens are reviewed elsewhere.[103] The ^{131}I anti-CD45 antibody has been successfully combined with targeted oral busulfan and cyclophosphamide or with fludarabine and low-dose TBI.[63,104]

Transplants for Acute Myelogenous Leukemia in First Complete Remission

Although multiple phase 2 studies have indicated that both allogeneic and autologous transplants benefit subsets of patients with AML in first CR, the conclusions from randomized trials are less clear.[105–108] The majority of studies indicate that allogeneic and autologous transplants are associated with lower relapse rates but also with higher mortality rates in CR (especially allogeneic HSCT). Nonrelapse mortality (death of all causes for patients in CR) traditionally has reduced the benefit of less relapses after allogeneic HSCT, and most randomized studies did not show statistically significant advantage in survival (Table 131.8). Furthermore, patients relapsing after HSCT may have shorter survival, although this is a controversial issue. The debate is far from resolved, given that newer preparative regimens (as discussed above) and improvements in supportive care are reducing nonrelapse mortality significantly. A common feature of these large clinical trials is the fact that while most patients assigned to chemotherapy will complete the intended treatment, a significant minority of those assigned will not receive an allogeneic or autologous HSCT.

Most studies indicate that use of consolidation chemotherapy prior to allogeneic HSCT in first remission does not influence survival after transplant.[107] In the autologous HSCT setting, however, another retrospective registry analysis concluded that consolidation may improve transplant outcomes. Patients receiving no consolidation (n = 146) were compared with patients receiving standard-dose (less than 1 gm/m^2) (n = 244) or high-dose (1 to 3 gm/m^2) (n = 249) ara-c prior to autologous HSCT. Leukemia-free and overall survival rates were improved for those who received consolidation. Number of consolidation cycles (one versus two) and cytarabine dose did not significantly affect transplantation outcome.[109]

The EORTC-LG/GIMEMA AML-10 trial set out to compare autologous and allogeneic HSCT for patients in first CR.[107] After one course of consolidation chemotherapy, patients younger than 46 years with an HLA-identical sibling donor were assigned to undergo allogeneic HSCT, while all others were to undergo autologous HSCT. The trial was conducted between 1993 and 1999. In the donor group, 68.9% received an allogeneic HSCT, while in the no-donor subset, an autologous transplant was performed in 55.8% of those eligible. DFS was improved in the former group, while death rate in first CR was decreased in the latter (17.4% vs. 5.3%). Overall survival was similar, but DFS was improved for patients with poor prognosis cytogenetics after allogeneic HSCT, especially for patients aged 15 to 35 years. Instead the MRC study, however, indicated an advantage in survival for allogeneic transplanted recipients with intermediate-risk disease.[106] In both the EORTC/GIMENA AML-8 and the MRC AML-10 trials the relapse-free survival was improved with autologous HSCT when compared to chemotherapy alone, without an overall survival benefit. Likelihood of achieving another remission after relapse was higher in the chemotherapy arms, which led to the similar survival.

TABLE 131.8

ACUTE MYELOID LEUKEMIA IN FIRST COMPLETE REMISSION: STUDIES COMPARING ALLOGENEIC AND AUTOLOGOUS HEMATOPOIETIC STEM CELL TRANSPLANTATION TO CHEMOTHERAPY

Clinical Study/ Type (Ref.)	No. of Patients and Age	Treatment Assignment	Proportion Completing Assigned Treatment	Risk of Relapse	Actuarial Progression-Free Survival	Preparative Regimen	Treatment-related Mortality	Actuarial Survival
United Kingdom Medical Research Council Acute Myeloid Leukemia 10 trial Prospective, genetic randomization (236)	N = 1,602 in CR1 <56 years Tissue typed = n = 1,063	**Donor** n = 419 **No donor** n = 868	61% (n = 257) (allogeneic HSCT) 93% (chemotherapy) 66% (autologous HSCT)	Donor vs. no donor 36% vs. 52% (*P* = .001) Auto vs. chemo only 37% vs. 58% (*P* = .0007)	Benefit for allogeneic HSCT in intermediate risk cytogenetics 50% vs. 39% (*P* = .004)	Cy-TBI for both autologous and allogeneic HSCT (BuCy in 43 patients)	**Donor:** allogeneic = 24% Chemo = 11% **No donor:** autologous* = 12% Chemo = 8%	Donor × No donor 55% × 50% (*P* = 0.1) Benefit for allogeneic HSCT in intermediate risk cytogenetics 55% × 44% (*P* = 0.02) Autologous × chemo 7-year: 57% × 45% (*P* = 0.2)
The European Organisation for Research and Treatment of Cancer Leukemia Group and Gruppo Italiano Malattie Ematologiche dell' Adulto (EORTC-LG/GIMEMA) Prospective, genetic randomization (107)	N = 734 in CR1 that received a single intensive consolidation chemotherapy <46 years	**Donor** n = 293 **No donor** n = 441	55.8% (autologous HSCT) 68.9% (allogeneic HSCT)	Donor vs. no donor 30% vs. 52% (*P* <.0001) **Poor risk cytogenetics: 43% vs. 18% (*P* = NS)**	4-year Donor vs. no donor 52% vs. 42% (*P* = 0.44)	Cy-TBI or BuCy	Death in CR1: Donor × no donor 17% × 5% (*P* <0.0001)	Donor × no donor 58% × 51% (*P* = 0.18)
Dutch-Belgian Hemato-Oncology Cooperative Group (HOVON) and the Swiss Group for Cancer Research (SAKK) Retrospective analysis of three prospective studies conducted from 1987 to 2004. Genetic randomization (111)	N = 1,032 patients in CR after two chemotherapy cycles Consolidation: either third cycle of chemotherapy, auto or allo HSCT Age <55 years Median follow-up from diagnosis is 63 months	**Donor** n = 326 patients (32%) **No donor** n = 706 (68%)	82% (n = 268) (allogeneic HSCT) 28% (n = 165) (autologous HSCT) No donor group: 8% received allogeneic HSCT from other donors, 65% went to receive a 3rd chemo cycle	Donor vs. no donor 32% vs. 59% (*P* <.001) **Reduction in risk of relapse was observed in all cytogenetics categories, including poor risk group**	Donor vs. no donor 48% vs. 27%, HR 0.7, 95% CI, 0.59–0.84 (*P* <.001) Improved DFS was observed in all cytogenetics categories, but was only significant in the intermediate and poor risk groups Age <40 years (HR 0.59, 95% CI, 0.46–0.77; *P* <.001) Age >40: HR 0.83, 95% CI, 0.64–1.07; *P* = NS)	BuCy	Death in CR1: Donor × no donor 21% × 4% (*P* <0.001)	Donor × no donor 4-year survival 54% × 46% (HR 0.85, CI 0. 70–1.03; P = 0.09)

NS, not statistically significant; HR, hazard ratio; CI, confidence interval; CR, complete remission; DFS, disease-free survival; HSCT, hematopoietic stem cell transplant; Cy-TBI, cyclophosphamide and total-body irradiation; BuCy, busulfan and cyclophosphamide.

[a]Two patients died after unrelated donor transplant.

Jourdan et al.[110] reported the long-term follow-up results of four studies investigating postremission consolidation strategies conducted by the Bordeaux Grenoble Marseille Toulouse (BGMT) cooperative group in Europe. The donor group (HLA-identical sibling) comprised 182 patients (38% of those who had achieved first CR); allogeneic HSCT was performed in 171 patients (94%). The no-donor group had 290 patients, of which 62% received an autologous HSCT. The intent-to-treat analysis (donor versus no donor) showed a statistically nonsignificant advantage in overall 10-year survival probability of 51% versus 43% for the donor group. Patients were stratified using the covariates WBC count at diagnosis, FAB subtype, cytogenetic risk, and number of induction courses to achieve CR. An intermediate risk group benefited from allogeneic HSCT, with longer survival, while small numbers precluded definitive conclusions in other subgroups.

Cornelissen et al.[111] updated follow-up and consolidated the results of three consecutive studies sponsored by the Dutch-Belgian Hemato-Oncology Cooperative Group (HOVON) and the Swiss Group for Cancer Research (SAKK) between 1987 and 2004. These studies investigated myeloablative allogeneic HSCT for young patients with AML in first CR, comparing results in patients with a transplant donor identified versus those with no donor who received conventional chemotherapy. Subsets of patients in the no-donor subgroup were eligible to receive autologous HSCT. The initial sample size was 2,287 patients. Patients younger than 55, without FAB M3 disease, who achieved first CR after a maximum of two cycles of chemotherapy and then received consolidation treatment were considered eligible for allogeneic HSCT (n = 1,032, 45% of the cohort). The donor group comprised 326 patients (32%), and the no-donor group comprised 599 patients (58%). Information was not available in 107 cases. In the donor group, 82% went on to allogeneic transplant. The outcome of the study showed that the donor group had fewer relapses and longer DFS. Patients with a donor younger than 40 years of age and with an intermediate or poor risk profile had statistically significantly improved DFS. The authors also presented a meta-analysis that included their patients and those enrolled in the MRC, BGMT, and EORTC studies described above. That meta-analysis suggested a 12% improvement in overall survival for young patients with a donor and without favorable cytogenetic abnormalities (hazard ratio [HR] 0.84; confidence interval [CI], 0.74 to 0.95).

It is likely that some subsets of patients in first CR will benefit more from HSCT than others. Older patients (older than 55 years) have an extremely poor outcome with conventional chemotherapy. Historically they have not been eligible for myeloablative allogeneic transplantation because of concern for toxicities. Recent studies indicate that this group may benefit from nonmyeloablative allogeneic HSCT. A recent feasibility study demonstrated a marked improvement in relapse-free survival with nonablative allogeneic transplants in elderly patients with AML in first CR compared to patients without a donor who received standard chemotherapy.[112] High-dose ara-C–containing chemotherapy regimens, on the other hand, have improved the outcome of young patients, particularly for patients with good risk cytogenetics [t(8;21) and inv16]; the consensus is to not perform allogeneic HSCT in these patients while in first CR. An HLA-compatible family donor (HLA identical sibling or a one-antigen mismatch relative) is available in less than 35% of the cases. Recent data indicate that unrelated donor transplants that are HLA matched using high resolution methods for the HLA-A, -B, -C and -DR loci fare comparably with matched sibling donors.[113]

Autologous HSCT has been proposed and extensively investigated as an option for first CR consolidation (Table 131.8). The role of autologous HSCT in first CR, however, remains controversial. Phase 2 and 3 studies demonstrate that some subgroups of AML patients may benefit from autologous HSCT, with reduction in relapse and improvement in leukemia-free survival. Patients with unfavorable cytogenetics do not appear to benefit, and allogeneic transplant is their preferred option. Peripheral blood has largely replaced bone marrow as the stem cell source of choice for autologous HSCT. Cells are collected upon recovery from consolidation chemotherapy. AML patients, however, are very often poor mobilizers of stem cells, possibly due to AML and treatment-related changes on the normal stem cell pool. Reinfusion of leukemia stem cells contained in the autologous graft is a possibility, and gene marking studies have demonstrated that malignant cells contained in the autograft may contribute to systemic relapse.[91] "Purging" describes the various *ex vivo* procedures that have been used to eliminate these residual leukemic cells from the graft.[114] Preclinical studies have suggested that this strategy reduces significantly the number of clonogenic progenitors. Chemotherapeutic agents have been extensively used for *ex vivo* purging. Most investigators in the United States used 4-hydroperoxycylophosphamide (4-HC), while mafosfamide, another cyclophosphamide derivative, was investigated chiefly in Europe. These agents affect normal and leukemic stem cells and typically are associated with delayed hematologic recovery posttransplant. None of the purging techniques has been tested in a randomized fashion, conclusive evidence of a contribution to improved DFS is lacking, and there is only indirect evidence of a possible benefit for purged grafts.

Most studies of autologous HSCT enrolled patients younger than 50 years old. However, autologous HSCT transplants have also been investigated for patients older than 60 years. The EORTC-GIMEMA AML-13 trial proposed collection of peripheral blood stem cells after induction therapy with mitoxantrone, etoposide, and cytarabine (MICE) with or without G-CSF, and consolidation chemotherapy with idarubicin, etoposide, and cytarabine (mini-ICE). Patients aged 61 to 70 years with good performance status were eligible. Fifty-four of 61 patients (88%) had peripheral blood stem cells harvested, but only 35 patients received autologous HSCT (57%). Median disease-free and overall survival was 1 years and 1.4 years, respectively. The 3-year disease-free and overall survival rates were 21% and 32%, respectively. The authors considered this a negative study that exemplified the limitations of dose intensification for patients with AML in this age range.[115]

In a recent meta-analysis of 24 trials comparing chemotherapy to autologous and allogeneic HSCT that involved 6,007 patients (3,638 patients with cytogenetics information), remission-free survival benefit was observed for poor-risk (HR 0.69; 95% CI, 0.57 to 0.84) and intermediate-risk AML (HR 0.76; 95% CI, 0.68 to 0.85) but not for good-risk disease (HR 1.06; 95% CI, 0.80 to 1.42). Similar results were obtained in the overall survival analysis. Allogeneic HSCT improved survival for poor-risk (HR 0.73; 95% CI, 0.59 to 0.90) and intermediate-risk AML (HR 0.83; 95% CI, 0.74 to 0.93) but not for good-risk AML (HR 1.07; 95% CI, 0.83 to 1.38). Use of autologous HSCT was not associated with improved outcomes.[116] Therefore, considering that TRM has decreased substantially in the context of allogeneic HSCT, this approach is considered in all adult patients up to age 75 years in first CR who do not have good risk cytogenetics if a sibling or a molecularly matched unrelated donor (HLA-A, -B, -C, -DRB1, -DQB1) is available (Table 131.7). At the M. D. Anderson Cancer Center the full dose busulfan-fludarabine regimen is used up to age 60 years and the reduced-intensity fludarabine-melphalan regimen is used for those over age 60 or those with serious comorbidities.

Transplantation for Acute Myelogenous Leukemia in Relapse and Primary Induction Failure

Outcomes of relapsing AML patients are influenced to a large extent by duration of the first CR. First remissions shorter than 6 months and failure to achieve a CR with initial therapy (primary induction failure) are associated with a likelihood of CR of less than 10% to 20%. Patients relapsing within the first year of remission that fail to respond to the first salvage attempt are for practical purposes incurable with standard chemotherapy regimens.

Autologous HSCT has been used to treat relapsed and refractory patients, but with poor results. Allogeneic HSCT is considered the treatment of choice for AML in primary induction failure or beyond first CR, resulting in long-term disease-free survival in 20% to 40% of patients.[117] Results of allogeneic and autologous HSCT are generally better if performed in second CR as opposed to active relapse. However, results were comparable in patients in early relapse versus second remission if one can proceed promptly with HSCT.[118]

Armistead et al.[119] performed a retrospective review to evaluate all relapsed AML patients treated at M. D. Anderson Cancer Center between 1995 and 2004. Median age was 58 years and 59% of the patients had poor risk cytogenetics. After removing patients who died from their initial salvage therapy or who received a stem cell transplant as their first salvage regimen, the survival outcomes from 490 patients (130 of whom were transplanted) were analyzed. This cohort was divided into the 113 patients who achieved a second CR and 377 who did not. In both groups the patients who underwent allogeneic HSCT had a statistically significant survival benefit compared to those who did not. In patients who achieved a second CR 2-year overall survival was 45% versus 20% for patients who did not undergo transplant after achieving a second CR (P = .005). For the relapsed refractory group, 2-year overall survival in the transplant cohort was 13% versus 0% for the nontransplanted patients (P <.001).[119]

The value of salvage chemotherapy prior to transplant is controversial. As indicated above, patients in second CR have a better prognosis after HSCT than those transplanted in relapse in most studies. On the other hand, early and more indolent relapses should probably be treated with allogeneic transplantation as soon as possible assuming that an acceptable donor is readily available. A patient who had a remission duration of 6 months or less is unlikely to enter second remission with chemotherapy, which may be needed, however, given the speed of progression or other problems that may preclude allogeneic HSCT in a timely fashion. Patients transplanted in second CR will have long-term disease control in 20% to 60% of the cases with HSCT, while patients transplanted in primary induction failure will benefit in 10% to 30% of the cases. The cure rate for patients in first and subsequent relapses is in the 10% to 30% range, and as expected, refractory relapses comprise the worse subgroup.

Reduced Intensity Conditioning and Preparative Regimen Intensity

Given the relative insensitivity of AML to the graft-versus-leukemia effect, chemotherapy or radiation intensity is an important component of HSCT. There is a tradeoff between nonrelapse mortality and dose intensity, which may negate the decrease in relapse rates associated with higher-dose regimens.[95,102]

The CIBMTR collects information on most transplants performed in North America. The most commonly used reduced-intensity regimens (for all indications) as reported to the CIBMTR are fludarabine combined with low-dose TBI[120], with cyclophosphamide[121], with busulfan[122], with melphalan,[123] or with other drugs. Antithymocyte globulin or alemtuzumab are commonly added to the regimen for *in vivo* depletion of T cells in order to reduce the risk of GVHD; this benefit may be offset by an increase the risk of leukemia relapse.[124]

The fludarabine-melphalan reduced intensity regimen has been used at the M. D. Anderson Cancer Center for approximately 10 years, and long-term follow-up demonstrates its ability to induce durable disease control in a significant fraction of AML patients. The authors have updated results of a cohort comprised of 112 patients. Most had high-risk AML/MDS (80% with active disease at transplantation). Median age was 55 years.[125] Donors were HLA-identical siblings and matched unrelated. Nonrelapse mortality was highly influenced by disease status: 100-day TRM of patients treated in CR was 0%, as opposed to 32% for heavily pretreated, relapsed subjects. After a median follow-up of 29 months, approximately 70% of patients transplanted in CR were alive in remission. Likewise, the Seattle group experience of treating AML in first CR (median age of 59 years) with a nonmyeloablative, low-dose TBI-based regimen achieved a low TRM rate. However, the 1-year progression-free survival was lower than that reported with more aggressive regimens (42%).[126]

Monoclonal antibodies may improve preparative regimens for AML. Gemtuzumab ozogamicin targets the CD33 antigen present on myeloid cells. The authors performed a phase 1 and 2 study at the M. D. Anderson Cancer Center adding gemtuzumab ozogamicin 2 mg/m^2 to the fludarabine/melphalan regimen, indicating prolongation of survival compared to historic controls receiving the fludarabine/melphalan regimen alone.[127]

A retrospective registry analysis from the European Group for Blood and Marrow Transplantation (EBMT) addressed the issue of preparative regimen intensity. Patients with AML (older than 50 years) treated with HLA identical sibling HSCT after regimens of reduced intensity were compared to recipients of myeloablative conditioning. Most reduced intensity regimens consisted of fludarabine with busulfan or low-dose TBI. Ablative regimens were those incorporating 10 Gy or greater TBI-based regimens or busulfan-based combinations with more than 8 mg/kg of the drug. The proportion of patients transplanted in remission was similar (approximately 70%), while 16% and 12%, respectively, of each group had poor prognosis cytogenetics. Recipients of reduced intensity transplants were older (57 vs. 54 years). The reduced intensity group had a decrease in transplant-related mortality rates, similar GVHD rates, and a statistically significant higher probability of relapse. Leukemia-free survival, however, was not statistically different in the two groups.[128,129]

There is controversy regarding which patients should receive myeloablative versus reduced-intensity preparative regimens. Improvements in supportive care and development of new myeloablative regimens may limit the applicability of these historic comparisons. The safety of myeloablative regimens is improving, and their use for "fit" patients aged 55 to 65 is now an attainable goal. Table 131.9 summarizes the results of studies that enrolled AML patients in the sixth and seventh decades of life treated with reduced-intensity allogeneic HSCT. Randomized clinical trials are necessary to resolve this question. It is recommended that older patients with AML be treated within clinical trials.

Stem Cell Transplantation for Acute Promyelocytic Leukemia

The introduction of ATRA and ATO has revolutionized the treatment of APL. The achievement of a molecular remission (as determined by a real-time quantitative PCR for the PML/RARα hybrid gene) is the therapeutic goal in the management of APL. Since the majority of patients now achieve prolonged remissions, there is no role for HSCT for patients in molecular remission after initial therapy and consolidation. Consideration is frequently given to storing autologous hematopoietic stem cells while in this minimal residual disease state, especially if no HLA-identical sibling is available. Allogeneic or autologous HSCT should be offered to patients without molecular remission or with recurrent disease.

PRACTICE OF ONCOLOGY

TABLE 131.9

ALLOGENEIC HEMATOPOIETIC STEM CELL TRANSPLANTATION FOR PATIENTS IN THE SIXTH AND SEVENTH DECADES OF LIFE

Study Type (Ref.)	Diagnosis (No. of Patients)	Median Age (Years; Range)	Disease Status at Transplant	Preparative Regimen	Donor	GVHD Prophylaxis	Median Follow-Up	aGVHD and cGVHD Rates	Nonrelapse Mortality	PFS/Relapse Rate	Survival
Phase 2, multicenter (126)	AML N = 122	57.5 (17–74)	CR1 = 51 CR2 = 39 Other = 32 High-risk cytogenetics = 17%	**Nonmyeloablative** 2 Gy total-body irradiation with or without fludarabine	HLA-identical sibling = 58 MUD = 64	CsA and mycophenolate mofetil	44 months (range, 26–79 months)	gd II–IV: 35% (related) and 46% (unrelated)	2-year 10% (related) 22% (unrelated)	2-year: disease-free survival 44%	2-year (all patients): 48% (CR1): 44% (related) 63% (unrelated)
Retrospective analysis, single center (102)	MDS: 26 AML: 68	FAI: 61 (27–74) FM: 54 (22–75)	Remission = 24 (26%) Not in remission = 70 (74%) Remission: FAI: 44% vs. FM: 16%	Reduced-intensity (FM) Fludarabine, and melphalan (n = 62) **Nonmyeloablative (FAI)** Fludarabine, ara-C, and idarubicin (n = 32)	HLA-identical sibling = 54% MUD or mismatched related = 46%	Tacrolimus and minimethotrexate	40 months	Gd II–IV = 34% gd III–IV = 16% cGVHD = 34%	100-day = 21% 3-year cumulative incidence = FAI =15.6% = FM = 39.2%	3-year cumulative incidence of relapse = FAI = 53.4% = FM =26%	Actuarial 3-year survival: 33%
Registry analysis, retrospective (128, 129)	AML age >50 years Reduced-intensity regimens (A): 315 Myeloablative regimens (B): 407	(A): 57 years (50–73) (B): 54 years (50–64)	CR: A = 223; B = 297 Relapse: A = 92; B = 110 Poor prognosis cytogenetics: A = 16%; B = 12%	**Reduced-intensity** Fludarabine combined to busulfan (53%) or low-dose TBI (24%) + various regimens	HLA-identical sibling 100%	Majority cyclosporine-based	13 months	Gd II–IV A = 22%; B = 31% (*P* = .003) cGVHD A = 48% ± 3%; B = 56% ± 3% (*P* = .64)	2-year cumulative incidence A = 18±2% B = 32 ± 2% (*P* <.0004)	2-year LFS A = 40 ± 3% B = 44 ± 3% (P = 0.8) Relapse incidence A = 41 ± 3% B = 24 ± 2% (P<0.0004)	2-year survival A = 47 ± 3% B = 46 ± 3% (P = 0.43)
Phase 2, multicenter (237)	MDS: 10 AML: 65	52.3 (18.5–65.8)	CR1 = 8 CR2 = 8 REL1–2 = 28 PIF = 21 Unt = 10	Chemotherapy with fludarabine, amsacrine, and ara-C, followed in 3 days by 4 Gy TBI, ATG, Cy (**Reduced-intensity**) Prophylactic DLI in 12 patients	HLA identical sibling (n = 31) MUD or mismatch related (n = 44)	CsA and MMF	35.1 months (13.6–47.6 months)	gd II–IV: 49% cGVHD: 45%	HLA-identical sibling donor: 22.6% MUD or mismatched related: 50%	2-year leukemia-free survival: 40%	2-year overall survival: 42%
Phase 2, single center (238)	MDS: 11 AML: 41	52 (17–71)	CR1 = 9 CR2 = 4 AML active disease = 28 MDS = 11	**Reduced-intensity** Fludarabine, melphalan, and alemtuzumab	HLA identical sibling (n = 23) MUD or mismatch related (n = 29)	Tacrolimus	18 months (2–34 months)	gd II–IV: 33% gd III–IV: 10% Ext cGVHD: 18%	1-year: 33%	Relapse rate: 27% 1-year PFS: 38%;	1-year survival: 48%

Retrospective, single center (125)	N = 112 AML: 82 Advanced MDS: 30	55 (22–74)	CR1 = 20 CR2 or 3 = 10 Active disease = 82 Poor prognosis cytogenetics: 43%	**Reduced-intensity (FM)** Fludarabine, and melphalan 100–180 mg/m^2	HLA identical sibling (n = 59) MUD or mismatch related (n = 53)	Tacrolimus and minimethotrexate	29.4 months (13.1–87.7 months)	gd II–IV: 39% cGVHD: 49%	**Patients in CR:** day-100 = 0% 1-year = 20% **Patients with active disease and MUD HSCT:** day-100 = 35% 1-year = 56%	2-year cumulative incidence of relapse: 25% (presence of circulating blasts at HSCT predicted worse DFS	2-year estimates of survival - **CR at HSCT:** 66% **Active disease with circulating blasts:** 23%
Registry analysis, retrospective (239)	AML **Allogeneic** HSCT = n = 361 **Autologous** N = 1,369 All older than 49 years	Autologous = 57 (50–78) Allogeneic = 58 (50–73)	**Allogeneic** CR1 = 59% CR2 = 17% Advanced = 23% Poor prognosis cytogenetics: 18% **Autologous** CR1 = 84% CR2 = 10% Advanced = 6% Poor prognosis cytogenetics: 8%	**Reduced-intensity regimens** **Allogeneic** Fludarabine-based (93%); 2 Gy TBI-based in 26% **Autologous** Busulfan-based (85%); TBI-based (15%)	HLA identical siblings	CsA-based in 96%	**Allogeneic:** 24 months (1–73) **Autologous:** 16 months (0.5–94)	Gd II–IV: 22% Gd III–IV: 9%	2-year **Allogeneic** = CR1: 17% CR2: 12% Advanced:9% **Autologous** = CR1: 10% CR2: 8% Advanced: 19% Allo > auto in CR1 (*P* = .001)	**Allo × Auto** CR1 36% × 50% (P = 0.001) Other disease status, **P = NS**	**Autologous** = 2-year = 54% **Allogeneic**= 2-year = 50% Allo>auto for CR2 and advanced patients (***P*** **< = 0.05**)
Registry analysis (240)	AML, n = 545	Age 40–54 (n = 201), age 55–59, n = 149; age 60–64, n = 132; age ≥ 65, n = 63	**CR1**	**Various; all reduced intensity or non-myeloablative**	HLA identical sibling or unrelated	Tacrolimus or cyclosporine-based in most transplants	**25–37 months**	Probability of acute GVHD: 31%–36% (similar in all age cohorts); chronic: 37%–45% (also similar incidence across age cohorts)	At 2 years: Age 40–54, 33%; age 55–59, 39%; age 60–64, 35%; age ≥ 65, 39%	Relapse at 2 years: Age 40–54, 28%; age 55–59, 29%; age 60–64, 29%; age >=65, 25%. Similar 2-year DFS across age cohorts	Survival at 2 years: Age 40–54, 42%; age 55–59, 35%; age 60–64, 45%; age >=65, 38%

PFS, progression-free survival; DFS, disease-free survival; aGVHD, acute graft-versus-host disease; cGVHD, chronic graft-versus-host disease; MDS, myelodysplastic syndrome; AML, acute myelogenous leukemia; CML, chronic myelogenous leukemia; CsA, cyclosporine; MMF, mycophenolate mophetyl; CR1, first complete remission; DLI, donor lymphocyte infusion; BuCy, busulfan and cyclophosphamide; Cy-TBI, cyclophosphamide and total-body irradiation; BuFlu, busulfan and cyclophosphamide; MUD, matched unrelated donor; gd, grade; REL1-2, first or second relapse; PIF, primary induction failure; Unt, untreated.

ATO salvage therapy induces a second remission in the majority of patients who relapse after ATRA-based treatment. It is, however, unclear which is the best approach for the patient with arsenic-induced second CR. Patients in molecular remission may be offered autologous HSCT. Long-term remission rates in the range of 50% to 80% have been reported with autologous HSCT in second CR. In regard to transplantation timing, Tallman[130] reported an update of the U.S. multicenter trial with arsenic as a single treatment agent for relapsed or refractory APL. The preliminary results indicate that autologous transplants done in second remission elicit better results than transplants done later when disease relapses. Allogeneic transplants are associated with higher treatment-related mortality and lower risk of relapse than autologous transplants. The EBMT reviewed 625 patients who received an autologous or allogeneic-HSCT after year 1993. The authors analyzed transplants performed in first or second CR. Five-year leukemia-free survival for patients in first CR was 69% (n = 149) and 68% (n = 144), respectively, for recipients of autografts and allografts.[131] Those transplanted in second CR achieved leukemia-free survival of 51% (n = 195) and 59% (n = 137), respectively, after autologous and allogeneic HSCT. The analysis also indicated that the number of transplants for patients in first CR decreased since 1998 but remained stable until 2002 for patients in second CR, after which the number of procedures decreased. Although limited by the lack of information on therapies that preceded HSCT or the PML/RARα status of the patients, it is reasonable to assume that these results reflect outcomes of transplants performed in the ATRA era, while some of the yearly trends may also reflect incorporation of arsenic trioxide in the treatment schemas. No large studies have compared transplantation approaches to continuing therapy with arsenic or other drugs, such as gemtuzumab ozogamicin.

Umbilical Cord Blood Transplantation

As discussed previously, many patients lack an HLA-compatible related or unrelated donor. It is often necessary to proceed to transplantation urgently, and unrelated donor searches typically require several months to identify a donor. Therefore, alternative approaches have been studied including unrelated umbilical cord blood transplants or related haploidentical grafts.

Cord blood is a rich source of hematopoietic stem cells for transplantation. Approximately 100 mL of cord blood can be collected from the placenta after delivery of a child. These units have been successfully used for transplantation. The number of cells is approximately one log fewer than in a typical bone marrow harvest. Cord blood is immunologically immature, and GVHD is less severe than after transplantation of bone marrow or peripheral blood progenitor cells from adult donors; this has allowed the successful use of cord blood transplants from donors mismatched for up to two of the HLA-A, -B, and -DR loci. Given the lower cell dose, cord blood transplants are associated with slower engraftment, particularly in adults. Results of recent studies are similar to those with unrelated donor bone marrow transplants in selected patient populations.[132] Although outcomes are better in pediatric patients, cord blood transplants have been used successfully in patients in the sixth and seventh decades of life.[133]

Haploidentical Transplantation

Individuals inherit one HLA haplotype from each parent, so almost all patients will have a haploidentical relative available. Haploidentical transplants are associated with a high risk of graft rejection and GVHD. The most successful approach has utilized extensive T-lymphocyte depletion in order to prevent GVHD, and immune recovery posttransplant is a major problem.[134] Engraftment is enhanced by transplantation of a large numbers of CD34+ cells. Another approach is the use of T-cell replete hematopoietic stem cell grafts followed by two doses of posttransplant cyclophosphamide, with or without additional immunosuppression.[135]

There is increasing preclinical and clinical evidence that NK cells mediate a potent antileukemia effect. Donor versus host NK-cell reactivity can thus be predicted by *KIR* gene expression in the donor, and the absence of inhibitory KIR ligands in the recipient (HLA BW4 and C alleles). AML patients who receive haploidentical HSCT in which donor NK cells were predicted to be alloreactive had significantly lower relapse rates and improved leukemia-free survival.[136]

Treatment of Relapse after Allogeneic Transplantation

AML recurrence is a major cause of treatment failure. Reduction of early TRM, leading to higher overall survivorship rates, and transplantation of patients at high risk for relapse have led to an increase in the number of recurrences after allogeneic HSCT. There is no homogeneity or consensus regarding treatment of this difficult clinical scenario. Donor lymphocyte infusion, second transplant, chemotherapy, and immunosuppression withdrawal are commonly used with low success rates. CR duration after HSCT is a major determinant of salvage success, as is response to treatment of relapse.[137] The biology of disease relapse is complex, and this is an area of active basic and clinical research.[138,139] Prevention of relapse may include immunologic or pharmacologic interventions, such as the use of leukemia-specific cytotoxic T lymphocytes or maintenance of remission with 5-azacitidine or other drugs.[140]

Future Directions in Stem Cell Transplantation

A major goal of allogeneic hematopoietic transplantation is separation of the beneficial graft-versus-leukemia activity from the adverse effects of GVHD. One approach is to specifically deplete or anergize alloreactive T cells that produce GVHD, leaving nonalloreactive cells to reconstitute immunity.

Separation of GVHD and graft-versus-leukemia may be attainable by targeting antigens restricted to hematopoietic cells or the malignancy, avoiding broadly reactive alloantigens expressed by visceral tissues. Potential targets include HA-1 and HA-2, minor histocompatibility antigens restricted to hematopoietic cells; elimination of host hematopoietic cells is acceptable, since these cells are replaced by donor stem cells.[141] Other antigens such as proteinase-3 and neutrophil elastase are aberrantly expressed by myeloid leukemia cells and serve as targets for T cell immunity. Molldrem et al.[81] detected PR1-specific cytotoxic T cells in leukemia patients and subsequently documented the contribution of these cells to remission in CML and AML patients. The Wilms' tumor antigen (WT1) is another potential leukemia antigen.[82] Both the PR1 and Wilms' tumor antigens are under active investigation. It is expected that vaccination approaches or adoptive cellular therapy targeting multiple antigens will be more successful than a single leukemia-associated antigen. One may also vaccinate the donor prior to stem cell donation, so immunity would be transferred with the transplant.

ACUTE LYMPHOBLASTIC LEUKEMIA

ALL is a heterogeneous disease with distinct biologic and prognostic groupings. Considerable progress has been made in understanding the biology of ALL has led to more precise disease prognostication and treatment strategies tailored to specific disease subgroups. This has resulted in dramatic improvements in the outcomes of children with ALL, with cure rates up to 80%. The therapeutic approach for adult ALL is modeled on pediatric regimens, and although initial remission rates range between 80% to 90%, only 25% to 50% of adults achieve long-term disease-free survival. This stark difference in outcome for adults as compared to children has been variously attributed to the greater incidence of adverse cytogenetic subgroups found in adults and possibly poorer tolerance and compliance of adults with intensive therapies required for the successful treatment of ALL. Continued research into the biology of this heterogeneous disease and further development of targeted therapies used in a risk-stratified manner will hopefully lead to comparable survival rates in the near future.

Epidemiology

ALL accounts for approximately 20% of acute leukemias in adults, with increasing incidence above 50 years of age. The incidence of ALL is more common in whites compared with African Americans, with an age-adjusted overall incidence in the United States of 1.5 per 100,000 in whites and 0.8 per 100,000 in blacks.[142] A higher incidence of ALL has been reported in industrialized countries and urban areas. Finally, ALL is slightly more common among men than among women (1.3 to 1.0).

Diagnosis and Evaluation

Historically, the FAB classification system distinguished three subtypes of ALL based on cell morphology.[10] L1 lymphoblasts, which were small to intermediate size, were the most common, followed by L2, which defined slightly larger-sized blasts, and finally L3, which defined large blasts, described as having a "starry sky" appearance, which were seen in Burkitt's leukemia or lymphoma. This classification system has been replaced by the WHO system, which is based on immunophenotypic, cytogenetic, and molecular information, and consequently provides more precise and clinically relevant disease subgroupings.[11] Phenotypic evaluation begins with cytochemical studies with a myeloperoxidase or Sudan black B reaction, as well as nonspecific esterase reactions (ANA, ANB) to exclude most cases of AML. Immunophenotypic analysis is then used to confirm the morphologic diagnosis of ALL and to subclassify cases into B- and T-lineage types, and further subtype groupings based on different levels of maturation in B- and thymic T-cell development. In some cases, ambiguous expression of myeloid markers (CD13, CD33, CD14, CD15, CDw65) may be noted concurrently with lymphoid markers; the presence of myeloid markers lacks prognostic significance,[143,144] but it can be used to distinguish leukemic cells from normal hematogones. Since there is no consensus on these differentiation schemes, the WHO classification system simply classifies cases as precursor-B and precursor-T ALL without additional categorization. A specific immunophenotype identified at diagnosis may also be used for evaluating MRD by flow cytometry at subsequent time points in disease treatment.

Eighty-five percent of cases of ALL are of B-cell lineage, and the most common form is the precursor-B phenotype (also called common precursor-B ALL or early precursor-B ALL); these cells express a B-cell immunophenotype (CD19, CD22), TdT, cytoplasmic CD79A, CD34, CD10 (CALLA), and lack cytoplasmic μ and surface immunoglobulin (sIg). It is found frequently in patients with the Philadelphia chromosome, t(9;22) (q34;q11). A less common type, termed pro-B ALL, lacks CD10 expression and may represent an earlier level of B-cell maturation. Mature B-cell lineage ALL has the immunophenotype of mature B cells with sIg expression and is seen with Burkitt's leukemia or lymphoma. T-lineage ALL accounts for 15% to 20% of cases. This "common thymocyte" type expresses pan T-cell markers, CD2, cytoplasmic CD3 (cCD3), CD7, CD5, and distinctively shows coexpression of CD4 and CD8 and expression of CD1a. A more primitive type called *prothymocyte* or *immature thymocyte* type has TdT, cCD3, and variable expression of CD5, CD2, and CD7, but lacks CD4, CD8, and CD1a. The mature T-lineage phenotype expresses the pan T-cell markers, variable TdT, but lacks CD1a.

Cytogenetic and Molecular Abnormalities

Specific and well-characterized recurring chromosomal abnormalities facilitate diagnosis, confirm subtype classification, and have major prognostic value for treatment planning. Abnormalities in chromosome number or structure are found in approximately 90% of children and 70% of adult ALL patients.[145–149] Differences in the frequency at which good- and poor-risk prognosis cytogenetic abnormalities occur in children versus adults may partially explain the differences in treatment outcomes between childhood and adult ALL (Table 131.10). These cytogenetic abnormalities are acquired somatic mutations that frequently result from translocations of chromosomal DNA and lead to new aberrant protein products presumed to be responsible for the cellular dysregulation that leads to the malignant state. Deletions or loss of DNA may eliminate genes that have tumor suppressor functions. Gains of additional chromosomes may lead to gene dosage effects that provide transformed cells with survival advantages. As in AML, cytogenetic abnormalities in ALL define unique prognostic groups, as listed in Table 131.10.

Molecular methods are increasingly used to better understand the genetic consequences of these cytogenetic abnormalities intrinsic to the pathophysiology of ALL, as well as to refine prognosis and identify novel therapeutic targets in ALL. Quantitative reverse transcription-polymerase chain reaction technology (RT-PCR) allows for quantification of MRD, which is an independent prognostic factor in both pediatric and adult ALL.[150,151] DNA microarray-based gene expression profiling has revealed distinct gene-expression patterns in subtypes of ALL, which may be used to yield insights into the biology of ALL and identify new therapeutic targets,[152–158] as well as further refine disease-risk stratification[159,160] and identify genetic markers associated with drug sensitivity and resistance pathways.[161] For example, activating *NOTCH1* mutations are present in up to 50% of T-ALL cases,[158] and the signaling pathways and target genes responsible for Notch1-induced neoplastic transformation are currently under investigation; the nuclear factor κB (NF-κB) pathway appears to be one of the major mediators, suggesting that the use of gamma-secretase inhibitors used in combination with NF-κB inhibitors, such as bortezomib, may have synergistic effects.[155]

Mechanisms for drug resistance are also affected by pharmacogenetics and pharmacogenomics.[162] For example, hyperdiploid cells accumulate more methotrexate polyglutamates as they possess extra copies of the gene-encoding reduced folate carrier, an active transporter of methotrexate.[163] Associations also have been identified between germline genetic characteristics (genes that encode drug-metabolizing enzymes, transporters, and drug targets) and drug metabolism and sensitivity to chemotherapy. Rocha et al.[164] studied 16 genetic polymorphisms that affected the pharmacodynamics of antileukemic agents and observed that, among 130 children with high-risk disease, the glutathione S-transferase μ1 (*GSTM1*) nonnull genotype was associated with a higher risk of recurrence, which

TABLE 131.10

COMMON KARYOTYPIC ABNORMALITIES IN PEDIATRIC AND ACUTE LYMPHOBLASTIC LEUKEMIA

				Frequency (%) in ALL		Overall Survival (%) at 3–5 Years	
Phenotype	Karyotype	Genes Involved	Function of Fusion Protein	Children	Adults	Children	Adults
Pro-B	t(4;11)(q21;q23)	*MLL, AF4*	Alters HOX gene expression	5–8	3–6	<10	10–24
Pre-B	t(1;19)(q23;p13)	*E2A, PBX1*	transcription factor; induction of cell differentiation arrest	5–6	1–3	70–80	30–60
B-lineage	t(9;22)(q34;q11)	*BCR, ABL*	tyrosine kinase	2–3	15–36	30–80[a]	45–75[a]
B-lineage	t(12;21)(p13;q22) or del 12p	*ETV6-RUNX1*	Alters HOX gene expression	20–25	1–3	85–90	40
T-lineage	14q11, 7q35, 7p14-15	Translocation of oncogenes to T-cell receptor genes	Overexpression of respective proteins	40–50	<5	65–75	30–60
B- or T-lineage	t(8;14), t(8;22), t(2;8)	*c-MYC*	MYC overexpression	2–5	3–7	75–85	20–45
B- or T-lineage	del 9p/9p abnormality	*MTAP, CDKN2, CDKN2B*	Tumor suppressor genes	10	<10	60	40–60
B- or T-lineage	del 6q	?	Tumor suppressor genes?	5	<10	>70	30–40
B- or T-lineage	<45 Chromosomes			5–7	4–10	25–50	10–20
B- or T-lineage	>50 Chromosomes			25–38	2–10	80–90	40–50

[a]These results include the use of imatinib with average 3-year follow-up.

was increased further by the thymidylate synthetase (*TYMS*) 3/3 genotype.

Finally, epigenetic changes, including hypermethylation of tumor-suppressor genes or microRNA genes, and hypomethylation of oncogenes have been identified in up to 80% of patients with ALL,[165,166] and insights into these mechanisms provide another area for therapeutic development.[167]

Therapy for Acute Lymphoblastic Leukemia

Treatment for adult ALL is modeled on therapy developed for childhood ALL and consists of remission induction, consolidation, and maintenance therapy and CNS prophylaxis, using a risk-stratified approach. Selecting therapy based on patient- and disease-specific prognostic factors has led to a significant improvement in outcomes for childhood ALL, and the adoption of this approach for adults has had a similarly favorable impact.

Prognostic Factors and Risk Assessment

Several classic evaluations of prognostic features in adult ALL have been made and have led to five widely accepted prognostic features: age, WBC count, leukemic cell immunophenotype, cytogenetic subtype, and time to achieve CR[168] (Table 131.11). The presence of any of these features portends a high risk for relapse following standard ALL therapy, and the remaining patients are considered standard risk. Up to 75% of adults with ALL are considered to be poor-risk patients, with an expected DFS rate of 25%, and 25% of adults with ALL constitute standard-risk patients, with a projected DFS rate of greater than 50%.[169] However, recent advances in ALL biology and therapy are changing the risk assignment of some of these features.

Age, WBC count, and treatment response during induction therapy remain classic prognostic features. Age is a continuous variable with overall survival (OS), decreasing with increasing age; OS ranges from 34% to 57% for patients younger than 30 years compared with only 15% to 17% for patients older than 50 years.[170] A high WBC count is also a continuous variable; generally, a WBC count greater than 30,000/mcL or 50,000/mcL for B-lineage ALL and greater than 100,000/mcL for T-lineage ALL predict for poor prognosis. Of note, while an increased WBC count holds prognostic significance independently as a measure of tumor burden, a high WBC count

TABLE 131.11

UNFAVORABLE PROGNOSTIC FEATURES IN ADULT ACUTE LYMPHOBLASTIC LEUKEMIA

Characteristic	High-Risk Factor(s)
Clinical Factors	
Age	>35 yr
Leukocytosis	>30 × 10^9/L (B-lineage); >100 × 10^9/L (T-lineage)
Karyotype	t(9;22), t(4;11), complex, hypodiploid
Treatment-related	
Therapy response	Time to morphologic CR >4 weeks Persistent MRD

CR, complete response; MRD, minimal residual disease.

may be also associated with increased risk of complications during induction therapy, increased risk of CNS relapse, and association with poor-risk cytogenetic subgroups [e.g., t(4;11) and t(9;22)]. Finally, the achievement of CR and time to CR after induction therapy carry significant prognostic implications, with patients who require more than 4 weeks to achieve a CR having a lower likelihood of being cured. The emergence of MRD monitoring provides an even more accurate assessment of disease response. In contrast to children, a decrease in MRD burden occurs more slowly in adults.[150] In general, the presence of MRD, defined as 10^{-4}, at any time after the start of consolidation is associated with an increased relapse risk, and the predictive value increases at later time points.[150] Patel et al.[151] prospectively analyzed MRD samples following induction, consolidation, and maintenance of 161 patients with non-T-lineage, Ph negative, ALL treated on the international Medical Research Council (MRC) UKALL XII/ECOG 2993 trial. MRD status best discriminated outcome after 10 weeks of therapy, when the relative risk of relapse was 8.95-fold higher in MRD positive patients and the 5-year relapse-free survival was 15% compared to 71% in MRD negative patients. The predictive value of MRD depends on the technical quality of the assay and the frequency of monitoring. Furthermore, there is not yet a consensus on standard methodology to measure MRD.

Specific cytogenetic abnormalities have a major impact on prognosis. The presence of the Ph chromosome and t(4;11)(q21;q23) has been associated with inferior survival in multiple large series.[144,147,169] Additionally, the presence of the t(8;14)(q24.1;q32) complex karyotype, defined as *five or more* chromosomal abnormalities or low hypodiploidy or near triploidy, was noted to result in poor survival in the analysis of patients treated on the UKALL XII/ECOG 2993 trial; in contrast, the presence of hyperdiploidy or del(9p) indicated a good prognosis.[144] Of note, the t(8;14) associated with a mature B ALL phenotype has a poor prognosis when treated with standard ALL regimens. However, modified ALL regimens, incorporating CD20-targeted therapy, now result in significantly better survival for this group.[171] Similarly, although the Ph chromosome has traditionally been considered a marker of high-risk disease, the outcome for this subset of patients has greatly changed with the incorporation of TKIs into classic ALL therapy. Reports from studies incorporating imatinib into their regimens show a greater proportion achieving CR and MRD negativity, and thus suggesting a better prognosis.[172–174] Finally, patients with T-lineage ALL formerly had inferior CR rates in comparison with precursor-B ALL. However, modification of the standard ALL therapy, to include cytarabine, cyclophosphamide, and CNS prophylaxis in T-lineage ALL regimens, now result in uniformly better outcomes for these patients as compared to their B-lineage ALL counterparts, with CR rates up to 80% and leukemia-free survival greater than 50%.[175]

Remission Induction

In the remission-induction phase of therapy, the goals are to eradicate 99% of the initial tumor burden and to restore normal hematopoiesis and performance status. Current induction regimens for adults consist of at least a glucocorticoid (prednisone, prednisolone, or dexamethasone), vincristine, and an anthracycline, with expected remission rates of 72% to 92% and median remission duration of 18 months (Table 131.12). Dexamethasone has replaced prednisone based on better *in vitro* antileukemic activity and higher drug levels in the CSF.[175] The German multicenter study group for ALL (GMALL) noted decreased early mortality when the dexamethasone was given in an interrupted schedule rather than continuously.[176] The most commonly used anthracycline is daunorubicin, and attempts have been made to increase the dosage, with no clear benefit noted, possibly due to the increased hematologic toxicity.[177] Intensification of the induction regimen has been attempted with the addition of cyclophosphamide, asparaginase, or cytarabine. Although no clear improvement in CR rates have been noted,[178,179] remission duration may be improved in some ALL subtypes (e.g., cytarabine in T-ALL, cyclophosphamide in mature B ALL). Additionally, treatment intensification specifically for patients in the adolescent age range (e.g., 15 to 20 years old) appears to result in better outcomes with survival rates nearing those of pediatric patients.[180] The use of targeted therapies during induction (e.g., rituximab for mature B ALL and imatinib for Ph+ ALL) has improved CR rates for these subtypes of ALL. Finally, supportive care is of great importance during this period. Treatment-related early deaths occur in up to 10% of patients, and significant comorbidities, such fungal infections, occur as a consequence of prolonged cytopenia. The

TABLE 131.12

SELECTED PROSPECTIVE TRIALS IN ADULT ACUTE LYMPHOBLASTIC LEUKEMIA

Study (Ref.)	Year	N	Median Age (Range)	SCT	CR (%)	Early Death (%)	Survival (%)
CALGB 8811, USA (184)	1995	197	32 (16–80)	—	85	9	50 (3 yr)
CALGB 9111, USA (181)	1998	198	35 (16–83)	Ph+	82	8	43 (3 yr)
LALA 87, France (188)	2000	572	33 (15–60)	D	76	9	27 (10 yr)
GMALL 05/93, Germany (186)	2001	1163	35 (15–65)	R	83	NR	35 (5 yr)
JALSG-ALL93, Japan (191)	2002	263	31 (15–59)	D	78	6	33 (6 yr)
GIMEMA 0288, Italy (177)	2002	778	28 (12–60)	—	82	11	27 (9 y)
M.D. Anderson, USA (241)	2004	288	40 (15–92)	Ph+	92	5	38 (5 yr)
EORTC ALL-3, Europe (192)	2004	340	33 (14–79)	D	74	NR	36 (6 yr)
LALA 94, France (189)	2004	922	33 (15–55)	R	84	5	36 (5 yr)
Pethema ALL-93, Spain (193)	2005	222	27 (15–50)	HR	82	6	34 (5 yr)
MRC XII/ECOG E 2993, UK-USA (190)	2008	1913	31 (15–65)	D	91	NR	39 (5 yr)

SCT, stem cell transplant; HSCT, hematopoietic stem cell transplantation; ALL, acute lymphoblastic leukemia; Ph+, HSCT in Philadelphia–positive ALL; D, prospective HSCT in all patients with donor; R, HSCT according to prospective risk model; HR, prospective HSCT in high-risk patients only; NR, not reported.
[a]Median survival in months.

use of growth factors lessens the regimen-induced myelosuppression and may allow timely administration of treatment. In a randomized trial, the use of G-CSF during induction was associated with faster recovery of neutrophils and decreased hospital stay.[181] In the G-CSF treated group, the CR rate was higher (90% vs. 81%; P = .10), and the rate of induction deaths was lower (4% vs. 11%; P = .04).

Consolidation Therapy

Once in remission, consolidation is administered at a relatively higher level of intensity in efforts to further reduce the leukemic burden and decrease the likelihood of relapse. Consolidation may include rotational consolidation programs, modified induction regimens, or HSCT. Most regimens include methotrexate, cytarabine, cyclophosphamide, and asparaginase. But it is difficult to compare regimens as the number and schedule of the chemotherapy agents used vary. Results from the UKALL XA, GIMEMA ALL 0288, and PETHEMA (Programa para el Estudio de la Terapéutica en Hemopatía Maligna) ALL-89 multicenter randomized trials failed to demonstrate a benefit for intensification in terms of prolonging OS and DFS.[177,182,183] However, more recent nonrandomized studies and regimens using a risk-adapted strategy indicate that intensive consolidation may improve outcome.

In the CALGB 8811 study the induction course consisted of a five-drug combination and was followed by early and late intensification courses with eight drugs.[184] This regimen improved the median duration of CR and median survival to 29 and 36 months, respectively, considerably better than results with earlier trials.[184] A dose-intense regimen of hyperfractionated cyclophosphamide, vincristine, doxorubicin, and dexamethasone (hyper-CVAD), alternating with high doses of cytarabine and methotrexate, led to significantly higher CR rates and survival (P <.01)[178] when compared to the less-intense vincristine, doxorubicin, dexamethasone (VAD) regimen,[185] with an OS of 38% at 5 years.

Finally, the GMALL 05/93 study intensified consolidation in a subtype-specific manner. High-dose methotrexate was used in standard-risk B-lineage ALL, high-dose methotrexate and high-dose cytarabine in high-risk B-linage ALL, and cyclophosphamide and cytarabine in T-linage ALL. The CR rate was 87% in standard-risk patients, with a 5-year OS of 55%.[186] Intensified induction and consolidation improved the CR and DFS rates in a subset of high-risk patients with the pro-B ALL immunophenotype, in whom a continuous CR rate of 41% was achieved as compared to 19% for the others.[186]

Hematopoietic Stem Cell Transplantation for Acute Lymphoblastic Leukemia in First Remission

Allogeneic hematopoietic transplantation has a major role in the treatment of ALL, particularly in patients who have recurrent disease or poor risk features. The role of allogeneic HSCT for ALL patients in first CR is controversial. A review of a number of small, phase 2 trials in high-risk adult ALL who underwent allogeneic HSCT in first CR suggests a higher DFS when compared with historic controls based on conventional chemotherapy, ranging broadly from 21% to 71%.[187] Several, multicenter, randomized, prospective studies have been conducted (Table 131.12). To minimize patient selection bias, these trials employed a "genetic" randomization method, offering allogeneic HSCT in first CR to all patients with a sibling donor and chemotherapy or autologous HSCT to patients without a donor. Results were then analyzed using intent-to-treat methods that compared patients with or without donors.

The multicenter French study group Leucemie Aigue Lymphoblastique de l'Adulte completed two large studies between 1986 and 1991 (LALA-87)[188] and 1994 and 2002 (LALA-94).[189] Using an intent-to-treat analysis, a significant DFS and OS benefit was observed for allogeneic HSCT in high-risk patients in both trials. High-risk was defined as having one or more of the following factors: presence of the Ph chromosome, null ALL, age older than 35 years, WBC count greater than 30×10^9/L, or time to CR greater than 4 weeks. The international MRC UKALL XII/ECOG E2993 trial also noted significantly improved survival (53% vs. 45%) for patients who received an allogeneic HSCT in first CR as compared to chemotherapy or autologous HSCT.[190] However, in contrast to the LALA studies, this advantage was confined to the standard-risk patient subset (OS 63% vs. 51%) due to the high TRM observed in the high-risk group (39%) as compared to the standard-risk group (20%). Of note, high risk in this study was defined as age older than 35 or a high WBC (greater than 30,000 for B-lineage or greater than 100,000 for T-ALL); Ph+ patients were excluded in this analysis. In contrast to these three studies, no survival advantage was noted for allogeneic HSCT in first CR in three other multicenter, prospective studies.[191–193] In the EORTC ALL-3 trial, although the donor group had a lower relapse rate (38% vs. 56%; P = .001), it also had a higher cumulative incidence of death in CR (23% vs. 7%; P = .0004), resulting in similar survival rates (41% vs. 39%).[192] Finally, no survival advantage has ever been shown for autologous HSCT as compared to chemotherapy for patients who do not have a matched related donor.[188–190,192,193]

In addition to the transplant donor, the transplant preparative regimen, source of stem cells, and immunosuppression prophylaxis all impact treatment outcome. TBI remains the standard backbone for myeloablative ALL transplant preparative regimens. The most widely used regimen remains the combination of TBI and cyclophosphamide, although a retrospective analysis of registry data from the CIBMTR suggests that the combination of TBI and etoposide may afford better survival for patients in second CR when compared to cyclophosphamide and TBI.[194] Nonradiation-containing regimens, most commonly busulfan and cyclophosphamide, have been investigated in hopes of decreasing radiation-related complications, with no significant differences noted in outcome.[101,195]

As illustrated in the MRC UKALL XII/ECOG 2993 study, an increasing TRM rate with age compromises the antileukemia benefit for older patients.[190] Since the incidence of ALL increases in adults over age 50 years, transplant approaches with reduced TRM are needed. Reduced-intensity preparative regimens are under evaluation with a goal to reduce toxicity.

The EBMT reported results from the largest series of 97 adult patients with ALL treated with reduced-intensity conditioning (RIC) HSCT and confirmed the benefit of RIC for patients in remission, with a 2-year OS of 52% versus 27% for patients transplanted with advanced disease.[196] Smaller studies have corroborated the benefit for RIC transplantation for older patients with early stage ALL.[197–199] Marks et al.[195] compared transplant conditioning regimen intensity, myeloablative versus RIC, within the limitations of a retrospective analysis in patients with Ph-ALL receiving an allogeneic HSCT in first CR and second CR. Although regimen intensity did not impact TRM or relapse risk in a multivariate analysis, a significantly older patient population was able to tolerate RIC versus myeloablative conditioning (median age 45 years vs. 28 years; P <.001). Thus, RIC merits further investigation in prospective studies.

Maintenance Therapy

Maintenance therapy is administered to patients in remission after consolidation therapy at a low level of intensity, but for a protracted period of time. It has experienced the least modification over time. It consists of a backbone of daily 6-mercaptopurine, weekly methotrexate, and monthly pulses of vincristine and prednisone, generally administered for 2 to 3 years.[200] Attempts to omit maintenance, or shorten its duration to 12 to 18 months, have led to inferior results.[168] However, maintenance therapy is not necessary in mature B ALL, in which a high cure rate is achieved with short-term, dose-intense regimens. The best maintenance regimen for Ph+ patients is not clear but should include a TKI.

Many investigators recommend maintaining the WBC count below 3,000/mcL during maintenance. Transaminitis is commonly observed during this period and appears to be caused by the methylated metabolites of mercaptopurine. It is not necessary to alter the regimen because of liver enzyme elevation, as the transaminitis promptly resolves with completion of therapy.

Central Nervous System Prophylaxis

CNS prophylaxis can consist of intrathecal (IT) chemotherapy (methotrexate, cytarabine, corticosteroids), high-dose systemic chemotherapy (methotrexate, cytarabine, L-asparaginase), and CNS irradiation. Despite aggressive systemic therapy, the CNS remains a sanctuary site, and without specific meningeal-directed therapy, CNS disease will develop in up to 50% of adult patients.[13] Risk factors for CNS disease include elevated WBC or lactate dehydrogenase (LDH) at diagnosis, traumatic lumbar puncture, and T-lineage ALL phenotypes. Although some trials still rely on CNS irradiation, most treatment regimens are adopting a risk-adapted approach[201] and attempting to omit CNS irradiation[168] due to its many acute and late complications, including endocrinopathy, neurocognitive deficits, and secondary cancers.

Treatment of Specific Acute Lymphoblastic Leukemia Subgroups

Philadelphia Chromosome Positive Acute Lymphoblastic Leukemia

Historically, patients with Ph+ ALL have had a poor prognosis, with long-term DFS rates of 10% to 20%.[202] Allogeneic transplantation from a related or unrelated donor was widely used for consolidation, with 30% to 65% long-term survival for patients receiving HSCT in first CR.[203–205] Beyond first remission, HSCT was curative in only a small fraction of patients, with DFS ranging between 5% and 17%.[206]

However, the development of potent TKI of the tyrosine kinase activity of the BCR-ABL fusion product, resulting from the Philadelphia chromosome translocation, has revolutionized therapy for Ph-associated leukemias. Imatinib mesylate was the first TKI to demonstrate significant activity in patients with CML and Ph+ ALL,[207] although response duration in Ph+ ALL was short, with a median time to progression and median overall survival of 2.2 and 4.9 months, respectively. However, synergistic effects have been observed *in vitro* when imatinib has been combined with commonly used chemotherapy agents, and a number of studies have investigated the benefit of concurrent or sequential administration of imatinib with chemotherapy. Results from these trials suggest that the incorporation of imatinib into standard ALL therapy results in significantly improved remission induction rates, more patients being able to receive transplant in first remission, and ultimately, better overall survival rates[172–174,208] (Table 131.13). Furthermore, some data suggest that TKI used as maintenance following transplant helps to improve outcome in patients who are free of transplant-related complications and are able to take TKIs.[209] Whether consolidation with HSCT in first CR will remain the standard of care for these patients will depend on the durability of the remission inductions, which is currently under investigation. A national multicenter trial is currently in progress in which patients with Ph+ ALL were prospectively randomized to continued chemotherapy or allogeneic transplants in an effort to determine the best route of consolidation for these patients.

The role of imatinib in the treatment of elderly patients with Ph+ ALL is of particular interest. This is a group with a historically poor outcome due to poor tolerance of the standard chemotherapy regimens and disease resistance. Several trials have examined various approaches in this population. Use of imatinib and methylprednisolone alternated with chemotherapy improved the CR rate and OS at 1 year in 30 patients older than 55 years as compared to historical controls (72% vs. 29% and 66% vs. 44%, respectively).[210] More impressive was a 100% CR noted among 29 patients, with median age 60 years, ranging from 61 to 83 years, who were treated with a combination of imatinib and prednisone only. The median survival from diagnosis was 20 months.[211] Finally, Ottmann et al.[212] conducted a randomized trial of imatinib monotherapy versus standard induction therapy followed by imatinib plus standard consolidation chemotherapy for all patients. Fifty-five patients with a median age of 67 years were treated. The imatinib-treated arm had a significantly higher CR rate (96% vs. 50%) with less regimen-related toxicity as compared to the standard induction arm, however, there was no significant difference in OS between the two arms (42% at 2 years).

The development of resistance to imatinib has led to the search for alternative, second generation TKI such as dasatinib and nilotinib.[213,214] Dasatinib is a dual Src and Abl kinase inhibitor that has shown significant activity in patients with

TABLE 131.13

SELECTED PROSPECTIVE TRIALS INCORPORATING IMATINIB THERAPY IN Ph+ ACUTE LYMPHOBLASTIC LEUKEMIA

Study Imatinib (IM) vs. No Imatinib (Ref.)	Year	N	Median Age (Range)	CR (%) (Historical)	Survival (%) (Historical)
IM vs. no IM (208)	2005	29	36 (18–55)	79 (82)	78, 3 yr (39)
JALSG-ALL202 (172) vs. JALSG-ALL93 (191)	2006	80	48 (15–63)	96 (51)	76, 1 yr (44)
GRAAPH 2003 (174) vs. LALA 94 (189)	2007	45	45 (16–59)	96 (71)	65, 1.5 yr (39)
HyperCVAD+IM (173, 242) vs. HyperCVAD (241)	2008	45	15 (17–84)	93 (92)	55, 3 yr (15)

CR, complete remission; HyperCVAD, fractionated cyclophosphamide, vincristine, doxorubican, dexamethasone.

imatinib-resistant disease.[215–217] The significant activity of dasatinib has prompted investigation of its use in front-line regimens. The follow-up of these trials is currently too short to make meaningful conclusions, but early response rates suggest a higher rate of molecular remissions when compared to imatinib.[218]

Mature B-Lineage Acute Lymphoblastic Leukemia

Treatment of Burkitt's leukemia or lymphoma with the conventional ALL regimens have been disappointing. Short-duration, intensive regimens that maintain serum drug concentrations and minimize treatment delays have demonstrated the greatest efficacy in this disease, mainly due to its high growth fraction.[219] These regimens incorporate strategies such as the use of fractionated cyclophosphamide, alternation of non–cross-resistant cytotoxic agents between treatment cycles, and aggressive CNS prophylaxis.[220] More recently, the addition of the anti-CD20 monoclonal antibody rituximab has further improved the outcome of patients with Burkitt's leukemia or lymphoma. Thomas et al.[221] administered rituximab in addition to the hyper-CVAD regimen and reported a CR rate of 86%, with 3-year OS of 89%. This was significantly better than the 19% 3-year survival reported for hyper-CVAD alone.

T-Cell Acute Lymphoblastic Leukemia and T-Lymphoblastic Lymphoma

The survival of patients with T-cell ALL and T-lymphoblastic lymphoma (T-LBL) has improved significantly using the regimens designed for ALL, with OS ranging from 50% to 70%.[222] Use of mediastinal radiation given after chemotherapy appears to reduce mediastinal relapse. A proportion of patients with relapsed disease can achieve a second CR and long-term survival with allogeneic stem cell transplant. Compared to patients with B-lineage ALL, the spectrum of genetic abnormalities in T-cell ALL is less well characterized; FISH or PCR testing is required to detect the higher rate of cryptic chromosomal translocations and gene mutations in T-cell ALL. Subset analysis of T-cell ALL patients treated on the MRC/UKALL trial revealed complex cytogenetics, CD13 positivity, and CD1a negativity to be associated with poorer outcome.[223] Greater understanding of the molecular pathogenesis of this subset of ALL has led to the development of novel therapies, such as nelarabine and forodesine,[224] developed specifically towards neoplastic T-cells, and gamma-secretase and TKIs developed specifically toward aberrant pathways.[155,157] In CALBG study 19801, 26 patients with relapsed T-cell ALL received nelarabine at 1.5 g/m^2/d on days 1, 3, and 5 repeated every 22 days, with a median number of two courses administered.[225] A relatively high CR rate of 31% was noted in this heavily treated group of patients, suggesting that nelarabine induces cytotoxicity through therapeutic pathways different from that of currently used standard drugs. Furthermore, the median DFS was 20 weeks, which should allow sufficient time for a select group of patients with a preserved performance status to proceed to transplant (approximately one-third of patients progressed to transplant in this study). The most common nonhematologic toxicity noted in the study was reversible peripheral sensory and motor neuropathy.[225] Unfortunately, many of the commonly used agents for ALL therapy, such as vincristine and methotrexate, also have neuropathic toxicities, so nelarabine use remains limited.

Treatment of Primary Refractory or Relapsed Adult Acute Lymphoblastic Leukemia

Most current induction regimens obtain complete responses in 72% to 92% of newly diagnosed patients. Early deaths account for some of the induction failures, but in most studies 5% to 10% of patients have disease that is resistant to the remission induction regimen. These patients often have poor prognostic factors at presentation, and additional attempts at induction chemotherapy may be unsuccessful. Several studies suggest that patients with an HLA-identical sibling benefit if they proceed directly to allogeneic transplantation without undergoing a second attempt at induction therapy.[117,226] In the largest of these studies, approximately 35% of these patients with primary refractory disease became long-term disease-free survivors.[227]

In addition to primary refractory patients, 60% to 70% of patients who achieve a complete response eventually relapse. Numerous regimens have been reported in the setting of relapsed ALL. These can be divided into two main groups: those that repeat the regimens used for newly diagnosed patients and those that involve high-dose, typically cytarabine-based regimens, with no superior reinduction therapy identified. Cytarabine has been used in combination with L-asparaginase, anthracyclines, or mitoxantrone, with responses as high as 72%.[228,229] However, these are transient, short-lived responses, and allogeneic HSCT remains the most effective modality for achieving durable remissions for patients in/or beyond second CR. Two large multicenter trials have best characterized prognosis and outcome following relapse. The outcome of 609 adults with relapsed ALL, all of whom were previously treated on the MRC UKALL12/ECOG 2993 study, was investigated.[230] The survival at 5 years after relapse was 7%. Factors predicting a good outcome after salvage therapy were young age (OS 12% for patients older than 20 years vs. 3% for patients older than 50 years) and duration of first remission greater than 2 years (OS 11% vs. 5%). When survival was evaluated based on treatment strategy, survival following HSCT ranged from 15% to 23% depending on donor type (15% for autograft, 16% for matched unrelated donor, 23% for matched related donor), and was significantly better than chemotherapy only at 4% ($P < .00005$).[230] Oriol et al.[231] reported on the outcome of 263 adults with relapsed ALL, all of whom were previously treated on four consecutive PETHEMA trials with similar induction therapies. Overall survival at 5 years was 10%. Factors predicting a good outcome were identical to the prior study: age less than 30 years (OS 21% vs. 10%) and duration of first remission greater than 2 years (OS 36% vs. 17%). Forty-five percent of patients achieved a second remission, with better outcome noted in the group who then proceeded to transplant. The best outcome was noted for patients younger than 30 years old with a long first remission duration transplanted in second CR, with an OS of 38% at 5 years. TRM was higher for patients who had received a prior transplant during first remission (TRM 45% vs. 23%), but there was no difference in OS. Similar long-term leukemia-free survival rates of 14% to 43% have been reported from other small series for patients who received HSCT in second CR. As expected, the primary cause of failure is relapse (greater than 50%).

CNS relapse occurs in approximately 2% to 10% of patients who have received appropriate prophylaxis. In the majority of patients, concurrent bone marrow relapse can be documented. Occasionally CNS relapse may occur without demonstrable systemic relapse; however, this event almost always predicts subsequent bone marrow relapse, and patients with isolated CNS relapse should first receive CNS-directed therapy and then systemic reinduction chemotherapy. Long-term outcome is poor, with 0% to 6% OS at 4 years.[230] Intensive treatment, with a combination of intrathecal or radiotherapy and systemic chemotherapy, followed by consolidation with HSCT may improve results.

Selected References

The full list of references for this chapter appears in the online version.

1. Fialkow PJ, Janssen JW, Bartram CR. Clonal remissions in acute nonlymphocytic leukemia: evidence for a multistep pathogenesis of the malignancy. *Blood* 1991;77(7):1415.
2. Reya T, et al. Stem cells, cancer, and cancer stem cells. *Nature* 2001;414 (6859):105.
4. Pui CH, et al. Acute myeloid leukemia in children treated with epipodophyllotoxins for acute lymphoblastic leukemia. *N Engl J Med* 1991;325 (24):1682.
9. Cheson BD, et al. Report of the National Cancer Institute–sponsored workshop on definitions of diagnosis and response in acute myeloid leukemia. *J Clin Oncol* 1990;8(5):813.
10. Bennett JM, et al. The morphological classification of acute lymphoblastic leukaemia: concordance among observers and clinical correlations. *Br J Haematol* 1981;47(4):553.
11. Harris NL, et al. World Health Organization classification of neoplastic diseases of the hematopoietic and lymphoid tissues: report of the Clinical Advisory Committee meeting, Airlie House, Virginia, November 1997. *J Clin Oncol* 1999;17(12):3835.
15. Downing JR. The core-binding factor leukemias: lessons learned from murine models. *Curr Opin Genet Dev* 2003;13(1):48.
17. Thiede C, et al. Analysis of FLT3-activating mutations in 979 patients with acute myelogenous leukemia: association with FAB subtypes and identification of subgroups with poor prognosis. *Blood* 2002;99(12):4326.
19. Falini B, et al. Cytoplasmic nucleophosmin in acute myelogenous leukemia with a normal karyotype. *N Engl J Med* 2005;352(3):254.
21. Schnittger S, et al. Nucleophosmin gene mutations are predictors of favorable prognosis in acute myelogenous leukemia with a normal karyotype. *Blood* 2005;106(12):3733.
24. Frohling S, et al. CEBPA mutations in younger adults with acute myeloid leukemia and normal cytogenetics: prognostic relevance and analysis of cooperating mutations. *J Clin Oncol* 2004;22(4):624.
25. Caligiuri MA, et al. Rearrangement of ALL1 (MLL) in acute myeloid leukemia with normal cytogenetics. *Cancer Res* 1998;58(1):55.
27. Marcucci G, et al. Overexpression of the ETS-related gene, ERG, predicts a worse outcome in acute myeloid leukemia with normal karyotype: a Cancer and Leukemia Group B study. *J Clin Oncol* 2005;23(36):9234.
28. Bullinger L, et al. Use of gene-expression profiling to identify prognostic subclasses in adult acute myeloid leukemia. *N Engl J Med* 2004;350(16):1605.
29. Appelbaum FR, et al. Age and acute myeloid leukemia. *Blood* 2006;107(9): 3481.
30. Cheson BD, et al. Revised recommendations of the International Working Group for Diagnosis, Standardization of Response Criteria, Treatment Outcomes, and Reporting Standards for Therapeutic Trials in Acute Myeloid Leukemia. *J Clin Oncol* 2003;21(24):4642.
31. Buchner T, et al. 6-Thioguanine, cytarabine, and daunorubicin (TAD) and high-dose cytarabine and mitoxantrone (HAM) for induction, TAD for consolidation, and either prolonged maintenance by reduced monthly TAD or TAD-HAM-TAD and one course of intensive consolidation by sequential HAM in adult patients at all ages with de novo acute myeloid leukemia (AML): a randomized trial of the German AML Cooperative Group. *J Clin Oncol* 2003;21(24):4496.
33. Fernandez HF, et al. Anthracycline dose intensification in acute myeloid leukemia. *N Engl J Med* 2009;361(13):1249.
34. Lowenberg B, et al. High-dose daunorubicin in older patients with acute myeloid leukemia. *N Engl J Med* 2009; 361(13):1235.
35. Bloomfield CD, et al. Frequency of prolonged remission duration after high-dose cytarabine intensification in acute myeloid leukemia varies by cytogenetic subtype. *Cancer Res* 1998;58(18):4173.
36. Grimwade D, et al. The importance of diagnostic cytogenetics on outcome in AML: analysis of 1,612 patients entered into the MRC AML 10 trial. The Medical Research Council Adult and Children's Leukaemia Working Parties. *Blood* 1998;92(7):2322.
38. Byrd JC, et al. Repetitive cycles of high-dose cytarabine benefit patients with acute myeloid leukemia and inv(16)(p13q22) or t(16;16)(p13;q22): results from CALGB 8461. *J Clin Oncol* 2004;22(6):1087.
39. Schlenk RF, et al. Individual patient data-based meta-analysis of patients aged 16 to 60 years with core binding factor acute myeloid leukemia: a survey of the German Acute Myeloid Leukemia Intergroup. *J Clin Oncol* 2004;22(18):3741.
41. Paschka P, et al. Adverse prognostic significance of KIT mutations in adult acute myeloid leukemia with inv(16) and t(8;21): a Cancer and Leukemia Group B study. *J Clin Oncol* 2006;24(24):3904.
43. Bradstock KF, et al. A randomized trial of high-versus conventional-dose cytarabine in consolidation chemotherapy for adult de novo acute myeloid leukemia in first remission after induction therapy containing high-dose cytarabine. *Blood* 2005;105(2):481.
45. Acute myeloid leukemia. Clinical practice guidelines in oncology. *J Natl Compr Canc Netw* 2003;1(4):520.
46. Farag SS, et al. Pretreatment cytogenetics add to other prognostic factors predicting complete remission and long-term outcome in patients 60 years of age or older with acute myeloid leukemia: results from Cancer and Leukemia Group B 8461. *Blood* 2006;108(1):63.
47. Estey EH, et al. Comparison of idarubicin + ara-C−, fludarabine + ara-C−, and topotecan + ara-C–based regimens in treatment of newly diagnosed acute myeloid leukemia, refractory anemia with excess blasts in transformation, or refractory anemia with excess blasts. *Blood* 2001;98(13):3575.
48. Mayer RJ, et al. Intensive postremission chemotherapy in adults with acute myeloid leukemia. Cancer and Leukemia Group B. *N Engl J Med* 1994;331(14):896.
50. Tilly H, et al. Low-dose cytarabine versus intensive chemotherapy in the treatment of acute nonlymphocytic leukemia in the elderly. *J Clin Oncol* 1990;8(2):272.
51. Estey EH, et al. Experience with gemtuzumab ozogamycin ("mylotarg") and all-trans retinoic acid in untreated acute promyelocytic leukemia. *Blood* 2002;99(11):4222.
57. Avvisati G, et al. Induction therapy with idarubicin alone significantly influences event-free survival duration in patients with newly diagnosed hypergranular acute promyelocytic leukemia: final results of the GIMEMA randomized study LAP 0389 with 7 years of minimal follow-up. *Blood* 2002;100(9):3141.
60. Asou N, et al. A randomized study with or without intensified maintenance chemotherapy in patients with acute promyelocytic leukemia who have become negative for PML-RARalpha transcript after consolidation therapy: the Japan Adult Leukemia Study Group (JALSG) APL97 study. *Blood* 2007;110(1):59.
65. Ravandi F, et al. Effective treatment of acute promyelocytic leukemia with all-trans-retinoic acid, arsenic trioxide, and gemtuzumab ozogamicin. *J Clin Oncol* 2009;27(4):504.
66. Faderl S, et al. Clofarabine and cytarabine combination as induction therapy for acute myeloid leukemia (AML) in patients 50 years of age or older. *Blood* 2006;108(1):45.
69. Egger G, et al. Epigenetics in human disease and prospects for epigenetic therapy. *Nature* 2004;429(6990):457.
83. Estey E, et al. A stratification system for evaluating and selecting therapies in patients with relapsed or primary refractory acute myelogenous leukemia. *Blood* 1996;88(2):756.
87. Schlenk RF, et al. Mutations and treatment outcome in cytogenetically normal acute myeloid leukemia. *N Engl J Med* 2008;358(18):1909.
89. Duval M, Klein JP, He W, et al. Hematopoietic stem cell transplantation for acute leukemia in relapse or primary induction failure. *J Clin Oncol* 2010;28(23):3730.
92. Thomas ED, et al. One hundred patients with acute leukemia treated by chemotherapy, total body irradiation, and allogeneic marrow transplantation. *Blood* 1977;49(4):511.
93. Santos GW, et al. Marrow transplantation for acute nonlymphocytic leukemia after treatment with busulfan and cyclophosphamide. *N Engl J Med* 1983;309(22):1347.
94. Andersson BS, et al. Once daily I.V. busulfan and fludarabine (I.V. Bu-Flu) compares favorably with I.V. busulfan and cyclophosphamide (I.V. BuCy2) as pretransplant conditioning therapy in AML/MDS. *Biol Blood Marrow Transplant* 2008;14(6):672.
96. Tutschka PJ, Copelan EA, Klein JP. Bone marrow transplantation for leukemia following a new busulfan and cyclophosphamide regimen. *Blood* 1987;70(5):1382.
97. Andersson BS, et al. Conditioning therapy with intravenous busulfan and cyclophosphamide (IV BuCy2) for hematologic malignancies prior to allogeneic stem cell transplantation: a phase II study. *Biol Blood Marrow Transplant* 2002;8(3):145.
99. Blaise D, et al. Long-term follow-up of a randomized trial comparing the combination of cyclophosphamide with total body irradiation or busulfan as conditioning regimen for patients receiving HLA-identical marrow grafts for acute myeloblastic leukemia in first complete remission. *Blood* 2001;97(11):3669.
101. Blume KG, et al. A prospective randomized comparison of total body irradiation-etoposide versus busulfan-cyclophosphamide as preparatory regimens for bone marrow transplantation in patients with leukemia who were not in first remission: a Southwest Oncology Group study. *Blood* 1993;81(8):2187.
102. de Lima M, et al. Nonablative versus reduced-intensity conditioning regimens in the treatment of acute myeloid leukemia and high-risk myelodysplastic syndrome: dose is relevant for long-term disease control after allogeneic hematopoietic stem cell transplantation. *Blood* 2004;104(3):865.
107. Suciu S, et al. Allogeneic compared with autologous stem cell transplantation in the treatment of patients younger than 46 years with acute myeloid leukemia (AML) in first complete remission (CR1): an intention-to-treat analysis of the EORTC/GIMEMAAML-10 trial. *Blood* 2003;102(4):1232.
111. Cornelissen JJ, et al. Results of a HOVON/SAKK donor versus no-donor analysis of myeloablative HLA-identical sibling stem cell transplantation

in first remission acute myeloid leukemia in young and middle-aged adults: benefits for whom? *Blood* 2007;109(9):3658.

112. Estey E, et al. Prospective feasibility analysis of reduced-intensity conditioning (RIC) regimens for hematopoietic stem cell transplantation (HSCT) in elderly patients with acute myeloid leukemia (AML) and high-risk myelodysplastic syndrome (MDS). *Blood* 2007;109(4):1395.
114. Champlin R. Purging: the separation of normal from malignant cells for autologous transplantation. *Transfusion* 1996;36(10):910.
116. Koreth J, et al. Allogeneic stem cell transplantation for acute myeloid leukemia in first complete remission: systematic review and meta-analysis of prospective clinical trials. *JAMA* 2009;301(22):2349.
119. Armistead PM, et al. Quantifying the survival benefit for allogeneic hematopoietic stem cell transplantation in relapsed acute myelogenous leukemia. *Biol Blood Marrow Transplant* 2009;15(11):1431.
122. Slavin S, et al. Nonmyeloablative stem cell transplantation and cell therapy as an alternative to conventional bone marrow transplantation with lethal cytoreduction for the treatment of malignant and nonmalignant hematologic diseases. *Blood* 1998;91(3):756.
123. Giralt S, et al. Melphalan and purine analog-containing preparative regimens: reduced-intensity conditioning for patients with hematologic malignancies undergoing allogeneic progenitor cell transplantation. *Blood* 2001;97(3):631.
125. Oran B, et al. Allogeneic hematopoietic stem cell transplantation for the treatment of high-risk acute myelogenous leukemia and myelodysplastic syndrome using reduced-intensity conditioning with fludarabine and melphalan. *Biol Blood Marrow Transplant* 2007;13(4):454.
127. de Lima M, Giralt S, Caldera Z, et al. Results of a phase I/II study of gemtuzumab ozogamicin added to fludarabine (F), melphalan (M) and allogeneic hematopoietic stem cell transplantation (HSCT) for relapsed myeloid leukemias [abstract]. *Blood (ASH Annual Meeting Abstracts)* 2005, 106: (abst 841).
132. Rocha V, et al. Transplants of umbilical-cord blood or bone marrow from unrelated donors in adults with acute leukemia. *N Engl J Med* 2004;351(22): 2276.
134. Aversa F, et al. Treatment of high-risk acute leukemia with T-cell-depleted stem cells from related donors with one fully mismatched HLA haplotype. *N Engl J Med* 1998;339(17):1186.
138. Vago L, et al. Loss of mismatched HLA in leukemia after stem-cell transplantation. *N Engl J Med* 2009;361(5):478.
139. Cairo MS, et al. NCI first international workshop on the biology, prevention, and treatment of relapse after allogeneic hematopoietic stem cell transplantation: report from the committee on the biological considerations of hematological relapse following allogeneic stem cell transplantation unrelated to graft-versus-tumor effects: state of the science. *Biol Blood Marrow Transplant* 2010;16(6):709.
146. Moorman AV, et al. Karyotype is an independent prognostic factor in adult acute lymphoblastic leukemia (ALL): analysis of cytogenetic data from patients treated on the Medical Research Council (MRC) UKALLXII/Eastern Cooperative Oncology Group (ECOG) 2993 trial. *Blood* 2007;109(8):3189.
149. Faderl S, et al. Clinical significance of cytogenetic abnormalities in adult acute lymphoblastic leukemia. *Blood* 1998;91(11):3995.
150. Bruggemann M, et al. Clinical significance of minimal residual disease quantification in adult patients with standard-risk acute lymphoblastic leukemia. *Blood* 2006;107(3):1116.
152. Ebert BL, Golub TR. Genomic approaches to hematologic malignancies. *Blood* 2004;104(4):923.
154. Mullighan CG, et al. Genome-wide analysis of genetic alterations in acute lymphoblastic leukaemia. *Nature* 2007;446(7137):758.
162. Evans WE, Relling MV. Moving towards individualized medicine with pharmacogenomics. *Nature* 2004;429(6990):464.
165. Garcia-Manero G, et al. Epigenetics of acute lymphocytic leukemia. *Semin Hematol* 2009;46(1):24.
167. Issa JP. DNA methylation as a therapeutic target in cancer. *Clin Cancer Res* 2007;13(6):1634.
168. Pui CH, Evans WE. Treatment of acute lymphoblastic leukemia. *N Engl J Med* 2006;354(2):166.
172. Yanada M, et al. High complete remission rate and promising outcome by combination of imatinib and chemotherapy for newly diagnosed BCR-ABL-positive acute lymphoblastic leukemia: a phase II study by the Japan Adult Leukemia Study Group. *J Clin Oncol* 2006;24(3):460.
173. Thomas DA, et al. Treatment of Philadelphia chromosome-positive acute lymphocytic leukemia with hyper-CVAD and imatinib mesylate. *Blood* 2004;103(12):4396.
174. de Labarthe A, et al. Imatinib combined with induction or consolidation chemotherapy in patients with de novo Philadelphia chromosome-positive acute lymphoblastic leukemia: results of the GRAAPH-2003 study. *Blood* 2007;109(4):1408.
177. Annino L, et al. Treatment of adult acute lymphoblastic leukemia (ALL): long-term follow-up of the GIMEMA ALL 0288 randomized study. *Blood* 2002;99(3):863.
180. DeAngelo DJ. The treatment of adolescents and young adults with acute lymphoblastic leukemia. *Hematol Am Soc Hematol Educ Program* 2005:123.
181. Larson RA, et al. A randomized controlled trial of filgrastim during remission induction and consolidation chemotherapy for adults with acute lymphoblastic leukemia: CALGB study 9111. *Blood* 1998;92(5):1556.
184. Larson RA, et al. A five-drug remission induction regimen with intensive consolidation for adults with acute lymphoblastic leukemia: Cancer and Leukemia Group B study 8811. *Blood* 1995;85(8):2025.
187. Chao NJ, et al. Allogeneic bone marrow transplantation for high-risk acute lymphoblastic leukemia during first complete remission. *Blood* 1991;78(8):1923.
189. Thomas X, et al. Outcome of treatment in adults with acute lymphoblastic leukemia: analysis of the LALA-94 trial. *J Clin Oncol* 2004;22(20):4075.
190. Goldstone AH, et al. In adults with standard-risk acute lymphoblastic leukemia, the greatest benefit is achieved from a matched sibling allogeneic transplantation in first complete remission, and an autologous transplantation is less effective than conventional consolidation/maintenance chemotherapy in all patients: final results of the International ALL Trial (MRC UKALL XII/ECOG E2993). *Blood* 2008;111(4):1827.
191. Takeuchi J, et al. Induction therapy by frequent administration of doxorubicin with four other drugs, followed by intensive consolidation and maintenance therapy for adult acute lymphoblastic leukemia: the JALSG-ALL93 study. *Leukemia* 2002;16(7):1259.
192. Labar B, et al. Allogeneic stem cell transplantation in acute lymphoblastic leukemia and non-Hodgkin's lymphoma for patients < or = 50 years old in first complete remission: results of the EORTC ALL-3 trial. *Haematologica* 2004;89(7):809.
195. Marks DI, et al. The outcome of full intensity and reduced intensity conditioning matched sibling or unrelated donor (URD) transplantation in adults with Philadelphia chromosome negative acute lymphoblastic leukemia (PH-ALL) in first and second complete remission (CR1 and CR2). *Blood* 2010;116(3):366.
196. Mohty M, et al. Reduced intensity conditioning allogeneic stem cell transplantation for adult patients with acute lymphoblastic leukemia: a retrospective study from the European Group for Blood and Marrow Transplantation. *Haematologica* 2008;93(2):303.
201. Cortes J, et al. The value of high-dose systemic chemotherapy and intrathecal therapy for central nervous system prophylaxis in different risk groups of adult acute lymphoblastic leukemia. *Blood* 1995;86(6):2091.
202. Wetzler M, et al. Prospective karyotype analysis in adult acute lymphoblastic leukemia: the Cancer and Leukemia Group B experience. *Blood* 1999;93(11):3983.
203. Laport GG, et al. Long-term remission of Philadelphia chromosome-positive acute lymphoblastic leukemia after allogeneic hematopoietic cell transplantation from matched sibling donors: a 20-year experience with the fractionated total body irradiation-etoposide regimen. *Blood* 2008;112(3):903.
210. Delannoy A, et al. Imatinib and methylprednisolone alternated with chemotherapy improve the outcome of elderly patients with Philadelphia-positive acute lymphoblastic leukemia: results of the GRAALL AFR09 study. *Leukemia* 2006;20(9):1526.
216. Ottmann O, et al. Dasatinib induces rapid hematologic and cytogenetic responses in adult patients with Philadelphia chromosome positive acute lymphoblastic leukemia with resistance or intolerance to imatinib: interim results of a phase 2 study. *Blood* 2007;110(7):2309.
218. Ravandi F, O'Brien S, Thomas D, et al. The first report of phase II study of combination of hyper-CVAD with dasatinib in frontline therapy of patients with Philadelphia chromosome positive acute lymphoblastic leukemia. *Blood* 2010;116(12):2070.
221. Thomas DA, et al. Chemoimmunotherapy with hyper-CVAD plus rituximab for the treatment of adult Burkitt and Burkitt-type lymphoma or acute lymphoblastic leukemia. *Cancer* 2006;106(7):1569.
223. Marks DI, et al. T-cell acute lymphoblastic leukemia in adults: clinical features, immunophenotype, cytogenetics, and outcome from the large randomized prospective trial (UKALL XII/ECOG 2993). *Blood* 2009;114 (25):5136.
224. Ravandi F, Gandhi V. Novel purine nucleoside analogues for T-cell-lineage acute lymphoblastic leukaemia and lymphoma. *Expert Opin Invest Drugs* 2006;15(12):1601.
225. DeAngelo DJ, et al. Nelarabine induces complete remissions in adults with relapsed or refractory T-lineage acute lymphoblastic leukemia or lymphoblastic lymphoma: Cancer and Leukemia Group B study 19801. *Blood* 2007;109(12):5136.
226. Terwey TH, et al. Allogeneic SCT in refractory or relapsed adult ALL is effective without prior reinduction chemotherapy. *Bone Marrow Transplant* 2008;42(12):791.
230. Fielding AK, et al. Outcome of 609 adults after relapse of acute lymphoblastic leukemia (ALL); an MRC UKALL12/ECOG 2993 study. *Blood* 2007;109(3):944.
231. Oriol A, et al. Outcome after relapse of acute lymphoblastic leukemia in adult patients included in four consecutive risk-adapted trials by the PETHEMA Study Group. *Haematologica* 2010;95(4):589.
235. Estey EH, et al. Gemtuzumab ozogamicin with or without interleukin 11 in patients 65 years of age or older with untreated acute myeloid leukemia and high-risk myelodysplastic syndrome: comparison with idarubicin plus continuous-infusion, high-dose cytosine arabinoside. *Blood* 2002;99(12):4343.
236. Burnett AK, et al. Randomised comparison of addition of autologous bone-marrow transplantation to intensive chemotherapy for acute myeloid leukaemia in first remission: results of MRC AML 10 trial. UK Medical Research Council Adult and Children's Leukaemia Working Parties. *Lancet* 1998;351(9104):700.

CHAPTER 132 MOLECULAR BIOLOGY OF CHRONIC LEUKEMIAS

ANUPRIYA AGARWAL, JOHN C. BYRD, AND MICHAEL W. DEININGER

Chronic myeloid leukemia (CML) and chronic lymphocytic leukemia (CLL) are very different diseases and yet share important clinical features. Both are usually diagnosed in an indolent stage characterized by expansion of differentiating cells that can last for several, sometimes many years. In both, the acquisition of additional mutations promotes progression to advanced therapy-refractory disease and both are incurable with currently available drug therapy. In this chapter, we will discuss the key pathogenetic mechanisms of CML and CLL, with emphasis on recent data and potential therapeutic implications.

CHRONIC MYELOID LEUKEMIA

CML is caused by BCR-ABL, a constitutively active tyrosine kinase generated as the result of a reciprocal translocation between chromosomes 9 and 22. The annual incidence of CML is 1.3 to $1.5/10^5$, with a slight male preponderance, but no significant differences across ethnicities. The only established CML risk factor is exposure to ionizing radiation, evident from studies in survivors of the nuclear explosions in Japan and patients exposed to thorotrast or radiotherapy. During the initial chronic phase (CP) cellular differentiation and function are largely maintained, therapy is effective and mortality is low. Without effective treatment the disease invariably progresses to blastic phase (BP), a rapidly fatal acute myeloid or lymphoid leukemia.

Pathogenesis

The first cases of what was probably CML were described by Bennett and Virchow in the mid 1840s.[1] In 1960, Philadelphia cytogeneticists Nowell and Hungerford[2] described a "minute" chromosome 22 in CML cells that became known as the *Philadelphia chromosome* (Ph). In 1973, Janet Rowley[3] discovered that Ph is in fact the result of a reciprocal translocation between chromosomes 9 and 22 [t(9;22) (q34;q11)]. The genes juxtaposed by the translocation were subsequently identified as *ABL* (Abelson) on 9q34[4] and breakpoint cluster region (*BCR*) on chromosome 22q11 (Fig. 132.1). The next critical discoveries were that the constitutive tyrosine kinase activity of BCR-ABL is required for cellular transformation and that the clinical disease was reproducible in a murine model.[5,6] According to the World Health Organization the presence of BCR-ABL in the context of a myeloproliferative neoplasm is diagnostic of CML, although the translocation is also found in a subset of patients with acute lymphoblastic leukemia (ALL) and rare cases of acute myeloid leukemia (AML).

Molecular Anatomy of the BCR-ABL Junction

The breakpoints within *ABL* occur upstream of exon 1b, downstream of exon 1a, or, more frequently, between the two. Regardless of the exact breakpoint location, splicing of the primary transcript yields an mRNA in which *BCR* sequences are fused to *ABL* exon a2. Breakpoints within *BCR* localize to one of three breakpoint cluster regions (*bcr*). More than 90% of CML patients and one-third of Ph+ ALL patients express the 210kDa isoform of BCR-ABL, in which the break occurs in the 5.8-kb major breakpoint cluster region (M-*bcr*), which spans exons e12-e16 (formerly exons b1-b5). Alternative splicing gives rise to either b2a2 (e13a2) or b3a2 (e14a2) transcripts.[5] In remaining Ph+ ALL patients and in rare CML cases, the breakpoints are further upstream in the 54.4-kb minor breakpoint cluster region (m-*bcr*), generating an e1a2 transcript that is translated into $p190^{BCR\text{-}ABL}$.[7] A third breakpoint downstream of exon 19 in the micro breakpoint cluster region (μ-*bcr*) gives rise to an e19a2 *BCR-ABL* mRNA and $p230^{BCR\text{-}ABL}$ and is associated with neutrophilia.

Other BCR-ABL variants, including b2a3, b3a3, e1a3, e6a2 or e2a2, have been observed in isolated cases.[8] Deletions flanking the breakpoints are detected in a subset of patients, which confer a poor prognosis to patients on interferon therapy, but probably not on imatinib.[9–11] The reciprocal ABL-BCR transcript, although detectable in approximately two-thirds of patients, does not seem to play any significant role in pathogenesis.[12]

Functional Domains of BCR-ABL and Kinase Activation

$p210^{BCR\text{-}ABL}$ contains several distinct domains (Fig. 132.2).[13] The N-terminal coiled-coil domain of BCR allows BCR-ABL dimerization, which is critical for kinase activation. The $p210^{BCR\text{-}ABL}$ protein also retains the serine/threonine kinase and Rho guanine nucleotide exchange factor homology (Rho-GEF) domains of BCR, which are deleted in $p190^{BCR\text{-}ABL}$, which may explain the differences in disease phenotype associated with the two variants. In contrast to BCR, the ABL sequence is almost completely retained, including SRC homology domains 2 and 3, the tyrosine kinase domain, a proline-rich sequence, and a large C terminus with nuclear localization signal, DNA-binding, and actin-binding domains. The N-terminal "cap" region of ABL negatively regulates kinase activity by binding to a hydrophobic pocket at the basis of the kinase domain, which in the Ib isoform is mediated by N-terminal myristoylation. It is believed that the replacement of the cap with BCR sequences contributes to constitutive kinase activation.

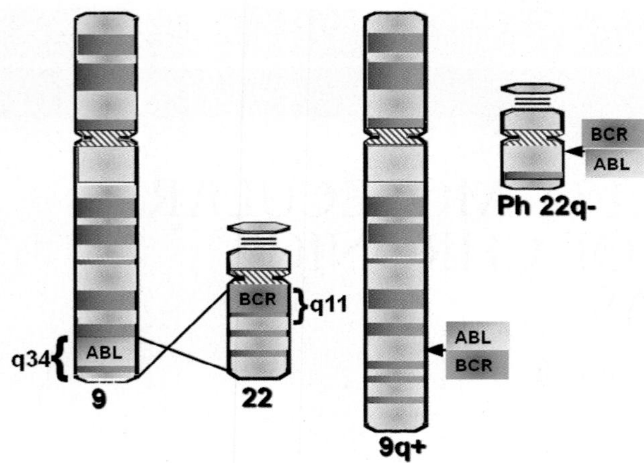

FIGURE 132.1 Schematic representation of the t(9;22)(q34;q11) translocation that creates the Philadelphia (Ph) chromosome. The *ABL* and *BCR* genes reside on the long arms of chromosome 9 and 22, respectively. As a result of the (9;22) translocation, the *BCR-ABL* gene is formed on the derivative of chromosome of 22 (22q–, Ph chromosome), while the reciprocal *ABL-BCR* resides on the derivative of 9q+.

Signal Transduction

Numerous substrates and binding partners of BCR-ABL have been identified (Fig. 132.2). Current efforts are directed at linking these pathways to the specific phenotypic defects that characterize CML, such as increased proliferation, decreased apoptosis, defective adhesion to bone marrow stroma, and genetic instability.[14] As comprehensive review of the multiple implicated pathways is beyond the scope of this chapter, we will focus on those for which strong evidence supports a rate-limiting role in disease pathogenesis.

Phosphatidylinositol-3 Kinase (PI3K)

PI3K is activated by autophosphorylation of tyrosine 177, which generates a high-affinity docking site for the SH2 domain of the GRB2 adapter, which in turn recruits GAB2 into a complex that activates PI3K.[15,16] Consistent with a critical role of the Y177/GRB2/GAB2 axis, mutation of tryosine 177 to phenylalanine or lack of GAB2 abrogates myeloid leukemia.[16] An alternative pathway of PI3K activation is complex formation between its p85 regulatory subunit, CBL, and CrkL,

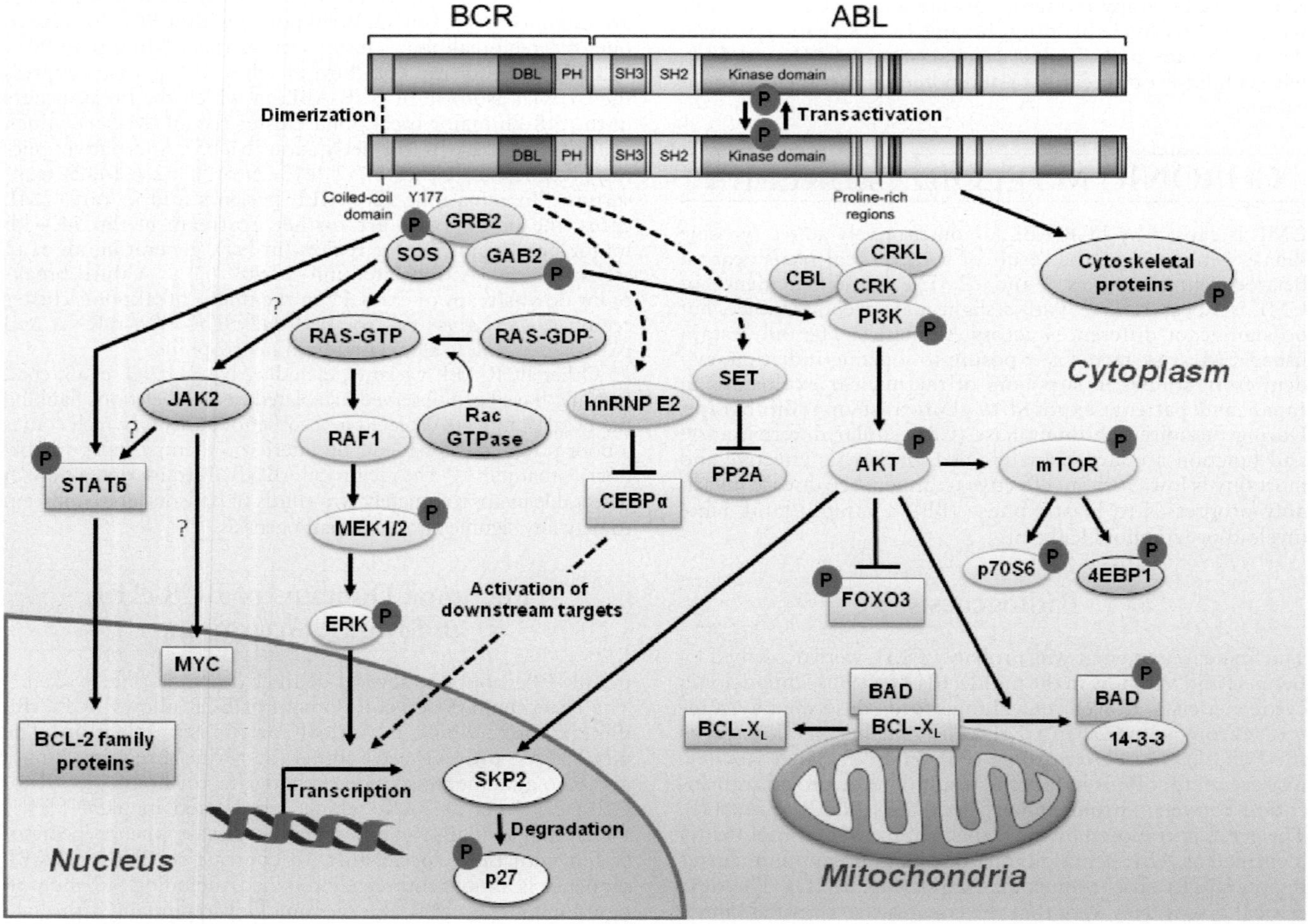

FIGURE 132.2 *BCR-ABL* domain structure and simplified representation of molecular signaling pathways activated in CML cells. Following dimerization of *BCR-ABL*, autophosphorylation generates docking sites on *BCR-ABL* that facilitate interaction with intermediary proteins such as GRB2. CrkL and CBL are also direct substrates of *BCR-ABL* that are part of a multimeric complex (*purple*). These *BCR-ABL*–dependent signaling complexes in turn lead to activation of multiple pathways whose net result is enhanced survival, inhibition of apoptosis, and perturbation of cell adhesion and migration. A subset of these pathways and their constituent transcription factors (*blue*), serine/threonine-specific kinases (*green*), cell-cycle regulatory protein (*yellow*), and apoptosis-related proteins (*red*) are shown. Several pathways were identified that are responsible for CML stem cell maintenance and/or *BCR-ABL*–mediated disease transformation (*orange*).

which bind to the SH2 and proline-rich domains of BCR-ABL.[17] PI3K activates the serine-threonine kinase AKT, which suppresses the activity of the forkhead O transcription factors (FOXO), thereby promoting survival.[18,19] Additionally PI3K enhances cell proliferation by promoting proteasomal degradation of p27 through up-regulation of SKP2, the F-Box recognition protein of the SCF^{SKP2} E3 ubiquitin ligase; absence of SKP2 from the leukemia cells prolongs survival in a murine CML model.[20] Another important outlet of PI3K signaling is AKT-dependent activation of mTOR, which leads to the constitutive phosphorylation of ribosomal protein p70S6 kinase and 4E-BP1, which enhance protein translation and cell proliferation.[21,22]

RAS/Mitogen-activated Protein Kinase (MAPK) Pathways

GRB2-mediated recruitment and activation of SOS promotes exchange of GTP for GDP on RAS.[15,23] GTP-RAS activates MAP kinase, promoting proliferation. Signaling from RAS to MAPK involves the serine-threonine kinase RAF-1[24,25] and RAC, another GTP–GDP exchange factor.[26] A crucial role for the latter is supported by the fact that lack of RAC1/2 delays BCR-ABL leukemia in a murine model.[27]

Janus Kinase (JAK) Signal Transducer and Activator of Transcription (STAT) Pathway

BCR-ABL activates STAT5 through direct phosphorylation or indirectly through phosphorylation by HCK, a SRC family kinase, or JAK2.[28,29] Active STAT5 induces the transcription of antiapoptotic proteins like MCL-1 and BCL-X_L.[30] Initial experiments in mice failed to demonstrate a critical role for STAT5.[31] However, it was subsequently established that the mice used in this study were not null for STAT5, but expressed an N terminally deleted protein with partially retained function. In contrast, complete lack of STAT5 abrogates both myeloid and lymphoid leukemogenesis.[32]

Cytoskeletal Proteins

BCR-ABL phosphorylates several proteins involved in adhesion and migration, including FAK, paxillin, p130CAS and HEF1. This and activation of RAS[15,33] are thought to impair integrin-mediated adhesion of CML progenitors to stroma and extracellular matrix, causing premature circulation as well as abnormal proliferation of Ph+ progenitors.[34]

DNA Repair

BCR-ABL impairs DNA damage surveillance by various mechanisms. For example, BCR-ABL has been shown to suppress checkpoint kinase 1 (CHK1) through inhibition of ATR[35] or down-regulation of BRCA1, a substrate of ataxia telangiectasia mutated (ATM).[36] Nonhomologous end-joining and homologous recombination, both critical double-strand break repair pathways, are defective in CML. BCR-ABL also up-regulates RAD51, inducing rapid but low-fidelity double-strand break repair on challenge with cytotoxic agents and induces reactive oxygen species that promote chronic oxidative DNA damage, double-strand breaks and point mutations. Lastly, telomere length decreases with disease progression from CP to BP.[37]

Although progress has been made to understand the extraordinary complexity of BCR-ABL signaling, a complete picture is still elusive. To overcome the limitations of investigating single pathway, quantitative proteomics is being used to establish a comprehensive picture of BCR-ABL signaling.[38] These results suggest that cellular processes in CML, rather than relying on a single pathway, use integrated networks to fully realize their leukemogenic potential.

Murine Models of CML

The most commonly used murine model of CML is retroviral expression of BCR-ABL in bone marrow followed by transplantation into lethally irradiated syngeneic recipients, which develop a CML-like myeloproliferative neoplasm.[39] Recently, an inducible transgenic mouse model has been developed, in which conditional BCR-ABL expression is under the control of the 3' enhancer of the murine stem cell leukemia (*SCL*) gene. This model serves as a promising new tool for studying leukemogenic mechanisms in hematopoietic stem cells during disease initiation and progression.[40] Lastly, xenograft models use various strains of immunodeficient mice for engraftment of primary CML cells.[41] The problem with xenograft models is that the engraftment of CP cells is low, probably because of their compromised interactions with the microenvironment as a result of species differences in cytokines and adhesion molecules. More promising results have been obtained by injecting CML cells directly into the livers of newborn mice.[42]

CML Stem Cell

The origin of CML in a pluripotent hematopoietic stem cell (HSC) was elegantly demonstrated in the late 1970s in studies showing clonality of granulocytes, erythrocytes, and platelets of female patients heterozygous for glucose-6-phosphate dehydrogenase, a polymorphic X-chromosomal gene.[43] BCR-ABL does not confer self-renewal, implying that Ph must be acquired by an HSC already endowed with this capacity.[44] For unknown reasons the main cellular expansion occurs in the progenitor cell compartment, while at least initially the majority of HSC are Ph-negative.[45] Serial xenograft studies have shown that CML leukemia stem cells (LSCs) reside within the quiescent CD34+38− fraction of bone marrow cells. Significant progress has recently been made by the identification of the IL-1 receptor–associated protein (IL-1RAP) as a surface marker specifically expressed on CD34+38− CML HSC.[45a] If confirmed, this will enable studies into the biology of these cells. Several genes were shown to have a critical role for leukemia-initiating cells maintenance in CML, including promyelocytic leukemia,[46] the hematopoietic-specific Rac2 GTPase,[47] smoothened, which is an essential component of the hedgehog pathway,[48] and β-catenin. The fact that these genes are also critical for maintenance and self-renewal of normal HSCs may be an obstacle to exploiting them as therapeutic targets.

Progression to Blastic Phase

Disease progression is believed to be due to the accumulation of molecular abnormalities that lead to a loss of terminal differentiation capacity of the leukemic clone, which however continues to depend on BCR-ABL activity. BCR-ABL mRNA and protein levels are higher in BP than in CP cells, including CD34+ granulocyte macrophage progenitors (GMPs), which are expanded in BP.[49] Another mechanism that enhances BCR-ABL activity in BP is inactivation of PP2A through up-regulation of SET, which in turn inhibits the PP2A phosphatase and its substrate protein tyrosine phosphatase I (SHP1). As SHP1 normally promotes BCR-ABL degradation through dephosphorylation, its reduced activity stabilizes BCR-ABL.[50]

The most striking feature of BP, the loss of differentiation capacity, suggests that the function of key myeloid transcription factors must be compromised. Occasionally, the differentiation block can be ascribed to mutations that result in the formation of dominant-negative transcription factors such as AML1-EVI or NUP98-HOXA9, which block differentiation or favor preferential growth of immature precursors.[51–53] Isolated cases of myeloid transformation have been associated with the acquisition of core binding factor mutations typical of AML. A more universal mechanism appears to be the BCR-ABL–induced down-regulation of CCAAT/enhancer binding protein-α (CEBPα) through the stabilization of the translational regulator heterogeneous nuclear ribonucleoprotein E2 (hnRNP E2), which is low or undetectable in CP but readily detectable in BP CML.[54] Interestingly, dominant-negative mutations of CEBPα are fairly common in AML,[55] but rare in CML-BP.[56]

Aberrant activation of Wnt/β-catenin signaling is believed to contribute to CML progression by conferring self-renewal capacity to GMPs. Activated β-catenin regulates self-renewal by undergoing translocation to the nucleus where it interacts with lymphoid enhancer factor/T-cell factor and regulates the transcription of genes such as *Myc* and *Cyclin D1*.[57] The acquisition of self-renewal by GMPs is expected to greatly increase the pool of LSCs in BP. Interestingly, expression microarray studies have implicated β-catenin activation not only in disease progression but also in resistance to tyrosine kinase inhibitors, supporting the view that drug resistance and disease progression share a common genetic basis.[58,59] This has implications for prognostication as well as for the development of strategies to prevent progression and overcome resistance.

Conclusions

BCR-ABL orchestrates an integrated network of signaling pathways that upend the physiological control of proliferation, cell death, DNA repair and microenvironment interaction, and lead to the clinical phenotype of CML. Cooperation with additional genetic events that accumulate over time inevitably leads to BP and drug resistance. Although significant progress has been made toward understanding transformation and disease progression, much remains to be learned. The availability of genome-wide scanning tools will undoubtedly accelerate this process and hopefully lead to the discovery of new therapeutic targets to eliminate CML LSC, overcome drug resistance unless effective therapy is initiated early on, and improve the prognosis of patients whose disease has progressed to BP.

CHRONIC LYMPHOCYTIC LEUKEMIA

CLL is one of the most common types of leukemia in adults and has a relatively consistent immunophenotype including dim-surface immunoglobulin expression, CD19, CD20, CD23 along with the pan T-cell marker CD5.[60] The impact on overall survival in young and elderly patients with CLL is quite substantial. Patients with a diagnosis under the age of 50 have a median expected lifespan of 12.3 years, which compares to 31.2 years in an age-matched control group.[61] Although younger patients have poor outcome and shortened survival with CLL, several recent studies have also identified elderly patients as a high-risk group for poor survival following treatment.[62–65] A small subset of CLL patients have indolent disease for many years and do not require therapy or intervention. Improving our understanding of the origin, biology, and progression of CLL will best help define both risk stratification of patients and also identify potential new treatments for this disease.

Origin of CLL

Attempts to identify the origin of CLL with respect to a normal B-cell counterpart has also occurred and remains a controversial area.[66–68] Unlike most other B-cell lymphomas and leukemia with the exception of mantle cell lymphoma, CLL expresses typical mature B-cell markers with coexpression of CD5. This prompted many to hypothesize that CLL may be derived from CD5+ B cells whose immunoglobulin (Ig)V_H is unmutated. However, the overall phenotype of CLL with expression of CD5, CD23, and CD19, and low levels of sIgM or IgD is not observed in any other type of normal B-cell counterpart. Additionally, investigators identified that approximately 40% of CLL cases are IgV_H unmutated, whereas the remainder are IgV_H mutated.[69,70] These two groups also were shown to have distinct clinical features, prompting the hypothesis that CLL may represent two distinct diseases.[69,70]

Two sentinel articles examining mRNA gene expression profiling in CLL and normal B cells provided similar findings, suggesting CLL is in fact one disease with a common CLL gene signature.[71,72] The first, by Klein et al.,[71] examined cDNA gene expression profiles derived from IgV_H unmutated, IgV_H mutated, and normal B cells derived from different stages of differentiation. A nonsupervised analysis of gene expression profile demonstrated that IgV_H mutated and unmutated CLL cases were not distinguished in any manner among a common profile typical of CLL. This CLL profile in the majority of samples had best resemblance to postgerminal center memory B cells and lacked any similarity to naive B cells, CD5+ B cells, and germinal center centroblasts. A supervised analysis of IgV_H unmutated and mutated CLL did demonstrate distinct genes that could separate these two clinical subsets of CLL.

A second article, published concurrently by Rosenwald et al.,[72] demonstrated similar findings of a common CLL phenotype described by Klein et al. as compared with other normal B cells and B-cell malignancies. In particular, the CLL gene phenotype was not shared by CD5+ normal B cells, thereby providing collaborating evidence that this is likely not the CLL cell of origin. Using a nonsupervised analysis of CLL samples, IgV_H unmutated and mutated samples were intermingled. However, supervised analysis of IgV_H unmutated and mutated CLL identified a number of genes differentially expressed in the former group related to B-cell receptor signaling and proliferation. In particular, ZAP-70 (zeta-chain associated protein kinase) overexpression was overexpressed in IgV_H unmutated CLL as compared with IgV_H mutated CLL.[73–76]

Subsequent studies have suggested that ZAP-70 expression may partly explain why IgV_H unmutated CLL patients have more active evidence of B-cell receptor signaling on ligation of the B-cell receptor.[77–79] Multiple studies confirming both the clinical prognostic significance of IgV_H mutational status and/or ZAP70 expression have subsequently been reported. IgV_H and/or ZAP70 represent very strong independent variables in predicting early disease progression, treatment remission duration, and survival of CLL patients. Unfortunately, the extreme variability in measurement of ZAP-70 expression among different investigators has limited full application of this biomarker clinically.

Chromosomal Abnormalities in the Pathogenesis of CLL

In CLL, conventional metaphase cytogenetics can identify chromosomal aberrations in only 20% to 50% of cases because of the low in vitro mitotic activity of CLL tumor cells.[80] Early nonstimulated metaphase karyotype studies of CLL demonstrated abnormalities in descending frequency of occurrence, including trisomy 12, deletions at 13q14, structural aberrations of 14q32, and deletions of 11q, 17p, and 6q.[81] In addition, complex karyotype (three or more abnormalities) occur in approximately 15% of patients and were noted in these early studies to predict for rapid disease progression, Richter's transformation, and inferior survival.[82–84] The use of CD40L or combination of interleukin (IL)-2 and cytosine-phosphate-guanosine (CpG) stimulation prior to metaphase analysis has also been reported with identification of translocations in 33 of 96 patients (34%) that were both balanced and unbalanced, which is associated with significantly shorter median time from diagnosis to requiring therapy and overall survival.[85] Subsequent comparative genomic hybridization (CGH) and global single nucleotide polymorphism (SNP) array studies in CLL have confirmed these deletions and also other chromosomal deletions in CLL.[86–88] Increasing aberrations in these same studies of CGH or SNP arrays have been associated with more aggressive disease.

Given the limitation of standard or stimulated karyotype analysis and inability to feasibly analyze patients by CGH or SNP arrays, interphase cytogenetics of known abnormalities are used to identify common, clinically significant aberrations in CLL. The largest study of interphase cytogenetics resulted in improved sensitivity to detect partial trisomies (12q12, 3q27, 8q24), deletions (13q14, 11q22-23, 6q21, 6q27, 17p13), and translocations (band 14q32) in more than 80% of all cases. In a large study of 325 patients by Dohner et al.,[89] a hierarchical model consisting of five genetic subgroups was constructed on the basis of regression analysis of CLL patients with chromosomal aberrations. The patients with a 17p deletion had the median survival time of 32 months and shortest treatment-free interval (TFI) of 9 months, whereas patients with 11q deletion followed closely with 79 months and 13 months, respectively.[89] The favorable 13q14 deletion group had a long TFI of 92 months and a median survival of 133 months, while the group without detectable chromosomal anomalies and those with trisomy 12 fell into the intermediate group with median survival of 111 and 114 months. Their TFI was 33 and 49 months, respectively. Based on this pivotal study, CLL patients are prioritized in a hierarchical order (deletion 17p13 > deletion 11q22-q23 > trisomy 12 > no aberration > deletion 13q14).[89] Of interest, patients with high-risk interphase cytogenetic abnormalities or other complex abnormalities are almost always found to have IgVH unmutated or ZAP-70–positive CLL.[90] The impact of high-risk interphase cytogenetics relative to disease progression, outside its association with IgVH unmutated CLL, remains uncertain.

Gene Mutation or Deletion Versus Epigenetic Silencing in the Pathogenesis of CLL

In many types of cancer including leukemia and lymphoma, the presence of activating mutations of specific oncogenes and also inactivating mutations and/or deletions of tumor suppressor genes directly contribute to the pathogenesis of the disease. In CLL only a few known tumor suppressor genes have been noted to be mutated or deleted in tumor cells. Of these, the p53 tumor suppressor gene has been the most rigorously studied based on it being one of the most commonly silenced genes in cancer. Deletions of the p53 gene are generally noted to occur in 3% to 10% of patients at diagnosis and generally occur as part of loss of large regions in del(17p13).[89,91] Mutations of p53 are also relatively uncommon and occur in a similar low proportion of CLL patients. The presence of deletion and mutation of p53 is more common but not uniform, with a proportion of patients having only one of the aberrations. Outcome in all studies is negatively influenced by the presence of a del(17p13.1), whereas only a subset of studies have shown that loss of p53 predicts aggressive disease course with rapid progression to time requiring therapy and inferior survival.[92–97] Both del(17p) and p53 mutations become more frequent as the disease progresses.[96] Overall, this suggests that loss of p53 function by mutation or deletion may be an important contributor to disease progression, but it likely does not contribute to the early pathogenesis of the disease. Indirect inactivation of p53 by mutation of ATM also occurs in CLL and correlates with more rapid disease progression.[93,98–100] Similar to p53, loss of ATM becomes more frequent with disease progression and also is likely a late event in the pathogenesis of this disease.

Whereas enhanced B-cell receptor signaling and ZAP-70 expression has been shown to contribute to the pathogenesis of CLL, efforts to identify mutations in this pathway have been limited. A screen of the tyrosine kinase kinome in selected exons that encode the kinase domain was reported from 95 CLL patients in whom 65 different kinases were examined based on relevance to B-cell biology.[101] No somatic tumor-associated mutations were found. The estimated frequency of mutations in the CLL genome based on this study was less than one mutation per 6.21 Mb DNA. The low proportion of mutations fall well under that observed in most solid tumors and also supports that gene mutations may not be a major contributor to the pathogenesis of this disease.

Finally, efforts to identify mutations in commonly deleted gene regions in CLL have been undertaken. Greatest attention has been placed on the most common del(13q14), where no protein coding gene mutation has been observed. However, the Croce group in 2002 identified that the microRNAs miR15 and miR16 resided in the minimally deleted region that was lost in approximately 70% of CLL patients.[102] MicroRNAs are small noncoding RNAs that effectively inhibit translation or induce degradation of numerous genes based on partial complementarity to site at the 3′ untranslated region of mRNA. Further support for the role of miR16.1 in the pathogenesis of CLL came from identification of both germ line mutations in a small number of CLL patients with a history of familial CLL.[103] Additionally, it was noted that New Zealand Black mice that develop both autoimmune disease and an indolent murine CLL and also have an acquired point mutation in the 3′ flanking sequence of microRNA mir-16-1.[104] The linkage of the mir-15a/16-1 complex to the development of murine CLL in a spontaneous mouse model suggests that mir-15a/16-1 is at least one of the molecular aberrations responsible for CLL. Klein et al.,[105] in a recent article, have demonstrated that a mouse with deletion of the miR15/miR16 region also develops a disease similar to human CLL, confirming the ultimate importance of this miR cluster in the development of CLL. These findings related to miRs and absent mutations suggest that miRs and other forms of epigenetic silencing, as opposed to mutational silencing of genes, are likely much more important in the pathogenesis and progression of CLL.

The role of microRNA and other noncoding genes in transcriptional and translational silencing of genes in CLL is now widely expanding. A subsequent study has demonstrated miR15 and miR16 target genes involved in disrupting apoptosis (bcl-2).[106] Multiple additional studies have demonstrated several other known important genes in the pathogenesis of CLL. Similarly, other forms of epigenetic silencing are also being shown to be relevant. Examples of alternative forms of epigenetic silencing can occur via promoter CpG methylation, recruitment of specific corepressor complexes, or recruitment of specific chromatin remodeling ATPase screening of CLL patients demonstrate distinct patterns of methylation by several groups.[107–110] Multiple oncogenes (*bcl-2, TCL1, ZAP70*)[111–113] have been shown to be aberrantly hypomethylated (hence expressed), whereas tumor suppressor genes (*DAPK1, SFRP1, ID4,* and *PTPRO*)[114–117] are hypermethylated (hence silenced), suggesting promoter methylation is one important key to gene regulation as part of malignant transformation. The current model for gene silencing likely involves loss of gene transcriptional activity followed by methylation.[118,119]

CLL and Proliferation

For many decades, CLL was viewed as a nonproliferating leukemia whose pathogenesis was driven solely by disrupted apoptosis and extended tumor cell survival. This paradigm was in part perpetuated based on the nonproliferating blood compartment. However, as with normal B cells, it has come to be recognized that CLL cell proliferation likely occurs in sites where microenvironment stimulation can occur, such as the lymph node and bone marrow. In such sites, proliferation centers are observed with a high proportion of dividing CLL cells that are often surrounded by either T cells or accessory stromal cells capable of providing cytokine costimulation.[120,121] Advances in technology including oral intake of heavy water have come forward to accurately measure all body compartments of CLL and assess the birth rate of CLL tumor cells *in vivo* in patients.[122] These studies have demonstrated a broad range of proliferation of CLL cells that varies based on disease state and also IgV_H mutational status.[123,124] As one might expect, this same proliferation rate identified through heavy water studies in CLL was also shown to be predictive of disease progression. Collectively, these studies have at least partially discredited the theory that CLL is purely an accumulative disease, and rather focused study on specific compartments of the body that have very different biologic features of proliferation.

CLL and Disrupted Apoptosis

As the normal cell from which the disease CLL is derived is uncertain, it is quite difficult to equivalently compare to know if a difference in spontaneous apoptosis exists. However, several studies derived from CLL do provide evidence that apoptosis at least *in vivo* is disrupted. Despite the rarity of *Bcl-2* gene rearrangement in B-CLL, overexpression of *Bcl-2* mRNA and bcl-2 protein expression is common and has been shown to contribute to both disrupted spontaneous apoptosis and also *ex vivo* drug resistance.[112,125–128] Similarly, other antiapoptotic bcl-2 family member proteins including MCL-1, A1, and BCL-XL have also been shown to be elevated either in resting CLL or in CLL cells exposed to soluble and contact factors present in the microenvironment and they also contribute to drug resistance.[129–131]

Finally, a host of transcription factors involving the NFκB,[132] WNT,[133] hedgehog,[134] and JAK/STAT[135] signaling pathway have been shown to be constitutively active and also to contribute to disrupted apoptosis and drug resistance in CLL. In particular, differential activation of NF-kappa B activation in CLL[119,136–139] as compared with normal resting B cells and its relevant prognostic significance[140–142] with respect to predicting outcome and also its positive role in regulating many of the antiapoptotic genes up-regulated in CLL has generated particular interest.

B-cell Receptor Signaling in CLL

Identification of the divergent natural history of CLL based on IgVH mutational status, ZAP-70 expression, and associated enhanced B-cell receptor signaling has raised interest in the role of this in the pathogenesis of CLL.[77–79,143] Activation of the proximal lyn kinase and also downstream syk has been demonstrated in CLL.[144–146] Additionally, increased activity of the PI3-kinase pathway as measured by both lipid kinase activity and also baseline phosphorylation of p-AKT has been preliminarily reported.[147,148] Complementing this finding, a recent study demonstrated that mature memory B-cell development was in great part dependent on the PI3-kinase pathway.[149] A recent study using the isoform-specific inhibitor of PI3-kinase-δ demonstrated that much of the survival protection generated by the microenvironment from stromal cells, cytokines (CD40L, IL-6, TNF-α), and fibronectin contact is mediated via PI3-Kinase δ isoform signaling.[150] Of great interest has been the transition of these B-cell receptor kinase pathway inhibitors to clinical trials. Here, with syk, PI3-kinase δ isoform inhibitors, and BTK inhibitors they have demonstrated dramatic and often rapid clinical responses with relatively favorable toxicity profile in CLL patients. The success of such therapeutics further emphasizes the importance of BCR signaling in the pathogenesis of CLL.

Progression of CLL: Role of Genomic Instability and Clonal Evolution

Two small studies of previously untreated patients have been examined for features associated with clonal evolution and have noted this to be more frequent in patients with IgVH unmutated status[151] or those expressing the surrogate marker for IgVH mutational status, ZAP70.[91] The smaller of these studies noted clonal evolution to occur more commonly among those patients with progression.[151] One recently published study in which patients with long telomere length were more likely to have IgVH mutated disease and del(13q14), whereas those with del(11q22.3), del(17p13.1), complex karyotype (more than abnormalities) and IgVH unmutated disease were likely to have extended telomeres.[152] Furthermore, one small study suggested long telomere length among patients with IgVH unmutated disease could identify patients with an expected extended progression-free survival.[153] The contribution of clonal evolution, telomere length, and global hypomethylation in CLL progression will require further study.

Conclusion

A significant amount of data has been produced concerning the pathogenesis of CLL. Emerging from such work is the importance of epigenetics in the progression of CLL from normal B cells and also enhanced B-cell receptor signaling. Murine mouse models have demonstrated the importance of NF-κB, Bcl-2, TCL1, and loss of miR 15, MiR 16, and Leu2 in the pathogenesis of CLL. It is likely that current lines of investigation, along with emerging technologies related to whole-genome signaling, global proteomic assessment, and miR profiling, will lead to further advances in risk stratification and improvement in CLL therapy.

Selected References

The full list of references for this chapter appears in the online version.

1. Deininger MW. Chronic myeloid leukemia: an historical perspective. *American Society of Hematology Education Program Book*, 50th Anniversary Review. 2008:418.
2. Nowell PC, Hungerford DA. Chromosome studies on normal and leukemic human leukocytes. *J Natl Cancer Inst* 1960;25:85.
3. Rowley JD. A new consistent chromosomal abnormality in chronic myelogenous leukaemia identified by quinacrine fluorescence and Giemsa staining. *Nature* 1973;243:290.
5. Groffen J, Stephenson JR, Heisterkamp N, et al. Philadelphia chromosomal breakpoints are clustered within a limited region, bcr, on chromosome 22. *Cell* 1984;36:93–99.

6. Daley GQ, Van Etten RA, Baltimore D. Induction of chronic myelogenous leukemia in mice by the P210bcr/abl gene of the Philadelphia chromosome. *Science* 1990;247:824–830.
7. Melo JV. The diversity of BCR-ABL fusion proteins and their relationship to leukemia phenotype. *Blood* 1996;88:2375–2384.
9. Huntly BJ, Guilhot F, Reid AG, et al. Imatinib improves but may not fully reverse the poor prognosis of patients with CML with derivative chromosome 9 deletions. *Blood* 2003;102:2205.
12. Melo JV, Gordon DE, Cross NC, et al. The ABL-BCR fusion gene is expressed in chronic myeloid leukemia. *Blood* 1993;81:158–165.
16. Sattler M, Mohi MG, Pride YB, et al. Critical role for Gab2 in transformation by BCR/ABL. *Cancer Cell* 2002;1:479–492.
18. Naka K, Hoshii T, Muraguchi T, et al. TGF-beta-FOXO signalling maintains leukaemia-initiating cells in chronic myeloid leukaemia. *Nature* 2010;463:676.
20. Agarwal A, Bumm TG, Corbin AS, et al. Absence of SKP2 expression attenuates BCR-ABL-induced myeloproliferative disease. *Blood* 2008;112:1960.
23. Kardinal C, Konkol B, Lin H, et al. Chronic myelogenous leukemia blast cell proliferation is inhibited by peptides that disrupt Grb2-SoS complexes. *Blood* 2001;98:1773–1781.
29. Ilaria RL, Jr., Van Etten RA. P210 and P190(BCR/ABL) induce the tyrosine phosphorylation and DNA binding activity of multiple specific STAT family members. *J Biol Chem* 1996;271:31704.
32. Hoelbl A, Schuster C, Kovacic B, et al. Stat5 is indispensable for the maintenance of bcr/abl-positive leukaemia. *EMBO Mol Med* 2010;2:98–110.
33. Verfaillie CM, Hurley R, Zhao RC, et al. Pathophysiology of CML: do defects in integrin function contribute to the premature circulation and massive expansion of the BCR/ABL positive clone? *J Lab Clin Med* 1997;129:584–591.
34. Ramaraj P, Singh H, Niu N, et al. Effect of mutational inactivation of tyrosine kinase activity on BCR/ABL-induced abnormalities in cell growth and adhesion in human hematopoietic progenitors. *Cancer Res* 2004;64:5322–5331.
35. Melo JV, Barnes DJ. Chronic myeloid leukaemia as a model of disease evolution in human cancer. *Nat Rev Cancer* 2007;7:441–453.
38. Brehme M, Hantschel O, Colinge J, et al. Charting the molecular network of the drug target Bcr-Abl. *Proc Natl Acad Sci U S A* 2009;106:7414.
39. Pear WS, Miller JP, Xu L, et al. Efficient and rapid induction of a chronic myelogenous leukemia-like myeloproliferative disease in mice receiving P210 bcr/abl-transduced bone marrow. *Blood* 1998;92:3780–3792.
40. Koschmieder S, Gottgens B, Zhang P, et al. Inducible chronic phase of myeloid leukemia with expansion of hematopoietic stem cells in a transgenic model of BCR-ABL leukemogenesis. *Blood* 2005;105:324–334.
41. Agliano A, Martin-Padura I, Mancuso P, et al. Human acute leukemia cells injected in NOD/LtSz-scid/IL-2Rgamma null mice generate a faster and more efficient disease compared to other NOD/scid-related strains. *Int J Cancer* 2008;123:2222–2227.
43. Fialkow PJ, Jacobson RJ, Papayannopoulou T. Chronic myelocytic leukemia: clonal origin in a stem cell common to the granulocyte, erythrocyte, platelet and monocyte/macrophage. *Am J Med* 1977;63:125–130.
44. Huntly BJ, Shigematsu H, Deguchi K, et al. MOZ-TIF2, but not BCR-ABL, confers properties of leukemic stem cells to committed murine hematopoietic progenitors. *Cancer Cell* 2004;6:587–596.
46. Ito K, Bernardi R, Morotti A, et al. PML targeting eradicates quiescent leukaemia-initiating cells. *Nature* 2008;453:1072.
48. Zhao C, Chen A, Jamieson CH, et al. Hedgehog signalling is essential for maintenance of cancer stem cells in myeloid leukaemia. *Nature* 2009;458:776–779.
50. Perrotti D, Neviani P. ReSETting PP2A tumour suppressor activity in blast crisis and imatinib-resistant chronic myelogenous leukaemia. *Br J Cancer* 2006;95:775–781.
57. Jamieson CH, Ailles LE, Dylla SJ, et al. Granulocyte-macrophage progenitors as candidate leukemic stem cells in blast-crisis CML. *N Engl J Med* 2004;351:657–667.
58. McWeeney SK, Pemberton LC, LoWWriaux MM, et al. A gene expression signature of CD34+ cells to predict major cytogenetic response in chronic-phase chronic myeloid leukemia patients treated with imatinib. *Blood* 2010;115:315–325.
59. Radich JP, Dai H, Mao M, et al. Gene expression changes associated with progression and response in chronic myeloid leukemia. *Proc Natl Acad Sci U S A* 2006;103:2794–2799.
60. Matutes E, Wotherspoon A, Catovsky D. Differential diagnosis in chronic lymphocytic leukaemia. *Best Pract Res Clin Haematol* 2007;20:367–384.
69. Hamblin TJ, Davis Z, Gardiner A, et al. Unmutated Ig V(H) genes are associated with a more aggressive form of chronic lymphocytic leukemia. *Blood* 1999;94:1848–1854.
70. Damle RN, Wasil T, Fais F, et al. Ig V gene mutation status and CD38 expression as novel prognostic indicators in chronic lymphocytic leukemia. *Blood* 1999;94:1840–1847.
71. Klein U, Tu Y, Stolovitzky GA, et al. Gene expression profiling of B cell chronic lymphocytic leukemia reveals a homogeneous phenotype related to memory B cells. *J Exp Med* 2001;194:1625–1638.
72. Rosenwald A, Alizadeh AA, Widhopf G, et al. Relation of gene expression phenotype to immunoglobulin mutation genotype in B cell chronic lymphocytic leukemia. *J Exp Med* 2001;194:1639.
75. Rassenti LZ, Huynh L, Toy TL, et al. ZAP-70 compared with immunoglobulin heavy-chain gene mutation status as a predictor of disease progression in chronic lymphocytic leukemia. *N Engl J Med* 2004;351:893–901.
77. Chen L, Apgar J, Huynh L, et al. ZAP-70 directly enhances IgM signaling in chronic lymphocytic leukemia. *Blood* 2005;105:2036–2041.
85. Mayr C, Speicher MR, Kofler DM, et al. Chromosomal translocations are associated with poor prognosis in chronic lymphocytic leukemia. *Blood* 2006;107:742–751.
89. Dohner H, Stilgenbauer S, Benner A, et al. Genomic aberrations and survival in chronic lymphocytic leukemia. *N Engl J Med* 2000;343:1910–1916.
91. Shanafelt TD, Witzig TE, Fink SR, et al. Prospective evaluation of clonal evolution during long-term follow-up of patients with untreated early-stage chronic lymphocytic leukemia. *J Clin Oncol* 2006;24:4634.
101. Brown JR, Levine RL, Thompson C, et al. Systematic genomic screen for tyrosine kinase mutations in CLL. *Leukemia* 2008;22:1966–1969.
102. Calin GA, Dumitru CD, Shimizu M, et al. Frequent deletions and down-regulation of micro- RNA genes miR15 and miR16 at 13q14 in chronic lymphocytic leukemia. *Proc Natl Acad Sci U S A* 2002;99:15524–15529.
103. Calin GA, Ferracin M, Cimmino A, et al. A MicroRNA signature associated with prognosis and progression in chronic lymphocytic leukemia. *N Engl J Med* 2005;353:1793–1801.
104. Raveche ES, Salerno E, Scaglione BJ, et al. Abnormal microRNA-16 locus with synteny to human 13q14 linked to CLL in NZB mice. *Blood* 2007;109:5079–5086.
105. Klein U, Lia M, Crespo M, et al. The DLEU2/miR-15a/16-1 cluster controls B cell proliferation and its deletion leads to chronic lymphocytic leukemia. *Cancer Cell* 2010;17:28–40.
116. Raval A, Tanner SM, Byrd JC, et al. Downregulation of death-associated protein kinase 1 (DAPK1) in chronic lymphocytic leukemia. *Cell* 2007;129:879.
119. Chen SS, Raval A, Johnson AJ, et al. Epigenetic changes during disease progression in a murine model of human chronic lymphocytic leukemia. *Proc Natl Acad Sci U S A* 2009;106:13433–13438.
124. Messmer BT, Messmer D, Allen SL, et al. In vivo measurements document the dynamic cellular kinetics of chronic lymphocytic leukemia B cells. *J Clin Invest* 2005;115:755-764.
132. Furman RR, Asgary Z, Mascarenhas JO, et al. Modulation of NF-kappa B activity and apoptosis in chronic lymphocytic leukemia B cells. *J Immunol* 2000;164:2200–2206.
150. Herman SE, Gordon AL, Wagner AJ, et al. The phosphatidylinositol 3-kinase-{delta} inhibitor CAL-101 demonstrates promising pre-clinical activity in chronic lymphocytic leukemia by antagonizing intrinsic and extrinsic cellular survival signals. *Blood* 2010;116:2078–2088.
151. Stilgenbauer S, Sander S, Bullinger L, et al. Clonal evolution in chronic lymphocytic leukemia: acquisition of high-risk genomic aberrations associated with unmutated VH, resistance to therapy, and short survival. *Haematologica* 2007;92:1242.

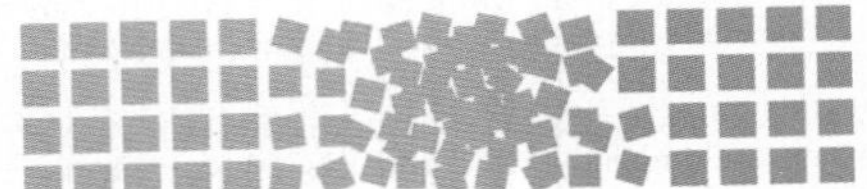

CHAPTER 133 CHRONIC MYELOGENOUS LEUKEMIA

BRIAN J. DRUKER AND STEPHANIE J. LEE

Chronic myelogenous leukemia (CML; also called *chronic myeloid leukemia* or *chronic granulocytic leukemia*) is a clonal hematopoietic disorder caused by an acquired genetic defect in a pluripotent stem cell. CML is a bi- or triphasic illness, with most patients diagnosed in a relatively indolent chronic or stable phase that is characterized by excessive numbers of myeloid lineage cells that fully mature. The disease progresses to a more aggressive leukemia as a malignant clone loses the capacity for terminal differentiation. This more aggressive or advanced phase can be further subdivided into an accelerated phase and a blastic phase, with survival in the blastic phase measured in months.

CML has become a paradigm for targeted drug development based on an understanding of the molecular pathogenesis of a disease. A series of discoveries led to the recognition that the BCR-ABL protein, which results from a reciprocal translocation involving chromosomes 9 and 22, has a central role in the pathogenesis of CML. The BCR-ABL protein functions as a constitutively activated tyrosine kinase and this knowledge led to the development of imatinib (Gleevec, Glivec), a drug that specifically inhibits the BCR-ABL tyrosine kinase.[1] New, improved potency BCR-ABL tyrosine kinase inhibitors have substantial activity in patients with imatinib resistance, and early results show improved outcomes when compared with imatinib for newly diagnosed patients. Despite good long-term disease control, tyrosine kinase inhibitor therapy is not considered a curative therapy. The only proven curative therapeutic option is allogeneic hematopoietic cell transplantation (HCT), but this procedure is associated with substantial morbidity and mortality. Integration of the various treatment modalities and determining optimal therapy or response to therapy is evolving rapidly.

EPIDEMIOLOGY

CML accounts for approximately 15% of all leukemias, with 4,000 to 5,000 new cases diagnosed in the United States annually. The incidence of CML is 1.6 to 2.0 cases per 100,000 persons per year, and the incidence is similar in all countries worldwide.[2,3] Although CML occurs in all age groups, its incidence increases with each decade of life, making it mainly a disease of adults. According to the Surveillance, Epidemiology, and End Results (SEER) program, the median age at diagnosis is 66 years,[2] which is much higher than reported in single-institutional series and clinical trials. [3] The disease has a slight male predominance (2.2:1.3).[2,3]

The only known risk factor for development of CML is exposure to radiation in high doses. This is evident from studies of survivors of the atom bomb explosions in Japan in 1945 and from follow-up of patients treated with radiation for ankylosing spondylitis and cervical cancer.[4–6] No known association has been found between CML and infectious agents or chemical exposures, and no familial predisposition has been implicated in CML.

PATHOGENESIS

The discovery of the Philadelphia (Ph) chromosome in 1960 made CML the first human neoplasm to be characterized by a consistent cytogenetic marker.[7] In 1973, the Ph chromosome, a shortened chromosome 22 (22q-), was shown to be the result of a balanced, reciprocal translocation between the long arms of chromosomes 9 and 22, t(9;22) (q34;q11) (Fig. 133.1).[8] In the 1980s, the *BCR-ABL* chimeric gene and protein formed as a result of the (9;22) translocation was characterized and its central role in the pathogenesis of CML was established.[9,10] The Ph chromosome and *BCR-ABL* are found in cells of the myeloid, erythroid, and megakaryocytic lineages, some B cells, and a small proportion of T cells, but not other cells of the body, establishing CML as a clonal disorder that originates in a pluripotent hematopoietic stem cell.

The (9;22) translocation transposes the *ABL* (Abelson) protooncogene from chromosome 9 into a relatively small, 5.8-kb genomic region on chromosome 22 named the *breakpoint cluster region* (*bcr*).[11] Although the genomic breakpoints in the *ABL* gene are highly variable, they almost always occur upstream of the second exon (a2), resulting in translocation of all but exon 1 of ABL. Two slightly different chimeric *BCR-ABL* genes are present in most patients with CML, depending on the precise location of the breakpoint in the *BCR* gene. Breaks can occur between exon 13 (also known as b2) and exon 14 (b3), yielding a b2a2 fusion messenger RNA (mRNA), whereas a break occurring between exons 14 and 15 produces a b3a2 fusion mRNA (Fig. 133.2).[10] Historically, b3a2 was referred to as the *major breakpoint cluster region* (*M-BCR*). In the majority of patients, either b2a2 or b3a2 transcripts are present, but occasionally patients have both transcripts in their leukemia cells. Although the b3a2 mRNA encodes a BCR-ABL protein that is 25 amino acids larger than that encoded by the b2a2 transcript, both are referred to as *p210BCR-ABL*. Patients with b2a2 or b3a2 transcripts have similar prognoses.

The Ph chromosome and the *BCR-ABL* fusion gene are not pathognomonic for CML, being found in 25% to 50% of adult patients with acute lymphoblastic leukemia (ALL) and rare cases of acute myeloid leukemia.[12] In adults with Ph chromosome–positive ALL, one-third have *BCR-ABL* transcripts indistinguishable from those found in CML. In two-thirds of these patients, the genomic breakpoint on chromosome 22 occurs in the first intron of the *BCR* gene (between e1 and e2) in an area termed the *minor breakpoint cluster region*

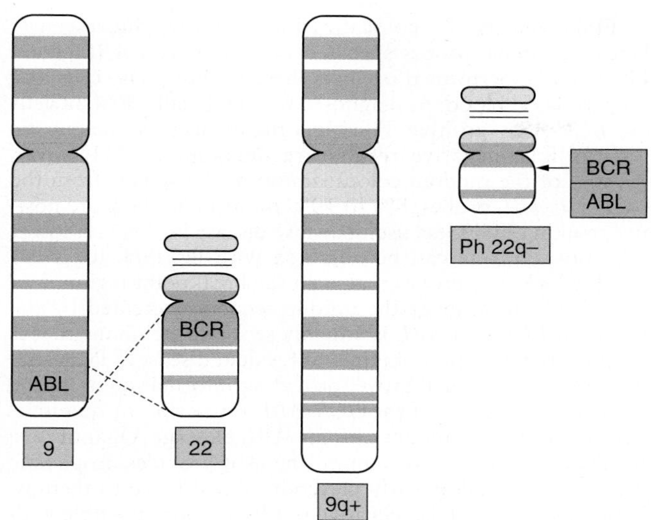

FIGURE 133.1 Diagrammatic representation of the formation of the Philadelphia (Ph) chromosome. The normal chromosomes 9 and 22 are shown, along with the derivative chromosomes 9q+ and 22q- (Ph). The approximate positions of the normal *ABL* gene at 9q34 and *BCR* at 22q11 and the *BCR-ABL* fusion gene formed as a result of the translocation are shown.

(*m-BCR*), resulting in a protein of 190 kD (p190), also referred to as *p185* (Fig. 133.2). Approximately 5% of children with ALL are Ph chromosome–positive, and 95% of these patients have the p190 form of BCR-ABL. The p190 transcript is rarely found in patients with CML. An uncommon Ph chromosome–positive chronic neutrophilic leukemia has also been described with an e19a2 *BCR-ABL* mRNA product that encodes a 230-kD protein (p230). Other types of fusions have been observed in isolated cases.

The BCR-ABL fusion protein resides in the cytoplasm and has constitutive tyrosine kinase activity compared to the tightly regulated activity of the normal *ABL* product (p145).[13,14] The BCR-ABL tyrosine kinase binds to and phosphorylates numerous intracellular proteins. The net effect of this is to induce all of the phenotypic abnormalities observed in patients with CML.[10] This includes increased proliferation or decreased apoptosis of hematopoietic stem or progenitor cells leading to a massive increase in myeloid cell numbers; premature release of immature myeloid cells into the circulation, postulated to be due to a defect in adherence of myeloid progenitors to marrow stroma; and genetic instability resulting in disease progression. Despite the complexity of BCR-ABL signal transduction, all of the transforming functions of BCR-ABL depend on its tyrosine kinase activity, making this disease an ideal candidate for therapy directed against this activity.

DIAGNOSIS

Clinical Manifestations

Ninety percent of patients with CML are diagnosed in the chronic or stable phase. Ten percent to 20% of patients in older studies and as many as 50% in more recent studies present without symptoms and are diagnosed as a result of finding an elevated white blood count on routine blood sampling. The most common presenting symptoms of CML are related to anemia, splenomegaly, and increased cell turnover. These symptoms include fatigue, left upper quadrant pain, abdominal distention or discomfort, early satiety, weight loss, and night sweats.[15]

Occasionally, patients may present with a hyperviscosity syndrome with manifestations such as stroke, priapism, stupor, or visual changes caused by retinal hemorrhage and require leukapheresis. The most common physical finding in patients with CML is splenomegaly, with the magnitude of splenomegaly correlating with the degree of leukocytosis. Ecchymoses are frequently observed, but spontaneous bleeding is uncommon. Lymphadenopathy is not usually seen in the chronic phase.

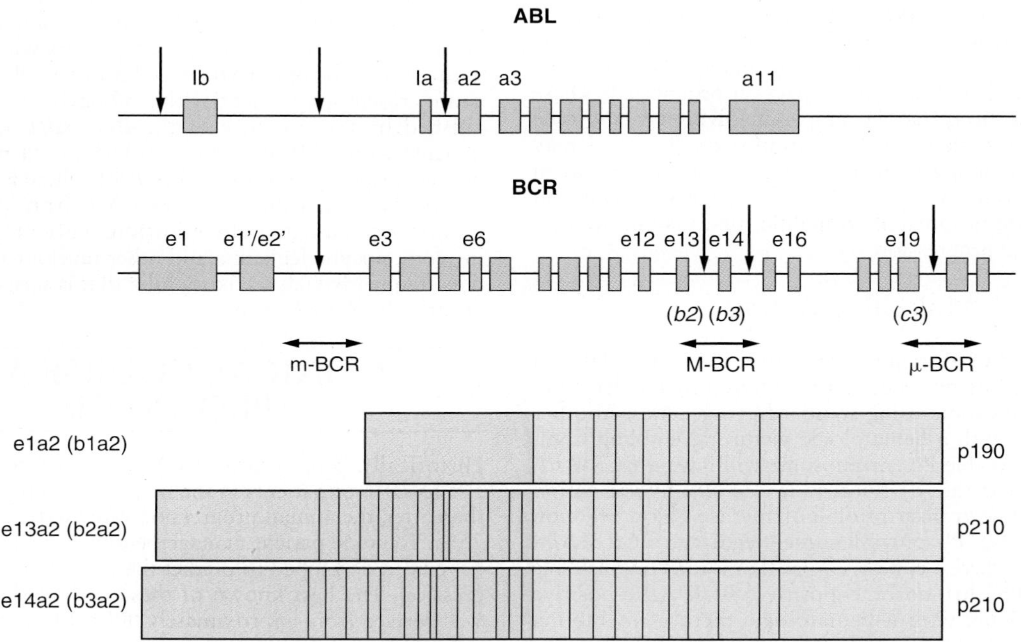

FIGURE 133.2 Schematic representation of the genomic structure of the normal *ABL* and *BCR* genes (*top*) and various fusion transcripts generated by the different *BCR-ABL* fusion genes (*bottom*). The b2a2 or the b3a2 transcript is found in the majority of patients with chronic myelogenous leukemia. See text for details.

Laboratory Tests

Peripheral Blood and Bone Marrow

The diagnosis of CML is frequently suspected from examination of the peripheral blood and bone marrow. The white blood cell (WBC) count in the chronic phase of CML usually exceeds 50×10^9/L at the time of diagnosis and can range up to 800×10^9/L. During the chronic phase, leukemic WBCs differentiate and function normally. The peripheral blood smear shows a full spectrum of myeloid cells from blasts to neutrophils, with blasts comprising less than 15% and usually less than 5% of the WBC differential. Basophilia is invariably present, and its absence should prompt consideration of other myeloproliferative disorders. Eosinophilia is also commonly present. The majority of patients have thrombocytosis, and on occasion, the platelet count may be more than 1000×10^9/L. Most patients with CML have a normochromic, normocytic anemia that is inversely proportional to the degree of leukocytosis.

Blood levels of leukocyte alkaline phosphatase are low or undetectable in most patients with CML. As transcobalamin I is produced by granulocytes, serum B_{12} levels are increased in proportion to the total WBC count. Uric acid and lactate dehydrogenase are also frequently elevated, reflecting the increased WBC mass and turnover.

The bone marrow in patients with chronic phase CML is markedly hypercellular, with a predominance of myeloid cells with full maturation. Blasts are less than 15% and most commonly less than 5%, and basophilia is also present. Megakaryocytes are usually increased in number and may form clusters. Occasional micromegakaryocytes may be present. Erythroid hypoplasia is frequently present and may seem exaggerated because of the increased myeloid-to-erythroid ratio. Erythroid precursors are otherwise morphologically unremarkable. Reticulin fibrosis is usually absent or mild but may become more prominent with disease progression.

Cytogenetics

Cytogenetic analysis of 20 bone marrow metaphases has been the standard method to detect the Ph chromosome, which is present in the majority of cells at diagnosis. Although most patients have a typical t(9;22), approximately 5% have variant translocations that have no impact on prognosis.[16] These variant translocations may be simple, involving chromosome 22 and a chromosome other than chromosome 9, or they may be complex, involving one or more other chromosomes in addition to chromosomes 9 and 22.[17] Cytogenetics can also detect other chromosomal abnormalities that may be an indication of disease progression.

Molecular Testing

The diagnosis of CML requires the presence of *BCR-ABL*. In 95% of patients, its presence can be inferred by the detection of the Ph chromosome using standard cytogenetics. Another 5% of patients with a hematologic picture resembling CML who lack a detectable Ph chromosome will have a *BCR-ABL* fusion gene detectable by fluorescence *in situ* hybridization (FISH) or reverse transcription–polymerase chain reaction (RT-PCR). These Ph chromosome–negative, *BCR-ABL*–positive patients have a clinical course that is indistinguishable from that of Ph chromosome–positive, *BCR-ABL*–positive patients.[18] Patients with a hematologic picture resembling CML but who are Ph chromosome–negative and *BCR-ABL*–negative are now classified as having atypical CML and may have a more aggressive clinical course.[19]

FISH detects the colocalization of large, fluorescently labeled genomic probes specific to the *BCR* and *ABL* genes. FISH can be performed on metaphase or interphase cells and on peripheral blood. At diagnosis, when typically 90% of cells are *BCR-ABL*–positive, FISH is a highly accurate diagnostic test, as false-negative results are uncommon.[20] However, because of the random colocalization of the signals from the *BCR* and *ABL* probes, 8% to 10% of normal cells score positive, making FISH less useful at low disease burdens. A lower false-positive rate can be obtained with D-FISH, for *dual*-FISH, which uses probes that span the breakpoint region.[21]

RT-PCR to amplify the unique sequences created by the fusion of *BCR* and *ABL* is a highly sensitive technique that is ideal for the detection of minimal residual disease.[20] PCR testing can either be qualitative, providing information as to the presence or absence of the *BCR-ABL* transcript, or quantitative, assessing the amount of *BCR-ABL* message. Quantitative RT-PCR is preferred for monitoring as it provides prognostic value and may allow early detection of resistance to therapy. False-positive and false-negative results are both possible with RT-PCR, and rigorous controls are required to detect these instances. False-negative results can be due to poor-quality RNA or failure of the reaction, whereas false-positive results are usually due to contamination of the sample.

Differential Diagnosis

Anyone presenting with a WBC count over 50×10^9/L with a peripheral blood smear showing a full spectrum of myeloid lineage cells plus basophilia should be suspected of having CML. The diagnosis of chronic phase CML can be confirmed by the presence of the *BCR-ABL* gene as described in "Cytogenetics" and "Molecular Testing" and by the absence of advanced phase features described later in "Advanced Phase Disease." The differential diagnosis includes a leukemoid reaction, which is typically seen in patients with underlying infections. In patients with a leukemoid reaction, the WBC count is usually less than 50×10^9/L and the peripheral blood smear consists predominantly of segmented neutrophils and bands, often with toxic granulations. Less mature myeloid cells are rarely seen; there is no basophilia; the leukocyte alkaline phosphatase is elevated; and the Ph chromosome and *BCR-ABL* are absent. Approximately 5% of patients with CML present with extreme thrombocytosis and a minimally elevated WBC count, resembling essential thrombocytosis, but are distinguished by the presence of the *BCR-ABL* gene. Although patients with CML may have an increase in monocyte numbers corresponding to the leukocytosis, there is relative monocytopenia, which differentiates CML from chronic myelomonocytic leukemia. In addition, patients with chronic myelomonocytic leukemia and other myeloproliferative disorders frequently lack the basophilia that is seen with CML and lack the *BCR-ABL* gene.

CLINICAL COURSE AND PROGNOSIS

Historically, progression of CML to blast crisis occurred in 5% to 10% of patients in the first 2 years after diagnosis, and thereafter, the annual progression rate increased from 20% to 25%. To guide patient management, various prognostic scales have been developed to predict the probability of disease progression. The best known of these is the Sokal score, which was derived from approximately 800 CML patients treated in the 1960s and 1970s.[22] Input of patient age, platelet count, peripheral blast count, and spleen size at diagnosis into an equation allows separation of the population into three groups: high, intermediate, and low risk of disease progression, with median survivals of 3, 4, and 5 years, respectively. Many of these patients received therapies not currently in use, such as busulfan, splenectomy, and intensive chemotherapy, but the Sokal risk score does have some value for predicting responses to imatinib therapy. Early data suggesting that genomic deletions in the *ABL* gene on chromosome 9q+ may have prognostic significance for patients treated with imatinib[23] have not been confirmed in larger studies.[24,25] Clonal cytogenetic abnormalities in addition to the Ph chromosome are present at diagnosis in some patients, with the most common being duplication of the Ph chromosome, trisomy 8, iso-17q, and trisomy 19. Although iso-17q has been associated with a poorer prognosis, the prognostic significance of the other chromosomal abnormalities is less clear.[26–28]

TREATMENT OF CHRONIC PHASE DISEASE

Currently available therapies for CML range from relatively nontoxic oral medications to high-dose chemoradiotherapy with allogeneic HCT. Although allogeneic HCT is regarded as the only curative therapy, the risks of this procedure combined with the ability of tyrosine kinase inhibitor therapy to achieve long-term disease control have made tyrosine kinase inhibitor therapy the treatment of choice for most newly diagnosed, chronic phase patients. Table 133.1 summarizes criteria for assessment of responses to therapy.

Nontransplant Therapies

Historically, busulfan, hydroxyurea, and interferon-α (IFN-α were the mainstays of therapy for CML. Hydroxyurea, a well-tolerated oral agent that inhibits DNA synthesis by inhibiting ribonucleotide reductase, remains in use as an initial therapy to control blood counts pending definitive diagnosis and therapy. Although the 5-year survival for IFN-α-treated patients (57%) is better than the 5-year survival of patients treated with hydroxyurea or busulfan (42%, $P < .00001$),[29] the clinical use of IFN-α is limited by its toxicity profile and has largely been supplanted by BCR-ABL kinase inhibitor therapy.

TABLE 133.1

CRITERIA FOR TREATMENT RESPONSES IN CHRONIC MYELOGENOUS LEUKEMIA

COMPLETE HEMATOLOGIC RESPONSE

WBC <10 × 10⁹/L, platelets <450 × 10⁹/L, basophils < 5%, no immature cells such as blasts, promyelocytes, or myelocytes, no palpable splenomegaly

CYTOGENETIC RESPONSE

Complete	0% Ph+	Major
Partial	1%–35% Ph+	Major
Minor	36%–65% Ph+	

MAJOR MOLECULAR RESPONSE

≥3-log reduction in BCR-ABL transcript level below median baseline value[38]

WBC, white blood cells; Ph+, Philadelphia chromosome–positive metaphases.

TYROSINE KINASE INHIBITORS

Imatinib

Imatinib (Gleevec) was the first tyrosine kinase inhibitor developed for CML and rapidly became the treatment of choice for patients with chronic phase CML after its was approved by the U.S. Food and Drug Administratin (FDA) in 2001.[1] Imatinib is an orally administered inhibitor of the BCR-ABL tyrosine kinase; thus, it targets the molecular pathogenetic event in CML. Other tyrosine kinases inhibited by imatinib are the platelet-derived growth factor receptors, KIT, and ARG (*ABL*-related gene). Based on remarkable activity in phase 1 and 2 clinical trials,[30,31] a phase 3 randomized study (n = 1,106) compared imatinib at 400 mg/d to IFN-α plus Ara-C in newly diagnosed patients with chronic phase CML. With a median follow-up of 19 months, patients randomized to imatinib had statistically significant better results than patients treated with IFN-α plus Ara-C in all parameters measured, including rates of complete hematologic response (CHR) (97% vs. 69%), major and complete cytogenetic responses (87% and 76% vs. 35% and 14%), discontinuation of assigned therapy because of intolerance (3% vs. 31%), and progression to accelerated phase or blast crisis (3% vs. 8.5%).[32] Quality of life was maintained on the imatinib arm and worsened on the IFN-α plus Ara-C arm.[33]

With 5 years of follow-up, the overall survival of patients randomized to imatinib as initial therapy is 89% and with 8 years, it is 85%.[34,35] At 5 years, an estimated 7% of patients have progressed to accelerated phase or blast crisis and an additional 8% of patients have relapsed either hematologically or cytogenetically.[34] The risk of relapse has trended down over time and was less than 1% per year in years 5 through 8.[35]

The current standard dose of imatinib is 400 mg/d. Several randomized studies have compared 400 mg/d to 800 mg/d in newly diagnosed patients. These studies demonstrate that more rapid responses are obtained with the higher doses, but with longer follow-up, the response rates to 400 mg/d and higher doses are similar. Toxicity of 800 mg/d is greater, with up to one-third of patients requiring dose reductions. Progression-free survival was not impacted by the higher doses.[36,37]

Cytogenetic responses on imatinib therapy have a statistically significant impact on disease progression. A landmark analysis of 350 newly diagnosed chronic phase patients who achieved a complete cytogenetic response within 12 months of initiating imatinib treatment revealed that at 60 months, 97% had not progressed to the accelerated phase or blast crisis. For patients with a partial cytogenetic response (n = 86), the estimate was 93%, and for patients who did not achieve a major cytogenetic response within 12 months (n = 73), the estimate was 81% (overall $P < 0.001$).[34] Patients with high-risk Sokal scores at diagnosis had a lower rate of complete cytogenetic responses, 69% versus 91% for patients with low risk Sokal scores. If, however, a complete cytogenetic response was obtained, there was no significant difference in the risk of disease progression at 5 years based on pretherapy Sokal risk score (4.6% high risk, 1.2% low risk, $P = .16$).[34]

Molecular responses also correlate with long-term outcomes. Of note, no patient with a complete cytogenetic response and a three-log or more reduction in BCR-ABL transcripts (termed *major molecular response* or *MMR*) at 12 or 18 months progressed to accelerated phase or blast crisis at 60 months.[34] MMR is defined as a decrease from a median baseline value established from newly diagnosed patients.[38] Thus, it corresponds to a specific value; an individual's baseline value is not necessary to determine this parameter.

Several factors have been shown to correlate with achievement of a complete cytogenetic response and MMR during imatinib therapy. These include trough imatinib levels greater than 1,000 ng/mL,[39] higher OCT-1 activity or expression,[40–42] a one-log decrease in quantitative RT-PCR for BCR-ABL at 3 months,[43,44] and drug compliance.[45] Because newer agents described in the following sections are less dependent on OCT-1 for cellular uptake, this prognostic factor may not apply to these drugs. Drug levels that are associated with response to the newer agents have also not been established. For all oral agents, compliance is an important factor, particularly with the requirement for prolonged therapy.

Dasatinib and Nilotinib

Two new tyrosine kinase inhibitors, dasatinib (Sprycel) and nilotinib (Tasigna), initially FDA-approved for patients with imatinib resistance or intolerance, have been compared to imatinib in newly diagnosed patients with chronic phase disease. Both dasatinib and nilotinib are significantly more potent ABL inhibitors than imatinib. Nilotinib, a structurally modified imatinib, inhibits a similar spectrum of kinases as imatinib.[46] In contrast, dasatinib is a distinct chemical compound that inhibits significantly more kinases, most notably, SRC family members.[47] Based on data demonstrating that cytogenetic response and MMR have prognostic significance, the randomized comparisons of imatinib to dasatinib and imatinib to nilotinib used these as primary end points. In both studies, with a median follow-up of approximately 14 months, dasatinib at 100 mg/d and nilotinib at 300 mg twice daily or 400 mg twice daily achieved higher rates of complete cytogenetic responses, MMR, and improvements in progression-free survival (Table 133.2).[48,49] Similar to the imatinib studies, no patients with MMR had disease progression to accelerated phase or blast crisis. Although longer follow-up will be required to confirm the durability of responses and safety, it is reasonable to consider dasatinib at 100 mg/d or nilotinib at 300 mg twice daily as initial therapy, particularly in patients with intermediate and high-risk Sokal scores. One additional tyrosine kinase inhibitor, bosutinib, which inhibits a similar spectra of kinases to dasatinib, has also been evaluated in newly diagnosed patients, with results expected to be reported soon.[50]

Responses and Side Effects

Responses with tyrosine kinase inhibitors are rapid, with noticeable decreases in the WBC count after 1 to 2 weeks and normalization within 4 to 6 weeks in the majority of patients. The decline in the platelet count is typically delayed by 1 to 2 weeks, with the majority of patients obtaining a CHR within 3 months. Bone marrow morphologies revert to normal in most patients, even patients without cytogenetic responses.

As shown in Table 133.2, the majority of patients will achieve a complete cytogenetic response. Despite the high response rates, only a fraction of patients treated with tyrosine kinase inhibitors will have undetectable levels of BCR-ABL transcripts by RT-PCR,[38,48,49] and the majority of these patients will relapse if therapy is discontinued. Thus, tyrosine kinase inhibitor therapy is currently viewed as a chronic, noncurative therapy.

The most common nonhematologic adverse events of the various tyrosine kinase inhibitors are shown in Table 133.3. As the 300 mg twice daily dose of nilotinib was generally better tolerated than the 400 mg twice daily dose with similar response rates, the 300 mg twice daily dose has been recommended as a starting dose for newly diagnosed patients. Only a minority of patients experience grade 3/4 toxicity, and most side effects can be managed successfully with supportive measures.[51–54] Specific side effects from nilotinib, including increases in bilirubin, amylase, or lipase, generally do not require specific intervention unless they progress to grade 3/4 toxicity or become symptomatic. Ten percent of patients treated with dasatinib will develop pleural effusions. These can generally be managed with diuretics or a short course of low-dose prednisone, and rarely require thoracentesis. Recurrent pleural effusions may also be less problematic with dose reductions to 70 mg/d.

Grade 3 or 4 myelosuppression is relatively common and is probably a therapeutic effect as the majority of hematopoiesis in patients with CML is derived from Ph chromosome–positive stem cells. As there is minimal suppression of normal hematopoiesis by imatinib, nilotinib, and dasatinib, dose reductions are unlikely to assist in the recovery of normal hematopoiesis. In the case of imatinib, doses lower than 300 mg/d may allow emergence of resistant leukemic clones, but the minimum adequate doses of dasatinib and nilotinib have not been established. For chronic phase patients, treatment should only be interrupted for an absolute neutrophil count of less than 1.0×10^9/L and a platelet count less than 50×10^9/L. These parameters can be modified for patients with more advanced disease. The use of myeloid or erythroid growth factors while continuing therapy with imatinib appears to be safe.

Disease Monitoring

Because of the risk of myelosuppression, patients should have complete blood counts checked weekly to every other week during the first 2 months of therapy. In the absence of significant myelosuppression, the frequency of hematologic monitoring can then be reduced. Liver function tests should also be monitored regularly during therapy, as should other laboratory tests to monitor for drug-specific adverse events.[51,52,54] Bone marrow cytogenetics should be monitored every 6 months until a complete cytogenetic response is obtained. Quantitative RT-PCR for *BCR-ABL*, should be monitored every 3 to 6 months on peripheral

TABLE 133.2

THERAPEUTIC MILESTONES WITH IMATINIB

	Time (mo)			
	3	6	12	18
Acceptable	CHR	<95% Ph+	< 35% Ph+	
Frequently observed	CHR	<35% Ph+	0% Ph+	MMR

CHR, complete hematologic response; Ph+, Philadelphia chromosome–positive metaphases; MMR, major molecular response.

TABLE 133.3

RANDOMIZED COMPARISONS OF IMATINIB TO NILOTINIB[49] AND IMATINIB TO DASATINIB[48]

	Imatinib 400 mg/d	Nilotinib 300 mg bid	Nilotinib 400 mg bid	*P* Value/ Comments
No. of patients	283	282	281	
CCyR at 12 mo	65%	80%	78%	<.001 for both comparisons
MMR at 12 mo[a]	22%	44%	43%	<.001 for both comparisons
Disease progression to AP/BC (median F/U 14 mo)	4%	<1%	<1%	
Adverse events	Nausea, diarrhea, vomiting, muscle spasms, and edema	Rash, headache, pruritus, alopecia, elevations of alanine aminotransferase, aspartate aminotransferase, and bilirubin, increased glucose		All grades, most being grade 1/2; adverse events were similar with both doses of nilotinib
Discontinuation for adverse events	7%	5%	9%	
Neutropenia	20%	12%	10%	Grade 3/4
Thrombocytopenia	9%	10%	12%	Grade 3/4
Anemia	5%	3%	3%	Grade 3/4

	Imatinib 400 mg/d	Dasatinib 100 mg/d	*P* Value/Comments
No. of patients	260	259	
CCyR at 12 mo[a]	72%	83%	.001
MMR at 12 mo	28%	46%	<.0001
Disease progression to AP/BC (median F/U 14 mo)	3.5%	1.9%	
Adverse events	Nausea, vomiting, diarrhea, muscle inflammation, rash, headache and fluid retention, hypophosphatemia	Nausea, vomiting, muscle inflammation, rash, and fluid retention Pleural effusions (10%)	All grades, most being grade 1/2; all except pleural effusions were more common with imatinib
Discontinuation for adverse events	4.3%	5%	
Neutropenia	20%	21%	Grade 3/4
Thrombocytopenia	10%	19%	Grade 3/4
Anemia	7%	10%	Grade 3/4

bid, twice daily; CCyR, complete cytogenetic response; MMR, major molecular response; AC/BP, accelerated phase/blastic crisis; F/U, follow-up.
[a]Primary end point.

blood as this provides a more sensitive assessment of residual disease and may allow earlier detection of relapse. In a small percentage of patients with a complete cytogenetic response, new cytogenetic abnormalities in Ph chromosome–negative clones have developed.[55] The significance of these abnormalities is unclear, but there have been rare reports of some of these patients developing myelodysplasia[56]; thus, bone marrow tests may still need to be performed on patients with complete cytogenetic responses but at less frequent intervals.

Defining Resistance and Optimal Responses

The loss of a CHR or the loss of a complete or major cytogenetic response on tyrosine kinase inhibitor therapy clearly signals resistance and should prompt a change in treatment strategy. Similarly, a rise in quantitative PCR may indicate resistance, but defining the fold-change that is consistent with resistance depends on the value and the sensitivity of the test. As a conservative estimate, a fivefold change should at least prompt repeat sampling, with further increases prompting additional evaluation, including bone marrow cytogenetics and ABL kinase mutational analysis. Defining suboptimal response is less clear, with two different sets of landmarks summarized in Table 133.2. Which of these guidelines is most appropriate depends on numerous factors, including goals of therapy, patient age, availability of a donor for HCT, and tolerance of therapy.[57,58] What is becoming increasingly clear is that achievement of a MMR results in the lowest risk of disease progression. Efforts to standardization BCR-ABL quantitation testing are ongoing to aid in determining whether patients achieve this landmark.

Management of Primary Treatment Resistance or Relapse

For patients treated with imatinib, loss of disease control in chronic phase patients occurs in approximately 15% in the first 5 years of therapy. In contrast, relapses have been a significant problem with single-agent imatinib for advanced phase disease. The most common mechanism mediating relapse is point mutations in the BCR-ABL kinase that render the kinase less sensitive to imatinib. The point mutations are scattered throughout the kinase domain and disrupt critical contact points between imatinib and the BCR-ABL protein or induce structural alterations that prevent imatinib binding.[1,59] Many of the mutations are highly imatinib-insensitive, whereas some may be amenable to increased doses of imatinib.[60,61] Other mechanisms of resistance include BCR-ABL amplification, drug efflux, and BCR-ABL–independent mechanisms, such as clonal evolution.[62,63]

Given that the majority of patients who relapse and have disease that remains dependent on the BCR-ABL kinase, it was logical to develop novel agents that inhibit imatinib-resistant mutations. As noted previously, dasatinib and nilotinib were initially developed for patients with imatinib resistance or intolerance, and others are in development. Both compounds inhibit the majority of imatinib-resistant mutations, with the exception of T315I.[46,47,61] Consistent with the preclinical profile, high response rates were seen in patients with all imatinib-resistant mutations except T315I. Responses were also seen in patients with resistance that was not caused by mutations.[64–67] The potency of dasatinib and nilotinib against imatinib-resistant mutation varies. Some mutations are less sensitive to nilotinib (Y253H, E255K/V, and F359V/C), whereas others are less sensitive to dasatinib (F317L and V299L).[61] T315I is the most common mutation that emerges in patients with resistance to dasatinib and nilotinib, although compound mutations that are highly drug-resistant have been seen on occasion.[68,69]

In phase 2 studies comparing various dose schedules of dasatinib (70 mg twice daily, 140 mg/d, 50 mg twice daily, and 100 mg/d), 100 mg/d yielded similar responses to higher doses or twice daily dosing, but had a lower incidence of pleural effusions.[70] In the phase 2 studies of nilotinib, it was found that despite the structural relation of nilotinib to imatinib, there was little, if any, cross intolerance.[66] Because of the desire to maximize activity against partially nilotinib-insensitive mutations, the recommended dose of nilotinib in patients with resistance to other drugs is 400 mg twice daily.

For patients who lose their response to one tyrosine kinase inhibitor or fail to achieve a desired response, available nontransplant treatment options include dose escalation (imatinib to 600 or 800 mg/d, nilotinib to 400 mg twice daily, or dasatinib to 140 mg/d) or using an alternate ABL kinase inhibitor. Responses in patients who relapse into chronic phase and achieve complete cytogenetic responses or MMR have been quite durable.[71,72] Patients not achieving at least a complete cytogenetic response or who progress on second-line therapy should be considered for HCT.[57] For patients who progress to accelerated phase or blast crisis, relapse rates for all nontransplant therapies are high, and alternate ABL kinase inhibitors should be considered only a bridge to transplant.

Mutational analysis may be useful in guiding selection of second-line therapies, but may not be the sole determining factor of response.[73–75] For example a patient with T315I would not be expected to respond to currently available kinase inhibitors. Available treatments besides HCT for patients with T315I include the plant alkaloid omacetaxine or clinical trials of oral inhibitors with activity against T315I. Subcutaneous administration of oxametacine in chronic phase patients with T315I achieved a high rate of hematologic response, with 15% of patients achieving a major cytogenetic response with a median durability of 6 months.[76] AP24534 is an orally available multiple tyrosine kinase inhibitor designed using a structure-based approach as a pan–BCR-ABL inhibitor with an inhibitory profile that includes T315I.[77] In a phase 1 dose-escalation clinical trial, activity was observed in patients with the T315I mutation,[78] and phase 2 studies are in progress. A third agent with activity against T315I in early-phase clinical trials is DCC-2036. This compound binds to a unique pocket of the ABL kinase formed in the transition between inactive and active states.[79]

HEMATOPOIETIC CELL TRANSPLANTATION

Despite the effectiveness of BCR-ABL kinase inhibitor therapy in controlling disease, allogeneic HCT remains the only therapy that can durably eradicate all evidence of CML. CML used to be the leading indication for allogeneic HCT until 1999, but with the widespread availability of imatinib, HCT rates for CML have fallen,[80] and the proportion proceeding to HCT with advanced-stage CML has increased.[81] If transplantation is performed with myeloablative conditioning during chronic phase using an HLA-matched sibling donor, 5-year survival rates are 60% to 80%, with a 10-year disease-free survival of 50% to 60%, and a 20-year survival of 38% (Table 133.4).

CML is rare in childhood, but 3-year survival rates with transplantation are 65% to 75% in first chronic phase.[82] For younger patients, HCT performed using unrelated donors early in the disease yields results similar to those obtained with HLA-matched siblings.[83] Better HLA matching to guide selection of unrelated donors,[84] consideration of non-HLA donor factors,[85] and general improvements in supportive care will likely result in continued improvement in the results of HCT.

Long-term quality of life after allogeneic HCT is quite good, although a subset of patients report physical limitations and many specific problems.[86,87] Approximately 50% to 60% of patients experience chronic graft-versus-host disease

TABLE 133.4

SUMMARY OF TRANSPLANT OUTCOMES USING MYELOABLATIVE CONDITIONING

	Related Donor		Unrelated Donor	
Phase	Hematologic Relapse (%)	5- to 15-Year Disease-Free Survival (%)	Hematologic Relapse (%)	5-Year Disease-Free Survival (%)
Chronic	5–15	40–80	5–7	40–70
Accelerated	10–25	20–40	15	20–40
Blast crisis	25–58	0–25	50	0–5

(GVHD), which is the leading cause of morbidity and nonrelapse mortality more than 2 years after HCT.[88]

Reduced-intensity conditioning regimens, otherwise known as *nonmyeloablative* or *mini* preparative regimens, emphasize immunosuppression rather than myeloablation to facilitate engraftment and can be performed in the outpatient setting. Cure relies on immune reconstitution from the donor, with or without additional lymphocyte infusions, to eradicate residual disease. Common preparative regimens include combinations of fludarabine, busulfan, low-dose total body irradiation, T-cell antibodies, and other immunosuppressive drugs. The reduced-intensity conditioning regimens avoid the high early mortality associated with myeloablative conditioning toxicity and prolonged neutropenia. However, infections and acute and chronic GVHD remain significant problems. Disease-free survival ranges from 40% to 85% at 3 to 5 years.[89,90] A large retrospective study conducted by the European Blood and Marrow Transplant group (EBMT) suggested that patients at low risk for transplant-related mortality did so well they should undergo conventional transplantation, whereas higher-risk patients might be best treated using reduced-intensity condition regimens because of their lower transplant-related mortality.[89]

Although CML is a stem cell disease, it arises from a somatic mutation, and normal progenitors are detectable in most patients with CML. This suggests that autologous HCT may be efficacious. However, a meta-analysis of six randomized studies showed no benefit to autologous HCT compared to interferon-based therapy.[91]

Timing of HCT

Most newly diagnosed patients with chronic phase CML receive a trial of BCR-ABL kinase inhibitor therapy. This approach should not preclude HLA typing of patients who are medically fit for HCT because some patients will not have adequate disease control with kinase inhibitor therapy, will be intolerant of therapy, or will have insufficient financial resources to continue medication indefinitely.[92] Pediatricians may be more aggressive about early HCT, particularly if an HLA-matched sibling donor is available.[93]

For the most part, factors that predict survival after HCT are different than those that predict response to imatinib. The EBMT identified five adverse prognostic factors for HCT: accelerated or blastic phase, disease duration greater than 12 months, patient age greater than 20 or 40 years, a female donor for a male patient, and transplantation from an unrelated donor (Fig. 133.3). The score was validated in independent cohorts of myeloablative and reduced-intensity conditioned patients.[89,94,95] Disease progression represents the major concern with deferring HCT while attempting an initial or subsequent trial of kinase inhibitor therapy as some patients will progress to accelerated phase or blast crisis. Stage of disease before transplantation is one of the most consistent predictors of outcome in related and unrelated donor HCT, with survival estimates roughly halving as the disease progresses from chronic phase to accelerated phase to blast crisis (Table 133.4).

A major controversy in HCT is whether to recommend an allogeneic HCT or second-line kinase inhibitor to patients who fail to attain a satisfactory response to imatinib or progress during treatment. Many considerations including risk of transplant-related mortality and aggressiveness of CML are being evaluated to help guide these decisions.[57,96,97]

Effect of Exposure to Tyrosine Kinase Inhibitors Prior to HCT

There are concerns that pretransplant exposure to BCR-ABL kinase inhibitor therapies could compromise the success of HCT. Poorer outcomes could result from direct drug toxicity, selection of resistant or more aggressive clones, or inability to undergo HCT later (e.g., because of disease progression, older age, comorbidities, inability to quickly find a donor, obtaining insurance coverage). The largest observational studies suggest similar[98] or better[99] outcomes if patients are exposed to imatinib prior to allogeneic HCT. A small case series suggested imatinib-resistant mutations are not associated with inferior HCT outcomes beyond what might be expected from clinically advanced disease.[100] Early reports about the outcomes of HCT after receipt of nilotinib or dasatinib suggest no adverse effects on HCT success.[101,102]

Disease Monitoring and Prophylaxis after Transplantation

A molecular remission achieved with allogeneic HCT appears more durable than one achieved with imatinib. Molecular

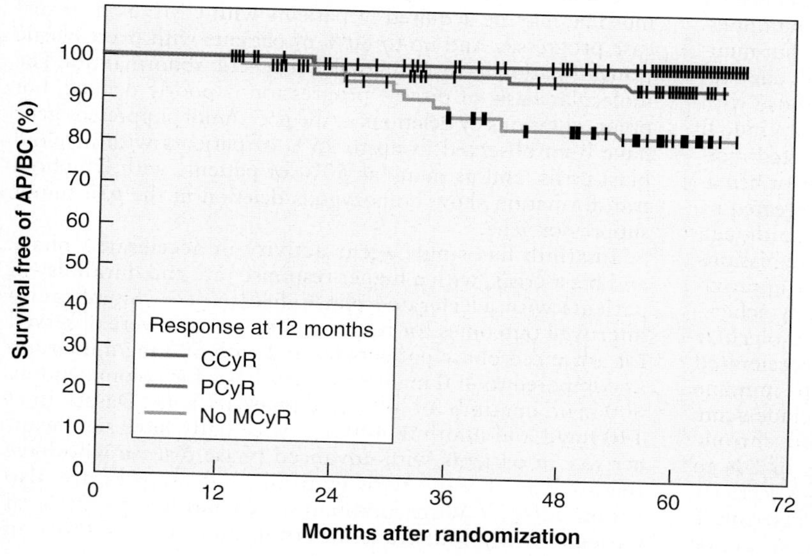

FIGURE 133.3 Survival of patients with chronic myelogenous leukemia undergoing allogeneic hematopoietic stem cell transplantation in the Center for International Bone Marrow Transplant Research validation set according to European Blood and Marrow Transplant risk score. The number of adverse prognostic factors correlates with survival.

PRACTICE OF ONCOLOGY

evidence of CML after myeloablative conditioning disappears with time in most patients; however, approximately 10% of patients remain RT-PCR–positive for years after HCT.[103] Quantitative PCR for the BCR-ABL transcript allows closer monitoring and detection of rising leukemia burden before cytogenetic or clinical relapse. A small study suggested that detection of BCR-ABL at day 100 after HCT is predictive of relapse.[104]

Imatinib has been used after HCT for prophylaxis against relapse. Small series suggest that therapeutic doses of imatinib can be safely administered from the time of engraftment through the first post-HCT year without serious cytopenias or exacerbation of GVHD.[105,106] Dasatinib and nilotinib post-HCT have also been used in a small number of patients.[107,108] These small numbers do not allow an assessment of the effectiveness of this approach in increasing long-term disease-free survival rates.

Management of Relapse after HCT

Most relapses occur early, with half during the first posttransplant year prior to imatinib and fewer than 5% occurring after 5 years. Early intervention for relapse offers the best chance of controlling disease, but overtreatment can result in serious toxicity or death. IFN, imatinib, withdrawal of immunosuppression, and/or donor lymphocyte infusion (DLI) from the original donor can all restore molecular remission. Patients may also undergo a second transplant from the same or different donor if sufficient time has elapsed to allow recovery from the first procedure. In recognition of the excellent prognosis of CML patients who re-enter remission after relapse, the current leukemia-free survival methodology allows them to be included on the disease-free survival curve.[109]

Imatinib as initial treatment for patients who relapse into chronic phase after allogeneic HCT restores complete molecular remission in 83% of patients in molecular relapse and 58% of those in cytogenetic relapse.[110] Approximately 10% to 25% of patients attaining complete molecular remissions are able to discontinue imatinib after 6 to 24 months and remain in remission, whereas the others required either reinstitution of imatinib or DLI.[111] Lower and less durable responses to imatinib are seen in patients relapsing into accelerated phase or blast crisis.[112] Early studies with dasatinib and nilotinib confirm their efficacy in this situation, but numbers are too small to draw firm conclusions.[107,113]

Of the hematologic malignancies, CML is uniquely sensitive to the graft-versus-leukemia (GVL) effect and has been a model for eradicating malignant disease through manipulation of the immune system. Patients with detectable but minimal (grade I) acute GVHD have the highest overall survival after HLA-matched sibling HCT compared with those with no GVHD (associated with increased relapse rates) or grade II to IV GVHD (associated with higher transplant-related mortality).[114] Of the patients who relapse cytogenetically or hematologically into chronic phase, 60% to 80% can be treated by DLI alone without further cytotoxic chemotherapy, although responses take several months to manifest. These remissions are durable, and 5-year disease-free survival rates are approximately 50%.[115] Some patients relapsing after initially achieving remission with DLI may achieve prolonged molecular remissions after additional DLI.[116] In contrast, accelerated phase and blast crisis are much less responsive to immune manipulations. Risks of DLI are significant and include acute GVHD, pancytopenia with infectious risks, and chronic GVHD resulting in a treatment-related mortality of 8% to 20%.[117] Efforts to decrease the toxicity of DLI by selectively infusing subsets of lymphocytes (CD8-depleted), inserting a suicide gene before infusion, minimizing the dose of donor lymphocytes, spreading out the dosing schedule, or expanding specific T-cell clones *ex vivo* before infusion appear to have some success. Combinations of imatinib and DLI are reported to have higher efficacy than either alone, although results are from a T-cell–depleted population.[118]

The biologic basis for the GVL effect, and whether it can be separated from a generalized GVHD phenomenon, is controversial. Because GVL responses can be observed without apparent GVHD, it is likely that leukemia-specific antigens can be recognized by the immune system. Hypothesized antigens include peptides derived from the BCR-ABL fusion protein; tissue-specific peptides, such as those derived from proteinase 3 or the Wilms tumor protein; or minor histocompatibility peptides.

Practically, the decision of how to manage relapse after allogeneic HCT depends on the kinetics of the CML relapse (molecular, hematologic, advanced phase), the likely sensitivity to kinase inhibitor therapy (previous resistance, known kinase mutations), the transplantation context (availability of donor lymphocytes, presence or absence of GVHD, whether the patient is on immunosuppressive medications), and the clinical status of the patient.

ADVANCED PHASE DISEASE

The transformation to advanced phase typically occurs gradually, with the disease becoming more difficult to control with medical therapy. In some patients, the disease transforms abruptly into an acute leukemia. This is called *blast crisis* or *blastic transformation*. Morphologically, the bone marrow of blastic-phase CML has greater than 30% blasts. Approximately 65% of patients evolve to blast crisis with myeloid lineage blasts; 30% have blasts of pre–B lymphoid origin; and 5% have undifferentiated or T-cell blasts. On occasion, an isolated blast phase of extramedullary origin may occur while the patient's blood and marrow otherwise meet criteria for chronic phase disease.

The intermediate period during which the patient is no longer in chronic phase but is not yet in blastic transformation has been termed the *accelerated phase*. The criteria for defining the accelerated phase are highly variable (Table 133.5), and only the M. D. Anderson criteria have been correlated with a median survival of 18 months or less. In some patients, a myelofibrotic picture characterizes the accelerated phase, where there is massive splenomegaly with extensive marrow fibrosis and extramedullary hematopoiesis.

Clonal cytogenetic abnormalities besides a single Ph chromosome may be acquired in patients with CML as their disease progresses, and up to 80% of patients with overt blastic transformation have additional cytogenetic abnormalities. The molecular basis of disease progression is poorly defined, but point mutations or deletions in the *p53* tumor suppressor gene have been observed in up to 25% of patients with myeloid blast crisis, and as many as 50% of patients with lymphoid transformation show homozygous deletion in the *p16* tumor suppressor gene.[119]

Imatinib has single-agent activity in accelerated phase and blast crisis, with a higher response rate and durability in patients with accelerated phase disease.[120,121] Significantly improved outcomes for response and survival were observed for advanced phase patients treated with 600 mg/d imatinib as compared to 400 mg/d and is the basis for recommending 600 mg/d imatinib for advanced phase patients. Dasatinib at 140 mg/d and nilotinib 400 mg twice daily have significant activity in patients with advanced phase disease who have relapsed on therapy with imatinib, but relapses are also common.[122–125] With combination chemotherapy, 20% of patients in myeloid transformation and 50% of those in

TABLE 133.5

CRITERIA FOR ACCELERATED PHASE OF CHRONIC MYELOGENOUS LEUKEMIA

International Bone Marrow Transplant Registry	M. D. Anderson Cancer Center
WBC difficult to control with busulfan or hydroxyurea	Peripheral blood blasts ≥15% but <30%
Rapid WBC doubling time (<5 d)	Peripheral blood blasts and promyelocytes ≥30%
Peripheral blood or marrow blasts ≥10% but <30%	Peripheral blood basophils ≥20%
Peripheral blood or marrow blasts and promyelocytes ≥20%	Platelet count <100 × 10^9/L unrelated to therapy
Peripheral blood basophils and eosinophils ≥20%	Clonal evolution
Anemia or thrombocytopenia unresponsive to busulfan or hydroxyurea	
Persistent thrombocytosis	
Clonal evolution	
Progressive splenomegaly and myelofibrosis	

WBC, white blood cell count.

lymphoid blast transformation achieve a second chronic phase, which is usually short-lived. The results for treatment of myeloid blast crisis with imatinib compare favorably to those of historical controls treated with chemotherapy. The high relapse rates suggest that kinase inhibitor therapy should be viewed as either a bridge to allogeneic HCT or patients should be enrolled in clinical trials combining kinase inhibitors or combining kinase inhibitor therapy with other agents. The results of allogeneic SCT in advanced phase disease are discussed in "Timing of HCT" and are summarized in Table 133.4.

FUTURE DIRECTIONS

There are now numerous treatment options available for patients with CML, and long-term disease control appears possible with current therapies. Ongoing studies will help to define the optimal treatment approach for newly diagnosed patients. As noted, there are two kinase inhibitors in clinical trials that appear to have activity against the recalcitrant T315I mutant. In addition, there are a variety of signal transduction inhibitors under development that impact pathways downstream of BCR-ABL. These include PI3-kinase, RAF, and MEK inhibitors.

Perhaps the most critical area for future development is minimal residual disease. As noted, the majority of patients being treated with tyrosine kinase inhibitors have disease that is well controlled but not eradicated. Although the molecular basis of disease persistence is poorly understood, studies of the mechanism are ongoing. Meanwhile, a variety of therapies based on manipulation of the immunologic system and signal transduction pathways are being investigated for their ability to impact CML stem cells.

PRACTICE OF ONCOLOGY

Selected References

The full list of references for this chapter appears in the online version.

1. Druker BJ. Translation of the Philadelphia chromosome into therapy for CML. *Blood* 2008;112:4808.
7. Nowell PC, Hungerford DA. A minute chromosome in human chronic granulocytic leukemia. *Science* 1960;132:1497.
8. Rowley JD. A new consistent abnormality in chronic myelogenous leukaemia identified by quinacrine fluorescence and giemsa staining. *Nature* 1973;243:290.
10. Deininger MW, Goldman JM, Melo JV. The molecular biology of chronic myeloid leukemia. *Blood* 2000;96:3343.
15. Savage DG, Szydlo RM, Goldman JM. Clinical features at diagnosis in 430 patients with chronic myeloid leukaemia seen at a referral centre over a 16-year period. *Br J Haematol* 1997;96:111.
22. Sokal JE, Cox EB, Baccarani M, et al. Prognostic discrimination in "good-risk" chronic granulocytic leukemia. *Blood* 1984;63:789.
29. Interferon alfa versus chemotherapy for chronic myeloid leukemia: a meta-analysis of seven randomized trials: Chronic Myeloid Leukemia Trialists' Collaborative Group. *J Natl Cancer Inst* 1997;89:1616.
30. Druker BJ, Talpaz M, Resta D, et al. Efficacy and safety of a specific inhibitor of the Bcr-Abl tyrosine kinase in chronic myeloid leukemia. *N Engl J Med* 2001;344:1031.
31. Kantarjian H, Sawyers C, Hochhaus A, et al. Hematologic and cytogenetic responses to imatinib mesylate in chronic myelogenous leukemia. *New Engl J Med* 2002;346:645.
32. O'Brien SG, Guilhot F, Larson RA, et al. Imatinib compared with interferon and low-dose cytarabine for newly diagnosed chronic-phase chronic myeloid leukemia. *N Engl J Med* 2003;348:994.
34. Druker BJ, Guilhot F, O'Brien SG, et al. Five-year follow-up of patients receiving imatinib for chronic myeloid leukemia. *N Engl J Med* 2006;355:2408.
38. Hughes TP, Kaeda J, Branford S, et al. Frequency of major molecular responses to imatinib or interferon alfa plus cytarabine in newly diagnosed chronic myeloid leukemia. *N Engl J Med* 2003;349:1423.
45. Marin D, Bazeos A, Mahon FX, et al. Adherence is the critical factor for achieving molecular responses in patients with chronic myeloid leukemia who achieve complete cytogenetic responses on imatinib. *J Clin Oncol* 2010;28:2381.
46. Weisberg E, Manley PW, Breitenstein W, et al. Characterization of AMN107, a selective inhibitor of native and mutant Bcr-Abl. *Cancer Cell* 2005;7:129.
47. Shah NP, Tran C, Lee FY, et al. Overriding imatinib resistance with a novel ABL kinase inhibitor. *Science* 2004;305:399.

48. Kantarjian H, Shah NP, Hochhaus A, et al. Dasatinib versus imatinib in newly diagnosed chronic-phase chronic myeloid leukemia. *N Engl J Med* 2010;362:2260.
49. Saglio G, Kim DW, Issaragrisil S, et al. Nilotinib versus imatinib for newly diagnosed chronic myeloid leukemia. *N Engl J Med* 2010;362:2251.
53. Quintas-Cardama A, Cortes JE, Kantarjian H. Practical management of toxicities associated with tyrosine kinase inhibitors in chronic myeloid leukemia. *Clin Lymphoma Myeloma* 2008;8(Suppl 3):S82.
57. Baccarani M, Cortes J, Pane F, et al. Chronic myeloid leukemia: an update of concepts and management recommendations of European LeukemiaNet. *J Clin Oncol* 2009;27:6041.
59. Shah NP, Nicoll JM, Nagar B, et al. Multiple BCR-ABL kinase domain mutations confer polyclonal resistance to the tyrosine kinase inhibitor imatinib (STI571) in chronic phase and blast crisis chronic myeloid leukemia. *Cancer Cell* 2002;2:117.
61. O'Hare T, Walters DK, Stoffregen EP, et al. In vitro activity of Bcr-Abl inhibitors AMN107 and BMS-354825 against clinically relevant imatinib-resistant Abl kinase domain mutants. *Cancer Res* 2005;65:4500.
65. Kantarjian H, Giles F, Wunderle L, et al. Nilotinib in imatinib-resistant CML and Philadelphia chromosome-positive ALL. *N Engl J Med* 2006; 354:2542.
67. Talpaz M, Shah NP, Kantarjian H, et al. Dasatinib in imatinib-resistant Philadelphia chromosome-positive leukemias. *N Engl J Med* 2006; 354:2531.
68. Shah NP, Skaggs BJ, Branford S, et al. Sequential ABL kinase inhibitor therapy selects for compound drug-resistant BCR-ABL mutations with altered oncogenic potency. *J Clin Invest* 2007;117:2562.
69. Soverini S, Gnani A, Colarossi S, et al. Philadelphia-positive patients who already harbor imatinib-resistant Bcr-Abl kinase domain mutations have a higher likelihood of developing additional mutations associated with resistance to second- or third-line tyrosine kinase inhibitors. *Blood* 2009; 114:2168.
70. Shah NP, Kantarjian HM, Kim DW, et al. Intermittent target inhibition with dasatinib 100 mg once daily preserves efficacy and improves tolerability in imatinib-resistant and —intolerant chronic-phase chronic myeloid leukemia. *J Clin Oncol* 2008;26:3204.
73. Hughes T, Saglio G, Branford S, et al. Impact of baseline BCR-ABL mutations on response to nilotinib in patients with chronic myeloid leukemia in chronic phase. *J Clin Oncol* 2009;27:4204.
74. Jabbour E, Jones D, Kantarjian HM, et al. Long-term outcome of patients with chronic myeloid leukemia treated with second-generation tyrosine kinase inhibitors after imatinib failure is predicted by the in vitro sensitivity of BCR-ABL kinase domain mutations. *Blood* 2009;114:2037.
75. Valent P. Standard treatment of Ph+ CML in 2010: how, when and where not to use what BCR/ABL1 kinase inhibitor? *Eur J Clin Invest* 2010; 40(10):918.
77. O'Hare T, Shakespeare WC, Zhu X, et al. AP24534, a pan-BCR-ABL inhibitor for chronic myeloid leukemia, potently inhibits the T315I mutant and overcomes mutation-based resistance. *Cancer Cell* 2009; 16:401.
80. Gratwohl A, Schwendener A, Baldomero H, et al. Changes in the use of hematopoietic stem cell transplantation: a model for diffusion of medical technology. *Haematologica* 2010;95:637.
81. Giralt SA, Arora M, Goldman JM, et al. Impact of imatinib therapy on the use of allogeneic haematopoietic progenitor cell transplantation for the treatment of chronic myeloid leukaemia. *Br J Haematol* 2007; 137:461.
83. Weisdorf DJ, Anasetti C, Antin JH, et al. Allogeneic bone marrow transplantation for chronic myelogenous leukemia: comparative analysis of unrelated versus matched sibling donor transplantation. *Blood* 2002;99: 1971.
84. Lee SJ, Klein J, Haagenson M, et al. High-resolution donor-recipient HLA matching contributes to the success of unrelated donor marrow transplantation. *Blood* 2007;110:4576.
88. Goldman JM, Majhail NS, Klein JP, et al. Relapse and late mortality in 5-year survivors of myeloablative allogeneic hematopoietic cell transplantation for chronic myeloid leukemia in first chronic phase. *J Clin Oncol* 2010;28:1888.
89. Crawley C, Szydlo R, Lalancette M, et al. Outcomes of reduced-intensity transplantation for chronic myeloid leukemia: an analysis of prognostic factors from the Chronic Leukemia Working Party of the EBMT. *Blood* 2005;106:2969.
90. Or R, Shapira MY, Resnick I, et al. Nonmyeloablative allogeneic stem cell transplantation for the treatment of chronic myeloid leukemia in first chronic phase. *Blood* 2003;101:441.
93. Lee SJ, Joffe S, Artz AS, et al. Individual physician practice variation in hematopoietic cell transplantation. *J Clin Oncol* 2008;26:2162.
94. Gratwohl A, Hermans J, Goldman JM, et al. Risk assessment for patients with chronic myeloid leukaemia before allogeneic blood or marrow transplantation. Chronic Leukemia Working Party of the European Group for Blood and Marrow Transplantation. *Lancet* 1998;352:1087.
95. Passweg JR, Walker I, Sobocinski KA, et al. Validation and extension of the EBMT Risk Score for patients with chronic myeloid leukaemia (CML) receiving allogeneic haematopoietic stem cell transplants. *Br J Haematol* 2004;125:613.
96. Pavlu J, Kew AK, Taylor-Roberts B, et al. Optimizing patient selection for myeloablative allogeneic hematopoietic cell transplantation in chronic myeloid leukemia in chronic phase. *Blood* 2010;115:4018.
97. Saussele S, Lauseker M, Gratwohl A, et al. Allogeneic hematopoietic stem cell transplantation (allo SCT) for chronic myeloid leukemia in the imatinib era: evaluation of its impact within a subgroup of the randomized German CML Study IV. *Blood* 2010;115:1880.
98. Oehler VG, Gooley T, Snyder DS, et al. The effects of imatinib mesylate treatment before allogeneic transplantation for chronic myeloid leukemia. *Blood* 2007;109:1782.
99. Lee SJ, Kukreja M, Wang T, et al. Impact of prior imatinib mesylate on the outcome of hematopoietic cell transplantation for chronic myeloid leukemia. *Blood* 2008;112:3500.
110. Hess G, Bunjes D, Siegert W, et al. Sustained complete molecular remissions after treatment with imatinib-mesylate in patients with failure after allogeneic stem cell transplantation for chronic myelogenous leukemia: results of a prospective phase II open-label multicenter study. *J Clin Oncol* 2005;23:7583.
119. Calabretta B, Perrotti D. The biology of CML blast crisis. *Blood* 2004;103: 4010.
120. Sawyers CL, Hochhaus A, Feldman E, et al. Imatinib induces hematologic and cytogenetic responses in patients with chronic myelogenous leukemia in myeloid blast crisis: results of a phase II study. *Blood* 2002;99:3530.
121. Talpaz M, Silver RT, Druker BJ, et al. Imatinib induces durable hematologic and cytogenetic responses in patients with accelerated phase chronic myeloid leukemia: results of a phase 2 study. *Blood* 2002;99:1928.
122. Cortes J, Kim DW, Raffoux E, et al. Efficacy and safety of dasatinib in imatinib-resistant or -intolerant patients with chronic myeloid leukemia in blast phase. *Leukemia* 2008;22:2176.
125. le Coutre P, Ottmann OG, Giles F, et al. Nilotinib (formerly AMN107), a highly selective BCR-ABL tyrosine kinase inhibitor, is active in patients with imatinib-resistant or -intolerant accelerated-phase chronic myelogenous leukemia. *Blood* 2008;111:1834.

CHAPTER 134 CHRONIC LYMPHOCYTIC LEUKEMIAS

WILLIAM G. WIERDA AND SUSAN O'BRIEN

Chronic lymphocytic leukemia (CLL) is a monoclonal hematopoietic disorder characterized by progressive expansion of B lymphocytes. These small, mature-appearing lymphocytes accumulate in the blood, bone marrow, lymph nodes, liver, and spleen. CLL is a common leukemia in the Western world, accounting for 25% to 30% of all adult leukemias.[1]

The 2003–2007 annual age-adjusted incidence of CLL in the United States was 4.2 per 100,000 per year; it was 5.7 per 100,000 for men and 3.0 per 100,000 for women.[2] The median age at diagnosis was 72 years, a nd the incidence increases with increasing age. For 2010, there were 14,990 estimated new cases, 8,870 men and 6,120 women. During the same year there were 4,390 estimated deaths, 2,650 men and 1,740 women, with a median age at death of 79.[3] The majority of patients have significant comorbidities owing to their advanced age. As a result, they tend to have health, geographic, and access limitations. Patients with CLL enrolled in clinical trials tend to be younger, with a median age of 58 to 62 years, thereby limiting the ability to generalize results from such trials to practice.

In Asian countries, CLL represents only 5% of leukemias, with T-cell phenotype predominating. Geographic and ethnic differences in incidence are most likely the result of genetic factors, since Japanese who settled in Hawaii do not have a higher incidence of CLL than native Japanese.[4] Population studies have not linked the development of CLL to known occupational or environmental risk factors.[5] CLL has a strong familial aggregation, with a two- to sevenfold higher prevalence among family clusters than in the general population.[6]

MOLECULAR BIOLOGY

Immunophenotype

Clonality of CLL is confirmed by restricted expression of either kappa or lambda light chain on the cell surface membrane.[1] The immunoglobulin (Ig) gene rearrangement is clonal, and therefore the CLL cells possess a unique idiotypic specificity and often have cytogenetic or molecular abnormalities.[7] With the use of sensitive techniques, monoclonal Ig can be detected in serum of many patients, although only 5% to 10% of patients produce large enough quantities to be detected by serum electrophoresis. CLL cells express the B-cell markers CD19, CD20, CD21, CD23, and CD24; most CLL cells are also positive for major histocompatibility complex (MHC) class II (DR and DQ) Fc receptors and have receptors for mouse erythrocytes (Table 134.1).[8] Some surface markers that are usually found on normal B cells, including CD22, are infrequently found on CLL cells. CLL cells characteristically express CD5, an antigen normally found on T cells. CD5 can be found in small numbers of normal polyclonal B cells, predominantly in fetal circulation or in tonsils of normal adults. They usually are not detected in peripheral blood using standard immunophenotyping techniques.

Unexpectedly, as high as 3.5% of otherwise normal individuals over age 40 may harbor a population of clonal (by light chain analysis) CD5+/19+/23+ B cells.[9] These asymptomatic individuals do not have an absolute lymphocytosis or clinical evidence of CLL and are referred to as having monoclonal B lymphocytosis (MBL). Furthermore, as many as 13% of family members of patients with familial CLL harbor a population of cells with an immunophenotype consistent with CLL, but do not fulfill diagnostic criteria. Therefore, the incidence of a monoclonal lymphoproliferative process is potentially much more common than previously appreciated. It is estimated that the rate of progression to reach a diagnosis of CLL in this population is 1% to 2% per year.[10] Currently, there is no indication for MBL screening.

Immunoglobulin Heavy Chain Variable Gene Mutation Status

Because CD5+ B cells are found in fetal spleen and because surface immunoglobulin D is present on cells that have not encountered antigen in the germinal center, it was long presumed that CLL cells are naive B cells. Normal B-cell development involves an antigen-independent phase and an antigen-dependent phase. During the antigen-independent phase, B cells undergo rearrangement of the V, D, and J genes in the bone marrow. Somatic mutation of the heavy- and light-chain variable gene occurs after encounter with antigen in the germinal center. Somatic mutations have occurred when there is less than 98% sequence homology with the germline gene. The figure of 98% is used because polymorphisms may account for lesser degrees of disparity.[11]

In the 1990s, data emerged that a significant percentage of patients had mutation of their immunoglobulin heavy chain variable gene (*IGHV*). Subsequently, it was confirmed that approximately 50% of patients have mutated IGHV and that this provides prognostic information; patients with an unmutated IGHV have significantly shorter survival.[12] The characterization of the IGHV sequence is labor intensive and has not been readily exportable to clinical laboratories. Thus, correlates with mutation status that may be more easily identified may be clinically relevant. A correlation between expression of CD38 and lack of somatic mutation has been described.[13] Although the correlation is significant and the presence of CD38, irrespective of mutation status, is associated with inferior survival, a significant minority of patients have mutated *IGHV* and yet express CD38, and vice versa. These patients may have an intermediate prognosis. Also, there may be variation in CD38 expression over time or by disease site in some patients.

TABLE 134.1

IMMUNOPHENOTYPING IN CHRONIC B-CELL LEUKEMIA

Disease	sIg	CD5	CD23	FMC7	CD22	CD79b	CD10
CLL	Weak	++	++	−/+	Weak/−	Weak/−	−
B-PLL	Strong	−/+	−/+	++	+	++	−
HCL	Strong	−	−	++	++	+	−
SLVL	Strong	−/+	−/+	++	++	++	−
FL	Strong	−	−	++	++	++	++
MCL	Strong	++	−/+	++	++	++	−/+

CLL, chronic lymphocytic leukemia; +, present; −, not present; B-PLL, B-cell prolymphocytic leukemia; FL, follicular lymphoma; HCL, hairy cell leukemia; MCL, mantle cell lymphoma; sIg, surface immunoglobulin; SLVL, splenic lymphoma with villous lymphocytes.

It was hypothesized that since patients with CLL can be segregated into two distinct prognostic categories based on IGHV mutation status that CLL may represent two separate disease entities, one derived from a naive B cell that expressed unmutated IGHV and the other derived from a memory B cell that had been exposed to antigen and displayed a mutated IGHV. This hypothesis has been examined using gene expression profiling.[14] Investigators found that mutated and unmutated CLL show a common pattern of expression that is clearly distinguishable from that of other lymphomas, as well as normal B cells. Nevertheless, although the overall profile was similar, many genes were differentially expressed between the two groups. The gene that was most differentially expressed in one series was *ZAP-70*, with unmutated cases having significant expression of ZAP-70. Interestingly, this protein is normally found in T cells, where it functions as an intracellular signal-transduction molecule for the T-cell receptor. It was subsequently shown that ligation of the B-cell receptor (BCR) in CLL cells that expressed ZAP-70 produced greater tyrosine phosphorylation of cytosolic proteins than did stimulation of CLL cells that did not express ZAP-70; therefore, it may function in activating CLL cells. Expression of ZAP-70 was analyzed in 56 patients with CLL. This expression correlated with mutational status, disease progression, and survival in retrospective analyses (Fig. 134.1).[15]

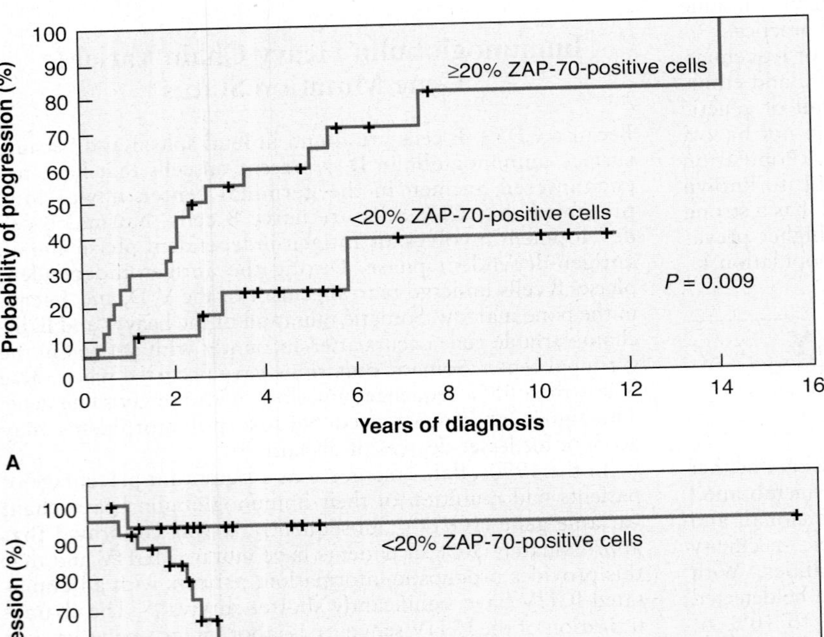

FIGURE 134.1 Kaplan-Meier estimates of the actuarial risk of disease progression (A) and the likelihood of survival (B) among patients with Binet stage A chronic lymphocytic leukemia, according to the level of expression of ZAP-70.

Molecular Abnormalities

Conventional chromosome banding identified cytogenetic abnormalities in 40% to 50% of CLL cases, with trisomy 12 being most common. This technique is hampered by the low mitotic activity of CLL cells. Fluorescence *in situ* hybridization (FISH), using genomic DNA probes, has enhanced the ability to detect molecular abnormalities. This technique can detect aberrations in interphase cells. The use of FISH has shown molecular abnormalities in over 80% of CLL cases.[7]

Deletion 13q is the most common genetic aberration in CLL; it is found by FISH as a sole abnormality in 55% of cases, followed by 11q deletion (18%), 12q trisomy (16%), and 17p deletion (7%).[7] Prognosis in CLL has been correlated with the presence of these chromosomal abnormalities. When divided into five hierarchical prognostic categories—17p deletion, 11q deletion, 12q trisomy, normal karyotype, and 13q deletion (sole abnormality)—the survival times were 32, 79, 114, 111, and 133 months, respectively. Patients with 17p or 11q deletion had more advanced disease with extensive lymphadenopathy.

The frequency of 13q deletion led to a search for a potentially new tumor suppressor gene in that location. At least eight genes were identified and screened for alterations at the DNA or RNA level, or both, but studies failed to find consistent involvement of any of those genes. However, two potentially relevant microRNA (miR) genes, miR15 and miR16, were identified in the critical minimal deleted region of 13q and were noted to be deleted or down-regulated in more than two-thirds of all CLL cases.[16] MicroRNAs are nontranslated small RNAs that function to regulate gene expression. Both miR15 and miR16 negatively regulate *BCL-2* transcript level, and absence of miR15 and miR16 in cases with 13q deletion may be responsible for Bcl-2 overexpression and resultant resistance to apoptosis.

Another important finding that may significantly aid in identifying factors that lead to the development of CLL is a *TCL-1* murine model whereby mice accumulate an expanded CD51 B-cell population, initially in the peritoneal cavity and then in the bone marrow; in addition, older mice develop a CLL-like disorder.[17] This transgenic mouse model was established with the T-cell leukemia-1 (*TCL-1*) gene under the control of an immunoglobulin promoter. This model may also be useful to test novel anti-CLL therapies in the future.

IMMUNE ABNORMALITIES

CLL cells disrupt immune function of patients with CLL. The most prominent manifestation of immune dysfunction is the increased risk and frequency of infections. Many patients with CLL succumb to infection or ineffectively treated autoimmunity. The treatments used for CLL, such as purine analogues, further immunosuppress patients and put them at increased risk for opportunistic infections and may exacerbate or unmask autoimmunity.

Early in the disease, the absolute number of T cells is increased in untreated CLL with inversion of the T helper–T suppressor cell ratio.[18,19] The CD4 to CD8 ratio continues to drop with disease progression or after therapy with nucleoside analogues or alemtuzumab. Qualitative functional assessment of T cells has been inconclusive. Normal and decreased CD4 cell function has been reported. Similarly, decreased, normal, or excessive CD8 cell function has been reported. Others have shown that T-cell functions may be impaired by immunosuppressive factors produced by CLL cells.[18] Hypogammaglobulinemia is a common and progressive immune defect in patients with CLL and is another factor that increases the risk for infection. The pathogenesis of hypogammaglobulinemia in CLL is poorly understood. Impaired B-cell function and regulatory abnormalities of T cells, including the reversal of the normal helper–suppressor cell ratio, may play a role. In addition, CLL-derived natural killer (NK) cells have been shown to suppress immunoglobulin secretion by normal B cells *in vitro*.

DIAGNOSIS

The International Workshop on CLL (IWCLL) recently updated the National Cancer Institute Working Group 1996 guidelines for diagnostic criteria and treatment for CLL.[20]

International Workshop on Chronic Lymphocytic Leukemia Revised Diagnostic Criteria

1. A peripheral blood B lymphocyte count greater than 5×10^9/L, with less than 55% of the cells being atypical (prolymphocytes).
2. The lymphocytes should be monoclonal (by light chain restriction) B lymphocytes expressing B-cell surface antigens (CD19, CD20, CD23), low-density surface immunoglobulin (M or D), and CD5.

A B-lymphocyte count greater than 5×10^9/L was specified to distinguish CLL from small lymphocytic lymphoma (SLL) in patients with palpable lymph nodes or splenomegaly. However, it is arguable as to whether that distinction is clinically relevant. Bone marrow aspirate will usually show greater than 30% lymphocytes, with flow cytometry confirming monoclonality in the CD19/CD20/CD23/CD5+ population; however, bone marrow evaluation is not required for diagnosis.

Other B-cell malignancies may also present with increased circulating lymphoid cells and should be differentiated from CLL. The diseases that may be confused with CLL are prolymphocytic leukemia (PLL), the leukemic phase of non-Hodgkin's lymphoma (mantle cell lymphoma, follicular lymphoma, or splenic lymphoma with circulating villous lymphocytes), and hairy cell leukemia (HCL). Immunophenotyping is helpful in differentiating these disorders (Figs. 134.2, 134.3, and 134.4; Table 134.1).

CLINICAL MANIFESTATIONS

Approximately half of CLL patients are asymptomatic and are diagnosed after routine blood counts. Some patients remain asymptomatic for a long period of time. In patients presenting with symptoms, the most common complaint is fatigue; this is generally mild. Sometimes enlarged lymph nodes or the

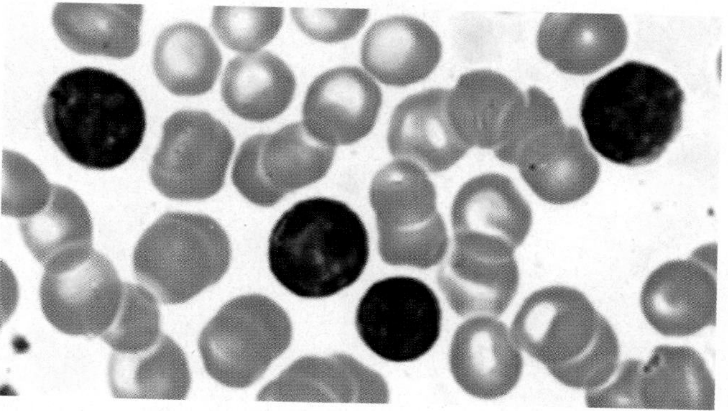

FIGURE 134.2 Chronic lymphocytic leukemia. Peripheral smear showing mature-appearing lymphocytes.

PRACTICE OF ONCOLOGY

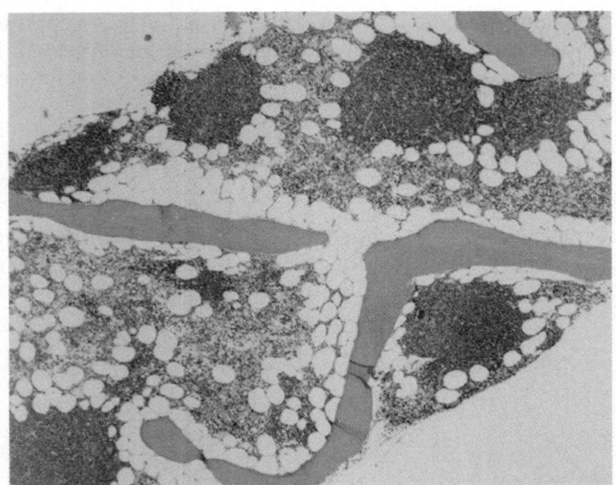

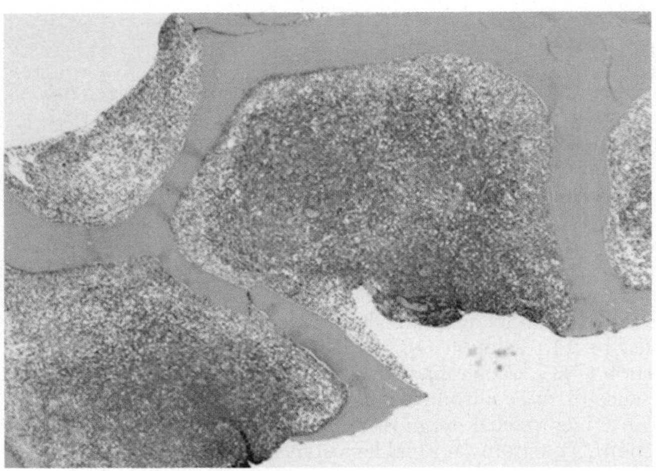

FIGURE 134.3 Chronic lymphocytic leukemia. Bone marrow infiltration may range from nodular/focal (A) to diffuse (B).

development of an infection is the initial manifestation of disease. Bacterial infections, such as pneumonia, are more common in patients who present with advanced-stage disease. Infections secondary to opportunistic organisms, particularly herpes zoster, may occur. An exaggerated skin reaction to a bee sting or an insect bite is frequent (Well syndrome). In contrast to the situation in lymphoma, fever in the absence of infection is rare in CLL. The lymph nodes, when enlarged, are usually discrete, freely movable, and nontender. Splenomegaly may occur, but massive splenomegaly is usually only seen in patients with end-stage disease. Splenic infarction is rare. Hepatomegaly occurs less frequently than splenomegaly. Skin involvement occurs in fewer than 5% of cases. Leptomeningeal leukemia is rare and, if present, is usually seen in patients with refractory disease. Malignant pleural effusions are also rare, and when present, are associated with aggressive disease.

Laboratory Findings

Absolute lymphocyte counts range from roughly 5×10^9/L to over 500×10^9/L. Unlike in acute myeloid leukemia, leukostasis is uncommon in CLL, probably because of the small size and pliability of the leukemia cells.

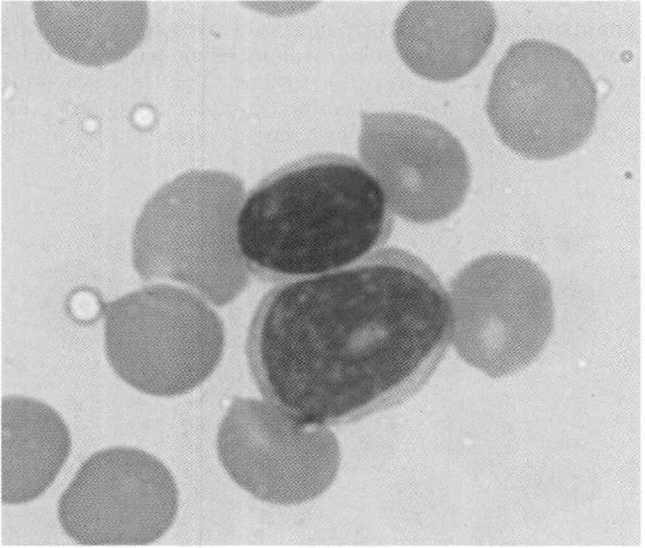

FIGURE 134.4 Prolymphocyte juxtaposed with a mature-appearing lymphocyte. Note larger size, less-condensed chromatin, and prominent nucleolus.

Marrow infiltration by lymphocytes is universal, affecting from 30% to 100% of the cellularity, with increased marrow cellularity. The lymphocyte count usually increases over time, but fluctuations in the lymphocyte counts of untreated patients may occur, particularly in the setting of infection. In most cases, the lymphocytes are small and mature appearing, but there may be variations in cell morphology, with some lymphocytes being larger or atypical, whereas others may be plasmacytoid or cleaved or there may be prolymphocytes. Ruptured lymphocytes or "smudge" cells are commonly seen in the peripheral smear, reflecting fragility and distortion during preparation of the peripheral smear on the glass slide. The patterns of lymphoid infiltration of the marrow seen in biopsy specimens include nodular, interstitial, diffuse, or a combination. Patients with diffuse infiltration typically have advanced disease and a worse prognosis. Nodular and interstitial patterns may be grouped together as "nondiffuse" and are associated with less advanced disease and better outcome.

Anemia (hemoglobin less than 11 g/dL) and thrombocytopenia (platelet count less than 100×10^9/L) are frequent with disease progression but are found in only a minority of patients at diagnosis. A positive direct antiglobulin test (Coombs') is seen in approximately 25% of cases, but overt autoimmune hemolytic anemia (AIHA) occurs less frequently. The incidence of a positive Coombs' test increases significantly with clinical stage.[21] Autoimmune thrombocytopenia is usually diagnosed on the basis of a low platelet count in the presence of adequate numbers of megakaryocytes in the bone marrow. Neutropenia may also be encountered. These cytopenias may be the result of bone marrow failure due to "packed" marrow by CLL or occur as a result of an immune-mediated process or hypersplenism. Hypogammaglobulinemia occurs in approximately 50% of patients with CLL. At diagnosis, it may be noted in fewer than 10% of patients, but its incidence increases significantly with disease progression. Usually, all three Ig classes (G, A, and M) are decreased, but in some patients, only one or two may be low. Significant hypogammaglobulinemia and neutropenia result in increased susceptibility to bacterial infections.

Autoimmune Complications

When autoantibodies are present in CLL, they are usually targeted against hematopoietic cells, resulting in AIHA, immune thrombocytopenia, immune-mediated granulocytopenia, and pure red cell aplasia, AIHA being the most frequent.[22] Several factors indicate that antibodies against blood cell antigens are not produced by the leukemic clone. The autoantibodies are polyclonal and are usually IgG.[23] The severity of the autoimmune phenomenon does not necessarily correlate with the severity of CLL, and such events may develop in patients whose disease is responding to therapy. Prednisone is the most commonly used treatment for autoimmune complications, with high initial response rates. It is usually given at a dose of 1 mg/kg orally and tapered once a response is noted. Relapses are not uncommon. Cyclosporin A is another effective therapy and can produce good results, even in steroid-refractory patients.[24] The monoclonal antibodies rituximab and alemtuzumab have been used in some patients in whom standard therapy fails and have produced responses. Splenectomy is also a viable therapeutic option for refractory cases.

Staging

The natural history of CLL is variable, with survival times ranging from 2 to over 20 years from diagnosis. In 1975, Rai et al.[25] developed a staging system consisting of five stages (Rai 0 to IV) based on Dameshek's model of orderly disease progression in CLL (Table 134.2). The Rai staging system was later modified into a three-stage system: low risk (Rai 0), intermediate risk (Rai I, II), and high risk (Rai III, IV). A similar staging system was developed in Europe by Binet et al.[26]; Binet stages A, B, and C generally correspond to low-risk, intermediate-risk, and high-risk disease in Rai staging. Both classifications reflect bulk of disease and extent of marrow compromise (i.e., anemia, thrombocytopenia). Both staging systems have been recognized as simple and accurate predictors of survival (Table 134.2). Although most patients in the high-risk group (Rai III, IV; Binet C) have a progressive clinical course and short survival, the course of the disease is not uniform. Patients in the low- and intermediate-risk groups may have an indolent disease course that spans years or even decades, or the course may be progressive and associated with a shortened survival. Thus, it is important to have prognostic factors associated with clinical outcomes in CLL in the low-risk groups. Several prognostic factors have been associated with shortened survival in CLL. These include a short lymphocyte doubling time (less than 6 months), a diffuse pattern of bone marrow infiltration, advanced age and male gender, abnormal karyotype, high serum levels of β_2-microglobulin and soluble CD23, and a CLL-PLL category (11% to 54% prolymphocytes in the blood).[27] Newer prognostic factors in CLL include IGHV mutation status, expression of CD38 and ZAP-70, as previously described.

TREATMENT AND RESPONSE CRITERIA

An unusual feature of CLL compared to other leukemias is that making the diagnosis is not necessarily an indication to initiate treatment. This is true for several reasons. CLL is a disease of the older population, it may be diagnosed in an asymptomatic patient and have a prolonged course, it is not curable with current treatment approaches, and a survival advantage was not demonstrated with early intervention clinical trials. Given that the majority of patients are older than 70 years, may have serious comorbid conditions associated with aging, and may have indolent disease, a significant fraction of patients will die of other causes and may never require therapy for CLL.

The IWCLL revised criteria for active disease, an indication to initiate treatment,[20] include constitutional symptoms attributable to CLL: weight loss (greater than 10% of baseline weight within the preceding 6 months), extreme fatigue (Eastern Cooperative Oncology Group performance status 2 or more), fever (temperature higher than 38°C or 100.5°F for at least 2 weeks) or night sweats without evidence of infection; evidence of progressive bone marrow failure characterized by the development or worsening anemia, thrombocytopenia, or both; AIHA or autoimmune thrombocytopenia, or both, poorly responsive to corticosteroid therapy; massive (greater than 6 cm below the left costal margin) or progressive splenomegaly; massive (greater than 10 cm in longest diameter) or progressive lymphadenopathy; progressive lymphocytosis defined as an increase in the absolute lymphocyte count by greater than 50% over a 2-month period, or a doubling time predicted to be less than 6 months.

Hypogammaglobulinemia or monoclonal gammopathy is not a sufficient criterion to initiate therapy.

Several European groups conducted trials in the 1980s to evaluate whether immediate treatment in patients with early stage disease could improve survival.[28] These large randomized trials of immediate chlorambucil (CLB) therapy versus a watch-and-wait approach were consistent in showing no survival benefit with early treatment. Nevertheless, given the significantly better therapies available in the 21st century, this question has been raised again. A limitation of randomizing all early stage patients is that approximately one-third of them may never require therapy for their disease, thus diluting any potential benefit to early treatment. The discovery of prognostic factors that can identify early stage patients with a high likelihood of developing progressive disease may now allow such randomized trials to be conducted.

The response criteria published in 1988 by the National Cancer Institute Working Group (NCI-WG) on CLL were

TABLE 134.2

STAGING OF CHRONIC LYMPHOCYTIC LEUKEMIA

Rai Stage	Modified Rai Stage	Description	Binet Stage	Description
0	Low risk	Lymphocytosis only	A	Two or fewer lymphoid-bearing areas
1	Intermediate risk	Lymphocytosis and lymphadenopathy	B	Three or more lymphoid-bearing areas
2	Intermediate risk	Lymphocytosis and splenomegaly with/without lymphadenopathy	—	—
3	High risk	Lymphocytosis and anemia (hemoglobin, <11 g/dL)	C	Anemia (hemoglobin, <10 g/dL) or thrombocytopenia (platelets, 100 × 10⁶/dL)
4	High risk	Lymphocytosis and thrombocytopenia (platelets, <100 × 10⁶/dL)	—	—

TABLE 134.3

2008 INTERNATIONAL WORKSHOP ON CHRONIC LYMPHOCYTIC LEUKEMIA REVISED NATIONAL CANCER INSTITUTE–SPONSORED WORKING GROUP RESPONSE CRITERIA FOR CHRONIC LYMPHOCYTIC LEUKEMIA

Parameter[a]	CR	PR
Lymphocytes	≤4,000/mcL[b]	≥50% ↓
Lymph nodes (liver, spleen)	No palpable disease (LN < 1.5 cm)[c]	≥50% ↓
Neutrophils	≥1,500/mcL	≥1,500/mcL or ≥50% improvement
Platelets	>100,000/mcL	>100,000/mcL or ≥50% improvement
Hemoglobin	>11 g/dL (untransfused)	>11 g/dL or ≥50% improvement
Bone marrow	<30% lymphocytes, no nodules[d]	NA
Constitutional symptoms	None	Variable

↓, decrease; CR, complete response; NA, not applicable; PR, partial response.
[a]Assessed at least 2 months after completion of therapy.
[b]Include minimal residual disease (MRD) assessed for clinical trials with reported sensitivity of method.
[c]Computed tomography scan of chest, abdomen, and pelvis desired for patients to confirm for patients on clinical trial.
[d]Less than 30% lymphocytes in marrow with residual nodules should have immunohistochemistry to characterize nodules.

revised in 1996 and most recently updated by the IWCLL (Table 134.3).[20] The recommendation was made that patients treated in a clinical trial have evaluation of the blood or bone marrow by sensitive tests for residual disease such as multi-color flow cytometry or allele-specific polymerase chain reaction (PCR) for the *IGHV* gene. In some patients who achieve complete remission by IWCLL criteria, one or both of these methods can demonstrate residual disease, referred to as minimal residual disease (MRD). Patients free of MRD following treatment have a longer remission duration and longer survival.[29] Therefore, in addition to improving complete remission rates, investigators are focusing on eliminating MRD.

A sensitive four-color flow cytometry assay was developed to differentiate CLL cells from normal B cells (CD5/CD19 with CD20/CD38, CD81/CD22, and CD79b/CD43).[30] The assay can detect one CLL cell in 10^4 to 10^5 leukocytes. PCR techniques can also be used to assess MRD. Consensus primers for rearrangement of *IGHV* can be used in 70% to 80% of patients and may detect 1 in 10^4 residual cells. Allele-specific oligonucleotide primers generated for individual patients are more sensitive, detecting 1 in 10^5 CLL cells. Development of quantitative PCR techniques may aid in following patients over time but are technically complicated and therefore not available for routine clinical use. The NCI-WG 1996 response criteria are undergoing revision at the time of this printing.

Chemotherapy with Alkylating Agents

For many decades, the mainstay of therapy for CLL was alkylating agents: CLB and cyclophosphamide (CTX). These alkylating agents may be given with or without corticosteroids. Various doses and schedules of oral CLB have been used. CLB is usually administered for several months, and the dose is adjusted to avoid its primary toxicity, myelosuppression. The overall response rate with either CLB or CTX is approximately 40% to 60%, with 3% to 5% complete remission. Alkylating agents have been combined with steroids to improve response rates.[31] Alkylating agent–based combinations have also included an anthracycline (CHOP). No superior alkylating-agent combination has been identified.

Purine Analogues

Purine analogues, including fludarabine monophosphate, 2-chlorodeoxyadenosine (2-CdA), and pentostatin (deoxycoformycin), all have major activity in the treatment of patients with CLL.[31]

In a phase 2 trial conducted at M. D. Anderson Cancer Center, fludarabine was given at a dose of 30 mg/m^2/d for 5 days. A response rate of 59% was observed in 68 previously treated patients, with 15% achieving complete remission. A subsequent study explored the combination of fludarabine and prednisone. Response rates were identical to those seen with single-agent fludarabine, but the addition of prednisone was associated with an increased incidence of *Pneumocystis jiroveci* and *Listeria monocytogenes* infections. The major side effects associated with fludarabine were myelosuppression and immunosuppression, with low CD4 counts lasting for several months to years after completion of treatment.[31]

Single-arm studies evaluated fludarabine in previously untreated patients. Response rates were higher at 70% to 80% and complete remission was seen in 10% to 25%.[31] An oral formulation of fludarabine was evaluated in relapsed patients with CLL. Seventy-eight patients received oral fludarabine, 40 mg/m^2/d for 5 days every 4 weeks for six to eight cycles. The overall response rate was 51%, almost identical to prior trials using the intravenous formulation as a salvage regimen. Furthermore, oral fludarabine was used in the frontline Leukemia Research Foundation (LRF) CLL4 trial[32] to compare fludarabine plus CTX versus fludarabine versus CLB, demonstrating efficacy and tolerability with the oral formulation, which is now approved by the U.S. Food and Drug Administration (FDA).

Comparative Studies

A randomized European trial compared six cycles of fludarabine versus six cycles of CAP (cyclophosphamide, doxorubicin, prednisone) in 196 patients with Binet stage B or C CLL (Table 134.4).[33] In previously treated patients, a significantly higher overall response rate was observed with fludarabine compared to CAP. In previously untreated patients (Table 134.4), the response rates with fludarabine were similar to those with CAP, but the duration of response was significantly longer with fludarabine. The French Cooperative Group on CLL randomized nearly 1,000 previously untreated patients to one of three treatment regimens: fludarabine, CHOP, or CAP.[34] Higher overall response rate and longer time to progression were seen for fludarabine. Infection rates were similar, but extramedullary toxicity was less with fludarabine.

TABLE 134.4

RANDOMIZED TRIALS OF MONOTHERAPY OR ALKYLATING AGENT–BASED COMBINATIONS AS INITIAL TREATMENT FOR CHRONIC LYMPHOCYTIC LEUKEMIA

Study (Ref.)	Agent	No. of Patients	CR (%)	OR (%)	Median RD	Median OS (mo)
Leporrier et al. (34)	Fludarabine vs.	341	40	71	32 mo (TTP)	69
	CAP vs.	240	15	58	28 mo (TTP)	70
	CHOP	357	30	72	30 mo (TTP)	67
Rai et al. (35)	Fludarabine + Chlorambucil vs.	123	20	61	NR	55
	Fludarabine vs.	170	20	63	25 mo (TTP)	66
	Chlorambucil	181	4	37	14 mo (TTP)	56
Johnson et al. (33)	Fludarabine vs.	52	23	71	NR	60%@4 yr
	CAP	48	17	60	7	60%@4 yr
Eichhorst et al.[a] (37)	Fludarabine vs.	87	7	72	19 (PFS)	46
	Chlorambucil	98	0	51	18 (PFS)	64
Knauf et al. (38)	Bendamustine vs.	162	31	68	21.6 (PFS)	NR
	Chlorambucil	157	2	31	8.3 (PFS)	NR
Hillmen et al. (49)	Alemtuzumab vs.	149	24	83	14.6	NR
	Chlorambucil	148	2	55	11.7	NR

CR, complete remission; OR, overall response; RD, remission duration; OS, overall survival; NR, not reached; TTP, time-to-progression; CAP, cyclophosphamide, doxorubicin, prednisone; CHOP, cyclophosphamide, doxorubicin, prednisone, vincristine.
[a]Age 65 years or older.

Results from an Intergroup trial with 509 previously untreated patients with CLL showed significantly higher complete and overall remission rates in patients treated with fludarabine versus those given CLB (Table 134.4).[35] A third arm, fludarabine plus CLB, was closed early because of infection-related toxicity. Crossover was allowed for patients with no response or early relapse. Although a longer duration of response and an improved progression-free survival were noted in patients treated with fludarabine, no difference in overall survival was found between the two groups in the initial report. Half of the patients who failed to respond to CLB responded to fludarabine, including a 14% complete remission rate; in contrast, only 7% of patients who failed to respond to fludarabine achieved partial response with CLB. A recent update of this trial with significantly longer follow-up reported improved overall survival for patients treated initially with fludarabine; this difference emerged after 6 years of follow-up.[36] The German CLL Study Group (GCLLSG) CLL5 evaluated fludarabine versus CLB monotherapy as initial treatment for patients older than 65 years (Table 134.4).[37] Surprisingly, while treatment with fludarabine was associated with superior complete (7% vs. 0%) and overall (72% vs. 51%) response rates, there was no associated improvement in progression-free or overall survival for these patients over age 65. Thus there is no clearly established standard first-line treatment for older patients with CLL.

Bendamustine has a benzimidazole (purinelike) ring structure with an alkylating group and has potent alkylating agent activity, inducing intra- and interstrand DNA crosslinks. Bendamustine was compared to CLB in a randomized phase 3 trial in previously untreated patients with CLL (Table 134.4).[38] Bendamustine was associated with superior progression-free survival (21.6 months vs. 8.3 months), and complete (31% vs. 2%) and overall (68% vs. 31%) response rates; this was the basis for FDA approval of this agent. Myelosuppression was mild but more frequent with bendamustine; this did not result in increased infection rate.

Fludarabine inhibits excision repair of DNA interstrand crosslinks induced by CTX, thereby potentiating activity and providing a rationale for combining these agents.[39] Phase 2 trials that combined fludarabine and cyclophosphamide (FC) suggested increased efficacy compared to that seen in historical patients treated with fludarabine alone.[40–42] Three large randomized trials evaluated efficacy of the FC combination versus fludarabine monotherapy in previously untreated patients (Table 134.5). In the GCLLSG CLL4 trial, previously untreated patients younger than 65 with indications for treatment were randomized to receive six cycles of FC or fludarabine.[43] The U.S. Intergroup E2997 trial[44] randomized previously untreated patients to receive standard dose fludarabine versus FC and the UK LRF CLL4 trial randomized patients to FC, fludarabine monotherapy, or CLB in a 1:1:2 randomization. All three trials demonstrated superior progression-free survival with FC treatment versus fludarabine or CLB, and this was associated with superior complete and overall response rates. There was more myelosuppression with the combination, yet there was no difference in the incidence of infections in any of the trials. None of these trials showed a difference in overall survival with the follow-up available. Patients with 17p deletion were confirmed to be high risk with lower response rates and shorter survival compared to patients with other chromosome abnormalities,

TABLE 134.5

RANDOMIZED TRIALS OF SINGLE-AGENT PURINE ANALOGUE VERSUS COMBINATIONS AS INITIAL TREATMENT FOR CHRONIC LYMPHOCYTIC LEUKEMIA

Study (Ref.)	Agent	No. of Patients	CR (%)	OR (%)	RD (PFS) (mo)
GCLLSG CLL4 (43)	FC vs.	164	24	95	48
	Fludarabine	164	7	83	20
E2997 (44)	FC vs.	137	23	74	32
	Fludarabine	132	6	60	19
LRF CLL4 (32)	FC vs.	196	38	94	43
	F vs.	194	15	80	23
	Chlorambucil	387	7	72	20
PALG CLL2 (46)	Cladribine vs.	166	21	77	24
	CC vs.	162	29	83	22
	CMC	151	36	80	24

GCLLSG, German CLL Study Group; CR, complete remission; OR, overall response; RD, remission duration; PFS, median progression-free survival; CC, cladribine + cyclophosphamide; CMC, cladribine + mitoxantrone + cyclophosphamide; FC, fludarabine + cyclophosphamide; PALG, Polish Adult Leukemia Group.

regardless of treatment. Patients with 11q deletion were high risk, but there appeared to be a large benefit for those patients treated with an alkylating agent combined with fludarabine. Patients with an unmutated *IGHV* gene had similar response rates to those with a mutated *IGHV*, however, their progression-free and overall survival was shorter.

Cladribine (2-CdA) and pentostatin (2-deoxycoformyin) also have activity in CLL.[45] Results of a large randomized trial that compared single-agent cladribine, cladribine with cyclophosphamide (CC), and cladribine with cyclophosphamide and mitoxantrone (CMC) as initial therapy demonstrated a higher complete response rate for CMC compared to the other treatments (Table 134.5).[46] Neutropenia was more common with CMC, as was infection. There were no significant differences in progression-free or overall survival rates among the three arms. There are no head-to-head comparisons available for single-agent purine analogues.

Monoclonal Antibodies

Alemtuzumab is a humanized monoclonal antibody (mAb) targeting CD52, an antigen that is highly expressed on CLL cells and normal T and B lymphocytes. Alemtuzumab was approved by the FDA based on the pivotal trial that demonstrated single-agent activity in fludarabine-refractory patients with CLL (Table 134.6).[47] Complete remission and partial remission were noted in 2% and 31% of 93 treated patients, respectively. Fifty-five patients (59%) had stable disease. Identical results were reported in a trial with a similar patient population treated with the same dose and duration of alemtuzumab administered subcutaneously.[48] Subcutaneous administration eliminates the infusion-related side effects, although local injection-site reactions occur. Alemtuzumab was very effective at eliminating disease in the peripheral blood and bone marrow; bulky lymphadenopathy was less effectively treated, a pattern observed in other studies with alemtuzumab. Infusion-related adverse events were seen with intravenous (IV) administration in the majority of patients. More concerning was the T-cell suppression that occurred with this agent. As a consequence, a significant incidence of infections (including cytomegalovirus reactivation) is associated with therapy. Antibacterial and antiviral prophylaxis should always be used with alemtuzumab. Other studies confirmed the activity of alemtuzumab in less heavily pretreated patients (Table 134.6). A randomized frontline trial demonstrated superior progression-free survival associated with alemtuzumab monotherapy compared to CLB, as well as higher complete and overall response rates (Table 134.4).[49]

The mechanism of action for alemtuzumab is independent of p53. *TP53* is a gene deleted in patients who have loss of chromosome 17p by FISH. Loss of p53 function by deletion or mutation confers resistance to treatment with standard antileukemia drugs such as CLB and purine analogue–based therapy. Alemtuzumab has been reported to have activity in patients with leukemia cells that lack p53 function.[50] Nevertheless, despite treatment with alemtuzumab, patients with 17p deletion have short remission duration and overall survival; new treatments are urgently needed for these patients.

Rituximab is a chimeric IgG1 CD20 mAb; CD20 is expressed on malignant and normal B cells.[51] Relatively low levels of CD20 are expressed on CLL cells compared to normal B or neoplastic B cells of other lymphomas. In addition, circulating CD20 has been demonstrated in plasma of patients with CLL; this may inhibit the capacity of rituximab to bind to CLL cells, resulting in rapid clearance and negatively affecting pharmacokinetics.[52] Rituximab binds to the large-loop domain of CD20 and mediates antileukemic activity predominantly through complement-dependent cytotoxicity (CDC) and antibody-dependent cellular cytotoxicity (ADCC). Standard-dose rituximab monotherapy has limited activity in treating patients with CLL (Table 134.6). Dose-intense[53] and dose-dense[54] single-agent rituximab increased efficacy (Table 134.6). In addition, greater efficacy was seen when rituximab was used as initial therapy for patients with CLL (Table 134.6).[55] Maintenance rituximab is not routine practice for patients with CLL.

The primary toxicity seen with rituximab is usually with the initial infusion and is predominantly fever and chills. These symptoms are generally mild to moderate and abate with subsequent infusions. Although normal B cells are also targeted by rituximab, trials to date have shown no decrease in Ig levels, and infection rates are low.

Rituximab has been combined with alemtuzumab based on the rationale of targeting two distinct antigens expressed on CLL cells as well as the differential effectiveness by disease site; rituximab has activity in treating lymph node disease, and

TABLE 134.6

MONOCLONAL ANTIBODY–BASED THERAPY FOR CHRONIC LYMPHOCYTIC LEUKEMIA

Study (Ref.)	Monoclonal Antibody	Prior Rx	No. Patients Evaluable	CR (%)	OR (%)	Median TTP (mo)
ALEMTUZUMAB						
Keating et al. (47)	30 mg IV TIW × 12 wk	Yes[a]	93	2	33	9
Osterborg et al. (98)	30 mg IV TIW × 12 wk	Yes	29	4	42	12
Rai et al. (99)	30 mg IV TIW × 16 wk	Yes	24	0	33	19.6
Ferrajoli et al. (100)	30 mg IV TIW × 12 wk	Yes	42	5	31	NA
Moreton et al. (29)	30 mg IV TIW × 16 wk	Yes	91	35	54	NA
Lundin et al. (101)	30 mg SC TIW × 18 wk	No	41	19	87	NR
Stilgenbauer et al. (48)	30 mg SC TIW × 12 wk	Yes[a]	103	4	34	7.7
RITUXIMAB						
McLaughlin et al. (102)	375 mg/m^2 IV weekly × 4	Yes	30	0	13	NA
Huhn et al. (103)	375 mg/m^2 IV weekly × 4	Yes	28	0	25	5
O'Brien et al.[b] (53)	500–825 mg/m^2 IV weekly × 4	Yes	24	0	21	—
	1,000–1,500 mg/m^2 IV weekly × 4	Yes	7	0	43	8
	2,250 mg/m^2 IV weekly × 4	Yes	8	0	75	
Byrd et al.[c] (54)	375 mg/m^2 IV TIW × 4 wk	No/Yes	29	4	52	11
Hainsworth (104)	375 mg/m^2 IV weekly × 4 then q6 mo for 2 yr	No	43	9	58	19
Ferrajoli (56)	375 mg/m^2 IV weekly × 4 GM-CSF 25 mcg SC TIW × 8	Yes	118	9	65	NA
Castro et al. (105)	375 mg/m^2 IV weekly × 4 + HDMP 1 gm/m^2 daily × 5	Yes[a]	14	36	93	15
Bowen et al. (106)	375 mg/m^2 IV weekly × 4 + HDMP 1 gm/m^2 daily × 5	Yes	37	22	78	21
Castro et al. (107)	375 mg/m^2 IV weekly × 4 + HDMP 1 gm/m^2 daily × 3	No	28	32	96	30
ALEMTUZUMAB + RITUXIMAB						
Faderl et al. (108)	A-30 mg IV TIW × 4 wk + R-375 mg/m^2 IV weekly × 4	Yes	48	8	52	6
Zent et al. (109)	A-30 mg SC TIW × 4 wk + R-375 mg/m^2 IV weekly × 4	No	30	37	90	12.5
OFATUMUMAB						
Coiffier et al. (57)	2,000 mg IV weekly × 4	Yes	26	0	50	NA
Wierda et al. (58)	2,000 mg IV weekly × 8, then monthly × 4	FA-ref	59	0	58	5.7
		BF-ref	79	1	47	5.9

Rx, treatment; CR, complete remission; OR, overall response; TTP, time-to-progression for responders; IV, intravenous; SC, subcutaneous; TIW, thrice weekly; NA, not available; NR, not reached; HDMP, high-dose methylprednisolone; FA-ref, refractory to both fludarabine and alemtuzumab; BF-ref, refractory to fludarabine with bulky (>5 cm) adenopathy

[a]Fludarabine refractory.

[b]Dose-intense regimen.

[c]Dose-dense regimen.

alemtuzumab is highly effective at clearing blood and bone marrow. Efficacy and tolerability were demonstrated in both untreated and previously treated CLL (Table 134.6). In addition, rituximab has been combined with high-dose methylprednisolone in an active regimen for untreated and previously treated patients (Table 134.6). Immunosuppression was seen with this combination, owing to use of high-dose steroids, and was effectively managed with prophylactic antibiotics. Finally, granulocyte-monophosphate colony-stimulating factor (GM-CSF) may enhance *in vivo* ADCC activity, thereby enhancing the therapeutic activity of rituximab. This formed the basis for a trial that combined these two agents, the final results of which will be compared to historic results with rituximab monotherapy (Table 134.6).[56]

Ofatumumab is a fully human IgG1 CD20 mAb that binds to an epitope encompassing both large- and small-loop domains of CD20 and is highly effective at CDC and also mediates ADCC (type I mAb). Ofatumumab monotherapy was first evaluated in a phase 1 and 2 trial of escalating doses of 4-weekly infusions. An overall response rate of 50% was reported in 26 patients who received the phase 2 dose of 2,000 mg weekly × 4 (Table 134.6).[57] The pivotal trial that led to regulatory approval of ofatumumab enrolled patients who were refractory to fludarabine and alemtuzumab (FA-ref) as well as fludarabine refractory patients with bulky (greater than 5 cm) lymph nodes (and therefore poor candidates for treatment with alemtuzumab) (BF-ref); regulatory approval was based on outcome for the FA-ref group. Patients received ofatumumab 2,000 mg IV weekly for 8 weeks, then monthly for 4 months. The overall response rate was 58% and 47% for the FA-ref and BF-ref group, respectively. The median progression-free and overall survival were 5.7 and 13.7 months in the FA-ref and 5.9 and 15.4 months in the BF-ref group, representing clinical benefit for these patients compared to historic outcomes with available treatment (Table 134.6).[58] First infusion-related toxicity was the most common side effect and was manageable with premedication. Infection was seen, but expected in these highly refractory, heavily pretreated patients. Combinations with ofatumumab are being investigated.

Chemoimmunotherapy

In vitro data demonstrate synergy between fludarabine and rituximab. Rituximab down-modulates levels of the antiapoptotic protein bcl-2 and may sensitize leukemia cells to fludarabine-induced apoptosis. Furthermore, fludarabine down-modulates expression of complement-resistance proteins, CD46, CD55, and CD59 on malignant B cells and renders them more susceptible to rituximab-induced CDC. The randomized phase 2 multi-institutional Cancer and Leukemia Group B (CALGB) 9712 trial evaluated the activity of concurrent versus sequential fludarabine and rituximab as initial treatment for patients with CLL (Table 134.7).[59] All patients in this study received rituximab, but the concurrent group received 2.5 times the cumulative dose given to the sequential group. This trial demonstrated a significantly higher complete remission rate of 47% in the concurrent group versus 28% in the sequential group. The overall response rate and progression-free survival were not significantly different between the two groups. Shorter progression-free survival was noted for patients with unmutated *IGHV* status; shorter progression-free survival and overall survival were noted for patients with 17p deletion or 11q deletion by FISH. Notably, the incidence of grade 3 to 4 neutropenia was increased in patients who received concurrent fludarabine and rituximab (77%), compared to the sequential patients who received fludarabine alone (41%). No significant difference was seen in the incidence of infection between the two arms. Subsequently, an analysis of all patients treated in the CALGB-9712 trial compared to a historical group of patients treated with frontline single-agent fludarabine in the randomized CALGB-9011 trial (no rituximab) demonstrated a statistically significantly higher complete remission rate, overall response rate, 2-year disease-free survival, and 2-year overall survival for patients who received fludarabine and rituximab.[60]

The combination of fludarabine, cyclophosphamide, and rituximab (FCR) was initially evaluated in phase 2 trials in previously treated and chemotherapy-naive patients with CLL (Table 134.7).[61–63] In 300 previously untreated patients with CLL, the complete remission rate with FCR was 72% and the overall response rate was 95%, with most patients having no detectable disease by two-color flow cytometry evaluation of the bone marrow at the end of therapy.[61] Over 40% of complete responders were free of disease in the bone marrow by PCR testing. The estimated median progression-free survival in a recent report was 80 months. This was the highest response rate reported for any regimen in previously untreated patients with CLL. The German CLL Study Group CLL8 trial was a randomized phase 3 clinical trial of FCR versus FC for previously untreated patients (Table 134.7).[64] This trial clearly demonstrated superior progression-free survival associated with FCR (median 52 months) versus FC (median 33 months) as well as superior complete and overall response rates at 44% and 95% versus 22% and 88%, respectively. FCR treatment was also associated with a higher incidence of grade 3 or 4 neutropenia (33.7% vs. 21%; $P < .0001$); however, there was no difference in the incidence of grade 3 or 4 infection (18.8% vs. 14.9%; $P = .14$). Most important, this trial demonstrated superior overall survival associated with frontline treatment with FCR (84% alive) versus FC (79% alive) at 38 months ($P = .01$). The largest benefit was seen for patients with Binet stage A and B disease and patients younger than 70. The REACH trial was an international randomized phase 3 trial with identical treatment arms as CLL8 and enrolled previously treated patients (Table 134.7).[65] Eligible patients could only have had one prior treatment that did not include rituximab or FC. The conclusions of this trial were consistent with those of CLL8, superior progression-free survival associated with superior complete and overall response rate for FCR versus FC. Thus far, no difference in overall survival between treatment arms has been observed in REACH.

Efforts to improve the efficacy of the FCR regimen have included adding mitoxantrone to the regimen in phase 2 clinical trials (Table 134.7).[66,67] There was no clear evidence that this addition represented a marked improvement over FCR. In addition, in an effort to reduce the myelosuppression of FCR and make the regimen more tolerable, a phase 2 trial was conducted with reduced doses of fludarabine and cyclophosphamide and with the addition of maintenance rituximab, referred to as "FCR-lite" (Table 134.7).[68] Impressive response rates were reported; important information will come from time to event end points with further follow-up. Rituximab has been combined with pentostatin and cyclophosphamide for previously treated and chemotherapy-naive patients with CLL (Table 134.7).[69,70] Both studies demonstrated that this regimen was active and well tolerated; the principal toxicity was myelosuppression; nausea and vomiting were the most common nonhematologic toxicities.

Results from a variety of clinical trials with chemoimmunotherapy regimens for CLL and non-Hodgkin's lymphomas generally indicate potential for synergy between the monoclonal antibodies and chemotherapy. Indeed, rituximab was also combined with bendamustine and evaluated in phase 2 trials for previously treated and chemotherapy-naive patients with CLL (Table 134.7).[71,72] Efficacy and tolerability were demonstrated with this regimen. Furthermore, the "FluCam" regimen is an active and safe regimen of fludarabine combined with alemtuzumab (Table 134.7).[73] Confirmation of a superior regimen to FCR for either frontline or salvage therapy will need supporting randomized phase 3 data. Currently the GCLLSG is conducting a phase 3 frontline noninferiority trial comparing FCR versus bendamustine, which will generate interesting data regarding the comparison of tolerability and myelosuppression of these regimens.

Eliminating Minimal Residual Disease

The clinical benefit of eliminating MRD was suggested in a report of 91 previously treated patients with CLL who received alemtuzumab; 20% had eradication of MRD in the blood and bone marrow evaluated by four-color flow cytometry.[29] MRD-free status was associated with longer progression-free and overall survival. The overall survival for the 18 patients who were MRD free was 84% at 60 months. Clinical trials focused on evaluating the impact of eliminating MRD on progression-free and overall survival continue.

For patients with residual disease after purine analogue–based therapy, the marrow is the usual site of involvement. Because alemtuzumab has significant activity in clearing blood and bone marrow, it has been evaluated in trials to eliminate MRD following chemotherapy.[74,75] These studies demonstrated the ability to improve responses and achieve MRD-free status in a percentage of patients treated with alemtuzumab, with anticipated associated risk for infection. Other studies have reported unacceptable toxicity with this strategy.[76,77]

TABLE 134.7

CHEMOIMMUNOTHERAPY FOR PATIENTS WITH CHRONIC LYMPHOCYTIC LEUKEMIA

Study (Ref.)	Treatment	Prior Treatment	No. Evaluable	CR (%)	OR (%)	PFS (mo)
FluCam (73)	F—30 mg/m² d1-3, c1-6 A—30 mg d1-3, c1-6	Yes	36	30	83	13 (TTP)
MDACC-FCR (62, 63)	F—25 mg/m² IV d2-4, c1; d1-3, c2-6	No (ref. 62)	300	72	95	80
	C—250 mg/m² IV d2-4, c1; d1-3, c2-6 R—375–500 mg/m² IV d1, c1-6	Yes (ref. 63)	177	25	73	28
Foon et al. (68)	F—20 mg/m² IV d2-4, c1; d2-3, c2-6 C—150 mg/m² IV d2-4, c1; d2-3, c2-6 R—375 mg/m² IV d1, c1; 500 mg/m² d14, c1; 500 mg/m² d1, c2-6; then 500 mg/m² q3 mo	No	50	79	100	NR
Bosch et al. (66)	F—25 mg/m² IV d1-3, c1-6 C—250 mg/m² IV d1-3, c1-6 M—6 mg/m² IV d1, c1-6 R—375–500 mg/m² IV d1, c1-6	No	71	83	96	NR
Faderl et al. (67)	F—25 mg/m² IV d2-4, c1; d1-3, c2-6 C—250 mg/m² IV d2-4, c1; d1-3, c2-6 M—6 mg/m² IV d1, c1-6 R—375–500 mg/m² IV d1, c1-6	No	30	83	96	NR
Kay et al. (69)	P—2 mg/m² IV d1, c1-6 C—600 mg/m² IV d1, c1-6 R—375 mg/m² IV d1, c2-6	No	64	41	91	33
Lamanna et al. (70)	P—4 mg/m² IV d1, c1-6 C—600 mg/m² IV d1, c1-6 R—375 mg/m² IV d1, c2-6	Yes	32	25	75	40 (TTF)
Fischer et al. (71)	B—70 mg/m² IV d1,2, c1-6 R—375–500 mg/m² IV d1, c1-6	Yes	62	15	77	NA
Fischer et al. (72)	B—90 mg/m² IV d1,2, c1-6 R—375–500 mg/m² IV d1, c1-6	No	110	33	91	NA
CALGB-9712 (59)	Randomized concurrent F—25 mg/m² IV d1-5, c1-6 R—375 mg/m² IV d1,4, c1; d1, c2-6 2 months observation then R—375 mg/m² IV weekly × 4 vs.	No	51	47	90	32
	Sequential F—25 mg/m² IV d1-5, c1-6 2 months observation then R—375 mg/m² IV weekly × 4	No	53	28	77	40
REACH (65)	Randomized F—25 mg/m² IV d2-4, c1; d1-3, c2-6 C—250 mg/m² IV d2-4, c1; d1-3, c2-6 R—375–500 mg/m² IV d1, c1-6 vs.	Yes	276	24	70	30.6
	F—25 mg/m² IV d1-3, c1-6 C—250 mg/m² IV d1-3, c1-6	Yes	276	13	58	20.6

(*continued*)

TABLE 134.7

(CONTINUED)

Study (Ref.)	Treatment	Prior Treatment	No. Evaluable	CR (%)	OR (%)	PFS (mo)
GCLLSG CLL8 (64)	Randomized F—25 mg/m² IV d2-4, c1; d1-3, c2-6 C—250 mg/m² IV d2-4, c1; d1-3, c2-6 R—375–500 mg/m² IV d1, c1-6	No	388	44	95	52
	vs. F—25 mg/m² IV d2-4, c1; d1-3, c2-6 C—250 mg/m² IV d2-4, c1; d1-3, c2-6	No	371	22	88	33

CR, complete remission; OR, overall response; A, alemtuzumab; B, bendamustine; M, mitoxantrone; R, rituximab; F, fludarabine; C, cyclophosphamide; P, pentostatin; d, day; c, course; wk, weeks; IV, intravenous; TTF, time to treatment failure.

NEW AND NOVEL AGENTS FOR TREATMENT OF CHRONIC LYMPHOCYTIC LEUKEMIA

A number of new therapeutic approaches are under development for patients with CLL. Important novel targets and pathways include targeting bcl-2 family members for inhibition with BH3 mimetics, inhibition of cyclin-dependent kinases, immune-modulating agents, and interfering with BCR signaling and leukemia cell–microenvironment interactions, among others.

CLL cells express high levels of antiapoptotic members of the bcl-2 family of proteins, rendering these cells long lived and resistant to senescence and death. Small molecule inhibitors of Bcl-2 family members are in therapeutic development. Navitoclax (ABT-263) is one small molecule inhibitor of Bcl-2, Bcl-w, and Bcl-xL. *In vitro* treatment of CLL cells with navitoclax induces cell death. A phase 1 and 2 trial of orally administered navitoclax is ongoing and has generated promising results thus far. Preliminary reports indicate the majority of patients treated in the phase 1 study had greater than 50% reduction in leukemia counts and some patients experienced reduction in lymph node size.[78] The maximum tolerated dose was 250 mg daily continuously; the dose-limiting toxicity was thrombocytopenia. The mechanism for thrombocytopenia is accelerated platelet senescence owing to inhibition of Bcl-xL in platelets. The phase 2 portion of this trial is ongoing. Phase 1 and 2 trials are ongoing with navitoclax in combination with chemoimmunotherapy and monoclonal antibodies. Obatoclax, another BH3 mimetic, is also under clinical development.[79]

Flavopiridol, a synthetic flavone, inhibits cyclin-dependent kinases 1, 2, 4, and 9, giving it antiproliferative and apoptosis-inducing properties. Induction of apoptosis is via a p53-independent mechanism of inhibition of gene transcription, preferentially and profoundly affecting proteins with short transcript half-lives like Mcl-1. Flavopiridol has substantial binding to human serum proteins, which makes the therapeutic activity of the drug highly dose and schedule dependent. As a result, pharmacologically based administration was developed and tested in a phase 1 trial consisting of a bolus loading dose followed by a 4-hour continuous infusion to maintain therapeutic drug levels to induce leukemia killing. In phase 1 and 2 studies response rates of up to 50% in heavily pretreated, refractory patients, including those with high-risk cytogenetic features, were achieved with associated tumor lysis syndrome, indicating therapeutic activity.[80] The pivotal trial with flavopiridol monotherapy is ongoing. Flavopiridol was also combined with fludarabine and rituximab for untreated and relapsed lymphoproliferative diseases and showed promising results, including in CLL.[81]

Lenalidomide, a thalidomide analogue, has immune-modulatory and antiangiogenic activities. The mechanisms of action and effects on the microenvironment are not well understood; lenalidomide monotherapy and combinations are being studied in patients with CLL. Phase 2 clinical trials in relapsed or refractory patients with CLL evaluated continuous and interrupted (21 of 28 days) administration of up to 25 mg daily and reported overall response rates of 32% to 47% with 7% to 9% achieving complete remission, including patients who achieved MRD-free status.[82,83] Furthermore, responses were noted in patients with high-risk features including 11q deletion and 17p deletion. Tumor-flare and tumor lysis syndrome were reported upon treatment initiation; fatigue and myelosuppression were associated with longer-term exposure. Lenalidomide remains a promising agent with unique properties and is being studied earlier in treatment and in combinations.

BCR signaling and interaction with the microenvironment involve complex biochemical cascades and protein interactions for intracellular signaling. Phosphatidylinositol 3-kinase (PI3K) is one protein complex involved in this cascade, upstream of a critical central mediator, Akt. There are four class I PI3K isoforms; PI3K-delta is expressed by leukocytes and participates in B-cell signaling, development, and survival. CAL-101 is a small molecule inhibitor of p110δ of the PI3K-delta complex; it has no significant inhibition of other class I isoforms and no significant off-target inhibition of PI3K class II or III isoforms, mammalian target of rapamycin (mTOR), or DNA protein kinases. A phase 1 trial of CAL-101 is being conducted in relapsed and refractory patients with low-grade lymphoproliferative diseases, including CLL. CAL-101 was well tolerated; elevated liver function test was the dose-limiting toxicity and treatment resulted in a 30% response rate in relapsed patients with CLL.[84] There was rapid and marked reduction in lymph node size and an initial increase followed by decrease in leukemia counts, indicating an initial redistribution of leukemia cells followed by cell death. Phase 2 studies are being planned with CAL-101 combinations. Bruton's tyrosine kinase (Btk) is another key proximal signaling protein of the BCR pathway. PCI-32765 is a potent, irreversible small molecule inhibitor of Btk. Preclinical studies with PCI-32765 demonstrated inhibition of BCR-stimulated activation of nuclear factor κB and extracellular signal-regulated protein kinase (ERK), resulting in death of malignant B cells; antitumor activity was also seen in animal models of B-cell malignancies. A phase 1 clinical trial with oral PCI-32765 is ongoing for patients with low-grade lymphoproliferative disorders, including CLL.[85] Preliminary reports indicate excellent tolerability with no dose-limiting toxicities and target inhibition associated with clinical reductions in tumor bulk. This interesting agent remains under investigation.

Stem Cell Transplantation

Myeloablative allogeneic stem cell transplantation was not a viable option in CLL in the past because of the prohibitive toxicity of this approach in elderly patients. The use of reduced-intensity conditioning or nonmyeloablative transplants has broadened the eligibility to include older patients and has made this approach available to increasing numbers of patients with CLL. The largest series was reported by the European Blood and Marrow Transplant Registry in patients with CLL younger than 60 years from 30 centers worldwide transplanted between 1984 and 1992.[86] Most patients received CTX and total body irradiation followed by HLA-matched marrow from siblings. The 3-year probability of survival was 46%, with a projected survival at 5 years of 30% to 40%. Chronic graft-versus-host disease developed in 16 of 27 evaluable patients. Smaller single-institution studies have shown impressive survival times given that most patients were chemorefractory before transplant.[87] Early data with nonmyeloablative allogeneic transplants indicate almost universal engraftment, although the development of chimerism was slower than with myeloablative transplants. Patients with sensitive disease who were transplanted had a better outcome than those who had resistant disease.[88] With the recognition that 60% of CLL patients younger than 55 years eventually develop progressive disease and have a median survival probability of only 5 years after therapy, innovative therapies with curative intent, including the use of stem cell transplantation, will play an increasing role in the future. Autologous bone marrow transplantation has also been evaluated.[87,89] The procedure appears to be safe, with a lower relapse rate in patients transplanted in first remission as an intensification procedure compared to those who received their transplant as a salvage regimen for active disease, but no cures are seen.

Splenectomy

Studies suggest hematologic and survival benefits from splenectomy in patients with CLL. Splenectomy may be beneficial in individuals with immune-mediated cytopenias such as AIHA and immune thrombocytopenia purpura (ITP) after corticosteroid failure or in improving blood counts in patients with hypersplenism. In a study from M. D. Anderson Cancer Center,[90] perioperative mortality among 55 patients was 9%, mostly related to poor preoperative performance status. Improvements in the platelet count, neutrophil count, and hemoglobin occurred in 81%, 59%, and 33% of patients, respectively. Among Rai stage IV patients, a trend for improved survival was observed using case-control analysis.

Therapeutic Considerations for Specific Problems in Patients with Chronic Lymphocytic Leukemia

The most common cause of morbidity in patients with CLL is infection. Because hypogammaglobulinemia is a contributing factor to patients' increased susceptibility to infections, a randomized double-blind study evaluated the use of intravenous immunoglobulin, 400 mg/kg, versus placebo given every 3 weeks for 1 year to 84 patients with CLL. A significant reduction in bacterial infections was seen in the group treated with intravenous immunoglobulin, but no statistically significant difference was observed in the number of life-threatening infections or nonbacterial infections. Because of the high cost of this therapy, monthly intravenous immunoglobulin therapy is best used in patients with hypogammaglobulinemia who experience repeated bacterial infections.

SECOND MALIGNANCIES AND TRANSFORMATION

Approximately 25% of patients with CLL develop second neoplasms, the most common being skin cancer. Second neoplasm is the cause of death in 7% to 10% of patients. In approximately 2% to 6% of patients, CLL may evolve into a high-grade lymphoma of the diffuse large cell type (Richter's transformation); less commonly Hodgkin's histology is diagnosed. Usually, Richter's transformation arises from the original CLL clone, and its onset is heralded by fever, weight loss, a rising lactate dehydrogenase, and an asymmetric rapid lymph node enlargement.[91] Because the lymphoma may be patchy, a gallium or positron emission tomography scan, usually negative in CLL, may aid in identifying a "hot" lymph node that can be targeted for biopsy. Transformation must be diagnosed by histology. The prognosis of Richter's transformation is poor, with a median survival of only 6 months. Prolymphocytic transformation develops in approximately 2% to 5% of CLL patients. This transformation is different immunophenotypically and clinically from primary or *de novo* PLL. Secondary PLL is marked by development of progressive refractory anemia and thrombocytopenia, progressive splenomegaly, and an increase in the percentage of prolymphocytes to greater than 30% of the leukemia cells. As with Richter's transformation, PLL transformation portends a poor prognosis despite aggressive therapy.

PROLYMPHOCYTIC LEUKEMIA

PLL is characterized by a high number of circulating prolymphocytes, splenomegaly, minimal lymphadenopathy, and a median survival of less than 3 years. This leukemia can be present at diagnosis or evolve from CLL.[92] Prolymphocytes are larger and less homogeneous than CLL cells and have abundant clear cytoplasm, clumped chromatin, and a prominent nucleolus. Prolymphocytes can be of either B- or T-cell type. B-PLL cells usually do not express CD5 but stain strongly for surface immunoglobulin and FMC7 (Table 134.1). In 20% of cases of PLL, T-cell markers are expressed.

Splenectomy and lymphomalike regimens have been used to treat PLL without much success. Nucleoside analogue–based regimens appear to be the most effective, and alemtuzumab has shown promising activity in T-PLL.[93]

LARGE GRANULAR LYMPHOCYTE LEUKEMIA

Large granular lymphocytes (LGLs) are larger than normal lymphocytes that contain azurophilic granules in their cytoplasm. LGLs comprise 10% to 15% of peripheral blood mononuclear cells and are predominantly of NK-cell phenotype, a smaller fraction being of T-cell phenotype. There are generally four lymphoproliferative disorders of LGL: reactive/transient LGL expansion, chronic LGL lymphocytosis, indolent LGL leukemia, and aggressive LGL leukemia.[94] Clonal expansion of LGL can be of NK-cell or T-cell phenotype; the T-cell phenotype comprises 80% of LGL leukemias. T-LGL cells have a

CD3+/CD57+/CD56− immunophenotype, and NK-LGL express CD3−/CD56+/CD57−. Clonality of T-LGL may be established by T-cell receptor gene rearrangement studies. T-LGL leukemia is usually indolent. Patients present with cytopenias, including neutropenia with accompanying infections, pure red cell aplasia, thrombocytopenia, and anemia. Serologic abnormalities, such as positive rheumatoid factor or antinuclear antibody, or both, hypergammaglobulinemia, and high β_2-microglobin are frequent. A small percentage of LGL leukemias have a more aggressive course, and these cases tend to have an NK-cell phenotype. Because lymphocyte counts are usually not elevated, diagnosis requires a high degree of suspicion and a careful examination of the peripheral blood smear and bone marrow. Although the disease is usually indolent, most patients require treatment for cytopenias. Various therapies, including low-dose methotrexate (10 mg/m^2 orally once weekly), cyclosporine (2 mg/kg orally every 12 hours), or CTX (100 mg orally daily) with or without oral prednisone (1 mg/kg orally daily), have all been effective. Complete remissions may be seen in up to 50% of cases. Lymphoma-type regimens, such as CHOP, have not been effective for aggressive disease.

HAIRY CELL LEUKEMIA

HCL is a rare B-cell lymphoproliferative disorder that affects adults and represents 2% of all leukemias. It has a marked preponderance in men. Most patients have cytopenias; splenomegaly is also frequent.[95] Hairy cells can be seen in the peripheral blood, but at low frequency, and therefore are easily missed. These cells are twice as large as normal lymphocytes, with the nuclei showing a loose chromatin pattern and villilike cytoplasmic projections (best viewed under phase contrast microscopy). Hairy cells infiltrate the bone marrow in an interstitial or focal pattern, with clear zones in between cells ("fried egg appearance"). Marrow reticulin is increased, and aspirates may result in a dry tap. Immunophenotypic analysis of hairy cells shows the presence of CD19, CD20, CD22, CD25, and CD103, and, in contrast to CLL, hairy cells are negative for CD5 and CD23. Hairy cells also stain strongly for surface immunoglobulin and FMC-7. Use of the CD103 antibody, which stains tartrate-resistant acid phosphatase, has obviated the need for cytochemical staining for tartrate-resistant acid phosphatase (TRAP).

HCL has no staging system. For many years the only effective therapy was splenectomy. Pentostatin (2′ deoxycoformycin) and cladribine (2-CdA) are the nucleoside analogues that are the mainstay of treatment of HCL.[96] Pentostatin is administered at 4 mg/m^2 every 2 weeks until maximum response, and 2-CdA is given at 0.1 mg/kg/d as a continuous intravenous infusion for 7 days; the same total dose can be administered as a 2-hour infusion over 5 days. Because 2-CdA involves a single course of therapy and produces remission rates comparable to those of pentostatin, 2-CdA is used more frequently in the United States for the treatment of HCL. Multiple series have reported high response rates, with patients remaining in remission for many years. The majority of relapsed patients achieve second remission when retreated with pentostatin or 2-CdA. The choice of agent may depend on the duration of the first remission: if less than 3 years, an alternate agent should be used; if greater than 5 years, the same agent should be given. The role of interferon alfa is currently limited to patients who are unresponsive to nucleoside analogues.

Adding Rituximab in Hairy Cell Leukemia

A percentage of patients may relapse with 2-CdA–resistant disease. In addition, 10% to 20% of patients have a variant form of HCL with high numbers of circulating hairy cells and a poor response to nucleoside analogues. Classic and variant hairy cells strongly express CD22, an adhesion molecule found on B cells. Data suggest marked efficacy of a recombinant immunotoxin, BL22, in the treatment of chemotherapy-resistant HCL.[97] This immunotoxin contains the variable domain of the anti-CD22 monoclonal antibody RFB4, which is fused to a fragment of *Pseudomonas* exotoxin called *PE38*; this fragment lacks the domain necessary for cell binding and contains only the domain responsible for cell death. Between 0.2 and 4.0 mg BL22 was administered intravenously over 30 minutes daily for 3 days. Patients were retreated at intervals of 3 weeks or more and could receive a total of 16 cycles of BL22 or two cycles beyond complete remission. Of 16 patients who were resistant to 2-CdA, 11 achieved a complete remission and 2 a partial remission with BL22. After a median follow-up of 16 months (range, 10 to 23), 3 of 11 patients in complete remission relapsed and were retreated; all 3 patients achieved a second complete remission. Common side effects included transient hypoalbuminemia and elevated aminotransferase levels. In 2 of 16 patients, a reversible hemolytic-uremic syndrome developed. This high complete remission rate in refractory patients has not been described with any other agent.

Selected References

The full list of references for this chapter appears in the online version.

3. Jemal A, Siegel R, Xu J, Ward E. Cancer statistics, 2010. *CA Cancer J Clin* 2010;60:277.
7. Dohner H, Stilgenbauer S, Dohner K, Bentz M, Lichter P. Chromosome aberrations in B-cell chronic lymphocytic leukemia: reassessment based on molecular cytogenetic analysis. *J Mol Med* 1999;77:266.
9. Rawstron AC, Green MJ, Kuzmicki A, et al. Monoclonal B lymphocytes with the characteristics of "indolent" chronic lymphocytic leukemia are present in 3.5% of adults with normal blood counts. *Blood* 2002;100:635.
10. Rawstron AC, Bennett FL, O'Connor SJ, et al. Monoclonal B-cell lymphocytosis and chronic lymphocytic leukemia. *N Engl J Med* 2008;359:575.
12. Hamblin TJ, Davis Z, Gardiner A, Oscier DG, Stevenson FK. Unmutated Ig V(H) genes are associated with a more aggressive form of chronic lymphocytic leukemia. *Blood* 1999;94:1848.
13. Damle RN, Wasil T, Fais F, et al. Ig V gene mutation status and CD38 expression as novel prognostic indicators in chronic lymphocytic leukemia. *Blood* 1999;94:1840.
14. Rosenwald A, Alizadeh AA, Widhopf G, et al. Relation of gene expression phenotype to immunoglobulin mutation genotype in B cell chronic lymphocytic leukemia. *J Exp Med* 2001;194:1639.
15. Crespo M, Bosch F, Villamor N, et al. ZAP-70 expression as a surrogate for immunoglobulin-variable-region mutations in chronic lymphocytic leukemia. *N Engl J Med* 2003;348:1764.
16. Calin GA, Dumitru CD, Shimizu M, et al. Frequent deletions and down-regulation of micro-RNA genes miR15 and miR16 at 13q14 in chronic lymphocytic leukemia. *Proc Natl Acad Sci U S A* 2002;99:15524.
20. Hallek M, Cheson BD, Catovsky D, et al. Guidelines for the diagnosis and treatment of chronic lymphocytic leukemia: a report from the International Workshop on Chronic Lymphocytic Leukemia updating the National Cancer Institute-Working Group 1996 guidelines. *Blood* 2008;111:5446.
24. Cortes J, O'Brien S, Loscertales J, et al. Cyclosporin A for the treatment of cytopenia associated with chronic lymphocytic leukemia. *Cancer* 2001;92:2016.
25. Rai KR, Sawitsky A, Cronkite EP, et al. Clinical staging of chronic lymphocytic leukemia. *Blood* 1975;46:219.
26. Binet JL, Auquier A, Dighiero G, et al. A new prognostic classification of chronic lymphocytic leukemia derived from a multivariate survival analysis. *Cancer* 1981;48:198.
35. Rai KR, Peterson BL, Appelbaum FR, et al. Fludarabine compared with chlorambucil as primary therapy for chronic lymphocytic leukemia. *N Engl J Med* 2000;343:1750.

36. Rai KR, Peterson BL, Appelbaum FR, et al. Long-term survival analysis of the North American Intergroup Study C9011 comparing fludarabine (F) and chlorambucil (C) in previously untreated patients with chronic lymphocytic leukemia (CLL). *Blood* 2009;114: (abst 536).
37. Eichhorst BF, Busch R, Stilgenbauer S, et al. First-line therapy with fludarabine compared with chlorambucil does not result in a major benefit for elderly patients with advanced chronic lymphocytic leukemia. *Blood* 2009; 114:3382.
38. Knauf WU, Lissichkov T, Aldaoud A, et al. Phase III randomized study of bendamustine compared with chlorambucil in previously untreated patients with chronic lymphocytic leukemia. *J Clin Oncol* 2009;27:4378.
43. Eichhorst BF, Busch R, Hopfinger G, et al. Fludarabine plus cyclophosphamide versus fludarabine alone in first-line therapy of younger patients with chronic lymphocytic leukemia. *Blood* 2006;107:885.
44. Flinn IW, Neuberg DS, Grever MR, et al. Phase III trial of fludarabine plus cyclophosphamide compared with fludarabine for patients with previously untreated chronic lymphocytic leukemia: US Intergroup Trial E2997. *J Clin Oncol* 2007;25:793.
46. Robak T, Blonski JZ, Gora-Tybor J, et al. Cladribine alone and in combination with cyclophosphamide or cyclophosphamide plus mitoxantrone in the treatment of progressive chronic lymphocytic leukemia: report of a prospective, multicenter, randomized trial of the Polish Adult Leukemia Group (PALG CLL2). *Blood* 2006;108:473.
47. Keating MJ, Flinn I, Jain V, et al. Therapeutic role of alemtuzumab (Campath-1H) in patients who have failed fludarabine: results of a large international study. *Blood* 2002;99:3554.
48. Stilgenbauer S, Zenz T, Winkler D, et al. Subcutaneous alemtuzumab in fludarabine-refractory chronic lymphocytic leukemia: clinical results and prognostic marker analyses from the CLL2H study of the German Chronic Lymphocytic Leukemia Study Group. *J Clin Oncol* 2009;27:3994.
49. Hillmen P, Skotnicki AB, Robak T, et al. Alemtuzumab compared with chlorambucil as first-line therapy for chronic lymphocytic leukemia. *J Clin Oncol* 2007;25:5616.
53. O'Brien SM, Kantarjian H, Thomas DA, et al. Rituximab dose-escalation trial in chronic lymphocytic leukemia. *J Clin Oncol* 2001;19:2165.
54. Byrd JC, Murphy T, Howard RS, et al. Rituximab using a thrice weekly dosing schedule in B-cell chronic lymphocytic leukemia and small lymphocytic lymphoma demonstrates clinical activity and acceptable toxicity. *J Clin Oncol* 2001;19:2153.
57. Coiffier B, Lepretre S, Pedersen LM, et al. Safety and efficacy of ofatumumab, a fully human monoclonal anti-CD20 antibody, in patients with relapsed or refractory B-cell chronic lymphocytic leukemia: a phase 1-2 study. *Blood* 2008;111:1094.
58. Wierda WG, Kipps TJ, Mayer J, et al. Ofatumumab as single-agent CD20 immunotherapy in fludarabine-refractory chronic lymphocytic leukemia. *J Clin Oncol* 2010;28:1749.
59. Byrd JC, Peterson BL, Morrison VA, et al. Randomized phase 2 study of fludarabine with concurrent versus sequential treatment with rituximab in symptomatic, untreated patients with B-cell chronic lymphocytic leukemia: results from Cancer and Leukemia Group B 9712 (CALGB 9712). *Blood* 2003;101:6.
60. Byrd JC, Rai K, Peterson BL, et al. Addition of rituximab to fludarabine may prolong progression-free survival and overall survival in patients with previously untreated chronic lymphocytic leukemia: an updated retrospective comparative analysis of CALGB 9712 and CALGB 9011. *Blood* 2005; 105:49.
61. Keating MJ, O'Brien S, Albitar M, et al. Early results of a chemoimmunotherapy regimen of fludarabine, cyclophosphamide, and rituximab as initial therapy for chronic lymphocytic leukemia. *J Clin Oncol* 2005;23:4079.
62. Tam CS, O'Brien S, Wierda W, et al. Long-term results of the fludarabine, cyclophosphamide, and rituximab regimen as initial therapy of chronic lymphocytic leukemia. *Blood* 2008;112:975.
63. Wierda W, O'Brien S, Wen S, et al. Chemoimmunotherapy with fludarabine, cyclophosphamide, and rituximab for relapsed and refractory chronic lymphocytic leukemia. *J Clin Oncol* 2005;23:4070.
64. Hallek M, Fingerle-Rowson G, Fink A-M, et al. First-line treatment with fludarabine (F), cyclophosphamide (C), and rituximab (R) (FCR) improves overall survival (OS) in previously untreated patients (pts) with advanced chronic lymphocytic leukemia (CLL): results of a randomized phase III trial on behalf of an international group of investigators and the German CLL Study Group. *Blood* 2009;114: (abst 535).
65. Robak T, Dmoszynska A, Solal-Celigny P, et al. Rituximab plus fludarabine and cyclophosphamide prolongs progression-free survival compared with fludarabine and cyclophosphamide alone in previously treated chronic lymphocytic leukemia. *J Clin Oncol* 2010;28:1756.
69. Kay NE, Geyer SM, Call TG, et al. Combination chemoimmunotherapy with pentostatin, cyclophosphamide, and rituximab shows significant clinical activity with low accompanying toxicity in previously untreated B chronic lymphocytic leukemia. *Blood* 2007;109:405.
70. Lamanna N, Kalaycio M, Maslak P, et al. Pentostatin, cyclophosphamide, and rituximab is an active, well-tolerated regimen for patients with previously treated chronic lymphocytic leukemia. *J Clin Oncol* 2006;24:1575.
71. Fischer K, Stilgenbauer S, Schweighofer CD, et al. Bendamustine in combination with rituximab (BR) for patients with relapsed chronic lymphocytic leukemia (CLL): a multicentre phase II trial of the German CLL Study Group (GCLLSG). *Blood* 2008;112: (abst 330).
72. Fischer K, Cramer P, Stilgenbauer S, et al. Bendamustine combined with rituximab (BR) in first-line therapy of advanced CLL: a multicenter phase II trial of the German CLL Study Group (GCLLSG). *Blood* 2009;114: (abst 205).
76. Schweighofer CD, Ritgen M, Eichhorst BF, et al. Consolidation with alemtuzumab improves progression-free survival in patients with chronic lymphocytic leukaemia (CLL) in first remission: long-term follow-up of a randomized phase III trial of the German CLL Study Group (GCLLSG). *Br J Haematol* 2009;144:95.
80. Byrd JC, Lin TS, Dalton JT, et al. Flavopiridol administered using a pharmacologically derived schedule is associated with marked clinical efficacy in refractory, genetically high-risk chronic lymphocytic leukemia. *Blood* 2007;109:399.
81. Lin TS, Blum KA, Fischer DB, et al. Flavopiridol, fludarabine, and rituximab in mantle cell lymphoma and indolent B-cell lymphoproliferative disorders. *J Clin Oncol* 2010;28:418.
82. Chanan-Khan A, Miller KC, Musial L, et al. Clinical efficacy of lenalidomide in patients with relapsed or refractory chronic lymphocytic leukemia: results of a phase II study. *J Clin Oncol* 2006;24:5343.
83. Ferrajoli A, Lee BN, Schlette EJ, et al. Lenalidomide induces complete and partial remissions in patients with relapsed and refractory chronic lymphocytic leukemia. *Blood* 2008;111:5291.
98. Osterborg A, Dyer MJ, Bunjes D, et al. Phase II multicenter study of human CD52 antibody in previously treated chronic lymphocytic leukemia. European Study Group of CAMPATH-1H treatment in chronic lymphocytic leukemia. *J Clin Oncol* 1997;15:1567.
101. Lundin J, Kimby E, Bjorkholm M, et al. Phase II trial of subcutaneous anti-CD52 monoclonal antibody alemtuzumab (Campath-1H) as first-line treatment for patients with B-cell chronic lymphocytic leukemia (B-CLL). *Blood* 2002;100:768.
102. McLaughlin P, Grillo-Lopez AJ, Link BK, et al. Rituximab chimeric anti-CD20 monoclonal antibody therapy for relapsed indolent lymphoma: half of patients respond to a four-dose treatment program. *J Clin Oncol* 1998; 16:2825.
105. Castro JE, Sandoval-Sus JD, Bole J, Rassenti L, Kipps TJ. Rituximab in combination with high-dose methylprednisolone for the treatment of fludarabine refractory high-risk chronic lymphocytic leukemia. *Leukemia* 2008;22:2048.
107. Castro JE, James DF, Sandoval-Sus JD, et al. Rituximab in combination with high-dose methylprednisolone for the treatment of chronic lymphocytic leukemia. *Leukemia* 2009;23:1779.
108. Faderl S, Thomas DA, O'Brien S, et al. Experience with alemtuzumab plus rituximab in patients with relapsed and refractory lymphoid malignancies. *Blood* 2003;101:3413.
109. Zent CS, Call TG, Shanafelt TD, et al. Early treatment of high-risk chronic lymphocytic leukemia with alemtuzumab and rituximab. *Cancer* 2008; 113:2110.

CHAPTER 135 MYELODYSPLASTIC SYNDROMES

STEFAN FADERL AND HAGOP M. KANTARJIAN

Myelodysplastic syndromes (MDSs) are a group of complex and heterogeneous clonal hematopoietic stem cell disorders whose defining characteristics are dysplasia of one or several hematopoietic cell lineages, hypercellular marrows, and blood cytopenias (Fig. 135.1).[1] Although historically considered as a preleukemic state, most patients with MDS do not transform into an acute myeloid leukemia (AML), but will instead succumb to complications of persistent cytopenias. Indeed, the pathophysiology of MDS extends from immune-mediated mechanisms and excessive apoptosis resulting in marrow failure to arrest of maturation and proliferation resembling the mechanisms at play in AML.[2] The diverse pathophysiology of factors that contribute to the development of MDS is reflected in vast differences of patients' prognosis, which is increasingly recognized and reflected in the design of more elaborate systems of diagnosis, classification, and prognostication.

Accordingly, the management of patients with MDS is becoming more complex and demanding. Several treatments are now available, including hematopoietic growth factors and iron chelation therapy, immunomodulation and immunomodulatory inhibitory derivatives (e.g., lenalidomide), epigenetic therapy (DNA methyltransferase and histone deacetylase inhibitors), nucleoside analogues and AML-type therapy, and allogeneic stem cell transplant (SCT). The challenge remains to identify a pathophysiologic basis for therapeutic intervention and to adapt the goals and intensity of therapy to the individual patient's stage of the disease.[3]

EPIDEMIOLOGY AND ETIOLOGY

The incidence of MDS in the United States is reported to be 3.4 per 100,000 persons.[4] MDS is rare in patients younger than 50 years, but can reach as high as 20 to 50 per 100,000 in individuals older than 70 years.[4] With around 15,000 new patients diagnosed every year in the United States, MDS has become one of the most common disorders in the section of leukemias. The increase in incidence that is currently observed may relate to increased reporting by clinicians and pathologists. Reasons for not diagnosing MDS in the past may have included little interest in pursuing this diagnosis, especially in older patients (perceived lack of effective therapy other than supportive, comorbidities), and overlap of MDS with other disorders (aplastic anemia, myeloproliferative diseases, and AML).

No etiologic factor is identified in most patients with MDS. MDS is more frequent in men than women by a factor of 1.8.[4] It has been associated with smoking and hair dyes, exposure to agricultural and industrial toxins, drugs (e.g., chloramphenicol), and occupational exposures to stone and cereal dusts. MDS has been associated with exposure to ionizing radiation (atomic bomb survivors in Japan, decontamination workers following the Chernobyl nuclear plant accident) and chronic exposure to low-dose radiation (radiopharmaceuticals).[5,6] Some inherited hematologic disorders (Fanconi anemia, dyskeratosis congenita, Shwachman-Diamond syndrome, Diamond- Blackfan syndrome) are also associated with a higher risk of MDS.

About 20% to 30% of patients with MDS have therapy-related MDS (t-MDS).[7] Distinct clinical features have been described based on the nature of the triggering event. t-MDS following exposure to alkylating agents has a longer latency period (3 to 8 years) and is often associated with abnormalities of chromosomes 5 and 7; the latency period following topoisomerase II inhibitors is shorter (2 to 3 years), and cytogenetic-molecular abnormalities tend to involve rearrangements of the *MLL* gene on chromosome 11q23. Risk factors associated with t-MDS include the cumulative dose of alkylating agents (e.g., cyclophosphamide, melphalan, procarbazine, chlorambucil) or topoisomerase II inhibitors (e.g., etoposide), previous radiation exposure, older age, and use of radiotherapy prior to transplantation.

The number of patients with t-MDS is increasing because of better outcome for tumors that formerly lacked effective therapy. The incidence of t-MDS following therapy for other hematologic (e.g., Hodgkin's disease, non–Hodgkin's lymphoma, chronic lymphocytic leukemia) or nonhematologic malignancies (e.g., breast or testicular cancers) is between 1% and 15% according to which particular study and malignancy is concerned.[8–12] Secondary and t-MDS are distinguishable from primary MDS by an earlier age of onset, more prominent dysplasia, more severe cytopenias, more rapid progression to AML, and worse outcome. The worse prognosis may be related to a higher frequency of poor-prognosis cytogenetic abnormalities in these cases.

PRESENTATION AND DIAGNOSIS

Clinical and Laboratory Features

Presenting features in MDS are variable. Anemia is most common; neutropenia and thrombocytopenia are less frequent. Blood monocytosis more than 1×10^9/L favors the diagnosis of chronic myelomonocytic leukemia (CMML). Symptoms arise due to cytopenias and include fatigue, pallor, exertional dyspnea, infections, easy bruising and bleeding. Lymphadenopathy and hepatosplenomegaly are uncommon (10% to 20%). Central nervous system involvement is rare. Patients with CMML and leukocytosis may present with organ infiltration (hepatomegaly and splenomegaly in 25% and 50%, respectively) and dysfunction including pulmonary insufficiency, cardiac decompensation, and renal failure. This may be exacerbated once treatment is started, and patients may develop bilateral lung infiltrates (leukemic cell necrosis and inflammation) and

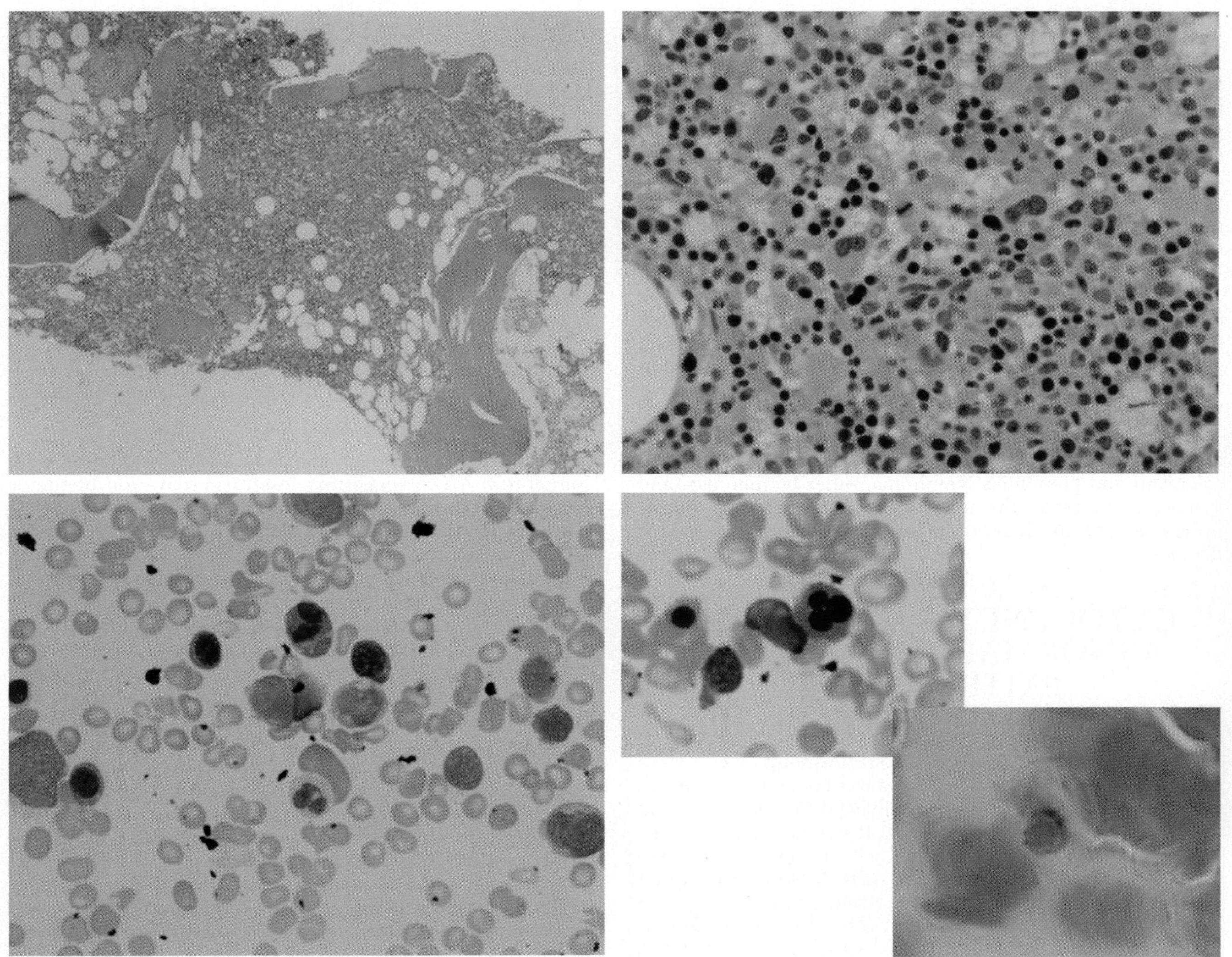

FIGURE 135.1 Composite illustrating ineffective hematopoiesis with hypercellular marrow including dysplastic megakaryocytes, smear with increased blasts (RAEB-1), dysgranulopoiesis, dyserythropoiesis, and ringed sideroblasts. (Courtesy of Carlos Bueso-Ramos, Department of Hematopathology, M. D. Anderson Cancer Center.)

a picture resembling adult respiratory distress syndrome. Worsening renal dysfunction and tumor lysis complications may also develop.

Morphology

Bone marrow biopsies or aspirates are usually normocellular or hypercellular, and only occasionally hypocellular. Hypocellular MDS is relevant in the context of immune-mediated mechanisms as, in these cases, there is an overlap with aplastic anemia, and immunomodulatory treatment strategies may be of benefit.

The minimal morphologic criterion for the diagnosis of MDS is dysplasia in at least 10% in one or more of the myeloid lineages.[13] Although cytopenias in the absence of dysplasia should not be diagnosed as MDS, a presumptive diagnosis of MDS can be made in the absence of dysplasia if certain cytogenetic abnormalities are present (see later discussion).

Blasts in MDS are myeloid in origin by histochemistry (myeloperoxidase-positive, positive monocytic stains) and by immunophenotyping (CD13, CD14, CD33 positivity), although some cases exhibit B-lineage lymphoid (CD19 or CD10) or mixed-lineage morphologies. Cytochemical stains of importance in the workup of MDS include stains for (1) iron to assess iron content and to identify ringed sideroblasts, (2) myeloperoxidase to identify abnormal granulation of myeloblasts, (3) periodic acid-Schiff to identify abnormal erythroblasts, (4) reticulin to define the degree of fibrosis, and (5) platelet antibodies to mark micromegakaryocytes.

Blood chemistries should include determination of vitamin B_{12} and folic acid levels to exclude vitamin deficiency–induced MDS-like changes. Iron studies are helpful to assess iron overload, but also to exclude iron deficiency anemia. Serum and urinary lysozymes may be increased in CMML; hypokalemia (lysozyme-induced renal tubular loss), renal dysfunction (leukemic involvement), and hyperuricemia may be present. Testing for the human immunodeficiency virus (HIV) will exclude MDS-like changes associated with HIV positivity.

Additional abnormalities observed in MDS include polyclonal gammopathies in up to one-third of patients, monoclonal gammopathies or hypogammaglobulinemia, the presence of autoimmune antibodies, and B- or T-cell abnormalities.

Differential Diagnosis

Dysplastic changes in the bone marrow are not pathognomonic for MDS and may occur with other conditions. One of the vexing problems of MDS is persistent cytopenias in the presence of only mild morphologic abnormalities of blood or marrow cells and lack of cytogenetic abnormalities. Dyserythropoiesis in particular is a common morphologic manifestation of secondary dysplasia, and every attempt should be made to identify other conditions associated with dysplasias and cytopenias. These other conditions include vitamin B_{12} or folic acid deficiencies; nutritional factors (anorexia nervosa); essential element deficiencies and exposure to heavy metal (e.g., arsenic), exposure to antibiotics, chemotherapy, ethanol, benzene, or lead; granulocyte colony-stimulating factor can result in hypergranularity and nuclear hypolobation of neutrophils; regenerating bone marrow following a hypoplastic phase induced by drugs or infections; HIV-positive disease; parvovirus B19 infections; chronic inflammation and tuberculosis; liver disorders; hypersplenism; and Hodgkin's lymphoma, other lymphomas, and metastatic disease to the marrow. In some situations, follow-up testing and an observation period will help to clarify the diagnosis.

CYTOGENETIC-MOLECULAR ABNORMALITIES AND MDS PATHOGENESIS

Cytogenetic abnormalities occur in 50% to 55% of primary MDS, and in 80% to 100% of t-MDS.[14] Although they help to establish clonality and in some instances clinch the diagnosis, they are particularly helpful clinically to define prognosis and to select the choice of therapy (e.g., lenalidomide in low-risk MDS with deletion 5q-; imatinib with t[5q33;X]). A large study of more than 2,000 patients with MDS identified 684 different cytogenetic categories.[15] Almost two-thirds of all abnormalities that were observed in about half of the patients were rare, with a frequency of less than 2%. The most frequent abnormalities were del(5q) (30%), monosomy 7/del(7q) (21%), trisomy 8 (16%), followed by monosomy 18/18q- (7%), 20q- (7%), and monosomy 5 (6%) (Fig. 135.2). The genetic profile in MDS differs from that of AML.[16] Whereas balanced structural abnormalities predominate in AML, loss

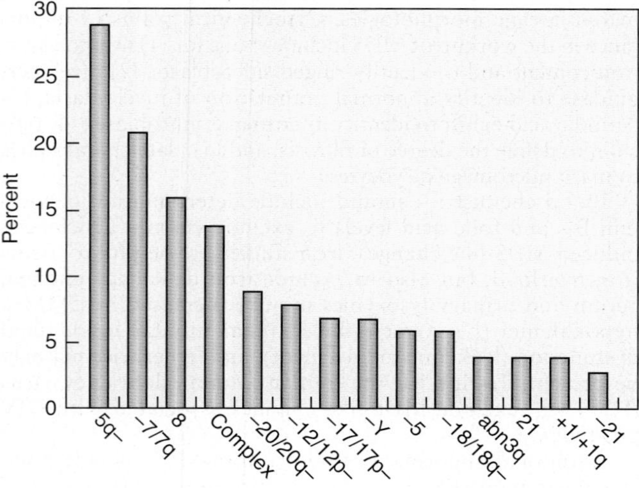

FIGURE 135.2 Distribution of cytogenetic abnormalities in myelodysplastic syndrome. (Modified from ref. 15.)

TABLE 135.1

CYTOGENETICS AND PROGNOSIS IN MYELODYSPLASTIC SYNDROMES

Cytogenetic Category	Median Survival (mo)
del(9q), del(15q), t(15q), del(12p), +21, del(5q), del(20q), diploid, +8, +1, t(1q), t(7q), t(11q), −21	32–108 and not reached
del(11q), +8, t(11q23), rea 3q, del(7q), del(11q), −5, −7, any 3 abnormalities	14–26.1
Complex, >3 abnormalities, t(5q)	5–8.7

Modified from ref. 15.

of genetic material through unbalanced translocations is more common in MDS, suggesting loss or inactivation of tumor suppressor genes as a prime molecular mechanism in MDS. The prognostic significance of cytogenetic abnormalities in MDS is substantial, not inferior to a high blast percentage, and has been underestimated in the International Prognostic Scoring System (IPSS, see later discussion).[15,17] Table 135.1 provides an overview of the cytogenetic abnormalities and the likelihood of survival based on karyotype alone.

Some cytogenetic abnormalities are associated with particular morphologic characteristics and clinical syndromes. The 5q- syndrome consists of an isolated abnormality involving deletions between bands q21 and q32 of the long arm of chromosome 5. The clinicopathologic characteristics are summarized in Table 135.2.[14] Prognosis is typically benign (prolonged survival, rare transformation to AML), but patients may require transfusions of blood products on a regular and longer-term basis, which is associated with its own problems (e.g., iron accumulation). Although identification of a critical gene has long evaded scientific inquiry, more recently decreased expression (haploinsufficiency) of a ribosomal protein, *RPS14*, was found to inhibit erythroid growth and promote megakaryocytic colony growth and erythroid apoptosis.[18] Reintroduction of the *RPS14* gene into 5q- MDS cells could

TABLE 135.2

CLINICAL AND PATHOLOGIC CHARACTERISTICS OF THE 5q- SYNDROME

Clinicopathologic features
- del(5)(q31-33) as the sole cytogenetic abnormality
- Macrocytosis, erythroid hypoplasia, mono- or hypolobated megakaryocytes
- Normal or increased platelet count

Demographics
- Younger females

Indolent disease course
- Low rate of AML transformation (5% to 10%)
- Long median survival (>5 y)
- Long-term PRBC transfusion needs (iron overload!)

Treatment
- Lenalidomide ± hematopoietic growth factors (ref. 90)
- High rate of transfusion independence (>60%)
- Durable median response duration (~2 y)

PRBC, packed red blood cells.

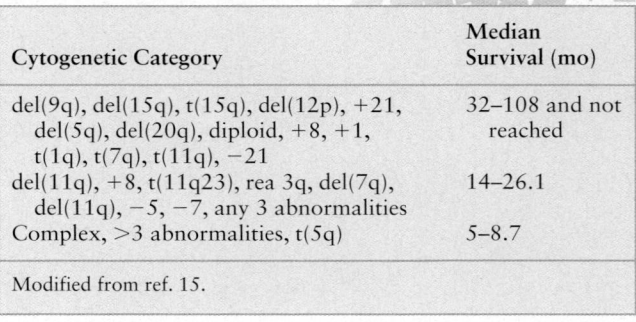

rescue the disease phenotype. Del(17q) has been associated with pseudo Pelger-Huët cells, small vacuolated neutrophils, and mutations of *TP53*. It is the most common abnormality in t-MDS and carries a high risk of leukemic transformation.[14] An isolated del(20q) and abnormalities of chromosome 3 have been described in the context of abnormal megakaryocytes. Complex karyotypes (i.e., three or more abnormalities) are generally associated with an unfavorable clinical outcome and often contain abnormalities of chromosomes 5 and/or 7.[14]

Although less is known about the molecular basis of MDS, a number of molecular lesions have been identified (*RAS, FLT3, KIT, PDGFRβ, FMS, JAK2, TET2, CDC25C*, and others). *SPARC*, another gene located on 5q31 and affected by haploinsufficiency, has been involved in responses to lenalidomide.[19] *CTNNA1* is also located on 5q31 and is part of the heme biosynthesis pathway linking mitochondrial iron regulation to some forms of MDS (such as refractory anemia with ringed sideroblasts [RARS]). It is epigenetically suppressed, and re-expression was shown to increase apoptosis and to decrease the proliferation rate of the affected cells.[1]

Abnormal methylation of DNA promoters and deacetylation of histone (protein complexes that form part of the chromatin structure of genes) have been linked to silencing of genomic regions, including tumor suppressor genes. Although large-scale methylation studies are pending, several gene-specific studies have been reported and have shown associations between progressive alterations in DNA methylation and transformation of MDS to AML.[3]

It is currently understood that MDS arises from a genetically transformed, primitive hematopoietic stem cell.[1] The initial insult remains elusive, but at least in some cases the phenotypic process may start with suppression of normal hematopoiesis by polyclonal, unaffected CD8-positive T cells and other cytokine suppressor cells through production of proapoptotic cytokines (e.g., tumor necrosis factor α, transforming growth factor-β, and Fas/Fas ligand).[20] An exaggerated immune response following injury to hematopoietic progenitors ensues, which provides the explanation for the actions of immunomodulators (e.g., antithymocyte globulins [ATG], cyclosporine A, steroids) or antiapoptotic mediators in early MDS therapy. In addition to abnormal immune and cytokine responses, an altered marrow stromal response in its interplay with hematopoietic elements has received heightened attention, which is supported by the success of immunomodulatory, antiangiogenic, and microenvironment-oriented therapies such as lenalidomide in at least some subtypes of MDS.

Cytogenetic and molecular abnormalities, haploinsufficiency, and epigenetic changes eventually shift the emphasis from excessive apoptosis toward arrest of maturation and increased proliferation as is more common in advanced stages of MDS and those patients whose disease transforms to AML.

CLASSIFICATION

Historically, the classification of MDS relied heavily on morphologic criteria (percentage of blasts and marrow-ringed sideroblasts, degree of blood monocytosis, and Auer rods) as these formed the backbone of the French-American-British (FAB) classification in the early 1980s.[21] Five subtypes were defined: refractory anemia, refractory anemia with ringed sideroblasts (RARS), refractory anemia with excess of blasts (RAEB), refractory anemia with excess of blasts in transformation (RAEB-t), and chronic myelomonocytic leukemia (CMML). Although time-tested, the FAB classification has a number of limitations, not least of which is its lack of inclusion of cytogenetic and molecular markers.

The World Health Organization (WHO) proposed a new classification in the 1990s, which was updated in 2008, with the goal to integrate biological, immunophenotypic, and genetic information[14,22] (Table 135.3). The WHO categories have correlated better with prognosis and with response to therapy

TABLE 135.3

THE WORLD HEALTH ORGANIZATION (WHO) CLASSIFICATION OF MDS

MDS Type	Blood	Marrow
Refractory cytopenia with unilineage dysplasia (RCUD) Refractory anemia (RA) Refractory neutropenia (RN) Refractory thrombocytopenia (RT)	Uni- or bicytopenia <1% blasts	Unilineage dysplasia <5% blasts <15% sideroblasts
Refractory anemia with ring sideroblasts (RARS)	Anemia No blasts	Erythroid dysplasia <5% blasts ≥15% sideroblasts
Refractory cytopenia with multilineage dysplasia (RCMD)	Cytopenia(s) <1% blasts $<1 \times 10^9$/L monocytes	Dysplasia in ≥2 lineages <5% blasts ±15% sideroblasts
Refractory anemia with excess blasts-1 (RAEB-1)	Cytopenia(s) <5% blasts $<1 \times 10^9$/L monocytes	Dysplasia 5%–9% blasts
Refractory anemia with excess blasts-2 (RAEB-2)	Cytopenia(s) 5%–19% blasts $<1 \times 10^9$/L monocytes	Dysplasia 10%–19% blasts
Myelodysplastic syndrome – unclassified (MDS-U)	Cytopenias ≤1% blasts	Dysplasia <5% blasts
MDS associated with isolated del(5q)	Anemia, normal or elevated platelets <1% blasts	<5% blasts Isolated del(5q)

From ref. 14.

TABLE 135.4

THE INTERNATIONAL PROGNOSTIC SCORING SYSTEM (IPSS) FOR MYELODYSPLASTIC SYNDROME

Prognostic Variable	Score Value				
	0	0.5	1	1.5	2.0
Marrow blasts (%)	<5	5–10	—	11–20	21–30
Karyotype[a]	Good	Intermediate	Poor		
Cytopenias[b]	0/1	2/3			

Combined Score	IPSS Risk Group	Survival (%)[c]	Progression to AML (%)[c]
0	Low	55	15
0.5–1	Int-1	35	30
1.5–2	Int-2	7	65
>2	High	0	100

AML, acute myeloid leukemia; Int, intermediate.
[a]Good: diploid, -Y, del(5q), del(20q); poor: complex, chr. 7 abnormalties; intermediate: others.
[b]Hemoglobin <10 g/dL, neutrophils $<1.5 \times 10^9$/L, platelets $<100 \times 10^9$/L.
[c]At 5 years.
(Modified from ref. 31.)

than the FAB system.[23] Attempts at a molecular classification of MDS and identification of genetic abnormalities in morphologic subgroups (e.g., *JAK2* mutations in RARS-T [refractory anemia with ringed sideroblasts and thrombocytosis]) are in early stages, but are likely to take a larger stage in the upcoming years and may lead to further revisions from the WHO.[24]

In about 10% of patients with MDS, marrow specimens are hypocellular rather than normocellular or hypercellular. Although not prognostic *per se*, hypoplastic MDS may be difficult to distinguish from aplastic anemia, toxic marrow insults, or autoimmune conditions.[25] Both aplastic anemia and hypoplastic MDS share common features such as T-cell–mediated myelosuppression, presence of paroxysmal nocturnal hemoglobinuria–type clones, and responsiveness to immunosuppressive therapy (e.g., steroids, cyclosporine A, or ATG). Distinctive features based on antigen expression patterns of CD34-positive cells by flow cytometry or immunohistochemistry may be helpful in the differential diagnosis.[26]

Significant degrees of myelofibrosis occur in about 10% of patients with MDS. Minimal diagnostic criteria require diffuse, coarse reticulin fibrosis and dysplasia in at least two cell lineages. Depending on blast percentage and other clinical features, the differential diagnostic considerations include acute panmyelosis with fibrosis, acute megakaryocytic leukemia (FAB M7), malignant lymphomas, or hairy cell leukemia. MDS with fibrosis identifies a subgroup of MDS with high transfusion requirements and poor prognosis.[27]

RARS-T is a fairly recently defined subgroup of MDS.[28] It is characterized by a dysplastic marrow associated with thrombocytosis and mutations of *JAK2*, which are typically found in patients with myeloproliferative disorders. RARS-T is a provisional entity in the group of myelodysplastic/myeloproliferative neoplasms. Myelodysplastic/myeloproliferative neoplasms are clonal myeloid neoplasms that possess both dysplastic and proliferative features, and are difficult to unambiguously assign to one or the other disease entity. This group contains, among others, CMML. As it is now considered separate from MDS, it will not be considered further in this chapter.

Different prognostic classifications exist to predict outcome of patients with MDS. The most commonly used is the IPSS.[29] The IPSS was developed in 1996 based on a multivariate analysis of 816 patients with *de novo* MDS who mostly (92%) did not receive any therapy other than supportive care. Three variables were significant for survival (calculated from diagnosis) and AML transformation: percentage of marrow blasts, cytogenetic abnormalities, and severity of cytopenias. It assigns points to each of the factors and divides patients into low, intermediate-1, intermediate-2, and high-risk groups with a corresponding decline of median survival times and increase of the risk of AML transformation, respectively (Table 135.4).

Given the characteristics of the patients based on whom the IPSS was developed, there are a few limitations of its application in daily clinical practice: (1) the expectations for survival and AML transformation do not apply to previously treated patients (i.e., the score needs to be calculated at the initial presentation) or those with secondary MDS and proliferative CMML; (2) the poor prognostic cytogenetic abnormalities are undervalued in their relation to the percentage of blasts; and (3) the prognostic significance of worse degrees of neutropenia and/or thrombocytopenia is not taken into account. To overcome these shortcomings, new models continue to be proposed. The WPSS (WHO-based prognostic scoring system) includes transfusion dependency (which has been associated with poorer prognosis in MDS), cytogenetic risk group, and criteria of the WHO classification.[30] The M. D. Anderson group designed a new prognostic model accounting for duration of MDS and prior therapy.[31] The so-called global M. D. Anderson Cancer Center model distinguishes four prognostic groups of patients whose outcome differs significantly. It can be calculated at any time during a patient's disease course and does not need to be referenced to the WHO classification, as is the case with the WPSS. Another model addresses the identification of different risk assignments within the lower-risk group of patients with MDS.[32] Although only partially validated and pending confirmation in larger studies, models such as these can have significant clinical implications for therapy selection of early-stage patients with MDS.

THERAPY

For many years, supportive care was the standard approach in MDS (except for those patients who were considered candidates for AML-type chemotherapy or SCT). Today there are vastly more therapeutic possibilities (Table 135.5). Supportive

TABLE 135.5

TREATMENT IN MYELODYSPLASTIC SYNDROME

Low Risk (IPSS Low and Intermediate-1; <10% Marrow Blasts)	High Risk (IPSS Intermediate-2 and High; ≥10% Marrow Blasts)

■ Iron chelation
■ Hematopoietic growth factors
  ■ Erythropoietin ± filgrastim
■ Immunomodulation
  ■ Antithymocyte globulins ± cyclosporine A, ± steroids
■ Lenalidomide for del(5q)
■ Imatinib mesylate for translocations involving 5q33, e.g., t(5;12)
■ DNMT inhibitors
  ■ Azacitidine
  ■ Decitabine
■ Investigational
	■ DNMT inhibitors
	  ■ Azacitidine
	  ■ Decitabine
	■ Intensive chemotherapy (younger patients, diploid cytogenetics)
	■ Allogeneic stem cell transplantation
	■ Investigational

IPSS, International Prognostic Scoring System; DNMT, DNA methyltransferase.

care and other forms of MDS-specific therapy are not mutually exclusive, are often combined, and may be synergistic. New guidelines have been published to establish algorithms in which patients are usually divided into those with lower- and those with higher-risk disease using the IPSS or occasionally marrow blasts of less than 10% versus 10% or more.[33]

Different treatment goals accompany different treatment strategies. Improvement of hematologic indices, quality of life, and disease-related complications are acknowledged as objective response criteria for lower-risk MDS. Given the poorer prognosis and higher risk of transformation to AML, changing the natural course of MDS by aiming for remissions remains the purpose of therapy in higher-risk MDS. Standardized response criteria for clinical trials in MDS facilitate reporting of responses and are crucial in the evaluation of patients with MDS on clinical trials[34] (Fig. 135.3).

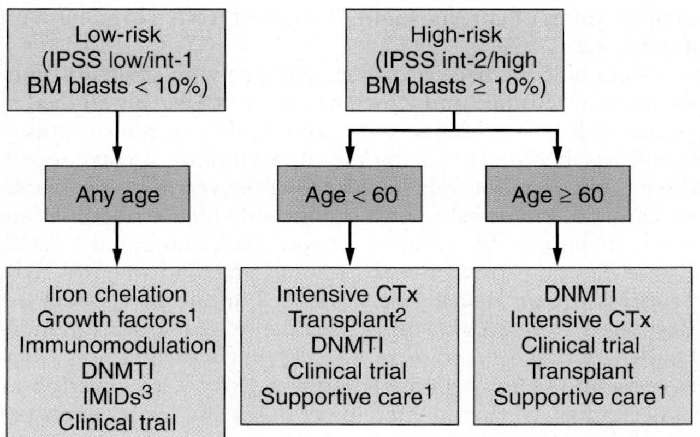

FIGURE 135.3 Treatment algorithm for myelodysplastic syndrome (MDS). Decision of low- versus high-intensity treatment based on the International Prognostic Scoring System (IPSS) score, age, and performance status: [1]consider growth factors/supportive care in patients with poor performance status; [2]consider stem cell transplant (SCT) especially in younger patients with availability of a matched-related sibling donor; [3]in patient with 5q- MDS. BM, bone marrow; DNMTI, DNA methyltransferase inhibitor (azacitidine, decitabine); IMiD, immunomodulatory inhibitory derivative (lenalidomide); intensive CTx, intensive chemotherapy.

Iron Chelation

Significant iron accumulation is likely once patients have received 5 g of iron or the equivalent of 20 to 25 units of packed red blood cells. As the body has no active mechanisms to clear excess iron, there is concern of iron accumulation in parenchymal organs (e.g., liver, heart, endocrine glands). Although there is limited evidence that iron causes organ damage in patients with MDS, iron overload and transfusions have been associated with worse survival and increased rates of AML transformation.[35] Iron accumulation is of particular concern in patients with more indolent forms of MDS who are likely to require transfusion support over several years (e.g., patients with 5q- syndrome or other forms of refractory anemia with likely long survival). Iron overload can be effectively managed with iron chelation therapy (e.g., desferrioxamine, deferasirox, deferiprone). Whether or not iron chelation therapy in MDS is able to prolong survival is not established yet. Although there has been an association between iron chelation therapy and better survival in some studies, these data need to be corroborated in larger randomized studies.[36,37]

Hematopoietic Growth Factors

Erythropoietic and myeloid growth factors are commonly used as supportive care measures in MDS. Some data from clinical trials also suggest a survival benefit for patients treated with erythropoietins and defined clinical characteristics.[38] Erythropoietin alone or with granulocyte colony-stimulating factor (filgrastim) achieves erythroid responses in 40% to 50% of patients, which can be durable for a median of 2 to 2.5 years. Low pretreatment serum erythropoietin levels (<200 to 500 mU/mL), low transfusion requirements (<2 units packed red blood cells per month), and favorable IPSS group have been predictive factors for response.[39]

Patients with predominantly neutropenia and thrombocytopenia present bigger challenges for growth factor therapy alone. Even in nonneutropenic patients, neutrophils may be dysfunctional and predispose patients to infections. Filgrastim, its pegylated variant pegfilgrastim, or granulocyte-monocyte colony-stimulating factor (sargramostim) should be used in patients with neutropenic fever or to improve response rates in combination with erythropoietins. Although neutropenia may be improved in up to 70% of patients, no data exist to indicate any impact on the number of infections, prolongation of survival, or the transformation rate to AML.

Severe thrombocytopenia (platelet count <20 × 10^9/L) is noted in almost 20% of patients with MDS, with hemorrhagic complications ranging from 3% to 53%, and the frequency of hemorrhagic deaths ranging from 14% to 24%.[40] Recently, two new thrombopoietic drugs have received U.S. Food and Drug Administration approval for use in idiopathic thrombocytopenic purpura: eltrombopag and romiplostim. Both act through stimulation of the thrombopoietin receptor (m-mpl). Although both are of interest in MDS therapy, their role remains undefined and under investigation.[41]

Immune Modulation Therapy

Immunosuppression

Some patients may benefit from immunosuppressive therapy such as with ATG or antilymphocyte globulins and cyclosporine A with or without steroids. Response rates to immunosuppressive therapy range from 16% to 50%[42] and responses may last for up to 1 year. Although some factors (expression of HLA-DR15, CD59-deficient [paroxysmal nocturnal hemoglobinuria] phenotype, hypocellular marrow, low-risk MDS) were thought to correlate with response to immunosuppression, recent larger studies have challenged the predictive value of these factors with the possible exception of marrow hypocellularity.[42,43] Better responses are generally achieved when ATG is combined with cyclosporine A.[42] As antithymocyte globulins are derived from horses, goats, and other animals, problems with serum sickness and other toxicities may be significant, especially in older patients. Selection of appropriate patients is therefore essential. That T-cell suppression has a role in some forms of MDS has recently been underlined in a small pilot study by surprisingly high response rates with the anti-CD52 monoclonal antibody alemtuzumab.[44]

Immunomodulatory Inhibitory Drugs

Lenalidomide is a second-generation immunomodulatory inhibitory drug that combines superior efficacy with better tolerability compared to its predecessor thalidomide.[45] In a series of 43 patients with transfusion-dependent or symptomatic anemia, lenalidomide at doses of 25 mg or 10 mg daily or 10 mg daily for 21 days with a 1-week rest achieved a response rate of 56% including 47% of patients with sustained independence from transfusions.[46] Significant differences in response were observed in select karyotypes. In patients with an interstitial deletion of chromosome 5q31, 83% responded. These results were confirmed in two subsequent multicenter trials.[47,48] Among 148 patients with lower risk MDS, transfusion dependence, and chromosome 5q deletion, 67% became transfusion-independent with a median time to response of 4.6 weeks and a median duration of transfusion independence of 2.2 years.[47] Cytogenetic responses were common (overall 73%, complete in 45%) and associated with transfusion independence, resolution of cytogenetic dysplasia, and possibly a survival advantage (compared with cytogenetic nonresponders). Response rates (including cytogenetic) and duration were lower in patients with MDS without del(5q).[48] Myelosuppression is common and more pronounced in patients with del(5q) in whom thrombocytopenia or the need for treatment interruption in the first 8 weeks were independent predictive variables for achievement of transfusion independence.

Lenalidomide has been approved by the U.S. Food and Drug Administration for patients with low-risk MDS who are transfusion-dependent and have a detectable del(5q) and should be considered standard of care in these situations. Its role in patients with non del(5q), higher-risk MDS or in combinations with other agents (e.g., DNA methyltransferase inhibitors, chemotherapy) remains investigational.

Epigenetic Therapy

Global and gene-specific methylation of promoter-associated CpG islands in combination with deacetylation and methylation of nucleosome-associated histone tails leads to inactivation of genes important for cell function and tumor suppressor genes.[49] Reversal of abnormal methylation patterns or inhibition of deacetylase activity of histone proteins allows a permissive gene expression state and therefore results in reactivation of silenced genes. Two DNA methyltransferase (DNMT) inhibitors are approved in the United States for treatment of patients with MDS, 5-azacitidine (azacitidine), and 5-aza-2′-deoxycytidine (decitabine).

In the randomized Cancer and Leukemia Group B (CALGB) 9221 study in high-risk MDS, patients receiving azacitidine (75 mg/m^2 subcutaneously daily × 7 days every 4 weeks) as opposed to best supportive care, achieved higher response rates (63% vs. 7%), better quality of life, a longer time to leukemia transformation (median, 21 vs. 13 months; $P < .01$), and a trend toward improved survival (median, 24 vs. 14 months).[50] Survival outcome was not significant because of the cross-over design of the study. In a more recent and larger multicenter study (AZA-001) 358 patients were randomized to receive azacitidine or conventional care regimens (best supportive care, low-dose cytarabine, "3+7"-type AML therapy).[51] The median age of the patients was 70 years; most had higher-risk disease. The median number of courses was nine for azacitidine, but only one to seven for the conventional care arm. With a median follow-up time of 21 months, median overall survival was 24.5 months for azacitidine versus 15 months for conventional care ($P = .0001$). This study was the first to demonstrate a survival advantage of any therapeutic intervention in MDS. The study also highlighted a couple of other points of interest: (1) there was no correlation between achieving complete response and survival and (2) patients with abnormalities of chromosome 7 benefited from treatment with azacitidine.

Decitabine is a deoxycytidine analogue with structural similarity to azacitidine and which has been extensively studied in similar types of patients, with comparable response rates.[52] Using a schedule of 15 mg/m^2 of decitabine intravenously three times daily for 3 days every 6 weeks versus best supportive care, decitabine achieved a significantly higher response rate (17% including 9% complete responders, compared to 0%; $P < .001$) and a trend toward a longer median time to AML progression or death (12.1 vs. 7.8 months; $P = .16$).[53] Responses were durable and associated with transfusion independence. Based on *in vitro* models that indicated less cytotoxicity and better hypomethylating activity with lower doses of decitabine, trials evaluated lower doses and longer exposure schedules of decitabine. In a single institution, randomized three-arm study, decitabine 20 mg/m^2 intravenously daily for 5 days every 4 weeks was found to be safe and effective with an overall response rate of 80%.[54] The efficacy of this schedule was confirmed in a single-arm multicenter study, albeit with a lower overall response rate than in the single institution trial (51% vs. 73%).[55] In contrast to azacitidine, treatment with decitabine was not associated with a survival benefit over supportive care in patients with higher-risk MDS.[56] Barring any significant differences of the biological activity of the two

DNMT inhibitors, explanations for this finding include the shorter dose exposure and less frequent schedule used (15 mg/m^2 intravenously every 8 hours × 3 days to be repeated every 6 to 8 weeks), the capping of the number of courses at eight (medium number of courses four versus nine in the azacitidine study), and the lower total patient number (N = 233). Compared with intensive cytarabine-based chemotherapy, decitabine appears to be superior according to a separate, retrospective comparison: given similar complete response rates (43% vs. 46%), mortality at 6 weeks (3% vs. 12%; $P = .002$) and 3 months (7% vs. 22%) and estimated 2-year survival (47% vs. 25%; $P < .001$) were in favor of decitabine-treated patients.[57]

Both azacitidine and decitabine need to be administered for a minimum of three to six cycles to be able and evaluate a clinical response. Several questions remain: (1) optimal dose and schedule: there are several studies looking at shorter exposure (less days) with either agents; (2) routes of administrations: recent phase 1 studies have evaluated oral azacitidine and subcutaneous and oral administration of decitabine; (3) combinations: many studies are assessing combinations with other agents, mainly histone deacetylase inhibitors; (4) duration of therapy: chronic uninterrupted therapy is currently recommended; (5) strategies for patients who fail to respond to or lose their response to DNMT inhibitors: this area represents a major focus of clinical research in MDS. This situation raises the necessity for intensive therapy (e.g., AML therapy, SCT) and other investigational drugs.

Stem Cell Transplant

Allogeneic SCT remains the only treatment modality that can lead to long-term disease-free survival.[58] Given the demographics of MDS, only few patients will ultimately benefit from SCT. Treatment-related morbidity and mortality remain substantial impediments to SCT. SCT with reduced intensity conditioning can decrease the toxicity of the procedure, but at the cost of higher relapse likelihood.[59] Matched unrelated donor transplants may overcome some of the shortage of suitable donors. Although effective, they carry a higher risk of toxicities.[60] Judicious selection of patients for SCT is therefore crucial, particularly in the context of therapies such as lenalidomide or DNMT inhibitors.

Outcome is generally most favorable in patients who may need transplant the least, such as younger patients with low-risk MDS.[61] In a study by the International Bone Marrow Transplant Registry, 452 recipients of HLA-identical sibling transplants with a median age of 34 years and high-risk MDS in two-thirds, overall survival at 3 years was 42%.[62] Survival was more favorable with young age and platelet counts less than 100 × 10^9/L. Relapse was highest in patients with high percentages of marrow blasts at transplantation, with high IPSS scores, and with T-cell depleted transplants. Diseases-free survival was 60% in the low-risk, 36% in the intermediate-1, and 28% in intermediate-2 risk groups. This compared to 5-year survival rates of 55%, 35%, and 7%, respectively, for unselected patients not receiving SCT, suggesting a benefit of SCT mostly for high-risk MDS patients.

A key issue remains the optimal timing of SCT. Using a Markov decision model, three transplant strategies were compared: (1) SCT at diagnosis, (2) SCT at the time of progression to leukemia; and (3) SCT some time after diagnosis but prior to leukemic progression.[63] Delaying transplant was most beneficial for patients in the low and intermediate-1 IPSS groups, an effect that was more noticeable in patients younger than 40 years. Earlier transplantation, on the other hand, improved survival in the intermediate-2 and high IPSS groups.

OUTLOOK

Although more treatments are available now than there have been 5 to 10 years ago, MDS remains incurable with non-SCT treatments. MDS therapy is currently defined by DNMT inhibitors. Lenalidomide is effective in the small subset of patients with PRBC transfusion-dependent low-risk MDS and del(5q) (3%–5% of patients). Hematopoietic growth factor and iron chelation therapy are considered supportive and adjunctive care measures, which by themselves are not likely to change the natural course of the disease. Current clinical research focuses on optimizing the use of DNMT inhibitors by (1) introducing oral therapy (e.g., azacitidine); (2) expansion of low-dose approaches with decitabine (e.g., lower dose schedules in low-risk MDS, subcutaneous and oral route); and (3) evaluating combinations with histone deacetylase inhibitors.[64–66] The glutathione analogue ezatiostat (TLK199), available by intravenous and oral route, is a novel small molecule with properties of a hematopoietic growth factor whose role in MDS therapy is being evaluated.[67] There is only limited experience with tyrosine kinase inhibitors whose activity remains restricted to the rare MDS cases with specific molecular abnormalities (e.g., fusion of the *PDGFRB* gene on chromosome 5q33 to the *ETV6* gene in translocation t[5;12]).

SCT is the only curative strategy available, but its benefits extend to only a small fraction of patients. One of the major challenges is represented by patients who fail epigenetic-based therapy and for whom SCT is not an option. New nucleoside analogues (e.g., sapacitabine, clofarabine) may provide strategies to achieve responses for some of these patients.[68] Combinations of the nucleoside analogues with epigenetic therapy are being explored in higher-risk MDS.

References

1. Tefferi A, Vardiman JW. Myelodysplastic syndromes. *N Engl J Med* 2009;361:1872.
2. Albitar M, Manshouri T, Shen Y, et al. Myelodysplastic syndrome is not merely "preleukemia." *Blood* 2002;100:791.
3. Garcia-Manero G. Progress in myelodysplastic syndromes. *Clin Lymph Myeloma Leuk* 2009;9(Suppl):S286.
4. Sekeres MA. Epidemiology, natural history, and practice patterns of patients with myelodysplastic syndromes in 2010. *J Natl Compr Canc Netw* 2011;9(1):57–63.
5. Nagata C, Shimizu H, Hirashima K, et al. Hair dye use and occupational exposure to organic solvents as risk factors for myelodysplastic syndrome. *Leuk Res* 1999;23:57.
6. Kimura A, Takeuchi Y, Tanaka H, et al. Atomic bomb radiation increases the risk of MDS. *Leuk Res* 2001;25:S13.
7. Leone G, Pagano L, Ben-Yehuda D, Voso MT. Therapy-related leukemia and myelodysplasia. *Haematologica* 2007;92:1389.
8. Delwail V, Jais JP, Colonna P, et al. Fifteen-year secondary leukemia risk observed in 761 patients with Hodgkin's disease prospectively treated by MOPP or ABVD chemotherapy plus high-dose irradiation. *Br J Haematol* 2002;118:189
9. Armitage JO, Carbone PP, Connors JM, et al. Treatment-related myelodysplasia and acute leukemia in non-Hodgkin's lymphoma patients. *J Clin Oncol* 2003;21:897.
10. McLaughlin P, Estey E, Glassman A, et al. Myelodysplasia and acute myeloid leukemia following therapy for indolent lymphoma with fludarabine, mitoxantrone, and dexamethasone (FND) plus rituximab and interferon α. *Blood* 2005;105:4573.
11. Le Deley MC, Suzan F, Cutuli B, et al. Anthracyclines, mitoxantrone, radiotherapy, and granulocyte colony-stimulating factor: risk factors for

leukemia and myelodysplastic syndrome after breast cancer. *J Clin Oncol* 2007; 25:292.
12. Houck W, Abonour R, Vance G, Einhorn LH. Secondary leukemias in refractory germ cell tumor patients undergoing autologous stem cell transplantation using high-dose etoposide. *J Clin Oncol* 2004;22:2155.
13. Bowen D, Culligan D, Jowitt S, et al of the UK MDS Guidelines Group. Guidelines for the diagnosis and therapy of adult myelodysplastic syndromes. *Br J Haematol* 2003;120:187.
14. Swerdlow SH, Campo E, Harris NL, et al., eds. *WHO Classification of Tumours of Haematopoietic and Lymphoid Tissues*. 4th ed. Lyon: International Agency for Research on Cancer, 2008.
15. Haase D, Germing U, Schanz J, et al. New insights into the prognostic impact of karyotype in MDS and correlation with subtypes: evidence from a core dataset of 2124 patients. *Blood* 2007;110:4385.
16. Haase D. Cytogenetic features in myelodysplastic syndromes. *Ann Hematol* 2008;87:515.
17. Pozdnyakova O, Miron PM, Tang G, et al. Cytogenetic abnormalities in a series of 1029 patients with primary myelodysplastic syndromes. *Cancer* 2008;113:3331.
18. Ebert B, Pretz J, Bosco J, et al. Identification of RPS14 as a 5q- syndrome gene by RNA interference screen. *Nature* 2008;451:335.
19. Pellagatti A, Jadersten M, Forsblom AM, et al. Lenalidomide inhibits the malignant clone and up-regulations the SPARC gene mapping to the commonly deleted region in 5q- syndrome patients. *Proc Natl Acad Sci U S A* 2007;104:11406.
20. Rosenfeld C, List A. A hypothesis for the pathogenesis of myelodysplastic syndromes: implications for new therapies. *Leukemia* 2000;14:2.
21. Bennett JM, Catovsky D, Daniel MT, et al. Proposals for the classification of the myelodysplastic syndromes. *Br J Haematol* 1982;51:189.
22. Vardiman JW, Harris NL, Brunning RD. The World Health Organization (WHO) classification of the myeloid neoplasms. *Blood* 2002;100:2292.
23. Germing U, Strupp C, Kuendgen A, et al. Prospective validation of the WHO proposals for the classification of myelodysplastic syndromes. *Haematologica* 2006;91:1596
24. Bruce Galili N, Mehdi M, Mumtaz J, et al. Can molecular profiling of cytogenetic subgroups draw a roadmap for individualizing therapy in myelodysplastic syndromes? *Future Oncol* 2006;2:407.
25. Wong KF, So CC. Hypoplastic myelodysplastic syndrome—a clinical, morphologic, or genetic diagnosis? *Cancer Genet Cytogenet* 2002;138:85.
26. Matsui WH, Brodsky RA, Smith BD, et al. Quantitative analysis of bone marrow CD34 cells in aplastic anemia and hypoplastic myelodysplastic syndromes. *Leukemia* 2006;20:458.
27. Della Porta MG, Malcovati, L, Boveri E, et al. Clinical clusters of bone marrow fibrosis and CD34-positive cell clusters in primary myelodysplastic syndromes. *J Clin Oncol* 2009;27:754.
28. Remacha AF, Nomdedéu JF, Puget G, et al. Occurrence of the *JAK2* V617F mutation in the WHO provisional entity: myelodysplastic/myeloproliferative disease, unclassifiable-refractory anemia with ringed sideroblasts associated with marked thrombocytosis. *Haematologica* 2006;91:719.
29. Greenberg P, Cox C, LeBeau MM, et al. International scoring system for evaluating prognosis in myelodysplastic syndromes. *Blood* 1997;89:2079.
30. Malcovati L, Germing U, Kuendgen A, et al. Time-dependent prognostic scoring system for predicting survival and leukemic evolution in myelodysplastic syndromes. *J Clin Oncol* 2007;25:3503.
31. Kantarjian H, O'Brien S, Ravandi F, et al. Proposal for a new risk model in myelodysplastic syndrome that accounts for events not considered in the original International Prognostic Scoring System. *Cancer* 2008;113:1351.
32. Garcia-Manero G, Shan J, Faderl S, et al. A prognostic score for patients with lower-risk myelodysplastic syndrome. *Leukemia* 2008;22:538.
33. Greenberg PL, Attar E, Battiwalla M, et al. Myelodysplastic syndromes. *J Natl Compr Cancer Netw* 2008;6:902.
34. Cheson BD, Greenberg PL, Bennett JM, et al. Clinical application and proposal for modification of the International Working Group (IWG) response criteria in myelodysplasia. *Blood* 2006;108:419.
35. Sanz G, Nomdedeu B, Such E, et al. Independent impact of iron overload and transfusion dependency on survival and leukemic evolution in patients with myelodysplastic syndrome. *Blood* 2000;112:640.
36. Leitch HA, Goodman TA, Wong KK, et al. Improved survival in patients with myelodysplastic syndrome (MDS) receiving iron chelation therapy. *Blood* 2006;108:78a.
37. Fox F, Kündgen A, Nachtkamp K, et al. Matched-pair analysis of 186 MDS patients receiving iron chelation therapy or transfusion therapy only. *Blood* 2009;114:1747
38. Jädersten M, Malcovati L, Dybedal I, et al. Erythropoietin and granulocyte-colony stimulating factor treatment associated with improved survival in myelodysplastic syndrome. *J Clin Oncol* 2008;26:3607.
39. Jädersten M, Montgomery SM, Dybedal I, et al. Long-term outcome of treatment of anemia in MDS with erythropoietin and G-CSF. *Blood* 2005; 106:803.
40. Kantarjian HM, Giles F, List AF, et al. The incidence and impact of thrombocytopenia in myelodysplastic syndrome (MDS). *Blood* 2006;108:739a.
41. Greenberg PL, Garcia-Manero G, Moore MR, et al. Efficacy and safety of romiplostim in patients with low or intermediate-risk myelodysplastic syndrome (MDS) receiving decitabine. *Blood* 2009;114:1769.
42. Sloand EM, Wu C, Greenberg P, et al. Factors affecting response and survival in patients with myelodysplasia treated with immunosuppressive therapy. *J Clin Oncol* 2008;26:2505.
43. Lim ZY, Killick S, Germing U, et al. Low IPSS score and bone marrow hypocellularity in MDS patients predict hematological responses to antithymocyte globulin. *Leukemia* 2007;21:1436.
44. Sloand EM, Olnes MJ, Weinstein B, et al. Alemtuzumab treatment of intermediate-1 (INT-1) myelodysplasia patients is associated with sustained improvement in blood counts and cytogenetic remissions. *Blood* 2009;114:116.
45. List A. Lenalidomide: a transforming therapeutic agent in myelodysplastic syndrome. *Clin Lymph Myeloma Leuk* 2009;9(Suppl):S302
46. List A, Kurtin S, Roe DJ, et al. Efficacy of lenalidomide in myelodysplastic syndromes. *N Engl J Med* 2005;352:549.
47. List A, Dewald G, Bennett J, et al. Lenalidomide in the myelodysplastic syndrome with chromosome 5q deletion. *N Engl J Med* 2006;355:1456.
48. Raza A, Reeves JA, Feldman EJ, et al. Phase 2 study of lenalidomide in transfusion-dependent, low-risk, and intermediate-1 risk myelodysplastic syndromes with karyotypes other than deletion 5q. *Blood* 2008;111:86.
49. Issa J-P. Optimizing therapy with methylation inhibitors in myelodysplastic syndromes: dose, duration, and patient selection. *Nat Clin Pract Oncol* 2005;2(Suppl 1):S24.
50. Silverman LR, Demakos EP, Peterson BL, et al. Randomized controlled trial of azacitidine in patients with the myelodysplastic syndrome: a study of the Cancer and Leukemia Group B. *J Clin Oncol* 2002;20:2429.
51. Fenaux P, Mufti GJ, Hellström-Lindberg E, et al. Efficacy of azacitidine compared with that of conventional care regimens in the treatment of higher-risk myelodysplastic syndromes: a randomized, open-label, phase III study. *Lancet Oncol* 2009;10:223.
52. Wijermans P, Lübbert M, Verhoef G, et al. Low-dose 5-aza-2′-deoxycytidine, a DNA hypomethylating agent, for the treatment of high-risk myelodysplastic syndrome: a multicenter phase II study in elderly patients. *J Clin Oncol* 2000;18:956.
53. Kantarjian H, Issa J-P, Rosenfeld CS, et al. Decitabine improves patient outcome in myelodysplastic syndrome. *Cancer* 2006;106:1794.
54. Kantarjian H, Oki Y, Garcia-Manero G, et al. Results of a randomized study of 3 schedules of low-dose decitabine in higher-risk myelodysplastic syndrome and chronic myelomonocytic leukemia. *Blood* 2007;109:52.
55. Steensma DP, Baer MR, Slack JL, et al. Multicenter study of decitabine administered daily for 5 days every 4 weeks to adults with myelodysplastic syndromes: the alternative dosing for outpatient treatment (ADOPT) trial. *J Clin Oncol* 2009;10;27(23):3842.
56. Wijermans P, Suciu S, Baila L, et al. Low dose decitabine versus best supportive care in elderly patients with intermediate or high risk MDS not eligible for intensive chemotherapy: final results of the randomized phase II study (06011) of the EORTC Leukemia and German MDS Study Groups. *Blood* 2009;112:226.
57. Kantarjian HM, O'Brien S, Huang X, et al. Survival advantage with decitabine versus intensive chemotherapy in patients with higher risk myelodysplastic syndrome: comparison with historical experience. *Cancer* 2007;109:1133.
58. Warlick ED, Cioc A, Defor T, et al. Allogeneic stem cell transplantation for adults with myelodysplastic syndromes: importance of pretransplant disease burden. *Biol Blood Marrow Transplant* 2009;15:30.
59. Martino R, Iacobelli S, Brand R, et al. Retrospective comparison of reduced-intensity conditioning and conventional high-dose conditioning for allogeneic hematopoietic stem cell transplantation using HLA-identical sibling donors in myelodysplastic syndromes. *Blood* 2006;108:836.
60. Deeg HJ, Storer B, Slattery JT, et al. Conditioning with targeted busulfan and cyclophosphamide from related and unrelated donors in patients with myelodysplastic syndrome. *Blood* 2002;100:1201.
61. Deeg HJ, Appelbaum FR. Hematopoietic stem cell transplantation in patients with myelodysplastic syndrome. *Leuk Res* 2000;24:653.
62. Sierra J, Perez WS, Rozman C, et al. Bone marrow transplantation from HLA-identical siblings as treatment for myelodysplasia. *Blood* 2002;200:1997.
63. Cutler CS, Lee SJ, Greenberg P, et al. A decision analysis of allogeneic bone marrow transplantation for the myelodysplastic syndromes: delayed transplantation for low-risk myelodysplasia is associated with improved outcome. *Blood* 2004;104:579.
64. Garcia-Manero G, Gore SD, Skikne B, et al. A phase 1, open-label, dose-escalation study to evaluate the safety, pharmacokinetics, and pharmacodynamics of oral azacitidine in patients with myelodysplastic syndromes (MDS) or acute myeloid leukemia (AML). *Blood* 2009;114:117.
65. Garcia-Manero G, Couriel DR, Tambaro FP, et al. A phase II randomized Bayesian study of very low dose subcutaneous decitabine administered daily or weekly times three in patients with lower risk myelodysplastic syndrome (MDS). *Blood* 2009;114:119.
66. Braiteh F, Soriano AO, Garcia-Manero G, et al. Phase I study of epigenetic modulation with 5-azacytidine and valproic acid in patients with advanced cancers. *Clin Cancer Res* 200814:6296.
67. Raza A, Galili N, Smith S, et al. Phase 1 multicenter dose-escalation study of ezatiostat hydrochloride (TLK199 tablets), a novel glutathione analog prodrug, in patients with myelodysplastic syndrome. *Blood* 2009;113:6533.
68. Faderl S, Garcia-Manero G, Estrov Z, et al. Oral clofarabine in the treatment of patients with higher-risk myelodysplastic syndrome. *J Clin Oncol* 2010;28(16):2755.

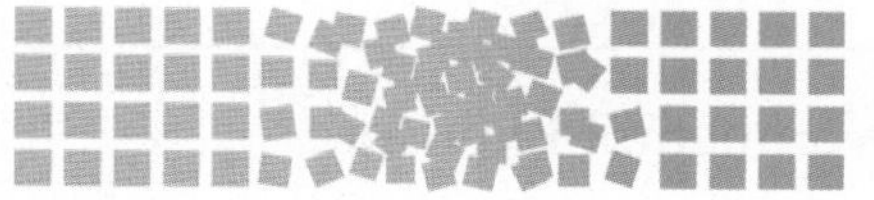

CHAPTER 136 PLASMA CELL NEOPLASMS

NIKHIL C. MUNSHI AND KENNETH C. ANDERSON

Plasma cell neoplasms represent a spectrum of diseases characterized by clonal proliferation and accumulation of immunoglobulin-producing terminally differentiated B cells. The spectrum includes clinically benign common conditions, such as monoclonal gammopathy of unknown significance (MGUS) as well as rare disorders such as Castleman disease and α heavy chain-disease; indolent conditions such as Waldenström macroglobulinemia; the more common malignant entity, plasma cell myeloma; and a more aggressive form, plasma cell leukemia, with circulating malignant plasma cells in the blood. All of these disorders share common features of plasma cell morphology, production of immunoglobulin molecules, and immune dysfunction. A plasma cell neoplasm is considered to originate from a single B cell, with resultant monoclonal protein secretion that characterizes its type. Occasional oligoclonal or polyclonal protein abnormalities are observed in conditions such as Castleman disease.

There are five major classes of immunoglobulins synthesized by normal B cells and plasma cells: immunoglobulin G (IgG), IgA, IgM, IgD, and IgE. The dysfunctional plasma cells secrete one of these intact immunoglobulin molecules; however, there may be a discrepancy in the production of the heavy and light chains leading to an imbalance with an excess of κ or λ light chain that is excreted in the urine (Bence Jones proteinuria); or in some instances, produce only κ or λ light chain molecules. Occasionally, plasma cells do not secrete any paraproteins (nonsecretory type myeloma); however, they usually have cytoplasmic immunoglobulin and produce low levels of immunoglobulins undetectable by current methods. Although myeloma can be associated with any of the immunoglobulin subtypes, the IgM type is predominately associated with other malignant conditions such as Waldenström macroglobulinemia and chronic lymphocytic leukemia.

HISTORY

The earliest evidence of myeloma has been reported from the Egyptian mummies; however, the first published clinical description of the disease was reported in 1850 in England. A patient, Thomas Alexander McBean, presented to Dr. William Macintrye of London in 1845 with symptoms of episodes of fatigue, diffuse bone pain, and urinary frequency. The urinalysis detected a urinary protein with a peculiar heat property and McIntyre called it "mollities and fragilitas ossium" based on the patient's bony symptoms.[1] Later that year, Dr. Henry Bence Jones also tested urine specimens provided by Macintyre and corroborated the heat properties of urinary light chains. Bence Jones thought that the protein was the "hydrated deuteroxide of albumin" (now called *Bence Jones proteins*) and published his findings several years before Macintyre published his case report.[2] After the patient died in 1846, a surgeon, Dr. John Dalrymple, examined several bones and his gross and microscopic observations are consistent with morphology of myeloma cells.

The term *multiple myeloma* was coined by Rustizky in 1873 following his independent observation in a similar patient with multiple bone lesions. Kahler in 1889 published a review on this condition and the disease became known, particularly in Europe, as Kahler disease.[3] Ellinger, in 1899, described the increased serum proteins and sedimentation rate in myeloma. In 1900, Wright described the involvement of plasma cells in this neoplasm and for the first time he described roentgenographic abnormality in myeloma, which to date remains one of the diagnostic tests.

The development of bone marrow aspiration in 1929,[4] electrophoresis to separate serum proteins in 1937,[5] and a later report of a specific spike in the γ globulin region enhanced the diagnosis and understanding of myeloma. Identification of the heavy and light chains in the monoclonal protein by immunoelectrophoresis was described by Grabar in 1953, confirming the monoclonality of immunoglobulin in this disease. Other developments in recent times include understanding of the role of bone marrow microenvironment in myeloma cell growth, survival, and development of drug resistance through cell–cell interaction and activation of cytokine networks.[6,7] The significance of chromosomal translocation in myeloma pathobiology, and more recently gene expression profiling and proteomics, are providing insights into the molecular pathogenesis of the disease.

No effective systemic therapy existed before 1947, when urethan was reported to show effect in a few patients. However, a subsequent randomized trial indicated that the survival of patients receiving urethan was inferior to that observed with a placebo.[8] The first successful use of chemotherapeutic agent in myeloma was reported in 1958 by Blokhin and colleagues with the use of a racemic mixture of D- and L-phenylalanine mustards (Sarcolysine). Subsequently, the D- and L-isomers of phenylalanine mustard were tested separately, and the antimyeloma activity was found to reside in the L-isomer, melphalan. In 1962, Bergsagel[9] and colleagues from the Southwest Oncology Group reported remissions in about one-third of myeloma patients treated with melphalan. Administration of high doses of glucocorticoid was first reported to induce remissions in relapsing or refractory myeloma in 1967.[10] The use of melphalan in combination with prednisone was then studied extensively.[11] The role of high-dose therapy (HDT) was investigated by McElwain and Powles[12] in 1983, and addition of bone marrow and subsequently stem cell transplantation with improved safety and further dose escalation was later evaluated. In the last 10 years, improved understanding of the role of the bone marrow microenvironment in myeloma biology and development of drug resistance has led to identification of novel agents, such as thalidomide and its immunomodulatory analogue lenalidomide, proteasome inhibitor bortezomib, and bisphosphonates, which target myeloma cells in their microenvironment and can overcome resistance to conventional therapy.

EPIDEMIOLOGY

According to the most recent data from the Surveillance, Epidemiology, and End Results (SEER) program, multiple myeloma (or, variably, MM throughout text) is a relatively uncommon malignancy in the United States, representing 1.0% of all malignancies in whites and 2.0% in African Americans. Among hematologic malignancies, it constitutes 10% of the tumors and ranks as the second most frequently occurring hematologic cancer in the United States after non–Hodgkin's lymphoma. The prevalence of myeloma in the United States in 2007 was over 61,600 and estimated new cases in 2010 were approximately 20,180; 10,650 patients died from myeloma in 2010. The disease is more common in men and has average annual age-adjusted (1970 U.S. standard) incidence rates per 100,000 among whites of 7.1 in men and 4.5 in women, whereas for African Americans the incidence is 14.3 in men and 10.0 in women. The increased incidence in African Americans is not explained by factors such as social or economic condition, household size, or family income.[13]

A recent study in black population from Ghana has demonstrated an incidence of MGUS similar to that of African American population in the United States, possibly implicating genetic risk factors.[23] The incidence data for other ethnic groups including native Hawaiians, female Hispanics, American Indians from New Mexico, and Alaskan natives also show higher myeloma rates relative to U.S. whites in the same geographic group; however, the Chinese and Japanese populations have a lower incidence than whites. The incidence of multiple myeloma has slowly increased in the U.S. white population since 1970; however, the incidence among African Americans has increased more prominently during the 1970s and 1980s and is still increasing in the 1990s. These observed differences in the prevalence have not been associated with any difference in the disease characteristics, response to therapy, and prognosis of myeloma worldwide.

The incidence of myeloma and other plasma cell disorders increases with advancing age. The median age at diagnosis is 70 years. The mortality pattern also closely follows the Incidence curves for age distribution, with median age at death is 75 years. As seen in Figure 136.1, fewer than 2% of patients are younger than 40 years and more than 50% of patients are older than 70 years. A similar age distribution is also observed in other related plasma cell disorders including MGUS and Waldenström macroglobulinemia.

ETIOLOGY

Environmental Exposure

Exposure to ionizing radiation is the strongest single factor linked to an increased risk of multiple myeloma.[14] This has been documented in atomic bomb survivors with a five times greater incidence than the control group and a latent period of approximately 20 years from exposure.[15] People exposed to low levels of radiation also demonstrate an increased incidence of myeloma, including radiologists, people employed in the nuclear industry, or those handling radioactive materials. An increase in myeloma risk with increasing numbers of diagnostic radiographs was demonstrated without an increased risk of leukemia or lymphoma, suggesting that even a low level of radiation may be a risk factor for myeloma. An association between exposure to various chemicals and the risk of multiple myeloma remains ill defined. Exposure to metals, especially nickel; agricultural chemicals; benzene and petroleum products; other aromatic hydrocarbons; agent orange; and silicon have been considered as potential risk factors.[14,16–18] Alcohol and tobacco consumption has not been clearly linked to myeloma. Among medications, only mineral oil used as a laxative has been reported to be associated with an increased risk of multiple myeloma in some patients.[19,20]

Hereditary and genetic factors may predispose to myeloma development.[21,22] Occurrence among siblings was reported in 25 of 37 families with at least two family members who had myeloma. However, direct genetic linkage has not been established. Myeloma risk also appears to be enhanced by the presence of HLA-Cw2 in both African American and white populations. In a study in 917 Ghanaian men, the prevalence of MGUS was twice that in white men, implicating race-related genetic susceptibility in the higher rates of MGUS in black populations.[23]

MGUS has been considered a premalignant condition; however, the rate of conversion to myeloma remains extremely low and often associated with additional genetic changes.[24,25] Repeated infections or antigenic stimulation of the plasma cell

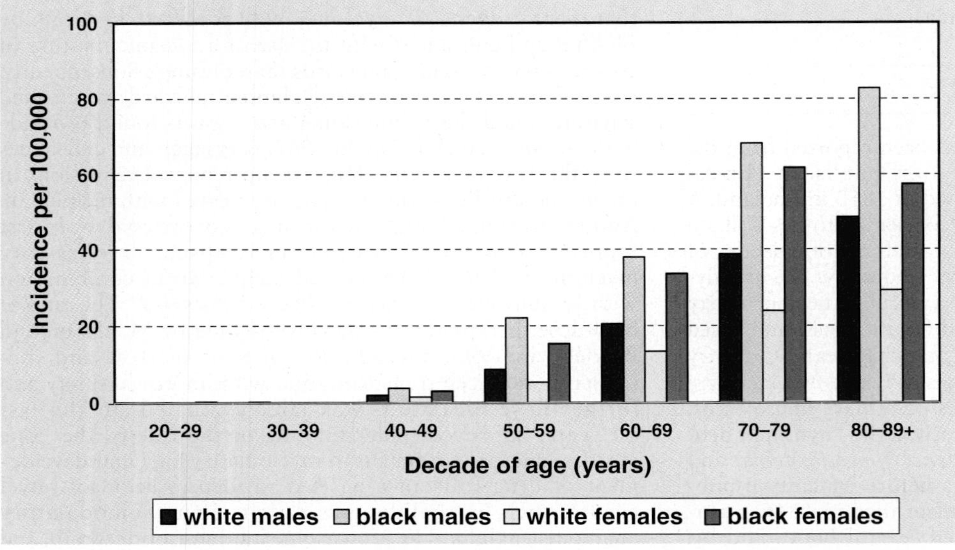

FIGURE 136.1 Multiple myeloma average annual age, sex, and race-specific incidence per 100,000 in United States, 1996 to 2000. Increase in incidence is noted with advancing age, and higher incidence is observed in male than female and in African American than white population.

compartment has also been proposed as a possible predisposing condition for myeloma. In one interesting patient report in the literature, a prior therapy with horse antiserum against tetanus led to subsequent development of MGUS, which lasted for 3 decades before conversion to multiple myeloma. At the time of myeloma diagnosis, the serum IgG component was found to react specifically against horse β-2 macroglobulin.[26] This report suggests an initial antigen-driven stimulation of monoclonal protein-producing plasma cells, eventually becoming malignant after acquiring additional genetic alterations. MGUS has been observed in mice, and in that species it depends on strain of mice, aging, pre-existing immune status, and antigenic stimulation. MGUS has been associated with immune disorders and infectious diseases. In one report of 57 patients with MGUS who had undergone evaluation for *Helicobacter pylori* infection for various gastrointestinal symptoms, 39 (68%) had evidence of *H. pylori* infection and 11 of these 39 patients (28%) had normalization of the serum paraproteins following eradication of *H. pylori* infection.[27] Seroprevalence of *H. pylori,* however, has not been consistently correlated with MGUS.[28] Development of MGUS has also been reported with T-cell deficiency disorders as in AIDS.[29] Importantly, a recent study indicates that the diagnosis of symptomatic multiple myeloma is always preceded by MGUS by 2 or more years.[30]

Although epidemiologic studies have not been able to conclusively establish an association between multiple myeloma and infectious or autoimmune diseases, a recent retrospective cohort study in United States veterans demonstrated significantly elevated risks of MM in patients with a history of autoimmune, infectious, and inflammatory disorders. Risks for MGUS were generally of similar magnitude. These results indicate that various types of immune-mediated conditions might act as triggers for MM/MGUS development.[31] Although an initial report suggested presence of the human herpes virus 8 (HHV8, Kaposi sarcoma herpes virus) in the bone marrow dendritic cells of the majority of patients with multiple myeloma,[32] analogous to its association with other lymphoproliferative diseases such as Castleman disease,[33] body-cavity lymphoma,[34] and Kaposi sarcoma,[35] other investigators have failed to identify HHV8 in myeloma cells or dendritic cells from various sources including mobilized peripheral blood stem cells.[36–39] Because HHV8 produces unique gene products, including possible growth-promoting factors for myeloma such as analogues of interleukin (IL)-6, insulinlike growth factor (IGF) 1, and an IL-8, the possible linkage of HHV8 to myeloma was intriguing. However, even antibodies against HHV8 have not been observed in multiple myeloma.[40]

PATHOGENESIS

Multiple myeloma is a germinal center-derived tumor with mainly postswitch B-cell phenotype characterized by extensive Ig gene hypermutation in a pattern suggesting antigen selection. This is reflected in the exceedingly rare occurrence of IgM myeloma. Somatic mutations of other loci, such as BCL-6, have also been reported in myeloma B cells, along with characteristic immunoglobulin gene rearrangement.[41] Similar mechanisms may be affecting other cell-cycle control genes whose products regulate cell proliferation and malignant transformation.

As in most malignancies, pathogenesis of multiple myeloma appears to be associated with dysregulated expression and function of multiple key cellular genes controlling apoptosis, cell growth, and proliferation. Understanding the evolution of myeloma from MGUS has provided a background for a multistep process involving alterations in various oncogenes and tumor suppressor genes.[42] In one study the presence of 14q32 abnormalities were reported in patients with MGUS, and the addition of chromosome 13 change was associated with a transformation to overt multiple myeloma.[43] This led to a theory that a subset of myeloma may derive from prior MGUS with a high incidence of monosomy 13 and a second group of *de novo* myeloma in which other genetic abnormalities may be involved.[43] However, a recent report suggests that all myelomas are preceded by MGUS[30] and that a small subset of MGUS carry del(13) along with t(4;14), which is not associated with increased rate of progression to myeloma.[44,45]

Myeloma occurs not only in humans but also in mice, canines, and hamsters. In fact, genetic susceptibility to plasma cell tumors has been demonstrated in an inbred strain of mice. A common factor in various species has been the prevalence of endogenous retroviruses.[46,47] Animal models are now providing a basis for understanding the role of activation of oncogenes and tumor suppressor genes, cytokines, and the role of the bone marrow microenvironment in promoting and sustaining myeloma cell growth.

Cytogenetic and Molecular Genetic Alterations

Myeloma karyotypes are complex with an average of 11 numeric and structural abnormalities per cell.[48,49] The relative incidence of gain or loss of various chromosomes with involved p and q arms are shown in Figure 136.2. The inherent problem in the low proliferative activity of the tumor cells and possible clonal evolution have been obstacles to identify specific chromosomal and molecular changes in myeloma. The frequency and complexity of the chromosomal aberration increases with advanced disease and is uniformly abnormal in plasma cell leukemia. Detection of a complex karyotype predicts for poor prognosis. The newer techniques of multicolor fluorescent *in situ* hybridization (FISH) and spectral karyotyping, along with refined G-banding techniques, have identified many nonrandom changes in a large number of patients.[50–52] Using these techniques, over 90% of patients are detected to have involvement of at least one chromosome. A substantial fraction of MGUS plasma cells are also reported to have aneuploidy. By FISH analysis, the incidence of trisomy for at least one chromosome was reported in over 40% of MGUS cells.[53] The characteristic numerical abnormalities are monosomy 13 and trisomies of chromosome 3, 5, 7, 9, 11, 15, and 19.

The most frequent structural abnormality involves chromosome 1 and the immunoglobulin heavy chain gene at 14q32. By conventional cytogenetics 14q32 region is involved in translocation in 20% to 40% of cases, and by molecular and FISH techniques, it is detectable at higher frequency ranging from 50% in MGUS to 90% in advanced myeloma.[48,49,54] The demonstration of this abnormality in MGUS suggests its involvement in the initial step of transformation.[43,55,56] Light chain translocations involving Igλ (22q11) or Igκ (2p12) are less commonly observed; only 20% even in advanced multiple myeloma. The most common translocation involving 14q32 results in overexpression of cyclins D1 (on 11q13) and D3 (on 6p21).[54,57] The other biologically important partner chromosomes are 4p16 (FGFR3 and MMSET), 16q23 (c-MAF), and 20q11 (MAFB) (Table 136.1).

Other recurrent partner loci less frequently identified include 8q24 (c-myc) in less than 5%, 18q21 (bcl-2), 11q23 (MLL-1), and 6p21.1. The 4p16 region contains fibroblast growth factor receptor III (*FGFR3*) and *MMSET* genes. *FGFR3* and its activating mutations trigger MAP kinase signaling and growth of myeloma cells.[58] Mutated *FGFR3* also confers resistance to caspase 3-related apoptosis.[59–61] This translocation also activates the *MMSET* gene, a homologue of *MLL1* which is also independently involved in 11q23 translocation. With the

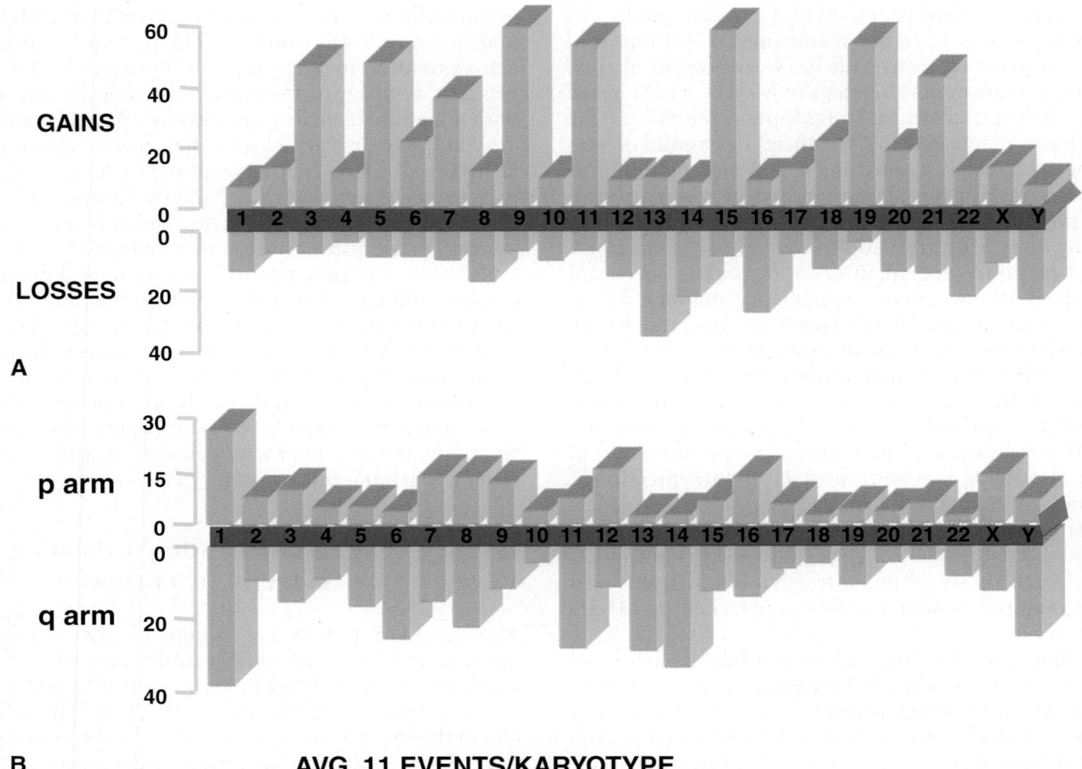

FIGURE 136.2 Summary karyotypic abnormalities in 158 patients with evaluable abnormal cytogenetics from a study of 492 patients demonstrating "chromosomal chaos." **A:** Numeric changes with trisomies (gain) and monosomies (loss). **B:** Structural changes involving short (p) and long (q) arm. (Courtesy of J. R. Sawyer.)

enhanced sensitivity of spectral karyotyping, a nonrandom involvement of t(14:16) (q32:q22–23) has recently been described. Molecular analysis of the locus at chromosome 16q22 shows fusion of immunoglobulin heavy chain with the sequence near the *cMAF* oncogene, a b-ZIP transcription factor.[62] Additionally, translocation partners t(9;14) involving *PAX-5* gene and t(6;14) involving *IRF4* genes have been described.[63,64] In the majority of cases, however, the translocating partner chromosome locus is not yet identified. Although 14q32 is one of the common translocations, its role in myeloma pathogenesis remains unclear because of the variety of partner chromosomes involved and its lack of prognostic significance.

Standard cytogenetics techniques did not identify rearrangements involving 8q24, which contains c-*MYC* oncogene and is commonly involved in murine plasmacytoma. However, FISH analyses in one study identified karyotypic abnormalities that involve c-*MYC* in 45% cases of advanced myeloma.[65] A recent study with interphase FISH confirmed c-*MYC* rearrangement in 15% of multiple myeloma, with increasing frequency correlated with severity of disease. Interestingly, c-MYC involvement was heterogeneous suggesting evolution of disease.[66] Changes in c-MYC in the form of either abnormal size transcript or high level of expression have also been reported in a majority of patients in one study.[67,68]

Partial or complete deletion of chromosome 13q arm confers a poor prognosis, even after HDT.[69] Using the *RB1* gene as a probe, FISH analysis reveals RB1 deletion in more than 40% of these patients.[70] In a detailed analysis of the 13q chromosome with an 11-probe FISH panel, more than 80% of 50 patients showed molecular deletions with 13q14 representing a critical region most frequently involved.[71] Additionally, constitutive phosphorylation of pRB in myeloma cells can be further enhanced by IL-6.[72] Cyclin D, cyclin-dependant kinases and cyclin-dependant kinase inhibitors p15 and p16 (ink), p21

TABLE 136.1

NONIMMUNOGLOBULIN SITES FOR ILLEGITIMATE SWITCH RECOMBINATION IN MULTIPLE MYELOMA

Chromosome	Frequency, % Patients	Gene(s)	Function
11q13	30	*Cyclin D1*	Induces growth
4p16	25	*FGFR3, MMSET*	Growth factor
8q24	5	*C-myc*	Growth/apoptosis
16q23	1	*C-maf*	Transcription factor
6p25	<1	*IRF4* Transcription factor	

and p27 (cip), and p57 (kip) have also been investigated in myeloma because of their effect on pRB phosphorylation. Abnormalities in p16 and p15 have been reported in 75% and 67% of myeloma patients, respectively, suggesting an important defect in the pRB regulatory pathway.[73–75]

Mutations involving Ras are observed in about 39% of newly diagnosed MM patients, and are more frequently observed following progressive disease. Activating mutations of the *ras* oncogenes may also result in growth factor independence and suppression of apoptosis in MM. One of the commonly altered genes in many malignancies is *p53*. In myeloma, abnormalities in *p53* are detected in fewer than 10% of patients with early-stage disease[76,77]; however, *p53* abnormalities represent an important late event associated with progression to an aggressive form of the disease. A study of *p53* gene mutations in 52 patients with myeloma showed 7 of 52 patients to have *p53* abnormalities, all with advanced clinically aggressive acute/leukemic stage of multiple myeloma.[76] One study showed poor prognosis in patients with *p53* gene deletion, as assessed by FISH, after standard-dose therapy.[78] In contrast to primary patient samples, mutations in *p53* are more commonly detected in myeloma cell lines, which are usually derived from patients with aggressive myeloma. MDM2, an important inhibitor of *p53* function, is overexpressed in the majority of myeloma cell lines; however, increased MDM2 expression is infrequently observed in primary myeloma cells.[79]

An important antiapoptotic gene, *BCL2*, is uniformly overexpressed in low-grade non–Hodgkin's lymphoma. In this family of genes, *BCL2* and *BCL-XL* are antiapoptotic genes, while *BAX*, *BAD*, and BCL_{XS} are proapoptotic genes. A balance between these genes determines cell survival. The t(14:18) translocation involving the *BCL2* gene is quite rare (2%–3%) in myeloma. However, numerous myeloma cells lines as well as primary cells express high levels of *BCL2*. [80,81] Its relationship to development of drug resistance, as well as radiation resistance, in myeloma cells is also well described.[82,83] One study of 63 patients showed a significant correlation between *BCL2* expression and resistance to therapy with interferon (IFN), but not melphalan and prednisone.[84] The association of *BCL2* expression with prognosis remains controversial, as one small study failed to show a correlation with short survival. *BCL-XL* is up-regulated in myeloma cells as a consequence of IL-6 induced activation of STAT-3.[85] It confers a drug-resistant phenotype and, in conjunction with bcl-2, leads to increased genetic instability. These molecular changes, coupled with abnormalities of gp130, NF-κB and STATs, promote progression of myeloma.[86] *Mcl-1,* another antiapoptotic gene, is overexpressed in MM and is upregulated by IL-6. Its overexpression mediates potent resistance to apoptosis, and conversely, its down-regulation by antisense oligonucleotide triggers apoptosis. High telomerase activity has also been demonstrated in myeloma cells, relative to normal cells and other malignant cell lines.[87] Although the clinical implication of this activity remains under investigation, telomerase activity confers growth and survival and is therefore an additional target for therapeutic intervention.

Transcriptional and Genomic Studies

Gene expression profiling as well as studies focused on relative gains or loss of genomic DNA have provided both prognostic and therapeutic information in MM. Molecular diagnostic tools and novel therapeutics now offer the potential for more accurate prognosis and personalized treatment.

The expression profiling studies in MM have provided insight into progression of MGUS to MM, and provided a basis to predict outcome as well as identify potential therapeutic targets.[42] Expression studies have identified subtypes within the nonhyperdiploid group associated with specific chromosomal translocations.[88] A comprehensive expression profiling survey of uniformly treated MM patients has identified 70 genes predictive of early disease-related death. Interestingly, one-third of these genes are located on chromosome 1, confirming potential significance of chromosome 1 in MM pathobiology.[89] Patients with high-risk scores using this gene signature had significantly shorter complete response (CR) duration (20% patients at 3 years) compared to those patients without such high-risk features (60% at 5 years). A multivariate discriminant analysis identified a 17-gene signature that performed as well as the 70-gene model.

A second large study by the Intergroupe Francophone du Myelome (IFM) group studied gene expression profiles in 182 newly diagnosed patients and developed a 15-gene model to calculate a risk score associated with overall survival (OS). In this study, high-risk group had overexpression of cell-cycle progression and its surveillance-related genes, while hyperdiploid signature and heterogeneous gene expression characterized low-risk patients. Overall survival at 3 years in the low-risk group was 91%, and it was only 47% in the high-risk groups. These results were independent of traditional prognostic factors.[90] It is intriguing that the 15- and 17-gene models do not share a single common gene, highlighting the redundancy and complexity of tumor cell biology.

In a recent study in 320 newly diagnosed myeloma patients from the Dutch-Belgian/German HOVON-65/GMMG-HD4 trial, gene expression profiling identified ten subgroups in multiple myeloma that may represent unique diagnostic entities with potential for unique therapeutic targeting.[91] Additional expression profile studies have begun to define subtypes of myeloma with different prognostic significance following various therapies. An apparent lack of uniformity in the genes identified by these investigations suggests that therapy-related factors may determine the influence of different classes of genes in MM. Based on cytogenetics as well as expression data, cyclin D dysregulation occurs in the early pathogenesis of MM.

A high-resolution analysis of recurrent copy number alterations, coupled with expression analysis in MM cell lines and primary MM cells using array comparative genomic hybridization, has identified distinct genomic subtypes. Additionally, this study has defined 87 discrete minimal common regions that have identified gene candidates that will allow targeted drug discovery, improve our understanding of MM initiation and progression, and predict clinical course (Fig. 136.3). A high-density, single-nucleotide polymorphism array analysis of myeloma cells from 192 newly diagnosed patients identified genomic copy number alteration in 98% of patients. Amplifications in 1q and deletions in 1p, 12p, 14q, 16q, and 22q were the most frequent lesions associated with adverse prognosis, whereas amplifications of chromosomes 5, 9, 11, 15, and 19 were linked to a favorable prognosis. Amp(1q23.3), amp(5q31.3), and del(12p13.31) have been identified in multivariate analysis as conferring independent prognostic features. This prognostic model was validated in an independent validation cohort of 273 patients with myeloma, and identified patients with amp(5q31.3) alone and low serum beta-2-M with an excellent prognosis (5-year OS, 87%) versus patients with del(12p13.31) alone or amp(5q31.3) and del(12p13.31) and high-serum beta-2-M with poor outcome (5-year OS, 20%).

Epigenetic changes modulating myeloma cell growth and survival genes are also reported. For example, methylation of *p16*, a negative cell-cycle regulator, is common and is reported as an early event even in MGUS. However, in a single large cohort study *p16* methylation was not predictive of OS.

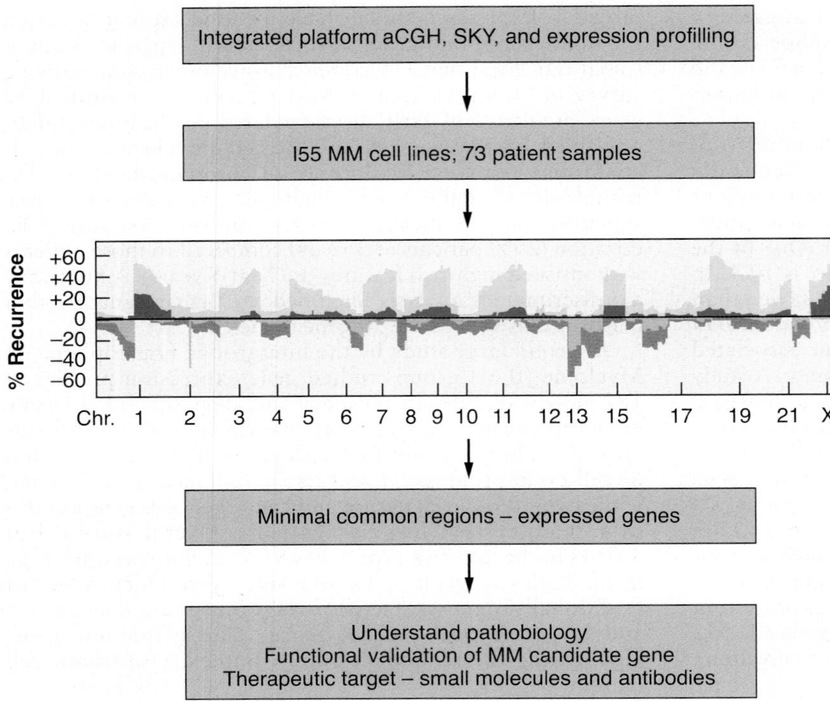

FIGURE 136.3 Array-based comparative genomic hybridization analysis evaluating 55 cell lines and 73 patient samples identified recurrent areas of gains and losses in multiple myeloma (MM) with potential for understanding biology and validating target genes, which will then be potential therapeutic targets.

A role of microRNAs (miRs), and potential therapeutic targeting multiple mRNAs, has recently been described in myeloma. An miRNA expression profile of MM and MGUS cell compared with normal donor plasma cells identified a signature with overexpression of miR-21, miR-106b, and miR-181a and b in MM and MGUS samples, as well as selective up-regulation of miR-32 and miR-17-92 in MM but not in MGUS.[92] Another study analyzed the expression level of miRs and the gene expression profile in 60 newly diagnosed myeloma patients, and identified significantly dysregulated miRs expression pattern in cytogenetically distinct subtypes.[93] The putative targets and their function are now being defined; for example, miR-192, 194, and 215, which are down-regulated in a subset of newly diagnosed myeloma, are transcriptionally activated by *p53* and then modulate *MDM2* expression. In addition, miR-192 and 215 target the IGF pathway, prevent enhanced migration of plasma cells into bone marrow, and are positive regulators of *p53*, suggesting that their down-regulation plays a key role in myeloma pathogenesis.[94]

Microenvironment and Cell Signalling

Myeloma cells express adhesion molecules, which mediate interaction with the microenvironment including both bone marrow stromal cell elements and extracellular matrix proteins (Table 136.2). These adhesion molecules mediate both homotypic and heterotypic adhesion. Adhesion not only plays a role in migration and localization of myeloma cells in the bone marrow, but also induces tumor cell growth and survival. For example Syndecan-1, a cell surface transmembrane heparan sulfate proteoglycan present on MM cells, interacts with type I collagen and regulates growth of MM cells; it also mediates increased osteoclast activity.[95–97] Elevated levels of syndecan-1 shed into serum correlate with increased tumor mass, decreased matrix metalloproteinase-9 activity in serum, and poor prognosis.[95]

The bone marrow (BM) microenvironment consists of a variety of cell types including stromal cells (BMSC), endothelial cells, osteoclasts, osteoblasts, as well as immune cells. The physical interaction between myeloma cells and these cells in the BM milieu plays a crucial role in MM pathogenesis both by direct adhesion-mediated signaling, as well as by secretion of growth and/or antiapoptotic factors, such as IL-6, IGF-1, vascular endothelial growth factor (VEGF), B-cell activating

TABLE 136.2

ADHESION MOLECULE EXPRESSION ON NORMAL PLASMA CELLS, MULTIPLE MYELOMA, AND PLASMA CELL LEUKEMIA CELLS

Molecule	Normal Plasma Cell	MM Cell	PCL Cell
Adhesion			
CD11[a]	+	−	−
CD11[b]	−	−	+
CD44	+	+	+
CD54	+	+	+
CD56	−	+	−
CD58	−	+	ND
LFA-1	−	−/+	+
VLA-4	+	+	ND
VLA-5	+	+	−
MPC-1	+	+	−
RHAMM	−	+	−/+
Syndecan-1	+	+	−
Surface			
CD19	+	−	−
CD28	−	−	+
CD38	+	+	+
CD40	+	+	+[a]
CD45	+	−[b]	−

MM, multiple myeloma; PCL, plasma cell leukemia.
[a]CD40 expression is enhanced on PCL cells relative to normal plasma cells and MM cells.
[b]CD45 on immature myeloma cells.

factor, fibroblast growth factor, stromal cell-derived factor (SDF) 1α, and tumor necrosis factor (TNF)-α, which mediate tumor cell growth, survival, drug resistance, and migration.[4,98–102] These interactions lead to activation of several proliferative/antiapoptotic signaling cascades in MM cells: phosphatidylinositol-3 kinase (PI3K)/Akt; Ras/Raf/mitogen-activated protein kinase (MAPK) kinase (MEK)/extracellular signal-related kinase (ERK); Janus kinase (JAK) 2/signal transducers and activators of transcription (STAT)-3; and NFκB pathways. These pathways lead to MM cell growth, survival, antiapoptosis, migration, and development of drug resistance. Additionally, adhesion as well as cytokines secreted from MM cells and accessory cells in turn further augment cytokine secretion from these cells.

Activation of NF-κB has been noted in myeloma cells, especially following their interaction with BMSC. A number of abnormalities contributing to the dysregulation of NF-κB and constitutive activation of the noncanonical NF-κB pathway have recently been described.[103] Elevated expression of NIK due to genomic alterations or protein stabilization, and inactivating mutations of TRAF3 are able to trigger the classic and alternative NF-κB pathways.[104] These alterations activating NF-κB pathway may allow MM cells to achieve autonomy from the bone marrow microenvironment. [105]

Each accessory cell in the BM milieu contributes differently to the overall effect of the microenvironment. The biologic and clinical relevance of increased angiogenesis, while established in solid tumors, has only recently been appreciated in hematologic malignancies. Increased bone marrow microvessel density (MVD) has been reported in MM patients compared to individuals with MGUS.[106–108] Moreover, in patients with myeloma the degree of MVD has been correlated with prognosis.[109,110] Immunohistochemical studies show that the angiogenic factor VEGF is expressed by MM cells.[111] Hepatocyte growth factor, which also promotes angiogenesis, is increased in serum of myeloma patients and predicts for poor outcome, especially in patients with increased β2 microglobulin levels.[112] Finally, novel agents such as thalidomide inhibit angiogenesis and can also overcome drug resistance in myeloma.

Role of Cytokines

Myeloma cells and BMSCs produce cytokines including IL-6,[98] IGF-1,[102] VEGF,[100] SDF-1,[101] TNF,[99] transforming growth factor-beta (TGF-β),[113] IL-21,[114] and others that mediate tumor cell growth, survival, antiapoptosis, migration, and development of drug resistance.

Interleukin 6

IL-6 is an essential growth and survival factor for myeloma. The IL-6 receptor expressed by myeloma cells is composed of two polypeptide components: the α chain (gp80, IL-6Rα) and the signal transducing element, the β chain (gp130). The gp130 component is shared by a family of cytokines including oncostatin M and leukemia inhibitory factor. Interaction of IL-6 with its receptor activates Ras/RAF/MEK/ERK, JAK/STAT, and PI3K/AKT signaling pathways, mediating growth, survival, and drug resistance (Fig. 136.4). IL-6 is mainly produced by stromal cells following binding of myeloma cells and is also triggered by other cytokines including TNF-α,[99] IL-1β, and VEGF in the BM milieu.[100] IL-6 mediates both autocrine and paracrine growth of myeloma cells. It increases the proportion of cells in S phase, prevents apoptosis of malignant plasma cells, and confers resistance to antitumor agents such as dexamethasone (Dex). Dex-induced apoptosis is mediated by cytochrome C, but not Smac, release from mitochondria into the cytosol, followed by caspase 9 and 3 activation[115]; IL-6 blocks caspase 9 activation, thereby protecting cells against Dex-induced apoptosis.[116] Soluble IL-6Rα, shed by myeloma cells into serum, can amplify the response of myeloma cells to IL-6; both high-serum IL-6Rα levels and high-serum IL-6 levels portend poor prognosis. IL-6 and soluble IL-6Rα also mediate enhanced bone resorption by osteoclasts.

To date IL-6 has been targeted therapeutically using antibodies specific for IL-6 or its receptor, as well as using IL-6 superantagonist (SANT-7), which binds IL-6R but does not trigger downstream signaling. These treatment approaches have produced only transient responses in a small number of patients. Neutralizing anti-IL-6 murine monoclonal antibodies have been administered either locally (malignant pleural effusions) or intravenously in patients with advanced MM; although clinical responses were not seen, therapy led to reduced survival and proliferation of malignant plasma cells, confirming a role for IL-6 in mediating myeloma growth *in vivo*.

Insulinlike Growth Factor 1

IGF-I is a growth and survival factor in human multiple myeloma that activates PI-3K and MAPK signaling pathways mediating proliferation and antiapoptosis.[117,118] It induces more potent protection against Dex than does IL-6. IGF-1 also up-regulates FLIP, XIAP, and A1/Bfl1[117] and increases telomerase activity, thereby further enhancing tumor cell growth and survival.[119] We have recently shown that IGF-1 mediates adhesion and migration of myeloma cells via β1-integrin.[102] These studies have identified IGF-1 as a novel therapeutic target; both antibodies and small-molecule inhibitors against IGF-1 show promise in preclinical studies.

Vascular Endothelial Growth Factor

VEGF has only modest proliferative effects on myeloma cells; however, it plays a more important role in triggering tumor cell migration and angiogenesis.[120,121] Its production in the BM milieu is up-regulated both by myeloma cell adhesion to BMSCs and by IL-6.[122] Because it is a specific endothelial cell mitogen, elevated levels in myeloma may account, at least in part, for increased angiogenesis.[111] Myeloma cells express Flt-1, and VEGF triggers its phosphorylation and activation of downstream MEK and PKCα signaling. These data have provided the preclinical rationale to evaluate VEGF as a therapeutic target. PTK787, a potent inhibitor of VEGF receptor, has shown antimyeloma activity *in vitro*,[123] and pazopanib, an anti-VEGFR antibody is under clinical evaluation.

Other Cytokines

TNF-α is secreted by myeloma cells and does not have any significant direct effect on myeloma cell growth and survival; however, it induces secretion of IL-6 by BMSCs. It is also a strong inducer of NFκB activation, thereby up-regulating adhesion molecules, with resultant binding of myeloma cells to BM, and related cell adhesion-mediated drug resistance. Although specific antibody inhibitors of TNF-α have not shown clinical response, thalidomide and its IMiD analogues have potent anti-TNF-α activity and can overcome cell adhesion-mediated drug resistance.

SDF-1 is expressed by BMSCs, and its receptor CXCR4 is expressed by myeloma cells. It induces only a minimal proliferative effect; however, it plays a more important role mediating migration.

TGF-β is produced by MM cells and induces secretion of IL-6 by BMSCs; it also contributes to immunosuppression characteristic of myeloma.

Increased levels of serum IL-17, IL-21, IL-22, and IL-23, the proinflammatory cytokine associated with Th17 cells, are also observed in myeloma. IL-17 promotes myeloma cell growth and colony formation as well as adhesion to BMSCs.

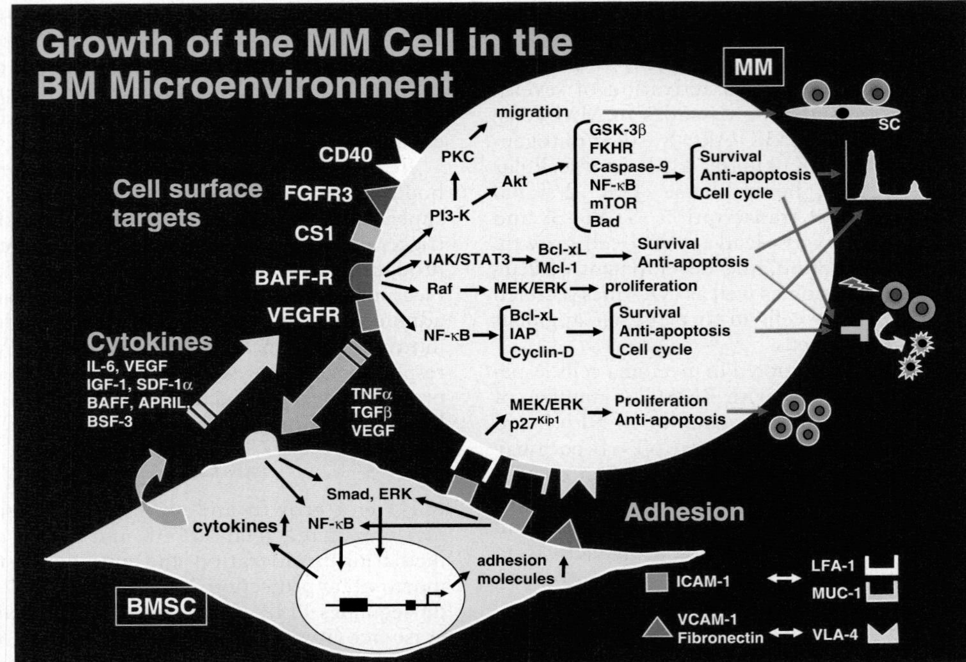

FIGURE 136.4 The interaction and adhesion of multiple myeloma (MM) cells to the bone marrow (BM) stromal cells (BMSCs) leads to adhesion- and cytokine-mediated signaling. MM cell binding to BMSCs induces the activation of p42/44 mitogen-activated protein kinase (MAPK) and nuclear factor κB (NFκB) in BMSCs. The activation of NFκB up-regulates adhesion molecules on BMSCs. Cytokines secreted through this interaction includes interleukin-6 (IL-6) secretion, tumor-necrosis factor-α (TNF-α), and vascular endothelial growth factor (VEGF) to activate the main signaling pathways (p42/44 MAPK, Janus kinase [JAK]/signal transducer and activator of transcription 3 (STAT3) and/or phosphatidylinositol 3-kinase (PI3K)/AKT) and their downstream targets, which triggers MM cell growth, survival, and migration.

The RAS/RAF/MAPK kinase (MEK)/MAPK pathway mediates proliferation of MM. JAK/STAT3 along with up-regulation of BCL-X_L and MCL1 mediates survival. Phosphatidylinositol 3-kinase (PI3K)/AKT through downstream activation of BAD and NFκB, and/or inactivation of caspase-9 mediates anti-apoptosis. NFκB and forkhead in rhabdomyosarcoma (FKHR) modulate cyclin D and KIP1, thereby regulating cell-cycle progression. Signaling through PI3K induces downstream protein kinase C (PKC) activity and MM cell migration. ICAM1; intercellular adhesion molecule 1; LFA1, lymphocyte function-associated antigen 1; muc1, mucin 1; VCAM1, vascular cell adhesion molecule 1; VLA4, very-late antigen 4; IGF1, insulinlike growth factor-1; IL, interleukin; SDF-1α, stromal-cell-derived factor-1α. (Adapted from Hideshima T, Mitsiades C, Tonon G, et al. Understanding multiple myeloma pathogenesis in the bone marrow to identify new therapeutic targets. *Nat Rev Cancer* 2007;7:585.)

In combination with IL-22, it inhibits the production of Th1-mediated cytokines, including IFN-gamma.[124] IL-21 induces proliferation and inhibits apoptosis independently of IL-6 signaling. It triggers phosphorylation of Jak1, Stat3, and Erk1/2 (p44/42 MAPK). TNF-α up-regulates expression of both IL-21 and of IL-21 receptor (IL-21R).

DRUG RESISTANCE

Intrinsic and acquired resistance of plasma cells to conventional chemotherapy is common, and as a result only 50% of patients achieve a partial response (PR), with few complete responses. Drug resistance is mediated by several mechanisms.[125] First, altered intracellular drug concentration may be due to overexpression of *MDR1* gene, encoding for P-glycoprotein, an integral membrane protein that functions as an ATP-dependent drug efflux pump. Cyclosporine A and verapamil inhibit Pgp function and have been tested as chemosensitizers, but achieved only modest short-term benefit.[126] PSC 833, a nonimmunosuppressive and nonnephrotoxic derivative of cyclosporine D, has also been evaluated in a phase 2 trial, with limited success.[127] Second, the multidrug resistance-associated protein (MRP), a member of the ATP-binding cassette transporter gene superfamily, may also confer clinical drug resistance.[128] Third, expression of lung resistance-related protein (LRP), a member of the class of major vault proteins, is associated with poor response and shortened survival.[129] Vault proteins are multisubunit proteins localized to the nuclear membrane, which are implicated in transport of substances such as alkylating agents to the nucleus. Dose intensification of melphalan has been shown to overcome the resistance due to increased LRP expression.[130] It may be possible to combine vault protein inhibitors with Pgp inhibitors to increase sensitivity of myeloma cells to chemotherapy.

Phenotype

Myeloma cells display heterogeneous cell surface phenotypes, with differences both between different patients and differences within the same patient at different disease stages. In general, all myeloma cells express high levels of CD38, with immature plasma cells additionally expressing CD45 and the IL-6 receptor.[131–133] More mature myeloma cells do not express CD45 and lack IL-6 receptor expression.[134] A subpopulation of myeloma cells may also express CD10, CD56, or CD49e (VLA-5).[134–136] CD28 expression is associated with more aggressive disease[137]; CD20 expression is present on 20% to 30% of myeloma patients, and can be further up-regulated with IFN-α.[138] The identity of the myeloma stem cell still remains an enigma. B cells expressing CD19 and CD11b can be induced to mature on stromal cells into monotypic plasma cells, suggesting that this cellular compartment may contain myeloma cell progenitors.[139,140] Using allele-specific oligonucleotide polymerase chain reaction and the SCID-hu model, the myeloma stem cell will be better defined in the future.

Immune Status

Myeloma patients present with suppressed immune function by a variety of factors. Most significant is suppression of uninvolved immunoglobulins; for example, in patients with IgG myeloma there is suppression of serum IgA and IgM levels.[141] The factors causing this suppression include a direct effect of monoclonal immunoglobulin, increased soluble Fc receptor or Fc expressing cells, suppression of helper cell functions, monoclonal Ig, and macrophage-related factors that affect B-cell maturation to plasma cells.[142] Recovery of uninvolved immunoglobulins to normal levels following effective therapy has been associated with both improved survival and protection from infectious complications.

The total T-cell count may be decreased; however, in a substantial number of patients it may be normal, with no significant changes in CD_8 cells.[143–145] A stage-dependent suppression of NK-cells has been observed.[146] Deficiency of CD4 helper cells is also pronounced.[147] In one study the proliferation and frequency of Epstein-Barr virus-negative and Inf A-specific T cells was significantly reduced in a cohort of 24 newly diagnosed or conventionally treated MM patients when compared with 19 healthy individuals, suggesting an impaired response of CD8+ T cells in MM patients.[148] Although a defect in NKT cell function has also been detected in patients with progressive myeloma compared to patients with MGUS or nonprogressive disease,[149] invariant NKT cells from myeloma patients can be activated and expanded *in vitro*.[150] Dysfunctional T-regulatory cells have been associated with disturbed immune homeostasis in both MGUS and MM.[151] Elevated levels of IL-17 producing Th17 cells, possibly related to high IL-6 and TGF-β expression, have also been described in myeloma, and promote myeloma cell growth, immune suppression, and osteoclast function.[124]

Anti-idiotype T-cell response has been demonstrated in the majority of patients, with higher Id-specific T-cell frequency in MGUS and early stage of myeloma compared to advanced disease.[152] This observation has led to a provocative hypothesis that immunologic response plays an important role in controlling proliferation of the malignant clone in early stages of the disease, whereas loss of immune regulation is associated with evolution to an overt or more aggressive form of the disease. These data also provide the scientific basis to develop idiotype-specific T-cell responses for therapeutic purpose through either vaccination *in vivo* or production of idiotype or myeloma-specific cytotoxic T lymphocytes *in vitro*.[153]

Murine Models

In C57BL/Ka strains of inbred mice, 16% spontaneously develop monoclonal gammopathies without tumor formation by 2 years.[46,47,154] Interestingly, however, the C57BL/Ka strain with a high incidence of spontaneous monoclonal gammopathies is relatively resistant to induction of plasmacytoma by mineral oil. In other strains, such as BALB/c, which have a low spontaneous incidence of monoclonal gammopathies, induction of plasmacytoma or myeloma is observed after intraperitoneal injection of mineral oil or its clinically defined component, pristane.[46] Production of such tumors can be blocked by administration of indomethacin and accelerated by subsequent infection of the mice with Abelson's virus. Plasmacytomas develop within the oil- or other foreign body-mediated granulomas and lymphoplasmacytic infiltration. Plasmacytoma progression is associated with dysregulated expression of *c-myc*, as a result of translocation analogous to t(8;14) in humans. These plasmacytomas produce IgA immunoglobulins, and a growth factor present in the peritoneal fluid has been confirmed to be IL-6. Additionally, when animals are raised in a germ-free environment, incidence of myeloma after mineral oil stimulation is markedly reduced, whereas that of other lymphoid neoplasms increases.[46] These studies suggest an important role of immune stimulation in myeloma development.

Human myeloma cell lines can grow and disseminate in a severe combined immunodeficiency (SCID) mouse model, providing a unique opportunity to study this disease in an *in vivo* setting.[155] The introduction of fetal human bone into SCID mice (SCID-hu) has allowed engraftment and proliferation of stromal cell-dependent human myeloma cell line[156] as well as primary human myeloma cells[157,158] in more than 80% of mice with detection of human myeloma-specific protein (soluble IL-6 receptor) or human Ig and light chains in murine blood samples, respectively. In this murine model of primary human disease, the fetal bone undergoes osteoporotic and osteolytic change as a consequence of clonotypic plasma cell proliferation and production of human cytokines. Of interest, the murine bones remain uninvolved at least in the early stages of the disease.[157]

This model provides a unique opportunity to study the importance of stromal cell myeloma cell interactions, genetic and molecular mechanisms critical for myeloma growth and dissemination *in vivo*; and may provide clues to the origin of myeloma stem cells, thereby providing the opportunity to evaluate new treatment approaches targeting the myeloma cell and its microenvironment, as well as bone disease, in myeloma. A transgenic Eu-directed X-box binding protein-1 (XBP-1) spliced isoform mouse model has been generated in which mice develop features of MGUS and progress to MM.[159] XBP-1 is a transcription factor that is required for plasma cell differentiation and is expressed at high levels in MM cells versus normal plasma cells.[160] The transgenic model demonstrates features diagnostic of human myeloma, including bone lytic lesions and subendothelial immunoglobulin deposition; additionally, the transcriptional profiles of lymphoid and MM cells from mice show deregulation of genes with known dysfunction in human myeloma including cyclin D1, IL-6R (gp80), gp130, MAF, MAFB, B-cell activating factor, and APRIL. This model provides unique opportunity to study the biology of human myeloma, and assess novel therapies *in vivo*. Recently, conditional *MYC* transgene expression has been demonstrated in Vk*MYC mice, which eventually develop an indolent multiple myeloma with features characteristics of human disease. This model serves to highlight the role of myc in myeloma and provides a unique animal model to test therapeutic or preventative strategies in myeloma.[160]

CLINICAL MANIFESTATIONS

Patients with multiple myeloma may be entirely asymptomatic and diagnosed on routine blood work or may present with a myriad of symptoms: hematologic manifestations, bone-related problems, infections, various organ dysfunctions, neurologic complaints, or bleeding tendencies (Table 136.3). These signs and symptoms result from direct tumor involvement in BM or extramedullary plasmacytomas, the effect of the protein produced by the tumor cells deposited in various organs, production of cytokines by the tumor cells or by the BM microenvironment, and effects on the immune system.

PRACTICE OF ONCOLOGY

TABLE 136.3

CLINICAL FEATURES OF MULTIPLE MYELOMA

Symptoms	Common Cause
Bone pain	Pathologic fracture
Easy fatigue	Anemia, high serum IL-6, therapy
Nausea and vomiting	Renal failure, hypercalcemia
Recurrent infections	Low uninvolved Ig, T-cell dysfunction, therapy
Paraplegia	Cord compression
Confusion and CNS symptoms	Hyperviscosity or hypercalcemia
Peripheral neuropathy	Nerve compression, amyloidosis, POEMS, immune-mediated effects, therapy induced

IL, interleukin; Ig, immunoglobin; POEMS, polyneuropathy, organomegaly, endocrinopathy, monoclonal gammopathy, and skin changes.

Anemia

A normochromic normocytic anemia is usually observed in myeloma patients because of tumor cell involvement of the marrow as well as inadequate erythropoietin responsiveness. The suppressive effects of various cytokines on erythropoiesis and the effect of renal dysfunction on erythropoietin production are also contributing factors. High immunoglobulin levels exacerbate the anemia by dilutional effects. Anemia gives rise to fatigue, weakness, and occasionally shortness of breath. Erythropoietin administration is therefore an important supportive care therapy for patients with symptomatic anemia. In one study, improvement in hemoglobin by more than 2 g/dL was observed in 60% of treated patients, and responses were more frequent in patients with low erythropoietin levels than in patients with normal or high levels (72% vs. 20%).

Renal Failure

Nephropathy is one of the serious adverse complications that can be observed at the time of clinical presentation. The etiology of renal failure can be multifactorial. The most common cause is development of light chain tubular casts leading to interstitial nephritis (myeloma kidney).[161] Another common cause of renal dysfunction is hypercalcemia leading to osmotic diuresis, volume depletion, and prerenal azotemia. Other modes of kidney involvement in myeloma include light chain deposition disease, which is more commonly associated with kappa light chain proteins and impaired glomerular filtration; AL amyloidosis, which is more frequently associated with lambda light chain (especially lambda light chain subtype VI) and may have an initial presentation as nephrotic range proteinuria; and renal calcium deposition, leading to interstitial nephritis.[162–164] The presence of lambda light chains in the urine is also more commonly associated with myeloma kidney. Bence Jones proteins bind to a common peptide segment of Tom-Horsfall glycoprotein to promote heterotypic aggregation and deposition in the kidney.[165]

Additional factors exacerbating renal failure in myeloma patients include use of nonsteroidal anti-inflammatory drugs for pain control, hyperuricemia, nephrotoxic chemotherapeutic agents, intravenous contrast for radiographic studies, bisphosphonate therapy, as well as calcium deposition and stones in the kidney. The proteinuria observed in patients with amyloidosis is more often nonspecific, which can help to differentiate it from typical myeloma-related kidney disease characterized by excessive light chain excretion.[166] Pathologic renal changes similar to human myeloma-related nephropathy develop in IL-6 transgenic mice expressing IL-6 under metallothionein-1 promoter, indicating a relationship between constitutive high IL-6 expression in the liver, dysproteinemia and long acute-phase response, and renal changes.[167]

Hypercalcemia and Bone Disease

The mechanism of bone abnormalities in myeloma, especially destruction, is an unbalanced process of increased osteoclast activity and suppressed osteoblast activity. These changes are due to an increase in osteoclast-activating factors produced predominantly by the BM microenvironment but also by myeloma cells.[168,169] These factors include IL-1β, TNF-β (lymphotoxin), IL-6, and MIP-1α.[170–173] The receptor activator of nuclear factor kappa B ligand (RANKL) plays an important role in osteoclast differentiation via its receptor located on the osteoclast membrane. A member of the TNF family, it was originally described as a factor secreted by T cells, which induces maturation of dendritic cells. RANKL is also secreted by stromal cells and osteoblasts and induces differentiation and maturation of osteoclast progenitors. Moreover, its production is elicited by factors such as parathyroid hormone (PTH), parathyroid hormone-related protein (PTHrP), and osteoclast-activating factors (OAFs).[169,174] Osteoprotegerin acts as a decoy receptor for RANKL,[175,176] and has been implicated in the development of bone changes in myeloma. Additionally, a recently identified soluble factor produced by myeloma cell, DKK-1, inhibits osteoblast activity and is being therapeutically targeted.[177,178] Similarly, activin A, a TGF-β family member that induces osteolysis by inhibiting osteoblast differentiation via SMAD2-dependent distal-less homeobox-5 down-regulation, is now being targeted therapeutically.[178a]

All of these factors contribute to the development of osteoporosis and lytic bone lesions. Radiographic findings of such destruction are shown in Figure 136.5. These bone changes frequently involve the vertebral column resulting in compression fractures, lytic bone lesions, and related pain.

A new onset of back pain or other bone pain is a frequent presenting symptom in myeloma patients. Changes in the cytokine milieu and bone destruction may also lead to development of hypercalcemia, which is observed in approximately 25% of patients at some stage of the disease. Symptoms of high calcium include mental status changes, lethargy, constipation, and vomiting. High paraprotein levels, low albumin levels, or both, commonly observed in patients with myeloma, require measurement of ionized calcium. Hypercalcemia may also contribute to renal failure and should therefore be considered an oncologic emergency requiring prompt intervention.

Infections

Myeloma patients are at risk for developing recurrent bacterial infections due to deficiencies in both humoral and cellular immunity.[142,179,180] Various factors including high monoclonal immunoglobulin levels, soluble Fc receptor in serum, and TGF-β lead to suppression of B-cell function, which in turn leads to depressed uninvolved immunoglobulins.[113,181] This impairment in patients' abilities to mount humoral responses predisposes patients to infections with bacteria that are ordinarily opsonized by antibodies specific against bacterial antigens. Patients also have profound T-cell dysfunction due to various immunosuppressive cytokines such as TGF-β and IL-6 secreted by the microenvironment and fas ligand present on

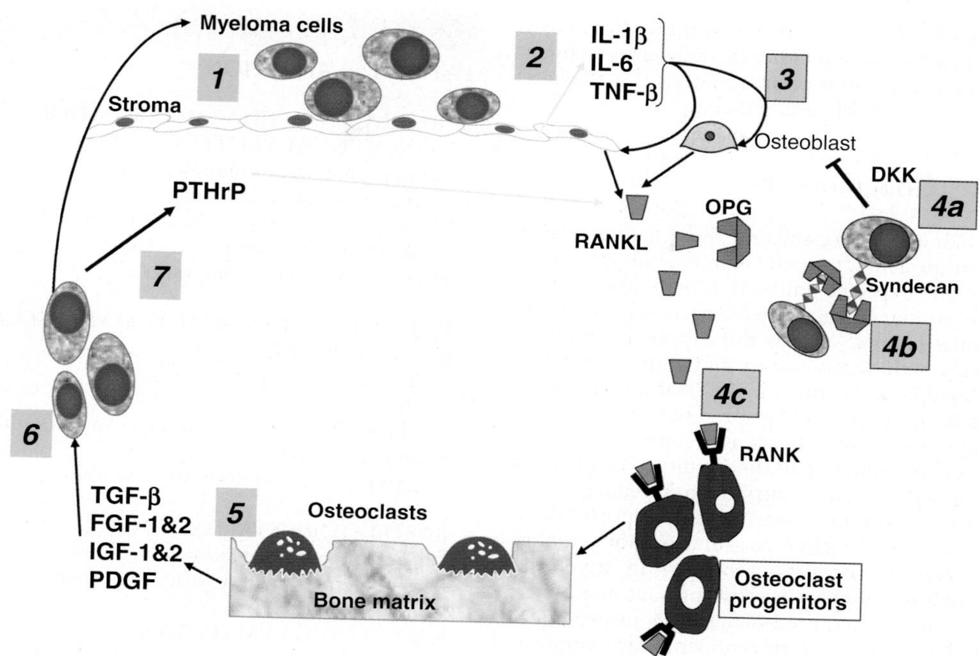

FIGURE 136.5 Biology of bone destruction in multiple myeloma (MM): 1. MM cells adhere to stroma. 2. Stromal cells secrete osteoclast-activating factors (OAFs). 3. OAFs elicit stroma and osteoblasts to secrete receptor activator of NFκB ligand (RANKL). 4a. DKK-1 produced by myeloma cells blocks osteoblast activity; 4b. RANKL is blocked by osteoprotegerin (OPG); OPG levels are reduced in MM due to syndecan trapping OPG; 4c. Excess RANKL is available to stimulate osteoclast differentiation and maturation. 5. Increased osteoclastic activity leads to increased cytokine release from the bone matrix. 6. These cytokines stimulate MM cell growth, which increases process number 1. 7. These cytokines also cause release of parathyroid hormone-related protein (PTHrP) from MM cells, which activate stromal cells to secrete additional RANKL. TGF, tumor growth factor; FGF, fibroblast growth factor; IGF, insulinlike growth factor; PDGF, platelet-derived growth factor; IL, interleukin; TNF, tumor necrosis factor.

the membrane of the myeloma cells. The therapy for myeloma, especially high-dose corticosteroids, increases infection-related risks in these patients. Therapy with bortezomib is also associated with a higher frequency of herpes zoster.[182] The highest risk of infection is within the first 2 months of initiation of therapy as well as in patients with renal failure and in those with relapsed and refractory disease. Recurrent bacterial, fungal, and viral infections in myeloma require prompt diagnosis and treatment with additional prophylactic measures while receiving immunosuppressive therapy. Infections are an important cause of morbidity and the most common cause of death in myeloma.[183]

Neurologic Symptoms

The most common cause of neurologic abnormalities is related to a tumor mass effect, especially compression of the spinal cord or cranial or spinal nerves. This may present as motor or, less frequently, sensory problem. An interesting constellation of symptoms described as POEMS syndrome (polyneuropathy, organomegaly, endocrinopathy, monoclonal gammopathy, and skin changes) is observed in osteosclerotic myeloma with prominent sensory neuropathy.[184–187] The biologic and cellular basis of these manifestations is not yet well understood. Additionally, neurologic symptoms may occur as a consequence of hypercalcemia or hyperviscosity. Leptomeningeal involvement in myeloma with manifestations involving the CNS has been described, usually in the late phase of the disease and is associated with high-risk chromosomal abnormalities, plasmablastic morphology, and extramedullary manifestations.[188,189]

Paraneoplastic CNS syndromes have also been described as possibly related to an immune mechanism directed at proteins present in the CNS, including the cerebellum. Peripheral neuropathy in myeloma may be due to an infiltrative process associated with deposition of amyloid protein in the paraneural or *vasa nervorum;* due to a metabolic abnormality such as hypercalcemia, uremia, or hyperviscosity; or mediated by autoimmune process or cytokines.[190] Peripheral neuropathy is also observed in patients with MGUS and is more frequently associated with IgM paraprotein. More recently, peripheral neuropathy has been observed frequently with newer therapeutics including thalidomide and bortezomib, especially with their prolonged use.

Hyperviscosity

The M components in myeloma can cause hyperviscosity and compromise circulation when the serum immunoglobulin levels exceed certain levels. The incidence is highest in Waldenström macroglobulinemia with IgM, followed by IgA myeloma (25% patients), and is least common in IgG myeloma (<10% patients).[191–193] It can also be observed when immunoglobulins have a self-aggregating property leading to increased viscosity: For example, the IgG3 subclass is more commonly associated with hyperviscosity.[194] The syndrome is usually observed when serum viscosity exceeds 4.0 cp units relative to normal serum and manifests with circulatory compromise involving the CNS, kidneys, and lungs; it may also be associated with bleeding complications. Because of varying characteristics of idiotypes, the same level of increased viscosity may produce different severity of symptoms in individual patients.

A high level of suspicion for this syndrome is important in any patient with paraproteinemia and either mental status changes or pulmonary distress, as prompt plasmapheresis can alleviate symptoms and avoid irreversible organ damage.

Coagulopathy

Myeloma patients may acquire coagulation abnormalities related to a high level of paraprotein interfering with the normal coagulation cascade or exhibit specific antibody activity leading to a clinical syndrome similar to acquired deficiency of factor VIII.[195,196] Additional factors, such as thrombosis in capillary circulation associated with hyperviscosity and anoxia, may lead to coagulation-related complications in 15% of patients with IgG myeloma and in more than 33% of the patients with IgA myeloma. Although platelet counts are not suppressed in the early stages of myeloma, functional abnormalities of platelets have been described and may also contribute to bleeding.

Acquired activated protein C resistance is reported as a common single transitory baseline coagulation abnormality associated with venous thromboembolism in myeloma patients.[197] Additionally, patients may also present in a hypercoagulable state related to acquired deficiencies in protein S, or lupus anticoagulants leading to thromboembolic complications.[198] The fab fragment of the myeloma protein binds to fibrin and may prevent its aggregation.[199] Factor X deficiency is reported in patients with systemic AL amyloidosis[200]; however, an inhibitor has not been demonstrated *in vitro* to account for this manifestation.

Therapy may also increase the hypercoagulable state in myeloma. An increased incidence of deep venous thrombosis (12%–24%) is observed in patients taking thalidomide and lenalidomide, especially along with dexamethasone or other combination chemotherapies. In one study 12 of 50 patients (24%) receiving thalidomide developed deep vein thrombosis (DVT), compared with 2 of 50 (4%) patients receiving identical therapy without thalidomide.[201] Activated protein C resistance in the absence of factor V Leiden mutation and high serum homocysteine levels are associated with an increased risk of thrombotic complications with thalidomide.[202]

Extramedullary Disease

Extramedullary disease manifestations are uncommon in patients with myeloma at presentation. However, such manifestations have been observed in the setting of advanced-stage disease or relapse following allogeneic transplantation. Solitary or multiple extramedullary plasmacytomas has been described in the liver, spleen, lymph nodes, kidneys, subcutaneous tissues, and brain parenchyma. Extramedullary involvement may be suspected in patients who have more aggressive features of myeloma including high lactate dehydrogenase levels, immunoblastic morphology, high tumor cell labeling index, and complex karyotypic features.[203]

Diagnosis

As myeloma patients present with a variety of symptoms not specific to the disease, the diagnosis of myeloma is quite often delayed. An older patient with a new onset of unexplained back pain or bone pain, recurrent infection, anemia, or renal insufficiency should be screened for myeloma. Additional findings such as hyperproteinemia or proteinuria, anemia, hypoalbuminemia, low immunoglobulin levels, or marked elevation of erythrocyte sedimentation rate should prompt a further complete evaluation for diagnosis of plasma cell myeloma.

TABLE 136.4

PATIENT EVALUATION

PRESENCE AND CHARACTERIZATION OF MONOCLONAL PROTEIN
Serum protein electrophoresis
Quantitative immunoglobulin
24-hour urine: total protein and Bence Jones protein
Immunofixation of urine and serum
Serum free light chain and ratio

DETECTION OF CLONAL PLASMA CELLS
BONE MARROW
- Aspirate and biopsy
- Histology
- Clonality by immunostaining—kappa/Lambda
- Flow cytometry
- Cytogenetics and fluorescent *in situ* hybridization

LABORATORY EVALUATION
Chemistry panel (renal, calcium, albumin, uric acid, LDH)
Beta-2 microglobulin, C-reactive protein

RADIOLOGIC EVALUATION
Skeletal Survey
MRI with STIR images
Bone densitometry

SPECIALIZED STUDIES FOR SELECTED PATIENTS
Abdominal fat pad or rectal biopsy for amyloid
Solitary lytic lesion biopsy
Serum viscosity if IgM component or high IgA levels or serum M-component >7 g/dL
Immunofixation for IgD or IgE in select cases

LDH, lactate dehydrogenase; MRI, magnetic resonance imaging; STIR, short tau inversion recovery; Ig, immunoglobin.

The first step in the evaluation includes tests to confirm the presence, type, and quantity of monoclonal protein, and detection and quantification of clonal plasma cells (Table 136.4). The second component to differentiate MGUS, smoldering and indolent myeloma (SMM) versus symptomatic myeloma is to identify end-organ damage by performing a hemogram to detect anemia, complete skeletal radiographic survey to detect bone lesions, and chemistry to detect renal dysfunction and hypercalcemia. The diagnostic criteria for MGUS, SMM, and multiple myeloma are shown in Table 136.5.

Protein Electrophoresis

Among patients with myeloma, 70% have IgG whereas 20% have IgA subtype, and an additional 5% to 10% have production of monoclonal light chains only. A small proportion, less than 1%, of patients produce monoclonal IgD, IgE, IgM, or have nonsecretory myeloma. Suppression of uninvolved immunoglobulins, (e.g., IgM and IgA in IgG myeloma) is present in the majority of the patients at diagnosis. Suppression of all of the three major classes of immunoglobulins should raise the possibility that the patient may have light chain-only disease, IgD or IgE myeloma, or nonsecretory disease. Patients producing intact immunoglobulin can also have excess light chain production and excretion in the urine (Fig. 136.6). The distribution of κ and λ light chains in the majority of myeloma cases is similar, except in IgD myeloma in which λ light chain is more common. Currently there is no difference in therapeutic

TABLE 136.5

DIAGNOSTIC CRITERIA FOR MULTIPLE MYELOMA, MYELOMA VARIANTS, AND MONOCLONAL GAMMOPATHY OF UNKNOWN SIGNIFICANCE (MGUS)

MGUS OR MONOCLONAL GAMMOPATHY, UNATTRIBUTED/UNASSOCIATED (MG[u])
M protein in serum <30 g/L
Bone marrow clonal plasma cells[a] <10%
No evidence of other B-cell proliferative disorders
No myeloma related organ or tissue impairment (no end-organ damage, including bone lesions)

ASYMPTOMATIC MYELOMA (SMOULDERING MYELOMA)
M protein in serum >30 g/L and/or
Bone marrow clonal plasma cell ≥10%
No related organ or tissue impairment (no end-organ damage, including bone lesions) or symptoms

SYMPTOMATIC MULTIPLE MYELOMA
M protein in serum and/or urine
Bone marrow (clonal) plasma cells[a] or plasmacytoma
Related organ or tissue impairment (end organ damage, including bone lesions)

SOLITARY PLASMACYTOMA OF BONE
No M protein in serum and/or urine[b]
Single area of bone destruction due to clonal plasma cells
Bone marrow not consistent with multiple myeloma
Normal skeletal survey (and MRI of spine and pelvis if done)
No related organ or tissue impairment (no end-organ damage other than solitary bone lesion)

NONSECRETORY MYELOMA
No M protein in serum and/or urine with immunofixation
Bone marrow clonal plasmacytosis ≥10% or plasmacytoma
Related organ or tissue impairment (end-organ damage, including bone lesions)

EXTRAMEDULLARY PLASMACYTOMA
No M protein in serum and/or urine[b]
Extramedullary tumour of clonal plasma cells
Normal bone marrow
Normal skeletal survey
No related organ or tissue impairment (end-organ damage including bone lesions)

MULTIPLE SOLITARY PLASMACYTOMAS (± RECURRENT)
No M protein in serum and/or urine[b]
More than one localized area of bone destruction or extramedullary tumour of clonal plasma cells, which may be recurrent
Normal bone marrow
Normal skeletal survey and MRI of spine and pelvis if done
No related organ or tissue impairment (no end-organ damage other than the localized bone lesions)

MYELOMA-RELATED ORGAN OR TISSUE IMPAIRMENT (END ORGAN DAMAGE) (ROTI)
Calcium levels increased: serum calcium >0–25 mmol/L above the upper limit of normal or >2–75 mmol/L
Renal insufficiency: creatinine >173 mmol/L
Anemia: hemoglobin 2 g/dL below the lower limit of normal or hemoglobin <10 g/dL
Bone lesions: lytic lesions or osteoporosis with compression fractures (MRI or CT may clarify)
Other: symptomatic hyperviscosity, amyloidosis, recurrent bacterial infections (more than two episodes in 12 months)

MRI, magnetic resonance imaging; CT, computed tomography.
[a]If flow cytometry is performed, most plasma cells (>90%) will show a neoplastic phenotype.
[b]A small M component may sometimes be present.
(From the International Myeloma Working Group. Criteria for the classification of monoclonal gammopathies, multiple myeloma and related disorders: a report of the International Myeloma Working Group. *Br J Haematol* 2003;121:749.)

approach between the different types of myeloma; however, patients with IgA myeloma, despite a higher initial response rate, have inferior survival.

Myeloma plasma cells usually produce a single, abnormal, unique, monoclonal antibody with a constant isotype and light-chain restriction. Rare occurrences of biclonal and triclonal cases have been reported at the time of diagnosis.[204] Occurrence of isotype switch and appearance of abnormal protein bands have, however, been reported in myeloma patients after therapy, especially HDT.[205] This appears to be related to recovery of normal immunoglobulin production rather than alteration in disease biology. This change is also associated with improved survival. Occasionally, patients with initial intact Ig production relapse with only Bence Jones proteinuria (light chain escape), or nonsecretory disease, and this change has been correlated with more aggressive disease.[206]

Further analysis of a unique variable region in the myeloma-related idiotype (e.g., CDRIII) provides information on the monoclonal nature of the protein and also provides a tool to investigate minimal residual disease by polymerase chain reaction using allele-specific oligonucleotide, thus allowing determination of molecular complete remissions.[207]

Serum Free Light Chain

Although its measurement has not yet been incorporated into diagnostic criteria for myeloma, it has become an important tool to follow the disease process including response to therapy. It is especially useful in patients with light chain-only disease, oligo- or nonsecretory myeloma, patients with renal disease, in amyloidosis, and as a prognostic marker in MGUS and SMM, where an abnormal kappa/lambda free light chain ratio predicts higher likelihood of progression to myeloma.[208–212]

Bone Marrow Examination

Various degrees of BM infiltration are observed in myeloma, with the majority of the patients having an excess number of plasma cells (>5%). The pattern of BM involvement (diffuse vs. nodular) is important, as patients with nodular disease seem to have poorer outcomes (in contrast to chronic lymphocytic leukemia).[213] The morphology of the plasma cell seems to be an important factor determining severity of the disease. This is based on histologic examination (Bartl grade) in which

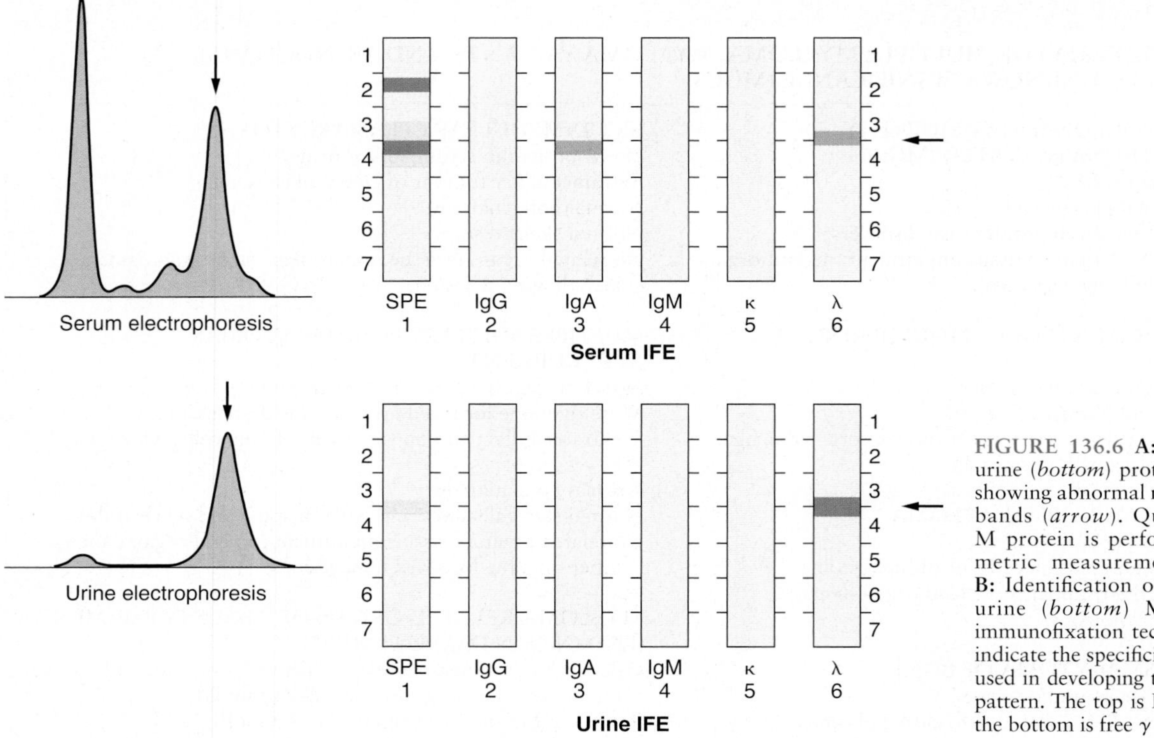

FIGURE 136.6 **A:** Serum (*top*) and urine (*bottom*) protein electrophoresis showing abnormal monoclonal protein bands (*arrow*). Quantitation of the M protein is performed by nephelometric measurement of the band. **B:** Identification of serum (*top*) and urine (*bottom*) M component by immunofixation technique. The labels indicate the specificity of the antiserum used in developing the immunofixation pattern. The top is IgA-γ in serum and the bottom is free γ light chain in urine.

grade I suggests a slow-growing disease, whereas grade III represents plasmablastic disease with an aggressive course.[214] There is also an increased incidence of cytogenetic abnormalities in patients with higher grade disease. Plasma cells contain cytoplasmic immunoglobulins with a constant heavy and light chain, which can be evaluated by flow cytometric analysis or immunohistochemical staining of plasma cells.[215] When coupled with DNA staining using propidium iodide, two-parameter analysis can detect changes in DNA content in myeloma cells (Fig. 136.7). DNA aneuploidy is observed in the BM of more

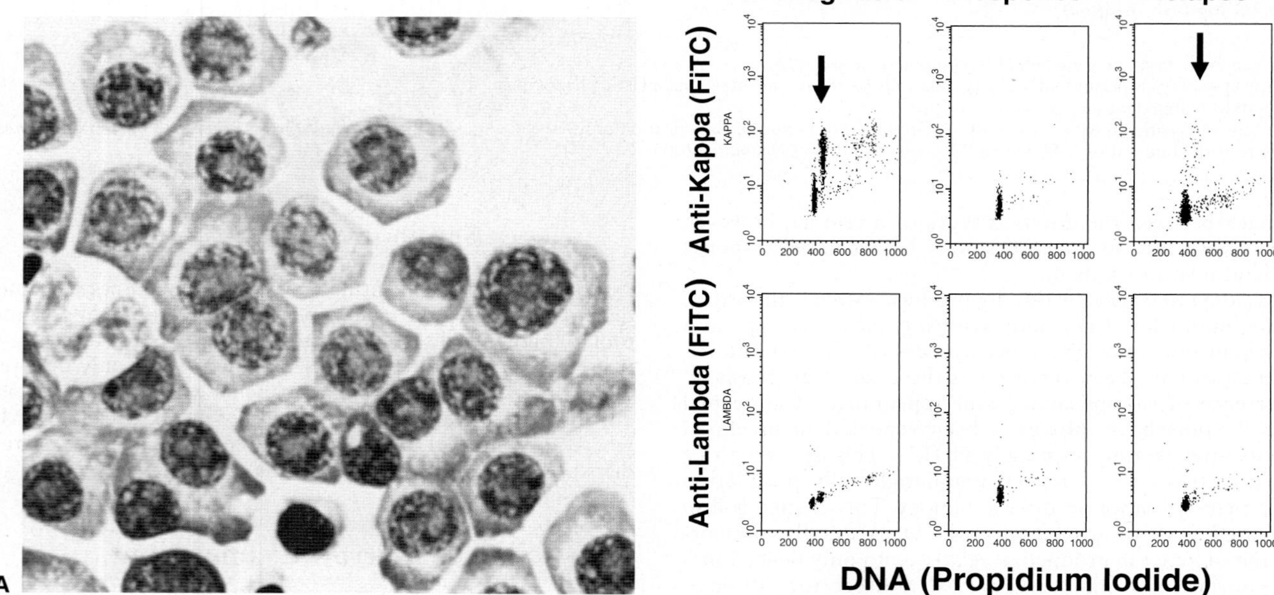

FIGURE 136.7 **A:** Bone marrow plasma cells in a patient with immunoglobulin G (IgG) myeloma showing neoplastic plasma cells at various stages of differentiation. **B:** Two-parameter flow cytometry of DNA content of bone marrow cells; abscissa (propidium iodide) and cytoplasmic immunoglobulin (ordinate, anti-κ or anti-γ fluorescein isothiocyanate [FiTC]). At diagnosis approximately 45% hyperdiploid tumor cells with κ light chain restriction (*left panel*); at the time of maximal response no hyperdiploid light chain restricted cells are seen (*middle panel*); at the time of early relapse reappearance of small hyperdiploid and κ light chain restricted population (<1%) is indicative of re-emergence of a small number of clonal cells, which may not yet be apparent on cytologic examination of the bone marrow (*right panel*). A population of κ restricted but diploid cell population (*small arrow*) may represent a second clone.

than 80% of patients, suggesting the existence of chromosomal abnormalities in the majority of patients.[215] This analysis also provides an objective marker to evaluate response to therapy and to distinguish reactive from clonal plasmacytosis, especially in nonsecretory disease. A hypodiploid tumor cell has also been associated with refractoriness to standard-dose therapy.

Staging and Risk Assessment

Following the diagnostic investigation, more detailed cellular and molecular studies are required to stage myeloma and evaluate prognostic variables that determine the patient's probable outcome.

Cytogenetics

As the myeloma cell represents a mature differentiated cell with low proliferative activity, cytogenetic abnormalities are not frequently detected. Abnormalities are observed in only one-third of the patients at the time of diagnosis; however, repeated analysis improves the yield to almost one-half of the patients. The normal karyotypic pattern observed in the remaining half most likely originates from dividing normal hematopoietic cells.[48]

As described previously, a complex karyotypic pattern is frequently observed, and its distribution is shown in Figure 136.2. Although a predominant single cytogenetic abnormality has not been described, certain recurrent changes have been noticed. These include the common B-cell tumor–related changes in the 14q32 region involving the *IGH* gene, chromosome 1q, and chromosome 13-related changes.[216–218] A longitudinal analysis in patients undergoing high-dose chemotherapy has shown cytogenetic evolution, which portends poor prognosis.[219] Detection of chromosome 13 deletion abnormalities at diagnosis, as well as after high-dose chemotherapy, has been reported to carry poor prognosis. However, recent reports suggest ability of bortezomib as well as lenalidomide to overcome adverse effects associated with chromosome 13 abnormality. The application of FISH technology has improved our ability to detect genetic changes by using interphase cells. The Rb-1 probe detects an abnormality in the 13q14 region, and its deletion detected by interphase FISH has been reported in more than 40% of patients and also predicts for poor outcome after standard-dose therapy and HDT.[220] Interphase FISH analysis for numeric chromosomal aberrations has identified trisomies of 7, 9, and 17 chromosomes predicting for favorable outcomes.[51] Plasma cell leukemia has been reported to frequently contain complex hypodiploid or pseudodiploid karyotypes with higher frequency of t(11:14) and monosomy 13; compared with patients with hypodiploid karyotypes and monosomy 13, significantly longer survival is observed in patients with t(11;14).[221]

Labeling Index

Early in the disease, the proportion of cycling myeloma cells is small; bromodeoxyuridine or tritiated thymidine methods show a median of 1% cycling cells at diagnosis. With progressive disease the labeling index increases, suggesting more proliferative phenotype. The labeling index has important prognostic significance, as patients with more than 1% cells in S phase in BM have worse outcomes[215,222,223]; however, lack of standardized reproducible methods to measure labeling index has limited its use as a prognostic marker.

Radiographic Evaluation

The radiographic survey of bone still remains a standard diagnostic evaluation, which shows osteopenia in an early phase of the disease and, with increasing tumor burden, lytic punched out lesions (Fig. 136.8). Osteosclerotic lesions are observed in POEMS syndrome.[184,186] Because of the predominant osteoclastic activity with osteoblastic inactivity, bone scans are seldom positive and are therefore not useful in the diagnosis of multiple myeloma.

As demineralization of bone (osteoporosis) is one of the common manifestations of myeloma, measurement of bone mineral density (BMD) by dual-energy x-ray absorptiometry (DEXA) is an important evaluation at diagnosis.[224] In a study of 66 patients at diagnosis, the majority of the patients had decreased BMD with lumbar mean BMD value (Z score) -1.24 ± 1.45. Following standard-dose therapy, lumbar BMD increased by 0.7%, while in a group treated with HDT the improvement was by 4.6% ($P = .02$).[225] Similar improvements in BMD have also been noted in patients undergoing HDT with addition of bisphosphonates.[226] Differential effects of pamidronate on cortical and cancellous bone have been described in patients with myeloma undergoing autotransplants.[225,226]

Magnetic resonance imaging (MRI) of bone marrow provides a better assessment of tumor burden. More than 95% of myeloma patients have MRI abnormalities: one-third each have diffuse involvement of the bone marrow, focal lesions, or heterogeneous focal and diffused marrow involvement (Fig. 136.9A). As myeloma is a macrofocal disease, random BM sampling may not be diagnostic or predictive of disease status and MRI short-τ inversion recovery images (STIR) may provide a better assessment of bone marrow involvement in myeloma.[227–229] An MRI of the spine and pelvis is required in all patients with a solitary plasmacytoma and SMM to detect occult lesions and to predict progression. In symptomatic myeloma, MRI can be considered as routine evaluation to detect unsuspected focal lesion, and plasmacytomas involving the spine and pelvis, to define patterns of bone marrow involvement (i.e., diffuse pattern or a high number of focal lesions), to obtain a detailed evaluation of a painful area of the skeleton, and to investigate suspicion of cord compression.[230,231] A focal marrow plasmacytoma can be further analyzed through computerized tomography (CT)-guided fine-needle aspiration (Fig. 136.8), allowing cytologic diagnosis. With effective therapy, the MRI pattern may change (Fig. 136.9B); diffuse involvement of the marrow may evolve into focal disease and normalization of MRI abnormalities may provide a better definition of complete responses.[229]

Positron emission tomography (PET) scanning has also been evaluated in a small number of studies and may provide a better functional definition of lesions observed on MRI or CT, as well as allowing selection of lesions for biopsy.[229,232] The PET-CT is used for detection of extraosseous soft tissue masses, as well as evaluation of rib and appendicular bone lesions. A combination of PET-CT and MRI may improve the diagnostic accuracy for solitary plasmacytoma.[230] A recent study has identified independent predictive value of baseline FDG-PET/CT and of FDG suppression before high-dose therapy.[233]

Differential Diagnosis

In the presence of end-organ damage associated with monoclonal protein and clonal plasma cells in bone marrow, the distinction of myeloma from SMM and MGUS can be readily established (Table 136.5). Conventional cytogenetic results are usually normal in MGUS; however, monoclonal plasma

PRACTICE OF ONCOLOGY

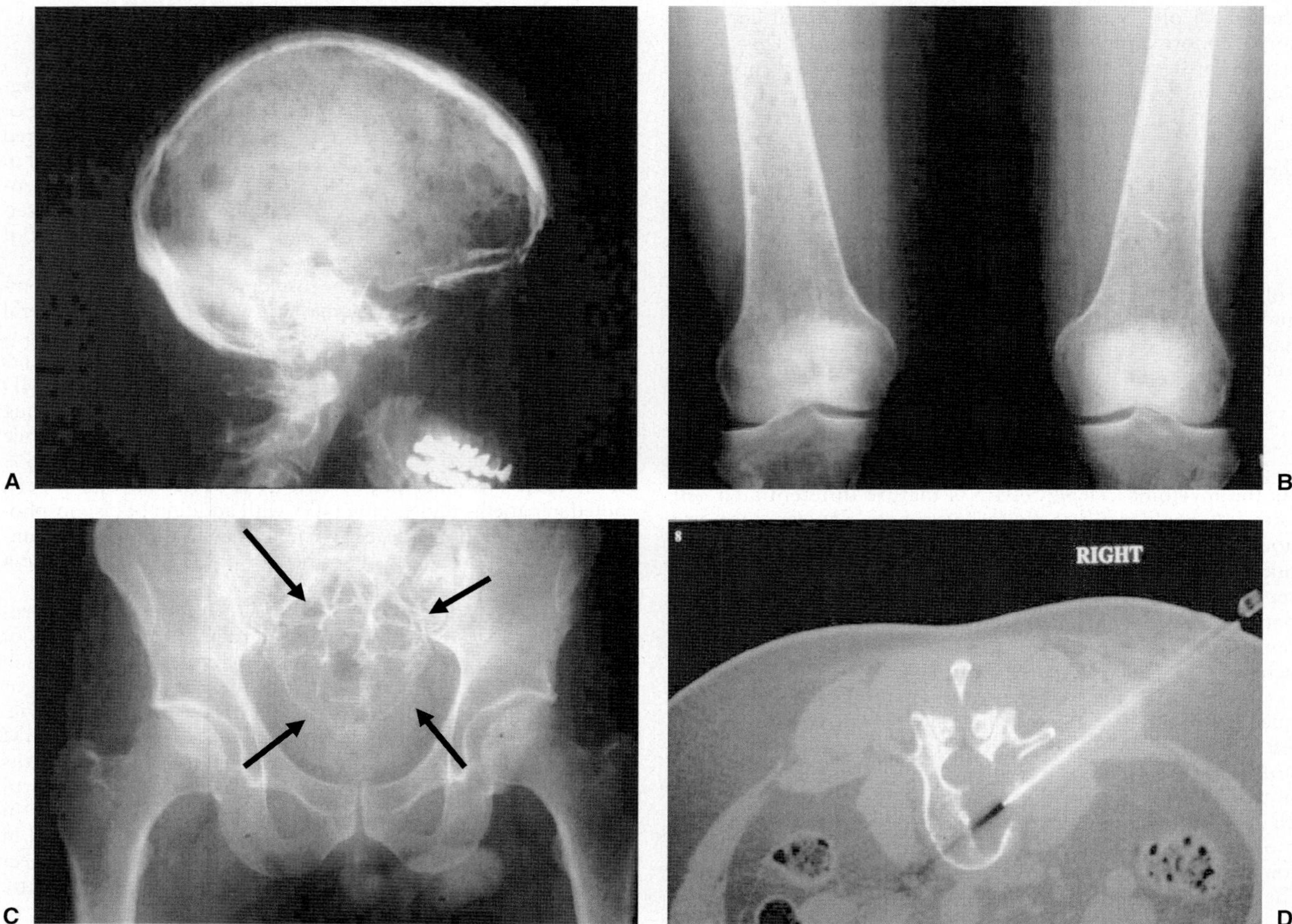

FIGURE 136.8 Typical skeletal changes on roentgenogram. A: Example of "punched-out" lytic lesions in skull. B: Small lytic lesions in the left femur. C: Large lytic lesion in sacrum. D: Fine-needle aspiration biopsy of the vertebral lesion. (Courtesy of Dr. Hemendra Shah.)

cells in some individuals with MGUS may be aneuploid and chromosomal abnormalities including IgH translocations and chromosome 13 deletions have been reported in MGUS with unclear prognostic significance. Patients with nonsecretory myeloma are diagnosed based on marrow plasmacytosis and presence of bone lesions. MRI abnormalities and CT- or MRI-guided fine-needle aspiration biopsy of involved anatomic sites are important for follow-up of the disease.

Diagnosis of solitary plasmacytoma of bone or soft tissue requires intense investigation to rule out systemic disease. Bone marrow examination in a true solitary lesion is normal, with no clonal cell population evidenced on DNA cytoplasmic immunoglobulin (cIg) examination. MRI evaluation for myelomatous involvement of the BM helps detect early lesions, before their detection by standard roentgenographic examination. Detection of such lesions and cytologic confirmation through CT- or MRI-guided fine-needle aspiration biopsy may help confirm solitary plasmacytoma and its genetic makeup. In case of MGUS, such detection may change the diagnosis to solitary plasmacytoma or multiple myeloma. It is important to note that patients with MGUS or solitary plasmacytoma seldom have suppression of uninvolved immunoglobulins.

Besides plasma cell neoplasms, various other conditions can present with monoclonal immunoglobulin secretion. These conditions include other B-cell neoplasms such as chronic lymphocytic leukemia and B-cell non–Hodgkin's lymphoma; autoimmune conditions such as cold agglutinin diseases, mixed cryoglobulinemia, hypergammaglobulinemia and Sjögren syndrome; inflammatory or storage diseases such as lichen myxedematous, Gaucher disease, sarcoidosis and cirrhosis; and rarely, other malignancies such as chronic myeloid leukemia, colon, breast, or prostate cancer.

Protein deposition disease involving various organs requires additional special diagnostic procedures. Deposition of amyloid protein (amyloidosis) can be clinically suspected based on macroglossia, vascular fragility (raccoon's eyes, periorbital subcutaneous hemorrhages), carpal tunnel syndrome, organomegaly, nephropathy, and cardiomegaly with arrhythmia. Detection of Congo red-positive amyloid in perivascular areas and subcutaneous fat, bone marrow or rectal biopsy specimens with classic apple-green birefringence when visualized under polarized light, are diagnostic of AL amyloid. Electrocardiography may reveal low voltage, and echocardiographic evaluation shows thickening of the interventricular septum or classic speckled pattern in myocardium. Endomyocardial biopsy may establish the diagnosis of cardiac amyloid, which is usually associated with elevated serum B-type natriuretic peptide (BNP) levels. Another manifestation of amyloid deposition includes autonomic dysfunction due to amyloid deposition in the vasa nervorum of the autonomic nerves leading to orthostatic hypotension. Deposition in adrenal glands leads to hypoadrenalism. Amyloid deposition in spleen may lead to

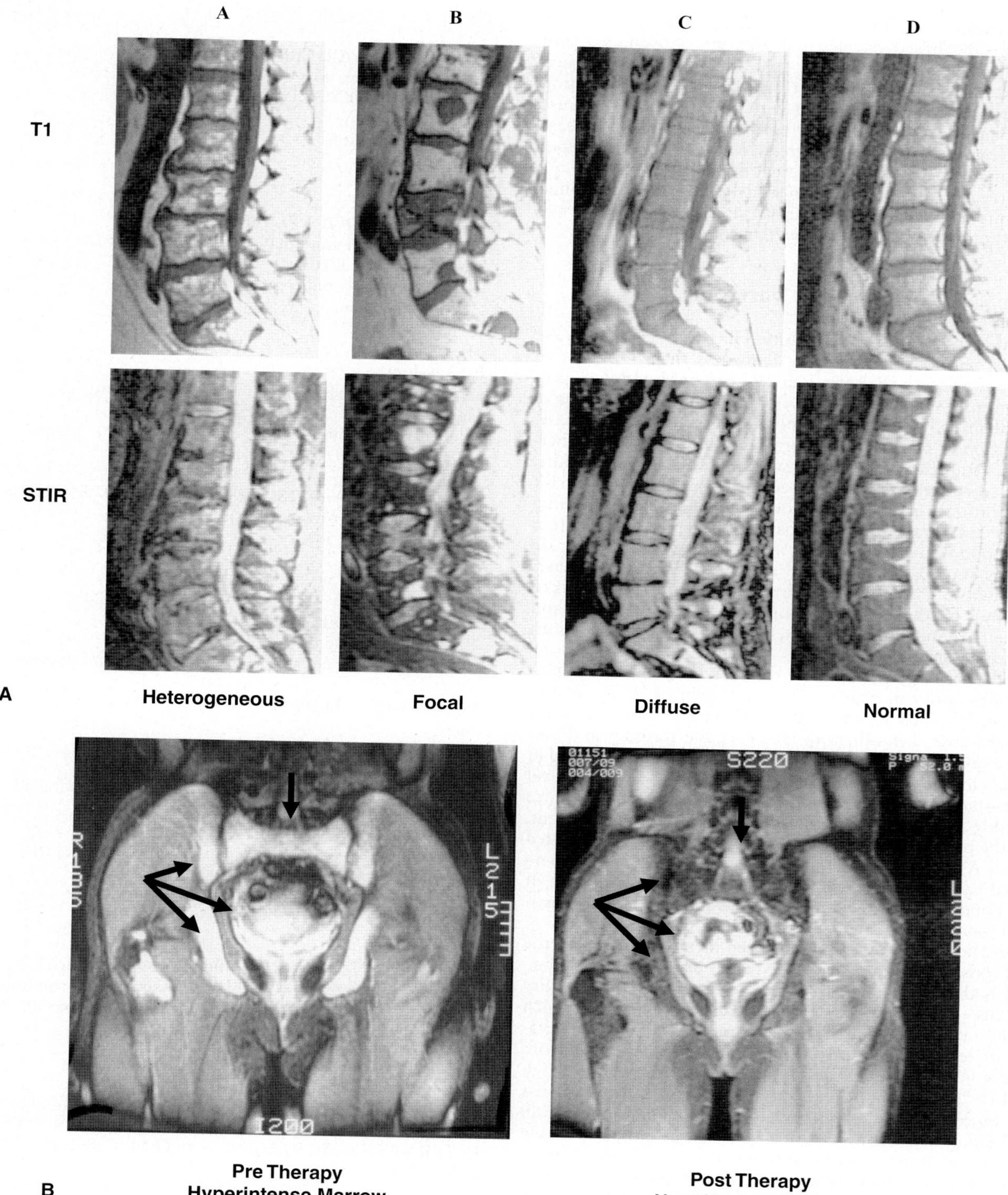

FIGURE 136.9 **A:** Magnetic resonance imaging (MRI) pattern in multiple myeloma at diagnosis: T1 weighted and STIR (short inversion-time inversion recovery) imaging shows approximately one-third of patients each presenting with heterogeneous pattern (*panel 1*), focal plasmacytoma lesions (*panel 2*), or diffuse homogeneous hyperintense marrow pattern (*panel 3*). Hyperintensity of marrow on STIR image is suggestive of uniform marrow involvement by myeloma. Few patients have a hypointense and homogenous pattern also seen in normal individuals (*panel 4*). **B:** The hyperintense marrow pattern suggestive of extensive marrow involvement pretherapy (*left; arrows*) changes to hypointense pattern following complete response and normalization of marrow (*right, arrows*); fine-needle aspiration examination in 72 patients with MRI-focal disease showed tumor in 92%, indicating that minimal-response focal lesions in myeloma represent tumor.

hyposplenism with thrombocytosis. Deposition in liver may be suspected based on elevated alkaline phosphatase and γ-glutamyl transpeptidase, and deposition in gastrointestinal tract may lead to malabsorption syndrome. Renal dysfunction must to be further investigated with a renal biopsy, because light chain cast nephropathy or light chain deposition disease may be reversible following aggressive therapy, whereas deposition of amyloid requires a different therapeutic approach. As deposition of immunoglobulin and light chain can mimic many manifestations of AL amyloid, immunofluorescence analysis of unfixed tissue is important for diagnosis.

Prognostic Variables

Patients with multiple myeloma have variable disease courses, with survival ranging from less than 1 year with aggressive disease to more than 10 years with indolent presentation or sensitive disease. Various characteristics have been identified to predict the possible course of the disease. Evaluation of prognostic factors is important to define therapeutic strategies, permit comparison of clinical trial results, and predict life expectancy after diagnosis. The current risk stratification is applicable to newly diagnosed patients using parameters obtained at diagnosis. On relapse there is often acquisition of additional or new risk features, in which case patients should be reclassified as having high-risk disease. As shown in Table 136.6, prognostic factors are related to the tumor burden, intrinsic property of the tumor, host and microenvironmental influences, and treatment/intervention-related factors.

A clinical staging system for multiple myeloma using standard laboratory measurement was developed by Durie and Salmon,[234] which was predictive of clinical outcomes after standard-dose chemotherapy. However, the accuracy and predictive value of the Durie-Salmon system is less pronounced in patients undergoing high-dose chemotherapy as well as novel agents–based therapy. These therapeutic interventions are probably able to reduce the disease burden to a greater extent, with the patient outcome depending on tumor biology–related factors. As the Durie-Salmon system considers tumor burden–related variables and depends on subjective interpretation of lytic bone lesions, additional parameters have been investigated to better assess patient prognosis.

β2-Microglobulin (β2M) has been identified as one of the most consistent predictors of survival in plasma cell myeloma. β2M is the light chain gene of the class I histocompatibility antigens expressed on the surface of all nucleated cells, which is shed into the blood. Its renal excretion explains its elevation in renal failure. In multiple myeloma β2M therefore reflects both tumor burden and renal function.[235,236] High β2M (>2.5 mg/L) levels carry a poor prognosis for treatment with both standard-dose and HDT.[237] Combination of serum β2M along with serum albumin has been proposed as a new three-stage International Staging System (Table 136.7). Although this system predicts outcome following both high-dose therapy as well as novel agents–based treatments, it lacks consideration of tumor biology–related factors such as cytogenetics or molecular markers.

Cytogenetic abnormalities have been identified as a major prognostic factor in plasma cell myeloma. Although detection of any cytogenetic abnormality is considered to suggest higher-risk disease, the specific abnormalities considered as poor risk are cytogenetically detected chromosomal 13 or 13q deletion, t(4;14) and del17p; and detection by FISH of t(4;14); t(14;16) and del17p. Del13 or 13q- detected only by FISH independently in the absence of other abnormality does not carry significantly higher risk, while t(11;14) does not predict superior outcome. Limited studies have shown that 1q+, and del1p may have clinical significance as a poor-risk feature. Importantly, bortezomib is able to overcome adverse outcome associated with chromosome 13 deletion, and to an extent t(4;14).

TABLE 136.6

PROGNOSTIC VARIABLE

TUMOR-BURDEN RELATED FACTORS
β-2 microglobulin
>3 lytic bone lesions
Hemoglobin
Serum calcium
TUMOR-BIOLOGY RELATED FACTORS
Cytogenetic/FISH abnormality (,t(4;14), t(14;16), del17p-); hypodiploidy
Gene expression profile pattern
Plasma cell labeling index
Bartl grade
Mitotic activity
IgA myeloma
C-reactive protein (CRP)
LDH
Soluble IL-6 receptor
Renal failure
TUMOR MICROENVIRONMENT-RELATED FACTORS
Bone marrow microvessel density
Serum syndecan-1 levels
MMP-9 levels
Soluble CD16
TREATMENT-RELATED FACTORS
Tandem transplant
Achieving complete response or very good partial response
PATIENT-RELATED FACTORS
Age
Albumin
Performance status
Other organ problems not related to myeloma or amyloid deposits

FISH, fluorescent *in situ* hybridization; Ig, immunoglobin; LDH, lactate dehydrogenase; IL, interleukin.

TABLE 136.7

INTERNATIONAL STAGING SYSTEM (GREIPP, 2005 #2861)

Stage[a]	Criteria	Median Survival (mo)
I	Serum β_2 microglobulin <3.5 mg/L Serum albumin ≥3.5 g/dL	62
II	Not stage I or III	44
III	Serum β_2 microglobulin ≥5.5 mg/L	29

[a]There are two categories for stage II: serum β_2 microglobulin <3.5 mg/L but serum albumin <3.5 g/dL; or serum β_2 microglobulin 3.5 to <5.5 mg/L irrespective of the serum albumin level.

Other independent factors associated with poor prognosis include elevated C-reactive protein (CRP), elevated serum lactate dehydrogenase (LDH) with extramedullary disease, serum IL-6, serum soluble IL-6 receptor, and IgA isotype.[238] As CRP levels reflect IL-6 activity and elevated CRP levels can be associated with acute-phase reactions including inflammation and infections, the predictive value of elevated CRP in myeloma is important only when other possible causes for its elevation are ruled out. The BM plasmacytosis reflects tumor burden, but does not predict survival. Peripheral blood monoclonal plasma cells predict for survival in myeloma: in a study of 254 patients, blood monoclonal plasma cell count 4% or more in 57% patients was associated with a median survival of 2.4 years versus 4.4 years in patients with less than 4% circulating plasma cells.[239]

Among the various other disease biology–related variables, plasma cell proliferation rate, as measured by the labeling index, is a valuable prognostic factor: labeling index more than 2% predicts inferior survival. One study combining β2M and labeling index identified a low-risk group with both parameters low, intermediate-risk group with one parameter high, and high-risk group with both parameters high to have median survivals of 71 months, 40 months, and 15 months, respectively.[223] Additional tumor-related factors predictive of inferior survival include increased soluble IL-6 receptor level, elevated serum LDH with extramedullary disease, and increased tumor cell mitotic activity (>1 per high power field).

Among the microenvironment-related factors, BM MVD has been identified as an important prognosticator. High MVD in BM ($\geq$4 per high power field) at diagnosis confers shorter event-free (2.7 vs. 4.3 years; $P = .03$) and overall (7.9+ vs. 4.3 years; $P = .006$) survival after high-dose chemotherapy.[240] An increased level of serum syndecan-1 as well as reduced levels of soluble CD16 have been described to portend poor prognosis.[241]

Among therapy- and intervention-related prognostic factors, type of response and length of response to prior therapy are additional risk stratification criteria; progression while on therapy and short duration of response to prior therapy are poor risk features. The speed of response does not suggest poor overall outcome with newer agents.

Availability of larger-scale expression profiling data in uniformly treated patient populations has provided the basis for RNA-based prognostic classification systems.[88] Moreover, a high-resolution array-based comparative genomic hybridization analyzing recurrent copy number alterations with integrated expression profiling data has allowed for further identification of DNA-based prognostic classification systems. These initial attempts at molecular classification and prognostication will need further validation and incorporation into more commonly available methods for larger application. Moreover, the high-risk features previously identified are highly dependent on the therapeutic intervention used. For example, the newer biologically based therapies such as lenalidomide and bortezomib are able to overcome drug resistance, and some traditional adverse prognostic factors are no longer predictive of survival. Additional molecular studies with FISH analysis, as well as proteomic and genomic analysis including single nucleotide polymorphism, may identify future uniformly applicable prognostic systems.

TREATMENT

The therapeutic intervention in plasma cell disorders depends on presenting condition. For example, individuals with diagnosis of MGUS do not require immediate treatment. Patients with solitary plasmacytomas can be treated with local therapy only, while those with indolent asymptomatic myeloma can smolder for a long period of time prior to becoming symptomatic and requiring treatment.

Solitary Plasmacytoma

Solitary plasmacytoma requires specialized techniques for accurate staging, including a CT scan and MRI to exclude more disseminated disease. Solitary plasmacytomas of bone involve vertebral bodies in one-third of patients and frequently affect men (70%) at a younger age (median, 56 years).[242] A monoclonal protein in the serum is observed in 24% to 54% of patients, but no detectable monoclonal protein is observed, even on immunofixation, in the remaining cases. Extramedullary plasmacytomas are diagnosed less frequently and require a workup including MRI and PET scanning to rule out additional sites or disseminated disease. The optimal therapy for true solitary plasmacytoma is curative-dose (40 to 50 Gy) radiotherapy.[243,244] With this dose, local tumor recurrence rate has been less than 10%; 30% of patients with solitary bone lesions versus more than 70% of patients with solitary extramedullary plasmacytomas achieve long disease-free survival.[245,246] Monoclonal protein disappears after radiotherapy in 25% to 50% of patients, suggesting possible eradication of disease; conversely, reappearance of monoclonal protein predicts for recurrence of disease. With better staging using MRI, true solitary plasmacytoma of the bone can be cured in a high proportion of patients.

MGUS and Smoldering Myeloma

Patents with MGUS or smoldering myeloma have a low tumor mass and indolent disease course presenting without specific symptoms. Such patients do not have end-organ damage. In patients with indolent light chain disease, Bence Jones proteinuria does not exceed more than 10 g/day. About 1% patients with MGUS per year progress to symptomatic myeloma. Non-IgG subtype, abnormal κ/λ free light chain ratio, and serum M protein more than 1.5 gm/dL are associated with higher incidence of progression of MGUS to myeloma. Patients with none of the risk features have 5% chance, while those with all three features have 60% chance of progression to myeloma in 20 years. The features responsible for higher risk of progression from smoldering myeloma to active MM are bone marrow plasmacytosis more than 30%, abnormal κ/λ free light chain ratio, and serum M protein more than 30 g/L (3.0 g/dL). Patients with all three adverse features have nearly 50% chance of progression in 2 years.[247,248] Typically, outside clinical studies, patients with MGUS require no therapy. Similarly patients with smoldering myeloma are also not treated routinely until disease progression or appearance of end-organ damage, such as development of bone lesions or anemia. However, ongoing studies have focused on evaluating role of early intervention to prevent progression to symptomatic myeloma. For example, a recent evaluation of thalidomide in 31 patients with indolent myeloma showed responses in 66% of patients, with potential to delay progression to symptomatic disease.[249] Similarly, in a recent study patients with SMM were randomized to lenalidomide with dexamethasone followed by lenalidomide maintenance versus no intervention.[249a] Overall response was 81% and time to progression to symptomatic MM was 19 months in control arm with 16 of 47 patients progressing, while no patient progressed in the treatment arm. In the future, gene expression profiling of tumor cells from these patients may provide important prognostic information and define the need for early intervention in selected patients.

Symptomatic Multiple Myeloma

Standard-Dose Therapy

Oral melphalan and prednisone was the first successful combination chemotherapy for myeloma; subsequently various other single agents and combination as well as high-dose chemotherapy regimens have been investigated and reported to have significant antimyeloma activity.

Melphalan and Prednisone. Treatment with oral melphalan and prednisone (MP), introduced 35 years ago, remained an important therapeutic option until recently, providing symptomatic relief as well as tumor mass reduction.[250] MP achieves a PR in 50% to 60% of patients, with 3% to 5% of patients achieving a CR. The median response duration is 18 months, and OS 24 to 36 months. The absorption of oral melphalan is unpredictable, requiring its ingestion on an empty stomach and an increase in dose if the patient does not develop cytopenia.[251] With availability of an intravenous formulation, dose and pharmacokinetics are now predictable. In patients receiving MP, a prompt response, reflecting a highly proliferative tumor, is associated with a poor survival. Frequent complications after MP therapy include the development of cytopenia, and with chronic administration there are myelodysplastic changes in the marrow. Melphalan and prednisone should not be used as induction therapy in patients eligible for HDT and stem cell transplant, as the ability to mobilize adequate numbers of stem cells decreases with use of melphalan, which damages stem cells. As described later, MP is now combined with one of the novel agents.

Other Alkylating Agent-Based Combinations. Various chemotherapeutic combinations have been investigated in myeloma, including vincristine (V), cyclophosphamide (C), BCNU (B), melphalan (M), Adriamycin (A), and prednisone (P). Commonly used combinations in the past include VBMCP or VMCP/VBAP.[252,253] These combinations in randomized studies achieved similar response rates, as well as event-free survival (EFS) and OS, as melphalan and prednisone. A meta-analysis of 18 published studies with 3,814 patients randomized to receive either melphalan and prednisone or various other chemotherapeutic combinations showed that outcome after melphalan and prednisone versus other chemotherapeutic combinations is equivalent. These combinations are no longer used.

VAD and High-Dose Dexamethasone. High-dose Dex (40 mg orally on days 1–4, 9–12, and 17–20) was evaluated in combination with 24 hours continuous infusion of vincristine (0.25 mg/m^2) and Adriamycin (9 mg/m^2; VAD) for 4 days with cycles repeated every 5 weeks.[254] This regimen achieved nearly 50% response rate with rapid and marked responses. In the past this regimen was used as induction therapy before transplant, as it does not affect stem cell mobilization. Addition of cyclophosphamide to VAD (CVAD) has been shown to achieve responses in up to 40% of VAD-refractory patients. However, with availability of novel agent-based combinations, VAD is no longer used as an induction regimen.[255] Studies using high-dose Dex alone given in doses similar to the VAD regimen have shown response rates similar to those observed with VAD in primary resistant myeloma, indicating that Dex is clearly an important agent in VAD.

Although effective, high-dose dexamethasone is associated with increased mortality and predisposition to systemic infections, as well as insomnia, hyperactivity, hyperglycemia, and psychiatric problems. Various dexamethasone dosage (20–40 mg) and schedules (once a week, 4 days every 2 weeks to 4 days on and 4 days of regimen) have been used. A clear dose-response relationship has not been established. A recent Eastern Cooperative Oncology Group study suggests that, in combination with lenalidomide, a once a week dexamethasone regimen may be less toxic and possibly more effective than a high-dose regimen.[256] Glucocorticoids down-regulate IL-6 production and induce apoptosis *in vitro*. The molecular mechanism of steroid-induced apoptosis in myeloma involves a decrease in NFκB activity through IκB activation. Interestingly, myeloma cells can be rescued from glucocorticoid-mediated killing by addition of IL-6 to *in vitro* cultures or by coculturing them with bone marrow stromal cells, which are a source of IL-6 *in vivo*.

Interferon. Interferon causes direct growth inhibition, as well as antiangiogenic and immunomodulatory activity. It has been shown to achieve up to 20% responses in relapsed myeloma patients. However, in combination with other chemotherapeutic regimens, it has failed to demonstrate beneficial effects.[257] In a meta-analysis of 16 trials involving 2,286 patients, response rate was 45.9% in patients treated with chemotherapy versus 54.4% for those receiving chemotherapy with IFN.[258] The difference in OS was 5 months. The role of IFN in maintenance therapy after standard-dose or HDT has remained unclear despite number of studies.[257,259] A meta-analysis of eight trials involving 929 patients showed prolongation of relapse-free survival by 7 months and OS by 5 months in patients receiving IFN. However, a large U.S. intergroup study failed to show benefit of IFN maintenance after HDT.[260] IFN is associated with flulike symptoms, weight loss, impotence, depression, mental status changes, and cytopenia; in addition, its prolonged use has been associated with inability to mobilize stem cells, so it is no longer used.

Radiation Therapy

Radiation therapy was considered the mainstay of treatment for myeloma prior to availability of chemotherapeutic options. However, with more effective therapy the role of radiation has now been limited.[261] A definitive role remains in patients with solitary bone and extramedullary plasmacytoma. Importantly, patients with solitary bone plasmacytoma treated with definitive radiation therapy (40–50 Gy) have progression-free survival (PFS) of 30%, compared with 70% in those with extramedullary plasmacytomas.[243–246,262] The indication for radiation therapy in multiple myeloma remains palliation, in cases of impending pathologic fracture, and to treat spinal cord compression. In patients with bone pain or symptomatic soft tissue masses, radiation is only considered when patients have failed chemotherapeutic options.[263,264] Radiation to BM-containing areas, such as the pelvic bone, should be used judiciously if there is need for collection of stem cells. The dose of palliative radiation therapy ranges from 15 to 25 Gy. Studies to date have failed to show any benefit of hemibody radiation in multiple myeloma. However, total-body radiation has been used prior to allogeneic and autologous transplantation. More recent studies have demonstrated that total-body radiation does not provide additional cytoreductive potential and, moreover when used with high-dose melphalan conditioning, it increases treatment-related morbidity and mortality, as well as delays immune recovery following HDT compared with high-dose melphalan alone. Recent studies with nonmyeloablative regimens followed by allogenic stem cell transplantation use low-dose radiation and achieve adequate engraftment, without myeloablation and attendant toxicity of TBI.

Novel Biologically Based Agents

Novel therapeutic agents specifically targeting the mechanisms whereby myeloma cells grow and survive in the BM milieu can overcome resistance to standard-dose and high-dose therapies.

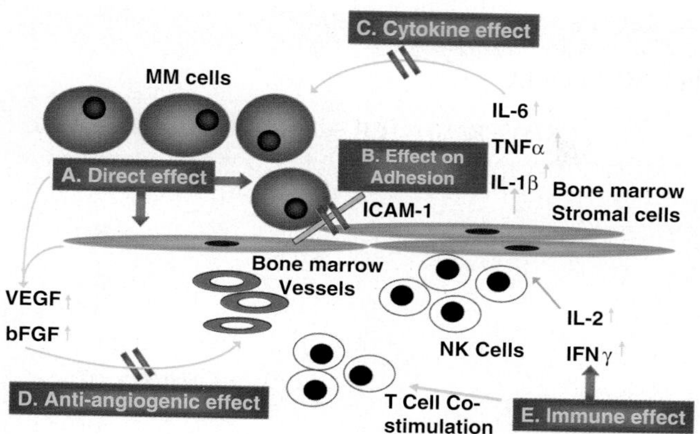

FIGURE 136.10 Potential mechanisms of action of thalidomide and its analogues. **A:** Direct effect on the myeloma cells. **B:** Inhibition of multiple myeloma (MM) cell–bone marrow stromal cell (BMSC) adhesion. **C:** Inhibition of cytokine production in the microenvironment. **D:** Antiangiogenic effects through inhibition of the proangiogenic cytokines. **E:** Modulation of immune function, especially natural killer cells and T cells. ICAM, intracellular adhesion molecule; IL, interleukin; TNF, tumor necrosis factor; VEGF, vascular endothelial growth factor; bFGF, basic fibroblast growth factor; IFN, interferon.

The immunomodulatory agents thalidomide and its analogue lenalidomide, as well as the proteasome inhibitor bortezomib, are the newer agents that have demonstrated efficacy in both relapsed and newly diagnosed myeloma and have now been integrated into standard algorithms for myeloma management.

Thalidomide. The initial rationale for use of thalidomide in myeloma was its known antiangiogenic activity, coupled with reports of increased angiogenesis in MM BM. Further investigations have shown that besides their direct effect on MM cells, thalidomide and other immunomodulatory agents (lenalidomide and pomalidomide) abrogate the adhesion of MM cells to BMSCs and block the secretion of MM growth and survival factors such as IL-6, TNF-α, VEGF, and fibroblast growth factor triggered by the binding of MM cells to BMSCs (Fig. 136.10).[265] Additionally, these agents significantly modulate immune responses by expanding the number and function of natural killer cells, improving dendritic cell (DC) function, and importantly, enhancing T-cell function by providing T-cell costimulatory signals through B7-CD28 pathway.[265]

Thalidomide was initially evaluated in a phase 2 study in 169 posttransplant-relapsed MM patients in incremental doses of 200 to 800 mg. A PR was observed in 26% patients, with an overall response rate (ORR) of 34%.[266,267] Subsequently, the efficacy of thalidomide has been confirmed in several phase 2 studies in relapsed MM (Table 136.8A). Based on *in vitro* results showing synergism as well as reversal of resistance, thalidomide has been combined with dexamethasone. This combination has achieved more than 50% responses in relapsed MM patients and 70% responses in newly diagnosed patients. Additional combinations of thalidomide with MP have improved overall response, as well as both EFS and OS, in newly diagnosed patients over age of 65 years (Table 136.8B). The major toxicities of thalidomide are somnolence, constipation, and neurologic symptoms including neuropathy, fatigue, and DVT.[201] Because of significant risk of DVT and pulmonary embolism when thalidomide is used in combination with dexamethasone, a prophylactic measure is warranted in all patients. Although aspirin has been used as prophylaxis in patients at low risk of DVT, in patients at higher risk of DVT either standard-dose Coumadin or low-molecular-weight heparin is indicated.[268]

Lenalidomide. Lenalidomide is a more active analogue of thalidomide, which demonstrated in a phase 1 clinical trial, at least a minimal response (at least a 25% reduction in paraproteins) in 15 of 24 (63%) patients, including 11 patients who had received prior thaidomide.[269] These results provided the basis for further evaluation of lenalidomide, in both relapsed and newly diagnosed MM. In a randomized study in patients with at least one prior therapy, combination of lenalidomide and dexamethasone was compared to dexamethasone alone; the PR or better rate (61% vs. 20%; $P < .001$), CR rate (14% vs. 0.6%; $P < .001$), median time to progression (11.1 vs. 4.7 months; $P < .001$), and median OS (29.6 vs. 20.2 months; $P < .001$) were superior in combination group compared to dexamethasone alone, respectively. In newly diagnosed patients, when combined with dexamethasone and used beyond four cycles, it achieves over 90% PR or better rate.[270] A similar study in Europe had almost identical results. Table 136.9A and

PRACTICE OF ONCOLOGY

TABLE 136.8A

THALIDOMIDE (THAL) REGIMENS IN RELAPSED/REFRACTORY MULTIPLE MYELOMA

Study (Ref.)	Phase	N	Regimen	Median No. of Prior Tx	Median TTP (mo)	CR/VGPR(%)	CR + PR(%)
Singhal et al. (267) *NEJM* 1999	2	84	Thal	N/R	3.0 (EFS)	17	25
Barlogie et al. (266) *Blood* 2001	2	169	Thal	N/R	~5 (EFS)	20	30
Palumbo (267a) *Haematol* 2001	2	77	Thal + Dex	2	12	18	41
Dimopoulos (267b) *Ann Oncol* 2001	2	44	Thal + Dex	3	4.2	30	55
Terpos[a] ASH 2006	2	53	VMD-T	2	9.5	37	60
Palumbo[b] ASH 2006	1/2	30	VMP-T	3	N/R	43	67

[a]Terpos E, et al. *Blood* 2006;108:3541a.
[b]Palumbo A, et al. *Blood* 2006;108:407a.
Tx, treatment; TTP, time to progression; CR, complete remission; VGPR, very good partial remission; N/R, not reported; EFS, event-free survival; Dex, dexamethasone; VMD-T, velcade, melphalan, dexamethasone, thalidomide; VMP-T, velcade, melphalan, prednisone, thalidomide.

TABLE 136.8B

THALIDOMIDE REGIMENS IN NEWLY DIAGNOSED MULTIPLE MYELOMA

Study (Ref.)	Phase	N	Regimen	CR/VGPR(%)	CR + PR(%)	1-yr Survival (%)
Rajkumar (Mayo) (281a) *JCO* 2002	2	50	Thal + Dex	N/R	64	N/R
Weber (MDACC) (281b) *JCO* 2003	2	28 40	Thal Thal + Dex	N/R 16	36 72	N/R
Cavo (255) *Hematologica* 2004	2	71	Thal + Dex	17	66	N/R
Rajkumar, E1A00 (281) *JCO* 2006	3	103	Thal + Dex	4 (CR)	63	80
Rajkumar, MM003 (281c) ASH 2006	3	470	Thal + Dex	44	69	80
Palumbo (281d) *Lancet* 2006	3	129	MP-T	36	76	87
Facon (281e) ASCO 2006	3	124	MP-T	50	81	88
Barlogie (281f) *NEJM* 2006	3	323	TT2 + Thal	69	83	92
Lockhorst (281h) *Haematologica* 2008	3	203	TAD	7	80	N/R
Offidani (281g) *Blood* 2006	2	50	ThaDD (Thal + PLD + Dex)	56	84	89
Borrello[a] ASH 2006	2	27	Thal + Bort	22	82	N/R
Wang[b] ASH 2005	2	36	Thal + Bort + Dex (VTD)	19	92	N/R

[a]Borello I, et al. *Blood* 2006;08:3528a.
[b]Wang M, et al. *Blood* 2005;106:784a.
N/R, not reported.

B lists selected major studies demonstrating its activity in both relapsed and newly diagnosed myeloma. Importantly, no significant somnolence, constipation, or neuropathy is observed with lenalidomide. However, myelosuppression was the dose-limiting toxicity and requires monitoring during therapy. Similar to thalidomide, it is associated with increased incidence of DVT and requires concurrent prophylactic measures for its prevention.[268] Because of its renal excretion, a dose modification is necessary when used in patients with renal dysfunction.

TABLE 136.9A

LENALIDOMIDE REGIMENS IN RELAPSED/REFRACTORY MULTIPLE MYELOMA

Study (Ref.)	Phase	N	Regimen	Median No. of Prior Tx	Median TTP (mo)	CR/VGPR(%)	CR + PR(%)
Richardson (269)	1/2	24	Len	3	N/R	13	30
Richardson (270a) *Blood* 2006	2	102	Len	>3	4.6	4	17
Weber (270) *NEJM* 2007	3	171	Len + Dex	3	11.1	13	59
Dimopoulos (270b) *NEJM* 2007	3	176	Len + Dex	3	11.3	15	59
Richardson (270c) *JCO* 2009	1	36	Len + Bort	5	N/R	6	39
Richardson (207d) *Blood* 2010	1/2	28	Len + Bort + Dex	5	N/R	6	31
Knop[a] ASH 2006	1/2	31	Len + AD (RAD)	3	N/R	5	84
Baz (270e) *Ann Oncol* 2006	1/2	52	Len + DVD (Len + PLD + Vd)	3	12	29	75
Morgan (270f) *Br J Haemat* 2007	2	20	RCD (Len + Cyclophos + Dex)	4	N/R	27	65

[a]Knop S, et al. *Blood* 2006;108;408a.
TTP, time to progression; N/R, not reported.

TABLE 136.9B

LENALIDOMIDE REGIMENS IN NEWLY DIAGNOSED MULTIPLE MYELOMA

Study (Ref.)	Phase	N	Regimen	CR/VGPR(%)	CR + PR(%)	1-yr Survival Rate (%)
Rajkumar (256a) *Blood* 2005; ASH 2005	2	34	Len + Dex	56	91	90
Niesvizky (256b) ASCO 2006	2	42	Len + Dex + clarithro	51	94	86
Rajkumar, E4A03 Arm A (256) *Lancet Oncol* 2010	3	223	Len + std-dose Dex	NA	NA	87
Rajkumar, E4A03 Arm B (256) *Lancet Oncol* 2010	3	222	Len + low-dose Dex	NA	NA	96
Palumbo[a] ASH 2009	1/2	21	Len + MP (MP-R)	48	81	100

[a]Palumbo A, et al. *Blood* 2009; 114:613a.
NA, not available.

Bortezomib. Bortezomib is the first in class proteasome inhibitor originally used in MM because of its blockade of NFκB activation and related paracrine IL-6 production by BMSCs. Bortezomib has been subsequently demonstrated to act directly on MM cells to induce apoptosis through both caspase 8 and 9 activation, and it overcomes the protective effects of IL-6 and adds to the anti-MM effects of Dex. Importantly, it acts in the microenvironment to inhibit the binding of MM cells to BMSCs, secretion of MM growth-promoting cytokines, and BM angiogenesis.[271–274] Based on efficacy and safety profile in a phase 1 study, a multicenter phase 2 trial in 193 evaluable patients showed 35% PR or greater response.[275] The median duration of response was 12 months and the median OS was 16 months. Grade 3 adverse events included thrombocytopenia (28%), fatigue (12%), peripheral neuropathy (12%), and neutropenia (11%). Addition of Dex in this study improved responses in 19% of patients, confirming synergism between these two agents.

A subsequent randomized study in 669 patients with relapsed myeloma comparing bortezomib versus dexamethasone reported a higher response rate (38% vs. 18%, respectively; $P < .001$), a longer time to progression (6.22 vs. 3.49 months, respectively; $P < .001$), and a longer survival (1-year survival rate, 80% vs. 66%, respectively; $P = .003$).[276] Table 136.10A and B lists selected major studies demonstrating its activity in both relapsed and newly diagnosed myeloma. In a recent randomized multicenter international study, the combination of bortezomib and pegylated

PRACTICE OF ONCOLOGY

TABLE 136.10A

BORTEZOMIB REGIMENS IN RELAPSED/REFRACTORY MULTIPLE MYELOMA

Study (Ref.)	Phase	N	Regimen	Median No. of Prior Tx	Median TTP (mo)	CR/VGPR(%)	CR + PR(%)
Richardson (276) *NEJM* 2003	2	193	Bort	>3	~7	10	27
Richardson (276) *NEJM* 2005; ASH 2005	3	333	Bort	2	6.2	4	43
Richardson (270d) *Blood* 2010	1/2	28	Len + Bort + Dex	5	N/R	6	31
Berenson (276a) *JCO* 2006	1/2	35	Bort + Mel	3	8	6	47
Harrousseau[a] ASCO 2007	3	324	Bort + PLD	≥2	9.3	36	48
Chanan-Khan[b] ASH 2006	2	23	Bort + PLD + Thal (VDT)	5	10.9	23	65
Terpos[c] ASH 2006	2	53	VMDT (Bort + Mel + Thal + Dex)	2	9.5	37	60
Morgan[d] ASH 2006	2	11	Bort + Cyclo + Dex	3	N/R	27	64
Palumbo[e] ASH 2006	1/2	30	Bort + MPT (VMPT)	3	N/R	43	67
Baz (276b) *Ann Oncol* 2006	1/2	52	Len + DVD	3	12	29	75

[a]Harousseau JL, et al. *Proc ASCO* 2007;25:8002.
[b]Chanan-Khan AA, et al. *Blood* 2006;108:3539a.
[c]Terpos E, et al. *Blood* 2006;108:3541a.
[d]Morgan GJ, et al *Blood* 2006;108:3555a.
[e]Blood 2006;108:407a.
TTP, time to progression; N/R, not reported.

TABLE 136.10B

BORTEZOMIB REGIMENS IN NEWLY DIAGNOSED MULTIPLE MYELOMA

Study (Ref.)	Phase	N	Regimen	CR/VGPR(%)	CR + PR(%)	1-yr Survival (%)
Richardson (277a) ASCO 2000	2	63	Bort	10	40	N/R
Jagannath (277b) *BrJH* 2005	2	48	Bort ± Dex	19	90	80
Harousseau (277c) Haem 2006	2	48	Bort + Dex	31	66	N/R
Harousseau (277d) JCO 2010	3	79	Bort + Dex	43	82	N/R
Rosinol (277e) JCO 2007	2	40	Alternating Bort/Dex	22	64	N/R
Cahosh (277f) *BrJH* 2011	2	27	Bort + Thal	22	82	N/R
Wang (277g) *Hematology* 2007	2	36	Bort/TD (VTD)	19	92	N/R
Mateos (277h) *Blood* 2006	1/2	60	MP-V	43	89	87
Oakervee (277i) *BrJH* 2005	2	21	PAD	29	95	N/R
Orlowski (277) *Blood* 2006	2	29	Bort + PLD	28	79	N/R
Jakubowiak (277j) *JCO* 2009	2	28	Bort + PLD + Dex	53	89	N/R
Barlogie *BrJH* 2007	2	303	TT3 with bort	80	90	92

N/R, not reported.

liposomal doxorubicin was shown to be superior to bortezomib alone for both overall response (50% vs. 42% respectively; *P* = .05) and time to progression (9.3 vs. 6.5 months, respectively; *P* <.0001) leading to approval of this combination in relapsed multiple myeloma by the U.S. Food and Drug Administration.[277] Bortezomib has been shown to overcome the adverse outcome associated with chromosome 13 abnormality,[278] can be given safely in patients with renal failure,[279] and improves osteoblastic activity.[280] The major toxicities include fatigue, diarrhea, reversible thrombocytopenia, and peripheral neuropathy.

Induction Therapy in Newly Diagnosed Patient

Decision about the induction regimen in newly diagnosed MM is partly influenced by whether or not the patient is a transplant candidate. Mainly, alkylating agents should be avoided in patients who are potential transplant candidates as these agents may affect stem cell collection. In newly diagnosed patients thalidomide and dexamethasone have been demonstrated to be superior to dexamethasone alone (ORR, 63% vs. 41%, respectively; *P* = .0017).[281] Based on these data thalidomide and dexamethasone combination is approved by the U.S. Food and Drug Administration as an induction regimen.

With the availability of lenalidomide and bortezomib, alternative combinations have been investigated. The Southwest Oncology Group compared lenalidomide plus dexamethasone (n = 97) to placebo plus high-dose Dex (n = 95) in newly diagnosed myeloma in a randomized study.[282] Overall response rate and 1-year PFS were superior with lenalidomide plus dexamethasone (78% vs. 48%, *P* <.001; and 78% vs. 52%, *P* =.002, respectively), while 1-year OS was similar (94% vs. 88%; *P* = .25). Toxicities were more pronounced with lenalidomide plus dexamethasone (neutropenia grade 3–4, 21% vs. 5%, *P* <.001; and DVT despite aspirin prophylaxis, 23.5% vs. 5%, *P* <.001). A randomized study performed by Eastern Cooperative Oncology Group compared lenalidomide at 25 mg daily for 3 of 4 weeks along with high-dose dexamethasone (40 mg days 1–4, 9–12, and 17–20) versus lenalidomide with low-dose dexamethasone (40 mg once a week).[256] With 445 patients randomized, 79% patients receiving high-dose and 68% patients on low-dose dexamethasone had CR or PR within four cycles (*P* = .008). However, OS at 1 year was 96% versus 87% in favor of the low-dose dexamethasone group (*P* = .0002) and toxicity was also higher in high-dose versus low-dose dexamethasone group (any grade 3 or 4 toxicity, 52% vs. 35%, respectively, *P* = .0001; early mortality, 5.4% vs. 0.5%, respectively, *P* = .003; and DVT, 26% vs. 12%, respectively, *P* = .0003).

Bortezomib-containing regimens have also been evaluated in newly diagnosed patients. Jagannath et al. have reported 18% CR and 88% ORR in a phase 2 study using combination of bortezomib and dexamethasone in newly diagnosed patients. The IFM group has randomized 242 newly diagnosed patients to VAD or bortezomib plus dexamethasone (VD) followed by DCEP consolidation and autologous stem cell transplantation.[283] CR plus near CR (CR/nCR) (15% vs. 6%), at least VGPR (38% vs. 15%), and overall response (79% vs. 63%) rates after four cycles of induction therapy were significantly higher with VD compared with VAD. Interestingly, the superior response after induction also translated into significantly improved response after transplant with CR/nCR (35% vs. 18%) and at least VGPR (54% vs. 37%) rates in favor of VD compared with VAD group. Median PFS was 36.0 months

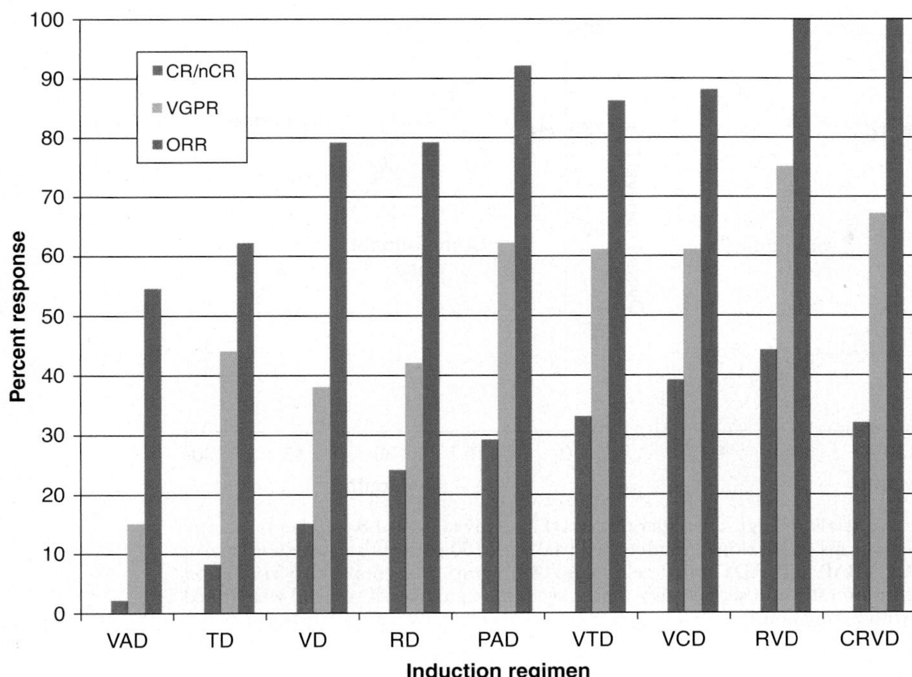

FIGURE 136.11 Progressive improvement in response to combination therapies incorporating newer agents. The near complete response (nCR/CR), very good partial remission (VGPR), and partial response (PR) or greater rates following induction therapy of newly diagnosed multiple myeloma patients is plotted for a common novel agent combinations selected from larger phase 3 and 2 studies and compared with VAD regimen. VAD: vincristine, Adriamycin, dexamethasone; T, thalidomide; D, dexamethasone; R, lenalidomide; P, bortezomib. V, bortezomib (except in VAD); A, Adriamycin; C, cyclophosphamide.

versus 29.7 months (P = .064) with VD versus VAD. The incidence of severe adverse events appeared similar between the groups. A short-term bortezomib induction has been reported to improve outcome of patients with t(4;14) but not the outcome of patients with del(17p).[284]

With the success of two-drug combinations, three-drug combinations have been investigated with demonstrated high response rates. Bortezomib and dexamethasone have been combined with thalidomide (VTD: CR, 32%; VGPR, 62%; ORR, 94%), Doxorubicin (VDD: CR/nCR, 31%; VGPR, 42%; ORR, 83%), cyclophosphamide[285] (VCD: CR/nCR, 39%; VGPR, 61%; ORR, 88%), and lenalidomide[286] (VRD: CR/nCr, 52%; VGPR, 74%; PR, 100%). Randomized comparison between these three-drug and two-drug combinations is ongoing. A four-drug combination combining VRD with cyclophosphamide has not shown clear benefit yet. These novel agent combinations have progressively improved responses, both frequency and depth, in patients newly diagnosed with myeloma (Fig. 136.11).

For patients who are not transplant candidates, the same regimen described here can be used. In addition, a regimen that incorporates melphalan and prednisone (MP) can also be considered. MP in combination with novel agents have significantly improved outcome. Five randomized studies have compared MP with thalidomide (MPT) versus MP (Table 136.11) and demonstrated both superior overall response and complete response rate, as well as event-free survival (four of five studies) and OS (two of five studies), suggesting MPT as a

TABLE 136.11

RANDOMIZED STUDIES COMPARING MELPHALAN AND PREDNISONE (MP)-RELATED REGIMENS: RESULTS

Authors (Ref.)	Regimen	Complete Response	Partial Response	PFS (Median mo)	OS (Median mo)
Palumbo et al./GIMEMA (268)	MPT vs. MP	16% vs. 4% (P <.001)	69% vs 48% (P <.0001)	21.8 vs. 14.5 (P = .0004)	45 vs 47.6 (P value NS)[b]
Facon et al./IFM 99-06 Laurel 2007 (268a)	MPT vs. MP	13% vs. 2% (P = .0008)	76% vs. 35% (P <.0001)	27.5 vs. 18 (P <.0001)	51.5 vs. 33 (P = .006)
Hulin et al./IFM 01-01 *JCO* 2009 (268b)	MPT vs. MP	7% vs. 1% (P <.001)	62% vs. 31% (P <.001)	24 vs. 18.5 (P = .001)	44 vs. 29 (P = .028)
Wijermans et al./HOVON *JCO* 2010 (268c)	MPT vs. MP	2% vs. 2%	66% vs. 45% (P <.001)	13 vs. 9 (P <.001)	40 vs. 32 (P = .05)
Waage et al./NMSG[a] *ASCO* 2010	MPT vs. MP	—	57% vs. 40% (P < 0.0001)	15 vs. 14 (P value NS)	29 vs. 32 (P value NS)
San Miguel et al./VISTA (287)	MPV vs. MP	30% vs. 4% (P <.001)	71% vs. 35% (P <.001)	*24 vs. 16.6 (P <.001)	Not reached vs. 43
Palumbo et al.[b] ASH 2009	MPRR vs. MP	18% vs. 5% (P <.001)	77% vs. 49% (P <.001)	Not reached vs. 13 (P = .002)	Not reached

[a]Waage A, et al. *Proc ASCO* 2010;28:8130.
[b]Palumbo A, et al. *Blood* 2009;114:613.
PFS, progression-free survival; OS, overall survival; MPT, MP with thalidomide; NS, significant difference; HOVON, Dutch-Belgian Hematology-Oncology Cooperative group; MPV, MPRR, MP followed by lenalidomide maintenance.

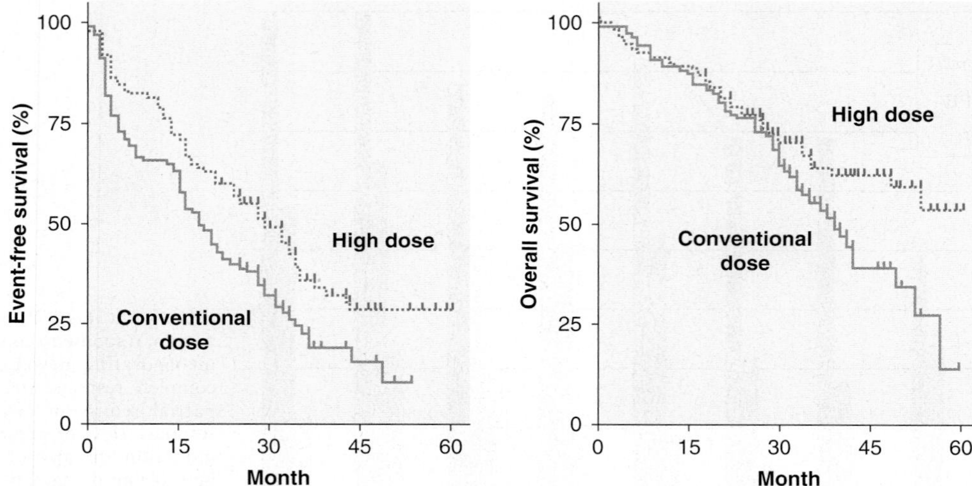

FIGURE 136.12 Comparative trials of high-dose therapy (HDT) versus standard-dose chemotherapy (SDT). IFM-90 (Intergroupe Francais de Myelome) randomized trial with 100 patients accrued to each arm comparing SDT with VMCP-VBAP and HDT with melphalan 140 mg/m² plus total-body irradiation (8 Gy). Higher complete remission rates and significantly longer event-free and overall survival were noted with HDT. (From ref. 292, with permission.)

standard regimen in this patient population. Combination of bortezomib with MP (VMP) has been compared with MP in a randomized study[287] demonstrating superior CR and PR rates for VMP regimen (71% vs. 35% and 30% vs, 4%, respectively; $P <.001$). The time to progression for VMP group was 24.0 months, as compared with 16.6 months for MP group ($P <.001$). More recently the combination of lenalidomide with MP followed by lenalidomide maintenance (MPRR) has been compared with MP, demonstrating higher response rate (CR, 18% vs. 5% and ORR, 76% vs. 49%; $P <.001$) and PFS (not reached vs. 13.2 months; $P = .002$) for MPRR. A four-drug combination combining MPT with bortezomib has not shown significant further improvement.

High-Dose Therapy with Peripheral Blood Stem Cell Support

To overcome resistance to standard-dose therapy, as evidenced by the low incidence of complete responses to induction chemotherapy even in newly diagnosed patients, a pilot study by the late Tim McElwain and his colleagues at the Royal Marsden Hospital evaluated the role of melphalan dose escalation (140 mg/m²).[12] They reported complete remissions in refractory patients; however, treatment-related mortality was high because of BM toxicity. Bone marrow support in subsequent studies improved the treatment-related mortality; and further dose escalation of melphalan to 200 mg/m² further improved response.

Transplant in Newly Diagnosed Patients

The initial demonstration of activity of high-dose melphalan therapy led to series of evaluations of the role of HDT with stem cell support in myeloma. These studies reported complete remissions in up to 50% of patients, with prolongation of EFS and OS to more than 3 years and more than 5 to 6 years, respectively.[288–292]

The superiority of high-dose chemotherapy with autologous BM support was confirmed in a randomized trial conducted by IFM. The response rate (≥50% reduction in myeloma protein) in 100 patients receiving HDT (Mel-140 + total-body irradiation [TBI]) was 81% (22% complete remission) compared with 57% (5% complete remission) in a similar number of patients receiving standard-dose chemotherapy consisting of VMCP (vincristine, melphalan, cyclophosphamide, and prednisone) alternating with BVAP (carmustine, vincristine, doxorubicin, and prednisone) regimen ($P <.001$). Significantly longer event-free (median, 28 vs. 18 months) and overall (median, 57 vs. 42 months) survival were reported after HDT (Fig. 136.12). The projected 5-year EFS and OS were 28% and 52% after HDT compared to 10% and 12% following standard-dose therapy, respectively.[293]

A similar response and survival benefit has been reported from the Medical Research Council VII trial, which randomized 407 patients to either standard-dose chemotherapy or HDT with transplantation.[294] A Spanish trial of 164 patients treated with HDT versus conventional therapy also showed a superior CR rate in the HDT arm, with a trend for prolonged EFS and OS in the HDT arm (Table 136.12).[295] In contrast, the Myelome Autogreffe Group (MAG) trial by Fermand et al.[296] in 190 newly diagnosed MM patients failed to show superiority of HDT. Most recently, the U.S. intergroup study randomizing patients between HDT versus conventional therapy followed by delayed HDT at relapse failed to show superiority of HDT for either achievement of CR or OS; EFS benefit was modest (4 months) in the HDT cohort.[260] A meta-analysis combining nine studies comprising 2,411 patients reported a combined hazard of death with HDT of 0.92 (95% (Confidence Interval [CI]: 0.74–1.13) and a combined hazard of progression with HDT of 0.75 (95% [CI]: 0.59–0.96). The analysis of the randomized data indicated PFS benefit but not OS benefit for HDT with single autologous transplantation in multiple myeloma.[297]

Although the responses to induction therapy have now significantly improved with the use of novel agent combination therapies (Fig. 136.11), some recent studies have indicated that HDT is able to further improve the depth of response (Fig. 136.13). These observations have raised questions about the role of HDT in newly diagnosed patients with myeloma receiving novel agent combination therapy. An ongoing study is evaluating the role of transplant in patients receiving RVD combination.

Tandem Transplants

Attempts to further improve the results of autotransplantation have included intensification with tandem transplants.

TABLE 136.12

RESULTS OF LARGE RANDOMIZED STUDY COMPARING STANDARD-DOSE THERAPY WITH HIGH-DOSE THERAPY

Study (Ref.)	Therapy	No. of Patients	CR (%)	EFS (Median mo)	OS (Median mo)
Attal et al. (274)	Conventional	100	5[b]	18[b]	37[b]
	HDT	100	22	27	52
Fermand et al. (277)	Conventional	96	—	18.7[b]	50.4[a]
	HDT	94	—	24.3	55.3
Blade et al. (280)	Conventional	83	11[b]	34.3[b]	66.9[a]
	HDT	81	30	42.5	67.4
Child et al. (275)	Conventional	200	8.5[b]	19.6[b]	42.3[b]
	HDT	201	44	31.6	54.8
Barlogie et al. (249)	Conventional	255	15[a]	21[a]	53[a]
	HDT	261	17	25	58

CR; complete remission; EFS, event-free survival; OS, overall survival; HDT, high-dose therapy.
[a]No significant difference.
[b]Significant difference.

Harousseau et al.[298] were the first to report feasibility of tandem autologous BM transplantation, with a 69% CR rate in small select group of patients. Barlogie et al.[299] investigated a sequential noncross-resistant remission induction regimen, followed by tandem autologous transplantations ("total therapy") in 231 newly diagnosed patients: 41% patients achieved CR after two transplants, and the median EFS and OS times were 43 months and 68 months, respectively.

Attal et al.[237] (IFM-94) reported a randomized comparison of single HDT (melphalan [140 mg/m^2] and TBI [8 Gy]) vs. double HDT (melphalan [200 mg/m^2], followed by melphalan [140 mg/m^2] and TBI [8 Gy]) in 399 newly diagnosed patients. This study reported no significant improvement in CR or very good PR rate between the two arms (42% vs. 50%, respectively, $P = .10$); however, there was a significant improvement in the double HDT arm in probability of EFS at 7 years (10% vs. 20%; $P = .03$) and estimated OS at 7 years (21% vs. 42%; $P = .01$) (Fig. 136.14). A similar study by the Dutch-Belgian Hematology-Oncology Cooperative group (HOVON; N = 255) showed superior CR rate (13% vs. 28%) and EFS (20 vs. 22 months) in favor of tandem transplants; however, it failed to show OS benefit. The MAG (N = 193) and Bologna (N = 178) trials, with a median follow-up of 27 to 30 months, have not yet shown a significant benefit for tandem transplantation (Table 136.13).

Various factors need special consideration in the management of myeloma with high-dose chemotherapy. These factors include source of stem cells, conditioning regimen, timing of transplant, and tumor-cell purging.

Timing of High-dose Therapy. To obtain high-quality hematopoietic stem cells, ideal timing for stem cell collection is early in the course of the induction treatment. Ability to collect adequate stem cells (≥2 × 10^6 CD34+ cells per kilogram) in patients with less than 12 months of prior therapy is 86% compared to 48% in patients with more than 24 months of prior therapy.[300] Prolonged lenalidomide induction therapy has been reported to affect stem cell mobilization. Patients undergoing peripheral blood stem cell (PBSC) mobilization with granulocyte colony-stimulating factor following lenalidomide induction had significant decrease in total CD34(+) cells collected, average daily collection, and increased number of aphereses.[301] However,

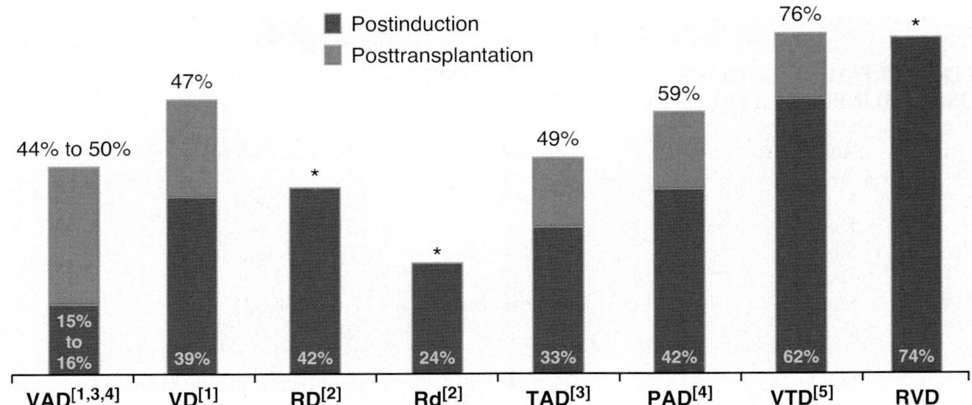

FIGURE 136.13 Despite improvements in response with novel agents, high-dose therapy further improves the depth of response. *Posttransplant intention-to-treat data not available. 1. Harousseau et al. Presented at: 50th Annual ASH Meeting; December 2008; San Francisco, California. 2. Rajkumar SV et al. *Lancet Oncol.* 2009; 3. Lokhorst HM et al. *Haematologica* 2008;93:124. 4. Sonneveld P et al. Presented at: XII IMW; February 2009; Washington, DC. Abstract 152. 5. Cavo M et al. Presented at: 50th Annual ASH Meeting; December 2008; San Francisco, California.

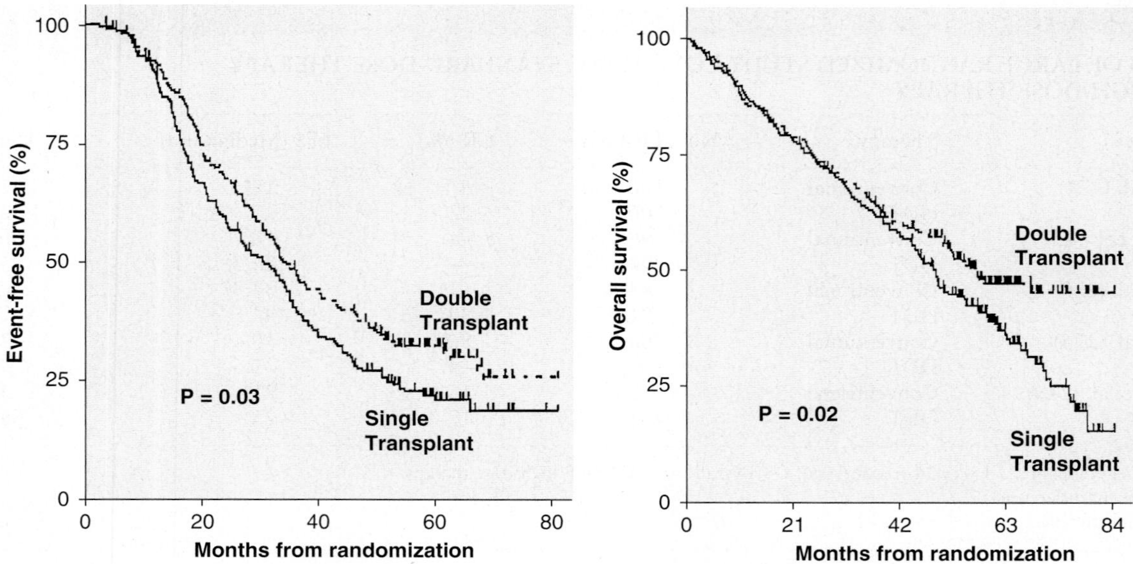

FIGURE 136.14 Comparative trial of single versus double high-dose therapy (HDT). Intergroupe Francophone du Myelome (IFM) 94 trial with 399 patients randomized to a single HDT with melphalan 140 mg/m² plus total-body irradiation (8 Gy) versus first HDT with melphalan 140 mg/m² and subsequent second HDT with melphalan 140 mg/m² plus total-body irradiation (8 Gy). Superior event-free and overall survival was noted with double HDT. (From ref. 237, with permission.)

there is no effect on quality of PBSC collected as indicated by similar engraftment across all groups. Based on these facts, collection within 6 months of lenalidomide therapy and with cyclophosphamide-based mobilization is recommended.[302,303]

Multi-institutional trials demonstrating that initial HDT prolongs remission duration and survival but is not curative has led to the exploration of whether HDT should be used early after diagnosis versus delayed as a treatment for relapsed myeloma. To evaluate this important question, Fermand et al.[296] randomized 185 newly diagnosed patients to undergo three to four cycles of VAMP (vinblastine, doxorubicin, methotrexate, and prednisone) followed by early HDT and autotransplantation (n = 91), versus conventional chemotherapy with VMCP for 1 year and HDT at relapse (n = 94). Although patients who underwent early transplantation had significantly longer EFS times (39 vs. 13 months), OS was identical in both arms (median, 64.6 and 64 months). Importantly, the time without symptoms and toxicity analysis reflecting quality of life (mean, 27.8 vs. 22.3 months) showed superior results for the early HDT arm (Table 136.14).

Vesole et al.[304] have confirmed effectiveness of high-dose chemotherapy as a salvage therapy achieving EFS and OS times of 21 and more than 43 months, respectively, in 135 patients with advanced refractory MM. In this study, patients with primary unresponsive disease had superior outcomes to patients with resistant relapse (progression on last-salvage chemotherapy), with EFS of 37 months versus 17 months, respectively (P = .0004), and OS of ≥43 months versus 21 months, respectively (P = .0003). Gertz et al.[305] from the Mayo Clinic have also reported a similar experience in 64 patients undergoing elective delayed transplant at the time of progression following standard therapy. Finally, the recently reported Intergroup trial in the United States randomizing patients to up-front HDT or standard therapy with HDT as a salvage treatment also confirms a similar modest EFS benefit for early versus late transplant.[260]

TABLE 136.13

SINGLE VERSUS DOUBLE AUTOLOGOUS STEM CELL TRANSPLANT (ASCT) FOR NEWLY DIAGNOSED MULTIPLE MYELOMA

Study (Ref.)	ASCT	N	CR (%)[a]	Median EFS (mo)	Median OS (mo)
Attal et al. (237)	Single	199	42[b] (P = NS)	25 (P = .03)	48 (P = .01)
(IFM-94)	Double	200	50[b]	30	58
Fermand et al. (296)	Single	94	42[a] (P = NS)	No difference	No difference
(MAG-95)	Double	99	37[a]		
Sonneveld et al. (296a)	Single	148	13 (P = .002)	20 (P = .02)	55 (P = NS)
(HOVON-24)	Double	155	28	22	50
Hematology 2007					
Cavo et al. (296b)	Single	115	35 (P = NS)	Significant prolongation of	59 (P = NS)
(Bologna 96) *JCO* 2007	Double	113	48	EFS with double SCT	73

CR, complete remission; EFS, event-free survival; OS, overall survival; NS, not significant; IFM, Intergroupe Francophone du Myelome MAG, Myelome Autogreffe Group; SCT, stem cell transplant, VGPR, very good partial remission.
[a]CR + minimum residual disease.
[b]CR + VGPR.

TABLE 136.14

STEM CELL TRANSPLANTATION AS UP-FRONT VERSUS RESCUE TREATMENT: RESULTS OF RANDOMIZED STUDY[a]

	Early Transplant (N = 91)	Late Transplant (N = 94)
CR	19%	5%
Med EFS	39 mo	13 mo
Med OS	64.6 mo	64 mo
TWISTT	27.8 mo	22.3 mo

CR, complete remission; EFS, event-free survival; TWISTT, time without symptoms or treatment toxicity.
[a]Median follow-up, 58 months.
Significant difference.

High-Dose Regimen. High-dose melphalan (140–200 mg/m^2), with or without TBI, is the most common conditioning regimen used in myeloma.[306–308] Melphalan's predominant myelotoxicity and metabolism independent of renal function is ideal for multiple myeloma patients who commonly have renal function abnormalities. Melphalan seems to be superior to thiotepa when given with TBI, with patients achieving longer relapse-free and OS duration.[308] A combination regimen containing high-dose carboplatin with etoposide and cytoxan, or a combination with cyclophosphamide, BCNU, VP-16 (CBV), has achieved only occasional responses in resistant patients.[309,310] No regimen has shown marked superiority over others. The addition of TBI has not been shown to improve cytoreduction, and in fact increases morbidity and treatment-related mortality. A poor outcome in one study using TBI was attributed to delayed immune recovery.

Stem Cell Purging. Myeloma cell contamination, as evaluated by polymerase chain reaction or sensitive immunofluorescence, is universally observed in stem cell products. Purging of tumor cells by positive selection of CD34+ cells leads to a 3 to 5 log reduction in contamination.[311,312] Negative selection using the monoclonal antibody cocktail containing CD10 (common acute lymphoblastic leukemia antigen); CD20 (a pan B-cell antigen); and PCA-1, (plasma cell-associated antigen) or peanut agglutinin (PNA) and anti-CD19 antibodies results in undetectable myeloma cells by conventional flow cytometry.[291] The early follow-up results from these studies have not revealed any significant advantage in responses or survival, but they consistently show a delay in engraftment posttransplantation. A multicenter, randomized study comparing CD34-selected PBSCs versus unselected PBSCs in 131 patients failed to show any significant difference in EFS or OS time.[313] Even when cells were purged using flourescence activated cell sorting of very early hematopoietic stem cells (CD34$^+$,Thy1$^+$, Lin), relapses were frequent and patients had delayed hematopoietic engraftment and suppressed immune status for prolonged periods of time.[314,315] Due to these data, emphasis is now on strategies to improve responses to HDT, rather than on purging autografts.

Hematopoietic Stem Cell Source. Mobilized PBSCs provide for more rapid engraftment compared to BM. Myeloma patients with less than 1 year of prior therapy had faster granulocyte and platelet recovery after peripheral blood stem cell transplants compared with BM autografts.[316] The duration of prior chemotherapy, especially with stem cell–damaging agents (melphalan, BCNU, and high doses of cyclophosphamide) along with radiation to BM-containing areas, significantly affects the ability to procure adequate quantities of PBSCs and engraftment kinetics post-transplant.[317] After mobilization with cyclophosphamide and GM-CSF, normal PBSCs are mobilized during the first 3 days of leukapheresis, while peak levels of contaminating myeloma cells are present on subsequent days. These myeloma cells show a higher labeling index and a more immature phenotype (CD19$^+$).[318]

Management of Older Patients

Unlike in the past, melphalan and prednisone is no longer a standard of care for older adults with myeloma. The combination of novel agents previously described for newly diagnosed patients remains an important option. In this age group, which most of the time is not considered eligible for transplant, combination of bortezomib or lenalidomide, or both, with dexamethasone is considered the preferred option. However, MP in combination with these novel agents also achieves high level of response and can be considered an alternative. To manage toxicity, dose of dexamethasone and thalidomide needs to be reduced in patients older than 75 years. As the incidence of myeloma increases with age, the role of HDT has also been evaluated in patients older than 65 years old. Older age does not impact stem cell mobilization or engraftment.[319] The feasibility and efficacy of HDT with PBSC transplant has been evaluated in 70 patients 70 or more years old (median age, 72 years; range, 70–83 years) treated with melphalan (200 or 140 mg/m^2).[320] Of note, treatment-related mortality was higher (16%) in the initial 25 patients receiving melphalan at 200 mg/m^2. CR was achieved in 27% of patients, but median CR duration was only 1.5 years, with 3-year EFS and OS rates projected at 20% and 31%, respectively. Although this study confirms the feasibility of HDT in older patients with MM, it also indicates a higher risk in this patient population, highlighting the need for strict patient selection based on clinical status.

Management of Patients with Renal Dysfunction

One-third of patients with overt MM present with renal insufficiency. With hydration, control of hypercalcemia, and effective therapy, it is reversible in 50% cases. Renal dysfunction of less than 6 months' duration and rapid initiation of therapy with reduction in monoclonal protein are associated with higher likelihood of improvement in renal function. Improved renal function is observed mainly in patients with light chain cast nephropathy and light chain deposition disease; therefore, renal biopsy is used to identify these reversible conditions and the need for aggressive treatment. A number of agents can be safely used in patients with renal dysfunction. This includes steroids, melphalan,[321] cyclophosphamide, bortezomib,[279,322] and thalidomide. Ease of administration, limited toxicity, and effectiveness make these novel agents the primary modes of therapy for myeloma patients with renal failure. In one retrospective analysis, 24 patients on dialysis were treated with bortezomib or bortezomib-based combinations. Of 20 patients with available response data, 75% patients achieved at least PR, with 30% patients achieving CR/nCR. One patient was spared dialysis, and three other patients became independent of dialysis following bortezomib-based treatment.[279,322] Lenalidomide has predominant renal excretion and requires dose modification if used in patients with renal failure based on creatinine claerance.[322] As the pharmacokinetics of melphalan are unaltered by renal failure, such patients are potentially candidates for HDT.[321]

Based on these observation, high-dose melphalan and PBSC transplantation was used to treat 81 patients with MM and renal dysfunction (creatinine >2 mg/dL).[323] In this setting, renal failure had no impact on the quality of stem cell collection and/or engraftment. However, treatment-related mortality rates were 6% and 13% after the first and second autologous stem cell transplants, respectively, and melphalan at 200 mg/m^2

TABLE 136.15

RANDOMIZED STUDIES COMPARING MAINTENANCE THERAPY IN MYELOMA

Study (Ref.)	Regimen	PFS (Median mo)	OS (Median mo)
Spencer et al. (326a)	Control vs. thalidomide/prednisone	23 vs. 42 (P <.001)	75 vs. 86 (P = .004)
Barlogie et al. (326b)	Control vs. thalidomide	44% vs. 57%[a] (P = .01)	Not reached
Attal et al. (326)	Control vs. thalidomide + pamidronate	36 vs. 52 (P = .009)	77 vs. 87 (P = .04)
Attal et al. (326)	Control vs. lenalidomide	24 vs. NA (P <.0001)	80% vs. 88%[b]
Palumbo et al.[d]	MPRR vs. MPR	Not reached vs. 13.2 (P = .002)	Not reached
McCarthy et al.[e]	Control vs. lenalidomide	Not reached vs. 25.5 (P <.001)[c]	Not reached
Mateos et al.[f]	VP vs. VT	32 vs. 24 (P = .01)	Not reached

PFS, progression-free survival; OS, overall survival; NS, significant difference
[a]Five-year PFS rate.
[b]Survival after 3 years.
[c]Time to progression.
[d]Palumbo A, et al. *Blood* 2010;116:1940a.
[e]McCarthy PL, et al. *Blood* 2010;116:37a.
[f]Mateos MV, et al. *Blood* 2009;114:3a.

caused excessive toxicity. Complete remission was achieved in 31 patients (38%) after tandem stem cell transplant, and the probabilities of EFS and OS to 3 years were 48% and 55%, respectively. Dose reduction and close monitoring are therefore needed to ensure the safety of the procedure, and the role of transplantation in the setting of renal failure remains investigational.

Maintenance Therapy

Despite improvements in remission rates, there is no clear plateau in the survival curves following conventional therapy or HDT. Although the proportion of patients achieving CRs has increased, all patients eventually relapse. Various maintenance therapies have been evaluated in MM in an effort to sustain remission. IFN-α is the most widely evaluated agent as maintenance therapy; however, randomized studies have only demonstrated modest improvements in EFS and OS times (5–12 months) in patients achieving remission with standard-dose therapy, and its role following HDT has not been confirmed.[324] Low-dose prednisone administered on alternate days has prolonged remission duration following standard-dose therapy in a single randomized study.[325] In last few years numbers of studies have evaluated novel agent–based maintenance regimen (Table 136.15). Attal et al.[326] from the IFM group reported improved probability of EFS and OS at 3 years in patients receiving thalidomide and pamidronate, compared with the patient cohorts receiving either pamidronate alone or no maintenance therapy following HDT (PFS, 52%, 37%, 36%, respectively, P <.009; OS, 87%, 74%, 77%, respectively, P <.04).In this study patients had not received thalidomide prior to its evaluation as maintenance therapy and the benefit was observed in those patients who had further evidence of response to thalidomide.

Prolonged use of thalidomide leads to development of neuropathy and in this regard lenalidomide, which has a more favorable toxicity profile, has been evaluated as maintenance therapy in the dose of 10 to 15 mg daily for 21 days of a 28-day cycle in three different studies, two posttransplantation and one following standard-dose MPR therapy. All three studies show clear evidence of benefit as observed by prolongation of PFS; however, OS in these studies with limited follow-up is not yet observed. These studies have confirmed lenalidomide as one of the standard of care for maintenance therapy in myeloma. A recent study has also highlighted use of Velcade-based maintenance regimen, especially in combination with low-dose thalidomide.[327] Additional immune manipulations such as idiotype vaccination and protein-pulsed dendritic cell-based vaccination are also strategies under evaluation as maintenance treatments to prolong EFS and OS in myeloma.

Allogeneic Transplantation

Syngeneic Transplantation

Bensinger et al.[328] have reported their experience with 11 patients receiving syngeneic transplants: five patients achieved CR and three achieved PR. The most recent update shows one patient from both groups alive 9 and 15 years after transplantation, respectively. A larger experience from the European Group for Blood and Marrow Transplantation Registry was reviewed by Gahrton et al.[329] Twenty-five patients undergoing syngeneic transplants were compared with 125 case-matched patients undergoing autotransplantation or allogeneic transplantation. The complete remission rate was not significantly different between the three grafts (twin, 68%; autologous, 48%; allogeneic, 58%). However, patients undergoing syngeneic transplantation had significantly superior median survival time compared with autologous (72 vs. 25 months; P = .009) or allogeneic (72 vs. 16 months; P = .008) transplant recipients.

Allogeneic Transplantation

Allogeneic transplantation has remained a difficult procedure for patients with myeloma. Older age population with limited donor availability, coupled with frequent renal impairment, has restricted the use of matched-sibling transplantation in MM. Additionally, almost 50% 1-year mortality has limited use of this procedure to only a high-risk patient population. Importantly, the allogeneic graft-versus-myeloma effect may result in a favorable long-term outcome after allogeneic transplantation. Results of three large studies are listed in Table 136.16. A retrospective review of case-matched analysis of European Group for Blood and Marrow Transplantation registry data compared 189 patients receiving allografts with an equal number of patients from the same period receiving autotransplants. This study showed a superior median survival outcome for patients undergoing autotransplants compared with allogeneic transplants (34 vs. 18 months, respectively).[330] The 1-year treatment-related mortality was significantly higher following allogeneic transplantation (41% with allotransplants and 13% with autotransplants). However, patients undergoing allogeneic transplantation and surviving the first year had a tendency for better PFS and OS.

TABLE 136.16

STUDIES OF ALLOGENEIC TRANSPLANTATION FOR NEWLY DIAGNOSED MYELOMA

Study (Ref.)	No. of Patients	TRM (%)	CR (%)	OS (Actuarial, mo)	EFS (Actuarial, mo)
Gahrton et al. (329)	162	41	44	28% at 84	45% at 60
Bensinger et al. (329a)	80	44	36	20% at 54	24% at 54
Alyea et al. (331)	61[a]	5	28	40% at 36	20% at 38

TRM, treatment-related mortality; CR, complete remission; OS, overall survival; EFS, event-free survival.
[a]T-cell depleted.

A very low transplant-related mortality of 10% has been reported from a single-center experience from the Dana-Farber Cancer Institute due to selective depletion of CD6+ T cells as the sole form of graft-versus-host disease (GVHD) prophylaxis.[331] However, the median PFS time was 12 months and the median OS time was 22 months, a result inferior to their previous experience of autologous transplantation. Case-matched comparative studies from other single institutions have also failed to show a survival advantage for allotransplants.[332]

Donor Lymphocyte Infusions

A graft-versus-myeloma effect has been demonstrated by the induction of CR with donor lymphocyte infusion (DLI) following relapse after allogeneic transplantation.[333] In a large study, Lokhorst et al.[334] have reported six CRs and eight PRs following DLI in 27 patients after allotransplant. Five of these patients remained disease-free more than 30 months after DLI. However, DLI was associated with acute GVHD in 55% and chronic GVHD in 26% of patients. Five patients experienced BM aplasia, which was fatal in two cases. A similar DLI experience has been reported by Salama et al.[335] Several strategies have been explored to reduce GVHD after DLI,[336,337] including lowering the number of T cells infused, selective depletion of CD8+ T cells, and use of herpes simplex virus thymidine kinase-gene transduction of DLI to allow for use of ganciclovir to deplete T cells if significant GVHD develops. Immunizing donors with idiotype vaccine may allow selective transfer of T cells specific for graft-versus-myeloma without increasing the incidence of GVHD.

Nonmyeloablative Transplants

Studies in a canine model showed that a nonmyeloablative dose of TBI could lead to successful engraftment when used in conjunction with a combination of cyclosporine and mycophenolate mofetil.[338] This animal experience, coupled with reduced day 100 transplant-related mortality in pilot studies in patients, has allowed for allogeneic-matched sibling transplantation in patients who were otherwise considered poor risk for the standard allogeneic preparative regimen. Results from larger published studies evaluating nonmyeloablative regimens with allogeneic transplantation are listed in Table 136.17 Badros et al.[339] first reported on 31 patients undergoing allogeneic transplants following nonmyeloablative conditioning with melphalan (100 mg/m^2). Transplant-related mortality in the first 120 days was low (10%). Nineteen (61%) patients achieved CR or near CR; however, acute GVHD developed in 18 patients (58%) and chronic GVHD was seen in 10 patients (35%). Giralt et al.[340] have used reduced intensity conditioning with fludarabine and melphalan in 16 patients; successful engraftment was observed in all patients; however, the 100-day mortality rate was 20% and the 1-year mortality rate was 40%, with only six patients alive after a median follow-up period of 15 months. Maloney et al.[341] have evaluated the combination of initial autotransplantation for tumor cytoreduction followed by nonmyeloablative matched-sibling transplantation in 54 patients. The treatment was performed in an outpatient setting with a low 100-day mortality (2%). The ORR was 83%, with 53% CRs. With a median follow-up of 552 days after allografting, OS is 78%. However,

TABLE 136.17

REPRESENTATIVE STUDIES OF MINIALLOGENEIC TRANSPLANTATION IN MYELOMA

Study (Ref.)	Conditioning	N	TRM at 1 Year (%)	Response (%)	Acute Grade II–IV GVHD (%)	Chronic Extensive GVHD (%)	PFS/EFS/DFS	OS
Lee et al. (342a)	Mel or Mel/ TBI/Flu	45	36	CR 64	36	36	3-y EFS 13%	Median 14 mo
Kroger et al. (342b)	PBSCT + Mel/ Flu/ATG	17	18	CR 73 PR 20	38	7	2-y DFS 56%	2-y 74%
Maloney et al. (341)	PBSCT + TBI/ MMF/cvc	54	7	CR 57 PR 26	39	46	2-y PFS 55%	18 mo 78%
Giralt et al. (340)	Mel/Flu	13	38	CR 54	38	15		
Bruno et al. (342)	PBSCT + TBI/ MMF/Cyc	58	7	CR 55 PR 31	43	36	Median 43 mo	Median >46 mo

TRM, treatment-related mortality; GVHD, graft versus host disease; PFS, progression-free survival; EFS, event-free survival; DFS, disease-free survival; OS, overall survival; CR, complete response; PBSCT, peripheral blood stem cell transplant; PR, partial response; TBI, total-body irradiation; MHF, mycophenolate mofetil; Flu, fludarabine, Cyc, cyclosporine.

GVHD continues to be a problem; 38% of patients developed acute GVHD and 46% had chronic GVHD requiring therapy.

In a recent evaluation, 162 consecutive patients less than 65 years of age with newly diagnosed myeloma received induction therapy with VAD, followed by either nonmyeloablative TBI and stem cells from the HLA-identical sibling after an initial autograft (N = 80) or two consecutive myeloablative doses of melphalan, each of which was followed by autologous stem cell rescue if HLA-identical donors were not available (N = 82). After a median follow-up of 45 months (range, 21 to 90 months), the median OS (80 vs. 54 months; *P* = .01) and EFS (35 vs. 29 months; *P* = .02) were longer in the patients with HLA-identical siblings than in the patients without HLA-identical siblings. Treatment-related mortality did not differ significantly between the two groups (*P* = .09), but disease-related mortality was significantly higher in the double-autologous transplant group (43% vs. 7%; *P* <.001). The cumulative incidence rates of higher than grades I and grade IV GVHD were 43% and 4%. These results suggest a role for allografting, especially in patients with high-risk disease where improvement in long-term outcome has been limited.[342] Although the early clinical results with nonmyeloablative transplants are encouraging, this strategy is associated with significant morbidity because of acute and chronic GVHD and a mortality rate of 10% to 20% at 1 year.

In another study, by Rosinol et al.,[343] 110 patients with multiple myeloma undergoing autologous stem cell transplantation received a second autologous stem cell transplantation (85 patients) or a reduced-intensity conditioning allograft (25 patients), depending on the HLA-matched–sibling donor availability. In this study, although there was a trend toward a longer PFS (median, 31 months vs. not reached; *P* = .08) in favor of reduced-intensity conditioning allograft, it was associated with a trend toward a higher transplantation-related mortality (16% vs. 5%; *P* = .07), and no statistical difference in EFS and OS.[343] Allogeneic transplantation should therefore only be used in the context of clinical trials attempting to improve patient outcome by both enhancing efficacy and reducing toxicity.[344]

Bisphosphonates

The second- and third-generation bisphosphonates, pamidronate and zoledronate, reduce skeletal complications and bone pain in myeloma (Table 136.18). [345,346] Their mechanism of action includes down-regulation of osteoclast activity, decreased IL-6 production, activation of gam/delta T cells with antimyeloma activity, and induction of apoptosis of osteoclasts through inhibition of farnesyl and geranyl-geranyl transferase activity.[347,348] Besides reducing bone-related problems, continued administration of pamidronate over 21 months showed some survival advantage (21 vs. 14 months; *P* = .041) in patients receiving salvage chemotherapy and pamidronate versus chemotherapy alone.[345,349] *In vitro* cytotoxic effects of bisphosphonates have been observed in myeloma cell lines,[350,351] patient cells *in vitro,* as well as in tumor specimens in the SCID-hu *in vivo* model. Preliminary reports of pamidronate administered alone frequently (every 2 weeks) have shown response or delay in disease progression in occasional patients.[352] Pamidronate 90 mg and zoledronic acid 4 mg are equipotent in reducing bone-related problems in myeloma; infusion time for zoledronic acid is 15 minutes compared to 1 to 2 hours for pamidronate.

Patients on long-term bisphosphonate therapy should be monitored for development of renal toxicity. Renal dysfunction induced by pamidronate affects mainly tubules and so it manifests first as proteinuria followed by rise in creatinine, while zoledronic acid affects glomeruli, which manifests as rise in creatinine without proteinuria. Even mild renal dysfunction requires bisphosphonate dose adjustment, and renal effects of bisphosphonates can be partly prevented by extending the duration of infusion. Osteonecrosis of the jaw (ONJ) is another complication of prolonged bisphosphonate therapy. It is observed in patients with dental procedures and in relationship to dental infection. In one study, 11 of 292 patients (3.8%) with MM had ONJ.[353] There is also some association between prolonged use and development of ONJ. With the increased detection of this complication, a prophylactic dental checkup and follow-up is recommended. After 2 years of administration, frequency of administration of bisphosphonate may be modified in patients achieving VGPR or CR.[354] In a recent large phase 3 study, antimyeloma activity of zoledronic acid has been described. Agents directed at novel bone-related targets are under investigation. Efficacy of denosumab, a RANKL targeting antibody, has been confirmed in phase 3 study in myeloma and breast cancer. An antibody targeting DKK-1 (BHQ-880), which improves osteoblastic activity, and a chimeric protein targeting activin A (ACE-011), are currently under phase 1/2 studies.

Therapy in Relapsed Patients

The options and therapeutic strategies for relapsed MM patients depend on the induction regimen used and whether

TABLE 136.18

SUMMARY OF PUBLISHED PLACEBO-CONTROLLED TRIALS OF BISPHOSPHONATES IN PATIENTS WITH MULTIPLE MYELOMA

Variable	Belch et al.	Lahtinen et al.	Berenson et al.
No. of evaluable patients	166	336	377
Bisphosphonate therapy	Etidronate 5 mg/kg daily (oral)	Clondronate 2.4 g/d (oral) for 24 mo	Pamidronate 90 mg (IV q 4 weeks × 9 cycles)
Lytic bone lesions	0	+	0
Pathologic fractures	0	0	+
Radiation therapy	NA	NA	+
Bone pain	0	0	+
Hypercalcemia	0	0	+
Survival	–	0	+

IV, intravenous; 0, no effect; +, beneficial effect; NA, not assessed.

the patients have undergone HDT and stem cell transplant. With the availability of four new agents that have been approved for clinical use in MM—thalidomide, bortezomib, lenalidomide, and liposomal doxorubicin—the choice will depend partly on the agent or combination not used as an induction and on the presence of existing toxicity such as neuropathy, cytopenia, or DVT.

The results of the international randomized phase 3 trial of bortezomib (1.3 mg/m^2 intravenously on days 1, 4, 8, and 11 every 3 weeks for eight cycles) have demonstrated its superiority over dexamethasone alone (40 mg orally on days 1–4, 9–12, and 17–20 every 5 weeks for four cycles) in terms of response rates (38% vs. 18%, respectively; $P < .001$), median time to progression (6.22 vs. 3.49 months, respectively; $P < .001$), and survival (1 year survival, 80% vs. 66%, respectively; $P = .003$) in 669 relapsed patients with multiple myeloma who had received one to three prior therapies.[276] Another open label study has further confirmed the ability of added dexamethasone to improve response in relapsed patients.

Various combinations of bortezomib with other agents such as doxorubicin, cyclophosphamide, and melphalan have been used to treat patients with multiple myeloma, and results of some larger representative studies are shown in Table 136.10B. For example, a randomized phase 3 multicenter international study has confirmed that the combination of bortezomib and pegylated liposomal doxorubicin is superior to bortezomib alone for both overall response (50% vs. 42%, respectively; $P = .05$), and time to progression (9.3 vs. 6.5 months, respectively; $P < .0001$) in relapsed MM patients. Additionally a combination of oral cyclophosphamide, dexamethasone, and bortezomib in 50 patients with relapsed/refractory multiple myeloma has been reported to achieve ORR in 88% of patients, with a median EFS of 10 months, and median OS not yet reached. The broader clinical benefit of other regimens remains to be determined.

Lenalidomide has been evaluated in two large phase 3 studies comparing it in combination with dexamethasone to high-dose dexamethasone and placebo. The combination of lenalidomide and dexamethasone showed significant advantages in response rate (CR + PR, 56% vs. 24%, respectively; $P < .001$) and in time to progression (14 vs. 5 months, respectively; $P < .01$) as well as OS (30 vs. 20 months, respectively; $P < .01$). Lenalidomide was equally active in patients with or without previous exposure to bortezomib or thalidomide. However, lenalidomide in combination with high-dose dexamethasone had significantly higher rates of DVT (14 vs. 5%, respectively; $P < .01$). Lenalidomide has been also assessed in combination with bortezomib and dexamethasone in a phase 1/2 trial in patients with relapsed or refractory multiple myeloma.

A pilot phase 1/2 study in relapsed refractory myeloma has evaluated combination of lenalidomide and bortezomib in 38 patients. A 61% minimal response or better was observed; with dexamethasone added, 83% achieved stable disease or better, which included patients who were resistant to either agents individually. Thalidomide has been an active agent, both alone and in combination with dexamethasone, in relapsed patients (Table 136.8B). Although lenalidomide activity has been demonstrated in patients relapsing after thalidomide, it is unclear whether patients relapsing after lenalidomide will respond to thalidomide. An ongoing Eastern Cooperative Oncology Group study will answer this important question. A combination of bortezomib (1.0–1.3 mg/m^2), thalidomide (50–200 mg/d), and dexamethasone (40 mg for 4 days) has been evaluated by Zangari et al. In 83 patients with relapsed/refractory disease (over 70% patients having previously received thalidomide), 80% overall response with 16% CRs was reported. In relapsed patients, combination of conventional chemotherapy not previously used with or without novel agents can be effective. Four-drug combinations DCEP (dexamethasone, cyclophosphamide, etoposide, and *cis*-platinum) have been reported to achieve high response rates in relapsed patients, especially with aggressive disease. A regimen incorporating thalidomide plus Adriamycin with DCEP (DTPACE) for relapsed/refractory patients (N = 236) prior to HDT/stem cell transplant achieved 32% partial remission rate after two cycles of DTPACE, with 16% attaining a CR or near CR.[355]

A number of newer agents have been investigated in relapsed and/or refractory myeloma. A thalidomide analogue, pomalidomide, has demonstrated activity even in patients resistant to lenalidomide. Thirty-four lenalidomide refractory patients were treated with combination of pomalidomide (2 mg orally daily) and dexamethasone (40 mg weekly). The best response achieved included VGPR in 9%, PR in 23%, and additional minimal response (MR) in 15% for an ORR of 47% and a response duration of 9.1 months. Toxicity was primarily hematologic and tolerable.[356] Ongoing phase 2 and phase 3 studies are evaluating a second generation of proteasome inhibitor, carfilzomib, which has demonstrated activity in patients refractory to bortezomib. As a single agent, 5 of 26 patients (19%) responded to carfilzomib, while response was 57% in bortezomib-naïve patients. In this early stage of its development, significant neuropathy has not been observed. Based on preclinical synergistic activity and phase 2 studies showing ability of HDAC inhibitors (vorinostat and panobinostat) to overcome bortezomib resistance, there are ongoing phase 3 studies comparing bortezomib with a combination of bortezomib with vorinostat and with panobinostat. Similarly, combination of bortezomib and AKT inhibitor perifosine is able to overcome bortezomib resistance, leading to a phase 3 study. Finally, an antibody targeting CS-1 cell surface molecule elotozumab has been shown to achiever over 80% response when combined with lenalidomide/dexamethasone in a relapsed patient population. This combination is now undergoing phase 3 evaluation in relapsed myeloma.

Other Potential Agents and Future Direction

Both *in vitro* systems and *in vivo* animal models have been developed to characterize mechanisms of MM cell homing to BM, as well as factors (MM cell-BM stromal cell interactions, cytokines, angiogenesis) promoting MM cell growth, survival, drug resistance, and migration in the BM milieu. These model systems have allowed for the development of several promising biologically based therapies that can target the MM cell and the BM microenvironment. This includes pomalidomide, the next generation of proteasome inhibitors (carfilzomib and NPI 0052), VEGF receptor kinase inhibitor PTK787, HDAC inhibitors, and heat shock protein 90 inhibitor (AUY 922); those that target MM cells directly, including telomerase inhibitor GRN 163L, antibodies directed at CD40, CS-1, CD70, IL-6, and IGK-1; and those that target only the BM microenvironment, including IκB kinase inhibitors and p38MAPK inhibitors, among others (Fig. 136.15). To optimize response, these agents will need to be combined in a rational biologically based fashion. Based on genomic and proteomic analysis, a number of combinations have been preclinically evaluated and are under evaluation in derived phase 2 and 3 clinical studies. As previously described, the combination of bortezomib, which inhibits DNA repair pathway, and liposomal doxorubicin, which damages DNA, has shown efficacy in relapsed MM. Based on cell signaling studies showing up-regulation of AKT activity in myeloma following *in vitro* exposure to bortezomib, preclinical studies were performed and demonstrated synergistic activity of

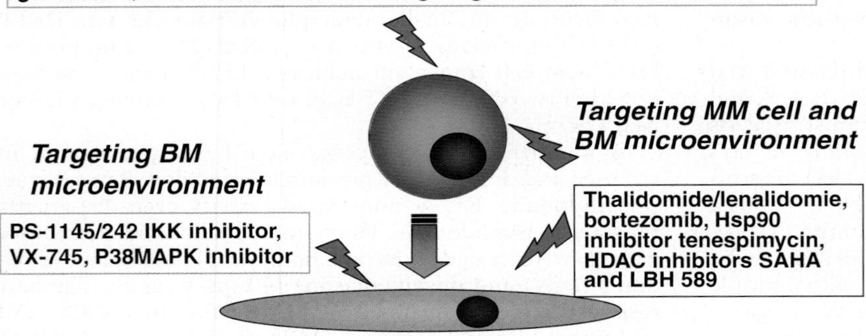

FIGURE 136.15 Novel therapies in preclinical or clinical development targeting the myeloma cells or their microenvironment or both. MM, multiple myeloma; BM, bone marrow.

bortezomib and Akt inhibitor perifosine. A derived clinical study has demonstrated that the combination can overcome bortezomib resistance. The detailed oncogenomic studies are identifying novel targets and pathways operative in myeloma, and ongoing studies are determining mechanisms of action of novel agents at a gene and protein level in order to provide the framework for rational combination clinical trials to overcome drug resistance and improve patient outcome.

Selected References

The full list of references for this chapter appears in the online version.

6. Chauhan D, Uchiyama H, Akbarali Y, et al. Multiple myeloma cell adhesion-induced interleukin-6 expression in bone marrow stromal cells involves activation of NF-kappa B. *Blood* 1996;87:1104.
24. Kyle RA, Therneau TM, Rajkumar SV, et al. A long-term study of prognosis in monoclonal gammopathy of undetermined significance. *N Engl J Med* 2002;346:564.
27. Malik AA, Ganti AK, Potti A, Levitt R, Hanley JF. Role of Helicobacter pylori infection in the incidence and clinical course of monoclonal gammopathy of undetermined significance. *Am J Gastroenterol* 2002;97:1371.
30. Landgren O, Kyle RA, Pfeiffer RM, et al. Monoclonal gammopathy of undetermined significance (MGUS) consistently precedes multiple myeloma: a prospective study. *Blood* 2009;113:5412.
31. Brown LM, Gridley G, Check D, Landgren O. Risk of multiple myeloma and monoclonal gammopathy of undetermined significance among white and black male United States veterans with prior autoimmune, infectious, inflammatory, and allergic disorders. *Blood* 2008;111:3388.
42. Davies FE, Dring AM, Li C, et al. Insights into the multistep transformation of MGUS to myeloma using microarray expression analysis. *Blood* 2003;102:4504.
45. Kaufmann H, Ackermann J, Baldia C, et al. Both IGH translocations and chromosome 13q deletions are early events in monoclonal gammopathy of undetermined significance and do not evolve during transition to multiple myeloma. *Leukemia* 2004;18:1879.
48. Sawyer J, Waldron J, Jagannath S, Barlogie B. Cytogenetics findings in 200 patients with multiple myeloma. *Cancer Genet Cytogenet* 1995;82:41.
51. Perez-Simon JA, Garcia-Sanz R, Tabernero MD, et al. Prognostic value of numerical chromosome aberrations in multiple myeloma: a FISH analysis of 15 different chromosomes. *Blood* 1998;91:3366.
55. Drach J, Angerler J, Schuster J, et al. Interphase fluorescence in situ hybridization identifies chromosomal abnormalities in plasma cells from patients with monoclonal gammopathy of undetermined significance. *Blood* 1995;86:3915.
59. Chesi M, Nardini E, Brents LA, et al. Frequent translocation t(4;14) (p16.3;q32.3) in multiple myeloma is associated with increased expression and activating mutations of fibroblast growth factor receptor 3. *Nat Genet* 1997;16:260.
62. Chesi M, Bergsagel PL, Shonukan OO, et al. Frequent dysregulation of the c-maf proto-oncogene at 16q23 by translocation to an Ig locus in multiple myeloma. *Blood* 1998;91:4457.
66. Avet-Loiseau H, Gerson F, Magrangeas F, Minvielle S, Harousseau JL, Bataille R. Rearrangements of the c-myc oncogene are present in 15% of primary human multiple myeloma tumors. *Blood* 2001;98:3082.
72. Urashima M, Ogata A, Chauhan D, et al. Interleukin-6 promotes multiple myeloma cell growth via phosphorylation of retinoblastoma protein. *Blood* 1996;88:2219.
87. Shammas MA, Shmookler Reis RJ, Akiyama M, et al. Telomerase inhibition and cell growth arrest by G-quadruplex interactive agent in multiple myeloma. *Mol Cancer Ther* 2003;2:825.
88. Bergsagel DE, Kuehl M, Zhan F, Sawyer J, Barlogie B, Shaughnessy J. Cyclin D dysregulation: an early and unifying pathogenic event in multiple myeloma. *Blood* 2005;106:296.
89. Shaughnessy JD Jr, Zhan F, Burington BE, et al. A validated gene expression model of high-risk multiple myeloma is defined by deregulated expression of genes mapping to chromosome 1. *Blood* 2007;109:2276.
90. Decaux O, Lode L, Magrangeas F, et al. Prediction of survival in multiple myeloma based on gene expression profiles reveals cell cycle and chromosomal instability signatures in high-risk patients and hyperdiploid signatures in low-risk patients: a study of the Intergroupe Francophone du Myelome. *J Clin Oncol* 2008;26:4798.
91. Broyl A, Hose D, Lokhorst H, et al. Gene expression profiling for molecular classification of multiple myeloma in newly diagnosed patients. *Blood* 2010;116:2543.
92. Pichiorri F, Suh SS, Ladetto M, et al. MicroRNAs regulate critical genes associated with multiple myeloma pathogenesis. *Proc Natl Acad Sci U S A* 2008;105:12885.
94. Pichiorri F, Suh SS, Rocci A, et al. Downregulation of p53-inducible microRNAs 192, 194, and 215 Impairs the p53/MDM2 Autoregulatory Loop in Multiple Myeloma Development. *Cancer Cell* 18:367.
95. Dhodapkar MV, Kelly T, Theus A, Athota AB, Barlogie B, Sanderson RD. Elevated levels of shed syndecan-1 correlate with tumour mass and decreased matrix metalloproteinase-9 activity in the serum of patients with multiple myeloma [published erratum appears in *Br J Haematol* 1998; 101(2):398]. *Br J Haematol* 1997;99:368.
99. Hideshima T, Chauhan D, Schlossman R, Richardson P, Anderson KC. The role of Tumor necrosis factor a in the pathophysiology of human multiple myeloma: therapeutic applications. *Oncogene* 2001;20:4519.
103. Keats JJ, Fonseca R, Chesi M, et al. Promiscuous mutations activate the noncanonical NF-kappaB pathway in multiple myeloma. *Cancer Cell* 2007;12:131.
104. Annunziata CM, Davis RE, Demchenko Y, et al. Frequent engagement of the classical and alternative NF-kappaB pathways by diverse genetic abnormalities in multiple myeloma. *Cancer Cell* 2007;12:115.
108. Rajkumar SV, Mesa RA, Fonseca R, et al. Bone marrow angiogenesis in 400 patients with monoclonal gammopathy of undetermined significance, multiple myeloma, and primary amyloidosis. *Clin Cancer Res* 2002;8:2210.

109. Munshi NC, Wilson C. Increased bone marrow microvessel density in newly diagnosed multiple myeloma carries a poor prognosis. *Semin Oncol* 2001;28:565.
117. Mitsiades CS, Mitsiades N, Poulaki V, et al. Activation of NF-kappaB and upregulation of intracellular anti-apoptotic proteins via the IGF-1/Akt signaling in human multiple myeloma cells: therapeutic implications. *Oncogene* 2002;21:5673.
119. Akiyama M, Hideshima T, Hayashi T, et al. Cytokines modulate telomerase activity in a human multiple myeloma cell line. *Cancer Res* 2002;62:3876.
122. Gupta D, Treon SP, Shima Y, et al. Adherence of multiple myeloma cells to bone marrow stromal cells upregulates vascular endothelial growth factor secretion: therapeutic applications. *Leukemia* 2001;15:1950.
124. Prabhala RH, Pelluru D, Fulciniti M, et al. Elevated IL-17 produced by TH17 cells promotes myeloma cell growth and inhibits immune function in multiple myeloma. *Blood* 2010;115:5385.
140. Matsui W, Huff CA, Wang Q, et al. Characterization of clonogenic multiple myeloma cells. *Blood* 2004;103:2332.
141. Pilarski LM, Andrews EJ, Mant MJ, Ruether BA. Humoral immune deficiency in multiple myeloma patients due to compromised B-cell function. *J Clin Immunol* 1986;6:491.
142. Munshi NC. Immunoregulatory mechanisms in multiple myeloma. *Hematol Oncol Clin North Am* 1997;11:51.
150. Song W, van der Vliet HJ, Tai YT, et al. Generation of antitumor invariant natural killer T cell lines in multiple myeloma and promotion of their functions via lenalidomide: a strategy for immunotherapy. *Clin Cancer Res* 2008;14:6955.
151. Prabhala RH, Neri P, Bae JE, et al. Dysfunctional T regulatory cells in multiple myeloma. *Blood* 2006;107:301.
152. Yi Q, Osterborg A, Bergenbrant S, Mellstedt H, Holm G, Lefvert AK. Idiotype-reactive T-cell subsets and tumor load in monoclonal gammopathies. *Blood* 1995;86:3043.
156. Tassone P, Neri P, Carrasco DR, et al. A clinically relevant SCID-hu in vivo model of human multiple myeloma. *Blood* 2005;106:713.
157. Urashima M, Chen BP, Chen S, et al. The development of a model for the homing of multiple myeloma cells to human bone marrow. *Blood* 1997; 90:754.
159. Carrasco DR, Sukhdeo K, Protopopova M, et al. The differentiation and stress response factor XBP-1 drives multiple myeloma pathogenesis. *Cancer Cell* 2007;11:349.
161. Solomon A, Weiss DT, Kattine AA. Nephrotoxic potential of Bence Jones proteins [see comments]. *N Engl J Med* 1991;324:1845.
185. Lacy MQ, Gertz MA, Hanson CA, Inwards DJ, Kyle RA. Multiple myeloma associated with diffuse osteosclerotic bone lesions: a clinical entity distinct from osteosclerotic myeloma (POEMS syndrome). *Am J Hematol* 1997;56:288.
186. Miralles GD, O'Fallon JR, Talley NJ. Plasma-cell dyscrasia with polyneuropathy. The spectrum of POEMS syndrome. *N Engl J Med* 1992;327: 1919.
189. Fassas AB, Muwalla F, Berryman T, et al. Myeloma of the central nervous system: association with high-risk chromosomal abnormalities, plasmablastic morphology and extramedullary manifestations. *Br J Haematol* 2002;117:103.
205. Zent CS, Wilson CS, Tricot G, et al. Oligoclonal protein bands and Ig isotype switching in multiple myeloma treated with high-dose therapy and hematopoietic cell transplantation. *Blood* 1998;91:3518.
208. Rajkumar SV, Kyle RA, Therneau TM, et al. Serum free light chain ratio is an independent risk factor for progression in monoclonal gammopathy of undetermined significance. *Blood* 2005;106:812.
209. Dispenzieri A, Lacy MQ, Katzmann JA, et al. Absolute values of immunoglobulin free light chains are prognostic in patients with primary systemic amyloidosis undergoing peripheral blood stem cell transplantation. *Blood* 2006;107:3378.
210. Mead GP, Carr-Smith HD, Drayson MT, Morgan GJ, Child JA, Bradwell AR. Serum free light chains for monitoring multiple myeloma. *Br J Haematol* 2004;126:348.
221. Avet-Loiseau H, Daviet A, Brigaudeau C, et al. Cytogenetic, interphase, and multicolor fluorescence in situ hybridization analyses in primary plasma cell leukemia: a study of 40 patients at diagnosis, on behalf of the Intergroupe Francophone du Myelome and the Groupe Francais de Cytogenetique Hematologique. *Blood* 2001;97:822.
229. Walker R, Barlogie B, Haessler J, et al. Magnetic resonance imaging in multiple myeloma: diagnostic and clinical implications. *J Clin Oncol* 2007;25:1121.
231. Dimopoulos M, Terpos E, Comenzo RL, et al. International myeloma working group consensus statement and guidelines regarding the current role of imaging techniques in the diagnosis and monitoring of multiple Myeloma. *Leukemia* 2009;23:1545.
237. Attal M, Harousseau JL, Facon T, et al. Single versus double autologous stem-cell transplantation for multiple myeloma. *N Engl J Med* 2003; 349:2495.
242. Dimopoulos MA, Moulopoulos A, Delasalle K, Alexanian R. Solitary plasmacytoma of bone and asymptomatic multiple myeloma. [Review] [29 refs]. *Hematol Oncol Clin North Am* 1992;6:359.
245. Corwin J, Lindberg RD. Solitary plasmacytoma of bone vs. extramedullary plasmacytoma. *Cancer* 1979;43:1007.
247. Kyle RA, Remstein ED, Therneau TM, et al. Clinical course and prognosis of smoldering (asymptomatic) multiple myeloma. *N Engl J Med* 2007; 356:2582.
248. Dispenzieri A, Kyle RA, Katzmann JA, et al. Immunoglobulin free light chain ratio is an independent risk factor for progression of smoldering (asymptomatic) multiple myeloma. *Blood* 2008;111:785.
256. Rajkumar SV, Jacobus S, Callander NS, et al. Lenalidomide plus high-dose dexamethasone versus lenalidomide plus low-dose dexamethasone as initial therapy for newly diagnosed multiple myeloma: an open-label randomised controlled trial. *Lancet Oncol* 2010;11:29.
260. Barlogie B, Kyle RA, Anderson KC, et al. Standard chemotherapy compared with high-dose chemoradiotherapy for multiple myeloma: final results of phase III US Intergroup Trial S9321. *J Clin Oncol* 2006;24:929.
266. Barlogie B, Desikan R, Eddlemon P, et al. Extended survival in advanced and refractory multiple myeloma after single-agent thalidomide: identification of prognostic factors in a phase 2 study of 169 patients. *Blood* 2001;98:492.
268. Palumbo A, Rajkumar SV, Dimopoulos MA, et al. Prevention of thalidomide-and lenalidomide-associated thrombosis in myeloma. *Leukemia* 2008; 22:414.
271. Hideshima T, Anderson KC. Molecular mechanisms of novel therapeutic approaches for multiple myeloma. *Nat Rev Cancer* 2002;2:927.
275. Richardson PG, Barlogie B, Berenson J, et al. A phase 2 study of bortezomib in relapsed, refractory myeloma. *N Engl J Med* 2003;348:2609.
276. Richardson PG, Sonneveld P, Schuster MW, et al. Bortezomib or high-dose dexamethasone for relapsed multiple myeloma. *N Engl J Med* 2005; 352:2487.
277. Orlowski RZ, Zhuang SH, Parekh T, Xiu L, Harousseau JL. The combination of pegylated liposomal doxorubicin and bortezomib significantly improves time to progression of patients with relapsed/refractory multiple myeloma compared with bortezomib alone: results from a planned interim analysis of a randomized phase III study. *Blood* 2006;108:404a.
282. Zonder JA, Crowley J, Hussein MA, et al. Lenalidomide and high-dose dexamethasone compared with dexamethasone as initial therapy for multiple myeloma: a randomized Southwest Oncology Group trial (S0232). *Blood* 2010;116:5838.
283. Harousseau JL, Attal M, Avet-Loiseau H, et al. Bortezomib plus dexamethasone is superior to vincristine plus doxorubicin plus dexamethasone as induction treatment prior to autologous stem-cell transplantation in newly diagnosed multiple myeloma: results of the IFM 2005-01 phase III trial. *J Clin Oncol* 2010;28:4621.
284. Avet-Loiseau H, Leleu X, Roussel M, et al. Bortezomib plus dexamethasone induction improves outcome of patients with t(4;14) myeloma but not outcome of patients with del(17p). *J Clin Oncol* 2010;28:4630.
285. Reeder CB, Reece DE, Kukreti V, et al. Cyclophosphamide, bortezomib and dexamethasone induction for newly diagnosed multiple myeloma: high response rates in a phase II clinical trial. *Leukemia* 2009;23:1337.
286. Richardson PG, Weller E, Lonial S, et al. Lenalidomide, bortezomib, and dexamethasone combination therapy in patients with newly diagnosed multiple myeloma. *Blood* 2010;116:679.
287. San Miguel JF, Schlag R, Khuageva NK, et al. Bortezomib plus melphalan and prednisone for initial treatment of multiple myeloma. *N Engl J Med* 2008;359:906.
293. Attal M, Harousseau JL, Stoppa AM, et al. A prospective, randomized trial of autologous bone marrow transplantation and chemotherapy in multiple myeloma. Intergroupe Francais du Myelome. *N Engl J Med* 1996;335:91.
294. Child JA, Morgan GJ, Davies FE, et al. High-dose chemotherapy with hematopoietic stem-cell rescue for multiple myeloma. *N Engl J Med* 2003; 348:1875.
296. Fermand JP, Ravaud P, Chevret S, et al. High-dose therapy and autologous peripheral blood stem cell transplantation in multiple myeloma: up-front or rescue treatment? Results of a multicenter sequential randomized clinical trial. *Blood* 1998;92:3131.
297. Koreth J, Cutler CS, Djulbegovic B, et al. High-dose therapy with single autologous transplantation versus chemotherapy for newly diagnosed multiple myeloma: A systematic review and meta-analysis of randomized controlled trials. *Biol Blood Marrow Transplant* 2007;13:183.
298. Harousseau JL, Milpied N, Laporte JP, et al. Double-intensive therapy in high-risk multiple myeloma. *Blood* 1992;79:2827.
301. Kumar S, Dispenzieri A, Lacy MQ, et al. Impact of lenalidomide therapy on stem cell mobilization and engraftment post-peripheral blood stem cell transplantation in patients with newly diagnosed myeloma. *Leukemia* 2007;21:2035.
309. Fermand JP, Levy Y, Gerota J, et al. Treatment of aggressive multiple myeloma by high-dose chemotherapy and total body irradiation followed by blood stem cells autologous graft. *Blood* 1989;73:20.
313. Stewart AK, Vescio R, Schiller G, et al. Purging of autologous peripheral-blood stem cells using CD34 selection does not improve overall or progression-free survival after high-dose chemotherapy for multiple myeloma: results of a multicenter randomized controlled trial. *J Clin Oncol* 2001;19:3771.

322. Dimopoulos MA, Terpos E, Chanan-Khan A, et al. Renal impairment in patients with multiple myeloma: a consensus statement on behalf of the International Myeloma Working Group. *J Clin Oncol* 2010.
327. Mateos MV, Oriol A, Martinez-Lopez J, et al. Bortezomib, melphalan, and prednisone versus bortezomib, thalidomide, and prednisone as induction therapy followed by maintenance treatment with bortezomib and thalidomide versus bortezomib and prednisone in elderly patients with untreated multiple myeloma: a randomised trial. *Lancet Oncol* 2010;11:934.
342. Bruno B, Rotta M, Patriarca F, et al. A comparison of allografting with autografting for newly diagnosed myeloma. *N Engl J Med* 2007;356:1110.
344. Lokhorst H, Einsele H, Vesole D, et al. International Myeloma Working Group consensus statement regarding the current status of allogeneic stem-cell transplantation for multiple myeloma. *J Clin Oncol* 2010;28:4521.
349. Berenson JR, Lichtenstein A, Porter L, et al. Long-term pamidronate treatment of advanced multiple myeloma patients reduces skeletal events. Myeloma Aredia Study Group. *J Clin Oncol* 1998;16:593.
354. Kyle RA, Yee GC, Somerfield MR, et al. American Society of Clinical Oncology 2007 clinical practice guideline update on the role of bisphosphonates in multiple myeloma. *J Clin Oncol* 2007;25:2464.
355. Lee CK, Barlogie B, Munshi N, et al. DTPACE: an effective, novel combination chemotherapy with thalidomide for previously treated patients with myeloma. *J Clin Oncol* 2003;21:2732.

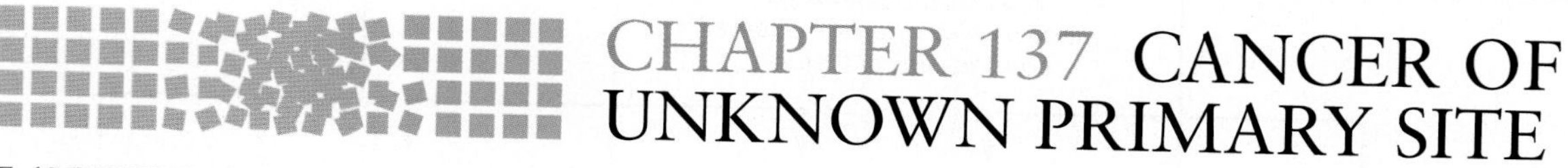

CHAPTER 137 CANCER OF UNKNOWN PRIMARY SITE

F. ANTHONY GRECO AND JOHN D. HAINSWORTH

Cancer of unknown primary (CUP) site is a clinical syndrome that represents many types of cancers. Patients are considered to have CUP if no primary site is identified after a standard clinical and pathological evaluation. As diagnostic techniques improve, the spectrum of patients with CUP continues to evolve.

Patients with CUP are common. The exact incidence is unknown because many of these patients are "assigned" other diagnoses and therefore are not accurately represented in tumor registries (see section "Carcinoma of Unknown Primary Site as a Distinct Clinical Syndrome"). Nonetheless, in the United States, CUP accounted for approximately 2% of all cancer diagnoses reported by Surveillance, Epidemiology, and End Results (SEER) registries.[1] International registries from seven other countries have reported incidences ranging from 2.3% to 7.8%.[2] The authors believe a more realistic estimate of the incidence of these patients is 5% of all invasive cancers, approximately 80,000 to 90,000 patients per year in the United States.

Within this heterogeneous patient group, there are a wide variety of clinical presentations and histologic tumor types. Most patients have metastatic carcinoma; however, some neoplasms are difficult to categorize using histologic features alone. Improvements in the evaluation of tumors using immunohistochemical (IHC) staining has aided in differential diagnosis, particularly in separating carcinomas from neoplasms of other lineages. The recent development of molecular gene profiling of tumors promises to aid in defining the tissue of origin of various metastatic adenocarcinomas.

Treatment for patients with CUP has improved slowly and has been the focus of only scattered clinical trials. Early autopsy studies, which showed a preponderance of primary sites considered at the time to be untreatable (lung, pancreas, stomach, colon, liver), have added to the negativity surrounding the diagnosis of CUP.[3] Nevertheless, several important patient subsets, identified either by clinical or pathologic features, are now known to benefit from specific first-line therapy. Also during the past 20 years, treatment has improved for many advanced solid tumors. Standard treatment now improves survival for patients with advanced cancers of the colon, lung, ovary, breast, stomach, kidney, gallbladder, and others. Novel agents for the treatment of cancer are being developed at an accelerated rate. Improved diagnosis of patients with CUP is therefore critical, so that site-specific treatments can be applied.

This chapter is divided into three major sections. The first section, greatly expanded in this edition, reviews the pathologic evaluation of patients with CUP. New information regarding the emerging role of molecular tumor profiling is included. In the second section, the clinical evaluation of CUP patients is summarized. Situations in which results from the pathologic evaluation direct the clinical evaluation are addressed. Finally, the treatment of patients with CUP is discussed, with special focus on specific treatable patient subsets.

PATHOLOGIC EVALUATION

Histologic examination of a biopsy tumor specimen remains the gold standard for initial evaluation and provides a practical classification system on which to base subsequent evaluation. In the broad category of CUP, there are five major light microscopic histologic diagnoses: (1) poorly differentiated neoplasm, (2) poorly differentiated carcinoma (with or without features of adenocarcinoma), (3) well-differentiated and moderately well-differentiated adenocarcinoma, (4) squamous cell carcinoma, and (5) neuroendocrine carcinoma. Sarcoma and melanoma are also occasionally diagnosed without an obvious primary tumor site, and management of these patients follows established guidelines.

These histologic diagnoses vary to some extent with respect to clinical characteristics, recommended diagnostic evaluation, treatment, and prognosis. The approximate size of the various groups and subsets of patients are illustrated in Figure 137.1.

Histologic Subtypes

Poorly Differentiated Neoplasms of Unknown Primary Site

If the pathologist cannot differentiate a general category of neoplasm (e.g., carcinoma, lymphoma, melanoma, sarcoma), the tumor is designated a poorly differentiated neoplasm. A more precise diagnosis is essential because many patients in this category have responsive tumors. Approximately 5% of all patients with CUP (4,000 patients annually in the United States) present with this diagnosis by routine hematoxylin and eosin (H&E) light microscopy, but few remain without a defined lineage after specialized pathologic study.[4–7] The most frequent tumor for which effective therapy is available is non-Hodgkin's lymphoma. In reported series, 35% to 65% of poorly differentiated neoplasms were found to be lymphomas after further pathologic study.[4,5] Most of the remaining tumors in this group are carcinomas, including poorly differentiated neuroendocrine tumors. Melanoma and sarcoma together account for less than 15% of all patients.

Immunohistochemical staining, electron microscopy, and genetic analysis are helpful in the differential diagnosis. The most common cause of a nonspecific light microscopic diagnosis is an inadequate or poorly handled biopsy specimen. If

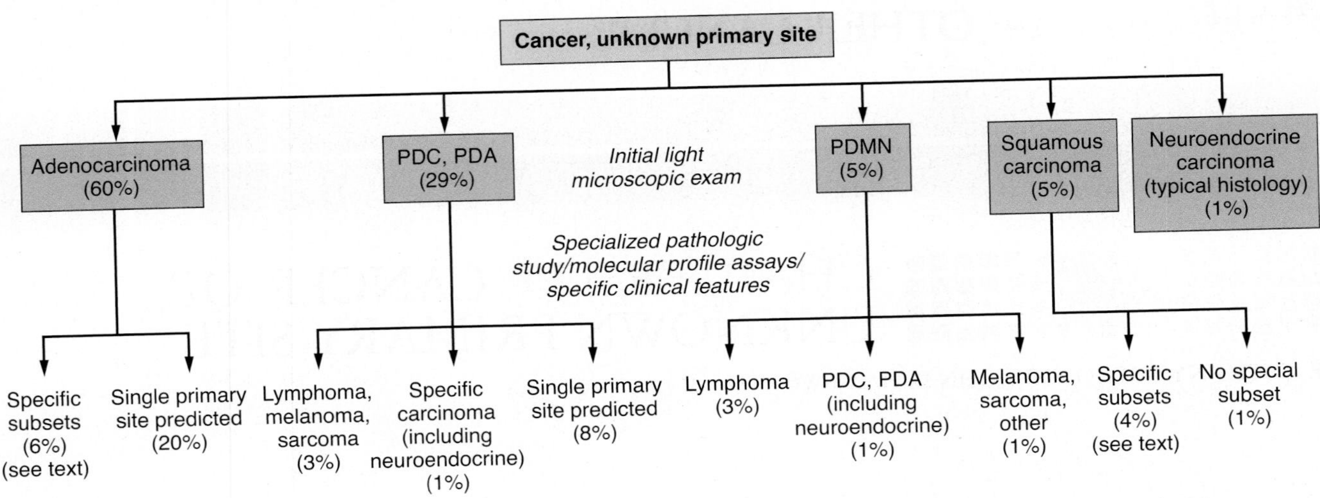

FIGURE 137.1 Relative size of various clinical and histologic subgroups of patients as determined by clinical and pathologic evaluations. PDC, poorly differentiated carcinoma; PDA, poorly differentiated adenocarcinoma; WD, well differentiated; PDMN, poorly differentiated malignant neoplasm.

possible, fine needle aspiration biopsy should not be performed as an *initial* diagnostic procedure because the histologic pattern is not preserved and the ability to perform special studies is limited.

Poorly Differentiated Carcinoma

Poorly differentiated carcinomas (PDC) account for approximately 30% of CUP (about 25,000 patients annually in the United States). In approximately one third of these patients, some features of adenocarcinomatous differentiation can be identified (poorly differentiated adenocarcinoma). Some patients have extremely responsive neoplasms, and therefore careful pathologic evaluation is crucial.

Histopathologic features that can differentiate chemotherapy-responsive tumors from nonresponsive tumors have not been identified.[8] Even with careful retrospective review of these tumors, responsive tumors of well-defined types (e.g., germ cell tumor, lymphoma) are only rarely identified.

All PDCs should undergo additional pathologic study with IHC staining (see section "Immunohistochemical Staining"). In selected tumors, electron microscopy, karyotypic/cytogenetic analysis, and gene expression profiling are also appropriate. Although site-directed or -tailored therapy based on these diagnoses seems reasonable now, there are still only preliminary data supporting an improved outcome with this approach for these patients.

Electron microscopy can be useful for a small minority of these carcinomas and should be reserved for tumors in which IHC is not contributory. Lymphoma can be diagnosed reliably in most instances in those tumors mistakenly believed to be carcinoma. In addition, sarcoma, melanoma, mesothelioma, and neuroendocrine tumors occasionally are defined by subcellular features.

Identification of cytogenetic abnormalities may be useful in patients with PDC. In reference to germ cell tumors, Motzer et al.[9] performed karyotypic analysis on tumors in 40 young men with extragonadal germ cell syndrome or midline carcinomas of uncertain histogenesis. In 12 of the 40 patients abnormalities of chromosome 12 (e.g., i[12p]; del [12p]; multiple copies of 12 p) were diagnostic of germ cell tumor. Other specific abnormalities were diagnostic of melanoma (two patients), lymphoma (one patient), peripheral neuroepithelioma (one patient), and desmoplastic small cell tumor (one patient). Of the germ cell tumors diagnosed on the basis of genetic analysis, five patients achieved a complete response to cisplatin-based chemotherapy. This confirms the authors' previously formulated hypothesis that some of these patients have histologically atypical germ cell tumors. These genetic findings can be diagnostic in these patients.

Autopsy data looking specifically at patients with PDC are limited. Based on the limited necropsy data the authors have accumulated, it appears that primary sites are found in only a minority of these patients (about 40%). These findings are contrary to those for well-differentiated or poorly differentiated adenocarcinoma of unknown primary site, in which the primary site is found in most patients (about 75%) at autopsy.[3,6]

Adenocarcinoma

Well-differentiated and moderately well-differentiated adenocarcinomas are the most common tumors identified by light microscopy and account for 60% of CUP diagnoses (about 50,000 patients annually in the United States). These are the patients that many physicians associate with the entity of CUP. Typically, patients with adenocarcinoma of unknown primary site are elderly and have metastatic tumors at multiple sites. The sites of tumor involvement frequently determine the clinical presentation; common metastatic sites include lymph nodes, liver, lung, and bone.

The diagnosis of well-differentiated or moderately well-differentiated adenocarcinoma is based on light microscopic features, particularly the formation of glandular structures by neoplastic cells. The authors have considered patients with well-differentiated or moderately well-differentiated adenocarcinoma as one group. All adenocarcinomas share histologic features, and the primary tumor site usually cannot be determined by histologic examination. Certain histologic features are typically associated with a particular tumor type (e.g., papillary features with ovarian cancer and signet ring cells with gastric cancer). However, these features are not specific enough to be used as definitive evidence of the primary site.

The identification of relatively cell-specific antigens by IHC staining has improved the ability to predict the site of origin in patients with adenocarcinoma of unknown primary site.[7,10] Panels of IHC stains are most useful and are often directed by clinical features (e.g., sites of metastases, gender). Molecular tumor profiling assays also appear relatively accurate and often provide additional diagnostic information. Both of these new diagnostic modalities should be considered in the pathologic evaluation of adenocarcinoma of unknown primary site (see sections "Immunohistochemical Staining" and "Gene Expression Profiling and Cancer of Unknown Primary Classification").

Squamous Carcinoma

Squamous carcinoma of unknown primary site represents approximately 5% of patients with CUP (about 4,000 patients annually in the United States). Effective treatment is available for patients with certain clinical syndromes (approximately 90% of patients), and appropriate clinical evaluation is important.

The diagnosis of squamous carcinoma is usually definitively made by examination of histology. Additional pathologic evaluation is usually not necessary. However, IHC staining or molecular studies should be considered in patients with poorly differentiated squamous carcinoma, particularly if the clinical presentation is atypical.

Neuroendocrine Carcinoma

Neuroendocrine carcinomas with widely varying clinical and histologic features are represented in patients with CUP. Neuroendocrine tumors account for approximately 3% of all CUP (about 3,500 patients annually in the United States). Improved pathologic methods for diagnosing neuroendocrine tumors have resulted in the recognition of an increased incidence and wider spectrum of these neoplasms.

Two subgroups of neuroendocrine carcinoma can be routinely recognized by histologic features. Well-differentiated or low-grade neuroendocrine tumors share the same histologic features as carcinoids and islet cell tumors and frequently secrete bioactive substances. A second histologic group (variously described as small-cell carcinoma, atypical carcinoid, or poorly differentiated neuroendocrine carcinoma) has typical neuroendocrine features and an aggressive histology.

A third group of neuroendocrine carcinomas appears histologically as a poorly differentiated neoplasm or poorly differentiated carcinoma. Accurate identification of these tumors requires IHC staining and occasionally electron microscopy or molecular tumor profiling.

Immunohistochemical Tumor Staining

Immunohistochemical staining is the most widely available specialized technique for the classification of neoplasms. Staining usually can be done on formalin-fixed, paraffin-embedded tissue, which broadens its applicability. Immunohistochemical antibodies are usually directed at normal cellular proteins. These proteins are commonly retained during neoplastic transformation. Many new antibodies are being developed against a variety of rather cell-specific proteins, making this area of diagnostic pathology a dynamic and evolving field.

Several important questions can usually be answered by IHC staining. The correct lineage of poorly differentiated neoplasms can be reliably identified in most instances[7,10–12] (Table 137.1). In particular, lymphomas (common leukocyte antigen

TABLE 137.1

IMMUNOHISTOCHEMICAL TUMOR STAINING PATTERNS IN THE DIFFERENTIAL DIAGNOSIS OF CANCER OF UNKNOWN PRIMARY

Tumor Type	Immunohistochemical Staining
Carcinomas	pan-cytokeratin AE1/3 (+), EMA (+), S100 (−), CLA (−), vimentin (−), CK7, 20 (variable)
Lymphomas	CLA (+), pan-cytokeratin AE1/3 (−), EMA (−), S100 (−)
Melanoma	S100 (+), HMB45 (+), melan-A (+), pan-cytokeratin (–), CLA (−)
Sarcoma	vimentin (+), desmin (+), CD117 (+), myogen (+), factor VIII antigen (+), pan-cytokeratin AE1/3 (usually–), S100 (usually –),CLA (−), HMB45 (−), melan-A (−)
Neuroendocrine	Epithelial stains (+), chromogranin (+), synaptophysin (+)
Specific Carcinomas	
Colorectal	CK20 (+), CK7 (−), CDX2 (+)
Lung: adenocarcinoma	CK7(+), CK20 (−), TTF1 (+)
Lung: squamous	CK7 (+), CK20 (−), P63 (+), CK5/6 (+)
Lung: neuroendocrine (small cell/large cell)	TTF1 (+), chromogranin (+), synaptophysin (+)
Breast	CK7 (+), ER (+), PR (+), GCDFP-15 (+), Her2/neu (+), mammogloblin (+)
Ovary	CK7 (+), ER(+), WT1 (+), mesothelin (+)
Bladder (transitional cell)	CK20(+), CK5/6(+), P63(+)
Prostate	PSA (+), CK7(−), CK20(−)
Pancreas	CK7(+), Ca19-9 (+), mesothelin (+)
Renal	RCC (+), CD10(+), pan-cytokeratin AE 1/3(+)
Liver	hepar1(+), CD10(+)
Adrenocortical	alpha-inhibin(+), melan-A(+), CK7(−), CK20(−)
Germ cell	PLAP(+), OCT4(+)
Thyroid/follicular/papillary	thyroglobulin(+), TTF1(+)

EMA, epithelial membrane antigen; S100, calcium binding protein expressed in melanocytes; CLA, common leukocyte antigen; CK, cytokeratin; HMB-45, anti-human melanosome antibody; melan-A, melanoma antigen; CD117, tyrosine kinase receptor (c-kit); CDX2, intestinal specific transcription factor; TTF-1, thyroid transcription factor-1; ER, estrogen receptor; PR, progesterone receptor; GCDFP-15, gross cystic fluid protein 15; WT1, Wilm's tumor transcription factor; p63, tumor suppression gene protein; PSA, prostate specific antigen; RCC, brush border of proximal kidney tubule antibody; CD10, common acute lymphocytic leukemia antigen; hepar1, hepatocyte paraffin 1 marker; PLAP, placental alkaline phosphatase; OCT4, octamen binding transcription factor-4.
(Derived from refs. 7, 10–16.)

staining) and poorly differentiated neuroendocrine carcinomas (chromogranin, synaptophysin staining) can be identified,[7,13] and staining for germ cell tumors (HCG, AFP, OCT4, PLAP) is suggestive in an appropriate clinical situation.

The ability of IHC staining to identify the origin of various adenocarcinomas has improved, but in most cases the staining results must be interpreted in the context of clinical and histologic features. An exception is the prostate-specific antigen (PSA) stain, which is very specific for prostate carcinoma.[7] Stains suggestive of other primary sites are summarized in Table 137.1; the use of panels improves specificity.[7,10–16]

Several problems are associated with the IHC stains. Technical expertise is required to perform these tests accurately and reproducibly, and proper interpretation requires an experienced pathologist. False-positive and false-negative results can occur with any of these stains. For example, some carcinomas stain with vimentin, some sarcomas stain with cytokeratins, and a wide variety of carcinomas do not always stain in the expected patterns.[7,17] The classic staining patterns as illustrated in Table 137.1 often overlap with staining patterns of other adenocarcinomas, forcing the pathologist to consider two or three possible primary sites. However, consideration of the clinical setting helps to direct the selection of the IHC stains and may narrow the spectrum of possibilities if staining patterns are not completely specific. For example, in a patient with mucin-positive adenocarcinoma and metastases limited to the liver, a CK20+/CK7− staining pattern provides strong evidence for the colon as a primary site. Conversely, IHC findings may lead to additional diagnostic procedures; in the above example, a colonoscopy should be performed and may result in the identification of a primary site.

In many cases, a single primary site cannot be identified with certainty even after histologic examination, IHC staining, and correlation with clinical features. Additional pathologic evaluation with either electron microscopy or a search for specific chromosomal abnormalities is useful in a few situations. In addition, molecular tumor profiling is a new technique that promises to be of broad importance in identifying the tissue of origin in patients with CUP.

Electron Microscopy

A diagnosis can be made by electron microscopy in some poorly differentiated neoplasms. Electron microscopy should be reserved for the study of neoplasms whose lineage is unclear after routine light microscopy and IHC staining. Electron microscopy is also reliable in undifferentiated sarcoma. Ultrastructural features such as neurosecretory granules (neuroendocrine tumors) or premelanosomes (melanoma) can suggest a particular tumor. Undifferentiated tumors can lose these specific ultrastructural features; therefore, the absence of a particular ultrastructural finding cannot be used to rule out a specific diagnosis. Electron microscopy is not able to distinguish among various adenocarcinomas and should not be used to identify a tissue of origin in patients with adenocarcinoma of unknown primary site.

Karyotypic or Cytogenetic Analysis

The existence of specific chromosomal abnormalities is well characterized in several hematopoietic neoplasms. Most B-cell non-Hodgkin's lymphomas are associated with tumor-specific immunoglobulin gene rearrangements, and typical chromosomal changes have been identified in some B-cell and T-cell lymphomas and in Hodgkin's lymphoma.[18,19] In the rare instance when the diagnosis of lymphoma cannot be definitively established by IHC staining, electron microscopy, molecular profiling, or chromosomal analysis [t(14:18); t(8:14); t(11:14) and others], the presence of an immunoglobulin gene rearrangement is diagnostic.

A few other nonrandom chromosomal rearrangements associated with nonlymphoid tumors have been identified and occasionally can be useful in the diagnosis of CUP. A chromosomal translocation, t(11:22), has been found in peripheral neuroepitheliomas, desmoplastic small round cell tumors, and frequently in Ewing's tumor.[20–22] A balanced translocation, t(15:19), resulting in the *BRDA-NUT* oncogene has been identified in children and young adults with carcinoma of midline structures of uncertain histogenesis.[23] An isochromosome of the short arm of chromosome 12 (i12p) and other chromosome 12 abnormalities are found in a large percentage of germ cell tumors.[24–26] A genomic hybridization technique has been developed that can detect extra 12p material in paraffin-embedded tissue specimens.[26]

Other nonrandom cytogenetic abnormalities include t(2:13) in alveolar rhabdomyosarcoma; 3p deletion in small-cell lung cancer; 1p deletion in neuroblastoma; t(X:18) in synovial sarcoma; and 11p deletion in Wilm's tumor. Epstein-Barr viral genomes have been identified in the tumor cells of patients with cervical lymph node metastases of unknown primary site, highly suggesting nasopharyngeal primaries.[27,28] The search for specific chromosomal abnormalities should be limited to patients with the histologic diagnoses of poorly differentiated neoplasm or poorly differentiated carcinoma, in whom IHC stains have failed to narrow the diagnostic spectrum. No specific chromosomal changes have been identified to aid in the evaluation of adenocarcinomas.

Gene Expression Profiling and Cancer of Unknown Primary Classification

Gene expression or molecular profiling of human neoplasms arose from DNA microarray analysis described about 15 years ago.[29,30] CUP patients represent a large group with a clinically undefined primary tumor site of origin and are ideal candidates for classification by molecular profiling.[31] Molecular profiling may identify the specific type of cancer present and, when used in concert with the clinical and pathological features, may be useful in predicting the primary tumor site of origin. Primary site identification in CUP will likely improve the therapeutic outcome by allowing site-specific therapy to be administered, rather than an empiric single regimen to all patients. In addition to defining the precise tumor type, molecular tumor profiling may aid in unraveling various gene-specific, cancer-activated, or overexpressed cellular pathways and in identifying new targets for therapy.[32,33]

A pivotal study in cancer classification and diagnosis was reported by Golub et al.[34] and demonstrated for the first time that patterns of gene expression alone could discriminate acute myeloid leukemia from acute lymphoblastic leukemia. Other investigators demonstrated that numerous cancer types could be classified accurately by measuring the differential expression of specific gene sets.[35–44] One basis of molecular profiling in recognizing specific cancer types is the identification of the genes responsible for the synthesis of proteins required for specific normal cellular functions (e.g., milk production in breast luminal duct cells, albumin production in hepatocytes, etc.) in the approximately 400 different normal cell types in humans. Cancer cells retain some normal cell-type specific functional characteristics in their gene expression profile, and usually their origin can be predicted, regardless of neoplastic differentiation.[42] Molecular profiling assays designed to determine the type of cancer are not measuring tumor-specific markers but, rather, gene expression dynamics in relation to cell lineage.

Retrospective Studies in Cancer of Unknown Primary Site

Molecular profiling assays have been validated in patients with metastatic tumors of known primary site. When applied to biopsy specimens from a metastatic site, various molecular assays have correctly predicted the primary site in 76% to 89 % of patients.[38–43] Correct identification of the primary tumor type in CUP is difficult to validate, since the primary tumor site is unknown and rarely becomes apparent during the subsequent clinical course of these patients. It would seem reasonable to assume a similar accuracy rate for these assays in predicting the primary tumor site by testing a metastasis in CUP, and this assumption is supported by the results of several retrospective studies in CUP patients (Table 137.2).[38,39,45–50] However, this validation has usually been indirect and is based on correlation with clinical features, pathology (including IHC stains), and response to treatment.

A complementary DNA microarray was utilized by Tothill et al.[38] on the biopsy specimens from 13 patients with CUP. The primary tumor site predictions were compared with clinicopathologic features. In 11 of 13 patients (85%) the molecular classification prediction was consistent with the most likely primary site as determined by the clinical and pathologic data.

Talantov et al.[39] included 33 patients with CUP in their tumor samples from 449 patients in a validation study of their reverse transcriptase polymerase chain reaction (RT-PCR) assay for known primary cancers. Twenty-two of 33 patients (77%) with CUP were assigned a primary tumor site, and 17 of those (85%) correlated with the prediction of the primary site made by IHC.

Varadhachary et al.[45] used a RT-PCR assay (same as Talantov et al.[39]) on biopsies of 120 patients with CUP. This assay was capable of recognizing only six primary cancer types. In 63 patients (61%), a primary site was predicted, and the clinicopathologic features and response to treatment were compatible with the predicted primary site in most patients. Twenty-three patients with colorectal profiles are of interest. Twelve patients who were retrospectively identified received empiric chemotherapy, usually with paclitaxel and carboplatin, and only two had an objective response. In contrast, 10 of the 11 prospectively identified patients received colorectal cancer regimens in either the first- or second-line setting, and 9 had objective responses to therapy.

A microarray assay was used by Bridgewater et al.[46] on biopsies from 21 CUP patients and results were correlated with clinical and pathologic features. The predicted primary site was "clinically feasible" in 18 (86%) based on clinicopathologic features. The authors felt the management of 12 patients would have been influenced had the assay results been available at the time of the initial diagnosis.

Horlings et al.[47] reported results of a microarray assay on biopsies from 38 patients. Sixteen of these patients had been given a diagnosis based on IHC results; molecular profiling results correlated with the IHC prediction in 15 of 16 patients. Twenty-two of the biopsies could not be classified by IHC staining results. However, molecular profiling predicted a primary site in 14 of these 22 patients (64%).

Monzon et al.[49] used a microarray assay on fresh-frozen biopsy specimens from 21 patients. The primary site of origin was predicted in 16 of 21 patients (76%) and was indeterminate in 5 (24%). In 10 of the 16 patients the assay predictions were consistent with the clinicopathologic suggestions of the primary site.

These small retrospective studies provide some indirect validation of the accuracy of the molecular assays. More direct evidence is now available from a study of CUP patients who had a primary site identified later during their clinical course (latent primary).[50] The authors identified 20 such patients who had primary sites identified 2 to 54 months (median 10 months) after the initial diagnosis of CUP. Four additional patients were later identified (unpublished data). The initial diagnostic biopsies were evaluated by an RT-PCR assay (Cancer Type ID, BioTheranostics, Inc.) capable of identifying

PRACTICE OF ONCOLOGY

TABLE 137.2

MOLECULAR PROFILE ASSAY VALIDATION STUDIES IN CANCER OF UNKNOWN PRIMARY

Study (Ref.)	Assay (Ref.)	Assay Validated Indirectly by Clinicopathological Correlation[a]	Assay Validated by Latent Primary Site[b]
Tothill et al. (38)	Microarray (38)	13 patients 11 correlated (85%)	Not done
Talantov et al. (39)	RT-PCR (39)	22 patients 17 correlated (85%)	Not done
Bridgewater et al. (46)	Microarray(43)	21 patients 18 correlated (86%)	Not done
Monzon et al. (49)	Microarray (41)	21 patients 16 patients correlated (76%)	Not done
Varadhachary et al. (45)	RT-PCR (39)	120 patients 63 correlated (61%)	Not done
Horlings et al. (47)	Microarray (43)	38 patients 29 correlated (76%)	Not done
Greco et al. (50) and unpublished data	RT-PCR (42)	Not applicable latent primary site known	24 patients 18 predicted accurately (75%)
Greco et al. (unpublished data)	RT-PCR (42)	147 patients (127 evaluable) 83 correlated (66%) 59 patients with single site suspected (52 evaluable) 40 correlated (77%)	Not done

RT-PCR, reverse transcriptase polymerase chain reaction.
[a]Clinical and pathologic (immunohistochemistry) features only; no primary tumor site documented.
[b]Primary tumor site of origin later definitely identified.

32 tumor types. In 18 of 24 biopsies (75%), the primary tumor was accurately predicted (matched the latent primary site identified), providing direct validation of the accuracy and confirming the usefulness of a molecular profiling assay in classifying the primary tumor site in CUP patients.

Comparison of Immunohistochemical and Molecular Profiling Predictions

The small retrospective studies summarized in Table 137.2 suggest that molecular tumor profiling adds to the information obtainable by standard pathologic evaluation. To examine this question more closely, the authors began a prospective study in March 2008 in which all new CUP patients and selected CUP patients already being followed had a molecular profiling assay (Cancer Type ID). Results were correlated with clinical features, pathologic evaluation (including IHC staining), and response to treatment. Although the study is ongoing, the results in 171 patients provide useful information regarding the role of molecular profiling in diagnosis. Molecular tumor profiling provided putative diagnoses in 144 of 171 patients (84%); 22 patients had insufficient tumor in the biopsy specimen to allow successful assay, while 5 tumors had molecular profiles that were unclassifiable. A total of 21 different primary sites were identified; primary sites accounting for 5% or more of patients included intestine (16%), non–small-cell lung (11%), breast (9%), liver (6%), pancreas (5%), and ovary (5%) cancers.

The large majority of patients also had complete IHC profiling. A specific diagnosis based on IHC staining results was predicted in 59 patients (35%). In this group of patients, summarized in Table 137.3, the molecular profiling diagnosis was obtainable in 52 patients and was identical to the IHC prediction in 40 patients (77%). The high level of correlation in lung-adeno/large cell (74%), intestinal (predominantly colorectal; 93%), and breast cancer (100%) is notable; molecular profiling may be superfluous in these patients when the diagnosis is predicted by IHC.

TABLE 137.3

SINGLE PRIMARY SITE SUSPECTED IN CANCER OF UNKNOWN PRIMARY BASED ON IHC STAINING FEATURES: CORRELATION WITH MOLECULAR PROFILE DIAGNOSIS (N = 59)[a]

		Molecular Assay Diagnosis: Agreement with Suspected Primary Site	
Suspected Primary Site	Number	Number	%
Lung-adeno/large cell	19	14	74
Lung-neuroendocrine	3	2	66
Intestine	16	15	93
Breast	5	5	100
Melanoma	3	2	66
Germ cell	2	1	50
Liver	1	1	100
Ovary	1	0	0
Prostate	1	0	0
Sarcoma	1	0	0
Insufficient cells/RNA (Inevaluable)		7	
Total Evaluable	52	40	77

[a]Seven of 59 with insufficient cells/RNA to perform the molecular assay (excluded from analysis).

However, the correlation is lower in other tumor types and further decreases when IHC results are less specific. Ninety-seven of these patients had sufficient tissue for molecular profiling assays; results matched one of the diagnoses suggested by IHC in 43 (44%). In 47 patients with 2 or 3 suggested diagnoses by IHC, the molecular profiling prediction matched one of the two suspected diagnoses in only 20 (43%).

Summary

An increasing body of data now indicates that molecular tumor profiling can accurately predict the tissue of origin in a majority of patients with CUP. The correlation between IHC and molecular profiling is good when IHC predicts a specific primary site; in these patients, molecular profiling may not be necessary. However, in the majority of patients with adenocarcinoma, IHC is less specific and molecular profiling can provide valuable additional information. However, there are few published data regarding the impact of these diagnoses on patient treatment results. Until such data exists, these patients should still be considered to have CUP when planning management. In some cases, consideration of treatment based on the predicted primary site is now appropriate (see the "Treatment" section).

CLINICAL FEATURES AND EVALUATION

Most patients with CUP develop signs or symptoms at the site of a metastatic lesion and are diagnosed with advanced cancer. The subsequent clinical course is usually dominated by symptoms related to metastases; the primary site becomes obvious in only 5% to 10% of patients during their lifetime. At autopsy, a primary site is identified in about 75% of patients.[3,6] Primary sites in the pancreas, lung, colorectum, and liver account for approximately 60% of those identified. Primary sites in the breast, ovary, and prostate are uncommon in autopsy series, but preliminary data from molecular profiling series suggest that breast and ovarian primaries may be more common than previously recognized.

Although some clinical differences exist, there is substantial overlap between the clinical features of patients with adenocarcinoma, poorly differentiated adenocarcinoma, and poorly differentiated carcinoma. Patients with poorly differentiated carcinoma have been a somewhat younger median age and usually exhibit rapid tumor growth. These patients may also have more frequent location of dominant metastatic sites in the mediastinum, retroperitoneum, and peripheral lymph nodes. Because of the similarities, the clinical evaluation of patients with these histologies should follow the same guidelines. Patients with neuroendocrine carcinoma and squamous carcinoma of unknown primary site are discussed separately.

Clinical Evaluation

The recommended clinical evaluation for all patients is summarized in Table 137.4. In actuality, many of these procedures are usually done in the process of diagnosing CUP. Positron emission tomography (PET) scanning should be considered routine in the initial CUP evaluation, although definitive data in large numbers of patients have not been published.[51] Further evaluation for subsets of patients should be directed by results of the initial clinical and pathologic evaluations. Further focused evaluation may (1) identify a primary site, (2)

TABLE 137.4

INITIAL DIAGNOSTIC EVALUATION

- Complete history: including detailed review of systems
- Complete physical examination: including pelvic examination, stool for occult blood
- Complete blood cell count, comprehensive metabolic panel, lactate dehydrogenase, urinalysis
- Computed tomography scans of chest, abdomen, and pelvis
- Mammography in women
- Serum prostate-specific antigen in men
- Positron emission tomography scan in selected patients
- Pathology-including screening immunohistochemistry marker stains (CK7, CK20, TTF-1, CDX2)

narrow the spectrum of possible primary sites, or (3) identify specific treatable subsets of patients (see section "Treatable Subsets").

Table 137.5 summarizes the additional evaluation indicated for several common clinical presentations. Additional evaluation should be triggered by either clinical findings or IHC results during the initial evaluation. Although molecular tumor profiling is not yet considered a standard component of the diagnostic workup and is not included in Table 137.5, the authors believe this test will become standard in the future and can be considered in selected patients.

Neuroendocrine Carcinoma

Although the initial clinical evaluation is the same (Table 137.4), patients with neuroendocrine carcinoma require special consideration in determining appropriate treatment. Of major importance is the separation of this group into tumors with low-grade histology and indolent clinical course versus those likely to have an aggressive clinical course. This distinction can usually be made by the pathologist: patients with classical carcinoid tumors typically have indolent histology, while those with small-cell neuroendocrine carcinoma or poorly differentiated carcinoma with positive neuroendocrine IHC stains have aggressive cancers.

Low grade neuroendocrine carcinomas, when presenting with an unknown primary site, most frequently involve the liver. Other metastatic sites include lymph nodes (usually abdominal or mediastinal) and bone. Some are associated with various syndromes caused by secretion of bioactive peptides (carcinoid syndrome, glucagonoma syndrome, VIPomas, Zollinger-Ellison syndrome). Additional clinical evaluation in these patients should include serum or urine screening for these substances. In addition to the evaluation listed in Table 137.4, upper and lower gastrointestinal endoscopy should be performed, since some of these patients have detectable primary sites in the gastrointestinal tract.

Aggressive neuroendocrine carcinomas of unknown primary site are usually found in multiple metastatic sites and rarely secrete bioactive peptides. Patients with a history of cigarette smoking should be suspected of having a lung primary, particularly if the tumor has a small-cell histology, and a fiberoptic bronchoscopy should be performed. Patients with a positive tumor cell IHC stain for thyroid transcription factor-1 (TTF-1) should also have a bronchoscopy. Extra pulmonary small-cell carcinomas arising from a variety of other sites (salivary glands, paranasal sinuses, esophagus, pancreas, colorectum, bladder, prostate, uterus, cervix) have been described and are occasionally identified during clinical evaluation. Colonoscopy should be considered in patients with tumor IHC staining for CDX2.

The origin of these aggressive neuroendocrine carcinomas remains unclear. It is likely that some patients, with small-cell histology, have small-cell lung cancer with an occult primary tumor. However, more than half of these patients have no smoking history, and the absence of overt pulmonary involvement makes this diagnosis unlikely. It is probable that some of these tumors are undifferentiated variants of well-recognized neuroendocrine tumors (e.g., carcinoid tumor) without a recognizable primary site. In the undifferentiated form, the clinical and pathologic characteristics no longer resemble the characteristics of the more differentiated counterpart.

TABLE 137.5

FOCUSED DIAGNOSTIC EVALUATION OF PATIENT SUBSETS DEFINED BY INITIAL CLINICOPATHOLOGIC EVALUATION

Initial Evaluation	Additional Evaluation
Women with features of breast cancer (bone, lung, liver metastases, CK7+)	Breast magnetic resonance imaging ER, GCDFP-15, HER2 stains
Women with features of ovarian cancer (pelvic/peritoneal metastases; CK7+)	Pelvic/intravaginal ultrasound WT-1 stain
Mediastinal/retroperitoneal mass	Testicular ultrasound Serum HCG, AFP PLAP, OCT4 stains; FISH for i(12p)
Features of lung cancer (hilar/mediastinal adenopathy; TTF-1+)	Bronchoscopy
Features of colon cancer (liver/peritoneal metastases; CK20+/CK7−, CDX2+)	Colonoscopy
Poorly differentiated carcinoma, with or without clear cell features	Stains for chromogranin, synaptophysin, RCC, Hepar-1, HMB-45 (If Hepar-1+, obtain serum AFP; if neuroendocrine stains +, obtain octreotide scan)

HCG, human chorionic gonadotropin; AFP, α-fetoprotein; FISH, fluorescence *in situ* hybridization.

Anaplastic or atypical carcinoid tumors arising in the gastrointestinal tract are responsive to platinum-based chemotherapy, whereas carcinoid tumors with typical histology are usually resistant.[52] A few reports of patients with extrapulmonary small-cell carcinoma of unknown primary site have also documented chemotherapy responsiveness and occasional long-term survival after systemic therapy.[53,54] However, the term extrapulmonary small-cell carcinoma implies the existence of a known primary site; the tumors discussed here are more aptly described as neuroendocrine carcinoma of unknown primary site.

Squamous Carcinoma

As opposed to unknown primary cancers of other histologies, squamous carcinoma almost always presents with isolated metastases in the cervical or inguinal lymph nodes. The cervical lymph nodes are the most common metastatic site. Patients are usually middle aged or elderly, and frequently they have abused tobacco or alcohol, although recently these lesions have also been associated with human papilloma virus infection. When the upper or middle cervical lymph nodes are involved, a primary tumor in the head and neck region should be suspected. Clinical evaluation should include an examination of the oropharynx, hypopharynx, nasopharynx, larynx, and upper esophagus by direct endoscopy, with biopsy of any suspicious areas. Computed tomography (CT) of the neck better defines the disease in the neck and occasionally identifies a primary site. PET scanning is indicated, as it can identify primary tumor sites in a large number of these patients.[55] Detection of Epstein-Barr virus genome in the tumor tissue is highly suggestive of a nasopharyngeal primary site,[27,28] particularly in poorly differentiated carcinomas. Other genetic studies of squamous cell carcinoma of the head and neck region have shown genetic alterations in "normal tissue" as a precursor of invasive carcinoma.[56] Further study is indicated, as these findings do not yet have a practical application. When the lower cervical or supraclavicular lymph nodes are involved, a primary lung cancer should be suspected. Fiberoptic bronchoscopy should be performed if the chest radiograph and head and neck examinations are normal, as this has a high yield, frequently identifying a lung primary.[57]

Ipsilateral tonsillectomy has been advocated as a diagnostic modality in patients with a single node involving the subdigastric, midjugulocarotid, or submandibular areas, and bilateral tonsillectomy has been advocated in patients presenting with bilateral subdigastric adenopathy.[58] In one series of 87 patients who had tonsillectomy as part of their workup for cervical node presentations, 26% had a tonsillar primary identified.[59] The advantages of identifying the primary are worthwhile in this group of patients and include more a specific treatment plan, determination of prognosis, reduction of radiation therapy ports, and perhaps easier follow-up.

Most patients with squamous carcinoma involving inguinal lymph nodes have a detectable primary site in the genital or anorectal areas. Careful examination of the anal canal, vulva, vagina, uterine cervix, penis, and scrotum is important, with biopsy of any suspicious areas. Digital examination and anoscopy should be performed to exclude lesions in the anorectal area. Identification of a primary site in these patients is important because curative therapy is available for carcinomas of the vulva, vagina, cervix, and anus, even after spread to regional lymph nodes.

Metastatic squamous carcinoma in areas other than the cervical or inguinal lymph nodes usually represents metastasis from an occult primary lung cancer. Fiberoptic bronchoscopy should be considered.

TREATMENT

The heterogeneous group of patients with CUP contains some patients who experience long-term survival after appropriate treatment and others for whom treatment makes little or no impact. Patients who have a primary site defined clinically during their initial evaluation should no longer be considered to have CUP and should be treated appropriately for their defined tumor type. A second group of patients can be identified as having specific treatable clinical syndromes, even if the primary site is not identified. The management of these subsets is detailed in this section. Finally, a large group of patients retain the diagnosis of CUP and do not fit into any subset, even after appropriate clinical and pathologic evaluation. Empiric chemotherapy remains the standard treatment for these patients, and this is summarized separately. Site-specific therapy directed by the molecular profiling diagnosis in these patients is a developing area, and it is also briefly reviewed.

Favorable Subsets

Women with Peritoneal Carcinomatosis

Adenocarcinoma, particularly serous adenocarcinoma, causing diffuse peritoneal involvement is typical of ovarian carcinoma, although carcinomas from the gastrointestinal tract, lung, or breast can occasionally produce this clinical syndrome (Table 137.6). On occasion, women with diffuse peritoneal carcinomatosis have no primary site found in the ovaries or elsewhere in the abdomen at the time of laparotomy. These patients frequently have histologic features typical of ovarian carcinoma, such as papillary serous configuration or psammoma bodies, and also share clinical features, such as elevated serum cancer antigen 125 (CA 125) levels. It is now clear that many of these patients have a primary peritoneal carcinoma. These tumors are more common in women with a family history of ovarian cancer, and prophylactic oophorectomy does not always protect them from this tumor.[60] Like ovarian carcinoma, the incidence of primary peritoneal carcinoma is increased in women with *BRCA1* mutations.[61]

The site of origin of some of these carcinomas is from the peritoneal surface (primary peritoneal carcinoma) or from the fimbriated end of the fallopian tubes.[62,63] Because ovarian epithelium is in part an extension of the mesothelial surface, some carcinomas arising from the peritoneal (mesothelial) surface or the uterine tubes share a similar lineage (müllerian derivation) and biology with ovarian carcinoma. Support for this hypothesis has been strengthened by the demonstration of gene expression profiles nearly identical to ovarian carcinoma.[50] Treatment of these women using guidelines for advanced ovarian cancer (surgical cytoreduction followed by taxane or platinum chemotherapy) produces results similar to those seen in comparable stages of ovarian cancer[64,65] and should be the standard approach. Therefore, optimal management of these patients should follow guidelines for the management of advanced ovarian cancer.

Papillary serous peritoneal carcinomatosis has also been reported in men[66]; however, it is difficult to confirm the precise biology, and some of these tumors may be metastatic from an occult primary from elsewhere. The study of gene expression patterns in these patients may be very revealing, particularly if they match those seen in women. A trial of chemotherapy should be administered to good performance status patients.

TABLE 137.6

CARCINOMA OF UNKNOWN PRIMARY SITE: SUMMARY OF EVALUATION AND THERAPY OF RESPONSIVE SUBSETS

Carcinoma	Clinical Evaluation[a]	Special Studies	Subsets	Therapy	Prognosis
Adenocarcinoma (well-differentiated or moderately differentiated)[b]	Chest, abdominal CT scan; PET scan Men: Serum PSA Women: Mammogram Additional studies to evaluate symptoms, signs	Men: PSA stain Women: ER, PR, Other IHC (see text) Molecular Profiling assay (see text)	1. Women, axillary node involvement[b] 2. Women, peritoneal carcinomatosis[b] 3. Men, blastic bone metastases, high serum PSA, or PSA tumor staining 4. Single metastatic site[b] 5. Colon cancer profile	1. Treat as primary breast cancer 2. Surgical cytoreduction plus chemotherapy 3. Hormonal therapy for prostate cancer 4. Lymph node dissection, radiotherapy 5. Treat as metastatic colon cancer	Survival improved with specific therapy
Squamous carcinoma	Cervical node presentation[b] Panendoscopy PET scan Supraclavicular presentation[b] Bronchoscopy PET scan Inguinal presentation[b] Pelvic, rectal examinations, anoscopy PET scan	Genetic Analysis	1. Cervical adenopathy; nasopharyngeal cancer identified by PCR for Epstein-Barr viral genes 2. Supraclavicular 3. Inguinal adenopathy	1. Radiation therapy, neck dissection, chemotherapy 2. Radiation therapy, chemotherapy 3. Inguinal node dissection, radiation therapy, chemotherapy	Survival improved 1. 25%–50% 5-y survival 2. 5%–15% 5-y survival 3. 15%–20% 5-y survival
Poorly differentiated carcinoma, poorly differentiated adenocarcinoma	Chest, abdominal CT scans, serum HCG, AFP; PET scan; additional studies to evaluate symptoms, signs	IHC; electron microscopy; genetic analysis; molecular profiling assay (see text)	1. Atypical germ cell tumors (identified by chromosome 12 abnormalities) 2. Extragonadal germ cell syndrome (two features) 3. Lymph node-predominant tumors (mediastinum, retroperitoneum, peripheral nodes) 4. Gastrointestinal stromal tumors (identified by CD117 stain) 5. Other groups (see text)	1. Treatment for germ cell tumor 2. Cisplatin/etoposide 3. Newer chemotherapy 4. Imatinib 5. Newer empiric chemotherapy/or site-specific therapy	1. 40%–50% cure rate 2. Survival improved (10%–20% cured) 3. Survival improved 4. Survival improved 5. Survival improved
Neuroendocrine carcinoma	Chest, abdominal CT	IHC Electron microscopy Genetic analysis including molecular assay (see text)	1. Low-grade 2. Small-cell carcinoma (or Ewing's family of tumors) 3. Poorly differentiated	1. Treat as advanced carcinoid 2, 3. Carboplatin/etoposide or platinum/etoposide (or other)	1. Indolent biology/long survival 2, 3. High response rate survival improved; rarely cured

CT, computed tomography; PET, positron emission tomography; IHC, immunohistochemistry; PSA, prostate-specific antigen; ER, estrogen receptor; PR, progesterone receptor; HCG, human chorionic gonadotropin; AFP, α-fetoprotein.

[a]In addition to history, physical examination, routine laboratory tests, and chest x-ray films.

[b]May also present with poorly differentiated carcinoma, and management and outcome are similar.

Women with Axillary Lymph Node Metastases

Breast cancer should be suspected in women who have metastatic carcinoma in an axillary lymph node.[67] Men with occult breast cancer can present in this fashion, but these are rare. The initial lymph node biopsy should be stained for IHC breast markers including estrogen receptors, progesterone receptors, and *HER2*. Elevated levels provide strong evidence for the diagnosis of breast cancer.[68]

If no other metastases are identified, these patients may have stage II breast cancer with an occult primary, which is potentially curable with appropriate therapy. PET and magnetic resonance imaging have identified occult breast cancer even with normal mammography.[69–71] Modified radical mastectomy has been recommended in such patients, even when physical examination and mammography are normal. An invasive occult breast primary has been identified after mastectomy in 44% to 80% of patients. Primary tumors are usually less than 2 cm in diameter and may measure only a few millimeters; in occasional patients, only noninvasive tumor is identified in the breast. Prognosis after primary therapy is similar to that of other patients with stage II breast cancer.[67] Radiation therapy to the breast after axillary lymph node dissection represents a reasonable alternative primary therapy.[72] Either neoadjuvant or adjuvant systemic chemotherapy is indicated in this setting, following guidelines established for the treatment of stage II breast cancer.

Women with metastatic sites in addition to the axillary lymph nodes should be managed as if they have metastatic breast cancer. Hormone receptor and *HER2* status are of particular importance in these patients because they may derive major palliative benefit from hormonal therapy, chemotherapy, and trastuzumab. In the experience of the authors, a molecular profiling assay usually predicts breast carcinoma in these patients.

Men with Elevated Serum Prostate-Specific Antigen or Prostate-Specific Antigen Tumor Staining

Serum PSA concentrations should be measured in men with adenocarcinoma of unknown primary site. These tumors can also be stained for PSA. Even when clinical features (i.e., metastatic pattern) do not suggest prostate cancer, a positive PSA (serum or tumor stain) is reason for a trial of androgen deprivation.[73,74] In most of these patients, a needle biopsy of the prostate would confirm the primary site but may not be necessary for optimal clinical management. Osteoblastic bone metastases in the absence of other metastatic sites are also an indication for an empiric hormone trial, regardless of the PSA findings.

Extragonadal Germ Cell Cancer Syndrome

The extragonadal germ cell cancer syndrome was first described in 1979.[75–77] The full syndrome, which is seen in only a minority of patients, has the following features: (1) occurrence in men less than 50 years of age, (2) predominant tumor location in the midline (mediastinum, retroperitoneum) or multiple pulmonary nodules, (3) short duration of symptoms (less than 3 months) and a history of rapid tumor growth, (4) elevated serum levels of human chorionic gonadotropin (HCG), α-fetoprotein (AFP), or both, and (5) good response to previously administered radiation therapy or chemotherapy. If possible, cytogenetic evaluation for chromosome 12 abnormalities should be obtained, as previously discussed. Because these patients may have atypical germ cell tumors, treatment with cisplatin-based chemotherapy, as used in advanced poor-prognosis testicular cancer, is recommended.

Single Site of Neoplasm

When only one site of neoplasm is identified (e.g., one node group, one mass), the possibility of an unusual primary tumor mimicking metastatic disease should be considered. Several unusual tumors could present in this fashion, including Merkel-cell neuroendocrine tumors; skin adnexal tumors (e.g., apocrine, eccrine, and sebaceous carcinomas); and even sarcomas, melanomas, or lymphomas that are mistakenly interpreted as metastatic carcinoma (pathologically and clinically). Patients with one site of involvement (brain, liver, adrenal, subcutaneous tissue, bone, intestine, lymph node, skin, or other sites) usually have metastatic carcinoma, and many other sites are present but are not detectable. Some of these patients may have a primary tumor at the single site that developed from embryonic rest cells or adult stem cells (see the section "Special Issues in Carcinoma of Unknown Primary Cancer-Biology of the Primary Tumor"). Before initiating local treatment, a PET scan is helpful to exclude other unsuspected metastatic sites.[78]

In the absence of any other documented metastatic disease, these patients should be treated with aggressive local therapy (i.e., resection, radiation therapy, or both) because a minority enjoy long-term, disease-free survival. In addition to definitive local therapy, the authors believe these patients should also receive either neoadjuvant or adjuvant chemotherapy with one of the newer regimens, but it is difficult to be certain if this treatment is superior to local therapy alone.

Patients with a single small site of metastasis frequently survive 1 year or longer and thus represent a favorable prognostic subgroup. In a reported group of patients presenting with single brain metastasis of unknown primary site, 15% remained progression free 5 years after definitive therapy.[79] The authors have treated and followed 36 patients with single site metastases (unpublished observations). All patients had local therapy (resection with or without radiotherapy) and most also received empiric chemotherapy regimens. The median survival in this group is 17 months; 1-, 2-, and 3-year survivals are 65%, 40%, and 28% respectively.

Squamous Carcinoma Involving Cervical or Supraclavicular Lymph Nodes

Squamous carcinoma of unknown primary site is unusual, but most frequently presents with unilateral involvement of the cervical lymph nodes. The clinical evaluation of these patients has been previously described. The recommended evaluation results in the identification of a head and neck primary site in almost 85% of patients.

When no primary site is identified, local treatment should be given to the involved neck. The reported results in more than 1,400 patients are derived primarily from retrospective single-institution experiences, often using a variety of local treatment modalities.[80] In many of these series, a large minority of patients had poorly differentiated carcinoma or adenocarcinoma. A substantial percentage, usually 30% to 40%, of patients achieved long-term, disease-free survival after local treatment modalities. The results obtained using radical neck dissection, high-dose radiation therapy, or a combination of these modalities have been similar. The volume of tumor in the involved neck influences outcome, with N1 or N2 disease having a significantly higher cure rate than N3 or massive neck involvement.[81] Poorly differentiated carcinoma also represents a poor prognostic factor in these patients. When resection alone is used as the primary treatment modality, a primary tumor in the head and neck subsequently becomes apparent in 20% to 40% of patients. Primary tumors surface less commonly when radiation therapy is used, presumably because of the eradication of occult head and neck primary sites within the radiation field. Radiation therapy dosages and techniques should be similar to those used in patients with primary head and neck cancer, and the nasopharynx, oropharynx, and hypopharynx may be included in the irradiated field.

The role of chemotherapy for metastatic squamous carcinoma in cervical lymph nodes is now generally accepted. A nonrandomized comparison of patients treated with local modalities alone or with local modalities combined with chemotherapy (cisplatin and 5-fluorouracil [5-FU]) showed a higher complete response rate (81% vs. 60%) and longer median survival time (more than 37 vs. 24 months) in patients receiving chemotherapy.[82] Combined modality treatment with concurrent chemotherapy and radiotherapy in locally advanced head and neck carcinoma is now standard and should be the treatment of choice for squamous cell carcinoma in cervical lymph nodes. In those who receive local therapy first, adjuvant platinum-based or taxane-based chemotherapy should be considered.

Patients with low cervical and supraclavicular nodes do not do as well because lung cancer is a frequent site of occult primary tumors, although skin, uterine, cervix, and anal canal are also possible primary sites. Molecular assays may be helpful in predicting the primary site. Patients with no detectable disease below the clavicle should be treated with aggressive local therapy because 10% to 15% of these patients have long-term, disease-free survival. Concurrent chemotherapy should also be considered for these patients.

Squamous Carcinoma Involving Inguinal Lymph Nodes

Most patients with squamous carcinoma involving inguinal lymph nodes have a detectable primary site in the genital or anorectal areas. For the unusual patient in whom no primary site is identified, inguinal lymph node dissection with or without radiation therapy to the inguinal area sometimes results in long-term survival.[83] These patients should also be considered for neoadjuvant or adjuvant chemotherapy.

Low-Grade Neuroendocrine Carcinoma

These tumors usually exhibit an indolent biology, and slow progression over years is likely. Management should follow guidelines established for metastatic carcinoid or islet cell tumors from known primary sites. Treatment with octreotide long-acting release (LAR) results in a marked increase in time to tumor progression and is a first-line treatment of low toxicity.[84] Depending on the clinical situation, appropriate management may also include local therapy (resection of isolated metastasis, hepatic artery ligation or embolization, cryotherapy, radiofrequency ablation). Several cytotoxic agents have some activity (streptozocin, doxorubicin, 5-fluorouracil, temozolomide), and preliminary results with targeted agents (sunitinib, everolimus) are promising. These neoplasms are usually refractory to intensive systemic chemotherapy, and cisplatin-based chemotherapy produces low response rates.[76]

Aggressive Neuroendocrine Carcinomas

Patients with aggressive neuroendocrine carcinoma of unknown primary site are those with either small-cell carcinoma or poorly differentiated carcinoma (often large cell) with neuroendocrine staining by IHC. Both of these histologies are initially responsive to combination chemotherapy, and all patients should be considered for a trial of treatment.

The authors initially reported a group of 29 patients with poorly differentiated neuroendocrine tumors[85] and have updated their experience to include 99 patients, 94 treated with combination chemotherapy. Most of these patients had clinical evidence of rapid tumor growth and metastases in multiple sites. Fifty-nine of 87 assessable patients (68%) responded to chemotherapy with a platinum-based combination regimen. Nineteen patients (22%) had complete responses, and 13 remained continuously disease free more than 2 years after completion of therapy.

The results of a prospective trial using the combination of paclitaxel, carboplatin, and oral etoposide in 48 patients (48 of the 99 previously listed) have been reported.[86] The majority of these patients were initially called poorly differentiated carcinoma (about 20% were small-cell carcinoma) but later defined as neuroendocrine tumors by IHC staining or electron microscopy. Most of these patients had several sites of metastasis, often with predominant tumor in the bones, liver, and nodes (particularly retroperitoneum and mediastinum). Patients received a maximum of four courses of chemotherapy with paclitaxel, carboplatin, and oral etoposide; stable or responding patients subsequently received weekly paclitaxel for 24 weeks. The overall response rate was 55% with six complete responses (13%). The median survival was 14 months and 12 patients remain alive from 15 to 45 months.

Data from clinical trials remain limited in this uncommon group of patients; however, current first-line chemotherapy should include the platinum-based regimens used for small-cell lung cancer. The addition of paclitaxel to a carboplatin and etoposide regimen increased toxicity, but did not appear to improve efficacy.[86] In the uncommon patient with a single site of involvement, radiation therapy with or without resection should be added to combination chemotherapy.

Poorly Differentiated Carcinoma

Although patients with poorly differentiated carcinoma form a relatively large and heterogeneous group, the inclusion of patients with highly treatable neoplasms within this group has been recognized since the late 1970s.[75–77] At that time, several young men with mediastinal tumors were reported who had complete response to combination chemotherapy. Elevated serum levels of HCG or AFP were common in these young men. Although the histology was not diagnostic, these patients were thought to have histologically atypical extragonadal germ cell tumors. Several other tumor lineages have subsequently been identified in some of these patients (i.e., thymic neoplasms, neuroendocrine tumors, midline carcinoma with t(15;19), sarcomas, melanomas, lymphomas), but others still defy precise classification.

Further evidence for the responsiveness of many other patients has accumulated since 1978. Based on the encouraging results in a few patients treated from 1976 to 1978, the authors prospectively studied the role of cisplatin-based therapy. In a series of reports, the authors documented a high overall response rate and long-term disease-free survival in a minority of these patients.[87–90] The 220 patients seen and treated, between 1978 and 1989, are of interest.[90] Most of the patients did not have clinical characteristics strongly suggestive of extragonadal germ cell tumor. However, involvement of the mediastinum, retroperitoneum, and peripheral lymph node groups was relatively common; these clinical features are now known to be associated with a more favorable prognosis. All patients who received initial treatment with two courses of cisplatin-based chemotherapy and responding patients received a total of four treatment courses. Major tumor responses were seen in 138 of 220 patients (62%), and 58 patients (26%) had complete response to treatment.

Of the 58 complete responders, 22 patients remained alive and relapse free (38%), representing 10% of the entire group of 220. These results in this large series of patients are historically important, since long-term survival in these patients had not been previously reported. At that time, the results also supported the notion that poorly differentiated histologic types represent more sensitive tumors than well-differentiated adenocarcinoma. Other investigators also demonstrated the responsiveness of selected poorly differentiated carcinomas.[91–96]

Complete responses were seen in a minority (10% to 20%) of these patients, and a small cohort (5% to 10%) comprised long-term, disease-free survivors. These results were usually seen with platinum-based chemotherapy.

The authors now are certain that their original prospective clinical trial of the 220 patients with PDC was heavily weighted with patients now known to represent favorable subsets, each with a relatively good prognosis. These subsets included (1) patients with two or more features of the extragonadal germ cell syndrome, (2) patients with poorly differentiated neoplasms otherwise not specified, (3) patients with anaplastic lymphoma diagnosed as carcinoma in years past but routinely diagnosed today by specialized pathology, (4) patients with primary peritoneal carcinoma, (5) patients with poorly differentiated neuroendocrine carcinoma, and (6) patients with predominant sites of tumor involving the retroperitoneum, mediastinum, and peripheral lymph nodes. The authors' more recent experience has excluded these now recognizable more favorable subsets of patients in their clinical trials. After these favorable subsets of patients are excluded, the remaining patients have a similar prognosis to the large majority of the well-differentiated adenocarcinoma group, and since 1996 the authors have included all these patients in new clinical trials.

Colorectal Cancer Profile

With the introduction of more effective cytotoxic agents and targeted therapies, the median survival of patients with metastatic colon cancer has increased from 9 to about 24 months.[97,98] It is therefore likely that the ability to identify the subset of CUP patients likely to have advanced colorectal cancer would lead to better treatment for these patients. The improved specificity of IHC staining for colon cancer, coupled with the recent availability of molecular tumor profiling assays, may now allow identification of this patient subset. Although results to date are derived from relatively few patients, the potential importance of this syndrome merits inclusion here.

Patients with typical clinical features (liver, peritoneal metastases), histology compatible with a lower gastrointestinal primary, and typical IHC staining (CK20+/CK7− and/or CDX2+) have been defined as having the "colon cancer profile." Several such patients described by Varadhachary et al.[99] had excellent responses to colorectal cancer regimens.

Preliminary data also indicate that a molecular profiling assay that confirms a colorectal origin may identify patients who respond to colon cancer therapy. The authors and colleagues performed a molecular assay (Veridex RT-PCR assay) on biopsies from 104 patients with CUP; in 23 patients, colon was predicted as the site of origin.[45] In 17 of 23 patients, colonscopy was negative (6 not done). Nine of 10 patients who received colorectal cancer regimens had objective responses. In contrast, 2 of 12 patients (retrospectively identified) had responded to empiric chemotherapy for CUP (usually with taxane- or carboplatin-based regimens).

The authors now have data on 21 additional CUP patients in whom molecular profiling assay (Cancer Type ID) predicted a colorectal origin. Table 137.7 shows the clinicopathologic features, treatment, and outcome of these 21 patients; similar data are also included regarding the 11 patients who received colorectal cancer treatment as reported in a previous publication.[45] Thirty of 32 patients had normal colonoscopy. Twenty-three of the 30 evaluable patients received standard first-line regimens for colorectal cancer, and 16 (69%) had objective responses. In addition, 7 of 13 patients (54%) responded to colon cancer regimens as second-line treatment. The median survival for the entire group was 20 months (range: 4–65+ months); the 2- and 4-year survivals were 59% and 30%, respectively.

Although these data are derived from a relatively small group of patients from two institutions with some of the patients identified retrospectively, the treatment results are similar to those achieved in patients with known metastatic colon cancer. Further prospective studies are essential to confirm these results. In the meantime, the authors feel these results are sufficient to recommend treatment with colorectal cancer regimens for CUP patients with a colorectal cancer profile defined by either IHC staining or molecular profiling assay.

Empiric Therapy for Metastatic Carcinoma of Unknown Primary Site

Chemotherapy

Approximately 80% of patients with carcinoma of unknown primary site are not represented in any of the favorable prognostic clinical subsets (Table 137.6). In the past, empiric chemotherapy of various types has produced low response rates, very few complete responses, and even fewer long-term survivals.[2,80] The results of chemotherapy in several reported series of 10 or more patients from 1964 to 2002 are briefly summarized as follows. A total of 1,515 patients were reported in 45 trials.[2,80] The only single agent studied adequately in previously untreated patients was 5-FU, with response rates ranging from 0% to 16%. Cisplatin was evaluated as a single drug in only one series, with a response rate of 19%. Methotrexate, doxorubicin, mitomycin C, vincristine, and semustine had single agent response rates ranging from 6% to 16%. The FAM regimen (5-FU, doxorubicin, mitomycin C) and various modifications were used often, based on the demonstrated activity of these combination regimens in some gastrointestinal cancers. The combination of 5-FU and leucovorin has not been evaluated adequately but does not appear active in CUP patients with liver metastasis, a group most likely to have gastrointestinal primaries.[100] The overall response rates from all these prospective clinical trials varied from 8% to 39% (mean: 20%); the complete response rate was less than 1%. The median survival ranged from 4 to 15 months (mean: 6 months), and survival beyond 2 years was rare (although rarely reported).

Cisplatin-based combination chemotherapy regimens were also evaluated several years ago. In two small, randomized comparisons (subject to many confounding factors) of doxorubicin with or without cisplatin, no difference in median survival was observed, but there was more toxicity in the cisplatin-containing arms.[101,102] A third small, randomized trial did show the superiority of cisplatin, epirubicin, and mitomycin C compared with mitomycin C alone (median survival: 9.4 vs. 5.4 months).[91]

The authors have reviewed several reports of survival for large groups of patients with CUP[103–110] in an attempt to have some historical control data and better define the natural history of this syndrome. These reports were retrospective; therefore, treatments were not uniform, and some patients received no systemic therapy. In addition, these series usually contained patients now known to fit into specific treatable or favorable subsets. These historical series represent 31,419 reported patients. The median survival was 5 months, with a 1-year survival of 22% and 5-year survival of 5%. It is very likely that survival at 1 year and beyond is largely represented by subsets of patients with a more favorable prognosis who received local therapy (surgery or radiotherapy) or those with indolent tumors (e.g., carcinoids). Squamous cell carcinoma (usually in neck nodes) and well-differentiated neuroendocrine carcinoma (carcinoid, islet cell–type histology) reported from some of these series (N = 2,971 patients) had median, 1-year, and 5-year survivals of 20 months, 66%, and 30%, respectively. All

TABLE 137.7

CANCER OF UNKNOWN PRIMARY WITH INTESTINAL/ MOLECULAR PROFILE DIAGNOSES: CLINICOPATHOLOGIC CHARACTERISTICS AND RESULTS/SURVIVAL OF SITE-SPECIFIC THERAPY IN FIRST- AND SECOND-LINE SETTING

Age	Sex	Histology	Sites of Metastases	IHC + Marker	First-line Treatment	Response	Second-Line Treatment	Response	Survival (Months)
75	M	PDA	Liver, lung, bone	CK7	Folfox	PR	Folfiri/Ce	PR	19
56	F	Adeno	Peritoneum, ovary	CK20, CDX2	Folfox/B	PR			9+
46	F	PDA	Ovary	CK20, CDX2	Folfox/B	CR			19+
61	F	Adeno	Lung, nodes	CK20, villin	PC	PD	Cape/RT	PR	8
42	M	PDA	Peritoneum, testes	CK20, CDX2	Folfox	PR	Iri/Ce	PR	31+
54	F	PDA	Peritoneum, ovary, bone	CK20, CDX2, CK7	FU	NA	D/B	SD	30
53	M	Adeno	Liver, peritoneum	CK7, CK20, CEA	PC	PR			7+
52	F	PDA	Peritoneum, abdominal nodes	CK20, chromogranin, CK7	NA	NA			6
70	F	Adeno	Liver	CK7, CK20, CEA	Gem/Cis	SD	Folfox	PR	10+
55	M	PDA	Liver, bone	CK20, CDX2, CEA	Folfox/B	PR	Iri/Ce	NA	12+
58	F	Adeno	Liver, peritoneum, ovary	CDX2	PC	PD	Folfox	PR	38+
61	M	Adeno	Mesentery, omentum	CK7, CK20	Folfox	PR			9
47	F	Adeno	Neck node, lung, retroperitoneum	CK 20	Folfox/B	PR			6
53	F	Adeno	Retroperitoneum, liver	CK7, CK20, CDX2	Capox/B	PR			4
78	M	PDC	Pelvic mass	CK20, CDX2	Folfox/B	PR			16
53	M	PDA	Liver, lung, brain	CK7, villin	Capox	PR			5
48	F	PDA	Liver, retroperitoneum, mediastinum	CK7, Her2-neu	PC/T	PR	Capox	PD	6
63	F	Adeno	Pelvic mass	CK20, CDX2	Folfox/B	PR	Cape/DC/C/RT		65+
63	M	Adeno	Peritoneal, ascites	CK7, CK20, CDX2	Capox	PR			10+
54	F	Adeno	CA Omentum, peritoneal	CK20, CDX2	CE	PR	Folfox/B	PR	60+
68	F	PDC	Peritoneum, retroperitoneum	CK20	PC	PR			4+
46	M	PDC	Mediastinum	CK20, CDX2	Folfox/Iri/B	PR			32+
81	F	Adeno	Liver, lung	CK20, CDX2	Folfox/B	PR			5+
49	F	Adeno	Liver, peritoneum	CDX2	PCE	PR	Gem/Iri	PD	10
49	M	Adeno	Peritoneal mass	CK7, CK20, CDX2	Folfox	PD	Folfiri/B	PD	6+
68	F	Adeno	Liver, peritoneum, mediastinum	CDX2	Cape/B	PR			7
69	M	Adeno	Pelvic mass, bone	CK20, CDX2	Cape/RT	CR			29+
64	F	Adeno	Ovary, omentum	CK20, CDX2	Folfox/B	CR	Folfiri	PD	13
51	M	Adeno	Retroperitoneum	CK20	Capox	NA			13
49	M	PDA	Liver	CK20, CDX2	Gem/Iri	SD			10
47	F	PDA	Liver, lung, mesentery	CK20, CDX2	Cape/Iri/B	PR			22
62	M	Adeno	Retroperitoneal mass	CK7, CK20	FU/P/C	PD			4

IHC, immunohistochemistry; PDA, poorly differentiated adenocarcinoma; PDC poorly differentiated carcinoma; Adeno, adenocarcinoma; Gem, gemcitabine; Folfox, fluorouracil/leucovorin/oxaliplatin; Folfiri, fluorouracil/leucovorin/irinotecan; Iri, irinotecan; FU, fluorouracil; D, docetaxel; B, bevacizumab; Cis, cisplatin; Cape, capecitabine; Capox, capecitabine/oxaliplatin; P, paclitaxel; C, carboplatin, E, etoposide; T, trastuzumab; RT, radiotherapy; Ce, cetuximab; M. male, F, female; PR, partial response; CR, complete response; SD, stable disease; NA, not accessible; PD, progressive disease.

the remaining patients in these series had median, 1-year, and 5-year survivals of 6 months, 20%, and 5%, respectively.

In the past decade, empiric chemotherapy has improved for patients with adenocarcinoma and poorly differentiated carcinoma who do not fit into any of the treatable subsets.[111,112] The introduction of several new drugs with rather broad-spectrum antineoplastic activity from 1990 to 2000 and later with targeted mechanism-based therapies changed the approach to treatment and prognosis for patients with several common epithelial cancers. These drugs include the taxanes, gemcitabine, vinorelbine, irinotecan, topotecan, oxaliplatin, and several targeted agents (e.g., bevacizumab and erlotinib).

Since 1996, the Minnie Pearl Cancer Research Network/Sarah Cannon Oncology Research Consortium(MPCRN/SCORC) has completed nine sequential prospective phase 2 trials incorporating paclitaxel,[113,114] docetaxel,[114,115] gemcitabine,[116,117] gemcitabine/irinotecan,[118,119] bevacizumab/erlotinib,[120] and oxaliplatin[121] into the first-line or second-line therapy for 692 patients. One additional phase 3 randomized prospective trial has been reported with 198 patients.[122] Only patients with CUP who were not included in a favorable subset were eligible for these trials. The first five phase 2 studies (396 previously untreated patients) have a minimum follow-up of 4 years. The total objective response rate for all patients treated in the first five clinical trials was 30% (107 of 353 evaluable patients), with 85 (24%) partial responders and 22 (6%) complete responders. With a minimum follow-up of 4 years and maximum follow-up of 11 years, the median survival was 9.1 months, and the 1-, 2-, 3-, 5-, 8-, and 10-year survivals were 38%, 19%, 12%, 10%, 8%, and 8%, respectively. The median progression-free survival was 5 months, and the 1-, 2-, 3-, 5-, 8-, and 10-year progression-free survivals were 17%, 7%, 5%, 4%, 3%, and 3%, respectively. The toxicity of these regimens was generally moderate, primarily myelosuppression, with a total of eight (2%) treatment-related deaths.

Long-term follow-up on the 264 patients in the first four trials is of interest since follow-up of this duration has not been previously reported from prospective trials. After a minimum follow-up of 6.5 years (range: 6.5 to 11 years); the median survival was 10.2 months; and the 1-, 2-, 3-, 5-, 8-, and 10-year survivals were 41%, 24%, 15%, 11%, 8%, and 8%, respectively. The actuarial survival curves for the 428 other patients treated in four additional phase 2 trials and the single phase 3 trial[122] look similar. There have been no significant survival differences when results from the phase 2 studies were compared. The phase 3 trial compared paclitaxel with carboplatin and oral etoposide to gemcitabine and irinotecan; stable and responding patients received follow-up treatment with gefitinib. The survival at 2 years was similar (15% vs. 18%), and gemcitabine and irinotecan was significantly less toxic.[122] Although both empiric regimens appear to improve the 2-year survival compared to historical controls, the modest efficacy underscores the need for newer therapeutic approaches for these patients.

Three second-line regimens have been recently evaluated in phase 2 trials, including gemcitabine[117] (39 patients), gemcitabine with irinotecan[118] (40 patients), and oxaliplatin with capecitabine[121] (48 patients). Modest activity was documented in this difficult patient group with clinical benefit seen in about 35%; median survivals were 4.0, 4.2, and 9.7 months, and 2-year survival rates were 20%, 12%, and 25%, respectively.

Analysis of all the previously untreated patients in the MPCRN/SCORC trials shows no difference in survival for adenocarcinoma versus PDC. Women survived significantly longer than men, and those with performance status 0 or 1 (Eastern Cooperative Oncology Group Scale) lived longer than those with performance status 2.

Several trials reported by others in the past decade[92,123–133] have substantiated the activity of the newer combination regimens (Table 137.8). These phase 2 trials usually contained combinations of newer broad spectrum cytotoxic drugs (paclitaxel, docetaxel, gemcitabine, irinotecan, vinorelbine, oxaliplatin). The primary end points of these trials were response rate or median survival. The 1-year survival was reported in 12 studies (532 patients), and survival at both 1 and 2 years was reported by eight of the studies (363 patients). The 1-year survival ranged from 25% to 52% (mean: 34.4%) and at 2 years from 5% to 18% (mean: 12.3%). Only one study reported a 3-year survival rate (11%). These survival results are very similar to the 396 patients reported by the previously detailed six MPCRN/SCORC studies. The survival of all 988 patients (532 from 12 studies plus 456 from 6 MPCRN/SCORC studies) are shown in Table 137.8. These survival data are unique, as survival at 2 years and beyond had not been previously appreciated.

The survival data reported with newer empiric regimens during the past decade appear superior to historical retrospective control survival data and to the combined data from multiple prospective clinical trials reported from 1964 to 2002.[2,80] Although the median survival of this group has not changed dramatically, a larger number of patients derive major benefit from treatment, as indicated by the number of 1- and 2-year survivors. The survival curve has been shifted to the right and the survival at 2 years is comparable to the 1-year survival of historical control patients. Comparison of the existing phase 2 trials does not allow definition of an optimum regimen; several

TABLE 137.8

SURVIVAL IN PATIENTS WITH CANCER OF UNKNOWN PRIMARY AND UNFAVORABLE PROGNOSTIC FACTORS: SELECTED PHASE 2 TRIALS IN THE PAST DECADE

Year of Publication (Ref.)	No. of Patients	Regimen	Median Survival (months)	1-Year Survival (%)	2-Year Survival (%)	3-Year Survival (%)
2000 (92)	33	PC	10	25	5	NR
2001 (123)	34	PFUL	8.3	26	NR	NR
	17	CE	6.4			
2003 (125)	30	GemCisE	7.2	36	14	NR
2004 (127)	37	PCis	11	38	11	NR
2004 (128)	35	GemD	10	43	7	NR
2004 (126)	102	CDoxE	9	35.3	18	11
2005 (130)	22	PC	6.5	27	NR	NR
2006 (131)	66	GemCis	13.6	52	NR	NR
	33	GemVCis	9.6	30	NR	NR
2006 (124)	51	GemC	7.8	26	12	NR
2007 (133)	42	PC	8.5	33	17	NR
2007 (129)	47	OxIri	9.5	40	NR	NR
2007 (132)	33	GemCapeC	7.6	35.6	14.2	NR
1997–2009 (113–119, 134)	456	Multiple regimens	9.1	38	19	12
Total	988		9.0	35[a]	14[a]	12[a]

Gem, gemcitabine; Cape, capecitabine; Ox, oxaliplatin; Iri, irinotecan; V, vinorelbine; Cis, cisplatin; B, bevacizumab; FU, fluorouracil; C, carboplatin; P, paclitaxel; L, leucovorin; Dox, doxorubicin; E, etoposide; Er, erlotinib; D. docetaxel; NR, not reported
[a]Mean survivals of all studies

two-drug combinations appear similar and are currently acceptable. Many patients with adenocarcinoma or poorly differentiated carcinoma who do not fit or conform to any recognized favorable subset can now attain substantial clinical benefit from the new drug combinations, and a trial of treatment should be considered in all patients with acceptable performance status.

However, we believe that the era of empiric chemotherapy for patients with CUP is nearing its end. Improved diagnosis using IHC stains and molecular tumor profiling are likely to provide a more rational framework for decision making regarding therapy. Increasing numbers of targeted agents are now available or in clinical development, and their utility will most likely be defined by the identification of critical molecular abnormalities.

Targeted Therapy

A number of agents targeting pathways critical to cancer cells have been incorporated into the standard therapy of various solid tumors. It is likely that some patients in the heterogeneous group of CUP patients would also benefit from these targeted agents. Although there has been limited clinical experience with targeted agents, definite activity has been documented.

The combination of bevacizumab and erlotinib was evaluated in a group of 51 patients.[120] Thirty-seven patients had received previous chemotherapy (24 patients, 1 regimen; 13 patients, 2 regimens), and 14 patients were previously untreated but with poor prognostic features (advanced liver metastasis, bone metastasis or three or more visceral sites of metastases). All patients received bevacizumab 10 mg/kg intravenously every 2 weeks and erlotinib 150 mg orally daily. Forty-seven of 51 patients received at least 8 weeks of therapy; 5 patients (10%) had a partial response, and 29 patients (61%) had stable disease (many with tumor shrinkage). The median survival was 7.4 months with 33% of patients alive at 1 year and 18% at 2 years. Patients tolerated this therapy well (grade 3 or 4 toxicity of any type less than 10%, except fatigue at 16%). Survival seemed superior to second-line chemotherapy previously reported and was similar to results of many first-line chemotherapy trials.

This trial was followed by a first-line phase 2 study evaluating standard chemotherapy (paclitaxel and carboplatin) plus targeted therapy (bevacizumab and erlotinib).[134] Sixty patients received four cycles of these four agents repeated at 21-day intervals, followed by bevacizumab and erlotinib continued until tumor progression. Forty-nine of 60 patients completed the induction therapy, and 44 (73%) received the maintenance targeted drugs. Thirty-two patients (53%) had objective responses to treatment, and 18 others were stable. At a median follow-up of 19 months, the median progression-free survival was 8 months; 38% of the patients were progression free at 1 year. The median survival was 12.6 months, and the 2-year survival was 27%. There was no unexpected severe toxicity. This empiric regimen was relatively effective, and further empiric approaches using targeted therapy with chemotherapy are reasonable to investigate.

Prognostic Factors

The identification of prognostic factors in the population of patients with CUP continues to evolve as the group is divided into an increasing number of subsets. By definition, patients who fit into the favorable treatment subsets (see section "Treatable Subsets") have favorable prognosis compared to the remaining patients. As new treatable subsets are identified, the clinical features of the remaining patients can be expected to change. Therefore, results of previous analyses of prognostic factors, conducted primarily in patients receiving empiric chemotherapy, may no longer apply to the current population.

At M. D. Anderson Cancer Center, a large heterogeneous group with various histologic subtypes was analyzed retrospectively.[135,136] Patients with clinical features of extragonadal germ cell tumors were excluded, and only a minority of patients with PDC received cisplatin-based treatment. Clinical and pathologic features identified as favorable prognostic features included limited number of metastatic sites, tumor location in lymph nodes (including mediastinum and retroperitoneum) other than the supraclavicular lymph nodes, and female sex. Adverse prognostic factors included adenocarcinoma histology (as compared to other histologies) and liver metastasis.

Van der Gaast et al.[137] evaluated 79 patients with PDC and found three groups with median survivals of 4 years, 10 months, and 4 months based on performance status and serum alkaline phosphatase levels. A minority of their patients were long-term survivors following chemotherapy.

Culine et al.[138] have also defined a prognostic model based on retrospective analysis of 150 patients with various histologies. Patients with several known favorable prognostic subsets were excluded. Patients with good performance status and normal serum lactate dehydrogenase (LDH) levels had significantly better median survival (11.7 vs. 3.9 months) and 1-year survival (45% vs. 11%) after cisplatin-based chemotherapy. The LDH level was more predictive of prognosis than was the presence of liver metastasis.

Seve et al.[139] investigated a population of 317 patients in a Canadian center seen from 1998 to 2004 and found low serum albumin and lymphopenia to be important prognostic factors. A group of good-risk patients (normal serum albumin and no liver metastasis) had a median survival of about 1 year compared to 3.5 months ($P < .0001$) for poor-risk patients (low serum albumin with or without liver metastasis). These findings were validated in a group of 81 patients seen at two French centers from 2000 to 2004. Only 116 of the 317 patients in the initial test series were treated with chemotherapy, raising the question of the usefulness in patients in a setting appropriate for chemotherapy. Nonetheless, a number of easily obtainable clinical parameters appear to offer important prognostic information.

The authors examined prognostic factors in a large group of patients with PDC who were treated with cisplatin-based chemotherapy.[90] In this group, favorable features included mediastinal or retroperitoneal tumor location, metastases at less than three sites, age less than 35 years, female gender, negative smoking history, and normal LDH and carcinoembryonic antigen (CEA) levels.

In summary, prognostic factors that have been repeatedly identified are related to tumor location, extent of tumor, performance status, and measures of general health status (serum albumin, lymphocyte count). None of these features is surprising, since most have been repeatedly identified as prognostic factors in patients with various solid tumors. These factors should be considered when designing, interpreting, or comparing results of clinical trials in patients with CUP.

Site-Specific Treatment Directed by Results of Molecular Tumor Profiling

The emergence of molecular tumor profiling, as well as IHC staining of improved specificity, raises the question as to whether treatment guided by these results is superior to empiric therapy for CUP. At present, there are insufficient clinical data available to answer this question. However, the authors believe that the fragmentary information now available suggests a future change in the paradigm of treatment.

Since the biology of CUP is different from that of other cancers (as evidenced by the fact that the primary site does not become apparent), there has been speculation that these cancers will also respond differently to treatment. If so, the ability to identify the tissue of origin may not lead to improved therapy. However, most clinical data suggest that CUP represents a collection of cancer types, which, if identified, will respond to site-specific therapy in a predictable way. The successful treatment of patients in several of the treatable subsets supports this argument. For example, women with adenocarcinoma that involves the peritoneum respond to ovarian cancer treatment, patients with squamous carcinoma that present in neck nodes have successful outcomes following treatment for head and neck cancer, and so forth. Furthermore, preliminary data now suggest that patients identified as having a colorectal primary site by molecular tumor profiling have good responses to site-specific therapy for colon cancer (see section "Colorectal Cancer Profile").

Prospective evaluation of site-specific therapy selected on the basis of molecular profiling or IHC results is urgently needed. Demonstration of the superiority of site-specific versus empiric therapy will be most likely in tumor types where treatment efficacy has improved and differs from empiric CUP therapy (e.g., colorectal, renal, hepatic, biliary tract). In other tumor types where site-specific and empiric CUP therapy are similar (e.g., ovary, non–small-cell lung) or in situations where all therapy is relatively ineffective (e.g., pancreas), such differences remain currently difficult to demonstrate. However, an acceptance of the site-specific treatment approach, based on prospective validation in selected tumor types, would allow generalization to additional tumor types as improved tumor-specific treatments are developed.

SPECIAL ISSUES IN CARCINOMA OF UNKNOWN PRIMARY SITE

Biology of the Primary Tumor

The biology of the primary tumor in CUP remains an enigma. The majority of patients harbor a clinically occult primary tumor site, as demonstrated by autopsy series.[3,6] It is remarkable that many of these invasive primary tumors measure less than 1 cm and some only a few millimeters. Rarely a latent primary tumor site is found many weeks or months after the initial diagnosis of CUP. The mechanism explaining very small clinically occult invasive primary tumor sites remains unknown but almost certainly will be clarified by a better understanding of the molecular mechanisms controlling primary tumor growth and metastasis. There are several other potential explanations for the apparent absence of a primary cancer in some of these patients. First, some of these primary cancers may inexplicably regress or involute entirely, despite the fact that metastasis already occurred. This theory is supported by the scarring seen occasionally in the testicle of male patients with metastatic germ cell neoplasms (i.e., "burned-out primary"). Second, some of these tumors may have arisen from embryonic epithelial "rest cells" that are fully differentiated but did not complete their appropriate migration *in utero* to their designated tissue or organ. Extragonadal germ cell tumors with primaries in the mediastinum, retroperitoneum, or undescended testicular cancer are known examples of this phenomenon. Third, some of these patients have unrecognized primary neoplasms such as an extragonadal germ cell tumors, thymic neoplasms, lymphomas, melanomas, or sarcomas, which arise from these lineages virtually anywhere in the body. Fourth, the pathogenesis of some of these carcinomas may result from a specific genetic lesion present in all cells, and these tumors might be expected to have a similar gene expression distinct from specific carcinomas of recognized primary sites, as is suggested by the unusual occurrence of metastatic adenocarcinoma of unknown primary site in monozygotic twin brothers with primary immunodeficiency disorder (X-linked hyperimmunoglobulin M syndrome).[140]

Finally, some of these neoplasms may arise from adult undifferentiated pluripotent stem cells with an ability to differentiate to multiple lineages.[141–145] Hematopoietic stem cells appear to be able to give rise to or transform into liver cells as well as muscle, gastrointestinal, skin, and brain cells.[141] Reserve precursor stem cells exist within the connective tissue compartments throughout postnatal life[144] and can form any lineage in any tissue if they undergo neoplastic transformation. Therefore, some tumors might continue to reflect the differentiation or transformation of adult stem cells and may be "tumors of adult stem cells." For example, seemingly metastatic adenocarcinoma in bone, liver, lymph node, or elsewhere may, in fact, arise in these sites from an adult stem cell with the capacity to become any type of cell and to develop as a "primary" neoplasm in any of these tissues.[142]

Although carcinomas of unknown primary share a metastatic phenotype, it is currently unknown whether these tumors share specific molecular abnormalities. Karyotypic analysis of unknown primary carcinomas demonstrates multiple chromosomal abnormalities, but these are not unique and are shared with advanced solid tumors of known primary sites (e.g., various chromosomal 1p abnormalities).[146] Similarly, overexpression of *p53*, *bcl-2*, *c-myc*, *ras*, and *HER2* has been observed in some CUP, but are not specific.[147–151] Although the search for a CUP-specific molecular profile continues, none has yet been identified. At present, most evidence suggests that CUP retains typical site-specific molecular abnormalities and can be identified by molecular tumor profiling; however, this does not preclude the coexistence of CUP-specific molecular abnormalities.

Carcinoma of Unknown Primary Site as a Distinct Clinical Syndrome

The authors have found it amazing over the past three decades how often patients and their referring physicians (often oncologists) are frustrated by CUP. Physicians are often somewhat obsessed with finding the primary site or at least with giving the patient a more specific diagnosis. There are many reasons underlying these feelings. Some patients think their oncologist may not be a very good diagnostician and seek the advice of others. Some oncologists feel relatively inadequate and wonder what other test(s) they might order; some have been relatively tentative, not feeling confident in recommending any therapy. Certainly a reasonable evaluation of these patients and their tumors is indicated, being aware of possible primary sites and the relevance in particular patients. However, once these considerations and evaluations are complete, the physician should stop, discuss the issue with the patient and family, and accept the clinical syndrome as CUP. Patients are better served, and physicians eventually feel more comfortable and therefore manage these patients more effectively once their patients accept and understand this diagnosis. The authors now believe improved diagnostic techniques, including more specific IHC marker stains and molecular profile assays, will change the nature of these conversations in the future. Nonetheless, these patients will still lack anatomically defined primary sites and will therefore remain a distinct population.

A second practical issue in the United States is the determination of reimbursement for chemotherapy by Medicare for cancer diagnoses. Other than U.S. Food and Drug Administration approval for a specific tumor type, reimbursement for chemotherapy is most typically determined by Medicare (and some other third-party insurers) by consulting compendia—Medicare Drug Policies or the National Comprehensive Cancer Network Compendium. The list of "approved" drugs is based on published literature showing "effectiveness" or clinical benefit in a specific tumor type. This is an arbitrary system. For many years CUP was not included in any of the listings. Four drugs are currently listed as indicated for these patients (paclitaxel, carboplatin, cisplatin, and etoposide).

Medicare usually does not pay for any drug not listed as being indicated. For this reason, many patients with CUP are coded by oncologists as having other diagnoses. These diagnoses usually represent a "good guess" or statistical probability, based on clinicopathologic features. For example, patients with lung lesions or mediastinal node involvement are often coded as having non–small-cell lung cancer; patients with liver metastases are coded as colon or pancreatic cancer. Furthermore, patients are at times assigned a diagnosis based on the pathology report alone (e.g., adenocarcinoma consistent with pancreatic or colon primary) or by cytokeratin-staining results. This activity causes the true incidence of unknown primary cancer to be underestimated but also allows for reimbursement for some drug costs by a system that otherwise has not "approved" therapies for these patients.

There are now enough clinical and pathologic data to classify patients confidently and global acceptance of this syndrome will help these patients establish an identity, stimulate more interest by physician investigators, and eventually improve the general understanding of these patients and their tumors.

Isolated Pleural Effusion

An isolated malignant pleural effusion is most frequently a manifestation of a peripheral lung carcinoma (usually adenocarcinoma). The diagnosis of mesothelioma, or, rarely, a metastatic tumor from other sites, should also be considered. In a series of 42 patients, a primary lung cancer was eventually found in 15 patients (36%).[152] The primary may not be apparent even after chest tube drainage. Cytology usually shows adenocarcinoma; positive TTF-1 and CK7 stains support a diagnosis of lung carcinoma. Other IHC stains (i.e., calretinin in mesothelioma) or a molecular profiling assay may also assist in defining a primary site. In one small series of patients,[152] chemotherapy produced symptomatic improvement in 29 of 37 patients, and 30 of 37 patients had their pleural effusion reduced by chemotherapy; median survival was 12 months (range: 3–60 months).

In evaluating a female patient with an isolated pleural effusion, the possibility of an occult ovarian carcinoma or primary peritoneal carcinoma should be considered. Although this presentation is rare, these tumors are often relatively sensitive to treatment. This diagnosis is possible even when CT and PET scans of the abdomen and pelvis are normal. In such cases, an elevated CA 125 level suggests the diagnosis.

Germ Cell Tumors with Metastases of Other Histologies

On occasion, patients with germ cell tumors, particularly extragonadal primaries, may have a metastatic lesion that consists of only somatic tumor cells. This is particularly true for neuroendocrine or sarcomatous differentiation but can include any histology. Patients therefore may be diagnosed as having a neuroendocrine tumor or sarcoma. In these rare instances, a primary germ cell tumor (usually extragonadal) is present elsewhere and subsequently is clinically apparent. It is difficult to make the diagnosis initially. An elevated plasma AFP or HCG level is suggestive. The presence of a mediastinal, retroperitoneal, or testicular mass supports this possibility. Chromosomal analysis, IHC staining, or a molecular assay may confirm the diagnosis of germ cell tumor. The treatment of choice is cisplatin-based chemotherapy. Surgical resection should be pursued if feasible. These patients have a worse prognosis than those with typical germ cell tumors, probably because the somatic cell tumors are less sensitive to chemotherapy.

Melanoma and Amelanotic Melanoma

Approximately 10% to 15% of all melanomas that present with an unknown primary site are believed to be amelanotic. The authors have viewed this diagnosis with considerable skepticism. At times, the only reason for the pathologic diagnosis is the similarity of the histologic pattern to melanoma, even though no pigment is demonstrated. In the authors' experience, detailed pathologic and molecular study has occasionally revealed a group of other specific diagnoses, including lymphomas, neuroendocrine tumors, germ cell tumors, sarcomas, and poorly differentiated carcinoma (not otherwise specified).

Melanosomes or premelanosomes seen on electron micrographs have been considered diagnostic of melanoma, but on rare occasion these structures are seen in other tumors. Some believe amelanotic melanomas do not always form premelanosomes, raising the question as to whether they are really melanomas. Immunohistochemical panels and a molecular profiling assay are also useful in supporting the diagnosis of melanoma. It is of interest that in the authors' original report of 220 patients with poorly differentiated carcinoma, 9 were later believed to be amelanotic melanoma on the basis of IHC stains or electron microscopy.[90] These particular patients generally responded well to cisplatin-based chemotherapy, and several had long-term survival, an unexpected result for melanoma.

The history of a resected, abraded, or frozen pigmented skin lesion would certainly favor a metastatic melanoma in an individual. In addition, the rare primary visceral melanoma should be considered (e.g., eye, adrenal, bowel, others) as the source of the disease in questionable cases. For patients with the diagnosis of amelanotic melanoma, particularly without diagnostic IHC stains and no history or clinical features to support this diagnosis, empiric treatment based on guidelines for CUP should be considered. Recently *BRAF* mutations have been found in approximately 50% of melanomas, and if present would also support a presumptive diagnosis of melanoma and consideration of a clinical trial with a *BRAF* inhibitor.

UNKNOWN PRIMARY CANCER IN CHILDREN

There are limited data in children, and, as expected, many of these neoplasms represent embryonal malignancies.[153] They are exceedingly rare. In those rare patients with carcinoma, not otherwise specified, the authors favor following the same management plan as for adults.

Midline Carcinoma in Young Adults and Children with t(15;19) and *BRD4-NUT* Oncogene

A few young patients have been recently described with carcinomas arising from midline locations and an associated chromosomal translocation t(15;19) (q13,p13.1).[23] Patients with this syndrome ranged in age from 3 to 35 years, most had PDC, and all had widespread metastasis. The primary tumor site was difficult to identify in many of these patients. The *NUT* (nuclear protein in testes) oncogene is common to all these tumors and supports their possible origin from a specific cell type, perhaps an early epithelial progenitor cell that is more common in the first two or three decades of life. Perhaps these tumors are an example of "stem cell tumors" (see section "Biology of the Primary Tumor in Special Issues in Carcinoma of Unknown Primary Site").

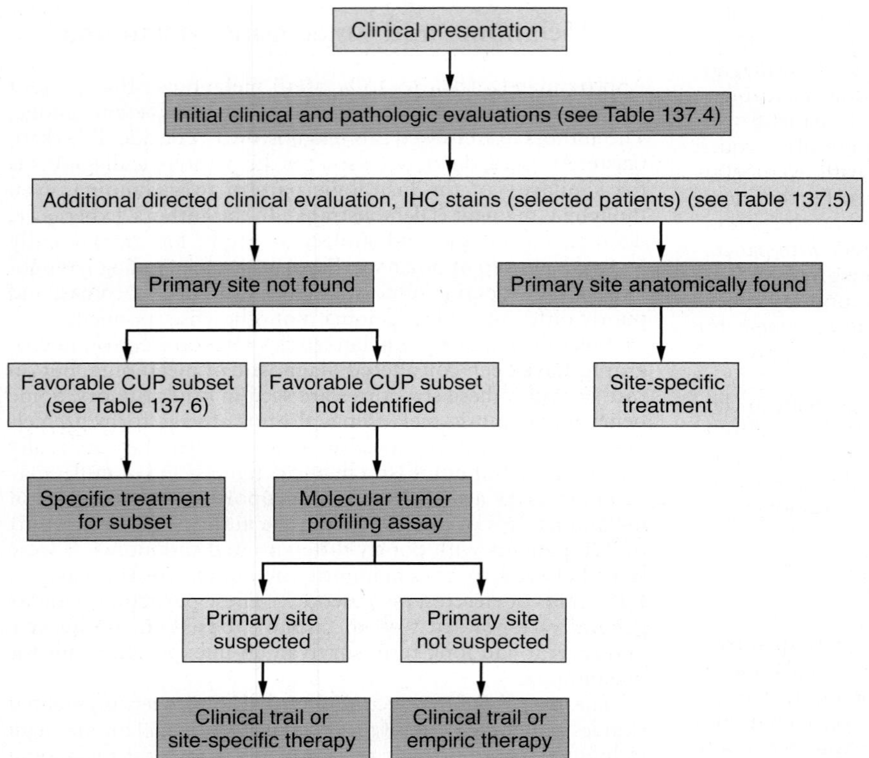

FIGURE 137.2 Suggested new management paradigm for the cancer of unknown primary site patient.

Despite intensive chemotherapies and radiation therapy, which produced initial good responses, all but one of these patients died from disease within 16 months (median: 7 months). Two additional patients were more recently reported: one patient with a tumor arising from the iliac bone (unknown primary site)[154] has been in complete remission for 13 years after combined modality therapy, and a second patient with mediastinal involvement (unknown primary site)[155] had a good response to secondary therapy with docetaxel and radiotherapy. They are clinically similar to the extragonadal germ cell cancer syndrome, and without a positive t(15;19), some of these patients could be included in that clinical syndrome and vice versa. Further knowledge of these *NUT*-rearranged carcinomas and improved treatment for these patients are likely to follow their more broad recognition.

FUTURE DIRECTIONS AND CHANGING TREATMENT PARADIGM

As described in this chapter, improving diagnostic methods are likely to change the diagnostic and therapeutic approach to patients with CUP in the near future. Although clinical data are currently incomplete, a change from empiric chemotherapy to site-specific therapy based on predictions from new diagnostic methods is predicted by both authors.

In Figure 137.2, we summarize what we believe to be the future management approach to patients with CUP. After standard initial clinical and pathologic evaluations, selected patients will have additional directed clinical evaluation or IHC staining of the tumor specimen. Patients with an identified primary site will be treated accordingly, and patients who fit into an identified favorable CUP subset will have appropriate subset-specific therapy (see section "Treatable Subset"). Patients in neither of these categories (i.e., patients who traditionally were candidates for empiric chemotherapy) will have molecular tumor profiling performed and will then be considered for site-specific therapy based on molecular profiling results interpreted in concert with clinical features and pathologic results.

The authors emphasize that the integration of molecular diagnostics into standard patient management is not yet supported unequivocally by clinical data. Continued clinical trials in this area are vital. Even with the ability to identify the tissue of origin, further improvements in the treatment of CUP are dependent on the development of improved treatments for advanced solid tumors.

Selected References

The full list of references for this chapter appears in the online version.

2. Pavlidis N, Briasoulis E, Hainsworth J, Greco FA. Diagnostic and therapeutic management of cancer of an unknown primary. *Eur J Cancer* 2003;39:1990.
5. Horning SJ, Carrier EK, Rouse RV, et al. Lymphomas presenting as histologically unclassified neoplasms: characteristics and response to treatment. *J Clin Oncol* 1989;7:1281.
6. Pentheroudakis G, Golfinopoulos V, Pavlidis N. Switching benchmarks in cancer of unknown primary: from autopsy to microarray. *Eur J Cancer* 2007;43:2026.
7. Owen KA. Pathologic evaluation of unknown primary cancer. *Semin Oncol* 2009;36:8.
8. Hainsworth JD, Wright EP, Gray GF Jr, Greco FA. Poorly differentiated carcinoma of unknown primary site: correlation of light microscopic

findings with response to cisplatin-based combination chemotherapy. *J Clin Oncol* 1987;5:1272.
9. Motzer RJ, Rodriguez E, Reuter VE, et al. Molecular and cytogenic studies in the diagnosis of patients with midline carcinomas of unknown primary site. *J Clin Oncol* 1995;13:274.
10. Dennis JL, Oien KA. Hunting the primary: novel strategies for defining the origin of tumours. *J Pathol* 2005;205:236.
23. French CA, Kutok JL, Faquin WC, et al. Midline carcinoma of children and young adults with NUT rearrangement. *J Clin Oncol* 2004;22:4135.
31. Greco FA, Erlander MG. Molecular classification of unknown primary cancer site. *Mol Diagn Ther* 2009;13:262.
32. Li X, Quigg RJ, Zhou J, et al. Clinical utility of microassays: current status, existing challenges and future outlook. *Curr Genomics* 2008;9:466.
34. Golub TR, Slonim DK, Tamayo P, et al. Molecular classification of cancer: class discovery and class prediction by gene expression monitoring. *Science* 1999;286:531.
35. Ramaswamy S, Tamayo P, Rifkin R, et al. Multiclass cancer diagnosis using tumor gene expression signatures. *Proc Natl Acad Sci U S A* 2001;98:15149.
41. Monzon FA, Lyons-Weiler M, Buturovic LJ, et al. Multicenter validation of a 1,550-gene expression profile for identification of tumor tissue of origin. *J Clin Oncol* 2009;27:2503.
42. Ma X-J, Pate R, Wang X, et al. Molecular classification of human cancers using a 92-gene real-time quantitative polymerase chain reaction array. *Arch Path Lab Med* 2006;130:465.
45. Varadhachary G, Talantov D, Raber M, et al. Molecular profiling of carcinoma of unknown primary and correlation with clinical evaluation. *J Clin Oncol* 2008:26:4442.
50. Greco FA, Spigel DR, Yardley DA, et al. Molecular profiling in unknown primary cancer: tissue of origin prediction. *Oncologist* 2010;15:500.
75. Richardson RL, Greco FA, Wolff S, et al. Extragonadal germ cell malignancy: value of tumor markers in metastatic carcinoma of young males. *Proc Am Assoc Clin Oncol Am Assoc Clin Res* 1979;20 (abstr 204).
76. Hainsworth JD, Greco FA. Poorly differentiated carcinoma of unknown primary site. In: Fer MF, Greco FA, Oldham R, eds. *Poorly differentiated neoplasms and tumors of unknown origin*. Orlando, FL: Grune Stratton, 1986:189.
80. Greco FA, Hainsworth JD. Cancer of unknown primary site. In: DeVita VT, Hellman S, Rosenberg SA, eds. *Cancer Principles and Practice of Oncology*, 7th ed. Philadelphia: Lippincott Williams & Wilkins, 2005: 2213.
85. Hainsworth JD, Johnson DH, Greco FA. Poorly differentiated neuroendocrine carcinoma of unknown primary site: a newly recognized clinicopathologic entity. *Ann Intern Med* 1988;109:364.
86. Hainsworth JD, Spigel DR, Litchy S, Greco FA. Phase II trial of paclitaxel, carboplatin, and etoposide in advanced poorly differentiated neuroendocrine carcinoma: a Minnie Pearl Cancer Research Network Study. *J Clin Oncol* 2006;24:3548.
87. Richardson RL, Schoumacher RA, Fer MF, et al. The unrecognized extragonadal germ cell cancer syndrome. *Ann Intern Med* 1981;94:181.
88. Greco FA, Vaughn WK, Hainsworth JD. Advanced poorly differentiated carcinoma of unknown primary site: recognition of a treatable syndrome. *Ann Intern Med* 1986;104:547.
89. Hainsworth JD, Greco FA. Treatment of patients with cancer of an unknown primary site. *N Engl J Med* 1995;329:257.
90. Hainsworth JD, Johnson DH, Greco FA. Cisplatin-based combination chemotherapy in the treatment of poorly differentiated carcinoma and poorly differentiated adenocarcinoma of unknown primary site: results of a 12 year experience at a single institution. *J Clin Oncol* 1992;10:912.
99. Varadhachary GR, Raber MN, Matamoros A, Abbruzzese JL. Carcinoma of unknown primary with a colon cancer-profile changing paradigm and emerging definitions. *Lancet Oncol* 2008;9(6):596.
104. Hess KR, Abbruzzese MC, Lenzi R, et al. Classification and regression free analysis of 1000 consecutive patients with unknown primary carcinoma. *Clin Cancer Res* 1999;5:3403.
111. Greco FA, Pavlidis N. Treatment for patients with unknown primary carcinoma and unfavorable prognostic factors. *Semin Oncol* 2009;36:74.
112. Greco FA. Therapy of adenocarcinoma of unknown primary: are we making progress? *J Natl Compr Canc Netw* 2008;6:1061.
113. Hainsworth JD, Erland JB, Kalman CA, et al. Carcinoma of unknown primary site: treatment with one-hour paclitaxel, carboplatin and extended schedule etoposide. *J Clin Oncol* 1997;15:2385.
114. Greco FA, Gray J, Burris HA, et al. Taxane-based chemotherapy with carcinoma of unknown primary site. *Cancer J* 2001;7:203.
115. Greco FA, Erland JB, Morrissey LH, et al. Phase II trials with docetaxel plus cisplatin or carboplatin. *Ann Oncol* 2000;11:211.
116. Greco FA, Burris HA, Litchy S, et al. Gemcitabine, carboplatin, and paclitaxel for patients with unknown primary site: a Minnie Pearl Cancer Research Network study. *J Clin Oncol* 2002;20:1651.
117. Hainsworth JD, Burris HA, Calvert SW, et al. Gemcitabine in the second-line therapy of patients with carcinoma of unknown primary site: a phase II trial of the Minnie Pearl Cancer Research Network. *Cancer Invest* 2001;19:335.
118. Hainsworth JD, Spigel DR, Raefsky EL, et al. Combination chemotherapy with gemcitabine and irinotecan in patients with previously treated carcinoma of an unknown primary site. *Cancer* 2005;104:1992.
119. Greco FA, Hainsworth JD, Yardley DA, et al. Sequential paclitaxel/carboplatin/etoposide followed by irinotecan/gemcitabine for patients with carcinoma of unknown primary site: a Minnie Pearl Cancer Research Network phase II trial. *Oncologist* 2004;9:644.
120. Hainsworth JD, Spigel DR, Farley C, et al. Bevacizumab and erlotinib in the treatment of patients with carcinoma of unknown primary site: a phase II trial of the Minnie Pearl Cancer Research Network. *J Clin Oncol* 2007;25:1747.
121. Hainsworth JD, Spigel DR, Burris HA 3rd, et al. Oxaliplatin and capecitabine in the treatment of patients with recurrent or refractory carcinoma of unknown primary site: a phase 2 trial of the Sarah Cannon Oncology Research Consortium. *Cancer* 2010;116:2948.
122. Hainsworth JD, Spigel DR, Clark BL, et al. Paclitaxel/carboplatin/etoposide versus gemcitabine/irinotecan in the first-line treatment of patients with carcinoma of unknown primary site: a randomized, phase III Sarah Cannon Oncology Research Consortium Trial. *Cancer J* 2010;16:70.
134. Hainsworth JD, Spigel DR, Thompson DS, et al. Paclitaxel/carboplatin plus bevacizumab/erlotinib in the first-line treatment of patients with carcinoma of unknown primary site. *Oncologist* 2009;14:1189.
135. Abbruzzese JL, Abbruzzese MC, Hess KR, et al. Unknown primary carcinoma: natural history and prognostic factors in 657 consecutive patients. *J Clin Oncol* 1994;12:1272.
139. Seve P, Ray-Coquard I, Trillet-Lenoir V, et al. Low serum albumin levels and liver metastasis are powerful prognostic markers for survival in patients with carcinomas of unknown primary site. *Cancer* 2006;107: 2698.
141. Korbling M, Katz RL, Khanna A, et al. Hepatocytes and epithelial cells of donor origin in recipients of peripheral blood stem cells. *N Engl J Med* 2002;346:738.
142. McCulloch EA. Stem cells and diversity. *Leukemia* 2003;17:1042.
143. Young HE, Duplaa C, Romera-Ramos M, et al. Adult reserve stem cells and their potential for tissue engineering. *Cell Biochem Bio Phys* 2004;40:1.
144. Dieterien-Lievre F. Lineage-switching by pluripotent cells derived from adults. *J Soc Biol* 2001;195:39.
147. Ramaswamy S, Ross KN, Lander ES, Golab TR. A molecular signature of metastasis in primary solid tumors. *Nat Genet* 2003;33:49.
151. Hainsworth JD, Lennington WJ, Greco FA. Overexpression of Her-2 in patients with poorly differentiated carcinoma or poorly differentiated adenocarcinoma of unknown primary site. *J Clin Oncol* 2000;18:632.
153. Kuttesch JF, Parham DM, Kaste SC, et al. Embryonal malignancies of unknown primary origin in children. *Cancer* 1995;75:115.
155. Englison J, Soller M, Panagopoulos I, et al. Midline carcinoma with t(15;19) and BRD4-NUT fusion oncogene in a 30-year-old female with response to docetaxel and radiotherapy. *BMC Cancer* 2006;16:69.

CHAPTER 138 BENIGN AND MALIGNANT MESOTHELIOMA

HARVEY I. PASS, NICHOLAS J. VOGELZANG, STEVEN M. HAHN, AND MICHELE CARBONE

Malignant mesotheliomas are highly aggressive neoplasms that arise primarily from the surface serosal cells of the pleural, peritoneal, and pericardial cavities.[1] Epidemiologic studies have established that exposure to asbestos fibers is the primary cause of malignant mesothelioma, and recent investigations have implicated simian virus 40 (SV40), genetic predisposition in the etiology of some malignant mesotheliomas, and possibly carbon nanotubes.[2] The disease is characterized by a long latency from the time of exposure to asbestos to the onset of disease, suggesting that multiple somatic genetic events are required for tumorigenic conversion of a normal mesothelial cell (see "Overview of Molecular Mechanisms in Mesothelioma"). Early evidence in support of this notion was provided by karyotypic analyses, which revealed multiple cytogenetic alterations in most human mesotheliomas. Although a specific chromosomal change is not shared by all malignant mesotheliomas, several prominent sites of chromosomal loss have been identified in this malignancy. Tumor suppressor genes (TSGs) residing in these deleted chromosomal regions may be responsible for the tumorigenic conversion of mesothelial cells, and recent studies have begun to identify the specific TSGs that contribute to the development and progression of malignant mesothelioma.

MECHANISM OF ASBESTOS-CARCINOGENESIS

Up to 5% of asbestos miners develop mesothelioma, and it is estimated that most mesothelioma patients have been exposed to asbestos.[3] Although this link is well accepted, the exact proportion of mesotheliomas linked to asbestos exposure and the relative carcinogenicity of the various fiber types, a dose-response relationship, remain controversial. There are six types of asbestos: amosite, crocidolite, anthophyllite, actinolite, tremolite, and chrysotile.[3] The five types other than chrysotile are termed *amphibole asbestos*. Chrysotile is a nonamphibole mineral that has a different texture, composition, and pathogenic behavior compared with amphibole asbestos.[3] Several nonasbestos minerals (e.g., erionite, wincherite) are very similar to asbestos structurally and chemically and are also capable of causing mesothelioma in humans. Numerous experimental models demonstrating asbestos carcinogenicity have been established in animals.[4] The mechanisms responsible for asbestos carcinogenicity are being elucidated and are linked to the secretion of tumor necrosis factor-alpha by mesothelial cells and macrophages exposed to asbestos that in turn leads to NFκB activation.[5] The activation of the NFκB pathway in mesothelial cells allows them to survive the toxic insult and the genetic damage caused by asbestos, and these damaged but viable cells may proliferate into a mesothelioma.[5] Asbestos has been shown to induce AP-1, which may enhance cell division and favor malignant growth. AP-1 activation is enhanced in mesothelial cells infected with SV40 and exposed to asbestos, and animal experiments have confirmed that asbestos and SV40 are cocarcinogens in causing mesothelioma.[6,7]

Exposure Quantification

The proportion of mesotheliomas that are thought to be associated with asbestos varies in the literature from 16% to 90%.[3] Although this wide range may reflect the distinct populations studied, it is more likely a result of the different methodologies used to determine exposure rates.[3] Rates determined by history are the most imprecise and appear to produce the greatest variation in results.[3] Even when exposure has been established in patients, such as in studies analyzing cohorts of asbestos workers, it is difficult to quantify the level of exposure by history.[3] In contrast, lung content analysis is a more reliable indicator of exposure because it allows the investigator to determine both the amount and type of exposure.[3] Nevertheless, these studies may also underestimate the number of chrysotile fibers that were originally deposited in the lungs because chrysotile fibers, but not amphiboles, are cleared from the lungs.[3] Aside from lung content analysis, a number of studies have reported pleural fiber content, which may be more biologically relevant for mesothelioma development. Pleural content studies demonstrate that chrysotile fibers are the predominant fiber type found in the pleura of asbestos-exposed individuals.[8] Higher lung asbestos burden is associated with cell-cycle gene methylation[9] and also associated with an increased risk of death from the disease.[10]

Animal Models of Asbestos Carcinogenicity

Mesotheliomas and sarcomas are induced in a dose-dependent fashion after intrapleural and intraperitoneal injection of asbestos into animals.[11–13] Chronic inhalational studies are thought to be the best representation of asbestos carcinogenicity. Because of the cost of these experiments, however, very few have been performed.

Asbestos Carcinogenicity in Humans

Although injection and inhalation studies in animals suggest that all forms of asbestos are equally carcinogenic and that there is a clear dose-response relationship between asbestos exposure and mesothelioma risk, epidemiologic studies in humans do not support these observations. Most human studies have indicated that amosite and crocidolite exposure carry a much greater risk than exposure to chrysotile.[14,15] Chrysotile, however, is frequently combined with tremolite, an amphibole, that may instead be responsible for mesothelioma development.[8] It is possible that the discrepancy between chrysotile carcinogenicity in animals and humans is related to the types of exposure in each group. In animal studies, exposure is usually intense and of a short duration, whereas humans tend to be exposed to asbestos in smaller concentrations over a longer period. Overall, at this time it is difficult to conclusively determine the relative carcinogenicities of different fiber types. Results of lung content analysis studies, which are the most reliable indicators of exposure to date, may underestimate the amount of chrysotile exposure because this mineral may dissolve over time.

In humans, there is no clear dose-response curve to asbestos, and a threshold level below which mesotheliomas do not develop has not been determined, although it is generally accepted in the scientific community that background levels of exposure, such as those found in the lungs of almost all individuals, do not increase the risk of mesothelioma. It is estimated that less than 5% of asbestos miners exposed to high levels of asbestos develop mesotheliomas.[3] However, wives of some of these workers have developed mesotheliomas after they were presumably exposed to lower levels of asbestos compared to their husbands while washing their clothes.[16,17] Similarly, mesothelioma development commonly occurs in workers in occupations in which asbestos exposure is higher than in the general population, but much lower than in asbestos miners. The carpenters, electricians, and construction workers who have developed mesotheliomas are a reflection of this.[18] These data suggest that high levels of exposure are not necessarily correlated with increased risk of malignancy compared to moderate asbestos exposure, arguing against a classic dose-response relationship.[3]

Mechanism of Asbestos Pathogenicity

It is thought that when fibers reach the alveoli after inhalation, smaller fibers are phagocytized and efficiently removed from the lung. Larger fibers are not easily engulfed and can usually only be removed if solubilized. However, amphiboles are not soluble and thus remain in the lung. These fibers may eventually reach the pleura via the lymphatics or direct extension, where they may lead to pleural plaques, fibrosis, and mesothelioma. In the pleura, asbestos fibers may cause mutagenic changes through hydroxy radical and superoxide anion production during phagocytosis, leading to DNA strand breaks and deletions. In hamster cells, asbestos fibers can also mechanically interfere with mitotic segregation to alter chromosome morphology and ploidy as well as to produce DNA strand breaks. In rat mesothelial cells, crocidolite asbestos was found to cause autophosphorylation of the epidermal growth factor receptor, which leads to ERKs kinase activation and AP-1 activity, which favors cell growth.

Two mouse models that recapitulate the genetic alterations found in human mesotheliomas have recently been developed and may help to dissect the exact mechanisms of asbestos carcinogenesis.[1,4] A critical mechanism of asbestos carcinogenesis is mediated by the secretion of tumor necrosis factor-alpha by mesothelial cells and macrophages exposed to asbestos that in turn leads to NFκB activation.[5] NFκB activity allows mesothelial cells that have encountered asbestos to survive the toxic insult of asbestos, and these genetically damaged mesothelial cells may grow into a malignancy. If NFκB activity is not induced, mesothelial cells die as a result of asbestos exposure. Most recently, data implicating necrosis, as opposed to apoptosis, in the genesis of mesothelioma have been reported in which the release of HMGB1 is necessary as a critical initial step in the pathogenesis of asbestos-related disease and provides a mechanistic link between asbestos-induced cell death, chronic inflammation, and mesothelial carcinogenesis (Fig. 138.1).[18a] Clinical trials are being prepared to test drugs that may be beneficial in the early stages of the disease or act as chemopreventive agents in high-risk individuals by interfering with this survival pathway.

It is difficult to reconcile what is known about the carcinogenic actions of asbestos and the long latency period between asbestos exposure and mesothelioma development. Lanphear and Buncher[19] reviewed 21 studies of 1,690 mesotheliomas and found that 96% occurred at least 20 years after exposure; the mean latency was 32 years. Several theories have been postulated to describe what happens during this latency period.[3] One

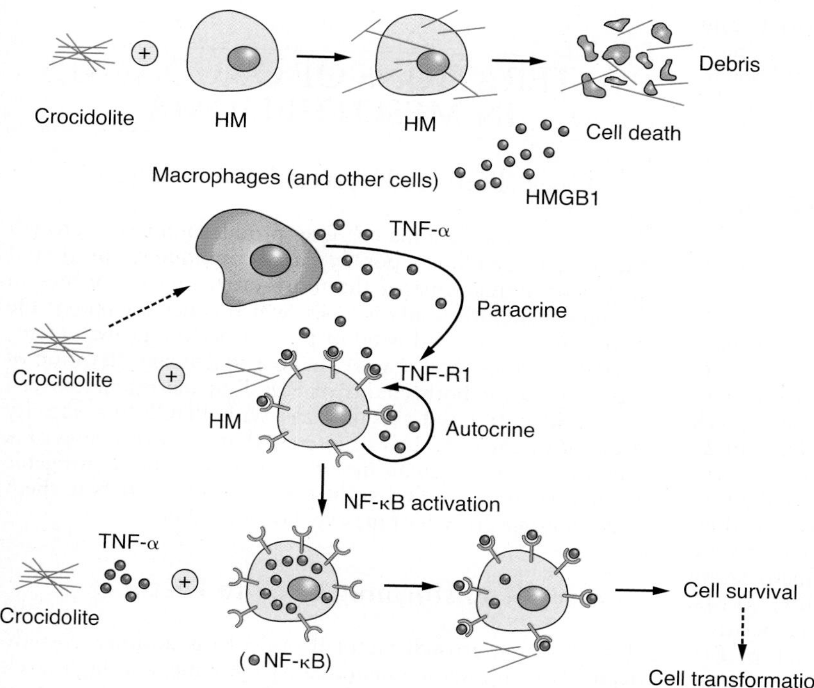

FIGURE 138.1 Asbestos causes necrotic cell death in human mesothelial (HM) cells, which leads to the release of HMGB1 into the extracellular space. HMGB1 release causes macrophages accumulation, inflammatory response, and especially the secretion of TNFαTNF-α activates the NF-κB pathway, which increases HM survival after asbestos exposure. This allows HM with asbestos-induced DNA damage to divide rather than die and, if key genetic alterations accumulate, to eventually develop into MM.

PRACTICE OF ONCOLOGY

theory suggests that malignant transformation of a mesothelial cell occurs soon after asbestos exposure and it then takes years for the tumor to grow. This is quite unlikely because malignant mesothelioma has no detectable preinvasive phase and is a rapidly growing tumor. A second hypothesis is that asbestos induces genetic alterations in mesothelial cells over a long period that eventually lead to malignant cells. This may occur if a key regulatory gene, such as the *INK4a/ARF* locus, is deleted or silenced. With loss of key regulatory genes, additional mutations could accumulate rapidly. INK4a/ARF codes for p16 (a cyclin-dependent kinase inhibitor) and for p14ARF, which promotes murine double minute-2 (MDM2) degradation, preventing MDM2 from neutralizing p53. Both p16 and p14ARF are often deleted in malignant mesotheliomas (see "Alterations of Specific Tumor Suppressor Genes in Mesothelioma"). Occasionally, this process may allow enough mutations to accumulate to lead to malignancy. Cell growth from this point would be rapid, leading to a clinically detectable tumor.[3]

OVERVIEW OF MOLECULAR MECHANISMS IN MESOTHELIOMA

Cytogenetic Assessment of Malignant Mesotheliomas

As previously mentioned, chromosome banding analyses have revealed that most malignant mesotheliomas have complex karyotypes. Deletions of specific chromosomal sites in the short (p) arms of chromosomes 1, 3, and 9 and long (q) arm of 6 are repeatedly observed in these tumors.[20] Using newer molecular platforms including array comparative genomic hybridization and representational oligonucleotide microarray analysis, deletions in chromosomes 22q12.2, 19q13.32, and 17p13.1 appear to be the most frequent events (55%–74%), followed by deletions in 1p, 9p, 9q, 4p, 3p, and gains in 5p, 18q, 8q, and 17q (23%–55%). Increasing numbers of copy number abnormalities in mesothelioma are associated with poor prognosis, especially when associated with deletions in 9p21.3 encompassing CDKN2A/ARF and CDKN2B as detailed later. Analysis of the minimal common areas of frequent gains and losses has pointed to novel potential TSGs including OSM (22q12.2), FUS1, PL6 (3p21.3), DNAJA1 (9p21.1), and CDH2 (18q11.2–q12.3).[21]

Alterations of Specific Tumor Suppressor Genes in Mesothelioma

p16

Cheng et al.[22] reported homozygous deletions of one or more of the three *p16* exons in 34 of 40 (85%) malignant mesothelioma cell lines and a point mutation in one cell line. Downregulation of *p16* was observed in four of the remaining cell lines. Homozygous deletions of *p16* were identified in 5 of 23 (22%) malignant mesothelioma tumor samples. Downregulation of *p16* in malignant mesothelioma cells may result from 5′CpG island hypermethylation, as has been demonstrated in other types of cancer. Recently it has been reported that *P16* inactivation by homozygous deletions or methylation is a frequent event in Japanese patients with MPMs. Homozygous deletion is the major cause of the *P16* inactivation, but methylation also leads to the inactivation of *P16* when the *P16* alleles are retained.[23] Homozygous deletions at this locus can lead to the inactivation of another putative TSG, *p14*^{ARF}, because *p16* and *p14*^{ARF} share exons 2 and 3 although their reading frames differ.[24,25] The prognostic significance of p16/CDKN2A loss in malignant mesotheliomas has been defined both by immunohistochemistry and fluorescence *in situ* hybridization (FISH). Both loss of p16 protein expression by immunohistochemistry and homozygous deletion of p16 by FISH are associated with an adverse prognosis.[26]

p53

Cell lines derived from murine models of asbestos-induced mesothelioma have reduced or absent expression of p53 messenger RNA (mRNA) compared to the RNA from nontumorigenic cell lines or reactive mesothelial cells.[27] In human cell lines derived from patients with malignant mesothelioma, attention has turned to specific mutations or genetic abnormalities in *p53*. In general, mutational analyses of *p53* in mesothelioma have not revealed reasons for its inactivation. As detailed later in "Simian Virus 40," a stronger candidate for such inactivation of *p53* is SV40 large tumor antigen.

Wilms Tumor Gene

The detection of Wilms tumor gene (*WT1*) mRNA or protein provides a specific molecular or immunohistochemical marker for differentiation of mesothelioma from other pleural tumors, in particular adenocarcinoma.[28] Vaccination protocols that exploit the selective presence of *WT1* in mesothelioma are under way at selected institutions.

Neurofibromatosis Gene

The tumor suppressor merlin is encoded by the neurofibromatosis type 2 gene (*NF2*), which is located on chromosome 22q12, and mutations in this gene have been found in 40% of mesothelioma and 50% of malignant mesothelioma cell lines.[29,30] Mutations including deletions and insertions lead to truncated and inactivated merlin. Experimental animal models indicate that disruption of the *NF2* signaling pathway, together with a deficiency in *ink4a*, is essential for mesothelioma development.

ALTERATIONS OF ONCOGENES IN MESOTHELIOMA

C-sis (Platelet-Derived Growth Factor)

Malignant mesothelioma cell lines produce numerous growth factors and cytokines, possibly as a consequence of altered oncogene status. One of the more intriguing oncogenes in malignant mesothelioma is C-sis, which codes for one of the two chains (alpha and beta) of platelet-derived growth factor (PDGF). Gerwin et al.[31] were the first to describe elevation of RNA levels for both chains of PDGF in mesothelioma cell lines and correlated the increase with PDGF-like activity secreted by the cells. It is of interest that overexpression of A chain transforms human mesothelial cells to the tumorigenic phenotype *in vitro* and that the use of antisense ODN to the A chain inhibits growth of mesothelioma cell lines.

Transforming Growth Factor

Transforming growth factor-B (TGF-B) is another growth-regulatory and immunomodulatory cytokine, and high levels of TGF-B have been described in several human and mouse malignant mesothelioma cell lines.[32,33] TGF-B may have a potential role in regulation of the differential PDGF receptor expression in malignant mesothelioma and thus have an effect on proliferation as well as other events. TGF-B production by tumors plays a significant role in blocking immune response by preventing T-cell infiltration into tumors, inhibition of T-cell activation/function, and mediation of T regulatory cell–induced immunosuppression. TGF-blockers (soluble receptors/antibodies) and receptor inhibitors have antitumor effects that, in several models, are due primarily to immunologic mechanisms. TGF blockade had antitumor effects that were CD8+ T-cell dependent in a murine malignant mesothelioma model.[34]

Insulin Growth Factor

Insulin growth factor (IGF) is another of the important autocrine loops in mesothelioma.[35] The IGF receptor-1 pathway is a significant regulator of mesothelioma growth acting through downstream kinases such as Akt. In humans, both normal mesothelium and mesothelioma cell lines express IGF-1 and IGF-1R RNAs (by Northern blot or reverse transcriptase polymerase chain reaction [RT-PCR]), and IGF-1 protein is detected in their conditioned media. These studies suggest that mesothelioma growth, both in human and animal models for the disease, may involve the IGFs, and trials using anti-IGF-1R antibodies or small-molecule IGF blockade are being formulated for mesothelioma.[36]

Angiogenic Mechanisms in Mesothelioma

The most relevant cytokines and growth factors in angiogenic pathways involve the interleukins (specifically IL-6 and IL-8), fibroblast growth factors (FGFs), vascular endothelial growth factors (VEGFs), platelet-derived endothelial growth factors, and IGFs. Moreover, mutational or posttranslational silencing of TSGs or their products, particularly *p53* and *p16*, has also been associated with increased angiogenic mechanisms.

IL-6 levels are elevated in the serum and pleural effusions of patients with mesothelioma, and there have been correlations seen between the IL-6 level and the degree of thrombocytosis in these patients.[37] IL-6 expression is elevated in tissues undergoing angiogenesis, but by itself it has a limited role in proliferation of endothelial cells. IL-6, however, induces angiogenesis by elevating the expression of VEGF, a specific mitogen for vascular endothelial cells. Serum VEGF and IL-6 levels are elevated in patients with mesothelioma, and their levels each correlate with platelet count.[38]

IL-8 is also an important angiogenic factor for the development of new capillaries *in vivo* and has direct growth-potentiating activity in mesothelioma. Pleural fluid from patients with mesothelioma has significantly higher IL-8 levels by enzyme-linked assay compared to patients with other malignant effusions.[39] Mesotheliomas present with a high intratumoral vessel density that also have prognostic relevance,[32,40,41] and, immunohistochemically, VEGF, FGF-1 and -2, and TGF-B immunoreactivity are present in 81%, 67%, 92%, and 96%, respectively, of mesotheliomas, and in 20%, 50%, 40%, and 10% of samples of the non-neoplastic mesothelium. Depending on the study, high immunohistochemical FGF-2 expression[41] or VEGF expression by RT-PCR correlate with more tumor aggressiveness and worse prognosis for mesothelioma.[40,42]

Simian Virus 40

SV40 is a DNA tumor virus that has been associated with the development of malignant mesothelioma.[7] Although this virus is endogenous in rhesus monkeys, epidemiologic studies have shown that it is also widespread among the human population. The mode by which the virus was transferred from monkey to human is uncertain, but the bulk of this transfer may have occurred from 1954 to 1963 through SV40-contaminated polio vaccines administered worldwide. Moreover, polio vaccines produced in the former Union of Soviet Socialist Republics (USSR) remained contaminated with infectious SV40 at least until 1978.[43]

Once inside its host, SV40 produces two proteins associated with its oncogenesis, the large and small tumor (T) antigens.[7] The large T antigen (Tag) is a 90-kD protein found predominantly in the nucleus of infected cells that is capable of inducing structural and numerical chromosomal alterations. Tag also induces IGF expression, inhibits *p53* and the pRB family, and induces c-met activity to stimulate cell proliferation.[7] The small T antigen (tag) is a 17-kD protein found in the cytoplasm of infected cells where it inhibits cellular phosphatase 2A and stimulates microtubule-associated protein (MAP) kinase and AP-1 activity. The small tag also works with Tag to bind and inhibit *p53* and pRB.[7] The combined activity of both the large Tag and the small tag induce Notch-1 and telomerase activity, which are required for malignant transformation and immortalization.[7]

The association of SV40 with mesothelioma started with the observation that when hamsters were injected with SV40 into the pleural space, all of the animals developed mesotheliomas within 6 months.[44] This finding prompted investigations into the possibility that some mesotheliomas in humans could be attributed to SV40 infection directly or with SV40 acting as a cocarcinogen with asbestos. Mesothelioma samples studied in 1994 showed that 60% of the samples contained SV40 DNA and expressed the SV40 large T antigen. The results were confirmed by numerous laboratories using a variety of techniques such as PCR, FISH, Western blot, immunohistochemistry, and laser dissection/PCR, but the percentage of positive samples varied from 6% to 83%, and a few studies were completely negative (reviewed in refs. 45 and 46). Technical and geographical differences may account for these variances.

Significant geographical differences in exposure to SV40 were confirmed by a recent study showing that the polio vaccines used in the former USSR and in the countries under its influence contained infectious SV40 until at least 1978.[43] These findings supported a previous conclusion of the Institute of Medicine of the National Academy of Sciences that the epidemiologic data were flawed and therefore it was not possible to accept or reject a causal association between SV40-containing polio vaccines and cancer. In fact, it was not possible to clearly distinguish exposed from nonexposed cohorts. Although the epidemiologic data are not available, mechanistic experiments in human mesothelial cells and animal experiments strongly support a pathogenic role of SV40 in mesothelioma. It is unlikely, however, that SV40 acts alone in mesothelioma development, as most cancers are multifactorial, and most mesotheliomas occur in asbestos-exposed individuals. Recently, SV40 has been shown to be a cocarcinogen in causing mesothelioma in animals and malignant transformation of mesothelial cells in tissue culture.[6] In addition, the data showed that in the presence of SV40 lower amounts of asbestos were sufficient to cause mesothelioma.[6] Cocarcinogenesis was mediated through the activation of the ERKs' kinases and AP-1 activity that led to cell proliferation and stromal invasion.[6]

Radiation and Mesothelioma

In the literature, there are a few studies reporting mesothelioma development in patients exposed to thorotrast (intravenously) or who had received radiation to the chest and abdomen.[3] In some of these cases, asbestos exposure could not be ruled out, and SV40 status was not investigated. However, in a few cases in which mesotheliomas developed in young adults who received radiotherapy (RT) because of Wilms tumor, radiation was the only likely causative factor. Studies in rats support a role for radiation as a causative factor. Although it appears that radiation may cause mesotheliomas, the number of mesotheliomas for which it is responsible is probably small.

Carbon Nanoparticles

Engineered single-wall carbon nanotubes (SWCNTs) are a class of nanoparticles being actively evaluated for myriad industrial and biomedical applications.[47] Exponential growth in the use of SWCNTs potentially can expose a large number of workers. Preliminary cellular and animal exposure investigations on the toxicity and pathogenicity of SWCNTs have demonstrated biological interactions, including toxicity, inflammatory reactions, oxidative stress, and fibroproliferative response.[48,49] SWCNTs are biopersistent and have the ability to distribute to subpleural areas after pharyngeal aspiration.[49] A recent report described the induction of mesothelioma in p53+/− mice by multiwall carbon nanotubes.[2] These earlier investigations compelled the present studies of potential interactions of SWCNTs with mesothelial cells. Exposure to SWCNTs induced reactive oxygen species generation, increased cell death, enhanced DNA damage, and H2AX phosphorylation, and activated poly(adenosine diphosphate-ribose) polymerase (PARP), AP-1, NFκB, p38, and Akt in a dose-dependent manner. These events recapitulate some of the key molecular events involved in mesothelioma development associated with asbestos exposure.[50,51]

Genetic Predisposition to Mesothelioma

Recent evidence indicates that genetic predisposition plays an important role in determining individual susceptibility to mineral fiber carcinogenesis and to the development of mesothelioma. In the villages of Karain (population ~600), Tuzkoy (population ~1,400), and Sarihidir (this village was abandoned) in Cappadocia, a region in Central Anatolia, Turkey, 50% or more of deaths are caused by malignant mesothelioma.[52] This epidemic has been linked to exposure to a mineral fiber called *erionite*. Erionite is a type of fibrous zeolite commonly found in the stones of the houses of Karain, Tuzkoy, and Sarihidir. Erionite induces mesothelioma in close to 100% of exposed animals, compared with 20% induction in parallel experiments when using crocidolite or other types of asbestos.[53] Thus, erionite is considered the most potent mineral fiber in causing mesothelioma. However, among Turkish villagers exposed to erionite, mesothelioma was more frequent in certain families than others. This observation prompted analyses that revealed that some families in Turkey were unusually susceptible to erionite carcinogenesis.[52]

Similar families have also been identified in other parts of the world[54] and in the United States, where they appear to be unusually susceptible to asbestos carcinogenesis. These findings indicate that genetics plays a role in influencing susceptibility to mineral fiber carcinogenesis.[52] Erionite is present in many parts of the world, including western American states such as North Dakota, but so far the contribution of erionite to the increased incidence of mesothelioma has not been studied except in Turkey. Recent analyses indicate that there are no differences among the erionite mineral found in the mesothelioma villages in Turkey and the erionite found in the United States.[55]

PATHOLOGY OF MESOTHELIOMA

Benign Mesotheliomas

True malignant mesothelioma is an aggressive malignancy with a dismal prognosis. There are, however, a number of benign mesothelial proliferations that must be distinguished from malignant mesothelioma. Multicystic mesothelioma, also called *multilocular peritoneal inclusion cyst*, is a benign mesothelial lesion, characteristically formed by multiple cysts arranged in grapelike clusters. Adenomatoid mesotheliomas are benign mesothelial lesions of the genital system. Mesothelioma of the atrioventricular node is neither a mesothelioma nor a tumor. This lesion represents congenital heterotopia of the endodermal sinus in the atrioventricular node. Well-differentiated papillary mesothelioma is found more often in the abdominal cavity of young women. Histologically, it is formed by multiple papillary structures covered by cytologically benign mesothelial cells. The lesion is benign, but there have been occasional cases in which several years after diagnosis the patient developed a true mesothelioma. Localized mesothelioma, better referred to as *localized fibrous tumor of the pleura* (FTP), is similar to other fibrous tumors found elsewhere in the body. The tumor cells have a benign appearance and are usually immersed in a fibrous and characteristically vascular stroma. FTPs are characteristically negative for cytokeratin (a marker of mesothelial cells) and positive for CD34, which suggests that these cells are not of mesothelial origin. The most important predictive factor in the prognosis of FTP is whether the tumor can be completely resected. Thus, pedunculated tumors have a much better prognosis than tumors that grow over a broad pleural area.

Tumor array studies comparing variant histologies with classic epithelial malignant mesothelioma may provide tools to identify these rare "benign malignant mesotheliomas" in the future. Thus far, the feasibility of using gene expression arrays to distinguish mesothelioma from adenocarcinoma has been reported. However, the majority of the markers that were significant in the expression arrays are already used as part of the standard immunohistochemical panel.[56]

Malignant Mesothelioma

Histologically, malignant mesothelioma can show an epithelial morphology (malignant mesothelioma epithelial type), a fibrous morphology (malignant mesothelioma fibrous type, also called sarcomatoid type), or a combination of both (mixed type or biphasic malignant mesothelioma) (Fig. 138.2). Most malignant mesotheliomas (50%–60%) are of the epithelial type, approximately 10% are sarcomatoid, and the remainder are biphasic malignant mesotheliomas. Correct identification of the histologic type is important, and tumors with a prevalently sarcomatous morphology are quite resistant to therapy and have median survivals of less than 1 year from diagnosis. In contrast, mostly epithelioid tumors, especially well-differentiated variants, are associated with prolonged survivals of up to 2 years from diagnosis. Unusual morphologic variants exist but are rare, and some malignant mesotheliomas cannot be subcategorized histologically and should be called poorly differentiated malignant mesothelioma.

The diagnosis of malignant mesothelioma is usually straightforward, in contrast to common belief, provided that the pathologist has extensive experience with this malignancy. Some epithelial mesotheliomas grow forming sheets of epithelioid cells. The experienced pathologist easily recognizes these tumors as mesothelial in origin. Some carcinomas, however, can look very much like a malignant mesothelioma, or a malignant mesothelioma can look so atypical that it resembles a metastatic

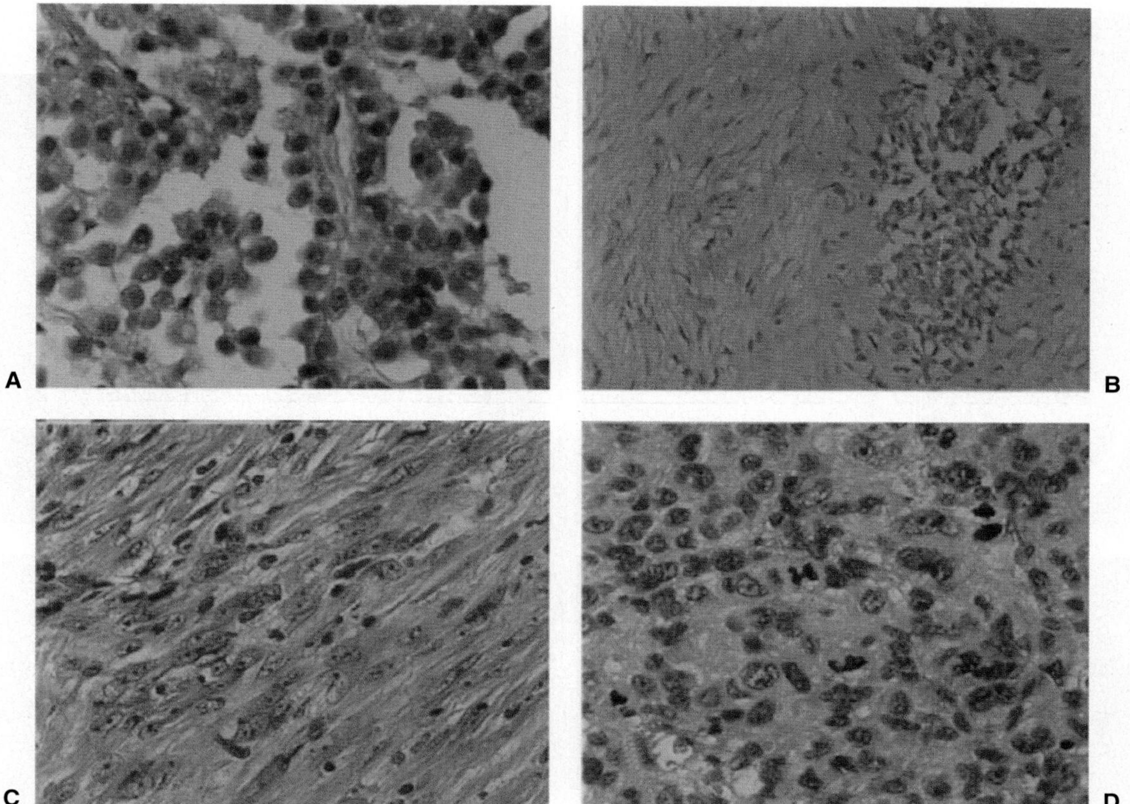

FIGURE 138.2 Histology of mesothelioma. **A:** Epithelioid mesothelioma. Note tubular structures and malignant mesothelioma cells showing a hobnail morphology with bland nuclei and abundant cytoplasm. **B:** Biphasic malignant mesothelioma, showing a nest of mesothelioma cells with epithelial differentiation within the sarcomatoid component. **C:** Sarcomatoid mesothelioma, positivity for pankeratin, and rare foci of cells suggestive of epithelioid differentiation indicated the diagnosis. **D:** High-grade sarcoma, a highly aggressive tumor that is vimentin-positive but vimentin-negative over 15 different immunostains for other markers and without distinctive electron microscopic features. In this case, the diagnosis of mesothelioma could not be confirmed. Original magnification: **A**, **C**, and **D**, ×400; **B**, ×200.

carcinoma. Therefore, to rule out these mimics, the diagnosis of malignant mesothelioma should be further confirmed by immunohistochemistry, which shows that the tumor cells are diffusively positive for pankeratin, keratin 5/6, calretinin, and WT-1, and negative for the epithelial markers such as CEA, CD15, Ber-EP4, Moc-31, TTF-1, and B72.3. For epithelial mesotheliomas, positive stainings for pankeratin and calretinin and negative stainings for three epithelial markers are considered sufficient for diagnosis. Occasionally, however, more stainings are required because some carcinomas are positive for calretinin or are negative for some of the epithelial markers. In these difficult cases, electron microscopy showing the classic long-branching microvilli of human mesothelial cells, compared to the short nonbranching microvilli of carcinomas, can still be considered the gold standard for a correct diagnosis.

Newer methods are under development for distinguishing mesothelioma from adenocarcinoma and include microRNA profiling of the tumors. Gee et al.[57] have described the use of seven miRNAs (miR-200c, miR-141, miR-200b, miR-200a, miR-429, miR-203, and miR-205) to distinguish lung adenocarcinoma from mesothelioma with a 10% misclassification error. Others have described a three microRNA profile (mir-205, mir-193a-3p, and mir-192) for the differential diagnosis of mesothelioma from colon, renal, lung, and breast cancer with a 95% specificity and 96% sensitivity.[58]

Biphasic mesotheliomas must be distinguished from carcinosarcomas metastasizing from various organs and from biphasic synovial sarcomas. Carcinosarcomas will stain negative or weakly and focally positive for calretinin and focally or diffusively positive for some epithelial markers. Mesotheliomas stain positive for pankeratin in both the epithelial and the fibrous component, whereas carcinosarcomas usually are positive mostly in the epithelial component. As mentioned, electron microscopy is very useful in identifying long-branching microvilli (mesothelioma) or short, thick microvilli (carcinosarcoma). Synovial sarcomas can be very difficult to distinguish from mesothelioma. Usually an ambiguous set of immunostains prompts the molecular testing for the X;18 translocation that is diagnostic.[59]

Fibrous mesotheliomas are more difficult to diagnose because they show a morphology that can be essentially identical to other primary or metastatic pleural sarcomas. Immunohistochemistry showing diffuse positive staining for pankeratin is useful to confirm the diagnosis. Only a fraction, which varies depending on the study, of sarcomatoid malignant mesothelioma is positive for calretinin, and WT-1.

Solitary Fibrous Tumors of Pleura

The solitary FTP is a mesenchymal growth that arises from the visceral or parietal pleura.[60–62] The benign variant is an encapsulated lobulated tumor that on microscopic examination may resemble a sarcomatoid mesothelioma with interweaving bundles of ovoid or spindle cells without atypia. A malignant variant characterized by high cellularity, marked pleomorphism, and a high mitotic activity is seen in approximately 10% of the cases. FTPs, unlike mesotheliomas, are immunohistochemically negative when stained for cytokeratins. Sixty percent of the patients

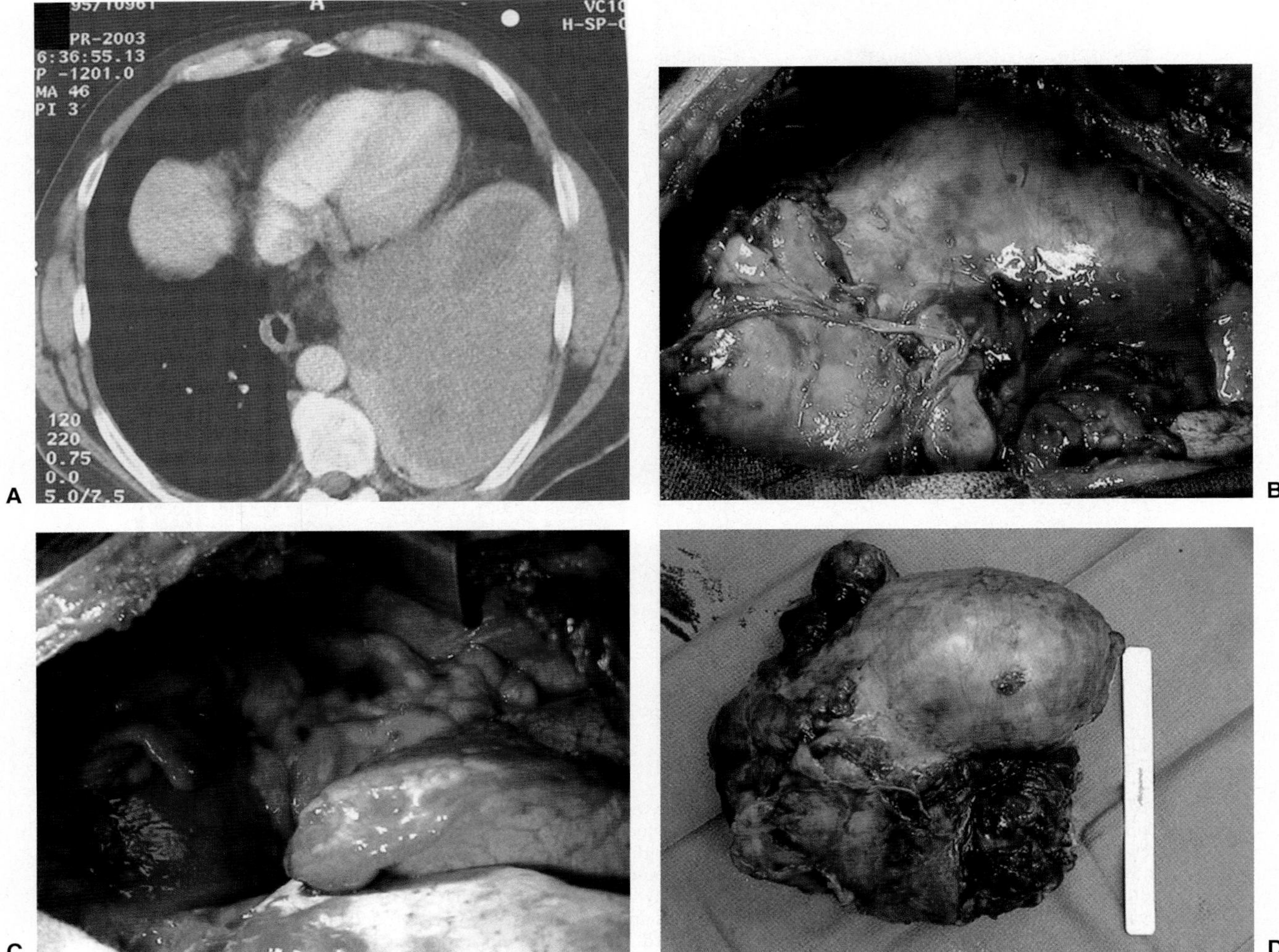

FIGURE 138.3 Fibrous tumor of pleura. **A:** Computed tomography reveals a large mass compressing the lower lobe of the lung. **B:** Intraoperative photograph. Tumor arose from a wide stalk on the diaphragm. **C:** Intraoperative photograph after resection of the mass revealing expansion of the lung and no other disease. **D:** Resected specimen.

have symptoms, and both male and female patients with FTP can present with dyspnea from compressive atelectasis, as well as with lower extremity edema from mediastinal compression. Clubbing and osteoarthropathy are present in 20% to 50% of cases versus only 6% in malignant mesothelioma. Hyponatremia attributed to inappropriate secretion of antidiuretic hormone and hypoglycemia has been described.

Plain chest radiograph reveals a well-circumscribed lobulated tumor that is heterogeneous-appearing on computed tomogram with a pedicle that is usually attached to the visceral pleura. Rarely, there are multiple tumors that are pedunculated on the visceral pleura. Effusions are seldom associated with FTPs, except with the malignant variety.

Benign FTPs can recur and transform to the malignant variant, and the malignant variants are usually not pedunculated, larger, and present in unusual locations.

Surgical resection (Fig. 138.3) is the treatment of choice, with complete resection of the tumor and its pedunculated portion along with the site of origin. Five-year survival rates as high as 97% have been reported. *En bloc* resection of the lung, chest wall, or diaphragm may be necessary. For recurrences, re-excision is the treatment of choice. Long-term survival with re-excision is possible, but with incomplete resection or malignant transformation the median survival is 24 to 36 months.

EPIDEMIOLOGY AND CLINICAL PRESENTATION

The death rates for mesothelioma parallel the consumption of asbestos by individual countries. When one considers mesothelioma death rates from 2000 to 2004 as a function of asbestos usage in the 1960s, Australia has the highest death rate for the disease in the world.[63] In addition, according to the World Health Organization database, the highest death rates per million population are seen in Australia, the United Kingdom, New Zealand, Canada, Western Europe and the United States. Moreover, it is predicted that between 2000 and 2049, over 400,000 lives will be lost in those countries from the disease. In the United States, there have been 2,500 deaths per year from the disease since 1999, with workers with industrial exposures in construction and shipbuilding being at highest risk, followed by plumbers, pipe fitters, and steamers. Mesothelioma affects men in their 50s, 60s, and 70s due to the aforementioned 25- to 40-year latency period between occupational asbestos exposure and the development of the tumor.[64] Women and children can have the disease, but the male-to-female ratio is approximately 5:3.[65]

Symptoms

The duration of symptoms varies from 2 weeks to 2 years, with most series having a median time to diagnosis from symptoms of 2 to 3 months. As many as 25% of patients with the disease have symptoms for 6 months or more before seeking medical attention. The right side is affected more than the left side (60% vs. 40%), most likely because of the right side's greater volume.

Approximately 60% of the patients present with nonpleuritic chest pain that classically is located posterolaterally and low in the thorax. Dyspnea is present in 50% to 70% of the cases, and, indeed, 80% of the patients present with dyspnea and effusion. The presence of a pleural effusion is documented at some time in the course of the disease in 95% of patients with malignant pleural mesothelioma (MPM). With the increasing use of positron emission tomography for pretreatment planning, between 5% and 25% of patients are found to have metastatic disease at presentation.[66]

Physical Examination

Physical examination reveals decreased breath sounds, dullness to percussion, or decreased motion of the involved chest wall. Failure to significantly relieve the dyspnea after thoracentesis may indicate that the lung is "trapped." In the late stages of the disease, there is often dramatic cachexia, marked contraction of the involved chest with narrowed interspaces, and hypertrophy of the contralateral hemithorax. A chest wall mass occurs in up to 25% of patients, often at the site(s) of prior thoracentesis, thoracotomy, or thoracoscopy wounds.

Laboratory Examination

Mesothelioma patients have nonspecific laboratory findings, including hypergammaglobulinemia, eosinophilia, and/or anemia of chronic disease. It has been recently noted that 14% to 15% of patients have elevated homocysteine levels, reflecting folic acid deficiency; 17% have biochemical evidence of vitamin B_{12} deficiency; and 32% have biochemical signs of vitamin B_6 deficiency.[67] The most striking laboratory abnormality is thrombocytosis (>400,000), which is seen in 60% to 90% of patients,[68] and approximately 15% of patients have platelet counts greater than 1,000,000.

Soluble mesothelin-related peptide (SMRP), osteopontin (OPN), and megakaryocyte potentiating factor are presently under investigation as early detection or therapy monitoring markers. Mesothelin, originally described by Chang et al.,[69] is a 40-kDa glycoprotein attached to the cell surface of mesotheliomas, ovarian cancers, and pancreatic cancers and is thought to have a role in cell adhesion and cell-to-cell recognition and signaling. Mesothelin is synthesized as a precursor 69 kDa protein and forms two proteins, the membrane-bound[70] and the soluble protein megakaryocyte potentiating factor. A third member of this family is SMRP. Robinson et al.[70] reported that determination of SMRP in serum is a marker of mesothelioma with a sensitivity of 83% and specificity of 95% in the first 48 MPM patients tested. These data have been validated by other laboratories in the United States[71,72] and internationally.[73] Changes in serum SMRP levels parallel clinical course/tumor size, and SMRP was elevated in 75% of patients at diagnosis.[74] Mesothelin assays (MesoMark, Fujirebio, Malvern, PA) are now available in Europe and Australia and are available for response monitoring in the United States through reference laboratories.

OPN is a glycoprotein overexpressed in many cancers that mediates cell-matrix interactions and is regulated by proteins in cell-signaling pathways that have been associated with asbestos-induced carcinogenesis.[75] In a study that compared serum OPN levels of patients with MPM to those of asbestos exposed individuals without cancer, serum OPN levels rose with duration of asbestos exposure (0–9 years vs. 10+ years; $P = .02$) and degree of radiographic abnormality (plaques and fibrosis vs. other lesser findings, $P = .004$).[76] The mean serum OPN level in individuals with mesothelioma (133 ± 10 ng/mL) was significantly higher than in the group exposed to asbestos (30 ± 3 ng/mL; $P < .001$). Using a cutpoint of 48.3 ng of OPN per milliliter results in 77.6% sensitivity and 85.5% specificity when comparing the group exposed to asbestos with the group with mesothelioma. Follow-up studies have demonstrated that serum OPN is not as robust a marker as SMRP because of the presence of a thrombin cleavage site, which causes degradation of the marker with time.[77] Plasma OPN, although not specific to mesothelioma, is being evaluated in the disease for both prognosis and early detection utility. A head-to-head comparison of markers by Creaney et al.[78] revealed that at a level of specificity of 95% relative to healthy controls and patients with benign asbestos-related disease, the sensitivity for mesothelioma was 34% for megakaryocyte potentiating factor, 47% for OPN, and 73% for mesothelin. Studies using SMRP in an attempt to diagnose early mesothelioma in high-risk cohorts have so far been disappointing, but follow-up is still short.[79]

Radiologic Examination

Malignant mesothelioma can have a diverse radiographic appearance. Many of the early changes are associated with a previous exposure to asbestos, consisting both of pleural and parenchymal changes, including pleural plaques or parenchymal pulmonary fibrosis.

Chest Radiography

The most common chest radiography features associated with mesothelioma progression and symptoms include the presence of a pleural effusion, diffuse pleural thickening, and nodularity. The involved hemithorax can eventually have smooth, lobular pleural masses that infiltrate the pleural space and fissures[80–82] in 45% to 60% of patients with contraction and fixation of the chest (Fig. 138.4). The lung becomes encased, and the mediastinum shifts because of volume loss. The effusion can be loculated, chiefly in the lower portion of the chest, completely obscuring a view of the diaphragm, lower lobes, and pericardium. In many of these instances, the lower lobe is viewed on computed tomography (CT) to be completely collapsed.

Chest Tomography

Pleural changes on chest tomography include pleural plaques, diffuse pleural thickening, and pleural effusion. Additional CT features of mesothelioma are localized nodular or plaquelike pleural thickening, possibly associated with pleural effusion. The lobulated pleural encasement frequently causes lower lobe collapse (Fig. 138.5). Intrapulmonary nodules can occur in 60% of patients, and infiltration into fissures along with enlarged hilar and mediastinal lymph nodes may be seen. The CT allows a better view of the involved pericardium, which is irregularly thickened and associated with infiltration to the pericardial fat pad. A clear fat plane between the inferior diaphragmatic surface and the adjacent abdominal organs as well as a smooth inferior diaphragmatic contour may imply resectability.[83] CT may reveal a hemidiaphragm encased by a mass or poor definition between the liver, stomach, and inferior diaphragmatic surface.

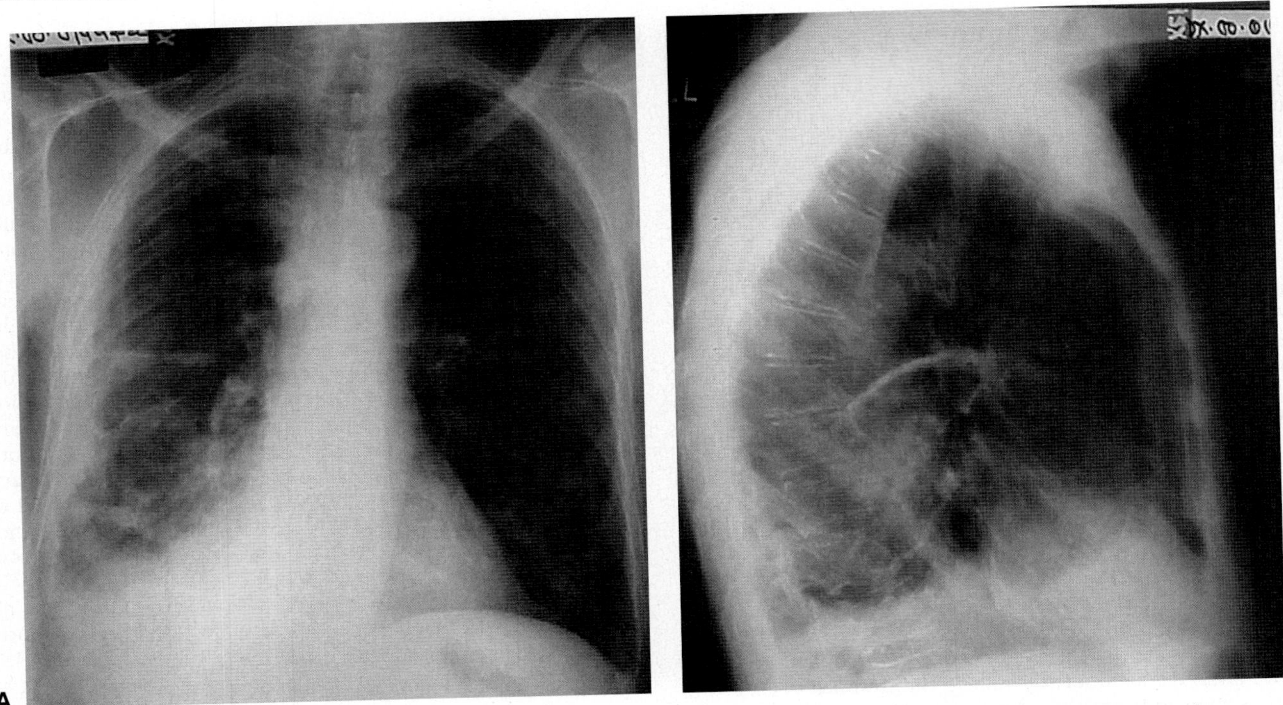

FIGURE 138.4 Chest radiography of malignant pleural mesothelioma. **A:** Anteroposterior view reveals a contracted right hemithorax with nodular scalloping of the pleura at the right base. There is fluid or tumor in the fissure, and the diaphragm and right heart border are obscured. **B:** Lateral view demonstrates fluid or tumor at the right base with thickened pleura and disease in the fissure.

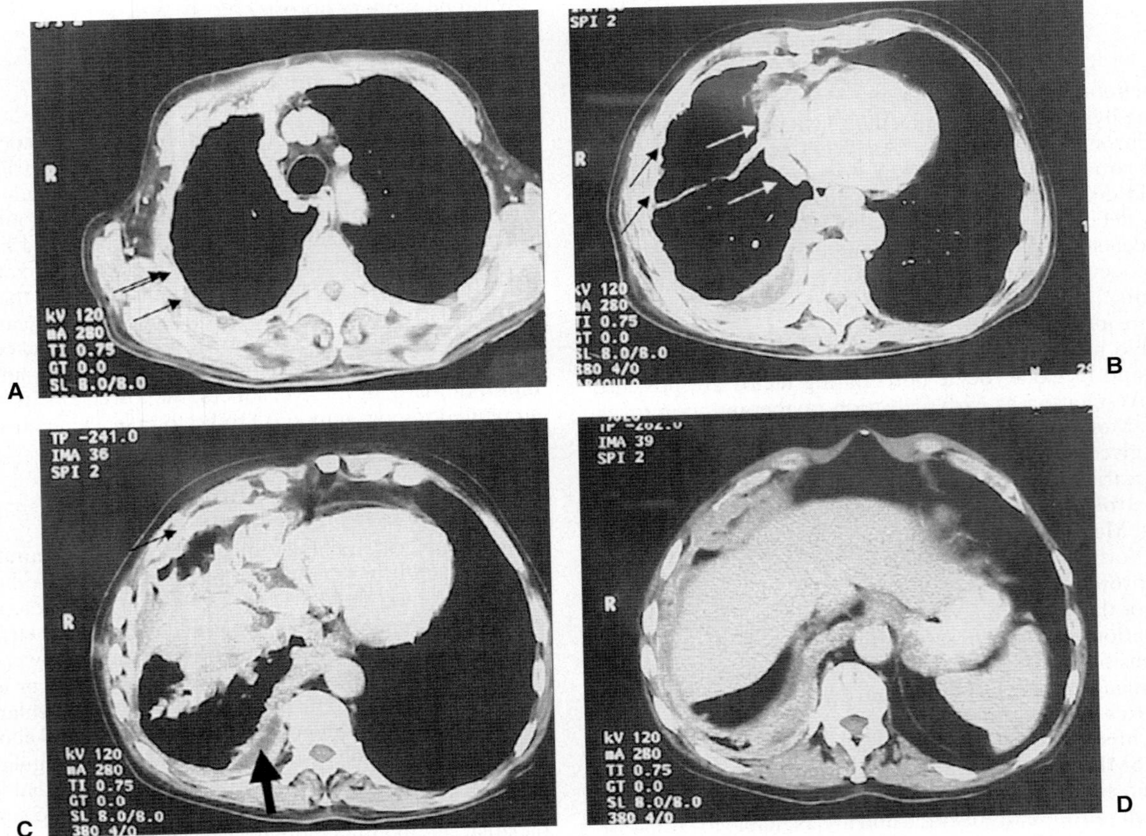

FIGURE 138.5 Computed tomography of a patient with a right-sided pleural mesothelioma. As one progresses from the apex (**A**) to the diaphragm (**D**), loculated fluid (*bold black arrow*), thickened pleura (*thin black arrows*), and thickened pericardium (*white arrows*) can be appreciated in panel C.

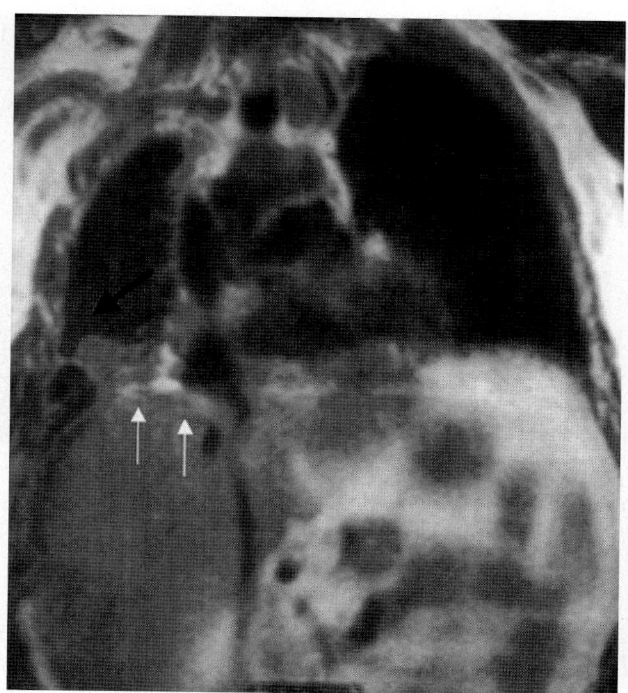
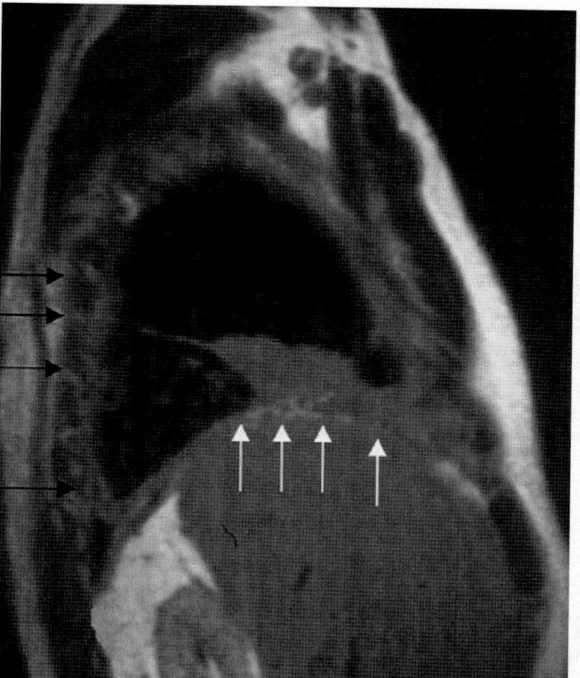

FIGURE 138.6 Magnetic resonance imaging and mesothelioma. **A:** Coronal magnetic resonance imaging of a right-sided pleural mesothelioma. *White arrows* indicate diaphragmatic involvement. *Black arrows* delineate fluid in fissure and associated mass. **B:** Sagittal magnetic resonance image of same patient reveals the thickened pleura (*thin black arrows*), involvement in the fissure (*thick black arrow*), and involvement of the diaphragm (*white arrows*).

Magnetic Resonance Imaging

Studies have suggested that gadolinium contrast enhancement magnetic resonance imaging (MRI) can improve mesothelioma staging (Fig. 138.6). Detection of diaphragm invasion and invasion of endothoracic fascia or a single chest wall focus may be better with MRI compared with CT.[83]

Positron Emission Tomography Imaging

There are a number of studies of positron emission tomography (PET) and the radionuclide imaging agent [^{18}F]fluorodeoxyglucose (FDG) in mesothelioma (Fig. 138.7). Early studies reported that FDG-PET was accurate in the diagnosis of pleural malignancies, specifically mesothelioma.[84–87] Recent studies

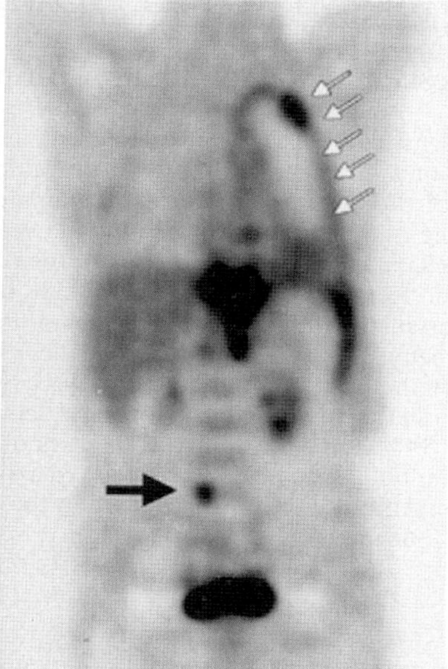
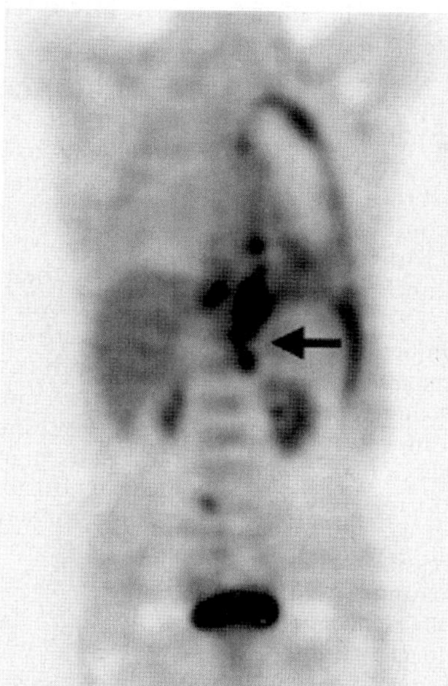
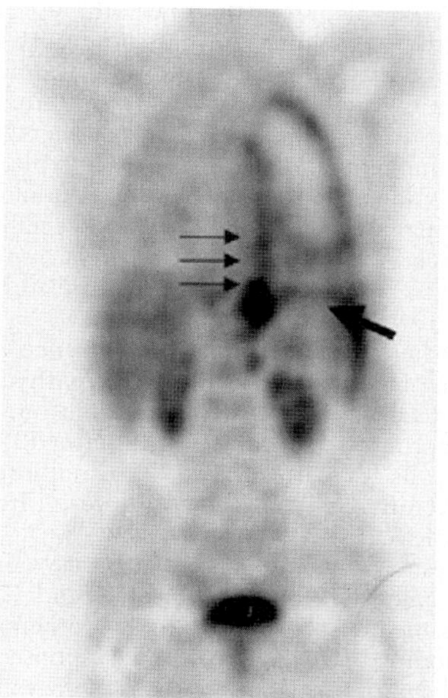

FIGURE 138.7 Positron emission tomography with [^{18}F]fluorodeoxyglucose in a patient with an unresectable stage IV mesothelioma. **A:** Short *white arrows* outline the involved pleura, with an area of bulky disease superiorly. *Bold black arrow* points out an occult metastasis in the abdomen. **B:** *Bold black arrow* depicts posterior infracrural mediastinal lymph node disease. **C:** Bold *black arrow* points out diaphragmatic involvement. *Thin black arrows* depict mesothelioma medially.

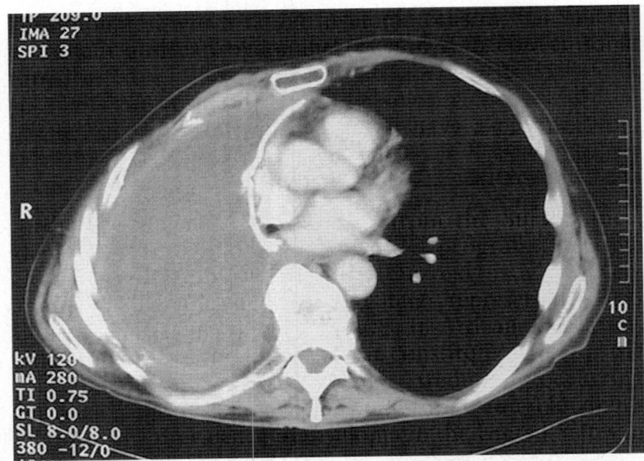

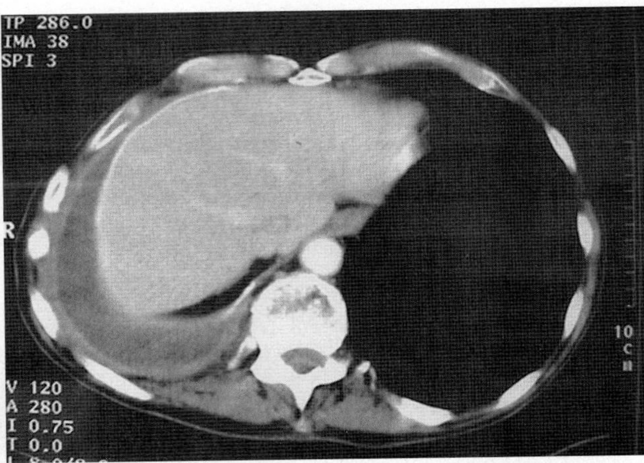

FIGURE 138.8 Appearance of computed tomogram after right extrapleural pneumonectomy. **A:** Smooth interior chest wall and intact pericardial patch. **B:** The new Gore-Tex diaphragm is seen as a white line at the edge of the liver. Note the smooth contour of the chest wall and lack of air in the hemithorax.

have concentrated on the accuracy of PET in defining lymph node metastases prior to surgical therapy. Flores et al.[84] reported a sensitivity of only 11% for PET imaging in the detection of nodal metastases in patients with MPM. Other studies in patients with N2 disease have demonstrated a sensitivity, specificity, positive predictive value, negative predictive value, and accuracy of CT-PET in lymph node staging of 38%, 78%, 60%, 58%, and 59%, respectively.[66] Because of the false-positive results in patients with FDG-avid pleural inflammatory/infectious etiologies, all FDG-avid nodes, if available, should be histologically confirmed in patients with MPM being considered for EPP. PET scanning may also have prognostic value in mesothelioma (see later discussion).

Follow-Up and Therapy Response Radiologic Assessment

After extrapleural pneumonectomy (EPP), CT scanning of the resected hemithorax reveals a smooth-walled, well-defined postoperative membrane lining the pneumonectomy space, which is usually concentrically smooth. As the interval from operation to follow-up lengthens, the membrane may actually become thicker (Fig. 138.8). Unexplained, irregular focal thickening at the base of the chest should alert the clinician to a recurrence of disease. This is especially pronounced in the pleurectomy patient in whom recurrent mesothelioma may start to thicken rapidly and infiltrate the underlying lung (Fig. 138.9).

Other presentations of recurrence include the development of new mediastinal adenopathy or ascites otherwise undetectable by physical examination. The development of asymptomatic abdominal fluid after EPP is an ominous sign and calls for paracentesis. CT usually reveals diaphragmatic thickening or diffuse mesenteric infiltration in these cases (Fig. 138.10).

Besides evaluation of postoperative progression, an important role of follow-up or sequential CT scanning is in the assessment of the response of mesothelioma to chemotherapy. A modified RECIST protocol (response evaluation criteria in solid tumors) has been used for the evaluation of response to therapy in mesothelioma.[88] The modified RECIST criteria use unidimensional measurement of tumor thickness perpendicular to the chest wall or mediastinum, measured in two sites at three different levels on CT scan. At reassessment, pleural thickness must be measured at the same position and level. A complete response requires disappearance of all target lesions with no evidence of tumor elsewhere, whereas a partial response requires at least a 30% reduction in the total tumor measurement with each of these responses being durable for at least 4 weeks. A 20% increase in the total tumor measurement or the appearance of one or more new lesions defines progressive disease.

PET scanning may have utility, however, in defining response after chemotherapy for mesothelioma.[89] PET scanning has been used in the early assessment of response of mesothelioma to chemotherapy, with an early metabolic response being significantly correlated to a longer median time-to-tumor progression than that seen in nonresponders. Moreover, patients with an early metabolic response had a trend toward longer overall survival.[90]

DIAGNOSTIC APPROACH FOR PRESUMED MESOTHELIOMA

Thoracentesis and Closed Pleural Biopsy

Patients who present with a large, unexplained pleural effusion and minimal or moderate evidence of pleural thickening should have initial thoracentesis and pleural biopsy. In the past, because of the difficulty in distinguishing between reactive mesothelial cells and tumor cells, the diagnosis of mesothelioma was made from pleural fluid in only 33% of cases. However, by preserving a cell block from the pleural fluid and using both histochemical and immunohistochemical staining techniques along with electron microscopic analysis, the diagnosis of mesothelioma can be obtained from the pleural effusion in as high as 84% of suspected cases. In cases of a large pleural effusion, multiple closed pleural biopsies to avoid sampling error with an Abrams or Cope needle aid in the diagnoses in 30% to 50% of cases.

Thoracoscopy

A video-assisted thoracoscopy is indicated for patients at risk for mesothelioma who (1) develop a large effusion and who have negative studies on thoracentesis and pleural biopsy or (2) who recur with effusion after initial thoracentesis. Thoracoscopy can be invaluable for estimating extent of disease with regard to the diaphragm, pericardium, chest wall,

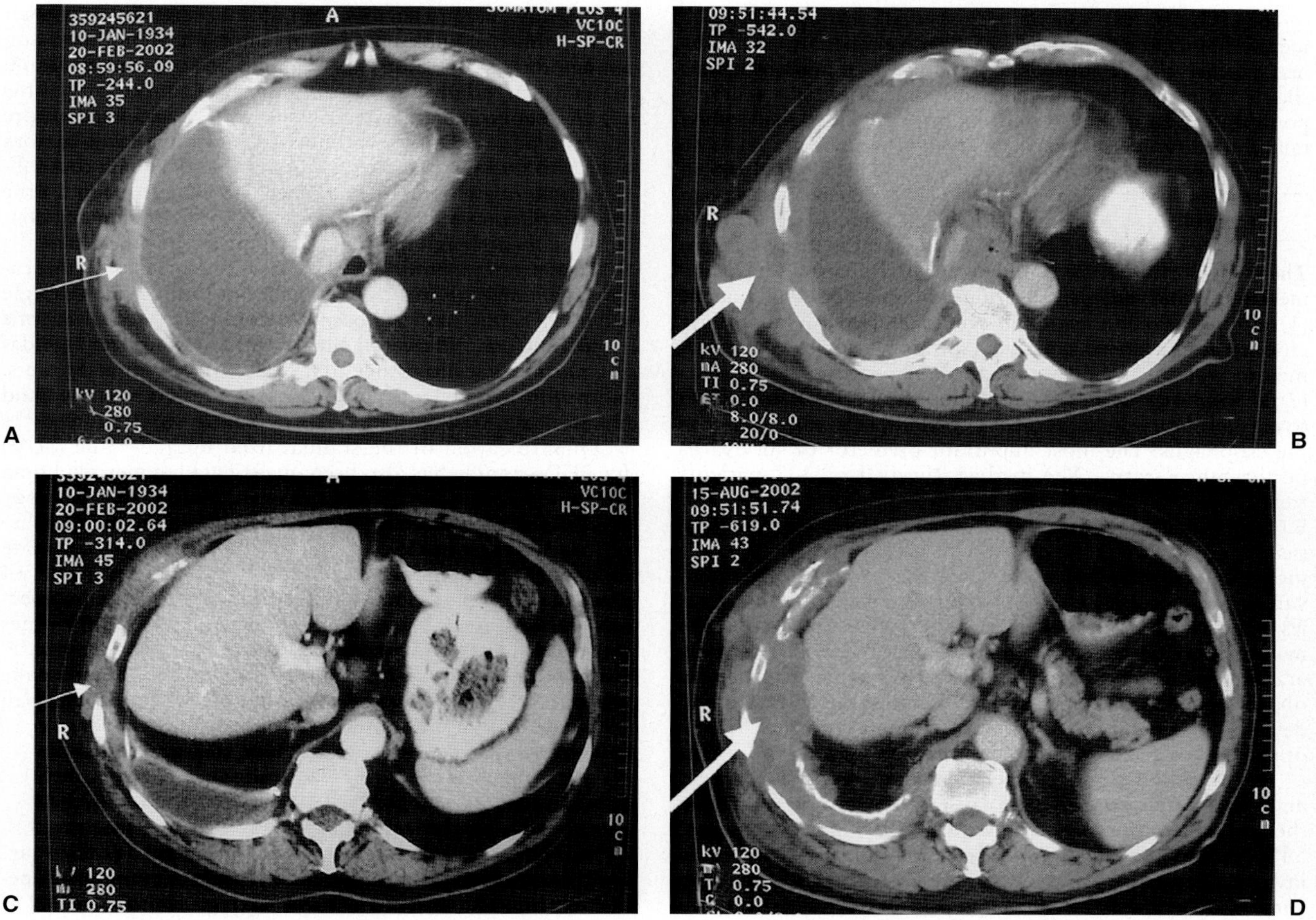

FIGURE 138.9 Progression of mesothelioma after extrapleural pneumonectomy. **A,C:** Minimal thickening in the soft tissues in the inferior portion of the right chest (*thin arrows*). **B,D:** Massive growth of subcutaneous and retroperitoneal and pleural tumor encasing the neodiaphragm (*thick arrows*).

and nodes. The compulsive use of thoracoscopy by Boutin et al.[91] led to the finding that patients with exclusive involvement of the diaphragmatic pleura and parietal pleura (stage IA) had a median survival of 31.2 months, whereas patients with visceral pleura invasion had a median survival of 6.75 months. The later development of chest wall masses from seeding of the biopsy site or surgical scar is an uncommon complication (approximately 10%) of any diagnostic procedure, but can usually be avoided by RT to the scar if appropriate.[92]

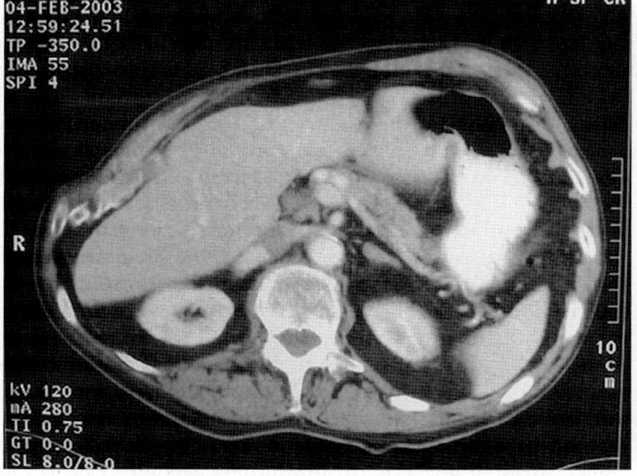

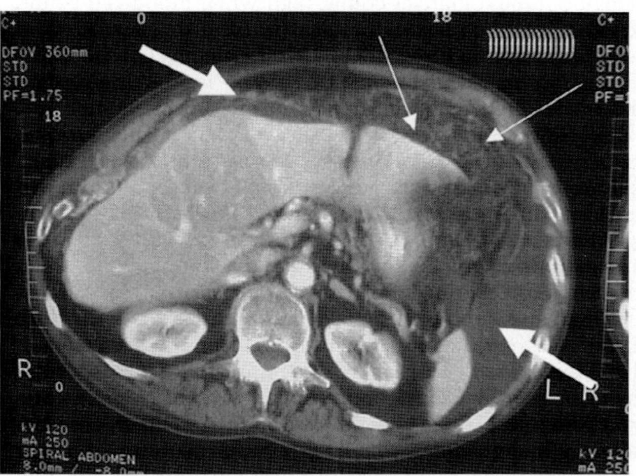

FIGURE 138.10 Progression of mesothelioma after resection. **A:** Normal-appearing upper abdomen without ascites and normal mesenteric fat. **B:** Ascites (*thick arrows*) surrounding the spleen and liver is present 3 months later, and there is diffuse infiltration of the mesentery with disease (*thin arrows*).

If there is no free pleural space because of previous treatment of pleural effusion and the bulk of the disease in the hemithorax is solid, open biopsy is required. Such a biopsy should be carefully planned such that the scar could be incorporated into the definitive incision if a major resection is entertained after definitive diagnosis.

NATURAL HISTORY

The majority of patients with treated or untreated pleural mesothelioma die of complications of local disease because of (1) increasing tumor bulk that eventually replaces the pleural effusion and causes progressive respiratory compromise, pneumonia, or myocardial dysfunction with arrhythmias; and/or (2) unrelenting chest wall pain requiring narcotics, which leads to cachexia; and/or (3) dysphagia from tumor compression of the esophagus. The most important predictor of survival is performance status. The median survival of 337 patients treated in ten clinical trials by the Cancer and Leukemia Group B (CALGB; all of whom were required to be performance status 0 to 2) was 7 months[68]; however, for those with performance status 0, the median survival was 13 to 14 months. In various series from single institutions the median survival varies from 4 to 18 months (range, weeks to 16 years), but performance status was rarely reported in older series. Patients generally die of respiratory failure or pneumonia. Small bowel obstruction from direct extension through the diaphragm develops in approximately one-third of patients, and 10% die of pericardial or myocardial involvement.[93]

Extrathoracic metastases occur late in the course of disease and are not usually the direct cause of the patient's death. In the largest series of patients with MPM who had autopsy, 54% to 82% had distant metastases, with the most frequently involved organs being the liver, adrenal gland, kidney, and contralateral lung.[94–96] Intracranial metastases are seen in approximately 3% of patients and are predominantly of the sarcomatous type.[95]

Prognostic Indicators

The best-known clinical prognostic scoring systems for MPM have originated from European Organisation for Research and Treatment of Cancer (EORTC) and CALGB, and use a combination of biological and clinical factors. Poor performance status, nonepithelioid histology, male gender, low hemoglobin, high platelet count, high white blood cell count, and high lactate dehydrogenase were found to be poor prognostic indicators in mesothelioma.[97] The EORTC model was validated at St. Bartholomew's Hospital in a group of 145 patients treated in sequential phase 2 chemotherapy trials.[98]

The molecular prognostication of mesothelioma has also been explored using gene expression array technology. Using the 12,000 U95 Affymetrix gene chip, Gordon et al.[99] developed a four-gene expression ratio test that was able to predict treatment-related patient outcome in mesothelioma independent of the histologic subtype of the tumor. In a follow-up publication, these MPM prognostic genes and gene ratio–based prognostic tests predicted clinical outcome in a separate cohort of 39 independent MPM tumor specimens in a statistically significant manner.[100,101] Using similar technology, Pass et al.[102] have reported a 27-gene expression array for mesothelioma prognostication. The groups predicted by the gene classifier recapitulated the actual time to progression and survival of the test set with 95.2% accuracy using tenfold cross-validation. There has, however, been variability in the gene sets and results of these prognostic tests when used in other MPM cohorts. Affymetrix U133A microarray analysis on 99 pleural mesotheliomas from Memorial Sloan-Kettering Cancer Center (MSKCC) revealed that advanced-stage, sarcomatous histology and P16/CDKN2A homozygous deletion were significant, independent, adverse prognostic factors. Examination of the gene expression correlates of survival showed that more aggressive mesotheliomas expressed higher levels of Aurora kinases A and B. Moreover, evaluation of three recently published microarray-based outcome prediction models in the MSKCC cohort revealed accuracies from 63% to 67%, consistently lower than reported.[103]

At present, there are no validated gene sets for prognostication of MPM. Most recently, the presence of a single microRNA, mir-29c* has been associated with improved time to progression and overall survival but needs further validation.[104] A variety of other tissue-based prognostic markers, including thymidylate synthase,[105] OPN,[106] MMP14,[107] and HAPLN1,[108] have been reported but require validation.

Quantification of the standardized uptake value (SUV) for PET scanning has also been investigated in mesothelioma as a prognostic marker. Low SUV and epithelial histology predict the best survival, whereas high SUV and nonepithelial histology indicate the worst survival. In a multivariate analysis of 65 patients with MPM, median survival was 14 and 24 months for the high and low SUV groups, respectively. High SUV tumors were associated with a 3.3 times greater risk of death than low SUV tumors (P = .03).[109] Gerbaudo et al.[110] reported that the intensity of FDG uptake by mesothelioma correlates poorly with histology, but well with surgical stage.

Staging

The original MPM staging system proposed by Butchart et al.[111] relied on pathologic generalizations instead of specific quantitative aspects of the disease and was designed at a time that was well before recognition of different prognostic implications of N1 and N2 nodes. The American Joint Committee on Cancer (AJCC) staging system for mesothelioma (Table 138.1) was adopted from that proposed by the International Mesothelioma Interest Group in 1995[112] and has been validated in a number of surgically based trials. The system evolved from a greater understanding of the relationships between the tumor (T) status and nodal (N) status and overall survival. There was a redefinition of the T categories, and the T1 lesions were divided into T1a (involvement of the parietal pleura only) and T1b (involvement of the visceral pleura), leading to a division of stage I into stage IA and IB. T3 is defined as a locally advanced but potentially resectable tumor, and T4 is defined as a locally advanced, technically unresectable tumor. A large international effort, sponsored by the International Association for the Study of Lung Cancer, to improve the AJCC staging system was launched in 2008. The Brigham and Women's Staging System has also been proposed for pleural mesothelioma and differs from the AJCC by defining intrapleural adenopathy as stage II disease and extrapleural adenopathy as stage III disease.[113] The AJCC system classifies any nodal involvement, either intrapleural or extrapleural, as stage III disease. An update of the Brigham and Women's Staging Classification has recently been reported incorporating surgical margins, emphasizing nodal status, and integrating the primary elements of Brigham and Women's Staging criteria into the previously published TNM framework. Regrouping of the T and N combinations based on relative hazard and Kaplan-Meier survival analysis of 368 patients having EPP resulted in improved stage distribution (stage I–IV: 8%, 43%, 33%, 16%, respectively) and survival stratification (51, 26, 15, 8 months, respectively).[114]

TABLE 138.1

INTERNATIONAL STAGING SYSTEM FOR DIFFUSE MALIGNANT PLEURAL MESOTHELIOMA

T1a
Tumor limited to the ipsilateral parietal ± mediastinal ± diaphragmatic pleura
No involvement of the visceral pleura

T1b
Tumor involving the ipsilateral parietal ± mediastinal ± diaphragmatic pleura
Tumor also involving the visceral pleura

T2
Tumor involving each of the ipsilateral pleural surfaces (parietal, mediastinal, diaphragmatic, and visceral pleura) with at least one of the following features:
- Involvement of diaphragmatic muscle
- Extension of tumor from visceral pleura into the underlying pulmonary parenchyma

T3
Describes locally advanced but potentially resectable tumor
Tumor involving all of the ipsilateral pleural surfaces (parietal, mediastinal, diaphragmatic, and visceral pleura) with at least one of the following features:
- Involvement of the endothoracic fascia
- Extension into the mediastinal fat
- Solitary, completely resectable focus of tumor extending into the soft tissues of the chest wall
- Nontransmural involvement of the pericardium

T4
Describes locally advanced technically unresectable tumor
Tumor involving all the ipsilateral pleural surfaces (parietal, mediastinal, diaphragmatic, and visceral pleura) with at least one of the following features:
- Diffuse extension or multifocal masses of tumor in the chest wall, with or without associated rib destruction
- Direct transdiaphragmatic extension of tumor to the peritoneum
- Direct extension of tumor to the contralateral pleura
- Direct extension of tumor to mediastinal organs
- Direct extension of tumor into the spine
- Tumor extending through to the internal surface of the pericardium with or without a pericardial effusion; or tumor involving the myocardium

N—LYMPH NODES
NX: Regional lymph nodes cannot be assessed
N0: No regional lymph node metastases
N1: Metastases in the ipsilateral bronchopulmonary or hilar lymph nodes
N2: Metastases in the subcarinal or the ipsilateral mediastinal lymph nodes, including the ipsilateral internal mammary nodes
N3: Metastases in the contralateral mediastinal, contralateral internal mammary, ipsilateral, or contralateral supraclavicular lymph nodes

M—METASTASES
MX: Presence of distant metastases cannot be assessed
M0: No distant metastasis
M1: Distant metastasis present

Stage I	Stage II	Stage III	Stage IV
Ia: T1aN0 M0	T2 N0 M0	Any T3 M0	Any T4
Ib: T1bN0 M0		Any N1 M0	Any N3
		Any N2 M0	Any M1

Based on Edge SB, Byrd DR, Compton CC, et al. *AJCC Cancer Staging Manual.* 7th ed. New York: Springer, 2010, and Rusch VW. A proposed new international TNM staging system for malignant pleural mesothelioma: from the International Mesothelioma Interest Group. *Chest* 1995;108(4):1122.

PRACTICE OF ONCOLOGY

TREATMENT

Overview

With the exception of the recently reported European Society for Medical Oncology recommendations for management of pleural mesothelioma,[115] there have been no published standards of care for the treatment of pleural mesothelioma. Treatment decisions are influenced not only by the functional evaluation of these often elderly individuals, but also by the philosophy of the treating physicians. The evolution of the use of surgery in MPM with or without intraoperative or postoperative innovative adjuvant therapies, or both, is being defined in general by centers that see more than 50 MPM patients per year, and innovative, multimodality protocols that incorporate surgery as part of the package are being explored in larger numbers of patients.

For unresectable patients who are candidates for chemotherapy, the well-powered phase 3 trial that showed a 3- to 4-month survival advantage for the two-drug regimen of pemetrexed and cisplatin compared with the one-drug regimen of cisplatin has defined the standard of care.[67]

Supportive Care

The median survival of MPM patients who select supportive care ranges only from 4[97] to 13 months.[93] This variation is likely due to variations in tumor biology, host response to tumor, detection bias, lead-time bias, and the use of ad hoc or unreported treatments by some patients and physicians.

There are a number of options for the control of pleural effusion, including repeated thoracenteses, talc pleurodesis, pleuroperitoneal shunting, or placement of a Pleur X (Denver Biomedical, Denver, CO) catheter. Talc pleurodesis is performed by instilling 2 to 5 g of asbestos-free, sterile talc over the lung and the parietal surfaces. Success rates in effusion control with talc, used either via thoracoscopy or via slurry, approach 90%. Failure of these techniques is usually associated with lung trapped by the tumor, a large solid tumor mass, a long history of effusion with multiple thoracenteses leading to loculations, age older than 70 years, or poor performance status. In such cases, the PleurX catheter with its one-way valve can be implanted under local anesthesia into pleural effusion, and patients can drain themselves at home using the available disposable drainage kits.[116] Internal drainage from the pleura to the abdomen can be accomplished using the Denver pleuroperitoneal shunt.

The chest pain of malignant mesothelioma requires narcotics, and these patients should be seen in consultation by a dedicated pain management team to assist in the optimization of the patient's quality of life. Subcutaneous tunneling of epidural catheters for long-term out-of-hospital use has also been used in selective cases. When only local RT has been delivered solely for chest wall pain or chest wall nodules, the median survival has been reported to be 4 to 5 months.[117,118]

Surgery

The protocols that use an aggressive approach to the treatment of mesothelioma incorporate surgery as part of the treatment package. The operations include thoracoscopy (usually for diagnosis and palliation only), PL/decortication, or EPP. The indications for each of these operations depend on the extent of disease, performance, and functional status of the patient, and the philosophy and experience of the treating institution. Basically, operative intervention in mesothelioma falls into one of three categories: (1) for primary effusion control, as described in "Supportive Care," (2) for cytoreduction before multimodal therapy, or (3) to deliver and monitor innovative intrapleural therapies.

Staging and Operative Therapy

The majority of patients seeking treatment for mesothelioma are middle- to older-aged individuals with a long latency period between asbestos exposure and tumor development. If surgical intervention is to be considered, a detailed physiologic and functional workup directed chiefly at the cardiopulmonary axis must be performed.

If patients are deemed medically operable from the cardiac and pulmonary standpoint, then surgery is indicated if a cytoreductive procedure can be performed that does not leave gross disease at its completion, or, in other words, leaves only microscopic residual disease. This would include all International Mesothelioma Interest Group (IMIG) clinically staged individuals from stages I to III, as the T3 category of stage III patients includes invasion of the endothoracic fascia or mediastinal fat, a solitary focus of tumor invading the soft tissues of the chest wall (i.e., at an old thoracoscopy site), and/or nontransmural involvement of the pericardium. When enlarged mediastinal lymph nodes are detected by CT or PET scan, a mediastinoscopy should be performed.[119] The yield from mediastinoscopy, however, may underestimate the extent of nodal involvement because the majority of mediastinal nodal involvement in mesothelioma is below the subcarinal level.[120] It is possible that FDG-PET scanning, as previously discussed, will help to at least define those patients with node-involved mesothelioma in the future.

Which Operation?

The role of surgery in mesothelioma, as well as what type of surgery, remain extraordinarily controversial as there is a lack of randomized controlled clinical trials, making it impossible to determine whether the use of EPP or pleurectomy (PL) improves survival or effectively palliates the symptoms of the disease.[121] Whether EPP should be performed at all is the critical question being examined by the Mesothelioma and Radical Surgery Trial (MARS) in the United Kingdom. The trial successfully met its accrual goal of 50 randomized patients after screening more than 300 patients at 11 participating centers. Only 45% of the patients eligible for surgery after chemotherapy underwent randomization. Surgery was performed by only five centers and RT was provided by only ten centers. No data regarding survival outcomes have been reported, yet plans for the next trial (i.e., MARS-2) apparently will be an evaluation of total PL,[122] with the implication that the morbidity of EPP fails to justify a limited survival advantage according to the MARS trial authors. Possibly influencing such a decision is that recent pooled data from MSKCC, the National Cancer Institute (NCI), and the Karmanos Cancer Institute demonstrate that for stage I patients, cytoreduction by PL may be as efficacious as EPP.[123]

Unfortunately, the majority of diffuse malignant mesotheliomas present in later stages, and cannot be surgically removed *en bloc* with truly negative histologic margins. This is because many of the patients have had a previous biopsy and there is invasion of the endothoracic fascia and intercostal muscles at that site and/or pleural effusion that, although cytologically negative, may be breached, leading to local permeation of tumor cells either into the residual cavity or into the abdomen. These cases can make the use of EPP mandatory as the cytoreductive operation. The importance of margin status has been emphasized by the Boston group and has been incorporated in their

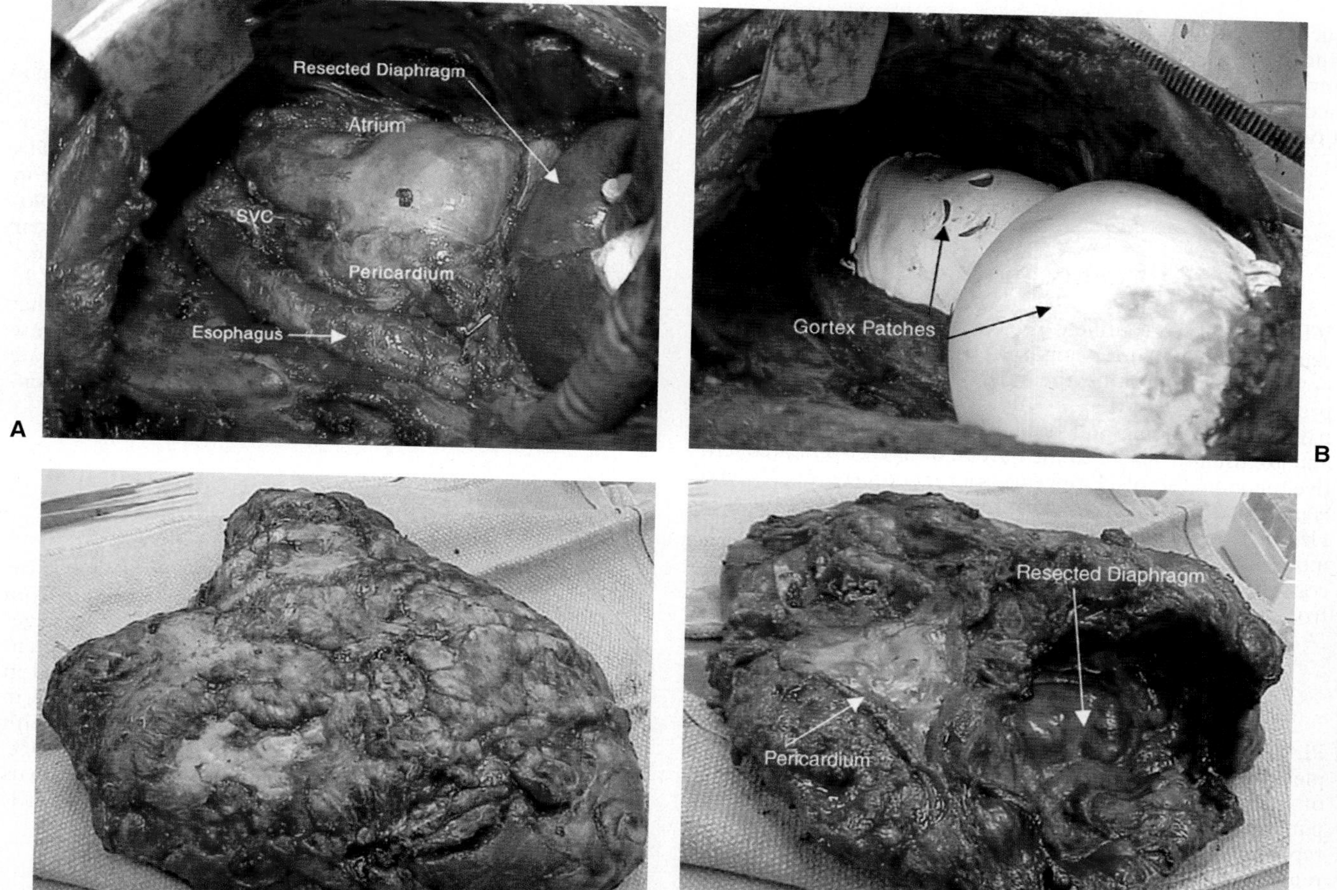

FIGURE 138.11 Intraoperative and specimen photography of the patient whose computed tomograms are seen in Figure 138.10. **A:** Right hemithorax after resection of lung, pleura, diaphragm, pericardium, and lymph nodes. **B:** Replacement of the diaphragm and pericardium with Gore-Tex material. **C:** View of lateral aspect of specimen, which reveals the entire lung coated with thickened, mesothelioma-involved pleura. **D:** Medial view of specimen revealing the resected pericardium and diaphragm, hilar structures, and lung. SVC, superior vena cava.

new staging update.[114] Because only a minority of patients is able to have a margin-free resection and because those patients who have margin-free resections usually have less bulky disease, it may be justifiable to spare the functioning lung if the visceral pleura is minimally involved (i.e., PL). Such "lung-preserving surgery" can potentially be accomplished by performing a radical parietal PL instead of EPP. Minimal visceral pleural disease is, however, an undefined entity, and there are no criteria for how many sites should be involved, the size of these involved sites, or whether involvement of the fissure is worse than nonfissural involvement. Suffice it to say that individual surgeons with expertise in the management of mesothelioma have different philosophies about the use of PL in this situation, and some make the decision regarding the type of operation in an individual patient at the time of the exploration.

There is no doubt that EPP is a more extensive dissection and may serve to remove more bulk disease than a PL, chiefly in the diaphragmatic and visceral pleural surfaces (Fig. 138.11). Some surgeons, however, include diaphragmatic resection and pericardial resection with their PLs to accomplish removal of "all gross disease." For EPP, it is almost a necessity to include pericardiotomy and partial pericardiectomy during the resection because the maneuver aids in the exposure of the vessels and allows intrapericardial control to prevent a surgical catastrophe. In many instances, the final decision as to whether PL or EPP is to be performed becomes an intraoperative decision unless a protocol calls specifically for one operation or the other.

Lymph node status has emerged as one of the most important prognostic indicators for patients having EPP. In a review from Canada, survival was significantly worse for patients with N2 disease than for those with no lymph node metastasis (median survival 10 months vs. 29 months, respectively; P = .005).[124] Recent data from the United Kingdom have also revealed that involvement of mediastinal or intrapulmonary lymph nodes is associated with decreased survival after EPP.[120] Retrospective data from selected small series suggest that for patients with nodal positivity, PL had a median survival of 16 months while for EPP median survival was 15 months.[125] One of the largest series commenting on lymph node status has recently been reported from MSKCC. From 1990 to 2006, EPP was performed in 223 cases and PL/decortication was performed in 125 cases. If lymph nodes were not involved or only involved within the visceral envelope, median survival was 19 months. For patients with N2 disease, or N2 and N1, the survival was 10 months. Survival was influenced by the number of involved N2 stations, and multivariate analysis grouping all N2 and internal thoracic versus N1and N0 demonstrated a hazard ratio for survival of 1.7 (P <.0001). Other independent prognostic factors included T3/T4 status, nonepithelioid histology, use of EPP and male gender. This study suggests that N1 only nodal involvement should be classified as lower stage disease and should be considered in the restaging IASLC studies mentioned earlier.[126]

PLEURECTOMY

Morbidity and Mortality

When performed routinely, PL for mesothelioma can be associated with few major complications. In the series that specify postoperative morbidity, the most common complication was prolonged air leak (i.e., >7 days) occurring in 10% of the patients. Pneumonia and respiratory insufficiency may occur and are usually related to the burden of disease and preoperative functional status. Empyema is a rare occurrence (2%) and is managed by prolonged chest tube drainage and antibiotics. Hemorrhage requiring re-exploration is rare (i.e., <1%). The modern-day mortality for PL for mesothelioma is generally considered to be 1.5% to 2.0%, with death resulting either from respiratory insufficiency or hemorrhage.[125,127,128]

Short- and Long-Term Results

PL and decortication are effective in controlling malignant pleural effusion. Law et al.[129] report effusion control in 88% of patients having decortication for mesothelioma. In 63 patients having partial decortication and PL, Ruffie et al.[130] reported 86% control of effusion, and Brancatisano et al.[131] reported a 98% control of effusion after PL in 50 cases of pleural mesothelioma.

There has recently been interest in the reporting of patients having alternative cytoreductive surgery procedures, including "debulking," as opposed to classic EPP. Neragi-Miandoab et al.[132] reported 64 patients who had PL as a palliative treatment for MPM. The 30-day mortality rate was 3.1%, and median survival was 9.4 months. Overall survival rates were 43%, 28%, and 10% at 1, 2, and 3 years, respectively. The overall median survival with epithelial histology was 21.7 months versus 5.8 months for the sarcomatoid or mixed type. Nakas et al.[133] reported 102 consecutive patients having a nonradical tumor decortication to obtain lung expansion or a radical PL/decortications to obtain macroscopic tumor clearance. Thirty-day mortality was 9.8% and 5.9%, respectively. Median survival for all cell types was significantly higher in the PL/decortications group (15.3 vs. 7.1 months; $P < .000$), and more patients in that group received chemotherapy. Survival rates at 1, 2, 3, and 4 years were 53%, 41%, 25%, and 13% for PL/decortications, respectively, while for the nonradical tumor decortication group they were 32%, 9.6%, 2%, and 0%, respectively. Radical PL followed by chemotherapy and radiation therapy could be completed in 32 of 35 patients by Bolukbas et al.,[134] with a surgical morbidity/mortality and trimodality treatment-related mortality of 20.0%, 2.9%, and 5.8%, respectively. Overall median survival was 30 months. One-, 2-, and 3-year survival were 69%, 50%, and 31%, respectively. Therefore, it appears that, if possible, a maximally cytoreductive PL decortication can be delivered in the majority of patients who are believed to be candidates for such an approach with less morbidity and mortality than for EPP. These data would tend to validate other large studies that have compared PL and EPP.[123] Survivals with such an approach are encouraging, but one must consider that these patients usually have less bulky disease to begin with and thus may benefit the most from their multimodal approach.

Extrapleural Pneumonectomy

Not all patients who are explored with the intent of undergoing an EPP are found to be truly cytoreducible at the time of the operation. In the review by Butchart et al.,[135] 29 of 46, or 63% of patients were eligible for EPP, and in a series of EPPs performed at Rush Presbyterian-St. Luke's Medical Center in Chicago, only 33 of 56 of patients undergoing surgical exploration for the intent of performing an EPP over a 27-year period (59%).[136] The Lung Cancer Study Group performed a pilot study of EPP from 1985 to 1988.[137] Only 20 of the 83 evaluated patients were resected with an EPP. The reasons that EPP could not be performed were chiefly the extent of disease not allowing complete gross resection (54%), inadequate respiratory reserve (33%), stage IV disease (11%), and concurrent medical illness (10%).

Complications of Extrapleural Pneumonectomy

Because of its magnitude, EPP has significantly greater morbidity than PL. The major complication rate ranges from 20% to 40%, and arrhythmia requiring medical management is the most common complication. In the most recent report of Sugarbaker et al.,[138] major morbidity occurred in 24% of the patients having EPP and minor morbidity in 41%. The rate for bronchopleural fistula is greater with right-sided EPPs, with an overall fistula rate of 3% to 20%. The bronchopleural fistula can be handled for the most part with open thoracostomy drainage with or without muscle flap interposition.

Mortality

The mortality rates after EPP were unacceptably high in the 1970s, with a 31% rate reported by Butchart et al.[135] Since then, however, there has been a steady decline in the operative mortality to consistent rates less than 10% in a series of 20 or more patients. Mortality occurs chiefly in older patients from respiratory failure, myocardial infarction, or pulmonary embolus. Rusch[139] and Rusch et al.[140] reported a perioperative mortality of 6% to 8% after EPP, and Sugarbaker et al.[138] reported a benchmark perioperative mortality of 3.4%.

Recurrence after Extrapleural Pneumonectomy

EPP is associated with distant sites of recurrence compared with locoregional sites of recurrence in patients having biopsy only or PL/decortication, and the local control for EPP is superior to that of the other modalities. Pass et al.[141] found that the pattern of recurrence was chiefly local progression after PL and systemic failures after EPP. In the series of patients operated on by Sugarbaker et al., Baldini et al.[142] have reported that the sites of first recurrence were local in 35% of patients, abdominal in 26%, in the contralateral thorax in 17%, and in other distant sites in 8%.

Survival

Long-term survival rates after EPP remain disappointing, with the median survival lengths ranging from 9.3 to 17.0 months for the majority of series. Rusch et al.[140] and Rusch and Venkatraman[143] reported a median survival of 10 months, and Pass et al.[141] reported the median survival after EPP (all histologies) to be 9.4 months. The majority of patients were pathologic stage II or III in these two series. Sugarbaker et al.[144] have reported a 17-month median survival for all patients in a series heavily weighted with stage I epithelial patients (n = 52 of 183) whose 2- and 5-year survivals were 68% and 46%, respectively. In the series by Rusch and Venkatraman,[143] the 2- and 5-year survivals of stage I patients (n = 16 of 131) were 65% and 30%, respectively.

RADIOTHERAPY FOR MESOTHELIOMA

Curative Radiation Therapy as a Single Modality

The limitation of potentially "curative" RT for treatment of MPM is the inability to treat a large volume of disease in the chest with a curative radiation dose (>60 Gy) because of the risks of severe damage to normal tissue. Law et al.[94,129] administered radiation using a rotational technique to deliver 50 to 55 Gy to the pleural space. Survival in this group of patients ranged from 3 to 10 months, with the exception of one patient who was alive and well 4 years after the completion of treatment. Ball and Cruickshank[145] treated 12 patients with 50 Gy to the entire hemithorax. Median survival of these patients was 17 months compared to 7 months for those offered palliative treatment only. This difference is likely the result of a selection bias, with those fit enough to undergo a full course of radiation likely to have a greater survival regardless of treatment given. Other studies[146] of definitive RT have had median survivals of less than 10 months.[130,146,147] In general, RT as a single modality alone in MPM patients is reserved for the palliative setting.

Combined Chemotherapy and Definitive Radiotherapy

The poor results reported for definitive RT alone have led to studies evaluating the combination of chemotherapy and radiation. Both Ruffie et al.[130] and Linden et al.[148] have reported that the median survival is increased in patients treated with combined modality therapy compared with RT alone. Some investigators have evaluated the addition of radiation sensitizers to definitive RT. Herscher et al.[149] from the NCI studied the use of a 5-day continuous infusion of paclitaxel with radical RT in patients with mesothelioma and non–small cell lung cancer. In mesothelioma patients, the hemithoracic radiation was delivered before the chemotherapy. Chen et al.[150] reported a 12% complete response rate and an 88% partial response rate when pulsed paclitaxel was delivered during RT in a phase 1 trial. Although these combination approaches are interesting, it is not likely that the addition of radiation sensitizers to radical RT will be curative, and as such, definitive chemoradiotherapy should be considered experimental for patients with mesothelioma.

Combined Surgical Resection and Definitive Radiotherapy

After an EPP, radical RT can be administered without concern for damage to the underlying ipsilateral lung because it has been removed surgically (Fig. 138.12). However, radical RT after a PL continues to place the ipsilateral lung at risk for substantial loss of function. In a retrospective review of patients having PL/decortication at MSKCC from 1974 to 2003, 123 patients received external-beam RT (median dose, 42.5 Gy; range, 7.2 to 67.8 Gy) to the ipsilateral hemithorax postoperatively. The median and 2-year overall survival for all patients was 13.5 months (range, 1 to 199 months) and 23%, respectively. Multivariate analysis for overall survival revealed a radiation dose less than 40 Gy (P = .001), nonepithelioid histology (P = .002), left-sided disease (P = .01), and the use of an implant (P = .02) to be unfavorable. These data reinforce the concept that residual disease cannot be eradicated with external RT with or without brachytherapy and that a more extensive surgery followed by external RT might be required to improve local control and overall survival.[151] Moreover, intraoperative RT for mesothelioma is associated with toxicity and failure to prolong survival.[152]

Radiation therapy after EPP, however, may be beneficial. Rusch et al.[140] at MSKCC completed a phase 2 trial of surgery followed by postoperative radiation in patients with pleural mesothelioma having EPP. Eighty-eight patients with biopsy-confirmed mesothelioma were treated. Twenty-one patients were unresectable and taken off the study. The majority of patients (n = 62) underwent an EPP followed by 54 Gy delivered through anterior and posterior fields in 30 fractions of 1.8 Gy. Five patients were treated with a PL, which was followed by intraoperative RT to a dose of 15 Gy using a high-dose iridium applicator. This was followed by 54 Gy to the hemithorax via anterior and posterior fields in the same fractionation schedule as those who underwent EPP. There were seven postoperative deaths, all primarily related to pulmonary complications in patients who had undergone an EPP. A total of 33 patients had some complications, with the most common being atrial arrhythmias (17 patients), respiratory failure (6 patients), pneumonia (5 patients), and empyema (5 patients). Only the patients who underwent EPP were considered for survival analysis. The median survival was 17 months, with an overall survival of 27% at 3 years. Only 13% had locoregional recurrence, with the majority of patients failing to respond and having distant metastases. The authors concluded that their approach of aggressive surgery with EPP followed by high-dose radiation to the entire hemithorax provided a favorable outcome for those patients who were able to complete the therapy when compared to historical data.

Lee et al.[153] retrospectively reviewed the efficacy and toxicity of surgery with intraoperative RT followed by chemotherapy. The median overall survival was 18.1 months, and the median progression-free interval was 12.2 months. Locoregional relapse was the most common site of failure. The authors concluded that this approach was a potential treatment option for adjuvant RT in patients who were unable to tolerate an EPP.

Newer RT techniques, notably intensity-modulated radiation therapy (IMRT), offer the potential for administering higher doses of RT with better target coverage to the hemithorax while minimizing normal tissue toxicities. Rice et al.[154] and Forster et al.[155] at the M. D. Anderson Cancer Center have treated MPM patients with IMRT after EPP. Recent data in 100 patients who underwent EPP 63 of whom were treated with IMRT reveal a median survival of 14.2 months and 3-year survival of 20% for IMRT patients. Recurrences in the irradiated field occurred in only three patients, and distant disease observed in 54% of patients was the major pattern of failure. Liver injury has been documented after hemithoracic IMRT.[156] However, pulmonary toxicity appears to be the most significant late toxicity observed in MPM patients after IMRT.[157–159] Allen et al.[157] reported fatal pulmonary complications in 6 of 13 MPM patients treated with IMRT to a dose

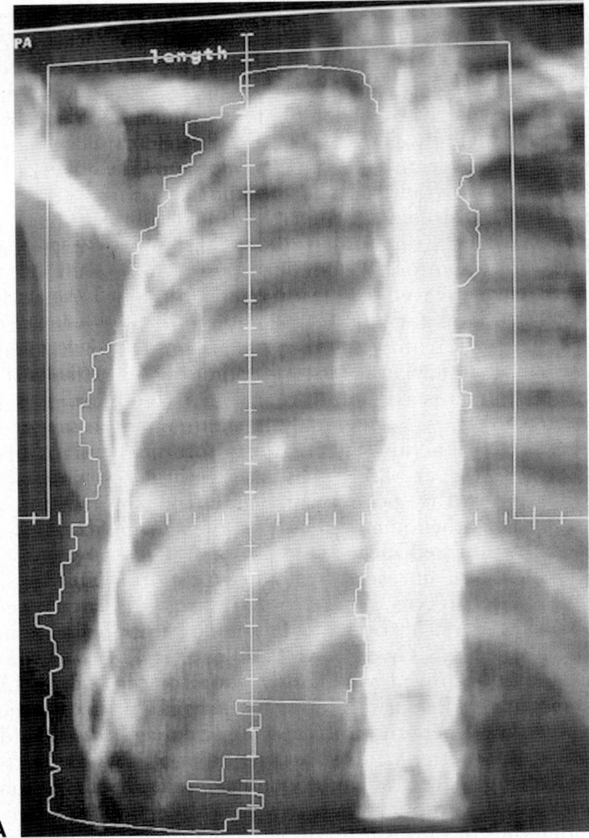

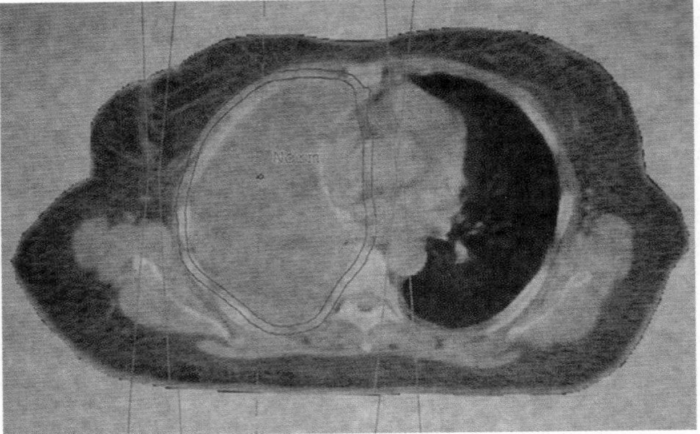

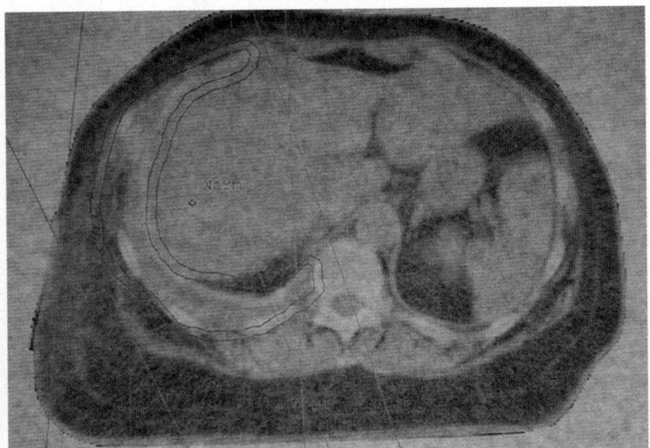

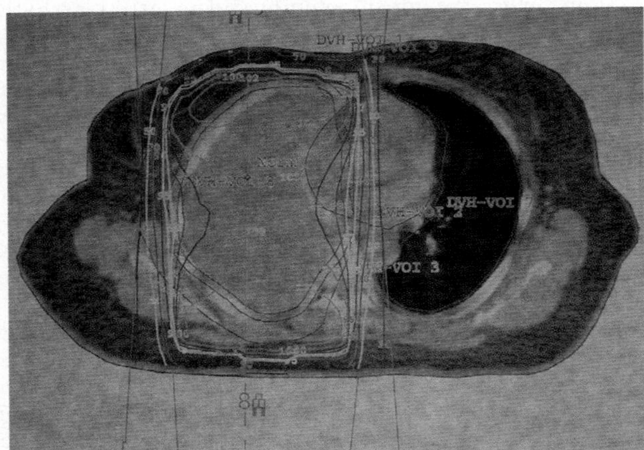

FIGURE 138.12 Postoperative radiation therapy for mesothelioma. **A:** Anterior projection of a typical field encompassing the right hemithorax. The hemithorax target volume is outlined. The target volume crosses midline and extends inferiorly to the diaphragmatic sulci. **B:** The target volume is shown on an axial projection. **C:** The complex geometry of the target volume at the inferior extent of the hemithorax is demonstrated on this axial projection. The target volume wraps around the liver. **D:** Isodose lines demonstrating the coverage of the target volume from anterior and posterior radiation fields.

of 54 Gy to the clinical target volume. The median time from completion of IMRT to the onset of radiation pneumonitis was 30 days (range, 5 to 57 days). Recent data from Kristensen et al.[159] showed fatal pulmonary toxicity in 4 of 26 (15%) of MPM patients treated with induction chemotherapy, EPP, and postoperative IMRT to a pleural surface dose of 50 Gy. These reports of pulmonary toxicity emphasize that care should be taken when planning and delivering IMRT to the hemithorax. An alternative technique using electrons and IMRT has been reported as an alternative to IMRT alone. However, it appears that better coverage of the target volume is achieved with IMRT.[160,161] If the use of IMRT after EPP is planned, doses of 45 to 50 Gy in 0.018 to 0.020 Gy fractions are typically recommended. In addition to other standard normal tissue constraints, a mean lung dose of 9 Gy or less and a V5 (volume of lung receiving ≥5 Gy) of 65% or less should be used during the planning process.

Prevention of Scar Recurrences

Malignant seeding in approximately 20% to 50% of mesothelioma patients along thoracentesis tracts, biopsy tracts, chest tube sites, and surgical incisions is a common complication of procedures in these patients.[92,162] Boutin et al.[92] randomized 40 patients after an invasive diagnostic procedure to either RT (7 Gy × three fractions) or no treatment. No patient in the radiation treatment group developed subcutaneous nodules. Alternatively, 8 of 20 patients in the untreated group developed metastases. Two additional small randomized trials have suggested that the use of short-course RT does not reduce the frequency of cutaneous seeding after invasive procedures.[163,164] These data are inconclusive and reviews of contemporary practice patterns suggest that radiation is commonly used to prevent scar recurrences.[165,166]

Palliation Using Radiation Therapy

RT is commonly used to palliate pain in patients with advanced mesothelioma,[117] and investigators from the Netherlands have reported using palliative RT to treat painful chest wall metastases in patients with mesothelioma. Ball and Cruickshank[145] reported a 72% rate of symptom improvement using palliative courses of RT. Ruffie et al.[130] and Davis et al.[167] reported the results of palliative RT in patients with mesothelioma. When doses greater than 45 Gy were used, pain relief was attained in more than 50% of the cases.

Adjuvant Therapy for Surgically Cytoreduced Mesothelioma Patients

Patients treated with surgery and postoperative adjuvant therapy have an apparently improved survival compared with those treated with palliative therapy alone in consecutively treated patients from single institutions. Yet there are no phase 3 trials of adjuvant therapy in mesothelioma. These results may be explained by selection bias or by a number of other factors. The possibility, however, remains that surgery and adjuvant therapy changes the course of the disease. Because it is unlikely that a phase 3 trial of adjuvant therapy will be conducted in this rare disease, strong consideration should be given to treating patients with postoperative chemotherapy (if PL was performed), or RT, or both (if EPP was performed).[168]

MULTIMODALITY TREATMENT

Pleurectomy/Intrapleural Chemotherapy ± Postoperative Chemotherapy

There has been interest in combining debulking surgery with intracavitary treatment of pleural mesothelioma since the first reports of intrapleural chemotherapy alone for malignant mesothelioma. Rusch et al.[169,170] used intrapleural chemotherapy with cisplatin and cytarabine after surgical debulking followed by systemic chemotherapy in ten patients. A subsequent report used an even more aggressive regimen of PL, immediate intracavitary cisplatin, and mitomycin C with two cycles of systemic cisplatin and mitomycin C. In the initial trial, there was one postoperative death, and the chemotherapy complications were reversible, making such an approach feasible. The most recent trial revealed an overall survival rate of 68% at 1 year and 44% at 2 years in the 27 patients who received the therapy, with a median survival of 17 months. Recurrences, however, were chiefly locoregional. A similar regimen combining PL or EPP with cisplatin and mitomycin C resulted in a disappointing median survival of 13 months, and only 50% of the chemotherapy treatments were delivered adjuvantly. In an Italian study of 20 patients, PL and diaphragmatic or pericardial resection were combined with intrapleural chemotherapy with cisplatin and cytarabine for 4 hours immediately after PL. This treatment followed by systemic chemotherapy with epirubicin and mitomycin C resulted in a median time to disease progression of 7.4 months and a median survival of only 11.5 months.[171]

The intrapleural route with standard agents or RT remains intriguing, but its efficacy remains unknown. Phase 2 studies with the following design principles continue to be performed and must use: (1) a tolerable regimen without chronic side effects, (2) a standard debulking approach with definition of the extent of residual disease, and (3) careful documentation of recurrence patterns. Intrapleural therapies for MPM have continued to be published and some are discussed in other sections of the chapter.[127,172–174]

Extrapleural Pneumonectomy/Intravenous Chemotherapy and Postoperative Radiotherapy

A multimodal approach to malignant mesothelioma using EPP, postoperative chemotherapy, and targeted postoperative RT has been the standard approach since 1980 at the Brigham and Women's Hospital in Boston.[113] The adjuvant therapy included two cycles of paclitaxel and carboplatin with concurrent radiation to a dose of 40.5 Gy. Over a 19-year period, 183 patients have been treated, with a perioperative mortality of 3.4%. The median survival in this group of patients was approximately 17 months, a significant improvement over other trials. Favorable subgroups include those with no mediastinal nodal involvement and with epithelial histology. Other trials of surgery and postoperative chemoradiation therapy have had median survival rates of 9.5 to 13 months.[175,176] This approach by the Boston group has now been generally replaced with novel trials of intrapleural hyperthermic perfusion (see later discussion).

Induction Chemotherapy Followed by Surgery

Induction or neoadjuvant therapy for pleural mesothelioma followed by surgery has been patterned after the use of such therapy with non–small cell lung cancer. With the improved efficacy of doublet chemotherapy (gemcitabine/cisplatin or pemetrexed/cisplatin), there has been renewed interest in investigating a neoadjuvant approach for mesothelioma. A Swiss neoadjuvant study used three cycles of cisplatin 80 mg/m^2 on day 1 and gemcitabine 1,000 mg/m^2 on days 1, 8, and 15 every 28 days followed by surgery. RT was considered after EPP to areas at risk. Nineteen patients with MPM were included in this pilot study. The response rate to neoadjuvant chemotherapy was 32%, and EPP was performed in 16 patients with no perioperative mortality. Thirteen patients received postoperative RT. The median survival time was 23 months and the 1-year survival rate was 77%.[177] This trial was then extended to the Swiss Group of Clinical Cancer Research (SAKK) and enrolled 58 eligible mesothelioma patients (45 of whom had EPP) who completed the chemotherapy regimen. Of the 37 patients who had complete resection, 36 received postoperative RT, and the mortality was 2%. Postoperative complications were observed in 62%, and two patients died within 30 days (3.2%).[178] For all patients, the 1-year survival was 69% with median survival of 19.8 months. For the 45 resected patients, 78% were alive at 1 year, with a median survival of 23 months.[179]

Flores[180] conducted a similar trial using four cycles of gemcitabine and cisplatin in 21 patients, but only 9 patients had cytoreductive surgery. Median survival of all patients was 19 months. A similar trial was performed by de Perrot et al.[181] that involved induction chemotherapy, surgery, and postoperative hemithorax RT, with a 6% operative mortality and 74% 1-year survival. A multicenter North American trial of four cycles of pemetrexed and cisplatin followed by EPP and postoperative hemithorax RT has been recently reported.[182] Of 77 patients initially enrolled, four cycles of chemotherapy could be delivered to 83% with a response rate of 33%, but only 55 had surgical exploration, of which 54 had an EPP. Of these 54, 44 completed RT. Operative morality was 4%, and 1-year survival was 68%, with a median survival of 16.8 months. Complete or partial radiologic response was associated with a significantly higher median survival of 26.0 months compared with 13.9 months for patients with stable disease or progressive disease.

When examining all these studies, one is impressed by the fact that only 50% of the patients end up having resection, fewer receive radiation, and the overall survival, although an improvement over previous surgical studies, remains less than ideal. In fact, a similar multi-institutional study (EORTC 08031) was presented at the 2009 annual meeting of the American Society of Clinical Oncology in which only 42% of the patients had "successful treatment," which was defined as a patient receiving the full protocol of pemetrexed (Alimta) and cisplatin and EPP followed by 54 Gy of postoperative radiation therapy.

NOVEL INTRAPLEURAL APPROACHES: NEW TECHNIQUES WITH NEW/OLD AGENTS

Intrapleural Photodynamic Therapy

Photodynamic therapy (PDT) involves the light-activated sensitization of malignant cells[183] using a photosensitizer, such as Photofrin II (Axcan Pharma US, Birmingham, AL), which is retained by malignant tissue *in vivo* in contrast to normal tissue (Fig. 138.13). The sensitizer is activated by 630-nm light and then interacts with molecular oxygen to produce an excited reactive oxygen species. After a series of phase 1 and 2 trials, a group of 63 patients with localized mesothelioma were randomized to surgery, with or without intraoperative PDT.[183] There were no significant differences in median survival (14.4 vs. 14.1 months) or median progression-free time (8.5 vs. 7.7 months), and sites of first recurrence were similar. Other phase 2 trials of PDT and mesothelioma have not demonstrated therapeutic efficacy,[184,185] and results using intrapleural PDT with meta-tetra (hydroxyphenyl) chlorin after EPP have revealed significant toxicities without survival benefit.[186]

Pleural Perfusion

Hyperthermic chemoperfusion of the pleura after resection of mesothelioma is based on the hypothesis that the treatment will provide increased local control and avoid systemic chemotherapy toxicity (Fig. 138.14). Ratto et al.,[187] who delivered cisplatin to the pleural space after PL or EPP in ten patients, and other small phase 2 studies using cisplatin or doxorubicin with cisplatin, have recorded morbidity rates of 33% to 65% using temperatures of 40°C to 42°C without impacting survival.[188,189] Richards et al.[190] reported a phase 1/2 trial using hyperthermic cisplatin (42°C) to perfuse both the abdomen and the pleura after PL/decortication. Operative mortality was 11%, and survival of all patients was 10.5 months. However, in the group of patients surviving surgery who

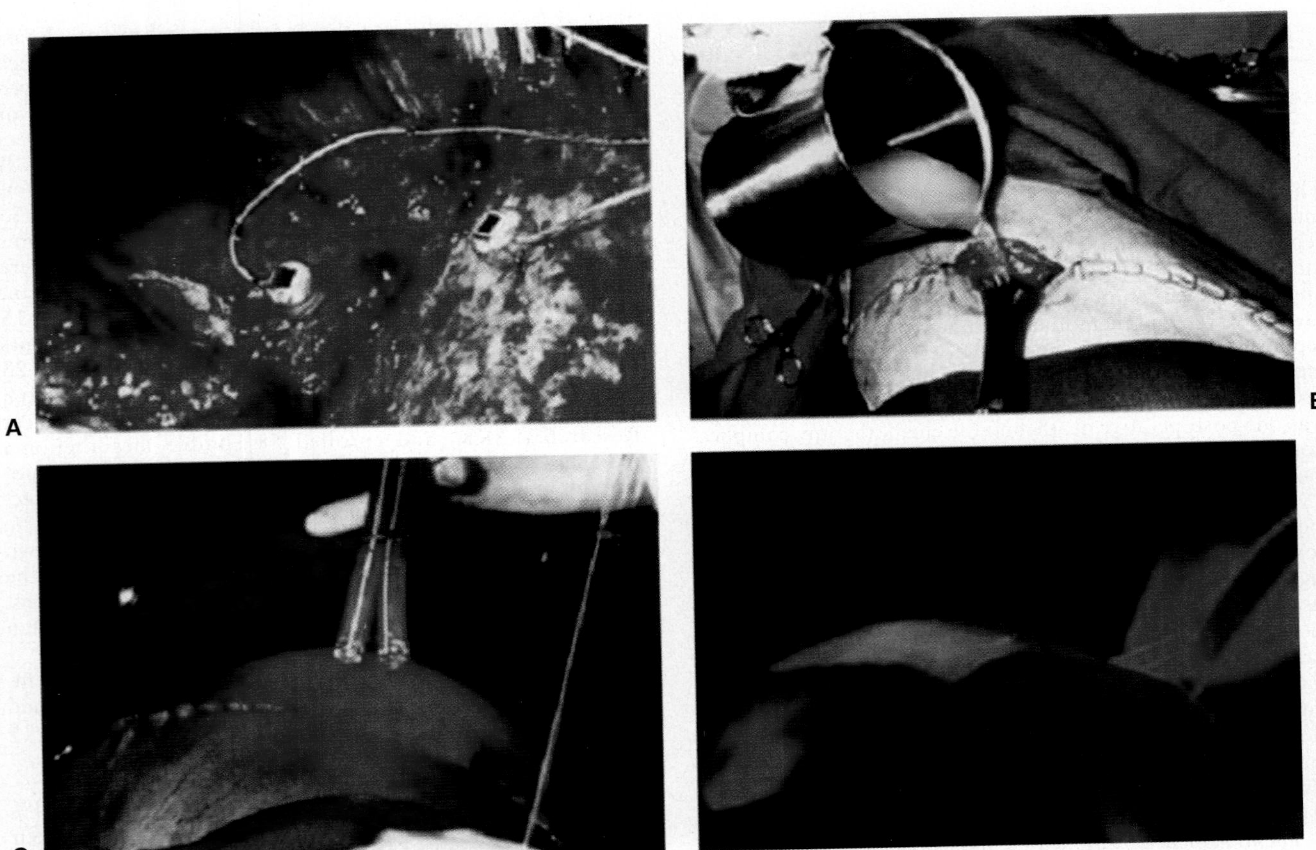

FIGURE 138.13 Intraoperative photodynamic therapy for mesothelioma. **A:** After pleurectomy or pneumonectomy, light-sensing diodes are placed in strategic areas of the chest for dosimetry measurements. **B:** Light-scattering solution, usually intralipid, is poured into the partially closed chest. **C:** Laser fibers housed in modified endotracheal tubes are then placed into the chest, illuminating the chest wall and remaining organs (**D**), which had received the photosensitizer 48 hours previously.

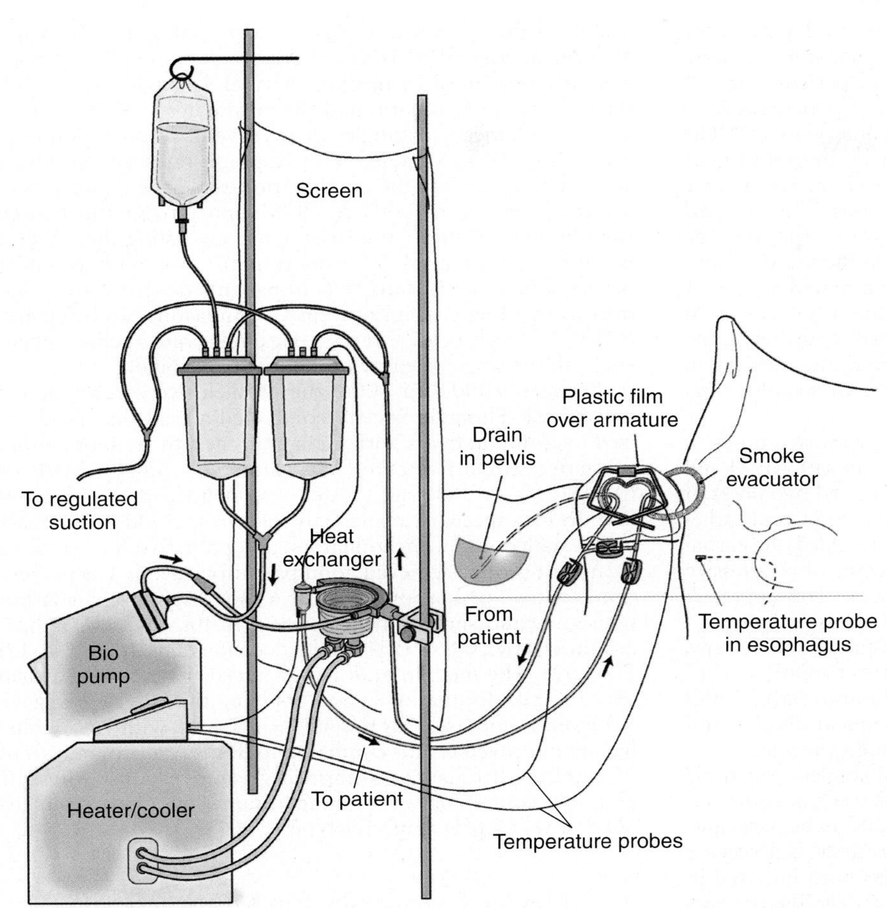

FIGURE 138.14 Intrathoracic chemoperfusion for mesothelioma. (From Jaktlitsch MT, Wiener D, Bueno R, Sugarbaker D. The development of the Brigham and Womens Multmodality Treatment Plan for Malignant Pleural Mesothelioma: a model for improving the treatment of rare diseases. In: Pass H, Vogelzang N, Carbone M, eds. *Malignant Mesothelioma: Advances in Pathogenesis, Diagnosis, and Translational Therapies.* New York: Springer, 2005.)

received 225 mg/m^2 of cisplatin, the median survival was 22 months, and disease-free survival was 20 months. This Boston group has also reported the maximum tolerated dose and toxicity of intraoperative intracavitary hyperthermic cisplatin perfusion with amifostine after EPP.[191] Forty-two patients were enrolled and 29 underwent resection (operative mortality 7%, 2 of 29). Overall median survival was 17 months (resected 20 months, unresected 10 months). Median survivals were 26 months for patients receiving higher cisplatin doses and 16 months for those receiving lower doses. A separate report detailed the entire EPP perfusion experience. Ninety-two (76%) of 121 enrolled patients underwent EPP and received hyperthermic intraoperative intracavitary cisplatin perfusion.[192] Hospital mortality was 4.3%. Nine patients had renal toxicity, which was attributable to cisplatin in eight of the patients. A disappointing recurrence rate of 51% was seen, with ipsilateral recurrence in 17.4% of patients; the median survival of the 121 enrolled patients was 12.8 months.

Novel Gene/Immunomodulatory Therapies

The use of intrapleural cytokine therapy by infusional techniques has chiefly been investigated in earlier-stage mesothelioma, and the effectiveness of interferon by this route has been documented by Boutin et al.,[193] Astoul et al.,[194] and Driesen et al.[195] Eight histologically confirmed complete responses and nine partial responses with at least a 50% reduction in tumor size were obtained. The overall response rate was 20%. The response rate for patients with stage I disease was 45%, with the main side effects being hyperthermia, liver toxicity, neutropenia, and catheter-related infection. Intrapleural IL-2–based regimens have also been exploited in mesothelioma.[196] Intrapleural IL-2 was given to 22 patients with mesothelioma over 5 days. There were 11 partial responses and 1 complete response. Stable disease occurred in three patients and disease progression in seven patients. The overall median survival time was 18 months, and the 24- and 36-month survival rates for responders were 58% and 41%. Lucchi et al.[127,197] have reported that from 1999 to 2004, 49 patients with IMIG stage II–III MPM underwent a protocol of multimodality treatment including: intrapleural preoperative IL-2, PL/decortication, intrapleural postoperative epidoxorubicin, IL-2, adjuvant RT (30 Gy), systemic chemotherapy (cisplatin, 80 mg/m^2 day 1; gemcitabine, 1,250 mg/m^2 days 1 and 8, up to six courses), and long-term subcutaneous IL-2. Of the 49 patients, there were only 9 patients with documented mediastinal disease. With a median follow-up of 59 months, the median actuarial survival was 26 months (31 and 21 months for stage II and III, respectively). Although promising, the complexity of the regimen, as well as the fact that only nine patients truly had a stage III poor prognosis (the rest were T3N0) mitigate the prospects for further studies by other investigators of the regimen's efficacy.

By transferring the herpes simplex virus thymidine kinase (*HSVtk*) gene to a tumor by infecting it with an adenovirus construct containing the TK gene (*AdHSVtk*), one essentially kills the tumor with the addition of ganciclovir. A phase 1 trial of intrapleural suicide gene therapy has been reported that delivered a replication-deficient adenovirus encoding *HSVtk*.[198] Gene transfer was demonstrated in 17 of 25 evaluable patients and was dose-dependent. There was 1 partial response, 3 of the first 18 patients remained stable for up to 2 years after treatment, and 1 early-stage patient was tumor-free for more than 31 months. The median survival of all patients was 11 months. Long-term follow-up of this series of patients reveals that there were two long-term (>6.5 years) survivors.[199] The investigators postulate that given the limited amount of gene transfer observed, the therapy may have been effective because of induction of antitumor immune responses. This has led them to pursue approaches aiming to augment the immune effects of adenovirus gene transfer (i.e., with the use of cytokines). Accordingly, these investigators have initiated a phase 1 adenovirus-interferon-beta immunogene therapy trial based on increased time to progression and greater cures using the adenovirus-interferon-beta along with debulking surgery in rats.[200] Preliminary data reveal consistent antimesothelioma humoral responses.

A phase 1 human trial[201] was conducted with two doses of adenovirus-interferon-beta vector in ten patients with MPM and seven with malignant pleural effusion who received two doses of adenovirus-interferon-beta through an indwelling pleural catheter. At 2 months, modified RECIST responses revealed one partial response, two cases of stable disease, nine cases of progressive disease, and two cases of nonmeasurable disease. This approach was safe and induced immune responses and disease stability.

Another approach uses mesothelin as a target for therapy, and presently three antimesothelin agents are currently in clinical trials for mesothelioma: SS1P (an immunotoxin) (PPO 49), Morab009 (an antimesothelin monoclonal antibody), and CRS-207 (a *Listeria monocytogene* mesothelin vaccine).[202–204] Both SS1P and Morab009 have completed single-agent trials and are now being investigated in phase 1/2 trials in combination with cisplatin and pemetrexed. CRS-207 is being evaluated as a single agent in phase 1 trials. A dendritic cell vaccine (pulsed with mesothelioma cell extracts) has been initiated in the Netherlands[205,206] based on preclinical models. Ten patients with MPM received three vaccinations of clinical-grade autologous dendritic cells intradermally and intravenously at 2-week intervals after chemotherapy. Each vaccine was composed of 50 × 10^6 mature dendritic cells pulsed with autologous tumor lysate and keyhole limpet hemocyanin as a surrogate marker. The study demonstrated that autologous tumor lysate-pulsed dendritic cell–based therapy is feasible, well tolerated, and capable of inducing immunologic response to tumor cells in mesothelioma patients. MSKCC has recently reported results from a pilot trial of a Wilms tumor 1 peptide vaccine, which demonstrated some activity against mesothelioma,[207] and an adjuvant clinical trial using the Wilms tumor 1 vaccine is currently under development.

Broomfield et al.[208] have reported that chemotherapy-induced cell killing that results in "immunogenic" cell death can deliver large amounts of tumor antigens that can be potentially used to prime the immune system. This principally occurs via apoptosis induction and the delivery of antigens into the cross-presentation pathway. By first treating mesothelioma tumors with gemcitabine (to release tumor antigens) and then activating the immune system with an agonistic anti-CD40 antibody, very strong antitumor immune responses can be generated, which induced tumor regressions and cured 50% to 80% of mice. Reviews detailing other novel strategies in mesothelioma have been recently published.[209,210]

CHEMOTHERAPY AND NEWER AGENTS

Chemotherapy for malignant mesothelioma has been used both as a single agent and in combination regimens. Most studies of malignant mesothelioma published in the past 2 decades evaluated the efficacy of chemotherapy predominantly in single-arm uncontrolled trials.[211] Most agents exhibited poor response rate and low median survival as single agents with the exception of cisplatin and the antifolates.[212,213] Owing to the lack of efficacy of single agents, several combination regimens have been examined with response rates and survivals generally greater for the combination regimens compared to single-agent regimens.[214] A 1998 report from the United Kingdom was somewhat encouraging, suggesting that clinical benefit (as measured by reduction in pain and dyspnea) occurred in up to 40% to 50% of patients treated with a regimen of three agents: mitomycin C, vinblastine, and cisplatin (MVP).[215] Steele et al.[216] reported a similar rate of clinical benefit with the single agent, vinorelbine (Navelbine).

Between 2000 and 2006, the Medical Research Council and British Thoracic Society conducted a trial that randomized over 400 patients with malignant mesothelioma to either (1) active supportive care (ASC) alone, (2) ASC + MVP, or (3) ASC + vinorelbine.[217] ASC was defined as regular follow-up in a specialist clinic, and treatment could include steroids, analgesics, bronchodilators, and palliative RT. All three treatment groups achieved good palliation (defined as prevention, control, or improvement) at 6 months, and a small, but nonsignificant, survival benefit was seen for ASC + CT (hazard ratio [HR], 0.89: 95% confidence interval [CI]: 0.72–1.12; P = .32). The median and 1-year survival for the ASC arm was 7.6 months and 30%, and applying the HR to this, gave 8.5 months and 34% for the ASC + CT arm, with vinorelbine having improved results compared to MVP. A meta-analysis of 59 published trials has confirmed greater response rates for platinum-containing versus nonplatinum-containing regimens (23.2% vs. 11.6%, respectively; P <.001).[213]

Newer Cytotoxics for Mesothelioma

Byrne et al.[218] first described the combination of cisplatin with a gemcitabine. Forty-seven percent of treated patients (10 of 21) had a 30% or greater reduction in the thickness of the pleural rind and improvement in symptoms. A follow-up multicenter trial from Australia in 53 patients reported a 26% rate of activity but with a median survival of only 7.5 months.[219] The activity of the combination in other multicenter phase 2 studies[220] in patients previously treated with other chemotherapy[221,222] has led to its widespread use. Gemcitabine,[223,224] cisplatin,[225–228] and carboplatin[229–231] all have independent but modest single-agent activity. Whether the cisplatin/gemcitabine doublet is superior to either single agent is not known, and no phase 3 studies are in progress examining the question. The antifolates pemetrexed and raltitrexed specifically inhibit one or several of the key enzymes involved in the synthesis of purines or pyrimidines.

Pemetrexed (Alimta) is an antifolate compound that has been in development over the past 10 years. Pemetrexed inhibits dihydrofolate reductase, thymidylate synthase, and glycinamide ribonucleotide formyltransferase, enzymes involved in purine and pyrimidine synthesis. Pemetrexed enters the cell primarily through the reduced folate carrier and undergoes extensive intracellular polyglutamation by folylpoly-gamma-glutammate synthetase. The polyglutamated forms, retained for long periods within the cell, have more than 100-fold greater affinity for thymidylate synthase and glycinamide ribonucleotide formyltransferase than the parent drug, pemetrexed monoglutamate.[232] Moreover, there is evidence that malignant mesothelioma cells overexpress the α-folate receptor and high levels of expression of this receptor may make malignant mesothelioma more susceptible to antifolate drugs.[233]

On the basis of the moderate-to-high activity observed with antifolates, investigators compared them in two randomized trials to cisplatin alone. In the first—and to date the largest—reported trial, Vogelzang et al.[67] randomized a total of 456 malignant mesothelioma patients; 226 received a combination of pemetrexed with cisplatin and 222 received cisplatin alone. Patients had measurable, histologically proven pleural malignant mesothelioma, a life expectancy of at least 12 weeks, a Karnofsky performance status of more than 70, and were not candidates for curative surgery. They were treated with pemetrexed 500 mg/m^2 intravenously followed by cisplatin 75 mg/m^2 on day 1 of a 21-day cycle, or with a normal saline infusion (to maintain single blinding) followed by the same dose of cisplatin alone. Median survival time in the pemetrexed/cisplatin arm was 12.1 months versus 9.3 months in the control arm (P = .020). The hazard ratio for death of patients in the pemetrexed/cisplatin arm versus those in the control arm was 0.77. Median time to progression was significantly longer in the pemetrexed/cisplatin arm: 5.7 months versus 3.9 months (P = .001), and response rates were 41.3% in the pemetrexed/cisplatin arm versus 16.7% in the control arm (P <.0001).

In preliminary studies, the combination of pemetrexed and cisplatinum had been found to be unexpectedly toxic and resulted in several treatment-related deaths. It was discovered that the toxicity was due to interference with homocysteine metabolism and could be prevented by the prophylactic use of folic acid and vitamin B_{12}. Both the control and experimental arms received supplementation in the phase 3 trial, resulting in a notable reduction of toxicity (Fig. 138.15). Interestingly, the cisplatin-alone arm also derived some benefit, possibly enabling patients to receive more cycles of chemotherapy. Altogether these results led to the licensing of the combination of cisplatin and pemetrexed for the treatment of malignant mesothelioma in several countries. In the second trial, by the EORTC, 250 malignant mesothelioma patients were randomized to raltitrexed in the presence or absence of cisplatin. Raltitrexed acts as a pure and specific thymidylate synthase inhibitor and costs significantly less than pemetrexed. Initial results showed that the combination of raltitrexed with cisplatin produced nonsignificant improvements in response rate (23.6% vs. 13.6%; P =.056), median survival (11.4 vs. 8.8 months; 95% CI: 7.8–10.8), and 1-year survival (46% vs. 40%; P = .048). However, significant improvement in efficacy and disease-related symptoms (pain and dyspnea) were observed with raltitrexed and cisplatin, and no significant serious additional toxicity was detected with this combination.[234] From these two pivotal randomized trials, it can be concluded that modern chemotherapy improves symptoms and has no deleterious effect on quality of life, despite the associated toxicity.

Taylor et al.[212] presented results for chemonaïve and pretreated malignant mesothelioma patients who received treatment with single-agent pemetrexed in an international Expanded Access Program (EAP). This program provided patients in 13 European countries with access to pemetrexed before its commercial availability. In this expanded access program, single-agent pemetrexed demonstrated promising activity in both chemonaïve and pretreated malignant mesothelioma patients. Of the chemonaïve patients evaluated for efficacy (n = 247), the overall response rate was 10.5%, median time to progressive disease was 6.0 months, and median survival was 14.1 months. Of the previously treated patients evaluated for efficacy (n = 396), the overall response rate was 12.1% and median time to progressive disease was 4.9 months. In this group, median survival could not be estimated because of a high censoring rate (78.9%); however, the 1-year survival was 54.7%. Regarding the safety of treatment, only myelotoxicity data were collected. Common terminology criteria grade 3/4 hematologic toxicity was mild in both groups, with neutropenia (17.3%) as the main toxicity.

In conclusion, the authors suggest single-agent pemetrexed as a possible option for patients not eligible for platinum-containing regimes.[212] Pemetrexed and cisplatin should be considered as the first choice for mesothelioma chemotherapeutic

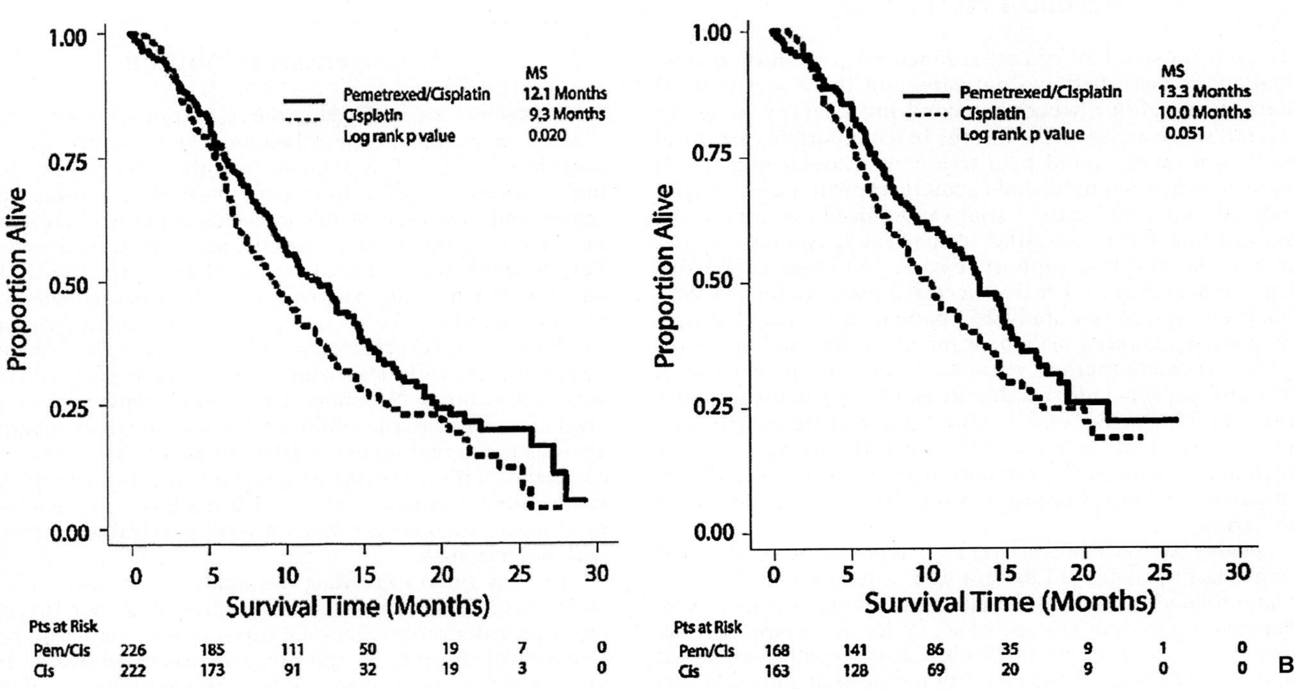

FIGURE 138.15 Results of the phase 3 trial of pemetrexed (Pem) and cisplatin (Cis) versus cisplatin alone. See text for details. MS, median survival; Pts, patients.

palliative treatment. Otherwise, in patients with contraindications to cisplatin treatment, the combination of carboplatin and pemetrexed could be considered. In a recent phase 2 trial, this regimen was shown to be moderately active with response rates of 25%, median survival of 14 months, and acceptable toxicity.[212] In patients unwilling or unable to use folic acid and vitamin B_{12}, or in the countries where pemetrexed is unavailable, raltitrexed should be used in combination with cisplatin. Moreover, the use of cisplatin or carboplatin together with gemcitabine can be considered as another alternative.

In two different phase 2 trials, the response rates and median survivals were assessed for both of these combinations. Gemcitabine with cisplatin showed response rate of 12% and median survival of 10 months, whereas combination with carboplatin revealed response rate of 26% and median survival of 15.4 months.[235,236] For patients who cannot tolerate *any* platinum-based regimen, a combination of pemetrexed and gemcitabine may be an option. A recent phase 2 trial assessed safety and efficacy of this combination in 20 chemonaïve patients with malignant mesothelioma. The response rate was 15% with promising time to disease progression (10.4 months) and overall survival (26.8 months). Conversely, this combination resulted in a notably high incidence of neutropenia (60%) with five patients discontinuing therapy because of unacceptable toxicities.[237] Evidence for a palliative benefit is also evident for vinorelbine, the only vinca alkaloid with proven single-agent activity for malignant mesothelioma. Treatment of 29 malignant mesothelioma patients with weekly vinorelbine alone gave a partial response rate of 24%, and the median overall survival from time of first treatment was 10.6 months and from time of first diagnosis was 13.8 months. Quality of life was improved in the majority of patients, and only one patient experienced neutropenic sepsis requiring hospital admission.[216] When vinorelbine was used with oxaliplatin in a phase 2 trial, however, oxaliplatin significantly increased toxicity and did not appear to be more effective than vinorelbine monotherapy.[238]

Second-Line Therapy

There is no standard of care regimen for previously treated malignant mesothelioma patients, and there are minimal data documenting whether second-line therapy increases overall survival. Nevertheless, the best supportive care, local radiation therapy, and pain treatment should be given to patients when required, and chemotherapy may also be considered. A recent phase 3 trial randomized patients in the second-line setting to either pemetrexed, vitamin supplementation, and best supportive care, or to best supportive care alone, failed to reveal a survival advantage for the combination arm. In this study 243 patients were enrolled with diagnosed advanced malignant mesothelioma and one prior systemic chemotherapy regimen (excluding pemetrexed). The authors conclude that despite an increase in the response rate (18.7% vs. 1.7%; $P < .0001$) and disease control rate (59.3% vs. 19.2%; $P < .0001$), overall survival was not increased significantly, possibly because of the significant imbalance in postdiscontinuation chemotherapy between the arms.[239]

In another study, Sorensen et al.[240] reported the efficacies of single-agent pemetrexed therapy and pemetrexed with carboplatin following platinum-based therapy without pemetrexed. Patients received an average of six cycles of therapy, and the response rates were 21% (95% CI: 8.3–40.9) with pemetrexed and 18% (95% CI: 2.3–51.8) with pemetrexed and carboplatin. Median times to progression were 4.9 months (95% CI: 1.0–21.5) and 7.4 months (95% CI: 1.7–30.0+), respectively, whereas median survival times were 9.8 months (95% CI: 1.0–23.3) and 8.6 months (95% CI: 2.4–30.0+).

NOVEL TREATMENT APPROACHES

Deregulated expression of growth factors and their receptors potentially contributes to chemoresistance and prognosis in mesothelioma.[214] As previously detailed in this chapter, autocrine circuits of activation have been identified in malignant mesothelioma for insulin growth factors,[241] hepatocyte growth factor,[242] and VEGF.[243] PDGF receptor signaling promotes tumor growth in short-term malignant mesothelioma survivors.[244] Other receptors such as c-Kit and endothelial growth factor receptor have been associated with malignant mesothelioma chemoresistance.[244,245] All these molecules are associated with downstream antiapoptotic pathways that have a prominent role in tumor cell survival, and inhibition of these downstream signals can increase cell susceptibility to cytotoxic drugs, allowing use of lower amounts to obtain the same effect. This was demonstrated in an *in vitro* study in which abrogation of PDGF receptor β (PDGFRβ) by imatinib mesylate increases sensitivity of malignant mesothelioma cell lines to gemcitabine and pemetrexed.[246]

Imatinib mesylate has no activity in malignant mesothelioma when used as single agent,[247,248] but because PDGFRβ receptor is also expressed in the tumor vasculature, the inhibition of this receptor has a combined effect on tumor shrinkage. An enhanced therapeutic effect of gemcitabine in human malignant mesothelioma xenografts by imatinib mesylate has also been described.[249] These studies have led to an ongoing phase 2 trial with imatinib mesylate combined with other agents in both chemonaïve and pretreated malignant mesothelioma patients. Tsao et al.[250] have reported that the combination of imatinib and pemetrexed cisplatin resulted in 2 partial responses, 2 mixed responses, 6 stable disease, and 3 progression of disease in 17 patients. Four patients were not evaluable for response.

Angiogenesis Inhibition

Several factors are involved in the regulation of tumor angiogenesis; in malignant mesothelioma the most important is thought to be VEGF. Malignant mesothelioma patients have higher levels of VEGF than patients with any other solid tumor, and inhibition of this molecule could play an important role in the future management of this disease.[40] Bevacizumab was examined in a phase 2 trial with 106 patients, in which 56 malignant mesothelioma patients were randomized to receive six cycles of gemcitabine and cisplatin combined with bevacizumab or placebo followed by maintenance therapy with bevacizumab or the same chemotherapy with a placebo.[251] No improvement in response rate or survival was seen with the addition of bevacizumab. A subgroup analysis noted that higher baseline plasma VEGF levels were correlated with a shorter progression-free and overall survival, and that patients with VEGF levels less than the median had longer progression-free and overall survival when treated with bevacizumab.

A recent report evaluating the addition of bevacizumab to pemetrexed-cisplatin in 43 patients enrolled at four U.S. centers achieved a progression-free survival of 6.9 months, a disease control rate of 81%, and a median overall survival of 14.8 months. These results compare favorably with historical controls of pemetrexed-cisplatin in mesothelioma patients.[252] The

French Intergroup IFCT is also testing pemetrexed/cisplatin with bevacizumab in a randomized phase 2/3 design at 53 French centers and 1 Belgian center. As of July 2009, 61 patients were enrolled and the triplet chemotherapy was relatively well tolerated and feasible, but was associated with a substantial increase in thromboembolic events.[253]

A multicenter phase 2 study has also assessed the efficacy of erlotinib plus bevacizumab in previously treated patients with malignant mesothelioma. The combination of erlotinib and bevacizumab was tolerated reasonably well, but there were no complete or partial responses, although 50% of patients achieved stable disease for at least two cycles of treatment.[254] Median time to progression was 2.2 months and median overall survival was 5.8 months. Previously, erlotinib was shown to be ineffective in patients with malignant mesothelioma when used as a single agent in a phase 2 study.[255] Another VEGF inhibitor, AZD2171, has been evaluated in 46 mesothelioma patients in a Southwest Oncology Group protocol with a 9% response rate and median survival of 9.8 months.[256]

There are other angiogenesis inhibitors that are currently being tested in clinical trials, including thalidomide, sunitinib, and sorafenib. Thalidomide has been shown to have antitumor activity against multiple myeloma, although the exact mechanism by which it acts is unclear.[257] As a single agent, thalidomide has been reported to achieve disease stabilization in 25% of mesothelioma patients for more than 6 months. The NAVLT (Nederlandse Vereniging van Artsen voor Longziekten en Tubercolose) is now recruiting patients for a phase 3 study to assess time to progression in malignant mesothelioma patients who do not have disease progression after four cycles of pemetrexed with carboplatin or cisplatin. Patients will be randomized to receive thalidomide or placebo.[258]

Sorafenib and sunitinib are able to inhibit several targets including receptors tyrosine kinase and intracellular kinases. Specifically, sorafenib inhibits the *Ras/Raf/MEK/ERK* and p38 signaling pathways, VEGFR2 and VEGFR3, and members of the PDGF receptor family, PDGFRβ and c-Kit. In a phase 1 trial, sorafenib in combination with doxorubicin was evaluated in patients with refractory solid tumors. In this study, one patient with pleural mesothelioma achieved a partial response and remained on therapy for 39.7 weeks.[259] A phase 2 trial (CALGB 30307) using sorafenib (targeting VEGFR-2, PDGFR, and Raf) at 400 mg twice daily for MPM that was chemonaïve or previously treated with pemetrexed found grade 3 to 4 adverse effects that included fatigue in 25% of patients and hand-foot syndrome in 13%. The overall response rate was only 4.4%, with a 38.8% disease-stabilization rate, median failure-free survival of 4.1 months, and median overall survival of 10.4 months. Chemonaïve patients had worse survival outcomes than the previously treated patients.[260]

Sunitinib malate (Sutent) acts only on receptors such as VEGFRs, PDGFRβ, and c-Kit and has shown promising activity in phase 3 trials with renal cell carcinoma and gastrointestinal stromal tumors. Nowak et al.[261] have reported a confirmed partial response rate of 18% and median survival of 8.2 months in 23 previously treated mesothelioma patients receiving sunitinib malate. Based on these promising results, the National Cancer Institute of Canada in conjunction with the U.S. NCI has initiated a phase 2 trial with sunitinib in patients with inoperable malignant mesothelioma.[262] In a phase 2 trial, vatalanib (targeting VEGFR-1, -2, and -3; PDGFR; and c-Kit) had an 11% response rate, a 66% stable-disease rate, median progression-free survival of 4.1 months, and median overall survival of 10 months.[263]

In a trial from the North Central Cancer Treatment Group pazopanib, or GW786034 (targeting VEGFR-1, -2, and -3 and PDGFR) at a dose of 800 mg daily for 21 days was tolerated very well; in the patients who received single-agent pazopanib as first-line treatment, a median overall survival of 14.4 months was achieved.[264]

OTHER AGENTS

Ribonuclease Inhibitors

Ranpirnase specifically targets tumor cell tRNA and inhibits protein synthesis, resulting in cell-cycle arrest at the G_1 phase. The adverse effect profile includes hypersensitivity, renal toxicity (proteinuria, azotemia), fatigue, and peripheral edema. Single-agent ranpirnase in a phase 2 MPM trial resulted in a 5% response rate, a 43% stable disease rate, and a median overall survival of 6 months.[265] A phase 3 trial (n = 105) compared ranpirnase (480 mg/m^2 weekly) with doxorubicin (60 mg/m^2 every 3 weeks) and showed no difference in overall survival in the intent-to-treat analysis. However, patients with CALGB prognostic groups 1 to 4 and EORTC risk criteria had a 2-month survival benefit when treated with ranpirnase over doxorubicin.[266]

A large international phase 3 trial (P30-302)[267] comparing doxorubicin (n = 210) with the combination of doxorubicin and ranpirnase (n = 203) revealed no significant difference in overall survival (median survival time: 11.1 vs. 10.7 months), but in a preplanned analysis including 130 pretreated patients, a significant advantage in survival in favor of Adriamycin and ranpirnase was found (median survival time: 10.5 vs. 9 months; HR, 1.49; 95% CI: 1.02–2.17). Further studies of the effect of ranpirnase on chemoresistance are being planned.

Histone Deacetylase Inhibitors

Histone acetylation regulates gene expression by allowing transcription factor access to genomic DNA. Deacetylation of histones leads to cell-cycle progression and unchecked growth. Histone deacetylase inhibitors are agents that prevent deacetylation and reinstate control over the cell cycle. Vorinostat, an oral agent that inhibits class I and II histone deacetylases, is a potent inhibitor of mesothelioma growth *in vitro*. In a phase 1 trial of vorinostat, two partial responses were observed in the 13 patients with mesothelioma. Decreased dyspnea or pain was observed in all patients who achieved at least stable disease.[268] An ongoing randomized phase 3 trial is comparing therapy with vorinostat with placebo in 660 previously treated patients.[269]

Proteasome Inhibitors

Proteasome complexes process ubiquitinated proteins and facilitate protein degradation. When proteasome activity is inhibited, nuclear factor-κB production is also inhibited, and tumor cells undergo apoptosis. Preclinical studies in cell lines and murine xenograft models showed antitumor activity against MPM.[270,271] Recent results of the All Ireland Cooperative Oncology Research Group revealed that bortezomib had only minimal clinical activity in relapsed MPM.[272] Gruppo Italiano Mesotelioma is presently investigating the combination of cisplatin and bortezomib (EORTC).

Selected References

The full list of references for this chapter appears in the online version.

5. Yang H, Bocchetta M, Kroczynska B, et al. TNF-alpha inhibits asbestos-induced cytotoxicity via a NF-kappaB-dependent pathway, a possible mechanism for asbestos-induced oncogenesis. *Proc Natl Acad Sci U S A* 2006;103:10397–402.
7. Gazdar AF, Butel JS, Carbone M. SV40 and human tumours: myth, association or causality? *Nat Rev Cancer* 2002;2:957.
10. Christensen BC, Godleski JJ, Roelofs CR, et al. Asbestos burden predicts survival in pleural mesothelioma. *Environ Health Perspect* 2008;116: 723–6.
11. Altomare DA, You H, Xiao GH, et al. Human and mouse mesotheliomas exhibit elevated AKT/PKB activity, which can be targeted pharmacologically to inhibit tumor cell growth. *Oncogene* 2005;24:6080–9.
12. Wagner JC, Berry G, Timbrell V. Mesotheliomata in rats after inoculation with asbestos and other materials. *Br J Cancer* 1973;28:173–85.
14. Stanton MF, Wrench C. Mechanisms of mesothelioma induction with asbestos and fibrous glass. *J Natl Cancer Inst* 1972;48:797.
21. Ivanov SV, Miller J, Lucito R, et al. Genomic events associated with progression of pleural malignant mesothelioma. *Int J Cancer* 2009;124: 589–99.
22. Cheng JQ, Jhanwar SC, Klein WM, et al. p16 alterations and deletion mapping of 9p21-p22 in malignant mesothelioma. *Cancer Res* 1994;54: 5547–51.
28. Amin KM, Litzky LA, Smythe WR, et al. Wilms' tumor 1 susceptibility (WT1) gene products are selectively expressed in malignant mesothelioma. *Am J Pathol* 1995;146:344–56.
29. Cheng JQ, Lee WC, Klein MA, Cheng GZ, Jhanwar SC, Testa JR. Frequent mutations of NF2 and allelic loss from chromosome band 22q12 in malignant mesothelioma: evidence for a two-hit mechanism of NF2 inactivation. *Genes Chromosomes Cancer* 1999;24:238–42.
31. Gerwin BI, Lechner JF, Reddel RR, et al. Comparison of production of transforming growth factor-beta and platelet-derived growth factor by normal human mesothelial cells and mesothelioma cell lines. *Cancer Res* 1987;47:6180.
34. Kim S, Buchlis G, Fridlender ZG, et al. Systemic blockade of transforming growth factor-beta signaling augments the efficacy of immunogene therapy. *Cancer Res* 2008;68:10247–56.
36. Pass HI, Mew DJ, Carbone M, et al. Inhibition of hamster mesothelioma tumorigenesis by an antisense expression plasmid to the insulin-like growth factor-1 receptor. *Cancer Res* 1996;56:4044.
40. Ohta Y, Shridhar V, Bright RK, et al. VEGF and VEGF type C play an important role in angiogenesis and lymphangiogenesis in human malignant mesothelioma tumours. *Br J Cancer* 1999;81:54–61.
41. Kumar-Singh S, Vermeulen PB, Weyler J, et al. Evaluation of tumour angiogenesis as a prognostic marker in malignant mesothelioma. *J Pathol* 1997;182:211–6.
43. Carbone M, Pass HI. Evolving aspects of mesothelioma carcinogenesis: SV40 and genetic predisposition. *J Thorac Oncol* 2006;1:169.
50. Pacurari M, Castranova V, Vallyathan V. Single- and multi-wall carbon nanotubes versus asbestos: are the carbon nanotubes a new health risk to humans? *J Toxicol Environ Health A* 2010;73:378.
52. Carbone M, Emri S, Dogan AU, et al. A mesothelioma epidemic in Cappadocia: scientific developments and unexpected social outcomes. *Nat Rev Cancer* 2007;7:147.
53. Wagner JC, Skidmore JW, Hill RJ, Griffiths DM. Erionite exposure and mesotheliomas in rats. *Br J Cancer* 1985;51:727–30.
59. Carbone M, Rizzo P, Powers A, Bocchetta M, Fresco R, Krausz T. Molecular analyses, morphology and immunohistochemistry together differentiate pleural synovial sarcomas from mesotheliomas: clinical implications. *Anticancer Res* 2002;22:3443.
64. Roggli VL, Sharma A, Butnor KJ, Sporn T, Vollmer RT. Malignant mesothelioma and occupational exposure to asbestos: a clinicopathological correlation of 1445 cases. *Ultrastruct Pathol* 2002;26:55.
66. Erasmus JJ, Truong MT, Smythe WR, et al. Integrated computed tomography-positron emission tomography in patients with potentially resectable malignant pleural mesothelioma: staging implications. *J Thorac Cardiovasc Surg* 2005;129:1364.
67. Vogelzang NJ, Rusthoven JJ, Symanowski J, et al. Phase III study of pemetrexed in combination with cisplatin versus cisplatin alone in patients with malignant pleural mesothelioma. *J Clin Oncol* 2003;21:2636–44.
68. Herndon JE, Green MR, Chahinian AP, Corson JM, Suzuki Y, Vogelzang NJ. Factors predictive of survival among 337 patients with mesothelioma treated between 1984 and 1994 by the Cancer and Leukemia Group B. *Chest* 1998;113:723–31.
70. Robinson BW, Creaney J, Lake R, et al. Mesothelin-family proteins and diagnosis of mesothelioma. *Lancet* 2003;362:1612–6.
72. Pass HI, Wali A, Tang N, et al. Soluble mesothelin-related peptide level elevation in mesothelioma serum and pleural effusions. *Ann Thorac Surg* 2008;85:265.
74. Creaney J, Robinson BW. Detection of malignant mesothelioma in asbestos-exposed individuals: the potential role of soluble mesothelin-related protein. *Hematol Oncol Clin North Am* 2005;19:1025–40, v.
76. Pass HI, Lott D, Lonardo F, et al. Asbestos exposure, pleural mesothelioma, and serum osteopontin levels. *N Engl J Med* 2005;353:1564–73.
77. Grigoriu BD, Grigoriu C, Chahine B, Gey T, Scherpereel A. Clinical utility of diagnostic markers for malignant pleural mesothelioma. *Monaldi Arch Chest Dis* 2009;71:31–8.
84. Flores RM, Akhurst T, Gonen M, Larson SM, Rusch VW. Positron emission tomography defines metastatic disease but not locoregional disease in patients with malignant pleural mesothelioma. *J Thorac Cardiovasc Surg* 2003;126:11–6.
88. Nowak AK. CT, RECIST, and malignant pleural mesothelioma. *Lung Cancer* 2005;49(Suppl 1):S37–S40.
90. Ceresoli GL, Chiti A, Zucali PA, et al. Early response evaluation in malignant pleural mesothelioma by positron emission tomography with [18F] fluorodeoxyglucose. *J Clin Oncol* 2006;24:4587–93.
97. Edwards JG, Abrams KR, Leverment JN, Spyt TJ, Waller DA, O'Byrne KJ. Prognostic factors for malignant mesothelioma in 142 patients: validation of CALGB and EORTC prognostic scoring systems. *Thorax* 2000;55: 731–5.
98. Fennell DA, Steele JP, Shamash J, et al. Efficacy and safety of first- or second-line irinotecan, cisplatin, and mitomycin in mesothelioma. *Cancer* 2007;109:93–9.
101. Gordon GJ, Dong L, Yeap BY, et al. Four-gene expression ratio test for survival in patients undergoing surgery for mesothelioma. *J Natl Cancer Inst* 2009;101:678.
102. Pass HI, Liu Z, Wali A, et al. Gene expression profiles predict survival and progression of pleural mesothelioma. *Clin Cancer Res* 2004;10:849–59.
104. Pass HI, Goparaju C, Ivanov S, et al. hsa-miR-29c* is linked to the prognosis of malignant pleural mesothelioma. *Cancer Res* 2010;70:1916–24.
105. Righi L, Papotti MG, Ceppi P, et al. Thymidylate synthase but not excision repair cross–complementation group 1 tumor expression predicts outcome in patients with malignant pleural mesothelioma treated with pemetrexed-based chemotherapy. *J Clin Oncol* 2010;28:1534–9.
106. Cappia S, Righi L, Mirabelli D, et al. Prognostic role of osteopontin expression in malignant pleural mesothelioma. *Am J Clin Pathol* 2008;130:58.
109. Flores RM, Akhurst T, Gonen M, et al. Positron emission tomography predicts survival in malignant pleural mesothelioma. *J Thorac Cardiovasc Surg* 2006;132:763–8.
111. Butchart EG, Ashcroft T, Barnsley WC, Hoden MP. The role of surgery in diffuse malignant mesothelioma of the pleura. *Semin Oncol* 1981;8: 321–8.
112. Rusch VW. A proposed new international TNM staging system for malignant pleural mesothelioma. From the International Mesothelioma Interest Group. *Chest* 1995;108:1122.
114. Richards WG, Godleski JJ, Yeap BY, et al. Proposed adjustments to pathologic staging of epithelial malignant pleural mesothelioma based on analysis of 354 cases. *Cancer* 2010;116:1510.
115. Stahel RA, Weder W, Felip E. Malignant pleural mesothelioma: ESMO clinical recommendations for diagnosis, treatment and follow-up. *Ann Oncol* 2009;20(Suppl 4):73–5.
120. Edwards JG, Stewart DJ, Martin-Ucar A, Muller S, Richards C, Waller DA. The pattern of lymph node involvement influences outcome after extrapleural pneumonectomy for malignant mesothelioma. *J Thorac Cardiovasc Surg* 2006;131:981.
122. Treasure T. Surgery for mesothelioma: MARS landing and future missions. *Eur J Cardiothorac Surg* 2010;37:509–10.
123. Flores RM, Pass HI, Seshan VE, et al. Extrapleural pneumonectomy versus pleurectomy/decortication in the surgical management of malignant pleural mesothelioma: results in 663 patients. *J Thorac Cardiovasc Surg* 2008; 135:620–6.
126. Flores RM, Routledge T, Seshan VE, et al. The impact of lymph node station on survival in 348 patients with surgically resected malignant pleural mesothelioma: implications for revision of the American Joint Committee on Cancer staging system. *J Thorac Cardiovasc Surg* 2008;136:605.
133. Nakas A, Trousse DS, Martin-Ucar AE, Waller DA. Open lung-sparing surgery for malignant pleural mesothelioma: the benefits of a radical approach within multimodality therapy. *Eur J Cardiothorac Surg* 2008; 34:886.
134. Bölükbas S, Manegold C, Eberlein M, et al. Survival after trimodality therapy for malignant pleural mesothelioma: radical pleurectomy, chemotherapy with cisplatin/permetrexed and radiotherapy. *Lung Cancer* 2011;71(1):75–81.
135. Butchart EG, Ashcroft T, Barnsley WC, Holden MP. Pleuropneumonectomy in the management of diffuse malignant mesothelioma of the pleura. Experience with 29 patients. *Thorax* 1976;31:15–24.
140. Rusch VW, Rosenzweig K, Venkatraman E, et al. A phase II trial of surgical resection and adjuvant high-dose hemithoracic radiation for malignant pleural mesothelioma. *J Thorac Cardiovasc Surg* 2001;122:788.

141. Pass HI, Kranda K, Temeck BK, Feuerstein I, Steinberg SM. Surgically debulked malignant pleural mesothelioma: results and prognostic factors. *Ann Surg Oncol* 1997;4:215.
142. Baldini EH, Recht A, Strauss GM, et al. Patterns of failure after trimodality therapy for malignant pleural mesothelioma. *Ann Thorac Surg* 1997;63:334–8.
144. Sugarbaker DJ, Flores RM, Jaklitsch MT, et al. Resection margins, extrapleural nodal status, and cell type determine postoperative long-term survival in trimodality therapy of malignant pleural mesothelioma: results in 183 patients. *J Thorac Cardiovasc Surg* 1999;117:54–63.
152. Rosenzweig KE, Fox JL, Zelefsky MJ, Raben A, Harrison LB, Rusch VW. A pilot trial of high-dose-rate intraoperative radiation therapy for malignant pleural mesothelioma. *Brachytherapy* 2005;4:30–3.
153. Lee TT, Everett DL, Shu HK, et al. Radical pleurectomy/decortication and intraoperative radiotherapy followed by conformal radiation with or without chemotherapy for malignant pleural mesothelioma. *J Thorac Cardiovasc Surg* 2002;124:1183.
154. Rice DC, Smythe WR, Liao Z, et al. Dose-dependent pulmonary toxicity after postoperative intensity-modulated radiotherapy for malignant pleural mesothelioma. *Int J Radiat Oncol Biol Phys* 2007;69:350.
155. Forster KM, Smythe WR, Starkschall G, et al. Intensity-modulated radiotherapy following extrapleural pneumonectomy for the treatment of malignant mesothelioma: clinical implementation. *Int J Radiat Oncol Biol Phys* 2003;55:606.
157. Allen AM, Czerminska M, Janne PA, et al. Fatal pneumonitis associated with intensity-modulated radiation therapy for mesothelioma. *Int J Radiat Oncol Biol Phys* 2006;65:640–5.
161. Gupta V, Krug LM, Laser B, et al. Patterns of local and nodal failure in malignant pleural mesothelioma after extrapleural pneumonectomy and photon-electron radiotherapy. *J Thorac Oncol* 2009;4:746.
166. Lee C, Bayman N, Swindell R, Faivre-Finn C. Prophylactic radiotherapy to intervention sites in mesothelioma: a systematic review and survey of UK practice. *Lung Cancer* 2009;66:150.
177. Weder W, Kestenholz P, Taverna C, et al. Neoadjuvant chemotherapy followed by extrapleural pneumonectomy in malignant pleural mesothelioma. *J Clin Oncol* 2004;22:3451–7.
178. Opitz I, Kestenholz P, Lardinois D, et al. Incidence and management of complications after neoadjuvant chemotherapy followed by extrapleural pneumonectomy for malignant pleural mesothelioma. *Eur J Cardiothorac Surg* 2006;29:579–84.
179. Weder W, Stahel RA, Bernhard J, et al. Multicenter trial of neo-adjuvant chemotherapy followed by extrapleural pneumonectomy in malignant pleural mesothelioma. *Ann Oncol* 2007;18:1196–202.
181. de Perrot M, Feld R, Cho BC, et al. Trimodality therapy with induction chemotherapy followed by extrapleural pneumonectomy and adjuvant high-dose hemithoracic radiation for malignant pleural mesothelioma. *J Clin Oncol* 2009;27:1413.
182. Krug LM, Pass HI, Rusch VW, et al. Multicenter phase II trial of neoadjuvant pemetrexed plus cisplatin followed by extrapleural pneumonectomy and radiation for malignant pleural mesothelioma. *J Clin Oncol* 2009;27:3007.
183. Pass HI, Temeck BK, Kranda K, et al. Phase III randomized trial of surgery with or without intraoperative photodynamic therapy and postoperative immunochemotherapy for malignant pleural mesothelioma. *Ann Surg Oncol* 1997;4:628.
190. Richards WG, Zellos L, Bueno R, et al. Phase I to II study of pleurectomy/decortication and intraoperative intracavitary hyperthermic cisplatin lavage for mesothelioma. *J Clin Oncol* 2006;24:1561–7.
191. Zellos L, Richards WG, Capalbo L, et al. A phase I study of extrapleural pneumonectomy and intracavitary intraoperative hyperthermic cisplatin with amifostine cytoprotection for malignant pleural mesothelioma. *J Thorac Cardiovasc Surg* 2009;137:453–8.
192. Tilleman TR, Richards WG, Zellos L, et al. Extrapleural pneumonectomy followed by intracavitary intraoperative hyperthermic cisplatin with pharmacologic cytoprotection for treatment of malignant pleural mesothelioma: a phase II prospective study. *J Thorac Cardiovasc Surg* 2009;138:405.
193. Boutin C, Nussbaum E, Monnet I, et al. Intrapleural treatment with recombinant gamma-interferon in early stage malignant pleural mesothelioma. *Cancer* 1994;74:2460.
194. Astoul P, Bertault-Peres P, Durand A, Catalin J, Vignal F, Boutin C. Pharmacokinetics of intrapleural recombinant interleukin-2 in immunotherapy for malignant pleural effusion. *Cancer* 1994;73:308.
198. Sterman DH, Treat J, Litzky LA, et al. Adenovirus-mediated herpes simplex virus thymidine kinase/ganciclovir gene therapy in patients with localized malignancy: results of a phase I clinical trial in malignant mesothelioma. *Hum Gene Ther* 1998;9:1083–92.
200. Kruklitis RJ, Singhal S, DeLong P, et al. Immuno–gene therapy with interferon-beta before surgical debulking delays recurrence and improves survival in a murine model of malignant mesothelioma. *J Thorac Cardiovasc Surg* 2004;127:123.
201. Sterman DH, Recio A, Haas AR, et al. A phase I trial of repeated intrapleural adenoviral-mediated interferon-beta gene transfer for mesothelioma and metastatic pleural effusions. *Mol Ther* 2010;18:852.
202. Hassan R, Ho M. Mesothelin targeted cancer immunotherapy. *Eur J Cancer* 2008;44:46–53.
204. Hassan R, Bullock S, Premkumar A, et al. Phase I study of SS1P, a recombinant anti-mesothelin immunotoxin given as a bolus I.V. infusion to patients with mesothelin-expressing mesothelioma, ovarian, and pancreatic cancers. *Clin Cancer Res* 2007;13:5144–9.
206. Hegmans JP, Veltman JD, Lambers ME, et al. Consolidative dendritic cell-based immunotherapy elicits cytotoxicity against malignant mesothelioma. *Am J Respir Crit Care Med* 2010.
207. Brown AB, Krug L, Maaslak P. Pilot trial of a Wilms tumor-1 (WT-1) peptide vaccine in patients with thoracic and myeloid neoplasms. *J Clin Oncol* 2008;26(1445).
208. Broomfield S, Currie A, van der Most RG, et al. Partial, but not complete, tumor-debulking surgery promotes protective antitumor memory when combined with chemotherapy and adjuvant immunotherapy. *Cancer Res* 2005;65:7580–4.
212. Taylor P, Castagneto B, Dark G, et al. Single-agent pemetrexed for chemonaive and pretreated patients with malignant pleural mesothelioma: results of an International Expanded Access Program. *J Thorac Oncol* 2008;3:764.
216. Steele JP, Shamash J, Evans MT, Gower NH, Tischkowitz MD, Rudd RM. Phase II study of vinorelbine in patients with malignant pleural mesothelioma. *J Clin Oncol* 2000;18:3912–7.
217. Muers MF, Stephens RJ, Fisher P, et al. Active symptom control with or without chemotherapy in the treatment of patients with malignant pleural mesothelioma (MS01): a multicentre randomised trial. *Lancet* 2008;371:1685–94.
219. Nowak AK, Byrne MJ, Williamson R, et al. A multicentre phase II study of cisplatin and gemcitabine for malignant mesothelioma. *Br J Cancer* 2002;87:491.
223. van Meerbeeck JP, Baas P, Debruyne C, et al. A phase II study of gemcitabine in patients with malignant pleural mesothelioma. European Organization for Research and Treatment of Cancer Lung Cancer Cooperative Group. *Cancer* 1999;85:2577–82.
234. van Meerbeeck JP, Gaafar R, Manegold C, et al. Randomized phase III study of cisplatin with or without raltitrexed in patients with malignant pleural mesothelioma: an intergroup study of the European Organisation for Research and Treatment of Cancer Lung Cancer Group and the National Cancer Institute of Canada. *J Clin Oncol* 2005;23:6881.
235. Kalmadi SR, Rankin C, Kraut MJ, et al. Gemcitabine and cisplatin in unresectable malignant mesothelioma of the pleura: a phase II study of the Southwest Oncology Group (SWOG 9810). *Lung Cancer* 2008;60:259–63.
237. Simon GR, Verschraegen CF, Janne PA, et al. Pemetrexed plus gemcitabine as first-line chemotherapy for patients with peritoneal mesothelioma: final report of a phase II trial. *J Clin Oncol* 2008;26:3567–72.
239. Jassem J, Ramlau R, Santoro A, et al. Phase III trial of pemetrexed plus best supportive care compared with best supportive care in previously treated patients with advanced malignant pleural mesothelioma. *J Clin Oncol* 2008;26:1698.
240. Sorensen JB, Sundstrom S, Perell K, Thielsen AK. Pemetrexed as second-line treatment in malignant pleural mesothelioma after platinum-based first-line treatment. *J Thorac Oncol* 2007;2:147.
248. Porta C, Mutti L, Tassi G. Negative results of an Italian Group for Mesothelioma (G.I.Me.) pilot study of single-agent imatinib mesylate in malignant pleural mesothelioma. *Cancer Chemother Pharmacol* 2007;59:149–50.
251. Karrison T. Final analysis of a multi-centre, double blind, placebo controlled, randomized phase II trial of gemcitabine/cisplatin plus bevacizumab or placebo in patients with malignant mesothelioma. *Proc Am Soc Clin Oncol* 2007;25(18S):7526.
255. Garland LL, Rankin C, Gandara DR, et al. Phase II study of erlotinib in patients with malignant pleural mesothelioma: a Southwest Oncology Group Study. *J Clin Oncol* 2007;25:2406–13.
256. Garland LL, Chansky A, Wozniak AJ, et al. A phase II study of novel oral antiangiogenic agent AZD2171 (NSC-732208) in malignant pleural mesothelioma. *J Clin Oncol* 2010;27(15S).
257. Baas P, Boogerd W, Dalesio O, Haringhuizen A, Custers F, van Zandwijk N. Thalidomide in patients with malignant pleural mesothelioma. *Lung Cancer* 2005;48:291.
260. Dubey S, Jänne PA, Krug L, et al. A phase II study of sorafenib in malignant mesothelioma: results of Cancer and Leukemia Group B 30307. *J Thorac Oncol* 2010;5(10):1655–1661.
261. Nowak AK, Millward M, Francis RJ, et al. Phase II study of sunitinib as second-line therapy in malignant pleural mesothelioma (MPM). *J Clin Oncol* 2008;28(15S):7036. Available at: http://meeting.ascopubs.org/cgi/content/abstract/28/15_suppl/7036.
263. Jahan TM, Gu L, Wang XF, et al. Vatalanib (V) for patients with previously untreated advanced malignant mesothelioma (MM): a phase II study

by the Cancer and Leukemia Group B (CALGB 30107). *J Clin Oncol* 2006;24(384 Suppl):226.

266. Beck AK, Pass HI, Carbone M, Yang H. Ranpirnase as a potential antitumor ribonuclease treatment for mesothelioma and other malignancies. *Future Oncol* 2008;4:341.
267. Reck M, Krzakowski M, Jassem J, et al. Randomized, multicentre phase IIIb study of ranpirnase + doxorubicin (DOX) versus DOX in patients with unresectable malignant mesothelioma (MM). *J Thorac Oncol* 2009; 4(9 Suppl 1):S319.
268. Krug LM, Curley T, Schwartz L, et al. Potential role of histone deacetylase inhibitors in mesothelioma: clinical experience with suberoylanilide hydroxamic acid. *Clin Lung Cancer* 2006;7:257–61.
269. Paik PK, Krug LM. Histone deacetylase inhibitors in malignant pleural mesothelioma: preclinical rationale and clinical trials. *J Thorac Oncol* 2010;5:275.
272. Fennell D, van Meerbeeck JP, O'Byrne K, et al. A pilot phase II clinical trial of the 20S proteasome inhibitor bortezomib in patients with relapsed malignant pleural mesothelioma. *J Thorac Oncol* 2009;4(9 Suppl 1):S457.

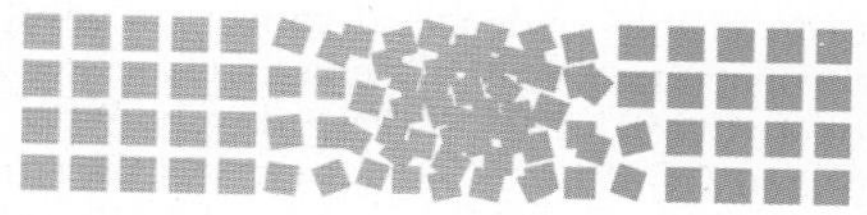

CHAPTER 139 PERITONEAL SURFACE MALIGNANCY

MARCELLO DERACO, DOMINIQUE ELIAS, OLIVIER GLEHEN, CYRIL W. HELM, PAUL H. SUGARBAKER, AND VIC J. VERWAAL

Peritoneal carcinomatosis, mesothelioma, and sarcomatosis are included in the group of diseases collectively referred to, in this chapter, as peritoneal surface malignancy. Over the past three decades there has emerged an increasing optimism concerning the management of cancer dissemination within the abdomen and pelvis. The clinical problem was originally defined by several important clinical studies that established the natural history of peritoneal surface malignancy.[1–3]

Concomitant with these manuscripts that identified the guarded prognosis of patients with peritoneal surface malignancy, isolated reports appeared concerning an emerging technology that described a new approach to management. This alternative treatment plan had two essential components. First, cytoreductive surgery (CRS) was used in an attempt to resect visible implants within the abdomen and pelvis. Peritonectomy along with visceral resections was developed to surgically deal with cancer on peritoneal surfaces.[4] The second component was local-regional chemotherapy (intraperitoneal chemotherapy) used in the operating room or within the early postoperative period. Chemotherapy used in the operating room with moderate heat has been referred to as hyperthermic intraperitoneal chemotherapy (HIPEC)[5]; chemotherapy used within the early postoperative period has been referred to as early perioperative intraperitoneal chemotherapy (EPIC).[6] The chemotherapy is used in an attempt to eradicate free cancer cells and minute attached nodules that remain following surgery.[7] The unique aspect of this new combination of treatments was the perioperative timing of the chemotherapy. It is not adjuvant chemotherapy and it is not neoadjuvant chemotherapy; it is chemotherapy used simultaneously with a major cytoreductive surgical procedure. Of course, all efforts to maintain benefits from systemic chemotherapy in patients with peritoneal carcinomatosis, mesothelioma, or sarcomatosis must continue.

RATIONALE FOR A COMBINED TREATMENT FOR PERITONEAL SURFACE MALIGNANCY

Lack of Clinical Evidence for Alternative Management Strategies

There are many reasons why this combined approach to the management of peritoneal surface malignancy has continued to grow. Perhaps the greatest impetus toward further development of CRS and perioperative chemotherapy (POC) is a near total lack of scientific data to support an alternative treatment plan. Level 1 data regarding the effectiveness of systemic chemotherapy for peritoneal carcinomatosis has not been published.[8] The response to systemic chemotherapy is not the same for all anatomic sites of metastatic disease. It must be concluded that no reliable data from the medical oncology literature regarding the benefits of systemic chemotherapy for peritoneal carcinomatosis from gastrointestinal cancer are available. In sharp contrast, over the past decade, multiple phase 2 and 3 studies with CRS and POC report a median survival benefit two to four times greater than survival using systemic chemotherapy.

Natural History Studies Document the Importance of Local-Regional Progression

A second strong rationale for the emergence of CRS and POC as a valid treatment option comes from natural history studies. In a proportion of patients, recurrence of the primary cancer isolated to the surfaces of the abdomen and pelvis is a reality. Patients with primary or recurrent disease at the resection site and on peritoneal surfaces in the absence of hepatic metastases or systemic metastases are appropriate for treatment by CRS and POC. Isolated peritoneal surface progression of abdominal or pelvic malignancy is not unusual.[9–13]

To fully understand the importance of cancer cells that gain access to the peritoneal space prior to or at the time of a cancer resection, one must appreciate the clinical manifestations of progression. Figure 139.1 illustrates the mechanism of local-regional progression. Cancer cells at low density result in peritoneal carcinomatosis at a distance from the primary cancer resection. Cancer cells at higher density become trapped within raw surfaces at the resection site. A fusiform layer of cancer that conforms to the anatomic structures within the bed of the primary resection site results from high density seeding.[14] The progression of cancer implants within the resection site and on peritoneal surfaces in the absence of liver metastases or systemic disease presents a major rationale for comprehensive local-regional treatments.[15]

VALIDATED QUANTITATIVE PROGNOSTIC INDICATORS

A third factor strongly recommending CRS and POC as a valid treatment option comes from well-established selection factors applied to this patient population. With some variations between diseases, the same group of quantitative prognostic indicators operates for all patients with peritoneal surface malignancy. Now, prognostic indicators are used to refine the selection of patients to those most likely to benefit and to exclude those who are unlikely to benefit.[16] Histopathology assessments, the peritoneal cancer index (PCI), the completeness of cytoreduction score (CC), and radiologic imaging by

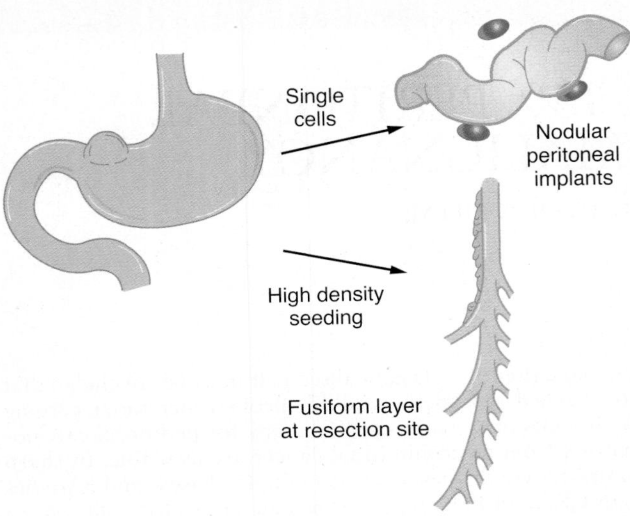

FIGURE 139.1 Intraoperative dissemination of gastric cancer cells. If cancer cells gain access to the peritoneal space either prior to or at the time of gastrectomy, two patterns of dissemination are observed. Low density of cancer cells into the free peritoneal space results in nodules as peritoneal implants. A high density of cancer cells that fall into the cancer resection site results in a layering of cancer.

computed tomography (CT) play a central role in refining patient selection.

Biological Aggressiveness as Measured by Histopathology

Epithelial Appendiceal Neoplasms

Mucinous appendiceal neoplasms have a broad spectrum of aggressiveness, and the histologic type of the appendiceal neoplasm has a profound effect on survival following treatment by CRS and POC.[17] Patients with adenomucinosis obtain maximal survival benefit, while those with mucinous carcinoma show survivals similar to that for peritoneal carcinomatosis of colorectal origin.[18]

Peritoneal Mesothelioma

Seven different histologic patterns of peritoneal mesothelioma contribute to three distinct histologic groups that have a very different prognosis following CRS with POC: poor prognosis for sarcomatoid, deciduoid, or biphasic type; intermediate prognosis for papillary and epithelial type; and excellent prognosis for low-grade or multicystic type.[19,20]

Extent of Disease as Measured by the Peritoneal Cancer Index

The PCI is an assessment combining lesion size (0 to 3) with tumor distribution (abdominopelvic regions 0 to 12) to quantify the extent of disease within the abdomen and pelvis as a numerical score (Fig. 139.2).[21] It is calculated from observations obtained at the time of surgical exploration of the abdomen and pelvis. The higher the PCI, the less likely CRS and POC will result in long-term survival for all the peritoneal surface malignancies discussed in this chapter.

The Completeness of Cytoreduction Score Performed after the Resection

The size of residual tumor nodules after CRS has been completed has a profound effect on outcome. The new definition of complete cytoreduction is no visible evidence of cancer or only minute nodules reliably penetrated by POC, a completeness of cytoreduction score of 0 (CC-0) or CC-1, respectively. With few exceptions an optimal CC-0 or CC-1 score is necessary for long-term benefit with CRS and POC.[21]

Preoperative Radiologic Imaging by Computed Tomography

CT of the chest, abdomen, and pelvis is an essential tool in the selection of patients for CRS with POC. Systemic metastases and spread to pleural surfaces can be identified. The location and quantity of mucinous carcinoma within the peritoneal cavity can be accurately determined.[22,23] If the small bowel and its mesentery are coated by tumor or a large mass of cancer occupies the epigastric region, the likelihood of achieving complete cytoreduction is small. The CT should be performed with maximal intravenous and oral contrast in order to identify patients who have small bowel compartmentalization versus diffuse involvement of the small bowel.

Pharmacokinetic Advantage of Perioperative Chemotherapy

A fourth argument in favor of CRS and POC as a treatment option for peritoneal surface malignancy is a well-studied pharmacologic rationale. As determined by physical properties, some chemotherapy agents are especially appropriate for hyperthermic use in the peritoneal cavity after a cytoreductive surgery has been completed. Other chemotherapy agents are more appropriate for early postoperative intraperitoneal chemotherapy. As experience with POC has accumulated, the use of multiple-agent chemotherapy has evolved and promises to be increasingly effective. Heat targeting of both the intravenous and intraperitoneal chemotherapy to the peritoneal surface cancer nodule is the goal of treatment.

Combined Use of Cytoreductive Surgery and Perioperative Chemotherapy as a Standard of Care

A fifth and final argument for use of CRS and POC as a treatment option for peritoneal surface malignancy concerns the well-defined management parameters that are currently in practice at experienced treatment centers. The cytoreductive surgical procedure involves visceral resections and peritonectomy procedures in an attempt to leave the abdomen visibly free of cancer. After the CRS is complete, tubes and drains are positioned to facilitate inflow and outflow of the chemotherapy solution. The chemotherapy solution circulates through roller pumps and a heat exchanger to maintain moderate hyperthermia (42°C/109°F) within the abdomen and pelvis. The skin edges are elevated on a self-retaining retractor (open method) or the skin closed (closed method) in order to create a reservoir for the hyperthermic chemotherapy solution. Following the HIPEC treatment, access to the abdomen and pelvis is re-established to perform the intestinal reconstruction.

The cancer resection, intraoperative chemotherapy washing, intestinal reconstruction sequence is important to optimize the destruction of small volumes of cancer cells and prevent suture line and abdominal incision recurrence. During the peritonectomy and visceral resections, large volumes of cancer

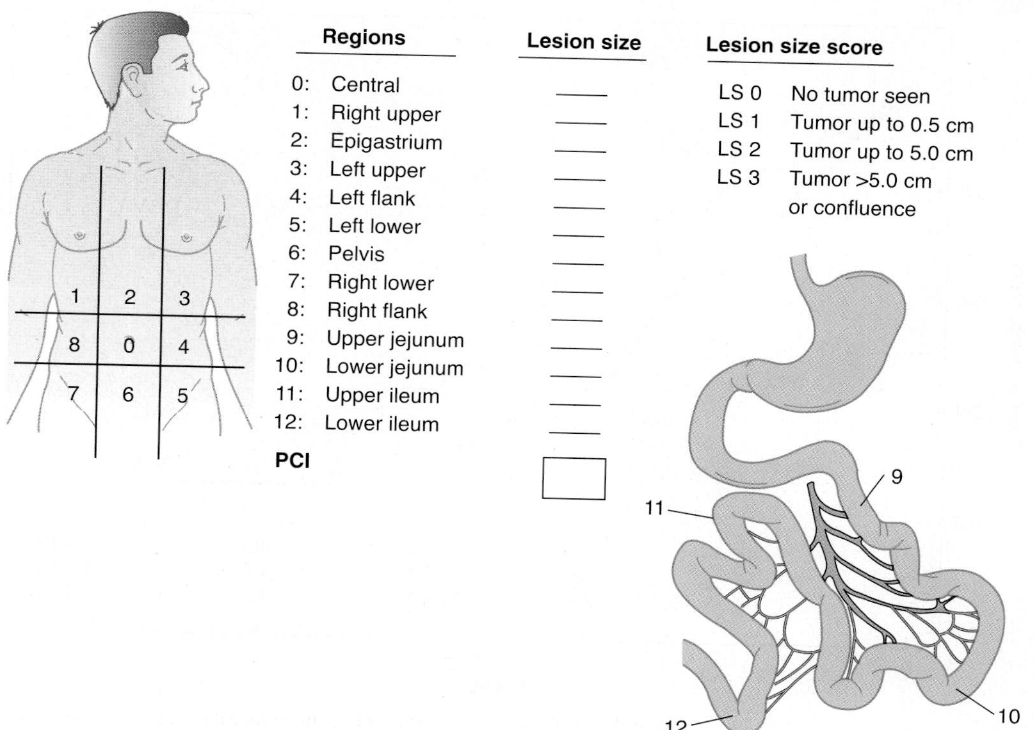

FIGURE 139.2 The peritoneal cancer index (PCI). This index combines a size and a distribution parameter to achieve a numerical score. The lesion size (LS) is used to quantitate the size of peritoneal nodules. The distribution of tumor is determined within the 13 abdominopelvic regions.

are removed; however, residual cancer cells remain especially within the raw surfaces created by the surgical dissection. Mechanical and chemical washing of the complete parietal and visceral surfaces by the warm chemotherapy solution will prevent a reimplantation of cancer cells following CRS. A review of the important recent contributions to the literature that critically assesses the benefits of CRS and POC constitutes the remainder of this chapter.

APPENDICEAL MALIGNANCY

Natural History

Although similarities exist, there are unique features of appendiceal malignancies as compared to colorectal adenocarcinoma. The first and probably the most obvious difference between the colon and the appendix malignancies is the diameter of the bowel lumen involved. A colon tumor grows as an intraluminal mass in the bowel and will invade through the wall. The intraluminal growth pattern causes the primary cancer to reach the serosa in a late stage. In contrast, the appendix is a small organ, up to 1 cm in diameter. A tumor obliterates the appendix lumen in an early stage. This may cause an early blowout of the appendix, resulting in spreading of tumor cells in the abdominal cavity or a perforation of the tumor through the wall the appendix. In both situations this results in an intra-abdominal seeding of tumor cells early in the natural history of the disease with neoplastic cells throughout the peritoneal cavity.[24,25]

Histologic Classification

The biology of appendiceal malignancies varies from simple mucinous adenoma to solid intestinal type adenocarcinoma. The histology of the primary tumor itself has a major influence on the outcome of the treatment by CRS and HIPEC. Ronnett et al.[26] and Bruin et al.[27] described three different types in their analyses of appendiceal malignancies. A tumor with more than 90% mucus, flat epithelial cells, no atypia, and no mitoses had a good prognosis despite extensive intra-abdominal spreading. At the other end of the spectrum, a primary tumor with much atypia, abundant mitoses, and less than 50% mucus has a prognosis similar to colorectal carcinomatosis, even with much less intra-abdominal spreading. It is called peritoneal carcinoma (PCA).

Outcome of Treatment of Peritoneal Dissemination by Cytoreductive Surgery Followed by Hyperthermic Intraperitoneal Chemotherapy

The survival outcome with peritoneal dissemination of appendiceal origin neoplasms is shown in Figure 139.3. The overall survival is shown according to the histologic classification. For the least aggressive form (disseminated peritoneal adenomucinosis) the median survival is not reached within 5 years.[27] Those patients who were affected by PCA had a much poorer prognosis. The median survival was only 14 months in these patients. These survival data compare with the median survival of peritoneal carcinomatosis of colorectal origin, 26 months, treated with cytoreduction followed by HIPEC. Accepting the fact that complete cytoreduction is always the goal of CRS, these data document that survival in peritoneal carcinomatosis from appendiceal malignancies is highly dependent upon the histopathological characteristics of the tumor.

The treatment of recurrence after primary treatment with cytoreduction followed by HIPEC depends largely on the

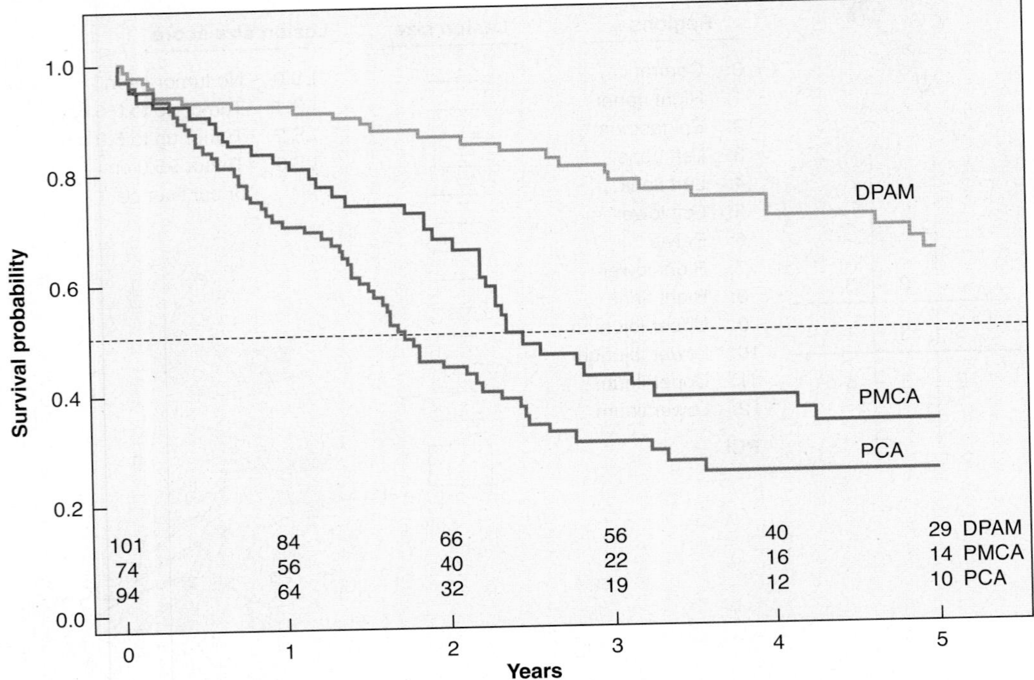

FIGURE 139.3 Survival of 269 patients with peritoneal dissemination of an appendiceal neoplasm by histologic classification. DPAM, disseminated peritoneal adenomucinosis; PMCA, peritoneal mucinous carcinoma; PCA, peritoneal carcinoma. (From ref. 27.)

number and location of tumor masses. With a limited number of locations the first choice is resection; if more diffuse disease is present and cytoreduction is complete, a second HIPEC can be performed. In patients in whom the pathology is more aggressive, systemic chemotherapy, with all it limitations, should be considered.[28]

Learning Curve

Cytoreduction followed by HIPEC is a complex treatment. The complexity originates from the treatment as well as from the management of the complications.[29,30] The peak of the learning curve in the study of Smeenk et al.[31] was reached after approximately 130 procedures. Surgical skill is undoubtedly the main component of this learning process, but experience in handling complications by the entire medical team has contributed to a decreased morbidity and mortality. Besides technical skill, the establishment of modified treatment strategy for an individual patient advanced treatment expertise.

COLORECTAL CARCINOMATOSIS: CURATIVE TREATMENT AND PREVENTION

Stage IV colorectal cancer is a very morbid disease, with a 5-year survival rate of 10% and a median survival of 14.4 months. The prognosis is significantly worse when peritoneal carcinomatosis (PC) is present, with a median survival of 6.7 months versus 18.1 months without PC ($P < .01$).[32] When colorectal PC is diagnosed, the crucial question for the physicians is whether curative or palliative therapy should be proposed to the patient.

Incidence of the Disease and Incidence of Peritoneal Carcinomatosis

At the initial diagnosis of colon cancer, the peritoneal surface is involved with tumor in 10% to 15% of patients.[12,33] Besides the liver, the peritoneal surfaces are the most common sites of cancer recurrence after "curative" colorectal cancer resections. Cancer progression occurs in as many as 50% of patients who had an R0 resection. In 10% to 35% of patients with recurrent disease, the anatomic site of treatment failure is confined to the peritoneal surface.[12,33] In patients with advanced or disseminated cancer at presentation, the peritoneal surface is involved at laparotomy in 30% to 50% of cases.[12,33] However, when PC is isolated or anatomically closely associated with the primary tumor, potentially curative treatment is possible.

Useful Prognostic Indicators for the Disease

The key issue is to determine whether palliative (systemic chemotherapy) or curative (complete cytoreductive surgery [CCRS] with HIPEC) treatment is indicated. Contraindications for this combined treatment are the presence of metastases at another site (although, up to three easily resectable liver metastases is not an absolute contraindication),[34] a poor general status (the combined treatment is rather aggressive), and extensive PC. Extensive PC is likely to be unresectable in its entirety. Even when a complete cytoreduction is possible, the prognosis is poor. Most of the series using CCRS with HIPEC report a poor survival rate when Sugarbaker's peritoneal cancer index is higher than 20.[35,36] Consequently, a score exceeding 20 can be considered a relative contraindication for the combined approach.

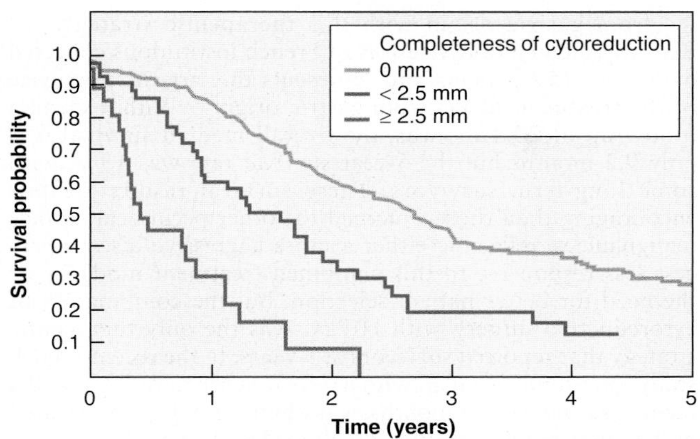

FIGURE 139.4 Overall survival according to the completeness of cytoreduction after cytoreductive surgery (CRS) and hyperthermic intraperitoneal chemotherapy (HIPEC) for peritoneal carcinomatosis. (From ref. 38.)

Results of Treatment

Figure 139.4 reports the survival rates according to the completeness of surgery in the 523 patients collected by the Association Française de Chirurgie.[36] Five years after surgery, no patient was alive if the size of the residual tumor nodules exceeded 2 mm after surgery, whereas 30% of the patients were alive if CCRS was possible (P <.0001).

The real impact of HIPEC alone in this situation is currently unknown for humans. In a randomized trial in rats, those treated with HIPEC survived longer than those treated with intraperitoneal chemotherapy alone or with intraperitoneal hyperthermia alone.[37] A recent retrospective study compared similar patients (all of whom underwent a laparotomy) with resectable PC treated with CCRS and HIPEC to patients who received standard systemic chemotherapy. Median survival was 63 months in the CCRS with HIPEC group versus 24 months in the systemic chemotherapy group.[38]

Summary of Important Results from Other Institutions, Including Morbidity/Mortality

This combined treatment (CCRS immediately followed by HIPEC) is effective. Benefits were definitively demonstrated by the randomized study of the Amsterdam group: 105 patients who presented with colorectal PC were randomized between surgery with HIPEC (and systemic chemotherapy) versus systemic chemotherapy alone.[39] In this study, close to 50% of the patients in the experimental arm were at presentation not good candidates for HIPEC because their PC could not be completely resected. In spite of this bias, the reported median survival was 22 months in the experimental arm versus 13 months in the control group (P = .032).

The results obtained with CCRS with HIPEC are interesting and promising: in the Association Française de Chirurgie study, the 5-year overall survival rate was 30%.[36] This result accepts clinical data over an 18-year interval and includes the learning curves of 28 different centers. It will be the worst ever to be reported by the authors' group. The results of experienced centers concerning patients who underwent CCRS with HIPEC are comparable, with 5-year overall survival rates close to 40%. It was 32% for the 70 patients in the study by da Silva et al.,[40] 43% for the 59 patients in the Verwaal et al.[41] study, and 48% for the 30 patients treated by Elias et al.[42] Such a survival rate has never been published before for colorectal PC, even if it includes only selected patients.

This is truly a therapeutic revolution. Furthermore, these results are identical to those obtained with hepatectomy for liver metastases. So the message appears to be that selected patients with PC should be treated with this combined therapy just as selected patients with liver metastases should be treated with hepatectomy given that similar results are achieved in terms of survival.[43]

Conclusion Regarding Current Practice and Future Application to Patients at High Risk for Local-Regional Recurrence

Unfortunately, early diagnosis of PC is not possible with imaging, but only with a laparotomy. This is why the authors proposed second-look surgery plus HIPEC in asymptomatic patients who presented with a primary exhibiting a high risk of developing PC.[44] High-risk patients were those who presented with a few (resected) peritoneal implants, ovarian metastases, or perforated tumors. Second-look surgery was performed 6 months after the end of the classic 6 months of systemic adjuvant chemotherapy. Among 47 patients, macroscopic PC was found and treated in 50% of them. In the remaining patients with no macroscopic PC, peritoneal recurrence occurred frequently in those who did not receive HIPEC, but rarely in those who did receive HIPEC (P = .02). Finally, only 17% of the patients treated with HIPEC developed a peritoneal recurrence.[45]

DIFFUSE MALIGNANT PERITONEAL MESOTHELIOMA

Clinical Presentation and Diagnosis

Diffuse malignant peritoneal mesothelioma (DMPM) is characterized by progressive peritoneal seeding, eventually leading to the patient's death due to tumor layering on peritoneal surfaces, bowel obstruction, and intractable malignant ascites. Patients are usually diagnosed with presenting signs and symptoms of advanced disease. In a recently published series of 81 patients with DMPM reported by an Italian group, ascites, abdominal pain, and asthenia were the most frequent symptoms present on 77%, 69%, and 43% of patients, respectively. CT scan shows ascites, peritoneal thickening, abdominal mass, and mesenteric thickening, respectively, on 80%, 63%, 32%, and 29% of cases. CT scan is used as an accurate prognostic radiologic test for patient selection for comprehensive treatment.[23]

Cytological diagnosis of ascitic fluid is often inconclusive, since cells frequently resemble elements with mesothelial hyperplasia. In the series of the Washington Cancer Institute, diagnosis was made by fluid sampling in 0 of 68 patients. Laparotomy was required in 44% of patients, laparoscopy in 52%, and ultrasound/CT-guided biopsy in 4%.[46] Recently, cytological and ultrastructural methods have enhanced the diagnostic accuracy of cytological assessment.[47]

Treatment and Results with Systemic Chemotherapy and Biological Therapies

Numerous single-drug and combination regimens have been tested over the past decades with modest results. Preliminary data also suggest a possible survival advantage for a combination of cisplatin and pemetrexed as compared to cisplatin alone. Other cytotoxic agents that have shown to be active in this setting include vinorelbine and gemcitabine, either alone or combined with platinum compounds. In historical case series, standard therapy with palliative surgery and systemic or intraperitoneal chemotherapy is associated with a median survival of about 1 year, ranging from 9 to 15 months.[48,49]

The combined approach consisting of CRS and HIPEC modified the natural history of DMPM with a dramatic improvement in outcomes in the authors' study and in a multi-institutional registry series.[11,19,50–53] Median survival grew from 12 months with a systemic chemotherapy treatment to 53 months with CRS with HIPEC, with 50% 5-year overall survival.[54]

GASTRIC CANCER

Prevention and Treatment of Carcinomatosis

Peritoneal dissemination is the most frequent pattern of metastasis and recurrence with gastric cancers. Also, it occurs in 5% to 20% of patients being explored for potentially curative resection.[55] In the past, gastric carcinomatosis has been regarded as a terminal disease, and most oncologists would regard it as a condition only to be palliated. Over the past two decades, novel therapeutic approaches to PC have emerged, combining cytoreductive surgery and peritonectomy procedures with perioperative intraperitoneal chemotherapy (PIC), including HIPEC and EPIC.[56] Because of the aggressive nature of gastric cancer, the question regarding the efficiency of this combined procedure remains controversial for carcinomatosis.

Natural History and Palliative Treatment

Traditionally, there has been mutual agreement in the oncologic community that those patients with peritoneal dissemination of gastric cancer were incurable. The studies that prospectively evaluated the prognosis indicated median survival of not more than 6 months.[2] Despite improvements in systemic chemotherapy with encouraging tumor response rates, there has been no improvement in survival.[57] Moreover, positive effects of palliative gastric cancer resection have been recently reported in patients with PC but without any long-term survivors.[55]

Curative Treatment: Cytoreductive Surgery and Hyperthermic Intraperitoneal Chemotherapy

The experience of a few single institution phase 2 studies showed encouraging survival results following treatment of PC from gastric origin with this therapeutic strategy.[58–63] Recently, a collaborative effort of French institutions collected data from 159 patients and represents the largest experience of the treatment of PC from gastric origin.[61] With a median follow-up of 20.4 months, the overall median survival was only 9.2 months but the 5-year survival rate was 13%, with some long-term survivors. These survival results are less encouraging than those obtained for other peritoneal surface malignancies, reflecting either a more aggressive disease process less responsive to this combined treatment modality or the need for better patient selection. But the combination of cytoreductive surgery with HIPEC was the only therapeutic strategy that reported survivors at 5 years. In the recent French study long-term survival, with a 5-year survival of 23% and a median survival of 15 months, was obtained in patients treated with complete macroscopic resection (Fig. 139.5).[61]

PC with localized or small tumor nodules seems to be the best indication for this combined procedure. In the French study, in patients who had undergone complete cytoreductive surgery, the extent of carcinomatosis represented the only strong prognostic factor.[61] When the PCI was more than 12, despite a complete cytoreductive surgery, no patient was alive at 3 years.

The institution in which the procedure was performed plays an important role for the postoperative course and for survival. It is also reasonable to assume that experience may provide better patient selection and greater surgical expertise with a higher rate of complete cytoreductive surgery and improved postoperative management. A learning curve has been reported by several authors and institutions who performed the combination of cytoreductive surgery with HIPEC for the management of PC.[31,64,65] All interventional complex procedures have an inherent risk and experience diminishes this risk, but they can never abolish it. The high rates of morbidity and mortality reported may reach 60% and 6.5%, respectively.[61] These high rates of morbidity and mortality emphasize the necessity for patient selection using strict criteria regarding physiologic age and general status.

Prevention of Gastric Carcinomatosis

For many Korean and Japanese researchers, HIPEC has been performed in an adjuvant setting in phase 3 trials. Most of them demonstrated the benefit of HIPEC, especially for T3, T4 and lymph node positive gastric tumors.[66–69] In Western countries, some small experiences also suggested the benefit of using HIPEC as adjuvant treatment for the prevention of PC recurrence in advanced gastric cancer.[70,71]

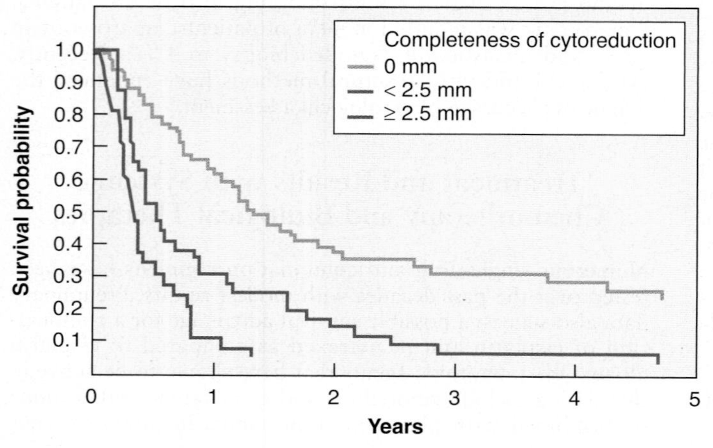

FIGURE 139.5 Overall survival of 159 patients with carcinomatosis from gastric cancer treated by cytoreductive surgery (CRS) and hyperthermic intraperitoneal chemotherapy (HIPEC) according to completeness of cytoreduction. (From ref. 61.)

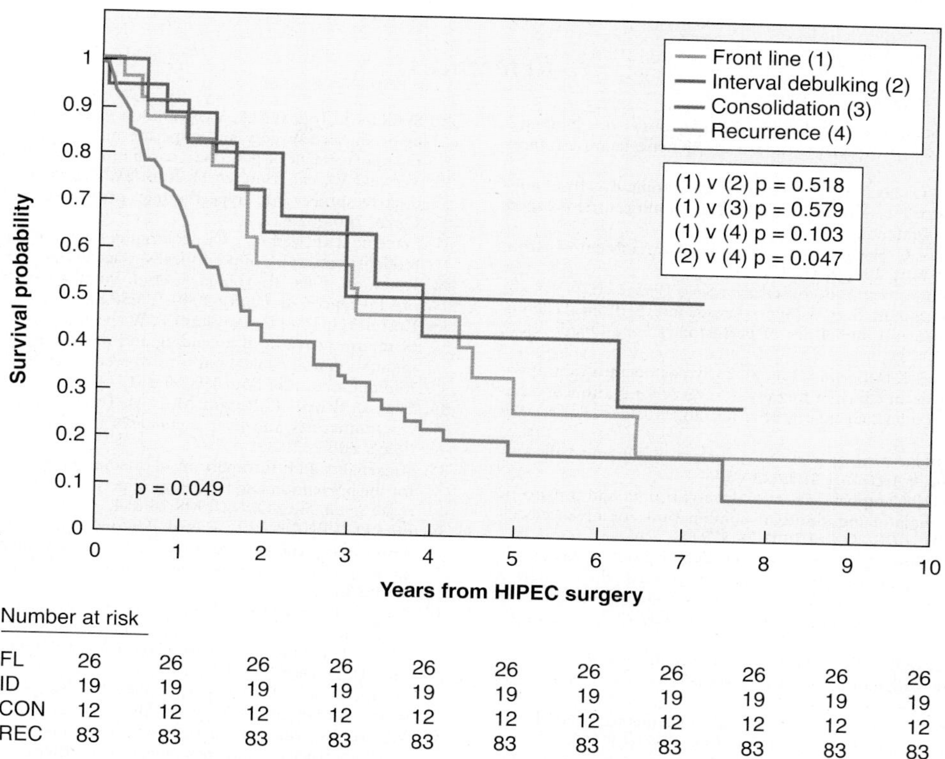

FIGURE 139.6 Kaplan-Meier survival curve by time for intervention in epithelial ovarian cancer (EOC) patients treated by cytoreductive surgery (CRS) and hyperthermic intraperitoneal chemotherapy (HIPEC). (From ref. 72.)

PERITONEAL CARCINOMATOSIS IN OVARIAN CANCER

Cytoreductive Surgery and Hyperthermic Intraperitoneal Chemotherapy in Epithelial Ovarian Cancer

An Internet-based registry was initiated to collect data from many centers in a format that can be analyzed for factors such as prognostic indicators, variations in technique, and outcomes.[72] Patient eligibility includes epithelial ovarian cancer, fallopian tube, or primary peritoneal carcinoma treated with HIPEC at some point in the natural history of the disease. Low malignant potential and nonepithelial ovarian cancer tumors are excluded. Each participating institution uses its own HIPEC technology regarding chemotherapy solutions, duration of perfusion, temperature, and technique of open or closed peritoneal perfusion. In the initial report, 141 women were analyzed who had been treated with either frontline (n = 26), at interval debulking (n = 19), for consolidation (n = 12), or for recurrence (n = 83).

The median overall survival was 30.3 months. Despite the size of data set as a whole, there were insufficient numbers who underwent frontline, interval debulking, and consolidation for reliable statistical comparisons at these time points. The 83 patients with recurrent disease represent the largest number yet analyzed as a single group. In multivariable analysis, the factors significant for increased survival were sensitivity to platinum response (P = .048), completeness of cytoreduction score of 1 or 0 (P = .025), carboplatin alone or combination (P = .011), and duration of hospital stays of 10 days or less (P = .021). Figure 139.6 shows the Kaplan-Meier survivals by timing of combined treatment.

There have been at least 18 reports including over 400 patients treated with HIPEC for recurrent epithelial ovarian cancer. Despite the numbers, there are great problems in interpreting the data because they represent heterogeneous groups, with data difficult to extract, and there is often no way of differentiating platinum-resistant from platinum-sensitive cases. The overall survival would suggest activity in patients with recurrent disease particularly if the prognostic factor composition were similar to those on the study. Notable papers in this setting included that of Rufian et al.,[73] who reported a 75% 5-year survival in those 55 years or less, with the best survival in those with no visible disease at the end of CRS.

SARCOMATOSIS

Soft tissue tumors of the viscera or retroperitoneum are associated with high rates of local-regional relapse. An attempt to achieve adequate margins of excision may be impossible because of anatomic constraints. Cancer cell seeding into the peritoneal cavity either prior to or at the time sarcoma resection combined with positive or narrow margins of excision result in this high likelihood of local-regional recurrence.[74] In patients with local-regional disease progression or sarcomatosis, the survival is limited to approximately 2 years.

If cytoreductive surgery is performed in this group of patients and combined with POC, the median survival is extended past 2 years. In four of the five studies referenced, an overall 5-year survival was greater than 30%.[75–80] A consensus statement has been published.[81]

References

1. Chu DZ, Lang NP, Thompson C, et al. Peritoneal carcinomatosis in nongynecologic malignancy. A prospective study of prognostic factors. *Cancer* 1989;63:364.
2. Sadeghi B, Arvieux C, Glehen O, et al. Peritoneal carcinomatosis from non-gynecologic malignancies: results of the EVOCAPE 1 multicentric prospective study. *Cancer* 2000;88:358.
3. Jayne DG, Fook S, Loi C, Seow-Choen F. Peritoneal carcinomatosis from colorectal cancer. *Br J Surg* 2002;89:1545.
4. Sugarbaker PH. Peritonectomy procedures. *Ann Surg* 1995;221:29.
5. Glehen O, Cotte E, Kusamura S, et al. Hyperthermic intraperitoneal chemotherapy: nomenclature and modalities of perfusion. *J Surg Oncol* 2008; 98:242.
6. Sugarbaker PH, Graves T, DeBruijn EA, et al. Early postoperative intraperitoneal chemotherapy as an adjuvant therapy to surgery for peritoneal carcinomatosis from gastrointestinal cancer: pharmacologic studies. *Cancer Res* 1990;50:5790.
7. Sugarbaker PH. Management of peritoneal surface malignancy: the surgeon's role. *Langenbeck Arch Surg* 1999;384:576.
8. Sanoff HK, Sargent DJ, Campbell ME, et al. Five-year data and prognostic factor analysis of oxaliplatin and irinotecan combinations for advanced colorectal cancer: N9741. *J Clin Oncol* 2008;26:5721.
9. Gonzalez-Moreno S, Brun E, Sugarbaker PH. Lymph node metastasis in epithelial malignancies of the appendix with peritoneal dissemination does not reduce survival in patients treated by cytoreductive surgery and perioperative intraperitoneal chemotherapy. *Ann Surg Oncol* 2005; 12:72.
10. Yan TD, Yoo D, Sugarbaker PH. Significance of lymph node metastasis in patients with diffuse malignant peritoneal mesothelioma. *Eur J Surg Oncol* 2006;32:948.
11. Baratti D, Kusamura S, Cabras AD, et al. Lymph node metastases in diffuse malignant peritoneal mesothelioma. *Ann Surg Oncol* 2010;17:45.
12. Dawson LE, Russell AH, Tong D, Wisbeck WM. Adenocarcinoma of the sigmoid colon: sites of initial dissemination and clinical patterns of recurrence following surgery alone. *J Surg Oncol* 1983;22:95.
13. Brodsky JT, Cohen AM. Peritoneal seeding following potentially curative resection of colonic carcinoma: implications for adjuvant therapy. *Dis Colon Rectum* 1991;34:723.
14. Carmignani CP, Sugarbaker TA, Bromley CM, Sugarbaker PH. Intraperitoneal cancer dissemination: mechanisms of the patterns of spread. *Cancer Metastasis Rev* 2003;22:465.
15. Weiss L. Metastatic inefficiency: causes and consequences. *Cancer Rev* 1986;3:1.
16. Gilly FN, Cotte E, Brigand C, et al. Quantitative prognostic indices in peritoneal carcinomatosis. *Eur J Surg Oncol* 2006;32:597.
17. Ronnett BM, Zahn CM, Kurman RJ, et al. Disseminated peritoneal adenomucinosis and peritoneal mucinous carcinomatosis. A clinicopathologic analysis of 109 cases with emphasis on distinguishing pathologic features, site of origin, prognosis, and relationship to "pseudomyxoma peritonei." *Am J Surg Pathol* 1995;19:1390.
18. Sugarbaker PH. Epithelial appendiceal neoplasms. *Cancer J* 2009;15:225.
19. Yan TD, Deraco M, Baratti D, et al. Cytoreductive surgery and hyperthermic intraperitoneal chemotherapy for malignant peritoneal mesothelioma: multi-institutional experience. *J Clin Oncol* 2009;27:6237.
20. Cerruto CA, Brun EA, Chang D, Sugarbaker PH. Prognostic significance of histomorphologic parameters in diffuse malignant peritoneal mesothelioma. *Arch Pathol Lab Med* 2006;130:1654.
21. Jacquet P, Sugarbaker PH. Current methodologies for clinical assessment of patients with peritoneal carcinomatosis. *J Exp Clin Cancer Res* 1996;15: 49.
22. Jacquet P, Jelinek JS, Chang D, et al. Abdominal computed tomographic scan in the selection of patients with mucinous peritoneal carcinomatosis for cytoreductive surgery. *J Am Coll Surg* 1995;181:530.
23. Yan TD, Haveric N, Carmignani CP, Bromley CM, Sugarbaker PH. Computed tomographic characterization of malignant peritoneal mesothelioma. *Tumori* 2005;91:394.
24. Smeenk RM, van Velthuysen ML, Verwaal VJ, Zoetmulder FA. Appendiceal neoplasms and pseudomyxoma peritonei: a population based study. *Eur J Surg Oncol* 2008;34:196.
25. Sugarbaker PH. Pseudomyxoma peritonei. A cancer whose biology is characterized by a redistribution phenomenon. *Ann Surg* 1994;219:109.
26. Ronnett BM, Shmookler BM, Sugarbaker PH, Kurman RJ. Pseudomyxoma peritonei: new concepts in diagnosis, origin, nomenclature, and relationship to mucinous borderline (low malignant potential) tumors of the ovary. *Anat Pathol* 1997;2:197.
27. Bruin S, Verwaal VJ, Vincent A, Veer LJ. A clinicopathologic analysis of peritoneal metastases from colorectal and appendiceal origin. *Ann Surg Oncol* 2010;17(9):2330.
28. Smeenk RM, Verwaal VJ, Antonini N, Zoetmulder FA. Progression of pseudomyxoma peritonei after combined modality treatment: management and outcome. *Ann Surg Oncol* 2007;14:493.
29. Spiliotis J, Rogdakis A, Vaxevanidou A, et al. Morbidity and mortality of cytoreductive surgery and hyperthermic intraperitoneal chemotherapy in the management of peritoneal carcinomatosis. *J BUON* 2009;14:259.
30. Verwaal VJ, van Tinteren H, Ruth SV, Zoetmulder FA. Toxicity of cytoreductive surgery and hyperthermic intra-peritoneal chemotherapy. *J Surg Oncol* 2004;85:61.
31. Smeenk RM, Verwaal VJ, Zoetmulder FA. Learning curve of combined modality treatment in peritoneal surface disease. *Br J Surg* 2007;94:1408.
32. Rosen SA, Buell JF, Yohida A, et al. Initial presentation with stage IV colorectal cancer. *Arch Surg* 2000;135:503.
33. Russel AH, Tong D, Dawson LE, Wisbeck W, Griffin TW. Adenocarcinoma of the retroperitoneal ascending and descending colon: sites of initial dissemination and clinical patterns of recurrence following surgery alone. *Int Radiat Oncol Biol Phys* 1983;9:361.
34. Elias D, Benizri E, Pocard M, et al. Treatment of synchronous peritoneal carcinomatosis and liver metastases from colorectal cancer. *Eur J Surg Oncol* 2006;32:632.
35. Sugarbaker PH. Intraperitoneal chemotherapy and cytoreductive surgery for the prevention and treatment of peritoneal carcinomatosis and sarcomatosis. *Semin Surg Oncol* 1998;14:254.
36. Elias D, Gilly F, Boutitie F, et al. Peritoneal colorectal carcinomatosis treated with surgery and perioperative intraperitoneal chemotherapy: retrospective analysis of 523 patients from a multicentric French study. *J Clin Oncol* 2010:28:63.
37. Koga S, Hamazoe R, Maeta M, et al. Treatment of implanted peritoneal cancer in rats by continuous hyperthermic peritoneal perfusion in combination with an anticancer drug. *Cancer Res* 1984;44:1840.
38. Elias D, Lefevre JH, Chevalier J, et al. Complete cytoreductive surgery plus intraperitoneal chemohyperthermia with oxaliplatin for peritoneal carcinomatosis of colorectal origin. *J Clin Oncol* 2009;27:681.
39. Verwaal VC, van Ruth S, de Bree E, et al. Randomized trial of cytoreduction and hyperthermic intraperitoneal chemotherapy versus systemic chemotherapy and palliative surgery in patients with peritoneal carcinomatosis from colorectal cancer. *J Clin Oncol* 2003;21:3737.
40. da Silva RG, Sugarbaker PH. Analysis of prognostic factors in seventy patients having a complete cytoreduction plus perioperative intraperitoneal chemotherapy for carcinomatosis from colorectal cancer. *J Am Coll Surg* 2006;203:878.
41. Verwaal VJ, van Ruth S, Witkamp A, et al. Long-term survival of peritoneal carcinomatosis of colorectal origin. *Ann Surg Oncol* 2005;12:65.
42. Elias D, Raynard B, Farkhondeh F, et al. Peritoneal carcinomatosis of colorectal origin. *Gastroenterol Clin Biol* 2006;30:1200.
43. Elias D. Peritoneal carcinomatosis or liver metastases from colorectal cancer: similar standards for a curative surgery? *Ann Surg Oncol* 2004;11:122.
44. Sugarbaker PH. Second-look sugery for colorectal cancer: revised selection factors and new treatment options for greater success. *Int J Surg Oncol* 2011.
45. Elias D, Goere D, Di Pietrantonio D, et al. Results of systematic second-look surgery in patients at high risk of developing colorectal peritoneal carcinomatosis. *Ann Surg* 2008;247:445.
46. Sugarbaker PH, Welch LS, Mohamed F, et al. A review of peritoneal mesothelioma at the Washington Cancer Institute. *Surg Oncol Clin North Am* 2003;12:605.
47. de Pangher Manzini V, Recchia L, Cafferata M, et al. Malignant peritoneal mesothelioma: a multicenter study on 81 cases. *Ann Oncol* 2010;21:348.
48. Carteni G, Manegold C, Martin Garcia G, et al. Malignant peritoneal mesothelioma. Results from the International Expanded Access Program using pemetrexed alone or in combination with a platinum agent. *Lung Cancer* 2009;64:211.
49. Garcia-Carbonero R, Paz-Ares L. Systemic chemotherapy in the management of malignant peritoneal mesothelioma. *Eur J Surg Oncol* 2006;32:676.
50. Feldman AL, Libutti SK, Pingpank JF, et al. Analysis of factors associated with outcome in patients with malignant peritoneal mesothelioma undergoing surgical debulking and intraperitoneal chemotherapy. *J Clin Oncol* 2003;21:4560.
51. Sugarbaker PH, Yan TD, Stuart OA, Yoo D. Comprehensive management of diffuse malignant peritoneal mesothelioma. *Eur J Surg Oncol* 2006; 32:686.
52. Deraco M, Nonaka D, Baratti D, et al. Prognostic analysis of clinicopathologic factors in 49 patients with diffuse malignant peritoneal mesothelioma treated with cytoreductive surgery and intraperitoneal hyperthermic perfusion. *Ann Surg Oncol* 2006;13:229.
53. Deraco M, Baratti D, Zaffaroni N, et al. Advances in clinical research and management of diffuse peritoneal mesothelioma. *Recent Results Cancer Res* 2007;169:137.
54. Deraco M, Bartlett D, Kusamura S, Baratti D. Consensus statement on peritoneal mesothelioma. *J Surg Oncol* 2008;98:268.
55. Hioki M, Gotohda N, Konishi M, et al. Predictive factors improving survival after gastrectomy in gastric cancer patients with peritoneal carcinomatosis. *World J Surg* 2010;34:555.

56. Glehen O, Mohamed F, Gilly FN. Peritoneal carcinomatosis from digestive tract cancer: new management by cytoreductive surgery and intraperitoneal chemohyperthermia. *Lancet Oncol* 2004;5:219.
57. Boku N. Chemotherapy for metastatic disease: review from JCOG trials. *Int J Clin Oncol* 2008;13:196.
58. Yonemura Y, Kawamura T, Bandou E, et al. Treatment of peritoneal dissemination from gastric cancer by peritonectomy and chemohyperthermic peritoneal perfusion. *Br J Surg* 2005;92:370.
59. Glehen O, Cotte E, Sayag-Beaujard AC, et al. Cytoreductive surgery and intraperitoneal chemohyperthermia for peritoneal carcinomatosis arising from gastric cancer. *Arch Surg* 2004;139:20.
60. Fujimoto S, Takahashi M, Mutou T, et al. Improved mortality rate of gastric carcinoma patients with peritoneal carcinomatosis treated with intraperitoneal hyperthermic chemoperfusion combined with surgery. *Cancer* 1997;79:884.
61. Glehen O, Gilly FN, Arvieux C, et al. Peritoneal carcinomatosis from gastric cancer: a multi-institutional study of 159 patients treated by cytoreductive surgery combined with perioperative intraperitoneal chemotherapy. *Ann Surg Oncol* 2010;17(9):2370.
62. Yonemura Y, Fujimura T, Nishimura G, et al. Effects of intraoperative chemohyperthermia in patients with gastric cancer with peritoneal dissemination. *Surgery* 1996;119:437.
63. Hall JJ, Loggie BW, Shen P, et al. Cytoreductive surgery with intraperitoneal hyperthermic chemotherapy for advanced gastric cancer. *J Gastrointest Surg* 2004;8:454.
64. Mohamed F, Moran BJ. Morbidity and mortality with cytoreductive surgery and intraperitoneal chemotherapy. *Cancer J* 2009;15:196.
65. Yan TD, Links M, Fransi S, et al. Learning curve for cytoreductive surgery and perioperative intraperitoneal chemotherapy for peritoneal surface malignancy—a journey to becoming a nationally funded peritonectomy center. *Ann Surg Oncol* 2007;14:2270.
66. Yonemura Y, de Aretxabala X, Fujimura T, et al. Intraoperative chemohyperthermic peritoneal perfusion as an adjuvant to gastric cancer: final results of a randomized controlled study. *Hepatogastroenterology* 2001; 48:1776.
67. Fujimoto S, Takahashi M, Mutou T, et al. Successful intraperitoneal hyperthermic chemoperfusion for the prevention of postoperative peritoneal recurrence in patients with advanced gastric carcinoma. *Cancer* 1999; 85: 529.
68. Kim JY, Bae HS. A controlled clinical study of serosa-invasive gastric carcinoma patients who underwent surgery plus intraperitoneal hyperthermo-chemo-perfusion (IHCP). *Gastric Cancer* 2001;4:27.
69. Zhu ZG, Tang R, Yan M, et al. Efficacy and safety of intraoperative peritoneal hyperthermic chemotherapy for advanced gastric cancer patients with serosal invasion. A long-term follow-up study. *Dig Surg* 2006;23:93.
70. Scaringi S, Kianmanesh R, Sabate JM, et al. Advanced gastric cancer with or without peritoneal carcinomatosis treated with hyperthermic intra-peritoneal-chemotherapy: a single Western center experience. *Eur J Surg Oncol* 2008; 34:1246.
71. De Roover A, Detroz B, Detry O, et al. Adjuvant hyperthermic intraperitoneal preoperative chemotherapy (HIPEC) associated with curative surgery for locally advanced gastric carcinoma. An initial experience. *Acta Chir Belg* 2006;106:297.
72. Helm CW, Richard SD, Pan J, et al. Hyperthermic intraperitoneal chemotherapy in ovarian cancer: first report of the HYPER-O registry. *Int J Gynecol Cancer* 2010;20:61.
73. Rufian S, Munoz-Casares FC, Briceno J, et al. Radical surgery-peritonectomy and intraoperative intraperitoneal chemotherapy for the treatment of peritoneal carcinomatosis in recurrent or primary ovarian cancer. *J Surg Oncol* 2006;94:316.
74. Karakousis CP, Kontzoglou K, Driscoll DL. Intraperitoneal chemotherapy in disseminated abdominal sarcoma. *Ann Surg Oncol* 1997;4:496.
75. Bilimoria MM, Holtz DJ, Mirza NQ, et al. Tumor volume as a prognostic factor for sarcomatosis. *Cancer* 2002;94:2441.
76. Berthet B, Sugarbaker TA, Chang D, et al. Quantitative methodologies for selection of patients with recurrent abdominopelvic sarcoma for treatment. *Eur J Cancer* 1999;35:413.
77. Eilber FC, Rosen G, Forscher C, et al. Surgical resection and intraperitoneal chemotherapy for recurrent abdominal sarcomas. *Ann Surg Oncol* 1999; 6:645.
78. Rossi CR, Deraco M, De Simone M, et al. Hyperthermic intraperitoneal intraoperative chemotherapy after cytoreductive surgery for the treatment of abdominal sarcomatosis: clinical outcome and prognostic factors in 60 consecutive patients. *Cancer* 2004;100:1943.
79. Bonvalot S, Cavalcanti A, Le Pechoux C, et al. Randomized trial of cytoreduction followed by intraperitoneal chemotherapy versus cytoreduction alone in patients with peritoneal sarcomatosis. *Eur J Surg Oncol* 2005;31:917.
80. Lim SJ, Cormier JN, Feig BW, et al. Toxicity and outcomes associated with surgical cytoreduction and hyperthermic intraperitoneal chemotherapy (HIPEC) for patients with sarcomatosis. *Ann Surg Oncol* 2007;14:2309.
81. Rossi CR, Casali P, Kusamura S, et al. The consensus statement on the locoregional treatment of abdominal sarcomatosis. *J Surg Oncol* 2008; 98: 291.

CHAPTER 140 INTRAOCULAR MELANOMA

DANIEL M. ALBERT AND AMOL D. KULKARNI

INCIDENCE AND ETIOLOGY

Melanomas are the most common primary intraocular malignancy in adults.[1] They represent 5% of all melanomas,[1] but, because of the high rate of metastases and poor response to treatment, they account for about 13% of melanoma deaths.[2] Choroidal and ciliary body melanomas constitute about 95% of all uveal melanomas.[3] Melanomas of the iris are rare, having an estimated European incidence of 0.02 to 0.08 per 100,000 per year.[4,5] The incidence of ocular melanomas for whites in the United States as tracked by the Surveillance, Epidemiology, and End Results (SEER) program was 0.69 per 100,000 person-years for males and 0.54 for females.[3,6] The incidence is several-fold lower for blacks and Hispanics. The incidence of ocular melanoma peaks in the seventh decade, and the mean age of patients was 60 years in the Collaborative Ocular Melanoma Study (COMS).[7]

Based on SEER data, white race is a significant risk factor for uveal melanoma.[8] Interestingly, increased choroidal pigmentation was found not to be protective but rather a risk factor for the development of posterior uveal melanoma in white patients.[9] The available data on sunlight as a cause of uveal melanoma reveal incomplete and conflicting results.[10] There is growing support for the hypothesis that cutaneous dysplastic nevus syndrome patients are at increased risk of developing uveal melanoma.[11] Ocular and oculodermal melanocytosis (i.e., nevus of Ota) clearly predisposes to the development of uveal melanomas.[12] Studies of families in which two or more members had a uveal melanoma have revealed no clear mode of inheritance.[13]

ANATOMY AND PATHOLOGY

Histology

In 1931 Callender recognized distinct cell types in the spectrum of cells that compose uveal melanomas (Table 140.1). According to Callender's cytologic characterization,[14] uveal melanomas are divided into three categories:

- Spindle cell melanomas (type A, B, or both), accounting for about 30% of intraocular tumors;
- Mixed-cell melanomas, when fewer than half of the cells in the sections examined are composed of epithelioid cells, accounting for about 65% of intraocular tumors;
- Epithelioid cell melanomas, when greater than half of the tumor sections are composed of epithelioid cells, accounting for 5% of intraocular tumors.[15]

The pathologist's designation of a particular cell type involves subjective judgment.

Microvascular Circulation

The microvascular circulation of uveal melanomas is a heterogenous mixture. It may contain pre-existing normal vessels engulfed by the lesion; new angiogenic vessels formed from pre-existing vessels; matrix-rich vascularlike networks of fluid-conducting channels, termed *vasculogenic mimicry*, which are formed by tumor cells; and mosaic vessels lined by both tumor cells and endothelium. According to Folberg and Maniotis,[16] there is a hierarchy of microvascular structures that they divide into nine patterns. It is theorized that vasculogenic mimicry's contribution to the microcirculation requires a highly invasive tumor cell phenotype, with deregulated expression of genes typical of vascular cells. Other investigators have expressed different opinions about the histogenesis, nature, and function of the structures defined as vasculogenic mimicry.[17]

Tumor Growth and Intraocular Spread

Uveal melanomas appear to develop through a multistep process. Among the changes that result are alterations in membrane receptors, enzymes, cytokines, cytoskeleton components, cell cycle proteins, and nuclear antigens.[18] These changes enable the melanoma cells to acquire self-sufficient growth signals, sensitivity to antigrowth signals, evasion of apoptosis, unlimited replication potential, sustained angiogenesis, tissue invasion, and metastasis.[19] In rapidly growing tumors, a high mitotic activity and the presence of epithelioid cells have been documented.[20]

From a clinical and histopathologic standpoint, small melanomas grow from a discoid to a hemispheric shape. They progressively obliterate the choriocapillaris and displace Bruch's membrane and the retina inward. When Bruch's membrane is disrupted, the tumor usually grows in the subretinal space in a mushroomlike configuration. The retinal pigment epithelium overlying the tumors undergoes early changes called *tumor-associated retinal pigment epitheliopathy*, which includes drusen formation and orange pigment (lipofuscin) accumulation. The neurosensory retina is frequently detached and, in some cases, infiltrated by tumor cells, which can seed into the vitreous. Anterior tumors are more likely to indent the lens and cause cataract. A secondary glaucoma may result from obstruction of the outflow pathways by tumor cells, cell debris, and phagocytic cells swollen with ingested cell debris. Scleral infiltration by tumor cells along ciliary vessels and nerves and along the vortex veins are frequent. Approximately 5% of melanomas grow diffusely in the plane of the uvea or circumferentially along the root of the iris. They induce a slight thickening of the uvea (3 to 5 mm) and are often unsuspected or diagnosed late when secondary glaucoma or extraocular spread occurs.

TABLE 140.1

DESIGNATION OF THE CELL TYPE BASED ON THE ARMED FORCES INSTITUTE OF PATHOLOGY MODIFICATION OF THE CALLENDER CLASSIFICATION

Callender Cell Type	Cell Size and Description	Cytoplasm	Nucleus	Nucleolus	Other
Spindle A	Elongated spindle or small and round, depending on plane of section; cell membrane not distinct; may appear more distinct in cross-section	Usually sparse but may be relatively abundant	Elongated, fine chromatin pattern; chromatin line characteristic but not necessary for diagnosis; plumper than in nevus cells	Indistinct or none	Cohesive; mitoses extremely rare
Spindle B	Plumper spindle or round, depending on plane of section; cell membrane not typically distinct (syncytial) but may be identified in cross-section	Relatively sparse	Larger, plumper than spindle A; coarser chromatin pattern; chromatin clumping	Sharper definition; deeply stained, small, and round; often eccentric	Less cohesive than spindle A; may form fascicular arrangements; occasional mitoses
Epithelioid	Larger, more pleomorphic, often polygonal; distinct cell border	Abundant; may be eosinophilic	Largest, round; pleomorphic; chromatin margination, often marked; can be multinucleated	Largest, may be multiple; eosinophilic; usually central; distinct	Loss of cohesiveness; cells possibly separated easily in sectioning; more mitoses

From ref. 15, with permission.

Extrascleral Extension

Extrascleral extension is more common in large tumors, with approximately 15% of ocular melanomas demonstrating extrascleral extension. Other less common paths of extraocular spread include the optic nerve and the lumen of vortex veins.[21]

Metastasis

Metastasis occurs in 31% of patients in 5 years, 45% of patients in 15 years, and almost 50% of patients in 25 years.[22,23] In the COMS, the liver was the most common site (89% in patients with metastasis); the death rate following the report of melanoma metastasis was 80% at 1 year and 92% at 2 years.[24]

Histopathology of Radiation-Treated Globes

The aim of treatment is to kill all tumor cells or to render them incapable of sustained proliferation. It is thought that this can be achieved through direct tumor necrosis or hypoxia secondary to blood supply damage. Unfortunately, histopathologic analysis of eyes enucleated for radiation-induced complications or poor tumor control may not reflect the radiation response of most treated cases.[25] In the COMS, pre-enucleation radiation significantly reduced, but did not eliminate, mitotic activity.[15] In successfully treated tumors, mitotic figures persist only for the first 30 months after treatment. Not surprisingly, tumor regrowth is correlated with significant mitotic activity. Good tumor response is linked with fewer mitotic figures and tumor and blood vessel damage. Other significant features of irradiated tumors include necrosis, fibrosis, and balloon cell formation. Recent histopathologic studies of the microvascular loops and networks in irradiated melanomas show that these structures are less common in tumors enucleated after irradiation.[26]

DIAGNOSIS

Clinical Examination

The diagnosis of choroidal and ciliary body melanomas has reached a high degree of accuracy (99.7%) among experienced clinicians and with modern ancillary testing facilities.[27] In a review of 12,000 patients referred because of a lesion believed to be a posterior uveal melanoma, Shields et al.[28] found that 1,739 (14%) had simulating conditions, 49% of which were choroidal nevi. In distinguishing choroidal melanomas from choroidal nevi, Shields et al.[29] suggest a thickness of greater than 2 mm, subretinal fluid, orange pigment, and a margin touching the optic disc are all critical indicators of a choroidal melanoma (Fig. 140.1*A*).

Ultrasonography

The combined use of A- and B-mode ultrasonographic techniques is of great value in confirming the clinical diagnosis of choroidal melanoma, especially in the presence of opaque media. The A-scan mode typically reveals a solid tumor with low to medium internal reflectivity (Fig. 140.1*B*). The B-mode ultrasonographic characteristics useful in differentiating melanomas from metastases or hemangiomas are acoustic hollowness, choroidal excavation, and orbital shadowing (Fig. 140.1C).[30,31] Small tumors elevated less than 2 to 3 mm cannot be evaluated accurately. In larger tumors, ultrasonography provides valuable size data for serial measurements and is an important follow-up tool after conservative treatment.

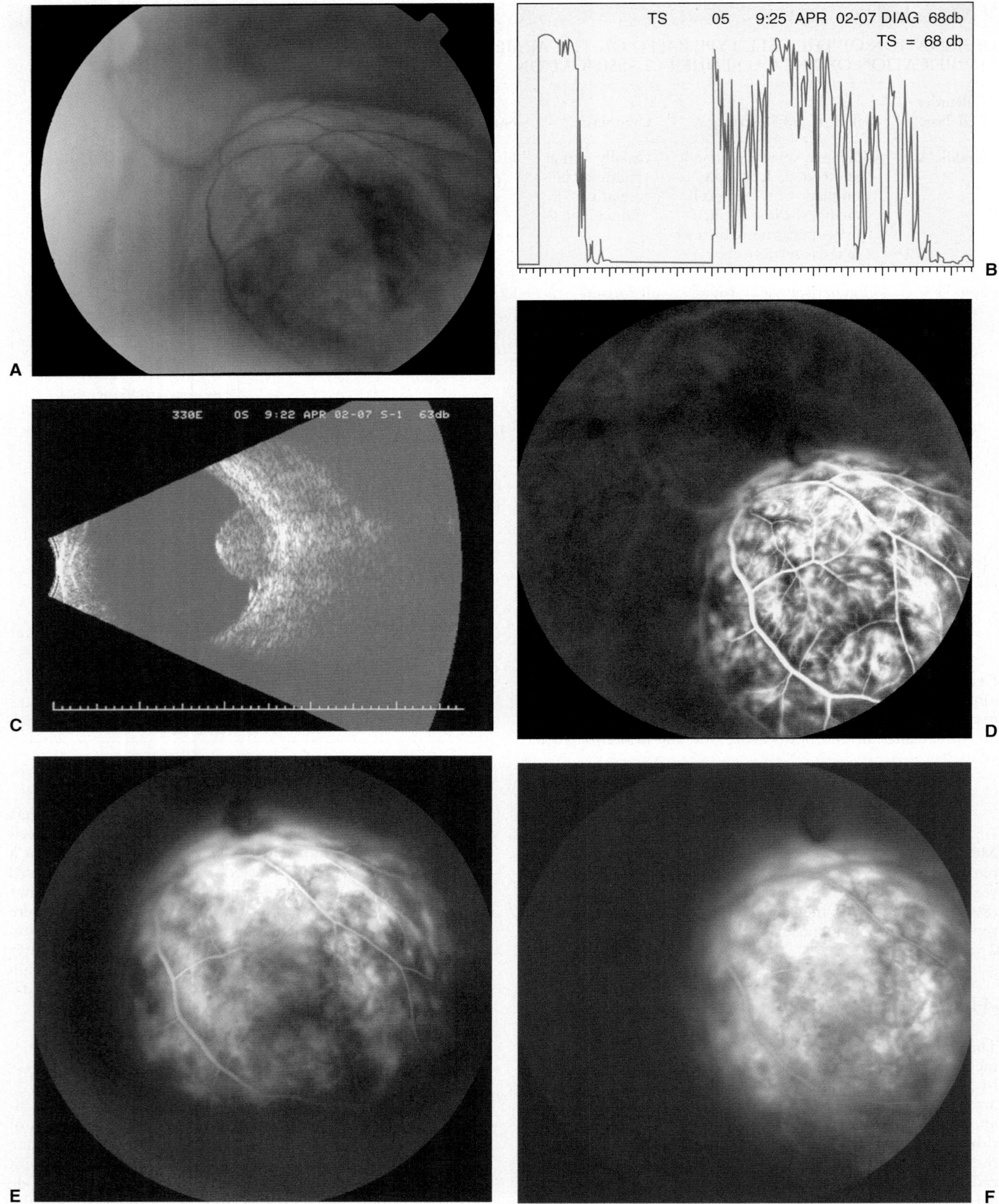

FIGURE 140.1 Choroidal melanoma. **A:** Fundus photograph of a large choroidal melanoma. **B:** A-scan ultrasonography with medium internal reflectivity. **C:** B-scan ultrasonogram of a choroidal melanoma with secondary retinal detachment. **D–F:** Fluorescein angiography showing dual circulation in early phases and mild hyperfluorescence due to leakage in late phases. (Courtesy of Suresh Chandra, M.D.)

Photography

Fluorescein angiography and monochromatic photography have proved useful in differentiating subretinal or choroidal hemorrhage and hemangioma from melanoma (Fig. 140.1*D–F*). Although no angiographic pattern is pathognomonic, features supporting melanoma include early mottling fluorescence, orange pigment over the margin of the tumor, progressive fluorescence of the lesion with late staining, and multiple pinpoint leaks that increase in size. Breaks in Bruch's membrane and retinal invasion can be detected from abnormalities such as a double circulation pattern (i.e., simultaneous visualization of retinal and choroidal circulation). Indocyanine green video angiography with high-resolution fundus digital imaging systems can be helpful in further differentiating amelanotic choroidal tumors (nevi or melanomas) from hemangiomas or metastases to the uvea.[32] This method has been also used to image microvascular patterns.[33]

Fine-Needle Aspiration Biopsy with Adjunct Studies

In choroidal tumors, which present a dilemma for conventional diagnostic procedures, fine-needle aspiration biopsy may be helpful. Some ocular oncologists recommend biopsies and cytogenetic studies prior to enucleation, radiation, or other treatment to obtain information about the aggressiveness of the tumor and risk of metastasis.[34] The routine use of biopsies, however, is controversial.[35,36]

Other Diagnostic Tools

Ocular coherence tomography can be helpful in the differential diagnosis of small choroidal lesions, particularly in distinguishing choroidal nevi from melanomas.[37] Magnetic resonance imaging (MRI) can provide contrast enhancement of intraocular lesions, which may be useful for indicating the degree of malignancy and for monitoring response to treatment.[38] Three-dimensional MRI can provide a high degree of accuracy for tumor volumes, as well as shape and tumor base.[39]

METASTATIC WORKUP

Patients with suspected intraocular melanoma should undergo a physical examination and metastatic workup. Clinical laboratory studies should include routine blood examination and liver function tests. Liver ultrasonography or tomography, chest radiography, and computed tomography (CT) of the head are useful in the initial workup and surveillance. The COMS study indicates that liver function test results, followed by diagnostic tests, have high specificity and predictive values but low sensitivity.[40] Although ocular oncologists in North America rely mainly on liver function tests and chest x-rays to screen for metastatic uveal melanoma, most European centers use liver ultrasonography at initial diagnosis of the primary tumor and continue to do so every 6 months.

Whole-body positron emission tomography/computed tomography imaging can be a sensitive tool for the detection and location of hepatic and extrahepatic metastatic melanoma.[41] The use of real-time reverse transcription-polymerase chain reaction to detect melanoma cells in the peripheral blood is currently under evaluation in several prospective randomized trials.[42] The presence of tyrosinase or *MelanA/MART1* transcripts have been reported to be an independent prognostic factor for the development of metastases.[43]

TABLE 140.2

CLASSIFICATION OF TUMOR SIZE ACCORDING TO BOUNDARY LINES

Type	Apical Height	Largest Basal Diameter
Small	1.0–2.5 mm	5 mm
Medium	2.5–10.0 mm	5–16 mm
Large	>10 mm	>16 mm

Adapted from ref. 44.

STAGING

For staging, tumor size classification that takes into account tumor thickness and basal diameter is currently in use in most centers and in the COMS (Table 140.2).[44] The current TNM (tumor, node, metastasis) staging by the American Joint Committee on Cancer draws somewhat different boundary lines for small, medium, and large tumors.[45] Hence, the COMS classification is probably more useful because it carries with it the results of the large randomized clinical studies.

MANAGEMENT

The therapy selected for choroidal melanoma currently depends on a number of factors, including patient age, tumor size and location, general health, and status of the fellow eye.

Small Choroidal Melanoma

In the management of suspected small choroidal melanomas, the key and very controversial issue is whether or not to treat immediately for clinical signs associated with presumptive malignant transformation before instituting definitive therapy. Curtin[46] advocated observational management until clinical signs of malignant transformation were seen. Shields,[47] however, argues for treatment of selected small choroidal melanomas that possess risk factors. There is general agreement that each case should be individualized. The therapies used to treat small choroidal melanoma include laser photocoagulation and transpupillary thermal therapy (TTT). Cryotherapy in combination with TTT may be also used. Plaque radiotherapy can also be customized to treat small uveal melanomas.[48]

Laser Photocoagulation Therapy

Xenon arc photocoagulation was initially used for the treatment of uveal melanoma by Meyer-Schwickerath in 1952.[49] It was subsequently replaced by argon laser photocoagulation, which showed fewer complications but less tumor control. Limitation of tissue penetration and the need for multiple treatment sessions are drawbacks. Laser therapy has been largely replaced by transpupillary thermal therapy, although it is still used on rare occasions.[50]

Transpupillary Thermal Therapy

TTT uses infrared light (diode laser, 810 mm) delivered as heat to induce necrosis in tumor tissues. In a consecutive series of 256 patients treated initially with TTT (mean of three treatments), Shields et al.[51] estimated tumor recurrence in 10% of cases at 3 years, with visual acuity worse than 20/200 in 32%. The addition of indocyanine green does not appear to enhance the efficacy of TTT. The tumors most suitable for TTT are

TABLE 140.3

CLINICAL OUTCOMES FROM THREE DIFFERENT RADIOTHERAPY TECHNIQUES

Treatment (Ref.)	Local Control (%)	Enucleation (%)	5-Year Overall Survival (%)	Distant Metastasis Rate (%)	Visual Acuity 20/200 or Better (%)
Proton beam (65)	95	10	80	16	49
Helium ion beam (62)	95	22	80	24	36
Plaque therapy (60,66–69)	82–94	6–17	83–87	5–22	44

small, heavily pigmented melanomas less than 3 mm thick with minimal or no subretinal fluid, located in the extramacular region but not touching the optic disc. Because of delayed recurrence and extrascleral extension, choroidal melanomas treated with TTT require long-term follow-up. TTT can also be used as a supplement to plaque radiotherapy.[52]

Medium-Sized Choroidal Melanoma

During the past decade, the century-old practice of enucleation has been largely replaced by plaque radiotherapy in the treatment of medium-sized choroidal melanomas due to the COMS findings that these two mechanisms result in equivalent survival.[53–57] Charged-particle radiotherapy and local resection continue to be used and reported on. Local sclerochorioretinal resection techniques for choroidal melanomas are designed to preserve vision and maintain a cosmetically normal-appearing eye.[58,59] Reports indicate, however, a relatively high rate of early complications. Most patients treated by local resection are also amenable to radiation therapy, and local resection has not been widely adopted.

Radiation Therapy

Radiotherapy is presently the most widely used treatment for medium-sized posterior uveal melanoma. Successful local control has been reported with a variety of radiotherapeutic modalities, including brachytherapy (plaque) techniques; external-beam radiation using photons or charged particles (protons and helium ions); and stereotactic radiosurgery with modified linear accelerators and multisource cobalt units.[60–64] The techniques with the most widely reported clinical experience to date are plaque therapy and charged-particle beam therapy. A comparison of clinical outcomes for these latter techniques is given in Table 140.3.

Episcleral Plaque Radiation Therapy

A concave plaque is constructed to house several small radioactive sources (or seeds) based on preoperative tumor measurements. This requires integration of data from clinical examination, ultrasonography, and occasionally CT or MRI scan. The custom-designed plaque is temporarily sutured to the sclera overlying the tumor, usually under retrobulbar or general anesthesia. Operative localization of the plaque placement is guided by transillumination, ophthalmoscopic observation, or ultrasonography. The plaque remains in place for 2 to 5 days, depending on the type and activity of the radioactive source, and it is then removed under similar operative conditions.

Iodine 125 (^{125}I) is the most commonly used radioisotope in the United States and was the only isotope permitted in the COMS trial. Ruthenium 106 (^{106}Ru) is frequently used in Europe; other isotopes include cobalt 60 (^{60}Co) and palladium 103 (^{103}Pd). Isotopes with lower photon and electron radiation (^{125}I, ^{106}Ru, ^{103}Pd) are more easily shielded to reduce the exposure to adjacent normal tissues in the patient, with a concomitant reduction in exposure risk to medical personnel. The choice of radioisotope has historically been based on availability, institutional experience, and physician preference. The radioisotope ^{103}Pd has dosimetric advantages based on its lower photon energy as compared to ^{125}I. Clinical trials of ^{103}Pd have been favorable.[60] A nonrandomized comparison of ^{125}I and ^{106}Ru plaques, however, showed better tumor control with the ^{125}I.[61]

The COMS group has published 12-year results of a landmark randomized trial comparing enucleation to ^{125}I plaque radiotherapy for medium-sized melanoma (Table 140.4).[57] It consisted of 1,317 patients from 43 centers in the United States and Canada randomly assigned to enucleation (660 patients) or ^{125}I plaque brachytherapy (657 patients). At 12 years, 471 of 1,317 enrolled patients had died. Of 515 patients evaluated at 12-year follow-up, 231 (45%) were alive and clinically cancer free. The 12-year all-cause mortality rate was 43% in the ^{125}I

TABLE 140.4

COLLABORATIVE ONCOLOGY MELANOMA STUDY GROUP RANDOMIZED TRIAL DATA FOR MEDIUM-SIZED MELANOMA: IODINE 125 PLAQUE BRACHYTHERAPY VERSUS ENUCLEATION

	Iodine 125 Plaque Brachytherapy	Enucleation
Eyes treated	657	660
Follow-up (y)	Minimum = 2; 81% of patients = 5; 32% of patients = 10	Minimum = 2; 81% of patients = 5; 32% of patients = 10
Enucleation	13%[a]	100%
Local control at 5 y	90%	100%
Visual acuity better than 20/200 (treated eye, at 3 y)	57%	0%
Overall survival	5 y = 82%	5 y = 81%
Death with metastatic disease	5 y = 9%	5 y = 11%

[a]Includes enucleations for plaque treatment failure and complications.
(Data from refs. 53–55.)

brachytherapy arm and 41% among those in the enucleation arm. Five-, 10-, and 12-year rates of death with histopathologically confirmed melanoma metastasis were 10%, 18%, and 21%, respectively, in the ^{125}I brachytherapy arm and 11%, 17%, and 17%, respectively, in the enucleation arm. No clinically or statistically significant difference was found in any survival- or melanoma-specific end point.

Charged-Particle Beam Therapy

Charged-particle beams (protons or helium ions) produced by a cyclotron or synchrotron are available at relatively few sites around the world. Charged-particle beams have specific dosimetric advantages in the delivery of a high dose of radiation to very precisely localized targets. A retrospective review of 218 patients treated with helium ion irradiation, with a minimum follow-up period of 10 years, demonstrated 95% local control.[62] Twenty-two percent of patients required enucleation, most often for anterior segment complications rather than tumor recurrence. The 10-year overall survival was 53%, with half of the deaths from metastatic melanoma. Significant impairment of visual acuity was noted for tumors 6 mm thick or greater and located within 3 mm of the optic nerve and fovea.

Randomized studies comparing proton beam therapy and enucleation have not been reported, and retrospective comparisons are difficult because of the need to balance the known prognostic factors between the treatment groups. A large single-institution retrospective comparison of proton beam–treated patients with those undergoing enucleation showed no apparent difference in long-term survival: an update on 1,922 patients with a median follow-up of 5.2 years showed 5- and 10-year local failure rates of 3.2% and 4.3%, respectively, following proton beam treatment. Approximately half of the failures were marginal, suggesting possible treatment planning or delivery errors.[63] In general, it appears that tumor control with charged-particle and plaque radiotherapy, as well as radiation complications, is similar.

More recent radiotherapy techniques have been suggested and include Gamma Knife (Elekta Corp, Stockholm) radiosurgery, linear accelerator–based radiosurgery, and the robot-controlled linear-accelerator radiosurgery CyberKnife (Accuray, Sunnyvale, California). But currently there are insufficient data for comparison with plaque or charged-particle beam therapy.[64]

Large Choroidal Melanoma

Enucleation is generally reserved now for advanced melanomas greater than 15 mm in diameter and more than 10 mm thick. It is also employed with resection of a long portion of optic nerve in cases where there is optic nerve invasion. Plaque radiotherapy can also be customized to treat large uveal melanomas. Patients with large tumors or with tumors at peripapillary and macular locations have a poorer visual outcome and lower local control that must be taken into account in the patient decision-making process.

Orbital Exenteration

Although in past years orbital exenteration was often done in cases of extrascleral extension, it now appears that it does not improve survival for patients with mild to moderate extrascleral extension. In cases of massive orbital extension occurring with a blind, painful eye, primary orbital exenteration appears justified.[70]

Pre-Enucleation External Beam Radiation

Radiotherapy of eyes with uveal melanoma prior to enucleation (pre-enucleation radiotherapy) was thought to possibly reduce enucleation-induced systemic metastasis. As part of the COMS, approximately 1,000 patients with large uveal melanomas were randomized into one of two groups, either receiving or not receiving external-beam radiation prior to enucleation.[7] Results indicated no survival advantage attributable to pre-enucleation radiation (Table 140.5).[71]

Management of Patients with Metastatic Disease

Uveal melanoma has a unique metastatic predilection for the liver (Fig. 140.2). According to various reports, the liver is involved in 71% to 94% of uveal melanoma patients with metastases and is the sole or initial site of metastases in more than 50% of these patients.[73] Hepatic metastases are recognized as a poor prognostic marker for response to treatment and survival. The overall 1-year survival after the development of metastasis is only 13%, and median survival estimates range from 2 to 9 months.[73] Surgical resection of liver metastases is not widely practiced because such surgery is considered a local therapy and of little value in the management of disseminated disease.[74] Systemic chemotherapy has been ineffective, with response rates reported to be 1% or less in most series, and cytokine therapy with interleukin-2 and interferon-γ have been similarly ineffective.[73] A variety of regional treatment modalities, such as hepatic arterial chemotherapy, hepatic artery chemoembolization, regional immunotherapy, isolated

TABLE 140.5

COLLABORATIVE OCULAR MELANOMA STUDY GROUP RANDOMIZED TRIAL OF PRE-ENUCLEATION RADIOTHERAPY FOR LARGE CHOROIDAL MELANOMAS

	Enucleation Alone	Pre-Enucleation Radiation Therapy	Statistic
Patients randomized (n)	506	497	—
Acute complications	4%	8%	$P = .03$
Severe ptosis	10%	5%	$P = .007$
Orbital recurrence	5 patients	None	$P = .03$
5-y overall survival	57% (CI, 52%–62%)[a]	62% (CI, 57%–66%)[a]	—
Death from metastatic melanoma (at 5 y)	26%	28%	—

[a]CI = 95% confidence interval.
(From ref. 72, with permission.)

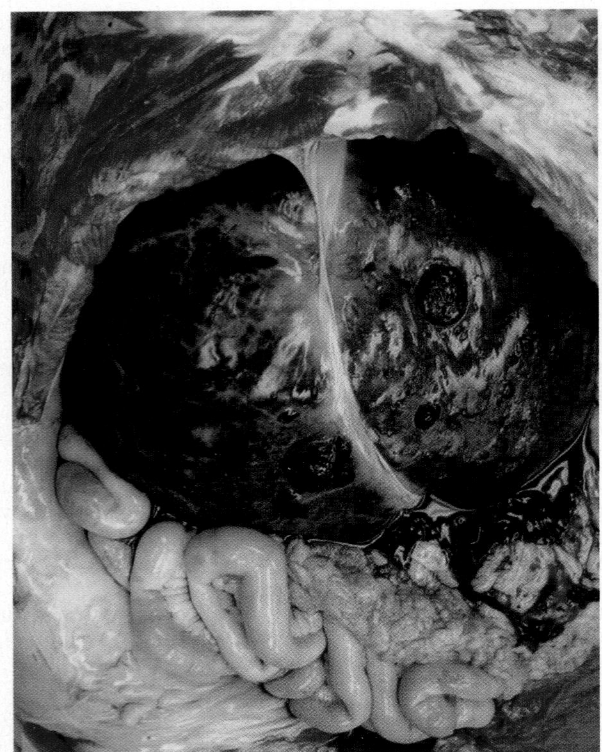

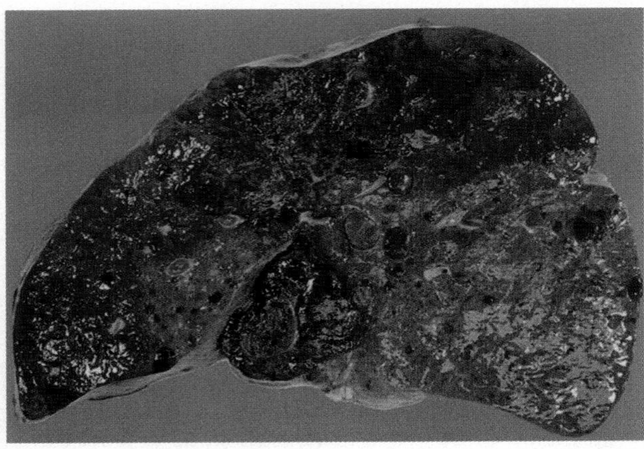

FIGURE 140.2 Metastatic choroidal melanoma to the liver. **A:** At autopsy, the liver weighed 4,500 g and was infiltrated with melanoma. **B:** Liver cross-section revealed complete loss of normal parenchyma, large (greater than 10 cm) metastasis and portal vein thrombosis. (Courtesy of David H. Abramson, M.D.)

hepatic perfusion, and percutaneous hepatic perfusion, are being used to control tumor progression in the liver.[75] These treatments are dealt with in detail in Chapters 64 and 149. Chemotherapeutic agents used to date include cisplatin, fotemustine, bleomycin, vincristine, lomustine, dacarbazine, melphalan, bendamustine, gemcitabine, and treosulfan. Most reports show at best a modest response rate, suggesting that selected patients with uveal melanoma may occasionally benefit from aggressive treatment. Kodjikian et al.[76] suggest that the two independent, favorable prognostic factors are (1) fewer than ten metastases at screening and (2) the absence of ciliary body involvement.

PROGNOSTIC AND PREDICTIVE FACTORS

Prognostic information is useful in predicting patient outcomes and offers potential for allowing patient stratification and recognition of sensitivity of tumors to new treatments.[77,78] However, the utility of prognostic information in uveal melanoma is limited because of the lack of effective treatment to prevent or delay metastasis, as well as the absence of effective treatment for metastatic disease itself.

Clinical Prognostic Factors

Anatomic Site

Iris melanomas have a ten times lower mortality rate than ciliary body and choroidal melanomas, with metastases developing in 5 years from iris lesions in approximately 3%. Most tumors that involve the ciliary body are thought to arise in the anterior choroid and secondarily invade the ciliary body. Tumors actually arising in the ciliary body are aggressive and have a 5-year mortality of 53%, compared with 14% for choroidal-based melanomas.[79] Invasion of the optic nerve carries with it a significantly higher all-cause and melanoma-related mortality than in other patients.[80] If a tumor extends outside the eye, the 10-year mortality rate is 75%.[79]

Tumor Size

Tumor size is an extremely useful prognostic factor because tumor measurements are available at the time of diagnosis. Large basal diameter is believed to be an important predictor of outcome. Diener-West et al.,[81] using selected data published from 1966 to 1988, performed a meta-analysis of 5-year mortality among enucleated patients, providing weighed estimates of 5-year mortality after enucleation: 16% for small tumors, 32% for medium-sized tumors, and 53% for large tumors.

Tumor Growth Pattern

Most choroidal melanomas have a dome-shaped or collar-button shape, but, as noted above, about 5% of posterior uveal melanomas grow in a diffuse pattern. Twenty-four percent of patients with diffuse melanoma have metastases at 5 years and 36% at 10 years.[82] Ring melanomas, which grow circumferentially along the trabecular meshwork and adjacent anterior angle structures, represent less than 0.2% of melanomas.[83] Demirici et al.[83] reported that distant metastases occurred in 25% at a mean follow-up of 6 years.

Postbrachytherapy Tumor Regression Rate

A recent study found that the risk of liver metastases correlated with the postbrachytherapy initial tumor regression rate.[84] The initial height regression rate was 6.1% per month in patients who later developed metastasis, as opposed to 4.3% per month in those who did not.

Histopathological Prognostic Factors

Cell Type

Cell type, as determined by the Callender classification, is predictive of outcome.[85] Paul et al.[86] reviewed 2,652 cases accessioned at the Armed Forces Institute of Pathology by 1959 and found that 95% of patients with spindle A tumors, 85% of those with spindle B tumors, 60% of those with mixed tumors, and 83% with epithelioid tumors were alive 5 years after enucleation. At 15 years after enucleation, the survival rates were 85% for spindle A, 80% for spindle B, 46% for mixed, and 34% for epithelioid. In the series by Jensen and Prause,[87] of 302 patients reported from Denmark who had been observed for 25 years, 150 (50%) died of metastatic melanoma. Less than 1% of patients with spindle A tumors died of metastatic disease; 63% with mixed tumors and 71% with epithelioid tumors died from metastatic melanoma.

Microvascular Patterns

As noted above, Folberg and Maniotis[16] have extensively studied the morphological characteristics of intratumoral vascular patterns in primary uveal melanomas. The presence of microvascular networks, defined as at least three back-to-back closed loops, is a feature strongly associated with the development of metastatic disease.

Tumor-Infiltrating Lymphocytes and Macrophages

Approximately 5% to 12% of uveal melanomas contain lymphocytes, and these are thought to represent an important component of the host's immune response to the tumor. In several studies, both T- and B-lymphocyte infiltration were associated with higher mortality.[78] In addition, tumor-infiltrating macrophages (CD68+ cells) are an independent prognostic factor with regard to survival.[88]

Cytogenetic and Molecular Prognostic Factors

A frequent and striking anomaly in uveal melanoma is the loss of an entire copy of chromosome 3.[89,90] Uveal melanomas characterized by monosomy 3 are associated with greater tumor size, ciliary body involvement, the presence of epithelioid cells, and closed loop vasculogenic mimicry.[89] These features denote aggressive tumor behavior and a poor prognosis for survival.[89] Conversely, metastasis in the absence of monosomy 3 is rare. However, partial deletions (long arm, short arm, or both) or isodisomy 3 may behave as functional equivalents to monosomy 3. Although long-term survival with monosomy 3 is probably rare, there is no significant difference in time until death between metastatic melanomas with and without monosomy 3.[91] Also important in uveal melanomas are abnormalities involving chromosomes 8, 6, 9, and 1.[89]

Recent studies of genetic pathways and global gene expression changes have provided insight into the molecular pathogenesis of uveal melanoma. Rb protein is expressed in virtually all melanomas, indicating a lack of *Rb* gene mutation.[92] In melanomas analyzed for microarray gene expression and comparative genomic hybridization, gain of chromosome 8q correlated strongly with expression of *DDEF1*, a gene located at 8q24. The authors concluded that *DDEF1* overexpression may be a pathogenetically relevant consequence of chromosome 8a amplification, commonly associated with aggressive uveal melanomas.[93] They concluded that *DDEF1* may act as an oncogene in uveal melanoma, and it may be a useful diagnostic marker. Also, it was found that expression of the Nijmegen breakage syndrome (*NBS1*) gene was a strong predictor of uveal melanoma survival.[94] Thus, several cytogenetic or chromosomal abnormalities, including loss of 1p, loss of chromosome 3 (monosomy 3), gain of 6p, loss of 6q, loss of 8p, and gain of 8q, have been linked to metastatic death in uveal melanoma. Among these markers, monosomy 3 seems to be the most significant predictor of metastatic risk.[95]

POSTTREATMENT QUALITY OF LIFE

The COMS group interviewed 209 patients enrolled in the COMS medium-sized tumor study, using several survey instruments plus additional questions about satisfaction with posttreatment appearance and concerns about cancer recurrence.[96] Patients who had brachytherapy reported significantly better visual function than patients who were treated with enucleation, with respect to driving and peripheral vision, for up to 2 years following treatment. Differences between treatments and visual function diminished by 3 to 5 years posttherapy, paralleling a decline in visual acuity in brachytherapy-treated eyes. Patients with brachytherapy were found to be more likely to have symptoms of anxiety during follow-up than patients treated with enucleation.[97] Since survival is equivalent between enucleation and radiotherapy, differences demonstrated in quality of life studies allow the patient and physician to make informed choices about treatment based on personal preferences.

Selected References

The full list of references for this chapter appears in the online version.

1. Singh AD, Bergman L, Seregard S. Uveal melanoma: epidemiological aspects. *Ophthalmol Clin North Am* 2005;18:75.
5. Starr OD, Patel DV, Allen JP, et al. Iris melanoma: pathology, prognosis and surgical intervention. *Clin Experiment Ophthalmol* 2004;32:294.
7. Collaborative Ocular Melanoma Study Group. The Collaborative Ocular Melanoma Study (COMS) randomized trial of pre-enucleation radiation of large choroidal melanoma. II: initial mortality findings. COMS report no. 10. *Am J Ophthalmol* 1998;125:779.
9. Harbour JW, Brantley MA, Hollingsworth H, et al. Association between choroidal pigmentation and posterior uveal melanoma in a white population. *Br J Ophthalmol* 2004;88:39.
10. Singh AD, Rennie IG, Seregard S, et al. Sunlight exposure and pathogenesis of uveal melanoma. *Surv Ophthalmol* 2004;49:419.
14. McLean IW, Foster WD, Zimmerman LE. Modifications of Callender's classification of uveal melanoma at the Armed Forces Institute of Pathology. *Am J Ophthalmol* 1983;96:502.
15. Collaborative Ocular Melanoma Study Group. Histopathologic characteristics of uveal melanomas in eyes enucleated from the Collaborative Ocular Melanoma Study: COMS report no. 6. *Am J Ophthalmol* 1998; 125:745.
16. Folberg R, Maniotis AJ. Vasculogenic mimicry. *APMIS* 2004;112:508.
17. Kivela T, Makitie T, Al-Jamal RT, et al. Microvascular loops and networks in uveal melanoma. *Can J Ophthalmol* 2004;39:409.
18. Saraiva VS, Edelstein C, Burnier MNJ. New prognostic factors in uveal melanomas: potential molecular targets for therapy. *Can J Ophthalmol* 2004;39:422.
20. Char DH, Kroll S, Phillips TL. Uveal melanoma. Growth rate and prognosis. *Arch Ophthalmol* 1997;115(8):1014.
23. Singh AD, Borden EC. Metastatic uveal melanoma. *Ophthalmol Clin North Am* 2005;18:143.
24. Diener-West M, Reynolds SM, Agugliaro DJ, et al. Collaborative Ocular Melanoma Study Group. Development of metastatic disease after enrollment in the COMS trials for treatment of choroidal melanoma: COMS report no. 26. *Arch Ophthalmol* 2005;123:1639.

25. Avery RB, Diener-West M, Reynolds SM, et al. Histopathologic characteristics of choroidal melanoma in eyes enucleated after iodine 125 brachytherapy in the collaborative ocular melanoma study. *Arch Ophthalmol* 2008;126(2):207.
26. Toivonen P, Mäkitie T, Kujala E, et al. Macrophages and microcirculation in regressed and partially regressed irradiated choroidal and ciliary body melanomas. *Curr Eye Res* 2003;27(4):237.
27. Collaborative Ocular Melanoma Study Group. Accuracy of diagnosis of choroidal melanoma in the Collaborative Ocular Melanoma Study. COMS report no. 1. *Arch Ophthalmol* 1990;108:1268.
29. Shields CL, Demirci H, Materin MA, et al. Clinical factors in the identification of small choroidal melanoma. *Can J Ophthalmol* 2004;39:351.
31. Collaborative Ocular Melanoma Study Group. Comparison of clinical, echographic, and histopathological measurements from eyes with medium-sized choroidal melanomas in the Collaborative Ocular Melanoma Study: COMS report no. 21. *Arch Ophthalmol* 2003;121:1163.
33. Mueller AJ, Bartsch DU, Folberg R, et al. Imaging the microvasculature of choroidal melanoma with confocal indocyanine green scanning laser ophthalmoscopy. *Arch Ophthalmol* 1998;116:31.
34. Faulkner-Jones BE, Foster WD, Harbour JW, et al. Fine needle aspiration biopsy with adjunct immunohistochemistry in intraocular tumor management. *Acta Cytol* 2005;49:297.
35. Kvanta A, Seregard S, Kopp ED, et al. Choroidal biopsies for intraocular tumors of indeterminate origin. *Am J Ophthalmol* 2005;140:1002.
40. Diener-West M, Reynolds SM, Agugliaro DJ, et al. Collaborative Ocular Melanoma Study Group. Screening for metastasis from choroidal melanoma: the Collaborative Ocular Melanoma Study Group: report no. 23. *J Clin Oncol* 2004;22:2438.
41. Kurli M, Reddy S, Tena LB, et al. Whole body positron emission tomography/computed tomography staging of metastatic choroidal melanoma. *Am J Ophthalmol* 2005;140:193.
43. Schuster R, Bechrakis NE, Stroux A, et al. Circulating tumor cells as prognostic factor for distant metastases and survival in patients with primary uveal melanoma. *Clin Cancer Res* 2007;13:1171.
44. Mortality in patients with small choroidal melanoma. COMS report no. 4. The Collaborative Ocular Melanoma Study Group. *Arch Ophthalmol* 1997;115:886.
45. Malignant melanoma of the uvea staging form. In: *AJCC cancer staging manual*. 7th ed. New York: Springer, 2010:555.
47. Shields JA. Treating some small melanocytic choroidal lesions without waiting for growth. *Arch Ophthalmol* 2006;124:1344.
50. Shields CL, Shields JA. Recent developments in the management of choroidal melanoma. *Curr Opin Ophthalmol* 2004;15:244.
51. Shields CL, Shields JA, Perez N, et al. Primary transpupillary thermotherapy for small choroidal melanoma in 256 consecutive cases: outcomes and limitations. *Ophthalmology* 2002;109:225.
52. Shields CL, Cater J, Shields JA, et al. Combined plaque radiotherapy and transpupillary thermotherapy for choroidal melanoma: tumor control and treatment complications in 270 consecutive patients. *Arch Ophthalmol* 2002;120:933.
53. Diener-West M, Earle J, Fine SL, et al. The COMS randomized trial of iodine 125 brachytherapy for choroidal melanoma. III: initial mortality findings. COMS report no. 18. *Arch Ophthalmol* 2001;119:969.
54. Melia M, Abramson DH, Albert DM, et al. Collaborative ocular melanoma study (COMS) randomized trial of I-125 brachytherapy for medium choroidal melanoma. I. Visual acuity after 3 years COMS report no. 16. *Ophthalmology* 2001;108:348.
55. Jampol LM, Moy CS, Murray TG, et al. The COMS randomized trial of iodine 125 brachytherapy for choroidal melanoma: IV. Local treatment failure and enucleation in the first 5 years after brachytherapy. COMS report no. 19. *Ophthalmology* 2002;109:2197.
57. Collaborative Ocular Melanoma Study Group. The COMS randomized trial of iodine 125 brachytherapy for choroidal melanoma: V. Twelve-year mortality rates and prognostic factors: COMS report no. 28. *Arch Ophthalmol* 2006;124:1684.
60. Finger PT, Berson A, Ng T, Szechter A. Palladium-103 plaque radiotherapy for choroidal melanoma: an 11-year study. *Int J Radiat Oncol Biol Phys* 2002;54:1438.
62. Char DH, Kroll SM, Castro J. Ten-year follow-up of helium ion therapy for uveal melanoma. *Am J Ophthalmol* 1998;125:81.
63. Gragoudas ES, Lane AM, Munzenrider J, et al. Long-term risk of local failure after proton therapy for choroidal/ciliary body melanoma. *Trans Am Ophthalmol Soc* 2002;100:43.
64. Daftari I, Petti PL, Shrieve DC, Phillips TL. Newer radiation modalities for choroidal tumors. *Int Ophthalmol Clin* 2006;46:69.
71. Hawkins BS, Collaborative Ocular Melanoma Study Group. The Collaborative Ocular Melanoma Study (COMS) randomized trial of pre-enucleation radiation of large choroidal melanoma: IV. Ten-year mortality findings and prognostic factors. COMS report no. 24. *Am J Ophthalmol* 2004;138:936.
72. Collaborative Ocular Melanoma Study Group. The Collaborative Ocular Melanoma Study (COMS) randomized trial of pre-enucleation radiation of large choroidal melanoma III: local complications and observations following enucleation. COMS report no. 11. *Am J Ophthalmol* 1998;126:362.
73. Agarwala SS, Panikkar R, Kirkwood JM. Phase I/II randomized trial of intrahepatic arterial infusion chemotherapy with cisplatin and chemoembolization with cisplatin and polyvinyl sponge in patients with ocular melanoma metastatic to the liver. *Melanoma Res* 2004;14:217.
77. Mudhar HS, Parsons MA, Sisley K, et al. A critical appraisal of the prognostic and predictive factors for uveal malignant melanoma. *Histopathology* 2004;45:1.
79. Seddon JM, Albert DM, Lavin PT, Robinson N. A prognostic factor study of disease-free interval and survival following enucleation for uveal melanoma. *Arch Ophthalmol* 1983;101:1894.
81. Diener-West M, Hawkins BS, Markowitz JA, Schachat AP. A review of mortality from choroidal melanoma. II: a meta-analysis of 5-year mortality rates following enucleation, 1966 through 1988. *Arch Ophthalmol* 1992;110:245.
86. Paul EV, Parnell BL, Fraker M. Prognosis of malignant melanomas of the choroid and ciliary body. *Int Ophthalmol Clin* 1968;5:387.
89. Singh AD, Damato B, Howard P, et al. Uveal melanoma: genetic aspects. *Ophthalmol Clin North Am* 2005;18:85.
90. Prescher G, Bornfeld N, Hirche H, et al. Prognostic implications of monosomy 3 in uveal melanoma. *Lancet* 1996;347:1222.
95. Harbour JW. Molecular prognostic testing and individualized patient care in uveal melanoma. *Am J Ophthalmol.* 2009;148:823.
96. Melia M, Moy CS, Reynolds SM, et al. Collaborative Ocular Melanoma Study—Quality of Life Study Group. Quality of life after iodine 125 brachytherapy vs enucleation for choroidal melanoma: 5-year results from the Collaborative Ocular Melanoma Study: COMS QOLS report no. 3. *Arch Ophthalmol* 2006;124:226.

SECTION 15: IMMUNOSUPPRESSION-RELATED MALIGNANCIES

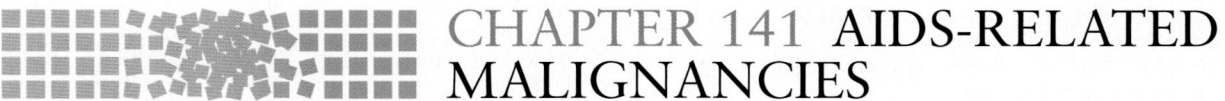

CHAPTER 141 AIDS-RELATED MALIGNANCIES

ROBERT YARCHOAN, THOMAS S. ULDRICK, AND RICHARD F. LITTLE

In 1981, the U.S. Centers for Disease Control (CDC) reported the first cases of Kaposi sarcoma (KS) and *Pneumocystis jiroveci* pneumonia (PCP) that heralded a pandemic now known as *acquired immune deficiency syndrome* (AIDS). AIDS was subsequently found to be caused by a novel retrovirus, *human immunodeficiency virus* (HIV). During the initial decade of the epidemic, patients often manifested KS or aggressive B-cell non-Hodgkin's lymphoma (NHL). Without therapy for HIV, they had an uncharacteristically high mortality. As the CDC formulated the initial definition of AIDS, KS in young men was AIDS-defining. Subsequently, the CDC definition evolved, and since 1993, three tumors have been considered AIDS-defining in the context of HIV: KS, certain NHL (Table 141.1), and invasive cervical cancer.[1]

With the development of nucleoside reverse transcriptase inhibitors in the 1980s[2] and protease inhibitors and nonnucleoside reverse transcript inhibitors in the 1990s, combination antiretroviral therapy (cART) involving three or more drugs became broadly available in 1996.[3] This approach leads to preserved CD4 lymphocyte counts, preserved immune function, decreased immune activation, decreased infectious complications, and decreased mortality,[4–8] transforming HIV infection into a manageable chronic disease. There are currently five classes of antiretroviral agents,[9] and various combinations can be individualized for control of HIV. During the Past 15 years, therapy for the major AIDS-associated cancers has also improved.[10]

The availability of cART has transformed cancer epidemiology in people with HIV. Although AIDS-defining tumors are still the most common cancers in people with HIV, incidence of KS and some NHL subtypes that occur at low CD4 counts has decreased. However, given the constant or increasing incidence of new HIV infections in the United States, and the decrease in deaths from AIDS since the introduction of cART, the number of persons living with HIV in the United States has increased by more than 50%. It is estimated that more than 1.1 million people in the United States are now infected with HIV.[11,12] With HIV-infected individuals living longer, the population at risk for malignant complications has increased and aged, and this pattern may continue into the future. In addition to AIDS-defining malignancies, HIV-infected patients are at increased risk of a number of other malignancies, including lung cancer, liver cancer, anal cancer, Hodgkin's lymphoma (HL), certain head and neck cancers, and Merkel cell carcinoma. Interestingly, other common cancers such as breast or colon cancer are not more frequent in HIV-infected patients, but the burden of these cancers is increasing as the HIV-infected population ages. As such, the cumulative risk of developing other malignancies, collectively known as *non-AIDS defining malignancies* (NADM) (Table 141.2), is an increasing public health concern.[6,13–17] Without effective HIV prevention or cure, cancer burden in patients with HIV/AIDS will likely increase substantially, and cancer has emerged as the leading cause of death in people with HIV.[6,18,19]

CANCER AND HIV: INCIDENCE AND ETIOLOGY

Cancer epidemiology has provided insights leading to discoveries regarding pathogenesis of HIV-associated tumors. KS in AIDS was a departure from the indolent form in elderly men described by Moritz Kaposi in 1872[20] in that it was clinically aggressive and occurring in young men who had sex with other men (MSM), but generally not in those infected by other transmission routes.[21,22] MSM without HIV also occasionally developed KS. This suggested that KS had an infectious cause other than HIV itself, and ultimately a novel gamma-herpesvirus, called *Kaposi sarcoma-associated herpes virus* (KSHV) or *human herpes virus-8*, was discovered in 1994.[23] Subsequent studies showed that KSHV was an essential causative agent for all forms of KS. Seroprevalence of KSHV parallels geographic incidence of KS.[24] In the United States, KSHV seroprevalence is elevated in MSM.[25]

Early in the AIDS epidemic, excess cases of aggressive B-cell NHL were also a departure from previous epidemiologic patterns. Certain NHLs were included in the AIDS-case definition in 1985.[26] In the CDC 1993 revision of the definition of AIDS, three NHLs were AIDS-defining: Burkitt (or equivalent), immunoblastic (or equivalent), or primary brain.[1] This terminology is now dated; however, it is appreciated that several histological lymphoma subtypes are associated with HIV. In this chapter, we use the term *AIDS-related lymphoma* (ARL) to encompass both AIDS-defining lymphomas and other HIV-associated NHLs (Table 141.1).[27] Cervical cancer was added to the CDC list of AIDS-defining conditions in 1993.[1] The increased incidence of AIDS-related malignancies was paralleled by high mortality. However, since the development of cART, epidemiologic and clinical patterns of the AIDS-defining tumors have changed. Incidence of KS and some ARL subtypes has fallen markedly, and survival has improved substantially.[28–30]

TABLE 141.1

HUMAN IMMUNODEFICIENCY VIRUS (HIV)-ASSOCIATED LYMPHOMAS[a]

Lymphomas also occurring in immunocompetent patients
- Burkitt lymphoma
- Diffuse large B-cell lymphoma
  - Germinal center subtype
  - Activated B-cell subtype
- Extranodal marginal zone B-cell lymphoma of mucosa-associated lymphoid tissue type (MALT lymphoma; rare, mainly in pediatric patients)
- Classic Hodgkin's lymphoma (commonly mixed cellularity or lymphocyte depleted forms)[b]

Lymphomas occurring more specifically in HIV+ patients
- Primary effusion lymphoma
- Large B-cell lymphoma arising in HHV-8 associated multicentric Castleman disease
- Plasmablastic lymphoma
- Primary diffuse large B-cell lymphoma of the central nervous system (in patients with AIDS, >95% EBV associated)

Lymphomas also occurring in other immunodeficiency states
- Polymorphic B-cell lymphoma (PTLD-like)

HHV, human herpes virus; EBV, Epstein-Barr virus; PTLD, posttransplant lymphoproliferative disorder.
[a]Adapted from the most current lymphoma nomenclature from (The 2008 World Health Organization Classification, Tumours of Haematopoietic and Lymphoid Tissues.[115])
The Centers for Disease Control definition of AIDS-defining lymphoma in 1993 as Burkitt (or equivalent term), immunoblastic (or equivalent term), and primary brain lymphoma is based on older terminology.
[b]In this chapter, as in general usage, Hodgkin's lymphoma will be considered as a separate entity and will not be encompassed in the term *AIDS-related lymphoma*.

TABLE 141.2

RISKS OF VARIOUS MALIGNANT CONDITIONS IN PATIENTS WITH AIDS[a]

		Standard Incidence Ratio	
	Tumor	Pre-cART (1980–1989)	cART (1996–2002)
AIDS-Defining	Kaposi sarcoma	52,900	3,640
	Non-Hodgkin's lymphoma	79.8	49.5
	Burkitt lymphoma	57.4	49.5
	DLBCL	98.1	29.6
	Immunoblastic	140.5	59.5
	Primary diffuse large B-cell lymphoma of the CNS	5,000	1,020
	Cervix	7.7	5.3
Non–AIDS-Defining	Hodgkin's lymphoma	7.0	13.6
	Oral cavity and pharynx	1.2 (NS)	2.1
	Anus	18.3	19.6
	Lung	2.5	2.6
	Vagina and vulva	0 (NS)	4.4 (NS)
	Seminoma	2.6	0.8 (NS)
	Penis	0 (NS)	8.0
	Renal cell carcinoma	0.8 (NS)	1.9
	Liver	2.4 (NS)	3.3
	Myeloma	2.7 (NS)	2.2
	Breast	0	0.8 (NS)
	Colon	0.9 (NS)	1.0 (NS)
	Prostate	0.9 (NS)	0.5

cART, combination antiretroviral therapy; NS, not significant.
[a]Identification of cancers in people with AIDS based on matches to the cancer registries in patients grouped according to AIDS onset as either prior to development of combination antiretroviral therapy (1980–1989) or following cART (1996–2002). Cancer risk was described using the standardized incidence ratio (SIR), which compares incidence to that in the general population. All SIRs in table are significant ($P < .05$) unless noted.
From ref. 28, with permission.

Prior to 1985, KS was the initial manifestation of AIDS in approximately 30% of cases,[31] but decreased as an index disease with revision of the CDC definition of AIDS in 1992.[32] After peaking in the early 1990s, KS incidence declined rapidly in developed countries, largely because of the use of nucleoside anti-HIV therapy and then cART. In the United States the incidence of AIDS-associated KS decreased by 83.5% in 1996 to 2002 compared with 1990 to 1995.[28] Nonetheless, KS risk remains markedly elevated in people with HIV, with an estimated incidence in the United States of 62 cases per 100,000 person-years, and a broad variability in incidence that is related to CD4 count.[16] It is now the second most common tumor in people with HIV/AIDS in the United States.[16] AIDS-associated KS remains a much more common cause of morbidity and mortality in some parts of the world with high prevalence of HIV and KSHV coinfection. In certain parts of sub-Saharan Africa, KS represents almost half of all cancer cases in men, is the second most frequent tumor in women, and is a growing public health problem because of limited access to cART.[33–35]

For ARL, the risk in HIV-infected patients in the pre-cART era was more than 250-fold greater than the general population. More than 80% of lymphomas that occur in HIV-infected patients are high-grade mature B-cell lymphomas,[36] including both germinal center (GC) and activated B-cell (ABC) subtypes of diffuse large B-cell lymphoma (DLBCL),[37] Burkitt lymphoma (BL), plasmablastic lymphoma, primary diffuse large B-cell lymphoma of the central nervous system (PCNSL), and primary effusion lymphoma (PEL). By contrast, these histologies make up only 22% to 26% of lymphomas in the general population.[38]

The epidemiologic effects of cART on ARL are complex. The risk of developing ARL increases with the degree and duration of immunosuppression, with risk inversely related to CD4 count.[39] Inflammation in the setting of uncontrolled HIV viremia may also contribute to the pathogenesis, as several inflammatory markers[40–42] as well as uncontrolled HIV viremia[43,44] are risk factors for the development of NHL. Since the advent of cART, the incidence of NHL has decreased by approximately 50%.[45] Nonetheless, with an estimated incidence in the United States of 97 per 100,000 person-years in the cART era, NHL is now the most common malignancy in HIV-infected individuals in the United States.[16] ARL survival has increased since introduction of cART by nearly twofold, due in part to the effect of cART on AIDS and its infectious complications, as well as a shift away from poor-prognosis immunoblastic histologies occurring more frequently in cases of advanced AIDS. This is most remarkable for PCNSL, which tends to occur in patients with less than 50 CD4 cells/mm^3, and whose incidence has fallen 80%.[28] For systemic ARL, immunoblastic subtypes predominated in the pre-cART era, but the predominant subtypes have become the GC variant of DLBCL and BL,[45–47] which are associated with longer survival.[48] Additionally, therapeutic advances have contributed to improved survival in ARL. With the best current regimens, treatment results for these high-grade B-cell NHLs now approach those obtained in the general population. Effects of improved therapy may be particularly apparent for DLBCL[47] and BL.[29]

Although the incidence of ARL and KS has decreased, the incidence of certain NADMs has increased. In fact, where cART is widely available, NADM now occurs as frequently as AIDS-defining malignancies in HIV/AIDS.[17,19] Recent studies indicate that where cART is widely used, cancer is the most common cause of death in patients with HIV, with about half of cancer-associated deaths caused by AIDS-defining malignancies and half by NADM.[6,49] Excess risk of certain NADMs is partly attributable to HIV-infected patients having increased infection with, and in some cases, poor immunologic control of, oncogenic pathogens, such as *human papillomavirus* (HPV), *hepatitis B virus*, and *hepatitis C virus*. It is possible that additional infectious agents will be discovered and found responsible for some of these tumors. For example, a novel virus, *Merkel cell polyomavirus*, was recently identified as the likely etiologic agent for Merkel cell carcinoma,[50] a rare skin cancer that occurs with increased frequency in immunosuppressed individuals, including those with HIV.[51] Other risk factors for some tumors include cigarette smoking or alcohol use, and aging of the HIV-infected population. However, risk of NADM does not always appear to be fully explained by known cofactors. For example, a nearly fivefold excessive lung cancer risk in HIV appears related to age and cART use, but not CD4 cell count, and the risk remains 2.5-fold greater than that of the general population even when adjusted for smoking.[52] Given these epidemiologic trends, cancer burden among HIV-infected individuals will likely continue to increase in coming years, and medical oncologists will be called on to manage such cases.

KAPOSI SARCOMA

Pathophysiology

KS is characterized by inflammatory angiogenic lesions that arise in multiple sites. It occurs predominantly on the skin, but can involve virtually any organ, perhaps except the brain (Fig. 141.1). KS was quite rare in most of the Western world prior to AIDS. The initially described form, now known as *classic KS*, predominantly involves lower extremities of elderly men, and is found mostly in Ashkenazi Jews or in individuals living near the Mediterranean Sea. A more aggressive form of KS, now called *endemic KS*, was subsequently recognized in Africa. This form can occur earlier in life, often in the third or fourth decades, frequently involves the lymph nodes, and occurs in a higher percentage of females than *classic* KS. Also, it can develop in children, causing severe morbidity. The term *epidemic KS* is used to describe KS arising in HIV-infected patients. It is generally more clinically aggressive than *classic* KS (Fig. 141.1). KS can also occur in transplant recipients. KSHV is the etiologic agent for all forms of KS.

KS lesions are characterized by vascular slits filled with blood that often extravasates and accounts for their purplish hue. Microscopically, tumors are heterogeneous but characterized by a predominance of KSHV-infected spindle-shaped cells with certain markers of lymphatic endothelial cells.[53,54] There

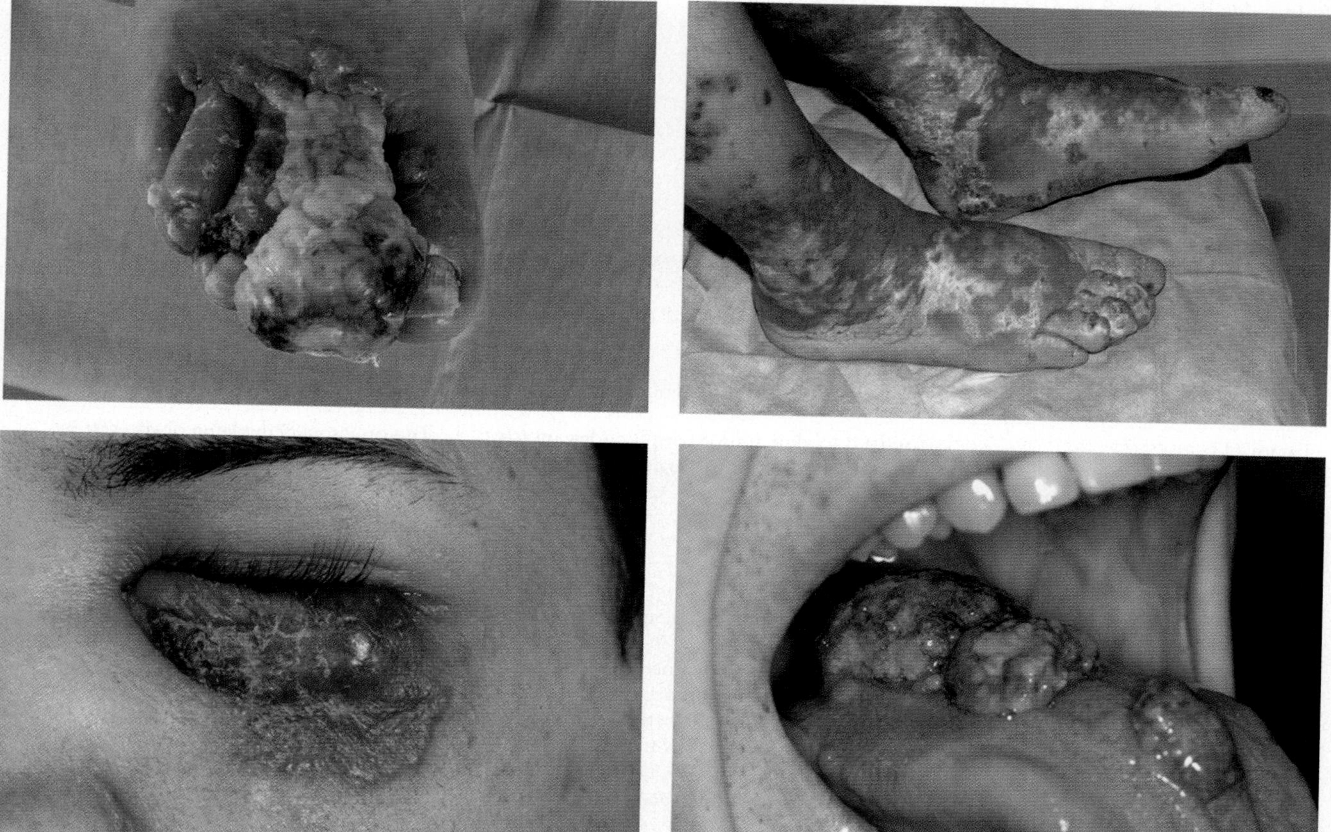

FIGURE 141.1 Mucocutaneous manifestations of AIDS-Kaposi sarcoma observed in the era of combination antiretroviral therapy.

are conflicting data regarding the monoclonality of KS lesions.[55,56] However, evidence indicates that hyperproliferation of endothelial-derived spindle cells is important in the pathogenesis of this disease.[54,57,58] Most of this hyperproliferation appears to be directly or indirectly induced by KSHV. KSHV encodes for a number of mimics of human genes, and several have direct angiogenesis activity that may be important in KS pathogenesis. Examples include a viral homologue to human IL-6 and three homologues of macrophage inhibitory protein that have been shown to have angiogenic activity.[54,57] Also, ORF74 of KSHV encodes for a constitutively active G-protein–coupled receptor (KSHV-GPCR) that induces production of vascular endothelial growth factor and other angiogenic factors.[58,59] Several mouse models suggest that ORF74 is a key factor in KS pathogenesis and can by itself induce lesions very similar to KS.[60,61] These and other viral genes and human cytokines and growth factors potentially stimulate spindle cell proliferation and angiogenesis. Indeed, of all tumors, autocrine and paracrine stimulation are arguably of greatest importance in the pathogenesis of KS and other tumors caused by KSHV. Furthermore, KSHV can be induced to undergo lytic replication by hypoxia,[62] and it is possible that the tendency of KS to arise in the feet, which are relatively hypoxic, is partly the result of hypoxia-induced KSHV reactivation.

KSHV transmission can occur by both sexual and nonsexual routes. Saliva of infected individuals has greater KSHV shedding than other body fluids, suggesting that culture-specific behaviors such as caretaker premastication of foods for infants or use of saliva as a sexual lubricant may play a role in transmission.[63–66] Blood-borne transmission is relatively inefficient,[63,67] but infection from donated solid organs into transplant recipients and subsequent development of KS has been documented.[68]

Individuals infected with KSHV but not HIV can develop KS, but it is rare and usually occurs after their fifth decade of life. KS risk is increased by as much as 500- to 10,000-fold in people with HIV/AIDS, suggesting an important role for immune surveillance of KSHV and the risk of KS. Identification of cellular immune responses to KSHV epitopes illustrates the importance of cellular immune function in protecting against KS.[69,70] Interestingly, decreased immune responsiveness to certain KSHV epitopes is found in patients with KS, regardless of HIV serostatus. Furthermore, HIV may promote KS by nonimmunologic mechanisms. For example, the Tat protein of HIV can enhance infection of target cells by KSHV.[71]

Staging and Prognosis

KS lesions arise simultaneously at multiple sites without an obvious primary site (Fig. 141.1). Multiple areas of skin involvement may not necessarily imply a worse prognosis than focal involvement. The term *metastatic* in relation to KS, as well as standard tumor staging, is not useful. The most widely used staging system for KS, devised prior to available cART, is the AIDS Clinical Trials Group Oncology Committee TIS staging system.[30] This system has been re-assessed and refined since the advent of cART[72] (Table 141.3). Patients are scored based on extent of tumor involvement (T), immune status (I), and systemic illness (S).[30] Risk is assigned as good or poor, depending on the presence or absence of localized tumor versus more extensive tumor with associated edema, ulceration, visceral disease, or extensive oral KS; CD4 more or less than 150 cells/mm^3; and the presence or absence of antecedent opportunistic infections, constitutional symptoms, other HIV-related illness, and Karnofsky performance status. Good risk is designated with a subscript 0, and poor risk by subscript 1, the summary taking the form T_0 or T_1, I_0 or I_1, or S_0 or S_1. Before the introduction of cART, a patient with poor risk in any single category was considered poor risk overall. In the era of cART, baseline CD4 level does not seem to provide prognostic information,[72] and two main risk categories have been identified: a good risk (T_0S_0, T_1S_0, or T_0S_1) and a poor risk (T_1S_1).

In assessing KS response to therapy, Response Evaluation Criteria in Solid Tumors (RECIST) criteria is not useful. Most clinical trials of KS use some modification of criteria established by the AIDS Clinical Trials Group Oncology Committee.[73] Criteria for a partial response include 50% decrease in the total number of lesions, 50% decrease in the area of measured cutaneous lesions, or flattening of 50% of nodular lesions in the absence of progressive disease.

TABLE 141.3

REVISED AND PROPOSED AIDS CLINICAL TRIALS GROUP STAGING CLASSIFICATION FOR KAPOSI SARCOMA (KS)[a]

Stage	Good Risk (0) (All of the Following)	Poor Risk (1) (Any of the Following)
Tumor (T)	Confined to skin and/or lymph nodes and/or non-nodular oral disease confined to the palate	Tumor-associated edema or ulceration Extensive oral KS Gastrointestinal KS KS in other nonnodal viscera
Immune system (I) (not included if HIV-sensitive to cART[49])	CD4 cells ≥150/mcL	CD4 cells <150/mcL
Systemic illness	No history of opportunistic infection or thrush No B symptoms (unexplained fever, night sweats, >10% involuntary weight loss, or diarrhea) persisting more than 2 weeks Performance status ≥70 (Karnofsky)	History of opportunistic infections and/or thrush; "B" symptoms present Performance status <70 Other HIV-related illness (e.g., neurologic disease, lymphoma)

HIV, human immunodeficiency virus; cART, combination antiretroviral therapy.
[a]Based on refs. 30 and 72. The revised CD4 cutoff of 150 cells/mcL[30] is lower than the original proposal of 200 cells/mcL. However, in the cART era, CD4 cells do not appear to confer prognostic information. Example of staging: in the pre-cART era, a patient with KS restricted to the skin, CD4 count of 10 cells/mcL, and a history of *Pneumocystis jiroveci* pneumonia would be $T_0I_1S_1$, and would be considered poor risk.[30] Suggested revision since cART would be staged as T_0S_1, and would be considered good risk.[72]

Treatment

Treatment with cART is fundamental to AIDS-KS therapy, and whenever possible should be the first therapeutic maneuver. Effective cART controls HIV viremia and generally leads to immune reconstitution. Additional therapy may also be required. Regression of KS with cART alone has been well documented; a pooled analysis of patients with early disease (T_0) who had not received cART previously suggests that up to 80% will have disease regression with cART alone, with median time to response ranging from 3 to 9 months.[74] In the setting of T_0 disease, chemotherapy can generally be avoided unless a patient has concurrent malignancies.[75] It has been suggested that HIV protease inhibitors may have a direct effect on KS,[76] and at least one ongoing study in Africa is looking at this parameter. However, in a retrospective study, response rates in KS were equivalent in patients receiving protease-sparing cART regimens as compared with those containing protease inhibitors.[77] It appears that control of HIV viremia itself and associated immune reconstitution are the more important requisites for KS effect. On the other hand, patients with advanced KS (T_1) generally do not have adequate responses with cART alone.

On occasion, KS patients have a sudden or dramatic progression of KS within the first 3 months of cART initiation, suggesting that an immune reconstitution inflammatory syndrome may be contributing to the KS progression.[78] Such patients should be considered for additional anti-KS therapy. Also, responses to cART may not be evident for many months, and patients who have substantial morbidity associated with the KS or are psychologically distressed by the visible lesions should be considered for additional therapy in addition to cART, so that a meaningful therapeutic benefit can be realized more quickly.

A number of local therapies have activity in KS patients with limited mucocutaneous disease. These include cryotherapy, photodynamic therapy, intralesional injections, radiation therapy, and topical application of various drugs. Surgical biopsy is important for making a definitive diagnosis of KS before chemotherapy is used. However, KS is a systemic disease, and clear surgical margins do not imply curative potential. At times, KS may develop in the site of surgical wounds. Therefore, surgery has a limited role as a treatment modality for KS. Topical 9-*cis*-retinoic acid (Panretin gel) is approved by the U.S. Food and Drug Administration (FDA) for use in KS and may result in responses in more than 45% of lesions, but can cause local inflammation and yield inadequate cosmesis. Intralesional injection or iontophoresis of low-dose vinblastine (0.1 mL of 0.1 mg/mL) or 3% sodium tetradodecyl sulfate injection (0.1 to 0.3 mL) are sometimes used. These cause a nonspecific necrosis or sclerosis of mucocutaneous tissue, but administration can be painful, and cosmetic results may be unsatisfactory. Radiation therapy is effective for local control. Short-term local toxicities are usually manageable, but radiation can lead to a "woody" skin and other long-term ill effects. For these reasons, it is generally reserved for disease that is limited, yet causing severe pain or distress. Doses range from an 8 Gy single dose to fractionated therapy to a total of 16 to 30 Gy, and are individualized for a given patient.

Systemic therapy in addition to cART should be considered in AIDS-KS if cART alone is thought to be insufficient or not rapid enough and if the tumor burden is not treatable by local modalities (Table 141.4). Although complete and long-lasting resolution of evident disease can be realized, this outcome does not imply cure. Treatment is palliative and may require chronic intermittent administration for long-term control. Indications for systemic therapy are imprecise and should be individualized. Systemic therapy is generally justified for patients with extensive cutaneous KS, life-threatening KS, symptomatic visceral KS, substantial pulmonary KS, ulcerating KS, extensive edema, or tumor-related pain; in such cases, it should be initiated as soon as safely possible. Social withdrawal due to KS is also an indication for systemic chemotherapy. Early initiation of cytotoxic chemotherapy in addition to cART is appropriate in patients in whom a rapid response is desired or who would not tolerate worsening KS.

TABLE 141.4

SYSTEMIC THERAPIES FOR PATIENTS WITH ADVANCED KAPOSI SARCOMA

Therapy Type	Response Rates (Ref.)
Commonly used standard therapy	
cART[a]	Variable; should be optimized in combination with other therapies
Liposomal doxorubicin	59%–76% (80,188)
Paclitaxel	59%–71% (84,189)
Alternative therapies	
Interferon-α	Variable, CD4 cell-dependent
Adriamycin/bleomycin/vinca alkaloids	24%–88% (higher response rates with higher doxorubicin doses, but greater toxicity)
Vincristine/vinblastine	45%
Bleomycin/vinca alkaloids	23%

[a]cART, combination antiretroviral therapy.
This should be administered to all patients with HIV-associated Kaposi sarcoma unless there is a clear contraindication.

Several cytotoxic agents have activity in KS, including vincristine, vinblastine, doxorubicin, etoposide, bleomycin, or dacarbazine. Early in the AIDS epidemic, high response rates were obtained with combination regimens of doxorubicin, bleomycin and vinblastine or vincristine (ABV), although toxicity was often substantial and limited dosing.[79] ABV has largely been replaced by monotherapy using liposomal anthracyclines.[79,80] Pegylated liposomal doxorubicin (Doxil) (20 mg/m^2 every 3 weeks) was shown in a randomized trial to yield better tumor responses and to be less toxic than ABV,[81] and is approved by the FDA in treating KS in patients whose disease has progressed on combination chemotherapy or who are intolerant to such therapy. In practice, it has become the standard of care first-line cytotoxic chemotherapy for KS. In the cART era, response rates of 80% or more may be anticipated, depending on the TIS stage.[82] A liposomal daunorubicin (DaunoXome) is approved as first-line therapy for advanced KS, but was used less than Doxil for KS, and is currently not available in the United States. Paclitaxel has activity in KS, with responses ranging from 59% to 71% demonstrated in phase 2 trials conducted prior to the use of cART.[83,84] Based on these findings, the FDA approved paclitaxel as second-line therapy for KS. Some oncologists recommend it as first-line therapy for life-threatening KS. Lastly, oral etoposide 50 mg/day on days 1 through 7 of a 14-day cycle is active, with an overall response rate of 36% in previously treated patients, the majority of whom were not receiving cART.[85] This approach may be particularly useful in resource-limited settings, although the association between etoposide and secondary myeloid leukemia raises concerns of long-term etoposide administration. Monitoring of complete blood counts is required.

In treating KS, a general strategy is to treat patients until a reasonable response plateau or remission is attained, then either stop or increase time between doses to maintain the response. The number of cycles of chemotherapy required varies and depends on the regimen used. In cases of advanced immune depletion or when HIV cannot be well controlled, KS generally progresses shortly after therapy is stopped. In such cases, a useful strategy can be to increase cycle length to the time just before KS starts to progress again (usually within 6 weeks) in an effort to maintain disease stability while administering the lowest dose intensity of therapy possible. Growth of KS after therapy with a given chemotherapy does not necessarily imply tumor resistance or treatment failure, so the same agent can often be used again. Patients with substantial immune reconstitution on cART are more likely to be able to stop chemotherapy after an early response, with maintained or even improved KS response with cART continuation. However, despite substantial cART benefit, some patients require ongoing antitumor therapy in addition to cART. Chronic chemotherapy can be associated with cumulative treatment-related toxicities that can limit the ability to continue therapy. In particular, patients should if at all possible not receive a cumulative lifetime anthracycline dose over 550 mg/m^2 because of the risk of severe, irreversible cardiotoxicity. The risk of this complication is believed to be somewhat less with a liposomal formulation; however, this dose should not be exceeded without careful cardiac monitoring and an awareness of the risks involved. Although cART has dramatically decreased the incidence and improved the overall survival, it is not a panacea for KS. The need for chronic intermittent chemotherapy in the management of KS in a subset of patients and the lifetime limit on anthracycline exposure reinforces the need to develop better therapies, including pathogenesis-based treatments.

Both immune modulating and antiangiogenic therapies have been explored in patients with KS. Interferon-α (IFN-α) was identified as active in KS in the early 1980s, particularly in patients with more than 200 CD4 cells/mm^3 and disease limited to the skin.[86,87] Most practitioners begin with IFN-α 1 to 5 $\times$ 10^6 units subcutaneous injection daily and gradually increase the dose as tolerated. IFN-α should be used in combination with cART, and when used with cART, may be effective even in patients with lower CD4 counts. However, IFN-α is associated with significant toxicities, including decreased white blood count, flulike symptoms, and sometimes depression and hypothyroidism. Additional compounds with antiangiogenic activity that have shown evidence of activity include thalidomide,[88,89] COL-3,[90] and IL-12,[91] and promising results have been demonstrated with the combination of IL-12 and cytotoxic chemotherapy for advanced KS.[92] Interestingly, agents such as IFN-α, IL-12, and thalidomide may have several mechanisms of action that are beneficial in the treatment of KS. Clinical studies targeting vascular endothelial growth factor pathways through the use of bevacizumab, sunitinib, or sorafenib are also under way. Several antiherpes drugs including ganciclovir and cidofovir block KSHV replication *in vitro*, and the question has been raised of whether they might have activity in KS. A randomized clinical trial of oral ganciclovir for *cytomegalovirus* infections showed that systemic administration was associated with a lower rate of KS development compared with ganciclovir ocular implants.[93] In spite of this activity in preventing KS, antiherpes drugs generally have not been found to be effective therapy for established disease. For example, in a small phase 2 trial of intermittent cidofovir in KS, each of seven patients had disease progression.[94] However, it may still be possible that other antiviral approaches may be developed for this disease. In this regard, it is of interest that zidovudine is activated to a toxic moiety by a KSHV-encoded thymidine kinase[95] and that several patients with HIV-KS had tumor regression on high doses of zidovudine in the initial phase 1 trial.[96]

KSHV-ASSOCIATED MULTICENTRIC CASTLEMAN DISEASE

There are several forms of Castleman disease: unicentric hyaline-vascular form, a multicentric plasma cell form, and a multicentric form associated with KSHV. Nearly all Castleman disease arising in the setting of HIV infection is KSHV-associated MCD (KSHV-MCD).[97] This polyclonal[98] hyperproliferative B-cell disorder is considered to be rare, although its incidence is not well defined. In contrast with KS, MCD may be more common since the advent of cART.[99]

KSHV-MCD is characterized by intermittent flares of inflammatory symptoms, including fevers, fatigue, and cachexia, and edema, together with lymphadenopathy and/or splenomegaly. Gastrointestinal symptoms and cough are also common. Flares can be severe and often fatal[100]; they are primarily caused by cytokine overproduction related to the highly lytic state of the KSHV in MCD.[101] In particular, a KSHV-encoded analogue of interleukin-6 (vIL-6) and/or overproduction of cellular IL-6 are believed to cause many of the symptoms of KSHV-MCD.[102]

There is no validated staging or prognostic system. KSHV-MCD should be considered in the differential diagnosis of patients with HIV and unexplained inflammatory symptoms or autoimmune phenomena, particularly anemia or thrombocytopenia. The clinical course waxes and wanes, but untreated, is frequently fatal within 2 years of diagnosis, with patients succumbing to severe inflammatory syndromes or progressing to large B-cell lymphoma arising in HHV-8 associated MCD.[100] Diagnosis of KSHV-MCD generally requires excisional lymph node biopsy and demonstration of KSHV-infected plasmablasts. Laboratory abnormalities include anemia, thrombocytopenia, hypoalbuminemia, hyponatremia, and elevated C-reactive protein. Patients with MCD should undergo computed tomography (CT) of neck, chest, abdomen, and pelvis. There is no standard therapy for KSHV-MCD. HIV-infected patients should receive cART, although intolerance to a number of drugs, including antiretrovirals, may occur until MCD is controlled.

Several agents have reported activity against MCD in case series or small studies. Perhaps best studied is the anti-CD20 monoclonal antibody rituximab.[103] Most patients respond initially to rituximab-containing regimens, although relapses are common. However, rituximab monotherapy may be insufficient in advanced disease, and has been associated with exacerbation of intercurrent KS.[103,104] Rituximab combined with liposomal doxorubicin appears promising in preliminary reports.[105] Other potentially active agents include ganciclovir,[106] IFN-α,[107] and high-dose zidovudine combined with ganciclovir.[108] Chemotherapy regimens used in NHL have also been employed.[100] Splenectomy[100,109] has sometimes been used to manage severe cytopenias in KSHV-MCD; however, recent studies suggest that this practice can usually be replaced by biochemotherapeutic approaches, sparing patients long-term infectious risks associated with splenectomy. With increased experience treating patients with MCD, as well as the availability of cART, survival of over 2 years is now relatively common, although this may partly reflect lead-time bias from higher clinical awareness and earlier diagnosis. However, given the many uncertainties in managing patients with KSHV-MCD, including length of treatment, role of maintenance therapy, and evaluation and management of concurrent malignancies, consideration should be given to referral to a clinical trial, and several pathogenesis-based regimens are currently under evaluation.

AIDS-ASSOCIATED LYMPHOMAS

Pathophysiology

Risk of ARL is inversely related to CD4 cell count, although the relationship varies among different lymphomas.[46,110] PCNSL and other immunoblastic phenotypes of ARL often develop in patients with very low CD4 counts, and are frequently associated with Epstein-Barr virus (EBV), while GC-DLBCL and BL generally present in patients with higher counts (Table 141.5).

TABLE 141.5

COMPARISON OF HUMAN IMMUNODEFICIENCY VIRUS–ASSOCIATED LYMPHOMAS

		Viral Associations (%)		Histogenetic Markers (%)		Pathobiologic Markers (%)						
Histogenetic Origin	**Histology**	**EBV**	**KSHV**	**MUM1**	**Syn-1**	**BCL-2**	**BCL-6**	**P53**	**c-MYC**	**CD4 Cells**	**Prospects for Chemosensitivity**	**Prognosis in cART Era**
Germinal center	Burkitt lymphoma	<50	0	<15	0	0	100	60	100	May be relatively well preserved	Favorable	Excellent
	DLBCL–GC	<30	0	<30	0	0	>75	Rare	0–50	Variable	Favorable	Excellent
Postgerminal center	DLBCL–ABC	>50	Rare	100	>50	30	0	0	0–20	Usually low	Intermediate	Improved
	PCNSL	>95	0	>50	<60	90	<50	0	0	<50/mm³	Unknown	Poor
	Primary effusion lymphoma	>80	100	100	>90	0	0	0	0	Variable	Unknown	Poor
	Plasmablastic lymphoma	>70	Rare	100	100	0	0	Rare	0	Variable	Unknown	Poor

EBV, Epstein-Barr virus; KSHV, Kaposi sarcoma-associated herpes virus; MUM1, multiple myeloma-1; cART, combination antiretroviral therapy; DLBCL, diffuse large B-cell lymphoma; GC, germinal center subtype; ABC, activated B-cell subtype.
Data from refs. 29, 46, 47, and 117.

Additional immune factors affect risk of ARL and provide insight into lymphomagenesis. Elevated cytokines, such as IL-6, IL-10,[41,111] and tumor necrosis factor-β along with frequent aberrant somatic hypermutation of immunoglobulin V genes suggest a role for immune stimulation in lympomagenesis.[112] Chemokine pathway polymorphisms also affect risk of ARL. For example, the 3′A variant of stromal cell-derived factor 1 doubles and quadruples NHL risk in heterozygotes and homozygotes, respectively.[113] Interestingly, the stromal cell-derived factor 1-1-3′A variant is carried by 37% of whites and 11% of blacks, and may contribute to the relatively lower risk of ARL in blacks. The HIV-coreceptor CCR5 deletion variant CCR5-Δ32 confers approximately a threefold protection against NHL, independent of its HIV protective effect.[114]

ARLs are a histologically heterogeneous group of aggressive mature B-cell neoplasms, and should be classified using current World Health Organization criteria.[115] Lymphomas associated with HIV-infection (Table 141.1) include lymphomas seen in immunocompetent patients as well as lymphomas more specifically associated with HIV infection. Classic HL, especially the mixed cellularity subtype,[116] occurs with increased frequency in people infected with HIV, but is categorized as an NADM. Polymorphic lymphoproliferative disorders resembling post-transplant-associated lymphoproliferative disease may also be seen in people with AIDS.

Immunohistochemical markers are helpful in categorizing ARLs (Table 141.5), and provide important prognostic information, especially for DLBCL.[48,117,118] It is increasingly recognized that ARL is not a single lymphoma type with one treatment for all, but rather treatment should be informed by histology. For example, treating all ARL with CHOP-like regimens regardless of histology may account for the relative lack of improved outcomes for BL compared to GC-DLBCL after cART was introduced.[29,47] Emerging data strongly support more dose-intensive approaches suitable to BL as is used in the background HIV-unrelated population.

Clinical Presentation and Staging of Peripheral Lymphomas

ARL frequently presents with either a rapidly growing mass or development of "B" symptoms (unexplained fever, drenching night sweats, or unexplained weight loss in excess of 10% of the normal body weight). Extranodal involvement is common, including bone marrow (25% to 40%), gastrointestinal tract (26%), and CNS (12% to 57%).[36] Staging should include CT of neck, chest, abdomen, and pelvis; fluorodeoxyglucose (^{18}F)-positron emission tomography (FDG-PET); lactate dehydrogenase; complete blood count with differential bone marrow biopsy; and lumbar puncture with evaluation of cerebral spinal fluid (CSF) by cytology and flow cytometry. Evaluation of cardiac function using echocardiography or multigated acquisition scan is recommended. Magnetic resonance imaging (MRI) of the brain with gadolinium should be strongly considered to evaluate for CNS involvement, or other CNS complications of AIDS in patients with low CD4 counts. HIV viral load, CD4 count, and hepatitis B (HBV) core antibody and surface antigen, as well as hepatitis C (HCV) serology should be evaluated. Patients with detectable HBV core antibody or surface antigen should be screened for quantitative HBV viral load.

Treatment of the More Common Peripheral Acquired Immunodeficiency Syndrome-Related Lymphomas

Prior to the cART era, the prognosis of ARL was determined primarily by CD4 cell count. ARL was treated as a single disease entity without regard to lymphoma subtype, often with reduced dose regimens. Patients with fewer than 100 CD4 cells/mm^3 had a median survival of about 4 months, and those with 100 or more CD4 cells/mm^3 had a median survival of 11 to 18 months.[119] However, clinical trials performed in the cART era have shown improved tolerance to standard-dose chemotherapy and improved survival. Moreover, it has become clear that lymphoma-specific features are important in prognosis and that the CD4 cell count, although still important, is not the predominant prognostic factor.[29,45,47,120]

Therapy with curative intent is indicated for nearly all patients with ARL. DA-EPOCH-R (rituximab, 96-hour continuous infusion etoposide, doxorubicin, and vincristine with oral prednisone and bolus cyclophosphamide, followed by filgrastim, dose-adjusted for tolerance), short-course DA-EPOCH with dose-dense rituximab (SC-EPOCH-RR), R-CHOP (rituximab, cyclophosphamide, doxorubicin, vincristine, and prednisone), and R-CDE (rituximab, 96-hour continuous infusion cyclophosphamide, doxorubicin, and etoposide, followed by filgrastim) have all been evaluated prospectively (Table 141.6), although never directly compared. Studies of these regimens have enrolled populations with widely differing characteristics, including immunologic and virologic parameters, different approaches to cART, varying numbers of chemotherapy cycles, as well as differing disease subtypes, including in some cases BL and unclassifiable NHL, as well as a varying or unknown proportion of GC and ABC DLBCL. Given the impact of these factors on prognosis, direct comparison between studies is difficult. Nonetheless, recent studies have clarified the role of rituximab, provided evidence that patients with ARL can tolerate full-dose regimens, and demonstrated that a high percentage of patients have good outcomes with the infusional regimen, DA-EPOCH combined with rituximab.[47,121,122]

The majority of ARLs express CD20, and a monoclonal antibody targeting CD20, rituximab, improves complete response rates and overall survival in a range of lymphomas in HIV-negative patients. Consensus exists that rituximab should also be used in CD20-expressing lymphomas in the setting of HIV. Early controversy regarding rituximab stemmed from a randomized trial comparing CHOP with R-CHOP, in which improvements in progression-free survival with the additional of rituximab were not statistically significant and 14% of patients receiving rituximab died of treatment-related infectious deaths, annulling any advantage to overall survival.[123] The majority of deaths occurred in patients with less than 50 CD4 cells/mm^3. However, the complete response rate was 22% higher in the group that received R-CHOP, although the study was not powered to show statistical significance. Moreover, 8% of the group receiving R-CHOP had disease progression, compared with 21.6% of those receiving CHOP. This is similar to rituximab benefit documented in non-AIDS lymphoma trials powered to show statistical significance with differences of this magnitude.[124] Subsequent studies have further evaluated the safety, toxicity, and efficacy of rituximab combined with several anthracycline-based regimens.

Two additional phase 2 trials of R-CHOP in ARL have been published. One found no excess in infectious deaths and documented, in evaluable patients, a complete response rate of 77% and 2-year overall survival rate of 75%.[125] Importantly, this trial included only those considered at good or intermediate prognosis by virtue of having no more than one of the following: CD4 less than 100 cells/mm^3, prior AIDS, or performance status less than 2. Most patients were on protease inhibitor–based therapies. In the other study, which did not limit eligibility to low-risk patients and required protease inhibitor–based cART, the complete response rate was 69%, although 23% of these patients relapsed, and the estimated 3-year overall survival was 56%. There were seven infectious deaths during treatment in this study (9%), and two additional patients died of opportunistic

TABLE 141.6

SELECTED REGIMENS AND OUTCOMES FOR AIDS-ASSOCIATED NON-HODGKIN'S LYMPHOMA

Regimen	Evaluable Patients/ Total Patients	Median Baseline CD4 cells/mm³	Complete Response Rate (%)	Percent Progression-Free 1 y	2 y	Study (Ref.)
Infusional CDE (cART-era patients only)	55/55	227	44		36	Sparano et al. (190)
Three pooled phase II trials of R-CDE	74/74	161	70		59	Spina et al. (127)
Dose-adjusted EPOCH (cART deferment until chemotherapy completion)	39/39	198	74		73	Little et al. (46)
Randomized						Sparano et al. (122)
R-DA-EPOCH	48/54	181	73	78	66	
vs. DA-EPOCH followed by rituximab	53/56	194	55	66	63	
Short-course dose-adjusted EPOCH-RR (cART deferment until chemotherapy completion)	33/33	208	91		84	Dunleavy et al. (47)
Subgroup analysis, GC	21				96	
Subgroup analysis, non-GC	8				38	
Randomized						Kaplan et al. (123)
R-CHOP	99/99	130	57.6	50	34	
vs. CHOP	50/51	147	47	48	38	
Phase 2 R-CHOP						
High-risk patients excluded	52/61	172	77		69	Boue et al. (125)
No exclusion of high-risk patients	80/86	158	69		55	Ribera et al. (126)

CDE, cyclophosphamide, doxorubicin, and etoposide; EPOCH, etoposide, doxorubicin, and vincristine with oral prednisone and bolus cyclophosphamide; cART, combination antiretroviral therapy; R-CDE, rituximab with CDE; R-CHOP, rituximab with cyclophosphamide, doxorubicin, vincristine, and prednisone (CHOP); R-DA-EPOCH, rituximab (R) with dose-adjusted (DA) EPOCH.
Patients enrolled in the short-course DA-EPOCH-RR study received cyclophosphamide 750 mg/m² compared to lower doses adjusted to CD4 counts in the other DA-EPOCH studies, as well as additional rituximab 375 mg/m² on day 6 of therapy. Only the studies in refs. 47 and 126 were limited to DLBCL.

infections during follow-up.[126] It is important to note that in both of these studies, filgrastim was not mandated on the first cycle but was required on subsequent cycles in 77% to 94% of patients. Furthermore, bone marrow toxicity was common when R-CHOP was used with protease inhibitor–based cART, and dose reductions or delays were required in 33% to 77% of patients.

A number of studies of rituximab combined with infusional regimens also clarify the role of rituximab in CD20-positive ARL. An early phase 2 trial of DA-EPOCH with suspension of cART reported a complete response rate of 74% and a disease-free survival and overall survival 92% and 60%, respectively, at a median follow-up of 53 months.[46] Two follow-up studies combining rituximab with DA-EPOCH have been recently reported. The first was a multicenter randomized phase 2 study of DA-EPOCH with concurrent versus sequential rituximab performed by the AIDS Malignancy Consortium. In this study, cyclophosphamide dosing was based on CD4 count, and cART was continued in 71% of patients. Patients with BL or Burkitt-like lymphoma (25% of patients) were included in the analysis. Therapeutic benefit of rituximab was demonstrated through a 73% complete response rate in the concurrent rituximab arm compared with 55% in the sequential rituximab arm.[122] Two-year progression-free survival was 66% in the combined arm versus 63% in the sequential arm, and 2-year overall survival was 70% versus 67%. There were no differences between arms in terms of treatment-related deaths (9% vs. 7%). In a study performed at the National Cancer Institute (NCI) intramural program, SC-EPOCH-RR with suspension of cART during therapy and no decrease in cyclophosphamide dosing based on CD4 count was evaluated in patients with DLBCL.[47] Number of cycles administered was adapted to response, with patients receiving one cycle beyond stable radiographic and negative ^{18}FDG-PET scans. Patients received a median of three cycles (range, three to five cycles). Ninety-one percent of patients had a complete response, and with 5-year median follow-up, progression-free and overall survival were 85% and 68%, respectively. Three patients died of AIDS-related opportunistic infections after completing therapy. Tumor histogenesis was the most important predictor of estimated 5-year progression-free survival, with 95% of patients with GC-DLBCL progression-free, compared with fewer than 40% with ABC-DLCBL. Intriguingly, this study of SC-EPOCH-RR demonstrates that many patients with HIV-associated GC-DLBCL may be cured with as few as three cycles, and can tolerate standard cyclophosphamide dosing. However, validation of the approach, particularly the generalizability of the use of interim ^{18}FDG-PET, is required. Although the study appears to show high negative predictive value of ^{18}FDG-PET, positive scans were insufficiently predictive, and the use of interim ^{18}FDG-PET should be reserved for clinical studies until this approach is better evaluated.

The third rituximab-based regimen that has been explored in ARL is R-CDE. In a pooled analysis from three phase

2 studies of rituximab with CDE every 4 weeks for a planned six cycles, a complete response rate of 70% and both disease-free and overall survival of 55% at a median follow-up of 23 months was observed.[127] In these studies, 76% of patients received concurrent cART. There was a 3% infection-related death rate during treatment, with additional deaths due to opportunistic infections following treatment.

Until recently, clinical trials of ARL generally included both DLBCL and BL. It is now appreciated that there are substantial differences between responses of these diseases to therapy and that they should be considered separately. Both CHOP-based[29] therapy and R-CDE given every 4 weeks[127] result in poor outcomes in AIDS-BL. However, improved outcomes appear achievable with other regimens. DA-EPOCH-R (with full-dose cyclophosphamide), combined with intrathecal methotrexate, appears to have excellent activity and is well tolerated in BL.[46] A report of 19 patients, including 6 with HIV, demonstrated a 100% complete response rate, with no relapses observed with a median 29 months of potential follow-up.[128] A prospective study is under way to further evaluate this regimen in BL. CODOX-M/IVAC (cyclophosphamide, vincristine, doxorubicin, methotrexate plus ifosfamide, etoposide, and cytarabine)[129] has also been used to treat HIV-associated BL,[130,131] with an estimated 70% complete response rate in retrospective studies, but with treatment-related mortality reaching 30% in one series.[131] Evaluation of this regimen combined with rituximab has completed accrual for patients with HIV-associated BL, and results from this study are forthcoming. However, owing to the toxicity of CODOX-M/IVAC, and other short-duration intensive multiagent regimens,[132] it is reasonable to consider DA-EPOCH-R with full-dose cyclophosphamide and intrathecal methotrexate for patients with AIDS-BL, preferably within a clinical trial.

A high percentage (12% to 57%) of ARLs have involvement of the CNS at presentation, especially BL.[36,46,47] Routine CNS prophylaxis is generally used, although some favor risk stratifying patients based on the presence of extranodal disease. Prophylaxis has varied between studies, but generally includes intrathecal methotrexate (12 mg) or cytosine arabinoside (ARA-C; 50 mg) for a total of four to eight doses. CNS involvement by DLBCL confers a poor prognosis. Several intensive intraventricular and intrathecal methotrexate schedules have shown activity. Most commonly, therapy is administered using an Ommaya reservoir twice weekly until 2 weeks after negative CSF flow cytometry is documented (for a minimum of eight doses), and then continued weekly for 6 to 8 weeks, then monthly for 6 months.

Outside the setting of HIV infection, high-dose chemotherapy with autologous peripheral stem cell transplant (HDT-PBSCT) is often used for patients with relapsed DLBCL or HL. Data increasingly support HDT-PBSCT feasibility and effectiveness in HIV-infected patients.[133–136] In the largest study of HDT-PBSCT limited to relapsed or refractory disease, the Italian GICAT group evaluated 50 patients, 31 with NHL and 19 with HL.[135] Twenty-seven patients completed debulking chemotherapy, had chemosensitive disease, underwent successful stem cell collection, and received transplantation. By intent-to-treat analysis with median follow-up of 44 months, overall and progression-free survival were each approximately 50%. These results are comparable with results in HIV-negative patients. Benefit appears limited to those with chemotherapy-sensitive disease. Across several conditioning regimens, treatment-related mortality is 3% to 5%,[133–136] and, as in the HIV-uninfected setting, there is the risk of secondary myelodysplastic syndrome.[136]

Even though effective cART for HIV has reduced the incidence of ARL and has improved survival, no randomized trial exists to clarify the utility of cART during lymphoma chemotherapy. On one hand, earlier control of HIV viremia and immune reconstitution may improve long-term infectious outcomes, especially in patients with low CD4 counts. However, physicians should be alert to potential pharmacokinetic interactions between cART and chemotherapeutic agents that have the possibility of compromising timely delivery of appropriately dosed chemotherapy. Consideration of holding cART in the face of treatment toxicity as a maneuver to maintain chemotherapy dose intensity is reasonable. As a class, protease inhibitors (especially ritonavir) inhibit CYP3A4 and clinicians must be aware of potential interactions with other drugs. Also, zidovudine should generally be avoided because of additive hematotoxicity, and stavudine should be avoided because of enhanced neurotoxicity with vincristine. A study performed early in the cART era to evaluate standard-dose CHOP for ARL included cART during the treatment period.[137] This study demonstrated that cART could be given with multiagent chemotherapy but also that pharmacokinetic interactions could occur. Compared with historic controls that received CHOP without cART, cyclophosphamide clearance was decreased by about 50% in the study patients. Doxorubicin elimination was similar to that in previous studies. Although there were no obvious clinical consequences related to these findings with either reduced-dose cyclophosphamide or full-dose cyclophosphamide and filgrastim support, the high rate of dose reductions in two phase 2 studies of R-CHOP in which the most patients received protease inhibitors suggests potential drug-drug interactions and supports the use of growth factor support in this setting.[125,126]

Substantial data from both large cohorts[138] and phase 2 studies that have included cART suggest that chemotherapy and cART can be concomitantly administered, as long as there is use of growth factor support and prophylaxis for opportunistic and bacterial infections. However, use of cART during chemotherapy for lymphoma is not essential, and phase 2 studies of DA-EPOCH (both with dose-dense rituximab and without rituximab) in HIV-associated lymphoma have achieved excellent results while withholding cART during the lymphoma treatment.[46,47] CD4 cell depletion and recovery mirrored that expected in patients without HIV who were similarly treated, with immune recovery 6 to 12 months following treatment.[46,47,139] Supportive care measures included PCP prophylaxis in all patients and *Mycobacterium avium* (MAI) prophylaxis for patients with CD4 counts less than 100 cell/mm^3. Nonetheless, patients with CD4 count less than 100 cells/mm^3 at baseline were at high risk from death from opportunistic infections after completion of therapy. The available data therefore support varied approaches with regard to cART. Often, physicians who treat ARL continue cART in patients on effective and tolerable regimens, but will not initiate cART while treating lymphoma.

Given risk of infections both during and after completion of chemotherapy, especially in patients with CD4 counts less than 100 cells/mm^3, detailed attention to supportive care measures is critically important. All patients with ARL, regardless of CD4 count at time of diagnosis, should receive prophylaxis against PCP, preferably with trimethoprim-sulfamethoxazole (one double strength tablet three times weekly throughout therapy and continued until CD4 counts recover to >200 cells/mm^3). Patients with CD4 count less than 50 to 100 cells/mm^3 also require azithromycin 1,200 mg weekly as prophylaxis against MAI. Prophylaxis against herpes simplex virus reactivation using valacyclovir should be considered for patients with a history of oral or anogenital herpes. Patients with detectable hepatitis B viremia require antiviral therapy for HBV. Care is required to ensure that therapy of intercurrent HBV avoids compromising HIV control, as single-agent therapy for HBV will increase the likelihood of a specific HIV mutation, M184V, which renders patients resistant to several important antiretroviral agents. Patients with mucosal Candida infections should not receive azoles concurrently with chemotherapy.

Rarer Peripheral ARLs: Plasmablastic Lymphoma and PEL

A number of rare lymphomas can occur in the setting of HIV infection (Table 141.1). Two are of special interest given their strong association with both HIV as well as gamma-herpesviruses. Plasmablastic lymphoma (PBL) is an EBV-associated B-cell NHL proposed as a new entity in 1997.[140] Although most common in the setting of HIV, PBL also occurs in organ transplantation patients and elderly individuals.[141–143] It often presents with disease within the oral cavity, but may occur at other extranodal or nodal sites. A review of 112 published cases summarized the spectrum of clinical presentations.[144] HIV-associated PBL usually presents as either stage I or stage IV disease and has a 7:1 male predominance. The median CD4 count at diagnosis was 178 cells/mm³. Ann Arbor staging does not appear prognostic, and patients with stage I disease should be treated the same as those with systemic disease. PBL is characterized by a high proliferative index and aggressive clinical course. Historically, the prognosis has been poor, with median survival less than 2 years. CHOP has often been used and results are often poor, but there are few clinical trial data at this time demonstrating superiority of other regimens. Also at this time, based on expert opinion, treatment with regimens effective in tumors with high proliferative rates, such as DA-EPOCH and CODOX-M/IVAC, are recommended.

PEL is a rare KSHV-associated aggressive mature B-cell lymphoma that usually presents as a lymphomatous effusion in serous body cavities; patients are at risk for other concomitant KSHV-associated malignancies. Many cases are pleural, but peritoneal, pericardial, and leptomeningeal presentations are seen. Extracavitary PEL is a KSHV-positive, clonal mature B-cell neoplasm with phenotypic and molecular similarities to PEL[145] that may present in a variety of locations, including lymph nodes, the gastrointestinal tract, or cutaneous tissues. Diagnosis of PEL depends on the demonstration of KSHV infection of tumor cells. In more than 70% of cases, tumor cells are coinfected with EBV. Common B-cell surface markers (CD19, CD20, CD79a) are absent, while activation markers (CD30, CD38, CD71, CD138) are often present; immunoglobulin gene rearrangements confirm B-cell monoclonality. Evaluation of the extent of disease should be performed following the guidelines for NHL staging. There are few data to guide therapy in PEL and the outcome is generally poor. Case series using doxorubicin-based regimens report initial complete response rates as high as 40%, but the clinical course is characterized by rapid relapse, with a median survival of less than 6 months.[146] However, it should be noted that there are a few case reports of patients having long-term remissions. The potential role of molecularly targeted therapies in PEL remains the subject of exploration. Given this paucity of data, patients should ideally be treated within clinical studies if possible.

Primary Diffuse Large B-Cell Lymphoma of the CNS

AIDS-related PCNSL almost always occurs in patients with a CD4 count of less than 50 cells/mm³ and can occur in the setting of other CNS pathology such as toxoplasmosis or cryptococcal meningitis. Contrast CT or MRI usually demonstrates single or multiple contrast-enhancing masses that are not reliably distinguishable from toxoplasmosis or other CNS processes. Definitive diagnosis requires stereotactic biopsy. In the pre-cART era, AIDS patients with brain masses, regardless of cause, had a very poor prognosis. Definitive treatment had little impact on survival, and diagnostic biopsy was often omitted. Therefore, empiric treatment was often standard. First, antitoxoplasmosis therapy would be administered for 2 to 3 weeks and assessment was made as to whether the disease responded or progressed. Progression of disease was empirically considered most likely to be PCNSL, and whole-brain radiotherapy would then be considered. Patients rarely survived more than 6 months, regardless of the cause or treatment.[147,148] However, this paradigm must be reconsidered in the cART era, as advanced AIDS can be successfully treated. Optimal outcome for such patients is predicated on prompt treatment of the underlying HIV infection and timely institution of appropriate therapy for the brain lesions. Treatment delays increase the likelihood of permanent residual neurologic disability, and the practice of instituting empiric antibiotic therapy for possible toxoplasmosis with a 2-week watch-and-wait period is no longer justified. As in patients without HIV infection, neurologic impairment with a brain mass should be viewed as a medical urgency requiring immediate diagnostic evaluations, so that prompt treatment can be initiated.

A major advance in diagnosis of CNS masses in AIDS patients was the incorporation of relatively noninvasive diagnostic methods.[149,150] Because essentially all AIDS-PCNSL is EBV-related,[151] detection of EBV DNA by polymerase chain reaction in the CSF combined with positive brain ^{201}Tl single-photon emission computed tomography (^{201}Tl-SPECT) has been shown to reliably predict the presence of PCNSL.[150] Increased ^{201}Tl-SPECT uptake combined with positive EBV-DNA had 100% sensitivity and 100% positive predictive value for PCNSL, whereas if both tests have negative results, negative predictive value is 100%. ^{18}FDG-PET is also highly specific for malignancy, and can also be used in combination with cerebrospinal fluid EBV-PCR evaluation in patients with fewer than 50 CD4 cells/mm³.[152,153] These diagnostic modalities should be incorporated in upfront evaluation of patients with AIDS and CNS masses; however, it should be noted that CSF evaluation alone of EBV-PCR is not specific for PCNSL, as EBV can be detected in CSF of HIV patients with systemic NHL[154] and nonmalignant conditions.[155] Also, brain ^{18}FDG-PET can detect other malignancies, and evaluation of HIV-infected patients with CNS masses must take into account immune status and the possibility of CNS involvement of a systemic NHL or metastatic NADM. Ideally, treatment of AIDS-PCNSL should be based on a tissue diagnosis. Nonetheless, in the context of CD4 count less than 50 cells/mm³, the combination of a high EBV viral load in the CSF, a ring-enhancing brain mass on MRI, and a positive ^{201}Tl-SPECT or CNS, ^{18}FDG-PET may be considered highly suggestive of AIDS-PCNSL, and if a tissue diagnosis cannot be obtained, it can be used as a basis to institute therapy for AIDS-PCNSL.

There is no standard therapy for AIDS-PCNSL, and patients should be considered for referral to a clinical trial. Treatment should include initiation of cART, which has been shown in retrospective studies to improve overall survival.[148,156] AIDS-PCNSL is highly responsive to whole-brain irradiation, and most patients can be expected to have initial clinical improvement. Estimates of long-term outcomes are more varied in analysis performed early in the cART era: 1-year overall survival with whole-brain irradiation and cART was only 20%.[148] In a subsequent Japanese report, the estimated 3-year overall survival in patients receiving more than 30 Gy whole-brain irradiation combined with focal boost in 57% of patients as well as cART was 64%.[157] However, given improved survival of AIDS patients with the availability of cART and the risk of devastating late neurotoxicity from radiation therapy to the CNS, especially when combined with chemotherapy,[46,158] radiation-sparing approaches may be preferable. The best therapeutic approach in such patients may be shown to be institution of cART to achieve rapid immune reconstitution that may potentially control the EBV-related lymphoproliferative process, along with T-cell–sparing cytotoxic chemotherapy (such as high-dose methotrexate with leucovorin rescue) for the lymphoma. Intriguingly, reports of sustained complete responses in select patients with primary CNS EBV-associated posttransplant lymphoproliferative disorder treated with rituximab alone have been reported.[159] Ongoing clinical trials are investigating the incorporation of rituximab into chemotherapy-based PCNSL treatments, and preliminary data suggest this to be useful.[160,161]

HODGKIN'S LYMPHOMA

Patients with HIV-associated HL generally present at a younger age, with higher-stage disease, less frequent mediastinal involvement, more frequent involvement of extranodal sites of disease, and more frequent "B" symptoms as compared with the general population. Immune status is often relatively good, with a median 275 or so CD4 cells/mm^3 in patients diagnosed with HIV-associated HL.[162] Mixed cellularity or lymphocyte-depleted histology is most commonly seen, in comparison with nodular sclerosis histology in cases developing in HIV-negative patients.[162,163]

In general, complete response rates in HIV-associated HL are relatively high with systemic chemotherapy (50% to >80%), but relapse is common. For patients successfully treated for HL, long-term control of HIV appears to improve overall survival.[163] There is no separate standard of care for HIV-HL, but conventional chemotherapy regimens such as ABVD (doxorubicin, bleomycin, vinblastine, and dacarbazine) or combined-modality therapy are used, as is autologous stem cell transplant in the second-line setting. CNS evaluation and prophylaxis are not indicated because the CNS is uncommonly involved.

HPV-ASSOCIATED CANCER IN HIV INFECTION

HIV-infected patients have an increased incidence of several cancers caused by HPV, including cancer of the cervix, anus, penis, vulva, oral pharynx, and tonsil.[164,165] Only cancer of the cervix is considered AIDS-defining, as cervical cancer was included in part to promote the integration of gynecologic care into the care of HIV-infected women.[1] The increase in these cancers is related both to an increased exposure to oncogenic strains of HPV and an impaired ability to clear these strains attributed to HIV-associated immunodeficiency. HIV-infected women have about a fivefold increased incidence of cervical cancer as compared with HIV-uninfected women,[165] as well as an increased risk of premalignant cervical,[166] vulvovaginal, and anal intraepithelial neoplasia.[167] Although not AIDS defining, people with HIV, especially women and MSM, have a markedly increased risk of anal cancer. The annual incidence of anal cancer in patients with HIV in the United States, estimated at 80 per 100,000 individuals, is much higher than that of the general population, and is increasing.[165] Other HPV-associated cancers, especially cancers of the oral pharynx and tonsil, have also increased in the past decade in HIV-infected individuals.

CERVICAL CANCER

Prevention of cervical cancer is an important part of care for women with HIV. HIV-infected women require regular periodic cervical Papanicolaou (Pap) testing.[168] The CDC and the U.S. Preventative Services Task Force recommend cytologic screening as part of the initial evaluation when HIV is diagnosed.[169] If the initial Pap smear is normal, additional evaluation should be repeated within 6 months. Thereafter women with normal PAP smears should be re-evaluated at least annually. Pap smears showing severe inflammation with reactive squamous cellular changes should be repeated within 3 months. Additional evaluation of HPV DNA, with a subsequent screening frequency of 6 months in women with detectable high-risk subtypes of HPV and yearly in those without high risk HPV, has been proposed as a more individualized screening algorithm.[170] If a Pap smear shows squamous intraepithelial lesions or atypical squamous cells of undetermined significance, cervical colposcopic examination with directed biopsies of mucosal abnormalities is indicated. Management of premalignant cervical lesions in woman with HIV, especially those with low CD4 counts, is more complicated than that in HIV-negative women because of higher rates of positive margins and recurrent cervical intraepithelial neoplasia (CIN).[171,172] Low-grade lesions (CIN1) are generally observed closely, and higher-grade lesions (CIN2-3) are generally treated. Initiation of cART and associated immune reconstitution has been associated with regression of lesions over time in certain cases, and may decrease the risk of recurrence.[173] Treatment options for CIN include ablative therapy, loop excision of the transformation zone, or conization procedures, and should be individualized based on lesion size and location.

Invasive cervical cancer should largely be approached using principles of oncologic management that guide treatment in HIV-negative patients. The International Federation of Gynecology and Obstetrics staging system, used for non–HIV-infected patients, is used in this population as well. More recently, ^{18}FDG-PET has been incorporated in the initial assessment of women with cervical cancer, largely because of the prognostic value of FDG-avid para-aortic lymph nodes. However, in women with HIV and cervical cancer, results should be interpreted with the understanding that uncontrolled HIV viremia is associated with lymph node ^{18}FDG-avidity.[174] Treatment is based on clinical stage. There are no clinical trials specific to HIV-infected women with cervical cancer. In the absence of information to the contrary, HIV-positive women with cervical cancer should be treated in the same manner as those without HIV infection, with cART integrated into the overall treatment plan.

ANAL CANCER

Given biologic similarities to cervical cancer and the effectiveness of cervical cancer screening, some experts have suggested that routine periodic cytologic examination of the anal mucosa should also be considered in high-risk individuals,[175] and programs to screen HIV-infected women and men for anal intraepithelial neoplasia and to treat high-grade lesions are being considered. This approach has the potential to prevent anal cancer by detecting and treating premalignant lesions. Modeled estimates of the clinical benefits and cost-effectiveness of screening HIV-positive MSM for anal squamous intraepithelial lesions and anal squamous cell cancer indicate that Pap screening every 1 to 2 years, beginning in early HIV disease, could potentially result in an incremental cost-effectiveness ratio of $13,000 to $16,000 per quality-adjusted life-year saved, offering quality-adjusted life expectancy benefits at a cost comparable with other accepted clinical preventive interventions.[176] However, this approach has not yet been tested in prospective studies, and it has not been determined what effect screening and treatment of precancerous lesions has on the development of anal cancer. Also, a major difference between anal and cervical cancer is the greater difficulty in doing preventive surgery on precancerous lesions of the anus. The primary tool to screen for anal cancer is cytology of the anal epithelium. Abnormal cytology should be followed up with high-resolution anoscopy if possible.

Treatment decisions are based on the grade of the lesion. Current options for high-grade anal intraepithelial neoplasia include local treatment with topical immune modulators (e.g., imiquimod)[177,178] or antiviral agents (e.g., cidofovir),[179] electrocautery, laser or infrared coagulation,[180,181] and surgery.

The standard of care for stages I–III anal cancer is concurrent chemoradiation, and patients with HIV should receive standard regimens. Given concern of hematologic toxicity associated with mitomycin-C–based chemoradiation in patients with HIV, cisplatin-based regimens have been advocated by some. In the pre-cART era, patients with CD4 counts less than 200 cells/mm^3 were more likely to suffer treatment-related toxicity including cytopenias, intractable diarrhea, moist desquamation requiring hospitalization, or a colostomy either for a therapy-related complication or for salvage, whereas patients with 200 or more CD4 cells/mm^3 appeared to have better disease control with acceptable morbidity.[182] However, with the availability of cART, as well as increasing use of intensity-modulated radiation therapy in the treatment of anal cancer over the past decade, toxicities associated with concurrent chemoradiation in this patient population may have decreased. Outcomes in patients with HIV receiving concurrent chemoradiation, including mitomycin-C–based therapy, appear comparable to that of the general population.[183] The alternative to chemoradiation is surgical abdominoperineal resection, leaving patients with a permanent colostomy. Abdominoperineal resection is an option for patients with poor performance status or who do not wish to undergo concurrent chemoradiation, but should generally be employed only for the management of locoregional recurrence.

FUTURE DIRECTIONS

Many HIV-associated cancers are associated with oncogenic viruses. In this regard, HIV can play a varied role. It can induce an immunosuppressed host in which oncogenic viral infection and opportunistic neoplasia can develop relatively unchecked. HIV can stimulate immune system cytokine production that promotes cellular proliferation and oligoclonal expansions of premalignant cells. Many HIV-associated cancers thus appear to be preventable, through measures to prevent or treat the infection with HIV or the specific oncogenic virus. The HBV and HPV vaccines, for example, hold the potential to dramatically reduce the incidence of hepatocellular, anogenital, and head and neck cancers. Also, studies of the biology of the oncogenic viruses may lead to more targeted treatment or prevention strategies.

The introduction of cART led to a marked decrease in the incidence of AIDS-associated tumors that are associated with very low CD4 counts. As the cART era enters its second decade, however, other trends are beginning to emerge. NADMs are an increasingly important cause of morbidity and mortality.[17,19] For some cancers, there are known biological differences between those that arise in HIV-infected patients and those that arise in HIV-uninfected patients. In HL, for example, HIV-infected patients are more likely than the general population to present with mixed cellularity and lymphocyte depleted subtypes. However, in other cancers, such biologic differences have not been established. Until recently, HIV-infected patients have been excluded from most clinical trials of non-HIV–related tumors, and there are few specific clinical trial data to guide therapy. The NCI recently started an initiative to permit and encourage enrollment of HIV-infected patients on NCI-funded cancer trials when there are not clear contraindications. In the absence of evidence for specialized cancer treatment regimens in patients with HIV, standard therapeutic approaches should be strongly considered, especially in patients with good performance status and who are free of other HIV infectious comorbidities.

With the availability of cART, many such patients are now able to tolerate standard cancer therapy, including allogeneic stem cell transplantation.[184] Special considerations in treating patients with HIV and cancer include whether to modify the standard treatment for the cancer, whether to continue or start cART, and whether prophylaxis is required for PCP or MAI. Special attention should be paid to potential drug-drug interactions between antiretroviral agents and chemotherapeutic agents. Additionally, oncologists should be aware that protease inhibitors, especially nelfinavir, may have radiosensitizing effects. Pharmacokinetic studies evaluating the effect of commonly used antiretroviral agents on chemotherapeutic agents are warranted.[185,186] For surgically managed tumors, cART use should follow Department of Health and Human Services guidelines. In patients for whom chemotherapy or radiation is required, most physicians with experience in this area recommend the use of cART in most cases unless there is a clear reason not to. Trimethoprim-sulfamethoxazole is recommended for patients with a CD4 count less than 200 cells/mm^3, but more liberal use may be warranted in patients undergoing chemotherapy and/or radiotherapy. It should be used in all patients receiving lymphotoxic regimens, regardless of baseline CD4 count.

Although increased knowledge about treatment outcomes for patients with HIV and cancer are required, it appears that with the better-studied tumors, treatment outcomes for those with HIV-related malignancies equivalent to that of HIV-seronegative patients may be attainable.[47,183] In order to promote the oncologic care of patients with HIV/AIDS, it will be important for clinical trials to include or focus on this population so that informative data become available.[187]

PRACTICE OF ONCOLOGY

Selected References

The full list of references for this chapter appears in the online version.

1. MMWR: 1993 Revised Classification System for HIV Infection and Expanded Surveillance Case Definition for AIDS Among Adolescents and Adults, MMWR. Atlanta, Centers for Disease Control, 1992.
3. Walensky RP, Paltiel AD, Losina E, et al. The survival benefits of AIDS treatment in the United States. *J Infect Dis* 2006;194:11.
4. Lundgren JD, Babiker A, El-Sadr W, et al. Inferior clinical outcome of the CD4+ cell count-guided antiretroviral treatment interruption strategy in the SMART study: role of CD4+ Cell counts and HIV RNA levels during follow-up. *J Infect Dis* 2008;197:1145.
6. Bonnet F, Burty C, Lewden C, et al. Changes in cancer mortality among HIV-infected patients: the Mortalite 2005 Survey. *Clin Infect Dis* 2009;48:633.
12. Yarchoan R, Tosato G, Little RF. Therapy insight: AIDS-related malignancies—the influence of antiviral therapy on pathogenesis and management. *Nat Clin Pract Oncol* 2005;2:406.
15. Burgi A, Brodine S, Wegner S, et al. Incidence and risk factors for the occurrence of non-AIDS-defining cancers among human immunodeficiency virus-infected individuals. *Cancer* 2005;104:1505.
16. Engels EA, Biggar RJ, Hall HI, et al. Cancer risk in people infected with human immunodeficiency virus in the United States. *Int J Cancer* 2008;123:187.
18. Lewden C, Salmon D, Morlat P, et al. Causes of death among human immunodeficiency virus (HIV)-infected adults in the era of potent antiretroviral therapy: emerging role of hepatitis and cancers, persistent role of AIDS. *Int J Epidemiol* 2005;34:121.
21. Hymes KB, Cheung T, Greene JB, et al. Kaposi's sarcoma in homosexual men—a report of eight cases. *Lancet* 1981;2:598.
23. Chang Y, Cesarman E, Pessin MS, et al. Identification of herpesvirus-like DNA sequences in AIDS-associated Kaposi's sarcoma. *Science* 1994;266:1865.
25. Martin JN, Ganem DE, Osmond DH, et al. Sexual transmission and the natural history of human herpesvirus 8 infection. *N Engl J Med* 1998;338:948.

30. Krown SE, Testa MA, Huang J. AIDS-related Kaposi's sarcoma: prospective validation of the AIDS Clinical Trials Group staging classification. AIDS Clinical Trials Group Oncology Committee. *J Clin Oncol* 1997;15:3085.
34. Mbulaiteye SM, Katabira ET, Wabinga H, et al. Spectrum of cancers among HIV-infected persons in Africa: the Uganda AIDS-Cancer Registry Match Study. *Int J Cancer* 2006;118:985.
43. Engels EA, Pfeiffer RM, Landgren O, et al. Immunologic and virologic predictors of AIDS-related non-Hodgkin lymphoma in the highly active antiretroviral therapy era. *J Acquir Immune Defic Syndr* 2010;54:78.
47. Dunleavy K, Little RF, Pittaluga S, et al. The role of tumor histogenesis, FDG-PET, and short course EPOCH with dose-dense rituximab (SC-EPOCH-RR) in HIV-associated diffuse large B-cell lymphoma. *Blood* 2010;115(15):3017.
50. Feng H, Shuda M, Chang Y, et al. Clonal integration of a polyomavirus in human Merkel cell carcinoma. *Science* 2008;319:1096.
54. Moore PS, Boshoff C, Weiss RA, et al. Molecular mimicry of human cytokine and cytokine response pathway genes by KSHV. *Science* 1996;274:1739.
57. Boshoff C, Endo Y, Collins PD, et al. Angiogenic and HIV-inhibitory functions of KSHV-encoded chemokines. *Science* 1997;278:290.
65. Butler LM, Osmond DH, Jones AG, et al. Use of saliva as a lubricant in anal sexual practices among homosexual men. *J Acquir Immune Defic Syndr* 2009;50:162.
68. Moore PS. Transplanting cancer: donor-cell transmission of Kaposi sarcoma. *Nat Med* 2003;9:506.
73. Krown SE, Metroka C, Wernz JC. Kaposi's sarcoma in the acquired immune deficiency syndrome: a proposal for uniform evaluation, response, and staging criteria. AIDS Clinical Trials Group Oncology Committee. *J Clin Oncol* 1989;7:1201.
75. Bower M, Weir J, Francis N, et al. The effect of HAART in 254 consecutive patients with AIDS-related Kaposi's sarcoma. *AIDS* 2009;23:1701.
77. Martinez V, Caumes E, Gambotti L, et al. Remission from Kaposi's sarcoma on HAART is associated with suppression of HIV replication and is independent of protease inhibitor therapy. *Br J Cancer* 2006;94:1000.
78. Bower M, Nelson M, Young AM, et al. Immune reconstitution inflammatory syndrome associated with Kaposi's sarcoma. *J Clin Oncol* 2005;23:5224.
79. Gill PS, Wernz J, Scadden DT, et al. Randomized phase III trial of liposomal daunorubicin versus doxorubicin, bleomycin, and vincristine in AIDS-related Kaposi's sarcoma. *J Clin Oncol* 1996;14:2353.
81. Northfelt DW, Dezube BJ, Thommes JA, et al. Pegylated-liposomal doxorubicin versus doxorubicin, bleomycin, and vincristine in the treatment of AIDS-related Kaposi's sarcoma: results of a randomized phase III clinical trial. *J Clin Oncol* 1998;16:2445.
83. Welles L, Saville MW, Lietzau J, et al. Phase II trial with dose titration of paclitaxel for the therapy of human immunodeficiency virus-associated Kaposi's sarcoma. *J Clin Oncol* 1998;16:1112.
84. Gill PS, Tulpule A, Espina BM, et al. Paclitaxel is safe and effective in the treatment of advanced AIDS- related Kaposi's sarcoma. *J Clin Oncol* 1999; 17:1876.
93. Martin DF, Kuppermann BD, Wolitz RA, et al. Oral ganciclovir for patients with cytomegalovirus retinitis treated with a ganciclovir implant. Roche Ganciclovir Study Group. *N Engl J Med* 1999;340:1063.
97. Soulier J, Grollet L, Oksenhendler E, et al. Kaposi's sarcoma-associated herpesvirus-like DNA sequences in multicentric Castleman's disease. *Blood* 1995;86:1276.
101. Oksenhendler E, Carcelain G, Aoki Y, et al. High levels of human herpesvirus 8 viral load, human interleukin-6, interleukin-10, and C reactive protein correlate with exacerbation of multicentric Castleman disease in HIV-infected patients. *Blood* 2000;96:2069.
102. Aoki Y, Yarchoan R, Wyvill K, et al. Detection of viral interleukin-6 in Kaposi sarcoma-associated herpesvirus-linked disorders. *Blood* 2001;97: 2173.
104. Gerard L, Berezne A, Galicier L, et al. Prospective study of rituximab in chemotherapy-dependent human immunodeficiency virus associated multicentric Castleman's disease: ANRS 117 CastlemaB Trial. *J Clin Oncol* 2007;25:3350.
106. Casper C, Nichols WG, Huang M-L, et al. Remission of HHV-8 and HIV-associated multicentric Castleman disease with ganciclovir treatment. *Blood* 2004;103:1632.
115. IARC: WHO Classification of Tumours of Haematopoetic and Lymphoid Tissues. 4th ed. Lyon: IARC, 2008.
116. Biggar RJ, Jaffe ES, Goedert JJ, et al. Hodgkin lymphoma and immunodeficiency in persons with HIV/AIDS. *Blood* 2006;108:3786.
117. Carbone A, Gloghini A, Larocca LM, et al. Expression profile of MUM1/IRF4, BCL-6, and CD138/syndecan-1 defines novel histogenetic subsets of human immunodeficiency virus-related lymphomas. *Blood* 2001;97:744.
120. Miralles P, Berenguer J, Ribera JM, et al. Prognosis of AIDS-related systemic non-Hodgkin lymphoma treated with chemotherapy and highly active antiretroviral therapy depends exclusively on tumor-related factors. *J Acquir Immune Defic Syndr* 2007;44:167.
122. Sparano JA, Lee JY, Kaplan LD, et al. Rituximab plus concurrent infusional EPOCH chemotherapy is highly effective in HIV-associated B-cell non-Hodgkin lymphoma. *Blood* 2010;115:3008.
123. Kaplan LD, Lee JY, Ambinder RF, et al. Rituximab does not improve clinical outcome in a randomized phase III trial of CHOP with or without rituximab in patients with HIV-associated non-Hodgkin's lymphoma: AIDS-malignancies consortium trial 010. *Blood* 2005;106(5)1538.
125. Boue F, Gabarre J, Gisselbrecht C, et al. Phase II trial of CHOP plus rituximab in patients with HIV-associated non-Hodgkin's lymphoma. *J Clin Oncol* 2006;24:4123.
127. Spina M, Jaeger U, Sparano JA, et al. Rituximab plus infusional cyclophosphamide, doxorubicin, and etoposide in HIV-associated non-Hodgkin lymphoma: pooled results from 3 phase 2 trials. *Blood* 2005;105:1891.
130. Wang ES, Straus DJ, Teruya-Feldstein J, et al. Intensive chemotherapy with cyclophosphamide, doxorubicin, high-dose methotrexate/ifosfamide, etoposide, and high-dose cytarabine (CODOX-M/IVAC) for human immunodeficiency virus-associated Burkitt lymphoma. *Cancer* 2003;98:1196.
140. Delecluse HJ, Anagnostopoulos I, Dallenbach F, et al. Plasmablastic lymphomas of the oral cavity: a new entity associated with the human immunodeficiency virus infection. *Blood* 1997;89:1413.
148. Newell ME, Hoy JF, Cooper SG, et al. Human immunodeficiency virus-related primary central nervous system lymphoma: factors influencing survival in 111 patients. *Cancer* 2004;100:2627.
155. Corcoran C, Rebe K, van der Plas H, et al. The predictive value of cerebrospinal fluid Epstein-Barr viral load as a marker of primary central nervous system lymphoma in HIV-infected persons. *J Clin Virol* 2008;42:433.
156. Diamond C, Taylor TH, Im T, et al. Highly active antiretroviral therapy is associated with improved survival among patients with AIDS-related primary central nervous system non-Hodgkin's lymphoma. *Curr HIV Res* 2006;4:375.
165. Chaturvedi AK, Madeleine MM, Biggar RJ, et al. Risk of human papillomavirus-associated cancers among persons with AIDS. *J Natl Cancer Inst* 2009;101:1120.
168. Heard I. Prevention of cervical cancer in women with HIV. *Curr Opin HIV AIDS* 2009;4:68.
169. Workowski RA, Benman SM. Sexually transmitted diseases treatment guidelines, 2006. *MMWR Morb Mortal Wkly Rep* 2006;55(RR11):1.
175. Palefsky JM. Anal cancer prevention in HIV-positive men and women. *Curr Opin Oncol* 2009;21:433.
190. Sparano JA, Lee S, Chen MG, et al. Phase II trial of infusional cyclophosphamide, doxorubicin, and etoposide in patients with HIV-associated non-Hodgkin's lymphoma: an Eastern Cooperative Oncology Group Trial (E1494). *J Clin Oncol* 2004;22:1491.

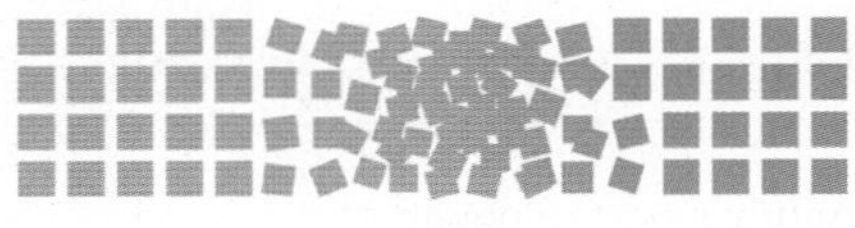

CHAPTER 142 TRANSPLANTATION-RELATED MALIGNANCIES

SMITA BHATIA AND RAVI BHATIA

An important and potentially devastating complication of hematopoietic cell transplantation (HCT) is the occurrence of subsequent malignant neoplasms (SMNs).[1–13] The magnitude of risk of SMNs after HCT ranges from 4-fold to 11-fold that of the general population. The estimated actuarial incidence is reported to be 3.5% at 10 years, increasing to 12.8% at 15 years among recipients of allogeneic HCT (Table 142.1).

Several host and clinical factors are associated with an increased risk of SMNs after HCT. These include age at HCT, exposure to chemotherapy and radiation prior to HCT, use of total-body irradiation (TBI) and high-dose chemotherapy for myeloablation, infection with viruses such as Epstein-Barr virus (EBV) and hepatitis B and C viruses, immunodeficiency after HCT aggravated by the use of immunosuppressive drugs for prophylaxis and treatment of graft-versus-host disease (GVHD), type of transplantation (autologous vs. allogeneic), source of hematopoietic stem cell, and primary malignancy.[1,2]

The heterogeneous nature of SMNs, with differing clinicopathologic characteristics, precludes assessment of risk factors in aggregate. It has become conventional practice to classify SMNs into three distinct groups[2]: (1) myelodysplasia (MDS) and acute myeloid leukemia (AML); (2) lymphoma, including lymphoproliferative disorders; and (3) solid tumors. Although secondary leukemia and lymphoma develop relatively early in the posttransplantation period, secondary solid tumors have a longer latency (Fig. 142.1). In this chapter the three broad categories of SMNs seen among patients undergoing HCT are discussed, with emphasis on clinical presentation, magnitude of risk and associated risk factors, current insights into pathogenesis, and treatment options and outcome of patients with these malignancies.

MYELODYSPLASIA AND ACUTE MYELOID LEUKEMIA

Therapy-related myelodysplasia (t-MDS) and therapy-related acute myeloid leukemia (t-AML) have emerged as the major cause of nonrelapse mortality in patients undergoing autologous HCT for Hodgkin's lymphoma (HL) and non-Hodgkin's lymphoma.[4,14] Depending on the size of study population and the completeness of follow-up, the cumulative probability of t-MDS/t-AML ranges from 1.1% at 20 months to 24.3% at 43 months after autologous HCT, with a median latency of 12 to 24 months after HCT (range, 4 months to 6 years).

Clinicopathologic Syndromes

Two types of t-MDS/t-AML are recognized in the World Health Organization classification, depending on the causative therapeutic exposure: alkylating agent/radiation and topoisomerase II inhibitor.[15]

Alkylating Agent/Radiation-Related t-MDS/t-AML

In patients exposed to alkylating agents, t-MDS/t-AML usually appears 4 to 7 years after exposure. Approximately two thirds of patients present with MDS and the remainder with AML with myelodysplastic features. Patients frequently present with cytopenias. Multilineage dysplasia is often present. There is a high prevalence of abnormalities involving chromosomes 5 (-5/del[5q]) and 7 (-7/del[7q]).

Topoisomerase II Inhibitor-Related AML

AML secondary to topoisomerase II inhibitors presents as overt leukemia, without a preceding myelodysplastic phase. The latency is brief, ranging from 6 months to 5 years, and is associated with balanced translocations involving chromosome bands 11q23 or 21q22. Other translocations including inv(18)(p13q22) or t(17,19)(q22;q12) have been reported.[16]

Clinical Diagnosis

The common and nonspecific nature of cytopenias after autologous HCT resulted in the development of criteria for diagnosing t-MDS/t-AML after HCT. These include (1) significant marrow dysplasia in at least two cell lines, (2) peripheral cytopenias without alternative explanations, and (3) blasts in the marrow defined by French-American-British classification.[17] Because many patients may not have an increase in blasts, presence of a clonal cytogenetic abnormality in addition to morphologic criteria of dysplasia may aid in making this diagnosis.

Risk Factors for t-MDS/t-AML after HCT

Several studies have described an increased risk of t-MDS/t-AML with host factors (older age at HCT),[1] pretransplantation therapy with alkylating agents, topoisomerase II inhibitors, and radiation therapy,[4] use of peripheral blood hematopoietic cells, method of stem cell mobilization (priming with etoposide), difficult stem cell harvests, conditioning with TBI, number of CD34$^+$ cells infused, and a history of multiple transplants (Table 142.1).[1,4,12,18,19]

The impact of pre-HCT chemotherapy and radiotherapy on the risk of t-MDS and t-AML after HCT points toward an origin of events prior to HCT. A role for pretransplantation exposures is further supported by the observation that specific cytogenetic abnormalities observed posttransplantation have

TABLE 142.1

RISK FACTORS FOR SUBSEQUENT MALIGNANT NEOPLASMS (SMNS) AFTER HEMATOPOIETIC CELL TRANSPLANTATION (HCT)

Study (Ref.)	Cohort Size/No. of SMNs	Time to (y, median)	Incidence (%)	Relative Risk	Risk Factors	Outcomes (% Alive)
ALL SUBSEQUENT MALIGNANT NEOPLASMS						
Witherspoon et al. (2)[a]	2,245/35	—	—	6.7	■ Antithymocyte globulin ■ Anti-CD3 monoclonal antibody ■ TBI	14
Bhatia et al. (1)[a]	2,150/53	—	9.9 (13 y)	11.6	—	32
Kolb et al. (11)[b]	1,036/53	—	11.5 (15 y)	3.8	Older age at HCT	81
THERAPY-RELATED MYELODYSPLASIA/ACUTE MYELOID LEUKEMIA AFTER AUTOLOGOUS HCT						
Krishnan et al. (4)	612/22	1.9	8.6 (6 y)	—	■ Etoposide (stem cell priming) ■ Peripheral blood stem cell transplant ■ Pretransplant radiation	32
Stone (18)	262/20	2.6	18 (6 y)	—	■ Number of chemotherapy regimens ■ Previous radiation ■ Age >38 y ■ Low platelet counts ■ Prolonged interval between diagnosis and HCT	—
Bhatia et al. (1)	258/10	3.0	13.5 (6 y)	—	■ Peripheral blood stem cell transplant ■ Age >35 y	20
Milligan et al. (12)	4,998/66	—	4.6 (5 y: HL) 3.0 (5 y: NHL)	—	■ Age at HCT ■ TBI ■ Number of transplants ■ Years from diagnosis to HCT	—
Friedberg et al. (19)	552/41	—	19.8 (10 y)	—	■ Fewer number of cells infused	17
LYMPHOMA AFTER ALLOGENEIC HCT						
EBV-associated posttransplant lymphoproliferative disorder						
Bhatia et al. (1)	2,150/22	0.2 years	1.6 (4 y)	105.6	■ Primary diagnosis of immunodeficiency ■ Antithymocyte globulin (preparative regimen or GVHD prophylaxis) ■ T-cell depletion	9
Curtis et al. (57)	42,349 (person-years at risk)/78	0.4 years	1 (10 y)	51.5	■ HLA mismatch ■ Unrelated donor transplantation ■ T-cell depletion of donor marrow ■ Antithymocyte globulin ■ Anti-CD3 monoclonal antibody ■ TBI ■ Acute GVHD (grades II to IV) ■ Chronic GVHD (extensive)	15
Landgren et al. (56)	26,901/127	83% within first year	Patients with no major risk factors: 0.2% Patients with 1, 2, or 3 or more risk factors: (1.1%, 3.6%, 8.1%, respectively)	—	■ T-cell depletion of donor marrow ■ ATG use ■ Unrelated/ donor mismatch grafts ■ Acute or chronic GVHD ■ Older age at HCT ■ Second HCTs	

(continued)

TABLE 142.1

(CONTINUED)

Study (Ref.)	Cohort Size/No. of SMNs	Time to (y, median)	Incidence (%)	Relative Risk	Risk Factors	Outcomes (% Alive)
Hodgkin's lymphoma after transplantation						
Rowlings et al. (5)	18,531/8	4.2 years	—	6.2	■ Acute GVHD (grade II to IV) ■ Chronic GVHD	75
SOLID TUMORS AFTER HCT						
Curtis et al. (3)[b]	19,229/80	—	6.7 (15 y)	2.7	■ TBI ■ Younger age at HCT ■ Chronic GVHD (squamous cell cancer)	55
Bhatia et al. (13)[a]	2,129/29	—	6.1 (10 y)	2.0	■ Younger age at HCT	90
Bhatia et al. (1)[a]	2,150/17	4	5.6 (13 y)	3.2	■ TBI	60
Rizzo et al. (6)[b]	28,874/ 189	—	3.3 (15y)	2.1	■ TBI ■ Young age at exposure ■ Chronic GVHD and male sex (squamous cell carcinoma)	—

TBI, total-body irradiation; HL, Hodgkin's lymphoma; NHL, non-Hodgkin's lymphoma; EBV, Epstein-Barr virus; GVHD, graft-versus-host disease; HLA, human leukocyte antigen.
[a]Allogeneic and autologous HCT.
[b]Allogeneic HCT only.

also been observed in the pretransplant marrow or peripheral blood graft among patients who develop t-MDS/t-AML after HCT, supporting a role for genetic abnormalities induced by prior cytotoxic chemotherapy in the etiology of t-MDS/t-AML.

The association of t-MDS/t-AML with TBI remains controversial. TBI at 12 Gy does not increase the risk, whereas an increased risk is observed with TBI at 13.2 Gy.[20] An association with TBI indicates that the disease may arise from residual stem cells that persist in the patient despite myeloablative treatment, rather than from reinfused stem cells, although TBI-induced alteration in the hematopoietic microenvironment may contribute to the development of t-MDS/t-AML. Whether t-MDS/t-AML arises from the graft, from residual cells in the patient, or as a result of a damaged microenvironment needs to be determined.

Recipients of CD34-enriched cells isolated from peripheral blood after chemotherapy priming and growth factors are at a higher risk of t-MDS/t-AML as compared with recipients of CD34+ cells from the bone marrow.[1,4] Potential explanations include harvesting of hematopoietic precursor cells damaged by chemotherapy at a time before they have completed DNA repair or an overrepresentation of damaged cells in the mobilized product. Supporting this hypothesis is the study[4] demonstrating an increased risk of t-AML with 11q23 abnormalities among patients mobilized with high doses of etoposide for collection of stem cells prior to autologous HCT.

Patients receiving a smaller number of reinfused cells, or those experiencing difficult stem cell harvests, have been reported to be at an increased risk of t-MDS.[19] Reconstitution of bone marrow clearly may result in a great proliferative stress in the setting of low stem cell numbers, increasing susceptibility

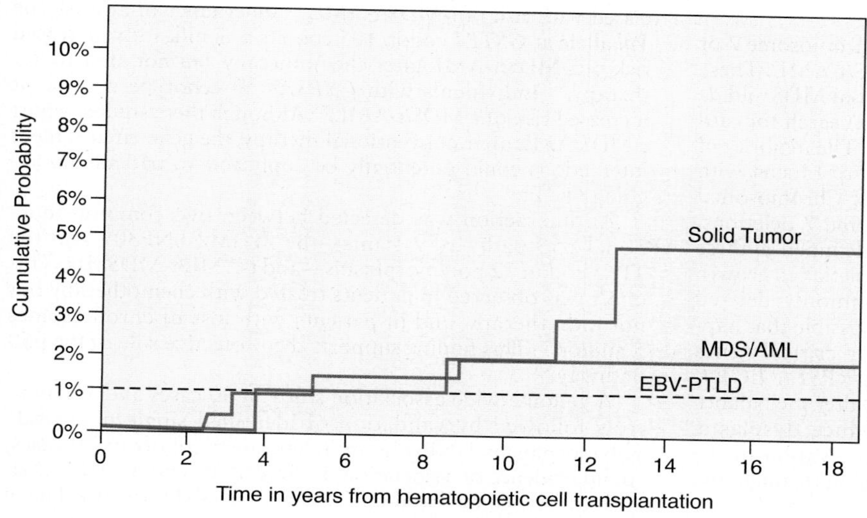

FIGURE 142.1 Cumulative probability of subsequent malignancies after hematopoietic cell transplantation. MDS, myelodysplasia; AML, acute myeloid leukemia; EBV, Epstein-Barr virus; PTLD, posttransplantation lymphoproliferative disorder. (Adapted from ref. 1.)

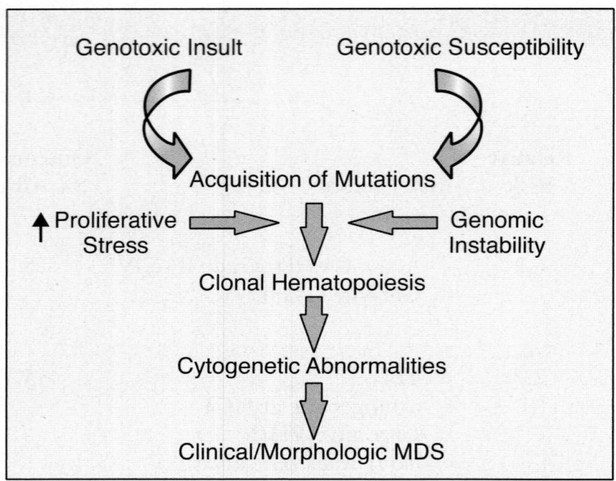

FIGURE 142.2 Proposed pathogenesis of therapy-related myelodysplasia (MDS)/acute myeloid leukemia after autologous hematopoietic cell transplantation.

to irreversible DNA damage associated with t-MDS. These observations are supported by *in vitro* data suggesting an increased proliferative stress placed on committed progenitors at the expense of the primitive progenitors.[21] Alternatively, reduced ability to harvest cells could indicate an existing defect in marrow function.

Pathogenesis of t-MDS/t-AML

t-MDS/t-AML is a clonal hematologic disorder that results from acquired genetic or epigenetic changes induced by cytotoxic therapy in hematopoietic stem cells. Improved understanding of the molecular pathogenesis of t-MDS/t-AML is required to allow development of strategies to identify populations at increased risk and of therapies to decrease the morbidity and mortality associated with this complication. Furthermore, t-MDS/t-AML offers a unique perspective on mutagen-induced carcinogenesis. The clinical and epidemiologic data previously discussed suggest that t-MDS/t-AML after autologous HCT results from genetic damage to the stem cell from pretransplant cytotoxic treatment, which may be potentiated by the transplant process itself. A hypothetical schema for the sequence of events leading to the development of t-MDS/t-AML after autologous HCT is shown in Figure 142.2.

Genetic Lesions associated with t-MDS/t-AML

Loss of chromosome 5 or del(5q) and loss of chromosome 7 or del(7q) are recurring abnormalities in t-MDS/t-AML. These abnormalities are also seen in AML evolving from MDS and *de novo* AML in elderly patients. This has led to a search for candidate tumor suppressor genes in these regions. The majority of patients with 5q deletions exhibit losses at the 5q31 locus, with deletions in 5q33 being seen in some patients. Chromosomal segment 7q22 is a common site of chromosome 7 deletions. Although several candidate genes have been identified in these regions, including genes that regulate hematopoietic cell growth and differentiation, identification of a commonly deleted tumor suppressor gene has been elusive. It is possible that haploinsufficiency and reduced gene dosage for critical genes involved in hematopoiesis on 5q, including *RPS14, EGR1, APC, NPM1*, and *CTNNA1*, may sufficiently alter the balance between growth and differentiation to induce dysplastic hematopoiesis.[22] Alternatively, epigenetic inactivation of the remaining allele or alterations in gene expression through loss of miRNA loci could play a role.

Another possibility is that these chromosomal abnormalities may be secondary events important for disease progression rather than initiation. Abnormalities in chromosome 7 are also associated with myeloid leukemias in genetically predisposed individuals, such as Fanconi anemia or neurofibromatosis type 1.[23] This observation raises the possibility that similar predisposition may be present in patients with t-MDS/t-AML with loss of chromosome 7, 5q, and 7q deletions in familial platelet disorder with leukemia are associated with mutations or deletions of a single *AML1* allele. Balanced translocations involving the *AML1* gene have also been associated with t-MDS/t-AML in patients exposed to topoisomerase II inhibitors. *AML1* point mutations were found in 26 of 110 patients (23.6%) with refractory anemia with excess blasts (RAEB), RAEB in transformation (RAEBt), and AML following MDS.[24] Transgenic expression of *AML1-ETO* leads to immortalization of murine myeloid progenitors but not overt leukemia; additional mutations are required for leukemogenesis.[25] Therefore, altered *AML1* function may have a major role in dysregulation of hematopoietic growth and genomic instability and predispose to leukemia through a multistep process.

The *MLL* gene located at chromosome band 11q23, frequently involved in translocations associated with topoisomerase II inhibitors, has a major role in developmental regulation. Altered *MLL* function, as with *AML1*, may dysregulate hematopoietic growth and genomic instability and predispose to leukemia through a multistep process. The long latency to leukemia in MLL-fusion gene knock-in mice suggests that additional genetic changes are required for evolution of t-AML. The role of *MLL* and *AML1* mutations as early events in the development of t-MDS/t-AML merits further investigation.

A second class of mutations in genes regulating cytokine signaling pathways has been recognized in AML patients. The *RAS* signaling pathway is activated downstream of several cytokine receptors. Constitutively activating point mutations of NRAS are detected in 10% to 15% of t-MDS/AML patients. In contrast mutations of the *FLT3* gene, (point mutations and internal tandem duplications), although commonly seen in *de novo* AML, are not seen in t-MDS/t-AML.[26]

Genetic Susceptibility

Several genetic polymorphisms of enzymes capable of metabolic activation or detoxification of anticancer drugs, such as NAD(P)H:quinone oxidoreductase (NQO1), glutathione-*S*-transferase-M1, -T1, and -P1, and CYP3A4, have been examined for their role in the development of t-MDS/t-AML.[27–30] *NQO1* polymorphism has been shown to be significantly associated with risk of t-MDS/t-AML.[31] Inheritance of at least one *Val* allele at *GSTP1* codon 105 confers a significantly increased risk of t-MDS/t-AML after chemotherapy, but not after radiotherapy.[30] Individuals with *CYP3A4-W* genotype may be at increased risk of t-MDS/t-AML.[28] Although these studies report t-MDS/AML after conventional therapy, the gene-environment interactions could potentially be applicable to patients undergoing HCT.

An interaction was detected between two common functional p53-pathway variants—the *MDM2* SNP309 and the TP53 codon 72 polymorphisms—and t-AML/t-MDS risk. This effect was observed in patients treated with chemotherapy but not radiotherapy, and in patients with loss of chromosomes 5 and/or 7. This finding supports the protective role of the p53 pathway.[32]

A genome-wide association study in 80 cases and 150 controls followed by validation of identified single nucleotide polymorphisms (SNPs) in an independent cohort of 70 cases, found evidence of association of three SNPs with t-MDS/AML with chromosome 5 and/or 7 lesions. The SNPs identified have not been previously studied in t-MDS/t-AML and their biological significance is unknown at this time.[33]

A study of genes that regulate t-MDS/t-AML susceptibility was performed by analyzing mouse strains resistant or susceptible to t-MDS/t-AML induced by the alkylator ethyl-N-nitrosourea. Mice in a PML-RARA background were used for these studies. Thirteen quantitative trait loci on 8 chromosomes were significantly associated with leukemia-free survival, white blood cell count, and spleen weight. The quantitative trait loci regions identified contained several genes with established roles in leukemogenesis. These results suggest that susceptibility to alkylator-induced leukemia in mice is a complex trait related to genes at multiple loci.[34]

Genetic Instability

Genetic instability is hypothesized to be an early event in the development of malignancy, allowing accumulation of multiple mutations in the same cell over time and evolution of a clonal malignant population. T cells from patients who have received chemotherapy for acute lymphoblastic leukemia demonstrate increased frequency of mutations in the hypoxanthine-guanine phosphoribosyltransferase (*HPRT*) reporter gene.[35] Multiple mutations were present in individually isolated mutant T-cell clones from 4 of 15 individuals with high frequency of *HPRT* mutations, consistent with genetic instability.[35] Therefore, treatment with cytotoxic agents can lead to genetic instability in some individuals, which could contribute to the induction of t-MDS/t-AML. The mechanism underlying genetic instability could be related to altered expression or function of cell cycle, apoptosis, or DNA repair regulatory genes.

Defective DNA Repair Mechanisms

DNA repair mechanisms play a major role in maintaining genomic integrity. The major repair pathways include mismatch repair, base excision repair, nucleotide excision repair, and DNA double-strand break repair.[36] Defects in repair proteins and proteins associated with the regulation of repair are connected to many different types of cancer, including t-MDS/t-AML. Defects in several proteins, in particular MSH2 or MLH1, impair the DNA mismatch repair system and result in a mutator phenotype seen in a variety of sporadic and inherited cancers. Ben-Yehuda et al.[37] demonstrated that 94% of the evaluable cases of t-MDS/t-AML had microsatellite instability (MSI), suggesting a role for an inherited defect of a DNA mismatch repair gene. However, another study failed to failed to demonstrate MSI in patients with t-MDS/t-AML.[38] A T>C transition polymorphism has been identified at position −6 of the 3′ splice acceptor site of exon 13 of hMSH2 and may alter the efficiency of RNA splicing. The variant (C) hMSH2 allele was significantly overrepresented in t-MDS/t-AML cases that had previously been treated with O^6-guanine alkylating agents, including cyclophosphamide and procarbazine.[39] It is suggested that this allele may confer moderate alkylation tolerance with concomitant susceptibility to t-MDS/t-AML. Therefore, MSI and defective DNA mismatch repair may contribute to development of t-MDS/t-AML in a subset of patients, but heterogeneity in mechanisms of susceptibility are likely to occur.

The xeroderma pigmentosum group D (*XPD*) gene encodes a DNA helicase that mediates DNA unwinding required for basal transcription and nucleotide excision DNA repair. Smith et al.[40] have shown that XPD codon 751 glutamine-encoding variant significantly associates with risk of developing AML with a chromosome 5q deletion or a chromosome 7q deletion. RAD51 and XRCC3 are involved in double-strand break repair via homologous recombination. The risk of t-MDS/t-AML was significantly increased in the presence of polymorphisms in both the *RAD51* (RAD51-G135C) and *XRCC3* (XRCC3-Thr241Met) genes.[41]

p53 Gene Mutations

The *p53* gene has a critical role in DNA damage response signaling, affecting cell cycle, cell death, and DNA repair pathways. Abnormal *p53* activity could lead to reduced ability to repair DNA damage, resulting in genomic instability and increased susceptibility to leukemogenesis. In patients with *de novo* MDS and AML, *p53* mutations are seen in less than 10% of patients, but are more common in patients with t-MDS/t-AML. Ben-Yehuda et al.[37] identified *p53* mutations in 38% of patients. Mutations were non–germ line and restricted to leukemic cells, and differed from *p53* mutations seen in the original tumors of individual patients.

Horiike et al.[42] identified *p53* mutations in 6 of 12 patients with t-MDS/t-AML with chromosome 5 and/or 7 losses, but did not observe any *p53* mutations in 9 other patients without chromosome 5 and/or 7 involvement. Christiansen et al.[43] observed *p53* mutations in 21 of 77 patients (27%) with t-MDS/t-AML, 19 of whom had received alkylating agents. The *p53* mutations were associated with deletion or loss of 5q and a complex karyotype, were more common in elderly patients, and were associated with an extremely poor prognosis.[43] These studies indicate that *p53* mutations may be observed in certain cytogenetic and prognostic subsets of patients with t-MDS/t-AML, but do not identify a clear role in the pathogenesis.

Telomeric Shortening

Telomeres are noncoding regions of DNA that provide a cap at the ends of chromosomes and prevent dicentric fusion and other chromosomal aberrations. Each somatic cell division is associated with a loss of telomere length. Cumulative telomere shortening can impose a limit on cell divisions and lead to cell senescence. Telomere shortening is also associated with genetic instability. Following HCT, the increased replicative demand on stem cells associated with hematopoietic regeneration can lead to accelerated telomere shortening. Telomere shortening could be an important issue in autologous HCT especially when telomere length in the transplanted cells is already short because of prior chemotherapy, older age at HCT, or increased replicative stress on the stem cells because of a small number of cells transplanted. Analysis of changes in telomere length revealed accelerated telomere shortening in t-MDS/AML patients when compared with matched controls who did not develop t-MDS/t-AML, preceding the onset of t-MDS/t-AML. Patients with t-MDS/t-AML also showed reduced generation of committed progenitors, suggesting that telomere alterations were related to reduced regenerative capacity of hematopoietic stem cells.[44]

Hematopoietic Abnormalities

Autologous HCT for lymphoma and HL is associated with hematopoietic abnormalities including marked and prolonged reduction in primitive progenitor long-term culture-initiating cells and committed progenitor colony-forming cell numbers, altered progenitor expansion potential, and microenvironmental defects. These abnormalities may be related in part to damage to hematopoietic cells from pretransplant chemotherapy because hematopoietic defects can also be seen in pretransplant samples.[21] Although committed progenitors recover to pretransplant levels, primitive progenitor capacity is further depleted and does not show evidence of recovery for up to 2 years after HCT, consistent with extensive proliferation and differentiation of the committed progenitors and subsequent depletion of primitive progenitors during hematopoietic regeneration post-HCT.[21] Pretransplant chemotherapy may also lead to reduced engraftment potential of primitive progenitor cells.[45] HCT may also be associated with defects in the marrow hematopoietic microenvironment, including reduction in stromal precursor growth and reduced capacity to support growth of myeloid progenitors and B progenitors. These microenvironmental defects may contribute to hematopoietic abnormalities posttransplantation. Extensive proliferation of stem cells bearing genotoxic damage posttransplant may have a role in establishment and amplification of an abnormal clone. Alternatively, the numerous replication cycles imposed on hematopoietic stem cells after HCT may result in excessive shortening of telomeres in descendent cells (as previously discussed).

Gene Expression Profiling

Gene expression profiling of acute lymphoblastic leukemia cells at diagnosis has been shown to be predictive of t-MDS/t-AML.[46] Gene expression profiling of $CD34^+$ hematopoietic progenitor cells from t-MDS/t-AML patients has identified different subtypes of t-MDS/t-AML with characteristic gene expression patterns.[47] Common to each subgroup were gene expression patterns characteristic of arrested differentiation in early progenitor cells. Extension of such studies may enhance our understanding of the molecular pathways involved in t-MDS/t-AML.

Outcomes of Patients with t-MDS/t-AML after Autologous HCT

The diagnosis of t-MDS/t-AML after autologous HCT confers a uniformly poor prognosis, with a median survival of 6 months in patients treated with conventional chemotherapy. Allogeneic HCT has been attempted with actuarial survival ranging from 0% to 24% at 3 years.[48] Older age (>37 years), male sex, positive recipient cytomegalovirus serology, absence of complete response at HCT, and intensive conditioning schedules were independently associated with poor outcome.[49] Among t-MDS/t-AML patients with balanced aberrations, 11q23 translocations are an independent adverse risk factor.[50] Treatment-related mortality (TRM) and relapse were reported to be 41% and 27% at 1 year and 48% and 31% at 5 years, respectively, in a large cohort of patients undergoing allogeneic HCT.[51] Disease-free survival (DFS) and overall survival were 32% and 37% at 1 year and 21% and 22% at 5 years, respectively. Age older than 35 years, poor-risk cytogenetics, t-AML not in remission or advanced t-MDS, and donor other than an HLA-identical sibling or a partially or well-matched unrelated donor had adverse impact on DFS and overall survival: 5-year survival for subjects with none, one, two, three, or four of these risk factors was 50%, 26%, 21%, 10%, and 4%, respectively. These studies indicate that in spite of the significant TRM, the DFS was better when transplantation was performed earlier in the evolution of disease because it resulted in a lower relapse rate.

These data also help identify subjects more likely to benefit from allogeneic transplantation. It is important to follow patients at risk for development of t-MDS/t-AML closely to identify the disease early. Prompt transplantation should be considered after diagnosis of t-MDS/t-AML. Innovative transplantation strategies are needed to reduce the high risk of relapse and nonrelapse mortality. Because the poor outcomes of allogeneic transplant for t-MDS/t-AML are related in part to the high risk of TRM, it is important to evaluate the role of reduced-intensity conditioning approaches in this setting. Preliminary reports suggest that allogeneic HCT using reduced-intensity conditioning is feasible and may result in improved outcomes.

Prediction of Risk of t-MDS/t-AML

Because of the poor prognosis associated with t-MDS/t-AML, attempts are underway to identify predictors or early biomarkers to decrease the morbidity associated with this disease. Several studies have attempted to correlate identification of genetically abnormal clones with subsequent risk of t-MDS/t-AML. Assessment of risk of t-MDS/t-AML after autologous HCT is complicated by the lack of a single underlying genetic abnormality. Development of t-MDS/t-AML requires acquisition of several mutations. Moreover, t-MDS/t-AML is a heterogeneous disorder with multiple subtypes characterized by different genetic abnormalities. Therefore, identification of a single genetic abnormality may not necessarily have predictive value for development of t-MDS/t-AML.

Standard Cytogenetics and Fluorescent *in situ* Hybridization

Abnormal clones are frequently detected after autologous HCT for lymphoma. Traweek et al.[52] reported the risk of developing a clonal cytogenetic abnormality typical of MDS to be 9% at 3 years. Five of 10 patients with the abnormal clone developed t-MDS. Stone[18] reported that 50% of sporadically tested posttransplant patients who were hematologically normal had clonal cytogenetic abnormalities. However, fewer than 30% of these patients developed t-MDS/t-AML. Evaluation by fluorescence *in situ* hybridization may enhance sensitivity of detection of chromosomal abnormalities. Significant levels of clonally abnormal cells could be detected by fluorescence *in situ* hybridization prior to high-dose therapy in samples obtained from 20 of 20 patients who developed t-MDS/t-AML, but only 3 of 24 patients did not.[53] However, this technique is locus-specific and requires prior selection of markers for analysis and has limited sensitivity of detection.

Clonality Analysis

The predictive value of clonal bone marrow hematopoiesis for the development of t-MDS/t-AML was investigated in a group of patients undergoing autologous HCT for non-Hodgkin's lymphoma. An X-inactivation–based clonality assay at the human androgen receptor locus (HUMARA) was used. Clonal hematopoiesis at the time of transplantation or after was predictive of t-MDS/t-AML.[54] Five of seven patients with clonal hematopoiesis also had a clonal cytogenetic abnormality involving 50% or more metaphases. This assay is limited by its low sensitivity, requiring a high proportion of monoclonal cells to be present prior to reaching the threshold for detection, and is applicable only to female patients.

Loss of Heterozygosity Analysis and Polymerase Chain Reaction Assays for Point Mutations

Loss of heterozygosity analysis and polymerase chain reaction (PCR) assays for point mutations may be useful for detection of evolution of clonal genetic abnormality after HCT.[55] In loss of heterozygosity analysis, loss of one allele at a particular locus is evaluated, most commonly by PCR. This method is specific and can be adapted to high-throughput strategies, but is relatively insensitive and requires prior selection of loci. This method has not been validated as being a useful predictor of t-MDS/t-AML.

PCR for point mutations and chromosomal translocations is another potentially useful tool. Mutations in genes such as *MLL* or *AML1* or gene rearrangements involving 11q23 gene may be useful markers for risk of subsequent t-MDS/t-AML. This method is highly sensitive but is locus-specific, and the specificity and predictive value of such assays is unknown at present. This test may be most helpful if performed using quantitative techniques that would allow assessment of increasing levels of abnormality.

Reducing Risk of t-MDS/t-AML after Autologous HCT

Our understanding of the etiology and pathogenesis should help develop potential risk-reduction strategies, such as minimization of pretransplant cytotoxic exposure by bringing high-risk patients to HCT earlier in the course of disease. Alteration in hematopoietic cell procurement and conditioning regimens could also be considered. If strategies to develop predictors for patients at high risk prior to HCT are realized, alternative treatment approaches such as allogeneic transplantation or nontransplant modalities may be considered for patients identified at increased risk. Finally, strategies for chemoprevention may be worth exploring in this population.

LYMPHOMAS

Posttransplantation Lymphoproliferative Disorders

Posttransplantation lymphoproliferative disorders (PTLD) is the most common SMN in the first year after allogeneic T-cell–depleted HCT, and is related to a compromised immune status and EBV infection.[56,57] Subgroups of patients at elevated risk of PTLD have been clearly defined for whom prospective monitoring of EBV activation and early therapeutic intervention may be particularly useful. The vast majority of PTLDs develop within the first year. The risk of PTLD is strongly associated with T-cell depletion of the donor marrow, antithymocyte globulin use, unrelated or HLA-mismatched grafts, presence of acute or chronic GVHD, older age at HCT, and multiple transplants. The cumulative incidence is low (0.2%) among patients with no major risk factors, but is increased to 1.1%, 3.6%, and 8.1% with one, two, and three or more major risk factors, respectively. The large majority of the PTLDs have a B-cell origin.

B-cell PTLD, a clinically and morphologically heterogeneous group of diseases, usually develops within the first 6 months after HCT, with a cumulative incidence of 1% to 2% at 10 years. Risk factors include *in vitro* T-cell depletion of the donor marrow, unrelated or HLA-mismatched related donor, use of antithymocyte globulin or anti-CD3 monoclonal antibody for acute GVHD prophylaxis or in the preparative regimen, TBI, and primary immunodeficiency (Table 142.1).[1] The risk of PTLD also depends on the method of T-cell depletion, being considerably higher when specific monoclonal antibodies are used for T-cell depletion (11% to 25%) rather than in patients in whom techniques removing both T and B lymphocytes, such as soybean agglutinin or Campath-1 (<1%), are used.[57] The more recent use of nonmyeloablative therapy coupled with highly immunosuppressive therapy needs close observation for the development of PTLD.

Pathogenesis of B-Cell PTLD

B-cell PTLD is commonly associated with T-cell dysfunction, occurs in the presence of EBV infection, and is thought to develop because of a combination of depressed EBV-specific cellular immunity and the inherent transforming capacities of EBV. EBV is a ubiquitous herpesvirus that infects 95% of individuals by adulthood. The virus persists as a latent infection in B lymphocytes, where reactivation and replication occur intermittently. The latent membrane protein 1 (LMP-1) is one of the EBV-encoded proteins believed to have an important role in B-cell immortalization by inducing the expression of *bcl-2*, which inhibits programmed death of infected cells. LMP-1 is also considered to be an oncogene, and deletions near the 3′end of the *LMP-1* gene, in a region that affects the half-life of the LMP-1 protein, have been reported in some PTLDs. Infection of B cells by EBV also induces high levels of cytokines such as interleukin (IL)-1, IL-5, IL-6, IL-10, CD23, and tumor necrosis factor. Some of these factors have been shown to act as autocrine growth factors, stimulating the proliferation of EBV-transformed B cells and inhibiting their susceptibility to apoptosis.[58]

Cytotoxic T-lymphocyte precursor frequencies are low at 3 months after allogeneic HCT, but appear to normalize at 9 to 12 months, thus correlating with the period when B-cell PTLD is most frequently observed. Moreover, the EBV-specific cytotoxic T lymphocytes home preferentially and induce selective regression of autologous EBV-induced B-cell lymphoproliferative lesions in xenografted severe combined immunodeficiency syndrome mice. These studies have formed the basis for clinical trials using adoptive transfer of EBV-specific cytotoxic T lymphocytes.[59]

Prediction of Risk of B-Cell PTLD

Quantitative competitive PCR is an effective technique for frequent monitoring of DNA load to predict development of PTLD. EBV-specific T lymphocytes are rapidly established following unmanipulated sibling allogeneic HCT. HLA class I tetramers complexed with viral peptides provide direct and rapid assessment of pathogen-specific immunity. However, patients undergoing T-cell–depleted or unrelated cord blood HCT have undetectable EBV-specific T cells, even in the presence of Epstein-Barr viremia.

Treatment of B-Cell PTLD

Close monitoring of patients at increased risk for PTLD allows for early institution of appropriate therapy prior to development of overt disease. Therapeutic approaches include B-cell–specific monoclonal antibodies, and cellular therapy. The efficacy of anti-CD20 monoclonal antibody (rituximab) in the treatment of PTLD has been reported. The drug is more efficacious in patients without mass lesions, forming the basis for recommendations to initiate treatment at an early stage, based on increasing EBV load. Because EBV-associated PTLD results from T-cell dysfunction, reconstitution of "at-risk" patients with EBV-specific cytotoxic T-lymphocyte lines reactivated and expanded *in vitro* has been shown to be efficacious in controlling PTLD, with a decrease in the EBV DNA concentrations and clinical remission.

Late-Onset Lymphoma

Late-occurring lymphoma represents an entity that is distinct from the early-occurring PTLD[60] and is associated with extensive chronic GVHD. HL has also been described after HCT.[5] Mixed cellularity is the most commonly reported subtype, and most of the cases contain the EBV genome. These cases differ from the EBV-PTLD by the absence of risk factors commonly associated with EBV-PTLD, by a later onset (>2.5 years), and relatively good prognosis.

SOLID TUMORS

Solid tumors develop after syngeneic, allogeneic, and autologous HCT, and the magnitude of risk exceeds twofold that of an age- and sex-matched general population.[3,6] The risk increases with time from HCT and, for those who survive 10 or more years after HCT, is reported to be eightfold that of the general population. The risk of solid tumors is higher among those exposed to radiation at a younger age, and rises with the dose of radiation (Table 142.1).[7] Types of solid tumors reported in excess among HCT recipients include melanoma, cancers of the oral cavity and salivary glands, brain, liver, uterine cervix, thyroid, breast, bone, and connective tissue.[3] The magnitude of risk and associated risk factors are detailed in the following sections.

Skin Cancer

The 20-year cumulative incidence of basal cell carcinoma (BCC) and squamous cell carcinoma (SCC) are reported to be 6.5% and 3.4%, respectively, after allogeneic HCT.[7] TBI is a risk factor of BCC particularly among patients younger than 18 years at HCT. Acute GVHD increased the risk of SCC, and chronic GVHD increased the risk of BCC and SCC.[8]

Breast Cancer

The 25-year cumulative incidence of breast cancer is reported to be 11% after allogeneic HCT; the incidence is higher among those exposed to TBI (17%) than among those who did not receive TBI (3%).[9] Allogeneic HCT survivors are at a 2.2-fold increased risk of developing breast cancer, when compared with age- and sex-matched general population. The median latency from HCT to diagnosis of breast cancer is 12.5 years. The risk is increased among those exposed to TBI at a younger age.

Thyroid Cancer

HCT recipients are at a 3.3-fold increased risk of thyroid cancer, when compared with age- and sex-matched general population.[10] Age younger than 10 years at HCT, neck radiation, female sex, and chronic GVHD are associated with an increased risk. Thyroid cancer develops after a latency of 8.5 years and is associated with an excellent outcome.

Pathogenesis of Solid Tumors after HCT

Radiation is the single most important risk factor for the development of solid tumors. These radiogenic cancers have a long latent period, and the risk is frequently high among patients undergoing irradiation at a young age. Immunologic alterations may predispose patients to SCC of the buccal cavity, particularly in view of the association with chronic GVHD.[7] In immunosuppressed patients, oncogenic viruses such as human papillomavirus may contribute to SCC of the skin and buccal mucosa after transplantation.

Patients with a family history of early-onset cancers have been shown to be at an increased risk for developing a SMN. The tumor types occurring in excess in close relatives were also observed as SMNs in patients (cancers of the breast, bone, joint, or soft tissue), indicating that the risk of SMN is associated with a familial predisposition. Genetic predisposition also has a substantial impact on risk of SMNs (e.g., sarcomas in patients with hereditary retinoblastoma). This risk is further increased by radiation and increases with the total dose of radiation.[61]

Chronic tissue stress due to interaction of alloreactive donor cells with host epithelium, may cause genomic alterations and increase the risk of SMNs. This hypothesis was tested by analyzing buccal cells from allotransplanted patients for MSI. MSI was observed in 52% of the allotransplant recipients, but not among healthy or autotransplanted controls.[62] SMNs were identified in five of the MSI-positive patients (14%) and only one of the MSI-negative patients. In an *in vitro* model of mutation analysis, significant induction of frameshift mutations and DNA strand breaks in HaCaT keratinocytes cocultured with mixed lymphocyte cultures were observed, but not after exposure to interferon gamma, tumor necrosis factor-alpha, transforming growth factor-beta, or phytohemagglutinin-stimulated peripheral blood mononuclear cells, suggesting a reactive oxygen species-mediated mechanism. These data indicate that alloreactions may induce genomic alterations in epithelium.

In summary, an interaction of cytotoxic therapy (radiation in particular), genetic predisposition, viral infection, and GVHD with the consequent antigenic stimulation and use of immunosuppressive therapy may play a role in the development of new solid tumors.

Treatment of Patients with Solid Tumors after HCT

Treatment strategies for patients developing solid tumors after HCT are not well defined. Small case series indicate both ends of the spectrum: favorable outcomes and hence a recommendation for an intensive approach and aggressive tumor growth, and early relapse after standard therapy. A comprehensive study of a large number of patients with second solid tumors will help determine the nature of these tumors and their outcomes as compared to *de novo* tumors. Until then, patients with solid tumors should be treated with the best available therapy for that tumor, unless there is compelling evidence that they will not be able to tolerate that therapy.

Screening for Solid Tumors after HCT

Extending the follow-up of HCT recipients beyond 10 years posttransplantation will help clarify the risks of radiation-associated cancers such as breast, lung, and colon cancers. These epithelial cancers typically develop at a median of 15 to 20 years after exposure to radiation therapy, suggesting that HCT survivors face an increasing risk of solid tumors with increasing time from HCT, thus supporting the need for lifelong surveillance.

Preventive measures that need to be considered include programs to educate clinicians and survivors about the risk of SMNs, and measures taken to decrease the morbidity associated with SMNs, such as adopting healthy lifestyle choices. Other measures include intervention programs for smoking cessation; periodic and aggressive screening for breast, lung, skin, colorectal, prostate, thyroid, and cervical cancers; chemoprevention for specific cancers; and avoidance of unnecessary exposure to sunlight, especially among patients who have received radiation. Health counseling should include guidance about smoking cessation, diet, and physical activity. By understanding the risk factors for secondary malignancies, and taking measures to avoid them, it may be possible to decrease the incidence of the most devastating consequences of surviving cancer while maintaining the high cure rates in this population.

Evidence-based guidelines for screening for early detection of cancer in HCT survivors are not available at present, but guidelines published by the American Cancer Society[63] and the National Comprehensive Cancer Network Practice Guidelines in Oncology[64–66] present a reasonable framework for the physicians taking care of this high-risk population. The recommended frequency and age at onset are based on the American Cancer Society recommendations for individuals identified to be at increased risk for the development of these cancers. Colon cancer screening should include colonoscopy with biopsy for dysplasia every 1 to 2 years beginning 10 years after TBI. Cervical screening is recommended annually, beginning at age 18 years, until the age of 45 years, and should be performed with conventional cervical cytology smears. The prostate-specific antigen test and digital rectal examination should be offered annually beginning at age 45. For female patients receiving radiation to the chest and/or TBI, screening recommendations include monthly breast self-examination, beginning at age 20 (or earlier, if the patients have received radiation to the chest at an earlier age), and clinical breast examination, beginning at age 20 (or earlier if needed), performed yearly until age 25, and then every 6 months. The National Comprehensive Cancer Network guidelines also recommend a baseline mammogram at 8 years after exposure to radiation, or at the attained age of 40, whichever occurs first, and then annually. Patients with a history of transfusions prior to 1993 should be screened for viral hepatitis. An examination for cancerous and precancerous lesions of the oral cavity should be in the periodic health examination of patients with oral chronic GVHD.

Selected References

The full list of references for this chapter appears in the online version.

1. Bhatia S, Ramsay NK, Steinbuch M, et al. Malignant neoplasms followin-bone marrow transplantation. *Blood* 1996;87:3633.
2. Witherspoon RP, Fisher LD, Schoch G, et al. Secondary cancers after bone marrow transplantation for leukemia or aplastic anemia. *N Engl J Med* 1989;321:784.
3. Curtis RE, Rowlings PA, Deeg HJ, et al. Solid cancers after bone marrow transplantation. *N Engl J Med* 1997;336:897.
4. Krishnan A, Bhatia S, Slovak ML, et al. Predictors of therapy-related leukemia and myelodysplasia following autologous transplantation for lymphoma: an assessment of risk factors. *Blood* 2000;95:1588.
5. Rowlings PA, Curtis RE, Passweg JR, et al. Increased incidence of Hodgkin's disease after allogeneic bone marrow transplantation. *J Clin Oncol* 1999;17:3122.
6. Rizzo JD, Curtis RE, Socie G, et al. Solid cancers after allogeneic hematopoietic cell transplantation. *Blood* 2009;113:1175.
7. Leisenring W, Friedman DL, Flowers ME, Schwartz JL, Deeg HJ. Nonmelanoma skin and mucosal cancers after hematopoietic cell transplantation. *J Clin Oncol* 2006;24:1119.
9. Friedman DL, Rovo A, Leisenring W, et al. Increased risk of breast cancer among survivors of allogeneic hematopoietic cell transplantation: a report from the FHCRC and the EBMT-Late Effect Working Party. *Blood* 2008;111:939.
10. Cohen A, Rovelli A, Merlo DF, et al. Risk for secondary thyroid carcinoma after hematopoietic stem-cell transplantation: an EBMT Late Effects Working Party Study. *J Clin Oncol* 2007;25:2449.
13. Bhatia S, Louie AD, Bhatia R, et al. Solid cancers after bone marrow transplantation. *J Clin Oncol* 2001;19:464.
14. Bhatia S, Robison LL, Francisco L, et al. Late mortality in survivors of autologous hematopoietic-cell transplantation: report from the Bone Marrow Transplant Survivor Study. *Blood* 2005;105:4215.
15. Vardiman JW, Harris NL, Brunning RD. The World Health Organization (WHO) classification of the myeloid neoplasms. *Blood* 2002;100:2292.
16. Pedersen-Bjergaard J, Andersen MK, Christiansen DH, Nerlov C. Genetic pathways in therapy-related myelodysplasia and acute myeloid leukemia. *Blood* 2002;99:1909.
17. Gilliland DG, Gribben JG. Evaluation of the risk of therapy-related MDS/AML after autologous stem cell transplantation. *Biol Blood Marrow Transplant* 2002;8:9.
19. Friedberg JW, Neuberg D, Stone RM, et al. Outcome in patients with myelodysplastic syndrome after autologous bone marrow transplantation for non-Hodgkin's lymphoma. *J Clin Oncol* 1999;17:3128.
20. Metayer C, Curtis RE, Vose J, et al. Myelodysplastic syndrome and acute myeloid leukemia after autotransplantation for lymphoma: a multicenter case-control study. *Blood* 2003;101:2015.
21. Bhatia R, Van Heijzen K, Palmer A, et al. Longitudinal assessment of hematopoietic abnormalities after autologous hematopoietic cell transplantation for lymphoma. *J Clin Oncol* 2005;23:6699.
22. Qian Z, Joslin JM, Tennant TR, et al. Cytogenetic and genetic pathways in therapy-related acute myeloid leukemia. *Chem Biol Interact* 2010;184:50.
23. Shannon KM, Turhan AG, Chang SS, et al. Familial bone marrow monosomy: 7. Evidence that the predisposing locus is not on the long arm of chromosome 7. *J Clin Invest* 1989;84:984.
24. Harada H, Harada Y, Niimi H, Kyo T, Kimura A, Inaba T. High incidence of somatic mutations in the AML1/RUNX1 gene in myelodysplastic syndrome and low blast percentage myeloid leukemia with myelodysplasia. *Blood* 2004;103:2316.
25. Downing JR. AML1/CBFbeta transcription complex: its role in normal hematopoiesis and leukemia. *Leukemia* 2001;15:664.
26. Side LE, Curtiss NP, Teel K, et al. RAS, FLT3, and TP53 mutations in therapy-related myeloid malignancies with abnormalities of chromosomes 5 and 7. *Genes Chromosomes Cancer* 2004;39:217.
27. Woo MH, Shuster JJ, Chen C, et al. Glutathione S-transferase genotypes in children who develop treatment-related acute myeloid malignancies. *Leukemia* 2000;14:232.
28. Felix CA, Walker AH, Lange BJ, et al. Association of CYP3A4 genotype with treatment-related leukemia. *Proc Natl Acad Sci U S A* 1998;95:13176.
29. Chen H, Sandler DP, Taylor JA, et al. Increased risk for myelodysplastic syndromes in individuals with glutathione transferase theta 1 (GSTT1) gene defect. *Lancet* 1996;347:295.
30. Allan JM, Wild CP, Rollinson S, et al. Polymorphism in glutathione S-transferase P1 is associated with susceptibility to chemotherapy-induced leukemia. *Proc Natl Acad Sci U S A* 2001;98:11592.
31. Naoe T, Takeyama K, Yokozawa T, et al. Analysis of genetic polymorphism in NQO1, GST-M1, GST-T1, and CYP3A4 in 469 Japanese patients with therapy-related leukemia/myelodysplastic syndrome and de novo acute myeloid leukemia. *Clin Cancer Res* 2000;6:4091.
32. Ellis NA, Huo D, Yildiz O, et al. MDM2 SNP309 and TP53 Arg72Pro interact to alter therapy-related acute myeloid leukemia susceptibility. *Blood* 2008;112:741.
35. Finette BA, Homans AC, Albertini RJ. Emergence of genetic instability in children treated for leukemia. *Science* 2000;288:514.
36. Das-Gupta EP, Seedhouse CH, Russell NH. DNA repair mechanisms and acute myeloblastic leukemia. *Hematol Oncol* 2000;18:99.
37. Ben-Yehuda D, Krichevsky S, Caspi O, et al. Microsatellite instability and p53 mutations in therapy-related leukemia suggest mutator phenotype. *Blood* 1996;88:4296.
38. Rimsza LM, Kopecky KJ, Ruschulte J, et al. Microsatellite instability is not a defining genetic feature of acute myeloid leukemogenesis in adults: results of a retrospective study of 132 patients and review of the literature. *Leukemia* 2000;14:1044.
40. Smith AG, Worrillow LJ, Allan JM. A common genetic variant in XPD associates with risk of 5q- and 7q-deleted acute myeloid leukemia. *Blood* 2007;109:1233.
41. Seedhouse C, Faulkner R, Ashraf N, Das-Gupta E, Russell N. Polymorphisms in genes involved in homologous recombination repair interact to increase the risk of developing acute myeloid leukemia. *Clin Cancer Res* 2004;10:2675.
43. Christiansen DH, Andersen MK, Pedersen-Bjergaard J. Mutations with loss of heterozygosity of p53 are common in therapy-related myelodysplasia and acute myeloid leukemia after exposure to alkylating agents and significantly associated with deletion or loss of 5q, a complex karyotype, and a poor prognosis. *J Clin Oncol* 2001;19:1405.
44. Chakraborty S, Sun CL, Francisco L, et al. Accelerated telomere shortening precedes development of therapy-related myelodysplasia or acute myelogenous leukemia after autologous transplantation for lymphoma. *J Clin Oncol* 2009;27:791.
46. Yeoh E-J, Williams K, Patel S, al. E. Expression profiling of pediatric acute lymphoblastic leukemia (ALL) blasts at diagnosis accurately predicts both the risk of relapse and of developing therapy-induced acute myelogenous leukemia (AML). *Blood* 2001;98:433A.
47. Qian Z, Fernald AA, Godley LA, Larson RA, Le Beau MM. Expression profiling of CD34+ hematopoietic stem/ progenitor cells reveals distinct subtypes of therapy-related acute myeloid leukemia. *Proc Natl Acad Sci U S A* 2002;99:14925.
48. Witherspoon RP, Deeg HJ. Allogeneic bone marrow transplantation for secondary leukemia or myelodysplasia. *Haematologica* 1999;84:1085.
50. Bloomfield CD, Archer KJ, Mrozek K, et al. 11q23 balanced chromosome aberrations in treatment-related myelodysplastic syndromes and acute

leukemia: report from an international workshop. *Genes Chromosomes Cancer* 2002;33:362.
51. Litzow MR, Tarima S, Perez WS, et al. Allogeneic transplantation for therapy-related myelodysplastic syndrome and acute myeloid leukemia. *Blood* 2010; 115:1850.
53. Lillington DM, Micallef IN, Carpenter E, et al. Detection of chromosome abnormalities pre-high-dose treatment in patients developing therapy-related myelodysplasia and secondary acute myelogenous leukemia after treatment for non-Hodgkin's lymphoma. *J Clin Oncol* 2001;19:2472.
56. Landgren O, Gilbert ES, Rizzo JD, et al. Risk factors for lymphoproliferative disorders after allogeneic hematopoietic cell transplantation. *Blood* 2009;113:4992.
57. Curtis RE, Travis LB, Rowlings PA, et al. Risk of lymphoproliferative disorders after bone marrow transplantation: a multi-institutional study. *Blood* 1999;94:2208.
59. Heslop HE, Ng CY, Li C, et al. Long-term restoration of immunity against Epstein-Barr virus infection by adoptive transfer of gene-modified virus-specific T lymphocytes. *Nat Med* 1996;2:551.
61. Wong FL, Boice JD, Jr., Abramson DH, et al. Cancer incidence after retinoblastoma. Radiation dose and sarcoma risk. *JAMA* 1997;278:1262.
63. Smith RA, Cokkinides V, von Eschenbach AC, et al. American Cancer Society guidelines for the early detection of cancer. *CA Cancer J Clin* 2002;52:8.
64. Kawachi MH, Bahnson RR, Barry M, et al. NCCN clinical practice guidelines in oncology: prostate cancer early detection. *J Natl Compr Canc Netw* 2010;8:240–262.
65. Burt RW, Barthel JS, Cunn KB, et al. NCCN clinical practice guidelines in oncology: colorect cancer screening. *J Natl Compr Canc Netw* 2010;8:8–61.
66. Bevers TB, Anderson BO, Bonaccio E, et al. NCCN clinical practice guidelines in oncology: breast cancer screening and diagnosis. *J Natl Compr Canc Netw* 2009;7:1160–1196.

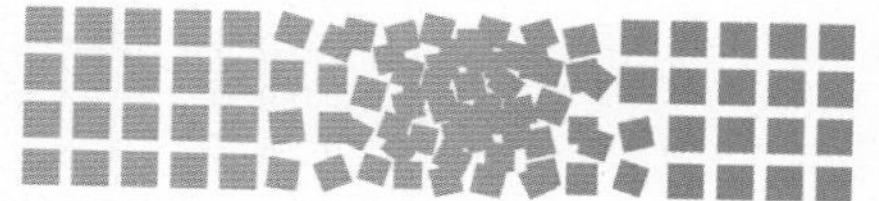

CHAPTER 143 SUPERIOR VENA CAVA SYNDROME

JOACHIM YAHALOM

Superior vena cava syndrome (SVCS) is the clinical expression of obstruction of blood flow through the SVC. Characteristic symptoms and signs may develop quickly or gradually when this thin-walled vessel is compressed, invaded, or thrombosed by processes in the superior mediastinum. Most cases reported in the past were due to syphilitic aneurysms or tuberculosis mediastinitis.[1,2] These entities have since virtually disappeared, and malignancy is now the most common underlying process in patients with SVCS.[3] More recently, thrombosis of the SVC caused by intravascular devices such as catheters and pacemakers is often the cause of SVCS.[4] It is estimated that SVCS develops in 15,000 people in the United States each year.[5]

ANATOMY AND PATHOPHYSIOLOGY

The SVC is the major vessel for drainage of venous blood from the head, neck, upper extremities, and upper thorax. It is located in the middle mediastinum and is surrounded by relatively rigid structures, such as the sternum, trachea, right bronchus, aorta, pulmonary artery, and perihilar and paratracheal lymph nodes. The SVC extends from the junction of the right and left innominate veins to the right atrium, for a distance of 6 to 8 cm. The distal 2 cm of the SVC is within the pericardial sac, with a point of relative fixation of the vena cava at the pericardial reflection. The azygos vein, the main auxiliary vessel, enters the SVC posteriorly, just above the pericardial reflection. The width of the SVC is 1.5 to 2.0 cm, and it maintains blood at a low pressure. The SVC is thin-walled, compliant, easily compressible, and vulnerable to any space-occupying process in its vicinity. The SVC is completely encircled by chains of lymph nodes that drain all the structures of the right thoracic cavity and the lower part of the left thorax. The auxiliary azygos vein is also threatened by enlargement of paratracheal nodes. Other critical structures in the mediastinum, such as the main bronchi, esophagus, and spinal cord, may be involved by the same process that led to obstruction of the SVC.[6,7]

When the SVC is fully or partially obstructed, an extensive venous collateral circulation may develop. The azygos venous system is the most important alternative pathway. Carlson[8] found that dogs could not survive sudden ligation of the SVC below the level of the azygos vein, but ligation of the SVC above it was tolerated well. He could, however, successfully obstruct the SVC and the azygos vein in operations performed in two stages, presumably by allowing time for collaterals to form. Other collateral systems are the internal mammary veins, lateral thoracic veins, paraspinous veins, and esophageal venous network. The subcutaneous veins are important pathways, and their engorgement in the neck and thorax is a typical physical finding in SVCS. Despite these collateral pathways, venous pressure is almost always elevated in the upper compartment if the SVC is obstructed. Venous pressures have been recorded as high as 200 to 500 cm H_2O in severe SVCS.[9]

ETIOLOGY AND NATURAL HISTORY

SVCS can develop gradually or abruptly.[3] Dyspnea is a common symptom, and sensation of fullness in the head and facial swelling is typical (Table 143.1).[10–12] The characteristic physical findings are venous distention of the neck (66%) and chest wall (54%), facial edema (46%), plethora (19%), and cyanosis (19%). These symptoms and signs may be aggravated by bending forward, stooping, or lying down. Malignant disease is the most common cause of SVCS, but SVCS from catheter-related thrombosis of the SVC has increasingly been observed.[4] The percentage of patients in different series with a confirmed diagnosis of malignancy varies from 60% to 86% (Table 143.2).[4,6,11–13] In large series of lung cancer, SVCS was identified in 2% to 4% of the patients.[10,14] Small cell lung cancer (SCLC) and squamous cell carcinoma are the most common histologic subtypes (Table 143.3).[14–20] Lymphoma involving the mediastinum was the cause of SVCS in 8% of patients reported in the series (Table 143.2). Most lymphoma patients with SVCS had either diffuse large cell lymphoma or lymphoblastic lymphoma.[21] In a series of patients with primary mediastinal B-cell lymphoma with sclerosis, SVCS was present in 57% of patients.[22] Hodgkin's lymphoma commonly involves the mediastinum, but it rarely causes SVCS. Other primary mediastinal malignancies that cause SVCS are thymoma and germ cell tumors. Breast cancer is the most common metastatic disease that causes SVCS.[6,11,13] In one report, breast cancer was the cause of SVCS in 11% of the cases.[23]

In recent years, nonmalignant conditions causing SVCS are more often observed. When the data were collected from general hospitals, as many as 40% of patients had noncancerous causes of SVCS.[4,6,11,12,24] Parish et al.[11] reported six patients with thrombosis of SVC, and in five, the thrombosis developed in the presence of central vein catheters or pacemakers. Sculier and Feld[25] reviewed 24 cases of central venous catheter–induced SVC. Of these, 18 were caused by pacemaker catheters.

TABLE 143.1

COMMON SYMPTOMS AND PHYSICAL FINDINGS OF SUPERIOR VENA CAVA SYNDROME

Symptoms	Patients Affected[a] (%)	Physical Findings	Patients Affected[a] (%)
Dyspnea	63	Venous distention of neck	66
Facial swelling and head fullness	50	Venous distention of chest wall	54
Cough	24	Facial edema	46
Arm swelling	18	Cyanosis	20
Chest pain	15	Plethora of face	19
Dysphagia	9	Edema of arms	14

[a]Analysis based on data from 370 patients.
(Adapted from refs. 10–12.)

LeVeen peritoneovenous shunts, Swan-Ganz catheters, and hyperalimentation catheters were also involved. The increasing use of these devices for the delivery of chemotherapy agents or for hyperalimentation contributes to the development of SVCS in the cancer patient.[26]

Obstruction of SVC in the pediatric age group is rare and has a different etiologic spectrum. The causative factors are mainly iatrogenic,[27] secondary to cardiovascular surgery for congenital heart disease, ventriculoatrial shunt for hydrocephalus, and SVC catheterization for parenteral nutrition. In a report of 175 children with SVCS, 70% were iatrogenic. Of the remaining 53 cases, 37 (70%) were caused by mediastinal tumors, 8 (15%) were caused by benign granuloma, and 4 (7.5%) by congenital anomalies of the cardiovascular system. Two-thirds of the tumors causing SVCS in childhood are lymphomas.[27–29] Issa et al.[28] reported that mediastinal fibrosis secondary to histoplasmosis caused SVCS in 7 (5%) of the 150 patients reviewed.

DIAGNOSTIC PROCEDURES

SVCS has long been considered to be a potentially life-threatening medical emergency.[7,24,30] It was common practice to immediately apply radiation therapy with initial high-dose fractions, sometimes even before the histologic diagnosis of the primary lesion was established.[24,30,31] Diagnostic procedures, such as bronchoscopy, mediastinoscopy, thoracotomy, or supraclavicular lymph node biopsy, were often avoided because they were considered to be hazardous in the presence of SVCS.[7,24] However, the safety of these invasive procedures in patients with SVCS has markedly improved, and the modern treatment of SVCS has become disease-specific from the outset.[3,6,32–34] Temporizing emergency mediastinal irradiation before biopsy is rarely used because it may preclude proper interpretation of the specimen in almost half of the patients.[35]

The clinical identification of SVCS is simple because the symptoms and signs are typical and unmistakable. The chest film shows a mass in most patients. The most common radiographic abnormalities are superior mediastinal widening and pleural effusion.

Computed tomography (CT) provides more detailed information about the SVC, its tributaries, and other critical structures, such as the bronchi and the cord.[36] The additional information is necessary because the involvement of these structures requires prompt action for relief of pressure.

CT phlebography provides excellent imaging information on the site and extent of obstruction and the status of collaterals.[37] Although not fully evaluated, FDG-PET (fluorodeoxyglucose-positron emission tomography) scanning is useful in patients with SVCS as it may influence the design of the radiotherapy field in lymphoma or lung cancer.[3] In 58% of 107 patients reported by Schraufnagel et al.,[6] the SVCS developed before the primary diagnosis was established. The diagnostic procedures used in different studies are summarized in Table 143.4. Sputum cytology established the diagnosis for almost half of the patients. Cytologic diagnosis is as accurate as tissue diagnosis in small cell carcinoma.[38] Bronchoscopy supplies the malignant cells for cytologic evaluation in most cases of small cell disease.[39] Transbronchial needle aspiration was reported to be highly effective.[40] Pleural effusions are common in SVCS. In one series effusions were detected in 60% of patients, both in those with malignant etiology and in those with a nonmalignant cause.[41] The majority are exudative and often chylous. In the presence of pleural effusion, thoracocentesis established the diagnosis of malignancy in 71% of patients with malignancy.[41] Biopsy of a palpable supraclavicular node was rewarding in two-thirds of the reported attempts. SCLC and non–Hodgkin's lymphoma (NHL) often involve the bone marrow. A biopsy of the bone marrow may provide the diagnosis and stage for these patients. Mediastinoscopy has a very high

TABLE 143.2

PRIMARY PATHOLOGIC DIAGNOSES FOR SUPERIOR VENA CAVA SYNDROME

Histologic Diagnosis	Bell et al.[12] 159 Patients (%)	Schraufnagel et al.[6] 107 Patients (%)	Parish et al.[11] 86 Patients (%)	Yellin et al.[13] 63 Patients (%)	Rice et al.[4] 78 Patients (%)
Lung cancer	129 (81)	67 (63)	45 (52)	30 (48)	36 (46)
Lymphoma	3 (2)	10 (9)	8 (9)	13 (21)	6 (8)
Other malignancies (primary or metastatic)	4 (3)	14 (13)	14 (16)	8 (13)	5 (6)
Nonneoplastic	2 (1)	16 (15)	19 (22)	11 (18)	31 (40)
Undiagnosed	21 (13)	—	—	—	—

TABLE 143.3

LUNG CANCER SUBTYPES ASSOCIATED WITH SUPERIOR VENA CAVA SYNDROME

Histology	No. of Patients	Percentage of Patients
Small cell	142	38
Squamous cell	97	26
Adenocarcinoma	52	14
Large cell	43	12
Unclassified	34	9
Total	370	10

(Adapted from refs. 10–12.)
See also refs 14–20.

success rate for providing a diagnosis and has a complication rate of approximately 5%.[42] Reports by several authors on using mediastinoscopy for patients with SVCS whose histologic diagnosis could not be established with less invasive techniques confirmed the safety and high diagnostic yield of mediastinoscopy.[34,42–44] No perioperative mortality was recorded, and the diagnosis yield was excellent.

Percutaneous transthoracic CT-guided fine-needle biopsy is an effective and safe alternative to an open biopsy or mediastinoscopy, with a sensitivity rate of 75%.[34,45] Successful diagnostic transluminal atherectomy also has been reported.[46] A thoracoscopic biopsy or thoracotomy is diagnostic if all other procedures have failed. In contrast to past opinions, there is little evidence to suggest that diagnostic procedures such as venographies, thoracotomies, bronchoscopies, mediastinoscopies, and lymph node biopsies carry an excessive risk in patients with SVCS.[3,47]

MANAGEMENT

The goals of treatment of SVCS are to relieve symptoms and to attempt the cure of the primary malignant process. SCLC, NHL, and germ cell tumors constitute almost half of the malignant causes of SVCS. These disorders are potentially curable, even in the presence of SVCS. The treatment of SVCS should be selected according to the histologic disorder and stage of the primary process. The prognosis of patients with SVCS strongly correlates with the prognosis of the underlying disease.

When the therapeutic goal is only palliation of SVCS, or when urgent treatment of the venous obstruction is required, direct opening of the occlusion should be considered. The newer techniques of endovascular stenting and angioplasty with possible thrombolysis should provide prompt relief of symptoms before more specific cancer therapy.[5,48–53]

SMALL CELL LUNG CANCER

Chemotherapy alone or in combination with thoracic irradiation therapy is the standard treatment for SCLC.[54] Chemotherapy and radiotherapy as initial treatments are effective in rapidly improving the symptoms of SVCS.[20] In an analysis of 50 patients with SCLC who presented with SVCS, response rate to chemotherapy was 93% and the response to radiation was 94%, and 70% of patients remained SVCS-free before death.[20] It is of interest that, when the total treatment of SCLC included chemotherapy and radiation, the risk of SVCS recurrence was significantly lower than when the treatment was chemotherapy alone.[20]

Among 643 patients with SCLC, Sculier et al.[16] identified 55 patients (8.5%) with SVCS. Symptomatic relief of SVCS was obtained in 73% of patients initially treated with chemotherapy and in 43% of those initially treated with radiation. Relief of SVCS occurred within 7 to 10 days after initiation of therapy. In SCLC patients with recurrent or persistent SVCS after initial chemotherapy, additional chemotherapy and/or radiotherapy is still likely to relieve symptoms.[20] It is of interest to note that some researchers found a higher incidence of brain metastases at the time of diagnosis in SCLC patients with SVCS compared with patients without SVCS.[18,]

NON–SMALL CELL LUNG CANCER

A review of SVCS in lung cancer by Rowell and Gleeson[48] indicated that chemotherapy relieved SVCS in 59% of patients with non-SCLC; radiotherapy relieved the obstruction in 63% of non-SCLC patients. Nevertheless, in almost 20% of the patients the obstruction has recurred. Response to radiotherapy was higher in patients who had received prior therapy (94% vs. 70%).[48] Another review indicated that the median survival of patients with non-SCLC was shorter in the presence of SVCS (only 6 months) than without SVCS (9 months).[55]

NON–HODGKIN'S LYMPHOMA

In report of patients with SVCS secondary to NHL whose treatment included chemotherapy alone, chemotherapy combined with irradiation, or radiotherapy alone,[21] all 30 patients achieved complete relief of SVCS symptoms within 2 weeks of

PRACTICE OF ONCOLOGY

TABLE 143.4

POSITIVE YIELD OF DIAGNOSTIC PROCEDURES FOR PATIENTS WITH SUPERIOR VENA CAVA SYNDROME

Procedure	No. of Procedures	No. Positive	Percent Positive
Sputum cytology	59	29	49
Thoracocentesis	14	10	71
Bone marrow biopsy	13	3	23
Lymph node biopsy	95	64	67
Bronchoscopy	124	65	52
Mediastinoscopy	105	95	90
Thoracotomy	49	48	98

(Adapted from ref. 10.)

the onset of any type of treatment. No treatment modality appeared to be superior in achieving clinical improvement. The presence of dysphagia, hoarseness, or stridor was a major adverse prognostic factor for patients with lymphoma who presented with SVCS. Eighteen of 22 patients (81%) with large cell lymphoma achieved complete response. However, relapse was common and the median survival was only 21 months.

It has become apparent that SVCS secondary to lymphoma is rarely an emergency that requires treatment before a histologic diagnosis is made. The choice of treatment should be based on the histologic diagnosis and that the patients should undergo, if possible, a complete staging workup before therapy. The primary treatment is chemotherapy, as it has both local and systemic activity.[56] Local consolidation with radiation therapy is beneficial in patients with early-stage diffuse large cell lymphoma, particularly if the mass is bulky.

NONMALIGNANT CAUSES

Patients with nonmalignant causes of SVCS differ significantly from patients with malignant disease. If the cause is not malignant, the patients often have symptoms long before they seek medical advice, it takes more time to establish the diagnosis, and their survival is markedly longer.[6] Schraufnagel et al.[6] reported that the average survival rate was 9 years if the primary process was benign, compared with an average survival of 5 months for patients with lung cancer. Mahajan et al.[57] reviewed the literature of benign SVCS and reported 16 new cases. Twelve (75%) of these 16 patients had a mediastinal granuloma that was attributed to histoplasmosis. Most patients had an insidious onset of SVCS and were relatively young. Ten patients who were available for a follow-up of 1 to 11 years were all doing well at the time of the report. It was suggested that the good prognosis of patients with benign SVCS caused by fibrosing mediastinitis does not provide a role for SVC bypass surgery.[57] However, Nieto and Doty[58] advocated surgery for SVCS caused by benign disorders if the syndrome develops suddenly, progresses, or persists after 6 to 12 months of observation for possible collateral development. In patients whose histoplasmosis complement fixation titers suggest active disease, ketoconazole treatment may prevent recurrent SVCS.[59]

CATHETER-INDUCED OBSTRUCTION

In catheter-induced SVCS, the mechanism of obstruction is usually thrombosis. Streptokinase, urokinase, or recombinant tissue-type plasminogen activator may cause lysis of the thrombus early in its formation.[25,60–63] Heparin and oral anticoagulants may reduce the extent of the thrombus and prevent its progression. Removal of the catheter, if possible, is another option and should be combined with anticoagulation to avoid embolization. In patients for whom electrodes of a pacemaker must be changed, the broken wire should be removed to prevent the risk of developing SVCS.[25,60,64] Percutaneous transluminal angioplasty, with or without thrombolytic therapy, and stent insertion have been successfully used to open catheter-induced SVC obstructions.[61,65–68]

TREATMENT

Radiation Therapy

In patients with SVCS as a result of non-SCLC, radiotherapy has long been the primary treatment. The likelihood of relieving the symptoms and signs of SVCS is high,[7,10] but the overall prognosis for these patients is poor.[5,7,10,26] More recently, the use of percutaneous metal stent insertion to improve blood flow through the SVC has been introduced as an alternative to palliative radiation therapy in malignant SVCS.[5,49,50,69] Radiotherapy is an optional treatment for most patients with SVCS.[24,30,31] It is also used as an effective initial treatment if a histologic diagnosis cannot be established and the clinical status of the patient is deteriorating. However, most experts agree that SVC obstruction alone rarely represents an absolute emergency that requires radiotherapy without a specific diagnosis, and endovascular stenting can be used as an alternative to radiotherapy for obtaining immediate relief of the obstructi on.[3,5,13,32,33,49,50,69] Yet, SVCS may be the earliest manifestation of invasive involvement of additional critical structures in the thorax (Table 143.5), such as the bronchi. Under such circumstances, prompt treatment with irradiation may be required without any delay.

The fractionation schedule of radiation that has been recommended includes two to four large initial fractions of 3 to 4 Gy, followed by conventional fractionation to a total dose of 30 to 50 Gy.[7,24,30] However, no data clearly support a particular fractionation scheme.[20]

A radiotherapy study evaluated the efficacy of treating patients with SVCS with a short course of hypofractionated irradiation.[70] The study compared a regimen of 8 Gy per fraction once a week to a total dose of 24 Gy to a program of delivering only two fractions of 8 Gy (total of 16 Gy) within 1 week. Transient dysphagia was the main side effect in almost half of the patients in both programs. The 24-Gy regimen resulted in a complete resolution of symptoms in 56% of patients and a partial response in another 40%. The 16-Gy regimen yielded a complete response in only 28% of patients. The mean time for SVCS recurrence and the median overall survival rate were longer in the higher-dose regimen (6 months and 9 months, respectively) compared with the low-dose regimen (3 months and 3 months, respectively). A more recent

TABLE 143.5

COMPLICATIONS OF MALIGNANT INVASION ASSOCIATED WITH SUPERIOR VENA CAVA SYNDROME

Complication	No. of Patients[a] (%)
ESOPHAGUS	
Symptoms of dysphagia or esophageal dysfunction	26 (24)
Anatomic evidence of esophageal invasion	6 (6)
TRACHEA	
Displaced on examination or roentgenogram	7 (7)
Compressed or invaded by lesion	14 (13)
VOCAL CORD PARALYSIS	
Unilateral	6 (6)
Bilateral	3 (3)
PERICARDIUM	
Tamponade	3 (3)
Neoplastic invasion at necropsy	6 (6)

[a]Some patients may have had more than one complication.
(Adapted from ref. 6.)

study reported the experience of using only two fractions, 6 Gy each, 1 week apart in 23 elderly (more than 71 years old) patients with malignancy-related SVCS.[71] Overall response was 87% with relatively minimal toxicity.

Serial venograms and autopsies suggest that the symptomatic improvement achieved by radiotherapy is not always due to improvement of flow through the SVC.[32] It is probably also a result of the development of collaterals after the pressure in the mediastinum is eased.

The field of radiation for SVCS induced by lung cancer should encompass the gross tumors with appropriate margins and mediastinal, hilar, and supraclavicular lymph nodes. In the series of Armstrong et al.,[10] supraclavicular failures occurred in 8 of 91 patients (9%) receiving radiation therapy to the supraclavicular fossae and in 2 of 6 patients (33%) not receiving therapy to these lymph nodes.

In general, when radiation is given as initial treatment, CT-based simulation and fractions of 1.8 to 2 Gy are recommended for lymphomas. For lung cancers, higher daily fractions of 2 to 3 Gy may be considered. The field and fractionation may be altered after administration of several fractions and achievement of symptomatic relief.[3]

Endovascular Stenting and Angioplasty

Percutaneous transluminal angioplasty using the balloon technique, insertion of expandable wire stents, or both have been successfully used to open and maintain the patency of SVC obstruction resulting from malignant and benign causes.[5,48–50,52,53,68,69,72] Thrombolysis is often an integral part of the endovascular management of SVCS because thrombosis is frequently a critical component of the obstruction and lysis is necessary to allow the passage of the wire. Balloon dilatation (angioplasty) can also be used before stenting. Most reports have emphasized the use of combination endovascular therapy: thrombolysis, angioplasty, and stent therapy.[5,50] Total occlusion of the SVC is not a contraindication to stent therapy, and a success rate of 85% in total occlusion situations has been reported.[73] The largest experience in using stents to open malignant obstruction of the SVC was reported by Nicholson et al.[69] in Great Britain. The British team used WALLSTENTs in 75 patients and obtained improvement of obstruction in all patients; 90% remained free of symptoms until death. This study retrospectively compared stent therapy with radiation therapy and found that only 12% of patients treated with radiation remained free of SVCS until death. However, long-term experience in maintaining patency after stent therapy in patients with SVCS from benign causes who are expected to have long survival is still limited.[68] Complication rates for endovascular therapy have ranged from 0% to 50% and include bleeding, stent migration, stent occlusion, and pulmonary embolus.[5] Most complications can be successfully treated with percutaneous methods.

Surgery

The experience with successful direct bypass graft for SVC obstruction is limited. It was recommended that autologous grafts of almost the same size as the SVC should be used.[74] Doty et al.[75] used a composite spiral graft, which was constructed from the patient's saphenous vein. They reported 23 years of experience with this procedure in 16 patients with benign obstruction of SVC; 14 patients maintained patency and 15 were relieved of symptoms of SVCS. Avashti and Moghissi[76] reported successful bypasses of obstructed SVCs using Dacron prostheses. Magnan et al.[77] used an expanded polytetrafluoroethylene prosthesis to reconstruct the SVC in nine patients with malignancy-induced SVCS and in one patient with chronic mediastinitis. In all patients the symptoms disappeared promptly after the operation, the grafts remained open, and survival rates at 1, 2, and 5 years were 70%, 25%, and 12.5%, respectively.[77] The preferred bypass route is between an innominate or jugular vein on the left side and the right atrial appendage, using an end-to-end anastomosis.[45] Piccione et al.[78] used the autologous pericardium to reconstruct the SVC after resection for malignant obstruction.

The most common surgical approach is sternotomy or thoracotomy with extensive resection of the tumor and reconstruction of the SVC. Case series indicate an operative mortality of approximately 5% and patency rates of 80% to 90%.[3] However, with malignancy-induced SVCS, surgical intervention should be considered only after other therapeutic maneuvers with irradiation, chemotherapy, and stenting have been exhausted. A recent series from Boston of 19 patients requiring SVC resection for mostly malignant disease reported a median survival of 45 months with 30% of lung cancer patients surviving 5 years.[79] Most patients with SVCS of benign origin have long survivals without surgical intervention.[58,59] However, if the process progresses rapidly or if there is a retrosternal goiter or aortic aneurysm, surgical intervention may relieve the obstruction.

Thrombolytic Therapy

Thrombolysis is an important component of comprehensive endovascular therapy.[5] Successful experience with thrombolytic agents was also obtained in the treatment of catheter-induced SVCS.[2,5,63,80] The higher yield of thrombolytic therapy in patients with catheters is probably related to the mechanism of obstruction, the ability to deliver the agent directly to the thrombus, and earlier recognition of SVCS in patients with malfunctioning catheters. Early intervention and use urokinase were associated with favorable results.[63] Favorable experience with recombinant tissue-type plasminogen activator has been reported.[61,62] Many patients who undergo stenting for SVCS receive thrombolytic therapy during or during and after the procedure.[48]

AREAS OF UNCERTAINTY

Standardized criteria to grade the severity of symptoms in the SVCS are still lacking. More recently, a grading system with an accompanying treatment algorithm has been proposed.[81] It emphasizes that in most patients (>85%) with SVCS, the symptoms are not severe (grades 0, 1, and 2) and cancer-specific treatment could follow appropriate diagnosis and staging. Only grade 3 (severe) patients who present with mild or moderate cerebral edema or mild/moderate laryngeal edema or diminished cardiac reserve should be considered for immediate stent intervention or early radiation therapy (if tumor is not chemoradiosensitive), otherwise they should receive disease-specific treatment. Only the rare (<5%) grade 4 (life-threatening) patients, who develop significant cerebral edema or laryngeal edema with stridor or have significant hemodynamic compromise, should be stented immediately.[81]

The benefit of either short- or long-term anticoagulation therapy for SVCS is unclear, although thrombolytic agents have been used effectively in patients with vena caval thrombosis.[3] Most experts recommend anticoagulation after thrombolysis (to prevent disease progression and recurrence) and aspirin after stent placement in the absence of thrombosis, but data are limited.[39] The optimal management of recurrent obstruction of the SVC is also controversial. Placement of a stent is often considered because of the limited benefit or the risk of excessive toxic effects from repeat chemotherapy or radiation, but data to guide decision making are limited.[82–84]

RECOMMENDATIONS

The clinical course of SVCS rarely represents an absolute emergency. In patients without a clear cause of SVCS who do not have life-threatening symptoms (like confusion, obtundation, stridor or syncope without precipitating factors, hypotension or renal insufficiency), an efficient diagnostic effort should be attempted before any oncologic treatment is given.[3,81] Percutaneous endovascular intervention should be considered in severe cases because it relieves symptoms rapidly without masking the diagnosis. If simple diagnostic efforts do not provide the histologic diagnosis of the primary process, percutaneous transthoracic fine-needle biopsy under CT is safe and highly effective.[34,36] If all the proposed testing has failed to establish the diagnosis, the location of the suspicious lesion in the chest and the experience of the surgical team should determine whether mediastinoscopy or thoracotomy is performed.

During the diagnostic process, the patient can benefit from bedrest and oxygen administration. Some clinicians advocate the use of diuretics and/or corticosteroids if the patient is uncomfortably symptomatic. Anticoagulation is of no proven benefit and may interfere with diagnostic procedures. After the cause of SVCS has been established, treatment of the primary process should promptly follow. Combination chemotherapy with an appropriate regimen is the treatment of choice for SCLC and NHL. Radiation therapy of the lesion and adjacent nodal areas may enhance control after initial response to chemotherapy. Non-SCLC causing SVCS is best treated with radiation therapy or endovascular stent insertion, or both.[3,81] The incorporation of CT scan and FDG-PET information into a carefully designed treatment plan may enable the administration of a total radiation dose of more than 50 Gy, which may provide long-term local control for some patients. Most patients with nonmalignant causes for SVCS have an indolent course and a good prognosis. Percutaneous transluminal angioplasty or stent insertion should be considered an effective alternative to surgery.[80,82–84] However, the long-term maintenance of patency with stent insertion is still unknown. Surgery is indicated only when the process is rapidly progressing or caused by a retrosternal goiter or an aortic aneurysm. If SVCS is induced by a catheter, the catheter should be removed if possible. Heparin should be administered during the removal of the catheter to prevent embolization. In catheter-induced SVCS, urokinase, streptokinase, or recombinant tissue-type plasminogen activator is of value if used early in the thrombotic process.[59–61,84]

Selected References

The full list of references for this chapter appears in the online version.

3. Wilson LD, Detterbeck FC, Yahalom J. Superior vena cava syndrome with malignant causes. *N Engl J Med* 2007;356:1862.
4. Rice TW, Rodriguez RM, Light RW. The superior vena cava syndrome, clinical characteristics and evolving etiology. *Medicine* 2006;85:37.
5. Schindler N, Vogelzang RL. Superior vena cava syndrome: experience with endovascular stents and surgical therapy. *Surg Clin North Am* 1999;79:683.
6. Schraufnagel DE, Hill R, Leech JA, Pare JAP. Superior vena caval obstruction: is it an emergency? *Am J Med* 1981;70:1169.
10. Armstrong BA, Perez CA, Simpson JR, Hederman MA. Role of irradiation in the management of superior vena cava syndrome. *Int J Radiat Oncol Biol Phys* 1987;13:531.
11. Parish JM, Marschke RF, Dines DE, Lee RE. Etiologic considerations in superior vena cava syndrome. *Mayo Clin Proc* 1981;56:407.
13. Yellin A, Rosen A, Reichert N, Lieberman Y. Superior vena cava syndrome: the myth—the facts. *Am Rev Respir Dis* 1990;141:1114.
19. Wurschmidt F, Bunemann H, Heilmann HP. Small cell lung cancer with and without superior vena cava syndrome: a multivariate analysis of prognostic factors in 408 cases. *Int J Radiat Oncol Biol Phys* 1995; 33:77.
20. Chan RH, Dar AR, Yu E, et al. Superior vena cava obstruction in small-cell lung cancer. *Int J Radiat Oncol Biol Phys* 1997;38:513.
21. Perez-Soler R, McLaughlin P, Velasquez WS, et al. Clinical features and results of management of superior vena cava syndrome secondary to lymphoma. *J Clin Oncol* 1984;2:260.
22. Lazzarino M, Orlandi E, Paulli M, et al. Primary mediastinal B-cell lymphoma with sclerosis: an aggressive tumor with distinctive clinical and pathologic features. *J Clin Oncol* 1993;11:2306.
29. Ingram L, Rivera GK, Shapiro DN. Superior vena cava syndrome associated with childhood malignancy: analysis of 24 cases. *Med Pediatr Oncol* 1990;18:476.
32. Ahmann FR. A reassessment of the clinical implications of the superior vena cava syndrome. *J Clin Oncol* 1984;2:961.
33. Shimm DS, Lugue GL, Tigsby LC. Evaluating the superior vena cava syndrome. *JAMA* 1981;245:951.
35. Loeffler JS, Leopold KA, Recht A, et al. Emergency prebiopsy radiation for mediastinal masses: impact on subsequent pathologic diagnosis and outcome. *J Clin Oncol* 1986;4:716.
36. Sheth S, Ebert MD, Fishman EK. Superior vena cava obstruction evaluation with MDCT. *AJR Am J Roentgenol* 2010;194:336.
40. Selcuk ZT, Firat P. The diagnostic yield of transbronchial needle aspiration in superior vena cava syndrome. *Lung Cancer* 2003;42:183.
41. Rice TW, Rodriguez RM, Barnette R, Light RW. Prevalence and characteristics of pleural effusions in superior vena cava syndrome. *Respirology* 2006;11:299.
42. Mineo TC, Ambrogi V, Nofroni I, et al. Mediastinoscopy in superior vena cava obstruction: analysis of 80 consecutive patients. *Ann Thorac Surg* 1999;68:223.
44. Dosios T, Nikolaos T, Chatziantoniou C. Cervical mediastinoscopy and anterior mediastinotomy in superior vena cava obstruction. *Chest* 2005;128:1551.
48. Rowell NP, Gleeson FV. Steroids, radiotherapy, chemotherapy and stents for superior vena caval obstruction in carcinoma of the bronchus: a systematic review. *Clin Oncol* 2002;14:338.
53. Greillier L, Barlesia F, Doddoli C, et al. Vascular stenting for palliation of superior vena cava obstruction in non-small cell lung cancer patients: a future "standard" procedure? *Respiration* 2004;71:178.
56. Yellin A, Mandel M, Rechavi G, et al. Superior vena cava syndrome associated with lymphoma. *Am J Dis Child* 1992;146:1060.
58. Nieto AF, Doty DB. Superior vena cava obstruction: clinical syndrome, etiology and treatment. *Curr Probl Cancer* 1986;10:442.
59. Urshel HC Jr, Razzuk MA, Netto GJ, Disiere J, Chung SY. Sclerosing mediastinitis: improved management with histoplasmosis titer and ketoconazole. *Ann Thorac Surg* 1990;50:215.
60. Goudevonos JA, Reid PG, Adams PC, Holden MP, Williams DO. Pacemaker-induced superior vena cava syndrome: report of four cases and review of the literature. *Pacing Clin Electrophysiol* 1989;12:1890.
62. Greenberg S, Kosinski R, Daniels J. Treatment of superior vena cava thrombosis with recombinant tissue type plasminogen activator. *Chest* 1991;99:1298.
63. Gray BH, Olin JW, Grador RA, et al. Safety and efficacy of thrombolytic therapy for superior vena cava syndrome. *Chest* 1991;99:54.
67. Sunder SK, Ekong EA, Sivalingam K, Kumar A. Superior vena cava thrombosis due to pacing electrodes: successful treatment with combined thrombolysis and angioplasty. *Am Heart J* 1992;123:790.
68. Kee ST, Kinoshita L, Razavi MK, et al. Superior vena cava syndrome: treatment with catheter-directed thrombolysis and endovascular stent placement. *Radiology* 1998;206:187.
69. Nicholson AA, Ettles DF, Arnold A, et al. Treatment of malignant superior vena cava obstruction: metal stents or radiation therapy. *J Vasc Interv Radiol* 1997;8:781.
70. Rodrigues CI, Njo KH, Karim ABMF. Hypofractionated radiation therapy in the treatment of superior vena cava syndrome. *Lung Cancer* 1993;10:221.
71. Lonardi F, Gioga G, Agus G, et al. Double-flash, large-fraction radiation therapy as palliative treatment of malignant superior vena cava syndrome in the elderly. *Support Care Cancer* 2002;10:156.

72. Shah R, Sabanathan S, Lowe RA, et al. Stenting in malignant obstruction of superior vena cava. *J Thorac Cardiovasc Surg* 1996;112:335.
73. Crowe MT, Davies CH, Gaines PA, et al. Percutaneous management of superior vena cava occlusions. *Cardiovasc Intervent Radiol* 1995;18:367.
75. Doty JR, Flores JH, Doty DB. Superior vena cava obstruction: bypass using spiral vein graft. *Ann Thorac Surg* 1999;67:1111.
77. Magnan PE, Thomas P, Giudicelli R, et al. Surgical reconstruction of the superior vena cava. *Cardiovasc Surg* 1994;2:598.
79. Lanuti M, De Delva PE, Henning A, et al. Review of superior vena cava resection in the management of benign disease and pulmonary or mediastinal malignancies. *Ann Thorac Surg* 2009:88;392
80. Uberoi R. Quality assurance guidelines for superior vena cava stenting in malignant disease. *Cardiovasc Intervent Radiol* 2006;29:319.
81. Yu JB, Wilson LD, Datterbeck FC. Superior vena cava syndrome: a proposed classification and algorithm for management. *J Thorac Oncol* 2008;3:811.
82. Comerota AJ. Safety and efficacy of thrombolytic therapy for superior vena caval syndrome. *Chest* 1991;99:3.
83. Nicholson AA, Ettles DF, Arnold A, Greenstone M, Dyet JF. Treatment of malignant superior vena cava obstruction: metal stents or radiation therapy. *J Vasc Interv Radiol* 1997;8:781.

CHAPTER 144 INCREASED INTRACRANIAL PRESSURE

KEVIN P. BECKER AND JOACHIM M. BAEHRING

An increase in intracranial pressure (ICP) is a common neurologic complication of patients with cancer involving the nervous system. Various pathomechanisms have to be considered in this patient population. Large cerebral metastases are the most common cause and can give rise to intracranial hemorrhage. Subependymal or leptomeningeal masses located at "bottlenecks" of spinal fluid pathways such as the foramen of Monro or the aqueduct of Sylvius raise pressure by obstructing spinal fluid flow. A cancer-related hypercoagulable state can lead to dural sinus thrombosis or extracranial venous outflow obstruction, and coagulopathies predispose to subdural bleeding. The cancer patient as an immunocompromised host is at risk for infections of the nervous system such as fungal or bacterial meningitis or a bacterial abscess resulting in increased ICP. Communicating hydrocephalus reflects decreased reabsorption of spinal fluid, which can be seen in leptomeningeal carcinomatosis. Dural venous sinus stenosis from dural metastases causes a syndrome resembling idiopathic intracranial hypertension.

This chapter provides an overview of the various mechanisms of increased ICP, the clinical manifestations, diagnosis, and treatment options.

PATHOPHYSIOLOGICAL CONSIDERATIONS

Intracranial volume is not expandable in an adult because of its containment by the skull and the dura. The brain itself has an average volume of 1,400 mL, spinal fluid of 52 to 160 mL, and blood 150 mL.[1] An increase in the volume of one compartment occurs at the expense of the other two (Monro-Kellie hypothesis).[2–4] If brain volume increases as a result of a brain tumor, the spinal fluid volume decreases as a compensatory mechanism. Up to an ICP of 200 to 250 mm cerebral spinal fluid (CSF) compartmental volume increase results in only minor increases in ICP as long as CSF flow is not obstructed, the rate between CSF production and reabsorption remains constant, and the dural venous sinuses remain open. However, intracranial compliance decreases with rising ICP (i.e., with rising pressure, increase in volume leads to a disproportionate increase in pressure). This is reflected in the occurrence of plateau waves, which are acute elevations of ICP up to 1,300 mm CSF lasting 5 to 20 minutes. These transient elevations are of pathogenic significance because they further compromise cerebral perfusion in patients with increased ICP.[5] Plateau waves have been suspected to cause intermittent symptoms with orthostasis in patients with brain tumors.[6]

Volume changes within the brain parenchyma that lead to increased ICP in cancer patients are caused by the direct mass effect of primary or secondary brain tumors, peritumoral edema, or indirect neurologic complications of cancer. Vasogenic edema results from increased leakage of plasma filtrate into brain tissue through leaky capillaries within a brain tumor or surrounding a brain abscess or cerebral hemorrhage. Cytotoxic edema occurs with the breakdown of the adenosine triphosphate–dependent transmembranous ion transport system that leads to the intracellular entrapment of water. This can be seen with ischemic injury, cytotoxic chemotherapy agents, or toxic metabolites in liver failure. Extra-axial mass lesions can arise from neoplastic growth (dural tumors such as metastases, meningioma, or lymphoma), infection (subdural empyema), or hemorrhage (subdural hematoma in the coagulopathic or thrombocytopenic patient).

Increased ICP can also be the consequence of an imbalance between CSF production and reabsorption. Spinal fluid is produced at an average rate of 21 to 22 mL/h or approximately 500 mL/day. CSF represents a plasma filtrate passively diffusing through the choroid plexus of the lateral, third, and fourth ventricles. It is reabsorbed within the arachnoid granulations overlying the cerebral hemispheres. Mass lesions in proximity to bottlenecks of CSF flow (foramen of Monro, cerebral aqueduct, medullary foramina, basilar subarachnoid cisterns) cause obstructive or noncommunicating hydrocephalus. Carcinomatosis or meningitis interferes with CSF reabsorption at the arachnoid granulations. Under chronic conditions, the spinal fluid pressure reaches a new equilibrium within the high normal range, and gives rise to a condition called *normal pressure hydrocephalus* (NPH) characterized by ventricular enlargement out of proportion to age-related cortical atrophy. Increased production of CSF is a rare cause of raised ICP. Idiopathic intracranial hypertension (IIH) or pseudotumor cerebri denotes a syndrome characterized by signs of increased ICP in the absence of mass lesions or hydrocephalus. Although poorly defined from a pathophysiologic standpoint, an increasing number of patients with IIH have been found to have partial obstruction of dural venous sinuses. Iatrogenic causes of IIH include isotretinoin, tetracycline antibiotics, and sulfonamides.

Acute increases in arterial and venous pressure result in an increase in ICP. Cerebral perfusion is kept constant over a wide arterial pressure range (50 to 160 mm Hg). Once this autoregulatory mechanism fails, further increase in arterial blood pressure passively increases ICP. Venous obstruction can be reproduced with the Queckenstedt maneuver (manual compression of both internal jugular veins). Dural venous sinus pressure fluctuates with intrathoracic pressure changes. Thus, coughing, sneezing, and straining (Valsalva maneuver) are accompanied by an increase in ICP. In a patient with increased ICP and decreased intracranial compliance, gagging or coughing can lead to transient decompensation and the acute onset of symptoms (syncope in patients with colloid cyst of the third ventricle, plateau waves).

Depending on the etiology and location of an increase in cerebral parenchymal or extra-axial volume, patients may have relatively few symptoms until herniation ensues. The faster the pathologic process evolves, the more likely is the patient to have symptoms. Cingulate or transfalcian herniation denotes lateral shift of a hemisphere underneath the falx cerebri. Vascular structures (ipsilateral anterior cerebral artery, internal cerebral vein, vein of Galen) can be compromised in this process. In transtentorial herniation, the diencephalon is forced through the tentorial notch as a consequence of a supratentorial mass lesion. Infratentorial masses can result in an upward herniation of posterior fossa structures. Uncal herniation, most often encountered in temporal lobe mass lesions, leads to compression of the midbrain at the level of the tentorial notch. When the ICP exceeds 40 to 50 mm Hg, cerebral blood flow is diminished, leading to irreversible brain damage.

EPIDEMIOLOGY AND PATHOGENESIS

Increase in Cerebral Parenchymal Pressure

Brain metastases are the most common cause of increased ICP in a cancer patient. In adults, lung cancer and melanoma are particularly prone to seeding to brain.[7] Cerebral metastasis can be further complicated by intratumoral hemorrhage. Although lung cancer is the most common primary tumor leading to hemorrhagic brain seeding, the relative incidence of hemorrhagic transformation of a cerebral metastasis is highest in melanoma, choriocarcinoma, renal cell carcinoma, and papillary thyroid cancer.[8] In children, the brain metastases most commonly associated with intracranial hemorrhage are Ewing sarcoma, rhabdomyosarcoma, and melanoma.[9] Primary brain tumors with a predilection for subependymal or intraventricular locations such as subependymal giant cell astrocytoma, lymphoma, subependymoma, choroid plexus papilloma, ependymoma, meningioma, colloid cyst, central neurocytoma, chordoid glioma of the third ventricle, or thalamic tumors can cause spinal fluid obstruction early in their course. Secondary cerebral volume increase in cancer patients results from hemorrhage, ischemia, infection, or autoimmune inflammatory processes. Cerebral hemorrhage from cancer-related coagulopathies typically occurs in patients with hematologic malignancies such as acute lymphocytic or myelocytic leukemia.[10] Diffuse cerebral edema and increased ICP in patients with leukemia can be the mere result of leukostasis and occurs at blast counts exceeding 4×10^5/mcL. Higher counts are usually required in lymphoblastic leukemia because cells are smaller and less adherent than myeloid blasts.[11] An increase in ICP can also be the consequence of diffuse cerebral hemorrhages in disseminated intravascular coagulopathy.

Herpes simplex encephalitis gives rise to extensive vasogenic edema affecting the medial temporal and inferior frontal lobe. Depending on disease burden, patients with cerebral toxoplasmosis, aspergillosis, or candidiasis can present with signs of increased ICP as well. Brain abscess complicates neurosurgical interventions for resection of metastases, drainage of cerebral hemorrhage, or placement of ventricular catheters. Autoimmune inflammatory encephalomyelitis has been described as a rare entity in patients after bone marrow transplantation.

Disorders Affecting Cerebral Spinal Fluid Production or Reabsorption

A syndrome resembling normal pressure hydrocephalus has been observed in long-term survivors of whole-brain or less commonly, partial-brain irradiation. Fibrosis of arachnoid granulations has been suspected to play a role in the pathogenesis of this entity that is also characterized by extensive white matter demyelination and frank necrosis. Selected patients seem to respond favorably to ventriculoperitoneal shunting.[12–14] An acute imbalance between CSF production and reabsorption occurs in neoplastic meningitis and opportunistic meningeal infections in the immunocompromised cancer patient. Cryptococcus neoformans meningitis is almost invariably associated with elevation of ICP. Patients after splenectomy are susceptible to meningitis with encapsulated bacteria. The pathogenesis of communicating hydrocephalus in patients with spinal cord tumors or nonobstructive masses of the cerebellopontine angle is not well understood. Most commonly ependymomas, but also Schwannoma, meningioma, neurofibroma, and glioma, might release protein degradation products or cells into CSF that obstruct the arachnoid granulations.[15,16] However, the protein level is rarely elevated in these patients. Others have suspected blockage of the lumbar CSF reservoir,[17–19] arachnoiditis, or increased fibrinogen levels[20] as the cause of this syndrome. Retinoic acid, a differentiating agent used for the treatment of promyelocytic leukemia, has been associated with episodes of communicating hydrocephalus, likely as a consequence of decreased CSF reabsorption.[21] Increased ICP is rarely caused by CSF overproduction. Patients with choroid plexus papilloma, especially if they are multifocal, are at risk.[22]

Venous Outflow Obstructions

A hypercoagulable state in cancer patients can manifest itself as dural venous sinus thrombosis (Fig. 144.1A). The incidence is increased in patients receiving L-asparaginase therapy. Increased ICP is the only manifestation of cerebral venous thrombosis in more than one-third of patients.[23] Nonthrombotic causes of dural sinus stenosis or occlusion are dural mass lesions such as meningioma or diffuse meningiomatosis of the convexity, metastases from breast or prostate cancer, non-Hodgkin's lymphoma, Ewing sarcoma, plasmocytoma, or neuroblastoma that either compress or invade the sinus.[24–26] Venous hypertension can also arise from metastases at the base of the skull, causing obstruction of the internal jugular vein or from compression of the superior vena cava by mediastinal masses. Lesions giving rise to IIH compromise the distal superior sagittal sinus or the torcula Herophili.[27]

CLINICAL PRESENTATION

Headache is the most common complaint of patients with increased ICP. In its classic form, the head pain is severe, resistant to common analgesics, and reaches maximum intensity on awakening in the morning.[28] Decreased venous drainage in the supine position likely accounts for this observation. Patients frequently report immediate relief from their headache by vomiting. However, the majority have nonspecific tension-type or migrainelike headaches. The patient with increased ICP falls easily, particularly backward. With rising pressure, nausea and vomiting ensue. The patient becomes increasingly somnolent and ultimately lapses into a coma.

Funduscopic examination reveals papilledema in about half of patients with increased ICP. Absence of venous pulsations within the center of the optic disc is an early finding, whereas papilledema with blurring of the disc margins or small hemorrhages characterizes later stages. The Foster-Kennedy syndrome—optic nerve atrophy as a result of a sphenoid wing meningioma and contralateral papilledema from

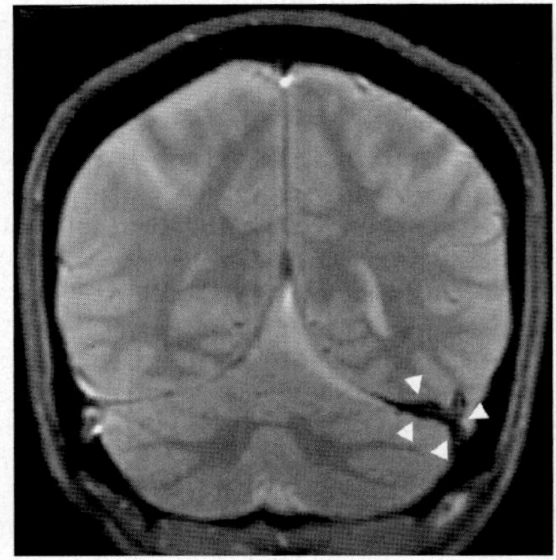
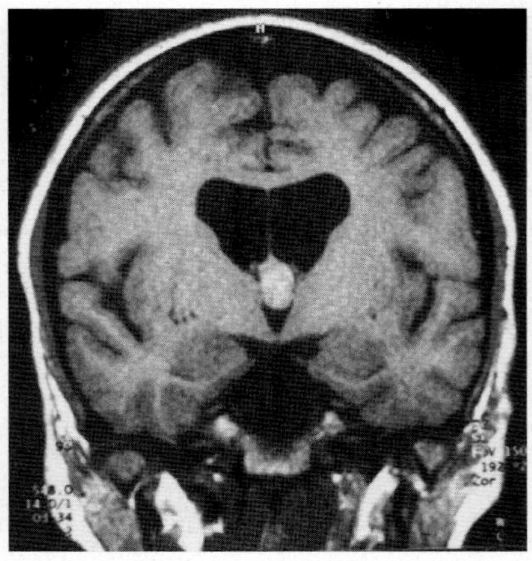
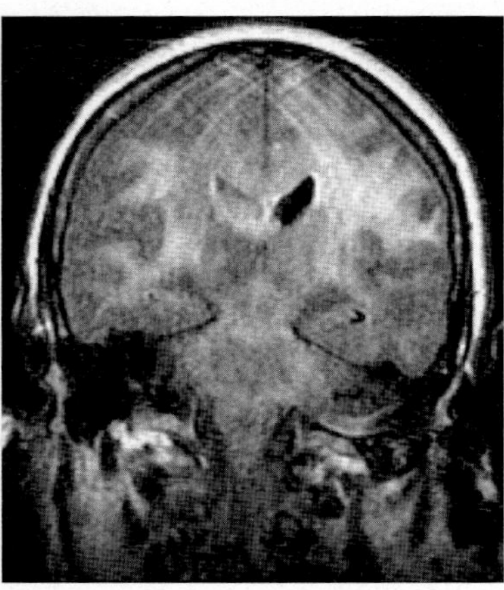

A,B C

FIGURE 144.1 **A:** Increased intracranial pressure caused by venous outflow obstruction. A 48-year-old woman with idiopathic myelofibrosis complained of a severe headache. Workup revealed a left transverse sinus thrombosis (gradient echo MRI, coronal section, intraluminal thrombus outlined by *arrowheads*). **C:** A 78-year-old woman with gliomatosis cerebri. Hyperintense signal on this coronal fluid attenuated inversion recovery (FLAIR) MRI demarcates the extent of cerebral infiltration by neoplastic cells and vasogenic edema. There is extensive effacement of the sulcal pattern and early transtentorial herniation. **B:** Intermittent obstructive hydrocephalus caused by the "pressure-valve" effect of a colloid cyst of the foramen of Monro. This 38-year-old patient had experienced several presyncopal episodes and was suffering from positional headaches. The lateral ventricles are dilated (unenhanced T1-weighted magnetic resonance image [MRI], coronal section).

increased ICP—is rarely seen in the days of improved neuroimaging methods and earlier diagnosis.

Focal neurologic deficits can help localize the mass accounting for the pressure increase. Cognitive complaints such as slowness to respond and inattentiveness reflect frontal lobe dysfunction. Gaze paresis to the side opposite the lesion indicates involvement of the frontal eye field. Posterior frontal masses cause contralateral hemiparesis. Hemianesthesia or complex neglect syndromes reflect parietal lobe pathology. Temporal and occipital lobe disease causes visual field deficits. An upward gaze paresis occurs in patients with tumors of the tectal region such as pineal neoplasms or metastases. Paresis of extraocular muscles results from stretch injury of the fourth or sixth nerve or uncal herniation with compression of the third nerve. However, the clinician must be aware of "false" localizing signs. Temporal lobe tumors can cause compression of the cerebral peduncle at the tentorial notch on the opposite side, resulting in a hemiparesis on the same side as the mass lesion (Kernohan syndrome).

Symptoms are aggravated by vasogenic edema surrounding intraparenchymal masses and partially or completely resolve with medical management. Hyponatremia as a result of inappropriate secretion of antidiuretic hormone is observed as a metabolic complication of increased ICP. Sphincter incontinence occurs in chronically elevated ICP. Patients with acute meningitis present with classic signs of meningeal irritation, including photophobia, phonophobia, and a Kernig or Brudzinski sign. In meningeal carcinomatosis, these signs are frequently absent.

Elevated ICP in infants results in increased head circumference. Chronic hydrocephalus can be recognized on plain radiographs of the skull as focal thinning of the tabula interna of the skull (Lückenschädel). This is accompanied by personality changes and loss of previously acquired motor skills. Herniation of one cerebellar tonsil causes a head tilt, neck stiffness, and unilateral forced eye closure.[29] Tectal masses result in upgaze inhibition, light-near dissociation of pupillary response, and convergence-retraction nystagmus (Parinaud syndrome). Pressure on the mesencephalic tegmentum leads to pathologic lid retraction and an upward gaze palsy (setting sun sign).

Slowly progressive static ICP changes are accompanied by little or no symptoms. On the other hand, clinical deterioration is profound when dynamic pressure changes such as plateau waves occur or abnormal intracranial compartmentalization or herniation ensues.[30] Signs and symptoms of increased ICP manifest earlier in patients with lesions of the posterior fossa because of the small size of this compartment. A brief bedside assessment including level of consciousness, pupillary size and reflexes, extraocular movements, blood pressure, heart rate, breathing pattern, and motor response to noxious stimuli enables the clinician to determine if herniation is present and which level of the central neuraxis is compromised. The triad of changes in breathing pattern, arterial hypertension, and bradycardia observed with rising ICP is known as the *Kocher-Cushing reflex*.[31] In uncal herniation from temporal lobe masses or herpes encephalitis, ipsilateral compression of the third nerve and associated parasympathetic nerve fibers leads to pupillary dilatation before extraocular dysmotility. With progression of shift of brain substance, complete third nerve palsy ensues and signs of midbrain dysfunction appear. Patients develop contralateral hemiparesis from pressure on the cerebral peduncle and ultimately become stuporous. Increasing pressure from hemispheric or diencephalic mass lesions results in central (transtentorial) herniation. This leads to a progressive syndrome reflecting sequential damage to brainstem structures in a rostrocaudal fashion. At the early diencephalic stage, mild changes in the patient's alertness are accompanied by periodic breathing, yawning, or hiccuping. Pupils are small but remain reactive to light. With further progression of central herniation, the patient becomes obtunded or stuporous. Roving eye movements reflect diffuse cortical dysfunction and preservation of lower brainstem gaze centers. Noxious stimuli elicit flexion of upper extremities and extension of lower extremities (decorticate posturing). Midsize pupils unresponsive to light indicate midbrain dysfunction. Damage to the mesencephalic reticular activating system produces coma. A fast and regular breathing pattern evolves (central neurogenic hyperventilation). Transition to the pontine stage of central herniation is accompanied by extensor posturing of all limbs to noxious stimulation (decerebrate posturing). Absence of the oculocephalic reflex (doll's head maneuver) and horizontal eye movements to caloric stimulation of the vestibular system indicate damage to pontine structures. Breathing becomes apneustic with pontine compression. When the cerebellar tonsils herniate through the foramen magnum, ataxic breathing is observed and the blood pressure drops.

The syndrome of raised ICP and cerebral herniation can evolve slowly over days to weeks or acutely over hours. Rapid progression usually indicates hemorrhage. Subdural hematomas in patients with coagulopathies can evolve so rapidly that signs of cerebral herniation are present before an imaging study can be obtained. Hemorrhage into a metastatic focus is typically characterized by the sudden onset of focal neurologic signs, including seizures. Intraparenchymal hemorrhage as a result of coagulopathy leads to slowly progressive neurologic deterioration.[10]

A peculiar syndrome is associated with tumors causing a pressure valve effect, such as a colloid cyst of the foramen of Monro (Fig. 144.1B). Patients, typically in their late childhood or early adulthood, report sudden onset of severe imbalance, headache, and nausea that is brought on by positional changes (bending down) or Valsalva maneuvers. Sudden deaths have occurred, stressing the need for close observation of these patients until appropriate therapy can be provided.[32,33]

IIH (pseudotumor cerebri) is mostly characterized by nocturnal or hypnopompic headaches aggravated by Valsalva maneuver. Nonspecific visual changes, diplopia due to sixth nerve palsy, or transient visual obscuration are less frequent manifestations. On physical examination, papilledema is the most striking abnormality.[34] The blind spot is enlarged. It is presumed that the disorder is due to decreased CSF absorption.

Another characteristic clinical syndrome is recognized in patients with chronic disturbance of spinal fluid reabsorption. These patients, or more likely their family members on their behalf, report a combination of cognitive decline, precipitate micturition, and gait apraxia.[35,36] Dementia is usually of the subcortical type. Precipitate micturition reflects dysfunction of the cortical center for bladder control (paracentral lobule). Minimal bladder filling results in the uncontrollable urge to urinate. The gait disturbance is characterized by difficulty initiating ambulation and postural instability with retropulsion. Strength is preserved.

DIAGNOSIS

The history and clinical examination detect the presence of increased ICP. Imaging studies are helpful in determining its cause and confirming the clinical impression. The most readily available imaging study is unenhanced computed tomography. The study is adequate to determine the presence of intraventricular and subarachnoid CSF flow obstruction (Fig. 144.2), as well as uncal, transfalcian, and transtentorial herniation (Fig. 144.3). The presence of intracranial hemorrhage or a neoplastic or infectious mass lesion can be identified and emergency treatment initiated. Transependymal edema is seen as periventricular hypodensity and indicates CSF flow obstruction.

More detailed neuroanatomic imaging and the distinction between a neoplastic, infectious, inflammatory, or ischemic process requires magnetic resonance imaging and magnetic resonance spectroscopy. The use of intravenous gadolinium is advised as most conditions associated with increased ICP in cancer patients cause breakdown of the blood–brain barrier and thus can be better visualized with contrast dye. The use of diffusion-weighted imaging can help identify evolving ischemia or high cellularity suggestive of malignant tumor growth. CSF flow studies (cine magnetic resonance imaging) are helpful to evaluate the functional significance of minute structural lesions within or surrounding the cerebral aqueduct. Slitlike ventricles in the correct clinical setting are indicative of IIH. Coronal images through the orbit may reveal dilatation of the optic nerve sheaths in this condition. *Ex vacuo* ventricular dilatation out of proportion to cortical atrophy is characteristic for NPH. Magnetic resonance imaging of the spine should be considered in patients with unexplained communicating hydrocephalus. Obstruction or infiltration of dural venous sinuses is best visualized with magnetic resonance venography.[37]

Scintigraphic cisternography can document spinal fluid circulation abnormalities such as NPH. Early ventricular filling with tracer substance after lumbar injection and delayed or absent demarcation of subarachnoid space overlying the cerebral hemispheres is indicative of decreased reabsorption of CSF through the arachnoid granulations.

A,B
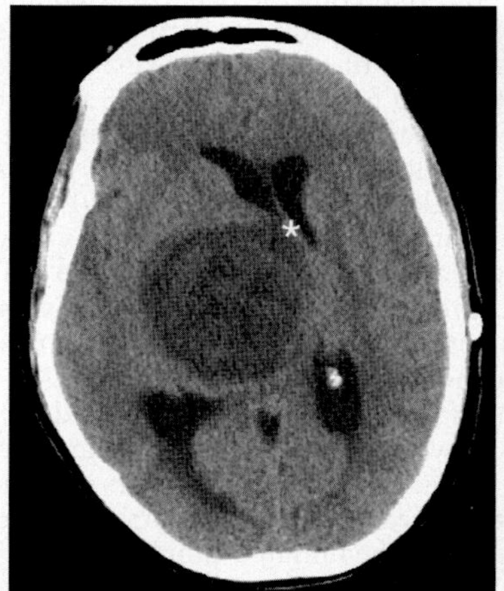

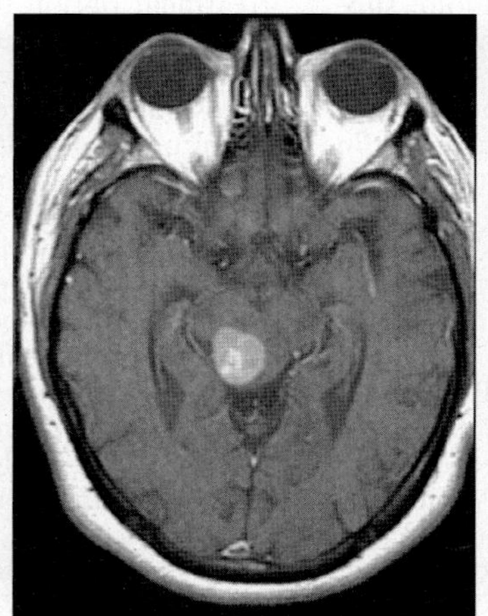
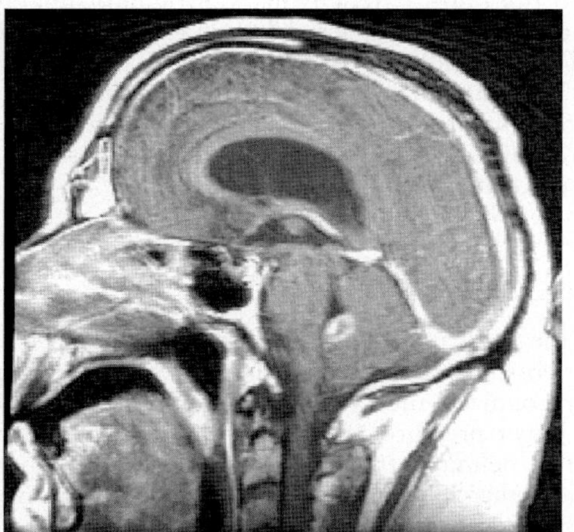
C

FIGURE 144.2 **A:** A 45-year-old patient with an anaplastic astrocytoma of the right thalamus. Computed tomography revealed obstruction at the level of the foramen of Monro (*asterisk*). **B:** A 55-year-old patient with a midbrain metastasis from an adenocarcinoma of the lung. There is partial obstruction at the level of the cerebral aqueduct. The temporal horns of the lateral ventricles are dilated (T1-weighted magnetic resonance image [MRI] with gadolinium). **C:** A 38-year-old patient with seeding of non–small cell lung cancer to the floor of the fourth ventricle. He presented with intractable headaches, nausea, vomiting, and severe back pain, indicative of obstructive hydrocephalus and leptomeningeal spread to the spinal canal (T1-weighted MRI with gadolinium, sagittal view).

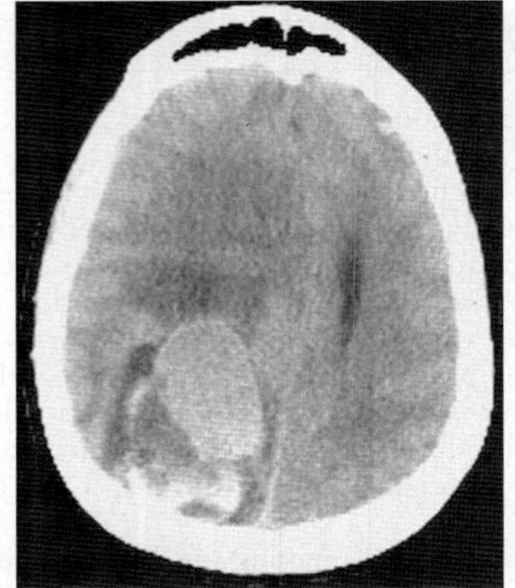
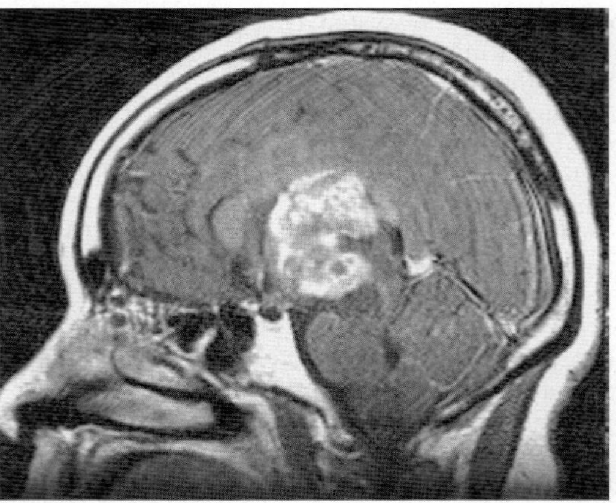
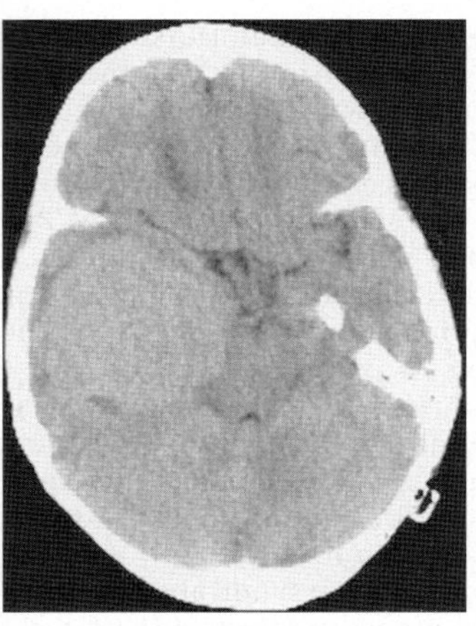

FIGURE 144.3 **A:** This unenhanced computed tomographic (CT) scan of the head shows a hemorrhagic brain metastasis in a 42-year-old woman with malignant melanoma. The metastasis exerts mass effect on the right lateral ventricle. There is transfalcian herniation of the right hemisphere. **B:** A 37-year-old woman with an anaplastic astrocytoma of the diencephalon. There is imminent transtentorial herniation (T1-weighted MRI with gadolinium, sagittal view). **C:** A 25-year-old woman who developed a large right temporal meningioma years after whole-brain radiation therapy for acute lymphoblastic leukemia in early childhood. The tumor compresses the cerebral peduncle and displaces the midbrain (unenhanced CT).

CSF pressure can be measured directly through a lumbar puncture performed in the lateral decubitus position. Puncture of the subarachnoid space below the level of spinal fluid obstruction bears the risk of initiating or aggravating cerebral herniation. The risk is considerable in mass lesions of the posterior fossa. A computed tomography scan should be obtained prior to lumbar puncture in patients with signs of increased ICP. Compartmentalization (obstructive hydrocephalus at the foramen of Monro or cerebral aqueduct, obliteration of basal cisterns as a result of transtentorial or transforaminal herniation) prohibits puncture of the subarachnoid space below the level of obstruction. When unperturbed communication between the intraventricular and subarachnoid spaces has been determined and the basal cisterns are patent, lumbar puncture should not be delayed if it is deemed necessary for accurate diagnosis, such as in cryptococcal meningitis.

Intracranial pressure can be monitored in the intensive care unit with a variety of strain gauge or fiberoptic devices placed into the brain parenchyma, ventricular, subarachnoid, subdural, or epidural space. All these methods require neurosurgical intervention.[38]

Transcranial Doppler sonography is helpful in the intensive care unit for monitoring cerebral perfusion and alteration in cerebrovascular resistance (e.g., in vasospasm or intra-arterial disease) in patients with increased ICP.[39]

TREATMENT

In the majority of cases, the onset of increased ICP in cancer patients is protracted over days to weeks. After increased ICP is recognized and symptomatic measures have been initiated to lower pressure, a diagnostic procedure can be performed before definitive treatment is provided. Fewer patients present as an emergency but the ones that do require immediate neurosurgical intervention.

The normovolemic patient with increased ICP and suspected decreased intracranial compliance is best positioned with head and upper trunk slightly elevated (~30 degrees). As fever above 100.5°F contributes to elevated ICP, it is common practice to use antipyretics such as acetaminophen above this threshold. Serum osmolality is kept in the high normal range. Isotonic saline solutions are recommended for intravenous hydration, while hypotonic fluids are avoided because free water shifts along an osmolar gradient further exacerbating increased ICP.

Corticosteroids are effective agents for the initial management of increased ICP caused by vasogenic edema. No benefit has been convincingly shown for cytotoxic edema of an acute ischemic stroke, intracranial hemorrhage secondary to remote effects of cancer, or spinal fluid obstruction. Moderate (6 to 10 mg dexamethasone every 6 hours) to high doses (up to 100 mg/d of dexamethasone) are used. A superior therapeutic effect has not been demonstrated for high doses, and the risk of adverse reactions, in particular gastroduodenal ulceration, is considerable. Corticosteroids should be avoided if CNS lymphoma is suspected before a tissue diagnosis has been established. Dexamethasone and related drugs induce lymphocytic apoptosis and may obscure morphologic diagnosis.

Osmotic diuresis through infusion of hyperosmolar agents such as mannitol or glycerol is an alternative or additional treatment option for the reduction of ICP. Most commonly used are intravenous infusions of 20% to 25% mannitol solutions given at an initial dose of 0.75 to 1 g/kg body weight followed by 0.25 to 0.5 g/kg body weight every 3 to 6 hours. Monitoring of serum osmolality is required. The osmotic effect is transient, and treatment should be stopped if the target serum osmolality is exceeded (~300 to 310 mOsm/L).

Monitoring in the neurologic intensive care unit is required in patients with depressed mental status secondary to ICP elevation. Careful blood pressure adjustment is needed to avoid blood pressure peaks without decreasing cerebral perfusion.

The most rapid method to decrease ICP is intubation with mechanical hyperventilation. The pCO_2 should be decreased to 25 to 30 mm Hg. Lower pCO_2 levels are avoided because cerebral perfusion is reduced. The effect of hyperventilation is transient and thus other measures such as corticosteroid use and osmotic diuresis need to be initiated simultaneously.

Obstructive hydrocephalus constitutes a neurosurgical emergency. Rapid neurologic deterioration with signs of cerebral herniation mandate the immediate placement of an external ventriculostomy. Permanent drainage of CSF through a ventriculoperitoneal shunt or endoscopic placement of a third ventriculostomy may be necessary when the cause of spinal fluid flow obstruction cannot be definitively treated. Although filter systems are available, ventriculoperitoneal shunting is avoided in patients with leptomeningeal tumor in order to prevent peritoneal seeding.

Normal pressure hydrocephalus responds favorably to ventriculoperitoneal shunting. It is the task of the clinician to carefully select patients who may benefit from this procedure. Patients with a short history of the classic clinical triad of gait apraxia, precipitate micturition, and cognitive decline are most likely to respond. Large-volume spinal fluid releases or scintigraphic cisternography have been used as objective means to predict outcome of a shunting procedure.

Disease-specific treatment of increased ICP in addition to symptomatic management with corticosteroids or osmotic diuresis is indicated in the majority of cases. Infectious complications are treated with antimicrobial therapy. Patients with a brain abscess undergo surgical drainage. A hematoma within a metastatic focus is resected if located in a noneloquent area of the brain and in the absence of widely metastatic disease. Subdural hematoma or empyema requires immediate surgical decompression. Leukostasis in leukemic diseases responds to hydration, leukapheresis, systemic chemotherapy, and whole-brain irradiation. Systemic intravenous anticoagulation with heparin or fractionated heparinoid is used in dural sinus thrombosis. When L-asparaginase therapy is involved in the pathogenesis of the prothrombotic stage, substitution with fresh-frozen plasma and antithrombin III is required prior to consideration of anticoagulant use. Petechial hemorrhages due to thrombocytopenia require transfusion of blood platelets. A coagulopathy can be corrected using transfusion of fresh-frozen plasma and substitution of vitamin K. Increased ICP secondary to medication requires discontinuation of the causative drug. IIH in the cancer patient is typically caused by malignant dural sinus compression and responds to local surgical treatment or irradiation. Leptomeningeal carcinomatosis is treated with irradiation and intrathecal chemotherapy. CSF flow obstruction prohibits intraventricular injection of cytotoxic agents as it can give rise to a severe, irreversible toxic encephalopathy.

References

1. Fishman RA. *Cerebrospinal Fluid in Diseases of the Nervous System.* Philadelphia: W.B. Saunders, 1992.
2. Monro A. *Observations on the Structure and Function of the Nervous System.* Edinburgh: Creech and Johnson, 1783.
3. Kelly G. Appearances observed in the dissection of two individuals; death from cold and congestion of the brain. *Trans Med Chir Sci Edinb* 1824;1:84.
4. Mokri B. The Monro-Kellie hypothesis: applications in CSF volume depletion. *Neurology* 2001;56(12):1746.
5. Lundberg N. Continuous recording and control of ventricular fluid pressure in neurosurgical practice. *Acta Psychiatrica Scand* 1960;36(Suppl 149):1960.
6. Watling CJ, Cairncross JG. Acetazolamide therapy for symptomatic plateau waves in patients with brain tumors: report of three cases. *J Neurosurg* 2002;97(1):224.
7. Lassman AB, DeAngelis LM. Brain metastases. *Neurol Clin* 2003;21(1):1.
8. Posner JB. *Neurologic Complications of Cancer.* Philadelphia: FA Davis,1995.
9. Kaste SC, Rodriguez-Galindo C, Furman WL, Langston J, Thompson SJ. Imaging aspects of neurologic emergencies in children treated for non-CNS malignancies. *Pediatr Radiol* 2000;30(8):558.
10. Quinn JA, DeAngelis LM. Neurologic emergencies in the cancer patient. *Semin Oncol* 2000;27(3):311.
11. Choo-Kang LR, Jones DM, Fehr JJ, Eskenazi AE, Toretsky JA. Cerebral edema and priapism in an adolescent with acute lymphoblastic leukemia. *Pediatr Emerg Care* 1999;15(2):110.
12. DeAngelis LM, Delattre JY, Posner JB. Radiation-induced dementia in patients cured of brain metastases. *Neurology* 1989;39(6):789.
13. Thiessen B, DeAngelis LM. Hydrocephalus in radiation leukoencephalopathy: results of ventriculoperitoneal shunting. *Arch Neurol* 1998;55(5):705.
14. Perrini P, Scollato A, Cioffi F, Mouchaty H, Conti R, Di Lorenzo N. Radiation leukoencephalopathy associated with moderate hydrocephalus: intracranial pressure monitoring and results of ventriculoperitoneal shunting. *Neurol Sci* 2002;23(5):237.
15. Caviness JA, Tucker MH, Pia SK, Tam DA. Hydrocephalus as a possible early symptom in a child with a spinal cord tumor. *Pediatr Neurol* 1998;18(2):169.
16. Rifkinson-Mann S, Wisoff JH, Epstein F. The association of hydrocephalus with intramedullary spinal cord tumors: a series of 25 patients. *Neurosurgery* 1990;27(5):749.
17. Phan TG, Krauss WE, Fealey RD. Recurrent lumbar ependymoma presenting as headache and communicating hydrocephalus. *Mayo Clin Proc* 2000;75(8):850.
18. Costello F, Kardon RH, Wall M, Kirby P, Ryken T, Lee AG. Papilledema as the presenting manifestation of spinal schwannoma. *J Neuro-Ophthalmol* 2002;22(3):199.
19. Kordas M, Czirjak S, Doczi T. The spinal tumour related hydrocephalus. *Acta Neurochir (Wien)* 1997;139(11):1049.
20. Pirouzmand F, Tator CH, Rutka J. Management of hydrocephalus associated with vestibular schwannoma and other cerebellopontine angle tumors. *Neurosurgery* 2001;48(6):1246.
21. Colucciello M. Pseudotumor cerebri induced by all-trans retinoic acid treatment of acute promyelocytic leukemia. *Arch Ophthalmol* 2003;121(7):1064.
22. Di Rocco C, Iannelli A. Poor outcome of bilateral congenital choroid plexus papillomas with extreme hydrocephalus. *Eur Neurol* 1997;37(1):33.
23. Biousse V, Ameri A, Bousser MG. Isolated intracranial hypertension as the only sign of cerebral venous thrombosis. *Neurology* 1999;53(7):1537.
24. Gironell A, Marti-Fabregas J, Bello J, Avila A. Non-Hodgkin's lymphoma as a new cause of non-thrombotic superior sagittal sinus occlusion. *J Neurol Neurosurg Psychiatr* 1997;63(1):121.
25. Kim AW, Trobe JD. Syndrome simulating pseudotumor cerebri caused by partial transverse venous sinus obstruction in metastatic prostate cancer. *Am J Ophthalmol* 2000;129(2):254.
26. Thomas DA, Trobe JD, Cornblath WT. Visual loss secondary to increased intracranial pressure in neurofibromatosis type 2. *Arch Ophthalmol* 1999;117(12):1650.
27. Goldsmith P, Burn DJ, Coulthard A, Jenkins A. Extrinsic cerebral venous sinus obstruction resulting in intracranial hypertension. *Postgrad Med J* 1999;75(887):550.
28. Forsyth PA, Posner JB. Headaches in patients with brain tumors: a study of 111 patients. *Neurology* 1993;43(9):1678.
29. Kelly KM, Lange B. Oncologic emergencies. *Pediatr Clin North Am* 1997;44(4):809.
30. Plum F, Posner JB. *The Diagnosis of Stupor and Coma.* Philadelphia: FA Davis, 1980.
31. Cushing HW. Some experimental and clinical observations concerning states of increased intracranial tension. *Am J Med Sci* 1902;124:375.
32. Aronica PA, Ahdab-Barmada M, Rozin L, Wecht CH. Sudden death in an adolescent boy due to a colloid cyst of the third ventricle. *Am J Forensic Med Pathol* 1998;19(2):119.
33. Jeffree RL, Besser M. Colloid cyst of the third ventricle: a clinical review of 39 cases. *J Clin Neurosci* 2001;8(4):328.
34. Foley J. Benign forms of intracranial hypertension; toxic and otitic hydrocephalus. *Brain* 1955;78(1):1.
35. Hakim S, Adams RD. The special clinical problem of symptomatic hydrocephalus with normal cerebrospinal fluid pressure. *J Neurol Sci* 1965;2:307.
36. Fisher CM. Hydrocephalus as a cause of disturbance of gait in the elderly. *Neurology* 1982;32:1358.
37. Chaudhuri R, Tarnawski M, Graves MJ, Graves PE, Cox TC. Dural sinus occlusion due to calvarial metastases: A CT blind spot. *J Comput Assist Tomogr* 1992;16(1):30.
38. Brain Trauma Foundation, American Association of Neurological Surgeons, Congress of Neurological Surgeons, et al. Guidelines for the management of severe traumatic brain injury: VIII. Intracranial pressure thresholds [erratum appears in *J Neurotrauma* 2008;25(3):276; note: multiple author names added]. *J Neurotrauma* 2007;24(Suppl 1):S55.
39. Rasulo FA, De Peri E, Lavinio A. Transcranial Doppler ultrasonography in intensive care. *Eur J Anaesthesiol Suppl* 2008;42:167.

CHAPTER 145 SPINAL CORD COMPRESSION

KEVIN P. BECKER AND JOACHIM M. BAEHRING

Compression of the spinal cord is one of the most devastating neurologic complications, affecting 5% to 10% of patients who have cancer.[1–3] The majority of cases result from spine metastases with extension into the epidural space. Pain is the most common initial clinical manifestation of metastases to the axial skeleton. Within weeks, neurologic impairment ensues and is irreversible if treatment is not initiated promptly. Malignant spinal cord compression (MSCC) is a diagnostic challenge, especially in patients without a history of cancer. Back pain is one of the most common ailments in the general population and, in most cases, results from degenerative changes of the spine. Early identification of patients at risk of MSCC is essential as limitation of workup, symptomatic management, and bed rest—common practice in patients with "benign" back pain—almost invariably leads to profound neurologic morbidity.

This chapter describes the clinical syndromes, diagnosis, and treatment of epidural cancer metastases. Metastases below the conus medullaris, corresponding to the level of the first lumbar vertebra in adults and giving rise to isolated radiculopathies or a cauda equina syndrome, are included.

EPIDEMIOLOGY

An estimated 20,000 patients are diagnosed with MSCC per year in the United States.[4,5] The lifetime incidence in cancer patients is 1% to 6%, although autopsy series have revealed higher numbers (5% to 10%).[6–9] The majority of patients with MSCC are older than 50 years of age. However, cumulative incidence decreases with age; 4.4% in 40- to 50-year olds, 3.8% in 50- to 60-year olds, 2.9% in 60- to 70-year olds, 1.7 % in 70- to 80-year olds, and 0.54% in patients older than 80 years.[10] The most common types of cancer that account for spinal cord compression are breast, prostate, lung cancer, and lymphoma.[1,6–8,11–14] The cumulative incidence of MSCC is disease specific and is highest in multiple myeloma (8%), prostate cancer (7%), nasopharyngeal cancer (6.5%), and breast cancer (5.5%).[7] The median interval between cancer diagnosis and manifestation of MSCC ranges from 6 to 12.5 months. Late axial bone metastases that cause cord compression are more common in breast cancer (43 months).[6] In only 1 in 500 cancer patients is spinal cord compression part of the presenting oncologic syndrome.[7] However, 20% of MSCC cases lack a history of cancer.[8,15] MSCC as the primary manifestation of a malignancy is more common in non-Hodgkin's lymphoma, myeloma, and lung cancer, especially the small-cell variant; it is almost unheard of in breast cancer.[16,17] Two-thirds of MSCC cases affect the thoracic spine and 20% the lumbar spine, whereas cervical and sacral spine are rarely involved (less than 10% for each site).[1,12,14,18,19] Colon and prostate cancers seem to have a predilection for the lumbosacral spine, whereas lung and breast cancers are more common in the thoracic spine. Multiple epidural metastases are detected on initial presentation in up to one-third of patients in whom the whole axial skeleton is investigated.[20] Local recurrence after irradiation is rare, but one in ten patients develops a second metastatic deposit that causes cord compression at a different spine level within 5 months of the first event.[1,12]

The tumor spectrum that causes cord compression in the pediatric population differs from adults and includes neuroblastoma, Ewing's sarcoma, and, less commonly, primary vertebral osteosarcoma, germ cell tumors, and lymphoma. Cord compression as an initial manifestation of the tumor in children occurs more frequently than in the adult population.[21,22]

PATHOPHYSIOLOGY

Bone, particularly the axial skeleton, is one of the most common organ systems involved by metastatic spread. Up to one-third of patients dying of cancer develop metastases to the spine at some point during their illness.[23] Release of bone-derived growth factors and cytokines, capillary structure, and peculiar blood flow phenomena may facilitate deposition and growth of metastases.[24,25] Venous blood from intra-abdominal and intrathoracic organs is not only drained through the vena cava but also through the vertebral and epidural venous plexus (Batson's plexus). This low-pressure circulation without valves and with frequent flow reversal, depending on intrathoracic and intra-abdominal pressure, would appear to be an ideal transportation system for cancer cells.

The most common mechanisms of spinal cord compression are the direct extension of tumor from a hematogenous metastasis to a vertebral body into the epidural space or the pathologic fracture of a vertebral body infiltrated by a metastatic deposit, resulting in cord injury by a bone fragment or spine instability (Fig. 145.1*A*). Involvement of posterior spine elements with nerve root impingement is less common.[26] Transforaminal progression of paravertebral tumor is encountered in lymphoma and neuroblastoma. Highly aggressive paravertebral tumors such as the Pancoast tumor of the lung apex simply grow through anatomic barriers, including bone, into the epidural space. Primary hematogenous seeding to the epidural space is rare.[11] Spinal cord compression can also result from intradural mass lesions (meningioma, nerve sheath tumors, large leptomeningeal metastases) (Fig. 145.2) or intraneural spread of neurogenic tumors. Nonmetastatic causes are epidural hematoma in patients with coagulopathy or abscess in an immunocompromised host.

The mechanism of cord injury is not entirely understood. The early myelopathy associated with MSCC may be due to impairment of venous drainage, leading to intramedullary vasogenic edema. When the interstitial pressure rises beyond a critical threshold, cord perfusion is compromised, resulting in

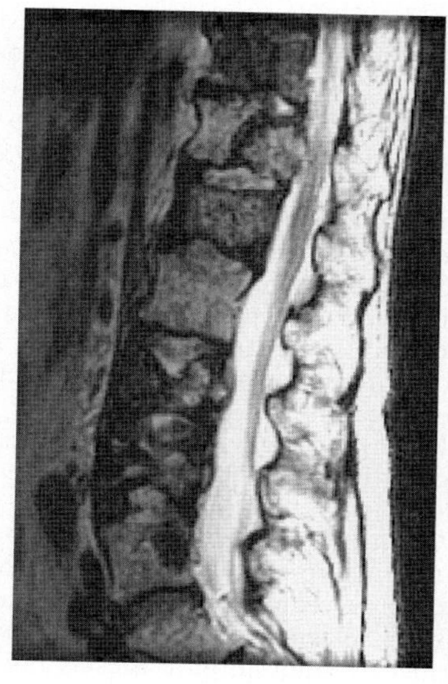

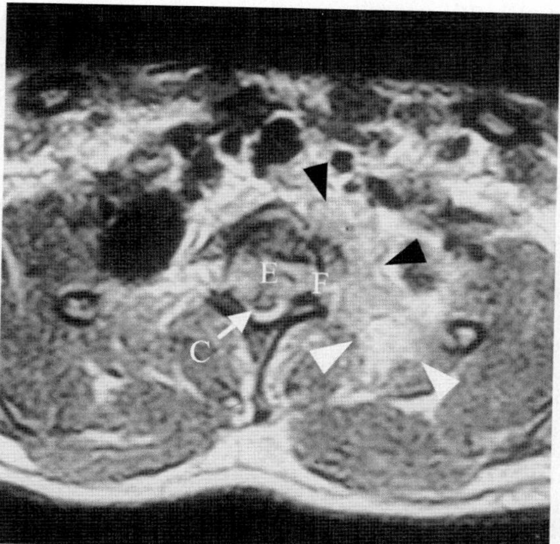

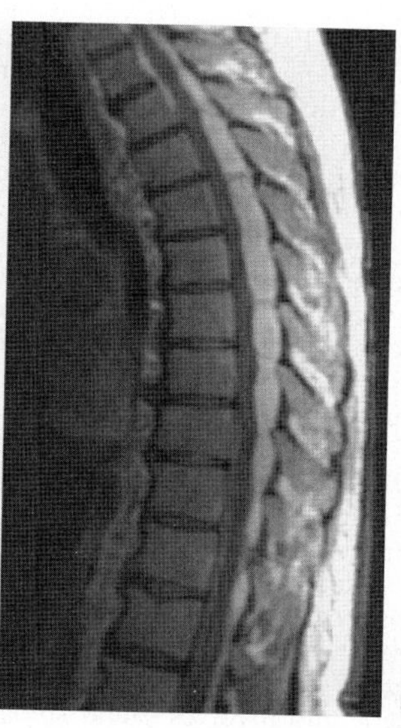

A, B C

FIGURE 145.1 **A:** A 53-year-old patient with metastatic renal cell cancer. T2-weighted magnetic resonance image (MRI; sagittal view) of the lumbosacral spine shows a pathologic fracture of the T12 vertebral body, posterior dislocation of a bone fragment, and compression of the spinal cord. **B:** T1-weighted MRI with gadolinium (axial view) of a 19-year-old patient with Ewing's sarcoma involving the T2 vertebral body. An enhancing soft tissue lesion is seen in the paravertebral space (*black and white arrowheads*), the intervertebral foramen (F) and the epidural space (E). The cord (*C, arrow*) is compressed and displaced posteriorly. The patient had noticed that his left pupil had become smaller (Horner's syndrome). He then started complaining of intermittent upper back pain aggravated by coughing, difficulty walking up stairs, and initiating urination. **C:** A 73-year-old man with polycythemia rubra vera complained of progressive leg weakness and back pain. An MRI of the thoracic spine (T1 without contrast dye) revealed a large hyperintense epidural mass lesion compressing the cord posteriorly. A biopsy confirmed the suspected diagnosis of extramedullary hematopoiesis.

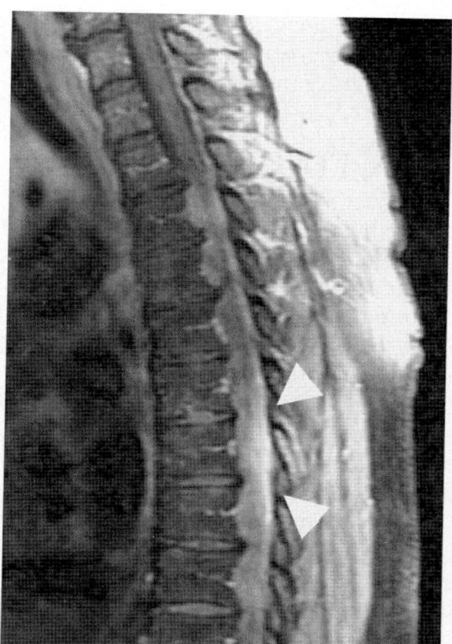

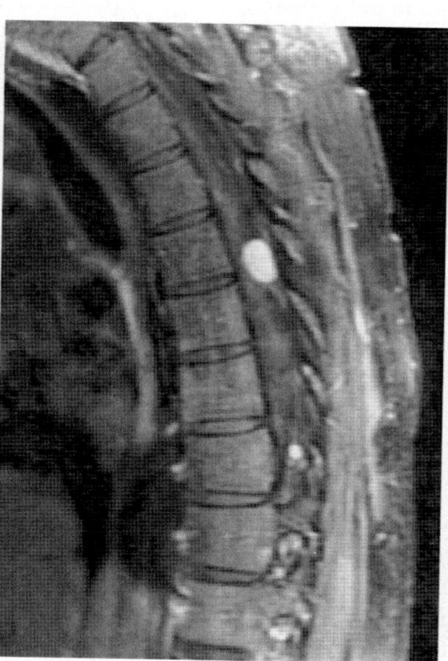

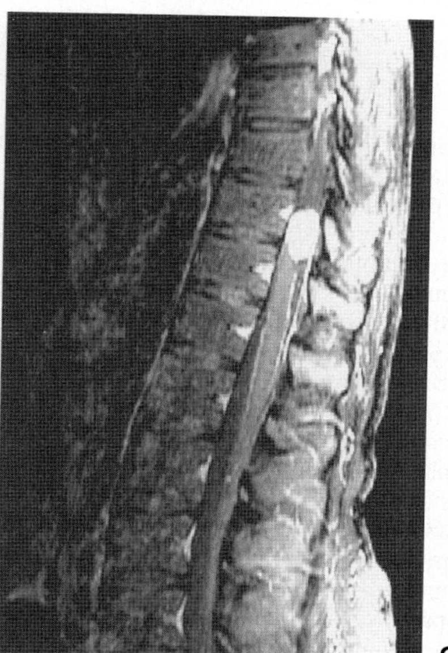

A, B C

FIGURE 145.2 Topical differential diagnosis of cord compression. **A:** Diffuse epidural infiltration by granulocytic sarcoma in a 65-year-old woman, causing cord compression in the lower thoracic spine (*arrowheads*). The tumor originated in the uterus and likely metastasized through the epidural venous plexus (Batson's plexus) into the spinal canal (T1-weighted magnetic resonance image [MRI] with gadolinium and fat suppression). **B:** A 32-year-old woman with neurofibromatosis type II and a meningioma of the spinal canal. This T1-weighted MRI with gadolinium and fat suppression (thoracic spine, sagittal view) demonstrates an intradural, extramedullary mass lesion with cord compression. **C:** Leptomeningeal metastasis with cord infiltration and compression at the level of the T10 vertebral body in a 27-year-old patient with leptomeningeal spread of a diencephalic yolk sac tumor. The tumor infiltrated the thoracic spinal cord, giving rise to a Brown-Sequard syndrome below the level of infiltration (T1-weighted MRI with gadolinium and fat suppression, lower spine, sagittal view).

necrosis. Pathologic fracture of a vertebral body and posterior displacement of bone fragments lead to mechanical cord destruction. On histopathologic examination, demyelination or necrosis of white matter is the predominant finding at the level of cord compression, whereas gray matter is relatively well preserved.[13]

The complex syndrome of back pain is composed of local, radicular, and referred components. Pain-sensitive structures of the spine are the vertebral periosteum, the posterior longitudinal ligament, and the synovia of the facet joints innervated by branches of segmental spinal nerves. Pain from metastatic tumor spread to the spine ensues when the cancer infiltrates the periosteum. Radicular pain results from compression or infiltration of a nerve root. Pain can also be the consequence of irritation of long tracts of the spinal cord (funicular pain) or paravertebral muscle spasm.

Micturition is frequently impaired in patients with MSCC. A brief review of the anatomy of bladder control may help to correctly interpret patients' symptoms. Excitatory input to the detrusor muscle that promotes bladder emptying is parasympathetic and involves sacral spinal cord segments. Relaxation of the internal sphincter is transmitted through the sympathetic nervous system. Preganglionic neurons originate from thoracic and upper lumbar cord segments. The external sphincter muscle is innervated by motor neurons located in the anterior horn of the sacral cord (nucleus of Onufrowicz). Voluntary bladder control requires sensory input from stretch receptors within the bladder wall. This is transmitted to the pontine micturition center that also receives descending input from the paracentral lobule of the frontal lobe. The coordinated inhibition of internal and external sphincter muscle is mediated through the pontine micturition center. Spinal cord compression above the conus results in lack of voluntary control of micturition. Reflex emptying is possible but incomplete. When the sacral spinal cord is destroyed, the patient suffers from external sphincter insufficiency, unawareness of bladder fullness, and overflow incontinence. The mechanisms for control of defecation are similar.

CLINICAL PRESENTATION

Pain is the most common presenting symptom in patients with metastases involving the axial skeleton.[6,8,18,19] Any back pain in a patient with cancer known to frequently seed to spine or epidural space should be considered of metastatic origin until proven otherwise. Pain ensues when the richly innervated periosteum is involved. In its early stage, it may be localized to the affected spine segment. The vertebral body is tender to percussion. Pain that results from epidural mass effect is typically exacerbated by sneezing, coughing, or the Valsalva maneuver. Because it is aggravated by the recumbent position, patients experience maximum pain intensity on awakening in the morning; they may even sleep in a sitting position. Compression of a nerve root is associated with lancinating pain in the corresponding radicular distribution provoked by Valsalva maneuver. Radicular pain in the thoracic region is usually bilateral, whereas cervical and lumbar radiculopathies are unilateral.[27] Paravertebral muscle spasm caused by nerve root irritation from a metastasis results in straightening of the physiologic cervical or lumbar lordosis. Straight-leg raising (Lasegue maneuver) or, more specifically, crossed straight-leg raising (passive elevation of the contralateral, pain-free leg), exacerbates a lumbosacral radiculopathy. Referred pain may mimic a radiculopathy. Especially with intraneural tumor spread, neuropathic features (allodynia, hyperpathia, hyperalgesia) may predominate.

Neurologic symptoms typically evolve within weeks to months of the onset of back pain.[15,19] Hyperacute presentation with the evolution of paraplegia within hours to days is not uncommon in bronchogenic carcinoma, while a much slower course is typical for metastases from breast cancer.[13] Motor dysfunction (weakness, spasticity) is the earliest sign and occurs before sensory disturbance. Only one-third of patients report lower extremity weakness as an initial symptom. However, at diagnosis, less than one-third of patients are ambulatory.[6,8,18] Typical early complaints are leg "heaviness" and difficulty climbing stairs or getting up from a chair. As the majority of malignancy-related cord compressions occur at the level of the thoracic spinal cord, most patients present with a paraparesis. The rare patient with a cervical spinal cord metastasis is expected to have quadriparesis of varying degree and, if the high cervical cord is compromised, respiratory insufficiency. Epidural progression of metastases to the upper lumbar spine results in conus medullaris syndrome with distal lower extremity weakness, saddle paresthesia, and overflow leakage from bladder and bowel.

Only few patients report diminished sensation below the level of compression at initial presentation. The level of hypesthesia is usually two to three segments below the metastatic lesion. Discrepancy of up to ten levels above or below the lesion has been described.[18] Tingling paresthesias radiating down the spine into the extremities on brisk flexion of the neck (Lhermitte's sign) indicates an intrinsic or extrinsic spinal cord process. Ataxia in a patient with MSCC reflects compression of spinocerebellar pathways.

Symptoms of neurogenic bladder dysfunction are less common at symptom onset but are frequently overlooked or "rationalized" by the patient. A detailed micturition history is indispensable as patients are unlikely to report their symptoms until their compensatory mechanisms fail. New onset of nocturia or pollakisuria in the correct clinical setting should alarm the physician, and a common explanation by the patient ("I've been drinking a lot") should be disregarded. Alarming symptoms of bladder dysfunction are hesitancy and urinary retention. At diagnosis, almost half of patients with MSCC are incontinent or require catheterization.[8]

Presence of a Horner's syndrome (the combination of miosis, ptosis, and enophthalmos) indicates transforaminal progression of tumors located at the level of the cervicothoracic junction and infiltration of the stellate ganglion.

DIFFERENTIAL DIAGNOSIS

Infiltration of the lumbosacral plexus or peripheral nerves originating from it (femoral, sciatic nerve) has to be distinguished from malignant epidural compression of a root or the cauda equina. With unilateral involvement, bladder and bowel symptoms are absent; however, bilateral infiltration of plexus or nerve, giving rise to incontinence, has been seen in neurolymphomatosis and perineural spread from pelvic malignancies. Herpes zoster is encountered at spinal levels previously or concurrently affected by cancer.[13,28]

The cauda equina syndrome is characterized by an asymmetric painful lumbosacral polyradiculopathy, a patchy sensory deficit corresponding to multiple lumbar and sacral nerve roots, and bladder and bowel incontinence. In a cancer patient, this syndrome raises suspicion for leptomeningeal carcinomatosis. The presence of signs and symptoms referable to intracranial disease (headache, asymmetric cranial neuropathies) facilitates the diagnosis.

Intraparenchymal spinal cord metastases and primary cord tumors are rare but may resemble epidural disease. Metastatic cord tumors predominantly arise from small-cell lung and breast cancers.[29] Infectious (herpes simplex, human T-lymphotropic virus) and autoimmune myelitis are examples of not directly cancer-related myelopathies that have to be distinguished from MSCC. Predominance of transverse myelopathic features in the absence of pain is indicative of an intraparenchymal process.

Spinal cord hemisyndromes indicate intrinsic spinal cord disease. A classic Brown-Sequard syndrome characterized by leg weakness and loss of proprioception on the side of cord infiltration and loss of pain and temperature sensation on the opposite side is rarely seen but incomplete variants exist. Leptomeningeal spread of highly aggressive tumors can lead to spinal cord infiltration, causing an overlap syndrome of extrinsic and intrinsic cord disease (Figure 145.2C).

DIAGNOSIS

The mere complaint of back pain in a cancer patient frequently does not lead to an immediate workup for vertebral metastases. Only the occurrence of more severe symptoms such as sphincter dysfunction or paraparesis sets off a comprehensive diagnostic procedure.[6] In spite of the availability of sensitive diagnostic tests, the average time between onset of symptoms and definitive diagnosis is still 3 months (range, 37 to 205 days). Two-thirds of this time passes after the patient reports the symptoms to a health professional.[18] An interesting pattern was observed in a Scottish study. The rate of cord compression diagnosis steadily increased throughout the course of the week and reached its peak on Friday.[18]

With the availability of magnetic resonance imaging (MRI), the diagnosis of MSCC has been simplified. The decision to use this tool depends on the clinical evaluation. New onset or change in character of preexisting back pain in a cancer patient or atypical back pain in the absence of a cancer history warrants measures beyond plain x-ray films and symptomatic therapy. Degenerative spine disease mostly affects the lower cervical and lower lumbar spine, the segments of largest motion. The pain waxes and wanes and responds to bed rest and symptomatic treatment with nonsteroidal anti-inflammatory agents. Pain located in the thoracic spine, progressive pain in spite of conservative measures, or pain aggravated by supine position should raise the suspicion for MSCC.

MRI of the entire spine is the most sensitive diagnostic test when MSCC is suspected in a cancer patient. The study can accurately identify the level of the metastatic lesion and guide the radiation oncologist in planning the treatment field. Multiple levels of involvement present in up to one-third of patients with metastatic spinal cord compression are recognized.[20,30] Vertebral metastases without protrusion into the epidural space are detected before a potentially irreversible cord syndrome ensues. Metastases can be distinguished from other pathologic processes, involving the axial skeleton, epi- and intradural space, and spinal cord. Bacterial abscesses typically cause end-plate destruction and invasion of the disc space, whereas metastatic deposits leave the latter intact. Leptomeningeal carcinomatosis appears as nodular or linear tumor deposits in the medullary pia and along intradural nerve roots. Intradural extramedullary tumors such as meningioma or nerve sheath tumors can be easily diagnosed by their characteristic appearance and enhancement with contrast dye. Intramedullary metastases or primary tumors cause enlargement of the cord and thus can be distinguished from infectious or inflammatory myelitis that does not expand its transverse diameter.

Plain x-ray films of the spine lack sufficient sensitivity. Series of the pre-MRI era found signs of vertebral metastasis at the level of cord compression on plain x-ray films in only 80% of patients, and multiple levels of involvement were missed.[19] The local extent of metastatic disease is frequently underestimated, and paraspinal tumors with transforaminal extension may be entirely overlooked.

Myelography after intrathecal injection of water-soluble contrast material with or without computed tomography (myelography, computed tomographic myelography) was the diagnostic procedure of choice in the pre-MRI era. Epidural lesions that result in complete block of the subarachnoid space obscure the extent of disease and require a second procedure with cervical or suboccipital injection of dye in order to characterize metastatic deposits rostral to the block. The study remains an option for patients in whom MRI is contraindicated.

Scintigraphic examination of the skeletal system is most useful as a screening procedure for bone metastases. Its resolution, specificity, and sensitivity are inadequate to evaluate a patient with signs or symptoms of epidural metastasis and predict the level of cord compromise.[18] Myeloma may completely evade scintigraphic detection.

Positron emission tomography is likewise most useful as a staging procedure and cannot substitute for more detailed anatomic imaging techniques.

If cancer initially presents with MSCC, a biopsy is mandatory prior to initiation of therapy. This can be done by excisional biopsy of the mass or by computed tomography–guided needle biopsy.

A lumbar puncture is of no diagnostic value in epidural cancer. Complete obliteration of the subarachnoid space by an epidural metastasis results in compartmentation of the spinal canal with the possibility of herniation ("coning") after pressure reduction in the compartment below the level of obstruction by a lumbar puncture. Although cord herniation is a rare event, an MRI scan of the spine is advisable whenever MSCC is suspected before a lumbar puncture is performed. Thrombocytopenic cancer patients are at risk of developing a spinal epidural hematoma at the site of a lumbar puncture. A platelet transfusion may be required before the procedure can be safely performed.

TREATMENT

Treatment with corticosteroids should be initiated immediately when MSCC is suspected. Corticosteroids not only facilitate pain management but also reduce vasogenic cord edema and may prevent additional damage to the spinal cord from decreased perfusion. After an initial intravenous bolus, doses of up to 10 mg every 6 hours are most commonly used. Oral bioavailability is excellent and intravenous application is required only in patients who cannot swallow. Protocols using higher doses (initial bolus of 100 mg followed by 96 mg divided into four doses for 3 days and a subsequent rapid taper) may achieve better pain control, but it remains unclear if their use leads to an improvement in neurologic recovery or preservation of motor function and sphincter control.[19,31,32] Complications of steroid use (gastroduodenal ulceration, hallucinations, euphoria, insomnia, generalized burning sensation) is more likely with use of higher doses.[33,34]

At the time of diagnosis, two-thirds of patients are treated with radiotherapy and one in five or six patients with surgical decompression. One-quarter of patients with MSCC are provided comfort care only when there is widespread disease and poor quality of life.[7]

Conventional external-beam radiation therapy is the most commonly used treatment modality for patients. Various schedules have been applied with comparable results. Protocols consist of five to ten applications of 3 to 4 Gy. Others have provided higher daily doses (5 Gy) during a 3-day induction phase followed by daily fractions of 3 Gy over 5 days for consolidation.[19] In the palliative situation, single fractions of 8 Gy may be preferable. Response to treatment depends on tumor histology. As one would anticipate, patients with relative radiosensitive tumors (breast cancer, lymphoma) have a higher chance of regaining or preserving motor function than patients with less radiosensitive tumors (non–small cell lung cancer, melanoma, renal cell carcinoma).[19]

Recently there has been an increase in the use of stereotactic radiosurgical techniques for spine metastases. A distinct advantage over conventional radiotherapy is the ability to deliver a higher radiation dose without exceeding the tolerance of the spinal cord. Various techniques and dosing schedules are available: linear-accelerator–based somatostatin receptor scintigraphy (SRS), proton beam radiosurgery, or image-guided radiosurgery. SRS is typically administered as a 8 to 24 Gy single fraction. Stereotactic radiation therapy (SRT) is given in three to five fractions of 4 to 9 Gy. To date, radiosurgery has largely been used as salvage therapy for tumor progression in patients who have already been treated with conventional radiotherapy or as an adjuvant therapy following surgery. A role for spinal radiosurgery as a primary modality is seen in patients who are unable to undergo surgery or those with tumors poorly responsive to conventional radiotherapy. Local control rates of 85% to 90% and durable responses even against radioresistant tumors have been reported.[35–37] In 2009, the Spine Oncology Study Group issued a "strong" recommendation to consider radiosurgery over conventional radiotherapy for patients with solid-tumor spinal metastases.[38] However, when spinal tumors abut the cord or if there is MSCC, SRS or SRT may not be feasible. Proper prospective evaluation of efficacy, morbidity, and cost-effectiveness as a function of tumor stage is pending and, considering the complexity of the patient population, may only become available for highly selected patient populations.

Strontium-89 is used as palliative treatment for widely metastatic bone metastases from prostate cancer. It provides pain control but cannot reverse the neurologic syndrome from epidural cord compression.

The role of surgical decompression in patients with MSCC remains a controversial subject. For the majority of patients, a benefit from surgical intervention has not been convincingly shown.[39] However, in carefully selected patients, tumor resection results in improved functional outcome compared with irradiation. In a prospective randomized trial, the ability to walk was preserved for a longer period of time after surgery compared with radiation therapy (122 days vs. 13 days). Patients were eligible only if they did not have certain radiosensitive tumors (lymphomas, leukemia, multiple myeloma, and germ-cell tumors) or concomitant neurologic problems not directly related to MSCC (e.g., brain metastases), the duration of paraplegia was less than 48 hours, MSCC occurred at one level, their general medical status rendered them acceptable surgical candidates, and their life expectancy exceeded 3 months.[40] Other commonly accepted indications for surgery are the lack of a recent history of cancer, involvement of a previously irradiated segment, progressive painful radiculopathy in spite of irradiation, cord compression resulting from pathologic fracture, and spinal instability.[6,26,30] Younger patients are more likely to undergo surgical debulking.[7] Posterior exposure with laminectomy at the level of cord compression has been a common approach. The metastatic focus, usually located within the vertebral body, cannot be completely visualized and thus at best is only partially removed. Laminectomy may increase the degree of instability in kyphotic deformities, resulting from pathologic fracture. Thus, an anterior approach for surgical decompression is favored in selected patients. This procedure, reserved for patients with the possibility of long-term survival, includes resection of the affected vertebral body and implantation of stabilizing instrumentation. Frequently, two surgical sessions are required.[26,41] Surgical morbidity is considerable. A posterolateral transpedicular approach with stabilizing instrumentation is a feasible alternative.[26]

Treatment guidelines are similar in the pediatric population. Surgical intervention is recommended for patients with rapid neurologic deterioration or a severe transverse myelopathy at initial presentation.[21]

Systemic chemotherapy is an appropriate treatment only for patients with MSCC caused by highly chemosensitive tumors such as non-Hodgkin's lymphoma. Radiation or surgical intervention may not be necessary.[16,42]

It is unclear if asymptomatic patients benefit from treatment of incidentally detected epidural metastases. The decision depends on tumor type and the patient's condition. Observation and serial MRI scans may be appropriate until pain ensues.

Bisphosphonates are now widely used, particularly in the treatment of breast cancer and multiple myeloma. Monthly provision of intravenous pamidronate at a dose of 90 mg in combination with other treatment modalities for the underlying cancer significantly reduces skeletal morbidity.[24]

PROGNOSIS

Naturally, the prognosis for the patient with epidural metastasis and cord compression depends on the type and extent of the underlying malignancy. Untreated, patients with MSCC succumb within a month of diagnosis. The median overall survival of patients with MSCC ranges from 3 to 16 months and most patients die of systemic tumor progression.[1,6–8,12,41,43] Patients with therapy-sensitive tumors such as lymphoma or myeloma live longer (lymphoma, 6 to 14 months) than patients with solid tumors.[6,7,12,44] The most important determinant of functional outcome is the severity of neurologic damage at the time treatment is initiated. Eighty percent of patients treated at a time when a significant neurologic deficit is absent, and 50% of those with mild transverse myelopathy, but only 5% of patients who are paraplegic when definitive treatment is initiated, remain ambulatory or regain the ability to walk after treatment.[1,8,11,12,14] Late return of function within 6 to 20 months of treatment has been observed in long-term survivors of MSCC in non-Hodgkin's lymphoma.[14,16] The faster the neurologic deficit evolves, the lower the chance for recovery of motor function after treatment.[44]

References

1. Helweg-Larsen S, Sorensen PS, Kreiner S. Prognostic factors in metastatic spinal cord compression: a prospective study using multivariate analysis of variables influencing survival and gait function in 153 patients. *Int J Radiat Oncol Biol Phys* 2000;46(5):1163.
2. Bilsky MH, Lis E, Raizer J, Lee H, Boland P. The diagnosis and treatment of metastatic spinal tumor. *Oncologist* 1999;4(6):459.
3. Klimo P Jr, Thompson CJ, Kestle JRW, Schmidt MH. A meta-analysis of surgery versus conventional radiotherapy for the treatment of metastatic spinal epidural disease. *Neuro-Oncology* 2005;7(1):64.
4. Nelson KA, Walsh D, Abdullah O, et al. Common complications of advanced cancer. *Sem Oncol* 2000;27(1):34.
5. Quinn JA, DeAngelis LM. Neurologic emergencies in the cancer patient. *Sem Oncol* 2000;27(3):311.
6. Kovner F, Spigel S, Rider I, et al. Radiation therapy of metastatic spinal cord compression. Multidisciplinary team diagnosis and treatment. *J Neurooncol* 1999;42(1):85.
7. Loblaw DA, Laperriere NJ, Mackillop WJ. A population-based study of malignant spinal cord compression in Ontario. *Clin Oncol (R Coll Radiol)* 2003;15(4):211.
8. Bach F, Larsen BH, Rohde K, et al. Metastatic spinal cord compression. *Acta Neurochir (Wien)* 1990;107:37.
9. Loblaw DA, Laperriere NJ. Emergency treatment of malignant extradural spinal cord compression: an evidence-based guideline. *J Clin Oncol* 1998;16(4):1613.
10. Prasad D, Schiff D. Malignant spinal-cord compression. *Lancet Oncol* 2005;6(1):15.

11. Posner JB. Back pain and epidural spinal cord compression. *Med Clin North Am* 1987;71(2):185.
12. Maranzano E, Latini P. Effectiveness of radiation therapy without surgery in metastatic spinal cord compression: final results from a prospective trial. *Int J Radiat Oncol Biol Phys* 1995;32(4):959.
13. Barron KD, Hirano A, Araki S, Terry RD. Experiences with metastatic neoplasms involving the spinal cord. *Neurology* 1959;9:91.
14. Helweg-Larsen S. Clinical outcome in metastatic spinal cord compression. A prospective study of 153 patients. *Acta Neurol Scand* 1996;94(4):269.
15. Schiff D, O'Neill BP, Suman VJ. Spinal epidural metastasis as the initial manifestation of malignancy. *Neurology* 1997;49:452.
16. McDonald AC, Nicoll JA, Rampling RP. Non-Hodgkin's lymphoma presenting with spinal cord compression; a clinicopathological review of 25 cases. *Eur J Cancer* 2000;36(2):207.
17. Bach F, Agerlin N, Sorensen JB, et al. Metastatic spinal cord compression secondary to lung cancer. *J Clin Oncol* 1992;10(11):1781.
18. Levack P, Graham J, Collie D, et al. Don't wait for a sensory level—listen to the symptoms: a prospective audit of the delays in diagnosis of malignant cord compression. *Clin Oncol (R Coll Radiol)* 2002;14(6):472.
19. Greenberg HS, Kim JH, Posner JB. Epidural spinal cord compression from metastatic tumor: results with a new treatment protocol. *Ann Neurol* 1980; 8(4):361.
20. Schiff D, O'Neill BP, Wang CH, O'Fallon JR. Neuroimaging and treatment implications of patients with multiple epidural spinal metastases. *Cancer* 1998;83(8):1593.
21. Bouffet E, Marec-Berard P, Thiesse P, et al. Spinal cord compression by secondary epi- and intradural metastases in childhood. *Childs Nerv Syst* 1997; 13(7):383.
22. Antunes NL. Acute neurologic complications in children with systemic cancer. *J Child Neurol* 2000;15(11):705.
23. Abrams HL, Spiro R, Goldstein N. Metastases in carcinoma. *Cancer 3* 1950;3:74.
24. Coleman RE. Metastatic bone disease: clinical features, pathophysiology and treatment strategies. *Cancer Treat Rev* 2001;27(3):165.
25. Coleman RE. Skeletal complications of malignancy. *Cancer* 1997;80(8 Suppl):1588.
26. Healey JH, Brown HK. Complications of bone metastases: surgical management. *Cancer* 2000;88(12 Suppl):2940.
27. Posner JB. Neurological complications of systemic cancer. *Med Clin North Am* 1971;55(3):625.
28. Mullins GM, Flynn JP, el-Mahdi AM, McQueen JD, Owens AH Jr. Malignant lymphoma of the spinal epidural space. *Ann Inter Med* 1971;74(3):416.
29. Schiff D, O'Neill BP. Intramedullary spinal cord metastases. *Neurology* 1996;47:906.
30. Hardy JR, Huddart R. Spinal cord compression–what are the treatment standards? *Clin Oncol (R Coll Radiol)* 2002;14(2):132.
31. Sorensen S, Helweg-Larsen S, Mouridsen H, Hansen HH. Effect of high-dose dexamethasone in carcinomatous metastatic spinal cord compression treated with radiotherapy: a randomised trial. *Eur J Cancer* 1994;30A(1):22.
32. Delattre JY, Arbit E, Rosenblum MK, et al. High dose versus low dose dexamethasone in experimental epidural spinal cord compression. *Neurosurgery* 1988;22:1005.
33. Heimdal K, Hirschberg H, Slettebo H, Watne K, Nome O. High incidence of serious side effects of high-dose dexamethasone treatment in patients with epidural spinal cord compression. *J Neurooncol* 1992;12(2):141.
34. Klimo P Jr, Kestle JR, Schmidt MH. Treatment of metastatic spinal epidural disease: a review of the literature. *Neurosurg Focus* 2003;15(5):E1.
35. Yamada Y, Lovelock DM, Yenice KM, et al. Multifractionated image-guided and stereotactic intensity-modulated radiotherapy of paraspinal tumors: a preliminary report. *Int J Radiat Oncol Biol Phys* 2005;62(1):53.
36. Gerszten PC, Burton SA, Ozhasoglu C, Welch WC. Radiosurgery for spinal metastases: clinical experience in 500 cases from a single institution. *Spine* 2007;32(2):193.
37. Yamada Y, Bilsky MH, Lovelock DM, et al. High-dose, single-fraction image-guided intensity-modulated radiotherapy for metastatic spinal lesions. *Int J Radiat Oncol Biol Phys* 2008;71(2):484.
38. Gerszten PC, Mendel E, Yamada Y. Radiotherapy and radiosurgery for metastatic spine disease: what are the options, indications, and outcomes? *Spine* 2009;34(22 Suppl):S78.
39. Young RF, Post EM, King GA. Treatment of spinal epidural metastases. Randomized prospective comparison of laminectomy and radiotherapy. *J Neurosurg* 1980;53(6):741.
40. Patchell RA, Tibbs PA, Regine WF, et al. Direct decompressive surgical resection in the treatment of spinal cord compression caused by metastatic cancer: a randomised trial. *Lancet* 2005;366(9486):643.
41. Sundaresan N, Sachdev VP, Holland JF, et al. Surgical treatment of spinal cord compression from epidural metastasis. *J Clin Oncol* 1995;13(9): 2330.
42. Wong ET, Portlock CS, O'Brien JP, DeAngelis LM. Chemosensitive epidural spinal cord disease in non-Hodgkins lymphoma. *Neurology* 1996;46(6): 1543.
43. Maranzano E, Latini P, Checcaglini F, et al. Radiation therapy in metastatic spinal cord compression. A prospective analysis of 105 consecutive patients. *Cancer* 1991;67(5):1311.
44. Rades D, Blach M, Nerreter V, Bremer M, Karstens JH. Metastatic spinal cord compression. Influence of time between onset of motoric deficits and start of irradiation on therapeutic effect. *Strahlenther Onkol* 1999;175(8): 378.

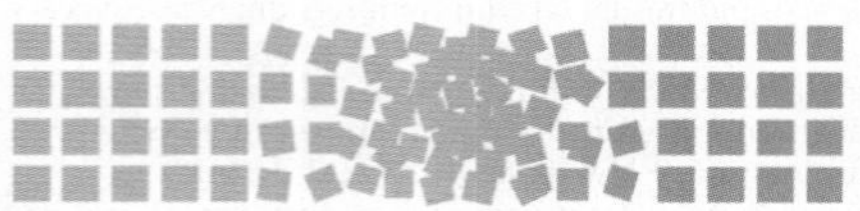

CHAPTER 146 METABOLIC EMERGENCIES

ANTONIO TITO FOJO

Despite improvements in the therapy of many cancers, metabolic emergencies, usually encountered in patients with advanced cancer, continue to present challenges to the practicing oncologist. Although the availability of better therapies has made these difficult problems increasingly manageable, prompt recognition and the institution of adequate therapy are essential.

TUMOR LYSIS SYNDROME

Spontaneous or treatment-induced cell death leads to a constellation of metabolic abnormalities that together comprise the tumor lysis syndrome (TLS) (Tables 146.1 and 146.2). Although TLS can occur as a result of cell death in a rapidly growing tumor, it occurs most frequently following administration of cytotoxic chemotherapy to patients with hematologic malignancies, where a large percentage of cells are proliferating and drug sensitive. In these patients, TLS occurs a few hours to a few days after the initiation of therapy. Cell death leads to the release of potassium, phosphate, uric acid, and other purine metabolites that overwhelm the kidneys' capacity for clearance with resultant hyperkalemia, hyperphosphatemia and secondary hypocalcemia, and hyperuricemia (discussed further below). Unchecked, TLS can progress to lactic acidosis and acute renal failure. Although established TLS is associated with a high morbidity and mortality, judicious prophylaxis can avoid these complications. A higher mortality among patients with solid tumors who develop TLS is likely a consequence of less prophylaxis and reduced awareness of its occurrence in solid tumors.

TLS occurs most frequently in rapidly growing, chemosensitive myelolymphoproliferative malignancies with either large bulky adenopathy or high white blood cell counts. The highest incidence of TLS occurs in patients with myeloproliferative diseases, acute leukemias, and high-grade non-Hodgkin's lymphomas (NHL), especially Burkitt lymphoma.[1–4] In high-grade NHL an incidence as high as 42% has been reported, although clinically significant TLS occurred in only 6% of patients.[5] The latter percentage is more in agreement with a pan-European retrospective chart review that identified TLS in 3.4%, 5.2%, and 6.1%, of patients with acute myeloid leukemia (AML), acute lymphoid leukemia (ALL), and NHL, respectively; with an overall mortality of 0.9% for all patients and 17.5% for patients who developed TLS.[6] By comparison, TLS occurs infrequently in solid tumors, most likely due to the longer doubling time, low growth fraction, and slow response to treatment compared to lymphoproliferative malignancies.[7] In solid tumors it usually occurs with tumors that are *highly or moderately* sensitive to chemotherapy, although less sensitive tumors may lead to TLS if bulky, metastatic disease is present, as evidenced by a high serum lactate dehydrogenase (LDH).[7] TLS has also been reported following ionizing radiation, including TBI in the transplant setting, embolization, radiofrequency ablation, monoclonal antibody therapy, glucocorticoids, interferon, and in the setting of hematopoietic stem cell transplantation. As new therapies emerge, TLS may occur in unanticipated settings, as seen in indolent chronic lymphocytic leukemia treated with flavopiridol.[8]

Risk factors include (1) bulky disease (hepatosplenomegaly, bulky adenopathy) or a high leucocyte count, often evidenced by elevated pretreatment LDH; (2) elevated pretreatment uric acid; (3) compromised renal function or decreased urine output; and (4) potentially nephrotoxic drugs. The clinical presentation can range from asymptomatic laboratory abnormalities, to clinical changes secondary to the electrolyte disturbances.[9]

Pathogenesis

Cell lysis with the release of contents at a rate exceeding the kidneys' clearance capacity is the most important etiologic factor in TLS (Table 146.1). Rapidly dividing cells have high nucleic acid turnover, and some cancer cells, particularly lymphoid cells, contain higher levels of phosphate than normal counterparts.

Hyperkalemia poses the greatest immediate threat. Although release of potassium from dying cells is the principal cause, falling adenosine triphosphate (ATP) levels before cell lysis may lead to potassium leakage, explaining why a rising serum potassium is often the first sign of TLS.

Hyperphosphatemia, like hyperkalemia, follows cell lysis. The initial adaptation involves increased urinary excretion and decreased tubular reabsorption of phosphate. However, as transport becomes saturated, phosphorus levels rise, the calcium phosphorus multiple exceeds 70, and calcium phosphate precipitates in tissues, resulting in hypocalcemia. Hypocalcemia leads to increased levels of parathyroid hormone, with decreased proximal tubule phosphate reabsorption, accentuating hyperphosphaturia and the risk of calcium phosphate crystals in renal tubules (nephrocalcinosis) with tubular obstruction.

Hyperuricemia (Fig. 146.1, discussed below), while not an acute threat, is the most common finding and contributes to renal failure, a complication that in the setting of tumor lysis is usually multifactorial.

Therapy

In approaching patients with potential TLS it is easier to stay out of trouble than get out of trouble (Table 146.1). In the modern era, laboratory abnormalities alert physicians and guide preventive management. In adults, preventive measures

TABLE 146.1

TUMOR LYSIS SYNDROME

Complication	Etiology	Manifestations	Management
Hyperkalemia	Release of intracellular potassium at a rate that exceeds renal clearance capacity; potassium leakage secondary to falling ATP levels	■ Electrocardiographic abnormalities ■ Muscle cramps, weakness, and paresthesias ■ Nausea, vomiting, and diarrhea	■ Aggressive hydration ■ Cation exchange resins ■ Calcium gluconate ■ Sodium bicarbonate ■ Hypertonic dextrose plus insulin ■ Loop diuretics
Hyperphosphatemia	Release of intracellular phosphate at rate that exceeds renal clearance capacity	■ Acute renal failure ■ Secondary hypocalcemia	■ Aggressive hydration ■ Hypertonic dextrose plus insulin ■ Oral phosphate binders
Hypocalcemia	Secondary to hyperphosphatemia and the ensuing tissue precipitation of calcium phosphate	■ Muscle twitches, cramps, carpopedal spasm, paresthesia, or tetany ■ Mental status changes, confusion, delirium, hallucinations ■ Rarely seizures ■ Exacerbation of hyperkalemia	■ Manage hyperphosphatemia
Hyperuricemia	Release of intracellular uric acid at rate that exceeds renal clearance capacity	■ Acute renal failure	■ Allopurinol ■ Urate oxidase ■ Conventional hemodialysis if patient develops acute renal failure
Lactic acidosis	Hypovolemia and acute renal failure	■ Acidemia	■ Volume replacement ■ Correct acidosis

include foremost hydration, allopurinol, and *oral phosphate binders*, beginning preferably 24 hours before chemotherapy administration.

Aggressive hydration, the most important intervention, should begin immediately, administering at least 3,000 mL/m^2/d. *When possible tumor therapy should be delayed so hydration can be administered.* Urine alkalinization remains controversial since it favors precipitation of calcium/phosphate complexes in renal tubules; calcium phosphate, unlike uric acid, becomes less soluble at an alkaline pH. Furthermore, metabolic alkalemia can worsen the neurological manifestations of hypocalcemia. Administration of 100 mEq sodium bicarbonate will maintain urine pH above 7.5, a pH that is needed not because of uric acid, which has a pKa of 5.4, but because of xanthine, which as a pKa of about 7.4. Thus alkalinization is not a means to avoid uric acid crystallization, since at pH 6.4 more than 90% already exists as sodium urate.

TABLE 146.2

CAIRO AND BISHOP CLASSIFICATION SYSTEM FOR TUMOR LYSIS SYNDROME

Laboratory TLS	Clinical TLS
Abnormality in two or more of the following, occurring within 3 days before or 7 days after chemotherapy: ■ Uric acid >8 mg/dL or 25% increase ■ Potassium >6 meq/L or 25% increase ■ Phosphate >4.5 mg/dL or 25% increase ■ Calcium <7 mg/dL or 25% decrease	Laboratory TLS plus one or more of the following: ■ Increased serum creatinine (1.5 times upper limit of normal) ■ Cardiac arrhythmia or sudden death ■ Seizure

TLS, tumor lysis syndrome.
(Adapted from Cairo MS, Bishop M. Tumor lysis syndrome: new therapeutic strategies and classification. *Br J Haematol* 2004;127:3–11.)

Hyperkalemia should be treated aggressively. Cation exchange resins should be used, recognizing their value will be delayed. Calcium gluconate antagonizes cardiac effects of hyperkalemia and can be especially helpful with concomitant hypocalcemia. Sodium bicarbonate corrects acidemia and shifts potassium back into cells; administering hypertonic dextrose and insulin can augment this. Loop diuretics can eliminate excess potassium in patients without renal failure; hemodialysis is indicated in renal impairment.

Hyperphosphatemia and its resultant hypocalcemia require oral phosphate binders. With the exception of managing hyperkalemia, avoid calcium administration because it can promote metastatic calcifications.

Given its central role in acute renal failure, hyperuricemia should be managed aggressively. Allopurinol, an analogue of the natural purine base hypoxanthine, lowers uric acid by inhibiting xanthine oxidase, the enzyme responsible for converting hypoxanthine to xanthine and in turn xanthine to uric acid (Fig. 146.1). Its active metabolite, oxypurinol, also inhibits xanthine oxidase. Because both allopurinol and oxypurinol inhibit uric acid synthesis but have no effect on pre-existing uric acid, uric acid levels usually do not fall until after 48 to 72 hours of treatment. Furthermore, inhibition of xanthine oxidase leads to increased plasma levels of hypoxanthine and xanthine, with increased renal excretion of both metabolic products. Like uric acid, xanthine (pKa = 7.4) but not

PRACTICE OF ONCOLOGY

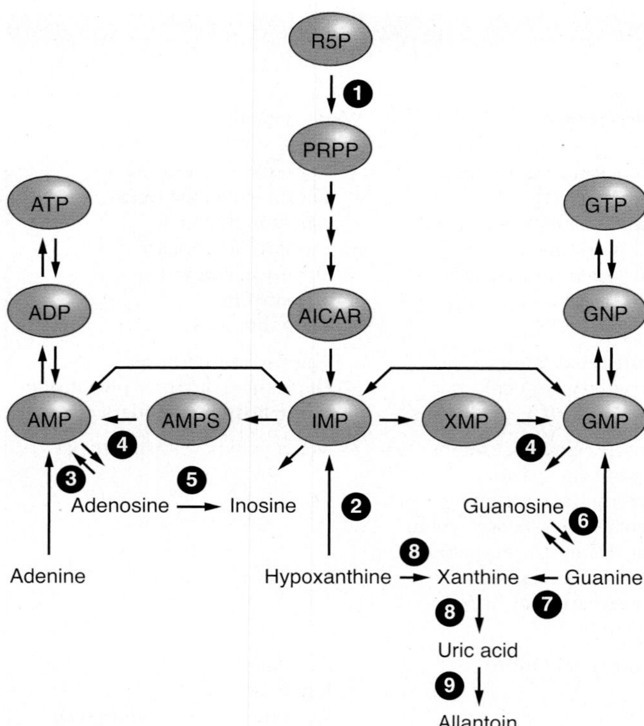

FIGURE 146.1 Purine metabolism pathways. The figure shows the pathways of purine metabolism in mammals with an emphasis on pathways involved in purine catabolism and generation of uric acid. The numbers enclosed in circles identify the enzymes involved in catalyzing the reaction. These are: (1) PRPP synthetase; (2) hypoxanthine phosphoribosyltransferase (HPRT); (3) adenosine kinase; (4) 5′ nucleotidase; (5) adenosine deaminase (ADA); (6) purine nucleoside phosphorylase (PNP); (7) guanase; (8) xanthine oxidase, which also catalyzes the conversion of allopurinol to oxypurinol; and (9) urate oxidase or uricase, an enzyme that is present in mammals with the exception of humans and many primates. R5P, ribose 5′ phosphate; PRPP, phosphoribosyl pyrophosphate; AICAR, aminoimidazole carboxamide ribonucleotide; IMP, inosine monophosphate; XMP, xanthosine monophosphate; GMP, guanosine monophosphate; guanosine diphosphate; GTP, guanosine triphosphate; AMPS, adenylosuccinate; AMP, adenosine monophosphate; ADP, adenosine diphosphate; ATP, adenosine triphosphate.

hypoxanthine (pKa = 1.98) may precipitate acute renal failure. Oral allopurinol has a bioavailability of 50%; alternately, intravenous allopurinol (Aloprim®) may be administered. Allopurinol should be discontinued if allergic reactions such as skin rashes and urticaria occur (incidence increased in patients who are given amoxicillin, ampicillin, or thiazides). Finally, the doses of allopurinol should be adjusted for creatinine clearance as follows:

Creatinine Clearance	Allopurinol Dose
>20 mL/min	300 mg/d
10–20 mL/min	200 mg/d
3–10 mL/min	100 mg/d
<3 mL/min	100 mg/36–48 hours

An alternate approach to the treatment of hyperuricemia involves the use of the enzyme urate oxidase (rasburicase [Elitek®]), discussed in greater detail under hyperuricemia.

If acute renal failure develops, immediate hemodialysis is recommended. Indeed, in patients presenting with TLS, hemodialysis should be started before cytotoxic therapy is administered. Conventional hemodialysis is more effective in eliminating uric acid and phosphate than peritoneal dialysis.

HYPERURICEMIA

Although hyperuricemia occurs in the setting of TLS, it is frequently an isolated finding in cancer patients. For example, a pan-European retrospective chart review that examined 755 patients with ALL, AML, or NHL identified hyperuricemia without TLS in 13.6% of cases, with TLS in an additional 5.3%.[6]

Pathogenesis

Within the cell there is continuous turnover and salvage of bases (Fig. 146.1). In humans, the end product of purine metabolism is uric acid. Adenine is catabolized to hypoxanthine, and this is converted by xanthine oxidase to xanthine and in turn to uric acid. Guanine forms xanthine that is converted to uric acid by xanthine oxidase. In most mammals *urate oxidase* catalyzes the uric acid oxidation to allantoin, a catabolite that is more soluble in urine. However, in humans a nonsense mutation in the coding region acquired during evolution precludes urate oxidase expression.[10] Thus, the final metabolite of purine metabolism is uric acid in humans and allantoin in other mammals.

Hyperuricemia occurs primarily as a result of accelerated cellular breakdown. Acute uric acid nephropathy occurs when urate and uric acid crystals obstruct renal tubules. Urate is filtered at high concentrations from the plasma and is further concentrated along the course of the tubular system. As the pH becomes more acidic, uric acid can precipitate, obstructing tubules and collecting ducts, even pelves and ureters. Crystal deposition increases tubular and intrarenal pressure with extrinsic compression of the vasa recta, an increase in renal vascular resistance, and a fall in renal blood flow. The elevated tubular pressure and decreased renal blood flow reduce glomerular filtration and can lead to acute renal failure.

Therapy

The use of allopurinol is described in the section dealing with treatment of TLS. Detractors point out allopurinol has no effect on pre-existing uric acid and, therefore, has a slow onset of action, is ineffective in many patients, elicits allergic reactions, and can interfere with metabolism of some chemotherapeutic agents. Supporters note it is easy to use and inexpensive, has been administered to millions with few severe toxicities (including an incidence of allergic reactions not too dissimilar to that of many drugs), and that *rasburicase* can result in serious hypersensitivity reactions, including anaphylaxis. Indeed in a recent trial drug-related adverse events, mainly immunoallergic in nature, occurred in 4% of patients receiving rasburicase, 5% of those receiving rasburicase plus allopurinol, and only 1% of those treated with allopurinol[11] (Table 146.3).

Uricozyme, a nonrecombinant urate oxidase extracted from *Aspergillus flavus*, has been available in France and Italy for over two decades for the treatment of hyperuricemia. Because of encouraging results and a 4.5% incidence of hypersensitivity reactions, recombinant urate oxidase, rasburicase (Fasturtec®/Elitek®) was developed. Rasburicase is produced in *Saccharomyces cerevisiae* using a urate oxidase cDNA from *Aspergillus flavus*. Because urate oxidase degrades uric acid rather than prevent its synthesis, as does allopurinol, rapid reduction in uric acid occurs following its administration

TABLE 146.3

A COMPARISON OF RASBURICASE AND ALLOPURINOL IN THE MANAGEMENT OF TUMOR LYSIS SYNDROME

	Patients Experiencing Event (%)		
Event	Rasburicase (n = 92)	Rasburicase + Allopurinol (n = 92)	Allopurinol (n = 91)
Clinical TLS[a]	3	3	4
Laboratory TLS[b]	21	27	41
Hyperuricemia	8	12	29
Hyperphosphatemia	49	58	57
Hypocalcemia	16	19	25
Hyperkalemia	21	14	17
Renal Events			
Increased blood creatinine	8	10	10
Renal failure/impairment	4	9	2
Acute renal failure	2	5	2

TLS, tumor lysis syndrome.
[a]Clinical TLS was defined by changes in two or more laboratory parameters for hyperuricemia, hyperkalemia, hyperphosphatemia, and hypocalcemia and at least one of the following events occurring within 7 days of treatment: renal failure/injury, need for renal dialysis and/or increase in serum creatinine greater than 1.5 times upper limit of normal, arrhythmia, or seizure. No formal statistical comparisons were performed because of the small number of patients experiencing the events.
[b]Two or more laboratory changes within 7 days after cytotoxic therapy according to the Cairo-Bishop definition.
(Adapted from ref. 11.)

without precursor accumulation. Studies in adults and children have shown uric acid levels falling to 0.5 to 1 mg/dL within 4 hours of rasburicase injection, with low levels maintained throughout treatment. Only a small percentage have required dialysis despite normalization of uric acid levels, an observation not unexpected, given the multifactorial nature of renal failure in TLS and the fact that rasburicase affects only one component, albeit the most significant one.

The manufacturer recommends a rasburicase dose 0.2 mg/kg for up to 5 days. However, except in rare patients with very high serum levels of uric acid, much less is usually sufficient. Side effects include skin rash, mild nausea and vomiting, and rarely a hypersensitivity reaction including anaphylaxis. Antibodies against rasburicase or its epitopes occur in about 10% to 20% of patients, and subsequent retreatment appears associated with a higher incidence of allergic reactions, without affecting efficacy, since to date the antibodies do not appear to have blocking activity.[12] *Patients of African or Mediterranean ancestry should be screened for G6PD deficiency prior to starting rasburicase, because hydrogen peroxide, a byproduct of the urate oxidase reaction, can lead to hemolysis.*

Although the efficacy of rasburicase over allopurinol in preventing acute renal failure secondary to hyperuricemia is less clear, its rapid onset of action and ability to lower pre-existing elevated uric acid levels are distinct advantages that rasburicase possesses over allopurinol. This may allow one to begin chemotherapy treatment without delay. However, one must remember that rasburicase has no effect on the other manifestations of TLS, and these must continue to be addressed. Because at the present time a 5-day course of therapy with rasburicase is about 15,000 times more expensive than a 5-day course of allopurinol and 15 to 30 times more than intravenous allopurinol, cost must be factored into the decision making. With a 2010 price of approximately $435 per mg (Bluebook average wholesale price is $1,957 for three vials containing 1.5 mg each), the 5-day cost for a 70-kg patient who receives the manufacturer's recommended dose of 0.2 mg/kg for 5 days exceeds $30,450. At this price rasburicase can be justified only if it will prevent acute renal failure, and the existing data are not compelling. Although some studies suggest rasburicase can reduce the need for dialysis, no differences or only clinically insignificant differences in serum creatinine have been reported in other studies, and at the present time the data do not definitively proof that less dialysis is required in rasburicase-treated patients.[11,13] Although it *appears* rasburicase therapy is beneficial in children with hematologic malignancies, randomized controlled trials in adults have been less convincing. Nevertheless, rasburicase was recently approved by the U.S. Food and Drug Administration (FDA) for use in adults based on a randomized phase 3 trial[11] (Table 146.3). Because outcomes other than laboratory parameters were not different, the authors could only conclude "the incidence of laboratory TLS, which can be regarded as an indicator of the risk of clinical TLS, was significantly lower with rasburicase than with allopurinol" and "the rapid reduction in uric acid to less than 1.0 mg/dL with rasburicase simplifies uric acid control by reducing the need for urinary alkalinization in patients who are often critically ill with compromised organ function."[11] An earlier pan-European multicenter economic evaluation of rasburicase in prevention and treatment of hyperuricemia and TLS in patients with hematological malignancies concluded rasburicase is economically attractive in the *treatment of hyperuricemia* both in adults and children while in the *prevention of hyperuricemia* it "has an attractive economic profile in children and is cost-effective in adults with ALL and NHL . . . whereas in adult AML patients, the short average life expectancy and the lower baseline risk of hyperuricemia and TLS limits the cost-effectiveness of rasburicase."[6]

In both children and adults it appears that the manufacturer's recommended dose of 0.2 mg/kg/d for up to 5 days is excessive.[14–17] Evidence indicates a single 3-mg dose is effective in the prophylaxis and treatment of hyperuricemia in adults with uric acid levels up to 12 mg/dL, with uric acid levels continuing to decline beyond 24 hours in most patients without additional treatment.[17] For a 70-kg patient, a 3-mg dose—approximately one-fifth the recommended dose of 0.2 mg/kg—is convenient since vials contain 1.5 mg rasburicase and more affordable (at the time of writing $1,305).

TABLE 146.4

TUMOR LYSIS SYNDROME PROPHYLAXIS BASED ON TUMOR LYSIS SYNDROME RISK[a]

Low-Risk Disease	Intermediate-Risk Disease	High-Risk Disease
All solid tumors except those specifically identified as intermediate risk disease (IRD)	■ Neuroblastoma ■ Germ cell tumors ■ Small cell lung cancer ■ Others with bulky or advanced stage disease	—
Multiple myeloma	—	—
CML	—	—
Indolent non-Hodgkin's lymphoma	—	—
Hodgkin's lymphoma	—	—
CLL	CLL treated with fludarabine, rituximab, and/or those with WBC ≥50 × 10⁹/l	—
AML + WBC <25 × 10⁹/l + LDH <2 × ULN	■ AML + WBC 25–100 × 10⁹/l ■ AML + WBC <25 × 10⁹/l and LDH ≥ 2 × ULN	AML + WBC ≥100 × 10⁹/l
Adult intermediate grade non-Hodgkin's lymphoma + LDH <2 × ULN	Adult intermediate grade non-Hodgkin's lymphoma + LDH ≥2 × ULN	—
Adult anaplastic large cell lymphoma	Stage III/IV childhood anaplastic large cell lymphoma	—
—	Stage III/IV childhood intermediate grade non-Hodgkin's lymphoma + LDH <2 × ULN	—
—	ALL and WBC <100 × 10⁹/l + LDH < 2 × ULN	ALL + WBC ≥100 × 10⁹/l ALL + LDH ≥2 × ULN
—	Burkitt's lymphoma + LDH <2 × ULN	■ Stage III/IV Burkitt's lymphoma ■ Any stage Burkitt's lymphoma + LDH ≥2 × ULN
—	Stage I/II lymphoblastic lymphoma + LDH <2 × ULN	■ Stage III/IV lymphoblastic lymphoma ■ Any stage lymphoblastic lymphoma + LDH ≥2 × ULN
—	—	■ Intermediate-risk disease with renal dysfunction and/or renal involvement ■ Intermediate-risk disease with uric acid, potassium and/or phosphate >ULN
Prophylaxis Recommendations		
Monitoring Hydration ± Allopurinol	Monitoring Hydration Allopurinol	Monitoring Hydration Rasburicase[b]

CML, chronic myeloid leukaemia; CLL, chronic lymphoid leukaemia; AML, acute myeloid leukaemia; ALL, acute lymphoblastic leukaemia; WBC, white blood cell count; LDH, lactate dehydrogenase; ULN, upper limit of normal.
[a]Adapted from Cairo MS, Coiffier B, Reiter A, et al. Recommendations for the evaluation of risk and prophylaxis of tumor lysis syndrome (TLS) in adults and children with malignant diseases: an expert TLS panel consensus. *Br J Haematol* 2010;149:578–586.
[b]Contraindicated in patients with a history consistent with glucose-6 phosphate dehydrogenase. In these patients, rasburicase should be substituted with allopurinol.

Note that since the half-life of rasburicase in serum is approximately 18 to 21 hours, about one-half of the administered dose is still present 24 hours after administration. If needed, faster reductions can be achieved using higher doses. Given this, a reasonable strategy to consider might be the following: (1) continue to rely on the triad of aggressive hydration, management of electrolyte disturbances, and institution of allopurinol beginning immediately upon presentation; (2) evaluate patients for their TLS risk (Table 146.4) and *administer a single 3-mg dose of rasburicase at presentation* to patients with "high risk disease"; (3) follow the levels of uric acid and administer additional rasburicase doses only to patients with uric acid levels above an arbitrary number such as 5 mg/dL 24 hours after a rasburicase dose. Remember, a few additional uric acid measurements are far less expensive than a dose of rasburicase. (*Important:* Because serum samples contain rasburicase, immediately cool samples obtained for uric acid to 0 to 4°C, so as to prevent *ex vivo* enzymatic uric acid degradation, which will falsely lower levels. Label test tubes as requiring chilling to avoid removal from ice upon arrival in the laboratory.)

CANCER AND HYPONATREMIA

Water and sodium homeostasis is frequently disordered in patients with cancer. Optimal homeostasis requires a delicate balance between renal free water clearance and renal sodium metabolism. Hyponatremia, commonly defined as serum sodium lower than 130 mEq/L, occurs with a reported incidence of 3.7% in medical cancer patients.[18] Clinical manifestations of hyponatremia range from none to impaired consciousness progressing to coma and generalized hypotonia or seizure activity, all secondary to cerebral edema. Less dramatic symptoms, including anorexia, nausea, and asthenia, are often difficult to ascribe to a single cause in cancer patients.

The differential of hyponatremia is extensive and includes among others head injuries, pulmonary infections, space-occupying intracranial lesions, recent surgical intervention or radiation therapy, gastrointestinal losses, cardiac failure, diabetes, hypothyroidism, as well as iatrogenic secondary to the administration of hypotonic fluids, or one of many drugs, including diuretics. Among medical cancer patients, inappropriate secretion of arginine vasopressin (AVP) (syndrome of inappropriate secretion of antidiuretic hormone [SIADH])[19] and sodium depletion secondary to reduced intake and gastrointestinal or renal losses each account for about one-third of cases (Table 146.5). Other etiologies more likely to occur in cancer patients rather than the general patient population include ectopic atrial natriuretic peptide (ANP) production, hyponatremia associated with third spacing of fluids (ascites), and "pseudohyponatremia" as might occur in a patient with multiple myeloma and hyperproteinemia; although one can argue the latter is in fact true, hyponatremia with the reduced sodium is an adaptation at electrical neutrality imposed by the increase in positively charged myeloma proteins.[20]

TABLE 146.5

DIAGNOSIS OF SYNDROME OF INAPPROPRIATE SECRETION OF ANTIDIURETIC HORMONE

Key Features:

1. Decreased effective osmolality (<275 mOsm/kg of water)
2. Urine osmolality >100 mOsm/kg of water
3. Clinical euvolemia
4. Urine sodium >40 mmol/L in the face of normal salt intake
5. Normal thyroid and adrenal function
6. No recent diuretic use

Ancillary Features:

1. Plasma uric acid <4 mg/dL
2. Blood urea nitrogen <10 mg/dL (0.357 mmols/L)
3. Fractional sodium excretion >1%
4. Fractional urea excretion >55%
5. Hyponatremia corrected by fluid restriction but not by normal saline
6. Urine concentration >100 mOsm/kg water—"abnormally high relative" to plasma osmolarity.
7. Elevated plasma arginine vasopressin levels despite hypotonicity and euvolemia

Adapted from ref. 19.

Pathogenesis

Under normal circumstances plasma osmolality is closely regulated in the range of 280 to 292 mOsm/kg through (1) thirst perception; (2) control of free water clearance in the kidney by antidiuretic hormone (ADH) also known as AVP; and (3) and renal sodium excretion regulated by ANP and the renin angiotensin system.

In cancer patients, hyponatremia secondary to inappropriate secretion of AVP (SIADH) occurs as a paraneoplastic syndrome or as a complication of therapy.[19] The inappropriate secretion of AVP can originate from its normal source, the hypothalamus, as a consequence of dysregulation, or can be ectopic in origin, arising from cancer cells themselves. In cases of ectopic production, AVP is detectable in plasma and correlates with detectable AVP messenger RNA (mRNA) or immunoreactive peptides in tumor cells. Although inappropriate AVP secretion can occur with any cancer, it is most frequently reported with small cell lung cancer, head and neck carcinomas, hematological malignancies, and non–small cell lung cancer (SCLC).[21] Drugs reported to cause SIADH include cyclophosphamide and its isomeric analogue, ifosfamide, the vinca alkaloids including vincristine, vinblastine, and vinorelbine, the proteasome inhibitor bortezomib (Velcade), as well as carboplatin and cisplatin, although the latter more frequently cause renal salt wasting. SIADH is defined as a hypo-osmolar or dilutional hyponatremia with excessive natriuresis (20 mEq/L or greater). Hyponatremia occurs because AVP secretion continues even after plasma osmolality falls below the threshold for AVP release. Key and ancillary features are summarized in Table 146.5.[19]

SCLC patients with hyponatremia without measurable AVP have also been reported.[21,22] In a fraction of these patients, ectopic production of ANP mRNA and a peptide similar to the bioactive 28-amino acid ANP form present in plasma has been shown in tumors. ANP is a 28 amino acid peptide produced, stored, and released by atrial myocytes that binds to a specific set of receptors, increasing renal sodium excretion. ANP has a 17 amino acid ring formed by an intramolecular disulfide bond and is closely related to BNP (brain natriuretic peptide) and CNP (C-type natriuretic peptide). Ectopically produced ANP leads to hyponatremia, in part through receptor binding and also possibly by suppressing an aldosterone response.

Besides SIADH and ANP there is increasing awareness of an alternate mechanism of cerebral-mediated salt losses referred to as the cerebral salt wasting syndrome (CSWS). Two major criteria must be met for a diagnosis of CSWS: (1) a cerebral lesion and (2) high urinary excretion of $Na+$ and $Cl-$ in a patient with contraction of the extracellular fluid volume. Although the frequency of CSWS is far less than SIADH or sodium depletion, it is important to make the correct diagnosis since the management is different.

Therapy

The first step in the treatment of hyponatremia in the cancer patient is to identify the cause—a step that in practice often focuses on deciding whether sodium depletion is secondary to either reduced intake, gastrointestinal losses, or renal losses (Table 146.6). After excluding the latter, physicians often proceed with a presumptive diagnosis of SIADH. In the case of SIADH, the aim of therapy is to restore serum sodium and osmolality to normal. If the hyponatremia is thought to be drug-induced, the offending agent(s) should be discontinued. The rapidity of correction is guided by the severity of the clinical presentation and the pace with which the hyponatremia developed. If the evidence suggests hyponatremia developed

TABLE 146.6

MANAGEMENT OF HYPONATREMIA

Initial Treatment of Hyponatremia:

1. Asymptomatic patients with serum sodium ≤125 mmol/L, who developed hyponatremia over weeks
   - Aim to increase serum sodium a maximum of 0.5 to 2 mmol/L/hr
   - Intravenous normal saline ± 20 to 40 mg furosemide
2. Symptomatic patients, or serum sodium ≤115 mmol/L
   - Aim to increase serum sodium 2 mmol/L/hr
   - 1 to 2 mL/kg/hr hypertonic (3%) saline, then 100 to 250 mL/hr normal saline
   - 20 to 40 mg oral or intravenous furosemide when patient is euvolemic

Treatment of Syndrome of Inappropriate of Antidiuretic Hormone (SIADH) Secretion or Syndrome of Inappropriate Secretion of Arginine Vasopressin (SIAVP) Secretion

1. 300 to 600 mg demeclocycline, twice daily
2. Aquaretic agents (AVP-receptor antagonists): intravenous conivaptan and oral tolvaptan
   www.samsca.com/pdf/Samsca_prescriber_brochure.pdf
   www.astellas.us/docs/raprisol.pdf

Treatment of Cerebral Salt Wasting Syndrome

1. Aggressive fluid and electrolyte replacement
2. Mineralocorticoid supplementation (fludrocortisone 100 to 400 mg/d)

slowly, it is likely that some equilibration has occurred and correction *can and should* proceed over several days. Patients in whom hyponatremia develops rapidly are more likely to present with severe clinical symptoms but can tolerate more rapid correction. Fortunately most cases present with mild hyponatremia and can be managed with judicious water restriction and intravenous or even oral salt administration. Management options are summarized in Table 146.6. If saline and furosemide prove inadequate so that the hyponatremia fails to improve or worsens after 72 to 96 hours of fluid restriction, plasma levels of *AVP and ANP* should be measured to discriminate between SIADH (SIAVP) and SIANP, especially in patients with SCLC. *Unlike patients with SIADH and hyponatremia, patients whose tumors produce ANP experience a persistent decline in serum sodium following fluid restriction, especially if sodium intake is not concomitantly increased.* If plasma levels of AVP support the diagnosis of SIADH, demeclocycline, a tetracycline antibiotic thought to produce a state of renal AVP resistance, may be used. Aquaretic agents, AVP-receptor antagonists, have demonstrated efficacy and safety in clinical trials and represent additional options for managing hyponatremia.[23,24] Conivaptan is a nonselective AVP antagonist available intravenously, and tolvaptan is a V2 selective AVP antagonist available as an oral tablet. However, given their high cost, additional studies are needed to determine benefits in terms of disease outcome and length of hospital stays to justify their use.

LACTIC ACIDOSIS AND CANCER

Among cancer patients, spontaneous lactic acidosis can occur with hematologic and lymphoid malignancies as well as solid tumors, having been described in patients with breast, colon, ovarian, and small cell lung cancer among others. In some patients with TLS a metabolic acidosis not accounted for by the degree of renal insufficiency can be caused by lactic acidosis. Although most patients with lactic acidosis present or evolve to a more severe acidosis, lactic acidosis is defined as a pH 7.35 or less, with a plasma lactate concentration of 5 meq/L or more.[25] Not surprisingly, the occurrence of metabolic acidosis in cancer patients portends a poor prognosis.

Pathogenesis

Lactic acid production normally occurs under conditions of hypoxia in all tissues, and following release into the circulation, 90% of lactic acid is metabolized in the liver, where it is converted to pyruvate, with the remaining 10% metabolized or excreted by the kidneys. Unlike normal cells, tumor cells rely on anaerobic glycolysis disproportionately, even in the presence of oxygen, producing large quantities of lactate that can lead to an imbalance between lactate production and its utilization by the liver. The essential role of liver in lactic acid metabolism explains why patients with compromised liver function are more likely to develop severe lactic acidosis. In patients with cancer, compromise of liver function can occur when extensive hepatic metastases replace a substantial portion of the liver parenchyma. In these patients, once established, lactic acidosis can progress inexorably.

Among patients with leukemias and lymphomas, lactic acidosis usually occurs in adults and has an extremely poor prognosis.[25] Liver involvement is frequently present and in a substantial proportion of patients contributes to hypoglycemia. Indeed the high frequency of liver involvement in adults with lymphoma and leukemia who develop lactic acidosis supports the possibility of reduced hepatic lactate utilization, which is necessary in the pathogenesis of lactic acidosis. Some have suggested the loss of mitochondrial membrane potential ($\Delta\Psi m$) during programmed cell death or apoptosis results in compensatory glycolysis with accumulation of lactic acid and acidosis.[26]

Therapy

Lactic acidosis usually develops in patients with extensive disease and frequently progresses rapidly. Even with maximal supportive therapy, mortality rates of 60% to 90% are common.[27] The developing acidosis can lead to cardiac arrhythmias and hypotension, with potential for cardiovascular collapse. Consequently, an aggressive therapeutic approach is indicated including: (1) aggressive blood pressure support with fluids and vasopressors to preclude generalized hypoperfusion, which will lead to further lactic acid accumulation; (2) possible sodium bicarbonate use, which is controversial, since no controlled study has shown improvement in outcome but can be supported with acidosis severe enough to impact hemodynamic function and the response to catecholamines; (3) hemodialysis and hemofiltration with a bicarbonate-based replacement fluid; and (4) correction of the underlying causes, which is essential but often very difficult, if not impossible, if the lactic acidosis is a complication of the patient's cancer.

HYPERCALCEMIA AND CANCER

Hypercalcemia is the most common paraneoplastic syndrome, occurring in about 10% to 30% of patients with advanced cancer.[28] Although hypercalcemia has been reported with most tumors, humoral hypercalcemia, discussed below, is most frequently encountered in patients with carcinomas of the breast, lung, kidney, and head and neck, while hypercalcemia with skeletal metastases is seen most often in patients with multiple myeloma.

Symptoms of hypercalcemia include nausea, vomiting, constipation, polyuria, and disorientation. Clinical evidence of volume contraction may be apparent. Severe hypercalcemia is a poor prognostic sign. In the past decade the early and widespread use of bisphosphonates has resulted in a decrease in the frequency and severity of hypercalcemia in cancer patients.

Pathogenesis

Hypercalcemia can occur as result of focal bone destruction (osteolytic) or more frequently as a humoral paraneoplastic syndrome. Focal bone destruction can be mediated by local (paracrine) factors secreted by tumor cells that infiltrate bone, including cytokines and growth factors that stimulate osteoclasts directly or indirectly via osteoblast-mediated up-regulation of osteoclast-activating factors (OAFs). Alternately, hypercalcemia can occur as a paraneoplastic syndrome caused by tumor-produced factors that affect bone resorption or tubular calcium reabsorption. The systemic factor most commonly secreted by tumor cells, parathyroid hormone related protein (PTHrP), mediates a humoral form of malignant hypercalcemia, often referred to as humoral hypercalcemia of malignancy (HHM). Circulating PTHrP is found in approximately 80% of hypercalcemic cancer patients. Although PTHrP shares only limited homology with PTH, the common amino terminus binds to the same cell surface receptor in bone and kidney and stimulates an increase in bone resorption together with an increase in renal tubular calcium reabsorption, leading to hypercalcemia. In addition, PTHrP can synergize local (paracrine) factors including interleukin-1 (IL-1), IL-6, and tumor necrosis factor-α (TNF-α), further contributing to hypercalcemia.[28,29] Finally, some lymphomas secrete the active form of vitamin D, 1,25 dihydroxyvitamin D (1,25$(OH)_2$D), enhancing osteoclastic bone resorption and intestinal calcium absorption.

Hypercalcemia induces an osmotic diuresis while inhibiting antidiuretic hormone. The resultant polyuria, together with nausea and vomiting, leads to progressive dehydration, reduced glomerular filtration, and increased calcium resorption, further worsening the hypercalcemia.

Therapy

Therapeutic interventions depend on the presentation. Asymptomatic patients with a serum calcium level of 3.25 mmol/L or less can be managed conservatively, whereas symptomatic patients or those with a serum calcium level above 3.25 mmol/L require immediate aggressive measures.

Although hydration results at most in only a mild 0.5 mmol/L (approximately 2 mg/dL) decrease in serum calcium levels, it is a simple, rapid, and effective intervention that can also preclude continued renal calcium reabsorption. After adequate hydration, 20 to 40 mg of intravenous furosemide can enhance calcium excretion by increasing delivery to and blocking transport of calcium and sodium from the loop of Henle.

Together with hydration the bisphosphonates are currently the cornerstone of therapy for malignancy-associated hypercalcemia. Bisphosphonates are based on a phosphorous-carbon-phosphorous backbone, similar to pyrophosphate. The carbon replacing the central oxygen renders the molecules resistant to hydrolysis but allows the retention of pyrophosphatelike inhibition of bone resorption. Their mechanism of action is complex. Bisphosphonates inhibit both normal and pathologic bone resorption via direct and indirect effects on osteoclasts. The affinity of bisphosphonates for hydroxyapatite leads to their concentration in bone at the interface, and they are internalized by osteoclasts at the time of bone resorption. Evidence indicates nonnitrogen-containing bisphosphonates such as clodronate resemble pyrophosphate and are metabolized intracellularly to nonhydrolyzable analogues of ATP that inhibit ATP-dependent intracellular enzymes and are thus cytotoxic; while nitrogen-containing bisphosphonates (aminobisphosphonates), including pamidronate, ibandronate, and zoledronate, inhibit protein prenylation and bone resorption by osteoclasts by inhibiting the mevalonate pathway, disrupting the signaling functions of key regulatory proteins.[30,31] As a group, the biphosphonates are well tolerated, with a small incidence of fever the most frequently reported adverse event. Transient hypocalcemia and hypophosphatemia and a reversible increase in serum creatinine can also occur. Because of poor oral absorption and gastrointestinal discomfort, most are administered intravenously. Several bisphosphonates have been used in the treatment of hypercalcemia of malignancy. Clodronate, a second-generation bisphosphonate of intermediate potency, is usually given orally and achieves normocalcemia in 80% of cases. One-fifth of those treated have an increase in creatinine.[32] In the palliative setting, clodronate can be given subcutaneously with mild local reaction in one-third as the principal side effect.[33] Pamidronate, a nitrogen-containing bisphosphonate, achieves normocalcemia in as many as 90% of patients for a longer period of time than clodronate.[32,34] Zoledronate, a third-generation bisphosphonate that contains a heterocyclic nitrogen, is considered the current best choice, with normalization of serum calcium in 4 to 10 days that lasts 4 to 6 weeks in 90% of patients.[35]

Bisphosphonates are most effective in the therapy of hypercalcemia associated with multiple myeloma but are also efficacious in solid tumors with skeletal metastases. They are somewhat less effective in the treatment of patients with humoral-mediated hypercalcemia because they have no effect on tubular calcium reabsorption mediated by humoral factors, including PTHrP. Although one study found a correlation between pretreatment PTHrP levels and time to reach normocalcemia after pamidronate, zoledronate was equally effective regardless of serum PTHrP, although in one study the time to relapse was shorter in patients with high PTHrP levels.[35–37] Other agents, including gallium nitrate,[38] plicamycin (mithramycin), and calcitonin, can be tried in hypercalcemia refractory to bisphosphonates. Plicamycin and calcitonin can effect rapid declines of serum calcium but require frequent administration.

Agents in development include osteoprotegerin (OPG), a naturally occurring soluble receptor that inhibits bone resorption by inhibiting osteoclast differentiation (Fig. 146.2). OPG is part of a cytokine system that belongs to the TNF superfamily.[39] The components include the ligand RANKL (receptor activator of nuclear factor-κB ligand), its specific receptor RANK (receptor activator of nuclear factor-κB) and OPG, a soluble "decoy" receptor. By binding to RANK, RANKL enhances bone resorption by increasing osteoclast formation from hematopoietic precursors and osteoclast activity, while inhibiting osteoclast apoptosis. The activity of RANKL, also known as osteoclast differentiation factor (ODF) or osteoprotegerin ligand (OPGL), is counterbalanced physiologically by circulating OPG, with the net effect dependent on the local ratio of ODF to OPG. By acting as a "decoy," intravenous administration of OPG has potent hypocalcemic effects in murine models of humoral hypercalcemia.

Denosumab (Prolia), a fully human monoclonal antibody with a high affinity and specificity for RANKL, is the first RANK ligand inhibitor to receive FDA approval, having been approved for treatment of postmenopausal women who have a high risk for osteoporotic fractures. Two recently completed phase 3 trials randomized patients with breast cancer or castration-resistant prostate cancer (CRPC) to receive either 120 mg denosumab subcutaneously every 4 weeks or intravenous zoledronic acid (Zometa) administered at a dose of 4 mg every four weeks.[40,41] Denosumab was superior both in delaying

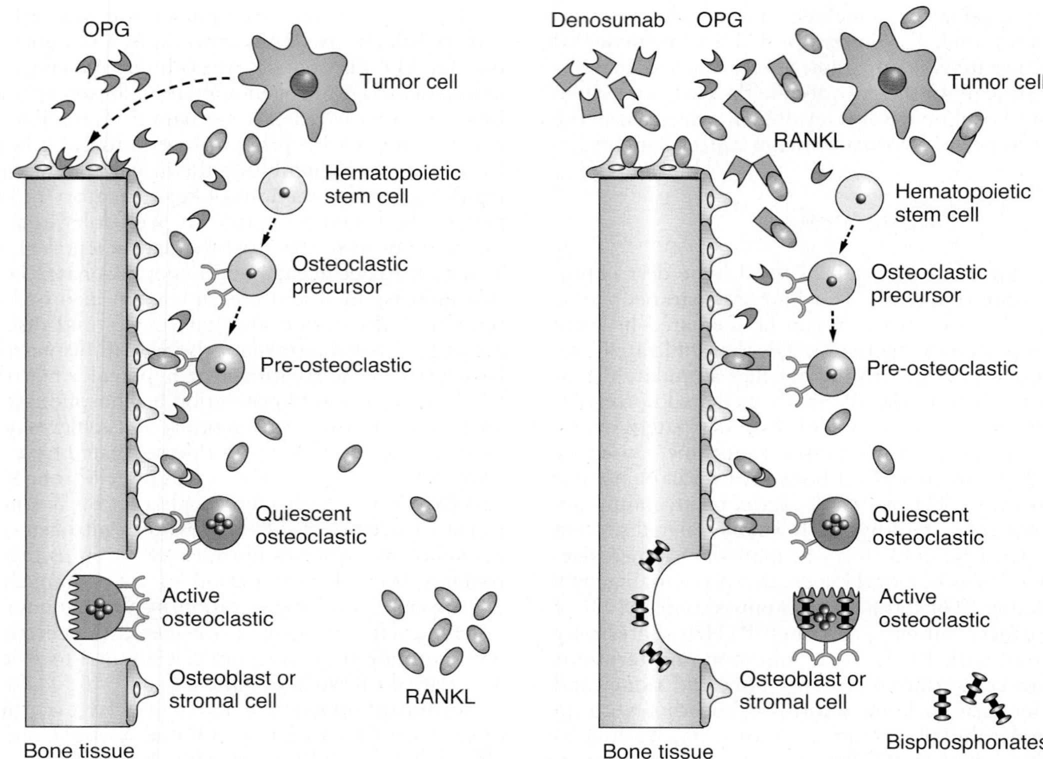

FIGURE 146.2 Bone remodeling involves complex interactions between osteoblasts and osteoclasts, as shown in the left panel. The RANK/RANKL signaling pathway mediates osteoclast-induced bone resorption. RANK (receptor activator of nuclear factor-kappa B), a transmembrane signaling receptor, is a member of the tumor necrosis factor (TNF) receptor superfamily. RANK is expressed on the surface of osteoclast precursors, while RANKL (receptor activator of nuclear factor-kappa B ligand) is expressed on the surface of osteoblasts and stromal cells. The interaction of RANKL with its receptor, RANK, induces osteoclast formation, increases bone resorption by osteoclasts, and enhances osteoclast survival. OPG (osteoprotegerin) is a soluble decoy receptor for RANKL. It is also a member of the TNF receptor superfamily and acts as an alternate receptor for RANKL. OPG is produced by osteoblasts and blocks the interaction of RANKL with RANK, limiting osteoclastogenesis. Normally, the RANKL/OPG ratio strongly favors OPG. Tumor cells can interact with stromal cells in a paracrine manner to up-regulate expression of RANKL and down-regulate expression of OPG, leading to increased osteoclast formation and activity. Tumor cells may also produce RANKL. The panel on the right shows the mechanism of action of current therapies. The affinity of bisphosphonates for hydroxyapatite leads to their concentration in bone at the bone resorption surface. From here they are released and internalized by osteoclasts at the time of bone resorption, inhibiting osteoclast function. Denosumab mimics the endogenous effects of OPG by binding to RANKL and inhibiting osteoclast maturation and bone degradation.

the time in the first study to "skeletal related events or SREs" (fracture, radiation to bone, surgery to bone, or spinal cord compression) and delaying the time to the first and subsequent SREs. In patients with CRPC overall adverse event (AE) rates were similar, with hypocalcemia in 13% and 6% of denosumab- and zoledronate-treated patients, respectively, and osteonecrosis of the jaw (ONJ) in 2.3% of patients receiving denosumab and 1.3% of patients treated with zoledronate (P = .09). Although denosumab will likely garner FDA approval for hypercalcemia associated with malignancy, it is likely that, as happened with the bisphosphonates, the optimal dose and schedule will evolve over time, mitigating an incidence of hypocalcemia and ONJ that is possibly higher than that observed with bisphosphonates.

CANCER-RELATED HEMOLYTIC UREMIC SYNDROME

The hemolytic uremic syndrome (HUS) is a microvascular disorder characterized histopathologically by disseminated microthrombi occluding the microvasculature. HUS is often associated with the presence of large von Willebrand factor multimers capable of agglutinating circulating platelets. The hallmark of a Coombs-negative hemolytic anemia with an elevated schistocyte count results from fragmentation of erythrocytes as they pass through clogged arterioles. The disseminated microthrombi lead to ischemic organ damage, most commonly in kidneys and brain, with renal insufficiency and a range of neurological symptoms. Although thrombotic thrombocytopenic purpura (TTP) and HUS represent a spectrum with considerable overlap, renal insufficiency invariably occurs in HUS but is often milder in TTP, where neurological symptoms often predominate.

Pathogenesis

In cancer patients, HUS has been reported (1) as a manifestation of the cancer itself; (2) as a complication of chemotherapy; (3) in the setting of bone marrow transplantation; and (4) more recently as a problem in patients who are receiving antibodies and immunotoxins. In untreated patients HUS has been described primarily with disseminated cancer, although occasionally as a manifestation of occult or early cancers.[42–44] Although HUS has been reported more frequently with adenocarcinomas of the breast, lung, pancreas, prostate, and stomach, it has also been reported in patients with lymphomas as well as other malignancies.[42] In treated patients, a diverse group of chemotherapeutic agents have been implicated in the etiology of HUS. A 1986 review of chemotherapy-related HUS implicated mitomycin-C and 5-fluoruracil as the most frequent culprits.[44] Subsequent reports of gemcitabine associated HUS reflect the widespread use of this agent.[45] Other agents that have been implicated in the etiology of this syndrome, include bleomycin, cisplatin, cytosine arabinoside, daunomycin, deoxycoformycin, estramustine, and methyl-CCNU. The incidence in patients undergoing bone marrow transplant is uncertain, given the difficulty in establishing a diagnosis.[46]

The clinical manifestations of fulminant HUS include the classic pentad of microangiopathic hemolytic anemia, thrombocytopenia, fever, rapidly progressive renal failure, and neurological deficits. Acute respiratory distress syndrome (ARDS) can also develop in some patients. In this setting a high mortality rate has been reported, because treatment is made even more difficult in a patient with a severe underlying disease. In some patients, a subacute presentation with microangiopathic changes, mild thrombocytopenia, and gradual deterioration of renal function have been described. The main differential is disseminated intravascular coagulopathy (DIC). In patients undergoing allogeneic stem cell transplantation, transplant-associated microangiopathy (TAM), defined as hemolysis and red blood cell (RBC) fragmentation, can be found in 25% to 38% of patients. Associated renal dysfunction and neurologic manifestations in patients with more severe forms of this syndrome demonstrate a spectrum of severity that may represent endothelial damage driven by donor-host interactions.[47]

Therapy

Although a definitive treatment approach for cancer associated HUS remains to be established, a consensus is emerging.[48–50] When a given therapy is implicated as causative, this should be discontinued. Blood pressure should be controlled. The value of steroids is uncertain precluding their routine use. Hemodialysis is indicated in patients with renal failure. Although the efficacies of therapeutic plasma exchange (TPE) using fresh frozen plasma (FFP) as the substitution fluid and of immunoadsorption chromatography are arguable, either or both should be initiated promptly at diagnosis in all patients. These therapies may need to be continued for months. Cryosupernatant plasma (CSP) has been reported to be at least as effective as FFP. Greater success can be expected in patients with smaller tumor burdens or those in whom anticancer therapy is effective, and in cases where vigilance has led to an early diagnosis. Some have also suggested that treatment may be more efficacious when HUS occurs as a manifestation of the underlying cancer rather than as a complication of therapy.

References

1. Cohen LF, Balow JE, Magrath IT, Poplack DG, Ziegler JL. Acute tumor lysis syndrome. A review of 37 patients with Burkitt's lymphoma. *Am J Med* 1980;68:486.
2. Altman A. Acute tumor lysis syndrome. *Semin Oncol* 2001;28(2 Suppl 5):3.
3. Sallan S. Management of acute tumor lysis syndrome. *Semin Oncol* 2001; 28(2 Suppl 5):9.
4. Fleming DR, Doukas MA. Acute tumor lysis syndrome in hematologic malignancies. *Leuk Lymphoma* 1992;8:315.
5. Hande KR, Garrow GC. Acute tumor lysis syndrome in patients with high-grade non-Hodgkin's lymphoma. *Am J Med* 1993;94:133.
6. Annemans L, Moeremans K, Lamotte M, et al. Pan-European multicentre economic evaluation of recombinant urate oxidase (rasburicase) in prevention and treatment of hyperuricaemia and tumour lysis syndrome in haematological cancer patients. *Support Care Cancer* 2003;11:249.
7. Baeksgaard L, Sorensen JB. Acute tumor lysis syndrome in solid tumors—a case report and review of the literature. *Cancer Chemother Pharmacol* 2003; 51:187.
8. Byrd JC, Lin TS, Dalton JT, et al. Flavopiridol administered using a pharmacologically derived schedule is associated with marked clinical efficacy in refractory, genetically high-risk chronic lymphocytic leukemia. *Blood* 2007;109:399.
9. Cairo MS, Coiffier B, Reiter A, Younes A, TLS Expert Panel. Recommendations for the evaluation of risk and prophylaxis of tumour lysis syndrome (TLS) in adults and children with malignant diseases: an expert TLS panel consensus. *Br J Haematol* 2010;149:578.
10. Yeldandi AV, Yeldandi V, Kumar S, et al. Molecular evolution of the urate oxidase-encoding gene in hominoid primates: nonsense mutations. *Gene* 1991;109:281.
11. Cortes J, Moore JO, Maziarz RT, et al. Control of plasma uric acid in adults at risk for tumor lysis syndrome: efficacy and safety of rasburicase alone and rasburicase followed by allopurinol compared with allopurinol alone—results of a multicenter phase III study. *J Clin Oncol* 2010;28:4207.
12. Navolanic PM, Pui CH, Larson RA, et al. Elitek-rasburicase: an effective means to prevent and treat hyperuricemia associated with tumor lysis syndrome. Meeting Report, Dallas, Texas, January 2002. *Leukemia* 2003; 17:499.
13. Goldman SC, Holcenberg JS, Finklestein JZ, et al. A randomized comparison between rasburicase and allopurinol in children with lymphoma or leukemia at high risk for tumor lysis. *Blood* 2001;97:2998.
14. Liu CY, Sims-McCallum RP, Schiffer CA. A single dose of rasburicase is sufficient for the treatment of hyperuricemia in patients receiving chemotherapy. *Leuk Res* 2005;29:463.
15. Hutcherson DA, Gammon DC, Bhatt MS, Faneuf M. Reduced-dose rasburicase in the treatment of adults with hyperuricemia associated with malignancy. *Pharmacotherapy* 2006;26:242.
16. Trifilio S, Gordon L, Singhal S, et al. Reduced-dose rasburicase (recombinant xanthine oxidase) in adult cancer patients with hyperuricemia. *Bone Marrow Transplant* 2006;37:997.
17. Trifilio SM, Pi J, Zook J, et al. Effectiveness of a single 3-mg rasburicase dose for the management of hyperuricemia in patients with hematological malignancies. *Bone Marrow Transplant* 2010.
18. Berghmans T, Paesmans M, Body JJ. A prospective study on hyponatraemia in medical cancer patients: epidemiology, aetiology and differential diagnosis. *Support Care Cancer* 2000;8:192.
19. Ellison DH, Berl T. Clinical practice. The syndrome of inappropriate antidiuresis. *N Engl J Med* 2007;356:2064.
20. Sachs J, Fredman B. The hyponatremia of multiple myeloma is true and not pseudohyponatremia. *Med Hypotheses* 2006;67:839.
21. Johnson BE, Chute JP, Rushin J, et al. A prospective study of patients with lung cancer and hyponatremia of malignancy. *Am J Respir Crit Care Med* 1997;156:1669.
22. Chute JP, Taylor E, Williams J, et al. A metabolic study of patients with lung cancer and hyponatremia of malignancy. *Clin Cancer Res* 2006;12(3 Pt 1): 888.
23. Palm C, Pistrosch F, Herbrig K, Gross P. Vasopressin antagonists as aquaretic agents for the treatment of hyponatremia. *Am J Med* 2006;119(7 Suppl 1):S87.
24. Veeraveedu PT, Palaniyandi SS, Yamaguchi K, et al. Arginine vasopressin receptor antagonists (vaptans): pharmacological tools and potential therapeutic agents. *Drug Discov Today* 2010;15:826.
25. Sillos EM, Shenep JL, Burghen GA, et al. Lactic acidosis: a metabolic complication of hematologic malignancies: case report and review of the literature. *Cancer* 2001;92:2237.
26. Tiefenthaler M, Amberger A, Bacher N, et al. Increased lactate production follows loss of mitochondrial membrane potential during apoptosis of human leukaemia cells. *Br J Haematol* 2001;114:574.
27. van der Beek A, de Meijer PH, Meinders AE. Lactic acidosis: pathophysiology, diagnosis and treatment. *Neth J Med* 2001;58:128.
28. Esbrit P. Hypercalcemia of malignancy—new insights into an old syndrome. *Clin Lab* 2001;47:67.
29. Stewart AF. Clinical practice. Hypercalcemia associated with cancer. *N Engl J Med* 2005;352:373.
30. Benford HL, Frith JC, Auriola S, Monkkonen J, Rogers MJ. Farnesol and geranylgeraniol prevent activation of caspases by aminobisphosphonates: biochemical evidence for two distinct pharmacological classes of bisphosphonate drugs. *Mol Pharmacol* 1999;56:131.

31. Luckman SP, Hughes DE, Coxon FP, et al. Nitrogen-containing bisphosphonates inhibit the mevalonate pathway and prevent post-translational prenylation of GTP-binding proteins, including Ras. *J Bone Miner Res* 1998;13: 581.
32. Purohit OP, Radstone CR, Anthony C, Kanis JA, Coleman RE. A randomised double-blind comparison of intravenous pamidronate and clodronate in the hypercalcaemia of malignancy. *Br J Cancer* 1995;72:1289.
33. Walker P, Watanabe S, Lawlor P, et al. Subcutaneous clodronate: a study evaluating efficacy in hypercalcemia of malignancy and local toxicity. *Ann Oncol* 1997;8:915.
34. Vinholes J, Guo CY, Purohit OP, Eastell R, Coleman RE. Evaluation of new bone resorption markers in a randomized comparison of pamidronate or clodronate for hypercalcemia of malignancy. *J Clin Oncol* 1997;15:131.
35. Major P, Lortholary A, Hon J, et al. Zoledronic acid is superior to pamidronate in the treatment of hypercalcemia of malignancy: a pooled analysis of two randomized, controlled clinical trials. *J Clin Oncol* 2001;19:558.
36. Walls J, Ratcliffe WA, Howell A, Bundred NJ. Response to intravenous bisphosphonate therapy in hypercalcaemic patients with and without bone metastases: the role of parathyroid hormone-related protein. *Br J Cancer* 1994;70:169.
37. Kawada K, Minami H, Okabe K, et al. A multicenter and open label clinical trial of zoledronic acid 4 mg in patients with hypercalcemia of malignancy. *Jpn J Clin Oncol* 2005;35:28.
38. Warrell RP Jr. Gallium nitrate for the treatment of bone metastases. *Cancer* 1997;80(8 Suppl):1680.
39. Hofbauer LC, Neubauer A, Heufelder AE. Receptor activator of nuclear factor-kappaB ligand and osteoprotegerin: potential implications for the pathogenesis and treatment of malignant bone diseases. *Cancer* 2001; 92:460.
40. Stopeck A, Fallowfield L, Patrick D, et al. Effects of denosumab versus zoledronic acid (ZA) on pain in patients (pts) with metastatic breast cancer: results from a phase III clinical trial. *J Clin Oncol* 2010;28(15s): (abst 1024).
41. Fizazi K, Carducci MA, Smith MR, et al. A randomized phase III trial of denosumab versus zoledronic acid in patients with bone metastases from castration-resistant prostate cancer. *J Clin Oncol* 2010;28(18s): (abst LBA4507).
42. Mungall S, Mathieson P. Hemolytic uremic syndrome in metastatic adenocarcinoma of the prostate. *Am J Kidney Dis* 2002;40:1334.
43. Gordon LI, Kwaan HC. Cancer- and drug-associated thrombotic thrombocytopenic purpura and hemolytic uremic syndrome. *Semin Hematol* 1997; 34:140.
44. Sheldon R, Slaughter D. A syndrome of microangiopathic hemolytic anemia, renal impairment, and pulmonary edema in chemotherapy-treated patients with adenocarcinoma. *Cancer* 1986;58:1428.
45. Walter RB, Joerger M, Pestalozzi BC. Gemcitabine-associated hemolytic-uremic syndrome. *Am J Kidney Dis* 2002;40:E16.
46. Verburgh CA, Vermeij CG, Zijlmans JM, van Veen S, van Es LA. Haemolytic uraemic syndrome following bone marrow transplantation. Case report and review of the literature. *Nephrol Dial Transplant* 1996;11:1332.
47. Martinez MT, Bucher Ch, Stussi G, et al. Transplant-associated microangiopathy (TAM) in recipients of allogeneic hematopoietic stem cell transplants. *Bone Marrow Transplant* 2005;36:993.
48. Snyder HW Jr, Mittelman A, Oral A, et al. Treatment of cancer chemotherapy-associated thrombotic thrombocytopenic purpura/hemolytic uremic syndrome by protein A immunoadsorption of plasma. *Cancer* 1993; 71:1882.
49. von Baeyer H. Plasmapheresis in thrombotic microangiopathy-associated syndromes: review of outcome data derived from clinical trials and open studies. *Ther Apher* 2002;6:320.
50. Kaplan AA. Therapeutic apheresis for cancer related hemolytic uremic syndrome. *Ther Apher* 2000;4:201.

CHAPTER 147 METASTATIC CANCER TO THE BRAIN

DAVID A. LARSON, JAMES L. RUBENSTEIN, MICHAEL W. McDERMOTT, AND IGOR BARANI

BRAIN METASTASIS

Brain metastases affect 10% to 30% of patients with cancer.[1] Most brain metastases are detected after the primary tumor has been diagnosed (metachronous metastases). Less frequently they are the first manifestation of disease or are diagnosed at the same time as the primary tumor (synchronous metastases). Brain metastases are symptomatic in 67% of patients.[2] Current posttreatment outcome data indicate that local control and good neurologic quality of life are commonly achieved with modern treatment techniques.

Epidemiology

Approximately 8.5% of cancer patients develop brain metastases,[3] with a 5-year cumulative incidence of brain metastases of 16%, 10%, 7%, 5%, and 1% for patients with lung cancer, renal cell cancer, melanoma, breast cancer, and colorectal carcinoma, respectively. These incidence estimates imply approximately 60,000 to 70,000 cases of brain metastases will be diagnosed within the United States in 2010.[4] However, autopsy-based incidence figures imply the expected number of cases of brain metastases may be as high as 170,000.[5] The interval from diagnosis of cancer to that of brain metastasis varies considerably (median 12 months).[6] Synchronous metastases, brain metastases that are diagnosed within 1 month of the primary cancer diagnosis, occur in up to one-third of patients.[3]

Clinical Presentation

Two-thirds of cancer patients found to have brain metastases at autopsy had experienced neurologic symptoms from the metastases.[7] The most common clinical presentations include headache (24% to 53%), focal weakness (16% to 40%), altered mental status (24% to 31%), seizures (15% to 16%), and ataxia (9% to 20%).[6,8] Data acquired during 1973 to 1993 indicate only 10% of patients diagnosed with brain metastases by computed tomography (CT) or magnetic resonance imaging (MRI) were asymptomatic.[6] It is likely that a smaller percentage of today's patients are symptomatic, since screening imaging is more frequently performed and imaging modalities are more sensitive.

Imaging and Diagnosis

MRI is more sensitive than CT for determining the number, distribution, and size of lesions.[8] Imaging characteristics, known cancer diagnosis, and multiplicity of lesions may aid in making a diagnosis. If the diagnosis of brain metastasis remains in doubt, biopsy should be considered. Patchell et al.[9] reported that of 54 patients with a single brain lesion who were enrolled on a formal study in which biopsy was required prior to therapy, 11% had nonmetastatic lesions, including glial tumor, abscess, and inflammatory process. A stereotactic biopsy series in 100 patients with multifocal brain lesions and no known primary cancer diagnosed malignant gliomas in 37% of patients, primary central nervous system (CNS) lymphoma in 15%, brain metastases in 15%, low-grade gliomas in 12%, infectious processes in 10%, and ischemic lesions in 6% of patients.[10]

Prognosis

The Radiation Therapy Oncology Group (RTOG) retrospective recursive partitioning analysis (RPA) was among the early prognostic systems proposed for application in patients with brain metastases. The RPA of prognostic factors was performed by Gaspar et al.[11] who studied 1,100 to 1,200 patients who received external beam radiotherapy after enrolling in various RTOG brain metastasis trials during 1979 to 1993. The radiotherapy fractionation and dose schedules varied over a broad range. By today's standards, and with today's imaging, only some of these patients would have been candidates for focal therapy. Gaspar et al. found that patients fell into three well-defined prognostic groups, with significantly different median survivals. For RPA class 1 patients (those less than 65 years old, with Karnofsky performance scores [KPS] 70 or greater, controlled primary tumor, and no extracranial metastases), median survival was 7.1 months. For RPA class 3 patients (those with KPS less than 70), median survival was 2.3 months. For the remaining patients, those in RPA class 2, median survival was 4.2 months (Fig. 147.1). This system provides a simple method to stratify patients and provides and excellent indication of the small subsets of patients with excellent or poor survival prognosis. The major disadvantage is the large size and heterogeneity of class 2 in studies of focal brain therapy (e.g., radiosurgery) with or without whole-brain radiotherapy (WBRT).[12,13]

More recently, Sperduto et al.[14] proposed the graded prognostic assessment (GPA). This system was developed by analysis of data selected from five prior RTOG studies. The GPA is the sum of scores (0, 0.5, or 1.0) for age, KPS score, known extracranial metastases, and number of metastases, stratified into four prognostic groups (Fig. 147.2). Of note, only 56% of the patients in the five RTOG studies that were used to develop this prognostic system could be scored; the majority of the patients used in the development of the GPA were treated with

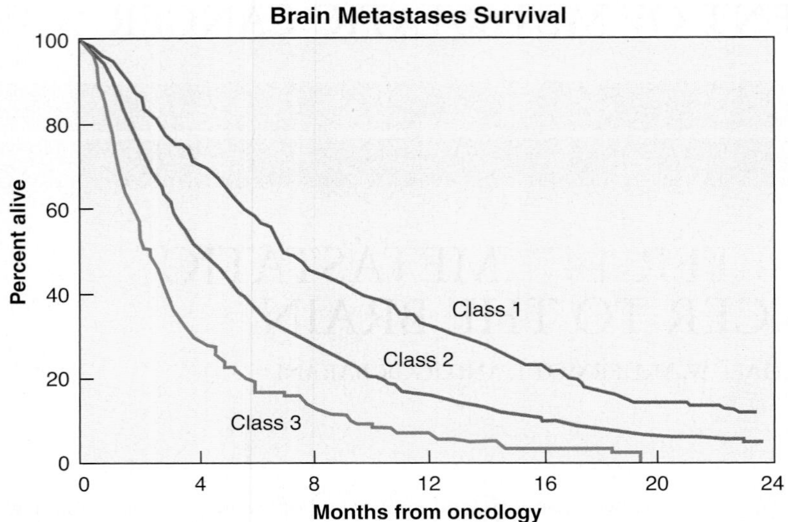

FIGURE 147.1 Median survival according to recursive partitioning analysis (RPA) class, based on analysis of 1,200 patients treated on three consecutive Radiation Therapy Oncology Group (RTOG) trials conducted between 1979 and 1993, testing several different fractionation schemes and radiation sensitizers. RPA class 1 comprises patients less than 65 years old, Karnofsky performance scores (KPS) 70 or greater, controlled primary tumor, and no extracranial metastases. RPA class 3 comprises patients with KPS less than 70. RPA class 2 comprises all other patients. (From ref. 11, with permission.)

WBRT, and only one of the five studies included an arm treated with WBRT and radiosurgery. The GPA can be applied during patient evaluation prior to radiosurgery, but the number of metastases may change after treatment planning with triple-dose gadolinium-enhanced MRI.[15] Therefore, the applicability of the GPA in patients imaged with highly sensitive techniques is uncertain.[16] Nevertheless, GPA was validated by Sperduto et al. in all patients with brain metastases.[17]

Today, many diagnoses of brain metastases are made relatively early, while patients are asymptomatic and when aggressive focal therapy, such as surgery or stereotactic radiosurgery (SRS), may be offered. Patients who satisfy selection criteria for focal therapy appear to have a more favorable prognosis. Sneed et al.[18] found that survival was substantially greater in patients who received SRS, with or without WBRT, than that found in patients in the RTOG WBRT trials, for each of the three RPA classes. Agboola et al.[19] found improved survival in all three RPA classes for patients who underwent surgery with WBRT. Tendulkar et al.[20] allowed for WBRT or SRS or both following resection and confirmed the prognostic significance of the RPA classification. These RPA prognostic data are summarized in Table 147.1. Several authors beyond those listed here have confirmed the prognostic importance of RPA. Similarly, Sperduto et al.[17] and Nieder et al.[21] performed similar validation studies of the GPA. Nieder and Mehta[22] performed a comprehensive comparison and review of the various prognostic indices for patients with brain metastases.

Symptom Management

Corticosteroids

Corticosteroids are generally instituted in brain metastasis patients with symptomatic peritumoral edema. The antiedemic effect of corticosteroids is usually attributed to a reduction in the permeability of abnormal tumor capillaries.[23] Dexamethasone is typically used, given its low mineralocorticoid activity and relatively low risk of cognitive impairment and infection. Typical dosing consists of a 10 mg loading dose followed by 16 mg/d in divided doses (e.g., 4 mg every 6 hours), though lower doses are often used. Patients commonly improve within hours after the first dose, attaining maximum benefit after approximately 3 to 7 days. After patients become asymptomatic or reach maximum benefit, steroids should be tapered as clinically indicated, with taper based primarily on clinical rather than imaging evaluation.

	Score		
	0	0.5	1.0
Age	>60	50–59	<50
KPS	<70	70–80	90–100
No. of CNS metastases	>3	2–3	1
Extracranial metastases	Present	—	None

Abbreviations: KPS = Karnofsky Performance Status; CNS = Central Nervous System.

A

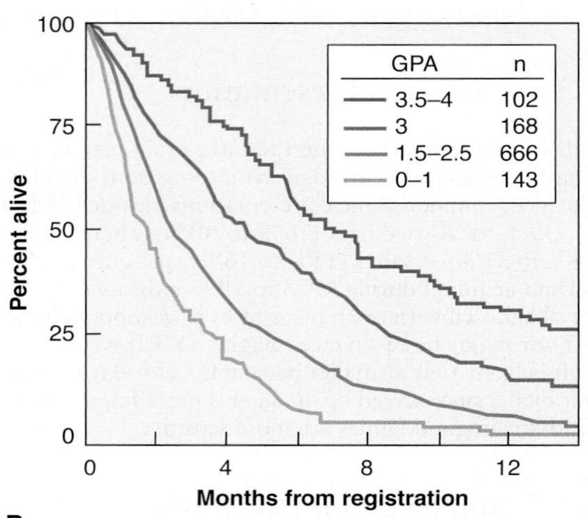

B

FIGURE 147.2 **Panel A:** Graded prognostic assessment (GPA). **Panel B:** Kaplan-Meier curves for overall survival time by GPA class and number of patients in each class. (From ref. 14 with permission.)

TABLE 147.1

MEDIAN SURVIVAL ACCORDING TO RECURSIVE PARTITION ANALYSIS CLASS AND SELECTED INITIAL BRAIN THERAPY[a]

Initial Treatment (Ref.)	No. of Patients	Median Survival by RPA Class (months)		
		Class 1	Class 2	Class 3
WBRT (RTOG phase III trials) (15)	1,176	7.1	4.2	2.3
Radiosurgery (16)	265	14.0	8.2	5.3
WBRT + radiosurgery (16)	295	15.2	7.0	5.5
Surgery + WBRT (17)	125	14.8	9.9	6.0
Surgery ± WBRT ± SRS (18)	271	21.4	9.0	8.9

WBRT, whole-brain radiotherapy; RTOG, Radiation Therapy Oncology Group; SRS, stereotactic radiosurgery, RPA, recursive partition analysis, KPS, Karnofsky performance scores.

[a]Patients who satisfied selection criteria for and received focal therapy according to various institutional policies appear to have better median survival than RTOG WBRT trial patients treated during 1977 to 1993. It is not known how many of the RTOG WBRT patients might have met current selection criteria for surgery or radiosurgery. RPA class 1 comprises patients less than 65 years with KPS 70 or greater and controlled primary tumor and without obvious extracranial metastases. RPA class 3 comprises patients with KPS less than 70. RPA class 2 comprises all other patients.

Common acute side effects include insomnia, increased appetite, fluid retention, mood changes, acne, and exacerbation of diabetes. Long-term side effects include significant weight gain, steroid myopathy, immunosuppression, myopathy, and femoral head aseptic necrosis.

Some early studies used radiation dose-fractionation regimens that are currently considered nonstandard. In particular, Harwood and Simson[24] found that 40% of patients treated with rapid fractionation (100 Gy single fraction) experienced acute signs or symptoms of increased intracranial pressure, now thought to be caused by dose-dependent, radiation-induced permeability of the blood–brain barrier.[25] These data lend support to the view of some that patients receiving SRS for brain metastases should receive a single loading dose of corticosteroids at the time of radiosurgery. However, there is little evidence to suggest that steroids have a role in standard WBRT for brain metastases in the absence of clinical symptoms.

Anticonvulsants

Seizures, which occur in 25% of patients with brain metastases, are the presenting symptom in 10% of cases.[26] Patients who present with seizures or who develop seizures during therapy should be started on antiseizure medications.[27] In the absence of seizures, prophylactic antiseizure medications are generally not started.[27,28]

Venous Thromboembolism

Venous thromboembolism occurs commonly in cancer patients, resulting in significant morbidity and mortality. Sorensen et al.[29] found the 1-year survival rate for cancer patients with thrombosis was only 12%, compared to 36% in cancer patients without thrombosis, possibly reflecting both thromboembolism and a more aggressive course of cancers associated with it. Other studies confirmed the negative impact of thromboembolic events on overall survival in patients with cancer.[30] American Society of Clinical Oncology (ASCO) recently published guidelines for prophylaxis and treatment of venous thromboembolism in patients with cancer.[31] Patients with brain tumors and thrombosis are thought to be at increased risk for intracranial hemorrhage with anticoagulation. Schiff and DeAngelis[32] provide data that suggest that anticoagulation may be safe for patients with those metastatic cancer pathologies that are thought to be less prone to hemorrhage.

Treatment

This section will emphasize the results of important randomized trials involving brain metastases, with less emphasis on retrospective studies. Concern for toxicity of WBRT motivates some practitioners to avoid initial WBRT and instead recommend focal therapy alone (SRS or surgery). Most patients who qualify for focal therapy are likely to be carefully followed, and most are likely to have salvage therapy at the time of brain recurrence. Several of the randomized trials do not evaluate neurocognitive function and quality-of-life outcomes nor do they fully report actuarial outcome analysis of initial *plus* salvage therapy. Sneed et al.,[33] in a retrospective study, found that omission of WBRT in patients who received initial SRS for up to four brain metastases did not compromise intracranial control provided response to salvage therapy was incorporated into the actuarial outcome analysis.

Whole-Brain Radiotherapy

The standard treatment for brain metastases consists of WBRT, covering the entire intracranial contents with shielding of the eyes. The benefits of WBRT were first described over 50 years ago, with symptomatic improvement noted in approximately 60% of patients and with median survival times of 3 to 6 months, compared to 1 to 2 months without treatment. Beginning in 1970, numerous WBRT randomized trials were conducted by the RTOG (Table 147.2).[34–38] These trials examined a wide variety of fractionation schemes and drew numerous conclusions. For example, RTOG-6901 and RTOG-7361, comprising more than 1,800 patients, found complete or partial clinical responses in 60% to 90% of symptomatic patients, with median duration of improvement 10 to 12 weeks, and with 75% to 80% of remaining survival time spent in an improved or stable neurologic state. However, brain metastases were reported to be the cause of death in 30% to 50% of patients. These trials did not show significant outcome differences with respect to survival times, symptomatic response rates, or duration of symptomatic response.

Studies of ultrarapid fractionated WBRT (10 Gy in one fraction, 12 Gy in two fractions, 15 Gy in two fractions over

TABLE 147.2

SELECTED RANDOMIZED TRIALS OF WHOLE-BRAIN RADIOTHERAPY ALONE FOR BRAIN METASTASES

Protocol (Ref.)	Years	No. of Patients	Fractionation Scheme	Median Survival Time (months)
RTOG-6901 (34,36)	1971–1973	233	30 Gy/10 fractions/2 wk	4.8
First study		217	30 Gy/15 fractions/3 wk	4.1
		233	40 Gy/15 fractions/3 wk	4.1
		227	40 Gy/20 fractions/4 wk	3.7
RTOG-7361 (34,36)	1973–1976	447	20 Gy/5 fractions/1 wk	3.4
Second study		228	30 Gy/10 fractions/2 wk	3.4
		227	40 Gy/15 fractions/3 wk	4.1
RTOG-6901 (35)	1971–1973	26	10 Gy/1 fractions/1 d	3.4
RTOG-7361 (35)	1973–1976	33	12 Gy/2 fractions/2 d	3.0
Ultra-rapid				
RTOG-7606 (37)	1976–1979	130	30 Gy/10 fractions/2 wk	4.1
Favorable patients		125	50 Gy/20 fractions/4 wk	3.9
RTOG-9104 (38)	1991–1995	213	30 Gy/10 fractions/2 wk	4.5
Accelerated hyperfx		216	54.4 Gy at 1.6 twice daily	4.5

RTOG, Radiation Therapy Oncology Group; hyperfx, hyperfractionation.

3 days), as carried out by RTOG and other investigators,[34–40] showed a possible increased risk of herniation and death within a few days of treatment and are generally avoided. Likewise, no advantage was seen with extended fractionation (50 Gy in 20 fractions or 54.4 Gy at 1.6 Gy twice daily) compared to the more commonly prescribed 30 Gy in 10 fractions.[37,38] Consequently, the most common WBRT fractionation schemes include 30 Gy in 10 fractions, 37.5 Gy in 15 fractions, and 40 Gy in 20 fractions. Regimens using ten or fewer fractions, which are thought to have increased toxicity, are used in patients with poor prognosis, since such patients are not expected to live long enough to experience serious side effects.

The most thorough imaging analysis of response rates to WBRT was performed by Nieder et al.,[41] who studied CT responses in 108 patients with 336 measurable lesions following WBRT (30 Gy in ten fractions). They found an overall response rate at up to 3 months of 59%, by lesion (complete response rate of 24%, partial response rate of 35%). Complete response rates by tumor type were 37% for small cell carcinoma, 35% for breast cancer, 25% for squamous cell carcinoma, 14% for nonbreast adenocarcinoma, 0% for renal cell carcinoma, and 0% for melanoma. Improved complete response rates were associated with smaller tumor volume and absence of necrosis. Complete response rates were 39% for solid metastases, 15% if less than 50% necrosis, and 11% if 50% or more necrosis, consistent with the notion that poorly oxygenated tumor cells respond less well to radiotherapy. Complete response rates were inversely related to volume, ranging stepwise from 52% for lesion volumes 0.5 mL or less to 0% for lesions greater than 10 mL, likewise consistent with general radiobiological principles. An MR-based treatment response study has not yet been done. In another study by the same group, there was a suggestion that a higher response rate was obtained with 40 Gy at 2 Gy per fraction with or without a partial boost to 50 or 60 Gy compared with 30 Gy at 3 Gy per fraction.[42] For the WBRT-only arm of a recent RTOG trial of WBRT with or without radiosurgery, the complete response rate was 8%, partial response rate 54%, stable disease rate 22%, and progression rate 17% among 78 patients with imaging follow-up.[12] Data on long-term control of brain metastases after WBRT alone are limited and highly variable. The 1-year actuarial local control probability by patient ranged from 0% to 14% in the WBRT-only arms of randomized trials reported by Kondziolka et al.[43] and Patchell et al.,[9] but as high as 71% in the WBRT-only arm of the RTOG randomized trial of WBRT with or without radiosurgery.[12] In aggregate, these data indicate that long-term control of gross brain metastases following WBRT is not likely.

The primary justification for WBRT in the setting of multiple brain metastases is control of presenting neurological symptoms, which can be achieved in 70% to 90% of cases without causing acute neurological side effects.[44] Side effects occurring during or shortly after WBRT include hair loss, mild skin reaction, fatigue, and, in some patients, ototoxicity. Hair usually regrows in 6 to 12 months, but alopecia may be permanent in a central strip on the top and back of the head from the reduced skin sparing of tangential radiation beams. Skin reactions resolve after several weeks, and fatigue improves after a few months. In occasional patients outpatient myringotomy may be required to relieve radiation-induced fluid buildup behind the tympanic membrane.

The long-term side effects of WBRT are still a controversial issue. Remarkably, they were often discounted in the treatment of brain metastases because of the relatively short survival of metastatic patients; however, as systemic therapy continues to improve, the number of long-term survivors who experience these late side effects will increase. The frequency of long-term side effects of WBRT is unclear. Radiologic effects include long-term white matter changes, often with uncertain clinical correlates. The most frequently referenced clinical study is that of DeAngelis et al.,[45] who reported a 1-year rate of dementia of 11% in patients with nonrecurrent brain metastases initially treated with WBRT. A separate report from the same group described 12 patients cured of brain metastases who developed severe radiation-induced dementia with associated ataxia and urinary incontinence.[46] Imaging with CT showed atrophy, ventricular dilation, and hypodense white matter. These reported complications must be viewed within the context of the study, which involved 47 patients, with 5 patients developing dementia. Each of the five received either daily dose fractions greater than 3 Gy or radiation sensitizing agents. Of 15 patients treated with "safe" radiation fractionation (less than

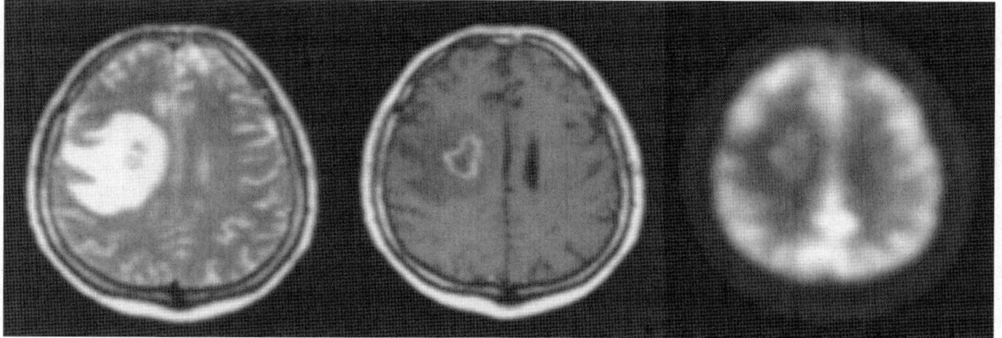

FIGURE 147.3 Example of renal cell metastasis treated with radiosurgery, with follow-up magnetic resonance imaging (MRI) and positron emission tomography (PET) studies at 15 weeks. From left to right the images are T2-weighted MRI, T1-weighted postgadolinium MRI, and fluorodeoxyglucose (FDG) positron emission tomography (PET). MRI was consistent with recurrence. PET was considered negative because only slight FDG accumulation was seen in the margin around the irradiated lesion, a common pattern after radiosurgery. At 41 weeks the patient showed clinical and radiological signs of regression. (From ref. 57, with permission.)

3 Gy per fraction), none had dementia at 1 year. Nieder et al.[47] reported a 42% 2-year actuarial probability of symptomatic mild, moderate, or severe late radiation toxicity in patients treated with resection of a single brain metastasis followed by WBRT to 30 Gy in 10 fractions or 40 Gy in 20 fractions, but no details were provided regarding the nature of the toxicity. Among 112 patients on the WBRT-only arm of a recent RTOG randomized trial, Andrews et al.[12] reported four grade 1, one grade 2, one grade 3, and one grade 4 late central neurological toxicities, two grade 1, two grade 2, and one grade 3 late ototoxicities, and eleven grade 1 and four grade 2 chronic skin toxicities. This RTOG trial did not include formal neurocognitive testing, but it is becoming more common to incorporate baseline and follow-up neurocognitive testing into prospective trials in patients with brain metastases. In an interesting study, Penitzka et al.[48] assessed intelligence, attention, and memory in 29 brain metastases patients prior to and following WBRT. They determined that neuropsychological capacity in small cell lung patients was impaired even prior to prophylactic cranial irradiation, possibly caused by previous chemotherapy. More important, they concluded that therapeutic WBRT delivered in patients with brain metastases other than from small cell lung cancer did not induce a significant decline in cognitive function. Although these two studies are small, they lend support to the notion that risk of brain radiation toxicity is dose and fractionation dependent, but relatively low provided today's standard fractionation schemes are used.

A recent randomized controlled trial from the M. D. Anderson Cancer Center by Chang et al.[49] stratified 58 patients by RPA class (class 1 vs. 2), number of brain metastases (1 or 2 vs. 3), and radioresistant histology (melanoma or renal cell carcinoma vs. other) and randomized patients in 1:1 fashion between SRS plus WBRT (group 1) and SRS alone (group 2). Patients in group 1 received upfront SRS followed by WBRT to 30 Gy (12 fractions, 2.5 Gy/d) that was completed within 3 weeks of randomization. Formal neurocognitive testing and quality-of-life instruments were administered at baseline (pretreatment) and at each follow-up visit (1, 2, 4, 6, 9, 12, 15, and 18 months following completion of the last radiation treatment). The battery of neurocognitive tests included HVLT-R (Hopkins Verbal Learning Test–Revised, which tests total recall, delayed recall, and delayed recognition), Wechsler Adult Intelligence Scale–III (WAIS-III) digit span and digit symbol, Trail Making Test parts A and B, Multilingual Aphasia Examination Controlled Oral Word Association (COWA), and the Lafayette Grooved Pegboard. The trial was stopped prematurely after recruitment of 58 patients based on the early stopping rules because it was determined that patients treated with SRS plus WBRT were at a greater risk of a significant decline in learning and memory function by 4 months, as shown by HVLT-R, compared with the group that received SRS alone. The study was highly criticized for basing its conclusions on neurocognitive outcomes at an early time point (4 months) when it has been suggested by prior longitudinal studies in long-term survivors of WBRT that an early decline in cognitive performance occurs at about the 2- to 4-month point, but subsequently rebounds.[50] Other criticisms of the study include a significant imbalance between the study groups, with the combined group (SRS with WBRT) having a worse prognosis at the outset. The combined therapy group included patients with a greater volume of disease, whereas the SRS alone group contained an excess of women, single metastasis, and RPA class I patients and an absence of patients with lung and abdominal metastases. Though the patients were well matched in terms of numbers of lesions, the disproportionately higher volume of disease in the combined therapy group biases the neurocognitive function performance in favor of the SRS alone group; the baseline neurocognitive function is highly correlated with volume of lesions, but not with number of metastases.[51] The comparison of the two treatment groups in terms of prognostic baseline characteristics is the basis of a valid randomized trial; however, the study by Chang et al.,[49] though randomized, is not likely to detect meaningful outcome differences between the two treated groups given the small numbers of evaluated patients.

Nonetheless, new approaches to deliver WBRT are currently being explored by delivering reduced doses to brain structures, such as the hippocampal formation[52–55] and neural stem cell compartments,[56,57] with low radiation tolerance (Fig. 147.3). These approaches are currently in feasibility trials and not yet ready for widespread use until the risks and benefits are properly evaluated in a proper phase 3 trial.

Prophylactic cranial irradiation (PCI) in patients with small cell lung cancer (SCLC) has been investigated as a strategy to prevent dissemination to the brain, given that the risk of developing multiple brain metastases is 45% to 54% at 2 and 3 years in patients treated without PCI. Patients who are most likely to benefit from PCI are those who achieve a complete response to induction chemotherapy. Two meta-analyses have been conducted to evaluate the efficacy of PCI. In the first, Prophylactic Cranial Irradiation Overview Collaborative Group[58] reported the results of 987 patients with complete response to systemic therapy in seven previously published PCI trials. This analysis demonstrated a statistically significant survival advantage favoring the patients treated with PCI, with a relative risk of death of 0.84. Additionally, there was a significant reduction in the incidence of new brain metastases (from 58.6% to 33.3% at 3 years). The second meta-analysis of PCI efficacy was conducted by Meert et al.,[59] who evaluated a total of 12 randomized trials published between 1977 and 1998; only 5 studies included in the analysis evaluated the role of PCI in SCLC patients who had a complete response after induction chemotherapy. The meta-analysis revealed a significant decrease in the incidence of brain metastases when all studies were considered (hazard ratio [HR] 0.48; 95% confidence interval [CI], 0.39 to 0.60) compared to when only patients with complete systemic response were considered (HR 0.49; 95% CI, 0.39 to 0.62). The meta-analysis of survival included 11 randomized trials and showed the absence of survival improvement (HR 0.94; 95% CI, 0.87 to 1.02) but revealed an improvement in survival when PCI was given only to patients who experienced a complete systemic response (HR 0.82; 95% CI, 0.71 to 0.96). In a recent randomized study, Slotman et al.[60] evaluated 286 extensive stage SCLC patients and reported that the use of PCI increased overall survival at 1 year from 13.3% to 27.1% ($P = .003$). In addition, the disease-free survival at 1 year was only 14.6% in the observation group compared to 40.4% in the treatment group ($P < .001$).

The cognitive effects of PCI in SCLC patients were prospectively studied by Arriagada[61] in an trial of 300 patients with SCLC controlled systemically who either received PCI or were observed. A neurocognitive assessment of these patients 2 years after PCI revealed no significant difference in cognitive status between the observation and PCI treated cohorts and from baseline measurements. Another study by Gregor et al.[62] demonstrated similar results in 136 patients seen at 1 year posttreatment. More data from studies with follow-up in excess of 2 years are needed to properly assess the long-term neurocognitive sequelae of PCI.

In aggregate, current data support the effectiveness of PCI in reducing brain recurrence and in prolonging survival in patients with SCLC, but toxicity data, particularly late neurocognitive sequelae, are not sufficient to generalize its use to all patients with complete response to systemic therapy.

Whole-Brain Radiotherapy with or without Radiation Sensitizers. Mehta et al.[63] reported on survival and neurologic outcomes in a randomized trial of WBRT (30 Gy in ten fractions) with or without daily injections of motexafin gadolinium (MGd). MGd is a redox mediator that selectively targets tumor cells, decreases local oxygen consumption, and is detectable by MRI. A total of 401 patients were enrolled. No significant differences were seen in median survival (5.2 months in the sensitizer arm compared to 4.9 months in the control arm) or median time to neurologic progression (9.5 months compared to 8.3 months). However, among 251 non–small cell lung cancer patients, MGd was found to improve median time to neurologic progression (not reached compared to 7.4 months; $P = .048$). A subsequent confirmatory trial, the Study of Neurologic Progression with Motexafin Gadolinium (MGd) with Radiation Therapy,[64] randomized 554 non–small cell lung cancer patients to WBRT plus MGd or WBRT alone. There was no significant difference in time to neurological progression; however, a subset analysis of patients treated in North America ($N = 348$) demonstrated a benefit that was thought to be related to an early initiation of WBRT (within 3 weeks of diagnosis).[64]

A randomized trial was conducted to compare WBRT (30 Gy in 10 fractions) and supplemental O_2 with WBRT following daily injections of RSR-13 (efaproxiral). RSR-13 is an allosteric modifier of hemoglobin that reduces hemoglobin O_2-binding affinity, facilitates O_2 release, and increases tissue pO_2. In a multicenter, phase 2 study, WBRT plus RSR-13 resulted in a median survival time of 6.4 months compared with 4.1 months published in the RTOG database ($P = .017$).[65] This led to a phase 3 trial with 538 RPA class 1 and 2 patients where no survival difference was detected between the two arms of the study (4.5 vs. 5.3 months; $P = .17$).[66] Among patients with breast cancer primaries, median survival was 8.7 months in the RSR-13 arm compared to 4.6 months in the control arm. In addition, an RSR-13 dose–response relationship was demonstrated. A confirmatory phase 3 trial in 360 women with brain metastases from breast cancer did not subsequently demonstrate a survival improvement.[67]

Surgery

Lang and Sawaya[68] summarized median survival following surgical resection of brain metastasis, according to primary tumor type, based on 46 published reports. They found the following average median survivals by tumor type: melanoma (7 months), lung cancer (12 months), renal cell cancer (10 months), breast cancer (12 months), and colon cancer (9 months). The rate of leptomeningeal dissemination appears to be higher after piecemeal rather than *en bloc* resection of metastases, although larger tumors cannot always be removed without some internal decompression.[69,70]

Patients with multiple metastases may be candidates for surgery provided each lesion is considered resectable. If all lesions are not considered resectable, surgery may be considered for those symptomatic lesions that are resectable. The most complete analysis of outcome following surgical resection of multiple lesions is that of Bindal et al.,[71] who reviewed 56 patients wo underwent resection for multiple brain metastases. Patients were retrospectively placed in one of two groups: 30 patients who had at least one unresected lesion (group A), and 26 patients who had all lesions resected (group B). A third group (group C), for comparison purposes, consisted of 26 matched controls with single surgically resected metastasis. Median survivals were 6, 14, and 14 months for groups A, B, and C, respectively. Surgical mortality was 3%, 4%, and 0%; surgical morbidity was 8%, 9%, and 8%, respectively. Among group B patients, 83% of symptomatic patients improved, 11% remained stable, and 6% worsened. These data imply that in patients with multiple brain metastases who are otherwise good surgical candidates, surgical resection of all lesions is as effective as surgical resection in patients with a single metastasis. An example of resection of multiple cerebral metastases is shown in Figure 147.4.

Whole-Brain Radiotherapy with or without Surgery. Patchell et al.[9] studied 48 patients with a single brain metastasis who were randomized to surgical resection and WBRT versus needle biopsy and WBRT (36 Gy in 12 fractions). Patients in the resection arm had significantly improved local control (80%) compared to those randomized to biopsy and WBRT (48%). Patients in the resection arm also had significantly increased median duration of functional independence (38 weeks vs. 8 weeks) and median survival (40 weeks vs. 15 weeks). Factors found to be associated with longer survival included younger age, no extracranial disease, surgical resection, and longer interval from primary diagnosis to diagnosis of brain metastasis.

Noordijk et al.[72] studied 63 patients with a single brain metastasis who were randomized to surgical resection and WBRT versus WBRT (40 Gy in 20 fractions). Patients in the resection arm had significantly longer functionally independent median survival (7.5 months vs. 3.5 months) and longer median survival (10 months vs. 6 months). However, there was no survival benefit for patients with active extracranial disease (5 months in each arm). For patients without active extracranial disease, the median survival time was significantly improved in the resection arm (12 months vs. 7 months).

Mintz and Cairncross[73] performed a similar trial on 84 patients but failed to find a benefit for surgical resection and

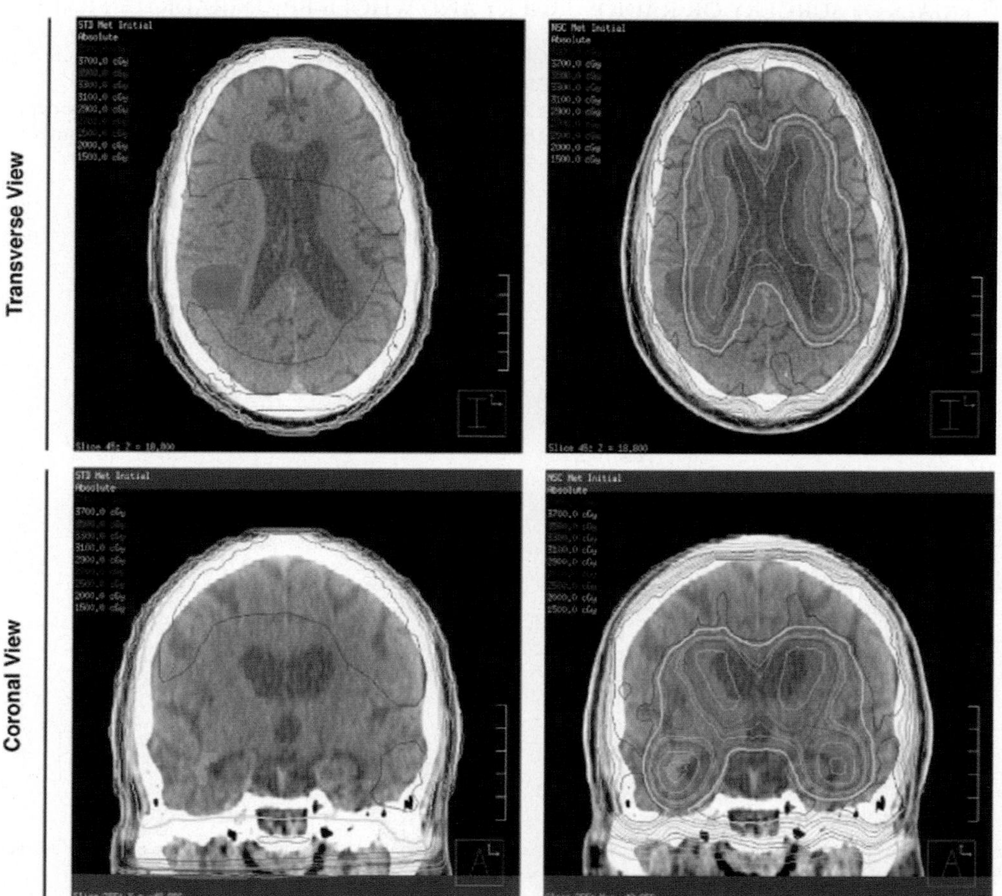

FIGURE 147.4 Isodose distributions of standard whole-brain radiotherapy (WBRT) compared with neural stem cell (NSC)-preserving whole-brain intensity-modulated radiotherapy treatment are shown in the three cardinal projections. The bold, yellow isodose line represents the prescription dose (3,750 cGy/15 daily fractions). The planning target volume (PTV_m) is shown in red, and NSC niches are shown in blue. Please note the dose gradient across PTV_m. This relative underdosing of PTV_m is due to its proximity to SVZ and SGZ niches that carry a high-dosimetric penalty. A stereotactic radiosurgery (SRS) boost of PTV_m can adequately compensate for this relative underdosing.

WBRT (30 Gy in ten fractions) compared to WBRT alone. The median survival times were 6.3 months in the WBRT alone arm and 5.6 months in the resection arm. The presence of extracranial metastases was found to be an important predictor of mortality. There were no significant differences in the 30-day mortality, morbidity, or causes of death. The presence of extracranial metastases was an important predictor of mortality (relative risk, 2.3). The mean proportion of days that the Karnofsky performance status was 70% or more did not differ between the two groups.

Surgery with or without Whole-Brain Radiotherapy. The benefit of WBRT following surgical resection was addressed in a randomized study by Patchell et al.[74] (Table 147.3). Ninety-five adults who had single metastases to the brain were treated with complete surgical resections and randomly assigned to observation versus postoperative WBRT (50.4 Gy in 28 fractions). The WBRT arm was found to have a significantly decreased risk of local failure (10% vs. 46% for observation), distant brain failure (14% vs. 37%), and any brain failure (18% vs. 70%), longer median time to local failure (more than 52 weeks vs. 27 weeks), and longer median time to any brain failure (more than 70 weeks vs. 26 weeks). Patients randomized to WBRT were significantly less likely to die neurologic deaths (14% vs. 44%), though they had similar median survival and length of functional independence. Topics not addressed in the report include the use or success of salvage therapy and acute and late toxicity of WBRT and salvage therapies.

Rades et al.[75] compared two radiotherapy schemes in a retrospective study of 33 patients who underwent resection of a solitary brain metastasis. Group A received 40 Gy WBRT following resection. Group B received 40 Gy WBRT plus a 10 Gy boost following resection. Actuarial analysis demonstrated significantly improved local control and survival in the group B patients ($P < .05$).

Radiosurgery

Shaw et al.[76] studied the relationship between maximum tolerated radiosurgery dose and tumor volume in an RTOG dose escalation trial involving patients with recurrent brain tumors. Flickinger et al.[77] calculated logistic dose–response curves fit to the RTOG data to demonstrate the relationship between target size and dose likely to produce a 10% risk of late toxicity: less than 2 cm (21.0 Gy), 2 to 3 cm (16.0 Gy), 3 to 4 cm (13.5 Gy). Most radiosurgery practitioners use the RTOG data as an approximate, volume-dependent, dose prescription guideline. However, for any given tumor size clinical reports vary considerably regarding dose actually prescribed, ratio of maximum to

TABLE 147.3

RANDOMIZED TRIALS OF SURGERY OR RADIOSURGERY AND WHOLE-BRAIN RADIOTHERAPY FOR BRAIN METASTASES

Study (Ref.)/Years	Treatment	No. of Patients	Patients with Extracranial Disease (%)	Median Local FFP (months)	Median fn. indep. Survival (months)	Median Survival (months)
Patchell (9)	Biopsy + WBRT	23	83	4.8	1.8	3.4
1985–1988	Surgery + WBRT	25	76	>13.6	8.7	9.2
	(36 Gy/12 fx)			(*P* <.0001)	(*P* <.005)	(*P* <.01)
Noordijk (72)	WBRT	31	68	—	3.5	6
1985–1990	Surgery + WBRT	32	69	—	7.5	10
	(40 Gy at 2 Gy twice a day)			—	(*P* = .06)	(*P* = .04)
Mintz (73)	WBRT	43	84	—	—	6.3
1989–1993	Surgery + WBRT	41	73	—	—	5.6
	(30 Gy/10 fx)			—	(*P* = NS)	(*P* = .24)
Patchell (74)	Surgery	46	65	6.2	8.0	9.9
1989–1997	Surgery + WBRT	49	63	>12.0	8.5	11.0
	(50.4 Gy/28 fx)			(*P* <.001)	(*P* = .61)	(*P* = .39)
Kondziolka (43)	WBRT	14	71	6	—	7.5
1985–1988	WBRT + RS	13	62	36	—	11.0
	(36 Gy/12 fx)			(*P* = .0005)	—	(*P* = .22)
Andrews (12)	WBRT	167	69	[71% 1-yr LC]	—	5.7
1996–2001	WBRT + RS	164	68	[82% 1-yr LC]	—	6.5
	(37.5 Gy/15 fx)			(*P* = .013)	—	(*P* = .136)
Aoyama (84)	RS	67	43	[73% @ 1 yr]	[27% @ 1 yr]	8.0
1999–2003	WBRT + RS	65	37	[89% 1-yr LC]	[34% @ 1 yr]	7.5
	(30 Gy/10 fx)			(*P* = .002)	(*P* = .53)	(*P* = .42)

WBRT, whole-brain radiotherapy; FFP, freedom from progression; fn. indep., functionally independent; fx, fractions; RS, radiosurgery; NS, not significant; LC, local control.

prescription dose, degree of dose conformity, and so forth. Because the risk of radiation injury increases with increasing volume, lower doses are generally prescribed for larger target volumes, and radiosurgery targets tend to be limited to about 2.5 to 3.0 cm in diameter. Reported rates of radiation necrosis are mostly in the 0% to 5% range (Table 147.4).

In the past decade scores of retrospective clinical investigations have addressed the outcome of radiosurgery for brain metastasis, with or without WBRT or surgery (Table 147.4), and reported results are relatively consistent: for median target volumes, in the range of 2 to 7 cc, and for median prescribed radiosurgery doses, in the range of 15 to 25 Gy, the 1-year local control rate is 80% to 90% and does not appear to depend strongly on the number of brain metastases treated, with median survival rates in the range of 6 to 12 months. Specific actuarial rates of freedom from progression depend on dose, volume, histology, and pattern of MRI or CT enhancement at the time of radiosurgery.[78,79]

Concerns of potential late WBRT toxicity have motivated some investigators to treat initially with radiosurgery alone. Sneed et al.[33] found that omission of WBRT in patients who received initial radiosurgery for up to four brain metastases did not compromise intracranial control, provided salvage therapy information was included in the actuarial outcome analysis, an analysis that is not usually reported. The main argument against initial omission of WBRT is that patients who recur could develop new neurologic deficits.

An issue faced by those who perform radiosurgery has to do with number of brain metastases: how many is too many to treat? In the absence of definitive data, many institutions individualize treatments. At others, institutional policy may allow any number to be treated by extending treatment to several days. The RTOG limits the number of metastases treated with radiosurgery to three.[12,76] To a large extent, this limitation was reflective of the technological and practical limitations of the radiosurgical equipment available in the 1990s. The development of automated patient positioning, image-guided treatment setup verification, and improved immobilization techniques dramatically reduced treatment times and made routine treatments of multiple metastatic lesions feasible and more practical. As a result, institutions equipped with modern radiosurgical tools tend to treat larger number of lesions than just three or fewer, as evidenced by a plethora of institutional reports (Table 147.4). Yamamoto et al.[80] analyzed dose distributions in 80 patients who were each treated with radiosurgery for more than ten lesions and concluded that cumulative brain doses did not exceed the threshold level for necrosis in normal brain.

Radiosurgery or Surgery

Auchter et al.[81] reported on 122 patients treated with radiosurgery and WBRT who met selection criteria similar to those used in randomized trials of WBRT with or without surgical resection. Local control, functional independence, and median survival were comparable to those of the surgery plus WBRT arms of the reported randomized trials.[9,72] Bindal et al.[82] reported 61% versus 87% crude local control rates for radiosurgery with or without WBRT versus surgery with or without WBRT, and median survival times of 7.5 months versus 16.4 months, respectively. O'Neill et al.[83] compared patients with single metastases who were candidates for either radiosurgery

TABLE 147.4

SELECTED RESULTS OF RADIOSURGERY WITH OR WITHOUT WHOLE-BRAIN RADIOTHERAPY FOR NEWLY DIAGNOSED OR RECURRENT BRAIN METASTASES

Study (Ref.)	No. of Metastases/ Patients	Mean or Median Dose (Gy)	Median Target Volume (mL)	Local Control (%) by Lesion (Crude[a] or 1-yr Actuarial[b])	Median Survival Time (months)	Necrosis (%)
SINGLE METASTASES						
Auchter (81)	122/122	17.0	2.7	86[a]/85[b]	12.9	0
Flickinger (77)	116/116	17.5	—	85[a]	11	4
Simonova (113)	237/237	21.5	7.5	95[a]	9	2.5
SINGLE OR MULTIPLE METASTASES						
Deinsberger (114)	161/110	18.3	3.1	89[a]	12.4	2
Flickinger (115)	229/157	16.0	3.0	89[a]	10	1
Fukuoka (116)	>215/130	>25	5.5	≥96[a]	8	5
Gerosa (117)	1307/804	20.6	4.8	94[b]	13.5	—
Goodman (78)	682/258	18.5	1.7	82[b]	9.1	—
Joseph (118)	189/120	26.6	5.3	94[a]	7.4	17
Kihlstrom (119)	235/160	27.0	4.5	94[a]	7	5
Petrovich (120)	1305/458	18	0.9	87[b]	9	4.7
Pirzkall (121)	311/236	20	—	92[a]	5.5	2
Sansur (122)	411/193	20	—	82% by pt.	7.5	2

or surgery, most of whom received WBRT in addition. One-year survival probabilities were not significantly different (56% for radiosurgery vs. 62% for surgery). It must be assumed that the differing results have to do with differences in selection factors or surgical or radiosurgical technique.

Whole-Brain Radiotherapy with or without Radiosurgery. Kondziolka et al.[43] performed the first randomized trial of WBRT with or without radiosurgery boost. Inclusion criteria included KPS 70 or more, two to four brain metastases 2.5 cm or less in diameter, and target more than 5 mm from the optic chiasm. WBRT consisted of 30 Gy delivered in 12 fractions. Radiosurgery was delivered at any time within 1 month before or after WBRT and consisted of a single dose of 16 Gy. Only 27 patients were enrolled based on early stopping rules. The two arms were well balanced with respect to age, KPS, and presence of extracranial disease. The radiosurgery arm was found to have significantly improved time to local failure (median, 36 months vs. 6 months; $P = .0005$) and time to any brain failure (median, 34 months vs. 5 months; $P = .002$). Nevertheless, survival was not found to differ significantly in the two arms (median, 7.5 months for WBRT vs. 11 months for WBRT plus radiosurgery; $P = 0.22$), although several patients who failed WBRT alone underwent salvage radiosurgery.

In 1996 the RTOG activated a phase 3 trial to study WBRT with or without radiosurgery boost (RTOG-9508).[12] Three hundred thirty-three patients with one to three newly diagnosed brain metastases were enrolled between January 1996 and June 2001, with balanced accrual in both arms. Single metastases had to be considered unresectable (based on location in deep gray matter or in eloquent cortex). Exclusions included patients with metastases to the brainstem or metastases located within 1 cm of the optic apparatus, RPA class 3 patients, and patients who had received systemic treatment within 1 month of enrollment. WBRT consisted of 37.5 Gy delivered in 3 weeks (15 fractions), and radiosurgery doses were based on tumor size according to RTOG-9005 toxicity information.[76] No survival benefit was seen in patients with multiple metastases. Univariate analysis demonstrated a significant survival advantage in the WBRT plus SRS group for the following patients: single brain metastases (median survival, 6.5 months vs. 4.9 months; $P = .039$), patients with tumor size greater than 2 cm (median survival, 6.5 months vs. 5.3 months; $P = .045$), and RPA class 1 patients (median survival, 11.6 months vs. 9.6 months; $P = .045$). Patients in the radiosurgery arm were more likely to have stable or improved KPS through 6 months (43% vs. 27%; $P = .03$). Multivariate analysis showed SRS improved survival only in patients with single metastases ($P < .0001$) or RPA 1 ($P < .0001$). No differences were noted between treatment groups when assessing time to intracranial tumor progression, although the risk of developing a local recurrence was 43% greater in the nonradiosurgery arm. Likewise, the neurologic death rate was similar in the two arms (approximately 34%). Patients in the radiosurgery arm had significantly improved KPS and decreased steroid use at 6 months, although no differences were seen when assessing mental status. No survival advantage was noted based on type of radiosurgery unit used (linear accelerator [LINAC] vs. GammaKnife, Elekta Corp, Stockholm). The authors concluded that WBRT plus radiosurgery improved performance for all patients with one to three metastases and survival for patients with a single unresectable brain metastasis.

Radiosurgery with or without Whole-Brain Radiotherapy. Between 1999 and 2003 Aoyama et al.[84] performed a randomized controlled trial at 11 hospitals in Japan of 132 patients with one to four brain metastases, each less than 3 cm. Patients were randomly assigned to receive WBRT and radiosurgery or radiosurgery alone. The primary end point was overall survival, and secondary end points included brain tumor recurrence, salvage brain treatment, functional preservation, toxicity, and cause of death. The median survival time and the 1-year actuarial survival rate were 7.5 months and 38.5% in the WBRT plus SRS group and 8 months and 28.4% for SRS alone ($P = .42$). The 12-month brain tumor recurrence rate was 46.8% in the WBRT plus SRS group and 76.4% for SRS alone group ($P < .001$). Salvage brain treatment was less frequently required in the WBRT plus SRS group (n = 10) than with SRS alone (n = 29) ($P < .001$). Death was attributed to neurologic causes in 22.8% of patients in the WBRT plus SRS group and in 19.3% of those treated with SRS alone ($P = .64$). There were no significant differences in systemic and neurologic functional preservation and toxic effects of radiation. The authors concluded that compared with SRS alone, the use of WBRT plus SRS did not improve survival for patients with one to four brain metastases. However, salvage therapy was frequently required in patients not receiving WBRT, because intracranial relapse occurred considerably more frequently in those patients.

As previously mentioned, Chang et al.[49] recently published results of a randomized trial to examine neurocognitive function (primary end point) in patients who underwent SRS treatment with or without WBRT. This study was criticized for the imbalance of the patient characteristics between the two treatment arms, the use of a 4-month neurocognitive endpoint, and an earlier and longer duration of chemotherapy in the SRS only arm. Not surprisingly, the median and 1-year survival outcomes favored the cohort of patients treated with SRS alone. It is difficult to extrapolate the results of this study to general clinical practice given these limitations.

Salvage Therapy

Patients who recur in the brain may be candidates for salvage therapy, particularly those in whom nonbrain systemic metastases are either currently of lesser clinical significance or absent. No matter what the initial therapy, patients who may benefit from possible future salvage therapy are followed at 3-month intervals with repeat brain MRI. Possible tumor enhancement seen after surgery must be distinguished from postsurgical changes, and any seen following WBRT, radiosurgery, or brachytherapy must be distinguished from radiation necrosis. Radiation necrosis can closely resemble recurrent tumor on anatomic ("conventional") MRI because of the following shared features: (1) focus at or close to the original tumor site, which is commonly the site of maximal radiation dose, (2) contrast enhancement, (3) progressive enlargement, at least over several months, (4) surrounding edema, and (5) exertion of mass effect. In cases where MRI shows progression, magnetic resonance spectroscopy (MRS),[85] diffusion-weighted imaging (DWI),[86–89] perfusion MRI,[90,91] fluorodeoxyglucose (FDG) positron emission tomography (PET),[92] amino acid PET,[93,94] and single photon emission CT (SPECT)[95] may be useful in making the distinction.

In general, the same array of therapeutic options available for initial treatment may be considered for salvage therapy, including chemotherapy. There are no reliable data that accurately describe the relative frequency of various combinations of first and second therapies. However, in patients who initially receive either WBRT or focal therapy, salvage is often performed focally, particularly in patients whose primary tumor remains controlled and who otherwise do not have extensive extracranial disease. WBRT is not usually repeated in patients who are expected to live more than 6 months because of concerns of radiation injury. However, in poor prognosis patients it may be repeated, usually by delivering lower doses and smaller fraction sizes, such as 20 to 25 Gy in 10 fractions or 30 Gy in 30 fractions (1 Gy twice a day). Treatments outcomes are similar to that obtained following initial WBRT for RPA class 2 or 3 patients, with symptomatic improvement in up to 75% of patients and mean or median survival times of 3 to 5 months.[96–98] The risk of serious radiation toxicity following repeat WBRT is thought to be low in patients who are unlikely to survive 6 months.

Surgery is not often repeated, although it certainly may be. The largest reported reoperation series is that of Bindal et al.,[99] who reported neurologic improvement in 75% of 48 patients, median survival following reoperation of 11.5 months, and no operative mortality or morbidity. Others have also reported favorable reoperation results, reflecting both the positive role for surgery and the need for careful patient selection.

Radiosurgery, on the other hand, is often repeated. Chen et al.[100] reviewed 45 patients with up to five new tumors, all remote from the initial radiosurgery sites, treated with repeat radiosurgery. Median time between first and second procedures was 17 weeks; median survival following the second procedure was 28 weeks. Ten of the 28 patients underwent two salvage radiotherapies and one underwent a third. The 1-year actuarial freedom from progression of treated tumors was 92%. Hillard et al.[101] studied ten patients who received two or more radiosurgeries to at least three isocenters and who were followed for toxicity for at least 6 months. One patient developed seizures in association with radiation necrosis, but no other significant focal or global neurotoxicities were seen.

CARCINOMATOUS MENINGITIS

Dissemination and growth of cancer cells within the leptomeningeal space are among the most serious complications faced by the cancer patient. Early diagnosis of these complications is often elusive, and management represents a significant challenge. The median survival for patients diagnosed with carcinomatous meningitis is 3 to 6 months.

Because carcinomatous meningitis from solid tumors is often associated with an advanced stage of systemic disease and often occurs with concomitant parenchymal brain metastases, therapeutic goals may be limited to the palliation of symptoms and to the prevention of further neurologic deterioration. The goals in treating leukemic and lymphomatous meningitis are more optimistic and include significant prolongation of survival and cure. In all cases, early aggressive intervention is critical to preserve neurologic function. Therapeutic intervention relies on traditional approaches with radiation with or without chemotherapy, with the goal of treating the entire neuroaxis.

Epidemiology

Approximately 5% of cancer patients are affected by neoplastic meningitis. Although the vast majority of tumor histologies have been associated with this phenotype, this complication occurs most commonly in particular subsets of both hematologic and solid tumor patients. Neoplastic meningitis is relatively common in patients with acute lymphoblastic leukemia and aggressive non-Hodgkin's lymphoma. This complication is extremely rare in patients with Hodgkin's lymphoma. Approximately 25% of patients with metastatic melanoma and small cell carcinoma develop leptomeningeal disease. In addition, approximately 2% to 5% of breast cancer patients develop carcinomatous meningitis. Leptomeningeal metastases have also been described in less common solid tumors, including germ cell tumors, sarcomas, gastrointestinal tumors, and squamous cell carcinoma. In addition, primary tumors of the CNS, such as medulloblastoma or ependymoma, often disseminate within the leptomeningeal space throughout the craniospinal axis. Overt leptomeningeal dissemination in patients with astrocytic neoplasms is relatively rare.

Clinical Presentation

Leptomeningeal tumor dissemination disrupts neurologic function by at least three distinct processes. Leptomeningeal tumor cell infiltration may result in altered mentation, incontinence, lower motor neuron weakness, back or radicular pain, cranial nerve deficits resulting in diplopia, hearing loss, hoarseness, alterations in taste, dysphagia, meningismus, and headache. Leptomeningeal tumor cell growth may also cause regional disturbances in blood flow in the affected nervous tissue, resulting in metabolic dysfunction that produces seizures, strokelike symptoms, and generalized encephalopathy. Finally, bulky leptomeningeal deposits may result in the obstruction of normal cerebrospinal fluid (CSF) flow pathways, leading to increased intracranial pressure and hydrocephalus.

Diagnostic Studies

A detailed examination of the CSF is usually required to make a diagnosis of neoplastic meningitis. Cytological evaluation of the CSF, the gold standard, is an extremely insensitive test; 40% to 50% of patients with neoplastic meningitis have negative CSF cytology.[102] Repetitive CSF cytological evaluations may result in increased diagnostic sensitivity. Unfortunately, conversion to positive cytology is usually a manifestation of tumor progression and resultant neurologic deterioration. Given the importance of early diagnosis and intervention in treating leptomeningeal disease, there has been significant effort to identify biomarkers for this complication. For example, in the 1980s it was demonstrated that the tumor antigen carcinoembryonic antigen as well as the enzymatic activity of β-glucuronidase could be detected in the CSF in patients with brain and leptomeningeal metastases.[103] These biomarkers could facilitate clinical detection of neoplastic meningitis and were shown to rise and fall in parallel with the clinical course. Unfortunately, to date no biomarker has emerged with adequate sensitivity and specificity, and the diagnosis of leptomeningeal cancer relies heavily on cytology and clinical impression.

Approximately 50% of patients with neoplastic meningitis and spinal symptoms have abnormal imaging studies using gadolinium-enhanced MRI.[102] Common radiographic presentations include hydrocephalus without an identifiable mass lesion as well as leptomeningeal contrast enhancement. Abnormal enhancement of the meninges is not specific, however, and may also be seen after lumbar puncture, with infection, trauma, inflammation, or following craniotomy.

Radiation Therapy

Effective palliation in most cases of carcinomatous meningitis relies on radiation therapy. Focal irradiation of symptomatic sites and regions where imaging studies have demonstrated bulk disease is a favorable strategy. It avoids the substantial acute toxicities of craniospinal axis irradiation. Craniospinal axis irradiation has a negative impact on bone marrow function, which may significantly compromise the ability to administer subsequent myelosuppressive chemotherapy. One strategy, therefore, is to selectively use external beam irradiation to treat symptomatic sites of disease and to rely on intrathecal chemotherapy to suppress the remainder of the disease in the neuroaxis. Examples include external beam irradiation to the base of the skull in patients with cranial nerve deficits or external beam irradiation to the lumbosacral plexus in patients with cauda equina syndrome.[104–106]

Intrathecal Chemotherapy

The most reliable means of administering chemotherapy within the leptomeningeal space is through an implanted subcutaneous reservoir and ventricular catheter (Ommaya reservoir). Retrospective analysis suggests that intraventricular administration may result in prolonged remission in patients with leptomeningeal leukemia compared with administration by lumbar puncture.[107] Chemotherapeutic agents administered into the ventricle disseminate through the neuroaxis by bulk CSF flow. CSF flow abnormalities are common in patients with leptomeningeal metastases who frequently present with hydrocephalus and increased intracranial pressure as a result of bulky disease, which obstructs CSF flow. Up to 70% of patients with neoplastic meningitis have obstruction in CSF pathways as detected by radionuclide ventriculography.[108] Obstruction in CSF flow may be reversed with local irradiation. A CSF flow study is therefore recommended for every patient beginning intrathecal chemotherapy via a ventricular catheter because of the potential risk of irreversible neurotoxicity from high sustained concentrations of intrathecal chemotherapy.[106]

Cytarabine and methotrexate are the most widely used agents for intrathecal administration in the prophylaxis and treatment of leptomeningeal cancer. Intraventricular administration of methotrexate achieves therapeutic concentrations (more than 1 mcmol/L) that persist for up to 48 hours. One approach to the treatment of active neoplastic meningitis is to use twice weekly intrathecal therapy until CSF clears followed by weekly and then monthly maintenance therapy until progression. Intrathecal methotrexate can cause myelosuppression as well as mucositis, toxicities that can be attenuated by oral leucovorin administration.

Cytarabine is also commonly used in the treatment of neoplastic meningitis. Cytarabine is metabolized by cytidine deaminase. Because of low CNS levels of cytidine deaminase, metabolism of cytarabine occurs relatively slowly in the CSF, resulting in an extended half-life of this drug in the leptomeningeal compartment.[104]

Treatment-Related Toxicity

Placement of an intraventricular catheter is associated with an approximate 1% risk of perioperative hemorrhage. Extended use of the device is associated with at least a 5% risk of infection, usually with gram-positive organisms. Ultimately the development of a necrotizing leukoencephalopathy is the most significant toxicity associated with the treatment of leptomeningeal carcinomatosis. This appears to occur most commonly in patients who receive intrathecal methotrexate following cranial irradiation. The clinical manifestations are initially radiographic: usually bilaterally symmetric abnormalities in white matter. Subsequently patients may develop progressive dementia that can progress to substantial debility and to death.[104]

Systemic Chemotherapy and New Approaches

Most water-soluble chemotherapy drugs are limited by the intact blood–brain barrier, and thus systemic therapy often fails to effectively treat microscopic, nonenhancing disease both in brain parenchyma and in the subarachnoid space. An important exception is the high-dose systemic administration of methotrexate, which results in therapeutic drug levels in the CSF; this therapeutic approach has been shown to be active in neoplastic meningitis both in lymphoma and in some solid tumors. Moreover, high-dose intravenous methotrexate administration overcomes problems associated with obstruction of CSF flow, which may compromise the subarachnoid administration of drugs. However, an important limitation of this approach is that high-dose methotrexate administration requires detailed inpatient monitoring of fluid status, renal function, urine alkalinization, and leucovorin rescue. Therefore, systemic administration of methotrexate at high doses is not appropriate or practical for all patients.[109]

Finally, there is increasing interest in the administration of targeted, biological therapies into the leptomeningeal compartment to treat brain and leptomeningeal tumors. There is mounting evidence that most water-soluble small molecules or monoclonal antibodies exhibit inefficient penetration into the brain or leptomeninges. For example, systemic administration of monoclonal antibodies, which target CD20 in B-cell lymphomas, or of some molecules that inhibit the bcr-abl tyrosine kinase (e.g., imatinib) results in low levels in the CSF.[110] The direct administration of biologic therapies within the leptomeningeal compartment to treat brain tumors and neoplastic meningitis is an area of current early phase clinical investigation.[111,112]

Selected References

The full list of references for this chapter appears in the online version.

3. Schouten LJ, Rutten J, Huveneers HA, Twijnstra A. Incidence of brain metastases in a cohort of patients with carcinoma of the breast, colon, kidney, and lung and melanoma. *Cancer* 2002;94:2698.
4. Jemal A, Siegel R, Xu J, Ward E. Cancer statistics, 2010. *CA Cancer J Clin* 2010;60:277.
6. Nussbaum ES, Djalilian HR, Cho KH, Hall WA. Brain metastases. Histology, multiplicity, surgery, and survival. *Cancer* 1996;78:1781.
8. Schellinger PD, Meinck HM, Thron A. Diagnostic accuracy of MRI compared to CCT in patients with brain metastases. *J Neurooncol* 1999;44:275.
9. Patchell RA, Tibbs PA, Walsh JW, et al. A randomized trial of surgery in the treatment of single metastases to the brain. *N Engl J Med* 1990;322:494.
10. Franzini A, Leocata F, Giorgi C, et al. Role of stereotactic biopsy in multifocal brain lesions: considerations on 100 consecutive cases. *J Neurol Neurosurg Psychiatry* 1994;57:957.
11. Gaspar L, Scott C, Rotman M, et al. Recursive partitioning analysis (RPA) of prognostic factors in three Radiation Therapy Oncology Group (RTOG) brain metastases trials. *Int J Radiat Oncol Biol Phys* 1997;37:745.
12. Andrews DW, Scott CB, Sperduto PW, et al. Whole brain radiation therapy with or without stereotactic radiosurgery boost for patients with one to three brain metastases: phase III results of the RTOG 9508 randomised trial. *Lancet* 2004;363:1665.
14. Sperduto PW, Berkey B, Gaspar LE, Mehta M, Curran W. A new prognostic index and comparison to three other indices for patients with brain metastases: an analysis of 1,960 patients in the RTOG database. *Int J Radiat Oncol Biol Phys* 2008;70:510.
15. Yuh WT, Fisher DJ, Runge VM, et al. Phase III multicenter trial of high-dose gadoteridol in MR evaluation of brain metastases. *AJNR Am J Neuroradiol* 1994;15:1037.
17. Sperduto CM, Watanabe Y, Mullan J, et al. A validation study of a new prognostic index for patients with brain metastases: the graded prognostic assessment. *J Neurosurg* 2008;109(Suppl):87.
18. Sneed PK, Suh JH, Goetsch SJ, et al. A multi-institutional review of radiosurgery alone vs. radiosurgery with whole brain radiotherapy as the initial management of brain metastases. *Int J Radiat Oncol Biol Phys* 2002;53:519.
19. Agboola O, Benoit B, Cross P, et al. Prognostic factors derived from recursive partition analysis (RPA) of Radiation Therapy Oncology Group (RTOG) brain metastases trials applied to surgically resected and irradiated brain metastatic cases. *Int J Radiat Oncol Biol Phys* 1998;42:155.
23. Batchelor T, DeAngelis LM. Medical management of cerebral metastases. *Neurosurg Clin North Am* 1996;7:435.
25. van Vulpen M, Kal HB, Taphoorn MJ, El-Sharouni SY. Changes in blood–brain barrier permeability induced by radiotherapy: implications for timing of chemotherapy? [review]. *Oncol Rep* 2002;9:683.
27. Glantz MJ, Cole BF, Forsyth PA, et al. Practice parameter: anticonvulsant prophylaxis in patients with newly diagnosed brain tumors. Report of the Quality Standards Subcommittee of the American Academy of Neurology. *Neurology* 2000;54:1886.
31. Lyman GH, Khorana AA, Falanga A, et al. American Society of Clinical Oncology guideline: recommendations for venous thromboembolism prophylaxis and treatment in patients with cancer. *J Clin Oncol* 2007;25:5490.
33. Sneed PK, Lamborn KR, Forstner JM, et al. Radiosurgery for brain metastases: is whole brain radiotherapy necessary? *Int J Radiat Oncol Biol Phys* 1999;43:549.
34. Borgelt B, Gelber R, Kramer S, et al. The palliation of brain metastases: final results of the first two studies by the Radiation Therapy Oncology Group. *Int J Radiat Oncol Biol Phys* 1980;6:1.
38. Murray KJ, Scott C, Greenberg HM, et al. A randomized phase III study of accelerated hyperfractionation versus standard in patients with unresected brain metastases: a report of the Radiation Therapy Oncology Group (RTOG) 9104. *Int J Radiat Oncol Biol Phys* 1997;39:571.
42. Nieder C, Nestle U, Walter K, Niewald M, Schnabel K. Dose/effect relationships for brain metastases. *J Cancer Res Clin Oncol* 1998;124:346.
47. Nieder C, Schwerdtfeger K, Steudel WI, Schnabel K. Patterns of relapse and late toxicity after resection and whole-brain radiotherapy for solitary brain metastases. *Strahlenther Onkol* 1998;174:275.
49. Chang EL, Wefel JS, Hess KR, et al. Neurocognition in patients with brain metastases treated with radiosurgery or radiosurgery plus whole-brain irradiation: a randomised controlled trial. *Lancet Oncol* 2009;10:1037.
51. Meyers CA, Smith JA, Bezjak A, et al. Neurocognitive function and progression in patients with brain metastases treated with whole-brain radiation and motexafin gadolinium: results of a randomized phase III trial. *J Clin Oncol* 2004;22:157.
53. Marsh JC, Gielda BT, Herskovic AM, Abrams RA. Cognitive sparing during the administration of whole brain radiotherapy and prophylactic cranial irradiation: current concepts and approaches. *J Oncol* 2010;2010:198208.
56. Barani IJ, Benedict SH, Lin PS. Neural stem cells: implications for the conventional radiotherapy of central nervous system malignancies. *Int J Radiat Oncol Biol Phys* 2007;68:324.
57. Barani IJ, Cuttino LW, Benedict SH, et al. Neural stem cell-preserving external-beam radiotherapy of central nervous system malignancies. *Int J Radiat Oncol Biol Phys* 2007;68:978.
60. Slotman B, Faivre-Finn C, Kramer G, et al. Prophylactic cranial irradiation in extensive small-cell lung cancer. *N Engl J Med* 2007;357:664.
61. Arriagada R. Re: prophylactic cranial irradiation for patients with small-cell lung cancer. *J Natl Cancer Inst* 1995;87:766.
69. Suki D, Abouassi H, Patel AJ, et al. Comparative risk of leptomeningeal disease after resection or stereotactic radiosurgery for solid tumor metastasis to the posterior fossa. *J Neurosurg* 2008;108:248.
70. Suki D, Hatiboglu MA, Patel AJ, et al. Comparative risk of leptomeningeal dissemination of cancer after surgery or stereotactic radiosurgery for a single supratentorial solid tumor metastasis. *Neurosurgery* 2009;64:664.
71. Bindal RK, Sawaya R, Leavens ME, Lee JJ. Surgical treatment of multiple brain metastases. *J Neurosurg* 1993;79:210.
74. Patchell RA, Tibbs PA, Regine WF, et al. Postoperative radiotherapy in the treatment of single metastases to the brain: a randomized trial. *JAMA* 1998;280:1485.
75. Rades D, Raabe A, Bajrovic A, Alberti W. Treatment of solitary brain metastasis. Resection followed by whole brain radiation therapy (WBRT) and a radiation boost to the metastatic site. *Strahlenther Onkol* 2004;180:144.
76. Shaw E, Scott C, Souhami L, et al. Single dose radiosurgical treatment of recurrent previously irradiated primary brain tumors and brain metastases: final report of RTOG protocol 90-05. *Int J Radiat Oncol Biol Phys* 2000;47:291.
77. Flickinger JC, Kondziolka D, Lunsford LD, et al. A multi-institutional experience with stereotactic radiosurgery for solitary brain metastasis. *Int J Radiat Oncol Biol Phys* 1994;28:797.
82. Bindal AK, Bindal RK, Hess KR, et al. Surgery versus radiosurgery in the treatment of brain metastasis. *J Neurosurg* 1996;84:748.
84. Aoyama H, Shirato H, Tago M, et al. Stereotactic radiosurgery plus whole-brain radiation therapy vs stereotactic radiosurgery alone for treatment of brain metastases: a randomized controlled trial. *JAMA* 2006;295:2483.
85. Law M, Cha S, Knopp EA, et al. High-grade gliomas and solitary metastases: differentiation by using perfusion and proton spectroscopic MR imaging. *Radiology* 2002;222:715.
88. Park SH, Chang KH, Song IC, et al. Diffusion-weighted MRI in cystic or necrotic intracranial lesions. *Neuroradiology* 2000;42:716.
90. Cha S, Lu S, Johnson G, Knopp EA. Dynamic susceptibility contrast MR imaging: correlation of signal intensity changes with cerebral blood volume measurements. *J Magn Reson Imaging* 2000;11:114.
92. Langleben DD, Segall GM. PET in differentiation of recurrent brain tumor from radiation injury. *J Nucl Med* 2000;41:1861.
93. Hustinx R, Pourdehnad M, Kaschten B, Alavi A. PET imaging for differentiating recurrent brain tumor from radiation necrosis. *Radiol Clin North Am* 2005;43:35.
95. Alexiou GA, Tsiouris S, Kyritsis AP, Polyzoidis KS, Fotopoulos AD. Brain SPECT by 99mTc-tetrofosmin for the differentiation of tumor recurrence from radiation injury. *J Nucl Med* 2008;49:1733.
97. Cooper JS, Steinfeld AD, Lerch IA. Cerebral metastases: value of reirradiation in selected patients. *Radiology* 1990;174:883.
99. Bindal RK, Sawaya R, Leavens ME, Hess KR, Taylor SH. Reoperation for recurrent metastatic brain tumors. *J Neurosurg* 1995;83:600.
104. DeAngelis LM, Posner JB, Posner JB. *Neurologic complications of cancer*. 2nd ed. New York: Oxford University Press, 2009.
110. Motl S, Zhuang Y, Waters CM, Stewart CF. Pharmacokinetic considerations in the treatment of CNS tumours. *Clin Pharmacokinet* 2006;45:871.
111. Laske DW, Muraszko KM, Oldfield EH, et al. Intraventricular immunotoxin therapy for leptomeningeal neoplasia. *Neurosurgery* 1997;41:1039.
112. Rubenstein JL, Fridlyand J, Abrey L, et al. Phase I study of intraventricular administration of rituximab in patients with recurrent CNS and intraocular lymphoma. *J Clin Oncol* 2007;25:1350.
120. Petrovich Z, Yu C, Giannotta SL, O'Day S, Apuzzo ML. Survival and pattern of failure in brain metastasis treated with stereotactic gamma knife radiosurgery. *J Neurosurg* 2002;97:499.

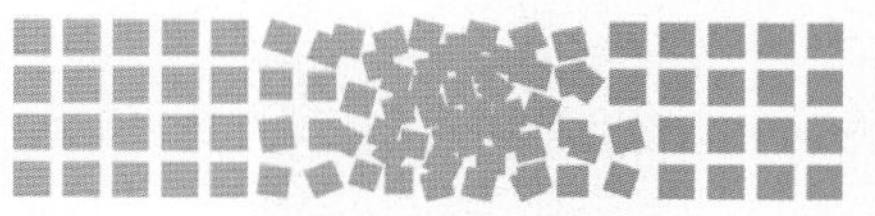

CHAPTER 148 METASTATIC CANCER TO THE LUNG

KING F. KWONG AND ROBERT TIMMERMAN

RATIONALE FOR LOCAL THERAPIES FOR LUNG METASTASES

Skeptics may argue that many (or most) patients with aggregates of gross tumor in the lungs detected by conventional imaging or even direct palpation (i.e., the "targets" for local therapy) are likely to also harbor microscopic tumor cell deposits within the residual lung or other organs and that upon completion of the local therapy, these microscopic deposits would soon replace those removed by the local therapy, making such local therapy a futile and possibly a costly adventure for the patient. In response to this critique, one can simply draw on the published literature, as discussed in this chapter, that shows long-term disease-free survivors among patients with lung metastases. Indeed, some long-term survivors are only treated with local therapy without any systemic therapy for disseminated disease. Even patients with multiple metastases, if all are removed or ablated, can experience long-term disease-free survival. As the natural history of these cancers is to progress to lethal tumor burden, it is logical to assume that the local intervention taken in long-term survivors altered the cancer's natural history and allowed for cure. So based on these observations and the fairly large clinical experience behind it, local therapies should be considered an integral option in formulating a treatment plan for patients with metastases to the lungs.

Clearly, the justification for local therapies in metastatic lung disease would be strengthened if results from well-controlled randomized clinical studies were available. At present, there are few phase 3 clinical trials to compare local therapy to no local therapy in patients with cancer metastases to the lungs. Instead, there is a large amount of lower level evidence, mostly in the form of registry databases and retrospective reports. For ablative therapies, phase 1 and 2 evidence is emerging, but again no phase 3 data. Similarly, renewed interest is emerging, based on past and ongoing work at the National Cancer Institute and other institutions, to better explore the role of surgery in the treatment of metastatic disease.

MODES OF METASTATIC SPREAD

Cancer cells may disseminate to the lung hematogenously or via the lymphatic. Metastatic cells will often grow as distinct tumors; however, widespread involvement of the intrapulmonary lymphatics can result in lymphangitic carcinomatosis (Fig. 148.1). From surgical experience, isolated lung metastases treated aggressively with resection can be associated with improved survival in select cancers. More recently, dramatic metastatic tumor regression has also been seen with several molecular-targeted agents and specific immunotherapy strategies, respectively. In responsive patients, these novel treatment strategies can ultimately change the tempo or the natural progression of metastatic disease, possibly creating new clinical windows for additional therapy or allowing for extirpation of residual isolated metastases.

DIAGNOSIS

Signs and Symptoms

Patients with pulmonary metastasis can present asymptomatically despite new lung lesions on radiologic examination. Alternatively, bulky hilar disease can result in dyspnea, protracted cough, or hemoptysis; whereas endobronchial metastasis can obstruct the airway, causing stridor, atelectasis, or postobstructive pneumonia, depending on the tumor's anatomic location and the degree of endoluminal obliteration. Cancers predisposed for endobronchial involvement include squamous cell lung cancer, colon cancer, renal cell cancer, breast cancer, and, less frequently, sarcoma and melanoma (Fig. 148.2). Hilar compression of the main pulmonary artery by tumor can also result in dyspnea due to severe physiologic shunting of pulmonary blood flow. Tumor invasion of the parietal pleura or chest wall usually causes localized pain. In many early cases, chest wall invasion is often equivocal on computed tomography (CT) scan, but the presence of localized chest wall pain experienced by the patient is virtually diagnostic of chest wall invasion.

Imaging Studies

Chest Radiography, Computed Tomography, and Magnetic Resonance Imaging

Although the plain chest x-ray is often the first to demonstrate features consistent with pulmonary metastasis, CT is the more sensitive method of imaging lung metastasis. Features such as new lung nodules, lobar or segmental collapse, hilar or mediastinal nodal fullness, lymphangitic spread, or pleural effusions can be seen on plain x-rays. However, the helical CT scan can detect subcentimeter tumors smaller than 5 mm and provide precise localization of tumors.[1] Intravenous contrast is recommended to allow better visualization of anatomy near vascular structures, unless contraindicated by severe renal impairment or severe contrast allergy. Magnetic resonance imaging (MRI) has only limited utility in patients with lung metastasis, especially when a high-resolution CT scan can be readily obtained.

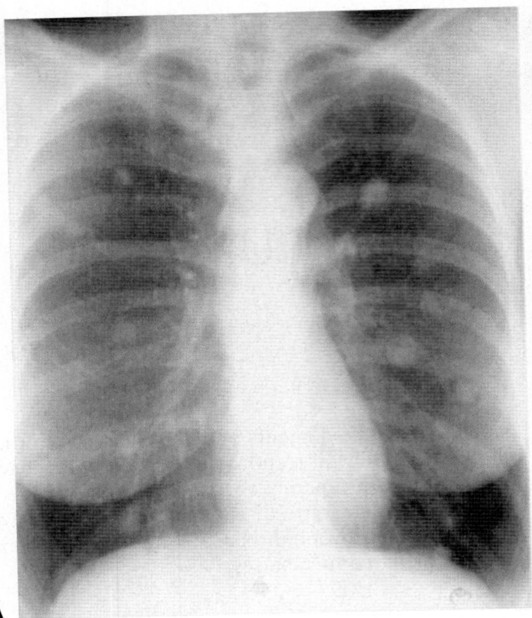

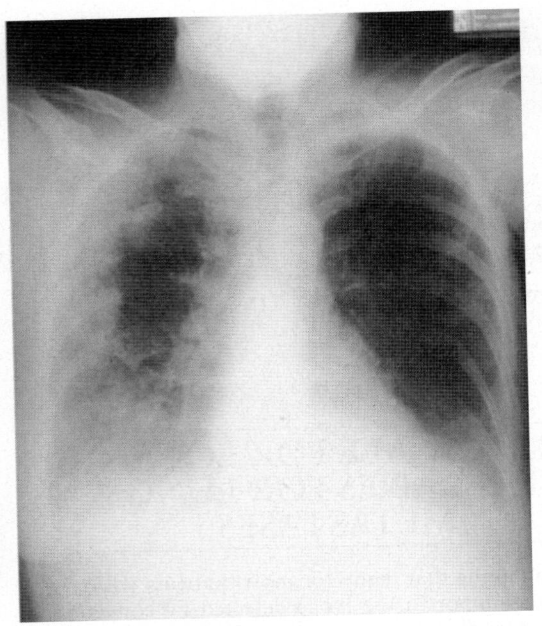

FIGURE 148.1 Chest radiographs of patients with lung metastasis. **A:** Hematogenous metastasis. **B:** Lymphangitic metastasis.

Positron Emission Tomography

The clinical application of positron emission tomography (PET) has increased widely over the past decade. PET utilizes ^{16}fluorodeoxyglucose (FDG), which enters glucose-dependent cells but is unable to undergo normal glucose metabolism; therefore, ^{16}FDG rapidly accumulates within cells that exhibit increased metabolic activity, such as many cancer cells. Tumor uptake of ^{16}FDG can be visualized due to the radioactive fluorine's beta-decay, an emission of positron particles. The combination of positrons with nearby electrons releases detectable gamma photons. Simultaneous 360-degree detection and ultrafast computerized data acquisition can then generate three-dimensional reconstructed images of focal FDG concentrations above background tissue levels. Because FDG-PET is dependent on normal glucose metabolism, diabetic patients must have good glucose regulation and withhold oral hypoglycemic medications prior to the PET examination. As well, increased FDG uptake can localize to normal bowel peristaltic activity, skeletal muscular contraction, in tissues with high glucose metabolism such as the heart and brain, and in anatomic structures of glucose metabolism and elimination such as the liver, kidneys, ureters, and bladder. Since increased FDG avidity can be found in inflammatory, infectious, or benign conditions as well, a multidisciplinary group review of a PET study can greatly aid correct interpretation of observed focal areas of FDG avidity. PET sensitivity is also highly related to the specific tumor type, so the input of clinicians experienced with the use of PET in a particular cancer is especially advantageous.

Tissue Diagnosis

Frequently the diagnosis of lung metastasis is commonly unequivocal from the clinical scenario, and obtaining confirmatory tissue is not needed, especially if the recommended treatment would be unaltered by the additional discovery of lung metastases. However, some cancer patients deserve a refreshed investigation when a new lung lesion is discovered. For example, a patient with a distant history of cancer and long-standing remission or the long-term cancer survivor with significant personal risk factors for also developing a primary bronchogenic carcinoma should receive an unbiased workup of new pulmonary lesions to guide appropriate treatment. Depending on the location of the tumor in the lung, diagnostic tissue biopsy can often be obtained by transthoracic needle aspiration or bronchoscopic transbronchial biopsy. In specific patients, surgical resection is needed to establish the histologic diagnosis.

Pretreatment Evaluation

Successful respiration involves the capacity to deliver adequate oxygen necessary for metabolism at the cellular level coupled with the elimination of carbon dioxide, a waste product of metabolism. Obviously, this function must be maintained at a tolerable physiologic level after local therapy. Pretreatment assessment of baseline function coupled with prediction of the posttreatment loss of function is required to evaluate the potential toxicity costs of treatment relative to the perceived benefit.

A direct measurement of pulmonary function is usually undertaken in patients who are being considered for resection or ablative therapies. Tidal volume exchange via inhalation and exhalation occurs as a result of physical forces exerted by the chest wall and diaphragmatic musculature upon the lung parenchyma. Dysfunction of tidal volume exchange can be profound in chronic obstructive pulmonary diseases (e.g., emphysema) and patients with secondary obstructions (e.g., bronchitis and pneumonia), but it is also present in patients prone to shallow breathing (e.g., generally frail patients, patients with phrenic nerve palsy, or patients with chest wall pain). Tidal volume exchange capacity can be quantified before or after a local therapy for lung metastases by spirometry (e.g., forced expiratory volume in 1 second [FEV-1]).

Gas exchange across the membranes between the terminal alveolus and corresponding pulmonary capillary endothelium follows along concentration gradients. Membrane transport (diffusion) can become dysfunctional through thickening of alveolar or capillary membranes associated with conditions such as pulmonary fibrosis. Furthermore, overall limitation of

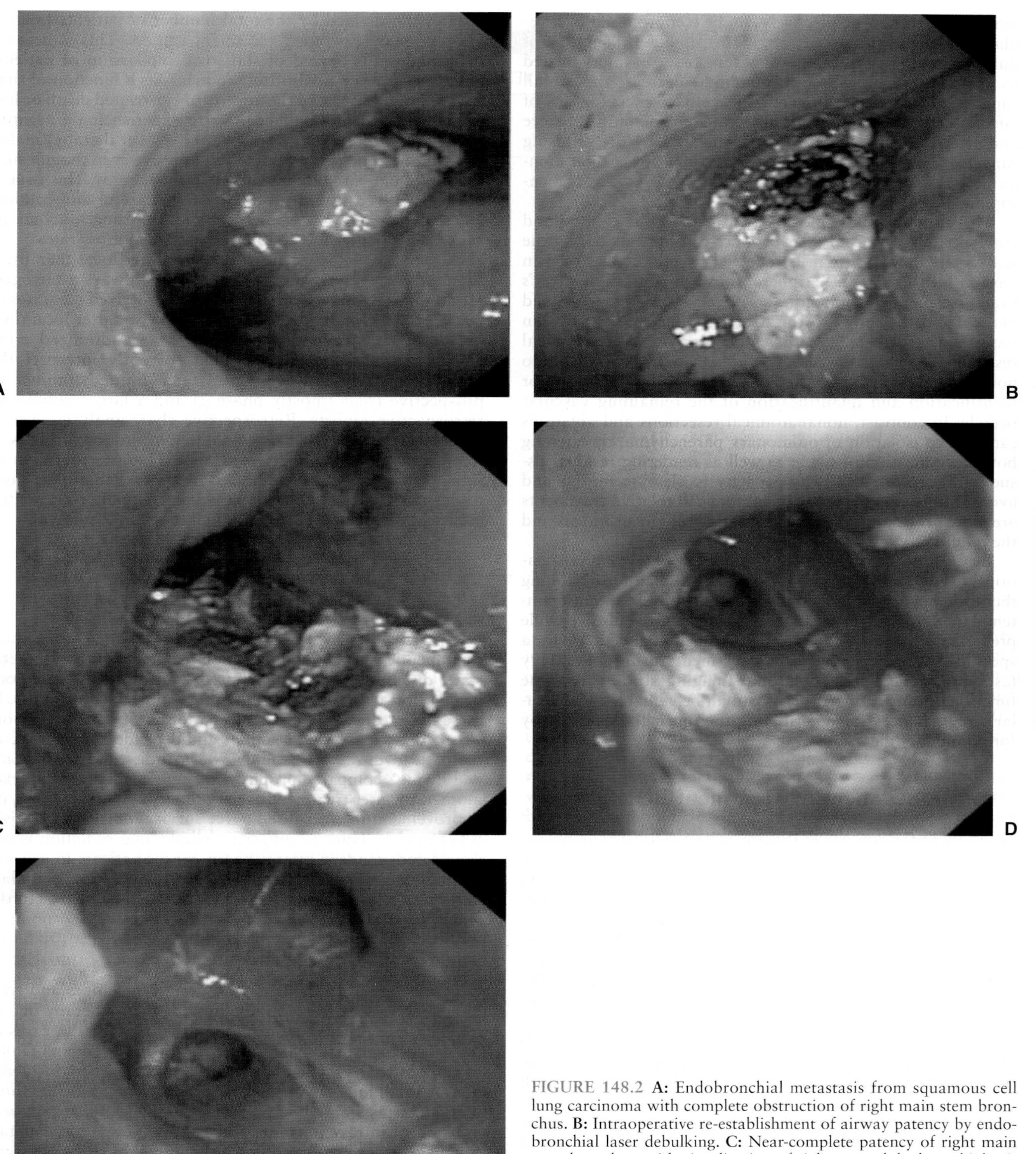

FIGURE 148.2 **A:** Endobronchial metastasis from squamous cell lung carcinoma with complete obstruction of right main stem bronchus. **B:** Intraoperative re-establishment of airway patency by endobronchial laser debulking. **C:** Near-complete patency of right main stem bronchus, with visualization of right upper lobe bronchial orifice and bronchus intermedius. **D:** Distal clearing of bronchus intermedius and visualization of middle lobe and lower lobe bronchial openings. **E:** Close-up examination reveals middle and lower lobe bronchi are not involved with cancer and immediate re-expansion of middle and lower lobes resulted in this patient. (Courtesy of King F. Kwong, MD, National Cancer Institute.)

(n = 74), 5-year disease-free and overall survival were a modest 7% and 18%, respectively.[23]

Repeat thoracotomy for pulmonary metastasectomy in both osteosarcoma and STS can be performed safely. Over the past decade, clinical experience with repeat thoracotomies for metastasectomy has become fairly widespread, and this approach has been reported with good results for select patients,[26–29] resulting in a median survival between 25 and 28 months after the second thoracotomy. Improved survival was associated with completeness of resection, a single lung metastasis, and a disease-free interval greater than 18 months.[26,27] In 86 patients who underwent lung reresection for metastatic STS, Weiser et al.[30] reported an estimated 5-year survival of 36%, while poor prognosis was associated with greater than three pulmonary nodules, nodules greater than 2 cm, and high-grade histology of the primary tumor.

Breast Cancer. Metastatic disease from breast cancer located solely in the lungs represents only a small fraction of all patients with metastatic breast cancer. The factors associated with improved survival after metastasectomy include solitary metastasis, disease-free interval before presenting with metastasis greater than 2 or 3 years, and ability to perform a complete resection of the metastasis.[31–36] A review of 467 patients from the International Registry of Lung Metastases reported survival rates of 38% after 5 years, 22% after 10 years, and 20% after 15 years.[36] Most of these patients had only one metastasis, which was completely resected. Favorable prognostic factors included complete resection, single metastasis, and disease-free interval of at least 3 years—in the subgroup of patients with favorable prognostic factors, the median survival was 59 months and 5-, 10-, and 15-year survival was 50%, 26%, and 26%, respectively. Incomplete resection was often attributed to positive lymph nodes or chest wall or diaphragmatic invasion. Patients with only one lung metastasis had a survival rate of 44% at 5 years and 23% at 10 and 15 years. Nineteen patients from this series underwent repeat surgery for recurrent lung metastasis, but showed no difference in survival when compared to patients who underwent a single surgical resection. Five-year survival was 37% after the first procedure and 40% after a second metastasectomy.

Colorectal Cancer. Since the early 1980s, metastasectomy for metastatic colorectal carcinoma (CRC) has been introduced into clinical practice and has even been extended to patients with lung and liver metastasis. Lung metastasis without other hematogenous metastases occurs in a minority of CRC patients. For example, in one series of 1,578 patients who underwent curative surgery for colorectal carcinoma, 137 (8.7%) developed lung metastasis and only 16 (1%) were candidates for metastasectomy. Although the incidence of liver metastasis was similar between colon and rectal carcinomas, lung metastasis appeared more frequently (11.5%) in rectal carcinoma than in colon carcinoma (3.6%).[37]

Several groups have reported more than 100 cases of pulmonary metastasectomy for colorectal cancer,[38–40] showing low operative mortality and 5-year survival between 31% and 37%. Favorable factors included solitary metastasis, carcinoembryonic antigen (CEA) less than 5 ng/mL, and disease-free interval greater than 3 years. Repeat resection of lung metastases was associated with increased survival as well.[41] In one series of 33 patients with repeat metastasectomies, the median survival was 73 months, and 5-year and 10-year survival rates of 54% and 21% were seen, respectively.[42] Metastases to mediastinal lymph nodes can be found in up to one-third of patients with resectable lung metastasis from colorectal carcinoma. In another series, 15 of 100 patients who underwent lung metastasectomy from colorectal carcinoma demonstrated histologically proven positive hilar or mediastinal lymph nodes.[43] Survival was significantly worse in mediastinal lymph node–positive patients. Inoue et al.[44] found a 5-year survival of 50% in patients with negative mediastinal or hilar lymph nodes, compared to only 14% in those with positive nodes.

More recently, patients with liver and lung metastasis from colorectal carcinoma have been considered for metastasectomy. Resection of synchronous liver and lung metastasis is rare and, despite complete surgical resection, is associated with an overall poor prognosis.[45–48] Resection of liver metastasis after a previous lung metastasectomy has been reported,[46] as well as resecting pulmonary metastasis after liver metastasis.[49] However, the occurrence of previous liver involvement appears to adversely impact survival independent of a potentially complete pulmonary metastasectomy.[50] Because much of the data that support pulmonary metastasectomy are based on retrospective data, some have argued that case selection alone may potentially account for the apparently favorable results. To address this criticism, a randomized prospective clinical trial, the Pulmonary Metastasectomy in Colorectal Cancer (PulMiCC) trial, recently opened in 2010 in the United Kingdom; the accrual success and outcomes data from this trial will likely redefine the use of pulmonary metastasectomy in CRC.[51]

Renal Cell Carcinoma. Metastatic disease develops in 60% to 70% patients with renal cell carcinoma (RCC) during the course of disease, with pulmonary metastasis frequently encountered in about one-third of RCC patients. In 141 RCC patients who presented with metastatic disease and underwent metastasectomy, an overall survival of 44% at 5 years was seen, compared to 14% for those with noncurative surgery and 11% for those treated medically.[52] Favorable variables include single site of metastasis, complete resection, and disease-free interval greater than 12 months. Other groups have reported similar results for lung resection for metastatic renal cell carcinoma, with 5-year survivals between 33% to 47%. Favorable prognostic factors included a disease-free interval greater than 1 to 4 years, solitary metastasis, and metachronous presentation of the lung metastasis. Metastatic involvement of mediastinal or hilar lymph nodes is usually associated with significantly worse survival. When systematic hilar and mediastinal lymph node dissection was performed at the time of lung metastasectomy in 191 patients, the 5-year survival rate fell from 42% to 24% with positive nodes.[53] Positive mediastinal or hilar lymph nodes remained statistically significant as a poor prognostic variable in multivariate analysis.[53]

Germ Cell Tumors. Nonseminomatous germ cell tumors (embryonal, teratocarcinoma, choriocarcinoma, and yolk sac tumors) disseminate widely, including to the lungs, but exhibit good sensitivity to chemotherapy. Cisplatin-based regimens have greatly improved cure rates from 30% or less to almost 90%.[54] Surgical resection of stable residual tumors after chemotherapy serves to remove chemoresistant disease and possibly direct additional chemotherapy as well as evaluation of indeterminate lesions. Often, benign teratoma is found in residual lesions as this element of the tumor is unresponsive to conventional chemotherapy.

Surgical resection of pulmonary lesions is indicated when there is (1) absence of response to chemotherapy; (2) partial response followed by recurrence on chemotherapy; (3) recurrence after standard and second-line chemotherapy; and (4) residual tumors after chemotherapy.

Kesler et al.[55] reported on 268 patients with nonseminomatous germ cell tumors of testicular origin who were treated with cisplatin-based chemotherapy followed by surgery to remove residual mediastinal disease. The 5- and 10-year overall survival rates were 86% and 74%, respectively. Survival was associated negatively with an elevated preoperative beta-human chorionic gonadotropin (β-hCG) and by the presence of residual malignant disease. In addition to elevated levels of β-hCG and incomplete resection, the number and size of lung metastases, as well as their persistence after chemotherapy, have been seen as adverse prognostic factors.[56]

Steyerberg et al.[57] evaluated the probability of necrosis, mature teratoma, and cancer in residual pulmonary masses after chemotherapy in 215 patients and found that resected specimens only contained necrosis in 54% of patients, mature teratoma in 33%, and residual cancer in 13%. Thus, a majority of resected lesions ultimately contain necrotic nonviable tumor or benign teratomatous tissue. Teratomas are chemoresistant and can degenerate into malignancy[58] or enlarge to produce growing teratoma syndrome,[59] so excision is often a prudent choice. However, no presurgical algorithm or variable exists to guide whether or not to perform resection of residual pulmonary lesions, and the precise contribution of pulmonary metastasectomy therefore remains unclear in these cancers.[60] Given the excellent survival rate with chemotherapy, it is not surprising that surgical resection of residual tumors is often advocated so as to definitively rid all disease from the patient while simultaneously obtaining important prognostic information from the histology of the resected tissues.

Melanoma. Historical reports of pulmonary metastasectomy in melanoma have been generally disappointing, with 5-year survival close to 10%. However, several modern series have reported more favorable 5-year survival around 20%[61,62] and as high as 33% for solitary pulmonary metastasectomy.[63] These outcomes compare favorably against best current therapies for metastatic melanoma (interleukin-2 and dacarbazine/DTIC), where response rates are between 7% and 20%, along with significant potential side effects.

Petersen et al.[62] reported on 1,720 patients who presented with melanoma lung metastasis, including 318 patients who underwent pulmonary metastasectomy. The 5-year survival was 21% in those with complete resection, compared to 13% for those incomplete resection. Four risk factors that adversely affected survival include nodular histology, two or more metastases, a disease-free interval of 5 years or less, and the presence of extrathoracic metastases. Patients with no risk factors had a 5-year survival of 26%, whereas there were few 5-year survivors with three or more risk factors. In 328 metastatic melanoma patients from the International Registry of Lung Metastases, a similar 5-year survival rate of 22% was found.[64] Factors correlating with improved survival were complete resection, longer disease-free interval, treatment with chemotherapy, one or two lung metastases only, and the absence of metastatic lymph nodes. Common to many patient series was a disease-free interval greater than 12 months, which was associated with better prognosis.

Head and Neck Cancer. Head and neck cancers, except for cancers of the lip, tonsil, and adenoid, metastasize early to the lung. A unique challenge in this patient population is distinguishing between a metastatic lesion and a primary lung carcinoma because many individuals in this group are smokers who are at high risk of developing other aerodigestive tract cancers. If both the lung tumor and head and neck tumor are squamous carcinomas, it is usually not possible based simply on light microscopy to distinguish between a metastasis and a primary lung cancer. More recently, DNA analysis of tumors has been used to identify common head and neck cancer patterns of loss of heterozygosity (LOH) and serves to verify the origin of the metastatic tumor.[65] The metastasectomy experience for head and neck carcinoma is still limited, but several reports suggest possible benefit if an aggressive surgical treatment is taken.

A review of 83 patients operated on between 1966 and 1995 showed an operative mortality of 2%, with complete resection in 86% of the patients and a 5-year survival of 50%.[66] Patients with glandular tumors had 64% survival compared to 34% survival at 5 years in squamous cell cancer. When patients with glandular tumors were analyzed in isolation, adenoid cystic carcinoma patients had a 5-year survival of 84%. Shiono et al.[67] recently reported on 237 patients who underwent pulmonary metastasectomy with an overall 5-year survival of 27%. Importantly, there were no 5-year survivors among the 17 men with oral cavity cancers. Winter et al.[68] reported on 67 patients with pathology-proven metastasis who achieved a 5-year survival of 20% with metastasectomy.

Gynecologic Cancers. Isolated lung metastasis from uterine or cervical carcinoma is fairly uncommon, and clinical experience with pulmonary metastasectomy with these cancers remains quite limited. Anraku et al.[69] reported on 133 patients who underwent pulmonary metastasectomy for uterine malignancies from 1984 to 2002 and found overall 5- and 10-year survivals of 55% and 45%, respectively. Clavero et al.[70] reported on 70 patients with metastatic disease confined to the lungs and pulmonary metastasectomy with overall 5- and 10-year survivals of 47% and 34%, respectively.

Chemotherapy is the primary treatment for metastatic choriocarcinoma, but occasionally pulmonary resection is needed to remove lung metastases that secrete hCG despite chemotherapy. In another series of 43 patients who underwent resection pulmonary metastasectomy for chemotherapy-resistant choriocarcinoma, a 5-year survival rate of 50% was observed.[71]

Ewing's Sarcoma Family of Tumors. Defined by common chromosomal rearrangement patterns, tumors such as Ewing's sarcoma, peripheral neuroectodermal tumor, Askin's tumor, and neuroepithelioma have been grouped collectively as the Ewing's sarcoma family of tumors (ESFT). ESFT is the second most common primary osseous malignancy in childhood and adolescence, and multimodality therapy is the current therapy standard in these patients. Metastatic disease occurs in one-quarter of patients. Approximately one-third of primary metastases are limited to the lung and pleura; patients with bone or bone marrow metastasis usually have worse outcomes clinically.

Modalities used to treat patients with metastatic ESFT include use of whole-lung radiation, dose-intensified chemotherapy, and high-dose therapy followed by autologous bone marrow or peripheral blood stem cell transplantation. The outcome of patients with ESFT and synchronous thoracic disease is influenced by the response of the primary tumor to chemotherapy, the extent of metastasis to the chest, and the use of whole-lung irradiation.[72] Pulmonary metastasectomy does not improve survival convincingly in these patients and should be limited to those with isolated pulmonary disease.[73,74]

Ablative Therapies

Although an ablative therapy may be considered any locally destructive therapy (in this case, destructive specifically of the lung metastases), this section will focus on the two more commonly used ablative therapies: radiofrequency ablation (RFA) and stereotactic ablative radiotherapy (SBRT), also known as stereotactic body radiation therapy.

Surgical versus Ablative Local Therapy

Given its established and specifically defined success and generally acceptable morbidity with long term follow-up in treating large numbers of patients with lung metastases, surgical resection should be considered the first-line therapy when indicated. Rather than dwell on the competition between surgical and nonsurgical therapies, it is also reasonable to consider when they are complementary. Surgical resection shows the most value when all gross tumor can be completely resected (called an R0 resection). Depending on tumor location and the health status of the patient, achieving an R0 resection may be problematic. This is especially evident with multiple metastases spaced diffusely throughout the lungs, where larger incision or bilateral surgeries might be required. In contrast, when metastatic lung tumors are aggregated in a limited area (e.g., a single lung or lobe), there could be little additional cost in toxicity for removing multiple lesions via a single thoracotomy. Physicians who treat lung metastases will encounter both circumstances. In such cases, it would be entirely legitimate, for example, to resect as many lesions via a unilateral thoracotomy while treating remaining lesions with RFA or SBRT, as demonstrated in Figure 148.3. In general, pneumonectomy should be avoided unless absolutely necessary for achieving an R0 resection in the absence of alternate therapies. In selected patients, combining local therapies might be most optimal and should be considered early in formulating a broad care plan.

Basis of Radiofrequency Ablation. Both extremes of heat and cold can lead to cellular destruction with necrosis known as thermal ablation. This section, however, will focus on the use of high temperatures delivered via the minimally invasive techniques of RFA, given its more widespread use and larger treatment experience in comparison to other thermal ablation methods. A conductive probe (electrode) is inserted into the tumor by image-guided or manual techniques.[75] High-frequency alternating current is transmitted from the tip or tips of the probe into the immediate tissue. This causes excitation of molecules and heating of tissue to a degree capable of causing coagulative necrosis. Tissues, including tumor and surrounding microvasculature, in the vicinity of temperatures greater than 60°C become significantly damaged. The amount of destruction is related to the impedance of the tissue and distance from the electrode. This effect may be modulated by cooling from an immediate heat sink such as a large blood vessel adjacent to the tumor.

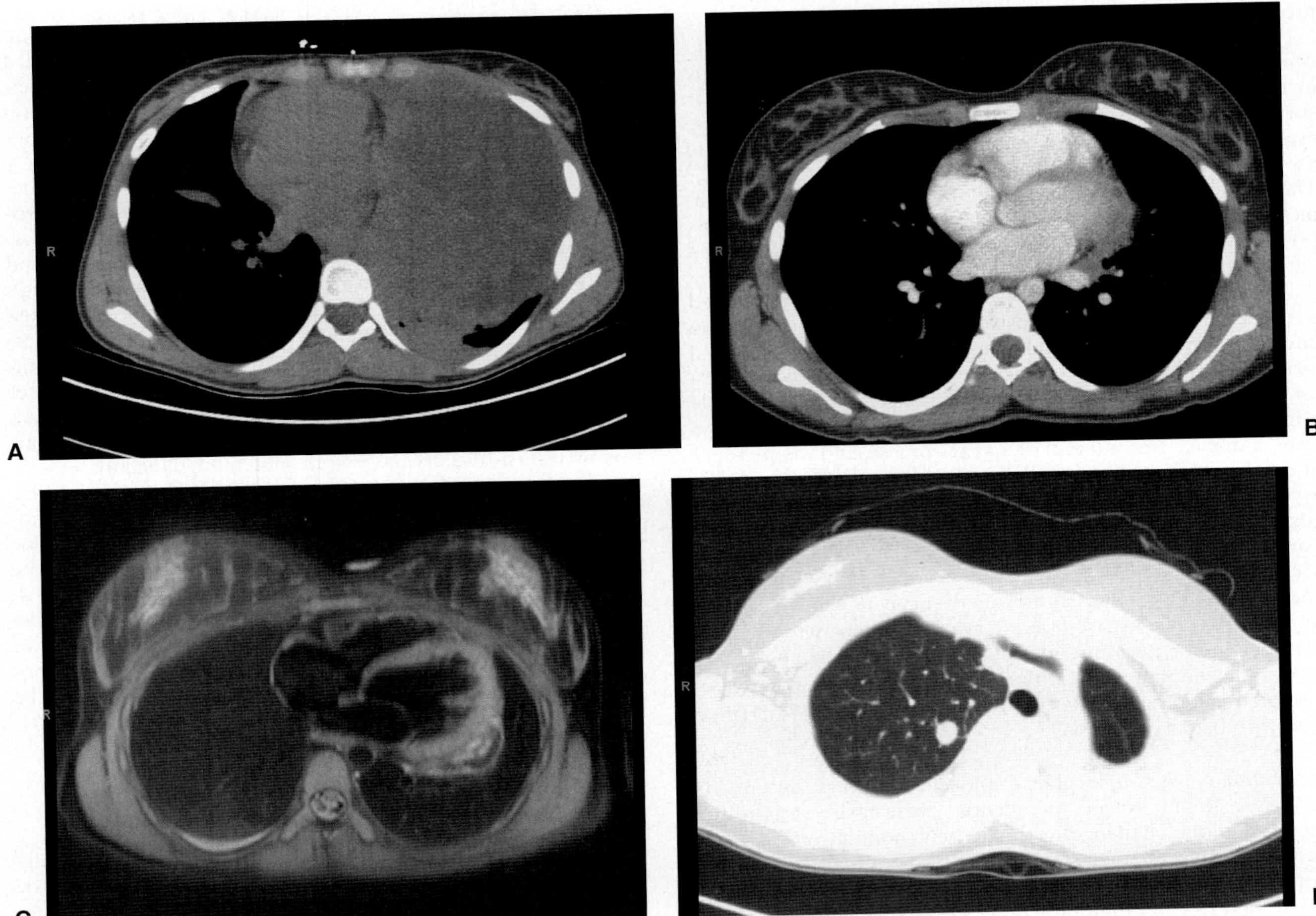

FIGURE 148.3 Fifteen-year-old female presented with shortness of breath and was noted to have an extremely large mass filling much of the left hemithorax as well as several other bilateral pulmonary masses. Biopsy was consistent with Ewing's sarcoma, and she was subsequently found to have a primary tumor located at the distal femoral shaft. She was started on chemotherapy. **A:** Axial computed tomography (CT) image shows a large mass filling much of the left hemithorax at diagnosis. **B:** After systemic therapy, the left lung mass shows dramatic response on CT with residual tumor adjacent to the left cardiac margin. **C:** Magnetic resonance imaging shows that the mass is distinct from the cardiac tissues. The other lung lesions had complete response from chemotherapy. Three months after diagnosis and having completed conventional radiation to the femur primary, she underwent an attempt at surgical resection of the residual left lung mass. Tumor was adherent to hilar structures at time of surgery such that a left pneumonectomy was required to achieve an R0 resection. She completed consolidation chemotherapy. **D:** Twenty-four months after diagnosis, a small apical metastasis reappeared in the right upper lobe. She began salvage chemotherapy with initial response and then stable disease for 12 months. At that point, the right upper lobe nodule showed progression. Now 18 years old, the patient elected to undergo stereotactic ablative radiotherapy (SBRT) for the remaining pulmonary nodule.

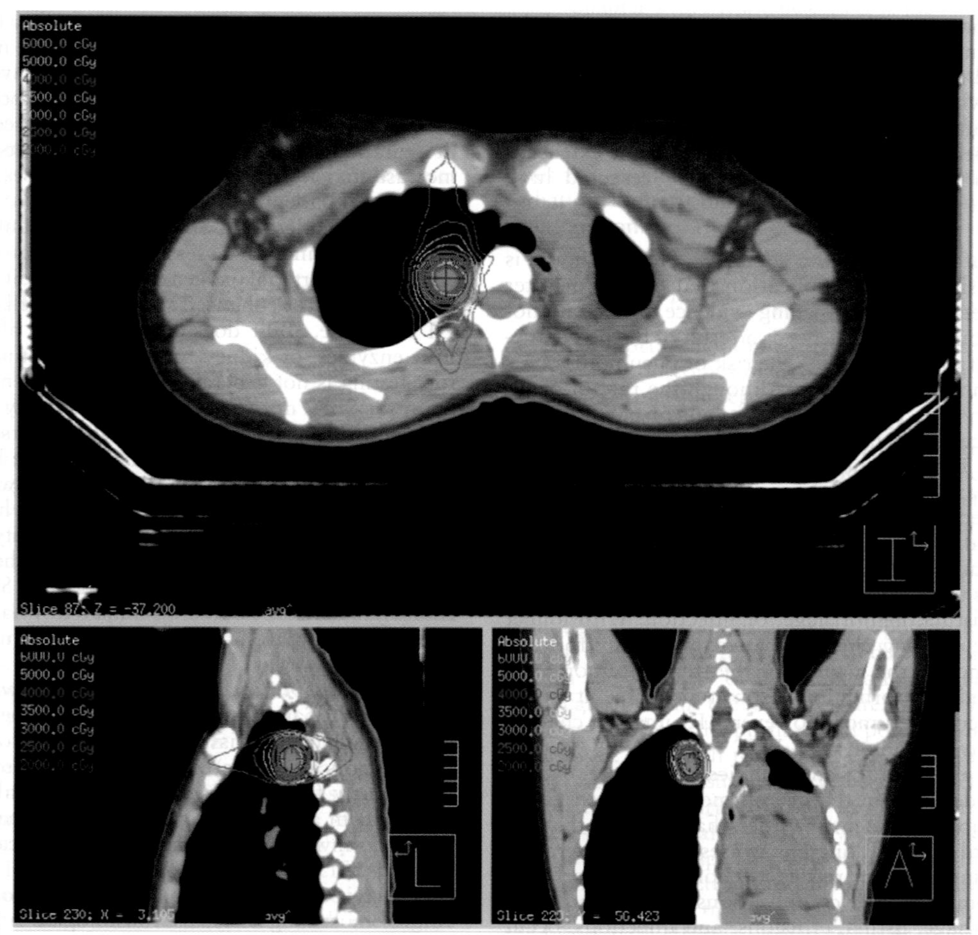

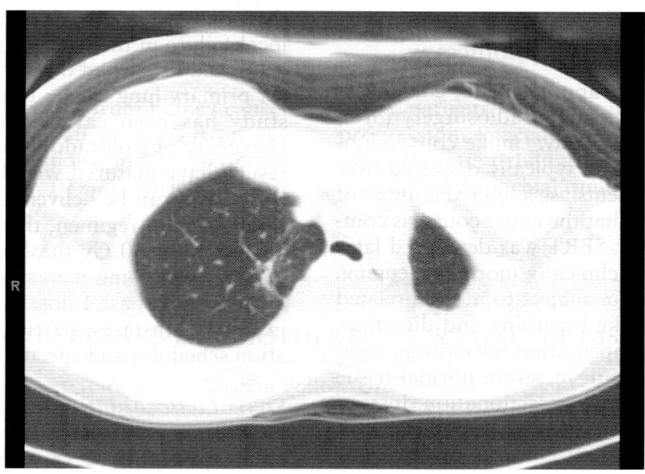

FIGURE 148.3 (*Continued*) **E:** Treatment planning dosimetry for SBRT using 10 noncoplanar beams to a dose of 40 Gy in five fractions. **F:** Follow-up CT image 16 months after SBRT (52 months after diagnosis) showing a linear scar within the treatment site (*arrow*). She remains disease free at last follow-up and is involved in a competitive soccer league. (Courtesy of Robert Timmerman, MD, University of Texas Southwestern.)

Evaluation and Treatment Using Radiofrequency Ablation. Proper selection and pretreatment evaluation is crucial for the success of RFA in treating lung metastases. The guidance needle would ideally not traverse large emphysematous blebs (predisposing pneumothorax) or vascular structures (predisposing hemorrhage). Although the exact number of pulmonary lesions appropriate for thermal ablation therapies has yet to be defined, it is considered reasonable to treat as many as four metastases. Likewise, the maximum size for effective treatment has also not been established, but adequate temperatures are difficult to achieve beyond 3.5 cm from the heat source,[76] indicating that lesions should not be much larger than 3 cm in diameter.

RFA in the lung is guided primarily by CT. In contrast to liver RFA, the surrounding mostly air-filled pulmonary parenchyma actually acts as a thermal insulator, protecting tissues

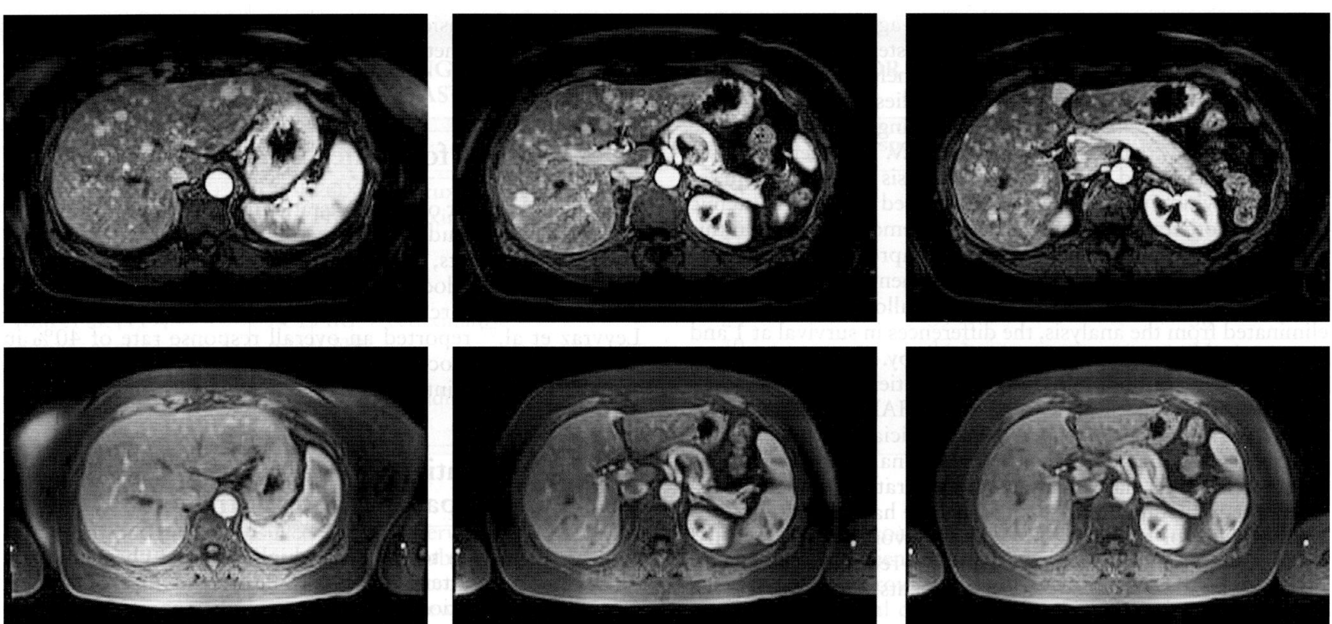

FIGURE 149.4 Magnetic resonance images of the liver showing diffuse metastatic ocular melanoma before (*top panels*) and corresponding images 1 year after percutaneous hepatic perfusion with melphalan.

operative procedure during which time the liver is extensively prepared to prevent leakage of systemic perfusate during treatment. Venous outflow is from a cannula positioned in an isolated segment of the retrohepatic inferior vena cava, and arterial inflow is through a cannula placed in the gastroduodenal artery.

There are data from three centers in Europe and the National Cancer Institute in Bethesda, Maryland, reporting results with IHP using tumor necrosis factor (TNF) and melphalan. Oldhafer et al.[81] reported a series of 12 patients of whom 6 received TNF and melphalan; there was an overall radiographic response rate of 50% and a median survival of 11 months. A Swedish group treated 11 patients and had an operative mortality of 18%. Antitumor activity was observed in three of six patients with ocular melanoma to liver and in zero of five patients with CRC. The modest antitumor activity may be secondary to the very low doses of agents used, only 0.2 to 0.3 mg of TNF and 0.5 mg/kg of melphalan, which are considerably lower than the maximum safe tolerated doses determined in phase 1 trials at the National Cancer Institute.[80,82] Investigators from the National Cancer Institute reported an overall radiographic response rate of 75% in 34 patients with metastatic unresectable cancers confined to liver using 1 mg of TNF and 1.5 mg/kg of melphalan.[83]

A series of patients with CRC liver metastases underwent IHP as second-line treatment after systemic chemotherapy.[16] The overall radiographic response rate was 60%, the median duration of response was 12 months, and the 2-year survival was 28%. Responses were markedly longer in those who also received HAI with floxuridine starting about 8 weeks after IHP (Table 149.9). The same group has reported results of hyperthermic IHP with melphalan alone in 29 patients with metastatic ocular melanoma to the liver.[84] There were 3 (10%) radiographic complete responses and 15 partial responses (52%). Median actuarial overall survival was 12.1 months.

Chemoembolization

Transarterial chemoembolization (TACE) delivers intra-arterial chemotherapeutic agent(s) usually mixed with Ethiodol followed by infusion of one of a number of embolic agents such as degradable starch microspheres, gelatin powders, polyvinyl chloride, or pledgets. More recently, a new class of embolic agent, drug-eluting beads, has been employed for TACE. These agents bind to the chemotherapeutic agent via ionic interactions. The largest body of work with TACE relates to the treatment of hepatocellular carcinoma (see Chapter 84).

TACE has been used to treat a wide variety of metastatic tumor types, including but not limited to cholangiocarcinoma, CRC, pancreatic NET, breast, sarcoma, melanoma, renal cell, and lung. A large body of evidence exists for the use of TACE in patients with carcinoid or NET. These tumors tend to metastasize to the liver early and often have liver-only or dominant disease for long periods. Long-term palliation is usually obtained in these patients because of the generally slow progression of disease. In addition, a reduction in overall tumor burden can provide substantial palliation for those who have symptoms resulting from an excess uncontrolled tumor-related hormone secretion. There are two recent large series that have reported results with TACE in patients with NET. Marrache et al.[85] performed 167 HACE procedures in 67 patients using either streptozotocin or doxorubicin. There was an overall response rate of 37%; factors independently associated with response and

TABLE 149.9

RESULTS OF ISOLATED HEPATIC PERFUSION IN 25 COLORECTAL CANCER PATIENTS WITH ISOLATED LIVER METASTASES AFTER TUMOR PROGRESSION ON IRINOTECAN

Group	N	RR	Mean Duration (mo)
Overall	25	15 (60%)	13.2 (5–35)
IHP alone	13	7 (54%)	8.6 (5–13)
IHP + HAI	12	8 (67%)	17.3 (11–35)

RR, recovery rate; IHP, isolated hepatic perfusion; HAI, hepatic artery infusion.

duration of response on multivariate analysis were increasing body mass index (assuming that low body mass index reflected high tumor burden) and tumor enhancement on the arterial phase of the CT scan (a measure of vascularity and relative tumor blood flow). The median overall survival was 61 months; the actuarial 5-year survival was 50%. Bloomston et al.[86] reported results on 122 patients with metastatic carcinoid tumor undergoing TACE. Complications were observed in 23% and periprocedural mortality was 5%. Significant palliation of symptoms was observed in over 90% of patients, with a median duration of 13 months; median overall survival was 33 months.

TACE has also been used for patients with CRC liver metastases. In contrast to NETs, most patients with metastatic CRC demonstrate a more aggressive disease progression within the liver and systemically and usually only present after progression on first- and often second-line systemic therapy. However, recent data derived from multiple phase 2 trials have shown encouraging results. For example, Salman et al.[87] demonstrated a 15-month survival following chemoembolization in patients who had failed first-line therapy. Further work is needed to clarify the role for this therapy in the treatment of CRC. A multicenter phase 3 trial investigating the use of irinotecan drug-eluting beads as a first-line therapy for stage IV CRC is currently accruing patients.

Local Ablative Therapy

Multiple techniques are currently available for percutaneous, laparoscopic, and open surgical ablation of liver metastases. These techniques generally fall under the headings of chemical ablation, thermal ablation, and, most recently, electroporation. Chemical ablation usually entails the percutaneous injection of toxic agents such as ethanol or acetic acid. Thermal ablative therapy includes radiofrequency, microwave, and cryoablation. A new entrant into the ablation field is irreversible electroporation, which causes cell death by inducing permanent cell membrane disruption.

The goal of local ablation is complete necrosis of a tumor with minimal injury to surrounding normal hepatic parenchyma. Currently its use is indicated in patients who are not surgical candidates, for those whose tumors are not amenable to resection because of distribution within the hepatic parenchyma, tumors arising in cirrhotic livers where preservation of parenchyma is imperative, small tumors straddling the interlobar plane for which an extended resection would be necessary, recurrent tumors after previous resection where further resection may be unsafe or anatomically impossible, and in combination with surgical resection to eradicate a solitary tumor deposit in the remnant liver. Limitations of local ablation therapy include its ineffectiveness in treating occult or microscopic metastases, difficulty in treating tumors greater than several centimeters in diameter, inability to treat tumors abutting major vascular structures, and difficulty in assessing the adequacy of tissue destruction during therapy. Success of treatment depends on patient selection and operator expertise in probe placement, use of appropriate treatment parameters, and adequate monitoring of the zone of tissue destruction.

Cryotherapy destroys tissue via a freeze–thaw process using a variety of cryogenic agents such as nitrous oxide, liquid nitrogen, or argon. Until recently cryoablation was by necessity performed as either a laparoscopic or open procedure as the probe sizes prohibited the percutaneous approach. However, newer argon probes have allowed the use of 11- to 17-guage probes that are amenable to percutaneous access. In addition, use of helium gas for active ice thawing has allowed for shorter freeze–thaw cycles. The probe is placed into the center of the lesion under ultrasound guidance; CT or MRI can be used for percutaneous procedures. Introduction of the cryogenic gas (or liquid) leads to cooling below −100°C. Cell death occurs during the thaw cycle. Repeated freeze–thaw cycles can improve tumor cell killing, and vascular inflow occlusion to the liver can improve the cooling rate and may allow successful freezing of larger tumors with smaller probes. Complications related to this technique include cracking of the liver parenchyma, hemorrhage, and abscesses related to biliary injuries. One advantage of this technique is that multiple probes can be used simultaneously, thus reducing procedure times.

Coagulative thermal ablation employs deposition of thermal energy into a tissue in order to achieve irreversible cellular damage. Most tissues with normal perfusion can withstand temperatures up to 45°C. However, tissues exposed to 50° to 55°C temperatures for 4 to 6 minutes will undergo irreversible damage. At temperatures in the 60° to 100°C range, there is almost immediate tissue coagulation. Above 100°C, there is near instantaneous vaporization of the cell with charring.[88] Radiofrequency ablation (RFA), the most commonly used ablation technique, uses alternating electrical current to agitate ions in adjacent tissue. This agitation generates frictional energy, which heats the tissue and extends into surrounding tissue by conduction. Current commercially available probes are designed to ablate 3 to 5 cm of tissue. Larger zones of ablation are achievable by performing overlapping ablations. A newer technique of thermal ablation, microwave ablation, uses high-frequency electromagnetic radiation to heat intracellular water molecules.[89]

Unlike RFA, which uses conduction to spread the heat throughout the ablation zone, microwaves uniformly and continuously distribute their energy throughout the ablation zone. Therefore, microwave ablations are less susceptible to heat-sink effects and produce shorter ablation times, and theoretically can produce larger ablation zones, although current commercial probes are in the 3 to 5 cm range.

RFA has become the most widely used technique for local ablation. Bilchik et al.[90] treated over 300 patients between 1992 and 1998 with cryotherapy, RFA, or a combination of the two. Although older-generation probes were used, they reported that the use of RFA was associated with less blood loss, thrombocytopenia, and shorter hospital stay compared with cryotherapy. Ablation site recurrences for tumors greater than 3 cm were higher with RFA; however, newer-generation RFA probe designs are associated with lower ablation site recurrences. Adam et al.[91] reported results in 64 patients undergoing percutaneous RFA or cryotherapy and found a higher incidence of ablation site recurrences in patients being treated with cryotherapy compared to RFA (71% vs. 19%, respectively). Curley et al.[92] treated 123 patients with RFA using either the percutaneous or open operative technique with ultrasound guidance. A total of 169 tumors ranging in size from 0.5 to 12 cm (median diameter, 3.4 cm) were ablated. Three-quarters of patients underwent open operative RFA, and there were no treatment-related deaths in the study. The authors report 3 tumor recurrences in 169 treated lesions (1.8%) at a median follow-up of 15 months. The low recurrence rate may be because many patients were treated operatively to facilitate probe placement and more reliably assess adequacy of therapy. In addition, the authors used inflow occlusion via the Pringle maneuver, which may have enhanced the effectiveness of the thermal ablation. (Table 149.10).

Kesmodel et al.[93] reported results in 51 patients with unresectable colorectal liver metastases who were treated with RFA and HAI using a floxuridine-based regimen. Despite this aggressive regional strategy, disease progression in liver was observed in over 60%. Overall median survival was 24 months, suggesting that combination therapy may be superior to HAI alone. In practice, the technologies behind the various local ablation therapies are evolving, and as smaller probe sizes are developed and techniques for monitoring adequacy of tissue destruction are refined, the advantages of one form of ablative therapy over another may become increasingly obscure.

TABLE 149.10

FACTORS WITH INDEPENDENT PROGNOSTIC SIGNIFICANCE IN COLORECTAL PATIENTS UNDERGOING ABLATIVE THERAPY OF HEPATIC METASTASES

1. Low pretreatment carcinoembryonic antigen value
2. Diameter largest lesion <3 cm
3. No extrahepatic disease
4. Node negative involvement of primary tumor
5. Metachronous (versus synchronous) liver metastases
6. Successful cryotherapy of all hepatic lesions

Adapted from ref. 101.

For decades it was realized that during experiments where electrical fields were applied to cell membranes to create reversible permeability, a large proportion of cells were permanently permeabilized. This permeability leads to large shifts in intracellular ions, which in turn lead to cell death. This phenomenon has now been adapted to create an *in vivo* ablation technology that induces cell death in a nonthermally dependent fashion. Recent animal and human studies suggest that irreversible electroporation allows effective tumor destruction while preserving underlying vascular, neural, and biliary structures.[94]

Percutaneous ethanol injections into malignant deposits in the liver have most broadly been applied to the treatment of patients with hepatocellular carcinomas. The density of tumors associated with hepatocellular carcinoma and the common occurrence of this malignancy in the setting of severe underlying hepatic disease lend themselves to this form of local therapy as opposed to surgical resection, which is often not possible in patients with severe underlying hepatic cirrhosis.[95] A more detailed presentation of its use is presented in Chapter 84.

RADIATION THERAPY FOR LIVER METASTASES

Whole-Liver Radiation Therapy

Historically, radiation therapy (RT) has played a limited role in the treatment of liver metastases. Given that the whole-liver tolerance to radiation is relatively low, clinically meaningful doses could not be delivered to liver tumors without consequent risk of liver toxicity in the form of radiation-induced liver disease. Radiation-induced liver disease has been formerly referred to in the historical literature as "radiation hepatitis," and represents the dose-limiting complication of RT treatment to the liver.[96] Radiation-induced liver disease is a clinical syndrome that consists of painful hepatomegaly anicteric ascites and elevated liver enzyme levels (particularly alkaline phosphatase, which is markedly elevated versus the typically modest increases in alanine aminotransferase, aspartate aminotransferase, and bilirubin), occurring 2 to 12 weeks after the completion of hepatic irradiation. There is no effective treatment for radiation-induced liver disease, and although it typically resolves in 1 to 2 months, 10% to 20% of patients develop overt liver failure and subsequent death.[97] The Radiation Therapy Oncology Group (RTOG) conducted a multicenter dose-escalation study of whole-liver RT in the palliation of liver metastases and found that the maximum tolerated dose was 33 Gy and conferred a median survival of only 4 months.[98] For colorectal and pancreatic cancer patients at high risk for development of liver metastases, prophylactic hepatic radiation combined with chemotherapy in cooperative group trials has resulted in increased toxicity without meaningful improvements in outcome.[99] Whole-liver RT has largely been abandoned in favor of modern techniques to treat liver metastases, such as yttrium-90 microspheres and stereotactic body radiation therapy (SBRT), which are more effective and better tolerated. Both of these modern RT techniques have arisen from a better understanding of partial liver tolerance to modern RT.

Highly Conformal Partial Liver Therapy

Investigators at the University of Michigan are largely credited for establishing modern models of liver tolerance in the context of highly conformal RT given cooperatively with chemotherapy. Based on 203 patients treated with conformal liver radiotherapy and concurrent hepatic arterial chemotherapy and followed for development of radiation-induced liver disease, Dawson et al.[100] generated a curve estimating the risk of liver disease based on volume of liver irradiated and total dose. It is now known that for a small effective liver volume irradiated, much higher and clinically effective doses of radiation can be safely delivered than previously estimated (Fig. 149.5). These data have been instrumental in laying the foundation for the recent emergence of highly conformal RT techniques for the treatment of focal liver lesions, such as SBRT and CyberKnife (Accuray, Sunnyvale, California). SBRT (also referred to as *extracranial radiosurgery*) and CyberKnife represent an emerging treatment paradigm whereby high doses of RT can be precisely delivered to a target while minimizing radiation dose to normal nearby anatomic tissues. Typically, plans are complex with multiple beam angles and/or arcs that are selected by the physician based on the region of the body being treated and the spatial relationship of the target volume to critical normal structures.

Studies of SBRT in the treatment of liver metastases have included both single-fraction and multifraction regimens[101,102]; two phase 1 studies have been reported in the past 3 years. Investigators at Heidelberg University conducted a phase 1 or 2 dose-escalation study in patients with primary and metastatic liver lesions and safely escalated single-dose treatments from 14 to 26 Gy.[103] Schefter et al.[104] conducted a phase 1 dose-escalation study of SBRT in patients with one to three liver metastases of tumor diameter less than 6 cm. All patients were treated with three fractions of RT, beginning at a total dose of 36 Gy and escalating safely to 60 Gy total. The maximum tolerated dose was not reached. The authors concluded that 60 Gy in three fractions could be delivered safely with SBRT in patients with adequate hepatic function and a minimum of 700 mL of uninvolved normal liver planned to receive less than 15 Gy total dose. In an interim analysis of the same phase 1 or 2 study, Kavanagh et al.[105] reported an 18-month actuarial local control rate of 93% for the 21 patients treated and followed for a minimum of 6 months. For institutions treating to a lower radiobiologic equivalent dose, the local control rates have not been as high, suggesting a dose–response phenomenon. Katz et al.[102] reported the outcome of 69 patients with liver metastases secondary to a variety of different primary tumors treated with SBRT to a median total dose of 48 Gy in fractionated doses of between 2 and 6 Gy dose per fraction. With a median follow-up of 14.5 months, they reported a 76% in-field local control rate at 10 months.

Highly conformal radiation treatment techniques appear promising in phase 1 or 2 single-institutional studies to date. They have been well tolerated, and when adequate doses are used, they result in excellent local control. Although the ideal fractionation schema has not yet been established, ongoing studies will help to define the optimal treatment regimen. Given

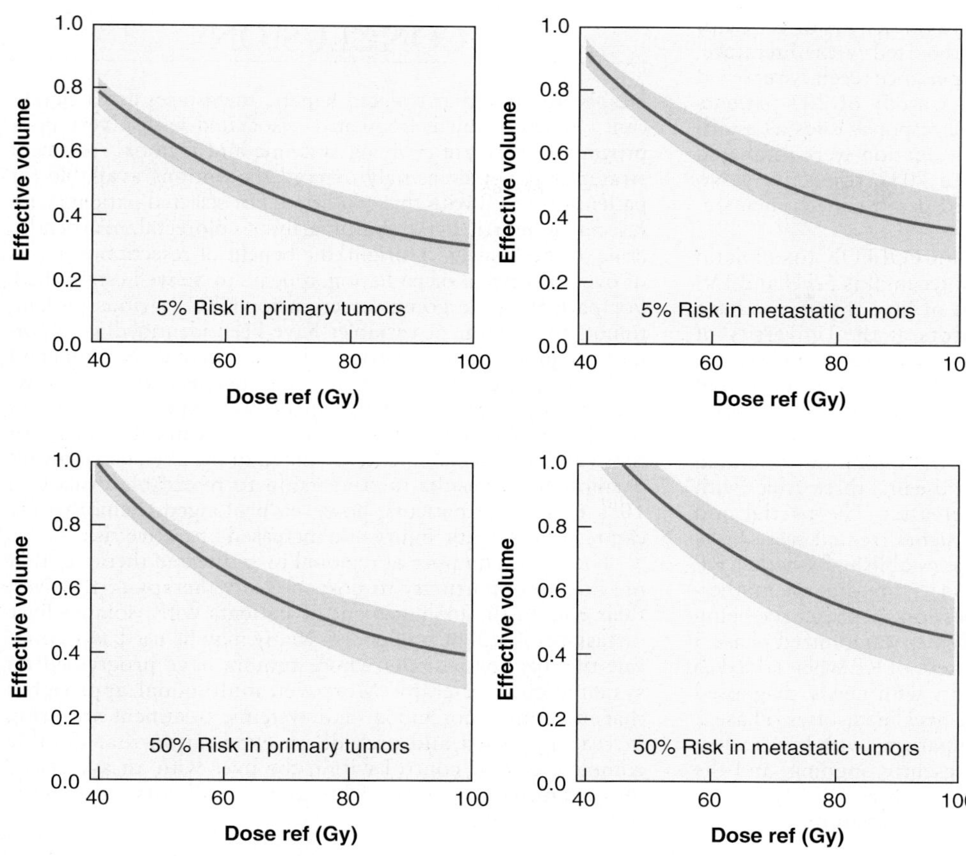

FIGURE 149.5 Partial liver tolerance to radiation therapy. The upper graphs demonstrate the dose conveying a 5% risk of liver toxicity for a given volume of liver radiated. The lower graphs demonstrate the dose conveying a 50% risk of liver toxicity for a given liver volume irradiated. (From ref. 100, with permission.)

the increasing interest in SBRT in the treatment of liver metastasis, a recent phase 1 cooperative group trial has recently been undertaken. Radiation Therapy Oncology Group 0438 is a phase 1 multicenter trial currently being conducted for patients with five or fewer liver lesions measuring 6 cm or less. Patients will be treated with two fractions of SBRT, beginning at 3.5 Gy per dose (total 35 Gy) up to 5.0 Gy per dose (total 50 Gy). As the data for SBRT and CyberKnife mature, it is likely that these therapies will compete directly with other locally ablative treatments, such as RFA for patients with a minimal number of liver lesions.

Yttrium-90 Microsphere Liver Treatment

Given the limitations and minimal benefit of historical efforts with conventional whole-liver RT, investigators have sought alternative radiotherapeutic approaches to patients with diffuse disease. Radioembolization (RE) with yttrium-90 microspheres is a novel microbrachytherapy approach to diffuse liver metastases that has been administered to more than 4,500 patients as of 2007.[106] The procedure involves the catheterization of the hepatic artery and subsequent injection of millions of radioactive embolic microspheres that contain yttrium-90, a pure β-emitter. Similar to chemoembolization, this approach takes advantage of the differential in vascular supply between the normal parenchyma of the liver and tumors within the liver. The radioactive microspheres are engineered to be several times larger than the diameter of a capillary so that they become permanently lodged in the tumor's vascular bed. The yttrium-90 particles have a half-life of 64 hours, an average energy of 0.9 MeV, and a range of 2.5 mm. This relatively short range allows for lethal doses of ionizing radiation to be delivered to the tumor by the cumulative "dose cloud" generated by the microspheres that become permanently trapped in the malignant microvasculature.[107] Because of the relatively short range of the yttrium-90 and the vascular differential, this approach minimizes the radiation exposure of the normal liver and has thus been referred to as *selective internal* RT.[108] *Ex vivo* studies of four explanted livers previously treated with yttrium-90 microspheres at the University of Maryland have helped to characterize the permanent *in vivo* distribution of radioactive microspheres.[109] Greater than 90% necrosis was noted in the pathologically examined tumor nodules in these previously treated patients, indicative of good treatment effect.

The clinical use of RE with yttrium-90 microspheres was approved in 2002 by the U.S. Food and Drug Administration for the treatment of hepatic metastases secondary to colorectal adenocarcinoma that have progressed after one chemotherapy regimen. The phase 3 clinical trial that led to U.S. Food and Drug Administration approval was reported by Gray et al.[110] and randomized 74 patients with liver-only colon cancer metastases to HAI chemotherapy administered as a 12-day infusion of floxuridine and repeated at monthly intervals versus HAI and RE with yttrium-90 microsphere treatment to the whole liver. The partial and complete response rates as measured by CT and CEA were significantly better for patients who received RE. The mean time to progression of disease in the liver increased significantly from 10.1 months to 19.2 months (P = .001), favoring the RE arm. Time to disease progression was 15.9 months in patients treated with RE versus 9.7 months for those who did not receive RE. Overall survival also favored the RE arm, with 1-, 2-, 3-, and 5-year survivals of 72%, 39%, 17%, and 3.5%, respectively, for patients receiving RE versus 68%, 29%, 6.5%, and 0% for those receiving HAC alone. Importantly, there was no significant difference in grade 3 or 4 treatment-related toxicity or quality of life for patients receiving RE in comparison to those who did not. Although most patients eventually died of disease progression, liver metastases were not the primary cause of death for most patients treated with RE.

Several large single-institutional experiences of RE with yttrium-90 microspheres have been reported in the literature, including a summarized large U.S. experience recently reported by Kennedy et al.[111] In the summary study of 203 patients treated with RE in the United States, response rates as established by CT, FDG-PET, and CEA evaluation were estimated to be approximately 40%, 90%, and 70%, respectively. No patient experienced treatment-related death or treatment-related veno-occlusive liver failure.

Phase 1 studies combining RE with FOLFOX (oxaliplatin plus 5-FU and LV) or FOLFIRI (irinotecan plus 5-FU and LV) in the first- or second-line treatment of liver metastases have recently been reported.[99] Investigators at the University of Oxford conducted a phase 1 study combining RE on cycle one (day 3) of FOLFOX4 chemotherapy in 20 previously untreated patients with liver metastases secondary to CRC. Oxaliplatin doses tested were 30, 60, and 85 mg/m^2. Dose-limiting toxicity was grade 3 or 4 neutropenia, and the maximum tolerated dose was 60 mg/m^2 of oxaliplatin for the first three cycles with full FOLFOX4 doses tolerated thereafter. The partial and complete liver response rate for patients treated were 90% and 5%, respectively. It has yet to be established whether RE improves survival when added to modern first-line chemotherapy for metastatic CRC. This question is presently being addressed by an international multicenter randomized phase 3 (SIRFLOX) trial investigating the benefit of RE when added to FOLFOX in the treatment of patients with newly diagnosed and previously untreated CRC with liver metastases. Phase 2 investigations of the benefit of RE in patients with liver metastases secondary to non-CRC are presently ongoing, and the role of RE in the treatment of liver metastases is likely to continue to expand and evolve as these studies mature.

CONCLUSIONS

Despite the fact that isolated hepatic metastases are a significant clinical problem frequently associated with a very poor prognosis, there are evolving systemic and regional treatment strategies that increasingly expand the options available for patients afflicted with this condition. For selected patients with resectable hepatic deposits primarily of colorectal, neuroendocrine, or genitourinary origin, the benefit of resection in terms of overall survival or palliation appears to be well established. For patients undergoing resection for CRC, various patient, tumor, and treatment variables have been identified as important prognostic factors associated with outcome. Neoadjuvant and adjuvant chemotherapy is being increasingly used; however, the optimal type of treatment and appropriate patient population has to be defined in additional clinical studies. For those with unresectable CRC confined to the liver, neoadjuvant chemotherapy results in conversion to resectable disease in 10% to 15% of patients; however, prolonged chemotherapy can result in hepatic injury and increased operative risk.

There are a number of regional liver-directed therapies that provide an opportunity to dose-intensify therapy to the liver; their role in the management of patients with isolated liver metastases is still being defined. Many may be used as second-line therapy for patients whose tumors have progressed on systemic chemotherapy. Moreover, multimodal approaches that integrate locoregional and systemic treatment are being increasingly used and provide an expectation that durable complete disease control within the liver with an associated improvement in quality of life and overall survival may be routinely achieved.[112,113]

Selected References

The full list of references for this chapter appears in the online version.

3. Yao KA, Talamonti MS, Nemcek A, et al. Indications and results of liver resection and hepatic chemoembolization for metastatic gastrointestinal neuroendocrine tumors. *Surgery* 2001;130:677.
8. Goldberg RM, Rothenberg ML, van Cutsem E, et al. The continuum of care: a paradigm for the management of metastatic colorectal cancer. *Oncologist* 2007;12:38.
16. Alexander HR Jr, Libutti SK, Pingpank JF, Bartlett DL, Helsabeck C, Beresneva T. Isolated hepatic perfusion for the treatment of patients with colorectal cancer liver metastases after irinotecan-based therapy. *Ann Surg Oncol* 2005;12:138.
19. Quaia E, D'Onofrio M, Palumbo A, Rossi S, Bruni S, Cova M. Comparison of contrast-enhanced ultrasonography versus baseline ultrasound and contrast-enhanced computed tomography in metastatic disease of the liver: diagnostic performance and confidence. *Eur Radiol* 2006;16:1599.
24. Wiering B, Krabbe PF, Jager GJ, Oyen WJ, Ruers TJ. The impact of fluor-18-deoxyglucose-positron emission tomography in the management of colorectal liver metastases. *Cancer* 2005;104:2658.
25. Hussain SM, Semelka RC. Hepatic imaging: comparison of modalities. *Radiol Clin North Am* 2005;43:929.
29. Jarnagin WR, Gonen M, Fong Y, et al. Improvement in perioperative outcome after hepatic resection: analysis of 1,803 consecutive cases over the past decade. *Ann Surg* 2002;236:397.
33. Vanounou T, Steel JL, Nguyen KT, et al. Comparing the clinical and economic impact of laparoscopic versus open liver resection. *Ann Surg Oncol* 2010;17:998.
35. Buell JF, Cherqui D, Geller DA, et al. The international position on laparoscopic liver surgery: The Louisville Statement, 2008. *Ann Surg* 2009;250: 825.
36. Choti MA, Sitzmann JV, Tiburi MF, et al. Trends in long-term survival following liver resection for hepatic colorectal metastases. *Ann Surg* 2002; 235:759.
37. Wei AC, Greig PD, Grant D, Taylor B, Langer B, Gallinger S. Survival after hepatic resection for colorectal metastases: a 10-year experience. *Ann Surg Oncol* 2006;13:668.
41. Antoniou A, Lovegrove RE, Tilney HS, et al. Meta-analysis of clinical outcome after first and second liver resection for colorectal metastases. *Surgery* 2007;141:9.
43. Adam R, Chiche L, Aloia T, et al. Hepatic resection for noncolorectal nonendocrine liver metastases: analysis of 1,452 patients and development of a prognostic model. *Ann Surg* 2006;244:524.
45. Reddy SK, Barbas AS, Marroquin CE, Morse MA, Kuo PC, Clary BM. Resection of noncolorectal nonneuroendocrine liver metastases: a comparative analysis. *J Am Coll Surg* 2007;204:372.
47. Kemeny NE, Gonen M. Hepatic arterial infusion after liver resection. *N Engl J Med* 2005;352:734.
50. Clancy TE, Dixon E, Perlis R, Sutherland FR, Zinner MJ. Hepatic arterial infusion after curative resection of colorectal cancer metastases: a meta-analysis of prospective clinical trials. *J Gastrointest Surg* 2005;9:198.
51. Power DG, Kemeny NE. Role of adjuvant therapy after resection of colorectal cancer liver metastases. *J Clin Oncol* 2010;28:2300.
52. Ychou M, Hohenberger W, Thezenas S, et al. A randomized phase III study comparing adjuvant 5-fluorouracil/folinic acid with FOLFIRI in patients following complete resection of liver metastases from colorectal cancer. *Ann Oncol* 2009;20:1964.
53. Mitry E, Fields AL, Bleiberg H, et al. Adjuvant chemotherapy after potentially curative resection of metastases from colorectal cancer: a pooled analysis of two randomized trials. *J Clin Oncol* 2008;26:4906.
56. Adam R, Delvart V, Pascal G, et al. Rescue surgery for unresectable colorectal liver metastases downstaged by chemotherapy: a model to predict long-term survival. *Ann Surg* 2004;240:644.
57. Adam R, Pascal G, Castaing D, et al. Tumor progression while on chemotherapy: a contraindication to liver resection for multiple colorectal metastases? *Ann Surg* 2004;240:1052.
60. Delaunoit T, Alberts SR, Sargent DJ, et al. Chemotherapy permits resection of metastatic colorectal cancer: experience from Intergroup N9741. *Ann Oncol* 2005;16:425.
61. Nordlinger B, van Cutsem E, Gruenberger T, et al. Combination of surgery and chemotherapy and the role of targeted agents in the treatment of patients with colorectal liver metastases: recommendations from an expert panel. *Ann Oncol.* 2009;20:985.
62. Kemeny NE, Melendez FD, Capanu M, et al. Conversion to resectability using hepatic artery infusion plus systemic chemotherapy for the treatment of unresectable liver metastases from colorectal carcinoma. *J Clin Oncol* 2009;27:3465.
63. Nordlinger B, Sorbye H, Glimelius B, et al. Perioperative chemotherapy with FOLFOX4 and surgery versus surgery alone for resectable liver

metastases from colorectal cancer (EORTC Intergroup trial 40983): a randomised controlled trial. *Lancet* 2008;371:1007.

64. Vauthey JN, Pawlik TM, Ribero D, et al. Chemotherapy regimen predicts steatohepatitis and an increase in 90-day mortality after surgery for hepatic colorectal metastases. *J Clin Oncol* 2006;24:2065.
65. Aloia T, Sebagh M, Plasse M, et al. Liver histology and surgical outcomes after preoperative chemotherapy with fluorouracil plus oxaliplatin in colorectal cancer liver metastases. *J Clin Oncol* 2006;24:4983.
67. Karoui M, Penna C, min-Hashem M, et al. Influence of preoperative chemotherapy on the risk of major hepatectomy for colorectal liver metastases. *Ann Surg* 2006;243:1.
68. Benoist S, Brouquet A, Penna C, et al. Complete response of colorectal liver metastases after chemotherapy: does it mean cure? *J Clin Oncol* 2006;24:3939.
69. Callahan MK, Kemeny NE. Implanted hepatic arterial infusion pumps. *Cancer J* 2010;16:142.
72. Kemeny NE, Niedzwiecki D, Hollis DR, et al. Hepatic arterial infusion versus systemic therapy for hepatic metastases from colorectal cancer: a randomized trial of efficacy, quality of life, and molecular markers (CALGB 9481). *J Clin Oncol* 2006;24:1395.
74. Ducreux M, Ychou M, LaPlanche A, et al. Hepatic arterial oxaliplatin infusion plus intravenous chemotherapy in colorectal cancer with inoperable hepatic metastases: a trial of the gastrointestinal group of the Federation Nationale des Centres de Lutte Contre le Cancer. *J Clin Oncol* 2005;23:4881.
77. Leyvraz S, Spataro V, Bauer J, et al. Treatment of ocular melanoma metastatic to the liver by hepatic arterial chemotherapy. *J Clin Oncol* 1997;15:2589.
79. Pingpank JF, Libutti SK, Chang R A, et al. A phase I study of hepatic arterial melphalan infusion with hepatic venous hemofiltration using percutaneously placed catheters in patients with unresectable hepatic malignancies. *J Clin Oncol* 2005;23:3465.
83. Alexander HR, Bartlett DL, Libutti SK, Fraker DL, Moser T, Rosenberg SA. Isolated hepatic perfusion with tumor necrosis factor and melphalan for unresectable cancers confined to the liver. *J Clin Oncol* 1998;16:1479.
86. Bloomston M, Al-Saif O, Klemanski D, et al. Hepatic artery chemoembolization in 122 patients with metastatic carcinoid tumor: lessons learned. *J Gastrointest Surg* 2007;11:264.
87. Salman HS, Cynamon J, Jagust M, et al. Randomized phase II trial of embolization therapy versus chemoembolization therapy in previously treated patients with colorectal carcinoma metastatic to the liver. *Clin Colorectal Cancer* 2002;2:173.
92. Curley SA, Izzo F, Delrio P, et al. Radiofrequency ablation of unresectable primary and metastatic hepatic malignancies: results in 123 patients. *Ann Surg* 1999;230:9.
94. Bertacchini C, Margotti PM, Bergamini E, Lodi A, Ronchetti M, Cadossi R. Design of an irreversible electroporation system for clinical use. *Technol Cancer Res Treat* 2007;6:313.
102. Katz AW, Carey-Sampson M, Muhs AG, Milano MT, Schell MC, Okunieff P. Hypofractionated stereotactic body radiation therapy (SBRT) for limited hepatic metastases. *Int J Radiat Oncol Biol Physics* 2007;67:793.
103. Herfarth KK, Debus J, Wannenmacher M. Stereotactic radiation therapy of liver metastases: update of the initial phase-I/II trial. *Front Radiat Ther Oncol* 2004;38:100.
105. Kavanagh BD, Schefter TE, Cardenes HR, et al. Interim analysis of a prospective phase I/II trial of SBRT for liver metastases. *Acta Oncol* 2006;45:848.
111. Kennedy AS, Coldwell D, Nutting C, et al. Resin 90Y-microsphere brachytherapy for unresectable colorectal liver metastases: modern USA experience. *Int J Radiat Oncol Biol Physics* 2006;65:412.
114. Kemeny N, Huang Y, Cohen AM, et al. Hepatic arterial infusion of chemotherapy after resection of hepatic metastases from colorectal cancer. *N Engl J Med* 1999;341:2039.
116. Folprecht G, Gruenberger T, Bechstein WO, et al. Tumour response and secondary resectability of colorectal liver metastases following neoadjuvant chemotherapy with cetuximab: the CELIM randomised phase 2 trial. *Lancet Oncol* 2010;11:38.
117. Skof E, Rebersek M, Hlebanja Z, Ocvirk J. Capecitabine plus irinotecan (XELIRI regimen) compared to 5-FU/LV plus irinotecan (FOLFIRI regimen) as neoadjuvant treatment for patients with unresectable liver-only metastases of metastatic colorectal cancer: a randomised prospective phase II trial. *BMC Cancer* 2009;9:120.
118. Ducreux M, Raoul JL, Marti P, et al. High-dose irinotecan plus LV5FU2 or simplified LV5FU (HD-FOLFIRI) for patients with untreated metastatic colorectal cancer: a new way to allow resection of liver metastases? *Oncology* 2008;74:17.
119. Min BS, Kim NK, Ahn JB, et al. Cetuximab in combination with 5-fluorouracil, leucovorin and irinotecan as a neoadjuvant chemotherapy in patients with initially unresectable colorectal liver metastases. *Onkologi* 2007;30:637.
120. Barone C, Nuzzo G, Cassano A, et al. Final analysis of colorectal cancer patients treated with irinotecan and 5-fluorouracil plus folinic acid neoadjuvant chemotherapy for unresectable liver metastases. *Br J Cancer* 2007;97:1035.
121. Alberts SR, Horvath WL, Sternfeld WC, et al. Oxaliplatin, fluorouracil, and leucovorin for patients with unresectable liver-only metastases from colorectal cancer: a North Central Cancer Treatment Group phase II study. *J Clin Oncol* 2005;23:9243.

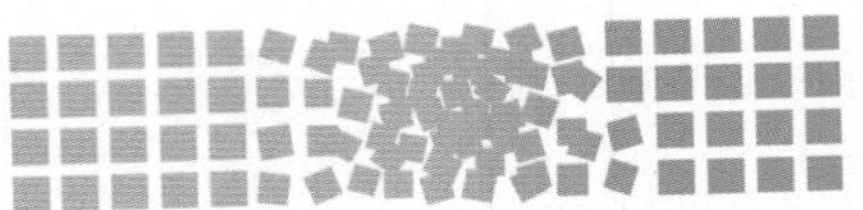

CHAPTER 150 METASTATIC CANCER TO THE BONE

EDWARD CHOW, JOEL A. FINKELSTEIN, ARJUN SAHGAL, AND ROBERT E. COLEMAN

Bone metastases are most frequent in breast and prostate carcinomas, and affect two-thirds to three-quarters of patients with advanced disease from these tumors. In addition, lung, thyroid, and renal carcinoma metastasize to bone in approximately 30% to 40% of cases.[1]

Survival prospects after metastases to bone vary greatly depending on tumor type and sites of involvement. Mean survival ranges from a low of 6 months for those with lung carcinoma, to several years for those with bone metastases from prostate, thyroid, or breast carcinoma.[1] If patients have skeletal metastases only, their average survival is even longer. With prolongation in survival, the main challenge is to improve the quality of the patient's remaining life.

PRESENTATION

The morbidity associated with metastatic bone disease, often referred to as skeletal-related events or SREs, includes pain that may require opiates, the need for radiotherapy and/or surgery, hypercalcemia, pathologic fractures, and spinal cord compression.

The most common symptom is pain. Pain initially may be either a well-localized focus of pain or a diffuse ache, typically worse at night and often not relieved by lying flat. Pain from extremity lesions tends to be well defined, in contrast to spine and pelvic sites, which produce vague, diffuse symptoms. Eventually the pain worsens with weight-bearing activity. Initially, pain results from the physical presence of tumor in the bone, with the release of inflammatory mediators, neuropeptides, and cytokines, as well as elevation of the intraosseous pressure from tumor mass effect, and causes irritation of intraosseous and periosteal nerve endings.[2] Functional pain is caused by the mechanical weakness of the bone, which can no longer support the normal stresses of daily activities. Mechanical pain is more typically associated with the focal bone loss within lytic lesions; however, radiographically blastic lesions may also weaken the bone through associated areas of osteolysis that are sufficient to compromise structural integrity. The development of functional pain may be a marker for bone at risk for fracture.

Pathologic fractures may be the first sign of metastatic bone disease. In breast carcinoma, as many as 35% of patients with bone disease experience a fracture.[3] Breast, lung, renal, and thyroid cancers have been the most common cancers with pathologic fracture, but even in endocrine-resistant prostate cancer where osteoblastic metastases are typical, annual fracture rates in excess of 20% may be seen.[1]

PATHOPHYSIOLOGY

Historically, Batson[1] described the high-flow, low-pressure, valveless plexus of veins that connects the visceral organs to the spine and pelvis. Recent research has focused on the multistep cellular process of metastases. First the cancer cell must disengage from its primary site. The loss of expression of E-cadherin, a cell-surface adhesion molecule, has been demonstrated in breast, prostate, colorectal, and pancreatic carcinoma as an early step in cellular disengagement. After invasion of the vascular or lymphatic system, the cancer cell must survive the immune system and then arrest at its final destination. At the distant site, the malignant cell must adhere to the basement membrane, invade the surrounding tissue, induce angiogenesis, and develop into a secondary mass.

However, in addition to these generic steps involved in metastases, tumor cells in the bone marrow require interaction with normal bone cells to establish a metastatic lesion in bone. The growth factor and cytokine expression of the tumor cells leads to an interaction with osteoclasts and osteoblasts, the balance of which determines the nature of the lesion and its corresponding radiographic appearance. Osteoclastic activity has been shown to be increased by tumor expression of interleukins 6 and 11 PTHrP (parathyroid hormone-related protein).[4] Bone resorption leads to the release of bone-derived growth factors, notable transforming growth factor beta (TGF-β) that in turn may react with receptors on the tumor cells. This sets up the so-called vicious cycle whereby the stimulation of bone cell activity produces a favorable microenvironment for the neighboring tumor cells and facilitates the metastatic process. The new bone formation associated with osteoblastic lesions has been associated with endothelin-1 and insulinlike growth factor stimulation of osteoblasts, but typically even in osteoblastic lesions there is also an associated increase in osteoclastic bone resorption.[5]

DIAGNOSTIC EVALUATION

In patients who are suspected of having metastatic disease because of pain to the spine or extremity with or without a known primary, radiographs and bone scanning are the first line of imaging. These are used to document the presence or absence of an osseous lesion, and to identify whether these are solitary or multiple lesions. In the spine, plain films classically show absence of a pedicle with the "winking owl sign" (Fig. 150.1).

A computed tomography (CT) scan is the best modality to define the size of an osseous lesion and to evaluate the extent of cortical involvement. In the spine, CT scanning is most useful to evaluate aspects of bony stability as measured by pedicle and/or posterior body wall integrity. These factors are important in establishing risk of burst fracture and for planning and assessing the safety of vertebroplasty as a treatment alternative.[6] CT-guided biopsy can be used for obtaining tissue samples.

Magnetic resonance imaging (MRI) is valuable for evaluating marrow disease and is most sensitive in identifying metastatic deposits in the spine and pelvis. In patients with

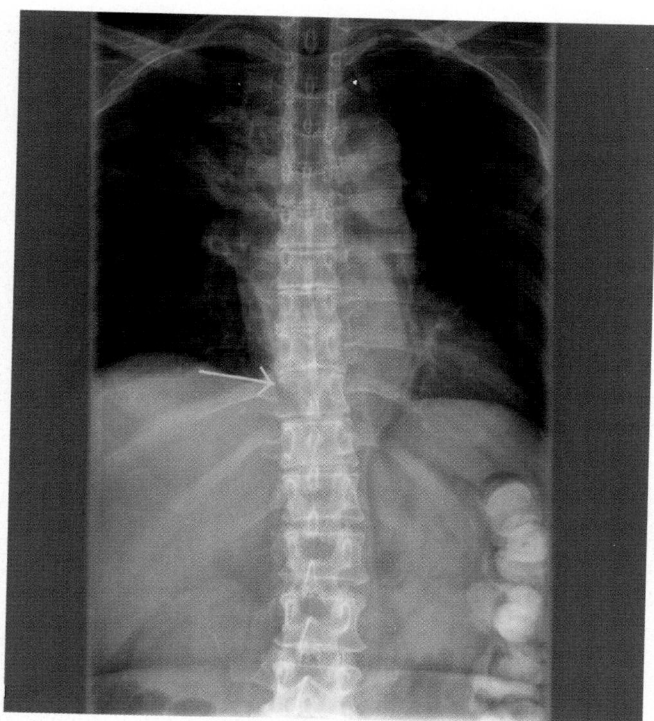

FIGURE 150.1 Anteroposterior radiograph of thoracolumbar spine. Right-sided T10 pedicle is absent giving appearance of a winking owl.

neurologic compromise, MRI is best for assessing epidural disease and extent of vertebral involvement (solitary vs. multifocal).

Positron emission tomography uses radioactive [^{18}F] fluorodeoxyglucose as a tracer to highlight metabolically active cells. This nonspecific study can be used to locate an unknown primary or to evaluate for multiple sites of metastatic disease. It is currently only an investigational tool for most cancers.

THERAPEUTIC MODALITIES

Optimal management requires a multidisciplinary team. Medical treatment, radiation therapy, surgery, and bone-targeted treatment with the bisphosphonates are combined depending on the biology of the disease, extent of the skeletal involvement, and the life expectancy of the patient.

Systemic Therapy

Systemic therapy for bone metastases can be targeted against the tumor cell itself to reduce tumor burden or, alternatively, directed toward blocking the effect of tumor-derived growth factors and cytokines on host cells. Chemotherapy, biologically targeted agents, and endocrine treatments have direct antitumor effects, whereas agents such as the bisphosphonates and denosumab are effective by preventing host cells (primarily osteoclasts) from reacting to tumor products. Systemic therapy, therefore, has either direct or indirect actions.

In general, the choice of systemic treatment for metastatic bone disease is based on the same criteria as those used for other metastatic manifestations of the malignancy.[7] Treatment must therefore be discussed according to tumor type. For a fuller discussion of systemic cancer management, the relevant site-specific chapters should be consulted.

For breast cancer, endocrine therapy is the treatment of choice for the initial treatment of metastatic disease unless the disease is known to be estrogen receptor-negative or there is extensive and/or aggressive visceral disease. Objectively responding patients usually gain relief of symptoms (including bone pain) and might become able to resume their previous activities. Although in general the median duration of response to endocrine therapy is around 15 months, prolonged responses to first-line hormone treatments lasting several years are not uncommon in patients with bone metastases.

There have been many recent developments in cytotoxic and biological treatments of relevance to the patient with metastatic bone disease from breast cancer. Response in bone to chemotherapy is nearly always only partial, with a median duration of response of 9 to 12 months. The precise choice of drugs and schedule of administration to obtain the best results will vary from one patient or clinical problem to another. Chemotherapy can be especially hazardous for patients with extensive bone disease, because of both poor bone marrow tolerance after replacement of functioning marrow by tumor and the effects of previous irradiation. Primary prophylaxis with hematopoietic growth factors may be required to enable chemotherapy to be administered safely.

In prostate cancer at least 80% of prostate tumors exhibit some degree of hormone responsiveness with a median duration of response of around 2 years. Patients with advanced prostate cancer tend to be elderly and often of poor performance status. Thus, their tolerance of chemotherapy regimens may be poor. Recently, docetaxel has been shown to improve survival in endocrine-resistant disease, and cautious use of this agent may be appropriate.

Skeletal morbidity is a major problem in multiple myeloma despite a high rate of response to chemotherapy. Despite the subjective improvement that is seen, bone healing is rare, with lytic lesions persisting despite control of the disease for months or years. Newer agents provide many more options and have transformed the clinical course of multiple myeloma in recent years into that of a chronic disease. Bone involvement in germ cell tumors and lymphoma conveys a worse prognosis, but despite this, cure with chemotherapy is frequent. For relatively chemotherapy-resistant solid tumors such as non–small cell lung cancer or melanoma the benefits of current chemotherapy regimens are limited and patients with skeletal metastases from these tumors derive most benefit from local radiotherapy and bisphosphonates. More effective treatments are emerging, notably the angiogenesis inhibitors in renal cell cancer and small molecules and antibodies are being developed at a rapid pace across a range of tumors.

Bisphosphonates for Metastatic Bone Disease

Over the past 10 years the bisphosphonates have become established as a valuable additional approach to the range of current treatments. Bisphosphonates are analogues of pyrophosphate, characterized by a P-C-P–containing central structure that binds to bone, and a variable side chain that determines the relative potency, side effects, and the precise mechanism of action.[8] After administration, bisphosphonates bind avidly to exposed bone mineral, and during bone resorption, bisphosphonates are internalized by the osteoclast and subsequently cause apoptotic cell death.

After intravenous administration of a bisphosphonate, approximately 25% to 40% of the injected dose is excreted by the kidney, and the remainder is taken up by bone where it is retained for months or even years. All bisphosphonates suffer from poor bioavailability when given by mouth and must be taken on an empty stomach, as they bind to calcium in the diet.

As indicated previously, it is now generally accepted that osteoclast activation is the key step in the establishment and growth of bone metastases. Biochemical data indicate that bone resorption is of importance not only in classic "lytic" diseases such as myeloma and breast cancer but also in prostate cancer.[5] As a result, the osteoclast is a key therapeutic target for skeletal metastases irrespective of the tissue of origin.

Although radiotherapy is the treatment of choice for localized bone pain, the bisphosphonates provide an additional treatment approach for the relief of bone pain across a range of tumor types. Additionally, the bisphosphonates have become the standard of care for the treatment and prevention of skeletal complications associated with bone metastases in patients with breast cancer and multiple myeloma. More recently, they have also demonstrated benefits in patients with bone metastases secondary to other cancers including prostate cancer, lung cancer, and other solid tumors.[9]

Oral Bisphosphonates

The absorption of bisphosphonates from the gut is poor, variable, and dramatically inhibited by food intake. Nevertheless, oral clodronate has been shown in randomized trials to have some clinical efficacy in breast cancer and multiple myeloma, while oral ibandronate is of value in advanced breast cancer.[9,10]

Intravenous Bisphosphonates

There is extensive experience with intravenous bisphosphonates in breast cancer with zoledronic acid, pamidronate, and ibandronate all showing useful clinical activity.[10] However, a double-blind randomized trial of 1,130 patients with advanced breast cancer showed a significant advantage to zoledronic acid with an additional 20% reduction in the risk of a skeletal-related events (SREs) over pamidronate ($P = .025$).[11] Ibandronate is licensed in Europe for the treatment of metastatic bone following a placebo-controlled trial of monthly infusions that showed a significant reduction in skeletal-related morbidity.[12] Additionally, improvements in pain and quality of life were demonstrated. However, the clinical value of intravenous ibandronate is unclear pending comparative trials with established bisphosphonates.

Intravenous bisphosphonates have become routine clinical management for most patients with multiple myeloma. Both zoledronic acid[11] and pamidronate,[13] but not ibandronate, have shown comparable efficacy with the choice of preferred agent depending largely on cost and convenience.

In advanced castrate-resistant prostate cancer, zoledronic acid was shown to reduce the overall risk of skeletal complications by 36%.[14] Additionally, zoledronic acid significantly reduced the risk for SRE(s) by about 30% ($P = .003$) in the management of bone metastases from solid tumors other than breast or prostate cancer.[15] However, to date other bisphosphonates have not shown clear evidence of benefit in either of these disease settings.

Optimum Use of Bisphosphonates in Metastatic Bone Disease

Despite the obvious clinical benefits of bisphosphonates, it is clear that only a proportion of events is prevented, and some patients do not experience a skeletal event despite the presence of metastatic bone disease. It is currently impossible to predict whether an individual patient needs or will benefit from a bisphosphonate. Criteria are needed as to when in the course of metastatic bone disease bisphosphonates should be started and stopped. Because of the logistics and cost of delivering monthly intravenous infusions for all patients with metastatic bone disease, certain empiric recommendations on who should receive treatment are needed. These should take into account the underlying disease type and extent, the life expectancy of the patient, the probability of the patient experiencing an SRE, and the ease with which the patient can attend for treatment (or be treated by a domiciliary service).

Consensus guidance recommendations indicate that all patients with multiple myeloma and radiologically confirmed bone metastases from breast cancer should receive bisphosphonates from the time of diagnosis and continue indefinitely.[16,17] The development of an SRE is not a sign of treatment failure or a signal to stop treatment; evidence is now available to confirm that bisphosphonates delay second and subsequent complications, not just the first event. However, there is evidence that switching to a more potent agent like zoledronic acid may be an appropriate option in patients in whom pamidronate or clodronate therapy prove unsatisfactory.[18]

Bisphosphonate treatment—specifically zoledronic acid—is also appropriate for patients with endocrine-resistant metastatic bone disease from prostate cancer. Patients with other tumors and symptomatic metastasis to bone should be considered for treatment with zoledronic acid if bone is the dominant site of metastasis, especially if the prognosis is reasonable (>6 months). Patients with renal cell cancer particularly appear to benefit from treatment.[11]

Bone resorption markers such as N-telopeptide of type 1 collagen (Ntx) may be useful to identify patients at high risk of skeletal complications.[5] Additionally, normalization of bone resorption is associated with improved clinical outcomes including fewer SREs and prolonged survival.[19] Thus, a more cost-effective use of bisphosphonates, particularly in patients with additional extensive visceral metastases or solid tumors associated with a short life expectancy, might be to reserve them until patients have raised Ntx levels, and to adjust the dose and schedule to maintain a normal rate of bone resorption. Randomized trials to assess this approach are planned.

NEW TARGETED THERAPIES IN THE TREATMENT OF METASTATIC BONE DISEASE

As our understanding of the signaling mechanisms between bone cells and tumor cells increases, a number of targeted agents have entered clinical development. These include inhibition of RANKL, cathepsin K, an osteoclast-derived enzyme that is essential for the resorption of bone, PTHrP, and Src kinase, a key molecule in osteoclastogenesis. Of all these, inhibition of RANKL currently shows the most promise.

Denosumab is a fully human monoclonal antibody that binds and neutralizes RANKL with high affinity and specificity,[20] thereby inhibiting osteoclast function and bone resorption. Denosumab could potentially be used to treat bone loss caused by bone metastases, multiple myeloma, or osteoporosis. Following a single subcutaneous dose, denosumab caused rapid and sustained suppression of bone turnover in multiple myeloma and breast cancer patients.[21] A subsequent dose-finding phase 2 study has defined a dose and schedule for phase 3 development of 120 mg given 4 weekly.

The results of a broad development program in metastatic disease have recently been reported. These indicate superiority over zoledronic acid in the time to first SRE in trials encompassing a broad range of solid tumors. The hazard rates for first SRE were 0.82 (95% confidence interval [CI]: 0.71–0.95),[22] 0.82

(95% CI: 0.71–0.95),[23] and 0.84 (95% CI: 0.71–0.98),[24] in the trials performed in breast cancer, castrate-resistant prostate cancer, and other solid tumors and myeloma patient groups, respectively. Denosumab has also been shown to prevent treatment-induced bone loss and reduce fragility fractures related to the use of androgen-deprivation therapy in prostate cancer.[25]

EXTERNAL-BEAM RADIATION THERAPY

About half of cancer patients will receive palliative radiation therapy during the course of their illness. Palliation of bone metastases comprises a significant workload in radiation oncology. Radiotherapy is effective in relieving bone pain, preventing impending fractures, and promoting healing in pathologic fractures. Hematologic or gastrointestinal side effects are usually mild and transient.

Numerous randomized trials have been conducted on dose-fractionation schedules of palliative radiotherapy. Despite that, there is still no uniform consensus on the optimal dose fractionation scheme. One of the first randomized studies on bone metastases was conducted by Radiation Therapy Oncology Group (RTOG 74-02).[26] Ninety percent of patients experienced some relief of pain and 54% achieved eventual complete pain relief. The trial concluded that the low-dose, short-course schedules were as effective as the high-dose protracted programs. However, this study was criticized for using physician-based pain assessment. A reanalysis of the same set of data, grouping solitary and multiple bone metastases, using the end point of pain relief and taking into account of analgesic intake and retreatment, concluded that the number of radiation fractions was statistically significant related to complete combined relief (absence of pain and use of narcotics). The conclusion was that protracted dose-fractionation schedules were more effective than short-course schedules.[27] This reanalysis was contrary to the initial report, highlighting the choice of end points are very important in defining the outcomes of clinical trials.[28]

Several large-scale prospective randomized trials were subsequently performed. The United Kingdom Bone Pain Trial Working Party randomized 765 patients with bone metastases to either an 8-Gy single fraction or a multifraction regimen (20 Gy per five fractions or 30 Gy per ten fractions).[29] There were no differences in the time to first improvement in pain, time to complete pain relief, or in time to first increase in pain at any time up to 12 months from randomization. Retreatment was twice as common after 8 Gy than after multifraction radiotherapy. There were no significant differences in the incidence of nausea, vomiting, spinal cord compression, or pathologic fracture between the two groups. The study concluded that a single fraction of 8 Gy is as safe and effective as a multifraction regimen for the palliation of metastatic bone pain for at least 12 months. The greater convenience and lower cost make 8-Gy single fraction the treatment of choice.

The Dutch Bone Metastases Study included 1,171 patients and found no difference in pain relief or the quality of life following a single 8-Gy or 24-Gy in six daily radiation treatments.[30] However, the retreatment rates were 25% in the single 8-Gy arm and 7% in the multiple-treatment arm, respectively. More pathologic fractures were observed in the single-fraction group, but the absolute percentage was low. In their cost-utility analysis of this randomized trial, there was no difference in life expectancy or quality-adjusted life expectancy. The estimated cost of radiotherapy, including retreatments and nonmedical costs, was statistically significantly lower for the single-fraction schedule than for the multiple-fraction schedule.[31]

One critical review included a systematic search for randomized trials of localized radiotherapy of bone metastases employing different dose fractionations.[32] The primary outcomes of interest were complete and overall pain relief. The authors suggested that protracted fractionated radiotherapy, given over 2 to 4 weeks, results in more complete and durable pain relief.

However, two earlier meta-analyses showed no significant difference in complete and overall pain relief between single fraction and multifraction palliative radiotherapy for bone metastases.[33,34] The meta-analysis reported that the complete response rates (absence of pain) were 33.4% and 32.3% after single fraction and multifraction radiation treatments, respectively, while the overall response rates were 62.1% and 58.7%, respectively. The latter became 72.7% and 72.5%, respectively, when the analysis was restricted to evaluated patients alone. Most patients will experience pain relief in the first 2 to 4 weeks after radiotherapy, be it single or multiple fractionations.[33] However, the retreatment and pathologic fracture rates were higher in single-fraction treatments.[34] Nevertheless, considerable controversy over the optimal treatment fractions still persists. There is reluctance among radiation oncologists worldwide to adopt single fraction as standard practice, even though it offers greater patient convenience and cost-effectiveness.

Since the publication of the two meta-analyses, seven more randomized trials on bone metastases have been reported. The Radiation Therapy Oncology Group (RTOG) repeated the randomized study in patients with breast or prostate cancer who had one to three sites of painful bone metastases and moderate to severe pain with patient self-assessment.[35] There were 455 patients in the single 8-Gy arm and 443 in the 30-Gy in ten fractions arm. Grade 2–4 acute toxicity was more frequent in the multiple arms (17%) than in the single arm (10%) ($P = .002$). Late toxicity was rare (4%) in both arms. The overall response rate was 66%. Complete and partial response rates were 15% and 50%, respectively, in the single-fraction arm compared with 18% and 48% in the multiple fractions arm ($P = .6$). Both regimens were equivalent in terms of pain and narcotic relief at 3 months. The single-fraction arm had a higher rate of retreatment (18% vs. 9%; $P < .001$).

Four Norwegian and six Swedish hospitals planned to recruit 1,000 patients with painful bone metastases. Patients were randomized to single 8 Gy or 30 Gy in ten fractions.[36] The data monitoring committee recommended closure of the study after 376 patients had been recruited because interim analyses indicated that, as in other recently published trials, the treatment groups had similar outcomes. Similar pain relief within the first 4 months was experienced in both groups and this was maintained throughout the 28-week follow-up. No differences were found for fatigue, global quality of life, and survival in both groups.

An updated meta-analysis reporting 16 randomized trials totaling 2,513 and 2,487 randomizations in single-fraction and multiple-fraction arms revealed the overall and complete response rates were 58% and 23%, respectively, in single-fraction arm versus 59% and 24% in multiple-fraction arms, again demonstrating equal efficacy.[37]

However, there is some evidence that certain groups of patients would benefit from a protracted schedule. Roos et al.[38] compared a single 8 Gy versus 20 Gy in five fractions for 272 patients with bone metastases causing pain with a neuropathic component (Trans-Tasman Radiation Oncology Group, TROG 96.05). They concluded that a single dose was not as effective as multiple fractions for the treatment of neuropathic pain; however, it was also not significantly worse. They recommended that 20 Gy in five fractions be used as standard radiotherapy for patients with neuropathic pain. However, in patients with short survival, poor performance status, where the cost/inconvenience of multiple treatments was a factor and in treatment centers with lengthy wait times, single fractions could be used instead.[38]

How, then, are radiation oncologists to prescribe treatment? The answer most likely resides within the clinical circumstances and individual wishes of each patient. There is no doubt that in patients with short life expectancy, protracted schedules are a burden. However, in patients with a longer expected survival, such as breast and prostate cancer patients with bone metastases only, other parameters need to be taken into account. Since retreatment rates are known to be higher following a single versus multiple fractions, about 25% versus 10%, respectively, patients with good performance status may wish to share in the decision-making process.

What should be an optimal dose for single fraction treatment then? A prospective randomized trial on 270 patients with painful bone metastases compared 4 Gy or 8 Gy single doses in its efficacy.[39] At 4 weeks, the actual response rates were 69% for 8 Gy and 44% for 4 Gy ($P < .001$), but there was no difference in complete response rates at 4 weeks or duration of response between the two arms. It is concluded that 8 Gy gives a higher probability of pain relief than 4 Gy, but that 4 Gy can be an effective alternative in situations of reduced tolerance. Another randomized trial of three single-dose radiation therapy regimens in the treatment of metastatic bone pain consisted of single 4 Gy, 6 Gy, or 8 Gy.[40] The authors confirmed that 8 Gy could be considered as probably "lowest" optimal single-fraction radiation treatment for painful bone metastases, although single fraction 4 Gy should not be easily discarded because of its applicability in specific cases. In their study, single 6 Gy achieved results not different from that obtained with 8 Gy, and they recommend further studies to define the "lowest" optimal single-fraction radiation in the treatment of painful bone metastases.

Wide-Field or Half-Body External-Beam Radiation

Wide-field or half-body irradiation (HBI) differs from localized external-beam radiation mainly in the volume of tissues and bone metastases covered as a single treatment field. It is more useful for patients with multiple painful bone metastases. HBI is usually delivered either to the upper half or to the lower half of the body.

Single-fraction HBI has been shown in retrospective and prospective phase 1 and 2 studies to provide pain relief in 70% to 80% of patients.[41,42] Pain relief is apparent within 24 to 48 hours, suggesting that cells of the inflammatory response pathway may be the initial target tissue, as tumor cell activities are unlikely to be halted so quickly. Toxicities include minor bone marrow suppression and gastrointestinal side effects such as nausea and vomiting in upper-abdominal radiation and may be controlled with Ondansetron or dexamethasone.

Pulmonary toxicity is minimal provided the lung dose is limited to 6 Gy.[43] Fractionated HBI was investigated in a randomized phase 2 study involving 29 patients, comparing a single fraction with fractionated HBI (25 to 30 Gy in a nine to ten fractions). Pain relief was achieved in over 94% of patients. At 1 year, 70% in the fractionated and 15% in the single-fraction group had pain control, and repeat radiation was required in 71% and 13% for the single and fractionated group.[44] Poulter et al.[45] reported results of a randomized trial of 499 patients comparing local radiation alone versus local radiation plus a single fraction of HBI. The study documented a lower incidence of new bone metastases (50% vs. 68%) and fewer patients requiring further local radiotherapy at 1 year after HBI (60% vs. 76%).

The choice of dose-fractionation schedule for HBI was explored by Salazar et al.[46] among 156 randomized patients from six countries. Among the three trial arms of 15 Gy in five fractions over 5 days, 8 Gy in two fractions over 1 one day, and 12 Gy in four fractions over 2 days, the 15 Gy/five fractions/5 days regimen not only provided pain relief as much as the other regimens, but also a longer survival duration in prostate cancer patients.

Reirradiation

As effective systemic treatment and better supportive care result in improved survival, certain subsets of patients with bone metastases have longer life expectancies than before. An increasing number of patients outlive the duration of the benefits of initial palliative radiotherapy for symptomatic bone metastases, requiring reirradiation of the previously treated sites. Additionally, some patients fail to respond initially but may benefit from reirradiation.

Among the radiation trials comparing single versus multiple fractionation schemes, reirradiation rates varied from 11% to 42% following single-fraction and 0% to 24% following multiple-fraction schedules. There are at least three scenarios of "failure" where reirradiation may be considered. Response to reirradiation may be different for each of these scenarios:

1. No pain relief or pain progression after initial radiotherapy,
2. Partial response with initial radiotherapy and the hope to achieve further pain reduction with more radiotherapy, and
3. Partial or complete response with initial radiotherapy but subsequent recurrence of pain.

Mithal et al.[47] reported a retrospective analysis of 105 patients treated with palliative radiotherapy for painful bone metastases. A total of 280 individual treatment sites were identified, of which 57 were retreated once and 8 were retreated twice. The overall response rate to initial treatment was 84% for pain relief, and at first retreatment this was 87%. Seven of the eight (88%) patients retreated a second time also achieved pain relief. A total of 17 of 23 (74%) patients responded to second radiation that used a number of single-fraction regimens, which was not significantly inferior to 31 of 34 (91%) obtained with more protracted regimens. No relation to radiation dose, primary tumor type, or site was seen.

Jeremic et al.[48] investigated the effectiveness of a single fraction of 4 Gy given for retreatment of bone metastasis after previous single-fraction radiotherapy. Of 135 patients retreated, 109 patients were retreated because of pain relapsing while 26 patients were reirradiated after initial nonresponse. Of the 109 patients who were reirradiated for pain relapse, 80 (74%) patients responded (complete response = 31%; partial response = 42%). Among the 26 patients who did not respond initially, there were 12 (46%) responses. The authors concluded that the lack of response to initial single-fraction radiotherapy should not deter repeat irradiation. Toxicity in their series was low and gastrointestinal only. Grade 1 or 2 diarrhea (RTOG acute toxicity criteria) was observed in 25 of 135 (19%) patients. No acute toxicity grade 3 or higher was reported. Pathologic fractures were reported in 3 of 135 (2%) patients and spinal cord compression in 3 of 135 (2%) patients in their series.

The same group recently reported the efficacy of the second single 4 Gy reirradiation for painful bone metastases following the previous two single fractions. The overall response rate of the 25 patients (19 responders and 6 nonresponders to the two prior single fractions) was 80%, with both complete response and partial response being 40%. No acute or late high-grade toxicity (≥ 3) was observed in their study. No pathologic fractures or spinal cord compression were seen in any of these patients during the follow-up.[49]

The Dutch Bone Metastases Study Group presented the efficacy of reirradiation of painful bone metastases.[50] For patients not responding to the initial radiation who were reirradiated, 66% of patients who initially received a single 8-Gy fraction responded to the retreatment versus 33% of patients who received the initial multifraction regimens. Retreatment for patients with progression was successful in 70% single fraction patients versus 57% multifraction patients. In general, retreatment was effective in 63% of all retreated patients.

In summary, available data support the reirradiation of sites of metastatic bone pain following initial irradiation, particularly where this follows an initial period of response. There is also limited evidence that a proportion of nonresponders would respond to a reirradiation. However, there remains a small group of patients who appear to be nonresponsive to any amount of palliative radiotherapy. Although the data do support the clinical practice of reirradiation, the preferred dose-fractionation at time of reirradiation is unknown. A phase 3 international randomized trial of single versus multiple fractions for reirradiation of painful bone metastases is ongoing and will help address the practical questions facing radiation oncologists when providing palliative radiation services.

SYSTEMIC RADIONUCLIDES

Patients with bone metastases often have diffuse bony disease. Administration of a systemic radionuclide has the advantage of targeting all bony lesions simultaneously, and can be given as a single administration on an outpatient basis. Osteoblastic bone metastases can be detected by a technetium-99 methylene-diphosphonate bone scan. Radionuclides react with bone mineral (hydroxyapatite), and the pattern of uptake mirrors that seen on the bone scan. Strontium-89 and samarium-153 are the agents most commonly used in clinical practice; phosphorus-32, rhenium-186, and tin-117 have also been used. These radionuclides emit beta particles with a mean range between 0.2 to 3 mm, thereby minimizing toxicity to surrounding tissue. Retention in the areas of bone metastases is greater than in the normal bone marrow, with a tumor-to-marrow ratio of 10:1. The average time to clinical response is 7 to 14 days, with a median duration of action of 18 weeks. Retreatment is possible, with an interval of 10 to 12 weeks for strontium-89 and 6 to 10 weeks for samarium-153, although a nonresponder is unlikely to respond to subsequent administration. The mechanism of pain reduction is unclear, but may include radiation-induced apoptosis of lymphocyte-secreting cytokines, and direct cell kill and reduction of mass effect.

Treatment-related toxicity consists mainly of reversible myelosuppression, especially thrombocytopenia. The nadir is 4 to 6 weeks after injection, recovery is completed by 6 to 10 weeks, with severity related to disease burden. Bone marrow toxicity is therefore of concern with the use of systemic chemotherapy. A small percentage of patients (10%–20%) may experience a pain flare shortly after administration. Contraindications to the use of radionuclides include poor performance status, less than 2 months projected survival, extensive soft tissue metastases, platelet count less than 60×10^9/L, recent rapid fall in platelet count even if more than 60×10^9/L, white count less than 2.5×10^9/L, and disseminated intravascular coagulation within 1 month of myelosuppressive chemotherapy and within 2 months of hemibody radiotherapy. Impending or actual pathologic fracture and cord compression are also contraindications for use.

The evidence for use of radionuclides has been reported in several phase 2 and 3 trials. Overall pain reduction rates for the various radionuclides are comparable and similar to localized and hemibody external-beam radiotherapy, with an overall response rate of 80% and complete response rate of 20%. The "Trans Canada" study reported on 126 patients with metastatic prostate cancer randomized to strontium-89 or placebo in addition to external-beam radiotherapy.[51] Patients receiving strontium showed a significant improvement at 3 months in analgesic use and an improved quality of life. Reduced lifetime requirements for radiotherapy and reduction in development of new painful bone metastases were seen. Hematologic toxicity was acceptable. A lifetime management cost savings of $5,800 in the group receiving strontium-89 was found.[52] A second multicenter trial in prostate cancer patients compared strontium-89 with either local field or wide-field radiotherapy and found no significant difference in analgesic efficacy, with a significant increase in time for further radiotherapy and development of new pain sites.[53] Samarium-153 is also licensed for use in the United States and has shown similar efficacy to strontium. Patients with a variety of primary malignancies had an 85% pain response rate, with breast cancer patients achieving the best palliation.

Radionuclides offer a method of delivering localized radiation to osteoblastic metastasis with similar response rates to external-beam radiotherapy. Advantages lie in the ability to treat all metastatic lesions simultaneously with a single injection administered on an outpatient basis. A reduction in the management costs has been found. Myelosuppression is the major toxicity, and may limit the use of radionuclides in patients managed with systemic chemotherapy.

Controlling Side Effects of Treatment

Radiation treatment planning is the most critical aspect of reducing radiation side effects. Management of the acute effects of radiotherapy requires attentive medical management that prevents expected side effect. Radiation side effects are specific to the area treated. Careful radiation treatment planning that avoids critical structures like mucosal surfaces can prevent most side effects.

Patients should be reassured that the unavoidable side effects that they experience will resolve following the completion of radiotherapy. Skin reactions are usually minimal during radiotherapy for bone metastases and are limited only to the radiation portal. Nausea and vomiting, resulting from a radiation portal that includes the abdomen, will usually respond to antiemetic therapy, but Ondansetron or dexamethasone also is commonly used, especially if patients have recently received emetogenic chemotherapy. Diarrhea, resulting from abdominopelvic radiation, will respond to antidiarrhea medications such as loperamide. Local irritation from mucositis of the oropharyngeal region may be relieved by soluble aspirin, analgesics, or benzydamine mouthwashes. Secondary infections, like *Candida*, should be treated.

The side effects of electron-beam radiation are more limited because they only treat superficial structures like the ribs, skin lesions, and superficial lymph nodes. Underlying structures are spared with the selection of the proper electron-beam energy. This characteristic is especially important with reirradiation to avoid injury to critical structures like the spinal cord. The most prominent side effect of electron-beam radiation is an erythematous skin reaction. Other side effects listed here do not occur with electron-beam radiation because the radiation beam does not penetrate to these structures.

No side effects, other than a possible flare of pain in the first 2 weeks after administration, are observed with systemic radioisotope therapy because all the radiation is localized to the bone. This is a significant consideration for patients who have significant symptoms of the disease or other treatments. Side effects from external-beam radiation also are more severe when the radiation fields are large because more normal tissues are treated. Pain flare is common after palliative radiotherapy for osseous metastases, and patients receiving single-fraction radiotherapy may be at higher risk.[54] Systemic radioisotopes can have significant advantage over large external-beam radiation fields by reducing risk for side effects like nausea and diarrhea.

RADIOTHERAPY FOR COMPLICATIONS OF BONE METASTASES: LOCALIZED EXTERNAL BEAM RADIOTHERAPY FOR PATHOLOGICAL FRACTURES AND SPINAL CORD COMPRESSION

Pathologic and Impending Fractures

Pathologic fractures are handled with orthopaedic stabilization whenever possible. Surgery rapidly controls pain and returns that patient to mobility. Elective orthopaedic stabilization has reportedly resulted in good pain relief and sustained mobility in up to 90% of patients. Early identification of patients with a high risk of fracture is especially important. A fracture of the weight-bearing long bones can be a devastating event even in a healthy person. Prophylactic orthopaedic fixation is often advised to avoid the trauma of a pathologic fracture. The operative procedure has fewer complications and less impact on functional outcome.

In the randomized Dutch Bone Metastasis Study on the palliative effect of a single fraction of 8 Gy versus six fractions of 4 Gy on painful bone metastases, 14 fractures occurred in 102 patients with femoral metastases. The authors analyzed the pretreatment radiographs of femoral metastases and concluded that fracturing of the femur mostly depended on the amount of axial cortical involvement of the metastases. They recommend treating femoral metastases with an axial cortical involvement of 30 mm or less with a single fraction of 8 Gy for relief of pain. If the axial cortical involvement is greater than 30 mm, prophylactic surgery should be considered to minimize the risk of pathologic fracturing or, if the patient's condition is limited, irradiation to a higher total dose.[55]

Although radiotherapy provides pain relief and tumor control, it does not restore bone stability. Postoperative radiotherapy is usually recommended after surgical stabilization of a pathologic fracture. Townsend et al.[56] reported normal use of extremity (with or without pain) in 53% for postoperative radiotherapy versus 11.5% for surgery alone. Second orthopaedic procedures to the same site were more frequent in the group that received surgery alone. The actuarial median survival for the surgery-alone group was 3.3 months, compared with 12.4 months for the postoperative radiotherapy group. However, this study needs to be interpreted with great caution because of its retrospective nature and possible unaccountable selection biases.

Patients who are without visceral metastases and who have a relatively long survival (e.g., >3 months) are more likely to benefit from postoperative radiotherapy. Because the entire bone is at risk for microscopic involvement and the procedure involved in rod placement may seed the bone at other sites, the length of the entire rod used for bone stabilization should be included in the radiation field. When the radiation fields are more limited, instability of the rod, resulting in pain and need for reoperation, can result from recurrent osteolytic metastases outside the radiation portal.

When a pathologic fracture has occurred, the primary goal is to provide pain relief. Secondary intentions are to achieve stability and restore function. Unless there are medical contraindications or extremely short life expectancy, surgery is usually recommended. Otherwise, radiotherapy alone may be considered.

Stereotactic Body Radiotherapy of Spinal Metastases

Technological advances in radiation oncology now permit spine stereotactic body radiotherapy (SBRT) defined as the precise delivery of high dose per fraction radiotherapy in one to five fractions to a spinal target.[57] The dose per fraction is typically greater than 5 Gy, and the total dose is not palliative in intent but a dose equivalent to those used in the curative setting. Typical doses prescribed include 16 to 24 Gy in a single fraction, 24 Gy in three fractions, and 30 to 35 Gy in five fractions. These doses are biologically equivalent to two to six times those investigated in the conventional radiotherapy literature that consist typically of 8 Gy in a single fraction, 20 Gy in five fractions, and 30 Gy in ten fractions, as discussed in this chapter.

Beyond the high-dose aspect of SBRT, the intent of spine SBRT is significantly different from that of conventional radiotherapy. The aim of spine SBRT is to target only those vertebrae (or disease within a vertebrae) involved with metastatic disease while sparing the spinal cord and surrounding normal tissues from the high tumor dose. This is achieved using sophisticated radiotherapy treatment planning and delivery units that allow for intensity-modulated radiotherapy, image guidance, and multiple beams of radiation centered on the target. Traditional practice would mandate at least one or two healthy vertebrae beyond the disease to be included in a simple one- or two-field conventional external-beam radiotherapy treatment. This ensures the entire target will receive the prescribed dose and compensates for the physical limitations of dose delivery when using a limited numbers of fields. This fundamental contrast in treatment approach is illustrated in Figures 150.2 and 150.3.

Spine SBRT is in its infancy and is currently being investigated as an alternative to conventional wide-field radiation in the initial management of spinal metastases in the reirradiation scenario, and in the postoperative patient.[57,58] Spine SBRT evidence is limited to retrospective reviews and a few phase 2 trials documenting prospective outcomes.[57] Clearly, follow-up in patients is premature and long-term data are required. This is challenging in this cohort of patients, given the presence of metastatic disease. However, actuarial data are still required in order to make firm conclusions. Crude local control is promising based on imaging follow-up. As to pain relief, the data are promising but no conclusion can be reached until there is uniformity in the pain assessment tool, consistent definitions of response, and actuarial data reported. The RTOG 0631 randomized study evaluating 8 Gy in a single fraction delivered conventionally to 16 Gy in a single fraction delivered with SBRT for painful spinal metastases will hopefully provide us insight as to the role of SBRT in patients with no prior radiation. However, randomized studies are also required dedicated to reirradiation and postoperative patients.

The treatment of spinal metastases with SBRT is not without risk to the patient given the high doses delivered millimeters away from tissues such as the spinal cord, esophagus, and kidneys. When considering that the risk of clinically significant late toxicities with conventional palliative radiotherapy regimens is negligible, spine SBRT has to prove itself as a safe technique for the palliative patient. The most devastating late toxicity associated with this technique is radiation myelopathy that can leave the palliative patient paralyzed, and is unacceptable considering the goals of treatment for this population. There are currently five known cases of radiation myelopathy in patients with no prior radiation and four known cases in patients treated with SBRT as reirradiation. Although analysis of these patients has yielded guidelines for safe practice,[59,60] there is an overall lack of data to make firm conclusions. With

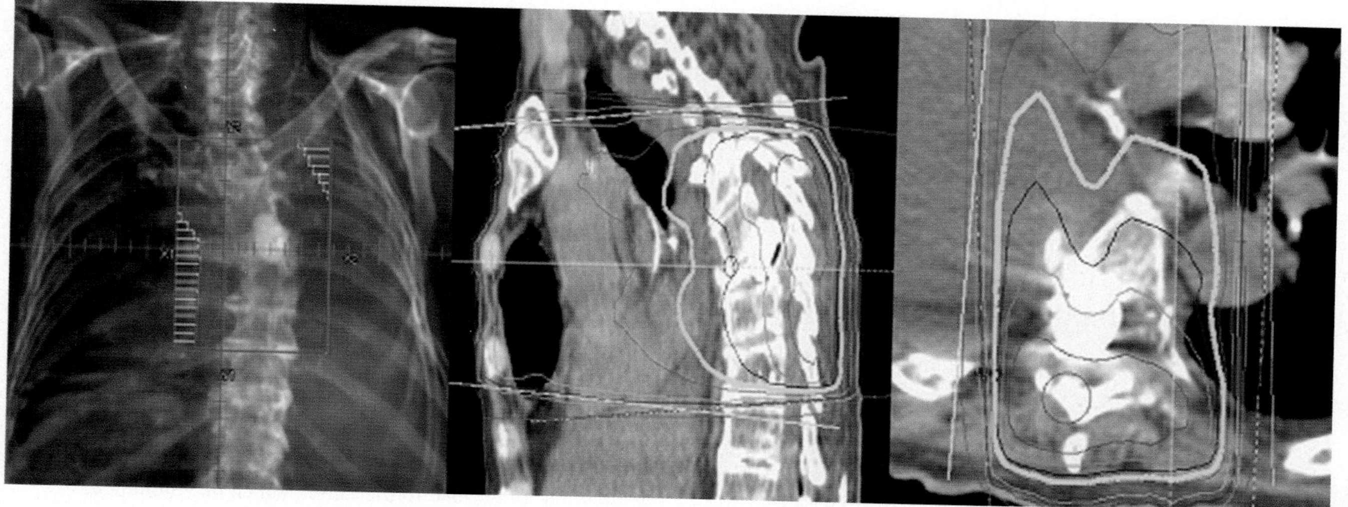

FIGURE 150.2 Illustrates a typical radiation field for a seventh thoracic vertebrae metastases where two vertebral bodies above and below the target are included in the radiotherapy field. This patient was treated with 8 Gy in a single fraction and one can appreciate the entire vertebral column within the field being encompassed by the 8-Gy isodose line in yellow.

such a high dose within the bone, recent data report a significant rate of new or progressive vertebral compression fracture with fracture progression occurring in 27 of 71 (38%) vertebrae treated with SBRT.[61] Other toxicities of fatal esophageal necrosis, bronchial stenosis requiring dilatation, and significant skin toxicities have also been reported.[62,63] These toxicities reflect the lack of understanding of normal tissue toxicity with an extreme high dose, as this approach has only become a possibility by the dramatic revolution in modern radiation technology (Table 150.1).

Spine SBRT is in its infancy as a therapeutic option for patients with spinal metastases. However, it is technically demanding, requires considerable skill, and there is potential for serious late toxicities that are not otherwise an issue with conventional radiotherapy. Although there is a significant potential to improve long-term pain relief and local control, this will only become apparent if these are dose-dependent outcomes and proven in randomized controlled trials.

MECHANICAL STABILITY AND FRACTURE RISK

Stability is an important concept to understand. In the spine this is the ability of the supporting structures of the spine to allow for physiological loading so to prevent pain and deformity. Spinal instability may not necessarily result in a catastrophic collapse and paralysis, but with a pathologic burst fracture this can occur. More commonly, the spine afflicted with malignancy will develop a gradual loss of architecture resulting in mechanical pain and/or rest pain. In the appendicular skeleton, instability results in

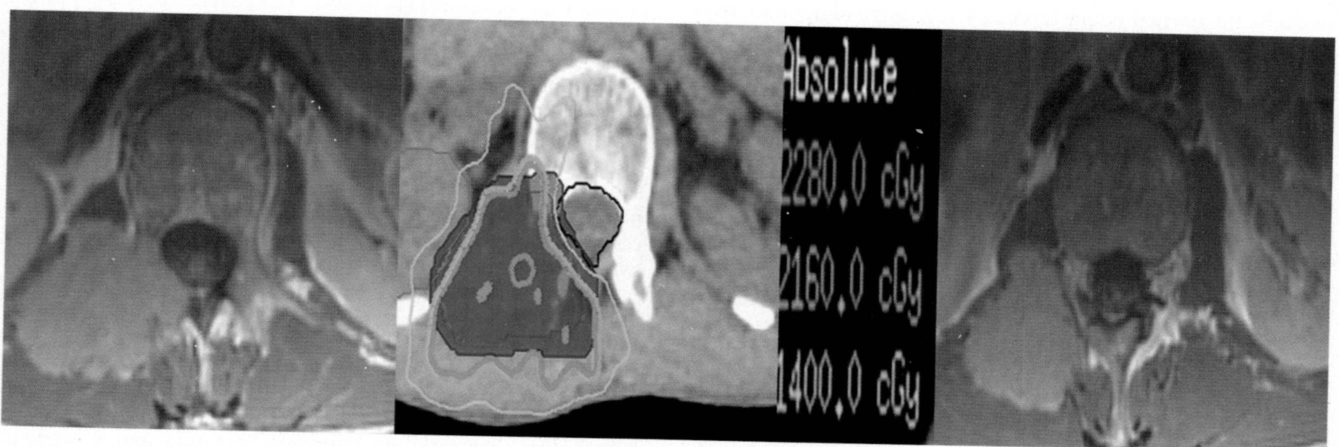

FIGURE 150.3 Illustrates a spine stereotactic body radiotherapy (SBRT) treatment plan for a patient with a first lumbar vertebrae hepatocellular paraspinal metastases that involves the ipsilateral pedicle and lamina. The location of this target is complicated as it is situated between the kidneys and, together with thecal sac sparing, the treatment planning is even more complex. This patient was treated with 24 Gy in three fractions and the high-dose isodose lines in green and orange conform tightly around the target while the thecal sac and kidneys are spared from the high dose. The lower 14-Gy isodose line skims the left kidney while sparing the spinal cord, hence, reflecting the highly shaped nature of the dose distribution at both the high and lower dose levels. Despite a radioresistant hepatocellular histology, the patient had an excellent response 4 months following therapy with significant regression of the disease as shown on the right-hand posttreatment axial image.

TABLE 150.1

SUMMARY OF KEY ISSUES COMPARING AND CONTRASTING CONVENTIONAL EXTERNAL-BEAM RADIOTHERAPY AS COMPARED WITH SPINE STEREOTACTIC BODY RADIOTHERAPY (SBRT) IN THE TREATMENT OF SPINAL METASTASES

Conventional External-Beam Radiotherapy	Stereotactic Body Radiotherapy
■ Low BED delivered to the tumor	■ 2–6 times the BED delivered to the tumor
■ Technique requires at least one or two healthy vertebral bodies to be treated	■ Targeted treatment to only those areas of disease
■ Low risk of long-term side effects due to low BED exposure to healthy tissues	■ Technical errors, or lack of proper dose constraints, can result in overdosing of critical structures and devastating late toxicity
■ Protracted regimes can include 5 to 20 fractions	■ Fewer treatment where by definition SBRT involves 1 to 5 fractions
■ May be less efficacious in radioresistant histologies like sarcoma and renal cell carcinoma	■ Greater dose may lead to better outcomes for radioresistant tumors
■ Greater volume of normal tissue exposed to the prescribed tumor dose and potential for greater acute toxicities	■ Dose to the normal surrounding nontumor tissue much lower than that prescribed to the tumor, which may limit acute toxicities
■ Short treatment times of 5 to 10 minutes, which are ideal for the patient in pain	■ Prolonged treatment times where each treatment takes 45–60 minutes and requires strict immobilization
■ If local failure occurs then likely dose- or biology-related as opposed to geographic miss	■ Potential for geographic miss and if within the epidural space then tumor regrowth can lead to cord compression
■ Limited doses apply in the retreatment patient, which may preclude efficacy	■ High doses still possible in the retreatment patient and data suggest efficacy[59]
■ Standard of care for patients with malignant epidural cord compression with level 1 evidence for efficacy[64]	■ Contraindicated in the patient with symptomatic malignant epidural spinal cord compression
■ Indicated for the patient with multiple level spinal metastatic disease	■ No more than three consecutive metastases to be treated at once
■ Deliverable in any radiotherapy department and low cost	■ Requires sophisticated radiation equipment and quality assurance
■ Level 1 evidence and well-defined outcomes supporting common palliative treatment regimens[65]	■ No level 1 evidence to indicate superiority over conventional radiotherapy

BED, biologically effective dose

mechanical pain from cortical loss creating symptoms with use of the extremity or with weight bearing. A pathologic fracture can result when loads applied are greater than the support provided by the normal boney trabeculae. An impending fracture is a bone at risk of fracture if not treated.

The biomechanical effects of osteolytic metastases are of two categories: stress risers and open-section defects.[66] Stress risers are perforations that are smaller than the cross-sectional diameter of the bone that decrease torsional rigidity by 60%. Open-section defects decrease bone strength by almost 90%.

Lower Extremity

Radiographic criteria for operative management of lytic metastases to bone are largely based on the femur. Pathologic fractures of the femur have profound morbidity for the patient as well as considerable issues related to stabilization that are preventable if treated prior to fracture. It has been recommended that femoral metastases can be treated nonoperatively if they are less than 2.5 cm, less than 50% of the diameter of the cortex, and are in a low-risk location (i.e., not in the subtrochanteric region of the femur).[67–69] The subtrochanteric segment of the femur extends from the lesser trochanter to the junction of the proximal and middle thirds of the diaphysis. This segment of the femur is subjected to very high axial loads of weight bearing and tremendous bending forces because of the eccentric load application to the femoral head. The medial cortex is loaded in compression and the lateral cortex in tension.

Ward et al.[70] compared the results of 97 impending fractures of the femur with 85 complete fractures. In the impending group, there was less blood loss (438 vs. 636 mL), shorter hospital stays (7 vs. 11 days), greater likelihood of discharge home as opposed to an extended-care facility (79% vs. 56%), and a greater likelihood of resuming support-free ambulation (35% vs. 12%).

For diaphyseal lesions of the femur, the loads are less and the threshold for surgical stabilization is higher. Each case needs to be individualized, taking into consideration the degree of functional impairment, pain, and radiosensitivity of the tumor. The same size lesion in the diaphysis is less of a risk for fracture than in the subtrochanteric region. Recent work at our center on remineralization of bone following radiation may allow us to avoid surgical intervention in the appropriate candidate.[71]

Operative Techniques

Proximal Femur. Impending or pathologic fractures of the femoral neck or head or intertrochanteric region are usually managed with hemiarthroplasty. If there is involvement of the acetabulum then total hip arthroplasty is indicated. Lesions in the intertrochanteric region can also be stabilized with a hip screw and side plate device with consideration for augmentation using polymethylmethacrylate (PMMA) cement. It is imperative to plan preoperatively with a full-length femur radiograph to ensure the plate is able to span the length of disease involvement. With associated diaphyseal or distal femur involvement, an intramedullary device is indicated in order to span the entire length of the femur. Second- and third-generation nails are most

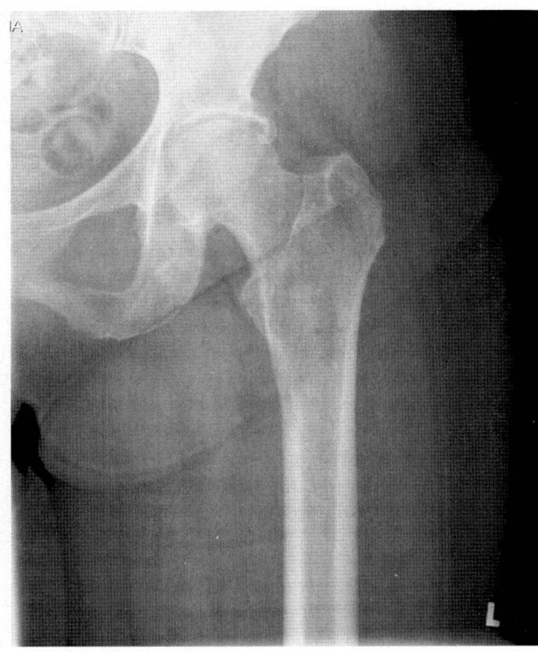

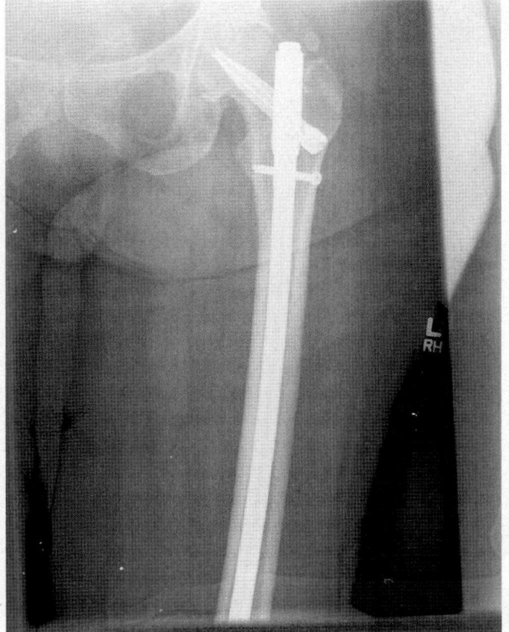

FIGURE 150.4 **A:** Plain AP radiograph of a lytic metastatic lesion with impending fracture of the peritrochanteric region of the femur. **B:** Plain AP radiograph after treatment with recontruction intramedullary nail providing fixation into the femural head.

commonly used in order to allow fixation into the femoral head[72] (Fig. 150.4).

Femoral Diaphysis. Similar to proximal femoral lesions, intramedullary devices are used for fixation. In the case of an impending fracture, a distal vent should be used to allow efflux of marrow contents in order to reduce the risk of fat emboli.[73,74]

Pelvis and Acetabulum. Reconstruction of the proximal part of the femur and the acetabulum is often technically demanding and hardware failure not uncommon. The implant is at risk of failure because the forces about the hip are extremely high for most normal activities. Forces on the proximal femur can be 3.5 times body weight during the midstance phase of gait and can increase to 7.7 times body weight during stair climbing.[75,76] Acetabular insufficiency secondary to bone metastasis is classified according to location and extent of bone loss. Where the acetabulum is structurally intact, a conventional total hip arthroplasty can be performed. PMMA is often used to provide added support in cases of perforations of the medial wall. When the medial wall has an unconstrained defect, techniques are required that transfer the stress of weight bearing away from the deficiency and onto the intact acetabular rim with use of a protrusion ring. With more extensive bone involvement including both the medial and lateral walls, reconstruction of the acetabular columns requires the use of implants such as Steinmann pins and PMMA to fix the protrusion ring into place.

Preoperative Embolization of Bone Metastases

Metastases from renal cell carcinoma are hypervascular as a result of neovascularization. Other primaries can also be associated with hypervascularity.[77] Historically, stabilization of spinal or appendicular lesions from renal cell carcinoma was associated with excessive bleeding requiring transfusion. Uncontrollable hemorrhage may even result in death. There is growing experience and evidence that preoperative embolization is a safe and reliable method of reducing intraoperative blood loss at the time of stabilization of bone metastases. The methods of embolization include the use of polyvinyl alcohol, coils, and gel foam. The procedure is performed in the angiography suite and surgery should be performed within 48 to 96 hours of embolization or revascularization will occur.

Roscoe et al.[78] reported on the use of embolization for renal cell carcinoma metastases to the spine before stabilization. Comparing 8 patients who underwent perioperative embolization with 20 patients who did not, the blood loss during stabilization for former group averaged 940 mL compared with 1,975 mL in the nonembolized group. Similar results have been reported by other authors on the safe and effective role of perioperative embolization prior to spinal decompression and stabilization[79,80] (Fig. 150.5).

Upper Extremity

In the upper extremity, the difference in management and patient outcome is less profound between an impending and pathologic fracture. Fractures of the humerus can be managed with plate fixation or with intramedullary devices. Recently, Atesok et al.[81] have shown that an unreamed humeral nail provides immediate stability and pain relief with minimum morbidity and early return of function to the arm. Similar conclusions were made by Dijkstra et al.[82] when comparing intramedullary nail with compression plating for humeral pathologic fractures.

Spine

Because of immunosuppression, poor nutritional status, and medical comorbidities, surgery to the spine may be associated with significant complications. Considerations in decision making are lifespan of the patient, general medical condition, number of spinal levels involved, age, cancer type, and radiation status.[83]

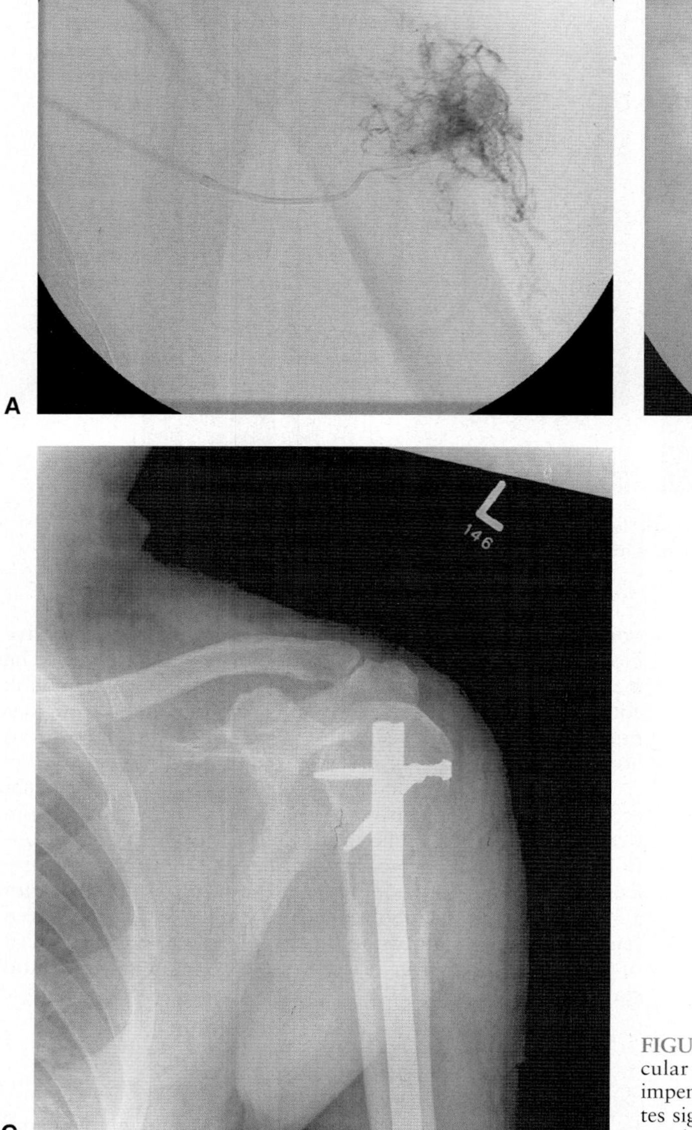

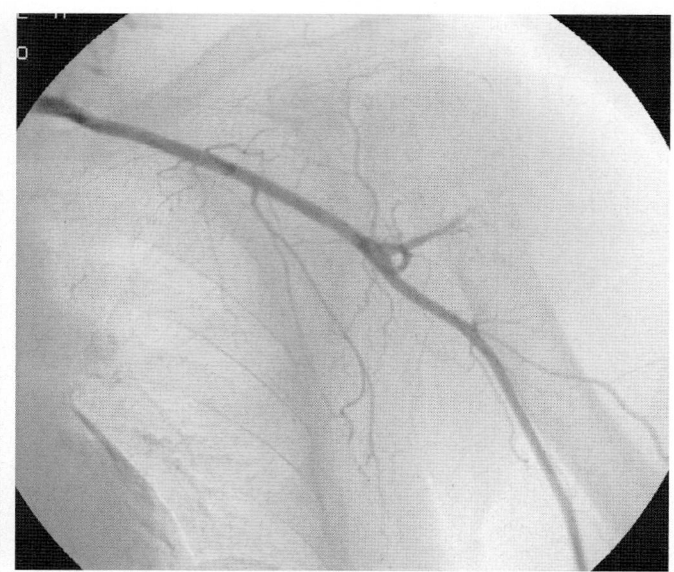

FIGURE 150.5 **A:** Pre-embolization angiogram demonstrating hypervascular renal cell tumor in the proximal humerus. Lytic metastases and impending fracture is present. **B:** Postembolization angiogram demonstrates significantly reduced neovascularization. **C:** Postoperative plain radiograph with fracture treated with an unreamed locked intramedullary nail.

The significance of the primary cancer type on survival is well established. After detection by bone scan of spine involvement, Tatsui et al.[84] reported a 1-year survival of 0% and 22% for gastric and pulmonary cancers and 78% and 83% for breast and prostate primaries.

In a population-based study, Finkelstein et al.[85] used Cox multivariate regression to model survival as a function of potential predictor variables in a cohort of 987 patients. This study also quantified postoperative complication rates and identified significant risk factors that were associated with poor survival and outcome. There was an overall 1- and 3-month mortality rate of 9% and 29%, respectively. Increasing age (1.04 relative risk per year) and primary lung cancer were significant risk factors for death within 30 days of surgery. For overall survival, each year of advancing age had a 1% increased risk of dying. Lung primary had a 2.65 relative risk of mortality within 30 days. The quantification of risks provides patients, families, and clinicians with objective data to help decide on treatment options and to better understand surgical risk and outcomes.

The effect of a preoperative neurologic deficit on survivorship has been evaluated by a number of authors. In a multicenter study by Argenson et al.,[86] patients with a preoperative deficit had significantly lower mean survival at 1 and 3 years after surgery. We have shown that patients with preoperative neurologic deficits were 71% more likely to get a postoperative infection, likely from the administration of preoperative radiation. Other authors have likewise found increased infection rates and poorer outcomes following surgery in the presence of preoperative radiation.[85,87–89]

Wai et al.[83] in 2003 prospectively evaluated the efficacy of surgery in patients with metastatic spinal disease with respect to quality of life using a validated outcome measure specific for palliative patients (Edmonton Symptom Assessment Scale). This study demonstrated the largest improvement to be in pain following surgery. There were significant improvements in six other domains and trends toward improvement in another one. There was no significant deterioration in any domain. The major benefit of surgery occurs within the first month and remained stable until death or at least 6 months (length of follow-up).

Principles of open surgical techniques and considerations are beyond the scope of this chapter. In general, tumor location within the vertebrae, spinal level, radiation status, neuron deficit, and number of levels involved affect decision making. Surgery can be from an anterior or posterior approach.

A more recent approach to management of metastatic spinal disease is percutaneous vertebroplasty (PV) and kyphoplasty. These are minimally invasive approachs and an alternative to open surgery for restoring stability to the spine.[90,91] PV may be applied to a greater number of candidates with pain due to instability. These same patients may not be suitable for invasive spinal surgery because of medical comorbidities, multilevel disease, or having a profound neurologic deficit.

PV is performed under intravenous sedation in the radiology suite or in the operating room. Real-time fluoroscopy is

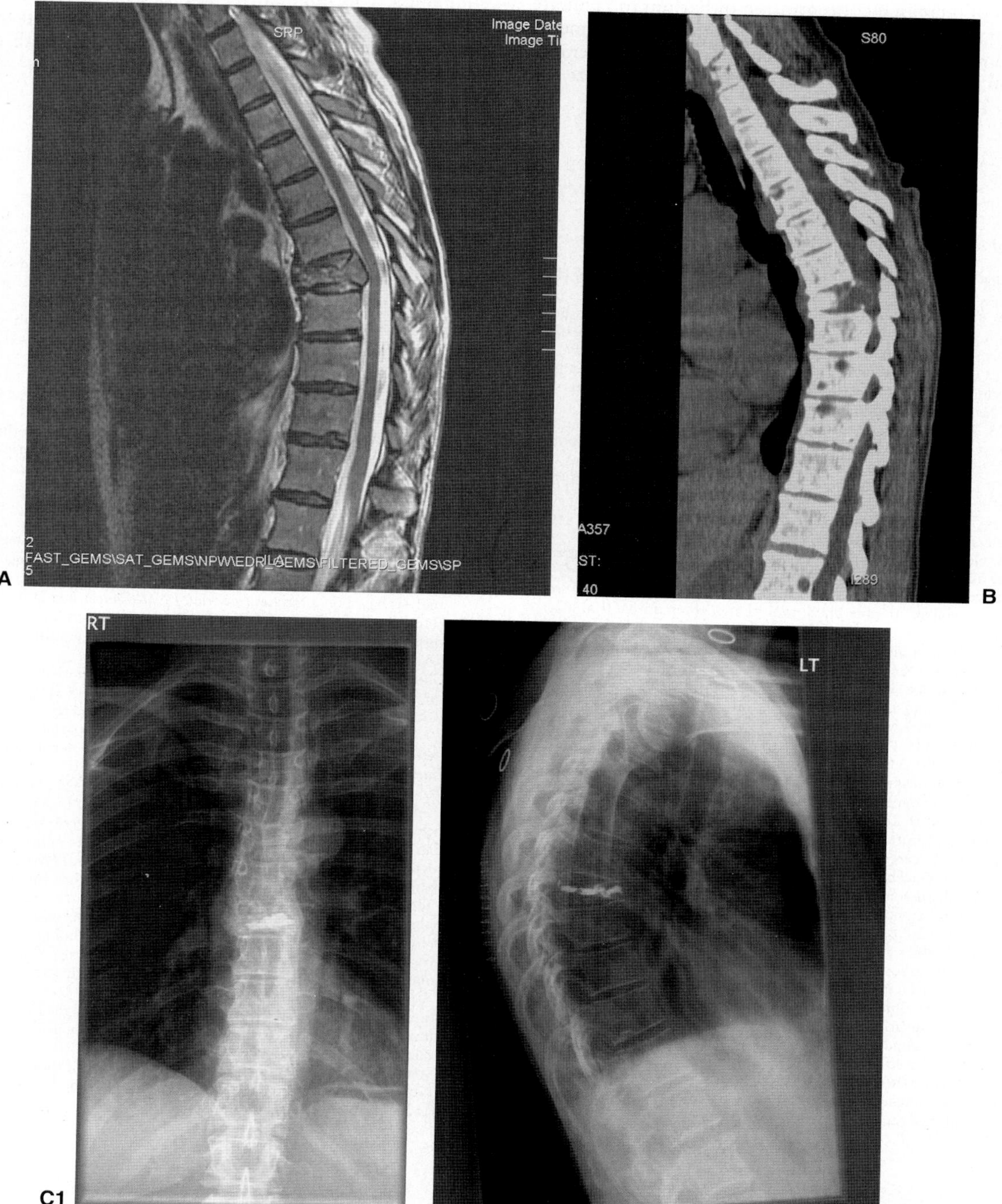

FIGURE 150.6 **A:** Magnetic resonance image of thoracic spine with T8 spinal cord compression. **B:** Computed tomographic sagittal reformat showing bony destruction of T8 and multiple level metastases. **C:** (1) Postoperative anteroposterior and (2) lateral radiographs following open posterolateral decompression and vertebroplasty of T8 vertebra.

PRACTICE OF ONCOLOGY

used to introduce bone cement (PMMA) into the vertebral body via a parapedicular or transpedicular approach. Commercially available PV kits contain bone cement, mixers, trocars, cannulas, and syringes. PMMA is injected in a semi-liquid state such that extravasation and intravertebral pressure is minimized.

Complication rates of PV have been reported to be around 10% in metastatic disease.[92] These complications include cement entering the nerve root foramen or spinal canal resulting in radiculopathy or spinal cord compression. Systemic complications include embolic events due to marrow fat, tumor fragments, or cement entering the circulation. The use of biplanar fluoroscopy and "live" imaging during injection, the addition of increased concentration of barium to facilitate visualization, intraosseous venogram, limiting the volume of fill, gentle and slow injection, and the use of viscous cement are technical details that have been described to minimize the complications of this procedure.[93] Despite these precautions, extrusion of cement has been commonly reported. The vast majority of extrusions, however, are minor and do not result in neurologic sequelae.[94]

Vertebroplasty and kyphoplasty more recently have been combined with decompression in an open technique (Fig. 150.6). PMMA is used to provide anterior column support following decompression and in some cases is able to replace the need for posterior instrumentation. In some candidates with or without previous radiation or in the high-risk/poor surgical candidate with multiple-level disease, unifocal decompression can be performed and stabilized in this technique. The concerns for hardware failure as previously noted are eliminated. This minimalistic approach is providing improved outcomes, allowing for greater numbers of patients to be operated on when previously the risks associated with multilevel fixations had unacceptable complication rates.

Selected References

The full list of references for this chapter appears in the online version.

1. Coleman RE. Clinical features of metastatic bone disease and risk of skeletal morbidity. *Clin Cancer Res* 2006;12(20 Suppl):6243.
4. Siclari, VA, Guise TA, Chirgwin JM. Molecular interactions between breast cancer cells and the bone microenvironment drive skeletal metastases. *Cancer Metastasis Rev* 2006;25:621.
5. Brown JE, Cook RJ, Major P, et al. Bone turnover markers as predictors of skeletal complications in prostate cancer, lung cancer, and other solid tumors. *J Natl Cancer Inst* 2005;97(10):59.
8. Roelofs AJ, Thompson K, Gordon S, Rogers MJ. Molecular mechanisms of action of bisphosphonates: current status. *Clin Cancer Res* 2006;12 (20 Pt 2):6222s–6230s.
9. Coleman RE. Risks and benefits of bisphosphonates. *Br J Cancer* 2008;98 (11):1736.
10. Pavlakis N, Schmidt R, Stockler M. Bisphosphonates for breast cancer. *Cochrane Database Syst Rev* 2005;3:CD003474.
11. Rosen LS, Gordon D, Kaminski M, et al. Long-term efficacy and safety of zoledronic acid compared with pamidronate disodium in treatment of skeletal complications in patients with advanced multiple myeloma or breast cancer: a randomized, double-blind, multicenter, comparative trial. *Cancer* 2003;98:1735.
12. Body JJ, Diel IJ, Lichinitser MR, et al. MF 4265 Study Group. Intravenous ibandronate reduces the incidence of skeletal complications in patients with breast cancer and bone metastases. *Ann Oncol* 2003;14(9):1399.
13. Berenson JR, Lichtenstein A, Porter L, et al. Efficacy of pamidronate in reducing skeletal events in patients with advanced multiple myeloma. *N Engl J Med* 1996;334:488.
14. Saad F, Gleason DM, Murray R, et al. Long-term efficacy of zoledronic acid for the prevention of skeletal complications in patients with advanced prostate cancer and bone metastasis. *J Natl Cancer Inst* 2004;96:879.
15. Rosen LS, Gordon D, Tchekmedyian S, et al. Long-term efficacy and safety of zoledronic acid in the treatment of skeletal metastases in patients with non small cell lung carcinoma and other solid tumors: a randomized, phase III, double-blind, placebo-controlled trial. *Cancer* 2004;100:2613.
16. Aapro M, Abrahamsson PA, Body JJ, et al. Guidance on the use of bisphosphonates in solid tumours: recommendations of an international expert panel. *Ann Oncol* 2008;19:420.
17. Berenson JR, Hillner BE, Kyle RA, et al. American Society of Clinical Oncology Bisphosphonates Expert Panel. American Society of Clinical Oncology clinical practice guidelines: the role of bisphosphonates in multiple myeloma. *J Clin Oncol* 2002;20:3719.
18. Clemons MJ, Dranitsaris G, Ooi WS, et al. Phase II trial evaluating the palliative benefit of second-line zoledronic acid in breast cancer patients with either a skeletal-related event or progressive bone metastases despite first-line bisphosphonate therapy. *J Clin Oncol* 2006;20:4895.
19. Lipton A, Cook R, Saad F, et al. Normalization of bone markers is associated with improved survival in patients with bone metastases from solid tumors and elevated bone resorption receiving zoledronic acid. *Cancer* 2008;113(1):193.
21. Lipton A, Steger GG, Figueroa J, et al. Extended efficacy and safety of denosumab in breast cancer patients with bone metastases not receiving prior bisphosphonate therapy. *Clin Cancer Res* 2008;14:6690.
25. Smith MR, Egerdie B, Hernandez Toriz N, et al. Denosumab in men receiving androgen-deprivation therapy for prostate cancer. *N Engl J Med* 2009; 361:745.
28. Chow E, Wu JS, Hoskin P, et al. International consensus on palliative radiotherapy endpoints for future clinical trials in bone metastases. *Radiother Oncol* 2002;64(3):275.
29. Bone Pain Trial Working Party. 8 Gy single fraction radiotherapy for the treatment of metastatic skeletal pain: randomized comparison with multifraction schedule over 12 months of patient follow-up. *Radiother Oncol* 1999;52:111.
30. Steenland E, Leer J, van Houwelingen H, et al. The effect of a single fraction compared to multiple fractions on painful bone metastases: a global analysis of the Dutch Bone Metastasis Study. *Radiother Oncol* 1999;52:101.
31. Van den Hout WB, van der Linden YM, Steenland, et al. Single- versus multiple-fraction radiotherapy in patients with painful bone metastases: cost-utility analysis based on a randomized trial. *J Natl Cancer Inst* 2003;95(3):222.
35. Hartsell WF, Scott CB, Watkins Bruner D, et al. Randomized trial of short- versus long-course radiotherapy for palliation of painful bone metastases. *J Natl Cancer Inst* 2005;97(11):798.
37. Chow E, Harris K, Fan G, Tsao M, Sze WM. Palliative radiotherapy trials for bone metastases: a systemic review. *J Clin Oncol* 2007;25(11):1423.
38. Roos DE, Turner SL, O'Brien PC, et al. Randomized trial of 8 Gy in 1 versus 20 Gy in 5 fractions of radiotherapy for neuropathic pain due to bone metastases (Trans-Tasman Radiation Oncology Group, TROG 96.05). *Radiother Oncol* 2005;75:54.
56. Townsend PW, Smalley SR, Cozad, SC, Rosenthal HG, Hassanein RE. Role of postoperative radiation therapy after stabilization of fractures caused by metastatic disease. *Int J Radiat Oncol Biol Phys* 1995;31(1):43.
57. Sahgal A, Larson DA, Chang EL. Stereotactic body radiosurgery for spinal metastases: a critical review. *Int J Radiat Oncol Biol Phys* 2008;71:652.
59. Sahgal A, Ma L, Gibbs I, et al. Spinal cord tolerance for stereotactic body radiotherapy. *Int J Radiat Oncol Biol Phys* 2009.
60. Sahgal A, Ma L, Weinberg V, et al. Re-treatment spinal cord tolerance for spine stereotactic body radiotherapy. *Int J Radiat Oncol Biol Phys* 2010;epub.
61. Rose PS, Laufer I, Boland PJ, et al. Risk of fracture after single fraction image-guided intensity-modulated radiation therapy to spinal metastases. *J Clin Oncol* 2009;27:5075.
62. Yamada Y, Bilsky MH, Lovelock DM, et al. High-dose, single-fraction image-guided intensity-modulated radiotherapy for metastatic spinal lesions. *Int J Radiat Oncol Biol Phys* 2008.
63. Gomez DR, Hunt MA, Jackson A, et al. Low rate of thoracic toxicity in palliative paraspinal single-fraction stereotactic body radiation therapy. *Radiother Oncol* 2009;93:414.

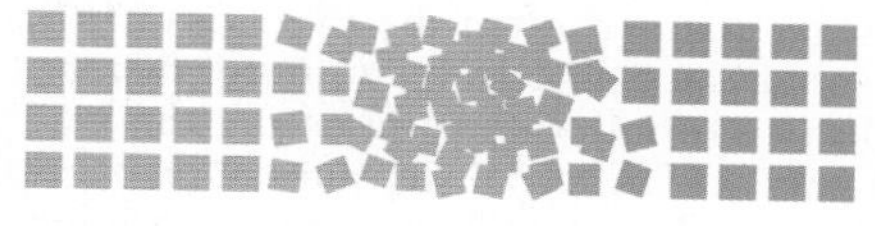

CHAPTER 151 MALIGNANT EFFUSIONS OF THE PLEURA AND THE PERICARDIUM

KING F. KWONG AND DAO M. NGUYEN

MALIGNANT PLEURAL EFFUSION

Over 150,000 cases of malignant pleural effusion (MPE) are estimated to occur annually in the United States.[1] MPE is the initial presenting sign in approximately 10% of cancer patients[2] and is commonly associated with the following cancers: bronchogenic carcinoma (40%), breast cancer (25%), lymphoma (10%), ovarian cancer (5%), and gastric cancer (5%).[3] Lung and breast cancers are the most common metastatic tumors to the pleura in men and women, respectively.[4] Ten percent of all MPE are due to primary cancers arising from the pleura, with malignant mesothelioma as the most common tumor. Cancer of unknown primary results in only 5% to 10% of MPE.[5,6]

Malignant pleural effusions arise predominantly from obstruction and disruption of lymphatic channels by malignant cells. Physiologically, the pleural space is a potential space formed by the parietal and visceral pleural linings of hemithorax. Between 5 and 10 liters of pleural fluid traverse the pleural space on a daily basis, with only 5 to 15 mL of pleural fluid present normally within the pleural space.[2,7] No significant differences in the quantity of pleural fluid are found between hemithoraces or genders.[7] Net accumulation of pleural fluid within the pleural space can result from increased pleural fluid production due to increased vascular permeability, reduced reabsorption of pleural fluid by lymphatics due to disrupted or occluded drainage channels, or contributions from multiple mechanisms.

The presence of MPE frequently indicates advanced disease, and the overall prognosis of patients with MPE depends largely on the underlying type of malignancy and the extent of primary disease. As life expectancy in patients with advanced cancer is often markedly reduced, the primary goal in the management of MPE should be palliation, with an emphasis on employing therapies that can be administered with minimal morbidity to the patient.

Clinical Presentation

Moderate to large MPEs are often symptomatic, with dyspnea being the predominant symptom. Chest discomfort can range from dull ache (characterized as heaviness or pressure) to sharp pleuritic pain. Physical examination usually reveals decreased breath sounds with dullness to percussion and diminished tactile fremitus. Tracheal deviation and low cardiac output related to mediastinal compression occasionally may be seen with massive effusions.

Diagnosis and Evaluation

Radiographic Examinations

As little as 200 mL of pleural fluid, resulting in blunting of the costophrenic angle, can be detected by standard chest radiographs. Upright and lateral decubitus chest radiographs are often performed initially and can demonstrate "free-flowing" pleural effusions. However, MPEs are best assessed radiographically with computer-assisted tomography (CT) scan of the chest performed with administration of intravenous contrast agents. Particularly in the setting of a newly diagnosed effusion, CT can define fluid loculations, mediastinal and/or hilar lymphadenopathy, pleural-based masses, and any associated parenchymal disease. Complete opacification of the hemithorax occurs in about 15% of MPEs. An opacified hemithorax with mediastinal shift toward the contralateral side indicates massive effusion, and raises concern for a tension hydrothorax, which requires urgent percutaneous drainage of the effusion to relieve the intrathoracic pressure. Opacification of the hemithorax from a massive effusion without mediastinal shift can also result—the etiology being the combined effects of pleural fluid accumulation and lung collapse secondary to proximal airway obstruction, or mediastinal fixation by malignant lymphadenopathy, or a diffuse malignant process involving the parietal pleura restricting mediastinal movement.

Invasive Diagnostic Maneuvers

After appropriate radiographic assessment of a newly presenting effusion, thoracentesis should be performed to obtain fluid for biochemical and cytologic analyses, to relieve symptoms, and to determine the extent of lung re-expansion following pleural fluid drainage. When a free-flowing effusion is found, thoracentesis can be safely performed at the level of the sixth or seventh intercostal space posteriorly.[8,9] In the presence of a large pleural effusion occupying more than 50% of the pleural cavity, gradual drainage of the fluid, vis-à-vis smaller volumes incrementally over time, has traditionally been advocated to avoid re-expansion pulmonary edema (RPE) and subsequent respiratory insufficiency.[10] However, the overall incidence of clinically significant RPE is low and thoracic surgeons routinely remove more than 1.5 liters of pleural effusion without serious sequelae during thoracoscopic procedures to treat various conditions. In a modern series of 185 patients in whom large-volume thoracentesis was performed in a single setting (>1 liter), only one patient (0.5%) manifested clinical RPE and another four patients (2.2%) exhibited radiographic RPE but without any clinical symptoms.[11] No association was found between the volume of effusion drained and the occurrence of clinical RPE. The occurrence of RPE is therefore rare, and its treatment often consists of a brief period of supportive measures including diuretic therapy and supplemental oxygen in a monitored hospital unit. Endotracheal intubation and mechanical ventilator support may be rarely required, especially in a patient with severely limited physiologic reserves or other clinically significant comorbidities. Recently, several groups have re-examined the arbitrary 1-liter cutoff limit for thoracentesis, as even large effusions ideally should be drained as completely as possible. Subsequent full re-expansion of the compressed lung can greatly relieve dyspnea, and alertness to monitor for the development of clinically symptomatic RPE and instituting early treatment can mitigate any RPE-related sequelae. If the pleural fluid collection is loculated, however, ultrasound or CT guidance may be necessary to direct drainage of accessible portions of the effusion.

Initial cytology from the pleural fluid is positive in approximately 66% of patients with MPE.[2] If initial cytology has negative results, repeat thoracentesis can be performed or the patient may proceed directly to thoracoscopic drainage. Repeat thoracentesis can improve the yield of confirming the diagnosis of MPE in an additional 20% of cases.[12] Thoracoscopy performed via direct pleuroscopy under local anesthesia with intravenous sedation or with video assistance under general anesthesia has a diagnostic yield of nearly 100% for malignant disease involving the pleura in cases in which CT identifies focal lesions on the parietal pleural to direct surgical biopsy.[13] In contrast, the likelihood of obtaining a successful diagnosis from a random biopsy of the pleura without radiographic or thoracoscopic visual evidence of focally abnormal pleura is considerably low.

Biochemical and Pathologic Analysis

If the diagnosis of MPE has not been previously confirmed cytologically, pleural fluid should routinely undergo biochemical analysis, cell counts, cultures, and cytopathology. Light's criteria remain the gold standard definition for exudative effusions such as MPE. Exudative effusions are defined by the presence of at least one of the following: pleural fluid lactic dehydrogenase (LDH) greater than two-thirds of the upper limit of normal serum value (approximately 200 U/mL), pleural fluid-to-serum LDH ratio greater than 0.6, or pleural fluid-to-serum protein ratio greater than 0.5.[14,15] To apply Light's criteria, however, simultaneous measurements of pleural fluid and serum levels of protein and LDH are necessary. Alternatively, meta-analysis of existing studies has identified parameter sets comparable in accuracy to Light's criteria: pleural fluid LDH greater than 0.45 of upper normal limit and pleural fluid cholesterol greater than 45 mg/dL or the combination of pleural fluid protein greater than 2.9 g/dL and pleural fluid LDH and cholesterol as previously defined.[16] The advantage of these alternative criteria sets is that only measurements performed on pleural fluid are needed.

Frequently, pleural fluid from an MPE is blood-tinged or grossly hemorrhagic because of disruption of capillaries or venules by direct tumor invasion or cytokine-mediated increased vascular permeability resulting in erythrocyte diapedesis. MPEs are typically hypercellular, populated with leukocytes (predominantly lymphocytes and monocytes), reactive mesothelial cells, and exfoliated tumor cells. About one-third of MPEs are acidic (pH $<$7.3) and with glucose-to-serum ratios less than 0.5. These biochemical parameters have been found to correlate with advanced disease, poor response to palliative pleurodesis maneuvers, and diminished survival in patients with MPE.[17,18] Identification of malignant cells within the cellular component of the effusion fluid (either via cell smears or cytospin cell blocks) or from a pleural biopsy specimen is diagnostic of the malignant nature of the pleural effusion.

Management and Treatment

Because advanced disease status is often the case with MPE, the overarching goal should be palliation by means of therapy associated with the least morbidity and preserving the best quality of life for the patient. The initial steps in the management of malignant effusions should be focused on confirming a diagnosis of MPE, within reasonable measures, and relieving to the extent possible the degree of symptoms associated with the newly identified pleural effusion. If the patient is asymptomatic from a respiratory standpoint and the corresponding effusion is small in size in a patient eligible to continue further effective anticancer treatment, then it may be prudent to closely observe the patient for the onset of pulmonary symptoms, deferring drainage of the effusion to a later time point, and thus avoiding delay to further anticancer therapy. In select patient series of non–small cell lung cancer and small cell lung cancer, a significant number of malignant effusions will regress by ongoing anticancer treatment alone or in conjunction with simple thoracentesis. The effusion regression response rate can be as high as 58% and 77% in the aforementioned cancers, respectively.[19,20]

In the patient with symptomatic or recurrent malignant effusion despite prior drainage procedures, intervention is warranted and the optimal choice of palliative treatment is primarily dependent on whether full lung re-expansion can occur after evacuation of the effusion to restore normal apposition of the visceral and parietal pleurae.

Thoracentesis

Thoracentesis is an appropriate treatment for MPE in those patients with very limited life expectancy or who cannot tolerate more invasive procedures. However, recurrent effusions are observed in many individuals following thoracentesis alone. In general, instillation of chemical pleurodesis agents into the chest without the placement of a pleural drainage catheter is ineffective because residual or reaccumulating pleural fluid will dilute the concentration of the sclerosing agent, thus diminishing its irritant effects on the pleura. Loculated effusions may also form after such treatment, making subsequent definitive therapy of the pleural effusion more complicated. In select patients presenting with MPE as the initial manifestation, thoracentesis alone followed by immediate systemic chemotherapy may successfully treat the pleural space as well, obviating the need for more invasive procedures in these patients. However, many other patients with MPE require additional intervention to prevent recurrence.

Complex multiloculated MPEs can pose a therapeutic challenge as they are frequently refractory to complete drainage by thoracentesis or chest tube drainage and thus unsuitable for percutaneous chemical pleurodesis. Some have reported that intrapleural instillation of fibrinolytics such as streptokinase or urokinase for loculated MPE can be effective in promoting lysis of fibrinous septations and facilitating complete pleural drainage and ultimately successful pleurodesis.[21,22] This noninvasive approach should be reserved for those patients with poor performance status or who may not tolerate surgical procedures to take down pleural loculations.

Tube Thoracostomy Pleurodesis

Following thoracentesis and re-expansion of the lung, the pleural space ideally should be completely evacuated with a chest tube or pleural catheter over several days to allow for full apposition of the visceral and parietal pleurae. Recurrent effusions occur in 60% to 100% of patients following chest tube drainage alone. In general, obliteration of the pleural space, either by intrapleural instillation of sclerosants or surgical parietal pleurectomy, to incite inflammation and subsequent pleural symphysis is required to provide durable relief and to minimize the recurrence of an uncontrolled MPE. Chemical pleurodesis is a preferred treatment for patients with MPE, and its efficacy is dependent on (1) complete drainage of the pleural space and full re-expansion of the lung to allow for apposition of the pleural surfaces, and (2) instillation of an effective sclerosing agent into the pleural space and retention of this agent in the chest for several hours to induce an intense inflammatory response from the pleurae to form pleural fusion. Such interventions aim to limit the subsequent expansive capacity of the pleural compartment.

To perform chest tube pleurodesis, chest tube insertion should be performed with a 32-Fr (or 28-Fr in a small patient) catheter at the level of the sixth or seventh intercostal space in the midaxillary line and directed posteriorly within the chest to a dependent portion of the pleural cavity. Smaller-caliber chest tubes or pigtail catheters are less ideal for pleurodesis given their propensity to be blocked by clotted blood, proteinaceous fluid, or cellular debris. Once complete drainage is achieved (as confirmed by chest radiograph and daily drainage <150 mL/day), the sclerosing agent (suspended or dissolved in 100–150 mL of normal saline) is instilled into the pleural space via the chest tube. The tube is then clamped for 1 to 2 hours to allow for retention of the sclerosant within the pleural space. Although many practitioners rotate the patient's positioning in bed (lateral decubitus, supine, and prone) to enhance distribution of the sclerosant while it is dwelling inside the pleural cavity, there is a paucity of objective data that support that such maneuvers are necessary for successful pleurodesis.[23] Concurrent intrapleural administration of lidocaine 3 mg/kg (up to 250 mg total) and the sclerosant of choice is recommended, as significant pleuritic chest pain occurs in 7% to 40% of patients having chemical pleurodesis as shown with talc or doxycycline, respectively.[24] Pain, discomfort, and anxiety associated with pleurodesis performed at bedside may also be alleviated with judicious use of intravenous sedatives and narcotics in a monitored setting. Subsequently, the tube is unclamped and the chest drain is connected to suction until the daily drainage is less than 150 mL, at which point the chest tube can be removed from the patient. This method of treatment typically requires hospitalization. However, more recent studies involving small numbers of patients have indicated that pigtail catheter drainage and chemical pleurodesis may be as successful as the more traditional chest tube–pleurodesis approach and associated with less discomfort and acceptable results.[25–27] Nonetheless, simple chest tube drainage of MPE *without* pleurodesis is unlikely to yield durable prevention of MPE recurrence.

Thoracoscopy

Thoracoscopy, also more commonly known as video-assisted thoracoscopic surgery (VATS), is a minimally invasive surgical procedure performed under general anesthesia, usually with single-lung isolation anesthetic technique. The advantages of thoracoscopy include complete drainage of pleural fluid, breakdown of fibrinous septations, evaluation for lung entrapment, biopsy of abnormal parietal pleura, and enhanced distribution of chemical pleurodesis via talc insufflation or instillation of other sclerosing agents such as doxycycline or bleomycin. VATS can be performed using a single 1-cm thoracic port site or several smaller 5-mm ports. When a single port and an operating thoracoscope are used, both pleural biopsy and instillation of the sclerosing agent can be accomplished through the inline working channel of the thoracoscope. As well, mechanical pleural abrasion or parietal pleurectomy can be performed concomitantly via a thoracoscopic approach that results in mechanically induced pleurodesis.

Complications of medical or surgical intervention for MPE include pleuritic pain, low-grade fever, soft tissue hematoma or hemothorax, empyema, RPE, and talc-induced acute respiratory distress syndrome. Moreover, particularly in malignant pleural mesothelioma, a high frequency of chest wall tumor recurrences occurs from seeding of cancer cells (up to 40% of cases) associated with pleural procedures (needle thoracentesis or pleural biopsy, tube thoracostomy, or thoracoscopy trocar site) performed in mesothelioma patients.

Pleurodesis Agents

The following sclerosants have been extensively evaluated in both randomized and nonrandomized clinical studies for their efficacy as pleurodesis agents. Among these agents, only bleomycin is known to possess antitumor activity. Overall, talc is perhaps the most effective sclerosant to date. All sclerosants share a common mechanism of inducing pleurodesis by causing intense pleural inflammation and subsequent adhesive fibrosis of the parietal and visceral pleurae.

Tetracycline and Doxycycline. Tetracycline has been extensively used as a sclerosant to treat pleural effusions of benign and malignant etiologies because of its efficacy, low cost, and safety. The overall efficacy of tetracycline in controlling MPE was 70%.[28,29] However, tetracycline is no longer commercially available for pleurodesis. The semisynthetic antibiotics, doxycycline and minocycline, are currently used in place of tetracycline in the United States. Response rates range from 67% to 88% following doxycycline pleurodesis.[30–32] The side effects are similar to those observed with tetracycline, but most patients require repeated doxycycline instillations for successful pleurodesis. In these reports, only 15% of patients responded to a single treatment, and 9% required more than four instillations. Doxycycline is administered intrapleural as 500 mg in 100 mL of normal saline; also, doxycycline is light-sensitive and care must be taken to avoid exposure of the drug to ambient light.

Bleomycin. Intrapleural administration of bleomycin (60 to 120 U) achieves pleurodesis in about 65% of patients with MPE (range 62%–81%).[33–35] Intrapleural bleomycin is well tolerated and associated with few side effects. In one multicenter randomized trial, bleomycin was found superior to tetracycline for pleurodesis; 70% of patients treated with bleomycin had successful control of their MPE compared with only 47% of patients treated with tetracycline.[28] Unfortunately, bleomycin can be considerably more expensive than its alternatives. Bleomycin has been compared with the less expensive talc in one prospective randomized study of 29 women with MPE secondary to breast cancer—all 10 patients (100%) treated with talc had complete control of their MPE compared with 10 of 15 patients (67%) receiving bleomycin.[35]

Talc. Asbestos-free, gas-sterilized, or heat-sterilized talc may be administered via chest tube as slurry (5 g in 100 mL of normal saline), or insufflated as aerosolized powder (4–8 g) during thoracoscopy or thoracotomy.[36] Talc pleurodesis is highly effective with overall response rates ranging from 80% to 100%.[37–42] Viallat et al.[41] reported on thoracoscopic talc poudrage (dusting of powder) pleurodesis for MPE in 360 cases (88 mesothelioma patients and 272 individuals with other malignancies). Approximately 3 to 4.5 g of heat-sterilized asbestos-free talc was insufflated via atomizer during thoracoscopy. Pleurodesis was successful in 90% of 327 evaluable patients at 1 month, and 82% of individuals had lifelong pleurodesis. Talc has been consistently shown to be superior to other commonly used sclerosing agents (tetracycline, doxycycline, or bleomycin). In a randomized controlled trial, talc poudrage was compared with tetracycline in 33 breast cancer patients with MPE[37]; 92% of patients receiving talc had successful pleurodesis compared with only 42% of patients receiving tetracycline. In another study, successful pleurodesis was observed in 97% of patients undergoing intrapleural talc insufflation by thoracoscopy compared with 70% and 47% of patients receiving bleomycin and tetracycline, respectively.[40] Thoracoscopic talc poudrage was also very effective in producing durable pleurodesis in patients with recalcitrant MPE who failed prior treatment with tetracycline.[43] Aelony et al.[43] reported a response rate of 88% with talc pleurodesis via thoracoscopy in patients whose pleural fluid pH was less than 7.2, contrasting the low response rate (57%) previously reported by Rodriguez-Panadero and Lopez.[18] Failure of talc thoracoscopic pleurodesis in this latter study was better correlated with the presence of entrapped lung rather than low pleural fluid pH per se. Many single-institution studies have similarly demonstrated the effectiveness of talc pleurodesis either by thoracoscopic insufflation of dry talc to the pleural cavity or by intrapleural instillation of talc slurry via chest tubes, but controversies still exist with respect to the cost-effectiveness and the clinical efficacy of each method. A random assignment phase 3 intergroup clinical trial led by the Cancer and Leukemia Group B (CALGB 9334) was initiated in 1993 to address this question.[44] The primary end point was 30-day freedom from radiographic MPE recurrence in surviving patients whose lungs initially re-expanded more than 90%. A total of 501 patients were accrued to this study that compared the efficacy, cost-effectiveness, and quality of life of talc pleurodesis for MPE using either talc slurry (TS) via chest tube or thoracoscopic talc insufflation (TTI). There was no difference between study arms in the percentage of patients with successful 30-day outcome (TS 71% vs. TTI 78%; $P = .169$). However, a subgroup of patients with primary lung or breast cancer had higher success with TTI than with TS (82% vs. 67%; $P = .022$). The 30-day survival rates were similar in both groups and respiratory complications were greater in the TTI group (13.5%) compared with TS group (5.6%; $P = .007$). Quality-of-life measurements demonstrated less fatigue with TTI than TS. Patient ratings for comfort and safety were also higher for TTI, but there were no differences on perceived value or convenience of the procedure.

The most commonly reported adverse effects of talc pleurodesis are fever (16%) and pain (7%). Less common complications include empyema, pneumonitis (similar to acute respiratory distress syndrome), and respiratory failure.[45–47] Pulmonary complications noted in earlier series have not been observed as frequently in modern trials involving large numbers of patients.[41,48–50] More precisely, the deleterious effects of talc appears related to the use of small rather than large particle-sized talc. Small particle-sized talc (<5 micron) is associated with increased pulmonary inflammation, damage, and impaired gas exchange while large particle-sized talc (5–70 micron) is not.[51–53] Thus, modern formulations of medicinal grade sterile size-calibrated talc should be considered safe in the treatment of MPE.

Long-term Indwelling Pleural Catheter

Malignant pleural effusions can be drained over an extended time using a small-caliber biocompatible silicone rubber indwelling catheter such as the Pleurx catheter (Surgimedics, Denver Biomaterials, Inc., Golden, Colorado). The Pleurx catheter is inserted percutaneously and tunneled subcutaneously under local anesthesia and mild intravenous sedation, which can be performed on an inpatient or outpatient basis. The external end of the Pleurx catheter has a unidirectional valve to allow for egress of pleural fluid when desired but prevents the inflow of air into the pleural space (Fig. 151.1). The patient or his or her caretaker can be taught to care for the catheter as the procedure for drainage is very simple and does not require complex nursing skills. The pleural fluid can be drained daily or less frequently as the amount of pleural fluid diminishes over time. The significant advantages of a chronic pleural catheter are the ease of insertion and minimal discomfort due to the catheter, allows for repeated rapid drainage of reaccumulating pleural fluid without additional invasive procedures, and minimal or no hospitalization required for catheter insertion and care. A long-term pleural catheter is indicated when the lung cannot re-expand fully and abut the chest wall despite complete drainage of an effusion; in such cases, pleurodesis is unlikely to be successful irrespective of the chosen sclerosant or approach to pleurodesis.

A prospective multi-institutional random-assignment clinical trial comparing the efficacy of the Pleurx pleural catheter versus chest tube and doxycycline sclerotherapy for recurrent symptomatic MPE in 144 patients was previously reported (randomization ratio of 2:1, 99 patients with indwelling catheter, 45 patients with doxycycline pleurodesis).[54]

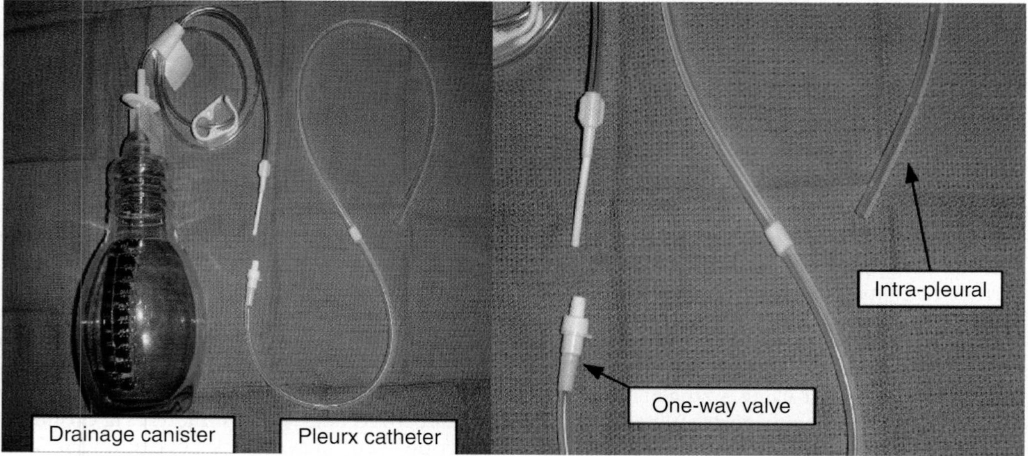

FIGURE 151.1 Pleurx catheter and disposable single-use vacuum drainage canister. The Pleurx catheter consists of a portion placed into the pleural space and an external portion with a one-way valve at the tip to allow for simple intermittent drainage of a malignant effusion.

The two groups in the study were equivalent with respect to performance status or initial dyspnea scores. After treatment, both groups showed similar improvements of respiratory symptoms and had similar morbidity. Because the study treatments differed markedly between the two arms, the most meaningful measure of success is the long-term absence of recurrent pleural effusion. In this study, there was no difference in the numbers of late failure as defined by recurrence of MPE between treatment groups (13% for pleural catheter group and 21% for doxycycline group, $x^2 = 0.23$; $P = .631$). Yet, this same study also demonstrates that long-term indwelling pleural catheters can exhibit safety and efficacy equivalent to chest tube and pleurodesis but requiring less hospitalization (median, 1 day) than chest tube and pleurodesis (median, 6.5 days). Outpatient management of MPE patients with Pleurx catheter was further evaluated by Putnam et al.[55] in whom 100 consecutive patients treated with Pleurx catheters (60 outpatients and 40 inpatients) were compared with 68 patients treated with chest tubes and pleurodesis (all inpatients), also showing that outpatient treatment of MPE with chronic indwelling catheter was safe and effective. Median duration of hospital stay was 7 days and 0 days for inpatient treatments (Pleurx or chest tube with pleurodesis) and outpatient Pleurx, respectively. The cost difference was significant: for patients treated in-hospital, mean charges ranged from $7,000 to $11,000 versus mean charges of $3,400 for outpatient treatments. Long-term indwelling pleural catheters are therefore effective and economical palliative measures for recurrent MPE refractory to pleurodesis or those associated with incomplete lung re-expansion and can decrease the overall in-hospital time for many cancer patients.

Other Surgical Procedures for Malignant Pleural Effusion

Pleurectomy, or resection of the parietal pleura, can be effective in controlling MPE; however, it requires a more invasive and extensive procedure and is not routinely performed because the associated morbidity (23%) and mortality (10%) is unjustifiable in debilitated patients for whom less invasive, and equally successful, treatment options may be available. The pleuroperitoneal shunt, introduced in 1982, has also been used in the treatment of MPE—historically used for recurrent effusions that are refractory to chest tube and pleurodesis or MPEs associated with incomplete lung re-expansion.[56] The shunt is a silicone rubber conduit consisting of a unidirectional valve pump chamber connecting to pleural and peritoneal portions of the catheter. The pumping chamber can be implanted in a subcutaneous pocket or exteriorized. In current practice, the Pleurx catheter has supplanted the pleuroperitoneal shunt in the vast majority of cases given the Pleurx's simpler placement technique and ease of care.

Summary

The prognosis of patients with MPE is primarily dependent on the histologic type of the primary tumor. In general, 65% of patients with MPE will succumb within 3 months and 80% within 6 months. As such, treatment of MPE should focus on expeditious and cost-efficient palliation. Our approach to patients with MPE with full lung re-expansion and good performance status is definitive talc pleurodesis via thoracoscopy. Long-term indwelling pleural catheters are safe and maintain good quality of life—they are especially indicated for patients with entrapped lung or severely limited life expectancies, requiring frequent intermittent drainage of the effusion.

MALIGNANT PERICARDIAL EFFUSION

Patients with malignant pericardial disease may be asymptomatic or may present with a number of manifestations, with pericardial effusion being the most common. Cardiac tamponade due to malignant pericardial effusion (MPCE) accounts for at least 50% of all reported cases of pericardial fluid that require intervention. Similar to malignant pleural effusions, MPCEs are frequently indicative of advanced incurable malignancy; and the overall median survival of patients with MPCE is often less than 6 months.

Clinical Presentation

In most cases, MPCE is observed in patients with an established diagnosis of cancer, typically at late stages of their disease. MPCE is rarely seen as the initial manifestation of extracardiac malignancy—only 90 such cases have been reported in the English literature over a 55-year period.[57] Nonspecific symptoms are frequent with MPE; as such, pericardial effusion may remain unsuspected in patients for whom nonspecific symptoms are otherwise attributed to overall disease progression. Whether cardiac tamponade presents as the initial manifestation of MPCE is highly variable and depends on the rate of fluid accumulation, volume of pericardial fluid, and the patient's underlying cardiac function. Normally, between 15 and 50 mL of fluid is found within the pericardial space, originating as a plasma ultrafiltrate from the visceral pericardium. Physiologic drainage is via the right pleural space in addition to the lymphatics on the parietal pericardium. Intrapericardial pressure rises steeply when the pericardial effusion volume exceeds 150 to 200 mL.[58] With slow accumulation of pericardial fluid, the pericardium undergoes "stress relaxation" and may distend over a period of time to accommodate large volumes of fluid (≥2 liters) prior to exhibiting tamponade physiology from impedance of right atrial and ventricular filling. Classic signs and symptoms of cardiac tamponade include dyspnea, orthopnea, low cardiac output (peripheral vasoconstriction, cold clammy extremities, poor capillary refill, and diaphoresis), jugular venous distention, distant heart sounds, pulsus paradoxus, and narrowed pulse pressure. An electrocardiogram may show low-voltage complexes across all monitoring leads and electrical alternans.

Diagnostic Modalities

Radiographic and Echocardiographic Studies

Pericardial effusion should be suspected in the asymptomatic cancer patient when an enlarged globular water-bottle pericardial silhouette is found on plain posteroanterior and lateral chest radiographs. Moreover, when pericardial effusion and tamponade are caused by malignancy, concomitant parenchymal involvement and/or pleural effusion are observed in 30% to 50% of cases, respectively.[59] CT scan can detect effusions as small as 50 mL of pericardial fluid (Fig. 151.2). However, CT is not the preferred diagnostic examination for pericardial effusion because motion artifacts from the heart and mediastinum can render inaccurate measurement and characterization of the effusion. Cardiac-gated magnetic resonance imaging is good for evaluating for intrapericardial masses as well as determining tumor invasiveness into the myocardium proper.

Once a pericardial effusion is suspected, echocardiography should be performed to confirm the presence and hemodynamic

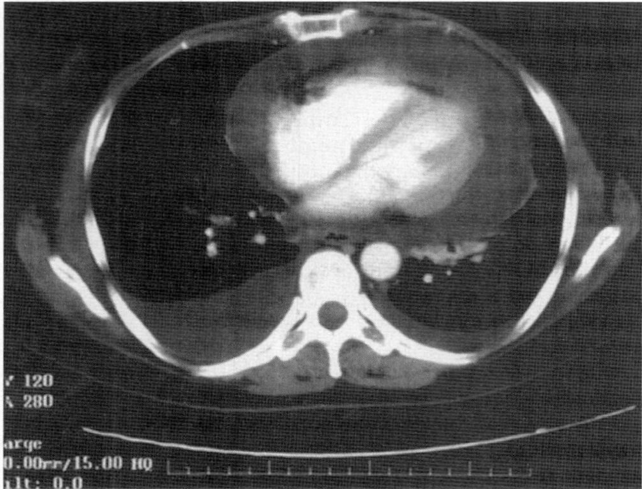

FIGURE 151.2 The chest computed tomographic scan of a patient with metastatic ovarian cancer shows a large pericardial effusion and bilateral pleural effusion (both effusions were proven to be malignant by cytologic and histopathologic examination of tissue obtained by subxiphoid pericardiostomy and tube thoracostomy).

significance of pericardial effusion (Fig. 151.3), and to define the anatomy and size of the effusion as well as the presence of pericardial or intracardiac masses. Right atrial and ventricular collapse are the classic echocardiographic signs of cardiac tamponade, with sensitivity ranging from 38% to 60% and specificity ranging from 50% to 100%.[60] Echocardiography-guided pericardiocentesis is a preferred method to percutaneously drain the effusion.[61]

Cytopathology and Histopathology

The cytology of a pericardial effusion determines definitively its benign or malignant nature. In a series of 95 cases of pericardial effusion,[62] malignant cells were identified in pericardial fluid from two-thirds of cancer patients, with the cytology correlating with histologic diagnosis of the underlying malignancy in 100% of these individuals. In another 190 cases of MPCE diagnosed by pericardiocentesis,[63] pericardial fluid was positive for malignant cells in 79% patients. In contrast, parietal pericardial biopsy is frequently nondiagnostic because the distribution of malignant involvement is not uniform.

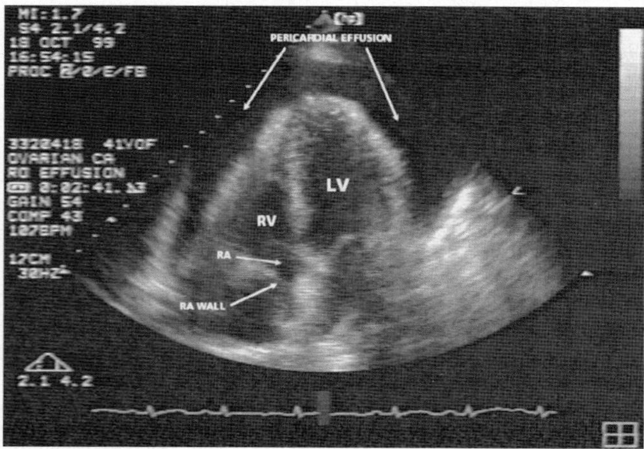

FIGURE 151.3 Two-dimensional echocardiography demonstrates a large pericardial effusion with circumferential fluid collection that resulted in a 1.5-cm separation of the visceral and parietal pericardium. Characteristic M-mode finding of ventricular collapse indicative of early cardiac tamponade. (Courtesy of Evans E. Tucker, MD; Clinical Center, National Institutes of Health, Bethesda, Maryland.)

Treatment

General goals of treatment for malignant pericardial effusion include relief of immediate symptoms, confirmation of the malignant nature of the fluid, and prevention of recurrence. Therapy for MPCE should be tailored to the performance status and prognosis of each patient. Although simple pericardiocentesis can be life-saving in cases of cardiac tamponade, more definitive treatment options for clinically significant MPCE include surgical procedures such as subxiphoid pericardiostomy (pericardial window), transthoracic pericardial window or pericardiectomy (either by VATS or thoracotomy), and medical interventions such as percutaneous tube pericardiostomy with or without intrapericardial instillation of sclerosing agents.

Subxiphoid Pericardiostomy (Subxiphoid Pericardial Window)

Subxiphoid pericardiostomy is the most commonly performed surgical procedure for benign as well as malignant pericardial effusions. This procedure can be performed under local anesthesia with intravenous sedation or general anesthesia. It can be performed as the initial procedure for MPCE in medically stable patients or following needle pericardiocentesis in unstable patients with signs and symptoms of significant cardiac tamponade. A comprehensive review of more than 800 patients with effusion of different etiologies who underwent subxiphoid pericardiostomy indicated an overall mortality rate of 0.62% (range, 0%–2%), an overall morbidity rate of 1.87% (range, 0%–7%), and a recurrence rate of 3.6% (range, 0%-9.1%).[64] These results compare favorably with percutaneous pericardiocentesis/pericardiostomy with or without sclerosis (1.03% mortality, 9.48% morbidity, and 13.8% recurrence (cumulative results from nine reported series including 427 patients).[64]

Partial Pericardiectomy or Pericardial Window via Thoracotomy

Pericardial window or pericardiectomy via thoracotomy is performed uncommonly today. Piehler et al.[65] reviewed surgical management of pericardial effusions in 145 patients and concluded that the extent of pericardial resection influenced incidence of recurrent effusions. However, several recent reports indicated no difference in recurrence rates of patients treated by subxiphoid pericardiostomy compared with those undergoing transthoracic drainage.[66,67] The postoperative complications (pneumonia, pleural effusion, respiratory failure, cardiac arrhythmia, deep vein thrombosis, and pulmonary embolism) are much less frequent following subxiphoid pericardial drainage compared with transthoracic pericardial resection (10% vs. 50%, respectively). Thus, transthoracic pericardial resection is rarely the initial recommended procedure for drainage of MPCE.

If a transthoracic approach is chosen, VATS[68,69] should be used if transthoracic pericardial resection is needed for the treatment of recurrent MPCE following subxiphoid pericardiostomy, or for diagnosis and treatment of simultaneous pleural/parenchymal pathology. Compared with thoracotomy, VATS approaches, when feasible, are more suitable interventions in the debilitated cancer patient. A potential limitation of

VATS pericardiectomy for patients is the need for general anesthesia and single-lung ventilation.

Pericardiocentesis

Pericardiocentesis can be life-saving when performed on patients with hemodynamically significant cardiac tamponade. Removal of as little as 50 mL of pericardial fluid can significantly improve signs and symptoms of acute cardiac tamponade. To perform pericardiocentesis following subcutaneous infiltration with local anesthetic, a needle is inserted at the patient's left subcostal angle of the xiphoid process and directed 45 degrees dorsally, aiming toward the tip of the left scapula. Attachment of an electrocardiogram lead to the aspirating needle during pericardiocentesis can help detect accidental contact of the needle with the myocardium. In cancer patients with symptomatic pericardial effusion, pericardiocentesis may be performed to stabilize the patient prior to additional drainage procedures, such as percutaneous tube pericardiostomy or subxiphoid pericardial window.

Echocardiography guidance during the procedure can reduce complications and improve the success of the pericardiocentesis by delineating the size and location of the effusion relative to cardiac structures. Overall rates of complication and success are approximately 2.4% and 100%, respectively, for echocardiography-guided pericardial drainage,[70] as compared with 4.8% and 90%, respectively, for unassisted pericardiocentesis.[71]

Percutaneous Tube Pericardiostomy and Pericardial Sclerotherapy

Following pericardiocentesis, the rate of fluid reaccumulation has been reported to range from 44% to 70%.[72] To improve these results, a 9-Fr pigtail draining catheter is now routinely placed into the pericardial space using Seldinger technique, following successful needle pericardiocentesis, to enable more complete evacuation of the effusion and provide access for sclerotherapy. Tetracycline and doxycycline have been most extensively evaluated as pericardial sclerosing agents. Maher et al.[72] reported 93 patients with MPCE treated by percutaneous pericardial drainage followed by tetracycline or doxycycline sclerosis. Successful placement of the pericardiostomy tube was achieved in 85 patients (92%). Pericardial effusion was controlled in 75 patients (88%); 10 patients (12%) did not respond to sclerosis, 8 of whom subsequently underwent surgical pericardiostomy. Successful sclerotherapy often requires multiple instillations of tetracycline or doxycycline (range, 1–8; median, 3); 50 patients required three or more instillations to control their effusions. Treatment-related complications (in decreasing order of frequency) included pain, catheter occlusion, fever, and atrial arrhythmias. The favorable results of this minimally invasive treatment strategy are offset by the need for repeated instillations of the sclerosing agent in order to achieve pericardial symphysis, but the procedure's minimal invasiveness confers great advantages over other therapeutic approaches in this patient population. Liu et al.[73] recently conducted a prospective study to evaluate the efficacy and toxicity of bleomycin versus doxycycline as sclerosing agents in MPCE. Bleomycin was found to be as effective as doxycycline in achieving satisfactory control of MPCE but with much less retrosternal pain. As a result, these authors recommend that bleomycin be considered the first-line chemical sclerosing agent for MPCE.

Percutaneous Balloon-Tube Pericardiostomy

Percutaneous balloon-tube pericardiostomy is an extension of the more commonly performed percutaneous tube pericardiostomy. In balloon-tube pericardiostomy, pericardiocentesis is performed as previously described but 150 to 200 mL of fluid is intentionally left in the pericardial space. Subsequently, dilatation of the needle tract is performed under fluoroscopy using a balloon catheter. Ziskind et al.[74] reported that this technique was effective in relieving pericardial effusions in 46 of 50 patients (92%). Procedure-related complications included fever (six patients), pleural effusion requiring chest tube placement or thoracentesis (eight patients), small pneumothorax (two patients), and right ventricular injury requiring surgery (one patient) for an overall clinically significant complication rate of 18%. This is an effective minimally invasive technique of pericardial drainage in experienced hands.

Local or Systemic Therapies for Malignant Pericardial Effusion

Radiotherapy is generally reserved for MPCE associated with lymphoma or breast carcinoma. Vaitkus et al.[75] reported 54 patients treated with radiotherapy as the primary mode of therapy for MPCE. Of these patients, 39 (72%) underwent initial pericardiocentesis. The majority received neither systemic nor other direct pericardial intervention. Radiation therapy was successful in controlling MPCE in 36 patients (66.7%). The highest success rates were noted in leukemia/lymphoma and breast cancer patients (93% and 71%, respectively). Forty-five percent of patients with other solid tumors had adequate control of their effusions as well. Although noninvasive radiotherapy requires repeated visits or even prolonged hospitalization and may theoretically cause acute pericarditis or myocarditis, these potential complications may not be as pertinent in many MPCE patients because of their limited survival.

Patients with MPCE secondary to lymphoma or breast carcinoma may have effusions that respond to systemic chemotherapy. Vaitkus et al.[75] also reported another 46 patients with breast (38 patients), lymphoma (2 patients), or other solid tumors (6 patients) treated with systemic chemotherapy. Of this group, 36 patients (78%) underwent initial therapeutic pericardiocentesis. Systemic chemotherapy prevented recurrence of effusion in 31 patients (67%); successful control of effusion was achieved in over two-thirds of these select individuals irrespective of whether or not pericardiocentesis preceded systemic therapy.

Summary

Malignant pericardial effusion is frequently an indication of advanced, incurable malignancy. Hence, the goals of intervention include relief of symptoms and prevention of recurrence if possible. The treatment of MPCE should proceed in a stepwise fashion. Surgical (subxiphoid pericardiostomy) or medical (ultrasound-guided percutaneous tube pericardiostomy and sclerotherapy) interventions have acceptable risks and provide excellent results. The choice of treatment for any particular patient should consider the individual's specific medical issues and overall life expectancy. In high-volume centers, the minimally invasive echocardiography-guided tube pericardiostomy procedure has become more popular and its use has greatly improved the quality of life for many cancer patients faced with incurable disease. Lastly, recurrent MPCE can be managed either by repeat pericardiostomy or pericardiectomy in select patients.

Selected References

The full list of references for this chapter appears in the online version.

1. Statement of the American Thoracic Society: Management of malignant pleural effusions. *Am J Respir Crit Care Med* 2000;162(5):1987.
2. Fenton KN, Richardson JD. Diagnosis and management of malignant pleural effusions. *Am J Surg* 1995;170:69.
3. Sahn SA. Malignant pleural effusions. *Semin Respir Crit Care Med* 2001;22(6):607.
4. Antunes G, Neville E. Management of malignant pleural effusions. *Thorax* 2000;55(12):981.
5. Chernow B, Sahn SA. Carcinomatous involvement of the pleura: an analysis of 96 patients. *Am J Med* 1977;63(5):695.
6. Johnston WW. The malignant pleural effusion: a review of cytopathologic diagnoses of 584 specimens from 472 consecutive patients. *Cancer* 198515;56(4):905.
7. Noppen M. Normal volume and cellular contents of pleural fluid. *Curr Opin Pulm Med* 2001;7(4):180.
8. Lombardi G, Zustovich F, Nicoletto MO, Donach M, Artioli G, Pastorelli D. Diagnosis and treatment of malignant pleural effusion: a systematic literature review and new approaches. *Am J Clin Oncol* 2010;33(4):420.
9. Putnam JB Jr. Malignant pleural effusions. *Surg Clin North Am* 2002;82:867.
10. Ratliff JL, Chavez CM, Jamchuk A, Forestner JE, Conn JH. Re-expansion pulmonary edema. *Chest* 1973;64:654.
11. Feller-Kopman D, Berkowitz D, Boiselle P, Ernst A. Large-volume thoracentesis and the risk of reexpansion pulmonary edema. *Ann Thorac Surg* 2007;84(5):1656.
12. Sahn SA. Pleural effusion in lung cancer. *Clin Chest Med* 1993;14(1):189.
13. DeCamp MM Jr, Jaklitsch MT, Mentzer SJ, Harpole DH Jr, Sugarbaker DJ. The safety and versatility of video-thoracoscopy: a prospective analysis of 895 consecutive cases. *J Am Coll Surg* 1995;181:113.
14. Light RW, Macgregor MI, Luchsinger PC, Ball WC Jr. Pleural effusions: the diagnostic separation of transudates and exudates. *Ann Intern Med* 1972;77 (4):507.
15. Assi Z, Caruso JL, Herndon J, Patz EF Jr. Cytologically proved malignant pleural effusions: distribution of transudates and exudates. *Chest* 1998;113:1302.
16. Heffner JE, Brown LK, Barbieri CA. Diagnostic value of tests that discriminate between exudative and transudative pleural effusions: Primary Study Investigators. *Chest* 1997;111(4):970.
17. Sahn SA, Good JT Jr. Pleural fluid pH in malignant effusions. Diagnostic, prognostic, and therapeutic implications. *Ann Intern Med* 1988;108:345.
18. Rodriguez-Panadero F, Lopez MJ. Low glucose and pH levels in malignant pleural effusions diagnostic significance and prognostic value in respect to pleurodesis. *Am Rev Respir Dis* 1989;139:663.
19. Fujita A, Takabatake H, Tagaki S, Sekine K. Combination chemotherapy in patients with malignant pleural effusions from non-small cell lung cancer: cisplatin, ifosfamide, and irinotecan with recombinant human granulocyte colony-stimulating factor support. *Chest* 2001;119(2):340.
20. Livingston RB, McCracken JD, Trauth CJ, Chen T. Isolated pleural effusion in small cell lung carcinoma: favorable prognosis: a review of the Southwest Oncology Group experience. *Chest* 1982;81(2):208.
21. Davies CW, Traill ZC, Gleeson FV, Davies RJ. Intrapleural streptokinase in the management of malignant multiloculated pleural effusions. *Chest* 1999;115:729.
22. Gilkeson RC, Silverman P, Haaga JR. Using urokinase to treat malignant pleural effusions. *AJR Am J Roentgenol* 1999;173:781.
23. Dryzer SR, Allen ML, Strange C, Sahn SA. A comparison of rotation and nonrotation in tetracycline pleurodesis. *Chest* 1993;104(6):1763.
24. Robinson LA, Fleming WH, Galbraith TA. Intrapleural doxycycline control of malignant pleural effusions. *Ann Thorac Surg* 1993;55:1115.
25. Morrison MC, Mueller PR, Lee MJ, et al. Sclerotherapy of malignant pleural effusion through sonographically placed small-bore catheters. *AJR Am J Roentgenol* 1992;158:41.
26. Clementsen P, Evald T, Grode G, et al. Treatment of malignant pleural effusion: pleurodesis using a small percutaneous catheter: a prospective randomized study. *Respir Med* 1998;92:593.
27. Patz EF Jr, McAdams HP, Erasmus JJ, et al. Sclerotherapy for malignant pleural effusions: a prospective randomized trial of bleomycin vs doxycycline with small-bore catheter drainage. *Chest* 1998;113:1305.
28. Ruckdeschel JC, Moores D, Lee JY, et al. Intrapleural therapy for malignant pleural effusions: a randomized comparison of bleomycin and tetracycline. *Chest* 1991;100:1528.
29. Gravelyn TR, Michelson MK, Gross BH, Sitrin RG. Tetracycline pleurodesis for malignant pleural effusions: a 10-year retrospective study. *Cancer* 1987;59:1973.
30. Heffner JE, Standerfer RJ, Torstveit J, Unruh L. Clinical efficacy of doxycycline for pleurodesis. *Chest* 1994;105:1743.
31. Mansson T. Treatment of malignant pleural effusion with doxycycline. *Scand J Infect Dis Suppl* 1988;53:29.
32. Kitamura S, Sugiyama Y, Izumi T. Intrapleural doxycycline for control of malignant pleural effusion. *Curr Ther Res* 1981;30:515.
33. Ostrowski MJ. An assessment of the long-term results of controlling the reaccumulation of malignant effusions using intracavity bleomycin. *Cancer* 1986;57:721.
34. Kessinger A, Wigton RS. Intracavitary bleomycin and tetracycline in the management of malignant pleural effusions: a randomized study. *J Surg Oncol* 1987;36:81.
35. Hamed H, Fentiman IS, Chaudary MA, Rubens RD. Comparison of intracavitary bleomycin and talc for control of pleural effusions secondary to carcinoma of the breast. *Br J Surg* 1989;76:1266.
36. Colt HG, Russack V, Chiu Y, et al. A comparison of thoracoscopic talc insufflation, slurry, and mechanical abrasion pleurodesis. *Chest* 1997; 111:442.
37. Fentiman IS, Rubens RD, Hayward JL. A comparison of intracavitary talc and tetracycline for the control of pleural effusions secondary to breast cancer. *Eur J Cancer Clin Oncol* 1986;22:1079.
38. Weissberg D, Ben Zeev I. Talc pleurodesis: experience with 360 patients. *J Thorac Cardiovasc Surg* 1993;106:689.
39. Sanchez-Armengol A, Rodriguez-Panadero F. Survival and talc pleurodesis in metastatic pleural carcinoma, revisited: report of 125 cases. *Chest* 1993;104:1482.
40. Hartman DL, Gaither JM, Kesler KA, et al. Comparison of insufflated talc under thoracoscopic guidance with standard tetracycline and bleomycin pleurodesis for control of malignant pleural effusions. *J Thorac Cardiovasc Surg* 1993;105:743.
41. Viallat JR, Rey F, Astoul P, Boutin C. Thoracoscopic talc poudrage pleurodesis for malignant effusions: a review of 360 cases. *Chest* 1996;110: 1387.
42. Webb WR, Ozmen V, Moulder PV, Shabahang B, Breaux J. Iodized talc pleurodesis for the treatment of pleural effusions. *J Thorac Cardiovasc Surg* 1992;103:881.
43. Aelony Y, King RR, Boutin C. Thoracoscopic talc poudrage in malignant pleural effusions: effective pleurodesis despite low pleural pH. *Chest* 1998;113:1007.
44. Dresler CM, Olak J, Herndon JE, et al. Phase III intergroup study of talc poudrage vs talc slurry sclerosis for malignant pleural effusion. *Chest* 2005;127:909.
45. Kennedy L, Rusch VW, Strange C, Ginsberg RJ, Sahn SA. Pleurodesis using talc slurry. *Chest* 1994;106:342.
46. Rinaldo JE, Owens GR, Rogers RM. Adult respiratory distress syndrome following intrapleural instillation of talc. *J Thorac Cardiovasc Surg* 1983; 85:523.
47. Bouchama A, Chastre J, Gaudichet A, Soler P, Gibert C. Acute pneumonitis with bilateral pleural effusion after talc pleurodesis. *Chest* 1984;86:795.
48. Weissberg D, Ben-Zeev I. Talc pleurodesis: experience with 360 patients. *J Thorac Cardiovasc Surg* 1993;106(4):689.
49. Cardillo G, Facciolo F, Carbone L, et al. Long-term follow-up of video-assisted talc pleurodesis in malignant recurrent pleural effusions. *Eur J Cardiothorac Surg*. 2002;21(2):302.
50. Janssen JP, Collier G, Astoul P, et al. Safety of pleurodesis with talc poudrage in malignant pleural effusion: a prospective cohort study. *Lancet* 2007; 369(9572):1535.
51. Ferrer J, Villarino MA, Tura JM, Traveria A, Light RW. Talc preparations used for pleurodesis vary markedly from one preparation to another. *Chest* 2001;119(6):1901.
52. Ferrer J, Montes JF, Villarino MA, Light RW, García-Valero J. Influence of particle size on extrapleural talc dissemination after talc slurry pleurodesis. *Chest* 2002;122(3):1018.
53. Maskell NA, Lee YC, Gleeson FV, Hedley EL, Pengelly G, Davies RJ. Randomized trials describing lung inflammation after pleurodesis with talc of varying particle size. *Am J Respir Crit Care Med* 200415; 170(4):377.
54. Putnam JB Jr, Light RW, Rodriguez RM, et al. A randomized comparison of indwelling pleural catheter and doxycycline pleurodesis in the management of malignant pleural effusions. *Cancer* 1999;86:1992.
55. Putnam JB Jr, Walsh GL, Swisher SG, et al. Outpatient management of malignant pleural effusion by a chronic indwelling pleural catheter. *Ann Thorac Surg* 2000;69:369.
56. Petrou M, Kaplan D, Goldstraw P. Management of recurrent malignant pleural effusions. The complementary role talc pleurodesis and pleuroperitoneal shunting. *Cancer* 1995;75:801.
57. Fincher RM. Case report: malignant pericardial effusion as the initial manifestation of malignancy. *Am J Med Sci* 1993;305:106.
58. Karam N, Patel P, deFilippi C. Diagnosis and management of chronic pericardial effusions. *Am J Med Sci* 2001;322(2):79.
59. Shepherd FA, Morgan C, Evans WK, et al. Medical management of malignant pericardial effusion by tetracycline sclerosis. *Am J Cardiol* 1987;60:1161.
60. Chong HH, Plotnick GD. Pericardial effusion and tamponade: evaluation, imaging modalities, and management. *Compr Ther* 1995;21:378.

61. Callahan JA, Seward JB, Tajik AJ, et al. Pericardiocentesis assisted by two-dimensional echocardiography. *J Thorac Cardiovasc Surg* 1983;85:877.
62. Wiener HG, Kristensen IB, Haubek A, Kristensen B, Baandrup U. The diagnostic value of pericardial cytology: an analysis of 95 cases. *Acta Cytol* 1991;35:149.
63. Press OW, Livingston R. Management of malignant pericardial effusion and tamponade. *JAMA* 1987;257:1088.
64. Allen KB, Faber LP, Warren WH, Shaar CJ. Pericardial effusion: subxiphoid pericardiostomy versus percutaneous catheter drainage. *Ann Thorac Surg* 1999;67:437.
65. Piehler JM, Pluth JR, Schaff HV, et al. Surgical management of effusive pericardial disease: influence of extent of pericardial resection on clinical course. *J Thorac Cardiovasc Surg* 1985;90:506.
66. Naunheim KS, Kesler KA, Fiore AC, et al. Pericardial drainage: subxiphoid vs. transthoracic approach. *Eur J Cardiothorac Surg* 1991;5:99.
67. Park JS, Rentschler R, Wilbur D. Surgical management of pericardial effusion in patients with malignancies: comparison of subxiphoid window versus pericardiectomy. *Cancer* 1991;67:76.
68. Liu HP, Chang CH, Lin PJ, et al. Thoracoscopic management of effusive pericardial disease: indications and technique. *Ann Thorac Surg* 1994;58:1695.
69. Mack MJ, Landreaneau RJ, Hazelrigg SR, Acuff TE. Videothoracoscopic management of benign and malignant pericardial effusion. *Chest* 1993;103:390.
70. Callahan JA, Seward JB, Nishimura RA, et al. Two-dimensional echocardiographically guided pericardiocentesis: experience in 117 consecutive patients. *Am J Cardiol* 1985;55:476.
71. Clarke DP, Cosgrove DO. Real-time ultrasound scanning in the planning and guidance of pericardiocentesis. *Clin Radiol* 1987;38:119.
72. Maher EA, Shepherd FA, Todd TJ. Pericardial sclerosis as the primary management of malignant pericardial effusion and cardiac tamponade. *J Thorac Cardiovasc Surg* 1996;112:637.
73. Liu G, Crump M, Goss PE, Dancey J, Shepherd FA. Prospective comparison of the sclerosing agents doxycycline and bleomycin for the primary management of malignant pericardial effusion and cardiac tamponade. *J Clin Oncol* 1996;14:3141.
74. Ziskind AA, Pearce AC, Lemmon CC, et al. Percutaneous balloon pericardiotomy for the treatment of cardiac tamponade and large pericardial effusions: description of technique and report of the first 50 cases. *J Am Coll Cardiol* 1993;21:1.
75. Vaitkus PT, Herrmann HC, LeWinter MM. Treatment of malignant pericardial effusion. *JAMA* 1994;272:59.

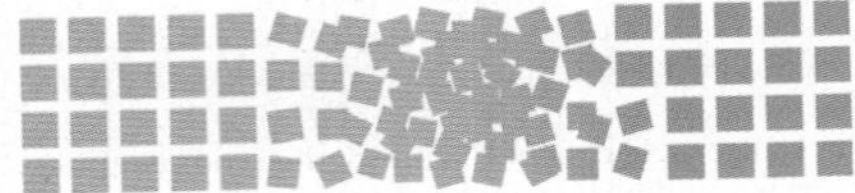

CHAPTER 152 MALIGNANT ASCITES

UDAI S. KAMMULA

Malignant ascites is generally defined as the abnormal accumulation of fluid within the peritoneal cavity as a consequence of advanced cancer. It is often associated with the terminal stage of a variety of neoplasms, including breast, colon, lung, ovarian, pancreatic, and gastric cancers. Although the term *malignant ascites* has been considered pathognomonic for the diffuse implantation and subsequent shedding of tumor cells in fluid throughout the peritoneal cavity, the actual tumor burden and location of the disease can vary quite dramatically. Only approximately two-thirds of patients with malignancy-related ascites have peritoneal carcinomatosis with cytologic evidence of tumor cells in the ascitic fluid.[1] The remaining one-third of patients have ascites secondary to portal hypertension or lymphatic obstruction, as in cases of massive liver metastases or lymphoma, respectively. Malignant ascites often present with challenging clinical symptoms that require thoughtful consideration of palliative options, as well as potentially innovative approaches to treating the underlying disease. For selected patients with cancers such as lymphoma and ovarian cancer, a meaningful therapeutic attempt is warranted with the goal of prolonging survival. The clinical end point for the majority of other patients with malignant ascites has traditionally been palliation of symptoms and improvement of quality of life given the poor prognosis at this stage of the disease. Future therapeutic efforts, however, will be dictated by a better understanding of the pathophysiology of malignant ascites formation and the development of novel regional and systemic treatments for the underlying malignancy. This chapter will summarize the known pathophysiology involved in the development of malignant ascites and provide an overview for the diagnosis and management of this condition.

PATHOPHYSIOLOGY

Normal peritoneal cavity fluid dynamics are governed by a balance of factors that influence peritoneal fluid production versus peritoneal fluid drainage. Malignancies that involve or metastasize to the peritoneum can directly and indirectly alter this balance and result in the accumulation of intra-abdominal ascites. Anatomically, the peritoneum consists of a single layer of mesothelial cells overlying five layers of connective tissue.[2] Mesothelial cells secrete a lubricant fluid consisting of phospholipids and glycosaminoglycans that allows free-sliding movement of the intra-abdominal viscera. The major intraperitoneal fluid production, however, is regulated by the capillaries of the peritoneal membrane, which consist of endothelial cells linked by impermeable tight junctions. This endothelium functions as a barrier that prevents plasma macromolecule loss, but allows highly controlled fluid and solute transport through intracellular pores.[3] The capillary endothelial cell surface also contains negatively charged glycoproteins that further protect against leakage of anionic macromolecules, such as albumin, into the interstitium. Thus, under normal physiologic conditions, a stable oncotic pressure is generated within the capillaries. Regulated flux of fluid between the plasma and the interstitium depends on homeostasis of the oncotic and hydraulic pressure gradients across the capillary bed, the permeability of the capillaries, and the surface area for filtration. The relationship between these parameters is described by Starling's law of capillary hemodynamics,[4]

$$\text{Net filtration} = \text{LpS} \times \left(\begin{array}{c} \text{capillary} \\ \text{hydraulic pressure} \\ \text{gradient} \end{array} - \begin{array}{c} \text{capillary} \\ \text{oncotic pressure} \\ \text{gradient} \end{array} \right)$$

where Lp is the capillary wall permeability (or porosity) and S is the surface area available for fluid movement.

Growing experimental data have suggested that intraperitoneal tumor cells can influence these Starling parameters and result in an increase in net capillary filtration and consequently increased intraperitoneal fluid production. In 1983, Senger et al.[5] described a glycoprotein, initially called *vascular permeability factor* (VPF), which was isolated from the tumor ascites of experimental animals. This tumor-secreted factor caused a rapid and completely reversible increase in microvascular permeability without causing mast cell degranulation or endothelial cell damage. They hypothesized that VPF may be responsible for the increased permeability that is commonly displayed by tumor vessels. Garrison et al.[6] further demonstrated in an experimental rat model of malignant ascites that the intraperitoneal infusion of cell-free malignant ascitic fluid into healthy animals caused an increase in omental edema formation and capillary permeability to protein. Independent studies by Leung et al.[7] described vascular endothelial growth factor (VEGF) as an important regulator of vascular growth and function. Subsequent observations led to the realization that VPF and VEGF were, in fact, the same glycoprotein. VPF/VEGF had the ability to stimulate endothelial cells to proliferate and migrate as well as render these same microvascular endothelial cells hyperpermeable to plasma proteins, leading to profound alterations in the extracellular matrix that favored angiogenesis.[8] Supporting a link between VEGF and malignant ascites was the observation in cancer patients that VEGF protein levels were markedly increased in ovarian, gastric, and colon cancer malignant ascites compared with levels in nonmalignant cirrhotic ascites.[9] Further, in mice engrafted with human ovarian cancer, a function-blocking VEGF antibody completely inhibited ascites production, but only partially inhibited intraperitoneal tumor growth. When the treatment was stopped, the mice rapidly developed ascites and became cachectic. The authors suggested that in ovarian cancer, tumor-derived VEGF was obligatory for ascites formation but not for intraperitoneal tumor growth.[10]

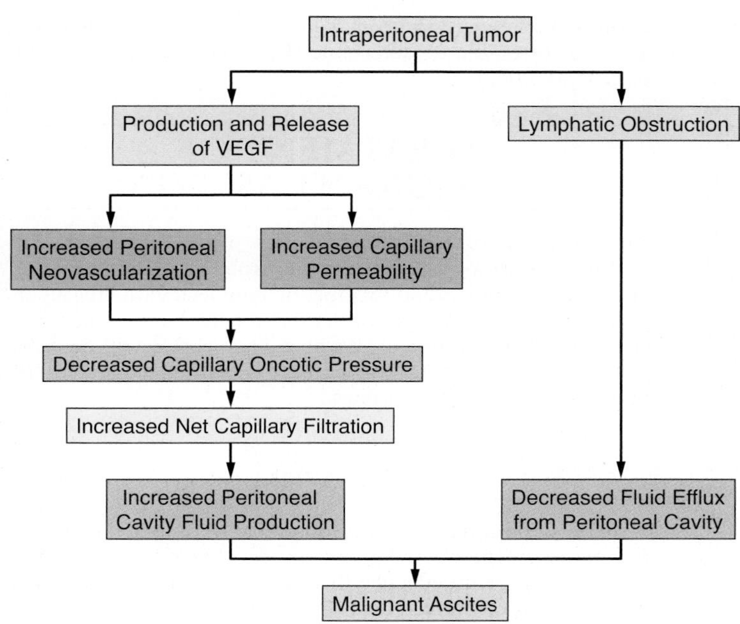

FIGURE 152.1 Proposed pathophysiology involved in malignant ascites development. VEGF, vascular endothelial growth factor.

Tamsma et al.[11] synthesized these observations with basic Starling physiology into a proposed mechanism for the development of malignant ascites. They theorized that tumor-derived factors such as VEGF could result in an increase in capillary permeability (Lp) and vascular surface area (S) through its neovascularization effects. These changes would, in turn, lead to extravasation of plasma proteins into the interstitial space and thereby decrease the capillary oncotic pressure. The alteration in these Starling forces would favor a net increase in capillary fluid filtration and result in the accumulation of intraperitoneal fluid.

$$\uparrow \text{Net filtration} = \uparrow \text{Lp} \uparrow \text{S} \times \left(\begin{array}{c}\text{capillary}\\ \text{hydraulic pressure}\\ \text{gradient}\end{array} - \uparrow \begin{array}{c}\text{capillary}\\ \text{oncotic pressure}\\ \text{gradient}\end{array} \right)$$

In the setting of massive liver metastases with the development of portal hypertension, Starling's formula would reflect an increase in capillary hydraulic pressure and consequently an increase in net filtration. The development of ascites in this situation would mimic the physiology associated with liver cirrhosis.

Intra-abdominal lymphatic obstruction with tumor would further contribute to the development of ascites by preventing compensatory drainage via normal lymphatic channels. Lymphoscintigraphy studies of patients with malignant ascites found that the majority of patients demonstrated diminished lymphatic flow through the major subdiaphragmatic channels.[12] A summary of the proposed pathophysiology involved in malignant ascites development is shown in Figure 152.1.

DIAGNOSIS AND WORKUP

The presence of ascites is established with a combination of history, physical examination, and an imaging test. A careful patient history may reveal subtle complaints of weight gain or an increase in abdominal girth associated with a noticeable difference in the fit of clothing. Patients with large amounts of ascites frequently present with increased abdominal pressure with symptoms of pain, dyspnea, early satiety, nausea, and fatigue. A history of cancer should further raise the suspicion for malignant ascites. Frequently, new-onset ascites is the first presenting sign of an advanced malignancy.[6] Physical examination can reveal abdominal distention with flank dullness to percussion. Classic signs of shifting dullness or a fluid wave can often be elicited if the volume of ascites is approximately 1,500 mL.[13] The accuracy of diagnosing ascites by physical examination in the presence of smaller amounts of fluid is highly variable.

Real-time ultrasonography is an easy and highly sensitive technique to detect volumes of free peritoneal fluid as small as 5 to 10 mL. Simple ascites appears as a homogenous, free-floating collection in the peritoneal cavity with deep acoustic enhancement. Free ascites typically do not displace organs but contour to organ margins. Small amounts of ascites can be visualized by the presence of fluid in Morison's pouch or around the liver as a sonolucent band. In the setting of massive ascites, the small bowel loops have a characteristic "lollipop" appearance due to fluid layering on either side of the floating mesentery. In malignant ascites due to carcinomatosis, the bowel loops often do not float freely but may be fixed to adjacent organs or tethered to intraperitoneal tumor deposits.

Computed tomography (CT) scanning is another effective method to diagnose ascites. Small amounts of ascitic fluid localize in the right perihepatic space, Morison's pouch, and the pouch of Douglas in the pelvis. Patients with malignant ascites may demonstrate a thickened cake of tumor involving the omentum and peritoneal surfaces. CT scanning provides excellent imaging of the pancreas, liver, and pelvic organs, and thus may also provide insight into the site of primary tumor.

The etiologies for newly diagnosed ascites include cirrhosis, congestive heart failure, nephrosis, pancreatitis, infectious processes, malignancy, and benign gynecologic conditions. Malignant ascites account for 10% of all cases of ascites.[14] Approximately one-third of patients with known malignancy and ascites will have nonmalignant causes for their ascites.[15] Differentiating between neoplastic and nonneoplastic causes of ascites can be challenging. Unless associated with overt evidence of peritoneal carcinomatosis, malignant ascites is indistinguishable by physical examination and radiographic appearance from ascites caused by benign conditions. Abdominal paracentesis with ascitic fluid analysis is the most effective way to determine the etiology of the ascites. It is a safe procedure with a low incidence of serious complications. Paracentesis is indicated in patients with new-onset ascites or in clinical situations in which a definitive diagnosis of malignant ascites will influence the staging and management of the patient.

The aspirated fluid appearance from a paracentesis procedure should be noted as it may be helpful in establishing the diagnosis. Normal ascitic fluid is translucent yellow. Infected fluid is frequently turbid or cloudy. A milky character would suggest an elevated triglyceride concentration and is referred to as *chylous ascites*. This type of ascites can be associated with obstruction or injury of the subdiaphragmatic lymphatic channels, as seen in intra-abdominal lymphomas or after surgery. Bloody fluid may result from a traumatic tap or recent intraperitoneal hemorrhage.

Generally, initial laboratory testing of ascitic fluid should mainly focus on establishing either the presence of infection, portal hypertension, or malignancy. The sample of fluid should be sent for cell count with differential, selected chemistries, cytology, and culture, if clinically indicated. Superfluous laboratory analysis is discouraged as it leads to unnecessary cost and irrelevant data for diagnosis. A neutrophil cell count greater than 250/mm^3 is highly suggestive of an intra-abdominal infection and can be obtained with a rapid turnaround. In this setting, a Gram stain and cultures for bacterial, fungal, and acid-fast organisms should be ordered to guide further management. The presence of portal hypertension is most accurately diagnosed by obtaining a serum and ascites level of albumin, rather than traditional total protein concentrations for transudate and exudate determination.[16] The serum-to-ascites albumin gradient can be calculated by subtracting the ascitic fluid albumin value from the serum albumin value. A serum to ascites albumin gradient value of 1.1 g/dL or greater is diagnostic of portal hypertension with 97% accuracy.[16] Conversely, if the serum-to-ascites albumin gradient value is less than 1.1 g/dL, the patient is very unlikely to have portal hypertension, and malignancy should be suspected. Additional select biochemical testing of ascitic fluid for total protein, glucose, lactate dehydrogenase, amylase, triglyceride, and bilirubin levels is warranted with suspicion for a particular etiology (e.g., chyle leak, perforation, pancreatitis).

Malignancy as a cause of ascites can be confirmed with the cytologic presence of tumor cells in the ascitic fluid. Runyon et al.[1] reported that approximately 97% of patients with peritoneal carcinomatosis had positive results for ascitic fluid cytology. However, patients with ascites due to advanced hepatocellular cancer, massive liver metastases, and lymphoma had uniformly negative cytology results. Two additional series report an overall diagnostic sensitivity of 50% to 60% for ascitic fluid cytology.[17,18] To further help differentiate between malignant versus nonmalignant ascites, a variety of ascitic fluid assays have been suggested, including sialic acid levels,[19] human chorionic gonadotropin-β levels,[20] VEGF levels,[9] telomerase activity,[21] fibronectin,[18] and cholesterol levels.[22] Although these reports suggest an improvement in the sensitivity and specificity for the diagnosis of malignant ascites, these tests have not been validated in large analyses to recommend their routine clinical use. Traditional serum tumor markers such as CA 125, carcinoembryonic antigen, and CA 19-9 may be helpful in linking the presence of ascites with an underlying primary malignancy, but the added benefit of measuring the levels of these markers directly in ascitic fluid is unclear.[23]

Among patients diagnosed with malignant ascites, 20% will have tumors of unknown primary origin.[24] For patients with a reasonable performance status, a search for the primary tumor should be pursued, as this may influence treatment strategies. This is especially important for female patients with malignant ascites in whom the most common primary tumor is ovarian cancer, which has effective therapeutic options.[25] Laparoscopy and biopsy have been demonstrated to be safe and minimally invasive techniques to help establish primary tumor diagnosis.[26] Chu et al.[27] performed laparoscopic evaluation of 129 patients with malignant ascites of unknown origin and were able to determine the cause of ascites in 111 patients (86.0%).

TREATMENT OF MALIGNANT ASCITES

The presence of malignant ascites often represents the advanced stage for a heterogeneous group of malignancies. A description of individual therapeutic regimens with efficacy in particular cancers will not be discussed here, but may be referenced in other chapters of this text. This section will describe general approaches to the palliation and management of patients with malignant ascites.

Diuretics

A survey of physician practices found that 61% used diuretics in the management of malignant ascites; however, only 45% believed it to be an effective therapy.[28] The role of diuretics is unclear given the limited data demonstrating their effectiveness and the lack of randomized trials comparing it with other palliative interventions. Becker et al.[29] reviewed the published literature and found that use of a loop diuretic or spironolactone in patients with malignant ascites was associated with symptomatic improvement in 43% of reported patients. Pockros et al.[30] reported in a prospective study that patients with malignant ascites due to massive liver metastases and who had evidence for portal hypertension were more likely to have a response to diuretics. In contrast, patients with ascites caused by peritoneal carcinomatosis or chylous ascites and who did not have portal hypertension were unlikely to have improvement of their ascites. Based on these findings, it has been proposed that diuretics be used in patients with malignant ascites who have evidence of portal hypertension as measured by an elevated serum-ascites albumin gradient 1.1 g/dL or higher. This approach, however, has not been validated in prospective studies.

Paracentesis

External drainage of tense ascites with a therapeutic paracentesis can provide immediate relief of pain and other symptoms for patients with malignant ascites. Drainage of up to 5 L of fluid per procedure has been reported to be well tolerated.[31] Although paracentesis represents the most popular and effective palliative intervention for malignant ascites, the results are short-lived, thus requiring repeated drainage of the reaccumulated fluid. Frequent drainage procedures can be associated with significant protein loss, electrolyte imbalance, hypotension, septic complications, and visceral or vascular injury. In an effort to minimize these complications and to provide greater patient comfort, indwelling percutaneous catheters, such as the Pleurx catheter (Denver Biomedical, Denver, Colorado), were developed to provide long-term access for repeated external drainage.[32] These catheters can be managed at home by the patient or his or her caregiver with drainage performed as needed for comfort. Complications associated with the use of these catheters include infection, catheter blockage, and malpositioning.

Peritoneovenous Shunting

Despite over 30 years of clinical experience, the use of peritoneovenous shunts in patients with malignant ascites is still controversial. The concept for palliative shunting of intractable ascitic

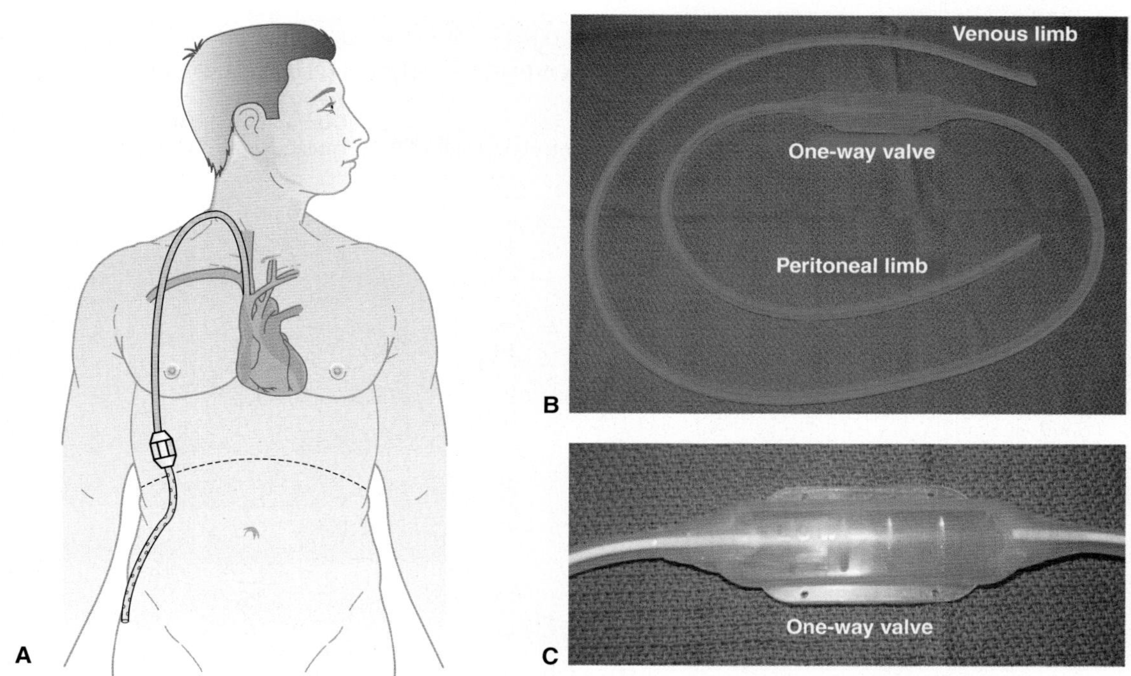

FIGURE 152.2 **A:** Peritoneovenous shunt placement. **B:** Example of Denver shunt components and **(C)** close-up view of compressible chamber and one-way valve. (Section A modified from ref. 44, with permission.)

fluid from the peritoneal cavity back into the intravascular space was introduced by Leveen et al.[33] in 1974. Although they initially introduced the peritoneovenous shunt for the management of nonmalignant ascites, it is now almost exclusively used in the setting of malignant fluid accumulation. The Laveen shunt is an indwelling silastic catheter that consists of an intraperitoneal portion of tubing with fenestrations, an intravascular portion that is commonly positioned in the superior vena cava, and a pressure sensitive one-way valve that regulates flow between the two limbs. The shunt was intended to provide relief by continuously draining and reinfusing accumulated ascites into the bloodstream, thereby avoiding the problems associated with frequent paracentesis, such as patient discomfort, risk of injury to viscera, and protein and fluid loss. The force required to pump the fluid from the peritoneal cavity into the superior vena cava is generated by the natural pressure differential between the abdominal and thoracic cavities. On inspiration, the negative pressure in the chest further increases, thus driving the intraperitoneal fluid through the shunt into the thoracic superior vena cava. The one-way valve allows only unidirectional flow of the ascites and prevents reflux. Another peritoneovenous shunt device, the Denver shunt (Denver Biomedical), uses the same flow mechanism as the Laveen shunt, but has an additional subcutaneous manual pump chamber that the patient or physician may use to clear debris from within the catheter (Fig. 152.2).[34] There are currently no prospective randomized studies comparing the efficacy, patency, and complication rates between these two shunt devices in the treatment of malignant ascites.

Patients are eligible for placement of a peritoneovenous shunt if they have intractable malignant ascites and have demonstrated transient symptomatic improvement with a trial of paracentesis. Traditionally, peritoneovenous shunts are placed in the operating room under local or general anesthesia. However, recently, minimally invasive techniques have allowed interventional radiologists to successfully place these shunts in the radiology suite under mild sedation.[35] Contraindications to peritoneovenous shunt placement include hemorrhagic ascites and chylous ascites, which are associated with high rates of shunt clotting and occlusion. Preoperatively, the ascites should also be evaluated for loculations that would impair effective drainage. Patients should not have cardiac, pulmonary, or renal insufficiency, which could be exacerbated by the increase in intravascular volume from the shunt. Eligible patients should have a life expectancy greater than a month to ensure that the palliative benefits from peritoneovenous shunt placement outweigh the potential complications, which are seen in about 50% of patients.[36,37] The most commonly reported complications are shunt occlusion/poor function, infection, disseminated intravascular coagulopathy, and congestive heart failure. Table 152.1 summarizes 21 recently published series using peritoneovenous shunts in 683 patients with malignant ascites.[38–56] Cumulatively, these studies demonstrate control of ascites in 72% of patients with a mean shunt patency of only 9.6 weeks. The median patient survival ranged from 5 to 33 weeks. Initial concerns for widespread systemic metastases due to the infusion of large numbers of malignant cells into the systemic circulation have not been substantiated in clinical experience or autopsy data from patients managed with peritoneovenous shunts.[57]

In summary, the decision to place a peritoneovenous shunt must take into account its short functional lifespan and the potential morbidities associated with its placement. Although it can provide relief of ascites in about 70% of patients, there have been no randomized trials comparing the palliative benefit of peritoneovenous shunt placement against simple repetitive paracentesis. Proper patient selection is critical to ensure that the overall palliation goals of the individual are met with the placement of these devices.

Intracavitary Chemotherapies

Intraperitoneal administration of chemotherapy attempts to target regional tumor cells in an effort to impact not only

TABLE 152.1

MANAGEMENT OF MALIGNANT ASCITES BY PERITONEOVENOUS SHUNTS (PUBLISHED SERIES SINCE 1985)

Year	Author (Ref.)	No. of Patients	Control of Ascites	Duration of Shunt Patency (mean wk)	Median Patient Survival (wk)
1985	Kostroff et al. (38)	31	—	—	8
1986	Campioni et al. (39)	42	—	—	5
1986	Sonnenfeld et al. (40)	27	21	11	8
1986	Roussel et al. (41)	36	21	14	13
1986	Soderlund (42)	24	—	—	7
1987	Timon et al. (43)	7	6	9	10
1988	Millard et al. (44)	11	10	11	11
1988	Li et al. (45)	7	6	10	4
1988	Shepherd et al. (46)	14	—	5	6
1989	Smith et al. (47)	50	—	10	22
1989	Edney et al. (48)	45	34	—	33
1989	Holm et al. (49)	13	—	—	—
1993	Gough et al. (50)	42	27	—	20
1994	Schumacher et al. (36)	89	57	12	10
1995	Faught et al. (51)	25	22	—	11
1997	Wickremesekera et al. (52)	19	16	—	22
2000	Tueche and Pector (53)	22	22	9	—
2001	Bieligk et al. (37)	51	—	—	7
2002	Zanon et al. (54)	42	37	—	19
2004	Clara et al. (55)	53	—	5	15
2006	Tomiyama et al. (56)	33	13	—	8
	Total	**683**	**292/405 72%**	**Mean 9.6 wk**	**Range, 5–33 wk**

ascites production, but also tumor burden and progression. This approach has the advantage of achieving high local concentrations of cytotoxic drug within the peritoneal cavity while minimizing systemic absorption and systemic toxicity. The choice of appropriate drug is dictated not only by the chemosensitivity of the target cancer, but also by peritoneal pharmacokinetics that limit systemic absorption and local peritoneal toxicities. Appelqvist et al.[58] reported on 23 patients with malignant ascites who were treated with intraperitoneal thiotepa. Temporary partial responses were seen in 8 of 23 (35%) patients. However, significant local toxicities were observed, including intestinal obstruction in five patients (22%). In 60% of autopsied patients there were abundant intestinal adhesions in the peritoneal cavity after the thiotepa administration. Better-tolerated intraperitoneal drugs include cisplatin, carboplatin, mitomycin-C, 5-fluorouracil, and bleomycin. With the exception of ovarian cancer, the effectiveness of intraperitoneal administration of these drugs is unclear given the lack of large randomized clinical studies.

Preclinical models have suggested that effective tumor absorption of locally administered cytotoxic drugs requires the deposits to be less than 10 mm in size.[59] This finding has served as the rationale behind aggressive surgical cytoreduction of intraperitoneal tumors followed by the intraperitoneal administration of chemotherapy. Yan et al.[60] have reported favorable survival in selected patients with colon cancer, appendiceal cancer, and mesothelioma undergoing radical tumor debulking and peritonectomy followed by intraperitoneal chemotherapy. Others have reported the intraoperative use of hyperthermic intraperitoneal chemotherapy delivered via continuous infusion using a roller pump and a heating element immediately after cytoreductive surgery.[61,62] Experimental data have demonstrated that hyperthermia can enhance the cytotoxicity of intraperitoneal chemotherapy.[63] Using this strategy, Ben-Ari et al.[64] reported complete resolution of malignant ascites in 38 of 41 patients with varying histologies. Park et al.[62] reported resolution of ascites in nine of ten patients with mesothelioma. Although encouraging, this aggressive combined approach should be reserved for selected patients with malignant ascites.

Biologic Therapies

A variety of biologic agents have been administered to patients with malignant ascites. Although some responses have been reported, their clinical use is still quite limited and considered investigational. One of the first biologic agents tested was OK-432, a preparation from the Su-strain of *Streptococcus pyogenes*. A single-institution experience of over 400 patients with malignant ascites treated with intraperitoneal OK-432 reported ascites reduction in approximately 60% of patients. Mean survival for patients receiving this therapy was 10.2 months compared with 3.1 months for a control group.[65] These results have not been validated by other investigators.

The first-generation metalloproteinase inhibitor batimastat has been studied in early-phase clinical trials of patients with malignant ascites.[66,67] The drug was well absorbed via the intraperitoneal route and associated with few side effects. Ascites prevention and reduction were reported, but larger trials are needed to define the actual clinical benefit of these inhibitors.

Based on the putative role of VEGF in the pathogenesis of malignant ascites, inhibitors of VEGF function have also been studied in preclinical models. Human clinical trial response data are still pending.

Direct intraperitoneal administration of cytokines including interferon-α,[68] interleukin-2,[69] and tumor necrosis factor[70] has been reported with variable effectiveness in small pilot studies.

References

1. Runyon BA, Hoefs JC, Morgan TR. Ascitic fluid analysis in malignancy-related ascites. *Hepatology* 1988;8:1104.
2. Baron MA. Structure of the intestinal peritoneum in man. *Am J Anat* 1941; 69:439.
3. Renkin EM. Some consequences of capillary permeability to macromolecules: Starling's hypothesis reconsidered. *Am J Physiol* 1986;250:706.
4. Starling E. On the absorption of fluids from the connective tissue spaces. *J Physiol* 1896;19:312.
5. Senger DR, Galli SJ, Dvorak AM, et al. Tumor cells secrete a vascular permeability factor that promotes accumulation of ascites fluid. *Science* 1983; 219:983.
6. Garrison RN, Kaelin LD, Galloway RH, et al. Malignant ascites: clinical and experimental observations. *Ann Surg* 1986;203:644.
7. Leung DW, Cachianes G, Kuang WJ, et al. Vascular endothelial growth factor is a secreted angiogenic mitogen. *Science* 1989;246:1306.
8. Dvorak HF, Brown LF, Detmar M, et al. Vascular permeability factor/vascular endothelial growth factor, microvascular hyperpermeability, and angiogenesis. *Am J Pathol* 1995;146:1029.
9. Zebrowski BK, Liu W, Ramirez K, et al. Markedly elevated levels of vascular endothelial growth factor in malignant ascites. *Ann Surg Oncol* 1999;6:373.
10. Mesiano S, Ferrara N, Jaffe RB. Role of vascular endothelial growth factor in ovarian cancer: inhibition of ascites formation by immunoneutralization. *Am J Pathol* 1998;153:1249.
11. Tamsma JT, Keizer HJ, Meinders AE. Pathogenesis of malignant ascites: Starling's law of capillary hemodynamics revisited. *Ann Oncol* 2001;12:1353.
12. Coates G, Bush RS, Aspin N. A study of ascites using lymphoscintigraphy with 99m Tc-sulfur colloid. *Radiology* 1973;107:577.
13. Cattau EL Jr, Benjamin SB, Knuff TE, et al. The accuracy of the physical examination in the diagnosis of suspected ascites. *JAMA* 1982;247:1164.
14. Runyon BA. Care of patients with ascites. *N Engl J Med* 1994;330:337.
15. Runyon BA. Malignancy-related ascites and ascitic fluid "humoral tests of malignancy." *J Clin Gastroenterol* 1994;18:94.
16. Runyon BA, Montano AA, Akriviadis EA, et al. The serum-ascites albumin gradient is superior to the exudate-transudate concept in the differential diagnosis of ascites. *Ann Intern Med* 1992;117:215.
17. DiBonito L, Falconieri G, Colautti I, et al. The positive peritoneal effusion: a retrospective study of cytopathologic diagnoses with autopsy confirmation. *Acta Cytol* 1993;37:483.
18. Siddiqui RA, Kochhar R, Singh V, et al. Evaluation of fibronectin as a marker of malignant ascites. *J Gastroenterol Hepatol* 1992;7:161.
19. Colli A, Buccino G, Cocciolo M, et al. Diagnostic accuracy of sialic acid in the diagnosis of malignant ascites. *Cancer* 1989;63:912.
20. Grossmann M, Hoermann R, Gocze PM, et al. Measurement of human chorionic gonadotropin-related immunoreactivity in serum, ascites and tumour cysts of patients with gynaecologic malignancies. *Eur J Clin Invest* 1995;25: 867.
21. Tangkijvanich P, Tresukosol D, Sampatanukul P, et al. Telomerase assay for differentiating between malignancy-related and nonmalignant ascites. *Clin Cancer Res* 1999;5:2470.
22. Rana SV, Babu SG, Kocchar R. Usefulness of ascitic fluid cholesterol as a marker for malignant ascites. *Med Sci Monit* 2005;11:136.
23. Torresini RJ, Prolla JC, Diehl AR, et al. Combined carcinoembryonic antigen and cytopathologic examination in ascites. *Acta Cytol* 2000;44:778.
24. Ringenberg QS, Doll DC, Loy TS, et al. Malignant ascites of unknown origin. *Cancer* 1989;64:753.
25. Wilailak S, Linasmita V, Srivannaboon S. Malignant ascites in female patients: a seven-year review. *J Med Assoc Thai* 1999;82:15.
26. Inadomi JM, Kapur S, Kinkhabwala M, et al. The laparoscopic evaluation of ascites. *Gastrointest Endosc Clin North Am* 2001;11:79.
27. Chu CM, Lin SM, Peng SM, et al. The role of laparoscopy in the evaluation of ascites of unknown origin. *Gastrointest Endosc* 1994;40:285.
28. Lee CW, Bociek G, Faught W. A survey of practice in management of malignant ascites. *J Pain Symptom Manage* 1998;16:96.
29. Becker G, Galandi D, Blum HE. Malignant ascites: systematic review and guideline for treatment. *Eur J Cancer* 2006;42:589.
30. Pockros PJ, Esrason KT, Nguyen C, et al. Mobilization of malignant ascites with diuretics is dependent on ascitic fluid characteristics. *Gastroenterology* 1992;103:1302.
31. Stephenson J, Gilbert J. The development of clinical guidelines on paracentesis for ascites related to malignancy. *Palliat Med* 2002;16:213.
32. Richard HM 3rd, Coldwell DM, Boyd-Kranis RL, et al. Pleurx tunneled catheter in the management of malignant ascites. *J Vasc Interv Radiol* 2001;12:373.
33. Leveen HH, Christoudias G, Ip M, et al. Peritoneo-venous shunting for ascites. *Ann Surg* 1974;180:5801.
34. Lund RH, Newkirk JB. Peritoneovenous shunting system for surgical management of ascites. *Contemp Surg* 1979;14:31.
35. Park JS, Won JY, Park SI, et al. Percutaneous peritoneovenous shunt creation for the treatment of benign and malignant refractory ascites. *J Vasc Interv Radiol* 2001;12:1445.
36. Schumacher DL, Saclarides TJ, Staren ED. Peritoneovenous shunts for palliation of the patient with malignant ascites. *Ann Surg Oncol* 1994;1:378.
37. Bieligk SC, Calvo BF, Coit DG. Peritoneovenous shunting for nongynecologic malignant ascites. *Cancer* 2001;91:1247.
38. Kostroff KM, Ross DW, Davis JM. Peritoneovenous shunting for cirrhotic versus malignant ascites. *Surg Gynecol Obstet* 1985;161:204.
39. Campioni N, Pasquali Lasagni R, Vitucci C, et al. Peritoneovenous shunt and neoplastic ascites: a 5-year experience report. *J Surg Oncol* 1986;33:31.
40. Sonnenfeld T, Tyden G. Peritoneovenous shunts for malignant ascites. *Acta Chir Scand* 1986;152:117.
41. Roussel JG, Kroon BB, Hart GA. The Denver type for peritoneovenous shunting of malignant ascites. *Surg Gynecol Obstet* 1986;162:235.
42. Soderlund C. Denver peritoneovenous shunting for malignant or cirrhotic ascites: a prospective consecutive series. *Scand J Gastroenterol* 1986;21:1161.
43. Timon C, Leahy A, Daly P, et al. Peritoneovenous shunts for malignant ascites. *Ir Med J* 1987;80:179.
44. Millard FC, Powis SJ. Management of intractable malignant ascites using the Denver peritoneovenous shunt. *J R Coll Surg Edinb* 1988;33:138.
45. Li MK, Shiu W, Li AK. The use of double valve Denver peritoneal venous shunt for malignant ascites. *Ann Acad Med Singapore* 1988;17:129.
46. Shepherd KE, Miller BJ. Peritoneovenous shunts—devices of last resort. *Can J Surg* 1988;31:444.
47. Smith DA, Weaver DW, Bouwman DL. Peritoneovenous shunt (PVS) for malignant ascites: an analysis of outcome. *Am Surg* 1989;55:445.
48. Edney JA, Hill A, Armstrong D. Peritoneovenous shunts palliate malignant ascites. *Am J Surg* 1989;158:598.
49. Holm A, Halpern NB, Aldrete JS. Peritoneovenous shunt for intractable ascites of hepatic, nephrogenic, and malignant causes. *Am J Surg* 1989;158:162.
50. Gough IR, Balderson GA. Malignant ascites. A comparison of peritoneovenous shunting and nonoperative management. *Cancer* 1993;71:2377.
51. Faught W, Kirkpatrick JR, Krepart GV, et al. Peritoneovenous shunt for palliation of gynecologic malignant ascites. *J Am Coll Surg* 1995;180:472.
52. Wickremesekera SK, Stubbs RS. Peritoneovenous shunting for malignant ascites. *N Z Med J* 1997;110:33.
53. Tueche SG, Pector JC. Peritoneovenous shunt in malignant ascites: the Bordet Institute experience from 1975–1998. *Hepatogastroenterology* 2000;47:1322.
54. Zanon C, Grosso M, Apra F, et al. Palliative treatment of malignant refractory ascites by positioning of Denver peritoneovenous shunt. *Tumori* 2002;88:123.
55. Clara R, Righi D, Bortolini M, et al. Role of different techniques for the placement of Denver peritoneovenous shunt (PVS) in malignant ascites. *Surg Laparosc Endosc Percutan Tech* 2004;14:222.
56. Tomiyama K, Takahashi M, Fujii T, et al. Improved quality of life for malignant ascites patients by Denver peritoneovenous shunts. *Anticancer Res* 2006;26:2393.
57. Tarin D, Price JE, Kettlewell MG, et al. Clinicopathological observations on metastasis in man studied in patients treated with peritoneovenous shunts. *Br Med J* 1984;288:749.
58. Appelqvist P, Silvo J, Salmela L, et al. On the treatment and prognosis of malignant ascites: is the survival time determined when the abdominal paracentesis is needed? *J Surg Oncol* 1982;20:238.
59. Los G, Mutsaers PH, van der Vijgh WJ, et al. Direct diffusion of cis-diamminedichloroplatinum (II) in intraperitoneal rat tumors after intraperitoneal chemotherapy: a comparison with systemic chemotherapy. *Cancer Res* 1989;49:3380.
60. Yan TD, Stuart OA, Yoo D, et al. Perioperative intraperitoneal chemotherapy for peritoneal surface malignancy. *J Transl Med* 2006;4:17.
61. Loggie BW, Fleming RA, McQuellon RP, et al. Cytoreductive surgery with intraperitoneal hyperthermic chemotherapy for disseminated peritoneal cancer of gastrointestinal origin. *Am Surg* 2000;66:561.
62. Park BJ, Alexander HR, Libutti SK, et al. Treatment of primary peritoneal mesothelioma by continuous hyperthermic peritoneal perfusion (CHPP). *Ann Surg Oncol* 1999;6:582.
63. Los G, Smals OA, van Vugt MJ, et al. A rationale for carboplatin treatment and abdominal hyperthermia in cancers restricted to the peritoneal cavity. *Cancer Res* 1992;52:1252.
64. Ben-Ari G, Scott D, Zippel D, et al. Continuous hyperthermic peritoneal perfusion (CHPP) for malignant ascites and irresectable intra-abdominal cancer. *Gan To Kagaku Ryoho* 2000;27:436.
65. Katano M, Morisaki T. The past, the present and future of the OK-432 therapy for patients with malignant effusions. *Anticancer Res* 1998;18:3917.
66. Beattie GJ, Smyth JF. Phase I study of intraperitoneal metalloproteinase inhibitor BB94 in patients with malignant ascites. *Clin Cancer Res* 1998;4:1899.
67. Parsons SL, Watson SA, Steele RJ. Phase I/II trial of batimastat, a matrix metalloproteinase inhibitor, in patients with malignant ascites. *Eur J Surg Oncol* 1997;23:526.
68. Stuart GC, Nation JG, Snider DD, et al. Intraperitoneal interferon in the management of malignant ascites. *Cancer* 1993;71:2027.
69. Lissoni P, Barni S, Tancini G, et al. Intracavitary therapy of neoplastic effusions with cytokines: comparison among interferon alpha, beta and interleukin-2. *Support Care Cancer* 1995;3:78.
70. Rath U, Kaufmann M, Schmid H, et al. Effect of intraperitoneal recombinant human tumour necrosis factor alpha on malignant ascites. *Eur J Cancer* 1991;27:121.

CHAPTER 153 PARANEOPLASTIC SYNDROMES

MICHAEL BOYIADZIS, FRANK S. LIEBERMAN, LARISA J. GESKIN, AND KENNETH A. FOON

Paraneoplastic syndromes are a group of clinical disorders associated with malignant diseases that are not directly related to the physical effects of the primary or metastatic tumor. The syndromes may be due to (1) tumor production of substances that directly or indirectly cause distant symptoms, (2) depletion of normal substances that leads to a paraneoplastic manifestation, or (3) host response to the tumor that results in the syndrome.

Paraneoplastic syndromes may parallel the underlying malignancy, and successful treatment of the tumor leads to disappearance of the syndrome. However, many paraneoplastic syndromes, especially those of an immune or neurologic etiology, do not predictably resolve with treatment of the underlying malignancy.

The paraneoplastic syndrome may be the first sign of a malignancy, and its recognition may be critical for early cancer detection. Proteins secreted in paraneoplastic syndromes may be used as tumor markers. In some situations, the underlying disease cannot be treated, but the symptoms and complications of the paraneoplastic syndrome can be successfully managed.

ENDOCRINOLOGIC MANIFESTATIONS OF CANCER

Cancers can produce endocrine syndromes or "ectopic" hormone syndromes through the production of cytokines, protein hormones, or hormone precursors by the tumor. Rarely, cancers can metabolize steroids to biologically active forms, which results in paraneoplastic syndromes. In general, treatment of the underlying malignancy results in resolution of the endocrinologic paraneoplastic syndrome.

Ectopic Adrenocorticotropic Hormone Syndrome

Cushing syndrome comprises a large group of signs and symptoms that reflect prolonged and inappropriately high exposure to glucocorticoids.[1] The differential diagnosis of a patient with hypercortisolism includes Cushing disease, adrenal dysfunction, ectopic ACTH (corticotropin) production, corticotropin-releasing hormone (CRH) overproduction, and exogenous ingestion of prescribed steroids, usually for nonendocrine disorders. Cushing disease is the most common cause of spontaneous Cushing syndrome, occurring in 60% to 70% of patients with Cushing disease. It results from the hypersecretion of ACTH by a pituitary corticotroph adenoma. Ectopic ACTH syndrome is responsible for 5% to 10% of the cases of spontaneous Cushing syndrome; it is caused by a variety of ACTH-secreting nonpituitary tumors. About 20% to 30% of spontaneous Cushing syndromes are independent of ACTH and are caused by primary adrenocortical tumors. Ectopic ACTH production is commonly associated with small cell lung cancer (SCLC) but can also be found in a variety of neoplasms including thyroid carcinomas, pancreatic cancer, pheochromocytomas, and thymic carcinomas.[2,3] Rarely, Cushing syndrome may results from the production of CRH from nonpituitary tumors.

The proopiomelanocortin (*POMC*) gene (chromosome 2p23) consists of three exons, with the first encoding a leader sequence, the second encoding the signal initiation sequence and the N-terminal portion of the POMC peptide, and the third encoding most of the mature peptide sequence, including ACTH and β-lipotropin.[4] The processing of POMC in nonpituitary tumors is often incomplete with the release into the circulation of POMC fragments with reduced biological activity. Thus, despite the high frequency of POMC in SCLC and carcinoid tumors, only a very small proportion of patients develop a clinical syndrome of ACTH excess. Signs and symptoms of classic hypercortisolism include truncal obesity, purple striae, hypertension, fatigue, moon facies, buffalo hump, weakness, depression, amenorrhea, hirsutism, decreased libido, osteopenia, osteoporosis, impaired wound healing, impaired glucose-tolerance diabetes, easy bruising, and edema. The signs of Cushing syndrome may be absent in the cancer patients because of rapid evolution of the clinical picture. Ectopic ACTH production from SCLC causes myopathy with weakness, muscle wasting, weight loss, hyperpigmentation, and hypokalemia. Carcinoid tumors that secrete ectopic ACTH may cause signs and symptoms that overlap those of pituitary-dependent Cushing disease and paraneoplastic ACTH overproduction.

Diagnosis

Distinguishing between pituitary adenoma, ectopic ACTH production, and primary adrenal disorders is the primary focus of the diagnostic workup.[5] Initial testing for Cushing syndrome includes one of the following tests: urine-free cortisol (at least two measurements), late-night salivary cortisol (two measurements), 1-mg overnight dexamethasone suppression test, and longer low-dose dexamethasone suppression test (2 mg/d for 48 hours). For subsequent evaluation of abnormal initial test results, the dexamethasone CRH test or the midnight serum cortisol test can be performed.

Once the diagnosis of ectopic ACTH production has been established, localization is the most important aspect of therapy. Because a major portion of patients with ectopic ACTH secretion have lung cancer, plain radiography followed by computed tomography (CT) detects more than 90% of the lung tumors associated with ACTH production.[6] The exception is bronchial carcinoid tumors, which are visualized on 36% of initial radiographs but are localized by CT scan in approximately 85% of cases.[7] Octreotide receptor scintigraphy has been used for localizing ACTH-producing tumors because many such tumors have octreotide receptors.[8] An additional advantage of localizing tumors with octreotide receptor scintigraphy is the suggestion of possible therapy with either somatostatin analogues or radiolabeled octreotide.

Treatment

The prognosis is dictated by the nature of the tumor and the severity of the hypercortisolism. Most patients with overt metastases at the time of presentation die of the cancer within 1 year, although patients with indolent tumors may survive for many years.[9–11] The optimal therapy of the ectopic ACTH syndrome is surgical excision of the tumor, thereby removing the source of ACTH and curing the metabolic disorder. For those patients with nonresectable tumors, the hypercortisolism can be controlled with adrenal enzyme inhibitors, such as *ketoconazole, metyrapone,* and *etomidate*. Primary suppression of ACTH production can be accomplished by cytotoxic chemotherapy for the primary malignancy or octreotide suppression of ACTH release. In general, chemotherapy alone is not associated with control of Cushing syndrome but is combined with adrenal suppression in most cases Although bilateral adrenal removal is effective in treating Cushing syndrome, the patient must have life-long glucocorticoid and mineralocorticoid replacement. The use of laparoscopic adrenalectomy has been reported to provide effective palliation in patients with Cushing syndrome, with minimal morbidity.[12] Some patients have indolent tumors and a long life expectancy but cannot be cured surgically. These patients can be treated with *mitotane* to achieve a medical adrenalectomy.

Syndrome of Inappropriate Antidiuretic Hormone Production

The principal malignancy associated with the syndrome of inappropriate antidiuretic hormone production (SIADH) is SCLC (75% of cases), although others have been described (non–small cell lung cancer, head and neck cancer, and other cancers are also associated with SIADH).[13]

Clinical Features and Diagnosis

The hyponatremia is initially mediated by antidiuretic hormone (ADH)–induced water retention. The ensuing volume expansion activates secondary natriuretic mechanisms, resulting in sodium and water loss and the restoration of near euvolemia. The combination of water retention due to inappropriate ADH secretion and secondary solute loss (sodium and potassium) accounts for the fall of the plasma sodium concentration. Thus, patients with SIADH have normal volume status, hyponatremia with hypo-osmolality, elevated renal excretion of sodium (>20 mEq/L), and urine osmolality greater than plasma osmolality.

Most patients are asymptomatic, but when symptoms develop they generally reflect central nervous system (CNS) toxicity. In the early stages, patients complain of fatigue, anorexia, headaches, and mildly altered mental status. As the syndrome progresses, patients may experience continued delirium, confusion, and seizures. Ultimately, patients develop refractory seizures, coma, and, in rare cases, death. Most patients, however, experience minimal symptoms and are discovered to have hyponatremia on routine laboratory evaluation.

In evaluating a patient with hyponatremia and cancer, other causes of hyponatremia need to be considered. In general, the first step in evaluating patients with hyponatremia is to assess volume status. SIADH is one of the euvolemic hyponatremic states. Therefore, it is necessary to rule out states associated with volume overload such as congestive heart failure, nephrotic syndrome, malignant ascites, and significant liver disease. It is also essential to exclude extrarenal volume depletion and renal sodium wasting. Once the patient is determined to be euvolemic, other causes of euvolemic hyponatremia must be ruled out, including hypothyroidism, renal dysfunction, and Addison disease. A careful review of medications is also essential including the current use of cytotoxic agents associated with SIADH (cyclophosphamide, ifosfamide, and vinca alkaloids).[14,15]

Once the diagnosis of SIADH is made, a wide variety of causes must be considered, including CNS diseases (stroke, acute psychosis, inflammatory and demyelinating disorders, seizures, infections, and hemorrhage), pulmonary diseases (pneumonia, tuberculosis, pulmonary abscess, acute respiratory failure), and drug effects (phenothiazines, tricyclic, antidepressants, chlorpropamide, clofibrate, oxytocin, desmopressin, opiate derivatives, serotonin reuptake inhibitors).[16]

Treatment

As with any syndrome associated with ectopic hormone production, treating the underlying disease is the most effective means of controlling SIADH. Chemotherapy treatment of the associated SCLC is generally associated with improvement in the syndrome. SIADH has not been shown to be a negative prognostic factor in terms of response to chemotherapy. In situations in which brain metastases are present, the addition of radiation therapy is important.

Correction of the hyponatremia is guided by the severity of the clinical presentation and the pace with which the hyponatremia developed. If it developed slowly, correction is safe over several days. The rate of correction should not exceed 8 to 10 mmol/L on any day of treatment. The initial rate of correction can be 1 to 2 mmol/L per hour for several hours in patients with severe symptoms of hyponatremia. Indications for stopping the rapid correction are the cessation of life-threatening manifestations or serum sodium of 125 to 130 mmol/L (or lower if the baseline serum sodium concentration is <100 mmol/L).

The mainstay in asymptomatic hyponatremia is water restriction (500 to 1,000 mL per 24 hours). The associated negative water balance raises the plasma sodium concentration toward normal. However, it can also lead to volume depletion due to unmasking of the sodium deficit.[17,18]

Severe, symptomatic, or resistant hyponatremia often requires the administration of salt. Although both sodium and water are retained in hypovolemia, sodium handling is intact in patients with SIADH. Thus, when isotonic saline is administered, the sodium is excreted in the urine, whereas some of the water may be retained, leading to possible worsening of hyponatremia. Consequently, to elevate the plasma sodium in patients with SIADH, 3% hypertonic saline may need to be administered. It is important not to raise the serum sodium level too rapidly because of the risk of central pontine myelinolysis.[19]

The effect of hypertonic saline can be enhanced if given with a loop diuretic. This lowers the urine osmolality and increases water excretion by impairing the renal responsiveness to ADH.

In the event that the serum sodium level does not normalize, pharmacologic agents such as demeclocycline that inhibit the effect of arginine vasopressin on the kidneys are indicated. Monitoring of renal function is required because demeclocycline has nephrotoxic effects. The arginine vasopressin (AVP)-receptor antagonists, a new class of agents, correct hyponatremia by directly blocking the binding of AVP with its receptors. In clinical trials AVP-receptor antagonists have increased serum osmolality and normalized the serum [Na(+)] in hyponatremia associated with SIADH, cirrhosis, or congestive heart failure. These drugs may have a therapeutic role in cancer-related hyponatremia.

Oncogenous Osteomalacia

Tumor-induced or oncogenous osteomalacia is a rare paraneoplastic syndrome characterized by osteomalacia with hypophosphatemia, hyperphosphaturia, and undetectable or inappropriately low circulating concentrations of 1,25-dihydroxyvitamin D_3. Mean age at diagnosis is approximately 35 years. Patients typically present with bone pain, phosphaturia, renal glycosuria, hypophosphatemia, normocalcemia with normal parathyroid hormone function, low levels of 1,25-dihydroxyvitamin D_3, and increased alkaline phosphatase levels. It is therefore important to monitor serum phosphate levels as well as to identify other biochemical features such as abnormally low circulating levels of $1,25(OH)_2D_3$ and low phosphate reabsorption per liter of glomerular filtrate.

Studies have isolated fibroblast growth factor 23 (FGF-23) as a possible phosphaturic substance that may be produced by tumors that induce osteomalacia.[20] FGF-23 genes are expressed at higher levels in tumors causing tumor-induced osteomalacia.[21] Its effect of inhibiting phosphorus transport across the proximal renal tubule epithelium has been demonstrated *in vitro*. FGF-23 levels are detectable in human serum and found to be elevated in patients with oncogenic osteomalacia.[22]

The majority of neoplasms causing this syndrome are benign, but the syndrome has also been described with carcinoma of the lung, multiple myeloma, and prostate cancer.[23,24] The typical tumor involves prominent giant cells, spindle cells, and a high degree of vascularity. Approximately half of the tumors are in the lower extremities, and the remaining tumors are divided between the head and neck and upper extremities, with some patients having tumors at multiple sites.

The definitive therapy is removal of the tumor, if possible, which leads to clinical and biochemical cure. Otherwise, treatment requires large doses of vitamin D and phosphate.

Hypoglycemia

Insulinomas frequently produce hypoglycemia; however, hypoglycemia associated with non–islet cell tumors is an unusual paraneoplastic syndrome. Mesenchymal tumors and hepatic carcinomas are responsible for two-thirds of cases associated with hypoglycemia. These tumors are typically large, often invade the liver, and have a protracted course. The patient may present with typical signs and symptoms of hypoglycemia, including generalized neurologic abnormalities. Gastrointestinal (GI) stromal tumors, lymphomas, and adrenal carcinomas are among the tumors that have been associated with hypoglycemia.[25–27]

The causes of paraneoplastic hypoglycemia are varied. Hypoglycemia is caused by increased secretion of insulinlike growth factor (IGF-II), altered IGF-II processing, and increased bioavailability. The serum from affected patients contains increased concentrations of IGF-II while tumor extracts have revealed high levels of IGF-II mRNA.[28,29] Characteristically, the fast-acting insulin and C-peptide levels are appropriately suppressed during hypoglycemia. In addition, hypermetabolism of glucose, production of substances stimulating ectopic insulin release, production of hepatic glucose inhibitor, insulin binding by a monoclonal protein, insulin receptor proliferation, or, rarely, ectopic insulin production are associative causes of hypoglycemia.[30–32]

The treatment of paraneoplastic hypoglycemia initially involves glucose infusion. After this, tumor debulking should be carried out, although the long-term effect of debulking is poorly understood. If treatment of the tumor is not possible, then the use of subcutaneous and long-acting intramuscular glucagons, high-dose corticosteroids, or somatostatin analogues may be considered.

HEMATOLOGIC MANIFESTATIONS OF CANCER

Erythrocytosis

The most common solid tumor leading to erythrocytosis is renal cell carcinoma, and hepatoma is the next common malignancy. Other tumors leading to erythrocytosis include Wilms tumor, hemangiomas, cerebellar hemangioblastoma, sarcomas, uterine fibroids, adrenal tumors, and pheochromocytomas.[33–36]

The causes of erythrocytosis are inappropriate production of erythropoietin by the neoplastic cells, decreased plasma volume, mechanical interference with renal blood supply, and functional interaction between aldosterone, rennin, and erythropoietin.[37]

It is important to rule out other causes of erythrocytosis, even in the presence of a tumor. There are obvious causes of polycythemia secondary to arterial desaturation associated with hemoglobinopathies, carboxyhemoglobinemia, and chronic hypoxic states. Paraneoplastic erythrocytosis rarely requires specific therapy other than control of the underlying neoplasm and occasional phlebotomy when required.

Granulocytosis

Granulocytosis with elevation of the white blood cell count above 15×10^9/L without infection or leukemia is common in neoplasms.[38–40] Neoplasms most commonly associated with granulocytosis include Hodgkin's lymphoma, lymphoma, and a variety of solid tumors, including gastric, lung, pancreatic, and brain cancers, and malignant melanoma. Paraneoplastic granulocytosis consists of mature neutrophils, in contrast to chronic myelogenous leukemia, in which more immature forms are seen, along with basophils and eosinophils, a decreased leukocyte alkaline phosphatase level, elevated vitamin B_{12} level and vitamin B_{12}–binding capacity, and the presence of the Philadelphia chromosome. The common mechanism associated with tumor-associated granulocytosis is tumor production of growth factors.

Granulocytopenia

Granulocytopenia is typically secondary to chemotherapy, radiation therapy, or tumor infiltration of bone marrow. Rarely, tumors may produce a factor that suppresses granulopoiesis by interfering with any number of growth factors. As well, there are rare reports of antibodies against granulocytes in patients with Hodgkin's lymphoma and non–chemotherapy-induced neutropenia.[41] Neutropenia associated with large granular lymphocytic leukemia and lymphoma may be caused by immune dysregulation of T cells. The preferred therapy for severe granulocytopenia is direct stimulation with growth factors, including granulocyte colony-stimulating factor or granulocyte-macrophage colony-stimulating factor.

Eosinophilia and Basophilia

Eosinophilia is associated with Hodgkin's lymphoma and mycosis fungoides and is rarely associated with other lymphomas and solid tumors. The tumor cells may be producing a factor that specifically stimulates eosinophil production, such as granulocyte-macrophage colony-stimulating factor, interleukin 3, or interleukin 5.[42–44] Extremely high eosinophil counts can cause symptoms similar to those of Löffler syndrome, which is associated with nodular pulmonary infiltrates with cough and fever in rare cases. Basophilia is associated with chronic myelogenous leukemia and a variety of other myeloproliferative disorders but does not typically give rise to symptoms.

Thrombocytosis

Thrombocytosis is quite common in cancer patients and may be associated with Hodgkin's lymphoma, lymphomas, and a variety of carcinomas and leukemias.[45] Thrombocytosis is expected early in the course of a variety of myeloproliferative neoplasms, including polycythemia vera and chronic myelogenous leukemia. In patients with cancer and thrombocytosis it is important to exclude underlying secondary causes such as inflammatory disorders, hemorrhage, iron deficiency, and hemolytic anemia. The thrombocytosis secondary to malignancies may be caused by tumor overproduction of thrombopoietin or interleukin 6.[46] Thrombosis and hemorrhage are rarely associated with this paraneoplastic syndrome, and treatment is not generally indicated.

Thrombophlebitis

Patients with cancer have a hypercoagulable state. The spectrum of homeostatic abnormalities in cancer patients ranges from abnormal coagulation tests in the absence of clinical manifestations to massive thromboembolism.

Clinical thromboembolism occurs in as many as 11% of patients with cancer and is the second leading cause of death in patients with overt malignant disease. Clearly, cancer-related thrombosis represents a complex imbalance of coagulation and fibrinolysis: increased fibrinogen and platelet catabolism; decreased levels of protein C, protein S, and antithrombin; direct generation of thrombin; and thrombocytosis all represent abnormalities associated with malignancy.[47] The activation of coagulation factors V, VII, IX, and XI as well as fibrinogen and fibrin-degradation products occurs. Increased secretion of plasminogen activators and a decrease in their inhibitors, activation of platelets, and increased platelet aggregation all contribute to thrombosis risk.[48]

The majority of cancers associated with thromboembolic events are clinically evident and have been previously diagnosed at the time of the event. However, thromboembolism can precede the diagnosis of malignancy.[49–51] The risk is highest for cancers of the ovary, pancreas, and liver. Patients with idiopathic first-time thromboembolism should not have an extensive workup beyond age-appropriate or symptom-directed cancer screening. Any abnormality observed on initial testing should then be further investigated. Patients with recurrent idiopathic deep venous thrombosis who represent a high-risk group may have more aggressive search for malignancy.

Patients with venous thromboembolism who are receiving chemotherapy or have active cancer or metastatic disease should receive anticoagulation for an indefinite period if there are no contraindications.[52–54] Patients should also be re-evaluated frequently for the individual risk–benefit ratio of ongoing anticoagulant therapy, taking into consideration the overall risk to the patient including the quality of life and life expectancy.

Nonbacterial Thrombotic Endocarditis

Nonbacterial thrombotic endocarditis may lead to thrombotic or hemorrhagic complications and may occur with or without disseminated intravascular coagulation. It is characterized by sterile, verrucous fibrin-platelet lesions on the heart valves. Although nonbacterial thrombotic endocarditis most commonly affects the aortic and mitral valves, any cardiac valve may be affected; vegetations on the atrioventricular valves are present on the atrial surface, while those involving the semilunar valves are found on the ventricular surface of the valve. Although the pathogenesis of nonbacterial thrombotic endocarditis is not fully understood, the most important predisposing factors appear to be an underlying coagulopathy (usually disseminated intravascular coagulation), microscopic edema, degeneration of valvular collagen, and perhaps a local valvular effect of mucin-producing carcinomas.

The diagnosis of nonbacterial thrombotic endocarditis is not easily made and is considerably more elusive than that of bacterial endocarditis. Not only is the marker of bloodstream infection lacking, but the small friable vegetations frequently embolize, leaving only small remnants to be identified on the valve. Indeed, cardiac murmurs, a hallmark of bacterial endocarditis, are frequently absent, and echocardiography is less sensitive for the detection of nonbacterial thrombotic endocarditis than it is for bacterial endocarditis. Nonbacterial endocarditis should be suspected in cancer patients who present with ischemic embolic events and is most commonly seen with adenocarcinomas of the lung and pancreas.[55]

Treatment of the underlying malignancy is the primary therapy. Anticoagulation therapy should be withheld from patients with disseminated cancer when there is no hope of tumor regression; in most instances, a diagnosis of nonbacterial thrombotic endocarditis warrants anticoagulation therapy. The most effective agent appears to be heparin, and recurrent thromboembolic complications have been reported after heparin therapy was discontinued.[56]

RENAL MANIFESTATIONS

Glomerular Disorders

Membranous nephropathy has been clearly associated with malignancy. Although the majority of cases are idiopathic, in the elderly as many as 22% may be associated with cancer. Various forms of malignancy have been described in patients with membranous nephropathy. The most common has been carcinomas of the lung, colon, and stomach. In 80% of cases of paraneoplastic nephrotic syndrome, the diagnosis is made concurrently or after that of the malignant disease. Nephrosis-range proteinuria, hypertension, and microscopic hematuria characterize the syndrome. Immune complexes are thought to play a role in malignancy-associated glomerular disease. A proposed mechanism is that deposition of tumor antigens in the glomeruli promotes antibody deposition and complement activation, leading to epithelial cell and glioblastoma multiforme injury and consequent proteinuria. The responsible antigens include fetal antigens, autologous nontumor antigens, tumor-associated antigens, and viral antigens.[57] Nephrotic syndrome may resolve with successful treatment of the underlying malignancy. Careful monitoring for the development of thrombosis, especially renal vein thrombosis, is warranted in severe protein wasting. Extensive workup beyond age-appropriate or symptom-directed cancer screening is not recommended in patients newly diagnosed with membranous nephropathy.

Other glomerular diseases include membranoproliferative glomerulonephritis[58] and minimal-change disease. Hodgkin's lymphoma is the cause of most cases of minimal-change disease, with lymphoproliferative disorders, pancreatic carcinoma, and mesothelioma also reported. Approximately 10%

PRACTICE OF ONCOLOGY

to 15% of cases precede the lymphoma, and 40% to 50% manifest after the tumor is diagnosed. There is a parallel relationship between the activity of the lymphoma and the degree of proteinuria. Curative treatment of Hodgkin's lymphoma is followed by remission of the disease, and curative surgery of the solid tumors can lead to resolution of the hematuria. The proteinuria tends to reappear with disease relapse or remits with secondary treatment.

Other cancer-associated glomerulopathies include focal and segmental glomerulosclerosis with chronic lymphocytic leukemia (CLL), T-cell lymphomas, and acute myelogenous leukemia; immunoglobulin A (IgA) nephropathy with lung, head and neck, and pancreatic cancers, mycosis fungoides, and liposarcoma; and membranoproliferative glomerulonephritis with CLL, Burkitt and other lymphomas, hairy cell leukemia, and malignant melanoma. Rarely, rapidly progressive glomerulonephritis has been associated with lymphoma and monoclonal gammopathies.[58]

Other tubular abnormalities, such as protein cast precipitation syndrome, paraprotein disease, uric acid nephropathy, and hypercalcemia and its treatment are discussed in Chapter 146.

CUTANEOUS MANIFESTATIONS OF CANCER

A wide variety of cutaneous syndromes is associated with malignancies and may precede, be concurrent with, or follow the discovery of the underlying malignancy. It is critical that, once a potential cutaneous paraneoplastic syndrome has been diagnosed, an appropriate systemic evaluation for a neoplasm be undertaken. The initial workup includes detailed medical history, physical examination, and routine screening laboratory tests, followed by focused studies, with emphasis on those malignancies most strongly associated with the particular skin lesion. Likewise, recognition of a particular diagnosis as a cutaneous paraneoplastic manifestation of malignancy is required to ensure an appropriate and timely therapy for the ailment. A true paraneoplastic process satisfies two main criteria: strong association of dermatosis with malignancy and its parallel course. Consequently, very common conditions frequently associated with a wide variety of common cancers may not represent true association, as in the case of the sign of the Leser-Trélat. It refers to the sudden appearance of seborrheic keratoses secondary to an occult malignancy,[59] and was described most commonly in adenocarcinoma of the stomach, but also in lymphoma, breast, colon cancers, and squamous cell carcinoma among many other cancers.[60]

DISORDERS OF EPIDERMAL PROLIFERATION AND KERATINIZATION (PAPULOSQUAMOUS DISORDERS)

Papulosquamous disorders are delineated in Table 153.1. Acquired ichthyosis is characterized by generalized dry, crackling skin, hyperkeratosis and rhomboidal scales of the extensor surfaces; histologically, it shows true hyperkeratosis (unlike simple dry skin or xerosis). It is most commonly associated with Hodgkin's lymphoma but may be seen with other lymphomas, multiple myeloma, Kaposi sarcoma,[61] and other malignancies. It tends to develop after the malignancy and runs a parallel course.

Palmar hyperkeratosis associated with internal malignancy may be diffuse (tylosis) or punctuate. Tylosis may be associated with higher incidence of esophageal (Howel-Evans syndrome),[62] breast, and ovarian carcinoma.[63] Punctuate hyperkeratosis patients present with discrete hyperkeratotic papules

TABLE 153.1

PAPULOSQUAMOUS ERUPTIONS

Disease	Description	Malignancy	Cause	Comments
Acrokeratosis paraneoplastica or Bazex disease[a]	Symmetric, psoriasiform acral hyperkeratosis	Squamous cell carcinoma of the esophagus, head and neck, lung	Unknown	Male predominance
Paget disease	Erythematous keratotic patch over areola/nipple, urogenital, or perianal area	Breast, uterine, ovarian, prostate, anal	Direct extension of underlying malignancy	Occurs in fewer than 3% of breast cancers; extramammary
Erythema gyratum repens[a]	Advancing concentric rings of erythema with trailing scales	Lung, breast, uterus, gastrointestinal cancers	Unknown	80% Associated with malignancies
Necrolytic migratory erythema[a]	Macules and papules progressing to epidermal necrolysis	Glucagonoma	Glucagon or metabolic product	Clinically similar to Zn deficiency; Somatostatin beneficial
Exfoliative dermatitis	Progressive erythema followed by scaling	Cutaneous T-cell and other lymphomas, Hodgkin's disease	Unknown	Accounts for 10%–20% of all exfoliative dermatitis
Acquired ichthyosis[a]	Generalized dry, crackling skin, hyperkeratosis, rhomboidal scales	Hodgkin's disease, other lymphomas, multiple myeloma, Kaposi sarcoma	Unknown	Should be differentiated from hereditary ichthyosis, which occurs before age 20 y
Dermatomyositis[a]	Erythema or telangiectasias of the knuckles, chest, periorbital region	Miscellaneous	Unknown	Malignant disease reported in up to 50%, precedes carcinoma by days to years

[a]True paraneoplastic syndrome.

on the palms and have higher incidence of cancers of the breast and uterus.[64] Arsenic exposure may play a role.

Acrokeratosis paraneoplastica (Bazex syndrome) is characterized by symmetric psoriasiform acral hyperkeratosis (usually on hands, feet, ears, and nose). It is associated with male gender and squamous cell carcinoma of the esophagus, head and neck, or lungs.[65] It precedes the tumor in 60% of cases. Cross-reaction between the basement membrane and tumor antigens as well as secretion of IGF-1 or transforming growth factor-α are postulated to cause this syndrome.[66]

Pachydermoperiostosis is subperiosteal new bone formation associated with acromegalic features. Patients develop painful bones and thickening of the skin with creation of new folds; thickened forehead and scalp, lips, ears, and lids (leonine facies); macroglossia; clubbing; and excessive sweating.[67] It is most often associated with bronchogenic carcinoma.

Exfoliative dermatitis is a progressive erythroderma with scaling (not in the setting of cutaneous T-cell lymphoma) that may be associated with lymphomas[68] and rarely with solid tumors (lung, liver, prostate, and others). It may resolve following dissection of the tumors.

Erythema gyratum repens presents as rapidly advancing (at a speed of 1 cm a day) concentric rings of erythematous plaques with trailing scales ("wood-grain" pattern) on the trunk and proximal extremities and precedes malignancy more than 80% of the time.[69] It is associated with lung, breast, uterine, cervix, prostate, and GI tract malignancies, as well as multiple myeloma.

Paget disease of the breast results from direct extension of the ductal carcinoma of the breast in 95% of the cases. It is characterized by erythematous keratotic patches over the areola, nipple, or accessory breast tissue.[70] Extramammary Paget disease can be primary or secondary, with the latter representing secondary involvement from an underlying carcinoma originating most commonly in the lower GI or urinary tract. As for the primary disease, skin adnexa (eccrine or apocrine glands), ectopic mammary glands, or pluripotential germinative cells in the epidermis and other structures have been implicated as a possible source of neoplastic cells. It presents as an erythematous exudative dermatitis located on the vulva in women, the genitals in men, and the perianal area in both sexes. Extramammary Paget disease is associated with an internal malignancy in 50% of cases, usually carcinoma of the uterus, rectum, bladder, vagina, or prostate gland. Most of these cancers are usually related to the site of the dermatosis.

DISORDERS OF CUTANEOUS DISCOLORATION AND DEPOSITION

Acanthosis nigricans is characterized by gray-brown hyperpigmented, velvety plaques that often affect the neck, flexor areas, and anogenital region (Table 153.2). The malignant and benign forms are similar in appearance, but the malignant form progresses rapidly, and pruritus is common. The malignant variety may precede the tumor, occur simultaneously, or follow the appearance of the tumor. It is typically associated with adenocarcinomas of the GI tract, predominantly gastric cancer, but has also been associated with a variety of other adenocarcinomas, including lung, breast, ovarian, and even hematologic malignancies.[71] The pathogenesis remains uncertain, but appears to be linked to overproduction of transforming growth factor by the tumor.[72] Tripe palms are often associated with acanthosis nigricans. Patients show thickened palms with exaggerated hyperkeratotic ridges, a velvety texture, and brown hyperpigmentation.[73] Tripe palms usually occur in patients with lung and gastric cancer.

Melanosis is caused by abnormal deposition of melanin, which results in diffuse gray-brown pigmentation in the skin.[74] Melanosis may appear before or after melanoma detection, and it is often accentuated in light-exposed areas of the upper body. Histopathologically, there are melanin granules in perivascular or interstitial melanophages, and free granules in the dermis. Melanosis can also be caused by ACTH-producing tumors.[75]

Generalized icterus is late manifestation of malignancy due to intrahepatic or extrahepatic obstruction (e.g., pancreatic cancer) or infiltration (e.g., amyloidosis due to multiple myeloma). Vitiligo is a variant of leukoderma (white discoloration of the skin) due to loss of skin pigment rarely associated with thyroid carcinoma and melanoma. New appearance of vitiligo in melanoma patients may signify appearance of developing of metastatic disease.

Plane xanthomas (lipid depositions) are large yellow-orange patches and plaques on the trunk most frequently

TABLE 153.2

DISORDER OF EPIDERMAL DISCOLORATION AND SKIN THICKENING

Disease	Description	Malignancy	Cause	Comments
Acanthosis nigricans	Gray-brown symmetric velvety plaques on the neck, axillae, flexor areas, and anogenital region	Adenocarcinomas; predominantly gastric	Unknown	Benign form is associated with syndrome X
Tripe palms	Hyperpigmented velvety thickened palms with hyperkeratotic ridges	Gastric, lung	Unknown	Often associated with acanthosis nigricans
Generalized melanosis	Diffuse gray-brown skin pigmentation	Melanoma, adrenocorticotrophic hormone–producing tumors	Melanin deposits in dermis	May be seen in benign conditions
Pachydermoperiostosis[a]	Thickening of skin, lips, ears, lids; forehead, scalp; clubbing; excessive sweating	Lung	Unknown	May be seen in lung abscess and benign tumors

[a]True neoplastic syndrome.

associated with multiple myeloma,[76] but also found in many other leukemias and lymphomas.

Amyloid deposits, which may manifest as macroglossia, superficial waxy yellow and pink elevated nodules on the skin, may be associated with multiple myeloma or Waldenström's macroglobulinemia.

NEUTROPHILIC DERMATOSES

Among the neutrophilic dermatoses (Table 153.3) is Sweet syndrome, which presents with acute onset of fever, neutrophilia, and the appearance of erythematous painful juicy cutaneous plaques on the face, neck, and upper extremities. Histopathologically, there is a dense dermal infiltration of well-differentiated neutrophils. Association with malignancy occurs in 20% of cases. Acute myelogenous leukemia is the most common malignancy, although association with myeloproliferative and lymphoproliferative disorders, myelodysplastic syndromes, and carcinomas has also been reported.[77] Sweet syndrome may precede the detection of malignancy by many years or occur concomitantly. The cause is thought to be hypersensitivity, and response to corticosteroids is usually prompt.

The lesions of pyoderma gangrenosum appear as painful papules that subsequently ulcerate and form nonhealing ulcers with violaceous irregular borders and a purulent, hemorrhagic exudate with a necrotic base. Histopathologic examination demonstrates a dense neutrophilic infiltrate. Pyoderma gangrenosum is associated with hematologic malignancies,[78] including cutaneous T-cell lymphomas,[79] as well as gastric carcinoma[80] and other GI abnormalities.

VASCULAR ABNORMALITIES

Vasculitis is observed in 4.5% to 8% of malignancies; it is found in solid tumors (most commonly lung non–small cell), squamous cell carcinoma of esophagus, and prostate, as well as in hematologic malignancies (hairy cell leukemia, lymphomas, and rarely multiple myeloma).[81,82]

Purpura secondary to underlying malignancy may have various causes such as thrombocytopenia, consumption coagulopathy, vascular injury, vasculitis, and immunoglobulin abnormalities. Hematologic paraneoplastic syndromes were previously discussed.

Cutaneous ischemia may be a manifestation of neoplasms of solid organs and blood. Etiology of ischemia varies depending on underlying cause and may include autoimmune phenomena (such as Raynaud), leukostasis (e.g., in leukemia with very high white blood cell count), and increased blood viscosity (e.g., polycythemia vera, cryoglobulinemia, multiple myeloma, or lymphoma).

Multifocal migratory thrombophlebitis has been associated with numerous malignancies especially in patients younger than 50 years of age. It is most commonly associated with GI, but also lung, prostate, and ovary cancers, as well as leukemias and lymphomas. It may be related to the hypercoagulable state associated with advance cancer. Specific syndrome of a cord-like thrombophlebitis of anterior chest (Mondor disease) may be associated with breast cancer.

ENDOCRINE AND METABOLIC DISORDERS

A variety of malignancies of endocrine organs result in metabolic disorders causing paraneoplastic manifestations in the skin. Systemic nodular panniculitis or subcutaneous fat necrosis is characterized by violaceous nodules, is associated with adenocarcinoma of the pancreas, and may be accompanied by polyarthralgia, fever, and eosinophilia.[83] Necrolytic migratory erythema is solely associated with glucagonoma and is characterized by erythema, papules, vesicles, and pustules that progress to blistering and epidermal necrosis on the central face, lower abdomen, perineum, and buttocks and other areas[84] (Table 153.1). The eruption clears after resection of the tumor, but in metastatic glucagonoma may wax and wane. Somatostatin is beneficial because of its suppression of glucagon secretion.[59]

Cushing syndrome is associated with broad purple striae, hyperpigmentation, telangiectasia, atrophy of the skin, facial plethora, acne vulgaris, ecchymosis, and mild hirsutism. Addison syndrome can occur with adrenocortical carcinoma and is characterized by generalized hyperpigmentation, especially in scars, pressure points, and points of friction. Hirsutism is associated with virilism and is caused by increased levels of glucocorticoids and testosterone, typically from adrenal and ovarian tumors. Carcinoid syndrome may cause telangiectasias and sclerodermalike and pellagralike skin changes. Many of these lesions resolve with treatment of the underlying malignancy.

Flushing is an episodic reddening of the face and neck, lasting a few minutes, typically associated with the carcinoid syndrome but also seen with leukemia, medullary carcinoma of the thyroid, renal cell carcinoma, and other malignancies (such as systemic mastocytosis and pheochromocytoma)[85–87] (Table 153.4). Harlequin syndrome is unilateral flushing and sweating due to ciliary ganglion destruction by cancer. Vasoactive peptides such as serotonin are thought to mediate this syndrome.[86] Isolated palmar erythema may be observed in liver failure caused by primary or secondary hepatic malignancy.

BULLOUS DISORDERS

Paraneoplastic pemphigus is most frequently seen in B-cell lymphoproliferative disorders, including lymphomas and CLL

TABLE 153.3

NEUTROPHILIC DERMATOSES

Disease	Description	Malignancy	Cause	Comments
Sweet syndrome	Erythematous painful raised cutaneous plaques	Hematologic malignancies, various carcinomas	Unknown	Responds to steroids; 10%–15% associated with cancer
Pyoderma gangrenosum	Painful papules, ulcers, violaceous borders, and purulent exudates	Multiple myeloma, squamous cell cancers; cutaneous T-cell non-Hodgkin's lymphoma	Unknown	Responds to steroids, may be associated with IBD, rheumatoid arthritis

IBD, inflammatory bowel disease.

TABLE 153.4

MISCELLANEOUS LESIONS

Disease	Description	Malignancy	Cause	Comments
Flushing[a]	Episodic reddening of face and neck	Carcinoids, medullary thyroid carcinoma	Serotonin or other vasoactive peptides	—
Hypertrichosis lanuginosa acquisita (malignant down)[a]	Rapid development of fine, long, silky hair, especially on ears and forehead	Lung, colon, bladder, uterus, gallbladder	Unknown	High association with cancer
Localized amyloidosis	Waxy yellow plaques and nodules	Multiple myeloma, Waldenström's macroglobulinemia	Unknown	Also associated with primary systemic amyloidosis
Pruritus[a]		Lymphomas, leukemias, multiple myeloma, CNS tumors, hepatic and other abdominal tumors	Unknown	Unexplained generalized pruritus necessitates an evaluation for an underlying systemic disease

[a]True paraneoplastic syndrome.

as well as Castleman disease, thymoma, Waldenström macroglobulinemia, and spindle cell neoplasms.[88] Patients develop painful oral (stomatitis) and conjunctival ulcers and erosive skin lesions. Internal organ involvement is common, and respiratory failure causes death in 30% of patients with this disorder.[89] In contrast to other types of pemphigus, severe mucosal involvement and distinct histopathologic features reminiscent of erythema multiforme and pemphigus with reactivity to numerous antigens simultaneously are hallmarks of paraneoplastic pemphigus[59,89,90]; the pathogenesis is not understood. The course of the disease is progressive and independent of the underlying malignancy, particularly the stomatitis. Corticosteroids and cyclosporine are beneficial.[88] Mycophenolate mofetil is added in patients with refractory disease.[91] It is extremely recalcitrant to therapy and prognosis is very poor.

COLLAGEN-VASCULAR DISEASES

Dermatomyositis (DM) may be idiopathic or paraneoplastic, and has been linked to malignancy in over 25% of cases. Clinical signs of DM include a heliotrope rash of the periorbital skin, shawl sign, V-neck erythema, periungual telangiectasias and erythema, and Gottron sign (pathognomonic erythematous papules on the extensor surfaces of joints).[92] Patients also exhibit progressive proximal muscle weakness. DM most commonly is associated with cancers of reproductive organs in women and respiratory tract in both genders.[59] Malignancy can precede, follow, or occur simultaneously with dermatomyositis; the most frequent pattern is onset of cancer within 1 year of the diagnosis of dermatomyositis.

Other collagen vascular disorders such as systemic lupus erythematosus may be rarely associated with leukemias or lymphomas. Pemphigus erythematosus is associated with thymoma and myasthenia gravis.

DISORDERS OF HAIR

Sudden change in pattern or quality of hair may be a sign of underlying malignancy. Diffuse hair loss may be present in advance cancers from numerous factors (besides chemotherapy-induced alopecia), including telogen effluvium and alopecia areata.[93] Increased hair growth has been associated with numerous malignancies,[94] including endocrinologic tumors, may be secondary to porphyria cutanea tarda, or as hypertrichosis lanuginosa acquisita (malignant down). Hypertrichosis lanuginosa acquisita is the sudden appearance of downy hair on the entire body. Lung cancer is the most commonly associated malignancy, followed by colon, bladder, ovarian, uterine, and pancreatic cancers.[95]

SKIN NEOPLASMS ASSOCIATED WITH INTERNAL MALIGNANCY

A Muir-Torre syndrome is autosomal dominant familial cancer syndrome (Table 153.5). A hallmark of Muir-Torre syndrome is the presence of numerous sebaceous gland neoplasms, including carcinomas that may precede, follow, or coexist with visceral cancers.[96] It is most often associated with GI tract adenocarcinoma of the colon or genitourinary tract, or lymphoma.

Cowden disease or multiple hamartoma syndrome is autosomal dominant syndrome with numerous tumors of the hair follicles called *tricholemmomas* located on the face. These patients have very high risk of breast and thyroid carcinoma. Bilateral mastectomies may be recommended. Mammography and other exposure of the breast tissue to radiation is contraindicated. Patients also have polyposis coli and are at increased risk for GI malignancy.[97]

Gardner syndrome is an autosomal dominant familial adenomatous polyposis, a colorectal cancer syndrome characterized by hundreds of adenomatous colorectal polyps, with an inevitable progression to colorectal cancer by age of 40. Cutaneous manifestations may be the presenting sign and include numerous epidermal cysts and soft tissue tumors. Desmoid tumors may be locally invasive and difficult to control. Other typical findings are congenital hypertrophy of the retinal pigment epithelium, osteomas, and dental anomalies.[98]

Mucosal neuroma syndrome is a variant of multiple endocrine neoplasia syndrome.[99] Children with multiple endocrine neoplasia type 2B have typical facies, marfanoid habitus, and characteristic mucosal neuromas. There is strong association with medullary thyroid carcinoma, and metastases are common. Pheochromocytomas are common as well, and are often bilateral.

Nevoid basal cell carcinoma syndrome (Gorlin-Goltz syndrome) is characterized by the presence of multiple basal cell

TABLE 153.5

HEREDITARY DISORDERS

Disease	Description	Malignancy	Heredity	Comments
Muir-Torre or syndrome[a]	Sebaceous gland neoplasm	Colon cancer, lymphomas	AD, mismatch repair genes defect hMLH1 and hMSH2	Part of HNPCC, or Lynch syndrome
Cowden syndrome (multiple hamartoma syndrome)	Fibromas of oral mucosa with "cobblestoning" of the tongue, facial trichilemmomas	Thyroid, breast, endometrial, renal cell carcinomas	AD, mutations in *PTEN* gene	Associated with multiple hamartomas, lipomas, neuromas, hemangiomas, thyroid adenomas. *No mammography for female carriers.*
Gardner syndrome FAP	Epidermal and sebaceous cysts, desmoid tumors, lipomas, fibromas, skull osteomas, CHRPE	Adenocarcinoma of large or small bowel in 100% of patients, thyroid cancer	AD, mutation in APC gene	Diagnosis is made by detection of multiple *impacted* and *supernumerary teeth,* multiple jaw osteomas ("cotton-wool" appearance) *odontomas*
Peutz-Jeghers syndrome	Hamartomatous polyps of the GI tract and mucocutaneous pigmentation of the lips, face, and oral mucosa	GI adenocarcinomas, pancreatic cancer, high risk for other cancers	AD, mutation in *STK11/LKB1* tumor suppressor gene	Colon with benign hamartomatous polyps, high risk of intussusceptions leading to death
Howel–Evans syndrome (palmoplantar keratoderma, or tylosis)	Hyperkeratosis of palms and soles around age 10	Esophageal carcinoma	AD, unidentified gene on chromosome 17	Incidence of carcinoma by 65 year is 95%
Neurofibromatosis type 1 (von Recklinghausen disease)	Neurofibromas, café-au-lait spots, freckling of axillae and groin	Pheochromocytoma, childhood leukemia, other (~7% risk lifetime)	AD, mutation in *NF1* gene	Associated with benign tumors (schwannomas, gliomas, Lisch nodules in eyes, other)
Nevoid basal cell carcinoma syndrome (Gorlin-Goltz syndrome)	Multiple basal cell carcinomas, pits on soles and palms, jaw cysts, skeletal abnormalities	Medulloblastoma, fibrosarcoma (jaw)	AD, mutation in *PTCH* gene	Infrequent association with internal malignancy
Tuberous sclerosis (Bourneville disease)	Facial angiofibromas, pigmented macules, adenomas, fibromas	Neurologic malignancies; overall low risk for malignancy	AD, mutations in *TSC1* and *TSC2* genes (hamartin and tuberin)	Numerous nonmalignant tumors of brain, kidneys, heart, eyes, lungs, and skin
Cerebelloretinal hemangioblastoma (von Hippel-Lindau syndrome)	Skin ecchymoses, retinal malformation, papilledema	Renal cell carcinoma, pheochromocytoma (20%)	AD, mutation in VHL tumor suppressor gene on chromosome 3	Angiomatosis, hemangioblastomas, renal angiomas
Encephalotrigeminal syndrome (Sturge-Weber syndrome)	Port-wine stains (capillary or cavernous hemangiomas) in the trigeminal nerve distribution	Rare neurologic malignancies	Possible somatic mutation in fibronectin gene	Glaucoma, seizures, mental retardation, ipsilateral leptomeningeal angioma
Ataxia-telangiectasia	Telangiectasias	Lymphomas, leukemias	Autosomal recessive, defect in double-stranded DNA repair gene	IgA ± IgE deficiency; sinopulmonary infections, tumors in <10%. No mammography.
Bloom syndrome	Photosensitivity, telangiectasias, butterfly erythema of face	Numerous leukemias, lymphomas, carcinomas	Autosomal recessive, defect in BLM gene, DNA helicase	Stunted growth, high incidence of pneumonias
Fanconi anemia	Patchy hyperpigmentation	Leukemias, esp. AML, bone marrow failure by age 40	Autosomal recessive, defect in DNA repair gene	High incidence in *Ashkenazi Jews* and *Afrikaans* in South Africa
Chédiak-Higashi syndrome	Recurrent pyoderma, giant melanosomes, partial albinism	Lymphomas	Autosomal recessive, *lysosomal trafficking regulator* gene, *LYST*	Anemia, hepatosplenomegaly High incidence of overwhelming infections
Werner syndrome (adult progeria)	Sclerodermalike changes, premature aging, leg ulcers, short stature	Sarcomas, meningiomas, other	Autosomal recessive, defect in DNA helicase WRN	Cancers in approximately 10%
Wiskott-Aldrich syndrome (eczema-thrombocytopenia-immunodeficiency syndrome)	Eczematous dermatitis, pyoderma	Lymphomas, leukemias	X-linked recessive (males affected)	Immunodeficiency, bloody diarrhea, thrombocytopenia *IgM* is reduced, *IgA* and *IgE* are elevated
Bruton's sex-linked agammaglobulinemia	Recurrent infections	Lymphomas, leukemias	X-linked, defect in Btk kinase	No B cells

AD, autosomal recessive; HNPCC, hereditary nonpolyposis colon cancer; FAP, familial adenomatous polyposis; CHRPE, congenital hypertrophy of the retinal pigment epithelium; GI, gastrointestinal; VHL, von-Hippel-Lindau; Ig, immunoglobulin.

carcinomas, numerous bony abnormalities, and a strong predisposition for malignancy. The most common malignant tumor is medulloblastoma, but there are also astrocytoma, meningioma, and craniopharyngioma.[100]

MISCELLANEOUS LESIONS

Multicentric reticulohistiocytosis is a disease that manifests as violaceous papules overlying joints with associated arthritis mutilans in 50% of patients. Patients develop malignancies in 28% of cases, including pancreatic and squamous cell lung carcinomas and melanoma. The disease results from the destructive effects of proteinases[101] and there is no effective therapy.

Pruritus may be the initial feature of an occult malignancy or the clinical manifestation of a previously diagnosed tumor. It is most frequently associated with Hodgkin's lymphoma but may be seen with polycythemia vera, cutaneous T-cell lymphomas, and a variety of other diseases.[102] Severe pruritus localized in the nostrils has been reported in some patients with advanced brain tumors.

There are other numerous additional hereditary disorders associated with cutaneous manifestations of malignancy.

NEUROLOGIC MANIFESTATIONS OF CANCER

Neurologic diseases are defined as paraneoplastic when they occur in increased frequency in patients with cancer and are not related to a direct effect of tumor, infection, metabolic abnormalities, or toxicity of therapy (Table 153.6).[103,104] Autoantibodies and evidence for cellular autoimmunity directed against neuronal, glial, or muscle cell antigens have been identified in a number of paraneoplastic neurologic disorders (Table 153.7).[104,105] This review follows the nosology used by Darnell and Posner.[104]

Paraneoplastic disorders are diagnosed by the identification of stereotypic clinical syndromes and confirmatory laboratory studies to demonstrate evidence of autoimmunity. Graus et al.[106] have proposed nosologic criteria for definite or possible paraneoplastic disorders incorporating the clinical syndrome, the detection of cancer, and antibodies to onconeural antigens. Autoantibodies against specific neural antigens characterize several neurologic disorders.[104,105] Cytotoxic T-cell populations, with limited Vbeta T-cell receptor repertoire, and B cells have been identified in the CNS of patients with CNS paraneoplastic syndromes, suggesting that these cellular mechanisms are producing cell injury.[107–109]

TABLE 153.6

ESTIMATED INCIDENCE OF NEUROLOGIC DISORDERS THAT ARE PARANEOPLASTIC SYNDROMES

Syndrome	% Paraneoplastic
Lambert-Eaton myasthenic syndrome	60
Subacute cerebellar degeneration	50
Subacute sensory neuronopathy	20
Opsoclonus-myoclonus (children)	50
Opsoclonus-myoclonus (adults)	20
Sensory motor peripheral neuropathy	10
Encephalomyelitis	10
Dermatomyositis	10

From Posner JB. Paraneoplastic syndromes. *Neurol Clin* 1991;9:919, with permission.

Subacute Sensory Neuronopathy and Encephalomyeloneuritis

Most frequently associated with SCLC, subacute sensory neuronopathy and encephalomyeloneuritis (SSN-EMN) may affect multiple sites within the central and peripheral nervous system.[110] When SSN-EMN occurs in patients with SCLC, antibodies called *anti-Hu* antibodies are usually present in the serum, and high titers of antibodies to the Hu antigen are almost never seen in patients without SCLC.[110] Diagnosis of SSN-EMN and documentation of anti-Hu antibody should lead to the search for an SCLC. Low-titer anti-Hu antibodies have been documented in patients with SCLC and no neurologic disease,[110] and the association with localized SCLC suggests that anti-Hu antibodies are a marker for systemic immune suppression of tumor progression.

The range of presentations in patients with paraneoplastic disorders associated with anti-Hu antibodies is quite broad. One presentation is a pure sensory neuropathy.[111,112] The disorder progresses relentlessly over days to weeks, and sensory nerve action potentials are lost.[111] The cerebrospinal fluid (CSF) usually demonstrates increased protein concentration and a lymphocytic pleocytosis, and in SSN associated with anti-Hu antibody, the dorsal root ganglia show lymphocytic infiltration and loss of neurons.[113] Most cases of SSN are associated with other autoimmune disorders rather than with cancer, and anti-Hu antibodies are absent. Treatment of the underlying SCLC may ameliorate signs of neurologic dysfunction,[114] and treatment of Hodgkin's lymphoma with chemotherapy was followed by clinical improvement in one patient. Immunosuppression may produce at least transient disease stabilization even in patients who did not receive treatment for the underlying tumor.[115,116]

LIMBIC ENCEPHALITIS

In the interval since the prior review, a series of clinical and immunopathologic studies have dramatically increased our understanding of the heterogeneity within the syndrome of limbic encephalitis (LE).[117,118] LE has been described with autoantibodies directed against a panoply of novel antigen targets.[119,120] The range of clinical presentations now includes rapid-onset psychotic symptoms and focal epilepsies including status epliepticus.[120,121] LE may be mistaken for herpes simplex encephalitis because it presents with memory disturbance, agitation, and seizures. Magnetic resonance imaging (MRI) may show mesial temporal contrast enhancement or T2 signal hyperintensities.[122–124] Fluorodeoxyglucose–positron emission tomography (FDG-PET) may show hypermetabolism in the affected temporal lobes.[125] The CSF shows increased protein concentration and a lymphocytic pleocytosis. Symptoms of SSN or involvement of brainstem or spinal cord may be present. Biopsy of temporal lobe may show perivascular lymphocytic infiltrates.[122,123]

Molecular characterization of target antigens divides this syndrome into distinguishable diseases. Most cases of LE are associated with SCLC, and anti-Hu antibodies are present in serum and CSF.[122,123] Patients with testicular cancer and LE harbor a different antibody.[126] In a series of 13 patients with testicular cancer and LE, 10 harbored antibodies against a novel onconeural antigen named Ma2. Ma2 is a 40-kD protein not found in normal testis, but expressed in the normal human CNS and dorsal root ganglia. Two other onconeural antigens, ANNA-3 and PCA2, have been reported in patients

TABLE 153.7

ANTINEURONAL ANTIBODIES AND ASSOCIATED PARANEOPLASTIC SYNDROMES AND CANCERS

Antibody	Site of Activity	Genes	Cellular Function	Clinical Syndrome	Cancers
Anti-Hu (ANNA-1)	Panneuronal	HuD, HuC, Hel-N1/N2	RNA binding	Paraneoplastic encephalomyelitis, paraneoplastic sensory neuronopathy, PCD, autonomic dysfunction	SCLC, sarcoma, neuroblastoma
Anti-Ri (ANNA-2)	Central nervous system neurons	Nova-1	RNA binding	Paraneoplastic opsoclonus-myoclonus, PCD	Breast, gynecologic, SCLC, bladder
Anti-Yo (APCA)	Purkinje cell	CDR34/62/3, PCD-17	Leucine zipper	PCD	Ovary, uterus, breast, SCLC
Anti-Tr	Purkinje cell	MAZ	Leucine zipper interacts with DCC gene product	PCD	Hodgkin's, non-Hodgkin's lymphoma
Anti-VGCC	Presynaptic neuromuscular junction	MysB, Synaptotagmin	Ach release	Lambert-Eaton myasthenic syndrome	SCLC, Hodgkin's lymphoma, thyroid
Anti-CAR	Photoreceptors	Recoverin	Calcium binding	Cancer-associated retinopathy	SCLC, melanoma
Antiamphiphysin	Synapse, CNS neurons	Amphiphysin	Synaptic vesicle protein	Stiff-person syndrome, encephalitis	Breast, SCLC
Anti-AChR	Postsynaptic neuromuscular junction	AChR	Ach receptor	Myasthenia	Thymoma
Anti-CV2, anti–CRMP-5	Oligodendrocyte	CRMP-5	Axonal growth factor	Neuropathy, uveitis, chorea, ataxia	SCLC, renal cell, breast, lymphoma
Anti-AChR (nicotinic)	Postsynaptic, ganglionic	Nicotinic AChR	AChR, nicotinic	Dysautonomia	SCLC, thymoma
Anti-Ta	Nucleus	Ma1, Ma2		Limbic encephalitis	Testis
Anti-NMDA	Cell surface	NMDA	Receptor	Limbic encephalitis	Ovarian teratoma
Anti-AMPAR	Cell surface	AMPA	Receptor	Limbic encephalitis	Lung, breast, thymus
Anti-GABAb	Cell surface	GABAb	Receptor	Limbic encephalitis	SCLC

Ach, acetylcholine; AChR, acetylcholine receptor; ANNA, antineuronal nuclear antibody; APCA, antiparietal cell antibody; CAR, carcinoma-associated retinal; CRMP, collapsin response mediator protein-2; MHC, major histocompatibility complex; PCD, paraneoplastic cerebellar degeneration; SCLC, small cell carcinoma of the lung; VGCC, voltage-gated calcium channel, NMDA, *N*-methyl-D-aspartate, GABAb, gamma aminobutyric acid receptor beta; AMPA, alpha-amino-3-hydroxy-5-methyl-4-isoxazolepropionic acid receptor.

with encephalomyelitis and SCLC.[127] A related onconeural antigen, Ma1, normally found in the testis, is associated with cerebellar or brainstem dysfunction in patients with lung, breast, parotid gland, or colon cancer.[128] Breast cancer is the underlying malignancy in about 5% of cases; anti-Ri antibodies have been reported in this setting.[129] A patient with thymoma and a novel autoantibody directed against synaptic vesicles has been reported.[121] LE has also been reported with Hodgkin's and non-Hodgkin's lymphoma.[130,131]

LE may be one of the more treatable forms of CNS paraneoplastic disorder.[122,123] More than 40% of patients followed for longer than 8 months in one series had some neurologic improvement. Treatment of the underlying tumor seems more effective than immunosuppression.[122,123] The distinction between anti-Ma2– and anti-Hu–associated LE is important clinically because anti-Ma2–associated LE appears to have a better prognosis. Orchiectomy and aggressive treatment of residual disease appear to be the most effective treatment for anti-Ma2–associated LE.[127] Immunosuppression has been less successful, but one patient improved after treatment with corticosteroids and intravenous immunoglobulin G (IgG). In a small, open-labeled study, rituximab produced clinical improvement in patients with various subtypes of LE.[132]

More recently, immunosuppression responsive forms of LE have been identified in association with anti–voltage-gated potassium channels, and less well-characterized antineutrophil antibodies.[124,133,134] The most common autoantibody associated with antineutrophil distribution of immunoreactivity appears to be anti-NMDA receptor,[117,119] with glutamic acid decarboxylase, GABAb, and AMPA receptor being the target antigen for autoantibodies in other cases.[120,121] These forms of LE may also occur in the absence of an identifiable cancer, in association with other autoimmune disorders.[135] These subtypes of LE may respond to immunotherapy while being resistant to antiepileptic drugs,[135] making the syndromes important to recognize. Successful treatment of anti-NMDA associated LE has been reported in a 22-month-old child.[136] MRI and FDG-PET demonstrated abnormalities on T2 and fluid-attenuated inversion recovery sequences, some patients also had diffusion abnormalities, as well as hypermetabolic regions on PET. In some patients, clinical improvement with immunosuppression and/or successful ablation of the tumor was associated with improvement in PET and MRI abnormalities. LE appearing in a young female should prompt search for an associated ovarian teratoma.[133]

Antibodies to voltage-gated potassium channels have been reported in patients with a syndrome similar to paraneoplastic

LE, but usually without identifiable cancer.[133,134] This syndrome appears to have a more favorable prognosis and response to immunosuppression. Rarely, small cell cancers of other organs, including the prostate, have been found as the only systemic cancer in patients with LE and anti-Hu antibodies.[137,138]

Brainstem encephalitis and myelitis usually occur together and in association with LE.[139] MRI scanning must exclude metastatic tumor. Most cases are associated with anti-Hu antibodies, but other autoantibodies may be present. Brainstem encephalitis and myelitis are usually rapidly and relentlessly progressive.

AUTONOMIC NEUROPATHY

A pure paraneoplastic autonomic neuropathy is rare, but approximately 25% of patients with anti-Hu syndrome and SSN-EMN have autonomic dysfunction.[109] Progressive paraneoplastic autonomic failure may rarely be the first manifestation of an occult malignancy. Bladder dysfunction, bowel immotility and obstipation, and postural hypotension may be disabling.[138] The disorder is usually associated with SCLC and autoantibodies that react with neurons in the myenteric plexus but other autoantibodies have been reported.[140] In a Mayo Clinic series, 42% of patients with subacute autonomic neuropathy demonstrated antibodies directed against the nicotinic acetylcholine receptor.[141,142] Autonomic dysfunction may occur in patients with myasthenia gravis; in some, gastroparesis was the only manifestation, but severe pandysautonomia has been reported.[143] In some, antibodies against the ganglionic nicotinic acetylcholine receptor or synaptophysin[144] were identified.[142,143] The intestinal dysmotility may respond to anticholinesterase inhibitors. Anti-CV2 and anti–voltage-gated potassium channels antibodies have also been associated with autonomic dysfunction.[104] GI dysmotility is usually a core complaint, with orthostatic hypotension, hypoventilation, sleep apnea, and cardiac dysrhythmias being variably present.[145] Treatment of the underlying tumor and/or immunosuppression is usually unable to reverse neurologic dysfunction, but may stabilize disease.[146,147]

PROGRESSIVE CEREBELLAR DEGENERATION

Darnell and Posner[104] have classified progressive cerebellar degeneration (PCD) into subcategories. Patients usually complain first of difficulty with walking, which progresses over weeks to months. Diplopia and vertigo may be early symptoms. Loss of dexterity, dysarthria, and oscillopsia associated with nystagmus appear. The disorder usually leaves patients incapacitated.[148] Subtle motor system or cognitive dysfunction may be present. Imaging may show diffuse cerebellar atrophy,[149] but contrast-enhancing lesions or lesions with mass effect are not part of PCD. CSF testing usually shows a lymphocytic pleocytosis and mildly elevated protein concentration during the early phase of the disorder, and oligoclonal bands have been reported.[148] Anti-Yo PCD is most commonly associated with ovarian or breast carcinoma. Frequently, the neurologic disorder antedates discovery of the tumor. The Yo antigen is one of a family of three cerebellar degeneration–related (cdr) antigens identified by expression cloning.[148,150–152] Only Yo, or CDR2, is transcribed in human tumors. The PCD renders patients unable to walk, and dysarthria is frequently severe. Once the disorder reaches this stage, treatment with immunosuppression or effective treatment of the underlying malignancy rarely produces significant improvement. Patients with PCD and Hodgkin's lymphoma are predominantly male and younger than the females with anti-Yo PCD.[153] The disorder frequently develops in patients who have already been treated for Hodgkin's lymphoma. This type of PCD also seems to be molecularly heterogeneous. Antibodies against a novel onconeural antigen named Tr have been found in patients with Hodgkin's lymphoma and PCD.[154,155]

PCD associated with Hodgkin's lymphoma appears to have a better prognosis for recovery.[153] Spontaneous improvement was seen in 15% of cases in one series, and one patient improved significantly with effective treatment of Hodgkin's lymphoma.[155] As the patient responded to treatment, the anti-Tr antibody declined tenfold in serum and disappeared from the CSF.[155] The target antigen for anti-Tr is a zinc finger protein MAZ.[154] Other patients with Hodgkin's lymphoma demonstrate antibodies against metabotropic glutamate receptor type 1. PCD may also be a component of more complex paraneoplastic syndromes; in some of these cases multiple antibodies are present. Approximately 15% of patients with anti-Hu antibodies develop PCD as the first manifestation of disease. In these patients, signs suggesting multisystem involvement are often present. Identification of the anti-Hu antibody directs the search for SCLC. In other patients with SCLC, antibodies against the voltage-gated calcium channel have been identified; some of these patients currently had Lambert-Eaton myasthenic syndrome, others did not.[156,157]

PCD may also be seen in association with anti Ma-1 antibodies, although these antibodies are more commonly associated with encephalomyelitis.[128] Anti-CRMP-5 (CV-2) and anti-Zic4 antibodies have been reported in patients with PCD.[158,159] Anti-CRMP antibodies are most commonly associated with thymoma, less commonly with SCLC or gynecologic tumors, and Zic4 most commonly with SCLC. Anti-Zic4 antibodies frequently are associated with anti-Hu or anti-CRMP-5 antibodies. Pure PCD is more common in patients with only Zic4. Treatment of patients with PCD has been disappointing; however, response of anti-Tr or anti-CRMP-5–associated PCD to antitumor treatment or systemic immunosuppression has been reported,[160,161] and one patient with anti-Yo PCD demonstrated rapid clinical improvement after treatment with high-dose corticosteroids and cyclophosphamide.[162] A study of 50 patients with PCD suggests that molecular characterization has prognostic significance.[160] Patients with anti-Ri had better functional outcomes and longer survival than patients seropositive for anti-Yo and anti-Hu antibodies. Effective antitumor treatment was the most important determinant of outcome and duration of survival.[160] Antibody-negative PCD may occur in conjunction with Lambert-Eaton myasthenic syndrome.[163] The most common associated tumor is SCLC. The PCD may not remit, even as the myasthenic syndrome responds to immunosuppression.

PARANEOPLASTIC VISUAL LOSS

Paraneoplastic disorders are a rare cause of vision loss in cancer patients.[164] Retinal disorders are the most common. Within this class, the photoreceptor degenerations are the best characterized.[165]

Patients with photoreceptor degeneration commonly note night blindness, photopsias, and blurred vision. If cones are involved, loss of color perception may occur. Electroretinograms are abnormal, and ophthalmoscopic examination may show retinal arteriolar attenuation.[165]

A number of different autoantibodies have been described in association with photoreceptor degeneration, but the most common is the anti–carcinoma-associated retinal antigen antibody. The target antigen is recoverin, a calcium-binding molecule involved in the transduction of light signaling in vertebrate photoreceptors.[166] The majority of patients with anti–carcinoma-associated retinal antigen have cancer, usually SCLC, but a similar syndrome has been reported in patients with no detectable cancer.[167] Usually the vision loss is relentlessly progressive and blindness is the ultimate result, but occasionally patients have responded to high-dose corticosteroids, plasmapheresis, or intravenous IgG.[167]

Antibodies directed against a variety of retinal antigens, including neurofilaments,[168] have been reported in patients with photoreceptor degeneration in addition to carcinoma-associated retinal antigen, including anti-HU antibodies. Most patients suffered from SCLC, non–small cell lung cancer, or breast cancer. Antibody against a photoreceptor antigen implicated in autosomal recessive retinitis pigmentosa, TLUP-1, has been reported in a patient with cancer-associated retinopathy and endometrial cancer.[169] Three cases of isolated cone dystrophy have been reported.[170]

Progressive vision loss with retinal pigmentary abnormalities has been separated into several syndromes. Most commonly associated with melanoma or adenocarcinomas of the gut,[170] these disorders have distinctive ophthalmoscopic appearances. Melanoma-associated retinopathy most commonly appears at the stage of metastatic melanoma and is more common in men than in women.[170] Autoantibodies against interphotoreceptor retinoid binding protein were identified in a patient with melanoma who developed multiple detachments of the neurosensory retina.[171] Only rods are affected, and progressive blindness is unusual. Autoantibodies against rod bipolar cells may be present.[172] Acquired night blindness may occur with melanoma.[170]

A small number of patients with paraneoplastic optic neuropathies have been reported.[173–176] Primary cancers include SCLC, lymphoma, neuroblastoma, glucagonoma, nasopharyngeal carcinoma, non–small cell lung cancer, thymoma, and myeloma.[170] Ophthalmoscopic examination may reveal optic disc pallor but not retinal pigmentary changes or vascular attenuation. Optic neuropathy may be associated with anti-CV2 antibodies.[173] Associated myelitis, mimicking Devic syndrome, was seen in three patients with paraneoplastic optic neuritis and anti-CV2 antibodies.[159] Electroretinograms are normal, but visual-evoked potentials are delayed. Patients do not complain of photopsia; instead, progressive scotomas related to optic nerve dysfunction develop. Neuromyelitis optica with antiaquaporin antibodies has been reported as well, in one patient with non–small cell lung cancer.[177] The autoimmune optic neuropathies seem to have a better visual prognosis as a class than the retinopathies.[170] Patients improve with immunosuppression, but most reports of recovery occurred with treatment of the cancer.[170] Steroids have been the most frequently used immunosuppressive treatment. For melanoma-associated retinopathy patients, aggressive multimodality antimelanoma therapy has improved vision.[178] A patient with multiple myeloma and an antibody directed against an antigen in retinal ganglion cells recovered completely after high-dose chemotherapy, and stem cell transplantation obliterated the autoantibody.[174]

OPSOCLONUS-MYOCLONUS

Opsoclonus-myoclonus (OM), a disorder of ocular motility and multifocal myoclonus, was first described in children with neuroblastoma. Probably only 5% of pediatric cases are associated with cancer. However, search for neuroblastoma is necessary in any child who develops OM. The peak age of onset for the disorder is 18 months, and girls are preferentially affected. Significant neurologic dysfunction frequently persists in children with OM and neuroblastoma.[179] Limited disease stage at diagnosis correlates with a higher risk of neurologic sequelae in pediatric patients with OM and neuroblastoma, but the presence of antineuronal antibodies does not.[180] Successful treatment of the neuroblastoma may be associated with a better neurologic outcome.[179] No one antigen seems to be common; antineurofilament[181] and anti-Hu antibodies have been reported.[182] OM has recently been reported as a component of anti-NMDA receptor LE.[183]

A novel antibody, anti-Ri, has been reported in several adult patients with opsoclonus and truncal ataxia or other cerebellar signs. These cases were associated with breast or gynecologic cancer.[184] It is unclear whether the neurologic prognosis is different for antibody-negative and anti-Ri–associated OM. The target antigen is Nova, an RNA-binding protein.

In a series of 24 adult patients with OM, 12 of 14 patients with paraneoplastic OM had no detectable autoantibodies. The ten idiopathic cases were monophasic, with good recovery in most patients. The paraneoplastic cases were relentlessly progressive despite administration of immunosuppressive therapy in five patients with refractory tumors, but at least partial recovery occurred in patients whose tumors were successfully treated.[185] In a series of 16 children with OM, rituximab treatment produced clinical improvement in 81%. An associated tumor was present in 50% of the cases, and was removed in all cases prior to initiation of treatment with rituximab.[186,187] Paraneoplastic OM, without Ri antibodies, has also been associated with Hodgkin's lymphoma.[188] In a study of 21 patients with OM, both with and without identified primary tumors, 25 putative targets were identified by probing a brainstem complementary DNA library.[189]

PARANEOPLASTIC MOTOR NEURON DISORDERS

Experienced neuromuscular clinicians discourage an extensive search for occult malignancy in patients with typical amyotrophic lateral sclerosis. However, paraneoplastic motor neuron disorders with a variable mixture of upper and lower motor neuron signs has been reported in association with both lymphoproliferative malignancies and solid tumors.[190–195] Diagnosis is important because patients may improve after tumor removal or immunosuppression.[194] Patients with paraneoplastic motor neuron disorders were separated into three groups in a series reported by Memorial Sloan-Kettering Cancer Center.[191] One group harbored anti-Hu antibodies[191,195] and a more complex presentation incorporating features of the anti-Hu syndrome. A second group of five women with primary lateral sclerosis and breast cancer were identified; none had anti-Hu antibodies or other autoantibodies. A third group of patients developed a syndrome resembling amyotrophic lateral sclerosis and had a variety of underlying solid tumors.

Patients with Hodgkin's or non-Hodgkin's lymphoma, paraproteinemia, and a mixed upper and lower motor neuron syndrome have been reported. Lower motor neuron syndromes, as well as a mixture of lower and upper motor neuron signs, have been reported in association with myeloproliferative disorders and paraproteinemia.[194] A rapidly progressive, painless lower motor neuron syndrome occurred in a patient with angiocentric lymphoma.

Case reports suggest that patients may improve substantially after effective treatment of the underlying malignancy or, less clearly, with immunosuppressive therapy. Remission of the motor neuron syndrome has been reported after nephrectomy in a patient with renal cell carcinoma[167] and after successful treatment of lung cancer.[192] Darnell and Posner[104] have suggested that the predominantly lower motor neuron disorder termed *subacute motor neuronopathy* or *spinal muscular atrophy* is an opportunistic viral syndrome. This syndrome has been reported with Hodgkin's and non-Hodgkin's lymphoma. Patients present with multifocal motor weakness.

Sensory complaints may be present. The CSF is usually acellular with mildly elevated protein levels. These patients often spontaneously stabilize neurologically. A subacute motor axonal neuropathy and ophthalmoplegia in a patient with melanoma treated with a MAGE (melanoma antigen) vaccine was associated with anti-GQ1b antibodies.[196]

One of the authors treated a patient who survived 15 years after diagnosis of metastatic adenocarcinoma of the colon and then developed a rapidly progressive motor neuron disorder and dementia (F. Lieberman, unpublished observation, 1998), which transiently responded to intravenous immunoglobulin. An antibody reactive with anterior horn cells in spinal cord and pyramidal cells in cortex was identified.

PARANEOPLASTIC PERIPHERAL NEUROPATHIES

Subacute sensorimotor neuropathy usually presents with progressive distal, symmetric sensory loss, and weakness, more severe in the legs.[197] Lung cancer is the most commonly associated malignancy. In approximately two-thirds of patients, the neuropathy precedes the diagnosis of cancer or is noted at the time of diagnosis. CSF is usually acellular, and protein concentration may be mildly elevated. Neurophysiologic studies usually indicate an axonal process, and nerve biopsy specimens show a mixture of axonal injury and demyelination. This disorder is usually relentlessly progressive, but some patients stabilize after tumor removal and some patients appear to benefit from corticosteroid therapy.[104] Women with breast cancer may develop a slowly progressive sensorimotor neuropathy with proximal weakness and upper motor neuron signs.[190–198] This disorder is frequently indolent.

Most patients with paraneoplastic sensorimotor neuropathies do not have antineuronal antibodies. Demyelinating neuropathies may respond to therapy with plasmapheresis, intravenous immunoglobulin, or corticosteroid immunosuppression; axonal neuropathies as a group respond unsatisfactorily to immunosuppression.[197]

A novel antigen, CV2, has been reported as the target antigen in a group of patients presenting with sensorimotor neuropathy, cerebellar degeneration, and uveitis.[199] Optic neuropathy may also occur. The CV2 antigen is a member of the Ulip/CRMP family of proteins. Anti-Hu antibodies were simultaneously present in 20% of the patients. Acute polyradiculoneuropathy (APN) appears to occur in increased frequency in patients with Hodgkin's lymphoma. The clinical features of APN in Hodgkin's lymphoma are similar to those of idiopathic Guillain-Barré syndrome.[200] Treatment of Hodgkin's lymphoma does not clearly modify the course of the neuropathy. No specific autoantibodies have been identified in these patients, but APN associated with Hodgkin's lymphoma may respond to plasmapheresis or intravenous gamma globulin.[201] APN has also been reported in association with leukemias, non-Hodgkin's lymphoma, and multiple myeloma.[201] Leukemic or lymphomatous infiltration of the peripheral nerves may be clinically indistinguishable from APN.[179] Relapsing and remitting forms of APN have also been reported in association with a variety of solid tumors, leukemia, and lymphoma.[201] A patient with hepatocellular carcinoma and APN demonstrated antineutrophil cytoplasmic antibodies.[199] Several cases of chronic inflammatory demyelinating polyneuropathy, sometimes with vitiligo, have been associated with melanoma.[202,203]

A number of different syndromes are associated with plasma cell dyscrasias.[196,197] Typical osteolytic multiple myeloma is only rarely associated with clinically significant peripheral neuropathy. Most commonly, the neuropathy is a sensorimotor neuropathy and is relatively mild. Pure sensory neuropathy has also been reported. Patients with osteolytic myeloma also develop more severe neuropathies that clinically resemble Guillain-Barré syndrome or chronic inflammatory demyelinating polyneuropathy.[204] Secondary amyloidosis may also cause a relentless, often painful, sensorimotor neuropathy in patients.

Unfortunately, the progressive neuropathies rarely respond to immunosuppressive therapy of any form.[204,205] Patients with Waldenström's macroglobulinemia and sensorimotor peripheral neuropathy may harbor antibodies against myelin-associated glycoprotein or other glycoproteins or lipids. Fludarabine, rituximab, and stem cell transplantation have produced improvement in some patients.

Sensorimotor neuropathies in patients with monoclonal gammopathy of unknown significance appear to respond to plasmapheresis if the paraprotein is IgG or IgA, but not IgM.[204] When the peripheral neuropathy mimics chronic inflammatory demyelinating neuropathy, patients respond to intravenous Ig, plasmapheresis, and corticosteroids. Current European Federation of Neurological Societies guidelines suggest intravenous immunoglobulin be considered as the initial treatment for demyelinating IgM monoclonal gammopathy of undetermined significance (MUGUS)-associated neuropathy based on level B evidence.[206]

Although osteosclerotic myeloma represents only 2% of cases of multiple myeloma, 50% of patients with osteosclerotic myeloma develop peripheral neuropathy.[204] This neuropathy frequently improves after radiation therapy or chemotherapy. M protein (IgG or IgA) may be missed unless immunoelectrophoresis or immunofixation is performed on the serum specimen and urine. A distinctive syndrome combining polyneuropathy, hepatosplenomegaly, endocrinopathy, skin changes, and paraproteinemia, known as the POEMS syndrome, is associated with osteosclerotic myeloma. The natural history and features of the neuropathy are the same as those for patients with osteosclerotic myeloma who do not meet all the diagnostic criteria for POEMS.[204] Elevated levels of serum vascular endothelial growth factor and erythropoietin have been reported with elevated expression of vascular endothelial growth factor and increased vascular density in peripheral nerve biopsy specimens.[207,208] High-dose chemotherapy and autologous stem cell transplantation have produced improvement in neuropathy within months of transplant.[209] Bevacizumab therapy has been effective in some patients,[210] but not others, even though vascular endothelial growth factor serum levels decreased.[211,212]

Painful mononeuritis multiplex due to small-vessel vasculitis has been linked to underlying malignancy. SCLC, prostate cancer, endometrial cancer, lymphoma, and renal cell carcinoma have been implicated.[194] In some patients, the mononeuritis multiplex is part of a more generalized vasculitis; in others, the vasculitis appears limited to the peripheral nerves. Nerve biopsy is necessary for diagnosis. Mononeuritis multiplex may be a presentation of the anti-Hu syndrome; the cases of prostate carcinoma associated with the vasculitic syndrome have been small cell, undifferentiated carcinomas. Immunosuppression or plasmapheresis may be beneficial, and removal of a resectable associated cancer has been followed by improvement as well.

Inflammatory brachial neuritis is usually not linked with malignancy, but when paraneoplastic, it is most frequently associated with Hodgkin's lymphoma.[104] Imaging studies should be performed to identify tumor infiltration of the plexus. Unlike radiation-induced plexopathy, the inflammatory disorder is frequently painful at onset.

NEUROMUSCULAR JUNCTION DISORDERS

Typical myasthenia gravis is associated with thymoma in approximately 15% of cases, and autoantibodies against contractile proteins of striated muscle are associated with increased probability of underlying thymoma.[194] All patients with myasthenia gravis should undergo CT scanning of the chest to identify thymic neoplasms. In patients with thymoma, the myasthenia gravis may remit after thymectomy.[194]

Lambert-Eaton myasthenic syndrome is one paraneoplastic neurologic disorder for which the immunobiology is clinically relevant.[213] In approximately 60% of patients with Lambert-Eaton myasthenic syndrome, the disorder is associated with an underlying cancer, usually SCLC.[194,214] Proximal weakness is a common presenting complaint, but bulbar symptoms are uncommon. In most patients, Lambert-Eaton myasthenic syndrome is not a pure motor syndrome. Paresthesias are frequently reported,[215] and patients may report dry mouth or erectile dysfunction. Characteristic electrophysiologic abnormalities include augmentation of the compound motor action potential with repetitive stimulation.[214]

Antibodies directed against protein epitopes in the voltage-gated calcium channel of presynaptic neurons are present in most patients with Lambert-Eaton myasthenic syndrome.[216] Most patients with Lambert-Eaton myasthenic syndrome benefit from plasmapheresis and immunosuppressive therapy.[214] Drugs that increase presynaptic acetylcholine release may also decrease symptoms; for example, 3,4-diaminopyridine. Current European Federation of Neurological Societies guidelines reiterate the importance of tumor ablation if possible, and immunosuppressive therapy is similar to that for non-paraneoplastic Lambert-Eaton myasthenic syndrome.[217]

PARANEOPLASTIC SYNDROMES WITH MUSCLE RIGIDITY

Stiff-person syndrome presents with muscle stiffness and rigidity, predominately in the paraspinal and abdominal muscles, and muscle spasms.[194] Stiff-person syndrome has been reported in association with breast cancer, Hodgkin's lymphoma, and colon cancer. Paraneoplastic stiff-person syndrome is associated with antibodies against amphiphysin or glutamic acid decarboxylase. Patients frequently improve with effective treatment for the underlying tumor, and steroids may also be beneficial.

Paraneoplastic neuromyotonia is a syndrome of spontaneous and continuous muscle fiber activity of peripheral origin.[194] The disorder frequently develops in association with myasthenia gravis in thymoma, and less commonly in Hodgkin's lymphoma, plasma cell dyscrasias, and SCLC. In 2002, Hart et al.[218] proposed that cramp fasciculation syndrome, undulating myokymia, syndrome of continuous muscle fiber activity, Isaac syndrome, neuromyotonia, and Morvan's fibrillary chorea can all be classified as peripheral nerve hyperexcitability disorders. The risk of peripheral nerve hyperexcitability being a paraneoplastic disorder was high when patients were over 40 years old and anti–voltage-gated potassium channel and acetylcholine receptor antibodies were identified. Corticosteroid, intravenous Ig, and plasma exchange may be effective in treating peripheral nerve hyperexcitability, and antiepileptic drugs such as phenytoin or carbamazepine may decrease nerve hyperexcitability while initiating immunotherapy.[194] Whether antineoplastic treatment benefits these patients in general is unclear.

DERMATOMYOSITIS

Although most patients with dermatomyositis do not have cancer, patients with the disorder do seem to be at higher risk for discovery of a cancer.[194] Breast cancer is the most commonly associated cancer in women, as are lung and GI cancer in men. Association with tumors of the pancreas, melanoma, germ cell tumors, nasopharyngeal carcinoma, and lymphoma has also been reported.

Immunosuppressive treatments effective in idiopathic dermatomyositis seem effective in the paraneoplastic disorder. It is unclear if antineoplastic therapy leads to improvement in the muscle disease in the absence of concomitant immunosuppression.

Necrotizing myopathy is characterized by rapidly progressive, predominantly proximal weakness and marked pain and tenderness of the muscles.[219] SCLC, breast cancer, and GI cancers have been reported with necrotizing myopathy. Although biopsy usually shows necrotic fibers without inflammatory infiltrates, immunosuppression has benefited some patients with this disorder.

MOVEMENT DISORDERS

Hyperkinetic syndromes predominate. Chorea has been reported in association with brainstem signs in patients with SCLC,[220–222] acute lymphocytic leukemia,[223] renal cell carcinoma,[224] and Hodgkin's lymphoma.[225] A normal MRI scan does not exclude paraneoplastic chorea.[226] Patients with chorea in association with CRMP-5 neuronal antibody may also manifest sensorimotor neuropathy, autonomic dysfunction, and visual symptoms.[227] Another similar patient improved clinically and radiologically after successful systemic chemotherapy.[228] Rubral tremor in an extremity has been described as a paraneoplastic syndrome.[229]

Paraneoplastic parkinsonian syndromes are extremely rare.[230] Rapidly progressive parkinsonism and autonomic failure have been reported in a man with multiple myeloma. The relationship between the myeloma and the movement disorder is unclear. Recently, hypokinetic parkinsonian-like features were reported associated with anti-MA2 receptor antibodies in a 40-year-old man with testicular seminoma.[231] Rapidly progressive multisystem degeneration resembling progressive supranuclear palsy, but associated with peripheral neuropathy and fever, has been reported in a patient with B-cell lymphoma.[232]

APPROACH TO THE PATIENT WITH PARANEOPLASTIC NEUROLOGIC DISEASE

Comprehensive neurologic history and examination remain the mainstay of diagnosis and characterization of paraneoplastic disorders. MRI, with and without gadolinium contrast, serves to identify intraparenchymal and leptomeningeal metastatic disease. MRI may also demonstrate structural abnormalities consistent with neuronal cell less and atrophy (e.g., in PCD), or evidence of inflammation (LE). In some settings, MRI and FDG-PET scan changes may help to monitor response to therapy. CSF examination identifies carcinomatous meningitis and opportunistic infections in the appropriate settings, and in paraneoplastic neurologic disease it may demonstrate pleocytosis and elevated protein, increased CSF IgG, increased IgG synthetic rate, and intrathecal production of specific antibodies. PET-CT appears to be the most sensitive imaging modality for identifying occult tumors.

Although the relative rarity of the syndromes has precluded definitive clinical trials for most syndromes, there is evolving consensus about approaches to treatment. Effective tumor ablation, either with surgery or systemic therapies, is more effective than immunosuppression in producing clinical neurologic improvement. However, recovery after effective tumor therapy is variable and frequently incomplete. Immunosuppression with corticosteroids, plasma exchange, intravenous IgG, and immunoadsorption is variably effective.[104,114–116,133,134,137] In a small and heterogeneous series of patients treated with extracorporeal immunoadsorption, there was a 75% response rate.[233] Humoral immunosuppression has been relatively ineffective in the treatment of central paraneoplastic neurologic diseases, although a series of patients with a variety of CNS paraneoplastic syndromes including LE reported clinical improvement after rituximab therapy.[132] The relative efficacy and safety of rituximab, corticosteroids, cyclophosphamide, cyclosporine, and tacrolimus remain to be established for the central paraneoplastic neurologic diseases. The ease and safety of intravenous IgG lead to its frequent choice as the first-line therapy for antibody-mediated or antibody-associated disorders.[234]

Selected References

The full list of references for this chapter appears in the online version.

5. Nieman LK, Biller BM, Findling JW, et al. The diagnosis of Cushing's syndrome: an Endocrine Society Clinical Practice Guideline. *J Clin Endocrinol Metab* 2008;93:1526.
9. Biller BM, Grossman AB, Stewart PM, et al. Treatment of adrenocorticotropin-dependent Cushing's syndrome: a consensus statement. *J Clin Endocrinol Metab* 2008;93:2454.
21. Shimada T, Mizutani S, Muto T, et al. Cloning and characterization of FGF23 as a causative factor of tumor-induced osteomalacia. *Proc Natl Acad Sci U S A* 2001;98:6500.
50. Prandoni P, Lensing AW, Buller HR, et al. Deep-vein thrombosis and the incidence of subsequent symptomatic cancer. *N Engl J Med* 1992;327:1128.
51. Sorensen HT, Mellemkjaer L, Steffensen FH, Olsen JH, Nielsen GL. The risk of a diagnosis of cancer after primary deep venous thrombosis or pulmonary embolism. *N Engl J Med* 1998;338:1169.
52. Kearon C, Kahn SR, Agnelli G, Goldhaber S, Raskob GE, Comerota AJ. Antithrombotic therapy for venous thromboembolic disease: American College of Chest Physicians Evidence-Based Clinical Practice Guidelines (8th Edition). *Chest* 2008;133:454S.
53. Lyman GH, Khorana AA, Falanga A, et al. American Society of Clinical Oncology guideline: recommendations for venous thromboembolism prophylaxis and treatment in patients with cancer. *J Clin Oncol* 2007;25:5490.
54. Noble SI, Shelley MD, Coles B, Williams SM, Wilcock A, Johnson MJ. Management of venous thromboembolism in patients with advanced cancer: a systematic review and meta-analysis. *Lancet Oncol* 2008;9:577.
56. Salem DN, O'Gara PT, Madias C, Pauker SG. Valvular and structural heart disease: American College of Chest Physicians Evidence-Based Clinical Practice Guidelines (8th Edition). *Chest* 2008;133:593S.
59. Boyce S, Harper J. Paraneoplastic dermatoses. *Dermatol Clin* 2002;20:523.
61. Young L, Steinman HK. Acquired ichthyosis in a patient with acquired immunodeficiency syndrome and Kaposi's sarcoma. *J Am Acad Dermatol* 1987;16:395.
62. Howel-Evans W, Mc Connell R, Clarke CA, Sheppard PM. Carcinoma of the oesophagus with keratosis palmaris et plantaris (tylosis): a study of two families. *Q J Med* 1958;27:413.
63. Blanchet-Bardon C, Nazzaro V, Chevrant-Breton J, Espie M, Kerbrat P, Le Marec B. Hereditary epidermolytic palmoplantar keratoderma associated with breast and ovarian cancer in a large kindred. *Br J Dermatol* 1987; 117:363.
66. Bolognia JL. Bazex' syndrome. *Clin Dermatol* 1993;11:37.
67. Vogl A, Goldfischer S. Pachydermoperiostosis: primary or idiopathic hypertrophic osteoarthropathy. *Am J Med* 1962;33:166.
69. Solomon H. Erythema gyratum repens. *Arch Dermatol* 1969;100:639.
70. Ashikari R, Park K, Huvos AG, Urban JA. Paget's disease of the breast. *Cancer* 1970;26:680.
74. Sexton M, Snyder CR. Generalized melanosis in occult primary melanoma. *J Am Acad Dermatol* 1989;20:261.
76. Bayer-Garner IB, Smoller BR. The spectrum of cutaneous disease in multiple myeloma. *J Am Acad Dermatol* 2003;48:497.
77. Cohen PR, Talpaz M, Kurzrock R. Malignancy-associated Sweet's syndrome: review of the world literature. *J Clin Oncol* 1988;6:1887.
79. Cohen PR, Kurzrock R. Mucocutaneous paraneoplastic syndromes. *Semin Oncol* 1997;24:334.
80. Gallo R, Parodi A, Rebora A. Pyoderma gangrenosum in a patient with gastric carcinoma. *Int J Dermatol* 1995;34:713.
82. Zurada JM, Ward KM, Grossman ME. Henoch-Schonlein purpura associated with malignancy in adults. *J Am Acad Dermatol* 2006;55:S65.
84. Hashizume T, Kiryu H, Noda K, Kano T, Nakano R. Glucagonoma syndrome. *J Am Acad Dermatol* 1988;19:377.
87. Izikson L, English JC 3rd, Zirwas MJ. The flushing patient: differential diagnosis, workup, and treatment. *J Am Acad Dermatol* 2006;55:193.
89. Nousari HC, Anhalt GJ. Pemphigus and bullous pemphigoid. *Lancet* 1999;354:667.
92. Sigurgeirsson B, Lindelof B, Edhag O, Allander E. Risk of cancer in patients with dermatomyositis or polymyositis. A population-based study. *N Engl J Med* 1992;326:363.
94. Slee PH, Verzijlbergen FJ, van Leeuwen JH, van der Waal RI. CASE 2. Acquired hypertrichosis: a rare paraneoplastic syndrome in various cancers. *J Clin Oncol* 2006;24:523.
97. Fistarol SK, Anliker MD, Itin PH. Cowden disease or multiple hamartoma syndrome–cutaneous clue to internal malignancy. *Eur J Dermatol* 2002; 12:411.
98. Galiatsatos P, Foulkes WD. Familial adenomatous polyposis. *Am J Gastroenterol* 2006;101:385.
100. Gorlin RJ. Nevoid basal cell carcinoma (Gorlin) syndrome. *Genet Med* 2004;6:530.
108. Hormigo A, Dalmau J, Rosenblum MK, River ME, Posner JB. Immunological and pathological study of anti-Ri-associated encephalopathy. *Ann Neurol* 1994;36:896.
110. Dalmau J, Graus F, Rosenblum MK, et al. Anti-Hu associated paraneoplastic encephalomyelitis/sensory neuronopathy: a clinical study of 71 patients. *Medicine (Baltimore)* 1992;71(2):59–72.
115. Keime-Guibert F, Graus F, Fleury A, et al. Treatment of paraneoplastic neurological syndromes with antineuronal antibodies (anti-Hu, anti-Yo) with a combination of immunoglobulins, cyclophosphamide, and methylprednisolone. *J Neurol Neurosurg Psychiatry* 2000;68:479.
117. Graus F, Saiz A, Dalmau J. Antibodies and neuronal autoimmune disorders of the CNS. *J Neurol* 2010;257:509.
123. Gultekin SH, Rosenfeld MR, Voltz R, Eichen J, Posner JB, Dalmau J. Paraneoplastic limbic encephalitis: neurological symptoms, immunological findings and tumour association in 50 patients. *Brain* 2000;123(Pt 7): 1481.
126. Voltz R, Gultekin SH, Rosenfeld MR, et al. A serologic marker of paraneoplastic limbic and brain-stem encephalitis in patients with testicular cancer. *N Engl J Med* 1999;340:1788.
129. Rojas-Marcos I, Rousseau A, Keime-Guibert F, et al. Spectrum of paraneoplastic neurologic disorders in women with breast and gynecologic cancer. *Medicine (Baltimore)* 2003;82:216.
133. Ances BM, Vitaliani R, Taylor RA, et al. Treatment-responsive limbic encephalitis identified by neuropil antibodies: MRI and PET correlates. *Brain* 2005;128:1764.
135. Vincent A, Irani SR, Lang B. The growing recognition of immunotherapy-responsive seizure disorders with autoantibodies to specific neuronal proteins. *Curr Opin Neurol* 2010;23:144.
140. Vernino S. Antibody testing as a diagnostic tool in autonomic disorders. *Clin Auton Res* 2009;19:13.
148. Peterson K, Rosenblum MK, Kotanides H, Posner JB. Paraneoplastic cerebellar degeneration. I: a clinical analysis of 55 anti-Yo antibody-positive patients. *Neurology* 1992;42:1931.
151. Fathallah-Shaykh H, Wolf S, Wong E, Posner JB, Furneaux HM. Cloning of a leucine-zipper protein recognized by the sera of patients with antibody-associated paraneoplastic cerebellar degeneration. *Proc Natl Acad Sci U S A* 1991;88:3451.
153. Hammack J, Kotanides H, Rosenblum MK, Posner JB. Paraneoplastic cerebellar degeneration: II. Clinical and immunologic findings in 21 patients with Hodgkin's disease. *Neurology* 1992;42:1938.
165. Thirkill CE, FitzGerald P, Sergott RC, Roth AM, Tyler NK, Keltner JL. Cancer-associated retinopathy (CAR syndrome) with antibodies reacting with retinal, optic-nerve, and cancer cells. *N Engl J Med* 1989;321:1589.
179. Russo C, Cohn SL, Petruzzi MJ, de Alarcon PA. Long-term neurologic outcome in children with opsoclonus-myoclonus associated with neuroblastoma: a report from the Pediatric Oncology Group. *Med Pediatr Oncol* 1997;28:284.
191. Forsyth PA, Dalmau J, Graus F, Cwik V, Rosenblum MK, Posner JB. Motor neuron syndromes in cancer patients. *Ann Neurol* 1997;41:722.
199. Yu Z, Kryzer TJ, Griesmann GE, Kim K, Benarroch EE, Lennon VA. CRMP-5 neuronal autoantibody: marker of lung cancer and thymoma-related autoimmunity. *Ann Neurol* 2001;49:146.
208. Scarlato M, Previtali SC, Carpo M, et al. Polyneuropathy in POEMS syndrome: role of angiogenic factors in the pathogenesis. *Brain* 2005;128: 1911.
209. Kuwabara S, Misawa S, Kanai K, et al. Autologous peripheral blood stem cell transplantation for POEMS syndrome. *Neurology* 2006;66:105.

CHAPTER 154 AUTOLOGOUS STEM CELL TRANSPLANTATION

JOHN MAGENAU, DALE BIXBY, AND JAMES FERRARA

The use of peripheral blood progenitor cells (PBPCs) in combination with hematopoietic growth factors has removed prolonged myelosuppression as a major barrier to high-dose chemotherapy. PBPC rescue after high-dose chemotherapy or autologous hematopoietic stem cell transplantation (AHSCT) shortens the duration of neutropenia and thrombocytopenia, so that it is now only slightly longer than that of aggressive standard chemotherapy. Because treatment-related mortality of AHSCT is only 1% to 2% at most centers, studies have begun of the use of AHSCT in treatment of nonmalignant diseases such as refractory autoimmune disorders.

Despite the relative safety and ease of current AHSCT, challenges remain. First, tumor cells are mobilized concomitantly with progenitor cells from the bone marrow. Second, a small percentage of patients still cannot achieve acceptable PBPC collections, although new agents such as plerixafor (AMD3100) have reduced this problem.[1] Third, late complications, including myelodysplastic syndrome (MDS) and acute myelogenous leukemia, occur in a small percentage of patients. Finally, the greatest challenge in AHSCT remains relapse after transplant.

HISTORY

In a landmark 1949 study, Jacobson showed that lead shielding of the spleen of mice protected against death from marrow aplasia after total body irradiation (TBI). Subsequent experiments confirmed the presence of circulating hematopoietic stem cells in mammals. The presence of pluripotential progenitor cells in the blood of humans was unequivocally demonstrated in 1975.[2]

The first successful PBPC autografts were reported in 1985 by Juttner et al.[3] when apheresis was timed to begin with neutrophil recovery after intensive myelosuppressive chemotherapy. Initially, use of PBPCs was limited by the inability to enumerate progenitor cells and thereby determine the number required for engraftment, and PBPC transplantation was reserved for patients who were not eligible for marrow harvest. Today, technology for same-day quantification of progenitor cells and more effective mobilization strategies have made PBPCs the standard of care for patients needing autologous hematopoietic stem cells rescue.

STEM CELL MOBILIZATION

Initially, mobilization following myelosuppressive chemotherapy occurred during the significant increase in PBPCs at the time of count recovery. In most early clinical trials, PBPCs were added to autologous bone marrow. These studies confirmed that neutrophil recovery was more rapid in patients who had been given PBPCs who also showed an additional improvement in platelet and red blood cell recovery,[4] providing the rationale for the use of mobilized PBPCs alone.

The discovery of the CD34 antigen as a progenitor cell marker represents a landmark in PBMC mobilization.[5] The "stemness" of CD34+ cells was first established by successful engraftment of lethally irradiated baboons and later humans with CD34+ selected cells. These studies suggested that both pluripotent and committed progenitor cells are contained within the small CD34+ fraction of bone marrow (1% to 2%) and peripheral blood mononuclear cells (0.05%).[6]

After 1991, a rapid flow cytometric assay for CD34+ cells replaced time-consuming *in vitro* assays for PBPC quantitation. This advance allowed apheresis to be timed to coincide with an increasing progenitor cell number rather than with neutrophil recovery. The correlation between CD34+ cells in peripheral blood and apheresis yields limited the number of collections required for each patient.[7–9]

The CD34+ cell count of the infused product is the most reliable predictive marker of engraftment. A large dose of 5.0×10^6 CD34+ cells/kg results in neutrophil and platelet recovery within 14 days in the majority of patients. An intermediate dose (2.5 to 5.0×10^6 CD34+ cells/kg) provides rapid neutrophil recovery, but platelet recovery may be delayed, particularly in heavily pretreated patients. The minimum dose of CD34+ cells/kg required for engraftment has not been defined because many regimens are not truly myeloablative. Lower CD34+ cell doses resulted in longer duration of hospitalization, greater use of antibiotics, and an increased need for transfusions.[10] However, the long-term impact of collection efficiency and CD34+ cell dose on AHSCT outcome is uncertain because infusion of large numbers of CD34+cells (greater than 8×10^6/kg) have not consistently correlated with improved survival.[11,12] Practically, a dose of 5.0×10^6 CD34+ cells/kg or greater is optimal, 2.5×10^6 CD34+ cells/kg or greater is acceptable, and less than 1.5×10^6 CD34 cells/kg requires an individualized decision as to whether to proceed to AHSCT.

PBPCs are mobilized in most patients with the use of chemotherapy followed by growth factors (granulocyte colony-stimulating factor [G-CSF] or granulocyte-macrophage colony-stimulating factor [GM-CSF]), although recent data suggest that plerixafor may assume an increasing role in the front-line setting for certain patients.[13,14] Combination therapy with chemotherapy and growth factors mobilizes greater numbers of CD34+ cells than the use of growth factors alone[15] and offers the advantage of providing additional treatment against the underlying disorder. The robust mobilization produced by this approach often requires only a single apheresis.[16] In most patients, standard disease-specific chemotherapy followed by

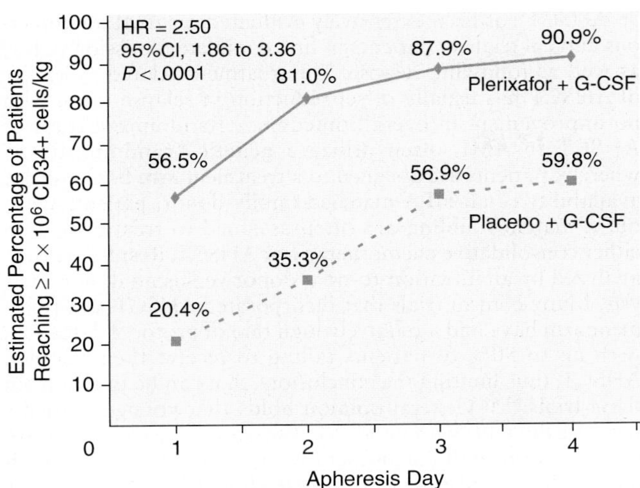

FIGURE 154.1 Addition of plerixafor to granulocyte colony-stimulating factor mobilization increases the proportion of patients achieving sufficient collection. Plerixafor treated patients collected 2×10^6 CD34+ cells/kg at a median of 1 day compared to 3 days for placebo-treated patients. (From ref. 13. Reprinted with permission. © 2008 American Society of Clinical Oncology. All rights reserved.)

G-CSF is sufficient to collect an adequate number of progenitor cells. Cyclophosphamide 2 g/m^2 followed by G-CSF 10 mcg/kg is a reliable and safe mobilization program for patients with non-Hodgkin's lymphoma and with multiple myeloma. VP-16 together with G-CSF is also an effective regimen, but this combination has been associated with increased rates of MDS or acute myelogenous leukemia (AML) in long-term survivors.[17]

Some centers routinely use growth factors alone for stem cell mobilization, which facilitates the secretion of neutrophil-associated proteases within the bone marrow niche, thereby releasing progenitor cells.[18] Two advantages of this approach are (1) apheresis can be scheduled ahead of time and (2) the absence of chemotherapy reduces morbidity. Although the yield of progenitor cells is lower, adequate numbers of PBPC can be collected, and engraftment is comparable to that observed after mobilization with the combination of chemotherapy and growth factors.

Several adhesive interactions mediate attachment of stem cells to the bone marrow microenvironment. Plerixafor is a small molecule that reversibly inhibits the binding of stromal cell–derived factor-1 (SDF-1) to its receptor CXCR4 and is synergistic with G-CSF in the mobilization of PBPC.[1] Because the mechanisms by which plerixafor and G-CSF mobilize are different, the populations of CD34+ cells may also be somewhat different.[19] Two recent randomized phase 3 trials have shown that addition of plerixafor to G-CSF increases the percentage of patients who mobilize sufficient numbers of CD34+ cells compared to G-CSF alone.[13,14] In both studies, plerixafor decreased the number of apheresis sessions needed for mobilization, and patients experienced rapid and durable engraftment (Fig. 154.1).

INADEQUATE MOBILIZATION OF STEM CELLS

The failure to mobilize adequate numbers of CD34+ cells is strongly associated with the type and number of previous therapies a patient has received. Patient age and disease stage (including degree of bone marrow involvement) also contribute to the effectiveness of mobilization. Higher CD34+cell numbers (greater than 20/mcL) correlate with successful collections, whereas the number of failures rises sharply below less than 10/mcL CD34+ cells.[20]

Prior chemotherapy exposure should be considered when selecting a mobilization regimen. Melphalan, nitrosourea agents, nitrogen mustard, and procarbazine are potent stem cell toxins, and fludarabine or cladribine are less so. Intensive combination chemotherapy, such as DT-PACE (cisplatin, doxorubicin, cyclophosphamide, and etoposide) or hyper-CVAD (cyclophosphamide, vincristine, doxorubicin, dexamethasone, methotrexate, cytarabine) may cause difficulty in mobilization after more than two or four cycles, respectively. The effect of newer induction agents such as thalidomide, lenalidomide, and bortezomib on mobilization is still under investigation.[21,22] Some investigators recommend that patients who receive more than four cycles of lenalidomide preferentially receive mobilization with cyclophosphamide and G-CSF.[23] The use of wide-field radiation also correlates with impaired progenitor cell mobilization, and interestingly, mediastinal radiation is as toxic as pelvic radiation in this regard.

No single approach consistently achieves adequate PBPC mobilization if the first approach fails. One-half of patients who achieve suboptimal collections with G-CSF alone may mobilize successfully with chemotherapy plus G-CSF. Higher doses of G-CSF (20 to 32 mcg/kg/d)[24,25] or the addition of GM-CSF to 10 mcg/kg/d of G-CSF may also be effective.[26] The harvest of bone marrow, particularly after stimulation with G-CSF, may be added to the peripheral blood stem cell harvest to increase the total cell number.[27]

Plerixafor has shown promise for patients whose initial mobilization fails. In one study, 64% of mobilization failures collected sufficient CD34+ cells (2×10^6 cells/kg) with plerixafor and G-CSF.[28] The majority (60% to 77%) of poor mobilizers with non-Hodgkin's lymphoma (NHL), Hodgkin's lymphoma (HL), and multiple myeloma (MM) were able to collect another 2.0×10^6 CD34+ cells in pilot studies.[29] Given the considerable cost of this agent, algorithms to select the optimal patients for whom plerixafor may be of benefit will likely be needed.

TUMOR CONTAMINATION

The clinical significance of administering tumor-contaminated progenitor cells remains unclear. Although gene marking studies show that infused tumor cells are present during relapse, there are few data to suggest that they are the sole or even principal cause of disease recurrence. In patients with breast cancer, two studies have shown comparable outcomes whether or not stem cell products contained occult tumor cells.[30,31] Sensitive detection techniques show that residual disease rather than contaminated reinfused stem cells was the major source of relapse in MM patients.[32] CD34+ cell selection (positive purging) reduced tumor cell contamination by over 1,000-fold in a randomized study of multiple myeloma patients, but did not increase disease-free or overall survival.[33] In NHL, contamination may be a significant issue in low-grade lymphoma[34] but probably not in intermediate- or high-grade lymphoma. The time, expense, marginal efficacy, and lack of a standardization process have diminished enthusiasm for purging. There is a theoretical concern of increased graft contamination following mobilization with plerixafor, but the viability and sensitivity of malignant cells to apoptosis following chemotherapy is unknown.[35]

INDICATION AND TIMING OF AUTOLOGOUS HEMATOPOIETIC STEM CELL TRANSPLANTATION

AHSCT enables the delivery of myeloablative doses of chemotherapy while protecting hematopoietic stem cells and thus enables the rescue of hematopoiesis. The ability to administer potentially curative doses of chemotherapy with AHSCT has been investigated in nearly all oncologic histologies but is currently indicated in only a handful of diseases. AHSCT improves event-free survival (EFS) and overall survival (OS) compared to conventional chemotherapy alone in patients with MM.[36,37] This improvement is most likely due to a larger proportion of patients achieving a complete remission (CR), which has been associated with significant prolongation in both EFS as well as OS.[38] The majority of patients diagnosed with MM are above the age of 65, and the use of AHSCT in this age group also improves EFS and OS compared to chemotherapy alone,[39] although not all trials have shown improvements in OS.[40] A recent systematic review of nine clinical trials that compared AHSCT to chemotherapy alone demonstrated an improvement in progression-free survival (PFS), but not OS.[41] Some trials that failed to demonstrate an advantage for AHSCT did not discriminate between AHSCT as initial therapy versus salvage following relapse. In MM there are, in general, two options regarding the timing of AHSCT: transplantation immediately after several cycles of induction versus observation and AHSCT after relapse (delayed transplant). In one randomized study, early transplant provided improved EFS, but there was no difference in OS.[42]

Several trials have evaluated the benefit of double versus single AHSCT in previously untreated MM patients.[43,44] A meta-analysis from six randomized controlled trials demonstrated an improved response rate in those who underwent double AHSCT but no OS advantage.[45] Many clinicians thus incorporate a second (tandem) AHSCT only for patients who do not achieve a CR or at least a very good partial response with the first transplant, although randomized data for this approach are limited. The availability of novel chemotherapeutics (bortezomib, thalidomide, lenalidomide, and liposomal doxorubicin) with significant response rates has recently raised questions of timing and even the need for AHSCT.[46] A few investigators favor AHSCT preoperative regimens that employ the newer agents in patients with high-risk cytogenetics, including t(4;14), t(14;16), or del17p13 as detected by fluorescence *in situ* hybridization (FISH) or karyotypic changes involving del13. The majority of centers still employ upfront AHSCT in most patients in the belief that maximizing the initial response will provide better disease control and long-term survival.[47]

NHL also incorporates AHSCT for significant numbers of patients. Many trials to evaluate early AHSCT in B-cell low-grade NHLs have demonstrated improved PFS, and equivalent OS.[48–51] As a result, AHSCT for the treatment of naïve low-grade B-cell NHLs patients has been reserved for clinical trials. AHSCT for relapsed low-grade B-cell NHL significantly improves both PFS as well as OS, but recent analyses may indicate less benefit of AHSCT if rituximab is included in the salvage regimen.[52,53] AHSCT is commonly used for aggressive B-cell NHLs, both early for high-risk disease (according to the International Prognostic Index) as well as for chemosensitive relapse of the bone marrow.[54,55] Indeed, recent trials have incorporated autologous transplantation as primary therapy for patients with mantle cell lymphoma, although randomized trials are not yet available.[56] Individuals with peripheral T-cell lymphomas not otherwise specified and Alk-negative anaplastic large cell lymphomas in complete remission may benefit from AHSCT in the upfront setting, although no randomized trials have tested this hypothesis.[57] In patients with relapsed HL, AHSCT is typically considered for early relapse (less than 12 months from completion of therapy) and for patients with chemotherapy resistant disease. Additionally, AHSCT can be beneficial in second relapse if conventional treatment was given for the first relapse.[58,59] AHSCT for high-risk HL in first remission has not demonstrated a survival advantage and therefore is not typically utilized in this setting outside of a clinical trial.[60]

AHSCT has been extensively evaluated for AML in numerous clinical trials in patients in first complete remission (CR1) as well as following relapse. The treatment-related mortality of AHSCT has usually offset reduction in relapse rates, with no improvement in overall outcome.[61] Randomized trials of AHSCT in AML often utilize a genetic "randomization" whereby patients are assigned to a treatment arm based on the availability of an HLA-matched family donor; patients without a matched sibling are often assigned to treatment with either consolidative chemotherapy or AHSCT. Results are then analyzed by an intention-to-treat donor versus no donor analysis. Many clinical trials that incorporated AHSCT as a treatment arm have had a relatively high rate of protocol deviation, with up to 50% of patients failing to receive their planned AHSCT, thus limiting the conclusions that can be drawn from these trials.[61,62] General opinion holds that younger patients (age less than 40) with good risk disease in CR1 should receive consolidation with chemotherapy alone, whereas those with intermediate- and poor-risk disease should be considered for an allogeneic transplant, especially if a matched related donor is available. The optimal consolidation for patients older than 40 years of age with intermediate- or poor-risk disease is not known. The recent incorporation of peripheral blood stem cells as a graft source may improve outcomes in those who receive consolidation with AHSCT.[63] An important exception is acute promyelocytic leukemia (APL) in second molecular remission, where AHSCT has been shown to produce better long-term survival rates than allogeneic hematopoietic stem cell transplantation HSCT if the patient is polymerase chain reaction–negative for PML/RAR-α.[64]

With regards to acute lymphoblastic leukemia (ALL), the majority of clinical trials have demonstrated that allogeneic stem cell transplant is superior to AHSCT or chemotherapy alone.[65] Many of these trials show no difference in ALL between AHSCT versus chemotherapy, and the use of AHSCT has thus largely fallen out of favor.

AHSCT has also been incorporated into the treatment of a number of nonhematologic malignancies, including pediatric solid tumor, such as neuroblastoma,[66] Ewing's sarcoma,[67] and sarcomas.[68] In testicular cancer, AHSCT can be curative in patients with relapsed or refractory disease.[69,70] However, the largest randomized trial showed no difference in OS between chemotherapy and chemotherapy with AHSCT.[71] The potential differences in outcomes may reflect the number of cycles of chemotherapy received prior to AHSCT. For metastatic breast cancer, although early trials were encouraging, AHSCT has largely fallen out of favor after randomized studies were negative.[72]

STANDARD INFECTION PROPHYLAXIS

AHSCT patients develop various infections after transplant due to profound immunosuppression, and infection prophylaxis is therefore routinely used, but it is not as extensive or well defined as that following allogeneic hematopoietic stem cell transplantation. Some heavily pretreated AHSCT patients, particularly those with lymphoma or MM, may be almost as immunosuppressed after AHSCT as after allogeneic hematopoietic stem cell transplantation and should receive special attention.

Oral antibiotics such as fluoroquinolones are recommended for adult AHSCT patients with anticipated neutropenic periods of 7 days or more, from the time of stem cell infusion until recovery from neutropenia.[73] For patients with repeated infections posttransplant, intravenous immunoglobulin (Ig) may be considered, particularly when the blood IgG level is lower than 400 mg/dL. For antiviral prophylaxis, acyclovir is routinely given at a dose of 200 to 800 mg twice a day orally for 12 months to prevent herpes simplex virus and varicella zoster virus infections.[74] Cytomegalovirus (CMV) prophylaxis and monitoring are not routinely performed in autologous bone marrow transplant recipients, however, these strategies may be considered in patients receiving TBI-based conditioning or prior alemtuzumab.

Patients who are heavily treated prior to transplant, who have received fludarabine or cladribine, who have a history of fungal infection, or who have prolonged neutropenia and mucosal damage from either intense conditioning regimens or graft manipulation may benefit from antifungal prophylaxis. The standard dose of fluconazole in allogeneic hematopoietic stem cell transplantation is 400 mg/d, but because of relatively high incidence of liver enzyme abnormalities, lower doses (100 to 200 mg/d) are commonly used.[75] *Pneumocystis carinii* pneumonia prophylaxis is also not standard after AHSCT except for patients who are heavily pretreated or have received chronic steroid therapy.

HIGH-DOSE CONDITIONING REGIMENS

In AHSCT, the intensity of conditioning regimens primarily provides antitumor activity. These regimens were therefore developed as the most effective combination of radiation and chemotherapeutic agents for a particular malignancy. Drugs with different spectra of side effects are usually combined to maximize their effectiveness at doses that exceed marrow tolerance.[76,77] Ideally, agents different from those used in the induction regimen are employed.

AHSCT conditioning regimens for acute and chronic leukemias are mainly cyclophosphamide and total body irradiation (CY-TBI) or bulsulphan and cyclophosphamide (Bu-CY),[78] the same regimens used in allogeneic hematopoietic stem cell transplantation. Other regimens, such as TBI/melphalan/etoposide[79] or carmustine/amsacrine/etoposide/cytarabine,[80] have been explored, but none has been shown to be advantageous. Conditioning regimens for lymphomas are more varied. Rituximab is frequently used in CD20+ B-cell lymphomas but not in T-cell lymphomas or HL. Cyclophosphamide/etoposide/carmustine with or without rituximab (CVB ± R) are often used together.[77] Similarly, the combination of carmustine/etoposide/ara-C/melphalan with or without rituximab (BEAM ± R) is effective.[76] A similar combination carmustine/etoposide/cytarabine/cyclophosphamide (BEAC) is also effective but is not widely used now because of cardiotoxicity.[34] TBI-containing regimens may be inferior to chemotherapy-only regimens for lymphomas.[81] In multiple myeloma, high-dose melphalan is used almost exclusively, as melphalan 200 mg/m^2 has been shown to be as effective and less toxic than melphalan 140 mg/m^2 plus TBI 8 Gy.[82] The usual melphalan dose of 200 mg/m^2 may be reduced to 140 mg/m^2 in older patients or patients with renal failure,[83] but some studies have explored doses greater than 200 mg/m^2 in order to increase efficacy.[84] In a recent prospective trail, patients receiving melphalan 200 mg/m^2 had superior PFS compared to those receiving 100 mg/m^2; mucositis and severe thrombocytopenia were more frequent at the higher dose, but nonrelapse mortality was equivalent.[85] The addition of bortezomib 1 mg/m^2 to melphalan 200 mg/m^2 has recently shown impressive activity without additional toxicity.[86]

For testicular cancer, carboplatin and etoposide are used most often,[70] and the addition of ifosfamide or cyclophosphamide may improve outcomes.[87] For neuroblastoma, the combination of melphalan, etoposide, and carboplatin is effective.[88] Regimens that contain thiotepa may also be used as a combination for pediatric solid tumors. Table 154.1 summarizes the common conditioning regimens for a variety of malignancies.

COMPLICATIONS OF AUTOLOGOUS HEMATOPOIETIC STEM CELL TRANSPLANTATION

The complications associated with AHSCT have been reduced in recent years, but they remain significant in multiple organ systems, including cardiac, pulmonary, gastrointestinal/hepatic, renal, and neurologic. Toxicities from chemotherapy intensify in older patients, particularly those with coexisting morbidities, and AHSCT is not usually offered to patients over the age of 70.

Acute cardiac toxicity is often associated with cyclophosphamide, especially in combination with cytarabine or mitoxantrone.[89] Toxicity may present as cardiomyopathy/heart failure, arrhythmia, or pericarditis. Treatment of pericarditis consists of steroids, as nonsteroidal anti-inflammatory drugs are usually contraindicated early after transplant because of low platelet counts.

During conditioning and immediately thereafter, nausea and vomiting are caused by the direct effect of chemotherapy. Delayed nausea and vomiting may be due to mucosal damage caused by chemotherapy or by gastroparesis[90] but have become much easier to control with newer and more effective antiemetics. Diarrhea is associated with high-dose melphalan, and in the rare instance when it persists for 4 to 6 weeks, total parenteral nutrition at home may be necessary.

Acute liver enzyme abnormalities after high-dose chemotherapy are common but are usually self-limited. Veno-occlusive disease (VOD) of the liver, also known as sinusoidal obstruction syndrome, consists of weight gain or ascites, increased bilirubin, and right upper quadrant tenderness; it is characterized by endothelial damage and low flow conditions and is usually seen within 30 days after AHSCT.[91] Risk factors for VOD include second transplant, prior abdominal radiation, busulfan, high doses of TBI, pre-existing liver disease, old age, and poor performance status.[91] High plasma levels of busulfan are associated with increased rates of VOD, and targeted busulfan dosing reduces this risk.[92] The use of gemtuzumab ozogamicin is also associated with the development of VOD,[93] but primarily when used prior to allogeneic hematopoietic stem cell transplantation. Severe VOD after AHSCT is rare with the exception of neuroblastoma.[94] Treatment of VOD is primarily supportive, including control of weight gain and maintenance of both intravascular volume and renal perfusion, while avoiding the accumulation of fluid in the extravascular compartment. Defibrotide, a polydispersed oligonucleotide mixture that protects vascular endothelium, has shown significant promise as treatment of severe VOD in multicenter phase 2 trials.[95,96] Defibrotide treatment increased day 100 survival in patients with severe VOD from historical rates of 10% to approximately 35% without increasing systemic bleeding.[97] A phase 3 trial of defibrotide as VOD prophylaxis is ongoing. Currently, ursodiol (Actigall) is often used as VOD prophylaxis because it is effective after allogeneic hematopoietic stem cell transplantation, but its utility in AHSCT is unknown.

Lung toxicity may be observed after AHSCT particularly if carmustine is part of the conditioning regimen.[98,99] Standard treatment for this complication is high-dose steroids (prednisone 1 to 2 mg/kg/d with a slow taper over several months), and recurrence is common particularly during the steroid taper.

TABLE 154.1

REPRESENTATIVE CONDITIONING REGIMENS FOR AUTOLOGOUS STEM CELL TRANSPLANTATION

Disease	Conditioning Regimen	Drugs and Representative Dose Schedules	Ref.
Leukemias	CY/TBI	Cyclophosphamide 60 mg/kg every day × 2 12 Gy	78
	BU/CY	Busulfan 1 mg/kg PO × 16 every 6 hours or 3.2 mg/kg IV every day × 4 Cyclophosphamide 60 mg/kg every day × 2	78
	TBI/melphalan/ etoposide	TBI 12 Gy in 6 fractions (other cases) Etoposide 60 mg/kg, melphalan 140 mg/m²	79
Hodgkin/NHL	BEAM ± R	Carmustine 300–600 mg/m² Etoposide 400–800 mg/m² Cytarabine 800–1,600 mg/m² Melphalan 140 mg/m² With or without rituximab 375 mg/m² × 1	76
	CVB ± R	Cyclophosphamide 6.0–7.2 g/m² Etoposide 600–2,400 mg/m² Carmustine 300–600 g/m² With or without rituximab 375 mg/m² × 1	77
	BEAC	Carmustine 300 mg/m² Etoposide 800 mg/m² Cytarabine 800 mg/m² Cyclophosphamide 140 mg/kg	34
Multiple myeloma	Melphalan	Melphalan 200 mg/m² × 1 With or without bortezomib 1 mg/m²	82, 85, 86
Testicular	CE CEI	Carboplatin 1,500 mg/m² Etoposide 1,200–1,500 mg/m² With or without iphosphamide 12,000 mg/m²	70, 87
Neuroblastoma		Melphalan 180 mg/m² Etoposide 40 mg/kg Carboplatin 1,500 mg/m²	88

TBI, total body irradiation; NHL, non-Hodgkin's lymphoma.

Renal toxicity associated with high-dose chemotherapy in AHSCT occurs less frequently than in myeloablative allogeneic transplantation due to the absence of calcineurin inhibitors and less frequent use of nephrotoxic antibiotics. Certain diseases such as MM are associated with pre-existing kidney damage and may predispose patients to further renal toxicity, but it is usually reversible after the offending agents are discontinued. Nevertheless, patients who require dialysis have poor outcomes.[100]

Hemorrhagic complications may occur during the period of thrombocytopenia prior to engraftment. Although idiopathic thrombocytopenic purpura and thrombotic thrombocytopenic purpura can occasionally occur after AHSCT, they occur significantly less frequently than after allogeneic hematopoietic stem cell transplantation.

Neurological complications are most often associated immediately following high-dose chemotherapy. Paresthesia in the hands and feet are common, especially when prior therapy has included vincristine or thalidomide. Occasionally, cerebral hemorrhage or infarction may be seen in older patients with atherosclerosis prior to AHSCT. Mental status changes in the peritransplant period are common, in the context of polypharmacy including antiemetics, sedatives, or narcotics for mucositis pain. This problem has become more prevalent as increased numbers of elderly patients are undergoing AHSCT, and it requires careful attention and close collaboration with the nursing staff.

Infectious complications are also common during the neutropenic period. Heavily pretreated patients are at especially high risk, as are patients in whom engraftment is delayed. Heavily pretreated lymphoma patients or myeloma patients may be almost as immunocompromised as those undergoing allogeneic hematopoietic stem cell transplantation and are at risk to develop viral infections even after engraftment. CMV and adenovirus must be considered in the differential diagnosis of unexplained fever for the first 100 days following AHSCT in these patients. Endocrine problems may often be encountered. TBI increases the incidence of hypothyroidism. Use of corticosteroid before or during transplant course will predispose adrenal insufficiency. In both cases replacement therapy is necessary and effective.

Deconditioning has become a serious problem as more elderly patients undergo AHSCT. Many elderly patients have medical comorbidities, predisposing them to functional decline from the transplant procedure. Appetite is often slow to return, and the attendant malnutrition delays recovery.

Second malignancies are the most frequent cause of latemortality following AHSCT. The risk of MDS or AML is greatest in the first 10 years following transplant and is associated with increasing age and high cumulative doses of alkylating therapy, including those administered prior to the transplantation.[101,102] No specific conditioning regimen has been implicated in post-AHSCT malignancies, but TBI may be a risk factor.[17,103,104]

In pediatric patients, retarded growth and development (including neurological development) is an important late toxicity. For children under age 2, TBI is avoided wherever possible because of damage to the developing brain. For patients of reproductive age, AHSCT may cause sterility, and this issue should be extensively discussed before transplant, with sperm (and embryo/oocyte) preservation performed if possible and available.

RECENT DEVELOPMENTS IN AUTOLOGOUS HEMATOPOIETIC STEM CELL TRANSPLANTATION

Targeted Therapy

The use of peripheral blood stem cells has significantly improved treatment-related mortality, but risk of relapse remains high. Many investigators have therefore focused on improving the therapies that are given either before or after AHSCT in order to minimize this relapse. Rituximab is frequently added to the conditioning regimens for B-cell NHL in an attempt to purge the graft of contaminating lymphoma cells.[56,105] However, the timing and the duration of the optimal strategy has not clearly been established.[106,107]

Radioimmunotherapy with iodine-131 tositumomab or yttrium-90–ibritumomabtiuxetan has also been evaluated.[108] High-dose myeloablative radioimmunotherapy prior to AHSCT is an attractive treatment option, but for patients unable to receive myeloablative chemotherapy, randomized studies are not yet available. A multicenter phase 3 study of Bexxar/BEAM (etoposide, cytosine arabinoside, melphalan) versus rituximab/BEAM followed by AHSCT in patients with relapsed or refractory diffuse large B-cell lymphomas (DLBCL) has recently completed accrual and will shed light on this important question. Radiolabeled iodine-131 metaiodobenzylguanidine has also been used to target neuroblastoma in pediatric patients with encouraging results.[109]

As noted previously, the use of molecularly targeted therapy in multiple myeloma has grown dramatically over the past 5 years. Incorporation of novel agents in the pretransplant setting has significantly improved response rates as well as survival, and these agents are now routinely employed together with AHSCT.[110–113]

Induction with bortezomib-containing regimens is encouraging, especially in patients with poor-risk cytogenetics.[114] The optimal regimen and duration of therapy prior to AHSCT have not yet been established. In a recently initiated randomized trial, patients will receive bortezomib, lenalidomide, and dexamethasone (VRD) followed by a randomization to either AHSCT versus VRD consolidation with AHSCT at relapse.

Posttransplant Therapy

Pretransplant therapies are aimed at treating systemic disease as well as clearing the stem cell graft prior to its use in the AHSCT. Posttransplant agents treat minimal residual disease that might persist despite prior myeloablative chemotherapy. In the setting of B-cell NHL, investigators have employed maintenance rituximab in an attempt to prolong the duration of remission.[115] Randomized trials of this approach in follicular lymphoma and in DLBCL have completed accrual, but final results have yet to be published. The use of maintenance rituximab following AHSCT as frontline therapy for high-risk DLBCL does not improve survival and is currently not routinely used.[116] Maintenance therapy with thalidomide following AHSCT in MM improves PFS as well as OS.[117,118] Investigations are ongoing using targeted agents in consolidation and maintenance. In patients in CR after single AHSCT, some clinicians proceed directly to maintenance therapy, given a lack of supportive evidence for the benefit of a second AHSCT in this population.[44,119]

Supportive Care

An important recent advance is improvement in supportive care to prevent mucositis, including the use of palifermin (recombinant human keratinocyte growth factor [rh-KGF]). Mucositis is a major dose-limiting toxicity of conditioning regimens, and rh-KGF has been shown to decrease both the incidence and severity of oral mucositis after AHSCT, particularly after TBI-containing regimens. In a large randomized phase 3 study, KGF improved patient well-being, shortened hospital stays, and decreased the use of total parenteral nutrition.[120] More recently, KGF was shown to reduce the incidence of intestinal mucositis.[121] Preclinical data also suggest that KGF, combined with androgen blockade given prior to conditioning, protects thymic epithelial cells and promotes T-cell reconstitution following allogeneic bone marrow transplant.[122] Despite these findings, KGF has yet to gain widespread use. With the shortened neutropenia and improved nutritional and fluid status, many AHSCT procedures now are safely performed on an outpatient basis.[123] There are both advantages and disadvantages to an outpatient approach, and many factors (including the types of health insurance) influence the decision for an individual patient. But AHSCT no longer necessarily means a commitment to a lengthy hospitalization.

FUTURE DIRECTIONS

With the development of targeted therapy, maintenance therapy, and new agents that reduce toxicities such as mucositis, AHSCTs are no longer limited to academic medical centers and are increasingly performed in large community hospitals, even on an outpatient basis. Indications for AHSCT are likely to grow (e.g., refractory autoimmune diseases). The rationale behind this approach is to eliminate autoreactive effector lymphocytes with high-dose chemotherapy and to reconstitute normal lymphopoiesis from autologous hematopoietic stem cells. Following AHSCT, there is some evidence of thymic regeneration of naïve CD4+ cells with greater T-cell receptor diversity, reduction of memory cells, and increased frequency of CD4+CD25^{bright}Foxp3+ regulatory T cells.[124,125] A pilot study with T-cell depleted AHSCT for severe scleroderma produced responses lasting as long as 5 to 7 years may lead to subsequent studies of AHSCT in several autoimmune diseases.[126,127] European registry data for AHSCT in severe refractory autoimmune diseases have reported a combined PFS up to 43% at 5 years.[128] Randomized phase 3 studies in North America and Europe are currently comparing AHSCT with standard therapy in systemic sclerosis, multiple sclerosis, Crohn disease, and systemic lupus erythematosus. AHSCT may thus eventually find a place in the treatment of nonmalignant as well as malignant diseases.

Selected References

The full list of references for this chapter appears in the online version.

1. Devine SM, Flomenberg N, Vesole DH, et al. Rapid mobilization of CD34+ cells following administration of the CXCR4 antagonist AMD3100 to patients with multiple myeloma and non-Hodgkin's lymphoma. *J Clin Oncol* 2004;22:1095.
2. Barr RD, Whang-Peng J, Perry S. Hemopoietic stem cells in human peripheral blood. *Science* 1975;190:284.
3. Juttner CA, To LB, Haylock DN, Branford A, Kimber RJ. Circulating autologous stem cells collected in very early remission from acute nonlymphoblastic leukaemia produce prompt but incomplete haemopoietic reconstitution after high dose melphalan or supralethal chemoradiotherapy. *Br J Haematol* 1985;61:739.
5. Civin CI, Strauss LC, Brovall C, et al. Antigenic analysis of hematopoiesis. III. A hematopoietic progenitor cell surface antigen defined by a monoclonal antibody raised against KG-1a cells. *J Immunol* 1984;133:157.
7. Fruehauf S, Haas R, Conradt C, et al. Peripheral blood progenitor cell (PBPC) counts during steady-state hematopoiesis allow to estimate the yield of mobilized PBPC after filgrastim (R-metHuG-CSF)-supported cytotoxic chemotherapy. *Blood* 1995;85:2619.
10. Ketterer N, Salles G, Raba M, et al. High CD34(+) cell counts decrease hematologic toxicity of autologous peripheral blood progenitor cell transplantation. *Blood* 1998;91:3148.
13. DiPersio JF, Micallef IN, Stiff PJ, et al. Phase III prospective randomized double-blind placebo-controlled trial of plerixafor plus granulocyte colony-stimulating factor compared with placebo plus granulocyte colony-stimulating factor for autologous stem-cell mobilization and transplantation for patients with non-Hodgkin's lymphoma. *J Clin Oncol* 2009;27:4767.
14. DiPersio JF, Stadtmauer EA, Nademanee A, et al. Plerixafor and G-CSF versus placebo and G-CSF to mobilize hematopoietic stem cells for autologous stem cell transplantation in patients with multiple myeloma. *Blood* 2009;113:5720.
16. Jones HM, Jones SA, Watts MJ, et al. Development of a simplified single-apheresis approach for peripheral-blood progenitor-cell transplantation in previously treated patients with lymphoma. *J Clin Oncol* 1994;12:1693.
20. Wuchter P, Ran D, Bruckner T, et al. Poor mobilization of hematopoietic stem cells-definitions, incidence, risk factors, and impact on outcome of autologous transplantation. *Biol Blood Marrow Transplant* 2010;16:490.
21. Kumar S, Dispenzieri A, Lacy MQ, et al. Impact of lenalidomide therapy on stem cell mobilization and engraftment post-peripheral blood stem cell transplantation in patients with newly diagnosed myeloma. *Leukemia* 2007;21:2035.
27. Phillips GL, Hale GA, Howard DS, et al. G-CSF primed autologous marrow harvest and transplantation in cytapheresis "mobilization failure" patients: a descriptive analysis; bone marrow transplantation. *Hematology* 2000;5:223.
28. Micallef IN, Stiff PJ, DiPersio JF, et al. Successful stem cell remobilization using plerixafor (Mozobil) plus granulocyte colony-stimulating factor in patients with non-Hodgkin lymphoma: results from the plerixafor NHL phase 3 study rescue protocol. *Biol Blood Marrow Transplant* 2009;15:1578.
29. Calandra G, McCarty J, McGuirk J, et al. AMD3100 plus G-CSF can successfully mobilize CD34+ cells from non-Hodgkin's lymphoma, Hodgkin's disease and multiple myeloma patients previously failing mobilization with chemotherapy and/or cytokine treatment: compassionate use data. *Bone Marrow Transplant* 2008;41:331.
32. Galimberti S, Morabito F, Guerrini F, et al. Peripheral blood stem cell contamination evaluated by a highly sensitive molecular method fails to predict outcome of autotransplanted multiple myeloma patients. *Br J Haematol* 2003;120:405.
33. Stewart AK, Vescio R, Schiller G, et al. Purging of autologous peripheral-blood stem cells using CD34 selection does not improve overall or progression-free survival after high-dose chemotherapy for multiple myeloma: results of a multicenter randomized controlled trial. *J Clin Oncol* 2001;19:3771.
36. Attal M, Harousseau JL, Stoppa AM, et al. A prospective, randomized trial of autologous bone marrow transplantation and chemotherapy in multiple myeloma. Intergroupe Francais du Myelome. *N Engl J Med* 1996;335:91.
37. Child JA, Morgan GJ, Davies FE, et al. High-dose chemotherapy with hematopoietic stem-cell rescue for multiple myeloma. *N Engl J Med* 2003;348:1875.
38. van de Velde HJ, Liu X, Chen G, et al. Complete response correlates with long-term survival and progression-free survival in high-dose therapy in multiple myeloma. *Haematologica* 2007;92:1399.
40. Barlogie B, Kyle RA, Anderson KC, et al. Standard chemotherapy compared with high-dose chemoradiotherapy for multiple myeloma: final results of phase III US Intergroup Trial S9321. *J Clin Oncol* 2006;24:929.
44. Attal M, Harousseau JL, Facon T, et al. Single versus double autologous stem-cell transplantation for multiple myeloma. *N Engl J Med* 2003;349:2495.
45. Kumar A, Kharfan-Dabaja MA, Glasmacher A, Djulbegovic B. Tandem versus single autologous hematopoietic cell transplantation for the treatment of multiple myeloma: a systematic review and meta-analysis. *J Natl Cancer Inst* 2009;101:100.
49. Deconinck E, Foussard C, Milpied N, et al. High-dose therapy followed by autologous purged stem-cell transplantation and doxorubicin-based chemotherapy in patients with advanced follicular lymphoma: a randomized multicenter study by GOELAMS. *Blood* 2005;105:3817.
54. Philip T, Guglielmi C, Hagenbeek A, et al. Autologous bone marrow transplantation as compared with salvage chemotherapy in relapses of chemotherapy-sensitive non-Hodgkin's lymphoma. *N Engl J Med* 1995;333:1540.
55. Blay J, Gomez F, Sebban C, et al. The International Prognostic Index correlates to survival in patients with aggressive lymphoma in relapse: analysis of the PARMA trial. Parma Group. *Blood* 1998;92:3562.
58. Yuen AR, Rosenberg SA, Hoppe RT, Halpern JD, Horning SJ. Comparison between conventional salvage therapy and high-dose therapy with autografting for recurrent or refractory Hodgkin's disease. *Blood* 1997;89:814.
61. Burnett AK, Goldstone AH, Stevens RM, et al. Randomised comparison of addition of autologous bone-marrow transplantation to intensive chemotherapy for acute myeloid leukaemia in first remission: results of MRC AML 10 trial. UK Medical Research Council Adult and Children's Leukaemia Working Parties. *Lancet* 1998;351:700.
62. Cassileth PA, Harrington DP, Appelbaum FR, et al. Chemotherapy compared with autologous or allogeneic bone marrow transplantation in the management of acute myeloid leukemia in first remission. *N Engl J Med* 1998;339:1649.
64. de Botton S, Fawaz A, Chevret S, et al. Autologous and allogeneic stem-cell transplantation as salvage treatment of acute promyelocytic leukemia initially treated with all-trans-retinoic acid: a retrospective analysis of the European Acute Promyelocytic Leukemia Group. *J Clin Oncol* 2005;23:120.
66. Matthay KK, Villablanca JG, Seeger RC, et al. Treatment of high-risk neuroblastoma with intensive chemotherapy, radiotherapy, autologous bone marrow transplantation, and 13-cis-retinoic acid. Children's Cancer Group. *N Engl J Med* 1999;341:1165.
70. Einhorn LH, Williams SD, Chamness A, et al. High-dose chemotherapy and stem-cell rescue for metastatic germ-cell tumors. *N Engl J Med* 2007;357:340.
72. Stadtmauer EA, O'Neill A, Goldstein LJ, et al. Conventional-dose chemotherapy compared with high-dose chemotherapy plus autologous hematopoietic stem-cell transplantation for metastatic breast cancer. Philadelphia Bone Marrow Transplant Group. *N Engl J Med* 2000;342:1069.
73. Tomblyn M, Chiller T, Einsele H, et al. Guidelines for preventing infectious complications among hematopoietic cell transplantation recipients: a global perspective. *Biol Blood Marrow Transplant* 2009;15:1143.
82. Moreau P, Facon T, Attal M, et al. Comparison of 200 mg/m(2) melphalan and 8 Gy total body irradiation plus 140 mg/m(2) melphalan as conditioning regimens for peripheral blood stem cell transplantation in patients with newly diagnosed multiple myeloma: final analysis of the Intergroupe Francophone du Myelome 9502 randomized trial. *Blood* 2002;99:731.
85. Palumbo A, Bringhen S, Bruno B, et al. Melphalan 200 mg/m(2) versus melphalan 100 mg/m(2) in newly diagnosed myeloma patients: a prospective, multicenter phase 3 study. *Blood* 2010;115:1873.
86. Roussel M, Moreau P, Huynh A, et al. Bortezomib and high-dose melphalan as conditioning regimen before autologous stem cell transplantation in patients with de novo multiple myeloma: a phase 2 study of the Intergroupe Francophone du Myelome (IFM). *Blood* 2010;115:32.
91. Carreras E. Veno-occlusive disease of the liver after hemopoietic cell transplantation. *Eur J Haematol* 2000;64:281.
93. Wadleigh M, Richardson PG, Zahrieh D, et al. Prior gemtuzumab ozogamicin exposure significantly increases the risk of veno-occlusive disease in patients who undergo myeloablative allogeneic stem cell transplantation. *Blood* 2003;102:1578.
96. Richardson PG, Murakami C, Jin Z, et al. Multi-institutional use of defibrotide in 88 patients after stem cell transplantation with severe veno-occlusive disease and multisystem organ failure: response without significant toxicity in a high-risk population and factors predictive of outcome. *Blood* 2002;100:4337.
97. Ho VT, Revta C, Richardson PG. Hepatic veno-occlusive disease after hematopoietic stem cell transplantation: update on defibrotide and other current investigational therapies. *Bone Marrow Transplant* 2008;41:229.
101. Govindarajan R, Jagannath S, Flick JT, et al. Preceding standard therapy is the likely cause of MDS after autotransplants for multiple myeloma. *Br J Haematol* 1996;95:349.
103. Pedersen-Bjergaard J, Andersen MK, Christiansen DH. Therapy-related acute myeloid leukemia and myelodysplasia after high-dose chemotherapy and autologous stem cell transplantation. *Blood* 2000;95:3273.
104. Curtis RE, Rowlings PA, Deeg HJ, et al. Solid cancers after bone marrow transplantation. *N Engl J Med* 1997;336:897.

105. Horwitz SM, Negrin RS, Blume KG, et al. Rituximab as adjuvant to high-dose therapy and autologous hematopoietic cell transplantation for aggressive non-Hodgkin lymphoma. *Blood* 2004;103:777.
109. Yanik GA, Levine JE, Matthay KK, et al. Pilot study of iodine-131-metaiodobenzylguanidine in combination with myeloablative chemotherapy and autologous stem-cell support for the treatment of neuroblastoma. *J Clin Oncol* 2002;20:2142.
110. Cavo M, Zamagni E, Tosi P, et al. Superiority of thalidomide and dexamethasone over vincristine-doxorubicin dexamethasone (VAD) as primary therapy in preparation for autologous transplantation for multiple myeloma. *Blood* 2005;106:35.
111. Barlogie B, Tricot G, Anaissie E, et al. Thalidomide and hematopoietic-cell transplantation for multiple myeloma. *N Engl J Med* 2006;354:1021.
117. Attal M, Harousseau JL, Leyvraz S, et al. Maintenance therapy with thalidomide improves survival in patients with multiple myeloma. *Blood* 2006;108:3289.
120. Spielberger R, Stiff P, Bensinger W, et al. Palifermin for oral mucositis after intensive therapy for hematologic cancers. *N Engl J Med* 2004;351:2590.
128. Farge D, Labopin M, Tyndall A, et al. Autologous hematopoietic stem cell transplantation for autoimmune diseases: an observational study on 12 years' experience from the European Group for Blood and Marrow Transplantation Working Party on Autoimmune Diseases. *Haematologica* 2010;95:284.

PRACTICE OF ONCOLOGY

CHAPTER 155 ALLOGENEIC STEM CELL TRANSPLANTATION

RICHARD W. CHILDS

Since the 1970s, allogeneic hematopoietic cell transplantation (HCT) has been used successfully as a therapeutic modality to treat patients with advanced hematological malignancies.[1] Despite its inherent risks, allogeneic transplantation offers many patients with treatment-resistant and treatment-refractory malignancies the only chance of a cure. The concept that cancer might be cured if high enough doses of cytotoxic agents were deliverable was based on the observation that some malignancies exhibit a steep dose–response effect to radiation and cytotoxic drugs. For total body irradiation (TBI) and for many classes of cytotoxic drugs, the permanent eradication of recipient bone marrow (BM) is the primary obstacle to dose intensification. For conventional transplant regimens, myeloablative dosages of chemoradiotherapy are given to maximally cytoreduce the malignancy, followed by an infusion of hematopoietic progenitor cells (either BM cells, cord blood cells, or progenitors mobilized into the blood by granulocyte colony-stimulating factor [G-CSF]) to rescue the patient from ensuing BM aplasia. However, even the most intense of conditioning regimens often fail to completely eradicate leukemic clones.[2] Rather, a powerful immune reaction generated from transplanted donor T cells against residual leukemia (called graft-versus-leukemia [GVL] effect or graft-versus tumor [GVT] effect) occurs in those who achieve durable disease-free survival.[3] It is through the combination of these two components, dose-intensive tumor killing followed by the donor immune–mediated GVL effect, that allogeneic HCT has its curative potential.

CONDITIONING REGIMENS

Conventional Myeloablative Conditioning

For conventional myeloablative transplantation of hematological malignancies, the preparative regimen serves two purposes: (1) to provide sufficient immunosuppression to prevent rejection while allowing for engraftment of transplanted donor hematopoietic or immune cells and (2) to eradicate malignant cells. Decisions regarding the choice of a specific preparative regimen are guided by following the sensitivity of the underlying malignancy to the drugs contained within that regimen, the age and performance status of the patient, the specific toxicities inherent to individual conditioning agents, and the HLA antigen compatibility between the recipient and donor. For many hematological malignancies, particularly those with rapid proliferation kinetics such as acute leukemia, cytoreduction through dose-intensive conditioning is required to optimize the induction of curative GVL effects. In general, myeloablative conditioning strategies can be divided into two categories: TBI-based or chemotherapy-based regimen.

Most TBI-based regimens are composed of high-dose cyclophosphamide given as 60 mg/kg intravenously (IV) on 2 consecutive days followed by varying doses of fractionated TBI to a cumulative dose of 120 to 150 Gy. Although evidence exists that the higher doses of TBI may have superior efficacy in preventing disease relapse, a concomitant increase in toxicity appears to negate a survival benefit.

Although a number of chemotherapy-based regimens without radiation have been used, the combination of cyclophosphamide (60 mg/kg IV on 2 consecutive days, total dose 120 mg/kg) and busulfan (3.2 mg/kg IV daily or 4 mg/kg orally daily both given on 4 consecutive days) has remained a popular conditioning strategy since its initial use in the early 1980s. More recently, investigators have shown that combining myeloablative doses of IV busulfan with the nucleoside analogue fludarabine is extremely well tolerated, achieving favorable outcome with a low risk of mortality in patients with a variety of hematological malignancies.[4] Similar to the experience with TBI, dose intensification of chemotherapy-based regimens usually results in a reduction in disease relapse, but this benefit is typically offset by an increase in toxicity and transplant-related mortality.

The decision guiding preparative regimen choice is often based on the disease-specific activity of the agents contained within the regimen. In general, radiation- and chemotherapy-based regimens have shown equivalence in disease-free survival in acute and chronic myelogenous leukemias. Two randomized trials evaluating cyclophosphamide and busulfan versus TBI and cyclophosphamide in patients with chronic myelogenous leukemia (CML) revealed equal efficacy between both regimens.[5] However, in acute lymphocytic leukemia (ALL), TBI-based regimens may be the treatment of choice, as two randomized trials reported a significantly increased risk of relapse in patients with ALL who received conditioning with chemotherapy alone (busulfan and etoposide or busulfan and cyclophosphamide) compared with regimens containing TBI (TBI and etoposide or TBI and cyclophosphamide).[6,7] In general, TBI-based regimens are associated with a higher risk of secondary malignancies, cataracts, hypothyroidism, and growth retardation, whereas chemotherapy-based regimens, particularly those containing busulfan, are associated with a higher risk of severe mucositis and veno-occlusive disease (VOD), with fewer effects on growth and development. A study from the Nordic Transplantation Group reported busulfan-treated patients to have a significantly higher incidence of VOD (12%) and death from graft-versus-host disease (GVHD) (22%) compared with patients receiving conditioning with TBI and cyclophosphamide (1%; P = .01 and 3%; P <.001, respectively).[8] Data exist showing patients with high busulfan area under the concentration–time curve levels are at greatest risk for the development of VOD and death.[9] The increasing use of IV busulfan now allows for more accurate targeting of busulfan drug levels in the therapeutic range without the need for drug level monitoring and has been reported to reduce the incidence of VOD, VOD-related death, and 100-day transplant-related mortality compared to regimens utilizing oral busulfan.[10]

Reduced-Intensity Conditioning Regimens

Over the past 15 years, investigators have increasingly explored the use of reduced-intensity (nonmyeloablative) preparative regimens in an effort to decrease the risk of regimen-related toxicity and mortality that occurs as a consequence of myeloablative conditioning. Reduced-intensity preparative regimens have less of a direct cytotoxic effect on malignant cells and are given primarily to induce immunosuppression of the recipient to allow for the engraftment of donor hematopoietic progenitor cells and immune cells, which mediate GVL effects. Such low-intensity transplants incorporate a number of strategies to enhance the GVL effect to eradicate the underlying malignancy, such as through early tapering of immunosuppression or the administration of escalating sequential doses of donor lymphocyte infusions. Furthermore, because host BM cells are not completely destroyed, autologous hematopoiesis may persist, resulting in mixed hematopoietic chimerism, which may shorten the time interval of neutropenia. In particular, reduced-intensity regimens utilizing low-dose TBI (2 to 3 Gy) frequently avoid conditioning-associated neutropenia altogether, which significantly decreases the risk of opportunistic infections in the first 30 days following transplantation, allowing for the transplant to occur in the outpatient setting.

Although reduced-intensity regimens vary considerably between institutions, results have been promising, showing high degrees of donor engraftment with a lower incidence of toxicities such as severe mucositis, pneumonitis, and VOD compared with those receiving conventional high-dose myeloablative regimens.[11] Furthermore, they have proven to be safe in older patients (e.g., older than 55 years) and in those with underlying medical comorbidities who would not be candidates for a myeloablative transplant due to an exceedingly high risk of transplant-related mortality.

GRAFT-VERSUS-LEUKEMIA EFFECT

Transplanted donor immune cells make an important contribution to the antileukemic effect of allogeneic BM transplant.[12] Seminal observations supporting the existence of a GVL effect in humans are shown in Table 155.1. A retrospective study of more than 2,000 recipients of HLA-matched sibling BM transplants confirmed acute GVHD and in particular chronic GVHD (CGVHD) were associated with a significant reduction in the risk of disease relapse, whereas T-cell depletion increased the risk of relapse.[13] Results from this study show the relationship of acute and chronic GVHD, T-cell depletion, and the sources of donor cells with relapse are shown in Figure 155.1. Data from this registry showed GVL effects vary according to the type of leukemia but were most evident in patients with chronic-phase CML undergoing transplant in the early chronic phase. Further indirect evidence for a donor immune-mediated antileukemic effect included the observation that up to 50% of patients who are ultimately cured after allogeneic transplantation have detectable CML BCR/ABL transcripts or small numbers of Philadelphia-positive chromosomes for months after allogeneic BM transplant; their delayed clearance is consistent with an active GVL effect.[14] In addition, abrupt discontinuation of cyclosporine after CML relapse has been associated with reinduction of cytogenetic remissions.[15]

TABLE 155.1

OBSERVATIONS SUPPORTING THE EXISTENCE OF A GRAFT-VS-LEUKEMIA EFFECT

- Leukemia relapse is decreased in patients who develop acute GVHD
- Leukemia relapse is decreased in patients who develop chronic GVHD
- Leukemic relapse is increased in identical twin transplants vs. HLA matched non-twin siblings
- Leukemic relapse is increased with use of T-cell depleted transplants to prevent acute GVHD
- Observation of delayed clearance of leukemia occurring months after transplantation
- Remission of leukemia following donor lymphocyte infusion

More recent data support chronic leukemias and lymphomas such as CLL, low-grade lymphomas, and mantle cell lymphoma as being exquisitely sensitive to the GVL effect.[16,17] The most compelling evidence supporting the curative nature of the GVL effect is the observation that durable molecular remissions can be induced in patients with CML in relapse after marrow transplant by the transfusion of donor lymphocytes in the absence of chemotherapy.[18] The efficacy of donor lymphocyte infusions (DLIs) for the treatment of relapsed leukemia is disease dependent, with remission induction occurring in a substantially higher percentage of patients with chronic-phase CML than patients with advanced CML or other acute leukemias. In general, 70% to 80% of patients with cytogenetic or hematological relapse of CML achieve a durable molecular remission after DLI. Remissions are usually not observed until months after DLI, consistent with the time required to expand antileukemic T-cell clones (Fig. 155.2).[19]

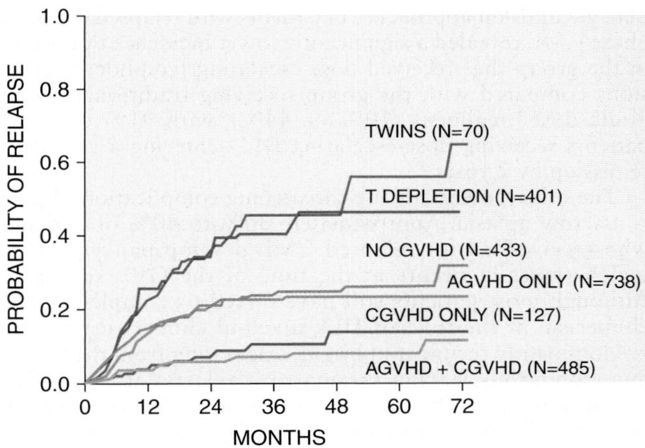

FIGURE 155.1 Actuarial probability of relapse after allogeneic bone marrow transplantation for early leukemia according to type of graft (T-cell replete vs T-cell depleted) and development of graft-versus-host disease (GVHD). AGVHD, acute GVHD; CGVHD, chronic GVHD. (From Horowitz MM, Gale RP, Sondel PM, et al. Graft-versus-leukemia reactions after bone marrow transplantation. *Blood* 1990;75:555, with permission.) Copyright © 2004 by Lippincott Williams & Wilkins.

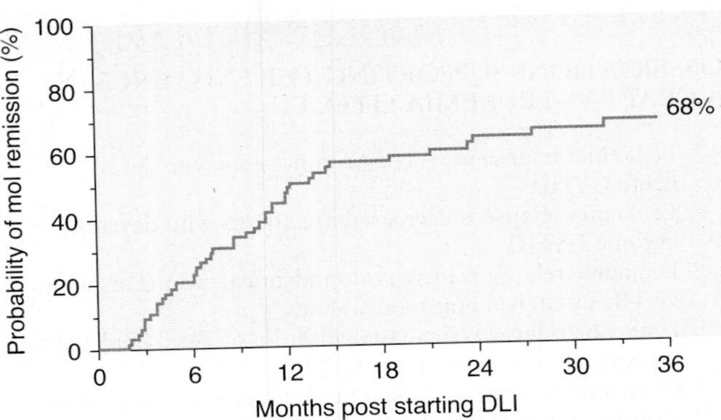

FIGURE 155.2 Probability of achieving a molecular remission after treatment with donor lymphocyte infusion (DLI) for 66 patients with chronic myelogenous leukemia in relapse after allogeneic stem cell transplantation. (From ref 19, with permission.) Copyright © 2004 by Lippincott Williams & Wilkins.

In contrast to the relatively high efficacy of DLI in relapsed chronic-phase CML, only a minority of patients with acute leukemias who relapse after allogeneic transplant achieve a durable remission after the infusion of donor lymphocytes.[20,21] Disease regression after DLI has also been described in patients with relapsed multiple myeloma, chronic lymphocytic leukemia (CLL), non-Hodgkin's lymphoma (NHL), and mycosis fungoides,[22] although too few have been treated to define the efficacy of this approach in these diseases.

The major complication associated with DLI is acute GVHD and CGVHD; up to 70% of patients develop acute GVHD after DLI that may be life-threatening (i.e., grades 3 to 4) in 15% to 20% of cases. The propensity for GVHD after DLI is likely impacted by the relatively large doses of T lymphocytes infused and the fact that these cells are usually given without GVHD prophylaxis.[23] The strategy of infusing donor lymphocytes in multiple aliquots, starting at low cell numbers and escalating the dosage at variable intervals until a GVL effect is achieved, has been reported to reduce the risk of DLI-associated GVHD.[24] A trial comparing these two lymphocyte infusion approaches in patients with relapsed chronic-phase CML revealed a significantly lower incidence of GVHD in the group that received dose-escalating lymphocyte infusions compared with the group receiving traditional single "bulk-dose" regimens (10% vs. 44%), with 91% of CML patients receiving dose-escalating DLI achieving a complete remission by 2 years.[25]

The other potentially life-threatening complication of DLI is marrow aplasia. Approximately 30% to 40% of patients who receive DLI for relapsed CML develop pancytopenia, which typically occurs at the time of the GVL response. Although most patients still have mixed or complete T-cell chimerism at the time of DLI, myeloid chimerism may be predominantly recipient in origin, originating from the leukemic clone, thus leaving the marrow aplastic after a GVH hematopoietic effect. Although in most cases, spontaneous reconstitution of marrow by donor cells usually occurs, some patients have persistent aplasia and may require a boost of donor CD34+ selected hematopoietic stem cells to rescue marrow function. Reconditioning before such stem cell infusions is not required, as most patients have predominant donor immunity and are therefore tolerant of donor hematopoietic progenitor cells. Although the infusion of donor lymphocytes with stem cells has been used successfully to treat relapsed leukemia, it is unclear if the incidence and severity of BM aplasia are mitigated.[26]

MECHANISMS OF GRAFT-VERSUS-LEUKEMIA EFFECT

Although evidence supporting the GVL effect is overwhelming, the target antigens on leukemic cells as well as the effector cells mediating these antileukemic effects are not fully understood.[27] Although the full nature of the effector cells mediating GVL are not entirely known, both CD4+ helper T cells and CD8+ cytotoxic T cells with direct antileukemic activity have been isolated from patients after allogeneic BM transplant.[28] The high incidence of leukemic relapse in syngeneic transplants suggests that a significant component of the GVL effect is the consequence of donor immune cells targeting allogeneic antigens. Minor histocompatibility antigens (major histocompatibility complex [MHC]-bound peptides derived from the degradation of cellular proteins with amino acid polymorphisms between the patient and donor) can lead to differential recognition by T cells and are likely the dominant targets for both GVHD and the GVL effect. The tissue-restricted pattern of minor histocompatibility antigens likely explains why some patients respond to DLI without the development of GVHD; T-cell populations mediating an antileukemia reaction against minor histocompatibility antigens restricted to hematopoietic cells would not be expected to cause GVHD, in contrast to T cells targeting antigens expressed broadly on both normal tissue and leukemic cells, where both GVHD and a GVL effect would occur. Indeed, T-cell clones have been generated *in vitro* that specifically recognize minor histocompatibility antigens restricted to leukemic cells and normal hematopoietic cells.[29] Minor histocompatibility antigens can be either MHC class I- or class II-restricted, thus evoking CD8+ and CD4+ alloreactive T-cell responses, respectively. Recently, investigators have shown that both CD8+ and CD4+ T-cell clones that recognize a number of different minor histocompatibility antigens expressed on hematopoietic cells emerge in the blood of some patients at the time of a GVL effect, further confirming minor antigens to be the dominant target of T cells mediating GVL effects.[30,31]

Donor T cells targeting tumor antigens restricted or overexpressed on malignant cells might also serve as targets for GVL.[32] Furthermore, the degradation of proteins restricted to tumor cells might result in the MHC binding and presentation of unique peptides from the region of fusion gene or mutated gene sequence. Although leukemia-restricted peptides would appear to be an attractive target for donor immune cells, there is very little evidence to implicate a specific antileukemic effect in most patients who have a GVL effect. However, patients with relapsed leukemia who achieve remission after DLI without GVHD lend credence to the notion that GVL may occasionally be a targeted antileukemic process. Furthermore, the recent identification of donor derived CD8+ T-cell clones targeting an antigen selectively expressed in kidney cancer cells in a patient who had tumor regression after an allogeneic transplant has provided evidence that donor immune–mediated GVT effects may in some cases be tumor specific.[32]

Recent data suggest natural killer (NK) cells may also play an important role in the GVL effect against myelogenous leukemia in the setting of haploidentical or partially mismatched allogeneic transplantation when killer immunoglobulin-like receptor (KIR) incompatibility exists in the direction of GVHD (defined as the absence of an MHC class I KIR ligand in the recipient that is present in the donor).[33] In the HLA-matched setting, the contribution that donor NK cells make to GVL is not known, although recent studies suggest alloreactive NK cells may also play a role in GVL in the setting of HLA-matched transplants.[34,35]

COMPLICATIONS OF ALLOGENEIC HEMATOPOIETIC STEM CELL TRANSPLANTATION

Allogeneic HCT is associated with a number of complications, many unique to this type of therapy, that can be divided into two general categories: (1) toxicities related to conditioning and (2) toxicities that occur as the consequence of transplanting allogeneic immune cells or tissue into the recipient, namely graft rejection, acute and chronic GVHD, and infectious complications associated with immunosuppression and immune dysregulation.

The complications associated with myeloablative dosages of chemoradiotherapy may occur as an immediate side effect, at or shortly after the preparative regimen, or in a delayed fashion years after transplantation. Commonly observed immediate toxicities include nausea and vomiting, mucositis, alopecia, and pancytopenia, including neutropenia associated with fever or opportunistic bacterial or invasive fungal infection.

High-dose cyclophosphamide may be associated with hemorrhagic cystitis or, more rarely, rapidly progressive heart failure. The routine use of mesna, hydration, and forced diuresis has largely eliminated early chemotherapy-associated hemorrhagic cystitis. In contrast, late hemorrhagic cystitis (occurring beyond 72 hours of cyclophosphamide) remains a continuing problem in allogeneic BM transplant and is usually viral in etiology (most commonly polyomavirus BK or adenovirus), occurring more frequently in profoundly immunosuppressed patients.[36] High-dose busulfan is associated with grand mal seizures; most busulfan-containing regimens use seizure prophylaxis with phenytoin, phenobarbital, benzodiazepenes, or more recently levetiracetam.[37]

Opportunistic infections as a consequence of preparative regimen-induced neutropenia remain a significant complication associated with allogeneic BM transplant. Neutropia-associated infections are particularly problematic for recipients of cord blood transplants, where neutropenia persists for an average 3 to 4 weeks following transplantation of the allograft. Most fungal and bacterial infections originate from micro-organisms colonizing the skin, oral cavity, perianal area, or gastrointestinal (GI) or respiratory tract. The most common life-threatening bacterial infections that occur during the neutropenic period include Gram-negative and aerobic Gram-positive bacteria. These pathogens gain entry into the host through indwelling vascular catheters or as a consequence of the breakdown of GI mucosa related to high-dose chemoradiotherapy. Decontamination of the gut with nonabsorbable antibiotics such as neomycin or vancomycin has met with mixed success, with poor patient compliance being a major drawback to this approach. Prophylactic oral quinolones such as levofloxacin, ciprofloxacin, or norfloxacin appear to decrease the incidence of febrile neutropenia and Gram-negative infections. Although consideration of the use of a fluoroquinolone as a bacterial prophylaxis should be considered in patients with an anticipated neutropenic period of more than 7 days, prophylactic antibiotics have not been shown to improve survival and they may come at the expense of more episodes of Gram-positive bacteremia.[38] *Candida* and *Aspergillus* species are the most common fungal pathogens, commonly causing infection during periods of neutropenia or systemic corticosteroid use for GVHD. Oral triazoles, such as fluconazole, have been shown in randomized trials to decrease the incidence of opportunistic Candidal infections but have no impact on the incidence of infections with resistant species such as *Aspergillus* or *Candida krusei*. The optimal duration of fluconazole prophylaxis has not yet been defined; one placebo-controlled randomized study showed patients who received prophylactic fluconazole for 75 days after the transplant not only had a lower incidence of invasive candidiasis (30 of 148 patients vs. 4 of 152 patients; $P < .001$) but also a significantly lower incidence of severe GVHD of the GI tract, resulting in an overall survival benefit.[39] Micafungin has been shown to be comparable to fluconazole for preventing fungal infections. Voriconazole (an orally available broad-spectrum triazole with high activity against *Aspergillus* species) has recently been shown to be the most effective agent for the treatment of acute invasive *Aspergillus* in immunocompromised patients; studies comparing prophylactic voriconazole with fluconazole are currently under way.[40] Patients who develop GVHD are at particularly high risk for developing invasive fungal infections as a consequence of being treated with corticosteroids and other immunosuppressive agents. A randomized trial comparing fluconazole versus posaconazole fungal prophylaxis in 600 patients with GVHD showed posaconazole was as effective as fluconazole in preventing all invasive fungal infections (incidence, 5.3% and 9.0%, respectively; $P = .07$) and was superior to fluconazole in preventing proven or probable invasive aspergillosis (2.3% vs. 7.0%; $P = .006$). Overall mortality was similar in the groups, but death from invasive fungal infections was lower in the posaconazole group (1% vs. 4%; $P = .046$).[41] Recently, a joint committee with representatives from the National Marrow Donor Program, Center for International Blood and Marrow Transplant Research, European Group for Blood and Marrow Transplantation, Centers for Disease Control and Prevention, and other committees, comprising international experts on infectious diseases, published guidelines for preventing and treating infections in hematopoietic cell transplant recipients.[38]

VENO-OCCLUSIVE DISEASE

One of the most serious life-threatening complications of dose-intensive chemoradiotherapy is hepatic VOD of the liver (also known as sinusoidal obstruction syndrome [SOS]). VOD produces a clinical syndrome of jaundice, tender hepatomegaly, and unexplained weight gain or ascites.[42] The incidence of transplant-associated VOD has dropped dramatically as oral busulfan-containing regimens have been used less often. For the minority 5% or less of patients who develop VOD, approximately 25% will have severe life-threatening disease, leading to progressive liver failure, hepatic encephalopathy, or hepatorenal syndrome. The pathogenesis of VOD is related to hepatic endothelial damage due to transplant conditioning, leading to fibrinogen and collagen deposition in vessel walls at the interface of hepatic sinusoids and terminal venules, which ultimately become obstructed; histologically, damage to zone 3 hepatocytes is present.[43] The diagnosis of VOD is based on the presence of clinical criteria (jaundice, tender hepatomegaly, and unexplained weight gain or ascites), in which there is a 90% correlation between the presence of all three criteria and a histologic confirmation by liver biopsy. Symptoms of VOD usually occur shortly after the conditioning regimen (less than 20 days), although late-onset VOD (symptoms developing 24 to 42 days after conditioning) has rarely been described in some patients. Therapy for established VOD is unsatisfactory and consists mostly of measures to support renal function, fluid balance, and coagulation status. Defibrotide, a polydeoxyribonucleotide with activity in several vascular disorders, has recently been used with success to treat patients with severe VOD after HCT[44,45] and is currently being investigated in an ongoing phase 3 trial for VOD treatment.[46] The therapeutic drug monitoring of oral busulfan, with appropriate dose adjustments, and the use of IV rather than oral busulfan appear to substantially reduce the incidence of VOD associated with this agent. Two randomized clinical trials have shown a significant reduction in the incidence of VOD in patients taking ursodiol prophylaxis versus those taking placebo (15% vs. 50% and 3% vs. 18.5%, respectively, in each study).[47,48] Because this agent is generally well tolerated, it has increasingly been used as prophylaxis in patients thought to be at high risk for VOD.

Pulmonary Complications

Pulmonary complications occur frequently after allogeneic BM transplant. Common life-threatening infectious etiologies include *Aspergillus* or other fungal organisms, respiratory syncytial virus, and cytomegalovirus (CMV). Late pneumonia from *Pneumocystis* may occur more than a year after transplantation and is usually related to the use of immunosuppressive drugs or prolonged CD4+ lymphopenia associated with T-cell depletion of the allograft or acute or CGVHD. Idiopathic pneumonia syndrome (IPS) is an inflammatory lung disease that is characterized by diffuse interstitial pneumonitis (IP) and alveolitis, sometimes leading to interstitial fibrosis. Clinically it is characterized by fever, hypoxia, and diffuse pulmonary infiltrates. Animal models have shown that lung irradiation appears to play an important role in the development of IPS after allogeneic BM transplant. The syndrome occurs in 10% to 20% of patients receiving myeloablative conditioning, usually within the first 3 months of transplantation, and is lethal in up to half of the cases.[49] Approximately 90% of the cases of IP are related to either CMV infection or have an idiopathic origin (such as IPS). The incidence of CMV pneumonitis has decreased significantly over the past 15 years, primarily as a result of more sensitive methods to detect early CMV reactivation (e.g., polymerase chain reaction [PCR] for CMV) weeks before clinical disease develops. Patient-specific risk factors for IPS include older age, prior history of exposure to pulmonary toxic drugs such as bleomycin, history of acute or CGVHD, dose intensity of the conditioning regimen, or the use of TBI.[50] Regimens that use a lower dose rate or total dose of TBI, lung shielding, as well as hyperfractionated TBI may be associated with a lower risk of IPS.[51]

Bronchoscopy with bronchoalveolar lavage should be performed in all patients with interstitial pneumonitis to differentiate IPS from infectious causes or diffuse alveolar hemorrhage (DAH). Empiric use of anti-CMV agents such as ganciclovir or foscarnet should be considered when bronchoalveolar lavage is not feasible. The prognosis of patients developing DAH is extremely poor, with mortality rates in the range of 48% to 80%; survival appears to be worse in those with DAH after allogeneic transplantation (versus autologous transplants) and in patients who develop this complication more than 30 days after transplant conditioning. High-dose corticosteroids and more recently recombinant factor VIIa may be effective in treating patients with DAH.[52,53] Although a mainstay of therapy, the effectiveness of corticosteroids for IPS remains equivocal. Donor T-cell derived tumor necrosis factor-α (TNF-α)-mediated endothelial apoptosis may play a role in the pathophysiology of IPS. Recently, a small number of case reports have suggested that etanercept, a dimeric tumor necrosis factor α (TNF-α)-binding protein, may be therapeutically effective for patients with IPS.[54]

Late Complications

Delayed complications associated with allogeneic HCT depend on patient age at transplantation and are primarily the consequence of the effects of long-term damage to normal tissues by either the preparative regimen or CGVHD. These effects include growth retardation, infertility, endocrine failure, avascular joint necrosis, osteopenia, hypertension, cataracts, renal insufficiency, restrictive or obstructive defects in pulmonary function, neurocognitive defects, and secondary malignancies.[55] A recent long-term follow-up study of 2,574 transplant patients surviving more than 5 years reported a four- to ninefold higher than expected mortality rate than the expected age-matched population for at least 30 years after transplantation, yielding an estimated 30% lower life expectancy compared with that in the general population, regardless of current age. In the order of their frequency, the leading causes of death were second malignancies and recurrent disease, followed by infections, CGVHD, respiratory illnesses, and cardiovascular disease.[56] The use of TBI in the conditioning regimen seems to be the factor associated with the greatest risk for secondary malignancies.[57] A long-term follow-up study of 1,036 patients undergoing BM transplant for a wide range of malignant and nonmalignant conditions reported a 12.6% incidence of secondary neoplasms at 15 years, a rate that was 3.8 times higher than an age-matched control population.[58] The most frequently observed secondary neoplasms are lymphomas, leukemias, and solid tumors (particularly oral cavity and skin). The characteristic time course for the development of secondary malignancies after allogeneic HCT is shown in Figure 155.3.[57] Increased solid tumor risk appears to be associated with younger patient age at transplantation and the use of radiation in the conditioning regimen. CGVHD and treatment for CGVHD are strongly associated with an increased risk of squamous cell carcinoma of the skin.

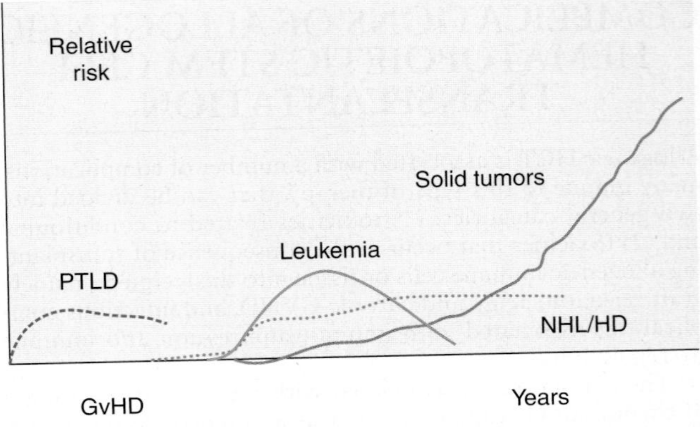

FIGURE 155.3 Scheme of time course and relative risk of second malignancies after allogeneic stem cell transplantation. GvHD, graft-versus-host disease; HD, Hodgkin's disease; NHL, non-Hodgkin's lymphoma; PTLD, posttransplant lymphoproliferative disorder. (From ref 57, with permission.) Copyright © 2004 by Lippincott Williams & Wilkins.

EPSTEIN-BARR VIRUS LYMPHOPROLIFERATIVE DISORDER

Posttransplant Epstein-Barr virus (EBV)-associated lymphoproliferative disorder (LPD) represents an aggressive and potentially fatal B-cell lymphoid proliferation that occurs after 5% to 30% of allogeneic transplants. This lymphoma originates from EBV-infected B cells, typically of donor origin, and usually stems from a deficiency of EBV-specific cytotoxic T cells associated with the use of immunosuppressive drugs or T-cell depletion of the allograft. EBV LPD was recently reported to occur with high frequency when antithymocyte globulin (ATG) is administered during transplant conditioning to recipients of cord blood transplants.[59] EBV LPD can be successfully treated by infusing donor lymphocytes that include (1) unmanipulated leukocytes from the donor, (2) donor lymphocytes that have been sensitized *in vitro* to irradiated EBV-transformed B-cell lines, or (3) donor lymphocytes that recognize and bind EBV peptides that have been isolated from the donor using magnetic beads.[60,61] Prophylactic infusion of *ex vivo*-generated EBV-specific T cells have been shown to prevent EBV LPD without causing acute GVHD in children receiving T-cell–depleted transplants from HLA-mismatched donors.[62] B-cell depletion of the allograft is another strategy that has been used to prevent this disorder. Rituximab, a monoclonal antibody to the B-cell antigen CD20, has also proven to be highly effective in treating established LPD.[59,63] Quantitative real-time PCR monitoring for EBV DNA can be used to identify patients at high risk for the development of posttransplant LPD. Furthermore, pre-emptive withdrawal of immunosuppression or therapy with rituximab in patients reactivating EBV by PCR may significantly reduce the risk of development of LPD.[63,64] Recently investigators have shown that EBV reactive T cells can be generated from cord blood cells with a naive phenotype; trials that investigate the adoptive transfer of these cells to prevent EBV LPD after cord blood transplantation will likely be forthcoming.[65,66]

Graft-versus-Host Disease

GVHD is the consequence of immunocompetent donor T cells targeting recipient tissues that possess antigens absent from the donor.[67] GVHD may manifest as either acute or chronic disease, each with characteristic clinical findings and a distinct pathophysiology. The major target tissues of acute GVHD are the skin, liver, and GI tract, although other tissues may be involved. The diagnosis of acute GVHD may be based on one or myriad characteristic clinical and laboratory findings.[68] Skin manifestations include a "sunburn-like" erythematous maculopapular rash that often involves the palms and soles (Fig. 155.4*A*), and under the most severe of circumstances, may be associated with desquamation. Hepatic involvement is characterized by a rise in alkaline phosphatase and total bilirubin, often in association with a mild to moderate increase in hepatic transaminases. GI GVHD predominantly involves the distal small bowel and colon and clinically is associated with abdominal pain or cramps and watery diarrhea, which may be voluminous and bloody under severe circumstances. Endoscopic findings are variable and may include a grossly normal-appearing bowel, bowel edema, and bowel ulcerations or total denuding of intestinal mucosa in severe cases; colonic biopsy usually reveals pathopneumonic features of crypt cell loss or necrosis with apoptotic bodies and lymphocytic infiltrates, although disease involvement is frequently patchy and can be missed on random biopsy. Upper GI involvement may be associated with recurrent nausea, vomiting, dyspepsia, and weight loss. Traditionally, acute GVHD has been divided into severity grades 1 to 4, depending on the extent of skin involvement, volume of diarrhea, or level of bilirubin elevation.[69]

Donor T cells are the principal mediators of GVHD. Antigens that are disparate between patient and donor that serve as targets for GVHD in the HLA-identical transplant setting are referred to as *minor histocompatibility antigens*.[70] Although

A
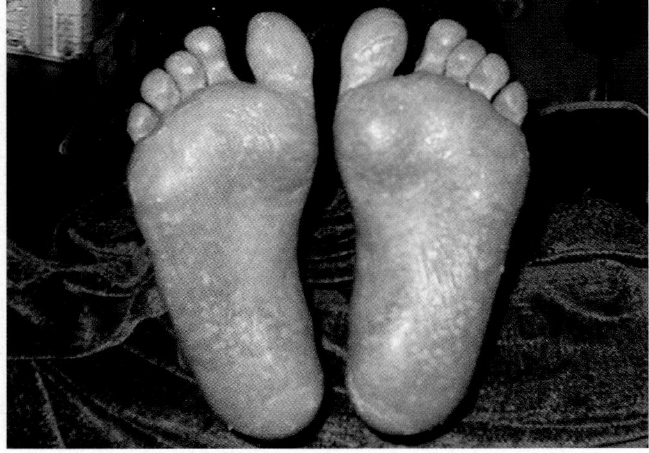
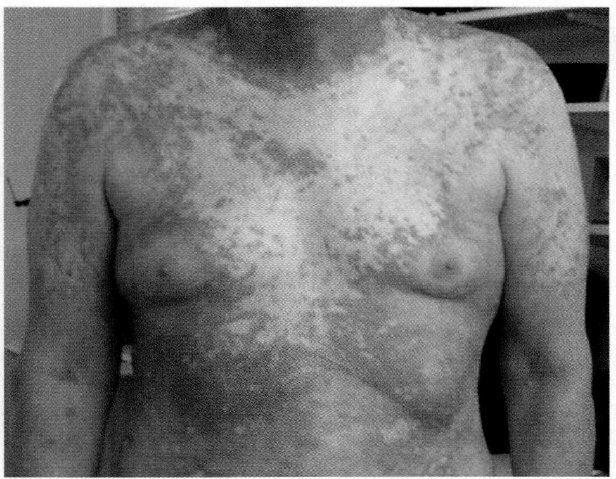
B

C
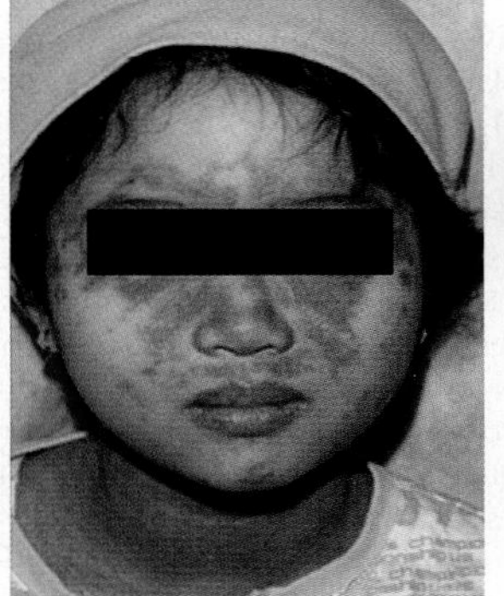
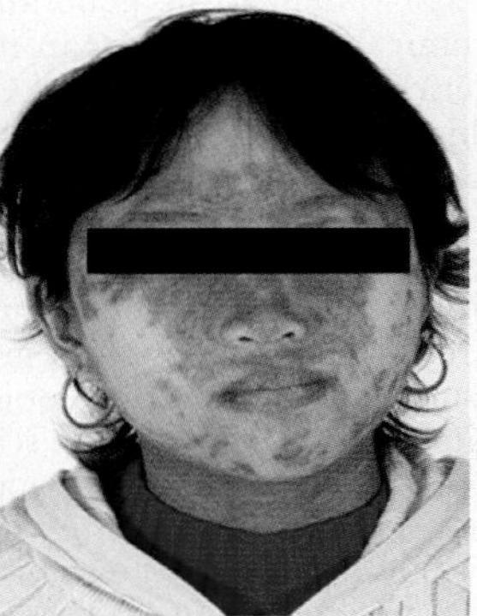
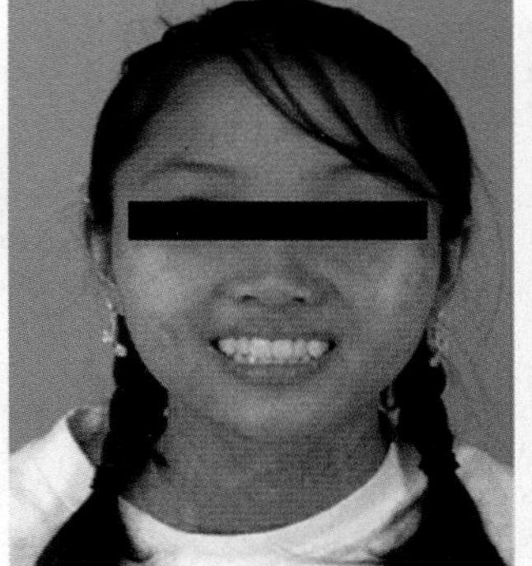
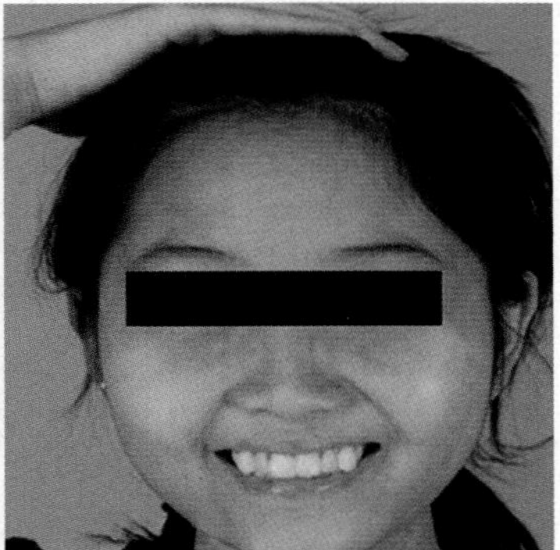

FIGURE 155.4 Typical appearance of skin rash from (**A**) acute GVHD involving soles of feet or from (**B**) sclerotic chronic GVHD of the skin. (**C**) Chronic GVHD of the skin resolving over years.

few minor histocompatibility antigens have been characterized to date, increasing evidence suggests the degree of disparity between recipient and donor minor histocompatibility antigens is a major determinant for the development of both acute GVHD and CGVHD.[71,72] The development of GVHD is a multistep process in which recipient tissues are recognized as foreign by the donor immune system; antigen-presenting cells present recipient alloantigens to donor T cells, resulting in the activation and expansion of GVHD effector populations, ultimately leading to T-cell–mediated cytotoxic damage of target tissues. Animal models suggest host antigen-presenting cells are the driving force behind the activation of donor CD8+ T cells that mediate acute GVHD.[73,74]

The incidence and severity of GVHD are determined by a number of variables, including degrees of HLA disparity between patient and donor, use of a T-cell–replete versus T-cell–depleted allograft, patient age, intensity of the conditioning regimen (e.g., myeloablative versus nonmyeloablative), and the agents used as prophylaxis for GVHD.[75] Furthermore, acute GVHD early after allogeneic BM transplant appears to be exacerbated by conditioning-induced cytokine release from damaged recipient tissues that mature and activate host antigen-presenting cells.

The incidence of clinically significant acute GVHD in patients undergoing T-cell–replete allogeneic HCT from an HLA-identical sibling using conventional GVHD prophylaxis (cyclosporin-A [CSA] or tacrolimus plus methotrexate) is on the order of 30% to 50%, with approximately 15% of patients developing severe grades 3 to 4 disease.[75] Several studies have suggested that the incidence of acute GVHD after unrelated transplantation is similar to HLA-identical sibling transplants when using high-resolution HLA-matched donors.[76] However, a recent Center for International Blood and Marrow Transplant Research analysis comparing transplant outcome in over 4,000 CML recipients of either an HLA-matched sibling transplant versus matched unrelated transplant reported significantly more acute and chronic GVHD in full 8/8 allele matched unrelated donors.[77,78] For recipients of partially matched related donors or partially matched unrelated donor transplants, acute GVHD occurs more frequently, affecting more than 70% of patients.

The two most common methods to prevent acute GVHD include the use of prophylactic immunosuppressive agents and the use of allografts in which donor T cells have been partially or completely depleted. Although the combined use of CSA and methotrexate has been found to be superior to either agent alone in the prevention of GVHD, the addition of prednisone to these agents does not appear to offer any additional benefit.[79] Furthermore, prolonging the time course that patients receive CSA (i.e., 24 months) as GVHD prophylaxis does not appear to significantly reduce the incidence of CGVHD compared with those receiving a shorter course (i.e., 6 months) of CSA.[80] In both HLA-identical sibling and unrelated transplants, T-cell depletion (both *in vitro* using CD34 selection or *in vivo* using drugs) is the most effective method for preventing GVHD but is associated with an increased risk of graft rejection, opportunistic viral infection, and leukemic relapse.[81] T-cell–depleted transplants that are followed by delayed scheduled infusions of donor lymphocytes appear to decrease acute GVHD without increasing the risk of disease relapse.[24,82]

The mainstay of therapy for the treatment of acute GVHD is corticosteroid therapy, usually in association with CSA or tacrolimus (FK506). Approximately 40% to 60% of patients with grades 2 to 4 GVHD can be expected to respond to these agents. A randomized trial of low-dose (2 mg/kg) versus high-dose (10 mg/kg) methylprednisolone for acute GVHD showed no difference in response rates with either regimen.[83] Response to steroids appears to predict survival. In particular, steroid refractory patients have a poor prognosis, with 60% to 80% dying from GVHD-related causes. At present, no effective standard first-line therapy exists for patients developing steroid-refractory disease. ATG has been used with minimal success (20% to 40% response rate), with no evidence that it improves survival in this setting.[84] Extracorporeal photopheresis and drugs such as continuous IV infusions of CSA or tacrolimus, IV or oral mycophenolate mofetil, and immunosuppressive monoclonal antibodies that target a variety of different T-cell antigens have been used with variable success.[85] At the National Heart, Lung, and Blood Institute, 20 of 23 patients with steroid refractory GVHD had complete resolution of GVHD after receiving treatment with the monoclonal antibody daclizumab (anti-CD25) in combination with infliximab (antitumor necrosis factor),[86] establishing a combined TNF-α/interleukin-2 (IL-2) blockade as a highly effective therapeutic option for patients with steroid refractory GVHD.[87]

Recently a few small case series have provided evidence that *in vitro* expanded BM-derived mesenchymal stromal cells (MSC) can improve severe GVHD when infused intravenously.[88,89] The results of a multicenter phase 3 trial in steroid refractory GVHD in which 260 patients were randomized to receive conventional second-line GVHD therapy plus MSCs versus second-line therapy plus placebo was recently reported in abstract form. A subgroup analysis showed MSC recipients with steroid refractory liver and GI GVHD had a significantly improved response rate compared to second-line therapy alone (76% vs. 47%; $P = .03$ and 82% vs. 68%; $P = .03$ respectively), although MSC therapy did not appear to improve overall GVHD response rates or overall survival.

CGVHD occurs in 15% to 50% of long-term survivors of allogeneic BM transplant and typically manifests with symptoms 3 months to 2 years after transplantation.[90] Risk factors for CGVHD include a prior history of acute GVHD, older patient age, use of mismatched or unrelated donors, and a history of DLI for relapsed malignancy. Furthermore, the use of peripheral blood (PB) stem cell allografts (in contrast to marrow) also appears to increase this risk.[91] Although extensive CGVHD is associated with an increase in transplant-related mortality, limited CGVHD appears to reduce the risk of disease relapse, which may offset the deleterious effects of this complication on survival.[92]

Patients with CGVHD are often severely immunocompromised, either as a consequence of the immunosuppressive therapy used to treat the disorder or from the underlying immune deregulation associated with the disease process. CGVHD is lethal in up to 20% of cases, with death predominantly being related to infectious causes. Patients with a particularly poor prognosis include those with hepatic involvement or thrombocytopenia. CGVHD is traditionally classified as either limited or extensive, limited disease being defined as localized skin involvement with or without mild hepatic involvement and extensive defined as generalized skin involvement with or without other target organ involvement. A newly proposed criterion for the diagnosis of CGVHD includes the integration of histopathology with clinical, laboratory, and radiographic information with chronic GVHD being scored as either mild, moderate, or severe.[93] The characteristic clinical manifestations of CGVHD are numerous and include lichenoid or sclerodermatous skin involvement (Fig. 155.4*B*), hepatic cholestasis, friable nails, dry eyes (Sjögren's syndrome), oral ulcerations, fasciitis, xerostomia, lichenoid buccal changes, bronchiolitis obliterans, vaginal dryness, serositis, malabsorption, diarrhea, GI dysmotility, and pancytopenia. Treatment depends on the extent of disease. Systemic disease is typically treated with alternate-day CSA or tacrolimus and low-dose corticosteroids. In general, approximately two-thirds of patients who develop CGVHD will have resolution of their symptoms, allowing for the eventual discontinuation of immunosuppressive therapy

(Fig. 155.4C). Patients not responding to standard therapy often benefit from alternative therapies, including mycophenolate mofetil, psoralen and ultraviolet A light (for skin involvement), oral thalidomide, imatinib, extracorporeal photophoresis or monoclonal antibodies targeting tumor necrosis factor, activation antigens on T cells, or rituximab targeting CD20 on B cells.[94–96] As infections are the main cause of death, prophylaxis for organisms such as *Pneumocystis* and encapsulated bacteria is usually warranted, particularly in those taking systemic immunosuppressive therapy.

Graft Failure

Failure to achieve or maintain sustained donor hematopoietic engraftment after allogeneic HCT is referred to as *graft failure*. Graft failure may manifest as persistent neutropenia, without evidence of engraftment (primary graft failure), or as initial engraftment followed by a delayed drop in blood count (late or secondary graft failure). *Graft rejection* is the term used to describe graft failure that occurs as a consequence of the active rejection of donor hematopoietic cells by immunocompetent host cells that survived the conditioning regimen. Graft rejection manifests as transient donor engraftment followed by a lymphocytosis of recipient origin, which ultimately leads to the rejection of donor hematopoietic cells and pancytopenia, or in some cases (e.g., following a reduced-intensity transplant), autologous hematopoietic recovery. The mediators of graft rejection include NK cells or residual recipient T cells that recognize donor mismatched MHC molecules, or in an HLA-matched setting, minor histocompatibility antigens.[97]

Primary graft failure is associated with a significant risk of death from hemorrhage or infection and should be suspected in all patients receiving a BM or peripheral blood transplant who remain pancytopenic for more than 3 to 4 weeks or in recipients of a cord blood transplant who remain pancytopenic for more than 7 weeks. Although graft failure occurs in less than 2% of patients undergoing myeloablative allogeneic HCT from an HLA-identical sibling, the incidence increases for recipients of T-cell–depleted transplants, particularly those from HLA-mismatched or unrelated donors. Other risk factors for graft rejection include the infusion of low stem cell numbers (i.e., less than 1×10^6 CD34+ cells/kg), history of multiple blood transfusions with or without alloimmunization, HLA disparity between the patient and donor, use of low-intensity or dose-reduced conditioning regimens, use of umbilical cord blood transplants, and transplantation for severe aplastic anemia.[98]

It is important to differentiate graft failure from pancytopenia related to other causes, including marrow suppression from infection, medications (i.e., ganciclovir), or CGVHD. Furthermore, it is important to give early consideration for a second donor stem cell infusion, given the high risk of opportunistic infection associated with prolonged periods of neutropenia and the difficult logistics of collecting more donor cells.

Cytomegalovirus Infection

CMV is a member of the herpes virus family that may cause serious and life-threatening pathology after allogeneic BM transplant. CMV disease occurs most commonly as the consequence of viral reactivation in patients who have a history of prior CMV infection. Disruption of cellular immunity associated with T-cell depletion (both *in vitro* and *in vivo*), GVHD, or immunosuppressive therapy can lead to CMV reactivation and subsequent disease. The clinical features of CMV disease may include pneumonitis, hepatitis, marrow suppression, upper GI involvement, and colitis. Reactivation tends to occur most commonly 3 weeks to 100 days after transplantation and is most strongly associated with acute GVHD and a positive pretransplant CMV serologic status of the recipient. Although 40% to 60% of patients who are serologically positive for CMV reactivate this virus after conventional allogeneic transplantation, the risk of reactivation in patients who are serologically negative before transplantation is extremely rare. *In vivo* T-cell depletion with alemtuzumab (anti-CD52) is associated with an increased incidence of CMV reactivation, as high as 85% in some studies.[99] Effective prevention of CMV reactivation in CMV seronegative patients can be achieved through the use of CMV-negative or leukocyte-filtered blood products. Because up to 60% of patients who are pretransplant seropositive for CMV (defined as "at risk for CMV") never reactivate CMV, ganciclovir or foscarnet therapy should be reserved for patients with detectable viral reactivation, most commonly utilizing PCR methods that detect CMV reactivation, usually several weeks before symptoms of CMV disease develop.[100,101] Several studies have shown that immunity to CMV after transplantation is mediated through donor CMV-specific T cells that are transplanted with the allograft. Therefore, for patients at risk for CMV reactivation (i.e., pretransplant CMV serologically positive), a donor who is serologically positive for CMV is actually desirable, as transference of donor immunity against this virus decreases the risk of CMV reactivation and may result in a reduction of CMV-associated morbidity.[102]

SOURCES OF ALLOGENEIC HEMATOPOIETIC STEM CELLS

Allogeneic Peripheral Blood Stem Cell Transplants

Allogeneic transplant regimens that use PB-derived stem cells, as opposed to marrow cells, have been used with increasing frequency over the past decade.[103] The recombinant growth factor G-CSF is usually given to donors for 4 to 6 consecutive days (10 to 15 mcg/kg/d) to mobilize hematopoietic progenitors into the circulation, followed by one or two leukapheresis procedures. G-CSF–mobilized PB stem cell transplants contain higher numbers of progenitor cells than marrow grafts, usually in the range of 5 to 10×10^6 CD34+ cells/kg. Higher volume apheresis procedures can improve the yield of hematopoietic stem cells[104]; one study showed a single 25-L apheresis procedure resulted in similar CD34+ cell yields compared with two consecutive daily 15-L procedures with less donor thrombocytopenia and inconvenience.[105]

The recovery of both neutrophils and platelets is faster with PB cells than with marrow. As a consequence, PB stem cell transplants are associated with a shorter period of neutropenia and red blood cell and platelet transfusion dependence. PB allografts contain a ten- to 20-fold higher T-cell dose compared to BM allografts. Although the incidence of acute GVHD is comparable with PB stem cell and BM transplants, most trials that compared allogeneic BM with PB stem cell transplantation have shown that PB stem cells are associated with a higher probability of chronic GVHD.[106–110]

A phase 3 trial of allogeneic HCT in 138 patients with hematological malignancies found that PB stem cell grafts were associated with more rapid engraftment and better disease-free survival and a trend toward improved overall survival than BM grafts, without a greater risk of acute GVHD.[111] Neutrophil engraftment occurred 6 days earlier (day 15 vs. 21), and platelet recovery occurred 8 days earlier (day 13 vs. 21) among those receiving PB stem cell transplants. The incidence of acute grade 2 to 4 GVHD was not significantly different between groups (64% with PB stem cell vs. 57% with BM), although there was a trend toward a higher cumulative incidence of CGVHD with PB stem cell compared to BM (46% vs. 35%). Two-year survival in the PB stem cell group was 66% versus 54% in the marrow group (P = .06), a finding that led to the early termination of this trial. A more recent study of long-term outcome in 413 recipients of BM versus PB stem cell transplants reported a higher incidence of CGVHD with PB stem cells compared to BM (risk ratio 1.65), yet relapse rates were similar in both groups. BM transplants may result in superior outcome for a subset of patients with chronic phase CML and for patients with BM failure syndromes such as aplastic anemia, where there is no need for a GVL effect occurring as a consequence of chronic GVHD.[106,112]

Unrelated Donors

Although allogeneic transplantation is potentially curative for a number of hematological malignancies, two-thirds of patients who would otherwise be candidates for the procedure lack an HLA-identical sibling to serve as a donor. Throughout the world, there are an estimated 14 million volunteer hematopoietic cell donors registered in numerous adult volunteer donor registries.[113] The National Marrow Donor Program (NMDP), the single largest volunteer registry, has a donor file containing HLA typing information on more than 7 million donors. Each NMDP search also evaluates millions of other donors listed in bone marrow donor registries worldwide.[114] In 2008, there were 10, 481 adult unrelated stem cell donations (3,221 BM and 7,260 PBSC donations) provided from stem cell donor registries in 38 countries and 3,529 cord blood products were provided from 21 countries[113] (Fig. 155.5). In 2009, the NMDP alone facilitated over 5,000 unrelated allogeneic stem cell transplants, including over 1,200 unrelated cord blood transplants. It is estimated that approximately 50% to 70% of white patients have an HLA-A–, HLA-B–, HLA-C–, and HLA-DR–matched (i.e., 8/8 match) unrelated donor. Because of the growing availability of volunteer unrelated donors, there has been a significant increase over the past 15 years in the number of unrelated transplants performed annually in adults (Fig. 155.5). The relative rarity of certain HLA haplotypes in ethnic or racial minorities makes finding a suitably matched unrelated donor particularly difficult for these patients.

The move from serologic- to molecular-based HLA typing has been associated with a significant improvement in outcome following unrelated transplants, including a decrease in life-threatening acute GVHD and CGVHD.[115–117] HLA class I antigen mismatches that are serologically detectable (including HLA-C) result in a significant increase in the risk of graft failure.[118] Likewise, high-resolution mismatches at HLA-A, -B, -C, and -DRB1 also adversely affect outcome, but less so than low-resolution mismatches.[119] Recent data show transplant outcome utilizing unrelated donors matched at an allele level for MHC classes I and II MHC loci results in similar albeit slightly inferior transplant outcomes compared to recipients of HLA matched sibling donors.[120] In a homogeneous cohort of good risk patients with CML, the risk of nonrelapse mortality was higher and the 5-year overall survival and leukemia-free survival (LFS) were modestly though significantly worse after receipt of a transplant from 8/8 allele-matched donors compared to patients who received a transplant from a matched sibling donor[78] (Fig. 155.6). In multivariate analysis, the risk of grades 2 to 4 acute GVHD was 2.44 times higher in 8/8 matched unrelated donor transplant recipients compared to matched sibling donor recipients.

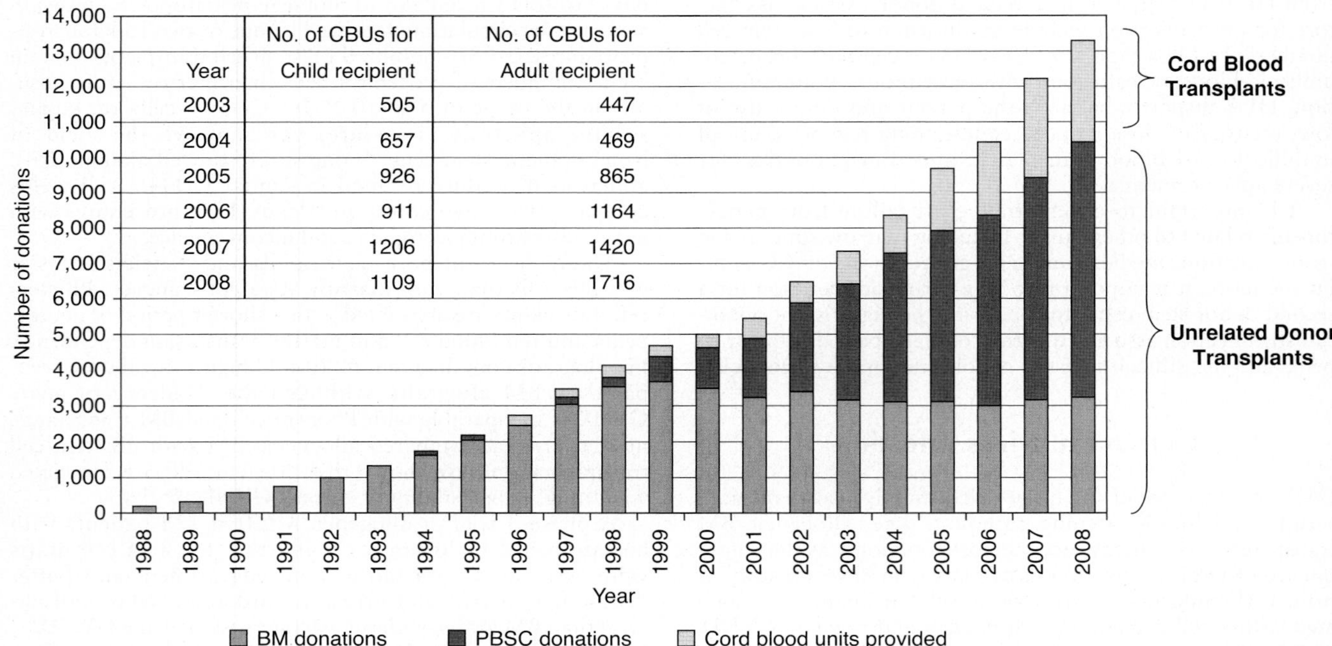

FIGURE 155.5 Monitoring the international use of unrelated donors for transplantation: the WMDA annual reports. (From Foeken LM, Green A, Hurley CK, et al. Monitoring the international use of unrelated donors for transplantation: the WMDA annual reports. *Bone Marrow Transplant* 2010;45:811, with permission.)

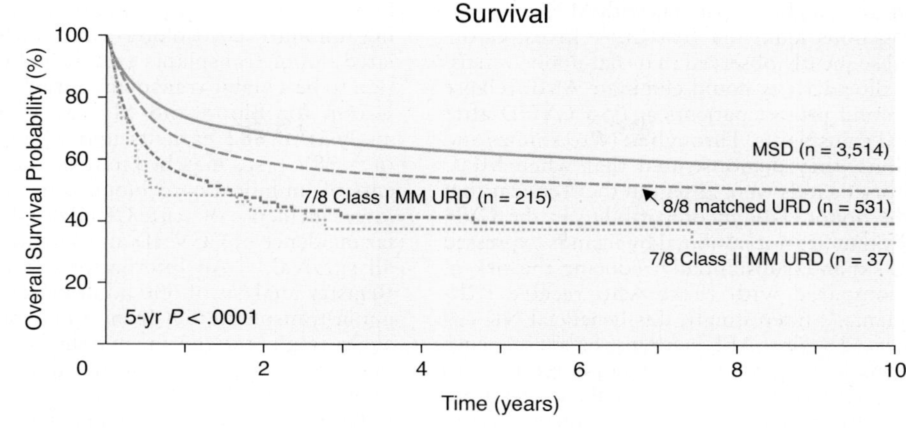

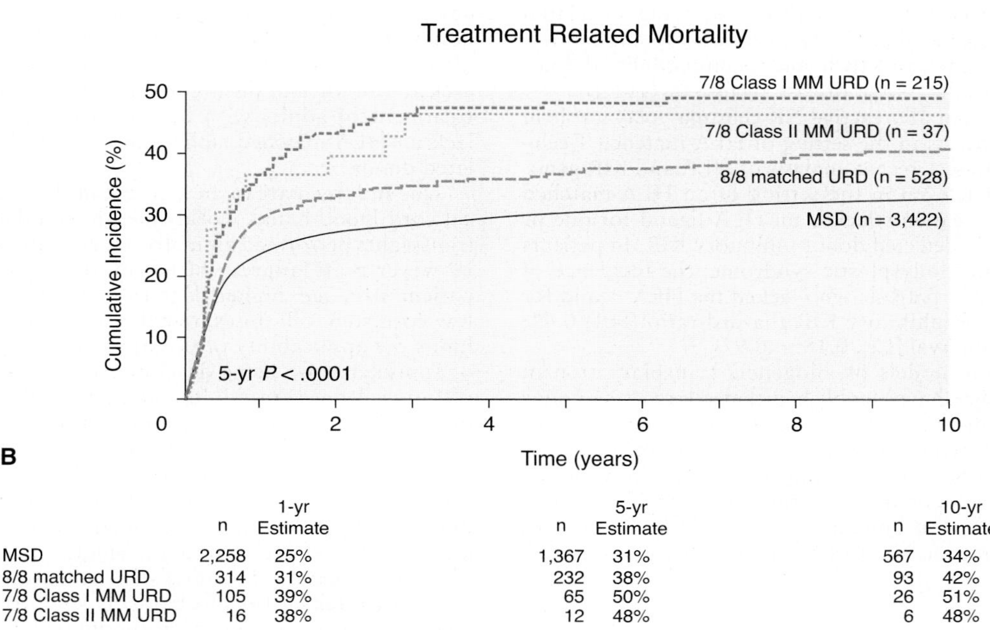

	1-yr n	1-yr Estimate	5-yr n	5-yr Estimate	10-yr n	10-yr Estimate
MSD	2,258	25%	1,367	31%	567	34%
8/8 matched URD	314	31%	232	38%	93	42%
7/8 Class I MM URD	105	39%	65	50%	26	51%
7/8 Class II MM URD	16	38%	12	48%	6	48%

FIGURE 155.6 Probability of overall survival (**A**) and transplant-related mortality (**B**) after BM transplantation from a matched sibling donor (MSD), 8/8 matched unrelated donor (URD), or a 7/8 matched URD mismatched at a single HLA class I or II allele. (From Arora M, Weisdorf DJ, Spellman SR, et al. HLA-identical sibling compared with 8/8 matched and mismatched unrelated donor bone marrow transplant for chronic phase chronic myeloid leukemia. *J Clin Oncol* 2009;27:1644, with permission.)

As observed with other studies, HLA mismatching in either the class I or II loci in unrelated donors was associated with a higher risk of GVHD, nonrelapse morality, and lower survival.

Mismatched-Related Transplants

Because the majority of patients in need of a hematopoietic stem cell transplant have at least a full-haplotype mismatched relative, haploidentical ("half-matched") or mismatched related donors have increasingly been used as an alternative source of stem cells for patients lacking an HLA-identical sibling. These donors may actually have a closer histocompatibility profile than matched unrelated donors, as the shared donor haplotype is genetically identical to the patient, which may be associated with better matching of minor histocompatibility antigens. Furthermore, potential family donors can usually be identified quickly and are usually more readily available than matched unrelated donors.

Graft rejection, GVHD, and ineffective immunity, leading to fatal opportunistic infection, are the major immune-mediated complications associated with HLA disparity; the greater the HLA disparity, the higher these risks. Trials comparing outcomes in patients receiving partially mismatched related versus matched sibling donor allografts have shown that engraftment, GVHD, and survival are inferior in the recipients of partially mismatched transplants.[115] Although opportunistic infections and disease relapse remain problematic, recent modifications in transplants using mismatched related donors, including the use of reduced-intensity conditioning regimens and high doses of donor CD34+ cells, have improved transplant outcomes with long-term disease-free survivals in the range of 20% to 40% being reported.[121–123] An analysis of 112 patients with hematological malignancies undergoing haploidentical transplantation showed the risk of disease relapse to be significantly higher in patients with ALL compared with acute myelogenous leukemia (AML).[124] Investigators from this group subsequently observed that that donor-versus-recipient NK cell alloreactivity could eliminate AML relapse and graft rejection and protect patients against GVHD after such haploidentical transplants. Through *in vitro* studies and clinical observations, they demonstrated that when MHC class I KIR inhibitory ligands were absent in the recipient that were present in the donor (KIR incompatibility in the GVH direction), NK cells that are not inhibited by ligands expressed on recipient AML expand, substantially reducing the risk of disease relapse compared with those who receive KIR-compatible transplants.[33] Interestingly, this beneficial NK cell effect was not observed against ALL, perhaps the consequence of these populations lacking activating ligands required to trigger NK cytolytic activity. The impact of KIR incompatibility when using partially mismatched unrelated donors has not yet been defined. One study reported disease-free survival in AML patients was superior in those receiving unrelated allografts with KIR incompatibility, in contrast to another retrospective analysis, where KIR ligand incompatibility did not appear to improve the risk of disease relapse or GVHD.[125,126] It is also possible that alloreactive NK cells may play a role in mediating GVL effects in the setting of HLA-matched T-cell–depleted transplants. A recent analysis of HLA and KIR genotypes revealed that even in the setting of an HLA-matched HCT, 63% of the patients lacked an HLA ligand for one or more genotypically detected donor-inhibitory KIR. In patients with AML and myelodysplastic syndrome, the incidence of relapse was lower in patients who lacked the HLA ligand for one or more donor-inhibitory KIR (hazard ratio [HR] 0.41; 95% confidence interval [CI], 0.18 to 0.97).[127]

MHC matched models of allogeneic transplantation in tumor bearing mice have established that alloreactive donor NK cells can mediate antitumor effects while simultaneously reducing GVHD, which together significantly prolong survival.[128] Furthermore, *in vitro* data now exists showing NK alloreactivity can occur in the setting of an MHC-matched allogeneic transplant in humans, which could lead to potentially powerful donor NK cell–mediated antitumor effects against cancer.[35,129]

Umbilical Cord Blood Transplantation

Umbilical cord blood offers an alternative source of hematopoietic progenitor cells for transplantation in both malignant and nonmalignant disorders for patients who lack an HLA-identical related or unrelated donor.[130] Cord blood contains primitive hematopoietic stem cells with remarkable proliferative potential, which may overcome the limitation of relatively low absolute cell numbers. Also, the immature and naive T cells in cord blood appear to decrease the risk and severity of acute GVHD and CGVHD, allowing greater HLA disparity and expanding donor availability. Currently, more than 500,000 blood units stored in 131 cord blood banks are available for unrelated donor HCT searches.[113,131] One major advantage of cord blood transplants over unrelated marrow is the speed with which cord blood units can be made available for transplantation (a median of only 13.5 days in one study).[132,133]

Higher degrees of HLA matching and higher cell doses significantly decrease the risk of transplant-related mortality after umbilical cord blood transplantation. Cord blood doses of greater than or equal to 2.5×10^7 nucleated cells/kg (recipient weight) or greater than or equal to 1.2×10^5 CD34+ cells/kg are associated with a higher probability of engraftment and a lower transplant-related mortality. Two seminal retrospective analyses comparing transplant outcome in adult patients with hematological malignancies undergoing umbilical cord blood transplants versus matched unrelated donor transplants established cord blood transplantation to be a viable transplant option for adults. In a European Group for Blood and Marrow Transplantation (EBMT) analysis of 682 patients undergoing umbilical cord blood (n = 98) versus matched unrelated donor transplants, recipients of umbilical cord blood transplants had a significantly lower incidence of acute GVHD (risk ratio 0.57) with a similar incidence of CGVHD and similar leukemia-free and overall survival.[134] An International Bone Marrow Transplant Registry analysis of 600 adult patients with leukemia undergoing transplantation from a matched unrelated donor versus a single antigen mismatched unrelated donor versus a one- or two-antigen mismatched umbilical cord blood transplant reported long-term leukemia-free and overall survival to be slightly superior with matched unrelated donors. In this analysis, leukemia-free and overall survival were similar among recipients of a single antigen mismatched unrelated donor transplant compared to umbilical cord blood transplant recipients.[135] These and other studies have now defined a clear role of umbilical cord blood transplantation in the treatment of adults with hematological malignancies who lack an HLA-matched sibling donor or fully matched unrelated donor.[136]

Due in large part to an increase in the number of umbilical cord blood banks worldwide, the number of cord blood transplants performed annually has steadily risen (Fig. 155.5) However, graft failure, which is most closely associated with patient size, age, higher degrees of HLA mismatching, and low cord stem cell doses, remains a significant problem that limits the applicability of this approach in adults. A number of approaches are being developed to overcome the obstacle of low-cell doses in adults, including the use of dual cord blood transplants in which umbilical cord blood grafts are combined from different cord donors to meet the minimum cell dose requirement. Such transplants usually result in early dual chimerism from both cord units with one cord unit eventually mediating a T-cell mediated graft-versus-graft immune effect, resulting in single unit chimerism.[137,138] The use of *ex vivo* expanded stem cells from umbilical cord blood through novel mechanisms such as Notch-ligand–mediated expansion has been shown in a recent pilot study to shorten the time of neutropenia associated with dual cord blood transplants by a median 1 week when one of the two cord blood units was expanded *in vitro* using this technique.[139,140]

RESULTS OF CONVENTIONAL ALLOGENEIC TRANSPLANTATION FOR HEMATOLOGIC MALIGNANCIES

Allogeneic HCT is potentially curative for a number of different hematological malignancies, including acute and chronic leukemias, myelodysplastic syndromes, myeloproliferative disorders, Hodgkin's and non-Hodgkin's lymphoma, and multiple myeloma. The indications for allogeneic HCT vary according to disease categories and are influenced by variables such as disease-specific prognostic factors (e.g., cytogenetic abnormalities), response to prior therapy, patient age and performance status, disease status (e.g., in remission versus relapsed refractory disease), and most important, availability of a suitable allogeneic donor to serve as a source for hematopoietic stem cells. For the majority who undergo this approach, allogeneic HCT remains the only therapy with established curative potential.

Chronic Myelogenous Leukemia

CML is a clonal myeloproliferative disease of hematopoietic stem cell origin that is characterized by an early chronic phase of 3 to 5 years' duration, followed by an accelerated phase of 3 to 6 months, which ultimately terminates in a fatal blastic phase. Over the past decade, the upfront use of imatinib mesylate has dramatically changed the method of management of chronic phase CML.[141] Five-year follow-up data show continuous treatment of chronic-phase CML with imatinib, as initial therapy induces durable responses and long-term survival in a high proportion of patients (89%).[142] Most institutes now use imatinib as first-line treatment for patients with chronic phase CML, reserving allogeneic transplant for those who are intolerant of the drug or who fail to achieve a cytogenetic remission. This has significantly reduced the number of allogeneic transplantations performed for this leukemia. Importantly, allogeneic HCT is capable of salvaging patients who are refractory or who develop resistance to imatinib. A retrospective analysis of outcome in chronic phase CML patients intolerant or failing to achieve an optimal response to imatinib reported no significant difference in survival, disease-free survival, or relapse and nonrelapse mortality after HCT compared to a historical CML cohort not treated with imatinib who underwent HCT as first-line therapy.[143] A recent transplant study reported excellent survival in imatinib failure patients with chronic phase disease; the 3-year survival of 56 patients in chronic phase was 91% (median follow-up: 30 months) with transplantation-related mortality of only 8%.[144] These data show allogeneic transplantation is an effective second-line therapy that maintains its ability to cure patients with CML who fail imatinib therapy without increasing the risk of an adverse outcome associated with transplantation.

Despite the success of imatinib and other newer and even more potent BCR-ABL tyrosine kinase inhibitors, allogeneic HCT remains the only treatment approach with proven curative potential in this leukemia. Patient age, disease status (chronic phase versus accelerated or blastic phase), and the time interval from diagnosis to transplant (i.e., less than 1 year versus more than 1 year) are the best predictors for long-term disease-free survival. In general, 65% to 80% of patients transplanted with chronic phase CML can expect to be cured, in contrast to a minority (10% to 20%) who undergo transplantation in the accelerated or blastic phase. Patients with chronic phase CML transplanted within a year from the time of diagnosis have the best outcome, with long-term disease-free survivals of 75% to 80%. A study from the Fred Hutchinson Cancer Center of 196 patients undergoing allogeneic HCT from matched unrelated donors reported a 5-year survival rate of 75%, which compared favorably to that institution's results using HLA-matched sibling donors.[116] However, a more recent study comparing outcomes in chronic phase CML patients who received a transplant from unrelated donors matched at an allele level for MHC classes I and II MHC loci compared to recipients of HLA-matched sibling donors reported the risk of nonrelapse mortality was higher and the 5-year overall survival and LFS were modestly worse in receipts of transplants from 8/8 allele-matched donors compared to transplants from an HLA-matched sibling donor.[78] Among hematological malignancies, CML appears most susceptible to the GVL effect. The majority of CML patients who relapse after an allogeneic HCT can be induced back into remission after treatment with a DLI.[20,25] The sensitivity of this leukemia to the GVL effect makes reduced-intensity transplants a viable treatment option for patients with CML, with durable molecular remissions reported in a number of transplant centers.[145] Notably, patients older than 60 have been successfully treated with minimal conditioning associated toxicity, an important finding given the median age of CML patients at diagnosis is 65.[146–148] Recent data suggest the combination of imatinib and DLI may be effective in achieving molecular remissions in patients with CML relapsing after transplant into blast crisis.[149] In contrast, when given alone, imatinib or donor-lymphocyte infusion rarely induces molecular remissions in blast-crisis CML.

Acute Myelogenous Leukemia

With the exception of those with favorable or low-risk cytogenetic abnormalities, such as t(8;21), t(15;17), inv, or del(16), most patients with AML have a high risk of relapse after chemotherapy-induced remission.[150] Compared with those who receive chemotherapy alone, patients undergoing an allogeneic HCT after first chemotherapy remission (CR1) have a lower probability of relapse, with 5-year disease-free survivals in the range of 46% to 62%.[151,152] Allogeneic transplantation represents a viable treatment option that should be considered for all patients who (1) have AML that is refractory to induction therapy, (2) have AML in two or more chemotherapy remissions, or (3) have AML in CR1 with high-risk cytogenetics, have secondary AML, or who do not have low-risk cytogenetics. AML patients with cytogenetic abnormalities associated with a poor prognosis in CR1 who are unlikely to be cured with chemotherapy alone may be cured after an allogeneic transplant.[153] Furthermore, patients in CR2 or those with untreated relapsed AML can only be cured by allogeneic HCT, albeit they are less likely to achieve long-term disease-free survival (22% to 30%). Retrospective studies have reported superior outcome with significantly improved to LSF and overall survival in cytogenetic high-risk AML patients consolidated with an allogeneic HCT in CR1 compared to consolidation with either conventional chemotherapy or autologous transplantation.[154] Based on these observations, it is reasonable to proceed to transplant in CR1 in patients who are at intermediate[155] or high risk of relapse, for example, in those with normal karyotype, abnormal chromosome 5, or 7,3q rearrangements, t(6;9), complex karyotype abnormalities, withholding the procedure until first relapse or CR2 in low-risk patients. For patients with normal cytogenetics, mutation analysis of several genes is increasingly being used to stratify patients who are most likely to benefit from an allogeneic transplant in CR1.[156] Patients with normal cytogenetics who appear to benefit from an allogeneic transplant in CR1 include those with an fms-related tyrosine kinase 3 gene internal tandem duplication (FLT3-ITD) or a genotype consisting of wild type nucleophosmin gene (NPM1) or the CCAAT/enhancer binding protein alpha gene (CEBPA) without a FLT3-ITD.[157] Patients with primary chemotherapy-refractory AML, associated with the worst prognosis, can still be salvaged by an allogeneic HCT in 10% to 25% of cases.

Acute Lymphoblastic Leukemia

Although 65% to 85% of adults with ALL achieve remission with primary chemotherapy, the majority (60% to 70%) eventually experience relapse that is rarely curable with salvage chemotherapy. Factors associated with a poor outcome (referred to as *high-risk ALL*) include age greater than 60 years; leukocyte count of more than 30,000 on presentation; and chromosomal translocations involving t(4;11), t(1;19), t(8;14), or the Philadelphia chromosome t(9;22) (found in approximately 15% to 30% of adult ALL cases).[158] In adults, allogeneic HCT in CR1 has traditionally been reserved for patients with high-risk features, where cure with chemotherapy is unlikely.[120,159]

Several studies of allogeneic HCT in high-risk patients transplanted in CR1 have reported long-term disease-free survival in the range of 40% to 60%, rates considerably higher than those observed with chemotherapy alone. Because some patients in CR1 (without high-risk features) are cured with chemotherapy alone, allogeneic HCT until recently had been reserved for ALL patients with disease relapse who were induced into remission with reinduction chemotherapy (e.g., CR2). Furthermore, long-term disease-free survival with allogeneic transplantation in CR2 is in the range of 35% to 40%, which is comparable to disease-free survival of patients undergoing transplantation in CR1. A recently reported Medical Research Council/Eastern Cooperative Oncology Group trial that randomized 1,980 adults with ALL in CR1 to consolidation with either conventional chemotherapy, autologous transplantation, or an allogeneic HCT (for those identified to have an HLA-identical sibling donor) reported superior outcomes in patients consolidated with up-front allogeneic transplantation; in an intention to treat analysis, recipients of an allogeneic HCT had an improvement in survival (53% vs. 45%), event-free survival (50% vs. 41%), and a lower incidence of disease relapse (29% vs. 54%) compared to those receiving conventional consolidation or autologous transplantation. A subgroup analysis revealed the benefits of allogeneic HCT in CR1 were limited to standard-risk patients with equivalent results to chemotherapy consolidation in high-risk patients due to a higher risk of transplant-related mortality in this older cohort.[160]

Because chemotherapy is considerably more effective in achieving durable remissions in children, allogeneic HCT is usually reserved for those who fail to be cured with primary therapy or have Philadelphia-positive ALL.

Myelodysplastic Syndrome

Allogeneic HCT is the only curative therapy available for patients with myelodysplastic syndrome (MDS). In general, approximately one third of myelodysplastic syndrome patients can be expected to achieve long-term disease-free survival, while one-third will die from complications of the procedure and another third will relapse after transplantation. Factors associated with improved outcome include younger age, lower pretransplant marrow blast percentage, shorter disease duration, and favorable cytogenetics.[161] A retrospective analysis of transplant events in relation to the International Prognostic Scoring System cytogenetic categories showed that cytogenetic abnormalities alone were highly predictive of posttransplant outcome.[162] The event-free survival for good-, intermediate-, and poor-risk cytogenetic subgroups were 51%, 40%, and 6%, respectively, with corresponding relapse rates of 19%, 12%, and 82%. International Prognostic Scoring System cytogenetic categories were defined as good risk if patients had normal karyotype, −Y alone, del(5q) alone, or del(20q) alone; poor risk if patients had anomalies of chromosome 7 or complex cytogenetics (three or more anomalies); and intermediate risk if other karyotypic anomalies were present that did not meet the criteria for good or poor risk. Numerous myeloablative and reduced-intensity conditioning regimens have been utilized to treat MDS patients, with no one ideal conditioning regimen emerging.[163] Although reduced-intensity transplants are associated with a lower risk of transplant-related mortality, retrospective studies suggest this benefit is offset by an increased risk of disease relapse compared to conventional myeloablative transplants.[164] A retrospective study from the EBMT of 1,333 MDS patients age 50 years or older who were transplanted was recently published summarizing transplant outcome based on patient age, conditioning regimen (myeloablative versus reduced intensity), and donor type (HLA-matched sibling versus HLA-matched unrelated donor).[165] The 4-year estimate for overall survival of the whole cohort was 31%, and on multivariate analysis, use of reduced-intensity conditioning (HR, 1.44; 95% CI, 1.13 to 1.84; $P < .01$) and advanced disease stage at transplantation (HR, 1.51; 95% CI, 1.18 to 1.93; $P < .01$) were associated with an increased relapse rate (Fig. 155.7). In contrast, advanced disease stage at transplantation (HR, 1.43; 95% CI, 1.13 to 1.79; $P = .01$) was associated with a higher risk of nonrelapse mortality and was the major independent variable associated with an inferior 4-year overall survival (HR, 1.55; 95% CI, 1.32 to 1.83; $P < .01$). When compared with the use of an HLA-matched sibling donor, HLA-matched and HLA partially–mismatched unrelated donors both had a higher risk of nonrelapse mortality (4-year estimate 34% vs. 40% vs. 54%, respectively; $P = .02$). In contrast, the use of reduced-intensity conditioning (HR, 0.79; 95% CI, 0.65 to 0.97; $P = .03$) was an independent variable associated with a lower risk of nonrelapse mortality (Fig. 155.7). In this analysis, disease stage at time of transplantation, but not recipient age or the intensity of the conditioning regimens, was the most important factor influencing outcomes.

Other Hematologic Malignancies

The role of allogeneic HCT in multiple myeloma, CLL, Hodgkin's and non-Hodgkin's lymphoma,[166] and myeloproliferative disorders is less well defined than with acute leukemias or chronic-phase CML. Most studies published to date have consisted of relatively small retrospective analyses. Nevertheless, reports of durable remissions in patients with relapsed or chemotherapy-refractory disease, often in association with GVHD or after DLI, provide strong evidence that these diseases are susceptible to a potentially curative GVL effect. Several trials of allogeneic transplantation in CLL have reported long-term disease-free survival rates in the range of 49% to 70%.[167,168] Allogeneic transplantation for CLL is usually reserved for patients who (1) are younger with relapsed disease, (2) have relapsed disease associated with a short response (i.e., less than 2 years) to chemotherapy, or (3) have disease refractory to conventional therapy. CLL with a chromosomal 17p deletion is associated with a particularly short progression-free and overall survival with conventional therapy. A recent EBMT report has provided evidence that allogeneic transplantation may offer potentially curative therapy for patients with 17p− CLL; 44 patients underwent an allogeneic transplant using predominantly reduced-intensity conditioning with 3-year survival and progression-free survival rates of 44% and 37%, respectively.[169] Although a number of patients with multiple myeloma have achieved long-term disease-free survival after myeloablative allogeneic HCT, transplant-related mortality limits the therapeutic potential of this approach. Regimens with reduced transplant-related toxicities, such as nonmyeloablative hematopoietic transplantation, avoid many conditioning-associated complications, reducing the risk of transplant-related mortality. An analysis of transplants performed in Europe for myeloma from 1998 to 2002 showed a significant move from myeloablative transplants toward the use of reduced-intensity transplants.[170]

Reduced-Intensity or Nonmyeloablative Allogeneic Hematopoietic Cell Transplantation

The disease-reducing antitumor effects of dose-intensive conditioning are often offset by their substantial and potentially life-threatening toxicities. Debilitated or older patients with hematological malignancies are at particularly high risk, thus limiting the applicability of this potentially curative treatment

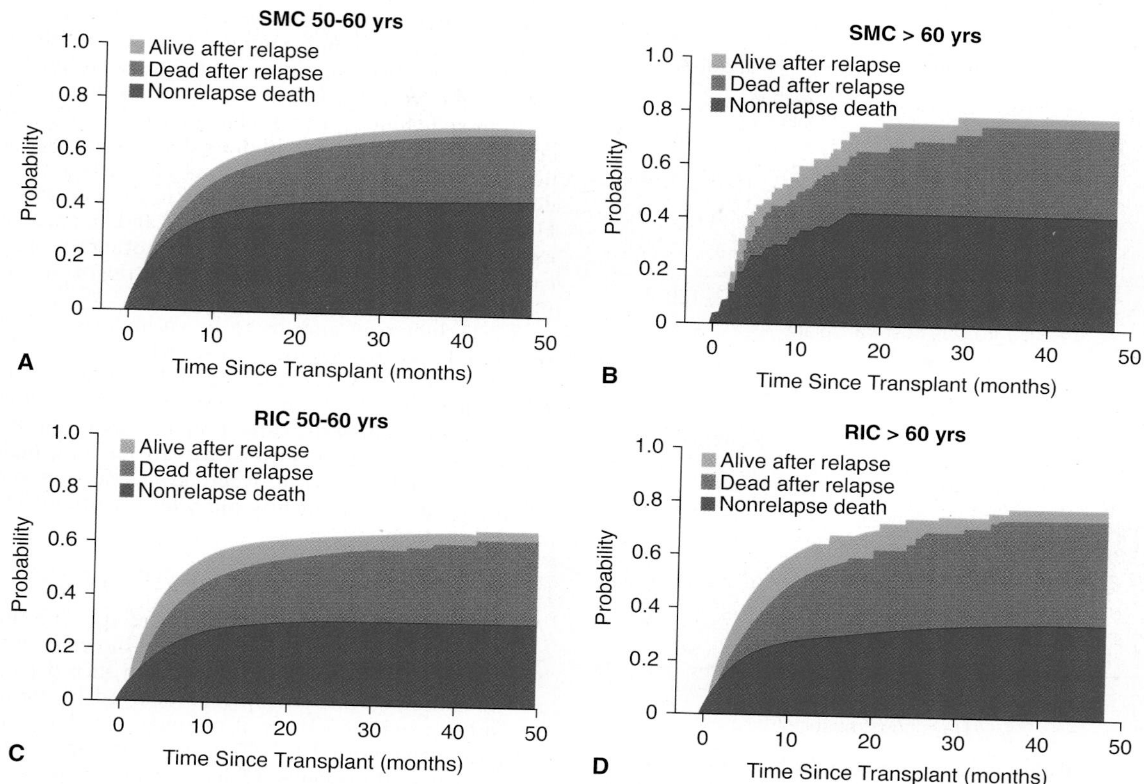

FIGURE 155.7 Stacked cumulative incidence curves from a competing risk model with relapse and death as competing risks, with the study population substratified according to (**A**) age 50 to 60 years, standard myeloablative conditioning (SMC), (**B**) age > years, SMC, (**C**) age 50 to 60 years, reduced intensity conditioning (RIC), and (**D**) age > 60 years, RIC. From Lim Z, Brand R, Martino R, et al. Allogeneic hematopoietic stem-cell transplantation for patients 50 years or older with myelodysplastic syndromes or secondary acute myeloid leukemia. *J Clin Oncol* 2010;28:405, with permission.

modality to relatively younger patients with a good performance status. Reduced-intensity or nonmyeloablative conditioning regimens utilize immunosuppressive conditioning to permit the engraftment of the donor immune system for the generation of GVL effects while sparing patients the toxicities associated with myeloablative therapy.[171,172] Importantly, regimen-related toxicity and mortality appear to be significantly decreased,[165] thus expanding eligibility for allotransplantation to include older or debilitated patients, as well as allowing for exploration of GVT effects in other treatment refractory or incurable malignancies.[173–175]

Reduced-Intensity Conditioning Regimens

A variety of low-intensity conditioning strategies have been successfully utilized to achieve donor lymphohematopoietic engraftment. Although regimens vary, most incorporate the nucleoside analogue fludarabine because of its profound immunosuppressive effects and low-toxicity profile. It is important to note that recipient hematopoietic stem cells that survive transplant conditioning in most cases are immunologically eradicated by donor T cells weeks to months after transplantation, a process referred to as graft-versus-marrow or *graft-versus-host lymphohematopoiesis*.[176,177]

Although randomized trials comparing myeloablative versus nonmyeloablative regimens have not yet been reported, retrospective studies comparing the safety of this approach to conventional HCT approaches have been encouraging,[178–180] with regimen-related mortality rates of less than 18% being reported in several reduced-intensity transplant studies. This mortality risk is remarkably low, given most patients in these trials were precluded from a myeloablative transplant because of a high risk (i.e., 40% or more) of regimen-related mortality related to heavy pretreatment or medical comorbidities such as poor performance status, debilitation, or advanced patient age.[175] Because reduced-intensity conditioning does not eradicate recipient hematopoietic progenitors, a mixture of both donor and patient myeloid and lymphoid cells is usually detectable at the time of neutrophil recovery.[176,181] This state of *mixed chimerism* can induce donor-immune tolerance to recipient antigens, leading to a reduction in the incidence of acute GVHD.[182] However, mixed chimerism may inhibit beneficial GVT effects, leading to a higher risk of disease relapse.[181] This negative aspect of mixed chimerism can be overcome by donor lymphocyte infusions, which induce GVH hematopoietic effects that shift chimerism from mixed to complete donor, thus breaking tolerance and enhancing a GVT effect (Fig. 155.8).[183]

Reduced-Intensity Transplant Toxicity

Compared with myeloablative approaches, conditioning-induced toxicity is relatively mild with nonmyeloablative regimens. In general, most patients tolerate the preparative regimen well, without the occurrence of mucositis, VOD, or the requirement for total parenteral nutrition.[172] Furthermore, retrospective data show transplant outcomes, including nonrelapse mortality rates, are similar among patients from the age of 40 to 65 years or older, establishing that older age alone should not be considered a contraindication to allogeneic stem

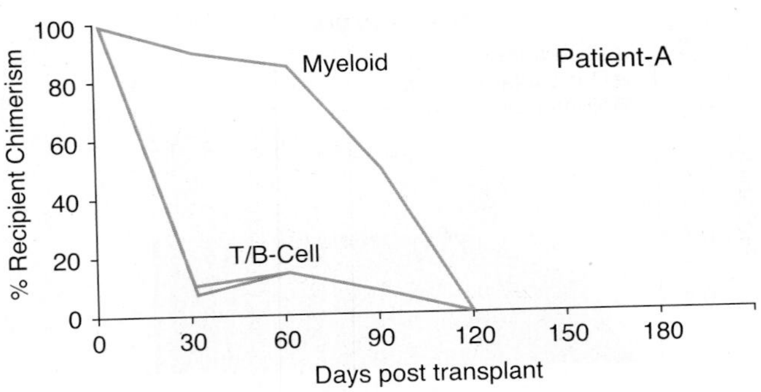

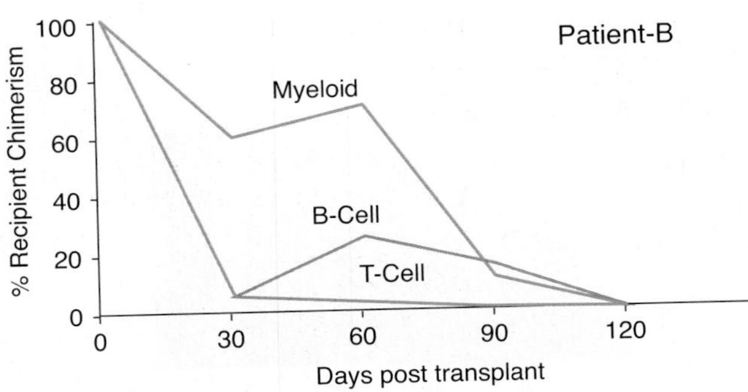

FIGURE 155.8 Patients receiving nonmyeloablative conditioning with cyclophosphamide and fludarabine have initial autologous recovery of lymphoid and hematopoietic cells. Recipient cells are gradually immunologically "ablated" as the consequence of a donor immune-mediated graft-versus-host hematopoietic or graft-vs-marrow effect.

cell transplantation.[184] Several retrospective studies comparing conventional myeloablative versus reduced-intensity HCT approaches have reported reduced-nonrelapse mortality in recipients of reduced-intensity approaches.[179,185] With the exception of low-dose TBI-based strategies, pancytopenia associated with the conditioning regimen is common.[173,175,186] However, the occurrence of partial autologous hematopoietic recovery shortens the overall depth and duration of neutropenia and reduces platelet and red blood cell transfusion requirements and the risk of opportunistic infections.[41,86,187–190]

Engraftment

The ability to establish engraftment of donor hematopoietic and lymphoid cells is directly related to the degree of host immunosuppression induced by the preparative regimen. Although graft rejection occurs with a higher frequency compared with myeloablative approaches, in general, more than 90% of patients can be expected to have durable donor engraftment. As with myeloablative transplants, *ex vivo* or *in vivo* T-cell depletion of the allograft is associated with lower degrees of donor T-cell chimerism and a higher risk of graft rejection. T-cell depletion with alemtuzumab is less commonly associated with graft rejection when DLIs are given after transplantation to patients with mixed chimerism.[181] Regimens that use low-dose TBI alone have a higher incidence of graft rejection (up to 20% in patients with chronic phase CML), although the addition of fludarabine significantly decreases this risk. Furthermore, the use of BM allografts after low-dose TBI appears to be associated with a greater risk of graft rejection compared with PB stem cells.[191]

The kinetics of donor engraftment after nonmyeloablative stem cell transplantation vary considerably depending on the type and intensity of agents used for conditioning.[176,177,192,193] Reduced-intensity conditioning frequently results in donor engraftment where significant differences in chimerism are observed between T cells and myeloid cells (Fig. 155.8).[176,192–194] In mixed chimeric states, characterized by high degrees of donor T-cell chimerism, withdrawal of posttransplant immunosuppression usually transitions chimerism to complete donor origin in all cellular lineages in the majority of cases. Higher doses of allograft CD34+ cells and, in particular, prior exposure to immunosuppressive chemotherapy may significantly facilitate and expedite the engraftment of donor lymphohematopoietic cells.[192]

T-cell chimerism appears to be an important determinant of multiple posttransplant events, including the risk of graft rejection, acute GVHD, and the ability to generate a GVL/GVT effect.[173,176,181,195] In general, patients with low degrees of donor T-cell chimerism are at higher risk for graft rejection and disease relapse, in contrast to patients with high degrees of donor T-cell chimerism, where graft rejection and disease relapse occur less frequently but where acute GVHD occurs more commonly.

Graft-versus-Host Disease

Acute GVHD remains the major nonrelapse life-threatening complication associated with reduced-intensity transplants. Furthermore, because conversion from mixed to predominantly donor chimerism may be delayed by months after transplantation, GVHD is also sometimes delayed in onset (i.e., occurring more than 100 days posttransplant) relative to myeloablative transplants. Older patient age, prior history of chemotherapy, and rapid T-cell engraftment appear to be associated with an increased risk of GVHD.[181,192,195] *Ex vivo* T-cell depletion of the allograft decreases the risk of GVHD but may significantly increase the risk of graft rejection. A more promising strategy involves *in vivo* T-cell depletion through the use of alemtuzumab.[196] A study of 129 patients undergoing fludarabine or melphalan-based conditioning reported a significant reduction in acute grades 2 to 4 GVHD in patients who received alemtuzumab plus CSA as GVHD prophylaxis (22%) compared with those receiving CSA plus methotrexate (45%; $P = .006$) with similar disease-free survival between cohorts.

Graft-versus-Leukemia Effect

GVL effects after nonmyeloablative stem cell transplantation have been observed in a heterogeneous group of hematological malignancies. Durable remissions lasting more than 12 years in patients transplanted with acute and chronic leukemias, myelodysplastic syndromes, multiple myeloma, lymphoid malignancies (e.g., Hodgkin's and non-Hodgkin's lymphomas), and myeloproliferative disorders now exist in the literature.[175]

A number of trials have shown that the GVT effects that follow nonmyeloablative transplantation are most effective against malignancies with slow growth kinetics, in particular chronic leukemias and indolent lymphomas. Indeed several studies have reported durable remissions of CML (see section "Chronic Myelogenous Leukemia"), low-grade NHL, CLL, mantle cell lymphoma, Hodgkin's lymphoma, and multiple myeloma after reduced-intensity allogeneic transplantation. In contrast, with diseases such as AML, ALL, myelodysplastic syndrome in transformation to leukemia, and lymphomas, induction of a remission before nonmyeloablative conditioning is required to optimize the chance of long-term disease-free survival.[197–199] Recent data suggest that patients with Hodgkin's lymphoma who relapse after autologous transplantation and who undergo reduced-intensity allogeneic transplantation have improved progression-free and overall survival compared to patients receiving conventional salvage therapy.[200]

Although retrospective data suggest reduced-intensity transplant approaches are associated with a lower risk of transplant-related mortality, conventional myeloablative conditioning results in greater cytoreduction of the underlying hematological malignancy, which may result in a lower incidence of disease relapse.[164] A retrospective study from the EBMT on 1,333 MDS patients age 50 years or older who received a myeloablative versus reduced-intensity allogeneic transplant reported the use of reduced-intensity conditioning was associated with a significantly higher risk of disease relapse (HR, 1.44; 95% CI, 1.13 to 1.84; $P < .01$), although the risk of nonrelapse mortality was significantly lower with reduced-intensity conditioning (Fig. 155.7; HR, 0.79; 95% CI, 0.65 to 0.97; $P = .03$). In this analysis, disease stage at time of transplantation, but not recipient age or the intensity of the conditioning regimens, was the most important factor influencing outcomes.[165] Similar to the above study, an analysis of 722 patients with AML over the age of 50 reported reduced transplant-related mortality associated with nonmyeloablative approaches, although the relapse rate was higher, resulting in similar overall survival between the two groups.[201] Until prospective trials are completed, data that show a higher risk of relapse with reduced-intensity conditioning suggest patients without a contraindication to myeloablative conditioning should not receive a reduced-intensity transplant outside the context of a clinical trial.

One strategy to reduce the risk of disease relapse associated with reduced-intensity conditioning is to first maximally cytoreduce the malignancy with an autologous transplant. This approach appears particularly successful for multiple myeloma.[202] A recently published trial of 162 patients with multiple myeloma comparing up-front autografting followed by consolidation with either a second autograft versus a nonmyeloablative HCT from an HLA-matched sibling reported a survival advantage for those who received an allogeneic transplant; at a median follow-up of nearly 4 years, the median overall survival (80 months vs. 54 months) and event-free survival (35 months vs. 29 months) were significantly longer in patients with an HLA-identical sibling donor assigned to allogeneic transplantation compared to those receiving a double autologous transplant.[203] This improvement in survival, previously not observed with conventional myeloablative transplants, was largely the consequence of the improved safety profile of the reduced-intensity transplant, where the 2-year cumulative incidence of treatment-related mortality was only 10%. The incorporation of newer myeloma drugs such as bortezomib and lenalidomide in the pretransplant cytoreductive phase of this regimen and posttransplant to potentiate a graft-versus-myeloma effect is currently being explored.[204]

Graft-versus-Solid Tumor

Case reports of disease regression in association with GVHD in the mid-1990s in a few patients with metastatic breast carcinoma undergoing myeloablative allogeneic transplantation lent credence to the concept that donor-immune cells might have activity against tumors of epithelial origin.[173,205–207] Since the first report of a graft-versus-renal cell carcinoma effect following nonmyeloablative HCT in 1999,[208] there has been a steady increase in the number of publications describing clinical outcome in patients with a variety of solid tumors undergoing mostly reduced-intensity transplantation, including 13 case series describing GVT effects in renal cell carcinoma (RCC) and four small series reporting breast cancer regression as a consequence of a GVT effect (Table 155.2).[205,206] Although partial responses have most often been observed, in some cases durable complete responses have been observed (Fig. 155.9).[32] Numerous case reports and a few case series that reported evidence for GVT effects in other solid tumors, including metastatic pancreatic carcinoma, colon carcinoma, ovarian carcinoma, and other tumors, have been described over the past 2 years.[173,209] Importantly, a number of series have reported significantly superior survival in patients having a GVT effect compared to nonresponders.

TABLE 155.2

PUBLISHED SERIES OF ALLOGENEIC HEMATOPOIETIC STEM CELL TRANSPLANTATION FOR METASTATIC RENAL CELL CARCINOMA

Authors (Reference)	N	Conditioning	GVHD Prophylaxis	aGVHD/(%)	cGVHD/(%)	TRM%	Overall Response (%)
Childs et al.	19	Flu+ Cy	CSA	53	21	11	53
Rini et al. Artz et al.	18	Flu + Cy	Tacro + MMF	22	39	14	22
Bregni et al.	7	Flu + TT	CSA + MTX	86	71	0	57
Pedrazzoli et al.	7	Flu + Cy	CSA + MTX	0	N/A	29	0
Blaise et al.	25	Flu + Bu + ATG	CSA	42	60	9	8
Nakagawa et al.	9	Flu/Cla + Bu +ATG	CSA	44	44	0	11
Ueno et al.	15	Flu + Mel	Tacro + MTX	47	27	33	20
Hentschke et al.	10	Flu + TBI +/–ATG	CSA + MMF	50	30	40	0
Massenkeil et al.	7	Flu + Cy + ATG	CSA +/–MMF	29	57	14	29
Tykodi et al.	8	Flu + TBI	CSA + MMF	50	50	13	13
Rinl et al.	22	Flu + Cy	Tacro + MTX	50	23	9	0
Barkholt et al.	124	Variable	CSA+/– MMF or MTX	40	33	16	32
Ishiyama et al.	7	Flu +/–Cy +/–TBI+/–Bu	CSA vs Tacro	71	50	42	57

Flu, fludarabine; cy, cyclophosphamide; TT, thiotepa: BU, busulfan: ATG, antithymocyte globulin; Cla, cladribine; Mel, melphalan; TBI, 200cGy total body irradiation; Tacro, tacrolimus: MMF, Mycophenolate mofetil; MTX, methotrexate; CSA, cyclosporine; TRM, transplantñrelated mortality; NA, not available.

[a]Mixed responses observed

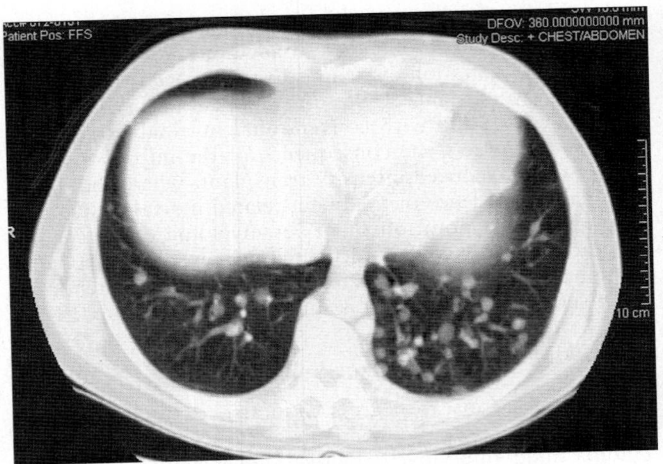

30 Days Post transplant

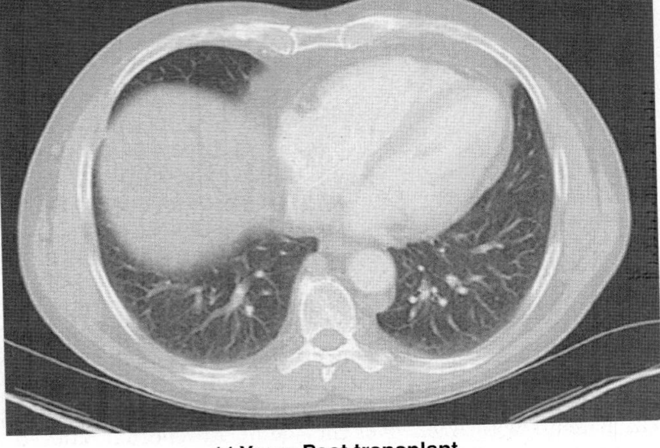

11 Years Post transplant

FIGURE 155.9 Graft-versus-tumor (GVT) effect resulting in a durable remission of metastatic RCC after nonmyeloablative allogeneic transplantation.

Disease regression compatible with a GVT effect in metastatic RCC has been observed in a subset of patients in 10 of 13 series (Table 155.2) published that investigated a variety of reduced intensity allogeneic transplant approaches.[32,205,206,210] The observation that disease regression is associated with acute GVHD, the withdrawal of immunosuppression, DLIs, and predominantly complete donor T-cell chimerism has provided compelling evidence that these disease responses occur as a consequence of a GVT effect.[161,211]

The identification of antigens expressed on RCC cells that serve as targets for donor immune cells remains an active area of investigation. Recently, T cells with *in vitro* tumor cytotoxicity patterns consistent with recognition of minor histocompatibility antigens and tumor restricted antigens have been identified in some responding patients.[32,209,212]

An innovative approach using tandem autologous followed by allogeneic HCT for patients with heavily pretreated metastatic breast cancer was reported by investigators from Italy. In 3 of 17 patients, durable complete responses lasting more than 1,320, 1,530, and 2,160 days post-HCT were observed.[213] Although proof of this concept has been established that shows GVT effects are inducible against select solid tumors, the overall response rate of most malignancies to this approach has been relatively low, with most responses only being partial. Although indubitably safer than conventional myeloablative transplantation, a 10% to 15% chance of transplant-related mortality further limits this approach. Therefore, "second-generation" transplant trials that focus on methods to target the alloimmune response specifically to the tumor through adoptive T/NK cell infusion or posttransplant tumor vaccination strategies are needed.[128]

FUTURE PROSPECTS

Exciting advances in the field of allogeneic HCT have significantly reduced the risks of morbidity and mortality associated with stem cell transplantation. The growing availability of volunteer donors in unrelated registries and the success of unrelated cord blood transplantation has led to a significant increase in the number of unrelated transplants being performed annually and has helped to make allogeneic transplantation an essential component to the treatment for an increasing number of malignant diseases. Furthermore, an expanded understanding of the requirements for the engraftment of donor cells, as well as the basic immunologic mechanisms involved in GVHD and GVL reactions, has greatly improved both the safety and efficacy of the procedure. The eventual identification of leukemia and tumor-specific antigens will likely lead to more targeted allogeneic immunotherapy approaches that avoid the morbidity associated with GVHD.

Selected References

The full list of references for this chapter appears in the online version.

12. Mathe G, Amiel JL, Schwarzenberg L, Cattan A, Schneider M. Adoptive immunotherapy of acute leukemia: experimental and clinical results. *Cancer Res* 1965;25:1525.
17. Khouri IF, McLaughlin P, Saliba RM, et al. Eight-year experience with allogeneic stem cell transplantation for relapsed follicular lymphoma after nonmyeloablative conditioning with fludarabine, cyclophosphamide, and rituximab. *Blood* 2008;111:5530.
20. Kolb HJ, Schattenberg A, Goldman JM, et al. Graft-versus-leukemia effect of donor lymphocyte transfusions in marrow grafted patients. European Group for Blood and Marrow Transplantation Working Party Chronic Leukemia. *Blood* 1995;86:2041.
25. Dazzi F, Szydlo RM, Craddock C, et al. Comparison of single-dose and escalating-dose regimens of donor lymphocyte infusion for relapse after allografting for chronic myeloid leukemia. *Blood* 2000;95:67.
32. Takahashi Y, Harashima N, Kajigaya S, et al. Regression of human kidney cancer following allogeneic stem cell transplantation is associated with recognition of an HERV-E antigen by T cells. *J Clin Invest* 2008;118:1099.
33. Ruggeri L, Capanni M, Urbani E, et al. Effectiveness of donor natural killer cell alloreactivity in mismatched hematopoietic transplants. *Science* 2002;295:2097.
41. Ullmann AJ, Lipton JH, Vesole DH, et al. Posaconazole or fluconazole for prophylaxis in severe graft-versus-host disease. *N Engl J Med* 2007;356:335.
63. Styczynski J, Einsele H, Gil L, Ljungman P. Outcome of treatment of Epstein-Barr virus-related post-transplant lymphoproliferative disorder in hematopoietic stem cell recipients: a comprehensive review of reported cases. *Transpl Infect Dis* 2009;11:383.
66. Hanley PJ, Cruz CR, Savoldo B, et al. Functionally active virus-specific T-cells that target CMV, adenovirus and EBV can be expanded from naive

T-cell populations in cord blood and will target a range of viral epitopes. *Blood* 2009;114:1958.
71. Goulmy E. Minor histocompatibility antigens: allo target molecules for tumor-specific immunotherapy. *Cancer J* 2004;10:1.
73. Shlomchik WD, Couzens MS, Tang CB, et al. Prevention of graft versus host disease by inactivation of host antigen-presenting cells. *Science* 1999;285:412.
77. Weisdorf DJ, Nelson G, Lee SJ, et al. Sibling versus unrelated donor allogeneic hematopoietic cell transplantation for chronic myelogenous leukemia: refined HLA matching reveals more graft-versus-host disease but not less relapse. *Biol Blood Marrow Transplant* 2009;15:1475.
78. Arora M, Weisdorf DJ, Spellman SR, et al. HLA-identical sibling compared with 8/8 matched and mismatched unrelated donor bone marrow transplant for chronic phase chronic myeloid leukemia. *J Clin Oncol* 2009; 27:1644.
86. Srinivasan R, Chakrabarti S, Walsh T, et al. Improved survival in steroid-refractory acute graft versus host disease after non-myeloablative allogeneic transplantation using a daclizumab-based strategy with comprehensive infection prophylaxis. *Br J Haematol* 2004;124:777.
93. Shulman HM, Kleiner D, Lee SJ. et al. Histopathologic diagnosis of chronic graft-versus-host disease: National Institutes of Health Consensus Development Project on Criteria for Clinical Trials in Chronic Graft-versus-Host Disease: II Pathology Working Group Report. *Biol Blood Marrow Transplant* 2006;12:31.
94. Couriel D, Carpenter PA, Cutler C, et al. Ancillary therapy and supportive care of chronic graft-versus-host disease: national institutes of health consensus development project on criteria for clinical trials in chronic Graft-versus-host disease: V. Ancillary Therapy and Supportive Care Working Group Report. *Biol Blood Marrow Transplant* 2006;12:375.
105. Bolan CD, Carter CS, Wesley RA, et al. Prospective evaluation of cell kinetics, yields and donor experiences during a single large-volume apheresis versus two smaller volume consecutive day collections of allogeneic peripheral blood stem cells. *Br J Haematol* 2003;120:801.
111. Bensinger WI, Martin PJ, Storer B, et al. Transplantation of bone marrow as compared with peripheral-blood cells from HLA-identical relatives in patients with hematologic cancers. *N Engl J Med* 2001;344:175.
113. Foeken LM, Green A, Hurley CK, et al. Monitoring the international use of unrelated donors for transplantation: the WMDA annual reports. *Bone Marrow Transplant* 2010;45:811.
118. Petersdorf EW, Hansen JA, Martin PJ, et al. Major-histocompatibility-complex class I alleles and antigens in hematopoietic-cell transplantation. *N Engl J Med* 2001;345:1794.
123. Rizzieri DA, Koh LP, Long GD, et al. Partially matched, nonmyeloablative allogeneic transplantation: clinical outcomes and immune reconstitution. *J Clin Oncol* 2007;25:690.
128. Lundqvist A, McCoy JP, Samsel L, Childs R. Reduction of GVHD and enhanced antitumor effects after adoptive infusion of alloreactive Ly49-mismatched NK cells from MHC-matched donors. *Blood* 2007;109:3603.
130. Gluckman E. Hematopoietic stem-cell transplants using umbilical-cord blood. *N Engl J Med* 2001;344:1860.
132. Wagner JE, Kernan NA, Steinbuch M, Broxmeyer HE, Gluckman E. Allogeneic sibling umbilical-cord-blood transplantation in children with malignant and non-malignant disease. *Lancet* 1995;346:214.
134. Rocha V, Labopin M, Sanz G, et al. Transplants of umbilical-cord blood or bone marrow from unrelated donors in adults with acute leukemia. *N Engl J Med* 2004;351:2276.
135. Laughlin MJ, Eapen M, Rubinstein P, et al. Outcomes after transplantation of cord blood or bone marrow from unrelated donors in adults with leukemia. *N Engl J Med* 2004;351:2265.
137. MacMillan ML, Weisdorf DJ, Brunstein CG, et al. Acute graft-versus-host disease after unrelated donor umbilical cord blood transplantation: analysis of risk factors. *Blood* 2009;113:2410.
156. Hill BT, Copelan EA. Acute myeloid leukemia: when to transplant in first complete remission. *Curr Hematol Malig Rep* 2010;5:101.
157. Schlenk RF, Dohner K, Krauter J, et al. Mutations and treatment outcome in cytogenetically normal acute myeloid leukemia. *N Engl J Med* 2008; 358:1909.
160. Goldstone AH, Richards SM, Lazarus HM, et al. In adults with standard-risk acute lymphoblastic leukemia, the greatest benefit is achieved from a matched sibling allogeneic transplantation in first complete remission, and an autologous transplantation is less effective than conventional consolidation/maintenance chemotherapy in all patients: final results of the International ALL Trial (MRC UKALL XII/ECOG E2993). *Blood* 2008;111:1827.
165. Lim Z, Brand R, Martino R, et al. Allogeneic hematopoietic stem-cell transplantation for patients 50 years or older with myelodysplastic syndromes or secondary acute myeloid leukemia. *J Clin Oncol* 2010;28:405.
169. Schetelig J, van Biezen A, Brand R, et al. Allogeneic hematopoietic stem-cell transplantation for chronic lymphocytic leukemia with 17p deletion: a retrospective European Group for Blood and Marrow Transplantation analysis. *J Clin Oncol* 2008;26:5094.
171. Giralt S, Estey E, Albitar M et al. Engraftment of allogeneic hematopoietic progenitor cells with purine analog-containing chemotherapy: harnessing graft versus leukemia without myeloablative therapy. *Blood* 1997;89: 4531.
172. Slavin S, Nagler A, Naparstek E, et al. Nonmyeloablative stem cell transplantation and cell therapy as an alternative to conventional bone marrow transplantation with lethal cytoreduction for the treatment of malignant and nonmalignant hematologic diseases. *Blood* 1998;91:756.
173. Sandmaier BM, Mackinnon S, Childs RW. Reduced intensity conditioning for allogeneic hematopoietic cell transplantation: current perspectives. *Biol Blood Marrow Transplant* 2007;13:87.
176. Childs R, Clave E, Contentin N, et al. Engraftment kinetics after nonmyeloablative allogeneic peripheral blood stem cell transplantation: full donor T-cell chimerism precedes alloimmune responses. *Blood* 1999;94: 3234.
181. Antin JH, Childs R, Filipovich AH, et al. Establishment of complete and mixed donor chimerism after allogeneic lymphohematopoietic transplantation: recommendations from a workshop at the 2001 Tandem Meetings of the International Bone Marrow Transplant Registry and the American Society of Blood and Marrow Transplantation. *Biol Blood Marrow Transplant* 2001;7:473.
184. McClune BL, Weisdorf DJ, Pedersen TL, et al. Effect of age on outcome of reduced-intensity hematopoietic cell transplantation for older patients with acute myeloid leukemia in first complete remission or with myelodysplastic syndrome. *J Clin Oncol* 2010;28:1878.
186. McSweeney PA, Niederwieser D, Shizuru JA, et al. Hematopoietic cell transplantation in older patients with hematologic malignancies: replacing high-dose cytotoxic therapy with graft-versus-tumor effects. *Blood* 2001;97:3390.
191. Maris MB, Niederwieser D, Sandmaier BM, et al. HLA-matched unrelated donor hematopoietic cell transplantation after nonmyeloablative conditioning for patients with hematologic malignancies. *Blood* 2003; 102:2021.
192. Carvallo C, Geller N, Kurlander R, et al. Prior chemotherapy and allograft CD34+ dose impact donor engraftment following nonmyeloablative allogeneic stem cell transplantation in patients with solid tumors. *Blood* 2004; 103:1560.
194. Storb RF, Lucarelli G, McSweeney PA, Childs RW. Hematopoietic cell transplantation for benign hematological disorders and solid tumors. *Hematology (Am Soc Hematol Educ Program)* 2003:372.
200. Sarina B, Castagna L, Farina L, et al. Allogeneic transplantation improves the overall and progression-free survival of Hodgkin's lymphoma patients relapsing after autologous transplantation: a retrospective study based on the time of HLA typing and donor availability. *Blood* 2010;115:3671.
202. Maloney DG, Molina AJ, Sahebi F, et al. Allografting with nonmyeloablative conditioning following cytoreductive autografts for the treatment of patients with multiple myeloma. *Blood* 2003;102:3447.
203. Bruno B, Rotta M, Patriarca F, et al. A comparison of allografting with autografting for newly diagnosed myeloma. *N Engl J Med* 2007;356: 1110.
204. Bruno B, Rotta M, Patriarca F, et al. Nonmyeloablative allografting for newly diagnosed multiple myeloma: the experience of the Gruppo Italiano Trapianti di Midollo. *Blood* 2009;113:3375.
206. Bregni M, Ueno NT, Childs R. The Second International Meeting on Allogeneic Transplantation in Solid Tumors. *Bone Marrow Transplant* 2006;38:527.
208. Childs RW, Clave E, Tisdale J, et al. Successful treatment of metastatic renal cell carcinoma with a nonmyeloablative allogeneic peripheral-blood progenitor-cell transplant: evidence for a graft-versus-tumor effect. *J Clin Oncol* 1999;17:2044.
210. Childs R, Chernoff A, Contentin N, et al. Regression of metastatic renal-cell carcinoma after nonmyeloablative allogeneic peripheral-blood stem-cell transplantation. *N Engl J Med* 2000;343:750.
213. Carella AM, Beltrami G, Corsetti MT, et al. Reduced intensity conditioning for allograft after cytoreductive autograft in metastatic breast cancer. *Lancet* 2005;366:318.

SECTION 19: MANAGEMENT OF ADVERSE EFFECTS OF TREATMENT

CHAPTER 156 INFECTIONS IN THE CANCER PATIENT

JUAN GEA-BANACLOCHE AND BRAHM H. SEGAL

RISK FACTORS FOR INFECTIONS IN PATIENTS WITH CANCER AND ANTIMICROBIAL PROPHYLAXIS

RISK FACTORS FOR INFECTION

Cancer patients are at increased risk for infection because of their disease and its treatment. Awareness of the risk factors present in the patient is important for diagnosis and empirical management. Selected host defense defects are presented on Tables 156.1 and 156.2.

Intrinsic Host Factors

Hematologic Malignancies

Some hematologic malignancies are associated with increased frequency of infections even in the absence of treatment. For instance, the rate of mycobacterial disease seems to be increased in hairy cell leukemia and Hodgkin's lymphoma. Multiple myeloma and chronic lymphocytic leukemia (CLL) are associated with a high risk of encapsulated bacterial infections due to impaired B-cell immunity.

Solid Tumors

Solid tumors may predispose to infection because of anatomic factors related to the cancer or its treatment. Tumor necrosis (either by spontaneous overgrow of the blood supply or therapeutic intervention like radiofrequency ablation) may facilitate a nidus for infection. Head and neck tumors may erode into the mouth, predisposing to serious infections by oral flora. Endobronchial tumors may cause postobstructive pneumonia. Obstruction of the genitourinary or hepatobiliary tracts may predispose to pyelonephritis and cholangitis, respectively. Direct invasion through the colonic mucosa is associated with local abscess formation and sepsis by enteric flora. Some other factors, less well understood, may contribute to the specific association of colon cancer with bacteremia caused by *Streptococcus gallolyticus* (formerly *Streptococcus bovis*), other streptococci, and anaerobes like *Clostridium septicum*. Breast tumors increase the risk of mastitis and abscess formation, usually by *Staphylococcus aureus*. Adrenal corticosteroid-producing tumors and ectopic adrenal corticotrophin hormone-secreting tumors are associated with an increased risk of bacterial and opportunistic infections. *Pneumocystis jirovecii* (formerly *Pneumocystis carinii*) and *Nocardia* infections have been reported in patients with Cushing disease.

Asplenia

The spleen is important for antigen presentation, production of opsonizing antibodies by B cells, and removal of opsonized and nonopsonized bacteria. This makes it essential for protection against encapsulated bacteria to which the person is not yet immune. Functional asplenia is present after splenectomy, splenic irradiation, and with chronic graft-versus-host disease (GVHD).[1] Functionally asplenic patients are at risk for overwhelming sepsis by encapsulated bacteria. The most common pathogen is *Streptococcus pneumoniae,* but other pathogens include *Hemophilus influenzae* and *Neisseria meningitidis*. Patients without a functional spleen who present with fever should be started promptly on antibiotics active against *S. pneumoniae* (e.g., ceftriaxone or a newer generation fluoroquinolone, such as levofloxacin or moxifloxacin). Vancomycin might be added in areas where high-level penicillin or cephalosporin resistance is common. If a history of exposure to dogs (bite, scratch) is present, *Capnocytophaga canimorsus* should be considered, and a beta-lactam with a beta-lactamase inhibitor or a carbapenem is preferred. Other pathogens of concern in asplenic individuals include babesiosis, malaria and *Salmonella* species.

The U.S. Centers for Disease Control and Prevention (CDC) recommends that asplenic persons be immunized with the pneumococcal polysaccharide and meningococcal vaccines. The conjugated meningococcal vaccine is preferred in adults 55 years of age or younger because it confers longer lasting immunity than the polysaccharide vaccine. Immunization of adults with the *H. influenzae* type B (Hib) vaccine is also recommended. Immunization is ideally performed at least 2 weeks in advance of splenectomy. If this is not feasible, immunization is still advisable after the procedure. One-time reimmunization with the pneumococcal vaccine is advised in asplenic persons 5 years after the time of initial vaccination. Penicillin prophylaxis is advised in asplenic patients to prevent pneumococcal disease.

TABLE 156.1

RISK FACTORS AND INFECTIOUS DISEASES ASSOCIATIONS IN CANCER PATIENTS

Risk Factors	Infection	Comment
MALIGNANCY-RELATED FACTORS		
Hematologic Malignancies		
Myelodysplastic syndrome and acute leukemia	Bacteria, viruses, and fungi	Infectious risk related to prolonged neutropenia
Acute lymphoblastic leukemia	*Pneumocystis jirovecii* pneumonia	Corticosteroid treatment possible confounding factor
Chronic lymphocytic leukemia	Encapsulated bacteria	Infectious risk linked to hypogammaglobulinemia
Multiple myeloma	Encapsulated bacteria	Impaired B-cell immunity, hypogammaglobulinemia
Hairy cell leukemia	Mycobacteria, herpes viruses	Defective T-cell immunity
Hodgkin's lymphoma	Mycobacteria, herpes viruses	Defective T-cell immunity
Adult T-cell lymphoma/leukemia	*P. jirovecii*, *Cryptococcus neoformans*, cytomegalovirus, *Strongyloides stercoralis*	Defective T-cell immunity
Solid Tumors		
Endobronchial tumors	Postobstructive pneumonia	Mechanical obstruction
Colon carcinoma	*Streptococcal bacteremia* *Clostridium bacteremia*	
Hepatobiliary tumors	Bacterial infection with enteric organisms	Mechanical obstruction plus abnormal liver function if underlying cirrhosis
Head and neck cancer	Infections with oral flora and anaerobes	Mechanical disruption
Genitourinary tumors	Gram-negative bacilli, *Enterococcus* sp.	Related to obstruction
Asplenia	*Streptococcus pneumoniae*, *Haemophilus influenzae*, and *Neisseria meningitidis* (encapsulated bacteria), *Salmonella*, *Capnocytophaga canimorsus*, *Babesia microti*, malaria	
TREATMENT-RELATED FACTORS		
Neutropenia	Bacterial and fungal infections (see Table 156.2)	
Mucositis	Bacterial infections caused by oral and enteric flora, candidiasis	
Corticosteroids	Bacteria, *P. jirovecii*, *C. neoformans*, molds, herpes viruses	Decrease signs and symptoms of inflammation.
Nucleoside analogues (e.g., fludarabine, 2-chlorodeoxyadenosine, and 2-deoxycoformycin)	Bacteria, *P. jirovecii*, *C. neoformans*, herpes viruses	Defective T-cell immunity by T-cell depletion
Alemtuzumab	Opportunistic and nonopportunistic infections, including bacteria, viruses (e.g., CMV, VZV), *P. jirovecii*, and fungi	Broad defect in host defense involving depletion of T, B, NK cells and monocytes
Rituximab	Bacterial infections, VZV, *P. jirovecii*	Occasional neutropenia Impaired B-cell immunity
Daclizumab	Bacterial sepsis	Infections in the setting of steroid-refractory GVHD
Antibodies inhibiting cytokine signaling (e.g., infliximab)	Bacterial infections, tuberculosis and other mycobacterial infections, mold infections in GVHD, other fungal infections (e.g., histoplasmosis)	Suppression of inflammation may allow infections to progress undetected
Calcineurin inhibitors	*P. jirovecii*, VZV	Defective T-cell immunity
Radiation therapy	Local and systemic bacterial infections, mucosal candidiasis and HSV infection	Damages mucosal surfaces, marrow suppression

CMV, cytomegalovirus; VZV, varicella-zoster virus; NK, natural killer; GVHD, graft-versus-host disease; HSV, herpes simplex virus.

Treatment-Related Factors

Mucositis

The mucosal linings of the gastrointestinal, respiratory, and genitourinary tracts constitute the first line of host defense against a variety of pathogens. Besides the physical barrier, mucosal epithelial cells secrete a variety of antimicrobial peptides, including lactoferrin, lysozyme, proteases, phospholipases, and defensins. Chemotherapy and radiation therapy impair mucosal immunity at several different levels. Chronic GVHD may further compromise mucosal immunity, including defective salivary immunoglobulin secretion. Compromise of

TABLE 156.2

PREDOMINANT IMMUNOLOGIC DEFECTS AND ASSOCIATED PATHOGENS IN PATIENTS WITH CANCER

Abnormality	Bacteria	Fungi	Protozoa	Viruses
Qualitative defect of phagocytic function or neutropenia	**Gram-positive:** *Staphylococcus aureus*, *Streptococcus* sp., *Nocardia* sp. **Gram-negative:** *Escherichia coli*, *Klebsiella* sp., *Enterobacter* sp., other Enterobacteriaceae *Pseudomonas aeruginosa*, *Stenotrophomonas maltophilia*, *Acinetobacter* sp.	Yeasts: *Candida* sp., *Trichosporon* sp. *Molds:* *Aspergillus* sp., *Fusarium* sp., dark-walled molds (phaeohyphomycosis), zygomycetes, others		Herpes simplex Community respiratory viruses (e.g., influenza, parainfluenza, RSV, adenovirus)
Defective cell-mediated immunity	*Mycobacterium* sp. *Nocardia* sp. *Listeria monocytogenes* *Salmonella* sp.	*Pneumocystis jirovecii* *Histoplasma capsulatum* *Coccidioides immitis* *Penicillium marneffei* *Cryptococcus neoformans*	*Toxoplasma gondii* *Strongyloides stercoralis*	Cytomegalovirus Epstein-Barr virus Varicella-zoster virus Herpes simplex virus Community respiratory viruses
Defective humoral immunity	*Streptococcus pneumoniae* *Haemophilus influenzae* *Neisseria meningitidis*			

RSV, respiratory syncytial virus.

the epithelial lining may result in invasion by local flora, and bacteremia and candidemia may result. Severe mucositis is a known risk factor for viridans-group streptococcal infections, but many pathogens, including oral anaerobes, may cause invasive disease in this setting. Preliminary studies suggest that the use of palifermin, a recombinant human keratinocyte growth factor, may result in decreased infections by reduction in severity of mucositis.[2]

Chemotherapy-Induced Neutropenia

Neutropenia is a major risk factor for infections in cancer patients. Lack of granulocytes facilitates bacterial and fungal infections, and blunts the inflammatory response, allowing infections to progress much faster. During neutropenia empirical treatment must be initiated in the presence of clinical markers of infection (e.g., fever, erythema, pain), which are frequently nonspecific. The risk of infection is proportional to the degree of neutropenia.[3] The source of bacterial infections is most commonly the commensal flora of the gastrointestinal tract. Fungal infections may be related to prior colonization in the case of *Candida* (skin or gastrointestinal flora) or inhalation in the case of molds. Risk of fungal diseases increases with the duration of neutropenia. Aspergillosis is uncommon during neutropenic periods of less than 10 days, but its incidence increases in direct proportion to the length of neutropenia after 14 days.[4]

Hematopoietic Stem Cell Transplantation

Autologous and allogeneic hematopoietic stem cell transplantation (HSCT) present different infectious disease problems. Autologous transplant may be considered a form of intensive chemotherapy. As such, it is typically associated with a few days or weeks of neutropenia and mucositis, followed by a few weeks or months of defective T-cell–mediated immunity. The duration of the defect in T-cell immunity varies depending on the type of cancer (longer in hematologic malignancies),[5] the manipulation of the stem cells preinfusion (longer with T-cell depletion), and the age of the recipients (shorter immunodeficiency in children).[6] Autologous transplants have fewer infections than allogeneic transplants, but T-cell depletion results in risk for cytomegalovirus (CMV) and other opportunistic infections similar to allogeneic HSCT recipients.[7]

Allogeneic transplant is a more complex procedure, and there are many variants: conditioning regimen (e.g., myeloablative, reduced intensity, nonmyeloablative), degree of HLA matching (e.g., matched sibling, matched unrelated, mismatched), source of stem cells (e.g., bone marrow, peripheral blood stem cells, umbilical cord cells) and GVHD prophylaxis (e.g., T-cell depletion or not, specific immunosuppressive regimen). Different combinations of these variables result in very different infectious disease risk profiles. Infections after HSCT tend to follow a time line associated with different predominant immune defects, presented schematically in Table 156.3. Early after HSCT, neutropenia is the principal host defense defect, predisposing mainly to bacterial and fungal infections. After myeloid engraftment (defined as the first day with absolute neutrophil count >500/mcL), a remaining risk factor for bacterial infection is the presence of a central venous catheter.

By far the most important risk factor for infection in allogeneic transplant following engraftment is the occurrence of severe GVHD and its treatment. Active GVHD is associated

TABLE 156.3

TIME LINE OF PRINCIPAL IMMUNE DEFECTS AND INFECTIOUS COMPLICATIONS IN ALLOGENEIC HEMATOPOIETIC STEM CELL TRANSPLANT RECIPIENTS (IN THE PRESENCE OF STANDARD PROPHYLAXES)

	Months after Transplantation		
Defect	<1	1–6	>6[a]
Principal immune defect	Neutropenia	T cell, humoral Phagocytic (qualitative)	Humoral
Bacterial pathogens	Staphylococci, enterococci, viridans group streptococci, Enterobacteriaceae, *Pseudomonas aeruginosa*	Catheter-related bacteremia occasionally enteric flora related to gut GVHD with translocation, encapsulated bacteria (generally after 3 months or more after HSCT), *Listeria monocytogenes*, mycobacteria, and nocardiosis,	Encapsulated bacteria (*Streptococcus pneumoniae, Haemophilus influenzae,* and *Neisseria meningitidis*) Respiratory viruses (e.g., influenza, parainfluenza, RSV, adenovirus)
Fungal pathogens	Non-albicans *Candida* species, *Aspergillus* sp., and other molds (e.g., zygomycetes, *Fusarium* sp., *Scedosporium* sp., dark-walled molds), *Staphylococcus* sp.	Same as <1 month plus *Pneumocystis jirovecii, Candida* sp., *Cryptococcus neoformans*, dimorphic fungi (e.g., histoplasmosis, coccidioidomycosis),	Risk of invasive fungal infections decreases after 6 months in absence of GVHD, varicella-zoster virus
Viral pathogens	Community respiratory viruses (e.g., influenza, parainfluenza, RSV, adenovirus, metapneumoviruses), acyclovir-resistant herpes simplex virus metapneumovirus), *Streptococcus* sp.	Cytomegalovirus, HHV-6, community respiratory viruses. If acyclovir/valacyclovir stopped, varicella-zoster virus, herpes simplex virus, *Candida* sp.	Varicella zoster virus, community respiratory viruses. Risk of other opportunistic viral infections decreases after 6 months in absence of GVHD.
Parasitic infections		Toxoplasmosis, strongyloidiasis	

GVHD, graft-versus-host disease; RSV, respiratory syncytial virus; HSCT, hematopoietic stem cell transplantation; HHV-6, human herpesvirus-6.
[a]Graft-versus-host disease necessitating intensive immunosuppressive therapy leads to lack of reconstitution of phagocytic (qualitative) and cell-mediated immunity, thus prolonging the period of risk for infection with both common bacteria and opportunistic pathogens (see text).

with immune dysregulation, may be accompanied by CMV reactivation or disease, and requires treatment with immunosuppressive agents (corticosteroids are the first-line agent), and is an independent risk factor for mold infection.[8] CMV disease delays immune reconstitution and is associated with an increased risk of bacterial and fungal infections.[9]

Defects in cell-mediated immunity persist for several months even in uncomplicated allogeneic HSCT recipients, predisposing to opportunistic infections, including candidiasis, *P. jirovecii*, CMV, and herpes zoster (Table 156.3). Repopulation of specific T-cell subsets occurs at different rates, resulting in a lower than normal CD4+ to CD8+ T-cell ratio for the first 6 months following engraftment.[10] In addition to low T-cell number, T-cell receptor diversity is reduced.[11] Whereas mature and cooperative T- and B-cell functions are usually reconstituted by 1 to 2 years after engraftment, chronic GVHD is associated with persistently depressed cell-mediated and humoral immunity.

Defective reconstitution of humoral immunity is a major factor contributing to increased infection susceptibility in the late transplant period. Invasive pneumococcal disease is relatively common after HSCT,[12] particularly in patients with chronic GVHD.[13]

Allografts from HLA-matched unrelated donors and partially mismatched related donors are at a higher risk of GVHD than allografts from HLA-matched siblings. T-cell depletion delays immune reconstitution and, consequently, carries a greater risk of infectious complications, most notably opportunistic viral[14] and fungal[15] pathogens. Cord blood transplant recipients have a higher risk of infections during the early transplant period because of slower myeloid engraftment. After engraftment, opportunistic infections still occur,[16,17] but seem to be no more common than in unmanipulated blood and bone marrow recipients, and generally less than in recipients of T-cell–depleted allografts.[18,19]

Immunomodulatory Agents and Infectious Risk

Corticosteroids

High-dose corticosteroids have profound effects on the distribution and function of neutrophils, monocytes, and lymphocytes. Corticosteroids blunt fever and local signs of infection such as peritonitis. Patients treated with corticosteroids have impaired phagocytic function (increasing risk of bacterial and fungal infections) and cell-mediated immunity (increasing risk of agents such as herpes zoster and *P. jirovecii*). The incidence of infectious complications increases when the adult equivalent of prednisone 20 mg per day is administered for longer than 4 to 6 weeks.[20] In allogeneic HSCT recipients, corticosteroid therapy for GVHD is a major risk factor for invasive fungal infections.

Fludarabine

Fludarabine is a fluorinated analogue of adenine that is lymphotoxic, primarily affecting CD4+ lymphocytes. The combination of fludarabine and corticosteroids is more immunosuppressive than either agent alone. Fludarabine plus prednisone results in a uniform depression of CD4+ cells that may persist for several months after completion of therapy, resulting in opportunistic infections like *P. jirovecii* pneumonia (PCP) or listeriosis, sometimes more than a year after treatment. Mycobacterial and herpes virus infections have also been described.

Interleukin-2

Patients receiving high dose interleukin-2 (IL-2) for malignancy have an increased risk of bacterial infections, mainly *S. aureus* and coagulase-negative staphylococci, possibly related to indwelling catheters. High-dose, continuous infusion IL-2 causes a profound but reversible defect in neutrophil chemotaxis that may account for the increased frequency of infections. Prophylactic oxacillin led to a reduction in central venous catheter-associated staphylococcal bacteremia in IL-2 recipients in one randomized trial.[21]

Monoclonal Antibodies

Alemtuzumab. Alemtuzumab (Campath-1H) is a humanized monoclonal antibody that targets CD52, a glycoprotein abundantly expressed on most B and T lymphocytes, macrophages, and natural killer cells. Alemtuzumab is Food and Drug Administration (FDA)-approved for refractory CLL and is increasingly used for a variety of hematologic malignancies. Alemtuzumab treatment results in prolonged and severe lymphopenia. It can also cause neutropenia in up to one-third of patients. Many infections have been reported in a significant fraction of patients receiving alemtuzumab.[22] Bacterial, viral, fungal mycobacterial and *P. jirovecii* infections are observed. CMV reactivation is seen in up to two-thirds of alemtuzumab recipients, although CMV disease seems to be uncommon. We recommend prophylaxis against herpes virus and *P. jirovecii* infections, and preemptive therapy for CMV reactivation in alemtuzumab recipients (specific recommendations by pathogen are presented in Table 156.4).

Rituximab. Rituximab is a chimeric human/murine monoclonal antibody directed against the B-cell marker CD20 and used in the treatment of B-cell malignancies. The increased risk of infection with rituximab seems to be low, related to repeated administration[23] and host cofactors (e.g., advanced human immunodeficiency virus [HIV] disease, HSCT, specific chemotherapeutic regimen).[24] Some patients develop persistent hypogammaglobulinemia after receiving this agent,[25] but the specific contribution of hypogammaglobulinemia to infection risk is unclear.[26] Hepatitis B reactivation may be more common in patients with lymphoma treated with rituximab–containing regimens.[27,28] Rarely, rituximab treatment for malignant and nonmalignant conditions can be complicated by progressive multifocal leukoencephalopathy (PML) a chronic encephalitis caused by the JC virus.[29]

Lymphocyte-depleting antibodies cause severe suppression of cellular immunity. Visilizumab (a humanized anti-CD3 monoclonal antibody) is associated with a high frequency of Epstein-Barr virus (EBV) reactivation and lymphoproliferative disease.[30] Anticytokine antibodies include the IL-2 receptor antagonist, daclizumab, and tumor necrosis factor (TNF)-α inhibiting agents, infliximab, etanercept, and adalimumab. Daclizumab in steroid-refractory GVHD is associated with a significant risk of bacterial sepsis. TNF-α is a principal mediator of neutrophil and monocyte activation and inflammation. In patients with autoimmune diseases, agents that deplete TNF-α or inhibit TNF-α signaling are principally associated with an increased risk of tuberculosis and histoplasmosis. In HSCT recipients with refractory GVHD, infliximab was associated with an increased risk of invasive molds.[31]

Bevacizumab, an inhibitor of vascular endothelial growth factor, has been associated with increased risk of gastrointestinal perforation. The risk seems to be highest in patients with colorectal carcinoma and renal cell cancer.

PREVENTION OF INFECTIONS

Infections may be prevented by avoidance of exposure, immunization, and chemoprophylaxis. A comprehensive guideline cosponsored by the Center for International Blood and Marrow Research, the National Marrow Donor program, the European Blood and Marrow Transplant Group, the American Society for Blood and Marrow Transplantation, the Canadian Blood and Marrow Transplant Group, the Infectious Diseases Society of America (IDSA), the Society for Healthcare Epidemiology of America, the Association of Medical Microbiology and Infectious Disease Canada, and the CDC makes evidence-based recommendations for HSCT that may be applicable to other cancer patients.[32] A summary of approaches for prophylaxis in this patient population is provided in Table 156.4.

In general, antimicrobial prophylaxis tends to reduce the number of episodes of the targeted infection. A different issue is whether this reduction in incidence of infection translates into an expected survival benefit or at least a reduction in a clinically meaningful outcome (e.g., sepsis, hospital admission, prolongation of hospitalization) that outweighs the toxicities or secondary effects (e.g., generation and spreading of resistant organisms) and cost. The number of subjects that need to be treated to prevent one episode of infection and the severity of the infection should be considered.

Prevention of Bacterial Infections

Antibacterial Prophylaxis in Afebrile Neutropenic Patients

Randomized controlled trials of antibacterial prophylaxis in neutropenic patients have often shown decreased number of episodes of fever and decreased infections, but no difference in mortality. Meta-analyses have confirmed these results and suggested possibly improved overall survival.[33,34] The effect is more marked in patients with prolonged neutropenia and it reflects mainly use or oral fluoroquinolones. In neutropenic patients with intermediate or higher risk of infection related to neutropenia, prophylactic levofloxacin led to a reduction in infections.[35] In contrast, the major benefit of prophylactic levofloxacin in lower risk neutropenic patients (e.g., those with solid tumors and short-duration neutropenia) relates to a modest but significant reduction in febrile episodes.[36] The potential risks of quinolone prophylaxis regarding selection for resistant organisms and *Clostridium difficile* colitis are important questions that remain unanswered. Other antibiotics may be effective, and some authorities would substitute trimethoprim/sulfamethoxazole (TMP/SMX) in specific patients at high risk for *P. jirovecii*. In patients with neutropenia expected to last 7 days or less and not receiving

TABLE 156.4

PROPHYLAXIS OF INFECTIONS IN CANCER PATIENTS

Intervention	Indication	Agent	Comments
PROPHYLAXIS FOR BACTERIAL INFECTIONS			
Prophylaxis for neutropenia	Patients who are expected to be neutropenic for >7 days	Levofloxacin 500 mg orally daily	Start the first day of ANC <1,000 and continue until resolution of neutropenia.
		TMP/SMX may be used	Other agents have been used, but there is less experience.
Prophylaxis for *Streptococcus pneumoniae*	Patients splenectomized	Penicillin V-K, 500 mg orally bid	Patient education related to early recognition of signs and symptoms of infection is imperative; consider having the patient keep systemic antibiotics (e.g., levofloxacin) at home for an emergency.
	Splenic irradiation Chronic GVHD	In penicillin-allergic: TMP/SMX 1 DS tablet daily or azithromycin 250 mg/d	
PROPHYLAXIS FOR FUNGAL INFECTIONS			
Antifungal prophylaxis	Induction therapy for AML and MDS	Posaconazole 200 mg orally tid is drug of choice. In patients unable to take oral medications or who are intolerant to posaconazole, alternatives include itraconazole, voriconazole, lipid formulation of amphotericin B, or an echinocandin.	Posaconazole was superior to fluconazole/itraconazole in a randomized controlled trial, but the risk of aspergillosis in this setting is variable and some institutions may choose to use fluconazole prophylaxis if their incidence of aspergillosis is low. If fluconazole prophylaxis is used, serial monitoring with serum galactomannan and/or β-D-glucan should be considered. Begin with initiation of chemotherapy and continue until resolution of neutropenia.
	Acute lymphoblastic leukemia receiving vinca alkaloid-containing regimen	Fluconazole[a] or an echinocandin	Mold-active azoles are potent inhibitors of cytochrome P-450 isoenzymes, and are expected to interfere with metabolism of vinca alkaloids. Continue prophylaxis for duration of neutropenia.
	Autologous HSCT recipient during neutropenia	Fluconazole[a] or echinocandin	Continue prophylaxis for duration of neutropenia. Consider no antifungal prophylaxis if regimen does not have significant mucosal toxicity.
	Allogeneic HSCT recipient during neutropenia	Fluconazole,[a] itraconazole, voriconazole, and micafungin have each been evaluated in this setting and are acceptable options. Posaconazole has not been evaluated in this setting, but is reasonable.	Continue prophylaxis for duration of neutropenia.
	Allogeneic HSCT with significant GVHD receiving intensive immunosuppressive therapy[b]	Posaconazole 200 mg orally tid is drug of choice. Alternatives include voriconazole, itraconazole, lipid formulation of amphotericin B, or an echinocandin.	Continue prophylaxis for 16 weeks and for at least the duration of intensive immunosuppressive therapy,[b] whichever occurs later

(*continued*)

TABLE 156.4

(CONTINUED)

Intervention	Indication	Agent	Comments
Prophylaxis against *Pneumocystis jirovecii*	Acute lymphocytic leukemia Allogeneic HSCT recipients Alemtuzumab recipients Fludarabine recipients Patients with gliomas receiving temozolomide and radiation or corticosteroids (≥20 mg of prednisone equivalent) for ≥1 month in the presence of other immunosuppression or myelotoxic chemotherapy	TMP/SMX 1 DS (TMP 160 mg + SMX 800 mg) orally daily or 3 days per week OR dapsone 100 mg orally daily OR inhaled pentamidine 300 mg every 4 weeks OR atovaquone 1,500 mg/d	TMP/SMX seems effective as long as three or four DS tablets are given every week; daily administration may be more effective In allo-HSCT, continue prophylaxis for 2 months after stopping immunosuppression. In patients treated with alemtuzumab, continue prophylaxis for 2 months after the last dose or until the CD4 count is >200, whichever occurs later.
PROPHYLAXIS FOR VIRAL INFECTIONS			
Prophylaxis for HSV	HSCT recipients (HSV-seropositive recipients) Induction chemotherapy for acute leukemia (HSV-seropositive) Consider in patients with recurrent HSV reactivation following chemotherapy, or patients receiving fludarabine and corticosteroids Patients treated with alemtuzumab	Acyclovir 400 mg orally bid or tid OR 800 mg orally bid OR 250 mg/m²/12 h or valacyclovir 500 mg orally once or twice (higher doses have been used up to 1,000 mg tid) or famciclovir 250 mg orally tid	In patients with acute leukemia and HSCT recipients, continue prophylaxis for HSV until resolution of neutropenia and mucositis. In patients treated with alemtuzumab, continue prophylaxis for 2 months after the last dose or until the CD4 count is >200, whichever occurs later.
Prophylaxis for VZV	Allogeneic HSCT recipients with a history of chicken pox or shingles	Acyclovir 800 mg orally bid OR valacyclovir 500 mg orally daily	
Prophylaxis for CMV (preemptive therapy)	Patients requiring CMV surveillance (1) Allogeneic HSCT recipients who are CMV+ or whose donor is CMV+ (standard of care) (2) Autologous SCT recipients receiving a CD34-enriched autograft (should be considered) (3) Patients treated with alemtuzumab (should be considered)	Induction for 1 week followed by maintenance for 1 week as follows: Ganciclovir 5 mg/kg IV q12h for 7 days (induction), followed by Ganciclovir 5 mg/kg IV daily 5 times a week (maintenance) OR Foscarnet[a] 60 mg/kg IV q12h times 7 days (induction) followed by Foscarnet[c] 60 mg/kg IV daily (maintenance) Oral valganciclovir (900 mg bid) is an acceptable alternative to IV formulations in patients who do not have severe gut GVHD (see text)	Time for CMV surveillance: (1) Allogeneic HSCT recipients: from day 30 to at least 6 months after allogeneic HSCT, during periods of GVHD, and until the CD4+ count is >100 mcL. (2) Recipients of CD34-enriched autologous grafts: from day 30 to day 100 and until the CD4+ count is >100 mcL. (3) Alemtuzumab recipients: from the time of initiation until at least 2 months after completion of therapy and until the CD4 count is >100 mcL, whichever occurs later.

TABLE 156.4

(CONTINUED)

Intervention	Indication	Agent	Comments
			The level of CMV reactivation that triggers preemptive therapy varies with the method. The CDC recommends any positive CMV antigenemia (pp65) or two consecutive qualitative PCR results within the first 100 days, and five cells per slide after the first 100 days. Some institutions initiate preemptive CMV therapy with any positive antigenemia result as late CMV disease is well established (see text). Institutions with quantitative PCR systems must establish their own standards, as the results are quite variable depending on the methodology.
Prophylaxis against CMV		Ganciclovir or foscarnet at the same dose as in preemptive regimen	Treatment is given for the first 100 days, then weekly or biweekly monitoring and preemptive management is initiated. Prophylaxis with ganciclovir is seldom used. The authors recommend preemptive therapy as described.
Prophylaxis against hepatitis B flare	Patients who are HBsAg+ or have detectable HBV DNA in the blood at high risk who are about to receive chemotherapy and are at high risk for hepatitis B reactivation	Lamivudine 100 mg/d	Start 7 days before chemotherapy and continue for 8 weeks after completing chemotherapy Not all cancer treatments are associated with the same risk; lymphoma therapy seems to be the highest risk.
	Patients who are HBsAg+ or have detectable HBV DNA in the blood who are about to receive hematopoietic stem cell transplant	Lamivudine 100 mg/d starting 2–3 weeks pretransplant and restart 2 weeks posttransplant	If the transplant may be delayed, start lamivudine and vaccinate the donor so anti-HBV immunity will be transplanted. It is not known how long to continue lamivudine.

ANC, absolute neutrophil count; TMP/SMX, trimethoprim/sulfamethoxazole; bid, twice daily; GVHD, graft-versus-host disease; DS, double strength; AML, acute myelogenous leukemia; MDS, myelodysplastic syndrome; tid, three times a day; HSCT, hematopoietic stem cell transplant; HSV, herpes simplex virus; VZV, varicella-zoster virus; SCT, stem cell transplant; CMV, cytomegalovirus; IV, intravenous; CDC, Centers for Disease Control and Prevention; PCR, polymerase chain reaction; HBsAg, hepatitis B surface antigen; HBV, hepatitis B virus; .

[a]Fluconazole is effective as prophylaxis against candidal, but not mold, infections. If prophylactic fluconazole is used in patients with prolonged neutropenia, the authors suggest a strategy of empirical modification to a mold-active drug in patients with persistent neutropenic fever (see text). The benefit vs. risk of surveillance laboratory markers for invasive fungal infection (e.g., serum galactomannan or β-glucan) coupled with preemptive antifungal therapy remains to be established (see text).

[b]In the pivotal randomized prophylactic trial by Ullmann et al.[49], eligibility criteria required either acute grade II to IV GVHD, or chronic extensive GVHD, or treatment with intensive immunosuppressive therapy consisting of either high-dose corticosteroids (1 mg/kg of body weight per day for patients with acute GVHD or 0.8 mg/kg every other day for patients with chronic GVHD), antithymocyte globulin, or a combination of two or more immunosuppressive agents or types of treatment.

[c]Doses apply to adults with normal renal function.

immunosuppressive regimens (e.g., systemic corticosteroids), we recommend avoiding antibiotic prophylaxis.[37]

Prophylaxis against Pneumococcal Infection

Pneumococcal prophylaxis should be considered in asplenic patients and in allogeneic HSCT recipients with chronic GVHD. Although most cases of pneumococcal sepsis occur within the first 2 years after splenectomy, a third may occur up to 5 years after, and cases of fulminant sepsis have been reported more than 20 years after splenectomy. The Working Party of the British Committee for Standards in Haematology recommend lifelong prophylactic antibiotics in patients who have had a splenectomy, and particularly in the first 2 years after splenectomy, in children up to age 16, and in patients with other immune impairment.[38]

Among allogeneic HSCT recipients, pneumococcal disease typically occurs in the later transplant period, from 3 months to years after transplant. Chronic GVHD is the major risk factor. Vaccination is recommended as in asplenic patients. Penicillin prophylaxis is also recommended.[39] Some experts recommend starting penicillin prophylaxis in all HSCT recipients 3 months after transplant, whereas others reserve it for patients with active chronic GVHD. In patients allergic to penicillin, prophylaxis with TMP/SMX or azithromycin should be considered. In areas with a significant frequency of penicillin-resistant pneumococcal isolates, alternative agents may be considered based on local susceptibility patterns, although the risk/benefit ratio is not well defined.

Prevention of Fungal Infections

Candida species and molds are the major fungal pathogens in patients with cancer. *Candida* species are endogenous flora; the major risk factors for candidemia in patients with cancer are chemotherapy-related mucositis (e.g., induction regimens for acute leukemia) and central venous catheters. Patients who have undergone gastrointestinal surgeries complicated by anastomotic leaks or prolonged care in the intensive care unit are also at risk for candidemia. In contrast, the risk of invasive mold infections is principally related to the duration of neutropenia, and, in allogeneic HSCT recipients, the intensity of immunosuppressive therapy used to treat GVHD.

The Transplant Associated Infections Surveillance Network (TRANSNET), composed of 23 U.S. transplant centers, prospectively analyzed HSCT recipients with proven and probable invasive fungal diseases.[40] Aspergillosis (43%), candidiasis (28%), and zygomycosis (8%) were the most common invasive fungal diseases. In HSCT patients with invasive aspergillosis, 239 of 415 patients (57.5%) died; independent poor prognostic factors in HSCT patients were neutropenia, renal insufficiency, hepatic insufficiency, early-onset invasive aspergillosis (IA), proven IA, and methylprednisolone use.[41]

Antifungal prophylaxis should be risk-based, targeting specific pathogens in different patient groups. Most patients with cancer do not require antifungal prophylaxis. Candidiasis during prolonged neutropenia is reduced by the use of fluconazole 400 mg/day.[42,43] Fluconazole prophylaxis may result in colonization by azole-resistant *Candida* strains.[44] Itraconazole results in similar efficacy and may reduce the risk of aspergillosis, but has higher toxicity (including drug-drug interactions) and gastrointestinal intolerance.[45,46] Micafungin, an echinocandin with activity against *Candida* and *Aspergillus*, was as effective as fluconazole to prevent candidiasis and showed a favorable trend to prevent aspergillosis in a randomized, double-blinded study in HSCT recipients.[47] Prevention of aspergillosis has been shown more convincingly with the newer azole, posaconazole. A randomized trial comparing standard prophylaxis (fluconazole or itraconazole) with posaconazole in patients receiving induction or reinduction therapy for acute myelogenous leukemia or myelodysplastic syndrome showed that posaconazole resulted in less fungal infections, including aspergillosis, and improved survival.[48] A similar study in HSCT recipients with severe GVHD showed that prophylactic posaconazole led to fewer cases of invasive aspergillosis than fluconazole, but no difference in overall survival.[49] A randomized trial comparing voriconazole and fluconazole prophylaxis coupled with serial serum galactomannan monitoring in allogeneic HSCT recipients showed a trend toward reduction of aspergillosis cases in voriconazole recipients, but no difference in overall or fungal infection–free survival.[50]

In summary, fluconazole is a safe and well-studied agent to prevent invasive candidiasis, but it has no activity against molds. When the risk of aspergillosis is significant, a mold-active drug should be considered, but different institutions may choose different agents.[51] Posaconazole is currently available only in an oral formulation (administration with food or enteral preparations is required to enhance bioavailability). The mold-active azoles (i.e., itraconazole, voriconazole, posaconazole) are potent inhibitors of certain cytochrome P-450 isoenzymes to a greater degree than fluconazole. This may lead to reduced clearance of other drugs, such as calcineurin inhibitors and vinca alkaloids. Careful monitoring of drug-drug interactions and appropriate dose modifications are required.

Prevention of *Pneumocystis Jirovecii*

Defective T-cell immunity is the principal risk factor for PCP. Recommendations for prophylaxis in the non-AIDS setting are based on the expected level of risk of PCP and consensus criteria rather than on randomized clinical trial data. The traditional groups of cancer patients at risk have been patients with acute lymphocytic leukemia and allogeneic HSCT recipients. In allogeneic HSCT recipients, we administer prophylaxis from day 30 to at least day 180 after transplant, and continue prophylaxis for 2 months after stopping all immunosuppression. PCP prophylaxis should be considered in patients with cancer who are receiving prolonged high-dose steroids (i.e., equivalent of prednisone 20 mg daily for ≥1 month), such as those with brain tumors.[52] Other candidates for prophylaxis include alemtuzumab recipients (package insert recommends prophylaxis until at least 2 months after completion of alemtuzumab and CD4 count ≥200/mcL, whichever occurs later), patients with CLL receiving fludarabine, and patients with gliomas receiving temozolomide and radiation or corticosteroids.

The most effective agent is TMP/SMX. A variety of dosages seem to be effective (from one double-strength tablet daily, to one double-strength tablet twice daily 2 days per week). When TMP/SMX cannot be administered because of marrow intolerance or hypersensitivity reaction, second-line agents include dapsone (50 mg twice daily or 100 mg orally daily), inhaled pentamidine (300 mg every 4 weeks), and atovaquone (1,500 mg daily) (Table 156.4). All the second-line agents are less effective than TMP/SMX, with the difference increasing with the degree of immune compromise. A retrospective study suggests dapsone may be more effective than inhaled pentamidine.[53]

Prophylaxis of Viral Infections

Prevention of Herpes Simplex Virus and Varicella Zoster Virus

Among seropositive patients, the incidence of herpes simplex virus (HSV) reactivation is approximately 70% to 80% following induction chemotherapy for leukemia or conditioning for HSCT. HSV and herpes zoster infections are common in alemtuzumab recipients. Antiviral prophylaxis (acyclovir, valacyclovir, or famciclovir) against HSV is advised in patients receiving chemotherapy for acute leukemia, in all HSV-seropositive allogeneic HSCT recipients, and in some autologous HSCT recipients at high risk for mucositis during the neutropenic period.[32,54] Prophylaxis is recommended until mucositis resolves and engraftment takes place. For alemtuzumab, the package insert recommends at least 2 months after completion of therapy and CD4 count 200/mcL or more, whichever occurs later. Prophylaxis may be considered for other patients (e.g., those with a history of consistent HSV reactivation following chemotherapy and patients with hematologic malignancies with prolonged neutropenia or receiving high-dose corticosteroids or T-cell–depleting agents like fludarabine), but it is unknown whether universal prophylaxis is a better strategy than episode-guided treatment.

A placebo-controlled trial showed that varicella zoster virus (VZV) reactivation after allogeneic transplantation was prevented by acyclovir 800 mg twice daily for 1 year,[55] but the effect was lost after stopping the drug. Additional patients at risk for HSV and/or VZV infections in whom prophylaxis should be considered include those receiving T-cell–depleting agents (e.g., fludarabine), calcineurin inhibitors, and the proteasomal inhibitor, bortezomib.

Prevention of Cytomegalovirus (CMV) Disease

CMV disease used to be the most important cause of infectious morbidity and mortality following allogeneic bone marrow transplantation, but with current practices it is much less common. Outside of transplantation, CMV disease has been reported mainly in patients receiving alemtuzumab, although asymptomatic reactivation without disease seems to be much more frequent. Nontransplanted patients receiving therapy for acute leukemia also occasionally develop CMV disease.

CMV infection happens early in life and results in viral latency. Most adults (60%–80%) are infected, as proven by the detection of CMV-specific immunoglobulin G in their serum. A transplant recipient is at risk for reactivation (if he or she is CMV seropositive) or for primary infection (from the allograft if the donor is CMV seropositive) or from blood products.).

Prevention of CMV Disease after Allogeneic Hematopoietic Stem Cell Transplantation.

Prevention of Primary CMV Infection. To prevent CMV primary infection, CMV-seronegative HSCT recipients receiving allografts from CMV-seronegative donors should receive transfusion products from only CMV-negative donors or leukocyte-depleted products. Filtered red blood cell transfusions from CMV-seropositive donors are associated with a small but significant increase in CMV transmission compared with restricting the transfusion product donor pool to CMV-seronegative persons.[56]

Prevention of CMV Disease Following Reactivation. In case of pre-existing CMV infection, CMV disease may be prevented by one of two approaches: prophylaxis or preemptive management. In prophylaxis, antiviral agents are administered for a variable period to all allogeneic HSCT recipients in which either the donor or recipient is CMV seropositive. In preemptive management, active surveillance of the patients at risk is followed by initiation of antiviral agents following detection of CMV reactivation.

Prophylaxis for CMV. When compared with placebo, ganciclovir prophylaxis for CMV-seropositive allogeneic transplant recipients was highly effective at suppressing CMV during the early transplant period, but was associated with higher rates of neutropenia, bacterial and opportunistic infections, and late CMV disease, without improvement in overall survival.[57,58] Reconstitution of CMV-specific T-cell responses was delayed in allogeneic HSCT recipients who received ganciclovir prophylaxis, conceivably predisposing such patients to late CMV disease.

Preemptive Therapy for Cmv. Highly sensitive methods for early CMV diagnosis include detection of the CMV pp65 antigen from peripheral blood leukocytes and CMV DNA by polymerase chain reaction (PCR). A single positive CMV antigenemia or two consecutive positive PCR results are triggers for preemptive antiviral therapy. When compared in a randomized controlled trial, preemptive therapy and prophylaxis resulted in equivalent overall survival, but with different complications: universal prophylaxis had less early CMV disease but more invasive fungal infections, more ganciclovir use, and more late CMV disease. Preemptive therapy (using pp65 antigenemia) resulted in more CMV disease by day 100.[59] Both strategies were considered appropriate and equivalent in the latest CDC/IDSA/American Society for Blood and Marrow Transplantation guidelines,[60] although the preemptive approach is more commonly used. Besides ganciclovir, foscarnet can also be used preemptively, with similar results but different toxicities (renal toxicity with foscarnet, myelosuppression with ganciclovir). Early studies suggest oral valganciclovir (a prodrug of ganciclovir with good oral bioavailability even in the presence of mild gut GVHD) is also safe and effective for this purpose, although it may result in increased exposure to ganciclovir and potentially more toxicity.[61,62]

Monitoring and Preventing Cmv Disease in Patients Treated with Alemtuzumab. CMV reactivation is common among alemtuzumab recipients and occurs most frequently between 3 and 6 weeks after initiation of therapy when T-cell counts reach a nadir. National Comprehensive Cancer Network (NCCN) guidelines advise that surveillance for CMV reactivation using PCR or antigen-based methods and preemptive therapy be performed in alemtuzumab recipients from the time of initiation until at least 2 months after completion of therapy and until the CD4 count is 100/mcL or more, whichever occurs later,[63] although this recommendation is not universally accepted.[64]

Prevention of Viral Hepatitis

Carriers of hepatitis B virus may develop severe hepatitis flare when they receive cytotoxic chemotherapy. The immunosuppressive effect of the chemotherapy allows virus reactivation in the liver, and the subsequent immune reconstitution may result in hepatocellular damage.[65] Patients with lymphoma seem to be at higher risk, but the phenomenon has been observed in solid tumors, particularly breast cancer.[66] A variety of risk factors have been identified: hepatitis B DNA at the time of initiation of chemotherapy, presence of hepatitis B surface antigen (HBsAg), hepatitis B "e" antigen (HBeAg), and, in some series, young age and male gender. Reactivation may also happen in patients with apparently resolved hepatitis B (HBsAg-negative, antisurface antibody-positive, and anticore-positive). There is no agreement in which is the best approach to this problem. Lamivudine 100 mg daily started 7 days before chemotherapy and continued for 8 weeks after completion of chemotherapy is safe and effective to prevent hepatitis B flares in this setting.[67] We recommend that all patients with hematologic malignancies and at least those breast cancer patients with known risk factors be screened for hepatitis B exposure before initiating chemotherapy, and those with HBsAg or detectable hepatitis B virus DNA should be considered for lamivudine prophylaxis.[68] In HSCT, some authorities recommend all recipients with markers of hepatitis B and all recipients of donors with any evidence of hepatitis B receive lamivudine. Unfortunately, there are not enough data to formulate guidelines to decide for how long to treat. Severe flares have been associated with discontinuation of antiviral treatment.[69]

During HSCT, HCV is universally transmitted from HCV RNA-positive donors to their recipients.[70] If an HCV-positive donor is the best available match, treatment of the donor with anti-HCV therapy before stem cell harvest may be considered to try to eliminate detectable viral replication and reduce the likelihood of HCV transmission. Interferon-alpha should be stopped at least 1 week before harvest to avoid problems with engraftment.[70] Significant acute hepatic dysfunction related to HCV reactivation is uncommon in nontransplant HCV-positive patients receiving chemotherapy for hematologic malignancies.

DIAGNOSIS AND MANAGEMENT OF INFECTIOUS DISEASES SYNDROMES

FEVER AND NEUTROPENIA

General Concepts

Fever: a single oral temperature of greater than 38.3°C (101°F) or 38.0°C (100.4°F) or greater for more than 1 hour. Neutropenia: absolute neutrophil count less than 500 mcL or less than 1,000 mcL with predicted rapid decline.[71]

Fever during neutropenia may be secondary to infection or to noninfectious causes. An infection is found in approximately half the episodes. The infection is documented microbiologically (e.g., positive blood cultures) in 30% of cases and clinically (e.g., pneumonia or cellulitis without an isolated pathogen) in 20%. Infections may develop and progress rapidly during neutropenia, so broad-spectrum antibiotics must be administered promptly even if other potential causes of fever (e.g., the malignancy itself, drugs, blood products, deep venous thrombosis) are present.

Initial Evaluation

The initial evaluation consists of a complete history and physical examination with special attention to the mouth, skin, catheter exit site, and perianal region. The oral cavity may show mucositis, gingivostomatitis caused by reactivation of HSV, and/or thrush. A black necrotic eschar in the palate of patients with prolonged neutropenia or high-dose corticosteroids may be a sign of mold infection. A detailed inspection of the skin, including the nails, may disclose a lesion suggestive of a possible portal of entry or of systemic infection. Catheter sites and sites of prior skin penetration (such as surgical wounds and biopsy sites) should be palpated. The perineum and perianal region need careful inspection and palpation.

Initial laboratory studies should include complete blood count and differential, serum chemistry including liver function tests, at least two sets of blood cultures, and a urine culture. An initial chest radiograph in the absence of symptoms or signs of pulmonary infection is of low yield in ambulatory adult patients with fever and neutropenia. We still advise obtaining a chest radiograph as part of the initial evaluation in patients requiring hospitalization and in patients at higher risk for infections (e.g., those with hematologic malignancies, anticipated prolonged neutropenia, and use of systemic corticosteroids).

Potential sites of infection, such as cutaneous lesions or sputum, should be sampled prior to instituting antibiotics. However, fever in neutropenic patients is a medical emergency, and prompt initiation of empirical antibiotics should not be delayed if cultures cannot be readily obtained.

Antibiotic Regimens

IDSA and the NCCN have published evidence-based guidelines on antibiotic therapy for neutropenic patients with fever.[54,71] In the absence of localizing symptoms, physical examination findings, or positive cultures several antibiotic regimens may be used.

Monotherapy with an Antipseudomonal Beta-Lactam

The cornerstone of the management of fever in neutropenic hosts is the prompt empirical administration of a broad-spectrum beta-lactam antibiotic with activity against *Pseudomonas aeruginosa* (see Table 156.5 for a summary of antibacterial agents). Standard intravenous monotherapy for stable patients with neutropenic fever of unknown etiology are ceftazidime, cefepime, imipenem, meropenem, and piperacillin/tazobactam. The choice of specific therapy should be guided by local antibiotic susceptibility patterns.

"Double Coverage" Against Gram-Negative Bacilli

Combination with an aminoglycoside has been shown in several meta-analyses to result in increased toxicity and similar overall survival[72,73]; therefore, the addition of an aminoglycoside, which used to be standard of care, should be limited to patients with hemodynamic instability (in whom it is imperative to administer agents effective against the causative pathogen) and when there is a high suspicion for antibiotic-resistant Gram-negative bacterial infections based on local susceptibility patterns or the individual patient's prior history. Ciprofloxacin may be an acceptable alternative to an aminoglycoside as part of a combination regimen.

Gram-Positive Coverage: Role of Vancomycin and Other Agents

Initial empirical addition of vancomycin has not been associated with improved outcome, results in increased toxicity, and cost and should be avoided in most patients.[63,71] Likewise, the addition of vancomycin solely for persistent fever after 48 to 72 hours of antibiotics is not associated with improved outcome.[74]

We suggest reserving vancomycin for specific settings during neutropenia, which include (1) clinically apparent catheter-related infection, (2) blood culture positive for a Gram-positive bacterium prior to identification and susceptibility testing (linezolid or daptomycin could be a better choice in an environment with high prevalence of vancomycin-resistant enterococcus [VRE], (3) known colonization with methicillin-resistant *Staphylococcus aureus* (MRSA) or penicillin-resistant *S. pneumoniae,* and (4) hypotension or septic shock without an identified pathogen (Fig. 156.1). Some experts add vancomycin in patients with neutropenic fever who are at high risk for viridans group streptococci (e.g., prior quinolone prophylaxis, severe mucositis), while others would choose to use a carbapenem or piperacillin/tazobactam, which have activity against oral flora. Empirical vancomycin should be discontinued after 2 to 3 days if the initial cultures are negative or show a pathogen for which other antibiotics can be used. In neutropenic-febrile patients with allergies to beta-lactams, vancomycin plus aztreonam is an acceptable regimen[75] (Table 156.6).

TABLE 156.5

ANTIBACTERIAL AGENTS COMMONLY USED TO TREAT PATIENTS WITH CANCER

Antibiotic	Spectrum	Usual Daily Dose[a]	Comments
Ceftazidime	Enterobacteriaceae *Pseudomonas aeruginosa* Less reliable activity than ceftriaxone, cefepime or carbapenems against Gram-positive bacteria (e.g., viridans group streptococci) Poor activity against anaerobes	2 g q8h	Used as monotherapy in F&N; inactivated by ESBLs and cephalosporinases
Cefepime	Enterobacteriaceae *P. aeruginosa* Most Gram-positive bacteria Poor activity against anaerobes	2 g q8h to q12h	Used as monotherapy in F&N, increased mortality for this indication in a meta-analysis not fully explained
			Active against most ESBL- and cephalosporinase-producing Gram-negative bacteria; active against most streptococci, except *Enterococcus* sp.
Piperacillin-tazobactam	Enterobacteriaceae *P. aeruginosa* Most Gram-positive bacteria (excluding MRSA) Anaerobes	4.5 g q6h	Used as monotherapy in F&N
Carbapenems	Enterobacteriaceae *P. aeruginosa* Most Gram-positive bacteria (excluding MRSA)	Imipenem: 500 mg q6h Meropenem: 1–2 g q8h Ertapenem: 1 g per day	Imipenem and meropenem may be used as monotherapy in F&N; broad spectrum of activity, including ESBL-producers; inactive against *Stenotrophomonas maltophilia* and KPC-producing strains (see text). Doripenem has a similar spectrum of activity, but experience is lacking in patients with cancer. Ertapenem is not active against *P. aeruginosa*
	Anaerobes		
Aztreonam	Enterobacteriaceae *P. aeruginosa*	2 g q8h	Limited spectrum requires pairing with an agent with Gram-positive activity for neutropenic fever and neutropenia; useful for persons with β-lactam allergies
Tigecycline	Gram-positive bacteria (including VRE)	100 mg loading dose, then 50 mg q12h	Approved for soft tissue and intra-abdominal infections; published experience in cancer patients is limited, but it may be a second-line agent for *Stenotrophomonas maltophilia* and VRE infections. Nausea and vomiting may be limiting side effects
	Gram-negative bacteria (excluding *P. aeruginosa*) Anaerobes		
Colistin	Gram-negative bacteria	Given IV as colistimethate sodium equivalent to colistin base 2.5 to 5 mg/kg daily in two to four divided doses; dose must be adjusted in renal failure, measuring levels may be helpful (peak plasma-colistin concentrations of 10 to 15 mcg/mL)	Used almost exclusively for multiresistant Gram-negative infections (*P. aeruginosa*, *Acinetobacter*) refractory to other treatments. Also used aerosolized in cases of multiresistant Gram-negative pneumonia.

(*continued*)

TABLE 156.5

(CONTINUED)

Antibiotic	Spectrum	Usual Daily Dose[a]	Comments
Vancomycin	Exclusively Gram-positive bacteria	1 g q12h	Growing frequency of resistance among *Enterococcus* sp.; rare cases of *Staphylococcus aureus* intermediately sensitive or resistant to vancomycin; *Leuconostoc*, *Pediococcus*, and *Lactobacillus* sp. are intrinsically resistant. Aim for high trough levels (15–20 mcg/mL) for MRSA pneumonia.
Fluoroquinolones	Enterobacteriaceae *P. aeruginosa* Newer-generation agents have increased activity against Gram-positive bacteria	—	Effective prophylaxis against aerobic Gram-negative rods during neutropenia; resistance is an important concern (see text).
Trimethoprim-sulfamethoxazole	Enterobacteriaceae (growing resistance) No activity against *P. aeruginosa* Active against *S. maltophilia*, *Burkholderia cepacia*, *Listeria monocytogenes*, *P. jirovecii*, *Nocardia* sp.	For serious infections (e.g., PJP or bacteremia) is trimethoprim 5 mg/kg IV q8h or oral two DS (160-mg) tablets 3 times daily. For prophylaxis against PJP, one single-strength (80 mg) or one DS tablet daily or one DS tablet 3 d/wk.	Effective prophylaxis against *P. jirovecii*; potential hypersensitivity and bone marrow toxicity
Aminoglycosides	Enterobacteriaceae *P. aeruginosa* Synergistic activity against sensitive Gram-positive organisms (e.g., *Enterococcus* sp.) when paired with a penicillin.	—	Should be paired with an antipseudomonal β-lactam agent if used for neutropenic fever or Gram-negative bacteremia. Once-daily dosing less nephrotoxic.
Metronidazole	Exclusively anaerobic activity	500 mg q6–8h	First-choice agent against *Clostridium difficile* (oral).
Linezolid	Exclusively Gram-positive activity, including MRSA and VRE	600 mg q12h	Seems at least as effective as vancomycin against MRSA. Excellent oral bioavailability; reversible marrow suppression and peripheral and optic neuropathy with long-term use; should be used with caution with adrenergic or serotonergic agents because of risk of serotonergic syndrome.
Quinupristin-dalfopristin	Similar spectrum as linezolid, but inactive against *Enterococcus faecalis*	7.5 mg/kg q8h	Toxicities include myalgias and reversible liver enzyme abnormalities (see text).
Daptomycin	Cyclic lipopeptide active against Gram-positive bacteria	6 mg/kg daily for bacteremia; 4 mg/kg daily for skin and soft tissue infections.	Effective for soft tissue infections by susceptible Gram-positive bacteria and for *S. aureus* bloodstream infections and endocarditis. As effective as vancomycin in MRSA bacteremia and endocarditis.

F&N, fever and neutropenia; ESBL, extended-spectrum β-lactamases; DS, double strength; MRSA, methicillin-resistant *Staphylococcus aureus*; KPC, *Klebsiella pneumoniae* carbapenemase; VRE, vancomycin-resistant enterococci; IV, intravenous; PJP, *Pneumocystis jirovecii* pneumonia.
[a]Doses apply to adults with normal renal function.

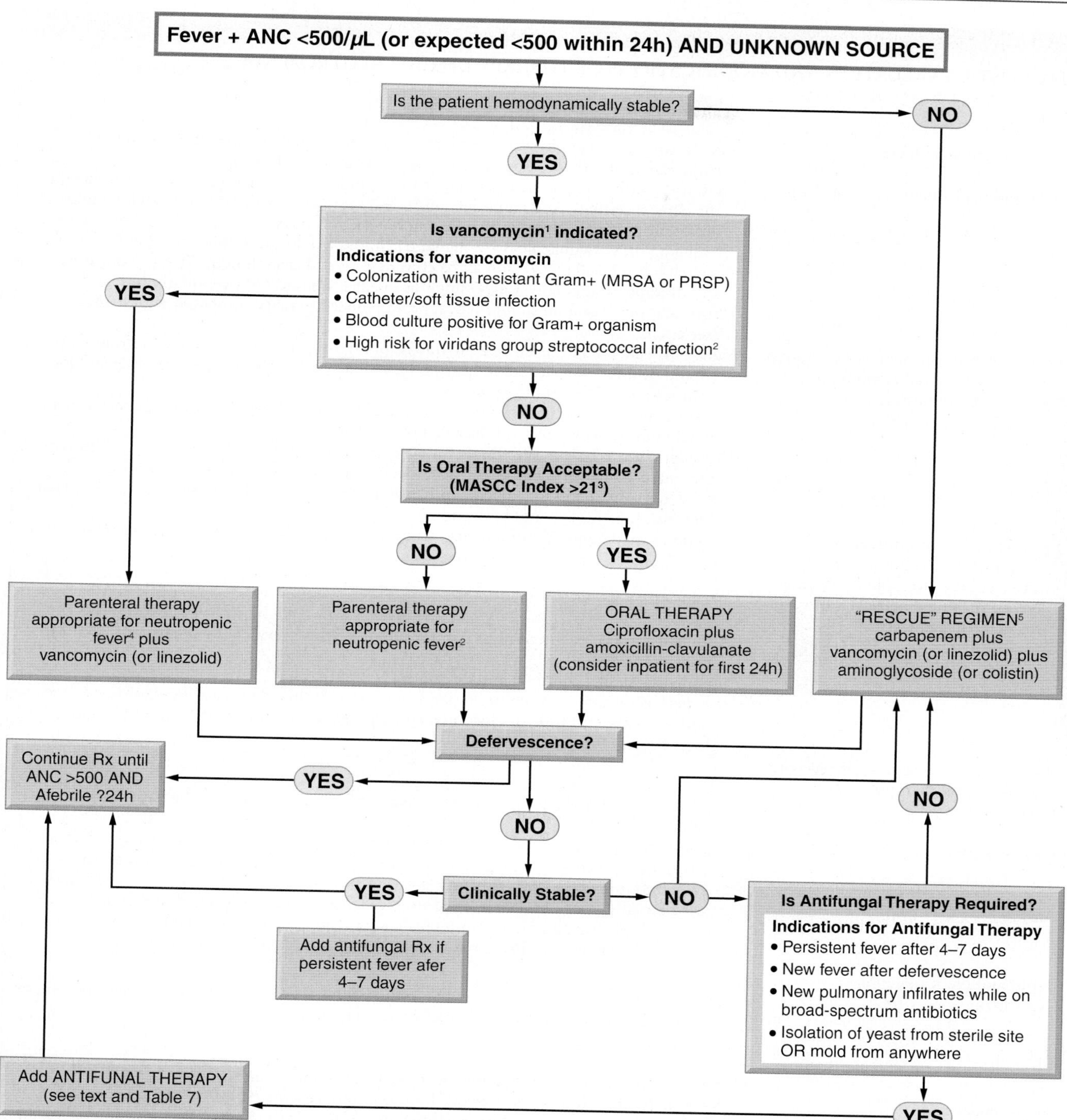

FIGURE 156.1 A general approach to patients with fever and neutropenia without a clinically or microbiologically documented infection. See text and Table 156.5 for more detailed descriptions. [1]Linezolid was comparable to vancomycin in this setting in a single randomized controlled trial. It may be considered instead of vancomycin for patients who are known carriers of vancomycin-resistant enterococcus (VRE), but experience is limited, and there are concerns about linezolid use (see text). [2]Some experts add vancomycin in patients with neutropenic fever at high risk for viridans streptococci (e.g., prior quinolone prophylaxis, severe mucositis associated with cytarabine-containing regimens); this must be weighed against the significant downside of selection for vancomycin-resistant pathogens. [3]Multinational Association for Supportive Care in Cancer (MASCC) index: burden of illness: no or mild symptoms, +5; moderate symptoms, +3; no hypotension, +5; no chronic obstructive pulmonary disease, +4; solid tumor or no previous fungal infection, +4; no dehydration, +3; outpatient status, +3; age less than 60 years, +2. A MASCC index of 21 or more has been associated with a relatively low frequency of severe complications. See text for a detailed discussion. [4]In a stable patient with undifferentiated neutropenic fever who does not require vancomycin, appropriate parenteral monotherapy consists of ceftazidime, cefepime, imipenem, meropenem, or piperacillin/tazobactam. For specific information on each of these agents, see text and Table 156.5. [5]This "rescue" antibacterial regimen will vary between institutions depending on the local patterns of antibiotic resistance. Carbapenem (imipenem or meropenem) plus vancomycin plus an aminoglycoside is a reasonable initial regimen that should be tailored once culture results are known. A fluoroquinolone may be used instead of an aminoglycoside in patients with significant renal impairment in institutions where fluoroquinolones retain significant activity against the local Gram-negative pathogens. In settings in which carbapenem-resistant *Acinetobacter* or carbapenemase-producing *Klebsiella* are prevalent, colistin or polymyxin B should be considered. ANC, absolute neutrophil count; MRSA, methicillin-resistant *Staphylococcus aureus*; PRSP, penicillin-resistant *Streptococcus pneumoniae*.

TABLE 156.6

DIAGNOSTIC EVALUATION AND MODIFICATIONS OF THERAPY DURING NEUTROPENIA

Findings	Evaluation and Modifications
Initial neutropenic fever	Take history, perform physical examination, and order appropriate cultures; initiate empirical antibiotic therapy promptly (see text and Fig. 156.1).
Persistent neutropenic fever (4–7 d)	Look for invasive fungal infection (chest CT recommended, serologic tests depending on the clinical setting). Add empirical antifungal therapy in patients not receiving mold-active prophylaxis. Options include amphotericin B deoxycholate (0.7 mg/kg/d), LAMB (3 mg/kg/d); voriconazole (IV 6 mg/kg q12h for two doses, followed by 3 mg/kg q12h; switch to oral 200 mg q12h may be considered); and caspofungin 70 mg × one dose, followed by 50 mg daily. Caspofungin is in general preferred over amphotericin B formulations based on similar efficacy and reduced toxicity compared with LAMB (see text).
Recurrent neutropenic fever without a source after initial response to empirical antibiotics	Signs of breakthrough sepsis (e.g., hypotension, rigors, tachypnea, decline in urine output) should prompt empirical modification of antibacterial regimen (see text). Repeat blood cultures and a chest radiograph. Consider modification of the antimicrobial regimen to include breakthrough bacterial and fungal infections while awaiting diagnostic results. Consider chest CT scan to evaluate for signs of mold infection. If a nodule or infiltrate is present, consider bronchoscopy or percutaneous biopsy depending on location. Galactomannan and ß-D-glucan antigenemia assays should be considered in patients at high risk for invasive mold infections
Persistent or recurrent fever without a source after ANC recovery	Infections are diagnosed infrequently. Consider chronic disseminated candidiasis (see text).
Positive culture from blood obtained before starting empirical antibiotics for neutropenic fever	
Gram-positive	Add vancomycin (or linezolid or daptomycin if VRE is prevalent or the patient is known to be colonized)
Gram-negative	If patient is stable, continue initial regimen. If patient is unstable, switch to imipenem or meropenem or piperacillin-tazobactam and add an aminoglycoside or ciprofloxacin. The selection of antibiotics should be guided by local susceptibility patterns.
Positive blood culture while receiving antibacterial therapy	
Gram-positive	Add vancomycin (or linezolid or daptomycin if VRE is prevalent or the patient is known to be colonized)
Gram-negative	Suspect a pathogen resistant to initial empirical regimen. If ceftazidime was used initially, suspect extended-spectrum β-lactamase or cephalosporinase-producing organisms; switch to imipenem or meropenem and add an aminoglycoside. If a carbapenem was used initially, consider *Stenotrophomonas maltophilia* or resistant *Pseudomonas* sp.; switch to piperacillin-tazobactam plus an aminoglycoside plus trimethoprim-sulfamethoxazole. Modify regimen once identification and sensitivity are known.
Head and Neck Infection	
Necrotizing gingivitis	If ceftazidime or cefepime was used in initial regimen, change to imipenem, meropenem, or piperacillin-tazobactam, or add metronidazole for anaerobic coverage. Culture for HSV.
Oral ulcerative or vesicular lesions	Culture for HSV. For documented or suspected mucocutaneous HSV infection, acyclovir 5 mg/kg q8h.
Sinus tenderness	Suspect aerobic Gram-negative rod (Enterobacteriaceae or *Pseudomonas aeruginosa*). Examine palate and nasal mucosa for signs of invasive infection. Perform sinus CT scan to evaluate extent of disease and to guide diagnostic and therapeutic drainage. With prolonged neutropenia or concomitant high-dose corticosteroids, invasive mold infections become more likely and initiation of empirical lipid formulation of amphotericin B (5 mg/kg/d) may be considered to cover both aspergillosis and zygomycosis.
Respiratory Tract	
Upper respiratory tract symptoms	Send nasopharyngeal washing for community respiratory viruses
New infiltrate after resolution of neutropenia	May be inflammatory response to old infection. Conservative management results in good outcome: If the patient is asymptomatic, observe; if symptomatic and not responding to antibacterial agents, consider BAL.[a]

TABLE 156.6

(CONTINUED)

Findings	Evaluation and Modifications
New infiltrate while neutropenic	Suspect resistant bacteria or mold infection. Perform chest CT scan to evaluate extent of disease and to detect other lesions. Perform sputum cultures and GM and BG antigenemia assay; if GM and BG assays are unavailable or nondiagnostic, bronchoscopy with BAL or percutaneous biopsy is warranted based on location of lesion. If pneumonia developed in hospital, broaden antibiotic regimen to cover nosocomial pathogens. Consider MRSA resistant Gram-negative pathogens and nosocomial legionellosis. Consider empirical addition of voriconazole (IV 6 mg/kg q12h for two doses followed by 4 mg/kg q12h). Diffuse infiltrates raise concern for community respiratory viruses (particularly during winter), *Pneumocystis jirovecii* (in setting of concomitant corticosteroid therapy), bacterial pneumonia, CMV (in acute leukemia, may infrequently be associated with neutropenia), and noninfectious causes (e.g., hemorrhage, aspiration, drug toxicity, respiratory distress syndrome, congestive heart failure). BAL recommended.
Gastrointestinal Tract	
Retrosternal burning, odynophagia	Consider esophagitis. Suspect *Candida* or HSV esophagitis. Bacterial esophagitis and CMV (primarily in allogeneic HSCT recipients) also possible. Add fluconazole (400 mg oral or IV) and acyclovir (5 mg/kg q8h IV) empirically. If no response in 3 d, consider endoscopy.
Acute abdominal pain	Differential diagnosis includes same causes as in nonneutropenic patient (e.g., cholecystitis, appendicitis) plus typhlitis (neutropenic colitis). Ensure that antibiotic regimen has adequate anaerobic activity (e.g., imipenem, meropenem, or piperacillin-tazobactam). Provide bowel rest. Abdominal and pelvic CT scan. Monitor for need for surgical intervention (see text).
Perianal cellulitis	Consider pelvic CT scan to evaluate extent of disease. Monitor need for surgical drainage. Broaden antibiotic regimen to include anaerobic activity. Provide local care.
Central Venous Catheter (surgically implanted)	
Exit-site cellulitis	Add vancomycin.
Tunnel infection	Add vancomycin; remove catheter.
Collection around catheter	Incise and drain; if infected, add appropriate antibiotics and remove catheter.
Infection by molds and mycobacteria	May require excision of tunnel tract.
Catheter-associated bacteremia	Add appropriate antibiotics. Remove catheter for infection by *Staphylococcus aureus*, *Candida* sp., and mycobacteria (see text) and for antibiotic-resistant pathogens

CT, computed tomography; LAMB, liposomal amphotericin B; IV, intravenous; ANC, absolute neutrophil count; VRE, vancomycin-resistant enterococcus; HSV, herpes simplex virus; BAL, bronchoalveolar lavage; GM, serum galactomannan; BG, β-glucan; MRSA, methicillin-resistant *Staphylococcus aureus;* CMV, cytomegalovirus; HSCT, hematopoietic stem cell transplant.

[a]The differential diagnosis of pneumonia in immunocompromised patients is broad, and the authors advise early BAL or percutaneous biopsy (depending on location of the lesion). Studies must be tailored to the individual patient. In highly immunocompromised patients perform Gram staining; culture for bacteria, mycobacteria, fungi, *Nocardia* sp., *Legionella* sp., herpes viruses, CMV, and community respiratory viruses (particularly during winter); and cytologic analysis for *P. jirovecii*.

There are a number of agents with activity against MRSA and VRE, including linezolid, quinupristin/dalfopristin (active against *Enterococcus faecium*, but not *Enterococcus faecalis*), daptomycin, tigecycline, and telavancin. In a randomized trial of patients with persistent neutropenic fever, linezolid and vancomycin had similar safety and efficacy.[76] The major concern regarding linezolid in patients with cancer relates to myelosuppression with prolonged use. In general, these agents with extended-spectrum Gram-positive activity should be reserved for patients with documented or suspected Gram-positive infections rather than as empirical therapy for neutropenic fever of unknown origin.

Modification of the Antibiotic Regimen

The initial antibiotic regimen needs to be modified 30% to 50% of the time, depending on clinical evolution and/or microbiological results. Daily evaluation of the patient is essential to search for new findings (e.g., tachypnea, tachycardia, hypotension, new skin lesions, pain, or tenderness) that may suggest persistent or breakthrough infection (see Table 156.6 for a detailed list of modifications). The median time to defervescence of neutropenic patients without documented infection in classic studies was 4 days.[77] Persistent fever of unknown origin in a clinically stable patient does not routinely require modification of the antibacterial regimen (see section on "Persistent Fever in the Neutropenic Patient and Addition of Empirical Antifungal Therapy," below).

Duration of Treatment

If fever resolves following initiation of empirical therapy, one should assume that an infection existed that has responded to antibiotics. The standard recommendation is to continue antibiotics until resolution of neutropenia. If the neutropenia persists, older studies showed that 7 days of treatment may not be enough, but 2 weeks may be adequate.[78,79] Some authorities may continue the initial intravenous antibiotics; it also may be acceptable to switch to an oral regimen like ciprofloxacin with amoxicillin/clavulanate in clinically stable patients.[71]

Persistent Fever in the Neutropenic Patient and Addition of Empirical Antifungal Therapy

The longer the fever persists without new findings, the higher the risk of fungal infection. The majority of persistently febrile neutropenic patients do not harbor an identifiable fungal infection, but several autopsy series in the 1970s documented occult fungal infection as a common cause of death in persistently neutropenic patients.[80] Delay in initiating antifungal therapy was associated with treatment failure and death,[81] The empirical addition of antifungal therapy in neutropenic patients with persistent fever was a logical response to these facts. The availability of newer antifungal agents resulted in several landmark studies that attempted to define which drug is safest and most effective in this setting. The availability of safer antifungal agents and better diagnostic adjuncts has resulted in a reevaluation of the best approach to this problem.[82] A summary of antifungal agents is presented in Table 156.7.

Empirical Addition of Amphotericin B Deoxycholate. Two randomized prospective studies showed that empirical amphotericin B deoxycholate (AmB-D) was associated with a trend toward fewer invasive fungal infections in antibiotic-treated neutropenic patients with persistent fever.[83,84] Although neither study showed a statistically significant benefit of empirical antifungal therapy in terms of preventing invasive fungal infections or overall mortality, both were underpowered and most experts agreed that the benefit of this strategy outweighed the risk. This practice became the standard of care, with a window of "4 to 7 days" as the time to initiate antifungals[71] based on the different timing chosen by the two mentioned studies.

Comparative Studies of Empirical Antifungal Therapy in Neutropenic Fever. Several major randomized trials over the past 10 years compared a variety of interventions: liposomal amphotericin B with AmB-D,[85] itraconazole (cyclodextrin formulation) with AmB-D,[86] and voriconazole[87] and caspofungin[88] with liposomal amphotericin B. In all these studies, patients were receiving either fluconazole or no antifungal prophylaxis. We consider liposomal amphotericin B, itraconazole, voriconazole, and caspofungin acceptable options as empirical antifungal therapy to be added on day 5 of persistent neutropenic fever. Given that no agent has shown higher overall efficacy than the others, the choice may be based on the concurrent medications and possible interactions as well as spectrum of toxicities.

Newer Approaches. The time-honored approach of adding empirical antifungal therapy at day 5 of persistent fever and neutropenia has been increasingly criticized, as it ignores newer diagnostic modalities and results in administering antifungal agents to many patients who do not need them. For example, in the empirical antifungal trial comparing caspofungin and liposomal amphotericin B, a baseline invasive fungal infection was documented in only approximately 5% of patients (almost 90% were candidiasis or invasive aspergillosis).[88] It is not known what the best approach is for persistent fever in the increasing proportion of patients who are receiving antifungal prophylaxis with agents active against molds.[82] There is also significant interest in "preemptive" antifungal therapy, defined as modification of the antifungal regimen based on radiologic and/or laboratory markers, in contrast to the empirical approach, in which persistent neutropenic fever is the trigger to modify the antifungal regimen. Maertens et al.[89] used serial serum galactomannan and chest computed tomographic (CT) scanning to detect early aspergillosis in high-risk neutropenic patients receiving fluconazole prophylaxis. The antifungal regimen was modified based on prespecified triggers that included CT scan, galactomannan, and bronchoalveolar lavage results, rather than persistent fever. This strategy reduced the use of empirical antifungal therapy and successfully identified early cases of invasive aspergillosis. In a randomized trial of a similar approach in high-risk febrile neutropenic patients comparing preemptive versus empirical antifungal treatment, however, preemptive treatment was associated with increased incidence of invasive fungal disease (without increasing mortality) and decreased costs of antifungal drugs.[90]

Persistent Fever after Resolution of Neutropenia. In most cases, an undiagnosed fever that has persisted during neutropenia will resolve around the time of myeloid recovery. In a minority of patients, a "fever of unknown origin" persists for several days. Evaluation of fever after myeloid recovery requires a methodical consideration of both noninfectious causes, such as engraftment syndrome, drug fever, transfusion reactions, and deep venous thrombosis, as well as infectious causes. A careful physical examination may show a site of infection that was inapparent during neutropenia, such as a perirectal process or a catheter exit site infection. A chest radiograph should be obtained as pulmonary infection may not be apparent radiographically during neutropenia. Pulmonary infiltrates identified after neutrophil recovery have a favorable prognosis and may be managed conservatively.[91] Blood and urine cultures, complete blood cell count, serum chemistry, and liver enzyme levels should be obtained. An elevated alkaline phosphatase should prompt consideration of hepatosplenic candidiasis (which is uncommon in patients receiving yeast-active antifungal prophylaxis) even if blood cultures were negative for *Candida* species. A CT scan, magnetic resonance imaging (MRI), and ultrasound are complementary imaging modalities, and may show discrete "bull's eye" lesions (see "Candidiasis").

In contrast to the neutropenic period, empirical antibiotics can be discontinued after resolution of neutropenia in patients who are stable with fever without apparent source, and cultures have negative findings. If a source of infection is identified, then antibiotic therapy targeted to the specific pathogen(s) is advised.

Immune Augmentation

Colony-Stimulating Factors

Multiple randomized clinical trials of prophylactic recombinant granulocyte colony-stimulating factor (G-CSF) and granulocyte-macrophage (GM)-CSF have shown the benefit of CSFs in reducing the time to neutrophil recovery, and duration of fever and hospitalization in patients with acute myelogenous leukemia.[92] A meta-analysis of randomized trials of prophylactic G-CSF and GM-CSF in autologous and allogenic HSCT recipients showed that CSFs were associated with a small reduction in the risk of documented infections but did not affect infection- or treatment-related mortality.[93] The American Society of Clinical Oncology has established authoritative guidelines related to the use of prophylactic CSFs in standard practice.[94]

The rationale to use for CSFs for established infections (as opposed to prophylaxis) stems from the quantitative and qualitative effects of these agents on phagocytic cells. In neutropenic patients with life-threatening infections, survival is strongly influenced by the rapidity of neutrophil recovery. Thus, CSFs and granulocyte transfusions could potentially be used in these settings to augment the number of circulating neutrophils. Randomized trials have not shown a benefit of CSFs as adjunct therapy for patients with newly diagnosed fever and neutropenia. Although the benefit of any CSF for established infections is unproven, it may be considered in selected cases of profound neutropenia (absolute neutrophil

TABLE 156.7

ANTIFUNGAL AGENTS

Antifungal Agent	Comments
AZOLES (TRIAZOLES)	Inhibit fungal cell membrane synthesis. Inhibit cytochrome P-450 isoenzymes, which may lead to impaired clearance of other drugs metabolized by this pathway; drug–drug interactions are common and need to be closely monitored (consult package inserts for details). Reversible liver enzyme elevations are observed. Liver failure rare.
Fluconazole	Acceptable alternative for candidemia in nonneutropenic patients at 400–800 mg/d; broad range of MICs to *Candida glabrata*; *Candida krusei* is resistant. Inactive against molds. Commonly used prophylactically in high-risk patients (e.g., acute leukemia during neutropenia, hematopoietic transplantation); maintenance therapy for cryptococcal meningitis. Standard dose in adults with normal renal function: 400 mg daily orally or IV.
Itraconazole	Active against *Candida* and *Aspergillus* sp., dimorphic fungi, dark-walled molds. Itraconazole has negative inotropic properties and is contraindicated in patients with significant cardiac systolic dysfunction or a history of heart failure. IV formulation should be used with caution in patients with significant renal dysfunction (e.g., creatinine clearance <50 mL/min). Standard dose: IV 200 mg q12h × four doses, followed by 200 mg daily; oral 400 mg daily (aim for trough of at least 0.25 mcg/mL after 7 days of therapy). IV formulation no longer marketed in the United States.
Voriconazole	Standard of care for invasive aspergillosis; treatment of other molds resistant to amphotericin B. No activity against zygomycetes. Effective in candidemia in nonneutropenic patients. Acceptable alternative to amphotericin B formulations as empirical therapy for neutropenic fever. Standard dose: IV 6 mg/kg q12h for two doses, then 4 mg/kg q12h; oral 200 mg (or 4 mg/kg) twice a day in adults. Pediatric dose (age ≤11 years: 7 mg/kg q12h) Blood levels achieved with normal dosing vary between individuals; the authors check levels in cases of suspected failure or toxicity. Levels above 2 mcg/mL have been associated with successful outcomes.
Posaconazole	Similar spectrum of activity to voriconazole but active against zygomycetes. Effective in salvage therapy of *Aspergillus* sp. and other refractory molds (*Fusarium* sp., *S. apiospermum*, and zygomycetes); it has not been evaluated as first-line therapy for invasive fungal diseases. Effective as antifungal prophylaxis in high-risk neutropenia[49] and during acute graft-versus- host disease. So far, only available as an oral formulation. Standard dose: 200 mg orally 3 times a day as prophylaxis. Salvage therapy (not FDA-approved): 200 mg orally 4 times a day followed by 400 mg orally twice a day once disease has stabilized.
AMPHOTERICIN B FORMULATIONS	Broad spectrum of antifungal activity. Significant infusion-related and renal toxicity, less so with lipid formulations. Infusion-related toxicity may be managed with antipyretics, an antihistamine, and meperidine (for rigors). Saline loading may reduce nephrotoxicity.
Amphotericin B deoxycholate (AMB-D)	Standard dose: varies based on indication, generally 0.5–1.5 mg/kg/d.
Liposomal amphotericin B	At least as effective and less toxic than AMB-D as empirical therapy for persistent fever during neutropenia; less infusion-related toxicity and nephrotoxicity than amphotericin B lipid complex as empirical therapy. For invasive aspergillosis 3 mg/kg/d is as effective as, but less toxic than 10 mg/kg/d.
Amphotericin B lipid complex	Standard dose for invasive mold infections: 5 mg/kg/d.
Amphotericin B colloidal dispersion	Substantial infusion-related toxicity; other lipid formulations of amphotericin B are generally preferred. Standard dose for invasive mold infections: 5 mg/kg/d.
5-FLUCYTOSINE	Used only in combination with AMB-D for cryptococcal meningitis; pyrimidine analogue with dose- and duration-dependent myelotoxicity and gastrointestinal toxicity; monitoring of serum levels and adjustment of dosing for azotemia required.
ECHINOCANDINS	Class of antifungal peptides that inhibit synthesis of glucan, a fungal cell wall constituent; potently fungicidal against *Candida* sp., including fluconazole-resistant strains; fungistatic against *Aspergillus* sp. No activity against other molds. Excellent safety profile. All three echinocandins have demonstrated efficacy as therapy for candidemia and invasive candidiasis in nonneutropenic patients. Potential for combination therapy with voriconazole or amphotericin formulations as therapy for invasive aspergillosis (see text).

(continued)

PRACTICE OF ONCOLOGY

TABLE 156.7

(CONTINUED)

Antifungal Agent	Comments
Caspofungin	Similar efficacy compared to AMB-D as primary therapy for candidemia and invasive candidiasis but significantly less toxicity. It is used as salvage therapy for invasive aspergillosis (not evaluated as first-line therapy). Similar efficacy, but less toxicity compared with LAMB as empirical therapy for persistent neutropenic fever. Dose: 70 mg in one dose, then 50 mg daily; can consider 70 mg daily as therapy for aspergillosis. Dose reduction may be considered in severe liver disease. Pediatric dose: 70 mg/m^2 once (maximum, 70 mg), then 50 mg/m^2 (maximum daily dose of 50 mg)
Micafungin	Similar efficacy compared to caspofungin and compared to LAMB as primary therapy for candidemia and invasive candidiasis. At least equivalent to fluconazole as prophylaxis during neutropenia in HSCT recipients. Dose: 100 mg/d for candidemia and 50 mg/d as prophylaxis.
Anidulafungin	At least as effective as fluconazole as primary therapy for candidemia and invasive candidiasis. Dose: 200 mg once, then 100 mg/d.

MICs, minimal inhibitory concentrations; IV, intravenous; FDA, U.S. Food and Drug Administration; LAMB, liposomal amphotericin B; HSCT, hematopoietic stem cell transplant.

count <100/mcL), uncontrolled primary disease, and in serious infections, such as pneumonia, hypotension, multiorgan dysfunction, and invasive fungal infection.

It is unclear whether CSFs are safe and effective as either prophylaxis or adjunctive therapy in nonleukopenic patients with severe impairment in phagocyte function. Intensive immunosuppressive corticosteroid-based regimens for GVHD cause global impairment of phagocyte effector functions and disable reconstitution of antigen-specific immunity, although circulating neutrophil counts are generally normal. In theory, GM-CSF may augment qualitative macrophage and neutrophil function that may protect against infections. However, there are no data to support prophylactic CSFs in nonneutropenic patients, and we advise against its use in this setting outside a clinical trial.

Granulocyte Transfusions

The rationale for granulocyte transfusions is to provide support for the neutropenic patient with a life-threatening infection by augmenting the number of circulating neutrophils until autologous myeloid regeneration occurs. In the 1970s, apheresis technology for harvesting large numbers of donor granulocytes became available. Controlled trials of granulocyte transfusions as adjuvant therapy in neutropenic patients at the time produced mixed results. In the 1980s, the enthusiasm for granulocyte transfusions waned as more effective antibiotics became available, survival from serious bacterial infections improved, and recombinant growth factors reduced the duration of neutropenia. In addition, concerns about the toxicity of granulocyte transfusions, including acute pulmonary reactions, HLA alloimmunization (which could render patients refractory to platelet transfusions and potentially impair myeloid engraftment following HSCT), and transfusion-associated infections (particularly CMV), outweighed the perceived benefits.

Today, the impetus to re-examine the role of granulocyte transfusions stems largely from improvements in donor mobilization methods (G-CSF). Currently, the mean absolute neutrophil yield per collection is in the range of 8×10^{10} cells, resulting in higher posttransfusion neutrophil counts that are sustained for 24 to 30 hours following transfusion.[95] The qualitative functions of G-CSF- and steroid-mobilized neutrophils are intact based on *in vitro* testing.

Successful outcomes using granulocyte transfusions have been described in patients with life-threatening fungal infections in small series and in case reports.[96–98] A Cochrane Review of eight randomized controlled trials found the data inconclusive.[99] We reserve granulocyte transfusions for patients with prolonged neutropenia and life-threatening infections refractory to conventional therapy, particularly when neutrophil recovery is anticipated. The majority of such refractory infections are likely to be caused by molds. Early reports of severe respiratory distress syndrome associated with granulocyte transfusions and infusions of amphotericin B[100] make it prudent to separate these by several hours, although the significance of this association is controversial. In some highly alloimmunized patients, transfused granulocytes are rapidly consumed and are likely to have more toxicity than benefit. In allogeneic transplants in which the donor and recipient are CMV-seronegative, using CMV-seronegative granulocyte donors is advised.[101]

Lower-Risk Patients with Fever and Neutropenia

Patients with fever and neutropenia can be stratified according to their risk of developing life-threatening infectious complications. Patients in the lowest risk group may be appropriate candidates for carefully monitored empirical outpatient antibiotic therapy.

The most sophisticated index for the stratification of risk for complications in febrile neutropenic patients is the Multinational Association for Supportive Care in Cancer (MASCC) index.[102] The prospective study of 756 febrile neutropenic adult cancer patients in the MASCC study identified the following independent factors that predicted a low risk of complications: (1) burden of illness characterized by low or moderate symptoms, (2) absence of hypotension, (3) absence of chronic obstructive pulmonary disease, (4) presence of solid tumor or absence of previous fungal infection in patients with hematologic malignancies, (6) outpatient status, (7) absence of dehydration, and (8) and age less than 60 years. These variables predicting low risk were assigned an integer weight, and a risk index score consisting of the sum of these integers was derived. In the validation set of 383 patients, the risk index accurately identified patients at low risk for complications. A score of 21 or greater identified low-risk patients with a positive predictive value of 91%, specificity of 68%, and sensitivity of 71% (Fig. 156.1).

Outpatient Management of Febrile Neutropenic Patients

The greatest concern about outpatient management of neutropenic fever relates to the possibility of life-threatening complications that may be reversible if detected and treated early (e.g., intravenous fluid, vasopressors, broadening of antibiotic coverage). Patients must live in close proximity to a facility that can provide emergency care (e.g., fluid resuscitation, intravenous antibiotics) should the need arise. Only centers with the required infrastructure, including the accessibility of trained staff 24 hours per day, should treat lower-risk febrile neutropenic patients in the outpatient setting. Several studies have supported the safety of outpatient antibiotic therapy for low-risk patients (reviewed in ref. 103), although each study was relatively small and meta-analysis is complicated by differences in eligibility criteria, choice of antibiotics, criteria for hospital admission, and criteria for a successful outcome.

Both the IDSA[71] and NCCN[54,63] support the use of outpatient oral antibiotic therapy in carefully selected lower-risk patients with neutropenic fever. In adults, ciprofloxacin plus amoxicillin/clavulanate is recommended. In patients allergic to penicillins, the NCCN guidelines recommend substituting amoxicillin/clavulanate with clindamycin.

For neutropenic pediatric patients, Klaassen et al.[104] prospectively derived a risk stratification model. Children with an absolute monocyte count 100/mcL or more were at the lowest risk for significant bacterial infections. In a retrospective series of 509 pediatric patients with neutropenic fever, lack of signs of sepsis on admission (chills, hypotension, requirement for intravenous hydration), absolute neutrophil count less than 100 mcL, and resolution of fever within 48 hours of therapy accurately distinguished patients who could be discharged on oral agents.[105]

Fluoroquinolones are the only class of oral antibiotics with activity against *P. aeruginosa*, and therefore have an important role in the outpatient management of febrile neutropenic adults. Fluoroquinolone use in pediatric patients is controversial because of the possible increased risk of arthropathy. Studies of lower-risk pediatric patients treated with outpatient ciprofloxacin-containing regimens have shown encouraging results. However, the number of patients studied is limited[106–109] and we think there are insufficient data to recommend initial outpatient oral therapy for neutropenic febrile pediatric patients.[71]

Bacteremia

Bacteremia is a common complication of antineoplastic cytotoxic chemotherapy. The dominant risk factor for bacteremia is the duration of neutropenia.[110,111] Common sources are the intravenous catheter and the digestive tract. Some Gram-positive bacteria, such as coagulase-negative *Staphylococcus* species and *Corynebacterium* ("diphtheroid") species are common blood culture contaminants, but they may also represent true bacteremia in the presence of intravenous catheters. The likelihood of true bloodstream infection caused by these organisms is increased when are isolated from more than one blood culture. Consequently we advise to always obtain at least two sets of blood cultures from separate sites, (which may include two or more catheter ports). *Corynebacterium jeikeium* is a virulent pathogen that causes catheter-associated bacteremia and disseminated organ infection; isolation of this organism from a single blood culture requires prompt initiation of vancomycin therapy. Similarly, isolation of *S. aureus* from a single blood culture (or from the urine in a febrile patient) should be considered hematogenous infection.

Intravascular Catheter-Associated Infections

Several types of catheter-related infections have been defined: exit site infection, tunnel infection (or pocket infection in the case of ports), and catheter-related bacteremia. Bacteremia may or may not be present in the first two types.[112] Exit and tunnel (or pocket) infections are clinical diagnoses based on whether pain, erythema, and tenderness extend more than 2 cm from the exit site (tunnel infection) or not (exit site infection). Most exit site infections may be treated without removal of the catheter. Purulence from the exit site may be present, although in neutropenic patients, local erythema and tenderness may be the only signs of infection, making it difficult to distinguish from sterile inflammation associated with mild trauma. Tunnel or pocket infections usually mandate removal of the catheter. The third major category, catheter-related bacteremia or fungemia, may occur with or without signs of localized infection. Determining whether an episode of bacteremia is associated to the catheter or not may be difficult, and it has important implications for management. Positive blood cultures drawn through the intravascular catheter are convincing evidence that the catheter is the source only if they became positive earlier than blood cultures simultaneously drawn simultaneously from the periphery. A differential time to positivity of 2 hours or more between the culture drawn through the catheter and the culture drawn peripherally has high sensitivity and specificity for the diagnosis of catheter-related bloodstream infection.[113] Septic thrombophlebitis is a complicated catheter-related bacteremia in which a catheter-associated venous thrombus is documented; it also mandates removal of the catheter.

In catheter-related bacteremia, we usually recommend removing infected nonpermanent (i.e., not surgically implanted) catheters. In the case of surgically implanted catheters, we attempt catheter salvage depending on the clinical scenario. The catheter should be removed for positive blood cultures for more than 3 days after starting appropriate therapy or recurrences of bacteremia by the same pathogen. Different recommendations exist regarding the need to remove the catheter depending on the pathogen. The IDSA guidelines suggest routine removal of catheters infected with fungi, mycobacteria, and *S. aureus*.[112,114] For other pathogens, consideration may be given to attempt to salvage the catheter with antibiotic lock or by rotating the infusion of antibiotics through all lumens.

For the prevention of these infections, we recommend following some of the proven protocols ("bundles") that include aseptic technique at insertion, hand hygiene, adequate preparation of the skin with chlorhexidine, gauze or transparent sterile dressing, disinfection of hubs with chlorhexidine or 70% alcohol, and daily assessment of the need for the catheter, with early removal.[115,116]

Skin Lesions and Soft Tissue Infections

Consider infectious and noninfectious causes for these lesions.[117] Some noninfectious causes include drug reactions (including chemotherapy-induced hand-foot syndrome), Sweet syndrome, erythema multiforme, vasculitis, leukemia cutis, and (in the case of allogeneic transplant) GVHD. Early biopsy of skin lesions for histology and culture is recommended.

Infections of the skin can either be localized or manifestations of systemic infection. Ecthyma gangrenosum is the most characteristic skin lesion associated with systemic *P. aeruginosa* infection, but can also be caused by *S. aureus*, enteric Gram-negative bacilli infection, and molds including *Aspergillus*, zygomycetes, and *Fusarium*. Ecthyma gangrenosum begins as a raised erythematous papule or nodule that progresses to a bluish-black necrotic lesion within 12 to 24 hours. A central area of necrosis surrounded by erythema is typical. Hemorrhagic bullae may occur. Pathologically, ecthyma gangrenosum is a necrotizing process in which masses of bacteria are often observed within the vessel wall, and infiltrating white cells are absent.

A needle aspirate of the lesion showing Gram-negative bacilli establishes the diagnosis of invasive infection, but a negative aspirate does not rule out the diagnosis. Parenteral antibiotics with activity against *P. aeruginosa*, MRSA, and anaerobes (e.g., carbapenem + vancomycin ± a second agent against Gram-negative bacteria) should be instituted emergently, pending culture results. The role for surgical debridement depends on type of lesion: necrotizing soft tissue infections require surgery and nonnecrotizing infections can be treated with antibiotics alone.[118] Sometimes surgical exploration is necessary to determine the extent of the infection.

Gram-positive bacteria that cause skin and soft tissue infections include *Streptococcus* (group A and B) and *S. aureus*. Besides *P. aeruginosa*, other Gram-negative bacilli with propensity to cause dermatologic infections include *Stenotrophomonas maltophilia* (mucocutaneous ulcerations, primary cellulitis, metastatic nodular cellulitis, and ecthyma gangrenosum), *Aeromonas hydrophila* and *Vibrio vulnificus* (septicemia with secondary cellulitis with hemorrhagic bullae after ingestion of contaminated seafood, most common in patients with underlying liver disease, or primary cellulitis with bacteremia when an open wound is exposed to seawater). *Clostridium* species are Gram-positive anaerobes that may cause deep soft tissue infection involving the fascia and muscle. In neutropenic patients, the typical presentation is disseminated soft tissue infection. Typically, a small dusky or purplish lesion on the leg or abdominal wall rapidly expands, and as infection progresses, the lesions may become necrotic, bullous, and hemorrhagic. Systemic toxicity including fever, malaise, and mental status changes occur early. Because the infection occurs in the deep soft tissue, tenderness and evidence of vascular compromise typically precede the development of cellulitis. A rapidly progressive deep soft tissue infection with gas formation suggests clostridial myonecrosis or polymicrobial necrotizing fascitis. Needle aspiration characteristically shows the organism in the setting of a mild or absent inflammatory response. Extensive surgical debridement may be life-saving if initiated early, but the mortality rate is high.[119] Polymicrobial sepsis with enteric flora is commonly observed in association with clostridial bloodstream infection. In neutropenic patients, metronidazole plus an antipseudomonal cephalosporin (such as ceftazidime or cefepime) or single-agent therapy with imipenem, meropenem, or piperacillin/tazobactam are reasonable regimens.

The characteristic skin lesions of disseminated candidiasis are raised erythematous discrete papules, measuring about 0.5 to 1 cm in diameter. In their earliest form the lesions resemble those of heat rash. They are usually not tender. Concurrent myalgias raise the possibility of *Candida myositis*. The yeast is cultured from skin lesions in only about half the cases. Biopsy and fungal staining of cutaneous lesions can provide an immediate clue to the diagnosis, prompting the early addition of antifungal therapy. Blood cultures are typically positive. Similar lesions may appear with disseminated trichosporonosis.[120]

Cutaneous infection by molds may be primary or result from systemic infection. The hematogenous lesions of *Aspergillus* and *Fusarium* usually begin as discrete subcutaneous nodules that may be tender, whereas traumatic inoculation appears as ulcerations. If a primary cutaneous lesion is isolated and surgically resectable, it has an excellent prognosis. In the neutropenic patient, the likelihood of systemic infection is high, and therefore systemic antifungal therapy is warranted. Clinically, these lesions resemble ecthyma gangrenosum. Histologically, hyphae are present with angioinvasion and infarction. Primary cutaneous fusariosis has a varied appearance, including cellulitis, paronychia, onychomycosis resembling dermatophyte infection, as well as papular and nodular lesions1[121]

Upper Respiratory Tract Infections

Most cancer patients with symptoms of a common cold have viral infections that remain undiagnosed and resolve spontaneously. Some viral infections like respiratory syncytial virus (RSV), parainfluenza, and influenza may cause high fever and systemic symptoms in immunocompromised patients (particularly after allogeneic HSCT). A nasopharyngeal wash should be obtained for diagnosis (by antigen detection, rapid culture, or PCR). During influenza season, the combination of fever and cough should prompt consideration of empirical anti-influenza treatment guided by susceptibility patterns.

Sinusitis

Congestion, sinus tenderness, and fever are common signs of sinusitis, but are nonspecific. In immunocompetent patients, respiratory bacterial pathogens, including *S. pneumoniae*, *H. influenzae*, and *Moraxella catarrhalis* predominate. In patients with neutropenia or who are otherwise highly immunocompromised, infections by *P. aeruginosa*, *S. aureus*, Enterobacteriaceae, and molds must be considered, and there should be a low threshold for CT imaging.

Treatment of sinusitis in immunocompetent patients with cancer involves a standard antibiotic regimen, such as amoxicillin-clavulanate, azithromycin, clarithromycin, or a cephalosporin with activity against respiratory pathogens. In cases of an obstructing tumor interfering with drainage from the maxillary sinuses, surgical creation of an antral window may be required to facilitate drainage.

In neutropenic patients with symptoms or signs of sinusitis, we start standard agents for fever and neutropenia, and promptly obtain a CT scan of the sinuses and otolaryngologist consultation to evaluate for endoscopy for aspiration and, in case of lesions suspicious for invasive mold (e.g., ischemia, necrotic eschar), biopsy.

There are no signs in the CT pathognomonic of invasive fungal sinusitis, but the presence of a heterogeneous mass or bony erosions is highly suggestive. Periorbital swelling and diplopia are late ominous signs. *Aspergillus* species is the most common isolate, but zygomycetes (e.g., mucor, rhizopus) as well as less common molds such as *Fusarium* spp., dark-walled molds like *Alternaria*, and *Scedosporium* species are being recognized more frequently. Pending microbiological identification, empirical therapy should include a lipid formulation of amphotericin B (5 mg/kg/d), to ensure treatment against *Aspergillus* species and zygomycetes. If the diagnosis of invasive fungal sinusitis is confirmed, surgical resection of involved tissue must be performed because medical therapy alone is unlikely to contain infection in the setting of neutropenia or severe immunosuppression. Antifungal therapy should be continued for weeks or months even if all of the visualized necrotic tissue is fully resected. An etiologic diagnosis is often obtained, and then the appropriate antifungal may be chosen (e.g., voriconazole for aspergillosis).

For zygomycosis, posaconazole may be a useful alternative to an amphotericin B formulation for long-term therapy (see "Zygomycosis").

Epiglottitis

Epiglottitis should be considered in patients with fever and throat pain, odynophagia, difficulty handling upper airway secretions, and signs of upper airway compromise. The combination of neutropenia and mucositis predisposes patients to epiglottitis. Pathogens include *S. pneumoniae* and *H. influenzae*, Gram-negative bacilli, and fungi. *Candida* epiglottitis, an unusual complication of neutropenia that simulates bacterial epiglottitis, may represent localized disease or disseminated infection.[122] If epiglottitis is considered, unnecessary manipulations of the upper airway should be avoided and urgent consultation with an otolaryngologist should be obtained.

Pulmonary Infiltrates

In addition to infection, numerous noninfectious processes should be considered in patients with pulmonary infiltrates: the malignancy, its treatment (drug toxicity, radiation pneumonitis), congestive heart failure, pulmonary hemorrhage, pulmonary embolism with infarction, cryptogenic organizing pneumonia (also known as bronchiolitis obliterans organizing pneumonia), and acute respiratory distress syndrome. Atypical radiographic appearances and several coexisting pulmonary processes are common in this patient population. The more immunocompromised the patient is, the more we would recommend early use of CT scans and invasive diagnostic procedures, including bronchoalveolar lavage, fine-needle aspiration, or lung biopsy if required.

Patients Who Are Not Neutropenic and Not Receiving Immunosuppressive Therapy

Community-Acquired Pneumonia. The history should include the time course of respiratory symptoms, sick contacts (e.g., community respiratory viral infections, tuberculosis), recent hospitalization, travel, animal exposures, and exposure to droplets from water distribution systems (*Legionella*). Community outbreaks of specific pathogens (e.g., influenza) should be considered in the differential diagnosis. Sputum and blood cultures should be collected prior to starting therapy if feasible. In patients with malignancies who do not require hospital admission based on a validated pneumonia severity index,[123] either a respiratory fluoroquinolone alone (levofloxacin, moxifloxacin) or a beta-lactam plus a macrolide (e.g., high-dose amoxicillin or amoxicillin-clavulanate and azithromycin) is advised. In patients requiring hospital admission, we use monotherapy with a respiratory fluoroquinolone or combine a macrolide with either ceftriaxone, cefotaxime, or, in selected cases, ertapenem. For cancer patients with severe community-acquired pneumonia (e.g., requiring admission to an intensive care unit), we usually institute broad-spectrum coverage with an antipseudomonal beta-lactam plus a newer fluoroquinolone. In patients with prior MRSA infection or known colonization with MRSA, addition of vancomycin or linezolid should be strongly considered. A parapneumonic effusion should be aspirated and submitted for microbiologic studies and cytologic examination.

Hospital-Acquired Pneumonia. Hospital-acquired pneumonia (HAP) is considered "early" when it happens within 4 days of admission or "late" when it occurs 5 days or more after admission. Late HAP is more likely to be caused by multidrug-resistant pathogens. Initial therapy for early-onset HAP is similar to that of community-acquired pneumonia, except when there are risk factors for colonization with multidrug resistant pathogens (e.g., prior antibiotics within the past 90 days, recent hospitalization, nursing home, dialysis center) in which case they should treated similar to patients with late-onset HAP. In late-onset HAP, the goal is to broadly cover nosocomial pathogens and then to de-escalate the antibiotic regimen once culture results and susceptibility are known. A reasonable initial regimen for late-onset HAP includes an antipseudomonal beta-lactam (e.g., ceftazidime, cefepime, imipenem, meropenem, or piperacillin/tazobactam) plus an antipseudomonal fluoroquinolone (e.g., ciprofloxacin or levofloxacin) or aminoglycoside, plus either linezolid or vancomycin (aim for trough vancomycin level of 15–20 mcg/mL).[124]

Pulmonary Infiltrates in Neutropenic Patients

In patients with less than 1 week of neutropenia, pulmonary infections are likely to be caused by Enterobacteriaceae, *P. aeruginosa*, and *S. aureus*. Particularly during winter months, community respiratory viruses should also be considered. Because of neutropenia, physical findings of consolidation and sputum production may be absent. Blood cultures, a chest radiograph, and, if possible, a sputum for Gram stain and culture should be obtained. Broad-spectrum antibiotics must be initiated immediately.

We recommend the early use of CT when suspicion of pneumonia arises in neutropenic patients. A CT scan of the chest may disclose lesions missed by the chest radiograph as well as findings characteristic of invasive fungal disease: well-circumscribed, dense infiltrates, the "halo sign" (Fig. 156.2), and/or cavitation. Cavitation may coincide with neutrophil recovery and does not indicate treatment failure. Other angioinvasive infections including *P. aeruginosa* may cavitate. A new or progressive infiltrate developing while on broad-spectrum antibacterial agents in patients with prolonged neutropenia (10 days or more) raises the concern about invasive mold infection,[91] and makes the need for definitive diagnosis more pressing.

In patients at risk for invasive mold diseases, a serum galactomannan and beta-D-glucan may be considered, although the interpretation of a single value of these tests (as opposed to trends) may be difficult. In a patient with a progressive pulmonary infiltrate despite initiation of broad-spectrum antibiotics in whom a diagnosis has not been made, an invasive diagnostic approach (bronchoalveolar lavage [BAL] or biopsy) must be considered.

In highly immunocompromised patients (e.g., chemotherapy for acute leukemia, HSCT receiving active treatment for GVHD), we suggest the following studies on BAL and lung biopsies: culture and stains for bacteria, including *Legionella*, mycobacteria, and *Nocardia* species as well as fungi; special stains or PCR for *P. jirovecii*; and rapid culture (shell vial) or PCR for virus (HSV, CMV, VZV, community respiratory viruses). Cytologic examination of the BAL may also be diagnostic of pneumocystis, nocardia, fungi, mycobacteria, CMV (characteristic viral inclusions), and can suggest diffuse alveolar hemorrhage. BAL galactomannan may be more sensitive than serum galactomannan, particularly in neutropenic patients, and should be considered in patients at risk for invasive aspergillosis.[125]

The yield of induced sputum for the diagnosis of PCP in non-HIV-infected patients may be only 60%,[126] and early consideration should be given to BAL. The yield of BAL is high for *P. jirovecii*, *M. tuberculosis*, and respiratory viruses. For focal lesions such as nodules, the diagnostic yield is much lower (15%–50%), and a percutaneous biopsy may be a better diagnostic choice.[127] Transbronchial biopsy may be helpful in diffuse processes. Video-assisted thoracic surgery has been used successfully in cases with diffuse involvement and with peripheral lesions. Open lung biopsy is the definitive diagnostic method, and it also allows for easier visualization and control of bleeding.

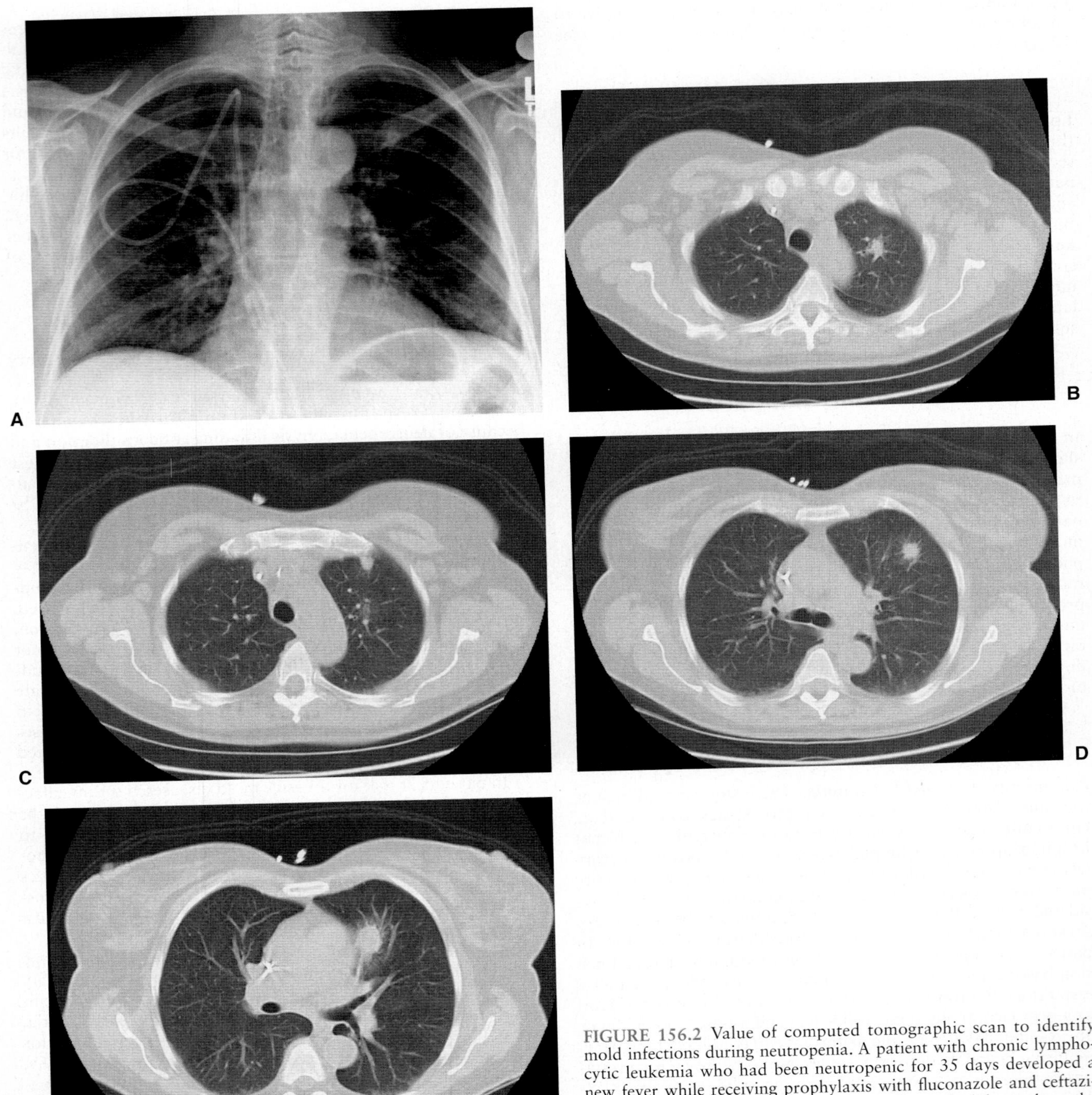

FIGURE 156.2 Value of computed tomographic scan to identify mold infections during neutropenia. A patient with chronic lymphocytic leukemia who had been neutropenic for 35 days developed a new fever while receiving prophylaxis with fluconazole and ceftazidime for neutropenic fever. The chest radiograph did not show the four nodules evident by computed tomography. Notice the "halo sign" in the largest nodule.

Initial Antimicrobial Therapy. The antibiotic regimen must include the standard antimicrobials used for fever and neutropenia and, if the pneumonia is community-acquired, a macrolide or fluoroquinolone to treat *Legionella* and agents of atypical pneumonia. Vancomycin or linezolid should be added for pneumonia in patients colonized with MRSA and for nosocomial pneumonia.

Depending on the clinical scenario and pre-existent antifungal prophylaxis, we may add voriconazole or a lipid formulation of amphotericin B (generally 3–5 mg/kg). There is disagreement between experts on which is the best antifungal strategy. *Aspergillus* species are by far the most common mold infections, but zygomycetes may be the cause in any individual case. Voriconazole is the drug of choice for invasive aspergillosis,[128] but is inactive against zygomycetes. Amphotericin B is active against both *Aspergillus* species (with the exception of *Aspergillus terreus*) and zygomycetes, but may be inferior to voriconazole in aspergillosis. In patients at high risk for invasive mold diseases with suspected pneumonia of unknown etiology, we advise initial antifungal therapy either with voriconazole or a lipid formulation of amphotericin B, with the decision about

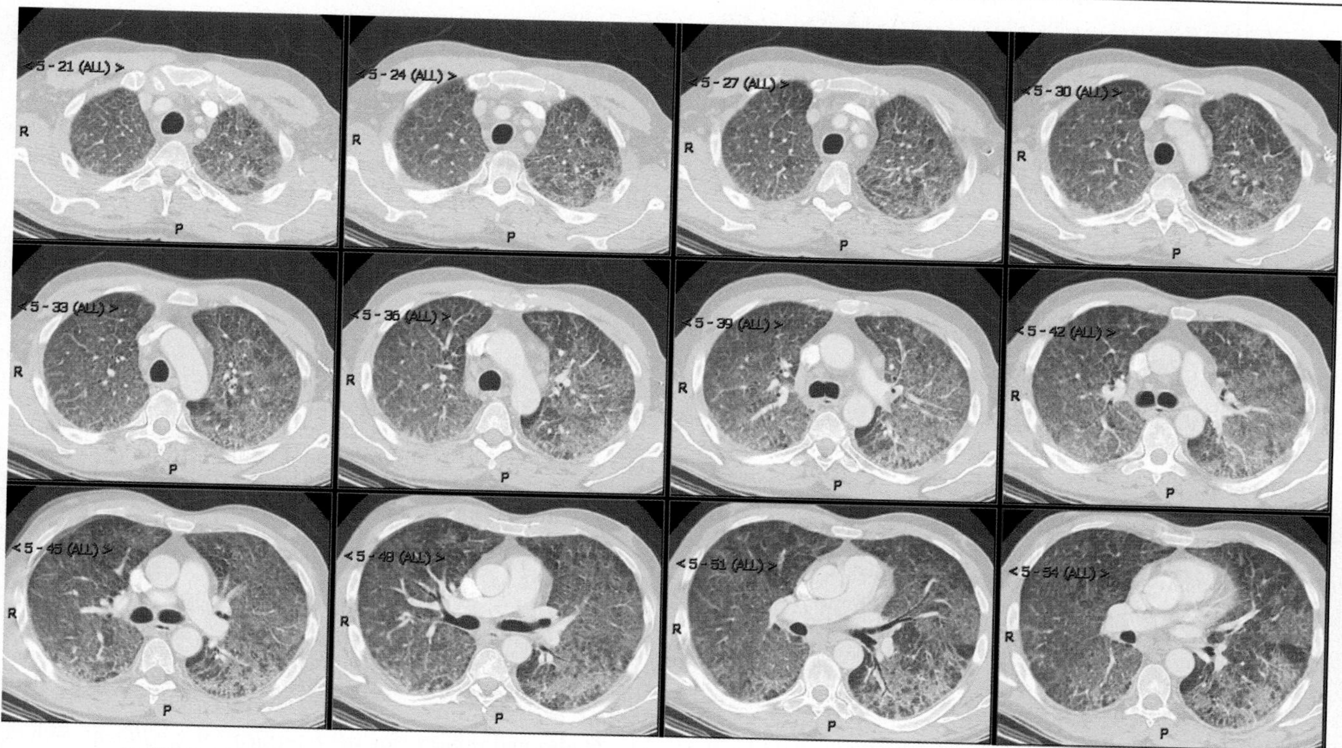

FIGURE 156.3 *Pneumocystis jirovecii* pneumonia (PCP). A patient with chronic lymphocytic leukemia developed fever, hypoxemia, and shortness of breath soon after tapering a prednisone course for hemolytic anemia. He had received multiple courses of fludarabine, rituximab, and corticosteroids. He was receiving inhaled pentamidine as PCP prophylaxis. His last treatment had taken place 3 weeks prior to this illness.

which agent being guided by local patterns of fungal diseases and drug toxicity.

Pulmonary Infiltrates in Patients with Defects in Cellular Immunity

Patients with impaired cellular immunity (Tables 156.1 and 156.2) and those taking corticosteroids are at increased risk for opportunistic infections, including fungi (*Cryptococcus neoformans*, dimorphic fungi, other molds), *Legionella* spp., *P. jirovecii* (Fig. 156.3), *M. tuberculosis*, nontuberculous mycobacteria, *Nocardia* spp., and viral pathogens. CMV pneumonia principally occurs in allogeneic HSCT recipients, but can uncommonly occur in other severely immunocompromised patients. Diffuse necrotizing pneumonia by varicella and HSV are also encountered in transplant recipients.

The diagnostic evaluation in patients with impaired cellular immunity and pulmonary infiltrates is similar to neutropenic patients, Typically broad-spectrum antibiotics for community-acquired pneumonia requiring hospitalization (see previous discussion) will be started, ideally after obtaining respiratory samples for diagnosis. The addition of TMP/SMX for PCP should be considered. We emphasize the need to establish a definitive diagnosis in patients with negative diagnostic results who are deteriorating clinically after a 2- to 3-day trial of broad-spectrum antibiotics.

Gastrointestinal Tract and Abdominal Infections

Oropharyngeal Infections

Oropharyngeal infections in patients with cancer usually result from the combination of neutropenia and mucositis. The distinction of chemotherapy-induced mucosal erosions and superimposed infection is difficult. HSV may produce mucosal ulcerations resembling chemotherapy-induced mucositis and necrotizing gingivitis, and it should be ruled out by culture or PCR. Oral mucosal candidiasis may present with typical thrush, but also with erosions and erythema; diagnosis is made by a wet mount or Gram stain preparation showing pseudohyphal forms (the culture is not of diagnostic value because *Candida* species are part of the normal oral flora). Molds (e.g., *Aspergillus* species and zygomycetes) can cause invasive disease of the hard palate and other oral cavity structures, principally in patients with prolonged neutropenia and allogeneic HSCT recipients with GVHD. Severe local bacterial infection may occur with spread to adjacent tissue structures (including paranasal sinusitis and septic thrombophlebitis) and bacteremia. The antibacterial regimen should cover both common oral flora (Gram-positive bacteria and anaerobes) and hospital-acquired Gram-negative bacilli.

Esophagitis

Gradual onset of retrosternal chest pain or burning and odynophagia are the most common symptoms of esophagitis. The infectious differential diagnosis includes candidiasis, HSV, CMV (principally in HSCT recipients), bacterial infections, and aspergillosis. *Candida* esophagitis is probably most common, but more than one infection may be present. Radiation therapy to the chest and chemotherapy-induced mucositis may produce an erosive esophagitis that is clinically indistinguishable from infection. The definitive diagnosis requires endoscopy with brushing or biopsy. The endoscopic appearance (ulcers suggesting viral etiologies and whitish plaques suggesting candidiasis) is often misleading. In neutropenic patients, we recommend empirical therapy with fluconazole, with or without high-dose acyclovir (10 mg/kg every 8 hours) for

Candida and HSV, respectively, followed by endoscopy if there is no improvement. In the setting of concurrent neutropenic fever, appropriate broad-spectrum antibacterial agents like imipenem, meropenem, or piperacillin/tazobactam should be added empirically. Esophagitis may be complicated by bacteremia by predominantly Gram-positive pathogens (viridans group streptococci, *S. aureus, Bacillus* sp.).

Intra-Abdominal Infections

Neutropenic Enterocolitis (Typhlitis)

Typhlitis ("inflammation of the cecum") results from a combination of neutropenia and defects in the bowel mucosa related to cytotoxic chemotherapy. Patients receiving chemotherapy for acute leukemia are at highest risk, but it is also observed in patients with solid tumors receiving taxanes.[129,130] Pathologically, typhlitis is characterized by ulceration and necrosis of the bowel wall, hemorrhage, and masses of organisms. Suggestive signs include fever, abdominal pain and tenderness, and radiologic evidence of right colonic inflammation. Nausea, vomiting, and diarrhea (sometimes bloody) are the most common associated symptoms. Abdominal distention, tenderness, and a right lower quadrant fullness or mass reflect thickened bowel. Bacteremia with bowel flora, *P. aeruginosa* and polymicrobial sepsis may occur. Clostridial species are the most common anaerobic pathogens.

A CT scan should be performed in patients with suspected typhlitis or undiagnosed abdominal pain in the setting of neutropenia. Positive CT scan findings are present in about 80% of cases of typhlitis,[131] and include a right lower quadrant inflammatory mass, pericecal fluid, soft tissue inflammatory changes, localized bowel wall thickening and mucosal edema, and a paralytic ileus (Fig. 156.4). Usually, disease is limited to the cecum, but more extensive involvement of the large bowel and disease of the terminal ileum may occur (hence, the more generic term *neutropenic enterocolitis*). The differential diagnosis includes *C. difficile* colitis, GVHD of the bowel, CMV colitis (rarely observed during neutropenia), and bowel ischemia.[132]

Treatment of typhlitis requires broad-spectrum antibiotics with activity against aerobic Gram-negative bacilli and anaerobes (e.g., ceftazidime plus metronidazole, imipenem, meropenem, or piperacillin/tazobactam) and supportive care, including intravenous fluids and bowel rest. Nasogastric decompression may be indicated. The majority of patients will respond to antibiotic therapy and supportive care without the need for surgery. The indications for surgery must be individualized, but include (1) persistent gastrointestinal bleeding after resolution of neutropenia, thrombocytopenia, and clotting abnormalities; (2) free intraperitoneal perforation; (3) uncontrolled sepsis despite fluid and vasopressor support; and (4) an intra-abdominal process (such as appendicitis) that would require surgery in the absence of neutropenia.[133]

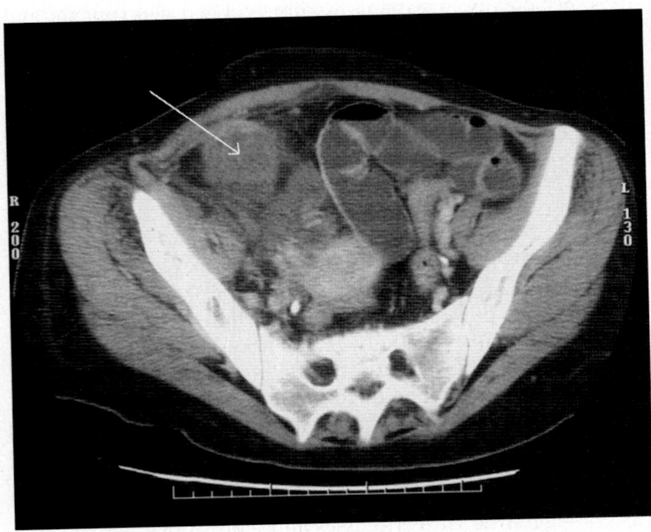

FIGURE 156.4 Typhlitis (neutropenic enterocolitis). The computed tomographic scan shows edema of the cecal wall and "stranding" of pericolic fat in a neutropenic patient with fever and abdominal pain.

Clostridium Difficile Colitis

Patients with cancer are at high risk for *C. difficile* colitis because of prolonged hospitalization and broad-spectrum antibiotics. The clinical spectrum includes asymptomatic carriage, colitis without pseudomembrane formation, pseudomembranous colitis, and fulminant colitis with toxic megacolon. In severe *C. difficile* disease, paralytic ileus, toxic dilatation of the colon, and bowel perforation may occur. An abdominal film may show a dilated colon with mucosal edema ("thumbprinting"), but is often nonspecific. The mainstay of diagnosis is detection of *C. difficile* toxin A, toxin B, or both, in the stool with a cytotoxin test, enzyme immunoassay, or PCR for the toxin gene. Enzyme immunoassays have variable sensitivity. The rate and severity of *C. difficile* colitis in the United States may be increasing, in part by the emergence of a more virulent strain.[134,135]

Traditional options for the treatment of *C. difficile* include oral or intravenous metronidazole and oral vancomycin. Metronidazole has been recommended as first choice as its efficacy seemed similar to oral vancomycin, and the selection pressure on other flora is less dangerous. Recently, the response rate without recurrence of *C. difficile* colitis to metronidazole has been reported to be in the 50% range, which is lower than historically expected.[136] A comparative trial suggests oral vancomycin may be more efficacious in severe *C. difficile* colitis,[137] and it is commonly the treatment of choice in the most severe cases. Successful management of refractory cases with tigecycline has been reported.[138] Nitazoxanide, which had efficacy similar to metronidazole in a randomized trial,[139] may be an option in milder cases. Patients in whom oral agents cannot be administered should receive intravenous metronidazole. In cases involving toxic dilatation of the colon or perforation, subtotal colectomy, diverting ileostomy, or colostomy may be required.

The safety and efficacy of probiotic agents in immunocompromised patients and patients with cancer is unknown, but it is worth noting that bloodstream infection with *Lactobacillus* or *Saccharomyces* has resulted occasionally from these preparations. Management of *C. difficile* recurrences is difficult, and many different strategies have been used (e.g., repeated courses of the same antibiotic, vancomycin "pulse" therapy, vancomycin taper).[140] Monoclonal antibodies against *C. difficile* toxins may become an option to reduce the recurrence of *C. difficile* infection in the future.[141]

Anorectal Infections. Anorectal infections may be life-threatening in patients who are receiving repeated courses of cytotoxic chemotherapy. Infection may follow the development of an anal fissure. Once anorectal infection is established, fascial extension to the external genitalia, pelvic floor, retroperitoneum, and peritoneal cavity may occur. Anorectal infections, with or without extensive regional spread, may lead to bacteremia. The most common pathogens in neutropenic patients are Enterobacteriaceae, anaerobes, enterococci and *P. aeruginosa*. In most cases, the infection is polymicrobial.[142]

Fever often precedes symptoms and signs suggestive of anorectal infection, and perirectal pain, often exacerbated by defecation, may initially occur in the absence of findings in the physical examination. Therefore, serial examinations of the perianal region are necessary, looking for point tenderness and poorly demarcated induration.[143] Perianal and perirectal infections are distinguished anatomically, clinically, and therapeutically. Among neutropenic patients, perianal infections are common and are usually managed medically, whereas perirectal infections are uncommon and often warrant surgical intervention. Visual inspection should assess for the presence of perianal fissures, fistulas, cellulitis, and induration. Digital rectal examination should be avoided during neutropenia. A CT scan should be obtained to show the extent of perirectal involvement and drainable collections. Stool softeners and analgesics should be provided. Most cases of anorectal infections can be managed with appropriate broad-spectrum antibiotics and supportive measures without surgical intervention.[142] Indications for surgery include progression of disease locally or continued sepsis despite adequate antibiotics.

Central Nervous System Infections

Central nervous system (CNS) infections in patients with cancer can be divided into surgical and nonsurgical. CNS infections unrelated to neurosurgical procedures are relatively uncommon in patients with cancer. Noninfectious disorders such as toxicity from drugs (e.g., cyclosporine and tacrolimus, intrathecal methotrexate), vasculitis, and malignancy may mimic infection; differentiating them from CNS infectious often requires brain biopsy.

Infections Related to Neurosurgical Procedures

Common surgical procedures include resection of tumor, insertion of a shunt for hydrocephalus, and insertion of a reservoir to facilitate delivery of chemotherapeutic agents and easy sampling of cerebrospinal fluid. Patients with cancer involving the brain typically receive high-dose corticosteroids and local radiation therapy, which may further increase the risk of infections.

Infection of a shunt or an Ommaya reservoir may manifest with malfunction of the device, fever, or abnormal mental status (alone or in combination). Overt signs of meningitis, such as meningismus and photophobia do not usually occur. A CT scan may suggest meningitis, ventriculitis, or a brain abscess if the device is infected at the proximal end. Evaluation of the cerebrospinal fluid (CSF), ideally from the reservoir, is required for a diagnosis. Infection may occur in the more distal region of the device manifesting as a soft tissue infection. In cases of ventriculoatrial shunts, a distal site of infection may cause persistently positive blood cultures, thrombophlebitis, right-sided endocarditis, or septic pulmonary emboli. Distal ventriculoperitoneal shunt infections are associated with peritonitis and intra-abdominal collections. A study comparing complications of ventriculoatrial and ventriculoperitoneal shunts did not demonstrate an appreciable difference in infection risk.[144]

Early postoperative infections after placement of intraventricular devices are usually caused by skin flora: coagulase-negative staphylococci, *S. aureus*, and streptococci and *Propionibacterium acnes*. However, Enterobacteriaceae and *P. aeruginosa* account for approximately 10% of infections. Coagulase-negative staphylococci and *P. acnes* usually cause indolent late postoperative infections.

Removal of the entire device plus systemic antibiotics is the most effective approach to eradicate infection. Use of parenteral and intraventricular instillation of antibiotics without hardware removal has met with variable success; however, recrudescence of infection is common, particularly those caused by *S. aureus*.[145] Antibiotic therapy should be tailored to the specific pathogen isolated. In an acutely ill patient with suspected meningitis related to prior neurosurgery, empirical therapy with parenteral vancomycin should be administered to cover *Staphylococcus*, *Streptococcus*, and *Propionibacterium* species in combination with an agent with activity against *Enterobacteriaceae* and *P. aeruginosa* such as ceftazidime or meropenem. Antibiotics may be safely stopped after 3 days if the CSF cultures (obtained prior to initiation of antibiotics) are negative.[146]

Meningitis/Meningoencephalitis

Meningitis and encephalitis in cancer patients are part of a clinical spectrum of CNS disorders causing fever and meningismus. Encephalitis may manifest with signs and symptoms of meningeal inflammation, but is distinguished by the predominance of alterations of consciousness and neurologic deficits. The IDSA has published guidelines on the management of bacterial meningitis[147] and encephalitis.[148]

Initial evaluation generally involves an MRI and lumbar puncture (assuming no contraindication). CSF studies should be tailored to specific host factors, epidemiologic exposures (e.g., travel history), and clinical presentation. At a minimum, cell count with differential, glucose, protein, and bacterial culture and Gram stain evaluation should be ordered. In patients with impaired cellular immunity, CSF cryptococcal antigen and fungal culture should be ordered. Noninfectious causes of meningitis include carcinomatous meningitis, nonsteroidal anti-inflammatory medications, TMP/SMX, and serum sickness (e.g., associated with antilymphocyte gammaglobulin or intravenous immunoglobulin [IVIG]).

A reasonable empirical regimen for suspected bacterial meningitis in patients with cancer is ceftriaxone (2 g every 12 hours in adults) plus ampicillin (2 g every 4 hours in adults with normal renal function) plus vancomycin (15 mg/kg every 8 to 12 hours in adults with normal renal function; maintain serum trough of 15 to 20 mcg/mL). This regimen will cover common causes of bacterial meningitis, including penicillin-resistant pneumococci and listeriosis. In the penicillin-allergic patient, the combination of vancomycin and TMP/SMX may be used. In patients at risk for *P. aeruginosa* meningitis (e.g., neutropenia, neurosurgery within the past 2 months, allogeneic HSCT, prior history of *P. aeruginosa* infection), cefepime or meropenem should be used instead of ceftriaxone.

In patients with suspected encephalitis (fever, mental status changes, CSF pleocytosis), intravenous acyclovir (10 to 12 mg/kg every 8 hours in patients with normal renal function) should be considered as empirical therapy for HSV. Additional CSF studies should include PCR for HSV and CSF cytology and, if available, flow cytometry. PCR for arboviruses should be considered in patients with exposure to endemic areas. The CSF should also be sent for nucleic acid amplification methods for the diagnosis of tuberculosis, adenosine deaminase level, and culture for tuberculosis in patients with known or suspected exposure to tuberculosis (e.g., residence in an endemic area, shelter, or prison, prior positive purified protein derivative test or other test for latent tuberculosis). In patients with severe impairment of cellular immunity (e.g., allogeneic HSCT recipient, advanced AIDS), additional CSF studies that should be considered include PCR for CMV, VZV, HHV-6, and toxoplasmosis, and culture for *Nocardia* species. Most cases of encephalitis occur in HSCT patients and are due to reactivation of latent viral, bacterial, or parasitic infections: herpesviruses (HSV, VZV, CMV, EBV, human herpes virus [HHV]-6), adenovirus, mycobacteria, and *Toxoplasma gondii*.

Herpesviruses. HSV meningoencephalitis has been associated with older age, steroid therapy, and brain irradiation. The diagnosis is usually made by viral PCR from the CSF and enhancement of the temporal lobe on MRI. Its treatment is summarized in Table 156.8. Other, less common herpesvirus infections can be diagnosed by PCR of viral DNA in the CSF.

TABLE 156.8

ANTIVIRAL AGENTS COMMONLY USED TO TREAT IMMUNOCOMPROMISED PATIENTS WITH CANCER

Disease	Antiviral Therapy[a]	Comments
Mucocutaneous herpes	Acyclovir, 5 mg/kg q8h (IV)	—
Acyclovir resistant	Foscarnet, 40 mg/kg q8h (IV)	Antiviral testing available at reference laboratories, takes too long to be helpful in clinical decision making.
Prophylaxis	Acyclovir, 400 mg tid (oral)	—
Herpes (disseminated or visceral organ involvement)	Acyclovir, 10 mg/kg q8h (IV)	—
Herpes encephalitis	Acyclovir, 10–12 mg/kg q8h (IV)	PCR of spinal fluid diagnostic method of choice.
Chickenpox	Acyclovir, 10 mg/kg q8h (IV)	—
Herpes zoster		
Single dermatome	Acyclovir, 800 mg 5 times daily or Valacyclovir, 1 g tid (oral) or Famciclovir, 500 mg tid (oral)	—
Less than one dermatome or disseminated	Acyclovir, 10 mg/kg q8h (IV)	—
CMV disease	Ganciclovir, 5 mg/kg q12h (IV) or	Add IV immunoglobulin in cases of pneumonia.
	Foscarnet, 60 mg/kg q8h (IV)	Use foscarnet for ganciclovir-resistant infection and consider in patients with borderline ANC (e.g., < 1,500 /mcL).
	Cidofovir, 5 mg/kg/wk	Limited experience outside of CMV retinitis in HIV+ patients. Probenecid and prehydration routinely used.
Influenza	Oseltamivir, 75 mg bid (oral)	Oseltamivir is the preferred agent for influenza infection because of its activity against both influenza A and B strains and safety profile.
	Zanamivir (two inhalations bid)	May cause bronchospasm.
	Rimantadine, 200 mg daily (oral) or	—
	Amantadine, 100 mg daily (oral)	—
Respiratory syncytial virus infection	Ribavirin, 6 g/300 mL water, by aerosol 12 h/d	The benefit of ribavirin for RSV infection in patients with cancer and in HSCT recipients is controversial. Some investigators add pooled intravenous immunoglobulin or palivizumab (see text).
Parainfluenza virus infection	Supportive care	—
Adenovirus infection	Cidofovir, 3–5 mg/kg weekly × 2, then every other week	Requires probenecid and hydration; gastroenteritis and cystitis are generally self-limiting and do not require therapy; consider for pneumonia or disseminated disease, although benefit not established.
Chronic hepatitis B	Lamivudine, 100 mg daily (oral)	Add or switch to tenofovir in cases of resistance.
Chronic hepatitis C	Pegylated interferon-α weekly (SC) and ribavirin bid (oral)	See package insert for dosing.
Parvovirus B19 infection	Intravenous immunoglobulin	—

IV, intravenous; tid, three times daily; PCR, polymerase chain reaction; SC, subcutaneous; CMV, cytomegalovirus; ANC, absolute neutrophil count; HIV, human immunodeficiency virus; bid, twice daily; RSV, respiratory syncytial virus; HSCT, hematopoietic stem cell transplant.
[a]Dosages are for adults with normal renal function.

Detection of high levels of EBV DNA should raise suspicion of EBV-related lymphoproliferative disorder, but encephalitis and myelitis have been described. In HSCT patents, HHV-6 has been associated with a characteristic syndrome consisting of confusion, lethargy, fever, rash, and hippocampal enhancement on T2-weighted MRI FLAIR images.[149] The presence of CSF pleocytosis is variable; the diagnosis is made by detection of HHV-6 DNA in the CSF by PCR.[150] Ganciclovir or foscarnet may be used, but there are no clinical data to choose one over the other. Adenovirus encephalitis also occurs in HSCT patients, and is usually part of disseminated adenoviral infection; treatment with cidofovir may be attempted.

Several uncommon but important causes of meningoencephalitis are due to new infections rather than reactivation. Advanced age and cancer are risk factors for devastating encephalitis from West Nile virus (WNV), which is transmitted by mosquito bites.[151] There is no proven treatment for WNV infection; clinical trials with IVIG from WNV-endemic countries are ongoing. *Nocardia* and *Acanthamoeba* are rare but treatable, and must generally be identified by brain biopsy.

Influenza rarely causes encephalitis, which is typically self-limited; the role of oseltamivir is unclear.

Brain Abscess

Brain abscesses usually manifest with headache, focal neurologic findings, or seizures. MRI typically shows single or multiple lesions with edema and ring enhancement. Bacterial abscesses in nonimmunocompromised patients are typically caused by dental flora. In cancer patients, brain abscesses unrelated to surgery occur primarily in patients with prolonged neutropenia or profoundly depressed cell-mediated immunity, and are frequently fungal (92% of 58 cases of brain abscesses following HSCT[152]). Almost all cases of CNS aspergillosis are associated with a pulmonary focus. Most cases of *Candida* brain abscess are associated with candidemia or neutropenia.

Manifestations of CNS aspergillosis include focal seizures, hemiparesis, cranial nerve palsies, and hemorrhagic infarcts due to vascular invasion.153 Serum galactomannan and B-glucan testing and CSF galactomannan testing are also useful to facilitate a diagnosis of CNS aspergillosis. Aspergillus brain abscesses are typically multiple, hypodense, and nonenhancing with little mass effect. CT scans with contrast enhancement initially may reveal no focal lesions, but usually evolve to focal ring-enhancing or hemorrhagic lesions. MRI may show varying patterns depending on the stage of the lesion. Other causes of CNS abscesses in patients with impaired cellular immunity include toxoplasmosis, nocardiosis, cryptococcosis, and mycobacterial infections. Noninfectious etiologies include CNS malignancies, including secondary lymphomas and EBV-associated posttransplant lymphoproliferative disease (PTLD) in patients with impaired cellular immunity. Given the broad differential diagnosis of new focal CNS lesions in the highly immunocompromised patient, a brain biopsy is recommended if feasible. Cultures and stains should include bacteria, fungi, mycobacteria, and *Nocardia* species.

In nonimmunocompromised patients with a bacterial brain abscess, initial therapy with ceftriaxone (2 g every 12 hours) plus metronidazole (7.5 mg/kg every 6 hours) is advised. In patients with prolonged neutropenia without corticosteroids or lymphocyte-depleting agents, a reasonable initial regimen consists of combination meropenem (2 g every 8 hours, or cefepime, 2 g every 8 hours plus metronidazole), and voriconazole (6 mg/kg every 12 hours intravenously for two doses, followed by 4 mg/kg every 12 hours in adults). Voriconazole (as well as itraconazole and posaconazole) has important drug–drug interactions with certain antiseizure agents (e.g., phenytoin). In allogeneic HSCT recipients and other patients with severe T-cell impairment, addition of high-dose TMP/SMX (trimethoprim component: 5 mg/kg every 8 hours) should be considered to cover toxoplasmosis and nocardiosis, pending a definitive diagnosis. In an analysis of 86 patients with CNS aspergillosis treated with voriconazole either as primary or salvage therapy, 34% had a complete or partial response.[154]

Toxoplasmosis

Reactivation of *Toxoplasma gondii* may cause life-threatening disease in patients with profound deficits in T-cell immunity. Risk factors include therapy with corticosteroids, alemtuzumab, cytotoxic agents and/or radiation therapy, and poorly controlled malignancy. Toxoplasmosis is an uncommon complication of HSCT, occurring in fewer than 1% of patients, nearly all seropositive prior to transplantation,.[155] It tends to occur in the presence of moderate to severe GVHD (median day of onset of disease was 64 days after HSCT).

CNS disease with altered mental status, coma, seizures, cranial nerve abnormalities, and motor weakness are the most common findings.[156] MRI typically shows two or more lesions that may be ring-enhancing (Fig. 156.5). The differential diagnosis includes bacterial infection, invasive aspergillosis, nocardiosis, and malignancy. Differentiating toxoplasmosis from lymphoma is particularly difficult; [18F]fluorodeoxyglucose positron emission tomography typically shows increased metabolism in lymphoma.[157] CSF in toxoplasmosis is usually normal; however, a mononuclear pleocytosis and elevated protein may be seen. Besides the CNS, other organs may also be involved (myocarditis, interstitial pneumonitis, culture-negative sepsis

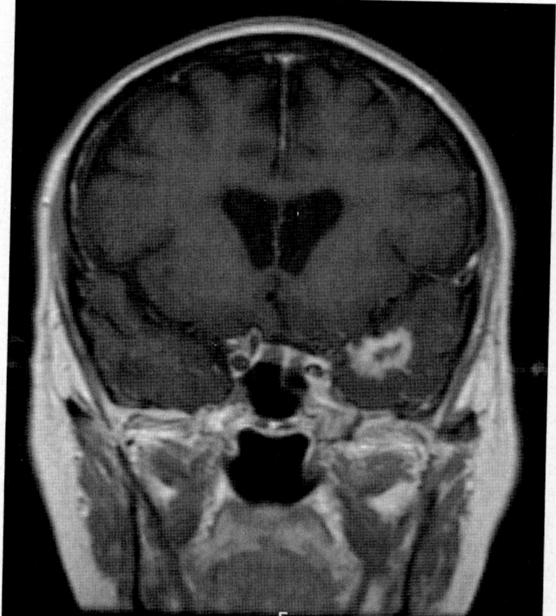

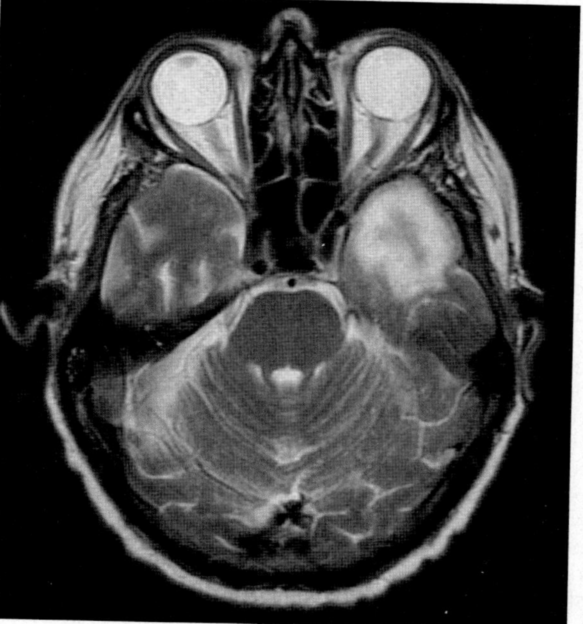

FIGURE 156.5 Toxoplasmosis. A 58-year-old man developed seizures and aphasia 8 months after allogeneic stem cell transplant for chronic Epstein-Barr virus lymphoproliferative disorder. Brain biopsy showed toxoplasmosis. **A:** Coronal T1-weighted image shows a necrotic lesion in the left anterior temporal lobe. **B:** Axial T2-weighted image shows significant edema. The magnetic resonance imaging differential diagnosis included infection, lymphoma, and glioma.

and hemophagocytic syndrome have been described). Although definitive diagnosis of toxoplasmosis relies on demonstration of tachyzoites and cysts in histopathologic sections, PCR applied to serum and CSF has become widely used and may facilitate earlier diagnosis.[155,158] The initial treatment of choice for toxoplasmosis is oral sulfadiazine 1 to 1.5 grams every 6 hours plus pyrimethamine (loading dose of 200 mg, followed by 75 mg daily). Folinic acid (10–20 mg daily) should be administered to reduce myeloid toxicity. At 4 to 6 weeks after resolution of symptoms and signs of infection and radiologic improvement, switching to a maintenance regimen (sulfadiazine 0.5 to 1 g 4 times daily plus pyrimethamine 50 mg/day) is reasonable. Maintenance therapy should be continued for the duration of immunosuppression and until radiologic resolution. In patients intolerant of sulfonamides, clindamycin and primaquine may be used instead after verifying normal glucose-6-phosphate dehydrogenase activity. Atovaquone has also been used after exhausting other options.

Dementias

Patients with cancer may develop a chronic dementia related to leukoencephalopathy, a debilitating complication of therapy for their malignancy. The combination of cranial radiation therapy and intrathecal or systemic methotrexate has been most closely linked with leukoencephalopathy, although other intrathecal regimens may produce similar findings.

PML is a demyelinating disease associated with lytic infection of oligodendrocytes by the human polyomavirus JC virus. Patients may develop rapidly progressive dementia as well as focal motor or cerebellar findings. Today this disease is most commonly seen in patients with advanced AIDS. Occasionally, PML is seen in severely immunocompromised persons with hematologic malignancies and in HSCT recipients. Several cases associated with the use of rituximab[29] have prompted an advisory by the FDA regarding a possible association. MRI typically shows unilateral or bilateral white matter disease without mass effect or enhancement. Diagnosis is generally established by detection of the JC virus in spinal fluid by PCR (90% sensitivity); PML can also be diagnosed by brain biopsy. There is no established therapy for PML. In patients with AIDS, highly active antiretroviral therapy is the best option. By extrapolation, it is logical to try to reduce immunosuppressive therapy in persons with cancer and PML as a means of augmenting cell-mediated immunity.

Genitourinary Infections

Neutropenic patients with a urinary tract infection are less likely to show pyuria, and are far more likely to become bacteremic compared with nonneutropenic patients. Asymptomatic candiduria is common in patients with bladder catheters. Removal of indwelling bladder catheters and cessation of antibacterial agents frequently leads to clearing of candiduria. Therefore, routine treatment of asymptomatic candiduria is not warranted. However, because of the risk of candidemia following genitourinary tract manipulations, candiduria should be treated before such procedures are performed. Patients with neutropenic fever and candiduria receive systemic antifungal therapy because of the potential of occult invasive candidiasis.

Hemorrhagic cystitis is a common consequence of some cytotoxic regimens, particularly cyclophosphamide. A viral etiology should be considered in HSCT recipients and other immunocompromised patients with unexplained hematuria. Adenovirus, the polyomavirus BK, and, rarely, CMV have been associated with hemorrhagic cystitis. Adenovirus hemorrhagic cystitis is usually self-limited, and the value of antiviral therapy is unclear. Low-dose cidofovir (1–3 mg/kg/week, without probenecid) is sometimes used with the aim of preventing disseminated adenovirus disease. BK virus commonly reactivates after allogeneic HSCT, but only a minority of patients develop hemorrhagic cystitis; high plasma viral load correlates with risk of BK-virus-associated hemorrhagic cystitis.[159] Although BK virus is an important cause of renal insufficiency following kidney transplant, only very few cases of BK virus-associated nephropathy have been described after allogeneic HSCT. A retrospective study suggested that low-dose cidofovir may be effective therapy for BK virus-associated hemorrhagic cystitis, but evidence supporting its use requires a randomized controlled trial, as the disease tends to be self-limited.[160]

Infections in Surgical Oncology

Patients undergoing surgery for malignancies are at risk for infections as a result of anatomic factors and impaired host defense. We agree with consensus guidelines on antimicrobial prophylaxis for surgery.[161] Ertapenem may be more effective than cefotetan in the prevention of surgical-site infection in patients undergoing elective colorectal surgery, but may be associated with an increase in *C. difficile* infection.[162]

Patients with head and neck cancers who undergo procedures that breach the upper aerodigestive tract mucosa are at significant risk for infection related to tumor stage, previous chemotherapy, duration of preoperative hospital stay, permanent tracheostomy, and type of cancer (hypopharyngeal and laryngeal cancers have increased risk of infection).[163] Preoperative radiotherapy was associated with more severe infections and late wound complications. Prolonged perioperative prophylaxis offers no benefit over standard 1-day regimens.[164,165] Among clean-contaminated procedures, factors affecting postoperative wound infection rates were performance of bilateral neck dissections, disease stage, type of laryngectomy, and prior tracheotomy.[165] Among clean procedures, radical neck dissection was associated with a higher rate of infections.

The highest frequency of postoperative infections is associated with surgery for gastrointestinal malignancies, esophageal, gastric, and pancreatic tumors.[166] Surgical procedures involving hepatobiliary tumors may be associated with severe and protracted infections. The biliary tract is usually sterile. However, patients with obstructive malignancies are usually treated with stents or diverting procedures that enable colonization of the biliary tract with intestinal flora, which increases the risk of postoperative infection. In a retrospective analysis of 170 therapeutic biliary drainage procedures in 90 patients with cancer, the overall infection rate was 61%, despite the fact that most patients received prophylactic antibiotics.[167] Cholangitis and bacteremia were the most common manifestations and Enterobacteriaceae, *Enterococcus* sp. and *Candida* sp. were the most frequent pathogens.

Chemoembolization and radiofrequency ablation of hepatic tumors are effective in reducing tumor bulk, but also create a necrotic bed that may be seeded by intestinal bacteria, predisposing to infection. The incidence of infection following these procedures is ~1%. Prior biliary enteric anastomosis seems to be the primary determinant for developing a liver abscess following chemoembolization.[168] Bowel preparation and systemic prophylactic antibiotics active against enteric flora should be considered in patients undergoing hepatic chemoembolization or radiofrequency ablation with a history of prior biliary stenting or reconstruction.[169]

Patients with cancer undergoing major abdominal surgery are also at risk for nosocomial candidiasis. Other risk factors for candidemia include triple-lumen catheters and need for parenteral nutrition.[170] In patients with gastrointestinal perforations or anastomotic leaks, prophylaxis with fluconazole reduced the frequency of peritoneal candidiasis, and may be warranted in this high-risk group.[171]

Malnutrition is an important and often overlooked condition predisposing to postoperative infections and morbidity. Randomized studies have shown the value of perioperative enteral nutrition in reducing serious postoperative infections and hospitalization days in patients with cancer.[172,173]

SELECTED PATHOGENS OF INTEREST IN ONCOLOGY

SELECTED BACTERIAL INFECTIONS IN PATIENTS WITH CANCER

Gram-Positive Bacteria

Staphylococcus aureus

Staphylococcus aureus colonizes the nares and the skin of 40% of individuals, and can cause both local (wound infection, cellulitis) and systemic disease (bacteremia and its complications, including endocarditis, septic arthritis and osteomyelitis). Removal of intravascular catheters should be considered in all patients with *S. aureus* bacteremia. The frequency of endocarditis following *S. aureus* bacteremia is high enough that a transesophageal echocardiogram is advised by the American Heart Association.[174] A 2-week course of intravenous antibiotics may be given for *S. aureus* bacteremia with negative results on transesophageal echocardiogram.[174] Nafcillin is superior to vancomycin in preventing recurrence of *S. aureus* bacteremia following initial therapy.[175] Vancomycin should be reserved for MRSA infections or patients with significant beta-lactam allergies.

The incidence of nosocomial MRSA bloodstream infections is increasing. MRSA isolates are resistant to all beta-lactam antibiotics, and often are cross-resistant to multiple classes of antibiotics. There has also been a dramatic increase in the incidence of community-acquired MRSA.[176] Community-acquired MRSA strains are generally susceptible to clindamycin and TMP/SMX. The standard treatment for MRSA is vancomycin. However, clinical infections caused by vancomycin-intermediate and vancomycin-resistant *S. aureus* have been reported sporadically, generally in patients receiving prolonged courses of vancomycin.[177] Failure of vancomycin in MRSA bacteremia has been associated with increasing vancomycin minimum inhibitory concentrations well within what is currently considered the susceptible range.[178] Based on these observations, new guidelines on vancomycin dosing and therapeutic monitoring have been published.[179] Minimum serum vancomycin trough concentrations should always be maintained above 10 mg/L to avoid development of resistance.

Linezolid seems at least as effective as vancomycin against MRSA in most published studies,[180,181] and American Thoracic Society guidelines consider both linezolid and high-dose vancomycin (trough level of vancomycin of 15–20 mcg/mL) to be acceptable options for suspected or proven MRSA pneumonia. The major concern of linezolid in patients with cancer relates to duration-dependent marrow suppression. Short courses of linezolid do not appear to delay myeloid recovery in neutropenic patients with cancer[76]; however, experience with long durations of therapy (e.g., >14 days) is limited. Peripheral and optic neuropathies have also been described with prolonged linezolid administration.

Daptomycin, a bactericidal lipopeptide (6 mg/kg daily) is an acceptable option for *S. aureus* bacteremia, based on the results of a randomized controlled trial.[182] Daptomycin is inactivated by lung surfactant and therefore should not be used to treat pneumonia.

Infection control programs that include judicious use of antibiotics, early identification of patients who are MRSA carriers by targeted surveillance testing, and initiation of appropriate contact precautions seem to result in decreased incidence of *S. aureus* infections.[183,184]

Vancomycin-Resistant *Enterococcus* Species

Enterococcus species are the third most common cause of bloodstream infection in the United States. Approximately 50% of *E. faecium* and the minority of *E. faecalis* isolates are resistant to vancomycin,[185] and are typically multiply resistant to penicillin, ampicillin, and aminoglycosides. VRE bloodstream infection is an important cause of morbidity in patients with cancer. The portal of entry for enterococcal bacteremia may be an indwelling central catheter or defects in the gut mucosa from chemotherapy or radiation toxicity. Risk factors for VRE include prolonged hospitalization, neutropenia, chemotherapy-induced mucositis, and use of vancomycin, cephalosporins, and metronidazole.[186] In patients with cancer, VRE bloodstream infection was associated with a significant reduction in survival and frequent microbiologic failure, despite treatment with linezolid and/or daptomycin.[187]

Few antibiotics are effective against VRE. Quinupristin/dalfopristin, linezolid, and daptomycin are typically considered first-line agents. Tigecycline often shows activity *in vitro*. Linezolid and daptomycin were discussed previously in the *Staphylococcus aureus* section above. Quinupristin/dalfopristin is a 30:70 mixture of these two semisynthetic streptogramin antibiotics. It has been shown to be safe and effective in serious vancomycin-resistant *E. faecium* infections, but is not active against *E. faecalis*. The common adverse effects are arthralgias, myalgias, and conjugated hyperbilirubinemia may limit its use in cancer patients.[188] One randomized controlled trial comparing treatments for VRE bacteremia showed that both quinupristin/dalfopristin and linezolid have similar (moderate) efficacy.[188] The reported results with daptomycin seem to be similar.[189]

We usually select linezolid or daptomycin as first-line agents for VRE. Persistent enterococcal bacteremia despite appropriate antibiotic therapy should prompt an evaluation for an endovascular nidus (e.g., catheter-associated infection, infected thrombus, endocarditis). In our experience, patients with severe bowel mucosal toxicity (e.g., from chemotherapy for acute leukemia or severe gut GVHD) may have refractory VRE bacteremia. In this setting, treatment is based on anecdotal observations or *in vitro* susceptibility data, and it includes tigecycline as well as combination regimens.

Other Gram-Positive Bacteria

Viridans group streptococci, part of the normal oral flora, are known causes of bacteremia in neutropenic patients with severe mucositis. Other risk factors include prophylaxis with TMP/SMX or fluoroquinolones and the use of histamine-2 blockers. Neutropenic patients with viridans streptococcal bacteremia may have a 24- to 48-hour prodrome of low-grade fever and facial flushing, followed by high fever and chills. In as many as 25% of cases, bacteremia is complicated by a toxic-shocklike syndrome characterized by hypotension, respiratory distress, renal failure, and a centrifugal maculopapular rash usually starting on the trunk with subsequent desquamation of the palms and soles. Septic shock may be more common in children than in adults.[190]

Resistance of viridans group streptococci to beta-lactams has been recognized. We use vancomycin as initial therapy for bloodstream infections by viridans group streptococci pending susceptibility testing.

Gram-Negative Bacteria

Pseudomonas aeruginosa

Infections caused by *P. aeruginosa* continue to be frequently documented during neutropenic fever.[191] Many cases of *P. aeruginosa* bacteremia now occur in outpatients.[192]

No single antimicrobial is effective against 100% of pseudomonas isolates, which is the reason most authorities recommend combining an antipseudomonal beta-lactam antibiotic and an aminoglycoside until the antibiogram is available. Serious infections due to strains of *P. aeruginosa* resistant to all common antipseudomonal agents are an increasingly serious problem.[193] Emergence of resistance to antibiotics during therapy may occur. Colistin administered parenterally[194] or aerosolized (in infections limited to the lung)[195,196] may be considered as salvage therapy. The continuous infusion of ceftazidime or other beta-lactam antibiotics has also been used in attempts to prevent or overcome the emergence of resistance during therapy.[197]

Other Resistant Gram-Negative Bacilli

The emergence of multidrug-resistant Gram-negative bacilli is an important challenge in the treatment of nosocomial infections, particularly in immunocompromised patient with cancer. *S. maltophilia* and *Klebsiella pneumoniae* carbapenemase–producing strains are resistant to carbapenems (e.g., imipenem, meropenem). There are also sporadic outbreaks of drug-resistant pathogens, such as *Acinetobacter* species. Their increasing incidence at several centers highlights the need for judicious use of antibiotics[198] and compliance with Infection Control policies. Knowledge of the local prevalence of these drug-resistant pathogens is essential to guide the initial selection of antibiotics.

Stenotrophomonas maltophilia colonizes hospital environments and establishes carriage in patients who have been treated with broad-spectrum antimicrobial agents. This organism has become an increasingly important cause of nosocomial infections in patients with cancer.[199] Clinical manifestations include catheter-associated cellulitis, bacteremia, pneumonia, endocarditis, mastoiditis, meningitis, and disseminated nodular soft tissue infection.[200] *Stenotrophomonas maltophilia* is resistant to carbapenems and often broadly resistant to other agents. The majority of strains are susceptible to TMP/SMX, which is the preferred initial antibiotic for this organism. If TMP/SMX cannot be used, there have been reports of success with ticarcillin-clavulanic acid and fluoroquinolones (particularly moxifloxacin). Tigecycline is active *in vitro*, and may be another option. Colistin is active against most isolates.

Acinetobacter species also colonize hospital environments, are a common cause of ventilator-associated pneumonia and catheter-related bacteremia, and have caused nosocomial outbreaks.[201] Infections caused by multidrug-resistant *Acinetobacter* (resistant to carbapenems) species may require intravenous colistin as a last resort. Resistance to tigecycline develops rapidly.

Legionella Species

Infection by *Legionella* species most commonly occurs following inhalation of contaminated droplets from water distribution systems. Nosocomial legionellosis has been linked to contamination of hospital water. *Legionella* infections are associated with compromised cellular immunity. In the cancer population, patients at highest risk include those receiving high-dose corticosteroids, T-cell–depleting agents, and allogeneic HSCT. The typical presentation is acute pneumonia with either a focal or diffuse infiltrate. Gastrointestinal symptoms (diarrhea) and myalgias (sometimes with elevated creatine phosphokinase) are common. There are no clinical or radiologic criteria that reliably distinguish legionellosis from pneumococcal pneumonia. A combination of culture (special culture medium required) and urinary antigen test is the optimal diagnostic combination in most situations.[202] The urine legionella antigen assay is sensitive and specific for *Legionella pneumophila* serogroup 1, the isolate responsible for up to 80% of clinical disease; however, it does not detect other serogroups or *Legionella* species. PCR on respiratory secretions is both sensitive and specific for *Legionella* detection, but standardized assays are not commercially available.[202] Azithromycin or fluoroquinolones (e.g., levofloxacin, moxifloxacin) are standard therapy for legionellosis.

Mycobacteria

Host defense against *Mycobacterium* species relies principally on cellular immunity. In the immunocompromised patient, the clinical manifestations of infection due to *Mycobacterium tuberculosis* may be atypical. Cavitary lung disease is less commonly observed. The chest radiograph may show an isolated nodule, an infiltrate, or a diffuse reticulonodular pattern. Disseminated disease is more common. The chest radiograph may be negative in patients with disseminated or extrapulmonary tuberculosis. Extrapulmonary manifestations may include meningitis, brain abscess, vertebral or paravertebral abscess, septic joint, hepatic and splenic disease, and bone marrow involvement. The tuberculin test may not be helpful in this patient population. Detection of mycobacterial DNA in clinical specimens by nucleic acid amplification methods may facilitate a more rapid diagnosis.

Systemic *Mycobacterium bovis* infection mimicking miliary tuberculosis may rarely occur following intravesicular therapy with *Bacille Calmette-Guerin* for bladder cancer.[203]

Infection with nontuberculous mycobacteria is well described among patients with cancer, particularly in patients with hematologic malignancies. Speciation of mycobacterial isolates is essential because nontuberculous mycobacteria are typically resistant to regimens for *M. tuberculosis*. Clinical manifestations include pneumonia, soft tissue or wound infections, and central catheter infections that may require surgical excision of the infected tunnel site. Pulmonary *Mycobacterium kansasii* infection is associated with significant chest radiographic findings, but relatively indolent symptoms, and responds well to rifampin-containing regimens.[204] The American Thoracic Society has published guidelines on the diagnosis and treatment of tuberculosis[205] and nontuberculous mycobacterial infections.[206]

Nocardia Species

Patients with hematologic malignancy, allogeneic HSCT recipients, lymphopenia, and receiving corticosteroids are at highest risk.[207] Bronchopneumonia, lobar pneumonia, nodules, or necrotizing abscesses with cavitation are observed. Empyema and extension to the chest wall may occur. Dissemination may include brain abscess, meningitis, osteomyelitis, soft tissue mass, cutaneous abscess, and liver abscess. It is important to alert the microbiology laboratory when nocardiosis is suspected so that a modified acid stain is performed, and appropriate culture conditions are used and culture plates are held for weeks instead of days. Treatment of nocardial infections is based on case series. Most experience is with TMP/SMX but other agents that have been used include carbapenems, minocycline, ceftriaxone, and linezolid.[208,209] Amikacin is active *in vitro* and may be used in combination. Surgical drainage or resection should be considered in cases refractory to medical therapy. Therapy should be continued for several months to a year.

Fungal Infections in Patients with Cancer

Pathogenic fungi include yeasts and molds. *Candida* species are yeasts that form part of the normal flora; they gain access to the bloodstream through disruption of anatomic barriers (mucositis or indwelling catheters). Molds are ubiquitous soil inhabitants whose conidia or spores are inhaled on a regular basis. Aspergillosis is the most common mold infection in cancer patients, but other pathogenic fungi (e.g., zygomycetes, *Fusarium* and *Scedosporium* species) have become more common over the past 20 years. Table 156.7 summarizes antifungal agents commonly used in patients with cancer. In-depth practice guidelines for the management of the different fungal diseases have been issued by the IDSA.[210–212]

Candidiasis

Oropharyngeal and Esophageal Candidiasis. Oral mucosal candidiasis ("thrush") is common with T-cell immunodeficiency. Cytotoxic chemotherapy, corticosteroids, and antibiotics predispose to oral candidiasis. The most common presentation is white adherent plaques on the palate, buccal mucosa, tongue, or gingiva. A wet mount or Gram stain showing pseudohyphae establishes the diagnosis. Therapy includes local treatments such as clotrimazole troches or oral fluconazole.

Esophageal candidiasis causes odynophagia. The differential diagnosis includes HSV, CMV (principally in HSCT recipients), and bacteria. Initial therapy with fluconazole is advised for esophageal candidiasis. Options for fluconazole-resistant mucosal candidiasis include an echinocandin, voriconazole, posaconazole, or amphotericin B formulation. Most fluconazole-resistant *Candida* isolates are susceptible to voriconazole and posaconazole, but cross-resistance may occur.

Candidemia. Candida species are the fourth most common cause of nosocomial bloodstream infections in the United States. Clinical findings vary from asymptomatic to full-blown septic shock. The species should be identified. *Candida albicans* is the most common, and it is usually susceptible to fluconazole, but the proportion of non-albicans *Candida* has been increasing. *Candida tropicalis* is highly virulent in neutropenic hosts but is susceptible to most agents. *Candida krusei* is always resistant to fluconazole and *Candida glabrata* has variable susceptibility. *Candida parapsilosis* is mostly associated with the vascular catheters and lipid formulations used for total parenteral nutrition, and is usually susceptible to fluconazole. A minority of *Candida lusitaniae* and *Candida guilliermondii* isolates are resistant to amphotericin B.

It is recommended to remove all intravascular catheters in patients with candidemia.[211] In neutropenic patients candidemia may arise from defects in the gut mucosa rather than the catheter,[213,214] so the need for catheter removal has been questioned.[215] In general, we remove the catheter where feasible, but sometimes attempt to conserve it when vascular access is limited and thrombocytopenia is present. We immediately remove all intravenous catheters in the setting of clinical instability, lack of resolution of fever within 2 to 3 days, or persistent candidemia after 2 days of appropriate antifungal therapy. Ophthalmologic examination to evaluate for retinitis is advised in patients with candidemia.

Chronic Disseminated Candidiasis. Chronic disseminated candidiasis (also called *hepatosplenic candidiasis*) is a complication of highly mucotoxic chemotherapy regimens, such as those used as induction therapy for acute leukemia. It has become less common with the widespread use of systemic antifungal prophylaxis with azoles. The typical picture is persistent fever after neutrophil recovery with elevation of liver enzymes (particularly alkaline phosphatase). Numerous target lesions in the liver and spleen become apparent by CT scan, ultrasonography, or MRI.

Frequently, the differential diagnosis includes the hematologic malignancy that was being treated. A liver biopsy is required for a definitive diagnosis, but because the lesions are discrete, a blind percutaneous biopsy may be falsely negative. Blood and biopsy cultures are almost always negative, but the pathology is diagnostic. We recommend surgical liver biopsy when the diagnosis is in question. Chronic disseminated candidiasis that is controlled with antifungal therapy is not a contraindication to subsequent chemotherapy or HSCT.[216]

Therapy for Invasive Candidiasis. An echinocandin (caspofungin, micafungin, or anidulafungin) or a lipid formulation of amphotericin B is recommended for candidemia in neutropenic patients.[211] In patients receiving an azole who develop breakthrough candidemia, an echinocandin is advised. Azoles (generally, fluconazole) can be used as step-down oral agents or as initial therapy in certain patients at lower risk for mortality and serious complications. Voriconazole does not have a demonstrated advantage over fluconazole, but can be considered for treatment of *C. krusei* (which is intrinsically fluconazole-resistant) infection and when a mold-active agent is warranted (e.g., as prophylaxis in a high-risk patient). We reserve amphotericin B products for unusual complicated cases, such as meningitis and endocarditis, in which data to support optimal therapy are lacking. Some authorities still prefer a lipid formulation of amphotericin B in neutropenic patients, particularly in the presence of hemodynamic instability.

Invasive *Aspergillosis*

Risk Factors and Clinical Manifestations. Prolonged and persistent neutropenia is a critical risk factor for IA.[4] In HSCT, most cases, however, take place during episodes of active GVHD treated with high doses of corticosteroids. Other risk factors for aspergillosis after allogeneic HSCT include T-cell–depleted transplant, lymphopenia, CMV disease, and respiratory virus infections.[8,15,217] Aspergillosis can involve virtually any organ in the immunocompromised host, but sinopulmonary disease is the most common. Angioinvasion of hyphae leading to vascular thrombosis and tissue infarction and coagulative necrosis is characteristic. Clinical manifestations of aspergillosis are quite variable. During neutropenia, persistent fever, chest pain and a pleural rub are common, although nonspecific, signs. When steroids are the only risk factor, the manifestations may be subtle, and sometimes a pulmonary infiltrate is found in the absence of symptoms.

Diagnosis of Invasive Aspergillosis. The most common finding on chest CT in early invasive pulmonary aspergillosis in patients with neutropenia and HSCT recipients is the presence of one or more well-circumscribed nodules.[218] These may be inapparent on chest radiographs (Fig. 156.2). Other characteristic findings include the halo sign, a haziness surrounding a nodule or infiltrate representing alveolar hemorrhage, and the "crescent sign" (cavitation that usually coincides with neutrophil recovery. These signs reflect different stages of hemorrhagic infarction secondary to angioinvasive organisms.[219] Sequential CT scans of neutropenic patients with invasive aspergillosis demonstrated that halo signs were common at diagnosis but decreased during the first week of infection as the frequency of the "air crescent sign" increased.[220] The median volume of lesions increased during the first week of therapy and remained stable during the second week.

BAL cultures have approximately 50% sensitivity in focal pulmonary lesions,[221] and definitive diagnosis often requires an invasive procedure and is usually made only when the disease is advanced. The use of galactomannan antigen seems to be much more sensitive.[125] Isolation of an *Aspergillus* species from sputum or BAL should be presumed to represent invasive disease in neutropenic patients.[222]

Both the serum *Aspergillus* galactomannan and beta-glucan assays,[223] immunoassays that detect fungal antigens in peripheral blood, have been accepted as diagnostic adjuncts of invasive fungal infections in the revised European Organisation for Research and Treatment of Cancer/Mycosis Study Group (EORTC/MSG) consensus criteria.[224] PCR-based detection is considered investigational. These immunoassays have three potential uses: (1) as a diagnostic adjunct, (2) as a surveillance tool in high-risk patients (e.g., allogeneic HSCT recipients) to detect early aspergillosis prior to clinically overt disease, and (3) in monitoring response to antifungal therapy.[225,226] The sensitivity of the galactomannan assay is significantly reduced by concomitant mold-active antifungal agents,[227] and false-positive results may be more common in allogeneic HSCT recipients[128] or with concomitant piperacillin/tazobactam.[228,229] A meta-analysis showed that the galactomannan assay had a sensitivity of 70% and specificity of 89% for proven IA, but that the accuracy of the test was variable among different patient populations.[230] A rising serum galactomannan correlates with failure of antifungal therapy and decreasing galactomannan correlates with a positive outcome in patients with IA.[231–236]

The serum beta-D-glucan assay has recently received FDA approval as a diagnostic adjunct. In patients with acute myeloid leukemia and myelodysplastic syndrome, the assay was highly sensitive and specific in detecting early invasive fungal infections, including candidiasis, fusariosis, trichosporonosis, and aspergillosis.[237] It does not detect zygomycosis.

Therapy for Invasive Aspergillosis. Voriconazole is currently the treatment of choice of invasive aspergillosis, because in a randomized controlled trial it was more effective than amphotericin B (successful outcomes: 53% vs. 32%) and was associated with significantly improved survival (71% vs. 58%).[128] Voriconazole led to a successful outcome in 34% of patients with CNS aspergillosis.[238] Voriconazole appears to have comparable safety and efficacy in children with invasive mold infections compared to adults.[239] Three different lipid formulations of amphotericin B are available: amphotericin B colloidal dispersion,[240] amphotericin B lipid complex,[241] and liposomal amphotericin B. The lipid formulations have less nephrotoxicity than conventional amphotericin B deoxycholate, and are therefore more suitable for long-term administration. A randomized controlled trial has shown that liposomal amphotericin B at a dose of 3 mg/kg per day is at least as effective, and less toxic, than 10 mg/kg per day[242] for invasive aspergillosis

Posaconazole is a broad-spectrum azole, so far only available in oral form, which has been used successfully as salvage therapy for a variety of invasive fungal infections refractory to standard therapy. The overall success rate of posaconazole in patients with IA refractory or intolerant of standard therapy was 42%.[243] Echinocandins have not been evaluated as initial monotherapy for invasive aspergillosis in controlled trials. Caspofungin as salvage therapy in patients with invasive aspergillosis led to a favorable response in 37 of 83 patients (45%).[244]

There has been significant interest in combination antifungal therapy pairing an echinocandin with either an amphotericin B preparation or a mold-active azole. The rationale is that echinocandins target a site (the beta-glucan constituent of the fungal cell wall) distinct from the polyenes and azoles that target the fungal cell membrane. *In vitro* and animal models data have been encouraging, and uncontrolled clinical studies suggest minimal toxicity and potentially improved outcome of aspergillosis.[245–248] The question of combination is far from settled, and a randomized prospective study comparing voriconazole plus anidulafungin versus voriconazole alone as primary therapy for invasive aspergillosis is underway.

Patients who recover from an episode of invasive aspergillosis are at risk for relapse of infection during subsequent immunosuppression.[249] Secondary prophylaxis with a mold-active agent is advised for the entire period of immunosuppression.

Zygomycosis ("Mucormycosis")

Risk factors for zygomycosis (commonly termed *mucormycosis*) include diabetic ketoacidosis, protein-calorie malnutrition, iron overload, desferrioxamine (but not other iron chelators), corticosteroid therapy, and prolonged neutropenia. Patients receiving potent cytotoxic chemotherapy for leukemia are at risk for locally invasive as well as disseminated disease.[250] Zygomycosis typically manifests as rhinocerebral or pulmonary disease following inhalation of spores. In rhinocerebral disease, fever, facial pain, and headache are common. Contiguous extension may lead to orbital involvement with proptosis and extraocular muscle paresis, involvement of hard palate, and spread to the brain. Several studies have noted an increased incidence of zygomycosis in patients receiving voriconazole.[251–253] Among patients with hematologic malignancies and allogeneic HSCT recipients, invasive sinus disease and use of voriconazole favored a diagnosis of zygomycosis over aspergillosis.[253]

Therapy for zygomycosis involves amphotericin B lipid formulation (5 mg/kg/d) plus early and aggressive surgical debridement in cases of localized cutaneous or sinus disease. Voriconazole and echinocandins are not active against zygomycetes. Posaconazole has shown promising results as salvage therapy.[254,255]

Less Common Molds

Fusarium species and *Scedosporium* species have become increasingly important causes of mortality in leukemia and in allogeneic HSCT recipients.[256] The likelihood of infection by a *Fusarium* species is increased by the presence of disseminated cutaneous lesions and isolation of a mold from blood culture.[121] Therapy for invasive fusariosis generally involves voriconazole, posaconazole, or a lipid formulation of amphotericin B. *Scedosporium* species are resistant to amphotericin B; therapy for *Scedosporium apiospermum* generally involves itraconazole, voriconazole, or posaconazole. Dark-walled molds can cause subcutaneous infection in immunocompetent persons following traumatic inoculation; pneumonia, CNS disease, and dissemination can occur in severely immunocompromised persons. Itraconazole, voriconazole, or posaconazole are appropriate initial therapy.

Adjunctive Therapy for Invasive Mold Infections

Corticosteroid therapy should be reduced or discontinued if possible. The use of G-CSF, GM-CSF, and granulocyte transfusions are discussed in the section "Fever and Neutropenia." Interferon-gamma, a cytokine produced by lymphocytes (CD4+, CD8+, natural killer cells) as well as macrophages and perhaps neutrophils, confers protection against a variety of experimental fungal infections in animals.[257] It has been used as adjunctive therapy in cases of refractory fungal disease,[258] even following allogeneic HCT.[259,260] We reserve recombinant interferon-gamma for patients with life-threatening invasive mold infections refractory to standard antifungal therapy. The efficacy of this approach is not established.

Cryptococcus Neoformans

Host defense against cryptococcal infection is principally dependent on cellular immunity. Among patients with cancer, those with hematologic malignancies, receiving high-dose corticosteroids, and allogeneic HSCT recipients are at highest risk for cryptococcosis. The principal portal of entry of this organism is likely via inhalation, with subsequent spread to the blood and then to the CNS.

Although meningitis is the most common presentation of cryptococcal infection, other manifestations include primary pneumonia, pulmonary nodules, fungemia, and cutaneous and visceral dissemination. Diagnosis in disseminated disease may be obtained by determining cryptococcal antigen in the peripheral blood; in cases of localized disease tissue must be obtained. In immunocompromised patients, the preferred regimen is amphotericin B (0.7 mg/kg daily) plus 5-flucytosine (100 mg/kg daily) for the first 2 weeks, followed by maintenance fluconazole therapy (400 mg daily). In neutropenic patients, reduction of the dosage of 5-flucytosine may be considered to avoid delay in myeloid recovery. Because fluconazole is well tolerated, continuing therapy with this agent for several months (or longer if intensive immunosuppressive therapy is continued) is reasonable.[210]

Endemic Dimorphic Fungi

These organisms include *Histoplasma capsulatum, Coccidioides immitis, Blastomyces dermatitidis*, and *Penicillium marneffei. P. marneffei* is endemic in Southeast Asia. These fungi are dimorphic, existing in nature in the fruiting mycelial stage and converting to the yeast stage at body temperature.

Endemic mycoses in the central United States (e.g., Ohio River valley) include histoplasmosis and blastomycosis. In the immunocompetent host, inhalation of *Histoplasma microconidia* is typically asymptomatic, but may manifest with acute fever, pulmonary infiltrates, and hypoxia. Immunocompromised patients have a higher risk of disseminated histoplasmosis involving the liver, spleen, lymph nodes, bone marrow, adrenal glands, mucocutaneous tissues, gastrointestinal tract, and CNS. The chest radiograph may show a miliary reticulonodular appearance, suggestive of tuberculosis. An acute sepsis syndrome with hypotension and disseminated intravascular coagulation, adrenal crisis, and meningitis are potentially lethal complications.

Blood culture (preferably lysis-centrifugation) may be positive in disseminated histoplasmosis. Antigen detection in blood, urine, and BAL is sensitive and specific.[261] Antibody detection may also be useful, but false-negative results may occur in immunocompromised patients.[262] Biopsy of specimens may show small intracellular or narrow budding yeasts suggestive of the diagnosis, which should be confirmed by culture. Severe pulmonary or disseminated histoplasmosis should be treated with an amphotericin B formulation.[263] Prolonged therapy with itraconazole may be initiated after stabilization of disease, and should probably be continued for the duration of immunosuppression.[263]

Coccidioides immitis is endemic in the southwestern United States. In healthy persons, infection is usually asymptomatic or self-limited. In patients with compromised cell-mediated immunity, *C. immitis* is more likely to cause disease. A large series in patients with hematologic malignancies reported a high rate of treatment failure and death.[264] Serology was positive in only 55% of the patients. The diagnosis was most often established by finding the fungus in BAL, sputum, or biopsies. Coccidioidomycosis can involve virtually any organ in disseminated disease but has a particular trophism for bone and the CNS. Therapy for disseminated disease generally requires amphotericin B followed by maintenance fluconazole. Intracisternal amphotericin B can be considered in cases of coccidioidal meningitis refractory to systemic treatment.[265]

Pneumocystis (Carinii) Jirovecii

Pneumocystis jirovecii (formerly *P. carinii*) is more appropriately classified as a fungus than a protozoan based on gene sequence data and cell wall constituents. Defective T-cell immunity is the principal risk factor for PCP. Corticosteroid use is the main risk factor in patients without AIDS.[266]

Pneumocystis jirovecii can have a more fulminant course in non-AIDS patients compared with AIDS patients, with more rapid progression to respiratory failure.[267] Patients treated with corticosteroids may develop initial clinical manifestations of PCP only during steroid taper. Bilateral interstitial infiltrates are most common in PCP, although unilateral or patchy infiltrates are also observed. Nodules, cavitary lesions, and pleural effusions are less common. In a minority of patients, the chest radiograph is normal. Extrapulmonary *P. jirovecii* infection is very rare in patients with cancer, and has for the most part been reported only in patients with AIDS.

Diagnosis of PCP relies on visualization of the organism microscopically, as it does not grow in culture. BAL is the standard diagnostic modality for PCP, but induced sputum has acceptable yield in some institutions.[268] Immunofluorescent staining using monoclonal antibodies is more sensitive than silver staining or Wright-Giemsa staining.[269] Patients with cancer have reduced organism burden compared with HIV-infected people, which decreases the sensitivity of every diagnostic modality. Quantitative PCR of respiratory samples may be the most sensitive test in this setting.[270] As pneumocystis is a fungus, PCP frequently results in a positive serum beta-glucan test.[271]

TMP/SMX (trimethoprim: 15 mg/kg daily in three divided doses) is the treatment of choice for *P. jirovecii*. If TMP/SMX is not feasible because of significant allergy or toxicity, intravenous pentamidine or pyrimethamine plus clindamycin can be used. In cases of mild or moderate PCP (which has been defined as room air $Pao_2 >70$ torr) in patients intolerant of TMP/SMX, dapsone-trimethoprim, clindamycin-primaquine, and atovaquone are acceptable options, but the efficacy of all these is less than that of TMP/SMX. In patients with moderate or severe PCP ($Pao_2 \leq 70$ torr), corticosteroids should be added based on studies of patients with AIDS-associated PCP. In patients who are not responding to therapy, repeat bronchoscopy should be considered to exclude additional pathogens.

Viral Infections

Table 156.8 summarizes common antiviral agents used in persons with cancer.

Herpes Viruses

Herpes Simplex Virus. The herpes viruses are DNA viruses that establish latency after primary infection. Host defense against these viruses is dependent on viral-specific helper and cytotoxic T lymphocytes. HSV disease is a common complication of prolonged chemotherapy-induced neutropenia in patients not receiving antiviral prophylaxis. Oropharyngeal HSV (mostly caused by HSV-1) during neutropenia may be severe, causing gingival disease, stomatitis, and cheilitis, clinically indistinguishable from mucositis following cytotoxic chemotherapy. HSV is usually diagnosed by culture or PCR. In immunocompromised patients with significant mucosal disease, we treat with intravenous acyclovir (5 mg/kg every 8 hours), switching to an oral regimen (e.g., valacyclovir or famciclovir) when the disease has improved. Disseminated HSV disease should be treated with intravenous acyclovir (10 mg/kg every 8 hours). Acyclovir-resistant HSV is occasionally observed in HSCT recipients.[272] When acyclovir resistance is suspected, the decision to switch therapy (generally to foscarnet) should be made on clinical grounds as antiviral susceptibility testing of the isolate at a reference laboratory takes weeks.

Cytomegalovirus. CMV disease is uncommon in cancer patients except following HSCT (either allogeneic or T-cell–depleted autologous) or after receiving alemtuzumab. An overview of the prevention of CMV disease was presented in the "Diagnosis and Management of Infectious Diseases Syndromes" section. Here we will discuss the most common syndromes caused by CMV.[273]

CMV Pneumonitis. Pulmonary disease typically manifests as bilateral infiltrates resembling PCP with hypoxia and progression to respiratory failure. In transplant patients the diagnosis is established by a compatible clinical syndrome with detection of CMV in BAL (by culture or cytopathology showing characteristic intracytoplasmic and intranuclear inclusions) or tissue (by culture or histologic diagnosis).[274] In nontransplant patients CMV pneumonia is rare, and the culture alone is not considered sufficient to make the diagnosis as CMV can be shed from pulmonary secretions without causing invasive disease. Demonstration of intracellular CMV inclusions on BAL is diagnostic of disease, but is uncommon. In many cases, other pathogens are found, including *P. aeruginosa, Legionella, Aspergillus* species, *Mycobacteria* species, *Nocardia* species, toxoplasmosis, or respiratory viruses.[275]

We treat CMV pneumonia with ganciclovir or foscarnet plus immunoglobulin (either regular IVIG or CMV-specific). The benefit of immunoglobulin is based on historical controls and has been questioned.[273] Cidofovir may be considered in cases of CMV disease after failure or intolerance to ganciclovir or foscarnet.[276]

CMV colitis. CMV disease can occur at any location within the gastrointestinal tract. In the esophagus, ulcerations may resemble HSV or candidal esophagitis. Definitive identification of CMV in these cases relies on biopsy or cytology. CMV colitis is associated with abdominal pain and diarrhea that clinically resembles GVHD. CMV involvement of enteric vessels may result in hemorrhage and infarction. For documented CMV infection of the gastrointestinal tract, we administer ganciclovir or foscarnet for 4 to 6 weeks.[273] There is no evidence that adding IVIG results in better outcome.

Other syndromes. CMV hepatitis should be considered in the setting of fever and elevations of liver enzymes. A liver biopsy documenting CMV inclusions is diagnostic. Less common sites of CMV disease in HSCT recipients include pancreas, brain, spinal cord (transverse myelitis), and adrenals. CMV retinitis, the most common complication in patients with AIDS, is uncommon in transplant recipients. A CMV syndrome associated with fever, pancytopenia, and CMV viremia may precede the development of organ-specific disease.

Varicella Zoster Virus. In immunocompromised patients, VZV infection may manifest with a multidermatomal or disseminated vesicular exanthem sometimes associated with hemorrhage and necrosis. Secondary bacterial infections, usually due to streptococci or *S. aureus*, may occur. Visceral involvement of VZV can manifest as hemorrhagic pneumonia, encephalitis, retinal necrosis, hepatitis, and small bowel disease. The diagnosis of cutaneous zoster can usually be made by visual inspection alone. Immunofluorescent staining of material from an unroofed skin lesion or from a skin biopsy can establish the diagnosis within hours. Disseminated zoster without skin lesions should be considered as a cause of severe abdominal pain, sometimes with concomitant syndrome of inadequate antidiuretic hormone secretion. Blood PCR may be diagnostic in this setting.

Intravenous acyclovir (10 mg/kg every 8 hours) is the established treatment for primary varicella (chicken pox) or disseminated zoster in immunocompromised patients. For localized dermatomal zoster, we use an oral regimen consisting of acyclovir (800 mg 5 times per day) or valacyclovir (1 g 3 times per day), or famciclovir (500 mg 3 times per day).

Nosocomial transmission of VZV is well documented. Patients with chicken pox, disseminated zoster, and immunocompromised patients with dermatomal zoster should be placed under contact and respiratory isolation. In the absence of varicella-zoster immune globulin, oral acyclovir for 2 weeks after exposure has been used successfully for postexposure prophylaxis.[277]

The two available live attenuated varicella vaccines are Varivax (used to induce immunity in persons who have not been exposed to varicella) and Zostavax (for older immunocompetent persons with prior exposure to varicella to augment immunity to prevent shingles). Neither vaccine should be used in highly immunosuppressed persons because of the risk of viral disease. Household contacts of immunocompromised patients and health care workers with no history of varicella and seronegative for VZV should receive the Varivax vaccine to prevent infection by wild type varicella.[32] If a rash occurs following vaccination, direct contact with immunocompromised persons should be avoided.

Epstein Barr Virus-Induced Posttransplant Lymphoproliferative Disorder. Most adults have been infected by EBV. Latent infection persists in B cells and produces no disease in the vast majority of people. EBV-specific cytotoxic T lymphocytes are the main controllers of the replication of EBV-infected B cells. EBV lymphoproliferative disorders are encountered in patients with severely impaired T-cell immunity, such as AIDS or intensive and prolonged immunosuppressive therapy. EBV-induced PTLD is defined as an abnormal proliferation of EBV-infected B cells in a transplant recipient. The lesions may be composed of polyclonal or monoclonal populations of transformed B cells. PTLD is most common between 1 and 6 months after allogeneic HSCT. Typically, the proliferating B cells are of donor origin. Immunosuppressive therapy for GVHD and T-cell–depleted allografts increases the risk of PTLD. Uncontrolled EBV infection may also cause a hemophagocytic syndrome that is characterized clinically by pancytopenia, hepatosplenomegaly, and fever.[278]

Clinical manifestations of PTLD are varied. Patients may have a mononucleosislike syndrome with fever and localized adenopathy. Disseminated disease may manifest with generalized adenopathy and extranodal organ involvement, including the bowel, liver, bone marrow, and CNS. A CT–positron emission tomography scan is useful in a high-risk patient with unexplained fever. Diagnosis of PTLD requires a biopsy showing the characteristic histology and evidence of EBV infection by immunohistochemistry or EBV DNA detection.

Whereas PTLD in organ transplant recipients typically responds to a reduction in the intensity of immunosuppression, PTLD in HSCT recipients may not respond to such conservative measures. Antiviral agents may attenuate the lytic cycle of EBV and reduce the frequency of new B-cell clones, but they will not affect the replication of EBV-transformed PTLD B cells, and are not useful. Other strategies include rituximab,[279] low-dose chemotherapy, anti-IL-6, donor lymphocyte infusions, and adoptive immunotherapy using donor-derived EBV-specific cytotoxic T-lymphocyte clones.[280] However, using alloreactive T cells in such unfractionated preparations may induce GVHD. A potentially safer approach involves transfer of EBV-specific donor CTL clones.[281,282] Adoptive transfer of EBV-specific CTLs has been generally safe and effective in controlling PTLD and in preventing EBV lymphoproliferative disorders when used prophylactically.[283]

Human Herpesvirus 6. HHV-6, the cause of roseola infantum, may also reactivate during immunosuppression. Reactivation is predictable after allogeneic transplant and more common with more intensive immunosuppression (peripheral HHV-6 levels are higher in recipients of allografts from unrelated donors[284] and cord blood[285]). Disease associations are difficult to establish, but there is convincing evidence HHV-6 may cause myelosuppression, pneumonitis, and encephalitis (see "Meningitis/Meningoencephalitis"). HHV-6 is susceptible *in vitro* to ganciclovir and foscarnet, and it is reasonable to initiate therapy with either of these agents when HHV-6 disease is proven or strongly suspected. Screening for asymptomatic HHV-6 infection and prophylaxis with antiviral agents is not advised.

Respiratory Viruses

Community respiratory viruses include influenza, parainfluenza, respiratory syncytial virus, human metapneumovirus, adenoviruses, rhinoviruses, and coronaviruses. Most respiratory viruses typically cause self-limited infection in healthy persons, but are important causes of morbidity and mortality in immunocompromised patients with hematologic malignancies and in HSCT recipients.[286] They may account for a significant proportion of undiagnosed or "idiopathic" pneumonias in HSCT recipients in older series. Immunocompromised persons with symptoms of respiratory infection should be evaluated for respiratory viruses, among other etiologies, and contact and respiratory precautions should be established. Rapid immunodiagnostic methods for common respiratory viruses are useful only to "rule in" these infections (i.e., a negative result of a rapid test may be falsely negative and cannot be used to rule out the disease).

Influenza Virus. During a winter outbreak period, influenza was diagnosed in ~30% of adult patients hospitalized for a respiratory illness at the M. D. Anderson Cancer Center.[287] Pneumonia occurred in 12 of 15 (80%) of patients with influenza, and 4 of these patients died. In other centers, the incidence of pneumonia and mortality associated with influenza virus infection was substantially lower.-[288]

Amantadine and rimantadine are active against influenza A, but not influenza B, and resistance to these agents may rapidly develop during therapy. The neuraminidase inhibitors, zanamivir and oseltamivir, are active against both influenza A and B. They are effective in reducing the duration of influenza illness if started early after onset of symptoms and they have a prophylactic benefit during community outbreaks.[289,290] Oseltamivir was safe and appeared to be effective in influenza infection in HSCT recipients.[291] We frequently administer oseltamivir to immunocompromised patients with influenza even if they have had symptoms for more than 48 hours based on the risk for developing complications.[292] Choice of drug should be based on the susceptibility patterns of the predominant influenza strain(s).

The CDC advises annual administration of the inactivated influenza vaccine to immunocompromised persons and their close contacts (e.g., health care workers and household members). Immunization should be provided ideally 2 weeks before chemotherapy, or if given during chemotherapy, immunization is preferably administered between cycles. The recently approved inhaled live attenuated influenza vaccine, FluMist, should not be used in the severely immunocompromised patient. Use of the injected inactivated vaccine is preferred among close contacts of the immunocompromised persons, including health care workers.

Respiratory Syncytial Virus. Respiratory syncytial virus infection is most virulent in patients with leukemia and in HSCT recipients.[293] Upper respiratory symptoms (sinusitis, coryza, rhinorrhea) usually precede lower respiratory tract involvement (dyspnea, wheezing) and pneumonia but may be absent. The historic mortality from RSV pneumonia in HSCT recipients is ~80%.[288] Uncontrolled studies suggest that aerosolized ribavirin and IVIG containing high RSV neutralizing titers for at least 24 hours prior to respiratory failure prevent respiratory failure and result in much better outcomes.[294] A randomized controlled trial of ribavirin in RSV upper respiratory infection ended early because of poor accrual and did not show a difference.[295] We only consider inhaled ribavirin and immunoglobulin in patients with RSV infection at highest risk for severe complications: allogeneic HSCT recipients and patients with acute leukemia and persistent neutropenia.

Parainfluenza. Parainfluenza viruses are important community respiratory viruses in leukemia and HSCT patients. Progression from upper respiratory infection to pneumonia is associated with a high frequency of respiratory failure and death. Nichols et al.[296] reported parainfluenza virus infections in 7% of HSCT recipients. Approximately 80% of these infections were community-acquired. Half the patients had coexistent pulmonary pathogens. Aerosolized ribavirin with or without immunoglobulin did not appear to affect clinical outcome in this study.

Human Metapneumovirus. Human metapneumovirus is a recently described paramyxovirus that causes upper and lower respiratory tract infection. It occurs mostly during the winter and spring. More severe disease is reported in young children, the elderly, and immunocompromised hosts.[297,298] The prevalence of human metapneumovirus is not completely elucidated, and very diverse rates have been reported, including fairly common asymptomatic carriage.[299] Initial symptoms are not distinctive: fever, cough, and upper respiratory symptoms. Severe disease was associated with respiratory failure, pulmonary hemorrhage, culture-negative septic shock, and a high mortality rate.[298] The treatment is supportive.

Adenovirus. The spectrum of adenovirus in immunocompromised patients extends from asymptomatic shedding to fatal multisystem disease with pneumonia and hepatitis, and includes upper respiratory tract infection, renal parenchymal disease, hemorrhagic cystitis, hepatitis, small and large bowel disease, and encephalitis.[300] Viral shedding from throat secretions, urine, and stool is common, occurring in ~5% to 20% of HSCT recipients, and should not be equated with disease. Gastroenteritis and hemorrhagic cystitis are usually self-limited, whereas pneumonia and disseminated disease are associated with a high mortality rate. Adenovirus is more common in T-cell–depleted transplants and in younger patients and recipients of stem cells from unrelated donors.[301] Cidofovir may be beneficial.[302,303]

Parvovirus B19

Parvovirus B19 is a DNA virus that is transmitted via respiratory secretions, blood products, and vertically from mother to fetus. It is the cause of erythema infectiosum (fifth disease), a common, self-limiting febrile exanthem of childhood. Infection in immunocompromised persons unable to mount a protective antibody response may cause prolonged fever, chronic pure red cell aplasia, thrombocytopenia, or pancytopenia. Predisposing conditions include acute and chronic leukemias, myelodysplastic syndrome, lymphoma, HSCT, potent antineoplastic chemotherapy, and systemic steroids.[304] Parvovirus B19 may also cause a virus-associated hemophagocytic syndrome that is characterized by fever, histiocytic hyperplasia, and cytopenia. Diagnosis of parvovirus B19 infection in the immunocompromised patient relies on PCR detection of viral DNA from serum; these patients may be incapable of antibody responses. Treatment consists of IVIG.

Parasitic Infections

Toxoplasmosis

For a discussion on toxoplasmosis, see "Central Nervous System Infections."

Strongyloides Stercoralis

Strongyloides stercoralis is an intestinal nematode that typically causes localized infection but can cause disseminated disease, "hyperinfection syndrome," in immunocompromised patients. *Strongyloides stercoralis* is endemic in tropical and subtropical regions, but it is also found in Europe and rural areas in the southeastern United States. *Strongyloides stercoralis* can establish an asymptomatic chronic gastrointestinal infection through autoinfection. The hyperinfection syndrome can occur years after the initial infection in the setting of immunosuppression. It results from penetration of filariform larvae through the intestinal mucosa, followed by dissemination. Secondary bacterial infection results from passage of enteric bacteria through the bowel or accompanying the migrating larvae, and may result in peritonitis, bacteremia, and meningitis. Polymicrobial bacteremia or meningitis with enteric bacteria are typical presentations Among reported cases of hyperinfection syndrome associated with cancer, ~90% of patients had a hematologic malignancy.[305]

Patients from endemic areas or with unexplained peripheral eosinophilia should be screened for *S. stercoralis* infection by serologic testing prior to receiving immunosuppressive agents. It is recommended to administer prophylaxis with ivermectin to potential HSCT recipients with a positive serology or unexplained eosinophilia despite a negative serology,[32] and this approach may be considered for other patients receiving potent immunosuppressive regimens. All infected patients should have at least three stools with negative findings after completion of treatment prior to beginning chemotherapy.

Selected References

The full list of references for this chapter appears in the online version.

3. Bodey GP, Buckley M, Sathe YS, et al. Quantitative relationships between circulating leukocytes and infection in patients with acute leukemia. *Ann Intern Med* 1966;64:328.
4. Gerson SL, Talbot GH, Hurwitz S, et al. Prolonged granulocytopenia: the major risk factor for invasive pulmonary aspergillosis in patients with acute leukemia. *Ann Intern Med* 1984;100:345.
7. Crippa F, Holmberg L, Carter RA, et al. Infectious complications after autologous CD34-selected peripheral blood stem cell transplantation. *Biol Blood Marrow Transplant* 2002;8:281.
8. Fukuda T, Boeckh M, Carter RA, et al. Invasive fungal infections in recipients of allogeneic hematopoietic stem cell transplantation after nonmyeloablative conditioning: risks and outcomes. *Blood* 2003;10:10.
13. Kulkarni S, Powles R, Treleaven J, et al. Chronic graft versus host disease is associated with long-term risk for pneumococcal infections in recipients of bone marrow transplants. *Blood* 2000;95:3683.
16. Rocha V, Labopin M, Sanz G, et al. Transplants of umbilical-cord blood or bone marrow from unrelated donors in adults with acute leukemia. *N Engl J Med* 2004;351:2276.
17. Laughlin MJ, Eapen M, Rubinstein P, et al. Outcomes after transplantation of cord blood or bone marrow from unrelated donors in adults with leukemia. *N Engl J Med* 2004;351:2265.
22. Martin SI, Marty FM, Fiumara K, et al. Infectious complications associated with alemtuzumab use for lymphoproliferative disorders. *Clin Infect Dis* 2006;43:16.
24. Gea-Banacloche JC. Rituximab-associated infections. *Semin Hematol* 47:187.
28. Yeo W, Chan TC, Leung NW, et al. Hepatitis B virus reactivation in lymphoma patients with prior resolved hepatitis B undergoing anticancer therapy with or without rituximab. *J Clin Oncol* 2009;27:605.
31. Couriel D, Saliba R, Hicks K, et al. Tumor necrosis factor-alpha blockade for the treatment of acute GVHD. *Blood* 2004;104:649.
32. Tomblyn M, Chiller T, Einsele H, et al. Guidelines for preventing infectious complications among hematopoietic cell transplantation recipients: a global perspective. *Biol Blood Marrow Transplant* 2009;15:1143.
33. Gafter-Gvili A, Fraser A, Paul M, et al. Meta-analysis: antibiotic prophylaxis reduces mortality in neutropenic patients. *Ann Intern Med* 2005;142:979.
37. Segal BH, Freifeld AG. Antibacterial prophylaxis in patients with neutropenia. *J Natl Compr Cancer Netw* 2007;5:235.
39. Couriel D, Carpenter PA, Cutler C, et al. Ancillary therapy and supportive care of chronic graft-versus-host disease: national institutes of health consensus development project on criteria for clinical trials in chronic Graft-versus-host disease: V. Ancillary Therapy and Supportive Care Working Group Report. *Biol Blood Marrow Transplant* 2006;12:375.
40. Kontoyiannis DP, Marr KA, Park BJ, et al. Prospective surveillance for invasive fungal infections in hematopoietic stem cell transplant recipients, 2001–2006: overview of the Transplant-Associated Infection Surveillance Network (TRANSNET) Database. *Clin Infect Dis* 2010;50:1091.
41. Baddley JW, Andes DR, Marr KA, et al. Factors Associated with Mortality in Transplant Patients with Invasive Aspergillosis. *Clin Infect Dis* 2010;50:1559–1567.
48. Cornely OA, Maertens J, Winston DJ, et al. Posaconazole vs. fluconazole or itraconazole prophylaxis in patients with neutropenia. *N Engl J Med* 2007;356:348.
51. De Pauw BE, Donnelly JP. Prophylaxis and aspergillosis—has the principle been proven? *N Engl J Med* 2007;356:409.
52. Sepkowitz KA. Pneumocystis carinii pneumonia without acquired immunodeficiency syndrome: who should receive prophylaxis? *Mayo Clin Proc* 1996;71:102.
54. Segal BH, Freifeld AG, Baden LR, et al. Prevention and treatment of cancer-related infections. *J Natl Compr Canc Netw* 2008;6:122.
55. Boeckh M, Kim HW, Flowers ME, et al. Long-term acyclovir for prevention of varicella zoster virus disease after allogeneic hematopoietic cell transplantation–a randomized double-blind placebo-controlled study. *Blood* 2006;107:1800.
64. Sandherr M, Einsele H, Hebart H, et al. Antiviral prophylaxis in patients with haematological malignancies and solid tumours: Guidelines of the Infectious Diseases Working Party (AGIHO) of the German Society for Hematology and Oncology (DGHO). *Ann Oncol* 2006;17:1051.
68. Lalazar G, Rund D, Shouval D. Screening, prevention and treatment of viral hepatitis B reactivation in patients with haematological malignancies. *Br J Haematol* 2007;136:699.
71. Hughes WT, Armstrong D, Bodey GP, et al. 2002 guidelines for the use of antimicrobial agents in neutropenic patients with cancer. *Clin Infect Dis* 2002;34:730.
76. Jaksic B, Martinelli G, Perez-Oteyza J, et al. Efficacy and safety of linezolid compared with vancomycin in a randomized, double-blind study of febrile neutropenic patients with cancer. *Clin Infect Dis* 2006;42:597.
82. Segal BH, Almyroudis NG, Battiwalla M, et al. Prevention and early treatment of invasive fungal infection in patients with cancer and neutropenia and in stem cell transplant recipients in the era of newer broad-spectrum antifungal agents and diagnostic adjuncts. *Clin Infect Dis* 2007;44:402.
89. Maertens J, Theunissen K, Verhoef G, et al. Galactomannan and computed tomography-based preemptive antifungal therapy in neutropenic patients at high risk for invasive fungal infection: a prospective feasibility study. *Clin Infect Dis* 2005;41:1242.
90. Cordonnier C, Pautas C, Maury S, et al. Empirical versus preemptive antifungal therapy for high-risk, febrile, neutropenic patients: a randomized, controlled trial. *Clin Infect Dis* 2009;48:1042.
93. Dekker A, Bulley S, Beyene J, et al. Meta-analysis of randomized controlled trials of prophylactic granulocyte colony-stimulating factor and granulocyte-macrophage colony-stimulating factor after autologous and allogeneic stem cell transplantation. *J Clin Oncol* 2006;24:5207.
102. Klastersky J, Paesmans M, Rubenstein EB, et al. The Multinational Association for Supportive Care in Cancer risk index: a multinational scoring system for identifying low-risk febrile neutropenic cancer patients. *J Clin Oncol* 2000;18:3038.
112. Mermel LA, Farr BM, Sherertz RJ, et al. Guidelines for the management of intravascular catheter-related infections. *Clin Infect Dis* 2001;32:1249.
113. Raad I, Hanna HA, Alakech B, et al. Differential time to positivity: a useful method for diagnosing catheter-related bloodstream infections. *Ann Intern Med* 2004;140:18.
114. Mermel LA, Allon M, Bouza E, et al. Clinical practice guidelines for the diagnosis and management of intravascular catheter-related infection: 2009 Update by the Infectious Diseases Society of America. *Clin Infect Dis* 2009;49:1.
115. Pronovost P, Needham D, Berenholtz S, et al. An intervention to decrease catheter-related bloodstream infections in the ICU. *N Engl J Med* 2006;355:2725.

118. Anaya DA, Dellinger EP. Necrotizing soft-tissue infection: diagnosis and management. *Clin Infect Dis* 2007;44:705.
123. Mandell LA, Wunderink RG, Anzueto A, et al. Infectious Diseases Society of America/American Thoracic Society consensus guidelines on the management of community-acquired pneumonia. *Clin Infect Dis* 2007;44:S27.
124. America ATSIDSo. Guidelines for the management of adults with hospital-acquired, ventilator-associated, and health-care associated pneumonia. *Am J Respir Crit Care Med* 2005;171:388.
125. Maertens J, Maertens V, Theunissen K, et al. Bronchoalveolar lavage fluid galactomannan for the diagnosis of invasive pulmonary aspergillosis in patients with hematologic diseases. *Clin Infect Dis* 2009;49:1688.
131. Sloas MM, Flynn PM, Kaste SC, et al. Typhlitis in children with cancer: a 30-year experience. *Clin Infect Dis* 1993;17:484.
132. Kirkpatrick ID, Greenberg HM. Gastrointestinal complications in the neutropenic patient: characterization and differentiation with abdominal CT. *Radiology* 2003;226:668.
140. Bartlett JG. Narrative review: the new epidemic of Clostridium difficile-associated enteric disease. *Ann Intern Med* 2006;145:758.
145. Brown EM, Edwards RJ, Pople IK. Conservative management of patients with cerebrospinal fluid shunt infections. *Neurosurgery* 2006;58:657; discussion 657.
147. Tunkel AR, Hartman BJ, Kaplan SL, et al. Practice guidelines for the management of bacterial meningitis. *Clin Infect Dis* 2004;39:1267.
148. Tunkel AR, Glaser CA, Bloch KC, et al. The management of encephalitis: clinical practice guidelines by the Infectious Diseases Society of America. *Clin Infect Dis* 2008;47:303.
149. Seeley WW, Marty FM, Holmes TM, et al. Post-transplant acute limbic encephalitis: clinical features and relationship to HHV6. *Neurology* 2007; 69:156.
150. Ljungman P, Singh N. Human herpesvirus-6 infection in solid organ and stem cell transplant recipients. *J Clin Virol* 2006;37 Suppl 1:S87.
155. Martino R, Maertens J, Bretagne S, et al. Toxoplasmosis after hematopoietic stem cell transplantation. *Clin Infect Dis* 2000;31:1188.
159. Erard V, Kim HW, Corey L, et al. BK DNA viral load in plasma: evidence for an association with hemorrhagic cystitis in allogeneic hematopoietic cell transplant recipients. *Blood* 2005;106:1130.
162. Itani KM, Wilson SE, Awad SS, Jensen EH, Finn TS, Abramson MA. Ertapenem versus cefotetan prophylaxis in elective colorectal surgery. *N Engl J Med* 2006;355:2640.
170. Blumberg HM, Jarvis WR, Soucie JM, et al. Risk factors for candidal bloodstream infections in surgical intensive care unit patients: the NEMIS prospective multicenter study. The National Epidemiology of Mycosis Survey. *Clin Infect Dis* 2001;33:177.
174. Baddour LM, Wilson WR, Bayer AS, et al. Infective endocarditis: diagnosis, antimicrobial therapy, and management of complications: a statement for healthcare professionals from the Committee on Rheumatic Fever, Endocarditis, and Kawasaki Disease, Council on Cardiovascular Disease in the Young, and the Councils on Clinical Cardiology, Stroke, and Cardiovascular Surgery and Anesthesia, American Heart Association: endorsed by the Infectious Diseases Society of America. *Circulation* 2005;111:e394.
179. Rybak M, Lomaestro B, Rotschafer JC, et al. Therapeutic monitoring of vancomycin in adult patients: a consensus review of the American Society of Health-System Pharmacists, the Infectious Diseases Society of America, and the Society of Infectious Diseases Pharmacists. *Am J Health Syst Pharm* 2009;66:82.
180. Wunderink RG, Rello J, Cammarata SK, et al. Linezolid vs vancomycin: analysis of two double-blind studies of patients with methicillin-resistant Staphylococcus aureus nosocomial pneumonia. *Chest* 2003;124:1789.
182. Fowler VG Jr, Boucher HW, Corey GR, et al. Daptomycin versus standard therapy for bacteremia and endocarditis caused by Staphylococcus aureus. *N Engl J Med* 2006;355:653.
190. Tunkell AR, Sepkowitz KA. Infections caused by viridans streptococci in patients with neutropenia. *Clin Infect Dis* 2002;34:1524.
192. Chatzinikolaou I, Abi-Said D, Bodey GP, Rolston KV, Tarrand JJ, Samonis G. Recent experience with Pseudomonas aeruginosa bacteremia in patients with cancer: retrospective analysis of 245 episodes. *Arch Intern Med* 2000; 160:501.
194. Levin AS, Barone AA, Penco J, et al. Intravenous colistin as therapy for nosocomial infections caused by multidrug-resistant Pseudomonas aeruginosa and Acinetobacter baumannii. *Clin Infect Dis* 1999;28:1008.
197. Alou L, Aguilar L, Sevillano D, et al. Is there a pharmacodynamic need for the use of continuous versus intermittent infusion with ceftazidime against Pseudomonas aeruginosa? An in vitro pharmacodynamic model. *J Antimicrob Chemother* 2005;55:209.
198. Dellit TH, Owens RC, McGowan JE Jr, et al. Infectious Diseases Society of America and the Society for Healthcare Epidemiology of America guidelines for developing an institutional program to enhance antimicrobial stewardship. *Clin Infect Dis* 2007;44:159.
205. Treatment of tuberculosis. American Thoracic Society, CDC, and Infectious Diseases Society of America. MMWR 2003;52(RR11):1.
206. Griffith DE, Aksamit T, Brown-Elliott BA, et al. An official ATS/IDSA statement: diagnosis, treatment, and prevention of nontuberculous mycobacterial diseases. *Am J Respir Crit Care Med* 2007;175:367.
207. Torres HA, Reddy BT, Raad II, et al. Nocardiosis in cancer patients. *Medicine (Baltimore)* 2002;81:388.
210. Perfect JR, Dismukes WE, Dromer F, et al. Clinical practice guidelines for the management of cryptococcal disease: 2010 update by the infectious diseases society of America. *Clin Infect Dis* 2010;50:291.
211. Pappas PG, Kauffman CA, Andes D, et al. Clinical practice guidelines for the management of candidiasis: 2009 update by the Infectious Diseases Society of America. *Clin Infect Dis* 2009;48:503.
212. Walsh TJ, Anaissie EJ, Denning DW, et al. Treatment of aspergillosis: clinical practice guidelines of the Infectious Diseases Society of America. *Clin Infect Dis* 2008;46:327.
218. Greene RE, Schlamm HT, Oestmann JW, et al. Imaging findings in acute invasive pulmonary aspergillosis: clinical significance of the halo sign. *Clin Infect Dis* 2007;44:373.
223. Ostrosky-Zeichner L, Alexander BD, Kett DH, et al. Multicenter clinical evaluation of the (1->3) beta-D-glucan assay as an aid to diagnosis of fungal infections in humans. *Clin Infect Dis* 2005;41:654.
224. De Pauw B, Walsh TJ, Donnelly JP, et al. Revised definitions of invasive fungal disease from the European Organization for Research and Treatment of Cancer/Invasive Fungal Infections Cooperative Group and the National Institute of Allergy and Infectious Diseases Mycoses Study Group (EORTC/MSG) Consensus Group. *Clin Infect Dis* 2008;46:1813.
225. Wheat LJ. Antigen detection, serology, and molecular diagnosis of invasive mycoses in the immunocompromised host. *Transpl Infect Dis* 2006;8:128.
250. Roden MM, Zaoutis TE, Buchanan WL, et al. Epidemiology and outcome of zygomycosis: a review of 929 reported cases. *Clin Infect Dis* 2005;41:634.
251. Marty FM, Cosimi LA, Baden LR. Breakthrough zygomycosis after voriconazole treatment in recipients of hematopoietic stem-cell transplants. *N Engl J Med* 2004;350:950.
255. van Burik JA, Hare RS, Solomon HF, et al. Posaconazole is effective as salvage therapy in zygomycosis: a retrospective summary of 91 cases. *Clin Infect Dis* 2006;42:e61.
257. Segal BH, Kwon-Chung J, Walsh TJ, et al. Immunotherapy for fungal infections. *Clin Infect Dis* 2006;42:507.
263. Wheat LJ, Freifeld AG, Kleiman MB, et al. Clinical practice guidelines for the management of patients with histoplasmosis: 2007 update by the Infectious Diseases Society of America. *Clin Infect Dis* 2007;45:807.
266. Sepkowitz KA, Brown AE, Armstrong D. Pneumocystis carinii pneumonia without acquired immunodeficiency syndrome. More patients, same risk [editorial]. *Arch Intern Med* 1995;155:1125.
270. Azoulay E, Bergeron A, Chevret S, et al. Polymerase chain reaction for diagnosing pneumocystis pneumonia in non-HIV immunocompromised patients with pulmonary infiltrates. *Chest* 2009;135:655
273. Boeckh M, Ljungman P. How we treat cytomegalovirus in hematopoietic cell transplant recipients. *Blood* 2009;113:5711.
278. Awaya N, Adachi A, Mori T, et al. Fulminant Epstein-Barr virus (EBV)-associated T-cell lymphoproliferative disorder with hemophagocytosis following autologous peripheral blood stem cell transplantation for relapsed angioimmunoblastic T-cell lymphoma. *Leuk Res* 2006;30:1059.
283. Heslop HE, Slobod KS, Pule MA, et al. Long-term outcome of EBV-specific T-cell infusions to prevent or treat EBV-related lymphoproliferative disease in transplant recipients. *Blood* 2010;115:925.
286. Martino R, Porras RP, Rabella N, et al. Prospective study of the incidence, clinical features, and outcome of symptomatic upper and lower respiratory tract infections by respiratory viruses in adult recipients of hematopoietic stem cell transplants for hematologic malignancies. *Biol Blood Marrow Transplant* 2005;11:781.
292. Casper C, Englund J, Boeckh M. How I treat influenza in patients with hematologic malignancies. *Blood* 2010;115:1331.
302. Neofytos D, Ojha A, Mookerjee B, et al. Treatment of adenovirus disease in stem cell transplant recipients with cidofovir. *Biol Blood Marrow Transplant* 2007;13:74.

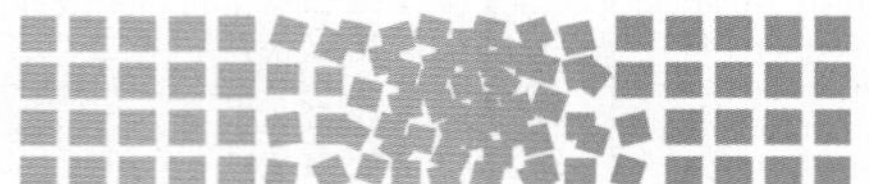

CHAPTER 157 LEUKOPENIA AND THROMBOCYTOPENIA

CARLA KURKJIAN AND HOWARD OZER

The term *hematopoietic growth factors* (HGFs) refers to cytokines that govern hematopoiesis by regulating the proliferation, differentiation, maturation, function, and viability of the cellular components of blood and their progenitor cells. The production of HGFs is primarily by the cells of the bone marrow, with the exception of erythropoietin (EPO), which is produced by the peritubular capillary endothelial cells of the kidney. Many other nonmarrow cells are capable of constitutive production of HGFs. Table 157.1 provides the endogenous cellular sources, inducers, and therapeutic roles of the four major HGFs currently used clinically: EPO, granulocyte colony-stimulating factor (G-CSF or CSF3), granulocyte-macrophage colony-stimulating factor (GM-CSF), and interleukin-11 (IL-11). Thrombopoietin is also included, although the currently available clinical agents are thrombopoietin mimetics due to antigenicity of the native cytokine.[1]

Recombinant human (rHu) HGFs are commonly used in oncology practice for a variety of purposes, including attenuation of chemotherapy-induced myelosuppression, treatment of hematopoietic malignancies, and management of decreased HGF production in malignancy. Six rHu HGFs are approved by the U.S. Food and Drug Administration (FDA) for use in the United States (Table 157.2). This chapter provides an evidence-based review of leukopenia and thrombocytopenia in the setting of cancer therapy with a focus on the appropriate use of recombinant HGFs.

OVERVIEW OF HEMATOPOIESIS AND HEMATOPOIETIC GROWTH FACTORS

The current model of hematopoiesis maintains that cellular components in blood (erythrocytes, leukocytes, and platelets) are derived from multipotent stem cells located primarily in the bone marrow (BM). These hematopoietic stem cells (HSC) s are responsible for the complex task of generating billions of blood cells each day.[2] However, it is believed that HSCs are largely quiescent, such that actively dividing progenitor cells with a more differentiated phenotype are derived from HSCs.[3–5] The ability of HSCs to undergo either symmetric cell division for self-propagation or asymmetric cell division to also produce a more differentiated daughter cell allows HSCs to maintain their niche within the BM.[6] Intracellular pathways activated by receptor-ligand interactions initiated by NOTCH ligand, bone morphogenic proteins, hedgehog proteins, and WNT proteins appear to play an important role in the self-renewal capacity of HSCs.[7] Pleiotrophin, a heparin binding growth factor and a neuron mitogen, has recently been shown to regulate HSC expansion.[8] Though the direct effects on HSC regeneration of pleiotrophin have been shown, its promotion of angiogenesis may play an important role in the maintenance of the bone marrow vascular environment, an important factor in bone marrow regeneration after insult.[9–12] HGFs regulate the proliferation, differentiation, and maturation of stem cells and multipotential progenitor cells. These include steel factor, FMS-like tyrosine kinase-3 (Flt-3) ligand, IL-2, -3, and -7, as well as GM-CSF (Fig. 157.1).[13]

The effects of HGFs are mediated through receptors located on both hematopoietic and nonhematopoietic cells. Thus, the physiologic effects of HGFs are numerous and not confined to hematopoiesis. Table 157.3 lists the various receptor locations and illustrates the pleiotropic effects of these proteins. Cell surface receptors for HGFs are transmembrane proteins with one or two extracellular cytokine-binding motifs and an intracellular domain that can bind cytoplasmic Janus kinases (JAKs). A single HGF molecule can induce a conformational change in the homodimeric HGF receptor, thereby bringing cytoplasmic JAKs into close proximity with resultant crossphorphorylation.[14] HGF-stimulated JAK activation then leads to subsequent phosphorylation of downstream proteins, promoting cell survival, differentiation, and proliferation. The downstream pathways most studied are those involving phosphoinositol-3 kinase, mitogen-activated protein kinase, and the signal transducer and activator of transcription (STAT).[14–16] Inhibition of the JAK-STAT pathway by suppressors of cytokine signaling (SOCS), of which there are eight members, appears to occur through a classic negative feedback mechanism.[17,18]

ERYTHROPOIETIN

Endogenous EPO is the primary regulator of red blood cell production, and both humans and mice deficient in EPO develop severe anemia. EPO is primarily produced in the kidney, likely by interstitial fibroblasts and proximal tubular cells, in response to hypoxia or decreased red cell oxygen-carrying capacity such that endogenous serum concentrations vary inversely with red cell oxygen–carrying capacity (Table 157.1).[19] Normal serum EPO levels range from approximately 4 to 30 U/L and rise when the hematocrit decreases below approximately 35%. Severe anemia can induce a 100- to 1,000-fold increase in EPO production. Endogenous EPO levels are depressed in cancer patients, which contributes to the chronic anemia detected in this patient population.[20]

A recombinant form of human EPO first became available in 1989, and currently three different forms are commercially available. In the United States, epoetin alfa and darbepoetin alfa are approved. Epoetin alfa contains the identical amino acid sequence to endogenous human EPO and has a half-life of approximately 3 to 10 hours in healthy volunteers after

TABLE 157.1

ENDOGENOUS SOURCES, INDUCERS, AND ROLES OF MAJOR HEMATOPOIETIC GROWTH FACTORS

Hematopoietic Growth Factor	Endogenous Sources	Physiologic States that Induce Production	Endogenous Substances that Induce Production	Endogenous Hematopoietic Role
EPO	Kidney Brain Uterus	Hypoxia	Estradiol (uterus)	Stimulates erythropoiesis
CSF3	Marrow stromal cells Neutrophils Monocytes/macrophages T cells Endothelial cells Fibroblasts Mesothelial cells Epithelial cells Various tumor cell lines	Infection Inflammation Tissue damage	Endotoxin Lipopolysaccharide TNF IL-1β IFN-γ GM-CSF M-CSF IL-3 IL-4	Regulates production, maturation, and function of neutrophil lineage
GM-CSF	Monocytes/macrophages T cells Endothelial cells Fibroblasts Mesothelial cells Epithelial cells Various tumor cell lines	Infection Inflammation Tissue damage	IL-1 IL-6 TNF Endotoxin	Regulates production, maturation, and function of myeloid lineage
IL-11	Bone marrow stromal cells Fibroblasts Chondrocytes Synoviocytes Osteoblasts Trophoblasts Epithelial cells	Thrombocytopenia Respiratory viruses	TGF-β IL-1 TNF Parathyroid hormone Calcium ionophores Phorbol esters	Regulates production and maturation of megakaryocytes Induces platelet production Stimulates erythropoiesis Regulates macrophage proliferation and differentiation

EPO, erythropoietin; CSF3, colony-stimulating factor 3; TNF, tumor necrosis factor; IL, interleukin; IFN, interferon; GM-CSF, granulocyte-macrophage colony-stimulating factor; M-CSF, macrophage colony-stimulating factor; TGF, transforming growth factor.

intravenous (IV) administration. Darbepoetin alfa is an rHu EPO modified by the addition of two *N*-glycosylation sites to produce a molecule with a longer half-life that is approximately threefold greater than epoetin alfa.[21] Outside the United States, epoetin beta is available, a protein with an identical amino acid sequence to endogenous human EPO but with a different glycosylation pattern than epoetin alfa. This difference in glycosylation does not appear to significantly alter efficacy compared with epoetin alfa.

Like their endogenous counterparts, rHu EPOs stimulate the proliferation, differentiation, and maturation of committed erythroid progenitors to mature erythrocytes. After administration of rHu EPOs, a rise in the red cell count does not begin to occur until 2 weeks of continuous dosing and may take up to 8 weeks.

The side effects of epoetin alfa or darbepoetin alfa are generally minimal. Some patients experience edema on epoetin alfa or darbepoetin alfa therapy. An increase in thrombotic events has been reported with recombinant EPO therapies; however, these appear to be more common in patients with chronic renal failure, particularly those with ischemic heart disease or congestive heart failure. Hypertension can also occur but is similarly more common in patients with chronic renal failure.[22]

GRANULOCYTE COLONY-STIMULATING FACTOR

Endogenous CSF3 regulates the production, maturation, and function of the neutrophil lineage. Serum concentrations vary inversely with blood neutrophil concentrations. Although mice deficient in CSF3 or CSF3 receptors display chronic neutropenia, trafficking of granulocytes from bone marrow to blood does not appear to be impaired. At steady state, CSF3 plays a critical role in the survival of granulocytes, but not in their transit time from the postmitotic bone marrow pool to peripheral blood.[23] CSF3 ranges from 20 to 100 pg/mL in healthy individuals and rises inversely with neutrophil concentration. Patients who are bacteremic and neutropenic can have serum levels of CSF3 exceeding 2,000 pg/mL.

rHu CSF3 is currently available commercially in four forms, of which filgrastim and pegfilgrastim are approved in the United States. Filgrastim, a recombinant protein produced in *Escherichia coli*, has an amino acid sequence identical to endogenous CSF3, with the exception of the addition of an N-terminal methionine and absence of glycosylation.[24] The half-life of rHu CSF3 is approximately 3.5 hours in both cancer patients and healthy subjects after either IV or subcutaneous

TABLE 157.2

HEMATOPOIETIC GROWTH FACTORS APPROVED FOR USE BY THE U.S. FOOD AND DRUG ADMINISTRATION WITH APPLICATIONS IN CANCER THERAPY

Hematopoietic Growth Factor	Generic Name	Brand Names	Molecular Description	Hematopoietic Effects	Applications in Cancer
EPO	Epoetin alfa	Epogen, Procrit	rHu EPO	Red cell lineage	Chemotherapy-induced anemia in nonmyeloid malignancies
	Darbepoetin	Aranesp	rHu EPO with altered glycosylation	Red cell lineage	Chemotherapy-induced anemia in nonmyeloid malignancies
CSF3	Filgrastim	Neupogen	rHu CSF3	Neutrophil lineage	Reduce febrile neutropenia in patients receiving myelosuppressive chemotherapy; reduce duration of neutropenia after bone marrow transplantation, mobilize progenitor cells
	Pegfilgrastim	Neulasta	Pegylated rHu CSF3	Neutrophil lineage	Reduce febrile neutropenia in patients receiving myelosuppressive chemotherapy
GM-CSF	Sargramostim	Leukine	rHu GM-CSF	Myeloid lineage	Reduce duration of neutropenia after bone marrow transplantation; mobilize progenitor cells
IL-11	Oprelvekin	Neumega	rHu IL-11	Megakaryocytes	Treatment of chemotherapy-associated thrombocytopenia

EPO, erythropoietin; rHu, recombinant human; CSF3, colony-stimulating factor 3; GM-CSF, granulocyte-macrophage colony-stimulating factor; IL-11, interleukin-11.

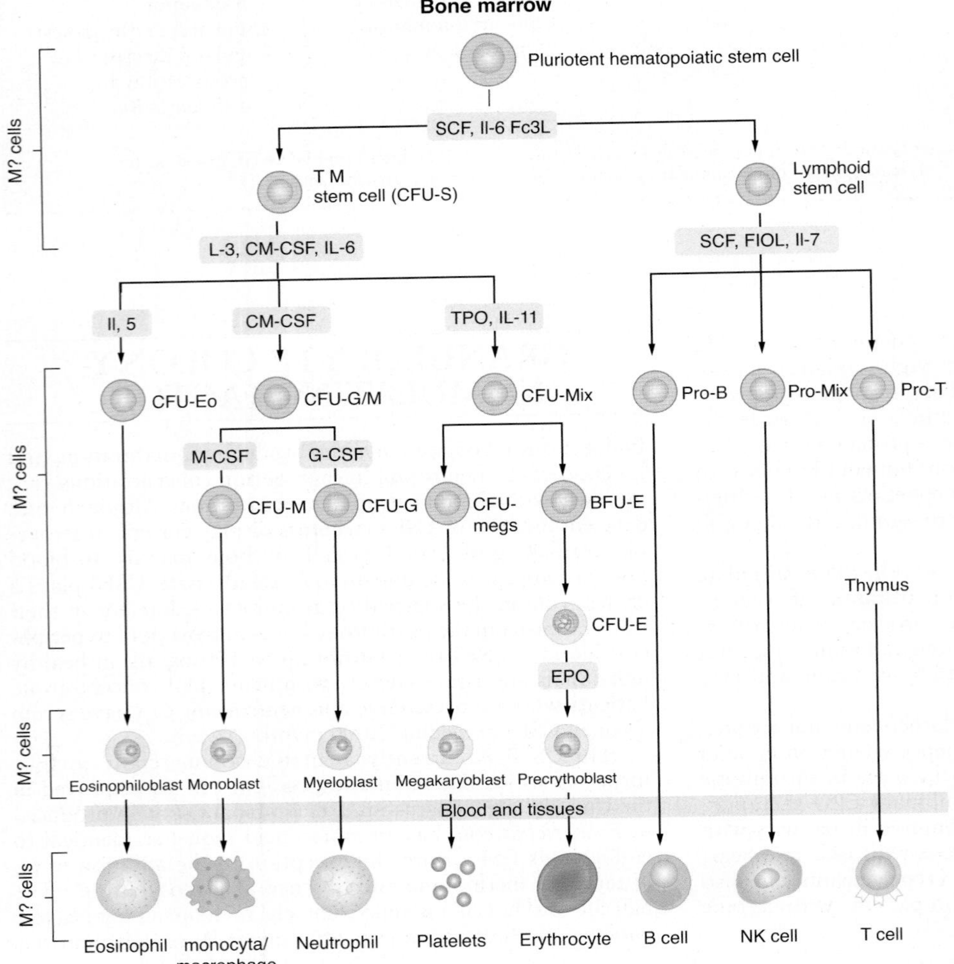

FIGURE 157.1 This schematic depiction of the hematopoietic cascade identifies the role of key hematopoietic growth factors and the maturation of blood cells in the process of hematopoiesis. SCF, stem cell factor; IL, interleukin; GM-CSF, granulocyte-macrophage colony-stimulating factor; SCF, stem cell factor; CFU, colony-forming unit; TPO, thrombopoietin; BFU, blast-forming unit; EPO, erythropoietin; CSF3, granulocyte colony-stimulating factor. (Adapted from Cotran RS, Kumar V, Collins T, eds. *Robbins pathologic basis of disease*. 6th ed. Philadelphia: WB Saunders, 1999: Figure 14-1.)

TABLE 157.3

RECEPTOR LOCATIONS AND PLEIOTROPIC EFFECTS OF MAJOR HEMATOPOIETIC GROWTH FACTORS

Hematopoietic Growth Factor	Receptor Locations	Potential Nonhematopoietic Effects
EPO	Breast tumor vasculature Neurons, astrocytes, endothelial cells, Leydig cells, gastric mucosal cells, vascular smooth muscle cells, cardiomyocytes, megakaryocytes, lymphocytes, myeloid cells	Neuroprotection Angiogenesis
	Colon adenocarcinoma, pancreatic adenocarcinoma, prostate carcinoma, bladder carcinoma, hepatoma, promyelocytic leukemia, erythroleukemia, AML, renal cell carcinoma, breast carcinoma, neuroblastoma, sarcoma, melanoma	Testosterone production Mucosal protection Hypertension
CSF3	Neutrophils and their progenitor cells, monocytes, platelets, endothelial and epithelial cells, myeloid and lymphocytic leukemic cells, small cell lung carcinoma, ovarian carcinoma, gastric adenocarcinoma, bladder cancer, B-cell lymphoma Placenta and endometrium	Anti-inflammatory activity Sensitization of malignant myeloid tumor cells to chemotherapy
GM-CSF	Myeloid cells, dendritic cells, endothelial cells Myeloid leukemias, ALL Endometrial carcinoma, renal cell carcinoma, skin carcinoma, glioma, non–small cell lung cancer, malignant plasma cells, prostate cancer, colon adenocarcinoma, melanoma, gastric carcinoma, osteosarcoma	Vaccine adjuvancy Mucosal protection Crohn's disease Wound healing
IL-11	Megakaryocyte progenitors, myeloid cells, lymphocytes, osteoclasts, osteoblasts, endometrial cells, ovarian epithelial cells, gastric mucosal cells, neurons, anterior pituitary cells	Mucosal protection and repair
	Chronic lymphocytic leukemia, ovarian cancer, prostate cancer, AML	Anti-inflammatory activity Increased bone resorption through osteoclast activation Inhibition of adipogenesis Regulation of neuronal differentiation Active in human reproduction

EPO, erythropoietin; CSF3, colony-stimulating factor 3; AML, acute myeloid leukemia; GM-CSF, granulocyte-macrophage colony-stimulating factor; ALL, acute lymphoblastic leukemia; IL-11, interleukin-11.

(SC) dosing; however, clearance appears to increase as blood neutrophil concentration increases, suggesting a negative feedback mechanism.[25] Pegfilgrastim is a polyethylene glycol-conjugated version of filgrastim designed for longer half-life, thereby necessitating fewer injections. In a study of ten cancer patients, the median half-life of pegfilgrastim was approximately 33 hours.[26] Serum clearance was directly related to blood neutrophil concentrations as in the case of filgrastim.[26] Outside the United States, rHu CSF3 is available as lenograstim, a glycosylated recombinant CSF3 derived from a mammalian cell system (Chinese hamster ovaries), and nartograstim, an N-terminal–mutated recombinant CSF3 produced in *E. coli*.

The administration of rHu CSF3 to humans increases the level of circulating neutrophils by accelerating production through reduction of transit time from stem cell to mature neutrophil and by inhibition of neutrophil apoptosis. These effects are associated with an increase in the number of neutrophil progenitors in the marrow and an increase in the percentage of myeloid progenitors in the S phase. Evidence suggests that rHu CSF3 may stimulate the entry of quiescent stem and progenitor cells into mitosis.[25]

After administration of CSF3, neutrophils show morphologic changes consistent with activation, including Döhle's inclusion bodies, toxic granulation, and an increase in band forms. At a minimum, these neutrophils are functionally normal as tested with standard assays of phagocytosis and respiratory burst. However, data suggest that CSF3 enhances chemotaxis, phagocytosis, and the oxidative burst of mature neutrophils *in vitro* and increases antibody-dependent cellular cytotoxicity *in vivo*.[27]

Marrow aspirates demonstrate a left shift in patients receiving CSF3 or other myeloid growth factors, and after IV administration, neutrophil counts may transiently drop. On discontinuation of recombinant CSF3, peripheral neutrophil counts decrease by approximately 50% per day and return to baseline in 4 to 6 days.[28] Lymphocytes and monocytes are also marginally increased with rHu CSF3 administration; however, the clinical significance of these changes is not established.

In addition to stimulating neutrophil production, CSF3 mobilizes hematopoietic progenitor cells (HPCs) into the peripheral circulation, the mechanism of which is not fully understood. It has been demonstrated that the presence of CSF3 receptors on HPCs is not required for mobilization by CSF3, suggesting that CSF3 may first activate a mature hematopoietic cell via a CSF3 receptor, and this activated cell in turn generates secondary signals, leading to HPC mobilization.[29]

The most common side effect from rHu CSF3 administration is mild-to-moderate bone pain.[30] Splenomegaly has been reported in chronic use as well as transient dyspnea and pulmonary infiltrates on chest radiography. IV administration is associated with a transient neutropenia thought to be secondary to up-regulation of neutrophil adhesion receptors, resulting in margination to endothelial surfaces. Regular white blood cell monitoring should be conducted during therapy to prevent leukocytosis; typically treatment is discontinued when the neutrophil count reaches 10,000 cells/mcL in the setting of chemotherapy-induced neutropenia. Rare, serious adverse events are reported, including allergic-type reactions (particularly with the first dose), splenic rupture in persons receiving recombinant CSF3 for peripheral blood stem cell mobilization (including healthy donors), and adult respiratory distress syndrome in neutropenic patients with infection.[31,32]

GRANULOCYTE-MACROPHAGE COLONY-STIMULATING FACTOR

Endogenous GM-CSF along with the receptors for IL-3 and IL-5 contribute to normal hematopoiesis. In fact, lymphoid progenitor cells can be redirected to myeloid differentiation through IL-2 and GM-CSF mediated stimulation.[33] Murine models deficient in GM-CSF do not develop hematopoietic abnormalities but demonstrate a syndrome similar to pulmonary alveolar proteinosis due to its role in pulmonary surfactant clearance by alveolar macrophages.[34–36] Though null animals demonstrate continued hematopoiesis, a systemic lupus erythematosus phenotype is displayed with evidence of macrophage dysfunction and a propensity for infection.[37,38] Activation of the JAK-STAT, ERK1/2, phosphatidylinositol 3-kinase (PI3K)/Akt, and inhibitor of κB/nuclear factor κB (IκB/NF-κB) pathways by GM-CSF in both normal and disease states has been well described.[39,40] Alternative mechanisms of GM-CSF receptor activation, specifically by Src-family kinases (SFK), have been proposed and demonstrate redundancy.[41] Activation of Lyn (of the SFK) in blasts from patients with AML and CML in blast crisis may be related to aberrant GM-CSF signaling.[42,43]

Three different rHu GM-CSFs exist, including sargramostim, molgramostim, and regramostim. Sargramostim, the only form available in the United States, is an rHu GM-CSF that has an amino acid sequence identical to endogenous GM-CSF, except for a substitution of leucine at position 23. The carbohydrate moiety may also differ from endogenous human GM-CSF. Sargramostim is derived from yeast (*Saccharomyces cerevisiae*) and is O-glycosylated. After SC administration in healthy subjects, the mean terminal half-life is approximately 2.7 hours. Outside the United States, rHu GM-CSF is available as molgramostim, a nonglycosylated rHu GM-CSF derived from *E. coli*, and regramostim, a fully glycosylated rHu GM-CSF derived from Chinese hamster ovary cells. The different formulations appear to have similar pharmacologic activity.

Administration of rHu GM-CSF increases levels of circulating neutrophils, eosinophils, and, to a lesser extent, macrophages and lymphocytes. In addition, rHu GM-CSF exerts immunomodulatory activity on cells of the granulocyte and macrophage lineages. Although endogenous GM-CSF is involved in erythropoiesis and megakaryocyte development, other growth factors are required for final maturation of these cell lines, and rHu GM-CSF has no significant clinical effect on erythrocyte or platelet levels.

The effects of rHu GM-CSF on neutrophils is similar to CSF3 in that it stimulates neutrophil progenitor proliferation; reduces neutrophil apoptosis; and enhances chemotaxis, phagocytosis, and respiratory burst.[44] Beyond these effects, rHu GM-CSF stimulates neutrophils and promotes their response to other stimuli.[45] Neutrophils exposed to rHu GM-CSF exhibit enhanced superoxide anion generation and expression of class II major histocompatibility complex molecules. As with rHu CSF3 administration, marrow aspirates show a left shift, and neutrophil counts may transiently drop after IV administration.

Typical side effects of sargramostim therapy include injection site reactions, low-grade fever, and myalgias.[46] Occasionally, patients experience dyspnea, likely resulting from sequestration of granulocytes in the pulmonary vasculature.[47] As with CSF3, patients can experience bone pain, and regular white blood cell monitoring should be conducted during therapy to prevent leukocytosis. Typically, treatment is discontinued when the neutrophil count reaches 10,000 cells/mcL. Rare adverse events include allergic-type reactions with the first dose and fluid retention. High doses induce weight gain, pericarditis, pleuritis, and capillary leak syndrome.[48,49]

That GM-CSF receptor propagates cell growth and survival signals induced by aberrant BCR-Abl expression[50] and mutations of JAK2[51] and its activation in acute myeloid leukemia[52] suggests a role for the receptor in the pathogenesis of malignant disease. GM-CSF appears to be a requirement in the biology of chronic myelomonocytic leukemia (CMML) and juvenile myelomonocytic leukemia (JMML).[53–55] The evolving understanding of the role of GM-CSF in disease provides an opportunity to exploit it with therapeutic intent. The GM-CSF receptor complex's physical structure is a hexameric complex with three interactive sites. E21R, a GM-CSF analogue that competitively binds at site 1, does not demonstrate activity against AML blasts *in vitro*.[56] Progenitor cells from patients with polycythemia vera demonstrate a nearly 50-fold increase in sensitivity in colony-forming assays after GM-CSF exposure when compared with normal progenitor cells.[57] Jak2V617F may act by stabilizing the GM-CSF dodecamer, thereby promoting the activation of downstream pathways.[58] The results of clinical studies investigating JAK2 inhibitors are eagerly awaited.

INTERLEUKIN-11

Endogenous IL-11 stimulates proliferation of megakaryocyte progenitor cells and induces megakaryocyte maturation, leading to increased platelet production.[59] Mice deficient in IL-11 have normal megakaryocyte development and platelet production, demonstrating that IL-11 alone does not regulate thrombopoiesis.[60] *In vitro* murine studies suggest that megakaryocytopoiesis is stimulated at very early developmental stages and that IL-11 is synergistic with stem cell factor and IL-3.[61] Like other cytokines, endogenous IL-11 has various sources and inducers (Table 157.1). Serum concentrations of IL-11 are typically undetectable or very low but are elevated in states of thrombocytopenia.[62]

Various thrombopoietic cytokines were tested in clinical trials, however, only oprelvekin, a rHu IL-11 produced in *E. coli*, which has an amino acid sequence nearly identical to endogenous IL-11, was granted FDA approval. This approval was given based on data from a randomized phase 2 trial in patients with chemotherapy-induced thrombocytopenia.[63] Patients with documented thrombocytopenia of 20,000/mcL or less with a previous chemotherapy cycle were randomized to rHu IL-11 or placebo once daily for 14 to 21 days beginning the day after chemotherapy. Thirty percent of patients who received the higher dose of rHu IL-11 were platelet transfusion independent compared with 4% in the placebo group. Adverse events in the treated patients included fatigue, atrial dysrthymias and syncope.

Recombinant human IL-11 stimulates megakaryocytopoiesis and thrombopoiesis through direct action on megakaryocytes and increases megakaryocyte ploidy.[64] The platelets produced are morphologically and functionally normal with no change in platelet reactivity and a normal lifespan. Platelet counts begin to rise 5 to 9 days after the initial dose, and after stopping therapy, platelet counts continue to rise for up to 7 days, then fall and return to normal in 14 days.

At doses indicated for thrombopoiesis, rHu IL-11 use is associated with several serious toxicities, including allergic reactions and anaphylaxis. Approximately two-thirds of patients who received rHu IL-11 in clinical trials experienced edema, and nearly half experienced dyspnea. Fluid retention has also resulted in exacerbation of existing pleural effusions and atrial arrhythmias. Many patients also become mildly anemic, primarily because of dilutional effects.[65] Papilledema has been reported. Preliminary data suggest that lower doses may be better tolerated with milder and less frequent toxicity.[66] As noted in Table 157.3, IL-11 receptors are located on cancer cell lines, including acute myeloid leukemia (AML) cells. *In vitro* studies with AML cells isolated from patients found IL-11 alone to have little effect on the cell cycle or AML blast apoptosis; however, IL-11 synergistically increased leukemic progenitor cell formation in combination with CSF3.[67]

THROMBOPOIETIN AGENTS

The isolation and characterization of thrombopoietin in 1994 eventually led to the development of recombinant human thrombopoietin (rhTPO) and pegylated human recombinant megakaryocyte growth and development factor (PEG-rHuMGDF).[68–73] Developed to have the same amino acid sequence as TPO, rhTPO was a glycosylated protein and was produced in Chinese hamster ovary cells.[74,75] Its administration was intravenous and resulted in a dose-dependent increase in platelet counts in patients with cancer. A rise in platelet counts was noted 5 days after administration and peaked 10 to 14 days later. PEG-rHuMGDF, a nonglycosylated protein, was made up of the amino-terminal 163 amino acids of TPO.[76] Administration of PEG-rHuMGDF was through the subcutaneous route. The agent demonstrated similar platelet kinetics as rhTPO in healthy volunteers.[77] Administration of PEG-rHuMGDF and rhTPO to patients undergoing stem cell transplant, as well as to those undergoing remission induction or consolidation therapy for acute leukemia, did not affect platelet recovery or number of platelet transfusions.[78–80] In contrast, when treated with either PEG-rHuMGDF or rhTPO, patients with solid tumors undergoing chemotherapy demonstrated shorter duration of thrombocytopenia and required fewer platelet transfusions.[74,81,82] The peak platelet count after administration of both agents occurred on day 12 to 18 in the various series.[75,83] This late effect was inadequate for those cytotoxic regimens in which the platelet nadir occurs at 10 to 14 days. However, in a trial of patients with ovarian cancer who were undergoing treatment with regimens that included high-dose carboplatin (known to have a late onset platelet nadir), administration of rhTPO with the second cycle resulted in a decrease in platelet transfusion requirement from 75% with cycle 1 to 25% with cycle 2.[74]

Initial trials of both agents yielded no serious adverse events until a randomized study in which approximately 1,000 healthy volunteers were given up to three doses of PEG-rHuMGDF or placebo.[1] Of the 13 patients who developed thrombocytopenia, 11 occurred with the third dose of the agent. Further investigation revealed a paucity of megakaryocytes in bone marrow aspirates from patients who developed low platelet counts after treatment. An immunoglobulin-G (IgG) antibody to PEG-rHuMGDF that cross reacted with the thrombopoietin receptor was detected, and quantitative analysis revealed an inverse relationship between platelet counts and IgG antibody concentration.[1] As a result of these findings, further development of PEG-rHuMGDF and rhTPO was halted.

CLINICAL USE OF ERYTHROPOIETIN-STIMULATING AGENTS IN CANCER THERAPY

Anemia secondary to malignancy or chemotherapy is a common and important clinical problem with a negative impact on quality of life (QOL). Anemia in the cancer patient can have a multitude of causes, including toxic effects to bone marrow by chemotherapy and radiation; tumor encroachment of the marrow; decreased red cell survival with hemolysis; hypersplenism and blood loss; or poor production secondary to iron, vitamin, or EPO deficiency. Important among the risk factors predictive of anemia in solid tumor patients is duration of chemotherapy.[84] The established negative impact of anemia on survival of patients with cancer prompted the development of novel agents to mitigate this negative risk factor.[85–88]

Until the 1990s, transfusion was the only treatment option for anemia. Transfusion, although necessary in acute situations, is a limited resource and carries the increased risk of transfusion-related infection. During the past decade, clinical trials with erythropoietin-stimulating agents (ESAs) have been conducted in a variety of settings in oncology. Some of these trials sought to establish a survival advantage in cancer patients with the use of these agents. The demonstration of a negative impact on survival with the use of ESAs, particularly when used in an attempt to normalize the hematocrit, resulted in the FDA's 2007 issuance of a black box warning outlining the risks of higher mortality, tumor progression, and thromboembolic events. In keeping with the FDA's recommendations, the American Society of Clinical Oncology (ASCO) and the American Society of Hematology (ASH) published updated guidelines for the appropriate use of recombinant EPO products.[89] These guidelines focus on chemotherapy-induced anemia and anemia associated with myeloid and lymphoproliferative disorders. The following sections discuss the changes to the guidelines as well as additional data that have been published since the 2007 guidelines were created.

Chemotherapy-Induced Anemia

Epoetin therapy in this setting improves clinical measures of efficacy, including hemoglobin (Hb) and the need for transfusions. Based on evidence from well-controlled trials, epoetin therapy produces significant hemoglobin increases compared with placebo when the baseline Hb concentration is 10 g/dL or less. In these trials, those receiving epoetin showed mean Hb increases of approximately 2 to 3 g/dL. Trials of patients with baseline Hb of more than 10 g/dL showed mixed results. The only well-controlled trial found no significant difference in Hb change. A meta-analysis of all randomized trials found that the use of epoetin decreased the relative odds of receiving a red blood cell transfusion by an average of 62% (odds ratio [OR], 0.38; 95% confidence interval [CI], 0.28 to 0.51). The meta-analysis did not test for effect stratified by baseline Hb. Based on these results, the updated ASCO/ASH guidelines recommend epoetin therapy for chemotherapy-induced anemia if the Hb has declined to 10 g/dL or less or is approaching 10 g/dL, with the intent of increasing Hb and reducing red blood cell transfusions. Epoetin use in patients with less severe anemia (i.e., Hb between 10 and 12 g/dL) is not clearly justified in all patients by the current evidence. Clinical judgment should be used to evaluate epoetin therapy in less severe anemia, with consideration being given to patients at risk for worse outcomes from anemia such as those with pre-existing cardiovascular morbidity. Transfusion remains an additional treatment option in severe clinical cases.[89]

Clinical Benefits of Erythropoietin-Stimulating Agents

The clinical benefits of the use of epoetin have been investigated in multiple clinical trials. Results of three open-label, randomized studies investigating the benefits of early or delayed ESA treatment did not demonstrate a statistically significant decrease in transfusion requirements with early institution of therapy.[90–92] Of the three trials, one demonstrated a statistically significant improvement in QOL measures with the early intervention arm, although the improvement was small.[91] A meta-analysis of five trials, including the three discussed above, sought to determine the clinical benefit of initiating ESA treatment with mild (greater than 10 g/dL) or moderate (less than 10 g/dL) anemia.[93] Although a statistically significant reduction in transfusion requirement (hazard ratio [HR] 0.55; 95% CI, 0.42 to 0.73; *P* = .0001)) was noted in this meta-analysis, it is difficult to draw reliable conclusions given the differences among the trials in transfusion thresholds such that widely variable proportions of patients did not receive ESA treatment.

Although ESAs have been thought to have a favorable impact on QOL, the magnitude of this impact has been difficult to determine. Given the difficulty of reliably measuring QOL, the potential for recall bias, as well as the large proportion of missing data, one can only interpret any purported QOL improvements with ESA therapy cautiously.

Thromboembolic Risk

In September 2003, Johnson & Johnson halted three ongoing clinical trials to investigate the use of epoetin alfa in cancer patients, with target Hb values of 13 g/dL up to 16 g/dL. The risk of thromboembolic event was found to be significantly higher in those patients who received ESA, and this appeared to be related to not only higher target Hb levels but also to rate of Hb rise. Published in 2008, Bennett et al.[94] analyzed over 8,000 patients enrolled on phase 3 randomized trials comparing ESAs with placebo in patients with cancer-associated anemia. The risk of venous thromboembolism (VTE) in patients who received ESAs was 7.9% compared with 4.9% in patients on placebo (relative risk 1.57; 95% CI, 1.31 to 1.87). In addition, survival rates were lower in patients on ESA treatment, relative risk of 1.10 (95% CI, 1.01 to 1.20). It appears from these data and others that the use of ESAs must be undertaken with caution, particularly regarding appropriate Hb targets, as well as taking into consideration thromboembolism risk factors.

Erythropoietin-Stimulating Agent Dosing

Guidance for dosing of epoetin and darbepoetin were most recently updated by the FDA in November 2007.[95] The clinical benefits of epoetin therapy noted earlier (improved Hb and reduced transfusion requirements) were primarily obtained in clinical trials that used weight-based dosing of epoetin.[89] As supported by data from clinical trials in chemotherapy-induced anemia, a starting dose of 150 U/kg three times weekly for a minimum of 4 weeks was included in the FDA guidelines. After 4 weeks, a dose increase to 300 U/kg for an additional 8 weeks in nonresponders (less than 1 g/dL improvement by week 4) can be considered.[29] However, weekly dosing (40,000 U/wk) is commonly applied in clinical practice, and based on the breadth of this clinical experience, weekly administration is included in the labeling as an option. The results of a randomized, double-blind trial of weekly dosing demonstrated statistically significant increases in Hb concentration and decreases in transfusions administered when compared with placebo.[96] In addition, a phase 3 randomized, double-blind trial of once-weekly dosing darbepoetin use resulted in significantly fewer patients requiring transfusions (27% vs. 52%; *P* <.01) and a significantly higher Hb response rate (66% vs. 24%; *P* <.001) compared with placebo in patients with chemotherapy-induced anemia.[97] In a randomized, noninferiority trial comparing darbepoetin alfa every 2 weeks with weekly epoetin alfa, comparable efficacy was noted for transfusion requirements, Hb increase, safety, as well as QOL measurements.[98] Important additions to the FDA-approved labeling include parameters by which to decrease the dose, particularly when a rise in Hb exceeds 1 g/dL in any 2-week period. Similarly, guidelines for withholding the dose of ESA when Hb reaches 12 g/dL were also included.[95] The optimal duration of therapy in patients who respond to epoetin therapy is not defined; however, it is recommended that Hb levels should be raised to or near 12 g/dL. No evidence exists for "normalization" of Hb above 12 g/dL. Once the Hb level approaches 12 g/dL, epoetin therapy should be dose-titrated down or discontinued and subsequently reinitiated if indicated. In nonresponders (defined as patients achieving a less than 1 to 2 g/dL rise in Hb), dosing beyond 6 to 8 weeks does not appear to be beneficial.[89]

Erythropoietin-Stimulating Agent Use in Nonmyeloid Malignancy

Since the ASCO/ASH 2002 guidelines on ESA therapy, multiple reviews have been undertaken to determine the benefits and risks of ESA use in patients with nonmyeloid hematological malignancies. The results of these reviews have provided additional evidence that there appears to be no statistically significant changes in mortality or survival with the use of epoetin or darbepoetin in patients with these hematological malignancies. Thus, the guidelines from 2002 remain unchanged.[89]

Erythropoietin-Stimulating Agent Use and Survival Impact

Safety concerns stemming from several randomized trials that suggested that survival outcomes were compromised by the use of ESAs prompted the FDA to convene the Oncology Drug Action Committee (ODAC) meetings in 2004 and again in 2007. Multiple randomized trials have suggested poorer survival rates or decreased tumor response in patients treated with ESAs.[99–101] Several meta-analyses have since been undertaken in an effort to define any negative impact on survival. In 2006 a Cochrane Collaborative Analysis of studies from 1985 until 2005[102,103] was published that included studies of ESA use in the setting of anemia associated with chemotherapy and radiotherapy alone as well as in combination. The increase in mortality risk, reported as an odds ratio, was not statistically significant (1.08; 95% CI, 0.99 to 1.18). As noted previously, Bennett et al.[94] published results of an analysis of over 13,611 patients from 51 randomized trials suggesting an increased mortality rate in those patients who received ESA (HR 1.10; 95% CI, 1.01 to 1.20; *P* = .03). These results did not appear to be influenced by data from a single study, as eight trials contributed 5% to 9% of the number of enrolled patients, respectively. Published in 2009, Bohlius et al.[104] obtained data on patients with cancer enrolled in randomized trials comparing transfusion alone with transfusion plus one of the following agents: epoetin alfa, epoetin beta, or darbepoetin. Data from nearly 14,000 patients enrolled in 53 trials were included in the analysis. Their findings demonstrated an increased risk of death during the study period (combined hazard ratio [cHR] 1.17; 95% CI, 1.06 to 1.30) as well as a decrease in overall survival (1.06; 94% CI, 1.00 to 1.12). It is of note that most of the studies included in the analysis did not adhere to current guidelines for ESA use and may have demonstrated a detrimental effect on survival by virtue of higher target Hb concentrations. In a comprehensive review of 60 trials with available survival data, Glaspy et al.[105] published a combined analysis of trials included in the Cochrane 2006 analysis, trials published since 2006, as well as unpublished data from Amgen, Centocor, and Ortho Biotech. The use of ESA did not appear to negatively impact survival (OR 1.06; 95% CI, 0.97 to 1.15). In the 26 studies evaluated for ESAs' impact on disease progression, no statistically significant impact was noted (OR 1.01; 95% CI, 0.90 to 1.14). The increased risk of VTE noted in other meta-analyses was confirmed in this meta-analysis of 44 studies for which data were available (OR 1.48; 95% CI, 1.28 to 1.72).

These and other meta-analyses have provided conflicting results on the true impact of ESA use on survival. To that end, the results of ongoing randomized trials of ESA use in the cancer patient population are awaited. In the interim, it is incumbent upon clinicians to approach the use of ESA's cautiously, particularly in those patients for whom treatment is intended to be curative.

CLINICAL USE OF RECOMBINANT GRANULOCYTE COLONY-STIMULATING FACTORS IN CANCER THERAPY

The CSF3s, rHu CSF3, and rHu GM-CSF have been applied in a variety of oncology settings, including the management of chemotherapy-induced neutropenia, hematopoietic reconstitution after stem cell transplant, mobilization and *ex vivo* expansion of HPCs, and as a priming agent in AML. However, research continues to identify the appropriate application of these growth factors within each setting. Key issues include optimizing outcomes and cost-effective use. The American Society of Clinical Oncology recently created updated recommendations for the use of CSFs; these guidelines are summarized in Table 157.4 and discussed in the following sections.[106]

TABLE 157.4

SUMMARY OF AMERICAN SOCIETY OF CLINICAL ONCOLOGY 2006 GUIDELINES FOR ADMINISTRATION OF GRANULOCYTE COLONY-STIMULATING FACTOR AND GRANULOCYTE-MACROPHAGE COLONY-STIMULATING FACTOR

Indication	Recommendation
Primary prophylactic CSF administration (administration of a CSF beginning with the first cycle of a treatment regimen)	Recommended if: 1. The chemotherapy regimen has an expected 20% or more incidence of FN. 2. A decrease in dose intensity would compromise long-term outcomes (survival/cure). 3. The patient is at increased risk for serious complications or death from FN (e.g., advanced age, prior treatment, low performance status, infection).
Secondary prophylactic CSF administration (administration of a CSF in all subsequent cycles after an episode of FN)	Use if a decrease in dose intensity would compromise long-term outcomes (survival/cure)
Treatment of established FN	Use with antibiotics in patients predicted to have a poor outcome (e.g., organ or intravenous site infection, hypotension, bacteremia, serious comorbidities)
Treatment of established neutropenia in afebrile patients	Not recommended
Use of CSF to increase dose intensity	Not recommended
Use of CSF to enable delivery of dose-dense chemotherapy regimens	Use with dose-dense ACT for lymph node–positive breast cancer; results inconclusive with other regimens
Adjuncts to stem cell transplantation	Use of CSF is warranted for PBSC mobilization and following PBSC or BM transplantation
Delayed engraftment-graft failure	Use of a CSF is warranted
Acute myeloid leukemia	Use after induction in patients older than 55 years if determined to be cost-effective based on shortened hospitalization secondary to shortened duration of neutropenia. Routine use in younger patients, postconsolidation, in relapsed disease, or for priming of leukemic cells is not recommended.
Acute lymphoblastic leukemia	Use with chemotherapy after initiation of induction or postremission chemotherapy in an effort to reduce the duration of neutropenia
Myelodysplastic syndromes	Routine use not recommended
Concurrent administration of CSFs with chemotherapy and radiation therapy	Avoid

CSF, colony-stimulating factor; FN, febrile neutropenia; ACT, doxorubin (Adriamycin), cyclophosphamide, paclitaxel; PBSC, peripheral blood stem cell; BM, bone marrow.

Neutropenia Associated with Standard-Dose Chemotherapy

Neutropenia and the associated complication of infection often manifest as febrile neutropenia (FN), lead to significant morbidity and mortality in patients receiving cancer chemotherapy, and are often dose-limiting. The incidence of infection directly correlates with the depth and duration of neutropenia. FN typically results in hospitalization for evaluation and initiation of IV broad-spectrum antibiotics, leading to reduced QOL, increased risk for iatrogenic complications, and increased health care utilization costs. Options for reducing the incidence of FN include use of CSFs, chemotherapy dose reduction or delay, and prophylactic antibiotic use. The latter option is used under limited circumstances because of the risk of promoting growth of resistant organisms. Thus, CSFs and reduction of chemotherapy dose intensity remain the two most frequently exercised alternatives.

Prophylactic Colony-Stimulating Factor Use

The decision to administer a CSF as primary prophylaxis (i.e., immediately after the first cycle of chemotherapy before any occurrence of neutropenia), secondary prophylaxis (i.e., immediately after subsequent cycles to reduce the risk of FN after the prior occurrence of FN), or therapeutically (i.e., treating severe neutropenia or FN once it is established) remains a challenge. In particular, the clinical benefit and economic value of routine primary prophylaxis have been extensively debated.

Current evidence indicates that primary prophylaxis with a CSF results in a relative risk reduction of FN by approximately 50% to 90%, depending on the type of cancer and chemotherapy regimen used.[106] A significant reduction in documented infections has also been demonstrated. In a meta-analysis including 17 randomized controlled trials of solid tumors as well as lymphoma, the relative risk reduction in the rate of FN was 46% ($P < .0001$) with the use of primary prophylactic CSF3. A relative risk reduction in infection-related mortality of 48% ($P < .01$) was found, with the absolute difference being 1.6%.[107] Data were not sufficient to determine growth factor impact on disease-free survival or overall survival. In a meta-analysis of 13 randomized trials involving more than 2,607 patients with lymphoma, prophylactic CSF use was associated with a significant reduction in the relative risk of severe neutropenia (relative risk, 0.67; 95% CI, 0.60 to 0.73) and febrile neutropenia (relative risk, 0.74; 95% CI, 0.62 to 0.89). However, CSFs did not appear to reduce the infection-related mortality (relative risk, 0.93; 95% CI, 0.51 to 1.71) or improve overall survival (HR 0.97; 95% CI, 0.87 to 1.09).[108] Clinical efficacy of CSFs in the prevention of neutropenia is well established. However, the appropriate indications for primary prophylactic therapy have evolved over the years.

Most recently, data support the use of primary prophylaxis in those chemotherapy regimens in which the risk of FN is approximately 20% or higher, a change from prior guidelines that supported its use if the risk of FN exceeded 40%. The use of CSFs in dose-dense chemotherapy regimens is essential and widely accepted. Oftentimes patient factors may result in a higher risk of neutropenia and support the use of primary prophylaxis even in regimens that do not have a risk of FN of greater than 20%. Such factors include age greater than 65 years, poor performance status, concurrent chemotherapy and radiation therapy, prior episodes of FN, extensive prior therapy, extensive bone marrow involvement by tumor, as well as other comorbidities.[106] It should be noted that current guidelines suggest the use of alternative chemotherapy regimens that do not result in elevated risk of FN if efficacy is not compromised.

The economic impact of primary prophylaxis has sparked an ongoing debate, particularly in light of recent guidelines allowing more liberal use of CSFs. The cost-effectiveness of CSFs has been well established in regimens in which the incidence of FN exceeded 40%; however, cost-analyses have suggested that their use in treatments, resulting in FN rates of 20% to 25%, also conferred a cost-benefit.[109] More recent analysis has suggested that the use of pegfilgrastim as prophylaxis may be not only cost-effective but also cost-saving.[110]

In the only prospective economic evaluation performed to date, the cost-effectiveness of primary prophylactic CSF3 was analyzed alongside a phase 3 trial involving small cell lung cancer patients in the Netherlands. This was one of the two trials that helped establish the current guidelines that allow the use of primary prophylaxis in those regimens with FN rates around 20%.[111] Although the use of CSF3 effected a significant reduction in the rate of FN in this cohort, economic analysis did not reveal that this approach was cost-saving. The 14% reduction in the incidence of FN was at a cost of €3,360. By average 2007 exchange rates, this would amount to approximately $4,400[112] (as of 2010 $4,334). This analysis did not address the potential savings associated with reduction of productivity loss due to FN, although this may not play a large role, given the advanced age of the cohort studied. Additionally, the apparent lack of cost-effectiveness may not be easily extrapolated to the use of CSF in the United States given our higher health care costs.

Alternatives to Primary Prophylaxis

Alternatives to primary prophylaxis include secondary prophylaxis, dose reduction or delay, or therapeutic use of CSFs. The panel recommended that secondary prophylaxis with CSFs should be considered in any patient who experiences a prior neutropenic complication in whom a recurrence would likely result in treatment delays or in any patient in whom dose reductions may compromise disease-free or overall survival or patient QOL. In settings such as palliative chemotherapy or others in which a reduction in dose intensity is not expected to compromise long-term outcomes, dose reduction or delay is considered the preferred option to CSF use.[106]

Therapeutic application of growth factors does not afford the benefit of reducing the incidence of hospitalization due to FN; however, treatment of FN with a CSF may reduce the risk of prolonged hospitalization, which accounts for a significant portion of hospitalization costs.[113] Routine treatment of FN with a CSF is not recommended but should be considered in any patient at increased risk for prolonged hospitalization, severe complications, or death. These populations include the elderly or those with uncontrolled cancer, serious comorbidities, absolute neutrophil count of less than 100/mcL, hospitalization at the time of fever development, hypotension, sepsis, or organ infection.[114,115] Current evidence does not support the treatment of afebrile neutropenia with a CSF.[116]

Neutropenia Associated with Dose-Intense or Dose-Dense Chemotherapy

Increasing the dose intensity of a chemotherapy regimen (i.e., increasing the total dose of one or more agents per cycle) or administering dose-dense chemotherapy (i.e., reducing the interval between chemotherapy cycles, resulting in an increased dose delivered per unit of time compared with standard-dose therapy) leads to an increased risk of neutropenia or reduces the amount of time a patient has for neutrophil recovery between cycles. The use of CSFs in these instances is considered necessary to be able to administer these regimens at the planned dose on schedule. However, the long-term benefits from using CSFs in this manner are still under investigation. Although *maintenance* of dose intensity of standard-dose regimens has been demonstrated to be necessary for optimal outcomes in certain settings, *increases* in dose intensity with or without CSF support have not been associated with improved outcomes.

Improvements in survival have been demonstrated using CSF support of the dose-dense approach, but a definitive benefit has been found to date only in the setting of dose-dense adjuvant chemotherapy for lymph node–positive breast cancer. The Cancer and Leukemia Group B trial 9741 evaluated four adjuvant chemotherapy regimens in 2005 in women with axillary node–positive breast cancer.[117] Patients received sequential doxorubicin 60 mg/m^2, paclitaxel 175 mg/m^2, and cyclophosphamide 600 mg/m^2, or concurrent doxorubicin and cyclophosphamide followed by paclitaxel. Each of these regimens was administered either every 3 weeks without CSF support or every 2 weeks with filgrastim support (dose-dense). The primary and secondary end points of the trial were disease-free survival (DFS) and overall survival (OS). Both DFS (relative risk 0.74; P = .010) and OS (relative risk 0.69; P = .013) were improved with the dose-dense regimens. At the San Antonio Breast Cancer Symposium in December 2005 the results were further updated now with 69 months of follow-up. These results showed a modest decline in the impact of dose-dense therapy on DFS and dramatic decline in the HR for OS for this regimen. The value of this therapy in estrogen receptor (ER) –positive disease is particularly questionable, with no significant impact on DFS and OS despite the fact that the trial has basically the same statistical power (a similar number of events) as in the ER-negative subgroup. Thus the value of the therapy is particularly questionable in ER-positive patients.[118]

CSF support of the dose-dense approach has been applied in other settings, with variable results. Two trials in small cell lung cancer found improved survival with dose-dense regimens of either doxorubicin, cyclophosphamide, and etoposide or ifosfamide, carboplatin, etoposide, and vincristine.[111,119] Lenograstim support enabled increased overall dose intensity in the dose-dense arm of doxorubicin, cyclophosphamide, and etoposide. Randomization to rHu GM-CSF or placebo was used in the trial of ifosfamide, carboplatin, etoposide, and vincristine; however, no benefit to therapy with rHu GM-CSF was demonstrated. Timmer-Bonte et al.[111] investigated intensified therapy to 171 patients with a diagnosis of small cell lung cancer. As already commented on previously, the rate of FN in the first cycle was reduced, as was the overall rate of FN. There appeared to be no survival effect. Conflicting data have been presented in the setting of non-Hodgkin's lymphoma (NHL). Although a survival advantage was found with 14-day cycles of cyclophosphamide, doxorubicin, vincristine, and prednisone (CHOP-14) compared with 21-day cycles in older patients with aggressive NHL, no such benefit was demonstrated in a trial enrolling a lower-risk group of younger patients with aggressive NHL.[120,121]

Based on these data, the panel stated that no justification exists for the use of CSFs to increase chemotherapy dose intensity outside a clinical trial. Dose-dense chemotherapy with doxorubicin, cyclophosphamide, and paclitaxel supported by filgrastim offers clinical benefit in lymph node–positive breast cancer; however, these results cannot be extrapolated to other regimens or settings without appropriate clinical investigation.

USE OF COLONY-STIMULATING FACTORS IN OTHER ONCOLOGY SETTINGS

CSFs have been applied for other purposes outside chemotherapy-induced neutropenia in oncology. Primarily, these settings include stem cell transplantation and hematologic malignancies.

Stem Cell Transplantation

Current use of CSFs in the setting of stem cell transplantation involves its administration in an effort to mobilize peripheral-blood progenitor cells (PBPC) as well as after autologous PBPC transplant to promote neutrophil recovery.

Although the use of CSFs in autologous PBPC transplantation has been demonstrated to diminish length of hospitalization as well as overall medical costs, the same advantages have not been shown in the allogeneic transplant setting.[122,123] In fact, in the setting of allogeneic BM transplant, the use of CSFs has been associated with increased incidence of graft-versus-host disease (GVHD). In a retrospective analysis of more than 1,700 patients, the rate of grade 2 to 4 GVHD was 50% in those who received CSF versus 39% in the cohort of patients who did not. The risk of transplant-related mortality was also higher in the group who received CSF3 (relative risk 1.73; P = .00016) as well as a lower overall survival (relative risk 0.59; P <.0001).[124] These risks were not observed in the approximately 400 patients also followed who had undergone PBSC transplant from HLA-identical siblings. Current evidence and guidelines support the use of CSFs to reduce the period of neutropenia after chemotherapy and PBPC transplantation.

The use of CSFs for stem cell mobilization in healthy donors is well tolerated, with bone pain being the most common side effect.[125–127] More serious adverse events, including splenic rupture, anaphylaxis, development of gouty arthritis, vasculitis, rash, capillary leak syndrome, stroke, and angina, have been reported, making cardiovascular, inflammatory, and cerebrovascular diseases relative contraindications.[125,128] The use of pegfilgrastim in healthy donors has shown similar results as when filgastrim is utilized. Kroschinsky et al.[129] administered a single 12-mg dose of pegfilgrastim to 25 healthy donors. Results demonstrated a similar increase in CD34+ cells as observed after filgastrim-stimulated mobilization. Stem cell harvest was successful in 80% of patients after a single apheresis procedure.[129] In a series of multiple myeloma patients who underwent autologous transplant, sufficient stem cell mobilization was possible after a single apheresis session in patients who received pegfilgasrim.[130] When compared with filgrastim, pegfilgrastim demonstrated equivalent bone marrow recovery at day 100 in this series of patients.

Acute Myeloid Leukemia

CSF use is recommended in the setting of induction chemotherapy as well as consolidation chemotherapy in patients with AML for the purposes of shortening the period of neutropenia as well as possibly reducing hospitalization length and incidence of infections. Generally, primary prophylactic postinduction CSF use has resulted in a decreased time to neutrophil recovery (500 cells/mcL) by 2 to 6 days, with resultant reductions in the duration of hospitalization and antibiotic use.[131–139] No consistent effects on complete response rates or patient survival have been demonstrated nor evidence of leukemia growth stimulation or enhanced drug resistance. Similarly, postconsolidation CSF use has resulted in a decreased duration of severe neutropenia with reduced infection rates but no effect on complete response rates or survival.[134,140] Current evidence does not support use of CSFs in the setting of relapsed AML; few data are available to confirm benefits in infection-related morbidity or absence of leukemic stimulation.

In vitro data exist suggesting that CSFs can sensitize leukemic cells to cell cycle–specific cytotoxic agents, such as cytarabine.[141–143] Clinical trial results have been mixed, with most trials demonstrating no benefit in terms of response rate, response duration, or survival.[136–138,144–146] However, a European multicenter, randomized trial of 640 previously untreated, nonelderly adults with AML found an improvement in disease-free survival, but no effect on complete response rates or overall survival.[147] Thomaset al.[148] recently published the results of a multicenter study to investigate the use of GM-CSF in patients with AML who had been treated with timed sequential chemotherapy.[148] Long-term follow-up demonstrated a statistically significant event-free survival (EFS) rate at 5 years of 43% in the GM-CSF cohort compared with 34% in the chemotherapy alone group ($P = .04$). The benefit was particularly apparent in the patients with poor prognostic features such as elevated white blood cell count at diagnosis or the presence of fms-like tyrosine kinase 3 internal tandem repeat (FLT-3 ITD) or mixed lineage leukemia (MLL) gene mutation. Patients with the presence of FLT-3 ITD or MLL gene mutation had a 5-year EFS rate of 39% with the addition of GM-CSF versus 8% in the chemotherapy alone group ($P < .007$). Patients with good prognosis features derived no appreciable benefit from the use of GM-CSF as part of induction therapy. These results warrant further study of this therapeutic approach, particularly in patients whose disease displays poor prognostic features.

Also of some increased interest has been the notion that CSF3 treatment could induce differentiation of AML blasts with resultant apoptosis.[149,150] Although interest in this approach has been tempered by the belief that eradication of the leukemic stem cell is likely necessary for durable remission, success with all-transretinoic acid in the treatment of acute promyelocytic leukemia supports differentiation induction as a potential area of interest.[151]

Acute Lymphoblastic Leukemia

Data supporting the clinical benefits of postinduction CSFs in both pediatric and adult acute lymphoblastic leukemia (ALL) are variable. Although typically CSFs do result in shortened durations of neutropenia, the impact on other clinical outcomes such as the incidence of infection or FN and the duration of hospitalization is variable.[152] No improvements in disease-free survival or overall survival have been demonstrated. A randomized pediatric study of patients with high-risk ALL receiving induction and consolidation therapy did not demonstrate an improvement in length of hospitalization, rate of FN, or development of severe infection in patients who received CSF3, although a faster time to neutrophil recovery was detected.[153] Current guidelines recommend CSF use after the first few days of the initial induction or first postremission course in an effort to diminish the duration of neutropenia. In a study of adults who received induction chemotherapy with a hyper-CVAD regimen (cyclophosphamide, doxorubicin, vincristine, and dexamethasone), patients who received CSF3 at day 5 were compared with those who received it on day 10.[154] Patient who received delayed treatment had a minimal increase in time to neutrophil recovery, but no increase in the risk of infection.

Myelodysplastic Syndromes

Although CSFs can increase neutrophil counts in patients with myelodysplastic syndrome (MDS), these counts decline on discontinuation of the CSF. A randomized trial compared rHu CSF3 with best supportive care and found overall survival to be shorter in patients with refractory anemia and excess blasts who received rHu CSF3.[155] *In vitro* evidence suggests a synergistic effect on erythropoiesis when CSF3 and erythropoietin are used simultaneously.[156,157] Clinical trials in patients with MDS have shown improvement in anemia with the concomitant use of erythropoietin and CSF3 in patients who have not responded to erythropoietin alone.[158–162] The use of myeloid colony-stimulating factors in patients with MDS in multiple studies has not been shown to impart an increased risk of transformation to AML.[163–165] Prolonged administration of CSF does not appear to confer any benefit in the natural history of MDS; however, its use may be recommended for those patients who suffer from repeated infections or in patients who do not have an adequate response to erythropoietin.

Use of Colony-Stimulating Factors in Older Patients

A significant addition to the American Society of Clinical Oncology 2006 guidelines on prophylactic CSF use included recommendations for its use in older patients.[106] Age above 65 represents a significant risk factor for neutropenia, as demonstrated in multiple studies.[166–171] The use of prophylactic CSF in multiple randomized studies of older patients with lymphoma receiving CHOP or similar regimens has demonstrated a more than 50% decrease in the incidence of FN or infection with a possible survival benefit, although the latter remains to be confirmed.[172–174] The current ASCO guidelines for the use of white blood cell growth factors call for prophylactic CSF to be used in patients aged 65 and older with diffuse aggressive lymphoma treated with curative intent.

Dosing and Timing of Colony-Stimulating Factors

The current recommendations for dosing and timing of CSFs are as follows: the recommended dose of filgrastim is 5 mcg/kg, and that of sargramostim is 250 mcg/m^2, each administered SC daily. For PBPC mobilization, a dose of 10 mcg/kg/d for filgrastim may provide an improved stem cell yield (Table 157.5).[175,176] The preferred route is subcutaneous.

The benefits documented in clinical trials were achieved with initiation of CSFs within 24 to 72 hours after chemotherapy, although after stem cell infusion, administration within 5 days has been demonstrated to maintain efficacy. For chemotherapy-induced neutropenia, daily injections of filgrastim are typically continued until an absolute neutrophil count of 2 to 3 $\times$ 10^9 cells/mcL.[106]

Currently approved to reduce the incidence of FN in patients with nonmyeloid malignancies who receive myelosuppressive chemotherapy, pegfilgrastim can be administered once during each chemotherapy cycle of 2 to 4 weeks. Clinical trials have demonstrated equivalent efficacy to filgrastim in this setting. Of interest is the use of pegfilgrastim to support dose-dense regimens. Feasibility studies in both small cell lung cancer as well as elderly patients with lymphoma who receive CHOP every 14 days have demonstrated safety and efficacy of pegfilgrastim, although its routine use in the dose-dense setting remains to be established.[177,178] The concern of administering

TABLE 157.5

RECOMMENDED DOSING AND TIMING OF COLONY-STIMULATING FACTORS

Agent	Recommended Dosing Schedule
Filgrastim	For neutropenia associated with myelosuppressive chemotherapy: 5 mcg/kg/d subcutaneous administration is preferred over intravenous until absolute neutrophil count is 2–3 × 10^9/mcL or up to 14 d. For peripheral blood stem cell collection: 10 mcg/kg/d to begin at least 4 d before the first leukopheresis and continue until the last leukopheresis. For bone marrow transplantation: 10 mcg/kg/d, subcutaneous route preferred. Doses may be increased by 5 mcg/kg based on duration and severity of neutropenia.
Pegylated filgrastim	6 mg subcutaneously once per chemotherapy cycle. Do not administer with 24 hr of administration of chemotherapy or within 14 d before administration of chemotherapy.
Sargramostim	Following chemotherapy in AML: 250 mcg/m²/d intravenously during 4 hr starting approximately 4 d after the completion of induction chemotherapy, if bone marrow biopsy at day 10 shows less than 5% blasts. Continue until the absolute neutrophil count is above 1,500/mcL or a maximum of 42 d. If severe adverse reaction occurs, reduce the dose by 50% or stop therapy. For peripheral blood stem cell collection: 250 mcg/m²/d intravenously during 24 hr or subcutaneously once daily. The optimal schedule for duration of administration has not been established.
rHu IL-11	For prevention of thrombocytopenia: 50 mcg/kg/d subcutaneously for 10 to 21 days or until postnadir platelet count exceeds 50,000/mcL. Administration should start 6 to 24 hr after initiation of chemotherapy and end 48 hr before the subsequent cycle.

AML, acute myeloid leukemia; rHu, recombinant human; IL, interleukin.

CSFs in either close proximity to or concurrent with cytotoxic chemotherapy or radiation therapy first arose with a trial of sargramostim in patients who received cisplatin, etoposide, and thoracic irradiation for small cell lung cancer.[179] Patients who received sargramostim concurrent with chemotherapy experienced an increase in thrombocytopenia. Since then, other trials have demonstrated worsened myelosuppression with concurrent filgrastim and chemotherapy.[180,181] At present, concomitant administration should be applied only in the setting of appropriately designed clinical trials.

The Association of Colony-Stimulating Factor Use and Myelodysplastic Syndrome/Acute Myeloid Leukemia

The potential for development of myeloid leukemia after CSF has been attributed to the antiapoptotic effect of CSF3 and GM-CSF, which rescues stem cells from death after lethal mutations induced by chemotherapy. Data from breast cancer patients 65 and older in the Surveillance, Epidemiology, and End Results-Medicare database who received adjuvant chemotherapy with CSF3 or GM-CSF and were diagnosed with MDS or AML before cancer recurrence were analyzed to assess the risk of leukemia.[182] The hazard ratio for AML or MDS in those who received CSF was 2.14 (95% CI, 1.12 to 4.08). The absolute risk within 48 months was 1.8% in patients who received growth factors versus 0.7% in those who did not. In a case-control study conducted in France including women treated for breast cancer during a 16-year period, the relative risk of AML or MDS was 6.3 in patients who received CSF3 support (95% CI, 1.9 to 21.0). This elevated risk was present even when controlled for topoisomerase-II inhibitor and radiotherapy exposure as well as chemotherapy dose intensity.[183] A meta-analysis of 25 randomized controlled trials to analyze data from over 12,000 patients with solid tumors or lymphoma who were randomly assigned to chemotherapy with or without CSF3 support was recently published.[184] The estimated relative risk of AML/MDS in the patients who received growth factor was 1.92, translating to an absolute risk of 0.4%. Interestingly, the patients assigned treatment with CSF3 demonstrated a benefit of survival with a relative risk of 0.897 (95% CI, 0.857 to 0.938; $P < .001$) and an absolute risk reduction of 3.4% (95% CI, 2.01% to 4.80%; $P < .001$). The survival benefit may be due to the ability to maintain chemotherapy dose intensity with the utilization of CSF3. The reported rates of AML/MDS in this meta-analysis are consistent with the results of prior studies.[183,185–189]

A causal relationship between CSF3 use and increased risk of MDS/AML cannot be definitively concluded in solid tumor patients. Maintenance of dose intensity with the use of CSF3 such that increased doses of chemotherapy agents with an inherent risk of leukemogenesis are administered may explain the above described findings. While the potential for an increased incidence of AML/MDS may exist with the use of CSF3 and chemotherapy, its positive impact on overall mortality should be taken into consideration when making treatment decisions.

CLINICAL USE OF THROMBOPOIETIN AGENTS

At present, platelet transfusion remains the primary therapeutic modality for treatment of thrombocytopenia in the oncology setting. Although rHu IL-11 (oprelvekin) is a therapeutic option, its use is limited by a high incidence of toxicity, prompting the search for other agents.

As previously discussed, the first-generation recombinant thrombopoietin agents, including recombinant human TPO (rh TPO) and pegylated recombinant human megakaryocyte growth and development factor (PEG-rHuMGDF), were studied in patients with chemotherapy-induced thrombocytopenia. Although a dose-dependent increase in platelet counts was observed,[190] these agents could not advance in clinical development after severe thrombocytopenia was observed due to the development of antibodies that neutralized endogenous TPO. However, important insight was gained from these studies for use in the development of subsequent agents.

Second-generation thrombopoietin mimetics include three agents currently used in the treatment of immune thrombocytopenia. Romiplostim, composed of a human TPO receptor-binding peptide joined by disulfide bonds to an immunoglobulin Fc fragment, has been shown to stimulate thrombopoiesis through binding and activation of the thrombopoietin receptor. It bears no homology to endogenous thrombopoietin, thereby eliminating the risk of cross-reactivity. It is administered subcutaneously and has demonstrated activity in patients with immune thrombocytopenic purpura without major adverse events.[107] Two double-blind, placebo controlled studies were conducted in which 125 patients with immune thrombocytopenic purpura (ITP) were randomized to receive treatment with romiplostim or placebo.[191] Prior to enrollment, patients were required to have had at least one prior therapy for ITP and have a platelet count of less than 30×10^9/L. The primary end point was the achievement of lasting platelet response defined as a platelet count above 50×10^9/L for any 6 weeks of the previous 8 weeks in the planned 24-week treatment period. The overall response rates in both studies were 87% and 38% in the romiplostim and placebo groups, respectively. Bleeding events in the patients who received romiplostim were less than half than in the patients who received the placebo treatment. Romiplostim gained FDA approval in August 2008 for patients with ITP who have had an insufficient response to corticosteroids, immunoglobulins, or splenectomy. The use of romiplostim in patients with chemotherapy-induced thrombocytopenia is currently being studied. An ongoing phase 1 and 2 study is investigating the use of romiplostim in patients with advanced disease who receive high-dose carboplatin or a combination of adriamycin and ifosfamide, regimens with late and early platelet nadirs, respectively.

Eltrombopag is an oral TPO agonist that was approved in November 2008 for the treatment of patients with ITP who have had an insufficient response to corticosteroids, immunoglobulins, or splenectomy. In a randomized trial of patients with refractory ITP, escalating doses of eltrombopag were shown to increase platelet count in a dose-dependent fashion.[192] Adverse event rates were similar in the treatment and placebo groups. Bleeding events decreased with platelet count increases, with the least number of events in the highest dose group. As with romiplostim, eltrombopag is undergoing investigation as a therapy for chemotherapy-induced thrombocytopenia. Results from a trial comparing its use to placebo in patients with cancer who are receiving carboplatin and taxol are awaited. Its use in sarcoma patients undergoing treatment with adriamycin and ifosfamide is open for recruitment.[193]

AKR-501 is another oral TPO receptor agonist that acts at the human TPO receptor.[194] It has demonstrated a dose-dependent increase in platelet response in healthy volunteers. The agent is currently undergoing investigation in patients with ITP.[195] ONO-7746 is currently recruiting healthy volunteers to investigate the safety and tolerability of this oral agent.[196]

Although the treatment of chemotherapy-induced thrombocytopenia remains largely limited to chemotherapy dose reductions and platelet transfusions, the development of novel thrombopoietin mimetics and TPO receptor agonists will hopefully provide feasible options to maintain dose intensity and avoid transfusions.

Selected References

The full list of references for this chapter appears in the online version.

1. Li J, Yang C, Xia Y, et al. Thrombocytopenia caused by the development of antibodies to thrombopoietin. *Blood* 2001;98(12):3241.
2. Ogawa M. Differentiation and proliferation of hematopoietic stem cells. *Blood* 1993;81(11):2844.
4. Cheshier SH, Morrison SJ, Liao X, Weissman IL. In vivo proliferation and cell cycle kinetics of long-term self-renewing hematopoietic stem cells. *Proc Natl Acad Sci U S A* 1999;96(6):3120.
6. Morrison SJ, Kimble J. Asymmetric and symmetric stem-cell divisions in development and cancer. *Nature* 2006;441(7097):1068.
7. Zon LI. Intrinsic and extrinsic control of haematopoietic stem-cell self-renewal. *Nature* 2008;453(7193):306.
11. Salter AB, Meadows SK, Muramoto GG, et al. Endothelial progenitor cell infusion induces hematopoietic stem cell reconstitution in vivo. *Blood* 2009;113(9):2104.
12. Hooper AT, Butler JM, Nolan DJ, et al. Engraftment and reconstitution of hematopoiesis is dependent on VEGFR2-mediated regeneration of sinusoidal endothelial cells. *Cell Stem Cell* 2009;4(3):263.
13. Kaushansky K. Lineage-specific hematopoietic growth factors. *N Engl J Med* 2006;354(19):2034.
18. Starr R, Willson TA, Viney EM, et al. A family of cytokine-inducible inhibitors of signalling. *Nature* 1997;387(6636):917.
29. Liu F, Poursine-Laurent J, Link DC. Expression of the G-CSF receptor on hematopoietic progenitor cells is not required for their mobilization by G-CSF. *Blood* 2000;95(10):3025.
30. Stroncek D, Clay M, Petzoldt M, et al. Treatment of normal individuals with granulocyte-colony-stimulating factor: donor experiences and the effects on peripheral blood CD34+ cell counts and on the collection of peripheral blood stem cells. *Transfusion* 1996;36:601.
33. Kondo M, Scherer DC, Miyamoto T, et al. Cell-fate conversion of lymphoid-committed progenitors by instructive actions of cytokines. *Nature* 2000;407(6802):383.
34. Dranoff G, Crawford A, Sadelain M, et al. Involvement of granulocyte-macrophage colony-stimulating factor in pulmonary homeostasis. *Science* 1994;264:713.
36. Stanley E, Lieschke GJ, Grail D, et al. Granulocyte/macrophage colony-stimulating factor-deficient mice show no major perturbation of hematopoiesis but develop a characteristic pulmonary pathology. *Proc Natl Acad Sci U S A* 1994;91(12):5592.
46. Jones SE, Schottstaedt MW, Duncan LA, et al. Randomized double-blind prospective trial to evaluate the effects of sargramostim versus placebo in a moderate-dose fluorouracil, doxorubicin, and cyclophosphamide adjuvant chemotherapy program for stage II and III breast cancer. *J Clin Oncol* 1996;14(11):2976.
49. Lieschke GJ, Burgess A. Granulocyte colony-stimulating factor and granulocyte-macrophage colony-stimulating factor (2). *N Engl J Med* 1992;327:99.
50. Wilson-Rawls J, Xie S, Liu J, Laneuville P, Arlinghaus RB. P210 Bcr-Abl interacts with the interleukin 3 receptor beta-C subunit and constitutively induces its tyrosine phosphorylation. *Cancer Res* 1996;56(15):3426.
51. James C, Ugo V, Le Couedic J-P, et al. A unique clonal JAK2 mutation leading to constitutive signalling causes polycythaemia vera. *Nature* 2005;434(7037):1144.
58. Hercus TR, Thomas D, Guthridge MA, et al. The granulocyte-macrophage colony-stimulating factor receptor: linking its structure to cell signaling and its role in disease. *Blood* 2009;114(7):1289.
69. Lok S, Kaushansky K, Holly R, et al. Cloning and expression of murine thrombopoietin cDNA and stimulation of platelet production in vivo. *Nature* 1994;369:565.
70. Kuter DJ, Beeler DL, Rosenberg RD. The purification of megapoietin: a physiological regulator of megakaryocyte growth and platelet production. *Proc Natl Acad Sci U S A* 1994;91(23):11104.
72. Sauvage Fd, Hass P, Spencer S, et al. Stimulation of megakaryocytopoiesis and thrombopoiesis by the c-Mpl ligand. *Nature* 1994;369:533.

89. Rizzo JD, Somerfield MR, Hagerty KL, et al. Use of epoetin and darbepoetin in patients with cancer: 2007 American Society of Clinical Oncology/American Society of Hematology Clinical Practice Guideline update. *J Clin Oncol* 2008;26(1):132.
91. Straus DJ, Testa MA, Sarokhan BJ, et al. Quality-of-life and health benefits of early treatment of mild anemia. *Cancer* 2006;107(8):1909.
94. Bennett CL, Silver SM, Djulbegovic B, et al. Venous thromboembolism and mortality associated with recombinant erythropoietin and darbepoetin administration for the treatment of cancer-associated anemia. *JAMA* 2008;299(8):914.
98. Glaspy J, Vadhan-Raj S, Patel R, et al. Randomized comparison of every-2-week darbepoetin alfa and weekly epoetin alfa for the treatment of chemotherapy-induced anemia: the 20030125 Study Group Trial. *J Clin Oncol* 2006;24(15):2290.
101. Henke M, Laszig R, Rübe C, et al. Erythropoietin to treat head and neck cancer patients with anaemia undergoing radiotherapy: randomised, double-blind, placebo-controlled trial. *Lancet* 2003;362(9392):1255.
102. Bohlius J, Langensiepen S, Schwarzer G, et al. Recombinant human erythropoietin and overall survival in cancer patients: results of a comprehensive meta-analysis. *J Natl Cancer Inst* 2005;97(7):489.
103. Bohlius J, Wilson J, Seidenfeld J, et al. Recombinant human erythropoietins and cancer patients: updated meta-analysis of 57 studies including 9353 patients. *J Natl Cancer Inst* 2006;98(10):708.
104. Bohlius J, Schmidlin K, Brillant C, et al. Recombinant human erythropoiesis-stimulating agents and mortality in patients with cancer: a meta-analysis of randomised trials. *Lancet* 2009;373(9674):1532.
106. Smith TJ, Khatcheressian J, Lyman GH, et al. 2006 update of recommendations for the use of white blood cell growth factors: an evidence-based clinical practice guideline. *J Clin Oncol* 2006;24(19):3187.
108. Bohlius J, Herbst C, Reiser M, Schwarzer G, Engert A. Granulopoiesis-stimulating factors to prevent adverse effects in the treatment of malignant lymphoma. *Cochrane Database Syst Rev* 2008;8:CD003189.
111. Timmer-Bonte JN, de Boo TM, Smit HJ, et al. Prevention of chemotherapy-induced febrile neutropenia by prophylactic antibiotics plus or minus granulocyte colony-stimulating factor in small-cell lung cancer: a Dutch randomized phase III study. *J Clin Oncol* 2005;23(31):7974.
112. Timmer-Bonte JNH, Adang EMM, Smit HJM, et al. Cost-effectiveness of adding granulocyte colony-stimulating factor to primary prophylaxis with antibiotics in small-cell lung cancer. *J Clin Oncol* 2006;24(19):2991.
113. Garcia-Carbonero R, Mayordomo JI, Tornamira MV, et al. Granulocyte colony-stimulating factor in the treatment of high-risk febrile neutropenia: a multicenter randomized trial. *J Natl Cancer Inst* 2001;93(1):31.
114. Klastersky J, Paesmans M, Rubenstein EB, et al. The multinational association for supportive care in cancer risk index: a multinational scoring system for identifying low-risk febrile neutropenic cancer patients. *J Clin Oncol* 2000;18(16):3038.
116. Hartmann LC, Tschetter LK, Habermann TM, et al. Granulocyte colony-stimulating factor in severe chemotherapy-induced afebrile neutropenia. *N Engl J Med* 1997;336(25):1776.
117. Citron ML, Berry DA, Cirrincione C, et al. Randomized trial of dose-dense versus conventionally scheduled and sequential versus concurrent combination chemotherapy as postoperative adjuvant treatment of node-positive primary breast cancer: first report of Intergroup Trial C9741/Cancer and Leukemia Group B Trial 9741. *J Clin Oncol* 2003;21(8):1431.
131. Dombret H, Chastang C, Fenaux P, et al. A controlled study of recombinant human granulocyte colony-stimulating factor in elderly patients after treatment for acute myelogenous leukemia. *N Engl J Med* 1995;332(25):1678.
133. Stone RM, Berg DT, George SL, et al. Granulocyte-macrophage colony-stimulating factor after initial chemotherapy for elderly patients with primary acute myelogenous leukemia. *N Engl J Med* 1995;332(25):1671.
147. Lowenberg B, van Putten W, Theobald M, et al. Effect of priming with granulocyte colony-stimulating factor on the outcome of chemotherapy for acute myeloid leukemia. *N Engl J Med* 2003;349(8):743.
150. Sachs L. The control of hematopoiesis and leukemia: from basic biology to the clinic. *Proc Natl Acad Sci U S A* 1996;93:4742.
151. Beekman R, Touw IP. G-CSF and its receptor in myeloid malignancy. *Blood* 2010;114:5131.
162. Greenberg PL, Sun Z, Miller KB, et al. Treatment of myelodysplastic syndrome patients with erythropoietin with or without granulocyte colony-stimulating factor: results of a prospective randomized phase 3 trial by the Eastern Cooperative Oncology Group (E1996). *Blood* 2009;114(12):2393.
178. Wolf M, Bentley M, Marlton P, et al. Pegfilgrastim to support CHOP-14 in elderly patients with non-Hodgkin's lymphoma. *Leuk Lymphoma* 2006;47(11):2344.
182. Hershman D, Neugut AI, Jacobson JS, et al. Acute myeloid leukemia or myelodysplastic syndrome following use of granulocyte colony-stimulating factors during breast cancer adjuvant chemotherapy. *J Natl Cancer Inst* 2007;99(3):196.
184. Lyman GH, Dale DC, Wolff DA, et al. Acute myeloid leukemia or myelodysplastic syndrome in randomized controlled clinical trials of cancer chemotherapy with granulocyte colony-stimulating factor: a systematic review. *J Clin Oncol* 2009;25:8723.
186. Praga C, Bergh J, Bliss J, et al. Risk of acute myeloid leukemia and myelodysplastic syndrome in trials of adjuvant epirubicin for early breast cancer: correlation with doses of epirubicin and cyclophosphamide. *J Clin Oncol* 2005;23(18):4179.
187. Leone G, Pagano L, Ben-Yehuda D, Voso MT. Therapy-related leukemia and myelodysplasia: susceptibility and incidence. *Haematologica* 2007;92(10):1389.
190. Somlo G, Sniecinski I, ter Veer A, et al. Recombinant human thrombopoietin in combination with granulocyte colony-stimulating factor enhances mobilization of peripheral blood progenitor cells, increases peripheral blood platelet concentration, and accelerates hematopoietic recovery following high-dose chemotherapy. *Blood* 1999;93(9):2798.
191. Kuter DJ, Bussel JB, Lyons RM, et al. Efficacy of romiplostim in patients with chronic immune thrombocytopenic purpura: a double-blind randomised controlled trial. *Lancet* 2008;371(9610):395.
192. Bussel JB, Cheng G, Saleh MN, et al. Eltrombopag for the treatment of chronic idiopathic thrombocytopenic purpura. *N Engl J Med* 2007;357(22):2237.

CHAPTER 158 CANCER-ASSOCIATED THROMBOSIS

AGNES Y. Y. LEE AND ALOK A. KHORANA

Cancer is a prothrombotic state. Cancer and anticancer therapies are frequently complicated by the development of vascular events, often with devastating clinical consequences. The most frequent vascular events include deep venous thrombosis (DVT) and pulmonary embolism (PE), together described as venous thromboembolism (VTE). Arterial events including stroke and myocardial infarction can also occur, particularly with regimens containing antiangiogenic agents. Subclinical abnormalities in the hemostatic system can be observed in up to 90% of cancer patients. Recent preclinical and translational data suggest that this prothrombotic state is driven by oncogenic events and the close linkage between regulation of angiogenesis and coagulation, and is integral to cancer growth and metastasis.

The association of cancer with thrombotic events is commonly linked to Armand Trousseau, who was the first to comprehensively describe the eponymous syndrome. In one of medical history's great ironies, Professor Trousseau himself developed thrombophlebitis prior to succumbing to gastric cancer. The past decade has seen a renewed emphasis in this area, owing to a rising incidence of cancer-associated thrombosis, particularly in the setting of chemotherapy and antiangiogenic therapy.[1,2]

The occurrence of vascular events has significant clinical consequences: VTE recurs at an annual risk of 21%, requires long-term anticoagulation with a 12% annual risk of major bleeding complications, impacts negatively on patients' quality of life, and consumes health care resources.[3] Most importantly, thrombosis is the second-leading cause of death in patients with cancer, accounting for 9% of deaths in a study of cancer outpatients.[4] Cancer patients with VTE have a twofold or greater increase in mortality compared with cancer patients without VTE, even after adjusting for stage.[5,6] This impact on prognosis likely reflects the close association between activation of coagulation and an unfavorable tumor biology. Consequently, development of cancer-associated thrombosis should prompt increased wariness on the part of health care providers. In this chapter, we will review the mechanisms underlying the prothrombotic state in cancer and the incidence, risk factors, prevention, and treatment of cancer-associated thrombosis.

MECHANISMS OF CANCER-ASSOCIATED THROMBOSIS

The pathogenesis of the prothrombotic state in cancer is complex, principally involving procoagulant molecules produced by tumor cells, suppression of fibrinolytic activity, and platelet activation. The genetic mechanisms responsible for malignant transformation such as oncogene activation (*RAS* or *MET*) or tumor suppressor gene inactivation (*P53* or *PTEN*) also directly induce the expression of genes regulating hemostasis.[7–9] Extrinsic factors such as antineoplastic therapy, surgery, and vascular access devices further exacerbate this prothrombotic state.

The most important procoagulant expressed by tumor cells is tissue factor (TF), a transmembrane glycoprotein and the physiologic initiator of coagulation. TF is present on neoplastic cells as well as tumor-associated endothelial cells in a variety of cancers. TF expression occurs early in neoplastic transformation, driven by oncogenic mutations in *KRAS* and *TP53* genes.[9] TF may contribute to tumor growth, metastasis, and angiogenesis through a variety of mechanisms including the formation of the TF/VIIa complex and activation of protease-activated receptor 2.[10] TF expression is associated with increased angiogenesis, tumor invasiveness, and worsened prognosis in various malignancies.[11] Secretion of TF-containing microvesicles into the circulation may also account for the systemic coagulopathy of cancer. Preliminary reports suggest that the degree of TF expression by tumor cells or elevated levels of circulating systemic TF may be predictive of VTE in select cancers, particularly pancreatic and ovarian cancers.[12]

Other factors that potentially influence the prothrombotic state of malignancy include cancer procoagulant, a cysteine protease that directly activates factor X. Tumor cells also express plasminogen activator inhibitor-1, a potent inhibitor of the fibrinolytic system that has prothrombotic properties and also promotes tumor growth and angiogenesis. Proinflammatory cytokines such as tumor necrosis factor, interleukins-1 and -6, and interferons are elevated in malignancy. Their enhanced expression results from activation of monocytes or direct release from tumor cells, and can in turn activate coagulation. Finally, interactions mediated by platelet P-selectin between circulating carcinoma mucins and platelets lead to platelet aggregation and platelet-rich thrombus formation without accompanying thrombin generation, and this may also contribute to the prothrombotic state in cancer.[13]

Antineoplastic therapy further exacerbates the prothrombotic state in cancer. Several studies have documented changes in the markers of thrombin generation within hours of chemotherapy administration.[14] Chemotherapy can induce endothelial cell activation leading to increased TF expression, elevated levels of plasma von Willebrand factor and factor VIII coagulant protein, and decreased levels of natural anticoagulants antithrombin and proteins C and S.[15] Induction of platelet aggregation and degranulation has been suggested as a mechanism for bevacizumab-induced thrombosis.[16]

EPIDEMIOLOGY OF CANCER-ASSOCIATED THROMBOSIS

Incidence and Prevalence

The incidence of VTE is increased several-fold in cancer patients when compared with noncancer patients.[17–19] The rates of VTE in cancer patients vary depending on the specific population analyzed and over time, with more contemporary studies demonstrating higher incidence. Among hospitalized cancer patients, overall VTE rates of 0.6% and 2% per hospitalization were reported in studies from 1988 to 1990 and 1979 to 1999, respectively; in the latter study, rates approached 4% in the late 1990s.[19] For hospitalized patients receiving chemotherapy, the rates of VTE rose from 3.9% to 5.7% per admission from 1995 to 2003, an increase of 47%.[1,20] Among ambulatory patients, the reported incidence of VTE varies from 7.8% during 26 months (0.3% per month) to 1.93% during a median follow-up of 2.4 months (0.8% per month) to 12% during 8 months (1.5% per month).[21,22] The cause of this recent increase in the rate of VTE is unclear but may be related to an increased awareness, improved diagnostic technologies, or a true increased incidence related to newer antineoplastic drugs and regimens. The advent of highly sensitive multidetector-row computed tomography scans for routine staging has led to an increased diagnosis of so-called incidental or unsuspected PE. However, retrospective studies show that these patients often have symptoms not recognized by their providers and that the consequences of incidentally discovered PE are no different than those following symptomatic VTE including mortality.[23,24]

Rates of arterial thromboembolism are less well studied. In a study of hospitalized neutropenic patients, 1.5% developed arterial events, with a proportional increase of 124% during the 6-year study period.[20] The use of bevacizumab-containing regimens is clearly associated with a high risk of arterial events. In a pooled analysis of five randomized studies, 4.4% of patients receiving bevacizumab and chemotherapy developed arterial events, compared with 1.9% of patients receiving chemotherapy alone. Rates were particularly high in older patients. Similarly high rates of thrombosis have been observed with other angiogenesis inhibitors still in development, suggesting that this may be a class effect; however, rates vary widely between specific agents and among various clinical trials.

TABLE 158.1

RISK FACTORS FOR CANCER-ASSOCIATED THROMBOSIS

Patient demographics
Older age
Race (higher in African Americans, lower in Asian-Pacific Islanders)
Patient comorbidities
Obesity, infection, renal disease, pulmonary disease, arterial thromboembolism
Prior history of VTE
Inherited prothrombotic mutations (e. g., factor V Leiden, prothrombin gene mutation)
Poor performance status
Cancer-related factors
Primary site of cancer (gastrointestinal, brain, lung, gynecologic, renal, bladder, lymphoma, myeloma)
Initial period after diagnosis
Histology
Metastatic disease
Treatment-related factors
Major surgery
Hospitalization
Antineoplastic therapy
Chemotherapy
Hormonal therapy
Antiangiogenic therapy (thalidomide, lenalidomide, bevacizumab)
Erythropoiesis-stimulating agents
Central venous catheters
Transfusions
Candidate biomarkers
Prechemotherapy leukocyte count >11,000/mm³
Prechemotherapy platelet count ≥350,000/mm³
Tissue factor (TF)
High grade of TF expression by tumor cells (immunohistochemistry)
Elevated systemic levels
D-dimer
C-reactive protein
Soluble P-selectin
Factor VIII

VTE, venous thromboembolism.

Risk Factors

Cancer patients comprise a heterogeneous group and include patients undergoing surgery, hospitalization, receiving antineoplastic therapy, or end-of-life care. The risk of VTE differs across these various cancer subpopulations as well as over the natural history of the disease. Table 158.1 provides a comprehensive list of risk factors for cancer-associated VTE. It is important to note that risk factors can change over time based on patient-, cancer-, and treatment-related variables (Fig. 158.1).

VTE is more likely to occur in the initial period after diagnosis. In a population-based study, the adjusted odds ratio (OR) for developing VTE in the first 3 months was 53.5 (95% confidence interval [CI]: 8.6–334.3), declining to 14.3 (95% CI: 5.8–35.2) and 3.6 (95% CI: 2.0–6.5) in the 3-month to 1-year and 1- to 3-year intervals, respectively.[17] Patients with metastatic disease have a 2- to 20-fold increased risk of VTE.[5,17] The primary site of cancer is strongly associated with the risk of VTE in multiple studies. Cancers of the pancreas, stomach, brain, ovary, kidney, and lung have long been associated with VTE; hematologic malignancies, particularly lymphomas, have in recent reports also been strongly associated with the highest risk of VTE.[17,19–22]

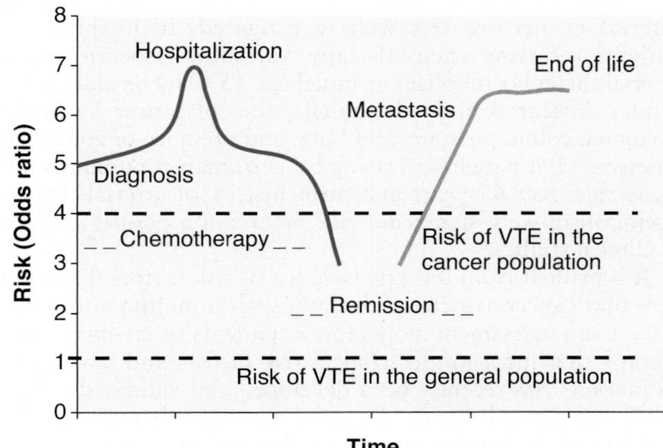

FIGURE 158.1 The risk for cancer-associated venous thromboembolism (VTE) changes over the natural history of cancer, based on patient-, cancer-, and treatment-related variables as shown in a hypothetical patient. (From Rao MV, Francis CW, Khorana AA. Who's at risk? Approaches to risk-stratifying cancer patients. In: Khorana AA, Francis CW, eds. *Cancer-Associated Thrombosis*. London: Taylor & Francis, 2007:169, with permission.)

Cancer patients undergoing surgery have a twofold increased risk of postoperative DVT and a threefold increased risk of fatal PE compared with noncancer patients. The risk of VTE increases significantly when cancer patients are hospitalized. Cancer patients on active therapy are at a greater risk for VTE. Specific chemotherapeutic agents are associated with higher rates of VTE. In a prospective study, platinum-based regimens were significantly associated with VTE.[25] Even within this class of agents, rates are higher in patients receiving cisplatin as compared with oxaliplatin.[26] Studies of newer cancer regimens that include antiangiogenic agents such as thalidomide, lenalidomide, and bevacizumab have reported very high rates of VTE. For thalidomide-containing regimens, rates of VTE up to 34% in myeloma patients have been reported.[27] Bevacizumab, an anti–vascular endothelial growth factor antibody, has been associated with an increased risk of VTE in a pooled analysis of randomized clinical trials as well (relative risk [RR], 1.33; 95% CI: 1.13–1.56).[2]

Hormonal therapy, particularly tamoxifen, has also been associated with an increased risk of VTE. Even supportive therapy drugs have been associated with increased VTE. In a large meta-analysis, erythropoiesis-stimulating agents were associated with a 1.7-fold increased risk of thromboembolism. In 2007, the U.S. Food and Drug Administration issued safety warnings regarding the risk of thrombosis and death in cancer patients receiving these agents. Some studies also suggest an increased risk of VTE with myeloid growth factors as well, but this has not been fully established. The presence of a central venous catheter increases the risk of upper extremity VTE.[28] Finally, comorbid illnesses strongly influence the risk of VTE. Those conditions most associated with VTE include infection, arterial thromboembolism, renal disease, pulmonary disease, and anemia.

Multiple recent studies have identified laboratory biomarkers, ranging from tests as simple as the complete blood count to novel assays that may be predictive of VTE in cancer.[29] Prechemotherapy platelet counts of 350,000/mm^3 or more (OR, 1.8; 95% CI: 1.1–3.2) and leukocyte counts above 11,000/mm^3 (OR, 2.2; 95% CI: 1.2–4.0) have been independently associated with VTE.[30] In preliminary studies, the degree of TF expression in tumor cells by immunohistochemistry, measuring systemic TF antigen levels, or TF activity have all been associated with the risk of VTE. Unfortunately, there is no currently accepted standard assay for measuring TF. Other candidate biomarkers predictive of VTE include D-dimer, soluble P-selectin, factor VIII, and C-reactive protein. Risk factors for arterial events are less well investigated. In hospitalized patients receiving chemotherapy, variables associated with arterial thromboembolism included age 65 years or older, male gender, African American ethnicity, sites of cancer including leukemia, colon, prostate, and lung, and presence of comorbid illnesses.[20] For patients receiving bevacizumab-containing regimens, age over 65 years and prior history of arterial thromboembolism were significant risk factors in a pooled analysis of clinical trials.

It is evident from the extensive list of risk factors discussed here that cancer-associated thrombosis is a multifactorial disease. A risk assessment model for outpatients receiving chemotherapy that incorporates clinical risk factors and laboratory biomarkers has recently been developed and validated.[30] Five predictive variables (site of cancer, prechemotherapy platelet and leukocyte counts, anemia and/or use of erythropoiesis-stimulating agents, and body mass index) are used to classify risk into three categories: low (score 0), intermediate (score 1–2), and high (score $\geq$3). Observed rates of VTE over median follow-up of 2.5 months in the development and validation cohorts were 0.8% and 0.3% for low-risk, 1.8% and 2% for intermediate-risk, and 7.1% and 6.7% for high-risk patients, respectively. This model was externally validated, with rates of 17.7% in the high-risk cohort as compared to 1.5% in low-risk patients, over a 6-month follow-up period.[31]

PREVENTION OF CANCER-ASSOCIATED THROMBOSIS

Prophylaxis in Major Surgery

Few clinical trials have been conducted to study the efficacy and safety of thromboprophylaxis specifically in cancer patients having major surgery. Randomized controlled trials of in-hospital prophylaxis in patients having major abdominal surgery for cancer have shown no difference in the incidence of DVT or major bleeding between unfractionated heparin (UFH) administered three times daily and a low-molecular-weight heparin (LMWH) enoxaparin given once daily.[32,33] Overall, up to 15% of cancer patients will develop DVT following surgery, despite standard prophylaxis with UFH or LMWH.[34] In addition to LMWH and UFH, fondaparinux is approved for prophylaxis following major abdominal surgery. This selective inhibitor of activated factor X is given once daily subcutaneously and is associated with a lower risk of heparin-induced thrombocytopenia compared with UFH and LMWH. In a phase 3 randomized trial, fondaparinux was found to be comparable to LMWH dalteparin in patients undergoing high-risk abdominal surgery.[35] A *post hoc* analysis of cancer patients suggested that fondaparinux was associated with a statistically significant reduction in VTE (4.7% vs. 7.7%; $P = .02$).

Mechanical methods of prophylaxis, such as graduated compression stockings or intermittent pneumatic calf compression devices, can lower the risk of VTE but are less effective than anticoagulants. Their use should be limited to patients in whom anticoagulation is contraindicated. There is weak evidence that combined mechanical and pharmacologic prophylaxis may further reduce VTE, especially in the patients who are at highest risk.

Extending prophylaxis beyond hospitalization can further reduce the risk of VTE in cancer patients. In a multicenter, placebo-controlled trial, patients undergoing elective, curative abdominal surgery for cancer received LMWH enoxaparin for the first 6 to 10 days after surgery and then were randomized to continue with enoxaparin or placebo injections for 4 weeks.[36] Extended prophylaxis with enoxaparin significantly reduced the rate of VTE by 60% (12.0% vs. 4.8%; $P = .02$) at 1 month and this benefit was maintained at 3 months. The absolute risk reduction of 7% means that 14 patients must be treated to avoid one case of DVT. Overall, there was no difference in bleeding during the treatment period and no difference in mortality up to 1 year of follow-up. Similar results were also reported in a subgroup analysis of an open-label randomized trial in which patients having abdominal surgery were randomized to receive LMWH dalteparin once daily and compression stockings, or to stockings alone for 21 days after hospital discharge.[37] Dalteparin significantly reduced the incidence of DVT from 19.6% to 8.8% ($P = .03$) as well as that of proximal DVT from 10.4% to 2.2% ($P = .02$). Accordingly, 9 patients must be treated to avoid 1 episode of DVT while 12 must be treated to avoid 1 episode of proximal DVT.

The increased risk of postdischarge symptomatic VTE has been shown to peak at 3 weeks after cancer surgery in two large prospective studies.[38,39] One study found that 46% of the deaths occurring within the first month after cancer surgery were due to fatal PE, and the other study reported that 1 in 85 women will develop VTE within the first 12 weeks after cancer surgery. The American Society of Clinical Oncology and the American College of Chest Physicians (ACCP) recommend that extended prophylaxis in patients undergoing cancer surgery should be considered, especially in patients with high-risk features.[34,40] These include previous history of VTE, anesthesia lasting 2 hours or longer, bed rest for 4 days or longer, advanced malignancy, and older age.[38]

Prophylaxis for Central Venous Catheters

Contemporary trials have provided evidence that neither warfarin (dose fixed at 1 mg daily or adjusted to an international normalized ratio [INR] between 1.5 and 1.9) nor prophylactic doses of LMWH is effective in reducing symptomatic catheter-related thrombosis.[41–43] With or without prophylaxis, symptomatic catheter-related thrombosis rates of approximately 4% were reported in these studies, and bleeding may be increased in those who received an anticoagulant. Based on these data, the ACCP guidelines have recommended against routine prophylaxis using LMWH and fixed-dose warfarin.[34] Although high-risk patients may still benefit from prophylaxis, the selection criteria of such patients and the optimal anticoagulant regimen are not defined.

Prophylaxis in Medical Patients

Randomized trials have studied the efficacy and safety of anticoagulant prophylaxis in outpatients receiving chemotherapy (Table 158.2).[44–49] One small randomized trial found that very low-dose warfarin was effective in reducing symptomatic DVT in women with stage IV breast cancer receiving multiagent chemotherapy,[46] while placebo-controlled trials in patients with a number of different solid tumors provided conflicting evidence for prophylactic doses of LMWH.[44,45,47–49] In contrast, two open-label studies in patients with advanced pancreatic cancer reported significant and dramatic reductions in clinically relevant VTE when therapeutic or half-therapeutic doses of LMWH were given in conjunction with standard chemotherapy. In one study, enoxaparin at 1 mg/kg daily for 3 months reduced the incidence of symptomatic VTE by 66% (from 14.5% to 5.0%; $P < .01$) while dalteparin at therapeutic dosing reduced the incidence from 31% to 12% (RR, 0.38; $P = .02$).[47,49] In the latter study, the risk of fatal PE was also significantly lowered (RR, 0.08; $P = .03$). Bleeding was not increased in the LMWH groups in these studies. Overall, the findings suggest that patients with specific tumor types benefit from anticoagulant prophylaxis but doses that are higher than what is used for standard primary prophylaxis are required. Identifying high-risk patients using a risk-assessment model will also improve the benefit-risk ratio of anticoagulant prophylaxis.

Another population in whom primary prophylaxis may be beneficial is patients with multiple myeloma who are receiving thalidomide or lenalidomide in combination with chemotherapy or high-dose steroids. Incidences of symptomatic VTE of 20% to 30% have been reported but the pathophysiologic mechanisms remain elusive. This high risk has prompted the use of aspirin, warfarin, and LMWH in uncontrolled settings and guidelines to recommend anticoagulation prophylaxis in patients receiving thalidomide- or lenalidomide-based regimens.[40] Randomized trials are urgently needed to identify a safe and effective prophylaxis regimen, given the potential for serious bleeding in this patient group.

Randomized trials in a cancer-specific population have not been done in acutely ill medical patients admitted to hospital. Recommendations regarding the efficacy and safety of thromboprophylaxis in these patients are based on three large randomized studies that included only a minority (5%–15%) of patients with cancer. However, given the known high risk of VTE during hospitalization for cancer patients and its attendant consequences, all of the guidelines recommend thromboprophylaxis in the absence of contraindications.[34,40] There continue to be ongoing concerns regarding the risk of bleeding in these patients, for which few cancer-specific data are available.

TREATMENT OF CANCER-ASSOCIATED THROMBOSIS

Anticoagulants are the cornerstone agents for the treatment of acute VTE. Although these agents are highly efficacious and have an acceptable safety profile in most patients, cancer patients have a threefold higher risk of recurrent VTE and

TABLE 158.2

RANDOMIZED CONTROLLED TRIALS OF PRIMARY PROPHYLAXIS IN PATIENTS WITH SOLID TUMORS

Study Population (Ref.)	No. of Patients	Anticoagulant Prophylaxis	VTE in Anticoagulant Group (%)	VTE in Control Group (%)	P Value
Stage IV breast cancer (46)		Warfarin 1 mg/d × 6 wk then INR 1.3–1.9	0.7	4.4	.03
Advanced breast cancer (45)	351	Certoparin 3,000 units once daily	4.0	3.9	NS
Advanced NSCLC (45)	532	Certoparin 3,000 units once daily	4.5	8.3	.07
Grade III/IV malignant glioma (48)	186	Dalteparin 5,000 units once daily	11.0	17.0	.3
Advanced cancer of breast, lung, GI, pancreas, ovary, head and neck (44)	1,150	Nadroparin 3,800 units once daily	2.0	3.9	.02
Advanced pancreatic cancer (49)	312	Enoxaparin 1 mg/kg once daily × 12 weeks then 40 mg once daily	14.5	5.0	<.01
Advanced pancreatic cancer (47)	123	Dalteparin 200 U/kg once daily × 4 wk then 150 U/kg × 8 wk	31.0	12.0	.02

VTE, venous thromboembolism; INR, international normalized ratio; NS, nonsignificant; NSCLC, non–small cell lung cancer; GI, gastrointestinal.

PRACTICE OF ONCOLOGY

twofold higher risk of anticoagulant-related bleeding compared with patients without cancer.[3] These complications likely reflect the prothrombotic state associated with malignant diseases and the multiple comorbidities in cancer patients that may alter their response to anticoagulant therapy and their risk of bleeding. LMWH is the preferred treatment for initial and long-term treatment because of its favorable efficacy, safety, and convenience profile compared with UFH and vitamin K antagonists (VKAs).

Initial Therapy

Formal comparisons of LMWH, UFH, and fondaparinux for initial treatment of VTE in cancer patients have not been conducted. Based on results extracted from randomized trials that evaluated these agents, LMWH and UFH appear equally effective in reducing recurrent thrombosis in cancer patients, but LMWH is associated with a 3-month survival benefit over UFH.[50] Furthermore, LMWH can be given safely as once-daily subcutaneous injections in an outpatient setting without the need for laboratory monitoring and have a lower risk of heparin-induced thrombocytopenia. Fondaparinux given once daily is also comparable to heparins for the initial treatment of VTE and may eliminate the risk of heparin-induced thrombocytopenia. However, a *post hoc* analysis of a randomized trial suggests that it is less effective than enoxaparin for outpatient treatment of DVT in patients with cancer.[51] New oral anticoagulants that inhibit activated factor X (e.g., rivaroxaban, apixaban) or thrombin (e.g., dabigatran) are now completing phase 3 evaluation for treatment of acute VTE. Because these trials included only a small number of cancer patients, further investigation is required to show efficacy and safety in this high-risk population. The major concerns about these new anticoagulants in cancer patients include potential interaction with chemotherapeutic agents, lack of antidote when patients are actively bleeding, and whether treatment doses in noncancer patients are as effective in these hypercoagulable patients.

Long-Term Therapy

Despite their pharmacologic and practical limitations, VKAs were the mainstay of long-term anticoagulant treatment for VTE in cancer patients for many years. Although VKAs are highly effectively in reducing recurrent thrombosis in the general population, treatment failures, serious bleeding, and difficulties with maintaining the INR within the therapeutic range are common problems in patients with cancer. A prospective cohort study reported that the 12-month cumulative incidence of recurrent VTE in cancer patients was 20.7%, versus 6.8% in patients without cancer, and the corresponding estimate for major bleeding was 12.4% versus 4.9%, respectively.[3] Patients with cancer also experience recurrent VTE despite having therapeutic INR levels and suffer serious bleeding complications even without receiving excessive anticoagulation.[52]

Clinical trials have now established LMWH as the preferred long-term treatment for VTE. The CLOT trial randomized 676 cancer patients with symptomatic proximal DVT, PE, or both, to receive usual treatment with dalteparin initially followed by 6 months of therapy with either VKA or dalteparin alone.[53] In the dalteparin group, patients self-injected therapeutic doses at 200 U/kg once daily for the first month followed by 75% to 80% of the full dose for the next 5 months. The VKA group was treated to maintain a therapeutic INR between 2.0 and 3.0. The cumulative risk of recurrent VTE at 6 months was reduced from 17% in the VKA group to 9% in the dalteparin group, resulting in a statistically significant risk reduction of 52% (P = .002; Fig. 158.2). Accordingly, one episode of recurrent VTE is prevented for every 13 patients treated with dalteparin. Overall, there were no differences in major or any bleeding between the groups. By 6 months, 39% of the patients had died in each group, with 90% of the deaths being from progressive cancer. A *post hoc* subgroup analysis showed that, among patients who had no known metastatic disease at randomization, those who were randomized to dalteparin had better survival compared with those who had received a VKA.[54] Whether this was the result of an anticoagulant or an anticancer effect remains uncertain. The observation that the separation of the survival curves occurred only after the discontinuation of dalteparin suggests that the survival benefit is not the result of a reduction in fatal PE. Ongoing research is being done to determine if LMWH offers antineoplastic effects in specific cancers and to explore the potential biological mechanisms. In contrast to the CLOT study, three randomized trials reported nonsignificant reductions in symptomatic VTE with LMWH compared with VKA therapy.[55–57] It is likely that these other trials were underpowered (two were terminated prematurely prior to achieving target sample size) or that the dosing of other LMWHs were inadequate. Fondaparinux has not been evaluated for long-term treatment in cancer patients.

There is also no evidence to guide the choice of anticoagulant after the first 6 months of treatment. For patients who have tolerated LMWH or VKA for the first 6 months, continuing

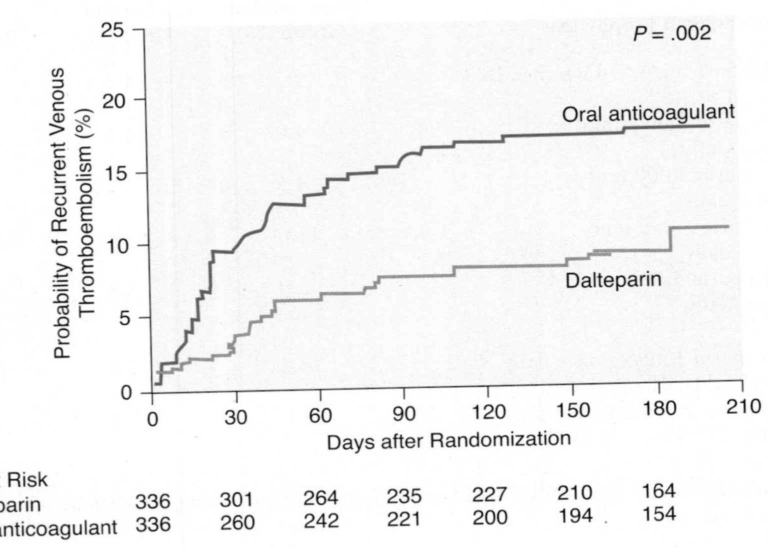

FIGURE 158.2 The cumulative risks of recurrent venous thromboembolism comparing 6 months of treatment with low-molecular-weight heparin dalteparin versus a vitamin K antagonist (hazard ratio, 0.48; 95% confidence interval: 0.30–0.77; P = .002). (From ref. 53, with permission.)

with the same anticoagulant is a sensible option if ongoing anticoagulation is needed. It is recommended that the risks and benefits of LMWH versus VKA therapy are discussed with the patient in order to individualize treatment. Besides the risk of bleeding, there does not appear to be any significant side effects associated with long-term use of LMWH or VKA. Although animal studies suggest that LMWH exposure may reduce bone density, this has not been shown to be a concern in patient populations (e.g., pregnant women with VTE) that also need extended treatment with LMWH.

Based on the evidence to date, long-term treatment with a LMWH for cancer patients with DVT is recommended by the ACCP Consensus Guidelines, the National Comprehensive Cancer Network Clinical Practice Guidelines in Oncology, and the American Society of Clinical Oncology.[40,58,59]

Therapy for Recurrent Venous Thromboembolism

Although recurrent VTE is frequent in cancer patients, optimal treatment has not been investigated in clinical trials. Insertion of an inferior vena cava filter is commonly used in patients with recurrent thrombosis despite anticoagulation, but evidence supporting this practice is lacking. In fact, studies have shown that patients with filters have a higher risk of recurrent DVT than those without the device, and fatal PE has been reported in cancer patients following filter insertion. It is recommended that the use of filters be limited to situations in which anticoagulant therapy cannot be used because of serious, active bleeding. Success has been reported with using LMWH in patients who break through VKA therapy and with using higher doses of LMWH in those who break through usual LMWH treatment doses. In a small series of cancer patients with recurrent thrombosis, 9% of patients treated with dose escalation of LMWH had a second thrombotic event and 1% had a major bleed over a 3-month follow-up period.[60] Mortality in patients who developed recurrent thrombosis was high, with a median time between recurrence and death at 11 months. This observation reinforces the concept that activation of coagulation is associated with unfavorable tumor biology.

Duration of Therapy

Although clinical trial evidence is lacking, it is generally recommended that patients with metastases should continue with "indefinite" anticoagulant therapy after a single thrombotic event because metastatic malignancy is a risk factor for recurrent thrombosis. In patients without metastases, anticoagulant treatment is recommended for as long as the cancer is "active" and while the patient is receiving antitumor therapy. Although this period is sometimes difficult to define, patients who have not experienced any complications often prefer to continue anticoagulant therapy to avoid recurrent thrombosis. Given the complex and changing clinical courses of most patients with cancer, periodic evaluation of the risk-benefit ratio of continuing anticoagulant therapy in individual patients is absolutely essential. The decision should take into consideration the patient's preference, the anticancer treatments, the comorbid conditions, and most importantly, the patient's quality of life and life expectancy.

Selected References

The full list of references for this chapter appears in the online version.

1. Khorana AA, Francis CW, Culakova E, Kuderer NM, Lyman GH. Frequency, risk factors, and trends for venous thromboembolism among hospitalized cancer patients. *Cancer* 2007;110:2339.
2. Nalluri SR, Chu D, Keresztes R, Zhu X, Wu S. Risk of venous thromboembolism with the angiogenesis inhibitor bevacizumab in cancer patients: a meta-analysis. *JAMA* 2008;300:2277.
3. Prandoni P, Lensing AW, Piccioli A, et al. Recurrent venous thromboembolism and bleeding complications during anticoagulant treatment in patients with cancer and venous thrombosis. *Blood* 2002;100:3484.
4. Khorana AA, Francis CW, Culakova E, Kuderer NM, Lyman GH. Thromboembolism is a leading cause of death in cancer patients receiving outpatient chemotherapy. *J Thromb Haemost* 2007;5:632.
5. Chew HK, Wun T, Harvey D, Zhou H, White RH. Incidence of venous thromboembolism and its effect on survival among patients with common cancers. *Arch Intern Med* 2006;166:458.
6. Sorensen HT, Mellemkjaer L, Olsen JH, Baron JA. Prognosis of cancers associated with venous thromboembolism. *N Engl J Med* 2000;343:1846.
7. Boccaccio C, Comoglio PM. Genetic link between cancer and thrombosis. *J Clin Oncol* 2009;27:4827.
8. Boccaccio C, Sabatino G, Medico E, et al. The MET oncogene drives a genetic programme linking cancer to haemostasis. *Nature* 2005;434:396.
9. Yu JL, May L, Lhotak V, et al. Oncogenic events regulate tissue factor expression in colorectal cancer cells: implications for tumor progression and angiogenesis. *Blood* 2005;105:1734.
10. Kasthuri RS, Taubman MB, Mackman N. Role of tissue factor in cancer. *J Clin Oncol* 2009;27:4834.
11. Belting M, Ahamed J, Ruf W. Signaling of the tissue factor coagulation pathway in angiogenesis and cancer. *Arterioscler Thromb Vasc Biol* 2005;25:1545.
13. Wahrenbrock M, Borsig L, Le D, Varki N, Varki A. Selectin-mucin interactions as a probable molecular explanation for the association of Trousseau syndrome with mucinous adenocarcinomas. *J Clin Invest* 2003;112:853.
14. Weitz IC, Israel VK, Waisman JR, et al. Chemotherapy-induced activation of hemostasis: effect of a low molecular weight heparin (dalteparin sodium) on plasma markers of hemostatic activation. *Thromb Haemost* 2002;88:213.
15. Lee AY, Levine MN. The thrombophilic state induced by therapeutic agents in the cancer patient. *Semin Thromb Hemost* 1999;25:137.
17. Blom JW, Doggen CJ, Osanto S, Rosendaal FR. Malignancies, prothrombotic mutations, and the risk of venous thrombosis. *JAMA* 2005;293:715.
19. Stein PD, Beemath A, Meyers FA, et al. Incidence of venous thromboembolism in patients hospitalized with cancer. *Am J Med* 2006;119:60.
20. Khorana AA, Francis CW, Culakova E, et al. Thromboembolism in hospitalized neutropenic cancer patients. *J Clin Oncol* 2006;24:484.
21. Khorana AA, Francis CW, Culakova E, Lyman GH. Risk factors for chemotherapy-associated venous thromboembolism in a prospective observational study. *Cancer* 2005;104:2822.
23. Gladish GW, Choe DH, Marom EM, et al. Incidental pulmonary emboli in oncology patients: prevalence, CT evaluation, and natural history. *Radiology* 2006;240:246.
24. O'Connell CL, Boswell WD, Duddalwar V, et al. Unsuspected pulmonary emboli in cancer patients: clinical correlates and relevance. *J Clin Oncol* 2006;24:4928.
27. Zangari M, Fink LM, Elice F, et al. Thrombotic events in patients with cancer receiving antiangiogenesis agents. *J Clin Oncol* 2009;27:4865.
28. Lee AY, Levine MN, Butler G, et al. Incidence, risk factors, and outcomes of catheter-related thrombosis in adult patients with cancer. *J Clin Oncol* 2006; 24:1404.
29. Khorana AA, Connolly GC. Assessing risk of venous thromboembolism in the patient with cancer. *J Clin Oncol* 2009;27:4839.
30. Khorana AA, Kuderer NM, Culakova E, Lyman GH, Francis CW. Development and validation of a predictive model for chemotherapy-associated thrombosis. *Blood* 2008;111:4902.
31. Ay C, Dunkler D, Maresi C, et al. Prediction of venous thromboembolism in cancer patients. *Blood* 2010;116:5377.
32. Efficacy and safety of enoxaparin versus unfractionated heparin for prevention of deep vein thrombosis in elective cancer surgery: a double-blind randomized multicentre trial with venographic assessment. ENOXACAN Study Group. *Br J Surg* 1997;84:1099.
33. McLeod RS, Geerts WH, Sniderman KW, et al. Subcutaneous heparin versus low-molecular-weight heparin as thromboprophylaxis in patients undergoing colorectal surgery: results of the Canadian colorectal DVT prophylaxis trial: a randomized, double-blind trial. *Ann Surg* 2001;233:438.
34. Geerts WH, Bergqvist D, Pineo GF, et al. Prevention of venous thromboembolism: American College of Chest Physicians Evidence-Based Clinical Practice Guidelines (8th Edition). *Chest* 2008;133:381S.
35. Agnelli G, Bergqvist D, Cohen AT, Gallus AS, Gent M. Randomized clinical trial of postoperative fondaparinux versus perioperative dalteparin for prevention of venous thromboembolism in high-risk abdominal surgery. *Br J Surg* 2005;92:1212.

36. Bergqvist D, Agnelli G, Cohen AT, et al. Duration of prophylaxis against venous thromboembolism with enoxaparin after surgery for cancer. *N Engl J Med* 2002;346:975.
38. Agnelli G, Bolis G, Capussotti L, et al. A clinical outcome-based prospective study on venous thromboembolism after cancer surgery: the @RISTOS project. *Ann Surg* 2006;243:89.
39. Sweetland S, Green J, Liu B, et al. Duration and magnitude of the postoperative risk of venous thromboembolism in middle aged women: prospective cohort study. *BMJ* 2009;339:b4583.
40. Lyman GH, Khorana AA, Falanga A, et al. American Society of Clinical Oncology guideline: recommendations for venous thromboembolism prophylaxis and treatment in patients with cancer. *J Clin Oncol* 2007;25:5490.
42. Verso M, Agnelli G, Bertoglio S, et al. Enoxaparin for the prevention of venous thromboembolism associated with central vein catheter: a double-blind, placebo-controlled, randomized study in cancer patients. *J Clin Oncol* 2005;23:4057.
43. Young AM, Billingham LJ, Begum G, et al. Warfarin thromboprophylaxis in cancer patients with central venous catheters (WARP): an open-label randomised trial. *Lancet* 2009;373:567.
44. Agnelli G, Gussoni G, Bianchini C, et al. Nadroparin for the prevention of thromboembolic events in ambulatory patients with metastatic or locally advanced solid cancer receiving chemotherapy: a randomised, placebo-controlled, double-blind study. *Lancet Oncol* 2009;10:943.
45. Haas SK, Kakkar AK, Kemkes-Matthes B, et al. Prevention of venous thromboembolism with low-molecular-weight heparin in patients with metastatic breast or lung cancer—results of the TOPIC Studies [abstract]. *J Thromb Haemost* 2005;3(Suppl 1):OR059.
46. Levine M, Hirsh J, Gent M, et al. Double-blind randomised trial of a very-low-dose warfarin for prevention of thromboembolism in stage IV breast cancer. *Lancet* 1994;343:886.
47. Maraveyas A, Waters J, Roy R, et al. Gemitabine with or without prophylactic weight-adjusted dalteparin in patients with advanced or metastatic pancreatic cancer (APC): a multicentre, randomised phase IIB trial (the UK FRAGEM study). *Eur Cancer Suppl* 2009;7:362.
48. Perry JR, Rogers L, Laperriere N, et al. PRODIGE: a phase III randomized placebo-controlled trial of thromboprophylaxis using dalteparin low molecular weight heparin (LMWH) in patients with newly diagnosed malignant glioma [abstract]. *J Clin Oncol* 2007;25:2011.
49. Riess H, Pelzer U, Deutschinoff G, et al. A prospective, randomized trial of chemotherapy with or without the low molecular weight heparin (LMWH) enoxaparin in patients (pts) with advanced pancreatic cancer (APC): results of the CONKO 004 trial. *J Clin Oncol* 2009;27:LBA4506.
50. Akl EA, Rohilla S, Barba M, et al. Anticoagulation for the initial treatment of venous thromboembolism in patients with cancer: a systematic review. *Cancer* 2008;113:1685.
51. van Doormaal FF, Raskob GE, Davidson BL, et al. Treatment of venous thromboembolism in patients with cancer: subgroup analysis of the Matisse clinical trials. *Thromb Haemost* 2009;101:762.
52. Hutten BA, Prins MH, Gent M, et al. Incidence of recurrent thromboembolic and bleeding complications among patients with venous thromboembolism in relation to both malignancy and achieved international normalized ratio: a retrospective analysis. *J Clin Oncol* 2000;18:3078.
53. Lee AY, Levine MN, Baker RI, et al. Low-molecular-weight heparin versus a coumarin for the prevention of recurrent venous thromboembolism in patients with cancer. *N Engl J Med* 2003;349:146.
54. Lee AY, Rickles FR, Julian JA, et al. Randomized comparison of low molecular weight heparin and coumarin derivatives on the survival of patients with cancer and venous thromboembolism. *J Clin Oncol* 2005; 23:2123.
56. Hull RD, Pineo GF, Brant RF, et al. Long-term low-molecular-weight heparin versus usual care in proximal-vein thrombosis patients with cancer. *Am J Med* 2006;119:1062.
57. Meyer G, Marjanovic Z, Valcke J, et al. Comparison of low-molecular-weight heparin and warfarin for the secondary prevention of venous thromboembolism in patients with cancer: a randomized controlled study. *Arch Intern Med* 2002;162:1729.
58. Wagman LD, Baird MF, Bennett CL, et al. Venous thromboembolic disease: clinical practice guidelines in oncology. *J Natl Compr Canc Netw* 2006;4: 838.
59. Kearon C, Kahn SR, Agnelli G, et al. Antithrombotic therapy for venous thromboembolic disease: American College of Chest Physicians Evidence-Based Clinical Practice Guidelines (8th Edition). *Chest* 2008;133:454S.

CHAPTER 159 NAUSEA AND VOMITING

ELIZABETH M. BLANCHARD AND PAUL J. HESKETH

Nausea and vomiting associated with cancer treatment have historically been among the most difficult side effects that patients face while being treated for cancer. Chemotherapy-induced nausea and vomiting (CINV) in particular remains one of the most dreaded side effects from a patient perspective. Patient surveys have consistently listed CINV as one of the most severe and troublesome adverse events related to treatment.[1] Although intuitive, nausea and vomiting related to chemotherapy have also been shown to negatively impact a patient's functional status as tested by objective measures.[2] In fact, CINV has been shown to negatively impact all aspects of quality of life for patients including emotional, social, and physical functioning as well as global quality of life.[3] The past 20 years have seen tremendous progress in this area, which has significant implications for patients in improving their quality of life as well as compliance with cancer treatment.

In the era before the use of newer antiemetics, nearly 80% of patients would experience an episode of nausea or vomiting during the 5 days following chemotherapy of moderate-to-high emetogenic potential.[2] The prevalence of CINV has been dramatically decreased with the introduction of the 5-hydroxytryptamine-3 (5-HT_3) receptor antagonists in the early 1990s and with the subsequent introduction of a new class of antiemetic, the neurokinin-1 (NK_1) antagonists. Despite the progress, CINV remains suboptimally controlled for a significant minority of patients. An important remaining challenge is the education of health care providers to fully recognize the magnitude of the unresolved problems, particularly the control of delayed emesis.[4]

Optimizing the control of treatment-induced nausea and vomiting should be a high priority for all health care providers involved in the care of patients with cancer. Knowledge of the extent of the problem, understanding the basic pathophysiologic principles, recognition of patients at risk, and applying available pharmacologic treatments in an evidence-based manner are all key elements in attaining this goal.

NAUSEA AND VOMITING SYNDROMES

CINV does not describe a single clinical entity but rather three relatively distinct clinical syndromes, including acute, delayed, and anticipatory nausea and vomiting. Although these distinctions have limitations and are somewhat arbitrary, they are nevertheless useful in terms of characterizing the problem and optimizing treatment. Acute CINV is defined as nausea and vomiting that develop within the first 24 hours after chemotherapy administration. With most emetogenic chemotherapy agents, in the absence of effective prophylactic therapy, nausea and vomiting will develop within a few hours of chemotherapy administration. Delayed CINV is defined as nausea and vomiting occurring more than 24 hours after chemotherapy administration. It is generally not as well understood as acute emesis and has been described in association with a number of chemotherapy agents such as cisplatin, carboplatin, cyclophosphamide, and the anthracyclines. It appears to be less severe than acute emesis but can last for a longer period of time.[5,6] Delayed CINV has been best characterized in relation to cisplatin.[7] In the absence of antiemetic treatment, it will develop in 90% or more of patients receiving this agent. It peaks between 24 and 72 hours after cisplatin and gradually dissipates during the next several days. Anticipatory nausea and vomiting occur as the result of a conditioned response to prior episodes of CINV. Symptoms occur after exposure to a variety of stimuli that remind the patients of their prior emetic experiences such as returning to the clinic and seeing health care personnel or the apparatus involved with chemotherapy administration.[8]

Unlike CINV, radiation-induced nausea and vomiting (RINV) has not been broken down into distinct clinical syndromes. Risk of nausea and vomiting is generally related to the body area exposed to treatment with fields encompassing small bowel and stomach associated with the greatest risk. This issue is further addressed in the section on defining the risk of nausea and vomiting.

PATHOPHYSIOLOGY OF TREATMENT-INDUCED NAUSEA AND VOMITING

The mechanisms underlying the control of nausea and vomiting are extraordinarily complex and still incompletely understood at the present time. The central nervous system (CNS) is thought to play a critical role in the physiology of nausea and vomiting, serving as the primary site where a variety of emetic stimuli are received and processed. The CNS is also believed to have the primary role in generating the efferent signals to a number of structures in the body that eventually result in the development of nausea and vomiting.

The mechanisms by which chemotherapy causes nausea and vomiting are only partially delineated. The current understanding of the pathophysiology of this process is based on the pioneering studies of Borison and Wang[9] conducted nearly 60 years ago and more recent insights provided during the development process of the newer antiemetic agents.[10] Borison and Wang proposed that two sites within the brainstem were critical in the control of emesis. The first of these sites is the area postrema, which is a circumventricular structure located at the caudal end of the fourth ventricle. It is positioned outside the blood–brain barrier and therefore is accessible to emetic substances borne in either blood or cerebral spinal fluid. Given its central role in processing a variety of emetogens, it has often been termed the *chemoreceptor trigger zone*. The area postrema cannot independently initiate the emetic process but does so indirectly through neural projections to a second site proposed by Borison and Wang, the vomiting center. According to their theory, a vomiting center located in the lateral reticular formation of the medulla is the final common pathway through which efferent signals are generated to initiate the emetic process. It is now appreciated that an anatomically distinct vomiting center does not exist and that the motor outputs are coordinated by a variety of brainstem nuclei such as the parvicellular reticular formation, the Botzinger complex, and the nucleus tractus solitarius.[11,12] These nuclei have been collectively referred to as the *vomiting center*.[10]

In addition to the area postrema, three other sources of afferent input to the vomiting center appear to have importance in the generation of the emetic response.[9,13] Of greatest importance with respect to CINV is the stomach and proximal small bowel. Chemotherapy agents can either directly or indirectly access the gut mucosa, causing release of local mediators from the enterochromaffin cells stimulating vagal and splanchnic afferent fibers within the bowel wall. These vagal afferents can then transmit afferent signals to the brainstem either directly to nuclei within the vomiting center, such as the nucleus tractus solitarius, or indirectly via the area postrema, initiating the emetic reflex. Direct stimuli arising within the limbic system in the CNS can also apparently trigger emesis by poorly defined mechanisms. This process may be operative in patients experiencing anticipatory emesis. Finally, input from the vestibular system may also induce emesis. This appears to be a predominant mechanism associated with motion sickness but is likely to have a modest role in CINV.

It is now appreciated that a number of neurotransmitters appear to have important roles in the emetic process. More than 30 neurotransmitters have been identified within the area postrema and nuclei of the vomiting center.[14] Some neurotransmitters such as histamine and acetylcholine, which have established roles in certain types of emesis such as motion sickness, appear to have minimal involvement in CINV. The most clinically relevant neurotransmitters involved in CINV include dopamine, serotonin (5-hydroxytryptamine [5-HT]), substance P, and the cannabinoids.[10,15] Much of the current understanding of the neurotransmitters relevant to CINV has come from preclinical studies that preceded the introduction of a number of the current antiemetics. The role of dopamine receptors in CINV forms the basis of some of the earliest interventions in the prevention of emesis related to chemotherapy. Dopamine D_2 receptors are found in the area postrema. Stimulation of these receptors has been shown to induce emesis in animal models.[12] Phenothiazines, which are dopamine antagonists, represented the first class of agents with antiemetic efficacy when introduced into clinical practice more than 40 years ago.

During the past two decades the role of 5-HT was gradually elucidated and ultimately surpassed dopamine as the most relevant neurotransmitter in the treatment of CINV. Of the more than a dozen known subtypes of 5-HT receptors, the type 3 (5-HT_3) receptor has been found to play the most important role in emesis, and antagonism of these receptors has had a significant impact on prevention of acute CINV.[10] The 5-HT_3 receptors are found on vagal afferent fibers, within the area postrema, and the nucleus tractus solitarius.[16–18] The precise mechanisms of 5-HT involvement in treatment-related emesis are incompletely understood. It appears that the most clinically relevant site of action of 5-HT occurs at the peripheral level by increasing afferent stimuli from the gut to the vomiting center and area postrema. Whether 5-HT has meaningful central activity is unclear.

Another neurotransmitter, substance P, has emerged during the past decade as playing a major role in the development of acute and delayed emesis. It is part of a class of regulatory peptides belonging to the tachykinins, which bind to NK receptors[19] and were first noted to cause emesis in animal models. Three tachykinin receptors have been identified, of which the NK_1 receptor is preferentially bound by substance P.[19] The NK_1 receptors are found in the gastrointestinal tract, the area postrema, and the nucleus tractus solitarius.[20] NK_1 receptor antagonists demonstrated wide-ranging antiemetic effects in ferrets, which prompted their development for clinical use.[21,22] Animal models have demonstrated that the site of action of substance P appears to be mainly central, as experimental NK_1 antagonists that do not cross the blood–brain barrier are ineffective in preventing cisplatin-induced emesis.[23]

Unlike dopamine, 5-HT and substance P, which all appear to have a "pro-emetic" role, other neurotransmitters such as the endogenous cannabinoids, enkephalins, and γ-amino butyric acid appear to exert an agonist antiemetic effect. This area of antiemetic research has received much less attention than efforts devoted to the development of neurotransmitter antagonist antiemetics. Of the endogenous neurotransmitters, only the cannabinoids have relevance in the treatment of CINV at present.[24]

There appear to be differences in the relative importance of the various neurotransmitters in the different emetic syndromes. Acute CINV as well as RINV are thought to be primarily due to 5-HT–mediated pathways. The effectiveness of the 5-HT_3 receptor antagonists in both of these settings is thought to be primarily secondary to the ability of these agents to antagonize the binding of 5-HT to the 5-HT_3 receptors on the afferent fibers of the vagus and splanchnic nerves, stimulating afferent nerves in the upper small intestine. Dopamine also appears to be most relevant to acute CINV and to a lesser extent in RINV given the utility of dopamine D_2 antagonists in these settings.

Dopamine and 5-HT appear to be less important in delayed CINV, given the limited clinical utility of the 5-HT_3 receptor antagonists and dopamine D_2 antagonists in this setting. The mechanisms underlying delayed CINV are very poorly defined. Changes in the gastrointestinal tract as a result of chemotherapy, such as altered gastrointestinal secretions and motility, may play a role. In addition, chemotherapy-induced enhanced cell breakdown and turnover with the resulting release of cytokines and inflammation may be important contributors to delayed CINV.[25] The clinical utility of the corticosteroids in delayed CINV may be partly due to their anti-inflammatory effect. Of the known clinically relevant neurotransmitters, substance P may have the most important role in the pathophysiology of delayed emesis. This is strongly supported by the unique preclinical and clinical efficacy of the NK_1 antagonists in the delayed emesis setting. In addition, an analysis of the time course of cisplatin-induced emesis demonstrated that 5-HT mechanisms appeared to predominate in the first 8 to 12 hours after cisplatin administration, but thereafter NK_1-dependent mechanisms appeared to be more important.[26]

The pathophysiology of RINV likely involves several mechanisms. If the gastrointestinal tract is included in the field of radiation, direct effects are likely with stimulation of afferent pathways in the upper gastrointestinal tract.[25,27] In addition, it is theorized that the chemoreceptor trigger zone in the area postrema may also be involved, possibly from radiation-induced tissue breakdown products.

DEFINING THE RISK OF NAUSEA AND VOMITING

There are a number of factors that can influence the development of CINV, including those related to the patient receiving therapy as well as the chemotherapy treatment itself. The most important patient-related factors include gender, age, history of ethanol consumption, and history of nausea or vomiting with prior chemotherapy treatment.[28–33] Gender is a strong and uniform predictor of difficulty with CINV, with women consistently experiencing poorer control of CINV than men.[28–32] Age is also an important risk factor, with younger patients having more difficulty than older patients.[28–32] A history of chronic alcohol consumption seems to decrease the risk of emesis.[28,30,31] Patients who have experienced CINV with prior chemotherapy treatment are also at greater risk of developing CINV with subsequent treatments.[33] A history of nausea and vomiting associated with pregnancy and a history of motion sickness have been suggested to predict for poor control of CINV, but definitive data are lacking. There is some genetic variation in the metabolism of 5-HT$_3$ receptor antagonists, and patients who are rapid metabolizers are at risk for more significant CINV.[34] In addition, genetic variations in the 5-HT$_3$ receptor may also predispose to a decreased response to this class of medication and more difficulty with CINV.[35]

TABLE 159.1

CLASSIFICATION OF EMETIC RISK OF INTRAVENOUS ANTINEOPLASTIC AGENTS

Emetic Risk (Estimated Incidence without Prophylaxis)	Antineoplastic Agent
High (>90%)	Cisplatin Mechlorethamine Streptozotocin Cyclophosphamide (≥1,500 mg/m^2) Carmustine Dacarbazine
Moderate (30% to 90%)	Oxaliplatin Cytarabine (>1 g/m^2) Carboplatin Ifosfamide Cyclophosphamide (<1,500 mg/m^2) Doxorubicin Daunorubicin Epirubicin Idarubicin Irinotecan Azacitadine Bendamustine Clofarabine Alemtuzumab
Low (10% to 30%)	Paclitaxel Docetaxel Mitoxantrone Doxorubicin HCl liposome injection Ixabepilone Topotecan Etoposide Pemetrexed Methotrexate Mitomycin Gemcitabine Cytarabine (≤100 mg/m^2) 5-Fluorouracil Bortezomib Cetuximab Trastuzumab Panitumumab Catumaxumab
Minimal (<10%)	Bleomycin Busulfan 2-Chlorodeoxydenosine Fludarabine Vinblastine Vincristine Vinorelbine Bevacizumab Rituximab

(From ref. 37, with permission.)

Treatment-related factors include the actual chemotherapy agent, its dose, rate, and route of administration. Of all the known predictive factors for CINV, clearly the most important is the intrinsic emetogenicity of the chemotherapeutic agent employed. The emetogenicity schema that is most widely used is modified from the Hesketh classification, which was first described in 1997.[36] This system, based on an extensive literature review, classifies chemotherapeutic agents according to their intrinsic emetogenicity and establishes a framework for the development of antiemetic treatment guidelines. What was originally described as five levels of emetogenicity has been subsequently modified to a four-level schema (Table 159.1), classifying agents as having a high, moderate, low, or minimal risk of inducing emesis.[38,39] Oral agents are considered separately and have been classified by emetic risk into four categories.[37,40]

Risk of radiation-induced nausea and vomiting is defined primarily by the anatomic area receiving treatment as well as the type of treatment.[39] The most commonly employed category includes four levels of risk: high, moderate, low, and minimal.[38,39] High-risk therapy consists of total-body irradiation. Moderate risk includes the upper abdomen, which carries a 60% to 90% risk of emesis without prophylaxis. Low risk includes the lower thoracic region and pelvis as well as the cranium (with radiosurgery) and craniospinal therapy. Minimal risk includes cranium, head and neck, extremities, and breast.

ANTIEMETIC AGENTS

Highest Therapeutic Index

There are several classes of drugs that are effective in the prevention of CINV (Table 159.2). Those of highest therapeutic index include the 5-HT$_3$ receptor antagonists, the NK$_1$ receptor antagonists, and corticosteroids. The most widely available first generation 5-HT$_3$ receptor antagonists include dolasetron, granisetron, ondansetron, and tropisetron. They have been shown to be superior to high-dose metoclopramide[41] and have replaced it as first-line therapy in prevention of acute emesis. They have proven to be most effective in the prevention of acute CINV in the settings of highly and moderately emetogenic chemotherapy. All first-generation 5-HT$_3$ receptor antagonists are considered therapeutically equivalent and are used interchangeably.[38,39,42] Oral formulations of the first-generation 5-HT$_3$ receptor antagonists have similar efficacy to intravenous formulations.[43]

Palonosetron is a second-generation 5-HT$_3$ antagonist that differs from other agents in this class by virtue of a longer half-life of 40 hours and a higher binding affinity to the 5-HT$_3$ receptor. It has been compared with first-generation 5-HT$_3$ antagonists in two randomized phase 3 trials in patients receiving moderately emetogenic chemotherapy.[44,45] Both trials were designed as noninferiority trials and met their primary end point. *Post hoc* analyses indicated superiority for palonosetron in a number of parameters to the comparator agents. In one trial, palonosetron 0.25 mg was superior to dolasetron 100 mg

PRACTICE OF ONCOLOGY

TABLE 159.2

DOSES OF COMMONLY USED ANTIEMETIC AGENTS

Drug	Prechemotherapy Dose (Day 1)	Postchemotherapy Dose
HIGHEST THERAPEUTIC INDEX		
Aprepitant	125 mg orally 110 mg IV	80 mg orally days 2 and 3
Dexamethasone		
With aprepitant	12 mg orally or IV	8 mg days 2–4[a]
Without aprepitant	20 mg orally or IV[a] 8 mg orally or IV[b]	8 mg bid days 2–4[a] 8 mg days 2 and 3[c]
Ondansetron	24 mg orally[a]; 8 mg orally bid[b] 8 mg or 0.15 mg/kg IV	8 mg bid days 2 and 3
Granisetron	2 mg orally 1 mg or 0.01 mg/kg IV	—
Tropisetron	5 mg orally or IV	—
Dolasetron	100 mg orally 100 mg or 1.8 mg/kg IV	—
Palonosetron	0.25 mg IV 0.5 mg orally	—
LOWER THERAPEUTIC INDEX		
Prochlorperazine	10 mg orally or IV	—
Dronabinol	5 mg/m^2 orally	5 mg/m^2 orally q2–4 hr prn
Nabilone	1–2 mg orally	1–2 mg bid or tid prn
Olanzapine	5 mg orally daily for 2 days preceding chemotherapy; 10 mg on day 1	10 mg days 2–4

IV, intravenously; bid, twice daily; q, every; tid, three times a day; prn, as needed.
[a]When used with highly emetic chemotherapy.
[b]With moderately emetic chemotherapy.
[c]When used with moderately emetic chemotherapy with potential for delayed emesis.

in complete response (no emesis or use of rescue medications) during the delayed (24 to 120 hours) and overall study periods.[44] In the other trial, palonosetron 0.25 mg was superior to ondansetron 32 mg in complete response during the first 24 hours, delayed period, and overall 5-day study period.[45] A third phase 3 trial in patients who received highly emetogenic chemotherapy also reached its end point of noninferiority in comparing palonosetron with ondansetron 32 mg.[46] Unlike the moderately emetogenic trials, there was no significant difference between palonosetron and ondansetron in the control of acute or delayed emesis. Approximately two thirds of patients also received corticosteroids at the discretion of the investigator in the highly emetogenic trial. A *post hoc* secondary subgroup analysis of the patients who received dexamethasone demonstrated superior control of acute and delayed emesis in the group receiving palonosetron. In a recently reported phase 3 trial,[47] patients who received either cisplatin or the combination of adriamycin or epirubicin and cyclophosphamide were randomized in a double-blind fashion to either a single dose of palonosetron at a dose of 0.75 mg or a single dose of granisetron (40 mcg/kg) on day 1 of chemotherapy. In this trial, steroids for acute and delayed emesis were mandated. Palonosetron was more efficacious than granisetron, with 56.8% of patients in the palonosetron group experiencing an overall complete response (no vomiting or use of rescue medications) compared with 44.5% in the granisetron group (P <.0001). This was also true for delayed emesis (56.8% vs. 44.5%; P <.0001). Palonosetron was found to be comparable to granisetron in the acute phase, with 75.3% complete response in the palonosetron group versus 73.3% in the granisetron group (difference of 2.29, 95% CI [confidence interval], −2.70 to 7.27). The results of the phase 3 trials with palonosetron suggest that this agent is superior in efficacy to the first-generation 5-HT_3 antagonists. Definitive conclusions await the completion of additional trials in which palonosetron is evaluated with regimens that incorporate NK_1 antagonists and first-generation 5-HT_3 antagonists are repetitively dosed throughout the study period. In 2008 an oral formulation of palonosetron at a dose of 0.5 mg was approved for use with moderately emetogenic chemotherapy based on the results of a trial demonstrating noninferiority with the 0.25 mg intravenous dose.[48]

Corticosteroids are a mainstay in the prevention of both acute and delayed CINV. In a large meta-analysis that included data from more than 5,000 patients, dexamethasone, the most commonly employed corticosteroid, was found to significantly improve the prevention of CINV compared with placebo or other antiemetics.[49] Most of the studies involved the use of highly emetogenic chemotherapy. In the acute phase, it was estimated to increase the chance of complete prevention of vomiting by 25% to 30% versus placebo. Similar results were seen with delayed emesis. With moderate to highly emetogenic chemotherapy regimens, corticosteroids are typically not used alone but rather in combination with other antiemetics. Single-agent use is appropriate with mildly emetogenic regimens. The appropriate doses of dexamethasone for use with highly and moderately emetogenic therapy (in the absence of a NK_1 antagonist) are 20 mg and 8 mg, respectively, based on the results of two large phase 3 trials.[50,51]

The most recent advance in CINV prevention has been the introduction of a selective antagonist of substance P's binding to the NK_1 receptor. Aprepitant is the first approved agent in this new class of antiemetics. In a phase 3 randomized study that included more than 500 patients, aprepitant significantly increased the overall 5-day complete response (no emesis or use of rescue) rate (72.7% vs. 52.3%) when added to the standard therapy of ondansetron and dexamethasone in patients receiving high-dose cisplatin chemotherapy.[52] Superiority for the aprepitant arm was demonstrated in both the control of acute and delayed emesis. Similar results were found in an identically designed phase 3 trial that enrolled patients from Latin America.[53] The addition of aprepitant may also improve the durability of antiemetic control over multiple cycles.[33]

One early series assessed the need for a 5-HT_3 receptor antagonist in an aprepitant-containing regimen.[54] More than 300 patients were included who were being treated with highly emetogenic chemotherapy. The group that received aprepitant, dexamethasone, and placebo did significantly worse in terms of vomiting compared with the arm receiving aprepitant, dexamethasone, and granisetron, with 80% of patients free of any vomiting in the group with aprepitant, dexamethasone, and granisetron compared with 57% in the group with aprepitant, dexamethasone, and placebo ($P < .01$). Aprepitant has also been shown to be beneficial in the prevention of CINV associated with moderately emetogenic chemotherapy. In a phase 3 trial in patients with breast cancer who received an anthracycline plus cyclophosphamide, patients were randomized to an aprepitant-containing regimen, which included dexamethasone and ondansetron, or a standard regimen that consisted of dexamethasone and ondansetron.[55] Aprepitant alone was used as delayed emesis prevention in the aprepitant arm, while ondansetron alone was used for delayed emesis protection in the comparison arm. A superior rate of complete response (50.8% vs. 42.5%) during the 5-day study period was noted on the aprepitant arm. Recently, Rapoport et al.[56] reported the results of another phase 3 trial evaluating aprepitant with a variety of moderately emetogenic chemotherapy regimens. Patients were treated with aprepitant or placebo plus ondansetron and dexamethasone on day 1 and either aprepitant (experimental arm) or ondansetron (control arm) for delayed emesis. Overall, patients randomized to the aprepitant-containing arm had significantly higher proportions of patients with complete response, including overall (62.8% vs. 47.1%; $P < .01$), in the acute setting (84.3% vs. 72.5%; $P < .01$), and the delayed setting (64.8% vs. 52.9%; $P < .01$). Retrospective analysis was done comparing patients receiving adriamycin and cyclophosphamide with other types of moderately emetogenic combinations, which confirmed the superiority of aprepitant in those patients treated with adriamycin and cyclophosphamide. For the nonadriamycin and cyclophosphamide arm, while the addition of aprepitant statistically improved the proportion of patients who did not experience vomiting, the overall complete response rate did not differ between the aprepitant-containing group and the nonaprepitant containing group. Citing the retrospective nature of this data set as well as the heterogeneity of cancer types studied, the most recent ESMO-MASCC (European Society of Medical Oncology and the Multinational Association of Supportive Care in Cancer) antiemetic consensus conference did not recommend the use of aprepitant in nonanthracycline-based moderately emetogenic chemotherapy.[37]

Of note, aprepitant is an inhibitor of the cytochrome P-450 enzyme CYP3A4, which is involved in the metabolism of many drugs, including dexamethasone and certain chemotherapeutic agents. A pharmacokinetic study demonstrated that the plasma concentration of dexamethasone as measured as the area under the curve was more than twofold higher with aprepitant compared with the same dose of dexamethasone without concomitant aprepitant.[57] A dose reduction of dexamethasone from 20 to 12 mg (day 1) and 8 to 4 mg (days 2 and 3) yielded similar plasma dexamethasone levels to those in patients not taking aprepitant. The slowed metabolism of dexamethasone in the presence of aprepitant accounts for the recommendation to reduce dexamethasone doses by approximately 50% when administered with aprepitant.[38] However, if the corticosteroids are given as part of the chemotherapeutic regimen rather than for antiemetic prophylaxis, the corticosteroid dose should not be adjusted.[38] There is also a theoretical concern that chemotherapeutic agents that are metabolized by CYP3A4 may have a slowed clearance, leading to higher drug exposure and increased toxicity. However, analysis of the completed phase 3 trials with aprepitant has not demonstrated a significant increase in adverse events in patients receiving aprepitant. In 2008 an intravenous formulation (fosaprepitant) of aprepitant received regulatory approval for use with moderately and highly emetogenic chemotherapy.

Casopitant is a novel NK_1 antagonist that has been tested in both highly emetogenic and moderately emetogenic chemotherapy. In a phase 3 trial, casopitant was given either at 50 mg daily for 3 days or 150 mg on day 1 with ondansetron and dexamethasone and was compared with ondansetron and dexamethasone alone in patients treated with cisplatin-based chemotherapy. The casopitant combination achieved a higher complete response compared with the noncasopitant arm. The 3-day casopitant regimen was similar to the single-day dosing in most of the parameters measured, including complete response (no vomiting or use of rescue medications) and total control (complete response plus no nausea).[58] Similarly, in a phase 3 trial of patients being treated with adriamycin and cyclophosphamide chemotherapy, single-day or 3-day dosing of casopitant resulted in a higher rate of complete response at 120 hours when compared with placebo, with 59% of patients in the control arm achieving complete response compared with 73% of patients receiving a single oral dose or 3-day oral dosing of casopitant ($P < .0001$). All patients received dexamethasone day 1 and ondansetron days 1 through 3.[59] Although regulatory approval is not being sought for casopitant, the reported clinical experience has added to the knowledge and principles of the use of NK_1 receptor antagonists in CINV.

Lower Therapeutic Index

Drugs of lower therapeutic index include metoclopramide, butyrophenones, phenothiazines, cannabinoids, and olanzapine (Table 159.2). These drugs in general are all associated with less efficacy than the high therapeutic index agents and can have troublesome adverse effects. These drugs are most commonly used in patients who are unable to tolerate or who do not respond to 5-HT_3 receptor antagonists, aprepitant, or dexamethasone. Of the lower therapeutic index agents, the phenothiazines are probably used most often either as monotherapy with patients receiving mildly emetogenic chemotherapy or as an as-needed agent in patients failing frontline antiemetics. Another class of agents that may have value in selected situations is the benzodiazepines. Although limited in their antiemetic efficacy, the antianxiety properties of these agents can be useful. The most commonly employed agent in the class is lorazepam, which has demonstrated value with anticipatory emesis and can be useful as an adjunct to other antiemetics in patients failing to completely respond to their frontline regimens. Olanzapine, which is an antagonist of multiple neurotransmitter receptors including those of dopamine and serotonin, may be effective in preventing both acute and delayed CINV. In a phase 2 trial that included patients who received both highly emetogenic and moderately emetogenic chemotherapy, olanzapine was found to be effective in controlling nausea and vomiting in both the acute and delayed settings when combined with granisetron and dexamethasone.[60] There is no available information on its use in combination with aprepitant.

ANTIEMETIC TREATMENT BY CLINICAL SETTING

In planning antiemetic therapy in cancer patients who receive chemotherapy it is important to consider a few basic principles: (1) the primary goal should be complete prevention; (2) to minimize the risk of anticipatory emesis, antiemetic therapy should be appropriately maximized from the initial cycle of chemotherapy; (3) antiemetic therapies should be chosen to match the intrinsic emetogenicity of the chemotherapy; and (4) consider prescribing antiemetics for use in the event breakthrough emesis develops. If emesis does develop in the patient who receives chemotherapy, an assessment should be made to exclude nonchemotherapy causes of the patient's nausea and vomiting. These include bowel obstruction or dysmotility; concomitant medications, particularly opioids; metabolic disturbances such as hyponatremia and hypercalcemia; and occult CNS metastasis.

For patients receiving single-day intravenously (IV) administered highly emetogenic chemotherapy such as cisplatin, recommended prophylaxis involves the use of a 5-HT_3 receptor antagonist on day 1, dexamethasone on days 1 to 4, and aprepitant on days 1 to 3 (Table 159.3). For moderately emetogenic chemotherapy given IV, excluding the combination of an anthracycline and cyclophosphamide, prophylaxis using palonosetron is recommended on day 1, along with dexamethasone on day 1. Patients should also receive either a 5-HT_3 antagonist or dexamethasone on days 2 to 3 after chemotherapy. For patients treated with an anthracycline and cyclophosphamide regimen, a 5-HT_3 receptor antagonist and dexamethasone and aprepitant should all be administered on day 1. In addition, patients should also receive aprepitant on days 2 and 3. For IV-administered chemotherapy of low emetogenic potential, dexamethasone is recommended on day 1 with no routine prophylaxis for delayed emesis. For minimal-risk chemotherapy agents, no routine antiemetic prophylaxis is indicated.

SPECIAL CHEMOTHERAPY-INDUCED NAUSEA AND VOMITING PROBLEMS

There are a number of situations in addition to single-day IV-administered chemotherapy that pose emetic challenges. Regimens containing highly emetogenic chemotherapy, such as cisplatin given on multiple days, require special attention. There are data supporting the use of a combination of a 5-HT_3 receptor antagonist plus dexamethasone during each day of chemotherapy administration, followed by dexamethasone for delayed emesis after the final day of chemotherapy.[61] There are no randomized data available on the use of aprepitant in multiple-day regimens, although a 3-day course would seem appropriate, based on the data from single-day regimens. In 2008 the U.S. Food and Drug Administration approved the use of a transdermal granisetron patch for use in patients receiving multiple-day regimens of chemotherapy based on a phase 3 multinational, double-blind, double-dummy, noninferiority study. In this trial 641 patients who received chemotherapy regimens of 3 to 5 days duration were randomized to the granisetron patch applied on the day prior to chemotherapy and kept on for 7 days or oral granisetron 2 mg daily prior to chemotherapy. The primary end point of this study was complete control: no vomiting, use of rescue medication, or more than mild nausea. The study met its primary end point of noninferiority with complete control in 59.8% of patients using the patch and 64.9% of patients taking single daily oral granisetron (difference of −5.51%, 95% CI, −13.6 to 2.5%).[62] A related problem is noted in patients who received high-dose chemotherapy in the setting of hematopoietic stem cell transplantation. Chemotherapy regimens are often administered during several days in sequence, and there are data supporting the value of daily 5-HT_3 receptor antagonist and dexamethasone in this setting as well.[61] A recently reported randomized trial in patients receiving preparative regimens for hematopoietic stem cell transplantation noted improved outcome with the addition of aprepitant to ondansetron and dexamethasone.[63] No emesis rates of 73.3% versus 22.5% were noted for the entire study period in the aprepitant and control arms, respectively. In addition complete response (no emesis and no or mild nausea) was seen in 48.9% versus 14.6% in the aprepitant and control arms, respectively.

Anticipatory nausea and vomiting pose additional special CINV challenges. These symptoms are often poorly responsive to common antiemetics. Fortunately, given the recent improvements noted in the control of CINV in general, anticipatory nausea and vomiting are much less commonly seen. Therapies that have been studied with some success include systemic desensitization and hypnosis. One series showed benefit for alprazolam when combined with a psychological support program.[64]

Oral chemotherapeutic agents are increasingly used in clinical oncology practices and also have a propensity to cause varying degrees of CINV. There is a scarcity of data on the

TABLE 159.3

RECOMMENDED ANTIEMETIC THERAPY FOR SINGLE-DAY INTRAVENOUS CHEMOTHERAPY

Emetic Risk Category	Prevention of Acute Emesis (Day 1 Prechemotherapy)	Prevention of Delayed Emesis
High	5-HT_3 receptor antagonist *plus* dexamethasone *plus* aprepitant	Dexamethasone days 2–4 *plus* aprepitant days 2 and 3
Moderate		
AC	5-HT_3 receptor antagonist *plus* dexamethasone *plus* aprepitant	Aprepitant days 2 and 3
Non-AC	Palonosetron *plus* dexamethasone	Dexamethasone days 2 and 3
Low	Dexamethasone *or* prochlorperazine	No preventive measures
Minimal	As needed	No preventive measures

AC, anthracycline and cyclophosphamide.

TABLE 159.4

RECOMMENDED ANTIEMETIC THERAPY FOR RADIOTHERAPY-INDUCED EMESIS

Risk Level	Irradiated Area	Antiemetic Guidelines
High (>90%)	Total body irradiation, total nodal irradiation	Prophylaxis with 5-HT$_3$ antagonists + DEX
Moderate (60–90%)	Upper abdomen, HBI, UBI	Prophylaxis with 5-HT$_3$ antagonists + optional DEX
Low (30–60%)	Cranium, craniospinal, H&N, lower thorax region, pelvis	Prophylaxis or rescue with 5-HT$_3$ antagonists
Minimal (<30)	Extremities, breast	Rescue with dopamine receptor antagonists or 5-HT$_3$ antagonists

HBI, half body irradiation; UBI, upper body irradiation; H&N, head and neck; DEX, dexamethasone.
Note: [a]In concomitant radiochemotherapy the antiemetic prophylaxis is according to the chemotherapy-related antiemetic guidelines of the corresponding risk category, unless the risk of emesis is higher with radiotherapy than chemotherapy.
(Adapted from ref. 42, with permission.)

emetogenicity of oral drugs; therefore, the risk of CINV has not been as well defined. The lack of clinical trials that address the issue of oral agent-induced CINV precludes definitive treatment recommendations.

Finally, if patients receive appropriate evidence-based prophylaxis for CINV and still develop so-called breakthrough emesis, this can also be a troublesome problem. As with oral chemotherapy, there are few prospective data evaluating treatment approaches for this problem. If other causes of nausea and vomiting are excluded, adjunctive medications such as benzodiazepines or dopaminergic antagonists can be added. One double-blind trial in patients who failed initial prophylaxis found that switching from one 5-HT$_3$ receptor antagonist to another afforded significantly higher rates of complete protection compared with those patients who remained on the original 5-HT$_3$ receptor antagonist.[65]

RADIOTHERAPY-INDUCED NAUSEA AND VOMITING

Radiotherapy can also clearly cause nausea and vomiting in a number of settings and warrants appropriate prophylactic therapy (Table 159.4). Updated recommendations were provided at the recent ESMO-MASCC consensus conference.[37] Optimal prophylaxis for total body or total nodal radiation is the use of a 5-HT$_3$ receptor antagonist plus dexamethasone. Reasonable prophylaxis for radiation of moderate emetic risk would be 5-HT$_3$ receptor antagonist before each fraction with dexamethasone use optional. Prophylaxis or rescue with 5-HT$_3$ antagonists is appropriate for low-risk radiation. Minimal-risk radiation is treated with 5-HT$_3$ receptor antagonists or dopamine antagonists as needed.

PRACTICE OF ONCOLOGY

Selected References

The full list of references for this chapter appears in the online version.

1. Griffin AM, Butow PN, Coates AS, et al. On the receiving end. V: Patient perceptions of the side effects of cancer chemotherapy in 1993. *Ann Oncol* 1996;7:189.
2. O'Brien BJ, Rusthoven J, Rocchi A, et al. Impact of chemotherapy-associated nausea and vomiting on patients' functional status and on costs: survey of five Canadian centers. *Can Med Assoc J* 1993;149:296.
4. Grunberg SM, Deuson RR, Mavros P, et al. Incidence of chemotherapy-induced nausea and emesis after modern antiemetics. *Cancer* 2004;100:2261.
5. Roila F, Donati D, Tamberi S, et al. Delayed emesis: Incidence, pattern, prognostic factors and optimal treatment. *Support Care Cancer* 2002;10:88.
7. Kris MG, Gralla RJ, Clark RA, et al. Incidence, course, and severity of delayed nausea and vomiting following the administration of high-dose cisplatin. *J Clin Oncol* 1985;3:1379.
9. Borison HL, Wang SC. Physiology and pharmacology of vomiting. *Pharmacol Rev* 1953;5:193.
10. Sanger GJ, Andrews PLR. Treatment of nausea and vomiting: gaps in our knowledge. *Auton Neurosci* 2006;129:3.
15. Hesketh PJ. Understanding the pathobiology of chemotherapy-induced nausea and vomiting. *Oncology* 2004;18:9.
19. Andrews PLR, Judd JA. The role of tachykinins and the tachykinin NK$_1$ receptor in nausea and emesis. In: Holzer P, ed. *Handbook of experimental pharmacology.* New York, Berlin: Springer, 2004;359.
20. Quartara L, Maggi CA. The tachykinin NK$_1$ receptor. Part II: distribution and pathophysiological roles. *Neuropeptides* 1998;32:1–49.
24. Tramer MR, Carroll D, Campbell FA. Cannabinoids for control of chemotherapy induced nausea and vomiting: quantitative systematic review. *BMJ* 2001;7:16.
26. Hesketh PJ, Van Bells S, Aapro M, et al. Differential involvement of neurotransmitters through the time course of cisplatin-induced emesis as revealed by therapy with specific receptor antagonists. *Eur J Cancer* 2003; 39:1074.
27. Endo T, Minami M, Hirafuji M, et al. Neurochemistry and neuropharmacology of emesis-the role of serotonin. *Toxicology* 2000;16:189.
28. Hesketh PJ, Plagge P, Bryson JC. Single-dose ondansetron for prevention of acute cisplatin-induced emesis: analysis of efficacy and prognostic factors. In: Bianchi AL, Grelot L, Miller AD, King GL, eds. *Mechanisms and control of emesis.* London: John Libbey, 1992:25.
29. du Bois A, Meerpohl HG, Vach W, et al. Course, patterns, and risk-factors for chemotherapy-induced emesis in cisplatin-pretreated patients: a study with ondansetron. *Eur J Cancer* 1992;28:450.
30. Osoba D, Zee B, Pater J, et al. Determinants of postchemotherapy nausea and vomiting in patients with cancer. *J Clin Oncol* 1997;15:116.
31. Hesketh P, Navari R, Grote T, et al. Double-blind, randomized comparison of the antiemetic efficacy of intravenous dolasetron mesylate and intravenous ondansetron in the prevention of acute cisplatin-induced emesis in patients with cancer. *J Clin Oncol* 1996;14:2242.
32. Pollera CF, Giannarelli D. Prognostic factors influencing cisplatin-induced emesis. *Cancer* 1989;64:1117.
33. de Wit R, Herrstedt J, Rapoport B, et al. Addition of the oral NK$_1$ antagonist aprepitant to standard antiemetics provides protection against nausea and vomiting during multiple cycles of cisplatin-based chemotherapy. *J Clin Oncol* 2003;21:4105.
34. Kaiser R, Sezer O, Papies A, et al. Patient-tailored antiemetic treatment with 5-hydroxytryptamine type 3 receptor antagonists according to cytochrome P-450 2D6 genotypes. *J Clin Oncol* 2002;20:2805.
35. Tremblay P, Kaiser R, Sezer O, et al. Variations in the 5-hydroxytryptamine type 3B receptor gene as predictors of the efficacy of antiemetic treatment in cancer patients. *J Clin Oncol* 2003;21:2147.
36. Hesketh PJ, Kris MG, Grunberg SM, et al. Proposal for classifying the acute emetogenicity of cancer chemotherapy. *J Clin Oncol* 1997;15:103.
37. Roila F, Herrstedt J, Aapro M, et al. Guideline update for MASCC and ESMO in the prevention of chemotherapy and radiotherapy-induced nausea and vomiting: results of the Perugia multinational consensus conference. *Annals Oncol* 2010;21(5):v232.

38. Kris MG, Hesketh PJ, Somerfield MR, et al. American Society of Clinical Oncology guideline for antiemetics in oncology: update 2006. *J Clin Oncol* 2006;24:2932.
39. The antiemetic subcommittee of the Multinational Association of Supportive Care in Cancer. Prevention of chemotherapy- and radiotherapy-induced emesis: results of the 2004 Perugia International Antiemetic Consensus Conference. *Ann Oncol* 2006;17:20.
40. Grunberg SM, Osoba D, Hesketh PJ, et al. Evaluation of new antiemetic agents and definition of antineoplastic agent emetogenicity—an update. *Support Care Cancer* 2005;13:80.
41. Bonneterre J, Chevallier B, Metz R, et al. A randomized double-blind comparison of ondansetron and metoclopramide in the prophylaxis of emesis induced by cyclophosphamide, fluorouracil, and doxorubicin or epirubicin chemotherapy. *J Clin Oncol* 1990;8:1063.
42. del Giglio A, Soares HP, Caparroz C, et al. Granisetron is equivalent to ondansetron for prophylaxis of chemotherapy-induced nausea and vomiting. *Cancer* 2000;89:2301.
43. Perez EA, Hesketh P, Sandbach J, et al. Comparison of single-dose oral granisetron versus intravenous ondansetron in the prevention of nausea and vomiting induced by moderately emetogenic chemotherapy: a multicenter, double-blind, randomized parallel study. *J Clin Oncol* 1998;16:754.
44. Eisenberg P, Figueroa-Vadillo J, Zamora R, et al. Improved prevention of moderately emetogenic chemotherapy-induced nausea and vomiting with palonosetron, a pharmacologically novel 5-HT3 receptor antagonist: results of a phase III, single-dose trail versus dolasetron. *Cancer* 2003;98:2473.
45. Gralla R, Lichinitser M, Van Der Vegt S, et al. Palonosetron improves prevention of chemotherapy-induced nausea and vomiting following moderately emetogenic chemotherapy: results of a double-blind randomized phase III trial comparing single doses of palonosetron with ondansetron. *Ann Oncol* 2003;14:1570.
46. Aapro MS, Grunberg SM, Manikhas GM, et al. A phase III double-blind, randomized trial of palonosetron compared with ondansetron in preventing chemotherapy-induced nausea and vomiting following highly emetogenic chemotherapy. *Ann Oncol* 2006;17:1441.
47. Saito M, Aogi K, Sekine I, et al. Palonosetron plus dexamethasone versus granisetron plus dexamethasone for prevention of nausea and vomiting during chemotherapy: a double-blind, double dummy, randomized, comparative phase III trial. *Lancet Oncol* 2009;10:115.
48. Grunberg S, Voisin E, Zufferli M, Piraccini G. Oral palonosetron is as effective as intravenous palonosetron: a phase 3 dose ranging trial in patients receiving moderately emetogenic chemotherapy. *EJC Suppl* 2007;5:155.
49. Ioannidis JPA, Hesketh PJ, Lau J. Contribution of dexamethasone to control of chemotherapy-induced nausea and vomiting: a meta-analysis of randomized evidence. *J Clin Oncol* 2000;18:3409.
50. Italian Group for Antiemetic Research: Double-blind, dose-finding study of four intravenous doses of dexamethasone in the prevention of cisplatin-induced acute emesis. *J Clin Oncol* 1998;16:2937.
51. Italian Group for Antiemetic Research. Randomized, double-blind, dose-finding study of dexamethasone in preventing acute emesis induced by anthracyclines, carboplatin, or cyclophosphamide. *J Clin Oncol* 2004;22:725.
52. Hesketh PJ, Grunberg SM, Gralla RJ, et al. The oral neurokinin-1 antagonists aprepitant for the prevention of chemotherapy-induced nausea and vomiting: a multinational, randomized, double-blind, placebo-controlled trial in patients receiving high-dose cisplatin—the aprepitant protocol 052 study group. *J Clin Oncol* 2003;21:4112.
53. Poli-Bigelli S, Rodrigues-Pereira J, Carides AD, et al. Addition of the neurokinin 1 receptor antagonist aprepitant to standard antiemetic therapy improves control of chemotherapy induced nausea and vomiting. *Cancer* 2003;97:3090.
54. Campos D, Pereira JR, Reinhardt RR, et al. Prevention of cisplatin-induced emesis by the oral neurokinin-1 antagonist, MK-869, in combination with granisetron and dexamethasone or with dexamethasone alone. *J Clin Oncol* 2001;19:1759.
55. Warr DG, Hesketh PJ, Gralla RJ, et al. Efficacy and tolerability of aprepitant for the prevention of chemotherapy-induced nausea and vomiting in patients with breast cancer after moderately emetogenic chemotherapy. *J Clin Oncol* 2005;23:2822.
56. Rapoport BL, Jordan K, Boice JA, et al. Aprepitant for the prevention of chemotherapy-induced nausea and vomiting associated with a broad range of moderately emetogenic chemotherapy and tumor types: a randomized, double blind study. *Support Care Cancer* 2010;18:423.
57. McCrea JB, Majumdar AK, Goldberg MR, et al. Effects of the neurokinin 1 receptor antagonist aprepitant on the pharmacokinetics of dexamethasone and methylprednisolone. *Clin Pharmacol Ther* 2003;74:17.
58. Grunberg SM, Rolski J, Strausz J, et al. Efficacy and safety of casopitant mesylate, a neurokinin 1 (NK1)-receptor antagonist, in prevention of chemotherapy-induced nausea and vomiting in patients receiving cisplatin-based highly emetogenic chemotherapy: a randomized, double blind, placebo controlled trial. *Lancet Oncol* 2009;10:549.
59. Herrstedt J, Apornwirat W, Shaharyar A, et al. Phase III trial of casopitant, a novel neurokinin-1 receptor antagonist, for the prevention of nausea and vomiting in patients receiving moderately emetogenic chemotherapy. *J Clin Oncol* 2009;27:5363.
60. Navari RM, Einhorn LH, Passik SD, et al. A phase II trial of olanzapine for the prevention of chemotherapy-induced nausea and vomiting: a Hoosier Oncology Group study. *Support Care Cancer* 2005;13:529.
61. Einhorn LH, Rapoport B, Koeller J, et al. Antiemetic therapy for multiple-day chemotherapy and high-dose chemotherapy with stem cell transplant: review and consensus statement. *Support Care Cancer* 2005;13:112.
62. Grunberg S, Gabrial N, Clark G. Phase III trial of transdermal granisetron patch (Sancuso) compared to oral granisetron (OG) for chemotherapy-induced nausea and vomiting (CINV) after multi-day moderately emetogenic (MEC) or highly emetogenic chemotherapy (HEC). Proceedings of the Multinational Association of Supportive Care in Cancer St Gallen, Switzerland. June 2007 (abstr P-18).
63. Stiff P, Fox-Geiman, M, Kiley K et al. Aprepitant vs. Placebo plus oral ondansetron and dexamethasone for the prevention of nausea and vomiting associated with highly emetogenic preparative regimens prior to hematopoietic stem cell transplantation; a prospective, randomized double-blind phase III trial. *Blood* (ASH Annual Meeting Abstracts) 2009;114: (abstr 2267).
65. de Wit R, de Boer AC, vd Linden GHM, et al. Effective cross-over to granisetron after failure to ondansetron, a randomized double blind study in patients failing ondansetron plus dexamethasone during the first 24 hours following highly emetogenic chemotherapy. *Br J Cancer* 2001;85:1099.

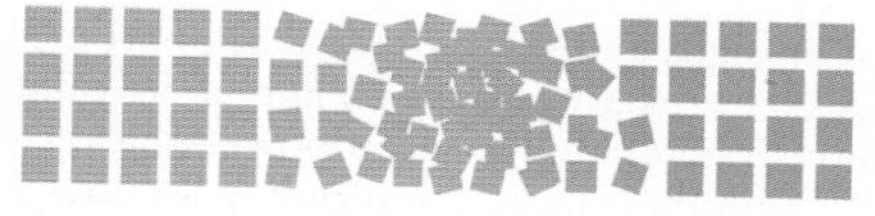

CHAPTER 160 DIARRHEA AND CONSTIPATION

NATHAN I. CHERNY

Constipation and diarrhea are both common problems in patients with advanced cancer. They are the sources of major morbidity and distress. Treatment-induced diarrhea can be severe and be associated with life-threatening dehydration and electrolyte abnormalities. Treatment-induced constipation is, as a result of very widespread use of opioid analgesics for cancer pain, more common that diarrhea. Oncologists must be familiar with the common causes of constipation and diarrhea among cancer patients and the strategies to evaluate and manage these common and distressing symptoms.

DIARRHEA

Diarrhea is defined as the frequent passage of loose stools with urgency. Objectively defined, it is the passage of more than three unformed stools in 24 hours. As with constipation, the patient's definition of diarrhea varies and needs to be clarified by medical staff.

Diarrhea is a common and significant problem among patients with advanced cancer. Increasingly it is seen as a major treatment complication particularly among patients who take fluoropyrimidines and irinotecan.[1] The causes of diarrhea among patients with advanced cancer are diverse, and some causes of diarrhea require specific therapies. Thus, careful evaluation of the underlying cause is necessary.

Severe diarrhea can be debilitating and at times even life-threatening.[1] It contributes to dehydration, electrolyte imbalance, malnutrition, declining immune function, and pressure ulcer formation.

Chemotherapy-Induced Diarrhea

The chemotherapy agents commonly causing diarrhea include 5-fluorouracil, capecitabine, and irinotecan (CPT-11).[1] This is usually a dose-related adverse effect and may be associated with other features of toxicity. Chemotherapy-induced diarrhea appears to be a multifactorial process whereby acute damage to the intestinal mucosa (including loss of intestinal epithelium, superficial necrosis, and inflammation of the bowel wall) causes an imbalance between absorption and secretion in the small bowel.

5-Fluorouracil

Mechanism. The chemotherapy agent 5-fluorouracil (5-FU) causes mitotic arrest of intestinal epithelial crypt cells, resulting in an increase in the ratio of immature secretory crypt cells to mature villous enterocytes. This results in abnormal absorption and secretion of fluids and electrolytes. Opportunistic infections, causing local inflammation, and factors released by necrosis secondary to chemotherapy directly stimulate intestinal secretion of fluids and electrolytes. The diarrhea associated with 5-FU therapy may be watery or bloody. Disruption of the integrity of the gut lining may permit access of enteric organisms into the bloodstream, with the potential for overwhelming sepsis, particularly if the granulocyte nadir coincides with diarrhea. Severity is variable but it may be severe and at times life threatening. Pathologic changes range in severity from a mild colitis to severe necrotizing enterocolitis with pneumocystic colitis.

Risk Factors. Diarrhea is most commonly observed when 5-FU is coadministered with leucovorin (LV). It is slightly more common with bolus rather than infusional administration of 5-FU/LV, in particular with high-dose LV (500 mg/m^2),[2,3] but it occurs with all administration schedules.[4] In the initial reports of weekly 5-FU/LV, diarrhea was seen in up to 50% of patients, with half of these requiring hospitalization for administration of intravenous fluids[2,3] and, in one study, a 5% mortality rate.[3] Other risk factors have been identified, including unresected primary tumor, previous episodes of chemotherapy induced diarrhea, and female gender.

Dihydropyrimidine Dehydrogenase Deficiency. 5-FU is normally metabolized to inactive dihydro-5-FU after an intravenous dose, and 80% of the drug is metabolized to the inactive dihydro-5-FU by dihydropyrimidine dehydrogenase (DPD) in the liver. Administration of 5-FU to patients with DPD deficiency can lead to life-threatening complications, including severe diarrhea, mucositis, and pancytopenia.[5] DPD deficiency is relatively common among whites (3% to 5%).[5] Although the diagnosis can be made by radioimmunometric assay for the DPD enzyme, this test is not readily available. More recently a simple breath test has been developed, and this may provide an effective screening tool.[5]

Irinotecan

Irinotecan can cause acute diarrhea (immediately after drug administration) or delayed diarrhea. Immediate-onset diarrhea is caused by acute cholinergic properties, and it is often accompanied by other symptoms of cholinergic excess, including abdominal cramping, rhinitis, lacrimation, and salivation. The mean duration of symptoms is 30 minutes and it usually responds rapidly to atropine.[6]

The delayed-onset diarrhea usually occurs at least 24 hours after drug administration and can be potentially life threatening, especially in combination chemotherapy regimens with bolus intravenous fluorouracil and leucovorin.[6] The late diarrhea associated with irinotecan is unpredictable, noncumulative, and occurs at all dose levels. It is more common with 3-weekly dose schedules than with lower weekly dosing.[6] The median time to onset is 6 to 14 days. The mechanism of irinotecan-induced delayed diarrhea is not known, but it is believed to result from the deconjugation of CPT's metabolite,

7-ethyl-10-hydroxycamptothecin (SN38) glucuronide by intestinal bacteria, thus enabling direct effect of the active agent on colonic epithelium. It is suggested that the active agent binds to topoisomerase I and induces apoptosis of intestinal epithelia, leading to the disturbance in the absorptive and secretory functions of mucosa. Additionally, both irinotecan and SN38 may also stimulate the production of proinflammatory cytokines and prostaglandins, thus contributing to an inflammatory or secretory diarrhea.[7]

Genetic factors may influence the glucuronidation of SN38 and thus increase this risk of diarrhea. Polymorphisms that alter UDP-glucuronosyltransferase (UGT) activities have been identified; the homozygous presence of the UGT1A1*28 polymorphism, which leads to less efficient glucuronidation of SN38, has been identified as a potential risk factor for the occurrence of delayed-type diarrhea and grade 3 or 4 neutropenia.[8] In one study, heterozygote had a double elevation of risk of severe diarrhea.[9]

Capecitabine

Capecitabine, a precursor of 5-FU, is an oral fluoropyrimidine cytotoxic agent developed with the aim of providing a more effective, less toxic alternative to 5-FU, with the added advantage of oral administration. Administered at usual doses (2,000 mg/m^2 per day for 14 of every 21 days) the prevalence of diarrheas is 30% to 40% and in 10% to 20% it is severe.[10]

Other Cytotoxics

The taxane, docetaxel, commonly causes a relatively mild diarrhea. Data from phase 2 and 3 studies indicate a prevalence of 25% to 24%.[11] In most cases the diarrhea is mild; however, cases of severe enteritis and colitis have been reported (discussed below).[12,13]

Similarly, the antifolate pemetrexed can also cause mild diarrhea. In phase 2 and 3 trials mild diarrhea was reported in about 10% to 15% of patients.[14]

Neutropenic Colitis

Neutropenic enterocolitis (also called necrotizing enterocolitis or typhlitis) is an acute life-threatening complication of chemotherapy that is most commonly observed with high-dose treatments in the setting of myeloablative therapies.[15,16] It is, however, also observed with nonmyeloablative therapies,[17,18] particularly with taxanes.[12,16,19]

Clinical Presentation

Neutropenic enterocolitis usually occurs when the absolute neutrophil count falls below 500 mcL. Patients present with fever, abdominal pain, nausea, vomiting, diarrhea, and, not uncommonly, sepsis. Abdominal pain may be diffuse or localized to the right lower quadrant. Sometimes pain is absent, particularly if the patient has received steroid therapy.

Pathogenesis

The pathogenesis of neutropenic enterocolitis is multifactorial: mucosal injury by cytotoxic drugs or other means, profound neutropenia, and impaired host defense to invasion by microorganisms.[16,20,21] The microbial infection leads to necrosis of various layers of the bowel wall. Anatomically, the cecum is almost always affected, and the process often extends into the ascending colon and terminal ileum. The predilection for the cecum is possibly related to its dispensability and its relatively diminished vascularization. Various bacterial or fungal organisms, including gram-negative rods, gram-positive cocci, anaerobes (e.g., *Clostridium septicum*), and *Candida* sp., are often seen infiltrating the bowel wall. Polymicrobial infection is frequent. Bacteremia or fungemia is also common, usually with enteric organisms such as pseudomonas or yeasts such as *Candida*.

Diagnostic Investigations

The diagnosis is based on signs and symptoms in the appropriate clinical setting as well as imaging studies. Plain abdominal radiographs may demonstrate dilated loops of bowel, thickening of the bowel wall, "thumbprinting," resulting from bowel wall edema, or indications of a right lower quadrant mass or phlegmon. Free intraperitoneal air indicates perforation of the bowel wall. Pneumatosis intestinalis is often seen.

Computed tomography (CT) scanning is the preferred imaging modality. CT scanning techniques can evaluate the entire abdomen for pathology, especially in patients with distended loops of bowel and ileus for whom ultrasound would not be possible. Scans commonly demonstrate concentric thickening of the bowel wall, a fluid filled cecum, pericolic fluid collections or abscesses, pneumatosis intestinalis, and free air if an underlying perforation exists. Bowel wall thickening of more than 3 to 5 mm is considered abnormal and is consistent with, but not diagnostic of, necrotizing enterocolitis.[22] Indeed, *Clostridium difficile*–related colitis in neutropenic patients may be associated with substantial or even greater wall thickening.[23] *Pneumatosis intestinalis* along with cecal and colonic wall thickening is very suggestive.[23]

Abdominal ultrasonography can identify thickening of the bowel wall that produces a target or halo sign. Indeed a bowel wall thickening of greater than 5 mm was associated with a higher mortality (29% vs. 0%). If one takes a cutoff of greater than 10 mm, the mortality was 60% versus 4.2%.[24] Ultrasound is useful as a follow-up tool to assess the gradual decrease in bowel wall thickening. Additionally signs of pericolic fluid and intramural or abdominal free air often indicate perforation.

Targeted Therapy-Associated Diarrhea

Almost all of the recently developed small molecule targeted therapies cause diarrhea as a side effect. Diarrhea, which can be severe, has been reported in 30% to 50% of patients who receive bortezomib,[25] erlotinib,[26] gefitinib,[27] sorafenib,[28] sunitinib,[29] and imatinib,[30] and the mammalian target of rapamycin (mTOR) inhibitors temsirolimus[31] and everolimus.[32]

The monoclonal therapies targeting epidermal growth factor receptor (EGFR), cetuximab[33] and panitumumab,[34,35] both cause diarrhea in 10% to 20% of patients, which may be severe in a small subset of patients.

Radiotherapy-Induced Diarrhea

Radiation injury to the lower intestine is usually encountered following treatment of cancers of the anus, rectum, cervix, uterus, prostate, urinary bladder, testes, and as part of total body irradiation. Radiotherapy of the abdomen or pelvis damages intestinal mucosa, causing prostaglandin release and bile salt malabsorption. These two factors increase intestinal peristalsis, causing diarrhea.

Acute radiation enteritis or proctitis occurs within 6 weeks of therapy. Symptoms include diarrhea, cramping, rectal urgency or tenesmus, and, uncommonly, bleeding. These symptoms usually resolve without specific therapy within 2 to 6 months.[36,37]

Late radiation enteritis or proctitis generally occurs 8 to 12 months after therapy, and in some cases it may be delayed by years.[38] It may manifest as malabsorption or diarrhea, with more rapid transit times occurring in the affected bowel. Bacterial overgrowth causes malabsorption and contributes to the nausea, abdominal pain, and diarrhea, and it should be suspected in patients with intestinal strictures or enterocolic fistulae.[38] Although the large intestine is less radiosensitive, some patients can develop a pancolitis that resembles inflammatory bowel disease.[39,40]

Other Causes of Treatment-Related Diarrhea

Clostridium Difficile Diarrhea

Clostridium difficile diarrhea occurs when the normal intestinal flora is altered, allowing *C. difficile* to flourish in the intestinal tract and produce a toxin that causes a watery diarrhea.[41] It can be triggered by repeated enemas, prolonged nasogastric tube insertion, gastrointestinal tract surgery, and the use of antibiotics, especially penicillin (ampicillin), clindamycin, and cephalosporins. Occasionally, however, it is reported after chemotherapy in the absence of antibiotic therapy.[42–44] The most common confirmatory study is an enzyme immunoassay for *C. difficile* toxins A and B, which yields results in 2 to 4 hours. Specificity of the assay is high (93% to 100%), but sensitivity ranges from 63% to 99%, and this limited sensitivity may require two to three repeat stool samples to document disease.[41] Recently, a polymerase chain reaction test, Xpert *C. difficile* test, has received U.S. Food and Drug Administration (FDA) approved. Limited data indicate that this may have greater sensitivity.[45]

Enteral Feeding

Tube feedings, either by nasogastric tube or gastrostomy or jejunostomy, may be associated with the development of diarrhea.[46,47] This is a common problem occurring in 10% to 60% of patients.[48] Many potential factors can contribute to the problem, and indeed it is often multifactorial.[49] Both formula osmolality and rate of delivery may be associated with diarrhea.[50] The use of fiber-containing formulas to control diarrhea related to tube feeding is controversial, and evidence of efficacy is mixed.[51,52]

Contamination of the enteral formula is often a contributing or causative factor.[53,54] Recommendations to reduce the risk of contamination include hand washing before handling the feeding system, use of clean equipment to prepare and mix feedings, bag and tubing change at least once a day, limitation of "hanging time" of individual bags to under 6 hours and refrigerated storage of prepared bags until use. Some data suggest that hypoalbuminemia predisposes patients to diarrhea by decreasing osmotic pressure and causing edema in the intestinal mucosa.[55]

Celiac Plexus Block

Celiac plexus block is commonly associated with a self-limiting acute diarrhea. Occasionally, diarrhea may be persistent.[56] This diarrhea may be amenable to treatment with atropine.[57]

Assessment

The National Cancer Institute grading for the severity of diarrhea is presented in Table 160.1. In the setting of chemotherapy-induced diarrhea it is an important consideration in treatment selection (discussed below).

Assessment includes a detailed medical history, dietary history, medication review, description of stools, and a physical examination focused on the identification of dehydration abdominal and rectal areas. When appropriate, abdominal radiographs can be ordered to evaluate for abdominal obstruction or fecal impaction. Biochemical parameters should be checked for evidence of dehydration, hypokalemia, or renal impairment. If enteric infections are suspected, stool samples should be sent for fecal leukocytes, *C. difficile* toxins A and B, and culture for organisms including *C. difficile*, *Salmonella*, *Escherichia coli*, *Campylobacter*, and infectious colitis.

As described above, when neutropenic enterocolitis is suspected, CT or ultrasound imaging of the abdomen should be undertaken and additional prognostic information may be obtained by ultrasound evaluation of bowel wall thickness.

General Principles in the Management of Diarrhea

Patients must be rehydrated either orally or, when appropriate, by parenteral infusion. In cases of large volume diarrhea there is the potential for very rapid dehydration with risk of prerenal impairment or even, in extreme cases, shock. Patients may suffer electrolyte imbalance particularly from hypokalemia. In general, milk products should be avoided if an infectious cause is suspected because a transient lactase deficiency may sometimes occur. Special attention should be given to patients who are incontinent of stool due to the risk of pressure ulcer

PRACTICE OF ONCOLOGY

TABLE 160.1

NATIONAL CANCER INSTITUTE COMMON TOXICITY CRITERIA FOR GRADING OF DIARRHEA

Toxicity	0	1	2	3	4
Patients without a colostomy	None	Increase of <4 stools/d over pretreatment	Increase of 4–6 stools/d or nocturnal stools	Increase of ≥7 stools/day	>10 stools/d
	None	None	Moderate cramping, not interfering with normal activity	Severe cramping and incontinence, interfering with daily activities	Grossly bloody diarrhea and need for parenteral support
Patients with a colostomy	None	Mild increase in loose, watery colostomy output compared with pretreatment	Moderate increase in loose, watery colostomy output compared with pretreatment, but not interfering with normal activity	Severe increase in loose, watery colostomy output compared with pretreatment, interfering with normal activity	Physiological consequences requiring intensive care; hemodynamic

Adapted from National Cancer Institute. Cancer Therapy Evaluation Program Common Toxicity Criteria, Version 2.0. 1999.

formation. Skin barriers should be used to prevent skin irritation caused by fecal material.

Antidiarrhea Medications

Opioids

Loperamide is generally the opioid of choice because it has local activity in the gut and is absorbed only minimally (this accounts for the lack of systemic effects). It reduces stool weight, frequency of bowel movements, urgency, and fecal incontinence in acute and chronic diarrhea. Loperamide can be started at an initial dose of 4 mg followed by 2 mg every 2 to 4 hours or after every unformed stool.[58,59] Other opioids, such as tincture of opium, morphine, or codeine, can be used.

Tincture of opium it is a widely used antidiarrheal agent. It is often recommended as an alternative to loperamide. Deodorized tincture of opium contains the equivalent of 10 mg/mL morphine and the recommended dose is 10 to 15 drops in water every 3 to 4 hours. It is important not to confuse this with paregoric, which is a camphorated (alcohol-based) tincture. The latter is a less-concentrated preparation that contains the equivalent of 0.4 mg/mL morphine. The recommended dose is 1 teaspoon (5 mL) in water every 3 to 4 hours.

Somatostatin Analogues

In cases of severe or persistent diarrhea, the somatostatin analogue octreotide should be considered. Octreotide has multiple antidiarrheal actions, including suppression of release of insulin, glucagon, vasoactive intestinal peptide (VIP), and gastric acid secretion, and it reduces motility and pancreatic exocrine function and alters increased absorption of water, electrolytes, and nutrients from the gastrointestinal (GI) tract. The usual starting dose for octreotide is 100 to 150 mcg subcutaneous or intravenous three times a day.[60] Since there is a dose–response relationship for its antidiarrheal effect, the dose can be titrated up to 500 mcg subcutaneous or intravenous three times a day or by continual intravenous infusion 25 to 50 mcg/h.[61] Recently, a microencapsulated, long-acting formulation of octreotide has been developed for once-monthly intramuscular dosing. This formulation has demonstrated efficacy in resolving severe diarrhea and preventing further episodes of diarrhea in patients who receive ongoing therapy.[62,63]

Other Agents

Budesonide is an orally administered, topically active steroid with high activity in inflammatory bowel disease (IBD), a 90% first-pass effect in the liver, and therefore low systemic availability. It is commonly used in the management of diarrhea in patients with low- to medium-grade IBD. A small study demonstrated efficacy of oral budesonide in the management of chemotherapy-induced diarrhea that was refractory to loperamide[64]; however, studies did not show benefit in prophylactic use to prevent CPT-11- or ipilimumab-induced diarrhea.[65,66]

Specific Management Guidelines

Chemotherapy-Induced Diarrhea

Chemotherapy-induced diarrhea is a major problem in the management of patients with gastrointestinal cancer in which the drugs irinotecan and fluorouracil are commonly used. Diarrhea can be severe and in some cases life threatening. The most recent American Society of Clinical Oncology (ASCO) guidelines for management of treatment-induced diarrhea were published in 2004.[61] Patients are classified as uncomplicated or complicated on the basis of clinical features, and this classification guides treatment approach.

Prevention. Although a randomized trial did not show any advantage of neomycin in the primary prevention of late irinotecan diarrhea,[9] there is limited evidence supporting its use as secondary prevention in selected patients.[67]

Uncomplicated Diarrhea. The first step in patients with grade 1 or 2 diarrhea with no other complicating signs or symptoms may be classified as "uncomplicated" and managed conservatively with oral hydration and loperamide. Initial management of mild to moderate diarrhea should include dietary modifications (e.g., eliminating all lactose-containing products and high-osmolar dietary supplements), and the patient should be instructed to record the number of stools and report symptoms of life-threatening sequelae (e.g., fever or dizziness on standing). Loperamide should be started at an initial dose of 4 mg followed by 2 mg every 4 hours or after every unformed stool (not to exceed 16 mg/d).

If diarrhea resolves with loperamide, the patients should be instructed to continue dietary modifications and to gradually add solid foods to their diet. In the case of chemotherapy-induced diarrhea, patients may discontinue loperamide when they have been diarrhea-free for at least 12 hours.

The second step, if mild to moderate diarrhea persists for more than 24 hours, is to increase the dose of loperamide to 2 mg every 2 hours, and oral antibiotics may be started as prophylaxis for infection.

The third step, if mild to moderate chemotherapy-induced diarrhea has not resolved after 24 hours on high-dose loperamide (48 hours total treatment with loperamide), is for the patient to be seen in the physician's office or outpatient center for further evaluation, including complete stool and blood workup. Stool workup should include evaluation for pathogens. Fluids and electrolytes should be replaced as needed. Loperamide should be discontinued and the patient should be started on a second-line antidiarrheal agent such as subcutaneous octreotide (100 to 150 mcg starting dose, with dose escalation as needed) or other second-line agents (e.g., oral budesonide or tincture of opium).

Complicated Chemotherapy-Induced Diarrhea. Patients with mild to moderate diarrhea complicated by moderate to severe cramping, nausea and vomiting, diminished performance status, fever, sepsis, neutropenia, bleeding, or dehydration and patients with severe diarrhea are classified as complicated and should be evaluated further, monitored closely, and treated aggressively.

Aggressive management of complicated cases usually necessitates admission and involves administering intravenous fluids, octreotide at a starting dose of 100 to 150 mcg subcutaneous three times a day or intravenous (25 to 50 mcg/h) if the patient is severely dehydrated, with dose escalation up to 500 mcg subcutaneous three times a day until diarrhea is controlled, and administration of antibiotics (e.g., fluoroquinolone). These patients should be evaluated with complete blood cell count and electrolyte profile and stool workup to evaluate for blood, fecal leukocytes, *C. difficile*, *Salmonella*, *E. coli*, *Campylobacter*, and infectious colitis.

Radiation Therapy-Induced Diarrhea

The most recent ASCO guidelines for management of treatment-induced diarrhea were published in 2004.[61] The initial management of uncomplicated radiation-induced diarrhea is the same as for chemotherapy-induced diarrhea: starting with low-dose loperamide and then progressing to high-dose loperamide if diarrhea persists beyond 24 hours.

If diarrhea has not resolved after a further 24 hours on high-dose loperamide, continue loperamide (2 mg every 2 hours). In such cases, the patient should be evaluated, and in severe cases, octreotide therapy may be indicated.

Patients with mild to moderate diarrhea complicated by moderate to severe cramping, nausea and vomiting, diminished performance status, fever, sepsis, neutropenia, bleeding, or dehydration and patients with sever diarrhea are classified as complicated. Complicated radiation-induced diarrhea needs intensive monitoring and aggressive management either in hospital or an intensive home care nursing program or an outpatient facility able to provide a high level of care. Patients with severe symptoms or features suggestive of sepsis should undergo complete stool and blood workup and should be treated with octreotide and intravenous antibiotics.

Management of Neutropenic Enterocolitis

Management of neutropenic enterocolitis is challenging and the risk of mortality is high. There are roles for both medical and surgical interventions.

The initial treatment for neutropenic enterocolitis is medical, with the administration of broad-spectrum antibiotics, granulocyte colony-stimulating factors, nasogastric decompression, intravenous fluids, bowel rest, and serial abdominal examinations.[16,21,68] In most patients, these measures are sufficient, and symptoms resolve after correction of the neutropenia. The administered antibiotics should have a broad spectrum of activity to cover enteric gram-negative organisms, gram-positive organisms, and anaerobes. Causative microorganisms include *Pseudomonas*, *S. aureus*, *E. coli*, and group A *Streptococcus*.[68] Reasonable initial choices include monotherapy with piperacillin-tazobactam or imipenem-cilastatin or duotherapy with cefepime or ceftazidime along with metronidazole.[15] In cases that do not respond to antibacterial agents, amphotericin should be considered because fungemia is common.[16] Blood transfusions may be necessary because the diarrhea is often bloody. Anticholinergic, antidiarrheal, and opioid agents should be avoided since they may aggravate the ileus.

The indications for and timing of surgical intervention are controversial. The mortality of patients who fail to respond to medical interventions is high, and many patients may not be salvageable. Nonetheless, in selected patients, surgery may be helpful to avoid progressive bowel necrosis and perforation and to help control sepsis. Commonly cited indications for surgery in include: (1) persistent GI bleeding after correction of thrombocytopenia and coagulopathy; (2) evidence of free intraperitoneal perforation; (3) abscess formation, (4) clinical deterioration despite aggressive supportive measures; and (5) to rule out other intra-abdominal processes such as bowel obstruction or acute appendicitis examinations.[16,21,68,69]

If exploratory surgery is performed, resection of grossly involved bowel is necessary. All necrotic material must be resected, usually by a right hemicolectomy, ileostomy, and mucous fistula. Failure to remove the necrotic focus in these severely immunocompromised patients is often fatal.[69] Primary anastomosis is not generally recommended in such severely immunocompromised patients because of the increased incidence of anastomotic leak.[69]

Diarrhea Prophylaxis

Prevention of Radiation Diarrhea

Several clinical trials have focused on prevention of diarrhea in patients who receive pelvic radiation, but, to date no evidence-based strategy has been found to be effective.

Sucralfate, a nonsystemically absorbed aluminum hydroxide complex, has been widely investigated. A recent meta-analysis found insufficient evidence of efficacy to support this approach.[70] Based on the hypothesis that prostaglandins play a role in the pathophysiology of diarrhea, the salicylates sulfasalazine and olsalazine have also been investigated for prevention of radiation-induced diarrhea. The results have been contradictory: the study of sulfasalazine suggested efficacy,[71] whereas the olsalazine study found increased diarrhea as compared with placebo.[72]

Prevention of Chemotherapy Diarrhea

Other than the use of atropine to prevent acute irinotecan diarrhea,[73] prophylactic antidiarrheal treatment is not a standard approach for any chemotherapy regimen. Small studies in the prevention of irinotecan-induced diarrhea have suggested the potential utility of oral alkalinization of the intestinal lumen[74] activated charcoal[75] and oral administration of probiotics microorganisms such as *Lactobacillus rhamnosus*.[76] Negative studies have been reported with prophylactic octreotide,[77] oral racecadotril,[78] and oral neomycin.[9]

CONSTIPATION

Definition

Constipation is the slow movement of feces through the large intestine, resulting in infrequent bowel movements and the passage of dry, hard stools. Constipation is a symptom, not a disease. It is usually a temporary condition and is not considered serious.

According to the Rome 2 Criteria proposed by a working group of gastroenterologists[79,80] the clinical definition of chronic constipation is the presence of any two of the following symptoms for at least 12 weeks (not necessarily consecutive) in the previous 12 months:

- straining during bowel movements;
- lumpy or hard stool;
- sensation of incomplete evacuation;
- sensation of anorectal blockage or obstruction;
- less than three bowel movements per week.

Prevalence

The prevalence of constipation in patients who have advanced cancer is approximately 40% to 60%[81]; the greatest prevalence occurs in the opioid-treated population.[82–84]

Treatment-Related Causes

Medications, in particular opioids, serotonin antagonist antiemetics, and vinca alkaloid chemotherapy agents, are the most common causes of constipation among patients with cancer.

Opioid Analgesics

All opioids cause constipation and tolerance to this effect is not observed over time. Importantly, the dose–response relationship to this effect is very flat and the severity does not appear to be strongly dose related. There are some data to indicate that the severity is less with fentanyl and, possibly, methadone[85,86] and with oxycodone/naloxone combined formulation tablets.[87,88] Other medications that are commonly implicated are listed in Table 160.2.

TABLE 160.2

DRUGS COMMONLY CAUSING CONSTIPATION IN CANCER PATIENTS

Opioids
Serotonin antagonists
Antidepressants
Aluminum- or calcium-containing antacids
Iron supplements
Diuretics
Antihypertensive medications
Anticonvulsants

Serotonin 5-HT_3 Receptor Antagonists

The 5-hydroxytryptamine (5-HT_3) receptor antagonist antiemetics slow colonic transit, increase fluid absorption, and increase left colon compliance.[89] Overall these agents are very well tolerated but 2% to 5% of patients do report constipation with use[90] and concurrent laxative therapy is often indicated.

Vinca Alkaloids

All the vinca alkaloids have pronounced neuropathic effects and reduce GI transit time. Severity appears to highest with vincristine and vindesine, less with vinblastine, and least with vinorelbine. Among patients who receive vincristine it is dose related and is more common and more severe among patients who receive doses greater than 2 mg per dose.[91,92] Severity can range from mild to severe and in one series of 392 patients, 2.8% required hospitalization for adynamic ileus.[93] Rarely, life-threatening ileus or megacolon have been reported.[94]

Thalidomide

Thalidomide is an antineoplastic agent with immunomodulatory and antiangiogenic activities used in multiple myeloma.[95] Other than sedation, constipation is the most common adverse effect.[96]

Other Medications

Other constipating drugs commonly used in the care of cancer include those with anticholinergic actions (antispasmodics, antidepressants, phenothiazines, haloperidol, antacids), some anticonvulsants or antihypertensive drugs, iron supplements, and diuretics.[84]

Differential Diagnosis

Other causes of constipation are also common among patients with advanced cancer. Among other causes that need to be considered are:

1. *Low-Fiber Diet*: A low-fiber diet or a diet rich in processed and low-fiber foods may exacerbate constipation.[97]
2. *Dehydration*: Liquids like water and juice add fluid to the colon and bulk to stools, making bowel movements softer and easier to pass. Liquids that contain caffeine and alcohol have a dehydrating effect.
3. *Lack of Exercise*: Lack of exercise can lead to constipation, although the reason is unclear.[97] For example, constipation often occurs after an injury or during an illness that promotes immobility.
4. *Colonic Pathology*: Many patients have coexisting irritable bowel syndrome or diverticular disease. In many instances constipation may be the first symptom of an impending obstruction due to tumor, adhesions, or a stricture.
5. *Neuromuscular Disorders*: Neurogenic factors may impair normal colonic function, including brain tumors, spinal cord compression, or the autonomic failure that is common in patients with far advanced cancer.[98] Neural integration of anal sphincter control and rectosigmoid propulsion occurs in the sacral segments of the spinal cord. Damage to sacral segments of the spinal cord or to efferent nerves may lead to severe constipation.[99]
6. *Metabolic Disorders*: Certain disorders of metabolism commonly seen in patients with cancer can lead to constipation and include the following: hypercalcemia, hyponatremia, hypokalemia, and uremia.[84]
7. *Psychological Disorders*: Constipation is a common manifestation of depression.[100]

Diagnosis

The medical history can assist in identifying the causes of constipation. An accurate history should elicit the change in bowel movements: frequency of bowel movements; whether defecation is associated with blood or mucus (suggestive of obstruction or hemorrhoids), pain, or straining; presence or absence of defecation urge (hard stool or rectal obstruction in former, colon inertia in latter); manual maneuvers by patient. Questions should also be aimed to determine the cause of the change in bowel movements, in particular eating and drinking habits, medication use, and level of physical activity.

The physical assessment could include a rectal examination to evaluate sphincter tone and detect tenderness, obstruction, or blood. Digital rectal examination may reveal:

1. hard, impacted feces
2. soft stool due to fecal leakage
3. complete absence of stool (colonic inertia, high obstruction, or impacted stools)
4. tumor masses
5. concomitant disease—hemorrhoids, anal fissure, perianal ulceration, rectocele or anal stenosis

If constipation manifests as part of a spinal cord compression syndrome, full neurological examination is necessary including assessment of anal sphincter tone (lax with colonic hypotonia) and rectal sensation.

Investigation

Investigations are not routinely necessary, however, plain abdominal radiography may be indicated to exclude bowel obstruction and to distinguish stool from tumor.[84] The former appears as rounded masses with entrapped gas and varying degrees of dilated bowel. Plain abdominal radiography is also the best way to assess the degree of constipation. If clinically suspected, corrected calcium levels and thyroid function should be checked. More extensive testing can proceed for patients with severe symptoms, for those with sudden changes in number and consistency of bowel movements or blood in the stool, and for older adults.

General Measures

Diet

All patients suffering from constipated should be advised as an initial measure to increase their dietary fiber intake as the simplest, most physiologic, and cheapest form of treatment. Patients should be encouraged to increase their intake of fiber-rich foods such as bran, fruits, vegetables, and nuts. Prune juice is commonly used to relieve constipation. The recommendation is to increase fiber intake gradually since adding fiber to the diet too quickly may cause excessive gas and bloating.

Fluid Intake

Dehydration or salt depletion is likely to lead to increased salt and water absorption by the large intestine, leading to the passage of small, hard stools. Children or adults with fever, or subjects in hot environments, should therefore be advised to consume plenty of fluid.

Physical Activity

Increasing physical activity is commonly recommended, though the evidence supporting efficacy of this recommendation is scant.

Laxatives

Bulk Laxatives

Bulk laxatives are a concentrated form of nonstarch polysaccharides useful for patients who cannot take adequate dietary fiber. Common formulations include ispaghula, sterculia, psyllium, and methylcellulose or carboxymethylcellulose. These agents are useful for patients who are able to ingest ample volumes of fluid, though their effect appears to wane with time.[101] Bulk laxatives are generally not recommended for opioid-induced constipation.[102]

Osmotic Laxatives

Polyethylene Glycol. Polyethylene glycol 3350 (Macrogol 3350) is an inert polymer that is not absorbed by the gut and is excreted unchanged in the feces. It is formulated with electrolytes to ensure that there is virtually no net gain or loss of sodium and potassium. It is generally well tolerated with a low tendency to gas formation. This is one of the approaches most strongly endorsed in recent systematic reviews of chronic constipation.[103,104]

Lactulose. Lactulose is a synthetic disaccharide that is not absorbed by the small bowel.[105] The recommended dose for adults is 15 to 30 mL of the syrup two to three times daily, reducing as necessary. It usually has a latency of 2 to 3 days before onset of effect. Some patients do not like the sweet taste, and others complain of abdominal distention or discomfort, presumably resulting from colonic gas production.

Magnesium and Sulfate Salts

Magnesium hydroxide, citrate, sulfate, and sodium sulfate are commonly used laxatives. The magnesium and sulfate ions are poorly absorbed from the gut and the action of these agents is mainly osmotic. In mildly constipated patients, regular magnesium hydroxide 1.2 to 3.6 g/d is a useful, safe laxative.[106] Magnesium sulfate (Epson salt) is a more potent laxative that tends to produce a large volume of liquid stool. Excessive doses of magnesium salts by mouth can lead to hypermagnesemia, and these medications should be used with caution in patients with renal impairment and in children.[107]

Stimulant Laxatives

Anthranoid Laxatives. Anthranoid laxatives, such as senna, aloe, cascara, and frangula, are plants compounds that are hydrolyzed by glycosidases of the colonic bacteria to yield the active molecules. The active compounds have both motor and secretory effects on the colon. The preparations available for clinical use vary from crude vegetable preparations through purified and standardized extracts to a synthetic compound. These preparations are best taken in the evening or at bedtime, with the aim of producing a normal stool next morning. The usual dose is 15 mg of sennosides at bedtime. There is wide variation in clinical effectiveness and some patients are not helped by this class of laxatives.

Polyphenolic (Diphenylmethane) Compounds. The effects of bisacodyl and sodium picosulfate on the colon are similar to those of the anthranoid laxatives.[108] Bisacodyl is available as enteric-coated 5-mg tablets, and the recommended adult dose is 5 to 10 mg taken at night. Sodium picosulfate is available as a liquid containing 5 mg per 5 mL. The recommended adult dose is 5 to 10 mL at night. These agents are generally recommended for short-term use in situations of refractory constipation.

Detergents or Stool Softeners

The detergent dioctyl sodium sulfosuccinate (docusate sodium) was developed as a stool softener. It stimulates fluid secretion by the small and large intestines. A Cochrane systematic review concluded that the use of docusate for constipation in palliative care is based on inadequate experimental evidence.[109]

Liquid Paraffin

Liquid paraffin is a commonly used mineral oil that softens and lubricates the stools. Aspiration may cause lipoid pneumonia,[110] and some patients suffer from anal seepage and a foreign body reaction if there is a break in the anorectal mucosa.[111]

Opioid Antagonists

Methylnaltrexone (MNTX) is a quaternary derivative of naltrexone that does not cross the blood–brain barrier in humans. As a result, MNTX antagonizes only peripherally located opioid receptors while sparing centrally mediated analgesic effects of opioid pain medications. There is evidence of very predictable effectiveness after administration by either the oral[112,113] or parenteral routes of administration,[114,115] with most patients achieving defecation within 90 minutes of administration.

An injectable formulation of methylnaltrexone was approved by the FDA in May 2008. It is administered as a subcutaneous injection, initially once every other day. The frequency of administration can be increased if needed to once daily. The approved dose is 8 mg for patients weighing 38 to 61 kg, and 12 mg for those weighing 62 to 114 kg; for those outside these ranges, the recommended dose is 0.15 mg/kg.

Enemas and Suppositories

Self-administration of enemas or suppositories is an alternative approach for patients who do not respond to oral laxatives. Compounds may be introduced into the rectum to stimulate contraction by distention or chemical action, to soften hard stools, or for both reasons. Since extravasation of the enema solution into the submucosal plane can damage the rectal mucosa, it is important to direct the enema nozzle posteriorly after passing the anal canal.

Osmotic microenemas are often useful when oral agents have not provided adequate laxation. Commercial preparations contain mainly sodium lauryl sulphoacetate (a stool softener similar to docusate) and osmotic agents and glycerol.

Saline or water enema act by distending the rectum and softening the feces. Large volume watery enemas risk water intoxication if the enema is retained. Alternatively polyethylene glycol can be used or incorporated into a suppository for its osmotic effect.

Hypertonic sodium phosphate enemas such as Fleet enema both distend and stimulate rectal motility. They are commonly used and side effects are uncommon. These enemas cause some superficial disruption of the surface epithelium, which heals rapidly. Rarely when phosphate enema are administered to patients who cannot evacuate promptly it can cause hyperphosphatemia and severe hypocalcemic tetany.[116,117]

Glycerin (suppositories), bisacodyl (suppositories or enema), and oxyphenisatin (Veripaque) are all stimulants to rectal motility. Likewise, they have been commonly used for short-term treatments and are often effective.

Managing Fecal Impaction

A fecal impaction is a large mass of dry, hard stool that can develop in the rectum due to chronic constipation.[118] This mass may be so hard that it cannot be excreted. Watery stool from higher in the bowel may move around the mass and leak.

Fecal impaction is a complication of chronic constipation. Patients may present with no bowel movement over a prolonged period or diarrhea resulting from overflow incontinence. The diagnosis is confirmed by rectal examination findings of hard, formed stool present in the rectal vault.

The complications of a fecal impaction are uncommon but include urinary tract obstruction, perforation of the colon, dehydration, electrolyte imbalance, renal insufficiency, fecal incontinence, decubitus ulcers, stercoral ulcers, and rectal bleeding.[119–121]

The treatment of a fecal impaction usually requires the digital fragmentation and extraction of the stool.[122] Lubricating enemas and suppositories may be helpful. Since this is a very uncomfortable procedure, sedation is generally recommended and anesthesia may occasionally be needed. Once the impaction is relieved, it is crucial that the patient start a prophylactic daily bowel regimen.

There is limited experience to suggest a noninvasive approach using a trial of high-dose polyethylene glycol (1 mg/kg) for 3 days.[123–125]

Selected References

The full list of references for this chapter appears in the online version.

1. Arnold RJ, Gabrail N, Raut M, et al. Clinical implications of chemotherapy-induced diarrhea in patients with cancer. *J Support Oncol* 2005;3(3):227.
4. Meta-Analysis Group In Cancer. Toxicity of fluorouracil in patients with advanced colorectal cancer: effect of administration schedule and prognostic factors. Meta-Analysis Group In Cancer. *J Clin Oncol* 1998;16(11):3537.
5. Mercier C, Ciccolini J. Profiling dihydropyrimidine dehydrogenase deficiency in patients with cancer undergoing 5-fluorouracil/capecitabine therapy. *Clin Colorectal Cancer* 2006;6(4):288.
6. Hecht JR. Gastrointestinal toxicity or irinotecan. *Oncology* 1998;12 (8 Suppl 6):72.
9. de Jong FA, Kehrer DF, Mathijssen RH, et al. Prophylaxis of irinotecan-induced diarrhea with neomycin and potential role for UGT1A1*28 genotype screening: a double-blind, randomized, placebo-controlled study. *Oncologist* 2006;11(8):944.
12. Rolston KV. Neutropenic enterocolitis associated with docetaxel therapy in a patient with breast cancer. *Clin Adv Hematol Oncol* 2009;7(8):527.
15. Cloutier RL. Neutropenic enterocolitis. *Emerg Med Clin North Am* 2009;27(3):415.
16. Bremer CT, Monahan BP. Necrotizing enterocolitis in neutropenia and chemotherapy: a clinical update and old lessons relearned. *Curr Gastroenterol Rep* 2006;8(4):333.
20. Ullery BW, Pieracci FM, Rodney JR, Barie PS. Neutropenic enterocolitis. *Surg Infect (Larchmt)* 2009;10(3):307.
22. Blijlevens NM. Neutropenic enterocolitis: challenges in diagnosis and treatment. *Clin Adv Hematol Oncol* 2009;7(8):528.
36. Babb RR. Radiation proctitis: a review. *Am J Gastroenterol* 1996;91(7):1309.
38. Theis VS, Sripadam R, Ramani V, Lal S. Chronic radiation enteritis. *Clin Oncol (R Coll Radiol)* 2010;22(1):70.
39. Kountouras J, Zavos C. Recent advances in the management of radiation colitis. *World J Gastroenterol* 2008;14(48):7289.
41. McFee RB, Abdelsayed GG. *Clostridium difficile. Dis Mon* 2009;55(7):439.
47. Reese JL, Means ME, Hanrahan K, et al. Diarrhea associated with nasogastric feedings. *Oncol Nurs Forum* 1996;23(1):59.
49. Burns PE, Jairath N. Diarrhea and the patient receiving enteral feedings: a multifactorial problem. *J Wound Ostomy Continence Nurs* 1994;21(6):257.
56. Chan VW. Chronic diarrhea: an uncommon side effect of celiac plexus block. *Anesth Analg* 1996;82(1):205.
58. Cascinu S, Bichisao E, Amadori D, et al. High-dose loperamide in the treatment of 5-fluorouracil-induced diarrhea in colorectal cancer patients. *Support Care Cancer* 2000;8(1):65.
59. Hanauer SB. The role of loperamide in gastrointestinal disorders. *Rev Gastroenterol Disord* 2008;8(1):15.
60. Topkan E, Karaoglu A. Octreotide in the management of chemoradiotherapy-induced diarrhea refractory to loperamide in patients with rectal carcinoma. *Oncology* 2006;71(5-6):354.
61. Benson AB 3rd, Ajani JA, Catalano RB, et al. Recommended guidelines for the treatment of cancer treatment-induced diarrhea. *J Clin Oncol* 2004;22(14):2918.
67. Blesa GMB, Candel VA, Marco VG, Castro CG, Pulido EG. Secondary prevention of CPT-11-induced delayed diarrhea with neomycin. *Cancer Ther* 2009;7:282.
73. Yumuk PF, Aydin SZ, Dane F, et al. The absence of early diarrhea with atropine premedication during irinotecan therapy in metastatic colorectal patients. *Int J Colorectal Dis* 2004;19(6):609.
80. Lembo A, Camilleri M. Chronic constipation. *N Engl J Med* 2003;349(14):1360.
81. Teunissen SC, Wesker W, Kruitwagen C, et al. Symptom prevalence in patients with incurable cancer: a systematic review. *J Pain Symptom Manage* 2007;34(1):94.
84. Mancini I, Bruera E. Constipation in advanced cancer patients. *Support Care Cancer* 1998;6(4):356.
85. Staats PS, Markowitz J, Schein J. Incidence of constipation associated with long-acting opioid therapy: a comparative study. *South Med J* 2004;97(2):129.
87. Holzer P, Ahmedzai SH, Niederle N, et al. Opioid-induced bowel dysfunction in cancer-related pain: causes, consequences, and a novel approach for its management. *J Opioid Manag* 2009;5(3):145.
88. Meissner W, Leyendecker P, Mueller-Lissner S, et al. A randomised controlled trial with prolonged-release oral oxycodone and naloxone to prevent and reverse opioid-induced constipation. *Eur J Pain* 2009;13(1):56.
103. Brandt LJ, Prather CM, Quigley EM, et al. Systematic review on the management of chronic constipation in North America. *Am J Gastroenterol* 2005;100(Suppl 1):S5.
104. Ramkumar D, Rao SS. Efficacy and safety of traditional medical therapies for chronic constipation: systematic review. *Am J Gastroenterol* 2005;100 (4):936.

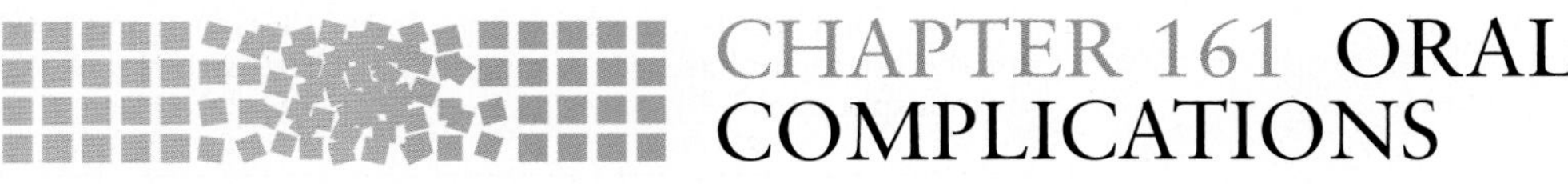

CHAPTER 161 ORAL COMPLICATIONS

ELIEZER SOTO, JANE M. FALL-DICKSON, AND ANN M. BERGER

The effectiveness of cancer therapies designed to improve cure rates and to extend survival time, including chemotherapy (CT), radiation therapy (RT), and conditioning regimens used for hematopoietic stem cell transplantation (HSCT), is tempered by intolerable or quality-of-life reducing side effects. Oral complications are one such side effect, including CT- and RT-related oral mucositis and oral chronic graft-versus-host disease (cGVHD) and related oropharyngeal pain, xerostomia, and oral infection. Pathogenesis of and management strategies for these oral complications, and future clinical research directions, are presented in this chapter.

ORAL MUCOSITIS

Oral mucositis is an inflammation of the mucous membranes of the oral cavity and oropharynx characterized by tissue erythema, edema, atrophy, often progressing to ulceration.[1] The clinical significance of CT- and RT-related oral mucositis as a dose- and treatment-limiting side effect is appreciated.[2] It is a painful and debilitating side effect that interferes with further treatment options and causes significant impairment in patient's quality of life and functional status.[3,4]

The frequency and severity of oral mucositis are influenced by numerous patient- and treatment-related risk factors (Table 161.1).[5,6] Risk factors for CT-related oral mucositis are complex. For example, although younger patients are considered at increased risk for oral mucositis, and women have been reported to have more frequent severe oral mucositis than men, Driezen[7] reported no age or gender risk for this oral condition. Children are three times more likely than adults to develop mucositis due to a higher proliferating fraction of basal cells. Results from 332 ambulatory CT patients showed no significant differences in oral mucositis incidence between outpatients who wore dental appliances, previously had oral lesions, used diverse oral hygiene and oral care practices, and had a history of smoking than those patients who did not.[6] Conflicting study results may be related to a lack of defined risk factors for those entering clinical trials.[5] Known risk factors include continuous CT infusion therapy for breast and colon cancer (5-fluorouracil [5-FU] and leucovorin); selected anthracyclines, alkylating agents, taxanes, vinca alkaloids, antimetabolites, and antitumor antibiotics; myeloablative conditioning regimens for HSCT (e.g., high-dose melphalan or carmustine, cytarabine, melphalan [BEAM])[8–10]; and RT to the head and neck. Individual drug metabolism affects oral mucositis incidence and severity.

CHEMOTHERAPY-INDUCED STOMATITIS

Approximately 40% of CT patients develop oral mucositis,[11] and approximately half of these patients develop painful lesions requiring parenteral analgesia or total parenteral nutrition that may lead to treatment modification.[12] Higher oral mucositis incidence rates of 60% are seen in the HSCT setting, with incidence rates of up to 78% for ulcerative oral mucositis.[13] Oral mucositis is also a risk factor for infections, which may be life-threatening for neutropenic patients. Oral infections, such as herpes simplex virus (HSV) may increase oral mucositis severity. There is a four times greater relative risk of septicemia in patients with oral mucositis and oral infections as compared with patients without oral mucositis. This greater risk is due to mucosal barrier injury, allowing pathogen entry into the peripheral circulation.

The relationship between severe oral mucositis and clinical outcomes in patients who receive conditioning chemotherapy has been reported in several studies.[14,15] McCann et al.[14] performed an observational study in 197 patients with multiple myeloma (MM) or non-Hodgkin's lymphoma (NHL) who underwent either high-dose melphalan or BEAM chemotherapy, respectively. Severe oral mucositis (World Health Organization [WHO] grades 3 and 4) increased the duration of total parenteral nutrition by 2.7 days, opiates by 4.6 days, and antibiotics by 2.4 days, prolonging the hospital stay for MM patients. Oral mucositis presents with asymptomatic erythema and progresses from solitary, white, elevated desquamative patches that are slightly painful to large, contiguous, pseudomembranous, painful lesions. Edema of the rete pegs and vascular changes are observed. Typical oral sequela of CT agents include epithelial hyperplasia, collagen and glandular degeneration, and epithelial dysplasia, atrophy, and localized or diffuse mucosal ulceration. Nonkeratinized mucosa areas are most affected: labial, buccal, and soft palate mucosa; floor of the mouth; and ventral surface of the tongue. The loss of basement membrane epithelial cells exposes underlying connective, innervated tissue stroma, which contributes to more severe oropharyngeal pain.

RADIATION-INDUCED STOMATITIS

Oral mucositis is virtually universal when RT targets the oropharyngeal area, with the severity dependent on type of ionizing radiation, volume of irradiated tissue, daily and cumulative dose, and duration. Oral mucositis is a dose- and rate-limiting toxicity of RT for head and neck cancer and of hyperfractionated RT and CT. Radiation interacts directly with DNA, leading to chromosome and cellular mitotic apparatus damage. Atrophic changes in the oral epithelium usually occur at total doses of 1600 to 2000 cGy, administered at a rate of 200 cGy/day.[16] Doses higher than 6000 cGy or concomitant CT place the patient at risk for permanent salivary gland changes.[16,17] The addition of total-body irradiation to HSCT increases oral mucositis severity through both direct mucosal damage and

PRACTICE OF ONCOLOGY

TABLE 161.1

CANCER TREATMENT- AND PATIENT-RELATED RISK FACTORS FOR STOMATITIS

PATIENT-RELATED
Age older than 65 or younger than 20
Gender
Inadequate oral health and hygiene practices
Periodontal diseases
Microbial flora
Chronic low-grade mouth infections
Salivary gland secretory dysfunction
Herpes simplex virus infection
Inborn inability to metabolize chemotherapeutic agents effectively
Inadequate nutritional status
Exposure to oral stressors including alcohol and smoking
Ill-fitting dental prostheses
TREATMENT-RELATED
Radiation therapy: dose, schedule
Chemotherapy: agent; dose, schedule
Myelosuppression
Neutropenia
Immunosuppression
Reduced secretory immunoglobulin A
Inadequate oral care during treatment
Infections of bacterial, viral, fungal origin
Use of antidepressants, opiates, antihypertensives, antihistamines, diuretics, and sedatives
Impairment of renal or hepatic function
Protein or calorie malnutrition, and dehydration
Xerostomia

Adapted from refs. 5 and 6, with permission.

xerostomia. CT-induced dental effects occur when the glands are within the treatment field and depend more on these effects then on direct irradiation of the teeth. Teeth in the irradiated field may be desensitized, leading to asymptomatic early caries. Therefore, daily fluoride application is necessary.

Health care costs associated with oral mucositis in head and neck cancer patients are significant.[18,19] In a prospective, longitudinal study with 75 patients with head and neck cancer receiving RT with or without CT,[19] 76% reported severe mouth and throat pain resulting in an increased number of visits to health care providers, 51% had a feeding tube placed, and 37% were hospitalized with a mean hospitalization stay of 4.9 days. These complications are directly correlated to a significant increase in resource use and excess costs.

RADIATION THERAPY-RELATED COMPLICATIONS

Long-term effects of head and neck RT include soft tissue fibrosis, trismus, nonhealing or slow-healing mucosal ulcerations, and slow healing of dental extraction sites. RT-induced fibrotic changes may occur in the masticatory muscles or the temporal mandibular joint up to 1 year posttherapy, becoming more serious over time. Early phases of fibrogenesis following RT may be viewed as wound healing characterized by up-regulation of tumor necrosis factor-alpha (TNF-α) and other proinflammatory cytokines.[20] As radiation fibrogenesis continues, it functions as a nonhealing wound.[20]

Osteoradionecrosis (ORN) is a relatively uncommon condition related to hypocellularity, hypovascularity, and tissue ischemia. Higher incidences are seen after total doses to the bone exceed 65 Gy.[21] ORN is usually related to trauma such as dental extraction and is reported following tooth extractions that were not timed to allow adequate extraction site healing for 10 to 14 days before the start of RT. Osteonecrosis of the jaw bone has been strongly associated with the use of bisphosphonate.[22,23]

PATHOGENESIS OF CHEMOTHERAPY- AND RADIATION-INDUCED ORAL MUCOSITIS

Current knowledge of oral mucositis pathogenesis is informed by translational research that applies advances in molecular-genetic technique and cell biology to this clinical condition.[24] Cancer therapy affects rapidly dividing cells, and the oral basal epithelium cell turnover rate is 7 to 14 days, thus placing them at risk for CT targeting. Sonis et al.[25] described a "burst" of cyclooxygenase-2 (COX-2) expression relative to RT-related oral mucositis progression, suggesting that COX-2 plays an amplifying role in this process. In a small pilot study the role of the cyclooxygenase pathway was investigated in three autologous HSCT patients.[26] Pain scores were significantly correlated with COX-1, microsomal prostaglandin-E synthase, and salivary prostaglandin, suggesting a role for the cyclooxygenase pathway in oral mucositis, possibly via up-regulation of proinflammatory prostaglandins.

Sonis[24] has described a five-phase oral mucositis pathogenesis model that includes initiation, message generation, signaling and amplification, ulceration, and healing. Initiation occurs after administration of cytotoxic CT as a result of DNA damage and the generation of reactive oxygen species. The relatively acute inflammatory or vascular phase occurs shortly after CT or RT administration.[12] Message generation involves the up-regulation of transcription factors, including nuclear factor κB (NF-κB) and activation of cytokines and stress response genes. Signaling and amplification involves the production of proinflammatory cytokines released from epithelial tissue, including TNF-α, which is related to tissue damage, and interleukin-1 (IL-1), which incites the inflammatory response and increases subepithelial vascularity that may lead to increased local CT levels. Logan et al.[27] reported preliminary results in a sample of 20 patients undergoing CT demonstrating elevated NF-κB and COX-2 after CT, even though histologically the tissue did not vary much pre- and post-CT. The epithelial phase shows reduced epithelial renewal and atrophy and typically begins 4 to 5 days after CT administration. The cell cycle S-phase specific agents, including methotrexate, 5-FU, and cytarabine, are most efficient for this phase. The ulcerative or bacterial phase begins approximately 1 week post-CT administration, occurring with maximum neutropenia.[12] This phase is the most complex, symptomatic phase, and probably not CT agent class-specific. Patients often experience acute oropharyngeal pain, leading to dysphagia, decreased oral intake, and difficulty speaking. Bacterial colonization of mucosal ulceration occurs, and gram-negative organisms release endotoxins that induce the release of IL-1 and TNF and production of nitric oxide that may increase local mucosal injury. RT and CT are likely to amplify and prolong this proinflammatory cytokine release, leading to exacerbated tissue response. Genetic expression of cytokines and enzymes critical in tissue damage may be modified by transcription factors.[12] Fall-Dickson et al.[28] described oropharyngeal pain related to oral mucositis in patients undergoing HSCT with CT and assessed the effectiveness of molecular biology methods for measuring TNF-α concentration in blood, saliva, and oral buccal brush biopsy samples. Oral mucositis severity was significantly associated with the overall intensity of oral pain. TNF-α RNA content in oral buccal brush biopsy samples also correlated with the worst intensity of oral pain with swallowing. Healing of oral lesions in the nonmyelosuppressed patient occurs within 2 to 3 weeks following cancer treatment. Mechanisms of healing include renewal of epithelial proliferation and differentiation in parallel with white blood cell recovery and re-establishment of normal local microbial flora. Oropharyngeal pain decreases in parallel with mucosal healing.

Avivi et al.[29] evaluated the salivary antioxidant and immunological capacities observed in MM patients with CT-induced oral mucositis. Twenty-five patients with MM who had received conditioning CT with melphalan followed by autologous HSCT were recruited. Salivary samples were collected and analyzed for secretory immunoglobulin-A (IgA) and antioxidant capacity, and mucosal damage was measured by salivary carbonyl and albumin (Alb) levels. Oral mucositis was associated with a reduction in secretory IgA and antioxidant activity. However, the increase in salivary Alb and carbonyl indicates mucosal and oxidative damage, respectively.

CHRONIC GRAFT-VERSUS-HOST DISEASE ORAL MANIFESTATIONS

Patients who have undergone allogeneic HSCT (alloHSCT) frequently develop GVHD, an alloimmune condition derived from an immune attack mediated by donor T cells recognizing antigens expressed on normal tissues. GVHD occurs following alloHSCT because of disparities in minor histocompatibility antigens between donor and recipient, inherited independently of HLA genes.[30] Acute GVHD occurs within the first 100 days after alloHSCT. Chronic GVHD begins as early as 70 days or as late as 15 months after alloHSCT. Increased incidence of cGVHD is related to changing patterns of alloHSCT.

The importance of oral cGVHD was recognized by the National Institutes of Health (NIH) Consensus Development Project on Criteria for Clinical Trials in cGVHD.[31] Consensus documents have been published, including response criteria guidelines to measure clinical progression over time. The Schubert Oral Mucositis Rating Scale was validated under the auspices of this NIH Consensus Development Project.[31] Treister et al.[32] analyzed inter- and intraobserver variability in the component and composite scores using the NIH oral cGVHD Activity Assessment Instrument. Twenty-four clinicians from six major HSCT centers scored high-quality intraoral photographs of 12 patients with a second evaluation 1 week later. Although mean interrater reliability was poor to moderate and unacceptable for the clinical trial setting, greater concordance among the oral medicine experts, high intrarater reliability, and participant feedback suggest that formal training may decrease variability.

Approximately 80% of patients with extensive cGVHD have some type of oral involvement[33] that is a major contributing factor to the morbidity seen with allogeneic HSCT. Although oral lesions are most common in patients with extensive cGVHD, patients may also present with limited disease involving only the oral cavity. Oral cGVHD presents with tissue atrophy and erythema, lichenoid changes, and pseudomembranous ulcerations, occurring typically on buccal and labial mucosa and the lateral tongue, angular stomatitis, and xerostomia.[33] Treister et al.[34] were able to correlate the distribution, type, and extent of lesions with patient-reported pain and discomfort. The buccal and labial mucosa and tongue were the sites of 93% of ulcerations, 72% of erythematous lesions, and 76% of reticular lesions. Ulcerations in the soft palate were uncommon but associated with increased pain. There was a statistically significant inverse relationship between the overall presence of ulceration and time since HSCT. Functional impact was significant as evidenced by restriction of oral intake due to discomfort. Decreased oral intake related to oral pain leads to weight loss and malnutrition, which remain serious problems. Despite the importance of oral cGVHD as one of the major long-term complications after alloHSCT, little is known about its pathogenesis. Imanguli et al.[35] has proposed a new model of cGVHD pathogenesis in which the production of type 1 interferon (IFN) by plasmacytoid dendritic cells plays a central role in the initiation and continuation of cGVHD. Fall-Dickson et al.[36] have analyzed the relationship among clinical characteristics of oral cGVHD and related oral pain and dryness, salivary proinflammatory cytokine IL-6, and IL-1α concentrations, and health-related quality of life. Salivary IL-6 was associated with oral cGVHD severity, oral ulceration, and erythema, suggesting its use as a potential biomarker of active oral cGVHD.

SEQUELAE OF ORAL COMPLICATIONS

Oropharyngeal Pain

Oral mucositis is the principal etiology of most pain experienced during the 3-week post–bone marrow transplant (BMT) time period. This oral pain is often described as the most unforgettable ordeal of BMT. McGuire et al.[37] reported in a sample of autologous and allogeneic BMT patients that pain was detected before observed mucositis, that pain intensity did not correlate directly with extent of mucosal injury, and that some patients reported limited or no pain after BMT. A descriptive, correlational, cross-sectional study of women with breast cancer undergoing autologous HSCT conducted by Fall-Dickson et al.[38] showed a significant positive correlation between oral pain and oral mucositis severity.

The sensory dimension of oral mucositis–related pain reported with general mucosal inflammation and breakdown ranges from mild discomfort to severe and debilitating pain requiring the use of opioids.[39] Immunocompromised cancer patients with HSV infections have larger, more painful lesions as compared with noncancer patients. Oral pain is associated strongly with cGVHD and has been described as severe, burning, and irritating, with dryness and loss of taste also reported. Mucositis-related oral pain reported with CT is usually of less than 3 months' duration, contrasting with the usually chronic oral pain accompanying oral cGVHD.

Research has demonstrated conflicting results regarding the association between age and pain perception, and intraethnic differences in pain perception. Gender differences have been reported for pain. For example, women in a study to test capsaicin efficacy for oral mucositis–related pain reported higher pain levels. Accomplishing pain control is critical to avoid suffering and psychological distress.[40] Adequate assessment of this oral pain experience requires a comprehensive pain assessment tool such as the Pain-O-Meter (Dola Health Systems, Baltimore, Maryland),[41] which assesses the overall intensity, sensory, and affective dimensions of pain.

Xerostomia

Xerostomia experienced by patients who receive head and neck RT is a major sequela, with severity dependent on RT dosage and location and volume of exposed salivary glands. Patients who have undergone HSCT may also develop xerostomia as a late oral complication. Brand et al.[42] reported in a cross-sectional study of patients with history of autologous or allogeneic HSCT significantly higher levels of xerostomia compared to the comparison group of age and gender-matched individuals. The severity of xerostomia was not significantly associated with RT given before HSCT or the type of HSCT. Xerostomia can affect taste, oral comfort, fit of prostheses, speech, and swallowing. Xerostomia-associated enzymes contribute to the growth of caries (decay)-producing organisms.

A recent cross-sectional study conducted by Imanguli et al.[43] evaluated sicca signs and symptoms in 101 cGVHD patients using tools from the studies of lacrimal and salivary gland dysfunction in Sjögren's syndrome. Xerostomia was reported in 77% of the patients. Those with salivary dysfunction showed histopathologic changes consisting of mononuclear infiltration and fibrosis or atrophy. These findings suggest that salivary gland involvement is a common manifestation in patients with cGVHD. A formal assessment tool is needed for further evaluation of salivary function in clinical trials. The salivary antioxidant capacity and function were assessed in 30 patients who had undergone HSCT in a study conducted by Nagler et al.[44] Salivary gland function was assessed, measuring total protein, secretory IgA, and the antioxidants peroxidase, uric acid, and total antioxidant status in a sample of saliva. In patients who developed GVHD, there was a significant decrease in salivary flow rate pre- and post-HSCT with no recovery and a reduction in salivary protein content and salivary antioxidant capacity. In patients who underwent HSCT without developing GVHD, salivary flow rates returned to normal in 3 to 5 months. This decreased salivary flow rate and related decrease in its protective functions for the oral mucosa may be contributing factors to oral cGVHD severity.

STRATEGIES FOR PREVENTION AND TREATMENT OF ORAL COMPLICATIONS

Pretherapy Dental Evaluation and Intervention

Oral or dental stabilization prior to CT and RT is critically important to avoid serious sequela and requires an experienced dental team and informed patients working together to provide adequate cleaning, eliminate sites of oral infection and trauma, and promote appropriate oral hygiene.[45]

Patients scheduled for CT or head and neck RT should receive dental screening at least 2 weeks before therapy starts to allow for proper healing of extraction sites, recovery of soft tissue manipulations, and restoration of teeth. These activities promote optimal mucosal health before, during, and following cancer treatment. Oral hygiene is one of the most important screening areas for all patients, regardless of type of cancer treatment modality. The initial dental appointment includes examination of the patient's dentition for carious lesions and defective restorations that may irritate the oral mucosa and necessitate replacement. The periodontium and pulp vitality must be evaluated. Periodontal status assessment includes measurement of pocket depth and assessment of furcation involvement. Denture fit assessment avoids ill-fitting dentures that may cause irritation of irradiated tissue and potential ulceration to underlying bone.[46]

A panoramic radiograph combined with intraoral radiographs as needed is necessary to detect periodontal disease, periapical infections, cysts, third-molar pathology, unerupted or partially erupted teeth, and residual root tips. Significant oral or dental problems that should be addressed before cancer treatment include inappropriate oral hygiene, periapical pathology, third-molar pathology, periodontal disease, defective restorations, dental caries, orthodontic appliances, and ill-fitting prostheses. Bacterial load should be reduced prior to cancer treatment via root planning, scaling, and prophylaxis, excluding visible tumor located at the site of anticipated dental manipulation. Comprehensive evaluation also includes assessment of the oral mucosa and the alveolar process to prepare for possible future prosthetic intervention and to assess for ulcerations, fibromas, irritation, hyperplasia, bony spicules, and tori. The decision to extract asymptomatic teeth prior to the commencement of RT is related to several important factors, including radiation exposure, type, portal field, fractionization, and total dosage in addition to tumor prognosis, and expediency of control of the cancer.[47] Lack of patient motivation regarding appropriate oral hygiene practices should lead to a decision to extract questionable teeth prior to RT. Teeth that are class II or III mobility without use as abutment teeth for prosthetic retention should also be considered for extraction before RT. Extractions of residual root tips and impacted teeth should be performed atraumatically. Alveolectomy and primary wound closure eliminate sharp ridges and bone spicules that could project to the overlying soft tissues. This is important for prosthetic consideration because negligible bone remodeling is predicted after RT.

Patients often receive their cancer treatment in the ambulatory setting and need specific written instructions for appropriate use of oral care agents and instruments for effective daily plaque removal, use of prescribed fluoride treatments, and reportable oral observations and symptoms.

Assessment of the Oral Mucosa

Consistent and frequent oral cavity assessment is needed to assess clinical signs before, during, and after treatment. No standard grading system for severity of oral complications of cancer treatment exists. Numerous available oral complications grading tools are based on two or more clinical parameters combined with functional status, such as eating ability. One commonly used tool is the National Cancer Institute Common Terminology Criteria for Adverse Events v. 3.0, which includes both descriptive terminology and a severity grading scale for each reportable adverse event.[48] Frequently used oral mucosal assessment tools include those that capture both objective and subjective data—the Oral Assessment Guide[49] and the World Health Organization Index[11,50]—and instruments that assess only the observed oral changes—the Oral Mucositis Rating Scale[39,51] the Oral Mucositis Index,[52] the Oral Mucositis Assessment Scale (OMAS).[53,54] The OMAS was developed as a scoring system for evaluating the anatomic extent and severity of oral mucositis in clinical research studies by an international team of oral medicine specialists, dentists, dental hygienists, oncologists, and oncology nurses.[53,54] Oral cavity regions assessed are lip (upper and lower), cheek (right and left), right and lateral tongue, left ventral and lateral tongue, floor of mouth, soft palate or fauces, and hard palate.[53] Erythema is rated on a scale from 0 to 2 (0 = none, 1 = not severe, and 2 = severe), and ulceration or pseudomembrane is a combined category rated on scores based on estimated surface area involved (0 = no lesion, 1 = less than 1 cm^2, 2 = 1 cm^2 to 3 cm^2, and 3 = more than 3 cm^2) and summed with a possible score range of 0 to 162.[47,55] Validity and reliability have been demonstrated for the OMAS through clinical research studies.[54,56]

TREATMENT STRATEGIES

The optimal treatment strategies for oral complications and related sequela are unknown. Treatment strategies for oral mucositis and related oropharyngeal pain are mainly empirical,

TABLE 161.2

FORMULARY OF COMMON TREATMENTS FOR ORAL COMPLICATIONS[a]

	Instructions
PREVENTION OF STOMATITIS	
Amifostine	200 mg/m² daily, as 3-minutes IV infusion 15 to 30 minutes preradiotherapy. Hydrate adequately, monitor blood pressure, and use antiemetics.
Cryotherapy	Place ice chips in mouth for 30 minutes beginning 5 minutes prior to bolus administration of chemotherapy.
Distilled water, 1 gallon	Rinse mouth twice a day for 30 s. Do not swallow.
$NAHCO_3$ powder, 3 tablespoons or 11.6 g NaCl powder, 3 tablespoons or 11.6 g	Combine all ingredients. Rinse mouth 2 to 4 times daily. Do not swallow.
Povidone iodine 0.5% oral rinse	Rinse mouth 2 to 4 times daily. Do not swallow.
TREATMENT OF STOMATITIS-RELATED PAIN	
Carafate suspension, 1 g	Rinse mouth 4 times daily. Do not swallow.
Diphenhydramine (Benadryl), 12.5 mg/5 mL; kaolin and pectin (Kaopectate)	Use equal amounts of each. Rinse mouth with 10–15 mL 4 to 6 times daily. Do not swallow.
Diphenhydramine (Benadryl), 12.5 mg/5 mL: 30 mL; Maalox, 30 mL; nystatin, 100,000 U/mL: 30 mL	Combine all ingredients. Rinse mouth with 15 mL 4 to 6 times per day. Do not swallow.
Diphenhydramine (Benadryl), 12.5 mg/5 mL: 30 mL; viscous lidocaine (Xylocaine) 2%, 30 mL; Maalox, 30 mL	Combine all ingredients. Rinse mouth with 15 mL 4 to 6 times per day. Do not swallow.
Diphenhydramine (Benadryl), 12.5 mg/5 mL: 30 mL; tetracycline, 125 mg/5 mL suspension 60 mL; nystatin oral suspension, 100,000 U/mL 45 mL; viscous lidocaine (Xylocaine) 2%, 30 mL; hydrocortisone suspension, 10 mg/5 mL: 30 mL; sterile water for irrigation, 45 mL	Combine all ingredients. Rinse mouth with 15 mL 4 to 6 times per day. Do not swallow.
Dyclonine hydrochloride 0.5% or 1.0% solution	Rinse mouth with 10–15 mL every 2–3h. Do not swallow.
Gelclair	Mix one Gelclair packet per manufacturer's directions with 40 mL or 3 tablespoons of water. Stir and rinse immediately for at least 1 minute, gargle, and spit out at least 3 times a day.
Opiates	Oral, transdermal or parenteral opiates may be used, such as PCA. Use tablet form of oral analgesics. Do not use elixir because alcohol exacerbates stomatitis.
Viscous lidocaine (Xylocaine) 2% solution	Rinse mouth with 10–15 mL every 2–3h. Do not swallow.
XEROSTOMIA	
Biotene chewing gum	Use as needed.
Pilocarpine	5 mg oral 3 times a day
Salivart synthetic saliva spray	Spray mouth 4 to 6 times per day.
Xerolube, salivary substitute	Rinse mouth 4 to 6 times per day

NaCl, sodium chloride; NAHCO3, sodium bicarbonate; PCA, patient-controlled analgesia.
[a]Many of the medications listed have been used alone or in combination to treat stomatitis.
(Adapted from Fall-Dickson JM, Berger AM. Oral manifestations and complications of cancer treatment. In: Shuster JL, Von Roenn JH, eds. *Principles and practice of palliative care and supportive oncology*. 3rd ed. Philadelphia: Lippincott Williams & Wilkins, 2006.)

and testing is needed in the randomized controlled clinical trial setting (Table 161.2). Zlotolow and Berger[57] presented a comprehensive review of clinical research regarding treatment strategies for oral complications of cancer strategies. Conflicting study results may be related to inappropriate design issues, use of limited oral assessment instruments unable to capture variations in oral cavity changes, and incorrect timing and dosage of interventions. The only standard forms of care are pretreatment oral or dental stabilization, saline mouthwashes, and oropharyngeal pain management.[58]

The need for standardized treatment for oral mucositis was appreciated by the Mucositis Study Section of the Multinational Association of Supportive Care in Cancer and the International Society for Oral Oncology through their formulation of the "Clinical Practice Guidelines for the Prevention and Treatment of Cancer Therapy-Induced Oral and Gastrointestinal Mucositis."[59] These guidelines are based on a comprehensive review of more than 8,000 English-language publications (1966 to 2001). Publications regarding alimentary tract mucositis were rated using criteria for level of evidence and quality of research design.[60]

A standardized approach for the prevention and treatment of CT- and RT-induced oral mucositis is essential. The prophylactic measures usually used for the prevention of oral mucositis include chlorhexidine gluconate, ice-cold water, saline rinses, sodium bicarbonate rinses, acyclovir, and amphotericin B. Regimens used commonly for the treatment of oral mucositis and related pain include a local anesthetic such as lidocaine or dyclonine hydrochloride, magnesium-based antacids, diphenhydramine hydrochloride, nystatin, or sucralfate. These agents are used either alone or in various combinations as a mouthwash formulation. Oral and parenteral opiates are used to relieve oral mucositis–related pain.

RADIOPROTECTORS

Vitamins and Other Antioxidants

Vitamin E has been tested in CT-induced oral mucositis because it can stabilize cellular membranes and may improve herpetic gingivitis, possibly through antioxidant activity. Wadleigh et al.[61] demonstrated the efficacy of vitamin E in 18 CT patients who were randomized to receive topical vitamin E or placebo. Statistically significant results showed that six of nine patients in the vitamin E group had complete oral mucositis resolution within 4 days of starting therapy, as compared with the placebo group, in which only one of nine had oral mucositis resolution during the 5-day study period.

Other antioxidants that have been tested for efficacy with oral mucositis include vitamin C and glutathione. Osaki et al.[62] reported findings from a study with a sample of 63 patients with head and neck cancer who were treated with chemoradiation. Twenty-six patients received regimen 1 (vitamins C and E and glutathione) and 37 patients received regimen 2 (regimen 1 plus azelastine). Study findings showed that in the azelastine arm, 21 patients remained at grade 1 or 2 oral mucositis, 6 patients had grade 3 oral mucositis, and 10 patients had grade 4 oral mucositis. In the control group, grade 3 or 4 oral mucositis was observed in more than half the patients. Azelastine may be useful to prevent CT-induced oral mucositis.[62] Polaprezinc (zinc L-carnosine), a zinc-containing molecule used for the therapy of gastric ulcers, has been shown to inhibit the induction of TNF-α. Watanabe et al.[63] investigated the effect of polaprezinc on CT- and RT-induced oral mucositis, pain, xerostomia, and taste disturbance in patients with head and neck cancer. Thirty-one patients were randomly assigned to polaprezinc or azulene solution as a control for 3 minutes four times a day until the end of the therapy. There was a marked decreased in the incidence of oral mucositis, pain, xerostomia, taste disturbance, and analgesic requirement as well as a significant increase in food intake in the polaprezinc group.

Amifostine

Amifostine is a thiol compound, selective cytoprotective agent that has been approved by the U.S. Food and Drug Administration for salivary gland protection in patient receiving RT. A retrospective study conducted by Kouloulias et al.[64] reported reduced severity of oral and esophageal toxicity. One hundred seventy-seven patients with a diversity of tumors were treated with amifostine before RT. Based on a meta-analysis that included patients who received amifostine before RT, there is a significant reduction in the severity of oral mucositis at doses above 300 mg/m^2.[65] A multicenter, open-label, randomized controlled trial analyzed the use of amifostine in MM patients who received conditioning CT with melphalan prior to autologous HSCT.[66] Ninety patients were randomized to receive or not receive amifostine (910 mg/m^2). The use of amifostine was associated with a reduction in the median grade and the frequency of severe (WHO grade 3 or 4) oral mucositis. However, there was no reduction in parenteral nutrition and analgesics use and no significant difference between the median progression-free or overall survival times.

Glutamine

Glutamine is an amino acid, immunomodulator, and mucosal protective agent that has been studied in multiple clinical trials with conflicting results. An extensive literature review performed by Savarese et al.[67] reported that glutamine supplementation may have an impact on incidence and severity of anthracycline-associated oral mucositis. A randomized, double-blind, placebo controlled trial on glutamine supplementation in patients who underwent autologous HSCT reported an increase in severe oral mucositis and opiate use as well as prolonged hospital stay.[68] Another randomized controlled study compared oral glutamine supplementation (30 g/d) versus placebo in 58 HSCT patients. There was no difference in length of hospitalization, nutrition, severity of oral mucositis, engraftment time, survival, relapse, or severity of diarrhea between both groups.[69]

Other clinical trials have reported more promising data on the use of glutamine.[70,71] In a double-blind, randomized, placebo-controlled trial of oral glutamine in the prevention of oral mucositis in children undergoing HSCT, 120 patients were randomized to receive glutamine or glycine twice a day until 28 days posttransplant. The glutamine group showed a significant reduction in days of intravenous opiates use and total parenteral nutrition but no difference in toxicity was observed between the two groups.[72]

A phase 3 study of topical AES-14, which is a novel drug system designed to concentrate delivery of L-glutamine to oral mucosa for ulceration treatment, was conducted with 121 patients at risk for oral mucositis.[73] Patients were randomized to either AES-14 or placebo and received protocol treatment from day 1 of CT until 2 weeks following the last CT dose or oral mucositis resolution. Results showed a potential 20% reduction of moderate-to-severe oral mucositis in the AES-14 group and a 10% increase in grade 0 oral mucositis.

Anti-Inflammatory Agents

Prostaglandins are a family of naturally occurring eicosanoids, some of which have shown cytoprotective activity. Topical dinoprostone was administered four times daily in a non-blinded study to ten patients with oral carcinomas who were receiving 5-FU and mitomycin with concomitant RT.[74] The control group comprised 14 patients who were receiving identical treatment. Eight of the ten patients who received dinoprostone were evaluable, and no patient developed severe oral mucositis as compared with six episodes in the control arm. A second pilot study was conducted with 15 patients who received RT to the head and neck, showing that an inflammatory reaction was detected in only five patients in the vicinity of their tumor when treated with topically applied PGE$_2$, and that no patients developed any bullous or desquamating inflammatory lesions.[75] A double-blind, placebo-controlled study of PGE$_2$ in 60 patients undergoing BMT revealed no significant differences in the incidence, severity, or duration of oral mucositis. The incidence of HSV was higher in those on the PGE$_2$ arm. There was an increase in oral mucositis severity in those patients who developed HSV.[76]

Benzydamine is a nonsteroidal anti-inflammatory drug with reported analgesic, anesthetic, and antimicrobial properties without activity on arachidonic acid metabolism. It has been shown to reduce the severity of oral mucositis and associated pain in patients who undergo RT. Epstein and Stevenson-Moore[77] reported in a double-blind, placebo-controlled trial that benzydamine produced statistically significant relief of pain from RT-induced oral mucositis and a reduction in both the total area and the size of ulceration. Positive responses to benzydamine have been reported in at least three other studies.[78–80] In a small prospective, double-blind, randomized study comparing the efficacy of chlorhexidine gluconate and benzydamine hydrochloride oral rinse in patients with head and neck cancer to prevent and treat RT-induced oropharyngeal mucositis, a trend emerged showing a decrease in mucositis, oropharyngeal pain, and dysphagia in those receiving benzydamine.[81]

Current evidence does not support the use of systemic steroids to reduce the frequency or severity of oral mucositis.[82]

BIOLOGICAL RESPONSE MODIFIERS

Epidermal Growth Factors

Studies on epidermal growth factor (EGF) as a potential treatment option for CT- and RT-induced oral mucositis have reported conflicting data. EGF may function as a marker of mucosal damage and could potentially facilitate the healing process.[83] In a phase 1 trial conducted by Girdler et al.,[84] EGF mouthwash was applied to patients treated with CT and showed a delay in onset and reduction in severity of recurrent ulcerations. However, no statistical difference was seen in resolution of established ulcers. A recent double-blind, placebo-controlled, prospective phase 2 study reported a potential benefit from EGF oral spray in the management of oral mucositis in patients undergoing RT for head and neck cancer. In this study, 113 patients were randomized into one of four arms: EGF-treatment groups (10, 50, 100 mcg/mL doses twice daily) and placebo. The 50 mcg/mL dose demonstrated the best efficacy for treatment of oral mucositis.[85] Further randomized controlled trials are needed to confirm these results.

Hematopoietic Growth Factors

Hematologic growth factors are currently the standard treatment for patients who are treated with high-dose CT because of their well-established efficacy to decrease the duration of CT-induced neutropenia. *In vitro* studies have demonstrated that epidermal growth factor is present in saliva and has the ability to affect growth, cell and migration, and repair mechanisms.[86] The development of increased oral toxicity or mucosal repair may be dependent on the timing of epidermal growth factor administration in relation to CT treatment.[87] Gabrilove et al.[88] reported from a sample of 27 patients with bladder cancer who received escalating doses of granulocyte-colony stimulating factor (G-CSF) during treatment with methotrexate, vinblastine, doxorubicin, and cisplatin. The patients received the G-CSF during the first of two cycles of CT. Although significantly less oral mucositis was seen during the first cycle with G-CSF, a limitation of this study is that positive results may be biased related to possible cumulative chemotherapeutic toxicity with resultant increase in oral mucositis severity. Conversely, Bronchud et al.[89] reported from a study of 17 patients with breast or ovarian carcinoma treated with escalating doses of doxorubicin with G-CSF that G-CSF did not prevent severe oral mucositis. A third study was conducted comparing clinical outcomes in a sample of 55 adult patients who received CT for non-Hodgkin's lymphoma and G-CSF with clinical outcomes in 39 patients who received CT alone. Patients who did not receive G-CSF had neutropenia as the primary cause of treatment delay, as compared with those patients who did receive G-CSF and experienced oral mucositis as the main cause of treatment delay.[90] Granulocyte-macrophage colony-stimulating factor (GM-CSF) has demonstrated conflicting results in patients who received diverse cancer treatments.[91–94] An open, randomized controlled phase 3 trial conducted by Masucci et al.[92] analyzed the efficacy of GM-CSF in head and neck cancer patients with RT-induced oral mucositis. A significant reduction in oral mucositis severity was observed in the GM-CSF treatment group. Conversely, results from a Radiation Therapy Oncology Group sponsored a double-blind, placebo-controlled, randomized study (N = 121) to analyze the efficacy and safety of GM-CSF in reducing severity and duration of oral mucositis and related pain in head and neck cancer patients receiving RT.[94] It showed GM-CSF had no significant effect on the severity or duration of oral mucositis. The use of CSFs in the treatment of oral mucositis remains investigational.

Keratinocyte Growth Factors

Recently, palifermin, which is a recombinant human keratinocyte growth factor and member of fibroblast growth factor family (FGF), has shown efficacy in the reduction of oral mucosal injury related to cytotoxic therapy.[95] Spielberger et al.[95] reported from a double-blind study that compared the effect of palifermin with a placebo for the development of oral mucositis in 212 patients with hematologic cancers. Palifermin or placebo was administered intravenously for 3 consecutive days immediately before initiating conditioning therapy. This conditioning therapy used fractionated total-body radiation plus high-dose CT. As compared with placebo, the palifermin group experienced significant reductions in grade 4 oral mucositis, soreness of the mouth and throat, use of opiate analgesics, and the incidence of total parenteral nutrition use. Luthi et al.[96] reported lower grade 3 or 4 oral mucositis in 34 patients who received melphalan or BEAM with HSCT and were treated with palifermin (0.06 mg/kg) injections 3 days before conditioning chemotherapy and 3 days following HSCT as compared with controls. Nasilowska-Adamska et al.[97] found palifermin 60 mcg/kg/d for 3 consecutive days before and after conditioning therapy for HSCT to significantly reduce the incidence, severity, and duration of oral mucositis in a sample of 106 patients. In a subsequent study,[98] 53 patients with hematological diseases were submitted to the same regimen, also showing a significant reduction in incidence and median duration of oral mucositis, decreased incidence of opiates use, and total parenteral nutrition as well as less prevalence of acute GVHD.

Palifermin has also been studied in patients with solid tumors. In a randomized controlled trial conducted by Rosen et al.,[99] 64 patients with metastatic colorectal cancer who received 5-FU and leucovorin were randomized to receive palifermin (40 mcg/kg) for 3 consecutive days before each of two cycles of chemotherapy. The incidence of oral mucositis WHO grade 2 or higher was significantly lower, and patients reported less severe symptoms in the treatment arm. Brizel et al.[100] compared palifermin (60 mcg/kg) versus placebo in patients with locally advanced head and neck cancer treated with chemoradiation. Patients were submitted to two types of RT—standard (total dose of 70 Gy delivered in 2 Gy daily fractions) and hyperfractionated (total dose 72 Gy delivered in 1.25 Gy fractions twice a day for 7 weeks)—and CT including cisplatin (20 mg/m^2 for 4 days) and continuous infusion of 5-FU (1,000 mg/m^2/d for 4 days on weeks 1 and 5 of RT). Palifermin was well tolerated and decreased the incidence of oral mucositis, dysphagia, and xerostomia in patients treated with hyperfractionated RT but not standard RT. However, palifermin did not reduce the morbidity of concurrent chemoradiotherapy.

Antimicrobials

Antimicrobial approaches have included systemic types such as antibiotics, antivirals (acyclovir, valacyclovir, ganciclovir), and the antifungal agent, fluconazole. Donnelly et al.[101] evaluated the evidence regarding the role of infection in the pathophysiology of oral mucositis via a comprehensive review of 31 prospective randomized trials. Conclusions were that there was no clear pattern of patient type, cancer treatment, or type of antimicrobial agent used, and that there is a lack of consistent oral mucositis assessment.

Oral candidiasis is a common acute and chronic oral sequela of head and neck RT, with lesions presenting as removable (whitish) chronic or hyperplastic (nonremovable) and chronic erythematous (diffused as patchy erythema), which frequently appear as angular cheilitis (first signs or symptoms). Treatment approaches for oral candidiasis include Mycostatin (troche), nystatin (liquid or ointment), or clotrimazole. Pseudomembranous candidiasis is successfully treated topically. Chronic candidiasis usually requires much longer treatment, and it may be necessary to use oral ketoconazole, fluconazole, or intravenous amphotericin B.

Acyclovir prophylaxis is the currently accepted treatment for HSV and cytomegalovirus seropositive HSCT patients. A randomized controlled clinical trial conducted in HSCT patients compared fluconazole with placebo. Results showed that fluconazole prevented systemic fungal infections (7% fluconazole vs. 18% placebo) and significantly reduced the incidence of mucosal infection and oropharyngeal colonization by *Candida albicans*.[102]

Conflicting reports have been published regarding the use of chlorhexidine mouthwash for alleviating oral mucositis and reducing oral colonization by gram-positive, gram-negative, and *Candida* species in patients receiving CT, RT, or HSCT. The majority of studies have not demonstrated efficacy of chlorhexidine mouthwash for oral mucositis reduction in patients receiving intensive CT.[103] Dodd et al.[104] tested the efficacy of the PRO-SELF Mouth Aware (PSMA) program combined with randomization to one of two mouthwashes (0.12% chlorhexidine or sterile water) for the prevention of CT-related oral mucositis in 222 patients. Although chlorhexidine was found to be no more effective than water regarding oral mucositis incidence, days to onset, and severity, the PSMA program appeared to reduce oral mucositis incidence. A double-blind, placebo-controlled, randomized study of chlorhexidine prophylaxis for 5-FU–based CT-induced oral mucositis in patients with gastrointestinal (GI) malignancies conducted by Sorensen et al.[105] suggested a role for chlorhexidine in the prevention of oral mucositis. Two hundred twenty-five patients were randomized to chlorhexidine mouth rinse three times a day for 3 weeks versus placebo or cryotherapy with ice 45 minutes during CT. The frequency and duration of oral mucositis were significantly improved in the chlorhexidine and cryotherapy arms.

Sutherland and Browman[106] reviewed 59 studies assessing prophylaxis of RT-induced oral mucositis in head and neck cancer patients. Interventions chosen based on the biological etiology of oral mucositis were effective. A study by Spijkervet et al.[107] evaluated the efficacy of lozenges containing polymyxin E_2 2 mg, tobramycin 1.8 mg, and amphotericin B 10 mg (PTA) taken four times daily for the oropharyngeal flora related to oral mucositis. These researchers compared 15 patients receiving RT using PTA and two other groups of 15 patients each, one of which was using 0.1% chlorhexidine and the other was using placebo. Results showed that the selectively decontaminated group had significantly reduced severity and oral mucositis extent when compared with the chlorhexidine and placebo groups.

Cryotherapy

Cryotherapy, which is administered as ice chips and frozen flavored ice products, has been used to prevent oral mucositis. Efficacy of cryotherapy for the reduction of 5-FU–induced oral mucositis severity was demonstrated through a North Central Cancer Treatment Group (NCCTG) and Mayo Clinic–sponsored controlled randomized trial.[108] A subsequent study with a sample of 178 patients who were randomized to receive 30 minutes versus 60 minutes of oral cryotherapy reported similar severity of oral mucositis in both groups.[109] The study recommended the use of 30 minutes of oral cryotherapy prior to bolus administration of 5-FU–based CT. Additional studies have confirmed these results.[110,111] Cryotherapy used to induce vasoconstriction should be considered for patients receiving 5-FU or melphalan[112] when these agents are administered during short infusion times.

Pain relief with intravenous opiates has become a common practice for patients with CT- and RT-induced oral mucositis. Cryotherapy is an important adjuvant technique to opiate analgesia. A randomized controlled trial conducted by Svanberg et al.[113] demonstrated that this technique may alleviate the development of oral mucositis and oral pain, resulting in a reduction in the number of days and total dose of intravenous opiates in patients treated with autologous BMT.

Laser

Several studies have confirmed the effectiveness of low energy laser for prevention and treatment of CT- or RT-induced oral mucositis.[114–119] A recent phase 3 double-blind, placebo-controlled randomized study compared two different low level GaA1As diode lasers (650 nm and 780 nm) to prevent oral mucositis in HSCT patients treated with either CT or chemoradiotherapy.[117] Seventy patients were randomized into treatment with 650 nm or 780 nm laser or placebo. Low-level laser therapy showed to be more effective for decreasing oral mucositis and related oral pain, and it was safe without side effects. The efficacy of low-energy He/Ne laser was studied in a sample of 30 and 24 patients in two randomized controlled clinical trial.[115,120] Low-energy He/Ne laser demonstrated a reduction in the severity and duration of oral mucositis.

Miscellaneous Agents

Mangoni et al.[121] analyzed the protective efficacy of a new heparan mimetic biopolymer, RGTA-OTR4131, alone or with amifostine, in the management of oral mucositis and evaluated its effects on tumor growth *in vitro* and *in vivo*. A single dose of 16.5 Gy was delivered to the snout of mice and the effects of OTR4131 were analyzed by macroscopic scoring and histology. OTR4131 was well tolerated and found to effectively reduce RT-induced oral mucositis without affecting tumor sensitivity to RT. These results need to be confirmed in clinical trials.

TREATMENT FOR ORAL CHRONIC GRAFT-VERSUS-HOST DISEASE

Almost all patients with extensive cGVHD require systemic immunosuppressive therapy. Therefore, there is a critical need for adjuvant therapies that are both efficacious and avoid the long-term consequences of these corticosteroid therapies. In general, advances in the treatment of cGVHD have been modest, and no standard therapy exists for cGVHD that fails to respond to initial therapy or recurs. Imanguli et al.[122] have presented a comprehensive review of the available therapies for cGVHD of the oral mucosa. Pharmacotherapy for oral cGVHD may be oral, topical, or injectable. The most common systemic therapy is corticosteroids with or without cyclosporine. Other agents such as tacrolimus, sirolimus, pentostatin, mycophenolate mofetil, and hydroxychloroquine have been used as salvage treatment.[122] Emerging systemic therapies include monoclonal antibodies such as infliximab, etanercept, daclizumab, and rituximab.[122,123] Extracorporeal photophoresis, a process that separates a patient's mononuclear cells through apheresis and exposes them to ultraviolet light A (UVA), has shown promise.

Topical and local therapy for oral cGVHD offers several advantages to systemic therapy, including fewer side effects.

There currently exists no evidence that one topical therapy is superior to another. Most trials have been open label with very small numbers of participants. Patients with symptomatic disease that is limited to the oral cavity have been found to benefit from topical steroids such as dexamethasone elixir (0.5 mg/5 mL) and budesonide rinse (3 mg/10 mL).[40,124] Dexamethasone elixir has shown efficacy when used as a mouth rinse (10 mL) for 2 to 3 minutes at least four times daily.[40,125] Topical steroids such as fluocinonide have also been tried. Clobetasol 0.05%, which is a topical high-potency steroid, has been administered four times daily for 2 to 3 weeks depending on the severity of the ulcerative oral cGVHD to decrease inflammation and oral pain. If local steroids alone are not adequate to control oral disease, then topical cyclosporine[126] or topical tacrolimus may be tried.[40,127,128] Intraoral psoralen plus ultraviolet A irradiation (PUVA) may be appropriate based on the patient's condition.[40,122] These treatments need evaluation in further randomized controlled clinical trials.

SYMPTOM MANAGEMENT

Oropharyngeal Pain

Oral mucositis is the principal etiology of most pain experienced during the 3-week post-HSCT time period. This pain is often described as the most unforgettable ordeal of HSCT. Oral mucositis–related oropharyngeal pain is multidimensional. The sensory dimension of oral mucositis–related pain has been described with general mucosal inflammation and breakdown as ranging from mild discomfort to severe and debilitating pain, requiring opiates for pain management.[50] Immunocompromised patients with cancer who are also human immunodeficiency virus (HIV)-positive develop larger, more painful lesions than those experienced by noncancer patients. Oral pain associated with cGVHD has been described as severe, with symptoms of burning, irritation, dryness, and loss of taste being reported. In contrast to the often long-lasting oral pain accompanying oral cGVHD, oral mucositis–related oral pain in the CT setting is usually of less than 3 months' duration.

Sucralfate

Sucralfate is an aluminum salt of a sulfated disaccharide that has shown efficacy in the treatment of GI ulcerations and has been tested as a mouthwash for the prevention and treatment of oral mucositis. Sucralfate creates a protective barrier at the ulcer site via the formation of an ionic bond to proteins. Study results with sucralfate are conflicting. A phase 3 study was conducted by the NCCTG to compare sucralfate suspension versus placebo for 5-FU–related oral mucositis. Results demonstrated that in the 50 patients who experienced oral mucositis, not only did the sucralfate suspension provide no beneficial reduction in 5-FU–induced oral mucositis severity or duration, but the sucralfate group also had considerable additional GI toxicity.[129] Additionally, no efficacy was demonstrated for a sucralfate mouthwash for prevention and treatment of 5-FU–induced oral mucositis in a randomized controlled clinical trial with 81 patients with colorectal cancer who received either sucralfate suspension or placebo four times daily during their first cycle of 5-FU and leucovorin.[130]

Sucralfate has also been tested in the head and neck RT population. A prospective, double-blind study compared the effectiveness of sucralfate suspension to a formulation of diphenhydramine hydrochloride syrup plus kaolin-pectin for RT-induced oral mucositis. Results showed no statistically significant differences between the two groups. In a study designed to compare outcomes in 21 patients who received standard oral care with 24 patients who received sucralfate suspension four times daily, the sucralfate group showed a significant difference in mucosal edema, oral pain, dysphagia, and weight loss.[131] Conversely, a double-blind, placebo-controlled study with sucralfate in 33 patients who received RT to the head and neck demonstrated no statistically significant differences in oral mucositis.[132] However, the sucralfate group did experience less oral pain and required a later start of topical and systemic analgesics throughout RT.[132] Dodd et al.[133] used a pilot randomized controlled clinical trial to evaluate the efficacy of a micronized sucralfate mouthwash compared with a salt and soda mouthwash in 30 patients who received RT. All patients also used PSMA, which is a systematic oral hygiene program. Results demonstrated no significant difference in efficacy between the two groups.

Gelclair

Gelclair (Sinclair Pharmaceuticals, Surrey, England) is a concentrated, bioadherent gel that has received U.S. Food and Drug Administration approval as a 510(k) medical device indicated for the management of oral mucositis–related pain. Gelclair adheres to the oral surface, creating a protective barrier for irritated tissue and sensitized nociceptors. The safety and efficacy have been evaluated in small clinical trials with mixed results. Innocenti et al.[134] reported a 92% decrease in oral pain from baseline 5 to 7 hours after Gelclair administration in patients with oral mucositis, severe diffuse oral aphthous lesions, and postoral surgery pain. More than half of these patients reported that the maximum effect of Gelclair lasted longer than 3 hours, and 87% of patients reported overall improvements from baseline for pain with swallowing food, liquids, and saliva following 1 week of treatment. DeCordi et al.[86] reported from a clinical study in which Gelclair was administered to patients with oral mucositis three times daily before meals as a 2- to 3-minute swish and spit for 3 to 10 days. Significant improvements were reported from baseline for pain, oral mucositis severity, and function. No adverse effects were reported during either trial. Patients reported that the taste, smell, texture, and use of Gelclair were acceptable. On the other hand, Barber et al.[135] conducted a prospective, randomized controlled trial comparing Gelclair versus standard therapy with sucralfate and oxethazaine (Mucaine) in patients with RT-induced oral mucositis. This study did not show any significant difference between both therapies in terms of general pain. Gelclair can be an important adjuvant to opiate therapy in the management of oral mucositis–related oral pain. However, more randomized controlled trials are needed to further support its use in the clinical setting.

Anesthetic Cocktails

Anesthetic cocktails, composed of agents such as viscous lidocaine or dyclonine hydrochloride, have been used with some success for oral mucositis–related oral pain but provide only temporary pain relief. Also, these agents may alter taste perception, which may decrease oral intake. Other analgesics and mucosal-coating agents used for pain control include kaolin-pectin, diphenhydramine, Orabase (Colgate), and Oratect Gel (MGI Pharma). Hospital-based pharmacies commonly formulate and dispense topical mixtures containing an analgesic, an anti-inflammatory agent, and a coating agent for use as an oral comfort measure for patients during cancer treatment. One large clinical research center uses a topical formulation that contains viscous lidocaine 2% (40 mL), diphenhydramine 12.5 mg/5 mL (40 mL), and Maalox (Norvartis, Basel,

Switzerland) 10 mg (40 mL) and prescribes its use every 3 to 4 hours as needed. Testing these various topical formulations through randomized controlled clinical trials is needed.

Doxepin

Doxepin is a tricyclic antidepressant that has been used for many years in the management of patients with chronic benign or malignant pain. Its topical application is prescribed for the management of pruritus and neuropathic pain. Pilot studies on topical doxepin rinse in patient with oral mucositis pain have shown adequate analgesia for up to 4 hours after application.[136,137] Epstein et al.[138] assessed the effectiveness of oral doxepin rinse for oral mucositis–related pain in head and neck cancer patients in the RT or HSCT setting. Nine patients rinsed with doxepin (5 mL) three to six times per day during a week and returned for a follow-up visit. Oral mucositis was scored using the OMAS and oral pain was assessed using a visual analog scale (VAS). There was a statistically significant reduction in VAS scores for 2 hours following doxepin rinse at the initial visit and also over a 1-week period, showing that repeated dosing continues to bring significant pain relief. Further randomized controlled trials are needed to confirm these results.

Opiates

Severe oral mucositis–related oropharyngeal pain may interfere with hydration and nutritional intake and affect quality of life. Management of this oropharyngeal pain may require use of opiates, often administered at high doses by patient-controlled analgesia pumps. Other routes of administration are oral, transmucosal, transdermal, and parenteral. The efficacy of oral transmucosal fentanyl citrate was compared with morphine sulfate immediate release in a randomized, controlled clinical trial for the treatment of breakthrough cancer pain in 134 adult ambulatory cancer patients.[139] Study results showed that oral transmucosal fentanyl was more effective than morphine sulfate immediate release in treating breakthrough pain. Darwish et al.[140] conducted a phase 1 open-label study to investigate the absorption profile of fentanyl buccal tablets in patients with or without oral mucositis. Sixteen patients (50% with oral mucositis), received a single 200 mcg dose of fentanyl buccal tablet, which was well tolerated and showed a similar absorption profile within both groups. Transdermal fentanyl has also shown to be an effective, convenient, and well-tolerated treatment in patients with oral mucositis pain in the RT and the HSCTsetting.[141,142]

Topical morphine for mucositis-related pain was evaluated in a sample of 26 patients following chemoradiation for head and neck cancer.[142] Patients were randomized to morphine mouthwash (1 mL 2% morphine solution) or magic mouthwash (equal parts of lidocaine, diphenhydramine, and magnesium aluminum hydroxide). Patients in the morphine group demonstrated both significantly shorter duration and lower intensity of oral pain than the magic mouthwash group. Swisher et al.[143] described an oral mucositis pain management algorithm to promote symptom management for HSCT patients who are transitioning from inpatient to ambulatory care. A key component of this successful program was the availability of a multidisciplinary team who could respond to the report of oral pain. At present, no standard treatment has been defined for the prevention or treatment of oral mucositis–related pain, and, therefore, it is essential to continue studies of the treatments already available and to develop promising new approaches. Other agents that are currently under investigation or have shown some potential in the management of oral mucositis–related oral pain are sublingual methadone, transdermal buprenorphine, and ketamine mouthwash.[144–146]

Xerostomia

Xerostomia is a major negative sequela for patients who receive RT to the head and neck. The severity of xerostomia depends on the radiation dosage, location, and volume of exposed salivary glands. Significant xerostomia has not been shown as a sequela in patients treated with CT alone. The degree of xerostomia is reported subjectively by both patients and clinicians and can affect oral comfort, fit of prostheses, speech, and swallowing. Many of the enzymes (mucin) found in patients who experience xerostomia contribute to the growth of caries-producing organisms. Oral hygiene regimens that include the use of water/saline and daily fluoride application along with brushing teeth at least three times daily may reduce colonization and proliferation of oral pathogens.

Treatment guidelines for the management of xerostomia have been designed to increase patient's comfort.[147] Sialagogues have been investigated as stimulants for the residual salivary parenchyma (pilocarpine, 5- and 10-mg doses), and subjective improvement has been reported in some patients.[148] However, extreme caution with the use of pilocarpine is warranted because of reported side effects of glaucoma and cardiac problems. A randomized, controlled trial tested the efficacy of amifostine in a sample of 315 patients with head and neck cancer.[149] The patients received standard fractionated radiation with or without amifostine, administered at 200 mg/m^2 as a 3-minute intravenous infusion 15 to 30 minutes before each fraction of radiation. Patient eligibility criteria required that the radiation field encompassed at least 75% of both parotid glands. The Radiation Therapy Oncology Group Acute and Late Morbidity Score and Criteria was used to rate the severity of xerostomia. The incidence of grade 2 or higher acute xerostomia (90 days from the start of radiotherapy) and late xerostomia (9 to 12 months after radiotherapy) was significantly reduced in patients receiving amifostine. Whole saliva collection 1 year following RT showed that in the amifostine group, more patients produced 0.1 g of saliva (72% vs. 49%) and that the median saliva production was greater (0.26 g vs. 0.1 g). Stimulated saliva collections showed no difference between the treatment arms. Supporting these improvements in saliva production were the patients' reports of oral dryness. Artificial saliva, which usually uses carboxymethylcellulose as a base, has not demonstrated increased oral cavity comfort. Patients have reported subjective improvement in comfort levels through the frequent use of sugarless gum, mints, or candies.

Selected References

The full list of references for this chapter appears in the online version.

2. National Institutes of Health Consensus Development Panel. Consensus statement: oral complications of cancer therapies. *NCI Monogr* 1989;9:3.

4. Elting LS, Keefe DM, Sonis ST, et al. Patient-reported measurements of oral mucositis in head and neck cancer patients treated with radiotherapy with or without chemotherapy. *Cancer* 2008;113:2704.

8. Grazziutti ML, Dong L, Miceli MH, et al. Oral mucositis in myeloma patients undergoing melphalan-based autologous stem cell transplantation:

incidence, risk factors and a severity predictive model. *Bone Marrow Transplant* 2006;38:501.
10. Blijlevens N, Schwenkglenks M, Bacon P, et al. Prospective oral mucositis audit: oral mucositis in patients receiving high-dose melphalan or BEAM conditioning chemotherapy—European Blood and Marrow Transplantation Mucositis Advisory Group. *J Clin Oncol* 2008;26:1519.
11. Sonis ST. Oral complications of cancer therapy. In: DeVita VT, Hellman S, Rosenberg SA, eds. *Cancer: principles and practice of oncology.* 4th ed. Philadelphia: JB Lippincott, 1993:2385.
12. Sonis ST. Mucositis as a biological process: a new hypothesis for the development of CT-induced stomatotoxicity. *Oral Oncol* 1998;34:39.
14. McCann S, Schwenkglenks M, Bacon P, et al. The prospective oral mucositis audit: relationship of severe oral mucositis with clinical and medical resource use outcomes in patients receiving high-dose melphalan or BEAM-conditioning chemotherapy and autologous SCT. *Bone Marrow Transplant* 2009;43:141.
15. Vera-Llonch M, Oster G, Ford CM, et al. Oral mucositis and outcomes of allogeneic hematopoietic stem-cell transplantation in patients with hematologic malignancies. *Support Care Cancer* 2007;15:491.
19. Murphy BA, Beaumont JL, Isitt J, et al. Mucositis-related morbidity and resource utilization in head and neck cancer patients receiving radiation therapy with or without chemotherapy. *J Pain Symptom Manage* 2009;38: 522.
24. Sonis ST. The pathobiology of mucositis. *Nat Rev Cancer* 2004;4:277.
25. Sonis ST, O'Donnell KE, Popat R, et al. The relationship between mucosal cyclooxygenase-2 (COX-2) expression and experimental radiation-induced mucositis. *Oral Oncol* 2004;40:170.
26. Lalla RV, Pilbeam CC, Walsh SJ, et al. Role of the cyclooxygenase pathway in chemotherapy-induced oral mucositis: a pilot study. *Support Care Cancer* 2010;18:95.
27. Logan RM, Gibson RJ, Sonis ST, Keefe DM. Nuclear factor-κB (NF-κB) and cyclooxygenase-2 (COX-2) expression in the oral mucosa following cancer CT. *Oral Oncol* 2007;43:395.
28. Fall-Dickson JM, Ramsay ES, Castro K, et al. Oral mucositis–related oropharyngeal pain and correlative tumor necrosis factor-α expression in adult oncology patients undergoing hematopoietic stem cell transplantation. *Clin Ther* 2007;29:2547.
29. Avivi I, Avraham S, Koren-Michowitz M, et al. Oral integrity and salivary profile in myeloma patients undergoing high-dose therapy followed by autologous SCT. *Bone Marrow Transplant* 2009;43:801.
31. Pavletic SZ, Martin P, Lee SJ, et al. Measuring therapeutic response in chronic graft-versus-host-disease: National Institutes of Health Consensus Development Project on Criteria for Clinical Trials in Chronic Graft-versus-Host Disease: IV. Response criteria working group report. *Biol Blood Marrow Transplant* 2006;12:252.
34. Treister NS, Cook EF, Antin J, et al. Clinical evaluation of oral chronic graft-versus-host disease. *Biol Blood Marrow Transplant* 2008;14:110.
35. Imanguli MM, Swaim WD, League SC, et al. Increased T-bet+ cytotoxic effectors and type interferon-mediated processes in chronic graft-versus-host disease of the oral mucosa. *Blood* 2009;113:3620.
36. Fall-Dickson JM, Mitchell SA, Marden S, et al. Oral symptom intensity, health-related quality of life, and correlative salivary cytokines in adult survivors of hematopoietic stem cell transplantation with oral chronic graft-versus-host disease. *Biol Blood Marrow Transplant* 2010;16(7):948.
38. Fall-Dickson JM, Mock V, Berk RA, et al. Stomatitis-related pain in women with breast cancer undergoing autologous hematopoietic stem cell transplant. *Cancer Nurs* 2008;31:452.
39. Schubert MM, Williams BE, Lloid ME, et al. Clinical scale for the rating of oral mucosal changes associated with bone marrow transplantation. Development of an oral mucositis index. *Cancer* 1992;69:2469.
43. Imanguli MM, Atkinson JC, Mitchell SA, et al. Salivary gland involvement by chronic graft-versus-host disease: prevalence, clinical significance and recommendations for evaluation. *Biol Blood Marrow Transplant* 2010;16 (10):1362.
45. Berger AM, Kilroy, TJ. Oral complications. In: DeVita VT, Hellman S, Rosenberg SA, eds. *Cancer: principles and practice of oncology.* 6th ed. Philadelphia: JB Lippincott, 1997:2714.
48. U.S. Department of Health and Human Services. Cancer Therapy Evaluation Program, *Common terminology criteria for adverse events*, version 3.0. Washington, DC: U.S. Department of Health and Human Services, National Cancer Institute, June 10, 2003.
50. World Health Organization. *WHO handbook for reporting results of cancer treatment.* Offset publication No. 48. Geneva: World Health Organization, 1979:15.
51. Schubert MM, Sullivan KM, Morton TH, et al. Oral manifestations of chronic graft-versus-host disease. *Arch Intern Med* 1984;144:1591.
52. McGuire DB, Peterson DE, Muller S, et al. The 20 item oral mucositis index: reliability and validity in bone marrow and stem cell transplant patients. *Cancer Invest* 2002;20:893.
53. Sonis ST, Eilers JP, Epstein JB, et al. Validation of a new scoring system for the assessment of clinical trial research of oral mucositis induced by radiation or CT. *Cancer* 1999;85:2103.
54. Sonis ST, Oster G, Fuchs H, et al. Oral mucositis and the clinical and economic outcomes of hematopoietic stem-cell transplantation. *J Clin Oncol* 2001;19:2201.
59. Rubenstein EB, Peterson DE, Schubert M, et al. Clinical practice guidelines for the prevention and treatment of cancer therapy-induced oral and gastrointestinal mucositis. *Cancer* 2004;100:2026.
65. Sasse AD, Clark LG, Sasse EC, et al. Amifostine reduces side effects and improves complete response rate during radiotherapy: results of a meta-analysis. *Int J Radiat Oncol Biol Phys* 2006;64:784.
66. Spencer A, Horvath N, Gibson J, et al. Prospective randomised trial of amifostine cytoprotection in myeloma patients undergoing high-dose melphalan conditioned autologous stem cell transplantation. *Bone Marrow Transplant* 2005;35:971.
71. Peterson DE, Jones JB, Pettit RG. Randomized, placebo-controlled trial of safaris for prevention and treatment of oral mucositis in breast cancer patients receiving anthracycline-based chemotherapy. *Cancer* 2007;109:322.
72. Aquino VM, Harvey AR, Garvin JH, et al. A double-blind randomized placebo-controlled study of oral glutamine in the prevention of mucositis in children undergoing hematopoietic stem cell transplantation: a pediatric blood and marrow transplant consortium study. *Bone Marrow Transplant* 2005;36:611.
80. Epstein JB, Silverman S, Paggiarino DA, et al. Benzydamine HCl for prophylaxis of radiation-induced oral mucositis: results from a multicenter, randomized, double-blind, placebo-controlled clinical trial. *Cancer* 2001;92:875.
82. Leborgne JH, Leborgne F, Zubizarreta E, et al. Corticosteroids and radiation mucositis in head and neck cancer: a double-blind placebo-controlled randomized trial. *Radiother Oncol* 1998;47:145.
85. Wu HG, Song SY, Kim YS, et al. Therapeutic effect of recombinant human epidermal growth factor (RhEGF) on mucositis in patients undergoing radiotherapy, with or without chemotherapy, for head and neck cancer: a double-blind, placebo-controlled prospective phase 2 multi-institutional clinical trial. *Cancer* 2009;115:3699.
87. Sonis ST, Costa JW Jr, Evitts SM, et al. Effect of epidermal growth factor on ulcerative mucositis in hamsters that receive cancer CT. *Oral Surg Oral Med Oral Pathol* 1992:74:749.
88. Gabrilove JL, Jakubowski A, Scher H, et al. Effect of granulocyte colony-stimulating factor on neutropenia and associated morbidity due to CT for transitional-cell carcinoma of the urothelium. *N Engl J Med* 1988;318: 1414.
94. Ryu JK, Swann S, LeVeque F, et al. The impact of concurrent granulocyte macrophage-colony stimulating factor on radiation-induced mucositis in head and neck cancer patients: a double-blind placebo-controlled prospective phase III study by Radiation Therapy Oncology Group 9901. *Int J Radiat Oncology Biol Phys* 2007;67:643.
97. Nasilowska-Adamska B, Rzepecki P, Manko J, et al. The significance of palifermin (Kepivance) in reduction of oral mucositis (OM) incidence and acute graft versus host disease (aGVHD) in a patient with hematological disease undergoing HSCT. *Blood* 2006;108:840.
98. Nasilowska-Adamska B, Rzepecki P, Manko J, et al. The influence of palifermin (Kepivance) on oral mucositis and acute graft versus host disease in patients with hematological diseases undergoing hematopoietic stem cell transplantation. *Bone Marrow Transplant* 2007;40:983.
100. Brizel DM, Murphy BA, Rosenthal DI, et al. Phase II study of palifermin and concurrent chemoradiation in head and neck squamous cell carcinoma. *J Clin Oncol* 2008;26:2489.
105. Sorensen JB, Skovsgaard T, Bork E, et al. Double-blind, placebo-controlled, randomized study of chlorhexidine prophylaxis for 5-fluorouracil-based chemotherapy-induced oral mucositis with nonblinded randomized comparison to oral cooling (cryotherapy) in gastrointestinal malignancies. *Cancer* 2008;112:1600.
114. Bensadoun RJ, Ciais G. Radiation- and chemotherapy-induced mucositis in oncology: results of multicenter phase III studies. *J Oral Laser Appl* 2002;2:115.
117. Schubert MM, Eduardo FP, Guthrie KA, et al. A phase III randomized double-blind placebo-controlled clinical trial to determine the efficacy of low level laser therapy for the prevention of oral mucositis in patients undergoing hematopoietic cell transplantation. *Support Care Cancer* 2007;15:1145.
121. Mangoni M, Yue X, Morin C, et al. Differential effect triggered by a heparin mimetic of the RGTA family preventing oral mucositis without tumor protection. *Int J Radiat Oncol Biol Phys* 2009;74:1242.
122. Imanguli M, Pavletic SZ, Guadagnini JP, Brahim JS, Atkinson JC. Chronic graft versus host disease of oral mucosa: review of available therapies. *Oral Surg Oral Med Oral Pathol Oral Radiol Endod* 2006;101:175.
147. Atkinson JC, Grisius M, Massey W. Salivary hypofunction and xerostomia: diagnosis and treatment. *Dent Clin North Am* 2005;49:309.
149. Brizel DM, Wasserman TH, Strnad V, et al. Final report of a phase III randomized trial of amifostine as a radioprotectant in head and neck cancer. Proceedings of the American Society for Therapeutic Radiology and Oncology 41st Annual Meeting. *Int J Red One Biol Phys* 1999, San Antonio, Texas, Oct. 31–Nov. 4, Texas. (abst).

CHAPTER 162 PULMONARY TOXICITY

DIANE E. STOVER AND ROBERT J. KANER

Pulmonary disease can be caused by a wide spectrum of pathogenetic mechanisms in patients with cancer. These include a variety of infectious agents and neoplastic disorders as well as pulmonary thromboembolic disease, pulmonary hemorrhage, pulmonary edema (cardiogenic and noncardiogenic), and leukocyte agglutinin reactions. Pulmonary toxicity caused by antineoplastic agents is being recognized more frequently, and the number of drugs known or suspected to cause lung disease is steadily increasing. Because continuing the offending agent may cause death and because withholding the agent may result in resolution of the pulmonary toxicity, it is important to recognize radiation- and drug-induced pulmonary disease. In this first section parenchymal lung disease caused by irradiation and chemotherapy is discussed. Mechanisms of lung injury, histopathologic findings, clinical and laboratory features, diagnosis, and treatment of the abnormalities produced by these agents are reviewed.

RADIATION-INDUCED PULMONARY TOXICITY

Mechanism of Lung Injury

Radiation can affect dividing and nondividing cells and can cause genetic and nongenetic damage. In the lung, a hypothetical reconstruction of radiation injury might be as follows.[1] Therapeutic radiation may result in nongenetic damage that is apparent in all cells, but capillary endothelial and type I cells (epithelial lining cells) appear most susceptible. Many of these cells, whether dividing or not, undergo early necrobiosis and slough. The apoptotic pathway appears to be an important mechanism of cellular destruction after radiation. Specific signal transduction pathways are activated by radiation, including sphingomyelin hydrolysis, which generates ceramide as a second messenger and leads to apoptotic DNA degradation. Nonlethal ionizing radiation also activates a stress response in cells, which leads to up-regulation of specific nuclear transcription factors such as nuclear factor κB and transcription of specific early-response genes such as *c-abl, c-jun, egr-1*, and *c-fos*. This cellular activation initiates a repair process that involves cytokines and growth factors, such as basic fibroblast growth factor, vascular endothelial growth factor, and platelet-derived growth factor, as well as tumor necrosis factor-α, interleukin-1, and transforming growth factor-β (TGF-β).

Prostaglandin synthesis is also up-regulated. Over time, capillaries regenerate, and the alveolar epithelium is repopulated by type II cells (surfactant-producing cells) because type I pneumocytes do not regenerate. Some of these type II cells redifferentiate into type I cells. In some animal models, bone marrow–derived stem cells also contribute to repopulation of the alveolar epithelium after radiation. If the initial injury is severe, damage to extracellular matrix components of the lung, such as basement membrane glycoproteins and proteoglycans, takes place. Consistent with this concept, ionizing radiation to lung epithelial cells *in vitro* stimulates production of matrix metalloproteinase, an enzyme capable of degrading the type IV basement membrane collagen.[2] This can impede reconstruction of the delicate three-dimensional structure of the alveolar-capillary unit and result in functional derangement and scar formation, even if the cellular components are able to regenerate. Additionally, extracellular matrix fragments generated by the activity of matrix metalloproteinases are chemotactic for neutrophils.

Genetic damage to dividing cells, such as endothelial cells or type II pneumocytes, can also occur. Depletion of these cells may result during successive mitoses, causing a loss of integrity of pulmonary capillaries and exudation of fluid into the alveoli. At the physiologic level, loss of compliance, abnormal gas exchange, and respiratory failure can occur as a result of leakage of plasma proteins into the alveolar space. This type of genetic damage may also explain why pneumonitis can happen so late after radiation. One might speculate that some endothelial cells initially remain normal but that in the course of the next four cell divisions, chromosomal aberrations prevent further reduplication, which leads to loss of integrity of the capillary. Alternatively or concurrently, a cellular infiltrate is observed in bronchoalveolar lavage fluid and lung tissue, which is interpreted as an inflammatory response to the radiation injury. In experimental animal models, systemic administration of corticosteroids can suppress this inflammatory response, yet does not abrogate the subsequent development of chronic fibrosis. Based on these pathophysiologic considerations, animal studies suggest that lung gene transfer of constructs encoding several superoxide dismutase genes confers protection against radiation pneumonitis. Similar protective effects have been observed with systemic administration of competitive inhibitors of nitric oxide synthase. Inhibition of endothelial cell apoptosis by therapeutic administration of basic fibroblast growth factor or vascular endothelial growth factor has been beneficial in some animal models, but no human trials have been attempted.

Certain factors are critical to the development of classic radiation pneumonitis. In general, damage to the lung increases as the volume of lung tissue irradiated increases. A threshold effect also appears to occur, such that irradiation of at least 10% of the lung is required to produce significant pulmonary toxicity. This threshold may be reached in the treatment of some patients with breast cancer, depending on the specifics of their individualized treatment program. Also, the toxic effects of radiation as measured by symptoms and signs, radiographic changes, and physiologic tests are proportionate to the total amount delivered to the lung. Radiation pneumonitis seldom occurs with fractionated total doses of less than 20 Gy but is more likely when doses exceed 60 Gy. Because local control of lung cancer is greater when higher doses are delivered to the tumor, methods have been devised to give high doses to the target tissue while sparing normal surrounding lung. One such technique is called *stereotactic body radiotherapy*, which is a noninvasive treatment that delivers small highly focused radiation beams in potent doses of one to five treatments to tumor targets. Studies have suggested that local control with this modality is comparable to surgery with minimal morbidity.[3,4]

Besides the total radiation dose, the number of fractions into which it is divided, and, to a lesser extent, the time span over which it is delivered are important factors. The greater the number of fractions in which the radiation is given, the lower is the damaging effect. However, the incidence of radiation pneumonitis still exhibits a threshold effect and a steep sigmoidal dose-response curve. Fractionation is different from dose rate, which refers to output of the machine during radiation therapy. Dose rate certainly has an effect on lung tolerance: radiation delivered as 0.05 Gy/min is less damaging than radiation delivered at 0.3 Gy/min, which in turn is less damaging than radiation delivered at 2 to 3 Gy/min. The incidence and severity of radiation damage to the lungs are thus related principally to the volume of lung tissue irradiated, the total dose, the fractions into which the total dose is divided, and the quality of the radiation.

Taking all of these considerations into account, stereotactic body radiotherapy offers the best strategy to reduce the risk of radiation pneumonitis while improving local control of the cancer.[5] Advances in the technology of positron emission tomography scanning have improved its usefulness for diagnosis and staging of lung cancer. Combined positron emission tomography/computed tomography (CT) imaging offers some advantages in designing the radiation port and in detecting metastases not evident on CT, thus changing the intent of the radiotherapy from curative to palliative.[6,7] Genetic factors also influence the severity of response to lung irradiation in animals and presumably may do so in humans as well, although there is no current method to evaluate this clinically.

A new technology for the curative treatment of early-stage medically inoperable lung cancer and palliation of small pulmonary metastases called *radiofrequency ablation* is emerging. Radiofrequency ablation is a minimally invasive technique that is performed percutaneously, under conscious sedation and as an outpatient or with a short hospital stay. The complication rates are low and early outcomes are acceptable compared with more aggressive procedures. Pneumothorax and pleural effusions are the major complications; radiation pneumonitis has not been reported with this technique. Other technologies such as protein beam therapy are being evaluated.

Histopathology

The histopathologic changes of radiation-induced pulmonary toxicity can be divided into early, intermediate, and late stages based on the time course and intensity of the radiation injury. Early radiation damage (0 to 2 months after radiation) is characterized by injury to small vessels and capillaries, with the development of vascular congestion and increased capillary permeability. At this stage, a fibrin-rich exudate is present in the alveolar spaces. Hyaline membranes form on the alveoli, probably from condensation of the intra-alveolar fibrin. After 1 month, there is also an inflammatory infiltrate, which may lead to a second course of increased permeability. Abnormalities in the intermediate stage (2 to 9 months after radiation) are characterized by obstruction of pulmonary capillaries by platelets, fibrin, and collagen. Alveolar-lining cells (primarily type II pneumocytes) become hyperplastic, and the alveolar walls become infiltrated with fibroblasts and mast cells. If the radiation injury is mild, these changes may subside entirely; however, when the injury is severe, a chronic phase (9 months or more after radiation) ensues that may persist or progress for months or years. In animal models, there is marked activation of genes that encode fibrillar collagens. The histopathologic appearance is then dominated by dense fibrosis, thickening of the alveolar walls, vascular subintimal fibrosis, and luminal narrowing. In some instances, the lung may shrink to less than half its original size, with a thickened adherent pleura and scarred hilar structures.

In addition to this classic pattern of radiation pneumonitis, another syndrome of out-of-field pneumonitis, characterized by a hypersensitivity pneumonitis in areas of lung not directly radiated, has been described. This syndrome, which occurs in a minority of patients, is characterized by a bilateral lymphocytic alveolitis of activated CD4+ T lymphocytes 4 to 6 weeks after strictly unilateral lung irradiation.

Clinical Features

Signs and Symptoms

The clinical syndrome of radiation pneumonitis develops in 5% to 15% of patients receiving high-dose external-beam radiation for treatment of lung cancer. Factors that can add to the development of radiation pneumonitis include concomitant chemotherapy, previous irradiation, and withdrawal of steroids. No significant difference is seen in the incidence of radiation pneumonitis between the young and elderly, but the pneumonitis is inclined to be more severe in the latter. Underlying chronic obstructive pulmonary disease does not appear to potentiate radiation damage.

Symptoms of acute radiation pneumonitis usually become evident 2 to 3 months after the completion of therapy; rarely, they occur within the first month and occasionally as late as 6 months after irradiation.[8] In general, the early onset of symptoms implies a more serious and more protracted clinical course. The cardinal symptom of radiation pneumonitis is dyspnea. It may be self-limited or may progress to severe respiratory distress depending on the extent and intensity of the injury. Patients may also have a nonproductive cough or a cough productive of small amounts of pinkish sputum. Frank hemoptysis early in the clinical course is distinctly uncommon; however, massive hemoptysis has been reported as a late complication of therapeutic pulmonary irradiation. Fever is unusual but can be high and spiking; in severe cases, other constitutional symptoms may occur. Chest pain, which is rarely a prominent feature, may be the result of fractured ribs, pleural changes, or coughing. Symptoms of airway obstruction can occur in the first few days of radiation therapy and are usually associated with swelling of a central bronchogenic carcinoma. Severe respiratory distress can result and may be prevented by the administration of steroids the day before and several days after the initiation of radiation therapy. Hemoptysis and other manifestations of radiation pneumonitis may also occur in patients given palliative endobronchial brachytherapy or after surgical implantation of radioactive seeds.

On physical examination, signs of pulmonary involvement are minimal. Occasionally, moist rales, a pleural friction rub, or evidence of pleural fluid may be heard over the area of irradiation. In severe cases, tachypnea and cyanosis may be present, and occasionally evidence of acute cor pulmonale appears, usually predicting a fatal outcome. Finger clubbing due to radiation is distinctly unusual and, if present, is most likely caused by the underlying malignancy. Skin changes corresponding to the ports of irradiation are often present but provide no clue as to the presence or severity of the pulmonary reaction beneath.

Although patients with acute pneumonitis may show complete resolution of signs and symptoms, most develop gradual progressive fibrosis. In some cases, patients present with radiation fibrosis without a previous history of acute pneumonitis.

The permanent changes of fibrosis take 6 to 24 months to evolve but usually remain stable after 2 years. Patients with fibrosis can be asymptomatic or can have varying degrees of dyspnea. The major complications of radiation pneumonitis occur late in the disease and are secondary to persistent fibrosis of a large volume of lung. These include cor pulmonale and respiratory failure.

Diagnostic Imaging

Although radiographic abnormalities are invariably found at the time clinical radiation pneumonitis is present, these changes may be seen in asymptomatic patients as well. Early radiographic changes include a ground-glass opacification, diffuse haziness, or indistinctness of the normal pulmonary markings over the irradiated area. Later, the chest radiograph may show alveolar infiltrates or dense consolidation with or without air bronchograms. As the pneumonitis progresses to fibrosis, the radiographic appearance changes to that of linear streaks radiating from the area of pneumonitis and of contraction toward the hilar, the perimediastinal, or the apical areas. Pleural effusions, if present, are usually small and always coincident with the pneumonitis. They can persist for long periods but often disappear spontaneously and never increase during a period of stability unless secondary complications occur, such as radiation-induced pericarditis. Mediastinal or hilar adenopathy and cavitation are almost always due to causes other than radiation pneumonitis. Pneumothorax is occasionally associated with radiation fibrosis but not with acute pneumonitis.

One of the most characteristic features of radiation pneumonitis and fibrosis is that the radiologic changes are confined to the outlines of the field of radiation. In a few cases, extensive changes outside the field, even in the contralateral lung, have been observed. This syndrome of out-of-field pneumonitis is thought to represent a hypersensitivity response to the radiation. Other possible explanations for this phenomenon include obstruction of lymphatic flow from radiation-induced mediastinal fibrosis and absorption of x-rays by regions outside the irradiated ports.

Some data suggest that CT scans of the chest and gallium-67 citrate imaging are more sensitive than chest radiography in the detection of radiation changes. Correlation of abnormalities seen in these tests with the development of physiologic dysfunction and clinical toxicity needs clarification.

Pulmonary Function Tests

Prediction of changes in pulmonary function after high-dose irradiation to the lung has proven to be problematic.[9] No gross physiologic changes occur in the lung until 4 to 8 weeks after completion of irradiation, usually coincident with the period of clinical pneumonitis. Then one sees a decrease in lung volumes, which can progress. These changes persist indefinitely, with little evidence of recovery. Gas exchange abnormalities, which include a decrease in diffusing capacity and arterial hypoxemia, especially with exercise, occur at approximately the same time but show some tendency toward recovery after 6 to 12 months. A fall in compliance coincident with the clinical pneumonitis is seen in most subjects. Accordingly, the elastic work of breathing is increased, and dyspnea, resulting from the increased workload, ensues. Air-flow parameters remain close to normal in most studies.

Diagnosis

The diagnosis of radiation pneumonitis can sometimes be made clinically based on the timing of irradiation in relation to symptoms and the typical chest radiographic appearance (i.e., infiltrates corresponding to the margins of the irradiated portal).[9] Differentiation from recurrent malignancy or infection often poses a problem, and then lung biopsy is necessary. Although histopathologic changes are nonspecific for radiation pneumonitis, when elements of the acute stages (fibrin exudate in the alveoli) are seen adjacent to the more chronic stages (alveolar fibrosis and subintimal sclerosis), this entity can be diagnosed with reasonable certainty.Biochemical markers that indicate radiation lung injury before the onset of clinical pathologic events would be valuable in the early diagnosis and management of patients with radiation toxicity. In irradiated animals, studies demonstrate that alveolar epithelial cell proteins such as KL-6 or surfactant apoproteins in addition to endothelial soluble intercellular adhesion molecule-1 or TGF-β found in the serum may be markers for later radiation pneumonitis.

Treatment

Corticosteroid administration during irradiation in mice markedly improves the physiologic abnormalities and decreases mortality without an effect on late pulmonary fibrosis. No controlled clinical trials in humans are available on the efficacy of steroid therapy in radiation pneumonitis. Rubin and Casarett[10] collected data from eight studies on humans and categorized them according to whether corticosteroids were used prophylactically or therapeutically. Corticosteroids given prophylactically failed to prevent radiation pneumonitis, but when they were administered as clinical pneumonitis occurred, an objective response was seen. In other reports, steroid therapy failed to ameliorate severe pneumonitis. Nonetheless, it is the authors' practice to begin prednisone, 1 mg/kg, as soon as the diagnosis is reasonably certain. The initial dose is maintained for several weeks and then reduced cautiously and slowly. It has been the authors' experience that symptoms can be exacerbated if steroids are tapered too rapidly, necessitating higher doses for longer periods. Similarly, if corticosteroids are part of a recent chemotherapeutic regimen, stopping them abruptly can precipitate clinically evident radiation pneumonitis. What parameters, if any, to follow during the tapering schedule are not known, and no studies are available. Generally, the authors follow symptoms. Most authors agree that corticosteroids have no place in the treatment of radiation fibrosis.

Pentoxifylline has been found to have some beneficial effects on radiation pneumonitis by inhibiting platelet aggregation and tumor necrosis factor. In a recent randomized trial, pentoxifylline, given prophylactically to breast and lung cancer patients receiving irradiation, showed a significant protective effect on both the early and late lung radiotoxicity.[11]

Radiation-Related Bronchiolitis Obliterans with Organizing Pneumonia

Although bronchiolitis obliterans with organizing pneumonia (BOOP) is an unusual histopathologic pattern for cancer therapy–related lung injury, radiation damage resulting in BOOP has been reported.[12] Patients with lung cancer usually receive the highest doses of radiation to the largest volume of lung tissue, which makes them more susceptible to radiation pulmonary injury compared with other irradiated patients. Most of the cases of radiation-related BOOP, however, have occurred in patients receiving radiation treatment to the breast. Whether the low dose or indirect radiation that these patients receive makes them more susceptible to this type of lung injury is not known. Besides the unusual pathologic pattern in these patients, there are clinical and radiologic differences, compared with conventional radiation pneumonitis. Whereas dyspnea is the hallmark of radiation-induced pneumonitis, fever and cough are the predominant features of radiation-related

BOOP. Radiographically, the pulmonary infiltrates can begin in radiated areas as with radiation pneumonitis, but they always progress outside the portal, and in approximately 40% of cases, infiltrates were observed on the side contralateral to the irradiated breast. Although patients respond dramatically to corticosteroid therapy with no obvious evidence of residual damage, there is a 67% relapse rate when the drug is tapered or discontinued. Similar to conventional radiation-induced pneumonitis, there are no studies available on the minimal effective dose or duration of therapy, but in view of the high relapse rate, it seems prudent to taper corticosteroid therapy very slowly, with meticulous vigilance for clinical signs of relapse.

CHEMOTHERAPY-INDUCED PULMONARY TOXICITY

The list of chemotherapeutic agents reported to cause cytotoxic drug-induced lung disease continues to grow. Recently some monoclonal antibodies used in cancer treatment have been associated with lung injury, the most common of which is bevacizumab. It has been associated with pulmonary hemorrhage and thromboembolic disease especially in patients with squamous cell carcinoma of the lung.[13,14] Other classes of drugs added to the list include tyrosine kinase inhibitors and the mammalian target of rapamycin (m-Tor) inhibitors (Table 162.1). There are also scattered reports of lung injury with ifosfamide, irinotecan/topotecan, oxaliplatin, temozolomide, and thalidomide.[13,15–20] A summary of the mechanisms of lung damage, the pathologic findings, common clinical, radiographic and physiologic features, and the diagnosis and treatment of the more common chemotherapeutic drugs that cause pulmonary toxicity are discussed in this section (Table 162.1).

Mechanisms of Pulmonary Injury

Except for a few chemotherapeutic agents (e.g., bleomycin), the details of the pathophysiology of lung injury are unknown. Various mechanisms of pulmonary toxicity have been proposed, including a direct toxic effect on alveolar epithelial cells, the induction of an inflammatory immunologic response, and endothelial cell injury or activation causing capillary leak syndrome. These events result in clinical presentations referred to as *nonspecific interstitial pneumonitis/fibrosis*, *hypersensitivity pneumonitis syndrome*, and *noncardiogenic pulmonary edema*.

Certain cytotoxic drugs may induce pulmonary injury by triggering the formation of reactive oxygen metabolites, including superoxide anions, hydrogen peroxide, and hydroxyl radicals, primarily from activated neutrophils.[21] Bleomycin induces reactive oxygen radicals by forming a complex with Fe^{3+}. Consistent with a direct pathologic role for this mechanism, iron chelators ameliorate the pulmonary toxicity of bleomycin in animal models.[22] Reactive oxygen species can produce direct toxicity through participation in redox reactions and subsequent fatty acid oxidation, which leads to membrane instability.[23] Oxidants can cause other inflammatory reactions within the lung. For example, the oxidation of arachidonic acid is an initial step in the metabolic cascade that produces active mediators, including prostaglandins and leukotrienes.[24] Cytokines such as interleukin-1, macrophage inflammatory protein-1, monocyte chemoattractant protein-1, and TGF-β are released from alveolar macrophages in animal models of bleomycin toxicity resulting in fibrosis.[21,25,26] Damage or activation of alveolar epithelial cells may result in release of cytokines and growth factors that stimulate proliferation of myofibroblasts and secretion of a pathologic extracellular matrix leading to fibrosis, as has been proposed for the pathophysiology of idiopathic pulmonary fibrosis.

Cytotoxic drugs may also affect the local immune system. Because the lung is exposed to so many substances that can activate its immune system, there appears to be a pulmonary immune tolerance state to avoid overreactions.[27] This tolerance state in part may be a result of an effector and suppressor cell balance. Cytotoxic drugs can alter the normal balance, which then may cause tissue damage.[27] For example, lymphocytic alveolitis is a consistent finding in methotrexate pneumonitis, with an imbalance of the CD4-to-CD8 ratio.[28] As clinical improvement occurs, the ratio normalizes.

Other homeostatic systems within the lung can be affected as well, such as the balance between collagen formation and collagenolysis.[27] Through modulation of fibroblast proliferation, excessive interstitial and intraalveolar collagen deposition may result in severe, irreversible pulmonary fibrosis. Bleomycin is one cytotoxic agent that has this potential.[26] In addition, bleomycin may up-regulate collagen synthesis in fibroblasts by stimulating transcription directly through a TGF-β response element in the procollagen (I)α promoter as well as by an autocrine loop involving extracellular release of TGF-β.[29] Imbalance between the protease and antiprotease system has also been implicated in a number of pulmonary disorders, including drug toxicities.[27] Bleomycin and cyclophosphamide produce substances that can inactivate the antiprotease system, enhancing the effects of proteolytic enzymes on the lung. Bleomycin also causes profound effects on the fibrinolytic system, altering the balance between fibrin deposition and fibrinolysis on the alveolar surface, leading to fibrin deposition. Drugs may damage the lung through a variety of other mechanisms, and considerable investigation needs to be done to define and clarify the exact mechanism of lung injury for each chemotherapeutic drug.

One of the potential determinants of bleomycin toxicity is the bleomycin hydrolase, which is the major enzyme responsible for metabolizing bleomycin to a nontoxic molecule.[30] Interestingly, the two organs that are the most common targets for bleomycin toxicity (lung and skin) have the lowest levels of the enzyme. With the possibility of cloning the gene that encodes bleomycin hydrolase, studies are now needed to determine if genetic variability of this enzyme accounts for individual susceptibility or immunity to bleomycin pulmonary toxicity in humans, as it does in animals.[31–33]

Histopathology

The histopathologic changes of drug-induced pulmonary toxicity show common features. Similar to radiation-induced damage, abnormalities are seen in endothelial and epithelial cells. The vascular damage is characterized by endothelial swelling with exudation of fluid into the interstitium and the intra-alveolar spaces. Destruction and desquamation of type I pneumocytes occur, with delamellation and proliferation of type II pneumocytes. Mononuclear cell infiltration and fibroblast proliferation with fibrosis are common findings; the character of the inflammatory cellular infiltrate may be a feature that distinguishes the toxicity of one drug from another. Bronchoalveolar lavage studies in patients with methotrexate pulmonary toxicity have shown the presence of a T-lymphocytic alveolitis, whereas studies on some patients with bleomycin toxicity have revealed a polymorphonuclear alveolitis.[28,34] Eosinophil infiltration and granulomatous inflammation have been associated with drugs that cause apparent hypersensitivity reactions, such as methotrexate, procarbazine, and sometimes bleomycin.[27,28,30]

Clinical Features

Combination chemotherapy, concurrent radiation treatments, oxygen therapy, renal dysfunction, pre-existing pulmonary

TABLE 162.1

CHARACTERISTICS OF PULMONARY TOXICITY CAUSED BY COMMONLY USED CHEMOTHERAPEUTIC AGENTS

Drug (Ref.)	Mechanism of Injury	Histopathology	Clinical Features	Chest Radiograph/ CT Scan	Diagnosis	Treatment
ALKYLATING AGENTS						
Busulfan (Myleran) (27,35,39,47)	No studies, but direct toxicity to epithelial lining cells suggested.	Pneumocyte dysplasia (degeneration of type I cells; atypical hyperplastic type II cells), mononuclear cell infiltration; fibrosis.	4% incidence; no direct dose-dependent toxicity but may be threshold dose (>500 mg); radiation and other alkylating agents may enhance toxicity; insidious onset after 4 y (8 mo–10 y). May contribute to toxicity after bone marrow transplant. Dyspnea, cough, weight loss, weakness, fever; crepitant basilar rales; pigmentation.	Most common bibasilar reticular pattern; rarely, pleural effusion, pulmonary ossification, normal chest radiograph.	Suggested by history and bizarre pneumocytes in sputum or lavage fluid. Definitive diagnosis by open lung biopsy.	Withdrawal of the drug; anecdotal reports of improvement with high-dose steroids. Prognosis poor. Mean survival after diagnosis is 5 mo.
Cyclophosphamide (Cytoxan) (35,39,48)	May be toxic through production of reactive oxygen species.	Endothelial swelling; pneumocyte dysplasia; lymphocytic and histiocytic infiltration; fibrosis.	<1% incidence; no direct dose dependence; synergy with oxygen and other agents possible. Acute symptoms occur early in course; subacute or chronic up to 8 y after initiation of therapy. Cough, dyspnea, fever; basilar rales.	Commonly bibasilar reticular pattern; diffuse pulmonary edema pattern also reported	As above.	Drug withdrawal; corticosteroids may hasten improvement but have no documented effect on mortality. Overall recovery approximately 65%.
Chlorambucil (27,35,49)	Unknown	Similar to busulfan; ranges from reversible interstitial to fatal fibrosis.	Rare reports; subacute onset (5 mo–10 y) after therapy. Cough, dyspnea, anorexia; bibasilar rales.	Bibasilar reticular pattern; rarely, normal radiograph; alveolar infiltrates not reported.	As above.	Half of reported patients died despite cessation of drug and administration of steroids. Anecdotal reports of response to steroids.
Melphalan (Alkeran) (27,50)	Unknown	Similar to busulfan; pneumocyte dysplasia more common than fibrosis.	Rare; appears (1–48 mo) after therapy. Progressive dyspnea, productive cough, fever, malaise; bibasilar rales.	Reticular and alveolar infiltrates.	As above.	Despite cessation of drug, three of five patients died of disease. In most cases, patients were receiving steroids for underlying disease.

ANTIBIOTICS						
Bleomycin (21–27,29–38, 44)	Possible mechanisms include direct toxicity through generation of reactive oxygen metabolites and activated neutrophils; inflammation caused by alveolar macrophages producing TNF-α and IL-1β; increased collagen synthesis directly and via TGF-β release	Endothelial blebbing; interstitial edema, necrosis of type 1 cells and metaplastic type II cells; inflammation with polymorphonuclear cells; fibroblast proliferation and fibrosis; occasionally eosinophilic infiltration.	Incidence up to 10%; common risk factors: increasing age, higher doses, renal dysfunction, oxygen therapy, thoracic irradiation. Occurs during and up to 6 mo after stopping therapy. Cough, dyspnea, fever; tachypnea, crepitant rales. Hypersensitivity pneumonitis variant.	Bibasilar reticular pattern; multiple nodules similar to metastatic disease; acinar pattern, especially with hypersensitivity reaction; rarely, localized infiltrate and cavitary nodules.	Bronchoalveolar lavage (BAL) might suggest diagnosis (polymorphonuclear alveolitis). Transbronchial or open lung biopsy required for diagnosis, especially to rule out other causes.	Drug withdrawal. Hypersensitivity reactions, definite role for steroids; in other forms of bleomycin toxicity, efficacy less clear. Mortality between 3% and 50%.
Mitomycin (27,35,41,51)	Endothelial injury by alkylation of DNA; alveolar macrophage activation and cytokine release.	Several patterns: similar to bleomycin; capillary leak with alveolar damage (especially with vinca alkaloid); capillary leak with thrombotic microangiopathy (related to total dose).	3%–14% incidence; usually not dose-related but possible synergy with oxygen, radiotherapy, and other agents. Dry cough, dyspnea; fever not seen; bibasilar rales. Acute dyspnea reaction with vinca alkaloids.	Diffuse interstitial and/or alveolar infiltrates; may be normal.	Clinical picture suggestive; lung biopsy for definitive diagnosis.	Drug withdrawal; steroids may alter outcome. Mortality between 14% and 50%.
Nitrosoureas[a]						
Carmustine (BCNU) (27,35–40)	Few studies; direct injury through generation of toxic oxidant molecules, perhaps due to depletion of the antioxidant glutathione.	Similar to bleomycin; fibrosis predominates.	20%–30% incidence; dose-related; increased risk with pre-existing lung disease and tobacco use; possible synergism with other agents; can be seen up to 17 y after drug stopped. Dry cough, dyspnea, bibasilar rales.	Bibasilar reticular pattern; >10-y posttreatment peripheral fibrosis pattern in upper lung zones; may be normal.	Lung biopsy for definitive diagnosis; no BAL studies reported.	Recognition and withdrawal of the drug; steroids not beneficial if patient already taking steroids for intracranial processes when toxicity develops. Mortality reported between 24% and 90%. Prognosis worse if patient treated before age 5 y. Steroids possibly beneficial acutely, after high-dose treatment.

(*continued*)

TABLE 162.1

(CONTINUED)

Drug (Ref.)	Mechanism of Injury	Histopathology	Clinical Features	Chest Radiograph/ CT Scan	Diagnosis	Treatment
ANTIMETABOLITES						
Methotrexate (27,28,35,52)	Direct toxic effect may play a role but mechanism not known; hypersensitivity suggested by occurrence of eosinophils and presence of increased T lymphocytes in lavage fluid	Interstitial and alveolar infiltration of lymphocytes, eosinophils, and plasma cells; occasionally poorly formed, noncaseating granuloma; fibrosis unusual.	2%–8% incidence; synergism with other agents possible; occurs usually days to weeks after beginning therapy; acute: fever, chills, cough, malaise, headache; subacute: dyspnea, cough; rales common. Skin rash in 17% and blood eosinophilia in 40%; progression to fibrosis in 10%.	Early interstitial infiltrates; later, alveolar infiltrates; hilar and mediastinal adenopathy, pleural effusions described; chest radiograph can be normal.	Clinical history suggestive; BAL might suggest diagnosis (increased T cells in fluid), but lung biopsy required for diagnosis.	Discontinue drug, but reports of reinstitution without recurrence of the abnormality. Dramatic responses to steroids reported. Mortality 1%; outlook favorable.
Cytosine arabinoside (53)	Unknown	Pulmonary edema; proteinaceous exudate with extravasation of red blood cells, no inflammatory cells.	Abrupt onset of dyspnea; gastrointestinal toxicity coexists.	Diffuse interstitial and alveolar pattern.	Clinical picture suggests diagnosis.	Supportive; no studies.
Gemcitabine (54,55,60)	—	Rare reports of diffuse alveolar damage; findings resemble ARDS.	Does not appear dose-dependent; dyspnea may be severe and progress to respiratory failure, chest tightness; dry cough, fine rales, low-grade fever.	Reticular nodular infiltrates or ground-glass opacities.	Clinical suspicion; other causes should be excluded.	Withdraw drug; usually brisk response to corticosteroids but fatalities reported.
Fludarabine (56)	—	Rare reports of granulomas; diffuse nonspecific inflammation.	Hypoxia, fever; produces decreases in CD4 cells.	Interstitial or nodular infiltrates	Associated with *Pneumocystis* so must rule out infection.	Discontinue drug; probable response to steroids.
TAXANES						
Paclitaxel (Taxol) (35,57–59)	Two types of reaction: "anaphylactoid hypersensitivity" (AH), direct mast-cell activation with histamine release; suspension vehicle (Cremophor El) causes, not the drug.	No data	AH: 3%–10% incidence; erythematous rash, urticaria, hypotension, dyspnea with or without bronchospasm in close proximity to infusion; rare reports and little data; no dose dependency known.	AH: normal chest radiograph.	AH: clinical picture highly suggestive.	AH: slow infusion; pretreatment with corticosteroid; H_1 and H_2 histamine blockers.

	Hypersensitivity pneumonitis (HP) mechanism not known, may be due to release of histamine or other vasoactive.	Little data; BAL Lymphocytic alveolitis; biopsy mononuclear cells with septal thickening.	HP: dyspnea and/or cough several days to weeks after treatment; fever may occur; crepitant rales or normal chest exam.	HP: patchy reticular or nodular infiltrates.	HP: clinical picture should raise suspicion; other causes (e.g., infection, progression of disease) should be excluded.	HP: can resolve on its own; if severe, corticosteroids; may not recur with rechallenge.
Docetaxel (Taxotere) (35,60,61)	—	Little data; diffuse alveolar damage.	Rare reports; fever, malaise, dyspnea.	Diffuse infiltrates	Clinical suspicion excludes other causes, especially infection.	Of four reported cases two patients died; two recovered with steroids.
TYROSINE KINASE INHIBITORS						
Epidermal Growth Factor Receptor (EGFR) Inhibitors						
Gefitinib/Erlotinib (Iressa/Tarceva) (35,62–67)	Unclear mechanism but augmentation of pulmonary fibrosis by decreasing EGFR phosphorylation resulting in a decrease in regenerative epithelial proliferation is a possibility.	Diffuse alveolar damage with hyaline membrane formation; interstitial inflammation with or without fibrosis, organizing pneumonia alveolar hemorrhage.	.3%–.8% incidence of lung toxicity in whites (higher in Asians, 2%–6%); usually occurs in first month; underlying pulmonary fibrosis significant risk factor; dyspnea with/without cough and fever sometimes progressing to respiratory failure.	Ground-glass opacities with or without airspace consolidation similar in both.	Diagnosis of exclusion; new or progressive symptoms of cough, dyspnea or fever should prompt diagnostic evaluation to exclude other causes such as progression of cancer or infection.	Discontinue the drug; steroids; small series report high mortality rate
Inhibitors of Kit/BCR-ABL Tyrosine Kinases						
Imatinib/Dasatinib (68–71)	Unknown but in one case of imatinib Hypersensitivity suggested by high number of lymphocytes with low CD4/CD8 ratio	Exudative pleural effusion/pulmonary edema; eosinophilic infiltration; interstitial inflammation/ fibrosis.	Low-grade fever; dry cough; dyspnea/with or without hypoxia.	Pleural effusions; ground glass; nodular opacities/ consolidation.	Clinical picture suggestive, especially if associated with pleural effusions; may see peripheral eosinophilia.	Discontinuation of drug; but most cases require steroids.

(*continued*)

TABLE 162.1

(CONTINUED)

Drug (Ref.)	Mechanism of Injury	Histopathology	Clinical Features	Chest Radiograph/ CT Scan	Diagnosis	Treatment
INHIBITORS OF MAMMALIAN TARGET OF RAPAMYCIN (M-TOR)						
Sirolimus (72–74)	Possibly may bind to plasma proteins evoking Th1 response and recruitment of an inflammatory response in lung.	Bronchiolitis obliterans organizing pneumonia lymphocytic alveolitis possibly a hypersensitivity response.	5%-15% incidence pneumonitis. Dyspnea, dry cough, fever, fatigue.	Air space consolidation; reticular and/or ground-glass opacities.	Risks factors include late switch to drug and/or renal impairment. Pulmonary symptoms and/or radiographic evidence of pneumonitis should raise suspicion.	Withdrawing the usually results in complete recovery.
Temsirolimus/ Everolimus (75–77)	As above	As above	.5%–5% incidence possibly higher (up to 25%). Dyspnea, cough, fatigue, fever.	Focal consolidation; ground-glass opacities.	Development of dyspnea and/or pneumonitis during therapy without other cause.	Withdrawal of drug recommended No data on effectiveness of steroids but recommended with severe or progressive symptoms.
MISCELLANEOUS						
Procarbazine (Matulane) (27,35)	Hypersensitivity	Mononuclear cell infiltration and scattered foci of eosinophils; fibrosis in one case.	Acute onset within hours to days of first dose. Nausea, fever, chills, arthralgias, urticaria, dry cough, and dyspnea. Blood eosinophilia.	Interstitial infiltrates; pleural effusion.	Clinical picture highly suggestive of diagnosis.	Rapid recovery after discontinuation of drug. Role of steroids not known.
Vinca alkaloids (vinblastine and vindesine) (27,41)	Unknown	Dysplasia of alveolar lining cells; interstitial and alveolar influx of inflammatory cells; fibrosis	Acute dyspnea during or shortly after the infusion, especially when given in combination with mitomycin. Wheezing may be prominent.	Diffuse interstitial and alveolar infiltrates with combination drugs; normal chest radiograph with vinca alkaloid alone	Clinical history suggests diagnosis.	Drug withdrawal; steroids probably beneficial. Prognosis poor if pulmonary infiltrates develop.
Etoposide (VP-16) (13,39)	Unknown	Alveolar hemorrhage	Case report of fatal toxicity after high-dose chemotherapy with bone marrow or stem cell transplant for breast cancer.	Interstitial and alveolar pattern; may be localized	Clinical picture suggestive.	Discontinue drug; some responses to steroids.

CT, computed tomography; TNF, tumor necrosis factor; IL, interleukin; TGF, transforming growth factor; ARDS, adult respiratory distress syndrome; Th1, T helper cell.
[a]Pulmonary toxicity has been reported with all other nitrosoureas, including lomustine (CCNU), semustine (methyl-CCNU), and chlorozotocin (DCNU).

TABLE 162.2

FACTORS ASSOCIATED WITH INCREASED RISK OF DRUG-INDUCED PULMONARY TOXICITY

Risk Factors	Drugs
Total dose	Bleomycin Carmustine
Advanced age	Bleomycin Carmustine Methotrexate
Oxygen therapy	Bleomycin Cyclophosphamide Mitomycin
Simultaneous or prior radiation therapy to lungs	Bleomycin Busulfan Mitomycin Gemcitabine
Increased toxicity when given with other drugs	Carmustine Mitomycin Cyclophosphamide Bleomycin Methotrexate Etoposide Gemcitabine Docetaxel
Pre-existing pulmonary disease	Carmustine
Renal dysfunction	Bleomycin

disease such as idiopathic pulmonary fibrosis, chronic obstructive pulmonary disease, radiation pneumonitis, extensive pulmonary metastases, and poor functional status and advanced age have been associated with increased pulmonary toxicity. Table 162.2 lists some of the drugs that have been associated with these predisposing factors.[27,35] Because bleomycin toxicity is relatively common, it deserves special mention. Although toxicity drastically increases with doses in excess of 450 to 500 mg, it can occur with much lower doses, especially when other risk factors are present. One study described 9 of 45 patients (20%) in whom lung toxicity developed when they received bleomycin after cisplatin infusion.[36] Renal damage after cisplatin administration, with subsequent accumulation of bleomycin, was a likely cause of the high pulmonary toxicity and mortality of 67%. Extreme caution is recommended in the administration of combined bleomycin and cisplatin chemotherapy; if possible, bleomycin should precede cisplatin infusion to minimize the risk. Some data suggest that continuous infusion of bleomycin may be associated with less pulmonary toxicity than bolus therapy; however, these data are inconclusive, and further studies are warranted.[27] Although supplemental oxygen has been a classic cofactor in bleomycin pulmonary toxicity, there are no large controlled studies.[27] An increased risk of pulmonary toxicity (4 of 12 patients, fatal in 3 of 4) was described in a small uncontrolled study of patients receiving granulocyte colony-stimulating factor in combination with bleomycin-containing chemotherapy (BACOP: bleomycin, doxorubicin, cyclophosphamide, vincristine, and prednisone) for non-Hodgkin's lymphoma.[37] Animal studies suggest that granulocyte colony-stimulating factor may enhance migration of neutrophils to vascular spaces and promote their adhesion to already injured endothelial cells potentiating proinflammatory cytokine expression.[38]

Interest in administration of several cycles of high-dose chemotherapy followed by peripheral stem cell rescue for treatment of breast cancer and lymphoma has led to reports of pulmonary toxicity for agents previously not thought to be highly toxic to the lung, such as etoposide.[39] Importantly, careful studies of pulmonary function after high-dose chemotherapy containing cyclophosphamide/cisplatin/BCNU (carmustine) followed by autologous bone marrow transplant for treatment of breast cancer show a delayed drop in diffusing capacity averaging 30% by week 18.[40] The majority of patients were symptomatic with dyspnea and responded well to systemic corticosteroids. More of this type of toxicity can be anticipated in the future as this treatment modality becomes more common and new regimens for high-dose chemotherapy are studied.

Long intervals between drug administration and onset of clinical toxicity have been described. Late-onset pulmonary fibrosis has been reported many years after cyclophosphamide and carmustine are discontinued.[27,35]

Signs and Symptoms

The cardinal symptom of drug-induced pulmonary toxicity is dyspnea. Nonproductive cough, fatigue, and malaise are other commonly associated complaints. Other characteristics of chemotherapy-induced pulmonary disease are outlined in Table 162.1. Although symptoms usually develop during a period of several weeks to months and sometimes years, hypersensitivity drug-induced lung disease can develop during a period of hours. Fever may be a common finding with this type of toxicity. Chest pain has been reported during infusion of bleomycin or immediately after therapy with methotrexate; however, it is an unusual manifestation of toxicity.[27,30] A syndrome of acute dyspnea, probably resulting from direct toxicity to the pulmonary vasculature, can occur during or shortly after vinca alkaloid infusion when given in combination with mitomycin for treatment of non–small cell lung cancer.[41] Because hemoptysis is an uncommon feature of drug-induced pulmonary toxicity, when it is present, other diagnoses should be considered. Physical examination of the lungs may be normal or may reveal end-inspiratory "Velcro" rales. Finger clubbing is distinctly unusual, but it may be related to the underlying malignancy.

All-*trans*-retinoic acid treatment of leukemias can induce the retinoic acid syndrome, which consists of fever; dyspnea; weight gain; pulmonary infiltrates; pleural or pericardial effusions, or both; hypotension; renal dysfunction; and leukocytosis.[42] The pulmonary disorder is thought to be mediated by newly differentiated leukemia cells marginating into the pulmonary circulation, increasing capillary permeability and releasing cytokines that induce neutrophil migration into the interstitium. High doses of corticosteroids are the most effective treatment, and steroid prophylaxis has been reported to be useful.

Diagnostic Imaging

The most common radiographic abnormality associated with drug-induced pulmonary toxicity is a reticulonodular or interstitial pattern, or both, which may be basilar or diffuse. Pleural effusions are uncommon but have occasionally been reported in association with mitomycin, busulfan, methotrexate, and procarbazine toxicity. Hypersensitivity lung disease associated with methotrexate and procarbazine may present with bilateral acinar infiltrates that clear rapidly.[27] In some instances, the chest radiograph is normal, even in the presence of histologically proven pulmonary infiltration and fibrosis.[27] Most commonly, methotrexate and carmustine toxicity have been reported, with normal chest radiographic findings. Hilar adenopathy is distinctly unusual and has been reported only with methotrexate toxicity.[27] Cavitating and noncavitating nodules, simulating metastatic disease, have been seen withbleomycin toxicity.[27]

High-resolution, thin-section CT chest scans and gallium scintigraphy have been shown to be more sensitive techniques than chest radiography to detect pulmonary parenchymal changes in association with drug toxicity. High-resolution chest CT scans can show diffuse areas of ground-glass opacities, poorly defined areas of nodular consolidation, and centrilobular nodules.[43] Although these changes can be seen when the radiograph is normal, they are not specific for drug-induced toxicity. Magnetic resonance spectrometry may eventually be useful to differentiate among fibrosis, edema, and hemorrhage in the lung, but at present it has not been helpful to diagnose interstitial lung disorders, including drug toxicity.

Pulmonary Function Tests

The most common abnormalities associated with chemotherapy-induced pulmonary toxicity are a reduced diffusing capacity for carbon monoxide and a restrictive ventilatory defect.[27] Isolated gas transport abnormalities manifested by a decrease in the diffusing capacity or arterial hypoxemia, or both, especially with exercise, have been seen. Screening pulmonary function tests to predict which patients receiving chemotherapy are likely to develop toxicity would be helpful but have not been established. In bleomycin toxicity, changes in the diffusing capacity may be transient, whereas decreases in total lung capacity seem to correlate better with radiographic abnormalities.[43,44]

Diagnosis

Although one might have a high clinical suspicion of drug-induced pulmonary toxicity, lung biopsy is usually necessary for a definitive diagnosis. Because pathognomonic pathologic changes associated with drug-induced pneumonitis are often not present, a biopsy is necessary to eliminate other specific diagnoses, such as opportunistic infection and malignancy. Through the use of bronchoalveolar lavage, several studies reported the presence of a characteristic or predominant cell associated with particular drugs.[28,32] Although these data might be of value in understanding the pathogenesis of drug-induced lung disorders, their usefulness in diagnosing drug toxicity is limited.

A serum marker for drug-induced pulmonary toxicity would be very useful, but none currently exists. Although elevated levels of TGF-β in plasma after high-dose chemotherapy for breast cancer predicted an increased risk of pulmonary toxicity after autologous bone marrow transplantation, its clinical applicability has been limited.[45]

Treatment

The most effective way to manage pulmonary toxicity associated with chemotherapeutic agents is to prevent it. Animal studies of bleomycin toxicity showed a beneficial preventive effect of dietary supplementation with taurine and niacin; no comparable human studies have been reported. If toxicity occurs, withdrawal of the offending agent is the cornerstone of therapy. Although no controlled studies in humans have systematically examined the efficacy of corticosteroids, a trial of these agents is probably warranted in most cases. The optimal dose and duration of therapy are not known; however, 1 mg/kg per day is usually initiated with a slow and careful tapering schedule because clinical deterioration after tapering has been reported. The use of lung transplant in the treatment of advanced drug-induced pulmonary fibrosis should be considered in appropriate patients. One report described the case of a 23-year-old male patient who underwent a single lung transplant because of presumed drug-induced pulmonary fibrosis 12 years after undergoing chemotherapy for acute lymphocytic leukemia.[46]

Selected References

The full list of references for this chapter appears in the online version.

3. Timmerman R, Paulus R, Galvin J, et al. Sterotactic body radiation therapy for inoperable early stage lung cancer. *JAMA* 2010;303:1070.
4. Fakiris AJ, McGarry RC, Yiannoutsos CT, et al. Stereotatic body radiation therapy for early stage non-small cell lung carcinoma: four year results of a prospective phase II study. *Int J Radiat Oncol Biol Phys* 2009;75:677.
8. McDonald S, Rubin P, Phillips TL, et al. Injury to the lung from cancer therapy: clinical syndromes, measurable endpoints, and potential scoring systems. *Int J Radiat Oncol Biol Phys* 1995;31:1187.
9. De Jaeger K, Seppenwoolde Y, Boersma LJ, et al. Pulmonary function following high-dose radiotherapy of non–small-cell lung cancer. *Int J Radiat Oncol Biol Phys* 2003;55:1331.
10. Rubin P, Casarett GW. *Clinical Radiation Pathology*. Philadelphia: WB Saunders, 1968.
11. Ozturk B, Egehan I, Atavci S, et al. Pentoxifylline in prevention of radiation induced lung toxicity in patients with breast and lung cancer; a double-blind randomized trial. *Int J Radiat Oncol Biol Phys* 2004;58:213.
12. Stover DE, Milite F, Zakowski M. A newly recognized syndrome—radiation related bronchiolitis obliterans and organizing pneumonia: a case report and literature review. *Respiration* 2001;68:540.
13. Vahid B, Marik P. Pulmonary complications of novel antineoplastic agents for solid tumors. *Chest* 2008;133:528.
14. Sandler AB, Schiller JH, Gray R, et al. Retrospective evaluation of the clinical and radiographic risk factors associated with severe pulmonary hemorrhage in first line advanced uresectable non-small cell lung cancer treated with Carboplatin and paclitaxel plus bevacizumab. *J Clin Oncol* 2009;27:3410.
15. Baker WJ, Fistel SJ, Jones RV, et al. Interstitial pneumonitis associated with ifosfamide therapy. *Cancer* 1990;65:2217.
16. Gagnadoux F, Roiron C, Carrie E, et al. Eosinophilic lung diseases under chemotherapy with oxaliplatin for colorectal cancer. *Am J Clin Oncol* 2002; 25:380.
17. Madarnas Y, Webster P, Shorter AM, et al. Irinotecan-associated pulmonary toxicity. *Anticancer Drugs* 2000;11:709.
18. Matland ML, Wilcox R, Hogarth DK, et al. Diffuse alveolar damage after a single dose of topotecan in a patient with pulmonary fibrosis and small cell cancer. *Lung Cancer* 2006;54:243.
19. Edgerton CC, Gilman M, Roth BJ. Topotecan-induced bronchiolitis. *South Med J* 2007;97:699.
20. Onozawa M, Hashino S, Sozobe S, et al. Side effects and good effects from new chemotherapeutic agents: case 2. Thalidomide-induced interstitial pneumonitis. *J Clin Oncol* 2005;23:2425.
26. Chandler DB. Possible mechanisms of bleomycin induced fibrosis. *Clin Chest Med* 1990;11:21.
27. Cooper JAD, White DA, Matthay RA. Drug-induced pulmonary disease. I. Cytotoxic drugs. *Am Rev Respir Dis* 1986;133:321.
28. White DA, Rankin JR, Stover DE, et al. Methotrexate pneumonitis: lavage findings suggest an immune mediated disorder. *Am Rev Respir Dis* 1989;139:18.
31. Ferrando AA, Pendas AM, Llano E, et al. Gene characterization, promoter analysis, and chromosomal localization of human bleomycin hydrolase. *J Biol Chem* 1997;272:33298.
34. White DA, Kris MG, Stover DE. Bronchoalveolar lavage cell populations in bleomycin-induced pulmonary toxicity. *Thorax* 1987;42:551.
35. Pulmonary toxicity associated with systemic antineoplastic therapy UptoDate. http://www.uptodate.com. Accessed September 2010.
37. Lei KI, Leung WT, Johnson PJ. Serious pulmonary complications in patients receiving recombinant granulocyte colony-stimulating factor during BACOP chemotherapy for aggressive non-Hodgkin's lymphoma. *Br J Cancer* 1994; 70:1009.
41. Rivera MP, Kris MG, Gralla RJ, et al. Syndrome of acute dyspnea related to combined mitomycin plus vinca alkaloid chemotherapy. *Am J Clin Oncol* 1995;18:245.
49. Khong AT, McCarthy J. Chlorambucil induced pulmonary disease: a case report and review of the literature. *Am Hematol* 1998;77:85.

51. Linette DC, McGee KH, McFarland JA. Mitomycin induced pulmonary toxicity: case report and review of the literature. *Ann Pharmacol Ther* 1992; 26:481.
52. Imokawa S, Colby TR, Leslie KO, Hemers RA. Methotrexate pneumonitis: review of the literature and histopathologic findings in nine patients. *Eur Respir J* 2000;15:373.
53. Haupt HM, Hutchins CM, Moore CW. Ara-C lung: noncardiogenic pulmonary edema complicating cytosine arabinoside therapy of leukemia. *Am J Med* 1981;70:256.
54. Gupta N, Ahmed I, Steinberg H, et al. Gemcitabine-induced pulmonary toxicity case report and review of the literature. *Am J Clin Oncol* 2002; 25:97.
56. Helman DL, Byrd JC, ales NC et al. Fludarabine-related pulmonary toxicity: a distinct clinical entity in chronic lymphoproliferative syndromes. *Chest* 2002;122:785.
57. Weiss RB, Donehower RC, Wiernik PH, et al. Hypersensitivity reactions from Taxol. *J Clin Oncol* 1990;8:1263.
58. Ramanathan RK, Reddy VU, Holbert JM, et al. Pulmonary infiltrates following administration of paclitaxel. *Chest* 1996;110:289.
60. Kouroussis C, Movroudis D, Kakolyris S, et al. High incidene of pulmonary toxicity of weekly docetaxel and gemcitabine in patients with non-small cell lung cancer: results of a dose-finding study. *Lung Cancer* 2004;44:363.
61. Read WL, Mortimer JE, Picus J. Severe interstitial pneumonitis associated with docetaxel administration. *Cancer* 2002;94:847.
62. Suzuki H, Aoshiba K, Yokohori N, et al. Epidermal growth factor receptor tyrosine kinase inhibition augments a murine model of pulmonary fibrosis. *Cancer Res* 2003;63:5054.
63. Okamoto I, Fujii K, Matsumoto M, et al. Diffuse alveolar damage after ZD1839 therapy in a patient with non-small cell lung cancer. *Lung Cancer* 2003;40:339.
65. Takano T, Ohe Y, Kusumoto M, et al. Risk factors for interstitial lung disease and predictive factors for tumor response in patients with advanced non-small cell lung cancer treated with gefitinib. *Lung Cancer* 2004;45:93.
66. Nagaria NC, Cogswell J, Choe JK, et al. Side effects and good effects from new chemotherapeutic agents: case 1. Gefibnib-induced insterstitial fibrosis. *J Clin Oncol* 2005;23:2423.
67. Vahid B, Esmaili A. Erlotinib-associated pneumonitis: report of two cases. *Can Respir J* 2007;14:167.
68. Lin JT, Yeh KT, Fang HY, et al. Fulminant, but reversible interstitial pneumonitis associated with imatinib mesylate. *Leuk Lymphoma* 2006;47:1693.
69. Grimison P, Goldstein D, Schneeweiss J, et al. Corticosteroid-responsive interstitial pneumonitis related to imatinib mesylate with successful rechallenge, and potential causative mechanisms. *Intern Med J* 2005;35:136.
71. Bergeron A, Bergot G, Vilela G, et al. Hypersensitivity pneumonitis related to imatinib mesylate. *J Clin Oncol* 2002;20:4271.
72. Champion L, Stern M, Israel-Biet D, et al. Brief communications: sirolimus-associated pneumonitis: 24 cases in renal transplant recipients. *Ann Intern Med* 2006;144:505.
73. Pham PT, Pham PC, Danovitch GM, et al. Sirolimus-associated pulmonary toxicity. *Transplantation* 2004;77:1215.
74. Chhajed PN, Dickenmann M, Bubendorf L, et al. Patterns of pulmonary complications associated with sirolimus. *Respiration* 2006;73:367.
75. Duran I, Sui LL, Oza AM, et al. Characteriztion of the lung toxicity of the cell cycle inhibitor temsirolimus. *Eur J Cancer* 2006;42:1875.
76. White DA, Schwartz LH, Dimitrijevic S, et al. Characterization of pneumonitis in patients with advanced non-small cell lung cancer treated with everolimus (RAD 001). *J Thor Oncol* 2009;4:1.
77. White DA, Camus P, Endo M, et al. Non-infectious pneumonitis after everolimus therapy in advanced renal cell carcinoma. *Am J Respir Crit Care Med* 010;182(10):396.

CHAPTER 163 CARDIAC TOXICITY

JOACHIM YAHALOM AND CAROL S. PORTLOCK

Ionizing radiation as well as many chemotherapeutic and biologic agents have been reported to have effects on the cardiovascular system.[1–4] The most important of these drugs (anthracyclines, mitoxantrone, cyclophosphamide, ifosfamide; paclitaxel, docetaxel; trastuzumab; 5-fluorouracil, capecitabine; and the tyrosine kinase inhibitors) will be discussed in detail. All others are listed in Table 163.1. The effects of radiotherapy on the cardiovascular system are detailed in the last part of this chapter.

ANTHRACYCLINES

There is both a rare but reversible acute cardiotoxicity, and a delayed but irreversible dilated cardiomyopathy with anthracycline therapy.[1,3] The acute toxicity presents as a myocarditis, with or without pericarditis, and may result in transient congestive heart failure (CHF)/arrhythmias. It is rarely a fatal complication of anthracycline therapy.

The delayed cardiomyopathy presents clinically as fatigue, dyspnea on exertion, orthopnea, sinus tachycardia, S3 gallop rhythm, pedal edema/pleural effusions, and elevated jugular venous distention. These classic features of CHF are late manifestations and may be quite subtle at onset. With awareness of the cardiac risk, anthracycline cardiomyopathy may be avoided by recognizing risk factors, early detection, limiting total cumulative dose, and more recently, using cardioprotective agents or modified/infusional drug regimens.

The risk of anthracycline cardiomyopathy depends on cumulative dose.[3] A 5% risk is seen at 400 to 450 mg/m^2 for doxorubicin, 900 mg/m^2 for daunorubicin, 800 to 935 mg/m^2 for epirubicin, and 223 mg/m^2 for idarubicin. Risk cofactors include mediastinal irradiation, older (>70 years) or younger (<15 years) age, coronary artery disease, other valvular or myocardial conditions, and hypertension. Concurrent trastuzumab appears to potentiate anthracycline cardiotoxicity (CD) and other agents that have independent cardiac effects may be additive.

CD diagnosis is generally made by comparing baseline with serial left ventricular function studies using radionuclide imaging and/or echocardiography. A left ventricular ejection fraction (LVEF) of 50% or more is considered within normal range by either method. A low LVEF is a contraindication for anthracycline therapy.

Echocardiograms can also evaluate other aspects of cardiac performance as well as anatomic changes. Typical findings are left ventricular diastolic dysfunction and, later, left ventricular systolic dysfunction, particularly affecting the septal motion. The left ventricle is initially not enlarged or only moderately enlarged; there may be a posteriorly directed mitral insufficiency jet and preservation of right ventricular function. With full development of cardiomyopathy, there is global hypokinesis and muscle wall thinning.

The electrocardiogram (ECG) findings associated with CD include sinus tachycardia, low voltage, poor R wave progression, and nonspecific T wave changes. Even sinus tachycardia alone is a relatively late finding, such that serial ECGs are of little value in early detection.

In pediatrics, it is important to be aware that conduction disturbances (second-degree atrioventricular block) and arrhythmias (both supraventricular and ventricular) may be detected during therapy, but have no known acute/chronic consequence; subclinical CD is probably more common than in adults at comparable doses (15.5% to 27.8% at more than 300 mg/m^2 doxorubicin); left ventricular fractional shortening is significantly reduced after doxorubicin and correlates with cumulative dose; although this may transiently improve, progressive loss of ventricular mass, reduced cardiac output, and restrictive cardiomyopathy are seen, and no threshold cumulative dose has been identified below which left ventricular dysfunction is not seen.[5–7]

Early detection of CD is important in preventing overt cardiomyopathy. In a small prospective study, Nousiainen et al.[8] reported that it was possible to distinguish patients likely to develop CD from others by LVEF measures at baseline and at 200 mg/m^2 doxorubicin. A fall of 10% or more at this low cumulative dose had 72% specificity and 90% sensitivity in detecting later CD. Mitani et al.[9] have examined the strategy of serial LVEF retrospectively and demonstrated that the overall costs of early detection were less than the medical costs of overt CHF management.

Serial diastolic pressures with gated radionuclide or echocardiogram function studies, serum cardiac troponin T levels (a measure of active myocardial myocyte necrosis), and levels of brain natriuretic peptide, a peptide synthesized in the ventricles correlate with degree of heart failure.[10] B-type natriuretic peptide levels and troponin T levels, appear to hold the greatest promise as these are simple plasma markers and may correlate with subclinical left ventricular diastolic dysfunction. Percutaneous endomyocardial biopsy of the right ventricle is rarely used.[10]

All patients should have a baseline measure of LVEF. For doxorubicin, poor-risk patients should have a repeat study at 200 mg/m^2, and all patients should have a follow-up study at 300 to 400 mg/m^2 and every 50 to 100 mg/m^2 thereafter.

Liposomal formulations[11,12] have been shown to permit higher cumulative anthracycline dosing and less CD at the same dose. Data remain limited, however, regarding tumor response and survival. The iron-chelating cardioprotectant dexrazoxane decreases the risk of clinical CD in patients who have received doxorubicin doses of 300 mg/m^2 or more.[13] The American Society of Clinical Oncology[14] recommends its use in this setting, but does not advocate dexrazoxane in the adjuvant setting, when doxorubicin cumulative dose is less than 300 mg/m^2, in pediatrics, or in high-risk patients. This organization also cautions against the use of dexrazoxane when doxorubicin

TABLE 163.1

OTHER CARDIOVASCULAR TOXICITIES

Drug	Incidence (%)	Cardiovascular Effects	Onset
Amsacrine	1	H, AR, VR, CHF	Acute, subacute
Arsenic trioxide	3–24	QT, VR	Acute
Bevacizumab	8–67; rare	HBP; CHF[a]	Acute, subacute
Bortezomib	2–5	CHF, H, QT	Acute, subacute
Busulfan	2	CHF	Late
Carmustine	Rare	H, AR, CP	Acute
Cisplatin	Rare	H, AR, VR, CP	Acute
Clofarabine	27	CHF, HBP, H	Acute, subacute
Cytarabine	Rare	AR, VR, CP, P, CHF	Acute, subacute
Dasatinib	<1–3	QT, CHF, HBP	Acute
Erlotinib	2.3	CP, MI	
Etoposide	1–2	H	Acute
	Rare	CP, MI	Acute
Gemcitabine	Rare	AR, CHF	Acute
Interferon	Rare	H, AR, CP, MI, CHF	Acute, subacute
Interleukin-2	Dose-dependent	H, AR, CP, MI	Acute, subacute
Lapatinib	Rare–16	QT	
Mechlorethamine	Rare	AR	Subacute
Mitomycin[a]	10	CHF	—
Nilotinib	1–10	QT	
Pentostatin	3–10	AR, VR, CP, MI, CHF	Subacute
Sorafenib	17–43	HBP	Acute, subacute
	2.7–3	CP, MI	
Sunitinib	5–47	HBP	Acute, subacute
	2.7–11	CHF, MI	
Teniposide	2	H	Acute
Tretinoin[b]	14–23	H, AR	Acute, subacute
	3–6	CP, MI, P, CHF	Acute, subacute
Vinca alkaloids	10; rare	H	Acute, subacute
		?MI	
Vorinostat	3.5–6	QT	

H, hypotension; AR, atrial arrhythmia; VR, ventricular arrhythmia; CHF, congestive heart failure; QT, prolonged QT; HBP, hypertension; CP, chest pain; P, pericarditis; MI, myocardial infarction.
[a]In association with anthracyclines.
[b]Retinoic acid syndrome.
(Data derived from refs. 1–4.)

therapy is anticipated to prolong survival. Clinical data are also insufficient to recommend dexrazoxane with other anthracyclines, except epirubicin in metastatic breast cancer. A pivotal study in pediatric acute lymphoblastic leukemia may serve to change these recommendations.[15] With a median follow-up of 5.7 years, this prospective trial revealed no significant impact on 5-year event-free survival while dexrazoxane reduced serial troponins during therapy. Late CD data from this trial is awaited.

The management of anthracycline CD is that of other causes of dilated cardiomyopathy.[1,10] Angiotensin-converting enzyme inhibitors, β-blockers, and diuretics are commonly used, but do not cure or permanently control CD. CD may progress in spite of these agents after more than 5 years. The only curative therapy at this time is cardiac transplantation.

The mechanism of anthracycline CD is not fully elucidated, but cardiomyocyte apoptosis is likely.[16] The production of free radicals generated during cardiomyocyte anthracycline metabolism results in membrane lipid peroxidation, with the consequent activation of the extrinsic and intrinsic apoptotic pathways. Free radicals are generated by enzymatic reduction of the anthracycline quinone ring and by formation of iron-anthracycline complexes. The intrinsic antioxidant defense of the cardiomyocyte is more limited than other organs, leading to its apparent selective toxicity profile. Miranda et al.[17] have reported a knockout mouse model suggesting that a deficiency of the *HFE* gene (associated with hereditary hemochromatosis) confers increased susceptibility to CD. They studied wild type, HFE (+/−), and HFE (−/−) mice that were chronically treated with doxorubicin. Survival was significantly decreased in the HFE-negative mice, and cardiac iron concentration was significantly elevated. Moreover, cardiac ultrastructural changes demonstrated iron-associated mitochondrial damage. A recent gene expression profile study in rats confirms the site of cardiac oxidative toxicity to be the cardiac cell mitochondria.[18]

Mitoxantrone

Mitoxantrone is an anthracenedione, structurally related to the anthracyclines. Mitoxantrone also causes a dose-related CD similar to anthracyclines. In cancer patients, the incidence of CHF or decrease in LVEF (below normal or 10% or more below baseline) is 2% to 4% of patients.[19,20] CD risk factors include prior exposure to anthracyclines and cumulative dose of mitoxantrone. In patients with multiple sclerosis[20] in whom mitoxantrone is used for relapsing/progressive disease, a retrospective review revealed 2 of 1,378 patients with symptomatic CHF and 2.18% with asymptomatic fall of LVEF below 50%.

As a single drug in anthracycline-naïve patients, mitoxantrone CD is rarely seen before 100 mg/m^2 cumulative dose. It is generally recommended that LVEF be monitored regularly thereafter and that a total dose of 140 mg/m^2 not be exceeded. When used after doxorubicin, CD is more frequent. An analysis by the Southwest Oncology Group[19] revealed a risk of 6% at 134 mg/m^2 prior doxorubicin and mitoxantrone 60 mg/m^2, rising to 15% risk at 120 mg/m^2 mitoxantrone. The mechanism of mitoxantrone CD appears to involve iron chelates as with anthracyclines.[16]

CYCLOPHOSPHAMIDE

The classic cardiac toxicity of cyclophosphamide (CTX) is an acute myopericarditis associated with high-dose therapy (HDT). In the era of stem cell transplantation and vigorous hydration, irreversible hemorrhagic myonecrosis is rare. More commonly, patients develop an acute/subacute CHF that is generally reversible with medical management.

CTX is hepatic-metabolized (cytochrome P-450–dependent) to the active drug, and it has been shown that more rapid CTX metabolism is associated with an increased risk of CHF. Ayash et al.[21] demonstrated an inverse correlation of CTX area under the curve with tumor response and CHF in the HDT of metastatic breast cancer. These investigators have suggested that CTX total dose, schedule of administration, and activation kinetics (affected by liver metabolism heterogeneity of cytochrome P-450 and/or concurrent drug exposures) all play a role in the development of CD.

Prospective monitoring of 16 patients during CTX high-dose administration (7 g/m^2) was reported by Morandi et al.[22] Serial enzymes (CPK, CPK-MB, and troponin I) did not become elevated using a fractionated drug administration schedule during 13 hours. The only positive findings were four cases of transient, mild diastolic and systolic left ventricular dysfunction. Moreover, Schrama et al.[23] reported their results of early and late cardiac toxicity with a CTX-based regimen. Six of 100 patients developed transient CHF. There were no acute cardiotoxic fatalities; late CD was not seen except in those patients requiring anthracycline salvage. Thus, with current administration guidelines used with HDT, CTX cardiotoxicity is uncommon (<10% of patients treated), generally transient, and reversible.

IFOSFAMIDE

Ifosfamide is a congener of CTX with similar alkylating agent properties. Because of potential chemical cystitis, it is always administered with mesna. Like CTX, ifosfamide may cause a dose-related CHF, which is generally transient and reversible. Quezado et al.[24] reported no CHF at 10 g/m^2, but CHF was more common at 16 g/m^2 or more. Clinical symptoms developed subacutely (mean, 12 days) and resolved with medical management. There is no evidence that mesna has any cardioprotective effect for CTX or ifosfamide. Cardinale et al.[25] prospectively studied high-dose CTX or ifosfamide-based regimens in 211 patients. The cardiac effects were similar with the two agents: troponin I became positive in 70 patients and remained negative in 141. LVEF fell significantly and continuously after the first month among the troponin I+ patients and the degree of dysfunction correlated with the troponin I level. Those who developed CHF had prior or concurrent exposure to anthracycline.

TAXANES

Paclitaxel, Docetaxel

The taxanes (paclitaxel and docetaxel) are important antimicrotubule agents and the taxine alkaloid fraction can affect cardiac conduction and automaticity. Although not fully proven, the mechanism of paclitaxel CD appears to be related to its taxane ring structural similarities to yew taxine.

The cardiovascular effects of paclitaxel are multiple: asymptomatic bradycardia may be documented in almost one-third of patients; hypersensitivity reactions associated with the Cremophor EL diluent (which can be ameliorated with corticosteroids, histamine H_1 and H_2 receptor antagonists); and most importantly, life-threatening atrial and/or ventricular rhythm disturbances and/or conduction abnormalities in approximately 0.5% of patients. Rare ischemic events have also been reported.

The life-threatening arrhythmias may occur acutely during infusion, or subacutely up to 14 days after treatment. These tend to occur after two or more treatment exposures, rather than with initial therapy. There does not appear to be a cumulative dosing threshold or limit, unlike that with anthracyclines.

In a summary review of adverse grade 4 and 5 cardiac events compiled by the National Cancer Institute,[26] atrial arrhythmias (tachycardia, flutter, and/or fibrillation) occurred in 0.24%, ventricular arrhythmias (tachycardia/fibrillation) in 0.26%, heart block in 0.11%, and ischemia in 0.29%. Paclitaxel does not appear to cause CHF. However, it has often been reported to potentiate doxorubicin-associated CHF.

Several groups have tested this question prospectively in metastatic breast cancer. Giordano et al.[27] studied 82 doxorubicin/taxane-naïve patients receiving doxorubicin 60 mg/m^2 followed by a 1- or 3-hour paclitaxel 200 mg/m^2 infusion. This AT regimen was administered every 21 days for six to seven cycles. The LVEF fell a median of 10% (to 52.5%) with a cumulative doxorubicin dose of 310 to 360 mg/m^2. Biganzoli et al.[28] studied AT, doxorubicin (60 mg/m^2) followed by paclitaxel (175 mg/m^2 in 3-hour infusion), versus AC, doxorubicin/CTX (60/600 mg/m^2) in 375 patients. Treatment was repeated every 3 weeks for six cycles (maximum doxorubicin, 360 mg/m^2). Overt CHF was not statistically different in the two study arms (3% vs. 1%; P =.62). However, a fall in LVEF was significantly more frequent for AT (27%) versus AC (14%). Moreover, the risk of LVEF fall was significantly greater for AT than AC at every cumulative doxorubicin dose level above 180 mg/m^2. In both these studies, paclitaxel was administered within 30 minutes of preceding doxorubicin. Other groups have reported minimal CD when the interval between doxorubicin was 4 to 24 hours or longer.[29,30]

The enhanced cardiac toxicity of doxorubicin-paclitaxel combinations has been attributed to an interaction that reduces doxorubicin elimination, resulting in a plasma exposure of up to 30% greater.[31] This effect on doxorubicin clearance is paclitaxel schedule-dependent, occurring most prominently when paclitaxel immediately precedes doxorubicin or follows it by less than 1 hour.

Salvatorelli et al.[32] have reported that paclitaxel appears to facilitate the metabolic conversion of doxorubicin to the toxic metabolite doxorubicinol in a human heart in vitro model. Docetaxel has a similar effect on doxorubicinol generation and both are attributed to allosteric interactions with cytoplasmic aldehyde reductases.

The taxane docetaxel has not been generally associated with clinical cardiac toxicity, CHF, or enhancement of doxorubicin cardiac dysfunction. However, recent data suggest this is due to lower cumulative anthracycline dosing rather than a different mechanism of drug interaction than paclitaxel.[33]

Both increase toxic cardiomyocyte doxorubicinol production *in vitro*. Therefore, the lack of docetaxel effect on doxorubicin clearance and the relatively lower doses of the drug used when combined with doxorubicin are now thought to be the explanation for the prior differences.

TRASTUZUMAB

Trastuzumab is a humanized monoclonal antibody that targets p185^{HER2} (ErbB2 or HER2 receptor), a transmembrane receptor tyrosine kinase of the epidermal growth factor family. This receptor protein is overexpressed or amplified in 20% to 30% of breast cancer and is associated with a poor clinical outcome. Trastuzumab is an important agent in the management of primary and metastatic breast cancer.[34]

Cardiac HER-2 is essential for normal embryonic and adult cardiac development and function, respectively. Using cardiac HER2-deficient conditional mutant mice, Crone et al.[35] and Ozcelik et al.[36] have reported the development of a dilated cardiomyopathy beginning in the second postnatal month and extending into adulthood of affected mice. Moreover, Crone et al.[35] have demonstrated that ErbB2-deficient cardiomyocytes from this mouse model are more susceptible to anthracycline toxicity.

HER2 and its coreceptor HER4 are localized to the T-tubule system of cardiomyocytes. Unfortunately, trastuzumab cannot be directly studied in the mouse because it is specific for the human HER2 receptor. A two-hit model has been proposed in HER2-deficient mice[37] in which hemodynamic overload or anthracycline exposure promotes the development of CHF. The finding of virtually no cardiac toxicity when trastuzumab preceded anthracycline-based adjuvant therapy in a prospective study supports this hypothesis.[38]

A retrospective meta-analysis[39] identified 112 patients with CD among 1,219 treated patients. Three studies used trastuzumab alone: 383 patients, of whom 17 (4%) had CD. Among 114 patients who received single-agent trastuzumab as first therapy for metastatic disease, 3% developed CD. In contrast, concurrent trastuzumab with anthracycline-based regimens or paclitaxel had an increased incidence of CD (27%; 13%) as compared with chemotherapy alone (11%; 1%) or antibody alone (3%).

The degree of cardiac functional impairment was greatest for patients receiving trastuzumab plus concurrent anthracycline (64%) as compared with 20% receiving trastuzumab plus paclitaxel. Moreover, all patients receiving trastuzumab plus paclitaxel had functional cardiac recovery with treatment as compared with only half the patients receiving trastuzumab plus concurrent anthracycline. Risk factors for CD included older age and cumulative doxorubicin 300 mg/m^2 or more. Concurrent anthracycline (doxorubicin or epirubicin) appeared to be more hazardous than temporally separated trastuzumab therapy.

The diagnosis of trastuzumab cardiac toxicity is often made by the detection of an asymptomatic fall in LVEF. Like anthracycline CD, tachycardia may be an early clinical indicator and the late constellation of dilated, hypokinetic CD is its late manifestation. Unlike anthracyclines, trastuzumab CD does not appear to be antibody-cumulative dose-dependent, and it appears to be both more treatable and more likely to be fully reversible. In one study of long-term follow-up echocardiography, the use of adjuvant trastuzumab had no additive adverse effect when used after anthracycline therapy.[40] It is not yet known how to prevent trastuzumab cardiac toxicity. As emphasized by Chien,[37] using trastuzumab prior to anthracycline is most likely to eliminate cardiac stress signals that precipitate toxicity. Avoidance of concurrent anthracycline exposure is essential. Sequential chemotherapy/trastuzumab schedules continue to be studied. Moreover, it is important to prospectively identify patients at high risk, such as those with low baseline LVEF. Guidelines, such as those developed in the United Kingdom,[41] are based on the observed safety of sequential therapy, delay of 1 to 2 months after cytotoxics, and restricting eligibility to those with LVEF of 55% or higher. Trastuzumab was discontinued in only 4.3% of such patients for CD. Monitoring of LVEF is recommended every 4 months during therapy and every 6 months thereafter for up to 2 years.

FLUOROPYRIMIDINES

5-Fluorouracil (5-FU) is a synthetic pyrimidine antimetabolite and an important agent in the treatment of many common solid tumors. Its cardiac toxicity is manifested as chest pain, anginal symptoms, atrial/ventricular arrhythmias, myocardial infarction (MI), and cardiogenic shock. Labianca et al.[42] reported the incidence of this potentially devastating complication to be 1.6% among 1,083 patients. Kosmas et al.[43] evaluated 644 patients, finding a 4% incidence of clinical and/or ECG findings among patients with no prior cardiac history. Continuous infusion had a higher incidence of CD (6.7%) as compared to daily schedules, and the addition of leucovorin to continuous infusion appeared to further increase risk. Schober et al.[44] did not find a higher incidence of toxicity with the addition of leucovorin in their study of 390 patients in which CD was noted in 3%. As others have noted, however, a prior history of cardiac disease significantly increases risk (15.1% vs. 1.5%, with no CD history).

A newer oral fluoropyrimidine, capecitabine, also appears to have associated CD similar to that reported for 5-FU.[43] Van Cutse et al.[45] retrospectively reviewed the cardiotoxic adverse events reported in four large trials: 593 patients receiving 5-FU/leuocovorin and 832 receiving capecitabine. The incidence of cardiotoxic events was 3%, with grade 3 to 4 adverse events in 1%. These authors cautioned that any fluoropyrimidine has the potential for CD and that treatment should be discontinued promptly for any clinical signs.

The mechanism of is not well understood and it is speculated that this is due to vascular spasm in reaction to the parent drug and its catabolites (fluoro-beta-alanine and fluoroacetate). In an *in vitro* model, 5-FU causes vasoconstriction in smooth muscle rings, which is reversible with nitrates[46]; on electron microscopy, the changes appear to be in the small arterial endothelium.[47] Coronary angiography following the 5-FU cardiotoxic syndrome has not revealed ongoing cardiac spasm, and an autopsy evaluation of two patients has suggested myocarditis.[48] A prospective study by Sudhoff et al.[49] used brachial artery ultrasound in 30 patients receiving 5-FU versus 30 receiving non–5-FU-containing regimens. Fifteen of 30 patients showed artery contraction with 5-FU and none with other therapy. Vessel tone recovered within 30 minutes and reoccurred with retreatment in most. Pretreatment with glyceroltrinitrate ablated the contractions among five patients studied.

Predisposing factors for fluoropyrimidine CD include a prior history of cardiac ischemia or arrhythmia, prior mediastinal irradiation, and prior/concurrent exposure to other cardiac toxic medications. There is no known prophylactic regimen that can be provided to prevent the CD, and vasodilators do not necessarily relieve the symptoms once they appear. It is best to discontinue the fluoropyrimidine and provide appropriate supportive measures, understanding the potential gravity of the syndrome. Excluding patients with risk factors may not always be possible, and if needed, such patients should be carefully monitored with available cardiac support.[50]

TYROSINE KINASE INHIBITORS

The tyrosine kinase inhibitors (TKIs) are a new class of anticancer agents with potential on- and off-target cardiac toxicity.[4] This was first described with imatinib, a small molecule that targets/inhibits the Bcr-Abl fusion protein associated with chronic myelogenous leukemia/Philadelphia chromosome. LVEF drop and symptomatic CHF were reported initially, but when critically examined in the prospective clinical trial databases, there were few significant differences in CD when comparing imatinib with the control arms. However, no standard monitoring for CD was employed during these trials. The related agents, dasatinib and nilotinib, have low and no CD incidence, respectively. Thus, although it has been demonstrated that the cardiomyocyte target is c-Abl in animal models, this on-target effect of imatinib and related drugs appears to have little clinical relevance.

On the other hand, some of the newer multitargeted TKIs appear to have off-target effects that include CD. Unlike imatinib, the potential mechanism of cardiomyocyte damage with sunitinib is not the direct inhibition of its anticancer targets (including vascular endothelial growth factor receptors 1 to 3 and platelet-derived growth factor), but rather, off-target inhibition of adenosine monophosphate-activated protein kinase, which regulates cardiomyocyte response to stress.[4] Prospective study of sunitinib CD[51] has revealed an approximate 10% incidence of LVEF decline, which is reversible with reduction in dose or discontinuance. Risk factors for CD include history of hypertension and coronary artery disease. Monitoring of blood pressure and LVEF during treatment is recommended.

Sorafenib, a related multitargeted TKI, whose targets include vascular endothelial growth factor receptor, platelet-derived growth factor receptor, RAF1 (v-raf-1 murine leukemia viral oncogene homolog 1), and others, is also associated with CD.[4] A recent animal study concluded that cardiomyocyte effects were not related to RAF inhibition.[52] The clinical cardiac effects of sunitinib and sorafenib appear similar.[53] With a cardiac event defined as increased enzymes, symptomatic arrhythmia, LV dysfunction, or acute coronary syndrome, 34% of treated patients experienced an event in one study. These cardiac events did not adversely affect survival when compared with patients not experiencing an event, and the TKIs could be reintroduced on recovery from the cardiac event.

Lapatinib is a TKI that targets epidermal growth factor receptor and *HER2* (as does trastuzumab).[54] Review of LVEF data in prospective clinical trials has reported low rates (1.5%–2.2%) of transient LVEF decline, which were predominantly asymptomatic and reversible. Two other TKIs that have no CD are gefitinib and erlotinib, both targeting epidermal growth factor receptor.[4] This would suggest that the CD of lapatinib is related to its on-target effect on *HER2*. Why CD is less severe with lapatinib than with trastuzumab is unknown.

RADIATION-INDUCED HEART DISEASE

Cardiac complications resulting from mediastinal irradiation were considered rare and insignificant for a long period in the history of radiotherapy.[55] Since the mid-1960s, when follow-up information on a large number of patients who had been cured of Hodgkin's lymphoma (HL) with higher doses of radiation became available, the heart has no longer been considered radioresistant.[56] Radiation-induced heart disease has now been characterized and investigated in experimental animals, and the pathologic features of the damage have been described with regard to the coronary arteries and all three layers of the heart.

Pericarditis and pericardial effusion have been regarded as the most common side effects of cardiac irradiation.[57] However, modern techniques of irradiation, dose fractionation, and reduction of the heart volume irradiated in most malignancies have substantially reduced the frequency of this complication. At the same time, evidence has accumulated to suggest that ischemic heart disease resulting from radiation-induced coronary heart disease (CHD) is the most concerning long-term risk of cardiac irradiation, particularly in high-risk patients.[58–69]

Pericardial Disease

The risk of radiation-induced pericardial disease depends on the dose given and on the volume of the heart irradiated.[57,58,63,70] Even when a large volume of the heart (60% or more) is irradiated at or below 40 Gy, the risk for mild pericarditis is below 5%, and severe pericarditis is rare.[71] Smaller heart volumes (20%–30%) may tolerate up to 60 Gy, with an expected 2% risk of mild pericarditis. When radiation of the mediastinum for HL no longer included the whole heart, the risk of pericarditis was reduced from 20% to below 2.5%.[60,72] With current radiotherapy techniques for HL and breast cancer, pericarditis is an infrequent event.

Acute Pericarditis During Radiation

Acute pericarditis during the course of radiotherapy is rare. It is almost always associated with massive mediastinal tumors adjacent to the heart. The signs and symptoms are of acute nonspecific pericarditis with chest pain, fever, and often ECG abnormalities. It does not lead to a significant risk of late pericardial damage and is not an indication for interrupting the radiation course.[58]

Delayed Pericarditis

Radiation-induced pericarditis typically occurs within the first year after mediastinal irradiation. Pericardial disease presents either as an acute pericarditis, as a pericardial effusion that may be asymptomatic, or as a combination of both. The symptoms of delayed acute pericarditis are indistinguishable from those of other types of pericarditis. Most cases of radiation-induced pericarditis and pericardial effusion resolve spontaneously, usually within 16 months.[73]

Treatment

Careful cardiac evaluation and monitoring with echocardiography and radionuclide ventriculography should be performed whenever radiation-induced heart disease is suspected.[74–76] Patients with mild symptoms and no hemodynamic compromise can be followed without treatment or can receive symptomatic therapy with salicylates or other nonsteroidal anti-inflammatory agents. Symptomatic pericardial effusion or clinical evidence for hemodynamic compromise warrants a drainage procedure. Pericardiocentesis with or without percutaneous placement of an indwelling catheter is successful in the majority of patients. Failure to relieve tamponade with pericardiocentesis, recurrence of effusion, or the presence of symptomatic constrictive pericarditis requires pericardiectomy. The mortality of this procedure in patients with postradiation pericarditis is high.[77] Occult constrictive pericarditis requires no surgical intervention and usually has a good prognosis.[57]

Myocardial Dysfunction

When myocardial dysfunction is detected after standard-dose mediastinal irradiation, it is typically mild or subclinical.[57,63,78,79] A study of asymptomatic patients who were treated with mediastinal irradiation for HL at a young age showed reduced average left ventricular dimension and mass suggestive of restricted cardiomyopathy in 42% of patients.[80] The majority of patients with abnormal ventricular function findings, however, do not have clinical heart failure.[80] The magnitude of the potential contribution of cardiac irradiation to the risk of doxorubicin-induced cardiomyopathy is not well established. Some data suggest potentiation of anthracycline-induced CD when combined with radiotherapy.[64,81] The histopathologies of radiation heart disease and anthracycline heart disease are different, and the combined effects are probably additive rather than synergistic. In programs of combined modality therapy for HL that included relatively low doses of doxorubicin (up to 300 mg/m^2) and mediastinal irradiation of 20 to 40 Gy, no significant clinical myocardial dysfunction was detected.[82] Further, in situations in which the addition of radiation allows for reduction in the cumulative dose of anthracyclines, as can be deducted from analysis of patients treated with or without RT for early-stage diffuse large B-cell lymphoma in the Surveillance, Epidemiology, and End Results database, using RT has actually decreased the rate of cardiac mortality.[83]

Symptomatic myocardial dysfunction after a radiation dose that does not exceed 60 Gy is rare.[56,57]

Valvular Disease

Clinically significant valvular heart disease resulting from mediastinal irradiation is relatively uncommon.[57,82] When echocardiographic studies were performed in asymptomatic HL patients more than 7 years after mediastinal irradiation, valvular abnormalities were detected in 25% to 33% of the patients, although there was rarely any clinical significance. An echocardiographic study of 294 asymptomatic patients who received mediastinal irradiation disclosed moderate or severe regurgitation of the aortic valve in 5.0% of patients, of the mitral valve in 3.4%, and of the tricuspid valve in 1.4%. Four percent of the patients had aortic stenosis.[84] Valvular disease, particularly involving the aortic valve, increased with time after irradiation.[85]

It is important to note that radiation dose, volumes, and technique of radiation delivery have markedly changed during the last 3 decades, and the lower prevalence of valvular disease in patients treated at less than 20 years may reflect those changes.[86] In a retrospective study of 415 patients that were irradiated from 1962 to 1998, 6.2% of patients developed clinically significant valvular dysfunction at a median of 22 years.[81] Of interest is a report from Norway that showed a significantly higher risk of cardiopulmonary complications for female subjects after radiation for HL.[86,87] The mean interval from irradiation to detection of valvular disease in asymptomatic and symptomatic patients was 11.5 and 16.5 years, respectively.[88] Patients that received mediastinal radiotherapy and an anthracycline-containing chemotherapy had significantly more valvular disorders than patients receiving radiation therapy (RT) with no anthracyclines.[64,89]

Electrical Abnormalities

Many ECG abnormalities were recorded years after mediastinal irradiation, the most common clinically significant abnormality being complete atrioventricular block.[76,90] Slama et al.[90] reported that radiation-related atrioventricular block was typically infranodal and occurred at long intervals (mean, 12 years), after radiation doses above 40 Gy, most frequently in patients with abnormal conduction on ECG before the advent of complete block, and in those who had other radiation-related cardiac abnormalities.

Another aspect of RT and heart disease relates to the management of patients with implanted cardiac pacemakers.[91–94] Placing the pacemaker in an unshielded radiotherapy field may cause cumulative damage to the pacemaker components.[91] The absorbed dose to the pacemaker should be estimated before treatment. If the total dose to the pacemaker might exceed 2 Gy, the pacemaker function should be checked weekly to detect any indicator of damage that may require replacement of the device.[91]

Coronary Heart Disease

Experiments in laboratory animals,[95–97] analysis of pathologic specimens,[98] clinical observations,[99,100] and since the 1990s, long-term risk analysis in large series of patients treated for HL[59–67] all indicate that mediastinal irradiation may facilitate the development of CHD.

Stenosis at the origin of the coronary arteries appears to be a common finding for radiation-associated CHD.[62,100–103] After mediastinal irradiation, there is a greater likelihood for right coronary or left main or left anterior descending coronary artery lesions as opposed to circumflex lesions, which might be because the former vessels, particularly at their origin, receive more radiation.[104] Coronary spasm after radiotherapy has also been documented in patients in whom acute MI developed with patent coronary arteries.[99]

The studies that analyzed the risk of mortality from MI in patients that were treated for HL are summarized in Table 163.2. Although only approximately 1% to 2% of HL patients in these series died of MI, the observed risk in all seven series was higher than expected.

Current involved field radiotherapy techniques, better fractionation schemes, and modern equipment deliver smaller doses of radiation to the coronary arteries and may have a lower risk of promoting CHD.[105] In a study by Boivin et al.,[104] the relative risk of acute MI was reduced from 6.33 for patients treated during the years 1940 to 1966 to 1.97 for patients irradiated from 1967 to 1985.

Hancock et al.[60,61] analyzed the risk of cardiac disease in patients with HL who received relatively high doses of radiation over a period of 30 years. The relative risk for death from acute MI was 3.2.[60] The study showed that patients younger than 20 years who received high-dose irradiation had the highest relative risk, that the risk decreases with increasing age, and that patients older than 50 years had no increased risk. However, these results contrast with data published by other investigators,[104] suggesting an increased risk of acute MI for the older age groups. The small number of patients in the Stanford study who received radiation doses of less than 30 Gy did not allow an adequate analysis of the dose effect. The average interval between HL treatment and death from acute MI was 10.3 years, but risk was already significant during the first 5 years after treatment and remained elevated throughout the follow-up period (more than 20 years).[60]

Several studies examined the interaction between recognized coronary risk factors and the risk of developing heart disease following mediastinal radiation for HL. A study from Rotterdam showed that increasing age, gender (male), and a pretreatment cardiac medical history were significant for developing ischemic heart disease. Treatment-related parameters did not affect the risk.[62] A recent registry-based study

TABLE 163.2

RELATIVE RISK OF MORTALITY FROM MYOCARDIAL INFARCTION AFTER MEDIASTINAL IRRADIATION FOR HODGKIN'S LYMPHOMA

Study (Ref.)	Center	No. of Patients	Lethal Myocardial Infarctions	Relative Risk	95% Confidence Interval
Boivin et al. (104)	Multiple	4,665	68	2.6	1.1–5.9
Hancock et al. (60)	Stanford (California)	2,232	55	3.2	1.5–5.8
Henry-Amar et al. (128)	European Organisation for Treatment and Research on Cancer	1,449	17	8.8	5.1–14.1
Mauch et al. (59)	Joint Center for Radiation Therapy (Boston)	636	15[a]	2.2[a]	1.2–3.6
Glanzmann et al. (63)	Zurich	352	8	4.2	1.8–8.3
Reinders et al. (62)	Rotterdam	258	12[b]	5.3	2.7–9.3
Swerdlow et al. (67)	Britain	7,033	168	2.5	2.1–2.9

[a]Includes one patient who died of cardiomyopathy.
[b]Myocardial infarction or sudden death.

from Ontario, Canada, analyzed the risk of cardiac hospitalizations in HL patients with pre-existing heart disease.[106] The investigators found that pre-existing heart disease was the strongest predictor for post-HL treatment cardiac hospitalizations. Other significant risk factors were older age at diagnosis and male sex. Combined doxorubicin chemotherapy plus mediastinal RT or mediastinal radiotherapy alone were associated with a higher risk than doxorubicin alone.[106] In a study from Zurich, a detailed analysis of the effect of other CHD risk factors on the radiation-induced risk was performed. The study showed that, although the risk of CHD after irradiation increased by 4.2 for all patients, in irradiated female patients and in all irradiated patients without other cardiovascular risk factors (smoking, hypertension, obesity, hypercholesterolemia, diabetes), the risk remained as expected in the normal population.[63] In a recent study of 1,474 HL survivors treated mostly with RT with or without chemotherapy, hypercholesterolemia was the most significant independent risk factor for developing CHD.[64] These data suggest that aggressive modification of CHD risk factors is warranted in patients who received mediastinal RT and/or anthracycline-containing chemotherapy.

Anthracycline-containing regimens like ABVD (doxorubicin, bleomycin, vinblastine, dacarbazine) and R-CHOP (rituximab, CTX, doxorubicin, vincristine, prednisone), with or without RT, are the mainstay of current treatment of HL and non-HL, respectively. Yet, only recently have serious concerns regarding anthracycline-related risks (with or without RT) to the coronary arteries been documented.[67,107] Aviles et al.[107] studied 476 patients with HL treated with anthracycline-containing chemotherapy and no RT. At a median follow-up of 11.5 years, 9% of patients who received ABVD had a clinical cardiac event and 7% had a cardiac-related death. The standard mortality ratio for cardiac death for patients who received doxorubicin was 46 and the absolute excess risk was 39.[107]

The largest and most recent analysis of MI mortality risk after treatment for HL is a collaborative British cohort study of 7,033 patients.[67] This study included 3,590 patients who received RT without anthracyclines, 3,052 patients who received chemotherapy with supradiaphragmatic RT, and 1,744 patients who received anthracycline regimens and no RT. For the whole group of HL survivors, the death from MI was statistically significantly more than expected: a standardized mortality ratio (SMR) of 2.5 with an absolute excess risk of 125.8. The relative risk of death from MI decreased sharply with older age at first treatment, but as expected, the absolute excess risk increased with age. The 20-year cumulative risk of MI mortality for patients treated at age younger than 35 years was 1.8%. The risk of death during the first year after treatment was fourfold compared with the general population and it was higher for patients treated before 1980.[67]

Of particular concern are the new data regarding chemotherapy alone.[67,107] In the British study,[67] the risk of death from MI was statistically significantly increased for patients who had received anthracyclines (SMR of 2.9) and especially those treated with ABVD (SMR of 9.5). These data remained significantly elevated for patients who received those chemotherapy regimens and no RT (ABVD, no RT; SMR of 7.8). The authors suggest that the risk was particularly high for ABVD (compared with other doxorubicin-containing regimens) because ABVD alone was virtually always given for the full six cycles. The increased risk for patients treated with anthracyclines was primarily during the first year after treatment and the highest risk was in young patients (35 years or less). MI mortality risk was also significantly increased for treatment with vincristine with or without radiation.[67]

Long-term mortality data from several trials, which randomized breast cancer patients to receive postmastectomy radiotherapy as opposed to no additional treatment, demonstrated a higher incidence of cardiac death in the irradiated group.[108,109] In one study, the increase in mortality risk was significant only in women who were irradiated for tumors in the left breast.[108] It was also increased in patients treated with orthovoltage irradiation, as opposed to those treated with more modern supervoltage equipment.[109]

A recent study from The Netherlands of 4,414 10-year breast cancer survivors who were treated from 1970 through 1986 recorded both cardiovascular morbidity and mortality events.[69] It showed that radiation to the breast alone is not associated with increased risk of cardiovascular disease. Similar to other studies,[110,111] it also documented that the increased risk of MI that was noted in patients treated prior to 1980 has disappeared with more recent RT techniques.

Prophylactic irradiation of the internal mammary nodes using a single anterior photon beam (hockey stick technique) or large tangents, which may deliver a high dosage to the heart,[112] is not indicated in most patients irradiated for breast conservation or postmastectomy.[113] Techniques that reduce the risk of irradiating the coronary arteries have been developed;

they include the prone breast technique[114] and use of three-dimensional CT planning and intensity-modulated RT, helical tomography, and using an image-guided deep inspiration breath hold technique in special cases.[115 117] Breast cancer patients irradiated with modern techniques are unlikely to receive a significant dose of radiation to the coronary arteries.

In breast cancer patients, conventional-dose doxorubicin-containing chemotherapy used as an adjuvant in combination with locoregional irradiation was not associated with a significant increase in the risk of cardiac events. However, higher doses of adjuvant doxorubicin were associated with a three- to fourfold increased risk of cardiac events. This appears to be especially true in patients treated with higher-dose volumes of cardiac irradiation.[118] Interestingly, in one recent large-scale study, breast cancer patients who were treated with CMF (CTX, methotrexate, 5-FU) and radiotherapy had a significantly higher risk of CHF compared with patients treated with radiotherapy alone.[110]

Monitoring and reduction of other contributing CHD risk factors in patients who received mediastinal irradiation should be part of the follow-up of patients who underwent mediastinal irradiation. However, the value of routine noninvasive or invasive cardiac studies in asymptomatic patients has not been fully determined.[62,118 121] In a recent screening study of 294 patients who received mediastinal radiation (median dose, 44 Gy) from 1960 to 1995, 21% of screened patients had abnormal ventricular images at rest.[66] During stress testing that included echocardiography and radionuclide perfusion, 14% showed abnormalities in one or both tests. Based on these tests, 40 patients underwent coronary angiography, and 55% of them (7% of the screened population) had 50% or more stenosis. The risk of a cardiac event in those patients was significantly related to abnormal stress testing, older age, radiotherapy given in early period, and to higher RT dose given to the mediastinum. More recently, new techniques to assess cardiac and particularly coronary disease in long-term survivors of HL included CT coronary angiography, coronary calcium scoring, and cardiac magnetic resonance.[122–124] The role of these technologies in surveillance patients who received mediastinal irradiation is still under investigation.

Early detection of coronary artery disease should be encouraged, particularly in patients irradiated with high RT dose (practiced mostly in the past) and/or those with other CHD risk factors[62,63] because angioplastic or surgical intervention may be indicated in special anatomic or clinical situations.[66] Successful treatment of radiation-induced coronary disease with bypass surgery and with stenting or angioplasty has been reported.[103,125–127] In some cases, surgery may be technically difficult because of mediastinal and pericardial fibrosis.[98]

FUTURE DIRECTIONS

It is hoped that increased awareness and knowledge about potential CD from chemotherapy and radiotherapy will enable physicians to adequately monitor patients and modify therapy so as to minimize serious acute and chronic cardiac sequelae. The growing information about late cardiac effects should facilitate early diagnosis and therapeutic intervention for the benefit of previously treated patients. Cardiologists and oncologists should work together in the management of survivors who are at risk for treatment-related cardiac damage.[128–130]

Selected References

The full list of references for this chapter appears in the online version.

3. Yeh ETH, Bickford CL. Cardiovascular complications of cancer therapy: incidence, pathogenesis, diagnosis and management. *J Am Coll Cardiol* 2009;53(24):2231.
4. Cheng H, Force T. Molecular mechanisms of cardiovascular toxicity of targeted cancer therapeutics. *Circ Res* 2010;106;21.
10. Barrett-Lee PJ, Dixon JM, Farrell C, et al. Expert opinion on the use of anthracyclines in patients with advanced breast cancer at cardiac risk. *Ann Oncol* 2009;20:816.
11. van Dalen EC, Michiels EMC, Caron HN, Kremer LCM. Different anthracycline derivates for reducing cardiotoxicity in cancer patients. *Cochrane Database Syst Rev* 2010;17;3:CD005006.
12. van Dalen EC, van der Pal HJH, Caron HN, Kremer LCM. Different dosage schedules for reducing cardiotoxicity in cancer patients receiving anthracycline chemotherapy. *Cochrane Database Syst Rev* 2009;7(4): CD005008.
13. van Dalen EC, Caron HN, Dickinson HO, et al. Cardioprotective inventions for cancer patients receiving anthracyclines. *Cochrane Database Syst Rev* 2008;(2):CD003917.
14. Hensley ML, Hagerty KL, Kewalramani T, et al. American Society of Clinical Oncology 2008 clinical practice guideline update: use of chemotherapy and radiation therapy protectants. *J Clin Oncol* 2009;27(1):127. Epub 2008 Nov 17.
21. Ayash LJ, Wright JE, Tretyakov O, et al. Cyclophosphamide pharmacokinetics: correlation with cardiac toxicity and tumor response. *J Clin Oncol* 1992;10(6):995.
29. Gianni L, Dombernowsky P, Sledge G, et al. Cardiac function following combination therapy with paclitaxel and doxorubicin: an analysis of 657 women with advanced breast cancer. *Ann Oncol* 2001;12:1067.
37. Chien KR. Herceptin and the heart—a molecular modifier of cardiac failure. *N Engl J Med* 2006;354(8):789.
39. Seidman A, Hudis C, Pierri MK, et al. Cardiac dysfunction in the trastuzumab clinical trials experience. *J Clin Oncol* 2002;20(5):1215.
41. Jones AL, Barlow M, Barrett-Lee PJ, et al. Management of cardiac health in trastuzumab-treated patients with breast cancer: updated United Kingdom National Cancer Research Institute recommendations for monitoring. *Br J Cancer* 2009;100(5):684.
50. Jensen SA, Sorensen JB. Risk factors and prevention of cardiotoxicity induced by 5-fluorouracil or capecitabine. *Cancer Chemother Pharmacol* 2006;58(4):487.
53. Schmidinger M, Zielinski CC, Vogl UM, et al. Cardiac toxicity of sunitinib and sorafenib in patients with metastatic renal cell carcinoma. *J Clin Oncol* 2008;26(32):5204.
60. Hancock SL, Tucker MA, Hoppe RT. Factors affecting late mortality from heart disease after treatment of Hodgkin's disease. *JAMA* 1993;270: 1949.
63. Glanzmann C, Kaufmann P, Jenni R, et al. Cardiac risk after mediastinal irradiation for Hodgkin's disease. *Radiother Oncol* 1998;46:51.
64. Aleman BM, van del Belt-Dusebout AW, De Bruin M, et al. Late cardiotoxicity after treatment for Hodgkin lymphoma. *Blood* 2007;109:1878.
66. Heidenreich PA, Schnittger I, Strauss HW, et al. Screening for coronary artery disease after mediastinal irradiation for Hodgkin's disease. *J Clin Oncol* 2007;25:43.
67. Swerdlow AJ, Higgins CD, Smith P, et al. Myocardial infarction mortality risk after treatment for Hodgkin disease: a collaborative British cohort study. *J Natl Cancer Inst* 2007;99:206.
69. Hooning MJ, Botma A, Aleman BMP, et al. Long-term risk of cardiovascular disease in 10-year survivors of breast cancer. *J Natl Cancer Inst* 2007; 99:365
85. Wethal T, Lund MB, Evardsen T, et al. Valvular dysfunction and left ventricular changes in Hodgkin's lymphoma survivors. A longitudinal study. *Br J Cancer* 2009;101:575
106. Myrehaug S, Pintilie m Yun L, et al. Population-based study of cardiac morbidity among Hodgkin lymphoma patients with pre-existing heart disease. *Blood* 2010 (prepublished online July 1, 2010)
110. Darby SC, McGale P, Taylor CW, Peto R. Long-term mortality from heart disease and lung cancer after radiotherapy breast cancer: prospective cohort study of about 300,000 women in US SEER registries. *Lancet Oncol* 2005; 6:539.
129. Albini A, Pennesi G, Donatelli F, et al. Cardiotoxicity of anticancer drugs: the need for cardio-oncology and cardio-oncological prevention. *J Natl Cancer Inst* 2010;102:14.
130. Bovelli D, Palataniotis G, Roila F. Cardiotoxicity of chemotherapeutic agents and radiotherapy-related heart disease: ESMO clinical practice guidelines. *Ann Oncol* 2010;21(Suppl 5);v277.

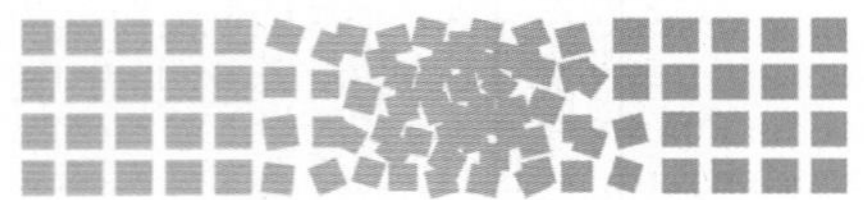

CHAPTER 164 HAIR LOSS

JOYSON J. KARAKUNNEL AND ANN M. BERGER

Hair is an important aspect of a person's self-image. Unfortunately, during many cancer treatments, hair is adversely affected. The incidence of alopecia is extremely high and is currently ranked third among the most common side effects of chemotherapy, directly behind nausea and vomiting.[1] In addition, cancer-related alopecia is not only due to chemotherapy but also to metastatic disease and presentations of different malignancies. Also, with the introduction of biologic agents, chemotherapy-induced alopecia is no longer limited to cytotoxics, but anecdotal reports of biologic agents inducing alopecia have been reported.[2] "The loss of hair is an extremely traumatic experience precisely because it is the symbolic precursor to the loss of self. This raises the psychological terror and consequent fear that the known self will no longer exist."[3]

Hair loss can be an immense burden psychologically and physically. Currently, there are modalities to help alleviate the physical and emotional issues that are involved with alopecia. In addition, several experimental treatments are being explored. This chapter focuses on chemotherapy-induced alopecia.

ANATOMY AND PHYSIOLOGY

Normal hair is divided into three parts: the infundibulum, the isthmus, and the inferior segment (deepest area). Other structures that are attached to the hair follicle are the sebaceous gland and arrector pili muscle. The hair follicle consists of the outer and inner sheath, cuticle, hair shaft, hair matrix, dermal papilla, and follicular sheath.

Hair growth is cyclical in nature. The three separate phases during the hair life cycle are anagen, telogen, and catagen. The majority of the time most hair is in the anagen phase. During this phase, hair undergoes mitotic changes and rapid cell growth. In the telogen phase, hair is dormant and mitotic activity is arrested. This phase lasts from 3 to 6 months. During the catagen phase, the hair root is separated from the hair bulb, pigment storage is terminated, and the club-shaped root end is pushed out from the bulb. Less than 1% of hair is in this phase at any time.[4]

Chemotherapy-induced alopecia frequently occurs during anagen. Hair that is exposed to chemotherapy during this phase is much thinner and more brittle because of the suppression of cell production.

Several types of alopecia are associated with problems in the transition between anagen and telogen. Hair lost during this period is called *telogen effluvium* or *hair breakage*. Normally, hair bulbs are released 4 to 6 weeks after the onset of anagen. The five functional mechanisms of telogen effluvium are immediate anagen release, delayed anagen release, short anagen syndrome, immediate telogen release, and delayed telogen release.[5] Immediate anagen release is the most important of all the mechanisms with respect to chemotherapy. The mechanism consists of hair being prematurely forced into telogen, leading to a greater amount of shedding. An example of this mechanism is seen during drug-induced alopecia and severe illness.

CLASSIFICATION

Classification for hair loss has been divided into several different categories. Telogen effluvium can be subdivided into three categories by the amount of time in which hair shedding occurs. These subcategories are acute telogen effluvium, chronic diffuse telogen effluvium, and chronic telogen effluvium. During acute telogen effluvium, hair loss begins to occur approximately 2 to 3 months after the insult. Some of the causes of this include fever, surgery, or hemorrhage. Hair growth begins again approximately 3 to 6 months after the insult has subsided. Chronic diffuse telogen effluvium is defined by shedding that is present for more than 6 months. Some of the causes are thyroid disease, acrodermatitis enteropathica, malnutrition, iron-deficiency anemia, pancreatic disease, zinc deficiency, and drug-induced alopecia. Hair loss associated with thyroid disease, zinc deficiency, and iron-deficiency anemia begins to resolve once therapy is begun. Finally, chronic telogen effluvium is a diagnosis of exclusion once the possibilities for chronic diffuse telogen effluvium have been considered. When evaluating a patient with a possible chronic telogen effluvium, androgenetic alopecia should be excluded.

Chemically induced alopecia is due to immediate anagen release and destruction known as *hair follicle dystrophy*. Intravenously administered chemotherapy usually leads to greater hair loss than does orally administered chemotherapy. Hair loss generally begins approximately 2 to 4 weeks after treatment; hair usually begins to return 3 to 6 months later.[1] There are several causes for alopecia, some of which are listed in Table 164.1. In addition, multiple other animal models are being developed to characterize alopecia that is associated with different chemotherapeutic agents.[6] Specifically, doxorubicin has been shown to inhibit angiogenesis in a mouse model, which may play a role in alopecia.

In addition, some malignancies specifically have been linked to alopecia. Mixed reports have appeared of the association of prostate cancer with male-pattern baldness. Some studies have indicated that the risk of prostate cancer is as high as 50% in men who have male-pattern baldness.[7] Conversely, other studies have found no association between male-pattern baldness and prostate cancer. In addition, follicular mycosis fungoides, a rare disease associated with a poor prognosis, should be differentiated from alopecia mucinosa when considered in the setting of alopecia. These illnesses as well as others should be carefully considered when a patient presents with hair loss.

TABLE 164.1

ETIOLOGIC CLASSIFICATION OF ALOPECIA

Telogen effluvium
Anagen effluvium
Follicular mucinosis (anecdotal reports)
Acute myeloid leukemia
Squamous cell cancer of tongue
T-cell lymphoma
Lung cancer
Alopecia neoplastica (anecdotal reports)
Breast cancer
Gastric cancer
Trophoblastic tumor
Androgenetic alopecia

DIAGNOSIS

The diagnosis of alopecia should begin with a thorough history and physical examination. Patients should be asked about the onset of alopecia. Drug-induced alopecia can be differentiated by considering the time elapsed since medication was initiated and alopecia started. In addition, the pattern of the hair loss should be considered as a physical finding that can help in etiology of the hair loss. Clinical examination revealing bitemporal recessions can help to narrow the diagnosis between telogen effluvium and androgenetic alopecia.

Several tests can be conducted if a diagnosis of telogen effluvium is being considered. A blood workup should include, but not be limited to, blood count, thyroid function studies, rapid plasma reagin, Venereal Disease Research Laboratory, antinuclear antibody, and zinc and other nutritional deficiencies. In addition, clinical tests can determine whether the patient exhibits telogen effluvium such as hair-pull test and phototrichogram.

The most important test that helps to differentiate chronic telogen effluvium and androgenetic alopecia is the 4-mm punch biopsy. Biopsy is used in obtaining a ratio of the amount of hair that is in anagen and telogen. This test has a diagnostic accuracy of 98%.[5] In addition, a biopsy helps to differentiate between a follicular mycosis fungoides and metastatic tumor.

TREATMENT

Several treatments in varying stages of research and with varying efficacies can be used in the treatment of chemotherapy-induced alopecia (Table 164.2). They include scalp cooling, minoxidil, immunomodulator AS101 (ammonium trichloro-9-dioxoethlyene-O,O′-tellurate), scalp tourniquet, α-tocopherol, pulsed electrostatic fields (ETG), and various immunomodulating compounds. The therapies fall into three general modes: decreasing blood flow to the scalp, pharmacologically protecting the hair bulb, and inactivating the chemotherapeutic agent locally.

The amount of chemotherapy that reaches the scalp can be reduced in two ways. These methods include using scalp tourniquet or scalp hypothermia. Both methods induce vasoconstriction of superficial scalp vessels. For these methods to be effective, the chemotherapeutic agents must have short half-lives and have a rapid clearance of the drug and its metabolites.

Scalp tourniquets were first attempted in 1966. They are pneumatic devices that are placed around the hairline and inflated to a pressure greater than the systolic blood pressure

TABLE 164.2

THERAPEUTIC INTERVENTIONS IN ALOPECIA

Decrease local delivery
Scalp tourniquet
Scalp hypothermia
Protection of the hair bulb
Topical minoxidil
AS101
α-Tocopherol
Inhibitors of cyclin-dependent kinase
Thiol solution
Inactivate chemotherapy locally
ImuVert
Epidermal growth factor and fibroblast growth factor
Topical cyclosporine
Interleukin-1
Topical calcitriol
Liposome-entrapped monoclonal antibody
Pulsed electrostatic field

while the patient is receiving the chemotherapy infusion. Several studies have been reported using scalp tourniquets that revealed their effectiveness in preventing hair loss; however, the studies are difficult to interpret because of inadequate sample size, different criteria of assessing alopecia, and differences in chemotherapy regimens. Side effects of the scalp tourniquet include nerve compression and headaches.[4]

Scalp hypothermia (i.e., scalp cooling), first used in 1978, decreases blood flow to the scalp and may slow uptake of the chemotherapeutic agent by the hair follicles. Several devices, such as bags of ice, molded gel packs, and thermocirculator devices, can be used to achieve scalp hypothermia; however, it is believed that the scalp temperature must be decreased to at least 24°C to effectively prevent alopecia. Side effects include cumbersome units and patient discomfort from heavy caps. Several concerns have been raised about the use of scalp hypothermia and its use in those with liver dysfunction or in hematologic malignancies including leukemia and lymphoma, as well as a concern about the possibility of developing scalp metastases. More recent studies have found that hypothermia was effective, and several studies found no increased incidence of scalp metastases.[8]

Several different medications may reduce or prevent alopecia by pharmacologically protecting the hair bulb from damaging effects of chemotherapy. These medications include AS101, topical minoxidil, α-tocopherol, thiol, and inhibitors of cyclin-dependent kinase (CDK).

AS101 is a synthetic compound that is structurally similar to cisplatin. Studies initially done with mice revealed that AS101 works as an immunomodulator by stimulating production of interleukin (IL)-1, IL-2, IL-6, colony-stimulating factor, and tumor necrosis factor, thereby potentially being used to minimize cytotoxicity. The mechanism of AS101 may be due to IL-1 because there is an inverse correlation between IL-1 and alopecia.[9] An open-label prospective randomized trial done with 44 patients who had unresectable or metastatic non–small cell lung cancer and were receiving carboplatin and etoposide revealed a significant reduction in neutropenia and thrombocytopenia as well as chemotherapy-induced alopecia.[10]

Topical minoxidil has been used for the treatment of androgenetic alopecia and alopecia areata. Two randomized trials have been performed in patients with cancer. The first trial was with 48 patients with many different solid tumors who were receiving doxorubicin-containing regimens. Minoxidil 2% twice a day did not prevent alopecia as compared with placebo.[11] A second randomized trial with 22 women being treated for breast cancer found that topical minoxidil did not prevent alopecia; however there was a statistically significant difference (favoring minoxidil) in the interval from maximal hair loss to first regrowth. Thus, the period of baldness was shortened in the minoxidil group.[12]

Oral α-tocopherol, initially tested in Angora rabbits, found that there was some degree of protection from doxorubicin-induced alopecia. α-Tocopherol was tested prospectively in two trials of patients with cancer who were receiving doxorubicin. In both trials oral α-tocopherol did not prevent alopecia.[13,14]

Several different immunomodulators have been studied for the treatment of alopecia by inactivating the chemotherapy locally. These include ImuVert, epidermal growth factor (EGF) and fibroblast growth factor (FGF), IL-1, topical calcitriol, topical cyclosporine, and liposome-entrapped monoclonal antibodies. All of these agents have been studied *in vitro* only and in animal models, with no translation into clinical practice.

ImuVert is a biologic response modifier that was initially developed to perform immunomodulating or immunorestorative properties for malignancies and other diseases in which immune system dysfunction is implicated. It is produced by the bacterium *Serratia marcescens*. The mechanism of action is unclear; however, it induces many cytokines, including IL-1, tumor necrosis factor, interferon-α, IL-6, granulocyte-macrophage colony-stimulating factor, and platelet-derived growth factor. In the laboratory with rats, ImuVert showed almost complete protection against ara-C (cytosine arabinoside) and doxorubicin-induced alopecia; however, it offered no protection against cyclophosphamide-induced alopecia. Dose-limiting side effects were hypotension and flulike symptoms. No human studies have been reported to date.[15]

Several studies in rat models have been done with other biologic response modifiers, including EGF, FGF, and IL-1. FGF given systemically provided relief only from cytarabine at the site of injection. Topical EGF provided protection in the treated area. EGF given systemically provided relief from cytarabine- but not cyclophosphamide-induced alopecia.[4] Animal studies with IL-1 revealed that it is a potent inhibitor of cytarabine-induced alopecia, in an action similar to that of ImuVert; however, there was no protective effect with IL-1 and cyclophosphamide-induced alopecia.[15] These results led to the hypothesis that there may be different mechanisms for inducing alopecia, depending on whether the chemotherapeutic agent is cell-cycle specific or cell-cycle nonspecific.

Cyclosporine A administered topically protected newborn rats from alopecia induced by cytarabine, etoposide, and a cyclophosphamide plus doxorubicin combination at the site of application. Cyclosporine is a potent inhibitor of P-glycoprotein, as well as a hypertrichotic agent. The mechanism of action is unknown; however, it is thought that it perhaps protects the hair follicle keratinocytes from chemotherapy by the expression of P-glycoprotein.[16]

A study done with a topical liposome-entrapped monoclonal antibody (MAD11) against doxorubicin-induced alopecia revealed that in 31 of 45 rats, alopecia was completely prevented.[17] No human studies have been done with this agent. In addition, this agent would have very little benefit in chemotherapy-induced alopecia from other agents.

Another area of interest that is being looked at is cell-cycle inhibition by inhibition of CDK2. Several preclinical models have explored the role of topical small-molecule inhibitors of CDK2. In the neonatal rat chemotherapy-induced alopecia model, the application of the topical CDK2 inhibitor led to areas of less hair loss in 33% to 50% of the animals.[18]

Topical calcitriol (1,25-dihydroxyvitamin D_3) has been evaluated in rat models and found to prevent alopecia from a cyclophosphamide-doxorubicin regimen or cyclophosphamide-etoposide regimen. At a dose of 0.2 mcg topical calcitriol, the protection was noted over the entire animal and not just at the site of topical application.[19]

A pilot project using ETGs was undertaken, with 13 women receiving chemotherapy with cyclophosphamide, methotrexate, and 5-fluorouracil for breast carcinoma. All patients were treated for 12 minutes twice weekly with an ETG. Twelve of the 13 women had good hair retention throughout the chemotherapy period and afterward. No side effects were reported. The mechanism of ETG is unknown. Randomized, double-blind control studies should be developed using ETG for chemotherapy-induced alopecia.[20]

Inhibition of apoptosis by p53 and caspase is another area of interest that is being explored in chemotherapy-induced alopecia. Unfortunately, there are drawbacks to each of these experimental theories. Inhibition of caspase has been tested only in etoposide animal models and p53 inhibition would not affect alopecia that is independent of p53. Further studies in this area may yield drugs that have a wider profile, which in the topical setting may be of greater benefit.[1]

Radiation-induced alopecia can be just as concerning for patients as chemotherapy-induced alopecia. One agent that is currently being explored for radiation-induced alopecia is Tempol gel. This is a topical agent that has shown efficacy in animal models. Specifically, this agent is a nitroxide that has protective properties *in vitro* against free radical compounds. In addition, there was no decrease in tumor control in mice.[20] The agent, applied prior to radiation treatments, has been shown to be well tolerated in a phase 1 trial in patients who were found to have metastatic lesions to the brain. Some of the patients in this study were found to have protection against radiation.[21] These results, however, will need to be further evaluated by ongoing phase 2 trials.

References

1. Wang J, Lu Z, Au JL. Protection against chemotherapy-induced alopecia. *Pharm Res* 2006;23(11):2505.
2. Tosti A, Pazzaglia M, Starace M, et al. Alopecia areata during treatment with biologic agents. *Arch Dermatol* 2006;142(12):1653.
3. Dorr VJ. A practitioner's guide to cancer-related alopecia. *Semin Oncol* 1998;25:562.
4. Hussein AM. Chemotherapy-induced alopecia: new developments. *South Med J* 1993;86:489.
5. Harrison S, Sinclair R. Telogen effluvium. *Clin Exp Dermatol* 2002; 27(5):389.
6. Amoh Y, Li L, Katsuoka K, Hoffman RM. Chemotherapy targets the hair-follicle vascular network but not the stem cells. *J Invest Dermatol* 2007;127(1):11.
7. Hawk E, Breslow RA, Graubard BI. Male pattern baldness and clinical prostate cancer in epidemiological follow-up of the first National Health and Nutrition Examination Survey. *Cancer Epidemiol Biomarkers Prev* 2000;9:523.
8. Protiere C, Katrin E, Camerlo J, et al. Efficacy and tolerance of a scalp-cooling system for prevention of hair loss and the experience of breast cancer patients treated by adjuvant chemotherapy. *Support Care Cancer* 2002;10:529.
9. Ridderheim M, Bjurberg M, Gustavsson A. Scalp hypothermia to prevent chemotherapy-induced alopecia is effective and safe: a pilot study of a new digitized scalp-cooling system used in 74 patients. *Support Care Cancer* 2003;11:371.

10. Sredni B, Xu RH, Albeck M, et al. The protective role of the immunomodulator AS101 against chemotherapy-induced alopecia studies on human and animal models. *Int J Cancer* 1996;65:97.
11. Sredni B, Albeck M, Tichler T, et al. Bone marrow-sparing and prevention of alopecia by AS101 in non–small-cell lung cancer patients treated with carboplatin and etoposide. *J Clin Oncol* 1995;13(9):2342.
12. Rodriguez R, Machiavelli M, Leone B, et al. Minoxidil (Mx) as a prophylaxis of doxorubicin-induced alopecia. *Ann Oncol* 1994;5:769.
13. Martin-Jiminez M, Diaz-Rubio E, Gonzalez L, Sangro B. Failure of high-dose tocopherol to prevent alopecia induced by doxorubicin [letter]. *N Engl J Med* 1986;315:894.
14. Perez JE, Macchiavelli M, Leone BA, et al. High-dose alpha-tocopherol as a preventative of doxorubicin-induced alopecia. *Cancer Treat Rep* 1986; 70:1213.
15. Hussein AM. Interleukin 1 protects against 1-beta-D-arabinofuranosylcytosine-induced alopecia in the newborn rat model. *Cancer Res* 1991;51:3329.
16. Hussein AM, Stuart A, Peters WP. Protection against chemotherapy induced alopecia by cyclosporine A in the newborn rat model. *Dermatology* 1995; 190:192.
17. Balsari AL, Morelli D, Menard S, et. al. Protections against doxorubicin induced alopecia in rats by liposome-entrapped monoclonal antibodies. *FASEB J* 1994;8:226.
18. Davis ST, Benson BG, Bramson HN, et al. Prevention of chemotherapy-induced alopecia in rats by CDK inhibitors. *Science* 2001;291:134.
19. Jimenenz JJ, Yunis AA. Protection from chemotherapy-induced alopecia by 1,25-dihydroxyvitamin D3. *Cancer Res* 1992;52:5123.
20. Benjamin B, Ziginskas D, Harman J, Meakin T. Pulsed electrostatic field (ETG) to reduce hair loss in women undergoing chemotherapy for breast carcinoma: a pilot study. *Psychooncology* 2002;11:244.
21. Metz JM, Smith D, Mick R, et al. A phase I study of topical Tempol for the prevention of alopecia induced by whole brain radiotherapy. *Clin Cancer Res* 2004;10(19):6411.

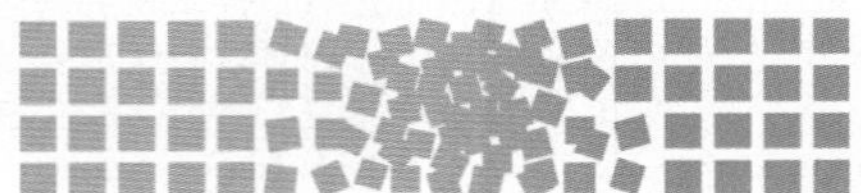

CHAPTER 165 GONADAL DYSFUNCTION

JOHN M. NORIAN, EVE C. FEINBERG, ALAN H. DECHERNEY, AND ALICIA Y. ARMSTRONG

The increased survival associated with oncologic treatment has made the late-term effects, such as gonadal failure, increasingly important. When the cancer is controlled, quality of life, which often includes the ability to have a normal child, then becomes a major issue.[1,2]

Both neoplastic disease and its treatment can interfere with normal sexual and reproductive function (Table 165.1). Testicular and ovarian cancers directly involve the gonad, and prostate, endometrial, and cervical cancers directly involve the reproductive tract. Surgical treatment for any of these diseases results in damage or loss of these important reproductive organs. Retroperitoneal lymph node dissection (RPLND) for testicular and colon cancer, prostatectomy, and surgery involving the bladder neck may result in loss of the ability to ejaculate. Primary and metastatic tumors in the hypothalamus and pituitary can directly affect gonadotropin secretion, resulting in secondary hypogonadism. Both chemotherapy and radiation cause toxic effects on the male and female gonads. Cytotoxic therapies delivered to women during pregnancy can have teratogenic effects on the fetus. If fertility is maintained or recovers, there remains the concern about the heritability of cancer and at least a theoretical risk of mutagenic alterations to germ cells caused by cytotoxic therapies.

The reproductive consequences of cancer therapy affect many people. In the United States, 17,000 men aged 15 to 45 years are diagnosed each year with Hodgkin's or other lymphoma, bone and soft tissue sarcomas, testicular cancer, or leukemia.[3,4] Of these, over 3,000 patients are treated with doses of alkylating agents, platinum drugs, or radiation that are sufficient to induce prolonged azoospermia. Similarly, 35,000 women aged 15 to 45 years are treated for breast cancer, ovarian cancer, Hodgkin's or other lymphoma, and leukemia; at least 80% of these patients receive radiation or alkylating agent–based cytotoxic therapies. These treatments cause not only sterility but also premature menopause in nearly 20,000 women. In addition, 12,000 children under 15 years are diagnosed each year with cancer, including leukemia, nervous system tumors, lymphomas, and renal and other solid tumors. Survival is approaching 80%, and because 85% of them receive chemotherapy or gonadal or pituitary irradiation, their subsequent reproductive function is a significant concern.[4]

EFFECTS OF CYTOTOXIC AGENTS ON ADULT MEN

Biologic Considerations

The testis consists of the seminiferous (or germinal) epithelium arranged in tubules and endocrine components (testosterone-producing Leydig cells) in the interstitial region between the tubules. The seminiferous tubules contain the germ cells, which consist of stem and differentiating spermatogonia, spermatocytes, spermatids, sperm, and the Sertoli cells, which support and regulate germ cell differentiation. The testicular vasculature is permeable, and drugs can freely reach the Leydig and Sertoli cells and the spermatogonia, which are at the outer rim of the tubules. Many chemotherapeutic drugs may penetrate the Sertoli cell barrier, albeit at a lower intensity, and damage late-stage germ cells.[5]

Among the germ cells, the differentiating spermatogonia proliferate most actively and are extremely susceptible to cytotoxic agents. In contrast, the Leydig and Sertoli cells, which do not proliferate in adults, survive most cytotoxic therapies. These cells, however, may suffer functional damage. Frequently, after cytotoxic therapies, germ cells appear to be absent and the tubules contain only Sertoli cells, a state described as *germinal aplasia*. This could be a result of killing of the spermatogenic stem cells, the loss of the ability of the somatic cells to support the differentiation of a few surviving stem cells, or a combination of the two.

After cytotoxic treatment, sperm count diminishes with a time course that depends on the sensitivities of the different spermatogenic cells and their kinetics of maturation to sperm.[6] Because the later-stage germ cells (spermatocytes onward) are relatively insensitive to killing and progress through spermatogenesis, sperm count is not immediately affected. However, these later-stage cells are susceptible to the induction of mutagenic damage, and studies in rodents have shown they can transmit mutations induced in their DNA to the next generation.[7] The eventual recovery of sperm production depends on the survival of the spermatogonial stem cells and their ability to differentiate. Surviving stem cells can remain in the testis but fail to differentiate to sperm for several years after cytotoxic insult.[8]

The loss of germ cells has secondary effects on the hypothalamic-pituitary-gonadal axis. Inhibin secretion by the Sertoli cells declines, and because inhibin limits follicle-stimulating hormone (FSH) secretion by the pituitary, serum FSH rises. Germinal aplasia reduces testis size, and testicular blood flow is consequently reduced, which results in distribution of less testosterone into the circulation[9] (Table 165.2). Because testosterone is a negative regulator of luteinizing hormone (LH) secretion by the pituitary, and LH is the primary stimulator of testosterone synthesis by the Leydig cells, LH increases to maintain constant serum testosterone levels.

Characteristics of Gonadal Toxicity

Although subnormal semen profiles, ejaculatory dysfunction, and low libido can often be results of cancer treatment, a thorough examination should be done to determine whether symptoms of these problems might have been present before

TABLE 165.1

IMPACT OF CANCER AND CANCER THERAPY ON THE REPRODUCTIVE SYSTEM

Tumor	Direct gonadal involvement Reproductive tract involvement Hypothalamic and pituitary involvement Concern about heritability of cancer susceptibility
Surgery	Removal of gonad Genital mutilation Failure of emission and retrograde ejaculation Impotence and loss of orgasm
Radiotherapy or chemotherapy	Germ cell depletion Loss of gonadal hormones Mutagenic changes in germ cells Teratogenic effects on fetus
Chemotherapy	Seminal transmission of drug
Radiotherapy (cranial)	Loss of gonadotropic hormones

treatment. A sexual and reproductive history should be taken, including information on developmental factors such as ages at testicular descent and puberty; surgery or injury to the genitals; diseases that might affect reproduction; drug, chemical, or heat exposure; and pretreatment fertility and libido status. A physical examination should consist of examination of the testicles and secondary sexual characteristics such as beard and hair distribution pattern. If there are indications, semen analysis and a hormone profile should be done and results compared with normal values (Table 165.2).

During the first 2 months of cytotoxic therapy, sperm counts may remain normal or be only moderately reduced. By 3 months after the initiation of therapy, which is the time required for differentiating spermatogonia to become sperm, azoospermia appears in patients who have been given highly gonadotoxic agents. Oligospermia or even normospermia may be maintained with less toxic regimens.[10]

The induced azoospermia can be either temporary or prolonged, depending on the survival of stem spermatogonia and their ability to proliferate, differentiate, and produce spermatozoa, which in turn depends on the nature of the cytotoxic agent and dose (Table 165.3).[11–14] If treatment is limited to the cytotoxic agents that do not kill stem spermatogonia or block their differentiation, normospermia is usually restored within 3 months after the cytotoxic therapy. However, if agents that kill stem spermatogonia or affect differentiation are used, longer periods of azoospermia ensue.[8,15]

To evaluate the effects of cytotoxic therapy, one must consider the initial gonadal status. Men with testicular germ cell tumors have impaired semen quality even before cytotoxic therapy is instituted. Approximately 65% are oligospermic (counts <20 million/mL) and approximately 20% are azoospermic,[16] whereas the values are 9% and 1%, respectively, in control populations. In half of the patients with reduced semen quality, this impaired testicular function is a result of abnormalities in the remaining gonad, such as carcinoma *in situ* or a history of cryptorchidism. In the other half, it may be a result of reversible factors such as chorionic gonadotropin production by the tumor with resulting increases in estradiol levels or the trauma of the recent orchiectomy.[17] In addition, emission and ejaculation may have been compromised by earlier RPLND so that the sperm density may not accurately reflect gonadal function.[18] In contrast to the severe dysfunction seen in cases of testicular cancer, in Hodgkin's lymphoma between 16% and 50% of patients are oligospermic, only 2% to 8% are azoospermic, and the distribution of counts in the remainder is not significantly different from normal.[19,20] Poor semen quality was more prevalent in patients with advanced than with early-stage Hodgkin's lymphoma, but specific risk factors have not been identified. In patients with other lymphomas and sarcomas, pretreatment sperm counts tend to be normal except for similar modest increases in the incidence of oligospermia.[8,15]

Age at treatment is not a major factor in recovery from gonadal damage in men. Most studies have failed to show any age effect,[8,15] but a few have indicated increased testicular damage after cytotoxic therapy in older men.[21]

Individual Drugs

The most sterilizing drugs are the alkylating agents (with the exception of dacarbazine) and cisplatin. The cumulative dose appears to be more important than the dose rate in determining whether or not sperm production will recover (Tables 165.3 and 165.4). Chlorambucil[22] and cyclophosphamide[23] induce prolonged azoospermia when given alone. The gonadal toxicities of other agents have generally been deduced from the effects of combination regimens; the doses given might be underestimates because there may be additive contributions from other drugs in the regimen. Procarbazine[24] and cisplatin in high doses[25] are also highly sterilizing. Busulfan has an additive effect on the sterility resulting from cyclophosphamide treatment.[26] Addition of high doses of ifosfamide (46 g/m^2) to cisplatin-containing chemotherapy regimens significantly reduced the recovery of spermatogenic function.[27] Carboplatin, an analogue of cisplatin, appeared in the same combination regimens to produce less sterility than cisplatin.[16] Treatment of boys with BCNU and CCNU produced prolonged

TABLE 165.2

TYPICAL CLINICAL AND LABORATORY FEATURES FOR DIAGNOSIS OF MALE REPRODUCTIVE DYSFUNCTION

	Testis Size		Serum Hormone Levels			
	Length × Width (cm)	Volume (mL)	Sperm Count (Millions/mL)	Follicle-Stimulating Hormone (mIU/mL)	Hormone (mIU/mL)	Testosterone (ng/dL)
Normal men	5.0 × 3.0	15–25	20 to >100	1–12	2–12	300–1,200
Germinal aplasia	3.7 × 2.3	8–15	0	>20	>12	200–700

PRACTICE OF ONCOLOGY

TABLE 165.3

EFFECTS OF DIFFERENT ANTITUMOR AGENTS ON SPERM PRODUCTION IN MEN

Agents (Cumulative Dose for Effect)	Effect
Radiation (2.5 Gy to testis) Chlorambucil (1.4 g/m²) Cyclophosphamide (19 g/m²) Procarbazine (4 g/m²) Melphalan (140 mg/m²) Cisplatin (500 mg/m²)	Prolonged azoospermia
BCNU (1 g/m²) CCNU (500 mg/m²)	Azoospermia in adulthood after treatment before puberty
Busulfan (600 mg/kg) Ifosfamide (42 g/m²) BCNU (300 mg/m²) Nitrogen mustard Actinomycin D	Azoospermia likely, but always given with other highly sterilizing agents
Carboplatin (2 g/m²)	Prolonged azoospermia not often observed at indicated dose
Doxorubicin (Adriamycin) (770 mg/m²) Thiotepa (400 mg/m²) Cytosine arabinoside (1 g/m²) Vinblastine (50 g/m²) Vincristine (8 g/m²)	Can be additive with above agents in causing prolonged azoospermia, but cause only temporary reductions in sperm count when not combined with above agents
Amsacrine, bleomycin, dacarbazine, daunorubicin, epirubicin, etoposide, fludarabine, 5-fluorouracil, 6-mercaptopurine, methotrexate, mitoxantrone, thioguanine	Only temporary reductions in sperm count at doses used in conventional regimens, but additive effects are possible
Prednisone	Unlikely to affect sperm production
Interferon-α	No effects on sperm production

azoospermia,[28] and it is likely, but not proven, that the same would occur in adults. The agents that have only temporary effects were also identified from single-agent and combination chemotherapy regimens.

Radiation Therapy

The effects of radiation on the testes depend on the fractionation regimen. Whereas in all other organ systems, fractionation of radiation reduces the damage, radiation doses to the germinal epithelium of the testis given in 3- to 7-week fractionated courses cause more gonadal damage than single doses.[29] In the usual fractionated regimens, doses to the testes above 0.15 Gy are required to produce any reduction in sperm count. Doses between 0.15 and 0.5 Gy cause oligospermia.[30] Above 0.6 Gy, azoospermia occurs. The duration of azoospermia is dose-dependent, and recovery can begin within 1 year after doses of less than 1 Gy, but not until more than 2 years after delivery of 2 Gy. Cumulative doses of fractionated radiotherapy of more than 2.5 Gy generally result in prolonged and likely permanent azoospermia. However, after a single dose of 8 Gy or fractionated doses of 10 to 13 Gy, given as total body irradiation in preparation for bone marrow transplantation, sometimes also with cyclophosphamide (4.5 g/m²), spermatogenesis eventually recovers in 15% of the patients.[14]

Testicular androgen production is relatively resistant to irradiation: doses of over 18 Gy are required before an effect is evident, and major damage does not occur until the dose exceeds 30 Gy.[31] The radiation-associated impotence after such treatments is likely a result of vascular damage.

Combination Regimens

The sterilizing potential of each combination chemotherapy or chemotherapy plus radiotherapy regimen is the additive effects of the doses of the individual agents given (Table 165.3); there is no evidence for synergistic interactions between the agents. Although it is impossible to predict whether sperm production in any given man will recover, the probability of prolonged azoospermia has been determined for many combinations (Table 165.4). The sterilizing potential of new regimens can be predicted from the information in Table 165.3 and the results found with similar combinations. The additive effects of agents can be seen in the case of cyclophosphamide: when cyclophosphamide is given alone, 19 g/m² is required to produce prolonged sterility in half the men, but only 15 g/m² is required when cyclophosphamide is given with a median doxorubicin dose of 450 mg/m² in the cyclophosphamide, doxorubicin, vincristine, and prednisone (CHOP) regimen, and only 11 mg/m² is required when it is given with a median doxorubicin dose of 880 mg/m² in the cyclophosphamide, vincristine, doxorubicin, and dacarbazine (CY[V]ADIC) regimen.[8,15]

EFFECTS OF CYTOTOXIC AGENTS ON ADULT WOMEN

Biologic Considerations

Gonadal cell kinetics in women are opposite to those in men: the germ cells are nonproliferative, whereas the somatic cells

TABLE 165.4

PROBABILITY OF GERMINAL APLASIA IN MEN TREATED WITH DIFFERENT COMBINATION CHEMOTHERAPY REGIMENS

Regimen	Disease	Courses or Dose	Patients with Prolonged Azoospermia (%)
HIGH-DOSE OR MODERATELY HIGH-DOSE ALKYLATING AGENTS			
MOPPd or MVPPd	Hodgkin's lymphoma	≥6 Courses	85
CyOPPd	Hodgkin's lymphoma	4–9 Courses	100
I, Pl, A, Mx	Osteosarcoma	I = 46 g/m^2 Pl = 560 mg/m^2	75
BuCy + HSCT BuTT + HSCT	Leukemia, lymphoma	Cy = 4.4 g/m^2 Bu = 600 mg/m^2 or TT = 400 mg/m^2	50
BcECaMl + HSCT	Lymphoma	Bc = 300 mg/m^2 Ml = 140 mg/m^2 + prior treatment	100
MOPPd/ABVD	Hodgkin's lymphoma	6–9 Courses	50
CyOPPd/ABVD, X	Hodgkin's lymphoma	6–9 Courses	85
ChlVPPd/EVA	Hodgkin's lymphoma	6–8 Courses	95
CyHOPd-Bleo	Lymphoma	Cy <9.5 g/m^2	17
		Cy >9.5 g/m^2	50
E, Ep, B, Cy, Pd (VEBEP)	Hodgkin's lymphoma	Cy = 8 g/m^2	40
CyVAD or CyAD	Sarcoma	Cy <7.5 g/m^2	30
		Cy >7.5 g/m^2	90
NONALKYLATING OR LOW-DOSE ALKYLATING AGENT			
Cy, A, Mx	Sarcoma	Cy = 5.6 g/m^2	20
MOPPd	Hodgkin's lymphoma	2 Courses	0
ABVD, X	Hodgkin's lymphoma	6 Courses	0
NOVPd, X	Hodgkin's lymphoma	3 Courses	0
Bc, Cy, Ca, L, Mp, TG	Leukemia	Cy = 5.1 g/m^2	0
Platinum			
PlVB	Testicular cancer	Pl ≤400 mg/m^2	10
		Pl >400 mg/m^2	50
PlVB-I	Testicular cancer	Pl = 400 mg/m^2 I = 30 g/m^2	55
PlEB	Testicular cancer	Pl ≤300 mg/m^2	0
		Pl = 400 mg/m^2	25
CbEB	Testicular cancer	Cb = 1.6 g/m^2	20
Pl, A, D	Osteosarcoma	Pl <600 mg/m^2	5
		Pl ≥600 mg/m^2	55

A, doxorubicin (Adriamycin); B, bleomycin; Bc, BCNU (carmustine); Bleo, bleomycin; Bu, busulfan; Ca, cytosine arabinoside; Cb, carboplatin; Chl, chlorambucil; Cy, cyclophosphamide; D, dacarbazine; E, etoposide; Ep, epirubicin; H, doxorubicin; HSCT, hematopoietic stem cell transplantation; I, ifosfamide; L, L-asparaginase; M, mechlorethamine (nitrogen mustard); Ml, melphalan; Mx, methotrexate; Mp, 6-mercaptopurine; N, mitoxantrone (Novantrone); O, vincristine (Oncovin); P, procarbazine; Pd, prednisone; Pl, cisplatin; TG, thioguanine; TT, thiotepa; V, vinblastine; X, radiotherapy.

proliferate. Female germ cells only proliferate prenatally and by birth are arrested at the oocyte stage. At birth there are 1 million oocytes, which are reduced to 300,000 at puberty and to fewer than 1,000 oocytes when menopause occurs at approximately age 50.[32]

Before recruitment to the process leading to ovulation, oocytes are found in primordial follicles with few pregranulosa cells, surrounded by thecal cells of the ovarian stroma. The stimulus for the initiation of follicular maturation depends on local growth factors, not the gonadotropic hormones. Once a follicle is recruited into growth, it develops until it either degenerates or ovulates. Follicular maturation is characterized by proliferation of granulosa cells and the development of steroidogenic potential of both the thecal and granulosa cells. Estrogen production involves the stimulation of both these cell types by LH and FSH and causes the LH surge that triggers ovulation. The cyclic variations in FSH, LH, and estradiol are essential for menstrual cycles and reproduction.

Because destruction of oocytes results in loss of follicles, germ cell loss leads directly to estrogen insufficiency. Radiation and chemotherapy appear to cause this germ cell loss by direct apoptotic action on the oocytes in mouse models.[33] When maturing follicles are destroyed by cytotoxic therapy, the result is oligomenorrhea or temporary amenorrhea. If the number of primordial follicles is reduced below the minimum necessary for menstrual cyclicity, irreversible *ovarian failure* and menopause (>12 months without a menstrual period) occur.

Characteristics of Gonadal Toxicity

Because the size of the germ cell population in women cannot be determined, menstrual and reproductive histories are important in assessing the effects of cytotoxic therapy on ovarian function. Information on the patient's sexual function and

TABLE 165.5

PERIODIC EVALUATION: CHILDREN'S ONCOLOGY GROUP

	Male	Female
History	Pubertal (onset, tempo) Sexual function (erections, nocturnal emissions, libido) Medication use impacting sexual function *Frequency:* Yearly	Pubertal (onset, tempo) Sexual function (vaginal dryness, libido) Medication use impacting sexual function Menstrual/pregnancy history *Frequency:* Yearly
Physical	Tanner staging Testicular volume by Prader orchidometry *Frequency:* Yearly until sexually mature	Tanner staging *Frequency:* Yearly until sexually mature
Screening	FSH LH Testosterone *Frequency:* Baseline at age 14 *and* as clinically indicated in patients with delayed puberty and/or clinical signs and symptoms of testosterone deficiency Semen analysis *Frequency:* As requested by patient and for evaluation of infertility. Periodic evaluation over time recommended as resumption of spermatogenesis can occur up to 10 years after therapy	FSH LH Estradiol *Frequency:* Baseline at age 13 *and* as clinically indicated in patients with delayed puberty, irregular menses, primary or secondary amenorrhea, and/or clinical signs and symptoms of estrogen deficiency

FSH, follicle-stimulating hormone; LH, luteinizing hormone.

menstrual histories during and after therapy is particularly useful (Table 165.5).[34] Because the mechanisms of temporary and irreversible treatment-related amenorrhea are different, posttreatment follow-up must be given to evaluate the significance of the outcome. To determine if effects are related to cytotoxic therapy, pretherapy ovarian function should be evaluated from the history of menarche, menses, pregnancies, and oral contraceptive use. The symptoms of recent primary ovarian failure, including hot flashes, night sweats, insomnia, mood swings, irritability, vaginal dryness, dyspareunia, decreased libido, and bladder infection, should be recorded. Laboratory measurements of hormone levels are most definitive in the diagnosis of primary ovarian failure. FSH level is the most sensitive, but LH and estradiol levels are also useful (Table 165.5). The physical symptoms and the changes in hormone levels associated with ovarian failure may be masked by oral contraceptive use or hormone replacement therapy.

Cytotoxic therapy often induces temporary amenorrhea, which may occasionally last several years.[35] Some patients with treatment-induced temporary amenorrhea do display menopausal symptoms. The permanent amenorrhea may begin during chemotherapy or subsequently, after several years of oligomenorrhea.[36] Factors resulting in temporary amenorrhea during treatment appear to be age-independent.[37] In contrast, the incidence of permanent treatment-induced amenorrhea (ovarian failure) dramatically and continuously increases with age at treatment (Tables 165.6 and 165.7), as expected from the decreasing number of follicles with increasing age.

TABLE 165.6

EFFECTS OF DIFFERENT CYTOTOXIC AGENTS ON OVARIAN FUNCTION

Agent	Prepuberty	Age 20 Y	Age 35 Y	Age 45 Y
CUMULATIVE DOSES TO CAUSE PERMANENT OVARIAN FAILURE				
Cyclophosphamide	>48 g	20–50 g	6–10 g	5 g
Melphalan	—	>240 mg/m²	>510 mg/m²	340 mg/m²
Busulfan	600 mg/m²	<600 mg/m²	<600 mg/m²	—
Chlorambucil	>3 g	>1.5 g	>1 g	1 g
Mitomycin C	—	—	≥30 g	≥30 g
Radiation	12 Gy	7 Gy	3 Gy	<2 Gy
INCIDENCE OF PERMANENT OVARIAN FAILURE (%)				
Cyclophosphamide (7.4 g/m²)	0	0	60	—
Radiation (pelvic) (4–5 Gy)	<10	40	90	95
Radiation (total body irradiation) (10 Gy)	40	75	100	100

TABLE 165.7

PROBABILITY OF OVARIAN FAILURE IN POSTMENARCHAL WOMEN TREATED WITH COMBINATION CHEMOTHERAPY REGIMENS CONTAINING ALKYLATING AGENTS

Regimen	Disease	Courses or Doses	Permanent Age (Y)	Incidence of Ovarian Failure (%)
MOPPd or MVPPd	Hodgkin's lymphoma	Approximately 6 courses P = approximately 6 g/m²	25 35	15 85
MOPPd/ABVD	Hodgkin's lymphoma	6 Courses P = 4.2 g/m²	25	0
CyOPPd	Hodgkin's lymphoma	Cy = 8 g/m² P = 8 g/m²	<24 >24	28 86
ChlVPPd/EVA	Hodgkin's lymphoma	6–8 courses P = 4 g/m² Chl = 300 mg/m²	25 36	0 100
Cy (alone) + HSCT	Aplastic anemia	Cy = 7.4 g/m²	13–58	50
BuCy + HSCT	Leukemia	Bu = 600 mg/m² Cy = 7.4 g/m²	14–57	99
BuMl + HSCT	Various	Bu = 600 mg/m² Ml = 140 mg/m²	9–17	100
FACy	Breast cancer	Cy = 13 g/m²	<34 >39	0 100
CyMxF	Breast cancer	Cy = 34 g/m²	<30 >35	0 100
CyAMx	Sarcoma	Cy = 5.3 g/m²	<35 >40	0 100

A, doxorubicin (Adriamycin); B, bleomycin; Bu, busulfan; Chl, chlorambucil; Cy, cyclophosphamide; D, dacarbazine; E, etoposide; F, 5-fluorouracil; HSCT, hematopoietic stem cell transplantation; M, mechlorethamine (nitrogen mustard); Ml, melphalan; Mx, methotrexate; O, vincristine (Oncovin); P, procarbazine; Pd, prednisone; V, vinblastine.

Childhood cancer survivors who retain ovarian function after treatment have a 13.21 relative risk of developing premature menopause.[38] When women aged 13 to 19 years are treated with alkylating agent chemotherapy and radiotherapy below the diaphragm, their median age at menopause is 32 years, compared with 44 years for women treated with either radiotherapy or chemotherapy alone and 49 years for controls.[39]

Cytotoxic therapy–induced ovarian failure accelerates bone density loss. However, when only chemotherapy is used, some residual ovarian function may be present despite the menopausal state, and the rate of bone density loss is less than when pelvic radiotherapy is used.[40]

Individual Drugs

In women, as in men, only alkylating agents appear to produce permanent gonadal failure (Table 165.6). The cumulative dose appears to be more important than the dose rate, as evidenced by similar incidences of ovarian failure in women who received similar total doses of cyclophosphamide, given either daily over several months[41] or within 4 days.[42] High doses of cisplatin (≥600 mg/m²) also produce permanent ovarian failure.[43] Procarbazine is likely to be highly sterilizing inasmuch as permanent ovarian failure is observed after treatment with several different procarbazine-containing combinations (Table 165.7).

Nonalkylating agents do not induce permanent ovarian failure. No ovarian failure was observed with 5-fluorouracil (30 g),[41] methotrexate (200 g) plus vincristine (40 g),[44] etoposide (5 g),[45] or cisplatin (<450 mg/m²) plus doxorubicin (<400 mg/m²)[43] in women aged 15 to 35 years. Doxorubicin (300 mg/m²), bleomycin, vincristine, and dacarbazine (ABVD) must not induce ovarian failure because none was observed after this treatment of women up to aged 41 years.[46]

Radiation Therapy

Radiation therapy induces permanent ovarian failure with marked age dependence in sensitivity (Table 165.6). Irradiation of the para-aortic nodes for Hodgkin's lymphoma results in cumulative ovarian doses of only 1.5 Gy and does not appear to interfere with menstruation in most patients.[47] Total nodal irradiation for Hodgkin's lymphoma or pelvic radiation for cervical cancer results in an ovarian dose of 4 to 5 Gy when proper transposition (oophoropexy) and shielding of the ovaries are performed, which preserves fertility in some younger women.[48] Total body irradiation in preparation for bone marrow transplantation delivers 8 to 12 Gy to the gonads, which destroys ovarian function in nearly all adult women.[42,49] Ovarian damage from radiation appears to be independent of whether it is given in one or six fractions.[26]

Combination Regimens

All combinations that include procarbazine and other alkylating agents (MOPP; CHOP; mechlorethamine, vinblastine, procarbazine, and prednisone [MVPP]; and chlorambucil, vinblastine, procarbazine, and prednisone [ChlVPP]) induce ovarian failure in almost all older women and even in some younger ones (Table 165.7). Ovarian function is maintained better by reducing the doses of these drugs through use of the MOPP/ABVD regimen.[50] Radiation and MOPP chemotherapy have additive, but not synergistic, effects, and the combination results in a higher incidence of ovarian failure than either modality alone.[51]

Similarly, regimens containing cyclophosphamide, as used in treatment of breast cancer (current average dose, approximately 3 g/m^2), also produce ovarian failure; however, the age dependence obscures any possible dose dependence. The treatments used for leukemia, which involve lower doses of cyclophosphamide and other agents that do not destroy primordial follicles, allow recovery of menses in women under age 35 years.[52] Combination chemotherapy regimens without alkylating agents do not produce ovarian failure.

EFFECTS OF CYTOTOXIC AGENTS ON CHILDREN

Extent of Gonadal Toxicity in Boys

The germinal epithelium in the prepubertal testis is not any more resistant to cytotoxic therapy than that in adults. When chemotherapy doses to boys are expressed appropriately on a per-meter-squared basis and radiation doses are calculated, the sterilizing effects of a variety of chemotherapy[53] and radiotherapy[54] regimens can be predicted on the basis of their effects on adult testes (Tables 165.3 and 165.4).

As in adults, radiation, alkylating agents such as procarbazine, cyclophosphamide, chlorambucil, BCNU, and CCNU, and cisplatin are the most sterilizing and produce prolonged and sometimes permanent azoospermia.[28,43] In addition, high doses of doxorubicin and cytosine arabinoside are additive with the aforementioned agents in producing gonadal damage.[55] Regimens lacking alkylating agents, such as some used for acute lymphocytic leukemia, can even allow pubertal progression of spermatogenesis during treatment.[56]

Most chemotherapy regimens do not affect Leydig cell function, and hence the timing of pubertal development and postpubertal testosterone levels are generally normal.[57] However, busulfan plus cyclophosphamide, used in preparation for hematopoietic stem cell transplantation, appears to delay puberty in approximately 30% of boys.[35]

Extent of Gonadal Toxicity in Girls

Prepubertal girls appear to be less susceptible than young postpubertal women to cytotoxic therapy–induced ovarian failure (Table 165.6). Furthermore, girls treated with radiation or alkylating agents, or both, between the ages of 0 and 12 years do not experience the premature menopause during their 20s and 30s that is observed in those treated at 13 to 19 years.[39]

Exposure of the ovaries to high-dose radiation, alkylating agents, and procarbazine are significant risk factors for acute ovarian failure in childhood cancer survivors.[58] Radiation is the most damaging agent to the prepubertal ovary: 20 to 30 Gy induces permanent ovarian failure in nearly all girls.[59] Doses of 8 to 15 Gy, usually with cyclophosphamide or melphalan in preparation for bone marrow transplantation, cause failure of ovarian function and pubertal development in 50% of girls,[60] with younger girls being less sensitive than older ones.[35] Radiation doses of up to 7 Gy do not cause ovarian failure or inhibit puberty[54] but can have additive effects if chemotherapy is also given.

Most chemotherapy regimens do not cause loss of primordial follicles or failure of pubertal development and menarche. This includes high doses of cyclophosphamide of up to 48 g,[61] various combination chemotherapy regimens used to treat leukemia, and the ABVD regimen for Hodgkin's lymphoma.[62] Even MOPP or nitrosourea chemotherapy does not affect pubertal and menstrual function development in 90% of the girls.[54,63] However, ChlVPP produces ovarian failure in 25% of girls[64] and busulfan plus cyclophosphamide inhibits puberty in 50% of girls.[35]

Besides causing ovarian damage, irradiation for solid tumors in the abdomen (20 Gy or more for Wilms' tumor) or in preparation for hematopoietic stem cell transplantation produces irreversible damage to uterine growth and blood flow in girls.[65] This damage affects achievement and outcome of pregnancy later in life.[66] If radiation doses are not too high (approximately 10 Gy, as in total body irradiation for transplantation), sex steroid replacement can improve uterine function.

GONADAL DYSFUNCTION AFTER CRANIAL IRRADIATION

Whereas gonadal irradiation causes primary hypogonadism, cranial irradiation is associated with secondary hypogonadism because of damage to the hypothalamus or the gonadotrophs in the pituitary, or both. In patients with pituitary or suprasellar lesions, gonadotropin deficiency is often present before antineoplastic therapy; however, patients with nasopharyngeal cancer or brain tumors have normal hypothalamic-pituitary-gonadal axes until they receive therapeutic irradiation with fields encompassing the hypothalamic–pituitary areas. In contrast, none of the cancer chemotherapeutic drugs directly impairs hypothalamic or anterior pituitary function.

In children, prophylactic cranial irradiation with 24 Gy for leukemia does not affect LH or FSH pulsatile secretion in the first 6 years,[67] but it does produce subtle effects that appear after puberty (Table 165.8).[68] However, in the shorter term, they may indirectly increase LH and FSH levels and cause precocious puberty in both boys and girls.[69] Because irradiation also produces growth hormone deficiency, precocious puberty further exacerbates the risk of adult shortness. Treatment with a gonadotropin-releasing hormone (GnRH) analogue to delay closure of the epiphysial growth plates and with growth hormone can be given to avoid growth stunting.

In adults, LH and FSH secretion decreases after cranial irradiation, and the decline becomes more severe with increasing treatment dose and time since treatment. This results in oligomenorrhea in women and low testosterone levels in men. Hyperprolactinemia might mediate the observed gonadal dysfunction in some cases.[70]

PRESERVATION OF FERTILITY, HORMONE LEVELS, AND SEXUAL FUNCTION

Choice of Regimens

It is sometimes possible to choose, among nearly equally curative regimens, one that minimizes the doses of the agents that are most sterilizing (Tables 165.3 and 165.6). The use of ABVD instead of MOPP to treat Hodgkin's lymphoma has dramatically reduced gonadal toxicity in a large group of patients.[10] In the treatment of non-Hodgkin's lymphoma, regimens that minimize the dose of cyclophosphamide, such as

TABLE 165.8

REPRODUCTIVE EFFECTS OF CRANIAL IRRADIATION

Radiation Dose to Pituitary/ Hypothalamus (Gy)	Disease	Reproductive Effects
CHILDHOOD CANCERS		
18–24	Leukemia	Slightly early puberty (girls)
		Subtle ovulatory disorder (after puberty)
25–49	Retinoblastoma, brain tumors, face and neck cancers	Some with precocious puberty (both genders)
		Higher doses: delay of puberty, gonadotropin deficiency at later times, failure of puberty
>50	Brain tumors, optic glioma	Some show gonadotropin deficiency (failure to undergo puberty)
CANCERS IN ADULTS		
10–13	Leukemia	No deficiencies at <5 y
20	Pituitary tumors	LH/FSH deficiency: 30% at 5 y; 40% at 10 y
35–40	Pituitary tumors	LH/FSH deficiency: 65% at 5 y, 90% at 10 y
40–70	Brain tumors	LH/FSH deficiency: 60% at 7 y
40–70	Nasopharyngeal, paranasal sinus tumors	LH/FSH deficiency: 15%–30% at 5 y, 45% at >10 y

FSH, follicle-stimulating hormone; LH, luteinizing hormone.

doxorubicin, cyclophosphamide, etoposide, vincristine, bleomycin, prednisone (VAPEC-B), produce gonadal failure less often in men than does CHOP with bleomycin.[71]

Gonadal Shielding and Oophoropexy

Except when the gonads must be irradiated because of actual or potential neoplastic involvement, they must be outside the field or shielded from the direct radiation beam. Nevertheless, an appreciable radiation dose from the accelerator head, collimator scatter, or internal lateral scatter may reach the gonads. Although moderately low radiation doses may be achieved, further reductions are desirable because of the possibilities of additive effects from chemotherapy and genetic damage to the sperm.

Gonadal dose depends on the distance from the field edge, field size, and photon energy. Pelvic radiation fields result in significant doses to the testis. Clamshell or other shields and beam blocking can reduce testicular doses two- to fivefold to 2 to 3 Gy for the inverted Y field used for Hodgkin's lymphoma and to 0.2 to 0.8 Gy for the hemipelvic field used for seminoma.[72]

To reduce ovarian dose, an oophoropexy, in which the ovaries are surgically translocated away from the direct beam, can be performed. That region is further shielded using lead blocks. Some investigators report reductions in cumulative ovarian doses to 4 to 5 Gy during total nodal irradiation,[54] which preserves fertility in younger women (Table 165.6).[48] There is convincing evidence that moving the ovaries outside the radiation field is beneficial in preserving ovarian function and future fertility in an adult population.[73,74] With advancement in the field of endoscopic surgery, these procedures can now be performed laparoscopically allowing for a shortened hospital stay, earlier mobilization, and earlier return to normal activity.[75,76]

Sperm Cryopreservation

Semen cryopreservation is an extremely important procedure for preserving the fertility potential of men after cytotoxic treatment for cancer.[77] The significance of notifying the patient of the potential risk of iatrogenic sterility as early as possible cannot be overemphasized.[78] Physicians often are aware early during the diagnostic process that the patient will most likely need to receive potentially sterilizing cytotoxic therapy, although the exact diagnosis, stage, and treatment regimen may not have yet been decided. This time should be used to initiate and complete the cryopreservation procedure. The number of samples to be banked may depend on how much time is available before starting therapy, sperm quality, and the cost of storing samples. Collection of three or four samples with approximately 48-hour periods of abstinence between sampling (a total of more than 5 days) is ideal. With current assisted reproductive technologies, however, success can be achieved with fewer samples, even with poor-quality semen. It is strongly advisable to complete sperm banking before starting therapy to avoid increased genetic damage in sperm collected after the start of therapy.[7] It is even possible to obtain semen with normal characteristics from 14- to 17-year-old boys by masturbation,[79] penile vibratory stimulation, or electroejaculation.[80] In addition, testicular sperm extraction is successful in 43% of pretreatment cancer patients who are azoospermic,[81] and the sperm obtained in this way can be cryopreserved and used in intracytoplasmic sperm injection (ICSI) procedures.[82] Testicular samples for sperm extraction can be obtained from orchiectomy or biopsy specimens that are routinely taken from testicular cancer patients if the surgeon is aware of the need and the processing procedures required for harvesting the sperm. Although a controversial topic, cryopreservation of immature testicular tissue in prepubertal boys with cancer may prove to be another suitable alternative.[83]

The success of *in vitro* fertilization (IVF) and ICSI makes cryopreservation of all samples containing any live sperm worthwhile. Even though 100% of oncologists in a study by Zapzalka et al.[84] reported discussing fertility issues with their patients, Schover et al.[77] found that only 60% of 900 male cancer patients surveyed who replied stated that they were informed about fertility issues and that only 51% stated they had been notified about sperm banking. The cost of sperm banking three samples, including analysis and storage for 5 years, is between $1,200 (at a university medical school clinic) and $2,500 (at some private sperm banks). Intrauterine insemination is the least expensive assisted reproductive technology method (cost per cycle, $200 to $500, plus $1,200 for superovulation of the female partner, if necessary), but the sperm count and quality after thawing must be high, and conception rates are lower than with IVF. If sperm count or motility is impaired or sample amounts are limited, IVF is necessary. The average cost of IVF, including the medications used, is $15,000 per cycle.

Optimization of Fertility after Treatment

If sperm count recovers after cancer therapy, it usually reaches normospermic levels. However, some men remain oligospermic for many years. Although controlled studies have not been done, men who have recovered sperm production appear to have normal fertility, and their incidence of infertility does not appear to be any higher than the 15% rate among couples in the general population. Furthermore, cancer patients with recovered sperm counts ranging from just below 1 million/mL to 10 million/mL are able to successfully father children.[13] Infertile patients with oligospermia should be managed in the same way as are those in the general population with male factor infertility, including the use of IVF with or without ICSI.[85]

Assisted Reproductive Technologies

Currently, the choices for preserving fertility in chemotherapy patients are limited (Table 165.9). Some are investigational, and all have demonstrated variable success. Fertility preservation can be attempted either with assisted reproductive technologies, gamete cryopreservation, or medical treatment. Assisted reproductive technology refers to *in vitro* handling of human oocytes and sperm or embryos for the purpose of establishing a pregnancy. Techniques for gamete preservation include sperm cryopreservation, oocyte cryopreservation, ovarian cortical cryopreservation, or whole ovary cryopreservation. Many advances are quickly developing in the arena of gamete preservation; however, these are still considered to be investigational. Medical therapy includes treatment with hormonal agents such as oral contraceptive pills, progesterone, and GnRH analogues.[86–99]

Assisted reproductive technology is still undergoing rapid advances and provides new options for cancer survivors with gonadal damage to achieve fertility. Previously, intrauterine insemination had been the only fertility preservation method available, and only 30% of men who had stored high-quality semen samples were able to achieve pregnancy.[100]

Currently, IVF with ICSI is the most successful method for achieving pregnancy from banked sperm. ICSI makes it possible to use a single spermatozoa to achieve oocyte fertilization through IVF. This technology has revolutionized the treatment of male infertility.[101] ICSI is also often used with frozen banked sperm. IVF can be performed to create embryos that can be frozen and stored for later use. Pregnancy outcomes vary by IVF center but overall are excellent with frozen embryo transfers. The downside of IVF is that a single cycle can take 2 to 3 weeks to complete and necessitates a delay in cancer treatment. Varying regimens can be used for ovarian stimulation.

Women with estrogen-responsive tumors can undergo ovulation induction with an aromatase inhibitor either as a solo agent or as an adjunct to standard stimulation protocols.[102,103] To avoid the potential risks of rising estradiol levels during ovarian stimulation (sometimes 10 to 20 times levels seen in natural cycles), an increasing number of fertility specialists are using aromatase inhibitors (letrozole or tamoxifen) for ovarian stimulation.[104] To date, the recurrence and survival rates of breast cancer patients undergoing such protocols were comparable with those of unstimulated control breast cancer patients.[105]

Clinical pregnancy rates of 30% to 50% per cycle and live birth rates of 25% to 50% can be expected at most fertility clinics. Cumulative live birth rates for three cycles have been reported as 63%.[106] Although fresh sperm is preferred to frozen sperm in intrauterine insemination and IVF cycles, studies have shown excellent outcomes using sperm that was frozen and banked prior to cancer treatment.[107] Although insemination with testicular sperm is an acceptable procedure, the use of

TABLE 165.9

OPTIONS FOR FERTILITY PRESERVATION

Males	Females
Sperm banking prior to chemotherapy Sperm collection via masturbation or surgical retrieval	**Medical treatment** GnRH analogues (agonists, antagonists)
Testicular cryopreservation and future transplantation	**Ovarian cryopreservation and future transplantation** Cortical strip Whole ovary
	Assisted reproductive technology Embryo banking (partner sperm or donor sperm) Oocyte banking (cryopreservation or vitrification)

GnRH, gonadotropin-releasing hormone.

nuclei from earlier stages (round spermatid nuclear injection) is not currently advisable.[108] Overall, embryo banking is the most successful form of fertility preservation and should be offered to all women who are either in a serious relationship, married, or who are open to the idea of using donor sperm.

Oocyte banking either via cryopreservation (slow freezing) or vitrification (rapid freezing) is an option for single women who are not interested in using donor sperm. Similar to IVF, this entails ovarian hyperstimulation followed by surgical oocyte retrieval and, similar to IVF, also necessitates a delay in treatment ranging from 2 to 6 weeks.[109] Oocyte cryopreservation and vitrification are still considered experimental procedures, although rapid advances are currently being made.[110,111]

Most studies indicate no increases in congenital malformations or developmental abnormalities in the offspring from pregnancies achieved with IVF or ICSI,[112] although there are occasional reports to the contrary.[113] However, there is an increased risk of approximately 3% for chromosomal abnormalities, mostly in the numbers of sex chromosomes, in offspring of ICSI procedures.[114] Most of the chromosome abnormalities were not caused by ICSI, however, but were already present in the sperm of the infertile male parent. These abnormalities, which are common in cases of primary male infertility, should not be present in cryopreserved sperm from cancer patients.

Female Germ Cell Cryopreservation and Development

In addition to cryopreservation of oocytes, cryopreservation of ovarian tissue can be undertaken (Table 165.9). One method entails surgical removal of ovarian tissue containing numerous primordial follicles, cryopreservation of tissue slices, and subsequent grafting back to the site of the ovary. This was initially successful in restoring ovarian endocrine function and fertility in sheep.[115] Restoration of hormone production and follicular growth in women after transplantation of fresh or cryopreserved ovarian tissue into heterotopic (forearm) sites has been reported and lasted up to 2 years after transplantation.[116] The true long-term success of this technique, including oocyte competence, remains to be determined. With some cancers, particularly leukemia, neuroblastoma, breast, and uterine carcinomas, there is also concern that malignant cells may be reintroduced to the host with subsequent transplantation of the ovarian tissue.[116]

A handful of reports have demonstrated the feasibility of this method. Poirot et al.[117] described 31 women, adolescents, and premenarchal girls who were referred by their oncologists for ovarian tissue cryopreservation. They evaluated the feasibility of long-term cryopreservation of ovarian tissue in women and young girls scheduled to undergo treatments that would probably render them sterile. Ages ranged from 2.7 to 34 years (16 were <18 years old) and most had received prior chemotherapy for different diseases. Ovarian cortical tissue was obtained by either laparotomy or laparoscopy. The procedure was well tolerated with no postsurgical complications reported. They analyzed numbers of primordial and primary follicles from one sample of ovarian cortex from each patient at the time of cryopreservation. The mean number of primordial and primary follicles per square millimeter was 20.36 ± 19.03 before 10 years of age, 4.13 ± 2.9 between 10 and 15 years of age, and 1.63 ± 3.35 after 15 years of age. An average mean number of 26 ± 8.2 ovarian fragments (range, 13 to 50) were cryopreserved per patient for future autografts or for *in vitro* growth of follicles. This enabled the patients to begin cancer treatment very quickly, especially when the ovarian collection was made by laparoscopy.[117] They showed that ovarian tissue cryopreservation was a viable option in patients exposed to chemotherapy and should result in higher fertility success rates in younger girls as their ovarian cortex contains many more primordial follicles compared with older patients. None of the cryopreserved ovarian tissue was transplanted, thus data regarding pregnancy success are unavailable.

Ovarian tissue cryopreservation is also an attractive alternative for fertility preservation and for restoring ovarian function in the pediatric population because ovarian stimulation is not required. Furthermore, patients do not need to have a partner at the time of treatment, there is no delay in treatment, and the tissue can remain frozen until the patient is ready for conception. Because of the large numbers of immature oocytes in the ovarian cortex, this is an excellent emerging method suitable for premenarchal girls.[116,118,119]

Does It Work?

Results in various animal models have been encouraging in demonstrating the efficacy of ovarian cryopreservation and reimplantation.[120–123] Further studies are needed to prove the efficacy of ovarian cryopreservation in humans.[98] To date there have a handful of reports of successful pregnancies after ovarian tissue cryopreservation and reimplantation. The first report was by Donnez et al.,[124] of a 25-year-old woman with Hodgkin's lymphoma. The patient had undergone removal of ovarian cortical strips prior to chemotherapy. The patient became newly amenorrheic and posttreatment ovarian failure was documented by FSH, LH, and estradiol levels. Although ovarian failure was documented on several occasions, the patient's ovaries remained *in situ*. After 9 months, the patient achieved a spontaneous conception and went on to deliver a healthy female infant at term. Critics of this work cite that it cannot be proven that ovulation occurred from the grafted tissue, which was in close proximity to the patient's ovaries as opposed to spontaneous ovulation from the ovary.[125]

Silber and Gosden[126] published a case series describing seven pairs of monozygotic twins discordant for ovarian function who underwent ovarian transplantation. Four of seven conceived and one patient conceived twice. On average, restoration of ovarian function ensued after 2 to 4 months after transplantation. Several other live births have been reported from ovarian cortical transplantation.[127–129] These cases are undoubtedly the first of many more to come. Ovarian cortical cryopreservation with subsequent reimplantation at this time is considered experimental and should only be performed in centers under institutional review board–approved protocols and necessary expertise. It can be anticipated that many more live births will occur as a result of this novel technique.

An alternate approach to ovarian preservation involves transplantation of the whole ovary as opposed to just cortical strips. The main obstacle facing ovarian cortical strip cryopreservation is the threat of ischemic damage prior to graft reimplantation.[121,130] To combat this threat, maintenance of blood supply via whole-ovary cryopreservation with preservation of vascular pedicles might offer a potential advantage in reduction of the large follicular loss. With the use of dimethylsulfoxide as a cryoprotectant, improved follicular preservation has been noted compared with glycerol, which had been used in the past. Furthermore, recent microsurgical advances to enhance intact ovarian freezing and transplantation have been successful in rodents. Nine of ten transplanted ovaries had successful restoration of ovarian function and six of ten transplanted rats became pregnant.[131] In sheep, whose ovarian structure is more comparable to that of humans, intact ovaries with vascular pedicles were cryopreserved and later autotransplanted with microvascular anastomosis of the ovarian artery and vein to the branches of deep inferior epigastric vessels.[132]

A recent study in sheep demonstrated ovarian function 6 years after transplantation of whole ovaries with the use of unidirectional solidification freezing technology.[133] The sheep underwent superovulation and the ovaries were found to have evidence of follicular growth and development.[133] More experience is needed with whole ovary transplantation for this to be a viable option for fertility preservation.

Another approach to oocyte preservation involves cryopreservation of immature oocytes in the germinal vesicle stage, followed by *in vitro* maturation (IVM) to meiotic metaphase II. These oocytes can then be fertilized *in vitro*. The first live birth from IVM was reported in 1991.[134] The application of IVM is becoming more widespread, ranging from retrieval of immature oocytes in unstimulated or minimally stimulated cycles to reduce the cost of IVF to retrieval of immature oocytes for fertility preservation.[135–137]

It is possible that in the future stem cells may be used to repopulate the ovary. The derivation of oocytes from mouse embryonic stem cells in culture suggests the eventual power of stem cell technology and nuclear transplantation for production of oocytes, perhaps even from somatic cell nuclei.[138] However, application of such techniques to human infertility is currently still under investigation.

Most women who continue to have menstrual function after cytotoxic therapy for cancer but are infertile should be treated in the same way as similar women in the general population. One important exception is women who have uterine damage from receiving more than 10 Gy of abdominal radiation in childhood. These patients have increased rates of adverse pregnancy outcomes, including fetal or neonatal death, premature delivery, and low-birthweight babies, and hence their pregnancies must be closely monitored.[66] In women with ovarian failure, the use of donor oocytes and hormonal treatment to maintain pregnancy has been successful.[130]

Immature Male Germ Cell Cryopreservation and Development

For restoration of spermatogenesis, the harvest and cryopreservation of spermatogonial stem cells, which are capable of proliferation, self-renewal, and repopulation of the seminiferous tubules, are under investigation. Transplantation of cryopreserved testicular germ cells from a donor mouse into the seminiferous tubules of a recipient mouse, in which endogenous stem spermatogonia were killed with busulfan, restored spermatogenesis and fertility.[139] There are preliminary indications that this technique might restore spermatogenesis in irradiated macaques.[140] Testicular cells have been harvested from men before sterilizing cytotoxic therapy and later injected back into the testicular tubules after the completion of radiotherapy or chemotherapy. This technique would be most valuable for prepubertal boys, who are too young to produce sperm but have testes enriched in spermatogonia. Similar to female cancer patients, there exists concern that cancer cells may be reintroduced into the recipients. This possibility is a contraindication in cases of leukemia or testicular cancer, but the risks with other cancers may not be high.[141] To date, there has not yet been a report of successful transplantation of testicular tissue in a male patient.

One way to circumvent the problem of the presence of tumor cells is to first transplant the tissue into a xenogeneic host. Human spermatogonial stem cells survive and proliferate in seminiferous tubules of mice.[142] Also, subcutaneous transplantation of cryopreserved testicular tissue from immature pigs and goats into nude mice results in the production of functional sperm.[143] However, the risks of transfer of animal DNA or viruses (especially retroviruses) from the host to the human spermatogonial cells must be evaluated before such techniques could be applied.

New experimental approaches to germ cell development could some day be applied to fertility preservation in men. The *in vitro* development of human round spermatids into elongated spermatids, which were used to produce normal embryos by ICSI, has been reported.[144] Development of an *in vitro* cell line derived from genetically modified mouse spermatogonia, which proliferates to produce more spermatogonia and can be stimulated to form haploid cells,[145] holds promise as a very useful resource for optimizing proliferation of spermatogonia and production of spermatids. Furthermore, the development of sperm from mouse embryonic stem cells by a combination of induction of differentiation *in vitro* and transplantation into host testes[146] might eventually lead to methods for development of sperm from other stem cell types obtained from a cancer patient.

PHARMACOLOGIC ATTEMPTS AT PRESERVING FERTILITY IN MEN

Hormone treatments have been investigated for their ability to enhance the survival of germ cells and promote recovery after cytotoxic treatments. Treatment of male rats with hormones that suppress testosterone levels or action (gonadal steroids, GnRH analogues, antiandrogens) before and during cytotoxic therapy with radiation or procarbazine enhances the subsequent recovery of spermatogenesis and fertility.[147] The original proposal that these treatments would protect the spermatogonia from killing by suppressing their proliferation is incorrect; rather, the suppression of testosterone levels protects the subsequent ability of the somatic cells of the testis to support the recovery of spermatogenesis from surviving stem spermatogonia.[148] The hormonal treatment can even be given several months after exposure to radiation or procarbazine and still restore spermatogenesis and fertility.[147]

Because stem spermatogonia are indeed present in regions of the testes of some cancer patients during prolonged periods of iatrogenic azoospermia, their recovery could possibly be stimulated. However, only one[149] of eight clinical trials has been able to demonstrate protection of spermatogenesis in humans by hormone treatment before and during cytotoxic therapy.[150] One attempt to restore spermatogenesis by steroid hormone treatment after cytotoxic therapy was unsuccessful[151]; however, the doses of cytotoxic therapy were very high, and the hormonal suppression was given many years after the anticancer treatment. More discouraging was the failure of GnRH antagonist treatment to enhance spermatogenic recovery in a controlled primate study,[152] which suggests that there are important differences in this process in rats and in primates.

PHARMACOLOGIC ATTEMPTS AT PRESERVING FERTILITY IN WOMEN

Although studies have been performed to assess the efficacy of oral contraceptive pills and GnRH analogues in girls, adolescents, and women, no comparative studies have been done using progestins in these age groups. Most studies do not support the use of hormonal therapy for the prevention of premature ovarian failure in girls and premenarchal adolescents receiving chemotherapy, because prior to the onset of menarche, the ovaries are thought to be quiescent and less likely to be subject to damage by cytotoxic agents. Therefore, there would be no additional benefit to giving hormonal therapy to an already suppressed hypothalamic-pituitary-ovarian axis. Furthermore, the use of estrogen may be associated with an increased risk of venous thrombosis. There is also concern regarding the side-effect profile of hormonal therapy in premenarchal girls.

Longhi et al.[86] performed a small, observational study that examined the effects of oral contraceptive pills on ovarian function in premenarchal girls and postmenarchal women undergoing neoadjuvant chemotherapy treatment for osteosarcoma. They concluded that age and alkylant dose were the most predictive factors for early menopause, and that oral contraceptives during high-dose alkylant-based chemotherapy did not prevent chemotherapy-induced premature ovarian failure. The follow-up time of this study was too short to rule out any positive long-term effects on the preservation of ovarian function. In addition, this study did show greater risk than benefit as two patients in the group receiving chemotherapy plus oral contraceptive pills developed thrombophlebitis. Similar findings have been observed in other studies.[87] The majority of the evidence suggests that children and premenarchal adolescents do not benefit from hormonal suppression to preserve their ovarian function while undergoing chemotherapy.

Contrary to oral contraceptives, GnRH analogues seem to be a promising therapy. Preservation of ovarian function with the use of GnRH analogues, specifically agonists, prior to cancer treatment, has been shown to be beneficial.[88,89] It has been proposed that GnRH agonist use prior to chemotherapy has a protective effect via two mechanisms. First, by down-regulating the hypothalamic-pituitary-ovarian axis, it might reduce the number of primordial follicles destroyed by toxic agents. Second, it may reduce the blood flow to the ovary and decrease the delivery of toxic chemotherapeutic agents.[90,91] This second theory may also explain the lack of a protective effect with GnRH analogues on ovarian function observed with increasing chemotherapeutic dosages and provide an explanation why this treatment has no effect with radiation therapy.[90,92]

Animal studies have provided very convincing evidence regarding the efficacy of GnRH analogues. Ataya et al.[88] conducted a prospective study looking at the effects of leuprolide on ovarian function in primates exposed to cyclophosphamide. Six adult female rhesus monkeys underwent unilateral oophorectomy and were divided into two groups. One group received cyclophosphamide and monthly injections of leuprolide, and the other received cyclophosphamide and placebo. At the end of treatment, the remaining ovary was removed and compared to the pretreated ovary. Ovarian follicle number and size were compared. As expected, there was a decline in follicle number with chemotherapy. Cyclophosphamide resulted in a significant reduction of nonprimordial follicles and primordial follicles compared to the leuprolide and cyclophosphamide group. The authors concluded that in rhesus monkeys, leuprolide protected the ovary against cyclophosphamide-induced damage.

Human studies have also provided evidence for the efficacy of GnRH analogues. Two recent randomized studies from patients with breast cancer demonstrated some evidence of protective effect of GnRH agonist treatment on the preservation of ovarian function.[153,154] However, these studies have been questioned[155–157] and will require larger study populations to definitively conclude the chemoprotective effects of GnRH analog therapy. Cancer patients are not the only population who routinely receive chemotherapy. In recent years, the use of cyclophosphamide has evolved to treat systemic lupus erythematosus (SLE) patients. Unfortunately, large numbers of affected patients are reproductive-aged women. Many of the studies using GnRH analogues were in women receiving chemotherapy either for cancer or SLE.

Blumenfeld et al.[89] have examined the use of GnRH agonists in both women with cancer and with SLE. In 1997, their group published a study using GnRH agonists in women with lymphoma and compared them to a historic control group. Eighteen cycling women with lymphoma, aged 15 to 40 years, were pretreated with leuprolide prior to chemotherapy until its conclusion, or for a maximum of 6 months. Most of the patients were treated with MOPP/ABVD combination chemotherapy followed by mantle field radiation, and were compared to a matched control group of 18 women who received MOPP/ABVD with or without mantle field radiotherapy. In the pretreated group 93.7% resumed spontaneous ovulation and menses compared with 39% in the control group. Sixty-one percent experienced premature ovarian failure in the control group. They concluded that GnRH agonist cotreatment with chemotherapy was protective from irreversible chemotherapy-induced ovarian damage. Although this study provides some convincing evidence, it is not without limitations. First, there were marked differences in the follow-up periods in the pretreated group compared to the controls (1.7 1 ± 0 years vs. 7.0 ± 4.9 years). Second, the treatment regimens varied greatly with the use of alkylating agents; only 4 of 16 in the study group received cyclophosphamide compared with 10 of 18 in the control group.[89,93]

Another study published by the same group in 2000 examined the preservation of fertility and ovarian function in young women with SLE treated with chemotherapy.[94] The investigators administered leuprolide to eight women with severe autoimmune connective tissue disease in parallel to chemotherapy, for up to 6 months. These women were compared with a control group of nine women similarly treated but who did not receive leuprolide. They found that those women who did not receive GnRH agonist suffered premature ovarian failure and had hypergonadotropic amenorrhea. Fifty-five percent of patients treated by alkylating agents experienced premature ovarian failure and had hypergonadotropic amenorrhea. However, two of these five women were 35 years old. Based on their data, they concluded that GnRH agonist cotreatment should be offered for preservation of future fertility and ovarian function in every young woman of reproductive age exposed to alkylating agents. This study also provides convincing data in support of the use of GnRH agonist treatment prior to the onset of chemotherapy.[94]

Although there is less evidence in the literature for the use of GnRH antagonists, the experience with ovulation induction and assisted reproductive technologies suggests it may have similar efficacy to GnRH agonists. On administration of GnRH agonists there is an initial stimulatory "flare" effect prior to pituitary desensitization that ensues after 7 to 14 days. GnRH antagonists work via rapid inhibition of gonadotropin and sex steroids secretion and have an almost immediate down-regulation of the pituitary gland. Because desensitization is so rapid, they have the advantage of not causing an initial flare effect. Gonadotropin deprivation halts follicular recruitment and decreases the size of the chemotherapy-sensitive pool.[90]

GnRH antagonists are beginning to be studied further in both animals and humans. Using a mouse model, Meirow et al.[90] administered a GnRH antagonist, cetrorelix, prior to exposure to increasing doses of cyclophosphamide. The aim of the study was to assess the number of surviving primordial follicles in the ovaries of young mice. In each treatment group, half of the females were injected daily with cetrorelix starting 9 days before and 7 days posttreatment of cyclophosphamide. After treatment, ovarian sections were taken and the total number of primordial follicles in both ovaries was counted.

A dose-response relationship was observed. Ovaries exposed to cyclophosphamide at dosages of 50 and 75 mg/kg had significantly fewer primordial follicles than those in the control group. In each of the cyclophosphamide groups that were pretreated with cetrorelix, there were higher numbers of primordial follicles compared to controls. Administration of GnRH antagonist cetrorelix to mice significantly decreased the extent of ovarian damage induced by the chemotherapeutic agent. Both GnRH agonists and antagonists have the added advantage of menstrual suppression and therefore can be used to avoid heavy uterine bleeding often seen with hematologic malignancies.

At this time, although the data seem promising with regard to GnRH analogues, the studies are plagued by low numbers and short follow-up periods. Thus, there is insufficient evidence to definitively recommend this therapy, and further study is greatly needed. For every study demonstrating a positive outcome, there is similarly a study with negative results.[93,98] It has also been theorized that GnRH agonists may counteract the effects of chemotherapeutic agents by two different mechanisms. First, they may potentially induce antioxidant enzymes that detoxify chemotherapeutics and render follicles more vulnerable to the effects of chemotherapy.[99] Alternatively, they may maintain tumor cells in the G0/G1 phase of the cell cycle, making them less responsive to chemotherapy. However, recent evidence has shown that disease-free survival and overall survival were not negatively impacted by the use of GnRH analogues.[158] A meta-analysis published in *The Lancet* based on data from 11,906 premenopausal women with early breast cancer randomized in 16 trials showed that the addition of GnRH-a to tamoxifen, chemotherapy, or both, reduced disease recurrence by 12.7% and death after recurrence by 15.1%.[159] The question of whether GnRH agonists and antagonists offer benefit needs to be answered by a randomized, controlled, double-blinded trial.

Ovarian suppression should be considered in all postmenarchal and reproductive-age women prior to initiating therapy, as it may help to preserve future fertility. There is no good evidence to support offering hormonal suppression to premenarchal girls. Patients who undergo chemotherapy and continue to menstruate should be closely followed for signs and symptoms of premature ovarian failure. Discussions regarding oocyte cryopreservation and ovarian cortical strip cryopreservation are needed and treatment offered if institutional review board protocols exist. Continuous developments will enable physicians to preserve and restore fertility in a growing number of cancer survivors. If these therapies are not available, or if they are offered and do not work, therapies such as oocyte donation are excellent alternatives.

FERTILITY PRESERVATION IN WOMEN WITH CERVICAL CANCER

Women with early-stage cervical cancer are most often treated with radical hysterectomy or radiotherapy to the pelvis. As women delay their childbearing and as screening programs have become more effective, an increasing number of patients with early-stage cervical cancer seek to preserve their future fertility.[160] Dargent et al.[161] first described a small group of patients who had undergone a radical vaginal excision of the cervix (radical trachelotomy) in whom they preserved the uterus and also performed a concomitant pelvic lymph node dissection. The incidence of recurrence of disease following radical vaginal trachelectomy is between 4.2% and 5.3% and there is a death rate of 2.5% to 3.2%,[162] not significantly different from historical controls.[163] Over 300 pregnancies with 195 live births have been reported but are at risk for premature rupture of membranes and preterm delivery.[160]

EVALUATION OF FERTILITY AFTER TREATMENT

Male and female cancer survivors should undergo timely evaluation when they are attempting conception. For males, it would be reasonable to obtain a semen analysis either before attempting conception or when conception fails to occur after 6 months of unprotected intercourse. Premature ovarian failure can be suspected based on a careful menstrual history. Shortening of the intermenstrual interval is an ominous sign that ovarian reserve is diminished. Evaluation of ovarian reserve with a gynecologist or reproductive endocrinologist is warranted for women who report amenorrhea, shortened menstrual cycles, irregular cycles, or for cancer survivors who have failed to conceive after 6 months of unprotected intercourse. There is no single best test available to measure ovarian reserve, but surrogate markers such as early follicular phase (cycle day 2–4) measures of antral follicles, ovarian volumes, FSH, estradiol, and antimüllerian hormone levels can been used. These tests, however, must be interpreted with caution, as the true utility is in predicting ovarian responsiveness and not reserve.

HORMONE REPLACEMENT THERAPY

New information that estrogen with or without progesterone given to postmenopausal women (aged 50 to 79 years) increases the cardiovascular risks[164] has led to the view that the risks of hormone replacement therapy for normal postmenopausal women (cardiovascular disease and breast cancer) outweigh the benefits (increased bone mineral density and reduced incidence of fracture). However, the physiologic replacement of ovarian hormones still remains appropriate for young, otherwise premenopausal girls who have developed premature ovarian failure as a result of their malignancy or cancer treatment. This is particularly true for adolescent girls and young women in whom bone mineral density is normally increasing.[165] In these cases, it is important to test for ovarian failure shortly after treatment and, if appropriate, to start hormone replacement therapy in a timely manner. If a woman has an intact uterus, estrogen should be combined with progesterone to prevent endometrial hyperplasia and cancer.[165]

In males, germinal aplasia is often associated with testosterone levels in the low to normal range, and such individuals may experience reduced bone mineral density and a slight reduction in sexual function.[166] However, a controlled trial failed to show any benefit of testosterone treatment on bone mineral density or sexual function, which indicates that this mild hypogonadism is not of clinical importance in most men.[166] Testosterone replacement is, nevertheless, very important in cases of overt Leydig cell failure in prepubertal boys to promote secondary sexual characteristics, growth, and bone density.

PREVENTION AND MANAGEMENT OF ERECTILE AND EJACULATORY DYSFUNCTION

Ejaculation of semen first requires emission (the deposition of semen in the posterior urethra by contractions of the vas deferens, seminal vesicles, and prostate) and then antegrade ejaculation, which involves coordinated tightening of the bladder neck, relaxation of the external sphincter, and expulsion of semen. Most of these processes are controlled by trunks of nerve fibers forming the hypogastric plexus overlying the aorta and sacrum below the origin of the inferior mesenteric artery.[167] Surgery for testicular, prostate, and bladder cancers can produce neurologic dysfunction, resulting in failure of emission, retrograde ejaculation, impotence, and loss of orgasm. However, improvements in surgical techniques have reduced these adverse outcomes without diminishing the efficacy of treating the cancer.[168] Newer RPLND techniques used for nonseminomatous testicular germ cell tumors in addition to bilateral nerve-sparing modification for patients undergoing radical prostatectomies preserves ejaculatory function compared with controls.[18,169] In cases in which the cavernous nerves cannot be spared, the technique of interposition sural nerve grafting has been shown to help preserve postoperative potency.[170]

For men experiencing erectile dysfunction, phosphodiesterase type 5 inhibitors, such as sildenafil, vardenafil, and tadalafil, are clinically effective and safe treatments.[171] For patients who are not responsive to oral administration of these drugs, other treatment options for improving erectile function include intracorporeal injection therapy with a prostaglandin or a mixture of a prostaglandin, an alkaloid, and an α-adrenergic blocker, or penile prosthetic surgery. A penile prosthesis is usually not offered to patients until 2 years after radical prostatectomy to allow for tissue healing and adequate monitoring of cancer control.

In patients who experience ejaculatory dysfunction after RPLND, the postmasturbation urine should be investigated for the presence of sperm cells.[172] Use of sympathomimetic agents may enhance seminal emission and partially or completely convert the patient to antegrade ejaculation.[173] Pseudoephedrine hydrochloride, ephedrine sulfate, phenylpropanolamine hydrochloride, or imipramine hydrochloride should be given sequentially in 2-week trials until improvements in semen volume and sperm count are observed.[172] Natural pregnancies have been reported, but use of assisted reproductive technologies is often needed. Even when retrograde ejaculation is present, sperm may be recovered from the bladder by direct voiding into a buffering medium or by catheterization and irrigation with a somewhat alkaline solution.[174] When no ejaculation is present, electroejaculation, using a rectal probe under general anesthesia, has been successful in most patients.[175] Although patients will have some antegrade ejaculate, catheterization should always be done to collect the retrograde semen. Sperm obtained by these methods can be used with IVF/ICSI procedures to achieve 15% pregnancy rates per cycle.

GENETIC CONCERNS

Biologic Considerations

Many anticancer agents damage DNA and interfere with its replication and repair and with chromosome segregation in both animal and human cells. These agents induce both single-gene and chromosomal mutations in germ cells of animals,[176] both of which cause genetic disease in offspring. Mutations induced in stem spermatogonia cause continued production of mutation-carrying sperm for the lifetime of the male, whereas those induced in later stages of spermatogenesis result in production of mutation-carrying sperm for only a few months. Radiation and several alkylating agents produce single-gene mutations in murine spermatogonia, whereas other tested chemotherapeutic drugs do not.[176] Radiation is the only agent that effectively induces stable reciprocal chromosomal translocations in stem spermatogonia that can be transmitted to offspring.[177]

In male rodents, meiotic and postmeiotic germ cells are more sensitive to induction and transmission of mutations than are stem spermatogonia.[7] Therefore, mutational risks are highest when a pregnancy occurs within one spermatogenic cycle (time required for stem cells to become sperm) after the male is exposed to the damaging agent. Clinical reports of outcomes of pregnancies in which conception occurred while the man was undergoing cytotoxic therapy are too limited to evaluate the risks, but animal experiments and gamete genetic analysis show a higher risk.[7] In men, this higher-risk period extends from the start of cytotoxic therapy until 3 months after the last course. Damage to sperm DNA for up to 2 years after completion of therapy has been reported in a patient undergoing radiation therapy and chemotherapy for testicular cancer and systemic therapy for Hodgkin's lymphoma.[178,179]

Fewer studies of the mutagenicity of cytotoxic agents have been done in female mice, but the limited results indicate induced mutation frequencies similar to those in male mice. Radiation induces single-gene and chromosomal mutations in developing oocytes.[180] Most alkylating agents and a variety of other chemotherapeutic drugs induce chromosome aberrations or other mutations in developing oocytes that result in embryonic death.[176] There are insufficient data to determine whether primordial or growing oocytes are more sensitive to induction of mutations.

Pregnancy Outcome

In humans, nearly all of the case reports, small series, and a few large retrospective case studies of the outcomes of pregnancies in, or produced by, survivors of cancer indicated no significant increase in birth defects or genetic disease in offspring conceived after cytotoxic treatment above the background level in the general population of approximately 4%.[180,181] No increase in genetic disease was observed in 630 offspring of patients who were children or adolescents at the time of treatment and received alkylating agents or radiation proximal to the gonads.[182] A study of 368 conceptions in adult women treated previously with methotrexate alone showed no significant adverse effects, as expected.[183] In males, 70 offspring of testicular cancer patients treated with radiotherapy or chemotherapy (most received cisplatin), or both, revealed no apparent increase in congenital malformations.[184] In a case-control study involving 45,000 children with congenital abnormalities, there was no higher incidence of parental exposure to alkylating agents or radiation proximal to the gonads in the parents of children with congenital abnormalities than in the parents of the control group of children.[185] The results from the atomic bomb studies in Japan also show no significant increase in genetic damage in 30,000 offspring born to radiation-exposed parents.[167]

These observations should reassure those who wish to have children after treatment for cancer. However, the power of these studies can only rule out twofold or higher increases in abnormalities; the possibility remains of a small genetic risk that would increase genetic abnormalities less than twofold over background levels. Also, these long-term studies do not include many patients receiving the newer chemotherapeutic agents.

There are significant teratogenic risks from cytotoxic therapy given to a woman during pregnancy. Radiation is highly damaging; doses as low as 0.1 to 0.2 Gy in the first trimester and doses higher than 0.7 Gy in the second trimester cause microcephaly.[186] Almost all cytotoxic chemotherapeutic agents are considered teratogenic; however, some may be safely given in the second and third trimesters of pregnancy.[187] Treatment with fluorouracil, doxorubicin, and cyclophosphamide during this period did not result in any adverse effects. Methotrexate, which is a documented teratogen in the first trimester, was excluded from the combination.

Gamete Genomic Analysis

Because epidemiologic studies of genetic damage in humans require large numbers of offspring, direct analyses of the genetic material of gametes have huge potential advantages for identifying heritable mutations in humans. Such analyses are used only in the male because harvest of female gametes is impractical. These analyses can be used to detect both single-gene and chromosomal mutations.

Chromosomal abnormalities are measured by sperm karyotyping after fusion with hamster eggs or by fluorescence *in situ* hybridization. Structural chromosomal aberrations were present in sperm more than 5 years after the end of MOPP or radiation therapy, or both, which indicates that they are induced in stem cells.[188] Numerical aberrations (aneuploidy) can show up to a fivefold increase during and shortly after chemotherapy with NOVP or bleomycin, etoposide, and cisplatin (BEP) and then return to baseline within 4 months or 2 years, depending on the study.[189,190] These results demonstrate that there can be significant genetic risks if conception or storage of sperm occurs during cytotoxic therapy, but that this risk declines after the end of such therapy.

Cancer patients should be informed by their physicians about the possibilities of sterility and genetic risk from their disease and its treatment. The probability that sterility will result from the planned cytotoxic therapy should be calculated from the cumulative doses of agents and combinations that cause prolonged azoospermia, ovarian failure, or pituitary damage (Tables 165.3, 165.4, and 165.6 through 165.8). They should also be told about psychological and physical effects on sexual desire, erectile function, and the ability to achieve orgasm. Now that a large percentage of reproductive-aged patients are surviving cancer, different methods of fertility preservation (Table 165.9) should be discussed with both male and female patients, and they should be given information about different education resources. Pretreatment gonadal function testing and referral to a reproductive endocrinologist should be considered.

Selected References

The full list of references for this chapter appears in the online version.

1. Lee SJ, Schover LR, Partridge AH, et al. American Society of Clinical Oncology recommendations on fertility preservation in cancer patients. *J Clin Oncol* 2006;24:2917.
7. Meistrich ML. Potential genetic risks of using semen collected during chemotherapy. *Hum Reprod* 1993;8:8.
8. Meistrich ML, Wilson G, Brown BW, da Cunha MF, Lipshultz LI. Impact of cyclophosphamide on long-term reduction in sperm count in men treated with combination chemotherapy for Ewing and soft tissue sarcomas. *Cancer* 1992;70:2703.
10. Viviani S, Santoro A, Ragni G, Bonfante V, Bestetti O, Bonadonna G. Gonadal toxicity after combination chemotherapy for Hodgkin's disease. Comparative results of MOPP vs ABVD. *Eur J Cancer Clin Oncol* 1985;21:601.
12. Brannigan RE. Fertility preservation in adult male cancer patients. *Cancer Treat Res* 2007;138:28.
13. Marmor D, Duyck F. Male reproductive potential after MOPP therapy for Hodgkin's disease: a long-term survey. *Andrologia* 1995;27:99.
14. Anserini P, Chiodi S, Spinelli S, et al. Semen analysis following allogeneic bone marrow transplantation. Additional data for evidence-based counselling. *Bone Marrow Transplant* 2002;30:447.
35. Sanders JE. Growth and development after hematopoietic cell transplantation. In: Thomas ED, Blume KG, Forman SJ, eds. *Hematopoietic cell transplantation.* Malden, MA: Blackwell Science, 1999.
38. Sklar CA, Mertens AC, Mitby P, et al. Premature menopause in survivors of childhood cancer: a report from the childhood cancer survivor study. *J Natl Cancer Inst* 2006;98:890.
48. Morice P, Juncker L, Rey A, El-Hassan J, Haie-Meder C, Castaigne D. Ovarian transposition for patients with cervical carcinoma treated by radiosurgical combination. *Fertil Steril* 2000;74:743.
58. Green DM, Sklar CA, Boice JD Jr, et al. Ovarian failure and reproductive outcomes after childhood cancer treatment: results from the Childhood Cancer Survivor Study. *J Clin Oncol* 2009;27:2374.
66. Critchley HO. Factors of importance for implantation and problems after treatment for childhood cancer. *Med Pediatr Oncol* 1999;33:9.
77. Schover LR, Brey K, Lichtin A, Lipshultz LI, Jeha S. Knowledge and experience regarding cancer, infertility, and sperm banking in younger male survivors. *J Clin Oncol* 2002;20:1880.
86. Longhi A, Pignotti E, Versari M, Asta S, Bacci G. Effect of oral contraceptive on ovarian function in young females undergoing neoadjuvant chemotherapy treatment for osteosarcoma. *Oncol Rep* 2003;10:151.
87. Whitehead E, Shalet SM, Blackledge G, Todd I, Crowther D, Beardwell CG. The effect of combination chemotherapy on ovarian function in women treated for Hodgkin's disease. *Cancer* 1983;52:988.
88. Ataya K, Rao LV, Lawrence E, Kimmel R. Luteinizing hormone-releasing hormone agonist inhibits cyclophosphamide-induced ovarian follicular depletion in rhesus monkeys. *Biol Reprod* 1995;52:365.
89. Blumenfeld Z, Avivi I, Linn S, Epelbaum R, Ben-Shahar M, Haim N. Prevention of irreversible chemotherapy-induced ovarian damage in young women with lymphoma by a gonadotrophin-releasing hormone agonist in parallel to chemotherapy. *Hum Reprod* 1996;11:1620.
100. Sanger WG, Olson JH, Sherman JK. Semen cryobanking for men with cancer–criteria change. *Fertil Steril* 1992;58:1024.
102. Azim AA, Costantini-Ferrando M, Lostritto K, Oktay K. Relative potencies of anastrozole and letrozole to suppress estradiol in breast cancer patients undergoing ovarian stimulation before in vitro fertilization. *J Clin Endocrinol Metab* 2007;92:2197.
107. Meseguer M, Molina N, Garcia-Velasco JA, Remohi J, Pellicer A, Garrido N. Sperm cryopreservation in oncological patients: a 14-year follow-up study. *Fertil Steril* 2006;85:640.
110. Noyes N, Knopman J, Labella P, McCaffrey C, Clark-Williams M, Grifo J. Oocyte cryopreservation outcomes including pre-cryopreservation and post-thaw meiotic spindle evaluation following slow cooling and vitrification of human oocytes. *Fertil Steril* 2010;94(6):2078–2082.
111. Ubaldi F, Anniballo R, Romano S, et al. Cumulative ongoing pregnancy rate achieved with oocyte vitrification and cleavage stage transfer without embryo selection in a standard infertility program. *Hum Reprod* 2010; 25:1199.
115. Baird DT, Webb R, Campbell BK, Harkness LM, Gosden RG. Long-term ovarian function in sheep after ovariectomy and transplantation of autografts stored at -196 C. *Endocrinology* 1999;140:462.
116. Oktay K. Ovarian tissue cryopreservation and transplantation: preliminary findings and implications for cancer patients. *Hum Reprod Update* 2001;7:526.
126. Silber SJ, Gosden RG. Ovarian transplantation in a series of monozygotic twins discordant for ovarian failure. *N Engl J Med* 2007;356:1382.
134. Cha KY, Koo JJ, Ko JJ, et al. Pregnancy after in vitro fertilization of human follicular oocytes collected from nonstimulated cycles, their culture in vitro and their transfer in a donor oocyte program. *Fertil Steril* 1991;55:109.
139. Avarbock MR, Brinster CJ, Brinster RL. Reconstitution of spermatogenesis from frozen spermatogonial stem cells. *Nat Med* 1996;2:693.
147. Meistrich ML, Shetty G. Suppression of testosterone stimulates recovery of spermatogenesis after cancer treatment. *Int J Androl* 2003;26:141.
167. Lange PH, Narayan P, Fraley EE. Fertility issues following therapy for testicular cancer. *Semin Urol* 1984;2:264.
172. Magelssen H, Brydoy M, Fossa SD. The effects of cancer and cancer treatments on male reproductive function. *Nat Clin Pract Urol* 2006;3:312.

CHAPTER 166 FATIGUE

SANDRA A. MITCHELL AND ANN M. BERGER

Fatigue is recognized as one of the most common symptoms in patients receiving treatment for cancer, often persisting beyond the conclusion of active treatment and at the end of life.[1–6] Longitudinal and comparative studies indicate that fatigue may also be a significant problem for cancer survivors, with many survivors reporting fatigue scores higher than that of an age-matched general population.[5,7–11] Prevalence estimates of fatigue vary from 25% to 90%, depending on how fatigue is defined and measured.[12] Fatigue is often a component of a cluster of symptoms such as depression, pain, sleep disturbance, and menopausal symptoms.[13–18]

Studies suggest that cancer-related fatigue (CRF) is a multifaceted condition characterized by diminished energy and an increased need to rest, disproportionate to any recent change in activity level, and accompanied by a range of other characteristics, including generalized weakness, diminished mental concentration, insomnia or hypersomnia, and emotional reactivity.[19] Consequences of CRF include decrements in physical, social, and vocational functioning[20–23]; mood[24] and sleep disturbances[9,25,26]; as well as emotional and spiritual distress for both the patient and the family members.[1,26–29]

This chapter reviews the state of the science concerning CRF and offers guidance for practice and continued research. Four major content areas relative to CRF are addressed: (1) definition and etiology, (2) explanatory models, (3) screening and evaluation of the patient with CRF, and (4) evidence-based pharmacologic and nonpharmacologic interventions to prevent and manage fatigue during and following cancer and its treatment.

DEFINITION AND ETIOLOGY OF CANCER-RELATED FATIGUE

The etiology and clinical expression of CRF is multidimensional. An inherently subjective condition, fatigue may be experienced and reported differently by each individual. Qualitative studies of fatigue underscore the fact that the cancer fatigue experience is unlike any other fatigue patients have previously experienced, and patients emphasize that its unpredictability and refractoriness to self-management strategies that were previously effective make fatigue a particularly distressing symptom.[30] Personality and coping style may also influence the experience of CRF.[31] Some patients complain of a loss of efficiency, mental fogginess, inertia, and that sleep is not restorative; others describe an excessive need to rest, the inability to recover promptly from exertion, or muscle heaviness and weakness. Whether these are features of CRF, the cause, or sequelae of fatigue, remains a focus of continued study.[32,33] Efforts continue to be directed toward clarifying the defining features of fatigue,[34] and determining how CRF may be distinguished from syndromes such as depression, cognitive dysfunction, or asthenia that have overlapping symptoms[35–40] or may share neurophysiologic mechanisms.[41,42]

Despite its complex etiology and presentation, fatigue may be defined quite simply as a distressing, persistent, subjective sense of physical, emotional, and/or cognitive tiredness or exhaustion related to cancer or cancer treatment that is not proportional to recent activity and that interferes with usual functioning.[43] The criteria for a diagnosis of CRF syndrome[19] are provided in Table 166.1.

The relationships between fatigue and treatment with radiation, chemotherapy, hematopoietic stem cell transplantation, and hormonal and biologic agents have been explored, but few relationships between treatment-related variables such as dose-intensity, radiation fractionation schedule, and time since treatment completion have been observed.[5] Associations between the occurrence and severity of CRF and demographic variables such as gender, age, marital status, and employment status have not been consistently identified. Studies do suggest that fatigue may be related to anemia; mood disorder; concurrent symptoms such as pain, sleep disturbances, electrolyte disturbances, cardiopulmonary, hepatic or renal dysfunction, hypothyroidism, hypogonadism, adrenal insufficiency, infection, malnutrition, and deconditioning; and the side effects of drugs that act on a central nervous system.[12,44–55] Accumulating evidence also suggests that gene polymorphisms, altered circadian rhythmicity, immune dysregulation, and proinflammatory cytokine activity[6,56–64] may directly or indirectly contribute to CRF.

CURRENT THEORIES OF CANCER-RELATED FATIGUE

Several different explanatory models of CRF have been proposed. Many of these models use similar constructs. Conceptual models can be organized into four thematic groups: (1) energy balance/energy analysis models, (2) fatigue as a stress response models, (3) neuroendocrine-based regulatory fatigue models, and (4) hybrid models.

Energy balance/energy analysis models depict energy as the major variable in fatigue and alterations in the balance among intake, metabolism, and expenditure of energy as factors in producing fatigue. Examples of this thematic group of models include the integrated fatigue model of Piper et al.,[65] the energy analysis model of Irvine et al.,[66] and the psychobiologic-entropy model of Winningham.[67] Fatigue as a stress response model posits that tiredness, fatigue, and exhaustion form an adaptational continuum of response to stress. Each state along this continuum from tiredness to exhaustion may be distinguished by different behavioral and symptom patterns. Examples of models included in this thematic class include

TABLE 166.1

INTERNATIONAL CLASSIFICATION OF DISEASES, 10TH REVISION, CRITERIA FOR CANCER-RELATED FATIGUE

Significant fatigue AND Five or more of these symptoms present every day or nearly every day during the same 2-week period in the past month AND	Significant fatigue, diminished energy, or increased need to rest, disproportionate to any recent change in activity in level ■ Complaints of generalized weakness or limb heaviness ■ Diminished concentration or attention ■ Decreased motivation or interest to engage in usual activities ■ Insomnia or hypersomnia ■ Experience of sleep as unrefreshing or nonrestorative ■ Perceived need to struggle to overcome inactivity ■ Marked emotional reactivity (e.g., sadness, frustration, irritability) to feeling fatigued ■ Difficulty completing daily tasks attributed to feeling fatigued ■ Perceived problems with short-term memory ■ Postexertional malaise lasting several hours
AND	The symptoms cause clinically significant distress or impairment in social, occupational, or other important areas of functioning.
AND	There is evidence from the history, physical examination, or laboratory findings that the symptoms are a consequence of cancer or cancer therapy.
AND	The symptoms are not primarily a consequence of comorbid psychiatric disorders such as major depression, somatization disorder, somatoform disorder, or delirium

Data derived from ref. 19.

fatigue models proposed by Aistars,[68] Rhoten,[69] Glaus,[70] and Olson.[71] Neuroendocrine-based regulatory fatigue models hypothesize that the multiple dimensions of fatigue are explained by dysregulation in the function of neuroendocrine-based regulatory systems including the hypothalamic-pituitary axis, circadian rhythms, and neuroimmune system transmitter secretion and function.[63] Examples of models based on neuroendocrine dysregulation include those that have been proposed by Lee et al.,[41] Payne,[72] and Schubert et al.[57] Models that represent *hybrid* conceptual approaches have also been proposed. Olson et al.[73] have recently proposed a model of CRF proposing that stressors associated with cancer and its treatment trigger declines in four systems—cognitive function, sleep quality, nutrition, and muscle endurance—and that these declines reduce one's ability to adapt. Al-Majid and Gray[74] have also proposed a hybrid model that incorporates biological, psychobehavioral, and functional variables implicated in the induction of fatigue, and illustrate the application of this model to define the mechanisms by which exercise may ameliorate cancer-related fatigue.

Models in all four thematic classes may be helpful in generating testable hypotheses for continued research into the problem of CRF and in guiding the development and evaluation of interventions to limit and manage fatigue, and to reduce its deleterious impact on health-related quality of life.

EVALUATION OF THE PATIENT WITH CANCER-RELATED FATIGUE

Studies suggest that CRF is underdiagnosed, that the assessment of fatigue in patients with cancer is suboptimal, and that health care professionals may not fully appreciate the degree of distress and functional loss that fatigue produces.[4,75–78] Identified barriers to communication between patients and their clinicians about fatigue include a tendency to view fatigue as an inevitable consequence of illness, clinicians' failure to offer interventions (47%), patients' lack of awareness of effective treatments for fatigue (43%), a desire on the patient's part to treat fatigue without medications (40%), and a tendency to be stoic about fatigue to avoid labeling as a "complainer" (28%) or a change in therapy toward less active/aggressive treatments.[20,75,79]

Identifying patients with CRF is the first step in improving fatigue evaluation and management. Although there is currently no consensus concerning the optimal method or frequency to screen for CRF in the clinical or research setting, evidence of the widespread occurrence of CRF support a conclusion that routine screening for CRF should occur at regular intervals throughout treatment, follow-up, and long-term follow-up. There is accumulating evidence that single-item measures to screen for fatigue are rapid and sensitive, and can be applied efficiently in the clinic to identify patients who would benefit from more systematic evaluation.[80–83] Based on National Comprehensive Cancer Network (NCCN) guidelines[43] fatigue should be assessed quantitatively on a 0 to 10 scale (0 = no fatigue and 10 = worst fatigue imaginable); those patients with a severity of more than 4 should be further evaluated by history and physical examination.

Although a single-item measure may provide rapid assessment of general fatigue or serve as a screening tool, evidence suggests that single-item measures do not fully capture all the dimensions of fatigue.[84] There is good consensus in the literature that fatigue generally consists of a sensory dimension (fatigue severity, persistence), a physiological dimension (e.g., leg weakness, diminished mental concentration), and a performance dimension (reduction in performance of needed or valued activities). More than 20 self-report measures (including single-item measures, multi-item unidimensional scales, and multidimensional inventories) have been developed to measure fatigue in patients with cancer.[85–87] Consideration of the measurement properties and strengths and limitations of these instruments including reliability, validity, specificity, sensitivity to change, recall period, respondent burden, translation in multiple languages, and the availability of normed values to aid interpretation should be used to guide decisions about the utility of a measure for specific clinical or research purposes.[40,50,88–94] Ecologic momentary assessment (a technique that offers real-time measurement of a phenomenon as it

TABLE 166.2

DIMENSIONS TO INCLUDE IN AN ASSESSMENT OF FATIGUE

- On a scale of 0 to 10, where zero is no fatigue and 10 is the worst fatigue imaginable, how severe has your fatigue been in the past 7 days:
- Would you say that your fatigue is mild, moderate, or severe?
- When did the fatigue start?____
- Duration of fatigue: ________________ days per week or hours per day ________________
- To what extent have you, because of fatigue, had to limit social activity, had difficulty getting things done, or thought that fatigue was making it difficult to maintain a positive outlook?
- To what extent does fatigue interfere with relationships or fulfilling responsibilities at work or in the home?
- What makes your fatigue better?
- What makes your fatigue worse?
- What do you do to help with fatigue or manage fatigue?
- Does rest relieve your fatigue?
- Do you have any trouble sleeping?
- Do you have other symptoms such as pain, difficulty breathing, nausea, and vomiting?
- Do you experience anxiety? If yes, how often?
- Do you feel discouraged, blue, or sad? If yes, how often?
- Have you discussed your fatigue with anyone on your health care team?
- Have you ever been given any recommendations for managing your fatigue?

occurs in a naturalistic setting) may overcome some of the methodologic limitations of fatigue assessment, including recall bias and the influence of current context on self-report of fatigue.[95]

A detailed history in patients with moderate or severe CRF includes the presence, intensity, and pervasiveness of fatigue, its course over time, the factors that exacerbate or relieve fatigue, and the impact of fatigue on functioning and level of distress. Clinicians can obtain valuable information about the consequences of CRF by exploring the effects of CRF on self-esteem, mood, and the ability to perform activities of daily living, fulfill important roles as parent, spouse, and worker, and relate to family and friends. Also important to the evaluation is an assessment of what interventions the patient is using to manage fatigue and the effectiveness of them. The dimensions of the fatigue experience that should be explored when evaluating a patient with CRF are listed in Table 166.2.

In evaluating the patient with CRF, it is important to screen for etiologic or potentiating factors including hypothyroidism, hypogonadism, adrenal insufficiency, cardiomyopathy, pulmonary dysfunction, anemia, sleep disturbance, fluid and electrolyte imbalances, emotional distress, and uncontrolled concurrent symptoms.[96–98] The medication profile should also be reviewed to identify specific classes of medications such as opiates, antidepressants, anticonvulsants, antiemetics, antihistamines, and β blockers, and drug–drug interactions that can also intensify fatigue.[43,55,99,100]

INTERVENTIONS FOR FATIGUE

Because fatigue typically has several different causes in any one patient, the treatment plan needs to be individualized. It is helpful to work with the patient and family caregivers to improve assessment of fatigue and identify management strategies. Open communication between the patient, family, and caregiving team will facilitate discussion about the experience of fatigue and its effects on daily life. General supportive care recommendations for patients with fatigue include encouraging a balanced diet with adequate intake of fluid, calories, protein, carbohydrates, fat, vitamins, minerals, and balancing rest with physical activity and attention-restoring activities such as exposure to natural environments, and pleasant distractions such as music.[43] There have been more than 170 empiric studies of pharmacologic and nonpharmacologic interventions to reduce or manage CRF, and several recent meta-analyses or systematic reviews.[101–107] These are summarized in Table 166.3 and selected findings are discussed here. Guidelines for the management of cancer-related fatigue have been disseminated by NCCN[43] and the Oncology Nursing Society.[108]

Pharmacologic Measures

Several pharmacologic agents (including paroxetine, venlafaxine, methylphenidate, donepezil, bupropion, and modafinil) have been evaluated for their effectiveness in reducing fatigue during and following cancer treatment.[103,109] Four trials have examined the effectiveness of paroxetine in treating fatigue during and following cancer treatment with mixed results. In three multicenter, randomized, double-blind, placebo-controlled trials, paroxetine 20 mg orally daily did not demonstrate a beneficial effect on fatigue outcomes, although improvements in depression and overall mood were noted in the paroxetine treatment group.[35,110,111] However, two small trials show a trend towards a possible benefit for either paroxetine[112] or venlafaxine[113] in treating fatigue in women experiencing hot flashes. The use of methylphenidate or dexmethylphenidate to reduce CRF has been evaluated in six open-label, single-arm trials with small samples, and in four randomized controlled trials (RCTs). In one RCT[114] and all six open-label, single-arm trials,[115–120] improvements in fatigue outcomes were observed. However, another RCT of patient-controlled methylphenidate dosing schedule for methylphenidate[121] and two RCTs of dexmethylphenidate[122,123] failed to demonstrate improvements in the outcome of fatigue. Moreover, in one study,[118] more than half of the patients experienced side effects such as insomnia, agitation, anorexia, nausea and vomiting, or dry mouth. However, a recent retrospective review suggests that the incidence of methylphenidate adverse effects may be less than 20% and concludes that some side effects improve spontaneously even with continued methylphenidate treatment.[124]

TABLE 166.3

EVIDENCE-BASED INTERVENTIONS FOR FATIGUE DURING AND FOLLOWING CANCER AND ITS TREATMENT

Interventions for Fatigue with Strong Evidence Supporting Effectiveness

- Exercise
- Education/information provision and supportive counseling
- Measures to optimize sleep quality
- Energy conservation and activity management

Interventions for Fatigue with Some Evidence Supporting Effectiveness

- Rehabilitation
- Cognitive-behavioral treatment for fatigue, depression or concurrent symptoms
- Acupuncture
- Massage
- Levocarnitine supplementation
- Mindfulness-based stress reduction
- Healing touch, hypnosis, relaxation, yoga

Interventions for Fatigue for Which Effectiveness Has Not Been Established

- Paroxetine, methylphenidate, donepezil, bupropion sustained release, modafinil, etanercept, infliximab, amisulpride, sertraline, venlafaxine
- Correction of anemia less than 10 g/dL with erythropoiesis-stimulating agents
- Essiac, Chinese medicinal herbs, ginseng, mistletoe extract
- High-dose vitamin C, multiple vitamin, omega-3 fatty acid supplementation
- Adenosine 5′-triphosphate infusion,
- Beta-hydroxyl beta-methyl butyrate, glutamine, and arginine mixture
- Individual and group psychotherapy
- Animal-assisted therapy, art therapy, expressive writing
- Reiki, aromatherapy, Qigong, distraction-virtual reality immersion
- Combination therapy: aromatherapy, foot soak, and reflexology
- Combination therapy: medroxyprogesterone, celecoxib, and enteral food supplementation
- Combination therapy: soy protein supplementation and nutrition counseling following discharge from hospital

Interventions for Fatigue Supported by Expert Opinion

- Work with patient and family to improve assessment of fatigue and identify management strategies.
- Promote open communication among patient, family, and caregiving team to facilitate discussions about the experience of fatigue and its effects on daily life.
- Consider attention-restoring activities such as exposure to natural environments, and pleasant distractions such as music.
- Encourage a balanced diet with adequate intake of fluid, calories, protein, carbohydrates, fat, vitamins, and minerals.

Data derived from refs. 101, 107, and 108.

Two small trials also suggest that donepezil 5 to 10 mg/day[125,126] or bupropion sustained release at a dose of 100 to 150 mg/day[127,128] may be effective in limiting fatigue. However, in a controlled-trial of donepezil, improvements in fatigue outcomes were not observed.[129] Several trials also suggest that modafinil at a dose of 100 mg twice daily may be effective in treating fatigue and improving daytime wakefulness and cognitive function in patients during and following cancer treatment.[130–133] Additional rigorously designed trials of donepezil, bupropion, and modafinil for fatigue appear warranted.

Several trials also suggest that levocarnitine supplementation in patients who have low serum carnitine levels[134–138] and treatment with ginseng[139] are safe and may be efficacious in treating CRF.

Treatment of Anemia with Erythropoiesis-Stimulating Agents

Although data from seven systematic reviews suggest that patients receiving erythropoiesis-stimulating agents (ESAs) to correct severe anemia (hemoglobin <10 g/dL) may experience diminished fatigue and increased vigor,[140–145] there is only limited evidence that ESAs improve fatigue when anemia is less severe. Moreover, the use of ESAs for fatigue must be considered in light of safety issues, including an increased risk of thrombotic events, hypertension, and pure red cell aplasia, and concerns that ESAs may decrease locoregional disease control and survival outcomes in particular tumor types.[146–150] Current national clinical practice guidelines[151] concluded that ESAs are not indicated for the treatment of fatigue, and restrict the use of ESAs to the treatment of anemia specifically related to myelosuppressive chemotherapy without curative intent.

National clinical practice guidelines[151,152] and product labeling from the United States Food and Drug Administration should direct individualized management of patients with cancer- or treatment-associated anemia, including an analysis of the risks and benefits of ESAs versus packed red blood cell transfusions based on cancer treatment goals, and decisions about patient monitoring, treatment thresholds, dose reductions, treatment discontinuation, and the use of supplemental iron in patients receiving ESAs.

Exercise

Meta-analyses of randomized trials support the benefits of exercise in the management of fatigue during and following cancer treatment in patients with breast cancer, solid tumors, or undergoing hematopoietic stem cell transplantation, although effect sizes are generally small and positive results for the outcome of fatigue have not been observed consistently across studies.[105,153–158] The exercise modalities that have been applied differ in content (walking, cycling, swimming, resistive exercise, or combined exercise), frequency (ranging from 2 times per week to 2 times daily), intensity (with most programs at 50% to 90% of the estimated VO_2 maximum heart rate), degree of supervision (fully supervised group vs. self-directed exercise), and duration (from 2 weeks up to 1 year). Knowledge about the type, intensity, and duration of physical exercise that is most beneficial in reducing fatigue at different stages of disease and treatment is not known,[159] and more research is needed to systematically assess the safety of exercise (both aerobic exercise and strength training) in cancer subpopulations.

Psychoeducational Supportive and Cognitive-Behavioral Interventions

Several adequately powered randomized controlled trials suggest that educational interventions, cognitive-behavioral treatment for fatigue, depression, and other depressing symptoms, and psychological support have a role in supporting positive coping in patients with fatigue.[102,104,106,158] Psychoeducational interventions that have been shown to be effective include anticipatory guidance about patterns of fatigue and recommendations for self-management, counseling and supportive psychotherapy, and coordination of care. Energy conservation and activity management (ECAM) is a self-management intervention that teaches patients to apply the principles of energy conservation and activity management and provides coaching to integrate these activities into their daily lifestyle. ECAM has been found to have a modest but significant effect in a large, multisite trial, and in a small pilot with historical controls.[107]

Studies indicate that cognitive-behavioral interventions designed to improve sleep quality also have a beneficial effect on fatigue.[160,161] In contrast, the impact on fatigue outcomes of pharmacologic therapies for chronic comorbid insomnia has had very little systematic study.[162] Cognitive-behavioral interventions to improve sleep quality can be delivered individually or in a group setting, and include relaxation training along with sleep-consolidation strategies (avoiding long or late afternoon naps, limiting time in bed to actual sleep time), stimulus control therapy (go to bed only when sleepy, use bed/bedroom for sleep and sexual activities only, consistent time to lie down and get up, avoid caffeine and stimulating activity in the evening), and strategies to reduce cognitive-emotional arousal (keep at least an hour to relax before going to bed and establish a presleep routine to be used every night).

Structured Rehabilitation

Several trials[163–166] and a systematic review[167] suggest that structured rehabilitation programs result in statistically significant and sustained improvements in fatigue, particularly in patients who have completed treatment and are in the survivorship phase. However, because at least one study suggests that programs that are too intensive[168] may actually worsen fatigue, tailoring of the program based on the patient's currently level of energy and stage along the treatment trajectory is important.

Integrative Therapies

There is preliminary evidence to support the efficacy of integrative approaches to the treatment of fatigue, including yoga, relaxation, mindfulness-based stress reduction, acupuncture, medical Qigong, massage, healing touch, and Reiki, and combined-modality interventions that include aromatherapy, lavender foot soak, and reflexology.[107,169] Studies of these interventions have utilized open-label and/or uncontrolled designs and had small sample sizes, making it difficult to draw firm conclusions about efficacy. Despite these limitations, and with acknowledgment that inclusion of controls such as double-blinding presents methodological challenges,[170] results suggest that these complementary therapies have potential in the treatment of fatigue in patients with cancer.

PRACTICE OF ONCOLOGY

Selected References

The full list of references for this chapter appears in the online version.

3. Cella D, Lai JS, Chang CH, Peterman A, Slavin M. Fatigue in cancer patients compared with fatigue in the general United States population. *Cancer* 2002;94(2):528.
5. Prue G, Rankin J, Allen J, Gracey J, Cramp F. Cancer-related fatigue: A critical appraisal. *Eur J Cancer* May 2006;42(7):846–863.
6. Bower JE. Behavioral symptoms in patients with breast cancer and survivors. *J Clin Oncol.* Feb 10 2008;26(5):768–777.
12. Servaes P, Verhagen C, Bleijenberg G. Fatigue in cancer patients during and after treatment: prevalence, correlates and interventions. *Eur J Cancer* Jan 2002;38(1):27–43.
19. Cella D, Peterman A, Passik S, Jacobsen P, Breitbart W. Progress toward guidelines for the management of fatigue. *Oncology (Williston Park, N.Y.)* 1998;12(11 A):369–377.
27. Servaes P, Verhagen S, Bleijenberg G. Determinants of chronic fatigue in disease-free breast cancer patients: a cross-sectional study. *Ann Oncol* Apr 2002;13(4):589–598.
29. Hofman M, Ryan JL, Figueroa-Moseley CD, Jean-Pierre P, Morrow GR. Cancer-related fatigue: the scale of the problem. *Oncologist* 2007;12 Suppl 1:4–10.
31. Andrykowski MA, Schmidt JE, Salsman JM, Beacham AO, Jacobsen PB. Use of a case definition approach to identify cancer-related fatigue in women undergoing adjuvant therapy for breast cancer. *J Clin Oncol* 2005;23(27):6613.
32. Sadler IJ, Jacobsen PB, Booth-Jones M, Belanger H, Weitzner MA, Fields KK. Preliminary evaluation of a clinical syndrome approach to assessing cancer-related fatigue. *J Pain Symptom Manage* 2002;23(5):406.
34. Jacobsen PB, Donovan KA, Weitzner MA. Distinguishing fatigue and depression in patients with cancer. *Semin Clin Neuropsychiatry* Oct 2003;8(4):229–240.
36. Reuter K, Harter M. The concepts of fatigue and depression in cancer. *Eur J Cancer Care (Engl)* May 2004;13(2):127–134.
41. Lee BN, Dantzer R, Langley KE, et al. A cytokine-based neuroimmunologic mechanism of cancer-related symptoms. *Neuroimmunomodulation* 2004;11(5):279.
42. Bower JE, Ganz PA, Aziz N. Altered cortisol response to psychologic stress in breast cancer survivors with persistent fatigue. *Psychosom Med* Mar-Apr 2005;67(2):277–280.
43. Cancer-related fatigue (version 1.2010). National Comprehensive Cancer Network; 2010. http://www.nccn.org/professionals/physician_gls/PDF/fatigue.pdf. Accessed June 6, 2010.
45. Wagner L, Cella D. Fatigue and cancer: causes, prevalence and treatment approaches. *Br J Cancer* Aug 31 2004;91(5):822–828.
53. Stone PC, Minton O. Cancer-related fatigue. *Eur J Cancer* Mar 30 2008.

54. Brown LF, Kroenke K. Cancer-related fatigue and its associations with depression and anxiety: a systematic review. *Psychosomatics* Sep–Oct 2009;50(5):440–447.
55. Dy SM, Lorenz KA, Naeim A, Sanati H, Walling A, Asch SM. Evidence-based recommendations for cancer fatigue, anorexia, depression, and dyspnea. *J Clin Oncol* Aug 10 2008;26(23):3886–3895.
57. Schubert C, Hong S, Natarajan L, Mills PJ, Dimsdale JE. The association between fatigue and inflammatory marker levels in cancer patients: A quantitative review. *Brain Behav Immun* May 2007;21(4):413–427.
59. Ancoli-Israel S, Liu L, Marler MR, et al. Fatigue, sleep, and circadian rhythms prior to chemotherapy for breast cancer. *Support Care Cancer* Mar 2006;14(3):201–209.
62. Berger AM, Farr LA, Kuhn BR, Fischer P, Agrawal S. Values of sleep/wake, activity/rest, circadian rhythms, and fatigue prior to adjuvant breast cancer chemotherapy. *Pain Sympt Manag* 2007;33(4):398–409.
63. Miller AH, Ancoli-Israel S, Bower JE, Capuron L, Irwin MR. Neuroendocrine-immune mechanisms of behavioral comorbidities in patients with cancer. *J Clin Oncol* Feb 20 2008;26(6):971–982.
64. Bower JE. Cancer-related fatigue: links with inflammation in cancer patients and survivors. *Brain Behav Immun* Oct 2007;21(7):863–871.
83. Butt Z, Wagner LI, Beaumont JL, et al. Use of a single-item screening tool to detect clinically significant fatigue, pain, distress, and anorexia in ambulatory cancer practice. *J Pain Symptom Manage* Jan 2008;35(1):20–30.
85. Mota DD, Pimenta CA. Self-report instruments for fatigue assessment: a systematic review. *Res Theory Nurs Pract* Spring 2006;20(1):49–78.
86. Wagner L, Cella D. Cancer related fatigue: Clinical screening, assessment and management. In: Marty M, Pecorelli S, eds. *ESO scientific updates: Fatigue, asthenia, exhuastion and cancer*. 5th ed. Oxford, England: Elsevier Science; 2001:201–214.
87. Whitehead L. The measurement of fatigue in chronic illness: a systematic review of unidimensional and multidimensional fatigue measures. *J Pain Symptom Manage* Jan 2009;37(1):107–128.
88. Meek PM, Nail LM, Barsevick A, et al. Psychometric testing of fatigue instruments for use with cancer patients. *Nurs Res* Jul-Aug 2000;49(4):181–190.
89. Schwartz A. Validity of cancer-related fatigue instruments. *Pharmacotherapy* 2002;22(11):1433.
92. Alexander S, Minton O, Stone PC. Evaluation of screening instruments for cancer-related fatigue syndrome in breast cancer survivors. *J Clin Oncol* Mar 10 2009;27(8):1197–1201.
96. Escalante CP, Kallen MA, Valdres RU, Morrow PK, Manzullo EF. Outcomes of a cancer-related fatigue clinic in a comprehensive cancer center. *J Pain Symptom Manage* Apr;39(4):691–701.
97. Cheville AL. Cancer-related fatigue. *Phys Med Rehabil Clin N Am* May 2009;20(2):405–416.
101. Mitchell S, Beck S, Hood L, Moore K, Tanner E. Putting evidence into practice (PEP): evidence-based interventions for fatigue during and following cancer and its treatment. *Clinical J Oncol Nurs* 2007;11:99.
102. Kangas M, Bovbjerg DH, Montgomery GH. Cancer-related fatigue: A systematic and meta-analytic review of non-pharmacological therapies for cancer patients. *Psychol Bull* Sep 2008;134(5):700–741.
103. Minton O, Richardson A, Sharpe M, Hotopf M, Stone P. A systematic review and meta-analysis of the pharmacological treatment of cancer-related fatigue. *J Natl Cancer Inst* Aug 20 2008;100(16):1155–1166.
104. Jacobsen PB, Donovan KA, Vadaparampil ST, Small BJ. Systematic review and meta-analysis of psychological and activity-based interventions for cancer-related fatigue. *Health Psychol* Nov 2007;26(6):660–667.
105. Cramp F, Daniel J. Exercise for the management of cancer-related fatigue in adults. *Cochrane Database Syst Rev* 2008(2):CD006145.
106. Goedendorp MM, Gielissen MF, Verhagen CA, Bleijenberg G. Psychosocial interventions for reducing fatigue during cancer treatment in adults. *Cochrane Database Syst Rev* 2009(1):CD006953.
107. Mitchell SA. Cancer-related fatigue: State of the science. *Phys Med Rehabil* 2010;2(5):364–383.
108. Mitchell SA, Beck SL, Eaton LH. ONS Putting Evidence Into Practice (PEP): fatigue. In: Eaton LH, Tipton JM, eds. *Putting evidence into practice*. Pittsburgh: Oncology Nursing Society, 2009.
109. Breitbart W, Alici Y. Pharmacologic treatment options for cancer-related fatigue: current state of clinical research. *Clin J Oncol Nurs* 2008;12 (5 Suppl):27.
148. Juneja V, Keegan P, Gootenberg JE, et al. Continuing reassessment of the risks of erythropoiesis-stimulating agents in patients with cancer. *Clin Cancer Res* Jun 1 2008;14(11):3242–3247.
149. Bohlius J, Schmidlin K, Brillant C, et al. Erythropoietin or Darbepoetin for patients with cancer–meta-analysis based on individual patient data. *Cochrane Database Syst Rev* 2009(3):CD007303.
151. Cancer- and chemotherapy-induced anemia (version 2.2010). National Comprehensive Cancer Network; 2010. http://www.nccn.org/professionals/physician_gls/PDF/anemia.pdf. Accessed June 6, 2010.
152. Rizzo JD, Somerfield MR, Hagerty KL, et al. Use of epoetin and darbepoetin in patients with cancer: 2007 American Society of Hematology/American Society of Clinical Oncology clinical practice guideline update. *Blood* 2008;111(1):25.
157. Velthuis MJ, Agasi-Idenburg SC, Aufdemkampe G, Wittink HM. The effect of physical exercise on cancer-related fatigue during cancer treatment: a meta-analysis of randomised controlled trials. *Clin Oncol (R Coll Radiol)* Apr;22(3):208–221.
158. Duijts SF, Faber MM, Oldenburg HS, van Beurden M, Aaronson NK. Effectiveness of behavioral techniques and physical exercise on psychosocial functioning and health-related quality of life in breast cancer patients and survivors-a meta-analysis. *Psychooncology* Mar 24.
160. Berger AM, Mitchell SA. Modifying cancer-related fatigue by optimizing sleep quality. *J Natl Compr Canc Netw* 2008;6(1):3.
161. Page MS, Berger AM, Eaton LH. Sleep-wake disturbances. In: Eaton LH, Tipton M, eds. *Putting evidence into practice*. Pittsburgh: Oncology Nursing Society, 2009:285.
169. Kwekkeboom KL, Cherwin CH, Lee JW, Wanta B. Mind-body treatments for the pain-fatigue-sleep disturbance symptom cluster in persons with cancer. *J Pain Symptom Manage* 2010;39(1):126.

CHAPTER 167 SECOND PRIMARY CANCERS

LOIS B. TRAVIS, SMITA BHATIA, JAMES M. ALLAN, KEVIN C. OEFFINGER, AND ANDREA NG

Given advances in early detection, supportive care, and therapy, the 5-year relative survival rate for all cancers combined has increased steadily over the past 3 decades.[1] As of January 1, 2007, there were approximately 12 million men and women with a history of cancer in the United States, representing about 3% of the population.[1] For some patients, gains in survival have come at a price in the form of the long-term physiologic effects of cancer and its therapy. One of the most serious events experienced by cancer survivors is the diagnosis of a new primary cancer. The number of patients with multiple primary cancers is growing, with independent malignancies comprising about 16% (or one in six) incident cancers reported to the National Cancer Institute's (NCI) Surveillance, Epidemiology and End Results (SEER) Program in 2007.[1] Moreover, solid tumors comprise a leading cause of mortality among several populations of long-term survivors, including patients with Hodgkin's lymphoma (HL).[2] Second cancers can reflect the late sequelae of treatment, as well as the effect of lifestyle choices, environmental exposures, host effects, and combinations of influences, including gene–environment interactions.[3] Travis et al.[4] grouped second primary cancers (SPCs) into three major categories according to predominant etiologic factors: treatment-related; syndromic; and those due to shared etiologic influences, emphasizing the nonexclusivity of these categories. The focus of this chapter will be treatment-associated malignancies. A comprehensive review of syndromic multiple primary cancers and those due to shared etiologic influences (e.g., alcohol and tobacco) was recently published.[5]

METHODS TO ASSESS SECOND CANCER RISK

Cohort and case-control epidemiology study designs have been successfully used to estimate second cancer risks (reviewed elsewhere).[6] In a cohort approach, cancer survivors identified through specified criteria are retrospectively or prospectively followed for the occurrence of second cancers. Cohort sources include population-based cancer registries such as the NCI SEER Program and nationwide registries. Registry strengths include the sizable number of patients, which allow quantification of even small second cancer risks and the ability to characterize in detail the influence of latency, gender, and age at first and second cancer diagnosis.[7] Further, the observed and expected number of second cancers is derived from the same source. Although the population-based nature of these registries avoids referral or selection bias, a major drawback is that treatment data are quite limited. Nonetheless, population-based registries permit a powerful assessment of site-specific second cancer risk according to a variety of parameters, including characterization of trends over time as cancer treatments evolve.[8]

Other patient cohorts in which second cancer risk can be evaluated include hospital-based tumor registries and clinical trials. Although the former source frequently includes detailed patient information, weaknesses include inconsistent follow-up, administration of a variety of treatments, and incomplete ascertainment of second cancers. Strengths of clinical trial data include the availability of detailed information for protocol therapies, and weaknesses include the lack of data regarding off-protocol therapy, limited follow-up, and incomplete ascertainment of second cancers.

Risk measures that can be estimated from cohort studies include the observed-to-expected ratio (or standardized incidence ratio, SIR) of second cancers. Person-years of observation in the cohort, grouped by age, gender, calendar year, or other factors, are used to estimate the expected number of second cancers, based on cancer incidence rates in the general population. A second calculation is the excess absolute risk (EAR), which is estimated by subtracting the expected number of second cancers from the observed number, dividing by the person-years at risk, and then multiplying by 10,000. Multivariable statistical methods have been used successfully to permit adjustment for the effects of age at first and second cancer diagnosis, latency, and calendar year.[7]

Even a large SIR can translate into a small absolute risk if the second cancer is rare. For example, in an international registry-based study of HL,[9] the EAR of acute myeloid leukemia (AML) was about 6 excess cases per 10,000 patients per year, whereas the SIR was over 20. Thus, the EAR is especially helpful to demonstrate which second cancers account for the greatest disease burden in a population and facilitates comparisons with the development of other late sequelae. Another measure of risk in cohort studies involves actuarial approaches in which censored data methods are used to evaluate in-cohort risk. A standard measure is the cumulative absolute risk, in which methods that allow for competing risks[10] should be used, because a patient may die of another cause before a second cancer can be diagnosed. Approaches that do not account for competing risks may overestimate the cumulative incidence of second cancers.

Nested case-control studies provide an efficient approach to address the role of therapy in second cancer risk, including quantification of the dose-response relation with radiation or total drug dose.[11,12] Here, the occurrence of second cancers (cases) is ascertained in a well-defined cohort of cancer survivors. Controls are a stratified, random matched sample of subjects without a second cancer identified in the same cohort. Therapies between cases and matched controls are then compared. A drawback of case-control studies is that statistical methods require identification of a reference category. Although an optimal group is nonexposed patients, this choice is usually unavailable. One approach is to select patients managed with surgery only or a low-dose exposure group, recognizing that with the latter choice, estimates may be diminished. An alternative approach is to use continuous variables (e.g., radiation dose) to model second cancer risk.[13] Recently, "counter-matching" as a technique to enhance the efficiency of case-control studies, in particular, with regard to evaluating the effect of gene-environment interactions,[14] has been successfully applied.

CARCINOGENICITY OF INDIVIDUAL TREATMENT MODALITIES

Radiation Therapy

The leukemogenic and carcinogenic effects of ionizing radiation have long been recognized, based on the elevated cancer risks in atomic bomb survivors[15–21] and the risk associated with occupational radiation exposure, historical use of low-dose radiation for benign conditions, and repeated diagnostic fluoroscopies.[22–26] The relation between radiation dose and cancer risk is well described in these low-dose ranges, with an approximately linear increase in risk with increasing radiation dose up to about 5 Gy for solid tumors,[18,27,28] and up to 1.5 to 2 Gy for leukemia.[19,29,30] *In vitro* studies as well as animal and epidemiologic studies of leukemia induction suggested that with increasing radiation doses above approximately 5 Gy, cell killing offsets the induction of malignancy, and the risk of developing leukemia declines.[30,31] The traditional view has been that increased cell killing occurs in the higher dose region and therefore a lowered cancer risk, while tissues exposed to intermediate doses are at highest risk for cancer development. A classic radiation dose-response curve plotting the incidence of cancer against the dose of radiation absorbed has a characteristic shape, with the incidence of malignancy increasing with dose up to a maximum of about 3 to 10 Gy, followed by a decrease in cancer risk with further increase in dose.

Therapeutic radiation for a number of primary cancers has been linked to subsequent malignancies. For a tumor to be classified as radiation-induced, the following criteria must be met: occurrence within the primary or secondary radiation beam, different histology than the original cancer, a latency period of several years, not present at the time of initial cancer diagnosis, and the lack of a cancer-prone syndrome in the patient.[32] In assessing radiation-related second malignancy among cancer survivors, it is important to take into consideration other potential contributing factors to cancer development. These include exposure to cytotoxic drugs (see "Chemotherapy"), genetic predisposition,[33–37] immunosuppression,[38,39] infections with specific agents,[39–41] environmental exposures,[42] and heightened surveillance in cancer survivors.[43] Additional factors can modify the effect of radiotherapy on second cancer risk. Patients with certain cancer-prone syndromes,[33,44–46] including hereditary retinoblastoma (RB), nevoid basal cell carcinoma syndrome, and neurofibromatosis-1 (NF1) are more susceptible to radiation-induced cancer. Tobacco history increases the risk of treatment-related lung cancer in a multiplicative manner as demonstrated in a case-control study of survivors of HL.[47] Younger age at irradiation is associated with a significantly increased risk of breast cancer[48–53] and thyroid cancer,[48,54] as shown in survivors of HL, breast cancer, and childhood cancer. On the other hand, early menopause has a protective effect on breast cancer after radiotherapy in survivors of HL,[11,12] suggesting that ovarian hormones play an important role in promoting tumorigenesis once an initiating event has been produced by radiation.

More recent studies have addressed the effect of radiation dose in the therapeutic range on second malignancy risk by estimation of radiation dose at the site of second cancer development. The risk of radiation-related cancer has been shown to increase with increasing dose for several malignancies, including breast cancer,[11,12,53,55] esophageal cancer,[56] lung cancer,[47,57] stomach cancer,[58] meningioma,[59] and sarcoma,[60–62] with no evidence of a downturn in risk at high doses within the therapeutic range. An exception is thyroid cancer risk, which has been shown to decrease after doses of greater than 30 Gy,[63] consistent with a cell-killing effect. The radiation dose-response relation in second malignancy development therefore appears to be tissue-specific. In addition to radiation dose, the radiotherapy fields, which directly reflect the volume of normal tissue exposed, can affect second cancer risk. The association between more extensive treatment fields and higher second malignancy risk has been shown in survivors of HL,[64,65] breast cancer,[66,67] and prostate cancer.[68]

Radiotherapy techniques and delivery systems have undergone major transformations over the past few decades. Earlier treatment machines based on kilovoltage x-rays and cobalt-60 gamma rays have been replaced by high-energy linear accelerators. Treatment techniques have also evolved from fluoroscopic-based two-dimensional therapy to three-dimensional conformal therapy. Because of the long latency between radiation exposure and cancer development, caution is needed when extrapolating existing epidemiologic data for radiation-related second malignancies to patients treated in the modern era.

In recent years, highly conformal radiation techniques including intensity-modulated radiation therapy (IMRT) have been increasingly adopted.[69] IMRT uses sophisticated computer technology and dose-optimization algorithms to produce precisely shaped dose distributions via multileaf collimator systems. By modulating photon fluence within a subset of the beams, improved dose conformality in the high-dose region is achieved, thus allowing the possibility of dose escalation for selected cancers. However, with the use of multiple modulated beams, a larger volume of normal tissue is exposed to low doses of radiation. In addition, more radiation output, or monitor units, are needed to deliver a specified dose to the target than for conventional treatments.[70] The treatment time is also longer, resulting in a higher total-body radiation dose by machine leakage.

There have been a number of studies using dosimetric plans of patients treated with IMRT versus conventional three-dimensional therapy to estimate second cancer risk using various dose-response risk models. Risks vary considerably depending on the models used. One study estimated the risk of fatal secondary malignancy associated with conventional radiotherapy and IMRT based on the treatment plans of ten early-stage prostate cancer patients.[71] Risk estimates were generated using dose equivalents to several sensitive organs and organ-specific risk coefficients. Estimated risks of second cancers with 18-mV conventional radiotherapy, and IMRT at 6, 10, 15, and 18 mV were 1.7%, 2.9%, 2.1%, 3.4%, and 5.1%, respectively. The IMRT plans were associated with higher estimated risks than the conventional plan largely because they required 3.5 to 4.9 times as many monitor units. The IMRT treatment associated with the lowest risk was the 10-mV treatment, partly because of its requirement for fewer monitor units than the 6-mV approach. The risk for the 10-mV treatment was lower than that of the 15- and 18-mV treatments because of the significant neutron contribution at higher energies. Other studies,[72,73] using a different model that included a plateau dose-response function for therapeutic doses more than 2 Gy, thereby taking into account cell killing at high doses, have estimated only modestly increased risk of second malignancies with IMRT. It is important to recognize that these risk estimates are associated with large uncertainties, depending on the model assumptions. Epidemiologic data for second malignancy risks in patients treated with IMRT for various types of primary cancers are currently lacking, and prolonged follow-up time is needed before true risk can be determined.

There is increasing momentum for the use of proton therapy, given the physical characteristics of the depth dose curve,[74,75] which peaks at the end of the particle range (Bragg peak). The beam has sharp edges with little side scatter, and the dose drops to zero after the Bragg peak. In addition, the integral dose, or the mean absorbed dose multiplied by the mass of irradiated tissue, is significantly lower with proton than photon beam. However, there have been concerns with regard to the second malignancy risk associated with ancillary neutron production, especially with the passive scattering technique, which results in dose exposure to the whole body.[76,77] In a modeling study of three prostate cancer patients, treatment plans for a passively scattered proton technique and 6-mV IMRT technique were compared.[78] Site-specific second malignancy risks of the two techniques were estimated, taking into account primary and secondary radiation exposures, including stray neutron exposures. Compared with photon IMRT, proton therapy was associated with a reduced risk of second malignancy (26% vs. 39%). The lower risk associated with proton therapy was attributed to the significantly reduced dose received by adjacent critical structures, including the rectum and bladder, when compared with photon IMRT (Fig. 167.1).

Preliminary epidemiologic data on second malignancy risks following proton beam therapy have recently become available. Patients (n = 503) treated at the Harvard Cyclotron with proton radiotherapy with passive scattering were matched to 1,591 photon-treated patients identified in the SEER database.[79] After adjusting for gender and age at treatment, treatment with photon therapy was associated with a significantly increased risk of second malignancy (hazard ratio, 2.73; $P < .0001$). The median duration of follow-up was 6.1 and 7.7 years, respectively, in the photon and proton cohorts. Additional observation time may be needed to fully assess the long-term second cancer risks following proton therapy. The newer beam scanning technique holds promise for reducing second cancer risk as a result of low neutron contamination.[76,80] This technique uses magnetically scanned pencil beams over the target volume, does not require scattering devices, collimation, or compensation, and therefore is associated with reduced secondary neutron production from the treatment head.

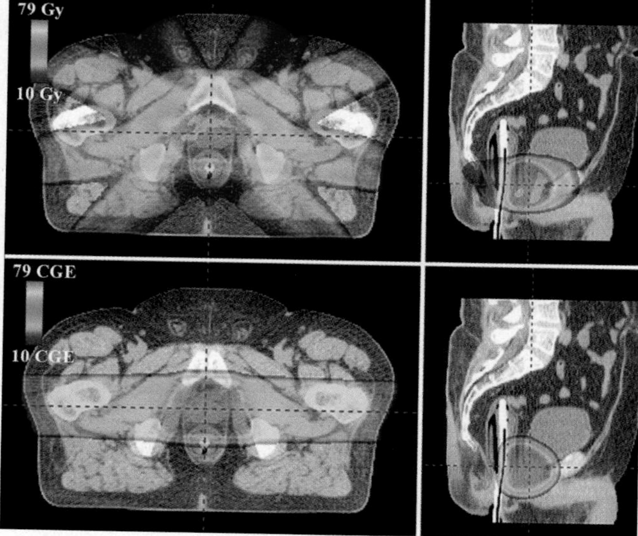

FIGURE 167.1 Comparison of dose distribution for intensity-modulated radiation therapy (*top*) versus proton therapy (*bottom*) plans for a prostate cancer patient, showing substantially lower doses at low-to-intermediate levels in the bladder and rectum in the proton therapy plan. (From ref. 78, with permission.)

Investigators have estimated a twofold or greater reduction in second malignancy risk with proton therapy when the scanning beam technique is used,[81] compared with photon therapy. However, epidemiologic studies with adequate follow-up time will be needed to confirm any reduction in second cancer risk.

Chemotherapy

The development of a second primary malignancy after chemotherapy was first reported in 1970 by Kyle et al.,[82] who described AML following alkylating agent therapy for multiple myeloma. Improvements in cancer prognosis have since contributed to the increasing incidence of therapy-related AML, such that this condition now represents 10% to 20% of all AML, and is a major life-threatening condition in some patient groups (see "Hodgkin's Lymphoma" and "Pediatric Malignancy"). Treatment-related leukemia represents a paradigm for the study of chemotherapy-induced malignancy. In contrast, the induction of solid tumors after chemotherapy is less well understood. To date, the causal link between cyclophosphamide and bladder cancer represents one of the few established relationships between a specific cytotoxic drug and a solid tumor (reviewed in "Non-Hodgkin's Lymphoma").[83] Elevated risks of bone sarcomas[84] and lung cancer[47] have also been observed after alkylating agent chemotherapy.

Therapy-related leukemias can be broadly classified based on the nature of the antecedent therapy and the molecular mechanisms underlying their development. For example, risk of leukemia after alkylating therapy peaks 5 to 8 years after the start of therapy and decreases thereafter.[50,85–87] The majority of such leukemias initially present as myelodysplastic syndrome (MDS) with a complex karyotype characterized by unbalanced chromosome aberrations often involving long-arm deletions or monosomy of chromosomes 5 and/or 7 (see "Pediatric Malignancy" and also Chapter 127).[88] These observations suggest the existence of an evolving genetically unstable clone. Indeed, microsatellite instability, a form of genomic instability characterized by the expansion or retraction of repetitive DNA sequences, is rare in *de novo* AML but is reported in up to 90% of therapy-related AML cases.[89,90]

Alkylating agents with known or suspected leukemogenic effects in humans include mechlorethamine, chlorambucil, cyclophosphamide, melphalan, semustine, lomustine, carmustine, procarbazine, prednimustine, busulfan, dihydroxy busulfan, and the platinating agents.[91–94] Of these, the platinating agents are among the most important cytotoxic drugs introduced in the past few decades, are widely used to treat numerous cancers including ovarian and testicular cancer, and are associated with significantly increased risks of secondary leukemia.[95,96] Like other alkylating agents, they can induce base lesions in DNA, demonstrate mutagenicity and clastogenicity *in vitro* and are carcinogenic in laboratory animals.[94] Moreover, the clastogenicity of the platinating agents, like other bifunctional alkylators, is largely the result of their ability to form cross-links in DNA. The risk of alkylating agent-related AML has been shown to increase with increasing cumulative dose, duration of therapy, and dose intensity.[91,93,95,97,98]

Chemotherapeutic topoisomerase II poisons, such as the epipodophyllotoxins (e.g., etoposide), the anthracyclines (e.g., epirubicin) and anthracenediones (e.g., mitoxantrone), are causative in the development of a clinically and cytogenetically distinct type of AML. AML that develops after treatment with these agents has a relatively short induction period (median, 2 to 3 years) and generally presents without preceding MDS (see "Pediatric Malignancy").[99–101] Further, this type of AML is characterized by balanced translocations often involving the *MLL*, *RARA*, and *RUNX1* loci at chromosome bands 11q23, 17q21, and 21q22, respectively,[102–104] but often with no major losses or gains of chromosomal material. These data indicate a comparatively simple mechanism of leukemogenesis, where the generation of chimeric fusion genes can in some cases be sufficient for transformation, although additional mutagenic events may also be required. Molecular mechanisms involved in the development of AML after administration of topoisomerase poisons are intrinsically dependent on the generation and misrepair of DNA strand breaks, described elsewhere[99–101] and in Chapter 130.

Treatment with azathioprine, a thiopurine prodrug related to 6-mercaptopurine and 6-thioguanine, is used as an immunosuppressant during organ transplant. It is associated with significantly increased risks of developing AML,[105] non-Hodgkin's lymphoma (NHL),[106] and skin cancer.[107] Reports of therapy-induced brain tumors in pediatric acute lymphoblastic leukemia (ALL) patients treated with combined-modality therapy that included thiopurines,[108] and of AML in patients treated with thiopurines for Crohn disease,[109,110] also support the carcinogenicity of this group of agents. The mechanism of thiopurine prodrug-induced malignancy is thought to involve immunosuppression (and the possible involvement of oncogenic viruses), selection for cells with a mutator phenotype, and the generation of reactive oxygen species when some thiopurine prodrugs are exposed to ultraviolet radiation.[111]

Clarification of the important interrelationships between putative risk factors, including host phenotype (e.g., age, gender), host genetics, and exposure-related variables (e.g., chemotherapy dose, regimen, cotreatment with radiotherapy), are critical to a better understanding of individual susceptibility to chemotherapy-induced cancers. For example, whether chemoprotectant agents and hematopoietic growth factors such as amifostine and granulocyte colony-stimulating factor, respectively, which are used to ameliorate the myelosuppressive effects of cytotoxic chemotherapies, might affect risks of secondary leukemia needs to be considered. Indeed, evidence suggests that granulocyte colony-stimulating factor, which is used in the treatment of lymphoblastic leukemia, breast, and other conditions, may be associated with an increased risk of therapy-related AML.[112–115] Likewise, as new classes of chemotherapy agents are developed and enter widespread clinical use, their potential impact on risk of second cancer must be considered. For example, there is evidence suggesting that the tyrosine kinase inhibitors, such as imatinib, which is used to treat Philadelphia chromosome-positive leukemia, might be leukemogenic.[116–119] The mechanisms underlying this association remain unclear, although the transient appearance of genetic abnormalities during imatinib treatment, such as trisomy 8, in Philadelphia chromosome-negative bone marrow cells suggests a causal role.[120]

Survival after chemotherapy-related AML is generally quite poor, typically only several months.[121] However, there are selected groups with a relatively favorable prognosis, such as acute promyelocytic leukemia with the t(15;17) translocation, that is often associated with epirubicin and mitoxantrone therapy for breast cancer.[122] The high frequency of poor-risk cytogenetics, including monosomy and long-arm deletions of chromosomes 5 and 7, may partly account for the poor prognosis of therapy-related disease in general, although evidence suggests that an etiology involving prior exposure to therapy is also associated with poor prognosis independent of karyotype.[123] For example, patients with postchemotherapy t(8;21)-positive leukemia have a worse outcome that patients with *de novo* disease displaying this translocation.[124] As such, the mechanisms underlying the poor prognosis of therapy-related AML remain to be fully elucidated, but it is plausible that some of the unique features of therapy-related disease may contribute to the poor outcome.

Although the study of chemotherapy-induced leukemia has yielded considerable insight into the molecular mechanisms underlying the etiology of SPC, it will be important determine whether these or other mechanisms are also operant in the development of solid SPC, for which there is a paucity of knowledge.

GENETIC SUSCEPTIBILITY TO SECOND PRIMARY CANCERS

Literature clearly supports the role of chemotherapy and radiation in the development of SPC[125]; however, the existence of considerable interindividual variability suggests a role for genetic variation. Proposed mechanisms for susceptibility to development of second cancers after exposure to genotoxic therapy in cancer survivors are summarized in Figure 167.2. The risk of SPC could potentially be modified by mutations in high-penetrance genes that lead to serious genetic diseases such as Li-Fraumeni syndrome,[126] Fanconi anemia,[127–130] and R\B (see "Pediatric Malignancy"). In fact, clues to the identification of loci important in affecting risk of SPC were initially suggested from studies of constitutional human cancer susceptibility syndromes (e.g., NF), many of which confer acute sensitivity to the mutagenic and cytotoxic effects of chemotherapy and radiotherapy, and where elevated risks of SPC is known or suspected.[44,131] However, because of their low frequency, these alleles appear to contribute to only a small fraction of SPC risk at the population level. Rather, evidence suggests that outside the context of familial cancer susceptibility syndromes, the genetic contribution to defining chemotherapy and radiotherapy-related cancer risk is multigenic, and likely related to common polymorphisms in low-penetrance genes that regulate the availability of active drug metabolites, or those responsible for DNA repair.

Genetic variation contributes 20% to 95% of the variability in cytotoxic drug disposition.[132] Polymorphisms in genes involved in drug metabolism and transport are relevant in determining both disease-free survival and drug toxicity.[133] Variation in DNA repair also plays a role in susceptibility to *de novo* cancer,[134,135] and likely modifies SPC risk after exposure to DNA-damaging agents, such as radiation and chemotherapy. Just as the pharmacology of cancer chemotherapy is impacted by underlying principles of pharmacokinetics and pharmacodynamics and is determined at least in part by host genetics, these influences likely also contribute to the risk of SPC. Many loci that influence risk of SPC encode proteins that metabolize and detoxify human carcinogens in an exposure-specific manner.[136–139]

Drug-Metabolizing Enzymes—Activation/ Detoxification Pathways

Metabolism of genotoxic agents occurs in two phases. Phase I involves activation of substrates into highly reactive electrophilic intermediates that can damage DNA, a reaction principally performed by the cytochrome P-450 family of enzymes. Phase II enzymes (conjugation) function to inactivate genotoxic substrates, and include glutathione S-transferase (GST), NAD(P)H:quinone oxidoreductase-1, and others. High activity of a phase I enzyme and low activity of a phase II enzyme can result in DNA damage from the excess resultant harmful products.

Cytochrome P-450 Enzymes

The chemotherapeutic substrates of cytochrome P-450 proteins include cyclophosphamide, ifosfamide, thiotepa, doxorubicin, and dacarbazine.[140] The expression of these enzymes is

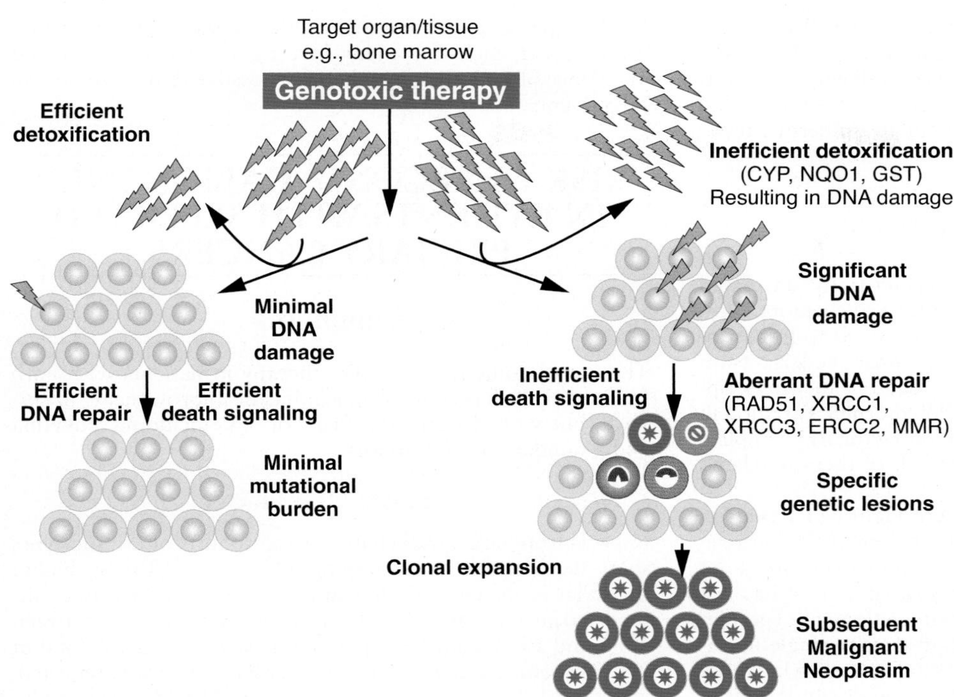

FIGURE 167.2 Proposed mechanisms for susceptibility to development of second cancers after exposure to genotoxic therapy in cancer survivors. (Adapted and modified from Seedhouse C, Russell N. Advances in the understanding of susceptibility to treatment-related acute myeloid leukemia. *Br J Haematol* 2007;137:513.)

highly variable among individuals because of several functionally relevant genetic polymorphisms.

Glutathione S-Transferases

Polymorphisms exist in cytosolic subfamilies such as μ [M], π [P), and Θ [T]. GSTs detoxify doxorubicin, lomustine, busulfan, chlorambucil, cisplatin, cyclophosphamide, melphalan, and others.[141] A common functional polymorphism in GSTP1 is associated with a significantly increased risk of developing therapy-related AML after prior exposure to chemotherapy that includes a leukemogenic GSTP1 substrate (chlorambucil, cyclophosphamide, melphalan, or doxorubicin) (odds ratio [OR], 4.34; 95% confidence limit [CI]: 1.43–13.20), but does not influence the risk of radiogenic leukemia.[142]

DNA Repair

Variants in pathways that mediate cellular response to genotoxic damage are also proposed to influence the risk of chemotherapy and radiotherapy-induced cancer, such as cell death signalling, cell proliferation, and DNA repair (*MLH1*,[143] *MSH2*,[90] XPD,[144] *XRCC1*,[145] *RAD51*,[146–148] and *P73*[149]). DNA repair mechanisms protect cells from mutations in tumor suppressor genes and oncogenes that can lead to cancer initiation and progression, with an individual's DNA repair capacity largely genetically determined.[150] A number of DNA repair genes contain polymorphic variants, resulting in large interindividual variation in DNA repair capacity, which could affect risk of SPC.[150] In support of this, a study of HL survivors suggested that those who developed a SPC had higher baseline levels of DNA damage than those who remained cancer-free.[151]

Mismatch Repair

Mismatch repair (MMR) functions to correct mismatched DNA base pairs that arise as a result of misincorporation errors that avoided polymerase proofreading during DNA replication.[152] Defects in the MMR pathway result in genetic instability or a mutator phenotype, manifested by an elevated rate of microsatellite instability. Up to 90% of therapy-related AML patients have microsatellite instability, associated with methylation of the MMR family member *MLH1*,[153,154] low expression of *MSH2*,[155] or polymorphisms in *MSH2*.[90,156]

Double-Strand Break Repair

High levels of double-strand breaks arise following ionizing radiation and chemotherapy exposures. Cellular pathways available to repair double-strand breaks include homologous recombination, nonhomologous end-joining, and single-strand annealing.[157] RAD51 is one of the central proteins in the homologous recombination pathway,[158] and a common variant in this gene (*G-135C*) is significantly overrepresented in patients with therapy-related AML compared with controls (C allele: OR, 2.7; 95% CI: 1.17–6.02).[146] XRCC3 also functions in the homologous recombination double-strand break repair pathway by directly interacting with, and stabilizing RAD51,[159] and functions to maintain genetic stability.[160,161] A polymorphism at codon 241 in the *XRCC3* gene results in a Thr→Met amino acid substitution.[162] The variant *Met*-encoding allele has been associated with a higher level of DNA damage, and has also been associated with increased levels of chromosome deletions in lymphocytes after exposure to radiation,[163] implying aberrant repair.[164] Although the XRCC3 Thr241Met variant was not an independent risk factor for t-MDS/AML, a synergistic interaction with the *RAD51*-135C variant resulting in an eightfold increased risk of therapy-related AML (OR, 8.1; 95% CI: 2.2–29.7) highlights the potential importance of gene-gene interactions in studies of SPC.[146]

Base Excision Repair

Base excision repair corrects individually damaged bases that result from ionizing radiation and exogenous xenobiotic exposure. A common variant at codon 399 of the XRCC1 protein, which is central to the base excision repair pathway and functions as a scaffold for other repair components,[165,166] was associated with an increased risk of developing t-AML,[145] and has also been implicated as a risk factor in numerous other cancers.

Nucleotide Excision Repair

Nucleotide excision repair removes structurally unrelated "bulky" DNA lesions induced by radiation and chemotherapy. The nucleotide excision repair pathway is linked to transcription, and components of the pathway comprise the basal transcription factor IIH complex, which is required for transcription initiation by RNA polymerase II. Polymorphic variation in ERCC2, a component of the transcription factor IIH complex, has been associated with an increased risk of therapy-related AML.[144]

The associations reported here were identified based on known gene-exposure interactions and analysis of loci in relevant pathways. Unfortunately, stratification by exposure is not always possible, particularly when a biological role has not been defined or when gene-exposure interactions are speculative. In this case, the application of high-density single nucleotide polymorphism arrays can prove useful in identifying those genetic variants and cellular pathways potentially important in causing chemotherapy- and radiotherapy-related cancer,[167–169] as have genome-wide studies in laboratory animals.[170]

Accurate estimates of the contribution of single gene variants in this context will also require large studies with sufficient power such that specific gene-exposure-dose interactions can be identified. Precise estimates are required in order to develop risk-adapted clinical strategies, including dose modification, alternative treatments, and posttherapy surveillance. Risk management could prove particularly important in children or young adults with primary cancers in whom cure rates are high and the risk of a subsequent cancer is associated with premature mortality.

In several instances, such as constitutional thiopurine methyltransferase (TPMT) activity and the risk of SPC, the stated goal has already been achieved. For example, children with ALL who received combined-modality therapy that included 6-mercaptopurine at a dose of 75 mg/m^2 and who had high TPMT activity (conferred by constitutional polymorphism in the *TMPT* gene) had an 8.3% cumulative risk of subsequently developing a brain tumor, while children who had low TPMT activity had a 42% risk of a posttherapy brain tumor (P = .0077).[108] It was hypothesized that the deficient TPMT activity resulted in higher exposures to thioguanine nucleotide metabolites of 6-mercaptopurine during the period of radiation. Likewise, patients with lower TPMT activity also had an increased risk of developing AML after high-dose thioguanine chemotherapy.[171,172] However, a reduction in 6-mercaptopurine dose (50 mg/m^2), along with other changes adopted as part of the Berlin-Frankfurt-Munster protocol for the treatment of childhood ALL, appeared to attenuate the effect of *TPMT* status on risk of developing AML after thioguanine-containing chemotherapy.[173]

Although it remains to be determined whether these data can be extended to other SPCs, dose and/or regimen modification has the potential to substantially reduce the risk of SPC in genetically susceptible individuals. Indeed, this principle has also applied to other populations at risk of therapy-induced SPC, such as patients with NF1. NF (caused by mutations in the *NF1* gene) is an autosomal dominantly inherited disorder characterized by a predisposition to benign tumours of the nerve sheath. There is evidence from studies of both laboratory animals[174] and humans[175] that constitutional heterozygosity for *NF1* pathogenic mutations confers susceptibility to radiogenic cancer, such that many investigators now recommend avoidance of radiotherapy wherever possible to treat tumors in NF patients.[176,177]

RISK OF SECOND MALIGNANCY IN PATIENTS WITH SELECTED PRIMARY CANCERS

Lymphoma

The use of combined-modality therapy in patients with both HL and NHL has resulted in significant improvements in survival, but with the attendant risk of SPC including leukemia and a number of solid tumors.

Hodgkin's Lymphoma

Reports from large, well-characterized cohorts of HL survivors show that the risk of developing SPC is 2 to 18 times higher than that in the general population.[9,49,50,86,178–184] Dores et al.[9] reported an analysis of 32,591 HL survivors diagnosed between 1935 and 1994 from 16 population-based registries. A total of 2,153 second cancers (relative risk [RR] = 2.3) was reported, including 1,726 solid tumors (RR = 2.0). The 25-year cumulative incidence of a solid tumor was 21.9%. Temporal trends for cancers of the female breast, thyroid, esophagus, stomach, rectum, bladder, and bone/connective tissue were suggestive of a radiogenic effect.

Survivors of childhood HL are at particularly high risk of second cancers. In the study by Dores et al.,[9] HL survivors diagnosed before the age of 21 had a 7.7-fold increased risk of a second cancer in comparison with the general population. Similarly, the risk of SPC in a cohort of 1,641 patients diagnosed before the age of 20 years in five Nordic countries was 7.7 times that of the general population.[181] The overall cumulative risk of SPC was 18% at 30 years. High risks were observed for breast cancer (RR = 17; 95% CI: 9.9–28), thyroid cancer (RR = 33; 95% CI: 15–62), secondary leukemia (RR = 17; 95% CI: 6.9–35), and NHL (RR = 15, 95% CI: 4.9–35). The Late Effects Study Group followed 1,380 children with HL in North America and Europe between 1955 and 1986.[185] The median age at last follow-up was 27.8 years, and the median length of follow-up was 17.0 years. The cohort's risk of developing SPC was 18.5 times higher than that of the general population. The cumulative incidence of any second malignancy was 26.3% at 30 years. Breast cancer was the most common solid tumor (SIR = 56.7). Other commonly occurring solid malignancies included cancers of the thyroid (SIR = 36.4), bone (SIR = 37.1), colorectal sites (SIR = 36.4), lung (SIR = 27.3), and stomach (SIR = 63.9). Risk factors for solid tumors included young age at HL diagnosis and radiotherapy. Thirty-two patients developed third neoplasms, with the cumulative incidence approaching 21% at 10 years from diagnosis of SPC.

In the last 15 to 20 years, the use, dose, and volume of radiation have been reduced in HL. It is anticipated that the incidence of SPC may decrease with contemporary therapy[186]; however, a potentially lower dose of radiation may still be highly carcinogenic, but associated with a longer latency period to induction of a second cancer. Illustrating this point, a small cohort (n = 112) of children with HL treated at a single institution with lower doses of involved-field radiation (up to 25.5 Gy) revealed a cumulative incidence of SPC of 17% at 20 years after HL diagnosis. The cohort was at 22.9-fold increased risk of developing SPC when compared with the general population, with an EAR of 9.4 cancers per 1,000 person-years of observation.[187] Finally, the cohort was at 72-fold increased risk of developing a second breast cancer when compared with the general population, with an EAR of 8.3 per 1,000 woman-years of observation. The authors concluded that the reduction in radiation dose was not associated with an appreciable decrease in risk of SPC, although these conclusions were based on a very small sample size.

Follow-up of large cohorts of HL survivors for extended periods of time documents the increasing occurrence of radiation-associated solid tumors, especially breast and thyroid cancers. In pediatric HL patients, the emergence of other cancers common in the adult population such as colon and lung cancer at younger ages than expected in the general population.

Non-Hodgkin's Lymphoma

Several population-based studies have provided estimates of the risk of second malignancies following NHL.[188–192] In the study by Dores et al.,[192] 5,490 subsequent cancers were observed among 73,958 2-month survivors of NHL, reflecting an overall elevated risk of 14% compared with the general population (observed/expected ratio [O/E], 1.14; 95% CI: 1.11–1.7; EAR, 19). The cumulative risk of second cancers reached 12.3% within 25 years. The risk of developing a new malignancy did not differ significantly by race or gender. Subsequent cancer risk was significantly elevated in patients age less than 30, 30 to 49, and 50 to 69 years at NHL diagnosis, with the largest excess among those ages 30 to 49 years (EAR = 35). The RR of all new cancers increased with time to reach 1.47% among 20-year NHL survivors (*P* trend <.0001). Significantly increased risks of new malignancies were observed for malignant melanoma (O/E = 1.57), Kaposi's sarcoma (O/E = 12.87), HL (O/E = 4.77), and AML (O/E = 3.22), as well as cancers of the buccal cavity (O/E = 1.76), lip (O/E = 1.76), salivary gland (O/E = 1.94), mouth (O/E = 1.39), lung (O/E = 1.32), vagina (O/E = 2.80), urinary bladder (O/E = 1.33), kidney parenchyma (O/E = 1.61), and bone (O/E = 3.53). Results from the SEER Program[192] corroborated findings in previous surveys of NHL, which have reported significant excesses of cutaneous melanoma, Kaposi sarcoma, HL, AML, and cancers of the buccal cavity, lip, lung, urinary bladder, and kidney.[188–190,193] Importantly, a SEER-based report by Tward et al.[191] also identified significantly increased risks of malignant mesothelioma among NHL patients initially given radiotherapy (O/E = 2.26), but not among those managed without irradiation (O/E = 0.86).

Lung cancer accounted for the largest excess of second cancers after NHL in the report by Dores et al.,[192] with overall increased risks noted in some—but not all—prior surveys.[188–191] A general upswing in the risk of lung cancer with time since NHL diagnosis was apparent, with 70% excesses among 20-year survivors (*P* trend <.01).[192] Given the overlap in treatment for NHL and HL, both therapy-related factors and tobacco use are likely involved in the observed lung cancer excesses.[47] In addition, tobacco use likely contributes to the excess risks observed for second cancers of the lip, mouth, urinary bladder, and kidney.

Radiotherapy for NHL appeared related to the increased risks for bladder cancer and bone sarcoma in the SEER Program.[192] Among NHL patients who initially received radiotherapy, significantly elevated risks of bladder cancer were confined to those surviving at least 10 years (O/E = 2.25), a pattern consistent with a prior analytic study[83] and with surveys of radiogenic bladder cancer in other populations.[194] In the analytic investigation of NHL patients,[83] cyclophosphamide increased the risk of bladder cancer in a dose-dependent manner and had an additive effect when combined with radiotherapy.

The immunosuppressive state associated with NHL[195] may contribute to excesses reported for cutaneous melanoma, HL, and lip cancer.[192,193,196,197] Although diagnostic misclassification of HL and NHL may affect risk estimates, one population-based study of NHL in which histopathologic materials for all cases were independently reviewed revealed a significant threefold excess of HL.[193] Epstein-Barr virus infection, an established cofactor in several subtypes of NHL and HL, may contribute to the fivefold increased risk of HL reported in the SEER Program.[192] The elevated 13-fold risk of Kaposi sarcoma based on 113 cases[192] probably reflects underlying HIV infection in some NHL patients, especially as significant excesses were not evident prior to 1980 (the pre-human immunodeficiency virus era). Individuals with AIDS have a 150- to 200-fold increased risk of NHL, which is associated with the degree of immune suppression.[198] In a reciprocal fashion, the significantly increased risks of NHL following HL, Kaposi sarcoma, and malignant melanoma in the SEER database point to the role of shared etiologic factors, possibly immune-related.

Survivors of childhood NHL are at fourfold increased risk of developing solid SPC when compared with the general population, with a cumulative incidence of 3% between 5 and 20 years from diagnosis.[199] The most common solid SPCs include cancers of breast, thyroid, brain, oropharynx, and musculoskeletal sites. Risk factors include female sex (threefold increased risk), mediastinal NHL (fivefold increased risk), and breast radiation (4.3-fold increased risk).

In summary, survivors of NHL are at increased risk for a number of second malignancies, although to a considerably smaller degree than are HL patients. The excess risks of AML and bladder cancer have been shown to be treatment-related. The persistent increase in the risk of all second cancers for more than 20 years after NHL treatment alerts clinicians to the importance of long-term surveillance. The elevated risk of lung cancer should encourage efforts aimed at smoking cessation. Health care providers should also be aware of the large risk of bladder cancer among patients treated with high-dose cyclophosphamide regimens of the past.[83]

Specific Cancers Following HL or NHL

Breast Cancer. Breast cancer is one of the most common solid tumors after HL. Studies have consistently shown that young age at radiotherapy is associated with a significantly higher risk of breast cancer.[48–51,200] In a population-based cohort study,[48] the absolute risks of breast cancer in women diagnosed with HL at ages 15 to 25 were higher than the absolute risks of women in the general population between 50 and 54 years, a standard age when mammography screening is recommended. Travis et al.[201] developed estimates of cumulative absolute risk of breast cancer, taking into account age and calendar year of HL diagnosis, current age, radiation dose, and competing causes of mortality. Thus, for an HL survivor who received a chest radiation dose of 40 Gy or more at age 25 years, the cumulative absolute risks of breast cancer at 10, 20, and 30 years are estimated to be 1.4%, 11%, and 29%, respectively.

There is a clear radiation dose-response relation for breast cancer risk after HL. In an international case-control study of breast cancer after HL that included 105 cases of breast cancer and 266 matched controls,[11] radiation dose to the area of the breast where the tumor developed in the case (and a comparable area in controls) was estimated. Breast cancer risk increased significantly with increasing radiation dose to reach eightfold for the highest category (median dose, 42 Gy) compared with the lowest-dose group (<4 Gy) (*P* trend for dose <.001) (Table 167.1).

A significant radiation dose-response relation was similarly demonstrated in a Dutch study that was included in the previous international investigation.[12] The Childhood Cancer Survivor Study (CCSS) published a case-control study of 120 cases of breast cancer (65% in survivors of HL) matched to 464 controls.[55] Again, a significant linear radiation dose-response was observed (*P* trend <.0001), with an estimated relative risk

TABLE 167.1

RELATIVE RISK OF BREAST CANCER AFTER CHEST RADIOTHERAPY, ACCORDING TO RADIATION DOSE TO AFFECTED SITE IN BREAST AND ALKYLATING CHEMOTHERAPY EXPOSURE

National Cancer Institute-International Study[a]				Childhood Cancer Survivor Study[b]			
Radiation Exposure							
Radiation Dose to Affected Site in Breast (Gy)	Cases/ Controls	Relative Risk	95% Confidence Interval	Radiation Dose to Affected Site in Breast (Gy)	Cases/ Controls	Relative Risk	95% Confidence Interval
0–3.9	15/76	1.0	(referent)	0	13/127	1.0	(referent)
4.0–6.9	13/30	1.8	0.7–4.5	>0–0.13	6/49	1.4	0.5–4.4
7.0–23.1	16/30	4.1	1.4–12.3	0.14–1.29	7/48	1.9	0.7–5.4
23.2–27.9	9/30	2.0	0.7–5.9	1.30–11.39	11/55	1.9	0.7–5.0
28.0–37.1	20/31	6.8	2.3–22.3	11.40–29.99	34/56	7.1	2.9–17
37.2–40.4	12/31	4.0	1.3–13.4	30.00–60.00	36/54	10.8	3.8–31
40.5–61.3	17/29	8.0	2.6–26.4	—	—	—	—
Alkylating Chemotherapy Exposure							
Number of Cycles of Alkylating Chemotherapy	Cases/ Controls	Relative Risk	95% Confidence Interval	Alkylating Agent Score[c]	Cases/ Controls	Relative Risk	95% Confidence Interval
0	68/132	1.0	(referent)	0	53/163	1.0	(referent)
1–4	10/20	0.7	0.3–1.7	1	12/63	0.67	0.3–1.5
5–8	17/55	0.6	0.3–1.1	2	12/36	1.40	0.6–3.4
≥9	4/29	0.2	0.1–0.7	3	17/37	1.15	0.6–2.4

[a](Adapted from ref. 13.) Population included women who were diagnosed with Hodgkin's lymphoma at age 30 or younger and who survived 1 or more years.
[b](Adapted from ref. 56.) Population included patients diagnosed with the following primary cancers at age younger than 21 and survived 5 or more years: Hodgkin's lymphoma (65%), soft tissue sarcoma (7.5%), leukemia (5.8%), non-Hodgkin's lymphoma (3.3%), central nervous system tumors (2.5%), kidney tumors (2.5%), and neuroblastoma (0.8%).
[c]Dose scores were assigned to individual alkylating agents on the basis of the distribution of dose (mg/m^2) of each agent, with scores then summed across agents.

of breast cancer of 6.4 at 20 Gy and 11.8 at 40 Gy (Table 167.1). Radiation field size for HL also affects breast cancer risk. A cohort study of 1,122 female HL 5-year survivors showed that mantle field irradiation (inclusion of mediastinum, bilateral axillae and neck) was associated with a 2.7-fold increased risk (95% CI: 1.1–6.9) of breast cancer compared with mediastinal irradiation alone.[64] A meta-analysis of SPC after HL found that extended field-radiotherapy was associated with a significantly higher breast cancer risk than involved-field radiotherapy (OR, 3.25; $P = .04$).[65] It is important to recognize that the high breast cancer risk in female HL survivors is largely based on women treated years ago with large radiation fields to doses in excess of 36 to 40 Gy. Indeed, a study using a validated radiobiological model estimated a 77% decrease in excess relative risk of breast cancer when 20 Gy of involved-field radiotherapy is used, compared with the historical standard of 35 Gy of mantle irradiation.[186]

Early menopause has been shown to be protective against breast cancer in HL survivors treated with radiotherapy. In particular, the Dutch study clearly documented that breast cancer risk reduction associated with chemotherapy was because of premature menopause.[12] In a more recent HL cohort study from the same group,[64] among women age less than 41 years at treatment, those women with more than 20 years of ovarian function posttreatment had a significantly higher risk of breast cancer compared with patients with 10 to 20 years of intact ovarian function after therapy (hazard ratio, 5.3; 95% CI: 2.9–9.9).

Studies have shown a reduced risk of breast cancer among NHL survivors compared with the general population, likely because of chemotherapy-related early menopause.[191,202,203] Although breast cancer risk after mediastinal irradiation for NHL has not been specifically assessed, indirect data suggested an increased risk with younger age at irradiation. In a SEER-based study of 77,876 NHL patients,[191] the relative risk of breast cancer was significantly increased among women irradiated at age less than 25 years (RR, 5.05; $P < .05$), whereas breast cancer excesses were not observed in the entire irradiated cohort. Similarly, in a Swedish Cancer Registry-based study of 29,134 patients with NHL,[204] the relative risk of breast cancer was significantly increased only among women diagnosed between ages 20 and 39 years (RR, 3.29; 95% CI: 1.91–5.67) and not in older patients. Presumably, the increased breast cancer risk in these young women was due to radiotherapy to the chest area, although this cannot be confirmed because sites of irradiation were not described.

Thyroid Cancer. Several population-based or multi-institutional cohort studies have reported an increased risk of thyroid cancer (papillary and follicular adenocarcinoma) among HL survivors treated with either mantle radiation field or an involved-neck field.[9,49,50,86] These studies had limited data or small sample sizes, thus the investigators were unable to examine modifying risk factors such as radiation dose, gender, and age at radiation exposure. In contrast, with many childhood cancers treated with radiation to the head/neck/chest region, these factors have been studied extensively and are discussed in the pediatric SPC section of this chapter.

Lung Cancer. Significantly elevated three- to sevenfold relative risks of lung cancer have been reported after HL,[9,47–50,57,86,205] with a dose-dependent relationship documented for antecedent alkylating agent chemotherapy[47,205] and for radiation dose to the area of lung in which cancer developed.[47] The modifying effect of smoking history on treatment-related lung cancer in HL survivors was investigated in a case-control study by Travis et al.[47] Using patients who had minimal radiation or alkylating chemotherapy exposure and who were nonsmokers as the reference group, exposure to more than 5 Gy of radiotherapy and/or alkylating agent chemotherapy was associated with a 4.3- to 7.2-fold increased risk of lung cancer. The relative risk increased to 16.8 and 20.2, respectively, in patients who had either one of the treatment exposures and who used tobacco. Moreover, the relative risk was 49.1 in patients who had more than 5 Gy of radiotherapy, received alkylating chemotherapy, and who used tobacco, consistent with a multiplicative effect of tobacco use on the risk of treatment-related lung cancer.

The risk of lung cancer is modestly increased after NHL, with most studies reporting a risk of less than twofold compared to the general population.[188,189,191,202–204,206,207] The increased risk appears to be associated with both chemotherapy and radiotherapy, with significantly increasing risk following higher cumulative doses of chemotherapy.[206] Male NHL survivors are at higher risk for lung cancer,[189,207] potentially because of a higher prevalence of tobacco use than among women with NHL.[207] The contribution of tobacco use to lung cancer risk after NHL therapy, however, has not been addressed in analytic studies. Increased risks for malignant mesothelioma have been reported in survivors of both HL and NHL, although the excesses appear limited to irradiated patients.[205,208,209]

Gastrointestinal Malignancies. Population-based and multi-institutional cohort studies have consistently reported an increased risk, compared with the general population, for cancers of esophagus, stomach, colon, and rectum among HL survivors.[9,49,50,183,185,210] Elevated risks first appear 10 to 15 years after HL treatment,[49,183,185] and then continue to increase with increasing follow-up time.[86,185] In a large international population-based study, Dores et al.[9] also reported an increased risk of pancreatic cancer among HL survivors compared with the general population, with the pattern of excesses consistent with a radiogenic effect.

van den Belt-Dusebout et al.[58] conducted a nested case-control study of 5,142 Dutch testicular cancer and HL survivors to examine the role of radiation dose and chemotherapy in the etiology of gastric cancer. Because demographic characteristics of the testicular cancer and HL patients were generally similar, these populations were pooled, although it should be kept in mind that the underlying cancers are distinctly different. Adenocarcinoma and signet ring cell carcinoma represented 52.1% and 28.6% of the gastric cancers, respectively; cancers were equally distributed throughout the stomach, with 35.7% occurring in the antrum. There was a 3.4-fold increased risk of gastric cancer compared with the general population. The risk increased with increasing mean radiation dose to the stomach, with an excess relative risk of 0.84 per Gy. Mean stomach doses of more than 20 Gy were associated with a relative risk of 9.9 compared with doses below 11 Gy. Adjusted for radiation, higher doses of procarbazine ($\geq$13,000 mg vs. $<$10,000 mg) were associated with a 5.4-fold increased risk of gastric cancer. Smoking more than ten cigarettes per day was associated with a 1.6-fold increased risk compared with survivors who did not smoke. Gender and age at radiation exposure did not modify risk.

Nonmelanoma Skin Cancer And Melanoma. The increased risks of malignant melanoma[9,49,50,210] and nonmelanoma skin cancer[210] following HL therapy are discussed in the pediatric section of this chapter.

Therapy-Related Leukemia. Therapy-related leukemia has been described after conventional chemotherapy and, to a lesser extent, radiotherapy for HL and NHL. The incidence of therapy-related leukemia following conventional chemotherapy or radiation for HL or NHL ranges from 0.8% at 30 years to 6.3% at 20 years.[185,188,211] In a large population-based study of 35,511 HL patients, the EAR of therapy-related AML was reported to be 0.6 per 1000 person-years of observation.[8] EAR was highest during the first 10 years after HL, and for patients diagnosed with HL at age 35 years and older. Further, the EAR declined significantly among HL patients treated after 1984, probably from modifications in therapeutic exposures, with replacement of the highly leukemogenic MOPP regimen (mechlorethamine, vincristine, procarbazine, prednisone) by ABVD (doxorubicin, bleomycin, vinblastine, dacarbazine).

Previous analytic studies of NHL patients have documented the leukemogenic effects of radiotherapy and alkylating agent chemotherapy, particularly mechlorethamine, procarbazine, and chlorambucil.[212,213] Numerous studies[214] report an increased risk of MDS/AML among patients receiving autologous bone marrow transplantation for lymphoma (described in Chapter 125).

The median time to development of therapy-related leukemia ranges from 3 to 5 years, with the risk decreasing markedly after the first decade. Factors associated with an increased risk of therapy-related leukemia include host factors (older age at diagnosis), exposure to alkylating agents, topoisomerase II inhibitors, and radiotherapy. The unique clinical characteristics of therapy-related leukemia associated with the two types of chemotherapeutic exposures (alkylating agents and topoisomerase II inhibitors) have been described in previous sections.

Breast Cancer

Women with breast cancer are at significantly elevated risk for developing subsequent malignancies. The largest amount of data have accrued on the risk of contralateral breast cancer (CBC), which is estimated to be increased two- to fivefold. Factors that may modify the increased risk include pre-existing breast cancer risk factors such as genetic predisposition, reproductive factors and health habits, as well as treatment exposures. The Women's Environmental, Cancer, and Radiation Epidemiology (WECARE) study is a population-based, multicenter, case-control study of 708 women with asynchronous bilateral breast cancer and 1,395 women with unilateral breast cancer. Reports from this data set have shown that age at menarche and parity,[215] which are established risk factors for first primary breast cancer, are also associated with CBC. Other known breast cancer risk factors including age at first full-term pregnancy and use of either oral contraceptives or hormonal replacement therapy[215,216] do not appear to increase risk of CBC. The WECARE group recently reported a significant association between regular alcohol consumption and risk for CBC.[217] Another population-based case-control study found that in addition to alcohol use, obesity and smoking significantly increased CBC risk,[218] highlighting the importance of lifestyle modifications among breast cancer survivors.

Treatment factors that influence the risk of CBC include tamoxifen use, which has been shown to reduce CBC risk by 30% to 40% in randomized trials.[219] The WECARE study documented that tamoxifen use was associated with a 34% reduction in CBC, and the association remained statistically significant for 5 years.[220] Chemotherapy lowered the risk of CBC by 43%, with the reduced risk persisting for up to 10 years after treatment.

Conflicting data exist on the contribution of radiotherapy to excess risks of CBC.[221–224] In a case-control study by Boice et al.,[223] the overall relative risk of CBC was not significantly increased after radiotherapy (RR, 1.19; 95% CI: 0.94–1.15).

Among women age less than 45 years at the time of irradiation, however, the relative risk was significantly elevated at 1.59 (95% CI: 1.07–2.36). Hooning et al.[52] assessed the long-term risk of CBC in 7,221 breast cancer survivors and found a 2.91-fold (95% CI: 2.66–3.18) increased risk compared with the general female population (EAR = 46.1/10,000 person-years). The risk of radiotherapy-related CBC also increased significantly with decreasing age at treatment; among women who received radiotherapy at age less than 35 years, the hazard ratio for CBC was 1.78 (95% CI: 0.85–3.72), whereas for women irradiated at age 45 or more years, risk decreased to 1.09 (95% CI: 0.82–1.45). Further, postlumpectomy radiotherapy was associated with a significantly higher risk of CBC compared with postmastectomy radiotherapy in which direct electron fields were typically used, resulting in lower radiation doses to the contralateral breast.

In a report from the WECARE group,[53] where absorbed doses to quadrants of the contralateral breast were estimated, women less than 40 years of age who received more than 1.0 Gy of absorbed dose to the specific quadrant of the contralateral breast had a significantly increased 2.5-fold greater risk for CBC than unexposed women. No excess risk was observed in women more than 40 years of age. Most recently, the WECARE group showed that breast cancer patients who carry rare deleterious *ATM* missense mutations and are treated with radiation may have an increased risk of CBC, noting however that the rarity of these variants would account for only a small percentage of CBC.[225]

The Early Breast Cancer Trialists' Collaborative Group reported a significantly increased risk of CBC with radiotherapy, mainly during the period 5 to 14 years after randomization (RR, 1.43; *P* = .00001), and the increased risk was significant even among women aged 50 years or more when randomized (RR, 1.25; *P* = .002).[226] In contrast, in an earlier large case-control study from Denmark, there was no significant difference in the risk of CBC in women who did and did not receive radiotherapy, regardless of age at treatment.[227] In the Danish study, it was found that the second breast cancers were evenly distributed in the medial, lateral, and central portions of the breast, which argued against a causal role of radiotherapy in tumorigenesis. A recent large-scale study from Institut Curie, which included 13,472 women, similarly failed to show an increased risk of CBC when comparing women who did or did not receive radiotherapy (RR, 1.1; 95% CI: 0.96–1.27). Analysis by age, however, was not performed in that study.[221] Available data therefore suggest that there is a modest but significant risk of CBC, mostly limited to younger women who receive radiotherapy.

Endometrial cancer is another malignancy in breast cancer survivors that can be linked with both shared etiologic factors and antecedent therapy, in particular, tamoxifen therapy. Several large studies have demonstrated a 2-4-fold increased risk of endometrial cancer after tamoxifen therapy.[26] Earlier studies indicated that endometrial cancer after tamoxifen use may have a more favorable prognosis, although recent data have raised the concern that tamoxifen-related endometrial cancers may have a more aggressive behavior.[228–230] In a study that included 732 women with endometrial carcinoma, 59 patients (8%) had a previous diagnosis of breast cancer, of whom 29 (49%) had used tamoxifen.[231] Breast cancer survivors were more likely to have high-risk endometrial cancer types (grade 3 endometrioid, papillary serous, or clear cell) than those without breast cancer (31% vs. 18%; *P* = .024). A longer duration of tamoxifen use was also associated with high-risk histologic type (60 vs. 46 months; *P* = .034). A Dutch study that examined endometrial cancer after tamoxifen treatment for breast cancer found that long-term tamoxifen use was associated with a higher proportion of nonendometrioid tumors than nonusers (32.7% vs. 17.4%; *P* = .004), especially serous adenocarcinomas and carcinosarcomas; a higher proportion of International Federation of Gynecology and Obstetrics stage III and IV tumors was also observed (20.0% vs. 11.3%; *P* = .049).[229] The differences in histologic and stage distributions translated to a significantly lower 3-year endometrial cancer-specific survival among long-term tamoxifen users (82% vs. 93%; *P* = .001).

Several other solid tumors have been linked to radiotherapy for breast cancer, including lung cancer, sarcoma, and esophageal cancer. Compared with women who did not receive radiotherapy, women given radiotherapy have a 1.5- to 3-fold increased risk of developing lung cancer.[221,232,233] The observation that lung cancer after breast cancer therapy is more frequently found in the ipsilateral lung also supports the contribution of radiotherapy to excess risk.[67] Several studies also show an enhancement of lung cancer risk among smokers treated with irradiation for breast cancer.[65,233] In a case-control study by Kaufman et al,[234] 113 breast cancer patients who developed lung cancer were matched to 364 controls without lung cancer; excess risks of lung cancer following postmastectomy radiotherapy were limited to ever-smokers. Compared with nonsmoking women who did not receive postmastectomy radiotherapy, the adjusted odds ratio for lung cancer among nonirradiated ever-smokers was 5.9 (95% CI: 27–12.8) and the adjusted odds ratio among ever-smokers who also received postmastectomy radiotherapy was 18.9 (95% CI: 7.9–45.4). Others have shown that the increased risks of lung cancer appeared more related to postmastectomy radiotherapy, in which the radiation target volume often also includes the supraclavicular, axillary, and/or internal mammary nodal regions, thus exposing a larger volume of lung tissue, while the risk after postlumpectomy radiotherapy is less clear.[66,67] Similarly, in a population-based study by Zablotska and Neugut[67] of squamous cell esophageal cancer after adjuvant radiotherapy for breast cancer, the relative risk was significantly increased only among women who received postmastectomy radiotherapy, but not among those who received postlumpectomy radiotherapy. In a Finnish population-based study of breast cancer patients treated with radiotherapy and followed for 15 years, the relative risk for esophageal cancer was 2.3 (95% CI: 1.4–5.4) compared with the general population, and no increase in risk was seen among women treated without radiotherapy.

Although the occurrence of sarcoma after breast cancer is a rare event, with a 15-year incidence rate of less than 0.5%, the relative risk has been estimated to be as high as 7 because of the low background incidence in the general population.[186,221,235,236] In a study by Rubino et al.,[62] all sarcomas occurred among women who had initially received radiotherapy, and in all cases, the sarcomas were located in the irradiated fields or in the upper extremity of the arm ipsilateral to the treated breast. Further, a significant dose-response relationship was demonstrated. By estimating the initial radiation dose to the site of sarcoma development, using a dose of 14 Gy or less to the site as reference, women who received 14 to 44 Gy had a 1.6-fold increased risk of sarcoma while those who received 45 Gy or more to the site had a 30.6-fold increased risk (*P* <.001). Angiosarcoma after breast cancer was initially associated with chronic lymphedema following radical mastectomy.[237]

With the increasing use of radiotherapy, there have been a growing number of reports of cutaneous angiosarcoma of the breast arising in the radiation field.[236,238–240] In a study from the SEER database of 563,155 breast cancer patients, women who received radiotherapy had a 1.5-fold risk (95% CI: 1.3–1.8) of all types of sarcomas, and a 7.6-fold risk (95% CI: 4.9–11.9) of angiosarcoma, compared with women who did not receive radiotherapy.[241] In addition to radiotherapy, partial mastectomies and lymph node dissections were also independent risk factors for the development of angiosarcoma. Unlike other radiation-related soft tissue sarcomas, angiosarcoma has a short latency and can occur in the first 5 years after therapy.

Breast cancer survivors are at risk for developing acute leukemia. Howard et al.[227] conducted a large international population-based study of 376,825 1-year survivors of breast cancer. Compared with the general population, the relative risk of all leukemias was 1.7 (95% CI: 1.6–1.8), and the corresponding EAR was 9.05 per 100,000 person-years (95% CI: 7.5–10.7). For women diagnosed with breast cancer after 1985, the 10-year cumulative risk of leukemia for those diagnosed before and after age 50 were 0.10% and 0.14%, respectively. Analytic studies show that the risk of leukemia following breast cancer is related to prior chemotherapy and radiotherapy.[91,242–244] In a case-control investigation by Curtis et al.[91] of women treated for breast cancer between 1973 and 1985, 90 women who developed leukemia and 264 matched controls were studied. Compared with women who did not receive alkylating chemotherapy or radiotherapy, the relative risk of AML after radiotherapy alone, alkylating chemotherapy alone, and both chemotherapy and radiotherapy were 2.4, 10, and 17.4, respectively. A significant dose-response effect was observed between cumulative doses of melphalan, cyclophosphamide, and radiation to the active bone marrow and subsequent leukemia risk. It should be noted that this study was conducted in an era when higher cumulative doses of chemotherapy and larger field radiotherapy were used. Moreover, the melphalan-containing regimens examined by Curtis et al.[91] are no longer used in the treatment of breast cancer. Indeed, in the large population-based study by Howard et al.,[227] decreasing leukemia risks were observed in women treated in more recent calendar years, likely reflecting these types of changes in treatment. Nonetheless, more modern systemic therapies for breast cancer can also contribute to leukemia risk. For example, an association between increasing cumulative doses of topoisomerase-II inhibitors and increasing leukemia risk after breast cancer has been demonstrated.[242,245] These findings are of particular relevance with the current routine use of anthracyclines as adjuvant therapy in breast cancer patients, and the trend toward use of dose-intensified regimens.

In addition to the evolution in systemic therapy for breast cancer that affects the risk of subsequent malignancies, recent advances in radiotherapy, including use of IMRT,[53] and the growing interest in partial breast irradiation,[227] will likely also influence risk. The risks associated with these newer radiotherapy approaches and techniques remain to be clarified.

Prostate Cancer

Although radiotherapy is an established treatment modality for patients with localized prostate cancer, evidence with regard to any increased site-specific risk of subsequent cancers is conflicting.[43,68,233,246–253] Whereas several studies have shown significantly increased risks of specific types of second cancers, including colorectal cancer, bladder cancer, soft tissue sarcoma, and lung cancer following radiotherapy,[43,233,246,248,249,251,252] other studies have not found significant associations.[68,250,253] The absolute risk of any associated SPC appears to be modest; Brenner et al.[246] estimated that radiation-associated malignancies after prostate cancer may affect 1 in 290 of all patients, 1 in 125 five-year survivors, and 1 in 70 ten-year survivors.

The findings of any association between radiotherapy for prostate cancer and increased subsequent cancer risk should be interpreted with caution. Following radiotherapy, treatment-related effects including proctitis, cystitis, and bleeding may lead to colonoscopies or cystoscopies, which in turn can result in an apparent increased incidence of colorectal or other urologic cancers.[43] In addition, patients with significant comorbid illnesses and/or heavy smoking histories are less likely to be selected for surgery and therefore more likely to undergo radiotherapy. Thus, selection bias may partly explain the observed increased lung cancer risk in prostate cancer patients treated with radiotherapy. This is highlighted by one study that showed that men selected for radical prostatectomy had a significantly lower risk of lung cancer mortality.[247]

Testicular Cancer

Significant excesses of solid tumors, leukemia, and contralateral testicular cancer (CTC) have been documented in testicular cancer survivors (TCS).[7,96,125,254–263] In an international population-based survey of 40,576 TCS,[7] significantly elevated 1.5- to fourfold relative risks were noted for malignant melanoma and cancers of lung, thyroid, esophagus, pleura, stomach, pancreas, colon, rectum, kidney, bladder, and connective tissue among 10-year survivors (Table 167.2). By age 75, men who were diagnosed with seminomas or nonseminomatous tumors at age 35 experienced cumulative risks of solid cancer of 36% and 31%, respectively. Among TCS treated with radiotherapy alone, relative risks of second malignant neoplasms (SMNs) at sites included in typical infradiaphragmatic radiotherapy fields were significantly larger than risks at nonexposed sites (RR, 2.7 vs. RR, 1.6; $P < .05$), and remained elevated for 35 or more years. No decrease in the risk of postradiotherapy in-site SMN was observed for seminoma patients diagnosed from 1975 to 2001, although a lowered risk was noted among nonseminoma patients. In a case-control investigation of 23 stomach cancers among TCS,[58] a significant relation with increasing radiation dose was observed. Mortality due to SMN after testicular cancer appears similar to that of matched first cancers.[264] In the international series,[7] the relative risk (RR = 1.8) of solid tumors was significantly elevated after chemotherapy alone, although information on specific cytotoxic drugs was not available. A subsequent investigation[254] showed that cisplatin-based chemotherapy was associated with a significantly elevated twofold risk of solid tumors, confirming other reports.[263]

Cytotoxic drugs used to treat testicular cancer that have been related with excess secondary leukemias include etoposide and cisplatin.[96,259,261,262] Kollmannsberger et al.[262] estimated that the cumulative risk of leukemia for TCS given etoposide at total doses of less than 2,000 and more than 2,000 mg/m^2 was 0.5% and 2%, respectively. A strong dose-response relation ($P < .001$) between cumulative dose of cisplatin and subsequent leukemia risk was reported by Travis et al.,[96] who also noted a nonsignificant threefold risk following involved-field radiotherapy.

In a population-based study of 29,515 TCS, the 15-year cumulative risk of CTC was 1.9%, representing a 12.4-fold higher risk than expected in the general population.[260] Chemotherapy may reduce the risk of CTC,[265,266] although the delaying effect and duration of cisplatin–based chemotherapy on the incidence of CTC should be examined further.

In the future, it will be important to determine whether the decrease in radiation dose and field size in the 1990s,[267,268] along with the use of carboplatin as adjuvant therapy in seminoma patients,[269] will be associated with a reduction in excess SMN. The long-term influence of cisplatin-based chemotherapy on the site-specific risk of solid tumors, temporal patterns, and the effect of age at exposure and attained age should also be addressed in analytic investigations that control for lifestyle factors, shared etiologic influences, and host determinants.[3,4] Screening strategies for selected SMN should be considered.

The risk of SMN in TCS initially treated with radiotherapy or chemotherapy should be compared with the risk in patients managed with surgery alone, as the development of cancer at a young age may itself indicate an underlying susceptibility for subsequent malignancy. Similarly, the incidence of SMN among TCS managed with surgical approaches alone should be contrasted with cancer incidence in the general male population in

TABLE 167.2

ESTIMATED RELATIVE RISK OF SECOND CANCERS ACCORDING TO TIME SINCE TESTICULAR CANCER DIAGNOSIS FOR PATIENTS DIAGNOSED WITH TESTICULAR CANCER AT AGE 35 YEARS[a]

	All ≥10 Y Intervals		Time since Testicular Cancer Diagnosis: 10–19 Y		20–29 Y		≥30 Y		Excess Number (%)[b]
	Obs.	RR (95% CI)	Obs.	RR (95% CI)	Obs.	RR (95% CI)	Obs.	RR (95% CI)	
CANCER SITE									
All solid tumors	1,694	1.9 (1.8–2.1)	802	2.1 (1.9–2.3)	563	2.0 (1.8–2.2)	329	1.7 (1.6–1.9)[c]	698 (100)[d]
Esophagus	26	1.7 (1.0–2.6)	13	2.0 (<1.0–3.8)	7	0.9 (<1.0–2.3)	6	2.1 (<1.0–4.0)	9 (1.3)
Stomach	129	4.0 (3.2–4.8)	64	4.9 (3.7–6.4)	49	4.5 (3.3–5.9)	16	1.9 (1.0–3.2)[e]	88 (12.6)
Colon	153	2.0 (1.7–2.5)	62	1.8 (1.3–2.6)	52	2.1 (1.5–2.8)	39	2.2 (1.6–3.0)	66 (9.5)
Rectum/anus	101	1.8 (1.4–2.3)	60	2.7 (1.9–3.8)	22	1.3 (<1.0–1.9)	19	1.7 (1.1–2.6)	39 (5.5)
Pancreas	95	3.6 (2.8–4.6)	44	4.1 (2.8–5.9)	38	4.3 (3.0–6.0)	13	2.3 (1.3–3.7)	63 (9.0)
Lung	256	1.5 (1.2–1.7)	148	2.2 (1.7–2.7)	73	1.4 (1.1–1.8)	35	1.0 (<1.0–1.4)[e]	65 (9.3)
Pleura	12	3.4 (1.7–5.9)	7	6.0 (2.3–12)	3	2.6 (0.5–6.6)	2	1.9 (0.4–6.1)	8 (1.1)
Prostate	249	1.4 (1.2–1.6)	88	1.1 (<1.0–1.6)	91	1.4 (1.1–1.8)	70	1.5 (1.2–1.8)	52 (7.4)
Kidney	80	2.4 (1.8–3.0)	29	1.7 (1.0–2.6)	30	2.5 (1.7–3.6)	21	3.0 (1.9–4.4)[f]	43 (6.2)
Bladder	211	2.7 (2.2–3.1)	75	2.0 (1.4–2.7)	85	3.2 (2.5–4.0)	51	2.6 (2.0–3.5)	115 (16.4)
Malignant melanoma	70	1.8 (1.3–2.3)	43	1.9 (1.3–2.6)	23	2.1 (1.4–3.1)	4	0.8 (0.3–1.7)	30 (4.2)
Thyroid	16	2.3 (1.0–4.4)	15	4.2 (1.8–8.2)	1	1.0 (<1.0–3.4)	0	—	9 (1.2)
Connective tissue	19	4.0 (2.3–6.3)	9	3.7 (1.7–7.0)	9	6.1 (2.8–11.0)	1	1.6 (<1.0–5.8)	14 (2.0)
Other solid tumors[g]	277	1.6 (1.4–1.9)	145	1.5 (1.2–1.9)	80	1.6 (1.3–2.0)	52	1.9 (1.4–2.4)	98 (14.1)
RADIOTHERAPY ONLY									
All solid tumors	892	2.0 (1.9–2.2)	399	2.2 (1.9–2.5)	300	2.0 (1.8–2.3)	193	1.8 (1.6–2.1)[h]	387 (100)[d]
Sites in-field[i]	445	2.7 (2.4–3.0)	174	2.6 (2.1–3.2)	165	2.9 (2.4–3.4)	106	2.5 (2.0–3.0)	246 (63.7)
Other sites	447	1.6 (1.4–1.8)	225	1.9 (1.6–2.3)	135	1.5 (1.3–1.8)	87	1.4 (1.1–1.7)[j]	141 (36.3)

Obs., observed number of cases; RR, relative risk; CI, confidence interval.
[a]The table is restricted to those sites for which significantly increased RR were observed in 10-year survivors of testicular cancer. The RR is a decreasing function of age at testicular cancer diagnosis; results are presented for age 35 years, which is the mean age of the cohort.
[b]Percentage contribution to the total excess is shown within the parentheses; percentages may not sum to 100 due to rounding.
[c]*P* trend (negative) = .007
[d]Obtained as sum of site-specific excesses.
[e]*P* trend (negative) <.001
[f]*P* trend (positive) = .02
[g]Includes 172 tumors for which site was specified and 105 tumors of unknown or ill-defined primary site.
[h]*P* trend (negative) = .013
[i]Restricted to those sites that are included in typical infradiaphragmatic radiotherapy fields for testicular cancer: stomach, small intestine, colon, rectum, liver, gallbladder and ducts, pancreas, kidney, and bladder.
[j]*P* trend (negative) = 0.005
(Modified from ref. 8.)

order to understand the evolution of cured testicular cancer, given its origin from a pluripotent stem cell and the presence of non–germ cell elements in nonseminomatous testicular cancer and their metastases.[270,271] Future research strategies for TCS, including detailed recommendations for the study of SPC, were recently published by Travis et al.,[272] with an overview provided in Table 167.3. These include evaluation of the role of genetic variants in the development of second cancers after testicular cancer and the development of site-specific risk prediction models.

Ovarian Cancer

In view of significant improvements in survival after a diagnosis of ovarian cancer in the last few decades,[1] quantification of second cancer risk has become increasingly important. The largest follow-up study to date included 41,489 two-month survivors of ovarian cancer reported to the SEER Program (1973–2001).[273] A total of 2,091 subsequent tumors was observed (O/E = 1.17). Cumulative incidence of second cancers was 9.4% within 25 years. Overall excesses were largely because of significantly increased risks of acute leukemia, as well as cancers of breast, colon, rectum, small intestine, bladder, renal pelvis, eye (ocular melanoma), and intrahepatic bile ducts. Reproductive and genetic factors predisposing to ovarian cancer may have contributed to the increased risk of breast, colorectal, and other neoplasms.[274,275] Significant excesses of subsequent cancers of bladder and soft tissue were restricted to SEER patients given radiotherapy.[273]

One analytic population-based investigation of over 28,000 ovarian cancer patients in whom 96 leukemias were diagnosed demonstrated that platinum-based combination chemotherapy was associated with a significantly increased fourfold risk of leukemia compared with women who received neither alkylating drugs nor radiotherapy.[95] Leukemia risk increased with increasing cumulative platinum dose (*P* trend <.001) and with increasing duration of platinum-based chemotherapy to reach

TABLE 167.3

SUMMARY OF MAJOR RESEARCH RECOMMENDATIONS—LATE EFFECTS OF TESTICULAR CANCER AND ITS TREATMENT

1. Overarching recommendation: lifelong follow-up of all testicular cancer survivors (TCS)
   - Integrate observational and analytic epidemiologic studies with molecular and genetic approaches to ascertain the risk of emerging toxicities and to understand the evolution of known late effects, especially with the aging of TCS.
   - Evaluate the influence of race and socioeconomic status on the late effects of testicular cancer and its treatment.
   - Characterize long-term tissue deposition of platinum (sites, reactivity), serum levels, and correlation with late effects.
   - Evaluate the lifelong burden of medical and psychosocial morbidity by treatment.
   - Use research findings to establish evidence-based, risk-adapted, long-term follow-up care.
2. Specific recommendations
   - Second malignant neoplasms (SMN) and late relapses
     - Determine the effect of reductions in field size and dose of radiotherapy, along with the use of carboplatin as adjuvant therapy in seminoma patients, on the risk of SMN.
     - Examine relation between platinum-based chemotherapy and site-specific risk of solid tumors, the associated temporal patterns, and the influence of age at exposure and attained age.
     - Compare risk of SMN in TCS managed with surgery alone to cancer incidence in the general male population.
     - Examine delaying influence of platinum-based chemotherapy (and duration and magnitude of effect) on development of contralateral testicular cancer.
     - Characterize the evolution of cured testicular cancer, in particular, the molecular underpinnings of late recurrences.
   - Cardiovascular disease (CVD)
     - Evaluate the contributions and interactions of subclinical hypogonadism, platinum-based chemotherapy, radiotherapy, lifestyle factors (diet, tobacco use, physical activity), body mass index, family history of CVD, race, socioeconomic status, abnormal laboratory values, and genetic modifiers (refer to text).
     - Develop comprehensive risk prediction models, considering the above variables, to stratify TCS into risk groups in order to customize follow-up strategies and develop evidence-based interventions.
   - Neurotoxicity
     - Evaluate evolution of neurotoxicity across TCS lifespan, role of genetic modifiers, and extent to which symptoms impact on work ability and quality of life.
   - Nephrotoxicity
     - Determine whether the natural decline in renal function associated with aging is accelerated in TCS, any influence of low-level platinum exposure, and the impact of decreased glomerular filtration rate on CVD and all-cause mortality.
     - Determine the incidence of hypomagnesemia, together with the role of modifying factors and resultant medical consequences, in long-term TCS.
   - Hypogonadism and decreased fertility
     - Address the incidence, course, and clinical effects of subclinical hypogonadism.
     - Evaluate effect of all levels of gonadal dysfunction in TCS on CVD, premature aging, fatigue, osteoporosis, mental health, quality of life, and sexuality.
   - Pulmonary function
     - Examine role of platinum compounds on long-term pulmonary damage in TCS, and interactions with other influences, including bleomycin, tobacco use, and occupational risk factors.
   - Psychosocial effects
     - Identify prevalence and predictors of depression, cancer-related anxiety, fatigue, infertility-related distress, problems with sexuality, and paired relationships and posttraumatic growth.
     - Examine the impact of different cultural backgrounds on posttreatment quality of life.
     - Evaluate TCS work ability throughout life.
     - Determine whether normal age-related declines in cognitive function are accelerated in TCS.
3. Interventions
   - Conduct targeted intervention trials aimed at promoting smoking cessation, healthy dietary habits, and an increase in physical activity.
   - Evaluate the role of information and communication technologies in promoting a healthy lifestyle among TCS.
   - Consider randomized, pharmacologic intervention trials among TCS with biochemical parameters approaching threshold values to avoid accelerated development into treatment-requiring CVD (see text).
   - Determine optimal schedule of testosterone replacement therapy among TCS with clinical hypogonadism.
   - Consider screening strategies for selected SMN.
4. Genetic and molecular considerations
   - Evaluate genetic risk factors (identified in the general male population) as modifiers for all late effects in TCS, in particular, CVD, SMN, neurotoxicity, nephrotoxicity, hypogonadism, and psychosocial effects.
   - Investigate the role of genome-wide association studies, epigenetics, mitochondrial DNA, microRNA, proteomics and related approaches in identifying genetic variants that contribute to the late effects of treatment.
   - Develop standardized procedures for biospecimen collection to support genetic and molecular studies, as reviewed previously.
5. Risk prediction models
   - Develop comprehensive risk prediction models that incorporate genetic modifiers of late sequelae (see text).

(From ref. 272, with permission.)

sevenfold in women treated for more than 12 months (P trend for duration = .001). A dose-response relation for platinum was apparent among women treated or not treated with radiotherapy, with larger risks in those receiving combined-modality therapy. Whether leukemia risk after treatment with platinum might be increased by radiotherapy, however, should be examined among patients with other cancers, especially cancers of the bladder and head and neck, given therapeutic approaches to increase dose intensities of both modalities in the management of these tumors.[276,277]

PEDIATRIC MALIGNANCIES

Survival rates for children with cancer have increased substantially over the past 3 decades, with this rapidly growing population at lifelong risk for the late effects of cancer treatment. In a British population-based study of 16,541 three-year survivors of childhood cancer diagnosed prior to age 15, the cumulative incidence of SPC was reported to be 4.2% at 25 years.[278] In a recent update of 14,359 five-year survivors (diagnosed prior to age 21) in the CCSS,[279] the 30-year cumulative incidence was 7.9% for invasive SPC, 9.1% for nonmelanoma skin cancers (NMSC), and 3.1% for meningiomas, with an overall 30-year incidence for all SPC of 20% (Fig. 167.3). Childhood cancer survivors have a three- to sixfold increased risk of developing an SPC compared with the general population, translating into an EAR ranging from 1 (in early life) to 6 per 1,000 patient-years of observation.[278–280] Further, survivors of childhood cancer have a persistent excess risk of a second (and subsequent) cancer throughout life, accompanied by continuous changes in the risk of cancers at specific sites.[278–280] The incidence and type of SPC differs with the primary diagnosis, type of therapy received, and presence of genetic conditions.

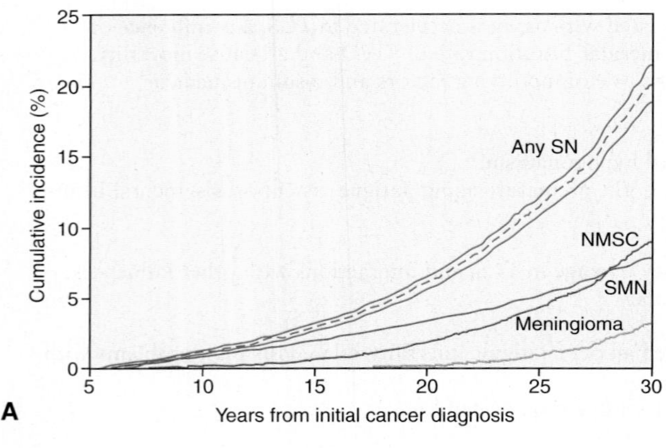

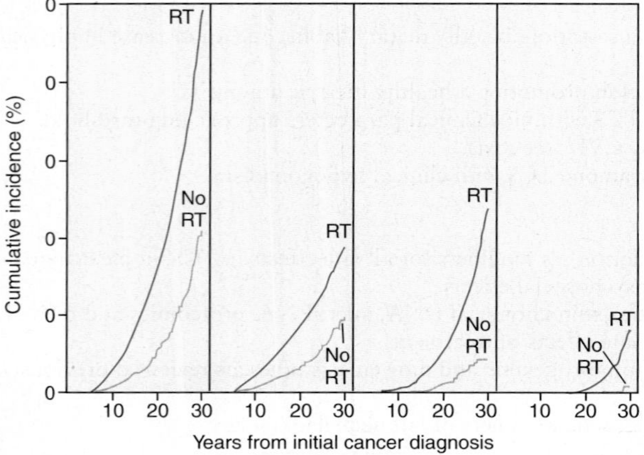

FIGURE 167.3 Cumulative incidence at 30 years for second neoplasms. **A:** All second malignant neoplasms. **B:** All second neoplasms by radiotherapy exposure. (From ref. 279, with permission.)

Influence of Primary Cancer

Among 5-year survivors in the CCSS, the 30-year cumulative incidence of SPC by primary cancer diagnosis was as follows: HL, 18.4%; Ewing sarcoma, 10.1%; soft tissue sarcoma, 8.8%; osteosarcoma, 6.0%; neuroblastoma, 5.9%; NHL, 5.8%; leukemia, 5.6%; CNS tumor, 5.5%; and kidney tumor, 4.0%. Hereditary RB, HL, and soft tissue sarcomas are overrepresented among patients who develop SPC relative to their incidence in the general population.[178,279,281] The 40- to 50-year cumulative incidence of a second cancer following RB ranges from 28% to 36%,[45,282] reflecting an interaction between genetic predisposition in patients with hereditary RB and radiotherapy,[44,281,283] as observed in familial soft tissue sarcoma. In individuals with other primary malignancies such as HL, it is not clear whether the primary cancer type is an independent risk factor for the development of SPC or whether the specific therapy needed to treat the primary cancer is the major contributor to the development of SPC.

Host-Related Risk Factors

Younger age at diagnosis of a primary cancer has been reported to be associated with a higher risk of radiation-associated solid tumors.[178-179, 284] Conversely for t-MDS/AML, which are strongly linked with specific chemotherapeutic agents, risk increases with age at treatment of primary cancer.[285,286]

Female sex is associated with a higher risk of SPC, contributed to primarily by the excess occurrence of secondary breast cancers among female cancer survivors. Moreover, some studies indicate a greater susceptibility of women to known carcinogens such as cigarette smoke, which has been postulated to account for differences in the risk of first primary lung cancers.[287] Possible mechanisms that underlie this greater susceptibility include greater activity of cytochrome P-450 enzymes, enhanced formation of DNA adducts, and the effects of hormones such as estrogen on tumor promotion.[287]

Radiation

Radiation is associated with the vast majority of SPC following therapy for childhood cancer, with a two- to threefold increased risk among irradiated patients compared with those treated with chemotherapy alone.[279,288–290] In order of decreasing prevalence, radiation-related SPC include NMSC, breast cancer, CNS tumors, bone and soft tissue sarcomas, and other carcinomas.[279,289]

Secondary Breast Cancer

Breast cancer following treatment for HL and NHL with chest irradiation is discussed previously. In addition, an excess risk of breast cancer has been noted following other chest radiation fields used in the treatment of childhood cancer, including whole lung, spinal, and chest wall radiation.[291] The cumulative incidence of breast cancer by 40 to 45 years of age is 13% to 20% among childhood cancer survivors treated with moderate to high-dose radiation to the chest.[64,185,292,293] In general, the characteristics of breast cancers in these women and their outcomes appear similar to *de novo* breast cancers. Further, second breast cancers can be detected by mammography, although sensitivity is limited. Based on this information, the Children's Oncology Group (COG) recommends annual surveillance mammography and breast magnetic resonance imaging, starting at age 25 or 8 years after completion of radiotherapy, whichever occurs last.[291,294] These recommendations are consistent with those of the American Cancer Society,[295] the United Kingdom Children's Cancer Study Group (UKCCSG),[296] and the Netherlands Cancer Institute.[297]

Secondary Thyroid Cancer

Childhood cancer survivors are at 11.3- to 18-fold increased risk of developing thyroid cancer when compared with the general population, with an EAR of 1.4 per 10,000 person-years.[178,289,298,299] Risk begins to increase about 8 to 10 years following radiation and the excess risk does not appear to plateau with age.[63,299] Histology of thyroid cancers is similar to that of the general population, with the vast majority of tumors either papillary or follicular carcinomas. Radiation-associated thyroid cancers are not more aggressive than thyroid cancer in the general population, with 5-year survival rates exceeding 95%.[300,301]

The most common primary diagnoses treated with radiation to the neck/thyroid region include HL, ALL, CNS tumors, NHL, and soft tissue sarcoma.[63,298,299]

In contrast to the linear dose-response relationship observed between radiation and risk of breast cancer[55] (Fig. 167.4A) or CNS tumors[59] (Fig. 167.4B), there is a linear exponential relation for the risk of thyroid cancer consistent with a cell-killing effect[63] (Fig. 167.4C). As illustrated in a nested case-control study conducted through the CCSS, Sigurdson et al.[63] reported a peak risk of thyroid cancer between 10 and 29 Gy with a fall in the dose-response relation at doses greater than 30 Gy. Risk was modified by age at diagnosis, with those treated before age 10 at highest risk.[63,299] Chemotherapy did not modify risk.[63,299] Although the majority of thyroid cancers occur in females, this reflects the same sex distribution of thyroid cancer seen in the general population. Taylor et al.[299] reported a higher SIR for males (26.2) compared with females (15.1; $P = .05$).

In an effort to reduce the incidence of serious late effects, including breast cancer and coronary artery disease, the dose of radiation has been lowered or omitted in contemporary risk-adapted therapy.[186,302] Although this may achieve these primary goals, the use of reduced radiation doses may in fact lead to an increased incidence of thyroid cancer among certain groups. From a small cohort of survivors of childhood HL who were treated with low-dose involved field radiation (15-25.5 Gy), O'Brien et al.[187] reported an SIR of 53.2 and an EAR of 22.9 per 10,000 person-years.

Given the indolent nature and excellent long-term survival rates among patients with a radiation-related thyroid cancer, the high incidence of thyroid nodules following radiation, and the high rate of false-positive findings with ultrasonography, neither the COG[294] nor the UKCCSG[296] recommend a screening thyroid ultrasound in the follow-up of asymptomatic survivors of pediatric or young adult cancer. Instead, both groups recommend a yearly neck examination. If a thyroid nodule is palpated, it should be further evaluated with an ultrasound and fine-needle aspiration.

Secondary Osteosarcoma and Soft Tissue Sarcoma

In a French-British cohort of 4,400 three-year survivors of a childhood solid tumor (including RB), the 20-year cumulative incidence of a secondary osteosarcoma and soft tissue sarcoma was 1% and 0.6%, respectively.[61,303] In an analysis of 5-year survivors in the CCSS (excluding RB), Henderson et al.[304] reported a 30-year cumulative incidence of a secondary sarcoma of 1.1% among those treated with radiation (any location) and 0.5% among those who did not receive radiation. There was a ninefold increased risk, in comparison with the general population, with an EAR of 3.3 cases per 10,000 person-years. Secondary osteosarcoma and soft tissue sarcoma begin to appear within 5 to 8 years after therapy, with risk remaining relatively stable with increasing interval from the primary cancer.[60,61,84,303,304]

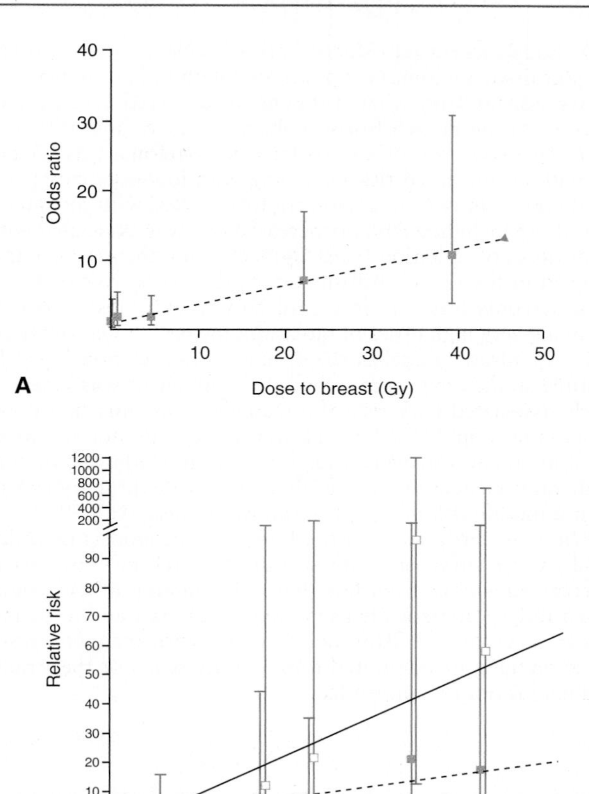

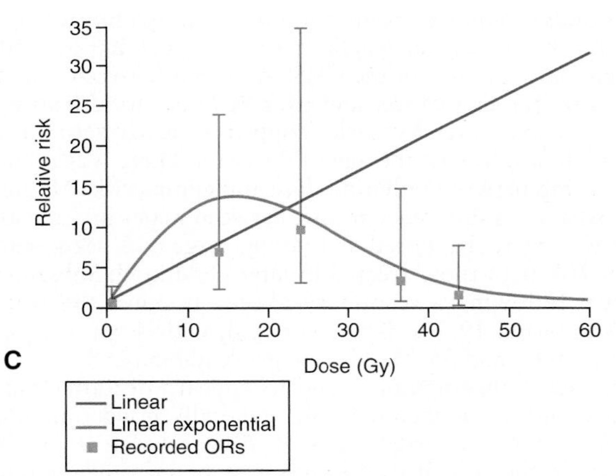

FIGURE 167.4 **A:** Breast cancer risk by radiation dose to the breast. (From ref. 55, with permission.) **B:** Relative risk of subsequent glioma and meningioma within the Childhood Cancer Survivor Study cohort by radiation dose (*open boxes*, mean observed relative risk for meningioma; *closed boxes*, mean observed relative risk for glioma; *solid line*, fitted line for meningioma risk; *hatched line*, fitted line for glioma risk). $P < .001$ (likelihood ratio test, two-sided). (From ref. 59, with permission.) **C:** Thyroid cancer risk by radiation dose in cases and controls after adjustment for first cancer. (From ref. 63, with permission.)

Although increased risks of both secondary osteosarcomas and soft tissue sarcomas are associated with radiation, patterns of risk appear somewhat different. In a nested case-control study from the French-British cohort (32 cases and 160 controls), the excess risk of a secondary osteosarcoma was 1.8 per Gy, with an increased risk beginning with low-dose exposures (1-10 Gy).[303] In two other case-control studies, with 59 and 64 cases (both including RB), no increased risk was associated with lower doses of radiation (<10 Gy).[60,84] In another case-control study from the French-British cohort, the excess risk of a soft tissue sarcoma was very low until 10 Gy, with most sarcomas following very high doses of radiation; the best fit was obtained with a quadratic model of the dose-response relationship.[61] In multiple studies, exposure to an alkylating agent was independently associated with risk of a secondary sarcoma in a dose-response fashion.[60,61,84,303,304] However, there did not appear to be an interaction between radiation and alkylating agent chemotherapy. Gender and age at diagnosis of the primary cancer did not modify risk in any of the above studies.[60,61,84,303,304]

There are little data on the long-term prognosis of childhood cancer survivors with secondary sarcoma, but 5-year survival rates have been less than 50% among other groups with a radiation-associated sarcoma (i.e., breast and testicular cancer survivors).[305] Routine screening with magnetic resonance imaging or computed tomography scans of the irradiated field is not recommended.[294,296]

Secondary CNS Tumors

Secondary gliomas and meningiomas are well-recognized late effects following cranial radiation. In the CCSS, there was an almost 11-fold increased risk of a second CNS tumor in comparison with the general population, with the vast majority of tumors occurring in patients treated with cranial radiation for another CNS tumor or ALL.

Secondary gliomas occur soon after completion of treatment for the first cancer. Neglia et al.[59] reported that over 50% of secondary gliomas in the CCSS occurred between 5 and 9 years after the first cancer and over 90% occurred before 15 years. The excess relative risk dropped to nearly zero among persons followed past the age of 25 years. There was a linear relationship between radiation dose and glioma risk. Although there was not a difference in risk between males and females, those who were diagnosed at a younger age (<5 years) had a higher risk than those treated in later childhood. Subsequent survival following a secondary glioma is poor: the British CCSS reported 19.5% 5-year survival, with 4.9% for high-grade gliomas and 38.9% for low-grade gliomas.[306]

Secondary meningiomas tend to appear later after radiotherapy and are associated with generally good outcomes. Taylor et al.[306] reported an 83% 5-year survival rate for patients in the British CCSS with a secondary meningioma. Most secondary meningiomas are benign,[279] but may be large or cause significant morbidity depending on location (e.g., seizures, hearing loss). Neglia et al.[59] reported that over 70% of the meningiomas occurring among CCSS survivors were diagnosed 15 years or more after the primary cancer. As with secondary gliomas, there was a strong radiation dose-response relation for meningioma risk with an excess relative risk per Gy of 1.06, translating to substantial excesses for the majority of CNS tumor survivors treated with 30 Gy or more to the whole brain. Gender did not modify risk. In contrast to the risk for secondary gliomas, children irradiated after the age of 5 years had a higher risk than those irradiated before 5 years. Genetic susceptibility may also increase the risk of radiation-induced meningiomas.[307]

Despite the poor outcomes associated with secondary gliomas and high frequency of secondary meningiomas following cranial irradiation, there is no evidence that surveillance improves outcomes. Consequently, neither the COG[294] nor the UKCCSG[296] recommend screening brain magnetic resonance imaging for asymptomatic patients. However, clinicians should have a heightened index of suspicion for childhood cancer survivors treated with cranial irradiation and who experience new neurologic signs or symptoms.

Secondary Melanoma and NMSC

Among the CCSS cohort, the risk of melanoma was 3.3-fold higher than the general population, with a median interval from primary cancer to melanoma of 18.9 years.[279] Similarly, in a Nordic population-based study, the risk of melanoma was 2.6-fold higher than the general population. Although many of these cases of melanoma occurred among patients who received irradiation, to date to our knowledge, there has not been a study assessing the radiation dose-relation or potentially modifying factors.

NMSC is common among childhood cancer survivors following irradiation, exceeding the incidence of all other second cancers combined.[279,280] Indeed, in the recent CCSS update, among 14,359 survivors, there were 1,574 cases of NMSC and 802 cases of invasive or *in situ* cancer.[279] The 30-year cumulative incidence of NMSC was 9.1%.[279] The vast majority of NMSC was basal cell carcinoma (97%), with a median age of 31 years at occurrence.[308] Ninety percent of the tumors occurred within the radiation field; radiotherapy was associated with a sixfold increase in risk. Gender did not appear to modify risk.[279,308] However, older age at radiation exposure (10–20 years of age) appeared to be associated with increased risk.[279] Among childhood cancer survivors who received hematopoietic cell transplantation, Leisenring et al.[309] reported that patients given either total-body irradiation or who were light-skinned had an increased risk of basal cell carcinoma. Acute graft-versus-host disease was associated with an increased risk of squamous cell carcinoma; chronic graft-versus-host disease was associated with an increased risk of both basal and squamous cell carcinoma. The COG[294] and the UKCCSG[296] recommend annual examination of the skin in irradiated fields.

Other Secondary Carcinomas

The risk of other carcinomas (besides breast, thyroid, and skin) appears to increase with age among childhood cancer survivors. Bassal et al.[310] from the CCSS reported that radiation was associated with a significantly increased risk for carcinomas in the following locations: head and neck, colorectal, other gastrointestinal sites, kidney, bladder, and lung. The risk for a secondary carcinoma (excluding breast, thyroid, and skin) was fivefold higher for survivors treated with radiation compared with the general population. In the CCSS update,[279] the number of these "other" carcinomas increased by 28% in just 4 years. As survivors in the CCSS and similar cohorts (e.g., British CCSS, Dutch LATER) enter midadulthood, this is an area that warrants further study to better understand modifying risk factors, quantify radiation dose-response relations, and identify surveillance approaches.

Genetic Conditions

RB is the prototype malignancy in which genetic factors are responsible for a substantial proportion of SPC. Familial RB is caused by inherited mutations of the *RB1* tumor suppressor gene, which has been localized to the long arm of chromosome 13q14.[311] Approximately 90% of hereditary RB patients have bilateral disease. In a large cohort of 1,601 RB survivors from Boston and New York, the risk of SPC was increased 19-fold in hereditary RB survivors; risk was not elevated in nonhereditary patients.[45] The 50-year cumulative incidence of an

SPC was 36% and 5.7% for hereditary and nonhereditary patients, respectively. Among the hereditary patients, radiotherapy increased the 50-year cumulative incidence of a second cancer to 38.2%, whereas the cumulative incidence was 21.0% for nonirradiated patients. Similar risks among hereditary RB survivors have been reported from the Dutch[282] and British[312] nationwide cohorts. The 50-year cumulative mortality from any SPC for hereditary RB survivors ranged from 17.3 to 25.5%.[313,314]

The majority of SPC are bone and soft tissue sarcomas occurring in the most heavily irradiated areas (head and neck region). There is a radiation dose-response relationship for sarcomas, with an almost 11-fold risk increase at doses of 60 Gy or greater.[281] Osteosarcomas and soft tissue sarcomas that develop after hereditary RB harbor similar *RB1* mutations as found in RB. Radiation is thus likely to cause somatic mutations needed to produce sarcomas in carriers of germline *RB1* mutations.

Importantly, hereditary RB survivors also have an increased risk in comparison with the general population of second (and third and fourth) cancers in sites distal to the radiation field suggesting a genetic predisposition independent of radiation exposure.[45,281,282,298,315] Sites for distal cancers include breast, lung, colon, bladder, uterus, and long bones. In particular, there is an excess risk of distal soft tissue sarcomas (leiomyosarcoma, fibrosarcoma, and rhabdomyosarcoma) and osteosarcoma (especially in the lower extremities), suggesting that carriers of an *RB1* mutation are predisposed to soft tissue sarcomas and osteosarcomas.[282,315,316]

Childhood sarcoma survivors also have an excess risk of nonradiation-related SPC, such as breast cancer.[279,292,317] Although many of these patients likely have a *p53* germ line mutation and are thus classified with Li-Fraumeni syndrome,[318] there may be other genetic factors affecting risk. These issues are discussed in detail elsewhere in the chapter.

Future Directions

Although the body of literature which documents the increased risk and patterns of SPC among childhood cancer survivors has grown considerably, only lifelong follow-up of these patients will reveal the true magnitude of late effects. Research efforts must target not only the impact of prevention strategies on the reduction in risk of SPC, but also the role of underlying genetic variation and modifying factors. One ultimate goal will be the development of biomarkers that might eventually help identify those patients who will develop SPC and other late effects, permitting opportunities for prevention.

COMMENT

There has been substantial progress in the description of treatment-related second cancers, but less so with regard to the quantification of dose-response relationships with radiation and chemotherapy. Moreover, fewer data exist with regard to underlying molecular mechanisms.[4] It would seem logical to be able to prospectively identify patient subgroups that might be at heightened susceptibility of developing therapy-associated second cancers (or other adverse effects) in order to modify planned treatment approaches or select alternative management strategies. The meticulous measurement and recording of potentially carcinogenic exposures (chemotherapy and radiotherapy) provide an ideal research setting for the investigation of gene–environment and gene–gene interactions. In 2006 Travis et al.[4] provided recommendations on the research agenda, study design considerations, and infrastructural requirements needed to further the knowledge of underlying genetic mechanisms of SPCs, and thus to also provide the foundation for evidence-based strategies for patient management and possible intervention measures. The recommendations were based on the proceedings of an NCI-sponsored workshop, which included a transdisciplinary group of experts in the fields of epidemiology, statistics, molecular genetics, clinical genetics, pharmacogenomics, informatics, radiation biology, medical oncology, pediatric oncology, and radiation oncology, and the advocacy community. The identified research priorities included (1) development of a national research infrastructure for studies of cancer survivorship; (2) creation of a coordinated system for biospecimen collection; (3) development of new technology, bioinformatics, and biomarkers; (4) design of new epidemiologic methods; and (5) development of evidence-based clinical practice guidelines. It was emphasized by workshop participants that many of the infrastructure resources and design strategies that would support second cancer research also provide an appropriate foundation for the investigation of other nonneoplastic adverse sequelae of cancer and its treatment. More recently, Bhatia and Robison[319] underscored the deficit in research in late effects, including SPC among survivors of adult-onset cancer.

Research progress over the past few decades has made it possible to identify those treatment regimens that are associated with high risks of second cancers. Although individual susceptibility factors remain largely unknown, groups of exposed patients can still be selected for close monitoring. Whenever effective screening methods (e.g., mammographic examination) are available, these should be included in patient follow-up (as described previously). Preventive strategies (e.g., smoking cessation, avoidance of ultraviolet light) may also diminish the risk of selected second cancers, and cancer survivors should be encouraged to adopt practices consistent with a healthy lifestyle. Although cancer treatment represents a double-edged sword, it should be kept in mind that many treatments have been accompanied by sizable improvements in patient survival. Thus, the benefits associated with many cancer treatments greatly exceed the risk of developing an SPC. Further, it should always be kept in mind that subsequent neoplasms may not necessarily be attributable solely to prior cancer treatment, but may also reflect the effect of shared etiologic factors, environmental exposures, host characteristics, and combinations of influences, including gene–environment and gene–gene interactions.[3,4]

Selected References

The full list of references for this chapter appears in the online version.

2. Ng AK, Bernardo MP, Weller E, et al. Long-term survival and competing causes of death in patients with early-stage Hodgkin's disease treated at age 50 or younger. *J Clin Oncol* 2002;20:2101.
4. Travis LB, Rabkin CS, Brown LM, et al. Cancer survivorship–genetic susceptibility and second primary cancers: research strategies and recommendations. *J Natl Cancer Inst* 2006;98:15.
7. Travis LB, Fossa SD, Schonfeld SJ, et al. Second cancers among 40,576 testicular cancer patients: focus on long-term survivors. *J Natl Cancer Inst* 2005;97:1354.
11. Travis LB, Hill DA, Dores GM, et al. Breast cancer following radiotherapy and chemotherapy among young women with Hodgkin disease. *JAMA* 2003;290:465.
48. Hodgson DC, Gilbert ES, Dores GM, et al. Long-term solid cancer risk among 5-year survivors of Hodgkin's lymphoma. *J Clin Oncol* 2007;25:1489.

52. Hooning MJ, Aleman BM, Hauptmann M, et al. Roles of radiotherapy and chemotherapy in the development of contralateral breast cancer. *J Clin Oncol* 2008;26:5561.
55. Inskip PD, Robison LL, Stovall M, et al. Radiation dose and breast cancer risk in the childhood cancer survivor study. *J Clin Oncol* 2009;27:3901.
63. Sigurdson AJ, Ronckers CM, Mertens AC, et al. Primary thyroid cancer after a first tumour in childhood (the Childhood Cancer Survivor Study): a nested case-control study. *Lancet* 2005;365:2014.
77. Hall EJ. Intensity-modulated radiation therapy, protons, and the risk of second cancers. *Int J Radiat Oncol Biol Phys* 2006;65:1.
85. Allan JM, Travis LB. Mechanisms of therapy-related carcinogenesis. *Nat Rev Cancer* 2005;5:943.
95. Travis LB, Holowaty EJ, Bergfeldt K, et al. Risk of leukemia after platinum-based chemotherapy for ovarian cancer. *N Engl J Med* 1999;340:351.
98. Bhatia S, Krailo MD, Chen Z, et al. Therapy-related myelodysplasia and acute myeloid leukemia after Ewing sarcoma and primitive neuroectodermal tumor of bone: a report from the Children's Oncology Group. *Blood* 2007;109:46.
101. Mistry AR, Felix CA, Whitmarsh RJ, et al. DNA topoisomerase II in therapy-related acute promyelocytic leukemia. *N Engl J Med* 2005;352:1529.
102. Mays AN, Osheroff N, Xiao Y, et al. Evidence for direct involvement of epirubicin in the formation of chromosomal translocations in t(15;17) therapy-related acute promyelocytic leukemia. *Blood* 2010;115:326.
105. Offman J, Opelz G, Doehler B, et al. Defective DNA mismatch repair in acute myeloid leukemia/myelodysplastic syndrome after organ transplantation. *Blood* 2004;104:822.
108. Relling MV, Rubnitz JE, Rivera GK, et al. High incidence of secondary brain tumours after radiotherapy and antimetabolites. *Lancet* 1999;354:34.
131. Allan JM. Genetic susceptibility to radiogenic cancer in humans. *Health Phys* 2008;95:677.
142. Allan JM, Wild CP, Rollinson S, et al. Polymorphism in glutathione S-transferase P1 is associated with susceptibility to chemotherapy-induced leukemia. *Proc Natl Acad Sci U S A* 2001;98:11592.
151. Lorenzo Y, Provencio M, Lombardia L, et al. Differential genetic and functional markers of second neoplasias in Hodgkin's disease patients. *Clin Cancer Res* 2009;15:4823.
167. Ellis NA, Huo D, Yildiz O, et al. MDM2 SNP309 and TP53 Arg72Pro interact to alter therapy-related acute myeloid leukemia susceptibility. *Blood* 2008;112:741.
168. Knight JA, Skol AD, Shinde A, et al. Genome-wide association study to identify novel loci associated with therapy-related myeloid leukemia susceptibility. *Blood* 2009;113:5575.
170. Funk RK, Maxwell TJ, Izumi M, et al. Quantitative trait loci associated with susceptibility to therapy-related acute murine promyelocytic leukemia in hCG-PML/RARA transgenic mice. *Blood* 2008;112:1434.
173. Stanulla M, Schaeffeler E, Moricke A, et al. Thiopurine methyltransferase genetics is not a major risk factor for secondary malignant neoplasms after treatment of childhood acute lymphoblastic leukemia on Berlin-Frankfurt-Munster protocols. *Blood* 2009;114:1314.
174. Chao RC, Pyzel U, Fridlyand J, et al. Therapy-induced malignant neoplasms in Nf1 mutant mice. *Cancer Cell* 2005;8:337.
175. Sharif S, Ferner R, Birch JM, et al. Second primary tumors in neurofibromatosis 1 patients treated for optic glioma: substantial risks after radiotherapy. *J Clin Oncol* 2006;24:2570.
186. Hodgson DC, Koh ES, Tran TH, et al. Individualized estimates of second cancer risks after contemporary radiation therapy for Hodgkin lymphoma. *Cancer* 2007;110:2576.
187. O'Brien MM, Donaldson SS, Balise RR, et al. Second Malignant Neoplasms in Survivors of Pediatric Hodgkin's Lymphoma Treated With Low-Dose Radiation and Chemotherapy. *J Clin Oncol* 2010;28:1232.
201. Travis LB, Hill D, Dores GM, et al. Cumulative absolute breast cancer risk for young women treated for Hodgkin lymphoma. *J Natl Cancer Inst* 2005;97:1428.
225. Bernstein JL, Haile RW, Stovall M, et al. Radiation Exposure, the ATM Gene, and Contralateral Breast Cancer in the Women's Environmental Cancer and Radiation Epidemiology Study. *J Natl Cancer Inst* 2010.
226. Clarke M, Collins R, Darby S, et al. Effects of radiotherapy and of differences in the extent of surgery for early breast cancer on local recurrence and 15-year survival: an overview of the randomised trials. *Lancet* 2005;366:2087.
227. Howard RA, Gilbert ES, Chen BE, et al. Leukemia following breast cancer: an international population-based study of 376,825 women. *Breast Cancer Res Treat* 2007;105:359.
234. Kaufman EL, Jacobson JS, Hershman DL, et al. Effect of breast cancer radiotherapy and cigarette smoking on risk of second primary lung cancer. *J Clin Oncol* 2008;26:392.
254. van den Belt-Dusebout AW, de Wit R, Gietema JA, et al. Treatment-specific risks of second malignancies and cardiovascular disease in 5-year survivors of testicular cancer. *J Clin Oncol* 2007;25:4370.
260. Fossa SD, Chen J, Schonfeld SJ, et al. Risk of contralateral testicular cancer: a population-based study of 29,515 U.S. men. *J Natl Cancer Inst* 2005;97:1056.
264. Schairer C, Hisada M, Chen BE, et al. Comparative mortality for 621 second cancers in 29356 testicular cancer survivors and 12420 matched first cancers. *J Natl Cancer Inst* 2007;99:1248.
272. Travis LB, Beard C, Allan JM, et al. Testicular cancer survivorship: research strategies and recommendations. *J Natl Cancer Inst* 2010;102:1114.
279. Friedman DL, Whitton J, Leisenring W, et al. Subsequent neoplasms in five year survivors of childhood cancer: the Childhood Cancer Survivor Study. *J Natl Cancer Inst* 2010;102:1083.
280. Olsen JH, Moller T, Anderson H, et al. Lifelong cancer incidence in 47,697 patients treated for childhood cancer in the Nordic countries. *J Natl Cancer Inst* 2009;101:806.
282. Marees T, Moll AC, Imhof SM, et al. Risk of second malignancies in survivors of retinoblastoma: more than 40 years of follow-up. *J Natl Cancer Inst* 2008;100:1771.
291. Henderson TO, Amsterdam A, Bhatia SB. Surveillance for breast cancer in women treated with chest radiation for a childhood, adolescent, or young adult cancer: a report from the Children's Oncology Group. *Ann Intern Med* 2010;152:444.
294. Long-term follow-up guidelines for survivors of childhood, adolescent, and young adult cancers, version 3. Accessed March 8, 2010: www.survivorshipguidelines.org.
296. Therapy-based long-term follow-up: practice statement. 2005. (Accessed March 8, 2010, at http://www.cclg.org.uk/researchandtreatment/content.php?3id=29&2id=19.)
301. Mertens AC, Liu Q, Neglia JP, et al. Cause-specific late mortality among 5-year survivors of childhood cancer: the Childhood Cancer Survivor Study. *J Natl Cancer Inst* 2008;100:1368.
304. Henderson TO, Whitton J, Stovall M, et al. Secondary sarcomas in childhood cancer survivors: a report from the Childhood Cancer Survivor Study. *J Natl Cancer Inst* 2007;99:300.
307. Flint-Richter P, Sadetzki S. Genetic predisposition for the development of radiation-associated meningioma: an epidemiological study. *Lancet Oncol* 2007;8:403.
308. Perkins JL, Liu Y, Mitby PA, et al. Nonmelanoma skin cancer in survivors of childhood and adolescent cancer: a report from the childhood cancer survivor study. *J Clin Oncol* 2005;23:3733.
314. Yu CL, Tucker MA, Abramson DH, et al. Cause-specific mortality in long-term survivors of retinoblastoma. *J Natl Cancer Inst* 2009;101:581.
316. Kleinerman RA, Tucker MA, Abramson DH, et al. Risk of soft tissue sarcomas by individual subtype in survivors of hereditary retinoblastoma. *J Natl Cancer Inst* 2007;99:24.
317. Ginsberg JP, Goodman P, Leisenring W, et al. Long-term follow-up among five-year survivors of childhood Ewing sarcoma: a report from the Childhood Cancer Survivor Study. *J Natl Cancer Inst* 2010;102:1272.
319. Bhatia S, Robison LL. Cancer survivorship research: opportunities and future needs for expanding the research base. *Cancer Epidemiol Biomarkers Prev* 2008;17:1551.

CHAPTER 168
NEUROCOGNITIVE EFFECTS

PAUL D. BROWN, NADIA N. I. LAACK, AND JEFFREY S. WEFEL

Patients with central nervous system (CNS) tumors frequently suffer from a number of adverse symptoms including cognitive impairment. Cognitive dysfunction occurs in most patients with brain tumors, often at presentation, and is frequently progressive even after aggressive treatment. In addition, recent advances in multimodality therapy have led to improvement in survival for many patients. As survival has improved, concerns have been raised regarding the effects these interventions have on cognitive function. Confounding any analyses of neurocognitive function are the number of factors such as surgery, chemotherapy, radiotherapy, tumor characteristics, tumor progression, concurrent medical illnesses, age (this chapter will focus on adult patients), neurologic comorbidity, and medications (e.g., antiepileptics) that can contribute to neurocognitive deficits. Because treatment options for neurocognitive deficits remain quite limited, a thorough understanding of the impact of brain tumor interventions (i.e., surgery, radiotherapy, chemotherapy) on cognitive function is necessary to help guide treatment decisions. In addition, an awareness of the neurocognitive function of adult brain tumor patients at presentation and over time is essential when making treatment recommendations, and this requires detailed neurocognitive assessments.

ASSESSMENT OF NEUROCOGNITIVE FUNCTION

Neurocognitive impairment in primary brain tumor patients is extremely common at presentation, before any interventions have been performed. Tucha et al.[1] reported that 91% of patients with lesions in the temporal or frontal lobes presented with at least one area of deficit compared with the normal population, and 71% demonstrated at least three deficits. Consistent with classical behavioral neuroanatomy, impairment in executive function occurred in 78% and memory and attention were impaired in 60%. Much of our understanding of behavioral neuroanatomy is derived from studies of patients suffering from stroke or epilepsy. These early investigations demonstrated that the nature of the cognitive impairments often relates to the location of a lesion. While tumor patients have shown typical lateralizing patterns of cognitive impairment (e.g., left hemisphere lesions frequently cause difficulties with verbal learning and memory and language functions),[2] these impairments are often more subtle and diffuse in tumor patients than are those observed in sudden-onset neurological conditions such as stroke.[3] Differences in the pathophysiology of these lesions are believed to underlie these observations; while a cerebrovascular accident may rapidly result in tissue destruction, tumors diffusely and often more slowly infiltrate the brain, thereby disrupting normal brain function in networks that are proximal to the visible tumor as well as more distant from the site through mechanisms such as diaschisis. Using magnetoencephalography, abnormal organization of widespread brain networks has been demonstrated in cognitively impaired brain tumor patients.[4]

Cognitive impairment is associated with difficulty in daily life more often than physical impairments, and caregivers cite cognitive problems as the most difficult problems to manage.[2] These deficits cause significant impairments in the daily life of the patient, including decreased independence, interference in academic or vocational pursuits, and increased caregiver distress and burden. Even subtle cognitive deficits can significantly limit a patient's ability to perform usual activities, but may not be evident on casual observation or detectable via routine medical examinations. If unrecognized, these cognitive deficits can lead to inaccurate judgment on the part of the medical team regarding the patient's ability for self-care and in the believed safety of the treatments themselves.

Neuropsychological assessment provides quantitative, objective measurement of potentially subtle, yet clinically significant changes in a patient's cognitive function. Neurocognitive testing involves the administration of standardized psychometric instruments (i.e., tests) that evaluate various aspects of brain function such as attention, learning and memory, information processing speed, expressive and receptive language function, executive function (e.g., abstract reasoning, planning, and decision making), visual perception and construction, and assessment of mood and personality. Test results are integrated with the patient's clinical history, observations of the patient's behavior, patient report, and reports of family members or caregivers. Interpretation of these psychometric instruments and assessments requires a trained neuropsychologist. Brief evaluation with screening instruments such as the Mini-Mental Status Examination is not recommended as these were not developed to assess cognition in brain tumor patients and provide limited information about domains of cognitive function frequently affected by brain tumors and their treatment (e.g., learning and memory, executive function, processing speed, and fine motor control).[5] Similarly, patient self-report does not routinely correlate with objectively measured cognitive function[6] or functional outcomes.[7]

Neuropsychological assessment allows for careful evaluation of the costs and benefits of a given treatment regimen or supportive therapy. Increasingly, neurocognitive outcomes are important end points in clinical trials of new agents; the U.S. Food and Drug Administration considers improvement in neurocognitive function or delay in expected decline approved end points in registration trials, as these end points directly relate to clinical benefit. The results of an appropriate cognitive assessment may also be used to identify and guide interventions for impaired patients, including compensatory strategy training (cognitive rehabilitation), pharmacotherapy, or psychotherapy. In addition, repeated assessments can track the patient's response to primary therapy (e.g., deterioration of cognitive function predicts tumor progression)[8] and to targeted interventions for cognitive dysfunction and facilitate designing realistic goals and future plans for patients with cognitive deficits.

IMPACT OF TREATMENT

Surgery

Nonbrain surgery is known to cause postoperative cognitive impairments, especially in the elderly. The deficits, particularly for memory, may be present for weeks or months.[9] Risk factors besides age include duration of anesthesia and postoperative complications. In contrast to nonbrain surgery, surgery for brain tumors may lead to focal neurocognitive deficits.[2] However, relief of mass effect and increased intracranial pressure frequently results in improvement in cognitive function. A study of 27 adult brain tumor patients that included extensive neurocognitive testing *before surgery* and after surgery found 84% improved in one or more cognitive domains, and 36% worsened in one or more cognitive domains. If memory was impaired at baseline, it was most likely to improve, while executive function was most likely to decline.[10] Potential adverse effects of surgery can be seen in patients with benign tumors, such as pituitary adenomas. Peace et al.[11] performed neuropsychological tests on a cohort of 69 patients treated for pituitary tumor and found that a transfrontal approach was associated with greater frequency (44% impaired) and severity of cognitive impairment when compared to the transsphenoidal approach (30% impaired) and even more so when compared to a nonsurgical control group with pituitary tumors.

The balance between attaining a maximal resection and at the same time preserving function has been difficult, especially because gliomas are infiltrative and invasive. However, that goal has been advanced by comprehensive evaluations, including neuropsychological assessment and technological advances such as intraoperative magnetic resonance imaging, functional neuroimaging techniques, white matter pathway mapping, and intraoperative stimulation.[12] Recent studies indicate that as many as 80% of patients with low-grade glioma will experience postoperative neurocognitive deficits even when using intraoperative guided imaging and functional mapping in patients with tumors in eloquent brain locations. However, most of these deficits resolve within a few months. In a report by Duffau,[12] 94% of patients returned to their preoperative functioning by 3 months, presumably owing to the plasticity of the normal brain and recovery from the acute effects of surgery.[13] Because the treatment of central nervous system tumors typically requires multimodality therapy, it has been difficult to assess the contribution of surgery to the cognitive dysfunction patients' experience. Further studies are necessary to evaluate patients, especially those receiving surgery alone, with formal neurocognitive testing *before* and after surgery to help address this issue.

Chemotherapy

The adverse effects of chemotherapy are usually presumed to be acute and reversible. The neurobehavioral effects of most cancer therapy agents tend to be nonspecific and diffuse, except for those that have a mechanism of action that is expected to affect focal brain regions[14] or immunologic agents that are known to affect particular inflammatory cytokines, neurotransmitters, and neuroendocrine hormones.[2] Neurocognitive dysfunction has been described in patients including those without CNS disease and frequently manifests as diminished memory, executive function, and attention and information processing speed.[15,16] Several risk factors have been identified that appear to increase the risk of developing neurotoxicity associated with chemotherapy, including (1) exposure to higher doses due to planned use of high-dose regimens or high concentrations due to impaired systemic clearance or pharmacogenetic modulation of drug pharmacokinetics[17]; (2) additive or synergistic effects of multiagent chemotherapy; (3) additive or synergistic effect of multimodality therapy that includes administration of chemotherapy either concurrent or subsequent to cerebral radiation[18,19]; (4) intra-arterial administration with blood–brain barrier disruption; and (5) intrathecal administration.[19–22]

Animal research has demonstrated that a number of antineoplastic agents can have adverse effects on cognitive function and have uncovered brain substrates that may be responsible for these cognitive alterations.[23] However, most of the preclinical studies involve investigations of hippocampal function and associated deficits in learning and memory, yet clinical experience with patients indicates that memory retrieval (generally mediated by frontal subcortical networks) and not memory consolidation (generally mediated by mesial temporal lobe structures including the hippocampus) is the more common cognitive abnormality on formal neuropsychological assessment. Han et al.[24] have found that administration of therapeutic levels of 5-fluorouracil is associated with delayed damage to myelin associated with altered transcriptional regulation in oligodendrocytes and extensive myelin pathology. In contrast, CNS inflammation and vascular damage were acute and did not appear to be related to the delayed effects on myelin. These findings support the notion of delayed white matter injury due to chemotherapy exposure that is consistent with the clinical syndrome observed in patients.

Methotrexate is a chemotherapeutic agent used in the treatment of primary CNS lymphoma as well other malignancies. It is often used in high doses and administered intravenously and intrathecally. Methotrexate therapy has been associated with cognitive dysfunction, including severe disseminated necrotizing leukoencephalopathy, which is more common in the elderly and in young children. Much of the toxicity of methotrexate has been attributed to alteration in normal blood–brain barrier and brain architecture secondary to tumor infiltration[25]; however, there have been reports of leukoencephalopathy after low-dose oral administration of methotrexate for benign disease such as rheumatoid arthritis.[26] Neurocognitive testing of primary CNS lymphoma patients after treatment with methotrexate (without cranial radiotherapy) has revealed conflicting results, with one small study of 10 patients observing mild cognitive dysfunction (although more pronounced than seen with "standard-dose chemotherapy").[27] However, two other investigations reported that treatment of primary central nervous system lymphoma with intravenous, intra-arterial, or intraventricular multiagent chemotherapy with blood–brain barrier disruption has been accomplished without induction of significant neurocognitive dysfunction.[28,29]

Unfortunately there has been only limited research to examine the neurocognitive effects of specific chemotherapy regimens in primary brain tumor patients. Agents such as temozolomide appear to increase survival without causing significant adverse symptoms.[30,31] Hilverda et al.[30] serially evaluated 13 glioblastoma patients before concomitant chemoradiation with temozolomide, shortly after completion of concurrent therapy and again after three cycles of adjuvant temozolomide. All patients were progression free with good performance status. At baseline the majority of patients had deficits in multiple cognitive domains. During the concomitant and adjuvant phases of treatment cognitive functioning remained generally stable with as many patients having improvement as worsening. In most cases, decline in neurocognitive function occurred in one domain, most frequently attention or psychomotor function. This small study suggests that nonprogressed glioblastoma patients with generally high performance status show limited adverse neurocognitive effects from concomitant temozolomide and three cycles of adjuvant temozolomide.

As mentioned, immunotherapy, particularly interferon-alfa (IFN), can cause significant cognitive impairments and organic mood disturbance. One prospective study of 30 chronic myelogenous leukemia patients examined before and during treatment with IFN-alfa alone or IFN-alfa and chemotherapy, found a significant decline in cognitive function in 53.3% of patients.[32] Several physiological mechanisms have been proposed for the neurotoxic effects of IFN, including actions mediated through neuroendocrine, neurotransmitter, and cytokine pathways. Patients with IFN neurotoxicity have been reported to exhibit mild-to-moderate symptoms of frontal-subcortical brain dysfunction, including cognitive and behavioral slowing, apathy, impaired executive functions, and decreased memory. The cognitive and behavioral symptoms of chronic IFN administration have been compared to Parkinson's disease.

Radiotherapy

Radiation therapy plays an important role in the treatment of primary and metastatic tumors located in the CNS. As more effective treatments for intracranial lesions have become available and long-term survival has increased, more attention has been placed on identifying and quantifying the adverse effects of radiation on neurocognitive function. Because of their relatively long progression-free and overall survival, patients with low-grade brain tumors are an ideal population to study when analyzing the potential cognitive deficits of radiotherapy since neurocognitive deficits can take years to develop. In addition, patients with low-grade brain tumors are often young and do not have underlying medical comorbidities that may confound the cognitive analysis. A number of retrospective studies have found increased neurocognitive difficulties after cranial radiotherapy for low-grade brain neoplasms. However, these studies have suffered from many deficiencies, besides the inherent weaknesses of retrospective studies, including outdated radiotherapy techniques (e.g., using whole-brain radiotherapy or large fraction sizes for low-grade glioma patients), patients being selected because of known cognitive deficits with an unknown number of patients treated but not studied (i.e., unidentified denominator), and, most important, the lack of baseline neurocognitive testing as the brain tumor itself is often the primary cause of cognitive difficulties.[33] A recent retrospective analysis by Douw et al.,[34] which is an update of a previously reported study of low-grade glioma patients followed longitudinally, highlights some of these shortcomings. With a median follow-up of 12 years, the authors report declines in attentional functioning in the patients who received radiotherapy, whereas the patients who were observed retained stable neurocognitive functioning. Although these data are valuable in that they provide long-term follow-up data on patients with low-grade glioma, the study has been criticized for lack of baseline testing, the inherent selection bias of patients who received radiotherapy generally having more aggressive disease (nearly 70% of the patients who had received radiotherapy in the first report had succumbed to their disease by the time of the second report compared to only 30% of the patients who did not receive radiotherapy), and excessive radiotherapy doses (mean dose of 56 Gy and as high as 69 Gy) and outdated techniques (such as whole-brain radiotherapy).[35]

In sharp contrast, a number of studies have prospectively performed extensive neuropsychological testing on adult patients with low-grade neoplasms before (baseline) and after radiotherapy (up to 6 years after radiotherapy) (Table 168.1) and have not found significant neurocognitive deterioration when compared to either baseline[36,40–43] or to a cohort of patients with low-grade brain neoplasms not treated with radiotherapy.[37,39] For example, a subset of 20 of the 203 adult low-grade glioma patients enrolled on an Intergroup prospective phase 3 trial that randomized patients to 50.4 or 64.8 Gy underwent psychometric testing before and up to 5 years after localized radiation therapy.[40] No significant losses in general intellectual function, new learning function, or memory function were seen. The groups' mean test scores were higher at follow-up evaluations than their initial performances on all

PRACTICE OF ONCOLOGY

TABLE 168.1

PROSPECTIVE TRIALS FOR LOW-GRADE NEOPLASMS WITH BASELINE AND SERIAL NEUROCOGNITIVE TESTING

Study (Ref.)	No. of Patients	RadiationTotal Dose/Fraction Size (Gy)	Mean Follow-Up (years)	Extensive Neurocognitive Assessment	Neurotoxicity After Radiotherapy
Glosser et al. (36)	17	Proton RT median 68.4 CGE/1.8	4	Yes	No; mild decline in psychomotor speed with high doses
Vigliani et al. (37)	17	Focal RT 54/1.8	4	Yes	No; transient decline in reaction time
Armstrong et al. (43)	26	Focal RT mean 54.6/1.8-2.0	3	Yes	No; mild decline in visual memory after 5 years
Brown et al. (38)	203	Focal RT 50.4/1.8 or 64.8/1.8	7.4 (median)	No (MMSE and NFS)	5.3% with MMSE decline at 5 years
Torres et al. (39)	15	Focal RT mean 54/1.8	2	Yes	No; decline in memory and attention only if tumor progression
Laack et al. (40)	20	Focal RT 50.4/1.8 or 64.8/1.8	3	Yes	No
Steinvorth et al. (41)	40	SRT median 57.6/1.8	1	Yes	No
Jalali et al. (42)	22	SRT median 54/1.8	2	Yes	No

RT, radiotherapy; CGE, centigray equivalent; MMSE, Folstein Mini-Mental State Examination; NFS, neurologic function scores; SRT, stereotactic radiotherapy.

psychometric measures, although the improvement was not statistically significant. However, four patients, all in the 64.8 Gy arm, had a mild decline in one or more of the domains assessed (i.e., immediate verbal memory, learning, and spatial problem solving). The results of this study are consistent with the weight of evidence that indicates a low incidence of neurocognitive difficulties after *focal*, conventionally fractionated (i.e., 1.8 to 2 Gy) radiotherapy using modern techniques to deliver moderate doses (i.e., 45 to 54 Gy) in adults.[33,44]

An extreme form of *focal* radiotherapy used to treat many benign and neoplastic cranial conditions is stereotactic radiosurgery (SRS). SRS uses multiple radiation beams and is able to encompass treatment volumes in the high-dose region with small margins because of the stereotactic imaging and immobilization. This results in rapid dose falloff, allowing greater sparing of normal brain tissues, and therefore minimizes risk to the surrounding structures. The neurocognitive impact of SRS was evaluated in a prospective trial assessing 95 patients with cerebral arteriovenous malformations with extensive neuropsychometric testing before and after SRS (median dose, 20 Gy in one fraction) and found all measures of cognitive function were stable or improved 3 years after SRS.[45]

The impact of whole-brain radiotherapy (WBRT) on cognitive function is best addressed by prophylactic cranial irradiation (PCI) trials because by definition these patients should not have brain metastases (and therefore tumor progression is less of a confounding variable). PCI has been shown to decrease the development of brain metastases and improve cure rates and survival for small-cell lung cancer patients because of the propensity of these patients to develop brain metastases. Similar to low-grade brain tumors, a number of retrospective studies have raised concerns of neurotoxicity after PCI, but these studies have been compromised by the use of large, unconventional fraction sizes, comorbid conditions (known brain metastasis), high total doses (up to 50 Gy), concomitant use of chemotherapy, and, most important, lack of baseline neuropsychological testing as prospective neurocognitive studies have shown up to 97% of limited stage small-cell lung cancer patients have evidence of cognitive dysfunction *prior* to PCI.[46,47] Two of the largest randomized trials of PCI did incorporate prospective neuropsychometric testing and both found a significant proportion of patients had cognitive dysfunction at baseline, but these studies found no differences in neurocognitive performance between the randomization arms of PCI or no PCI.[48,49]

More recently, there have also been prospective trials with extensive neurocognitive testing for patients with brain metastases treated with WBRT (Table 168.2). One of these studies, an international phase 3 trial, prospectively evaluated neurocognitive function in 135 patients with brain metastases before and after WBRT and found tumor progression was the predominant cause of cognitive decline, with stable or improving cognitive function in long-term (i.e., 15-month) survivors.[57] A smaller German trial assessed 15 brain metastases patients with a 90-minute battery of neuropsychometric tests before and after WBRT (40 Gy in 2-Gy daily fractions) and found stable cognitive function more than 9 months after cranial irradiation.[51] On the other hand, in a recent study comparing SRS alone to SRS and WBRT for 58 patients with up to up to three brain metastasis, 49% of patients in the WBRT group experienced declines in learning and memory at 4 months compared to only 23% in the SRS group.[50] Critics note the small size of the *single-institutional* study and a substantial difference in survival in the two groups, strongly suggesting the patients may not have been well matched for prognostic factors.[35] Additionally, at 4 months cognitive function after radiotherapy is at a nadir due to subacute or early delayed effects of radiotherapy that gradually resolve over time.[58] The measurement of cognitive function also occurred right before death in the WBRT arm (median survival 5.7 months). Previous studies confirm cognitive function declines significantly before death and is predictive of tumor progression.[58,59] The majority of other prospective and retrospective studies have found progression of brain metastases to be a much greater cause of neurocognitive dysfunction than WBRT. For example, in a similar but much larger (132 patients) multi-institutional trial of SRS with or without WBRT, neurocognitive function again correlated with tumor progression and found better preservation of

TABLE 168.2

COGNITIVE OUTCOMES AFTER WHOLE-BRAIN RADIOTHERAPY FOR BRAIN METASTASES IN PROSPECTIVE TRIALS WITH BASELINE TESTING

Study (Ref.)	No. of Patients	Radiation Total Dose/Fraction Size (Gy)	Extensive Neurocognitive Assessment	Neurotoxicity After WBRT
Regine et al. (50)	445	30/10 or 54.4/1.6 bid	No (MMSE)	No: Significant decrease MMSE for patients with progressive disease
Penitzka et al. (51)	64	40/20	Yes	No
Meyers et al. (52)	401	30/10	Yes	No: NCF measured at 2 months post-RT correlated with tumor progression
Li et al. (57)	208	30/10	Yes	No: 15-month survivors had stable or improving NCF
Aoyama et al. (54)	132 total; 65 received WBRT	30/10 with SRS boost vs. SRS alone	No (MMSE)	WBRT improved time until MMSE decline over SRS alone (7.6 mo vs. 16.5 mo, $P = .05$)
Corn et al. (55)	156	37.5/15 +/− thalidomide	No (MMSE)	Yes: 12% MMSE < 23 at 12 months post-WBRT[a]
Chang et al. (56)	58 total; 28 received WBRT	30/12 with SRS boost vs. SRS alone	Yes	Yes: HVLT decline at 4 months more frequent after WBRT+SRS than SRS alone (49% vs. 23%)

MMSE, Folstein Mini-Mental State Examination; RT, radiotherapy; WBRT, whole-brain radiotherapy; NCF, neurocognitive function; SRS, stereotactic radiosurgery; HVLT, Hopkins Verbal Learning Test.
[a]Data acquired from figure.

cognitive function with adjuvant WBRT.[54] Although cognitive effects are difficult to document in most modern studies, using large fraction sizes, as was done on many historical studies, is associated with dementia and cognitive decline in long-term survivors after WBRT; therefore, dose-fractionation schedules should be determined by the patient's estimated prognosis, with more protracted schedules used for patients with the possibility of long-term survival.[47]

In summary, although these prospective trials do not rule out detrimental neurocognitive effects of WBRT or even individual patient declines after WBRT (or PCI), they do suggest on the whole any detrimental effects on cognitive function seem to be balanced by the beneficial neurocognitive effects of improved tumor control in the brain, and taken together the evidence supports the safety of WBRT and PCI in adults when administered properly.

IMPACT OF TUMOR

Whether the *predominant* cause of cognitive decline in patients with brain tumors is the treatment or the tumor itself is an important question and has a significant impact on treatment recommendations. Older studies have emphasized the late neurotoxicity of treatment, especially radiotherapy.[59] However, these studies have suffered from many of the same deficiencies previously outlined, but most importantly they have lacked baseline neurocognitive testing as the brain tumor itself is often the primary cause of cognitive difficulties. The importance of baseline testing cannot be overemphasized because large prospective studies with baseline evaluations have found, for example, more than 90% of patients with brain metastases have significant cognitive impairment in one or more neurocognitive domains at the time of diagnosis (i.e., before WBRT).[52] More recent studies that have included prospective baseline and serial neurocognitive testing have found tumor to be the dominant cause of cognitive decline in patients with brain metastases[52,53] or low-grade[39] and high-grade glioma.[59] For example, Li et al.[57] grouped 135 patients with brain metastases into poor responders and good responders based on the response of their brain metastases on magnetic resonance imaging 2 months after WBRT. For all tests, the median time to cognitive deterioration was longer in good than in poor responders and was statistically significant in a number of domains. In long-term survivors, tumor shrinkage was significantly correlated with preservation of executive function and fine motor coordination.

There is also mounting evidence that cognitive decline in brain tumor patients after therapy may frequently reflect subclinical tumor progression rather than neurotoxicity as a result of treatment. In a North Central Cancer Treatment Group study of 1,244 high-grade glioma patients prospectively treated with radiation and nitrosourea-based chemotherapy, cognitive deterioration was noted at evaluations prior to radiographic failure; in contrast, patients without tumor progression had stable cognitive function.[59] In an M. D. Anderson Cancer Center study of 56 patients with recurrent high-grade gliomas treated on phase 1 and phase 2 trials, cognitive deterioration occurred 6 weeks prior to radiographic failure, highlighting the sensitivity and predictive value of neurocognitive assessments.[60]

TREATMENT OF COGNITIVE DYSFUNCTION

If cognitive impairment is identified in a patient, it is essential to evaluate for reversible causes such as depression, medications (e.g., changing or if possible discontinuing antiepileptics), or endocrine disturbances (i.e., hypothyroidism). The most common reversible cause of cognitive dysfunction is tumor progression because a number of studies have shown effective treatment of the tumor can result in improvement in cognitive function.[61]

Besides tumor-directed treatments, there are few proven therapies for cognitive dysfunction in brain tumor patients, although there are a number of small trials with interesting findings. Methylphenidate is a psychostimulant that has generated clinical and research interest for some time, and several small studies have suggested a benefit for patients with psychomotor slowing, decline in executive functioning, or general apathy.[62] Unfortunately, a phase 3, placebo-controlled trial did not confirm a benefit in cognitive function or quality of life in patients receiving radiotherapy for brain tumors.[63,64]

Another treatment option is brain injury rehabilitation, using methods developed for traumatic brain injury survivors. Shaw et al.[65] conducted a phase 3 trial of 140 adult brain tumor patients. Patients were randomly assigned to an intervention group or to a waiting-list control group. The intervention involved 6 weekly 2-hour sessions, self-study for reinforcement, and at 3 months a telephone-based booster session. The sessions incorporated both computer-based attention retraining and compensatory skills training of attention, memory, and executive functioning. At the 6-month follow-up, the intervention group performed significantly better in attention and verbal memory than the control group and reported less mental fatigue.

There is also interest in therapeutic agents that are frequently used in the treatment of Alzheimer's disease (e.g., donepezil, vitamin E), especially to treat radiation-induced injury, as in some aspects radiation-induced injury is clinically and radiographically similar to Alzheimer's dementia. In a trial from Wake Forest University, 24 previously irradiated brain tumor patients were treated for 24 weeks with the acetylcholinesterase inhibitor donepezil.[65] Cognitive functioning, mood, and health-related quality of life were significantly improved as well. A phase 3, placebo-controlled trial is currently enrolling patients to confirm this finding. Vitamin E has also been studied, including a trial from Queen Elizabeth Hospital in Hong Kong for 29 patients with temporal lobe radionecrosis.[66] Researchers treated 19 patients with a daily megadose of vitamin E for 1 year, whereas the other 10 patients served as controls (treatment assignment was decided on a voluntary basis). Significant improvement in global cognitive ability, memory, and executive function occurred among patients in the treatment group. However, as noted by the authors, the patients were not randomly assigned or blinded to treatment, and therefore the results should be considered preliminary.

Histologic evidence supports a role for vascular injury as a cause of late radiation injury. Hyperbaric oxygen (HBO) has been reported to improve radiation fibrosis and vascular injury at other anatomic sites.[67] Unfortunately, a phase 1 and 2 trial of HBO for seven patients with cognitive deficits after cranial radiation did not support a benefit for these patients.[68]

Although treatments for cognitive dysfunction are limited at this time, brain tumor patients actually represent an ideal population for research in neuroprotection because, unlike stroke patients, brain tumor patients typically have "planned" injurious events (i.e., surgery, chemotherapy, radiotherapy) to their brain, providing a golden opportunity for prophylactic treatment. For example, hippocampal-dependent functions of learning, memory, and spatial information processing seem to be preferentially affected by radiotherapy. Advances in radiotherapy treatment delivery and target localization allow delineation of hippocampus and avoidance of high doses of radiotherapy to that region, allowing "hippocampal-sparing radiotherapy."[69–71] The threshold dose for radiation injury to the hippocampus is unknown, so it is unclear whether the doses achievable will result in clinically significant improvements in cognitive function.

There are also a multitude of studies looking at novel agents (the majority currently laboratory based), and it is hoped that further elucidation of the cellular interactions between the different CNS cell types will lead to a better understanding of the CNS response to traumatic events and thereby more effective treatment regimens. Erythropoietin has been shown to be a CNS protectant in a number of studies, including a blinded, randomized trial of erythropoietin that found significantly less motor impairment in erythropoietin-treated rats after 100 Gy was delivered to the right striatum.[62] A similar study found that erythropoietin delivered 1 hour after WBRT was neuroprotective in mice.[62] Because of the positive results of these studies and others, there are ongoing trials assessing the neuroprotective properties of erythropoietin and its derivatives (typically without the hematogenic properties of erythropoietin).[47] The Radiation Therapy Oncology Group (RTOG) is currently conducting a prospective randomized trial evaluating memantine for the prevention of cognitive dysfunction after whole-brain radiotherapy. Memantine, an *N*-methyl-D-aspartate (NMDA)-receptor channel blocker,[72] has been shown to prevent propagation of vascular injury in mouse stroke models[73] and has been shown to improve cognitive function in vascular dementia patients.[36,75] Until time-proven treatment regimens for cognitive impairment are available, prevention of the development of cognitive dysfunction or worsening cognitive function will remain imperative. This requires a thorough understanding of the cognitive risks of all treatment modalities, balanced with the risks of uncontrolled tumor. For radiotherapy, there are many treatment variables to take into account (e.g., treatment volume, daily fraction size, total dose, beam arrangement) that can all have a significant impact on the therapeutic ratio. The same is true with surgery and, to a lesser extent, chemotherapy. However, it is important to recognize that as long as brain tumors and tumor progression remain the predominant causes of cognitive decline in brain tumor patients, physicians must primarily focus on durable tumor control.[59]

Selected References

The full list of references for this chapter appears in the online version.

1. Tucha O, Smely C, Preier M, et al. Cognitive deficits before treatment among patients with brain tumors. *Neurosurgery* 2000;47:324; discussion 333.
2. Scheibel RS, Meyers CA, Levin VA. Cognitive dysfunction following surgery for intracerebral glioma: influence of histopathology, lesion location, and treatment. *J Neurooncol* 1996;30:61–69.
5. Meyers CA, Wefel JS. The use of the Mini-Mental Status Examination to assess cognitive functioning in cancer trials: no ifs, ands, buts, or Sensitivity. *J Clin Oncol* 2003;21;3557–3558.
8. Meyers CA, Hess KR. Multifaceted end points in brain tumor clinical trials: cognitive deterioration precedes MRI progression. *Neurooncology* 2003;5:89.
10. Farace E, Sheehan JM, Shaffrey ME. Majority of patients show neurocognitive improvement after initial surgical resection of primary brain tumors. *Neurooncology* 2006;8:478 (abstr QL-417).
12. Duffau H. New concepts in surgery of WHO grade II gliomas: functional brain mapping, connectionism and plasticity—a review. *J Neurooncol* 2006;79:77.
13. Robles SG, Gatignol P, Lehericy S, et al. Long-term brain plasticity allowing multistage surgical approach to World Health Organization grade II gliomas in eloquent areas. *J Neurosurg* 2008;109:615.
15. Dietrich J, Monje M, Wefel J, et al. Clinical patterns and biological correlates of cognitive dysfunction associated with cancer therapy. *Oncologist* 2008;13:1285.
16. Wefel JS, Kayl AE, Meyers CA. Neuropsychological dysfunction associated with cancer and cancer therapies: a conceptual review of an emerging target. *Br J Cancer* 2004;90:1691.
17. Shah GD, DeAngelis LM. Treatment of primary central nervous system lymphoma. *Hematol Oncol Clin North Am* 2005;19:611.
19. Sul JK, Deangelis LM. Neurologic complications of cancer chemotherapy. *Semin Oncol* 2006;33:324.
21. Keime-Guibert F, Napolitano M, Delattre JY. Neurological complications of radiotherapy and chemotherapy. *J Neurol* 1998;245:695.
23. Dietrich J, Han R, Yang Y, et al. CNS progenitor cells and oligodendrocytes are targets of chemotherapeutic agents in vitro and in vivo. *J Biol* 2006;5:22.
25. Laack NN, Ballman KV, Brown PB, et al. Whole-brain radiotherapy and high-dose methylprednisolone for elderly patients with primary central nervous system lymphoma: Results of North Central Cancer Treatment Group (NCCTG) 96-73-51. *Int J Radiat Oncol Biol Phys* 2006;65:1429.
27. Correa DD, DeAngelis LM, Shi W, et al. Cognitive functions in survivors of primary central nervous system lymphoma [comment]. *Neurology* 2004;62:548.
30. Hilverda K, Bosma I, Heimans JJ, et al. Cognitive functioning in glioblastoma patients during radiotherapy and temozolomide treatment: initial findings. *J Neurooncol* 2010;97:89.
31. Macdonald DR, Kiebert G, Prados M, et al. Benefit of temozolomide compared to procarbazine in treatment of glioblastoma multiforme at first relapse: effect on neurological functioning, performance status, and health related quality of life. *Cancer Invest* 2005;23:138.
33. Brown PD. Low-grade gliomas: the debate continues. *Curr Oncol Rep* 2006;8:71.
34. Douw L, Klein M, Fagel SSAA, et al. Cognitive and radiological follow-up in low-grade glioma patients 12 years after primary treatment: a cross-sectional study. *Lancet Neurol* 2009;8:810.
35. Brown PD, Cerhan JH. Same, better, or worse? Neurocognitive effects of radiotherapy for low-grade gliomas remain unknown. *Lancet Neurol* 2009;8:779.
37. Vigliani MC, Sichez N, Poisson M, et al. A prospective study of cognitive functions following conventional radiotherapy for supratentorial gliomas in young adults: 4-year results. *Int J Radiat Oncol Biol Phys* 1996;35:527.
38. Brown PD, Buckner JC, O'Fallon JR, et al. Importance of baseline mini-mental state examination as a prognostic factor for patients with low-grade glioma. *Int J Radiat Oncol Biol Phys* 2004;59:117.
39. Torres IJ, Mundt AJ, Sweeney PJ, et al. A longitudinal neuropsychological study of partial brain radiation in adults with brain tumors. *Neurology* 2003;60:1113.
40. Laack NN, Brown PD, Ivnik RJ, et al. Cognitive function after radiotherapy for supratentorial low-grade glioma: a North Central Cancer Treatment Group prospective study. *Int J Radiat Oncol Biol Phys* 2005;63:1175.
41. Steinvorth S, Welzel G, Fuss M, et al. Neuropsychological outcome after fractionated stereotactic radiotherapy (FSRT) for base of skull meningiomas: a prospective 1-year follow-up. *Radiother Oncol* 2003;69:177.
42. Jalali R, Goswami S, Sarin R, et al. Neuropsychological status in children and young adults with benign and low-grade brain tumors treated prospectively with focal stereotactic conformal radiotherapy. *Int J Radiat Oncol Biol Phys* 2006;66:S14.
44. Brown PD, Buckner JC, Uhm JH, et al. The neurocognitive effects of radiation in adult low-grade glioma patients. *Neurooncology* 2003;5:161.
46. Komaki R, Meyers CA, Shin DM, et al. Evaluation of cognitive function in patients with limited small cell lung cancer prior to and shortly following prophylactic cranial irradiation. *Int J Radiat Oncol Biol Phys* 1995; 33:179.
47. Laack NN, Brown PD. Cognitive sequelae of brain radiation in adults. *Sem Oncol* 2004;31:702.
48. Arriagada R, Le Chevalier T, Borie F, et al. Prophylactic cranial irradiation for patients with small-cell lung cancer in complete remission. *J Natl Cancer Inst* 1995;87:183.
49. Gregor A, Cull A, Stephens RJ, et al. Prophylactic cranial irradiation is indicated following complete response to induction therapy in small cell lung cancer: results of a multicentre randomised trial. United Kingdom Coordinating Committee for Cancer Research (UKCCCR) and the European Organization for Research and Treatment of Cancer (EORTC)[see comment]. *Eur J Cancer* 1997;33:1752.
50. Regine WF, Scott C, Murray K, et al. Neurocognitive outcome in brain metastases patients treated with accelerated-fractionation vs. accelerated-hyperfractionated radiotherapy: an analysis from Radiation Therapy Oncology Group Study 91-04. *Int J Radiat Oncol Biol Phys* 2001; 51:711.
51. Penitzka S, Steinvorth S, Sehlleier S, et al. Assessment of cognitive function after preventive and therapeutic whole brain irradiation using neuropsychological testing. *Strahlenther Onkol* 2002;178:252.
52. Meyers CA, Smith JA, Bezjak A, et al. Neurocognitive function and progression in patients with brain metastases treated with whole-brain radiation and motexafin gadolinium: results of a randomized phase III trial. *J Clin Oncol* 2004;22:157.

54. Aoyama H, Tago M, Kato N, et al. Neurocognitive function of patients with brain metastasis who received either whole brain radiotherapy plus stereotactic radiosurgery or radiosurgery alone. *Int J Radiat Oncol Biol Phys* 2007;68:1388.
55. Corn BW, Moughan J, Knisely JP, et al. Prospective evaluation of quality of life and neurocognitive effects in patients with multiple brain metastases receiving whole-brain radiotherapy with or without thalidomide on Radiation Therapy Oncology Group (RTOG) trial 0118. *Int J Radiat Oncol Biol Phys* 2008;71:71–78.
56. Chang EL, Wefel JS, Hess KR, et al. Neurocognition in patients with brain metastases treated with radiosurgery or radiosurgery plus whole-brain irradiation: a randomised controlled trial. *Lancet Oncol* 2009;10:1037.
57. Li J, Bentzen SM, Renschler M, et al. Regression after whole-brain radiation therapy for brain metastases correlates with survival and improved neurocognitive function. *J Clin Oncol* 2007;25:1260.
58. Mahmood U, Kwok Y, Regine WF, et al. Whole-brain irradiation for patients with brain metastases: still the standard of care. *Lancet Oncol*;11:221; author reply 223.
59. Brown PD, Jensen AW, Felten SJ, et al. Detrimental effects of tumor progression on cognitive function of patients with high-grade glioma. *J Clin Oncol* 2006;24:5427.
60. Brown PD, Buckner JC, O'Fallon JR, et al. Effects of radiotherapy on cognitive function in patients with low-grade glioma measured by the Folstein Mini-Mental State Examination. *J Clin Oncol* 2003;21:2519.
61. Khuntia D, Brown P, Li J, et al. Whole-brain radiotherapy in the management of brain metastasis. *J Clin Oncol* 2006;24:1295.
64. Gehring K, Sitskoorn MM, Gundy CM, et al. Cognitive rehabilitation in patients with gliomas: a randomized, controlled trial. *J Clin Oncol* 2009; 27:3712.
65. Shaw EG, Rosdhal R, D'Agostino RB Jr, et al. Phase II study of donepezil in irradiated brain tumor patients: effect on cognitive function, mood, and quality of life. *J Clin Oncol* 2006;24:1415.
69. Barani IJ, Cuttino LW, Benedict SH, et al. Neural stem cell-preserving external-beam radiotherapy of central nervous system malignancies. *Int J Radiat Oncol Biol Phys* 2007;68:978.
70. Ghia A, Tome WA, Thomas S, et al. Distribution of brain metastases in relation to the hippocampus: implications for neurocognitive functional preservation. *Int J Radiat Oncol Biol Phys* 2007;68:971.
71. Gutierrez AN, Westerly DC, Tome WA, et al. Whole brain radiotherapy with hippocampal avoidance and simultaneously integrated brain metastases boost: a planning study. *Int J Radiat Oncol Biol Phys* 2007;69: 589.

CHAPTER 169 CANCER SURVIVORSHIP

WENDY LANDIER, CRAIG C. EARLE, SMITA BHATIA, MELISSA M. HUDSON, KEVIN OEFFINGER, PATRICIA A. GANZ, AND LOUIS S. CONSTINE

Living beyond cancer should be cause for celebration for the growing population of patients who have prevailed over cancer and survived its treatment. Although the war on cancer was formally declared in 1971, and the last 3 decades have seen several successful skirmishes, the battle is hardly won.

The challenge for oncologists and other involved clinicians is to understand and meet the complex interplay of biological, psychological, and socioeconomic needs of our surviving patients. Biological sequelae disrupt organ function and cause tissue-specific and systemic comorbidities, which can compromise quality of life (e.g., fatigue, infertility) or cause death (e.g., cardiovascular disease and second malignancies). Psychological sequelae, including depression and distress from fear of cancer recurrence, failure to work effectively, and socially engage with others, are clear detriments to life satisfaction. Socioeconomic consequences such as insufficient income and insurance compound any difficulties associated with daily living.

The multifaceted needs of patients demand a spectrum of actions from clinicians in order to provide them with a life worth living. It is necessary that clinicians diagnose and treat the chronic physical effects of cancer and its therapy, promote adaptive and rehabilitative lifestyle changes, and campaign for fair socioeconomic treatment by society. The process begins with communication between the clinician and patient regarding details of the treatment, potential sequelae in all the various domains, and an outline for ongoing care. Table 169.1 outlines the essential components of survivorship care as discerned by the Committee on Cancer Survivorship from the Institute of Medicine (IOM), and Table 169.2 states their ten recommendations.[1] In their report, specific goals were defined to ensure optimal outcomes for cancer survivors as follows:

- Raise awareness of the medical and psychosocial problems faced by cancer survivors and establish cancer survivorship as a distinct phase of the cancer trajectory during which specific clinical interventions are needed
- Define quality health care for cancer survivors and identify strategies to achieve it
- Improve quality of life through policies to ensure cancer survivors' access to psychosocial services, fair employment practices, and health insurance.

There are many unanswered questions about surveillance strategies, models of health care delivery, research strategies, and education of both patients and health care providers. This chapter is designed to serve as an introduction to understanding the scope of the survivorship problem.

DEFINITION OF SURVIVORSHIP AND SCOPE OF THE PROBLEM

Cancer survivorship is an evolving concept with multiple definitions. Prior to the recent evolution of curative cancer therapy, "cancer survivors" were defined as family members left behind after a loved one had succumbed to the disease.[2] In the latter half of the twentieth century, as survival rates increased, the dramatic impact of life-saving but potentially toxic therapies began to emerge. Izsak and Medalie[3(p 179)] are credited with first describing the "costs" of cancer survivorship: "Survival rates . . . do not relate to how the patient survives, at what cost to his physical functioning, how he adapted to his condition from a psychological point of view, and how he is fulfilling his roles in his family, at work, among friends, and in the wider society." Two decades ago, Fitzhugh Mullan,[4] a young physician and cancer survivor, challenged the binary concept of illness versus cure and suggested that survivorship was a process with predictable stages, ranging from the acute diagnosis and treatment phase, through the posttherapy phase of watchful waiting, and finally to the phase of permanent survival, when the focus shifts from concerns about risk of recurrence to those impacting long-term quality of survival. Soon after, the National Coalition for Cancer Survivorship (NCCS) was founded, raising awareness of the importance of the survivorship experience and setting the stage for recognition of survivorship as a distinct phase along the cancer control continuum.[5] In the mid-1990s, the National Cancer Institute established the Office of Cancer Survivorship, charged with directing and supporting research, training, and education regarding issues relating to cancer survivorship. More recently, the IOM[1] and the President's Cancer Panel[6] have released reports on issues relating to cancer survivorship. For the purposes of this chapter, the IOM's definition of cancer survivorship will be used, which focuses on the phases of cancer care following completion of primary treatment and lasting until cancer recurrence or end of life.[1]

The number of cancer survivors has increased more than threefold over the past 30 years by improvements in early detection and therapeutic successes (Fig. 169.1).[7] There are currently nearly 12 million cancer survivors in the United States[7] and more than 25 million worldwide.[8] The 5-year relative survival rate has also continued to increase steadily, and has now reached 66% for adults and 80% for children.[9] The number of cancer survivors is expected to increase dramatically over the next few decades, because of the general population growth and the increasing proportion of older adults in the population for whom cancer prevalence rates are the highest. More than six million cancer survivors in the United States are age 65 or older, representing 60% of all cancer survivors.[7]

TABLE 169.1

ESSENTIAL COMPONENTS OF SURVIVORSHIP CARE

1. **Education** of the cancer survivor, family, health care providers
   - A plan for care based on the treatment administered and future health risks
   - Promotion of healthy lifestyles
   - Information to assist health care providers in understanding future risks and to foster an effective interaction with the oncology team
2. **Surveillance** for cancer spread, recurrence, or second cancers and for long-term adverse physical, psychosocial, socioeconomic effects
3. **Intervention** to prevent or treat consequences of cancer or its therapy
4. **Communication** between specialists and primary care providers to ensure that the survivor's health needs are met and detailed records are kept about treatment history
5. **Research** focused on understanding, preventing, treating adverse consequences of cancer or its therapy
6. **Patient advocacy** to address problems related to employment, insurance, and disability

(Modified from ref. 1.)

Among male survivors, the most common diagnosis is prostate cancer (44%), followed by other genitourinary cancers (12%) and colorectal cancer (11%). Among female survivors, the most common diagnosis is breast cancer (43%), followed by gynecologic cancers (17%) and colorectal cancer (10%).[7] Survivors of hematologic malignancies, melanoma, lung, and other cancers each represent less than 10% of the population of cancer survivors.[10] Dramatic improvements in childhood cancer survival has resulted in a growing population that now exceeds 325,000 in the United States alone,[11] and multiple studies regarding the impact of cancer therapy on health-related outcomes in this population have been reported.[12] In a retrospective cohort of 10,397 childhood cancer survivors diagnosed between 1970 and 1986 (the Childhood Cancer Survivor Study), Oeffinger et al.[13] reported that 62.3% experienced at least one treatment-related late effect, 37.6% developed multiple late effects, and 27.5% developed a late effect that was severe or life-threatening. The impact of cancer therapy on health-related outcomes in the rapidly growing population of adult cancer survivors is largely unknown, but the need for ongoing follow-up care and late effects surveillance for all cancer survivors is clear.[1]

GOALS OF SURVIVORSHIP HEALTH CARE

Identifying Late Effects of Cancer Therapy

The modern era of cancer therapy is predicated on the safe intensification of radiation, chemotherapy, and biologic adjuvants. Malignancies resistant to therapy have demanded an aggressive treatment approach that often resides on the edge of normal tissue tolerance, or even exceeds tolerance to some "acceptable" degree. The potential to ameliorate or prevent such normal tissue damage, or to manage and rehabilitate affected patients, requires an understanding of these late or

TABLE 169.2

TEN RECOMMENDATIONS FOR CANCER SURVIVORSHIP CARE

1. Health care providers, patient advocates, and other stakeholders should work to raise awareness of the needs of cancer survivors, establish cancer survivorship as a distinct phase of cancer care, and act to ensure the delivery of appropriate survivorship care.
2. Patients completing primary treatment should be provided with a comprehensive care summary and follow-up plan that is clearly and effectively explained. This Survivorship Care Plan should be written by the principal provider(s) who coordinated the oncology treatment. This service should be reimbursed by third-party payors of health care.
3. Health care providers should use systematically developed evidence-based clinical practice guidelines, assessment tools, and screening instruments to help identify and manage late effects of cancer and its treatment. Existing guidelines should be refined and new evidence-based guidelines should be developed through public and private sector efforts.
4. Quality of survivorship care measures should be developed through public/private partnerships and quality assurance programs implemented by health systems to monitor and improve the care that all survivors receive.
5. The Centers for Medicare and Medicaid Services (CMS), National Cancer Institute (NCI), Agency for Healthcare Research and Quality (AHRQ), the Department of Veterans Affairs (VA), and other qualified organizations should support demonstration programs to test models of coordinated, interdisciplinary survivorship care in diverse communities and across systems of care.
6. Congress should support Centers for Disease Control and Prevention (CDC), other collaborating institutions, and the states in developing comprehensive cancer control plans that include consideration of survivorship care, and promoting the implementation, evaluation, and refinement of existing state cancer control plans.
7. The NCI, professional associations, and voluntary organizations should expand and coordinate their efforts to provide educational opportunities to health care providers to equip them to address the health care and quality of life issues facing cancer survivors.
8. Employers, legal advocates, health care providers, sponsors of support services, and government agencies should act to eliminate discrimination and minimize adverse effects of cancer on employment, while supporting cancer survivors with short-term and long-term limitations in ability to work.
9. Federal and state policy makers should act to ensure that all cancer survivors have access to adequate and affordable health insurance. Insurers and payors of health care should recognize survivorship care as an essential part of cancer care and design benefits, payment policies, and reimbursement mechanisms to facilitate coverage for evidence-based aspects of care.
10. The NCI, CDC, AHRQ, CMS, VA, private voluntary organizations such as the ACS, and private health insurers and plans should increase their support of survivorship research and expand mechanisms for its conduct. New research initiatives focused on cancer patient follow-up are urgently needed to guide effective survivorship care.

(Modified from ref. 1.)

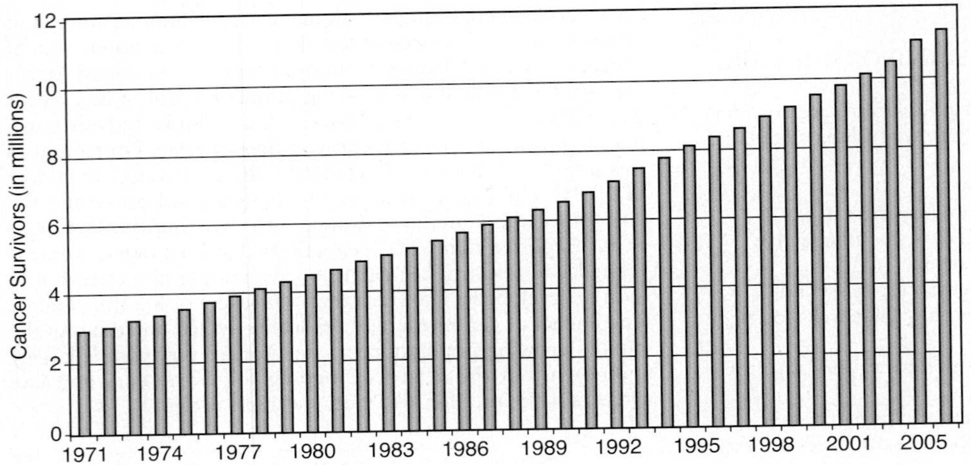

FIGURE 169.1 Estimated number of cancer survivors in the United States over time. (From http://dccps.nci.nih.gov/ocs/prevalence/prevalence.html, based on November 2008 SEER data submission. accessed 4-24-10.)

chronic effects. Because "late effects" can manifest months or years after cessation of treatment, therapeutic decisions intended to obviate such effects can be based only on the probability, not the certainty, that such effects will develop.

Determining the frequency and pathogenesis of late effects is difficult for several reasons: (1) patients must survive long enough for damage to develop, (2) the number of patients both affected and unaffected by therapy must be known, and (3) the latent period to the manifestation of damage compromises discernment of the responsible component of multimodality therapy. Further complicating our understanding of organ tolerance to therapy is that tumor and host factors interact with therapy in the causation of late effects. Tumor factors include direct tissue effects (e.g., from organ invasion such as the lung), systemic effects of tumor-induced organ damage (e.g., hepatic dysfunction), and indirect mechanical effects (e.g., renal or airway obstruction). Host factors include genetic (e.g., ataxia-telangiectasia) and comedical (e.g., vascular disease, diabetes) predispositions, the developmental status when children are treated, and underlying structural abnormalities (e.g., cardiac). The previously mentioned report by Oeffinger et al.[13] documents the high frequency of chronic health conditions in adult survivors of childhood cancer, many of which are severe or life-threatening. At 30 years, almost three-fourths of survivors had a chronic health condition, more than 40% had a serious health problem, and one-third had multiple conditions. Additionally, Yeh et al.[14] have recently developed a model based on Childhood Cancer Survivor Study data to estimate cumulative excess mortality in a simulated cohort of 5-year survivors of childhood cancer. These investigators predict a substantial decrement in life expectancy of 10.4 years (range, 4-17.8 years) for the childhood cancer survivors, compared with the general population.[14,15] Moreover the model estimates that the reduction in life expectancy is up to 28%, and that approximately one in four survivors will die of either a late recurrence or late effects related to secondary cancer and cardiopulmonary conditions. These data underscore the importance of understanding the toxic effects of our therapy. Several chapters in this text provide detailed information on the long-term physical effects of cancer therapy for each organ system.

Surveillance/Guidelines for Late Effects

Treatment-related sequelae can manifest at any time during or after therapy, and may be clinically silent at times when diagnosis might lead to effective interventions. Some chronic or late effects can evolve during normal development or aging. Health care providers need to anticipate these effects as well as evaluate those that are overt in order to optimize measures that can enhance quality of life. The need for standardized guidelines to direct follow-up care after cancer treatment and surveillance for late effects of therapy has been recognized as an important component of cancer care for over a decade.[1,5,16,17] However, the development of evidence-based long-term follow-up guidelines has proven to be a challenging endeavor. Following an IOM meeting in 2002, the Children's Oncology Group (COG) developed the Children's *Oncology Group Long-Term Follow-Up Guidelines for Survivors of Childhood, Adolescent, and Young Adult Cancers*, which was first published in 2003.[18] These guidelines consist of a set of risk-based, exposure-related screening recommendations to guide the long-term follow-up care of pediatric cancer survivors with the goals of improving quality of life and decreasing complication-related healthcare costs.

The COG guidelines (available at www.survivorshipguidelines.org)[19] exemplify a hybrid of evidence-based and consensus-driven approaches to guideline development. The strength of the evidence linking specific therapeutic exposures with adverse outcomes is considered for inclusion of a therapeutic agent or modality. Even though evidence from randomized controlled trials on which to base recommendations for periodic screening evaluations in childhood cancer survivors is presently not available or immediately forthcoming, lower levels of evidence exist and form the basis for the screening recommendations determined by consensus from a panel of experts in the late effects of pediatric cancer treatment. The screening recommendations outlined in the COG guidelines are organized by therapeutic exposure and appropriate for asymptomatic survivors presenting for routine exposure-based medical follow-up 2 or more years following completion of therapy for a pediatric malignancy. More extensive evaluations are appropriate, as clinically indicated, for survivors presenting with signs and symptoms suggesting illness or organ dysfunction. Recommendations for follow-up from the COG guidelines can be customized for individual patients based on age, gender, and treatment history.

Additional guidelines for follow-up of pediatric cancer survivors include the evidence-based Scottish Intercollegiate Guidelines Network (*Long Term Follow Up Care of Survivors of Childhood CancerSIGN 76*, available at www.sign.ac.uk/guidelines/fulltext/76/index.html), and the clinically focused *Therapy-Based Long Term Follow-up Practice Statement* from the United Kingdom Children's Cancer Study Group (available at www.ukccsg.org/public/followup/PracticeStatement/index.html). Guidelines for follow-up of long-term survivors of hematopoietic cell transplantation (*Recommended Screening and Preventive Practices for Long-term Survivors after*

Hematopoietic Cell Transplantation) have been developed jointly by the European Group for Blood and Marrow Transplantation, the Center for International Blood and Marrow Transplant Research, and the American Society of Blood and Marrow Transplantation, and were released in 2006.[20]

Comprehensive guidelines to direct the care of adult cancer survivors are increasingly becoming a focus of interest, particularly following the IOM's recommendation for development of such guidelines in their 2006 report.[1] As a result, the National Comprehensive Cancer Network now includes recommendations for surveillance as part of their 'evidence-informed consensus' guidelines (www.nccn.org), and the American Society of Clinical Oncology (ASCO) formed a Survivorship Task Force and instituted a Patient and Survivor Care Track at its annual meeting. The ASCO Health Services Committee released the ASCO *Recommendations on Fertility Preservation in Cancer Patients* in 2006.[21] However, illustrating the lack of high-quality data available to guide the care of adult cancer survivors, ASCO was unable to produce evidence-based guidelines for cardiopulmonary late effects, and instead published only an evidence summary.[22]

Intervention to Prevent Potential Late Effects

In the past decade, a growing number of studies have been designed and conducted with the intent of treating health conditions that are identified during or after the completion of therapy as well as preventing later occurring conditions. Randomized clinical trials have tested the effectiveness of a wide range of interventions, including ones aimed at increasing levels of physical activity, promoting healthy diets and smoking cessation, and reducing adverse psychosocial outcomes.

To illustrate the transition from observation to intervention studies and the evolution of survivor-focused intervention studies, one can look at studies of breast cancer survivors. In the general population, it has been well documented that physical inactivity and obesity are associated with an increased risk of all-cause mortality, several cancers, cardiovascular disease, insulin resistance, hypertension, osteoporosis, and diminished quality of life. Women with pre- or postmenopausal breast cancer and who are obese and physically inactive usually experience lower 5-year survival rates, increased rates of recurrence, and increased all-cause and cancer-related mortalities. Several randomized clinical trials conducted in breast cancer survivors have demonstrated that increasing levels of physical activity are associated with improved cardiorespiratory fitness, weight management, decreased fatigue, and quality of life.[23] Similar physical activity interventions are also being tested in other populations of cancer survivors.[24]

Recognizing that cancer survivors often have more than one risky health behavior, several behavior-based multicomponent interventions aimed at promoting a healthy lifestyle are underway. Morey et al.[25] recently described results from a study in which older long-term survivors of breast, colorectal, and prostate cancer reported reduced rates of functional decline following a 12-month home-based tailored diet and exercise intervention.

Although many interventions have been found to be effective in reducing psychosocial morbidity such as depression and anxiety in patients undergoing therapy for cancer, Stanton[26] notes that relatively few studies have focused on long-term survivors. Kazak et al.,[27] Pai and Kazak,[28] and Alderfer et al.[29] have published an elegant series of studies describing posttraumatic stress symptoms experienced by childhood and adolescent cancer survivors, and testing interventions to reduce these symptoms.

With this experience in survivor intervention studies, a growing survivor-based data set foundation and increased sophistication in study design have resulted in more standardized outcomes. Important challenges remain, including the ability to test specific interventions in survivor populations there are relatively small in numbers, and to recruit and retain long-term survivors in these studies.[30] Several potentially helpful interventions have yet to be studied, such as the use of statins to reduce the progression of radiation-associated atherosclerosis or chemoprevention to reduce the incidence of breast cancer in women who were treated with chest radiation.

Promotion of Adjustment and Healthy Lifestyles

The importance of providing appropriate support to facilitate positive psychosocial adjustment following treatment for cancer has been a central facet of the survivorship movement since its inception.[17] The rates of depression and other types of psychosocial distress in cancer survivors (such as anxiety, anger, and feelings of isolation) have been found to exceed those in the general population, and unmet psychosocial needs often persist following completion of cancer treatment.[26] The oncology health care provider should play a key role in screening for psychosocial distress in cancer survivors, and appropriate referrals to psychosocial professionals or other resources should be provided. Numerous print and online materials are available to address patient concerns, including: *Facing Forward: Life after Cancer Treatment*, from the National Cancer Institute (www.cancer.gov/cancertopics/life-after-treatment.pdf); the *Cancer Survivor Toolbox*, from the NCCS (www.cancersurvivaltoolbox.org); and online resources from the Office of Cancer Survivorship (http://dccps.nci.nih.gov/ocs/) and the American Cancer Society's (ACS) Cancer Survivors Network (http://csn.cancer.org/).

The potential for positive modification of lifestyle behaviors following a cancer diagnosis and treatment in adulthood has recently been recognized as a window of opportunity during which cancer survivors may be open to making significant changes in their health habits in an attempt to decrease the likelihood of cancer recurrence and to enhance their overall health status.[31] In a study of more than 1.2 million records from the Surveillance, Epidemiology, and End Results Program, cancer-specific death rates were found to underestimate the mortality associated with a cancer diagnosis; death rates from noncancer-related causes were noted to be higher among persons with a history of cancer than among the general population.[32] Taking advantage of the "teachable moment," which occurs when patients transit from active cancer therapy to follow-up care, is an important role for oncology health care professionals who are poised to serve as powerful catalysts in promoting behavioral change and the importance of reducing health risks.[33] Although a substantial proportion of cancer survivors may be willing to initiate positive lifestyle changes at this juncture, there are known groups of survivors who are less likely to adopt healthy lifestyle changes, including males, those with lower educational levels, and those who live in urban areas.[34] Additional support and intervention may be required in order to achieve positive lifestyle modification in these subgroups.

Survivors of childhood cancer often lack a distinct teachable moment for lifestyle modification such as that experienced by survivors of adult-onset cancers, given the wide variety of ages and developmental stages of patients treated for pediatric malignancies. They are known to be at increased risk for multiple chronic health conditions such as obesity and cardiovascular disease.[13] Several suboptimal health behaviors, including smoking and unhealthful dietary and exercise habits, have been observed in subsets of these survivors.[34] The importance of health promotion in this population should be emphasized, and attention should be given to providing targeted health counseling appropriate to each patient's cancer history, therapeutic exposures, age, gender, and developmental stage.

CARE PLANS

Providing high-quality care for cancer survivors presents several challenges. Cancer care is often fragmented among many different specialists, and traditionally there has been inadequate communication between physicians about the diagnosis and treatments a patient received. Primary care providers (PCPs) often have limited contact with patients undergoing active cancer treatment and lack details regarding their experience at its completion. Furthermore, there is limited information about the types and severity of potential long-term and late effects from cancer treatments, and a paucity of guidelines for surveillance for both recurrence and late effects. Most nononcology physicians will only have a handful of cancer survivors in their practice, and each survivor will likely have had a different disease and exposures. Consequently, it is not reasonable to expect PCPs to have knowledge of all of the potential survivorship scenarios these patients could face in the future.

The IOM[1] recommended that "upon discharge from cancer treatment . . . every patient should be given a record of all care received and important disease characteristics" (Table 169.3). This treatment summary would also be sent to all involved physicians, and would outline the primary site, histology, stage, and any surgery, radiation, and systemic therapy the patient received. The chemotherapy component would include the name of the regimen, component drugs, and starting dosages. It would indicate the number of cycles, the finishing doses (cumulative doses, when appropriate), and any major toxicities that necessitated any dose delays or reductions.

The IOM went on to assert that every patient should receive "a follow-up plan that is clearly and effectively explained." Such a *survivorship care plan* should include information about the likely course of recovery from acute treatment toxicities, as well as the need for ongoing health maintenance or adjuvant therapy such as hormonal therapy after breast cancer. It should also detail the plan for surveillance for recurrence or development of new cancers. It should designate the common late effects of treatment that need to be monitored, and identify which providers will be responsible for ongoing cancer follow-up, noncancer care, and psychosocial and supportive issues. Explicit identification of providers is important not only to minimize duplication of effort, but also to optimize coordination so that necessary care does not fall through the cracks from unclear expectations.[35] The survivor should receive a copy of this treatment summary and care plan as a record that can be used for consultation and coordination with future physicians. Discussion of the plan with the patient has been shown to increase clarity around different providers' roles.[36]

Several organizations have developed standardized treatment summaries and survivorship care plans to guide posttherapy follow-up care. Important components include surveillance for recurrence of the primary cancer, identification of potential long-term complications resulting from specific therapies employed during treatment of the primary cancer, and a plan for psychosocial support and coordination of cancer survivorship care.[1] Downloadable survivorship care plan templates are available from ASCO (www.asco.org/treatmentsummary), COG (www.survivorshipguidelines.org), Journey Forward (www.journeyforward.org), and the LiveSTRONG Survivorship Network (www.livestrongcareplan.org).

No single organizational model exists that must be adopted to deliver high-quality care to survivors. PCPs given explicit

TABLE 169.3

THE INSTITUTE OF MEDICINE SURVIVORSHIP CARE PLAN

On discharge from cancer treatment, every patient should be given a record including:

1. Contact information for each treating institution and key individual providers
2. Dates of treatment initiation and completion
3. Diagnostic tests and results
4. Tumor characteristics
5. Surgery or other therapies provided, including specific agents, regimens, dosage, number and title of clinical trials (if any), treatment response, and toxicities experienced
6. Psychosocial and nutritional services provided
7. Identification of a coordinator of continuing care

On discharge from cancer treatment, every patient and his or her primary health care provider should receive a written follow-up care plan including:

1. The likely course of recovery from treatment
2. Recommended periodic testing and examinations by whom and on what schedule
3. Possible late and long-term effects of treatment and symptoms
4. Possible signs of recurrence and second tumors
5. Possible effects of cancer on daily life (personal relationships, work, mental health) and available resources for support
6. Potential insurance, employment, and financial consequences of cancer and referrals to counseling, legal aid, and financial assistance if needed
7. Recommendations for healthy behaviors that should also be shared with first-degree relatives to minimize their potential risk of cancer
8. As appropriate, information on genetic counseling and testing to identify high-risk individuals who could benefit from more comprehensive cancer surveillance
9. As appropriate, information on known effective chemoprevention strategies for secondary prevention (e.g., tamoxifen for breast cancer; aspirin for colorectal cancer)
10. Referrals to specific follow-up care providers
11. A listing of cancer-related print or online information resources and support organizations

(Modified from ref. 1.)

instructions about the necessary components of surveillance and follow-up have been shown to produce the same outcomes as specialist follow-up.[37] Similarly, oncologists are able to provide primary noncancer care to patients,[31] although only a minority appear to want to regularly assume this role.[38] Most survivors experience some form of shared care, in which PCPs collaborate with cancer specialists. The role of oncologists in a shared care model is to provide or guide periodic surveillance and to be available to evaluate patients when potential cancer-related concerns arise. The PCP continues to carry out routine prevention and health maintenance interventions and manage comorbid conditions.[39–41]

Specialized survivorship clinics were proposed many years ago by the NCCS and have more recently been funded in several academic and community sites by the Lance Armstrong Foundation (LAF). These programs are effectively exploring different models of providing survivorship care.[42] Each provides a different menu of services: assuming all surveillance, providing primary care, health promotion, psychological support, consultations focused on detection of late effects, and/or transition visits with provision of treatment summaries and survivorship care plans. Whether follow-up is provided by oncologists, PCPs, or specialized survivor clinics is not important as long as there are identifiable providers with clear roles who are able to recognize and address issues as they arise and who communicate with each other about the care of the patient.

Creating a survivorship care plan as outlined here requires time and energy. Despite the barriers this presents, leading groups such as the IOM, LAF, COG, and ASCO are promoting the idea that treatment summaries and survivorship care plans should be the standard of care in oncology. This is now a specific quality metric in the ASCO quality of care certification program (Quality Oncology Practice Initiative). The information contained within well-developed care plans can greatly facilitate necessary communication among physicians, thereby maximizing the likelihood that high-quality survivor care can occur.

DELIVERY OF FOLLOW-UP CARE AND BEST-PRACTICE MODELS

There is no consensus on the best strategy for providing follow-up care to the growing number of cancer survivors. Most children with cancer are treated at pediatric oncology referral centers where, on termination of cancer therapy, they are seen in a follow-up clinic or program. Because of the diverse ages at diagnosis (infancy to adolescence), childhood cancer survivors may be under the care of pediatric oncologists for more than a decade. However, once they become young adults and leave home for college or work, they may need to transition to care outside the pediatric referral center.[43] This poses a substantial challenge, as few PCPs will be knowledgeable about the exposures and risks from prior cancer therapy. Thus, arming the young adult survivor with a treatment summary and care plan with specific surveillance recommendations can facilitate subsequent care with generalist physicians.

For adult survivors of cancer, most care is currently not coordinated and is divided among surgical, radiation, and medical oncologists with parallel care provided by the primary care physician. Based on the IOM report, better coordination is needed and direct communication among providers is critical to ensure that that appropriate follow-up care is provided. Currently available models are in development, but consist of tertiary care centers with consultative services, free-standing cancer centers that integrate survivorship care within their disease-oriented teams using advanced practice nurses and/or PCPs, and hybrid models. The LIVESTRONG Network of Survivorship Centers of Excellence is working to develop and evaluate these models.[42] This remains a work in progress.

EDUCATIONAL CONSIDERATIONS

Educating the cancer survivor, health care provider, and family is critical to promoting cancer survivorship. Studies evaluating health knowledge among childhood cancer survivors have revealed significant knowledge deficits and misconceptions regarding diagnosis, treatment, and therapy-related health risks.[44] Studies of survivors of adult cancers report similar knowledge deficits regarding risks of and surveillance for disease recurrence or therapy-related late effects, such as risks for infertility or second malignancies.[1] Many health care professionals are also ill-equipped to provide cancer survivorship care, primarily because of the lack of experience in caring for cancer survivors and a deficit of relevant information in professional and/or continuing education curricula.[1]

COG has developed a set of health education materials specifically targeted to childhood cancer survivors.[45] These materials, known as "Health Links," address 42 key topics within the *COG Long-Term Follow-Up Guidelines* and are designed to enhance health knowledge and improve compliance with guideline-specific recommendations. Each Health Link provides an overview of the potential therapy-related complication, a review of relevant risk factors, recommendations for screening, and an explanation of applicable health-protective behaviors. They are designed to be used in conjunction with the *COG Long-Term Follow-Up Guidelines* and are available for downloading from www.survivorshipguidelines.org.

COG is currently working with Baylor College of Medicine to develop an Internet-based decision support system that will provide childhood cancer survivors with up-to-date screening and health information from the COG guidelines that are individually tailored to each patient's specific treatment exposures.[46] It is hoped that this technology-driven Web portal, known as "Passport for Care," will empower survivors to assume greater control of their own health care by providing them with direct access to information that will assist in making decisions regarding individual lifestyle behaviors and follow-up care. When comprehensive guidelines for follow-up care are available for adult cancer survivors, similar Internet-based systems may prove valuable in disseminating this information to survivors and their health care providers. In addition to providing education to cancer survivors, incorporation of cancer survivorship care into the objectives for medical school core curricula, along with development and dissemination of continuing education programs for practicing health care professionals, are imperative in order to optimize care for survivors.[1]

ENHANCING RESEARCH

The growing and rather heterogeneous population of cancer survivors provides novel opportunities for research in many domains including the etiopathogenesis, screening, and early detection of adverse outcomes and their impact on quality of life. This population lends itself to research regarding these issues because of the ability to assess therapeutic exposures accurately, both in terms of the type of exposure and its timing, and to examine the role of host characteristics.

Reports demonstrating that childhood cancer survivors are at risk for developing adverse outcomes began more than 3 decades ago, and have subsequently proliferated.[47–59] Outcomes include premature death, second neoplasms, organ dysfunction, impaired growth and development, decreased fertility, impaired intellectual function, and overall reduced quality of life. Extended follow-up of large cohorts of survivors has demonstrated the emergence of adverse outcomes at a younger age than would be expected in the general population. There remains a critical need for systematic follow-up of large cohorts of adult cancer survivors to identify the role of host and clinical characteristics along with comorbidities in the health and well-being of this rapidly growing population.

The focus of investigation thus far has been on the magnitude of risk and identification of demographic and treatment-related risk factors. Attention needs to be devoted to understanding the underlying etiopathogenesis, such as the role of genetic susceptibility, or the mechanism of action of specific therapeutic exposures associated with the development of the adverse event. In addition, specific research initiatives focusing on the utility of surveillance and interventional strategies need to be mounted. These include efficacy of agents designed to protect normal tissues from the toxic effects of specific therapeutic agents (e.g., amifostine and cisplatin-induced ototoxicity, dexrazoxane and anthracycline-induced cardiomyopathy), use of chemopreventive agents for prevention of second malignancies, use of afterload reducing agents for prevention of further progression of myocardial dysfunction, lifestyle and behavior modifications, and education to increase awareness of the need for screening. Follow-up for extended periods of time is required to assess the efficacy of these strategies. The efficiency and cost-effectiveness of competing models of survivorship care and community-based services require study.

Several challenges persist in the conduct of survivorship research. The multifactorial nature of the etiology of long-term sequelae often demands large sample sizes in order to address the research questions effectively. Because of the mobility of the survivor population, incompleteness of follow-up of cancer survivors results in surveillance bias, which can significantly compromise the quality of research. Resources are therefore needed to establish the necessary infrastructure to conduct cancer survivorship research effectively.

SURVIVORSHIP ADVOCACY

Employment

Cancer survivors face challenges that go beyond strictly medical issues. Work and insurance are primary areas of difficulty, and not just in the United States. A study based on the 2000 National Health Interview Survey found that 18% of cancer survivors were unable to work because of residual health problems, compared with only 10% of matched controls.[60] A further 27% were limited in the amount or kind of work they could do. Such employment problems can impact many other people if the survivor was the main breadwinner. A recent prospective cohort study similarly showed that long-term labor force departures attributable to cancer occurred in 17% of lung and colorectal cancer survivors who were employed at diagnosis.[61] Even among those who are able to return to work, there may be discrimination that is either overt or an unstated undercurrent based on a perception by others that the cancer survivor is not well enough to perform his or her job at the highest level or would be unable to tolerate the added responsibilities entailed by a promotion. The situation has definitely improved over the years as federal laws like the Americans with Disabilities Act (1990) and the Family and Medical Leave Act (1993), and several state regulations have done much to protect the rights of workers such as those with a history of cancer.

Insurance

To be effective, health insurance options must be available, affordable, and adequate in coverage.[1] Unfortunately, health insurance options for cancer survivors are often deficient on one or more of these criteria. Cancer survivors over age 65 are almost all covered by Medicare, although there are still gaps in outpatient medication coverage. Moreover, certain services of particular relevance to survivors, such as fertility preservation, are not consistently covered.[62] Approximately 11% of nonelderly survivors are uninsured, and this rises to 19% when limited to those aged 25 to 44 years. Minority survivors are more likely to be uninsured than whites.[1] Although this is not greater than the overall rate of uninsured in the nonelderly general population (16%), the potential implications for patients who generally have clear need for ongoing care and monitoring are enormous. Unfortunately, private health insurance is usually impossible to purchase for a cancer survivor. Depending on state laws, if not rejected outright, survivors will often face exorbitant premiums or exclusions of anything related to the pre-existing condition. Even survivors with established insurance may find such aids as prostheses or mental health services uncovered. Life insurance applications by people with a personal history of cancer are often rejected or the plans come with very high premiums unless it is part of an employer-based group insurance.

Employed survivors who receive their health insurance through work are often reluctant to leave a job because of a fear of losing this benefit. Some protections are in place for workers who would like to change jobs, but these safeguards are generally considered lacking because of the unrealistic financial burden they entail. The Consolidated Omnibus Budget Reconciliation Act (COBRA) of 1986 allows workers to maintain their health insurance for 18 months after losing or leaving a job, but this comes at a great and often unmanageable expense as they become responsible for the full premium after leaving their job, not just the proportion (usually around 20%) they were previously paying. If the worker finds a new job, the Health Insurance Portability and Accountability Act (HIPAA) established in 1996 prohibits selective eligibility for employer-provided health insurance benefits based on health status considerations, such as a prior history of cancer. If survivors remain unemployed once COBRA benefits have been exhausted, HIPAA mandates that workers can purchase a new health insurance policy and insurers are prohibited from denying or limiting coverage because of the pre-existing conditions. Once again, the premium surcharges are not controlled and can be insurmountable for most patients who are unemployed.[63] At the time of this writing it is hoped that health care reform will ameliorate many of these problems, but the reality of its implementation remains to be seen.

Advocacy

Several nonprofit organizations have formed to provide advocacy for the issues that affect cancer survivors. Some, like the ACS and CancerCare, are not exclusively for survivors of cancer but have survivorship as one of their main areas of interest; while the NCCS and the LAF clearly make it their focus. In addition to advocating for more research funds and resources for survivor care, several of these organizations provide education, counseling, and links to legal contacts and other types of assistance to help survivors with employment, insurance, or economic issues. They also provide assistance in navigating the Social Security Disability system. The ACS reports that about 13% of the calls to an information line it operates are about employment concerns.[1] The NCCS produces a "Cancer Survival Toolbox" and publishes *What Cancer Survivors Need to Know About Health Insurance*. These resources are necessary because many survivors are not aware of their rights under COBRA and HIPAA and the time windows in which they must act in order to take advantage of these opportunities.

There are a few programs of limited financial assistance run through government and charitable organizations that assist with expenses incurred during cancer treatment or transportation to medical appointments. Programs are also offered by several pharmaceutical companies to help provide expensive long-term outpatient medications to cancer patients and survivors. Providing information about resources available to cancer survivors to help them deal with these nonmedical issues is a recommended component of the survivorship care plans discussed earlier in this chapter.

References

The full list of references for this chapter appears in the online version.

1. Hewitt M, Greenfield S, Stovall E, eds. *From Cancer Patient to Cancer Survivor: Lost in Transition.* Washington, D.C.: National Academies Press, 2006.
2. Leigh S. Cancer survivorship: a consumer movement. *Semin Oncol* 1994;21(6):783.
4. Mullan F. Seasons of survival: reflections of a physician with cancer. *N Engl J Med* 1985;313(4):270.
5. Rowland JH, Hewitt M, Ganz PA. Cancer survivorship: a new challenge in delivering quality cancer care. *J Clin Oncol* 2006;24(32):51013.
6. Reuben SH. Living beyond cancer: finding a new balance; President's Cancer Panel 2003-2004 annual report. May 2004. Washington, D.C.: National Cancer Institute, 2004.
7. Horner MJ, Ries LAG, Krapcho M, et al., eds. *SEER Cancer Statistics Review, 1975–2006.* Bethesda, MD: National Cancer Institute, 2009.
9. Jemal A, Siegel R, Ward E, Hao Y, Xu J, Thun MJ. Cancer statistics, 2009. *CA Cancer J Clin* 2009;59(4):225.
11. Mariotto AB, Rowland JH, Yabroff KR, et al. Long-term survivors of childhood cancers in the United States. *Cancer Epidemiol Biomarkers Prev* 2009;18(4):1033.
12. Hewitt M, Weiner S, Simone J. *Childhood Cancer Survivorship: Improving Care and Quality of Life.* Washington, DC: The National Academies Press, 2003.
13. Oeffinger KC, Mertens AC, Sklar CA, et al. Chronic health conditions in adult survivors of childhood cancer. *N Engl J Med* 2006;355:1572.
17. Clark EJ, Stovall EL, Leigh S, Siu AL, Austin DK, Rowland JH, eds. *Imperatives for Quality Cancer Care: Access, Advocacy, Action and Accountability.* Silver Spring, MD: National Coalition for Cancer Survivorship, 1995.
18. Landier W, Bhatia S, Eshelman DA, et al. Development of risk-based guidelines for pediatric cancer survivors: the Children's Oncology Group Long-Term Follow-Up Guidelines from the Children's Oncology Group Late Effects Committee and Nursing Discipline. *J Clin Oncol* 2004;22:4979–90.
19. Children's Oncology Group. *Long-term follow-up guidelines for survivors of childhood, adolescent, and young adult cancers,* Version 3.0. Arcadia, CA: Children's Oncology Group, 2008.
20. Rizzo JD, Wingard JR, Tichelli A, et al. Recommended screening and preventive practices for long-term survivors after hematopoietic cell transplantation: joint recommendations of the European Group for Blood and Marrow Transplantation, the Center for International Blood and Marrow Transplant Research, and the American Society of Blood and Marrow Transplantation. *Biol Blood Marrow Transplant* 2006;12:138.
21. Lee SJ, Schover LR, Partridge AH, et al. American Society of Clinical Oncology recommendations on fertility preservation in cancer patients. *J Clin Oncol* 2006;24:2917.
22. Carver JR, Shapiro CL, Ng A, et al. American Society of Clinical Oncology clinical evidence review on the ongoing care of adult cancer survivors: cardiac and pulmonary late effects. *J Clin Oncol* 2007;25(25):3991.
24. Schmitz K, Holtzman J, Courneya K, Masse L, Duval S, Kane R. Controlled physical activity trials in cancer survivors: a systematic review and meta-analysis. *Cancer Epidemiol Biomarkers Prev* 2005;14:1588.
25. Morey MC, Snyder DC, Sloane R, et al. Effects of home-based diet and exercise on functional outcomes among older, overweight long-term cancer survivors: RENEW: a randomized controlled trial. *JAMA* 2009;301(18):1883.
26. Stanton A. Psychosocial concerns and interventions for cancer survivors. *J Clin Oncol* 2006;24:5132.
27. Kazak A, Alderfer M, Streisand R, et al. Treatment of posttraumatic stress symptoms in adolescent survivors of childhood cancer and their families: a randomized clinical trial. *J Fam Psychol* 2004;18:493.
30. Sears S, Stanton A, Kwan L, et al. Recruitment and retention challenges in breast cancer survivorship research: results from a multisite, randomized intervention trial in women with early stage breast cancer. *Cancer Epidemiol Biomarkers Prev* 2003;12:1087.
31. Ganz P. A teachable moment for oncologists: cancer survivors, 10 million strong and growing! *J Clin Oncol* 2005;23:5458.
32. Brown B, Brauner C, Minnotte M. Noncancer deaths in white adult cancer patients. *J Natl Cancer Inst* 1993;85:979.
34. Demark-Wahnefried W, Aziz NM, Rowland JH, Pinto BM. Riding the crest of the teachable moment: promoting long-term health after the diagnosis of cancer. *J Clin Oncol* 2005;23:5814.
35. Cheung WY, Neville BA, Cameron DB, Cook EF, Earle CC. Comparisons of patient and physician expectations for cancer survivorship care. *J Clin Oncol* 2009;27(15):2489.
36. Cheung WY, Neville BA, Earle CC. associations among cancer survivorship discussions, patient and physician expectations, and receipt of follow-up care. *J Clin Oncol* 2010;28(15):2577.
37. Grunfeld E, Levine M, Julian J, et al. Randomized trial of long-term follow-up for early-stage breast cancer: a comparison of family physician versus specialist care. *J Clin Oncol* 2006;24:848.
39. Ganz PA. Survivorship: adult cancer survivors. *Prim Care* 2009;36(4):721.
40. Oeffinger KC, Hudson MM, Landier W. Survivorship: childhood cancer survivors. *Prim Care* 2009;36(4):743.
41. American Academy of Pediatrics Section on Hematology/Oncology Children's Oncology G. Long-term follow-up care for pediatric cancer survivors. *Pediatrics* 2009;123(3):906.
42. Shapiro CL, McCabe MS, Syrjala KL, et al. The LIVESTRONG Survivorship Center of Excellence Network. *J Cancer Surviv* 2009;3(1):4.
43. Freyer DR. Transition of Care for Young Adult Survivors of Childhood and Adolescent Cancer: Rationale and Approaches. *J Clin Oncol* 2010;28(32):4810.
44. Kadan-Lottick NS, Robison LL, Gurney JG, et al. Childhood cancer survivors' knowledge about their past diagnosis and treatment: Childhood Cancer Survivor Study. *JAMA* 2002;287(14):1832.
45. Eshelman D, Landier W, Sweeney T, et al. Facilitating care for childhood cancer survivors: integrating children's oncology group long-term follow-up guidelines and health links in clinical practice. *J Pediatr Oncol Nurs* 2004;21:271.
46. Poplack D, Fordis M, Horowitz M, et al. Improving the lives of childhood cancer survivors: development of a novel Internet resource for managing long-term health risks. Washington, DC: National Academies Press, 2007.
47. Bhatia S, Yasui Y, Robison L, et al. High risk of subsequent neoplasms continues with extended follow-up of childhood Hodgkin's disease: report from the Late Effects Study Group. *J Clin Oncol* 2003;21:4386.
48. Bhatia S, Sather HN, Pabustan OB, Trigg ME, Gaynon PS, Robison LL. Low incidence of second neoplasms among children diagnosed with acute lymphoblastic leukemia after 1983. *Blood* 2002;99:4257.
49. Bokemeyer C, Schmoll HJ, van Rhee J, Kuczyk M, Schuppert F, Poliwoda H. Long-term gonadal toxicity after therapy for Hodgkin's and non-Hodgkin's lymphoma. *Ann Hematol* 1994;68:105.
50. Christie D, Leiper A, Chessells J, et al. Intellectual performance after presymptomatic cranial radiotherapy for leukaemia: effects of age and sex. *Arch Dis Child* 1995(73):136.
51. Hancock S, Cox R, McDougall I. Thyroid diseases after treatment of Hodgkin's disease. *N Engl J Med* 1991;325:599.
52. Haupt R, Fears T, Robison L, et al. Educational attainment in long-term survivors of childhood acute lymphoblastic leukemia: a report from the NIH and the CCG. *JAMA* 1994;272:1427.
53. Kremer L, van der Pal H, Offringa M, et al. Frequency and risk factors of subclinical cardiotoxicity after anthracycline therapy in children: a systematic review. *Ann Oncol* 2002;13:819.
54. Mulrooney DA, Yeazel MW, Kawashima T, et al. Cardiac outcomes in a cohort of adult survivors of childhood and adolescent cancer: retrospective analysis of the Childhood Cancer Survivor Study cohort. *BMJ* 2009;339:b4606.
55. Mattano L, Sather H, Trigg M, et al. Osteonecrosis as a complication of treating acute lymphoblastic leukemia in children: a report from the Children's Cancer Group. *J Clin Oncol* 2000;18:3262.
56. Neglia J, Friedman D, Yutaka Y, et al. Second malignant neoplasms in five-year survivors of childhood cancer: Childhood Cancer Survivor Study. *J Natl Cancer Inst* 2001;93:618.
57. Gurney J, Kadan-Lottick N, Packer R, et al. Endocrine and cardiovascular late effects among adult survivors of childhood brain tumors: Childhood Cancer Survivor Study. *Cancer* 2003;97:663.
58. Sklar C, Mertens A, Mitby P, et al. Risk of disease recurrence and second neoplasms in survivors of childhood cancer treated with growth hormone: a report from the Childhood Cancer Survivor Study. *J Clin Endocrinol Metab* 2002;87:3136.
60. Yabroff K, Lawrence W, Clauser S, et al. Burden of illness in cancer survivors: findings from a population-based national sample. *J Natl Cancer Inst* 2004;96:1322.
61. Earle CC, Chretien Y, Morris C, et al. Employment among survivors of lung cancer and colorectal cancer. *J Clin Oncol* 2010;28(10):1700.
62. Campo-Engelstein L. Consistency in insurance coverage for iatrogenic conditions resulting from cancer treatment including fertility preservation. *J Clin Oncol* 2010;28(8):1284.

CHAPTER 170 MANAGEMENT OF CANCER PAIN

AMY ABERNATHY AND KATHLEEN M. FOLEY

Advances in the diagnosis and treatment of cancer, coupled with advances in understanding the anatomy, physiology, pharmacology, and psychology of pain perception, have led to improved care of the patient with pain of malignant origin. Specialized methods of cancer diagnosis and treatment provide the most direct approach to treating cancer pain by treating the cause of the pain. However, before the introduction of successful antitumor therapy, when treatment of the cause of the pain has failed, or when injury to bone, soft tissue, or nerve has occurred as a result of therapy, appropriate pain management is essential. Patients with cancer are managed most effectively by a multidisciplinary approach that draws on the expertise of a wide range of health care professionals.[1–3] The goal of pain therapy for patients receiving active treatment is to provide them with sufficient relief to tolerate the diagnostic and therapeutic approaches required to treat their cancer. For patients with advanced disease, pain control should be sufficient to allow them to function at a level they choose and to die relatively free of pain.

The management of the symptom of pain is only one component of a broad palliative care approach for cancer patients.[4–8] Control of other symptoms, treatment of psychological distress, and attention to the religious, spiritual, and existential dimensions of the patient's illness experience should be concurrently addressed to maintain the patient's quality of life throughout the cancer illness course from diagnosis to death. The World Health Organization (WHO) has published international guidelines for cancer pain relief and palliative care.[6–8] In the United States, the National Comprehensive Cancer Network has published specific guidelines that provide a best practice approach for both the provision of pain treatment and palliative care and the American Pain Society, the British Pain Society, and the European Society of Medical Oncology (ESMO) have also published specific pain guidelines.[9–13]

EPIDEMIOLOGY

Existing studies based on numerous national and international surveys and WHO estimates suggest that moderate to severe pain is experienced by one-third of cancer patients who receive active therapy and by 60% to 90% of patients with advanced disease.[14] There are 19 million new cases of cancer diagnosed worldwide each year and more than 7 million cancer deaths, which accounts for large numbers of patients who suffer from cancer pain.[15] Pain associated with direct tumor involvement is the most common cause of cancer pain, occurring in as many as 85% of patients as reported in a pain service study, to 65% as demonstrated by an outpatient cancer center pain clinic survey.[16–18] Bone pain is the most common type, with tumor infiltration of nerve and hollow viscus as the second and third most common pain sources. Cancer therapy causes pain in 15% to 25% of patients receiving chemotherapy, surgery, or radiation therapy. Three percent to 10% of patients with cancer have pain caused by non–cancer-related problems, with pain syndromes reflecting the common causes of pain in the general population. Chronic pain is also prevalent in cancer survivors, with prevalence rates ranging from 5% to 40% of patients and varying by tumor type and cancer treatment.[19,20]

Patients with cancer often have multiple causes of pain and multiple sites of pain.[21–28] Based on a variety of survey data, up to one-third of patients had more than one type of pain and 81% of patients reported two or more distinct pain complaints; 34% reported three types of pain.

Studies have focused not only on the prevalence of pain but also on its intensity, the degree of pain relief, and the effect of pain on quality of life in patients with various cancers, including lung, colon, and ovarian cancers.[21–25] These studies point out that pain is prevalent in ambulatory patients as well as hospitalized patients and compromises function in approximately one-half of the patients who experience it.

A series of studies have focused on the seriously ill and nursing home cancer population and have identified a high prevalence of pain in these populations. The Study to Understand Prognoses and Preferences for Outcomes and Risks of Treatments showed that 50% of adults who die in the hospital experience moderate to severe pain in their last 3 days of life.[26] A study of 4,000 elderly nursing home residents with cancer revealed that 24%, 29%, and 38% of those over age 85 years, 75 to 84 years, and 65 to 74 years, respectively, reported daily pain.[27] Twenty-six percent of these elderly in daily pain did not receive any medication. Those older than 85 years who reported pain were most likely to receive no analgesic. Similar studies of children report that 54% to 85% of pediatric inpatients and 26% to 35% of pediatric outpatients experience pain. Up to 62% to 90% of children experience pain at the end of life.[28]

Such studies have led to an assessment of the factors that influence the prevalence of cancer pain. Primary tumor type is one factor. Tumors that commonly metastasize to bone such as breast or prostate are associated with a higher incidence of pain (60% to 80%) than lymphoma and leukemia.[16] Stage of disease is a contributing factor, with pain prevalence increasing as disease progresses. For example, fewer than 15% of patients with nonmetastatic disease report pain, while pain is the most common symptom in patients in the last months of life.[29,30]

Tumors that occur in close proximity to neural structures also produce a higher incidence of pain. Patient variables such as anxiety, depression, and history of previous substance abuse influence the patient's report and experience of pain.[31,32]

DEFINITION OF PAIN

The definition of pain proposed by the International Association for the Study of Pain is "an unpleasant sensory and emotional experience associated with actual or potential tissue damage or described in terms of such damage."[33] Because pain is a subjective complaint, there is no definitive way to distinguish pain that occurs in the absence of tissue damage from pain that results from such damage. Pain as a somatic delusion or masked depression is rare in cancer patients; the presence of pain usually implies a pathologic process.

Types of Pain

Three types of pain have been described based on the neuroanatomy and neurophysiology of pain pathways: somatic, visceral, and neuropathic pain. Each type results from activation and sensitization of nociceptors and mechanoreceptors in the periphery by either mechanical stimuli (e.g., tumor compression or infiltration) or chemical stimuli (e.g., epinephrine, serotonin, bradykinin, prostaglandin, or histamine).

Somatic Pain

When nociceptors are activated in cutaneous or deep tissues, somatic pain results, typically characterized by a dull or aching but well-localized pain. Metastatic bone pain, postsurgical incisional pain, and myofascial and musculoskeletal pain are common examples of somatic pain.

Visceral Pain

Visceral pain results from activation of nociceptors from infiltration, compression, extension, or stretching of the thoracic, abdominal, or pelvic viscera. This typically occurs in patients with intraperitoneal metastases and is common with pancreatic cancer. This type of pain is poorly localized; is often described as deep, squeezing, and pressurelike; and when acute is often associated with significant autonomic dysfunction, including nausea, vomiting, and diaphoresis. Visceral pain is often referred to cutaneous sites that may be remote from the site of the lesion (e.g., shoulder pain with diaphragmatic irritation). It may be associated with tenderness in the referred cutaneous site. Increasing data have demonstrated the role of kappa-opioid receptors in modulating visceral pain.[34]

Neuropathic Pain

Neuropathic pain results from injury to the peripheral or central nervous system as a consequence of tumor compression or infiltration of peripheral nerves or the spinal cord or from chemical injury to the peripheral nerve or spinal cord caused by surgery, radiation therapy, or chemotherapy. Examples of neuropathic pain include both metastatic and radiation-induced brachial and lumbosacral plexopathies, chemotherapy-induced peripheral neuropathies, paraneoplastic peripheral neuropathies, and postmastectomy, postthoracotomy, and phantom limb pain.[35] Pain from nerve injury is often severe and is described as burning or dysesthetic, with a viselike quality. The pain is typically most common in the site of sensory loss and may be associated with hypersensitivity to nonnoxious (allodynia) and noxious stimuli. Intermittently, patients complain of paroxysms of burning or electric shock–like sensations. The latter symptoms result from the phenomenon of central sensitization.

These three types of pain may occur alone or combined in the same patient. Experimental models of bone and nerve pain have provided greater insight into the mechanisms underlying these clinical pain states. Clohisy and Mantyh,[36] Lindsay et al.,[37] and Peters et al.[38] have developed both a bone tumor model and a chemotherapy-induced peripheral neuropathy model in animals that have helped to elucidate the mechanisms of pain and their biologic correlates. These correlative studies with animal models provide the opportunity to test both bone and nerve pain model responses to clinical treatments. For example, opioids, gabapentin, and nonsteroidal anti-inflammatory agents produce analgesic efficacy in the bone tumor model.[36]

Temporal Aspects of Pain

Acute Pain

Acute pain is characterized by a well-defined temporal pattern of pain onset, generally associated with subjective and objective physical signs and with hyperactivity of the autonomic nervous system. These signs provide the physician with objective evidence that substantiates the patient's complaint of pain. Acute pain is usually self-limited and responds to treatment with analgesic drug therapy and to treatment of its precipitating cause. This type of pain can be further subdivided into subacute and episodic. Subacute pain comes on over several days, often with increasing intensity, and represents a pattern of progressive pain symptomatology. Episodic or intermittent pain occurs during confined periods of time on a regular or irregular basis. All of the pain in this category of acute pain have associated autonomic hyperactivity.

Chronic Pain

Chronic pain is pain that persists for more than 3 months, with a less well-defined temporal onset. The autonomic nervous system adapts, and chronic pain patients lack the objective signs common to those with acute pain. Chronic pain leads to significant changes in personality, lifestyle, and functional ability. Treatment of chronic pain in the cancer patient is especially challenging because it requires a careful assessment of not only the intensity of the pain but its broad multidimensional aspects. Evidence suggests that the persistence of pain has a major negative effect on patients' quality of life.

Investigators have developed a nomenclature to describe a series of specific pains in cancer patients with both acute and chronic pain states. *Baseline pain* is the average pain intensity experienced for 12 or more hours during a 24-hour period. *Breakthrough pain* is a transient increase in pain to greater than moderate intensity that occurs on a baseline pain of moderate intensity or less. Various epidemiologic studies provide a range of prevalence of breakthrough pain from 23% to as high as 90% of cancer patients.[39–42] Breakthrough pain has a diversity of characteristics. In this and other series, the transitory increase in pain marks the onset or worsening of pain at the end of the dosing interval or the regularly scheduled analgesic. In other patients, it is caused by an action of the patient, referred to as *incident pain*. Sometimes the incident pain has a nonvolitional precipitant, such as flatulence. Clinical trials have focused attention on the clinical management of breakthrough pain and dosing guidelines.[42]

Intensity of Pain

Pain may also be defined on the basis of intensity, but there are limitations to a concept of pain based solely on intensity. Specific categoric scales of pain intensity have been used in which patients are asked to describe their pain as mild, moderate, severe, or excruciating. Visual analog scales (VASs) have also been used. These are often a 10-cm line anchored on either end by two points, signifying *no pain* and *worst possible pain*. The patient is asked to mark the intensity of the pain on the line. Numeric scales are also commonly used, and patients are asked to rate their pain between 1 (no pain) and 10 (worst possible pain). These scales have their limitations, but they are part of a series of validated instruments that include a measure of pain intensity as one of the components of the pain experience to be defined.

Measurement of Pain

Multidimensional pain assessment is the recommended approach to the study of pain prevalence and pain intervention. Several validated instruments for pain measurement attempt to look at it in a multidimensional way. The use of such methods can provide rapid evaluation in clinical settings of the major aspects of the pain experienced by cancer patients. The Joint Commission for the Accreditation of Healthcare Organizations require the use of pain scales in routine clinical care.[43]

Brief Pain Inventory

The Wisconsin Brief Pain Inventory (BPI) is a self-administered, easily understood, brief method to assess pain.[44] It addresses the relevant aspects of pain (history, intensity, location, and quality) and the ability of the pain to interfere with the patient's activities and helps to provide an understanding of its cause. The history of pain and its relation to the patient's disease are assessed initially. If the patient admits to pain in the past month, he or she answers questions about current manifestations of pain. If the patient has no pain, he or she skips to the end of the questionnaire to complete demographic information. For patients with pain, a human figure drawing is provided on which the patients shade the area corresponding to the pain. Patients are asked to rate their pain at its worst, their usual pain, and their pain at the time they are completing the questionnaire. The pain scales consist of numbers from 0 to 10; 0 is labeled *no pain* and 10 is labeled *pain as bad as you can imagine*. Patients are asked to report the medications or treatments they receive for pain, the percentage relief that these medications or treatment provide, and their belief about the cause of their pain. Finally, they are asked to rate how much the pain interferes with their mood, relations with other people, and functional ability (walking, sleeping, working, enjoying life). All patients, including those without pain, are asked for basic demographic information about marital status, education, occupation, spouse's occupation, and months since diagnosis. This inventory has been translated into numerous languages and has been used to assess pain in cancer patients in diverse altered settings.

McGill Pain Questionnaire

The McGill Pain Questionnaire (MPQ) is an extensively used pain assessment instrument that produces scores on four empirically derived dimensions, as well as several summary scores.[45] The instrument consists of 78 adjectives that cluster in 20 categories. Within each category, the adjectives are arranged in order of intensity from low to high. The categories are divided into four dimensions: sensory, affective, evaluative, and miscellaneous. The patient is asked to choose one adjective from each applicable category that describes an aspect of his or her current pain, and the score for each dimension is obtained by adding the rank values of the selected adjectives. A total summary score is derived by adding the scores across the four dimensions, and a total word count is also obtained. Finally, a rating of present pain intensity is made on a five-point scale. Studies with this instrument have demonstrated that the factors derived reflect specific sensory qualities and combined emotional and sensory dimensions. This tool has also been used to assess distinct score profiles according to the nature of pain. For instance, patients with acute pain tend to use more sensory words, but patients with chronic pain tend to use more affective and reaction word subgroups. The MPQ offers a methodologic approach to assess the sensory, affective, and evaluative components of pain, but it may be more difficult and cumbersome for patients to understand and complete than some other pain assessment tools and may be limited by its language constraints.

Memorial Pain Assessment Card

The Memorial Pain Assessment Card (MPAC) (Fig. 170.1) was initially developed by the Analgesic Studies Section of the Memorial Sloan-Kettering Cancer Center to assess the relative potency of new and standard analgesic drugs. In that context, this method was found repeatedly to be a valid, reliable, efficient, and sensitive measure.[46] The MPAC consists of three VASs that measure pain intensity, pain relief, and mood and a set of pain severity descriptors adapted from the Tursky rating scale. The card is 8.5 by 11.0 inches and is folded in the middle so that the four sides can be quickly presented to the patient. Three sides are imprinted with the 100-mm-long VAS scale; the fourth side is the set of Tursky adjectives. The pain intensity VAS is anchored by the terms *least possible pain* and *worst possible pain*. The patient is asked to place a mark along the line to indicate his or her subjective judgment of pain intensity. The score on this and the other VASs is obtained by measuring the distance in millimeters between the left end of the line and the patient's mark. The Tursky pain adjective scale is a categorical measure of pain intensity. Eight intensity

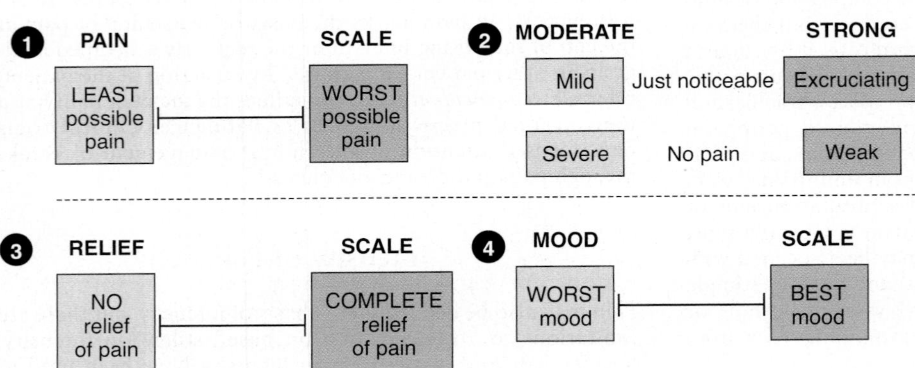

FIGURE 170.1 Memorial Pain Assessment Card, front (1 and 4) and back (2 and 3) sides. The card is folded along the broken line, and each measure is presented to the patient separately, in the numbered order. (1) Visual analog scale (VAS) for pain intensity; (2) modified Tursky pain descriptors scale; (3) VAS for pain relief; and (4) VAS for mood. (From ref. 46, with permission.)

descriptors, ranging from *no pain* to *excruciating*, are printed in a random arrangement and the patient is asked to circle the adjective that describes his or her subjective experience of pain severity. Side three of the MPAC is a pain-relief VAS. Patients are asked to indicate with a mark the degree of pain reduction they experienced after the most recent intervention, which is usually the administration of an analgesic drug. On side four, the VAS measures the subjective experience of mood; on this side patients are asked to rate their current feeling, from *worst* to *best*. The instructions for administration of these scales are simple and readily understood, and an experienced patient can complete the four ratings in less than 20 seconds.

The MPAC has been compared with the MPQ, the Profile of Mood States Questionnaire (a standardized self-report instrument that measures six dimensions of mood, reflecting degree and type of psychological distress), the Hamilton Rating Scale for Depression (an interviewer-rated scale evaluating the presence and severity of 17 symptoms typical of clinical depression), and the Zung Anxiety Scale (a standardized self-report scale that evaluates the presence and severity of various symptoms of anxiety). The MPAC and the MPQ provide reasonably equivalent assessments of the intensity dimension of pain. However, scores on the evaluative scales of the MPQ did not correlate significantly with any of the measures of the MPAC, which suggests that the cognitive-judgmental dimension of pain may be independent of the experiences of intensity, relief, and mood. None of the MPQ subscale ratings correlated significantly with the VAS ratings of mood and pain relief.

These observations have led to the conclusion that the VAS mood scale on the MPAC represents a global assessment of general psychological distress rather than a specific pain-related effect. This would suggest that the MPAC provides a broader assessment of the patient by its use of the mood scale, whereas the MPQ has a more narrow focus of simply representing pain-related emotional distress. The MPAC provides valid, multidimensional information for the evaluation of pain and distress in cancer patients. It can distinguish pain intensity from pain relief and from global suffering, and it can be used to study the subtle interactions of these factors. With repeated administration, it has now been demonstrated to be valid, reliable, easy to use, and nondisruptive. The MPAC and the BPI are the tools recommended for use in the clinical evaluation of individual patients and as outcome measures in clinical trials.

Memorial Symptom Assessment Scale

The Memorial Symptom Assessment Scale (MSAS) is a validated, patient-rated measure that provides multidimensional information about a diverse group of common symptoms.[47] Thirty-two physical and psychological symptoms are characterized in terms of intensity, frequency, and distress. The MSAS provides a Global Distress Index (MSAS-GDI), a ten-item subscale that reflects global symptom distress and separate subscales that measure physical (MSAS-Phys) and psychological (MSAS-Psych) symptom distress. Ongoing studies have confirmed its value in patients with various types of cancer, and studies of its reliability and validity with repeated administration are currently under way. The use of the MSAS allows the concurrent measurement of pain and various other symptoms, psychological distress, and psychological factors; overall, it represents a useful, patient-accepted method to measure the multidimensional issues facing cancer patients with pain. Newer studies have identified the usefulness of a short form for rapid assessment.[48]

European Organisation for Research and Treatment of Cancer Quality of Life Questionnaire-C30

The European Organisation for Research and Treatment of Cancer has included specific pain questions in its Quality of Life Questionnaire-C30 (QLQ-C30) scale. The pain scale measures pain intensity and interference with function. The pain scale has a four-level verbal rating scale (*not at all*, *a little*, *quite a bit*, *very much*), measuring the presence of pain and pain interference with daily activities. The responses are summed to a composite score and transformed to a 0 to 100 pain scale of severity. The pain severity composite score better represents the cancer pain experience than the intensity score alone. In published studies, it has been shown to reliably predict functional status, toxicity, and chemotherapy response. Because of its multiple scales, the QLQ-C30 requires more time, attention, and cooperation on the part of patients, which makes it less useful as a routine measurement tool.[49]

Edmonton Symptom Assessment Scale

The Edmonton Symptom Assessment Scale (ESAS) is a nine-item patient-reported symptom visual analog scale developed to assess symptoms in patients who receive palliative care. The scale has been validated in cancer patients and correlated closely with the MSAS and BPI measurement tools.[50]

COMMON PAIN SYNDROMES

Pain in the cancer patient results from direct tumor infiltration and from the various cancer treatments and can occur unrelated to the cancer and cancer therapy. Tables 170.1 and 170.2 list the common wide range of both acute and chronic pain syndromes in patients with cancer. These lists are a compendium of various sources and serve to summarize the broad and now well-recognized literature pain syndromes that occur often uniquely in this population of patients.[4,5,16–18,25]

Clinical Assessment of Pain

Certain general principles should be followed in evaluating cancer patients who complain of pain.[51] Lack of attention to these general principles is the major cause for misdiagnosis of a specific pain syndrome. Adequate assessment is a critical component for defining the appropriate therapeutic strategy for each patient. The general principles are the following:

- Believe the patient's complaint of pain.
- Take a careful history of the patient's pain complaint.
- Evaluate the patient's psychological state.
- Perform a careful medical and neurologic examinations.
- Order the appropriate diagnostic studies and personally review the results.
- Treat the pain to facilitate the appropriate workup.
- Reassess the patient's response to therapy.
- Individualize the diagnostic and therapeutic approaches.
- Discuss advance directives with the patient and family.

Critical to the management of the patient with cancer pain is the establishment of a trusting relationship with the physician. The complaint of pain is a symptom, not a diagnosis. Pain perception is not simply a function of the amount of physical injury sustained by the patient but is a complex state determined by multiple factors. The diagnosis of a specific pain syndrome and a complete understanding of the patient's psychological state is not always accomplished during the initial evaluation. In fact, it may take several weeks to define its nature because of the lack of radiologic or pathologic verification. It may take a similar period to fully comprehend each patient's psychological makeup. Numerous examples in the assessment of patients with pain and cancer highlight the limitations of the diagnostic process.

PRACTICE OF ONCOLOGY

TABLE 170.1

TUMOR-RELATED CHRONIC PAIN SYNDROMES

Bone Pain	**Tumor Involvement of the Peripheral Nervous System**
Multifocal or generalized bone pain	Tumor-related radiculopathy
Multiple bony metastases	Cervical plexopathy
Marrow expansion	Brachial plexopathy
Vertebral syndromes	Malignant brachial plexopathy
Atlantoaxial destruction and odontoid fractures	Idiopathic brachial plexopathy associated with Hodgkin's lymphoma
C7 to T1 syndrome	Malignant lumbosacral plexopathy
T12 to L1 syndrome	Tumor-related mononeuropathy
Sacral syndrome	Paraneoplastic painful peripheral neuropathy
Back pain and epidural compression	Subacute sensory neuropathy
Pain syndromes of the bony pelvis and hip	Sensorimotor peripheral neuropathy
Hip joint syndrome	
Headache and Facial Pain	**Pain Syndromes of the Viscera And Miscellaneous Tumor-Related Syndromes**
Intracerebral tumor	Hepatic distention syndrome
Leptomeningeal metastases	Midline retroperitoneal syndrome
Base of skull metastases	Chronic intestinal obstruction
Orbital syndrome	Peritoneal carcinomatosis
Parasellar syndrome	Malignant perineal pain
Middle cranial fossa syndrome	Malignant pelvic floor myalgia
Jugular foramen syndrome	Ureteric obstruction
Clivus syndrome	
Sphenoid sinus syndrome	**Paraneoplastic Nociceptive Pain Syndromes**
Painful cranial neuralgias	Tumor-related gynecomastia
Glossopharyngeal neuralgia	
Trigeminal neuralgia	

From ref. 25, with permission.

Take a Careful History of the Patient's Pain Complaint

A careful history of the patient's pain complaint should include the patient's description of site of pain, quality of pain, exacerbating and relieving factors, temporal pattern, exact onset, associated symptoms and signs, interference with activities of daily living, effect on the patient's psychological state, and response to previous and current analgesic therapies.[51] Patients should be asked to describe the intensity, frequency, and severity of their baseline pain and episodes of breakthrough pain. Routine pain assessment tools should be provided to patients and families to record the patient's pain experience and provide easy recording of analgesic drug use and the use of rescue medications. Multiple pain complaints are common in patients with advanced disease and must be ranked, classified, and recoded.

Evaluate the Patient's Psychological State

The patient's current level of anxiety and depression must be clarified and his or her past history of such symptoms must be defined. Knowledge of the patient's previous psychiatric history and need for past hospitalization for psychiatric care helps to clarify the patient's potential psychological risk.

TABLE 170.2

TREATMENT-RELATED CHRONIC PAIN SYNDROMES

Postchemotherapy Pain Syndromes	Phantom breast pain
Chronic painful peripheral neuropathy	Phantom anus pain
Avascular necrosis of femoral or humeral head	Phantom bladder pain
Plexopathy associated with intraarterial infusion	Stump pain
Chronic Pain Associated with Hormonal Therapy	Postsurgical pelvic floor myalgia
Gynecomastia with hormonal therapy for prostate cancer	**Chronic Postradiation Pain Syndromes**
Chronic Postsurgical Pain Syndromes	Radiation-induced brachial and lumbosacral plexopathies
Postmastectomy pain syndrome	Radiation-induced peripheral nerve tumors
Postradical neck dissection pain	Chronic radiation myelopathy
Postthoracotomy pain	Chronic radiation enteritis and proctitis
Postoperative frozen shoulder	Burning perineum syndrome
Phantom pain syndromes	Osteoradionecrosis
Phantom limb pain	

Adapted from ref. 25.

Information on how the patient has handled previous painful events may provide insight into whether the patient has demonstrated chronic illness behavior or has a past history of a chronic pain syndrome. It is important to know about a personal or family history of alcohol or drug dependence to understand why the patient may be fearful of taking or refuse to take opioid drugs.

Because each patient has his or her own understanding of the meaning of pain, it is useful to have the patient elaborate this meaning.[52–55] Does he or she think it represents recurrent tumor, or is he or she convinced it is simply arthritis? Evidence suggests that when patients have a clear understanding of the meaning of their pain as representing recurrent tumor, they have increased psychological distress.

The importance of defining the psychological makeup of the patient with pain is supported by a variety of studies that have focused on the effect of suffering in patients with pain.[52–57] Psychological factors play a significant role in accounting for the differences in pain experiences in cancer patients. A series of psychiatric syndromes have been described for cancer patients, with depression occurring in as many as 25% of patients.[53,56] The depression presents either as an acute stress response or as a major depression. Awareness of the common psychiatric syndromes when evaluating the pain complaint expands the physician's understanding of such a complaint.

Although it is critical to know as much as possible about each patient with pain, some information may not be readily available in the first interview; in some instances it may never be available because of the lack of intellectual competence on the patient's part to define clearly the various components of the pain complaint. It is often necessary to verify the history by consulting a family member who may provide information that the patient is unable or unwilling to provide. The family may be more objective in assessing a disability of a patient who underreports his or her symptoms. Similarly, in a patient who is a poor historian, the family member may be able to provide essential information that may alter the diagnostic approach. All attempts should be made to compile a careful history and define the medical, neurologic, and psychological profile of the pain complaint. In geriatric patients with compromised cognitive function, the use of geriatric pain and symptom scales should be integrated.[27]

It is also useful to define for the patient the goal of treatment. Some patients may have unreasonable expectations for adequate pain control, whereas others fail to critically consider the various options available to them. Before starting any new procedure, review carefully with patients the risks and benefits to provide them with their expectation of the potential outcome of the therapeutic approach. As patients become more active in defining advance directives and as they focus on the quality of life, it is critical to ask patients to define what they would do if the pain were intractable or intolerable.[56] Did the patient have a family member who died a painful death? In the authors' experience, patients who have had such an experience are particularly fearful of their own deaths. Does the patient have suicidal thoughts or a pact with a family member? Does the patient have a family history of suicide? Does the patient have drugs in reserve or a gun in the house that he or she might use in desperation? In a study by Chochinov et al.,[56] pain alone did not correlate with patients' suicidal ideation. Significant depression appeared to be the major correlating factor, although pain clearly played a role in the development of depression in some patients. This series of questions allows patients to discuss openly their fears of death and their intention to take matters into their own hands rather than trust the health care professional. Such open discussions can allow the physician to better define for the patient the options for care and to reassure the patient of the physician's commitment to care. Because patients rarely offer this information unless requested, it is critical to develop specific questions that can be readily integrated into the initial history taking by the physician. Discussing with the patient how he or she would die and engaging the patient in a discussion of his or her concerns and desires can address the commonly heard comment of patients, "I have never died before, how do I do it?"

Perform Careful Medical and Neurologic Examinations

Medical and neurologic examinations help provide the necessary data to substantiate the history. They also provide a direct assessment of the cognitive status of the patient. Knowledge of the referral patterns of pain and the common cancer pain syndromes can direct the examinations. The commonly described pain syndromes in cancer patients associated with postmastectomy pain can readily be defined as separate from tumor infiltration of the brachial plexus.[58]

The physical and neurologic examinations allow the physician to visually inspect and palpate the site of pain and to look for the associated physical and neurologic signs that might help to better define the nature of the pain symptom. Defining the degree of motor or sensory changes can help identify the specific site in the nervous system that may be involved. Similarly, in patients with sensory loss, the presence of allodynia and hyperesthesia can further identify the nature of the sensory problem and define a neuropathic pain syndrome. Moreover, the degree of muscle spasm, gait instability, and impaired coordination can only be fully assessed by such an evaluation. In patients with neuropathic pain, the use of quantitative sensory testing can help define the underlying mechanism and determine selection of drug therapy.

Order the Appropriate Diagnostic Studies and Personally Review the Results

Diagnostic studies confirm the diagnosis and define in patients with metastatic disease the site and extent of tumor infiltration. Computed tomography and magnetic resonance imaging (MRI) are the most useful diagnostic procedures for evaluating cancer patients with pain. Positron emission tomography helps to further define tumor and differentiate tumor from radiation injury and postsurgical injury. The bone scan is a useful screening device and is more sensitive for demonstrating abnormalities in the bone before changes appear on a plain radiograph. However, a negative finding on bone scan does not rule out bony metastatic disease, nor does a positive finding on bone scan confirm the diagnosis of metastatic tumor. In patients with collapsed vertebral bodies, MRI can distinguish osteoporotic from tumor-induced bony changes. The physician should review the results personally with the radiologist to correlate any pathologic change with the site of pain. As well, the measurement of tumor markers such as carcinoembryonic antigen, cancer antigen (CA) 125, CA 15-3, and prostate-specific antigen can be useful in a patient in whom recurrent tumor is suspected. The use of radiolabeled carcinoembryonic antigen to scan for tumor recurrence may be helpful to differentiate recurrent colon and other gastrointestinal tumors and recurrent lung tumors from postoperative changes. In certain pain syndromes, the presence of recurrent disease is closely associated with the onset of pain (e.g., the appearance of late postthoracotomy pain syndrome in a patient after initial resolution of the postoperative pain).[16]

Treat the Pain to Facilitate the Appropriate Workup

No patient should be evaluated inadequately because they are in severe pain. Early management of the pain while the source is investigated markedly improves the patient's ability to participate in the necessary diagnostic procedures. During the initial evaluation of the pain complaint, early consideration of the use of alternative methods of pain control, including anesthetic and neurosurgical approaches, should be considered (e.g., the temporary use of a local anesthetic via an epidural catheter to manage sacral pain).

Reassess the Patient's Response to Therapy

Continual reassessment of the response of the patient's pain complaint to the prescribed therapy provides the best method to validate the initial diagnosis as correct. If relief is less than predicted or if the pain worsens, reassessment of the treatment approach or a search for a new cause of the pain should be considered.

Individualize the Diagnostic and Therapeutic Approaches

Evaluation of the patient must be closely linked to the patient's level of function, ability to participate in the diagnostic workup, willingness to undergo the necessary diagnostic approaches, objective evidence that treatment approaches may be beneficial, and life expectancy. Careful judgment is required to select diagnostic approaches that will have a direct effect on the choice of the therapeutic strategy or will answer a specific question. The random use of diagnostic procedures in these patients, particularly those with advanced cancer and significant pain, is inappropriate. Open discussion with the patient about the need for assessment as well as the therapeutic options is critical to allow the patient to be part of the decision-making process. For some patients, diagnostic procedures such as MRI are inappropriate because they simply confirm the existence of a disease for which no treatment is available or for which the treatment would be a major surgical procedure (e.g., vertebral body resection) that would be inappropriate for a dying patient. Patient refusal of evaluation or treatment must be respected when the physician has fully explained the options and is convinced that the patient has an accurate understanding of the implications of undertaking no further workup or treatment.

Discuss Advance Directives with the Patient and Family

When approaches for treatment are being developed, there must be an open discussion about advance directives so that the physician has a clear understanding of the patient's goal for therapy or his or her ambivalence in developing a therapeutic strategy. The physician must have unconditional positive regard for the patient, placing the control of symptoms of pain and treatment of psychological distress in the highest regard. Knowledge of the patient's decisions about resuscitation, living wills, and symptom management should he or she become incompetent improves the physician's ability to appropriately and humanely care for the dying patient with advanced disease.[54]

MANAGEMENT OF CANCER PAIN

Evidence-based cancer pain management follows a systematic strategy of applying demonstrated interventions in the context of individual needs, circumstances, and preferences. The basic approach employs three categories of agents: opioid analgesics, nonopioid analgesics, and adjuvant therapies. The foundation of this approach is an individualized combination of opioid and nonopioid drugs; to this foundation is added tailored care that selects from a broad array of adjuvant interventions to achieve maximum comfort for the individual patient. Guidelines are available to assist the clinician in determining a foundation treatment plan (the reader is referred to the National Comprehensive Cancer Network, American Pain Society guidelines, ESMO guidelines, and British Pain Society as excellent sources of cancer pain management guidelines).[8–13] To enhance the effectiveness of this foundation, many pharmacologic and nonpharmacologic options exist for tailoring adjuvant care to individual exigencies.

The sections that follow will emphasize the principles of pharmacologic, nonpharmacologic, procedural, and manual management of cancer pain and briefly describe anesthesia and neurosurgical approaches to pain management to which the oncologist might refer a patient for specialized procedures.

Pharmacologic Management of Cancer Pain

Analgesic Drug Therapy: The Mainstay of Cancer Pain Management

Cancer pain management combines treatment of the primary disease with (1) analgesic drug therapy and (2) specific approaches that may include anesthetic, neurosurgical, rehabilitative, psychological (cognitive-behavioral), psychiatric, or complementary and alternative methods. The clinician begins with determining a patient-specific appropriate analgesic drug plan. Titration to effective pain relief and individualization of treatment represent hallmarks at this stage in the therapeutic approach. In recent years, standard analgesic drug therapy has become more effective due to increased sophistication in the use of analgesic drugs, coupled with research to understand the underlying mechanisms of pain. These new and more effective analgesic practices include the use of novel means of drug administration, particularly transdermal and transmucosal delivery; novel methods, such as the use of bisphosphonates and calcitonin for bone pain, and novel approaches to neuropathic pain, such as antidepressants and anticonvulsants; and anesthetic, neurosurgical, psychological, and psychiatric approaches concurrently applied in the overall continuum of care.

As noted above, numerous guidelines for the management of cancer pain have been issued by various organizations and researchers.[8–13] All of these guidelines have defined analgesic drug therapy as the mainstay of treatment and have articulated the aims of drug therapy as achievement of adequate pain relief safely within an acceptable time frame, minimization of side effects of treatment, and ongoing analgesia by the most convenient and least noxious means available. Yet, despite available guidelines and an agreed-upon approach to cancer pain management, determination of the best treatment path for the individual patient remains a complex, individualized process.

The World Health Organization Cancer Pain Guidelines

The WHO guidelines on cancer pain continue to provide a framework approach for pharmacologic management of cancer pain management. Field testing of these guidelines, as well as clinical experience, has shown that 70% to 90% of cancer patients' pain can be controlled using a simple and inexpensive method described as the *three-step analgesic ladder*.[59,60] The ladder describes a process for combining nonopioid, opioid, and adjuvant drugs, titrated to meet the individual needs of the patient according to the severity of pain and its pathophysiology A randomized controlled trial of an algorithm based on the WHO ladder demonstrated that a standardized approach to cancer pain management using the algorithm provided more effective analgesia than routine oncology care.[61] These new studies suggest that a two-step ladder is equally effective for cancer pain management, and the WHO is beginning a process of guideline revision and updates.[62]

Step 1 of the WHO ladder focuses on analgesic drug therapy for patients with mild to moderate cancer pain. Such patients should be treated with a nonopioid analgesic that may or may not be combined with an adjuvant drug, depending on the specific pain pathophysiology. For example, in a patient with mild pain from a peripheral neuropathy, the combination of a nonopioid with a tricyclic antidepressant or an anticonvulsant drug would be appropriate.

Step 2 of the WHO ladder focuses on patients with moderate pain who do not experience adequate pain relief from a nonopioid analgesic. These patients are candidates for a combination of a nonopioid, such as aspirin, acetaminophen, cyclooxygenase 2 (COX-2) inhibitors, or other nonsteroidal anti-inflammatory drug (NSAID), and low doses of opioid analgesics, such as codeine, oxycodone, or morphine, usually dosed at less than 60 mg oral morphine equivalents (OME) daily. These patients often require adjuvant drugs, depending on the pain pathophysiology.

Step 3 pertains to patients who report either severe pain (often gauged as greater than 7 to 10 on a 0 to 10 scale) or moderate pain that is inadequately managed after appropriate administration of drugs at the second step of the WHO ladder. For these patients, nonopioids are often used in combination with more potent doses of opioids to mitigate the opioid effect, and adjuvants are administered depending on the pain pathophysiology or need to control other concurrent symptoms in the individual patient. Opioid doses on step 3 are commonly greater than 60 mg OME daily.

In short, the analgesic drug ladder of the WHO defines a method for using drug combinations in three categories: nonopioids, opioids, and adjuvants; it is based on previously well-tested pharmacologic principles. However, controversy in the application of the WHO ladder continues to surround the choice of analgesic drug for the individual patient.[63–66] For example, a meta-analysis of the role of NSAIDs in bone pain found them to be no more or less effective than opioids.[67]

Cancer Pain Management Using the World Health Organization Three-Step Analgesic Ladder

Nonopioid Analgesics for Cancer Pain Management. The nonopioid analgesics include acetaminophen and the NSAIDs, of which aspirin is the prototypic agent. These compounds are most commonly administered orally. Their analgesia is limited by a ceiling effect, such that increasing the dose beyond a certain level (900 to 1,300 mg per dose of aspirin) produces no increase in peak effect. Tolerance and physical dependence do not occur with repeated administration. Aspirin and the other NSAIDs have analgesic, antipyretic, anti-inflammatory, and antiplatelet actions. Some NSAIDs, such as choline magnesium trisalicylate, lack the antiplatelet effects of aspirin and may have less collateral toxicity in cancer patients already at risk of bleeding. Others (e.g., ibuprofen) appear to produce fewer gastrointestinal side effects than aspirin. The COX-2 inhibitors potentially offer less gastrointestinal (GI) toxicity and without affecting platelet function. However, the drug currently marketed as a COX-2 inhibitor—celecoxib—has not been systematically studied in cancer patients to define its particular role in pain management; concerns regarding cardiovascular side effects have limited use of this class of agents.[68] Acetaminophen, an analgesic and antipyretic agent equipotent to aspirin, is much less effective as an anti-inflammatory agent but does not interfere with platelet function.

The nonopioid analgesics are generally thought to produce analgesia by inhibiting activation of peripheral nociceptors through their prevention of the formation of prostaglandin E_2, a known sensitizer of peripheral receptors to nociceptive stimulation from tissue injury. The NSAIDs differ from one another both in duration of their analgesic action and in their pharmacokinetic profile. Ibuprofen and fenoprofen have short half-lives and the same duration of action as aspirin, whereas diflunisal and naproxen have longer half-lives and are longer acting. Because clinical experience has found that some patients respond better to one NSAID than to another, each patient should be given an adequate trial of one drug on a regular basis before switching to another. Survey data from the WHO demonstration projects suggest that 20% to 40% of patients obtain pain relief with the use of nonopioid analgesics alone.[69]

These drugs are thought to play a special role in the management of bone pain because numerous studies have shown that aspirin inhibits tumor growth in an animal model of metastatic bone tumor. A meta-analysis of studies using NSAIDs to treat bone pain did not demonstrate them to be more effective than weak opioids such as codeine, oxycodone, and propoxyphene.[67] Recent data that detail cancer-related bone pain as a neuropathic pain model have challenged the dogma of NSAIDs for bone pain.[36]

Numerous studies have elucidated the major risk factors for GI toxicity, particularly ulcerative complications, associated with NSAIDs. These risk factors include advanced age, higher doses, concomitant administration of corticosteroids, and history of either ulcer disease or previous GI complications from NSAIDs. Various prophylactic therapies are administered to prevent GI complications. Misoprostol is the only U.S. Food and Drug Administration (FDA)–approved medication for this indication; a Cochrane systematic review supports its use for prevention of NSAID-induced GI complications.[70] More commonly, proton-pump inhibitors are prescribed, which have been associated with significantly decreased frequency of NSAID-related dyspepsia and fewer ulcers diagnosed by endoscopy.[71] Whether this leads to fewer GI bleeds and reduced health care utilization is still being debated. An empiric approach at this time is to administer misoprostol or a proton-pump inhibitor to all patients who are receiving NSAIDs with significant risk factors for GI complications.[72]

Nonopioid drugs represent the front-line approach for cancer pain management, but the choice and use of nonopioids need to be individualized. Although several NSAIDs have been approved by the FDA for use as analgesics for mild to moderate pain (Table 170.3), guidelines for the use of NSAIDs in patients with cancer are largely empirical. According to a 2004 Cochrane systematic review of 42 trials involving cancer pain patients, the evidence demonstrated at best a non-statistically significant trends toward improvements when NSAIDs and opioids were combined; conclusions were limited by the short duration of the studies.[73] The clinician must select an agent based on evidence, individual patient history, and patient-specific considerations, and then must give the patient an adequate trial of that nonopioid analgesic before switching to an alternative one. Such a trial should include administration of the drug to maximum levels at regular intervals. Because there is a great variability among patient responses to different drugs, patients may require trials with several NSAIDs before finding an effective drug and dose regimen. If pain relief is not obtained, adding an opioid to a nonopioid provides additive analgesia.

Combinations containing codeine, oxycodone, and propoxyphene are available, but these combinations often contain less than the full dose of 650 mg of aspirin or acetaminophen. Prescribing each drug separately provides a better method for individualizing pain control; this is particularly important when the patient requires escalation of the combination to provide analgesia, in which case the additional amount of the NSAID or acetaminophen may become excessive.

TABLE 170.3

NONOPIOID ANALGESICS FOR MILD TO MODERATE PAIN

Class	Generic Name	Half-Life (h)	Dosing Schedule	Recommended Starting Dose (mg)	Maximum Starting Dose (mg)
Salicylates	Aspirin	3–12	q4–6h	2,600	6,000
	Choline magnesium trisalicylate	9–17	q12h	200	600
	Diflunisal	8–12	q12h	1,500 mg × 1, then 1,000 q12h	4,000
p-Aminophenol derivative	Acetaminophen (paracetamol)	2–4	q4–6h	2,600	4,000
Propionic acids	Ibuprofen	1.8–2	q4–8h	1,200	3,200
	Fenoprofen	2–3	q4–6h	800	3,200
	Ketoprofen	2–3	q6–8h	150	300
	Naproxen	13	q12h	550	1,100
	Naproxen sodium	13	q12h	550	1,100
Acetic acids	Etodolac	7	q6–8h	600	1,200
	Ketorolac	4–7	q6h	15–30 q6h IV, IM 10 q6h PO	120 IV, IM 40 PO
Fenamates	Meclofenamic acid	1.3	q6–8h	150	400
	Mefenamic acid	2	q6h	500 × 1, then 250 q6h	1,000
COX-2 inhibitor	Celecoxib	11	qd–q12	100	200

IV, intravenous; IM, intramuscular; PO, by mouth; COX-2, cyclooxygenase 2.

Opioid Drugs for Cancer Pain Management. The opioid analgesics, of which morphine is the prototype, vary in potency, efficacy, and adverse effects. These drugs produce their analgesic effects by binding to discrete opiate receptors in the peripheral and central nervous systems. In contrast to the nonopioid analgesics, opioid analgesics, at least the opioid pure agonists, do not appear to have a ceiling effect (i.e., as the dose is escalated on a log scale, the increment in analgesia is linear to the point of loss of consciousness). There are also series of drugs that are pure antagonists (i.e., they block the effect of morphine at the receptor). The antagonist drug most commonly used in clinical practice is naloxone, which is administered to reverse respiratory depression and other complications associated with opioid overdose.

Effective use of the opioid drugs requires the balancing of the most desirable effects of pain relief with the undesirable effects of nausea, vomiting, mental clouding, sedation, constipation, tolerance, and physical dependence. These undesirable effects impose a practical limit on the dose useful for a particular patient and have led to the concept of opioid responsiveness.

The use of opioids in the management of cancer pain remains a controversial issue.[5,63–66,74–83] Some of the controversies include their role in the management of neuropathic pain, which has been suggested to be *opioid resistant*, the specific choice of opioid drug, the use of sequential trials of opioids, routes of administration, development of tolerance, risk of addiction, economic factors influencing these controversies, and the concern that opioids are agents of physician-assisted suicide and euthanasia. The following principles take account of these controversies while laying out a basic approach to the use of opioids in cancer pain management (Table 170.4).

1. *Start with a specific drug for a specific type of pain.* As defined by the WHO three-step analgesic ladder, the specific drug chosen depends in part on the degree of pain intensity and the type of pain. Cancer patients commonly have multiple sites and types of pain. A continuum of opioid responsiveness, rather than an all-or-none phenomenon, has been clearly observed. *Opioid responsiveness* is defined as the degree of analgesia achieved during dose escalation to either intolerable side effects or adequate analgesia. Patient characteristics and pain-related factors, as well as drug-selective effects, influence this variable response.[65]

It has been suggested that neuropathic pain, which accounts for 15% to 20% of pain problems that are difficult to manage, is opioid-resistant and that opioid drugs should not be used in this patient population.[84] In fact studies that explored reasons for inadequate pain treatment have identified that up to two-thirds of cancer pain patients have some contribution of neuropathic pain to their global pain syndrome[61]; when the concept of bone pain as a neuropathic pain syndrome is included, this number jumps again.[36] Studies of cancer patients with both nociceptive and neuropathic pain, as well as controlled studies of nonmalignant neuropathic pain, demonstrate the variable responsiveness of neuropathic pain to opioid analgesics. Hence, the contribution of neuropathic pain must be considered when assessing opioid responsiveness.

A wide range of adjuvant analgesics has been suggested to provide analgesia alone or in combination with opioid drug therapy, and there are specific adjuvants for bone pain and neuropathic pain. The choice of a specific drug is dictated not only by pain intensity and type of pain, but also by the patient's prior opioid exposure, history of allergy, and history of side effects.

The WHO's Cancer Pain Relief Program has developed cancer pain guidelines that designate morphine as the drug of choice based on practical, not scientific, considerations. The introduction of the WHO program rapidly demonstrated the limited availability of morphine worldwide for oral treatment of chronic cancer pain.[6,14] Morphine consumption worldwide is now used as an indicator of the success of the WHO Cancer Pain Relief Program.[15] Controlled-release oral morphine is currently available in a wide range of doses from 15 to 200 mg; differing products provide options for every 8-, 12-, and 24-hour administration. These preparations provide analgesia comparable to that of immediate-release forms and offer increased convenience, improved compliance, and a reduction in duration of pain. Historically, the dogma was to titrate patients to adequate pain relief using 4-hourly doses and then

TABLE 170.4

GUIDELINES FOR THE RATIONAL USE OF ANALGESICS IN THE MANAGEMENT OF CANCER PAIN

Start with a Specific Drug for a Specific Type of Pain
Know the pharmacology of the drug prescribed
Know the relative potency of the drug
Know the duration of the analgesic effect
Know the pharmacokinetics of the drug
Know the equianalgesic doses for the drug and its route of administration

Administer Analgesic on a Regular Basis
Gear the route of administration to the patient's needs
Oral
Buccal
Rectal
Subcutaneous
Intrathecal
Sublingual
Transmucosal
Transdermal
Intravenous
Intraventricular

Use a Combination of Drugs to Provide Additive Analgesia
Narcotic plus nonnarcotic (aspirin, acetaminophen, nonsteroidal anti-inflammatory drugs)
Narcotic plus adjuvants

Anticipate and Treat Side Effects
Sedation
Respiratory depression
Nausea and vomiting
Constipation
Multifocal myoclonus and seizures

Management of the Tolerant Patient
Use combinations of nonopioid and opioid drugs
Use combinations of drug therapy, anesthetic, and neurosurgical procedures
Switch to an alternative opioid analgesic, starting with one-half the equianalgesic dose
Use epidural local anesthetics
Reassess the nature of the pain

Prevent and Treat Acute Withdrawal
Taper drugs slowly

Anticipate Complications
Overdose
Psychological dependence

combine into sustained-release doses that provide an equal amount of opioid in 24 hours. In a recent randomized clinical trial it was demonstrated that for cancer pain patients receiving greater than 60 mg OME daily, titration with sustained release product was equally efficacious and yielded fewer side effects.[85]

The clinician's armamentarium for managing cancer pain now encompasses a series of opioid alternatives to morphine, including congeners of morphine—hydromorphone, oxycodone, oxymorphone—as well as methadone, levorphanol, fentanyl, and buprenorphine. The choice of agent depends on the clinician's knowledge about how to use the drug, patient factors such as age and renal function, route of delivery, opioid availability, and cost (Tables 170.5 and 170.6). Recently, new formulations of these drugs have been marketed with various combinations to deter tampering and to reduce their diversion.[86]

Hydromorphone has poor oral availability and a short half-life. Its high solubility and availability in high-potency parenteral form (10 mg/mL) make it a useful choice for chronic subcutaneous administration. Because of its short half-life, it is commonly used in the elderly patient. Myoclonus has been reported after high doses, possibly due to accumulation of its metabolites (3-0 methyl-glucuronide and hydromorphone-6-glucuronide).[87] When compared in a double-blind trial of patient-controlled analgesia, no differences in analgesia or side effects were noted between morphine and hydromorphone; these findings have been confirmed in several settings.[88,89] Although cognitive performance was poor in the hydromorphone group, patients reported better mood than those who received morphine.

Oxycodone, which is commonly administered in a 5-mg dose at the second step of the WHO analgesic ladder, can also be used in the third step at higher doses. It is available in a

TABLE 170.5

RELATIVE SINGLE-DOSE POTENCIES OF COMMONLY USED OPIOID DRUGS FOR PAIN AND THEIR ORAL-INTRAVENOUS RATIOS

Drug	Equianalgesic Intravenous or Intramuscular Dose (mg)	Oral-Intravenous Ratios
Morphine	10	3
Oxycodone	Not available	Not available
Oxymorphone	1	10
Hydromorphone	1.5	5
Methadone[a]	10	1–2
Levorphanol	2	2
Fentanyl	250 mcg	1 (transdermal intravenous)

This table should be used as a guide only. Individual dosing and drug selection depend on each patient's particular situation and comprehensive assessment.
[a]Refer to Table 170.6 for rotation to methadone for long-term administration.

PRACTICE OF ONCOLOGY

TABLE 170.6

VARIABILITY IN DOSE RATIOS WHEN SWITCHING ORAL MORPHINE, ORAL HYDROMORPHONE, AND TRANSDERMAL FENTANYL TO METHADONE

Dose	Morphine–Methadone Ratio
Morphine (mg/24 h)	
30–90	4:1
91–300	9:1
≥300	12:1
Hydromorphone (mg/24 h)	Hydromorphone–methadone ratio
<330	0.95:1
≥330	1.6:1
Fentanyl	Fentanyl–methadone ratio
50–2500 [mu]g/h	250 [mu]g/h:1 mg/h

Based on direct morphine to methadone, hydromorphone to methadone, and fentanyl to methadone conversion studies, when the clinician needs to rotate to methadone convert all opioids first to intravenous (IV) morphine (see Table 170.5 for equianalgesic dose ratios) and then convert the IV morphine dose to an IV methadone dose using a 10:1 ratio. The resulting methadone dose may be higher in less opioid-tolerant patients and lower in highly opioid-tolerant patients. (See ref. 5.)

slow-release preparation.[90] Its half-life is 3 to 4 hours. Oxymorphone is its active metabolite. Oxymorphone is currently available in oral sustained release, intravenous, and rectal preparations and serves as an alternative to morphine and its other congeners. Oxymorphone has a reduced histamine effect and may be of use in patients who complain of headache or itch after administration of other opioids.

Levorphanol has high bioavailability but a long plasma half-life (12 to 16 hours). It should be used cautiously because, with repeated administration, accumulation may occur.

The role of methadone in managing cancer pain also remains controversial.[5,75–78] Methadone represents a second-line drug for cancer pain patients who have had prior exposure to opioids. It is a relatively inexpensive oral analgesic, but its name has negative connotations for cancer patients, who view methadone as a drug used to treat addicts. The bioavailability of methadone is higher than that of morphine (85% vs. 35%, respectively). Its analgesic potency also differs, with a parenteral to oral ratio of 1:2 in contrast to 1:6 for morphine. Moreover, the plasma half-life of methadone is 17 to 24 hours, with reports of up to 50 hours in some cancer patients, but with a duration of analgesia of only 4 to 8 hours. Significant adverse effects have been reported in cancer patients receiving methadone by various routes. Most notably, recent reports of drug-induced long QT syndrome have increased concern, especially in cancer patients who may be on multiple agents that can prolong the QT interval.[91–93] The discrepancy between the analgesic duration and plasma half-life of methadone has made it a difficult drug to use in the naive patient because of the need for careful titration. In a randomized trial, initial treatment of cancer pain with morphine versus methadone provided equal analgesic efficacy.[94]

A number of case reports have highlighted the possibly greater analgesic potency of methadone than the often quoted 1:1 equivalency with morphine.[75–78] Studies of interindividual differences in response to opioid analgesics have demonstrated that dramatically reduced dosages of methadone are required to produce analgesia in patients chronically taking morphine or hydromorphone. Several authors have shown marked reductions in the equianalgesic dose of methadone when patients with either uncontrolled pain or extreme side effects were switched to methadone.[5,76] These clinical survey studies suggested up to a 75% reduction in the methadone equianalgesic dose when switching from hydromorphone to methadone (Table 170.6).

In the only prospective study, Ripamonti et al.[76] developed a specific dose ratio based on the patients' morphine doses. For patients taking 30 to 90 mg of morphine, the dose ratio is 4:1; for those taking 90 to 300 mg daily, the dose ratio is 6:1; and for those taking 300 mg or more, the dose ratio is 8:1. Bruera et al.[75] developed a similar ratio for hydromorphone based on survey data. In patients who received more than 330 mg of hydromorphone, the dose ratio is 1.6:1.0; and in those who received less than 300 mg, the dose ratio is 0.95:1.0.

Studies of the use of methadone by experienced clinicians in caring for advanced cancer patients at home report fewer dose escalations and good pain control, which supports the use of methadone in home settings.[78] Methadone can be administered by a variety of routes, but the subcutaneous route is associated with adverse effects, including cutaneous hypersensitivity.[95] Due to its long half-life, some offer the suggestion that methadone be administered every 8 to 12 hours, whereas others have demonstrated analgesic efficacy and safety in acute 3- to 4-hour dosing intervals.[96] Ongoing studies are attempting to elucidate better the clinical pharmacology of methadone to facilitate its broader use.

Meperidine is a drug that should not be used chronically in the management of patients with cancer pain. Meperidine has a poor parenteral to oral ratio (1:4). It is available in oral and intramuscular preparations, but repetitive intramuscular administration is associated with local tissue fibrosis and sterile abscess. Repetitive dosing of meperidine (more than 250 mg/d) can lead to accumulation of normeperidine, an active metabolite that can produce central nervous system hyperexcitability.[97] This hyperirritability is characterized by subtle mood effects followed by tremors, multifocal myoclonus, and occasional seizures. It occurs most commonly in patients with renal disease but can also occur after repeated administration in patients with normal renal function. Naloxone does not reverse meperidine-induced seizures, and its use in meperidine toxicity is controversial. There have been some case reports that the use of naloxone has precipitated generalized seizures in individual patients. In rare instances, central nervous system toxicity characterized by hyperpyrexia, muscle rigidity, and seizure has been reported after the administration of a single dose of meperidine to patients receiving treatment with monoamine oxidase inhibitors.

With the development of a novel transdermal patch for administration and various transmucosal preparations, fentanyl is an opioid analgesic used effectively in cancer patients for management of both acute and chronic pain.[98] The half-life of fentanyl is 1 to 2 hours. Guidelines for fentanyl use are available that summarize all of the current data.[79] In chronic cancer pain management, relative potency comparisons have not been fully established, but the common dosing guideline is that 4 mg of intravenous morphine is equivalent to 100 mcg of intravenous fentanyl. The uniqueness of this preparation facilitates the management of patients who are unable to take drugs by mouth by providing them with continuous opioid analgesia. Patches are currently available in 12.5 to 100 mcg/h doses and are changed every 72 hours. When a patient is started on the fentanyl patch, there is up to a 12- to 15-hour delay in the onset of analgesia, and alternate approaches must be used to maintain patients' pain control during this period. Specific guidelines for switching to the fentanyl patch after an intravenous infusion of fentanyl have been developed and are based on use of a 1:1 conversion ratio.[79] Fentanyl can also be used as an anesthetic premedication, as well as intravenously for pain control. Oral transmucosal and sublingual formulations have demonstrated effectiveness in treating breakthrough pain in cancer patients.[79,99,100]

Buprenorphine, a mixed agonist/antagonist opioid drug, is used to treat chronic noncancer pain and drug addiction and is also available in a transdermal preparation for cancer pain management. It is reported to be a useful agent in patients with moderate to severe pain, and it does not accumulate in patients with renal dysfunction. Its place in the management of cancer pain among the other opioids is not yet fully clarified.[101]

2. *Know the equianalgesic dose of the drug and its route of administration.* Knowing the equianalgesic dose (i.e., the dose of one analgesic drug that is equivalent in the pain-relieving potential of another analgesic drug) can ensure more appropriate drug use. The equianalgesic dose guides the recommended starting dose, with the optimal dose for each patient determined by dose adjustment. *Relative potency* is the ratio of the doses of two analgesics required to produce the same effect. Estimates of relative potency allow calculation of the equianalgesic dose, which provides the basis for selecting the appropriate dose when switching drugs or changing the route of administration of the same drug. The values in Table 170.5 are based on studies using 10 mg of morphine as the standard dose.[102] There is now evidence to suggest that relative potency may differ in single-dose and repeated-dose studies. For example, for morphine, a 1:6 relative analgesic potency ratio should be used for patients with acute pain, whereas a 1:2 or 1:3 ratio is more appropriate in patients treated with repeated doses on a chronic basis. Lack of attention to differences in drug dose is the most common cause of undermedication of pain patients.

3. *Administer analgesics regularly after initial titration.* Medication should be given regularly to maintain the plasma level of the drug above the minimum effective concentration for pain relief. In the initial titration, patients should be advised to take their medication as needed to determine their total 24-hour requirements. During this time, the patient should reach the steady-state level of drug, which depends on the drug's half-life. For morphine, steady state can be reached in 24 hours; with methadone, it may take up to 5 to 7 days to reach steady state. In patients on a fixed schedule, rescue medications equivalent to one-half of the standing dose should be available for breakthrough pain.

Continuous intravenous and subcutaneous opioid infusions to manage both acute and chronic cancer pain are commonly administered using a patient-controlled analgesic pump programmed to the patient's need with a set *lock-out time* to prevent overdosing. This method of drug administration is especially useful in managing patients with breakthrough pain. It is a significant advance in facilitating adequate titration of analgesics in chronic cancer patients, allowing discharge to home and hospice settings.

4. *Gear the route of administration to the patient's needs.* Various methods of opioid drug delivery have been developed in order to maximize pharmacologic effects and minimize side effects. Most patients require at least two routes of drug administration, and 20% need up to four approaches during the course of their cancer pain treatment.

The oral route is preferable and easy. Orally administered drugs have a slower onset of action, delayed peak time, and longer duration of effect. Drugs given parenterally have a rapid onset of action but a shorter duration of effect. Slow-release preparations of morphine, hydromorphone, and oxycodone allow more convenient dosing of cancer pain patients every 8 to 12 hours or every 24 hours.

For cancer pain management by the sublingual route, there are drugs that are well absorbed sublingually, including both fentanyl and methadone.[103] The oral transmucosal fentanyl citrate preparations have been widely studied for the management of breakthrough pain and are absorbed transmucosally.

For the rectal route, oxymorphone, hydromorphone, and morphine are available in suppository form. Oxymorphone suppositories produce analgesia equivalent to 10 mg of parenteral morphine. Slow-release oxycodone and morphine preparations have also been demonstrated to be effective rectally, and ongoing studies with rectal methadone suggest that this drug is well absorbed by the rectal route.

The transdermal route is a convenient way to deliver a potent short-acting opioid on a continuous basis. Drug is released through the skin patch at a nearly constant amount per unit time with a concentration gradient from patch to skin. Serum fentanyl concentrations increase and steady-state levels that are approached at 12 to 24 hours.[99] After patch removal, the drug persists in the skin, with falling blood levels over 24 hours. For calculation of the equianalgesic dose, 4 mg of intravenous morphine is equivalent to 100 mcg of fentanyl transdermally. Innovative transdermal delivery systems are in phase 3 testing, which include systems for immediate-dose delivery using iontophoresis and drug reservoirs. Iontophoresis is the transfer of ionic solutes through biologic membranes under the influence of an electric field. It offers an alternative system for parenteral administration and has been shown to allow for comparatively rapid achievement of fentanyl dose levels using a transdermal system.

Various parenteral routes include intermittent and continuous subcutaneous, intravenous, epidural, intraventricular, and intrathecal infusions. The use of intermittent and continuous subcutaneous infusions is most useful in patients who cannot tolerate oral analgesics because of GI obstruction or intractable nausea and vomiting and for those who do not have intravenous access. The usefulness of this technique has been demonstrated using morphine, heroin, hydromorphone, levorphanol, and fentanyl. Administration of methadone by this route is associated with the development of a cutaneous hypersensitivity syndrome.[95]

Patient-controlled analgesic pumps designed to infuse continuously but with options for bolus administration are connected to a 27-gauge butterfly needle that the patient can insert into a new subcutaneous site every 3rd to 6th day. Limited pharmacokinetic studies have demonstrated that, for example, systemic absorption of the drug at steady state reaches 87% bioavailability from subcutaneous infusion of hydromorphone.[88]

Intermittent and continuous intravenous infusions are used if intravenous access is available and more commonly in patients who are hospitalized. Specific guidelines for the use of continuous infusions have been developed.[5,104]

Use of intermittent and continuous epidural and intrathecal opioid infusions is based on the demonstration of opioid receptors in the dorsal horn of the spinal cord and the availability of opioid drugs to suppress noxious stimuli at the spinal cord level. Localized selective analgesia is produced without motor or sensory blockade. Analysis of the pharmacokinetics of epidural opioid administration demonstrates that there is significant systemic uptake after epidural injection, comparable with that after an intramuscular injection of the same drug and dose. However, distribution of the drug directly into the cerebrospinal fluid is 10 to 100 times greater. Existing studies demonstrate that this approach is used with approximately 10% of cancer patients to maximize analgesia and minimize side effects. This technique is commonly used in patients who have mixed nociceptive neuropathic pain syndromes and in whom combinations of local anesthetics and opioids are administered epidurally. A 3-year retrospective outcome study of the use of epidural catheters in the management of chronic cancer pain identified the occurrence of technical problems and infection, including epidural abscesses, in a significant number of patients. The study suggests that epidural catheters be used in patients with limited life expectancy.[105]

Smith et al.[106] completed a randomized clinical trial in which an implantable drug delivery system was compared to comprehensive medical management of refractory cancer pain. The patients using the implantable system reported better pain relief with fewer drug side effects and improved survival. Cost-effectiveness studies have not been done, but there is clearly the added cost of the pump, and the costs of the system need to be compared to the costs of nonpump medicines, with the potential savings from prevention of hospitalizations for pain management analyzed. Rarely, intraventricular opioid infusion has been used to manage patients with pain in the cervical and craniofacial region from tumor infiltration.[107] Doses between 1.0 and 7.5 mg per 24 hours have been used, and excellent results have been reported in 70% of patients. At present, there is not a clear indication that this intraventricular route offers special advantages over systemic approaches.

5. *Use a combination of drugs.* By using a combination of drugs, the physician can increase analgesic effects without escalating the opioid dose. Combinations that produce additive analgesic effects include an opioid plus a nonopioid, an opioid plus an antihistamine (100 mg of intramuscular hydroxyzine), and an opioid plus an amphetamine (10 mg of intramuscular dextroamphetamine).[108–111]

6. *Anticipate and treat side effects.* The side effects of the opioid analgesics often limit their effective use. The most common side effects are sedation, respiratory depression, nausea, vomiting, constipation, and multifocal myoclonus and seizures.

Sedation and drowsiness vary with the drug and dose and may occur after both single and repeated administration. They are mediated through activation of opiate receptors in the reticular formation and diffusely throughout the cortex. Management of these effects includes reducing the individual drug dose but giving the drug more frequently or switching to an analgesic with a shorter plasma half-life. In controlled trials, amphetamine, methylphenidate, and caffeine have been demonstrated to counteract opioid-induced sedative effects. It is important to discontinue all other drugs that might exacerbate the sedative effects of opioid analgesics, including a wide variety of medications such as cimetidine, barbiturates, and other anxiolytic medications.

Respiratory depression is the most serious adverse effect of the opioid drugs. It occurs most commonly after short-term administration of an opioid and is usually associated with other signs of central nervous system depression, including sedation and drowsiness. The opioid agonist drugs act on brainstem respiratory centers to produce, as a function of dose, increasing respiratory depression to the point of apnea. Tolerance to this effect develops rapidly with repeated drug administration, which allows prolonged use without significant risk of respiratory depression. Respiratory depression can be reversed by giving the short-acting opioid antagonist naloxone (suggested dose, 0.4 mg/mL). Repeated administration, including an intravenous drip, may be necessary to prevent respiratory arrest in such patients. In patients receiving opioids for prolonged periods who develop respiratory depression, diluted doses of naloxone (0.4 mg in 10 mL of saline) should be titrated carefully to prevent the precipitation of severe withdrawal symptoms while reversing the respiratory depression. A useful dosing nomogram for continuous intravenous infusion of naloxone has been developed in which two-thirds of the initial bolus is started on an hourly basis and titrated against the patient's symptoms.[112]

In some patients, the use of naloxone to reverse drug-induced respiratory depression can be dangerous. An endotracheal tube should be placed in the comatose patient before giving naloxone to prevent aspiration from excessive salivation and bronchial spasm induced by naloxone administration. In patients receiving meperidine over a longer period, naloxone may precipitate seizures by lowering the seizure threshold and by allowing the convulsant activity of the active metabolite, normeperidine, to become evident. In this instance, special attention must be given to the potential seizure effect of naloxone. If naloxone is used, diluted doses, slow titration, and appropriate seizure precautions are advised. There is insufficient clinical evidence to make more specific recommendations. If respiratory support can be effected by other means (i.e., continuous stimulation to maintain the patient's wakefulness), such an approach may place the patient at less risk and clearly in less discomfort.

The opioid analgesics produce nausea and vomiting by an action limited to the medullary chemoreceptor trigger zone. The incidence of nausea and vomiting is markedly increased in ambulatory patients. Tolerance develops to these side effects with repeated administration. The occurrence of nausea with one drug does not mean that all drugs will produce it. Switching to alternative opioid analgesics and using an antiemetic together with the opioid analgesic are ways to obviate this effect. Lack of controlled trials to identify a specific first-line agent has supported the practice of using sequential trials of agents, beginning with prochlorperazine concurrently with the opioid, to clarify a useful regimen. Droperidol has also been noted to be effective against opioid-induced nausea and vomiting.[113]

Constipation results from the action of these drugs at multiple sites in the GI tract and in the spinal cord to produce a decrease in the intestinal secretions and peristalsis, which leads to a dry stool and constipation. When opioid analgesics are started, a regular bowel regimen, including use of cathartics and stool softeners, should also be instituted. Laxative bowel regimens have been suggested because of their specific ability to counteract the effects of the opioid drugs, but none has been studied in a controlled way. Anecdotal surveys suggest that doses far above those used for routine bowel management are needed, that senna derivatives are effective, and that careful attention to dietary factors along with the use of a bowel regimen can reduce patient complaints dramatically. Tolerance to this effect develops over time, but relatively slowly. Oral naloxone has been shown to be effective in treating constipation, but its use is variable depending on the degree of opioid exposure of the patient; oral naloxone may reverse the analgesic effect of the opioid.[113] Clinical trials of two peripherally acting opioid antagonists, methylnaltrexone and alvimopan, have proved the concept that these drugs prevent opioid-induced constipation by targeting mu opioid receptors in the gut without interfering with analgesia and are available for clinical use in selected patients.[114,115]

Multifocal myoclonus may occur with high doses of all of the opioid drugs. Multifocal myoclonus and seizures have been reported in patients receiving multiple doses of meperidine (250 mg or more per day), although signs and symptoms of central nervous system hyperirritability may occur with toxic doses of all the opioid analgesics. In a series of cancer patients receiving meperidine, accumulation of the active metabolite normeperidine was associated with these neurologic signs and symptoms. However, in a similar group of cancer patients with pain, subtle mood effects were noted after meperidine administration, which suggests a spectrum of central nervous system effects. Management of this hyperirritability includes discontinuing the meperidine, using intravenous diazepam if seizures occur, and substituting morphine to control the persistent pain. Because the half-life of normeperidine is 16 hours, it may take 2 or 3 days for the signs of central nervous system hyperirritability to clear completely. Meperidine use is contraindicated in patients with chronic renal disease, but these complications as noted in cancer pain treatment occurred in patients with normal renal function.[97] Morphine and hydromorphone at high doses produce myoclonus, which has not been directly associated with their known active metabolite such as M6G and hydromorphone-6-glucuronide. In dying patients with myoclonus, the use of benzodiazepines or barbiturates has been reported anecdotally to suppress this sign, improving the patient's comfort.

Opioid hyperexcitability have been reported with the use of increasing opioid doses by the parenteral and epidural routes. They have most often been observed in patients on high doses of morphine and hydromorphone and are characterized by uncontrolled pain, hypervigilance, total body hyperalgesia, and allodynia. They are best managed by rapid dose reduction and substitution with an alternative opioid such as methadone. The mechanism of action is unclear.

7. *Manage tolerance.* The earliest sign of developing tolerance is the patient's complaint that the duration of effective analgesia has decreased. For reasons not yet understood, cancer patients develop tolerance at vastly different rates. Some demonstrate tolerance within days of initiating opioid therapy; others experience pain control for many months on the same dosage. Studies in an outpatient clinic population, a hospitalized population, and a home care population revealed three patterns of drug use: rapid increase in opioid requirements, stabilization at one dose for several weeks or months, and decrease or elimination of opioids.[116] Increased opioid requirements are most commonly associated with disease progression rather than with tolerance alone. With the development of tolerance, increases in the frequency of the dose of the opioid are required to provide continued pain relief. Because the analgesic effect is a logarithmic function of the dose of opioid, a doubling of the dose may be needed to restore full analgesia. There appears to be no limit to the development of tolerance, and with appropriate dose adjustments patients can continue to obtain pain relief. Tolerance to the respiratory effects of opioid doses occurs. This degree of tolerance makes it safe for patients to increase their opioid doses for analgesia.

Tolerance to one opioid does not lead to complete tolerance to another opioid. This phenomenon of incomplete cross-tolerance is best exemplified in the dramatic reduction in dosages needed to provide analgesia when patients are switched from, for example, morphine or hydromorphone to methadone, as previously discussed.[75–78] Further data elucidating the mechanism of opioid tolerance demonstrate that the *N*-methyl-D-aspartate (NMDA) receptor plays a critical role in opioid tolerance and analgesia.[117] These findings have focused new attention on methadone's opioid and nonopioid mechanisms of action and its potential role in the management of neuropathic pain. The use of analgesic combinations can reduce the amount of opioid required. Similarly, the use of bolus or continuous epidural local anesthetics in patients with perineal pain can dramatically reduce the need for systemic opioids and reverse tolerance.

8. *Taper drugs slowly.* The long-term administration of opioid analgesics is associated with the development of physical dependence; thereafter, the sudden cessation of the opioid analgesic produces signs and symptoms of withdrawal: agitation, tremors, insomnia, fear, marked autonomic nervous system hyperexcitability, and exacerbation of pain. Slowly tapering the dose of the opioid analgesic prevents such symptoms. The appearance of abstinence symptoms from the time of drug withdrawal is related to the elimination half-life for the particular drug. For example, with morphine, withdrawal symptoms occur within 6 to 12 hours after drug cessation. Reinstituting the drug in doses of approximately 25% of the previous daily dose suppresses these symptoms.

9. *Anticipate complications.* Overdose with opioid analgesics occurs either intentionally, when a patient takes an excessive amount of drug in a suicide attempt, or unintentionally, when the recommended dose accidentally produces excessive sedation and respiratory depression. In both instances, the complication can be treated effectively with naloxone. Intentional overdose in cancer patients occurs rarely, and concern for this is overemphasized. Overdose in patients previously stabilized on an opioid regimen for cancer pain rarely is caused by drug intake alone. More commonly, the cause is the medical deterioration of the patient with a superimposed metabolic encephalopathy. Reducing the opioid drug dosage and carefully assessing the patient's metabolic status usually provide the differential diagnosis.

Psychological dependence or addiction is characterized by a concomitant behavioral pattern of drug abuse evidenced by craving a drug for other than pain relief and overwhelming involvement in the use and procurement of the drug. This is a state distinct from tolerance and physical dependence, which are responses to the pharmacologic effects of long-term opioid administration. The profound fear of causing psychological dependence plays a major role in a physician's reluctance to prescribe opioid analgesics, particularly in cancer patients in the early phase of their disease. Patients may share this fear, consistently taking less analgesic drug than is effective to control their pain. Increasing evidence suggests that cancer patients with pain can take opioid analgesics for prolonged periods but can discontinue such drugs when adequate pain relief is achieved using other approaches. In almost all instances, dramatic escalation of drug intake is associated with progression of disease and subsequent death. Few patients with cancer and pain become psychologically dependent on the drugs and participate in drug seeking and illicit drug use. Careful evaluation of patients who might be at risk for this complication is necessary, but such concern should not be punitive to the patient with severe cancer pain.

Out-of-control aberrant drug taking among oncology patients with or without a prior history of substance abuse represents a serious and complex clinical occurrence. Passik and Portenoy[32] have developed guidelines for management of such patients. The most difficult situations present themselves in the patient who is actively abusing illicit or prescription drugs or alcohol while concurrently receiving medical therapies. Such patients need a multidisciplinary approach usually focused on a harm-reduction concept that attempts to enhance social support for the patient to maximize treatment compliance. Passik and Portenoy have outlined a series of approaches to maximize effectiveness of strategies for promoting compliance, including the consideration of a written contract between the team and patient, the inclusion of spot urine toxicology screens to assess compliance, set expectations regarding attendance at the clinic, and the patient's management of medication supplies. It is often most useful to see the patient on a regular basis, often every several days, and to limit prescribing of opioids on that basis until the patient has demonstrated his or her willingness to be compliant and to follow an appropriate drug regimen. In an inpatient setting when patients demonstrate manipulative behaviors in the inappropriate use of medication, direct discussion with the patient about the drug use in an open manner is a first step. Providing the patient with a private room near the nurses' station to monitor the patient, discouraging attempts to leave the hospital for purchase of illicit drugs, and requiring visitors to check in with the nursing staff before visitation are additional steps. Underlying all of this is the attempt to provide the patient with a supportive environment that respects the patient's pain symptomatology and serious medical illness and attempts to limit harm to the patient or others by the aberrant drug use and behaviors.

Adjuvant Drugs

Adjuvant drugs are used to enhance opioid analgesia, provide analgesia for certain types of pain (e.g., neuropathic pain, bone pain, and visceral pain), and treat opioid side effects or other symptoms associated with pain.[118] They are an integral part of the WHO three-step analgesic ladder. Because of the lack of well-defined guidelines for their use, sequential drug trials are necessary to identify the most useful drug and dose titration to find a safe and effective dose.

Adjuvants to Enhance Analgesia

Adjuvants to enhance analgesia have been previously discussed in this chapter. Acetaminophen, NSAIDs, hydroxyzine, and dextroamphetamine have been demonstrated to provide additive analgesia to patients chronically receiving opioids.

Adjuvant Analgesics for Neuropathic Pain

The common neuropathic pain syndromes in patients with cancer include injury to peripheral nerves and plexus by tumor invasion, chemotherapy, surgery, or viral agents. Cancer-related bone pain may be a neuropathic pain syndrome as well.[36] Depending on the intensity of pain, nonopioid and opioid analgesics are the first-line agents. However, neuropathic pain has a variable responsiveness to opioid drug regimens and may be less responsive than other types of pain.[65] Some of the commonly used adjuvant drugs for managing this population of patients are described in the following sections.

Antidepressants

The tricyclic antidepressants continue to be the most useful group of psychotropic drugs applied in pain management.[119,120] Their analgesic effects are mediated by enhancement of serotonin activity. Data from controlled trials indicate that both the tertiary amine tricyclic antidepressants (amitriptyline, doxepin, imipramine, and clomipramine) and the secondary amine compounds (desipramine and nortriptyline) have analgesic effects. One of the serotonin selective reuptake inhibitors, paroxetine, has also been shown to have analgesic properties in patients with neuropathic pain.[121] Similarly, duloxetine, a balanced and potent dual reuptake inhibitor of serotonin and norepinephrine, has recently been demonstrated to be an active analgesic for the management of diabetic peripheral neuropathic pain.[122]

These drugs have been reported to be effective in treating continuous dysesthesias as well as intermittent lancinating dysesthetic pain. The doses used for analgesia are far below those needed to produce an antidepressant effect, and the analgesic properties appear to be independent of the mood-altering effects. Patients should be started on low doses, for example amitriptyline at 25 mg nightly, and the dose titrated up to achieve adequate analgesia in a 2- to 4-week trial. Blood levels should be measured to determine both patient compliance and drug absorption because of wide individual variation. Patients who are unable to tolerate amitriptyline or who are predisposed to experiencing its sedative, anticholinergic, or hypotensive effects should be considered for a trial with a secondary amine tricyclic antidepressant, a serotonin selective reuptake inhibitor such as paroxetine, or duloxetine. In the management of cancer patients with pain, the antidepressant drugs are the first-line therapeutic approach for neuropathic pain, and every attempt should be made to provide the patient with a several-week trial before discontinuing these drugs.

Anticonvulsants

The role of anticonvulsants in the management of patients with neuropathic pain is based, in part, on the fact that the mode of action is to stabilize membranes and alter sodium and calcium influx.[123] Many patients with neuropathic pain complain of paroxysmal, brief, lancinating pains. To date, clinical experience with the anticonvulsants has been positive. The drugs most commonly used include gabapentin, carbamazepine, and phenytoin and pregabalin. Survey studies have suggested the usefulness of valproic acid, clonazepam, lamotrigine, topiramate, and oxycarbazepine.[124] Systematic review confirms these findings.[125,126] Gabapentin is considered the first-line anticonvulsant to manage neuropathic pain, although some meta-analyses suggest that it is equivocal with the other anticonvulsants.[126] Controlled trials in patients with diabetic neuropathy, postherpetic neuralgia, and acquired immunodeficiency syndrome neuropathy demonstrate the effectiveness of this agent in reducing pain. Dosages range from 900 to 1,800 mg/d.[125] The major drug side effect is sedation. Patients should be started at 300 mg/d and rapidly titrated to 900 mg/d; some patients may need to start at even lower doses, such as 100 mg/d, to avoid sedation. Pain relief in up to 30% to 50% of patients has been suggested. Clinical studies with carbamazepine demonstrate efficacy, but the usefulness of this drug in the cancer population is limited by its potential to produce bone marrow suppression, particularly leukopenia. The dosing guidelines used for the treatment of seizures are suggested in managing neuropathic pain. Each of the drugs should be initiated at low doses and gradually titrated upward. There is anecdotal experience to suggest that administering intravenous loading doses of phenytoin to patients in an acute crisis with severe lancinating pain may be of clinical value. Both valproate and clonazepam have been reported anecdotally to be useful in managing neuropathic pain, but these are considered third-line agents in this patient population.[124] Currently, there are no data to relate the plasma level and pain relief for any of these drugs. In patients with persistent neuropathic cancer-related pain, pregabalin is another option; in a randomized controlled trial of patients with noncancer neuropathic pain, over half of the patients treated with pregabalin experienced a decrease in their mean pain intensity over 50%.[127] Sequential trials of different agents are necessary to identify the most useful agent for an individual patient.[120]

Local Anesthetics

The use of both brief intravenous local anesthetic infusions (lidocaine) and maintenance oral anesthetic drugs has demonstrated some efficacy in the management of chronic neuropathic pain, particularly in those patients with both lancinating and continuous dysesthesias. Mexiletine is the oral local anesthetic for which there are pilot data to support analgesic efficacy.[128] The initial dosage of mexiletine is low, at 150 mg/d, with gradual upward dose titration. Electrocardiograms should be monitored at higher doses, and measurement of blood levels of mexiletine may be useful to prevent toxicity. Currently, there are no good data available to predict which patients might respond to the use of oral local or intravenous anesthetics.

Epidural local anesthetics (bupivacaine, lidocaine) have been most widely used to manage neuropathic pain, either alone or in combination with an opioid. Alternatively, the use of brief intravenous infusions of lidocaine may be helpful in patients who have an opioid-refractory continuous dysesthesia that has not responded to an antidepressant or anticonvulsant.[129] These drugs clearly serve as a second-line approach, with individualized therapy the rule.

Cutaneous Local Anesthetics

The use of cutaneous anesthesia has been suggested to be most helpful in patients who have significant allodynia and marked hyperesthesia. The topical application of a local anesthetic, such as an eutectic mixture of local anesthetics, has been demonstrated to be efficacious in patients who undergo painful procedures, especially children.[130] The cream should be applied under an occlusive dressing to increase skin penetration and augment analgesic efficacy. The use of high-concentration lidocaine (5% and 10%) has also been reported to be effective in patients with significant allodynia associated with postherpetic neuralgia.[131] Current indications for its use include peripheral nerve injury, peripheral neuropathy, ischemic pain, peripheral vascular disease, and unstable angina. Few cancer patients have been treated using this approach and, therefore, it is not possible to fully assess its role in cancer pain management.

Corticosteroids

A series of controlled and uncontrolled surveys have demonstrated that the use of chronic corticosteroid therapy to reduce pain in patients with breast and prostate cancer improves quality of life.[132,133] In a controlled study of corticosteroid use in patients with far-advanced disease, transient improvement in appetite, analgesia, and mood were noted, but they were not sustained after the initial effect. The major indications for corticosteroid use include refractory neuropathic pain, bone pain, pain associated with capsular expansion or duct obstruction, and headache due to increased intracranial pressure. In certain cancer pain syndromes, such as epidural cord compression, 85% of patients who received 100 mg of dexamethasone as part of their radiation therapy protocol reported significant pain relief associated with marked reduction in analgesic requirements.[79] Similarly, in patients with tumor infiltration of the brachial and lumbosacral plexus, corticosteroids provided additive analgesic effects. The risk of adverse effects associated with corticosteroid therapy varies with the duration. Long-term use may be associated with GI toxicity and acute psychosis. A wide range of dosages has been suggested, including a dose of 30 mg/d in patients with prostate cancer, which was effective in providing improved quality of life and reduced pain. With epidural cord compression, initial doses of 100 mg of dexamethasone with maintenance doses of 16 mg have been associated with effective analgesia. In the authors' experience, the use of 16 mg as a loading bolus and rapid titration to lower dosages of approximately 4 mg/d is one approach commonly used in the management of refractory chronic pain in patients with advanced disease.

Other Adjuvant Drugs

A wide variety of other drugs have been used to manage neuropathic pain, including benzodiazepines, neuroleptics, α_2-adrenergic agonist drugs, NMDA antagonists, and peptides. Of the benzodiazepines, clonazepam is commonly used in patients with lancinating or paroxysmal pain. The use of these drugs must be balanced with their potential to cause somnolence and cognitive impairment. They serve as second- to third-line therapy in patients who have not responded to antidepressant or anticonvulsant drug therapy. Of the neuroleptics, pimozide has been reported to be analgesic in patients with trigeminal neuralgia.[134] Methotrimeprazine has been demonstrated to have analgesic properties comparable to those of morphine.[135] This drug has sedative, anxiolytic, and antiemetic properties and is commonly used in patients who have excessive opioid side effects. It provides analgesia by a nonopioid mechanism.

Coadministration of these drugs with opioids can often be effective in patients with neuropathic pain. Of the α_2-adrenergic agonist drugs, clonidine has been demonstrated to be analgesic in controlled trials.[136] It can be administered by either the oral or transdermal route and has been reported to be specifically effective in patients with dysesthetic pain, who demonstrate sympathetic hyperactivity. After intrathecal administration, clonidine was reported to improve pain in patients with intolerable neuropathic pain. Dextromethorphan and ketamine are two commercially available NMDA antagonists. The mechanism of action relates to the fact that the NMDA receptor reduces the development of the windup phenomenon, which occurs as a result of changes in the response of central dorsal horn neurons with neuropathic pain. Ketamine has demonstrated analgesic effects in observational studies.[137–140] The use of ketamine infusions have been previously well established to produce analgesia, and they have been reintroduced into clinical use as brief infusions for the management of patients with refractory neuropathic pain; further studies are necessary. In a small randomized trial, oral ketamine had demonstrated efficacy as an adjuvant with opioid therapy.[141]

Calcitonin has been reported to provide analgesia in patients with sympathetically maintained pain and in patients with acute phantom pain.[142] The mechanism underlying these analgesic effects is unknown, but it has suggested the empiric use of calcitonin in patients with refractory neuropathic pain.

Adjuvant Drugs for Bone Pain

Metastatic disease to bone is the most common cause of pain in patients with cancer. Analgesic drug therapy is commonly used to manage pain during the initial treatment with either chemotherapy or radiation therapy. Numerous investigators have identified a management approach for bone pain, which includes the use of specific surgical palliative approaches, radiotherapeutic approaches, hormonal therapies, and bone resorption inhibitors. Patients with multifocal metastatic bone disease that is refractory to routine treatments may benefit from the use of a series of agents, including the bisphosphonate compounds, gallium nitrate, calcitonin, and radiopharmaceuticals. The newer models of metastatic bone pain as neuropathic pain imply that more traditional neuropathic pain drugs may have an important role in managing bone pain.[36] For example, in a murine bone pain model, opioids and tricyclic antidepressants demonstrated analgesic efficacy.[143] The selection of any one of these treatments to manage metastatic bone pain needs to be individualized.

Bisphosphonate drugs such as pamidronate, zoledronate, clodronate, and etidronate bind to bone hydroxyapatite, inhibiting osteoclast activity, and are highly effective in the management of bony metastatic disease and in multiple myeloma.[144–148] The major indication for these drugs is to prevent skeletal morbidity, with data in breast cancer patients and patients with multiple myeloma showing efficacy in reduction of fractures and reduction in bone pain. Pamidronate is usually administered as a brief infusion in a starting dose of 60 to 120 mg. Analgesia, if it occurs, usually appears within days but may accrue for many weeks with repeated infusions. In two studies, pamidronate at dosages of 30 to 60 mg every 2 weeks produced relief of pain in 30% to 60% of patients.[147,148] The analgesic effect of bisphosphonates appears to be dose dependent. Current recommendations include a regimen of intravenous pamidronate, 60 mg every 2 weeks for at least two or three treatments. If no response is obtained, therapy can be discontinued. If the drug is effective, a biweekly regimen can be continued. Zoledronate is administered at 4 mg intravenously over 15 minutes every 3 to 4 weeks. Systematic review suggests that it may be the most effective bisphosphonate in prostate cancer.[145] Clodronate may be administered orally (1,600 mg/d) and has been demonstrated to be efficacious in patients with breast cancer and multiple myeloma.

Calcitonin has also been reported anecdotally to be useful in patients with malignant bone pain, but the appropriate dose and dosing frequency have not been well defined.[149] Gallium nitrate has also been used with some efficacy in patients with metastatic bone pain, but due to limited experience, appropriate dosing guidelines have not been well defined, and nephrotoxicity has been reported.[150]

Strontium-89 and samarium-153 are bone-seeking radiopharmaceuticals that have been recognized as useful in the treatment of bone pain secondary to metastatic disease.[151–153] Use is indicated in patients with refractory multifocal pain due to osteoblastic lesions who have a life expectancy of longer than 3 months, who have sufficient bone marrow reserve (i.e., a platelet count above 60,000 and a white blood cell count above 2,400), and for whom there is no further planned myelosuppressive chemotherapy. The onset of effect is slow and may require several weeks, with peak effects at 2 to 3 months. Bone marrow suppression is the major adverse effect, with irreversible thrombocytopenia. Both radiopharmaceuticals have similar analgesic efficacy and side effects.

Adjuvants to Treat Side Effects

Nausea and vomiting, confusion, sedation, and constipation are common opioid-induced side effects. Side effects should be managed expectantly, rather than waiting until patients are experiencing negative consequences of analgesic therapy that aggravate the pain and suffering of cancer. The use of drugs to manage these effects has been discussed previously. The use of caffeine, methylphenidate, and dextroamphetamine to reduce opioid-induced sedation have all been demonstrated in clinical trials. Haloperidol is the treatment of choice to manage hallucinations and agitated delirium in patients receiving opioid analgesics. The use of bowel regimens to manage depressed GI motility is critical; since nearly all patients have some constipation when receiving opioids, a bowel regimen should be coprescribed with opioid therapy.

PSYCHOLOGICAL APPROACHES

Psychological approaches should be an integral part of the care of the cancer patient with pain.[154] Studies strongly support an association between cancer pain and psychological distress, predominantly manifested as mood disturbance, anxiety, and depression.[155] Pain catastrophizing (i.e., the tendency to ruminate about pain and negatively evaluate one's ability to deal with pain) leads to increased pain intensity, pain interference, and anxiety. Similarly, patients who lack confidence in their ability to control pain experience lower quality of life and higher psychological distress. Worse pain leads to decreased social interactions, reduced social functioning, and poor social networks. At the other end of the spectrum, increased self-efficacy and active coping manifested by the sense of ability to control or decrease pain is associated with improved pain control. Given these psychological factors, it follows that psychological approaches would be effective adjuvant interventions for cancer pain.

Established behavioral therapies for cancer pain fall into three categories: (1) comprehensive cognitive behavioral therapy (CBT); (2) hypnosis and imagery-based CBT; and, (3) psychoeducational interventions.[156] Comprehensive CBT comprises varied packages of adaptive strategies taught to a patient to maximize coping. There are several basic components, namely: (1) providing patients with a rationale that emphasizes pain as a complex experience influenced by thoughts, feelings, and behavior; (2) providing systematic training in one or more cognitive or behavioral strategies for controlling pain (e.g., progressive relaxation, imagery, goal setting, activity pacing) typically carried out over a series of sessions; and (3) emphasizing that the skills can only be mastered through home practice. In hypnosis-based CBT, a trained therapist helps the patient achieve a relaxed state and then actively provides specific hypnotic suggestions designed to enhance pain control and relaxation. In imagery-based CBT, also called *guided imagery*, the patient is taught how to intentionally focus attention on specific mental images so as to divert attention from pain. Psychoeducational interventions combine patient education with behavioral techniques such a skills training, personal interaction with the learner, and repeat visits to reinforce key messages and skills. Biofeedback and caregiver-assisted approaches have been advocated and studied as well, but to date, all evaluations of these methods have been uncontrolled or preliminary.[154]

Behavioral therapies have a defined role in the management of nonmalignant pain,[157] but their role in cancer pain is less clear. A systematic review of behavioral interventions for cancer pain that compared their relative efficacy was conducted in 2005.[156] Cognitive behavioral interventions were effective in the management of cancer-related pain. Imagery and hypnosis-based interventions were most effective. Education-focused interventions with brief CBT were intermediate with 56% of the studies positive. Comprehensive CBT interventions were least effective, with less than half of studies positive and no obvious relationships between components of the comprehensive CBT package, intensity of the intervention, and outcome. It appears that psychological approaches that incorporate therapeutic hypnosis and guided imagery have a role in the management of cancer-related pain, especially pain associated with acute situations such as a lumbar puncture or oral mucositis in the setting of bone marrow transplant. Psychoeducational interventions may have a role, especially nursing-based education programs with skills training for the patient and caregivers. Clearly, more studies are needed to better define when these approaches are indicated.

ANESTHETIC AND NEUROSURGICAL APPROACHES

Anesthetic and neurosurgical approaches are most effective in treating patients with well-defined localized pain. Tables 170.7 and 170.8 outline the indications for their use. Ten percent to 20% of cancer pain patients require these approaches, together with pharmacologic approaches, to obtain adequate analgesia.

TABLE 170.7

TYPES OF ANESTHETIC PROCEDURES COMMONLY USED IN CANCER PAIN

Type of Procedure	Most Common Indications
Inhalation therapy with nitrous oxide	Breakthrough pain, incidental pain in patients with diffuse poorly controlled pain
Intravenous barbiturates (sodium pentobarbital)	Diffuse body pain and suffering inadequately controlled by systemic opioids
Local anesthetic by intravenous, subcutaneous, or transdermal application	Neuropathic pain in any site with local application to the area of hyperesthesia or allodynia
Trigger point injections	Focal muscle pain
Nerve Block	
Peripheral	Pain in discrete dermatomes in chest and abdomen or in distal extremities
Epidural	Unilateral lumbar or sacral pain; midline perineal pain; bilateral lumbosacral pain
Intrathecal	Midline perineal pain; bilateral lumbosacral pain
Autonomic	
Stellate ganglion	Reflex sympathetic dystrophy
Lumbar sympathetic vascular insufficiency of the lower extremity	Reflex sympathetic dystrophy of the lower extremities; lumbosacral plexopathy
Celiac plexus	Midabdominal pain from tumor infiltration
Intermittent or continuous epidural infusion with local anesthetics	Unilateral and bilateral lumbosacral pain; midline perineal pain; neuropathic pain from the midthoracic region down
Intermittent or continuous epidural or intrathecal with local opioid analgesics	Unilateral and bilateral pain below the midthoracic region; often combined with local anesthetics
Intermittent or continuous intraventricular infusions with opioid analgesics	Head and neck pain and upper chest pain
Chemical hypophysectomy	Diffuse bone pain

PRACTICE OF ONCOLOGY

TABLE 170.8

NEUROABLATIVE AND NEUROSTIMULATORY PROCEDURES FOR RELIEF OF PAIN FROM CANCER

Site	Procedure	Indications
Neuroablative Procedures		
Nerve root	Rhizotomy	Useful in somatic and neuropathic pain from tumor infiltration of the cranial and, rarely, intercostal nerves.
Spinal cord	Dorsal root entry zone lesion	Useful in unilateral neuropathic pain from brachial, intercostal, and lumbosacral plexopathy and postherpetic neuralgia.
	Cordotomy	Useful in unilateral pain below the waist. Often combined with local neurolytic blocks in perineal and bilateral lumbosacral plexopathy; may be performed bilaterally.
	Myelotomy	Useful in midline pain below the waist but rarely used because it involves extensive surgery.
Brainstem	Mesencephalic tractomy	Useful in pain in the nasopharynx and trigeminal region.
Thalamus	Thalamotomy	Useful in unilateral neuropathic pain in the chest and lower extremity.
Cortex	Cingulotomy	Useful through a stereotactic approach for diffuse pain.
Pituitary	Transsphenoidal hypophysectomy	Useful in pain control of bone metastases in endocrine-dependent tumors, breast, and prostate.
Neurostimulatory Procedures		
Peripheral nerve	Transcutaneous and percutaneous electrical nerve stimulation	Useful in reducing painful dysesthesias from tumor infiltration of nerve or trauma (e.g., neuroma).
Spinal cord	Dorsal column stimulation	Of limited use in neuropathic pain in the chest, midline, and lower extremities.
Thalamus	Thalamic stimulation	Of rare use in neuropathic pain in the chest, midline, or lower extremity.

Several factors are important in selecting the appropriate procedure for each patient. Because diffuse pain problems are common in cancer patients, while most neurosurgical and anesthetic procedures are useful for management of well-defined localized pain, the role of these approaches is limited at best. Further complicating their use is the limited number of professionals who have expertise in these procedures. As patients become more cognizant of their disease and treatment options, they are often hesitant to undergo neurodestructive procedures. Patients often consider their pain to be an important marker for their disease and are frightened of the potential, although unlikely, complications of these procedures. As a result, these procedures are often performed late in the illness, and full evaluation of their effectiveness and duration of action is limited by patients' overriding medical problems.

Local Anesthetics

Anecdotal reports and several controlled studies support the use of cutaneous, subcutaneous, intravenous, intrapleural, and epidural local anesthetics in the management of patients with somatic, visceral, and neuropathic pain.

Intravenous lidocaine can be considered as both a diagnostic and therapeutic approach in patients with neuropathic pain.[158] If such patients obtain an analgesic response, a trial of oral mexiletine or the use of continuous subcutaneous lidocaine should be considered to determine whether prolonged relief may be possible, as previously discussed. Case reports suggest that continuous subcutaneous infusions of lidocaine may have a role in improving neuropathic cancer pain, but a small randomized study did not support these findings.[159]

Intrapleural local anesthetics have been used for acute pain in the chest wall and have been adapted for the management of chronic cancer pain.[160] Anesthetic delivered via a subcutaneously tunneled intrapleural catheter offered long-term relief of right upper-quadrant pain from hepatic metastases in a patient with significant pain from tumor infiltration of the liver. This novel method offers an alternative approach for patients with local or regional pain in the pleural and abdominal regions.

Epidural local anesthetics are used to manage localized pain syndromes, usually below the waist. Intermittent and continuous epidural infusions of local anesthetics have been used to manage the difficult chronic pain associated with metastatic disease below the waist, often involving the sacrum and lumbosacral plexus.[161] This method consists of infusing a local anesthetic via a subcutaneous infusion pump or reservoir to a catheter temporarily or permanently placed in the epidural space. If the amount and concentration of the anesthetic are varied, effective pain relief can be achieved without interrupting significant motor or autonomic function. The risk of infection is minimized because local anesthetics have antimicrobial effects. The use of continuous low-dose infusions of local anesthetics is associated with minimal systemic side effects. Further studies on the use of this technique in comparison with standard therapies are needed to define its place in the management of the cancer patient. Its major advantages are that the resultant analgesia is not cross-tolerant with the analgesia produced by the opioid analgesics, and that temporary use of this technique allows for reducing the amount of systemic opiate drugs and therefore partially reversing tolerance. This has been a useful preliminary approach in patients for whom the use of spinal opiate analgesia is considered but who have developed tolerance from large doses of systemic opiates. This approach is also most useful in patients who experience an acute pain crisis, such as the patient with a pathologic hip fracture who is not a surgical candidate; this approach would allow the patient to move about in bed.

Peripheral Nerve Block

Peripheral nerve blocks are used both diagnostically to localize the nerve distribution and therapeutically to interrupt pain transmission within a determined nerve distribution. This technique is limited to areas of the body in which the interruption of both motor and sensory function will not interfere with the patient's functional status. It is most commonly used in patients who have pain in the head, chest, or abdomen.[162] This technique is also limited by the fact that each peripheral nerve subserves sensory function over many levels, and usually several nerves must be blocked to provide adequate analgesia. These techniques are most useful in patients with somatic pain; neuropathic pain is rarely controlled by peripheral nerve blocks alone. Examples of successful blocks include gasserian ganglion block for craniofacial pain, intercostal blocks for chest wall infiltration from tumor, and paravertebral blocks for radicular pain. In patients with somatic pain who respond to a local anesthetic block, neurolytic blockade with either alcohol or phenol may provide more prolonged relief. A block produced by phenol tends to be less profound and of shorter duration than that produced by alcohol. Phenol has local anesthetic as well as neurolytic effects.

The most common peripheral neurolytic block is a paravertebral block for localized intercostal pain. Fluoroscopic, ultrasonic, or computed tomographic localization assist in more accurately interrupting the individual intercostal nerve.

Epidural and intrathecal neurolytic blocks have been used primarily to manage patients with far-advanced disease whose pain is either unilateral in the chest or abdomen or midline in the perineum. These approaches are less useful in managing upper and lower limb pain associated with brachial and lumbosacral plexopathy because of the high risk of motor weakness associated with effective neurolytic blockade by this route. Epidural phenol blocks are useful in management of chest wall pain over several dermatomes. Such an approach obviates the need for multiple paravertebral injections. Phenol is injected in small increments (1 to 2 mL/segment) over 2 or 3 days by an epidural catheter, and preliminary data demonstrate 80% pain relief in patients with documented somatic pain. Epidural and intrathecal phenol blocks have been used to manage perineal pain, but no studies have delineated the superiority of one approach over the other. Case series reviews suggest that an average of 60% of patients experience good relief, 21% achieve fair relief, and 18% obtain poor relief.[161] The duration of pain relief is poorly documented; the overall estimate for relief of pain with both subarachnoid alcohol and phenol blocks suggests a mean duration of pain relief of between 2 weeks and 3 months.

The selection of patients for management with epidural or intrathecal neurolytic agents is based on the following criteria: exhaustion of appropriate antitumor approaches; clear clinical and radiologic definition of the pain; poor candidacy for percutaneous cordotomy; failure of nonopioid, opioid, and adjuvant analgesics to produce adequate analgesia without significant side effects; a favorable response to diagnostic or epidural or intrathecal blocks, producing at least 75% pain relief; and MRI of the spine or myelography done before the procedure that rules out tumor infiltration of the subarachnoid space. Complications are of two kinds. With intrathecal injection, a self-limiting spinal headache may occur. Complications that result from the action of neurolytic substances on nerve fibers include motor paresis, loss of sphincter function, impairment of touch and proprioception, and troublesome dysesthesias. Injection in the thoracic region has a lower complication rate. If a patient already has both motor and autonomic dysfunction before the use of neurolytic blockade, these often remain the same or may worsen. Patients should be informed of the risk of these procedures, with particular attention given to the fact that they may develop motor paresis and bladder dysfunction, specifically incontinence, after the blockade.

Celiac Plexus Block

Sympathetic block is effective in conditions with vasomotor or visceromotor hyperactivity. This hyperactivity accompanies many of the cancer-related pain syndromes such as visceral pain or plexopathies. The most commonly used sympathetic block is that of the celiac ganglion for pain due to abdominal malignancy, including cancer of the pancreas, stomach, duodenum, liver, gallbladder, adrenal gland, and colon. Nociceptive fibers of the splanchnic, sympathetic, vagal, phrenic, and somatic nerves converge on the celiac ganglion, which is amenable to a regional block; this block is successful in 70% to 85% of patients treated.[163]

Standardized approaches for the use of this technique have been described using computed tomographic monitoring or fluoroscopic control. After placement of the needle, 25 mg of absolute alcohol mixed with local anesthetic and contrast is injected. The major side effect of the procedure is transient hypotension; patients must be well hydrated and monitored carefully during the procedure and for 4 to 6 hours afterward. Significant neurologic complications occur in fewer than 1% of patients if proper technique is used. Complications include paraparesis, postural hypotension, and urinary difficulties.

Although there has been debate about the usefulness of this procedure in patients with pancreatic cancer, it should be considered as one option, together with pharmacologic approaches, in managing these patients. A recent systematic review of five randomized trials of celiac plexus block for advanced pancreatic cancer demonstrated that overall the procedure led to less pain, opioid use, and constipation, albeit with small effect size of questionable clinical significance.[164] The use of thoracic endoscopy to perform sympathetic blockade in patients with cancer may replace the standard celiac plexus approach.

Lumbar Sympathetic Block

Lumbar sympathetic block may provide significant relief of intractable urogenital pain or pain due to carcinomatous invasion of local nerves and plexus in the perineum and lower extremity.[165] This ganglion conveys visceral nociceptive afferents from the pelvic viscera. Pain caused by cancer of the sigmoid colon or rectum may be relieved by bilateral lumbar sympathetic block if the disease is confined to those viscera. Similarly, pain caused by cancer of the seminal vesicles or prostate, and pain caused by uterine cancer confined to the body of the uterus, may be relieved by this block. In many instances, however, the block must be extended to the T12 ganglion. Lumbar sympathetic block alone is usually not useful in patients with lumbosacral plexopathy; therefore, the role of this procedure is limited to management of pain at specific anatomic sites.

Stellate Ganglion Block

Stellate ganglion block may sometimes be useful for pain in the face, upper neck, ear, and hemicranium. However, the potential complications of stellate ganglion block limit the use of neurolytic solution with this technique, because there is a high risk of spillage of the neurolytic material into the brachial plexus, with secondary nerve injury and focal pain.

NEUROPHARMACOLOGIC APPROACHES

Epidural and Interspinal Approach

Epidural and intraspinal analgesia, using opioids alone or in combination with (1) local anesthetics, (2) clonidine, (3) both local anesthetics and clonidine, or (4) experimental agents, is used to manage chronic cancer pain in patients with a reasonable (1-year) expected survival.[166] In all instances, patients should have a trial of an epidural or intraspinal drug combination before permanent implementation is considered. It is advised that patients have a continuous intrathecal trial lasting as long as possible before permanent implementation. A wide array of external and implantable catheters and pumps is available with specific indications and uses. Both computer-controlled battery-operated pumps and continuous fixed-infusion pumps are used. Cost of the pump, the patient's psychosocial status and social support systems, and the patient's ability to care for the pump and port are important considerations in the decision to use such devices. As discussed previously, a randomized clinical trial of intrathecal opioids compared to comprehensive medical management reported improved pain relief, less drug toxicity, and improved survival.[106]

NEUROABLATIVE AND NEUROSTIMULATORY PROCEDURES FOR THE RELIEF OF PAIN

Table 170.8 summarizes the commonly used neurosurgical approaches to cancer pain. A detailed review of these procedures is beyond the scope of this chapter. A review of the current literature suggests limited use of most of these ablative and stimulatory procedures. The integration of these procedures is often dependent on the specific training of the consultant neurosurgeon, and medical oncologists need to work effectively in a team to decide the optimal use of these approaches.[167–168]

TRIGGER POINT INJECTION AND ACUPUNCTURE

Patients with significant musculoskeletal pain often identify specific tender trigger point areas, and injection of these trigger points with either saline or local anesthetic is associated with significant pain relief. Effective relief of pain from trigger point injections is not by itself diagnostic of musculoskeletal pain, however, and an evaluation of the cause of the pain is still necessary to rule out other specific sources.

Acupuncture has been used to treat both acute and chronic pain. The selected acupuncture points are manually or electrically stimulated with a needle until the patient feels the sensation. A wide variety of acupuncture techniques are available, ranging from a traditional Chinese approach to a Western adaptation. Laser acupuncture with external laser probes has also been used. Randomized and systematic data are emerging in support of acupuncture to manage pain; however, a lack of detailed pain assessment with specific acupuncture techniques and lack of a critical review of the patient population make it difficult to interpret these observations.[169,170] Based on its current empiric use, this approach is relatively safe, but its benefit in cancer patients with pain remains undefined.

PHYSIATRIC APPROACHES

Rehabilitation medicine plays an important role in the multidisciplinary approach to the patient with cancer pain.[171] Physiatrists are concerned with a patient's physical functioning and provide expertise in assessing how impairment in a patient's physical capacity affects his or her ability to function. A wide variety of interventions are available, including transcutaneous electrical nerve stimulation (TENS), diathermy (heating pads, ultrasound treatments, hydrotherapy), and cryotherapy (ice and vapocoolants). Assistive devices and braces, as well as therapeutic exercise and massage, are important. Trigger point injections and acupuncture have also been used. These interventions are commonly used in combination with other pain therapy approaches, particularly behavioral and pharmacologic approaches. Rehabilitation approaches are discussed throughout the text specific to cancer patients' needs. A large body of data supports the use of rehabilitative interventions in acute and chronic nonmalignant pain, but similar studies have not addressed the rehabilitation needs of the cancer pain patient. Neurologic dysfunction is one of the common components in patients with cancer pain, and aggressive neurorehabilitation is necessary to promote ambulation in these patients and provide them with functional independence.

ALGORITHM FOR CANCER PAIN MANAGEMENT

An algorithm has been developed that integrates all of these management approaches for cancer pain. It attempts to integrate assessment techniques, drug therapy, behavioral approaches, and anesthetic and neurosurgical approaches and stresses continuity of care. Treatment begins with a diagnostic evaluation that addresses the medical, psychological, and social components of pain. A plan is developed to treat the cancer and pain. If the anticancer treatment is effective, pain relief usually occurs and the drugs used for analgesia can be discontinued without difficulty. Pain treatment begins with the use of analgesic drugs, starting with nonopioid drugs alone or in combination. If these drugs are successful, no further therapy is necessary. If severe, persistent pain does not respond to analgesic drugs or if the side effects of the drugs are not tolerated, the physician should consider switching analgesics (e.g., from oral morphine to methadone), changing the route of administration (e.g., from oral to subcutaneous), or performing a cordotomy for localized pain. A trial of an adjuvant drug together with the opioid and nonopioid drug would also be appropriate. In patients with excessive sedation or confusion, the use of a neurostimulant or haloperidol provides adequate treatment of the side effects of the opioid drugs and maintains the patient's analgesia while markedly reducing concurrent side effects. Alternatively, epidural or intrathecal opioids may be considered if systemic analgesics produce excessive side effects such as confusion or sedation. If the pain is localized (e.g., intercostal pain from tumor infiltration of the chest wall), neurolytic blocks are indicated. If the pain is unilateral and below the waist, cordotomy should be considered. For diffuse pain, nitrous oxide inhalation may be tried. Behavioral approaches including guided imagery should be integrated from the onset of treatment and used along with the medical and surgical approaches.

FUTURE DIRECTIONS

The study of pain in cancer patients offers a unique opportunity to use clinical observations to advance biologic knowledge. There is a critical need to expand both the research and educational efforts in cancer pain to improve the control of pain in these patients. Information on the basic mechanisms of pain modulation can be culled only from a careful study of these clinical pain problems. These studies can teach us the physiologic and psychological differences between acute and chronic pain problems, the importance of the evolution of psychological factors, the difference between pain and suffering, the clinical pharmacology of analgesic drugs, and the behavioral mechanisms humans use to suppress pain. The use of innovative approaches based on sound scientific principles and advances in research technology offers the opportunity to understand the complex phenomenon of pain. The development of animal models to test new therapies, the new insights learned from the molecular genetics of opioid receptors, and the increasing knowledge base of the molecular mechanisms of neuropathic pain, bone pain, and visceral pain offer the promise for translating these discoveries into the improved care of the patient with pain.

Selected References

The full list of references for this chapter appears in the online version.

1. Foley K, Gelband H, eds. *Institute of Medicine. National Cancer Policy Board. Improving palliative care for cancer*. Washington, DC: National Academies Press, 2001.
3. Foley KM. Advances in cancer pain. *Arch Neurol* 1999;56(4):413.
4. Foley KM. Clinical crossroads: a 44-year-old woman with severe pain at the end of life. *JAMA* 1999;281:1937.
5. Moryl N, Foley K, Coyle N. Perspectives on care at the close of life. Managing an acute pain crisis in patients with advanced cancer: this is as much of a crisis as a code. *JAMA* 2008;299(12):1457.
6. Stjernsward J, Foley KM, Ferris FD. The public health strategy for palliative care. *J Pain Symptom Manage* 2007;22(5):486.
7. World Health Organization. *Cancer pain relief and palliative care*. Report of WHO Expert Committee. Geneva: WHO, 1990.
8. World Health Organization. *Cancer pain relief*. 2nd ed. Geneva: WHO, 1996.
9. Swarm R, Anghelescu DL, Benedetti C, et al. NCCN practice guidelines for adult cancer pain. *J Natl Comp Cancer Ntw* 2007;5(8):726.
10. Sanft TB, Von Roenn JH. Palliative care across the continuum of care. NCCN Guidelines and Clinical Resources. *J Natl Comp Cancer Ntw* 2009;7:481.
11. Gordon DB, Dahl JL, Miaskowski C, et al. American Pain Society recommendations for improving the quality of acute and cancer pain management. American Pain Society Quality of Care Task Force. *Arch Inter Med* 2005;165(14):1574.
12. Raphael J, Ahmedazi S, Hester J, et al. Cancer pain; part 1: pathophysiology; oncological, pharmacological and psychological treatments: a perspective from the British Pain Society endorsed by the UK Association of Palliative Medicine and the Royal College of General Practitioners. *Pain Med* 2010;11(5):535.
13. Jost L, Rolla F. ESMO Working Guidelines Group. Management of cancer pain: ESMO Clinical Practice Guidelines. *Ann Oncol* 2010;5(Suppl):257.
14. Foley KM, Wagner JL, Joranson DE, Gelband H. Pain control for the people with cancer and AIDS. In: *Disease control priorities in developing countries*, 2nd ed. New York: Oxford University Press, 2006:981.
15. Foley KM. How well is cancer pain treated? *J Palliat Med* 2011; (in press).
16. Foley K. Acute and chronic cancer pain syndromes. In: Doyle D, Hanks G, Cherny N, Calman K, eds. *Oxford textbook of palliative medicine*, 3rd ed. New York: Oxford University Press, 2004:298.
22. Portenoy RK, Kornblith AB, Wong G, et al. Pain in ovarian cancer patients. Prevalence, characteristics, and associated symptoms. *Cancer* 1994; 74(3):907.

24. Cleeland CS, Gonin R, Hatfield AK, et al. Pain and its treatment in outpatients with metastatic cancer. *N Engl J Med* 1994;330(9):592.
25. Cherny NI, Portenoy RK. Cancer pain: principles of assessment and syndromes. In: Wall PK, Melzak R, eds. *Textbook of pain*. London: Churchill Livingstone, 1994:797.
28. Ellis JA, McCarthy P, Hershon L, et al. Pain practices: a cross-Canada survey of pediatric oncology centers. *J Pediatr Oncol Nurs* 2003;20(1):26.
31. Chochinov H, Breithart W, eds. *Handbook of psychiatry in palliative medicine*. New York: Oxford University Press, 2009.
32. Passik S, Portenoy R. Substance abuse issues in palliative care. In: Berger A, Portenoy RK, Weissman DE, eds. *Principles and practices of supportive oncology*. Philadelphia: Lippincott-Raven Publishers, 1998:513.
39. Portenoy RK, Hagen NA. Breakthrough pain: definition, prevalence and characteristics. *Pain* 1990;41(3):273.
46. Fishman B, Pasternak S, Wallenstein SL, et al. The Memorial Pain Assessment Card. A valid instrument for the evaluation of cancer pain. *Cancer* 1987;60(5):1151.
51. Foley KM. The treatment of cancer pain. *N Engl J Med* 1985;313(2):84.
53. Block SD. Perspectives on care at the close of life. Psychological considerations, growth, and transcendence at the end of life: the art of the possible. *JAMA* 2001;285(22):2898.
54. Cherny NI, Coyle N, Foley KM. Guidelines in the care of the dying cancer patient. *Hematol Oncol Clin North Am* 1996;10(1):261.
56. Chochinov HM, Wilson KG, Enns M, et al. Desire for death in the terminally ill. *Am J Psychiatry* 1995;152(8):1185.
65. Portenoy RK, Foley KM, Inturrisi CE. The nature of opioid responsiveness and its implications for neuropathic pain: new hypotheses derived from studies of opioid infusions. *Pain* 1990;43(3):273.
74. Cherny N, Chang V, Frager G, et al. Opioid pharmacotherapy in the management of cancer pain: a survey of strategies used by pain physicians for the selection of analgesic drugs and routes of administration. *Cancer Treat Rep* 1986;70(5):575.
75. Bruera E, Pereira J, Watanabe S, et al. Opioid rotation in patients with cancer pain. A retrospective comparison of dose ratios between methadone, hydromorphone, and morphine. *Cancer* 1996;78(4):852.
76. Ripamonti C, Groff L, Brunelli C, et al. Switching from morphine to oral methadone in treating cancer pain: what is the equianalgesic dose ratio? *J Clin Oncol* 1998;16(10):3216.
79. Kornick CA, Santiago-Palma J, Schulman G, et al. A safe and effective method for converting patients from transdermal to intravenous fentanyl for the treatment of acute cancer-related pain. *Cancer* 2003;97(12):3121.
80. Foley KM. Changing concepts of tolerance to opioids. What the cancer patient has taught us. In: Chapman C, Foley K, eds. *Current and emerging issues in cancer pain: research and practice*. New York: Raven Press, 1993:331.
81. Foley KM. Competent care for the dying instead of physician-assisted suicide [comment]. *N Engl J Med* 1997;336(1):54.
84. Joranson D, Ryan KM, Maurer MA. Opioid policy, availability and access in developing and non industrialized countries. In: Fishman S, Ballantyne J, Rathmell JP, eds. *Bonica's management of pain*. Philadelphia: Walters Kluwer, Lippincott, Williams & Williams, 2010:192.
92. Fredheim OMS, Borchgrevink PC, Hegrenaes L, et al. Opioid switching from morphine to methadone causes a minor but not clinically significant increase in QTc time: a prospective 9-month follow-up study. *J Pain Symptom Manage* 2006;32(2):180.
94. Bruera E, Palmer JL, Bosnjak S, et al. Methadone versus morphine as a first-line strong opioid for cancer pain: a randomized, double-blind study. *J Clin Oncol* 2004;22(1):185.
100. Coluzzi PH, Schwartzberg L, Conroy JD, et al. Breakthrough cancer pain: a randomized trial comparing oral transmucosal fentanyl citrate (OTFC) and morphine sulfate immediate release (MSIR). *Pain* 2001;91 (1–2):123.
101. Pergolizzi JV, Mercandante S, Echabru AV, et al. The role of transdermal buprenorphine in the treatment of cancer pain: an expert panel consensus. *Curr Med Res Opin* 2009;25(6):1517.
106. Smith TJ, Staats PS, Deer T, et al. Randomized clinical trial of an implantable drug delivery system compared with comprehensive medical management for refractory cancer pain: impact on pain, drug-related toxicity, and survival. *J Clin Oncol* 2002;20(19):4040.
107. Dennis GC, DeWitty RL. Long-term intraventricular infusion of morphine for intractable pain in cancer of the head and neck. *Neurosurgery* 1990;26(3):404.
112. Apfel CC, Cakmakkaya OS, Frings G, et al. Droperidol has comparable clinical efficacy against both nausea and vomiting. *Br J Anaesth* 2009; 103(3):369.
114. Holzer P. Opioid antagonists for prevention and treatment of opioid induced gastrointestinal effects. *Curr Opin Anaesthesiol* 2010;23(5):616.
115. Kanner RM, Foley KM. Patterns of narcotic drug use in a cancer pain clinic. *Ann N Y Acad Sci* 1981;362:161.
119. Finnerup NB, Otto M, McQuay HJ, et al. Algorithm for neuropathic pain treatment: an evidence based proposal. *Pain* 2005;118(3):289.
125. Wiffen PJ, McQuay HJ, Edwards JE, et al. Gabapentin for acute and chronic pain. *Cochrane Database System Rev* 2005;3:CD005452.
126. Wiffen P, Collins S, McQuay H, et al. Anticonvulsant drugs for acute and chronic pain. *Cochrane Database System Rev* 2005;3:CD001133.
148. Gralow J, Tripathy D. Managing metastatic bone pain: the role of bisphosphonates. *J Pain Symptom Manage* 2007;33(4):462.
156. Abernethy AP, Keefe FJ, McCrory DC, Scipio CD, Matchar DB. *Technology assessment on the use of behavioral therapies for treatment of medical disorders: part 2—impact on management of patients with cancer pain*. Report to the US Agency for Healthcare Research and Quality. Durham, NC: Duke Center for Clinical Health Policy Research, 2005.
168. Rasian AM, Burchiel KJ. Neurosurgical advances in cancer pain management. *Curr Pain Headache Rep* 2010;14(6):477.
171. Sliwa JA, Marciniak C. Physical rehabilitation of the cancer patient. In: Von Gunten C, ed. *Palliative care and rehabilitation of cancer patients*. Boston: Kluwer Academic, 1998:76.

CHAPTER 171 NUTRITIONAL SUPPORT

ALESSANDRO LAVIANO, ROBERT A. MEGUID, AND MICHAEL M. MEGUID

Many tumors can now be treated. However, toxicity associated with planned antineoplastic regimens remains a limiting factor in completing such planned schedule, since it may enhance or worsen a precarious nutritional status, often leading to malnutrition. This in turn favors the onset of adverse side effects, delays surgical procedures, and impedes the initiation or completion of radiation and chemotherapy. It must be emphasized that malnutrition *per se* is a disease, and the expected norm is the use of specific adjuvant nutrition therapy. Consequently, a working knowledge of nutritional therapy is mandatory for oncologists who aim to deliver antineoplastic therapies effectively and to maintain quality of life during cancer treatment and palliative care.

Malnutrition is frequently observed in cancer patients.[1] However, weight loss caused by cancer differs from that observed during simple starvation. The latter is characterized by preservation of lean body mass. Weight loss in cancer patients does not solely result from anorexia and reduced food intake, but largely due to the catastrophic derangements in metabolism induced by the inflammatory response to tumor growth[1] (Table 171.1), which in turn, prevents optimal nutrient utilization.

The etiology of cancer-associated malnutrition is related to the pathological loss of inhibitory control of central and peripheral catabolic pathways, whose increased activities are not counterbalanced by the increased central and peripheral anabolic drive.[1] The molecular mechanisms responsible for these metabolic derangements are increasingly being elucidated, leading to novel, pathogenesis-based therapeutic approaches currently being tested.[2]

The critical goals of nutrition therapy in cancer are (1) to maintain or improve nutritional status to allow for initiation and completion of aggressive anticancer therapies and (2) to increase the functional capacity and quality of life of patients, even in advanced cases. The issue of quality of life is of paramount importance because patients are more concerned with their ability to function as close to normal as possible and to maintain a good quality of life than being preoccupied with their ultimate mortality.[3] In this respect, it should be emphasized that when body weight and particularly lean body mass is lost, function and quality of life suffer.[4] In cancer patients an impressive 50% of the quality of life function scores are determined by nutritional intake and weight loss.[5]

Not only tumor growth but also cancer treatments, including surgery, chemotherapy, and radiation therapy, interfere with the patient's ability to taste, ingest, swallow, or digest food. Surgery and radiation of the gastrointestinal tract may affect the digestion and absorption of nutrients. Drugs may cause nausea and diarrhea. Although many new drugs exist to combat these symptoms, the prevalence of nausea and diarrhea remains high.

In summary, cancer-associated malnutrition is the result of a *deadly* combination of anorexia, with its attendant reduced food intake, and profound biochemical alterations of host metabolism, exacerbating weight loss and impeding its reversal with adjuvant nutrient therapy.

ANOREXIA

One of the most distressing symptoms presenting a significant challenge to the cancer patient is the progressive development of anorexia and reduced food intake.[6,7] Anorexia is defined as the loss of the desire to eat[8] and may result from the occurrence of changes in smell, generalized alterations of taste (i.e., dysgeusia), specific alterations of taste (e.g., meat aversion), early satiety, or nausea and vomiting. Anorexia may be the presenting symptom of cancer, occurring independently from cancer treatment, but it is frequently associated with antineoplastic therapy as a side effect of chemo- and radiation therapy. The pathogenesis of cancer-associated anorexia appears to be related to the inability of the neuroregulation of energy homeostasis due to locoregional inflammation.[9,10] As a result, the brain is persistently set in an anorexigenic mode, which induces the suppression of appetite, and is not influenced by the usual peripheral signals indicating the progressive depletion of energy stores.[2]

The diagnosis of anorexia can either be made by assessing the presence of specific symptoms (i.e., changes in taste and smell, meat aversion, nausea and vomiting, early satiety)[11] or by using specific questionnaires (e.g., the North Central Cancer Treatment Group and the Functional Assessment of Anorexia Cachexia Therapy questionnaires).[12,13] Recently, the European Society for Clinical Nutrition and Metabolism (ESPEN) has proposed an anorexia score allowing a qualitative and quantitative assessment of anorexia.[8]

When anorexia develops as a side effect of cancer treatment, it frequently results from the occurrence of nausea, vomiting, and dysgeusia. Drug-related toxicity is associated with the presence of malnutrition and is responsible for the nausea and vomiting that occurs with chemotherapy, but a strong psychological component has also been reported. Indeed, patient expectation of developing nausea and vomiting during chemotherapy is a strong predictor of actual severe nausea.[14] Thus, interventions designed to reduce the expectation of nausea by patients should be developed. Also, food aversion patterning may develop during chemo- and radiation therapy (i.e., the distressing emotional association of specific tastes and smells with negative psychological experiences).[9] Food aversion patterning may be responsible for vomiting when odors or tastes associated with chemotherapy are perceived. In this respect, during anorexigenic cancer treatments, it is important to suggest to patients not to eat their favorite foods to prevent the development of aversion to those foods.

Drugs such as vincristine and the taxanes have the strongest associations with dysgeusia. The pathogenesis of chemotherapy-induced dysgeusia is related to the excretion or secretion of drugs in saliva, thereby markedly altering taste and leading to

TABLE 171.1

METABOLIC DIFFERENCES BETWEEN THE RESPONSE TO SIMPLE STARVATION AND ADVANCED MALIGNANT DISEASE

Parameter	Simple Starvation	Advanced Malignant Disease
Basal metabolic rate	0 or −	0 or − or +
Presence of mediators	0	++
Hepatic ureagenesis	+	++
Negative nitrogen balance	+	++
Gluconeogenesis	+	++
Muscle proteolysis	+	++
Hepatic protein synthesis	+	++
Lipolysis	+	++

0, normal; −, decreased; +, slightly increased; ++, a substantial increase.

food revulsion and avoidance. Not only may certain tastes be affected, but food consistency or texture may be a factor as well, requiring more chewing, which may increase saliva production, perpetuating the cycle. Multiple other mechanisms may be involved in dysgeusia, including zinc deficiency, morphologic changes in the lingual papillae, and even neuropathy. Dysgeusia may also be caused by depression, which may initially go unrecognized in cancer patients.[15]

Various attempts at treatment of dysgeusia have been made, but with little success. Each patient must experiment to find foods that are associated with the least alteration in taste. Different tastes can be tested using sugar for sweet, lemon juice for sour, salt (for salt), and aspirin or quinine for bitter. Usually, foods that can be swallowed with little chewing and therefore little saliva production are tolerated best. Attempts at dietary supplementation with elements such as zinc, folic acid, alpha-lipoic acid, and the B vitamins may alleviate some metallic tastes but are only mildly helpful. Zinc seems to work best with a "sweet" dysgeusia, but drugs often give a more metallic taste, and the best treatment for dysgeusia remains withdrawal of the offending drug. After drug cessation, the taste usually returns to normal over a 2-month period. Perhaps a more effective regimen is nutritional counseling to give patients a goal of their necessary daily protein and calorie intake. This allows them to overcome the dysgeusia and avoid weight loss and muscle depletion and maintain an element of control in their management. Patients, with the aid of caregivers, must continually experiment to find foods that are palatable and provide the necessary amounts of nutrients.

CHANGES IN HOST METABOLISM: WEIGHT LOSS AND CACHEXIA

Most cancer patients lose weight as a result of their disease, exacerbated by aggressive antineoplastic therapeutic regimens. The amount of weight loss varies with the type of cancer.[16] Loss in excess of 10% of baseline body weight over 6 months is defined as critical weight loss.

In cancer patients, weight loss is secondary to the inflammation changes brought about by the tumor's presence, which impacts host metabolism and eating behavior[10,17] (Table 171.2). Direct effects of cytokines and other inflammatory mediators, the acute-phase response, and proteolysis are difficult to reverse with traditional nutritional support because the ensuing weight loss is not the result of starvation. This peculiar malnutrition syndrome is known as *cancer cachexia*. Lundholm et al.[18] highlighted the negative role of inflammation and metabolic derangement in cancer cachexia and showed that integrated metabolic support, including nutritional support, anti-inflammatory drugs, and erythropoietin, improves survival in advanced cancer patients.

An operational definition of cachexia has been recently proposed. Cachexia should be considered as a "complex metabolic syndrome associated with underlying illness and characterized by loss of muscle with or without loss of fat mass."[19] Therefore, cachexia can be diagnosed in a patient with involuntary weight loss of at least 5% in 12 months or less with at least three of the following symptoms: (1) decreased muscle strength, (2) fatigue, (3) anorexia, (4) low fat-free mass index, and (5) abnormal biochemistry (i.e., increased inflammatory markers, such as C-reactive protein, interleukin-6, tumor necrosis factor-alpha [TNF-α]), anemia (Hb less than 12 g/dL), or low serum albumin (less than 32 g/L).[19] The clinical relevance of the diagnostic criteria of cachexia has been highlighted by Fearon et al.,[20] who showed that the association of weight loss, reduced food intake, and systemic inflammation, as defined by increased levels of C-reactive protein, identifies patients with *both* adverse function and prognosis.

The presence of overt cachexia limits the efficacy of nutrition therapy. Therefore, the identification of symptoms related to the early phases of cachexia, or precachexia, helps to identify higher risk patients and may favor a prompt start of nutrition therapy. To this end, Bozzetti et al.[21] placed 1,307 cancer patients into four groups based on combinations of body weight loss (less than 10% signifying precachexia; greater than or equal to 10%, indicating cachexia) and the presence or absence of at least one symptom of either anorexia, fatigue, or early satiation. Moving from "asymptomatic precachexia" (group 1) to "symptomatic cachexia" (group 4), there were statistically significant trends in the percentage of gastrointestinal versus nongastrointestinal tumors, severity of cancer stage, percentage of weight loss, number of symptoms per patient, Eastern Cooperative Oncology Group (ECOG) performance status, and nutritional risk score. More recently, ESPEN proposed that precachexia could be diagnosed in the simultaneous presence of underlying chronic disease, unintentional weight loss 5% or less of usual

TABLE 171.2

METABOLIC ABNORMALITIES IN ANIMAL AND HUMAN CANCER CACHEXIA

Substrate	Clinical Parameter	Observation
Water	Total body water	Increased
Energy	Energy balance	Negative
	Energy stores	Decreased
Lipid	Body fat mass	Decreased
	Lipoprotein lipase activity	Decreased
	Fat breakdown	Increased
	Serum lipid levels	Increased
Carbohydrate	Gluconeogenesis	Increased
	Insulin resistance	Present
	Body glucose consumption	Increased
	Hepatic glucose production	Increased
Protein	Muscle mass	Decreased
	Muscle proteolysis	Increased
	Muscle amino acid release	Increased
	Hepatic protein synthesis	Increased
	Hepatic amino acid transport	Increased
	Nitrogen balance	Negative

body weight during the last 6 months, chronic or recurrent systemic inflammatory response, and anorexia or anorexia-related symptoms.[8] Prospective clinical trials are under way to validate such critical and fundamental advances in the operational definitions of cachexia and precachexia.

Multiple factors interact to produce cancer cachexia, including tumor products, hormones, and inflammatory mediators.[22] This interaction promotes gluconeogenesis, limits anabolism, and increases catabolism. The pathogenesis of cancer cachexia is mediated by the induction of an inflammatory response to the growing tumor.[10] Many host-derived inflammatory mediators involved in cancer cachexia have been identified. The cytokines TNF-α, interleukin-1, interleukin-6, and interferon-γ appear to play a significant role in this.[23] Because elevated levels of these cytokines are rarely found in the blood of cancer patients, the effect may be caused more from paracrine than from systemic production.

Additional mediators of cancer cachexia include two peptides produced by the tumor and known to influence protein and lipid metabolism: the proteolysis-inducing factor[24] and the lipid-mobilizing factor,[25] respectively. Proteolysis-inducing factor activates the ubiquitin proteolytic pathway, resulting in proteolysis; while lipid-mobilizing factor promotes breakdown of adipose tissue into fatty acids.[17] It should be acknowledged that concerns have been raised as to the yet undetected, but likely, human homologue to an existing murine proteolysis-inducing factor.[26]

The synergy between host-derived and tumor-derived factors increases the activity of the muscle ubiquitin-proteasome system,[22] which is not counterbalanced by a similar increase of protein synthesis, with the net result of progressive muscle wasting.

NUTRITION THERAPY FOR CANCER CACHEXIA

Nutritional interventions are valuable to cancer patients when they are easily user-friendly, promote preservation of lean body mass, and aim to maintain function and quality of life. Several new reports have examined supplements and additives for use in cancer patients to maintain lean body mass.

The best therapeutic option for cancer cachexia is effective treatment of the underlying disease.[27] If this cannot be achieved, then specialized nutritional therapy should be developed that aims at maintaining body weight, in particular lean body mass, by counteracting the negative effects on metabolism and eating behavior of the increased inflammatory response. Indeed, preserving lean body mass in cancer patients influences not only their morbidity but also their quality of life.[28]

The first step in the multimodal nutritional therapy of cancer patients is nutritional counseling. Early, intensive, individualized nutritional counseling has consistently been shown to be effective in preserving body weight and physical function in cancer patients.[29,30] It should be emphasized that the key to success of this approach is strict adherence to patients' needs and frequent monitoring of results. Therefore, the efficacy of nutritional counseling in cancer patients relies on the presence of a well-trained and specialized nutrition support team, particularly when considering that in many cancer patients body weight stabilization cannot be achieved by a daily energy intake lower than 30 kcal/kg of body weight.[6]

Pharmacologic agents, such as the steroid megestrol acetate, have been used to increase appetite but are associated with fat gain rather than increase in lean body mass.[31] Likewise, corticosteroids may also increase appetite but are actually catabolic agents that induce muscle breakdown, especially in inactive, fatigued cancer patients.[31] Dronabinol, a derivative of cannabis, which stimulates the endocannabinoid system, has not been proven effective in improving appetite in cancer patients.[32]

The identification of the prophagic effects of the peptide hormone ghrelin and the increased understanding of the role in cancer cachexia of the hypothalamic anorexigenic melanocortin system suggest the use of exogenous ghrelin or antimelanocortin peptides as anticachexia agents. Preliminary experimental and clinical studies appear promising,[33–35] but larger trials are needed before their use can be routinely applied. Considering the central role of proteolysis-inducing factor and cytokines in triggering muscle wasting, it has been postulated that inhibition of their synthesis and activity may decrease proteolysis. The omega-3 fatty acid eicosapentaenoic acid (EPA) has been shown to have antitumor and anticachectic effects. Although the available clinical data are not sufficient to draw definitive recommendations, it appears that the impact of supplemental fish oil capsules on cancer cachexia is minimal.[36,37] In contrast, the use of oral nutritional supplements enriched with EPA, at a dose of 2 to 3 g/d, appears to ameliorate lean body mass wasting,[28,38,39] but more high-quality clinical trials are needed to confirm these results.

The supplementation of essential amino acids, and particularly of branched-chain amino acids (BCAAs), has been shown to ameliorate cancer anorexia and stimulate protein synthesis, thereby maintaining muscle and lean body mass.[40] These effects appear to be secondary to the inhibitory influence of BCAAs, and in particular of leucine, on brain serotonergic neurotransmission, yielding to improved appetite, and on the ubiquitin–proteasome system, the main proteolytic system involved in cancer cachexia.[40] Similar to the results observed with the supplementation of leucine, the use of β-hydroxy-β-methylbutyrate, a leucine metabolite, promotes deposition of lean body mass in cancer patients.[41]

In patients who undergo surgery for gastrointestinal cancer, even in the absence of malnutrition, perioperative supplementation of immune-enhancing nutrients (i.e., arginine, omega-3 fatty acids, and nucleotides) is recommended to reduce postoperative complications. This emphasizes the relevance of priming the metabolism of cancer patients with specific nutrients prior to surgery.[42] Due to conflicting results and potential adverse effects, the use of anabolic agents in cancer patients is not generally recommended.

Branched-chain amino acids, EPA, and arginine represent a class of nutrients that has received much attention because of their influence on deranged host metabolism when administered at pharmacologic doses. These nutrients with pharmacologic properties have been termed *nutraceuticals*, and their identification is progressively changing and enhancing the nutrition–metabolic support of cancer patients.[43]

Based on the available evidence, it appears advisable to use a hypercaloric (30 to 35 kcal/kg of body weight), high-protein diet (1 to 1.5 g/kg of body weight) rich in BCAAs (approximately 10 to 15 g/d, 50% of which should be leucine), and EPA (2 to 3 g/d) for patients with cachexia who can tolerate oral feeding. These nutrients can easily be incorporated into a daily routine with appropriate nutritional counseling, which should also include regular mild to moderate physical exercise. In many cancer patients, swallowing liquids is often easier than chewing solid foods. Commercial oral nutritional supplements are also available that provide energy, protein, EPA, and amino acids in ready-to-drink cans.

NUTRITION AND TUMOR GROWTH

Supplementing cancer patients with therapeutic nutrients may raise the long feared, but yet unfounded, concern of stimulating tumor growth. The available evidence does not provide a definitive answer as to whether nutrition therapy stimulates tumor growth, but it is reasonable to assume that the biological risk of stimulating tumor growth by nutrition therapy exists.[44] However, the sensitivity of tumor cells to caloric restriction is related to specific mutations in the insulin pathway.[45] Therefore, it appears clinically unwise and ethically questionable to starve cancer patients in the absence of genetic evidence of potential efficacy. Also, it has been shown that glucose deprivation promotes the acquisition by cancer cells of mutations, rendering them more aggressive.[46] Finally, the tumor may be able to divert nutrient availability from the host for its own metabolism, regardless of nutrition support. It should be noted that specialized nutrition–metabolic support, aimed at providing nutrients and interfering with the metabolic changes induced by the tumor, has been demonstrated to yield significant clinical benefits.[18,28,38,39]

NUTRITIONAL ASSESSMENT OF THE CANCER PATIENT

To determine the best strategies for treatment, the nutritional status of the cancer patient must first be determined. Because there are different components of the human body (lean body mass, fat mass, bone, interstitial fluid, etc.), the assessment of nutritional status is a complex procedure that should be performed by trained individuals.[47] Determination starts with a careful history and physical examination followed by additional tests to confirm the clinical impression. The history should include inquiries regarding appetite, taste changes, swallowing and digestive problems, preferred foods, and weight loss.

The preservation of lean body mass is of paramount importance in cancer patients. Therefore, the evaluation of lean body mass should represent the main goal of any nutritional assessment procedure.[48] Bioimpedance analysis is an easily available tool to assess muscle mass in patients, but it is heavily influenced by water retention. Dual energy x-ray absorptiometry has proven very sensitive in detecting lean body mass but is not used routinely due to its high cost. Considering that all cancer patients undergo total body computerized tomography (CT) scan, it has been recently shown that evaluation of muscle mass on CT strata via specifically developed computerized software reliably measures lean body mass.[49]

To facilitate the identification of malnourished cancer patients or patients at risk of malnutrition, a screening procedure should be implemented in all cancer patients via validated tools,[50,51] followed by thorough nutritional assessment only when malnutrition or the risk of malnutrition is found.

Indications for Nutrition Therapy

Increased proteolysis has been demonstrated in gastric cancer patients who exhibit no weight loss.[52,53] Therefore, it is becoming widely accepted that all cancer patients should be screened and regularly monitored for their nutritional status, and that nutritional and metabolic therapy should be considered in cancer patients with precachexia and provided for patients with cachexia. In particular, it is critical that any support, either nutritional (i.e., providing macronutrients and micronutrients), or metabolic (i.e., providing nutraceuticals or drugs that interfere with tumor-induced metabolic change), or a combination thereof, should be started concomitantly with anticancer treatment.[54]

TABLE 171.3

PROPOSED BENEFITS OF ORAL AND ENTERAL NUTRITION VERSUS PARENTERAL NUTRITION

Maintains gut mucosal mass
Maintains brush border enzyme activity
Supports gut immune function
Preserves gut mucosal barrier function
Maintains balanced luminal microfloral environment
Improves outcome after chemo- and radiation therapy

PARENTERAL VERSUS ENTERAL NUTRITION IN CANCER PATIENTS

In cancer patients with an accessible and functional gastrointestinal tract, oral or enteral nutrition should be used (Table 171.3). Patients who can maintain adequate oral intake through food and dietary supplements may be able to avoid feeding tube placement. Close monitoring is also necessary to detect failure of oral feeding early so that tube feeding can begin in a timely manner. In this regard, ESPEN has recently issued guidelines for the use of enteral nutrition in adult cancer patients.[55]

Specific Indications for the Use of Total Parenteral Nutrition in Cancer Patients

Considering the higher cost and potential for severe complications associated with the use of parenteral nutrition, its use should be limited to those cancer patients whose gastrointestinal tracts are not functional (Table 171.4). The indications for the use of parenteral nutrition in cancer patients have been recently published by ESPEN.[56] In particular, the following clinical conditions may require the use of parenteral nutrition.

Acute Radiation and Chemotherapy Enteritis

Although parenteral nutrition is not routinely indicated during chemioradiotherapy,[56] cancer patients who receive abdominal or pelvic irradiation or chemotherapy and develop severe and prolonged mucositis and enterocolitis may benefit from total parenteral nutrition until the enteritis resolves and oral feeding can be resumed.

Indeed, during active treatment, nausea, vomiting, mucositis, xerostomia, dysphagia, diarrhea, and anorexia can develop, reducing or impeding oral intake. Whenever feasible and accepted by patients, enteral nutritional support is preferable, and patients undergoing irradiation of the head, neck, or chest need to be considered for early feeding tube placement.[57] However, in cases involving severe and prolonged dysfunction of the gastrointestinal tract, total parenteral nutrition or supplemental parenteral nutrition is indicated to fill the calorie and protein gaps between nutritional requirements and actual intake. If the time to resumption to normal oral intake does not exceed 7 to 10 days, then peripheral parenteral nutrition may be indicated. However, peripheral cannulae should be regularly changed every 48 to 72 hours to prevent the development of phlebitis. In this respect, the use of midterm peripheral catheters (i.e., Midline) is preferable since its replacement is not necessary if it is used less than 3 months.

Patients with Short Bowel Syndrome

Short bowel syndrome may develop in cancer patients secondary to multiple bowel resections or massive resection of

TABLE 171.4

INDICATIONS AND CONTRAINDICATIONS FOR THE USE OF TOTAL PARENTERAL NUTRITION IN THE CANCER PATIENT

A. TPN for anticipated brief, in-hospital periods (>5 days)
   1. TPN is not indicated:
      a. In well-nourished or mildly malnourished patients undergoing chemotherapy, radiation therapy, or surgery.
      b. In patients with rapidly progressive malignant disease who fail to respond to treatment.
      c. In patients who have evidence of terminal disease and are not candidates for further antitumor therapy.
   2. TPN is indicated:
      a. In severely malnourished patients who are responding to chemotherapy and in whom gastrointestinal or other toxicities preclude adequate enteral intake for 7 to 10 days or longer.[a]

B. Prolonged periods of in-hospital TPN or home TPN
   1. TPN is not indicated:
      a. In patients with rapidly progressive tumor growth that is unresponsive to therapy.
   2. TPN is indicated:
      a. In those patients for whom treatment-associated toxicities preclude the use of enteral nutrition and represent the primary impediment to the restoration of performance status. Such patients usually respond to antitumor therapy.
      b. In selected malnourished cancer patients in whom the natural history of the disease can be expected to permit a period of normal or near normal performance status. Such patients should be receiving antitumor therapy with a reasonable anticipation of response, or the natural history of the untreated tumor is such that a reasonable quality of life can be expected (survival longer than 6 to 12 months).

TPN, total parenteral nutrition.
[a]Available evidence would suggest that patients who are candidates for TPN under these circumstances should, when feasible, receive TPN before or in conjunction with the initiation of therapy.

infarcted bowel. Most of these individuals, if cured of their cancer, can now survive for long periods on home total parenteral nutrition. Due to the duration of therapy involved, these patients are at risk for development of long-term problems, including micronutrient deficiency, bone demineralization, and catheter sepsis. Gut rehabilitation could be enhanced and total parenteral nutrition dependency could be reduced by the use of growth hormone, glutamine, and an optimal diet.[58,59]

Composition of Total Parenteral Nutrition Formulations

Total parenteral nutrition solutions are administered through a central venous catheter that is generally inserted into the subclavian vein. Total parenteral nutrition solutions are hyperosmolar and calorie dense and usually comprised of amino acid, glucose, and lipid formulations. As a general rule, approximately 65% of total nonprotein calories are provided as dextrose and the remaining 35% as lipids.

Calories are provided at a daily dose greater than 30 kcal/kg body weight. Proteins are provided at a dose of 1 to 1.5 g/kg of body weight, but this dose should be reduced in the presence of hepatic or renal failure. The addition of minerals, vitamins, and electrolytes completes the basic composition of the solution. Solutions must be prepared under sterile conditions. Because of the hyperosmolarity of such solutions, they must be delivered into a high-flow venous system to prevent venous sclerosis, subsequent thrombosis, and distal embolization.

Potential Complications of Total Parenteral Nutrition

Advances in technology, including patient monitoring and catheter care, have greatly reduced the incidence of complications associated with the use of total parenteral nutrition. Complications of total parenteral nutrition that occur in cancer patients can be divided into four types: (1) mechanical (pneumothorax, laceration of the subclavian artery, air embolism, catheter embolism), (2) metabolic (hyperglycemia, electrolyte abnormalities, abnormalities in liver enzymes), (3) infectious (catheter sepsis), and (4) thrombotic (catheter occlusion, superior vena caval thrombosis). Catheter sepsis is a frequent cause of febrile neutropenia and must be excluded as a cause in these patients.

Patients receiving total parenteral nutrition should be monitored regularly by measuring blood glucose (initially every 6 hours, then daily once stable), serum electrolytes (daily to weekly), triglycerides, and liver function test results (weekly to monthly). Careful monitoring is critical as complications during aggressive feedings include electrolyte derangements such as severe hypokalemia or hypophosphatemia. Hypophosphatemia may develop in the chronically malnourished cachectic cancer patient given a dextrose infusion. This stems from the use of phosphate to make adenosine triphosphate, depleting phosphate stores rapidly. This is referred to as *refeeding syndrome* and was originally seen in starved refugees who were suddenly given high-calorie diets. These electrolyte disturbances can develop rapidly and are much more likely to become life-threatening than hyponatremia or hyperglycemia.

Effects of Total Parenteral Nutrition on the Gastrointestinal Tract

Disuse of the gastrointestinal tract, either via starvation or nutritional therapy by total parenteral nutrition, may lead to numerous physiologic derangements as well as changes in gut microflora, impaired gut immune function, and potential disruption of mucosal barrier integrity. Whether these effects mediate bacterial translocation and thus septic complications, as demonstrated in animal models, or by absorption of endotoxins or cytokines is still matter of debate. Regardless of mechanism, it appears that maintaining gut function in the cancer patient who is receiving vigorous therapy may be essential to minimize septic complications and organ failure.

Consequently, enteral nutrition should always be used preferentially over parenteral nutrition. In patients who cannot tolerate enteral nutrition, minimal enteral feeding should be maintained to preserve gut integrity.

Improving the Efficacy of Current Feeding Regimens

Role of Physical Exercise

Recent data indicate that physical exercise plays a relevant role in the multimodal approach to cancer cachexia.[60,61] These results underline the importance of starting nutrition therapy early in the clinical course of the disease, when fatigue, which may severely limit exercise capacity, has not yet developed. Therefore, cancer patients should be encouraged to ambulate or even perform isometric exercises in bed as much as is feasible. Exercise increases functional aerobic capacity, stimulates skeletal muscle amino acid uptake, and reduces proteolysis in normal individuals Additionally, increased motor activity has a positive influence on quality of life.[62]

Pharmacologic and Hormonal Therapy

The use of anti-inflammatory drugs and erythropoietin in combination with nutritional support reduces mortality in advanced cancer patients.[18] However, the use of erythropoietin should be cautiously considered due to the potential stimulatory effects on cancer cells.[63] Recombinant human growth hormone has anabolic effects in humans and is beneficial in cancer patients with cachexia. However, its use may also promote tumor growth. To minimize this risk, new strategies to deliver growth hormone directly in the muscle have been developed, including gene therapy. Preliminary animal studies show that this approach holds promise.[64,65]

Progestagens, including megestrol acetate, improve appetite and body weight in cancer patients, although most of the weight gain is due to water retention.[31] Current recommendations for megestrol acetate are 160 to 480 mg/d in conjunction with nutritional support.

Use of Glutamine and Arginine

Under physiologic conditions, a sufficient amount of glutamine is endogenously produced to meet the body's demand. In conditions of stress, the amount of glutamine produced is no longer sufficient, and a glutamine deficit may occur without supplementation. Therefore, glutamine is considered a conditionally essential amino acid. Glutamine is the preferential substrate of rapidly dividing cells, including bone marrow and gut mucosa. Therefore, its supplementation may be beneficial in patients receiving high-dose chemotherapy who develop mucositis. Clinical studies indicate that provision of glutamine, either orally or parenterally, in patients undergoing bone marrow transplantation, improves nitrogen balance and reduces complications.[66]

The enthusiasm over the potential beneficial role of glutamine supplementation in cancer patients has been recently challenged by *in vitro* evidence showing that glutamine may enhance energy metabolism of tumor cells.[67,68] Whether this experimental evidence may translate into negative clinical results remains to be tested. However, clinical trials that test for the impact of glutamine on cancer patients' outcome did not report major adverse effects,[69] although survival was not a primary end point in many studies.

Arginine has immunomodulatory effects that are beneficial to cancer patients. Arginine supplementation in combination with omega-3 fatty acids is effective in reducing surgical morbidity and hospitalization costs.[42] However, concern exists that as a precursor to nitric oxide, its use in septic patients may be contraindicated. However, no specific studies have tested this.

Techniques of Providing Enteral Nutrition

Transnasal (Nasogastric and Nasoduodenal) Feeding Tubes

The use of transnasal feeding catheters for intragastric or duodenal feeding is a popular adjunct for providing nutritional support enterally. The stomach is easily accessed by the passage of a soft flexible (8 French) feeding (nasogastric) tube. Intragastric feedings provide several advantages for the patient. The stomach has the capacity for bolus feedings that more closely mimic human meal patterns. Feeding into the stomach results in the stimulation of the biliary–pancreatic axis, which is probably trophic for the small bowel, and gastric secretions have a dilutional effect on the osmolarity of the feedings, reducing the risk of diarrhea. The major risk of intragastric feeding is the regurgitation of gastric contents, resulting in tracheal aspiration. This risk is highest in patients who have altered mental sensorium or who are paralyzed. The placement of the feeding tube past the pylorus into the fourth portion of the duodenum reduces the risk of regurgitation and aspiration.

Gastrostomy Feeding Tube

In patients with an unresectable head and neck or esophageal carcinoma who are not surgical candidates or in individuals who are unable to maintain caloric needs or require long-term enteral nutrition, a permanent feeding gastrostomy should be considered. Percutaneous endoscopic gastrostomy (PEG), providing access for gastric feedings, can be performed, avoiding a laparotomy and anesthesia (local, sedation, or general). The issues related to the use of PEG have been recently reviewed by ESPEN.[57]

Jejunostomy Placement and Witzel Jejunostomy

A feeding catheter jejunostomy should be placed after any major upper abdominal oncologic procedure if prolonged enteral nutrition support is anticipated, especially after gastric or pancreatic cancer surgery. The simplest method is a needle catheter jejunostomy, which can be performed fairly quickly at the end of the definitive operation. The needle catheter jejunostomy is generally removed 2 to 4 weeks postoperatively when no longer needed.

A more permanent form of feeding jejunostomy uses a 14-French red rubber catheter for feeding. The placement technique starts with construction of a simple Witzel tunnel and usually takes 10 to 15 minutes. Jejunal feeding catheters can be used immediately for feeding purposes after the operation. Catheter care is essential to maintain patency, and the catheter needs to be flushed with 30 mL of 0.9% saline every 8 hours to ensure adequate patency. The catheter can be removed at the patient's bedside at the desired time by simple traction, and the resulting fistula usually closes quickly. Gastrostomies and jejunostomies can now be done laparoscopically using anchors inserted across the abdominal wall to secure the wall of the stomach or jejunum to the parietal peritoneum.

Ordering or Prescribing Enteral Nutrition

Table 171.5 outlines the most important factors to be considered when ordering enteral nutrition, and commercial formulations are available. Specific instructions pertain to route of administration, feeding schedule, and infusion rate. In general, feeds are advanced by 10 mL every 2 to 6 hours until goal infusion volume is reached. Bolus feeds are reserved for gastric

TABLE 171.5

FACTORS TO BE CONSIDERED WHEN ORDERING ENTERAL NUTRITION

Route of administration (nasogastric, gastrostomy, etc.)
Industrial product available
Feeding schedule (continuous or bolus) and infusion rate
Nursing care of the feeding tube
Nutritional monitoring
Biochemical monitoring

TABLE 171.6

FACTORS TO BE CONSIDERED WHEN ORDERING PARENTERAL NUTRITION

Patient's dry body weight and nutritional requirements
Reason for parenteral nutrition
Standardized or individual mixture
Infusion rate
Additives (vitamins, trace elements, electrolytes)
Clinical and biochemical monitoring

delivery and not used with jejunostomy delivery of enteral nutrition. Selection of commercial enteral nutrition preparations should be tailored to the individual patient and based on a combination of caloric and protein requirements, accounting for issues such as renal insufficiency, ventilator dependency, and electrolyte derangements.

Central Venous Total Parenteral Nutrition

The preferred method of access to the superior vena cava is by percutaneous cannulation of the subclavian vein. Alternate sites include the internal and external jugular veins, but it is more difficult to maintain a sterile dressing with these positions. A long-term indwelling catheter should be placed over the chest wall due to the reduced risk of catheter infections associated with this position. In addition, percutaneous catheters and subcutaneous "ports" can be placed over the pectoral region for ease of access and repeated use.

When a peripherally inserted central catheter (PICC) is used, central total parenteral nutrition can be administered even if the subclavian or jugular veins are unavailable for use. PICC lines are usually inserted with the aid of ultrasonography through an antecubital location and then threaded into central veins. A PICC should not be used for infusing long-term (i.e., longer than 3 months) total parenteral nutrition. In such cases, long-term central catheters (tunneled or port) should be used.

Complications from long-term central venous catheterization in the cancer patient population include venous thrombosis and catheter-related infections. Thrombosis of the central vessels is a complication that may often be overlooked. Clinical suspicion of subclavian venous thrombosis is appropriate in approximately 3% of patients with central venous catheters, whereas studies using phlebography or radionuclide venography indicate that incidence is as high as 35%. With increased use of internal jugular veins for long-term indwelling catheters and ports, more patients are presenting with the signs of superior vena caval syndrome (swelling in the head, neck, and arms).

Febrile episodes are not uncommon in the cancer patient population, particularly in the neutropenic individual. Blood culture may not reveal a pathogen. However, if primary catheter sepsis is confirmed, the catheter must be removed immediately. The intradermal portion of the catheter should be sent to the laboratory for culture and compared with two blood cultures drawn from the patient at remote sites. Appropriate antibiotics should be administered and a new catheter inserted when the patient's repeat blood culture results are confirmed negative. If the patient has an indwelling port or long-term percutaneous catheter or is at high risk of developing complications during the insertion procedure, an attempt to sterilize the catheter with antibiotics (i.e., lock therapy) can be made, although results vary.

Ordering or Prescribing Parenteral Nutrition

Table 171.6 outlines the most important factors to consider when prescribing parenteral nutrition. Standardized formulations are provided on the order form, as well as custom formulations and options to include additives such as electrolytes, vitamins, trace elements, and medications. Care must be taken in patients with renal insufficiency, ventilator dependency, and electrolyte derangements. To order individualized parenteral nutrition formulations, the following steps should be taken: (1) the patient's daily caloric and protein requirements must be calculated; this is 30 to 35 kcal/kg of body weight and 1 to 1.5 g/kg of body weight, respectively, for most patients; (2) the caloric requirement must be distributed between macronutrients; (3) the amount of each macronutrient must be calculated; (4) the volume of each macronutrient must be calculated; finally (5) the total volume is calculated, including electrolyte, vitamin, and mineral additives, and then divided by the desired number of hours of infusion to calculate the hourly infusion rate. All parenteral nutrition orders are confirmed by a dietitian certified in nutrition therapy.

ETHICAL AND LEGAL ASPECTS OF NUTRITION THERAPY

Finally, when involved in the treatment plan for nutrition of a cancer patient, the benefit of providing nutrition should outweigh the burden of doing harm. A time may come when nutrition support during palliative care may no longer be necessary or the competent patient refuses further treatment. Consideration of withholding or withdrawing nutrition support is governed by the same laws and mandates a frank discussion as to its continued benefit with patient and family alike.[70]

Selected References

The full list of references for this chapter appears in the online version.

1. Laviano A, Meguid MM, Inui A, et al. Therapy insight: cancer anorexia-cachexia syndrome-when all you can eat is yourself. *Nat Clin Pract Oncol* 2005;2:158.
2. Laviano A, Inui A, Marks DL, et al. Neural control of the anorexia-cachexia syndrome. *Am J Physiol Endocrinol Metab* 2008;295:E1000.
4. Marin Caro MM, Laviano A, Pichard C. Nutritional intervention and quality of life in adult oncology patients. *Clin Nutr* 2007;26:289.

5. Ravasco P, Monteiro-Grillo I, Marques Vidal P, et al. Cancer: disease and nutrition are key determinants of patients' quality of life. *Support Care Cancer* 2004;12:246.
6. Hutton JL, Martin L, Field CJ, et al. Dietary patterns in patients with advanced cancer: implications for anorexia-cachexia therapy. *Am J Clin Nutr* 2006;84:1163.
8. Muscaritoli M, Anker SD, Argiles J, et al. Consensus definition of sarcopenia, cachexia and pre-cachexia: joint document elaborated by Special Interest Groups (SIG) "cachexa-anorexia in chronic wasting diseases" and "nutrition in geriatrics." *Clin Nutr* 2010;29:154.
9. Laviano A, Meguid MM, Rossi Fanelli F. Cancer anorexia: clinical implications, pathogenesis, and therapeutic strategies. *Lancet Oncol* 2003;4:686.
10. Seruga B, Zhang H, Bernstein LJ, Tannock IF. Cytokines and their relationship to the symptoms and outcome of cancer. *Nat Rev Cancer* 2008;8:887.
16. Laviano A, Meguid MM. Nutritional issues in cancer management. *Nutrition* 1996;12:358.
17. Tisdale MJ. Cachexia in cancer patients. *Nat Rev Cancer* 2002;2:862.
18. Lundholm K, Daneryd P, Bosaeus I, et al. Palliative nutritional intervention in addition to cyclooxigenase and erythropoietin treatment for patients with malignant disease: effects on survival, metabolism, and function. *Cancer* 2004;100:1967.
19. Evans WJ, Morley JE, Argiles J, et al. Cachexia: a new definition. *Clin Nutr* 2008;27:793.
20. Fearon KC, Voss AC, Hustead DS, et al. Definition of cancer cachexia: effect of weight loss, reduced food intake, and systemic inflammation on functional status and prognosis. *Am J Clin Nutr* 2006;83:1345.
21. Bozzetti F, Mariani L. Defining and classifying cancer cachexia: a proposal by the SCRINIO Working Group. *JPEN J Parenter Enteral Nutr* 2009; 33:361.
22. Baracos VE. Cancer-associated cachexia and underlying biological mechanisms. *Annu Rev Nutr* 2006;26:435.
23. Argiles JM, Busquets S, Lopez-Soriano FJ. Cytokines as mediators and targets for cancer cachexia. *Cancer Treat Res* 2006;130:199.
26. Wieland BM, Stewart GD, Skipworth RJ, et al. Is there a human homologue to the murine proteolysis-inducing factor? *Clin Cancer Res* 2007;13:4984.
28. Read JA, Beale PJ, Volker DH, et al. Nutrition intervention using an eicosapentaenoic acid (EPA)-containing supplement in patients with advanced colorectal cancer. Effects on nutritional and inflammatory status: a phase II trial. *Support Care Cancer* 2007;15:301.
29. Ravasco P, Monteiro Grillo I, Camilo M. Cancer wasting and quality of life react to early individualized nutritional counselling! *Clin Nutr* 2007;26:7.
30. van den Berg MG, Rasmussen-Conrad EL, Wei KH, et al. Comparison of the effect of individual dietary counselling and of standard nutritional care on weight loss in patients with head and neck cancer undergoing radiotherapy. *Br J Nutr* 2010;104:872–877.
31. Inui A. Cancer anorexia-cachexia syndrome: current issues in research and management. *CA Cancer J Clin* 2002;52:72.
32. Cannabis in Cachexia Study Group, Strasser F, Luftner D, et al. Comparison of orally administered cannabis extract and delta-9-tetrahydrocannabinol in treating patients with cancer-related anorexia-cachexia syndrome: a multicenter, phase III, randomized, double-blind, placebo-controlled clinical trial from the Cannabis in Cachexia Study Group. *J Clin Oncol* 2006;24:3394.
33. Neary NM, Small CJ, Wren AM, et al. Ghrelin increases energy intake in cancer patients with impaired appetite: acute, randomized, placebo-controlled trial. *J Clin Endocrinol Metab* 2004;89:2832.
34. DeBoer MD, Marks DL. Therapy insight: use of melanocortin antagonists in the treatment of cachexia in chronic diseases. *Nat Clin Pract Endocrinol Metab* 2006;2:459.
35. Lundholm K, Gunnebo L, Korner U, et al. Effects by daily long term provision of ghrelin to unselected weight-losing cancer patients: a randomized double blind study. *Cancer* 2010;116:2044.
36. Fearon KC, Barber MD, Moses AG, et al. Double-blind, placebo-controlled, randomized study of eicosapentaenoic acid diester in patients with cancer cachexia. *J Clin Oncol* 2006;24:3401.
37. Dewey A, Baughan C, Dean T, et al. Eicosapentaenoic acid (EPA, an omega-3 fatty acid from fish oils) for the treatment of cancer cachexia. *Cochrane Database Syst Rev* 2007;1:CD004597.
38. Fearon KC, von Meyenfeldt MF, Moses AG, et al. Effect of a protein and energy dense N-3 fatty acid enriched oral supplement on loss of weight and lean tissue in cancer cachexia: a randomised double blind trial. *Gut* 2003; 52:1479.
40. Laviano A, Muscaritoli M, Cascino A, et al. BCAA: the best compromise to achieve anabolism? *Curr Opin Clin Nutr Metab Care* 2005;8:408.
41. Berk L, James J, Schwartz A, et al. A randomized, double-blind, placebo-controlled trial of beta-hydroxyl beta-methyl butyrate, glutamine, and arginine mixture for the treatment of cancer cachexia (RTOG 0122). *Support Care Cancer* 2008;16:1179.
42. Weimann A, Braga M, Harsanyi L, et al. ESPEN guidelines on enteral nutrition: surgery including organ transplantation. *Clin Nutr* 2006;25:224.
44. Bozzetti F, Mori V. Nutritional support and tumour growth in humans: a narrative review of the literature. *Clin Nutr* 2009;28:226.
45. Kalaany NY, Sabatini DM. Tumours with PI3K activation are resistant to dietary restriction. *Nature* 2009;458:725.
46. Yun J, Rago C, Cheong I, et al. Glucose deprivation contributes to the development of KRAS pathway mutations in tumor cells. *Science* 2009;325:1555.
49. Baracos VE, Reiman T, Mourtzakis M, et al. Body composition in patients with non-small cell lung cancer: a contemporary view of cancer cachexia with the use of computed tomography image analysis. *Am J Clin Nutr* 2010; 91:1133S.
51. Kondrup J, Allison SP, Elia M, et al. ESPEN guidelines for nutrition screening 2002. *Clin Nutr* 2003;22:415.
52. Bossola M, Muscaritoli M, Costelli P, et al. Increased muscle ubiquitin mRNA levels in gastric cancer patients. *Am J Physiol Regul Integr Comp Physiol* 2001;280:R1518.
53. Bossola M, Muscaritoli M, Costelli P, et al. Increased muscle proteasome activity correlates with disease severity in gastric cancer patients. *Ann Surg* 2003;237:384.
55. Arends J, Bodoky G, Bozzetti F, et al. ESPEN guidelines on enteral nutrition: non-surgical oncology. *Clin Nutr* 2006;25:245.
56. Bozzetti F, Arends J, Lundholm K, et al. ESPEN guidelines on parenteral nutrition: non-surgical oncology. *Clin Nutr* 2009;28:445.
57. Loser C, Aschl G, Hebutherne X, et al. ESPEN guidelines on artificial enteral nutrition—percutaneous endoscopic gastrostomy (PEG). *Clin Nutr* 2005; 24:848.
59. Messing B, Blethen S, DiBaise JK, et al. Treatment of adult short bowel syndrome with recombinant human growth hormone: a review of clinical studies. *J Clin Gastroenterol* 2006;40(5 Suppl 2):S75.
60. Lira FS, Rosa JC, Zanchi NE, et al. Regulation of inflammation in the adipose tissue in cancer cachexia: effect of exercise. *Cell Biochem Funct* 2009;27:71.
61. Glare P, Jongs W, Zafiropoulos B. Establishing a cancer nutrition rehabilitation program (CNRP) for ambulatory patients attending an Australian cancer center. *Support Care Cancer* 2010 (in press).
62. Thorsen L, Skovlund E, Stromme SB, et al. Effectiveness of physical activity on cardiorespiratory fitness and health-related quality of life in young and middle-aged cancer patients shortly after chemotherapy. *J Clin Oncol* 2005; 23:2378.
66. Murray SM, Pindoria S, Nutrition support for bone marrow transplant patients. *Cochrane Database Syst Rev* 2009;1:CD002920.
67. Kaadige MR, Looper RE, Kamalanaadhan S, et al. Glutamine-dependent anapleurosis dictates glucose uptake and cell growth by regulating MondoA transcriptional activity. *Proc Natl Acad Sci U S A* 2009;106:14878.
68. Dang CV. PKM2 tyrosine phosphorylation and glutamine metabolism signal a different view of the Warburg effect. *Sci Signal* 2009;2:pe75.
69. Kuhn KS, Muscaritoli M, Wischmeyer P, et al. Glutamine as indispensable nutrient in oncology: experimental and clinical evidence. *Eur J Nutr* 2010; 49:197.
70. Korner U, Bondolfi A, Buhler E, et al. Ethical and legal aspects of enteral nutrition. *Clin Nutr* 2006;25:196.

CHAPTER 172 SEXUAL PROBLEMS

VERONICA SANCHEZ VARELA, CHRISTIAN J. NELSON, AND SHARON L. BOBER

Rapid and recent advances in cancer care now mean that the majority of newly diagnosed cancer patients will "live beyond cancer." This shift has resulted in a consistently increasing focus on maintaining and/or restoring quality of life. Yet despite the widespread acknowledgment that quality of life is often profoundly disrupted by changes in sexual function after cancer treatment, there is still a deafening silence when it comes to addressing the topic of sexuality for a majority of cancer patients and survivors. For example, in the recent Institute of Medicine report, *Cancer Care for the Whole Patient: Meeting Psychosocial Health Needs*, which calls for new standards of psychosocial care, sexual functioning was not even mentioned. Often, oncologists do not feel comfortable addressing sexual problems, preferring instead to focus on treatment outcomes related to survivorship rather than quality of life.[1] However, several studies have shown that patients, both male and female across diseases, are often disappointed by the lack of information, support, and practical strategies provided by their clinicians to help manage the sexual changes secondary to cancer and cancer treatments.[2–4]

Although there are real barriers to bringing frank conversation about sexuality into the routine clinical oncology encounter, the authors would like to begin this chapter by clarifying why these conversations are important. Sexuality and intimacy have been shown to help lessen emotional distress and improve psychosocial adjustment in the face of cancer.[5] Physical pleasure and emotional intimacy provide a life-affirming experience, and such experience can provide enormous stress relief and calm in the midst of a tenuous and often pressured time. In fact, acknowledging the importance of sexuality to patients' quality of life, the World Health Organization has recently declared that maintaining sexual health indeed falls under the purview of physicians. For patients who endure so many losses as a result of cancer, including social, financial, physical and emotional disruptions, the additional loss of sexual function adds a profound burden that is only magnified by the shame and embarrassment that this aspect of life is not only changed but also feels unspeakable. Moreover, patients worry that their experience of "damage" cannot be undone and often wrongly assume that sexual dysfunction cannot be adequately addressed. Many of these assumptions are unwittingly reinforced by clinicians who, by not addressing the topic, mistakenly give patients the message that "nothing can be done," an unfortunate occurrence because the majority of typical sexual problems facing cancer patients and cancer survivors can indeed be effectively treated.

Several studies have examined medical professionals' barriers to communication about sexual health needs with their patients. It has recently been suggested that these barriers appear to fall into three categories: issues related to patient characteristics, provider characteristics, and systems issues.[6] Patient characteristics refer to a range of assumptions about a patients' sexuality based on age, gender, partner status, sexual orientation, prognosis, and economic and social class, as well as religious, cultural, and ethnic background that may deter clinicians from asking about sexual health. For example, doctors may assume that an older person who is widowed or divorced is no longer sexually active or that if a patient is from another culture it would be inappropriate to ask about sexual concerns. Provider characteristics refer to the training, experience, knowledge, and attitudes of the provider that may either deter or facilitate conversations about sexuality after cancer. Lack of experience and lack of knowledge have repeatedly been shown to explain why sexuality is not addressed[7,8] with cancer patients and survivors. Moreover, clinicians will also report lack of clarity regarding whose role it is to initiate this conversation and clinicians will also report a lack of confidence and competence to move ahead toward this topic. Finally, systems issues are often reported as major barriers to this topic. Oncologists will aver that there is no time to address a topic like sexuality when there is barely enough time to manage more pressing concerns.[7] Further, oncologists may be concerned about lack of available resources for patients if a patient were to endorse a problem.[1]

The aim of this chapter is threefold: (1) to familiarize clinicians with the most common sexual problems for men and women that are related to specific cancers and their particular treatments, (2) to review intervention options for sexual problems including acknowledgment of current resources that are readily available to both clinicians and patients, and (3) to provide clear and straightforward language that clinicians can use to initiate a brief discussion about sexuality with their patients as well as to overview some brief and previously validated measures of sexual dysfunction that can be incorporated into standard practice in order to assess sexual dysfunction more systematically.

CANCER IN MEN

Prostate Cancer

The American Cancer Society estimates that prostate cancer is the second most common type of cancer and the second leading cause of cancer death in American men.[9] Over the past 2.5 decades prostate cancer rates have dramatically increased from 50,000 new cases diagnosed in 1981 to over 192,000 in 2009. If diagnosed in the early stages, the survival rates for prostate cancer are particularly encouraging. The relative 5-year survival rate has increased in the past 20 years from 67% to 99%.[9] The combination of the increase in diagnosed cases, the increasing survival rates, and the decreasing age at diagnosis has made sexual dysfunction following prostate cancer treatments a progressively more important issue.

Surgery

One of the primary treatment options for men diagnosed with early-stage prostate cancer is a prostatectomy, which can have a major impact on the sexual functioning of the patient. First, when removing the prostate, the seminal vesicles are also removed, which results in the inability for a man to ejaculate semen during orgasm. Most men report that at first a dry orgasm is a "little strange," but state that they quickly become used to the experience and report equal enjoyment as compared to presurgery orgasm. Second, the cavernous nerves that are responsible for erectile function run bilaterally along the prostate. If these nerves are removed or damaged during surgery to the point that they atrophy, a man will experience erectile dysfunction (ED). A wide variation in rates of ED following prostatectomy has been reported in the literature and range from 14% to 90%.[10,11] This range is due in large part to the numerous ways sexual function has been assessed.[11] Despite the wide variation in rates of ED, the general conclusion is that radical prostatectomy has a severe impact on erectile function. In a review, Dubbelman et al.[12] concluded that the ED rate after radical prostatectomy in the general urologic population is 81%.

As a result, physicians have developed a "nerve-sparing" surgical technique that has proven to be effective in helping patients sustain erectile function postsurgery.[12] Of note, the data suggest that even when the nerves are sparred during surgery, it may take at least 18 to 24 months for the nerves to fully heal[13] and therefore for the erections to be recovered. The ED rates following a nerve-sparing procedure also vary considerably. However, studies report a positive association between the number of neurovascular bundles and erectile function.[12] The rates of recovery of erections in men who had bilateral nerve-sparing surgery range from 31% to 86%,[14,15] while those who had unilateral nerve-sparing surgery report recovery of erections in 13% to 56% of the cases.[15,16]

There appear to be several predictors of erectile functioning after surgery. Younger men are more likely to retain erections after surgery,[17,18] and although there seems to be a clear association between age and ED, a number of physicians believe a reasonable cutoff point to consider is 65 or less years of age.[19] Erectile function presurgery is also an important predictor, with those who report poor functioning presurgery being more likely to develop severe ED after surgery.[13,20] Another important factor in the recovery of erections after prostatectomy is the use of erectogenic medications in the 24-month postoperative period when the cavernous nerves are healing. There is good evidence to suggest that the use of erectogenic therapy immediately after surgery reduces tissue fibrosis of the corporeal smooth muscle by increasing corporeal oxygenation.[21] In men following radical prostatectomy where spontaneous and nocturnal erectile function is poor or absent, the penile tissue may fail to achieve proper oxygenation. As a result, permanent structural alterations may occur, which is followed by the development of venous leak. Therefore, although debated, the current concept is that men after radical prostatectomy should be treated with early postoperative vasoactive therapy in whatever form is successful and acceptable to the individual patient.[20,22–24]

There are currently a variety of treatments for erectile dysfunction. With the advent of sildenafil, the first-line treatment for ED is oral medications.[25] Most patients prefer oral medication to other forms of ED treatment because these medications are less invasive and easier to use. Unfortunately, oral medications may not be effective immediately after prostatectomy and during the 18 to 24 months when the cavernous nerves are healing. Oral medications enhance the effects of nitric oxide (NO). The NO that impacts erectile function is secreted from the cavernous nerves that run bilaterally along the prostate. If these nerves are injured intraoperatively, the amount of NO secreted is dramatically reduced and oral medications will have little positive effect on increasing NO or enhancing erectile function.

Because oral medications may not be effective for 18 to 24 months after surgery, penile injection therapy is considered by many as a second-line treatment option for men in this period. This treatment delivers intracavernosal vasodilators at the base of the penis. This direct application produces consistent results and has found to be effective for 94% of injection users.[26] The primary concern with this treatment is that the thought of penile injections is anxiety-provoking and many patients worry that this type of therapy will disrupt the "mood" of a sexual experience. However, with appropriate training it is possible for many couples to use this treatment successfully. Mulhall et al.[27] reported that 69% of couples were still using injection therapy on average 38 months after initiation.

Other treatments are available, including suppositories administered into the urethra, vacuum devices, and prostheses. The suppositories produce inconsistent results, the vacuum devices can be cumbersome, and neither of these treatments rate high on patient satisfaction.[28] Conversely, the prosthesis is an effective and consistent solution, with patient satisfaction rates between 92% and 96% in one study.[29–31] However, this involves an invasive procedure that is irreversible.

Radiation

External-beam radiation and brachytherapy are also treatment options for men with early-stage prostate cancer. Many patients believe that radiation therapy will have less of a negative impact on erections, and oftentimes may choose radiation therapy over surgery as a way to preserve sexual function. However, the data suggest that the rates of ED are similar between the radiation and surgery groups at 3 to 5 years posttreatment.[32] What is often confusing to patients is that the course of ED is different in each treatment. As stated previously with surgery, rates of ED are highest after treatment and then improve slightly up to approximately 2 years after surgery. For radiation therapy, rates of ED are lowest directly after treatment and then slowly increase up to 3 years after treatment. The mechanism for this decline in function is that fibrosis continues to develop up to approximately 3 years after radiation and interfere with the neurovascular bundles and blood vessels adjacent to the prostate and necessary for erections.[32] As a result, men who have undergone radiation therapy have equivalent rates of ED to those undergoing nerve-sparing surgery at a 5-year medical follow-up.[32] The decline in potency rates can been seen in data presented by Mantz et al.,[33] who noted potency rates of 96%, 75%, 59%, and 53% at 1, 20, 40, and 60 months after external-beam radiation therapy.

Brachytherapy, or seed implants, also impacts sexual function. Although there are some data suggesting that brachytherapy may have less of an impact on sexual function, these data are still relatively limited. Brandees et al.[34] noted that there was no difference at 3 to 17 months follow-up between brachytherapy and surgery. However, reports presented from the Cancer of the Prostate Strategic Urologic Research Endeavor database suggest that brachytherapy patients reported better sexual functioning as compared with surgery or external-beam radiation patients at 3 to 4 years after treatment.[35] It is important to note that the brachytherapy patients still reported a significant decline in sexual function from their baseline scores.

The options for ED treatments after radiation are similar to those stated previously, and the first-line therapy continues to be oral treatment. However, the scar tissue that builds up over time on the nerves may block the secretion of NO, limiting the effectiveness of oral medication, and many patients may achieve potency after radiation therapy but then see a slow decline in erections. Although there are currently no data on the potential for erectile rehabilitation during this period after radiation, oxygenation of the penile tissue remains greatly important, and consistent erectile function during the 3-year period after radiation is in line with sustaining penile health.

Hormone Therapy

The primary treatment for men diagnosed with late-stage prostate cancer is androgen ablation therapy. Androgen deprivation therapy is accompanied with a number of side effects and quality of life implications. In addition to loss of libido and ED, this therapy has been associated with hot flashes, osteoporosis, anemia, fatigue, sarcopenia, gynecomastia, and emotional distress.[36–39]

The treatments for ED associated with hormone therapy remain oral medication for first-line therapy and a secondary line of therapies if oral medications fail. The more difficult sexual dysfunction to treat is the low libido. Clearly, enhancing testosterone would be counter to androgen deprivation therapy. Oftentimes the potential solutions are behavioral in nature. Because the man's desire to initiate sexual contact is virtually eliminated with the testosterone, the potential options are working with the couple to set specific times for sexual relations or encouraging the partner in the relationship to be more assertive with sexual initiation.

Quality of Life Implications of Erectile Dysfunction

ED has been found to impact quality of life in men in the healthy population as well as in prostate cancer patients. Lauman et al.[40] report that ED negatively impacts physical satisfaction, emotional satisfaction, and overall happiness with life. These findings have been replicated in men with prostate cancer. The Prostate Cancer Outcomes Study has provided data supporting that 2 years following the diagnosis of prostate cancer, ED is independently associated with lower quality of life.[41] In addition to the quality of life implications, there may be specific psychological implications to struggling with ED. And although little, if any, data exist on the association between ED and depression specifically in men with prostate cancer, it is clear from studies conducted in other settings that there is a relationship between these two variables.[42–44] Additionally, Nelson et al.[45] conducted a study assessing sexual bother after radical prostatectomy and found that many men were considerably "bothered" by their ED after prostatectomy, and that frustration with ED increases within the 24 months after surgery.

Testicular Cancer

Testicular cancer is the most common cancer type in men between 20 and 34 years of age.[9] These statistics signal to the fact that these men are in their sexual prime and at a likely age to start a family, making the sexual and fertility aspects of testicular cancer treatment an important topic. In general, there is paucity of research investigating the impact of testicular cancer and its treatment on sexual function. Surprisingly, only a small percentage of men report difficulty with sexual desire, erections, or enjoyment of the sexual experience.[46] Hartmann et al.[47] assessed 98 men who had undergone a variety of treatments for testicular cancer and concluded that the impact of these treatments on sexual function was minimal for these patients. The one possible exception is that dry orgasm was reported in 21% of patients. Other authors have suggested that sexual function after chemotherapy treatment for testicular cancer returns within the first year after treatment.[48]

The primary concern for men with testicular cancer is fertility. Although the data suggest a wide variation, abnormal sperm concentrations can be seen in as many as 50% of the patients.[46,49] Fortunately, cryopreservation of sperm allows for the banking of sperm, giving the potential to start a family for those patients with a desire to have children. This, in addition to new technology of intracytoplasmatic sperm injection that only needs one sperm to fertilize an egg, allows for those patients with low sperm count to provide adequate sperm for *in vitro* fertilization.[50,51] Kuczyk et al.[46] suggest that one of the most important aspects of treating these patients is providing proper education on the available reproductive technology.

CANCERS THAT AFFECT MEN AND WOMEN

Bladder Cancer

The most common presentation of bladder cancer is in the form of transitional cell carcinoma, and although most cases tend to be superficial when first diagnosed, repeated treatments may be required to treat recurrences. Treatments for bladder cancer mainly include surgery, radiation therapy, immunotherapy, and chemotherapy, with surgery used in most of the cases.[52] From a sexual health perspective, however, treatment of bladder cancer by radical cystectomy is the procedure that has received the most attention given its likely negative implications on sexual functioning.

Considerations for Men

A standard radical cystectomy for treating bladder cancer in men involves the removal of the bladder as well as the prostate, seminal vesicles, vasa deferentia, and the removal or damage of the neurovascular bundles, leaving the patient with the likely consequent loss of sexual function. The high prevalence of ED after radical cystectomy has fueled a number of studies examining whether potency-sparing cystectomy can be safely used as an alternative to the standard procedure for the treatment of bladder cancer. These studies have reported impressive rates, with a majority of patients reporting being postoperatively potent.[53–55] But with regard to the safety of the procedures, it is argued that the cancer outcome following potency-sparing cystectomy is significantly worse than results from the standard radical treatment, and that the 10% to 15% higher treatment failure rate is too high of a price to pay in exchange for the advantage of preserving sexual functioning.[56]

For men who are treated with radical or nerve-sparing cystectomy, ED prevails at similar rates to those seen after prostatectomy or nerve-sparing prostatectomy, respectively, and its treatment follows the standard of care for ED in men treated with prostatectomy. For instance, in a study examining sexual function after male radical cystectomy in a sexually active population, the authors found that, consistent with previous reports, ED was prevalent in 86% of their sample[57] and that those who recovered sexual functioning (either naturally or by using sildenafil citrate) were those who had undergone a nerve-sparing procedure. Of note, the authors found that a large number (47%) of men in their sample did not seek treatment for sexual dysfunction after surgery, and argued that preoperative counseling and consultation after surgery may be crucial in assisting patients in seeking treatment for sexual dysfunction.[57] Moreover, sexual counseling might also be useful to a number of men and women under surveillance for non–muscle-invasive bladder cancer, some of whom mistakenly report being afraid of harming their partner through sexual contact.[58]

Considerations for Women

The standard radical cystectomy for bladder cancer in women involves the removal of the bladder, urethra, anterior vaginal wall, uterus, and ovaries and it is likely to result in sexual dysfunction. The large prevalence of sexual dysfunction in women after radical cystectomy has also sparked a search for alternative procedures, and the literature that is available documents promising results for women undergoing nerve-sparing cystectomy.[59] However, very little has been reported on these procedures and their impact on sexual functioning versus their oncologic risks. Symptoms of sexual dysfunction reported by women after radical cystectomy include diminished ability or inability to achieve orgasm, decreased lubrication, decreased sexual desire, and dyspareunia.[60] In addition, research suggests that women who undergo ileal conduit or cutaneous Koch pouch diversion after radical cystectomy tend to report more body image concerns and worse sexual desire when compared with men with the same type of urinary diversion.[61] Therapies for sexual problems in women bladder cancer survivors follow many of the same recommendations for women survivors of breast, gynecologic, and colorectal cancer described in other sections of this chapter.

Head and Neck Cancer

Head and neck cancers account for approximately 3% to 5% of cancers diagnosed in the United States and are most common in men and women over the age of 50. These cancers tend to present as squamous cell carcinoma mostly linked to tobacco and alcohol use.[62] Although their prevalence is low compared with other malignancies, head and neck cancers are considered to be among the most impactful with regard to the patient's posttreatment quality of life.[63] Given the likely consequences of head and neck cancer treatments in a patient's daily functioning, rehabilitation tends to play an important role in posttreatment care. Rehabilitation efforts may include physical therapy, speech therapy, and learning how to take care of a stoma; depending on the extent of the treatment and disfigurement, patients may also require plastic surgery to rebuild some of the affected structures and facilitate recovery of functioning.

Despite the obvious toll that head and neck cancer may take on any patient's quality of life, research documenting sexual problems after treatment for these malignancies is noticeably scarce. Available reports suggest that approximately one-third to one-half of head and neck cancer patients complain of a detriment in their sexual lives including feeling less sexual interest and less sexual enjoyment.[64,65] Not surprisingly, it has also been documented that head and neck cancer patients with more extensive disfigurement secondary to surgery tend to experience a greater detriment in their sexual lives, greater social isolation, and worsened relationship with their partners than those with less disfigurement.[66] Other issues such as the loss of saliva and its impact on the ability to engage in sexual activities such as kissing, as well as the psychological distress associated with alcohol and tobacco withdrawal and/or the stigma of a diagnosis often perceived as "self-inflicted," are common in this population. Although rehabilitation efforts are a very important part of the treatment process for head and neck cancer patients, sexual rehabilitation has not been specifically studied in this population, and it generally follows some of the same recommendations made when sexual functioning is impacted by body image concerns and physical functioning impairments secondary to treatment for other cancers.

Blood, Bone Marrow, and Lymphatic System

Treatment of systemic disease often involves intense interventions with chemotherapy, whole-body irradiation, and/or bone marrow transplant, and may cause side effects including sexual dysfunction. In particular, preparative regimes of high-dose chemotherapy and total-body irradiation may result in ovarian failure and low estrogen levels for women, and gonadal and cavernosal arterial insufficiency in men.[67] Sexual problems in bone marrow transplant patients may still be present several years after the procedure and include difficulty obtaining an erection, ejaculation, and orgasm for men, and concerns about body appearance, vaginal dryness, and painful intercourse and orgasm for women.[68] Moreover, a longitudinal study of sexual function in long-term survivors of hematopoietic cell transplantation documented that at 5 years after treatment sexual dysfunction is a major problem for this population, with male survivors continuing to have lower sexual function and female survivors having lower scores for sexual activity and function, compared with controls.[69]

Another important issue that often develops for females after transplant is genital graft-versus-host disease (GVHD). Female genital GVHD after transplant is a complication that tends to receive little attention despite the significant impact it has on the survivor's quality of life. Female tract GVHD may manifest in several forms, from irritation of the vagina or the vulva to ulceration and vaginal stenosis, and it has been found to be present in at least 25% of the transplant survivor population.[70,71] Research studies suggest that early detection of genital GVHD is highly treatable with steroids and vaginal dilators, and therefore education on active self-surveillance should be given to patients, in addition to a plan for regular gynecologic follow-up posttransplant.[71]

Studies that investigate the effectiveness of interventions for sexual dysfunction in women after bone marrow transplantation are scarce, but therapies including vaginal lubricants, dilators, and vibrators can be recommended to improve some of the sexual side effects of treatment. In men, there is evidence to support that a number of patients recover sexual function over time,[69] and that testosterone cypionate and sildenafil have shown to improve ED in this population.[67] More importantly, many survivors and their partners may feel hesitant or even fearful to resume sexual activity after bone marrow transplantation given concerns about immunosuppression, such as coming in contact with germs. These concerns may prevail even after survivors have been cleared by their medical team to resume sexual activity. It is therefore important to anticipate and openly discuss these concerns with survivors and their partners while offering gentle guidance and reassurance about their eligibility to resume sexual activity.

Colorectal Cancer

Colorectal cancer is the third most common cancer among men and women in the United States. It typically affects people who are age 50 years and older, and prognosis varies depending on the extent of the disease, with a 5-year overall survival rate of 64% and a 5-year survival rate of 90% for localized disease.[72] Treatments for colorectal cancer mainly include surgery, radiation therapy, and chemotherapy, with surgery used in most of the cases.[52] Colorectal cancer surgery often causes damage to the sympathetic and parasympathetic nerves and results in erectile and ejaculatory disorders in men, and dyspareunia, decreased libido, and changes in the orgasm experience in women.[73] Even though the impact of radiotherapy in colorectal cancer survivors has rarely been addressed, the available research suggests that radiation is associated with sexual dysfunction in both men and women.[74]

Previous studies have documented a number of sexual problems in colorectal cancer survivors, but the prevalence of these problems varies from study to study, with some of this variance partly attributable to the modality of treatment and partly to methodologic differences between studies.[74] Because most colorectal cancer patients are over age 50 and may presumably have a higher incidence of non–cancer-related sexual dysfunction, studies that use a longitudinal design to assess the prevalence of sexual dysfunction in these survivors are of particular interest. In a longitudinal study by Jayne et al.,[75] the authors compared treatment outcomes in patients who underwent a laparoscopic-assisted surgery versus open surgery for colorectal cancer, including quality of life and sexual functioning. The authors assessed functioning preoperatively, and at 2 weeks and 3, 6, 18, and 36 months after surgery and found that although there was no change from baseline in sexual functioning or enjoyment for men and women in both arms, men tended to report more sexual problems from 3 months onward in the laparoscopic arm and from 6 months onward in the open surgery arm. The authors also found that body image was worse than at baseline from 2 weeks onward for all patients. Therapies to manage sexual side effects of colorectal cancer treatment in men and women have rarely been studied.[74] However, therapies recommended for prostate cancer survivors, such as the use of sildenafil,[76] appear to be adequate for a number of male colorectal cancer survivors who suffer from ED following treatment.

Therapies recommended for breast and gynecologic cancer survivors, such as the use of water-based lubricants, vaginal moisturizers, and vaginal dilators, can also be recommended for female colorectal cancer survivors who suffer from vaginal dryness and/or stenosis after radiation.[74] More specific to colorectal cancer survivors are the negative emotional reactions to the colostomy, such as poor body image and reduced self-esteem, which are commonly present and may negatively impact intimacy. But patients and their partners can and do learn how to manage the impact of an ostomy on sexuality and there are resources available for this purpose. Patients with ostomies should receive information on deodorants to minimize odor, as well as on foods that are likely to cause stronger odors, gas, or diarrhea. Patients should also receive information on pouch covers, and suggestions such as changing positions to avoid pain during intercourse and emptying the stoma before sexual activity.[77] Additional information for patients and their partners can also be found free of charge through the United Ostomy Associations of America, Inc.

CANCER IN WOMEN

Breast Cancer

Difficulty with sexual function, loss of desire, changes in body image, and disruption of emotional relationships are primary sexual complications of breast cancer from diagnosis through all stages of treatment and into survivorship. Chemotherapy, radiation, surgery, and adjunctive hormonal therapy, whether delivered alone or in combination with each other, all have the potential to negatively impact sexual function. Although breast cancer accounts for approximately one-third of new cancers diagnosed in North American women,[78] the survival rates of breast cancer for localized disease continue to improve and are now 95% or better.[79] Not only will the great majority of breast cancer survivors go on to become long-term cancer survivors, but studies have also shown that the majority of partnered women will remain sexually active either after diagnosis or at the end of treatment.[80,81] Thus, clinicians ought to better understand the range of sexual problems related to breast cancer treatment as well as the interventions available to address them.

A number of factors have been identified regarding who is at risk for developing sexual problems after breast cancer. Women who have premorbid sexual dysfunction,[82] negative self-concept,[83] depression and relationship discord[84] are all more likely to struggle with sexual problems. In one recent prospective study assessing the impact of breast cancer on women's sexuality, younger age was found to be the most salient predictor of lower sexual function in addition to lack of partner status.[85] Unfortunately, there is a wide range of sexual problems that are related to breast cancer, and reports of sexual problems range from 30% to 100%.[86] More specifically, 23% to 64% of women report problems with desire, 20% to 48% report arousal or lubrication problems, 16% to 36% report problems with orgasm, and 35% to 38% report problems with pain or dyspareunia.[87–89] Problems with body image are also quite common both during and after treatment, although there is some evidence that certain areas of distress such as feeling feminine or perceived attractiveness tend to improve over time.[78,80,90]

Surgery

Conceptually, losing one or both breasts would seem to be one of the most dramatic ways to damage a woman's core sense of femininity, body integrity, and attractiveness. In Western culture, the breast is highly sexualized, and images of breasts are often used to symbolize and epitomize sexual vitality and beauty. Concern about body image in the face of breast surgery and potential breast changes and breast loss is prevalent with approximately 30% to 67% of women reporting concern with body image.[84,91] Breast-conserving surgical procedures and reconstructive surgery have become a standard part of breast cancer care and it is generally assumed that breast-conserving surgery (lumpectomy vs. mastectomy) as well as breast reconstruction is essential in helping women maintain a positive body image.[92] Several studies have shown that women who undergo modified radical mastectomies have poorer body image than those who have had breast-conserving procedures. In Moyer's[93] meta-analysis of 40 studies comparing quality-of-life differences between breast-conserving surgery and mastectomy between 1980 and 1995, it was shown that patients undergoing breast conservation had a better body image compared with mastectomy patients.

However, aside from body image and maintaining body integrity, breast surgery can still have a significantly negative impact on sexuality. In particular, women who undergo breast reconstruction are typically left with complete lack of sensation, including nipple sensation. The nipple has been shown to be the most sensitive area of the breast and loss of nipple sensation is akin to losing a key erogenous zone for many women.[94] Although their breast shape may be restored, the loss of feeling is not. In addition to the use of saline-filled or silicone gel-filled implants, women may also have tissue flap procedures where tissue from a woman's body may be harvested from her abdomen, back, thighs, or buttocks in order to reconstruct a breast. These surgeries, although more intensive than implant surgery, offer the advantage of reconstruction that often feels and looks more natural without the concern about implant rupture or the need to replace implants over time. However, flap procedures necessitate a second surgical site and additional scars.

There is growing attention now being paid to the use of nipple-sparing mastectomy; however, although the nipple and areola may be left in place when breast tissue is removed, sensation is no longer intact. In the one largest study to date looking at patient satisfaction following nipple-sparing mastectomy, it was found that although the majority of women were satisfied with the appearance of their breasts and would choose this option again, over 90% reported only fair or poor sensation.[95]

Chemotherapy

Disruption of sexual function after breast cancer seems to be significantly related to whether a woman undergoes chemotherapy as part of her treatment.[78,80,84,86,87,96] Ganz et al.[81] looked at the impact of breast cancer treatment on sexual function and found that women who had either lumpectomy or mastectomy followed by chemotherapy were more likely to report negative sexual outcomes than patients who had surgery alone. Schover[96] has noted that younger women who undergo abrupt chemotherapy-related menopause are at the highest risk for sexual problems and that the rates of sexual dysfunction in these women are clearly higher than would be expected in a healthy, community-based sample. In particular, the intensive estrogen deficiency that comes with chemotherapy-induced menopause often leads to severe vaginal dryness and vaginal atrophy, which makes penetration painful. Painful intercourse due to vaginal dryness is one of the most common sexual problems after breast cancer and it is one of the primary factors also implicated in women's experience of decreased desire, another common and often vexing problem for breast cancer survivors.[96,97]

Testosterone deficiency related to premature ovarian failure has also been discussed as a factor related to loss of desire after breast cancer but research has not uniformly supported this hypothesis.[98] In one randomized placebo-controlled trial of transdermal testosterone with mostly breast cancer survivors who reported low desire, no benefit was found.[99] Loss of desire appears to be multidimensional with causes that span a biopsychosocial continuum. Changes in body image and body integrity, vaginal dryness, and painful intercourse as well as emotional dynamics and role changes are factors that are likely just as important as changes in androgen levels when it comes to affecting desire after breast cancer.

Hormonal Therapy

Endocrine therapy, including selective estrogen receptor modifiers and aromatase inhibitors (AIs), now play an important role in breast cancer treatment for both premenopausal as well as postmenopausal women. Tamoxifen has been used as systemic adjuvant treatment for over 20 years, and primary side effects are hot flashes, fatigue, and nausea. Regarding sexual function, tamoxifen use has been associated with vaginal dryness and low desire,[100] although in the large-scale Breast Cancer Prevention Trial there were no differences found in frequency of sexual activity between those using tamoxifen versus placebo.[101] Raloxifene, another selective estrogen receptor modifier, does not appear to confer significant difference from tamoxifen in patient-reported outcomes on physical health and depression, but sexual function has been reported as being slightly better than in women taking tamoxifen.[102] More recently, sexual side effects of raloxifene treatment have been examined and no deleterious effects were found.[103] The third-generation AIs (anastrozole, letrozole, and exemestane) have become an integral component in the care of postmenopausal women with estrogen-receptor–positive breast cancer and are currently being evaluated for use in chemoprevention.[104] The exacerbation of postmenopausal gynecologic symptoms such as vaginal dryness and dyspareunia has been reported in several studies investigating the quality of life of women taking AIs, including in the first and largest Arimidex and Tamoxifen Alone or in Combination (ATAC) trial with over 9,000 participants.[105] It has been noted that as use of AIs has become the gold standard of care for postmenopausal breast cancer survivors, it is imperative to explore comprehensive management of these gynecologic symptoms that impair sexual function.[106]

Radiotherapy

Radiation therapy for breast cancer is generally localized to the breast. Radiation can result in skin fibrosis, additional loss of sensitivity in the skin, and fatigue, all which can contribute to low desire. Some women talk about the psychological effects of radiation tattoos on their breasts and how these markings always serve as a reminder of their cancer long after treatment ends. Other effects such as skin irritations and burns are more short term. However, there has hardly been any research conducted that specifically examines the effects of breast cancer-related radiotherapy on sexuality.

Intervention

Several approaches for addressing sexual problems after breast cancer have been identified. Most approaches focus on individually based information and education about management of sexual side effects, such as vaginal dryness, and a minority of interventions have been developed aimed at working with couples around establishing new norms for intimacy after cancer. Ganz et al.[107] demonstrated that nurse-delivered, individually based counseling was more successful in managing menopausal and sexual side effects from treatment over a 4-month period than usual-care. Alternatively, it has been suggested that interventions need to actively involve women's partners in order to produce lasting benefits on sexual functioning.[108] It is the perspective of the authors that optimal intervention is essentially based on "two-tracks" and addresses sexuality in both an individual and relational context.

Track 1: Focus on the Individual. It is imperative that women receive information and education about how to maintain and restore good sexual health in the context of maintaining good vaginal health as well as overall well-being after breast cancer. In anticipation of the common side effects of both chemotherapy-induced menopause as well as adjuvant hormonal therapies, the authors believe that all women should receive information as part of their overall treatment planning about (1) nonhormonal vaginal moisturizers, (2) water-based vaginal lubricants, (3) pelvic floor strengthening (Kegel) exercises, and (4) the value of maintaining blood flow to vaginal tissue to prevent vaginal atrophy. This kind of information is readily available to patients through a number of resources including a free booklet by the American Cancer Society called *Sexuality and Cancer: For the Woman Who Has Cancer and Her Partner* (2007). This booklet is free to patients and can be obtained in a hard copy or online edition. In addition, the National Cancer Institute as well as the Lance Armstrong Foundation Websites also have information about sexuality.

It is also important to note that the use of systemic hormone replacement for relief of menopausal and sexual side effects is almost always contraindicated after breast cancer. However, the use of minimally absorbed local vaginal estrogen that may be delivered by tablet, cream, or ring is an individual decision that must be made between a woman and her oncology team. Long-term safety data are lacking regarding the use of local vaginal estrogen to combat vulvovaginal atrophy after breast cancer, and therefore this practice is still considered to be experimental.

Track 2: Focus on the Relational Context. For the majority of breast cancer patients who are in a partnered relationship, it may also be important to acknowledge that sexuality is experienced in a context. Patients often do not realize that partners may benefit from looking at some of the same educational resources, and many popular books and Websites about sexuality after breast cancer actually have sections that are specifically written for partners. It can be a great relief to patients to get the message that not only are sexual problems common after breast cancer, but that although the majority of partners want to be helpful when it comes to reconnecting sexually they too may be unsure of how to proceed and may need guidance. When clinicians convey this message to patients and partners, it can help promote vital and less fraught communication between a patient and partner because both partners have a greater sense of empathy for the other. Moreover, for patients who are not currently in a relationship, sexuality is partly still a relational experience whether based on past relationships or in the context of hopes for future relationships. Patients who are not partnered are frequently unsure of how to proceed in terms of dating and lack confidence initiating new sexual relationships after their treatment. These patients often gain enormous benefit from being able to talk about these challenges and strategize about communication with a new potential partner.

Gynecologic Cancers

Treatments for gynecologic cancer often result in sexual dysfunction that may affect a substantial number of patients and can persist for many years after diagnosis. The effect of surgeries on the genitals can impact a patient's self-esteem and body image and create significant physical barriers, such as pain, to satisfactory sexual experiences. In addition, women who receive radiation therapy may develop vaginal stenosis, and hormonal interventions are likely to result in an abrupt development of menopausal symptoms, all of which can considerably disrupt sexual functioning.[109]

Endometrial Cancer

Endometrial cancer is the most common gynecologic cancer, and it is highly curable if diagnosed early.[72] Treatment may include surgery, radiotherapy, hormonal therapy, and chemotherapy. However, and despite its high prevalence, there is limited information on the sexual outcomes associated with endometrial cancer treatment specifically as studies that include women with this diagnosis more often than not do so in combination with other gynecologic cancer patients and survivors.

Ovarian Cancer

Ovarian cancer is the second most common gynecologic cancer. It causes the most deaths compared with other cancers of the female reproductive system and has a survival relative rate that varies greatly by age.[72] Treatment options for ovarian cancer may consist of surgery, chemotherapy, and radiation with surgery often including the removal of one or both ovaries, the fallopian tubes, and the uterus.

Research studies on the specific sexual outcomes of ovarian cancer treatment are rare. The earliest results by Stewart et al.[110] indicated that the majority of their sample (57%) reported that their sex lives had been negatively impacted by the cancer, with women treated with radiation reporting more frequent and severe sexual problems, and women under the age of 55 reporting a greater sense of loss about their sexuality compared with older women.

Similarly, Carmack et al.[111] found that sexual problems were quite prevalent in ovarian cancer patients, with 80% reporting problems with vaginal dryness, 75% reporting problems reaching orgasm, and 62% reporting pain or discomfort during penetration. Moreover, research has found that ovarian cancer survivors report significantly less sexual pleasure than disease-free controls.[112]

Cervical Cancer

With Pap screenings becoming more common, preinvasive lesions are detected more frequently and the current 5-year relative survival rate for cervical cancer is 92% for localized disease and 71% overall.[72] Treatment options for cervical cancer include surgery, radiotherapy, and/or chemotherapy. Surgery may involve total hysterectomy, with or without salpingo-oophorectomy, or radical hysterectomy.

In a cross-sectional study of women diagnosed with early-stage cervical carcinoma, Bergmark et al.[113] noted that long-term survivors reported sexual function changes that appear to persist over time including decreased lubrication and genital swelling during arousal, reduced perceived elasticity during intercourse, as well as distress over these changes. Moreover, the authors found that the changes in sexual function reported by the survivors were associated with the effects of surgery, whether or not the treatment included radiotherapy.[113] Later results obtained by Jensen et al.,[114] who studied early-stage cervical cancer survivors longitudinally, suggest that while low sexual interest and vaginal dryness seem to persist for years after radical hysterectomy, other changes such as distress by a reduced vaginal size and problems completing sexual intercourse after surgery are likely to resolve over time. In contrast, research also suggests that women treated with radiation for advanced, recurrent, or persistent cervical cancer report sexual problems including low sexual interest, lack of lubrication, dyspareunia, and inability to complete sexual intercourse throughout the first 2 years after treatment and with little improvement over time.[115]

Even though most women who are diagnosed with cervical cancer are younger, Bergmark et al.[113] found that women of all ages included in their study are likely to consider sexuality an important aspect of their lives, and therefore providers should feel particularly encouraged to discuss with their patients possible disease- and treatment-related sexual changes that may occur.

Vulvar Cancer

Vulvar cancer is rare, affecting mostly women over 50 years old, and it is highly curable when detected early. There is limited information of the sexual outcomes associated with vulvar cancer treatment. However, the available research suggests that vulvar cancer survivors experience significant sexual dysfunction.[116,117]

Intervention

Research studies on interventions that may be used for women treated for gynecologic cancers and who experience subsequent sexual dysfunction are limited, and mostly focus on information-giving and suggestions to manage specific symptoms.[118] For instance, for women who experience vaginal dryness, silicone-based or water-based lubricants may be recommended. The use of vaginal dilators a few times per week, and even in combination with Kegel exercises, help stretch the vaginal tissue after radiation. As a general recommendation, vaginal dilation should start as soon as the woman is comfortable but usually within 4 weeks after completion of radiotherapy.[118] Of note, research suggests that psychoeducational interventions that combine information with motivational and behavioral skills are more effective than information alone in improving adherence to the use of vaginal dilators in younger women treated for gynecologic cancer.[119] Moreover, psychoeducation may be particularly useful in decreasing some of the distress associated with sexual changes following gynecologic cancer treatment.[120] For women who experience vaginismus after radiation therapy, a combined approach of pharmacotherapy and sex therapy should be recommended.[118] In addition, information should be given to patients on techniques to restore the blood flow to the clitoris[121] and the vagina. It is important to also consider that sexuality is more than the ability to complete sexual intercourse. For survivors who feel unable to have intercourse, either because of physical or psychological factors, counseling may facilitate the exploration and broadening of sexual and intimate interactions that feel comfortable to the survivors and their partners.

BRCA Mutation Carriers

Related to the sexual problems that both breast and gynecologic cancer patients face, women with a *BRCA1* or *BRCA2* mutation represent a vulnerable population that has received very little attention regarding sexual dysfunction. The hereditary cancer genes, *BRCA1* and *BRCA2*, confer a remarkably high lifetime risk of both breast (55%–85%) and/or ovarian cancer (15%–44%).[122] Prophylactic bilateral mastectomy (PBM) has been shown to reduce the risk of breast cancer in mutation carriers by over 90%,[123] and prophylactic bilateral salpingo-oophorectomy (BSO) significantly reduces both ovarian cancer risk over 80% and the risk of breast cancer by at least 50%.[124] Although BSO and PBM are the most effective options to reduce cancer risk in *BRCA* carriers, their impact on sexual functioning should not be underestimated. It is recommended that female *BRCA1* carriers have their ovaries and fallopian tubes removed prophylactically by age 35 to 40, whereas *BRCA2* carriers may be able to defer this surgery until their mid-40s, because the average age of developing ovarian cancer in *BRCA2* carriers is somewhat later. However, for both groups, recommendations for BSO is long before the average age of natural menopause, meaning that these women will face an abrupt surgically induced onset of menopause with all of the related sexual side effects such as vaginal dryness and irritation, pain with penetration, decreased arousal, and loss of desire. Like breast cancer patients who undergo breast surgery, mutation carriers who opt for PBM will face similar issues regarding surgical scars, loss of sensation, and changes in perceived self-image secondary to potentially significant body changes. However, unlike other cancer patients, *BRCA* carriers often identify their genetic mutation in a context in which they themselves do not have cancer, and may have to wrestle with the decisions about surveillance versus risk-reducing surgery with moderate to little support and a paucity of adequate counseling and guidance, including regarding management of sexual side effects of surgery.[125]

Regarding intervention, *BRCA* carriers should receive the same information and education regarding management of premature menopause as is given to other cancer patients, including recommendations for managing vaginal dryness using vaginal moisturizers and water-based lubricants. In contrast to women who have already had breast cancer, it has been shown that short-term hormone replacement therapy does not appear to negate the risk-reduction benefit gained by prophylactic surgery,[126] thus making systemic hormone replacement as well as localized vaginal estrogen both reasonable options to be explored. Thinking about sexuality in a larger sociocultural context, a further point to consider is that a social support for risk-reduction surgery may be compromised as partners and family members may not appreciate the significant imperative to "choose" surgery. As genetic testing is becoming progressively more widespread and a growing number of younger women have access to their genetic information, *BRCA* carriers often have to make decisions about PBM and BSO and wrestle with subsequent consequences in the context of being single, dating, and exploring new sexual relationships.

CANCER IN CHILDREN AND YOUNG ADULTS

Childhood cancers and their treatments can also have an impact on the sexual development and function of adolescents and young adults. Zebrack et al.[127] found that although most survivors report doing well with regard to their sexual functioning, a number of young adult cancer survivors report sexual dysfunction that appears to be related with overall psychological distress and poor quality of life. Experiencing a life-threatening illness in childhood may impair normal psychosexual development, with childhood cancer survivors appearing to have a risk for psychosexual problems such as feeling sexually unattractive and dissatisfied with their sexual lives.[128] Moreover, Bober et al.[129] recently found in a study of 291 childhood cancer survivors that approximately 30% endorsed having significant problems in at least two areas of sexual function (e.g., arousal, desire, achieving orgasm), with female survivors significantly more likely to experience marked sexual dysfunction.

RELEVANT SOCIOCULTURAL CONSIDERATIONS

It is now well documented that specific racial and ethnic groups in the United States have a higher risk for developing certain cancer diagnoses that directly affect sexual organs. For instance, African American men have a higher risk of developing prostate cancer compared with whites,[130] and Latinas have twice the risk of developing cervical cancer compared to non-Hispanic whites.[131] Moreover, minority groups in the United States, and particularly individuals who are poor, are often diagnosed at more advanced stages of the disease, treated with more aggressive therapies, and are more likely to have worse treatment outcomes.[132] But beyond gaining knowledge on the cancer facts and figures for different racial and ethnic groups, becoming aware of the impact that culture has on the development of sexual beliefs, attitudes, and practices may be one of the best tools for providers when understanding and helping cancer patients of diverse backgrounds who are coping with sexual dysfunction.

Guidelines for what constitute normative sexual behaviors and gender-specific role prescriptions are greatly influenced by consensus within particular communities,[133] and it has been found that certain prescribed gender roles can intensify sexual problems.[134] Although some of the sexual side effects and long-term effects of cancer treatment may be found across racial and ethnic groups, the following are some of the differences that have been observed in sexual attitudes and quality of life in cancer patients and survivors of diverse ethnicities and their implications for medical practice.

Special Considerations for Male Patients

Research studies on how sexual outcomes in cancer treatment for men may differ by race and ethnicity are scarce. However, recent findings on issues related to sexual functioning for African American prostate cancer patients report results that are worth noting. Even though having ED is likely to lead to psychological consequences for men across races and cultures, it has been found that African American men are significantly more likely than white men to consider sexual side effects when choosing treatment for prostate cancer.[135] In the same study by Jenkins et al.,[135] African American men were more likely than their white counterparts to indicate that an erection is an essential element to sex, and to seek help for sexual problems. According to Johnson et al.,[136] African American men, in spite of showing better recovery of sexual function at 12 and 60 months after diagnosis and treatment with prostatectomy, were more likely than non-Hispanic whites to report that sexual function continued to be a moderate to big problem. Knowledge of these reported differences may assist providers in framing a culturally sensitive discussion with prostate cancer patients of African American origin with regard to their options for treatment and management of sexual side effects. In particular, the fact that African American prostate cancer patients seem likely to have positive attitudes about seeking treatment for an erectile problem could be regarded as invaluable in that it allows providers to effectively generate discussions and provide psychoeducation around safe decision making about treatment options and available therapies for sexual problems.

Special Considerations for Female Patients

A few studies document special considerations for minority, female cancer patients and survivors with regard to their sexual functioning. For African American breast cancer survivors particular concerns about body image are reported, such as keloid formation and total-body hair loss,[137] and body image concerns in general appear to be greater for African American than for white women.[138] Although findings suggest that African American breast cancer survivors view their sex lives as less disrupted by cancer compared with their white counterparts,[139] feeling sexually attractive has been found to be predictive of subsequent psychological well-being for this population.[140] Similar to breast cancer survivors of other ethnicities, African American breast cancer survivors report a need to receive more information from their health care providers regarding sexual dysfunction as a possible side effect of treatment.[137] However, research suggests that African American women may prefer to address their sexual health concerns in a one-to-one context rather than in group settings.[137,140] Moreover, a randomized trial of peer counseling in African American breast cancer survivors documented that brief psychoeducational interventions can be effective in addressing informational needs on sexual health for this population.[141]

For Latina, Asian, and Native American women, the literature on sexual outcomes in cancer treatment and appropriate interventions for treatment-related sexual dysfunction continues to be limited. However, Asian and Latina cervical cancer survivors have reported great concern with the effects of treatment on their appearance, with Latinas expressing more negative feelings about the impact of treatment on their bodies and their relationships compared with Asian, African American, and white survivors.[142] Moreover, cultural factors such as the language barrier for Latinas[142] and the perception of sex as taboo for women from many Asian societies[143] ought to be considered as prevalent impediments in accessing services and to address treatment-related sexual dysfunction. In spite of these challenges, however, the available research findings suggest that psychoeducational interventions may be appropriate for Latinas[144] and factual information on sexuality after cancer, preferably delivered by nurses or doctors, is often sufficient and acceptable to Asian and African American women cancer survivors as a way to address their concerns.[137,145]

DISRUPTION OF INTIMACY AND RELATIONAL CONSIDERATIONS

In addition to the myriad of physiological changes that can disrupt sexual function after cancer diagnosis, it is important to acknowledge the significant interpersonal shifts that may take place and subsequently affect sexuality. For instance, although changes in body image are readily acknowledged and often anticipated when thinking about the effects of breast cancer, it is critical to understand that body image does not occur in isolation and that it is an experience that is contextually and relationally based. Women's perceptions of their partner's reactions to their appearance after cancer consistently predict their own acceptance of their self-image and of their sense of femininity.[146] Moreover, results from a study on the psychosexual adjustment of women treated for breast cancer suggest that a woman's perception of her partner as emotionally involved in the relationship consistently predicted the woman's sexual, marital, and emotional adjustment.[147] Women often do not feel comfortable voicing this aspect of their cancer experience with their partners out of a fear of rejection, and partners are afraid to broach the subject out of fear of causing distress. Similarly, male patients tend to avoid conversations with their wives about their sexual challenges that result from cancer treatment[148] and speculate how their wives feel about their sexual functioning.[149]

This interpersonal silence can quickly become the "elephant in the room" and over time disruptions in intimate functioning can become more difficult to address, with either one or both partners misperceiving each other's feelings and intentions. Consistent with this understanding, levels of relationship distress and emotional well-being have been found to be more related to variables such as arousal, orgasm, and sexual satisfaction than hormonal levels in women.[150] From a provider perspective, what seems most relevant is that providers are particularly well positioned to assist couples in communicating more openly about their fears and to answer questions regarding sexual dysfunction by providing them with available resources on social support and information on cancer treatments that affect sexuality.[151] Research shows that psychoeducational group interventions targeting communication-training and sex therapy show promise in improving women breast cancer survivors' relationships and sexual functioning even without including a partner in the intervention.[152] Moreover, Manne and Badr[153] have proposed an integrative theoretical framework to understanding and addressing the challenges that couples face during and after cancer. By focusing on relationship processes that contribute to intimacy, this framework can help providers facilitate a discussion of the illness as something that happens to the relationship, rather than to individual partners. Based on this approach, couples should be encouraged to perform "relationship-enhancing" behaviors such as reciprocal self-disclosure of fears and concerns, partner responsiveness, and relationship engagement, while discouraging "relationship-compromising" behaviors such as avoidance and criticism.[153]

Communication About Sexual Problems

Although the optimal time to initiate discussion about sexual concerns may vary, it is essential that clinicians prepare patients for potential changes that may be encountered and let them know that discussion about sexual health concerns is welcome. Many patients report that much of their distress often starts with the observation that they were not prepared for changes in sexual function. In the same way that clinicians overview a wide range of potential side effects from any course of cancer treatment, knowledge about potential cancer-related sexual side effects needs to be acknowledged. This allows patients to prepare for managing side effects and potentially may help make better informed decisions about treatment options. It is the belief of the authors that clinicians should learn to address this topic as though they would any other topic. Along with setting expectations, practical information should be provided and this information can be offered at multiple time points across the continuum of cancer care.

Asking About Sexual Problems

One straightforward model that has been proposed is the BETTER model,[154] which stands for (1) Bring up the topic;

(2) Explain that you are concerned with quality of life, including sexual health; (3) Tell patients that you will help find appropriate resources as needed; (4) Timing needs to be taken into consideration, including letting patients know that they can ask for information at any time point; (5) Educate patients about expected sexual side effects; and (6) Record your assessment in the patient's medical record. Specific language that clinicians can use to "bring up the topic" includes phrases such as, "How has your treatment affected your sexual health?" or "Tell me how your sexual function has been since you started treatment." Although clinicians often worry that patients will be offended or embarrassed if asked about sexual health, it is important to remember that multiple studies clearly indicate that patients want to talk about this topic with their doctors and that they desire more information about possible sexual side effects of treatment. Furthermore, it is notable that patients will rarely initiate conversation on this topic for fear of embarrassing their doctor and also out of concern that their symptoms are not treatable. For a majority of patients, it is invaluable to receive a brief yet clear message that serves to normalize their symptoms and reassures them that they are not alone and that resources are available. It is our belief that all patients should be queried about sexual function at multiple time points during treatment and into the survivorship phase of care, and such inquiry should be parallel to any other issue assessed in an ongoing general review of systems.

Use of Validated Assessment Tools

The overwhelming majority of cancer patients do not receive any kind of standardized screening for sexual dysfunction. One method of gaining information and assessing how patients are doing relative to others is to use a brief screening inventory in one's oncology practice. There are a number of measures that have been developed; some are specific to disease type and others are meant for cancer patients in general. Recently, Jeffery et al.[155] published a large-scale review article of sexual function measures to be used with cancer patients. The large majority of published articles relevant to measurements were focused on prostate cancer (76%), followed by breast (9%) and then gynecologic cancer (7%). On review, the authors identified three measures that, after undergoing extensive psychometric testing including trial administration in a clinical oncology setting, were deemed psychometrically valid for broad use. These measures are the University of California, Los Angeles Prostate Cancer Index/Expanded Prostate Cancer Index Composite (UCLA PCI/EPIC),[156] the International Index of Erectile Function (IIEF),[157] and the Female Sexual Function Index (FSFI).[158] The 20-item UCLA PCI is a measure of quality of life after prostate cancer and the IIEF is a measure specifically of sexual function after prostate cancer. Both are available at no cost, but the IIEF is self-administered in 5 to 10 minutes and may be easiest to use in a clinic setting. The 19-item FSFI is a general measure of sexual functioning for women, and it was the only measure for women that met the authors' criteria for being a "standard-setting" instrument. The FSFI is also readily available, free of charge, and takes less than 15 minutes to complete. This measure has been used with a broad range of female cancer patients, including breast, gynecologic, urologic, and rectal cancer.

Intervention

For the majority of cancer patients, a moderate amount of information and education, such as getting information about personal lubricants and vaginal moisturizers, is often adequate to address their needs. For others, more intensive consultation and/or referral may be necessary. For example, oncology practices often have "tip sheets" about managing fatigue, diet, and emotional changes that offer some basic information and usually give additional resource information; it is reasonable to add sexual health to such a roster. A sexual health tip sheet may begin by saying, for example, "Sexuality means different things for every individual but one thing we know for sure is that sexual problems are common both during and after treatment. The good news is that these changes can be addressed and there are lots of strategies for making intimacy pleasurable and exciting again." An educational sheet might also note that sexual problems are common during and after cancer treatment, and it may include general suggestions such as:

- Make a date for sexual activity and talk about sexual concerns beforehand.
- Focus on pleasure first! Take the pressure off of "sex" and start gradually by putting the focus on introducing sensual pleasure into daily life, such as nonsexual massages.
- This is the ideal time to "expand one's repertoire" such as using fantasy, relaxation exercises and extending foreplay in order to reconnect with desire.
- Get moving! Simple regular movement like walking, dancing, or gentle yoga is key for increasing total energy and sexual vitality.
- If you are dealing with body pain in general, plan ahead for the time of day when pain is lowest and you have more energy.
- Change your position! Try different positions that may be more comfortable.
- If you are using pain medications, use them strategically and take them about an hour prior to sexual activity.
- Sometimes medications such as pain medications, antidepressants, and antinausea drugs can affect desire. Talk to your doctor about possibly trying other medications.
- Also counseling, either alone or with a partner, can help.

For some patients, it may be valuable and/or necessary to make a referral for more intensive therapy. Additional intervention may include counseling with a licensed therapist who specializes in sex therapy and/or couples counseling. Other relevant referrals may be for urology, gynecology, endocrinology, psychiatry, and physical therapy including pelvic physical therapy in particular. Collaborative relationships should be developed across disciplines and within the community so that when a problem is identified, established resources are available. Often it can be useful within an oncology practice to identify one clinician, either a physician, nurse, social worker, or psychologist, who can serve as the primary resource person for sexual health issues and who can be responsible for updating available resources and maintaining relevant contacts with community referral sources. It is important to note that several professional organizations such as the American Psychosocial Oncology Society (APOS, www.apos-society.org), the Society for Sex Therapy and Research (SSTAR, www.sstarnet.org), and the American Association of Sexual Educators, Counselors and Therapists (AASECT, www.aasect.org) all have directories and resources for locating professionals who specialize in working with sexual dysfunction.

Without a doubt, it is imperative for oncologists to raise the topic of sexual heath after cancer. However, the authors do recognize that it is not easy to feel comfortable or competent bringing attention to a problem when next steps are unclear. It is rare that oncologists receive any kind of formal training in talking about sexual problems with their patients, and although both doctors and patients live in a culture saturated with graphic sexual images and content, frank and honest conversation about sexuality is not common. Fortunately, as cancer survivorship continues to garner more attention, it is likely that sexual functioning after cancer will also gain more professional focus and opportunity for additional training will become available. In terms of continuing medical education in this area, for example, the American Society for Clinical

Oncology and APOS have recently offered extended preconference workshops and symposia on sexuality and cancer. Moreover, when professionals in the oncology community invest the time and effort, they become more comfortable asking about sexual health after cancer and more competent addressing the issues when they arise. Like any other skill, such communication takes practice but with repeated effort comes mastery.

Selected References

The full list of references for this chapter appears in the online version.

1. Mercadante S, Vitrano V, Catania V. Sexual issues in early and late stage cancer: a review. *Support Care Cancer* 2010;18(6):659.
2. Hordern AJ, Street A. Issues of intimacy and sexuality in the face of cancer: the patient perspective. *Cancer Nurs* 2007;30:E11.
4. Feldman-Stewart D, Brundage M, Hayter C, et al. What questions do patients with curable prostate cancer want answered? *Med Decis Making* 2000;20:7.
6. Park ER, Norris RL, Bober SL. Sexual health communication during cancer care: barriers and recommendations. *Cancer J* 2009;15:74.
10. Schover LR, Fouladi RT, Warneke CL, et al. Defining sexual outcomes after treatment for localized prostate carcinoma.[see comment]. *Cancer* 2002;95:1773.
12. Dubbelman YD, Dohle GR, Schroder FH. Sexual function before and after radical retropubic prostatectomy: a systematic review of prognostic indicators for a successful outcome. *Eur Urol* 2006;50:711.
20. McCullough AR. Prevention and management of erectile dysfunction following radical prostatectomy. *Urol Clin North Am* 2001;28:613.
21. Schwartz EJ, Wong P, Graydon RJ. Sildenafil preserves intracorporeal smooth muscle after radical retropubic prostatectomy. *J Urol* 2004;171:771.
25. Hatzichristou DG. Current treatment and future perspectives for erectile dysfunction. *Int J Impot Res* 1998;10(Suppl 1):S3.
26. Linet OI, Neff LL. Intracavernous prostaglandin E1 in erectile dysfunction. *Clin Invest* 1994;72:139.
32. Potosky AL, Davis WW, Hoffman RM, et al. Five-year outcomes after prostatectomy or radiotherapy for prostate cancer: the prostate cancer outcomes study. *J Natl Cancer Inst* 2004;96:1358.
38. Herr HW, O'Sullivan M. Quality of life of asymptomatic men with nonmetastatic prostate cancer on androgen deprivation therapy. *J Urol* 2000; 163:1743.
40. Laumann EO, Paik A, Rosen RC. Sexual dysfunction in the United States: prevalence and predictors. *JAMA* 1999;281:537.
41. Penson DF, McLerran D, Feng Z, et al. 5-year Urinary and Sexual Outcomes after Radical Prostatectomy: Results from the Prostate Cancer Outcomes Study. *J Urol* 2008;179(5 Suppl):S40.
45. Nelson CJ, Deveci S, Stasi J, et al. Sexual bother following radical prostatectomyjsm. *J Sex Med* 2010;7:129.
47. Hartmann JT, Albrecht C, Schmoll HJ, et al. Long-term effects on sexual function and fertility after treatment of testicular cancer. *Br J Cancer* 1999; 80:801.
53. Spitz A, Stein JP, Lieskovsky G, et al. Orthotopic urinary diversion with preservation of erectile and ejaculatory function in men requiring radical cystectomy for non-urothelial malignancy: a new technique. *J Urol* 1999; 161(6):1761.
56. Hautmann RE, Stein JP. Neobladder with prostatic capsule and seminal-sparing cystectomy for bladder cancer: a step in the wrong direction. *Urol Clin North Am* 2005;32(2):177.
57. Zippe CD, Raina R, Massanyi EZ, et al. Sexual function after male radical cystectomy in a sexually active population. *Urology* 2004;64(4):685.
60. Zippe CD, Raina R, Shah AD, et al. Female sexual dysfunction after radical cystectomy: a new outcome measure. *Urology* 2004;63(6):1153.
65. Low C, Fullarton M, Parkinson E, et al. Issues of intimacy and sexual dysfunction following major head and neck cancer treatment. *Oral Oncol* 2009;45(10):898.
66. Gamba A, Romano M, Grosso IM, et al. Psychosocial adjustment of patients surgically treated for head and neck cancer. *Head Neck* 1992; 14(3):218.
67. Chatterjee R, Kottaridis PD, McGarrigle HH, et al. Management of erectile dysfunction by combination therapy with testosterone and sildenafil in recipients of high-dose therapy for haematological malignancies. *Bone Marrow Transplant* 2002;29(7):607.
68. Humphreys CT, Tallman B, Altmaier EM, et al. Sexual functioning in patients undergoing bone marrow transplantation: a longitudinal study. *Bone Marrow Transplant* 2007;39(8):491.
69. Syrjala KL, Kurland BF, Abrams JR, et al. Sexual function changes during the 5 years after high-dose treatment and hematopoietic cell transplantation for malignancy, with case-matched controls at 5 years. *Blood* 2008; 111(3):989.
71. Zantomio D, Grigg AP, MacGregor L, et al. Female genital tract graft-versus-host disease: incidence, risk factors and recommendations for management. *Bone Marrow Transplant* 2006;38(8):567.
73. Havenga K, Maas CP, DeRuiter MC, et al. Avoiding long-term disturbance to bladder and sexual function in pelvic surgery, particularly with rectal cancer. *Semin Surg Oncol* 2000;18(3):235.
74. Donovan KA, Thompson LMA, Hoffe SE. Sexual function in colorectal cancer survivors. *Cancer Control* 2010;17(1):44.
77. Sprunk E, Alteneder RR. The impact of an ostomy on sexuality. *Clin J Oncol Nurs* 2000;4(2):85.
81. Ganz PA, Kwan L, Stanton AL, et al. Quality of life at the end of primary treatment of breast cancer: first results from the moving beyond cancer randomized trial. *J Natl Cancer Inst* 2004;96:376.
89. Burwell SR, Case LD, Kaelin C, et al. Sexual problems in younger women after breast cancer surgery. *J Clin Oncol* 2006;24:2815.
93. Moyer A. Psychosocial outcomes of breast-conserving surgery versus mastectomy: a meta-analytic review. *Health Psychol* 1997;16:284.
96. Schover LR. Premature ovarian failure and its consequences: vasomotor symptoms, sexuality and fertility. *J Clin Oncol* 2008;26:753.
99. Barton DL, Wender DB, Sloan JA, et al. Randomized controlled trial to evaluate transdermal testosterone in female cancer survivors with decreased libido. North Central Cancer Treatment Group Protocol NO2C3. *J Natl Cancer Inst* 2007;99:672.
105. Cella D, Fallowfield L, Barker P, et al. Quality of Life of Postmenopausal Women in the ATAC ("Arimidex," Tamoxifen, Alone or in Combination) Trial after completion of 5 years' adjuvant treatment for early breast cancer. *Breast Cancer Res Treat* 2006;100:273.
109. Ratner ES, Foran KA, Schwartz PE, et al. Sexuality and intimacy after gynecological cancer. *Maturitas* 2010;66(1):23.
111. Carmack Taylor CL, Basen-Engquist K, Shinn EH, et al. Predictors of sexual functioning in ovarian cancer patients. *J Clin Oncol* 2004;22(5): 881.
113. Bergmark K, Avall-Lundovist E, Dickman PW, et al. Vaginal changes and sexuality in women with a history of cervical cancer. *N Engl J Med* 1999; 340(18):1383.
117. Likes WM, Stegbauer C, Tillmanns T, et al. Correlates of sexual function following vulvar excision. *Gynecol Oncol* 2007;105(3):600.
118. Katz A. Interventions for sexuality after pelvic radiation therapy and gynecologic cancer. *Cancer J* 2009;15(1):45.
125. Matloff ET, Barnett RE, Bober SL. Unraveling the next chapter: Sexual development, body image and sexual functioning in female BRCA carriers. *Cancer J* 2009;15:15.
127. Zebrack BJ, Foley S, Wittmann D, et al. Sexual functioning in young adult survivors of childhood cancer. *Psycho-oncology* 2009;19(8):814.
135. Jenkins R, Schover LR, Fouladi RT, et al. Sexuality and health-related quality of life after prostate cancer in African-American and White men treated for localized disease. *J Sex Marital Ther* 2004;30(2):79.
137. Wilmoth MC, Sanders D. Accept me for myself: African American women's issues after breast cancer. *Oncol Nurs Forum* 2001;28(5):875.
142. Ashing-Giwa KT, Kagawa-Singer M, Padilla GV, et al. The impact of cervical cancer and dysplasia: a qualitative multiethnic study. *Psycho-oncology* 2004;13(10):709.
147. Wimberly SR, Carver CS, Laurenceau JP, et al. Perceived partner reactions to diagnosis and treatment of breast cancer: impact on psychosocial and psychosexual adjustment. *J Consult Clin Psychol* 2005;73(2):300.
148. Boehmer U, Clark JA. Communication about prostate cancer between men and their wives. *J Fam Pract* 2001;50(3):226.
153. Manne S, Badr H. Intimacy and relationship processes in couples' psychosocial adaptation to cancer. *Cancer* 2008;112(11 Suppl):2541.
154. Mick J, Hughes M, Cohen MZ. Using the BETTER model to assess sexuality. *Clin J Oncol Nurs* 2004;8:84.
155. Jeffery DD, Tzeng JP, Keefe FJ, et al. Initial report of the cancer Patient-Reported Outcomes Measurement Information System (PROMIS) sexual function committee: review of sexual function measures and domains used in oncology. *Cancer* 2009;115:1142.

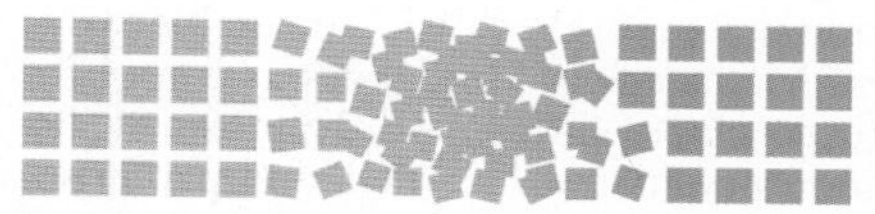

CHAPTER 173 PSYCHOLOGICAL ISSUES IN CANCER

DAVID SPIEGEL AND MICHELLE B. RIBA

Coping, distress, and support are crucial psychological issues that every cancer patient faces with his or her health care team. The diagnosis of cancer is a life-altering experience for anyone. The nature of the patient's response to it will affect mood, adherence to treatment, and the quality of his or her social support. Effective coping with the disease involves dealing with its direct and indirect effects, ranging from managing the details of medical appointments to handling existential dread. Facing the illness and its consequences requires acknowledging and managing strong but inevitable emotions that can interfere with medical care,[1] family and vocational engagement, sleep, diet, and exercise.[2]

A wide range and prevalence of psychiatric and psychological problem affect patients and families before, during, and after cancer care and treatment. Recent studies in adults treated in outpatient cancer clinics demonstrate a 40% to 50% clinically relevant level of distress.[3–4] Some of the more important factors are listed in Table 173.1.

In addition, there are also physical symptoms of the cancer and its treatments that overlap with the somatic symptoms that are included in many psychiatric conditions. For example, it is often very difficult for even skilled clinicians to determine the extent to which fatigue, decreased appetite, or sleep problems are related to depression or anxiety versus certain types of cancer and targeted therapies. It is thus easy to misattribute the symptoms of a mood disorder to the cancer itself and fail to notice important opportunities for treatment. Despite the complexity involved in coping with serious medical and psychiatric problems, there are some guiding principles for understanding patient dynamics and potential psychological issues.

UNDERSTANDING CANCER AS A TRAUMA

Although many would like to maintain a positive view of the diagnosis and treatment for cancer, it still is for many a trauma analogous to experiencing an assault, accident, or natural disaster. Patients can often remember the date and time they received their cancer diagnosis. They can remember exactly where it was discussed, who said it, the specific words that were used, and how they felt. These are life-altering, life-changing moments that are, psychologically, often transformative. In the initial stages of diagnosis and early treatment, the use of the term *acute stress disorder* (ASD) or *posttraumatic stress disorder* (PTSD) may best encapsulate the psychological problems that occur. In one study of breast cancer patients after treatment, 5% to 10% met diagnostic criteria for posttraumatic stress disorder,[5] and there was little change in their status over the ensuing year.[6] Often patients experience disbelief, inability to sleep, fears, and so forth. Lives and schedules change from the mundane routine of going to work or school, to being in a whirlwind of doctors' appointments, receiving news and data in technical language, making appointments for surgery, blood draws, chemotherapy, and radiotherapy.

As patients move through the various stages of cancer care, so too does the trauma response—from acute stress to a more chronic PTSD.[7–9] The adjustment to the trauma can also become chronic. Even cessation of acute treatment can be fraught with anxiety about recurrence.

COMMON PSYCHIATRIC CONDITIONS

Although there are many psychiatric conditions that occur in patients with cancer, the more commonly diagnosed are depression, anxiety (panic, PTSD, phobias), adjustment disorders, and delirium.

Often patients have mixed states or combinations of symptoms, such as depression and anxiety. Further, there are symptoms that often are not diagnosed but are quite difficult for patients to manage, such as difficulties with falling asleep and staying asleep and problems adhering to complex and lengthy medication regimens. This is especially difficult when patients have cognitive changes related to the underlying cancer (as in brain tumors) or to the chemotherapeutic agents (cisplatin, steroids). Some of these regimens alter the efficiency with which the brain processes information storage and retrieval.[10]

SCREENING FOR PSYCHOLOGICAL PROBLEMS

As part of good, routine clinical care, it is important to obtain a working diagnosis and treatment plan for each patient regarding psychiatric problems. There are numerous screening tools that are available for clinical as well as research purposes.[11–13] Regular, ongoing evaluation of emotional distress affects management and treatment of psychiatric issues and contributes to better patient outcome, satisfaction, doctor–patient communication, and improved overall oncologic care.[14] Approximately one third of patients in outpatient oncology clinics experience significant levels of distress, with greater degrees of distress in patients who have tumors with poorer prognosis and outcomes.[15] This means that any screening tool must include a routine, systematized method for busy clinicians to review the measures and provide clinical assessment, treatment, and referral as

TABLE 173.1

FACTORS IN PSYCHOLOGICAL ASSESSMENT

Past psychiatric history
Age at diagnosis
Gender
Type of cancer
Stage of cancer
Location of cancer
How the cancer was diagnosed
Types of cancer treatment
Family coherence
Marital/partner status
Behavioral/previous coping strategies
Religion/spirituality
Job/employment status
Medical/psychiatric insurance
Substance use or abuse
Pain
Finances
Genetic risks and testing
Survivorship resources

appropriate. The patient data should be included in the medical record and should provide sufficient diagnostic information to guide mental health care. The diagnostic criteria in the American Psychiatric Association's *Diagnostic and Statistical Manual* (DSM-IV-TR) provide the essential definitions of specific mental disorders utilized in practice.[16]

In 1997 the National Comprehensive Cancer Network published the Distress Management Guidelines as a tool for oncology clinicians to develop a differential diagnosis of distress, including common psychiatric disorders and psychosocial and spiritual problems. The panel addressed the issue of the difficulty of psychiatric symptoms that overlap with underlying oncologic disease and treatments and noted that using the term "distress" was a good starting point for clinicians, patients, and families to talk about problems. Using an algorithmic approach, clinicians are guided by the presenting symptoms, possible interventions, evaluation, and treatment options. As a self-report method of measuring and screening for distress, patients are asked to mark their level of distress on a visual analog tool, called the distress thermometer (Fig. 173.1). Along with the distress thermometer is a problem list the patient uses to indicate possible causes of distress such as practical, emotional, family, spiritual, or physical. Using a cutoff of 4 or 5 of a possible score of 10 provides an indication of distress and has been validated against other screening tools for psychological distress.[4] Psychosocial screening provides an

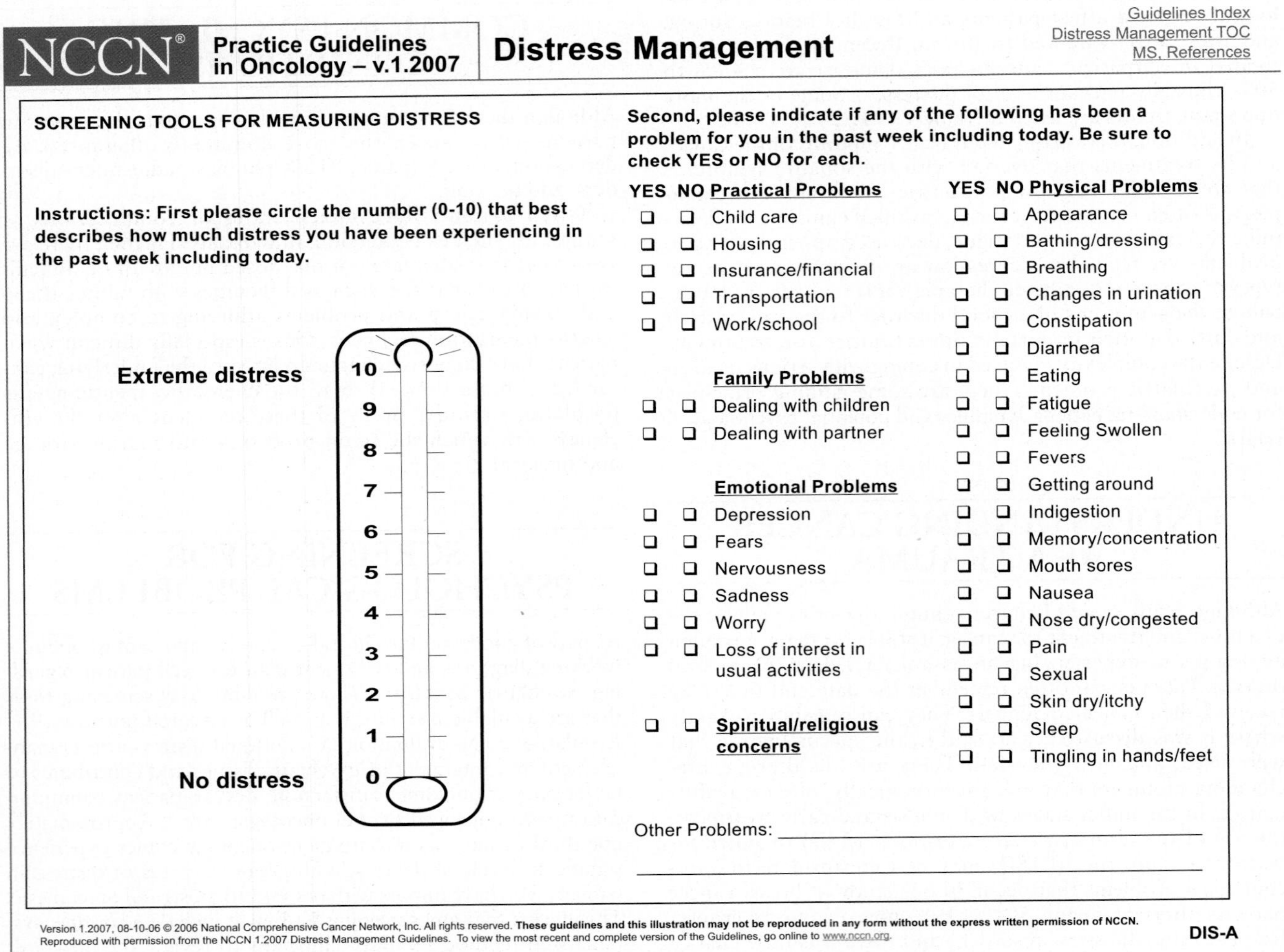

NCCN® Practice Guidelines in Oncology – v.1.2007 **Distress Management**

Guidelines Index
Distress Management TOC
MS, References

SCREENING TOOLS FOR MEASURING DISTRESS

Instructions: First please circle the number (0-10) that best describes how much distress you have been experiencing in the past week including today.

Extreme distress 10 9 8 7 6 5 4 3 2 1 0 **No distress**

Second, please indicate if any of the following has been a problem for you in the past week including today. Be sure to check YES or NO for each.

YES	NO	Practical Problems
❑	❑	Child care
❑	❑	Housing
❑	❑	Insurance/financial
❑	❑	Transportation
❑	❑	Work/school
		Family Problems
❑	❑	Dealing with children
❑	❑	Dealing with partner
		Emotional Problems
❑	❑	Depression
❑	❑	Fears
❑	❑	Nervousness
❑	❑	Sadness
❑	❑	Worry
❑	❑	Loss of interest in usual activities
❑	❑	**Spiritual/religious concerns**

YES	NO	Physical Problems
❑	❑	Appearance
❑	❑	Bathing/dressing
❑	❑	Breathing
❑	❑	Changes in urination
❑	❑	Constipation
❑	❑	Diarrhea
❑	❑	Eating
❑	❑	Fatigue
❑	❑	Feeling Swollen
❑	❑	Fevers
❑	❑	Getting around
❑	❑	Indigestion
❑	❑	Memory/concentration
❑	❑	Mouth sores
❑	❑	Nausea
❑	❑	Nose dry/congested
❑	❑	Pain
❑	❑	Sexual
❑	❑	Skin dry/itchy
❑	❑	Sleep
❑	❑	Tingling in hands/feet

Other Problems: ______________________

DIS-A

FIGURE 173.1 National Comprehensive Cancer Network Distress Thermometer.

TABLE 173.2

PRINCIPLES OF ADAPTIVE COPING WITH CANCER

Stressors are best handled by:
Facing rather than fleeing
Altering perception
Coping actively
Expressing emotion
Social support

opportunity to determine baseline distress and then prospectively evaluate response to psychosocial treatments.[17]

COPING

Cancer patients and their families are confronted with new situations arising from the illness itself or from the demands of the treatment (Table 173.2). Moos and Schaeffer[18] summarize these challenges as the need to preserve a reasonable emotional balance, maintain a sense of competence and mastery, sustain relationships with family and friends, and prepare for an uncertain future. Cancer patients benefit from help in improving their coping skills or in learning new and more adaptive ones. Previous coping strategies may no longer be appropriate to the new situation. Social support directed at expression of emotion helps cancer patients to maintain realistic optimism and mitigate distress.[19–23] The adaptive tasks that are necessary in order to adjust to the illness involve several different kinds of coping skills: evaluation of novel information, decision making, learning to express emotions, mobilizing social support, and increasing role flexibility. Adaptive coping has been divided into three types: information-focused, emotion-focused, and problem-focused.[24,25] Problem-focused coping skills are important to help the cancer patient live with the illness and manage its treatment. However, emotional adjustment to the illness is also essential. Some studies have shown that avoidant strategies may be less adaptive in the long run than task-oriented and approach strategies,[26] although in the context of medical illness coping is situation specific.[27,28] A broad coping-skills repertoire, consisting of both problem- and emotion-focused strategies, increases the probability of matching the response to the particular demands of a given stressful medical situation (Table 173.3).

TREATMENT INTERVENTIONS

Psychosocial

The appropriate treatment for psychological symptoms associated with cancer can be determined by clarifying the nature of emotional distress (anxiety, depression, psychosis), the use of pharmacotherapy to relieve acute and chronic symptoms, and the selection of appropriate psychosocial interventions for treating problems related to anxiety, depression, existential concerns, somatic symptoms, and social or communication problems.[2,27,28] The efficacy of psychosocial treatments for depression and anxiety in medically ill patients, particularly brief psychodynamic, educational, supportive, and interpersonal therapies, hypnosis, and behavioral and cognitive-behavioral methods, has been supported by numerous outcome studies.[29–33]

Psychoeducational Interventions

Principles of Psychoeducational Intervention

Medical knowledge enhances the sense of control and mastery a person has over his or her disease, and educational interventions generally yield positive outcomes. Interventions for medical patients are usually more effective when they provide patients with cues for using the knowledge related to their disease and daily management[24] or with some emotion-focused components, which helps them to adjust and live through the different phases of the illness. Anticipatory guidance is an important component of these interventions, helping patients to prepare to respond to future as well as current

TABLE 173.3

STAGE-SPECIFIC COPING CHALLENGES AND MEDICAL RESPONSES

Stage of Cancer	Coping Challenge	Physician Response
Initial diagnosis	Existential anxiety	Rapid and clear evaluation
Acute treatment	Helplessness	Invite participation in treatment decisions
	Fatigue/disruption of social roles	Invite involvement of family/friends
End of acute treatment	Increased sense of vulnerability/anxiety about relapse and long-term treatment effects Medical isolation	Treatment summary and long-term follow-up plan Survivorship program
Relapse	Anxiety about disease progression/treatment effects Truncated future Loss of social contacts	Clear communication Compassion Commitment to providing care Reordering priorities Group and other support

disease-related problems. The evaluation of outcomes of psychoeducational interventions indicates consistent if modest improvement.[32,34–40]

Coping Skills Training

Education-based group interventions that provide informational support can facilitate the initial adjustment of early stage breast cancer patients by improving self-esteem, body image, and perceived control and by reducing uncertainty about the illness.[41,42] Women who lack personal resources and support benefit the most. Many of these approaches have demonstrated benefit in controlled trials. One cognitive-behavioral stress management group program proposed a multimodal type of intervention combining 20 therapy hours of relaxation training, coping skills training, cognitive restructuring, assertiveness and anger management training, and social support for women with breast cancer. Patients improved in self-reports of benefits from cancer, but no improvement on the distress measures was found.[43] In this study, the greatest changes in positive benefits were reported by women who were low in optimism. An eight-session educational intervention, providing training in stress management, problem solving, goal setting, and assertiveness, produced improvements in general quality of life, as well as specific competence in managing emotional, financial, and legal problems.[44] A five-session family intervention for women with recurrent breast cancer, designed to improve communication, enhance information seeking, improve coping, and manage symptoms, did not affect overall quality of life but did reduce negative appraisal of the cancer and reduced hopelessness.[45] A multidimensional cancer rehabilitation program produced improvements in physical functioning and reductions in distress.[46] A more existentially oriented approach emphasized finding ways to develop a sense of meaning and has been shown to enhance self-efficacy, optimism, and self-esteem among breast and colorectal cancer patients.[47] It is quite clear that facing the existential threat posed by cancer in a supportive way improves coping and reduces distress rather than demoralizing cancer patients.[2,48–50]

Mindfulness Training

Mindfulness-based stress reduction is an adaptation of Zen Buddhist meditation techniques taught in weekly courses. The focus is on enhancing the ability to live in the moment and to tolerate stresses as real but transient phenomena, while more comfortably relating to one's body. Such techniques have been used to good effect with cancer patients. A meta-analysis of ten studies documented a significant (moderate effect size $d = .48$) overall improvement in quality of life and possible benefit for various aspects of physical health.[51] A seven-week group training for patients with a variety of cancers resulted in significantly reduced distress.[52] Other studies have shown that a combination of such techniques with more traditional group therapy produced reductions in intrusive thinking and other posttraumatic stress symptoms[53] as well as reduced depression and fear of recurrence and produced higher energy[54] among women with breast cancer. Such intervention has also been shown to result in lower cortisol, reduced Th1 (proinflammatory) cytokines, and lower systolic blood pressure[1,55] as well as improved natural killer cell cytotoxicity.[56]

Electronic Technology-Based Interventions

Technology-assisted interventions have proven highly effective. A peer-modeling videotape shown to patients shortly after diagnosis produced increases in vitality and posttraumatic growth and decreases in depression and intrusive thoughts.[57] A combined home visiting and telephone intervention resulted in reduced pain.[58] Computer-based patient support tools provided information, decision support, and interaction with other patients and produced not only increments in knowledge but better patient–doctor interactions and enhanced social support.[59] Support groups have been adapted to the Internet with remarkably good effect. Real-time leader-conducted groups for breast cancer patients have produced significant reductions in depression and pain.[60]

TABLE 173.4

USEFUL CANCER INFORMATION WEB SITES

American Cancer Society	www.cancer.org
Association of Cancer Online Resources	www.acor.org
Association of European Cancer Leagues	www.europeancancerleagues.eu
Breast Cancer Action	www.bcaction.org
LIVESTRONG: Lance Armstrong Foundation	www.livestrong.org
National Cancer Childhood Foundation	www.nccf.org
National Cancer Institute	www.cancer.gov
National Coalition for Cancer Survivorship	www.canceradvocacy.org
Stanford Survivorship Program	www.cancersupportivecare.com
Susan G. Komen Foundation	ww5.komen.org

Excellent Internet resources for information about various types of cancer and their treatments, as well as supportive services, are now available. These include the National Cancer Institute's Web site its database of cancer treatments, and its associated phone information line. Websites with authoritative information about supportive care services include those sponsored by the American Cancer Society. The Wellness Community Web site is maintained by the Cancer Support Community, a collaboration of the Wellness Community and Gilda's Clubs, which maintain a network of facilities that provide free community supportive services, including classes and support groups. Another excellent example is Breast Cancer Connections Web site.

Cognitive-Behavioral Therapy

The cognitive-behavioral approach[61] is built on the assumption that previous social learning, developmental history, and significant experiences lead people to form a unique set of meanings and assumptions, or cognitive schemas, about themselves, the world, and their future. These schemas are then used to organize perception and to govern and evaluate behavior.[62] When specific schemas are activated, they directly influence the content of a person's perceptions, interpretations, associations, and memories from a given time. Cognitive-behavioral therapy (CBT) was developed as a short-term (12 to 20 sessions) intervention for depression, targeting patients' thoughts and their relation to behavior and affect. CBT for cancer patients generally features a multicomponent intervention integrating coping skills training, stress management, and an intervention designed to enhance cognitive and behavioral processes that will be useful in adjusting to illness.[30] The CBT therapist seeks to identify maladaptive cognitions, turn them into testable hypotheses, and submit them to empirical investigation, so the patient can then reject, modify, or retain these thoughts based on the evidence. Alternatively, more adaptive cognitions and behaviors are similarly examined and tested. In the early sessions, the goal of CBT is to establish a therapeutic relationship, identify primary problems, produce symptom relief, and educate the patient about the process of psychotherapy, CBT, and the role of thoughts, images, and beliefs on emotions and behavior. Together, the therapist and patient decide on the treatment goal, a plan for subsequent therapy sessions, and homework assignments intended to augment the therapy and direct structured practice. The initial homework might require the patient to identify and record maladaptive cognitions (e.g., automatic thoughts). As therapy progresses, verbal techniques are employed to trigger automatic thoughts and associated assumptions and reveal core beliefs or schemas. In an environment of collaborative empiricism, the patient learns to identify, logically and empirically evaluate, and justify the usefulness of systematic biases, cognitive distortions and dysfunctional assumptions, and thoughts, images, and beliefs that underlie emotional distress. The therapist helps the patient challenge cognitive distortions such as overgeneralization, catastrophizing, "should" statements, magnification, minimization, dichotomous thinking, and the fallacies of control, worry, fairness, and attachment. Cognitive restructuring techniques and guided discovery help the patient choose more adaptive cognitions and behaviors. Cognitive techniques used in CBT include thought-stopping, self-instruction, distraction, direct disputation, labeling distortions, and development of replacement imagery. Behavioral techniques such as activity scheduling, relaxation training, social skills training, mastery and pleasure ratings, assertiveness training, bibliotherapy, homework, behavioral rehearsal, and *in vivo* exposure are also employed.

The efficacy of CBT as a treatment for depression is well established.[63] A review of empirically supported treatments for psychosomatic disorders determined that CBT is efficacious for chronic pain management and some cancers.[30]

Group Psychotherapy

Group intervention in a variety of forms has become an increasingly popular, effective, and efficient means of providing psychosocial support for cancer patients.[64] Groups of different types may encompass theoretical approaches that include the psychodynamic, existential, educational, and cognitive-behavioral, among others.[63] Although some cancer patients are disinclined to join a support group, most are initially reluctant to undertake other aspects of cancer treatment as well. Factors associated with reluctance include less favorable views of such groups, feeling less control over their cancer, using less active coping styles, and having less distress.[65,66] Although men may initially be more reluctant than women to openly discuss emotional problems relating to cancer, cognitive aspects of coping can be a good starting point, and men with prostate cancer report information sharing with other patients as a helpful aspect of group experience. Although reactions to catastrophic illness may differ for individuals with preexisting psychopathology, most cancer patients share with their emotionally healthy counterparts the need for support in dealing with diagnosis and treatment, changes wrought by disease, social isolation, and existential issues.

Common elements of group psychotherapeutic intervention include the following[64]:

1. *Social support.* Psychotherapy, especially in groups, can provide a new social network with the common bond of facing similar problems. At a time when the illness makes a person feel removed from the flow of life, when many others withdraw out of awkwardness or fear, group psychotherapeutic support provides a new and important social connection. Indeed, the very thing that damages other social relationships is the ticket of admission to such groups, providing a surprising intensity of caring among members from the very beginning. Furthermore, members find that the process of giving help to others enhances their own sense of mastery of the role of "patient" and increases their self-esteem, imbuing the experience of illness with a new meaning.
2. *Emotional expression.* The expression of emotion is important in reducing social isolation and improving coping. Yet patients often believe that they are controlling the psychological and even physical impact of the disease by suppressing their emotional reaction to it. This attitude is often reinforced by friends and family who are made anxious by a display of appropriate fear or sadness in the patient, and by medical professionals as well, who perceive a patient's sadness as an indication of nihilism about treatment or loss of hope. Persistent negative affect, as is seen in depression, often elicits anger in those involved with the patient, since the patient seems unwilling rather than unable to modulate their feelings. However, normal anxiety and sadness related to having cancer is phasic and is better managed through expression and discussion. Indeed there is evidence that emotional expression actually facilitates the resolution of long-term negative emotion.[20,48] Encouragement of emotional expression can enhance intimacy in families, providing opportunities for direct expression of affection and concern. The use of the psychotherapeutic setting to deal with painful affect also provides an organizing context for handling its intrusion. When unbidden thoughts involving fears of dying and death intrude, they can be better managed by patients who know that there is a time and a place during which such feelings will be expressed, acknowledged, and dealt with. Furthermore, disease-related dysphoria is more intense when amplified by isolation, leaving the patient to feel that he or she is deservedly alone with the sense of anxiety, loss, and fear that he or she experiences. Being in a group where many others express similar distress normalizes their reactions, making them feel less alien and overwhelming.
3. *Detoxifying dying.* Processing existential concerns by facing rather than avoiding issues such as dying and death, which could be considered likely to exacerbate depression, actually helps to reduce it. This approach encourages patients to face what they most fear and find some aspect of it they can do something about (e.g., control the process of dying when death is unavoidable). This helps patients to feel more active and less helpless, even in the face of dying. Others have combined principles of cognitive therapy with a focus on existential concerns,[64] finding it an effective approach to reduce symptoms of distress. Death anxiety in particular is intensified by isolation, in part because patients often conceptualize death in terms of separation from loved ones. This can be powerfully addressed by psychotherapeutic techniques that directly confront such concerns in a supportive social setting. Yalom[67] has described the ultimate existential concerns as death, freedom, isolation, and meaninglessness. Rather than avoiding painful or anxiety-provoking topics in attempts to "stay positive," this form of group therapy addresses these concerns head-on with the intent of helping group members make better use of the time they have left. The goal is to help those facing the threat of death to see it from a new point of view. Facing even life-threatening issues can directly help patients shift from emotion-focused to problem-focused coping.[24,25] The process of dying is

often more threatening than death itself. Direct discussion of death anxiety can help to divide the fear of death into a series of problems: loss of control over treatment decisions, fear of separation from loved ones, anxiety about pain, and control of the manner of one's own dying. Discussion of these concerns can lead to means of addressing if not completely resolving each of these issues. Even the process of grieving can be reassuring at the same time that it is threatening. The experience of grieving for others who have died of the same condition constitutes a deeply personal experience of the depth of loss that will be experienced by others after one's own death.

4. *Reorganizing life priorities and living in the present.* The acceptance of the possibility of illness shortening life carries with it an opportunity for reevaluating life's priorities. Facing the threat of death in a way that facilitates a sense of active coping can aid in making the most of what remains in life.[68] This can help patients take control of those aspects of their lives they can influence, while grieving and relinquishing those they cannot. Progress in life goal reappraisal, reorganization of priorities, and perception of benefits may also mediate improvement in symptoms and enhance quality of life.[69]
5. *Enhancing family support.* Psychotherapeutic interventions can also be quite helpful in improving communication, identifying needs, increasing role flexibility, and adjusting to new medical social, vocational, and financial realities.[70] The group format is especially helpful for such a task, in that problems expressing needs and wishes can be examined among group members as a model for clarifying communication in the family.
6. *Improving communication with physicians.* Support groups can be quite useful in facilitating better communication with physicians and other health care professionals.[2,71] Groups provide mutual encouragement to get questions answered, to participate actively in treatment decisions, and to consider alternatives carefully.
7. *Symptom control.* Many group and individual psychotherapy programs teach specific coping skills designed to help patients reduce cancer-related symptoms such as anxiety, anticipatory nausea and vomiting, and pain. Techniques used include specific self-regulation skills such as self-hypnosis, meditation, biofeedback, and progressive muscle relaxation. Hypnosis is widely used for pain and anxiety control in cancer to attenuate the experience of pain and suffering and to allow painful emotional material to be examined.[72] Group sessions that involve instruction in self-hypnosis provide an effective means of reducing pain and anxiety and consolidate the major themes of discussion in the group.[2,73,74] Hypnosis is an altered state of consciousness, composed of heightened absorption in focal attention, dissociation of peripheral awareness, and enhanced responsiveness to social cues.[75] It has a long tradition of effectiveness in controlling somatic symptoms such as pain and anxiety. Patients with the requisite hypnotic capacity can be taught to utilize self-hypnosis to reduce or eliminate pain and the tension that accompanies it. Hypnotic techniques have been shown to effectively reduce cancer pain[75] and to facilitate medical procedures. Hypnotic intervention actually alters perceptual processing in the brain, with reduced response to painful stimuli as measured by event-related potentials[76] and positron emission tomography.[77]

OUTCOME

Clinical trials have demonstrated the benefit of group therapy for breast cancer patients,[36,48,78] with notable reductions in pain[2,73] and emotional distress.[77] A systematic review of the literature that included two meta-analyses and nine well-designed randomized controlled trials indicated that psychoeducational interventions not only enhance patient knowledge about their cancer and its treatments, but also reduce depression, anxiety, nausea, and pain.[32]

IMPLICATIONS FOR CANCER PROGRESSION AND MORTALITY

There is a small base of literature that raises the possibility that psychotherapeutic intervention may affect survival time as well as quality of life.[79–83] Six of 13 published randomized trials demonstrate such an effect.[20] Spiegel et al.[79] reported that a year (minimum) of supportive-expressive group psychotherapy resulted in a significant 18-month increase in survival time in metastatic breast cancer patients. A 6-week cognitive behavioral group intervention composed of education, stress management, coping skills training, and psychological support for malignant melanoma patients found significantly lower death rates at 10-year follow-up in the treatment group.[81] A study of individual psychotherapeutic support offered at the bedside early in the course of disease to a group of gastrointestinal cancer inpatients also had favorable results on survival[82] that has been confirmed at ten-year follow-up.[84] A randomized replication trial of supportive-expressive group psychotherapy among 125 women with metastatic breast cancer found positive effects on mood[4,49] but no overall survival advantage,[85] although there was a significant interaction with tumor type, such that women with estrogen receptor–negative tumors who had been randomized to the group condition lived significantly longer than estrogen receptor–negative controls. A randomized trial among 227 women with primary breast cancer demonstrated that those who received group support had significantly lower rates of relapse and mortality at 11-year follow-up.[86]

However, six other trials found no effect of psychosocial intervention on survival time.[49,78,87–90] One large multicenter trial that utilized supportive-expressive group psychotherapy with metastatic breast cancer patients showed reduced distress and pain but no survival advantage.[78] A major randomized clinical trial of palliative care involving an average of four visits that focused on choices about resuscitation preference, pain control, and quality of life for patients with non-small cell lung cancer found that those who received this care lived longer than those who were provided standard anticancer care (median survival, 11.85 vs. 8.9 months; $p = 0.02$).[91] Taken together, these studies suggest that psychosocial effects on survival time are most pronounced when medical treatments have become less effective.[92] No study has found that psychotherapy, even involving direct confrontation with dying and death, shortens survival. Any potential benefit of psychotherapeutic support on cancer progression remains an open research question.

SURVIVORSHIP

Survivorship is becoming an increasingly important aspect of comprehensive cancer care as cancer survival improves. There are now some 12 million cancer survivors in the United States.[93] Provision of supportive services should continue after active oncologic treatment is completed.[94] Domains of intervention include surveillance for recurrence and late effects of treatment, genetic issues, overall health maintenance, attention to psychiatric, social, behavioral, and financial problems, and other factors that affect quality of life (Table 173.5). For many survivorship programs this involves preparation of a treatment summary and posttreatment surveillance planning, navigators to help patients and their

TABLE 173.5

SURVIVORSHIP CONCERNS

Screening Protocols for Recurrence
- Developing a screening calendar
- Dealing with relapse anxiety

Surveillance for Late Effects of Cancer Treatment
- Cardiotoxicity
- Cognitive decline
- Second cancers

Communication with Primary Care Clinicians

Genetic Issues
- Implications for patient's progeny
- Implications for extended family

General Health Maintenance
- Tobacco control
- Substance abuse
- Diet
- Exercise
- Sleep
- Regular Medical Checkups

Psychiatric Late Effects
- Depression
- PTSD/anxiety disorders
- Marital disruption
- Sexual dysfunction
- Infertility
- Social isolation

Financial/Vocational Problems
- Insurance discrimination
- Financial strain
- Disability
- Work limitations
- Educational disruption

families deal with the aftermath of treatment, as well as classes, group support, nutritional consultation, social services, and psychiatric support.

PSYCHOTROPIC MEDICATION

Antidepressants

It is becoming increasingly clear that, as is the case with major depression in general, depression that arises in the context of cancer is responsive to antidepressant treatment.[95] Using various measures of depression and outcome, studies indicate that paroxetine,[95] mianserin,[96] fluoxetine,[97] amitriptyline,[95] and desipramine[98] are useful in treating depression in patients with cancer (Table 173.6). Antidepressants decrease depressive symptoms, improve functional capacity, reduce cachexia, ameliorate some menopausal symptoms, and reduce pain.[99]

Fisch et al.[100] found that treatment with fluoxetine significantly improved depressive symptoms and some measures of quality of life when compared to placebo in cancer patients with a variety of tumors with an expected survival of 3 to 24 months. Importantly, these patients were recruited based on reporting that they were bothered by depressed mood at a

TABLE 173.6

ANTIDEPRESSANTS: SELECTIVE SEROTONIN REUPTAKE INHIBITORS AND NEWER ANTIDEPRESSANTS

Generic	Brand Names	Starting Dose	Maximal Suggested Dose (24 h)	Sedating	Forms Available	Comments
Bupropion	Wellbutrin, Zyban	75 mg	300 mg	√	SR (b.i.d.); XL	Use <150 mg per dose except XL; fewer sexual side effects; risk of seizures; also for smoking cessation
Citalopram	Celexa	10 mg	40 mg		soltabs	
Duloxetine	Cymbalta	20 mg	60 mg	√		Also for neuropathic pain; taper slowly
Escitalopram	Lexapro	5 mg	20 mg			Isomer of citalopram
Fluoxetine	Prozac, Sarafem	5 mg	60 mg			Moderate benefit for hot flashes, premenstrual syndrome
Mirtazapine	Remeron	15 mg	45 mg	√√	soltabs	Very sedating; stimulates appetite
Paroxetine	Paxil	5 mg	40 mg	√		Also for hot flashes; slow taper
Sertraline	Zoloft	25 mg	200 mg			
Trazodone	Desyrel	50 mg	300 mg	√		Primarily for insomnia
Venlafaxine	Effexor	25–37.5 mg	375 mg		XR	Also for hot flashes and neuropathic pain; slow taper

SR, sustained release; XL, extended release; XR, sustained release.

(Adapted from Holland JC, Greenberg DB, Hughes MK, et al., eds. *Quick reference for oncology clinicians: the psychiatric and psychological dimensions of cancer symptom management.* AOIS Institute for Research and Education (AIRE), IPOS Press, 2006, with permission.)

severity of "somewhat" or greater and not by meeting criteria for full major depression. Another large trial compared paroxetine to placebo in cancer patients with fatigue and found that the antidepressant significantly lowered depressive (but not fatigue) symptom scores.[101]

In double-blind trials fluoxetine, paroxetine, and venlafaxine have been shown to reduce hot flashes,[102] and mirtazapine and the anticonvulsant gabapentin have been reported to decrease pruritus in cancer patients.[103] Venlafaxine, bupropion, and the tricyclic antidepressants have been shown to relieve neuropathic pain, which frequently accompanies cancer and its treatment.[104] Trazodone, a tetracyclic antidepressant, which in low doses (50 to 150 mg) is often used as a sedative-hypnotic that does not produce dependency, has also been used to treat a variety of adjustment disorders among breast cancer patients.[105]

Cancer patients treated with cytokines such as interferon-alfa often become significantly depressed, with a substantial increase in suicidal ideation and acts.[106] Pretreatment of such patients with selective serotonin reuptake inhibitors (SSRIs) actually reduces the risk of developing depression.[107] There are increasing data that suggest that depression-specific symptoms may disproportionately contribute to the relationship between depression and morbidity or mortality in the context of medical illness.[108–110]

These findings may also provide an explanation for the oft-repeated observation that agents with catecholaminergic activity are generally more effective than SSRIs in the treatment of neurovegetative and somatic symptoms, such as pain and fatigue, even when these symptoms occur outside the context of a diagnosable mood disorder.[101] Combination treatment may also be especially helpful in more severe depressions.[111] Evidence that proinflammatory cytokines contribute to the development of depression, even in medically healthy individuals,[112] may explain the utility of combined serotonin-norepinephrine or dopamine treatment, such as adding desipramine or bupropion with an SSRI or using a serotonin-norepinephrine reuptake inhibitor, such as venlafaxine or duloxetine. These approaches may be more effective than selective serotonergic agents alone in the treatment of major depression, especially when comorbid pain is present. Stimulants such as amphetamine, methylphenidate, and modafinil can also be used effectively either alone or in combination with antidepressants, especially to provide more rapid onset. They rarely trigger anorexia in this population,[113] and they are also agents of choice for cancer patients with short expected survival periods.

Tamoxifen and Selective Serotonin Reuptake Inhibitors

Tamoxifen continues to be used as an important selective estrogen receptor modulator (SERM) to reduce the risk of recurrence in estrogen receptor–positive postmenopausal breast cancer patients. In order to be clinically active, tamoxifen is converted to 4-hydroxy-tamoxifen (endoxifen) and other active metabolites by cytochrome P450 (CYP) enzymes. Over 80 different major alleles of CYP2D6 genes have been identified, many of which confer decreased or absent CYP2D6 activity, and patients can be divided into poor, intermediate, extensive, and ultrarapid metabolizers based on their genotype.[114]

Breast cancer patients treated with tamoxifen who were homozygous for a poor metabolizer genotype had significantly lower serum concentrations of endoxifen than those with an active genotype.[115] In a review of retrospective studies evaluating the effect of CYP2D6 genotype on breast cancer outcomes, Goetz et al.[116] found that patients with estrogen receptor–positive breast cancer, homozygous for the poor metabolizer genotype and treated with tamoxifen monotherapy, were more likely to experience a recurrence of breast cancer than those patients who carried an allele coding for active enzyme. Stearns et al.,[117] in a prospective clinical trial, evaluated the effects of the coadministration of tamoxifen and paroxetine, a selective serotonin reuptake inhibitor, at the time, commonly used to treat depression and hot flashes. The authors found that the use of paroxetine, which inhibits CYP2D6, decreased the plasma concentration of endoxifen, suggesting that the CYP2D6 genotype and drug interactions should be considered in patients treated with tamoxifen.

More recently, Kelly et al.,[118] in a population-based cohort study, studied postmenopausal women aged 66 or older living in Ontario who had been treated between 1993 and 2005 with tamoxifen for breast cancer and overlapping treatment with a single SSRI, finding that after adjustment for age, duration of tamoxifen treatment, and other potential confounders, absolute increases of 25%, 50%, and 75% in the proportion of time on tamoxifen with overlapping use of paroxetine were significantly associated with 24%, 54%, and 91% increases in the risk of death from breast cancer, respectively. The authors concluded that paroxetine use during tamoxifen treatment is associated with an increased risk of death from breast cancer, supporting the hypothesis that "paroxetine can reduce or abolish the benefit of tamoxifen in women with breast cancer."

In addition to paroxetine, sertraline and venlafaxine have also been noted to reduce the metabolism of tamoxifen.[115] Lash et al.[119] found no reduction of tamoxifen effectiveness among patients using citalopram.[119] With the accumulation of studies, Desmarais et al.,[120] in an important review, provide recommendations that clinicians who are treating patients with breast cancer should carefully evaluate the best and safest options for treatment of depression, reviewing pharmacologic profiles, while being very mindful of the risks of untreated depression.[120]

TABLE 173.7

ANTIDEPRESSANTS: TRICYCLICS

Generic	Brand Name	Starting Dose	Maximal Suggested Dose (24 h)	Comments
Amitriptyline	Elavil	10 mg	300 mg	25–50 mg for pain
Desipramine	Norpramin	10 mg	300 mg	
Doxepin	Sinequan	10 mg	150 mg	Very antihistaminic; sedating; also for itching
Imipramine	Tofranil	10 mg	300 mg	
Nortriptyline	Pamelor	10 mg	150 mg	25 mg for pain

Adapted from Holland JC, Greenberg DB, Hughes MK, et al., eds. *Quick reference for oncology clinicians: the psychiatric and psychological dimensions of cancer symptom management.* AOIS Institute for Research and Education (AIRE), IPOS Press, 2006, with permission.

TABLE 173.8

HYPNOTICS

Generic	Brand Name	Starting Dose	Maximal Suggested Dose (24 h)	Half-Life Short/Med	Comments
Eszopiclone	Lunesta	1 mg	3 mg	Half-life short	For sleep
Oxazapam	Serax	10 mg	30 mg	Half-life short	For sleep, also for alcohol withdrawal
Temazepam	Restoril	7.5 mg	30 mg	Med	For insomnia
Triazolam	Halcion	0.125 mg	0.5 mg	Half-life short	For insomnia
Zaleplon	Sonata	5 mg	20 mg	Half-life short	For sleep
Zolpidem	Ambien	2.5 mg	10 mg	Half-life short	For sleep, technically nonbenzodiazapine but shares properties (dependence, withdrawal)

Adapted from Holland JC, Greenberg DB, Hughes MK, et al., eds. *Quick reference for oncology clinicians: the psychiatric and psychological dimensions of cancer symptom management*. AOIS Institute for Research and Education (AIRE), IPOS Press, 2006, with permission.

Antianxiety Agents

It is becoming increasingly clear that the antidepressants, as discussed above, have antianxiety properties as well and can be utilized effectively for the frequent problem of mixed anxiety and depression. Benzodiazepines can provide immediate short-term relief of anxiety symptoms, but generally are not a good strategy for long-term treatment, in part because of the problem of habituation and a tendency to produce dependence. Withdrawal from high doses can be a serious medical problem. Although many of the newer benzodiazepines such as lorazepam are relatively short acting, the problem of symptom recurrence may be addressed in the future with longer acting formulations.[121] In addition, many of the antianxiety agents are used for insomnia with good effect and are after used in the short term for symptom management (Tables 173.7 and 173.8).

Antipsychotics

Neuroleptics are rarely used among cancer patients, but they can be highly effective in managing symptoms of delirium, which can occur during worsening of medical status, with metabolic disequilibrium associated with cachexia, mood disorders, and psychosis associated with steroid treatment and as a preterminal event (Table 173.9). Disorientation to time, place, and person coupled with agitation can be misunderstood as a sign of poor pain management, but increases in opiates and other analgesics, which can be very useful when pain is the problem, may contribute to further delirium. Initially small but increasing doses of antipsychotics such as haloperidol either orally or intravenously can be very helpful in controlling delirium and agitation.[122]

TABLE 173.9

ANTIPSYCHOTIC MEDICATIONS: MAJOR TRANQUILIZERS

Generic	Brand Name	Starting Dose	Maximal Dose	Forms Available	Administration Routes	Comments
Chlorpromazine	Thorazine	10 mg	200 mg			Parenteral; postural hypotension; sedation; hiccups
Haloperidol	Haldol	0.25 mg	30 mg	IV, PO	IV, PO	Antiemetic; risk of extrapyramidal side effects; parenteral
Olanzapine	Zyprexa (Zydis)	2.5 mg	20 mg	Wafer, PO		Wafer form (Zydis); weight gain; antiemetic sedation; long-term risk of diabetes; can cause restlessness
Perphenazine	Trilafon	2 mg	32 mg			
Quetiapine	Seroquel	25 mg	500 mg		PO	Antihistamine associated somnolence; 5-hour half-life
Risperidone	Risperdal	0.25 mg	8 mg			Postural hypotension; smaller risk of Parkinson's than typical agents

IV, intravenous; PO, by mouth.
Adapted from Holland JC, Greenberg DB, Hughes MK, et al., eds. *Quick reference for oncology clinicians: the psychiatric and psychological dimensions of cancer symptom management*. AOIS Institute for Research and Education (AIRE), IPOS Press, 2006, with permission.

Selected References

The full list of references for this chapter appears in the online version.

1. Grube M. Compliance and coping potential of cancer patients treated in liaison-consultation psychiatry. *Int J Psychiatry Med* 2006;36:211.
2. Spiegel D. A 43-year-old woman coping with cancer [comments]. *JAMA* 1999;282:371.
3. Hoffman BM, Zevon MA, DíArrigo MC, et al. Screening for distress in cancer patients: the NCCN rapid-screening measure. *Psychooncology* 2004;13:792.
4. Jacobsen PB, Donovan KA, Trask PC, et al. Screening for psychologic distress in ambulatory cancer patients. *Cancer* 2005;103:1494.
8. Koopman C, Butler LD, Classen C, et al. Traumatic stress symptoms among women with recently diagnosed primary breast cancer. *J Trauma Stress* 2002;15(4):277.
10. Kesler SR, Bennett FC, Mahaffey ML, et al. Regional brain activation during verbal declarative memory in metastatic breast cancer. *Clin Cancer Res* 2009;15:6665.
14. Holland JC, Andersen B, Breitbart WS, et al. Distress management. *J Natl Compr Cancer Netw* 2010;8:448.
15. Zabora J, BrintzenhofeSzoc K, Jacobsen P, et al. A new psychosocial screening instrument for use with cancer patients. *Psychosomatics* 2001;42:241.
20. Giese-Davis J, Koopman C, Butler L, et al. Change in emotion-regulation strategy for women with metastatic breast cancer following supportive-expressive group therapy. *J Consult Clin Psychol* 2002;70:916.
21. Cordova MJ, Andrykowski MA. Responses to cancer diagnosis and treatment: posttraumatic stress and posttraumatic growth. *Semin Clin Neuropsychiatr* 2003;8:286.
33. Grunfeld E. Looking beyond survival: how are we looking at survivorship? *J Clin Oncol* 2006;24:5166.
43. Antoni MH, Lehman JM, Kilbourn KM, et al. Cognitive-behavioral stress management intervention decreases the prevalence of depression and enhances benefit finding among women under treatment for early-stage breast cancer. *Health Psychol* 2001;20:20.
44. Rummans TA, Clark MM, Sloan JA, et al. Impacting quality of life for patients with advanced cancer with a structured multidisciplinary intervention: a randomized controlled trial. *J Clin Oncol* 2006;24:635.
45. Northouse L, Kershaw T, Mood D, et al. Effects of a family intervention on the quality of life of women with recurrent breast cancer and their family caregivers. *Psychooncology* 2005;14:478.
46. van Weert E, Hoekstra-Weebers J, Grol B, et al. A multidimensional cancer rehabilitation program for cancer survivors: effectiveness on health-related quality of life. *J Psychosom Res* 2005;58:485.
48. Classen C, Butler LD, Koopman C, et al. Supportive-expressive group therapy reduces distress in metastatic breast cancer patients: a randomized clinical intervention trial. *Arch Gen Psychiatry* 2001;58:494.
49. Kissane DW, Love A, Hatton A, et al. Effect of cognitive-existential group therapy on survival in early-stage breast cancer. *J Clin Oncol* 2004;22:4255.
51. Ledesma D, Kumano H. Mindfulness-based stress reduction and cancer: a meta-analysis. *Psychooncology* 2009;18:571.
53. Levine EG, Eckhardt J, Targ E. Change in post-traumatic stress symptoms following psychosocial treatment for breast cancer. *Psychooncology* 2005;14:618.
56. Witek-Janusek L, Albuquerque K, Chroniak KR, et al. Effect of mindfulness based stress reduction on immune function, quality of life and coping in women newly diagnosed with early stage breast cancer. *Brain Behav Immun* 2008;22:969.
57. Stanton AL, Ganz PA, Kwan L, et al. Outcomes from the Moving Beyond Cancer psychoeducational, randomized, controlled trial with breast cancer patients. *J Clin Oncol* 2005;23:6009.
58. Miaskowski C, Dodd M, West C, et al. Randomized clinical trial of the effectiveness of a self-care intervention to improve cancer pain management. *J Clin Oncol* 2004;22:1713.
60. Lieberman MA, Golant M, Giese-Davis J, et al. Electronic support groups for breast carcinoma: a clinical trial of effectiveness. *Cancer* 2003;97:920.
64. Spiegel D, Classen C. *Group therapy for cancer patients: a research based handbook of psychosocial care*. New York: Basic Books, 2000.
65. Grande GE, Myers LB, Sutton SR. How do patients who participate in cancer support groups differ from those who do not? *Psychooncology* 2006;15:321.
68. Kinsinger DP, Penedo FJ, Antoni MH, et al. Psychosocial and sociodemographic correlates of benefit-finding in men treated for localized prostate cancer. *Psychooncology* 2006;15:954.
69. Andrykowski MA, Beacham AO, Schmidt JE, et al. Application of the theory of planned behavior to understand intentions to engage in physical and psychosocial health behaviors after cancer diagnosis. *Psychooncology* 2006;15:759.
74. Butler LD, Koopman C, Neri E, et al. Effects of supportive-expressive group therapy on pain in women with metastatic breast cancer. *Health Psychol* 2009;28:579.
78. Goodwin PJ, Leszcz M, Ennis M, et al. The effect of group psychosocial support on survival in metastatic breast cancer. *N Engl J Med* 2001;345:1719.
79. Spiegel D, Bloom JR, Kraemer HC, et al. Effect of psychosocial treatment on survival of patients with metastatic breast cancer. *Lancet* 1989;2:888.
81. Fawzy FI, Canada AL, Fawzy NW. Malignant melanoma: effects of a brief, structured psychiatric intervention on survival and recurrence at 10-year follow-up. *Arch Gen Psychiatry* 2003;60:100.
84. Kuchler T, Bestmann B, Rappat S, et al. Impact of psychotherapeutic support for patients with gastrointestinal cancer undergoing surgery: 10-year survival results of a randomized trial. *J Clin Oncol* 2007;25:2702.
85. Spiegel D, Butler LD, Giese-Davis J, et al. Effects of supportive-expressive group therapy on survival of patients with metastatic breast cancer: a randomized prospective trial. *Cancer* 2007;110:1130.
86. Andersen BL, Yang HC, Farrar WB, et al. Psychologic intervention improves survival for breast cancer patients: a randomized clinical trial. *Cancer* 2008;113:3450.
94. Institute of Medicine. *From Cancer Patient to Cancer Survivor: Lost in Transition*. Washington, DC: National Academies Press, 2005.
101. Morrow GR, Hickok JT, Roscoe JA, et al. Differential effects of paroxetine on fatigue and depression: a randomized, double-blind trial from the University of Rochester Cancer Center Community Clinical Oncology Program. *J Clin Oncol* 2003;21:4635.
102. Barton DL, Loprinzi CL, Novotny P, et al. Pilot evaluation of citalopram for the relief of hot flashes. *J Support Oncol* 2003;1:47.
104. McDonald AA, Portenoy RK. How to use antidepressants and anticonvulsants as adjuvant analgesics in the treatment of neuropathic cancer pain. *J Support Oncol* 2006;4:43.
106. Capuron L, Gumnick JF, Musselman DL, et al. Neurobehavioral effects of interferon-alpha in cancer patients: phenomenology and paroxetine responsiveness of symptom dimensions. *Neuropsychopharmacology* 2002;26:643.
107. Musselman DL, Lawson DH, Gumnick JF, et al. Paroxetine for the prevention of depression induced by high-dose interferon alfa. *N Engl J Med* 2001;344:961.
109. Spiegel D, Giese-Davis J. Depression and cancer: mechanisms and disease progression. *Biolog Psychiatry* 2003;54:269.
112. Raison CL, Miller AH. Depression in cancer: new developments regarding diagnosis and treatment. *Biol Psychiatry* 2003;54:283.
114. Henry NL, Stearns V, Flockhart DA, et al. Drug interactions and pharmacogenomics in the treatment of breast cancer and depression. *Am J Psychiatry* 2008;165:1251.
115. Jin Y, Desta Z, Stearns V, et al. CYP2D6 genotype, antidepressant use, and tamoxifen metabolism during adjuvant breast cancer treatment. *J Natl Cancer Inst* 2005;97:30.
117. Stearns V, Johnson MD, Rae JM, et al. Active tamoxifen metabolite plasma concentrations after coadministration of tamoxifen and the selective serotonin reuptake inhibitor paroxetine. *J Natl Cancer Inst* 2003;95:1758.
118. Kelly CM, Juurlink DN, Gomes T, et al. Selective serotonin reuptake inhibitors and breast cancer mortality in women receiving tamoxifen: a population based cohort study. *BMJ* 2010;340:c693.

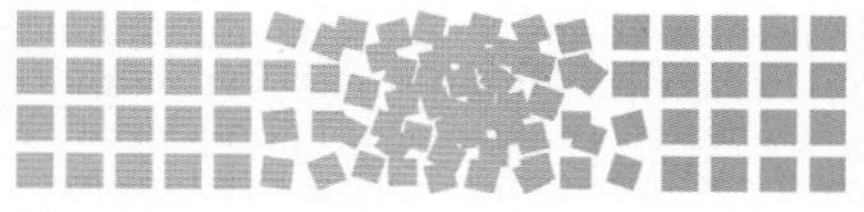

CHAPTER 174 COMMUNICATING NEWS TO THE CANCER PATIENT

ERIC J. CASSELL

Helene Fink was a 56-year-old woman with stage IV breast cancer. Toward the end of the course of the disease, her bone marrow was filled with tumor cells, with all the usual hematologic sequelae. Her pain was well-controlled and she continued an active life in seeming disregard of her disease. Her oncologist was concerned that Mrs. Fink did not appreciate the gravity of her situation, so she explained to the patient in detail what was happening and how serious it was. The patient stopped her activities and became bedridden. The oncologist explained to me at length that she believed in telling patients the truth and that truth-telling was essential for the patient's well-being, especially in the contemporary scene. She also called the patient's husband to explain the importance of telling the truth. It took considerable effort to get the patient back to her previous level of activity, which continued until shortly before her death 3 months later.

This scenario is quite common. Apparently, the physician's goal in such settings is to make sure the patient knows the truth. The emphasis is on telling the truth. All clinical actions, all actions meant to have an impact on the patient—in oncology, as elsewhere—should have a goal. For example, diagnostic actions have a goal-specific therapy; chemotherapy, radiation, or other modalities have a goal, usually curative, palliative, or local control of disease. The goal of cancer treatment in general has long been to improve survival. Recently, this has been modified by the addition of the goal to treat without decreasing quality of life. A general statement of these goals is that they are meant to help the patient.

Patient communication—talking with patients—is a clinical action. Therefore, talking with patients should also have a goal: as with the other clinical acts, it should help the patient be better. In the case of Helene Fink, the communication of her oncologist had a negative impact. Truth-telling is not a primary goal; telling the truth is a moral imperative. With rare exceptions, it is obvious that you should tell the truth. Put another way, your communication with the patient should be truthful, but that should be only one of several functions that that communication serves.

PREVENTING ILLNESS

The goal of increasing length of survival in the treatment of cancer has achieved considerable prominence over the past several decades. Although this is understandable, people do not get up in the morning just to survive; when they do—like soldiers in battle—survival is in the service of living a life. People get up in the morning to live their lives, to work, to play, to take care of their families, to become famous, or to achieve their goals in life, just like you and your family. Perhaps you believe your patients cannot do that because they are too sick. It is true that many patients with advanced disease are sick. By *sick,* the author means requiring care in bed, or, if out of bed, requiring regular skilled care. Most people (including doctors) think patients are sick because of the symptoms or because of their advanced disease. Symptoms are often very unpleasant, but the medical community has become very good at symptom relief; still, the patients are sick. Ask them, and they will tell you (whatever their other symptoms may be) that they are "weak," that they have "no energy," or that they have "run out of gas." They have all the characteristics of the sick: They are disconnected from their world, they have the feeling that they have no control over their lives, they have lost the normal feeling of indestructibility, their cognitive function is not what it was, they are filled with uncertainties, and they do not really understand (as hard as they try) what is happening to them. These features and others characterize the phenomenon called *the state of illness.*

The state of illness is usually brought on by the symptoms and presence of serious disease, but the state of illness is an independent phenomenon. It is not a necessary accompaniment of serious disease. Many clinicians have known patients with serious disease who are not as sick as described here. This was true of Mrs. Fink before the conversation about her bone marrow. They have also known others who were similarly sick, but in whom the disease and symptoms were not serious. The state of illness is an independent phenomenon. It is a state of being. The *Oxford English Dictionary* definition of a state is, "A combination of circumstances or attributes belonging for the time being to a person . . . a particular manner of existing as defined by the presence of certain circumstances or attributes; a condition." (For example, the state of love, the state of grief, or a state of helplessness.) States of being are not psychological or physical alone. States of being are physical, psychological, social, and personal. States of being are pervasive, with effects ranging from the molecular to the social. The state of illness can be worsened independently of the disease, and it can be improved independently of the disease. A state of illness is aggravated by pain and other symptoms, but particularly by inadequately controlled pain. The state is also activated or worsened by uncertainty and fear (the two are often related), and it is made worse by actions that remove independence or increase dependence on the staff. (Like the ubiquitous intravenous bag and pole.) Patients can leave the state of illness even though the disease is not better. An important therapeutic goal is ending a state of illness. The primary modalities for the relief of the state of illness are symptom relief and talking with the patient—communication.

COMMUNICATION

The spoken language is the most important tool in medicine; almost nothing happens in its absence. Physicians commonly train themselves to meet very high standards of expertise, but this everyday tool gets about as much respect and training in its use as paperwork.[1,2] Yet the most common complaint that patients have now and have had for decades past is that doctors do not talk to them. It has been repeatedly shown that patients who understand what is happening to them and why, are more cooperative and compliant with physician's suggested regimens. The implication is that what you say to patients really matters. Every word matters. Sometimes physicians say, "I can't watch every word," but that would be like a surgeon saying, "I can't watch my scalpel every moment." Physicians are all so accustomed to talking and using words in their everyday life that they forget the impact of words on the listener. And they forget that doctor–patient communication is not ordinary conversation. The spoken language acts on the person, and what acts on the person acts on every part of the person. In talking with patients, physicians themselves are the primary therapeutic agent. The vehicle through which virtually everything that physicians do to and with patients is the relationship between the patient and the physician. That relationship is best that is built on trust, and trust is best engendered by the truth. That is not the end of the story; it is the beginning.

Talking to patients necessarily transmits information, and in communication it is the information that counts; therefore, physicians should be aware that they are involved in information control. There are specific tasks that should be accomplished by information flowing to patients. First, it should reduce uncertainty. Second, it should improve the patient's ability to act. Finally, it should improve the relationship between physician and patient. It follows that information that you provide to patients should meet certain tests. Does it reduce the patient's uncertainty now or in the future? Does it improve the patient's ability act? Does it improve your relationship with the patient (now or in the future)? If information wisely used can do those things, then information poorly used can create uncertainty, paralyze action, and destroy the relationship. Going back to the example of the patient Helene Fink, explaining to her the entire nature of her disease had all those negative effects, *even though it was true*.

Here follows a small tangent about death and the issue of denial. Most patients receiving treatment for cancer are aware of the possibility of dying. It has been on their minds since their diagnosis, but not always within awareness. They are often afraid of the subject, or of talking about it; like many people (maybe even you), patients are afraid of dying. It is usually not dying (ceasing to be) that they are afraid of; instead, the author believes it is separation from others. One way in which worries about death are handled is denial. Is denial in and of itself a bad thing? This author personally does not believe that it is, especially as the opposite face of denial may be panic. The important question is whether the denial is getting in the way of anything else important; for example, treatment or family relationships. Further, the author thinks you should be very cautious if you decide to break through denial. For this reason the author usually does not tell people things, but rather answers their questions. When they do not ask the questions, the author can usually stimulate the question wanting to be answered. Telling Helene Fink the truth scared her and got her angry at her physician.

In giving information to a patient, a statement is only complete when it includes (1) what it is (the facts), (2) what it means, and (3) what is to be done about it. Here is an example:

What it is: "Your platelet count is lower today, which is why you are not getting your chemotherapy."

This is what it means: "The platelet count drops because of the action of the chemotherapy on your body. Today's platelet count is the expected reaction to the drugs and will cause you no harm. There is nothing unusual about it. It will not reduce the effect of your treatment if you do not get chemotherapy today."

This is what we are going to do about it: "There is no need to do anything about your platelet count. Because the platelet count is one way we decide how much medicine you should get, we will be testing it regularly. It usually comes back to a point where you can get your chemotherapy in about a week."

Patients frequently ask questions about what something is—for example, a pain, a new symptom, something on their skin, or a swelling somewhere. Physicians commonly give an "it is a this or that" answer. For example, "Oh that is a bruise," or "The swelling is some edema in your foot." The same rule applies as above, the answer should not be it is a this or a that, but this is what it is, this is what it means, and this is what is going to be done about it. "The black and blue mark is just a bruise. Because your platelet count is low from the chemotherapy you are going to bruise more easily than you used to. When your platelet count is normal again after the chemotherapy, that will stop happening. We don't have to do anything because it doesn't require any treatment."

EXPLANATIONS

Explanations should be brief, clear, unambiguous, and jargon-free. The test of the adequacy is not what you say, but what the patient understands. The best way to find that out is to ask the patient to repeat what you just said. Remember, explanation is focused on the patient's need for information. And the enemy of clarity is ambiguity.

Here is an example from an actual interaction (with a physician who prided himself on his communication skills). "It looks as though we'll probably get out of the woods. Most of the bad stuff seems pretty well gone and I doubt if we'll have trouble again if things hold the way they are."

Think what these phrases really mean:

- ". . . probably get out of the woods." Will we or won't we?
- ". . . most of the bad stuff . . ." Is it gone or is it not? And what about the rest?
- ". . . I doubt if we'll . . ." Do you believe it or not?

This is the way physicians commonly talk to patients. This is supposedly done this way because physicians do not want to commit themselves. If challenged, physicians may say, "I'm not God. I don't know what is going to happen." Or, "I don't have a crystal ball." Patients know both statements are true. But they are beside the point. The physician may not have a crystal ball, but he or she knows better than the patient what can happen and what will probably happen. It has been shown repeatedly that people do not understand clearly what percentages mean such as, "You have a 30% chance of recurrence." Cognitive psychologists have demonstrated that people understand information better if it has been translated into natural frequencies. (You have a three in ten chance of recurrence, or there is a seven in ten chance that you will not have a recurrence.) It is not necessary to pretend or lie. Here is a possible way to say the same thing that does not suggest omniscience, but that at the same time is reassuring. "These tests show regression of your cancer. You are getting a very good response to treatment and I believe you're going to do well." You can stop there; there is no reason to express doubt. If you believe you are not being truthful because you have not shared the whole truth, ask whether the patient has any questions. If there are questions, answer them honestly but briefly and wait for more questions. Do not answer a question that has not been asked. If the patient wonders whether things could turn bad again, here is a possible response. "You and I both know that I can't promise that this good response will keep up, but I expect it to. And even though that may leave you with some doubt or maybe you find it worrisome, don't make bad news out of good news. This is good news. We're doing well. Let's keep it up."

UNCOMFORTABLE QUESTIONS

If the patient asks a question that you do not want to answer, you can buy some time to find out what the patient is really asking by, "What do you mean by that?" Or, "I'm not sure I understand what you're asking me, say it again in a different way." If it is a direct difficult question that does not mince words, then answer it in the same manner in clear, unambiguous, spare, jargon-free, truthful language. Say no more than you must say to answer the question, and then wait for the next question. The same rules apply here as outlined previously: Say what it is, say what it means, and say what you are going to do about it. Do not leave the patient hanging in the air with statements like, "Let's wait a month and see how things stand." Be more specific. "In a month, we will repeat your CT scan. I expect that it will still show a good response. If you've had some growth of your tumor, we will decide what that means and then, if necessary, modify your treatment." You will notice that the author has repeatedly used the words "we," "we'll," "we're," and "let's" (as in, "let us"). In each instance you are telling the patient that you and the patient are a team; that the patient is not alone and that you are right there with him or her.

Earlier the author said that he did not believe that fear of death is a fear of ceasing to exist, but a fear of separation from others. He does not know if that is a correct interpretation, but he does know that patients greatly fear being abandoned by or distanced from their doctors. It does not take many words to express your continued connection to the patient, no matter what happens.

INFORMATION

Information can be conveyed in different quantities ranging from terse to fulsome. It has degrees of detail, complexity, or sophistication and should be tailored to the patient's ability to understand. It has timing. There is a big difference between conveying information to a patient in a recovery room or to someone who has come to the office specifically to discuss a diagnosis or treatment. It has timing. Choose your place and choose your time. If the patient wants information before you are ready, tell him or her that you are going to discuss this in detail at such and such a time and ask if that will be alright. If the patient insists on talking at that moment, then be brief and again refer to future discussion. Information has relevance; stay on the subject. And, finally, information has truth content.

Information is flowing all the time from multiple sources. Information comes to the patient from the environment. For example, a patient in a radiation suite in most hospitals is getting a lot more information than you may wish from simply looking around the waiting area. He or she gets information from knowledge stored in memory. Needs, wishes, desires, fears, or fantasies are another source of information. Other people: family, friends, nurses, attendants, technicians, and other doctors. Everybody! And everybody is talking all the time. Patients get information from their bodies as they interpret the feelings they have as well as what they see. Remember, you are only one source of information among many. Information is flowing all the time. Even no information is information.

The Internet represents a special problem. It seems that everyone goes to the Internet to find out about their disease, treatment, doctors, and the institutions in which they get care. Whatever the question, the Internet overflows with information. As of the time of this writing, if you enter "ingrown toenail" into Google, more than 440,000 sites become accessible. If you search Google about cancer of the breast, more than 59 million sites become accessible. Diverse sources of information inevitably bring conflict, and disagreement between sources of information produces uncertainty. The more pressing the need to act, the less tolerable is uncertainty.

Increased uncertainty often makes patients more fearful. Their fear increases the difficulty they experience when decisions have to be made, which also increases fearfulness. Uncertainty and fear reinforce the state of illness. One solution to the problem of uncertainty is increased trust in doctors. That is one of the reasons why patients put so much faith in their doctors' words and actions. This may make it uncomfortable for physicians who know that they are far from invulnerable, but it is much easier for patients. Also, it is one of the reasons that it is so important to maintain strong doctor–patient relationships. Too many times, doctors react to the amount of trust that patients lay on them by insisting that the patient make his or her own decision (see later discussion). This makes it more difficult for the patients in situations wherein they need support and they need to invest their trust. "Thank you—together we'll do the best we can," is much better than, "You know that I'm not infallible and that I can't make your decisions for you."

MEANING

The topic of meaning, in general, is complicated but some things about it are straightforward. Physicians do not act directly because of events, objects, or relations; they act because of the meaning of these things. Information does its work because it acts on meaning. Meaning has two characteristics that are important to this discussion. The first is significance. For example, "Dark clouds signify rain" or "Postmenopausal bleeding means I have cancer." Meaning also conveys importance. For example, "Rain will ruin the picnic" or "I could die from that kind of cancer." Importance is another way of saying value. And values, although they may be shared, are always personal; importance is always importance to someone. These two characteristics of meaning are present whenever you are talking and whenever the patient is listening. That is why it is so important to find out what significance the patient is giving to your explanation and what its importance is to the patient.

Another characteristic of meaning is that it can be changed. Sometimes, when you can do nothing else for a patient, you can change the meaning that the patient has assigned to objects, relations, events, or the words that you have used. For example, when someone presented in 1950 with what we now identify as stage I Hodgkin's lymphoma, after the diagnosis he or she was met with lies and pessimism. Now, the same patient is met with smiles and optimism. But for the individual patient, on first being diagnosed, death is still possible because you do not know for sure what the outcome will be. Why the smiles? For this patient, on first diagnosis, only the meaning of the disease has changed, but that is enough to change the physician's attitude and hearten both patient and family. To change the significance of the events, you must change the patient's meaning, the patient's objective knowledge of the world. To change the importance of events, you must address their impact on the patient, how they will affect the patient in the present and in the future.

Meaning is also used here in the sense of purpose. This was popularized by Viktor Frankl[3] in his book, *Man's Search for Meaning*. Here, patients may search for the meaning of the fact of their cancer, or use the disease as a spur to finding a new meaning in their life. This not the sense in which the author has been using the word. Meaning is important to physicians because words do not simply have a denotation, a dictionary meaning, or a personal or connotative meaning, but because every meaning has cognitive, emotional, physical, and spiritual dimensions. Words act on the body to the molecular level. As a simple example, if somebody tells you something with a meaning that induces fear in you, the fear may be felt like a gripping in the chest and may be accompanied by all the physiological manifestations of fear.[4] The words do not cause the fear; rather, the fear is part of the meaning of the words. In the same way, the physiological events are not caused by fear; they are part of fear itself.

CAFETERIA EXPLANATIONS

It cannot be said too strongly: Give up, get past, eschew, and forget about cafeteria information and decision making. Simply laying out the information and asking the patient to make the decisions is not fair to the patient and it takes away from you one of your important therapeutic options: control of the information. Cafeteria decisions abandon the patient when he or she needs you most. You can honor the patient's autonomy and honor the realistic need for clinicians to maintain the control of the case by helping patients make decisions that you believe are in their best interests as they know those interests. Ask yourself how well you would be able to make a decision if you were frightened, uncertain, and fundamentally ignorant about the issues involved in the decision. If just knowing the medical facts was enough to make decisions, doctors, when they are patients, would be the best decision makers of all. Doctors know that that is not true. Sick people need help expressing their best interests.

Communication, as with all other therapeutic agents, should be goal-directed. The goal is to help the patient be better, whatever the outcome. The spoken language is a powerful tool toward that end and worth learning how to use effectively.

References

1. Cassell EJ. *Talking with patients. Vol 1. The theory of doctor-patient interaction.* Cambridge, MA: MIT Press, 1985.
2. Cassell EJ. *Talking with patients. Vol. 2. Clinical technique.* Cambridge, MA: MIT Press, 1985.
3. Frankl V. *Man's search for meaning.* New York: Pocket Book, 1959.
4. Cassell EJ. *Mind and body: The nature of suffering and the goals of medicine.* 2nd ed. New York: Oxford University Press, 2004;221.

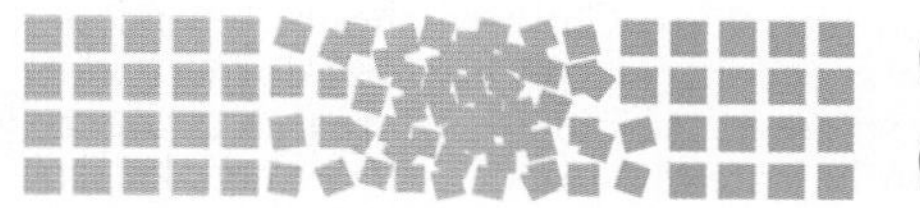

CHAPTER 175 SPECIALIZED CARE OF THE TERMINALLY ILL

KRISTEN G. SCHAEFER, KATHY SELVAGGI, AND JANET L. ABRAHM

Providing expert care to patients who are terminally ill presents new challenges to the oncology team. To do this, the team must engage in new types of conversations with patients and their families and among themselves and broaden their assessments to be able to ensure physical comfort, address psychological needs, and identify goals of care and social and spiritual sources of distress.[1]

DISCUSSING PROGNOSIS

When the disease is far advanced but the patient is still receiving antineoplastic therapy, the team faces a difficult choice: impart the best estimate of prognosis, which is usually only months, or continue therapy without "the talk." The cultural norms of medicine mitigate against offering realistic prognoses and they support optimism.[2] Even physicians who refer patients to a hospice program do not usually tell them the most likely prognostic estimate.[3] In one study, patients' actual median survival was 26 days, but the physicians' median formulated prognosis of survival was 75 days, and what they would have told the patient was 90 days. More experienced clinicians favored no disclosure. Female physicians and those physicians who referred more often to hospice programs were more likely to favor pessimistically discrepant disclosure.

Physicians may assume that patients who want to know their prognoses will raise the subject with them, and in one study 48% of oncologists specifically describe communicating terminal prognoses to patients only when specific preferences for prognosis information were expressed.[4] Although most patients report wanting prognostic information from their oncologist,[5] patients with advanced refractory disease may not ask about their prognosis or express their true feelings about their advanced illness.[6]

Discussions of prognosis can be very painful for clinicians, because they may cause feelings of guilt, failure, or sadness. Clinicians interested in improving their skills may refer to practical educational handbooks[7–9] and articles that outline how to discuss these issues both with patients who want to know their prognosis[10] and with those who do not or are ambivalent.[11]

Before beginning this difficult conversation, clinicians may find it helpful to examine their own feelings about the news they have to impart and identify any feelings of frustration, grief, or sadness they may be experiencing. After the meeting, other team members can remain behind to help patients and their families cope with the news and answer questions not previously raised. Paradoxically, the discussion is likely to lessen fears of abandonment and strengthen the trust patients have in the oncology team.[12] It will not eliminate their hope, though it may alter what they were hoping for and redirect their hope into accomplishing these new goals.

DISCUSSING END OF LIFE

Nearly all hospitalized patients do not like talking about advance directives with their oncologist, but the majority believe that the discussion is important, they are willing to talk with their doctors, and they prefer to have these conversations with their oncologists (48% chose their medical oncologist, 34% chose their primary care physician, 11% chose the admitting physician at the hospital). However, oncologists often do not often initiate the discussion.[13,14]

Having a discussion about end-of-life wishes with one's doctor has been shown to result in less aggressive medical care near death, earlier hospice referrals, cost-savings at end of life, and improved bereavement adjustment for caregivers.[15,16] Furthermore, having conversations about end-of-life wishes is not associated with higher rates of major depressive disorder or more worry. Patients who consider themselves very religious individuals and black and Hispanic patients often prefer aggressive life-extending measures.[17,18]

Discussions about resuscitation should begin with the larger exploration of the patients' hopes and fears, goals for their remaining life, and values about how they want to live that life.[19] Reviewing the patients' activities at home, their coping mechanisms, their fears and hopes, and what quality of life means to them naturally leads to a discussion of resuscitation and reliance on life-support machines. Using standardized advance directive forms, such as the POLST (Physician's Order for Life Sustaining Treatment) form, can also be a useful way to clarify and record the patient's wishes in the medical chart.[20]

Patients' beliefs about their likelihood of successful resuscitation and about the quality and length of their survival have a significant impact on their wishes regarding DNR (do not resuscitate) orders. Patients who have had a bone marrow transplant for hematologic malignancies and who required mechanical ventilation and more than 4 hours of pressor support or have had renal or hepatic failure did not survive the intensive care unit stay.[21] Patients with metastatic cancer with an observed in-hospital arrest have a 13% to 50% resuscitation rate, but all died during the hospitalization.[22,23] Patients who think their chance of surviving 6 months is as little as 10% often want resuscitation and ongoing life-prolonging care.[24] Not until they thought the odds of surviving 6 months were less than 10% did patients overwhelmingly choose comfort care and decline resuscitation.[24] Giving accurate prognoses also helps their caregivers; they are also usually unaware that the patient is incurable or would benefit from hospice care until their physician tells them directly.[25,26]

Phrasing the questions clearly can also help patients give answers that reflect their feelings accurately. Advance directive discussions that begin, "Do you want everything done?" will almost always lead to an affirmative response. Rephrasing to ask, rather, "If you *died*, would you want to be resuscitated?"

may lead to a very different answer, especially if the oncologist reviews the data about the efficacy of resuscitation.

HOPE

Discussions like the ones outlined above need not eliminate hope. Most patients with advanced disease do not hope for a cure, but hope their lives will be prolonged as much as possible. Most patients also hope for a pain-free death, one that is in accord with their wishes.[27]

Before they began treatment, most patients had a variety of plans for the future that filled up the calendars (holidays, family events, daily activities) by which they ran their lives. After the initiation of chemotherapy, however, the "treatment calendar" (in which patients vest magical powers to bring about a cure) supersedes all these.[28] Oncology teams can help patients with advanced disease develop new kinds of hope by deemphasizing the treatment calendar and encouraging patients to reintegrate into activities that were meaningful before treatment began.

There are patients, however, who, despite refractory disease, cling to the hope of further treatment "should their counts recover." The oncology team can help these patients and families enlarge the scope of their goals by encouraging them to work on projects and valued relationships while they are waiting for the next therapy.

HEALING VERSUS CURING

In discussing their lives, their hopes, and their fears with the oncology team, patients begin to understand that they are cared for as people, not just patients. Some may reveal fears that the team can dispel, such as a fear of dying in uncontrolled pain, of suffocating, or of being abandoned. Others identify problems best addressed by chaplains, social workers, and psychiatrists to whom the team can refer. Complementary medicine approaches, such as mindfulness-based cognitive therapy, can also facilitate this process.[29,30] Healing (i.e., a return to wholeness that includes body, mind, and spirit) can still occur even in patients who never achieve another remission.

HOW TO TELL THE CHILDREN

The oncology team can play an important role in helping parents tell their children about their illness, their prognosis, and even that they will die. The following techniques are recommended[31]:

1. *Learn about the children.* Ask the parents to tell you about their children, including their ages and how they coped with problems in the past.
2. *Maximize the child's support system.* Help the parents determine who among their family and friends can help keep the children's schedules as close to normal as possible.
3. *Facilitate honest communication about the illness.* Parents should avoid euphemisms and name the cancer specifically. In response to "How much should we share with the children?" Dr. Rauch recommends: "Everything." Assume that what adults are discussing children will hear, and that they will feel more frightened by being left to interpret the information alone than if they are present and able to be comforted should they show distress. Parents need to answer all their questions in an age-appropriate manner. Children from 3 to 7 years old may believe that they caused their parent's illness and feel guilty about it. These children do not understand that death is permanent, and so it does not help to prepare them for the death itself ahead of time. Older children (7 to 12) may also fear that their behavior contributed to the cancer, and they also need to be reassured that they cannot catch it, and that their parent did not do anything to acquire it. They do know that death is permanent, and so may need to discuss their fears and concerns about their parent leaving them.
4. *Address common questions.* Children should be encouraged to share any stories they have heard but do not understand and to ask whatever questions occur to them. Parents, however, have to be careful to understand what the real question is, and should feel free not to answer every question right away. Saying "That is an important question. Let me think about it," is acceptable, provided that the question is answered at a later time. "Are you going to die?" is the question parents most commonly fear.[31] In reply, ask about particular concerns, such as whom they will live with. Even when admitting they might die, parents need to add that they are doing all they can to live as long and as well as possible.
5. *Prepare for hospital visits* Children should be allowed to visit the hospital if they want to, except when a parent is confused or agitated, which a young child is unlikely to understand. But children need special preparation for what they are about to see, including a discussion of their fears and expectations. After the visit, the child should be asked to discuss any parts that were difficult or enjoyable or were different from what they expected. Children who do not want to visit can be helped to communicate by preparing letters, drawings, videotapes, or talking on the phone.
6. *Saying goodbye.* Rauch writes, "If one's children know they are loved, and why they are loved, there is usually no need to say the word 'goodbye.'" But she encourages parents and their children to say a last "I love you" in person whenever possible. Children should also be given "a road map for the grief process ahead"[31] and helped to feel all right about going on with school and other activities after the death by asking about them. Although they face their deaths with undiminished sadness, parents may be able to say what their children need to hear. Some parents with refractory cancer will see that choosing not to be resuscitated is actually a last gift to their children, not a betrayal.

CULTURAL AND RELIGIOUS CONSIDERATIONS

Ethnicity, culture, socioeconomic status, religion, and religious background all affect the ways patients experience illness and face death.[25,32–34] The best way to show respect for patient and family views is to individualize the approach with attention to language, religious beliefs or concerns, cultural context, health beliefs, decision-making patterns, and social support and resources.[32,35] Autonomy may be expressed in a number of ways. For example, patients from Asian, Bosnian, or Italian American cultures, depending on level of acculturation to the United States,[36] may feel that the frank disclosure of a serious illness or short prognosis is "at a minimum, disrespectful, and more significantly, inhumane."[37] And non Hispanic whites prefer to have only immediate family present, while African Americans want their extended family, friends, and pastor. They are also more interested in spiritual concerns, lack of trust, concerns about DNR orders and hospice, allowing adequate time for decisions and not feeling pressure to make them.[38,39] Non-Hispanic whites are more likely to want to discuss durable power of attorney, living wills, and hospice programs, the patient's prognosis, irreversibility of the illness, quality of life, financial concerns, and medical choices.[37–40] Qualified interpreters should also be provided whenever the clinician is not fluent in the patient's language.[37]

CARE WITHOUT CHEMOTHERAPY

There are some patients for whom the oncologist believes treatment would do more harm than good.[41] How can this be expressed to patients? The key is in the words used and their implications, not just their literal meanings.[42] If the oncologist says, "I could offer you a 5-FU-containing regimen," the patient and family think it would be of benefit. But if the oncologist adds, "but it is very unlikely to help you live longer or better," they clearly understand that the physician does not want to continue treatment. Most patients hear "There is nothing more I can offer you" and feel hopeless and abandoned. But what the oncologist actually means is more likely to be conveyed by saying, "There are no other treatments against the cancer that would help you live longer or more comfortably. But there are many ways I can care for you and help you achieve other goals. And we will ensure that no symptoms, such as pain, get in your way."

PALLIATIVE CARE PROGRAMS

Most oncologists and their nursing colleagues have not been trained, either in medical or nursing school or in postgraduate training, to help dying patients and their families make the transition to care directed at comfort rather than prolonging life.[43] For particularly complex situations, therefore, the primary oncology team can consult a palliative care team.[44] In 2006, hospice and palliative medicine was accepted as a specialty by the American Board of Medical Specialties. The Accreditation Counsel for Graduate Medical Education began accrediting fellowship programs in 2007 and the first qualifying examination in hospice and palliative medicine was given in 2008.

In addition to assistance with care at the end of life, palliative care teams assist oncology patients with symptom management; advance care planning; emotional, psychological, spiritual, or existential suffering; and closure and legacies.[43] They provide patient and family education and counseling, problem solving, and support at any point along their disease trajectory (diagnosis, relapse, or terminal care). Evidence suggests that patient and family satisfaction scores increase with palliative care consult team involvement.[45,46] Organizations wishing to start a palliative care team can obtain the logistical and financial information needed from the Center for Advancing Palliative Care.

HOSPICE PROGRAMS

Pain Control

The Medicare Hospice Benefit was established in 1982 as part of the Tax Equity and Fiscal Responsibility Act,[47,48] and the use of hospice services in the United States is increasing, more than doubling from 540,000 patients served in 1998 to 1.3 million in 2006.[49] Then, as now, both the attending physician and the hospice medical director were required to certify that the patient was terminally ill with a prognosis of 6 months or less, if the disease followed its usual course. There are no other mandated criteria for cancer patients. Patients need not be DNR, and they need not have a live-in caregiver to qualify for hospice care.[50]

Hospice teams (including nurses, medical directors, social workers, chaplains, and volunteers) are especially valuable partners in caring for patients who are dying from cancer. In addition to assessing and managing the patient's physical problems, the hospice team offers patient and family education, practical support, and psychological and spiritual counseling.[51,52]

Hospice programs provide a continuum of care, from home to the inpatient setting. While by law, 80% of days of patient care must take place in the home, all Medicare-certified hospices are required to provide four levels of care: routine home care, continuous home care, respite care in nursing homes, and inpatient care.[48] Hospice programs also provide all medications, durable medical equipment, supplies, and oxygen for needs related to the terminal diagnosis; laboratory and diagnostic procedures related to the terminal diagnosis; and transportation when medically necessary for changes in the patient's level of care. Hospice programs also prepare families for their losses and offer bereavement programs for a year after the death. The Medicare hospice benefit is a capitated program that reimburses a hospice *per diem* based on the patient's level of care (approximately $150/d for routine or respite care, approximately $600/d for inpatient acute care).[53] Benefits offered by other forms of insurance are modeled on Medicare's hospice program. Aggressive palliation, including transfusion, palliative radiation, and chemotherapeutic or hematopoietic agents, can be provided by large hospices (i.e., with an average daily census of more than 300 patients). Given this reimbursement schedule, however, such care is often prohibitively expensive for small to moderate size hospices (i.e., an average daily census of less than 50 patients). Hospices can work with insurers other than Medicare to "carve out" provision of the more costly therapies while allowing patients to receive hospice services.

RELIEF OF SUFFERING

Control of physical and psychological suffering is a prerequisite for both patients and caregivers to address the social and spiritual or existential dimensions of their lives and to minimize the suffering of bereaved survivors.[54] Clinical practice guidelines on how to provide this palliative care have been proposed by both the National Comprehensive Cancer Network for oncology patients, and as a consensus document from the National Consensus Project for Quality Palliative Care.[55–58]

Fatigue

Fatigue is common in the last weeks of life, and refeeding does not ameliorate the weakness. Caffeine, dextroamphetamine, or methylphenidate increase alertness.[59] Modafinil, approved for narcolepsy, is helpful for fatigue and opioid-induced sedation.[60,61]

Insomnia

Insomnia in dying patients may result from undertreated pain, depression, anxiety, delirium, dyspnea, nocturnal hypoxia, nausea and vomiting, or rarely, pruritus. The two most common and important mediating variables are pain and depression. Medications that can cause insomnia include corticosteroids and antiemetics (prochlorperazine, metoclopramide, 5-hydroxytryptamine 3 receptor antagonists).[62] In addition, patients' sleep–wake cycle may be reversed because they are inactive and napping much of the day.[63]

Data from controlled trials indicate that benzodiazepines (oxazepam, 10 to 20 mg, or temazepam, 15 to 30 mg), antidepressants, and zolpidem (Ambien) are effective agents. Trazodone (25 to 100 mg orally at bedtime) may be useful for patients with paradoxical reactions to benzodiazepines. For patients with nighttime delirium, oral quetiapine 25 to 50 mg orally at bedtime (for elderly patients), olanzapine 2.5 to 5.0 mg orally at bedtime, or haloperidol (beginning at 0.5 to 2.0 mg orally and increasing as needed to 5 mg) will be needed. Use clonazepam 0.5 to 1.0 mg orally for patients with restless-leg syndrome. Patients who resist taking these medications may fear that they will not reawaken. Exploring these concerns helps patients take the drugs and be less fatigued during the day.[64]

Using World Health Organization guidelines for cancer pain relief, 50% of cancer patients near death will have no pain, 25% mild to moderate pain, and only 3% severe pain.[65] Even in the last months or weeks, interventional anesthetic and neurolytic techniques, described elsewhere, should be considered for that small minority of patients whose pain cannot be relieved by any other method short of sedation.[66]

When patients have not previously received opioids, patient and family misconceptions about opioids must often be overcome first: fear of becoming an addict, "feeling high," "using up" the effective agents and having nothing left if the pain gets worse, or fear that the opioid is "killing" the patient.

Frequent pain assessment, including the patient's satisfaction with the pain level, remains the cornerstone of an effective management strategy. Some patients who lose the ability to use the numerical scales to describe their pain may be able to use the scales designed for children such as the Faces Pain Scale.[67] If the patient has impaired memory or poor concentration but can still report pain accurately, repeat assessments should be done when the peak pain relief is expected (e.g., 15 minutes after a parenteral dose, 60 minutes after an oral dose). If the patient becomes nonverbal, it may be necessary to monitor for expressions of apparent discomfort when the patient is moved or when a part of the body known to have been painful in the past is touched. Behavioral scales have been developed for nonverbal demented patients,[68] but they have not been validated for nonverbal dying patients.

Not all patients who exhibit distress are in pain. Delirium may present as pain. Patients who moan without any apparent provocation or in response to nonpainful stimuli such as having their lips moistened may be delirious. Delirium is especially likely in patients with these behaviors who have not reported pain before they became nonverbal.

Even in patients on stable drug regimens, physiologic changes in patients at the end of life make it necessary to monitor them carefully for the appearance of opioid-related side effects such as respiratory depression, myoclonus, or delirium. If the respiratory rate declines to less than 6 breaths per minute and opioids are thought to be the cause, opioid doses should be decreased 25% and the patient should be monitored carefully for increasing discomfort. Naloxone is almost never indicated. If a sedated patient has a dangerous reduction of the respiratory rate, both thought to be caused by opioids, the 1 mL ampule of naloxone can be diluted in 9 mL of saline and given 1 mL at a time every 2 to 3 minutes until the respiratory rate recovers to greater than 8 per minute. If the naloxone is given undiluted, the patient is likely to experience severe opioid withdrawal.

If the patient becomes unable to take pills, substitute a liquid, transmucosal,[69–70] rectal,[71,72] transdermal, or pelleted opioid. Kadian® and Avinza® are morphine sustained-release pellets packaged into capsules that can be opened. The pellets can be sprinkled on food or suspended in liquid and either swallowed or placed into feeding tubes every 12 to 24 hours. Patients whose opioid dose is too large to be delivered by sublingual, transdermal or rectal routes need a subcutaneous or intravenous opioid infusion, with or without Patient-Controlled Analgesia.

Changes in opioid route or agent require meticulous calculations using a table or a conversion program, which can be found online. Anesthesia pain or palliative care teams or clinical pharmacists can assist in performing these conversions if questions arise. First, the total daily dose of the current opioid being taken is calculated. Next, that dose is converted to the equianalgesic dose of the new opioid given in the new route. For patients with well-controlled pain, that equianalgesic dose of the new opioid is reduced by 25% to 33% because of incomplete cross-tolerance among opioids. If the patient has uncontrolled pain, no dose reduction should be taken. Finally, the total daily dose is divided into the desired oral or parenteral schedule.

For example, a patient with well-controlled pain on 300 mg MS Contin orally every eight hours develops hallucinations and becomes unable to take pills. The hospice nurse suggests replacing the oral morphine with a parenteral (SC) hydromorphone (Dilaudid) infusion. Oral morphine (900 mg/24h) is equivalent to $900/30 = X/1.5$, or 45 mg/24h of hydromorphone, because 30 mg of oral morphine is equivalent to 1.5 mg IV/SC hydromorphone. Decreasing by one-third for incomplete cross tolerance results in the total daily hydromorphone dose of 30 mg. The SC infusion rate is 30 mg/24h, or 1.25 mg/h of hydromorphone. If the patient had uncontrolled pain, the daily hydromorphone dose would be 45 mg and the hydromorphone infusion rate would be 45 mg/24h, or 1.8 mg/h SC.

Adjuvants for bone and nerve pain should be continued if they have been effective. For bone pain, both a liquid (e.g., ibuprofen) and a rectal nonsteroidal anti-inflammatory drug (NSAID) (e.g., indomethacin) are available.[51] In addition, parenteral ketorolac tromethamine (Toradol) offers the pain-relieving potency of parenteral morphine (30 mg parenteral ketorolac approximately equivalent to 12 mg parenteral morphine). Ketorolac has all the side effects of the NSAIDs, however, and is not recommended for long-term use. Adjuvants for neuropathic pain can also be given subcutaneously (e.g., dexamethasone) or rectally (e.g., doxepin to replace an oral tricyclic antidepressant).

Therapy to prevent and treat constipation in dying patients should be continued because constipation can cause delirium in this population. All patients on opioids should receive a scheduled, not an as-needed stool softener and laxative (e.g., colace plus senna) with an as-needed osmotic agent (e.g., sorbitol or polyethylene glycol) while they can still take liquids and oral medications. Patients who are nonverbal but appear uncomfortable and have not had a stool for more than 72 hours should be assessed for impaction and treated with appropriate enemas (e.g., mineral oil retention enema followed by a soap suds enema), disimpaction when needed, and suppositories. Subcutaneous methylnaltrexone is now available for the treatment of opioid-induced constipation in patients with advanced illness.[73]

Psychological Disorders

Among the most problematic psychological disorders are depression, anxiety, and delirium.[74–76]

Depression in terminally ill patients can be due to poorly controlled pain, drugs (e.g., opioids, corticosteroids), central nervous system tumor, metabolic abnormalities (e.g., hypercalcemia, hyponatremia), vitamin deficiency, or anemia. It may recur in patients with past histories of depression.

Symptoms and signs that are specific for depression in patients with advanced illness include feelings of sadness, crying, anhedonia, or feelings of worthlessness, guilt, hopelessness, or helplessness.[74] Comprehensive evaluation of terminally ill patients who answer yes when asked if they are depressed is very likely to confirm that the patients are depressed.[77] Treatment of depression, including counseling and medications, is worthwhile even when patients have only weeks to live. The psychostimulants dextroamphetamine and methylphenidate (2.5 to 5 mg 8 a.m. and noon, maximum dose 60 to 90 mg) often act within a few days.[78] If the patient is expected to live longer than weeks to a few months, a trial of a stimulant and a selective serotonin reuptake inhibitor (SSRI) should be initiated.

A psychiatric consult should be obtained for patients who do not respond to first-line agents, when unsure of the diagnosis, when the patient previously had a major psychiatric disorder, when there are complicating psychiatric disorders or the patient is suicidal or requesting assisted suicide, or when there are dysfunctional family dynamics.[74]

Anxiety in this population is often situational, involving concerns related to the terminal illness.[79,80] Fear of death, impairment, or pain and concerns about the past all contribute.

Hospitalization can add a sense of isolation, loneliness, uselessness, and concerns about lack of information or misinformation about what is happening. Other causes include drugs (corticosteroids, metoclopramide, opioid neurotoxicity, withdrawal from benzodiazepines or alcohol), uncontrolled pain or other symptoms, hypoxia, dyspnea, metabolic abnormalities (sepsis, hypoglycemia), insomnia, delirium, and preexisting psychiatric disorders.[60]

Anxious patients may present with uncontrolled worry, a sense of impending doom, motor tension, restlessness, autonomic hyperactivity (e.g., palpitations, sweating, dry mouth, tightness in the chest), nausea, vomiting, or diarrhea, feeling on edge, difficulty concentrating or relaxing, insomnia, or irritability. They often feel out of control and helpless, yet the anxiety can interfere with their ability to receive care.[81]

Finding a physiologic cause of the anxiety (e.g., hypoxia) in a dying patient should not stop the search for additional contributing psychological, social, or spiritual problems. Counseling from social work, psychiatry, or chaplaincy may be needed to identify and when possible allay the underlying cause(s).[54,79] For dying patients, empiric therapy with lorazepam (0.5 to 2 mg SL every 3 hours as needed) or clonazepam (0.5 to 2 mg orally twice a day) may offer significant benefit.

Delirium has been reported in up to 80% of dying patients and can be a significant source of stress and anxiety for family caregivers.[82–84] Etiologies of delirium include medications (especially opioids, NSAIDs, benzodiazepines, and high-dose corticosteroids), metabolic abnormalities (hypercalcemia, hyperglycemia, uremia), constipation, bladder outlet obstruction, dehydration, hypoxia, fever, infection, uncontrolled pain, hepatic failure, brain tumors, and brain metastases.[85–87] Opioid-related central nervous system toxicities occur more frequently in patients with renal dysfunction or with impaired cognition before the opioids began as well as in those who have been on high doses of opioids for months, have dehydration, or are taking other psychoactive drugs.[88]

Delirious patients may appear agitated or hypoactive or vacillate between these states.[86] Symptoms of delirium include insomnia and daytime somnolence, nightmares, restlessness or agitation (which mimics uncontrolled pain), irritability, distractibility, hypersensitivity to light and sound, anxiety, difficulty in concentrating, fleeting illusions, paranoia, hallucinations and delusions, emotional liability, attention deficits, and memory disturbances. The exact cause of delirium is found in only about 43% of cases,[86] and the etiology is often multifactorial.[83–89] Empiric therapy may be sufficient.

Treatment for delirium should be initiated as soon as the diagnosis is made, even in patients who are undergoing efforts to eliminate the underlying cause(s). Ask family members, friends, or well-known caregivers to be present. Make the patient's surroundings as familiar as possible, restore hearing aids and glasses, and reorient the patient frequently. Begin medications from those listed in Table 175.1. Olanzapine 2.5 to 5.0 mg orally twice a day and as needed every 4 hours or haloperidol 1 mg IV or 2 mg orally every 4 hours and every 2 hours as needed (up to 20 mg in 24 h) are most commonly used. Olanzapine is available in a wafer that dissolves in the mouth (Zydis®). For patients with advanced cancer and a hypoactive delirium not felt to be metabolic or drug-induced, consider using methylphenidate (10 mg orally day 1, then 10 mg orally at 8 a.m. and noon).[90]

Respiratory Disorders

The prevalence of cancer-related dyspnea in dying patients is approximately 70%.[91] Causes include anxiety, tumor infiltration, underlying cardiac and pulmonary conditions, anemia, and pleural and pericardial effusions. Dyspnea is often present in the absence of tachypnea in the hospice population: 77% of patients reported dyspnea, but only 39% had tachypnea charted.[92]

Terminally ill patients benefit from the same specific therapies recommended for patients with less advanced disease. For panic due to perceived breathlessness, an oral opioid, chlorpromazine, or, for refractory panic, midazolam, may be needed (Table 175.1). For patients with less anxiety, empiric opioids and anxiolytics are also used (Table 175.1).

Patients with continuous dyspnea often benefit from sustained-release opioid preparations with immediate-release rescue doses every 2 hours are useful. If a patient is already receiving an opioid for pain or cough suppression, the same opioid can be used to ameliorate the dyspnea. For patients unable to take oral medications, or furosemide,[93] opioid drips with a patient-controlled analgesia (PCA) option can be very effective. If an opioid drip is begun for dyspnea, hospital staff, patients, and families must be carefully educated that the purpose is to control the symptom of dyspnea, not to hasten death. Dosing is titrated to comfort, which is usually achieved without significant changes in respiratory rate or blood gases. Patients who resist use of the opioid may fear going to sleep and not reawakening. Exploring these concerns can facilitate patients' opioid use at night to improve their alertness and energy during the day.

Cough, which is present in about 40% of patients with advanced cancer, is caused by postnasal drip, infection, pleural effusions, heart failure, asthma or chronic obstructive pulmonary disease, esophageal reflux, angiotensin-converting enzyme inhibitors, obstruction of the airway, and disorders of swallowing. Patients respond to oral opioids, sweet elixirs containing dextromethorphan, opioid elixirs, or methadone syrup. For more resistant coughs, higher doses of oral or nebulized opioids (morphine or hydromorphone often combined with dexamethasone every 4 hours through a nebulizer using room air or oxygen through an open facemask) may be helpful. In addition, nebulized anesthetics (e.g., 2 mL of 2% lidocaine in 1 mL of normal saline for 10 minutes) can be given up to three times a day.[60] For patients who have tenacious mucous, nebulized saline, albuterol (0.5 mg in 2.5 mg normal saline) or terbutaline are helpful,[60] while expectorants and mucolytics are not. Ipratropium exacerbates this problem and should be discontinued when possible.

Hiccups interfere with a patient's ability to eat, drink, and sleep. In patients with cancer, they are most commonly caused by gastric compression, injury to vagus or phrenic nerves, uremia, hyponatremia, hypocalcemia, benzodiazepines, barbiturates, intravenous corticosteroids, or rarely ear infections, pharyngitis, esophagitis, or pneumonia. Pharmacologic therapies are listed in Table 175.1. Chlorpromazine is effective but causes significant postural hypotension, which may not be a problem in this population. Metoclopramide, baclofen, haloperidol, gabapentin, and nifedipine are probably equally effective and safer in older more ambulatory patients.[94,95] If tumor is compressing surrounding structures, dexamethasone (8 mg orally every morning) may reduce peritumor edema, relieve pressure, and control the hiccups. If sedation is not a concern, midazolam can be used.[96]

Massive hemoptysis from a tumor eroding into a major vessel is rare but can be horrifying to observe. If the patient is likely to develop such a complication, dark-colored sheets, towels, and blankets can be used to mask the blood. Consider insertion of a peripherally inserted central catheter line for patients without an indwelling venous access device to provide emergency intravenous access for patient sedation. For patients at home in hospice programs, hospice nurses provide instruction to those family members who feel able to administer an infusion of morphine intravenously and a benzodiazepine IV (e.g., midazolam 1.0 to 2.5 mg load followed by 0.4 mg/h IV initial infusion), or rectally (diazepam 10 mg or lorazepam 2 mg) while waiting for the nurse to arrive.[60] Inpatients must have these medications available on the hospital unit to be used immediately when needed. When the event occurs, the patient is placed bleeding

TABLE 175.1

PHYSICAL SOURCES OF DISTRESS NEAR THE END OF LIFE AND APPLICABLE MEDICATIONS

Source	Medication(s)	Dose and Route (PO/SL/IV/SC/PR)
Fatigue	Methylphenidate	2.5–5 mg PO 8am/noon; can increase as needed
Insomnia	Temazepam	7.5–30 PO hs (lower dose in elderly)
	Zoldipem	5–10 mg PO hs
	Trazadone	25–100 mg PO hs
Pain (continuous)	Opioid (morphine, oxycodone hydromorphone)	Oral concentrates or IV or SQ infusion
	Fentanyl	Transdermal
Pain (intermittent)	Morphine, oxycodone	SL oral concentrates
	Hydromorphone	PR
Depression	Methylphenidate	2.5–5 mg PO qam or qam and noon
Anxiety	Lorazepam	0.5–2 mg SL q2h
	Clonazepam	0.5–2 mg PO bid
Delirium	Haloperidol	1–5 mg PO, SQ, IV, PR q2–12h
	Chlorpromazine	12.5–50 mg PO, IV, PR q4–8h
	Olanzapine	2.5–5 mg SL qhs or bid; 2.5 mg SL prn q4h prn
Hypoactive delirium	Methylphenidate	10 mg PO day 1; then 10 mg 8am and noon PO
Agitated delirium	Midazolam	1–2.5 mg IV/SQ load; 0.5–1.5 mg/h IV/SQ or 25% of loading dose; increase as needed
Dyspnea (anxiety)	Lorazepam	1 mg PO, SL q2h
Dyspnea (other)	Opioid	For example, morphine 5–10 mg PO, IV q2h prn
	Chlorpromazine	25–50 mg PO, PR q4–12h
Cough	Opioid	Nebulized with dexamethasone, e.g. morphine 5–10 mg PO, IV or by nebulizer q2h
	Lidocaine	2 mL of 2% lidocaine in 1 mL of nl saline for 10″
	Albuterol/terbutaline	Nebulized
Hiccups	Baclofen	10–20 mg PO tid
	Metoclopramide	10–20 mg PO/IV/SQ/PR qid
	Nifedipine	10–20 mg PO tid
	Haloperidol	1–4 mg PO/SQ/PR tid
	Chlorpromazine	25–50 mg PO/IV qd-qid
"Death rattle"	Scopolamine	Transderm Scop patch 1–3 q3d
	Hyoscyamine	0.125–0.25 SL tid–qid
	Glycopyrrolate	0.2–0.6 mg PO/SQ/IV tid
Nausea	Olanzapine	2.5–5 mg SL hs to bid
	Lorazepam, metoclopramide, dexamethasone, or haloperidol	IV or compounded suppositories with desired agents (depending on presumed cause of nausea) q6 PR
Palliative sedation	Midazolam	1–2.5 mg IV/SC load; 0.4 mg/h IV/SQ drip; increase as needed
Refractory symptoms	Pentobarbital	2–3 mg/kg IV load; 1–2 mg/kg/h IV drip
	Lorazepam	0.5–1 mg/h IV
	Propofol	2.5–5 mcg/kg/min IV

PO, oral; SL, sublingual; IV, intravenous; SQ, subcutaneous; PR, per rectum.
(From ref. 60.)

side down, in the Trendelenburg position if possible, and the medications are given.

Gastrointestinal Disorders

Patients at the end of life are unlikely to be thirsty or hungry,[97] even if they voluntarily refuse food and fluids to hasten their deaths.[98] Families may equate not eating with "giving up" and may urge placement of a feeding tube or parenteral nutrition or hydration. Asking the caregiver what he or she hopes the patient will be able to do if given nutrition through a feeding tube may reveal that the patient or family has an unrealistic expectation of how much the intervention will improve the patient's function. Explain that these interventions are likely to be harmful. Parenteral hydration in dying patients causes nausea and vomiting from increased gastric secretions; dyspnea from ascites, upper airway secretions, and pulmonary edema; and pain from ascites and peripheral edema.[97] Feeding tubes may leak and lead to aspiration.

The xerostomia that is common in this population is usually due to opioids, not to dehydration.[99] There is no correlation

TABLE 175.2

NAUSEA AND VOMITING CAUSES AND APPLICABLE MEDICATIONS

Etiology	Drug	Initial Dose[a]
Initiation or escalation of opioid therapy	Prochlorperazine Olanzapine	10 mg PO or 25 mg PR bid/tid 2.5–5 mg PO/SL once daily
CNS disease	Dexamethasone	2–4 mg PO/PR bid
Vertigo	Hyoscyamine Scopolamine	0.125–0.25 mg PO/SQ tid Transdermal patch
Candidal mucositis	Fluconazole	100 mg PO qd
Liver/renal failure	Haloperidol Olanzapine	1.5–5 mg PO/IV tid 2.5 to 5 mg PO/SL bid
Constipation	Senna; polyethylene Glycol; Dulcolax	
Opioid-induced constipation	Methylnaltrexone	0.15 mg/kg SQ ×1 No more than 2 doses in a 24-hour period
Gastritis	Proton pump inhibitor	20 mg PO qd
Delayed gastric emptying	Metoclopramide	10–20 mg PO/PR bid; 1–3 mg/h IV/SQ
Bowel obstruction[b]	Octreotide	150–300 mcg SQ bid-tid

PO, oral; SL, sublingual; IV, intravenous; SQ, subcutaneous; PR, per rectum.
[a]For nausea, initial steps should be: (1) treat cause, if identified, (2) consider changing to a different opioid agent.
[b]For symptomatic therapy when surgery is not indicated.
(From refs. 78, 79, 128.)

between reports of thirst or dry mouth and hydration status,[100] and no controlled studies have shown that rehydration is effective. Moistening the mouth with swabs or offering sips of water or ice chips usually ameliorates the xerostomia.

Nausea or vomiting in the dying patient is due to initiation or escalation of opioids; disease of the central nervous system or the inner ear; oral infections; hepatic or renal failure; metabolic abnormalities (hypercalcemia, hyponatremia, hyper or hypoglycemia); constipation; gastritis; and functional or mechanical obstruction of the gastrointestinal tract. Therapy should be directed at the underlying etiology[60,101–103] (Table 175.2).

Social Sources of Distress

With increasing debility, patients may lose their roles in the community, the workplace, and in the family.[104] They may have concerns about who will care for their parents or children when they have died and who will provide financially. Worries about burdening the family or that the family will fail them when they really need them may lead patients to request physician-assisted suicide[105] or hastened death.[106] Social workers are the key team members who can help alleviate or at least ameliorate these sources of distress.

Caregivers of patients with advanced disease are themselves at increased risk of physical and psychological deterioration.[107,108] Virtually all caregivers are family members (96%), most of them women (72%).[107] Caregivers may have increased responsibilities for childcare, care of elderly family members, management of household tasks, as well as the care of the patient.[109] Spouses are at the greatest risk, with increased mortality and suicide rates following the spouse's death.[108] Caregivers at the highest risk for deterioration are in the lower socioeconomic groups,[110] are ill themselves, have a prior history of depression, are people of color,[108,110] or have been caring for patients for longer periods of time (more than 6 months).[111] Unrelieved symptoms and high physical caregiving needs also increase caregiver burden.[88] Caregiver education; communication among the health care team, patient, and family; and Internet, print, and telephone-based resources of support and information (e.g., Cancer Care, Inc.), all address caregiver needs.[108,112]

Ongoing communication with the oncology team, even when the patient can no longer go to see the physician, is crucial to the success of a home care program for the dying patient. The oncology team needs to provide orders to hospice or other home care services, explain to the family how to change from cheerleader to companion, teach them how to recognize when the patient's last days are approaching, and tell them what to expect as the patient dies.

Spiritual or Existential Distress

Spiritual or existential concerns of dying patients include making meaning of their lives; in creating and sharing the narratives of their lives, patients prioritize, order, celebrate, grow, heal, and mourn and transmit their legacies.[54,113] Some patients want to reconnect with religious traditions and carry out the rituals that surround dying in their culture or religion.[34] Clinicians can help patients find solace and closure at the end of life by exploring religious and spiritual beliefs and listening empathetically,[25,54,114] and by validating the need for religious or spiritual counseling.[115] For some patients and families, discussing Byock's[113] "Five Things" together will bring healing and closure: "Forgive me; I forgive you; Thank you; I love you, and Goodbye."

Palliative Sedation

Palliative sedation is "the monitored use of medications to relieve refractory and unendurable symptoms by inducing varying degrees of unconsciousness but not death."[116] It is considered when, despite expert multidisciplinary evaluation and management, a patient who is near death continues to experience intolerable physical, psychological, or spiritual or existential symptoms.[117,118] Fewer than 5% of patients will fall into

PRACTICE OF ONCOLOGY

this category. Those patients who do most commonly suffer from refractory pain, cough, dyspnea, seizures, or delirium. In these cases, the high doses of opioid, benzodiazepine, or neuroleptic needed to control symptoms may cause intolerable or paradoxical side effects (e.g., myoclonus or hyperalgesia), such that sedation is the only option to control the symptom. In other cases, the request for sedation for refractory symptoms arises when psychological or spiritual or existential concerns coexist with physical problems.[118] Patients with distress refractory to usual therapies should be referred to palliative care consultations teams, whose expertise includes assessment for and implementation of this rarely used, but immensely valuable, mode of relieving the suffering of patients who are imminently dying.[60,119–123]

THE FINAL DAYS

Signs that the patient is entering the last 10 to 14 days include[124,125]:

- Minimal intake progressing to no intake, tachycardia, followed by decrease in heart rate and blood pressure, perspiration, clammy skin, mottling
- Diminished breath sounds, irregular breathing pattern with periods of apnea or full Cheyne-Stokes respiration; grunting or moaning with exhalation
- Difficulty swallowing; loss of gag reflex with pooling of secretions causing "death rattle"
- Incontinence of bladder or rectum
- Agitation with or without hallucinations; decreasing level of consciousness; difficult to arouse

Comfort Measures Only versus Intensive Comfort Measures

When a patient is no longer improving from antibiotics or transfusions and is in the last weeks of life, neither families nor house staff intuitively understands that these formerly effective manifestations of care now are no longer relevant or useful. Statements such as "We are going to *stop* the antibiotics" or "Transfusions are not indicated" suggest that the treatment would be effective but is being withheld for an unclear reason. Offering intensive comfort measures instead of comfort measures only indicates the team's ongoing commitment to care. House staff can be redirected to make daily visits to monitor for pain, dyspnea, anxiety, delirium, urinary retention, constipation, myoclonus, and excessive upper airway secretions ("death rattle"). Family and friends should be invited to report their observations and encouraged to ask questions. Both family and visitors need to be encouraged to feel free to touch and speak with the patient. They may be afraid to do so, particularly when the patient is in an intensive care unit attached to a number of machines and intravenous lines.

Discussions should also begin with the family to learn whether their religious or cultural tradition has any specific requirements for the days immediately preceding or immediately following the death. The family can then begin to assemble the group who will perform the rituals and begin to explain to the unit staff what they will need.

Support for House Staff

House staff rarely review with the medical team their reactions to the care of dying patients and to the death itself.[126] Interns are in special need of emotional support following a patient's death.[127] Reviewing each death on the next morning's rounds in the intensive care unit or other unit provides the needed debriefing and shows respect for the patient who has died. When possible and it feels appropriate, clinicians can write a card or attend the funeral or memorial service, which may facilitate closure.[128]

AFTER THE DEATH

After the patient dies, the nurses usually will wash the body and remove intravenous lines, catheters, or any other equipment, unless the case will be reviewed by the medical examiner or such care is inconsistent with the family's religious or cultural practices.[125] Physicians called to confirm the death should first confer with the nurses regarding the circumstances of the death, offer them condolences, and ask if a hospital chaplain is needed to support the family or unit staff. After the physician verifies that the patient has died, the death is documented in the medical record, and a death certificate is completed. The family should not be asked to leave the room during the confirmation of death.

The physicians who are present at the death, or who have been asked to verify the patient's death, should offer condolences to the others present and offer to answer questions, as this can aid the coping of survivors and minimize anger at physicians.[129] If invited to participate in a prayer, it is appropriate to do so. Allowing those present to spend as much time as they need to, to say or do whatever they feel they need to do, including touching the body, improves their ability to cope with their acute grief.[128]

GRIEF AND BEREAVEMENT

Even before the patient dies, patients, family members, and loved ones may suffer from anticipatory grief, which can include "anger, guilt, anxiety, irritability, sadness, feelings of loss, and decreased ability to function at usual tasks."[130] Openly acknowledging their grief and providing counseling and support through social work, psychiatry, or chaplaincy staff is recommended.[130]

After the patient's death, the grief of the survivors has been described as a "process of experiencing the psychological, behavioral, social, and physical reactions to the perception of loss."[131] Their initial grief may manifest as "denial, intense crying spells, anxiety, numbness," and other physical, psychological, emotional, and spiritual manifestations.[130] Six months or so after the death, most survivors find they are suffering less from these symptoms.[129] They accept the reality of the death; they are able to be involved emotionally with family and friends; and they accommodate to the new demands of life without the person who has died.[129,131] "Pangs of grief," which are "intrusive, time-limited intense yearning and pining for the deceased,"[129] can occur at anniversaries or when an unexpected reminder of the deceased appears and may continue to occur for years.

Clinicians can help identify those families who need help through this process by contacting the family several weeks to a month after the death to ask about (1) how they have been responding to their loss ("Is there anything that has been especially troubling to you?"), (2) their current social support and coping strategies, and (3) practical concerns (e.g., finances).[130] Oncologists report varied contact with families after the death of their patients.[132]

Families of patients who had been enrolled in hospice programs will receive bereavement services for a year after the patient's death, including calls and cards after the death, and assessment of need for individual bereavement counseling,[133] invitations to bereavement support groups and memorial services, and letters at regular intervals offering practical advice. Oncology practices often offer similar programs.[134]

About 10% to 20% of survivors suffer either from depression, "complicated grief," or prolonged grief disorder. Patients with depression have "somatic distress, sleep and appetite disturbances, decreased concentration, social withdrawal and sighing,"[54] and "symptoms of sadness, impassivity, and psychomotor retardation."[135] They cannot enjoy anything, and these feelings are "constant, unremitting."[54] Depressed survivors, however, do not yearn for the deceased, and they can accept the death, yet they still can benefit from counseling and consideration of pharmacologic treatment, such as bupropion or paroxetine.[54,129,135,136]

On the other hand, the grief of survivors with prolonged grief disorder[137,138] causes serious functional impairments. They yearn for the deceased and have feelings of "numbness, feeling that part of oneself has died, assuming symptoms of the deceased, disbelief, or bitterness."[135,136] These survivors are at increased risk of medical and psychiatric illness[139] and substance abuse problems[129] and should be referred for psychiatric or spiritual counseling. Survivors with a history of attachment disorders (childhood abuse, childhood separation anxiety), aversion to lifestyle changes, being unprepared for the death and unsupported after it are at higher risk of developing prolonged grief disorders. Additional risks include a "dependent, close, confiding" relationship with the deceased.[135] Pharmacotherapy does not relieve these extreme grief symptoms,[135,140] but a new form of psychotherapy developed specifically for this disorder may be superior to standard interpersonal psychotherapy.[141]

Selected References

The full list of references for this chapter appears in the online version.

3. Lamont EB, Christakis NA. Prognostic disclosure to patients with cancer near the end of life. *Ann Intern Med* 2001;134:1096.
4. Daugherty CK, Hlubocky FJ. What are terminally ill cancer patients told about their expected deaths? A study of cancer physicians' self-reports of prognosis disclosure. *J Clin Oncol* 2008;26(36):5988.
5. Back AL, Anderson WG, Bunch L, et al. Communication about cancer near the end of life. *Cancer* 2008;113(7 Suppl):1897.
7. Buckman RR. *How to break bad news: a guide for health care professionals.* Baltimore: Johns Hopkins University Press, 1992.
9. Back A, Arnold R., Tulsky J. *Mastering communication with seriously ill patients: balancing honesty with empathy and hope.* New York: Cambridge University Press, 2009.
12. Finlay E, Casarett D. Making difficult discussions easier: using prognosis to facilitate transitions to hospice. *CA Cancer J Clin* 2009;59:250.
14. Dow LA, Matsuyama RK, Ramakrishnan V, et al. Paradoxes in advance care planning: the complex relationship of oncology patients, their physicians, and advance medical directives. *J Clin Oncol* 2010;28:299.
15. Wright AA, Zhang B, Ray A, et al: Associations between EOL discussions, patient mental health, medical care near death, and caregiver bereavement adjustment. *JAMA* 2008;300:1665.
17. Balboni TA, Vanderwerker LC, Block SD, et al. Religiousness and spiritual support among advanced cancer patients and associations with end-of-life treatment preferences and quality of life. *J Clin Oncol* 2007;25:555.
18. Smith AK, McCarthy EP, Paulk E, et al. Racial and ethnic differences in advance care planning among patients with cancer: impact of terminal illness acknowledgment, religiousness, and treatment preferences. *J Clin Oncol* 2008;26:4131.
24. Weeks JC, Cook EF, O'Day SSJ, et al. Relationship between cancer patients' predictions of prognosis and their treatment preferences. *JAMA* 1998; 279:1709.
26. Hebert RS, Schulz R, Copeland VC, Arnold RM. Preparing family caregivers for death and bereavement. Insights from caregivers of terminally ill patients. *J Pain Symptom Manage* 2009;37(1):3.
27. Curtis JR, Patrick DL. How to discuss dying and death in an ICU. In: Curtis JR, Rubenfeld GD, eds. *Managing death in the intensive care unit.* Oxford: Oxford University Press, 2001:85.
28. Schou KC, Hewison J. *Experiencing cancer: quality of life in cancer treatment.* Buckingham, England: Open University Press, 1999.
31. Muriel AC, Rauch PK. Talking with families and children about the death of a parent. In: Hanks G, Cherny NI, Christakis NA, et al., eds. *The Oxford textbook of palliative medicine*, 4th ed. Oxford: Oxford University Press, 2009
33. Crawley LM, Marshall PA, Lo B, et al. Strategies for culturally effective end-of-life. *Ann Intern Med* 2002;27(136):673.
38. Phipps E, True G, Harris D, et al. Approaching the end of life: attitudes, preferences and behaviors of African-American and white patients and their family caregivers. *J Clin Oncol* 2003;21:549.
40. Hwang SS, Chang VT, Cogswell J, et al. Knowledge and attitudes towards end-of-life care in veterans with symptomatic metastatic cancer. *J Palliat Support Care* 2003:1:221.
41. Harrington SE, Smith TJ. The role of chemotherapy at the end of life: "When is enough, enough?" *JAMA* 2008;299:2667.
42. Evans WG, Tulsky JA, Back AL et al. Communication at times of transitions: how to help patients cope with loss and re-define hope. *Cancer J* 2006;12:417.
43. Abrahm JL. The palliative care consultation team as a model for palliative care education. In: Portenoy RK, Bruera E, eds. *Topics in palliative care*, Vol. 4. Oxford: Oxford University Press, 2000:147.
45. Gelfman LP, Meier DE, Morrison RS. Does palliative care improve quality? A survey of bereaved family members. *J Pain Symptom Manage* 2008;36:22.
50. Casarett DJ, Quill TE. "I'm not ready for hospice": strategies for timely and effective hospice discussions. *Ann Intern Med* 2007;146:443.
54. Block SD. Psychological considerations, growth, and transcendence at the end of life: the art of the possible. *JAMA* 2001;285:2898.
55. Ferrell B, Connor SR, Cordes A, et al. The national agenda for quality palliative care: the National Consensus Project and the National Quality Forum. *Pain Symptom Manage* 2007;33(6):737.
56. Ferrell B, Paice, J, Koczywas M. New standards and implications for improving the quality of supportive oncology practice. *J Clin Oncol* 2008 26:3824.
57. Ferris FD, Bruera E, Cherny N, et al. Palliative cancer care a decade later: accomplishments, the need, next steps—from the American Society of Clinical Oncology. *J Clin Oncol* 2009;27(18):3052.
59. Miaskowski C, Cleary J, Burney R, et al. *Guideline for the management of cancer pain in adults and children.* APS Clinical Practice Guidelines Series, No. 3. Glenview, IL: American Pain Society, 2005.
60. Abrahm JL. *A physician's guide to pain and symptom management in cancer patients*, 2nd ed. Baltimore: Johns Hopkins University Press, 2005.
61. Morrow GR, Shelke AR, Roscoe JA, et al. Management of cancer-related fatigue. *Cancer Invest* 2005;23:229.
62. Savard J, Marin CM. Insomnia in the context of cancer: a review of a neglected problem. *J Clin Oncol* 2001;19:895.
66. Mannes A, Kim PS, Lonser RR. Neurosurgical interventional approaches to pain. In: Berger AM, Portenoy RK, Weissman DE, eds. *Principles and practice of supportive oncology*, 3rd ed. Philadelphia: Lippincott-Raven, 2006:87.
73. Thomas J, Karver S, Cooney GA, et al. Methylnaltrexone for opioid-induced constipation in advanced illness. *N Engl J Med* 2008;358(22):2332.
74. Block SD. Psychological issues in End-of-Life care. *J Palliat Med* 2006; 9:751.
76. Miovic M, Block S. Psychiatric disorders in advanced cancer. *Cancer* 2007;110(8):1665.
78. Rozans M, Dreisbach A, Lertora JJL, et al. Palliative uses of methylphenidate in patients with cancer: a review. *J Clin Oncol* 2002;20:335.
81. Spencer R, Nilsson M, Wright A, Pirl W, Prigerson H. Anxiety disorders in advanced cancer patients: correlates and predictors of end-of-life outcomes. *Cancer* 2010;116(7):1810.
82. Bush SH, Bruera E. The assessment and management of delirium in cancer patients. *Oncologist* 2009;14(10):1039.
91. Ben-Aharon I, Gafter-Gvili A, Leibovici PM, Stemmer SM. Interventions for alleviating cancer-related dyspnea: a systematic review. *J Clin Oncol* 2008;26(14):2396.
97. McCann RM, Hall WJ, Groth-Juncker A. Comfort care for terminally ill patients; the appropriate use of nutrition and hydration. *JAMA* 1994;272: 1263.
102. Wood GJ, Shega JW, Lynch B et al. Management of intractable nausea and vomiting in patients at the end of life. *JAMA* 2007;298:1196.
103. Ripamonte C, Mercadante S. How to use octreotide for malignant bowel obstruction. *J Support Oncol* 2004;2:357.
105. Block SD, Billings JA. Patient requests to hasten death: evaluation and management in terminal care. *Arch Intern Med* 1994;154:2039.
108. Hebert RS, Schulz R. Caregiving at the end of life. *J Palliat Med* 2006;9:1174.
115. Balboni TA, Paulk ME, Balboni MJ, et al. Provision of spiritual care to patients with advanced cancer: associations with medical care and quality of life near death. *J Clin Oncol* 2010;28(3):445.
120. De Graeff A, Dean M. Palliative sedation therapy in the last weeks of life: a literature review and recommendations for standards. *J Palliat Med* 2007;10(1):67.
124. Hallenbeck J. Palliative care in the final days of life. *JAMA* 2005;293:2265.

132. Chau NG, Zimmermann C, Ma C, Taback N, Krzyzanowska MK. Bereavement practices of physicians in oncology and palliative care. *Arch Intern Med* 2009;169(10):963.
137. Prigerson HG, Vanderwerker LC, Maciejewski PK. Prolonged grief disorder: a case for inclusion in DSMV. In: Stroebe M, Hansson R, Schut H, Stroebe W., eds. *Handbook of bereavement research and practice: 21st century perspectives*, . Washington, DC: Psychological Press, 2008: 165.
138. Greer S. Bereavement care: some clinical observations. *Psychooncology* 2010;19:1156–1160.

Consensus Statements

1. American Society of Clinical Oncology. ASCO-ESMO consensus statement on quality cancer care. *J Clin Oncol* 2006;24:3498.
2. World Health Assembly. WHA58.22 Cancer Prevention and Control, 2005. http://www.who.int/gb/ebwha/pdf_files/WHA58/WHA58_22-en.pdf.
3. National Quality Forum. *A national framework and preferred practices for palliative and hospice care quality*. Washington, DC: National Quality Forum, 2006; http://www.qualityforum.org/publications/reports/palliative.asp.
4. National Comprehensive Cancer Network. http://www.nccn.org.
5. National Consensus Project for Quality Palliative Care, 2009. http://www.nationalconsensusproject.org.
6. American Pain Society. Guidelines for the management of cancer pain in adult and children, 2005.

Online Resources

1. EPEC-Oncology at NCI.gov. http://www.cancer.gov/aboutnci/epeco.
   EPEC-Oncology Last Hours of Living Module on Medscape. http://www.medscape.com/viewprogram/5808.
   EPEC-Oncology Hydration and Nutrition Module on Medscape. http://www.medscape.com/viewprogram/8617.
2. National Consensus Project. www.nationalconsensusproject.org
3. Center to Advance Palliative Care. http://www.capc.org/
4. National Quality Forum. www.qualityforum.org
5. Education in Palliative and End-of-Life care for Oncology (EPEC-O) CD-ROM and DVD Self-Study Modules and Materials for Trainers. National Cancer Institute, U.S. Department of Health and Human Services.

Other Resources

Buckman R, Baile W. A Practical Guide to Communication Skills in Cancer Care. 2000. *Distributed by* Cinemedic Distributors, Inc. www.cinemedic.com

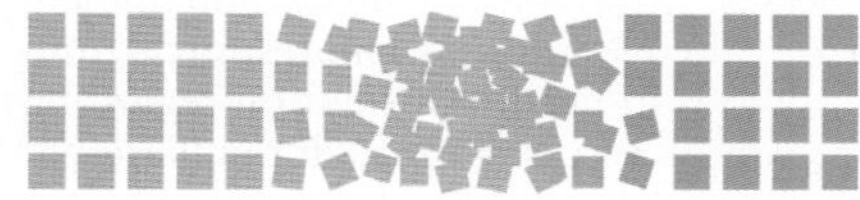

CHAPTER 176 COMMUNITY RESOURCES

BONNIE A. INDECK AND NORA RIGHTMER

COMMUNITY RESOURCES FOR THE CANCER PATIENT AND FAMILY

The latest statistics reveal that on January 1, 2007, there were close to 12,000,000 people alive in the United States, who had a history of cancer of all sites.[1] Cancer remains the second major cause of mortality, resulting in the deaths of over half a million people in the United States in 2009. Although advances in health care and medicine have made cancers more treatable, the individual diagnosed with cancer undergoes a personal crisis of such significant proportions that his or her entire social system is severely affected. Whether cancer be curable or fatal, the journey through treatment will be arduous, frightening, and time-consuming. Because of advances in medicine and the constraints of insurance reimbursement, more and more patients continue to be treated in the outpatient setting, requiring ongoing trips to medical providers, often by patients not well enough to navigate on their own. Personal and financial resources are often inadequate, increasingly necessitating the community to provide services for this vulnerable population.[2] Although more and more communities are attempting to provide these needed ancillary services, gaps still exist, leaving patients struggling to meet their own needs, either because there is no service available or more often because the patient is unaware of or unable to access the information or service.

Cancer patients report a moderate to high need for help regarding their ability to cope with their illness and its treatment, emotional support, information provision, and relations with staff at treatment centers.[3] Additionally, patients often report informational needs, with a strong preference for gaining access to information through the Internet. Health care professionals should be familiar with Internet as well as local resources to improve patient access and ability to cope with cancer.[4] This chapter will discuss patients' and families' psychosocial, informational, and instrumental needs and the resources available to meet those needs, followed by a comprehensive list of accessible resources.

THE CANCER PATIENT

Responses to a cancer diagnosis vary widely based on disease type, stage, location; treatment selected; treatment outcomes; and age, sex, and education. This also is mediated by previous experience, social support, hope, and coping strategies used.[5] However, a diagnosis of cancer places huge psychological and physical demands on individuals. Early-stage cancer patients will frequently experience depression and elevated levels of anxiety. Diagnosis is without a doubt the most difficult time, with external stressors and internal existential issues. Weisman and Worden,[6] in their seminal article "The Existential Plight in Cancer," describe the patient's experienced threat to life and well-being in which the patient focuses on life/death concerns, as well as worries about health or physical symptoms. They found the level of psychosocial distress to be predictive of a patient's ability to cope. An assessment of the patient's past coping, including strategies used, can be particularly helpful in evaluation of the patient's current needs for social, emotional, and informational support, and is useful to provide the most successful treatment. Characteristics such as rigidity of behavior, morose outlook, pessimism, and high emotional distress, should be noted, as well as substance abuse, recent losses, social isolation, family disturbances, and other debilitating illnesses, so that specialized or individualized support or counseling may be provided for these patients to cope with their diagnosis and successfully participate in treatment.[7]

Communication, therefore, becomes key to the relationship between patient and provider as the lack thereof may decrease patient disclosure, decrease satisfaction with care, increase anxiety, and result in noncompliance.[8] The management of some cancers presents difficult decisions because the impact of treatment on quality of life might overshadow its survival efficacy, and patients' preferences are not always in accord with those of clinicians. Unless patients' preferences are explicitly sought and incorporated into clinical decision making, patients may not receive the treatment that is best for them.[9] To this end, the physician may call on members of the health care team to assist in clarifying the patient's values and aid in understanding the psychosocial needs. The oncology social worker or oncology nurse can be instrumental both in providing the emotional support and counseling and in clarifying the patient understanding of the meaning of the diagnosis.

SOCIAL AND EMOTIONAL SUPPORT

Social Support Network

Cancer literature has consistently identified and recognized the importance of a social support network for patients. Social support is a critical ingredient to physical and mental health when facing cancer.[10] Research has shown that support networks, both formal and informal, play a significant role in assisting patients in coping with their cancer. A social support network may consist of professionals from the community, family members, friends, significant others, religious or fraternal organizations, support groups (formal or informal), and/or other agencies.[11] A social support network consisting of any of these has a strong positive impact on the psychological well-being of the cancer patient,[12] and as such, is able to assist that patient in coping with whatever barriers might interfere with the ability to comply with treatment. The constructs of the social support system identified as emotional, informational, and instrumental as defined by Wortman will be the structure with which we define support and resources for the person with cancer.[13]

Family as Emotional Support

As the newly diagnosed person enters the health care system, it is important for the health care professionals to recognize that this individual rarely functions alone. He or she is part of a relational system, and those closest are summoned to form the immediate support system. It is also helpful to be aware that the definition of family has been widened to include anyone the patient deems to be the significant persons in his or her life. As health care professionals, we must recognize the importance of including the family not only at time of diagnosis, but also whenever it is necessary to have a serious conversation such as on recurrence or change in treatment plans and certainly at the terminal phase. The family system is irrevocably changed at diagnosis, and all who interact with the patient must be aware of the impact on the entire system.[14,15]

The patient's family will provide support within the context of their sociocultural belief system and in accord with their familial and possibly religious values. Understanding the context of the patient's system will allow for better provision of service.[16] The family has many tasks, often including reorganization of roles and creative allocation of family resources. Family or "informal" caregivers provide the equivalent of more than $250 billion in caregiving services each year.[17] In a study of over 2,000 families caring for a family member with a serious illness, nearly 20% of family caregivers quit work or made major life rearrangements to provide care. In addition to the economic impact, long-term caregiving has been shown to have adverse effects on physical and mental health.[17] Many caregivers of advanced cancer patients either meet criteria or are being treated for psychiatric problems. Discussing mental health issues positively and preventively is one thing that health care professionals can do to promote better outcomes for this vulnerable population.[17]

Emotional Support Outside the Family

In addition to the family, there are other sources of support. Support may come from a variety of sources that the patient feels comfortable using, and this may mitigate a patient's distress.[18] One important component of support outside the family is that there should be a perceived commonality in the support system. Patients are reassured by speaking with people undergoing similar experiences. This kind of support is offered through various kinds of programs or groups.

Person-to-Person Programs

The American Cancer Society (ACS) has many programs maintained by trained volunteers who have themselves been cancer patients. Reach to Recovery, Man to Man, Cansurmount, and the ostomy programs all provide person-to-person contact for patients. Other organizations provide similar programs as well for specific cancers such as the Leukemia Lymphoma Society's First Connection program, and more recently, Cancer Buddies and Breast Cancer Buddies, which are online and e-mail person-to-person support programs. Cancer patients feel understood, validated, and hopeful when able to compare notes with other cancer survivors.

Support Groups

Self-Help Groups

Self-help groups are formed by people who have similar concerns, problems, or illnesses. Although not professionally led, they are often a source of valuable information, resources, and support for the patient who is in need. Information regarding specific self-help groups can be accessed through the National Self Help Network.

Face-to-Face Groups

Traditional support groups are available in most communities and are facilitated by health care professionals. The professional can assist group members in being cohesive and supportive to one another, as well as assuring that any information and resources brought into the group are appropriate and accurate.

Online Support

Recently there has been an explosion of the use of online support. A survey by Manhattan Research found that about 35% of adults use online support sites and other health-related social media. In just 2 years, the ACS has developed a following of more than 16,000 people on Twitter and nearly 170,000 on Facebook.[19] Additional advantages over traditional groups are the ease with which patients can connect despite impediments of ill health, lack of transportation, or scheduling.

Complementary and Alternative Medicine

Complementary and alternative medicine (CAM) includes forms of treatment that are used in addition to, or instead of, standard regimens. They may be biologically based (substances such as herbs, diets, or vitamins) energy-based (the use of energy fields, therapeutic touch, or electromagnetic therapy), manipulative and body-based (spinal manipulation and massage), and/or mind–body-based (using techniques designed to enhance the mind's ability to affect bodily functions (meditation, prayer, art, music and dance therapy). Many people with cancer use CAM to cope with the emotional distress of a cancer diagnosis and to assist in managing symptoms. According to the National Center for Complementary and Alternative Medicine, 38% of American adults use some form of CAM.[20] A major concern is that patients do not necessarily tell their physician about CAM use or their CAM practitioner about the traditional treatment they are undergoing, which can lead to unfavorable reactions or outcomes.[21] It is therefore imperative for the medical team to include questions about the use of these services in their comprehensive evaluation of the patient so that contraindications can be explained and adverse treatment interactions can be avoided.

INFORMATIONAL SUPPORT

It is axiomatic that knowledge is power. Cancer patients and families who know more about their illness and are actively involved in treatment decisions cope better than those who are more passive. Having the information also helps patients to feel less powerless and more in control. In a Canadian Survey of cancer patients' experiences, respondents reported that when trying to find information on symptoms, the most helpful sources were nurses, specialists, and other cancer patients.[22] Communication between the health care team and the patient/family is crucial to meet the informational needs of the patient.

As desire for information differs, it is important to first assess the patient's readiness to receive information, and as ability to receive information differs, it is important to review their cultural, literacy, educational, psychological, socioeconomic, and personal preferences. Cultural influences, values, and beliefs must be understood as they influence the very meaning of the disease to the individual. Culturally sensitive material should be developed with input from the community, as "they are more powerful than those that come from outside sources."[23]

Finally, knowledge of the patient's educational level and literacy is crucial to maximizing comprehension and retention of the material while encouraging greater participation in decision making and dialogue with the health care team. The ability to read, understand, and act on information can often be dangerously low. More than 40% of patients with chronic illnesses are functionally illiterate.[24] Ninety million Americans have difficulty understanding and acting on health information according to an Institute of Medicine report on health literacy.[25] Patients with low health literacy who may not understand medical instructions will be less likely to comply with treatment and follow-up. This can result in poor outcomes and increased cost.

Although health literacy cannot be improved by the health care professional, it can be addressed by modifying the delivery of care to improve communication, use of tools to ensure comprehension, simplifying health care situations such as check-in or referrals, development of simpler paperwork and educational materials, and empowering patients to ask questions.[26]

Internet, E-mail, Instant Messaging, and Electronic Records

Literature on health communication supports the need for multiple ways of accessing health information as a more comprehensive way of reaching more individuals. Internet usage continues to increase across all demographic variables. Eighty percent of American homes had a computer as of August 2008, and of those, 92% had Internet access.[27] Eighty percent of Americans have used the Web to seek health information. Many surveyed said the information had an impact on how they care for themselves or someone else, and that the information led them to ask different questions or seek a second opinion.[28] Additionally, respondents reported a strong preference for gaining access to information through resources such as the Internet.[29] Although some providers worry about misinformation, and potential misinterpretation of information obtained, patients report greater patient satisfaction when doctors showed interest and involvement in the information presented.[4,30]

As patients become more technologically sophisticated, their personal health management needs will be served better by access to their electronic medical records, in which they will be able to electronically pull copies of their personal health records from each provider to create their complete medical record. Newer personal health records include features that enable users to share their medical records; Microsoft's Health Vault has sophisticated privacy features that allows users to decide who has read or write access for each part of their record, and Google Health allows users to share read access on their entire record.[31]

The face of health care will continue to change as new technologies are incorporated into routine clinical use not only impacting diagnosis and treatment, but also impacting and improving patient–provider communication.[32]

INSTRUMENTAL SUPPORT

More and more cancer care is provided on an outpatient basis, which can create additional stressors and needs for the patient and their support system. Finances, transportation, medical equipment, prescriptions, home health care, and hospice care are all part of the cost of the illness.[33]

The direct cost of the illness as well as all ancillary expenses can overwhelm patients and their support system. For those on fixed incomes, the unemployed, uninsured, and underinsured, these expenses can become significant barriers to compliance with treatment. Patients who are often reluctant to disclose their financial difficulties can be assessed by the social worker who can recognize gaps in coverage, services, and resources that will be needed, thus preventing barriers to treatment by identifying resources at the onset and assisting with putting this instrumental support into place.

Resources for instrumental support as well as informational support and social/emotional support are listed in the following sections.

COMMON COMMUNITY RESOURCES

This section lists the most commonly used and helpful resources, but is not all-inclusive. They should be checked prior to referring patients as they may change without notice.

Health Literacy

The following health literacy resources may be helpful in simplifying communication.

Cultural Health	https://www.thinkculturalhealth.org/
Harvard School of Public Health	www.hsph.harvard.edu/healthliteracy
Literacy and Health Outcomes	www.ahrq.gov/clinic/epcsums/litsum.htm
Literacy Volunteers of America	www.literacyvolunteers.org
Medical Library Association	http://www.mlanet.org/resources/healthlit/
National Institute for Literacy	www.nifl.gov

Bone Marrow/Stem Cell Transplantation

- BMT Information Network: 1-888-597-7674, www.bmtinfonet.org. Provides a newsletter, resource directory, and support services via e-mail or telephone. Access to a list of attorneys who advocate for patients who have insurance difficulties.
- BMT Support Online: www.bmtsupport.org. Provides online support and education.
- Caitlin Raymond International Registry: 1-800-726-2824, www.crir.org. International search coordinating center that assists individuals in finding compatible donors.
- Cancer Care: 1-800-813-HOPE, www.cancercare.org. Provides information, counseling, and support in addition to limited financial aid.
- Center for International Bone Marrow Transplant Research: 1-414-456-8325, www.cibmtr.org. Provides statistical information on transplantation.
- Children's Organ Transplant Association: 1-800-366-2682, www.cota.org. Provides fund-raising assistance and promotes organ, marrow, and tissue donation.
- Leukemia and Lymphoma Society: 1-800-955-4572, www.lls.org. Provides publications, support, education, and limited financial aid.

- National Bone Marrow Transplant Link: 1-800-LINK-BMT, www.nbmtlink.org. A reference for your treatment process. Provides publications to help cope with logistics, finances, and medical insurance as well as peer support.
- National Children's Cancer Society: 1-800-882-6227, www.children-cancer.org. Provides financial assistance for children as well as emotional support, education information, and advocacy in addition to a parents' network.
- National Marrow Donor Program: 1-800-654-1247, www.marrow.org. Central registry facilitating searches and matches of unrelated donors and recipients.
- National Transplant Assistance Fund: 1-800-642-8399, www.transplantfund.org. Helps individuals raise funds for transplant expenses. Financial grants to eligible patients.

Care Facilities

Care facilities provide for the continuous health-related care of patients who are unable to manage living at home. Different levels of care are available, and patients should speak with a member of the health care team to ascertain the appropriate level needed. Patients should also confer with their insurance company to determine coverage.

- Hospice: Provides supportive, palliative, and terminal care.
- Rehabilitation: Provides services to patients with the goal of restoring them to an optimal level of functioning. This may include subacute or acute rehabilitation.
- Skilled nursing facility: A facility that provides skilled nursing care and other health-related services. Visit www.medicare.gov or www.ahca.org to begin a search.

Children's Camps

- Camps for siblings who are grieving a loss, often organized through a local Hospice. http://www.acor.org/ped-onc/cfissues/camps.html.
- Cancer Information Service: 1-800-4-CANCER, www.cancer.gov. Can help to guide you to local resources.
- Candlelighters Childhood Cancer Foundation: 1-800-366-2223, www.candlelighters.org. Provides a list of camps.
- Children's Oncology Camping Association: www.cocai.org. Camps categorized by state.
- Kids Camps, a listing by state: www.kidscamps.com. Use directory for "special needs."
- Therapy/Respite Camps for Kids: www.wmoore.net/therapy.html. Information about camps for children with special needs and/or respite, categorized by region.

Childhood Resources

- Candlelighters Childhood Cancer Foundation: 1-800-366-2223, www.candlelighters.org. Bibliography, resource guide, quarterly newsletter, youth newsletter, and handbooks.
- Captain Chemo and the Chemo Command, video game: www.royalmarsden.org/captchemo/index.asp. Website is based on comic strips by a cancer survivor. Involves interactive computer games.
- Children's Cancer Association: 1-503-244-3141, www.childrenscancerassociation.org. Provides programs and resources for children with cancer.
- Children's Hospice International: 1-800-242-4453, www.chionline.org. Ensures medical, psychological, social, and spiritual support to children and their families.
- Children's Organ Transplant Association: 1-800-366-2682, www.cota.org. Provides fund-raising assistance and promotes organ, marrow, and tissue donation.
- Compassionate Friends: 1-630-990-0010, www.compassionatefriends.org. Assists families toward the positive resolution of grief following the death of a child and to provide information to help others be supportive.
- Famous Phone Friends: 1-310-204-5683, www.thenancyshow.com/html/volunteer/volunteer_fff.html. Links children who are confined to the home or hospital by telephone with entertainers and athletes.
- National Childhood Cancer Foundation: 1-626-447-1674, www.curesearch.org. Provides information on new treatments and psychosocial support as well as newsletter.
- Pediatric Brain Tumor Foundation of the US: 1-800-253-6530, www.pbtfus.org. Provides educational and emotional support for children and families.
- Starbright Foundation: 1-310-479-1212, www.starbright.org. Creates media-based programs that help seriously ill children and teens better cope with their disease and enhance their quality of life.
- The National Children's Cancer Society: 1-314-241-1600, www.children-cancer.org. To improve the quality of life of children with cancer and their families.
- The Neuroblastoma Children's Cancer Society: 1-800-532-5162, www.neuroblastomacancer.org.

Complementary Therapy

ACS	http://www.cancer.org/docroot/ETO/ETO_5.asp
American Association of Integrative Medicine	www.aaimedicine.com/
Medline Plus	http://www.nlm.nih.gov/medlineplus/complementaryandalternativemedicine.html
Memorial Sloan-Kettering: Herbs, botanicals, and other products	www.mskcc.org/mskcc/html/11570.cfm?herbsaccept=yes
National Cancer Institute (NCI)—Office of Cancer Complementary and Alternative Medicine (OCCAM)	www.cancer.gov/cam/health_index.html
NCI—Comp. Therapies A-Z	www.cancer.gov/cam/health_camaz.html
NIH—National Center for Complementary and Alternative Medicine (NCCAM)	http://nccam.nih.gov
NIH—To see videos	http://nihseniorhealth.gov/videolist.html#cam

Emotional Support

This section will list common agencies, and most of the organizations that provide support will be listed in the "Internet" section.

- American Cancer Society: 1-800-ACS-2345, www.cancer.org
  - Cancer Survivors Network: Individuals supporting one another and sharing personal experiences with cancer.
  - I Can Cope: Educational program for people facing cancer, whether personally, or as friend or family caregiver.

- Look Good...Feel Better: A free service for women with cancer that teaches beauty techniques to help enhance appearance and self-image during treatment.
- Look Good Feel Better for Teens: A free program that assists teenage patients with the effects of cancer, similar to the program for adults.
- Man to Man: Helps men and their families cope with prostate cancer by providing education and support.
- Reach to Recovery: Support, information and comfort provided by trained volunteers before, during, and after breast cancer treatment.
- Road to Recovery: Volunteer driver program for medical appointments.
- Taking Charge of Money: A workshop for patients and families regarding financial concerns that arise during or after cancer treatment.

- Cancer Care: 1-800-813-HOPE, www.cancercare.org. Provides free professional help through counseling, education, information, referral, and direct financial assistance.
- Coping Magazine: 1-615-791-3859, www.copingmag.com. Practical tips for living with cancer.
- Cure Magazine: 1-800-210-2873, www.curetoday.com. A magazine that combines science with humanity, making cancer understandable.
- Family Service Agencies: Provides information, emotional and psychological assistance.
- Leukemia, Lymphoma Society: 1-800-955-4572, www.lls.org. Funds blood cancer research, education, and patient services for leukemia, lymphoma, Hodgkin's lymphoma, and myeloma.
- Mental Health Centers: Provides emotional support and psychological interventions.
- National Cancer Institute: www.cancer.gov. PDQ, the database of the NCI, is a comprehensive cancer information database. PDQ contains the most current information about cancer treatment, supportive care, screening, prevention, genetics, and complementary and alternative medicine and clinical trials.

The Cancer Information Service can provide the most up-to-date and accurate information from the NCI. 1–800–4–CANCER (1–800–422–6237). English and Spanish. By TTY: 1–800–332–8615. Over the Internet (instant messaging): If you have Internet access, you can get live, online assistance through *Live Help*'s instant-messaging service. By e-mail: If you have questions or comments or are unable to find what you need on the Website, you can send an e-mail using the online contact form.

- Private Practitioners: Emotional support and psychological interventions often partially covered through insurance reimbursement.
- Religious Organizations: Emotional support, pastoral care, and spiritual guidance.
- Su Familia: 1-866-783-2645. National Hispanic Family Health Helpline. Basic information to help prevent and manage chronic conditions and refer them to local health providers and federally supported programs.
- Well Spouse Foundation: 1-800-838-0879, www.wellspouse.org. Provides support to the spouses and partners of the chronically ill through groups and newsletters.
- Breast Cancer Network of Strength: 1-800-221-2141 (English), 1-800-986-9505 (Spanish), www.networkofstrength.org. Provides information, empowerment, and peer support for people with breast cancer.

Fertility

Often, the chances of having children may be decreased or eliminated by the effects of cancer treatment. There are several medically assisted ways that may keep your options open, but please explore insurance coverage as they are not always reimbursable.

- Sperm banking
- Intrauterine insemination
- Freezing embryos
- Cryopreservation of ovaries
- *In vitro* fertilization
- Donor sperm, eggs, and embryos
- Medications that preserve ovarian function by "shutting down" the ovaries during chemotherapy
- American Society for Reproductive Medicine: 1-205-978-5000, www.asrm.org
- Fertile Hope: 1-888-994-HOPE, www.fertilehope.org
- The National Infertility Association: www.resolve.org
- The Organization of Parents Through Surrogacy: 1-847-782-0224, www.opts.com
- Adoptive Families of America: 1-800-372-3300, www.adoptivefamilies.com

Financial Assistance

Income-Related

- Food Stamps: Designed to assist eligible individuals or families to purchase food.
- Short-term disability income is sometimes offered through an employer. Explore with the benefits office.
- Social Security Administration: 1-800-772-1213, www.ssa.gov. The governmental agency that oversees:
  - Supplemental Security Income: Supplements income for individuals who are aged, blind, or disabled with limited income.
  - Social Security Disability: Pays benefits for the long-term totally disabled person who has worked enough "quarters," and certain family members.

Treatment-Related

- AVONCares: www.avoncrusade.com. A special assistance fund for underserved women who are in need of diagnostic services and/or treatment for cancer.
- Cancer Care: 1-800-813-HOPE, www.cancercare.org. Limited grants for some people in need in some regions.
- Cancer Financial Assistance Coalition: www.cancerfac.org. Resource information by diagnosis or type of resource needed.
- Cancer Fund of America: 1-800-578-5284, www.cfoa.org. Assists patients by sending products such as Boost, adult diapers, bed pads, gloves, and hygiene kits.
- Children's Health Insurance Program; 1-877-543-7669, www.insurekidsnow.gov. Provides health insurance to children of eligible low income families.
- General Assistance: provides for medical expenses for those individuals with limited income and assets. Contact your local Department of Social Service for eligibility criteria.
- Hill-Burton Funds: www.hrsa.gov. Health facilities that provide free or low-cost care to individuals who cannot afford to pay. Eligibility is based on income and assets.
- Income Tax Deductions: www.irs.ustreas.gov. Medical costs that are not covered by insurance can sometimes be deducted.
- Lazarex Cancer Foundation; 1-877-866-9523, www.lazarex.org. Financial assistance to defray the costs associated with patient participation in U.S. Food and Drug Administration clinical trials.
- Leukemia-Lymphoma Society: 1-800-955-4572, www.lls.org. Limited financial aid to patients with leukemia,

lymphoma, Hodgkin's lymphoma, and myeloma, for specific items.

- Medicaid: Department of Social Service: www.cms.hhs.gov. A jointly funded, federal–state health insurance program for certain low-income and needy people.
- Medicare "D": 1-800-772-1213, www.medicare.gov. Prescription drug coverage.
- Pharmaceutical Assistance Programs:
  - Cancer Care Co-Payment Assistance: 1-866-552-6729, www.cancercarecopayment.org. Assists with copayments for oral or intravenous medication (chemotherapy).
  - Chronic Disease Fund: 1-877-968-7233, www.cdfund.org. Helps underinsured patients obtain medication.
  - Pharmaceutical companies offers drugs at no or low cost to eligible individuals. Application can be made directly to the company or access can be through www.needymeds.com or www.rxassist.org.
  - The Healthwell Foundation: 1-800-675-8416, www.healthwellfoundation.org. The Foundation provides financial assistance to eligible patients to cover certain out-of-pocket health care costs, including prescription drug coinsurance, copayments, and deductibles; health insurance premiums; and funds available for specific illnesses.
  - National Association of Rare Disorders: 1-800-999-6673, www.rarediseases.org. Assists under- or uninsured individuals to obtain medications.
  - Partnership for Prescription Assistance: 1-888-477-2669, www.pparx.org. Programs that provide single point of access for assistance.
  - Patient Advocate Foundation: 1-866-512-3861, www.copays.org. Copay assistance.
  - Patient Access Network: 1-866-366-7263, www.panfoundation.org. Provides support for out-of-pocket costs so patients can afford medical treatments.
  - Patient Services Incorporated: 1-800-366-7741, www.uneedpsi.org. Provides health insurance premium assistance, pharmacy copay, and copay waivers.
  - State Pharmaceutical Assistance Program: Some states offer programs that assist with the cost of prescriptions for the elderly or disabled.
- Transportation: Some agencies may provide services through a volunteer program such as the ACS or your local church or synagogue. Reimbursement may sometimes be obtained through various agencies such as the Leukemia-Lymphoma Society or Cancer Care.

American Society of Clinical Onology Cancer Net, Managing the cost of care	www.cancer.net/managingcostofcare
Cancer Financial Assistance Coalition	www.cancerfac.org/reading/advocacy-orgs.php
Colorectal Care Line	www.colorectalcareline.org
Myria:-Assistance with genetic testing thru Myriad Labs	www.myriadtests.com
National Breast & Cervical Cancer Early Detection Program	www.cdc.gov/cancer/nbccedp
National Children's Cancer Society (scholarships for survivors)	www.children-cancer.org
National Transplant Assistance Fund & Catastrophic Injury Program	www.ntafund.org
Surviving & Moving Forward: The SAM Fund for Young Adult Survivors of Cancer	www.thesamfund.org

Home Health Care

Resource guidance can be provided through your physician's office or through hospital departments of social work or discharge planning. The following require physician orders and, often, preauthorization.

- Durable medical equipment: Equipment that is available through certified local suppliers, such as wheelchairs or walkers.
- Hospice: Comprehensive home care services to individuals with a limited prognosis.
- Visiting nurse/Public health nurse: Provides skilled care, aides, and ancillary services to eligible individuals for limited periods of time
- Proprietary home care agencies: Provides highly technical care at home such as intravenous antibiotics or chemotherapy.

Housing

- American Cancer Society: 1-800-ACS-2345, www.cancer.org. Provides a resource list of free housing opportunities in various geographic locations.
- Joe's House: www.joeshouse.org. A lodging guide for cancer patients.
- National Association of Hospital Hospitality Houses: 1-800-542-9730, www.nahhh.org. Provides a resource list of hospitality houses.
- Ronald McDonald House: www.rmhc.com. Provides housing for families of out-of-town pediatric patients. Contact your physician's office or hospital social work department.

INTERNET RESOURCES

The following is a list of common, but not all-inclusive, Internet sites for people with cancer, their families, and caregivers. Resource books that list Internet sites, such as "A Helping Hand" by Cancer Care may also be helpful. A majority of states have 211 (information) lines that help pinpoint specific agencies that can assist; they can be accessed by dialing 211 or checking the internet at www.211.org.

Aim at Melanoma	www.aimatmelanoma.org
Alliance for Lung Cancer Advocacy Support and Education	www.alcase.org
American Brain Tumor Association	www.abta.org
American Cancer Society	www.cancer.org
American Head and Neck Society	www.headandneckcancer.org
American Institute for Cancer research	www.aicr.org
American Pain Society	www.ampainsoc.org
American Society of Clinical Oncology	www.asco.org
Association of Cancer Online Resources	www.acor.org
American Society for Radiation Oncology	www.astro.org
Blood and Marrow Transplant Newsletter	www.bmtnews.org
Breast Cancer Network of Strength	www.networkofstrength.org

Cancer Care	www.cancercare.org
Cancer Hope Network	www.cancerhopenetwork.org
Cancer Information Service	www.cancer.gov
Cancer Guide	www.cancerguide.org
Cancer Monthly	www.cancermonthly.com
Cancer Network Podcasts	www.cancernetwork.com
Cancer News on the Net	www.cancernews.com
Candlelighters Childhood Cancer Foundation	www.candlelighters.org
Caring Bridge	www.caringbridge.org
ChemoCare	www.chemocare.com
Children's Hospice International	www.chionline.org
Cleaning for a Reason	www.cleaningforareason.org
Clinical Trial Information	www.centerwatch.com
Coalition of Cancer Cooperative Groups	www.cancertrialshelp.org
Colon Cancer Alliance	www.ccalliance.org
Colorectal Care Line	www.colorectalcareline.org
Compassionate Friends	www.compassionatefriends.org
Corporate Angel Network	www.corpangelnetwork.org
Dream Foundation	www.dreamfoundation.com
Gilda's Club International/The Wellness Community	www.gildasclub.org
GIST (Gastrointestinal Stromal Tumor)	www.liferaftgroup.org
Government Benefits	www.govbenefits.gov
Hospice Education Institute	www.hospiceworld.org
I'm Too Young For This	http://i2y.com
Info Line	www.211.org
International Association of Laryngectomees	www.larynxlink.com
International Cancer Information Service Group	www.icisg.org
International Myeloma Foundation	www.myeloma.org
Kids Konnected	www.kidskonnected.org
Lance Armstrong Foundation	www.laf.org
LGBTQ	www.cancer.ca/lgbtq
LGBTQ	www.outwithcancer.com
Leukemia Lymphoma Society	www.lls.org
Living and Working with Cancer (Women)	www.cancerandcareers.org
Living Beyond Breast Cancer	www.lbbc.org
Lotsa Helping Hands	www.lotsahelpinghands.com
Lung Cancer Alliance	www.lungcanceralliance.org
Lymphoma Research Foundation	www.lymphoma.org
Make A Wish Foundation	www.wish.org
Male Care	www.malecare.org
Melanoma Foundation of New England	www.melanomafoundationne.org
Melanoma International Foundation	www.melanomaintl.org
Melanoma Resources	www.melanomaresources.info
National Association for Home Care and Hospice	www.nahc.org
National Association of Insurance Commissioners	www.naic.org
National Bone Marrow Transplant Link	www.nbmtlink.org
National Brain Tumor Society	www.braintumor.org
National Breast Cancer Coalition	www.natlbcc.org
National Childhood Cancer Foundation	www.curesearch.org
National Coalition for Cancer Survivorship	www.canceradvocacy.org
National Comprehensive Cancer Network	www.nccn.com
National Hospice & Palliative Care Organization	www.nhpco.org
National Kidney Cancer Association	www.nkca.org
National Lymphedema Network	www.lymphnet.org
National Marrow Donor Program	www.marrow.org
National Organization of Rare Disorders	www.raredisorders.org
National Ovarian Cancer Coalition	www.ovarian.org
National Prostate Cancer Coalition	www.centerwatch.com/ctrc/npcc
Office of Complementary and Alternative Medicine	www.cancer.gov/cam
Ovarian Cancer National Alliance	www.ovariancancer.org
Pancreatic Cancer Action Network	www.pancan.org
Patient Advocate Foundation	www.patientadvocate.org
Patient Power	www.patientpower.info
People Living with Cancer	www.plwc.org
Planet Cancer	www.planetcancer.org
Prostate Cancer Foundation	www.capcure.org
Prostate Cancer Support	www.malecare.org
Radiology	www.radiologyinfo.org
Ronald McDonald House	www.rmhc.com
Sarcoma Alliance	www.sarcomaalliance.org
Society for Integrative Oncology	www.integrativeonc.org
Society of Gynecologic Oncologists	www.sgo.org
Support for People with Oral & Head & Neck Cancer	www.spohnc.org
Susan G. Komen Breast Cancer Foundation	www.komen.org
The Brian Tumor Society	www.tbts.org
The Multiple Myeloma Research Foundation	www.multiplemyeloma.org
The Oral Cancer Foundation	www.oralcancerfoundation.org
The Skin Cancer Foundation	www.skincancer.org
The Ulman Cancer Fund for Young Adults	www.ulmanfund.org
The Wellness Community	www.thewellnesscommunity.org
Thyroid Cancer Survivors' Association	www.thyca.org
United Ostomy Association	www.uoa.org
Us Too	www.ustoo.com
Vital Options International	www.vitaloptions.org

Proprietary Internet Resources

www.cancereducation.com
www.cancerfacts.com
www.cancernews.com
www.cancerpage.com
www.oncolink.com

LANGUAGE RESOURCES

American Cancer Society	www.cancer.org	Spanish, Asian, Pacific Islander
American Society of Clinical Oncology	www.asco.org	Spanish
Breast Cancer Network of Strength	www.networkofstrength.org	Multilingual
Canadian Breast Cancer Network	www.cbcn.ca/en/	French
Canadian Cancer Society	www.cancer.ca/	French
Cancer Care	www.cancercare.org	Spanish
Cancer Council	www.cancervic.org.au/other_languages	Multilingual
Compassionate Friends	www.compassionatefriends.org	Spanish
Co-Pay Assistance	www.copays.org	Spanish
Danish Cancer Society	www.cancer.dk/Cancer/forside+cancerdk.htm	Danish
Dutch Cancer Society	www.kwfkankerbestrijding.nl/index.jsp	Dutch
Finnish Cancer Society	www.cancer.fi/	Finnish
General Cancer Information	www.cancer.net	Spanish
Germany	www.krebsliga.ch/de/index.cfm	German, French, Italian
Hellenic Cancer Society	www.add.gr/org/hc/index.html	Greek
Hong Kong Cancer Fund	www.cancer-fund.org/en/	Chinese
Israel Cancer Society	www.cancer.org.il/template/default.asp?maincat=26	Hebrew, Russian, Arabic
Leukemia Lymphoma Society	www.lls.org	Spanish
Male Care—Prostate Cancer Support	www.malecare.org	Spanish, French, Hebrew, Italian, Portuguese, Russian, Asian
Maria Sklodowska-Curie Memorial Cancer Center & Institute of Oncology	www.coi.pl/	Polish
National Braile Press	www.nbp.org/	Braile – Prostate
National Cancer Institute	www.cancer.gov	Spanish
National Center of Cancer	www.ligue-cancer.net/	French
Portuguese Cancer Office	www.ligacontracancro.pt/	Portuguese
U PENN—Oncolink	www.oncolink.com	Spanish

LEGAL RESOURCES

- The Cancer Legal Resource Center: 1-866-843-2572, www.CancerLegalResourceCenter.org. Provides free and confidential information on cancer-related legal issues, including health insurance, access to health care, navigating managed care, employment, estate planning, disability insurance, and more.
- LawHelp.org: www.lawhelp.org. Provides basic legal information to people on low incomes. Links to resources in every state, on a state-by-state basis are included.
- American Bar Association: www.findlegalhelp.org.
- Local bar associations typically coordinate pro bono work. Call your local bar association and tell them exactly your issue and ask for a referral. Some even have special projects or sections that can help you.

PALLIATIVE CARE

Focuses on the prevention and relief of physical, emotional, and spiritual pain and suffering, often occurring toward the end of life.

Center to Advance Palliative Care	www.capc.org
Growth House	www.growthhouse.org
Hospice Patients Alliance	www.hospicepatients.org
Last Acts	www.lastacts.org
National Hospice and Palliative Care Organization	www.nhpco.org
Promoting Excellence in End of Life Care	www.promotingexcellence.org

PERSONAL WEBSITES THAT FACILITATE COMMUNICATION

Care Pages	www.carepages.com
Caring Bridge	www.caringbridge.org
My Hope Space	www.myhopespace.com/
My Life Line	www.mylifeline.org

SURVIVORSHIP

Beyond the Cure	www.beyondthecure.org
Lance Armstrong Foundation	www.livestrong.org
National Coalition for Cancer Survivorship	www.canceradvocacy.org
Surviving & Moving Forward: The SAMFund for Young Adult Survivors of Cancer	www.thesamfund.org

TRANSPORTATION

- Air Charity Network: 1-877-621-7177, www.aircharitynetwork.org. Provides access to people in need seeking free air transportation to specialized health care facilities or distant destinations due to family, community, or national crisis.
- Angel Flight: 1-877-621-7177, www.angelflightne.org. Volunteer pilots provide transportation to those in medical and financial need on general aviation aircraft.
- Corporate Angel Network: 1-800-328-1313, www.corpangelnetwork.org. Free air transportation for patients traveling to treatment using empty seats on corporate jets.

- Midwest Miracle Miles: 1-414-570-3644, www.midwestairlines.com. Medical transportation for those in medical and financial need through a registered organization (e.g., hospital). See Website for details about organizational access.
- Miracle Flight: 1-800-359-1711, www.miracleflights.org. Provides medical air transportation to those in medical and financial need.
- National Patient Travel Center: 1-800-296-1217, www.patienttravel.org. Facilitates patient access to appropriate charitable air transportation.
- Operation Liftoff: 1-888-354-5757, www.operationliftoff.com. Provides medical transportation to those children 18 and under with a life-threatening illness. One person may accompany the child, and a discount may be given for the second adult.

WISH FOUNDATIONS

- A Wish with Wings: 1-817-469-9474, www.awishwithwings.com. Grants wishes to children with life-threatening diseases.
- Dream Foundation: 1-805-564-2131, www.dreamfoundation.com. Grants dreams to terminally ill adults.
- Make A Wish Foundation: 1-800-722-9474, www.makeawish.org. Grants wishes to children with life-threatening illnesses.
- Sunshine Foundation: 215-396-4770, www.sunshinefoundation.org. Grants wishes to chronically/terminally ill children whose families are in financial strain.

Selected References

The full list of references for this chapter appears in the online version.

5. Wortman, CB. Social support and the cancer patient. *Cancer* 1984;5(Supp 1): 2339.
11. Guidry JJ, Aday LA, Zhang D, Winn, RJ. The role of informal and formal social support networks for patients with cancer. *Cancer Pract* 1998; 6:31.
12. Cwikel JG, Behar LC, Zabora JR. Psychosocial factors that affect the survival of adult cancer patients: a review of research. *J Psychosoc Oncol* 1997;15:1.
17. Vanderwerker LC, Laff RE, Kadan-Lottick NS, McColl,S., Prigerson, HG. Psychiatric disorders and mental health service use among caregivers of advanced cancer patients. *J Clin Oncol* 2005;23:6899.
21. Hsiao A, Ryan GW, Hayes RD. Variations in provider conceptions of integrative medicine. *Soc Sci Med* 2006;62(12):2973.
23. Marks JP, Reed W, Colby K, et al. A culturally competent approach to cancer news and education in an inner city community; focus group findings. *J Health Commun* 2004;9:143.
24. Institute for Safe Medication Practices. To promote understanding, assume every patient has a literacy problem. www.ismp.org/MSAarticles/promote.html. 2001.
29. Bright MA, Fleisher L, Thomsen C, et al. Exploring e-Health usage and interest among cancer information service users: the need for personalized interactions and multiple channels remains. *J Health Commun* 2005;10:35.
33. Sittig D. Potential impact of advanced clinical information technology on care in 2015. *Cancer Causes Control* 2006;17:813.

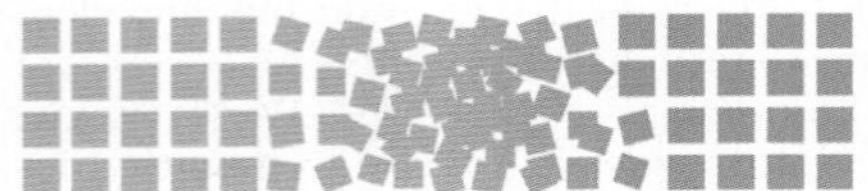

CHAPTER 177 REHABILITATION OF THE CANCER PATIENT

MICHAEL D. STUBBLEFIELD

Physical medicine and rehabilitation, also known as rehabilitation medicine or physiatry, is the medical specialty concerned with restoring and/or maintaining the highest possible level of function, independence, and quality of life. This relatively new specialty has evolved into a number of subspecialties to meet the needs of patients from all age groups and whose primary medical issues may be cardiac, pulmonary, amputation, spinal cord injury, traumatic brain injury, sports injury, or pain, just to name a few. The field of cancer rehabilitation is a rapidly emerging subspecialty of rehabilitation medicine whose primary focus is the evaluation and treatment of functional and pain disorders in cancer patients and survivors. These disorders can result directly or indirectly from cancer, or as importantly, from cancer treatments including surgery, chemotherapy, and radiation. Disorders commonly addressed by the cancer rehabilitation specialist include but are by no means limited to neuromuscular and musculoskeletal pain and dysfunction, spasticity, stroke, hemiplegia, myopathy, neuropathy, spinal cord injury, bowl and bladder dysfunction, amputation, and abnormalities of gait. This chapter will discuss the principles of safe and effective evaluation and rehabilitation of many of the common neuromuscular, musculoskeletal, and functional disorders faced by the cancer patient and survivor. A full accounting of all aspects of rehabilitation of the cancer patient is beyond the scope of this chapter because of space limitations; however, a recent comprehensive reference on the topic of cancer rehabilitation is available.[1]

There is a large but still developing role for rehabilitation medicine in the care of cancer survivors. This need is based not only on the clinical benefits offered by the specialized diagnosis and treatment skills of the physiatrist and other cancer rehabilitation specialists, but also on the vast numbers of patients who are joining the ranks of cancer survivors. As of 2010, there were estimated to be nearly 14 million persons in the United States living with a previously diagnosed cancer.[2] This compares with fewer than 300,000 survivors of spinal cord injury and represents a threefold increase from the estimated 3 million persons who were living with cancer in 1971.[3,4] This increase in cancer survivorship, largely attributable to advances in early detection and treatment, has led to a paradigm shift in how the diagnosis of cancer is perceived, with patients increasingly described as "cancer survivors" as opposed to "cancer victims."[3] The cost of cancer survivorship is high. Patients with cancer may look forward to various combinations of disfiguring surgery, toxic chemotherapy, and the insidious fibrotic effects of radiotherapy. All of these potentially lifesaving or prolonging treatments can result in marked impairments in every aspect of function and quality of life.

Dr. J. Herbert Dietz Jr.[5] can be considered the father of cancer rehabilitation. He noted that the goals for rehabilitation of cancer patients "must be set with realism" and that "individual goals depend on the aggregate variables for each patient."[6] Rehabilitation efforts are usually directed at maximizing function. *Function* is broadly defined as the ability to perform daily routines and includes elements from physical, psychological, social, and vocational domains. Deficits requiring rehabilitation have traditionally been conceptualized into three domains including *impairment* (anatomic or physiologic abnormality), *disability* (functional limitation), and *handicap* (limitation in ability to carry out individual or societal roles).

THE REHABILITATION TEAM

Successful rehabilitation generally benefits from an interdisciplinary team approach.[7] What constitutes an optimal cancer rehabilitation team varies based on the specific needs of a given patient. The core of the rehabilitation team is usually the physiatrist as well as the physical and occupational therapist. The importance of contributions from allied physicians (e.g., medical oncology, radiation oncology, surgical oncology, internal medicine) to maximizing the function and quality of life of cancer patients and survivors cannot be overstated. Similarly, nursing, speech and language pathology, recreational therapy, nutrition, social work, psychiatry or psychology, orthotics, prosthetics, and chaplaincy as well as vocational counselors, hospice liaisons, home care agencies, support groups, and educational outreach programs and many others often play a critical role. Successful rehabilitation of cancer patients and survivors also relies on meaningful contribution to rehabilitation efforts by the patient and, where appropriate, his or her family. Clear, consistent, and effective communication between members of the oncology team, rehabilitation team, patient, and family members is essential. Such communication is especially vital during periods when the patient's clinical status, prognosis, and treatment strategies are changing and it helps that realistic goals and expectations for rehabilitation can be set.[8]

Physiatrist

The *physiatrist* (or rehabilitation medicine specialist) is a neuromuscular and musculoskeletal physician specializing in the assessment and treatment of functional disability. Physiatrists specializing in cancer rehabilitation should also have expertise in the evaluation and treatment of medical comorbidities such as cardiac, pulmonary, and rheumatologic disorders. In addition, they should possess considerable knowledge of oncology and the various oncologic treatments as such information will impact heavily on their ability to safely and effectively restore function and quality of life to their patients. The ability to safely and effectively prescribe medications, modalities, orthotic, prosthetic and assistive devices, and so forth in a way that accounts all the competing medical and psychosocial issues faced by the patient is key to the success of a cancer rehabilitation specialist. The physiatrist serves as the link between the clinical oncology team and the multidisciplinary rehabilitation team to coordinate and optimize rehabilitation efforts. The physiatrist prepares a comprehensive plan for treatment and follow-up in order to increase function, reduce pain, and prevent disability.[9]

Assessment of functional limitations is a primary and critical function of the cancer rehabilitation physician. Functional assessment can be qualitative and geared toward specific limitations of concern to the patient such as steadiness of gait, difficulties with activities of daily living (ADLs), or pain. Several functional assessment tools have utility in the cancer rehabilitation setting including the Karnofsky Performance Scale, Functional Assessment of Cancer Therapy-General Scale, and the Functional Independence Measure.[10–12] Accuracy and specificity in diagnosis is imperative so that rehabilitative treatments can be targeted to provide the maximal clinical benefit while minimizing potential complications of treatment. Accuracy in diagnosing the specific cause of a given disorder starts with a comprehensive clinical evaluation. The key components of such an assessment are the history and physical examination. Physiatrists have extensive training in the use of physical examination to diagnose the multitude of neuromuscular and musculoskeletal disorders common to cancer patients and survivors. Imaging often plays a critical role in evaluation of pain and functional deficits in the cancer setting and may include radiographs, computed tomography (CT), and magnetic resonance imaging (MRI). Imaging, although often invaluable, can be misleading in the accurate diagnosis of a given disorder. The clinician should always strive to demonstrate congruence between the patient's symptoms, physical examination findings, and imaging. Electrodiagnostic testing can be an extremely valuable diagnostic and prognostic tool in the cancer population for evaluation and treatment of neuromuscular and musculoskeletal disorders. A well-designed study can help clarify the etiology of a patient's symptoms, localize peripheral nerve lesions, exclude competing diagnostic possibilities, predict neurologic prognosis, and assist in chemotherapeutic decision making.[8]

Physical and Occupational Therapist

The *physical therapist* generally concentrates on maintenance and/or restoration of the patient's strength, stamina, flexibility, gross motor function, and mobility. Therapy may include training the patient in the proper use of orthotics, prosthetics, and gait aids such as walkers, canes, or crutches. The *occupational therapist* focuses on the restoration of ADLs, emphasizing fine motor function, upper extremity strength, self-care, adapted equipment, orthotic fabrication and fitting, home safety, and cognitive function, among other issues. The physical and occupational therapists are often invaluable in the effective management of pain disorders of all types. Similarly, physical and occupational therapists with specialized training in the use of contemporary decongestive techniques are on the front line of lymphedema management.

Speech and language pathologists are specialized in the evaluation and treatment of dysphagia and communication disorders. The *prosthetists* and *orthotists* assist the physiatrist and therapist in the evaluation of gait and functional deficits including impaired ADLs and then construct and fit braces and prostheses designed to aid mobility and function. The *recreational therapist* provides leisure activities and facilitates community reintegration including independence at school, work, and other social settings. *Vocational rehabilitation* involvement would allow persons with physical disabilities to engage in gainful employment. The role of *psychologist*, *social worker*, and *nutritionist* are described in other chapters.

COMPLICATIONS OF CANCER AND ITS TREATMENT

The complications of cancer and its treatment represent a broad and diverse group of disorders that are covered in detail throughout this textbook. In the context of cancer rehabilitation, several specific disorders are of interest as they can impact heavily on the safety and effectiveness of rehabilitative efforts. It is imperative for the clinician to fully understand that there are no absolutes in oncology and that every decision made with or on behalf of a patient has an implicit cost-benefit analysis underlying it. This is as true of the for the physical or occupational therapist deciding if it is safe to ambulate a patient as it is for the neurosurgeon deciding whether or not to attempt resection of metastatic disease compressing the spinal cord. Bad outcomes are common in cancer and can happen at any time unexpectedly and occasionally dramatically. Our charge as rehabilitation specialists is to maximize function and quality of life while minimizing, to the best of our ability and knowledge, the potential adverse outcomes. Unfortunately we are often met with choosing between two very daunting options. For instance, do we attempt to ambulate a patient with a recently diagnosed deep vein thrombosis (DVT) who cannot be anticoagulated, or have an inferior vena cava filter placed because of competing medical conditions or because the patient refused it? This scenario and other equally challenging situations are not uncommon in oncology. The unknown risk of precipitating a pulmonary embolus (PE) and potentially contributing to a patient's death must be carefully weighed against the equally unknown and potentially deadly risk of maintaining the patient on bed rest indefinitely. This decision making carries no less gravity than subjecting a patient to a surgical procedure that carries a high mortality rate. The potential risks and benefits, when known, must be carefully considered, not in isolation but with input from other members of the clinical staff, the patient, and the family. All persons involved in this decision-making process should understand that the ultimate outcome in advanced cancer is invariably bad and that courses of action carefully considered and made with the best interest of the patient in mind were likely the correct decision regardless of the outcome.

Direct Effects of Cancer

The direct effects of cancer are often obvious, with clinical impact on function being dependent largely on the location and extent of disease. For instance, a large lung mass compromising pulmonary function and subsequently endurance and stamina, or an epidural metastasis to the spine compressing the spinal cord causing weakness and pain. A working understanding of several of the direct complications of cancer including its effects on the central and peripheral nervous system and on bony integrity are of great importance in cancer rehabilitation and will be discussed in detail in subsequent sections.

Paraneoplastic Effects

Paraneoplastic syndromes (PNS) are rare disorders ($<1\%$ of cancer patients) that cause tissue or organ damage via remote effects of a primary or metastatic cancer.[13] Most PNS occur because the tumor secretes a substance that mimics normal hormones or that interferes with circulating proteins. Systemic paraneoplastic disorders include cancer cachexia, hypercalcemia, Cushing syndrome, and Trousseau syndrome.[14–17] A number of PNS affect the central (limbic encephalitis, encephalomyelitis, cerebellar degeneration, opsoclonus-myoclonus, optic neuropathy/retinopathy, brainstem encephalitis, stiff person syndrome, motor neuron disease, necrotizing myopathy) and peripheral (sensory neuronopathy, acute sensorimotor neuropathy, chronic sensorimotor neuropathy, neuromyotonia, chronic gastrointestinal pseudo-obstruction/autonomic neuropathy, Lambert-Eaton myasthenic syndrome, myasthenia gravis, inflammatory myopathy) nervous system with potentially devastating impact on function and quality of life.[18] These disorders, although relatively rare, represent a significant therapeutic challenge to the rehabilitation specialist.

Chemotherapy

Chemotherapy is a cornerstone of cancer treatment for many malignancies and may be given either with intent to cure or to prolong life. The myriad complications of the ever-growing number of agents are discussed at length in other chapters. The impact of these complications on function and quality of life depends on the specific derangement or complications induced by the agent. Anemia, neutropenia, thrombocytopenia, myopathy, cardiomyopathy, neuropathy, contracture, fatigue, thromboembolism, nausea, and edema are just a few of the common disorders resulting from chemotherapy that can have a major impact on rehabilitation efforts. Several of these complications and their specific implications for rehabilitation will be discussed in subsequent sections.

Radiotherapy

Approximately 50% of cancer patients will be subjected to radiation therapy at some point during the course of their disease, and radiation may play a critical role in as many as 25% of cancer cures.[19] Despite the important beneficial effects of radiation in cancer care, its adverse effects on normal tissue are a major source of disability for both patients with active cancer and cancer survivors. Evaluation and treatment of the long-term complications of radiation are an extremely important component of the clinical activities of cancer rehabilitation specialist and will be discussed in detail later.

Surgery

Postsurgical impairments depend not only on the anatomic site and extent of the procedure but also on any medical comorbidity the patient may have. Surgical complications are common in the cancer setting and impact heavily on overall outcome as well as rehabilitation needs. Rehabilitation is often instrumental in returning function and quality of life to patients following surgery. Efforts may be directed at the restoration of functional disorders ranging from diminished stamina following prolonged bed rest to restoration of a limb following hemipelvectomy. The postsurgical rehabilitation needs of any given patient are unique.

Thromboembolism

There are considerable and high-quality data available on the prevention and treatment of thromboembolism, including comprehensive guidelines specific to the cancer setting.[20] There are comparatively little data concerning the safe and effective rehabilitation of patients with thromboembolism. The dogma from the not-too-distant past was to immobilize patients with DVT and range of motion (ROM) exercises for 2 to 10 days, presumably to allow the clot to mature by the formation of fibrin cross-links and thereby decrease the risk of it breaking free to become a PE. This commonly followed, long-held, and non–evidence-based recommendation was ultimately supported by a limited study suggesting that immobilization of the affected limb for at least 48 to 72 hours while the patient is anticoagulated was justified and prudent to prevent PE.[21] The development of low-molecular-weight heparin (LMWH) prompted a re-evaluation of 48- to 72-hour bed rest recommendation as patients with acute DVT treated with LMWH injections at home did at least as well in terms of recurrent thromboembolism and bleeding as did patients treated in the hospital with unfractionated heparin delivered intravenously.[22,23] Although not directly applicable to patients in either the inpatient or outpatient rehabilitation setting, the realization that no increase in morbidity or mortality was seen in patients with acute DVT treated with LMWH injections served as justification for liberalization of the bed rest recommendation that had inhibited rehabilitation efforts, particularly on inpatient rehabilitation wards.

Although the question of when a patient with lower extremity DVT can begin to ambulate has not been answered with the same evidence-based rigor as other questions concerning thromboembolism, there is a growing body of clinical trials on the topic that that support the safety and potential benefits of early mobilization.[24–29] Several reviews and one meta-analysis are also available and support the safety and benefits of early mobilization following both DVT and PE while dispelling the recommendation for bed rest as part of the early management of thromboembolism.[30–35]

Upper extremity DVT (UEDVT) represents about 10% of DVTs and can be idiopathic but is more often associated with central venous catheter use, pacemakers, or cancer.[36] The relative incidence of UEDVT may be rising because of increased use of central venous catheters and is associated with PE in up to one-third of patients. Other conditions associated with UEDVT include postthrombotic syndrome, superior vena cava syndrome, septic thrombophlebitis, thoracic duct obstruction, and brachial plexopathy.[37] Despite the high incidence of conversion of UEDVT to PE, no studies are available to address the multitude of questions concerning the rehabilitation of patients with UEDVT. This lack of data concerns such basic issues as the safe timing and type of exercise that can safely done following diagnosis of UEDVT as well as if and when decongestive therapy (massage, wrapping, pumps) for upper extremity swelling disorders such as lymphedema can be performed. Lack of even basic data on these matters represents a major shortcoming in our overall knowledge on the topic of cancer rehabilitation and challenges our ability to guide risk-benefit analyses for patients with UEDVT who will likely benefit from physical, occupational, or decongestive therapy.

Although not strictly evidence-based because of major shortcomings in the literature concerning the rehabilitation of patients with thromboembolism, the guidance developed by the author and used at the Memorial Sloan-Kettering Cancer Center is presented in Table 177.1. It is critical to remember that each patient and situation is unique and that these recommendations are only starting points that should not supersede clinical judgment and assessment of the risks and benefits to the patient of engaging in a given activity.

Other Medical Disorders

The evidence base for the safe and effective rehabilitation for rehabilitation of patients with a variety of general medical disorders is also limited. Despite this limitation, guidance with widespread clinical use has evolved on such issues as thrombocytopenia, anemia, neutropenia, cardiac dysfunction, pulmonary dysfunction, and electrolyte abnormalities. In general, these recommendations that are thought applied

TABLE 177.1

GUIDELINES FOR PHYSICAL, OCCUPATIONAL, AND LYMPHEDEMA THERAPY IN PATIENTS WITH VENOUS THROMBOEMBOLISM

- Lower extremities
  1. For patients with acute lower extremity deep vein thrombosis (DVT), with or without pulmonary embolism (PE), and no inferior vena cava (IVC) filter, therapy (including physical, occupational, and lymphedema with bandaging and manual lymphatic drainage) can be initiated once they are *therapeutic* on an anticoagulant. Resistive exercises should generally be deferred for 48–72 hours. Definition of therapeutic anticoagulation by modality:
     - Low-molecular-weight heparin (LMWH) preparations are preferred as they are therapeutic immediately following the first injection. Monitoring is not required. Common preparations include: enoxaparin (Lovenox), dalteparin (Fragmin), and tinzaparin (Innohep).
     - Unfractionated heparin may take 1 to 2 days to become therapeutic and is more prone to bleeding complications than LMWH. The adjusted partial thromboplastin time should be monitored and therapy can begin when it is between 50 and 70.
     - Warfarin (Coumadin) may take several days to become therapeutic. The international normalized ratio should be monitored and therapy can begin when it is between 2 and 3.
  2. For patients with acute lower extremity DVT (with or without PE) and an IVC filter, therapy can be initiated *immediately* regardless of their anticoagulation status.
  3. For patients with acute lower extremity DVT who cannot be anticoagulated and an IVC filter cannot be placed, therapy can be started immediately but should be *functional* in nature (ambulation, balance, activities of daily living [ADLs] training) and avoid resistive and repetitive exercises. Such patients are at very high risk for PE and death. Therapists are advised to discuss therapy interventions with the patient's primary or rehabilitation medicine physician so that the relative risks and benefits of therapy can be better delineated.
- Upper extremities
  1. Upper extremity DVT carries the same risk for PE and death as lower extremity DVT. IVC filters are not protective. For patients with acute upper extremity DVT with or without PE, therapy (including physical, occupational, and lymphedema with bandaging and manual lymphatic drainage) can be initiated once they are *therapeutic* on an anticoagulant. Resistive exercises should generally be deferred for 48–72 hours. (See above anticoagulation guidelines.)
  2. For patients with acute upper extremity DVT who cannot be anticoagulated, therapy should be *functional* in nature (ambulation, balance, ADLs training) and avoid resistive and repetitive exercises. Such patients are at very high risk for PE and death. Therapists are advised to discuss therapy interventions with the patient's primary or rehabilitation medicine physician so that the relative risks and benefits of therapy can be better delineated.

to rehabilitation are based on indirect evidence from the medical literature. Exercise precautions for cancer patients with a variety of disorders are presented in Table 177.2. Again, the potential risks and benefits of pursuing any course of therapy must be carefully weighed.

NEUROMUSCULAR COMPLICATIONS OF CANCER AND CANCER TREATMENT

The treatment of neuromuscular complications of cancer is a major component of the services offered by both the rehabilitation medicine physician and the physical and occupational therapists. Such disorders include those of the brain, spinal cord, nerve roots, plexus, peripheral nerve, and muscle.[38]

Brain Dysfunction

The brain, along with the myriad cognitive and physical functions that it serves, is often compromised in the cancer setting. Such dysfunction can result from direct effects of tumor, from paraneoplastic effects, from treatment or other medical disorders.

Brain tumors vary widely in aggressiveness and in prognosis. Even a benign or relatively low-grade lesion may have severe functional consequences depending on location. It is unclear to what extent tumor type or location impacts rehabilitation prognosis; however, some studies suggest a tendency for better gains in meningioma patients and in those with left hemispheric lesions.[39,40]

The most common neurologic deficits in brain tumor patients undergoing acute rehabilitation include impaired cognition (80%), weakness (78%), and visual-perceptual impairment (53%), with most patients have multiple impairments.[41] Although overall prognosis may be a factor, most rehabilitation disposition decisions are guided by the patient's neurologic status, clinical course, and activity tolerance. A patient whose neurologic status is actively worsening will likely not benefit from intensive rehabilitation.

Specific rehabilitation interventions depend on the combination of deficits and are generally similar to measures used for patients with other etiologies of brain disorders, such as traumatic brain injury or stroke. Rehabilitation efforts are directed toward such goals as the improvement of bed mobility, transfers, self-care, ambulation, and, if necessary, wheelchair training. Strategies are employed to promote functional cognition, clear communication, bowel and bladder continence, safe swallowing, adequate nutritional intake, optimal sensory input (including vision and hearing), and restorative sleep. Attention must be paid to prevention of complications of impaired mobility such as skin breakdown or DVT. Similarly, complications related to the primary tumor and other comorbidities such as pain, neurologic decline, seizure, and depression should be evaluated and treated. The hemiplegic patient will generally benefit from gait training with an assistive device and a brace such as an ankle-foot orthosis (AFO) when appropriate. Proper arm positioning, with support of the shoulder to prevent pain in a flaccid or spastic limb, should be used. A variety of adaptive equipment is available for individuals who

TABLE 177.2

EXERCISE PRECAUTIONS FOR CANCER PATIENTS

Medical Problem	Laboratory Values	Recommendations
THROMBOCYTOPENIA Normal values: platelets 150,000–450,000/m^3	30,000–50,000/m^3	ROM, aerobic activity, light weights (1–2 lb; no heavy resistance or isokinetic exercise); ambulation
	20,000–30,000/m^3	Self-care, gentle passive/active ROM, aerobic activity, ambulation
	<20,000/m^3	Ambulation and self-care with assistance as needed for safety; minimal/cautious activity; essential ADLs only
ANEMIA Normal values: hematocrit 37%–47%; hemoglobin 12–16 g/dL	Hematocrit <25%, hemoglobin <8 g/dL	ROM exercise, isometrics; avoid aerobic or progressive programs
	Hematocrit 25%–35%; hemoglobin 8–10 g/dL	Light aerobics, light weights (1–2 lb)
	Hematocrit >35%; hemoglobin >10 g/dL	Activity as tolerated
NEUTROPENIA Normal values: ANC <1,500/mm^3.	ANC 500–1,000/mm^3	Infection risk moderate; consider increased hygiene procedures and limited contact with other patients, particularly if further nadir anticipated
	ANC <500/mm^3	Infection risk high; strict hygiene and limit contact with other persons
PULMONARY DYSFUNCTION Pulmonary function tests, chest radiograph	Maintain pulse oximetry >90%	Titrate O_2 supplementation
	50%–75% of predicted FEV_1 or diffusion capacity	Light aerobic exercise
	75%+ of predicted FEV_1 or diffusion capacity	Most programs fine
	Large plural effusions or pericardial effusions or multiple metastases to lungs	ROM; few submaximal isometrics; consult cardiologist and oncologist
CARDIAC DYSFUNCTION Ejection fraction, electrocardiogram	Recent PVCs; fast atrial arrhythmia; ventricular arrhythmia; ischemic pattern	No aerobics; consult cardiologist
ELECTROLYTE ABNORMALITIES Na	Below 130	No exercise
K^+	Below 3.0 or above 6.0 requires treatment	No exercise

ROM, range of motion; ADLs, activities of daily living; ANC, absolute neutrophil count; FEV_1, forced expiratory volume in 1 second; PVCs, premature ventricular contractions.

must perform tasks one-handed, such as reachers, sock donners, and elastic shoelaces.

Cognitive strategies often rely on compensations such as keeping a regular routine and maintaining a journal or "memory notebook." The patient's insight into cognitive deficits may be impaired, and education regarding these deficits can allow the patient to more effectively compensate and allow the family, friends, and caregivers to have appropriate expectations. In some cases, especially those in which cognitive status is anticipated to remain fairly stable, in which functional expectations are high, or where conflict or confusion exists about the patient's abilities, neuropsychological testing helps to more fully define the extent of cognitive deficits and also to elucidate cognitive strengths. For example, determining whether an individual learns best with auditory, written, or nonverbal presentations can facilitate the most efficient compensation for cognitive deficits. Pharmacologic and nonpharmacologic therapies to address pain, spasticity, mood, bowel/bladder, and sleep/wake issues are often indicated.

Functional recovery is similar in patients with brain tumors as compared with acute stroke.[42] Better functional improvement is a significant predictor of longer survival in patients with brain metastases and glioblastoma multiforme. The literature suggests that the length of stay for inpatient rehabilitation in brain tumor patients is generally shorter than patients with other brain disorders such as traumatic brain injury and stroke.[39,40] This may relate to better initial functional status; other possible contributing factors include fewer behavioral sequelae, better social supports, and expedited discharge planning because of prognostic factors.[43] In one study, although functional status improved during rehabilitation, quality-of-life scores did not improve until discharge home. The Functional Independence Measure and the disability rating scale are more sensitive than the Karnofsky Performance Status Scale in detecting change in functional status.[44]

Spinal Cord Dysfunction

Symptomatic spinal cord injury (SCI) due to spinal metastasis occurs in up to 5% of all cancer patients.[45] Patients with cancer can develop SCI as a direct result of their cancer, its treatment, and other pre-existing or acquired conditions. SCI in the cancer setting often presents a significant decision-making and management challenge.[46] This challenge is compounded as cancer-related SCI most often occurs as a late complication when poor overall prognosis and declining medical status can significantly and adversely impact rehabilitation interventions and functional prognosis.

Life expectancy following spinal surgery varies with cancer type. One study demonstrated a median survival of 7.7 months for all cancer types combined, with colon cancer patients surviving only 3.3 months and lung cancer patients only 3.6 months. Sarcoma, prostate, renal cell, and breast carcinoma did better, with median survival ranging from 7.8 to 15.4 months.[47] A retrospective evaluation of patients with neoplastic SCI admitted for inpatient rehabilitation demonstrated a combined median overall survival time of only 4.1 months from the date of rehabilitation admission to death. Patients with gastrointestinal cancer had an even poorer prognosis, with a median survival of only 0.6 months.[48] The phase of cancer treatment can have a profound impact on survival and prognosis for functional recovery. A patient with metastatic prostate or breast cancer, for instance, whose initial presentation is with SCI and has not received systemic therapy, can be expected to have a much better prognosis for survival and functional restoration than a patient who has undergone and failed multiple treatment options.

SCI in the cancer setting can result directly from the cancer (epidural, leptomeningeal, or intramedullary tumor) (Fig. 177.1), indirectly from the cancer (paraneoplastic phenomenon), or from treatment of the cancer (radiation, chemotherapy, surgery). Other causes of SCI in the cancer setting may include infection (meningitis, epidural abscess, diskitis/osteomyelitis), vascular disorders (hemorrhage, infarct), degenerative disorders (cervical spinal stenosis), and even metabolic disorders (osteoporotic compression fractures).

The vertebral body is the most common site of metastasis within the spine, largely reflecting its volume relative to other spinal structures. Metastatic tumors of the spine are more common than primary spine tumors. Cancers that commonly metastasize to the spine are those of breast, lung, prostate, and kidney.[49] Epidural tumor is the most common cause of SCI in cancer and can arise from the vertebra, enter the spinal canal through the neural foramen, or be deposited hematogenously in the epidural space. Leptomeningeal metastases

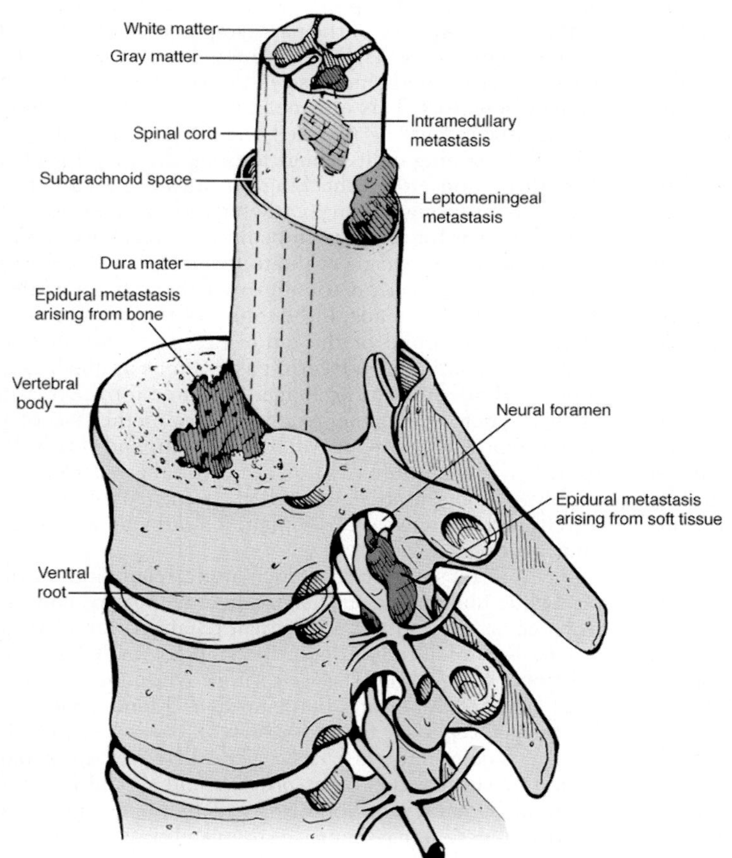

FIGURE 177.1 The spinal cord and nerve roots can be affected by metastatic or primary tumors arising from epidural, intramedullary, or leptomeningeal spaces. (From ref. 1, with permission.)

occur in 3% to 8% of all cancer patients and can be associated with significant neurologic dysfunction. The most common tumors that metastasize to the leptomeninges include leukemia, lymphoma, melanoma, breast, and lung cancer.[50] Intramedullary tumors are the rarest of the tumors that affect the central nervous system (CNS) but can produce profound neurologic deficits that vary depending on the location and pathology of the tumor.

SCIs are classified according to the level and completeness of the motor and sensory dysfunction using the American Spinal Injury Association (ASIA) impairment scale.[51] The ASIA impairment scale includes five letter grades (A to E) denoting impairment and ranging from complete paresis (ASIA-A) to normal (ASIA-E). The neurologic level of injury is described as the most distal level at which motor function or sensation is preserved. Although most neoplastic SCI is from circumferential compression by epidural-based tumor, other syndromes may occur. These include the anterior cord, central cord, conus medullaris, cauda equina, and Brown-Séquard syndromes. Selective damage to the dorsal spinal columns (posterior cord syndrome) or the spinocerebellar tracts are rare but may be seen.

SCI from epidural-based tumor generally affects all spinal tracts either completely or to varying degrees. Asymmetric compression does occur and can have unpredictable patterns in early compression but generally progresses to affect all components of the spinal cord. Clinically, such patients present with weakness, bowel and bladder dysfunction, and multimodal sensory loss including light touch, pain, vibration, and proprioception. Pain, if present, is usually local.

The level of injury significantly affects the potential for functional recovery. It should be noted that the degree of functional recovery anticipated in a patient with a nonmalignant cause of SCI (such as trauma from a motor vehicle accident) is generally greater than that anticipated in malignant SCI. This is because patients with cancer tend to develop SCI later in their disease and usually progress in their cancer and other medical comorbidities.

Some general guidelines from the nonmalignant population of patients with SCI at 1 year postinjury based on the level of SCI, however, may be illustrative of the maximal potential recovery anticipated for patients with cancer.[52] Persons with a C3 injury or above usually require long-term ventilation. Those with a C4 level injury may be able to wean off the ventilator. Persons with a C5 level of injury may be partially independent, with skills such as feeding and grooming with the aid of orthoses. A patient with C6 injury maintains active wrist extension, and, thus, these patients can use tenodesis to improve their grasp. Persons with a C6 level of injury are usually independent, with feeding, grooming, and upper extremity hygiene after assistance with setting up the utensils. They also have the potential to independently transfer with a transfer board. The C7 injury is the key level for becoming independent in most activities at the wheelchair level. Persons with a C7 level of injury should be able to transfer without a transfer board and drive a custom-adapted van or car. Those with C8 and T1 injuries have improved hand function. The preserved thoracic levels provide the ability to maintain trunk stability. They should all be independent, with ADLs and mobility skills at the wheelchair level. Persons with thoracic levels of injury have the potential to stand with the aid of orthoses and assistive devices for therapeutic benefit. The person with lower thoracic and high lumbar levels of injury may be able to stand and ambulate with lower extremity orthoses and assistive devices. This is generally for therapeutic endeavors and short household distances only because of the high cost of energy required to perform these activities. Persons with injuries at the L3 level or lower have the potential to ambulate in the community with the use of orthoses and assistive devices such as canes or walkers. In general, the more caudal the level of injury, the greater the potential for rehabilitation and functional independence.

The care of patients with acute SCI includes maintenance of ventilation in those with high levels of injury. It also includes treatment of pain, autonomic dysregulation, and bowel and bladder dysfunction. Patients are at risk of developing DVT, PE, pulmonary and urinary tract infections, fecal impaction, decubiti, immobilization hypocalcemia, spasticity, contractures, and osteoporosis. A comprehensive treatment plan includes DVT and PE prophylaxis, spirometry and chest physiotherapy; initiation of intermittent urinary catheterization every 4 to 6 hours when urine volumes are less than 2,000 mL/d; initiation of a bowel program; turning every 2 hours; and use of high-airflow mattresses, use of heel protectors, and daily physical therapy and ROM.[53]

The use of LMWH is currently recommended for DVT and PE prophylaxis during the acute management phase of SCI. The independent use of low-dose unfractionated heparin, elastic compression stockings, and intermittent pneumatic compression devices is not recommended. When used alone, they appear to be relatively ineffective. It is recommended that LMWH be continued or converted to full-dose oral anticoagulation for a minimum of 3 months or at least until completion of the rehabilitation phase.[54]

Patients with injuries above the T6 level are at risk of developing autonomic dysreflexia, which is defined as an increase in blood pressure of greater than 20 mm Hg above baseline. It results from stimulation of the splanchnic division of the sympathetic nervous system by a noxious stimulus below the level of the lesion and causes the sympathetic responses of vasoconstriction and hypertension. The body's autoregulation mechanisms are interrupted because of the spinal cord lesion, and the uncontrolled blood pressure continues. Classically, the patient's heart rate decreases because of the intact response of the parasympathetic nervous system via the vagus nerve. The patient may develop a severe headache, experience an increase in spasticity, and describe a vague discomfort. This is a medical emergency and immediate treatment must be initiated, including sitting the person upright, loosening tight-fitting clothing, checking for bladder distention, and either checking an indwelling catheter for kinks or initiating urinary catheterization. A urine sample should be sent for analysis and culture. A rectal examination should be performed to evaluate for and treat fecal impaction and an inspection for ingrown toenails and infected decubiti should be made. If the source of the autonomic stimulation is not found or the blood pressure continues to be elevated, or both, nitroglycerin paste can be applied. Oral or sublingual nifedipine is no longer indicated for the treatment of this hypertensive emergency because of the risk of profound hypotension, myocardial infarction, and death. If the source of the stimulus is not found or the blood pressure continues to be elevated, or both, the patient should be transferred to the intensive care unit for treatment with intravenous nitroprusside.[52]

The patient's ability to participate in rehabilitation therapies while undergoing further treatments must be considered when an acute or subacute inpatient rehabilitation program is sought. Rehabilitation programs for those with SCI due to spinal tumors have been shown to improve mobility and self-care.[55] Research indicates that clinical and functional status is a valuable prognostic factor for survival of those with SCI due to metastatic tumor disease.[56] The rehabilitation program should be started as early as possible and should be of short duration.[48] Thus, selection of patients who have potential to improve function may improve survivability as well as quality of life and ability to perform ADLs and mobility.

Peripheral Nervous System Dysfunction

Radiculopathy can result from any of a number of disorders that affect the nerve root; it is a very common cause of pain and disability in the cancer setting. Radiculopathy can occur from compressive or rarer noncompressive etiologies. The incidence of radiculopathy in the cancer patients and survivors is unknown but it is likely that the most nerve root pathology results from the same degenerative disorders, largely spondyloarthropathies, that affect the general population with a prevalence of 3% to 5%.[57] One large study on the epidemiology of cervical radiculopathy in a population of patients in Rochester, Minnesota, placed the average annual age-adjusted incidence at 83.2 per 100,000.[58] Degenerative causes of radiculopathy can be discogenic (i.e., herniated nucleus pulposus), from hypertrophy of ligaments and other soft tissues (i.e., ligamentum flavum), or from excess bone formation (i.e., osteoarthritis). The narrowing of the spinal canal or neural foramen with subsequent compression of neural and vascular structures resulting from one or more degenerative processes is called *spinal stenosis*. Lumbar spinal stenosis is estimated to affect 1 in 1,000 persons older than 65 years of age.[59]

Compressive radiculopathy resulting directly from cancer most commonly results from epidural tumor that can arise from the vertebral body, paravertebral structures, or epidural space itself.[60] Intradular tumor including leptomeningeal and intramedullary disease can also cause compressive radiculopathy. Of these, compression by leptomeningeal disease is far more common, affecting 5% to 8% of patients with cancer.[60]

Noncompressive causes of radiculopathy include radiation, chemotherapy, and paraneoplastic syndromes as well disorders such as acute idiopathic polyradiculoneuropathy, a subtype of Guillain-Barré syndrome (GBS), chronic idiopathic demyelinating polyradiculoneuropathy (CIDP), amyloidosis, sarcoidosis, diabetes mellitus, and rheumatologic disorders (Fig. 177.2).[1] *Herpes zoster* is also a common cause of radiculopathy in the cancer setting causing a dermatomal vesicular rash known as shingles (Fig. 177.3).[61] Herpes zoster causing dermatomal pain without a rash is termed *zoster sine herpete*.[62] Eruption of herpes zoster is related to immunosuppression from cancer, steroids, and chemotherapy, with 1% to 2% of cancer patients having at least one infection during the course of their disease.[63] Polyradiculopathy from radiation may mimic leptomeningeal tumor as the cauda equina may demonstrate enhancement on MRI (Fig. 177.2).[64]

Although relatively uncommon, radiculopathy from radiation has been reported as sequelae of testicular cancer, vertebral metastases, and lymphoma.[65–70] In the author's clinical experience radiation-induced radiculopathy is most commonly seen in Hodgkin's lymphoma (HL) survivors who have

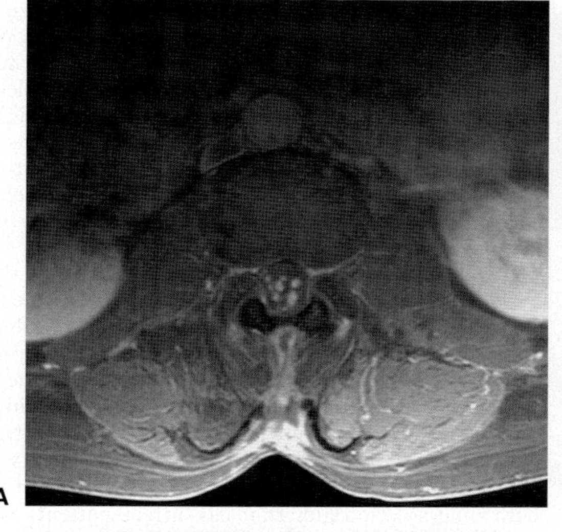

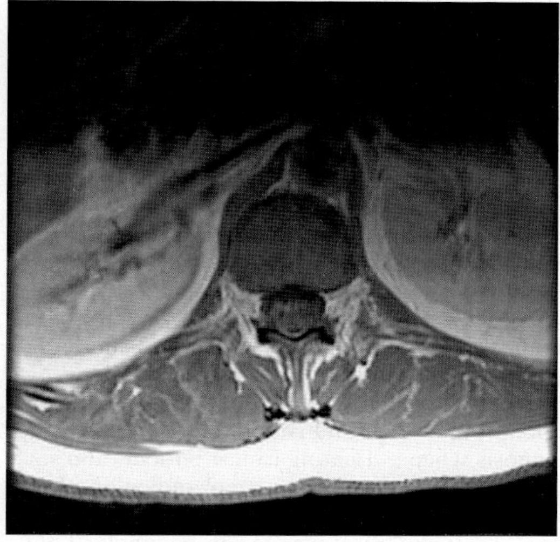

FIGURE 177.2 Radiculopathy can result from variety of etiologies and may demonstrate gadolinium enhancement on magnetic resonance imaging (MRI). **A:** Radiation-induced cauda equina enhancement in a patient with testicular cancer. **B:** Cauda equina enhancement from a chronic idiopathic demyelinating polyradiculoneuropathy from Waldenström's macroglobulinemia. **C:** Cauda equina enhancement from leptomeningeal metastases in a patient with breast cancer.

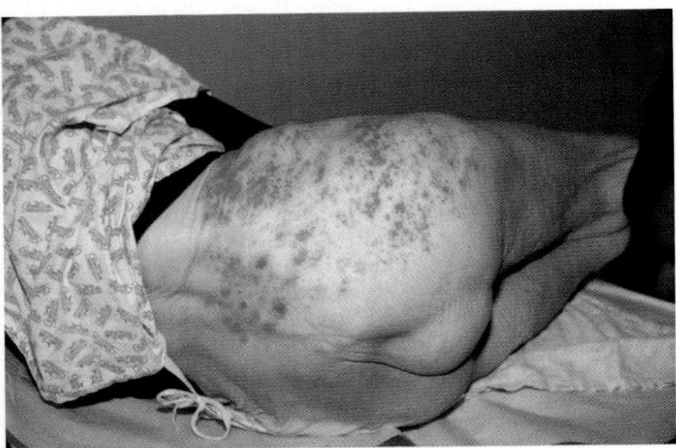

FIGURE 177.3 Shingles eruption in the distribution of multiple lumbar dermatomes in a patient with metastatic breast cancer. Reactivation and eruption of herpes zoster is common in the cancer setting because of immunosuppression and should be considered in the evaluation of patients presenting with neuropathic pain in a dermatomal distribution. Reactivation with pain but without a rash can occur and is known as *zoster sine herpete*.

received mantle field (MF) or periaortic radiation, and head and neck cancer patients often in conjunction with plexopathy. Neurotoxic chemotherapy can also adversely affect the nerve root as part of a more generalized neuropathy. Patients with pre-existing radiculopathy from a degenerative or other cause may be particularly predisposed to the adverse effects of neurotoxic chemotherapy.[71] Subacute motor neuronopathy is a paraneoplastic disorder described in patients with HL, non-Hodgkin's lymphoma, and thymoma as a subacute lower motor neuron syndrome that involves primarily the lower extremities without pain, significant sensory loss, or upper motor neuron findings. Secondary thinning of the ventral nerve roots and widespread patch segmental demyelination of spinal nerve roots, brachial, and lumbosacral plexus can be seen histologically in addition to patchy degeneration and loss of anterior horn cells and occasional inflammatory infiltrates.[72] Non–cancer-related causes of noncompressive radiculopathy including diabetes, rheumatologic disorders, and idiopathic radiculoneuropathies such as GBS and CIDP are not uncommon in the general population and should be included in the differential diagnosis when evaluating cancer patients and survivors with signs and symptoms suggestive of radiculopathy.

Plexopathy affects as many as 1% of cancer patients.[73] The cervical, brachial, or lumbosacral plexus can be involved and the etiology can be neoplastic or radiation-induced as well as idiopathic (idiopathic brachial neuritis, CIDP, GBS), diabetic (diabetic radiculoplexus neuropathy), or traumatic (surgery). Malignancy most commonly affects the brachial plexus followed by the lumbosacral plexus, and least commonly the cervical plexus.[74] Benign tumors of the plexus are usually reported to be more common than malignant ones.[75–77] Radiation plexopathy is a common component of the radiation fibrosis syndrome that is characterized by insidious fibrosis with axonal demyelination and ultimately axonal loss. Radiation plexopathy is commonly seen with radiculopathy. Radiation to the plexus can rarely cause a mild reversible syndrome but is more commonly a delayed and progressive one.[78] Delayed radiation-induced brachial plexopathy usually occurs after a latent interval that can vary from a few months to several years with a peak onset of neurologic symptoms occurring between 2 and 4 years after radiation.[79] The upper plexus is commonly affected preferentially in HL survivors treated with MF radiation and head and neck cancer patients, possibly because of the longer course of the upper trunk and lateral cord of the brachial plexus through the neck as well as the pyramidal shape of the thorax, providing less protective tissue. Additionally, the upper plexus may represent the most caudal extend of radiation delivered for some head and neck cancer patients. Differentiating radiation-induced from malignant plexopathy is a diagnostic challenge and both etiologies may be present together. Imaging with contrast MRI is the diagnostic test of choice.[80] Malignant etiologies of plexopathy are generally more painful than radiation-induced plexopathy, although either can manifest severe pain.[81] Myokymia on needle electromyography is suggestive of a radiation-induced etiology but does not exclude a malignant component.[82]

Idiopathic brachial neuritis (IBN), also known as neuralgic amyotrophy, Parsonage-Turner syndrome, and other synonyms, has an incidence of approximately 2 to 3 per 100,000 person-years.[83] The disorder can be idiopathic or hereditary. The idiopathic form is often precipitated by antecedent events such as infection, immunization, strenuous exercise, surgery, and a variety of other causes.[83] Clinically, IBN is classically characterized by severe and acute burning pain in the shoulder and arm that may last for several days or weeks and is followed by muscle weakness, atrophy, and sensory loss, and then the pain diminishes. IBN may go unrecognized in cancer patients if only the obvious cancer and treatment-related causes of brachial plexopathy are considered. Similarly, diabetic radiculoplexus neuropathies can affect the cervical, thoracic, and lumbosacral nerve roots as well as the brachial and lumbosacral plexus. Perhaps the best known of these disorders is diabetic lumbosacral radiculoplexus neuropathy, also known as diabetic amyotrophy among other synonyms. Diabetic lumbosacral radiculoplexus neuropathy usually presents clinically with unilateral acute to subacute and severe lower extremity pain in the thigh or leg that may spread to the entire extremity.[84] Like IBN, diabetic lumbosacral radiculoplexus neuropathy may go unrecognized in the cancer setting if only neoplastic or treatment-related etiologies are considered and can occur even with relatively low blood glucose levels, as might be seen with steroid-induced hyperglycemia.

Neuropathy is any condition arising from the damage and dysfunction of the peripheral nerves, including the motor, sensory, and autonomic nerves that connect the CNS (brain and spinal cord) to the rest of the body.[85] The peripheral nerve includes the nerve root and plexus as well as the peripheral nerve proper. Peripheral neuropathy is common in the cancer setting as a result of neurotoxic chemotherapy or radiation as well as from direct and paraneoplastic effects of cancer. Neuropathy is also very common in the general population with diverse etiologies that can affect patients with cancer even if unrelated to malignancy or its treatment. Such etiologies include toxic or metabolic derangements (diabetes mellitus, vitamin B_{12} deficiency, alcoholism), inherited disorders (Charcot-Marie-Tooth syndrome), paraprotein disorders (monoclonal gammopathy of unknown significance [MGUS]), critical illness neuropathy, and idiopathic disorders such as CIDP or GBS, just to name a few.[86] The clinical manifestations of neuropathy may include any combination of weakness, sensory deficits, pain, and autonomic dysfunction with resultant gait and other functional deficits. Often, multiple peripheral nervous system disorders such as radiculopathy and neuropathy coexist, compounding the clinical features of each disorder. It is important to remember that, as previously described, any pre-existing pathology at any part of the neuron (nerve root, plexus, or peripheral nerve), even if asymptomatic, may predispose the patient to development of weakness, paresthesias, pain, and other signs and symptoms commonly described as "neuropathy" when challenged with a neurotoxic chemotherapy or another insult to the peripheral nervous system. This phenomenon is termed *neuronal predisposition*.[71]

Peripheral neuropathy is one of the most common chronic complications of cancer and its treatment. It may be caused by a variety of chemotherapeutic agents including the taxanes (paclitaxel, docetaxel), the vinca alkaloids (vincristine, vinorelbine, vinblastine), the platinum analogues (cisplatin, carboplatin, oxaliplatin), bortezomib, thalidomide, and others.[71,87–89] The clinical, pathophysiologic, and electrodiagnostic features of the various neurotoxic chemotherapeutics vary significantly. The taxanes and vinca alkaloids are tubulin inhibitors and cause a predominately length-dependent motor and sensory axonal polyneuropathy in a distal symmetric distribution.[87] Clinically, this causes paresthesias, pain, sensory ataxia, and potentially weakness during and immediately following treatment that usually improves when the treatment is stopped. The platinum analogues, however, damage the cell body of the sensory nerves in the dorsal root ganglion, and at higher doses can damage the anterior horn cell within the spinal cord. It is the accumulation of the platinum analogues within neuron cell body with subsequent DNA damage and altered cellular activities that underlies the toxicity.[90] The clinical manifestations include severe sensory deficits including sensory ataxia and pain usually without significant weakness. Because the platinum analogues accumulate in the cell body, the deficits can progress for months following treatment, a phenomenon known as *coasting*. Electrophysiologically, neuropathy due to platinum analogues may demonstrate a widespread decrease in sensory nerve action potential amplitudes *without* a proximal to distal gradient. In such cases of non–length-dependent neuropathy it is possible to see an electrophysiologic pattern wherein the sensory nerve action potential amplitudes in the upper extremities (shorter nerves) are lower than those in the lower extremity nerves (longer nerves).[91] This pattern is useful not only in differentiating non–length-dependent from length-dependent neuropathies associated with tubulin inhibitors, but also from other causes of peripheral nervous system dysfunction likely to be encountered in the oncology setting, including radiculopathy, chronic idiopathic demyelinating polyradiculopathy, and diabetic neuropathy.

The need for evaluation of neuropathy is largely dependent on the context in which a patient develops neuropathic signs and symptoms. If a patient develops the expected signs and symptoms from chemotherapy or other treatment that is expected to produce those symptoms, then no further investigation is generally indicated. It is when a patient develops signs and/or symptoms that exceed what is generally anticipated or at a time when they would not have been expected to have complications of treatment that a workup is indicated. For instance, a patient with metastatic prostate cancer who develops lower extremity pain and weakness on hormonal therapy needs evaluation, as opposed to one who develops the same symptoms on paclitaxel. In the former case, it is prudent to consider a very broad differential diagnosis and eliminate possibilities systematically and logically as many of the causes of such symptoms are curable or highly treatable. Oncologic causes such as epidural spinal cord compression, leptomeningeal metastases, intramedullary metastases, and paraneoplastic disorders should be considered along with degenerative causes of lower extremity pain and weakness such as spinal stenosis, disk herniation, facet arthropathy, and compression fracture. Similarly, idiopathic and acquired causes of neuropathy should be considered including disorders like diabetic amyotrophy, vitamin B_{12} deficiency, Lyme disease, alcoholism, paraprotein neuropathies (MGUS), and CIDP. As with the nerve root and plexus, radiation can cause damage to any peripheral nerve in the radiation field. Such damage is usually obvious when it affects one or more named nerves in an extremity but may be less obvious when it affects nerves on the trunk such as the dorsal scapular nerve to the rhomboid muscles or the supraspinous nerve to the supra and infraspinatus muscles. These nerves are commonly affected by MF radiation and radiation for head and neck cancer. Radiculopathy mimicking peripheral neuropathy is an extremely common cause of lower extremity symptoms in cancer patients because of their often advanced age and predisposition to spinal degenerative disease. Acquired neuropathy including MGUS and CIDP are also relatively common and should be considered in the evaluation of patients with idiopathic neuropathies.[86,92]

Myopathy

Myopathy in the cancer setting can occur as a result of a variety of processes including direct invasion by primary or metastatic tumor, paraneoplastic disorders, inflammatory disorders (polymyositis, dermatomyositis, inclusion body myositis), infiltrative disorders (amyloid), toxins, or more commonly as a result of corticosteroid use or critical illness. Radiation can cause a focal nemaline rod myopathy.[93] Skeletal muscle metastases are relatively rare but can occur from a variety of tumor types including lung, breast, melanoma, thyroid, and liver.[94] Paraneoplastic necrotizing myopathy characterized by rapidly progressive proximal muscle weakness that occurs over months can be seen in association with breast, small cell lung, gastrointestinal, genitourinary, bladder, ovarian, and prostate carcinomas as well as melanoma, multiple myeloma, and head and neck cancer.[95] Each of the inflammatory myopathies has a distinct clinical phenotype and unique myopathologic features.[96] Amyloid myopathy is rare but can be seen as a complication of multiple myeloma or primary amyloidosis.[97,98] Vincristine, alcohol, and a variety of other agents can cause a toxic myopathy.[99]

By far the most common therapy-induced myopathy is steroid myopathy from glucocorticoid use. Steroid-induced myopathy is characterized by fast-twitch or type II muscle fiber atrophy with decreased fiber cross-sectional area and reduced myofibrillar protein content.[100] Steroid use is associated with a variety of adverse side effects that are related to the total and daily dose, duration of therapy, and poorly understood patient susceptibility facors.[101] In one small prospective study, glucocorticoid use was found to contribute to proximal muscle weakness in 9 of 15 (60%) patients and was severe enough to interfere with ADLs in 6 of 15 (40%) treated patients.[102] The development of steroid myopathy was rapid, occurring within 15 days in eight of nine patients who developed weakness. Ten of 16 (63%) patients also demonstrated a significant decline in respiratory function. Steroid myopathy is painless and usually demonstrates proximal weakness most evident on physical examination to affect the shoulder and hip girdle muscles with relative preservation of distal muscle strength. This pattern of weakness helps differentiate steroid myopathy from most types of neuropathy that cause distal relative to proximal weakness. In addition, sensation and reflexes should be preserved in steroid myopathy and abnormal in neuropathy. Although most cases of steroid myopathy are mild to moderate, at its extreme measure it can cause complete tetraplegia and respirator dependence. Most patients with steroid myopathy recover, some completely; the course of resolution can be on the order of months to years.

Critical illness myopathy is not unique to the cancer setting but because of the nature of cancer it is commonly seen. Critical illness myopathy is often associated with critical illness polyneuropathy. The first sign of these disorders is often difficulty in weaning a patient from a ventilator that is not explained by pulmonary, cardiovascular, or other disorder.[103] The clinical features and time course for resolution of critical illness myopathy are similar to those of steroid myopathy.

Evaluation of Neuromuscular Disorders

The key components of evaluation of neuromuscular disorders are history and physical examination. The etiology of most disorders can be elucidated with confidence by a skilled clinician in the majority of cases as most disorders, even in the cancer setting, have an obvious cause. More extensive evaluation with imaging, electrodiagnostic testing, and other laboratory studies is indicated when competing diagnoses are in consideration and require exclusion. Imaging is extremely useful when compressive etiologies of peripheral nervous system dysfunction are possible such as tumor or degenerative changes. Although a variety of tests have utility in select situations, MRI is usually the modality of choice for imaging the peripheral nervous system.[104,105] Intravenous gadolinium is useful in the identification of peripheral nerve and plexus tumors, leptomeningeal disease, and intramedullary spinal cord tumors as well as to differentiate scar from tumor, exclude infection, and identify radiation changes.[50,106] Nerve roots may be seen to enhance with gadolinium in acute idiopathic polyradiculoneuropathy and CIDP as well as radiation-induced radiculopathy (Fig. 177.2).[65–70,86]

Electrodiagnostic testing with nerve conduction studies and needle electromyography is often extremely useful in clarifying the etiology of symptoms (radiculopathy vs. plexopathy vs. neuropathy vs. myopathy), clarifying the type of neuropathy (i.e., axonal vs. demyelinating, polyneuropathy vs. mononeuropathy multiplex vs. mononeuropathy), and localizing a lesion (i.e., femoral mononeuropathy at the inguinal ligament vs. intrapelvic). Electrodiagnostic testing can also assist in chemotherapeutic or radiotherapeutic decision making, predict neurologic prognosis, and exclude disorders in the differential diagnosis. Specialized expertise is often needed in the electrophysiological assessment of cancer patients and survivors that may not be available at all centers.[85] Laboratory tests are often useful in evaluation of peripheral nervous system dysfunction, particularly neuropathy. Such tests may include complete blood count, erythrocyte sedimentation rate or C-reactive protein, vitamin B_{12}, folate (methylmalonic acid with or without homocysteine for low-normal vitamin B_{12} levels), comprehensive metabolic panel (fasting blood glucose, renal function, liver function), thyroid function tests, serum protein immunofixation electrophoresis, glucose tolerance test if indicated to evaluate for impaired glucose tolerance, and urine protein electrophoresis with immunofixation.[107] Specialized laboratory investigations may also be indicated depending on other clinical features exhibited or expressed by the patient. Evaluations may include but are not limited to those for connective tissue diseases with vasculitis (antinuclear antigen profile, rheumatoid factor, anti-Ro/SSA, anti-La/SSB, antineutrophil cytoplasmic antigen antibody, cryoglobulins), infections (hepatitis B and C, human immunodeficiency virus, cytomegalovirus), sarcoidosis (serum angiotensin converting enzyme), dysimmune disorders (antiganglioside antibody profile [GM1, GDla, GDlb, GD3, GQ1b, GT1b, antimyelin-associated glycoprotein]), and a paraneoplastic panel (anti-Hu, anti-CV2).[107]

Treatment of Neuromuscular Disorders

The treatment of peripheral nervous system disorders can be highly specific (injection of a median mononeuropathy at the wrist) or extremely general (prescription of opioids for pain). The most common impairments experienced by patients with peripheral nervous system dysfunction include pain and weakness with subsequent disorders of mobility and ADLs. Skin breakdown, secondary musculoskeletal derangements (i.e., Charcot joint, rotator cuff tendonitis/adhesive capsulitis), contracture, osteoporosis, and other conditions can also result. Dysfunction of the peripheral components of the autonomic nervous system can cause orthostatic hypotension, gastroparesis, constipation, urinary retention, erectile difficulties, and a variety of other autonomic derangements.

Specific treatments depend largely on accuracy of diagnosis of the underlying disorder. For instance, severe and disabling hand pain may be from a CNS cause (thalamic or funicular pain), radiculopathy, plexopathy, a polyneuropathy, or a mononeuropathy such as the median mononeuropathy responsible for carpel tunnel syndrome. In addition to neuromuscular causes of pain, a variety of musculoskeletal disorders such as osteoarthritis and tenosynovitis as well as infections and neoplasms should be considered in the differential diagnosis as they can coexist with or mimic neuromuscular dysfunction.

A primary responsibility of the cancer rehabilitation physician is as diagnostician. Accurate diagnosis of pain and functional disorders is often instrumental in guiding other clinicians in the care of patients, including on such important matters as whether or not to give or stop chemotherapy or which lesion to radiate. For instance, the treatment of hand pain that is due to carpel tunnel syndrome is very different from the treatment offered for a metastasis to the brachial plexus. A guide to the expected physical examination findings (pain/sensory abnormalities, weakness pattern, reflex abnormalities) anticipated from the various common central and peripheral nervous system abnormalities is listed in Table 177.3. A full accounting of the specific treatments for each of these disorders is beyond the scope of this chapter because of space limitations.

A comprehensive discussion on the management of neuropathic pain is discussed in elsewhere in this textbook. Again, the first step in effective treatment of neuropathic pain is its identification. Treatment may include behavior modification, physical and/or occupational therapy, modalities such as transcutaneous electric nerve stimulation (TENS) or ultrasound, splints and braces, injections and other procedures, and finally medications. Weakness and difficulties with ADLs can often be improved with physical and/or occupational therapy. Bracing may be required to compensate for certain weakened muscles, particularly the foot dorsiflexors, where an AFO is often indicated. Discussions on nonpharmacologic pain management and orthotic use are presented in the following sections.

MUSCULOSKELETAL COMPLICATIONS OF CANCER AND CANCER TREATMENT

Musculoskeletal disorders represent a diverse group that includes derangement of muscle, ligament, tendon, joint, cartilage, bone, and associated tissues. Included are arthritis, tendonitis, tenosynovitis, bursitis, myofascial pain, and countless other disorders. The pain associated with musculoskeletal disorders is somatic from activation of nociceptors in affected structures as opposed to neuropathic. There may be considerable overlap as when neuromuscular disorders (i.e., C5 radiculopathy) play a causal role in the development of musculoskeletal disorders (i.e., rotator cuff tendonitis).[108] As with neuromuscular disorders, musculoskeletal disorders are extremely common in the general population as well as the cancer setting. The accurate assessment of musculoskeletal disorders, including the differentiation of benign from malignant etiologies of pain, is an important component of the cancer rehabilitation physician's duties. It is often the case that benign musculoskeletal disorders cause as much morbidity as malignant ones. Successful identification and treatment of these disorders can help improve the function and quality of life of cancer patients and survivors. A full accounting of the

TABLE 177.3

PHYSICAL EXAMINATION FINDINGS IN PAINFUL NEUROLOGIC DISORDERS

Location	Pain/Sensory Abnormalities	Weakness Distribution	Reflex Abnormality
CENTRAL NERVOUS SYSTEM			
Thalamus	Contralateral to lesion, varies from discrete (i.e., arm only) to entire side of body	None (unless other structures involved)	None (unless other structures involved)
SPINAL CORD			
Ascending spino-thalamic tracts	Contralateral if small lesion or bilateral if larger lesion, varies from discrete (i.e., arm only) to entire side of body	None (unless other structures involved)	None (unless other structures involved)
ROOT			
C5	Posterior-lateral shoulder, lateral arm, lateral forearm	Rotator cuff, shoulder abduction < elbow flexion	Biceps tendon < brachio-radialis tendon
C6	Posterior-lateral shoulder, lateral arm, lateral forearm, thumb, index finger	Rotator cuff, shoulder abduction < elbow flexion, forearm pronation, wrist extension	Biceps tendon < brachio-radialis tendon, pronator teres tendon
C7	Posterior arm, posterior forearm, index/middle fingers	Elbow extension, wrist extension, finger extension	Triceps tendon
C8	Posterior-medial arm, posterior-medial forearm, little/ring fingers	Long finger extensors, long finger flexors < hand intrinsics	Finger flexors
T1	Anterior-medial arm, anterior-medial forearm (little/ring fingers generally spared)	Long finger extensors, long finger flexors < hand intrinsics	Finger flexors
T2 to T12	Corresponding thoracic dermatome (i.e., T4 nipples, T10 navel)	Corresponding thoracic myotome (rarely clinically evident)	None
L1	Upper low back, lateral hip, groin	None	None
L2	Upper/middle low back, lateral hip, groin, high anterior and medial thigh	Hip flexion < knee extension	Patellar tendon
L3	Middle low back, lateral hip, middle anterior and medial thigh	Hip flexion < knee extension, hip adduction	Patellar tendon
L4	Middle/low back, lateral hip, lateral thigh, knee, medial leg	Knee extension < ankle dorsiflexion	Patellar tendon
L5	Low back, buttock, lateral hip, posterior/lateral thigh, lateral leg, dorsal foot, big toe	Hip abduction, knee flexion, ankle and toe dorsiflexion, foot inversion and eversion	Medial hamstring tendon
S1	Low back, buttock, lateral hip, posterior thigh, posterior leg, lateral and plantar foot	Hip extension, knee flexion, plantar flexion, toe flexion	Achilles tendon, lateral hamstring tendon
S2 to S5	Posterior leg (S2), saddle anesthesia	None	None
Cauda equina syndrome	Varies, all lumbar roots possible, saddle anesthesia common	Varies, all lumbar roots possible	Varies, all lumbar roots possible
Conus medullaris	Varies, all lumbar roots possible, loss of bladder function common	Varies, all lumbar roots possible	Varies, all lumbar roots possible
PLEXUS			
Anterior cervical	Anterior neck	None	None
Upper trunk brachial	Shoulder, lateral arm, lateral forearm, lateral hand	Rotator cuff, shoulder abduction, elbow flexion, radial wrist extension (rhomboid and serratus anterior spared)	Biceps tendon, brachio-radialis tendon
Middle trunk brachial	Posterior arm and hand	Elbow extension (partial), wrist extension, finger extension (brachioradialis spared)	Triceps tendon
Posterior cord brachial	Posterior arm and hand	Shoulder abduction (past first 30 degrees), elbow extension, wrist extension, finger extension	Triceps tendon
Lower trunk brachial	Medial arm, medial forearm, little/ring fingers	Long finger extensors, long finger flexors, hand intrinsics	Finger flexors
Lumbar	Anterior thigh	Hip flexors, knee extensors, leg adductors	Patellar tendon

(*continued*)

TABLE 177.3

(CONTINUED)

Location	Pain/Sensory Abnormalities	Weakness Distribution	Reflex Abnormality
Lumbosacral trunk	Buttock, lateral leg, dorsum of foot	Hip extensors (variable), knee flexors (variable), dorsiflexion, ankle inversion, ankle inversion, toe flexion	Medial hamstring tendon
Sacral	Buttock, lateral hip, posterior thigh, posterior leg, lateral and plantar foot	Anal sphincter (variable), hip extensors, knee flexors, plantar flexors	Achilles tendon
NERVE			
Occipital	Posterior head	None	None
Trigeminal	Face	Masticatory muscles (rarely clinically evident)	None
Intercostobrachial	Axilla, medial arm	None	None
Axillary	Lateral arm	Shoulder abduction, external rotation	None
Musculocutaneous	Lateral forearm	Elbow flexion, supination	Biceps tendon
Radial	Distal posterior arm, posterior forearm, posterior-lateral hand	Elbow extension (spared if lesion below spiral groove), wrist extension, finger extension, supination	Triceps tendon (if above spiral groove), none (if below spiral groove)
Ulnar	Anterior-medial hand, posterior-medial hand	Finger flexion (4th–5th digits), Finger abduction (spares thumb abduction)	Finger flexors
Median	Anterior-lateral hand	Forearm pronation, wrist flexion, finger flexion (2nd–3rd digits), Thumb abduction (spares finger abduction)	None
Lateral femoral cutaneous	Anterior-lateral thigh (spares medial thigh)	None	None
Femoral	Anterior-medial thigh (spares lateral thigh), medial leg, medial foot	Hip flexion (if intrapelvic lesion, spared if at inguinal ligament), knee extension	Patellar tendon
Sciatic	Posterior buttock, posterior thigh, posterior-lateral leg, plantar foot	Hip extension < knee flexion, dorsiflexion, plantar flexion, foot eversion and inversion, toe flexion	Achilles tendon, hamstring tendons
Peroneal	Anterior-lateral leg, dorsum of foot	Dorsiflexion, foot eversion	None
Tibial	Plantar foot	Plantar flexion, foot inversion	None
Polyneuropathy	Generally distal symmetric in a "stocking and glove" distribution	Generally in distal muscle groups	Varies, generally distal tendon reflexes
Mononeuropathy multiplex	Varies by nerves affected	Varies by nerves affected	Varies by nerves affected
Small-fiber neuropathy	Generally distal symmetric in a stocking and glove distribution (affects pain/pinprick and temperature sensation but spares light touch, vibration and proprioception)	None	None

assessment and treatment of the countless musculoskeletal disorders is not possible because of space limitations.

Bony Metastases

Bone metastases are a common complication of cancer, found to occur in 69% of patients with advanced breast cancer in one study.[109] Of those, 85% had widespread skeletal involvement. The primary risk of bony metastases is fracture, with subsequent pain and disability. Long-bone fracture, in particular, poses a significant risk to the patient as pain may be severe and ambulation and ADLs compromised. Patients with bony metastatic disease may require protected weight bearing, either to avoid further bony injury (e.g., in the healing phase after radiation therapy and/or surgical stabilization of pathologic fracture) or to assist in pain control. Thus, if rehabilitation management is to include progressive mobility, assistive devices, ADL training, or other activities that place the patient at risk for pathologic fracture, the patient should be assessed for bony integrity at known sites of bony metastases. Additionally, the patient should be screened for occult sites of bony metastases that might present a fracture risk at the time of treatment or in the future.

Various criteria have been developed to quantify the risk of sustaining a pathologic fracture but none are useful except in long bones.[110] Mirels[111] proposed a scoring system to quantify the risk of sustaining a pathologic fracture through a metastatic lesion in a long bone based on the site (upper limb, lower limb, peritrochanteric), pain (mild, moderate, functional), lesion type (blastic, mixed, lytic), and size relative to the diameter of affected bone (less than one-third, one-third to two-thirds, greater than two-thirds). Each of these four variables was given a score of 1, 2, or 3 according to the degree of risk. It was determined that lesions with a cumulative score of 7 or lower could be safely irradiated without risk of fracture, but lesions with a score of 8 or higher required prophylactic internal fixation prior to irradiation. A recent study comparing various methods found only axial cortical involvement of more than 30 mm and circumferential cortical involvement as predictive of fracture; the former measure has the advantage of being accessible via plain radiograph.[112] In practice, the actual lesion size may be difficult to delineate because of infiltrative, permeating pattern and surrounding osteopenia. Factors such as histology (with highly vascular or lytic lesions perhaps at highest risk) and location (importance to weight bearing) are also considerations.[113] A walker or crutches are needed for complete non-weight bearing of a lower limb. A single cane can be used in cases of smaller, but painful, lesions. For somewhat larger or more symptomatic lesions, a forearm crutch permits approximately 25% more force transmission through the device than a conventional cane.

The three-column model of Denis[114] is often used in assessing stability. This model divides the spine into anterior (anterior longitudinal ligament, anterior half of vertebral body and disk), middle (posterior half of vertebral body and disk, and posterior longitudinal ligament), and posterior (posterior elements) columns. The lesion is considered unstable if two or more columns are involved or, in some cases, if the middle column alone is involved. Bilsky[115] has developed a conceptual framework to guide therapeutic decision making with respect to surgical, radiotherapeutic, and chemotherapeutic options for spine tumors. This tool for individual patient assessment is known as the "NOMS" criteria and is based on an evaluation of the neurologic (N), oncologic (O), mechanical instability (M), and systemic disease (S) status of the patient. In this model, mechanical instability is defined simply as movement-related pain referable to a focus of tumor. Instability pain is distinguished from biologic or tumor-related pain in that is does not respond to steroids. Tumor involving the atlantoaxial complex (C1-2) usually presents with rotational pain. Such patients are considered unstable if they have a fracture subluxation greater than 5 mm or angulation greater than 11 degrees with greater than 3.5 mm subluxation. Patients meeting these radiographic criteria are generally offered operation at presentation, while those with less than 5 mm subluxation can be irradiated in a hard collar (usually a Miami J design as it comes in a variety of sizes, is more adjustable, and more comfortable than other designs) and weaned 6 weeks following completion of radiation. Bracing is rarely used to treat instability of the subaxial cervical, thoracic, and lumbar spine as operation is the treatment of choice in those instances. In cases where surgery is indicated but unable to be performed because of other clinical contraindications or patient refusal, a thoracolumbar corset can provide limited support and pain relief. Use in combination with gait aids, such as a walker, minimizes torque across the spine. Bed rest should be avoided because additional functional loss will occur, and thromboembolic disease may complicate the course.

RADIATION FIBROSIS SYNDROME

Radiation therapy uses high-energy radiation to kill proliferating tumor cells with relative sparing of the surrounding normal cells, which are typically less active. The primary effect of radiation on tissues is the induction of apoptosis or mitotic cell death from free radical-mediated DNA damage. A variety of secondary effects occur that are mediated by cytokines, chemokines, and growth factors including activation of the coagulation system, inflammation, epithelial regeneration, and tissue remodeling. Radiation causes endothelial cell apoptosis, increased endothelial permeability, expression of chemokines, and expression of adhesion molecules with the subsequent loss of vascular thromboresistance. The loss of vascular thromboresistance is a result of decreased fibrinolysis, increased expression of tissue factor and von Willebrand factor, and decreased expression of prostacyclin and thrombomodulin. The increased expression of tissue factors and increased local thrombin formation occurs both intravascularly and in the perivascular areas and extracellular matrix by increased vascular permeability. It is the accumulation of thrombin in the intravascular and extravascular compartments that results in progressive fibrotic sclerosis of radiation affected tissues and thus fibrosis.[116]

Radiation fibrosis can damage any tissue type including skin, muscle, ligament, tendon, nerve, viscera, and even bone.[117] The effects of radiation can be experienced acutely during or immediately following treatment. Radiation effects can also be early-delayed (up to 3 months) or late-delayed (more than 3 months) following completion of treatment.[118] Fatigue is generally an acute or early-delayed complication of radiation therapy. Radiation fibrosis is generally a late complication, and may manifest years after treatment, progress rapidly or insidiously, and is not reversible.[116]

The term *radiation fibrosis syndrome* (RFS) describes the clinical manifestations that result from the progressive fibrotic sclerosis that follows radiation treatment. RFS results locally at the treated site, and may also cause distant effects when a neural structure passing through a radiation field is damaged.[119] The radiation field can be sharply localized; however, some radiation fields are quite extensive.[120] The mantle radiation field used to treat supradiaphragmatic HL, for instance, involves all lymph nodes in the neck, chest, and axilla, while the inverted-Y radiation field involves the periaortic and ilioinguinal lymph nodes. The combination of mantle and inverted-Y radiation is known as *total nodal irradiation* (Fig. 177.4). Such broad radiation fields can result in widespread sequelae including radiculopathy, plexopathy, neuropathy, myelopathy, cardiomyopathy, and pulmonary fibrosis.[121]

Radiation damage to the CNS is also classified temporally: acute, early delayed, and late delayed. Acute encephalopathy occurs days to weeks after initiation of treatment, and early-delayed encephalopathy at 1 to 6 months likely represents transient demyelination. Clinical manifestations include irritability, loss of appetite, exacerbation of tumorlike symptoms, Lhermitte's sign, and in children, somnolence syndrome.[116,118] Late-delayed encephalopathy, caused by irreversible white matter necrosis, may rarely occur. Early-delayed encephalopathy usually responds well to corticosteroids, but late-delayed encephalopathies respond less consistently. Memory loss or cognitive dysfunction may result from brain atrophy after whole-brain irradiation. Other side effects of cranial irradiation include fatigue, loss of taste, decreased salivation, impaired gag reflex, and decreased hearing.[122]

Radiation-induced myelopathy is usually of insidious onset several months or years after treatment. Clinical manifestations include progressive paresis, proprioceptive and other sensory deficits, spasticity, incontinence, and, occasionally, pain. Patients may have gait dysfunction from weakness, sensory loss, or spinal ataxia. Involvement of spinal tracks can be asymmetric and present as a Brown-Séquard syndrome. Unfortunately radiation-induced myelopathy that becomes clinically evident will usually progress.

Radiation fibrosis can damage any peripheral nervous system structure. Such injury can cause focal paraspinal muscle spasms, distant muscle spasms, referred pain, local pain, and weakness.[108] The upper brachial plexus may be more prone to

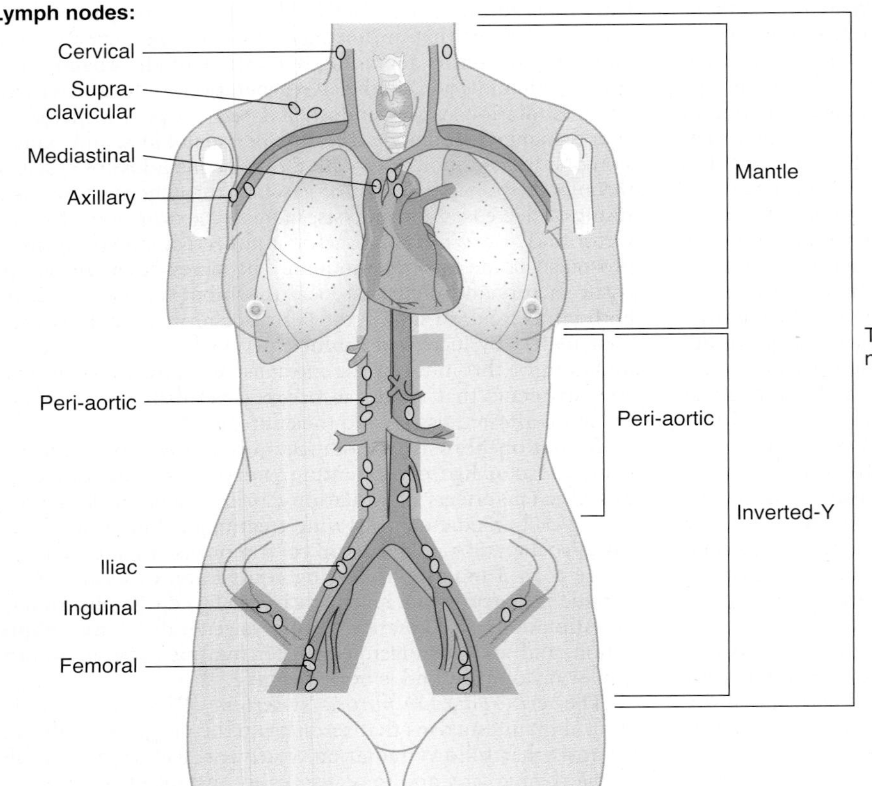

FIGURE 177.4 Radiation fields commonly used in the treatment of Hodgkin's lymphoma include the mantle, periaortic, and inverted-Y, among others. When all nodes are radiated it is known as *total nodal irradiation*. The late-term morbidity experienced by Hodgkin's lymphoma survivors often depends on the extent of their radiation treatment. (From ref. 1, with permission.)

damage than other plexus structures because of its superior location within the pyramid shaped chest where it is less protected by overlying tissue.[73] Muscle cramps commonly occur as a result of radiation damage, and are thought to arise from spontaneous discharges at any level of the motor nerve with resultant volleys of neural activity being sent to and across the neuromuscular junction. thereby involuntarily activating the muscle.[123] Myokymic discharges are common (but not pathognomonic) in radiation damage to the peripheral nervous system and are responsible for some of the muscle spasm seen in the RFS. Myokymia is seen clinically as vermiculations (wormlike movements under the skin) and have a characteristic sound and appearance on needle electromyography. Myokymia is thought to result from ephaptic cross-talk between motor nerves that have been focally demyelinated. Progressive fibrosis in muscle fibers within the radiation field can cause a focal myopathy that is associated with nemaline rods.[93] Myopathic muscles are weak relative to normal muscle and prone to spasm and pain. Myelopathy, radiculopathy, plexopathy, neuropathy, and myopathy (myelo-radiculo-plexo-neuro-myopathy) any clinical combination of these disorders (i.e., radiculo-plexo-neuro-myopathy) may be seen together with devastating functional effects such as severe head drop (Fig. 177.5).

Although RFS can potentially result from treatment with radiation for any cancer type, it is commonly encountered in head and neck cancer and HL patients and survivors.

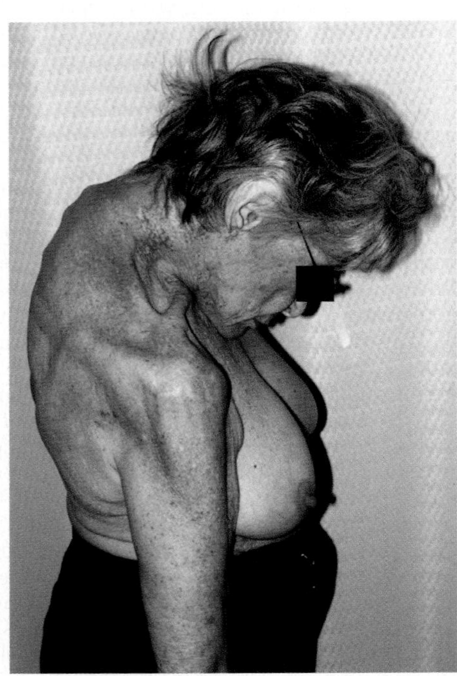

FIGURE 177.5 Head drop in a woman treated with resection and radiation for nasopharyngeal carcinoma. Severe atrophy of the right deltoid, biceps, supraspinatus, infraspinatus, and trapezius muscles is present. The woman has electromyographically documented cervical polyradiculopathy, brachial plexopathy involving predominately the upper plexus, mononeuropathies of several nerves within the radiation field, and myopathy of the cervical paraspinal musculature. (From Stubblefield MD. Radiation fibrosis syndrome. In: Cooper G, ed. *Therapeutic Uses of Botox*. 1st ed. Totowa, NJ: Humana Press, 2007:19, with permission.)

RFS in Head and Neck Cancer

Treatment-related musculoskeletal and neuromuscular complications are common in head and neck cancer. Surgical complications of radical neck dissection include facial lymphedema, wound infection and dehiscence, injury to cranial nerves V, VII, X, and XII, and carotid injury. Complications of RFS include focal neuropathic pain, weakness, muscle spasm, and bone necrosis, with vulnerable structures including muscles, cervical nerve roots, brachial plexus, and peripheral nerves, including the dorsal scapular nerve to the rhomboids, cranial nerve V to the masseter, trigeminal divisions of cranial nerve V, the anterior cervical plexus, C5, C6, and the upper brachial plexus. Muscle directly in the radiation field may weaken from a progressive nemaline rod myopathy. Muscle spasm is common from myopathy, compromised neural innervation, ectopic activity from damaged neural structures, and even ectopy within the muscle itself. Trismus and radiation-induced cervical dystonia are common. The effects of radiation and surgery often compound one another to devastating effect.

Asymmetric neck motion results from removal of the sternocleidomastoid, scalene, platysma, and other muscles.[124] Shoulder depression and protraction may result from sacrifice of the spinal accessory nerve with loss of trapezius muscle function. The rhomboids and levator scapula muscles become overstretched and the pectoralis major muscle is shortened. The sternoclavicular joint bears increased weight, leading to clavicle subluxation and potentially arthritic changes. This malalignment of the shoulder is often painful and leads to further dysfunction by impingement of the rotator cuff with tendonitis and even adhesive capsulitis.[108] Treatment should emphasize maintenance of neck and shoulder ROM and avoidance of excessive internal rotation at the shoulder and scapular protraction (the "sling" position). Stretching the pectoralis major muscle and strengthening of the remaining scapular stabilizer muscles should be pursued. Immediate postsurgical rehabilitation after radical neck dissection and other surgeries for head and neck cancer should involve guidance from the surgeon, taking into account skin, vascular, and bone integrity. In general, however, the therapy involves passive neck ROM, emphasizing flexion and rotation, beginning when the sutures are removed, to the limits of graft or suture line stretch, progressing to active ROM and isometric strengthening by week 4. Some patients may experience dyspnea because of loss of the sternocleidomastoid and platysmas muscles for accessory respiration, and they will benefit from instruction in breathing exercises and energy conservation techniques.

Trismus is a common complication of head and neck cancer and its treatment with a prevalence estimated range from 5% to 38%.[125] Impairment in mouth opening may have an adverse effect on quality of life by compromising functions such as chewing, swallowing, and breathing.[126,127] Maintenance of oral health and surveillance of cancer recurrence can also be compromised. Normal mouth opening for an adult ranges from 23 to 71 mm as measured between the incisors.[128] The wide variation in reported incidence reflects the lack of uniform criteria for the definition of trismus.[129] Trismus in the head and neck cancer setting can result from tumor invasion into critical structures of mastication including the masseter and pterygoid muscles and/or their neural innervation, the temporal mandibular joint, and/or other supportive tissues.[130] Surgery and radiation therapy are well known causes of trismus. Radiation can result in trismus in up to 45% of patients who received curative doses.[131] Trismus evolves most rapidly 1 to 9 months after completion of radiation therapy.[132] Mandibular opening worsens as the dose of radiation delivered to the pterygoid muscles increases, and the probability of developing trismus is reported to increase 24% for every 10 Gy of additional radiation delivered to the pterygoid muscles.[133,134] Noncancer and cancer treatment-related causes of trismus are also common in the cancer setting and include infection, trauma, and osteoradionecrosis of the jaw.[135]

Multiple modalities have been used in the treatment of trismus. Physical therapy is the mainstay of trismus treatment and is often used alone or in combination with other modalities. Despite widespread and accepted use, the use of physical therapy to treat trismus in the head and neck cancer population has not demonstrated significant efficacy in the literature.[136–138] Hyperbaric oxygen and pentoxifylline have shown no and modest efficacy, respectively.[139,140] Forced mouth opening under general anesthesia can improve trismus but the effect is often short-lived and potentially complicated by alveolus fracture and rupture of adjacent soft tissues. Surgical coronoidectomy has demonstrated significant efficacy in a noncontrolled study of head and neck cancer patients who had failed physical therapy but is not in widespread clinical use.[141] Botulinum toxin injection has been reported to have potential benefit in treating selected complications of the RFS, including trismus.[142] A study on the efficacy of botulin toxin injection into the masseter muscles of head and neck cancer patients with radiation-induced pain and trismus did not demonstrate significant improvement of trismus but did demonstrate significantly reduced local pain.[143]

A variety of jaw-opening devices are available to treat trismus (Fig. 177.6).[144] Devices currently in clinical use include stacked tongue depressors, corkscrew devices, the TheraBite Jaw Motion Rehabilitation System (TB) (Atos Medical AB, Hörby, Sweden), and the Dynasplint Trismus System (DTS) (Dynasplint Systems Inc., Severna Park, Maryland). The TB demonstrated efficacy in a small trial (seven patients) when used within 6 weeks of surgery for oropharyngeal carcinoma.[145] TB combined with unassisted exercise also demonstrated efficacy in patients who had undergone radiation therapy within the preceding 5 years (most within the preceding year) when compared with unassisted exercise and when compared to mechanically assisted mandibular mobilization using stacked tongue depressors combined with unassisted exercise.[138] The fabrication and/or use of dynamic jaw-opening devices to treat both benign and oncologic causes of trismus have been detailed in numerous reports as early as 1968.[146–151] The DTS is a commercially available dynamic jaw-opening device that operates on the principle of low-torque, prolonged-duration stretch. It has demonstrated efficacy in achieving improved jaw opening in a retrospective evaluation of 48 patients with trismus from four cohort groups including radiation therapy for head and neck cancer, dental treatment, oral surgery, and stroke.[152] Although the 20 patients in the head and neck cancer cohort improved their maximal interincisal distance by a mean of 13.6 mm, little demographic and oncologic information was given, except that they all received radiation therapy.

In clinical practice, the devices of choice are the TB and DTS. Stacked tongue depressors and corkscrew devices are relatively ineffective. The TB may be effective early in the course of trismus development and is inexpensive, easy and intuitive to use, and readily available. The device is inserted in the mouth and activated to near tolerance by squeezing leveraged handles for seven repetitions of 7 seconds. This is usually repeated 7 times per day. Although often effective in improving mouth opening, this regimen may cause rebound spasm of the masseter and pterygoid muscles. If the patient has had trismus for more then 3 months, the DTS may be a better option because it works on the principle of low-torque, prolonged stretch, which has been demonstrated to be more effective at improving range of motion in an experimental model involving contracted rat knees than high-torque, short-duration stretching.[153] A custom bite plate is fabricated for the device and it is use progressed until the patient is able to tolerate the device for 30 minutes 3 times per day. Physical therapy is usually used in collaboration with a jaw-stretching device to ensure its proper use, provide and teach muscle massage techniques, and to address other neuromuscular and musculoskeletal issues such as neck pain, stiffness, or weakness, that often accompany trismus. Pain medications may be necessary to diminish the pain and spasm of the muscles of mastication. Generally, nerve-stabilizing agents such as pregabalin, gabapentin, or duloxetine are used initially. Botulinum toxin injections will no improve oral opening in isolation but may decrease the dynamic muscle spasm that are contributing to

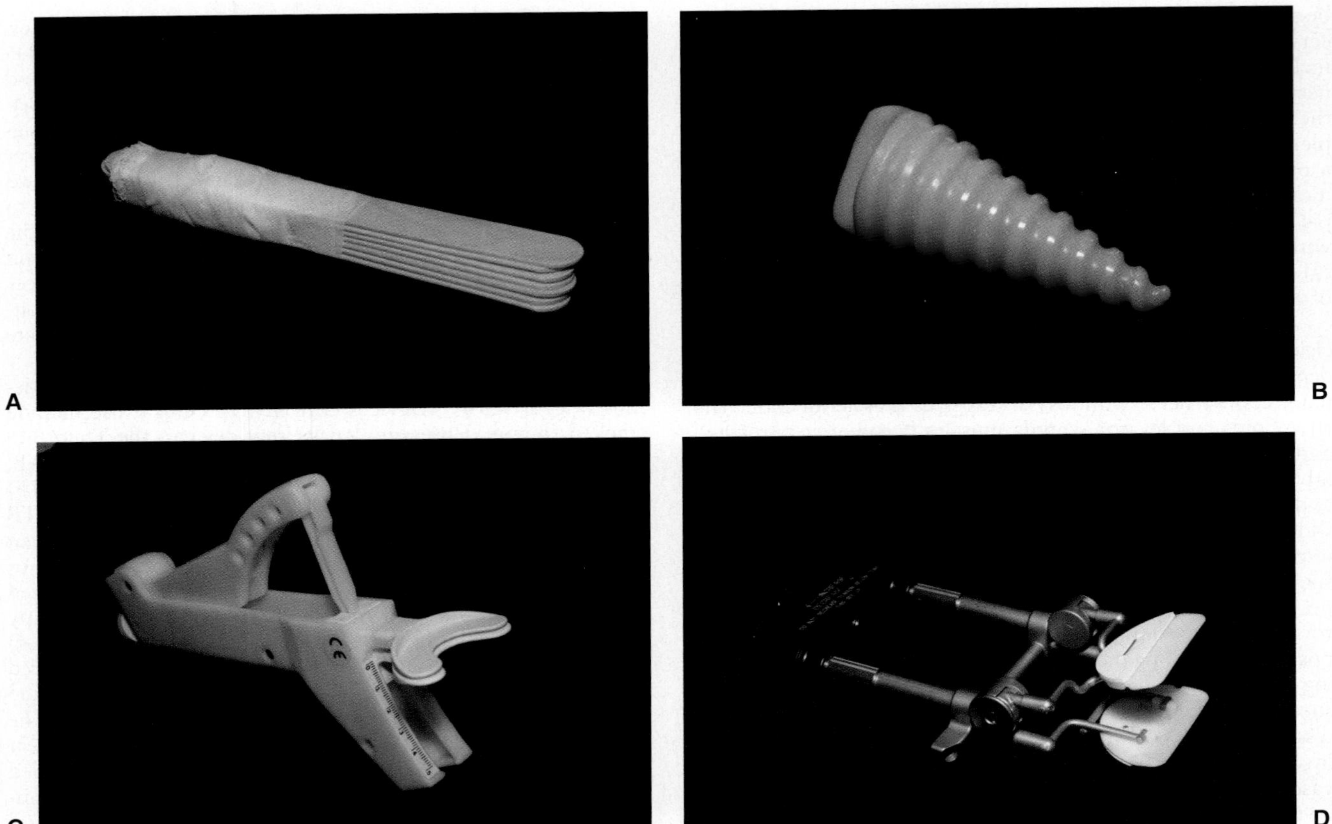

FIGURE 177.6 Jaw-stretching devices used to treat trismus include (**A**) stacked tongue depressors, (**B**) corkscrew devices, (**C**) the TheraBite Jaw Motion Rehabilitation System (TB), and (**D**) the *Dynasplint Trismus System* (DTS). (From ref. 1, with permission.)

trismus and make other therapeutic interventions including physical therapy and jaw-opening devices more effective.

Radiation-induced cervical dystonia can result not only from the treatment of head and neck cancers, but from treatment of any tumor treated with radiation that involves occiput, cervical spine, or upper thoracic spine including metastatic disease from any cancer type, sarcomas, lymphomas such as HL, thyroid cancer, and so forth.[154] Idiopathic cervical dystonia is broadly defined as a movement disorder characterized by involuntary contractions of the head and shoulders, which may be twisted into abnormal positions including torticollis, laterocollis, retrocollis, and anterocollis.[155] In radiation-induced cervical dystonia, radiation fibrosis likely contributes to ectopic activity in the distribution of the spinal accessory nerve and cervical nerve roots. This ectopic activity may be asymmetric or contribute to pain, soreness, tightness, or aberrant positioning of the head and neck characteristic of cervical dystonia. More often, symptoms are at least partially bilateral. As radiation fibrosis progresses, posturing of the head and neck becomes less pronounced and fixed contractures can develop. Most patients complain of neck tightness that progresses slowly and insidiously and is almost always accompanied by varying degrees of pain. Inability to position the head because of progressive fibrosis can affect swallowing, phonation, and ADLs such as driving and work-related tasks as well as other functions important to quality of life.

The natural history of radiation-induced cervical dystonia is usually one of progression. Aggressive physical therapy with emphasis on a lifelong home exercise program designed to maintain head and neck range of motion is critical. It is usually easier to prevent a contracture than to treat one. Medications may be useful in treating the symptoms of radiation-induced cervical dystonia but are not a substitute for ROM exercises. Medications of potential benefit include muscle relaxants such as baclofen, nerve stabilizers such as pregabalin, and analgesics.

Botulinum toxin injections can be effective in treating the pain and spasms associated with radiation-induced cervical dystonia. Botulinum toxin injections will not directly treat fixed contracture but may facilitate the progression of ROM through physical therapy and a home exercise program. Techniques used in the treatment of radiation-induced cervical dystonia are very similar to those used to idiopathic cervical dystonia. Clinical evaluation with particular emphasis on the patient's anatomy, which may have been compromised by neck dissection, and the patient's historical account of symptoms as well as physical examination are instrumental in choosing targets and dosing for botulinum toxin injection therapy. The dosages and technique are often modified on subsequent injection visits to maximize efficacy. Potential complications of botulinum toxin injection include bleeding and infection, especially if injections are near recent or active injection, spinal stabilization hardware, or tumor. Neck drop can occur when injecting weak or liminal cervical paraspinal muscles or the trapezius muscle. Precipitation or worsening of dysphagia is particularly problematic as patients with RFS that involves the neck often have pre-existing deficits. Overtreatment with botulinum toxin can potentially result in aspiration or the need for a feeding tube.

RFS in Hodgkin's Lymphoma

No group of cancer survivors better typifies the potential for long-term radiation complications than those treated for HL. The high doses of radiation used in this group of patients are responsible for a myriad of complications that can affect almost any organ system. Mantle field radiation is the most common port encountered in HL survivors, but a variety of other ports including inverted-Y and total nodal irradiation are important because the complications likely to be encountered in these patients depends largely on the structures involved by radiation. Although most of the complications are from radiation exposure, many are related to toxic chemotherapeutics such as doxorubicin, which can cause cardiomyopathy. Visceral complications of HL treatment include but are by no means limited to heart disease (cardiomyopathy, constrictive pericarditis, pericardial effusion, valvular heart disease, accelerated coronary artery disease, conduction abnormalities), lung disease (pulmonary fibrosis, pulmonary hypertension, chest wall restriction), vascular disease (carotid stenosis, carotid barrow receptor dysfunction), endocrine dysfunction (hypothyroidism) as well as a variety of gastrointestinal, genitourinary, and sexual disorders (infertility, impotence). Cardiac disease and secondary malignancies are the most ominous late complication of HL and significant causes of mortality.[156] The clinician who evaluates and treats HL survivors should be acutely aware of the vast potential for individual variation in the presenting symptoms and disorders in this complex group of patients.

Subacute myelopathy is estimated to occur in as many as 15% of patients treated with MF irradiation for HL.[122] Complete paraplegia or quadriplegia rarely results. Detrusor-sphincter dyssynergia, bowel dysfunction, spasticity, weakness, sensory abnormalities, ataxia, movement disorders, disordered gait, and funicular pain have all been seen in the author's clinical practice as likely myelopathic manifestations of distant radiation. Myelopathy is a likely contributing factor to the fatigue seen in many HL survivors. Myelopathy in HL rarely occurs in isolation and is usually part of a myelo-radiculo-plexo-neuro-myopathy. MRI of the spinal cord rarely demonstrates parenchymal abnormalities, although degenerative changes are often seen spine of older patients.

Radiculopathy in HL survivors is often part of a myelo-radiculo-plexo-neuro-myopathy but it is more commonly seen without clinically evident myelopathy. Neuronal predisposition from pre-existing or emergent degenerative spine disease is likely an extremity important as an etiologic factor in the development of radiculopathy. Radiculopathy can be seen in isolation, particularly when degenerative spinal disease at the affected level is present, but is more commonly as part of a radiculoplexopathy or a radiculo-plexo-neuro-myopathy. Patients treated with MF irradiation generally develop radiculopathy in the upper (C5, C6) roots but may have more widespread or patchy involvement. Patients treated with periaortic or inverted-Y radiation may develop radiculopathy at any lumbosacral root, but the L5 or S1 levels are most frequently involved, likely because of their coexistence with degenerative changes such as disk herniations and central or neuroforaminal spinal stenosis. A diffuse polyradiculopathy is commonly seen. Radiation-induced cauda equina syndrome should be suspected when no degenerative or other compressive etiologies are present on MRI to explain the nerve root dysfunction documented clinically and/or on electrophysiologic testing.

The electrophysiologic pattern of radiculopathy resulting from radiation is similar if not identical to radiculopathy seen from other causes. If the entire cauda equina is involved, the findings are more widespread and involve the distribution multiple nerve roots. Myokymia may or may not be present and its absence does not exclude radiation as an etiologic contributor. Electrophysiological assessment of radiculopathy in HL survivors treated with radiation may be complicated by the coexistence of plexopathy, neuropathy, and/or myopathy.

Plexopathy can affect both the brachial and lumbosacral plexus in HL survivors depending on the extent of radiation they received (i.e., MF, inverted-Y, total nodal). Brachial plexopathy is rarely seen without a component of radiculopathy, neuropathy of the nerves within the radiation field, and localized myopathy. Plexopathy seems less common in the author's clinical experience than radiculopathy. One possible reason for this observation is that the plexus is not directly affected by degenerative changes. Plexopathy from MF irradiation generally affects the upper brachial plexus (upper trunk and/or lateral cord) more severely than the rest of the plexus but a panplexopathy can be seen. The pyramidal shape of the thorax providing less protection from radiation and the longer anatomic course of the upper plexus relative to other plexus structures may explain this phenomenon. Lumbosacral plexopathy form peri-aortic and inverted-Y radiation may be seen, usually in combination with the polyradiculopathy of cauda equina syndrome. As with radiculopathy, the electrophysiological assessment of plexopathy in HL survivors is usually complicated by the presence of other neuromuscular disorders.

Neuropathy associated with MF radiation affects only proximal nerves confined within the field. A polyneuropathy from prior treatment with neurotoxic chemotherapy or other causes such as diabetes may be present and may predispose the patient to the peripheral nervous system dysfunction caused by radiation. Radiation-induced mononeuropathy from MF radiation affects nerves arising directly form the brachial plexus. Nerves originating from the proximal and superior plexus are most commonly involved clinically and include the dorsal scapular nerve to the rhomboids and the suprascapular nerve to the supraspinatus and infraspinatus. Other commonly affected nerves include the long thoracic nerve to the serratus anterior, the intercostal nerves, and the phrenic nerve. Nerves originating from the more distal brachial plexus such as the pectoral nerves are rarely involved clinically. Nerves originating from the lumbosacral plexus including the femoral nerve and lateral femoral cutaneous nerve can be affected from inverted-Y and total nodal radiation. Again, the electrophysiologic assessment of proximal mononeuropathies in HL survivors is usually complicated by the presence of coexistent pathology such as radiculopathy, plexopathy, and focal myopathy.

Focal myopathy is a commonly seen neuromuscular complication of radiation seen in HL survivors. Given enough time, it likely develops to at least some degree in most if not all patients and is likely the major cause of neck extensor weakness seen in this population. The myopathy is characterized by nemaline rods and is sharply localized to muscle fibers within the radiation field such as the cervical and thoracic paraspinal, rhomboid, supraspinatus, and infraspinatus muscles.

One of the most clinically obvious, ubiquitous, and disabling disorders afflicting HL survivors is neck atrophy and weakness (Fig. 177.7). At its worst, this usually painful condition can result in inability to maintain the head in a normal upright posture long enough to participate meaningfully in ADLs, or even complete neck drop. The atrophy of cervical musculature that precedes neck weakness is essentially universal in HL survivors treated with MF radiation. The underlying pathophysiology is the myelo-radiculo-plexo-neuro-myopathy described above but myopathy is likely a major component.

Even though there is no way to reverse the fibrosis and resultant cervical and thoracic atrophy that results from MF radiation, the function and quality of life of these patients can be meaningfully improved with physical therapy to improve core as well as neck strength, posture, body mechanics, and endurance. Emphasis on a lifelong home exercise program is of paramount importance if a durable benefit is to be achieved. In cases in which neck weakness and pain impair ADLs despite adequate physical therapy, the use of a cervical collar to assist elevation of the chin is recommended. The Headmaster Cervical Collar manufactured by Symmetric Designs in Salt

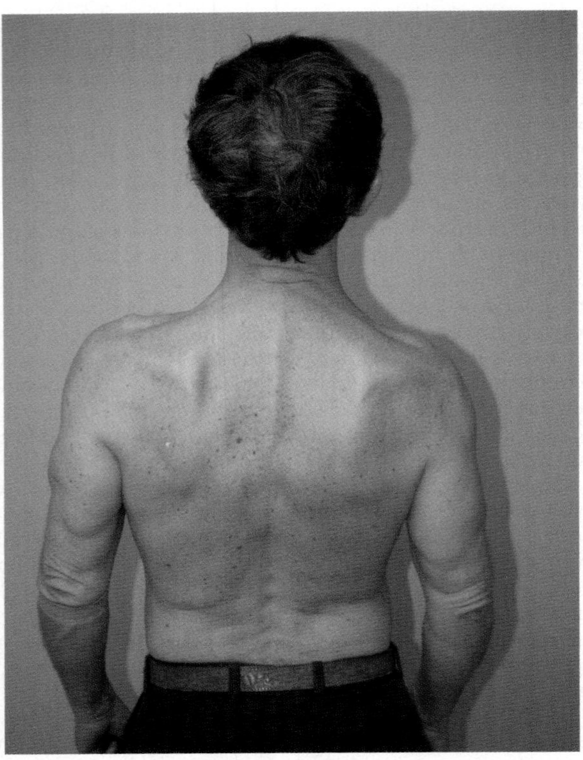

FIGURE 177.7 A 58-year-old man 25 years following mantle field radiation treatment for Hodgkin's lymphoma. Note the marked atrophy of the cervical and thoracic paraspinal, supraspinatus, infraspinatus, rhomboid, and trapezius muscles in this otherwise well-developed man. The patient suffers from a variety of neuromuscular and musculoskeletal disorders resulting in neck extensor weakness and shoulder/upper extremity pain.

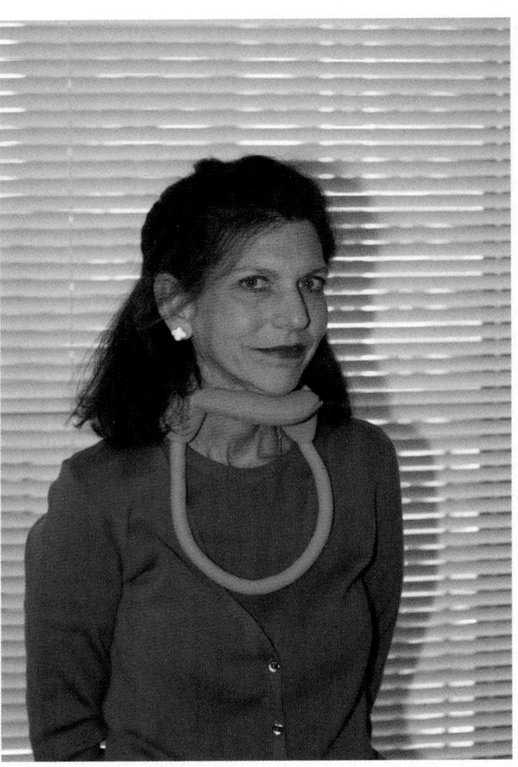

FIGURE 177.8 The Headmaster Cervical Collar is a simple and comfortable way to support the head in patients with weakened cervical paraspinal muscles from radiation and other cancer-associated causes.

Spring Island, British Columbia, Canada, is generally smaller, lighter, and more comfortable than other collars (Fig. 177.8). Some patients (i.e., those with anterior chest wall abnormalities) may prefer other designs such as a soft cervical collar and their preferences should be accommodated whenever possible. The cervical collar is not generally intended to be used at all times but as an energy-conservation device. Patients who experience pain from cervicothoracic muscle overload and/or fatigue as the day progresses are encouraged to use a collar whenever possible and convenient. Such activities may include house work, meals, time spent in front of the computer, watching television, and reading. Use of the collar during such activities may rest the neck muscles so the patient can tolerate and enjoy activates that occur later in the day without wearing the collar. For instance, using the collar during work might make it possible to comfortably attend and enjoy dinner with family or friends after work without the aid of the collar.

Shoulder pain and dysfunction in HL survivors and is usually causally related to their radiation treatment. Although the shoulder joint is largely outside the direct effects of the radiation field, the nerves and muscles that actuate the shoulder are not. Directly radiated structures include the cervical nerve roots, brachial plexus, rotator cuff muscles, and the nerves such as the suprascapular nerve that innervate the rotator cuff. Any damage to the C5 or C6 cervical nerve roots or upper brachial plexus can denervate and weaken the rotator cuff muscles and referred neuropathic pain to the lateral shoulder and arm. If rotator cuff weakness results in anterior translation of the humerus within the glenohumeral joint, then impingement of the rotator cuff tendons may develop and cause a secondary rotator cuff tendonitis and potentially a tertiary adhesive capsulitis due to the local inflammation within the shoulder capsule.[108,157]

Imaging of the rotator cuff is only necessary if clinical assessment including physical examination is not consistent with what is expected. For instance, MRI is indicated if a palpable mass is present or the pain elicited is atypical (i.e., sharply localized to the spine of the scapula, suggesting malignancy or fracture). Imaging is also useful if a patient has not responded to initial treatment measures and surgical intervention is contemplated. As a general rule, shoulder surgery should be avoided RFS patients as it is unlikely to impact the progressive neuromuscular disorders that precipitated the shoulder dysfunction and will continue to drive the shoulder pathology. Conservative measures are the mainstay of treatment for shoulder pathology in HL survivors. Physical therapy is the primary modality and is the only treatment to confer a durable benefit. Therapy should address, among other disorders, rotator cuff weakness and tightness of the pectoral girdle with the goal of restoring the normal anatomic alignment of the shoulder at the glenohumeral joint and thus the rotator cuff tendons within the coracoacromial arch. Anti-inflammatory medications and/or nerve-stabilizing agents are often indicated. Subacromial injection, although not curative, may facilitate physical therapy efforts and comfort.

LYMPHEDEMA

Lymphedema is the abnormal accumulation of protein-rich lymph in an extremity, the trunk, or face. If untreated, the accumulation of protein-rich lymphatic fluid can result in fibrotic deposition with progressive sclerosis further worsening the lymphedema and ultimately resulting in elephantiasis.[158] Primary lymphedema is due to aplastic or hypoplastic development of the lymphatics, whereas secondary lymphedema is usually the result of infection, tumor, or lymphatic injury. Lymphedema is not usually a painful condition but can cause a feeling of extremity heaviness or constriction. Increased weight, traction, and altered biomechanics can contribute to secondary neuromuscular and musculoskeletal pain disorders in patients with lymphedema.[108]

Lymphedema is most commonly seen in breast cancer patients following axillary dissection (including sentinel lymph node dissection), radiation, or tumor recurrence. Lymphedema can be seen in any other malignancy in which lymphatic flow is perturbed by tumor, surgery, scar, or radiation. Reports on the incidence of lymphedema vary depending on the type and extent of surgery and radiation as well as on the method of measurement.[159] Swelling that occurs immediately after surgery and resolves spontaneously is often due to axillary cording (superficial thrombophlebitis) and does not necessarily prognosticate the future development of lymphedema. New-onset lymphedema that develops after the acute treatment phase of the primary disease should prompt evaluation for recurrence. Imaging is the modality of choice to exclude a recurrence and should generally include an MRI with gadolinium and/or positron emission tomography alone or with a CT. A duplex Doppler ultrasound may be indicated to exclude DVT.[158] CT scans of the chest, abdomen, and pelvis commonly used by the primary oncologist as screening for visceral recurrences will likely miss an axillary or brachial plexus recurrence

Peripheral edema from fluid overload, heart failure, pulmonary hypertension, hypoalbuminemia, and other causes are common in the cancer setting and require differentiation from lymphedema. This differentiation is made on clinical grounds by history, physical examination, and laboratory evaluation when necessary. Typically, lower extremity lymphedema will involve the dorsal foot and spare the metatarsal-phalangeal joints and will not have peripheral vascular disease stigmata, vascular distention, or ulceration. Studies such as lymphoscintigraphy, which evaluates lymphatic transport and abnormalities, can clarify the etiology of venous edema from mixed or lymphatic edema. Lymphoscintigraphy is rarely done as it is very dependent on the skill of the examiner and carries considerable morbidity without providing significant information over a comprehensive clinical evaluation. Impedance plethysmography is a noninvasive technique that uses small changes in electrical resistance to evaluate and follow lymphedema.[160]

Improved cancer treatment approaches diminish but do not prevent the development of lymphedema.[161,162] Thus, at-risk patients should be educated about lymphedema and its complications, including cellulitis. Risk-reduction strategies include skin care and protection, avoiding venipuncture, blood pressure measurements, or constricting clothing to the affected region. The current research regarding airline travel in "at-risk" individuals is limited and controversial. One recent study concluded that domestic air travel (<4.5 hours) is low risk and that compression devices may actually contribute to increased swelling.[163]

Manual therapies are the standard of care for lymphedema.[161] Complex decongestive therapy (CDT), a combination of manual therapies, is performed by certified lymphedema therapists who have specialty training beyond their core therapy backgrounds. Phase I CDT is used to treat the initial edema and exacerbations. It combines manual lymphatic drainage and compression bandaging. Manual lymphatic drainage is a highly specialized gentle message technique to enhance the distal to proximal lymph transport. This is performed 5 to 7 days a week. Following each session, the limb/region is wrapped with multiple layers of short-stretch bandages and exercises are performed. The bandages are worn approximately 21 to 23 hours per day, until the next session. Phase I continues until maximal volume reduction is achieved.

A compression garment is prescribed during the period of transitioning from phase I to phase II of CDT. Garments vary in pressure, design, and price. Patients with minimal residual edema may use off-the-shelf designs. Those with more problematic swelling and fibrous tissue need custom-fitted garments. The expense is medically justifiable because an untreated cellulitis may become severe and require hospitalization for intravenous antibiotic therapy. The use of sports bras and custom-made compression bras are available for chest wall lymphedema. Foam may be used to provide additional compression to difficult areas such as the axilla, ankle, and dorsum of the hand and foot. Abdominal or genital swelling may be addressed with Lycra (Invista, Wilmington, Delaware) running shorts or custom garments. Static-gradient compression devices are available for patients who are unable to apply the short-stretch compressive bandages because of obesity, neuromuscular weakness, or inability to master the bandaging technique. They include the Circaid (CircAid Medical Products Inc., San Diego, California), the Reid (Peninsula Medical, Inc., Scotts Valley, California), and Mediassist (Mediassist, Port Richey, Florida) sleeves. External pneumatic compression pumping alone or in combination with CDT is controversial.[161]

The question of whether or not patients with lymphedema could exercise or lift weights has long been controversial. Considerable high-quality data are now available to affirm that resistance exercise including weight lifting does not increase the risk of or exacerbate symptoms of lymphedema.[164–166] In contradiction to the long-held dogma that weight lifting is not safe for patients with lymphedema, those in the weight lifting group of the study by Schmitz et al.[166] enjoyed a decreased incidence of exacerbations of lymphedema as well as reduced symptoms and increased strength. It is advisable that resistive strength training programs should be performed while wearing a compression garment. Comprehensive treatment of lymphedema should address weight control because of the association between increased body mass and lymphedema.[161,164,165]

Diuretics may have a role in treating lymphedema of mixed origin (i.e., cardiogenic and lymphedema) but are not recommended for long-term use because even though they may effect an intravascular fluid volume reduction they cannot effectively remove the elevated interstitial protein that characterizes lymphedema, resulting in an osmotic gradient that facilitates rapid fluid reaccumulation. The benzopyrones (e.g., coumarin [5,6-benzo-[[*a*]]-pyrone], or 1,2-benzopyrone) have had controversial findings and are not currently approved by the U.S. Food and Drug Administration in the United States.[167] Flavonoids have been reported to reduce stage 2 and 3 lymphedema; however, trials have been limited and they are not widely used in clinical practice.[168] Antibiotics including second-generation cephalosporins and penicillins are commonly used to treat cellulitis associated with lymphedema. Patients who have had multiple cellulitic infections may need to receive prophylactic antibiotics. Surgeries including debulking, bridging, and recreation of lymphatic channels are not commonly performed because of limited success rates and/or high rates of recurrence or complications.[161]

REHABILITTION INTERVENTIONS

Therapeutic Exercise

The benefits of exercise in cancer patients during and after treatment as well as for cancer survivors are perhaps the best studied topic in cancer rehabilitation.[169–172] The primary rationale for exercise in the setting of cancer is to avoid effects of deconditioning, which include muscle weakness and atrophy, loss of cardiopulmonary fitness, and decreased efficiency of energy metabolism at a cellular level. Improved immune effects have also been reported with exercise in cancer survivors, including increases in natural killer cell cytolytic activity, monocyte function, proportion of circulating granulocytes, and decrease in duration of neutropenia.[173] Appropriate precautions should be incorporated into the exercise program (Tables 177.1 and 177.2). A physician recommendation to exercise improves compliance.[174] The program should incorporate interventions for strength, endurance, and flexibility, and should be individualized. When possible, the form of exercise should be one that is enjoyable and sustainable.

From a rehabilitation standpoint, effects of exercise in improving physical performance is usually the primary goal. A multitude of other benefits are conferred by exercise, even among patients in the midst of active treatment. Such benefits include improved quality of life, decreased depression and anxiety, reduced fatigue and body weight, enhanced cellular function and cell counts, and even decreased hospital length of stay.[175–177] Studies measuring physical performance show benefit in parameters such as exercise time, functional capacity, heart rate, workload intensity, and timed walk distance. Aerobic exercise, at moderate levels, has been most thoroughly studied. Effect on fatigue is favorable but variable.[178] Patients treated with cardiotoxic agents such as anthracyclines (in doses of >100 mg/m^2) sustain permanent cardiac damage, resulting in reduced maximal oxygen uptake and lack of normal heart rate and stroke volume responses.[179] Despite these impairments, exercise time, peak oxygen uptake, and ventilatory anaerobic threshold improve with exercise via peripheral adaptation effects.[179]

A strong justification for exercise in cancer patients is weight reduction. Body mass index is directly proportional to tumor recurrence rates and all-cause mortality.[180] Obesity is also a risk factor for lymphedema.[181] Weight control and weight reduction require limitation of caloric intake, but patients in the active treatment phase may have side effects that interfere with adequate nutrition, and in this setting, promoting increased caloric intake may be an integral part of management. The use of anabolic steroids has been described to augment weight gain and the building of muscle mass.[14] Hydration must be adequate to prevent orthostatic hypotension.

The issue of an appropriate exercise program should be visited in all cancer patients, with the exception of those with cachexia. Cachexia is defined as more than 25% loss of lean bone mass or a body mass index 10% or less below normal range. Most cachectic patients are not consuming adequate amounts of protein or calories to meet basal needs, and rehabilitation efforts should focus on maintaining basic functional skills and quality-of-life priorities. Any activity program that is attempted should be individualized, take into account the patient's comfortable tolerance, and incorporate rest periods.

Multiple factors can lead to fatigue, which must be approached in an individualized manner. Common problems include cytokine effects (either endogenous or due to treatment), anemia, pain, depression, medication side effects, poor nutrition, and coexisting endocrine disturbances such as hypothyroidism. Physical deconditioning itself leads to fatigue. According to one recent study of patients with hematologic malignancy, fatigue correlated with depression and poor performance status, but not with thyroid, liver, or kidney function, anemia, albumin level, or immune markers, suggesting a primary treatment role for exercise in fatigue management.[182] Low- to moderate-intensity home-based aerobic exercise is associated with reduced fatigue in women receiving chemotherapy for breast cancer; however, the effect of exercise on fatigue may be more immediate (same day) than sustained.[183] Stimulant medication has also been employed to counteract fatigue, the dose-limiting drowsiness from opioids, and to accelerate response to tricyclic agents.[184,185]

Therapeutic Modalities

Physical modalities are nonpharmacologic agents used to produce a therapeutic effect in tissues.[186] They include heat, cold, and electrotherapy. They are frequently used to reduce pain, facilitate stretch, aid in wound care, and introduce medications such as corticosteroids.

Heat includes superficial and deep-heating modalities. Superficial heat is applied to the surface of the skin to achieve the maximum tissue temperatures in skin and subcutaneous fat. Heat should not be applied to an area of acute trauma and inflammation and in patients with bleeding diatheses, edema, peripheral vascular disease, large scars, impaired sensation, or cognitive or communication deficits that impair their ability to report pain. Superficial heat is applied using heating pads, moist compresses, hydrocollator packs, paraffin baths, and whirlpool baths. Deep heat is directed to heat muscle, tendons, ligaments, or bone. It is most commonly applied using ultrasound waves. Deep-heat modalities are generally avoided to an area where active regional malignancy exists for fear of causing tumor growth.[187–189] This recommendation, however, is based on *in vitro* studies of tumor growth in mice subjected to ultrasound at intensities 10 times higher than are possible by standard machines.[190] There is contradictory evidence that ultrasound at various intensities can actually have an antitumor effect.[188] It is unclear if this phenomenon represents a real clinical concern and if it can be extrapolated to other heating modalities such as laser or moist heat. Because of the reported risk of increasing tumor growth with such modalities they are generally avoided, particularly in primary tumors subject to potentially curative treatment, unless the potential benefit is substantial and outweighs the unknown risks. In patients with metastatic disease and in areas well away from a primary tumor, the risks of contributing significantly to tumor growth or spread, if any, are likely minimal.

Medication such as 1% lidocaine or corticosteroids can be applied using ultrasound. This technique is known as *phonophoresis,* and is often used to treat tendonitis, bursitis, scar tissue, neuromas, and adhesions that may be complications associated with cancer or its treatment.[191]

Cold modalities, also known as *cryotherapy*, are often used to treat acute pain and inflammation associated with musculoskeletal disorders, as well as myofascial pain, spasticity, and emergent care of minor burns. Cryotherapy is the treatment of choice for acute trauma and inflammation. It can also be used in patients with bleeding diathesis and large scars. Cryotherapy should not be used in cold-intolerant patients or those with cryoglobulins, cold hypersensitivity, and Raynaud disease.

TENS is the most common form of electroanalgesia and enjoys widespread use although its effectiveness in both acute and chronic pain conditions remains controversial in both benign and malignant conditons.[192–194] It has been used to help reduce neuropathic and nociceptive pain conditions, depending on the type of TENS unit and parameters chosen. It is applied by placing one to four electrode pads surrounding the area of pain. A small stimulating unit is connected and specific frequency, pulse width, and amplitude settings are selected based on the type of pain and the patient's response. The analgesic effect of TENS may be the result of a combination of mechanisms, including acting as a counterirritant in the CNS to inhibit activity of dorsal horn nociceptive neurons, activating the production of endogenous opioids, and possibly activating other neurotransmitter systems, including the serotonergic and substance P systems. As with deep-heating modalities such as ultrasound, it is recommended that

TENS not be delivered over or near a malignancy unless it is being used in patients with terminal cancer. However, as with ultrasound there is little evidence to support this recommendation.

Orthotics and Prosthetics

Patients with weakness or impaired balance often need equipment such as assistive devices for ambulation, bath equipment such as tub bench and raised toilet seat, and other equipment for self-care such as reachers. A wheeled walker usually suffices for individuals with balance impairment or with mild weakness and allows a quicker cadence than a standard walker, which must be manually lifted between steps. However, a standard walker is needed when more severe weakness is present or when protected weight bearing is needed.

Footdrop (weakness of dorsiflexion) is often seen in the cancer setting as a result of a brain, spinal cord, cauda equina, L-5 root, lumbosacral trunk, sciatic nerve, or, most commonly, a peroneal nerve injury. Patients with foot drop will often benefit from an AFO, which helps to restore a more normal gait pattern by allowing the foot to clear the ground without hiking the hip. A number of AFO designs exist. If the patient has some residual dorsiflexor strength, a relatively normal-shaped limb, and normal skin integrity, a prefabricated posterior leaf-spring orthosis may be adequate. For most patients, a custom-molded AFO or posterior leaf-spring orthosis is the brace of choice because of its better fit and more durable design. For patients with weakness of plantarflexion as well as dorsiflexion, a higher medial-lateral trim line will increase medial-lateral stability and help prevent ankle sprain. This modified AFO design may compromise optimal gait, however, as it is generally too stiff to allow for passive dorsiflexion in the terminal stance phase of the gait cycle. This can be overcome by using a hinged AFO design with free dorsiflexion or a dorsiflexion stop at 15 degrees and a plantarflexion stop at neutral. This will provide excellent medial-lateral stability without significantly affecting terminal stance. For patients with severe spasticity or pain on ankle motion, a solid AFO is indicated. For most patients, a plastic orthotic is preferred as it is relatively aesthetic, light weight, and can be used with different pairs of shoes. In instances in which lower extremity pain, fluctuating edema, skin fragility, deformity, or other circumstances prohibit the use of a plastic molded AFO, a double-metal upright AFO may be an option. There are a variety of other orthotics available to optimize deficits arising from other peripheral nervous system dysfunctions. Knee immobilizers, for instance, are often useful to control knee flexion in patients with femoral neuropathy or lumbar plexopathy.[63]

NONPHARMACOLOGIC PAIN MANAGEMENT

Rehabilitation medicine typically emphasizes nonpharmacologic interventions in addition to medications to address pain associated with musculoskeletal and neuromuscular syndromes. The primary goal of this approach is to limit the impact of pain on function and minimize disability. The emphasis of nonpharmacologic pain management may be of particular benefit in elderly patients who may not tolerate medications well. Historically, direct tumor spread is thought to account for most cancer pain.[184] As treatments for cancer have improved and emphasis placed on cancer survivorship, progressively more of the pain disorders encountered in the cancer setting are related to causes other than direct effects of tumor. These disorders include treatment effects and degenerative diseases of various types.

The appropriate treatment depends on the nature and type of pain. The identification and treatment of depression, anxiety, fatigue, quality of sleep, and mood can have a marked impact on pain and should be considered as part of multimodal treatment when appropriate in all patients.[195,196] Psychological strategies, such as guided imagery, hypnotherapy, biofeedback, and deep breathing, can be effective.[197] Pain may respond to physical therapy to improve muscle strength and condition as well as improve joint ROM. Physical modalities including heat, cold, and electrotherapy may be of benefit where appropriate.[186] Aerobic exercise has been shown to improve mental outlook and may result in an improved ability to cope with pain in a variety of clinical settings including cancer.[198] Pain of muscle or bone etiology is usually worse on weight bearing or other mechanical stress and improves with relative rest. Splinting or assistive devices may help achieve protected weight bearing. Neuropathic pain may benefit from desensitization measures such as vibration or tapping. Topical agents such as anesthetic (lidocaine) patches or chili pepper extract–based ointments (capsaicin) can be tried (the latter should not be applied to the face). Local injection of anesthetic into trigger or tender points can be effective at relieving pain in select patients although there is no clear evidence to support either the benefit or ineffectiveness of such procedures.[199] Similarly, injection of corticosteroid or viscosupplements into arthritic or inflamed joints may help decrease pain and improve function in some patients.[200] Complementary therapies such as acupuncture, mind-body techniques, and massage therapy may help with a variety of cancer and cancer treatment-related symptoms including pain.[201,202] In severe cases, neurosurgical procedures, such as intrathecal pumps, dorsal column stimulation, and neuroablative procedures (neurectomy, rhizotomy, cordotomy) can be considered.

PRACTICE OF ONCOLOGY

Selected References

The full list of references for this chapter appears in the online version.

1. Stubblefield MD, O'Dell MW. *Cancer Rehabilitation Principles and Practice*. New York: Demos Medical Pub, 2009.
6. Dietz JH. Rehabilitation oncology. New York: Wiley, 1981.
8. Stubblefield MD, Custodio CM, Franklin DJ. Cardiopulmonary rehabilitation and cancer rehabilitation. 3. Cancer rehabilitation. *Arch Phys Med Rehabil* 2006;87(3):S65.
9. DeLisa JA. A history of cancer rehabilitation. *Cancer* 2001;92(4):970.
13. Darnell RB, Posner JB. Paraneoplastic syndromes involving the nervous system. *N Engl J Med* 2003;349(16):1543.
18. Toothaker TB, Rubin M. Paraneoplastic neurological syndromes: a review. *Neurologist* 2009;15(1):21.
19. Hauer-Jensen M, Fink LM, Wang J. Radiation injury and the protein C pathway. *Crit Care Med* 2004;32(5 Suppl):S325.
20. NCCN Clinical Practice Guidelines in Oncology™ Venous thromboembolic Disease V.1.2010 2010 [cited ©2010 April 16, 2010]. Available from: URL: http://www.nccn.org. Accessed February 15, 2011.
21. Kiser TS, Stefans VA. Pulmonary embolism in rehabilitation patients: relation to time before return to physical therapy after diagnosis of deep vein thrombosis. *Arch Phys Med Rehabil* 1997;78(9):942.
24. Partsch H, Kechavarz B, Kohn H, Mostbeck A. The effect of mobilisation of patients during treatment of thromboembolic disorders with low-molecular-weight heparin. *Int Angiol* 1997;16(3):189.
27. Aschwanden M, Labs KH, Engel H, et al. Acute deep vein thrombosis: early mobilization does not increase the frequency of pulmonary embolism. *Thromb Haemost* 2001;85(1):42.
29. Junger M, Diehm C, Storiko H, et al. Mobilization versus immobilization in the treatment of acute proximal deep venous thrombosis: a prospective, randomized, open, multicentre trial. *Curr Med Res Opin* 2006;22(3):593.

33. Kahn SR, Shrier I, Kearon C. Physical activity in patients with deep venous thrombosis: a systematic review. *Thromb Res* 2008;122(6):763.
34. Gay V, Hamilton R, Heiskell S, Sparks AM. Influence of bedrest or ambulation in the clinical treatment of acute deep vein thrombosis on patient outcomes: a review and synthesis of the literature. *Medsurg Nurs* 2009; 18(5):293.
35. Aissaoui N, Martins E, Mouly S, Weber S, Meune C. A meta-analysis of bed rest versus early ambulation in the management of pulmonary embolism, deep vein thrombosis, or both. *Int J Cardiol* 2009;137(1):37.
38. Custodio CM. Neuromuscular complications of cancer and cancer treatments. *Phys Med Rehabil Clin N Am* 2008;19(1):27, v–vi.
39. Greenberg E, Treger I, Ring H. Rehabilitation outcomes in patients with brain tumors and acute stroke - comparative study of inpatient rehabilitation. *Am J Phys Med Rehab* 2006;85(7):568.
40. O'Dell MW, Barr K, Spanier D, Warnick RE. Functional outcome of inpatient rehabilitation in persons with brain tumors. *Arch Phys Med Rehab* 1998;79(12):1530.
41. Mukand JA, Blackinton DD, Crincoli MG, Lee JJ, Santos BB. Incidence of neurologic deficits and rehabilitation sd patients with brain tumors. *Am J Phys Med Rehab* 2001;80(5):346.
42. Geler-Kulcu D, Gulsen G, Buyukbaba E, Ozkan D. Functional recovery of patients with brain tumor or acute stroke after rehabilitation: a comparative study. *J Clin Neurosci* 2009;16(1):74.
43. Huang ME, Wartella JE, Kreutzer JS. Functional outcomes and quality of life in patients with brain tumors: A preliminary report. *Arch Phys Med Rehab* 2001;82(11):1540.
44. Kirshblum S, O'Dell MW, Ho C, Barr K. Rehabilitation of persons with central nervous system tumors. *Cancer* 2001;92(4):1029.
45. Parsch D, Mikut R, Abel R. Postacute management of patients with spinal cord injury due to metastatic tumour disease: survival and efficacy of rehabilitation. *Spinal Cord* 2003;41(4):205.
46. Stubblefield MD, Bilsky MH. Barriers to rehabilitation of the neurosurgical spine cancer patient. *J Surg Oncol* 2007;95(5):419.
48. Guo Y, Young B, Palmer JL, Mun Y, Bruera E. Prognostic factors for survival in metastatic spinal cord compression: a retrospective study in a rehabilitation setting. *Am J Phys Med Rehabil* 2003;82(9):665.
50. DeAngelis LM, Boutros D. Leptomeningeal metastasis. *Cancer Invest* 2005;23(2):145.
51. International standards for neurological classification of spinal cord injury, revised 2002. Chicago, IL: American Spinal Injury Association, 2002.
52. Kirshblum SC, Priebe MM, Ho CH, Scelza WM, Chiodo AE, Wuermser LA. Spinal cord injury medicine. 3. Rehabilitation phase after acute spinal cord injury. *Arch Phys Med Rehabil* 2007;88(3 Suppl 1):S62.
53. Wuermser LA, Ho CH, Chiodo AE, Priebe MM, Kirshblum SC, Scelza WM. Spinal cord injury medicine. 2. Acute care management of traumatic and nontraumatic injury. *Arch Phys Med Rehabil* 2007;88(3 Suppl 1): S55.
55. McKinley WO, Conti-Wyneken AR, Vokac CW, Cifu DX. Rehabilitative functional outcome of patients with neoplastic spinal cord compressions. *Arch Phys Med Rehabil* 1996;77(9):892.
60. Posner JB. *Neurologic Complications of Cancer.* Philadelphia: F.A. Davis Co, 1995.
71. Stubblefield MD, Slovin S, MacGregor-Cortelli B, et al. An electrodiagnostic evaluation of the effect of pre-existing peripheral nervous system disorders in patients treated with the novel proteasome inhibitor bortezomib. *Clin Oncol (R Coll Radiol)* 2006;18(5):410.
72. Dropcho EJ. Remote neurologic manifestations of cancer. *Neurol Clin* 2002;20(1):85.
73. Jaeckle KA. Neurological manifestations of neoplastic and radiation-induced plexopathies. *Semin Neurol* 2004;24(4):385.
78. Dropcho EJ. Neurotoxicity of radiation therapy. *Neurol Clin* 2010; 28(1):217.
79. Kori SH, Foley KM, Posner JB. Brachial plexus lesions in patients with cancer: 100 cases. *Neurology* 1981;31(1):45.
86. Vallat JM, Sommer C, Magy L. Chronic inflammatory demyelinating polyradiculoneuropathy: diagnostic and therapeutic challenges for a treatable condition. *Lancet Neurol* 2010;9(4):402.
87. Lee JJ, Swain SM. Peripheral neuropathy induced by microtubule-stabilizing agents. *J Clin Oncol* 2006;24(10):1633.
90. Quasthoff S, Hartung HP. Chemotherapy-induced peripheral neuropathy. *J Neurol* 2002;249(1):9.
93. Portlock CS, Boland P, Hays AP, Antonescu CR, Rosenblum MK. Nemaline myopathy: a possible late complication of Hodgkin's disease therapy. *Hum Pathol* 2003;34(8):816.
102. Batchelor TT, Taylor LP, Thaler HT, Posner JB, DeAngelis LM. Steroid myopathy in cancer patients. *Neurology* 1997;48(5):1234.
108. Stubblefield MD, Custodio CM. Upper-extremity pain disorders in breast cancer. *Arch Phys Med Rehabil* 2006;87(3 Suppl 1):S96–S100.
110. Bunting RW, Shea B. Bone metastasis and rehabilitation. *Cancer* 2001;92 (4 Suppl):1020.
111. Mirels H. Metastatic disease in long bones. A proposed scoring system for diagnosing impending pathologic fractures. *Clin Orthop Relat Res* 1989(249):256.
115. Bilsky MH. New therapeutics in spine metastases. *Expert Rev Neurother* 2005;5(6):831.
118. New P. Radiation injury to the nervous system. *Curr Opin Neurol* 2001;14(6):725.
119. Stone HB, Coleman CN, Anscher MS, McBride WH. Effects of radiation on normal tissue: consequences and mechanisms. *Lancet Oncol* 2003;4(9): 529.
121. Abrahamsen AF, Loge JH, Hannisdal E, et al. Late medical sequelae after therapy for supradiaphragmatic Hodgkin's disease. *Acta Oncol* 1999;38(4): 511.
122. Cross NE, Glantz MJ. Neurologic complications of radiation therapy. *Neurol Clin* 2003;21(1):249.
125. Dijkstra PU, Kalk WW, Roodenburg JL. Trismus in head and neck oncology: a systematic review. *Oral Oncol* 2004;40(9):879.
132. Wang CJ, Huang EY, Hsu HC, Chen HC, Fang FM, Hsiung CY. The degree and time-course assessment of radiation-induced trismus occurring after radiotherapy for nasopharyngeal cancer. *Laryngoscope* 2005;115(8): 1458.
136. Dijkstra PU, Sterken MW, Pater R, Spijkervet FK, Roodenburg JL. Exercise therapy for trismus in head and neck cancer. *Oral Oncol* 2007;43(4):389.
137. Grandi G, Silva ML, Streit C, Wagner JC. A mobilization regimen to prevent mandibular hypomobility in irradiated patients: an analysis and comparison of two techniques. *Med Oral Patol Oral Cir Bucal* 2007;12(2): E105.
138. Buchbinder D, Currivan RB, Kaplan AJ, Urken ML. Mobilization regimens for the prevention of jaw hypomobility in the radiated patient: a comparison of three techniques. *J Oral Maxillofac Surg* 1993;51(8):863.
142. Stubblefield MD, Levine A, Custodio CM, Fitzpatrick T. The role of botulinum toxin type a in the radiation fibrosis syndrome: a preliminary report. *Arch Phys Med Rehabil* 2008;89(3):417.
143. Hartl DM, Cohen M, Julieron M, Marandas P, Janot F, Bourhis J. Botulinum toxin for radiation-induced facial pain and trismus. *Otolaryngol Head Neck Surg* 2008;138(4):459.
145. Cohen EG, Deschler DG, Walsh K, Hayden RE. Early use of a mechanical stretching device to improve mandibular mobility after composite resection: a pilot study. *Arch Phys Med Rehabil* 2005;86(7):1416.
152. Shulman DH, Shipman B, Willis FB. Treating trismus with dynamic splinting: a cohort, case series. *Adv Ther* 2008;25(1):9.
153. Usuba M, Akai M, Shirasaki Y, Miyakawa S. Experimental joint contracture correction with low torque--long duration repeated stretching. *Clin Orthop Relat Res* 2007;456:70.
155. Costa J, Espirito-Santo C, Borges A, et al. Botulinum toxin type A therapy for cervical dystonia. *Cochrane Database Syst Rev* 2005(1):CD003633.
157. Herrera JE, Stubblefield MD. Rotator cuff tendonitis in lymphedema: a retrospective case series. *Arch Phys Med Rehabil* 2004;85(12):1939.
161. Cheville AL, McGarvey CL, Petrek JA, Russo SA, Taylor ME, Thiadens SR. Lymphedema management. *Semin Radiat Oncol* 2003;13(3):290.
164. Ahmed RL, Thomas W, Yee D, Schmitz KH. Randomized controlled trial of weight training and lymphedema in breast cancer survivors. *J Clin Oncol* 2006;24(18):2765.
165. Sagen A, Karesen R, Risberg MA. Physical activity for the affected limb and arm lymphedema after breast cancer surgery: a prospective, randomized controlled trial with two years follow-up. *Acta Oncol* 2009;48(8): 1102.
166. Schmitz KH, Ahmed RL, Troxel A, et al. Weight lifting in women with breast-cancer-related lymphedema. *N Engl J Med* 2009;361(7):664.
169. Spence RR, Heesch KC, Brown WJ. Exercise and cancer rehabilitation: a systematic review. *Cancer Treat Rev* 2010;36(2):185.
171. Knols R, Aaronson NK, Uebelhart D, Fransen J, Aufdemkampe G. Physical exercise in cancer patients during and after medical treatment: a systematic review of randomized and controlled clinical trials. *J Clin Oncol* 2005; 23(16):3830.
184. Cheville AL. Pain management in cancer rehabilitation. *Arch Phys Med Rehabil* 2001;82(3 Suppl 1):S84.
186. Allen RJ. Physical agents used in the management of chronic pain by physical therapists. *Phys Med Rehabil Clin N Am* 2006;17(2):315.
187. Sicard-Rosenbaum L, Danoff J. Cancer and ultrasound: a warning. *Phys Ther* 1993;73(6):404.
190. Robertson VJ, Ward AR. Dangers in extrapolating in vitro uses of therapeutic ultrasound. *Phys Ther* 1996;76(1):78.
191. Chapman BL, Liebert RB, Lininger MR, Groth JJ. An introduction to physical therapy modalities. *Adolesc Med State Art Rev* 2007;18(1): 11–23.
192. Carroll D, Moore RA, McQuay HJ, Fairman F, Tramer M, Leijon G. Transcutaneous electrical nerve stimulation (TENS) for chronic pain. *Cochrane Database Syst Rev* 2001(3):CD003222.
196. Tang MF, Liou TH, Lin CC. Improving sleep quality for cancer patients: benefits of a home-based exercise intervention. *Support Care Cancer* 2009;18:1329–1339.
198. Griffith K, Wenzel J, Shang J, Thompson C, Stewart K, Mock V. Impact of a walking intervention on cardiorespiratory fitness, self-reported physical function, and pain in patients undergoing treatment for solid tumors. *Cancer* 2009;115(20):4874.
201. Deng G, Cassileth BR, Yeung KS. Complementary therapies for cancer-related symptoms. *J Support Oncol* 2004;2(5):419.
202. Cassileth BR, Deng G. Complementary and alternative therapies for cancer. *Oncologist* 2004;9(1):80.

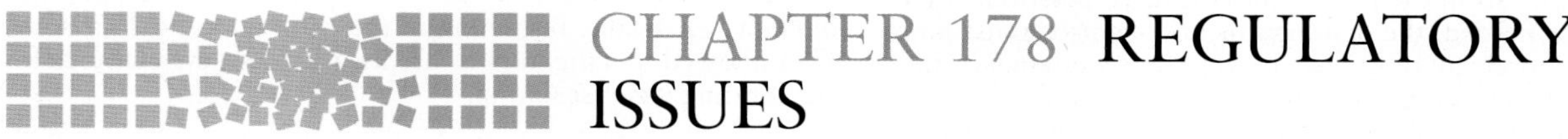

CHAPTER 178 REGULATORY ISSUES

ANN T. FARRELL, GRANT A. WILLIAMS, AND RICHARD PAZDUR

The U.S. Food and Drug Administration (FDA) plays important roles in the development and approval of drugs, biologics, and devices for treating cancer. These roles vary with the stage of product development and include subject protection, guidance on clinical trial design, verification of results in marketing applications, and determination of which products should be marketed. Cancer therapies are regulated by FDA centers. The Center for Drug Evaluation and Research regulates drugs and biotechnology-derived biologic products; the Center for Biologics Evaluation and Research regulates vaccines and cell-derived biologic products; and the Center for Devices and Radiological Health (CDRH) regulates medical devices. The regulatory requirements for cancer drugs and biologics are similar and will be summarized together throughout the following section. Cancer device regulation is discussed separately in a later section.

THE HISTORY OF FOOD AND DRUG ADMINISTRATION REGULATION OF DRUGS AND BIOLOGICS

The FDA's responsibility for regulating new drugs is derived largely from three laws. The Pure Food and Drug Act of 1906 authorized the FDA to regulate drugs only with regard to labeled claims of strength and purity. Two medical catastrophes led to FDA regulation of drug safety and efficacy. The Federal Food, Drug and Cosmetic Act of 1938 (FD&C Act), passed in response to deaths caused by a toxic vehicle in a sulfonamide elixir, required demonstration of drug safety before marketing. The effectiveness requirement was added in 1962 after birth defects were associated with the use of thalidomide. This law required substantial evidence of effectiveness and specified that this evidence must be derived from "adequate and well-controlled clinical investigations." Separate laws that pertain to medical devices are discussed in the section "Regulation of Devices for Cancer Treatment and Diagnosis."

The regulation of biologic products began with the 1902 Biologics Control Act, which was passed in response to the deaths of children from contaminated antitoxins and vaccines. This law provided federal authority to regulate all aspects of commercial production of vaccines, serums, toxins, and antitoxins and similar products with the objective of ensuring their safety, purity, and potency. The Biologics Control Act was subsequently incorporated into the 1944 Public Health Services Act, which defined biologic products as "any virus, therapeutic serum, toxin, antitoxin, vaccine, blood, blood component or derivative, allergenic product or analogous product, or arsphenamine." Regulatory oversight of biologic products was formally transferred from the National Institutes of Health to the FDA Bureau of Biologics in 1972. Appropriate provisions of both the Biologics Control Act and the 1938 FD&C Act are used to guide the regulation of biologic products.

Detailed regulations published in the *Federal Register* and codified in the Code of Federal Regulations (CFR) outline the regulatory requirements for investigational drugs and biologic products (21 CFR 312), licensure of biologic products under a Biologics License Application (BLA) (21 CFR 601), and drug marketing for New Drug Applications (NDAs) (21 CFR 314). Several regulations were specifically intended to improve or speed development of drugs for serious and life-threatening diseases such as cancer. In 1988, Subpart E of the investigational new drug (IND) regulations set the philosophical tone for cancer drug regulation, to "exercise the broadest flexibility in applying the statutory standards, while preserving appropriate guarantees for safety and effectiveness." Subpart E also outlines procedures to improve communication and facilitate early meetings between the FDA and drug sponsors. In 1992, the accelerated approval (AA) regulations (Subpart H of the NDA regulations or Subpart E of the BLA regulations) outlined standards for early approval of drugs for serious and life-threatening disease when they provide an advantage over available therapy, allowing reliance on surrogate end points reasonably likely to predict clinical benefit.

FOOD AND DRUG ADMINISTRATION OVERSIGHT OF CLINICAL TRIALS FOR DRUGS AND BIOLOGICS

Investigational drugs must be administered under an IND application submitted to the FDA. The regulations describe two parties involved in IND submission, the *sponsor*, who is responsible for reporting to the FDA, and the *investigator*, who performs the trial. The sponsor may be a pharmaceutical company, an academic institution, or an individual (e.g., the sponsor/investigator). Sponsors are to select only investigators "qualified by training and experience as appropriate experts to investigate the drug." For a cancer drug IND, one of the investigators is generally a licensed physician with training and experience in treating cancer.

The Initial Investigational New Drug Submission

When an IND is submitted to the FDA, a team of scientific reviewers evaluates the safety data from animals or other sources, evaluates the proposed phase 1 study, and judges whether patients would be exposed to an unreasonable and significant risk. These issues are discussed individually in the sections below.

The Need to Submit an Investigational New Drug Application

All studies of nonapproved drugs must be done under an IND. For approved drugs, however, some studies require an IND and some are exempt from the IND requirement. To determine that an IND is not needed, the investigator and sponsor must find that the study meets all of the five exemption requirements: the study (1) is not intended to support approval of a new indication or a significant change in the product labeling, (2) is not intended to support a significant change in advertising, (3) does not involve a route of administration or dosage level or use in a patient population or other factor *that significantly increases the risks* (or decreases the acceptability of the risks) associated with the use of the drug product, (4) is conducted in compliance with institutional review board (IRB) and informed consent regulations, *and* (5) will not be used to promote unapproved indications. Oncologists frequently use cancer drugs in doses and in combinations not yet described in the label. Such "off-label" use, when safety has been demonstrated by published data or past clinical experience, is not considered an increased risk and would not require an IND for study. The cancer IND exemption guidance provides examples to clarify FDA interpretation.[1]

The Investigational New Drug Application Process

The IND process spans the entire time of drug investigation. It includes the initial IND application and later IND amendments to provide safety reports or submit additional protocols. The initial IND application usually consists of a phase 1 clinical protocol and data to support the safety of the proposal. The latter would include *in vitro*, animal, or human evidence describing drug toxicity and allowing prediction of a safe starting dosage, and manufacturing data describing the composition, manufacture, and control of the drug substance and drug product. After the FDA receives the initial IND, sponsors are required to wait 30 days before initiating the proposed study unless they request and receive a waiver of the 30-day review period from the FDA. A multidisciplinary team of FDA scientists, including oncologists, animal toxicologists, chemists, and clinical pharmacologists, determine whether the study is safe to proceed. The FDA may put an IND "on hold" if it believes subjects would be exposed to unreasonable and significant risk of injury or if there is insufficient information to assess the risks. The most common reason for a hold is insufficient information to support the safety of the proposed dose or regimen.

The FDA frequently meets with sponsors and investigators in pre-IND meetings to review proposed IND plans and to clarify IND requirements. The FDA has provided guidance on the design of preclinical studies needed to support the proposed phase 1 study.[2,3] For oncology drugs, at least two studies are usually needed, one in a rodent and one in a nonrodent species. Animal studies should use the same schedule and administration proposed for the phase 1 clinical study. The starting dose for investigational drugs used in human studies is usually one tenth of the mouse STD[10] (dose in which 10% of animals have severe toxicity) calculated on a milligrams per meter squared basis, provided this dose does not cause irreversible toxicity in nonrodents. If this dose causes irreversible toxicity, one sixth of the highest dose that does not produce irreversible toxicity is selected for the starting dose.[2,3] The approach to establishing safe starting doses for protein therapeutics with agonistic properties differs, and the selection of the starting dose should consider the minimally anticipated biologic effect level.[2] Phase 1 oncology trials are seldom performed in healthy volunteers. Oncology drugs are usually toxic (often genotoxic), and phase 1 oncology studies usually escalate until the occurrence of severe toxicities. Limited phase 1 or pharmacokinetic studies may be performed in healthy volunteers for oncology drugs that are relatively nontoxic.

Phase 1 Trial Design

The FDA has accepted a variety of phase 1 trial designs for cancer drugs. In the 1980s and early 1990s, the modified Fibonacci scheme was commonly used. Pharmacologically guided dosing was evaluated in the early 1990s with some success, but was difficult logistically. Beginning in the early and mid-1990s, the FDA allowed investigators to use a variety of new methods for accelerating dose escalation.[4]

Food and Drug Administration Involvement in Clinical Trial Design

The FDA meets frequently with commercial IND sponsors throughout drug development. Prior to IND submission, the FDA and trial sponsor discuss the adequacy of preclinical studies and the design of proposed phase 1 clinical studies in "pre-IND meetings." A critical FDA role in drug development is to meet with sponsors to provide advice on the design of phase 3 (and sometimes phase 2) clinical trials that will support NDA or BLA marketing applications. Recent legislation allows sponsors to submit protocols subsequent to these meetings and request a "Special Protocol Assessment" that provides for a binding agreement.[5] After the clinical trials have been conducted and trial results are available, sponsors again meet with the FDA in "pre-NDA" meetings to discuss whether an NDA may be warranted and, if so, to discuss details of an NDA submission.

Food and Drug Administration and the Drug Approval Process

After clinical trials have been completed and an NDA has been submitted, the FDA verifies data quality and judges whether trial results demonstrate that the drug is safe and effective for the proposed use. After approval, the FDA continues to evaluate drug safety and regulate drug marketing.

The package insert describes clinical trial results from data that have been carefully reviewed and validated by FDA review teams. Regulations require that NDAs contain all relevant information about manufacturing, preclinical pharmacology and toxicology, human pharmacokinetics and bioavailability, clinical data, and statistical analyses. The FDA review of the NDA involves a multidisciplinary team. The FDA scientific reviewers evaluate the primary data, available in the form of case report forms or electronic data, verify analyses, and, where appropriate, perform additional analyses. The FDA field inspectors verify that information on case report forms is supported by source data, such as hospital charts. This NDA review process leads to a high level of confidence in the information that supports NDA approval and that is described in the package insert. This information not only documents the basis of drug approval but can be used in drug marketing, which is an incentive for manufacturers to submit additional NDA applications (supplemental NDAs) to update their labels.

Applications are prioritized for review according to their importance. Based on the Prescription Drug User Fee Act, the FDA performs NDA review with either a 6- or a 10-month goal. Applications representing a significant improvement compared with marketed products are assigned *priority* status and a 6-month review goal; whereas, *standard* applications have a 10-month review goal.

The FDA routinely seeks external advice on the design, analysis, and interpretation of clinical trials. Consultants are screened to exclude conflicts of interest. Individual consultants advise the FDA during the design of clinical trials and early stages of NDA review. After initial NDA review, the FDA presents selected NDAs to the Oncologic Drugs Advisory Committee (ODAC).[5] This group is composed of oncologists, statisticians, patient advocates, consumer representatives, and a nonvoting industry representative. At the public meetings of ODAC, the NDA applicant summarizes the results in an initial presentation, the FDA presents review findings, the ODAC discusses the issues, and then the ODAC votes on questions submitted by the FDA. The FDA is not obligated to adhere to the advice provided.[6] Information about ODAC meetings (including background packages, presentation slides, and meeting transcripts) and on drug approvals (including FDA review documents and approved labeling) may be found on the FDA Internet site.[7,8]

After reviewing the NDA, the FDA takes an action, which is communicated to the company by one of two types of letters: an approval letter that allows the sponsor to market the drug and a complete response letter that identifies deficiencies that must be corrected before drug marketing. At the time of an approval decision, the FDA may require companies to undertake certain actions to ensure the safe use of marketed drugs.

Under the Amendments Act of 2007 (FDAAA), the FDA may require a Risk Evaluation and Mitigation Strategy (REMS) for NDAs or for previously marketed drugs if the FDA determines that a REMS is necessary to ensure that the benefits of a drug outweigh its risks. An applicant may voluntarily submit a proposed REMS without having been required to do so. The FDA will determine which elements of a REMS are necessary and will approve the REMS after review. Elements of REMS are subject to inspection and are enforceable. A drug may be deemed misbranded if the sponsor fails to comply with a requirement of the approved strategy.

The REMS should have specific goals associated with pragmatic, specific, and measurable program objectives that result in processes or behaviors. Specific elements that may be included in a REMS include a patient package insert if patient labeling could help prevent serious adverse effects and communication plans for health care providers. In some cases programs may require special elements to ensure safe use, including required participation in a patient registry or certification of knowledge and training or experience of the health care provider.[9]

THE BASIS FOR CANCER DRUG APPROVAL

When determining whether to approve an NDA, the FDA evaluates whether the overall evidence supporting safety and efficacy meets the regulatory requirements for drug approval. The FDA has published guidance to assist sponsors on end points for cancer clinical trials to support effectiveness claims in NDAs, BLAs, or supplemental applications.[10] The following sections discuss the regulatory requirements, study end points (in the context of regular approval or accelerated approval), trial designs, and the number of studies needed for the approval of cancer drugs.

Regulatory Requirements for New Drug Approval

As previously discussed, sponsors must demonstrate that drugs are safe and must provide substantial evidence of effectiveness from "adequate and well-controlled clinical investigations." Such effects could include important clinical outcomes (e.g., survival), symptomatic improvement, or effects on established surrogate end points, such as blood sugar, blood pressure, or blood cholesterol, and all of these end points have often been used as a basis for approval.[11] In 1992, new regulations allowed AA for drugs intended for serious or life-threatening diseases and that showed an improvement over available therapy. In this setting, the FDA may grant marketing approval based on an effect on a surrogate end point that is reasonably likely ("based on epidemiologic, therapeutic, pathophysiologic, or other evidence") to predict clinical benefit. These surrogates were explicitly less well established than the ones in regular use (blood pressure, cholesterol). A drug is approved under the AA rule on condition that the manufacturer conducts clinical studies to verify and describe the actual benefit. If the postmarketing studies fail to demonstrate clinical benefit or if the applicant does not demonstrate due diligence in conducting the required studies, the drug may be removed from the market under an expedited process. In the following discussions the term *regular approval* (RA) will be used to designate the usual route of drug approval to distinguish it from *accelerated approval* (AA) associated with a postmarketing commitment to demonstrate clinical benefit. End points for RA and AA are described in the following sections.

End Points for Regular Approval of Cancer Drugs

RA requires evidence of clinical benefit or improvement in an established surrogate of benefit. In oncology, survival is obviously the gold standard for clinical benefit, but the FDA has accepted other end points for cancer drug approval. In the 1970s, the FDA usually approved cancer drugs based on objective response rates (ORR). In the early 1980s, after discussion with the ODAC, the FDA determined that ORR was generally not sufficient evidence for approval.[12] Given the toxicity of cancer drugs, to obtain approval evidence was needed of improvement in survival or in a patient's quality of life, for example, improved physical functioning or improved tumor-related symptoms. Potentially acceptable end points were described in a 1991 FDA/National Cancer Institute (NCI) publication.[13] Disease-free survival has been accepted as an adequate end point for adjuvant cancer treatment when a large proportion of patients with recurrence were symptomatic. Durable complete response was considered an acceptable end point in testicular cancer and acute leukemia because the untreated conditions were quickly lethal, or even in some chronic leukemias and lymphomas, in which it was clear that remission would lead to less infection, bleeding, and blood product support. The authors proposed that ORR alone might sometimes support drug approval, but that response duration, relief of tumor-related symptoms, and drug toxicity should also be evaluated. As discussed in the following sections, ORR alone with adequate response duration has sometimes supported both RA and AA, especially in patients with heavily pretreated or refractory disease.

Accelerated Approval of Cancer Drugs

The intent of the 1992 AA regulations was to speed access to promising new drugs for patients with serious or life-threatening disease who lacked satisfactory treatment. The AA regulations allow approval based on a surrogate end point "reasonably likely to predict clinical benefit." Because of the long-accepted role of tumor responses in guiding cancer treatment, ORR has been the main surrogate end point supporting cancer drug AA. Drugs approved under AA regulations must provide a benefit over available therapy. To satisfy this requirement, most sponsors have designed single-arm studies in patients with tumors refractory to available therapy. In the refractory setting, where by definition no available therapy exists, an acceptable ORR and response duration have served as evidence of benefit over available therapy, and thus the basis for AA. AA can also be achieved by demonstrating an improvement in a surrogate end point compared with a standard drug in a randomized trial. This approach will test drug activity in less refractory tumors and will provide a toxicity comparison relative to standard therapy.

The FDA recently concluded that more than one drug could be approved under AA for a given indication. Drugs approved only under AA will not be considered to be "available therapy." Thus, if a new drug (drug A) receives AA in a "refractory setting," that setting would still be considered a "refractory setting" until drug A wins RA.[14]

The AA initiative has clearly been successful in making cancer drugs available. Since the first cancer AA in 1995, AA has been the initial approval mechanism for 43 new indications for 34 cancer drugs and biologics.[15] New approvals under AA have predominantly relied on confirmed responses as surrogate end points, including tumor response, hematologic response, cytogenetic response, and cytologic response.

After gaining AA based on a surrogate end point, the drug manufacturer is responsible for completing phase 4 (postmarketing) commitments to determine whether the drug provides clinical benefit. The regulations allow the FDA to remove the drug from the market if sponsors do not demonstrate "due diligence" in completing these commitments or if the drug does not provide clinical benefit. In oncology, phase 4 studies have often targeted a slightly different population than the AA indication; for example, the AA may be for refractory colon cancer and the confirmatory study for first-line treatment of colon cancer. In 2003 and 2005, special sessions of ODAC discussed how the planning and conduct of oncology AA confirmatory studies could be improved. ODAC consensus was that phase 4 trials need to be planned early in oncology drug development, consistent with the AA regulations that state that phase 4 trials are generally expected to begin before drug approval. One strategy that may ensure completion of the confirmatory study is to target AA based on an interim analysis of a surrogate end point (e.g., response rate or time to progression [TTP]) in a randomized trial, with the ultimate clinical benefit (e.g., survival) to be demonstrated at the trial's completion. This design led to the AA of oxaliplatin in combination with 5-fluorouracil with leucovorin for advanced colorectal cancer.

Clinical Trials Supporting Drug Approval

Evidence from clinical trials is central to cancer drug approval. By law, the FDA must base approval decisions on substantial evidence of efficacy from "adequate and well-controlled investigations." Regulations describe the meaning of "adequate and well-controlled investigations" (21 CFR 314.126). Studies must allow a valid comparison to a control and must provide a quantitative assessment of the drug's effect. This section describes the type of evidence (clinical trial design) and the amount of evidence (number of trials) that have been required for cancer drug approval.

Single-Arm Studies

The most reliable method for demonstrating efficacy is to show a statistically significant improvement in a clinically meaningful end point in blinded randomized controlled trials. Other approaches have also been successful in certain settings. In single-arm studies, in which major tumor regressions occur infrequently in the absence of treatment (a kind of historical control), ORR and response duration have sometimes been accepted as substantial evidence supporting AA or even RA in settings where there is no effective alternative therapy. In contrast to the success of this approach, evidence from historically controlled trials that have attempted to show improvement in survival or TTP has seldom been adequate to support drug approval. These outcomes vary among study populations in ways that cannot always be predicted, such as changes in concomitant supportive care that may differ by location or may change over time.[16] Consequently, comparisons of time-to-event end points such as TTP or survival generally need a direct comparison to a control in a randomized trial, unless the effect is very large (e.g., testicular cancer or acute leukemia).

Studies Designed to Demonstrate Superiority

Placebo control (i.e., no treatment at all) is often considered unethical in cancer trials but, in some settings, may be acceptable. For instance, in early stage cancer, when standard practice is to give no treatment, comparing a relatively nontoxic treatment to a placebo would be reasonable. Placebo controls are not an ethical problem, however, if a new treatment is compared to placebo, with each added to standard therapy, a so-called add-on study. It is also possible to compare new therapy to standard therapy, where the benefit of standard therapy is unknown or marginal. In that case, the new therapy would need to show superiority.

Studies Designed to Demonstrate Noninferiority

The goal of noninferiority (NI) trials is to demonstrate that a new drug is effective by showing that it is not less effective, by some defined amount, than a standard drug. NI studies involve direct comparison to a control, but are based on historical assumptions about the control drug's efficacy, and usually assume that at least a substantial fraction of the control drug's historically documented effect is retained by the new drug. There are difficulties with NI trials. NI trials need to rely on historical data to establish the expected size of treatment effect of the active control. A critical assumption is that the treatment effect of the active control that was observed historically will also be observed in the current population in the new study. This assumption is difficult to support, as results of trials are almost never identical. Optimally, the estimated size of the treatment effect of the active control will be based on a comprehensive meta-analysis of historical studies that reproducibly demonstrates the effectiveness of the control agent. The variability in the meta-analysis will be reflected in the choice of the NI margin.[17] NI designs generally require a large patient cohort in order to provide meaningful results. Given the complex issues involved, sponsors who design NI trials should consult early with the FDA.[17,18]

Isolating Drug Effect in Combinations

Because marketing approval is for a drug product rather than for a drug combination, trials that support regulatory approval need to isolate the effectiveness of the proposed agent. Evidence is needed to show not only the effectiveness of the regimen but also to establish the contribution of the new drug to that regimen. The simplest way to demonstrate the individual contribution of a new drug in a regimen is to use an "add-on" design, as previously mentioned. There may be exceptional cases in which an effect of a combination is so dramatic that studies to isolate each component's contribution would be difficult or impossible to conduct. Approval of the component might nonetheless be possible if there were support for a contribution of each component (e.g., animal data, other human data).

Trial Designs for Radiotherapy Protectants and Chemotherapy Protectants

Radiotherapy protectants and chemotherapy protectants are drugs designed to ameliorate the toxicities of radiotherapy or chemotherapy. Trials to evaluate these agents usually have two objectives. The first objective is to assess whether the protecting drug achieves its intended purpose of ameliorating the cancer treatment toxicity. Unless the mechanism of protection is clearly unrelated to the mechanism of antitumor activity (e.g., antinausea agents that ameliorate nausea via central nervous system receptors), a second trial objective is to determine whether anticancer efficacy is compromised by the protectant. Because the comparison of antitumor activity between the two arms of the trial is an NI comparison, a large number of patients may be required to achieve this objective.[19]

Independent Substantiation of Clinical Trial Results

The legal basis for FDA efficacy requirements is the 1962 efficacy amendment to the FD&C Act that requires substantial evidence of effectiveness derived from "adequate and well-controlled clinical investigations." This led to the FDA's interpretation, supported by judicial decisions, that at least two studies are generally required for drug approval.[20] Results from a single trial may provide a false impression for reasons that include unrecognized trial bias and chance (associated with occasional spurious findings when trials are repeated multiple times). In most cases the FDA has required at least two well-controlled clinical trials. At other times, the FDA has found that evidence from a single trial was sufficient, but "generally only in cases in which a single multicenter study of excellent design provided highly reliable and statistically strong evidence of an important clinical benefit, such as an effect on survival, and a confirmatory study would have been difficult to conduct on ethical grounds." In many cases, however, the FDA has relied on one study of a specific condition, together with other studies of different stages of disease or in other populations.[20] Thus, as detailed in an FDA guidance document, for approved cancer drugs, often only a single study may be needed to support additional marketing indications.[21] The legal basis for drug approval based on a single trial plus other supporting evidence was written into law in the 1997 FDA Modernization Act (FDAMA).

DRUG SAFETY REPORTING AND EVALUATION

For studies conducted under an IND, investigators are required to promptly report drug-associated adverse experiences to the IND sponsor. Sponsors subsequently must report in writing to the FDA within 15 days events that are both serious and unexpected (e.g., events not described in the investigators' brochure) and to notify the FDA by telephone or facsimile within 7 days for fatal or life-threatening drug-associated events. At the time of drug approval, safety information collected during IND investigations is summarized in the package insert. After drug approval, additional drug safety information is collected through a mandatory system for drug manufacturers and a voluntary system for health providers and patients (MEDWatch). Manufacturers must promptly report information to the FDA about adverse experiences that are serious and unexpected (events not described in the package insert). MEDWatch reports may be submitted via the Internet.[22] Through the MEDWatch program, the FDA solicits information on serious adverse events, defined as those that involve death, a life-threatening condition, hospitalization, disability, a congenital anomaly, or medically important events that require an intervention to prevent one of these serious outcomes. These postmarketing reports are useful for identifying rare adverse events not detected in clinical trials. They are less useful for evaluating known toxicities because a precise toxicity event rate cannot be determined.

EXPANDED ACCESS TO INVESTIGATIONAL DRUGS

The FDA strongly endorses participation in clinical trials; however, situations exist when investigational drugs are made available under an IND primarily to treat a disease or condition rather than to study the drug's safety and effectiveness. Since the early 1970s, the FDA has facilitated access to drugs under investigation for serious and life-threatening diseases, including cardiovascular, antiviral, and oncology drugs, to thousands of patients. Through a collaborative agreement with the FDA, in the past the NCI has provided expanded access to approximately 20 investigation agents through a mechanism called Group C. The Group C mechanism was superseded by the Treatment IND regulations of 1987 and FDAMA of 1997, which codified longstanding FDA practices by providing guiding criteria for treatment access. FDAMA stated that a physician may seek to obtain a drug for an individual patient for treatment use when the patient's physician has determined that no comparable or satisfactory alternative therapy exists. The FDA must then determine (1) that there is sufficient evidence of safety and effectiveness to support the use of the investigational drug; (2) that provision of the investigational drug will not interfere with the initiation, conduct, or completion of clinical investigations to support marketing approval; and (3) that the sponsor or clinical investigator has submitted information sufficient to satisfy the IND requirements. Despite FDAMA's attempt to improve access to investigational agents for patients with serious or immediately life-threatening disease or condition, the FDA recognized that further clarity regarding access was necessary in order to provide broader use.

On August 12, 2009, the *Federal Register* published changes to these regulations (21 CFR 312.300-320) know as Subpart I-Expanded Access to Investigational Drugs for Treatment Use.[23,24] The new regulations define terms such as a serious or immediately life-threatening disease or condition, clarify that the patient being considered for access to an investigational agent must have no comparable or satisfactory alternative, and the potential patient benefit justifies the potential risks and those risks are not unreasonable. Treatment use of experimental drugs was broadened into three categories according to the number of people treated: expanded access (large numbers), single patient treatment, including emergency use, and a new category for intermediate-sized populations. Safeguards exist for expanded access use and vary by treatment population. For individual patient use, including emergency use, treatment is generally limited to a single course of therapy for a specified duration unless the FDA expressly authorizes multiple courses or chronic therapy. Regardless of the category of treatment use, all applications for investigational treatment require an IND submission. Expanded access protocols outline a treatment regimen that will be used for a predefined patient group. Information to be provided should include the name of the investigator, informed consent, a sponsor who accepts responsibility for the study and communicates with the FDA, a drug supplier (who may also be the sponsor), pharmacology and toxicology information adequate to conclude the drug is reasonably safe at the dose and duration proposed, and a protocol. For expanded access use under the individual patient emergency use provision, use may begin when it is authorized by the FDA reviewing official.[24,25] In other situations, expanded access use under a protocol submitted under an existing IND may begin as described provided the protocol has been submitted to the FDA and that the protocol has been approved by the IRB with responsibility for review and approval of the study. Otherwise if the expanded use is under a treatment IND or protocol, expanded access use under may begin 30 days after the FDA receives the protocol or upon earlier notification by the FDA that use may begin. In all cases, the FDA may place any expanded access IND or protocol on clinical hold if the need arises.

Charging for Investigational Drugs Under an Investigational New Drug

In 2009, the FDA revised the general requirements and conditions for charging for investigational new drugs under an IND (21 CFR 312.8). Sponsors and investigators who must obtain an approved drug from another entity for use in a clinical trial do not need to obtain FDA approval to charge for the approved drug. However, if they are using an unapproved drug and wish to charge, the new rule provides a mechanism for application to the FDA. The FDA will need to review the sponsor's written justification for charging, including potential for clinical benefit, evidence that the data to be obtained from the clinical trial would be essential for approval or support significant change in the labeling of an approved drug, demonstrating that the clinical trial could not be conducted without charging because the cost of the drug is extraordinary to the sponsor, and providing information on the duration of charging in a clinical trial. The sponsor must obtain written authorization from the FDA prior to charging.

REGULATION OF DEVICES FOR CANCER TREATMENT AND DIAGNOSIS

Many of the laws and regulations for medical devices differ from those guiding the regulation of drugs and biologics. The following sections review the history of medical device regulation, the types of investigational device applications, and CDRH review of device marketing applications.

The History of Food and Drug Administration Device Regulation

The medical device laws were enacted following a catastrophe associated with a female contraceptive implant. Congress gave the FDA authority for premarket regulation of devices on May 26, 1976, by passing the Medical Device Amendments (the 1976 amendments) to the FD&C Act. Under Section 513 of the FD&C Act, the FDA must classify devices into one of three regulatory classes: class I, class II, or class III. FDA classification of a device is determined by the amount of regulatory oversight needed to provide reasonable assurance of safety and effectiveness. The devices are classified as follows.

- Class I (general controls): Sufficient information exists showing that the general controls described in the act are sufficient.
- Class II (special controls): General controls by themselves are insufficient, but there is sufficient information to establish special controls to provide such assurance. The Safe Medical Devices Act of 1990 broadened the definition of class II devices to include devices where special controls can provide such assurance, including performance standards, postmarketing surveillance, patient registries, development and dissemination of guidelines, recommendations, and any other appropriate actions the agency deems necessary.
- Class III (premarket approval [PMA]): There is insufficient information to qualify for class I or class II, and the device meets one of the following conditions:
    - The device is life-sustaining or life-supporting,
    - The device use is of substantial importance in preventing impairment of human health, or
    - The proposed use presents a potentially unreasonable risk of illness.

In the late 1970s, the FDA held expert panel meetings to assist in classifying medical devices marketed in the United States. Subsequently, most preamendment devices (devices marketed before May 28, 1976, the date of the 1976 amendments) were classified by the FDA through regulations into one of the three regulatory classes. Devices introduced into interstate commerce for the first time on or after May 28, 1976, are classified through the *premarket notification* or *510(k) process*. Section 510(k) of the FD&C Act provides that persons who intend to market a new device without submitting a PMA (because they believe the device is "substantially equivalent" to a legally marketed predicate device) must submit a premarket notification (a 510(k) application) that will allow the FDA to verify whether the new device is substantially equivalent to a legally marketed device.[26] In 1998, based on FDAMA, the FDA published in the *Federal Register* (63 FR 3142) a list of each type of class II device that does not require a 510(k). Many devices were exempted from 510(k) requirements by this law. In summary, devices can be regulated as class I (exempt from any specific controls), class I reserved and class II requiring a 510(k), class II exempt from 510(k) requirements with special controls, and class III requiring a PMA.

Congress charged the FDA with development and implementation of the Mammography Quality Standards Act (MQSA) regulations in 1992. Interim regulations, issued in December 1993, became effective in February 1994. In 1995, the FDA began enforcing MQSA when it initiated an inspection program. Congress enacted MQSA to ensure that all women have access to quality mammography for the detection of breast cancer in its earliest, most treatable stages.

Food and Drug Administration Oversight of Device Investigations

The investigational device exemption (IDE) allows sponsors to ship their devices in interstate commerce for the purposes of investigational human use.[26] IDEs are required for studies of devices that are not yet marketed for use by the medical specialty that would use the device and when the studies involve significant risks to subjects.[27] The IDE does not provide marketing approval or clearance for a device. The focus of the IDE is to protect subjects participating in studies of investigational devices. The IDE is analogous to the IND required for drug investigations, with similar requirements for reporting adverse events.[28] The CDRH actively participates in device clinical trial design with the pre-IDE program. Pre-IDE submissions can be submitted to CDRH for consultation and for review of proposed clinical trials. CDRH reviewers work with the sponsor to define reasonable inclusion and exclusion criteria, outcome measures, follow-up details, and statistical analysis plans.[29]

Several mechanisms exist for use of investigational devices outside an approved IDE. These include emergency use of unapproved medical devices, individual patient access to investigational devices intended for serious diseases, treatment use of investigational devices, continued access to investigational devices, and expanded access mechanisms for unapproved devices. Additional information is available at CDRH Internet sites.[26–28]

Food and Drug Administration Review of Device Marketing Applications for Cancer

Device applications are reviewed by two CDRH offices, the Office of In Vitro Diagnostic Device Evaluation and Safety (OIVD) and the Office of Device Evaluation (ODE). OIVD was created in 2003 to regulate *in vitro* diagnostic devices, including the marketing of devices that detect and diagnosis cancer. OIVD uses the same general review mechanisms, regulations, and criteria as ODE to review and approve devices (21 CFR parts 862, 864, and 866). The ODE in the CDRH conducts the premarket reviews for all other devices. Most devices labeled for cancer treatments are marketed through the 510(k) process (class II) or PMA process (class III).

The 510(k) Submission: Equivalence to a Predicate Device

Under the 510(k) process, the applicant compares testing, design, and labeling of a new device to a predicate device.[30] On review of the application, the FDA can find the new device to be equivalent to the predicate device based solely on technical comparisons. One problem encountered in device review is the broad indications for use previously cleared for some predicate devices. For example, prior to the 1976 amendments, cryosurgery devices were cleared for uses such as for "oncology," "tumor destruction," or "prostate tumors." Thus, 510(k) applications that are approved based on technical arguments that the new device has the same performance characteristics as cryosurgery devices may have the same broad labeling indications previously granted for cryosurgery devices.

Devices for cancer treatment can be labeled in two ways: as a tool (e.g., to cut, coagulate, or ablate) or as a specific treatment (e.g., to treat melanoma). For example, a scalpel, a laser, and an electrosurgical device all cut soft tissues in surgery. However, if the applicant plans to market these devices for a specific use, then a specific equivalent predicate (with labeling) or clinical data that demonstrate that capability would be required.

The Premarket Approval Process and Product Development Plan

For devices requiring a PMA, the applicant must establish with valid scientific evidence that there is *reasonable assurance* the device is safe and effective under the conditions of use prescribed, recommended, or suggested in the proposed labeling (21 U.S.C. 360e). Effectiveness is to be determined with respect to the persons for whose use the device is represented or intended, with respect to the conditions of use prescribed, recommended, or suggested in the labeling of the device, and weighing any probable benefit to health from the use of the device against probable risk of injury or illness from such use. PMAs are to be reviewed in 180 days after FDA receipt of a PMA that meets established content requirements. Typically, the PMA review includes a detailed analysis of the device (including device design, performance, and manufacture) and a detailed analysis of the clinical study.[31] The amount of evidence necessary to establish that a device is safe and effective for its intended use depends on the particular study, the types of data involved, and the other evidence available to support the indication for use. PMA submissions rarely involve a comparison to other marketed devices, and usually compare the performance of the new device to no treatment or to standard of care in a randomized prospective study. The PMA review processes are similar to the NDA review process described in the section "Food and Drug Administration and the Drug Approval Process."[32]

Humanitarian Device Exemptions and Humanitarian Use Designations

The humanitarian device exemption (HDE) and humanitarian use designation (HUD) are mechanisms for early marketing of devices. HUD is determined by the Office of Orphan Products and is defined as a device intended to benefit patients in the treatment and diagnosis of diseases or conditions that affect fewer than 4,000 individuals in the United States per year.[33] After the HUD is granted, the sponsor may submit an HDE application to ODE for review of safety and probable benefit in the target patient population. There must be no comparable device available to treat the disease or condition, other than devices available under an HDE or being studied under an IDE. The ODE has 75 days from the date of receipt to review an HDE application.[34]

Evidence Needed for Cancer-Specific Device Applications

In vitro diagnostic devices (reviewed by OVID) and treatment and *in vivo* diagnostics devices (reviewed by ODE) are critical to the care of cancer patients. Devices are regulated according to the use(s) for which they are labeled and according to device design. An electrosurgical device can be labeled for cutting soft tissues, for coagulation necrosis of tumors, or for treating lung cancer. An x-ray machine can be for diagnostic or therapeutic use. The amount of evidence needed to support each indication is different, based on the predicate devices available, the degree of similarity of the new device to the predicate device(s), and the risks to the patients associated with the indication for use and the technology involved. For a surgical device with a "cutting soft tissues" indication for use, the ODE requires that the applicant demonstrate substantially equivalent performance of their device. Typically, if a surgical device is not marketed in the United States, *ex vivo* tissue comparison data are required to show equivalence. For a "coagulation necrosis of tumor" indication, sufficient information is required to show the device can reliably cause necrosis of a given volume of tumor tissue. For an indication for treatment of cancer or for the necrosis of a cancer that is not typically managed with necrosis, clinical evidence of benefit would be expected. The burden of demonstrating safety and effectiveness or substantial equivalence remains with the sponsor.

Food and Drug Administration Initiatives and Guidance Expediting Approval of Cancer Drugs, Biologics, and Devices

Numerous initiatives exist to expedite the availability, development, and approval of cancer drugs, biologics, and devices. These initiatives include Subpart E, Fast Track,[35] Orphan Drug Designation,[36] HUD,[33] HDE,[34] Expanded Access to Investigational Agents for Treatment Use,[23,24] priority review for NDA applications that appear to provide an advantage over existing therapy, and through publication of helpful guidance such as one that provides clarity on minimizing unnecessary data collection.[37]

Orphan Drugs

Cancer drug development has benefited from the Orphan Drug Act of 1983. This law provides for financial incentives to promote the development of drugs for rare diseases. For drugs intended to treat rare cancers (affecting less than 200,000 U.S. patients), sponsors may apply for Orphan Drug designation, which affords the potential for 7 years of marketing exclusivity on drug approval, tax incentives, and eligibility for orphan drug research grants.[36]

Food and Drug Administration Modernization Act and Fast Track

The FDAMA attempted to facilitate the review process by the "Fast Track" program. The FDA designates development plans as Fast Track if the drug is intended to treat a serious or life-threatening condition and if it demonstrates the potential to address an unmet medical need.[35] An advantage of Fast Track designation is that sponsors may submit portions of an application early, such as the chemistry section or the animal toxicology section, prior to submission of the complete NDA. The FDA review could provide early feedback on application deficiencies, thus speeding the overall process.

Special Protocol Assessments

The FDAMA also introduced the Special Protocol Assessment (SPA) to improve the quality of final protocols.[5] The SPA, usually submitted after an end of phase 2 meeting, provides for a 45-day FDA protocol review. The FDA responses to protocol-related SPA questions are binding unless new, previously unrecognized public health issues emerge. The FDA strongly encourages oncology sponsors to request an SPA when submitting phase 3 protocols.

Pediatrics

Recent initiatives have sought to improve drug development in children. These initiatives include the Pediatric Research Equity Act, which requires study of the drugs and biologics in children in the approved treatment indication and the Best Pharmaceuticals for Children Act, which provides an incentive to study drugs in children in all potentially useful indications.[38]

References

1. Guidance for industry: IND exemptions for studies of lawfully marketed drug or biological products for the treatment of cancer. Food and Drug Administration Web site. World Wide Web URL: http://www.fda.gov/downloads/RegulatoryInformation/Guidances/UCM126837.pdf.
2. Guidance for industry: International Conference on Harmonization (ICH) Topic S9, nonclinical evaluation for anticancer pharmaceuticals. Food and Drug Administration Web site. World Wide URL: http://www.fda.gov/downloads/RegulatoryInformation/Guidances/UCM129110.pdf, March 2010.
3. DeGeorge J, Ahn C, Andrews P, et al. Regulatory considerations for preclinical development of anticancer drugs. *Cancer Chemother Pharmacol* 1998;41:173.
4. Simon R, Freidlin B, Rubinstein L, et al. Accelerated titration designs for phase I clinical trials in oncology. *J Natl Cancer Inst* 1997;89:1138.
5. Guidance for industry: special protocol assessment. Food and Drug Administration Web site. World Wide Web URL: http://www.fda.gov/downloads/Drugs/GuidanceComplianceRegulatoryInformation/Guidances/ucm080571.pdf, May 2002.
6. Farrell AT, Papadouli I, Hori A, et al. The advisory process for anticancer drug regulation: a global perspective. *Ann Oncol* 2006;17(6):889.
7. Oncologic Drugs Advisory Committee, Food and Drug Administration Web site. World Wide Web URL: http://www.fda.gov/AdvisoryCommittees/CommitteesMeetingMaterials/Drugs/OncologicDrugsAdvisoryCommittee/default.htm.
8. New drug and biological product approval information, Food and Drug Administration Web site. World Wide Web URL: http://www.accessdata.fda.gov/scripts/cder/drugsatfda/index.cfm.
9. Draft Guidance for Industry: Format and Content of Proposed Risk Evaluation and Mitigation Strategies (REMS), REMS Assessments, and Proposed REMS Modifications. Food and Drug Administration Web site. World Wide Web URL: http://www.fda.gov/downloads/Drugs/GuidanceComplianceRegulatoryInformation/Guidances/UCM184128.pdf, September 2009.
10. Guidance for industry: clinical trial endpoints for approval of cancer drugs and biologics. Food and Drug Administration Web site. World Wide Web URL: http://www.fda.gov/downloads/Drugs/GuidanceComplianceRegulatoryInformation/Guidances/ucm071590.pdf, May 2007.
11. Temple R. Development of drug law, regulations, and guidance in the United States. In: Munson PL, Mueller RA, Breese GR, eds. *Principles of pharmacology: basis concepts and clinical applications.* New York: Chapman & Hall, 1996:1643.
12. Johnson JR, Temple R. Food and Drug Administration requirements for approval of anticancer drugs. *Cancer Treat Rep* 1985;69:1155.
13. O'Shaughnessy J, Wittes R, Burke G, et al. Commentary concerning demonstration of safety and efficacy of investigational anticancer agents in clinical trials. *J Clin Oncol* 1991;9:2225.
14. Dagher R, Johnson J, Williams G, Keegan P, Pazdur R. Accelerated approval of oncology products: a decade of experience. *J Natl Cancer Inst* 2004;96(20):1500.
15. Ning YM, Johnson JR, Farrell AT, et al. FDA accelerated approval of anticancer agents. 2010 Annual Meeting of the American Society of Clinical Oncology June 4–8, 2010. *J Clin Oncol* 2010;28(15s) (abstr 6065).
16. Guidance for industry: International Conference on Harmonization (ICH) Topic E10, choice of control group and related issues in clinical trials. Food and Drug Administration Web site. World Wide Web URL: http://www.fda.gov/downloads/RegulatoryInformation/Guidances/ucm125912.pdf, 2001.
17. Rothmann M, Li N, Chen G, et al. Design and analysis of non-inferiority mortality trials in oncology. *Stat Med* 2003;22:239.
18. Ibrahim A, Scher N, Williams G, et al. Approval summary for zoledronic acid in treatment of multiple myeloma and cancer bone metastases. *Clin Cancer Res* 2003;9(7):2394.
19. Williams G, Cortazar P, Pazdur R. Developing drugs to decrease the toxicity of chemotherapy. *J Clin Oncol* 2001;19(14):3439.
20. Guidance for industry: providing clinical evidence of effectiveness for human drug and biological products. Food and Drug Administration Web site. World Wide Web URL: http://www.fda.gov/downloads/Drugs/GuidanceComplianceRegulatoryInformation/Guidances/UCM078749.pdf, 1998.
21. Guidance for industry: FDA approval of new cancer treatment uses for marketed drug and biological products, Food and Drug Administration Web site. World Wide Web URL: http://www.fda.gov/downloads/Drugs/GuidanceComplianceRegulatoryInformation/Guidances/ucm071657.pdf, 1998.
22. MedWatch information is available at Food and Drug Administration Web site. World Wide Web URL: http://www.fda.gov/safety/MedWatch/default.htm.
23. Information at Food and Drug Administration Web site. World Wide Web URL: http://www.fda.gov/ForConsumers/ConsumerUpdates/ucm176845.htm, 2009.
24. Information on Subpart I Expanded Access is available at Food and Drug Administration Web site. World Wide Web URL: http://www.accessdata.fda.gov/scripts/cdrh/cfdocs/cfCFR/CFRSearch.cfm?CFRPart=314&showFR=1&subpartNode=21:5.0.1.1.4.9.
25. IND application information is available at Food and Drug Administration Web site. World Wide Web URL: http://www.fda.gov/Drugs/DevelopmentApprovalProcess/HowDrugsareDevelopedandApproved/ApprovalApplications/InvestigationalNewDrugINDApplication/ucm107434.htm.
26. Food Drug and Cosmetic Act, USC 21 360C §513(I).
27. IDE regulation information is available at Food and Drug Administration Web site. World Wide Web URL: http://www.fda.gov/MedicalDevices/DeviceRegulationandGuidance/default.htm.
28. Information on investigational device exemption policy is available at Food and Drug Administration Web site. World Wide Web URL: http://www.fda.gov/MedicalDevices/DeviceRegulationandGuidance/HowtoMarketYourDevice/InvestigationalDeviceExemptionIDE/default.htm.
29. Information on early collaboration for device exemptions is available at Food and Drug Administration Web site. World Wide Web URL: http://www.fda.gov/MedicalDevices/DeviceRegulationandGuidance/HowtoMarketYourDevice/InvestigationalDeviceExemptionIDE/ucm051480.htm.
30. Information on 510(k)s is available at Food and Drug Administration Web site. World Wide Web URL: http://www.fda.gov/MedicalDevices/DeviceRegulationandGuidance/Overview/default.htm#510k.
31. Information on the premarket approval process review process is available at Food and Drug Administration Web site. World Wide Web URL: http://www.fda.gov/MedicalDevices/DeviceRegulationandGuidance/Overview/default.htm#510k.
32. Information on premarket approval and product development is available at Food and Drug Administration Web site. World Wide Web URL: http://www.fda.gov/MedicalDevices/DeviceRegulationandGuidance/HowtoMarketYourDevice/PremarketSubmissions/PremarketApprovalPMA/default.htm.
33. Information on humanitarian use designation is available at Food and Drug Administration Web site. World Wide Web URL: http://www.fda.gov/MedicalDevices/DeviceRegulationandGuidance/GuidanceDocuments/ucm071473.htm.
34. Information on humanitarian device exemption is available at Food and Drug Administration Web site. World Wide Web URL: http://www.fda.gov/MedicalDevices/DeviceRegulationandGuidance/HowtoMarketYourDevice/PremarketSubmissions/HumanitarianDeviceExemption/default.htm.

35. Guidance for industry: Fast Track Drug Development programs—Designation, Development, and Application Review. Food and Drug Administration Web site. World Wide Web URL: http://www.fda.gov/downloads/RegulatoryInformation/Guidances/UCM126637.pdf, 2004.
36. Information on Orphan Product Development is available at Food and Drug Administration Web site. World Wide Web URL: http://www.fda.gov/ForIndustry/DevelopingProductsforRareDiseasesConditions/default.htm.
37. Guidance for industry: Cancer Drug and Biological Products—Clinical Data in Marketing Applications. Food and Drug Administration Web site. World Wide Web URL: http://www.fda.gov/downloads/Drugs/GuidanceCompliance-RegulatoryInformation/Guidances/ucm071323.pdf, October 2001.
38. Information on pediatric drug development is available at Food and Drug Administration Web site. World Wide Web URL: http://www.fda.gov/Drugs/DevelopmentApprovalProcess/DevelopmentResources/ucm049867.htm.

CHAPTER 179 HEALTH DISPARITIES IN CANCER

HAROLD P. FREEMAN

In 1971, President Richard Nixon declared a war on cancer and signed the National Cancer Act. During the past several decades since this declaration, the nation has made extraordinary progress toward a far better understanding of the molecular, cellular, and genetic changes resulting in cancer. We have also seen dramatic advances in the development of various therapeutic moralities resulting in more effective, more targeted, and less destructive treatments. Since the early 1990s, there have been declines in overall cancer mortality and for a number of specific cancers such as breast, colorectal, prostate, and lung cancers.[1] These declines have been attributed to cancer prevention, screening, and early detection measures as well as more effective cancer treatments.

The single most effective cause of the decline in cancer mortality is the marked reduction, during the past half century, in the percentage of adults who smoke cigarettes and, hence, a reduction in tobacco-related deaths. Note, for example, that the lung cancer death rate among men has decreased 2% per year from 1994 to 2006. Despite this decline, lung cancer remains as the number one cause of cancer deaths in both males and females.

Examples of effective cancer screening tests are mammography for breast cancer, colorectal cancer screening, and Pap smears for cervical cancer. The effectiveness of the use of the prostate-specific antigen blood test for prostate cancer screening is currently undergoing reassessment by the scientific community.

However, not everyone in the United States has shared sufficiently in this progress. Some populations have not benefited as well, as measured, in particular, by persistent differences in cancer mortality rates.[1] These findings suggest that there is a disconnect between the nation's discovery and delivery enterprises; between what we know and what we do. This discovery/delivery disconnect is believed to a principal determinant of the unequal burden of cancer and resultant cancer health disparities.[2] Another way of saying this is that disparities result when proven educational and medical interventions are not shared by everyone.[3] This unequal burden of cancer is a challenge to science and, perhaps more importantly, a moral and ethical dilemma for this nation.[4]

It is critical to accurately identify subgroups of Americans who do not fare as well and to determine the precise underlying reasons for the disparities. It might then be possible to design and implement targeted interventions that could lead to correction of the disparities.

Since the early 1970s the scientific community has documented racial disparities in cancer incidence, mortality, and survival by focusing mainly on black and white differences.[5] Data from the Surveillance, Epidemiology and End Results Program have consistently shown that black Americans experience higher cancer incidence rates, higher mortality rates, and lower survival than white Americans. African Americans have the highest death rate from all sites combined and from specific sites such as cancers of the lung, colorectum, breast, prostate, and cervix, compared with all other racial and ethnic groups in the United States. For example, the overall death rate for cancer among African American males is 34% higher than among white males; for African American females it is 17% higher than among white females.[6]

Figure 179.1 illustrates cancer incidence according to race, ethnicity, and sex.[6] Note that African American men have the highest overall incidence in males, followed by white males. White women have the highest overall cancer incidence in women, followed by African American women. Note that all other racial and ethnic groups have a lower overall cancer incidence compared with black and white males and females. All other race and ethnic groups have a lower cancer mortality compared with African American and white males and females.

One gross indicator of health disparities is relative life expectancy. African American men have the shortest life expectancy compared with all other sex/race groups. Specifically, on average, white men live 7 years longer than African American men. It should be noted, too, that white women, on average live 7 years longer than African American women (Fig. 179.2).

A landmark report in 1986 issued by the American Cancer Society Subcommittee on Cancer in the Economically Disadvantaged concluded that controlling for socioeconomic status greatly reduces and sometimes nearly eliminates, the apparent incidence, mortality, and survival disparities between black and white Americans. The report further concluded that racial disparities in cancer are largely secondary to socioeconomic factors.[7] Subsequent studies have supported this conclusion. Persons with lower socioeconomic status have disproportionately higher cancer death rates than those with higher socioeconomic status, irrespective of race and ethnicity.[1,8]

Health disparities arise from a complex interplay of economic, social and cultural factors. The model presented in Figure 179.3 illustrates the overlapping factors of poverty, culture, and social injustice as principal causes of health disparities.[9] These causal factors impact all aspects of the cancer continuum from prevention, detection, diagnosis, treatment, and survival to the end of life. Disparities occur principally in people who experience one or more of the following circumstances: insufficient resources, risk-promoting lifestyle and behavior, and social inequities. Approaches to reducing or eliminating disparities must necessarily take these factors into consideration.

For a better understanding of these issues the interrelationships between race, poverty, culture, and cancer will be considered.

Incidence
Mortality
Rate per 100,000
600
500
400
300
200
100
0
1975 1980 1985 1990 1995 2000 2007
Year of diagnosis
White
Black
API^b
AI/AN^c
Hispanic^d

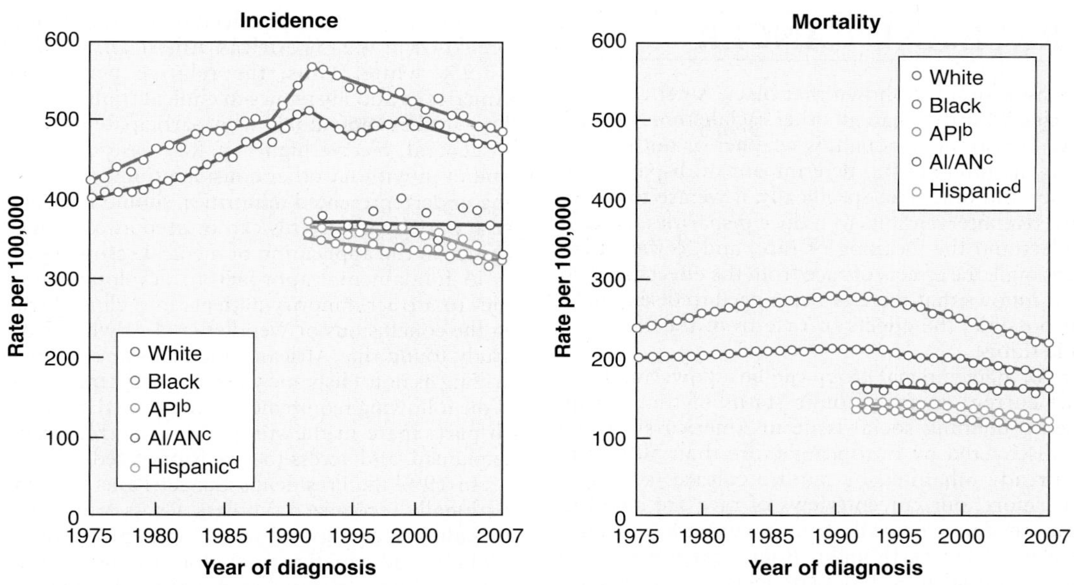

FIGURE 179.1 Surveillance, Epidemiology, and End Results incidence and U.S. death rates, 2010. All cancer sites of both sexes.

Years of age
85
80
75
70
65
60
0
White female
Black female
White male
Black male
1970 1975 1980 1985 1990 1995 2000 2003
Year

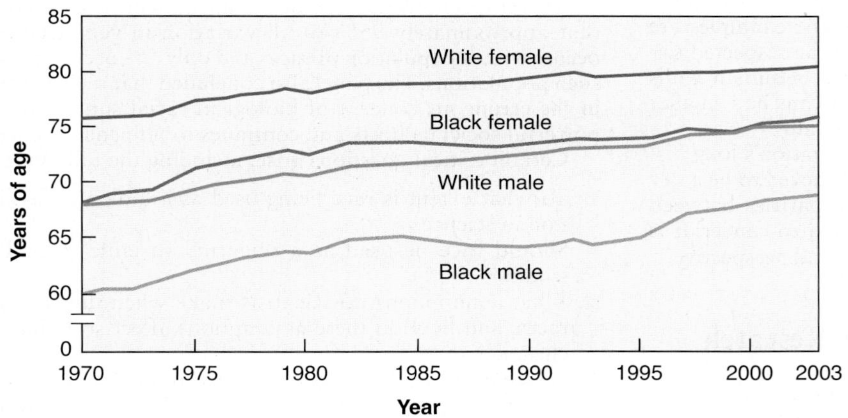

FIGURE 179.2 Life expectancy at birth.

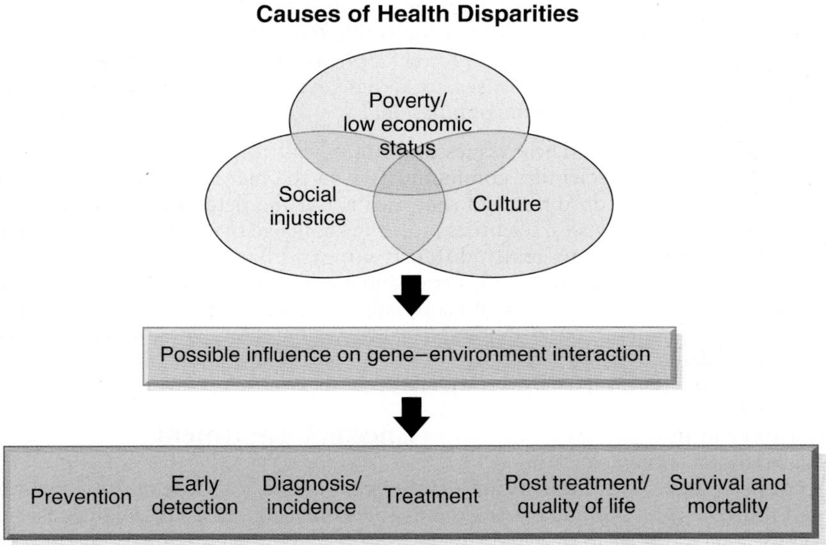

Causes of Health Disparities
Poverty/ low economic status
Social injustice
Culture
Possible influence on gene–environment interaction
Prevention
Early detection
Diagnosis/ incidence
Treatment
Post treatment/ quality of life
Survival and mortality

FIGURE 179.3 Causes of health disparities.

RACE AND CANCER

The previous discussion has shown that black Americans suffer a heavier cancer burden than all other racial/ethnic groups. Of substantive importance, though, is whether or not race, in and of itself, is the fundamental determinant of disparities in cancer incidence and outcome. Specifically, if we are to derive and apply effective interventions to reduce disparities, there is a need to understand the meaning of race, and to the extent possible, disentangle the effects of race from the effects of sociology status. It follows that there is also a need to disentangle, to the extent possible, the effects of race from the effects of socioeconomic status.

The history of a given racial group can be a powerful determinant of the current socioeconomic status of that group. Race has been a defining social issue in America since the country was discovered by Europeans more than 500 years ago, a land already inhabited by mature cultures of native people. Furthermore, our current views of race are based in conceptualizations derived mainly from nineteenth and early twentieth century scientific thought. Racial categories were based on visible traits such as skin color, facial characteristics, and the shape and size of the head and body. It was presumed that certain visible traits were immutable and could produce the measure of all other traits in an individual or population. Furthermore, in the past, scientific observations of racial difference were exploited to support racist doctrines, such as the superiority of one race over another. Dramatic examples are the studies in the mid-nineteenth century of the respected scientist Samuel Morton, who measured the sizes of human skulls and concluded that blacks and Native Americans had smaller brains, and therefore less intelligence, than whites.

The negative socioeconomic effect of this nation's long history of slavery and legalized segregation is believed to be a key factor in explaining many of the health disparities between races that still persist, including those related to cancer. It is apparent, then, that race is very real from social perspective.[4]

The Use of Race in Scientific Research

Racial classifications in America are determined by the Office of Management of the Budget (OMB). OMB racial categories are used to monitor civil rights-related progress in population groups that have historically experienced discrimination. OMB Directive Number 15, revised in 1997, sets forth the racial/ethnic categories used in the census and in medical and other research. The directive states that racial and ethnic categories are social-political constructs and should not be interpreted as being scientific and anthropologic in nature. The directive goes on to say that "the collection of this information and use of these categories is required for research that meets the National Institutes of Health (NIH) definition of clinical research."[9]

To place this issue in perspective, let us consider the status of NIH-sponsored clinical trial research with respect to minority participation. Clinical trial research is the component of the discovery process that determines by strict scientific criteria whether a specific intervention is effective in a given population. Thus, clinical trials are the principal method of determining if and how cancer treatment and prevention modalities should be applied to population as well as to individuals. An estimated 3% of adult patients diagnosed with cancer in this country are treated on clinical trials. To illustrate the racial/ethnic distribution of cancer patients in clinical trials, we refer to the 2005 National Cancer Institute Aggregate Enrollment Data for Extramural Phase 3 Research Protocols using the 1997 OMB standards. There were 90 such protocols with enrollment data that reflected the following racial/ethnic breakdown: 4.21% African American, 4.3% Hispanic, and 83.9% white. Thus, the relative percentage of African Americans and Hispanics in clinical trials is very low. It is well known that individuals who participate in clinical trials will, in general, receive higher-quality treatment. For this reason, and even without other considerations, all Americans, including underrepresented minorities, should have access to clinical trial participation. This can be seen as a matter of equity and justice in the application of medical resources in this nation.[10]

A fundamental approach to developing successful strategies to attract minority patients into clinical trials is provided in the conclusions of Wendler et al.,[11] who, in a large national study found that African Americans and Hispanics are just as willing as non-Hispanic whites to participate in health research if the following requirements are satisfied: minorities are invited to participate in the study, the study requirements are fully explained, and access to care is provided.

In 1997 the President's Cancer Panel convened a group of nationally recognized scholars across a number of disciplines including sociology, anthropology, epidemiology, philosophy, biology, and genetics to explore the meaning of race in science.[12] The panel concluded that the biologic concept of race is untenable and that racial categories are a product of the nation's social and political history. The report went on to say that racial classification has no basis in science. Neither is there a genetic basis for racial classification.

Modern technologies for measuring human variation reveal that approximately 95% of all variation in gene frequency occurs within population or races and only 5% occurs between such populations. The panel also concluded that racism, rooted in the erroneous concept of biological racial superiority, has powerful societal effects and continues to influence science.

Certain critical questions arise, including the following:

- To what extent is race being used as a biologic classification in science?
- Should race be used as a scientific variable in biologic studies?
- What assumptions do scientists make when they compare races, and how do these assumptions affect scientific conclusions?
- To what extent do societal and institutional values related to race shape the approach to scientific investigation in terms of selection of problems considered worthy of research and the development of hypotheses to be tested?
- In an increasingly mixed-race society, how is multiracial identity accounted for in the design, interpretation, and application of scientific research?
- How can race be applied validly to research studies that in many cases are designed to improve health conditions for specific populations?

These issues and others call for a serious dialogue in the scientific community. Given the fact that human populations do differ and that race is not the determinant of such differences, scientists faces the challenge of elucidating how populations really differ. It appears that expanded knowledge of population genetics and a more fundamental understanding of the effects of economic status and culture will be keys to this progress and essential to evaluating any use of race as variable in scientific research.[12]

Unequal Treatment

The Institute of Medicine issued a report in 2003 that concluded that even at the same economic and health insurance status, Africans Americans are less likely to receive the most curative treatment for cancer. There is convincing evidence to show that blacks are less likely to receive curative surgery for early-stage lung, colon, and breast cancer.[13,14]

Particularly troubling is the finding that the lower survival rate among black as compared to white patients with early-stage lung cancer is largely the result of a lower rate of potentially curative surgery among blacks. The two groups did not differ significantly with respect to socioeconomic status, insurance coverage, or access to care.[15]

Bach et al.[16] concluded that white patients and black patients are to a large extent treated by different physicians. The physicians treating black patients may be less well trained clinically and may have less access to significant clinical resources than physicians treating white patients. The extent to which these racial differences in treatment may be a cause of cancer disparities needs further investigation.

Furthermore, blacks with chronic renal failure are less likely to be referred for renal transplantation and are less likely to undergo transplantation than whites. These racial differences persist after adjustments for patient preferences, sociodemographic characteristics, the cause of renal failure, and the presence or absence of coexisting illness. Blacks are also not as likely as whites to undergo thorough diagnostic evaluation for symptoms that suggest the presence of life-threatening coronary artery disease. The Institute of Medicine concluded that "bias, stereotyping, prejudice, and clinical uncertainty among providers in the current health care system may contribute to racial and ethnic disparities in healthcare."[13,14]

RELATIONSHIPS BETWEEN CULTURE AND CANCER

Culture may be a significant determinant of cancer incidence and outcome. Culture is not synonymous with race. Many cultures exist within and across so-called racial groups. People who are in a particular culture often have common ancestors and are likely to have a similar social and physical environment and a shared communication system. Furthermore, members of culture tend to have similar values, traditions, beliefs, and world view. These shared elements lead to common lifestyle, attitude, and behavior. Such cultural factors deeply influence health status. Any successful intervention must necessarily take these powerful cultural realities into account.

For a better understanding of these issues the interrelationships between race, poverty, culture, and cancer will be considered. For example, if people of a certain culture such as Seventh Day Adventists do not smoke, do not drink alcoholic beverages, and are vegetarian, they gain a degree of protection from developing certain cancers. In contrast, people of other cultures, such as black Americans living in Harlem, New York, or whites living in Harlan, Kentucky, smoke heavily, have a heavy intake of alcohol, and a diet high in animal fat. The incidence of a number of cancers associated with these lifestyle factors is relatively high.

POVERTY AS A CAUSE OF CANCER DISPARITIES

Poverty is associated with low educational level, substandard living conditions, inadequate social support, unemployment, risk-promoting lifestyle, poor nutrition, and diminished access to health care. Diminished access is often manifested by low-quality and inadequate continuity of health care as well as insufficient access to methods of disease detection, diagnosis, treatment, and rehabilitation. Moreover, poor people tend to concentrate on day-to-day survival, often develop a sense of hopelessness and powerlessness, and may become socially isolated[3] (Fig. 179.4).

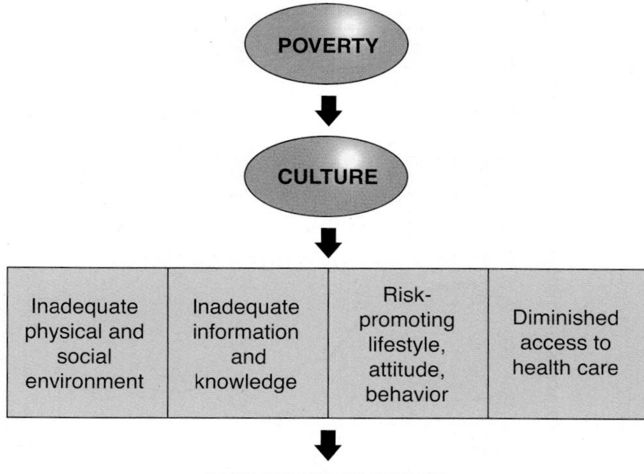

FIGURE 179.4 Poverty, culture, and decreased survival.

Who Are the Poor in America?

According to the 2010 U.S. Census Bureau report, in 2009 there were 43.6 million or 14.3% poor Americans.[17] This represents an increase of 4 million poor Americans compared to 2008 (Fig. 179.5). A disproportionate percentage of African Americans (25%) and Hispanic Americans (25%) live below the poverty line compared with 9.4% of white Americans. Note that of the total number of poor in America (46.4 million), 44% (18.5 million are white (Fig. 179.6).

Among all men and women the 5-year survival for all cancers combined is 10% lower in the poor than in more affluent Americans.

In addition, in the same year, 2009, an estimated 50.7 million Americans (16.7%) were without health insurance coverage.[17] This represents an increase of 4 million uninsured compared to 2008 (Fig. 179.7). According to race and ethnicity, 32% of Hispanics, 21% of blacks, and 12% of whites are uninsured (Fig. 179.8). Individuals with no health insurance are more likely to be diagnosed with late-stage cancer and are more likely to die from the disease.

Poverty also affects the quality of health care provided by physicians. Studies show that poor communities have fewer well-trained physicians, as measured by percentage of board-certified physicians. Such physicians are less likely to be reimbursed appropriately for services rendered.[16]

PATIENT NAVIGATION

Patient navigation is a community-based intervention designed to promote access to timely diagnosis and treatment of cancer and other chronic diseases.[18] The development of the concept of patient navigation was related to the findings of a of the American Cancer Society National Hearings on Cancer in the Poor. The hearings were conducted in 1989 in seven American cities. The testimony was primarily by poor Americans of all races and ethnicities who had been diagnosed with cancer.

Based on these hearings, the American Cancer Society issued its Report to the Nation on Cancer in the Poor in 1989.[19] The report indicated that one of the most critical issues leading to late cancer diagnosis is that poor people meet significant barriers when they attempt to seek diagnosis and treatment of cancer. The report also concluded that poor people experience more pain and suffering, often make sacrifices in seeking to obtain care, and frequently become fatalistic.

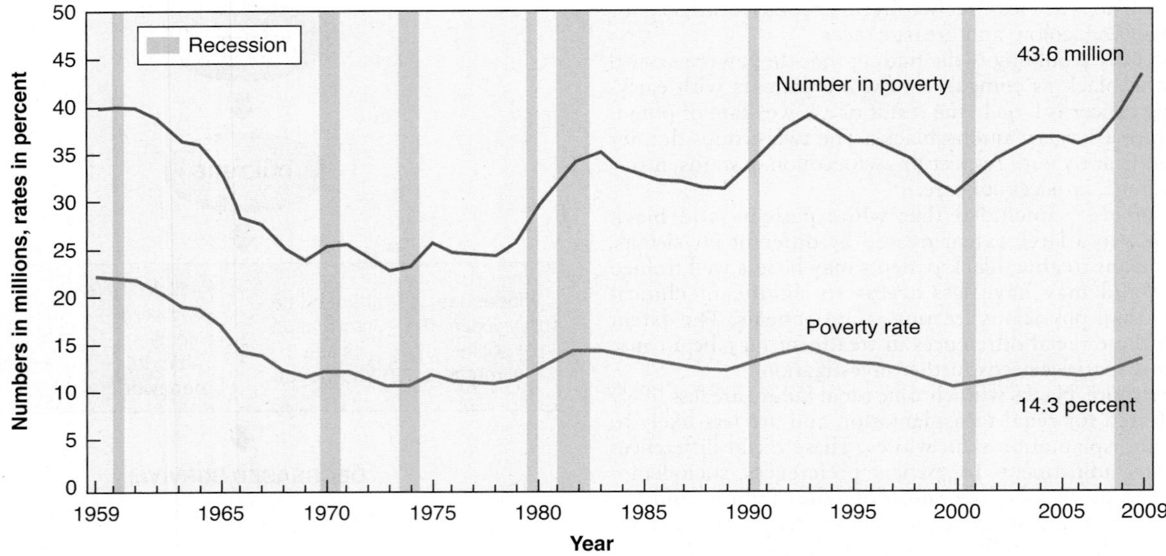

FIGURE 179.5 Number in poverty according to the 2010 Census.

Based on these findings, the nation's first "Patient Navigation Program" was initiated in 1990 at Harlem Hospital Center in New York City. The Harlem patient navigation program focused on the "critical window of opportunity" to save lives from cancer between the point of a suspicious finding and the resolution of the finding by further diagnosis and treatment. Subsequently, the scope of patient navigation has been expanded and is being applied across the entire health care continuum including prevention, detection, diagnosis, treatment, and survivorship to the end of life (Fig. 179.9).

Patient navigators provide one-on-one assistance to individuals by eliminating barriers to timely care and by serving to virtually integrate an often fragmented health care system for individual patients. Patients may experience many barriers to timely care. The most frequent barriers are financial barriers, communication and information barriers, medical system barriers, and barriers related to fear and distrust. Nonprofessional (lay) navigators may have a key role in eliminating nonmedical barriers. Professionally trained health care workers such as nurses and social workers increasingly are more likely to be assigned the role of navigating patients who confront medical and/or severe social barriers.

THE HARLEM BREAST CANCER EXPERIENCE

Before intervention, in a 22-year period ending in 1986, 606 patients (94% black) with breast cancer were treated at Harlem Hospital Center in New York City. Almost all patients were of low socioeconomic status and half had no medical insurance on initial visit. The results were as follows.

Only 6% of these patients had stage I disease. 49% had stage III and IV disease. The 5-year survival of these patients was 39% compared with a 75% in American white women and a 62% in American black women at that time.[20]

After intervention the results were dramatically improved. The intervention consisted of two elements: providing free or low-cost breast examinations/mammography according to guidelines and patient navigation to assure that all patients received timely diagnosis and treatment. In a 6-year time period between 1995 and 2000, 324 patients with breast

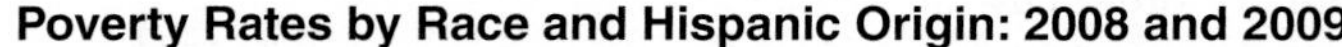

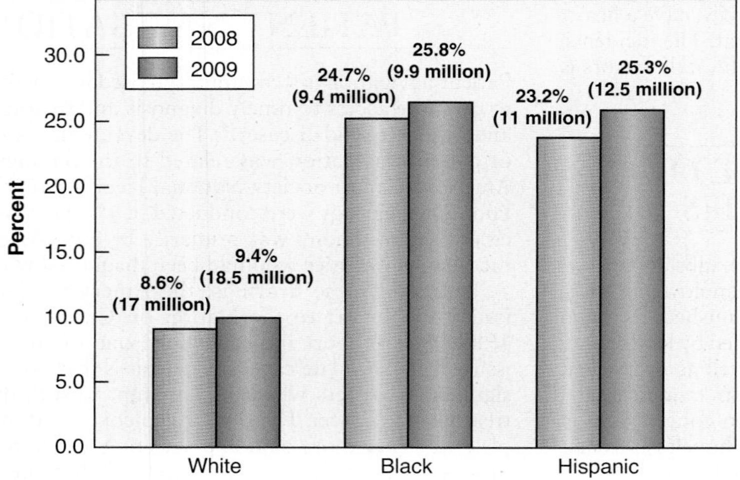

FIGURE 179.6 Poverty by race.

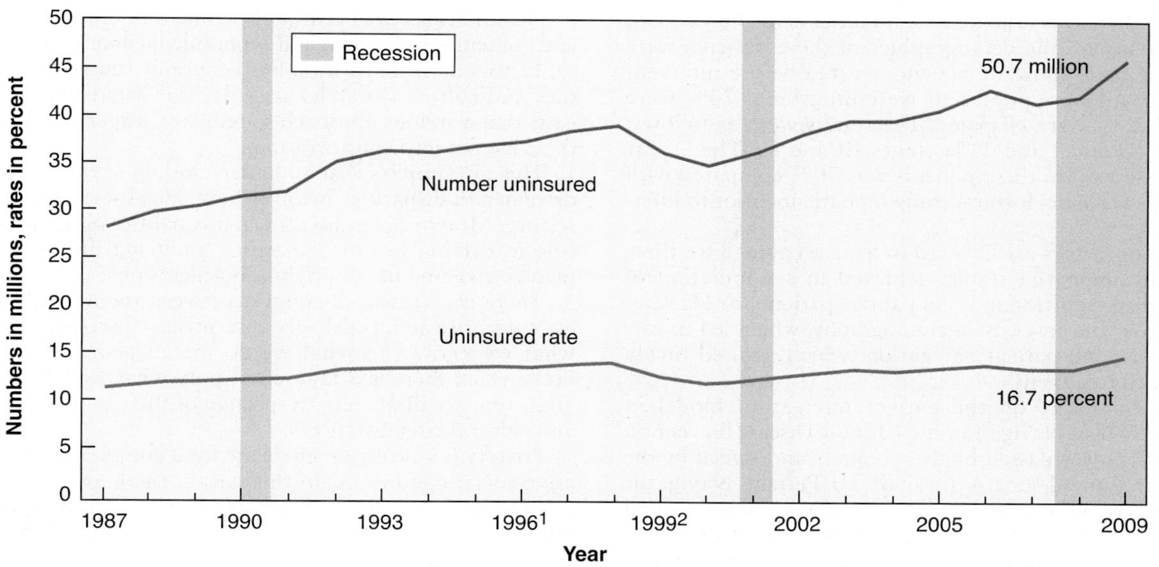

[1]The data for 1996 through 2003 were revised using an approximation method for consistency with the revision to the 2004 and 2005 estimates.
[2]Implementtation of Census 200-based population controls occured for the 2000 ASEC, which collected data for 1999. These estimates also reflect the results of follow-up verification questions, which were asked of people who responded "no" to all questions about specific types of health insurance coverage in order to verify whether they were actually uninsured. This change increased the number and percentage of people covered by health insurance, bringing the CPS more in line with estimates from other national surveys.

FIGURE 179.7 Number of uninsured according to the 2010 Census.

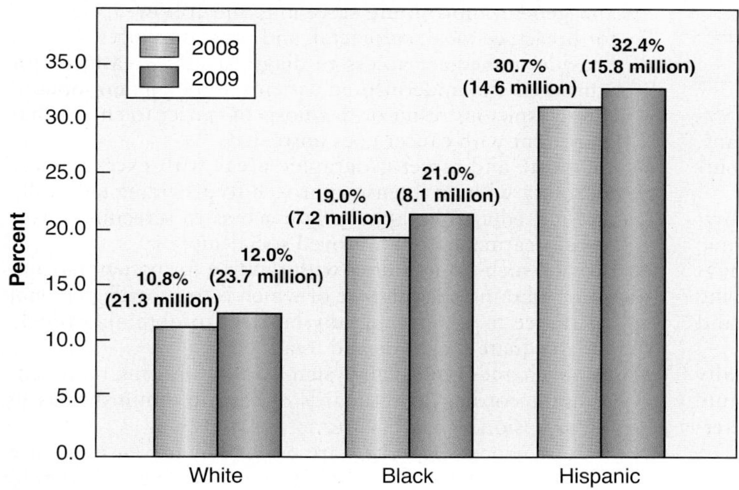

FIGURE 179.8 Percent of population without health insurance by race.

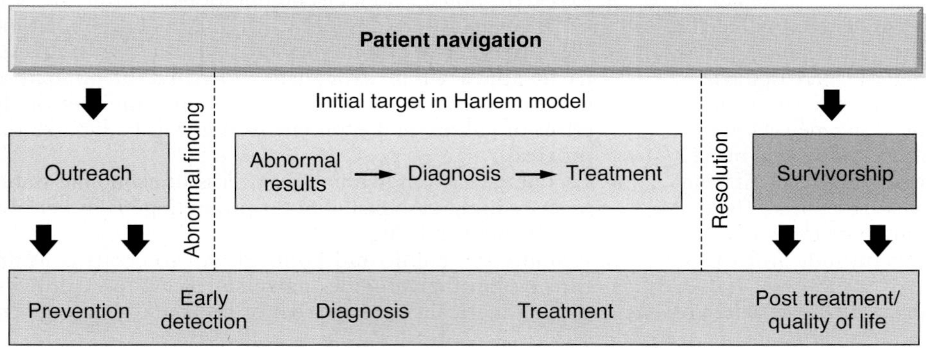

FIGURE 179.9 Patient navigation.

PRACTICE OF ONCOLOGY

cancer were diagnosed and treated at Harlem Hospital Center, after intervention. The demographics of these patients were no different from those of patients treated before intervention. Nearly all were poor, half were uninsured, 70% were black, and 26% were Hispanic. The results were as follows: 41% stages 0 and I and 21% stages III and IV. The 5-year results for survival of these patients was 70% compared with the previous Harlem Hospital study on patients prior to intervention.[21]

Two major factors are believed to have accounted for these dramatically improved results achieved in a population of poor and disproportionately uninsured patients in Harlem: providing free and low-cost mammography, which led to earlier diagnosis, and patient navigation, which assured timely diagnosis and treatment.

Based principally on the patient navigation model in Harlem, the Patient Navigation and Chronic Disease Prevention Act (HR 1812) was passed by the Congress and signed by the President in June 2005. A total of 20 Patient Navigator Demonstration Sites were funded by three separate federal agencies, the National Cancer Institute, the Centers for Medicare and Medicaid, and the Health Resources and Services Administration. In addition nongovernment organizations such as the American Cancer Society and the Komen Foundation are funding a significant number of patient navigation programs throughout the nation. The American College of Surgeons recently determined that patient navigation will soon be a required standard for its cancer center approval. It is estimated that there are currently more than 2,000 patient navigation programs at health care sites in America.

The early results of patient navigation are promising. Further research needs to be conducted to determine the level of benefits and cost-effectiveness of patient navigation.

DISCUSSION

African Americans and poor Americans have a 10% to 15% lower 5-year cancer survival compared with other Americans. Uninsured Americans also have a relatively lower 5-year survival rate.

African Americans have the highest mortality and the lowest 5-year survival rate compared to all other racial and ethnic groups. Evidence shows that disproportionate degree of poverty and relative lack of health insurance is the key underlying cause of the mortality and survival gap between black and white Americans.

Racial classification in America is socially and politically determined and has no basis in science. However, the Institute of Medicine has concluded that race is an independent determinant of black and white differences in cancer outcome.

There has been considerable discussion and writing about the role that genetics plays in racial disparities. It is true that genetic factors may explain some of the differences in cancer incidence in some population groups. For example, women from population groups with an increased frequency of *BRCA1* and *BRCA2* genes such as women of Ashkenazi Jewish descent have an increased risk of breast and ovarian cancer. Genetic factors may play a role in the increased risk of prostate cancer in black men and the increased rate of more aggressive forms of breast cancer in black women. However, genetic differences associated with race are thought to make a minor contribution to cancer disparities between different racial and ethnic populations. In considering the effect of genetic differences in groups of people, ancestry may be important. But race has very limited value as an indicator of the genetics of a group or an individual.

Poverty is a proxy or surrogate for a complex variety of negative social conditions.

Health disparities occur in the context of broader historical and contemporary social and economic inequality. Three critical factors drive disparities: low economic status, social injustice, and culture (lifestyle, attitude, and behavior). This suggests that a serious approach to reducing disparities must take these factors into consideration.

This also implies that an understanding of the factors that drive health disparities involves biomedical science and social science. Moreover, because social inequalities play a dominant role in driving health disparities, reducing disparities may involve civil and human rights considerations.

There is a critical disconnect between the nation's discovery enterprise and its delivery enterprise, a disconnect between what we know and what we do for all people. Disparities occur when there is a failure to apply what we know at any given time to all people irrespective of their economic, social, and cultural circumstances.

Poverty is a proxy or surrogate for a complex series of negative social conditions. In this nation there are known geographic areas of excess cancer mortality. The principal determinant of cancer mortality in such geographic areas is low socioeconomic status. This knowledge could be used to designate areas in the country that could be targeted for special assistance.

WHAT MUST BE DONE TO DIMINISH CANCER DISPARITIES

Reducing cancer health disparities will at a minimum require the following actions:

- Ensure that populations at highest risk have access to age- and gender-appropriate screening and follow-up services for breast, cervical, colorectal, and prostate cancer.
- Provide immediate access to diagnosis and treatment for uninsured and underinsured patients at the point of obtaining a suspicious result or diagnosis of cancer to ensure that no patient with cancer goes untreated.
- Delineate and target geographic areas with excess cancer mortality with an intense approach to providing culturally relevant education, appropriate access to screening, diagnosis, treatment, and improved social support.
- Provide such communities with funding for patient navigation programs, the purpose of which is to provide personal assistance in eliminating any barriers to obtaining timely and adequate diagnosis and treatment.
- Establish and implement systems for monitoring treatment equity according to standards of care to diminish bias in the provision of health care.
- Because cancer disparities are principally driven by failure to apply what we know at a given time, research should focus on determining how to close the gap between discovery and delivery of education and access to care for all Americans.
- Research should also focus on questions regarding how to make finer distinctions in identifying which populations are not faring as well and the precise reasons for the disparity. It appears that expanded knowledge of population genetics and a more fundamental understanding of the effect of culture and economic status will be keys to this progress.
- Encourage each individual, regardless of economic status, to share in the responsibility for promoting his or her own health and well-being.
- Promote the public and political will to create a health care system that provides universal access to health care of all Americans, irrespective of their ability to pay for services.

Americans who are poor or of low economic class constitute a high-risk group for developing and dying from cancer. The concentration of medical and educational resources on high-risk groups is an accepted medical principle. Accordingly, substantial resources should be directed toward education, prevention, detection, diagnosis, and treatment of cancer in Americans of low economic status.

There is a need for the entire scientific community to review the social values that shape its scientific perspectives with respect to race and to examine the biases and fundamental assumptions that scientists have made about the meaning of race in scientific investigation. At issue is the need to disentangle the social and political meaning of race from assumptions about its biological meaning. It is certain that future advances in scientific knowledge gained from the human genome and population genetics studies will further challenge us to re-examine how we group persons for biologic study.

To win the war against cancer we must continue to increase the nation's investment in the funding of research. However, the war cannot be won unless there is dramatic reduction cancer mortality and an increase in cancer survival of poor and uninsured Americans. In order to accomplish this we must apply what we know at any given time in an equitable manner to all Americans. We must tear down the economic and cultural barriers to prevention, detection, and treatment of cancer and achieve justice in the distribution of medical resources.

References

1. *Cancer facts and figures 2010*. Atlanta, GA: American Cancer Society, 2010.
2. Freeman HP. Poverty, culture, and social injustice: determinants of cancer disparities. *CA Cancer J Clin* 2004;54(2):72.
3. Freeman HP. Cancer in the socioeconomically disadvantaged. *CA Cancer J Clin* 1989:39(5):266.
4. Freeman HP. Commentary on the meaning of race in science and society. *Cancer Epidemiol Biomarkers Prev* 2003;12(Suppl):232S.
5. Henschke UK, Leffall LD Jr, Mason CH, Reinhold AW, Schneider RL, White JE. Alarming increase of cancer mortality in the US black population (1950–1967). *Cancer* 1973;31:763.
6. National Cancer Institute. SEER incidence and U.S. death rates, all cancer sites, both sexes. Worldwide URL: seer.cancer.gov/csr/1975_2007/results_merged/topic_race_ethnicity.
7. American Cancer Society special report on cancer in the economically disadvantaged. Atlanta, GA: American Cancer Society, 1986.
8. Ward E, Jemel A, Cokkinides V. Cancer disparities by race/ethnicity and socioeconomic status. *CA Cancer J Clin* 2004;54:78.
9. US Office of Management and Budget. Statistical Policy Directive No. 15, *Race and ethnic standards for federal statistics and administrative reporting*. 1977; Revised 1997. http://clinton4.nara.gov/OMB/fedreg/ombdir15.html.
10. Freeman HP. Considerations on the use on internet as a tool for minority recruitment into clinical trials. *Cancer J* 2006;12(6):459.
11. Wendler D, Kingston R, Madans J, et al. Are racial and ethnic minorities less willing to participate in health research? *Plos Med* 2006;3(2):E19.
12. Freeman HP. The meaning of race in science: considerations for cancer research. *Cancer* 1998;82:219.
13. Institute of Medicine. *The unequal burden of cancer.* Washington, DC: National Academy Press, 1999.
14. Institute of Medicine. *Unequal treatment: Confronting racial and ethnic disparities in healthcare.* Washington, DC: National Academy Press, 2003.
15. Bach PB, Cramer LD, Warren JL, Begg CB. Racial differences in the treatment of early stage lung cancer. *N Engl J Med* 1999;341:1198.
16. Bach PB, Pham HH, Schrag D. Primary care physicians who treat blacks and whites. *N Engl J Med* 2004;351:375.
17. Bureau of the Census. Income poverty and health 2010. www.census.gov/prod 2010/p 60-238, pdf.
18. Freeman HP, Muth BJ, Kerner JF. Expanding access to cancer screening and clinical follow up among medically underserved. *Cancer Pract* 1995:3:19.
19. *Report to the nation on cancer in the poor.* Atlanta, GA: American Cancer Society, 1989.
20. Freeman HP, Wasfie TJ. Cancer of the breast in poor black women. *Cancer* 1989;63:2562.
21. Oluwole SF. Impact of a cancer screening program on breast cancer stage at diagnosis in a medically underserved community. *J Am Coll Surg* 2003; 196(2):180.

CHAPTER 180 CANCER INFORMATION ON THE INTERNET

SHERRI L. PLACE AND J . ROBERT BECK

BACKGROUND

Internet use is now part of everyday life: in 2000, less than half of American adults had access to the Internet; by 2009, 74% of American adults were online.[1] Individuals have come to rely on the Internet to find health information: eight in ten Internet users seek health-related information, but only 9% claim to do so at least once per week.[1] Patients search online to find a variety of information resources to assist with decision making or to understand cancer diagnoses and treatment options, as well as to connect with medical professionals and support groups. Although mobile access and social networking are expanding the ways in which patients can find and discuss health-related information, most seek expert advice from health care professionals.

Individuals seek health information not only for themselves, but for others as well: 48% surveyed for the Pew Internet & American Life Project claimed their search for information was for someone else.[2] One in ten health-related queries have some impact on the information seeker's own care or how he or she would care for someone else.[1] Of those who thought the information found had any impact, 60% said what they found affected a decision relating to treatment and 53% reported that what they found helped them formulate new questions for their doctor or to get a second opinion.[1]

Data from 2003 Health Information National Trends Survey shows that cancer information seekers tend to have a personal or family history of cancer.[3] Of these seekers, 48.4% used the Internet, 34.5% used print materials, and 10.9% used their health care professional.[3] In searching for information on cancer, site-specific cancers were most frequently searched, with breast, prostate, and skin cancers at the topping the list.[3] A study by Basch et al.[4] found that patients with cancer often consulted both print and Internet resources and usually relied on more than one source. Of those using the Internet to find information, most searched for information on diagnosis and treatment as well as treatment side effects, clinical trials, drugs, hospitals, and physicians.[4]

Patients often come to health care providers with information gathered online, which may or may not be from authoritative sources. Many cancer patients seek information online because they want to be actively involved in their care and want to ask better questions when they do meet with physicians.[5] Hesse et al.[6] found that when individuals surveyed began their search for information about cancer, 48% started with an Internet search as opposed to 10% going to their health care provider first. Age also makes a difference: those in the 18- to 34-year age range were more likely to search the Internet before going to a health care provider. Even though an Internet search may be the first stop on a patient's search for information, most patients are using what they find on the Internet as a supplement to rather than a replacement for physician advice. One study found that Internet searches actually increase the likelihood that an individual will contact a health professional for more information as a well as an office visit.[7] However, cancer patients may or may not discuss their findings with physicians: 62% of respondents in a 2009 study reported not discussing with their doctors information they found online, even if they thought the information was important.[5]

The Internet is a powerful tool for finding and connecting people with information. Not only does it provide physicians with access to the latest information, but it can also help improve patient care. One Harris Interactive study found that consumers, as time-crunched as their doctors, would like personalized information delivered to them in an efficient and effective manner: face-to-face, by phone, or through the Internet.[8] By providing information via the Internet (by e-mail or linking patients with authoritative Websites), physicians can guide cancer patients to appropriate resources. The Websites listed in the Appendix at the end of this chapter provide Web-based information for both clinicians and patients.

TOOLS FOR FINDING INFORMATION

Many more health information seekers start their search with a search engine rather than a health-related site.[2] Doctors themselves are using Google as a tool to help diagnose difficult cases.[9] Because so many information seekers turn to search engines as their first source for finding information on the Web, it is important to note that overlap among search engines is not very common. Searching only one engine, such as Google, misses content that could be found by trying the same query on other search engines or professional resources such as MEDLINE.[10] To produce the best results while searching for information, it is often useful to query multiple engines rather than relying on the same source every time. It is also important to remember that not everything on the Internet can be found using a search engine. The invisible, or deep, Web includes content that cannot be "crawled," or found, by a search engine. Information may exist in a database or can only be accessed through a form.[11] Additionally, not everything on the Internet is freely available; although some biomedical information is available for free, much of it may be available by subscription only.

TABLE 180.1

HEALTH ON THE NET FOUNDATION HONCODE[a]

Criteria	Provides
Authoritative	Indicates the qualifications of the authors.
Complementarity	Information should support, not replace, the doctor-patient relationship.
Privacy	Information should support, not replace, the doctor-patient relationship.
Attribution	Cites the source(s) of published information, date, and medical and health pages.
Justifiability	Site must back up claims relating to benefits and performance.
Transparency	Provides accessible presentation, accurate e-mail contact.
Financial disclosure	Identifies funding sources.
Sponsorship	Clearly distinguishes advertising from editorial content.

[a]Available at http://www.hon.ch/HONcode/Conduct.html.

EVALUATING INFORMATION

Many information seekers do not check the source or date of the health information they find.[2] Critically evaluating information found online is important as out-of-date or incorrect information could be potentially harmful. Because most information seekers start their search on an engine rather than from an authoritative subject-specific site, it is important to evaluate a Website's authority, accuracy, objectivity, and currency. Patients may need guidance in finding trustworthy sites and appraising and filtering the information they do find. The Health on the Net Foundation's HONcode provides a list of evaluation criteria for health and medical Websites (Table 180.1).[12] Eysenbach[13] reports that the quality of cancer information on the Web is similar to what is found in other media, including print.

Search Engines

Different kinds of search engines exist: full-text engines like Google and searchable subject directories such as the ilp2 Website (http://www.ipl.org/) and the Open Directory Project (http://www.dmoz.org/). Full-text engines attempt to index the entire content of a Web page, whereas a subject index does not. Subject indexes are indexed and categorized by humans, while full-text engines are not. Some full-text engines also have searchable subject directories, while some subject directories have an option to search a full-text engine. Because of their degree of organization, searchable subject directories may be a useful place for patients to start their search for information. No matter what type of resource is used to find information, creating an effective search strategy will improve results. Quality keywords improve search results and influence the type of information found.

Google's popularity continues to eclipse all other search engines and dominates the search landscape.[14] Because of Google's ubiquitous presence on the Internet and for simplicity, features of Google and tips for using this engine will be discussed here. This is not an endorsement for Google: many other useful search engines exist and some provide specialized access to content that Google may not. Table 180.2 provides uniform resource locators (URLs) for alternatives to Google.

Search engines are useful starting points while seeking information, but subject-specific Websites target information to alleviate information overload. Sites such as MedlinePlus (http://

TABLE 180.2

BEYOND GOOGLE

Search Engine	Web Address	Information
Yahoo	http://www.yahoo.com/	Second most popular search engine.
Bing	http://www.bing.com/	Third most popular search engine.
IPL2	http://www.ipl.org/	Subject directory developed and managed by librarians.
Open Directory Project	http://www.dmoz.org/	Large subject directory constructed and managed by a global community of volunteers.
BioMedSearch	http://www.biomedsearch.com/	Specialized biomedical search engine that searches PubMed plus dissertations and other documents not found in PubMed.
OmniMedicalSearch	http://www.omnimedicalsearch.com/	Specialized search engine focusing on medical information for both consumers and health care professionals.
WolframAlpha	http://www.wolframalpha.com/	Specialized search engine focusing on computational information including medical test data, medical computations, and statistical data.
Zuula	http://www.zuula.com/	Searches several engines at once including the top three: Google, Yahoo, and Bing.

TABLE 180.3

GOOGLE SHORTCUTS[a]

To obtain:	*Try this:*
Definitions	Define: oncology
Exact phrase search	"To be or not to be"
Exclude adult content	Safesearch:breast
Exclude terms	Skin cancer–melanoma
File type search	NCI report filetype:pdf
Include terms	EGFR + inhibitors
Site search	Patients site:www.fccc.edu
Synonyms	~Cancer

[a]Available at: http://www.google.com/help/cheatsheet.html.

medlineplus.gov/) offer focused searching with access to multiple authoritative Websites. Sometimes, subject-specific article databases, such as PubMed (the free version of MEDLINE), are better places to start. An effective search strategy begins with an assessment of the types of information sought. Using the right tool along with the right search terms actually saves time.

Google ranks search results by use of a proprietary algorithm based on several factors including word frequency, advertising, and location of terms within Website titles or headers. Whether searching the Web as a whole, there are a few ways to get the most out of a search. Table 180.3 provides a few shortcuts. In addition to shortcuts, strategic use of advanced search features focuses searches to target the most useful information. Advanced search features allow searchers to create complex Boolean searches quite easily.

Google also provides the e-mail-based Google Alerts (http://www.google.com/alerts) service to track news articles about medical advances. Keyword searches may be run against news, blogs, the Web, Google Groups, or all four at once. Any new content will be sent to the specified e-mail address within the chosen timeframe.

Specialty Search Engines: Google Scholar

Google Scholar (http://scholar.google.com) offers full-text searching of scholarly literature including peer-reviewed articles, books, and theses. Unlike PubMed, Google Scholar culls information from a variety of disciplines and is an effective tool for finding gray literature as well as some meeting abstracts. In addition, results display "cited by" information, (i.e., links to articles citing the reference found), although accuracy about this information is not easily confirmed. Adjusting Google Scholar's preferences allows for the display of home library information as well as a link to import citations into bibliographic management software. Just like its parent, Google, this full-text engine allows some advanced searching (+, −, OR, phrase) and searches can be limited by author, publication, date, or subject area. Also available is an option to search for terms in the titles rather than in the full text, which focuses the search and narrows results.

Google Scholar provides the option to create e-mailbased alerts to facilitate keeping current with new content indexed in Google Scholar. Using the advanced search option allows the most tailored alert as searches can be limited to a particular author and a set of keywords. However, alerts cannot be created using the publication field in the advanced Google Scholar search. To limit to a particular publication, try searching the publication's title as an exact phrase. Once the search is performed, click on the envelope icon preceding the search results to create the alert.

Google Scholar also provides a way to track new citations to specific papers. After searching for a specific article, click on the "Cited by" link to display the results. From this display screen, create the alert by clicking on the envelope icon (Fig. 180.1).

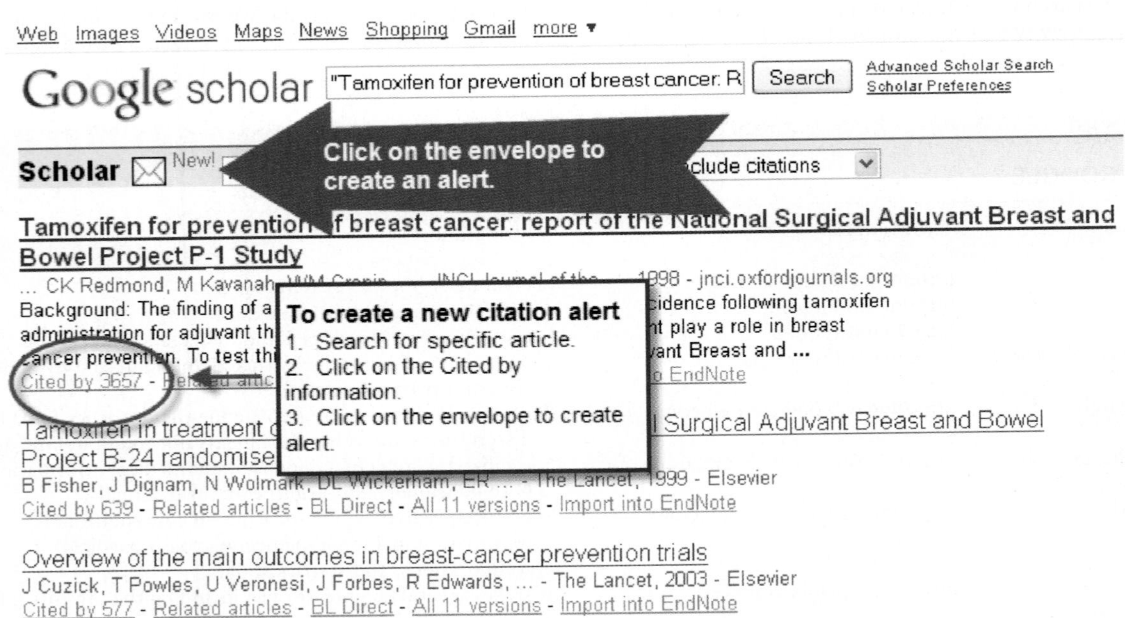

FIGURE 180.1 Google Scholar alerts.

SEARCH STRATEGIES

Boolean

The concepts used in Boolean searches can be employed not only in databases such as PubMed but may also be used in search engines such as Google. However, not all search engines allow use of Boolean operators, such as AND, OR, NOT. Many engines default to AND, which means it will search for all of the terms entered in the search box. A few may default to OR, which will look for the occurrence of any term, thus increasing results. The defaults may change, so entering multiple terms can clarify what algorithm the engine uses. If results increase, then it defaults to OR; if they decrease, it defaults to AND. The best place to do a Boolean search is to use the engine's advanced search options. In Google's advanced search (Fig. 180.2), all of the words = AND, at least one of the words = OR, and without the words = NOT.

Although some engines allow for nested Boolean searches, full nested searches can interfere with the engine's relevance rankings.[11] Google allows phrase searching either from the advanced search page or by simply enclosing terms in quotes. Phrase searching can narrow results significantly.

Truncation and Wild Cards

Unlike article databases such as PubMed, truncation is not often an option in search engines. However, it may be useful to consider searching both singular and plural forms of words. Google does support full-word wild card searches. An asterisk (*) is used to take the place of whole words.

TABLE 180.4

FIELD SEARCHING IN GOOGLE

Field	Provides
Site:	Restricts to specific domain or top-level domain
Intitle:	Restricts to Web page titles
Link:	Finds pages that link to the page

Field Searching

Field searching can be done using shortcuts or through the advanced search page. It allows specification of where matches to a term should occur. For example, in Google Scholar's advanced search, it is easy to specify whether a term occurs in a title or in the full text of a document. Specific syntax for field searching can be found on an engine's help page; prefixes can vary from engine to engine (Table 180.4).

Limits

Again, limits are available in the advanced search page. Restricting by language, date, or file format can be helpful in narrowing a search. However, the date limit only looks at when a page was last updated, not its creation date. Pages are updated for a number of reasons, not just for updating content.

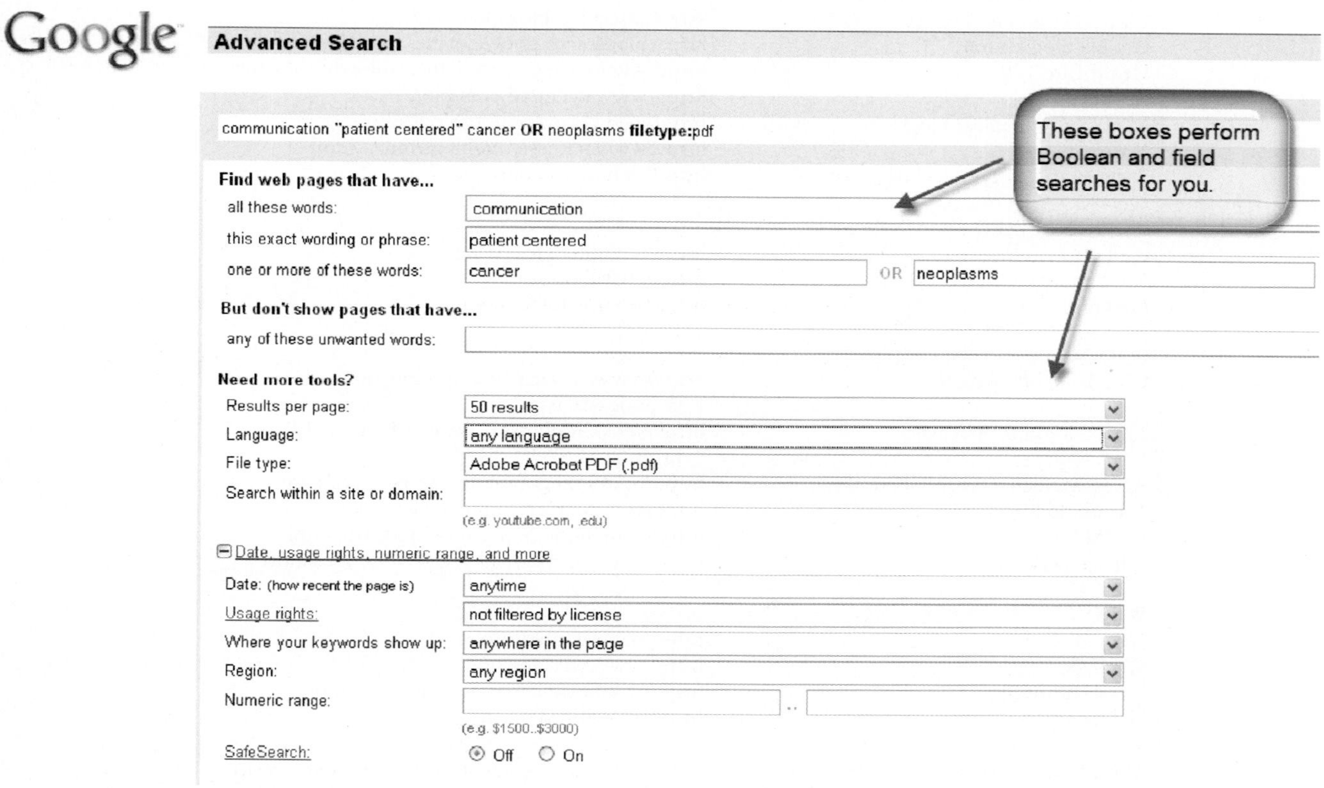

FIGURE 180.2 Google advanced search screen.

USEFUL TOOLS FOR KEEPING UP

Staying on top of the medical literature need not be time-consuming. Many Web-based tools make it easier to keep up with new developments in medicine. E-mail alerts, RSS feeds (see later discussion), and Weblogs (blogs) are a few of the tools that can help monitor trends and developments in oncology (Table 180.5). These types of resources will be described in the following sections.

PubMed

PubMed, a free bibliographic database from the National Library of Medicine, provides access to citations and abstracts to over 5,000 biomedical journals published in the United States and around the world. Coverage dates back to the 1950s and provides links to some free full-text publications as well as links to participating publishers' Web sites. PubMed includes MEDLINE and OLDMEDLINE as well as new items that have not yet been indexed by MEDLINE. New material is added Tuesday through Saturday.

PubMed offers a variety of powerful search options. Keyword searching is enhanced by automatic term mapping, which translates terms and looks for matches not only in the MeSH (Medical Subject Heading) terms and subheadings but also in the See-Reference terms and National Library of Medicine's Unified Medical Language System (UMLS). UMLS can be used in the development of systems that "understand" the language of health and biomedicine. Also matched are journals and authors. Using the limits feature allows a search

TABLE 180.5

TOOLS FOR KEEPING UP

Site	Web Address
RSS READERS AND FEEDS	
Bloglines	http://www.bloglines.com
Google Reader	http://reader.google.com
JAMA RSS feeds	http://pubs.ama-assn.org/misc/rssfeed.dtl?home
MedWorm	http://www.medworm.com
NCI Cancer Bulletin	http://feeds.feedburner.com/ncicancerbulletin
NEJM online feeds	http://content.nejm.org/rss/
Nature Web reeds	http://www.nature.com/webfeeds/index.html
RSS compendium	http://www.allrss.com
Science RSS feeds	http://www.sciencemag.org/rss/
BLOGS AND BLOG SEARCH	
Clinical cases and images	http://casesblog.blogspot.com/
Google blog search	http://blogsearch.google.com
Healthcare 100	http://www.edrugsearch.com/edsblog/healthcare100/
KevinMD	http://www.kevinmd.com/blog/
MedWorm: medical blogs	http://medworm.com/rss/blogs.php
Nature blogs	http://www.nature.com/blogs/index.html
Technorati	http://technorati.com/
PERSONALIZED HOME PAGES	
iGoogle	http://www.google.com/ig
My Yahoo!	http://my.yahoo.com/
Netvibes	http://www.netvibes.com
PODCASTS	
CR Magazine (AACR)	http://www.crmagazine.org/home/magazine/cr-podcasts.aspx
Johns Hopkins podcasts	http://www.hopkinsmedicine.org/mediaII/Podcasts.html
AccessMedicine Weekly Podcasts	http://books.mcgraw-hill.com/podcast/acm/
Nature podcasts	http://www.nature.com/podcast/index.html
NEJM	http://content.nejm.org/misc/podcast.shtml
Science podcast	http://www.sciencemag.org/about/podcast.dtl
WIKIS	
Ganfyd	http://www.ganfyd.org
WikiDoc	http://www.wikidoc.org
WikiHealthCare	http://wikihealthcare.jointcommission.org
Wikipedia	http://en.wikipedia.org

AMA, *Journal of the American Medical Association*; RSS, really simple syndication; NCI, National Cancer Institute; NEJM, *New England Journal of Medicine*; AACR, American Association for Cancer Research.

to be focused a number of ways, including by date, publication type, age range, journal group or topic (such as cancer), and language. PubMed supports nested Boolean searching as well as phrase searching and truncation.

In addition to being a powerful tool for finding medical literature, PubMed can also help keep an oncologist up-to-date with changes and trends. By creating a free "MyNCBI" account, searchers can save a search to be sent as an e-mail alert. MyNCBI accounts also allow for customization of PubMed results: setting filters to group results, and highlighting search terms, setting display options are all ways to make PubMed fit specific needs. Newer features of MyNCBI include the option to create collections, which allows the results of multiple searches to be combined. Users can share these results by making the collection "public" and sharing the URL with colleagues.

RSS Feeds

Although there is some debate on what RSS really stands for, here it will be referred to as really simple syndication. RSS uses XML (Extensible Markup Language) to format Web-based content. Feed readers, or aggregators, are software that read and display content. Whenever an RSS feed sends out notification of new content, the feed reader picks it up, thus making it easier to stay on top of medical literature, oncology news, or a favorite blog. Information is "pushed," eliminating the need to rerun a search or continually visit a site or group of sites. Because bloggers (people who write Web logs) and news organizations often create RSS feeds, RSS search engines can help find information as soon as it becomes available.

Many publisher Websites offer news and other information as RSS-based subscriptions. Resources such as PubMed allow the creation of keyword-based feeds to target specific topics. Journal sites may offer tables of contents alerts as a feed. Managing all these subscriptions can be streamlined in a number of ways, but the essential tool for using RSS is an aggregator. Most are Web-based, which means that they are accessible from any computer with Internet access. Integrating an aggregator, such as Google Reader, with a personalized home page allows multiple tools to be available at a glance, similar to a dashboard. Table 180.5 lists options for both RSS aggregators as well as personalized home pages.

Blogs, Wikis, and Podcasts

Blogs, which are a lot like an online journal or diary, are dated entries displayed in reverse chronological order on a particular topic. Often they are written by one person or a group of contributors and can contain commentary, links to other Websites, news, and images. Readers may post responses, allowing for discussion of particular topics. Blogs are an excellent way to keep current on a multitude of topics. Many bloggers consume vast amounts of information and then distill that information on their site. Most blogs offer the option to subscribe via RSS so that it is not necessary to visit the blog regularly.

Various tools exist for finding blogs. Keyword searches in general blog search engines, such as Technorati, will yield a wide variety of hits, which could retrieve a fair number of low-quality blogs. Subject-specific blog search engines, such as MedWorm, will allow for a more focused search as well as more authoritative content. Another way to find useful blogs is to explore the blogrolls on the blogs you already visit. Blogrolls, usually found in a sidebar on the site, imply that the author recommends the sites.

As social media evolves, the lines between blogging and social networking continue to blur. Twitter mixes blogging with social networking, and many sites, including publishers, have added Twitter as a method for linking consumers with information. Twitter is fast becoming a useful current awareness tool. Posting on the site is not a requirement for an account. Accounts allow a searcher to subscribe to, or "follow," tweets (posts by other users). The personalized home pages in Table 180.5 offer Twitter gadgets, making it easy to keep watch over both RSS feeds and Twitter updates.

Wikis provide a place for collaborative authoring and can refer to a Website or the collaborative software that facilitates the website.[15] The ability for visitors to add or change content provides a useful medium for sharing knowledge.

Podcasts, media files that can be played on mobile devices (MP3 players, cell phones) or computers, provide for learning

TABLE 180.6

SOCIAL MEDIA

Site	Web Address	Information
SOCIAL BOOKMARKING AND ANNOTATION		
CiteULike	http://www.citeulike.org/	Free site for managing and sharing scholarly references. Allows storing and searching of PDFs.
Connotea	http://www.connotea.org/	Free online tool for managing and sharing references tailored specifically to clinicians and researchers.
Delicious	http://delicious.com/	Free site for storing, sharing, and tagging bookmarks.
Zotero	http://www.zotero.org/	Free browser extension for managing, storing, and sharing research sources.
SOCIAL NETWORKS		
Facebook	http://www.facebook.com/	Most popular social networking site, open to all.
LinkedIn	http://www.linkedin.com/	Social networking site for professionals.
Ning	http://www.ning.com/	Fee-based service allows participants to create a private network.
Ozmosis	https://www.ozmosis.com/	Social network that only allows U.S. licensed physicians to join.
Sermo	http://www.sermo.com/	Free online physician community open to MDs and DOs in the U.S.
Twitter	http://twitter.com/	Free real-time information sharing tool.

PDFs, portable document format; MD, medical doctor; DO, doctor of osteopathic medicine.

anytime, anywhere. Both audio and video podcasts are available automatically through RSS.[16]

Social Bookmarking and Annotation Tools

Keeping track of Websites using a browser's bookmarks feature can be cumbersome. Web-based social bookmarking tools, such as Delicious, provide easy access to sites found on the Web. As an added benefit, these sites can be "tagged": users can choose keywords to describe the sites and then share what is found with others. Other resources such as Connotea, geared towards clinicians and scientists, takes social bookmarking a step further to include bibliographic management tools. Not only can searchers organize links to journal articles as well as Websites, but they can share what they find as well.

Social Networking

The Internet has long since been a place to collaborate and share resources and information. Many use the Internet to maintain ties and connect with their social network.[17] Social networking Websites, such as Facebook, allow groups of individuals come together to share ideas and information. Since 2007, time spent on social media use has increased 82% and users typically spend almost 6 hours per month on Facebook, the number one social networking site.[18] With its large market share, Facebook may seem like the ideal venue for oncologists to connect with colleagues and patients. However, physicians using Facebook should carefully consider the implications of "friending" patients. Dual relationships could be problematic as well as unethical, and physicians may violate a patient's privacy.[19] Additionally, physicians should carefully examine a site's privacy settings and exercise caution when posting any personal information.[19]

Sites such as Sermo offer a place for physicians to exchange information and insights and opportunities to collaborate with colleagues and network with other physicians from around the country. Other sites, such as Ning, allow users to create their own "private" social networks that allow gadgets such as RSS feeds and wikis. Table 180.6 provides links to other social networks.

References

1. Fox S, Jones S. The social life of health information, 2009. http://www.pewinternet.org/~/media//Files/Reports/2009/PIP_Health_2009.pdf.
2. Fox S. Online health search, 2006. http://207.21.232.103/pdfs/PIP_Online_Health_2006.pdf.
3. Rutten LJ, Squiers L, Hesse B. Cancer-related information seeking: hints from the 2003 Health Information National Trends Survey (HINTS). *J Hhealth Ccommun* 2006;11(Suppl 1):147.
4. Basch EM, Thaler HT, Shi W, Yakren S, Schrag D. Use of information resources by patients with cancer and their companions. *Cancer* 2004;100(11):2476.
5. Bylund C, Gueguen J, D'Agostino T, Imes R, Sonet E. Cancer patients' decisions about discussing Internet information with their doctors. *Psycho-oncology* 2009;18(11):1139.
6. Hesse BW, Nelson DE, Kreps GL, et al. Trust and sources of health information: the impact of the Internet and its implications for health care providers: findings from the first Health Information National Trends Survey. *Arch Intern Med* 2005;165(22):2618.
7. Lee C. Does the Internet displace health professionals? *J Health Commun* 2008;13(5):450.
8. Harris Interactive. Consumers demand combination of "high tech" and "high touch" personalized services to manage healthcare needs, 2000. http://www.harrisinteractive.com/news/index.asp?NewsID=166&HI.
9. Tang H, Ng JH. Googling for a diagnosisóuse of Google as a diagnostic aid: internet based study. *BMJ* 2006;333(7579):1143.
10. Sherman C. Search engine results continuing to diverge, 2005. http://searchenginewatch.com/showPage.html?page=3524411.
11. Notess GR. *Teaching Web Search Skills: Techniques and Strategies of Top Trainers*. Medford, NJ: Information Today, 2006.
12. HON Code of Conduct (HONcode) for medical and health Websites, 2007. http://www.hon.ch/HONcode/Conduct.html.
13. Eysenbach G. The impact of the Internet on cancer outcomes. *CA: Cancer J Clin.* 2003;53(6):356.
14. *NielsenWire*. U.S. search rankings, Nielsen reports February 2010. [http://blog.nielsen.com/nielsenwire/online_mobile/nielsen-reports-february-2010-u-s-search-rankings/.
15. Wikipedia. http://en.wikipedia.org/wiki/Wiki.
16. Podcast. http://en.wikipedia.org/wiki/Podcasts.
17. Boase J, Horrigan J, Wellman B, Rainie L. The strength of Internet ties, 2006. http://www.pewinternet.org/pdfs/PIP_Internet_ties.pdf.
18. *NielsenWire*. Led by Facebook, Twitter, global time spent on social media sites up 82% year over year,, 2010. http://blog.nielsen.com/nielsenwire/global/led-by-facebook-twitter-global-time-spent-on-social-media-sites-up-82-year-over-year/.
19. Guseh J, Brendel R, Brendel D. Medical professionalism in the age of online social networking. *BMJ* 2009;35(9):584.

APPENDIX

WEBSITES

Site	Web Address
COMPREHENSIVE	
American Cancer Society	http://www.cancer.org
National Cancer Institute (NCI)	http://www.cancer.gov/
National Comprehensive Cancer Network	http://www.nccn.org/
OncoLink	http://www.oncolink.com/
PDQ: NCI's Comprehensive Cancer Database	http://www.cancer.gov/cancertopics/pdq
CANCER LITERATURE	
American Association for Cancer Research (AACR)	http://www.aacr.org/
BioMed Central (includes RSS feed)	http://www.biomedcentral.com/
Cancernews (e-mail updates)	http://www.cancernews.com
Medscape (RSS news feed and e-mail alerts)	http://www.medscape.com/
Nation Cancer Institute Publications Locator	https://cissecure.nci.nih.gov/ncipubs/
PubMed (RSS and email updates)	http://www.pubmed.gov
CLINICAL TRIALS	
CenterWatch	http://www.centerwatch.com/
Clinical Trials (NCI)	http://www.cancer.gov/clinical_trials/
ClinicalTrials.gov	http://www.clinicaltrials.gov/
ORGANIZATIONS	
AACR	http://www.aacr.org/
American Joint Committee on Cancer	http://www.cancerstaging.org/
American Society of Clinical Oncology	http://www.asco.org
Association of American Cancer Institutes	http://www.aaci-cancer.org/
American Society for Therapeutic Radiology and Oncology	http://www.astro.org/
International Union Against Cancer	http://www.uicc.org/
Oncology Nursing Society	http://www.ons.org/
NATIONAL CANCER COOPERATIVE GROUPS	
American College of Surgeons Oncology Group	http://www.acosog.org/
Cancer and Leukemia Group B	http://www.calgb.org/
Children's Oncology Group	http://www.childrensoncologygroup.org/
Coalition of National Cancer Cooperative Groups	http://www.cancertrialshelp.org
Eastern Cooperative Oncology Group	http://www.ecog.org/
Gynecologic Oncology Group	http://www.gog.org/
National Surgical Adjuvant Breast and Bowel Project	http://www.nsabp.pitt.edu/
North Central Cancer Treatment Group	http://ncctg.mayo.edu/
Radiation Therapy Oncology Group	http://www.rtog.org/
STATISTICS	
American Cancer Society statistics	http://www.cancer.org/docroot/stt/stt_0.asp
CANCER*Modial* Statistical Information System (international)	http://www-dep.iarc.fr/
National Cancer Data Base	http://www.facs.org/cancer/ncdb/index.html
National Center for Health Statistics FastStats	http://www.cdc.gov/nchs/fastats/cancer.htm
National Program of Cancer Registries	http://www.cdc.gov/cancer/npcr/
North American Association of Central Cancer Registries	http://www.naaccr.org
SEER (Surveillance, Epidemiology, and End Results)	http://seer.cancer.gov/
State cancer profiles	http://statecancerprofiles.cancer.gov/
EVIDENCE-BASED RESOURCES	
Centre for Evidence-Based Medicine	http://www.cebm.net/
Centre for Health Evidence	http://www.cche.net/
National Guideline Clearinghouse	http://www.guideline.gov/
Netting the Evidence	http://www.shef.ac.uk/scharr/ir/netting/
The Cochrane Collaboration	http://www.cochrane.org/
SITES FOR PATIENTS	
Association of Cancer Online Resources	http://www.acor.org
Cancer Care (includes Spanish language materials)	http://www.cancercare.org/
Cancer Information Service (NCI)	http://cis.nci.nih.gov/
Cancer Prevention and Control (CDC)	http://www.cdc.gov/cancer/
Cancer.Net	http://www.cancer.net
The Cancer Journey	http://www.thecancerjourney.org/

(*continued*)

APPENDIX

(CONTINUED)

Site	Web Address
Cancerfacts.com	http://www.cancerfacts.com/
Healthfinder	http://www.healthfinder.gov/
Hospice Education Institute	http://hospiceworld.org/
MedlinePlus	http://medlineplus.gov/
National Hospice and Palliative Care Organization	http://www.nhpco.org
WebMD	http://www.webmd.com
CANCER RISK SITES	
Breast Cancer Risk Assessment Tool	http://www.cancer.gov/bcrisktool/
Cancer Awareness and Risk Program	http://pennstatehershey.org/web/cpog/home/communityoutreach/risktest
Cancer Risk Quiz	http://www.fccc.edu/cancer/risk-quiz.html
Cancer Risk: Understanding the Puzzle	http://understandingrisk.cancer.gov/
Cancer Risk: What the Numbers Mean	http://www.mayoclinic.com/health/cancer/CA00053
Lung Cancer Risk Assessment	http://www.mskcc.org/mskcc/html/12463.cfm
Melanoma Risk Assessment Tool	http://www.cancer.gov/melanomarisktool/
Risk Assessment Quiz: Prostate Cancer	http://www.prostatecancer.ca/Prostate-Cancer/Risk-Assessment-Quiz.aspx
Women's Cancer Network: Cancer Risk Assessment Survey	http://www.wcn.org/risk_assessment/
Your Disease Risk	http://www.yourdiseaserisk.wustl.edu/
SPECIFIC CANCERS	
Bladder	
Bladder Cancer Advocacy Network	http://www.bcan.org/
UrologyChannel	http://www.urologychannel.com/
UrologyHealth.org	http://www.urologyhealth.org/
Bone	
Bone & Cancer Foundation	http://www.boneandcancerfoundation.org/
Bonetumor.org	http://www.bonetumor.org/
Brain	
American Brain Tumor Association	http://hope.abta.org/
National Brain Tumor Society	http://www.braintumor.org/
Neuro-Oncology Branch	http://home.ccr.cancer.gov/nob/default.asp
Breast	
American Breast Cancer Foundation	http://www.abcf.org/
Breast Cancer Online	http://www.bco.org/
BreastCancer.org	http://www.breastcancer.org/
FORCE: Facing Our Risk of Cancer Empowered	http://www.facingourrisk.org/
Imagines	http://www.imaginis.com/
National Breast Cancer Coalition	http://www.natlbcc.org/
Program on Breast Cancer and Environmental Risk Factors	http://envirocancer.cornell.edu/
Susan G. Komen for the Cure	http://ww5.komen.org/
Breast Cancer Network of Strength	http://www.networkofstrength.org/
Colorectal	
American Gastroenterological Association	http://www.gastro.org/
Colon Cancer Alliance	http://www.ccalliance.org/
Colorectal Cancer Coalition	http://www.fightcolorectalcancer.org/
Eye	
Eye Cancer Network	http://www.eyecancer.com/
Gynecologic	
American College of Obstetricians and Gynecologists	http://www.acog.org/
FORCE: Facing Our Risk of Cancer Empowered	http://www.facingourrisk.org/
Gynecologic Cancer Foundation	http://www.thegcf.org/
National Cervical Cancer Coalition	http://www.nccc-online.org/
National Ovarian Cancer Coalition	http://www.ovarian.org/
Women's Cancer Network	http://www.wcn.org/

APPENDIX

(CONTINUED)

Site	Web Address
SPECIFIC CANCERS (*continued*)	
Head and Neck (Including Mouth and Throat)	
American Academy of Otolaryngology–Head and Neck Surgery	http://www.entnet.org/
International Association of Laryngectomees	http://www.theial.com/ial/
Let's Face It	http://www.dent.umich.edu/faceit/
National Institute of Dental and Craniofacial Research	http://www.nidcr.nih.gov/
Oral Cancer Foundation	http://www.oralcancerfoundation.org/
Support for People with Oral and Head and Neck Cancer	http://www.spohnc.org/
Kidney	
Kidney Cancer Association	http://www.curekidneycancer.org/
National Kidney Foundation	http://www.kidney.org/
Leukemia and Lymphoma	
Leukemia and Lymphoma Society	http://www.leukemia-lymphoma.org/
LymphomaInfo.net	http://www.lymphomainfo.net/
Lymphoma Research Foundation	http://www.lymphoma.org
Liver	
LiverTumor.org	http://www.livertumor.org/
Lung	
American Lung Association	http://www.lungusa.org
Lung Cancer.org	http://www.lungcancer.org/
Lung Cancer Alliance	http://www.lungcanceralliance.org/
Myeloma	
International Myeloma Foundation	http://www.myeloma.org/
Multiple Myeloma Research Foundation	http://www.multiplemyeloma.org/
Pancreatic Cancer	
Hirshberg Foundation for Pancreatic Cancer	http://www.pancreatic.org
Pancreatic Cancer Action Network	http://www.pancan.org/
Pediatric	
Candlelighters Childhood Cancer Foundation	http://www.candlelighters.org/
Children's Hospice International	http://www.chionline.org/
Children's Oncology Group	http://www.childrensoncologygroup.org/
Children's Tumor Foundation	http://www.ctf.org/
National Children's Cancer Society	http://www.nationalchildrenscancersociety.org/
Osteosarcoma Online	http://cancer.iu.edu/osteosarcoma/
Prostate	
Prostate Cancer Education Council	http://www.pcaw.com/
Prostate Cancer Foundation	http://www.prostatecancerfoundation.org/
UrologyHealth.org	http://www.urologyhealth.org
Us TOO International	http://www.ustoo.org/
Skin	
American Academy of Dermatology	http://www.aad.org/
Melanoma Education Foundation	http://www.skincheck.org/
Melanoma Patients' Information Page	http://www.mpip.org/
Skin Cancer Foundation	http://www.skincancer.org/

RSS, really simple syndication; CDC, Centers for Disease Control and Prevention.

SECTION 22: COMPLEMENTARY, ALTERNATIVE, AND INTEGRATIVE THERAPIES

CHAPTER 181 COMPLEMENTARY, ALTERNATIVE, AND INTEGRATIVE THERAPIES IN CANCER CARE

CATHERINE ULBRICHT, LORENZO COHEN, AND RICHARD LEE

BACKGROUND

Definitions

In the United States, complementary and alternative medicine (CAM) is defined by the National Center for Complementary and Alternative Medicine (NCCAM) as a group of diverse medical and health care systems, practices, and products that are not normally considered to be conventional medicine.[1] Other terms used to refer to CAM include folkloric, holistic, irregular, nonconventional, non-Western, traditional, unconventional, unorthodox, and unproven medicine. NCCAM classifies CAM therapies into five categories, or domains: alternative medical systems, mind–body interventions, biologically based therapies, manipulative and body-based methods, and energy therapies (Table 181.1).[1–3]

Recently, the term "integrative medicine" has come into common use. The Consortium of Academic Health Centers for Integrative Medicine has defined this term as the practice of medicine that reaffirms the importance of the relationship between practitioner and patient, focuses on the whole person, is informed by evidence, and makes use of all appropriate therapeutic approaches, providers, and disciplines to achieve optimal health and healing.

Prevalence

In the United States, an estimated 44% of the population used at least one CAM therapy in 1997.[2,4–6] According to the 2007 National Health Interview Survey (NHIS), the prevalence of CAM use in the United States was approximately 38% for adults and 12% for children.[7]

Surveys published since 1999 suggest that between 25% and 83% of U.S. adult cancer patients have used CAM therapies at some point after diagnosis, with variations in utilization rates depending on geographic area and type of cancer.[8–25] Earlier studies generally report lower overall prevalence of CAM use (9% to 54%), possibly due to increasing rates of use or broadening of the definition of CAM.[26,27] Initial studies of CAM prevalence during the 1970s and 1980s focused on the toxicity of the anticancer therapy laetrile. Reported prevalence of CAM was 9% to 16%,[27] but surveys within the past decade estimated the prevalence of use in pediatric oncology to be 31% to 87%; moreover, in many cases the treating physician was unaware that their patients were using CAM.[28–31] Use of CAM is also prevalent among cancer patients outside the United States in all regions of the world, with significantly varying use among different regions.[26,32,33]

In the West, CAM use appears to be more common among those with higher education levels and higher incomes. CAM use is also higher among young females who have had surgery, used chemotherapy, or had a history of CAM use before diagnosis.[19,32,34,35]

ESTABLISHING AN INTEGRATIVE ONCOLOGY APPROACH WITH PATIENTS

Integrative Oncology Model

The process of creating an integrative approach for cancer should address several principles: comprehensive, personalized, evidence based, and safety. The conventional model of cancer treatment involves three different disciplines (surgery, radiation, chemotherapy), and integrative oncology aims to expand the interdisciplinary approach to include therapies such as acupuncture, yoga, meditation, diet, exercise, and other modalities. This is in response to the concept of treating the whole patient in all domains. Engel's biopsychosocial model of health care, first published in *Science* more than 30 years ago, describes one conceptual model of these domains of patient care and its importance in the treatment of all patients.[36] The Integrative Medicine Program at M. D. Anderson Cancer Center provides one example of how this framework may assist in creating comprehensive integrative care plans (Fig. 181.1). Without comprehensive assessment and appropriate attention given to their needs, patients may perceive gaps in their care. Although symptoms such as severe pain or nausea are typically thought of as purely physical symptoms, if symptoms remain severe and chronic they will often impact the psychosocial dimensions of health as patients may become more irritable, socially inactive, and fatigued due to insomnia. With comprehensive care plans, patients will have cancer treatments that address all of their needs in a more seamless manner. These plans will also have the greatest

TABLE 181.1

NATIONAL INSTITUTES OF HEALTH: NATIONAL CENTER FOR COMPLEMENTARY AND ALTERNATIVE MEDICINE CATEGORIES

Whole medical systems	Traditional Chinese medicine, Ayurvedic medicine
Biologically based therapies	Herbs, supplements, special diets
Mind–body therapies	Meditation, prayer, yoga
Body manipulation	Chiropractic, massage
Energy therapies	Qi gong, reiki, magnetic

potential for improving the overall health and well-being of cancer patients. These basic comprehensive evaluations are aggregates of many different components; by addressing issues of nutrition, physical activity, symptom control, and other factors, these plans will help improve the performance of cancer patients throughout the continuum of care.

Physical Well-Being

Growing evidence supports the important role of physical activity and nutrition in the health of cancer patients, and these factors have been correlated with improved clinical outcomes. Moreover, several phytochemicals demonstrate pharmacological effects on molecular targets in known cancer signaling pathways.[37] The Women's Intervention Study reported that a 24% reduction in fat intake resulted in lower cancer recurrence rates.[38] The Women's Health Eating and Living randomized women to increase fruit and vegetable intake and reduce dietary fat, but did not find a significant reduction in breast cancer events; however, when secondary analyses were performed, including physical activity, an increased survival of approximately 50% was found among women who were physically active and maintained a diet high in fruits and vegetables.[39,40] Similar associations are beginning to be reported in colon cancer.[39–42] The American Institute for Cancer Research (AICR) and the World Cancer Research Fund (WCRF) have created a combined report for guidelines regarding nutrition and physical activity to prevent cancer; the American Cancer Society (ACS) has also published guidelines for those with cancer.[43–48] Additionally, a recent study examining obesity during neoadjuvant chemotherapy for breast cancer patients found obesity was correlated with decreased survival,[49] and a different study found that obesity predicts a second primary tumor on the contralateral breast.[50] Patients need to be encouraged to follow the ACS guidelines and the AICS/WCRF guidelines for cancer prevention; they are also encouraged to adopt healthful behaviors in regard to physical activity and diet.

Psychosocial Well-Being: The Mind–Body Connection

The mind–body connection is an important aspect of integrative oncology, as emphasized in the recent Institute of Medicine (IOM) report "Cancer Care for the Whole Patient."[51] This comprehensive report states that "cancer care today often provides state-of-the-science biomedical treatment, but fails to address the psychological and social (psychosocial) problems associated with the illness. These problems—including . . . anxiety, depression or other emotional problems . . .—cause additional suffering, weaken adherence to prescribed treatments, and threaten patients' return to health." Extensive research has documented that mind–body interventions appear to address many of the issues mentioned in the IOM report.

The belief that what we think and feel can influence our health and healing dates back thousands of years.[52] The importance of the role of the mind, emotions, and behaviors in health and well-being has been a part of medical traditions of the world, such as Chinese, Tibetan, and Ayurvedic medicine. Many patients with cancer turn to CAM therapies as a way to reduce stress; substantial evidence now shows the negative health consequences of sustained stress on health and well-being. The profound psychological and behavioral effects of stress may include posttraumatic stress disorder, increased health-impairing behaviors (e.g., poor diet, lack of exercise, or substance abuse), poor sleep, and decreased quality of life.[53–57]

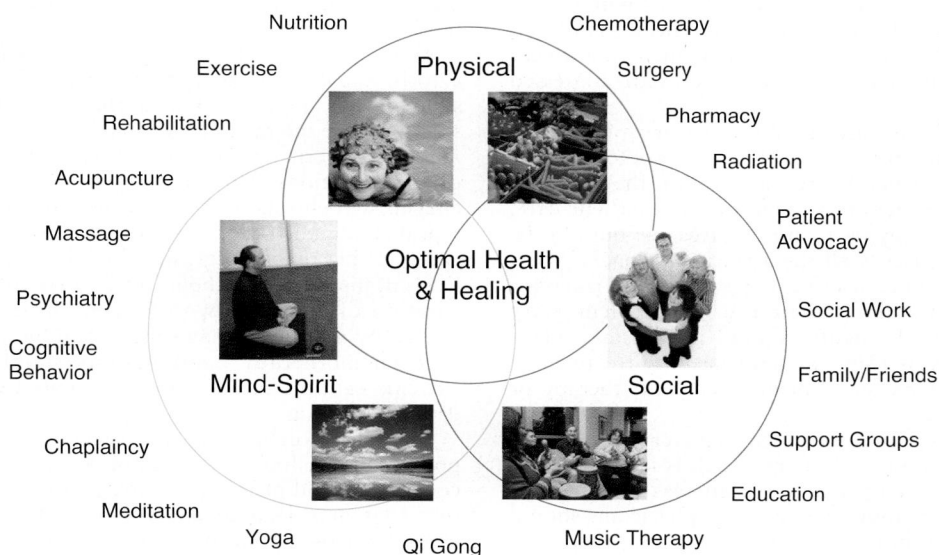

FIGURE 181.1 Guiding model for integrative medicine at M. D. Anderson Cancer Center.

Research has shown that stress can also decrease compliance with regular health screening.[58,59]

Many stress-induced physiological changes can have direct effects on health, including persistent increases in sympathetic nervous system activity and the hypothalamic–pituitary axis that can cause increased blood pressure, heart rate, catecholamine secretion, and platelet aggregation.[60–65] Furthermore, research has associated stress with increased latent viral reactivation, upper respiratory tract infections, and wound-healing time.[66–70] Stress also deregulates a variety of immune indices, as shown in both healthy subjects and cancer patients.[71] Such stress-induced physiological changes can affect cancer progression, treatment, recovery, recurrence, and survival.[72,73] Spiegel et al.[76] first published on the possible impact of a psychosocial intervention on breast cancer survival, but subsequent studies have not consistently reproduced these results.[74,75,77] However, recently Anderson et al.[78] demonstrated a survival advantage among breast cancer patients who received psychological intervention with more than 10 years of follow-up.[79] These studies underscore the importance of psychosocial intervention in cancer treatment.

Patient–Clinician Communication Regarding Complementary and Alternative Medicine

Research indicates that neither adult nor pediatric patients receive sufficient information or discuss CAM therapies with physicians, pharmacists, nurses, or CAM practitioners.[21,28] Most patients do not bring up the topic of CAM because no one asks; thus, patients may believe it is unimportant. It is estimated that 38% to 60% of patients with cancer are taking complementary medicines without informing their health care team.[8,80] This lack of discussion is of grave concern because biologically based therapies (such as herbs) may interact with cancer treatments. Patients are commonly unaware of the differences between U.S. Food and Drug Administration (FDA)–approved medications (which require evidence of efficacy, safety, and quality control manufacturing) and supplements, which are governed not by the FDA but by the Dietary Supplement Health and Education Act (DSHEA) of 1994. Supplements under this legislation are exempt from the same scrutiny the FDA imposes on medications; furthermore, these supplements are not intended to treat, prevent, or cure diseases. The common belief by patients that "natural" means safe needs to be addressed with education as some herbs and supplements have been associated with multiple drug interactions[81] as well as increased cancer risk and organ toxicity. These specific concerns are addressed later in this chapter.

Existing research suggests that the majority of cancer patients desire communication with their doctors about CAM,[82] and there is general agreement within the oncology community that in order to provide optimal patient care, oncologists must not only be aware of CAM use but also be willing and able to discuss all therapeutic approaches with their patients.[83,84] It is the health care professional's responsibility to ask patients about their use of complementary medicines,[85] and the discussion should ideally take place before the patient starts using a complementary treatment—whether it is a nutritional supplement, mind–body therapy, or other CAM approach.

A number of strategies can be used to increase the chance of a worthwhile dialogue.[86] One approach is to include the topic of CAM as part of a new patient assessment. For example, when asking about medications, physicians should inquire about everything the patient ingests—including over-the-counter products, vitamins, minerals, herbs, and even the patient's diet. Physicians may consider having the patients bring in the actual bottles of herbs and supplements for evaluation. When asking about a patient's past medical history, physicians may ask other health care professionals to determine if the patient has visited with naturopathic or chiropractic practitioners. If the issue of CAM arises, clinicians need to develop an empathic communication strategy that addresses the patient's needs while maintaining an understanding of the current state of the science. In other words, this strategy needs to be balanced between clinical objectivity and bonding with the patient so that it can benefit both the patient and the health care provider. These patients need reliable information on CAM from reliable resources, as well as adequate time to discuss this information with their oncologists.

Safety Concerns

Many CAM therapies can potentially cause adverse outcomes, and are thus a major concern among health care professionals.[87–90] Nonbiologically based CAM therapies, such as massage or acupuncture, often have minimal risks when performed by trained health professionals. In contrast, herbs and supplements should be considered more similar to prescription medications in that they have the potential to have powerful effects on the natural biological processes of the body. This is especially true when natural plants are processed into concentrated powders, liquids, or pills. The pathways by which CAM therapies may lead to negative clinical outcomes include metabolic interactions, treatment interactions, direct organ toxicity, direct biological effects on the cancer, and unregulated manufacturing of biologically based CAM. Some of these topics are briefly reviewed here.

Metabolic Interactions

Many botanical agents are pharmacologically active, raising concerns about pharmacodynamic effects that can lead to changes with conventional therapy, such as cytotoxic agents.[87] Limited published data are available regarding potential interactions between specific herbs or vitamins and prescription drugs.[87,88,91–97] Overall, there is substantial clinical evidence of herb–drug interactions in general.[81] Therefore, negative interactions should be considered prior to integrating herbs, vitamins, or nutritional supplements during chemotherapy.

Common chemotherapy agents metabolized through the cytochrome P-450 system and the specific isoenzymes responsible for their metabolism are at times a starting point to consider possible interactions. St. John's wort (*Hypericum perforatum*) is of particular concern, with multiple well-documented drug interactions. This herb appears to inhibit the hepatic enzyme cytochrome P-450 3A4 acutely, then induce it with repeated administration. A study of individuals given irinotecan (CPT11) reports a greater than 50% reduction in serum levels of the active metabolite SN38 after concomitant administration of St. John's wort.[98] Imatinib levels appear to be altered by similar mechanisms.[99] St. John's wort and similar herb–chemotherapy combinations should be used with extreme caution because of the potential for alterations in drug metabolism.

The common practice by patients of combining compounds, in which there is a lack of data regarding the pharmacodynamics and pharmacokinetics, creates a dangerous situation that may lead to inadvertent detrimental impact on clinical outcomes. This possible negative impact must be evaluated and discussed with patients whenever considering the use of untested natural products with other therapies.

Treatment Interactions

Antioxidant Interference with Chemotherapy or Radiation

Because oxidative damage to cells may increase the risk of cancer, the use of antioxidant herbs and vitamins has been proposed for cancer treatment or prevention. Examples include vitamins A, C, and E, as well as lycopene, green tea, soy, grape seed extract, melatonin, and selenium. Concern has been raised that antioxidants may interfere with radiation therapy or some chemotherapy agents (e.g., alkylating agents, anthracyclines, or platinums), which themselves can depend on oxidative damage to tumor cells for their cytotoxic effects. Studies of the effects of antioxidants on cancer therapies have yielded mixed results, with some reporting antagonistic effects, others noting synergism (i.e., benefits), and most suggesting no significant interaction.[89,90,100,101] A large randomized trial of head and neck cancer patients evaluated the use of beta carotene and vitamin E for the reduction of radiation side effects.[102] Results found a reduction in side effects, but also found decreased survival among patients taking beta carotene and vitamin E. Additionally, the use of these antioxidants seemed to correlate to an increase in second primary cancer.[103] Whether antioxidants are beneficial or harmful is a critical question without a clear scientific answer at this time; rather, it remains an area of continuing study and controversy.[104,105]

Direct Organ Toxicity

Hepatotoxicity and Nephrotoxicity

The long-term use of concentrated natural products is an increasing concern. A recent report evaluating the risk for end-stage renal disease in Taiwan found that chronic use of traditional Chinese medicine herbs carried an increased risk of kidney failure.[106] Multiple herbs and supplements may cause hepatotoxicity or transaminitis, based on human research or known hepatotoxic constituents, and should be used cautiously in combination with other hepatotoxic agents (Table 181.2).

Hematologic Toxicity

Many herbs and supplements carry an increased risk of bleeding. Multiple case studies have reported clinically significant bleeding with the use of *Ginkgo biloba* (either alone or with aspirin or warfarin), and isolated case reports of bleeding with the use of saw palmetto (*Serenoa repens*), fish oil, and garlic (*Allium sativum*).[81] The suspected mechanism for increased bleeding is interference with platelet function. Because herbal supplementation is common among cancer patients, surgical staff should screen patients presurgically for use of herbal and other dietary supplements. These agents should be discontinued before surgical procedures, and should be used cautiously with other agents that increase the risk of bleeding. Clinicians should also be cautious about combining natural products concurrently with warfarin, which is known to be sensitive to vitamin K intake and possible drug interactions. Numerous other herbs and vitamins may increase bleeding risk based on known constituents, preclinical data, or traditional use (Table 181.3).

Direct Biological Effects on Cancer

A common concern is the potential for herbs and supplements to have procancerous effects. One clear example comes from Sidney Farber from Harvard University and the discovery of antifolate agents such as methotrexate, which came from the observation that folic acid supplementation actually promoted disease progression.[107] Until appropriate clinical trials have been completed on herbs and supplements for individual types of cancer, the resulting impact, either beneficial, harmful, or neither, will remain unknown, and thus caution will always be considered a prudent approach.

Phytoestrogens

Phytoestrogens are plant-based compounds structurally similar to estradiol, and capable of binding to estrogen receptors as agonists or antagonists. Multiple popular herbs contain phytoestrogens, such as black cohosh (*Cimicifuga racemosa*), red clover (*Trifolium pratense*), and soy (*Glycine max*) (Table 181.4). Effects of these agents in hormone-sensitive cancers remain unclear, and use in patients with estrogen receptor–positive breast cancer is controversial (see "Soy" below for further discussion).

PRACTICE OF ONCOLOGY

TABLE 181.2

HERBS AND SUPPLEMENTS WITH POTENTIAL HEPATOTOXIC EFFECTS

Ackee (*Blighia sapida*), *Alkanna* spp., American (false) pennyroyal (*Hedeoma pulegioides*), antineoplastons, bee pollen, birch oil (*Betula lenta*), blessed thistle (*Cnicus Benedictus*)[a], boldo (*Peumus boldus*), borage (*Borago officinalis*), bush tea (*Crotalaria* spp.)[b], butterbur (*Petasites hybridus*), chaparral (*Larrea tridentata*), coltsfoot (*Tussilago farfara*), comfrey (*Symphytum* spp.), creatine, dehydroepiandrosterone (DHEA), echinacea (*Echinacea purpurea*), *Echium* spp.[b], germander (*Teucrium* spp.), greater celandine (*Chelidonium majus*), groundsel (*Senecio* spp.)[b], heliotrope (*Heliotropium* spp.), horse chestnut (*Aesculus hippocastanum*), jequirity (*Abrus precatorius*), jin-bu-huan (*Lycopodium serratum*), kava (*Piper methysticum*), lesser celandine (*Ranunculus ficaria*), lobelia (*Lobelia inflata*), L-tetrahydropalmatine (THP), mistletoe (*Viscum album*), niacin (vitamin B_3), niacinamide, nux vomica (*Strychnos nux-vomica*), Paraguay tea/yerba mate (*Ilex paraguariensis*)[b], periwinkle (*Catharanthus roseus*), plantain (*Plantago* spp.)[a], pride of Madeira (*Echium fastuosum*)[b], polysaccharide K (PSK) (*Trametes versicolor*, formerly *Coriolus versicolor*), ragwort (*Senecio* spp.)[b], rooibos (*Aspalathus linearis*), rosy periwinkle (*Catharanthus roseus*), rue (*Ruta graveolens*), sassafras (*Sassafras albidum*), skullcap (*Scutellaria* spp.), sorrel (*Rumex acetosa*), tea (*Camellia sinensis*), turmeric (*Curcuma longa*), tu-san-chi (*Gynura segetum*)[b], uva ursi (*Arctostaphylos uva-ursi*), valerian (*Valeriana officinalis*), white chameleon (*Atractylis gummifera*), white oak (*Quercus alba*), yerba mate (*Ilex paraguariensis*)[b]

[a]Contains tannins and may be hepatotoxic in large quantities.
[b]Contains pyrrolizidine alkaloids.

TABLE 181.3

HERBS AND SUPPLEMENTS THAT MAY INCREASE THE RISK OF BLEEDING OR CLOTTING

Agents Reported to Cause Clinically Significant Bleeding in Case Report(s)
Garlic (*Allium sativum*), *Ginkgo biloba*, saw palmetto (*Serenoa repens*)

Agents that May Increase the Risk of Bleeding, Based on Mechanism of Action, Preclinical Data, or Traditional Use
Acacia (*Acacia* spp.), acerola (*Malpighia emarginata*), aconite (*Aconitum* spp.), agrimony (*Agrimonia* spp.), alfalfa (*Medicago sativa*)[a], aloe (*Aloe vera*), alpha-linolenic acid, alpinia (*Alpinia* spp.), American ginseng (*Panax quinquefolius*), andrographis (*Andrographis paniculata*), angelica (*Angelica archangelica*)[a], angel's trumpet (*Brugmansia* and *Datura* spp.), anise (*Pimpinella anisum*)[a], annatto (*Bixa orellana*), aortic acid, arabinogalactan, arginine (L-arginine), aristolochia (*Aristolochia* spp.), arnica (*Arnica montana*), asafoetida (*Ferula foetida*)[a], ashwagandha (*Withania somnifera*), aspen (*Populus* spp.)[b], astragalus (*Astragalus membranaceus*), avocado (*Persea americana*), babassu (*Attalea speciosa*), banaba (*Lagerstroemia speciosa*), barley (*Hordeum vulgare*), bear's garlic (*Allium ursinum*), beta-sitosterol, bilberry (*Vaccinium myrtillus*), birch (*Betula barosma*)[b], black cohosh (*Cimicifuga racemosa*)[b], black currant (*Ribes nigrum*), bladderwrack (*Fucus vesiculosus*), blessed thistle (*Cnicus benedictus*), bogbean (*Menyanthes trifoliata*), boldo (*Peumus boldus*), borage seed oil (*Borago officinalis*), bromelain (*Ananas comosus*), bupleurum (*Bupleurum*), burdock (*Arctium lappa*), calamus (*Acorus calamus*), calendula (*Calendula* spp.), capsicum (*Capsicum* spp.), cat's claw (*Uncaria tomentosa*), celery (*Apium graveolens*)[a], chamomile (*Matricaria recutita*)[a], chaparral (*Larrea tridentata*), chia (*Salvia hispanica*), chlorella (*Chlorella* spp.), chondroitin sulfate, cinnamon (*Cinnamomum* spp.)[a], clove (*Eugenia aromaticum*), codonopsis (*Codonopsis* spp.), coenzyme Q10, coleus (*Coleus forskohlii*), coltsfoot (*Tussilago farfara*), cordyceps (*Cordyceps sinensis*), cowhage (*Mucuna pruriens*), cranberry (*Vaccinium* spp.), daisy (*Bellis perennis*), dandelion (*Taraxacum officinale*)[a], danshen (*Salvia miltiorrhiza*), datura (*Datura* spp.), dehydroepiandrosterone (DHEA), desert parsley (*Lomatium dissectum*), devil's claw (*Harpagophytum procumbens*), diallyl trisulfide, dong quai (*Angelica sinensis*), echistatin, eicosapentaenoic acid (EPA), elder (*Sambucus* spp.), evening primrose oil (*Oenothera biennis*)[c], fennel (*Foeniculum vulgare*), fenugreek (*Trigonella foenum-graecum*)[a], feverfew (*Tanacetum parthenium*)[c], fig (*Ficus carica*), fisetin, fish oil, flavonoids, flaxseed (*Linum usitatissimum*), gamma-linolenic acid, gamma-oryzanol, garlic (*Allium sativum*)[c], genistein, ginger (*Zingiber officinalis*)[c], ginkgo (*Ginkgo biloba*)[c], ginseng (*Panax* spp.)[c], globe artichoke (*Cynara scolymus*), goldenseal (*Hydrastis canadensis*), grape seed (*Vitis vinifera*), grapefruit (*Citrus* x *paradisi*), ground ivy (*Glechoma hederacea*), guarana (*Paullinia cupana*), guggul (*Commiphora mukul*), gymnema (*Gymnema sylvestre*), hawthorn (*Crataegus* spp.), heartsease (*Viola tricolor*)[b], hirudin, holy basil (*Ocimum tenuiflorum*), horny goat weed (*Epimedium* spp.), horse chestnut (*Aesculus hippocastanum*)[a], horseradish (*Radicula armoracia*), jackfruit (*Artocarpus heterophyllus*), jequirity (*Abrus precatorius*), jiaogulan (*Gynostemma pentaphyllum*), juniper (*Juniperus* spp.), kava (*Piper methysticum*), kelp (Laminariales), kinetin, kiwi (*Actinidia deliciosa*), kudzu (*Pueraria lobata*), lady's mantle (*Alchemilla* spp.), lavender (*Lavandula* spp.), lemongrass (*Cymbopogon* spp.), licorice (liquorice) (*Glycyrrhiza glabra*)[c], lotus (*Nelumbo* spp.), lovage (*Levisticum officinale*) , male fern (*Dryopteris filix-mas*), marjoram (*Origanum majorana*), meadowsweet (*Spirea/Filipendula ulmaria*)[b], melatonin (N-acetyl-5-methoxytryptamine), methylsulfonylmethane (MSM), mistletoe (*Viscum album*), modified citrus pectin, mugwort (*Artemisia vulgaris*), mullein (*Verbascum* spp.), nettle (*Urtica dioica*), niacin (vitamin B3), nopal (*Opuntia* spp.), nordihydroguaiaretic acid (NDGA), octacosanol, omega-3 fatty acids, onion (*Allium cepa*), oregano (*Origanum vulgare*), pagoda tree (*Styphnolobium* spp.), pantethine, papain, papaya (*Carica papaya*), parsley (*Petroselinum crispum*), passion flower (*Passiflora incarnata*), pawpaw (*Asimina* spp.), PC-SPES®, peony (*Paeonia* spp.), policosanol, polypodium (*Polypodium* spp.), poplar (*Populus* spp.)[b], prickly ash (*Zanthoxylum* spp.)[a], propolis, polysaccharide K (PSK) (*Trametes versicolor*, formerly *Coriolus versicolor*), Pycnogenol® (*Pinus pinaster* subsp. *atlantica*), quassia (*Picrasma excelsa*)[a], quercetin, quinine, red clover (*Trifolium pratense*)[a], red yeast (*Monascus purpureus*) rice, rehmannia (*Rehmannia* spp.), reishi (*Ganodermas* spp.), resveratrol, rhubarb (*Rheum rhabarbarum*), Roman chamomile (*Anthemis nobilis*), rose hip (*Rosa* spp.), rosemary (*Rosmarinus officinalis*), rue (*Ruta* spp.), rutin, safflower (*Carthamus tinctorius*), sage (*Salvia officinalis*), sarsaparilla (*Smilax regelii*)[b], sassafras (*Sassafras* spp.), savory (*Satureja* spp.), saw palmetto (*Serenoa repens*), schisandra (*Schisandra* spp.), scotch broom (*Cytisus scoparius*, syn. *Sarothamnus scoparius*), sea buckthorn (*Hippophae* spp.), seaweed, selenium, shea (*Vitellaria paradoxa*, syn. *Butyrospermum parkii*, *B. paradoxa*), shiitake mushroom (*Lentinula edodes*), Siberian ginseng (*Eleutherococcus senticosus*), skullcap (*Scutellaria* spp.), sorrel (*Rumex acetosa*), soy (*Glycine max*)[c], Spanish bayonet (*Yucca* spp.), spirulina (*Arthrospira* spp.) St. John's wort (*Hypericum perforatum*), star anise (*Illicium verum*), stinging nettle (*Urtica dioica*), strawberry (*Fragaria* x *ananassa*), sweet birch (*Betula lenta*)[b], sweet clover (*Melilotus* spp.)[a], sweet pea (*Lathyrus* spp.), sweet woodruff (*Galium odoratum*), tamanu (*Calophyllum inophyllum*), tamarind (*Tamarindus indica*), tarragon (*Artemisia dracunculus*), taurine, tea (*Camellia sinensis*), thyme (*Thymus vulgaris*), tonka bean (*Dipteryx odorata*), turmeric (*Curcuma longa*), usnea (*Usnea* spp.), vanilla (*Vanilla* spp.), verbena (*Verbena* spp.), vitamin A, vitamin C[c], vitamin E[c], wasabi (*Wasabia japonica*), watercress (*Nasturtium officinale*), wheatgrass (*Triticum aestivum*), wild carrot (*Daucus carota*), wild lettuce (*Lactuca virosa*), willow (*Salix* spp.)[b], wintergreen (*Gaultheria* spp.)[b], yarrow (*Achillea millefolium*), yew (*Taxus* spp.), yohimbe (*Pausinystalia yohimbe*, formerly *Corynanthe yohimbe*).

Possible Procoagulant Agents
Abuta (*Abuta* spp.), acerola (*Malpighia emarginata*), aconite (*Aconitum* spp.), African wild potato (*Hypoxis hemerocallidea*), agrimony (*Agrimonia* spp.), alfalfa (*Medicago sativa*), annatto (*Bixa orellana*), apricot (*Prunus armeniaca*), arnica (*Arnica montana*), astragalus (*Astragalus membranaceus*), bael (*Aegle marmelos*), bilberry (*Vaccinium myrtillus*), black haw (*Viburnum prunifolium*), blessed thistle (*Cnicus benedictus*), cat's claw (*Uncaria tomentosa*), chlorella (*Chlorella* spp.), coenzyme Q10, *cordyceps (Cordyceps sinensis)*, DHEA (dehydroepiandrosterone), dong quai (*Angelica sinensis*), ginseng (*Panax* spp.), goldenrod (*Solidago* spp.), goldenseal (*Hydrastis canadensis*), guggul (*Commiphora mukul*), horsetail (*Equisetum* spp.), jequirity (*Abrus precatorius*), jiaogulan (*Gynostemma pentaphyllum*), lime (*Citrus aurantifolia*), melatonin, milk thistle (*Silybum marianum*), mistletoe (*Viscum album*), myrcia (*Myrcia* spp.), nopal (*Opuntia* spp.), ginseng (*Panax ginseng*), psyllium (*Plantago* spp.), raspberry (*Rubus* spp.), rhubarb (*Rheum rhabarbarum*), sage (*Salvia officinalis*), Scotch broom (*Cytisus scoparius*, syn. *Sarothamnus scoparius*), shepherd's purse (*Capsella bursa-pastoris*), skunk cabbage (*Symplocarpus foetidus*), stinging nettle (*Urtica dioica*), tamanu (*Calophyllum inophyllum*), tea (*Camellia sinensis*), white oak (*Quercus alba*), white water lily (*Nymphaea alba*), yarrow (*Achillea millefolium*)

[a]Agents with coumarin constituents.
[b]Agents with salicylate constituents.
[c]Agents that inhibit platelets.
Note: This is not an all-inclusive list. Because passionflower, hydroalcoholic extracts, juniper, spinach, plants in the cabbage family (Brassicaceae, such as kale and broccoli), and verbena supply variable quantities of vitamin K, they may lessen the effect of oral anticoagulant therapy.

TABLE 181.4

HERBS AND SUPPLEMENTS WITH POTENTIAL PHYTOESTROGENS OR PHYTOPROGESTINS

Herbs Containing Potential Phytoestrogens (constituents reported to act as estrogen receptor agonists and/or to exhibit estrogenic properties in basic science studies, animal research, or human trials)

Aconite (*Aconitum* spp.), agrimony (*Agrimonia* spp.), alfalfa (*Medicago sativa*), alizarin (1,2-dihydroxyanthraquinone), allspice (*Pimenta dioica*), alpha-linolenic acid, amaranth (*Amaranth* spp.), anise (*Pimpinella anisum*), apple cider vinegar, arabinogalactan, arginine (L-arginine), arnica (*Arnica* spp.), ashwagandha (*Withania somnifera*), astragalus (*Astragalus* spp.), avocado (*Persea americana*), bay leaf (*Laurus nobilis*), bee pollen, belladonna (*Atropa belladonna*), beta-sitosterol, betel nut (*Areca catechu*), betony (*Stachys* spp.), bilberry (*Vaccinium* spp.), black cohosh (*Cimicifuga racemosa*)[c], black currant (*Ribes nigrum*), black haw (*Viburnum prunifolium*), black hellebore (*Veratrum nigrum*), black horehound (*Ballota nigra*), black seed (*Nigella sativa*), bladderwrack (*Fucus vesiculosus*), blessed thistle (*Cnicus benedictus*), bloodroot (*Sanguinaria canadensis*), blue cohosh (*Caulophyllum thalictroides*), blue flag (*Iris versicolor*), boldo (*Peumus boldus*), boneset (*Eupatorium* spp.), borage (*Borago officinalis*), boron, boswellia (*Boswellia* spp.), bromelain, bugleweed (*Lycopus* spp.), bupleurum (*Bupleurum* spp.), burdock (*Arctium lappa*), butterbur (*Petasites* spp.), calabar bean (*Physostigma venenosum*), calendula (*Calendula* spp.), camphor, Canada balsam (*Abies balsamea*), cannabis (*Cannabis indica*), carrot (*Daucus carota*), cat's claw (*Uncaria tomentosa*), chamomile (*Matricaria recutita*), chasteberry (*Vitex agnus-castus*), cherry (*Prunus* spp.), chia (*Salvia hispanica*), chicory (*Cichorium intybus*), cinnamon (*Cinnamomum* spp.), cleavers (*Galium aparine*), comfrey (*Symphytum* spp.), cordyceps (*Cordyceps* spp.), cornflower (*Centaurea cyanus*), daisy (*Bellis perennis*), damiana (*Turnera diffusa*), dandelion (*Taraxacum officinale*), danshen (*Salvia miltiorrhiza*), deer velvet, devil's claw (*Harpagophytum procumbens*), dill (*Anethum graveolens*), dogwood (*Cornus* spp.), dong quai (*Angelica sinensis*), echinacea (*Echinacea* spp.), Essiac®, eucalyptus (*Eucalyptus* spp.), evening primrose oil (*Oenothera biennis*), false pennyroyal (*Hedeoma* spp.), fennel (*Foeniculum vulgare*), fenugreek (*Trigonella foenum-graecum*), feverfew (*Tanacetum parthenium*), flax (*Linum usitatissimum*), fo-ti (*Polygonum multiflorum*), gamma-linolenic acid, gamma-oryzanol, garcinia (*Garcinia* spp.), garlic (*Allium sativum*), ginger (*Zingiber officinale*), ginkgo (*Ginkgo biloba*), ginseng (*Panax* spp.), goji (*Lycium barbarum*), goldenseal (*Hydrastis canadensis*), gotu kola (*Centella asiatica*), ground ivy (*Glechoma hederacea*), guggul (*Commiphora wightii*), hawthorn (*Crataegus* spp.), hop (*Humulus lupulus*)[a], horny goat weed (*Epimedium* spp.), horse chestnut (*Aesculus hippocastanum*), horsetail (Equisetum spp.), hyssop (*Hyssopus* spp.), ignatia (*Strychnos ignatia*), jointed flatsedge (*Cyperus articulatus*), kava (*Piper methysticum*), kelp (Laminariales), kudzu (*Pueraria lobata*)[b], lady's mantle (*Alchemilla* spp.), lady's slipper (*Cypripedium* spp.), lavender (*Lavandula spica*), lemongrass (*Cymbopogon* spp.), licorice (liquorice) (*Glycyrrhiza glabra*)[a], lotus (*Nelumbo nucifera*), lovage (*Levisticum officinale*), maca (*Lepidium meyenii*), meadowsweet (*Spirea/Filipendula ulmaria*), melatonin (*N*-acetyl-5-methoxytryptamine), milk thistle (*Silybum marianum*), mistletoe (*Viscum album*), mugwort (*Artemisia vulgaris*), muira puama (*Ptychopetalum olacoides*), mullein (*Verbascum thapsus*), neem (*Azadirachta indica*), niacin, noni (*Morinda citrifolia*), nux vomica (*Strychnos nux-vomica*), oleander (*Nerium oleander*, *Thevetia peruviana*), oregano (*Origanum vulgare*), ovaraden, passion flower (*Passiflora incarnata*), peony (*Paeonia* spp.), peppermint (*Mentha* x *piperita*), pleurisy (*Asclepias tuberosa*), pokeweed (*Phytolacca americana*), pomegranate (*Punica granatum*)[a], Pycnogenol®, pygeum (*Pygeum spp.*), quassia (*Quassia* spp.), quercetin, raspberry (*Rubus idaeus*), red clover (*Trifolium pratense*)[b], rehmannia (*Rehmannia* spp.), resveratrol, rhodiola (*Rhodiola* spp.), rhubarb (*Rheum officinale*), rose hip (*Rosa* spp.), rosemary (*Rosmarinus officinalis*), safflower (*Carthamus tinctorius*), sage (*Salvia officinalis*), sarsaparilla (*Smilax regelii*), saw palmetto (*Serenoa repens*), schisandra (*Schisandra chinensis*), Scotch broom (*Cytisus scoparius*, syn. *Sarothamnus scoparius*), sea buckthorn (*Hippophae* spp.), seaweed, shepherd's purse (*Capsella bursa-pastoris*), Siberian ginseng (*Eleutherococcus senticosus*, formerly *Acanthopanax senticosus*), sitosterol, skullcap (*Scutellaria* spp.), slippery elm (*Ulmus rubra*), soy (*Glycine max*)[b], St. John's wort (*Hypericum perforatum*), star anise (*Illicium verum*), stinging nettle (*Urtica dioica*), sweet almond (*Prunus amygdalus dulcis*), sweet marjoram (*Origanum majorana*), sweet woodruff (*Galium odoratum*), tansy (*Tanacetum vulgare*), tea (*Camellia sinensis*), thyme (*Thymus vulgaris*), tribulus (*Tribulus* spp.), turmeric (*Curcuma longa*), verbena (*Verbena* spp.), white horehound (*Marrubium vulgare*), wild ginger (*Asarum* spp.), yucca (*Yucca* spp.)

Herbs And Supplements Containing Potential Phytoprogestins (constituents reported to exhibit progestin-like activity in basic science and/or animal studies)

Bloodroot (*Sanguinaria canadensis*), chasteberry (*Vitex agnus-castus*), damiana (*Turnera diffusa*), ephedra/ma huang (*Ephedra sinica*), oregano (*Origanum vulgare*), PC-SPES®, saw palmetto (*Serenoa repens*), wild yam (*Dioscorea villosa*), yohimbe (*Pausinystalia yohimbe*, formerly *Corynanthe yohimbe*), yucca (*Yucca* spp.)

[a]Estriol, estrone, estradiol, or estrogen constituents.
[b]Isoflavone constituents.
[c]Estrogen and isoflavone constituents.

STANDARDIZATION AND QUALITY

Preparation of herbs and supplements can vary from manufacturer to manufacturer and from batch to batch within one manufacturer. Because the active components of a product are often not clear, standardization may not be possible, and the clinical effects of different brands may not be comparable. There may also be harmful contaminants in products not manufactured under good manufacturing practice (GMP). One example includes PC-SPES, an herbal formula for the treatment of prostate cancer. This product was taken off the market in 2002 by the FDA because different lots were found to contain warfarin, indomethacin, and estrogen diethylstilbestrol.[108]

SPECIFIC COMPLEMENTARY AND ALTERNATIVE MEDICINE THERAPIES

Many cancer therapies used are the same as those used in the general population for common noncancer indications such as St. John's wort (*Hypericum perforatum*) for depression, kava (*Piper methysticum*) for anxiety, *Echinacea purpurea* for common cold symptoms, or yoga/massage/tai chi for overall well-being. This chapter lists some of the more common therapies about which oncologists might be questioned by their patients; this only represents a small sample of therapies. Several resources are available that can provide a summary of the available evidence regarding CAM therapies.

Biologically Based Therapies Used for Cancer Treatment and Secondary Prevention

Beta Carotene

Two large randomized trials have been completed for the prevention of lung cancer: the Alpha-Tocopherol and Beta-Carotene Cancer Prevention Trial (ATBC) and the Beta-Carotene and Retinol Efficacy Trial (CARET).[109] Neither trial showed any efficacy of beta carotene to prevent lung cancer among patients at elevated risk, primarily smokers or those with secondhand smoke exposure. Additionally, the ATBC study showed a trend toward increased risk for lung cancer. Both trials found a higher mortality rate among those randomized to beta carotene supplementation. A meta-analysis of nine randomized clinical trials of beta carotene supplement also indicated an increase in stomach cancer with daily supplementation of 20 mg or higher.[110] Supplementation with beta carotene is generally discouraged as a result of these studies.

Coenzyme Q10 (Ubiquinol/Ubiquinone)

Clinical Studies. Coenzyme Q10 (CoQ10) has been studied for the prevention of anthracycline cardiotoxicity based on purported antioxidant effects, but without conclusive results. Cortes et al.[111] observed ten patients who received adriamycin and received CoQ10 at a dose of 50 mg/d. This was reported to show a decreased incidence of cardiac dysfunction. In another study, 20 children with acute lymphoblastic leukemia (ALL) or non-Hodgkin's lymphoma (NHL) who were treated with anthracyclines were randomized to CoQ10 therapy.[112] There was decreased fractional shortening in both the CoQ10-treated and untreated groups, but no comparison was made between these two groups. The small sample size and poor study design limit any ability to draw firm conclusions.

Safety. High doses (greater than 300 mg/d) for long periods may elevate liver enzymes (aspartate aminotransferase and lactate dehydrogenase).[113] Concern also exists when CoQ10 is used with antihyperglycemic,[114,115] psychiatric, cardiovascular agents, and warfarin or anticoagulants,[116,117] based on conflicting evidence and secondary sources.[118–120]

Polysaccharide K

Clinical Studies. An uncontrolled trial of polysaccharide K (PSK; *Trametes versicolor*, formerly *Coriolus versicolor*) reported improved survival in cancer patients compared with historical controls.[121] PSK has been reported to improve survival in colorectal,[122] gastric,[123,124] breast,[125–128] esophageal,[129–131] lung,[132–134] hepatocellular,[135] nasopharyngeal carcinoma,[121,136] and in acute leukemia.[137,138] However, other studies have reported no survival benefit with PSK as an adjuvant therapy.[121,128,137,138] Preoperative CEA, PPD, HLA-A2, and HLA-B40 have been reported to be associated with response to PSK therapy.[125,139–146]

Safety. PSK generally seems to have a low incidence of mild and tolerable side effects.[122,127] Cases of liver impairment and toxicity have been noted with PSK use, and gastrointestinal upset, darkening of the fingernails, leucopenia, thrombocytopenia, and coughing have been reported with extended use of PSK.[136,147–149] Theoretically, concomitant use of PSK with anticoagulants or antiplatelets could increase the risk of bleeding, although clinical evidence of this interaction is lacking.

Essiac Herbal Combination Tea

Clinical Studies. The original proprietary formula of Essiac® contained burdock root (*Arctium lappa*), sheep sorrel (*Rumex acetosella*), slippery elm inner bark (*Ulmus fulva*), and Turkish rhubarb (*Rheum palmatum*). There is a lack of reliable research on Essiac in the published literature. Mouse studies at Memorial Sloan-Kettering Cancer Center in the 1970s were not formally published, and 86 human case reports collected retrospectively in 1988 by the Canadian Department of National Health and Welfare yielded unclear results.[150]

Safety. Concern has been raised about Essiac herbal tonic's potential to stimulate the growth of human breast cancer cells through estrogen receptor–mediated as well as estrogen receptor–independent mechanisms of action. A 2004 systematic review did not identify any published clinical trials to evaluate this herbal complex in patients with cancer.[150] Despite this lack of evidence, Essiac and Essiac-like products (which may contain additional herbs) remain popular among cancer patients. Rhubarb and sheep sorrel contain oxalic acid, which is known to cause hepatic and renal damage in high doses.

Ginger

Clinical Studies. Although some evidence supports the use of ginger (*Zingiber officinale*) for nausea or emesis during pregnancy,[151–160] ginger's effects on other types of nausea or emesis, such as chemotherapy-induced postoperative nausea or motion sickness, remain undetermined.[161–167] Several randomized trials that utilized different doses of ginger along with standard antiemetics have found mixed results,[164,167,168] though overall the studies suggest that ginger is more effective than placebo.[169] Thus, more studies are needed to further examine ginger therapy for chemotherapy-induced nausea and vomiting.

Safety. The most frequent side effects associated with ginger use are gastrointestinal upset, heartburn, gas, and bloating. Estrogen receptor–positive patients should be cautious as ginger may also exert high estrogenic potency, based on *in vitro* evidence.[170] Ginger may inhibit platelet aggregation or decrease platelet thromboxane production, thus theoretically increasing bleeding risk. When ginger was used in patients who were taking nifedipine, antiplatelet aggregation was increased, which suggests a synergistic effect on the inhibition of platelet aggregation.[171]

Ginseng

Clinical Studies. Ginseng (*Panax ginseng*, *Panax quinquefolius*) is a common ingredient in traditional Chinese medicine herbal formulas, but few clinical trials have evaluated the use of ginseng alone as an anticancer agent. A clinical trial evaluating American ginseng to treat cancer-related fatigue found nonsignificant trends toward benefit in higher doses compared to placebo.[171,172] Similarly, an improvement in quality of life was found in another smaller randomized clinical trial utilizing sun ginseng.[173] A small study utilizing an American ginseng extract found a decreased length of respiratory symptoms.[174] Further clinical trials are needed to determine if ginseng will be beneficial for cancer patients without interfering with cancer treatments.

Safety. The most frequent side effects associated with ginseng include headache, insomnia, and gastrointestinal toxicities.[175] Concern exists when used in combination with diabetes medications (due to possible hypoglycemic properties), anticoagulants (due to increased risk of bleeding), monoamine oxidase inhibitors, and stimulants. Caution should be used when ginseng is taken with medications that are metabolized by cytochrome P-450 2D6.

Green Tea

Clinical Studies. Several large case-control and cohort studies have mainly focused on prevention of gastrointestinal and breast cancers with green tea (*Camellia sinensis*). Results are variable, with some suggesting chronic tea consumption may decrease cancer risk and others reporting no benefits.[176–187] Overall, the epidemiologic evidence suggests that green tea consumption may protect against cancer; however, these studies have been mostly observational, and other lifestyle choices of tea drinkers may confound these results. A few studies of green tea have shown some clinical benefits. A decreased occurrence of prostate cancer was reported among healthy men treated with green tea extract (GTE) versus placebo in a recent randomized, placebo-controlled study in 60 volunteers with high-grade prostate intraepithelial neoplasia.[188] The study reported a reduction in tumor development (9 of 30 vs. 1 of 30) after 1 year of therapy compared to placebo. GTE has also been evaluated to treat premalignant oral lesions. Patients were randomized to three doses of GTE or placebo for 12 weeks. The two higher dose levels were associated with a higher response rate.[176] In a breast cancer study, green tea ingestion was associated with improved prognosis in stage I and II cancers, but no effect was seen on grade III cancers.[181] Additional human research is needed before a recommendation can be made for or against the use of green tea in cancer prevention or treatment.

Safety. Studies of the specific side effects of green tea are limited. However, green tea, a source of caffeine, is known to act as a central nervous system (CNS) stimulant and diuretic; it may also increase the production of stomach acid, worsen ulcer symptoms, increase heart rate, and raise blood pressure. One cup of green tea contains approximately 30 to 50 mg of caffeine, and excessive tea consumption may lead to adverse effects or toxicity. Green tea supplement capsules usually contain less caffeine (approximately 5 mg of caffeine per 500 mg extract).

Lycopene

Lycopene is a carotenoid present in human serum, liver, adrenal glands, lungs, prostate, colon, and skin at higher levels than other carotenoids. Most dietary lycopene is derived from tomatoes and tomato-based products. Lycopene is also present in many other fruits and plant products, including apricots, pink grapefruit, guava, rose hip, palm oil, and watermelon. Antioxidant and antiproliferative properties have been reported in preclinical research, and there are more than 75 case-control or cohort studies of the association between increased tomato/tomato-based product intake or serum lycopene levels with cancer risk. Approximately two-thirds of these studies suggest benefits in the range of 40% risk reduction, although fewer than half of the studies are statistically significant, and numerous studies provide negative results.[189] A recent study that evaluated the association between intake of lycopene and specific tomato products and prostate cancer risk among 29,361 men during an average of 4.2 years of follow-up reported that lycopene intake was associated with reduction of prostate cancer risk among men with a family history of prostate cancer, but not in the male population overall.[190]

Maitake

Clinical Studies. In a small 2002 case series, therapy with Maitake (*Grifola frondosa*) powder and a proprietary Maitake extract ("MD fraction") was associated with tumor regression in greater than 50% of patients with stages II to IV breast, lung, and liver cancer, whereas no improvements were observed in leukemia, gastric cancer, or brain tumors.[191] This series had limited information, particularly regarding patient baseline characteristics. A recent report from Memorial Sloan-Kettering Cancer Center found that Maitake mushrooms had a mixed response on a profile of immune cells; thus, the belief that these mushrooms are purely immunostimulatory is likely incorrect.[192]

Safety. Although Maitake has not been well studied, a long history of dietary use suggests that it is safe in low doses. Possible adverse effects of concentrated extracts, based on animal research, include hypoglycemia and hypotension. It is not clear if this agent interacts with chemotherapy regimens.

Milk Thistle

Clinical Studies. One randomized clinical trial in children with acute lymphoblastic leukemia found a lower incidence of liver toxicity among children randomized to milk thistle (*Silybum marianum*) therapy.[193] Several other trials have evaluated milk thistle, but in combination with several other herbs or supplements; therefore, further study using milk thistle alone is needed before it can be recommended as an anticancer treatment.

Safety. Milk thistle has been investigated for anticancer effects in preclinical and clinical trials; the pharmacokinetics and its mechanisms, effectiveness, and adverse effects reported to date have been reviewed.[194] In clinical trials and traditional use, oral milk thistle has generally been reported as well tolerated in recommended doses for up to 6 years of use. Several studies report mild gastrointestinal symptoms, including nausea, heartburn, diarrhea, epigastric pain, abdominal discomfort, dyspepsia, flatulence, and loss of appetite. Urticaria, eczema, and headache have also been reported. Hypersensitivity and anaphylactic reactions have been associated with milk thistle ingestion in case reports. Because many patients in available clinical trials have liver conditions, it is unclear whether adverse effects are caused by milk thistle or by the underlying liver condition; the rates of adverse effects are often similar to placebo. Data from *in vivo* and *in vitro* studies suggest inhibition of cytochrome p-450 (CPY450) 3A4 and 2C9 to varying levels.

Mistletoe

Clinical Studies. Multiple case series, retrospective analyses, and prospective trials of mistletoe (*Viscum album*, Iscador®)

extracts in humans have been published; these studies were largely conducted in Europe and have examined patients with breast, lung, cervical, colorectal, gastric, ovarian, and pancreatic cancers, as well as renal cell carcinoma and glioma. A 1994 systematic review included 11 controlled clinical trials, not all randomized, and concluded that overall methodological quality of studies was poor and results indeterminate.[195] Subsequent publications have not provided definitive evidence of efficacy but have suggested survival advantages in patients with colorectal, gastric, or breast cancer.[196–198] Negative results have been reported in patients with melanoma.[199] According to a 2006 reanalysis of previously published nonrandomized studies on mistletoe therapy, breast cancer patients showed increased survival; however, this required further evaluation in a well-designed randomized controlled trial[200] In another randomized trial of mistletoe, researchers evaluated potential side effects from chemotherapy among breast cancer patients and concluded that patients randomized to mistletoe reported fewer side effects. No long-term evaluation was performed to explore the impact on efficacy of treatment.[201]

Safety. Mistletoe is contraindicated in patients with protein hypersensitivity or chronic progressive infections (e.g., tuberculosis). The most common reactions are erythema and hyperemia.[195] Other possible side effects include anorexia, general malaise, depressive moods, fever, local skin inflammation or pain at injection site, mydriasis and myosis/myalgia, and elevated liver enzymes.

Omega-3 Fatty Acids

Clinical Studies. Several population (epidemiologic) studies report that dietary omega-3 fatty acids (alpha-linolenic acid) or fish oil may reduce the risk of developing breast, colon, or prostate cancer.[202–208] There is evidence from epidemiologic studies and randomized controlled trials that intake of recommended amounts of docosahexaenoic acid (DHA) and eicosapentaenoic acid (EPA) in the form of dietary fish or fish oil supplements lowers triglycerides and reduces the risk of death from cardiovascular disease. Two randomized controlled trials report no significant benefits of supplementation with omega-3 fatty acids or fish oil in cancer patients with cachexia.[209,210] Questions have been raised, however, about the proportion of DHA to EPA used in these trials. An ongoing National Cancer Institute (NCI) –sponsored clinical trial is examining the effects of fish oil alone or in combination with vitamin D_3 in cancer prevention.

Safety. The FDA classifies intake of up to 3 g/d of omega-3 fatty acids from fish as "generally recognized as safe." Caution may be warranted in diabetic patients (due to potential hyperglycemic effects), patients at risk of bleeding, or those with low blood pressure or high low-density lipoprotein (LDL) cholesterol levels.[211] DHA may have greater effects than EPA.

An increased risk of bleeding is one of the primary concerns with fish oil supplementation.[211] Diets containing salmon oil, mackerel, or cod liver oil have been reported to prolong bleeding times significantly in healthy volunteers. However, in other studies of omega-3 fatty acid supplementation, no adverse effects on bleeding time have been observed. Increased bleeding time is suggested to result from either less thromboxane or higher prostacyclin levels. It is unclear if omega-3 fatty acids affect coagulation. Anecdotal evidence suggests that fish oil may increase international normalized ratio, a measure of bleeding time. However, clinical evidence suggests that fish oil does not affect coagulation, even when taken with anticoagulant therapy. Nevertheless, caution is warranted when omega-3 fatty acids (from plant or fish) are taken with anticoagulant agents. Some species of fish carry a higher risk of environmental contaminants, such as with methylmercury or other heavy metals.

Reishi

Clinical Studies. Treatment with reishi (*Ganoderma lucidum*) mushroom extract (Ganopoly) for 12 weeks resulted in a significant increase in plasma levels of interleukin 2 (IL-2), IL-6, and interferon-γ (IFN-γ), decreased IL-1 and tumor necrosis factor-alpha (TNF-α) levels, and increased natural killer (NK) cells in advanced-stage cancer patients.[212,213] Well-designed, long-term studies are needed to confirm these results and to examine potential side effects.

Safety. Caution is recommended when reishi is used in patients with bleeding disorders/coagulopathies or in those taking anticoagulants, as reishi mushroom may alter platelet aggregation and prolong bleeding time.[214] Caution is also advised in patients with low blood pressure, diabetes, or in those taking antidiabetic agents or antihypertensives.

Resveratrol

Clinical Studies. Resveratrol is a naturally occurring hydroxystilbene identified in more than 70 plant species, including nuts, grapes, pine trees, and certain vines, as well as in red wine. Although there are several observational studies that correlate the consumption of wine with a decrease in cancer or cardiovascular disease risk,[215,216] high-quality human trials supporting the efficacy of resveratrol for any indication are currently lacking in the available literature. Ongoing research is examining resveratrol and a possible role in increasing longevity and how it interacts with sirtuens.

Safety. Laboratory study suggests that resveratrol has antiaggregating and antithrombin activity, and may have additive effects when taken with other agents with the same actions[217]; thus, use of resveratrol with antiplatelets could cause increased risk of bleeding, although clinical reports of drug interactions are lacking. Resveratrol apparently has the potential to act as an estrogen agonist or antagonist, depending on such factors as cell type and estrogen receptor isoform (ER-α or ER-β).[218–220] Resveratrol has also been shown to inhibit vitamin D_3 receptor expression through estrogenic regulation.[221] Clinical evidence of estrogen interactions is lacking. Some *in vitro* and *in vivo* studies suggest that resveratrol might interfere with paclitaxel.[222] Resveratrol inhibited all of the cytochrome P-450 (CYP) tested (1A1, 1A2, 1B1, 2A6, 2B6, 2E1, 3A4, 4A), except for 2E1.[223]

Selenium

Clinical Studies. Initial evidence has suggested that selenium supplementation reduces the risk of developing prostate cancer in men with normal baseline prostate specific antigen (PSA) levels and low selenium blood levels. This is the subject of large, well-designed studies, including the Nutritional Prevention of Cancer Trial (NPC) and the Selenium and Vitamin E Cancer Prevention Trial (SELECT),[224–238] as well as prior population and case-control studies.[239,240]

The NPC trial with 1,312 Americans reported that 200 mg of daily selenium reduces the overall incidence of prostate cancer, although these protective effects only occurred in men with baseline PSA levels less than or equal to 4 ng/mL and those with low baseline blood selenium levels (less than 123.2 ng/mL).[227–229,241] The NPC trial was primarily designed to measure the development of nonmelanoma skin cancers and not other types of cancers; therefore, these prostate cancer results cannot be considered definitive.

SELECT was started in 2001 with 32,400 men with serum PSA levels less than or equal to 4 ng/mL. The study was ended early due to an interim analysis that determined the study could not meet its expected end point of a 25% reduction in prostate cancer. Subset analyses indicated selenium supplementation was associated with increased development of diabetes mellitus.

Safety. The level of selenium exposure that will cause chronic toxicity is not clear. Selenium toxicity may cause gastrointestinal symptoms (nausea, vomiting, abdominal pain, diarrhea, garliclike breath odor, and metallic taste), neuromuscular-psychiatric disturbances (weakness/fatigue, lightheadedness, irritability, hyperreflexia, muscle tenderness, tremor, and peripheral neuropathy), dermatologic changes (skin rash/dermatitis/flushing, fingernail loss/thickening/blotching/streaking/paronychia, and hair changes/loss), liver dysfunction, kidney dysfunction, thrombocytopenia (low blood platelets), immune alterations (natural killer cell impairment), thyroid dysfunction (decreased T3), reduced sperm motility, or growth retardation.

Soy

Clinical Studies. Preliminary research using soy (*Glycine max*) to control hot flashes in women with breast cancer suggests that it is possibly safe,[242] although the pending results of ongoing research in this area may provide more definitive safety data. Recent studies have indicated that moderate dietary soy intake (observed in most traditional Asian diets—no more than three servings daily) shows no risk and may have possible benefits to breast cancer patients, even among women with estrogen-positive breast cancers.[243,244] However, because higher doses of soy may have estrogenic effects, which clearly increase the risk for progression of estrogen receptor–positive breast cancer, it is prudent for breast cancer survivors to avoid the high doses of soy and soy isoflavones that are provided by more concentrated sources (such as soy powders and isoflavone supplements).[43] Preliminary clinical evidence suggests that short-term use of soy isoflavones does not elicit endometrial hypertrophy.

Safety. Soy is "generally regarded as safe" according to the FDA, and has long been a staple of Asian diets. Current epidemiological and laboratory evidence suggests there are unlikely to be harmful effects when soy is provided in the diet consistent with amounts in a typical Asian diet.[243]

Turmeric

Clinical Studies. A Phase I trial found limited toxicity with doses of tumeric (*Curcuma longa*, curcumin) as high as 8 g daily. A Phase II clinical trial in pancreatic cancer found a limited response rate with 3 of 25 patients with either stable disease or reduction in tumor size.[245] Multiple clinical trials are ongoing to evaluate the use of turmeric and associated compounds for the treatment of cancer.

Safety. The most common side effect with turmeric reported in humans is gastrointestinal upset, including epigastric burning, dyspepsia, nausea, and diarrhea.[245,246] High doses of turmeric are thought to be safe based on toxicology studies.[247] The turmeric constituent curcumin has been reported to induce liver function test abnormalities in rats, and may be mildly hepatotoxic in high doses.[246] Caution is warranted when using turmeric with hepatotoxic agents. Increased bleeding risk is a concern with high doses of curcumin.[246] There is evidence that turmeric may interfere with cytochrome P-450 (CYP450) enzymes, which are responsible for breaking down various agents in the liver.[248]

Vitamin A

Vitamin A is comprised of retinol and its carotenoid precursors. All-*trans*retinoic acid, a retinol analogue, is well established as a differentiation agent in patients with acute promyelocytic leukemia.[249] However, there is little evidence to support the use of nonprescription vitamin A supplements for cancer treatment or prevention. Trials have yielded variable results, suggesting no reduction in prostate cancer risk and possible increased risk of lung cancer in high-risk patients.[250] Due to the possibility of hypervitaminosis A with supplementation of this fat-soluble vitamin, chronic intake of large doses is discouraged.

Vitamin C

Limited clinical research has been conducted on vitamin C (ascorbic acid) for cancer prevention. In the 1980s, there was initial excitement over epidemiologic evidence correlating high dietary vitamin C intake with reduced rates of cancer, although use of vitamin C in observed populations may have correlated with other healthy lifestyle choices (diet, exercise) that confounded findings. A subsequent prospective trial found no reduction in rates of breast cancer. Preclinical evidence of reduced platelet aggregation suggests that risks may outweigh potential benefits. Patients may experience scurvy symptoms after abrupt withdrawal of chronic megadoses. Two randomized controlled trials of high-dose intravenous vitamin C in cancer patients found no benefits.[251,252]

Vitamin D

Vitamin D is one of four fat-soluble vitamins, and is traditionally linked with calcium metabolism and bone health. Vitamin D_2 (ergocalciferol) and vitamin D_3 (cholecalciferol) are precursors to calcitriol, the active form of vitamin D. Exposing skin to natural sunlight is the most common manner by which the body produces vitamin D. Growing evidence indicates the importance of vitamin D for immune processes. Additionally, studies in cancer populations indicate a possible worse outcome in those with vitamin D deficiency.[253–255] Appropriate supplementation should be considered for those with documented deficiency or those at risk for bone fractures due to poor bone health (i.e., osteoporosis). Prolonged high-dose use of vitamin D may lead to hypercalcemia.

Vitamin E

Vitamin E (α-tocopherol) is a fat-soluble vitamin with antioxidant properties. Epidemiologic studies suggest a possible reduced breast, lung, and prostate cancer risk with intake. However, prevention trials report no reduction in risk of lung, breast, or colon cancer. Several reviews and meta-analyses have also found a higher mortality rate in doses of 400 IU or less daily.[256–259] Additionally, a large randomized trial among head and neck cancer patients investigated vitamin E and beta carotene and found these agents were associated with decreased survival among subjects taking both. Some have hypothesized that the agents may have acted as an antioxidant and thus reduced the efficacy of the radiation treatment, leading to increased recurrence rates and ultimately decreased survival. Several studies have evaluated the potential to protect again chemotherapy-induced peripheral neuropathy with such agents as platinums and taxanes with positive results.[260–264] However, these studies were not designed to assess for alterations in chemotherapy effectiveness. Preclinical evidence of reduced platelet aggregation has been shown.

Other Therapies

Other herbs and supplements that are used in cancer treatment without reliable evidence include aloe, antineoplastons, barley, bitter melon, bladderwrack, bromelain, calendula, chamomile, clay, danshen, dehydroepiandrosterone (DHEA), echinacea, evening primrose oil, eyebright, flaxseed, Gerson therapy and coffee enemas, ginseng, ginkgo, goldenseal, guggul, gymnema, hops, horsetail, kava, lactobacillus, laetrile, lavender, marshmallow, passion flower, pennyroyal, peppermint, propolis, red clover, sorrel, St. John's wort, sweet almond, white horehound, and numerous types of mushroom extracts.

Numerous therapies have also been used for cancer prevention, but they have not been well studied. These include aloe, black tea, bromelain, cranberry, eucalyptus oil, ginseng, grape seed extract, lactobacillus (colon cancer risk reduction), oleander, omega-3 fatty acids/fish oil, psyllium (colon cancer risk reduction), red clover, and spirulina.

Nonbiologically Based Therapies

Nonbiologically based therapies generally fall into the categories of mind–body techniques, massage, acupuncture, and energy techniques. These techniques are generally used to support overall well-being or specific treatment-related side effects.[265–274]

Mind–Body Techniques

Background. Mind–body modalities, including meditation, hypnosis, relaxation techniques, cognitive-behavioral therapy, biofeedback, yoga, tai chi, qi gong, and guided imagery, are increasingly becoming part of mainstream care over the years. Mind–body practices are defined as a variety of techniques designed to enhance the mind's capacity to affect bodily function and symptoms[1]

Clinical Studies. Techniques of stress management that may be helpful include progressive muscle relaxation,[275,276] diaphragmatic breathing,[277,278] guided imagery,[279–281] social support,[282,283] and meditation.[284,285] Participating in stress management programs prior to treatment has enabled patients to tolerate therapy with fewer reported side effects.[286–289] Supportive expressive group therapy has also been found to be useful for patients with cancer.[290–292] Psychosocial interventions have been shown to specifically decrease depression and anxiety and increase self-esteem and active-approach coping strategies.[293–296]

There is some evidence that when incorporated into cancer care, yoga, tai chi, and meditation may help to improve aspects of quality of life, including improved mood, sleep quality, physical functioning, and overall well-being.[294,297–299] Hypnosis, and especially self-hypnosis, has been found to be beneficial in reducing distress and discomfort during difficult medical procedures.[279] A National Institutes of Health (NIH) Technology Assessment Panel found strong evidence for hypnosis in alleviating cancer-related pain.[300] Hypnosis effectively treats anticipatory nausea in pediatric[301] and adult cancer patients,[302] reduces postoperative nausea and vomiting,[303] and improves adjustment to invasive medical procedures.[304–306]

A meta-analysis of 116 studies found that mind–body therapies may reduce anxiety, depression, and mood disturbance in cancer patients and aid their coping skills.[307] Newell et al.[308] reviewed psychological therapies for cancer patients and concluded that interventions involving self-practice and hypnosis for managing nausea and vomiting may be recommended. More recently, Ernst et al.[309] examined the change in the state of the evidence for mind–body therapies for various medical conditions between 2000 and 2005 and found that there is now maximal evidence for the use of relaxation techniques for anxiety, hypertension, insomnia, and nausea due to chemotherapy.

Massage

Clinical Studies. Research to date suggests that massage is helpful for increasing relaxation and relieving pain, anxiety, fatigue, and distress.[267,310–312] The obvious challenge in conducting massage therapy research is the difficulty achieving a placebo control group. It is therefore not clear what the exact mechanisms are for the benefits of massage in an oncology setting. Despite some of the imperfections in research design, the current findings are encouraging.

Safety. Massage therapy is generally safe when practiced by credentialed practitioners who have also had some training in cancer patient care. Serious adverse events are rare and tend to be associated with exotic types of massage or untrained or inexperienced practitioners.[313] In general, cancer patients should not receive deep tissue massage, and patients with bleeding tendencies should only receive light touch. Obviously, areas that have recently had surgery or radiation should be avoided. Therapeutic benefit may also be derived from simply receiving a massage to the feet, hands, and head, as these areas are especially sensitive to tactile stimulation and may result in providing relaxation and an increase in general well-being.[314]

Acupuncture

Background. Acupuncture is a common treatment modality in many cultures. It is a form of traditional Chinese medicine (TCM) and has been practiced in China for thousands of years. Acupuncture is one of the most popular TCM therapies outside of China and is used in at least 78 countries[315] According to traditional theory, the placement of needles, heat, or pressure at specific places on the body can help to regulate the flow of qi (vital energy). The most common form of acupuncture involves the placement of solid, sterile, stainless steel needles into various points on the body.[316,317] Different techniques can be used to stimulate the needles, including manual manipulation or electrical stimulation.[316–318]

Clinical Studies. There is good scientific evidence that acupuncture is effective for managing both postoperative and chemotherapy-related nausea and vomiting.[44–47] An NIH consensus statement in 1998 supported this use, stating that the level of evidence was sufficient.[319] Further research has substantiated this claim, and the American Cancer Society now states that clinical studies have found acupuncture may help treat nausea caused by chemotherapy drugs and surgical anesthesia. There is also good evidence that certain types of acupuncture are effective for both postoperative and chronic pain in cancer patients.[319–321]

A growing number of clinical trials, both controlled and uncontrolled, suggest that acupuncture is beneficial for radiation-induced xerostomia, hot flashes, and aromatase-induced arthralgias.[322–325] For the management of other treatment- or cancer-related symptoms, the evidence is not as strong. Nevertheless, there is some preliminary and anecdotal evidence to suggest that acupuncture may be useful in the treatment of anxiety, depression, fatigue, constipation, loss of appetite, peripheral neuropathy, insomnia, dyspnea, and leucopenia.[326,327] However, the overall quality of the evidence for these symptoms remains weak, and further studies are needed.

Safety. When performed correctly, acupuncture has been shown to be a safe, minimally invasive procedure with very few side effects. The most commonly reported complications are fainting, bruising, and mild pain. Infection is also a potential risk, although very uncommon.[328,329] Acupuncture should only be performed by a health care professional with an appropriate license and preferably one who has had experience in treating patients with malignant diseases.

Selected References

The full list of references for this chapter appears in the online version.

1. National Center for Complementary and Alternative Medicine (NCCAM). What is complementary and alternative medicine? NCCAM Publication D347 2010. World Wide Web URL: http://nccam.nih.gov/health/whatiscam/.
2. Eisenberg DM, Davis RB, Ettner SL, et al. Trends in alternative medicine use in the United States, 1990–1997: results of a follow-up national survey. *JAMA* 1998;280(18):1569.
7. Barnes PM, Bloom B, Nahin RL. Complementary and alternative medicine use among adults and children: United States, 2007. *Natl Health Stat Rep* 2008;12:1.
8. Richardson MA, Sanders T, Palmer JL, Greisinger A, Singletary SE. Complementary/alternative medicine use in a comprehensive cancer center and the implications for oncology. *J Clin Oncol* 2000;18(13):2505.
32. Paltiel O, Avitzour M, Peretz T, et al. Determinants of the use of complementary therapies by patients with cancer. *J Clin Oncol* 2001;19(9):2439.
36. Engel GL. The need for a new medical model: a challenge for biomedicine. *Science* 1977;196(4286):129.
37. Aggarwal BB, Shishodia S. Molecular targets of dietary agents for prevention and therapy of cancer. *Biochem Pharmacol* 2006;71(10):1397.
38. Chlebowski RT, Blackburn GL, Thomson CA, et al. Dietary fat reduction and breast cancer outcome: interim efficacy results from the Women's Intervention Nutrition Study. *J Natl Cancer Inst* 2006;98(24):1767.
39. Pierce JP, Natarajan L, Caan BJ, et al. Influence of a diet very high in vegetables, fruit, and fiber and low in fat on prognosis following treatment for breast cancer: the Women's Healthy Eating and Living (WHEL) randomized trial. *JAMA* 2007;298(3):289.
43. Doyle C, Kushi LH, Byers T, et al. Nutrition and physical activity during and after cancer treatment: an American Cancer Society guide for informed choices. *CA Cancer J Clin* 2006;56(6):323.
44. Vickers AJ. Can acupuncture have specific effects on health? A systematic review of acupuncture antiemesis trials. *J R Soc Med* 1996;89(6):303.
49. Litton JK, Gonzalez-Angulo AM, Warneke CL, et al. Relationship between obesity and pathologic response to neoadjuvant chemotherapy among women with operable breast cancer. *J Clin Oncol* 2008;26(25):4072.
50. Li CI, Daling JR, Porter PL, Tang MT, Malone KE. Relationship between potentially modifiable lifestyle factors and risk of second primary contralateral breast cancer among women diagnosed with estrogen receptor-positive invasive breast cancer. *J Clin Oncol* 2009;27(32):5312.
51. Adler NE, Page AEK, National Institute of Medicine. *Cancer care for the whole patient: meeting psychosocial health needs*. Washington, DC: National Academies Press, 2008.
71. Glaser R, Kiecolt-Glaser JK. Stress-induced immune dysfunction: implications for health. *Nat Rev Immunol* 2005;5(3):243.
72. Antoni MH, Lutgendorf SK, Cole SW, et al. The influence of bio-behavioural factors on tumour biology: pathways and mechanisms. *Nat Rev Cancer* 2006;6(3):240.
73. Lutgendorf SK, Sood AK, Antoni MH. Host factors and cancer progression: biobehavioral signaling pathways and interventions. *J Clin Oncol* 2010; 28(29):4094.
78. Andersen BL, Yang HC, Farrar WB, et al. Psychologic intervention improves survival for breast cancer patients: a randomized clinical trial. *Cancer* 2008;113(12):3450.
81. Ulbricht C, Chao W, Costa D, et al. Clinical evidence of herb-drug interactions: a systematic review by the natural standard research collaboration. *Curr Drug Metab* 2008;9(10):1063.
86. Frenkel M, Ben Arye E, Baldwin CD, Sierpina V. Approach to communicating with patients about the use of nutritional supplements in cancer care. *South Med J* 2005;98(3):289.
87. Palmer ME, Haller C, McKinney PE, et al. Adverse events associated with dietary supplements: an observational study. *Lancet* 2003;361(9352):101.
88. Fugh-Berman A. Herb-drug interactions. *Lancet* 2000;355(9198):134.
102. Bairati I, Meyer F, Gelinas M, et al. A randomized trial of antioxidant vitamins to prevent second primary cancers in head and neck cancer patients. *J Natl Cancer Inst* 2005;97(7):481.
103. Bairati I, Meyer F, Jobin E, et al. Antioxidant vitamins supplementation and mortality: a randomized trial in head and neck cancer patients. *Int J Cancer* 2006;119(9):2221.
104. Block KI, Koch AC, Mead MN, et al. Impact of antioxidant supplementation on chemotherapeutic efficacy: a systematic review of the evidence from randomized controlled trials. *Cancer Treat Rev* 2007;33(5):407.
105. Lawenda BD, Kelly KM, Ladas EJ, et al. Should supplemental antioxidant administration be avoided during chemotherapy and radiation therapy? *J Natl Cancer Inst* 2008;100(11):773.
117. van Dalen EC, Caron HN, Dickinson HO, Kremer LC. Cardioprotective interventions for cancer patients receiving anthracyclines. *Cochrane Database Syst Rev* 2005;(1):CD003917.
151. Bryer E. A literature review of the effectiveness of ginger in alleviating mild-to-moderate nausea and vomiting of pregnancy. *J Midwifery Womens Health* 2005;50(1):e1.
169. Ernst E, Pittler MH. Efficacy of ginger for nausea and vomiting: a systematic review of randomized clinical trials. *Br J Anaesth* 2000;84(3):367.
172. Barton DL, Soori GS, Bauer BA, et al. Pilot study of *Panax quinquefolius* (American ginseng) to improve cancer-related fatigue: a randomized, double-blind, dose-finding evaluation: NCCTG trial N03CA. *Support Care Cancer* 2010;18(2):179.
180. Tsubono Y, Nishino Y, Komatsu S, et al. Green tea and the risk of gastric cancer in Japan. *N Engl J Med* 2001;344(9):632.
189. Giovannucci E. Tomatoes, tomato-based products, lycopene, and cancer: review of the epidemiologic literature. *J Natl Cancer Inst* 1999;91(4):317.
191. Kodama N, Komuta K, Nanba H. Can Maitake MD-fraction aid cancer patients? *Altern Med Rev* 2002;7(3):236.
192. Deng G, Lin H, Seidman A, et al. A phase I/II trial of a polysaccharide extract from Grifola frondosa (Maitake mushroom) in breast cancer patients: immunological effects. *J Cancer Res Clin Oncol* 2009;135(9):1215.
198. Schaefermeyer G, Schaefermeyer H. Treatment of pancreatic cancer with *Viscum album* (iscador): a retrospective study of 292 patients 1986–1996. *Comp Ther Med* 1998;6(4):172.
203. Rose DP, Connolly JM. Omega-3 fatty acids as cancer chemopreventive agents. *Pharmacol Ther* 1999;83(3):217.
208. Terry P, Lichtenstein P, Feychting M, Ahlbom A, Wolk A. Fatty fish consumption and risk of prostate cancer. *Lancet* 2001;357(9270):1764.
243. Shu XO, Zheng Y, Cai H, et al. Soy food intake and breast cancer survival. *JAMA* 2009;302(22):2437.
245. Dhillon N, Aggarwal BB, Newman RA, et al. Phase II trial of curcumin in patients with advanced pancreatic cancer. *Clin Cancer Res* 2008;14(14):4491.
250. The Alpha-Tocopherol and Beta Carotene Cancer Prevention Study Group. The effect of vitamin E and beta carotene on the incidence of lung cancer and other cancers in male smokers. *N Engl J Med* 1994;330(15):1029.
253. Goodwin PJ, Ennis M, Pritchard KI, Koo J, Hood N. Prognostic effects of 25-hydroxyvitamin D levels in early breast cancer. *J Clin Oncol* 2009; 27(23):3757.
254. Mezawa H, Sugiura T, Watanabe M, et al. Serum vitamin D levels and survival of patients with colorectal cancer: post-hoc analysis of a prospective cohort study. *BMC Cancer* 2010;10:347.
284. Coker KH. Meditation and prostate cancer: integrating a mind/body intervention with traditional therapies. *Semin Urol Oncol* 1999;17(2):111.
297. Bower JE, Woolery A, Sternlieb B, Garet D. Yoga for cancer patients and survivors. *Cancer Control* 2005;12(3):165.
298. Chandwani KD, Thornton B, Perkins GH, et al. Yoga improves quality of life and benefit finding in women undergoing radiotherapy for breast cancer. *J Soc Integr Oncol* 2010;8(2):43.
304. Lang EV, Benotsch EG, Fick LJ, et al. Adjunctive non-pharmacological analgesia for invasive medical procedures: a randomised trial. *Lancet* 2000;355(9214):1486.
308. Newell SA, Sanson-Fisher RW, Savolainen NJ. Systematic review of psychological therapies for cancer patients: overview and recommendations for future research. *J Natl Cancer Inst* 2002;94(8):558.
309. Ernst E, Pittler MH, Wider B, Boddy K. Mind-body therapies: are the trial data getting stronger? *Altern Ther Health Med* 2007;13(5):62.
310. Ahles TA, Tope DM, Pinkson B, et al. Massage therapy for patients undergoing autologous bone marrow transplantation. *J Pain Symptom Manage* 1999;18(3):157.
326. Filshie J, Hester J. Guidelines for providing acupuncture treatment for cancer patients–a peer-reviewed sample policy document. *Acupunct Med* 2006;24(4):172.

INDEX

Note: Page locators followed by *f* and *t* indicate figure and table, respectively.

E

P

T